AMERICAN MEDICAL
ASSOCIATION

MW01042332

ICD-10-CM 2023
The Complete Official Codebook

AMA publications fund initiatives that drive improvements in
patient health, practice innovation and medical education.

[Handwritten at top: L Skin. S: Injury]

Publisher's Notice

The *ICD-10-CM: The Complete Official Codebook* is designed to be an accurate and authoritative source regarding coding and every reasonable effort has been made to ensure accuracy and completeness of the content. However, the American Medical Association (AMA) makes no guarantee, warranty, or representation that this publication is accurate, complete, or without errors. It is understood that the AMA is not rendering any legal or other professional services or advice in this publication and that the AMA bears no liability for any results or consequences that may arise from the use of this book.

Our Commitment to Accuracy

The AMA is committed to producing accurate and reliable materials.

AMA product updates, errata, and addenda can be found at amaproductupdates.org.

To report corrections, please call the AMA Unified Service Center at (800) 621-8335.

To purchase additional copies, visit the AMA store at amastore.com. Refer to product number OP201423.

Acknowledgments

Marianne Randall, CPC, *Product Manager*
Anita Schmidt, BS, RHIA, AHIMA-approved ICD-10-CM/PCS Trainer, *Subject Matter Expert*
Leanne Patterson, CPC, *Subject Matter Expert*
LaJuana Green, RHIA, CCS, *Subject Matter Expert*
Jacqueline R. Petersen, BS, RHIA, CHDA, CPC, *Subject Matter Expert*
Stacy Perry, *Manager, Desktop Publishing*
Tracy Betzler, *Senior Desktop Publishing Specialist*
Hope M. Dunn, *Senior Desktop Publishing Specialist*
Katie Russell, *Desktop Publishing Specialist*
Kate Holden, *Editor*

Leanne Patterson, CPC

Ms. Patterson has more than 15 years of experience in the healthcare profession. She has an extensive background in professional component coding, with expertise in E/M coding and auditing, and HIPAA compliance. Her experience includes general surgery coding, serving as Director of Compliance, conducting chart-to-claim audits, and physician education. She has been responsible for coding and denial management in large multi-specialty physician practices, and most recently has been part of a team developing content for educational products related to ICD-10-CM. Ms. Patterson is credentialed by the American Academy of Professional Coders (AAPC) as a Certified Professional Coder (CPC).

LaJuana Green, RHIA, CCS

Ms. Green is a Registered Health Information Administrator with over 35 years of experience in multiple areas of information management. She has proven expertise in the analysis of medical record documentation, assignment of ICD-10-CM and PCS codes, DRG validation, and CPT code assignment in ambulatory surgery units and the hospital outpatient setting. Her experience includes serving as a director of a health information management department, clinical technical editing, new technology research and writing, medical record management, utilization review activities, quality assurance, tumor registry, medical library services, and chargemaster maintenance. Ms. Green is an active member of the American Health Information Management Association (AHIMA).

[Handwritten notes]

L80–L99 other skin disorder
M70–M79 other soft tissue disorder
N60–N65 Disorder of breast
S00–S09 injuries to the head
S10–S19 neck injury
S20–S29 thorax —
S30–S39 abdomen. lower back lumbar. pelvic. genital
S40–S49 shoulder. upper arm
S50–S59 elbow. forearm
S60–S69 wrist. hand. finger
S70–S79 hip. tight.
S80–S89 knee. lower leg
S90–S99 ankle. foot
T20–T25 Burn. corrosions. external
T26–T28 — internal. Ey
T30–T32. multiple. unspecified body region

Neoplasm table Page 342
C43–C44 Melanoma
C45–C49 Melanoma. mesothelial
C50 malignant neoplasm of breast
L00–L08 Skin. subcutaneous infection
L10–L14 Bullous disorder
L20–L30 Dermatitis and eczema
L40–L45 Urticaria. erythema
L55–L59 Radiation Related Skin
L60–L75 Skin Appendages

Contents

Contents

How to Use ICD-10-CM: The Complete Official Codebook 2023

Introduction

ICD-10-CM: The Complete Official Codebook 2023 is your definitive coding resource, combining the work of the National Center for Health Statistics (NCHS), Centers for Medicare and Medicaid Services (CMS), American Hospital Association (AHA), and Publisher experts to provide the information you need for coding accuracy.

The International Classification of Diseases, 10th Revision, Clinical Modification (ICD-10-CM), is an adaptation of ICD-10, copyrighted by the World Health Organization (WHO). The development and maintenance of this clinical modification (CM) is the responsibility of the NCHS as authorized by WHO. Any new concepts added to ICD-10-CM are based on an established update process through the collaboration of WHO's Update and Revision Committee and the ICD-10-CM Coordination and Maintenance Committee.

In addition to the ICD-10-CM classification, other official government source information has been included in this manual. Depending on the source, updates to information may be annual or quarterly. This manual provides the most current information that was available at the time of publication. For updates to the source documents that may have occurred after this manual was published, please refer to the following:

- **NCHS, International Classification of Diseases, Tenth Revision, Clinical Modification (ICD-10-CM)**

  https://www.cms.gov/medicare/icd-10/2023-icd-10-cm

- **CMS Integrated Outpatient Code Editor (IOCE), version 23.2**

  https://www.cms.gov/Medicare/Coding/OutpatientCodeEdit/OCEQtrReleaseSpecs.html

- **CMS-HCC Risk Adjustment Model, version 24**

- **CMS ESRD-HCC Risk Adjustment Model, version 24**

- **CMS RxHCC Risk Adjustment Model, version 08**

  https://www.cms.gov/Medicare/Health-Plans/MedicareAdvtgSpecRateStats/Risk-Adjustors.html

- **HHS-HCC Commercial Risk Adjustment Model, version 07**

  https://www.cms.gov/CCIIO/Resources/Regulations-and-Guidance

- **CMS Quality Payment Program (QPP)**

  https://qpp.cms.gov/mips/explore-measures/quality-measures?tab=qualityMeasures&py=2022

- **AHA Coding Clinics**

  https://www.codingclinicadvisor.com/

The official NCHS ICD-10-CM classification includes three main sections: the guidelines, the indexes, and the tabular list, all of which make up the bulk of this coding manual. To complement the classification, Optum's coding experts have incorporated Medicare-related coding edits and proprietary features, such as supplementary notations, coding tools, and appendixes, into a comprehensive and easy-to-use reference. This publication is organized as follows:

What's New for 2023

This section provides a high-level overview of the code changes made for fiscal 2023. The list of codes provided identifies new, revised, and deleted codes. Asterisked codes identify prior midyear changes that were made to the classification, effective April 1, 2022. All changes are based on official addenda, provided by the National Center for Health Statistics (NCHS), the agency charged with maintaining and updating ICD-10-CM. NCHS is part of the Centers for Disease Control and Prevention (CDC).

Conversion Table

The conversion table was developed by National Center for Healthcare Statistics (NCHS) to help facilitate data retrieval as new codes are added to the ICD-10-CM classification. This table provides a crosswalk from each fiscal 2023 new code to the equivalent code(s) assigned, prior to October 1, 2022, for that diagnosis or condition. Asterisked codes identify prior midyear additions, effective April 1, 2022. For the full conversion table, refer to the Conversion Table zip file at https://www.cms.gov/medicare/icd-10/2023-icd-10-cm.

10 Steps to Correct Coding

This step-by-step tutorial walks the coder through the process of finding the correct code — from locating the code in the official indexes to verifying the code in the tabular section — while following applicable conventions, guidelines, and instructional notes. Specific examples are provided with detailed explanations of each coding step along with advice for proper sequencing.

Official ICD-10-CM Guidelines for Coding and Reporting

This section provides the full official conventions and guidelines regulating the appropriate assignment and reporting of ICD-10-CM codes. These conventions and guidelines are published by the U.S. Department of Health and Human Services (DHHS) and approved by the cooperating parties (American Health Information Management Association [AHIMA], National Center for Health Statistics [NCHS], Centers for Disease Control and Prevention [CDC], and the American Hospital Association [AHA]).

Indexes

Index to Diseases and Injuries

The Index to Diseases and Injuries is arranged in alphabetic order by terms specific to a disease, condition, illness, injury, eponym, or abbreviation as well as terms that describe circumstances other than a disease or injury that may require attention from a health care professional.

Neoplasm Table

The Neoplasm Table is arranged in alphabetic order by anatomical site. Codes are then listed in individual columns based upon the histological behavior (malignant, in situ, benign, uncertain, or unspecified) of the neoplasm.

Table of Drugs and Chemicals

The Table of Drugs and Chemicals is arranged in alphabetic order by the specific drug or chemical name. Codes are listed in individual columns based upon the associated intent (poisoning, adverse effect, or underdosing). Drugs with an asterisk identify substances added to the table by Optum subject matter experts.

External Causes Index

The External Causes Index is arranged in alphabetic order by main terms that describe the cause, the intent, the place of occurrence, the activity, and the status of the patient at the time the injury occurred or health condition arose.

Index Notations

With

The word "with" or "in" should be interpreted to mean "associated with" or "due to." The classification presumes a causal relationship between the two conditions linked by these terms in the index. These conditions should be coded as related even in the absence of provider documentation explicitly linking them unless the documentation clearly states the conditions are unrelated or when another guideline specifically requires a documented linkage between two conditions (e.g., the sepsis guideline for "acute organ dysfunction that is not clearly associated with the sepsis"). For conditions not specifically linked by these relational terms in the classification or when a guideline requires explicit documentation of a linkage between two conditions, provider documentation must link the conditions to code them as related.

The word "with" in the index is sequenced immediately following the main term, not in alphabetical order.

> **Dermatopolymyositis** M33.90
> > with
> > > myopathy M33.92
> > > respiratory involvement M33.91
> > > specified organ involvement NEC M33.99
> > amyopathic M33.93

See
When the instruction "see" follows a term in the index, it indicates that another term must be referenced to locate the correct code.

> **Hematoperitoneum** — *see* Hemoperitoneum

See Also
The instructional note "see also" simply provides alternative terms the coder may reference that may be useful in determining the correct code but are not necessary to follow if the main term supplies the appropriate code.

> **Hematinuria** — *see also* Hemaglobinuria
> > malarial B50.8

Default Codes
In the index, the default code is the code listed next to the main term and represents the condition most commonly associated with that main term. This code may be assigned when documentation does not support reporting a more specific code. Alternatively, it may provide an unspecified code for the condition.

> **Hemiatrophy** R68.89
> > cerebellar G31.9
> > face, facial, progressive (Romberg) G51.8
> > tongue K14.8

Parentheses
Parentheses in the indexes enclose nonessential modifiers, supplementary words that may be present or absent in the statement of a disease without affecting the code.

> **Pseudomeningocele** (cerebral) (infective) (post-traumatic)
> > G96.198
> > postprocedural (spinal) G97.82

Brackets
ICD-10-CM has a coding convention addressing code assignment for manifestations that occur as a result of an underlying condition. This convention requires the underlying condition to be sequenced first, followed by the code or codes for the associated manifestation. In the index, italicized codes in brackets identify manifestation codes.

> **Polyneuropathy** (peripheral) G62.9
> > alcoholic G62.1
> > amyloid (Portuguese) E85.1 *[G63]*
> > > transthyretin-related (ATTR) familial E85.1 *[G63]*

Shaded Guides
Exclusive vertical shaded guides in the Index to Diseases and Injuries and External Causes Index help the user easily follow the indent levels for the subentries under a main term. Sequencing rules may apply depending on the level of indent for separate subentries.

> **Hemicrania**
> > congenital malformation Q00.0
> > continua G44.51
> > meaning migraine — *see also* Migraine G43.909
> > paroxysmal G44.039
> > > chronic G44.049
> > > > intractable G44.041
> > > > not intractable G44.049
> > > episodic G44.039
> > > > intractable G44.031
> > > > not intractable G44.039
> > > intractable G44.031
> > > not intractable G44.039

Following References
The Index to Diseases and Injuries includes "following" references to assist in locating out-of-sequence codes in the tabular list. Out-of-sequence codes contain an alphabetic character (letter) in the third- or fourth-character position. These codes are placed according to the classification rules — according to condition — not according to alphabetic or numeric sequencing rules.

> **Carcinoma** (malignant) — *see also* Neoplasm, by site, malignant
> > neuroendocrine — *see also* Tumor, neuroendocrine
> > > high grade, any site C7A.1 (*following* C75)
> > > poorly differentiated, any site C7A.1 (*following* C75)

Additional Character Required
The Index to Diseases and Injuries, Neoplasm Table, and External Causes Index provide an icon after certain codes to signify to the user that additional characters are required to make the code valid. The tabular list should be consulted for appropriate character selection.

> **Fall, falling** (accidental) W19 ☑
> > building W20.1 ☑

Tabular List of Diseases
ICD-10-CM codes and descriptions are arranged numerically within the tabular list of diseases with 19 separate chapters providing codes associated with a particular body system or nature of injury or disease. There is also a chapter providing codes for external causes of an injury or health conditions, a chapter for codes that address encounters with healthcare facilities for circumstances other than a disease or injury, and finally, a chapter for codes that capture special circumstances such as new diseases of uncertain etiology or emergency use codes..

Code and Code Descriptions
ICD-10-CM is an alphanumeric classification system that contains categories, subcategories, and valid codes. The first character is always a letter with any additional characters represented by either a letter or number. A three-character category without further subclassification is equivalent to a valid three-character code. Valid codes may be three, four, five, six, or seven characters in length, with each level of subdivision after a three-character category representing a subcategory. The final level of subdivision is a valid code.

Boldface
Boldface type is used for all codes and descriptions in the tabular list.

Italics
Italicized type is used to identify manifestation codes, those codes that should not be reported as first-listed diagnoses.

Deleted Text
~~Strikethrough~~ on a code and code description indicates a deletion from the classification for the current year.

Key Word

Green font is used throughout the Tabular List of Diseases to differentiate the key words that appear in similar code descriptions in a given category or subcategory. The key word convention is used only in those categories in which there are multiple codes with very similar descriptions with only a few words that differentiate them.

For example, refer to the list of codes below from category H55:

> ☑4ᵗʰ **H55** **Nystagmus and other** irregular eye movements
>   ☑5ᵗʰ **H55.0** **Nystagmus**
>   **H55.00** Unspecified **nystagmus**
>   **H55.01** Congenital **nystagmus**
>   **H55.02** Latent **nystagmus**
>   **H55.03** Visual deprivation **nystagmus**
>   **H55.04** Dissociated **nystagmus**
>   **H55.09** **Other forms of nystagmus**

The portion of the code description that appears in **green font** in the tabular list helps the coder quickly identify the key terms and the correct code. This convention is especially useful when the codes describe laterality, such as the following codes from subcategory H40.22:

> ☑6ᵗʰ **H40.22** Chronic **angle-closure glaucoma**
>   Chronic primary angle closure glaucoma
>   ☑7ᵗʰ **H40.221** **Chronic angle-closure glaucoma,** right eye
>   ☑7ᵗʰ **H40.222** **Chronic angle-closure glaucoma,** left eye
>   ☑7ᵗʰ **H40.223** **Chronic angle-closure glaucoma,** bilateral
>   ☑7ᵗʰ **H40.229** **Chronic angle-closure glaucoma, unspecified eye**

Tabular Notations

Official parenthetical notes as well as Optum's supplementary notations are provided at the chapter, code block, category, subcategory, and individual code level to help the user assign proper codes. The information in the notation can apply to one or more codes depending on where the citation is placed.

Official Notations

Includes Notes

The word INCLUDES appears immediately under certain categories to further define, clarify, or give examples of the content of a code category.

Inclusion Terms

Lists of inclusion terms are included under certain codes. These terms indicate some of the conditions for which that code number may be used. Inclusion terms may be synonyms with the code title, or, in the case of "other specified" codes, the terms may also provide a list of various conditions included within a classification code. The inclusion terms are not exhaustive. The index may provide additional terms that may also be assigned to a given code.

Excludes Notes

ICD-10-CM has two types of excludes notes. Each note has a different definition for use. However, they are similar in that they both indicate that codes excluded from each other are independent of each other.

Excludes 1

An EXCLUDES 1 note is a "pure" excludes. It means "NOT CODED HERE!" An Excludes 1 note indicates mutually exclusive codes: two conditions that cannot be reported together. An Excludes1 note indicates that the code excluded should never be used at the same time as the code above the Excludes1 note. An Excludes1 is used when two conditions cannot occur together, such as a congenital form versus an acquired form of the same condition.

An exception to the Excludes 1 definition is when the two conditions are unrelated to each other. If it is not clear whether the two conditions involving an Excludes 1 note are related or not, query the provider. For example, code F45.8 Other somatoform disorders, has an Excludes 1 note

for "sleep related teeth grinding (G47.63)" because "teeth grinding" is an inclusion term under F45.8. Only one of these two codes should be assigned for teeth grinding. However psychogenic dysmenorrhea is also an inclusion term under F45.8, and a patient could have both this condition and sleep-related teeth grinding. In this case, the two conditions are clearly unrelated to each other, so it would be appropriate to report F45.8 and G47.63 together.

Excludes 2

An EXCLUDES 2 note means "NOT INCLUDED HERE." An Excludes 2 note indicates that although the excluded condition is not part of the condition it is excluded from, a patient may have both conditions at the same time. Therefore, when an Excludes 2 note appears under a code, it may be acceptable to use both the code and the excluded code together if supported by the medical documentation.

Note

The term "NOTE" appears as an icon and precedes the instructional information. These notes function as alerts to highlight coding instructions within the text.

Code First/Use additional code

These instructional notes provide sequencing instruction. They may appear independently of each other or to designate certain etiology/manifestation paired codes. These instructions signal the coder that an additional code should be reported to provide a more complete picture of that diagnosis.

In etiology/manifestation coding, ICD-10-CM requires the underlying condition to be sequenced first, followed by the manifestation. In these situations, codes with "In diseases classified elsewhere" in the code description are never permitted as a first-listed or principal diagnosis code and must be sequenced following the underlying condition code.

Code Also

A "code also" note alerts the coder that more than one code may be required to fully describe the condition. The sequencing depends on the circumstances of the encounter. Factors that may determine sequencing include severity and reason for the encounter.

Revised Text

The revised text ▶◀ "bow ties" alert the user to changes in official notations for the current year. Revised text may include the following:

- A change in a current parenthetical description

- A change in the code(s) associated with a current parenthetical note

- A change in how a current parenthetical note is classified (e.g., an Excludes 1 note that changed to an Excludes 2 note)

- Addition of a new parenthetical note(s) to a code

Deleted Text

~~Strikethrough~~ on official notations indicate a deletion from the classification for the current year.

Publisher Notations

AHA Coding Clinic Citations

Coding Clinics are official American Hospital Association (AHA) publications that provide coding advice specific to ICD-10-CM and ICD-10-PCS.

Coding Clinic citations included in this manual are current up to the second quarter of 2022.

These citations identify the year, quarter, and page number of one or more Coding Clinic publications that may have coding advice relevant to a particular code or group of codes. With the most current citation listed first, these notations are preceded by the symbol **AHA:** and appear in purple type.

> **I15.1** **Hypertension secondary to other renal disorders**
>   **AHA:** 2016, 3Q, 22

Definitions

Definitions explain a specific term, condition, or disease process in layman's terms. These notations are preceded by the symbol **DEF:** and appear in purple type.

> √5ᵗʰ **M51.4 Schmorl's nodes**
> **DEF:** Irregular bone defect in the margin of the vertebral body that causes herniation into the end plate of the vertebral body.

Coding Tips

The tips in the tabular list offer coding advice that is not readily available within the ICD-10-CM classification. It may relate official coding guidelines, indexing nuances, or advice from *AHA's Coding Clinic for ICD-10-CM/PCS*. These notations are preceded by the symbol **TIP:** and appear in brown type.

> √5ᵗʰ **B97.2 Coronavirus as the cause of diseases classified elsewhere**
> **TIP:** Do not report a code from this subcategory for COVID-19, refer to U07.1.

Icons

Note: The following icons are placed to the left of the code.

Changes to ICD-10-CM codes, since the last published edition of this manual, are highlighted in two ways:

The following green icons identify new or revised codes effective April 1, 2022:

● **New Code – Midyear**

▲ **Revised Code – Midyear**

The following black icons identify new or revised codes effective October 1, 2022:

● **New Code**

▲ **Revised Code**

☑ **Additional Characters Required**

√4ᵗʰ This symbol indicates that the code requires a 4th character.

√5ᵗʰ This symbol indicates that the code requires a 5th character.

√6ᵗʰ This symbol indicates that the code requires a 6th character.

√7ᵗʰ This symbol indicates that the code requires a 7th character.

> √5ᵗʰ **H60.3 Other** infective **otitis externa**
> √6ᵗʰ **H60.31** Diffuse **otitis externa**
> **H60.311 Diffuse otitis externa,** right **ear**
> **H60.312 Diffuse otitis externa,** left **ear**
> **H60.313 Diffuse otitis externa,** bilateral
> **H60.319 Diffuse otitis externa, unspecified ear**

√x7ᵗʰ **Placeholder Alert**
This symbol indicates that the code requires a 7th character following the placeholder "X". Codes with fewer than six characters that require a 7th character must contain placeholder "X" to fill in the empty character(s).

> √x7ᵗʰ **T16.1 Foreign body in** right **ear**

This manual provides the most current information that was available at the time of publication. Except where otherwise noted, the icons and/or color bars reflect edits provided in the Integrated Outpatient Code Editor (IOCE) quarterly files utilized under the outpatient prospective payment system (OPPS). Because the October 2022 quarterly files were not available at the time this book was printed, the edits in this manual are based on the July 2022 quarterly files.

The following is a list of IOCE edits specifically identified in this manual:

- Age
- Sex
- Manifestation
- Unacceptable principal diagnosis

Note: The following icons are placed at the end of the code description.

Age Edits

Ⓝ **Newborn Age: 0**
These diagnoses are intended for newborns and neonates and the patient's age must be 0 years.

> **N47.0 Adherent prepuce, newborn** Ⓝ♂

Ⓟ **Pediatric Age: 0-17**
These diagnoses are intended for children and the patient's age must be between 0 and 17 years.

> **L21.1 Seborrheic** infantile dermatitis Ⓟ

Ⓜ **Maternity Age: 9-64**
These diagnoses are intended for childbearing patients between the age of 9 and 64 years.

> **O02.9 Abnormal product of conception, unspecified** Ⓜ♀

Ⓐ **Adult Age: 15-124**
These diagnoses are intended for patients between the age of 15 and 124 years.

> **R54 Age-related physical debility** Ⓐ
> Frailty
> Old age
> Senescence
> Senile asthenia
> Senile debility
> *EXCLUDES 1* age-related cognitive decline (R41.81)
> sarcopenia (M62.84)
> senile psychosis (F03)
> senility NOS (R41.81)

Sex Edits

♂ **Male diagnosis only**

> **Q98.0 Klinefelter syndrome karyotype 47, XXY** ♂

♀ **Female diagnosis only**

> **N35.12 Postinfective urethral stricture, not elsewhere classified,** female ♀

UPD **Unacceptable Principal Diagnosis**
This icon identifies codes that are not appropriate as a first-listed code for *outpatient* encounters. These codes describe circumstances that influence an individual's health status but are not a current illness or injury, or that are not specifically manifestations but may be due to an underlying cause.

> √7ᵗʰ **T48.5X5** Adverse effect **of other anti-common-cold drugs** UPD

CMS-HCC Condition

This icon identifies codes that are considered a CMS-HCC (hierarchical condition category) diagnosis.

The HCC codes represented in this manual have been updated to reflect the 2023 Initial ICD-10-CM Mappings for CMS-HCC Model v24. Midyear final mappings were not available at the time this publication went to print; refer to the following CMS website for final mappings: https://www.cms.gov/Medicare/Health-Plans/MedicareAdvtgSpecRateStats/Risk-Adjustors.html.

Y62.2	**Failure of sterile precautions during** kidney dialysis and other perfusion `HCC`

Rx-HCC Condition

This icon identifies codes that are included in the Rx-HCC risk-adjustment model, which covers the Part D (prescription drug) benefit.

The Rx-HCC codes represented in this manual have been updated to reflect the 2023 Initial ICD-10-CM Mappings for CMS Rx-HCC Model v08. Midyear final mappings were not available at the time this publication went to print; refer to the following CMS website for final mappings: https://www.cms.gov/Medicare/Health-Plans/MedicareAdvtgSpecRateStats/Risk-Adjustors.html.

Z21	**Asymptomatic human immunodeficiency virus [HIV] infection status** `HCC` `Rx` `ESR` `COM`

ESRD HCC Condition

This icon identifies codes that are included in the end-stage renal disease (ESRD) HCC risk-adjustment model.

The ESRD HCC codes represented in this manual have been updated to reflect the 2023 Initial ICD-10-CM Mappings for CMS ESRD HCC Model v24. Midyear final mappings were not available at the time this publication went to print; refer to the following CMS website for final mappings: https://www.cms.gov/Medicare/Health-Plans/MedicareAdvtgSpecRateStats/Risk-Adjustors.html.

Z21	**Asymptomatic human immunodeficiency virus [HIV] infection status** `HCC` `Rx` `ESR` `COM`

Commercial HCC Condition

This icon identifies codes that are included in the commercial HHS-HCC risk-adjustment model.

The commercial HCC codes represented in this manual are based on the commercial HCC Model v07. These mappings can be found at the following: https://www.cms.gov/CCIIO/Resources/Regulations-and-Guidance.

Z21	**Asymptomatic human immunodeficiency virus [HIV] infection status** `HCC` `Rx` `ESR` `COM`

QPP Condition

This icon identifies codes recognized as a quality measure for claims-based reporting under CMS's Merit-based Incentive Payment System (MIPS) Claims Single Source v6.0.

G44.52	New daily persistent headache (NDPH) `Q`

Z-code as First-Listed Diagnosis

Section IV of the official guidelines states that the term "first-listed diagnosis" is used instead of principal diagnosis in the outpatient setting and represents the diagnosis that is chiefly responsible for the services provided during the encounter. This icon identifies Z codes that, in general, may be reported only as a first-listed diagnosis. According to guideline I.C.21.c.16, these are the only Z codes that are specifically meant to be utilized as a first-listed diagnosis; all other Z codes may be either first-listed or secondary diagnoses, depending upon the circumstances of the encounter, coding instructions, and guidelines.

Note: The codes identified with this icon may be used as a secondary diagnosis if the patient has multiple encounters on the same day and those medical records are combined.

A comprehensive list of all Z codes primarily used as first-listed diagnoses appears in appendix D of this book.

Z51.12	**Encounter for antineoplastic** immunotherapy `PDx`

Color Bars

Manifestation Code

Codes defined as manifestation codes appear in italic type, with a blue color bar over the code description. A manifestation cannot be reported as a first-listed code; it is sequenced as a secondary diagnosis with the underlying disease code listed first.

G32.89	*Other specified degenerative disorders of nervous system in diseases classified elsewhere* Degenerative encephalopathy in diseases classified elsewhere

Unspecified Diagnosis

Codes that appear with a gray color bar over the alphanumeric code identify unspecified diagnoses. These codes should be used in limited circumstances, when neither the diagnostic statement nor the documentation provides enough information to assign a more specific diagnosis code. The abbreviation NOS, "not otherwise specified," in the tabular list may be interpreted as "unspecified."

G03.9	**Meningitis, unspecified** Arachnoiditis (spinal) NOS

Footnotes

Certain codes in the tabular section have a numerical superscript located to the upper left of the code. This numerical superscript corresponds to a specific footnote description.

For example:

[1] `√7th` **M48.51**	**Collapsed vertebra, not elsewhere classified, occipito-atlanto-axial region** `HCC`

For convenience, the footnote descriptions are provided on the front cover.

The following list also provides the footnote descriptions of all numerical superscripts found in the Tabular List of Diseases:

1   These codes are considered an HCC when reported as an initial encounter (7th character A, B, or C).

2   These codes are considered an HCC when reported as an initial encounter (7th character A or B) OR sequela (7th character S).

3   These codes are considered an HCC when reported as a sequela (7th character S).

Chapter-Level Notations

Chapter-specific Guidelines with Coding Examples
Each chapter begins with the Official Guidelines for Coding and Reporting specific to that chapter, where provided. Coding examples specific to outpatient care settings have been provided to illustrate the coding and/or sequencing guidance in these guidelines.

Muscle and Tendon Table
ICD-10-CM categorizes certain muscles and tendons in the upper and lower extremities by their action (e.g., extension or flexion) as well as their anatomical location. The Muscle/Tendon table is provided at the beginning of chapter 13 and chapter 19 to help users when code selection depends on the action of the muscle and/or tendon.

Note: This table is not all-inclusive, and proper code assignment should be based on the provider's documentation.

Appendixes
The additional resources described below have been included as appendixes for this book. These resources further instruct the professional coder on the appropriate application of the ICD-10-CM code set.

Appendix A: Valid 3-character ICD-10-CM Codes
The user may consult this table to confirm that no further specificity, such as the use of 4th, 5th, 6th, or 7th characters or placeholders (X), is necessary. All ICD-10-CM codes that are valid at the three-character level are listed.

Appendix B: Pharmacology List 2023
This reference is a comprehensive but not all-inclusive list of pharmacological agents used to treat acute and/or chronic conditions. Drugs are listed in alphabetical order by their brand and/or generic names along with their drug action and indications for which they may commonly be prescribed. Some drugs have also been mapped to their appropriate Z code for long-term drug use.

Appendix C: Z Codes for Long-Term Drug Use with Associated Drugs
This resource correlates Z codes that are used to identify current long-term drug use with a list of drugs that are typically categorized to that class of drug.

Note: These tables are not all-inclusive but list some of the more commonly used drugs.

Appendix D: Z Codes Only as Principal/First-Listed Diagnosis
This resource provides a comprehensive list of Z codes that are primarily used as first-listed diagnoses for outpatient encounters.

Appendix E: Centers for Medicare & Medicaid Services Hierarchical Condition Categories (CMS-HCC)
This resource provides the framework behind the Centers for Medicare and Medicaid Services' (CMS) Medicare Advantage (MA) program, a risk-adjustment model developed as a means of compensating health care plans with large numbers of Medicare Part C beneficiaries. It includes a brief synopsis of the evolution of the program from its inception; insight into the various elements needed to predict risk, including the principles used to develop the hierarchical condition categories (HCCs), which make up one of the fundamental components of the risk-adjustment model. This appendix also outlines the audit process used to ensure the accuracy of payments made to MA plans.

Appendix F: Centers for Medicare & Medicaid Services Quality Payment Program
This resource provides an overview of the Medicare Access and CHIP Reauthorization Act (MACRA), which replaced Medicare's sustainable growth rate (SGR) methodology with the Quality Payment Program (QPP). It summarizes the Merit-based Incentive Payment System (MIPS) track used by those who opt to participate in traditional Medicare and not an advanced alternative payment model (APM). This includes eligibility requirements and an overview of the four performance categories that combine to make up the MIPS.

Illustrations
This section includes illustrations of normal anatomy with ICD-10-CM-specific terminology.

What's New for 2023

Official Updates

A summary of changes to the official ICD-10-CM code set is provided below, identifying changes made for fiscal 2023, effective October 1, 2022, to September 30, 2023. Asterisked codes identify prior midyear changes that were made to the classification, effective April 1, 2022. All code changes were made by the agency charged with maintaining and updating the ICD-10-CM code set, the National Center for Health Statistics (NCHS), a section of the Centers for Disease Control and Prevention (CDC).

1179 New Codes

B37.31	B37.32	D59.30	D59.31	D59.32
D59.39	D68.00	D68.01	D68.020	D68.021
D68.022	D68.023	D68.029	D68.03	D68.04
D68.09	D75.821	D75.822	D75.828	D75.829
D75.84	D81.82	E34.30	E34.31	E34.321
E34.322	E34.328	E34.329	E34.39	E87.20
E87.21	E87.22	E87.29	F01.511	F01.518
F01.52	F01.53	F01.54	F01.A0	F01.A11
F01.A18	F01.A2	F01.A3	F01.A4	F01.B0
F01.B11	F01.B18	F01.B2	F01.B3	F01.B4
F01.C0	F01.C11	F01.C18	F01.C2	F01.C3
F01.C4	F02.811	F02.818	F02.82	F02.83
F02.84	F02.A0	F02.A11	F02.A18	F02.A2
F02.A3	F02.A4	F02.B0	F02.B11	F02.B18
F02.B2	F02.B3	F02.B4	F02.C0	F02.C11
F02.C18	F02.C2	F02.C3	F02.C4	F03.911
F03.918	F03.92	F03.93	F03.94	F03.A0
F03.A11	F03.A18	F03.A2	F03.A3	F03.A4
F03.B0	F03.B11	F03.B18	F03.B2	F03.B3
F03.B4	F03.C0	F03.C11	F03.C18	F03.C2
F03.C3	F03.C4	F06.70	F06.71	F10.90
F10.91	F11.91	F12.91	F13.91	F14.91
F15.91	F16.91	F18.91	F19.91	F43.81
F43.89	G71.031	G71.032	G71.033	G71.0340
G71.0341	G71.0342	G71.0349	G71.035	G71.038
G71.039	G90.A	G93.31	G93.32	G93.39
I20.2	I25.112	I25.702	I25.712	I25.722
I25.732	I25.752	I25.762	I25.792	I31.31
I31.39	I34.81	I34.89	I47.20	I47.21
I47.29	I71.010	I71.011	I71.012	I71.019
I71.10	I71.11	I71.12	I71.13	I71.20
I71.21	I71.22	I71.23	I71.30	I71.31
I71.32	I71.33	I71.40	I71.41	I71.42
I71.43	I71.50	I71.51	I71.52	I71.60
I71.61	I71.62	I77.82	J95.87	K76.82
M51.A0	M51.A1	M51.A2	M51.A3	M51.A4
M51.A5	M62.5A0	M62.5A1	M62.5A2	M62.5A9
M93.004	M93.014	M93.024	M93.034	M93.041
M93.042	M93.043	M93.044	M93.051	M93.052
M93.053	M93.054	M93.061	M93.062	M93.063
M93.064	M93.071	M93.072	M93.073	M93.074
M96.A1	M96.A2	M96.A3	M96.A4	M96.A9
N14.11	N14.19	N76.82	N80.00	N80.01
N80.02	N80.03	N80.101	N80.102	N80.103
N80.109	N80.111	N80.112	N80.113	N80.119
N80.121	N80.122	N80.123	N80.129	N80.201
N80.202	N80.203	N80.209	N80.211	N80.212
N80.213	N80.219	N80.221	N80.222	N80.223
N80.229	N80.30	N80.311	N80.312	N80.319
N80.321	N80.322	N80.329	N80.331	N80.332
N80.333	N80.339	N80.341	N80.342	N80.343
N80.349	N80.351	N80.352	N80.353	N80.359
N80.361	N80.362	N80.363	N80.369	N80.371
N80.372	N80.373	N80.379	N80.381	N80.382
N80.383	N80.389	N80.391	N80.392	N80.399
N80.3A1	N80.3A2	N80.3A3	N80.3A9	N80.3B1
N80.3B2	N80.3B3	N80.3B9	N80.3C1	N80.3C2
N80.3C3	N80.3C9	N80.40	N80.41	N80.42
N80.50	N80.511	N80.512	N80.519	N80.521
N80.522	N80.529	N80.531	N80.532	N80.539
N80.541	N80.542	N80.549	N80.551	N80.552
N80.559	N80.561	N80.562	N80.569	N80.A0
N80.A1	N80.A2	N80.A41	N80.A42	N80.A43
N80.A49	N80.A51	N80.A52	N80.A53	N80.A59
N80.A61	N80.A62	N80.A63	N80.A69	N80.B1
N80.B2	N80.B31	N80.B32	N80.B39	N80.B4
N80.B5	N80.B6	N80.C0	N80.C10	N80.C11
N80.C19	N80.C2	N80.C3	N80.C4	N80.C9
N80.D0	N80.D1	N80.D2	N80.D3	N80.D4
N80.D5	N80.D6	N80.D9	N85.A	O35.00X0
O35.00X1	O35.00X2	O35.00X3	O35.00X4	O35.00X5
O35.00X9	O35.01X0	O35.01X1	O35.01X2	O35.01X3
O35.01X4	O35.01X5	O35.01X9	O35.02X0	O35.02X1
O35.02X2	O35.02X3	O35.02X4	O35.02X5	O35.02X9
O35.03X0	O35.03X1	O35.03X2	O35.03X3	O35.03X4
O35.03X5	O35.03X9	O35.04X0	O35.04X1	O35.04X2
O35.04X3	O35.04X4	O35.04X5	O35.04X9	O35.05X0
O35.05X1	O35.05X2	O35.05X3	O35.05X4	O35.05X5
O35.05X9	O35.06X0	O35.06X1	O35.06X2	O35.06X3
O35.06X4	O35.06X5	O35.06X9	O35.07X0	O35.07X1
O35.07X2	O35.07X3	O35.07X4	O35.07X5	O35.07X9
O35.08X0	O35.08X1	O35.08X2	O35.08X3	O35.08X4
O35.08X5	O35.08X9	O35.09X0	O35.09X1	O35.09X2
O35.09X3	O35.09X4	O35.09X5	O35.09X9	O35.10X0
O35.10X1	O35.10X2	O35.10X3	O35.10X4	O35.10X5
O35.10X9	O35.11X0	O35.11X1	O35.11X2	O35.11X3
O35.11X4	O35.11X5	O35.11X9	O35.12X0	O35.12X1
O35.12X2	O35.12X3	O35.12X4	O35.12X5	O35.12X9
O35.13X0	O35.13X1	O35.13X2	O35.13X3	O35.13X4
O35.13X5	O35.13X9	O35.14X0	O35.14X1	O35.14X2
O35.14X3	O35.14X4	O35.14X5	O35.14X9	O35.15X0
O35.15X1	O35.15X2	O35.15X3	O35.15X4	O35.15X5
O35.15X9	O35.19X0	O35.19X1	O35.19X2	O35.19X3
O35.19X4	O35.19X5	O35.19X9	O35.AXX0	O35.AXX1
O35.AXX2	O35.AXX3	O35.AXX4	O35.AXX5	O35.AXX9
O35.BXX0	O35.BXX1	O35.BXX2	O35.BXX3	O35.BXX4
O35.BXX5	O35.BXX9	O35.CXX0	O35.CXX1	O35.CXX2
O35.CXX3	O35.CXX4	O35.CXX5	O35.CXX9	O35.DXX0
O35.DXX1	O35.DXX2	O35.DXX3	O35.DXX4	O35.DXX5
O35.DXX9	O35.EXX0	O35.EXX1	O35.EXX2	O35.EXX3
O35.EXX4	O35.EXX5	O35.EXX9	O35.FXX0	O35.FXX1
O35.FXX2	O35.FXX3	O35.FXX4	O35.FXX5	O35.FXX9
O35.GXX0	O35.GXX1	O35.GXX2	O35.GXX3	O35.GXX4
O35.GXX5	O35.GXX9	O35.HXX0	O35.HXX1	O35.HXX2
O35.HXX3	O35.HXX4	O35.HXX5	O35.HXX9	P28.30
P28.31	P28.32	P28.33	P28.39	P28.40
P28.41	P28.42	P28.43	P28.49	Q21.10
Q21.11	Q21.12	Q21.13	Q21.14	Q21.15
Q21.16	Q21.19	Q21.20	Q21.21	Q21.22
Q21.23	Q85.81	Q85.82	Q85.83	Q85.89
S06.0XAA	S06.0XAD	S06.0XAS	S06.1XAA	S06.1XAD
S06.1XAS	S06.2XAA	S06.2XAD	S06.2XAS	S06.30AA
S06.30AD	S06.30AS	S06.31AA	S06.31AD	S06.31AS
S06.32AA	S06.32AD	S06.32AS	S06.33AA	S06.33AD
S06.33AS	S06.34AA	S06.34AD	S06.34AS	S06.35AA
S06.35AD	S06.35AS	S06.36AA	S06.36AD	S06.36AS
S06.37AA	S06.37AD	S06.37AS	S06.38AA	S06.38AD
S06.38AS	S06.4XAA	S06.4XAD	S06.4XAS	S06.5XAA

What's New for 2023 *(side tab)*

S06.5XAD	S06.5XAS	S06.6XAA	S06.6XAD	S06.6XAS
S06.81AA	S06.81AD	S06.81AS	S06.82AA	S06.82AD
S06.82AS	S06.89AA	S06.89AD	S06.89AS	S06.8A0A
S06.8A0D	S06.8A0S	S06.8A1A	S06.8A1D	S06.8A1S
S06.8A2A	S06.8A2D	S06.8A2S	S06.8A3A	S06.8A3D
S06.8A3S	S06.8A4A	S06.8A4D	S06.8A4S	S06.8A5A
S06.8A5D	S06.8A5S	S06.8A6A	S06.8A6D	S06.8A6S
S06.8A7A	S06.8A8A	S06.8A9A	S06.8A9D	S06.8A9S
S06.8AAA	S06.8AAD	S06.8AAS	S06.9XAA	S06.9XAD
S06.9XAS	T43.651A	T43.651D	T43.651S	T43.652A
T43.652D	T43.652S	T43.653A	T43.653D	T43.653S
T43.654A	T43.654D	T43.654S	T43.655A	T43.655D
T43.655S	T43.656A	T43.656D	T43.656S	V20.01XA
V20.01XD	V20.01XS	V20.09XA	V20.09XD	V20.09XS
V20.11XA	V20.11XD	V20.11XS	V20.19XA	V20.19XD
V20.19XS	V20.21XA	V20.21XD	V20.21XS	V20.29XA
V20.29XD	V20.29XS	V20.31XA	V20.31XD	V20.31XS
V20.39XA	V20.39XD	V20.39XS	V20.41XA	V20.41XD
V20.41XS	V20.49XA	V20.49XD	V20.49XS	V20.51XA
V20.51XD	V20.51XS	V20.59XA	V20.59XD	V20.59XS
V20.91XA	V20.91XD	V20.91XS	V20.99XA	V20.99XD
V20.99XS	V21.01XA	V21.01XD	V21.01XS	V21.09XA
V21.09XD	V21.09XS	V21.11XA	V21.11XD	V21.11XS
V21.19XA	V21.19XD	V21.19XS	V21.21XA	V21.21XD
V21.21XS	V21.29XA	V21.29XD	V21.29XS	V21.31XA
V21.31XD	V21.31XS	V21.39XA	V21.39XD	V21.39XS
V21.41XA	V21.41XD	V21.41XS	V21.49XA	V21.49XD
V21.49XS	V21.51XA	V21.51XD	V21.51XS	V21.59XA
V21.59XD	V21.59XS	V21.91XA	V21.91XD	V21.91XS
V21.99XA	V21.99XD	V21.99XS	V22.01XA	V22.01XD
V22.01XS	V22.09XA	V22.09XD	V22.09XS	V22.11XA
V22.11XD	V22.11XS	V22.19XA	V22.19XD	V22.19XS
V22.21XA	V22.21XD	V22.21XS	V22.29XA	V22.29XD
V22.29XS	V22.31XA	V22.31XD	V22.31XS	V22.39XA
V22.39XD	V22.39XS	V22.41XA	V22.41XD	V22.41XS
V22.49XA	V22.49XD	V22.49XS	V22.51XA	V22.51XD
V22.51XS	V22.59XA	V22.59XD	V22.59XS	V22.91XA
V22.91XD	V22.91XS	V22.99XA	V22.99XD	V22.99XS
V23.01XA	V23.01XD	V23.01XS	V23.09XA	V23.09XD
V23.09XS	V23.11XA	V23.11XD	V23.11XS	V23.19XA
V23.19XD	V23.19XS	V23.21XA	V23.21XD	V23.21XS
V23.29XA	V23.29XD	V23.29XS	V23.31XA	V23.31XD
V23.31XS	V23.39XA	V23.39XD	V23.39XS	V23.41XA
V23.41XD	V23.41XS	V23.49XA	V23.49XD	V23.49XS
V23.51XA	V23.51XD	V23.51XS	V23.59XA	V23.59XD
V23.59XS	V23.91XA	V23.91XD	V23.91XS	V23.99XA
V23.99XD	V23.99XS	V24.01XA	V24.01XD	V24.01XS
V24.09XA	V24.09XD	V24.09XS	V24.11XA	V24.11XD
V24.11XS	V24.19XA	V24.19XD	V24.19XS	V24.21XA
V24.21XD	V24.21XS	V24.29XA	V24.29XD	V24.29XS
V24.31XA	V24.31XD	V24.31XS	V24.39XA	V24.39XD
V24.39XS	V24.41XA	V24.41XD	V24.41XS	V24.49XA
V24.49XD	V24.49XS	V24.51XA	V24.51XD	V24.51XS
V24.59XA	V24.59XD	V24.59XS	V24.91XA	V24.91XD
V24.91XS	V24.99XA	V24.99XD	V24.99XS	V25.01XA
V25.01XD	V25.01XS	V25.09XA	V25.09XD	V25.09XS
V25.11XA	V25.11XD	V25.11XS	V25.19XA	V25.19XD
V25.19XS	V25.21XA	V25.21XD	V25.21XS	V25.29XA
V25.29XD	V25.29XS	V25.31XA	V25.31XD	V25.31XS
V25.39XA	V25.39XD	V25.39XS	V25.41XA	V25.41XD
V25.41XS	V25.49XA	V25.49XD	V25.49XS	V25.51XA
V25.51XD	V25.51XS	V25.59XA	V25.59XD	V25.59XS
V25.91XA	V25.91XD	V25.91XS	V25.99XA	V25.99XD
V25.99XS	V26.01XA	V26.01XD	V26.01XS	V26.09XA
V26.09XD	V26.09XS	V26.11XA	V26.11XD	V26.11XS
V26.19XA	V26.19XD	V26.19XS	V26.21XA	V26.21XD
V26.21XS	V26.29XA	V26.29XD	V26.29XS	V26.31XA

V26.31XD	V26.31XS	V26.39XA	V26.39XD	V26.39XS
V26.41XA	V26.41XD	V26.41XS	V26.49XA	V26.49XD
V26.49XS	V26.51XA	V26.51XD	V26.51XS	V26.59XA
V26.59XD	V26.59XS	V26.91XA	V26.91XD	V26.91XS
V26.99XA	V26.99XD	V26.99XS	V27.01XA	V27.01XD
V27.01XS	V27.09XA	V27.09XD	V27.09XS	V27.11XA
V27.11XD	V27.11XS	V27.19XA	V27.19XD	V27.19XS
V27.21XA	V27.21XD	V27.21XS	V27.29XA	V27.29XD
V27.29XS	V27.31XA	V27.31XD	V27.31XS	V27.39XA
V27.39XD	V27.39XS	V27.41XA	V27.41XD	V27.41XS
V27.49XA	V27.49XD	V27.49XS	V27.51XA	V27.51XD
V27.51XS	V27.59XA	V27.59XD	V27.59XS	V27.91XA
V27.91XD	V27.91XS	V27.99XA	V27.99XD	V27.99XS
V28.01XA	V28.01XD	V28.01XS	V28.09XA	V28.09XD
V28.09XS	V28.11XA	V28.11XD	V28.11XS	V28.19XA
V28.19XD	V28.19XS	V28.21XA	V28.21XD	V28.21XS
V28.29XA	V28.29XD	V28.29XS	V28.31XA	V28.31XD
V28.31XS	V28.39XA	V28.39XD	V28.39XS	V28.41XA
V28.41XD	V28.41XS	V28.49XA	V28.49XD	V28.49XS
V28.51XA	V28.51XD	V28.51XS	V28.59XA	V28.59XD
V28.59XS	V28.91XA	V28.91XD	V28.91XS	V28.99XA
V28.99XD	V28.99XS	V29.001A	V29.001D	V29.001S
V29.008A	V29.008D	V29.008S	V29.091A	V29.091D
V29.091S	V29.098A	V29.098D	V29.098S	V29.101A
V29.101D	V29.101S	V29.108A	V29.108D	V29.108S
V29.191A	V29.191D	V29.191S	V29.198A	V29.198D
V29.198S	V29.201A	V29.201D	V29.201S	V29.208A
V29.208D	V29.208S	V29.291A	V29.291D	V29.291S
V29.298A	V29.298D	V29.298S	V29.31XA	V29.31XD
V29.31XS	V29.39XA	V29.39XD	V29.39XS	V29.401A
V29.401D	V29.401S	V29.408A	V29.408D	V29.408S
V29.491A	V29.491D	V29.491S	V29.498A	V29.498D
V29.498S	V29.501A	V29.501D	V29.501S	V29.508A
V29.508D	V29.508S	V29.591A	V29.591D	V29.591S
V29.598A	V29.598D	V29.598S	V29.601A	V29.601D
V29.601S	V29.608A	V29.608D	V29.608S	V29.691A
V29.691D	V29.691S	V29.698A	V29.698D	V29.698S
V29.811A	V29.811D	V29.811S	V29.818A	V29.818D
V29.818S	V29.881A	V29.881D	V29.881S	V29.888A
V29.888D	V29.888S	V29.91XA	V29.91XD	V29.91XS
V29.99XA	V29.99XD	V29.99XS	W23.2XXA	W23.2XXD
W23.2XXS	Z03.83	*Z28.310	*Z28.311	*Z28.39
Z59.82	Z59.86	Z59.87	Z71.87	Z71.88
Z72.823	Z79.60	Z79.61	Z79.620	Z79.621
Z79.622	Z79.623	Z79.624	Z79.630	Z79.631
Z79.632	Z79.633	Z79.634	Z79.64	Z79.69
Z79.85	Z87.61	Z87.68	Z87.731	Z87.732
Z87.760	Z87.761	Z87.762	Z87.763	Z87.768
Z91.110	Z91.118	Z91.119	Z91.190	Z91.198
Z91.199	Z91.A10	Z91.A18	Z91.A20	Z91.A28
Z91.A3	Z91.A4	Z91.A5	Z91.A9	

28 Revised Codes
Note: Each code is listed with its revised description only.

C84.40	Peripheral T-cell lymphoma, not elsewhere classified, unspecified site
C84.41	Peripheral T-cell lymphoma, not elsewhere classified, lymph nodes of head, face, and neck
C84.42	Peripheral T-cell lymphoma, not elsewhere classified, intrathoracic lymph nodes
C84.43	Peripheral T-cell lymphoma, not elsewhere classified, intra-abdominal lymph nodes
C84.44	Peripheral T-cell lymphoma, not elsewhere classified, lymph nodes of axilla and upper limb
C84.45	Peripheral T-cell lymphoma, not elsewhere classified, lymph nodes of inguinal region and lower limb

C84.46	Peripheral T-cell lymphoma, not elsewhere classified, intrapelvic lymph nodes
C84.47	Peripheral T-cell lymphoma, not elsewhere classified, spleen
C84.48	Peripheral T-cell lymphoma, not elsewhere classified, lymph nodes of multiple sites
C84.49	Peripheral T-cell lymphoma, not elsewhere classified, extranodal and solid organ sites
C94.6	Myelodysplastic disease, not elsewhere classified
F01.50	Vascular dementia, unspecified severity, without behavioral disturbance, psychotic disturbance, mood disturbance, and anxiety
F02.80	Dementia in other diseases classified elsewhere, unspecified severity, without behavioral disturbance, psychotic disturbance, mood disturbance, and anxiety
F03.90	Unspecified dementia, unspecified severity, without behavioral disturbance, psychotic disturbance, mood disturbance, and anxiety
G31.09	Other frontotemporal neurocognitive disorder
G31.83	Neurocognitive disorder with Lewy bodies
G31.84	Mild cognitive impairment of uncertain or unknown etiology
K35.32	Acute appendicitis with perforation, localized peritonitis, and gangrene, without abscess
K35.33	Acute appendicitis with perforation, localized peritonitis, and gangrene, with abscess
M93.011	Acute slipped upper femoral epiphysis, stable (nontraumatic), right hip
M93.012	Acute slipped upper femoral epiphysis, stable (nontraumatic), left hip
M93.013	Acute slipped upper femoral epiphysis, stable (nontraumatic), unspecified hip
M93.021	Chronic slipped upper femoral epiphysis, stable (nontraumatic), right hip
M93.022	Chronic slipped upper femoral epiphysis, stable (nontraumatic), left hip
M93.023	Chronic slipped upper femoral epiphysis, stable (nontraumatic), unspecified hip
M93.031	Acute on chronic slipped upper femoral epiphysis, stable (nontraumatic), right hip
M93.032	Acute on chronic slipped upper femoral epiphysis, stable (nontraumatic), left hip
M93.033	Acute on chronic slipped upper femoral epiphysis, stable (nontraumatic), unspecified hip

0 Deleted Codes

288 Codes with a Change in Validity

Note: Validity changes are the result of codes being added to or deleted from the classification. Codes that change from valid to invalid allow the creation of a new subcategory to which new codes can be assigned that provide greater detail about the condition. Codes that change from invalid to valid are the result of codes being deleted from a subcategory in the classification, when the detail provided in those codes is no longer required.

Valid to Invalid

B37.3	D59.3	D68.0	D75.82	E34.3
E87.2	F01.51	F02.81	F03.91	F43.8
G93.3	I31.3	I34.8	I47.2	I71.01
I71.1	I71.2	I71.3	I71.4	I71.5
I71.6	N14.1	N80.0	N80.1	N80.2
N80.3	N80.4	N80.5	O35.0XX0	O35.0XX1

O35.0XX2	O35.0XX3	O35.0XX4	O35.0XX5	O35.0XX9
O35.1XX0	O35.1XX1	O35.1XX2	O35.1XX3	O35.1XX4
O35.1XX5	O35.1XX9	P28.3	P28.4	Q21.1
Q21.2	Q85.8	V20.0XXA	V20.0XXD	V20.0XXS
V20.1XXA	V20.1XXD	V20.1XXS	V20.2XXA	V20.2XXD
V20.2XXS	V20.3XXA	V20.3XXD	V20.3XXS	V20.4XXA
V20.4XXD	V20.4XXS	V20.5XXA	V20.5XXD	V20.5XXS
V20.9XXA	V20.9XXD	V20.9XXS	V21.0XXA	V21.0XXD
V21.0XXS	V21.1XXA	V21.1XXD	V21.1XXS	V21.2XXA
V21.2XXD	V21.2XXS	V21.3XXA	V21.3XXD	V21.3XXS
V21.4XXA	V21.4XXD	V21.4XXS	V21.5XXA	V21.5XXD
V21.5XXS	V21.9XXA	V21.9XXD	V21.9XXS	V22.0XXA
V22.0XXD	V22.0XXS	V22.1XXA	V22.1XXD	V22.1XXS
V22.2XXA	V22.2XXD	V22.2XXS	V22.3XXA	V22.3XXD
V22.3XXS	V22.4XXA	V22.4XXD	V22.4XXS	V22.5XXA
V22.5XXD	V22.5XXS	V22.9XXA	V22.9XXD	V22.9XXS
V23.0XXA	V23.0XXD	V23.0XXS	V23.1XXA	V23.1XXD
V23.1XXS	V23.2XXA	V23.2XXD	V23.2XXS	V23.3XXA
V23.3XXD	V23.3XXS	V23.4XXA	V23.4XXD	V23.4XXS
V23.5XXA	V23.5XXD	V23.5XXS	V23.9XXA	V23.9XXD
V23.9XXS	V24.0XXA	V24.0XXD	V24.0XXS	V24.1XXA
V24.1XXD	V24.1XXS	V24.2XXA	V24.2XXD	V24.2XXS
V24.3XXA	V24.3XXD	V24.3XXS	V24.4XXA	V24.4XXD
V24.4XXS	V24.5XXA	V24.5XXD	V24.5XXS	V24.9XXA
V24.9XXD	V24.9XXS	V25.0XXA	V25.0XXD	V25.0XXS
V25.1XXA	V25.1XXD	V25.1XXS	V25.2XXA	V25.2XXD
V25.2XXS	V25.3XXA	V25.3XXD	V25.3XXS	V25.4XXA
V25.4XXD	V25.4XXS	V25.5XXA	V25.5XXD	V25.5XXS
V25.9XXA	V25.9XXD	V25.9XXS	V26.0XXA	V26.0XXD
V26.0XXS	V26.1XXA	V26.1XXD	V26.1XXS	V26.2XXA
V26.2XXD	V26.2XXS	V26.3XXA	V26.3XXD	V26.3XXS
V26.4XXA	V26.4XXD	V26.4XXS	V26.5XXA	V26.5XXD
V26.5XXS	V26.9XXA	V26.9XXD	V26.9XXS	V27.0XXA
V27.0XXD	V27.0XXS	V27.1XXA	V27.1XXD	V27.1XXS
V27.2XXA	V27.2XXD	V27.2XXS	V27.3XXA	V27.3XXD
V27.3XXS	V27.4XXA	V27.4XXD	V27.4XXS	V27.5XXA
V27.5XXD	V27.5XXS	V27.9XXA	V27.9XXD	V27.9XXS
V28.0XXA	V28.0XXD	V28.0XXS	V28.1XXA	V28.1XXD
V28.1XXS	V28.2XXA	V28.2XXD	V28.2XXS	V28.3XXA
V28.3XXD	V28.3XXS	V28.4XXA	V28.4XXD	V28.4XXS
V28.5XXA	V28.5XXD	V28.5XXS	V28.9XXA	V28.9XXD
V28.9XXS	V29.00XA	V29.00XD	V29.00XS	V29.09XA
V29.09XD	V29.09XS	V29.10XA	V29.10XD	V29.10XS
V29.19XA	V29.19XD	V29.19XS	V29.20XA	V29.20XD
V29.20XS	V29.29XA	V29.29XD	V29.29XS	V29.3XXA
V29.3XXD	V29.3XXS	V29.40XA	V29.40XD	V29.40XS
V29.49XA	V29.49XD	V29.49XS	V29.50XA	V29.50XD
V29.50XS	V29.59XA	V29.59XD	V29.59XS	V29.60XA
V29.60XD	V29.60XS	V29.69XA	V29.69XD	V29.69XS
V29.81XA	V29.81XD	V29.81XS	V29.88XA	V29.88XD
V29.88XS	V29.9XXA	V29.9XXD	V29.9XXS	*Z28.3
Z87.76	Z91.11	Z91.19		

Invalid to Valid
No applicable codes

Proprietary Updates
The following proprietary features have also been added:

- New definitions that describe, in lay terms, a specific condition or disease process

- New coding tips that provide coding advice beyond the code classification

- Updated *AHA Coding Clinic* references through second quarter 2022

Conversion Table of ICD-10-CM Codes

The fiscal 2023 (October 1, 2022–September 30, 2023) Conversion Table for new ICD-10-CM codes is provided to assist users in data retrieval. For each new code the table shows its previously assigned code equivalent. Asterisks identify new codes added to the classification April 1, 2022.

Code Assignment Beginning 10/1/2022	Previous Code(s) Assignment
B37.31	B37.3
B37.32	B37.3
D59.30	D59.3
D59.31	D59.3
D59.32	D59.3
D59.39	D59.3
D68.00	D68.0
D68.01	D68.0
D68.020	D68.0
D68.021	D68.0
D68.022	D68.0
D68.023	D68.0
D68.029	D68.0
D68.03	D68.0
D68.04	D68.0
D68.09	D68.0
D75.821	D75.82
D75.822	D75.82
D75.828	D75.82
D75.829	D75.82
D75.84	D75.89
D81.82	D81.89
E34.30	E34.3
E34.31	E34.3
E34.321	E34.3
E34.322	E34.3
E34.328	E34.3
E34.329	E34.3
E34.39	E34.3
E87.20	E87.2
E87.21	E87.2
E87.22	E87.2
E87.29	E87.2
F01.511	F01.51
F01.518	F01.51
F01.52	F01.51
F01.53	F01.51
F01.54	F01.51
F01.A0	F01.50
F01.A11	F01.51
F01.A18	F01.51
F01.A2	F01.51
F01.A3	F01.51
F01.A4	F01.51
F01.B0	F01.50
F01.B11	F01.51
F01.B18	F01.51
F01.B2	F01.51
F01.B3	F01.51
F01.B4	F01.51
F01.C0	F01.50
F01.C11	F01.51
F01.C18	F01.51
F01.C2	F01.51
F01.C3	F01.51
F01.C4	F01.51
F02.811	F02.81
F02.818	F02.81
F02.82	F02.81
F02.83	F02.81
F02.84	F02.81
F02.A0	F02.80
F02.A11	F02.81
F02.A18	F02.81
F02.A2	F02.81
F02.A3	F02.81
F02.A4	F02.81
F02.B0	F02.80
F02.B11	F02.81
F02.B18	F02.81
F02.B2	F02.81
F02.B3	F02.81
F02.B4	F02.81
F02.C0	F02.80
F02.C11	F02.81
F02.C18	F02.81
F02.C2	F02.81
F02.C3	F02.81
F02.C4	F02.81
F03.911	F03.91
F03.918	F03.91
F03.92	F03.91
F03.93	F03.91
F03.94	F03.91
F03.A0	F03.90
F03.A11	F03.91
F03.A18	F03.91
F03.A2	F03.91
F03.A3	F03.91
F03.A4	F03.91
F03.B0	F03.90
F03.B11	F03.91
F03.B18	F03.91
F03.B2	F03.91
F03.B3	F03.91
F03.B4	F03.91
F03.C0	F03.90
F03.C11	F03.91
F03.C18	F03.91
F03.C2	F03.91
F03.C3	F03.91
F03.C4	F03.91
F06.70	G31.84
F06.71	G31.84
F10.90	Z72.89
F10.91	Z72.89
F11.91	F11.90
F12.91	F12.90
F13.91	F13.90
F14.91	F14.90
F15.91	F15.90
F16.91	F16.90
F18.91	F18.90
F19.91	F19.90
F43.81	F43.8
F43.89	F43.8
G71.031	G71.09
G71.032	G71.09
G71.033	G71.09
G71.0340	G71.09
G71.0341	G71.09
G71.0342	G71.09
G71.0349	G71.09
G71.035	G71.09
G71.038	G71.09
G71.039	G71.09
G90.A	I49.8
G93.31	G93.3
G93.32	G93.3; R53.82
G93.39	G93.3
I20.2	I20.0-I20.1; I20.8
I25.112	I25.110-I25.111; I25.118
I25.702	I25.700-I25.701; I25.708
I25.712	I25.710-I25.711; I25.718
I25.722	I25.720-I25.721; I25.728
I25.732	I25.730-I25.731; I25.738
I25.752	I25.750-I25.751; I25.758
I25.762	I25.760-I25.761; I25.768
I25.792	I25.790-I25.791; I25.798
I31.31	I31.3
I31.39	I31.3
I34.81	I34.8
I34.89	I34.8
I47.20	I47.2
I47.21	I47.2
I47.29	I47.2
I71.010	I71.01
I71.011	I71.01
I71.012	I71.01
I71.019	I71.01
I71.10	I71.1
I71.11	I71.1
I71.12	I71.1
I71.13	I71.1
I71.20	I71.2
I71.21	I71.2
I71.22	I71.2
I71.23	I71.2
I71.30	I71.3
I71.31	I71.3
I71.32	I71.3
I71.33	I71.3
I71.40	I71.4
I71.41	I71.4
I71.42	I71.4
I71.43	I71.4
I71.50	I71.5
I71.51	I71.5
I71.52	I71.5
I71.60	I71.6
I71.61	I71.6
I71.62	I71.6
I77.82	I77.89
J95.87	J95.89
K76.82	K72.90-K72.91
M51.A0	M51.86
M51.A1	M51.86
M51.A2	M51.86
M51.A3	M51.87
M51.A4	M51.87
M51.A5	M51.87
M62.5A0	M62.58
M62.5A1	M62.58
M62.5A2	M62.58
M62.5A9	M62.58
M93.004	M93.001 & M93.002
M93.014	M93.011 & M93.012
M93.024	M93.021 & M93.022
M93.034	M93.031 & M93.032
M93.041	M93.011
M93.042	M93.012
M93.043	M93.013
M93.044	M93.011 & M93.012
M93.051	M93.031
M93.052	M93.032
M93.053	M93.033
M93.054	M93.031 & M93.032
M93.061	M93.011
M93.062	M93.012
M93.063	M93.013
M93.064	M93.011 & M93.012
M93.071	M93.031
M93.072	M93.032
M93.073	M93.033
M93.074	M93.031 & M93.032
M96.A1	M96.89 & Y84.8
M96.A2	M96.89 & Y84.8
M96.A3	M96.89 & Y84.8
M96.A4	M96.89 & Y84.8
M96.A9	M96.89 & Y84.8
N14.11	N14.1
N14.19	N14.1
N76.82	N76.89
N80.00	N80.0
N80.01	N80.0
N80.02	N80.0
N80.03	N80.0
N80.101	N80.1
N80.102	N80.1
N80.103	N80.1
N80.109	N80.1
N80.111	N80.1
N80.112	N80.1
N80.113	N80.1
N80.119	N80.1
N80.121	N80.1
N80.122	N80.1
N80.123	N80.1
N80.129	N80.1
N80.201	N80.2
N80.202	N80.2
N80.203	N80.2
N80.209	N80.2
N80.211	N80.2
N80.212	N80.2
N80.213	N80.2
N80.219	N80.2
N80.221	N80.2
N80.222	N80.2
N80.223	N80.2
N80.229	N80.2
N80.30	N80.3
N80.311	N80.3
N80.312	N80.3
N80.319	N80.3
N80.321	N80.3
N80.322	N80.3
N80.329	N80.3
N80.331	N80.3
N80.332	N80.3
N80.333	N80.3
N80.339	N80.3
N80.341	N80.3
N80.342	N80.3
N80.343	N80.3
N80.349	N80.3
N80.351	N80.3
N80.352	N80.3
N80.353	N80.3
N80.359	N80.3
N80.361	N80.3
N80.362	N80.3
N80.363	N80.3
N80.369	N80.3
N80.371	N80.3
N80.372	N80.3
N80.373	N80.3
N80.379	N80.3
N80.381	N80.3
N80.382	N80.3
N80.383	N80.3
N80.389	N80.3
N80.3A1	N80.3
N80.3A2	N80.3
N80.3A3	N80.3
N80.3A9	N80.3
N80.3B1	N80.3
N80.3B2	N80.3
N80.3B3	N80.3
N80.3B9	N80.3
N80.3C1	N80.3
N80.3C2	N80.3
N80.3C3	N80.3
N80.3C9	N80.3
N80.391	N80.3
N80.392	N80.3
N80.399	N80.3
N80.40	N80.3
N80.41	N80.4
N80.42	N80.4
N80.50	N80.5
N80.511	N80.5
N80.512	N80.5
N80.519	N80.5
N80.521	N80.5
N80.522	N80.5
N80.529	N80.5
N80.531	N80.5
N80.532	N80.5
N80.539	N80.5

Conversion Table of ICD-10-CM Codes

Code Assignment Beginning 10/1/2022	Previous Code(s) Assignment	Code Assignment Beginning 10/1/2022	Previous Code(s) Assignment	Code Assignment Beginning 10/1/2022	Previous Code(s) Assignment	Code Assignment Beginning 10/1/2022	Previous Code(s) Assignment	Code Assignment Beginning 10/1/2022	Previous Code(s) Assignment	Code Assignment Beginning 10/1/2022	Previous Code(s) Assignment
N80.541	N80.5	O35.01X3	O35.0XX3	O35.09X9	O35.0XX9	O35.BXX2	O35.8XX2	Q21.12	Q21.1	S06.81AA	S06.819A
N80.542	N80.5	O35.01X4	O35.0XX4	O35.10X0	O35.1XX0	O35.BXX3	O35.8XX3	Q21.13	Q21.1	S06.81AD	S06.819D
N80.549	N80.5	O35.01X5	O35.0XX5	O35.10X1	O35.1XX1	O35.BXX4	O35.8XX4	Q21.14	Q21.1	S06.81AS	S06.819S
N80.551	N80.5	O35.01X9	O35.0XX9	O35.10X2	O35.1XX2	O35.BXX5	O35.8XX5	Q21.15	Q21.1	S06.82AA	S06.829A
N80.552	N80.5	O35.02X0	O35.0XX0	O35.10X3	O35.1XX3	O35.BXX9	O35.8XX9	Q21.16	Q21.1	S06.82AD	S06.829D
N80.559	N80.5	O35.02X1	O35.0XX1	O35.10X4	O35.1XX4	O35.CXX0	O35.8XX0	Q21.19	Q21.1	S06.82AS	S06.829S
N80.561	N80.5	O35.02X2	O35.0XX2	O35.10X5	O35.1XX5	O35.CXX1	O35.8XX1	Q21.20	Q21.2	S06.8A0A	S06.0X0A
N80.562	N80.5	O35.02X3	O35.0XX3	O35.10X9	O35.1XX9	O35.CXX2	O35.8XX2	Q21.21	Q21.2	S06.8A0D	S06.0X0D
N80.569	N80.5	O35.02X4	O35.0XX4	O35.11X0	O35.1XX0	O35.CXX3	O35.8XX3	Q21.22	Q21.2	S06.8A0S	S06.0X0S
N80.A0	N80.8	O35.02X5	O35.0XX5	O35.11X1	O35.1XX1	O35.CXX4	O35.8XX4	Q21.23	Q21.2	S06.8A1A	S06.0X9A
N80.A1	N80.8	O35.02X9	O35.0XX9	O35.11X2	O35.1XX2	O35.CXX5	O35.8XX5	Q85.81	Q85.8	S06.8A1D	S06.0X9D
N80.A2	N80.8	O35.03X0	O35.0XX0	O35.11X3	O35.1XX3	O35.CXX9	O35.8XX9	Q85.82	Q85.8	S06.8A1S	S06.0X9S
N80.A41	N80.8	O35.03X1	O35.0XX1	O35.11X4	O35.1XX4	O35.DXX0	O35.8XX0	Q85.83	Q85.8	S06.8A2A	S06.0X9A
N80.A42	N80.8	O35.03X2	O35.0XX2	O35.11X5	O35.1XX5	O35.DXX1	O35.8XX1	Q85.89	Q85.8	S06.8A2D	S06.0X9D
N80.A43	N80.8	O35.03X3	O35.0XX3	O35.11X9	O35.1XX9	O35.DXX2	O35.8XX2	S06.0XAA	S06.0X9A	S06.8A2S	S06.0X9S
N80.A49	N80.8	O35.03X4	O35.0XX4	O35.12X0	O35.1XX0	O35.DXX3	O35.8XX3	S06.0XAD	S06.0X9D	S06.8A3A	S06.0X9A
N80.A51	N80.8	O35.03X5	O35.0XX5	O35.12X1	O35.1XX1	O35.DXX4	O35.8XX4	S06.0XAS	S06.0X9S	S06.8A3D	S06.0X9D
N80.A52	N80.8	O35.03X9	O35.0XX9	O35.12X2	O35.1XX2	O35.DXX5	O35.8XX5	S06.1XAA	S06.1X9A	S06.8A3S	S06.0X9S
N80.A53	N80.8	O35.04X0	O35.0XX0	O35.12X3	O35.1XX3	O35.DXX9	O35.8XX9	S06.1XAD	S06.1X9D	S06.8A4A	S06.0X9A
N80.A59	N80.8	O35.04X1	O35.0XX1	O35.12X4	O35.1XX4	O35.EXX0	O35.8XX0	S06.1XAS	S06.1X9S	S06.8A4D	S06.0X9D
N80.A61	N80.8	O35.04X2	O35.0XX2	O35.12X5	O35.1XX5	O35.EXX1	O35.8XX1	S06.2XAA	S06.2X9A	S06.8A4S	S06.0X9S
N80.A62	N80.8	O35.04X3	O35.0XX3	O35.12X9	O35.1XX9	O35.EXX2	O35.8XX2	S06.2XAD	S06.2X9D	S06.8A5A	S06.0X9A
N80.A63	N80.8	O35.04X4	O35.0XX4	O35.13X0	O35.1XX0	O35.EXX3	O35.8XX3	S06.2XAS	S06.2X9S	S06.8A5D	S06.0X9D
N80.A69	N80.8	O35.04X5	O35.0XX5	O35.13X1	O35.1XX1	O35.EXX4	O35.8XX4	S06.30AA	S06.309A	S06.8A5S	S06.0X9S
N80.B1	N80.8	O35.04X9	O35.0XX9	O35.13X2	O35.1XX2	O35.EXX5	O35.8XX5	S06.30AD	S06.309D	S06.8A6A	S06.0X9A
N80.B2	N80.8	O35.05X0	O35.0XX0	O35.13X3	O35.1XX3	O35.EXX9	O35.8XX9	S06.30AS	S06.309S	S06.8A6D	S06.0X9D
N80.B31	N80.8	O35.05X1	O35.0XX1	O35.13X4	O35.1XX4	O35.FXX0	O35.8XX0	S06.31AA	S06.319A	S06.8A6S	S06.0X9S
N80.B32	N80.8	O35.05X2	O35.0XX2	O35.13X5	O35.1XX5	O35.FXX1	O35.8XX1	S06.31AD	S06.319D	S06.8A7A	S06.0X9A
N80.B39	N80.8	O35.05X3	O35.0XX3	O35.13X9	O35.1XX9	O35.FXX2	O35.8XX2	S06.31AS	S06.319S	S06.8A8A	S06.0X9A
N80.B4	N80.8	O35.05X4	O35.0XX4	O35.14X0	O35.1XX0	O35.FXX3	O35.8XX3	S06.32AA	S06.329A	S06.8AAA	S06.0X9A
N80.B5	N80.8	O35.05X5	O35.0XX5	O35.14X1	O35.1XX1	O35.FXX4	O35.8XX4	S06.32AD	S06.329D	S06.8AAD	S06.0X9D
N80.B6	N80.8	O35.05X9	O35.0XX9	O35.14X2	O35.1XX2	O35.FXX5	O35.8XX5	S06.32AS	S06.329S	S06.8AAS	S06.0X9S
N80.C0	N80.8	O35.06X0	O35.0XX0	O35.14X3	O35.1XX3	O35.FXX9	O35.8XX9	S06.33AA	S06.339A	S06.8A9A	S06.0X9A
N80.C10	N80.8	O35.06X1	O35.0XX1	O35.14X4	O35.1XX4	O35.GXX0	O35.8XX0	S06.33AD	S06.339D	S06.8A9D	S06.0X9D
N80.C11	N80.8	O35.06X2	O35.0XX2	O35.14X5	O35.1XX5	O35.GXX1	O35.8XX1	S06.33AS	S06.339S	S06.8A9S	S06.0X9S
N80.C19	N80.8	O35.06X3	O35.0XX3	O35.14X9	O35.1XX9	O35.GXX2	O35.8XX2	S06.34AA	S06.349A	S06.89AA	S06.0X9A
N80.C2	N80.8	O35.06X4	O35.0XX4	O35.15X0	O35.1XX0	O35.GXX3	O35.8XX3	S06.34AD	S06.349D	S06.89AD	S06.0X9D
N80.C3	N80.8	O35.06X5	O35.0XX5	O35.15X1	O35.1XX1	O35.GXX4	O35.8XX4	S06.34AS	S06.349S	S06.89AS	S06.0X9S
N80.C4	N80.8	O35.06X9	O35.0XX9	O35.15X2	O35.1XX2	O35.GXX5	O35.8XX5	S06.35AA	S06.359A	S06.9XAA	S06.9X9A
N80.C9	N80.8	O35.07X0	O35.0XX0	O35.15X3	O35.1XX3	O35.GXX9	O35.8XX9	S06.35AD	S06.359D	S06.9XAD	S06.9X9D
N80.D0	N80.8	O35.07X1	O35.0XX1	O35.15X4	O35.1XX4	O35.HXX0	O35.8XX0	S06.35AS	S06.359S	S06.9XAS	S06.9X9S
N80.D1	N80.8	O35.07X2	O35.0XX2	O35.15X5	O35.1XX5	O35.HXX1	O35.8XX1	S06.36AA	S06.369A	T43.651A	T43.621A
N80.D2	N80.8	O35.07X3	O35.0XX3	O35.15X9	O35.1XX9	O35.HXX2	O35.8XX2	S06.36AD	S06.369D	T43.651D	T43.621D
N80.D3	N80.8	O35.07X4	O35.0XX4	O35.19X0	O35.1XX0	O35.HXX3	O35.8XX3	S06.36AS	S06.369S	T43.651S	T43.621S
N80.D4	N80.8	O35.07X5	O35.0XX5	O35.19X1	O35.1XX1	O35.HXX4	O35.8XX4	S06.37AA	S06.379A	T43.652A	T43.622A
N80.D5	N80.8	O35.07X9	O35.0XX9	O35.19X2	O35.1XX2	O35.HXX5	O35.8XX5	S06.37AD	S06.379D	T43.652D	T43.621D
N80.D6	N80.8	O35.08X0	O35.0XX0	O35.19X3	O35.1XX3	O35.HXX9	O35.8XX9	S06.37AS	S06.379S	T43.652S	T43.621S
N80.D9	N80.8	O35.08X1	O35.0XX1	O35.19X4	O35.1XX4	P28.30	P28.3	S06.38AA	S06.389A	T43.653A	T43.623A
N85.A	N85.8	O35.08X2	O35.0XX2	O35.19X5	O35.1XX5	P28.31	P28.3	S06.38AD	S06.389D	T43.653D	T43.623D
O35.00X0	O35.0XX0	O35.08X3	O35.0XX3	O35.19X9	O35.1XX9	P28.32	P28.3	S06.38AS	S06.389S	T43.653S	T43.623S
O35.00X1	O35.0XX1	O35.08X4	O35.0XX4	O35.AXX0	O35.8XX0	P28.33	P28.3	S06.4XAA	S06.4X9A	T43.654A	T43.624A
O35.00X2	O35.0XX2	O35.08X5	O35.0XX5	O35.AXX1	O35.8XX1	P28.39	P28.3	S06.4XAD	S06.4X9D	T43.654D	T43.624D
O35.00X3	O35.0XX3	O35.08X9	O35.0XX9	O35.AXX2	O35.8XX2	P28.40	P28.4	S06.4XAS	S06.4X9S	T43.654S	T43.624S
O35.00X4	O35.0XX4	O35.09X0	O35.0XX0	O35.AXX3	O35.8XX3	P28.41	P28.4	S06.5XAA	S06.5X9A	T43.655A	T43.625A
O35.00X5	O35.0XX5	O35.09X1	O35.0XX1	O35.AXX4	O35.8XX4	P28.42	P28.4	S06.5XAD	S06.5X9D	T43.655D	T43.625D
O35.00X9	O35.0XX9	O35.09X2	O35.0XX2	O35.AXX5	O35.8XX5	P28.43	P28.4	S06.5XAS	S06.5X9S	T43.655S	T43.625S
O35.01X0	O35.0XX0	O35.09X3	O35.0XX3	O35.AXX9	O35.8XX9	P28.49	P28.4	S06.6XAA	S06.6X9A	T43.656A	T43.626A
O35.01X1	O35.0XX1	O35.09X4	O35.0XX4	O35.BXX0	O35.8XX0	Q21.10	Q21.1	S06.6XAD	S06.6X9D	T43.656D	T43.626D
O35.01X2	O35.0XX2	O35.09X5	O35.0XX5	O35.BXX1	O35.8XX1	Q21.11	Q21.1	S06.6XAS	S06.6X9S	T43.656S	T43.626S

Code Assignment Beginning 10/1/2022	Previous Code(s) Assignment	Code Assignment Beginning 10/1/2022	Previous Code(s) Assignment	Code Assignment Beginning 10/1/2022	Previous Code(s) Assignment	Code Assignment Beginning 10/1/2022	Previous Code(s) Assignment	Code Assignment Beginning 10/1/2022	Previous Code(s) Assignment	Code Assignment Beginning 10/1/2022	Previous Code(s) Assignment
V20.01XA	V20.0XXA	V21.29XS	V21.2XXS	V22.59XD	V22.5XXD	V24.19XA	V24.1XXA	V25.41XS	V25.4XXS	V27.01XD	V27.0XXD
V20.01XD	V20.0XXD	V21.31XA	V21.3XXA	V22.59XS	V22.5XXS	V24.19XD	V24.1XXD	V25.49XA	V25.4XXA	V27.01XS	V27.0XXS
V20.01XS	V20.0XXS	V21.31XD	V21.3XXD	V22.91XA	V22.9XXA	V24.19XS	V24.1XXS	V25.49XD	V25.4XXD	V27.09XA	V27.0XXA
V20.09XA	V20.0XXA	V21.31XS	V21.3XXS	V22.91XD	V22.9XXD	V24.21XA	V24.2XXA	V25.49XS	V25.4XXS	V27.09XD	V27.0XXD
V20.09XD	V20.0XXD	V21.39XA	V21.3XXA	V22.91XS	V22.9XXS	V24.21XD	V24.2XXD	V25.51XA	V25.5XXA	V27.09XS	V27.0XXS
V20.09XS	V20.0XXS	V21.39XD	V21.3XXD	V22.99XA	V22.9XXA	V24.21XS	V24.2XXS	V25.51XD	V25.5XXD	V27.11XA	V27.1XXA
V20.11XA	V20.1XXA	V21.39XS	V21.3XXS	V22.99XD	V22.9XXD	V24.29XA	V24.2XXA	V25.51XS	V25.5XXS	V27.11XD	V27.1XXD
V20.11XD	V20.1XXD	V21.41XA	V21.4XXA	V22.99XS	V22.9XXS	V24.29XD	V24.2XXD	V25.59XA	V25.5XXA	V27.11XS	V27.1XXS
V20.11XS	V20.1XXS	V21.41XD	V21.4XXD	V23.01XA	V23.0XXA	V24.29XS	V24.2XXS	V25.59XD	V25.5XXD	V27.19XA	V27.1XXA
V20.19XA	V20.1XXA	V21.41XS	V21.4XXS	V23.01XD	V23.0XXD	V24.31XA	V24.3XXA	V25.59XS	V25.5XXS	V27.19XD	V27.1XXD
V20.19XD	V20.1XXD	V21.49XA	V21.4XXA	V23.01XS	V23.0XXS	V24.31XD	V24.3XXD	V25.91XA	V25.9XXA	V27.19XS	V27.1XXS
V20.19XS	V20.1XXS	V21.49XD	V21.4XXD	V23.09XA	V23.0XXA	V24.31XS	V24.3XXS	V25.91XD	V25.9XXD	V27.21XA	V27.2XXA
V20.21XA	V20.2XXA	V21.49XS	V21.4XXS	V23.09XD	V23.0XXD	V24.39XA	V24.3XXA	V25.91XS	V25.9XXS	V27.21XD	V27.2XXD
V20.21XD	V20.2XXD	V21.51XA	V21.5XXA	V23.09XS	V23.0XXS	V24.39XD	V24.3XXD	V25.99XA	V25.9XXA	V27.21XS	V27.2XXS
V20.21XS	V20.2XXS	V21.51XD	V21.5XXD	V23.11XA	V23.1XXA	V24.39XS	V24.3XXS	V25.99XD	V25.9XXD	V27.29XA	V27.2XXA
V20.29XA	V20.2XXA	V21.51XS	V21.5XXS	V23.11XD	V23.1XXD	V24.41XA	V24.4XXA	V25.99XS	V25.9XXS	V27.29XD	V27.2XXD
V20.29XD	V20.2XXD	V21.59XA	V21.5XXA	V23.11XS	V23.1XXS	V24.41XD	V24.4XXD	V26.01XA	V26.0XXA	V27.29XS	V27.2XXS
V20.29XS	V20.2XXS	V21.59XD	V21.5XXD	V23.19XA	V23.1XXA	V24.41XS	V24.4XXS	V26.01XD	V26.0XXD	V27.31XA	V27.3XXA
V20.31XA	V20.3XXA	V21.59XS	V21.5XXS	V23.19XD	V23.1XXD	V24.49XA	V24.4XXA	V26.01XS	V26.0XXS	V27.31XD	V27.3XXD
V20.31XD	V20.3XXD	V21.91XA	V21.9XXA	V23.19XS	V23.1XXS	V24.49XD	V24.4XXD	V26.09XA	V26.0XXA	V27.31XS	V27.3XXS
V20.31XS	V20.3XXS	V21.91XD	V21.9XXD	V23.21XA	V23.2XXA	V24.49XS	V24.4XXS	V26.09XD	V26.0XXD	V27.39XA	V27.3XXA
V20.39XA	V20.3XXA	V21.91XS	V21.9XXS	V23.21XD	V23.2XXD	V24.51XA	V24.5XXA	V26.09XS	V26.0XXS	V27.39XD	V27.3XXD
V20.39XD	V20.3XXD	V21.99XA	V21.9XXA	V23.21XS	V23.2XXS	V24.51XD	V24.5XXD	V26.11XA	V26.1XXA	V27.39XS	V27.3XXS
V20.39XS	V20.3XXS	V21.99XD	V21.9XXD	V23.29XA	V23.2XXA	V24.51XS	V24.5XXS	V26.11XD	V26.1XXD	V27.41XA	V27.4XXA
V20.41XA	V20.4XXA	V21.99XS	V21.9XXS	V23.29XD	V23.2XXD	V24.59XA	V24.5XXA	V26.11XS	V26.1XXS	V27.41XD	V27.4XXD
V20.41XD	V20.4XXD	V22.01XA	V22.0XXA	V23.29XS	V23.2XXS	V24.59XD	V24.5XXD	V26.19XA	V26.1XXA	V27.41XS	V27.4XXS
V20.41XS	V20.4XXS	V22.01XD	V22.0XXD	V23.31XA	V23.3XXA	V24.59XS	V24.5XXS	V26.19XD	V26.1XXD	V27.49XA	V27.4XXA
V20.49XA	V20.4XXA	V22.01XS	V22.0XXS	V23.31XD	V23.3XXD	V24.91XA	V24.9XXA	V26.19XS	V26.1XXS	V27.49XD	V27.4XXD
V20.49XD	V20.4XXD	V22.09XA	V22.0XXA	V23.31XS	V23.3XXS	V24.91XD	V24.9XXD	V26.21XA	V26.2XXA	V27.49XS	V27.4XXS
V20.49XS	V20.4XXS	V22.09XD	V22.0XXD	V23.39XA	V23.3XXA	V24.91XS	V24.9XXS	V26.21XD	V26.2XXD	V27.51XA	V27.5XXA
V20.51XA	V20.5XXA	V22.09XS	V22.0XXS	V23.39XD	V23.3XXD	V24.99XA	V24.9XXA	V26.21XS	V26.2XXS	V27.51XD	V27.5XXD
V20.51XD	V20.5XXD	V22.11XA	V22.1XXA	V23.39XS	V23.3XXS	V24.99XD	V24.9XXD	V26.29XA	V26.2XXA	V27.51XS	V27.5XXS
V20.51XS	V20.5XXS	V22.11XD	V22.1XXD	V23.41XA	V23.4XXA	V24.99XS	V24.9XXS	V26.29XD	V26.2XXD	V27.59XA	V27.5XXA
V20.59XA	V20.5XXA	V22.11XS	V22.1XXS	V23.41XD	V23.4XXD	V25.01XA	V25.0XXA	V26.29XS	V26.2XXS	V27.59XD	V27.5XXD
V20.59XD	V20.5XXD	V22.19XA	V22.1XXA	V23.41XS	V23.4XXS	V25.01XD	V25.0XXD	V26.31XA	V26.3XXA	V27.59XS	V27.5XXS
V20.59XS	V20.5XXS	V22.19XD	V22.1XXD	V23.49XA	V23.4XXA	V25.01XS	V25.0XXS	V26.31XD	V26.3XXD	V27.91XA	V27.9XXA
V20.91XA	V20.9XXA	V22.19XS	V22.1XXS	V23.49XD	V23.4XXD	V25.09XA	V25.0XXA	V26.31XS	V26.3XXS	V27.91XD	V27.9XXD
V20.91XD	V20.9XXD	V22.21XA	V22.2XXA	V23.49XS	V23.4XXS	V25.09XD	V25.0XXD	V26.39XA	V26.3XXA	V27.91XS	V27.9XXS
V20.91XS	V20.9XXS	V22.21XD	V22.2XXD	V23.51XA	V23.5XXA	V25.09XS	V25.0XXS	V26.39XD	V26.3XXD	V27.99XA	V27.9XXA
V20.99XA	V20.9XXA	V22.21XS	V22.2XXS	V23.51XD	V23.5XXD	V25.11XA	V25.1XXA	V26.39XS	V26.3XXS	V27.99XD	V27.9XXD
V20.99XD	V20.9XXD	V22.29XA	V22.2XXA	V23.51XS	V23.5XXS	V25.11XD	V25.1XXD	V26.41XA	V26.4XXA	V27.99XS	V27.9XXS
V20.99XS	V20.9XXS	V22.29XD	V22.2XXD	V23.59XA	V23.5XXA	V25.11XS	V25.1XXS	V26.41XD	V26.4XXD	V28.01XA	V28.0XXA
V21.01XA	V21.0XXA	V22.29XS	V22.2XXS	V23.59XD	V23.5XXD	V25.19XA	V25.1XXA	V26.41XS	V26.4XXS	V28.01XD	V28.0XXD
V21.01XD	V21.0XXD	V22.31XA	V22.3XXA	V23.59XS	V23.5XXS	V25.19XD	V25.1XXD	V26.49XA	V26.4XXA	V28.01XS	V28.0XXS
V21.01XS	V21.0XXS	V22.31XD	V22.3XXD	V23.91XA	V23.9XXA	V25.19XS	V25.1XXS	V26.49XD	V26.4XXD	V28.09XA	V28.0XXA
V21.09XA	V21.0XXA	V22.31XS	V22.3XXS	V23.91XD	V23.9XXD	V25.21XA	V25.2XXA	V26.49XS	V26.4XXS	V28.09XD	V28.0XXD
V21.09XD	V21.0XXD	V22.39XA	V22.3XXA	V23.91XS	V23.9XXS	V25.21XD	V25.2XXD	V26.51XA	V26.5XXA	V28.09XS	V28.0XXS
V21.09XS	V21.0XXS	V22.39XD	V22.3XXD	V23.99XA	V23.9XXA	V25.21XS	V25.2XXS	V26.51XD	V26.5XXD	V28.11XA	V28.1XXA
V21.11XA	V21.1XXA	V22.39XS	V22.3XXS	V23.99XD	V23.9XXD	V25.29XA	V25.2XXA	V26.51XS	V26.5XXS	V28.11XD	V28.1XXD
V21.11XD	V21.1XXD	V22.41XA	V22.4XXA	V23.99XS	V23.9XXS	V25.29XD	V25.2XXD	V26.59XA	V26.5XXA	V28.11XS	V28.1XXS
V21.11XS	V21.1XXS	V22.41XD	V22.4XXD	V24.01XA	V24.0XXA	V25.29XS	V25.2XXS	V26.59XD	V26.5XXD	V28.19XA	V28.1XXA
V21.19XA	V21.1XXA	V22.41XS	V22.4XXS	V24.01XD	V24.0XXD	V25.31XA	V25.3XXA	V26.59XS	V26.5XXS	V28.19XD	V28.1XXD
V21.19XD	V21.1XXD	V22.49XA	V22.4XXA	V24.01XS	V24.0XXS	V25.31XD	V25.3XXD	V26.91XA	V26.9XXA	V28.19XS	V28.1XXS
V21.19XS	V21.1XXS	V22.49XD	V22.4XXD	V24.09XA	V24.0XXA	V25.31XS	V25.3XXS	V26.91XD	V26.9XXD	V28.21XA	V28.2XXA
V21.21XA	V21.2XXA	V22.49XS	V22.4XXS	V24.09XD	V24.0XXD	V25.39XA	V25.3XXA	V26.91XS	V26.9XXS	V28.21XD	V28.2XXD
V21.21XD	V21.2XXD	V22.51XA	V22.5XXA	V24.09XS	V24.0XXS	V25.39XD	V25.3XXD	V26.99XA	V26.9XXA	V28.21XS	V28.2XXS
V21.21XS	V21.2XXS	V22.51XD	V22.5XXD	V24.11XA	V24.1XXA	V25.39XS	V25.3XXS	V26.99XD	V26.9XXD	V28.29XA	V28.2XXA
V21.29XA	V21.2XXA	V22.51XS	V22.5XXS	V24.11XD	V24.1XXD	V25.41XA	V25.4XXA	V26.99XS	V26.9XXS	V28.29XD	V28.2XXD
V21.29XD	V21.2XXD	V22.59XA	V22.5XXA	V24.11XS	V24.1XXS	V25.41XD	V25.4XXD	V27.01XA	V27.0XXA	V28.29XS	V28.2XXS

Conversion Table of ICD-10-CM Codes

Code Assignment Beginning 10/1/2022	Previous Code(s) Assignment	Code Assignment Beginning 10/1/2022	Previous Code(s) Assignment	Code Assignment Beginning 10/1/2022	Previous Code(s) Assignment	Code Assignment Beginning 10/1/2022	Previous Code(s) Assignment	Code Assignment Beginning 10/1/2022	Previous Code(s) Assignment	Code Assignment Beginning 10/1/2022	Previous Code(s) Assignment
V28.31XA	V28.3XXA	V29.091A	V29.09XA	V29.31XA	V29.3XXA	V29.601A	V29.60XA	W23.2XXA	W23.0XXA & W23.1XXA	Z79.64	Z79.899
V28.31XD	V28.3XXD	V29.091D	V29.09XD	V29.31XD	V29.3XXD	V29.601D	V29.60XD			Z79.69	Z79.899
V28.31XS	V28.3XXS	V29.091S	V29.09XS	V29.31XS	V29.3XXS	V29.601S	V29.60XS	W23.2XXD	W23.0XXD & W23.1XXD	Z79.85	Z79.899
V28.39XA	V28.3XXA	V29.098A	V29.09XA	V29.39XA	V29.3XXA	V29.608A	V29.60XA			Z87.61	Z87.898
V28.39XD	V28.3XXD	V29.098D	V29.09XD	V29.39XD	V29.3XXD	V29.608D	V29.60XD	W23.2XXS	W23.0XXS & W23.1XXS	Z87.68	Z87.898
V28.39XS	V28.3XXS	V29.098S	V29.09XS	V29.39XS	V29.3XXS	V29.608S	V29.60XS			Z87.731	Z87.738
V28.41XA	V28.4XXA	V29.101A	V29.10XA	V29.401A	V29.40XA	V29.691A	V29.69XA	Z03.83	Z03.89	Z87.732	Z87.738
V28.41XD	V28.4XXD	V29.101D	V29.10XD	V29.401D	V29.40XD	V29.691D	V29.69XD	*Z28.310	Z28.3	Z87.760	Z87.76
V28.41XS	V28.4XXS	V29.101S	V29.10XS	V29.401S	V29.40XS	V29.691S	V29.69XS	*Z28.311	Z28.3	Z87.761	Z87.76
V28.49XA	V28.4XXA	V29.108A	V29.10XA	V29.408A	V29.40XA	V29.698A	V29.69XA	*Z28.39	Z28.3	Z87.762	Z87.76
V28.49XD	V28.4XXD	V29.108D	V29.10XD	V29.408D	V29.40XD	V29.698D	V29.69XD	Z59.82	Z59.89	Z87.763	Z87.76
V28.49XS	V28.4XXS	V29.108S	V29.10XS	V29.408S	V29.40XS	V29.698S	V29.69XS	Z59.86	Z59.89	Z87.768	Z87.76
V28.51XA	V28.5XXA	V29.191A	V29.19XA	V29.491A	V29.49XA	V29.811A	V29.80XA	Z59.87	Z59.89	Z91.110	Z91.11
V28.51XD	V28.5XXD	V29.191D	V29.19XD	V29.491D	V29.49XD	V29.811D	V29.80XD	Z71.87	Z71.89	Z91.118	Z91.11
V28.51XS	V28.5XXS	V29.191S	V29.19XS	V29.491S	V29.49XS	V29.811S	V29.80XS	Z71.88	Z71.89	Z91.119	Z91.11
V28.59XA	V28.5XXA	V29.198A	V29.19XA	V29.498A	V29.49XA	V29.818A	V29.80XA	Z72.823	Z72.89	Z91.190	Z91.19
V28.59XD	V28.5XXD	V29.198D	V29.19XD	V29.498D	V29.49XD	V29.818D	V29.80XD	Z79.60	Z79.899	Z91.198	Z91.19
V28.59XS	V28.5XXS	V29.198S	V29.19XS	V29.498S	V29.49XS	V29.818S	V29.80XS	Z79.61	Z79.899	Z91.199	Z91.19
V28.91XA	V28.9XXA	V29.201A	V29.20XA	V29.501A	V29.50XA	V29.881A	V29.89XA	Z79.620	Z79.899	Z91.A10	Z91.19
V28.91XD	V28.9XXD	V29.201D	V29.20XD	V29.501D	V29.50XD	V29.881D	V29.89XD	Z79.621	Z79.899	Z91.A18	Z91.19
V28.91XS	V28.9XXS	V29.201S	V29.20XS	V29.501S	V29.50XS	V29.881S	V29.89XS	Z79.622	Z79.899	Z91.A20	Z91.19
V28.99XA	V28.9XXA	V29.208A	V29.20XA	V29.508A	V29.50XA	V29.888A	V29.89XA	Z79.623	Z79.899	Z91.A28	Z91.19
V28.99XD	V28.9XXD	V29.208D	V29.20XD	V29.508D	V29.50XD	V29.888D	V29.89XD	Z79.624	Z79.899	Z91.A3	Z91.19
V28.99XS	V28.9XXS	V29.208S	V29.20XS	V29.508S	V29.50XS	V29.888S	V29.89XS	Z79.630	Z79.899	Z91.A4	Z91.19
V29.001A	V29.00XA	V29.291A	V29.29XA	V29.591A	V29.59XA	V29.91XA	V29.9XXA	Z79.631	Z79.899	Z91.A5	Z91.19
V29.001D	V29.00XD	V29.291D	V29.29XD	V29.591D	V29.59XD	V29.91XD	V29.9XXD	Z79.632	Z79.899	Z91.A9	Z91.19
V29.001S	V29.00XS	V29.291S	V29.29XS	V29.591S	V29.59XS	V29.91XS	V29.9XXS	Z79.633	Z79.899		
V29.008A	V29.00XA	V29.298A	V29.29XA	V29.598A	V29.59XA	V29.99XA	V29.9XXA	Z79.634	Z79.899		
V29.008D	V29.00XD	V29.298D	V29.29XD	V29.598D	V29.59XD	V29.99XD	V29.9XXD				
V29.008S	V29.00XS	V29.298S	V29.29XS	V29.598S	V29.59XS	V29.99XS	V29.9XXS				

10 Steps to Correct Coding

Follow the 10 steps below to correctly code encounters for health care services.

Step 1: Identify the reason for the visit or encounter (i.e., a sign, symptom, diagnosis and/or condition).
The medical record documentation should accurately reflect the patient's condition, using terminology that includes specific diagnoses and symptoms or clearly states the reasons for the encounter.

Choosing the main term that best describes the reason chiefly responsible for the service provided is the most important step in coding. If symptoms are present and documented but a definitive diagnosis has not yet been determined, code the symptoms. *For outpatient cases, do not code conditions that are referred to as "rule out," "suspected," "probable," or "questionable."* Diagnoses often are not established at the time of the initial encounter/visit and may require two or more visits to be established. Code only what is documented in the available outpatient records and only to the highest degree of certainty known at the time of the patient's visit. For inpatient medical records, uncertain diagnoses may be reported if documented at the time of discharge.

Step 2: After selecting the reason for the encounter, consult the alphabetic index.
The most critical rule is to begin code selection in the alphabetic index. Never turn first to the tabular list. The index provides cross-references, essential and nonessential modifiers, and other instructional notations that may not be found in the tabular list.

Step 3: Locate the main term entry.
The alphabetic index lists conditions, which may be expressed as nouns or eponyms, with critical use of adjectives. Some conditions known by several names have multiple main entries. Reasons for encounters may be located under general terms such as admission, encounter, and examination. Other general terms such as history, status (post), or presence (of) can be used to locate other factors influencing health.

Step 4: Scan subterm entries.
Scan the subterm entries, as appropriate, being sure to review continued lines and additional subterms that may appear in the next column or on the next page. Shaded vertical guidelines in the index indicate the indentation level for each subterm in relation to the main terms.

Step 5: Pay close attention to index instructions.
- Parentheses ( ) enclose nonessential modifiers, terms that are supplementary words or explanatory information that may or may not appear in the diagnostic statement and do not affect code selection.

- Brackets [ ] enclose manifestation codes that can be used only as secondary codes to the underlying condition code immediately preceding it. If used, manifestation codes must be reported with the appropriate etiology codes.

- Default codes are listed next to the main term and represent the condition most commonly associated with the main term or the unspecified code for the main term.

- *"See"* cross-references, identified by italicized type and "code by" cross-references indicate that another term *must be referenced* to locate the correct code.

- *"See also"* cross-references, identified by italicized type, provide alternative terms that may be useful to look up but *are not mandatory*.

- "Omit code" cross-references identify instances when a code is not applicable depending on the condition being coded.

- "With" subterms are listed out of alphabetic order and identify a presumed causal relationship between the two conditions they link.

- "Due to" subterms identify a relationship between the two conditions they link.

- "NEC," abbreviation for "not elsewhere classified," follows some main terms or subterms and indicates that there is no specific code for the condition even though the medical documentation may be very specific.

- "NOS," abbreviation for "not otherwise specified," follows some main terms or subterms and is the equivalent of unspecified; NOS signifies that the information in the medical record is insufficient for assigning a more specific code.

- *Following* references help coders locate alphanumeric codes that are out of sequence in the tabular section.

- Check-additional-character symbols flag codes that require additional characters to make the code valid; the characters available to complete the code should be verified in the tabular section.

Step 6: Choose a potential code and locate it in the tabular list.
To prevent coding errors, always use both the alphabetic index (to identify a code) and the tabular list (to verify a code), as the index does not include the important instructional notes found in the tabular list. An added benefit of using the tabular list, which groups like things together, is that while looking at one code in the list, a coder might see a more specific one that would have been missed had the coder relied solely on the alphabetic index. Additionally, many of the codes require a fourth, fifth, sixth, or seventh character to be valid, and many of these characters can be found only in the tabular list.

Step 7: Read all instructional material in the tabular section.
The coder must follow any Includes, Excludes 1 and Excludes 2 notes, and other instructional notes, such as "Code first" and "Use additional code," listed in the tabular list for the chapter, category, subcategory, and subclassification levels of code selection that direct the coder to use a different or additional code. Any codes in the tabular range A00.0- through T88.9- may be used to identify the diagnostic reason for the encounter. The tabular list encompasses many codes describing disease and injury classifications (e.g., infectious and parasitic diseases, neoplasms, symptoms, nervous and circulatory system etc.).

Codes that describe symptoms and signs, as opposed to definitive diagnoses, should be reported when an established diagnosis has not been made (confirmed) by the physician. Chapter 18 of the ICD-10-CM code book, "Symptoms, Signs, and Abnormal Clinical and Laboratory Findings, Not Elsewhere Classified" (codes R00–R99), contains many, but not all, codes for symptoms.

ICD-10-CM classifies encounters with health care providers for circumstances other than a disease or injury in chapter 21, "Factors Influencing Health Status and Contact with Health Services" (codes Z00–Z99). Circumstances other than a disease or injury often are recorded as chiefly responsible for the encounter.

A code is invalid if it does not include the full number of characters (greatest level of specificity) required. Codes in ICD-10-CM can contain from three to seven alphanumeric characters. A three-character code is to be used only if the category is not further subdivided into four-, five-, six-, or seven-character codes. Placeholder character X is used as part of an alphanumeric code to allow for future expansion and as a placeholder for empty characters in a code that requires a seventh character but has no fourth, fifth, or sixth character. Note that certain categories require seventh characters that apply to all codes in that category. Always check the category level for applicable seventh characters for that category.

Step 8: Consult the official ICD-10-CM conventions and guidelines.
The *ICD-10-CM Official Guidelines for Coding and Reporting* govern the use of certain codes. These guidelines provide both general and chapter-specific coding guidance.

Step 9: Confirm and assign the code.

Having reviewed all relevant information concerning the possible code choices, assign the code that most completely describes the condition.

Repeat steps 1 through 9 for all additional documented conditions that meet the following criteria:

- They exist at the time of the visit *AND*
- They require or affect patient care, treatment, or management

Step 10: Sequence codes correctly.

Sequencing is the order in which the codes are listed on the claim. List first the ICD-10-CM code for the diagnosis, condition, problem, or other reason for the encounter/visit that is shown in the medical record to be chiefly responsible for the services provided. List additional codes that describe any coexisting conditions. Follow the official coding guidelines (see the guidelines, section II, "Selection of Principal Diagnosis"; section III, "Reporting Additional Diagnoses"; and section IV, "Diagnostic Coding and Reporting Guidelines for Outpatient Services") on proper sequencing of codes.

Coding Examples

Diagnosis: Anorexia

Step 1: The reason for the encounter was the condition, anorexia.

Step 2: Consult the alphabetic index.

Step 3: Locate the main term "Anorexia."

Step 4: Two possible subterms are available, "hysterical" and "nervosa." Neither is documented in this instance, however, so they cannot be used in code selection.

Step 5: The code listed next to the main term is called the default code selection. Because the two subentries (essential modifiers) do not apply in this instance, the default code (R63.0) should be used.

Step 6: Turn to code R63.0 in the tabular list and read all instructional notes.

Step 7: The Excludes 1 note at code R63.0 indicates that anorexia nervosa and loss of appetite determined to be of nonorganic origin should be reported with a code from chapter 5. The diagnostic statement does not describe the condition as anorexia nervosa, however, and does not indicate that the anorexia is of a nonorganic origin. There is no further division of the category past the fourth-character subcategory. Therefore, code R63.0 is at the highest level of specificity.

Step 8: Review of official guideline I.C.18 indicates that a symptom code is appropriate when a more definitive diagnosis is not documented.

Step 9: The default code, R63.0 Anorexia, is the correct code selection.

Repeat steps 1 through 9 for any concomitant diagnoses.

Step 10: Since anorexia is listed as the chief reason for the health care encounter, the first-listed, or principal, diagnosis is R63.0. Note that this is a chapter 18 symptom code but can be assigned for both inpatient and outpatient records since the provider did not establish a more definitive diagnosis, according to sections II.A and IV.D.

Diagnosis: Acute bronchitis

Step 1: The reason for the encounter was the condition, acute bronchitis.

Step 2: Consult the alphabetic index.

Step 3: Locate the main term "Bronchitis."

Step 4: There is a subterm for "acute or subacute." Additional subterms are not included in the diagnostic statement.

Step 5: Nonessential modifiers (with bronchospasm or obstruction) are terms that do not affect code assignment. Since no other subterms indented under "acute" apply here, the code listed next to this subentry—in this case J20.9—should be chosen.

Step 6: Turn to code J20.9 in the tabular list and read all instructional notes.

Step 7: The Includes note under category J20 lists alternative terms for acute bronchitis. Note that the list is not exhaustive but is only a representative selection of diagnoses that are included in the subcategory. The Excludes 1 note refers to category J40 for bronchitis and tracheobronchitis NOS. There are several conditions in the Excludes 2 notes that, if applicable, can be coded in addition to this code.

Note that the codes included in J20 represent acute bronchitis due to various infectious organisms that could be selected if identified in the documentation. In this case, the organism was not identified and there is no further division of the category past the fourth character subcategory. Therefore, code J20.9 is at the highest level of specificity.

Step 8: Review of official guideline I.C.10 provides no additional information affecting the code selected.

Step 9: Assign code J20.9 Acute bronchitis, unspecified.

Repeat steps 1 through 9 for any concomitant diagnoses.

Step 10: In the absence of additional diagnoses that may affect sequencing, code J20.9 should be sequenced as the first-listed, or principal, diagnosis.

Diagnosis: Cerebellar ataxia in myxedema

Step 1: The reason for the encounter was the condition, cerebellar ataxia.

Step 2: Consult the alphabetic index.

Step 3: Locate the main term "Ataxia."

Step 4: Available subterms include "cerebellar (hereditary)," with additional indented subterms for "in" and "myxedema," all essential modifiers that are included in the diagnostic statement. Two codes are provided, E03.9 and G13.2, the latter of which is in brackets.

Step 5: Note the nonessential modifier (in parentheses) after the subterm cerebellar includes the term "hereditary." Because it is in parentheses, this term is not required in the diagnostic statement for this subentry to apply. The brackets around G13.2 identify this code as a manifestation of the condition described by code E03.9 and indicate that the two must be reported together and sequencing rules apply.

Step 6: Locate codes E03.9 and G13.2 in the tabular list, and read all instructional notes.

Step 7: For code E03.9, there are no instructional notes in the tabular list at the category E03 or code level that indicate that this condition should be coded elsewhere in the classification or that additional codes are required. Without further information from the diagnostic statement, myxedema, not otherwise specified (NOS), is appropriately reported with code E03.9 Hypothyroidism, unspecified, according to the inclusion term at this code.

Code G13.2 in the tabular list has an instructional note to "Code first underlying disease," which includes conditions found in category E03.-. Based on this note, codes E03.9 and G13.2 are to be coded together, with G13.2 listed only as a secondary diagnosis. This correlates with what the alphabetic index indicated. As there is no further division of codes in category G13 beyond the fourth character, G13.2 is at the highest level of specificity.

Step 8: Although there are some general conventions, such as how to interpret brackets in the alphabetic index, no chapter-specific guidelines apply to this coding scenario.

Step 9: Assign codes E03.9 Hypothyroidism, unspecified, and G13.2 Systemic atrophy primarily affecting the central nervous system in myxedema.

Repeat steps 1 through 9 for any concomitant diagnoses.

Step 10: Based on the alphabetic index and tabular instructional notations, code E03.9 should be sequenced as the first-listed, or principal, diagnosis followed by G13.2 as a secondary diagnosis.

Diagnosis: Decubitus ulcer of right elbow with skin loss and necrosis of subcutaneous tissue

Step 1: The reason for the encounter was the condition, decubitus ulcer.

Step 2: Consult the alphabetic index.

Step 3: Locate the main term "Ulcer."

Step 4: For the subterm "decubitus," there is no code provided or additional subterms indented, but a cross-reference is listed.

Step 5: The italicized cross-reference instructs the coder to "*see* Ulcer, pressure, by site."

Repeat steps 3 through 5 for the cross-reference:

Step 3: Locate the main term "Ulcer."

Step 4: Review the subentries for the subterm "pressure." The next level of indent lists either the site of the ulcer or the specific stage of the ulcer (stage 1–4, unstageable, and unspecified stages). The diagnostic statement provides the site, right elbow, and the extent of tissue damage (skin loss and necrosis of subcutaneous tissue) but does not specifically state that the ulcer is stage 1, stage 2, etc. Nonessential modifiers (in parentheses) at each stage include a description of the typical extent of damage at each stage. For example, stage 1 describes "pre-ulcer skin changes limited to persistent focal edema." Based on the documentation in the record, the coder can correlate the documentation to the nonessential modifiers and choose the specific stage from the index. The coder can also go directly to the body site, choosing the stage of the ulcer after reviewing the code options and instructional notations in the tabular list.

The diagnostic statement indicates that the extent of the damage to the elbow includes skin loss and necrosis of subcutaneous tissue, coinciding with the nonessential modifier next to the subentry "stage 3." The body site of elbow (L89.0-) is listed as another level of indent with other body sites.

Step 5: Note that code L89.0 is followed by a dash and an additional-character-required icon, which indicate that more characters are needed to complete the code. From here, the tabular listing for L89.0- can be consulted.

Step 6: Locate code L89.0- in the tabular list and read all instructional notes.

Step 7: The tabular listing at category L89 has an Includes note for "decubitus ulcer," which confirms that category L89 is the appropriate category to represent what is documented in the diagnostic statement.

Several Excludes 2 notes are also listed at the category level. Excludes 2 notes represent conditions that can occur concomitantly with the decubitus ulcer and can be coded in addition to code L89, if supported by the documentation.

The subcategory codes under L89.0 indicate that the fifth character describes laterality. Locate the right elbow at subcategory L89.01. See that an additional sixth character to specify the stage of the ulcer is now needed to complete the code. The stage can be determined either by the specific documentation of the stage (e.g., stage 1, stage 2) or, in this case, a description that matches one of the inclusion terms that follow each stage code. For example, the diagnostic description in this case of "skin loss and necrosis of the subcutaneous tissue" matches the inclusion term under L89.013 Pressure ulcer of right elbow, stage 3. No additional characters are required because code L89.013 is at its highest level of specificity.

Step 8: The official guidelines contain quite a bit of information relating to pressure ulcers in chapter-specific guideline I.C.12 as well as information in general guideline I.B.14. These and any other pertinent guidelines should be reviewed to ensure appropriate code assignment.

Step 9: Assign code L89.013 Pressure ulcer of right elbow, stage 3.

Repeat steps 1 through 9 for any concomitant diagnoses.

Step 10: Since the decubitus ulcer is listed as the chief reason for the health care encounter, the first-listed, or principal, diagnosis is L89.013.

However, according to the code first instructional note at the L89 category level, gangrene (I96) would be sequenced before the pressure ulcer if it were documented.

Diagnosis: Emergency department visit for bimalleolar fracture of the right ankle due to trauma

Step 1: The reason for the encounter was the condition, bimalleolar fracture.

Step 2: Consult the alphabetic index.

Step 3: Locate the main term "Fracture." Note that many main terms represent fractures: "Fracture, burst," "Fracture, chronic," "Fracture, insufficiency," "Fracture, nontraumatic NEC," "Fracture, pathological," and "Fracture, traumatic." Since the diagnostic statement specifically states that this fracture was the result of trauma, the main term "Fracture, traumatic" should be used.

Step 4: Subterms that should be referenced are "ankle" and "bimalleolar (displaced)," which lists code S82.84-.

Step 5: A nonessential modifier (in parentheses) next to the term bimalleolar for "displaced" indicates that S82.84- is the default category unless the fracture is specifically identified as "nondisplaced."

Note that code S82.84- is followed by a dash and an additional-character icon, both of which indicate that more characters are required. From here, the tabular list can be consulted.

Step 6: Locate code S82.84- in the tabular list and read all instructional notes.

Step: 7: The instructional notes at category S82 indicate that fractures not specified as displaced or nondisplaced default to displaced and that fractures not designated as open or closed default to closed. Additional instructional notes can be found at the category level but none pertain to the current scenario.

Read through the subcategory codes under S82.84, and note that the sixth character specifies displaced or nondisplaced and laterality. Based on the index nonessential modifier (displaced) and the code note at category S82, code selection should identify a displaced fracture of the right side. A displaced bimalleolar fracture of the right lower leg is coded to S82.841.

To complete the code, a seventh character must be assigned to identify the type of encounter (initial, subsequent, or sequela) and whether the fracture is open or closed. Most of the codes in category S82 require a seventh character represented in the list at the category level. However, it is important to note that some subcategories have their own specific set of seventh characters. In this instance, subcategory S82.84- does not have a unique set of seventh characters and the list provided at the category level should be used. Without documentation of the fracture being open, the tabular notation indicates that the default is closed. Character A, representing "initial encounter for closed fracture," listed in the box at the category level is the most appropriate option.

Step 8: Assign code S82.841A Displaced bimalleolar fracture of right lower leg, initial encounter for closed fracture.

Repeat steps 1 through 9 for any concomitant diagnoses.

Step 9: Review chapter-specific guideline I.C.19. and any other official conventions or guidelines to ensure appropriate code assignment.

Step 10: Additional codes can be applied to relate the specific cause of the injury, the place of occurrence, the activity of the patient at the time of the injury, and the patient's status, when this information is available in the record. However, coding this information is voluntary and reporting requirements depend on state mandates and/or facility-specific reporting requirements. If assigned, the external cause codes should be reported as secondary diagnoses only with the injury (fracture) sequenced first. Most codes in chapter 20, "External Causes of Morbidity," require a seventh character to identify the type of encounter. The seventh character assigned to an external cause code should match the seventh character of the code assigned for the associated injury or condition for the encounter.

Notes

Notes

Notes

2023 ICD-10-CM Official Guidelines for Coding and Reporting

Narrative changes effective October 1, 2022 appear in **bold** text

Narrative changes effective April 1, 2022 appear in shaded text

Items underlined have been moved within the guidelines since the FY 2022 version

Italics are used to indicate revisions to heading changes

The Centers for Medicare and Medicaid Services (CMS) and the National Center for Health Statistics (NCHS), two departments within the U.S. Federal Government's Department of Health and Human Services (DHHS) provide the following guidelines for coding and reporting using the International Classification of Diseases, 10th Revision, Clinical Modification (ICD-10-CM). These guidelines should be used as a companion document to the official version of the ICD-10-CM as published on the NCHS website. The ICD-10-CM is a morbidity classification published by the United States for classifying diagnoses and reason for visits in all health care settings. The ICD-10-CM is based on the ICD-10, the statistical classification of disease published by the World Health Organization (WHO).

These guidelines have been approved by the four organizations that make up the Cooperating Parties for the ICD-10-CM: the American Hospital Association (AHA), the American Health Information Management Association (AHIMA), CMS, and NCHS.

These guidelines are a set of rules that have been developed to accompany and complement the official conventions and instructions provided within the ICD-10-CM itself. The instructions and conventions of the classification take precedence over guidelines. These guidelines are based on the coding and sequencing instructions in the Tabular List and Alphabetic Index of ICD-10-CM, but provide additional instruction. Adherence to these guidelines when assigning ICD-10-CM diagnosis codes is required under the Health Insurance Portability and Accountability Act (HIPAA). The diagnosis codes (Tabular List and Alphabetic Index) have been adopted under HIPAA for all healthcare settings. A joint effort between the healthcare provider and the coder is essential to achieve complete and accurate documentation, code assignment, and reporting of diagnoses and procedures. These guidelines have been developed to assist both the healthcare provider and the coder in identifying those diagnoses that are to be reported. The importance of consistent, complete documentation in the medical record cannot be overemphasized. Without such documentation accurate coding cannot be achieved. The entire record should be reviewed to determine the specific reason for the encounter and the conditions treated.

The term encounter is used for all settings, including hospital admissions. In the context of these guidelines, the term provider is used throughout the guidelines to mean physician or any qualified health care practitioner who is legally accountable for establishing the patient's diagnosis. Only this set of guidelines, approved by the Cooperating Parties, is official.

The guidelines are organized into sections. Section I includes the structure and conventions of the classification and general guidelines that apply to the entire classification, and chapter-specific guidelines that correspond to the chapters as they are arranged in the classification. Section II includes guidelines for selection of principal diagnosis for non-outpatient settings. Section III includes guidelines for reporting additional diagnoses in non-outpatient settings. Section IV is for outpatient coding and reporting. It is necessary to review all sections of the guidelines to fully understand all of the rules and instructions needed to code properly.

Section I. Conventions, general coding guidelines and chapter specific guidelines

The conventions, general guidelines and chapter-specific guidelines are applicable to all health care settings unless otherwise indicated. The conventions and instructions of the classification take precedence over guidelines.

A. Conventions for the ICD-10-CM

The conventions for the ICD-10-CM are the general rules for use of the classification independent of the guidelines. These conventions are incorporated within the Alphabetic Index and Tabular List of the ICD-10-CM as instructional notes.

1. **The Alphabetic Index and Tabular List**
   The ICD-10-CM is divided into the Alphabetic Index, an alphabetical list of terms and their corresponding code, and the Tabular List, a structured list of codes divided into chapters based on body system or condition. The Alphabetic Index consists of the following parts: the Index of Diseases and Injury, the Index of External Causes of Injury, the Table of Neoplasms and the Table of Drugs and Chemicals.
   See Section I.C.2. Neoplasms
   See Section I.C.19. Adverse effects, poisoning, underdosing and toxic effects

2. **Format and Structure:**
   The ICD-10-CM Tabular List contains categories, subcategories and codes. Characters for categories, subcategories and codes may be either a letter or a number. All categories are 3 characters. A three-character category that has no further subdivision is equivalent to a code. Subcategories are either 4 or 5 characters. Codes may be 3, 4, 5, 6 or 7 characters. That is, each level of subdivision after a category is a subcategory. The final level of subdivision is a code. Codes that have applicable 7th characters are still referred to as codes, not subcategories. A code that has an applicable 7th character is considered invalid without the 7th character.
   The ICD-10-CM uses an indented format for ease in reference.

3. **Use of codes for reporting purposes**
   For reporting purposes only codes are permissible, not categories or subcategories, and any applicable 7th character is required.

4. **Placeholder character**
   The ICD-10-CM utilizes a placeholder character "X". The "X" is used as a placeholder at certain codes to allow for future expansion. An example of this is at the poisoning, adverse effect and underdosing codes, categories T36-T50. Where a placeholder exists, the X must be used in order for the code to be considered a valid code.

5. **7th Characters**
   Certain ICD-10-CM categories have applicable 7th characters. The applicable 7th character is required for all codes within the category, or as the notes in the Tabular List instruct. The 7th character must always be the 7th character in the data field. If a code that requires a 7th character is not 6 characters, a placeholder X must be used to fill in the empty characters.

6. **Abbreviations**
   a. **Alphabetic Index abbreviations**
      NEC "Not elsewhere classifiable"
      This abbreviation in the Alphabetic Index represents "other specified." When a specific code is not available for a condition, the Alphabetic Index directs the coder to the "other specified" code in the Tabular List.
      NOS "Not otherwise specified"
      This abbreviation is the equivalent of unspecified.
   b. **Tabular List abbreviations**
      NEC "Not elsewhere classifiable"
      This abbreviation in the Tabular List represents "other specified". When a specific code is not available for a condition, the Tabular List includes an NEC entry under a code to identify the code as the "other specified" code.
      NOS "Not otherwise specified"
      This abbreviation is the equivalent of unspecified.

7. **Punctuation**
   [ ] Brackets are used in the Tabular List to enclose synonyms, alternative wording or explanatory phrases. Brackets are used in the Alphabetic Index to identify manifestation codes.
   ( ) Parentheses are used in both the Alphabetic Index and Tabular List to enclose supplementary words that may be present or absent in the statement of a disease or procedure without affecting the code number to which it is assigned. The terms within the parentheses are referred to as nonessential modifiers. The nonessential modifiers in the Alphabetic Index to Diseases apply to subterms following a main term except when a nonessential modifier and a subentry are

mutually exclusive, the subentry takes precedence. For example, in the ICD-10-CM Alphabetic Index under the main term Enteritis, "acute" is a nonessential modifier and "chronic" is a subentry. In this case, the nonessential modifier "acute" does not apply to the subentry "chronic".
   : Colons are used in the Tabular List after an incomplete term which needs one or more of the modifiers following the colon to make it assignable to a given category.

8. **Use of "and".**
   See Section I.A.14. Use of the term "And"

9. **Other and Unspecified codes**
   a. **"Other" codes**
      Codes titled "other" or "other specified" are for use when the information in the medical record provides detail for which a specific code does not exist. Alphabetic Index entries with NEC in the line designate "other" codes in the Tabular List. These Alphabetic Index entries represent specific disease entities for which no specific code exists, so the term is included within an "other" code.
   b. **"Unspecified" codes**
      Codes titled "unspecified" are for use when the information in the medical record is insufficient to assign a more specific code. For those categories for which an unspecified code is not provided, the "other specified" code may represent both other and unspecified.
      See Section I.B.18. Use of Signs/Symptom/Unspecified Codes

10. **Includes Notes**
    This note appears immediately under a three-character code title to further define, or give examples of, the content of the category.

11. **Inclusion terms**
    List of terms is included under some codes. These terms are the conditions for which that code is to be used. The terms may be synonyms of the code title, or, in the case of "other specified" codes, the terms are a list of the various conditions assigned to that code. The inclusion terms are not necessarily exhaustive. Additional terms found only in the Alphabetic Index may also be assigned to a code.

12. **Excludes Notes**
    The ICD-10-CM has two types of excludes notes. Each type of note has a different definition for use, but they are all similar in that they indicate that codes excluded from each other are independent of each other.
    a. **Excludes1**
       A type 1 Excludes note is a pure excludes note. It means "NOT CODED HERE!" An Excludes1 note indicates that the code excluded should never be used at the same time as the code above the Excludes1 note. An Excludes1 is used when two conditions cannot occur together, such as a congenital form versus an acquired form of the same condition.
       An exception to the Excludes1 definition is the circumstance when the two conditions are unrelated to each other. If it is not clear whether the two conditions involving an Excludes1 note are related or not, query the provider. For example, code F45.8, Other somatoform disorders, has an Excludes1 note for "sleep related teeth grinding (G47.63)," because "teeth grinding" is an inclusion term under F45.8. Only one of these two codes should be assigned for teeth grinding. However psychogenic dysmenorrhea is also an inclusion term under F45.8, and a patient could have both this condition and sleep related teeth grinding. In this case, the two conditions are clearly unrelated to each other, and so it would be appropriate to report F45.8 and G47.63 together.
    b. **Excludes2**
       A type 2 Excludes note represents "Not included here." An excludes2 note indicates that the condition excluded is not part of the condition represented by the code, but a patient may have both conditions at the same time. When an Excludes2 note appears under a code, it is acceptable to use both the code and the excluded code together, when appropriate.

13. **Etiology/manifestation convention ("code first", "use additional code" and "in diseases classified elsewhere" notes)**
    Certain conditions have both an underlying etiology and multiple body system manifestations due to the underlying etiology. For such conditions, the ICD-10-CM has a coding convention that requires the underlying condition be sequenced first, if applicable, followed by the manifestation. Wherever such a combination exists, there is a "use additional code" note at the etiology code, and a "code first" note at the manifestation code. These instructional notes indicate the proper sequencing order of the codes, etiology followed by manifestation.

    In most cases the manifestation codes will have in the code title, "in diseases classified elsewhere." Codes with this title are a component of the etiology/ manifestation convention. The code title indicates that it is a manifestation code. "In diseases classified elsewhere" codes are never permitted to be used as first listed or principal diagnosis codes. They must be used in conjunction with an underlying condition code and they must be listed following the underlying condition. See category F02, Dementia in other diseases classified elsewhere, for an example of this convention.

There are manifestation codes that do not have "in diseases classified elsewhere" in the title. For such codes, there is a "use additional code" note at the etiology code and a "code first" note at the manifestation code, and the rules for sequencing apply.

In addition to the notes in the Tabular List, these conditions also have a specific Alphabetic Index entry structure. In the Alphabetic Index both conditions are listed together with the etiology code first followed by the manifestation codes in brackets. The code in brackets is always to be sequenced second.

An example of the etiology/manifestation convention is dementia **with** Parkinson's disease. In the Alphabetic Index, code G20 is listed first, followed by code F02.80 or F02.81- in brackets. Code G20 represents the underlying etiology, Parkinson's disease, and must be sequenced first, whereas code**s** F02.80 and F02.81- represent the manifestation of dementia in diseases classified elsewhere, with or without behavioral disturbance.

"Code first" and "Use additional code" notes are also used as sequencing rules in the classification for certain codes that are not part of an etiology/ manifestation combination.

See Section I.B.7. Multiple coding for a single condition.

14. **"And"**
The word "and" should be interpreted to mean either "and" or "or" when it appears in a title.

For example, cases of "tuberculosis of bones", "tuberculosis of joints" and "tuberculosis of bones and joints" are classified to subcategory A18.0, Tuberculosis of bones and joints.

15. **"With"**
The word "with" or "in" should be interpreted to mean "associated with" or "due to" when it appears in a code title, the Alphabetic Index (either under a main term or subterm), or an instructional note in the Tabular List. The classification presumes a causal relationship between the two conditions linked by these terms in the Alphabetic Index or Tabular List. These conditions should be coded as related even in the absence of provider documentation explicitly linking them, unless the documentation clearly states the conditions are unrelated or when another guideline exists that specifically requires a documented linkage between two conditions (e.g., sepsis guideline for "acute organ dysfunction that is not clearly associated with the sepsis").

For conditions not specifically linked by these relational terms in the classification or when a guideline requires that a linkage between two conditions be explicitly documented, provider documentation must link the conditions in order to code them as related.

The word "with" in the Alphabetic Index is sequenced immediately following the main term or subterm, not in alphabetical order.

16. **"See" and "See Also"**
The "see" instruction following a main term in the Alphabetic Index indicates that another term should be referenced. It is necessary to go to the main term referenced with the "see" note to locate the correct code.

A "see also" instruction following a main term in the Alphabetic Index instructs that there is another main term that may also be referenced that may provide additional Alphabetic Index entries that may be useful. It is not necessary to follow the "see also" note when the original main term provides the necessary code.

17. **"Code also" note**
A "code also" note instructs that two codes may be required to fully describe a condition, but this note does not provide sequencing direction. The sequencing depends on the circumstances of the encounter.

18. **Default codes**
A code listed next to a main term in the ICD-10-CM Alphabetic Index is referred to as a default code. The default code represents that condition that is most commonly associated with the main term or is the unspecified code for the condition. If a condition is documented in a medical record (for example, appendicitis) without any additional information, such as acute or chronic, the default code should be assigned.

19. **Code assignment and Clinical Criteria**
The assignment of a diagnosis code is based on the provider's diagnostic statement that the condition exists. The provider's statement that the patient has a particular condition is sufficient. Code assignment is not based on clinical criteria used by the provider to establish the diagnosis. **If**

there is conflicting medical record documentation, query the provider.

B. General Coding Guidelines

1. **Locating a code in the ICD-10-CM**
To select a code in the classification that corresponds to a diagnosis or reason for visit documented in a medical record, first locate the term in the Alphabetic Index, and then verify the code in the Tabular List. Read and be guided by instructional notations that appear in both the Alphabetic Index and the Tabular List.

It is essential to use both the Alphabetic Index and Tabular List when locating and assigning a code. The Alphabetic Index does not always provide the full code. Selection of the full code, including laterality and any applicable 7th character can only be done in the Tabular List. A dash (-) at the end of an Alphabetic Index entry indicates that additional characters are required. Even if a dash is not included at the Alphabetic Index entry, it is necessary to refer to the Tabular List to verify that no 7th character is required.

2. **Level of Detail in Coding**
Diagnosis codes are to be used and reported at their highest number of characters available and to the highest level of specificity documented in the medical record.

ICD-10-CM diagnosis codes are composed of codes with 3, 4, 5, 6 or 7 characters. Codes with three characters are included in ICD-10-CM as the heading of a category of codes that may be further subdivided by the use of fourth and/or fifth characters and/or sixth characters, which provide greater detail.

A three-character code is to be used only if it is not further subdivided. A code is invalid if it has not been coded to the full number of characters required for that code, including the 7th character, if applicable.

3. **Code or codes from A00.0 through T88.9, Z00-Z99.8, U00-U85**
The appropriate code or codes from A00.0 through T88.9, Z00-Z99.8, and U00-U85 must be used to identify diagnoses, symptoms, conditions, problems, complaints or other reason(s) for the encounter/visit.

4. **Signs and symptoms**
Codes that describe symptoms and signs, as opposed to diagnoses, are acceptable for reporting purposes when a related definitive diagnosis has not been established (confirmed) by the provider. Chapter 18 of ICD-10-CM, Symptoms, Signs, and Abnormal Clinical and Laboratory Findings, Not Elsewhere Classified (codes R00.0-R99) contains many, but not all, codes for symptoms.

See Section I.B.18. Use of Signs/Symptom/Unspecified Codes

5. **Conditions that are an integral part of a disease process**
Signs and symptoms that are associated routinely with a disease process should not be assigned as additional codes, unless otherwise instructed by the classification.

6. **Conditions that are not an integral part of a disease process**
Additional signs and symptoms that may not be associated routinely with a disease process should be coded when present.

7. **Multiple coding for a single condition**
In addition to the etiology/manifestation convention that requires two codes to fully describe a single condition that affects multiple body systems, there are other single conditions that also require more than one code. "Use additional code" notes are found in the Tabular List at codes that are not part of an etiology/manifestation pair where a secondary code is useful to fully describe a condition. The sequencing rule is the same as the etiology/manifestation pair, "use additional code" indicates that a secondary code should be added, if known.

For example, for bacterial infections that are not included in chapter 1, a secondary code from category B95, Streptococcus, Staphylococcus, and Enterococcus, as the cause of diseases classified elsewhere, or B96, Other bacterial agents as the cause of diseases classified elsewhere, may be required to identify the bacterial organism causing the infection. A "use additional code" note will normally be found at the infectious disease code, indicating a need for the organism code to be added as a secondary code.

"Code first" notes are also under certain codes that are not specifically manifestation codes but may be due to an underlying cause. When there is a "code first" note and an underlying condition is present, the underlying condition should be sequenced first, if known.

"Code, if applicable, any causal condition first" notes indicate that this code may be assigned as a principal diagnosis when the causal condition is unknown or not applicable. If a causal condition is known, then the code for that condition should be sequenced as the principal or first-listed diagnosis.

Multiple codes may be needed for sequela, complication codes and obstetric codes to more fully describe a condition. See the specific guidelines for these conditions for further instruction.

8. **Acute and Chronic Conditions**

   If the same condition is described as both acute (subacute) and chronic, and separate subentries exist in the Alphabetic Index at the same indentation level, code both and sequence the acute (subacute) code first.

9. **Combination Code**

   A combination code is a single code used to classify:

   Two diagnoses, or

   A diagnosis with an associated secondary process (manifestation)

   A diagnosis with an associated complication

   Combination codes are identified by referring to subterm entries in the Alphabetic Index and by reading the inclusion and exclusion notes in the Tabular List.

   Assign only the combination code when that code fully identifies the diagnostic conditions involved or when the Alphabetic Index so directs. Multiple coding should not be used when the classification provides a combination code that clearly identifies all of the elements documented in the diagnosis. When the combination code lacks necessary specificity in describing the manifestation or complication, an additional code should be used as a secondary code.

10. **Sequela (Late Effects)**

    A sequela is the residual effect (condition produced) after the acute phase of an illness or injury has terminated. There is no time limit on when a sequela code can be used. The residual may be apparent early, such as in cerebral infarction, or it may occur months or years later, such as that due to a previous injury. Examples of sequela include: scar formation resulting from a burn, deviated septum due to a nasal fracture, and infertility due to tubal occlusion from old tuberculosis. Coding of sequela generally requires two codes sequenced in the following order: the condition or nature of the sequela is sequenced first. The sequela code is sequenced second.

    An exception to the above guidelines are those instances where the code for the sequela is followed by a manifestation code identified in the Tabular List and title, or the sequela code has been expanded (at the fourth, fifth or sixth character levels) to include the manifestation(s). The code for the acute phase of an illness or injury that led to the sequela is never used with a code for the late effect.

    See Section I.C.9. Sequelae of cerebrovascular disease

    See Section I.C.15. Sequelae of complication of pregnancy, childbirth and the puerperium

    See Section I.C.19. Application of 7th characters for Chapter 19

11. **Impending or Threatened Condition**

    Code any condition described at the time of discharge as "impending" or "threatened" as follows:

    If it did occur, code as confirmed diagnosis.

    If it did not occur, reference the Alphabetic Index to determine if the condition has a subentry term for "impending" or "threatened" and also reference main term entries for "Impending" and for "Threatened."

    If the subterms are listed, assign the given code.

    If the subterms are not listed, code the existing underlying condition(s) and not the condition described as impending or threatened.

12. **Reporting Same Diagnosis Code More than Once**

    Each unique ICD-10-CM diagnosis code may be reported only once for an encounter. This applies to bilateral conditions when there are no distinct codes identifying laterality or two different conditions classified to the same ICD-10-CM diagnosis code.

13. **Laterality**

    Some ICD-10-CM codes indicate laterality, specifying whether the condition occurs on the left, right or is bilateral. If no bilateral code is provided and the condition is bilateral, assign separate codes for both the left and right side. If the side is not identified in the medical record, assign the code for the unspecified side.

    When a patient has a bilateral condition and each side is treated during separate encounters, assign the "bilateral" code (as the condition still exists on both sides), including for the encounter to treat the first side. For the second encounter for treatment after one side has previously been treated and the condition no longer exists on that side, assign the appropriate unilateral code for the side where the condition still exists (e.g., cataract surgery performed on each eye in separate encounters). The bilateral code would not be assigned for the subsequent encounter, as the patient no longer has the condition in the previously-treated site. If the treatment on the first side did not completely resolve the condition, then the bilateral code would still be appropriate.

    When laterality is not documented by the patient's provider, code assignment for the affected side may be based on medical record documentation from other clinicians. If there is conflicting medical record documentation regarding the affected side, the patient's attending provider should be queried for clarification. Codes for "unspecified" side should rarely be used, such as when the documentation in the record is insufficient to determine the affected side and it is not possible to obtain clarification.

14. **Documentation by Clinicians Other than the Patient's Provider**

    Code assignment is based on the documentation by the patient's provider (i.e., physician or other qualified healthcare practitioner legally accountable for establishing the patient's diagnosis). There are a few exceptions when code assignment may be based on medical record documentation from clinicians who are not the patient's provider (i.e., physician or other qualified healthcare practitioner legally accountable for establishing the patient's diagnosis). In this context, "clinicians" other than the patient's provider refer to healthcare professionals permitted, based on regulatory or accreditation requirements or internal hospital policies, to document in a patient's official medical record.

    These exceptions include codes for:

    - Body Mass Index (BMI)
    - Depth of non-pressure chronic ulcers
    - Pressure ulcer stage
    - Coma scale
    - NIH stroke scale (NIHSS)
    - Social determinants of health (SDOH)
    - Laterality
    - Blood alcohol level
    - **Underimmunization status**

    This information is typically, or may be, documented by other clinicians involved in the care of the patient (e.g., a dietitian often documents the BMI, a nurse often documents the pressure ulcer stages, and an emergency medical technician often documents the coma scale). However, the associated diagnosis (such as overweight, obesity, acute stroke, pressure ulcer, or a condition classifiable to category F1Ø, Alcohol related disorders) must be documented by the patient's provider. If there is conflicting medical record documentation, either from the same clinician or different clinicians, the patient's attending provider should be queried for clarification.

    The BMI, coma scale, NIHSS, blood alcohol level codes, codes for social determinants of health **and underimmunization status** should only be reported as secondary diagnoses.

    See Section I.C.21.c.17. for additional information regarding coding social determinants of health.

15. **Syndromes**

    Follow the Alphabetic Index guidance when coding syndromes. In the absence of Alphabetic Index guidance, assign codes for the documented manifestations of the syndrome. Additional codes for manifestations that are not an integral part of the disease process may also be assigned when the condition does not have a unique code.

16. **Documentation of Complications of Care**

    Code assignment is based on the provider's documentation of the relationship between the condition and the care or procedure, unless otherwise instructed by the classification. The guideline extends to any complications of care, regardless of the chapter the code is located in. It is important to note that not all conditions that occur during or following medical care or surgery are classified as complications. There must be a cause-and-effect relationship between the care provided and the condition, and **the documentation must support that the condition is clinically significant. It is not necessary for the provider to explicitly document the term "complication." For example, if the condition alters the course of the surgery as documented in the operative report, then it would be appropriate to report a complication code.** Query the provider for clarification **if the documentation is not clear as to the relationship between the condition and the care or procedure.**

17. **Borderline Diagnosis**

    If the provider documents a "borderline" diagnosis at the time of discharge, the diagnosis is coded as confirmed, unless the classification provides a specific entry (e.g., borderline diabetes). If a borderline condition has a specific index entry in ICD-10-CM, it should be coded as such. Since borderline conditions are not uncertain diagnoses, no distinction is made between the care setting (inpatient versus outpatient). Whenever the documentation is unclear regarding a borderline condition, coders are encouraged to query for clarification.

18. Use of Sign/Symptom/Unspecified Codes

Sign/symptom and "unspecified" codes have acceptable, even necessary, uses. While specific diagnosis codes should be reported when they are supported by the available medical record documentation and clinical knowledge of the patient's health condition, there are instances when signs/symptoms or unspecified codes are the best choices for accurately reflecting the healthcare encounter. Each healthcare encounter should be coded to the level of certainty known for that encounter.

As stated in the introductory section of these official coding guidelines, a joint effort between the healthcare provider and the coder is essential to achieve complete and accurate documentation, code assignment, and reporting of diagnoses and procedures. The importance of consistent, complete documentation in the medical record cannot be overemphasized. Without such documentation accurate coding cannot be achieved. The entire record should be reviewed to determine the specific reason for the encounter and the conditions treated.

If a definitive diagnosis has not been established by the end of the encounter, it is appropriate to report codes for sign(s) and/or symptom(s) in lieu of a definitive diagnosis. When sufficient clinical information isn't known or available about a particular health condition to assign a more specific code, it is acceptable to report the appropriate "unspecified" code (e.g., a diagnosis of pneumonia has been determined, but not the specific type). Unspecified codes should be reported when they are the codes that most accurately reflect what is known about the patient's condition at the time of that particular encounter. It would be inappropriate to select a specific code that is not supported by the medical record documentation or conduct medically unnecessary diagnostic testing in order to determine a more specific code.

19. Coding for Healthcare Encounters in Hurricane Aftermath

a. Use of External Cause of Morbidity Codes

An external cause of morbidity code should be assigned to identify the cause of the injury(ies) incurred as a result of the hurricane. The use of external cause of morbidity codes is supplemental to the application of ICD-10-CM codes. External cause of morbidity codes are never to be recorded as a principal diagnosis (first-listed in non-inpatient settings). The appropriate injury code should be sequenced before any external cause codes. The external cause of morbidity codes capture how the injury or health condition happened (cause), the intent (unintentional or accidental; or intentional, such as suicide or assault), the place where the event occurred, the activity of the patient at the time of the event, and the person's status (e.g., civilian, military). They should not be assigned for encounters to treat hurricane victims' medical conditions when no injury, adverse effect or poisoning is involved. External cause of morbidity codes should be assigned for each encounter for care and treatment of the injury. External cause of morbidity codes may be assigned in all health care settings. For the purpose of capturing complete and accurate ICD-10-CM data in the aftermath of the hurricane, a healthcare setting should be considered as any location where medical care is provided by licensed healthcare professionals.

b. Sequencing of External Causes of Morbidity Codes

Codes for cataclysmic events, such as a hurricane, take priority over all other external cause codes except child and adult abuse and terrorism and should be sequenced before other external cause of injury codes. Assign as many external cause of morbidity codes as necessary to fully explain each cause. For example, if an injury occurs as a result of a building collapse during the hurricane, external cause codes for both the hurricane and the building collapse should be assigned, with the external causes code for hurricane being sequenced as the first external cause code. For injuries incurred as a direct result of the hurricane, assign the appropriate code(s) for the injuries, followed by the code X37.0-, Hurricane (with the appropriate 7th character), and any other applicable external cause of injury codes. Code X37.0- also should be assigned when an injury is incurred as a result of flooding caused by a levee breaking related to the hurricane. Code X38.-, Flood (with the appropriate 7th character), should be assigned when an injury is from flooding resulting directly from the storm. Code X36.0.-, Collapse of dam or man-made structure, should not be assigned when the cause of the collapse is due to the hurricane. Use of code X36.0- is limited to collapses of man-made structures due to earth surface movements, not due to storm surges directly from a hurricane.

c. Other External Causes of Morbidity Code Issues

For injuries that are not a direct result of the hurricane, such as an evacuee that has incurred an injury as a result of a motor vehicle accident, assign the appropriate external cause of morbidity code(s) to describe the cause of the injury, but do not assign code X37.0-, Hurricane. If it is not clear whether the injury was a direct result of the hurricane, assume the injury is due to the hurricane and assign code

X37.0-, Hurricane, as well as any other applicable external cause of morbidity codes. In addition to code X37.0-, Hurricane, other possible applicable external cause of morbidity codes include:

- X30-, Exposure to excessive natural heat
- X31-, Exposure to excessive natural cold
- X38-, Flood

d. Use of Z codes

Z codes (other reasons for healthcare encounters) may be assigned as appropriate to further explain the reasons for presenting for healthcare services, including transfers between healthcare facilities, or provide additional information relevant to a patient encounter. The ICD-10-CM Official Guidelines for Coding and Reporting identify which codes maybe assigned as principal or first-listed diagnosis only, secondary diagnosis only, or principal/first-listed or secondary (depending on the circumstances). Possible applicable Z codes include:

- Z59.0-, Homelessness
- Z59.1, Inadequate housing
- Z59.5, Extreme poverty
- Z75.1, Person awaiting admission to adequate facility elsewhere
- Z75.3, Unavailability and inaccessibility of health-care facilities
- Z75.4, Unavailability and inaccessibility of other helping agencies
- Z76.2, Encounter for health supervision and care of other healthy infant and child
- Z99.12, Encounter for respirator [ventilator] dependence during power failure

The external cause of morbidity codes and the Z codes listed above are not an all-inclusive list. Other codes may be applicable to the encounter based upon the documentation. Assign as many codes as necessary to fully explain each healthcare encounter. Since patient history information may be very limited, use any available documentation to assign the appropriate external cause of morbidity and Z codes.

C. Chapter-Specific Coding Guidelines

In addition to general coding guidelines, there are guidelines for specific diagnoses and/or conditions in the classification. Unless otherwise indicated, these guidelines apply to all health care settings. Please refer to Section II for guidelines on the selection of principal diagnosis.

1. Chapter 1: Certain Infectious and Parasitic Diseases (A00-B99), U07.1, U09.9

a. Human Immunodeficiency Virus (HIV) Infections

1) Code only confirmed cases

Code only confirmed cases of HIV infection/illness. This is an exception to the hospital inpatient guideline Section II, H.

In this context, "confirmation" does not require documentation of positive serology or culture for HIV; the provider's diagnostic statement that the patient is HIV positive or has an HIV-related illness is sufficient.

2) Selection and sequencing of HIV codes

(a) Patient admitted for HIV-related condition

If a patient is admitted for an HIV-related condition, the principal diagnosis should be B20, Human immunodeficiency virus [HIV] disease followed by additional diagnosis codes for all reported HIV-related conditions.

An exception to this guideline is if the reason for admission is hemolytic-uremic syndrome associated with HIV disease. Assign code D59.31, Infection-associated hemolytic-uremic syndrome, followed by code B20, Human immunodeficiency virus [HIV] disease.

(b) Patient with HIV disease admitted for unrelated condition

If a patient with HIV disease is admitted for an unrelated condition (such as a traumatic injury), the code for the unrelated condition (e.g., the nature of injury code) should be the principal diagnosis. Other diagnoses would be B20 followed by additional diagnosis codes for all reported HIV-related conditions.

(c) Whether the patient is newly diagnosed

Whether the patient is newly diagnosed or has had previous admissions/encounters for HIV conditions is irrelevant to the sequencing decision.

(d) Asymptomatic human immunodeficiency virus

Z21, Asymptomatic human immunodeficiency virus [HIV] infection status, is to be applied when the patient without any documentation of symptoms is listed as being "HIV positive," "known HIV," "HIV test positive," or similar terminology. Do not use this code if the term "AIDS" or "HIV disease" is used or if the patient is treated for any HIV-related illness or is described as having any condition(s) resulting from his/her HIV positive status; use B20 in these cases.

(e) Patients with inconclusive HIV serology
Patients with inconclusive HIV serology, but no definitive diagnosis or manifestations of the illness, may be assigned code R75, Inconclusive laboratory evidence of human immunodeficiency virus [HIV].

(f) Previously diagnosed HIV-related illness
Patients with any known prior diagnosis of an HIV-related illness should be coded to B20. Once a patient has developed an HIV-related illness, the patient should always be assigned code B20 on every subsequent admission/encounter. Patients previously diagnosed with any HIV illness (B20) should never be assigned to R75 or Z21, Asymptomatic human immunodeficiency virus [HIV] infection status.

(g) HIV Infection in Pregnancy, Childbirth and the Puerperium
During pregnancy, childbirth or the puerperium, a patient admitted (or presenting for a health care encounter) because of an HIV-related illness should receive a principal diagnosis code of O98.7-, Human immunodeficiency [HIV] disease complicating pregnancy, childbirth and the puerperium, followed by B20 and the code(s) for the HIV-related illness(es). Codes from Chapter 15 always take sequencing priority.

Patients with asymptomatic HIV infection status admitted (or presenting for a health care encounter) during pregnancy, childbirth, or the puerperium should receive codes of O98.7- and Z21.

(h) Encounters for testing for HIV
If a patient is being seen to determine his/her HIV status, use code Z11.4, Encounter for screening for human immunodeficiency virus [HIV]. Use additional codes for any associated high-risk behavior, if applicable.

If a patient with signs or symptoms is being seen for HIV testing, code the signs and symptoms. An additional counseling code Z71.7, Human immunodeficiency virus [HIV] counseling, may be used if counseling is provided during the encounter for the test.

When a patient returns to be informed of his/her HIV test results and the test result is negative, use code Z71.7, Human immunodeficiency virus [HIV] counseling.

If the results are positive, see previous guidelines and assign codes as appropriate.

(i) HIV managed by antiretroviral medication
If a patient with documented HIV disease, **HIV-related illness or AIDS** is currently managed on antiretroviral medications, assign code B20, Human immunodeficiency virus [HIV] disease. Code Z79.899, Other long term (current) drug therapy, may be assigned as an additional code to identify the long-term (current) use of antiretroviral medications.

b. Infectious agents as the cause of diseases classified to other chapters
Certain infections are classified in chapters other than Chapter 1 and no organism is identified as part of the infection code. In these instances, it is necessary to use an additional code from Chapter 1 to identify the organism. A code from category B95, Streptococcus, Staphylococcus, and Enterococcus as the cause of diseases classified to other chapters, B96, Other bacterial agents as the cause of diseases classified to other chapters, or B97, Viral agents as the cause of diseases classified to other chapters, is to be used as an additional code to identify the organism. An instructional note will be found at the infection code advising that an additional organism code is required.

c. Infections resistant to antibiotics
Many bacterial infections are resistant to current antibiotics. It is necessary to identify all infections documented as antibiotic resistant. Assign a code from category Z16, Resistance to antimicrobial drugs, following the infection code only if the infection code does not identify drug resistance.

d. Sepsis, Severe Sepsis, and Septic Shock Infections resistant to antibiotics
1) Coding of Sepsis and Severe Sepsis
(a) Sepsis
For a diagnosis of sepsis, assign the appropriate code for the underlying systemic infection. If the type of infection or causal organism is not further specified, assign code A41.9, Sepsis, unspecified organism.

A code from subcategory R65.2, Severe sepsis, should not be assigned unless severe sepsis or an associated acute organ dysfunction is documented.

(i) Negative or inconclusive blood cultures and sepsis
Negative or inconclusive blood cultures do not preclude a diagnosis of sepsis in patients with clinical evidence of the condition; however, the provider should be queried.

(ii) Urosepsis
The term urosepsis is a nonspecific term. It is not to be considered synonymous with sepsis. It has no default code in the Alphabetic Index. Should a provider use this term, he/she must be queried for clarification.

(iii) Sepsis with organ dysfunction
If a patient has sepsis and associated acute organ dysfunction or multiple organ dysfunction (MOD), follow the instructions for coding severe sepsis.

(iv) Acute organ dysfunction that is not clearly associated with the sepsis
If a patient has sepsis and an acute organ dysfunction, but the medical record documentation indicates that the acute organ dysfunction is related to a medical condition other than the sepsis, do not assign a code from subcategory R65.2, Severe sepsis. An acute organ dysfunction must be associated with the sepsis in order to assign the severe sepsis code. If the documentation is not clear as to whether an acute organ dysfunction is related to the sepsis or another medical condition, query the provider.

(b) Severe sepsis
The coding of severe sepsis requires a minimum of 2 codes: first a code for the underlying systemic infection, followed by a code from subcategory R65.2, Severe sepsis. If the causal organism is not documented, assign code A41.9, Sepsis, unspecified organism, for the infection. Additional code(s) for the associated acute organ dysfunction are also required.

Due to the complex nature of severe sepsis, some cases may require querying the provider prior to assignment of the codes.

2) Septic shock
Septic shock generally refers to circulatory failure associated with severe sepsis, and therefore, it represents a type of acute organ dysfunction.

For cases of septic shock, the code for the systemic infection should be sequenced first, followed by code R65.21, Severe sepsis with septic shock or code T81.12, Postprocedural septic shock.

Any additional codes for the other acute organ dysfunctions should also be assigned. As noted in the sequencing instructions in the Tabular List, the code for septic shock cannot be assigned as a principal diagnosis.

3) Sequencing of severe sepsis
If severe sepsis is present on admission, and meets the definition of principal diagnosis, the underlying systemic infection should be assigned as principal diagnosis followed by the appropriate code from subcategory R65.2 as required by the sequencing rules in the Tabular List. A code from subcategory R65.2 can never be assigned as a principal diagnosis.

When severe sepsis develops during an encounter (it was not present on admission), the underlying systemic infection and the appropriate code from subcategory R65.2 should be assigned as secondary diagnoses.

Severe sepsis may be present on admission, but the diagnosis may not be confirmed until sometime after admission. If the documentation is not clear whether severe sepsis was present on admission, the provider should be queried.

For infection-associated hemolytic-uremic syndrome with severe sepsis, see guideline I.C.1.d.9.

4) **Sepsis or severe sepsis with a localized infection**
If the reason for admission is sepsis or severe sepsis and a localized infection, such as pneumonia or cellulitis, a code(s) for the underlying systemic infection should be assigned first and the code for the localized infection should be assigned as a secondary diagnosis. If the patient has severe sepsis, a code from subcategory R65.2 should also be assigned as a secondary diagnosis. If the patient is admitted with a localized infection, such as pneumonia, and sepsis/severe sepsis doesn't develop until after admission, the localized infection should be assigned first, followed by the appropriate sepsis/severe sepsis codes.

For hemolytic-uremic syndrome associated with sepsis, see guideline I.C.1.d.9.

5) **Sepsis due to a postprocedural infection**
(a) **Documentation of causal relationship**
As with all postprocedural complications, code assignment is based on the provider's documentation of the relationship between the infection and the procedure.

(b) **Sepsis due to a postprocedural infection**
For infections following a procedure, a code from T81.40, to T81.43 Infection following a procedure, or a code from O86.00 to O86.03, Infection of obstetric surgical wound, that identifies the site of the infection should be coded first, if known. Assign an additional code for sepsis following a procedure (T81.44) or sepsis following an obstetrical procedure (O86.04). Use an additional code to identify the infectious agent. If the patient has severe sepsis, the appropriate code from subcategory R65.2 should also be assigned with the additional code(s) for any acute organ dysfunction.

For infections following infusion, transfusion, therapeutic injection, or immunization, a code from subcategory T80.2, Infections following infusion, transfusion, and therapeutic injection, or code T88.0-, Infection following immunization, should be coded first, followed by the code for the specific infection. If the patient has severe sepsis, the appropriate code from subcategory R65.2 should also be assigned, with the additional codes(s) for any acute organ dysfunction.

(c) **Postprocedural infection and postprocedural septic shock**
If a postprocedural infection has resulted in postprocedural septic shock, assign the codes indicated above for sepsis due to a postprocedural infection, followed by code T81.12-, Postprocedural septic shock. Do not assign code R65.21, Severe sepsis with septic shock. Additional code(s) should be assigned for any acute organ dysfunction.

6) **Sepsis and severe sepsis associated with a noninfectious process (condition)**
In some cases, a noninfectious process (condition) such as trauma, may lead to an infection which can result in sepsis or severe sepsis. If sepsis or severe sepsis is documented as associated with a noninfectious condition, such as a burn or serious injury, and this condition meets the definition for principal diagnosis, the code for the noninfectious condition should be sequenced first, followed by the code for the resulting infection. If severe sepsis is present, a code from subcategory R65.2 should also be assigned with any associated organ dysfunction(s) codes. It is not necessary to assign a code from subcategory R65.1, Systemic inflammatory response syndrome (SIRS) of non-infectious origin, for these cases.

If the infection meets the definition of principal diagnosis, it should be sequenced before the non-infectious condition. When both the associated non-infectious condition and the infection meet the definition of principal diagnosis, either may be assigned as principal diagnosis.

Only one code from category R65, Symptoms and signs specifically associated with systemic inflammation and infection, should be assigned. Therefore, when a non-infectious condition leads to an infection resulting in severe sepsis, assign the appropriate code from subcategory R65.2, Severe sepsis. Do not additionally assign a code from subcategory R65.1, Systemic inflammatory response syndrome (SIRS) of non-infectious origin.

See Section I.C.18. SIRS due to non-infectious process

7) **Sepsis and septic shock complicating abortion, pregnancy, childbirth, and the puerperium**
See Section I.C.15. Sepsis and septic shock complicating abortion, pregnancy, childbirth and the puerperium

8) **Newborn sepsis**
See Section I.C.16. f. Bacterial sepsis of Newborn

9) **Hemolytic-uremic syndrome associated with sepsis**
If the reason for admission is hemolytic-uremic syndrome that is associated with sepsis, assign code D59.31, Infection-associated hemolytic-uremic syndrome, as the principal diagnosis. Codes for the underlying systemic infection and any other conditions (such as severe sepsis) should be assigned as secondary diagnoses.

e. **Methicillin Resistant Staphylococcus aureus (MRSA) Conditions**
1) **Selection and sequencing of MRSA codes**
(a) **Combination codes for MRSA infection**
When a patient is diagnosed with an infection that is due to methicillin resistant *Staphylococcus aureus* (MRSA), and that infection has a combination code that includes the causal organism (e.g., sepsis, pneumonia) assign the appropriate combination code for the condition (e.g., code A41.02, Sepsis due to Methicillin resistant Staphylococcus aureus or code J15.212, Pneumonia due to Methicillin resistant Staphylococcus aureus). Do not assign code B95.62, Methicillin resistant Staphylococcus aureus infection as the cause of diseases classified elsewhere, as an additional code, because the combination code includes the type of infection and the MRSA organism. Do not assign a code from subcategory Z16.11, Resistance to penicillins, as an additional diagnosis.

See Section C.1. for instructions on coding and sequencing of sepsis and severe sepsis.

(b) **Other codes for MRSA infection**
When there is documentation of a current infection (e.g., wound infection, stitch abscess, urinary tract infection) due to MRSA, and that infection does not have a combination code that includes the causal organism, assign the appropriate code to identify the condition along with code B95.62, Methicillin resistant Staphylococcus aureus infection as the cause of diseases classified elsewhere for the MRSA infection. Do not assign a code from subcategory Z16.11, Resistance to penicillins.

(c) **Methicillin susceptible Staphylococcus aureus (MSSA) and MRSA colonization**
The condition or state of being colonized or carrying MSSA or MRSA is called colonization or carriage, while an individual person is described as being colonized or being a carrier.

Colonization means that MSSA or MSRA is present on or in the body without necessarily causing illness. A positive MRSA colonization test might be documented by the provider as "MRSA screen positive" or "MRSA nasal swab positive".

Assign code Z22.322, Carrier or suspected carrier of Methicillin resistant Staphylococcus aureus, for patients documented as having MRSA colonization. Assign code Z22.321, Carrier or suspected carrier of Methicillin susceptible Staphylococcus aureus, for patients documented as having MSSA colonization. Colonization is not necessarily indicative of a disease process or as the cause of a specific condition the patient may have unless documented as such by the provider.

(d) **MRSA colonization and infection**
If a patient is documented as having both MRSA colonization and infection during a hospital admission, code Z22.322, Carrier or suspected carrier of Methicillin resistant Staphylococcus aureus, and a code for the MRSA infection may both be assigned.

f. **Zika virus infections**
1) **Code only confirmed cases**
Code only a confirmed diagnosis of Zika virus (A92.5, Zika virus disease) as documented by the provider. This is an exception to the hospital inpatient guideline Section II, H. In this context, "confirmation" does not require documentation of the type of test performed; the provider's diagnostic statement that the condition is confirmed is sufficient. This code should be assigned regardless of the stated mode of transmission.

If the provider documents "suspected", "possible" or "probable" Zika, do not assign code A92.5. Assign a code(s) explaining the reason for encounter (such as fever, rash, or joint pain) or Z20.821, Contact with and (suspected) exposure to Zika virus.

g. **Coronavirus infections**
1) **COVID-19 infection (infection due to SARS-CoV-2)**
   (a) **Code only confirmed cases**

   Code only a confirmed diagnosis of the 2019 novel coronavirus disease (COVID-19) as documented by the provider, or documentation of a positive COVID-19 test result. For a confirmed diagnosis, assign code U07.1, COVID-19. This is an exception to the hospital inpatient guideline Section II, H. In this context, "confirmation" does not require documentation of a positive test result for COVID-19; the provider's documentation that the individual has COVID-19 is sufficient.

   If the provider documents "suspected," "possible," "probable," or "inconclusive" COVID-19, do not assign code U07.1. Instead, code the signs and symptoms reported. See guideline I.C.1.g.1.g.

   (b) **Sequencing of codes**

   When COVID-19 meets the definition of principal diagnosis, code U07.1, COVID-19, should be sequenced first, followed by the appropriate codes for associated manifestations, except when another guideline requires that certain codes be sequenced first, such as obstetrics, sepsis, or transplant complications.

   For a COVID-19 infection that progresses to sepsis, see Section I.C.1.d. Sepsis, Severe Sepsis, and Septic Shock

   See Section I.C.15.s. for COVID-19 infection in pregnancy, childbirth, and the puerperium

   See Section I.C.16.h. for COVID-19 infection in newborn

   For a COVID-19 infection in a lung transplant patient, see Section I.C.19.g.3.a. Transplant complications other than kidney.

   (c) **Acute respiratory manifestations of COVID-19**

   When the reason for the encounter/admission is a respiratory manifestation of COVID-19, assign code U07.1, COVID-19, as the principal/first-listed diagnosis and assign code(s) for the respiratory manifestation(s) as additional diagnoses.

   The following conditions are examples of common respiratory manifestations of COVID-19.

   (i) **Pneumonia**

   For a patient with pneumonia confirmed as due to COVID-19, assign codes U07.1, COVID-19, and J12.82, Pneumonia due to coronavirus disease 2019.

   (ii) **Acute bronchitis**

   For a patient with acute bronchitis confirmed as due to COVID-19, assign codes U07.1, and J20.8, Acute bronchitis due to other specified organisms.

   Bronchitis not otherwise specified (NOS) due to COVID-19 should be coded using code U07.1 and J40, Bronchitis, not specified as acute or chronic.

   (iii) **Lower respiratory infection**

   If the COVID-19 is documented as being associated with a lower respiratory infection, not otherwise specified (NOS), or an acute respiratory infection, NOS, codes U07.1 and J22, Unspecified acute lower respiratory infection, should be assigned.

   If the COVID-19 is documented as being associated with a respiratory infection, NOS, codes U07.1 and J98.8, Other specified respiratory disorders, should be assigned.

   (iv) **Acute respiratory distress syndrome**

   For acute respiratory distress syndrome (ARDS) due to COVID-19, assign codes U07.1, and J80, Acute respiratory distress syndrome.

   (v) **Acute respiratory failure**

   For acute respiratory failure due to COVID-19, assign code U07.1, and code J96.0-, Acute respiratory failure.

   (d) **Non-respiratory manifestations of COVID-19**

   When the reason for the encounter/admission is a non-respiratory manifestation (e.g., viral enteritis) of COVID-19, assign code U07.1, COVID-19, as the principal/first-listed diagnosis and assign code(s) for the manifestation(s) as additional diagnoses.

   (e) **Exposure to COVID-19**

   For asymptomatic individuals with actual or suspected exposure to COVID-19, assign code Z20.822, Contact with and (suspected) exposure to COVID-19.

   For symptomatic individuals with actual or suspected exposure to COVID-19 and the infection has been ruled out, or test results are inconclusive or unknown, assign code Z20.822, Contact with and (suspected) exposure to COVID-19. See guideline I.C.21.c.1, Contact/Exposure, for additional guidance regarding the use of category Z20 codes.

   If COVID-19 is confirmed, see guideline I.C.1.g.1.a.

   (f) **Screening for COVID-19**

   During the COVID-19 pandemic, a screening code is generally not appropriate. Do not assign code Z11.52, Encounter for screening for COVID-19. For encounters for COVID-19 testing, including preoperative testing, code as exposure to COVID-19 (guideline I.C.1.g.1.e).

   Coding guidance will be updated as new information concerning any changes in the pandemic status becomes available.

   (g) **Signs and symptoms without definitive diagnosis of COVID-19**

   For patients presenting with any signs/symptoms associated with COVID-19 (such as fever, etc.) but a definitive diagnosis has not been established, assign the appropriate code(s) for each of the presenting signs and symptoms such as:

   - R05.1, Acute cough, or R05.9, Cough, unspecified
   - R06.02 Shortness of breath
   - R50.9 Fever, unspecified

   If a patient with signs/symptoms associated with COVID-19 also has an actual or suspected contact with or exposure to COVID-19, assign Z20.822, Contact with and (suspected) exposure to COVID-19, as an additional code.

   (h) **Asymptomatic individuals who test positive for COVID-19**

   For asymptomatic individuals who test positive for COVID-19, see guideline I.C.1.g.1.a. Although the individual is asymptomatic, the individual has tested positive and is considered to have the COVID-19 infection.

   (i) **Personal history of COVID-19**

   For patients with a history of COVID-19, assign code Z86.16, Personal history of COVID-19.

   (j) **Follow-up visits after COVID-19 infection has resolved**

   For individuals who previously had COVID-19, without residual symptom(s) or condition(s), and are being seen for follow-up evaluation, and COVID-19 test results are negative, assign codes Z09, Encounter for follow-up examination after completed treatment for conditions other than malignant neoplasm, and Z86.16, Personal history of COVID-19.

   For follow-up visits for individuals with symptom(s) or condition(s) related to a previous COVID-19 infection, see guideline I.C.1.g.1.m.

   See Section I.C.21.c.8, Factors influencing health states and contact with health services, Follow-up

   (k) **Encounter for antibody testing**

   For an encounter for antibody testing that is not being performed to confirm a current COVID-19 infection, nor is a follow-up test after resolution of COVID-19, assign Z01.84, Encounter for antibody response examination.

   Follow the applicable guidelines above if the individual is being tested to confirm a current COVID-19 infection.

   For follow-up testing after a COVID-19 infection, see guideline I.C.1.g.1.j.

   (l) **Multisystem Inflammatory Syndrome**

   For individuals with multisystem inflammatory syndrome (MIS) and COVID-19, assign code U07.1, COVID-19, as the principal/first-listed diagnosis and assign code M35.81, Multisystem inflammatory syndrome, as an additional diagnosis.

   If an individual with a history of COVID-19 develops MIS, assign codes M35.81, Multisystem inflammatory syndrome, and U09.9, Post COVID-19 condition, unspecified.

   If an individual with a known or suspected exposure to COVID-19, and no current COVID-19 infection or history of

COVID-19, develops MIS, assign codes M35.81, Multisystem inflammatory syndrome, and Z20.822, Contact with and (suspected) exposure to COVID-19.

Additional codes should be assigned for any associated complications of MIS.

(m) Post COVID-19 Condition

For sequela of COVID-19, or associated symptoms or conditions that develop following a previous COVID-19 infection, assign a code(s) for the specific symptom(s) or condition(s) related to the previous COVID-19 infection, if known, and code U09.9, Post COVID-19 condition, unspecified.

Code U09.9 should not be assigned for manifestations of an active (current) COVID-19 infection.

If a patient has a condition(s) associated with a previous COVID-19 infection and develops a new active (current) COVID-19 infection, code U09.9 may be assigned in conjunction with code U07.1, COVID-19, to identify that the patient also has a condition(s) associated with a previous COVID-19 infection. Code(s) for the specific condition(s) associated with the previous COVID-19 infection and code(s) for manifestation(s) of the new active (current) COVID-19 infection should also be assigned.

(n) Underimmunization for COVID-19 Status

Code Z28.310, Unvaccinated for COVID-19, may be assigned when the patient has not received a COVID-19 vaccine of any type. Code Z28.311, Partially vaccinated for COVID-19, may be assigned when the patient has been partially vaccinated for COVID-19 as per the recommendations of the Centers for Disease Control and Prevention (CDC) in place at the time of the encounter. For information, visit the CDC's website https://www.cdc.gov/coronavirus/2019-ncov/vaccines/.

See Section I.B.14. for underimmunization documentation by clinicians other than patient's provider.

2. Chapter 2: Neoplasms (C00-D49)
General Guidelines

Chapter 2 of the ICD-10-CM contains the codes for most benign and all malignant neoplasms. Certain benign neoplasms, such as prostatic adenomas, may be found in the specific body system chapters. To properly code a neoplasm, it is necessary to determine from the record if the neoplasm is benign, in-situ, malignant, or of uncertain histologic behavior. If malignant, any secondary (metastatic) sites should also be determined.

Primary malignant neoplasms overlapping site boundaries

A primary malignant neoplasm that overlaps two or more contiguous (next to each other) sites should be classified to the subcategory/code .8 ('overlapping lesion'), unless the combination is specifically indexed elsewhere. For multiple neoplasms of the same site that are not contiguous such as tumors in different quadrants of the same breast, codes for each site should be assigned.

Malignant neoplasm of ectopic tissue

Malignant neoplasms of ectopic tissue are to be coded to the site of origin mentioned, e.g., ectopic pancreatic malignant neoplasms involving the stomach are coded to malignant neoplasm of pancreas, unspecified (C25.9).

The neoplasm table in the Alphabetic Index should be referenced first. However, if the histological term is documented, that term should be referenced first, rather than going immediately to the Neoplasm Table, in order to determine which column in the Neoplasm Table is appropriate. For example, if the documentation indicates "adenoma," refer to the term in the Alphabetic Index to review the entries under this term and the instructional note to "see also neoplasm, by site, benign." The table provides the proper code based on the type of neoplasm and the site. It is important to select the proper column in the table that corresponds to the type of neoplasm. The Tabular List should then be referenced to verify that the correct code has been selected from the table and that a more specific site code does not exist.

See Section I.C.21. Factors influencing health status and contact with health services, Status, for information regarding Z15.0, codes for genetic susceptibility to cancer.

a. Admission/Encounter for treatment of primary site

If the malignancy is chiefly responsible for occasioning the patient admission/encounter and treatment is directed at the primary site, designate the primary malignancy as the principal/first-listed diagnosis.

The only exception to this guideline is if the administration of chemotherapy, immunotherapy or external beam radiation therapy is chiefly responsible for occasioning the admission/encounter. In that case, assign the appropriate Z51.-- code as the first-listed or principal diagnosis, and the underlying diagnosis or problem for which the service is being performed as a secondary diagnosis.

b. Admission/Encounter for treatment of secondary site

When a patient is admitted because of a primary neoplasm with metastasis and treatment is directed toward the secondary site only, the secondary neoplasm is designated as the principal diagnosis even though the primary malignancy is still present.

c. Coding and sequencing of complications

Coding and sequencing of complications associated with the malignancies or with the therapy thereof are subject to the following guidelines:

1) Anemia associated with malignancy

When admission/encounter is for management of an anemia associated with the malignancy, and the treatment is only for anemia, the appropriate code for the malignancy is sequenced as the principal or first-listed diagnosis followed by the appropriate code for the anemia (such as code D63.0, Anemia in neoplastic disease).

2) Anemia associated with chemotherapy, immunotherapy and radiation therapy

When the admission/encounter is for management of an anemia associated with an adverse effect of the administration of chemotherapy or immunotherapy and the only treatment is for the anemia, the anemia code is sequenced first followed by the appropriate codes for the neoplasm and the adverse effect (T45.1X5-, Adverse effect of antineoplastic and immunosuppressive drugs).

When the admission/encounter is for management of an anemia associated with an adverse effect of radiotherapy, the anemia code should be sequenced first, followed by the appropriate neoplasm code and code Y84.2, Radiological procedure and radiotherapy as the cause of abnormal reaction of the patient, or of later complication, without mention of misadventure at the time of the procedure.

3) Management of dehydration due to the malignancy

When the admission/encounter is for management of dehydration due to the malignancy and only the dehydration is being treated (intravenous rehydration), the dehydration is sequenced first, followed by the code(s) for the malignancy.

4) Treatment of a complication resulting from a surgical procedure

When the admission/encounter is for treatment of a complication resulting from a surgical procedure, designate the complication as the principal or first-listed diagnosis if treatment is directed at resolving the complication.

d. Primary malignancy previously excised

When a primary malignancy has been previously excised or eradicated from its site and there is no further treatment directed to that site and there is no evidence of any existing primary malignancy at that site, a code from category Z85, Personal history of malignant neoplasm, should be used to indicate the former site of the malignancy. Any mention of extension, invasion, or metastasis to another site is coded as a secondary malignant neoplasm to that site. The secondary site may be the principal or first-listed diagnosis with the Z85 code used as a secondary code.

See section I.C.2.t. Secondary malignant neoplasm of lymphoid tissue.

e. Admissions/Encounters involving chemotherapy, immunotherapy and radiation therapy

1) Episode of care involves surgical removal of neoplasm

When an episode of care involves the surgical removal of a neoplasm, primary or secondary site, followed by adjunct chemotherapy or radiation treatment during the same episode of care, the code for the neoplasm should be assigned as principal or first-listed diagnosis.

2) Patient admission/encounter solely for administration of chemotherapy, immunotherapy and radiation therapy

If a patient admission/encounter is solely for the administration of chemotherapy, immunotherapy or external beam radiation therapy assign code Z51.0, Encounter for antineoplastic radiation therapy, or Z51.11, Encounter for antineoplastic chemotherapy, or Z51.12, Encounter for antineoplastic immunotherapy as the first-listed or principal diagnosis. If a patient receives more than one of these therapies during the same admission more than one of these codes may be assigned, in any sequence.

The malignancy for which the therapy is being administered should be assigned as a secondary diagnosis.

If a patient admission/encounter is for the insertion or implantation of radioactive elements (e.g., brachytherapy) the appropriate code for the malignancy is sequenced as the principal or first-listed diagnosis. Code Z51.0 should not be assigned.

3) **Patient admitted for radiation therapy, chemotherapy or immunotherapy and develops complications**
When a patient is admitted for the purpose of external beam radiotherapy, immunotherapy or chemotherapy and develops complications such as uncontrolled nausea and vomiting or dehydration, the principal or first-listed diagnosis is Z51.0, Encounter for antineoplastic radiation therapy, or Z51.11, Encounter for antineoplastic chemotherapy, or Z51.12, Encounter for antineoplastic immunotherapy followed by any codes for the complications.

When a patient is admitted for the purpose of insertion or implantation of radioactive elements (e.g., brachytherapy) and develops complications such as uncontrolled nausea and vomiting or dehydration, the principal or first-listed diagnosis is the appropriate code for the malignancy followed by any codes for the complications.

f. **Admission/encounter to determine extent of malignancy**
When the reason for admission/encounter is to determine the extent of the malignancy, or for a procedure such as paracentesis or thoracentesis, the primary malignancy or appropriate metastatic site is designated as the principal or first-listed diagnosis, even though chemotherapy or radiotherapy is administered.

g. **Symptoms, signs, and abnormal findings listed in Chapter 18 associated with neoplasms**
Symptoms, signs, and ill-defined conditions listed in Chapter 18 characteristic of, or associated with, an existing primary or secondary site malignancy cannot be used to replace the malignancy as principal or first-listed diagnosis, regardless of the number of admissions or encounters for treatment and care of the neoplasm.

See section I.C.21. Factors influencing health status and contact with health services, Encounter for prophylactic organ removal.

h. **Admission/encounter for pain control/management**
See Section I.C.6. for information on coding admission/encounter for pain control/management.

i. **Malignancy in two or more noncontiguous sites**
A patient may have more than one malignant tumor in the same organ. These tumors may represent different primaries or metastatic disease, depending on the site. Should the documentation be unclear, the provider should be queried as to the status of each tumor so that the correct codes can be assigned.

j. **Disseminated malignant neoplasm, unspecified**
Code C80.0, Disseminated malignant neoplasm, unspecified, is for use only in those cases where the patient has advanced metastatic disease and no known primary or secondary sites are specified. It should not be used in place of assigning codes for the primary site and all known secondary sites.

k. **Malignant neoplasm without specification of site**
Code C80.1, Malignant (primary) neoplasm, unspecified, equates to Cancer, unspecified. This code should only be used when no determination can be made as to the primary site of a malignancy. This code should rarely be used in the inpatient setting.

l. **Sequencing of neoplasm codes**
1) **Encounter for treatment of primary malignancy**
If the reason for the encounter is for treatment of a primary malignancy, assign the malignancy as the principal/first-listed diagnosis. The primary site is to be sequenced first, followed by any metastatic sites.

2) **Encounter for treatment of secondary malignancy**
When an encounter is for a primary malignancy with metastasis and treatment is directed toward the metastatic (secondary) site(s) only, the metastatic site(s) is designated as the principal/first-listed diagnosis. The primary malignancy is coded as an additional code.

3) **Malignant neoplasm in a pregnant patient**
When a pregnant patient has a malignant neoplasm, a code from subcategory O9A.1-, Malignant neoplasm complicating pregnancy, childbirth, and the puerperium, should be sequenced first, followed by the appropriate code from Chapter 2 to indicate the type of neoplasm.

4) **Encounter for complication associated with a neoplasm**
When an encounter is for management of a complication associated with a neoplasm, such as dehydration, and the treatment is only for the complication, the complication is coded first, followed by the appropriate code(s) for the neoplasm.

The exception to this guideline is anemia. When the admission/encounter is for management of an anemia associated with the malignancy, and the treatment is only for anemia, the appropriate code for the malignancy is sequenced as the principal or first-listed diagnosis followed by code D63.0, Anemia in neoplastic disease.

5) **Complication from surgical procedure for treatment of a neoplasm**
When an encounter is for treatment of a complication resulting from a surgical procedure performed for the treatment of the neoplasm, designate the complication as the principal/first-listed diagnosis. See the guideline regarding the coding of a current malignancy versus personal history to determine if the code for the neoplasm should also be assigned.

6) **Pathologic fracture due to a neoplasm**
When an encounter is for a pathological fracture due to a neoplasm, and the focus of treatment is the fracture, a code from subcategory M84.5, Pathological fracture in neoplastic disease, should be sequenced first, followed by the code for the neoplasm.

If the focus of treatment is the neoplasm with an associated pathological fracture, the neoplasm code should be sequenced first, followed by a code from M84.5 for the pathological fracture.

m. **Current malignancy versus personal history of malignancy**
When a primary malignancy has been excised but further treatment, such as an additional surgery for the malignancy, radiation therapy or chemotherapy is directed to that site, the primary malignancy code should be used until treatment is completed.

When a primary malignancy has been previously excised or eradicated from its site, there is no further treatment (of the malignancy) directed to that site, and there is no evidence of any existing primary malignancy at that site, a code from category Z85, Personal history of malignant neoplasm, should be used to indicate the former site of the malignancy.

Codes from subcategories Z85.0 – Z85.85 should only be assigned for the former site of a primary malignancy, not the site of a secondary malignancy. Code Z85.89 may be assigned for the former site(s) of either a primary or secondary malignancy.

See Section I.C.21. Factors influencing health status and contact with health services, History (of)

n. **Leukemia, Multiple Myeloma, and Malignant Plasma Cell Neoplasms in remission versus personal history**
The categories for leukemia, and category C90, Multiple myeloma and malignant plasma cell neoplasms, have codes indicating whether or not the leukemia has achieved remission. There are also codes Z85.6, Personal history of leukemia, and Z85.79, Personal history of other malignant neoplasms of lymphoid, hematopoietic and related tissues. If the documentation is unclear as to whether the leukemia has achieved remission, the provider should be queried.

See Section I.C.21. Factors influencing health status and contact with health services, History (of)

o. **Aftercare following surgery for neoplasm**
See Section I.C.21. Factors influencing health status and contact with health services, Aftercare

p. **Follow-up care for completed treatment of a malignancy**
See Section I.C.21. Factors influencing health status and contact with health services, Follow-up

q. **Prophylactic organ removal for prevention of malignancy**
See Section I.C.21, Factors influencing health status and contact with health services, Prophylactic organ removal

r. **Malignant neoplasm associated with transplanted organ**
A malignant neoplasm of a transplanted organ should be coded as a transplant complication. Assign first the appropriate code from category T86.-, Complications of transplanted organs and tissue, followed by code C80.2, Malignant neoplasm associated with transplanted organ. Use an additional code for the specific malignancy.

s. **Breast Implant Associated Anaplastic Large Cell Lymphoma**
Breast implant associated anaplastic large cell lymphoma (BIA-ALCL) is a type of lymphoma that can develop around breast implants. Assign code C84.7A, Anaplastic large cell lymphoma, ALK-negative, breast, for BIA-ALCL. Do not assign a complication code from chapter 19.

t. **Secondary malignant neoplasm of lymphoid tissue**
When a malignant neoplasm of lymphoid tissue metastasizes beyond the lymph nodes, a code from categories C81-C85 with a final character "9" should be assigned identifying "extranodal and solid organ sites" rather than a code for the secondary neoplasm of the affected solid organ. For example, for metastasis of B-cell lymphoma to the lung, brain and left adrenal gland, assign code C83.39, Diffuse large B-cell lymphoma, extranodal and solid organ sites.

3. **Chapter 3: Disease of the blood and blood-forming organs and certain disorders involving the immune mechanism (D50-D89)**
Reserved for future guideline expansion

4. **Chapter 4: Endocrine, Nutritional, and Metabolic Diseases (E00-E89)**
a. **Diabetes mellitus**
The diabetes mellitus codes are combination codes that include the type of diabetes mellitus, the body system affected, and the complications affecting that body system. As many codes within a particular category as are necessary to describe all of the complications of the disease may be used. They should be sequenced based on the reason for a particular encounter. Assign as many codes from categories E08 – E13 as needed to identify all of the associated conditions that the patient has.

1) **Type of diabetes**
The age of a patient is not the sole determining factor, though most type 1 diabetics develop the condition before reaching puberty. For this reason, type 1 diabetes mellitus is also referred to as juvenile diabetes.

2) **Type of diabetes mellitus not documented**
If the type of diabetes mellitus is not documented in the medical record the default is E11.-, Type 2 diabetes mellitus.

3) **Diabetes mellitus and the use of insulin, oral hypoglycemics, and injectable non-insulin drugs**
If the documentation in a medical record does not indicate the type of diabetes but does indicate that the patient uses insulin, code E11-, Type 2 diabetes mellitus, should be assigned. Additional code(s) should be assigned from category Z79 to identify the long-term (current) use of insulin, oral hypoglycemic drugs, or injectable non-insulin antidiabetic, as follows:

If the patient is treated with both oral **hypoglycemic drugs** and insulin, both code Z79.4, Long term (current) use of insulin, and code Z79.84, Long term (current) use of oral hypoglycemic drugs, should be assigned.

If the patient is treated with both insulin and an injectable non-insulin antidiabetic drug, assign codes Z79.4, Long term (current) use of insulin, and **Z79.85, Long-term (current) use of injectable non-insulin antidiabetic drugs.**

If the patient is treated with both oral hypoglycemic drugs and an injectable non-insulin antidiabetic drug, assign codes Z79.84, Long term (current) use of oral hypoglycemic drugs, and **Z79.85, Long-term (current) use of injectable non-insulin antidiabetic drugs.**

Code Z79.4 should not be assigned if insulin is given temporarily to bring a type 2 patient's blood sugar under control during an encounter.

4) **Diabetes mellitus in pregnancy and gestational diabetes**
See Section I.C.15. Diabetes mellitus in pregnancy.
See Section I.C.15. Gestational (pregnancy induced) diabetes

5) **Complications due to insulin pump malfunction**
(a) **Underdose of insulin due to insulin pump failure**
An underdose of insulin due to an insulin pump failure should be assigned to a code from subcategory T85.6, Mechanical complication of other specified internal and external prosthetic devices, implants and grafts, that specifies the type of pump malfunction, as the principal or first-listed code, followed by code T38.3X6-, Underdosing of insulin and oral hypoglycemic [antidiabetic] drugs. Additional codes for the type of diabetes mellitus and any associated complications due to the underdosing should also be assigned.

(b) **Overdose of insulin due to insulin pump failure**
The principal or first-listed code for an encounter due to an insulin pump malfunction resulting in an overdose of insulin, should also be T85.6-, Mechanical complication of other specified internal and external prosthetic devices, implants and grafts, followed by code T38.3X1-, Poisoning by insulin and oral hypoglycemic [antidiabetic] drugs, accidental (unintentional).

6) **Secondary diabetes mellitus**
Codes under categories E08, Diabetes mellitus due to underlying condition, E09, Drug or chemical induced diabetes mellitus, and E13, Other specified diabetes mellitus, identify complications/manifestations associated with secondary diabetes mellitus. Secondary diabetes is always caused by another condition or event (e.g., cystic fibrosis, malignant neoplasm of pancreas, pancreatectomy, adverse effect of drug, or poisoning).

(a) **Secondary diabetes mellitus and the use of insulin, oral hypoglycemic drugs, or injectable non-insulin drugs**
For patients with secondary diabetes mellitus who routinely use insulin, oral hypoglycemic drugs, or injectable non-insulin drugs, additional code(s) from category Z79 should be assigned to identify the long-term (current) use of insulin, oral hypoglycemic drugs, or non-injectable non-insulin drugs as follows:

If the patient is treated with both oral **hypoglycemic drugs** and insulin, both code Z79.4, Long term (current) use of insulin, and code Z79.84, Long term (current) use of oral hypoglycemic drugs, should be assigned.

If the patient is treated with both insulin and an injectable non-insulin antidiabetic drug, assign codes Z79.4, Long-term (current) use of insulin, and **Z79.85, Long-term (current) use of injectable non-insulin antidiabetic drugs**.

If the patient is treated with both oral hypoglycemic drugs and an injectable non-insulin antidiabetic drug, assign codes Z79.84, Long-term (current) use of oral hypoglycemic drugs, and **Z79.85, Long-term (current) use of injectable non-insulin antidiabetic drugs.**

Code Z79.4 should not be assigned if insulin is given temporarily to bring a secondary diabetic patient's blood sugar under control during an encounter.

(b) **Assigning and sequencing secondary diabetes codes and its causes**
The sequencing of the secondary diabetes codes in relationship to codes for the cause of the diabetes is based on the Tabular List instructions for categories E08, E09 and E13.

(i) **Secondary diabetes mellitus due to pancreatectomy**
For postpancreatectomy diabetes mellitus (lack of insulin due to the surgical removal of all or part of the pancreas), assign code E89.1, Postprocedural hypoinsulinemia.

Assign a code from category E13 and a code from subcategory Z90.41, Acquired absence of pancreas, as additional codes.

(ii) **Secondary diabetes due to drugs**
Secondary diabetes may be caused by an adverse effect of correctly administered medications, poisoning or sequela of poisoning.

See section I.C.19.e. for coding of adverse effects and poisoning, and section I.C.20 for external cause code reporting.

5. **Chapter 5: Mental, Behavioral and Neurodevelopmental disorders (F01-F99)**
a. **Pain disorders related to psychological factors**
Assign code F45.41, for pain that is exclusively related to psychological disorders. As indicated by the Excludes 1 note under category G89, a code from category G89 should not be assigned with code F45.41.

Code F45.42, Pain disorders with related psychological factors, should be used with a code from category G89, Pain, not elsewhere classified, if there is documentation of a psychological component for a patient with acute or chronic pain.

See Section I.C.6. Pain

b.　Mental and behavioral disorders due to psychoactive substance use

1)　In Remission

Selection of codes **describing** "in remission" for categories F1Ø-F19, Mental and behavioral disorders due to psychoactive substance use (categories F1Ø-F19 with -.11, -.21, **-.91**) requires the provider's clinical judgment **and** are assigned only on the basis of provider documentation (as defined in the Official Guidelines for Coding and Reporting), unless otherwise instructed by the classification.

Mild substance use disorders in early or sustained remission are classified to the appropriate codes for substance abuse in remission, and moderate or severe substance use disorders in early or sustained remission are classified to the appropriate codes for substance dependence in remission.

2)　Psychoactive Substance Use, Abuse and Dependence

When the provider documentation refers to use, abuse and dependence of the same substance (e.g. alcohol, opioid, cannabis, etc.), only one code should be assigned to identify the pattern of use based on the following hierarchy:

- If both use and abuse are documented, assign only the code for abuse
- If both abuse and dependence are documented, assign only the code for dependence
- If use, abuse and dependence are all documented, assign only the code for dependence
- If both use and dependence are documented, assign only the code for dependence.

3)　Psychoactive Substance Use, Unspecified

As with all other unspecified diagnoses, the codes for unspecified psychoactive substance use (F1Ø.9-, F11.9-, F12.9-, F13.9-, F14.9-, F15.9-, F16.9-, F18.9-, F19.9-) should only be assigned based on provider documentation and when they meet the definition of a reportable diagnosis (see Section III, Reporting Additional Diagnoses). These codes are to be used only when the psychoactive substance use is associated with a substance related disorder (chapter 5 disorders such as sexual dysfunction, sleep disorder, or a mental or behavioral disorder) or medical condition, and such a relationship is documented by the provider.

4)　Medical Conditions Due to Psychoactive Substance Use, Abuse and Dependence

Medical conditions due to substance use, abuse, and dependence are not classified as substance-induced disorders. Assign the diagnosis code for the medical condition as directed by the Alphabetical Index along with the appropriate psychoactive substance use, abuse or dependence code. For example, for alcoholic pancreatitis due to alcohol dependence, assign the appropriate code from subcategory K85.2, Alcohol induced acute pancreatitis, and the appropriate code from subcategory F1Ø.2, such as code F1Ø.2Ø, Alcohol dependence, uncomplicated. It would not be appropriate to assign code F1Ø.288, Alcohol dependence with other alcohol-induced disorder.

5)　Blood Alcohol Level

A code from category Y9Ø, Evidence of alcohol involvement determined by blood alcohol level, may be assigned when this information is documented and the patient's provider has documented a condition classifiable to category F1Ø, Alcohol related disorders. The blood alcohol level does not need to be documented by the patient's provider in order for it to be coded.

See Section I.B.14. for blood alcohol level documentation by clinicians other than patient's provider.

c.　Factitious Disorder

Factitious disorder imposed on self or Munchausen's syndrome is a disorder in which a person falsely reports or causes his or her own physical or psychological signs or symptoms. For patients with documented factitious disorder on self or Munchausen's syndrome, assign the appropriate code from subcategory F68.1-, Factitious disorder imposed on self.

Munchausen's syndrome by proxy (MSBP) is a disorder in which a caregiver (perpetrator) falsely reports or causes an illness or injury in another person (victim) under his or her care, such as a child, an elderly adult, or a person who has a disability. The condition is also referred to as "factitious disorder imposed on another" or "factitious disorder by proxy." The perpetrator, not the victim, receives this diagnosis. Assign code F68.A, Factitious disorder imposed on another, to the perpetrator's record. For the victim of a patient suffering from MSBP, assign the appropriate code from categories T74, Adult and child abuse, neglect and other maltreatment, confirmed, or T76, Adult and child abuse, neglect and other maltreatment, suspected.

See Section I.C.19.f. Adult and child abuse, neglect and other maltreatment

d.　Dementia

The ICD-10-CM classifies dementia (categories FØ1, FØ2, and FØ3) on the basis of the etiology and severity (unspecified, mild, moderate or severe). Selection of the appropriate severity level requires the provider's clinical judgment and codes should be assigned only on the basis of provider documentation (as defined in the *Official Guidelines for Coding and Reporting*), unless otherwise instructed by the classification. If the documentation does not provide information about the severity of the dementia, assign the appropriate code for unspecified severity.

If a patient is admitted to an inpatient acute care hospital or other inpatient facility setting with dementia at one severity level and it progresses to a higher severity level, assign one code for the highest severity level reported during the stay.

6.　Chapter 6: Diseases of the Nervous System (GØØ-G99)

a.　Dominant/nondominant side

Codes from category G81, Hemiplegia and hemiparesis, and subcategories G83.1, Monoplegia of lower limb, G83.2, Monoplegia of upper limb, and G83.3, Monoplegia, unspecified, identify whether the dominant or nondominant side is affected. Should the affected side be documented, but not specified as dominant or nondominant, and the classification system does not indicate a default, code selection is as follows:

- For ambidextrous patients, the default should be dominant.
- If the left side is affected, the default is non-dominant.
- If the right side is affected, the default is dominant.

b.　Pain - Category G89

1)　General coding information

Codes in category G89, Pain, not elsewhere classified, may be used in conjunction with codes from other categories and chapters to provide more detail about acute or chronic pain and neoplasm-related pain, unless otherwise indicated below.

If the pain is not specified as acute or chronic, post-thoracotomy, postprocedural, or neoplasm-related, do not assign codes from category G89.

A code from category G89 should not be assigned if the underlying (definitive) diagnosis is known, unless the reason for the encounter is pain control/ management and not management of the underlying condition.

When an admission or encounter is for a procedure aimed at treating the underlying condition (e.g., spinal fusion, kyphoplasty), a code for the underlying condition (e.g., vertebral fracture, spinal stenosis) should be assigned as the principal diagnosis. No code from category G89 should be assigned.

(a)　Category G89 Codes as Principal or First-Listed Diagnosis

Category G89 codes are acceptable as principal diagnosis or the first-listed code:

- When pain control or pain management is the reason for the admission/encounter (e.g., a patient with displaced intervertebral disc, nerve impingement and severe back pain presents for injection of steroid into the spinal canal). The underlying cause of the pain should be reported as an additional diagnosis, if known.
- When a patient is admitted for the insertion of a neurostimulator for pain control, assign the appropriate pain code as the principal or first-listed diagnosis. When an admission or encounter is for a procedure aimed at treating the underlying condition and a neurostimulator is inserted for pain control during the same admission/encounter, a code for the underlying condition should be assigned as the principal diagnosis and the appropriate pain code should be assigned as a secondary diagnosis.

(b) Use of Category G89 Codes in Conjunction with Site Specific Pain Codes

(i) Assigning Category G89 and Site-Specific Pain Codes

Codes from category G89 may be used in conjunction with codes that identify the site of pain (including codes from chapter 18) if the category G89 code provides additional information. For example, if the code describes the site of the pain, but does not fully describe whether the pain is acute or chronic, then both codes should be assigned.

(ii) Sequencing of Category G89 Codes with Site-Specific Pain Codes

The sequencing of category G89 codes with site-specific pain codes (including chapter 18 codes), is dependent on the circumstances of the encounter/admission as follows:

- If the encounter is for pain control or pain management, assign the code from category G89 followed by the code identifying the specific site of pain (e.g., encounter for pain management for acute neck pain from trauma is assigned code G89.11, Acute pain due to trauma, followed by code M54.2, Cervicalgia, to identify the site of pain).

- If the encounter is for any other reason except pain control or pain management, and a related definitive diagnosis has not been established (confirmed) by the provider, assign the code for the specific site of pain first, followed by the appropriate code from category G89.

2) Pain due to devices, implants and grafts

See Section I.C.19. Pain due to medical devices

3) Postoperative Pain

The provider's documentation should be used to guide the coding of postoperative pain, as well as *Section III. Reporting Additional Diagnoses* and *Section IV. Diagnostic Coding and Reporting in the Outpatient Setting.*

The default for post-thoracotomy and other postoperative pain not specified as acute or chronic is the code for the acute form.

Routine or expected postoperative pain immediately after surgery should not be coded.

(a) Postoperative pain not associated with specific postoperative complication

Postoperative pain not associated with a specific postoperative complication is assigned to the appropriate postoperative pain code in category G89.

(b) Postoperative pain associated with specific postoperative complication

Postoperative pain associated with a specific postoperative complication (such as painful wire sutures) is assigned to the appropriate code(s) found in Chapter 19, Injury, poisoning, and certain other consequences of external causes. If appropriate, use additional code(s) from category G89 to identify acute or chronic pain (G89.18 or G89.28).

4) Chronic pain

Chronic pain is classified to subcategory G89.2. There is no time frame defining when pain becomes chronic pain. The provider's documentation should be used to guide use of these codes.

5) Neoplasm Related Pain

Code G89.3 is assigned to pain documented as being related, associated or due to cancer, primary or secondary malignancy, or tumor. This code is assigned regardless of whether the pain is acute or chronic.

This code may be assigned as the principal or first-listed code when the stated reason for the admission/encounter is documented as pain control/pain management. The underlying neoplasm should be reported as an additional diagnosis.

When the reason for the admission/encounter is management of the neoplasm and the pain associated with the neoplasm is also documented, code G89.3 may be assigned as an additional diagnosis. It is not necessary to assign an additional code for the site of the pain.

See Section I.C.2. for instructions on the sequencing of neoplasms for all other stated reasons for the admission/encounter (except for pain control/pain management).

6) Chronic pain syndrome

Central pain syndrome (G89.0) and chronic pain syndrome (G89.4) are different than the term "chronic pain," and therefore codes should only be used when the provider has specifically documented this condition.

See Section I.C.5. Pain disorders related to psychological factors

7. Chapter 7: Diseases of the Eye and Adnexa (H00-H59)

a. Glaucoma

1) Assigning Glaucoma Codes

Assign as many codes from category H40, Glaucoma, as needed to identify the type of glaucoma, the affected eye, and the glaucoma stage.

2) Bilateral glaucoma with same type and stage

When a patient has bilateral glaucoma and both eyes are documented as being the same type and stage, and there is a code for bilateral glaucoma, report only the code for the type of glaucoma, bilateral, with the seventh character for the stage.

When a patient has bilateral glaucoma and both eyes are documented as being the same type and stage, and the classification does not provide a code for bilateral glaucoma (i.e. subcategories H40.10, and H40.20) report only one code for the type of glaucoma with the appropriate seventh character for the stage.

3) Bilateral glaucoma stage with different types or stages

When a patient has bilateral glaucoma and each eye is documented as having a different type or stage, and the classification distinguishes laterality, assign the appropriate code for each eye rather than the code for bilateral glaucoma.

When a patient has bilateral glaucoma and each eye is documented as having a different type, and the classification does not distinguish laterality (i.e., subcategories H40.10, and H40.20), assign one code for each type of glaucoma with the appropriate seventh character for the stage.

When a patient has bilateral glaucoma and each eye is documented as having the same type, but different stage, and the classification does not distinguish laterality (i.e., subcategories H40.10 and H40.20), assign a code for the type of glaucoma for each eye with the seventh character for the specific glaucoma stage documented for each eye.

4) Patient admitted with glaucoma and stage evolves during the admission

If a patient is admitted with glaucoma and the stage progresses during the admission, assign the code for highest stage documented.

5) Indeterminate stage glaucoma

Assignment of the seventh character "4" for "indeterminate stage" should be based on the clinical documentation. The seventh character "4" is used for glaucomas whose stage cannot be clinically determined. This seventh character should not be confused with the seventh character "0", unspecified, which should be assigned when there is no documentation regarding the stage of the glaucoma.

b. Blindness

If "blindness" or "low vision" of both eyes is documented but the visual impairment category is not documented, assign code H54.3, Unqualified visual loss, both eyes. If "blindness" or "low vision" in one eye is documented but the visual impairment category is not documented, assign a code from H54.6-, Unqualified visual loss, one eye. If "blindness" or "visual loss" is documented without any information about whether one or both eyes are affected, assign code H54.7, Unspecified visual loss.

8. Chapter 8: Diseases of the Ear and Mastoid Process (H60-H95)

Reserved for future guideline expansion

9. Chapter 9: Diseases of the Circulatory System (I00-I99)

a. Hypertension

The classification presumes a causal relationship between hypertension and heart involvement and between hypertension and kidney involvement, as the two conditions are linked by the term "with" in the Alphabetic Index. These conditions should be coded as related even in the absence of provider documentation explicitly linking them, unless the documentation clearly states the conditions are unrelated.

For hypertension and conditions not specifically linked by relational terms such as "with," "associated with" or "due to" in the classification, provider documentation must link the conditions in order to code them as related.

1) **Hypertension with Heart Disease**
Hypertension with heart conditions classified to I50.- or I51.4-I51.7, I51.89, I51.9, are assigned to a code from category I11, Hypertensive heart disease. Use additional code(s) from category I50, Heart failure, to identify the type(s) of heart failure in those patients with heart failure.

The same heart conditions (I50.-, I51.4-I51.7, I51.89, I51.9) with hypertension are coded separately if the provider has documented they are unrelated to the hypertension. Sequence according to the circumstances of the admission/encounter.

2) **Hypertensive Chronic Kidney Disease**
Assign codes from category I12, Hypertensive chronic kidney disease, when both hypertension and a condition classifiable to category N18, Chronic kidney disease (CKD), are present. CKD should not be coded as hypertensive if the provider indicates the CKD is not related to the hypertension.

The appropriate code from category N18 should be used as a secondary code with a code from category I12 to identify the stage of chronic kidney disease.

See Section I.C.14. Chronic kidney disease.

If a patient has hypertensive chronic kidney disease and acute renal failure, the acute renal failure should also be coded. Sequence according to the circumstances of the admission/encounter.

3) **Hypertensive Heart and Chronic Kidney Disease**
Assign codes from combination category I13, Hypertensive heart and chronic kidney disease, when there is hypertension with both heart and kidney involvement. If heart failure is present, assign an additional code from category I50 to identify the type of heart failure.

The appropriate code from category N18, Chronic kidney disease, should be used as a secondary code with a code from category I13 to identify the stage of chronic kidney disease.

See Section I.C.14. Chronic kidney disease.

The codes in category I13, Hypertensive heart and chronic kidney disease, are combination codes that include hypertension, heart disease and chronic kidney disease. The Includes note at I13 specifies that the conditions included at I11 and I12 are included together in I13. If a patient has hypertension, heart disease and chronic kidney disease, then a code from I13 should be used, not individual codes for hypertension, heart disease and chronic kidney disease, or codes from I11 or I12.

For patients with both acute renal failure and chronic kidney disease, the acute renal failure should also be coded. Sequence according to the circumstances of the admission/encounter.

4) **Hypertensive Cerebrovascular Disease**
For hypertensive cerebrovascular disease, first assign the appropriate code from categories I60-I69, followed by the appropriate hypertension code.

5) **Hypertensive Retinopathy**
Subcategory H35.0, Background retinopathy and retinal vascular changes, should be used along with a code from categories I10-I15, in the Hypertensive diseases section, to include the systemic hypertension. The sequencing is based on the reason for the encounter.

6) **Hypertension, Secondary**
Secondary hypertension is due to an underlying condition. Two codes are required: one to identify the underlying etiology and one from category I15 to identify the hypertension. Sequencing of codes is determined by the reason for admission/encounter.

7) **Hypertension, Transient**
Assign code R03.0, Elevated blood pressure reading without diagnosis of hypertension, unless patient has an established diagnosis of hypertension. Assign code O13.-, Gestational [pregnancy-induced] hypertension without significant proteinuria, or O14.-, Pre-eclampsia, for transient hypertension of pregnancy.

8) **Hypertension, Controlled**
This diagnostic statement usually refers to an existing state of hypertension under control by therapy. Assign the appropriate code from categories I10-I15, Hypertensive diseases.

9) **Hypertension, Uncontrolled**
Uncontrolled hypertension may refer to untreated hypertension or hypertension not responding to current therapeutic regimen.

In either case, assign the appropriate code from categories I10-I15, Hypertensive diseases.

10) **Hypertensive Crisis**
Assign a code from category I16, Hypertensive crisis, for documented hypertensive urgency, hypertensive emergency or unspecified hypertensive crisis. Code also any identified hypertensive disease (I10-I15). The sequencing is based on the reason for the encounter.

11) **Pulmonary Hypertension**
Pulmonary hypertension is classified to category I27, Other pulmonary heart diseases. For secondary pulmonary hypertension (I27.1, I27.2-), code also any associated conditions or adverse effects of drugs or toxins. The sequencing is based on the reason for the encounter, except for adverse effects of drugs (See Section I.C.19.e.).

b. **Atherosclerotic Coronary Artery Disease and Angina**
ICD-10-CM has combination codes for atherosclerotic heart disease with angina pectoris. The subcategories for these codes are I25.11, Atherosclerotic heart disease of native coronary artery with angina pectoris and I25.7, Atherosclerosis of coronary artery bypass graft(s) and coronary artery of transplanted heart with angina pectoris.

When using one of these combination codes it is not necessary to use an additional code for angina pectoris. A causal relationship can be assumed in a patient with both atherosclerosis and angina pectoris, unless the documentation indicates the angina is due to something other than the atherosclerosis.

If a patient with coronary artery disease is admitted due to an acute myocardial infarction (AMI), the AMI should be sequenced before the coronary artery disease.

See Section I.C.9. Acute myocardial infarction (AMI)

c. **Intraoperative and Postprocedural Cerebrovascular Accident**
Medical record documentation should clearly specify the cause-and-effect relationship between the medical intervention and the cerebrovascular accident in order to assign a code for intraoperative or postprocedural cerebrovascular accident.

Proper code assignment depends on whether it was an infarction or hemorrhage and whether it occurred intraoperatively or postoperatively. If it was a cerebral hemorrhage, code assignment depends on the type of procedure performed.

d. **Sequelae of Cerebrovascular Disease**
1) **Category I69, Sequelae of Cerebrovascular disease**
Category I69 is used to indicate conditions classifiable to categories I60-I67 as the causes of sequela (neurologic deficits), themselves classified elsewhere. These "late effects" include neurologic deficits that persist after initial onset of conditions classifiable to categories I60-I67. The neurologic deficits caused by cerebrovascular disease may be present from the onset or may arise at any time after the onset of the condition classifiable to categories I60-I67.

Codes from category I69, Sequelae of cerebrovascular disease, that specify hemiplegia, hemiparesis and monoplegia identify whether the dominant or nondominant side is affected. Should the affected side be documented, but not specified as dominant or nondominant, and the classification system does not indicate a default, code selection is as follows:

- For ambidextrous patients, the default should be dominant.
- If the left side is affected, the default is non-dominant.
- If the right side is affected, the default is dominant.

2) **Codes from category I69 with codes from I60-I67**
Codes from category I69 may be assigned on a health care record with codes from I60-I67, if the patient has a current cerebrovascular disease and deficits from an old cerebrovascular disease.

3) **Codes from category I69 and Personal history of transient ischemic attack (TIA) and cerebral infarction (Z86.73)**
Codes from category I69 should not be assigned if the patient does not have neurologic deficits.

See Section I.C.21.4. History (of) for use of personal history codes

e. **Acute myocardial infarction (AMI)**
1) **Type 1 ST elevation myocardial infarction (STEMI) and non-ST elevation myocardial infarction (NSTEMI)**
The ICD-10-CM codes for type 1 acute myocardial infarction (AMI) identify the site, such as anterolateral wall or true posterior wall. Subcategories I21.0-I21.2 and code I21.3 are used for type 1 ST elevation myocardial infarction (STEMI). Code I21.4, Non-ST

elevation (NSTEMI) myocardial infarction, is used for type 1 non-ST elevation myocardial infarction (NSTEMI) and nontransmural MIs.

If a type 1 NSTEMI evolves to STEMI, assign the STEMI code. If a type 1 STEMI converts to NSTEMI due to thrombolytic therapy, it is still coded as STEMI.

For encounters occurring while the myocardial infarction is equal to, or less than, four weeks old, including transfers to another acute setting or a postacute setting, and the myocardial infarction meets the definition for "other diagnoses" (see Section III, Reporting Additional Diagnoses), codes from category I21 may continue to be reported. For encounters after the 4-week time frame and the patient is still receiving care related to the myocardial infarction, the appropriate aftercare code should be assigned, rather than a code from category I21. For old or healed myocardial infarctions not requiring further care, code I25.2, Old myocardial infarction, may be assigned.

2) Acute myocardial infarction, unspecified
Code I21.9, Acute myocardial infarction, unspecified, is the default for unspecified acute myocardial infarction or unspecified type. If only type 1 STEMI or transmural MI without the site is documented, assign code I21.3, ST elevation (STEMI) myocardial infarction of unspecified site.

3) AMI documented as nontransmural or subendocardial but site provided
If an AMI is documented as nontransmural or subendocardial, but the site is provided, it is still coded as a subendocardial AMI.

See Section I.C.21.3. for information on coding status post administration of tPA in a different facility within the last 24 hours.

4) Subsequent acute myocardial infarction
A code from category I22, Subsequent ST elevation (STEMI) and non-ST elevation (NSTEMI) myocardial infarction, is to be used when a patient who has suffered a type 1 or unspecified AMI has a new AMI within the 4 week time frame of the initial AMI. A code from category I22 must be used in conjunction with a code from category I21. The sequencing of the I22 and I21 codes depends on the circumstances of the encounter.

Do not assign code I22 for subsequent myocardial infarctions other than type 1 or unspecified. For subsequent type 2 AMI assign only code I21.A1. For subsequent type 4 or type 5 AMI, assign only code I21.A9.

If a subsequent myocardial infarction of one type occurs within 4 weeks of a myocardial infarction of a different type, assign the appropriate codes from category I21 to identify each type. Do not assign a code from I22. Codes from category I22 should only be assigned if both the initial and subsequent myocardial infarctions are type 1 or unspecified.

5) Other Types of Myocardial Infarction
The ICD-10-CM provides codes for different types of myocardial infarction. Type 1 myocardial infarctions are assigned to codes I21.0-I21.4.

Type 2 myocardial infarction (myocardial infarction due to demand ischemia or secondary to ischemic imbalance) is assigned to code I21.A1, Myocardial infarction type 2 with the underlying cause coded first. Do not assign code I24.8, Other forms of acute ischemic heart disease, for the demand ischemia. If a type 2 AMI is described as NSTEMI or STEMI, only assign code I21.A1. Codes I21.01-I21.4 should only be assigned for type 1 AMIs.

Acute myocardial infarctions type 3, 4a, 4b, 4c and 5 are assigned to code I21.A9, Other myocardial infarction type.

The "Code also" and "Code first" notes should be followed related to complications, and for coding of postprocedural myocardial infarctions during or following cardiac surgery.

10. Chapter 10: Diseases of the Respiratory System (J00-J99), U07.0
a. Chronic Obstructive Pulmonary Disease [COPD] and Asthma
1) Acute exacerbation of chronic obstructive bronchitis and asthma
The codes in categories J44 and J45 distinguish between uncomplicated cases and those in acute exacerbation. An acute exacerbation is a worsening or a decompensation of a chronic condition. An acute exacerbation is not equivalent to an infection superimposed on a chronic condition, though an exacerbation may be triggered by an infection.

b. Acute Respiratory Failure
1) Acute respiratory failure as principal diagnosis
A code from subcategory J96.0, Acute respiratory failure, or subcategory J96.2, Acute and chronic respiratory failure, may be assigned as a principal diagnosis when it is the condition established after study to be chiefly responsible for occasioning the admission to the hospital, and the selection is supported by the Alphabetic Index and Tabular List. However, chapter-specific coding guidelines (such as obstetrics, poisoning, HIV, newborn) that provide sequencing direction take precedence.

2) Acute respiratory failure as secondary diagnosis
Respiratory failure may be listed as a secondary diagnosis if it occurs after admission, or if it is present on admission, but does not meet the definition of principal diagnosis.

3) Sequencing of acute respiratory failure and another acute condition
When a patient is admitted with respiratory failure and another acute condition, (e.g., myocardial infarction, cerebrovascular accident, aspiration pneumonia), the principal diagnosis will not be the same in every situation. This applies whether the other acute condition is a respiratory or nonrespiratory condition. Selection of the principal diagnosis will be dependent on the circumstances of admission. If both the respiratory failure and the other acute condition are equally responsible for occasioning the admission to the hospital, and there are no chapter-specific sequencing rules, the guideline regarding two or more diagnoses that equally meet the definition for principal diagnosis (Section II, C.) may be applied in these situations.

If the documentation is not clear as to whether acute respiratory failure and another condition are equally responsible for occasioning the admission, query the provider for clarification.

c. Influenza due to certain identified influenza viruses
Code only confirmed cases of influenza due to certain identified influenza viruses (category J09), and due to other identified influenza virus (category J10). This is an exception to the hospital inpatient guideline Section II, H. (Uncertain Diagnosis).

In this context, "confirmation" does not require documentation of positive laboratory testing specific for avian or other novel influenza A or other identified influenza virus. However, coding should be based on the provider's diagnostic statement that the patient has avian influenza, or other novel influenza A, for category J09, or has another particular identified strain of influenza, such as H1N1 or H3N2, but not identified as novel or variant, for category J10.

If the provider records "suspected" or "possible" or "probable" avian influenza, or novel influenza, or other identified influenza, then the appropriate influenza code from category J11, Influenza due to unidentified influenza virus, should be assigned. A code from category J09, Influenza due to certain identified influenza viruses, should not be assigned nor should a code from category J10, Influenza due to other identified influenza virus.

d. Ventilator associated Pneumonia
1) Documentation of Ventilator associated Pneumonia
As with all procedural or postprocedural complications, code assignment is based on the provider's documentation of the relationship between the condition and the procedure.

Code J95.851, Ventilator associated pneumonia, should be assigned only when the provider has documented ventilator associated pneumonia (VAP). An additional code to identify the organism (e.g., Pseudomonas aeruginosa, code B96.5) should also be assigned. Do not assign an additional code from categories J12-J18 to identify the type of pneumonia.

Code J95.851 should not be assigned for cases where the patient has pneumonia and is on a mechanical ventilator and the provider has not specifically stated that the pneumonia is ventilator-associated pneumonia. If the documentation is unclear as to whether the patient has a pneumonia that is a complication attributable to the mechanical ventilator, query the provider.

2) Ventilator associated Pneumonia Develops after Admission
A patient may be admitted with one type of pneumonia (e.g., code J13, Pneumonia due to Streptococcus pneumonia) and subsequently develop VAP. In this instance, the principal diagnosis would be the appropriate code from categories J12-J18 for the pneumonia diagnosed at the time of admission. Code J95.851, Ventilator associated pneumonia, would be assigned as an additional diagnosis when the provider has also documented the presence of ventilator associated pneumonia.

e. **Vaping-related disorders**
For patients presenting with condition(s) related to vaping, assign code U07.0, Vaping-related disorder, as the principal diagnosis. For lung injury due to vaping, assign only code U07.0. Assign additional codes for other manifestations, such as acute respiratory failure (subcategory J96.0-) or pneumonitis (code J68.0).

Associated respiratory signs and symptoms due to vaping, such as cough, shortness of breath, etc., are not coded separately, when a definitive diagnosis has been established. However, it would be appropriate to code separately any gastrointestinal symptoms, such as diarrhea and abdominal pain.

See Section I.C.1.g.1.c.i. for Pneumonia confirmed as due to COVID-19

11. **Chapter 11: Diseases of the Digestive System (K00-K95)**
Reserved for future guideline expansion

12. **Chapter 12: Diseases of the Skin and Subcutaneous Tissue (L00-L99)**
a. **Pressure ulcer stage codes**
1) **Pressure ulcer stages**
Codes in category L89, Pressure ulcer, identify the site and stage of the pressure ulcer.

The ICD-10-CM classifies pressure ulcer stages based on severity, which is designated by stages 1-4, deep tissue pressure injury, unspecified stage, and unstageable.

Assign as many codes from category L89 as needed to identify all the pressure ulcers the patient has, if applicable.

See Section I.B.14. for pressure ulcer stage documentation by clinicians other than patient's provider.

2) **Unstageable pressure ulcers**
Assignment of the code for unstageable pressure ulcer (L89.--0) should be based on the clinical documentation. These codes are used for pressure ulcers whose stage cannot be clinically determined (e.g., the ulcer is covered by eschar or has been treated with a skin or muscle graft). This code should not be confused with the codes for unspecified stage (L89.--9). When there is no documentation regarding the stage of the pressure ulcer, assign the appropriate code for unspecified stage (L89.-- 9).

If during an encounter, the stage of an unstageable pressure ulcer is revealed after debridement, assign only the code for the stage revealed following debridement.

3) **Documented pressure ulcer stage**
Assignment of the pressure ulcer stage code should be guided by clinical documentation of the stage or documentation of the terms found in the Alphabetic Index. For clinical terms describing the stage that are not found in the Alphabetic Index, and there is no documentation of the stage, the provider should be queried.

4) **Patients admitted with pressure ulcers documented as healed**
No code is assigned if the documentation states that the pressure ulcer is completely healed at the time of admission.

5) **Pressure ulcers documented as healing**
Pressure ulcers described as healing should be assigned the appropriate pressure ulcer stage code based on the documentation in the medical record. If the documentation does not provide information about the stage of the healing pressure ulcer, assign the appropriate code for unspecified stage.

If the documentation is unclear as to whether the patient has a current (new) pressure ulcer or if the patient is being treated for a healing pressure ulcer, query the provider.

For ulcers that were present on admission but healed at the time of discharge, assign the code for the site and stage of the pressure ulcer at the time of admission.

6) **Patient admitted with pressure ulcer evolving into another stage during the admission**
If a patient is admitted to an inpatient hospital with a pressure ulcer at one stage and it progresses to a higher stage, two separate codes should be assigned: one code for the site and stage of the ulcer on admission and a second code for the same ulcer site and the highest stage reported during the stay.

7) **Pressure-induced deep tissue damage**
For pressure-induced deep tissue damage or deep tissue pressure injury, assign only the appropriate code for pressure-induced deep tissue damage (L89.--6).

b. **Non-Pressure Chronic Ulcers**
1) **Patients admitted with non-pressure ulcers documented as healed**
No code is assigned if the documentation states that the non-pressure ulcer is completely healed at the time of admission.

2) **Non-pressure ulcers documented as healing**
Non-pressure ulcers described as healing should be assigned the appropriate non-pressure ulcer code based on the documentation in the medical record. If the documentation does not provide information about the severity of the healing non-pressure ulcer, assign the appropriate code for unspecified severity.

If the documentation is unclear as to whether the patient has a current (new) non-pressure ulcer or if the patient is being treated for a healing non-pressure ulcer, query the provider.

For ulcers that were present on admission but healed at the time of discharge, assign the code for the site and severity of the non-pressure ulcer at the time of admission.

3) **Patient admitted with non-pressure ulcer that progresses to another severity level during the admission**
If a patient is admitted to an inpatient hospital with a non-pressure ulcer at one severity level and it progresses to a higher severity level, two separate codes should be assigned: one code for the site and severity level of the ulcer on admission and a second code for the same ulcer site and the highest severity level reported during the stay.

See Section I.B.14. for pressure ulcer stage documentation by clinicians other than patient's provider

13. **Chapter 13: Diseases of the Musculoskeletal System and Connective Tissue (M00-M99)**
a. **Site and laterality**
Most of the codes within Chapter 13 have site and laterality designations. The site represents the bone, joint or the muscle involved. For some conditions where more than one bone, joint or muscle is usually involved, such as osteoarthritis, there is a "multiple sites" code available. For categories where no multiple site code is provided and more than one bone, joint or muscle is involved, multiple codes should be used to indicate the different sites involved.

1) **Bone versus joint**
For certain conditions, the bone may be affected at the upper or lower end, (e.g., avascular necrosis of bone, M87, Osteoporosis, M80, M81). Though the portion of the bone affected may be at the joint, the site designation will be the bone, not the joint.

b. **Acute traumatic versus chronic or recurrent musculoskeletal conditions**
Many musculoskeletal conditions are a result of previous injury or trauma to a site, or are recurrent conditions. Bone, joint or muscle conditions that are the result of a healed injury are usually found in chapter 13. Recurrent bone, joint or muscle conditions are also usually found in chapter 13. Any current, acute injury should be coded to the appropriate injury code from chapter 19. Chronic or recurrent conditions should generally be coded with a code from chapter 13. If it is difficult to determine from the documentation in the record which code is best to describe a condition, query the provider.

c. **Coding of Pathologic Fractures**
7th character A is for use as long as the patient is receiving active treatment for the fracture. While the patient may be seen by a new or different provider over the course of treatment for a pathological fracture, assignment of the 7th character is based on whether the patient is undergoing active treatment and not whether the provider is seeing the patient for the first time.

7th character D is to be used for encounters after the patient has completed active treatment for the fracture and is receiving routine care for the fracture during the healing or recovery phase. The other 7th characters, listed under each subcategory in the Tabular List, are to be used for subsequent encounters for treatment of problems associated with the healing, such as malunions, nonunions, and sequelae.

Care for complications of surgical treatment for fracture repairs during the healing or recovery phase should be coded with the appropriate complication codes.

See Section I.C.19. Coding of traumatic fractures.

d. **Osteoporosis**
Osteoporosis is a systemic condition, meaning that all bones of the musculoskeletal system are affected. Therefore, site is not a component of the codes under category M81, Osteoporosis without

current pathological fracture. The site codes under category M80, Osteoporosis with current pathological fracture, identify the site of the fracture, not the osteoporosis.

1) **Osteoporosis without pathological fracture**
Category M81, Osteoporosis without current pathological fracture, is for use for patients with osteoporosis who do not currently have a pathologic fracture due to the osteoporosis, even if they have had a fracture in the past. For patients with a history of osteoporosis fractures, status code Z87.310, Personal history of (healed) osteoporosis fracture, should follow the code from M81.

2) **Osteoporosis with current pathological fracture**
Category M80, Osteoporosis with current pathological fracture, is for patients who have a current pathologic fracture at the time of an encounter. The codes under M80 identify the site of the fracture. A code from category M80, not a traumatic fracture code, should be used for any patient with known osteoporosis who suffers a fracture, even if the patient had a minor fall or trauma, if that fall or trauma would not usually break a normal, healthy bone.

e. **Multisystem Inflammatory Syndrome**
See Section I.C.1.g.1.l. for Multisystem Inflammatory Syndrome

14. **Chapter 14: Diseases of Genitourinary System (N00-N99)**
a. **Chronic kidney disease**
1) **Stages of chronic kidney disease (CKD)**
The ICD-10-CM classifies CKD based on severity. The severity of CKD is designated by stages 1-5. Stage 2, code N18.2, equates to mild CKD; stage 3, codes N18.30-N18.32, equate to moderate CKD; and stage 4, code N18.4, equates to severe CKD. Code N18.6, End stage renal disease (ESRD), is assigned when the provider has documented end-stage renal disease (ESRD).

If both a stage of CKD and ESRD are documented, assign code N18.6 only.

2) **Chronic kidney disease and kidney transplant status**
Patients who have undergone kidney transplant may still have some form of chronic kidney disease (CKD) because the kidney transplant may not fully restore kidney function. Therefore, the presence of CKD alone does not constitute a transplant complication. Assign the appropriate N18 code for the patient's stage of CKD and code Z94.0, Kidney transplant status. If a transplant complication such as failure or rejection or other transplant complication is documented, see section I.C.19.g for information on coding complications of a kidney transplant. If the documentation is unclear as to whether the patient has a complication of the transplant, query the provider.

3) **Chronic kidney disease with other conditions**
Patients with CKD may also suffer from other serious conditions, most commonly diabetes mellitus and hypertension. The sequencing of the CKD code in relationship to codes for other contributing conditions is based on the conventions in the Tabular List.

See I.C.9. Hypertensive chronic kidney disease.

See I.C.19. Chronic kidney disease and kidney transplant complications.

15. **Chapter 15: Pregnancy, Childbirth, and the Puerperium (O00-O9A)**
a. **General Rules for Obstetric Cases**
1) **Codes from chapter 15 and sequencing priority**
Obstetric cases require codes from chapter 15, codes in the range O00-O9A, Pregnancy, Childbirth, and the Puerperium. Chapter 15 codes have sequencing priority over codes from other chapters. Additional codes from other chapters may be used in conjunction with chapter 15 codes to further specify conditions. Should the provider document that the pregnancy is incidental to the encounter, then code Z33.1, Pregnant state, incidental, should be used in place of any chapter 15 codes. It is the provider's responsibility to state that the condition being treated is not affecting the pregnancy.

2) **Chapter 15 codes used only on the maternal record**
Chapter 15 codes are to be used only on the maternal record, never on the record of the newborn.

3) **Final character for trimester**
The majority of codes in Chapter 15 have a final character indicating the trimester of pregnancy. The timeframes for the trimesters are indicated at the beginning of the chapter. If trimester is not a component of a code, it is because the condition always occurs in a specific trimester, or the concept of trimester of

pregnancy is not applicable. Certain codes have characters for only certain trimesters because the condition does not occur in all trimesters, but it may occur in more than just one.

Assignment of the final character for trimester should be based on the provider's documentation of the trimester (or number of weeks) for the current admission/encounter. This applies to the assignment of trimester for pre-existing conditions as well as those that develop during or are due to the pregnancy. The provider's documentation of the number of weeks may be used to assign the appropriate code identifying the trimester.

Whenever delivery occurs during the current admission, and there is an "in childbirth" option for the obstetric complication being coded, the "in childbirth" code should be assigned. When the classification does not provide an obstetric code with an "in childbirth" option, it is appropriate to assign a code describing the current trimester.

4) **Selection of trimester for inpatient admissions that encompass more than one trimester**
In instances when a patient is admitted to a hospital for complications of pregnancy during one trimester and remains in the hospital into a subsequent trimester, the trimester character for the antepartum complication code should be assigned on the basis of the trimester when the complication developed, not the trimester of the discharge. If the condition developed prior to the current admission/encounter or represents a pre-existing condition, the trimester character for the trimester at the time of the admission/encounter should be assigned.

5) **Unspecified trimester**
Each category that includes codes for trimester has a code for "unspecified trimester." The "unspecified trimester" code should rarely be used, such as when the documentation in the record is insufficient to determine the trimester and it is not possible to obtain clarification.

6) **7th character for fetus identification**
Where applicable, a 7th character is to be assigned for certain categories (O31, O32, O33.3-O33.6, O35, O36, O40, O41, O60.1, O60.2, O64, and O69) to identify the fetus for which the complication code applies.

Assign 7th character "0":

• For single gestations
• When the documentation in the record is insufficient to determine the fetus affected and it is not possible to obtain clarification.
• When it is not possible to clinically determine which fetus is affected.

7) **Completed weeks of gestation**
In ICD-10-CM, "completed" weeks of gestation refers to full weeks. For example, if the provider documents gestation at 39 weeks and 6 days, the code for 39 weeks of gestation should be assigned, as the patient has not yet reached 40 completed weeks.

b. **Selection of OB Principal or First-listed Diagnosis**
1) **Routine outpatient prenatal visits**
For routine outpatient prenatal visits when no complications are present, a code from category Z34, Encounter for supervision of normal pregnancy, should be used as the first-listed diagnosis. These codes should not be used in conjunction with chapter 15 codes.

2) **Supervision of High-Risk Pregnancy**
Codes from category O09, Supervision of high-risk pregnancy, are intended for use only during the prenatal period. For complications during the labor or delivery episode as a result of a high-risk pregnancy, assign the applicable complication codes from Chapter 15. If there are no complications during the labor or delivery episode, assign code O80, Encounter for full-term uncomplicated delivery.

For routine prenatal outpatient visits for patients with high-risk pregnancies, a code from category O09, Supervision of high-risk pregnancy, should be used as the first-listed diagnosis. Secondary chapter 15 codes may be used in conjunction with these codes if appropriate.

3) **Episodes when no delivery occurs**
In episodes when no delivery occurs, the principal diagnosis should correspond to the principal complication of the pregnancy which necessitated the encounter. Should more than one

complication exist, all of which are treated or monitored, any of the complication codes may be sequenced first.

4) When a delivery occurs
When an obstetric patient is admitted and delivers during that admission, the condition that prompted the admission should be sequenced as the principal diagnosis. If multiple conditions prompted the admission, sequence the one most related to the delivery as the principal diagnosis. A code for any complication of the delivery should be assigned as an additional diagnosis. In cases of cesarean delivery, if the patient was admitted with a condition that resulted in the performance of a cesarean procedure, that condition should be selected as the principal diagnosis. If the reason for the admission was unrelated to the condition resulting in the cesarean delivery, the condition related to the reason for the admission should be selected as the principal diagnosis.

5) Outcome of delivery
A code from category Z37, Outcome of delivery, should be included on every maternal record when a delivery has occurred. These codes are not to be used on subsequent records or on the newborn record.

c. Pre-existing conditions versus conditions due to the pregnancy
Certain categories in Chapter 15 distinguish between conditions of the mother that existed prior to pregnancy (pre-existing) and those that are a direct result of pregnancy. When assigning codes from Chapter 15, it is important to assess if a condition was pre-existing prior to pregnancy or developed during or due to the pregnancy in order to assign the correct code.

Categories that do not distinguish between pre-existing and pregnancy-related conditions may be used for either. It is acceptable to use codes specifically for the puerperium with codes complicating pregnancy and childbirth if a condition arises postpartum during the delivery encounter.

d. Pre-existing hypertension in pregnancy
Category O10, Pre-existing hypertension complicating pregnancy, childbirth and the puerperium, includes codes for hypertensive heart and hypertensive chronic kidney disease. When assigning one of the O10 codes that includes hypertensive heart disease or hypertensive chronic kidney disease, it is necessary to add a secondary code from the appropriate hypertension category to specify the type of heart failure or chronic kidney disease.
See Section I.C.9. Hypertension.

e. Fetal Conditions Affecting the Management of the Mother
1) Codes from categories O35 and O36
Codes from categories O35, Maternal care for known or suspected fetal abnormality and damage, and O36, Maternal care for other fetal problems, are assigned only when the fetal condition is actually responsible for modifying the management of the mother, i.e., by requiring diagnostic studies, additional observation, special care, or termination of pregnancy. The fact that the fetal condition exists does not justify assigning a code from this series to the mother's record.

2) In utero surgery
In cases when surgery is performed on the fetus, a diagnosis code from category O35, Maternal care for known or suspected fetal abnormality and damage, should be assigned identifying the fetal condition. Assign the appropriate procedure code for the procedure performed.

No code from Chapter 16, the perinatal codes, should be used on the mother's record to identify fetal conditions. Surgery performed in utero on a fetus is still to be coded as an obstetric encounter.

f. HIV Infection in Pregnancy, Childbirth and the Puerperium
During pregnancy, childbirth or the puerperium, a patient admitted because of an HIV-related illness should receive a principal diagnosis from subcategory O98.7-, Human immunodeficiency [HIV] disease complicating pregnancy, childbirth and the puerperium, followed by the code(s) for the HIV-related illness(es).

Patients with asymptomatic HIV infection status admitted during pregnancy, childbirth, or the puerperium should receive codes of O98.7- and Z21, Asymptomatic human immunodeficiency virus [HIV] infection status.

g. Diabetes mellitus in pregnancy
Diabetes mellitus is a significant complicating factor in pregnancy. Pregnant patients who are diabetic should be assigned a code from category O24, Diabetes mellitus in pregnancy, childbirth, and the

puerperium, first, followed by the appropriate diabetes code(s) (E08-E13) from Chapter 4.

h. Long term use of insulin and oral hypoglycemics
See section I.C.4.a.3 for information on the long-term use of insulin and oral hypoglycemics.

i. Gestational (pregnancy induced) diabetes
Gestational (pregnancy induced) diabetes can occur during the second and third trimester of pregnancy in patients who were not diabetic prior to pregnancy. Gestational diabetes can cause complications in the pregnancy similar to those of pre-existing diabetes mellitus. It also puts the patient at greater risk of developing diabetes after the pregnancy.

Codes for gestational diabetes are in subcategory O24.4, Gestational diabetes mellitus. No other code from category O24, Diabetes mellitus in pregnancy, childbirth, and the puerperium, should be used with a code from O24.4.

The codes under subcategory O24.4 include diet controlled, insulin controlled, and controlled by oral hypoglycemic drugs. If a patient with gestational diabetes is treated with both diet and insulin, only the code for insulin-controlled is required. If a patient with gestational diabetes is treated with both diet and oral hypoglycemic medications, only the code for "controlled by oral hypoglycemic drugs" is required. Codes Z79.4, Long-term (current) use of insulin, Z79.84, Long-term (current) use of oral hypoglycemic drugs, **and Z79.85, Long-term (current) use of injectable non-insulin antidiabetic drugs,** should not be assigned with codes from subcategory O24.4.

An abnormal glucose tolerance in pregnancy is assigned a code from subcategory O99.81, Abnormal glucose complicating pregnancy, childbirth, and the puerperium.

j. Sepsis and septic shock complicating abortion, pregnancy, childbirth and the puerperium
When assigning a chapter 15 code for sepsis complicating abortion, pregnancy, childbirth, and the puerperium, a code for the specific type of infection should be assigned as an additional diagnosis. If severe sepsis is present, a code from subcategory R65.2, Severe sepsis, and code(s) for associated organ dysfunction(s) should also be assigned as additional diagnoses.

k. Puerperal sepsis
Code O85, Puerperal sepsis, should be assigned with a secondary code to identify the causal organism (e.g., for a bacterial infection, assign a code from category B95-B96, Bacterial infections in conditions classified elsewhere). A code from category A40, Streptococcal sepsis, or A41, Other sepsis, should not be used for puerperal sepsis. If applicable, use additional codes to identify severe sepsis (R65.2-) and any associated acute organ dysfunction.

Code O85 should not be assigned for sepsis following an obstetrical procedure (See Section I.C.1.d.5.b., Sepsis due to a postprocedural infection).

l. Alcohol, tobacco and drug use during pregnancy, childbirth and the puerperium
1) Alcohol use during pregnancy, childbirth and the puerperium
Codes under subcategory O99.31, Alcohol use complicating pregnancy, childbirth, and the puerperium, should be assigned for any pregnancy case when a patient uses alcohol during the pregnancy or postpartum. A secondary code from category F10, Alcohol related disorders, should also be assigned to identify manifestations of the alcohol use.

2) Tobacco use during pregnancy, childbirth and the puerperium
Codes under subcategory O99.33, Smoking (tobacco) complicating pregnancy, childbirth, and the puerperium, should be assigned for any pregnancy case when a patient uses any type of tobacco product during the pregnancy or postpartum.

A secondary code from category F17, Nicotine dependence, should also be assigned to identify the type of nicotine dependence.

3) Drug use during pregnancy, childbirth and the puerperium
Codes under subcategory O99.32, Drug use complicating pregnancy, childbirth, and the puerperium, should be assigned for any pregnancy case when a patient uses drugs during the pregnancy or postpartum. This can involve illegal drugs, or inappropriate use or abuse of prescription drugs. Secondary code(s) from categories F11-F16 and F18-F19 should also be assigned to identify manifestations of the drug use.

m. Poisoning, toxic effects, adverse effects and underdosing in a pregnant patient

A code from subcategory O9A.2, Injury, poisoning and certain other consequences of external causes complicating pregnancy, childbirth, and the puerperium, should be sequenced first, followed by the appropriate injury, poisoning, toxic effect, adverse effect or underdosing code, and then the additional code(s) that specifies the condition caused by the poisoning, toxic effect, adverse effect or underdosing.

See Section I.C.19. Adverse effects, poisoning, underdosing and toxic effects.

n. Normal Delivery, Code O80

1) Encounter for full term uncomplicated delivery

Code O80 should be assigned when a patient is admitted for a full-term normal delivery and delivers a single, healthy infant without any complications antepartum, during the delivery, or postpartum during the delivery episode. Code O80 is always a principal diagnosis. It is not to be used if any other code from chapter 15 is needed to describe a current complication of the antenatal, delivery, or postnatal period. Additional codes from other chapters may be used with code O80 if they are not related to or are in any way complicating the pregnancy.

2) Uncomplicated delivery with resolved antepartum complication

Code O80 may be used if the patient had a complication at some point during the pregnancy, but the complication is not present at the time of the admission for delivery.

3) Outcome of delivery for O80

Z37.0, Single live birth, is the only outcome of delivery code appropriate for use with O80.

o. The Peripartum and Postpartum Periods

1) Peripartum and Postpartum periods

The postpartum period begins immediately after delivery and continues for six weeks following delivery. The peripartum period is defined as the last month of pregnancy to five months postpartum.

2) Peripartum and postpartum complication

A postpartum complication is any complication occurring within the six-week period.

3) Pregnancy-related complications after 6-week period

Chapter 15 codes may also be used to describe pregnancy-related complications after the peripartum or postpartum period if the provider documents that a condition is pregnancy related.

4) Admission for routine postpartum care following delivery outside hospital

When the mother delivers outside the hospital prior to admission and is admitted for routine postpartum care and no complications are noted, code Z39.0, Encounter for care and examination of mother immediately after delivery, should be assigned as the principal diagnosis.

5) Pregnancy associated cardiomyopathy

Pregnancy associated cardiomyopathy, code O90.3, is unique in that it may be diagnosed in the third trimester of pregnancy but may continue to progress months after delivery. For this reason, it is referred to as peripartum cardiomyopathy. Code O90.3 is only for use when the cardiomyopathy develops as a result of pregnancy in a patient who did not have pre-existing heart disease.

p. Code O94, Sequelae of complication of pregnancy, childbirth, and the puerperium

1) Code O94

Code O94, Sequelae of complication of pregnancy, childbirth, and the puerperium, is for use in those cases when an initial complication of a pregnancy develops a sequela or sequelae requiring care or treatment at a future date.

2) After the initial postpartum period

This code may be used at any time after the initial postpartum period.

3) Sequencing of Code O94

This code, like all sequela codes, is to be sequenced following the code describing the sequelae of the complication.

q. Termination of Pregnancy and Spontaneous abortions

1) Abortion with Liveborn Fetus

When an attempted termination of pregnancy results in a liveborn fetus, assign code Z33.2, Encounter for elective

termination of pregnancy and a code from category Z37, Outcome of Delivery.

2) Retained Products of Conception following an abortion

Subsequent encounters for retained products of conception following a spontaneous abortion or elective termination of pregnancy, without complications are assigned O03.4, Incomplete spontaneous abortion without complication, or code O07.4, Failed attempted termination of pregnancy without complication. This advice is appropriate even when the patient was discharged previously with a discharge diagnosis of complete abortion. If the patient has a specific complication associated with the spontaneous abortion or elective termination of pregnancy in addition to retained products of conception, assign the appropriate complication code (e.g., O03.-, O04.-, O07.-) instead of code O03.4 or O07.4.

3) Complications leading to abortion

Codes from Chapter 15 may be used as additional codes to identify any documented complications of the pregnancy in conjunction with codes in categories in O04, O07 and O08.

4) Hemorrhage following elective abortion

For hemorrhage post elective abortion, assign code O04.6, Delayed or excessive hemorrhage following (induced) termination of pregnancy. Do not assign code O72.1, Other immediate postpartum hemorrhage, as this code should not be assigned for post abortion conditions. Do not assign code Z33.2, Encounter for elective termination of pregnancy, when the patient experiences a complication post elective abortion.

r. Abuse in a pregnant patient

For suspected or confirmed cases of abuse of a pregnant patient, a code(s) from subcategories O9A.3, Physical abuse complicating pregnancy, childbirth, and the puerperium, O9A.4, Sexual abuse complicating pregnancy, childbirth, and the puerperium, and O9A.5, Psychological abuse complicating pregnancy, childbirth, and the puerperium, should be sequenced first, followed by the appropriate codes (if applicable) to identify any associated current injury due to physical abuse, sexual abuse, and the perpetrator of abuse.

See Section I.C.19. Adult and child abuse, neglect and other maltreatment.

s. COVID-19 infection in pregnancy, childbirth, and the puerperium

During pregnancy, childbirth or the puerperium, when COVID-19 is the reason for admission/encounter , code O98.5-, Other viral diseases complicating pregnancy, childbirth and the puerperium, should be sequenced as the principal/first-listed diagnosis, and code U07.1, COVID-19, and the appropriate codes for associated manifestation(s) should be assigned as additional diagnoses. Codes from Chapter 15 always take sequencing priority.

If the reason for admission/encounter is unrelated to COVID-19 but the patient tests positive for COVID-19 during the admission/encounter, the appropriate code for the reason for admission/encounter should be sequenced as the principal/first-listed diagnosis, and codes O98.5- and U07.1, as well as the appropriate codes for associated COVID-19 manifestations, should be assigned as additional diagnoses.

16. Chapter 16: Certain Conditions Originating in the Perinatal Period (P00-P96)

For coding and reporting purposes the perinatal period is defined as before birth through the 28th day following birth. The following guidelines are provided for reporting purposes.

a. General Perinatal Rules

1) Use of Chapter 16 Codes

Codes in this chapter are <u>never</u> for use on the maternal record. Codes from Chapter 15, the obstetric chapter, are never permitted on the newborn record. Chapter 16 codes may be used throughout the life of the patient if the condition is still present.

2) Principal Diagnosis for Birth Record

When coding the birth episode in a newborn record, assign a code from category Z38, Liveborn infants according to place of birth and type of delivery, as the principal diagnosis. A code from category Z38 is assigned only once, to a newborn at the time of birth. If a newborn is transferred to another institution, a code from category Z38 should not be used at the receiving hospital.

A code from category Z38 is used only on the newborn record, not on the mother's record.

3) **Use of Codes from other Chapters with Codes from Chapter 16**

Codes from other chapters may be used with codes from chapter 16 if the codes from the other chapters provide more specific detail. Codes for signs and symptoms may be assigned when a definitive diagnosis has not been established. If the reason for the encounter is a perinatal condition, the code from chapter 16 should be sequenced first.

4) **Use of Chapter 16 Codes after the Perinatal Period**

Should a condition originate in the perinatal period, and continue throughout the life of the patient, the perinatal code should continue to be used regardless of the patient's age.

5) **Birth process or community acquired conditions**

If a newborn has a condition that may be either due to the birth process or community acquired and the documentation does not indicate which it is, the default is due to the birth process and the code from Chapter 16 should be used. If the condition is community-acquired, a code from Chapter 16 should not be assigned.

For COVID-19 infection in a newborn, see guideline I.C.16.h.

6) **Code all clinically significant conditions**

All clinically significant conditions noted on routine newborn examination should be coded. A condition is clinically significant if it requires:

- clinical evaluation; or
- therapeutic treatment; or
- diagnostic procedures; or
- extended length of hospital stay; or
- increased nursing care and/or monitoring; or
- has implications for future health care needs

Note: The perinatal guidelines listed above are the same as the general coding guidelines for "additional diagnoses," except for the final point regarding implications for future health care needs. Codes should be assigned for conditions that have been specified by the provider as having implications for future health care needs.

b. **Observation and Evaluation of Newborns for Suspected Conditions not Found**

1) **Use of Z05 codes**

Assign a code from category Z05, Observation and evaluation of newborn for suspected **diseases and** conditions ruled out, to identify those instances when a healthy newborn is evaluated for a suspected condition/**disease** that is determined after study not to be present. Do not use a code from category Z05 when the patient **is documented to have** signs or symptoms of a suspected problem; in such cases code the sign or symptom.

2) **Z05 on other than the birth record**

A code from category Z05 may also be assigned as a principal or first-listed code for readmissions or encounters when the code from category Z38 code no longer applies. Codes from category Z05 are for use only for healthy newborns and infants for which no condition after study is found to be present.

3) **Z05 on a birth record**

A code from category Z05 is to be used as a secondary code after the code from category Z38, Liveborn infants according to place of birth and type of delivery.

c. **Coding Additional Perinatal Diagnoses**

1) **Assigning codes for conditions that require treatment**

Assign codes for conditions that require treatment or further investigation, prolong the length of stay, or require resource utilization.

2) **Codes for conditions specified as having implications for future health care needs**

Assign codes for conditions that have been specified by the provider as having implications for future health care needs.

Note: This guideline should not be used for adult patients.

d. **Prematurity and Fetal Growth Retardation**

Providers utilize different criteria in determining prematurity. A code for prematurity should not be assigned unless it is documented. Assignment of codes in categories P05, Disorders of newborn related to slow fetal growth and fetal malnutrition, and P07, Disorders of newborn related to short gestation and low birth weight, not elsewhere classified, should be based on the recorded birth weight and estimated gestational age.

When both birth weight and gestational age are available, two codes from category P07 should be assigned, with the code for birth weight sequenced before the code for gestational age.

e. **Low birth weight and immaturity status**

Codes from category P07, Disorders of newborn related to short gestation and low birth weight, not elsewhere classified, are for use for a child or adult who was premature or had a low birth weight as a newborn and this is affecting the patient's current health status.

See Section I.C.21. Factors influencing health status and contact with health services, Status.

f. **Bacterial Sepsis of Newborn**

Category P36, Bacterial sepsis of newborn, includes congenital sepsis. If a perinate is documented as having sepsis without documentation of congenital or community acquired, the default is congenital and a code from category P36 should be assigned. If the P36 code includes the causal organism, an additional code from category B95, Streptococcus, Staphylococcus, and Enterococcus as the cause of diseases classified elsewhere, or B96, Other bacterial agents as the cause of diseases classified elsewhere, should not be assigned. If the P36 code does not include the causal organism, assign an additional code from category B96. If applicable, use additional codes to identify severe sepsis (R65.2-) and any associated acute organ dysfunction.

g. **Stillbirth**

Code P95, Stillbirth, is only for use in institutions that maintain separate records for stillbirths. No other code should be used with P95. Code P95 should not be used on the mother's record.

h. **COVID-19 Infection in Newborn**

For a newborn that tests positive for COVID-19, assign code U07.1, COVID-19, and the appropriate codes for associated manifestation(s) in neonates/newborns in the absence of documentation indicating a specific type of transmission. For a newborn that tests positive for COVID-19 and the provider documents the condition was contracted in utero or during the birth process, assign codes P35.8, Other congenital viral diseases, and U07.1, COVID-19. When coding the birth episode in a newborn record, the appropriate code from category Z38, Liveborn infants according to place of birth and type of delivery, should be assigned as the principal diagnosis.

17. **Chapter 17: Congenital malformations, deformations, and chromosomal abnormalities (Q00-Q99)**

Assign an appropriate code(s) from categories Q00-Q99, Congenital malformations, deformations, and chromosomal abnormalities when a malformation/deformation or chromosomal abnormality is documented. A malformation/deformation/or chromosomal abnormality may be the principal/first-listed diagnosis on a record or a secondary diagnosis.

When a malformation/deformation or chromosomal abnormality does not have a unique code assignment, assign additional code(s) for any manifestations that may be present.

When the code assignment specifically identifies the malformation/deformation or chromosomal abnormality, manifestations that are an inherent component of the anomaly should not be coded separately. Additional codes should be assigned for manifestations that are not an inherent component.

Codes from Chapter 17 may be used throughout the life of the patient. If a congenital malformation or deformity has been corrected, a personal history code should be used to identify the history of the malformation or deformity. Although present at birth, a malformation/deformation/or chromosomal abnormality may not be identified until later in life. Whenever the condition is diagnosed by the provider, it is appropriate to assign a code from codes Q00-Q99. For the birth admission, the appropriate code from category Z38, Liveborn infants, according to place of birth and type of delivery, should be sequenced as the principal diagnosis, followed by any congenital anomaly codes, Q00-Q99.

18. **Chapter 18: Symptoms, signs, and abnormal clinical and laboratory findings, not elsewhere classified (R00-R99)**

Chapter 18 includes symptoms, signs, abnormal results of clinical or other investigative procedures, and ill-defined conditions regarding which no diagnosis classifiable elsewhere is recorded. Signs and symptoms that point to a specific diagnosis have been assigned to a category in other chapters of the classification.

a. **Use of symptom codes**

Codes that describe symptoms and signs are acceptable for reporting purposes when a related definitive diagnosis has not been established (confirmed) by the provider.

b. **Use of a symptom code with a definitive diagnosis code**

Codes for signs and symptoms may be reported in addition to a related definitive diagnosis when the sign or symptom is not routinely associated with that diagnosis, such as the various signs and symptoms associated with complex syndromes. The definitive diagnosis code should be sequenced before the symptom code.

Signs or symptoms that are associated routinely with a disease process should not be assigned as additional codes, unless otherwise instructed by the classification.

c. **Combination codes that include symptoms**
ICD-10-CM contains a number of combination codes that identify both the definitive diagnosis and common symptoms of that diagnosis. When using one of these combination codes, an additional code should not be assigned for the symptom.

d. **Repeated falls**
Code R29.6, Repeated falls, is for use for encounters when a patient has recently fallen and the reason for the fall is being investigated.

Code Z91.81, History of falling, is for use when a patient has fallen in the past and is at risk for future falls. When appropriate, both codes R29.6 and Z91.81 may be assigned together.

e. **Coma**
Code R40.20, Unspecified coma, may be assigned in conjunction with codes for any medical condition.

Do not report codes for unspecified coma, individual or total Glasgow coma scale scores for a patient with a medically induced coma or a sedated patient.

1) **Coma Scale**
The coma scale codes (R40.21- to R40.24-) can be used in conjunction with traumatic brain injury codes. These codes are primarily for use by trauma registries, but they may be used in any setting where this information is collected. The coma scale codes should be sequenced after the diagnosis code(s).

These codes, one from each subcategory, are needed to complete the scale. The 7th character indicates when the scale was recorded. The 7th character should match for all three codes.

At a minimum, report the initial score documented on presentation at your facility. This may be a score from the emergency medicine technician (EMT) or in the emergency department. If desired, a facility may choose to capture multiple coma scale scores.

Assign code R40.24-, Glasgow coma scale, total score, when only the total score is documented in the medical record and not the individual score(s).

If multiple coma scores are captured within the first 24 hours after hospital admission, assign only the code for the score at the time of admission. ICD-10-CM does not classify coma scores that are reported after admission but less than 24 hours later.

See Section I.B.14. for coma scale documentation by clinicians other than patient's provider

f. **Functional quadriplegia**
GUIDELINE HAS BEEN DELETED EFFECTIVE OCTOBER 1, 2017

g. **SIRS due to Non-Infectious Process**
The systemic inflammatory response syndrome (SIRS) can develop as a result of certain non-infectious disease processes, such as trauma, malignant neoplasm, or pancreatitis. When SIRS is documented with a noninfectious condition, and no subsequent infection is documented, the code for the underlying condition, such as an injury, should be assigned, followed by code R65.10, Systemic inflammatory response syndrome (SIRS) of non-infectious origin without acute organ dysfunction, or code R65.11, Systemic inflammatory response syndrome (SIRS) of non-infectious origin with acute organ dysfunction. If an associated acute organ dysfunction is documented, the appropriate code(s) for the specific type of organ dysfunction(s) should be assigned in addition to code R65.11. If acute organ dysfunction is documented, but it cannot be determined if the acute organ dysfunction is associated with SIRS or due to another condition (e.g., directly due to the trauma), the provider should be queried.

h. **Death NOS**
Code R99, Ill-defined and unknown cause of mortality, is only for use in the very limited circumstance when a patient who has already died is brought into an emergency department or other healthcare facility and is pronounced dead upon arrival. It does not represent the discharge disposition of death.

i. **NIHSS Stroke Scale**
The NIH stroke scale (NIHSS) codes (R29.7- -) can be used in conjunction with acute stroke codes (I63) to identify the patient's neurological status and the severity of the stroke. The stroke scale codes should be sequenced after the acute stroke diagnosis code(s).

At a minimum, report the initial score documented. If desired, a facility may choose to capture multiple stroke scale scores.

See Section I.B.14. for NIHSS stroke scale documentation by clinicians other than patient's provider

19. **Chapter 19: Injury, poisoning, and certain other consequences of external causes (S00-T88)**

a. **Application of 7th Characters in Chapter 19**
Most categories in chapter 19 have a 7th character requirement for each applicable code. Most categories in this chapter have three 7th character values (with the exception of fractures): A, initial encounter, D, subsequent encounter and S, sequela. Categories for traumatic fractures have additional 7th character values. While the patient may be seen by a new or different provider over the course of treatment for an injury, assignment of the 7th character is based on whether the patient is undergoing active treatment and not whether the provider is seeing the patient for the first time.

For complication codes, active treatment refers to treatment for the condition described by the code, even though it may be related to an earlier precipitating problem. For example, code T84.50XA, Infection and inflammatory reaction due to unspecified internal joint prosthesis, initial encounter, is used when active treatment is provided for the infection, even though the condition relates to the prosthetic device, implant or graft that was placed at a previous encounter.

7th character "A", initial encounter is used for each encounter where the patient is receiving active treatment for the condition.

7th character "D" subsequent encounter is used for encounters after the patient has completed active treatment of the condition and is receiving routine care for the condition during the healing or recovery phase.

The aftercare Z codes should not be used for aftercare for conditions such as injuries or poisonings, where 7th characters are provided to identify subsequent care. For example, for aftercare of an injury, assign the acute injury code with the 7th character "D" (subsequent encounter).

7th character "S", sequela, is for use for complications or conditions that arise as a direct result of a condition, such as scar formation after a burn. The scars are sequelae of the burn. When using 7th character "S", it is necessary to use both the injury code that precipitated the sequela and the code for the sequela itself. The "S" is added only to the injury code, not the sequela code. The 7th character "S" identifies the injury responsible for the sequela. The specific type of sequela (e.g. scar) is sequenced first, followed by the injury code.

See Section I.B.10. Sequelae, (Late Effects)

b. **Coding of Injuries**
When coding injuries, assign separate codes for each injury unless a combination code is provided, in which case the combination code is assigned. Codes from category T07, Unspecified multiple injuries should not be assigned in the inpatient setting unless information for a more specific code is not available. Traumatic injury codes (S00-T14.9) are not to be used for normal, healing surgical wounds or to identify complications of surgical wounds.

The code for the most serious injury, as determined by the provider and the focus of treatment, is sequenced first.

1) **Superficial injuries**
Superficial injuries such as abrasions or contusions are not coded when associated with more severe injuries of the same site.

2) **Primary injury with damage to nerves/blood vessels**
When a primary injury results in minor damage to peripheral nerves or blood vessels, the primary injury is sequenced first with additional code(s) for injuries to nerves and spinal cord (such as category S04), and/or injury to blood vessels (such as category S15). When the primary injury is to the blood vessels or nerves, that injury should be sequenced first.

3) **Iatrogenic injuries**
Injury codes from Chapter 19 should not be assigned for injuries that occur during, or as a result of, a medical intervention. Assign the appropriate complication code(s).

c. **Coding of Traumatic Fractures**
The principles of multiple coding of injuries should be followed in coding fractures. Fractures of specified sites are coded individually by site in accordance with both the provisions within categories S02, S12, S22, S32, S42, S49, S52, S59, S62, S72, S79, S82, S89, S92 and the level of detail furnished by medical record content.

A fracture not indicated as open or closed should be coded to closed. A fracture not indicated whether displaced or not displaced should be coded to displaced.

More specific guidelines are as follows:

1) **Initial vs. subsequent encounter for fractures**

   Traumatic fractures are coded using the appropriate 7th character for initial encounter (A, B, C) for each encounter where the patient is receiving active treatment for the fracture. The appropriate 7th character for initial encounter should also be assigned for a patient who delayed seeking treatment for the fracture or nonunion.

   Fractures are coded using the appropriate 7th character for subsequent care for encounters after the patient has completed active treatment of the fracture and is receiving routine care for the fracture during the healing or recovery phase.

   Care for complications of surgical treatment for fracture repairs during the healing or recovery phase should be coded with the appropriate complication codes.

   Care of complications of fractures, such as malunion and nonunion, should be reported with the appropriate 7th character for subsequent care with nonunion (K, M, N,) or subsequent care with malunion (P, Q, R).

   Malunion/nonunion: The appropriate 7th character for initial encounter should also be assigned for a patient who delayed seeking treatment for the fracture or nonunion.

   The open fracture designations in the assignment of the 7th character for fractures of the forearm, femur and lower leg, including ankle are based on the Gustilo open fracture classification. When the Gustilo classification type is not specified for an open fracture, the 7th character for open fracture type I or II should be assigned (B, E, H, M, Q).

   A code from category M80, not a traumatic fracture code, should be used for any patient with known osteoporosis who suffers a fracture, even if the patient had a minor fall or trauma, if that fall or trauma would not usually break a normal, healthy bone.

   See Section I.C.13. Osteoporosis.

   The aftercare Z codes should not be used for aftercare for traumatic fractures. For aftercare of a traumatic fracture, assign the acute fracture code with the appropriate 7th character.

2) **Multiple fractures sequencing**

   Multiple fractures are sequenced in accordance with the severity of the fracture.

3) **Physeal fractures**

   For physeal fractures, assign only the code identifying the type of physeal fracture. Do not assign a separate code to identify the specific bone that is fractured.

d. **Coding of Burns and Corrosions**

   The ICD-10-CM makes a distinction between burns and corrosions. The burn codes are for thermal burns, except sunburns, that come from a heat source, such as a fire or hot appliance. The burn codes are also for burns resulting from electricity and radiation. Corrosions are burns due to chemicals. The guidelines are the same for burns and corrosions.

   Current burns (T20-T25) are classified by depth, extent and by agent (X code). Burns are classified by depth as first degree (erythema), second degree (blistering), and third degree (full-thickness involvement). Burns of the eye and internal organs (T26-T28) are classified by site, but not by degree.

   1) **Sequencing of burn and related condition codes**

      Sequence first the code that reflects the highest degree of burn when more than one burn is present.

      a. When the reason for the admission or encounter is for treatment of external multiple burns, sequence first the code that reflects the burn of the highest degree.

      b. When a patient has both internal and external burns, the circumstances of admission govern the selection of the principal diagnosis or first-listed diagnosis.

      c. When a patient is admitted for burn injuries and other related conditions such as smoke inhalation and/or respiratory failure, the circumstances of admission govern the selection of the principal or first-listed diagnosis.

   2) **Burns of the same anatomic site**

      Classify burns of the same anatomic site and on the same side but of different degrees to the subcategory identifying the highest

degree recorded in the diagnosis (e.g., for second and third degree burns of right thigh, assign only code T24.311-).

3) **Non-healing burns**

   Non-healing burns are coded as acute burns.

   Necrosis of burned skin should be coded as a non-healed burn.

4) **Infected burn**

   For any documented infected burn site, use an additional code for the infection.

5) **Assign separate codes for each burn site**

   When coding burns, assign separate codes for each burn site. Category T30, Burn and corrosion, body region unspecified is extremely vague and should rarely be used.

   Codes for burns of "multiple sites" should only be assigned when the medical record documentation does not specify the individual sites.

6) **Burns and corrosions classified according to extent of body surface involved**

   Assign codes from category T31, Burns classified according to extent of body surface involved, or T32, Corrosions classified according to extent of body surface involved, for acute burns or corrosions when the site of the burn or corrosion is not specified or when there is a need for additional data. It is advisable to use category T31 as additional coding when needed to provide data for evaluating burn mortality, such as that needed by burn units. It is also advisable to use category T31 as an additional code for reporting purposes when there is mention of a third-degree burn involving 20 percent or more of the body surface. Codes from categories T31 and T32 should not be used for sequelae of burns or corrosions.

   Categories T31 and T32 are based on the classic "rule of nines" in estimating body surface involved: head and neck are assigned nine percent, each arm nine percent, each leg 18 percent, the anterior trunk 18 percent, posterior trunk 18 percent, and genitalia one percent. Providers may change these percentage assignments where necessary to accommodate infants and children who have proportionally larger heads than adults, and patients who have large buttocks, thighs, or abdomen that involve burns.

7) **Encounters for treatment of sequela of burns**

   Encounters for the treatment of the late effects of burns or corrosions (i.e., scars or joint contractures) should be coded with a burn or corrosion code with the 7th character "S" for sequela.

8) **Sequelae with a late effect code and current burn**

   When appropriate, both a code for a current burn or corrosion with 7th character "A" or "D" and a burn or corrosion code with 7th character "S" may be assigned on the same record (when both a current burn and sequelae of an old burn exist). Burns and corrosions do not heal at the same rate and a current healing wound may still exist with sequela of a healed burn or corrosion.

   See Section I.B.10. Sequela (Late Effects)

9) **Use of an external cause code with burns and corrosions**

   An external cause code should be used with burns and corrosions to identify the source and intent of the burn, as well as the place where it occurred.

e. **Adverse Effects, Poisoning, Underdosing and Toxic Effects**

   Codes in categories T36-T65 are combination codes that include the substance that was taken as well as the intent. No additional external cause code is required for poisonings, toxic effects, adverse effects and underdosing codes.

   1) **Do not code directly from the Table of Drugs**

      Do not code directly from the Table of Drugs and Chemicals. Always refer back to the Tabular List.

   2) **Use as many codes as necessary to describe**

      Use as many codes as necessary to describe completely all drugs, medicinal or biological substances.

   3) **If the same code would describe the causative agent**

      If the same code would describe the causative agent for more than one adverse reaction, poisoning, toxic effect or underdosing, assign the code only once.

   4) **If two or more drugs, medicinal or biological substances**

      If two or more drugs, medicinal or biological substances are taken, code each individually unless a combination code is listed in the Table of Drugs and Chemicals.

      If multiple unspecified drugs, medicinal or biological substances were taken, assign the appropriate code from subcategory

T50.91, Poisoning by, adverse effect of and underdosing of multiple unspecified drugs, medicaments and biological substances.

5) **The occurrence of drug toxicity is classified in ICD-10-CM as follows:**

   (a) **Adverse Effect**

   When coding an adverse effect of a drug that has been correctly prescribed and properly administered, assign the appropriate code for the nature of the adverse effect followed by the appropriate code for the adverse effect of the drug (T36-T50). The code for the drug should have a 5th or 6th character "5" (for example T36.0X5-) Examples of the nature of an adverse effect are tachycardia, delirium, gastrointestinal hemorrhaging, vomiting, hypokalemia, hepatitis, renal failure, or respiratory failure.

   (b) **Poisoning**

   When coding a poisoning or reaction to the improper use of a medication (e.g., overdose, wrong substance given or taken in error, wrong route of administration), first assign the appropriate code from categories T36-T50. The poisoning codes have an associated intent as their 5th or 6th character (accidental, intentional self-harm, assault and undetermined). If the intent of the poisoning is unknown or unspecified, code the intent as accidental intent. The undetermined intent is only for use if the documentation in the record specifies that the intent cannot be determined. Use additional code(s) for all manifestations of poisonings.

   If there is also a diagnosis of abuse or dependence of the substance, the abuse or dependence is assigned as an additional code.

   Examples of poisoning include:

   (i) Error was made in drug prescription
   Errors made in drug prescription or in the administration of the drug by provider, nurse, patient, or other person.

   (ii) Overdose of a drug intentionally taken
   If an overdose of a drug was intentionally taken or administered and resulted in drug toxicity, it would be coded as a poisoning.

   (iii) Nonprescribed drug taken with correctly prescribed and properly administered drug
   If a nonprescribed drug or medicinal agent was taken in combination with a correctly prescribed and properly administered drug, any drug toxicity or other reaction resulting from the interaction of the two drugs would be classified as a poisoning.

   (iv) Interaction of drug(s) and alcohol
   When a reaction results from the interaction of a drug(s) and alcohol, this would be classified as poisoning.

   See Section I.C.4. if poisoning is the result of insulin pump malfunctions.

   (c) **Underdosing**

   Underdosing refers to taking less of a medication than is prescribed by a provider or a manufacturer's instruction. Discontinuing the use of a prescribed medication on the patient's own initiative (not directed by the patient's provider) is also classified as an underdosing. For underdosing, assign the code from categories T36-T50 (fifth or sixth character "6"). **Documentation of a change in the patient's condition is not required in order to assign an underdosing code. Documentation that the patient is taking less of a medication than is prescribed or discontinued the prescribed medication is sufficient for code assignment.**

   Codes for underdosing should never be assigned as principal or first-listed codes. If a patient has a relapse or exacerbation of the medical condition for which the drug is prescribed because of the reduction in dose, then the medical condition itself should be coded.

   Noncompliance (Z91.12-, Z91.13- and Z91.14-) or complication of care (Y63.6-Y63.9) codes are to be used with an underdosing code to indicate intent, if known.

   (d) **Toxic Effects**

   When a harmful substance is ingested or comes in contact with a person, this is classified as a toxic effect. The toxic effect codes are in categories T51-T65.

Toxic effect codes have an associated intent: accidental, intentional self-harm, assault and undetermined.

f. **Adult and child abuse, neglect and other maltreatment**

Sequence first the appropriate code from categories T74, Adult and child abuse, neglect and other maltreatment, confirmed, or T76, Adult and child abuse, neglect and other maltreatment, suspected, for abuse, neglect and other maltreatment, followed by any accompanying mental health or injury code(s).

If the documentation in the medical record states abuse or neglect, it is coded as confirmed (T74.-). It is coded as suspected if it is documented as suspected (T76.-).

For cases of confirmed abuse or neglect an external cause code from the assault section (X92-Y09) should be added to identify the cause of any physical injuries. A perpetrator code (Y07) should be added when the perpetrator of the abuse is known. For suspected cases of abuse or neglect, do not report external cause or perpetrator code.

If a suspected case of abuse, neglect or mistreatment is ruled out during an encounter code Z04.71, Encounter for examination and observation following alleged physical adult abuse, ruled out, or code Z04.72, Encounter for examination and observation following alleged child physical abuse, ruled out, should be used, not a code from T76.

If a suspected case of alleged rape or sexual abuse is ruled out during an encounter code Z04.41, Encounter for examination and observation following alleged adult rape or code Z04.42, Encounter for examination and observation following alleged child rape, should be used, not a code from T76.

If a suspected case of forced sexual exploitation or forced labor exploitation is ruled out during an encounter, code Z04.81, Encounter for examination and observation of victim following forced sexual exploitation, or code Z04.82, Encounter for examination and observation of victim following forced labor exploitation, should be used, not a code from T76.

See Section I.C.15. Abuse in a pregnant patient.

g. **Complications of care**

1) **General guidelines for complications of care**

   (a) **Documentation of complications of care**
   See Section I.B.16. for information on documentation of complications of care.

2) **Pain due to medical devices**

   Pain associated with devices, implants or grafts left in a surgical site (for example painful hip prosthesis) is assigned to the appropriate code(s) found in Chapter 19, Injury, poisoning, and certain other consequences of external causes. Specific codes for pain due to medical devices are found in the T code section of the ICD-10-CM. Use additional code(s) from category G89 to identify acute or chronic pain due to presence of the device, implant or graft (G89.18 or G89.28).

3) **Transplant complications**

   (a) **Transplant complications other than kidney**

   Codes under category T86, Complications of transplanted organs and tissues, are for use for both complications and rejection of transplanted organs. A transplant complication code is only assigned if the complication affects the function of the transplanted organ. Two codes are required to fully describe a transplant complication: the appropriate code from category T86 and a secondary code that identifies the complication.

   Pre-existing conditions or conditions that develop after the transplant are not coded as complications unless they affect the function of the transplanted organs.

   See I.C.21. for transplant organ removal status

   See I.C.2. for malignant neoplasm associated with transplanted organ.

   (b) **Kidney transplant complications**

   Patients who have undergone kidney transplant may still have some form of chronic kidney disease (CKD) because the kidney transplant may not fully restore kidney function. Code T86.1- should be assigned for documented complications of a kidney transplant, such as transplant failure or rejection or other transplant complication. Code T86.1- should not be assigned for post kidney transplant patients who have chronic kidney (CKD) unless a transplant complication such as transplant failure or rejection is documented. If the documentation is unclear as to whether the patient has a complication of the transplant, query the provider.

Conditions that affect the function of the transplanted kidney, other than CKD, should be assigned a code from subcategory T86.1, Complications of transplanted organ, Kidney, and a secondary code that identifies the complication.

For patients with CKD following a kidney transplant, but who do not have a complication such as failure or rejection, *see section I.C.14. Chronic kidney disease and kidney transplant status.*

4) **Complication codes that include the external cause**
As with certain other T codes, some of the complications of care codes have the external cause included in the code. The code includes the nature of the complication as well as the type of procedure that caused the complication. No external cause code indicating the type of procedure is necessary for these codes.

5) **Complications of care codes within the body system chapters**
Intraoperative and postprocedural complication codes are found within the body system chapters with codes specific to the organs and structures of that body system. These codes should be sequenced first, followed by a code(s) for the specific complication, if applicable.

Complication codes from the body system chapters should be assigned for intraoperative and postprocedural complications (e.g., the appropriate complication code from chapter 9 would be assigned for a vascular intraoperative or postprocedural complication) unless the complication is specifically indexed to a T code in chapter 19.

20. **Chapter 20: External Causes of Morbidity (V00-Y99)**
The external causes of morbidity codes should never be sequenced as the first-listed or principal diagnosis.

External cause codes are intended to provide data for injury research and evaluation of injury prevention strategies. These codes capture how the injury or health condition happened (cause), the intent (unintentional or accidental; or intentional, such as suicide or assault), the place where the event occurred the activity of the patient at the time of the event, and the person's status (e.g., civilian, military).

There is no national requirement for mandatory ICD-10-CM external cause code reporting. Unless a provider is subject to a state-based external cause code reporting mandate or these codes are required by a particular payer, reporting of ICD-10-CM codes in Chapter 20, External Causes of Morbidity, is not required. In the absence of a mandatory reporting requirement, providers are encouraged to voluntarily report external cause codes, as they provide valuable data for injury research and evaluation of injury prevention strategies.

a. **General External Cause Coding Guidelines**
1) **Used with any code in the range of A00.0-T88.9, Z00-Z99**
An external cause code may be used with any code in the range of A00.0-T88.9, Z00-Z99, classification that represents a health condition due to an external cause. Though they are most applicable to injuries, they are also valid for use with such things as infections or diseases due to an external source, and other health conditions, such as a heart attack that occurs during strenuous physical activity.

2) **External cause code used for length of treatment**
Assign the external cause code, with the appropriate 7th character (initial encounter, subsequent encounter or sequela) for each encounter for which the injury or condition is being treated.

Most categories in chapter 20 have a 7th character requirement for each applicable code. Most categories in this chapter have three 7th character values: A, initial encounter, D, subsequent encounter and S, sequela. While the patient may be seen by a new or different provider over the course of treatment for an injury or condition, assignment of the 7th character for external cause should match the 7th character of the code assigned for the associated injury or condition for the encounter.

3) **Use the full range of external cause codes**
Use the full range of external cause codes to completely describe the cause, the intent, the place of occurrence, and if applicable, the activity of the patient at the time of the event, and the patient's status, for all injuries, and other health conditions due to an external cause.

4) **Assign as many external cause codes as necessary**
Assign as many external cause codes as necessary to fully explain each cause. If only one external code can be recorded, assign the code most related to the principal diagnosis.

5) **The selection of the appropriate external cause code**
The selection of the appropriate external cause code is guided by the Alphabetic Index of External Causes and by Inclusion and Exclusion notes in the Tabular List.

6) **External cause code can never be a principal diagnosis**
An external cause code can never be a principal (first-listed) diagnosis.

7) **Combination external cause codes**
Certain of the external cause codes are combination codes that identify sequential events that result in an injury, such as a fall which results in striking against an object. The injury may be due to either event or both. The combination external cause code used should correspond to the sequence of events regardless of which caused the most serious injury.

8) **No external cause code needed in certain circumstances**
No external cause code from Chapter 20 is needed if the external cause and intent are included in a code from another chapter (e.g., T36.0X1-, Poisoning by penicillins, accidental (unintentional)).

b. **Place of Occurrence Guideline**
Codes from category Y92, Place of occurrence of the external cause, are secondary codes for use after other external cause codes to identify the location of the patient at the time of injury or other condition.

Generally, a place of occurrence code is assigned only once, at the initial encounter for treatment. However, in the rare instance that a new injury occurs during hospitalization, an additional place of occurrence code may be assigned. No 7th characters are used for Y92.

Do not use place of occurrence code Y92.9 if the place is not stated or is not applicable.

c. **Activity Code**
Assign a code from category Y93, Activity code, to describe the activity of the patient at the time the injury or other health condition occurred.

An activity code is used only once, at the initial encounter for treatment. Only one code from Y93 should be recorded on a medical record.

The activity codes are not applicable to poisonings, adverse effects, misadventures or sequela.

Do not assign Y93.9, Unspecified activity, if the activity is not stated.

A code from category Y93 is appropriate for use with external cause and intent codes if identifying the activity provides additional information about the event.

d. **Place of Occurrence, Activity, and Status Codes Used with other External Cause Code**
When applicable, place of occurrence, activity, and external cause status codes are sequenced after the main external cause code(s). Regardless of the number of external cause codes assigned, generally there should be only one place of occurrence code, one activity code, and one external cause status code assigned to an encounter. However, in the rare instance that a new injury occurs during hospitalization, an additional place of occurrence code may be assigned.

e. **If the Reporting Format Limits the Number of External Cause Codes**
If the reporting format limits the number of external cause codes that can be used in reporting clinical data, report the code for the cause/intent most related to the principal diagnosis. If the format permits capture of additional external cause codes, the cause/intent, including medical misadventures, of the additional events should be reported rather than the codes for place, activity, or external status.

f. **Multiple External Cause Coding Guidelines**
More than one external cause code is required to fully describe the external cause of an illness or injury. The assignment of external cause codes should be sequenced in the following priority:

If two or more events cause separate injuries, an external cause code should be assigned for each cause. The first-listed external cause code will be selected in the following order:

External codes for child and adult abuse take priority over all other external cause codes.

See Section I.C.19., Child and Adult abuse guidelines.

External cause codes for terrorism events take priority over all other external cause codes except child and adult abuse.

External cause codes for cataclysmic events take priority over all other external cause codes except child and adult abuse and terrorism.

External cause codes for transport accidents take priority over all other external cause codes except cataclysmic events, child and adult abuse and terrorism.

Activity and external cause status codes are assigned following all causal (intent) external cause codes.

The first-listed external cause code should correspond to the cause of the most serious diagnosis due to an assault, accident, or self-harm, following the order of hierarchy listed above.

g. Child and Adult Abuse Guideline

Adult and child abuse, neglect and maltreatment are classified as assault. Any of the assault codes may be used to indicate the external cause of any injury resulting from the confirmed abuse.

For confirmed cases of abuse, neglect and maltreatment, when the perpetrator is known, a code from Y07, Perpetrator of maltreatment and neglect, should accompany any other assault codes.

See Section I.C.19. Adult and child abuse, neglect and other maltreatment

h. Unknown or Undetermined Intent Guideline

If the intent (accident, self-harm, assault) of the cause of an injury or other condition is unknown or unspecified, code the intent as accidental intent. All transport accident categories assume accidental intent.

1) Use of undetermined intent

External cause codes for events of undetermined intent are only for use if the documentation in the record specifies that the intent cannot be determined.

i. Sequelae (Late Effects) of External Cause Guidelines

1) Sequelae external cause codes

Sequela are reported using the external cause code with the 7th character "S" for sequela. These codes should be used with any report of a late effect or sequela resulting from a previous injury.

See Section I.B.10. Sequela (Late Effects)

2) Sequela external cause code with a related current injury

A sequela external cause code should never be used with a related current nature of injury code.

3) Use of sequela external cause codes for subsequent visits

Use a late effect external cause code for subsequent visits when a late effect of the initial injury is being treated. Do not use a late effect external cause code for subsequent visits for follow-up care (e.g., to assess healing, to receive rehabilitative therapy) of the injury when no late effect of the injury has been documented.

j. Terrorism Guidelines

1) Cause of injury identified by the Federal Government (FBI) as terrorism

When the cause of an injury is identified by the Federal Government (FBI) as terrorism, the first-listed external cause code should be a code from category Y38, Terrorism. The definition of terrorism employed by the FBI is found at the inclusion note at the beginning of category Y38. Use additional code for place of occurrence (Y92.-). More than one Y38 code may be assigned if the injury is the result of more than one mechanism of terrorism.

2) Cause of an injury is suspected to be the result of terrorism

When the cause of an injury is suspected to be the result of terrorism a code from category Y38 should not be assigned. Suspected cases should be classified as assault.

3) Code Y38.9, Terrorism, secondary effects

Assign code Y38.9, Terrorism, secondary effects, for conditions occurring subsequent to the terrorist event. This code should not be assigned for conditions that are due to the initial terrorist act.

It is acceptable to assign code Y38.9 with another code from Y38 if there is an injury due to the initial terrorist event and an injury that is a subsequent result of the terrorist event.

k. External Cause Status

A code from category Y99, External cause status, should be assigned whenever any other external cause code is assigned for an encounter, including an Activity code, except for the events noted below. Assign a code from category Y99, External cause status, to indicate the work status of the person at the time the event occurred. The status code indicates whether the event occurred during military activity, whether a non-military person was at work, whether an individual including a student or volunteer was involved in a non-work activity at the time of the causal event.

A code from Y99, External cause status, should be assigned, when applicable, with other external cause codes, such as transport accidents and falls. The external cause status codes are not applicable to poisonings, adverse effects, misadventures or late effects.

Do not assign a code from category Y99 if no other external cause codes (cause, activity) are applicable for the encounter.

An external cause status code is used only once, at the initial encounter for treatment. Only one code from Y99 should be recorded on a medical record.

Do not assign code Y99.9, Unspecified external cause status, if the status is not stated.

21. Chapter 21: Factors influencing health status and contact with health services (Z00-Z99)

Note: The chapter specific guidelines provide additional information about the use of Z codes for specified encounters.

a. Use of Z Codes in Any Healthcare Setting

Z codes are for use in any healthcare setting. Z codes may be used as either first-listed (principal diagnosis code in the inpatient setting) or secondary code, depending on the circumstances of the encounter. Certain Z codes may only be used as first-listed or principal diagnosis.

b. Z Codes Indicate a Reason for an Encounter or Provide Additional Information about a Patient Encounter

Z codes are not procedure codes. A corresponding procedure code must accompany a Z code to describe any procedure performed.

c. Categories of Z Codes

1) Contact/Exposure

Category Z20 indicates contact with, and suspected exposure to, communicable diseases. These codes are for patients who are suspected to have been exposed to a disease by close personal contact with an infected individual or are in an area where a disease is epidemic.

Category Z77, Other contact with and (suspected) exposures hazardous to health, indicates contact with and suspected exposures hazardous to health.

Contact/exposure codes may be used as a first-listed code to explain an encounter for testing, or, more commonly, as a secondary code to identify a potential risk.

2) Inoculations and vaccinations

Code Z23 is for encounters for inoculations and vaccinations. It indicates that a patient is being seen to receive a prophylactic inoculation against a disease. Procedure codes are required to identify the actual administration of the injection and the type(s) of immunizations given. Code Z23 may be used as a secondary code if the inoculation is given as a routine part of preventive health care, such as a well-baby visit.

3) Status

Status codes indicate that a patient is either a carrier of a disease or has the sequelae or residual of a past disease or condition. This includes such things as the presence of prosthetic or mechanical devices resulting from past treatment. A status code is informative, because the status may affect the course of treatment and its outcome. A status code is distinct from a history code. The history code indicates that the patient no longer has the condition.

A status code should not be used with a diagnosis code from one of the body system chapters, if the diagnosis code includes the information provided by the status code. For example, code Z94.1, Heart transplant status, should not be used with a code from subcategory T86.2, Complications of heart transplant. The status code does not provide additional information. The complication code indicates that the patient is a heart transplant patient.

For encounters for weaning from a mechanical ventilator, assign a code from subcategory J96.1, Chronic respiratory failure, followed by code Z99.11, Dependence on respirator [ventilator] status.

The status Z codes/categories are:

Z14   Genetic carrier
        Genetic carrier status indicates that a person carries a gene, associated with a particular disease, which may be passed to offspring who may develop that disease. The person does not have the disease and is not at risk of developing the disease.

Z15   Genetic susceptibility to disease
        Genetic susceptibility indicates that a person has a gene that increases the risk of that person developing the disease.
        Codes from category Z15 should not be used as principal or first-listed codes. If the patient has the condition to which he/she is susceptible, and that condition is the

reason for the encounter, the code for the current condition should be sequenced first. If the patient is being seen for follow-up after completed treatment for this condition, and the condition no longer exists, a follow-up code should be sequenced first, followed by the appropriate personal history and genetic susceptibility codes. If the purpose of the encounter is genetic counseling associated with procreative management, code Z31.5, Encounter for genetic counseling, should be assigned as the first-listed code, followed by a code from category Z15. Additional codes should be assigned for any applicable family or personal history.

Z16 Resistance to antimicrobial drugs
This code indicates that a patient has a condition that is resistant to antimicrobial drug treatment. Sequence the infection code first.

Z17 Estrogen receptor status
Z18 Retained foreign body fragments
Z19 Hormone sensitivity malignancy status
Z21 Asymptomatic HIV infection status
This code indicates that a patient has tested positive for HIV but has manifested no signs or symptoms of the disease.

Z22 Carrier of infectious disease
Carrier status indicates that a person harbors the specific organisms of a disease without manifest symptoms and is capable of transmitting the infection.

Z28.3 Underimmunization status
See Section I.B.14. for underimmunization documentation by clinicians other than the patient's provider.

Z33.1 Pregnant state, incidental
This code is a secondary code only for use when the pregnancy is in no way complicating the reason for visit. Otherwise, a code from the obstetric chapter is required.

Z66 Do not resuscitate
This code may be used when it is documented by the provider that a patient is on do not resuscitate status at any time during the stay.

Z67 Blood type
Z68 Body mass index (BMI)
BMI codes should only be assigned when there is an associated, reportable diagnosis (such as obesity). Do not assign BMI codes during pregnancy.
See Section I.B.14. for BMI documentation by clinicians other than the patient's provider.

Z74.01 Bed confinement status
Z76.82 Awaiting organ transplant status
Z78 Other specified health status
Code Z78.1, Physical restraint status, may be used when it is documented by the provider that a patient has been put in restraints during the current encounter. Please note that this code should not be reported when it is documented by the provider that a patient is temporarily restrained during a procedure.

Z79 Long-term (current) drug therapy
Codes from this category indicate a patient's continuous use of a prescribed drug (including such things as aspirin therapy) for the long-term treatment of a condition or for prophylactic use. It is not for use for patients who have addictions to drugs. This subcategory is not for use of medications for detoxification or maintenance programs to prevent withdrawal symptoms (e.g., methadone maintenance for opiate dependence). Assign the appropriate code for the drug use, abuse, or dependence instead.
Assign a code from Z79 if the patient is receiving a medication for an extended period as a prophylactic measure (such as for the prevention of deep vein thrombosis) or as treatment of a chronic condition (such as arthritis) or a disease requiring a lengthy course of treatment (such as cancer). Do not assign a code from category Z79 for medication being administered for a brief period of time to treat an acute illness or injury (such as a course of antibiotics to treat acute bronchitis).

Z88 Allergy status to drugs, medicaments and biological substances
Except: Z88.9, Allergy status to unspecified drugs, medicaments and biological substances status

Z89 Acquired absence of limb
Z90 Acquired absence of organs, not elsewhere classified
Z91.0- Allergy status, other than to drugs and biological substances
Z92.82 Status post administration of tPA (rtPA) in a different facility within the last 24 hours prior to admission to a current facility
Assign code Z92.82, Status post administration of tPA (rtPA) in a different facility within the last 24 hours prior to admission to current facility, as a secondary diagnosis when a patient is received by transfer into a facility and documentation indicates they were administered tissue plasminogen activator (tPA) within the last 24 hours prior to admission to the current facility.
This guideline applies even if the patient is still receiving the tPA at the time they are received into the current facility.
The appropriate code for the condition for which the tPA was administered (such as cerebrovascular disease or myocardial infarction) should be assigned first.
Code Z92.82 is only applicable to the receiving facility record and not to the transferring facility record.

Z93 Artificial opening status
Z94 Transplanted organ and tissue status
Z95 Presence of cardiac and vascular implants and grafts
Z96 Presence of other functional implants
Z97 Presence of other devices
Z98 Other postprocedural states
Assign code Z98.85, Transplanted organ removal status, to indicate that a transplanted organ has been previously removed. This code should not be assigned for the encounter in which the transplanted organ is removed. The complication necessitating removal of the transplant organ should be assigned for that encounter.
See section I.C.19. for information on the coding of organ transplant complications.

Z99 Dependence on enabling machines and devices, not elsewhere classified
Note: Categories Z89-Z90 and Z93-Z99 are for use only if there are no complications or malfunctions of the organ or tissue replaced, the amputation site or the equipment on which the patient is dependent.

4) **History (of)**
There are two types of history Z codes, personal and family. Personal history codes explain a patient's past medical condition that no longer exists and is not receiving any treatment, but that has the potential for recurrence, and therefore may require continued monitoring.

Family history codes are for use when a patient has a family member(s) who has had a particular disease that causes the patient to be at higher risk of also contracting the disease.

Personal history codes may be used in conjunction with follow-up codes and family history codes may be used in conjunction with screening codes to explain the need for a test or procedure. History codes are also acceptable on any medical record regardless of the reason for visit. A history of an illness, even if no longer present, is important information that may alter the type of treatment ordered.

The reason for the encounter (for example, screening or counseling) should be sequenced first and the appropriate personal and/or family history code(s) should be assigned as additional diagnos(es).

The history Z code categories are:

Z80 Family history of primary malignant neoplasm
Z81 Family history of mental and behavioral disorders
Z82 Family history of certain disabilities and chronic diseases (leading to disablement)
Z83 Family history of other specific disorders
Z84 Family history of other conditions
Z85 Personal history of malignant neoplasm
Z86 Personal history of certain other diseases

Z87   Personal history of other diseases and conditions

Z91.4-   Personal history of psychological trauma, not elsewhere classified

Z91.5-   Personal history of self-harm

Z91.81   History of falling

Z91.82   Personal history of military deployment

Z92   Personal history of medical treatment
Except: Z92.0, Personal history of contraception
Except: Z92.82, Status post administration of tPA (rtPA) in a different facility within the last 24 hours prior to admission to a current facility

5) Screening

Screening is the testing for disease or disease precursors in seemingly well individuals so that early detection and treatment can be provided for those who test positive for the disease (e.g., screening mammogram).

The testing of a person to rule out or confirm a suspected diagnosis because the patient has some sign or symptom is a diagnostic examination, not a screening. In these cases, the sign or symptom is used to explain the reason for the test.

A screening code may be a first-listed code if the reason for the visit is specifically the screening exam. It may also be used as an additional code if the screening is done during an office visit for other health problems. A screening code is not necessary if the screening is inherent to a routine examination, such as a pap smear done during a routine pelvic examination.

Should a condition be discovered during the screening then the code for the condition may be assigned as an additional diagnosis.

The Z code indicates that a screening exam is planned. A procedure code is required to confirm that the screening was performed.

The screening Z codes/categories:

Z11   Encounter for screening for infectious and parasitic diseases

Z12   Encounter for screening for malignant neoplasms

Z13   Encounter for screening for other diseases and disorders
Except: Z13.9, Encounter for screening, unspecified

Z36   Encounter for antenatal screening for mother

6) Observation

There are three observation Z code categories. They are for use in very limited circumstances when a person is being observed for a suspected condition that is ruled out. The observation codes are not for use if an injury or illness or any signs or symptoms related to the suspected condition are present. In such cases the diagnosis/symptom code is used with the corresponding external cause code.

The observation codes are primarily to be used as a principal/first-listed diagnosis. An observation code may be assigned as a secondary diagnosis code when the patient is being observed for a condition that is ruled out and is unrelated to the principal/first-listed diagnosis. Also, when the principal diagnosis is required to be a code from category Z38, Liveborn infants according to place of birth and type of delivery, then a code from category Z05, Encounter for observation and evaluation of newborn for suspected diseases and conditions ruled out, is sequenced after the Z38 code. Additional codes may be used in addition to the observation code, but only if they are unrelated to the suspected condition being observed.

Codes from subcategory Z03.7, Encounter for suspected maternal and fetal conditions ruled out, may either be used as a first-listed or as an additional code assignment depending on the case. They are for use in very limited circumstances on a maternal record when an encounter is for a suspected maternal or fetal condition that is ruled out during that encounter (for example, a maternal or fetal condition may be suspected due to an abnormal test result). These codes should not be used when the condition is confirmed. In those cases, the confirmed condition should be coded. In addition, these codes are not for use if an illness or any signs or symptoms related to the suspected condition or problem are present. In such cases the diagnosis/symptom code is used.

Additional codes may be used in addition to the code from subcategory Z03.7, but only if they are unrelated to the suspected condition being evaluated.

Codes from subcategory Z03.7 may not be used for encounters for antenatal screening of mother. *See Section I.C.21. Screening.*

For encounters for suspected fetal condition that are inconclusive following testing and evaluation, assign the appropriate code from category O35, O36, O40 or O41.

The observation Z code categories:

Z03   Encounter for medical observation for suspected diseases and conditions ruled out

Z04   Encounter for examination and observation for other reasons Except: Z04.9, Encounter for examination and observation for unspecified reason

Z05   Encounter for observation and evaluation of newborn for suspected diseases and conditions ruled out

7) Aftercare

Aftercare visit codes cover situations when the initial treatment of a disease has been performed and the patient requires continued care during the healing or recovery phase, or for the long-term consequences of the disease. The aftercare Z code should not be used if treatment is directed at a current, acute disease. The diagnosis code is to be used in these cases. Exceptions to this rule are codes Z51.0, Encounter for antineoplastic radiation therapy, and codes from subcategory Z51.1, Encounter for antineoplastic chemotherapy and immunotherapy. These codes are to be first listed, followed by the diagnosis code when a patient's encounter is solely to receive radiation therapy, chemotherapy, or immunotherapy for the treatment of a neoplasm. If the reason for the encounter is more than one type of antineoplastic therapy, code Z51.0 and a code from subcategory Z51.1 may be assigned together, in which case one of these codes would be reported as a secondary diagnosis.

The aftercare Z codes should also not be used for aftercare for injuries. For aftercare of an injury, assign the acute injury code with the appropriate 7th character (for subsequent encounter).

The aftercare codes are generally first listed to explain the specific reason for the encounter. An aftercare code may be used as an additional code when some type of aftercare is provided in addition to the reason for admission and no diagnosis code is applicable. An example of this would be the closure of a colostomy during an encounter for treatment of another condition.

Aftercare codes should be used in conjunction with other aftercare codes or diagnosis codes to provide better detail on the specifics of an aftercare encounter visit, unless otherwise directed by the classification. The sequencing of multiple aftercare codes depends on the circumstances of the encounter.

Certain aftercare Z code categories need a secondary diagnosis code to describe the resolving condition or sequelae. For others, the condition is included in the code title.

Additional Z code aftercare category terms include fitting and adjustment, and attention to artificial openings.

Status Z codes may be used with aftercare Z codes to indicate the nature of the aftercare. For example, code Z95.1, Presence of aortocoronary bypass graft, may be used with code Z48.812, Encounter for surgical aftercare following surgery on the circulatory system, to indicate the surgery for which the aftercare is being performed. A status code should not be used when the aftercare code indicates the type of status, such as using Z43.0, Encounter for attention to tracheostomy, with Z93.0, Tracheostomy status.

The aftercare Z category/codes:

Z42   Encounter for plastic and reconstructive surgery following medical procedure or healed injury

Z43   Encounter for attention to artificial openings

Z44   Encounter for fitting and adjustment of external prosthetic device

Z45   Encounter for adjustment and management of implanted device

Z46   Encounter for fitting and adjustment of other devices

Z47   Orthopedic aftercare

Z48   Encounter for other postprocedural aftercare

Z49   Encounter for care involving renal dialysis

Z51   Encounter for other aftercare and medical care

8) Follow-up

The follow-up codes are used to explain continuing surveillance following completed treatment of a disease, condition, or injury. They imply that the condition has been fully treated and no longer exists. They should not be confused with aftercare codes, or injury codes with a 7th character for subsequent encounter, that explain ongoing care of a healing condition or its sequelae. Follow-up codes may be used in conjunction with history codes to provide the full picture of the healed condition and its treatment. The follow-up code is sequenced first, followed by the history code.

A follow-up code may be used to explain multiple visits. Should a condition be found to have recurred on the follow-up visit, then the diagnosis code for the condition should be assigned in place of the follow-up code.

The follow-up Z code categories:

Z08   Encounter for follow-up examination after completed treatment for malignant neoplasm

Z09   Encounter for follow-up examination after completed treatment for conditions other than malignant neoplasm

Z39   Encounter for maternal postpartum care and examination

9) Donor

Codes in category Z52, Donors of organs and tissues, are used for living individuals who are donating blood or other body tissue. These codes are for individuals donating for others, as well as for self-donations. They are not used to identify cadaveric donations.

10) Counseling

Counseling Z codes are used when a patient or family member receives assistance in the aftermath of an illness or injury, or when support is required in coping with family or social problems.

The counseling Z codes/categories:

Z30.0- Encounter for general counseling and advice on contraception

Z31.5   Encounter for procreative genetic counseling

Z31.6- Encounter for general counseling and advice on procreation

Z32.2   Encounter for childbirth instruction

Z32.3   Encounter for childcare instruction

Z69   Encounter for mental health services for victim and perpetrator of abuse

Z70   Counseling related to sexual attitude, behavior and orientation

Z71   Persons encountering health services for other counseling and medical advice, not elsewhere classified
Note: Code Z71.84, Encounter for health counseling related to travel, is to be used for health risk and safety counseling for future travel purposes.

Code Z71.85, Encounter for immunization safety counseling, is to be used for counseling of the patient or caregiver regarding the safety of a vaccine. This code should not be used for the provision of general information regarding risks and potential side effects during routine encounters for the administration of vaccines.

Code Z71.87, Encounter for pediatric-to-adult transition counseling, should be assigned when pediatric-to-adult transition counseling is the sole reason for the encounter or when this counseling is provided in addition to other services, such as treatment of a chronic condition. If both transition counseling and treatment of a medical condition are provided during the same encounter, the code(s) for the medical condition(s) treated and code Z71.87 should be assigned, with sequencing depending on the circumstances of the encounter.

Z76.81 Expectant mother prebirth pediatrician visit

11) Encounters for Obstetrical and Reproductive Services

See Section I.C.15. Pregnancy, Childbirth, and the Puerperium, for further instruction on the use of these codes.

Z codes for pregnancy are for use in those circumstances when none of the problems or complications included in the codes from the Obstetrics chapter exist (a routine prenatal visit or postpartum care). Codes in category Z34, Encounter for supervision of normal pregnancy, are always first listed and are not to be used with any other code from the OB chapter.

Codes in category Z3A, Weeks of gestation, may be assigned to provide additional information about the pregnancy. Category Z3A codes should not be assigned for pregnancies with abortive outcomes (categories O00-O08), elective termination of pregnancy (code Z33.2), nor for postpartum conditions, as

category Z3A is not applicable to these conditions. The date of the admission should be used to determine weeks of gestation for inpatient admissions that encompass more than one gestational week.

The outcome of delivery, category Z37, should be included on all maternal delivery records. It is always a secondary code.

Codes in category Z37 should not be used on the newborn record.

Z codes for family planning (contraceptive) or procreative management and counseling should be included on an obstetric record either during the pregnancy or the postpartum stage, if applicable.

Z codes/categories for obstetrical and reproductive services:

Z30   Encounter for contraceptive management

Z31   Encounter for procreative management

Z32.2   Encounter for childbirth instruction

Z32.3   Encounter for childcare instruction

Z33   Pregnant state

Z34   Encounter for supervision of normal pregnancy

Z36   Encounter for antenatal screening of mother

Z3A   Weeks of gestation

Z37   Outcome of delivery

Z39   Encounter for maternal postpartum care and examination

Z76.81 Expectant mother prebirth pediatrician visit

12) Newborns and Infants

See Section I.C.16. Newborn (Perinatal) Guidelines, for further instruction on the use of these codes.

Newborn Z codes/categories:

Z76.1   Encounter for health supervision and care of foundling

Z00.1- Encounter for routine child health examination

Z38   Liveborn infants according to place of birth and type of delivery

13) Routine and Administrative Examinations

The Z codes allow for the description of encounters for routine examinations, such as, a general check-up, or, examinations for administrative purposes, such as, a pre-employment physical. The codes are not to be used if the examination is for diagnosis of a suspected condition or for treatment purposes. In such cases the diagnosis code is used. During a routine exam, should a diagnosis or condition be discovered, it should be coded as an additional code. Pre-existing and chronic conditions and history codes may also be included as additional codes as long as the examination is for administrative purposes and not focused on any particular condition.

Some of the codes for routine health examinations distinguish between "with" and "without" abnormal findings. Code assignment depends on the information that is known at the time the encounter is being coded. For example, if no abnormal findings were found during the examination, but the encounter is being coded before test results are back, it is acceptable to assign the code for "without abnormal findings." When assigning a code for "with abnormal findings," additional code(s) should be assigned to identify the specific abnormal finding(s).

Pre-operative examination and pre-procedural laboratory examination Z codes are for use only in those situations when a patient is being cleared for a procedure or surgery and no treatment is given.

The Z codes/categories for routine and administrative examinations:

Z00   Encounter for general examination without complaint, suspected or reported diagnosis

Z01   Encounter for other special examination without complaint, suspected or reported diagnosis

Z02   Encounter for administrative examination
Except: Z02.9, Encounter for administrative examinations, unspecified

Z32.0- Encounter for pregnancy test

14) Miscellaneous Z Codes

The miscellaneous Z codes capture a number of other health care encounters that do not fall into one of the other categories. Some of these codes identify the reason for the encounter; others are for use as additional codes that provide useful information on circumstances that may affect a patient's care and treatment.

Prophylactic Organ Removal

For encounters specifically for prophylactic removal of an organ (such as prophylactic removal of breasts due to a genetic susceptibility to cancer or a family history of cancer), the principal or first-listed code should be a code from category Z40, Encounter for prophylactic surgery, followed by the appropriate codes to identify the associated risk factor (such as genetic susceptibility or family history).

If the patient has a malignancy of one site and is having prophylactic removal at another site to prevent either a new primary malignancy or metastatic disease, a code for the malignancy should also be assigned in addition to a code from subcategory Z40.0, Encounter for prophylactic surgery for risk factors related to malignant neoplasms. A Z40.0 code should not be assigned if the patient is having organ removal for treatment of a malignancy, such as the removal of the testes for the treatment of prostate cancer.

Miscellaneous Z codes/categories:

Z28	Immunization not carried out Except: Z28.3-, Underimmunization status
Z29	Encounter for other prophylactic measures
Z40	Encounter for prophylactic surgery
Z41	Encounter for procedures for purposes other than remedying health state Except: Z41.9, Encounter for procedure for purposes other than remedying health state, unspecified
Z53	Persons encountering health services for specific procedures and treatment, not carried out
Z72	Problems related to lifestyle Note: These codes should be assigned only when the documentation specifies that the patient has an associated problem
Z73	Problems related to life management difficulty **Note: These codes should be assigned only when the documentation specifies that the patient has an associated problem.**
Z74	Problems related to care provider dependency Except: Z74.01, Bed confinement status
Z75	Problems related to medical facilities and other health care
Z76.0	Encounter for issue of repeat prescription
Z76.3	Healthy person accompanying sick person
Z76.4	Other boarder to healthcare facility
Z76.5	Malingerer [conscious simulation]
Z91.1-	Patient's noncompliance with medical treatment and regimen
Z91.83	Wandering in diseases classified elsewhere
Z91.84-	Oral health risk factors
Z91.89	Other specified personal risk factors, not elsewhere classified

See Section I.B.14. for Z55-Z65 Persons with potential health hazards related to socioeconomic and psychosocial circumstances, documentation by clinicians other than the patient's provider

15) Nonspecific Z Codes

Certain Z codes are so non-specific, or potentially redundant with other codes in the classification, that there can be little justification for their use in the inpatient setting. Their use in the outpatient setting should be limited to those instances when there is no further documentation to permit more precise coding. Otherwise, any sign or symptom or any other reason for visit that is captured in another code should be used.

Nonspecific Z codes/categories:

Z02.9	Encounter for administrative examinations, unspecified
Z04.9	Encounter for examination and observation for unspecified reason
Z13.9	Encounter for screening, unspecified
Z41.9	Encounter for procedure for purposes other than remedying health state, unspecified
Z52.9	Donor of unspecified organ or tissue
Z86.59	Personal history of other mental and behavioral disorders
Z88.9	Allergy status to unspecified drugs, medicaments and biological substances status
Z92.0	Personal history of contraception

16) Z Codes That May Only be Principal/First-Listed Diagnosis

The following Z codes/categories may only be reported as the principal/first-listed diagnosis, except when there are multiple encounters on the same day and the medical records for the encounters are combined:

Z00	Encounter for general examination without complaint, suspected or reported diagnosis Except: Z00.6
Z01	Encounter for other special examination without complaint, suspected or reported diagnosis
Z02	Encounter for administrative examination
Z04	Encounter for examination and observation for other reasons
Z33.2	Encounter for elective termination of pregnancy
Z31.81	Encounter for male factor infertility in female patient
Z31.83	Encounter for assisted reproductive fertility procedure cycle
Z31.84	Encounter for fertility preservation procedure
Z34	Encounter for supervision of normal pregnancy
Z39	Encounter for maternal postpartum care and examination
Z38	Liveborn infants according to place of birth and type of delivery
Z40	Encounter for prophylactic surgery
Z42	Encounter for plastic and reconstructive surgery following medical procedure or healed injury
Z51.0	Encounter for antineoplastic radiation therapy
Z51.1-	Encounter for antineoplastic chemotherapy and immunotherapy
Z52	Donors of organs and tissues Except: Z52.9, Donor of unspecified organ or tissue
Z76.1	Encounter for health supervision and care of foundling
Z76.2	Encounter for health supervision and care of other healthy infant and child
Z99.12	Encounter for respirator [ventilator] dependence during power failure

17) Social Determinants of Health

Codes describing **problems or risk factors related to** social determinants of health (SDOH) should be assigned when this information is documented. **Assign as many SDOH codes as are necessary to describe all of the problems or risk factors. These codes should be assigned only when the documentation specifies that the patient has an associated problem or risk factor. For example, not every individual living alone would be assigned code Z60.2, Problems related to living alone.**

For social determinants of health, such as information found in categories Z55-Z65, Persons with potential health hazards related to socioeconomic and psychosocial circumstances, code assignment may be based on medical record documentation from clinicians involved in the care of the patient who are not the patient's provider since this information represents social information, rather than medical diagnoses.

For example, coding professionals may utilize documentation of social information from social workers, community health workers, case managers, or nurses, if their documentation is included in the official medical record.

Patient self-reported documentation may be used to assign codes for social determinants of health, as long as the patient self-reported information is signed-off by and incorporated into the medical record by either a clinician or provider.

Social determinants of health codes are located primarily in these Z code categories:

Z55	Problems related to education and literacy
Z56	Problems related to employment and unemployment
Z57	Occupational exposure to risk factors
Z58	Problems related to physical environment
Z59	Problems related to housing and economic circumstances
Z60	Problems related to social environment
Z62	Problems related to upbringing
Z63	Other problems related to primary support group, including family circumstances
Z64	Problems related to certain psychosocial circumstances
Z65	Problems related to other psychosocial circumstances

See Section I.B.14. Documentation by Clinicians Other than the Patient's Provider.

22. **Chapter 22: Codes for Special Purposes (U00-U85)**
  U07.0 Vaping-related disorder (see Section I.C.10.e., Vaping-related disorders)
  U07.1 COVID-19 (see Section I.C.1.g.1., COVID-19 infection)
  U09.9 Post COVID-19 condition, unspecified (see Section I.C.1.g.1.m.)

Section II. Selection of Principal Diagnosis

The circumstances of inpatient admission always govern the selection of principal diagnosis. The principal diagnosis is defined in the Uniform Hospital Discharge Data Set (UHDDS) as "that condition established after study to be chiefly responsible for occasioning the admission of the patient to the hospital for care."

The UHDDS definitions are used by hospitals to report inpatient data elements in a standardized manner. These data elements and their definitions can be found in the July 31, 1985, Federal Register (Vol. 50, No, 147), pp. 31038-40.

Since that time, the application of the UHDDS definitions has been expanded to include all non-outpatient settings (acute care, short term, long term care and psychiatric hospitals; home health agencies; rehab facilities; nursing homes, etc.). The UHDDS definitions also apply to hospice services (all levels of care).

In determining principal diagnosis, coding conventions in the ICD-10-CM, the Tabular List and Alphabetic Index take precedence over these official coding guidelines.

(See Section I.A., Conventions for the ICD-10-CM)

The importance of consistent, complete documentation in the medical record cannot be overemphasized. Without such documentation the application of all coding guidelines is a difficult, if not impossible, task.

A. **Codes for symptoms, signs, and ill-defined conditions**
   Codes for symptoms, signs, and ill-defined conditions from Chapter 18 are not to be used as principal diagnosis when a related definitive diagnosis has been established.

B. **Two or more interrelated conditions, each potentially meeting the definition for principal diagnosis.**
   When there are two or more interrelated conditions (such as diseases in the same ICD-10-CM chapter or manifestations characteristically associated with a certain disease) potentially meeting the definition of principal diagnosis, either condition may be sequenced first, unless the circumstances of the admission, the therapy provided, the Tabular List, or the Alphabetic Index indicate otherwise.

C. **Two or more diagnoses that equally meet the definition for principal diagnosis**
   In the unusual instance when two or more diagnoses equally meet the criteria for principal diagnosis as determined by the circumstances of admission, diagnostic workup and/or therapy provided, and the Alphabetic Index, Tabular List, or another coding guidelines does not provide sequencing direction, any one of the diagnoses may be sequenced first.

D. **Two or more comparative or contrasting conditions**
   In those rare instances when two or more contrasting or comparative diagnoses are documented as "either/or" (or similar terminology), they are coded as if the diagnoses were confirmed and the diagnoses are sequenced according to the circumstances of the admission. If no further determination can be made as to which diagnosis should be principal, either diagnosis may be sequenced first.

E. **A symptom(s) followed by contrasting/comparative diagnoses**
   GUIDELINE HAS BEEN DELETED EFFECTIVE OCTOBER 1, 2014

F. **Original treatment plan not carried out**
   Sequence as the principal diagnosis the condition, which after study occasioned the admission to the hospital, even though treatment may not have been carried out due to unforeseen circumstances.

G. **Complications of surgery and other medical care**
   When the admission is for treatment of a complication resulting from surgery or other medical care, the complication code is sequenced as the principal diagnosis. If the complication is classified to the T80-T88 series and the code lacks the necessary specificity in describing the complication, an additional code for the specific complication should be assigned.

H. **Uncertain Diagnosis**
   If the diagnosis documented at the time of discharge is qualified as "probable," "suspected," "likely," "questionable," "possible," or "still to be ruled out," "compatible with," "consistent with," or other similar terms indicating uncertainty, code the condition as if it existed or was established. The bases for these guidelines are the diagnostic workup, arrangements for further workup or observation, and initial therapeutic approach that correspond most closely with the established diagnosis.

Note: This guideline is applicable only to inpatient admissions to short-term, acute, long-term care and psychiatric hospitals.

I. **Admission from Observation Unit**
   1. **Admission Following Medical Observation**
      When a patient is admitted to an observation unit for a medical condition, which either worsens or does not improve, and is subsequently admitted as an inpatient of the same hospital for this same medical condition, the principal diagnosis would be the medical condition which led to the hospital admission.
   2. **Admission Following Post-Operative Observation**
      When a patient is admitted to an observation unit to monitor a condition (or complication) that develops following outpatient surgery, and then is subsequently admitted as an inpatient of the same hospital, hospitals should apply the Uniform Hospital Discharge Data Set (UHDDS) definition of principal diagnosis as "that condition established after study to be chiefly responsible for occasioning the admission of the patient to the hospital for care."

J. **Admission from Outpatient Surgery**
   When a patient receives surgery in the hospital's outpatient surgery department and is subsequently admitted for continuing inpatient care at the same hospital, the following guidelines should be followed in selecting the principal diagnosis for the inpatient admission:
   - If the reason for the inpatient admission is a complication, assign the complication as the principal diagnosis.
   - If no complication, or other condition, is documented as the reason for the inpatient admission, assign the reason for the outpatient surgery as the principal diagnosis.
   - If the reason for the inpatient admission is another condition unrelated to the surgery, assign the unrelated condition as the principal diagnosis.

K. **Admissions/Encounters for Rehabilitation**
   When the purpose for the admission/encounter is rehabilitation, sequence first the code for the condition for which the service is being performed. For example, for an admission/encounter for rehabilitation for right-sided dominant hemiplegia following a cerebrovascular infarction, report code I69.351, Hemiplegia and hemiparesis following cerebral infarction affecting right dominant side, as the first-listed or principal diagnosis.

   If the condition for which the rehabilitation service is being provided is no longer present, report the appropriate aftercare code as the first-listed or principal diagnosis, unless the rehabilitation service is being provided following an injury. For rehabilitation services following active treatment of an injury, assign the injury code with the appropriate seventh character for subsequent encounter as the first-listed or principal diagnosis. For example, if a patient with severe degenerative osteoarthritis of the hip, underwent hip replacement and the current encounter/admission is for rehabilitation, report code Z47.1, Aftercare following joint replacement surgery, as the first-listed or principal diagnosis. If the patient requires rehabilitation post hip replacement for right intertrochanteric femur fracture, report code S72.141D, Displaced intertrochanteric fracture of right femur, subsequent encounter for closed fracture with routine healing, as the first-listed or principal diagnosis.

   See Section I.C.21.c.7., Factors influencing health states and contact with health services, Aftercare.

   See Section I.C.19.a., for additional information about the use of 7th characters for injury codes.

Section III. Reporting Additional Diagnoses

GENERAL RULES FOR OTHER (ADDITIONAL) DIAGNOSES

For reporting purposes, the definition for "other diagnoses" is interpreted as additional conditions that affect patient care in terms of requiring:

  clinical evaluation; or

  therapeutic treatment; or

  diagnostic procedures; or

  extended length of hospital stay; or

  increased nursing care and/or monitoring.

The UHDDS item #11-b defines Other Diagnoses as "all conditions that coexist at the time of admission, that develop subsequently, or that affect the treatment received and/or the length of stay. Diagnoses that relate to an earlier episode which have no bearing on the current hospital stay are to be excluded." UHDDS definitions apply to inpatients in acute care, short-term, long term care and psychiatric hospital setting. The UHDDS definitions are used by acute care short-term hospitals to report inpatient data elements in a standardized manner. These data elements and their definitions can be found in the July 31, 1985, Federal Register (Vol. 50, No, 147), pp. 31038-40.

Since that time, the application of the UHDDS definitions has been expanded to include all non-outpatient settings (acute care, short term, long term care and psychiatric hospitals; home health agencies; rehab facilities; nursing homes, etc.). The UHDDS definitions also apply to hospice services (all levels of care).

The following guidelines are to be applied in designating "other diagnoses" when neither the Alphabetic Index nor the Tabular List in ICD-10-CM provide direction. The listing of the diagnoses in the patient record is the responsibility of the attending provider.

A. Previous conditions

If the provider has included a diagnosis in the final diagnostic statement, such as the discharge summary or the face sheet, it should ordinarily be coded. Some providers include in the diagnostic statement resolved conditions or diagnoses and status-post procedures from previous admissions that have no bearing on the current stay. Such conditions are not to be reported and are coded only if required by hospital policy.

However, history codes (categories Z80-Z87) may be used as secondary codes if the historical condition or family history has an impact on current care or influences treatment.

B. Abnormal findings

Abnormal findings (laboratory, x-ray, pathologic, and other diagnostic results) are not coded and reported unless the provider indicates their clinical significance. If the findings are outside the normal range and the attending provider has ordered other tests to evaluate the condition or prescribed treatment, it is appropriate to ask the provider whether the abnormal finding should be added.

Please note: This differs from the coding practices in the outpatient setting for coding encounters for diagnostic tests that have been interpreted by a provider.

C. Uncertain Diagnosis

If the diagnosis documented at the time of discharge is qualified as "probable," "suspected," "likely," "questionable," "possible," or "still to be ruled out," "compatible with," "consistent with," or other similar terms indicating uncertainty, code the condition as if it existed or was established. The bases for these guidelines are the diagnostic workup, arrangements for further workup or observation, and initial therapeutic approach that correspond most closely with the established diagnosis.

Note: This guideline is applicable only to inpatient admissions to short-term, acute, long-term care and psychiatric hospitals.

Section IV. Diagnostic Coding and Reporting Guidelines for Outpatient Services

These coding guidelines for outpatient diagnoses have been approved for use by hospitals/ providers in coding and reporting hospital-based outpatient services and provider-based office visits. Guidelines in Section I, Conventions, general coding guidelines and chapter-specific guidelines, should also be applied for outpatient services and office visits.

Information about the use of certain abbreviations, punctuation, symbols, and other conventions used in the ICD-10-CM Tabular List (code numbers and titles), can be found in Section IA of these guidelines, under "Conventions Used in the Tabular List." Section I.B. contains general guidelines that apply to the entire classification. Section I.C. contains chapter-specific guidelines that correspond to the chapters as they are arranged in the classification. Information about the correct sequence to use in finding a code is also described in Section I.

The terms encounter and visit are often used interchangeably in describing outpatient service contacts and, therefore, appear together in these guidelines without distinguishing one from the other.

Though the conventions and general guidelines apply to all settings, coding guidelines for outpatient and provider reporting of diagnoses will vary in a number of instances from those for inpatient diagnoses, recognizing that:

The Uniform Hospital Discharge Data Set (UHDDS) definition of principal diagnosis does not apply to hospital-based outpatient services and provider-based office visits.

Coding guidelines for inconclusive diagnoses (probable, suspected, rule out, etc.) were developed for inpatient reporting and do not apply to outpatients.

A. Selection of first-listed condition

In the outpatient setting, the term first-listed diagnosis is used in lieu of principal diagnosis.

In determining the first-listed diagnosis the coding conventions of ICD-10-CM, as well as the general and disease specific guidelines take precedence over the outpatient guidelines.

Diagnoses often are not established at the time of the initial encounter/visit. It may take two or more visits before the diagnosis is confirmed.

The most critical rule involves beginning the search for the correct code assignment through the Alphabetic Index. Never begin searching initially in the Tabular List as this will lead to coding errors.

1. **Outpatient Surgery**

   When a patient presents for outpatient surgery (same day surgery), code the reason for the surgery as the first-listed diagnosis (reason for the encounter), even if the surgery is not performed due to a contraindication.

2. **Observation Stay**

   When a patient is admitted for observation for a medical condition, assign a code for the medical condition as the first-listed diagnosis.

   When a patient presents for outpatient surgery and develops complications requiring admission to observation, code the reason for the surgery as the first reported diagnosis (reason for the encounter), followed by codes for the complications as secondary diagnoses.

B. Codes from A00.0 through T88.9, Z00-Z99, U00-U85

The appropriate code(s) from A00.0 through T88.9, Z00-Z99 and U00-U85 must be used to identify diagnoses, symptoms, conditions, problems, complaints, or other reason(s) for the encounter/visit.

C. Accurate reporting of ICD-10-CM diagnosis codes

For accurate reporting of ICD-10-CM diagnosis codes, the documentation should describe the patient's condition, using terminology which includes specific diagnoses as well as symptoms, problems, or reasons for the encounter. There are ICD-10-CM codes to describe all of these.

D. Codes that describe symptoms and signs

Codes that describe symptoms and signs, as opposed to diagnoses, are acceptable for reporting purposes when a diagnosis has not been established (confirmed) by the provider. Chapter 18 of ICD-10-CM, Symptoms, Signs, and Abnormal Clinical and Laboratory Findings Not Elsewhere Classified (codes R00-R99) contain many, but not all codes for symptoms.

E. Encounters for circumstances other than a disease or injury

ICD-10-CM provides codes to deal with encounters for circumstances other than a disease or injury. The Factors Influencing Health Status and Contact with Health Services codes (Z00-Z99) are provided to deal with occasions when circumstances other than a disease or injury are recorded as diagnosis or problems.

See Section I.C.21. Factors influencing health status and contact with health services.

F. Level of Detail in Coding

1. **ICD-10-CM codes with 3, 4, 5, 6 or 7 characters**

   ICD-10-CM is composed of codes with 3, 4, 5, 6 or 7 characters. Codes with three characters are included in ICD-10-CM as the heading of a category of codes that may be further subdivided by the use of fourth, fifth, sixth or seventh characters to provide greater specificity.

2. **Use of full number of characters required for a code**

   A three-character code is to be used only if it is not further subdivided. A code is invalid if it has not been coded to the full number of characters required for that code, including the 7th character, if applicable.

3. **Highest level of specificity**

   Code to the highest level of specificity when supported by the medical record documentation.

G. ICD-10-CM code for the diagnosis, condition, problem, or other reason for encounter/visit

List first the ICD-10-CM code for the diagnosis, condition, problem, or other reason for encounter/visit shown in the medical record to be chiefly responsible for the services provided. List additional codes that describe any coexisting conditions. In some cases, the first-listed diagnosis may be a symptom when a diagnosis has not been established (confirmed) by the provider.

H. Uncertain diagnosis

Do not code diagnoses documented as "probable", "suspected," "questionable," "rule out," "compatible with," "consistent with," or "working diagnosis" or other similar terms indicating uncertainty. Rather, code the condition(s) to the highest degree of certainty for that encounter/visit, such as symptoms, signs, abnormal test results, or other reason for the visit.

Please note: This differs from the coding practices used by short-term, acute care, long-term care and psychiatric hospitals.

I. Chronic diseases

Chronic diseases treated on an ongoing basis may be coded and reported as many times as the patient receives treatment and care for the condition(s)

J. Code all documented conditions that coexist

Code all documented conditions that coexist at the time of the encounter/visit and that require or affect patient care, treatment or management. Do not code conditions that were previously treated and no longer exist. However, history codes (categories Z80-Z87) may be used as secondary codes if the historical condition or family history has an impact on current care or influences treatment.

K. Patients receiving diagnostic services only

For patients receiving diagnostic services only during an encounter/visit, sequence first the diagnosis, condition, problem, or other reason for encounter/visit shown in the medical record to be chiefly responsible for the outpatient services provided during the encounter/visit. Codes for other diagnoses (e.g., chronic conditions) may be sequenced as additional diagnoses.

For encounters for routine laboratory/radiology testing in the absence of any signs, symptoms, or associated diagnosis, assign Z01.89, Encounter for other specified special examinations. If routine testing is performed during the same encounter as a test to evaluate a sign, symptom, or diagnosis, it is appropriate to assign both the Z code and the code describing the reason for the non-routine test.

For outpatient encounters for diagnostic tests that have been interpreted by a physician, and the final report is available at the time of coding, code any confirmed or definitive diagnosis(es) documented in the interpretation. Do not code related signs and symptoms as additional diagnoses.

Please note: This differs from the coding practice in the hospital inpatient setting regarding abnormal findings on test results.

L. Patients receiving therapeutic services only

For patients receiving therapeutic services only during an encounter/visit, sequence first the diagnosis, condition, problem, or other reason for encounter/visit shown in the medical record to be chiefly responsible for the outpatient services provided during the encounter/visit. Codes for other diagnoses (e.g., chronic conditions) may be sequenced as additional diagnoses.

The only exception to this rule is that when the primary reason for the admission/encounter is chemotherapy or radiation therapy, the appropriate Z code for the service is listed first, and the diagnosis or problem for which the service is being performed listed second.

M. Patients receiving preoperative evaluations only

For patients receiving preoperative evaluations only, sequence first a code from subcategory Z01.81, Encounter for pre-procedural examinations, to describe the pre-op consultations. Assign a code for the condition to describe the reason for the surgery as an additional diagnosis. Code also any findings related to the pre-op evaluation.

N. Ambulatory surgery

For ambulatory surgery, code the diagnosis for which the surgery was performed. If the postoperative diagnosis is known to be different from the preoperative diagnosis at the time the diagnosis is confirmed, select the postoperative diagnosis for coding, since it is the most definitive.

O. Routine outpatient prenatal visits

See Section I.C.15. Routine outpatient prenatal visits.

P. Encounters for general medical examinations with abnormal findings

The subcategories for encounters for general medical examinations, Z00.0- and encounter for routine child health examination, Z00.12-, provide codes for with and without abnormal findings. Should a general medical examination result in an abnormal finding, the code for general medical examination with abnormal finding should be assigned as the first-listed diagnosis. An examination with abnormal findings refers to a condition/diagnosis that is newly identified or a change in severity of a chronic condition (such as uncontrolled hypertension, or an acute exacerbation of chronic obstructive pulmonary disease) during a routine physical examination. A secondary code for the abnormal finding should also be coded.

Q. Encounters for routine health screenings

See Section I.C.21. Factors influencing health status and contact with health services, Screening

Appendix I. Present on Admission Reporting Guidelines

Introduction

These guidelines are to be used as a supplement to the *ICD-10-CM Official Guidelines for Coding and Reporting* to facilitate the assignment of the Present on Admission (POA) indicator for each diagnosis and external cause of injury code reported on claim forms (UB-04 and 837 Institutional).

These guidelines are not intended to replace any guidelines in the main body of the *ICD-10-CM Official Guidelines for Coding and Reporting*. The POA guidelines are not intended to provide guidance on when a condition should be coded, but rather, how to apply the POA indicator to the final set of diagnosis codes that have been assigned in accordance with Sections I, II, and III of the official coding guidelines. Subsequent to the assignment of the ICD-10-CM codes, the POA indicator should then be assigned to those conditions that have been coded.

As stated in the Introduction to the *ICD-10-CM Official Guidelines for Coding and Reporting*, a joint effort between the healthcare provider and the coder is essential to achieve complete and accurate documentation, code assignment, and reporting of diagnoses and procedures. The importance of consistent, complete documentation in the medical record cannot be overemphasized. Medical record documentation from any provider involved in the care and treatment of the patient may be used to support the determination of whether a condition was present on admission or not. In the context of the official coding guidelines, the term "provider" means a physician or any qualified healthcare practitioner who is legally accountable for establishing the patient's diagnosis.

These guidelines are not a substitute for the provider's clinical judgment as to the determination of whether a condition was/was not present on admission. The provider should be queried regarding issues related to the linking of signs/symptoms, timing of test results, and the timing of findings.

Please see the CDC website for the detailed list of ICD-10-CM codes that do not require the use of a POA indicator (https://www.cdc.gov/nchs/icd/icd10cm.htm). The codes and categories on this exempt list are for circumstances regarding the healthcare encounter or factors influencing health status that do not represent a current disease or injury or that describe conditions that are always present on admission.

General Reporting Requirements

All claims involving inpatient admissions to general acute care hospitals or other facilities that are subject to a law or regulation mandating collection of present on admission information.

Present on admission is defined as present at the time the order for inpatient admission occurs -- conditions that develop during an outpatient encounter, including emergency department, observation, or outpatient surgery, are considered as present on admission.

POA indicator is assigned to principal and secondary diagnoses (as defined in Section II of the Official Guidelines for Coding and Reporting) and the external cause of injury codes.

Issues related to inconsistent, missing, conflicting or unclear documentation must still be resolved by the provider.

If a condition would not be coded and reported based on UHDDS definitions and current official coding guidelines, then the POA indicator would not be reported.

> Reporting Options
>> Y – Yes
>> N – No
>> U – Unknown
>> W – Clinically undetermined
>> Unreported/Not used – (Exempt from POA reporting)
>
> Reporting Definitions
>> Y = present at the time of inpatient admission
>> N = not present at the time of inpatient admission
>> U = documentation is insufficient to determine if condition is present on admission
>> W = provider is unable to clinically determine whether condition was present on admission or not

Timeframe for POA Identification and Documentation

There is no required timeframe as to when a provider (per the definition of "provider" used in these guidelines) must identify or document a condition to be present on admission. In some clinical situations, it may not be possible for a provider to make a definitive diagnosis (or a condition may not be recognized or reported by the patient) for a period of time after admission. In some cases, it may be several days before the provider arrives at a definitive diagnosis. This does not mean that the condition was not present on admission. Determination of whether the condition was present on admission or not will be based on the applicable POA guideline as identified in this document, or on the provider's best clinical judgment.

If at the time of code assignment the documentation is unclear as to whether a condition was present on admission or not, it is appropriate to query the provider for clarification.

Assigning the POA Indicator

Condition is on the "Exempt from Reporting" list

Leave the "present on admission" field blank if the condition is on the list of ICD-10-CM codes for which this field is not applicable. This is the only circumstance in which the field may be left blank.

POA Explicitly Documented

Assign Y for any condition the provider explicitly documents as being present on admission.

Assign N for any condition the provider explicitly documents as not present at the time of admission.

Conditions diagnosed prior to inpatient admission

Assign "Y" for conditions that were diagnosed prior to admission (example: hypertension, diabetes mellitus, asthma)

Conditions diagnosed during the admission but clearly present before admission

Assign "Y" for conditions diagnosed during the admission that were clearly present but not diagnosed until after admission occurred.

Diagnoses subsequently confirmed after admission are considered present on admission if at the time of admission they are documented as suspected, possible, rule out, differential diagnosis, or constitute an underlying cause of a symptom that is present at the time of admission.

Condition develops during outpatient encounter prior to inpatient admission

Assign Y for any condition that develops during an outpatient encounter prior to a written order for inpatient admission.

Documentation does not indicate whether condition was present on admission

Assign "U" when the medical record documentation is unclear as to whether the condition was present on admission. "U" should not be routinely assigned and used only in very limited circumstances. Coders are encouraged to query the providers when the documentation is unclear.

Documentation states that it cannot be determined whether the condition was or was not present on admission

Assign "W" when the medical record documentation indicates that it cannot be clinically determined whether or not the condition was present on admission.

Chronic condition with acute exacerbation during the admission

If a single code identifies both the chronic condition and the acute exacerbation, see POA guidelines pertaining to codes that contain multiple clinical concepts.

If a single code only identifies the chronic condition and not the acute exacerbation (e.g., acute exacerbation of chronic leukemia), assign "Y."

Conditions documented as possible, probable, suspected, or rule out at the time of discharge

If the final diagnosis contains a possible, probable, suspected, or rule out diagnosis, and this diagnosis was based on signs, symptoms or clinical findings suspected at the time of inpatient admission, assign "Y."

If the final diagnosis contains a possible, probable, suspected, or rule out diagnosis, and this diagnosis was based on signs, symptoms or clinical findings that were not present on admission, assign "N".

Conditions documented as impending or threatened at the time of discharge

If the final diagnosis contains an impending or threatened diagnosis, and this diagnosis is based on symptoms or clinical findings that were present on admission, assign "Y".

If the final diagnosis contains an impending or threatened diagnosis, and this diagnosis is based on symptoms or clinical findings that were not present on admission, assign "N".

Acute and Chronic Conditions

Assign "Y" for acute conditions that are present at time of admission and N for acute conditions that are not present at time of admission.

Assign "Y" for chronic conditions, even though the condition may not be diagnosed until after admission.

If a single code identifies both an acute and chronic condition, see the POA guidelines for codes that contain multiple clinical concepts.

Codes That Contain Multiple Clinical Concepts

Assign "N" if at least one of the clinical concepts included in the code was not present on admission (e.g., COPD with acute exacerbation and the exacerbation was not present on admission; gastric ulcer that does not

start bleeding until after admission; asthma patient develops status asthmaticus after admission).

Assign "Y" if all of the clinical concepts included in the code were present on admission (e.g., duodenal ulcer that perforates prior to admission).

For infection codes that include the causal organism, assign "Y" if the infection (or signs of the infection) were present on admission, even though the culture results may not be known until after admission (e.g., patient is admitted with pneumonia and the provider documents Pseudomonas as the causal organism a few days later).

Same Diagnosis Code for Two or More Conditions

When the same ICD-10-CM diagnosis code applies to two or more conditions during the same encounter (e.g. two separate conditions classified to the same ICD-10-CM diagnosis code):

Assign "Y" if all conditions represented by the single ICD-10-CM code were present on admission (e.g. bilateral unspecified age-related cataracts).

Assign "N" if any of the conditions represented by the single ICD-10-CM code was not present on admission (e.g. traumatic secondary and recurrent hemorrhage and seroma is assigned to a single code T79.2, but only one of the conditions was present on admission).

Obstetrical conditions

Whether or not the patient delivers during the current hospitalization does not affect assignment of the POA indicator. The determining factor for POA assignment is whether the pregnancy complication or obstetrical condition described by the code was present at the time of admission or not.

If the pregnancy complication or obstetrical condition was present on admission (e.g., patient admitted in preterm labor), assign "Y".

If the pregnancy complication or obstetrical condition was not present on admission (e.g., 2nd degree laceration during delivery, postpartum hemorrhage that occurred during current hospitalization, fetal distress develops after admission), assign "N".

If the obstetrical code includes more than one diagnosis and any of the diagnoses identified by the code were not present on admission assign "N". (e.g., Category O11, Pre-existing hypertension with pre-eclampsia)

Perinatal conditions

Newborns are not considered to be admitted until after birth. Therefore, any condition present at birth or that developed in utero is considered present at admission and should be assigned "Y". This includes conditions that occur during delivery (e.g., injury during delivery, meconium aspiration, exposure to streptococcus B in the vaginal canal).

Congenital conditions and anomalies

Assign "Y" for congenital conditions and anomalies except for categories Q00-Q99, Congenital anomalies, which are on the exempt list. Congenital conditions are always considered present on admission.

External cause of injury codes

Assign "Y" for any external cause code representing an external cause of morbidity that occurred prior to inpatient admission (e.g., patient fell out of bed at home, patient fell out of bed in emergency room prior to admission)

Assign "N" for any external cause code representing an external cause of morbidity that occurred during inpatient hospitalization (e.g., patient fell out of hospital bed during hospital stay, patient experienced an adverse reaction to a medication administered after inpatient admission).

A

Aarskog's syndrome Q87.19
Abandonment — *see* Maltreatment
Abasia (-astasia) (hysterical) F44.4
Abderhalden-Kaufmann-Lignac syndrome (cystinosis) E72.04
Abdomen, abdominal — *see also* condition
  muscle deficiency syndrome Q79.4
  angina K55.1
  acute R10.0
Abdominalgia — *see* Pain, abdominal
Abduction contracture, hip or other joint — *see* Contraction, joint
Aberrant (congenital) — *see also* Malposition, congenital
  adrenal gland Q89.1
  artery (peripheral) Q27.8
    basilar NEC Q28.1
    cerebral Q28.3
    coronary Q24.5
    digestive system Q27.8
    eye Q15.8
    lower limb Q27.8
    precerebral Q28.1
    pulmonary Q25.79
    renal Q27.2
    retina Q14.1
    specified site NEC Q27.8
    subclavian Q27.8
    upper limb Q27.8
    vertebral Q28.1
  breast Q83.8
  endocrine gland NEC Q89.2
  hepatic duct Q44.5
  pancreas Q45.3
  parathyroid gland Q89.2
  pituitary gland Q89.2
  sebaceous glands, mucous membrane, mouth, congenital Q38.6
  spleen Q89.09
  subclavian artery Q27.8
  thymus (gland) Q89.2
  thyroid gland Q89.2
  vein (peripheral) NEC Q27.8
    cerebral Q28.3
    digestive system Q27.8
    lower limb Q27.8
    precerebral Q28.1
    specified site NEC Q27.8
    upper limb Q27.8
Aberration
  distantial — *see* Disturbance, visual
  mental F99
Abetalipoproteinemia E78.6
Abiotrophy R68.89
Ablatio, ablation
  retinae — *see* Detachment, retina
Ablepharia, ablepharon Q10.3
Abnormal, abnormality, abnormalities — *see also* Anomaly
  acid-base balance (mixed) E87.4
  albumin R77.0
  alphafetoprotein R77.2
  alveolar ridge K08.9
  anatomical relationship Q89.9
  apertures, congenital, diaphragm Q79.1
  atrial septal, specified NEC Q21.19
  auditory perception H93.29- ☑
    diplacusis — *see* Diplacusis
    hyperacusis — *see* Hyperacusis
    recruitment — *see* Recruitment, auditory
    threshold shift — *see* Shift, auditory threshold
  autosomes Q99.9
    fragile site Q95.5
  basal metabolic rate R94.8
  biosynthesis, testicular androgen E29.1
  bleeding time R79.1
  blood amino-acid level R79.83
  blood level (of)
    cobalt R79.0
    copper R79.0
    iron R79.0

Abnormal, abnormality, abnormalities — *continued*
  blood level — *continued*
    lithium R78.89
    magnesium R79.0
    mineral NEC R79.0
    zinc R79.0
  blood pressure
    elevated R03.0
    low reading (nonspecific) R03.1
  blood sugar R73.09
  blood-gas level R79.81
  bowel sounds R19.15
    absent R19.11
    hyperactive R19.12
  brain scan R94.02
  breathing R06.9
  caloric test R94.138
  cerebrospinal fluid R83.9
    cytology R83.6
    drug level R83.2
    enzyme level R83.0
    hormones R83.1
    immunology R83.4
    microbiology R83.5
    nonmedicinal level R83.3
    specified type NEC R83.8
  chemistry, blood R79.9
    C-reactive protein R79.82
    drugs — *see* Findings, abnormal, in blood
    gas level R79.81
    minerals R79.0
    pancytopenia D61.818
    PTT R79.1
    specified NEC R79.89
    toxins — *see* Findings, abnormal, in blood
  chest sounds (friction) (rales) R09.89
  chromosome, chromosomal Q99.9
    with more than three X chromosomes, female Q97.1
    analysis result R89.8
      bronchial washings R84.8
      cerebrospinal fluid R83.8
      cervix uteri NEC R87.89
      nasal secretions R84.8
      nipple discharge R89.8
      peritoneal fluid R85.89
      pleural fluid R84.8
      prostatic secretions R86.8
      saliva R85.89
      seminal fluid R86.8
      sputum R84.8
      synovial fluid R89.8
      throat scrapings R84.8
      vagina R87.89
      vulva R87.89
      wound secretions R89.8
    dicentric replacement Q93.2
    ring replacement Q93.2
    sex Q99.8
      female phenotype Q97.9
        specified NEC Q97.8
      male phenotype Q98.9
        specified NEC Q98.8
      structural male Q98.6
    specified NEC Q99.8
  clinical findings NEC R68.89
  coagulation D68.9
    newborn, transient P61.6
    profile R79.1
    time R79.1
  communication — *see* Fistula
  conjunctiva, vascular H11.41- ☑
  coronary artery Q24.5
  cortisol-binding globulin E27.8
  course, eustachian tube Q17.8
  creatinine clearance R94.4
  cytology
    anus R85.619
      atypical squamous cells cannot exclude high grade squamous intraepithelial lesion (ASC-H) R85.611
      atypical squamous cells of undetermined significance (ASC-US) R85.610

Abnormal, abnormality, abnormalities — *continued*
  cytology — *continued*
    anus — *continued*
      cytologic evidence of malignancy R85.614
      high grade squamous intraepithelial lesion (HGSIL) R85.613
      human papillomavirus (HPV) DNA test
        high risk positive R85.81
        low risk postive R85.82
      inadequate smear R85.615
      low grade squamous intraepithelial lesion (LGSIL) R85.612
      satisfactory anal smear but lacking transformation zone R85.616
      specified NEC R85.618
      unsatisfactory smear R85.615
    female genital organs — *see* Abnormal, Papanicolaou (smear)
  dark adaptation curve H53.61
  dentofacial NEC — *see* Anomaly, dentofacial
  development, developmental Q89.9
    central nervous system Q07.9
  diagnostic imaging
    abdomen, abdominal region NEC R93.5
    biliary tract R93.2
    bladder R93.41
    breast R92.8
    central nervous system NEC R90.89
    cerebrovascular NEC R90.89
    coronary circulation R93.1
    digestive tract NEC R93.3
    gastrointestinal (tract) R93.3
    genitourinary organs R93.89
    head R93.0
    heart R93.1
    intrathoracic organ NEC R93.89
    kidney R93.42- ☑
    limbs R93.6
    liver R93.2
    lung (field) R91.8
    musculoskeletal system NEC R93.7
    renal pelvis R93.41
    retroperitoneum R93.5
    site specified NEC R93.89
    skin and subcutaneous tissue R93.89
    skull R93.0
    testis R93.81- ☑
    ureter R93.41
    urinary organs specified NEC R93.49
  direction, teeth, fully erupted M26.30
  ear ossicles, acquired NEC H74.39- ☑
    ankylosis — *see* Ankylosis, ear ossicles
    discontinuity — *see* Discontinuity, ossicles, ear
    partial loss — *see* Loss, ossicles, ear (partial)
  Ebstein Q22.5
  echocardiogram R93.1
  echoencephalogram R90.81
  echogram — *see* Abnormal, diagnostic imaging
  electrocardiogram [ECG] [EKG] R94.31
  electroencephalogram [EEG] R94.01
  electrolyte — *see* Imbalance, electrolyte
  electromyogram [EMG] R94.131
  electro-oculogram [EOG] R94.110
  electrophysiological intracardiac studies R94.39
  electroretinogram [ERG] R94.111
  erythrocytes
    congenital, with perinatal jaundice D58.9
  feces (color) (contents) (mucus) R19.5
  finding — *see* Findings, abnormal, without diagnosis
  fluid
    amniotic — *see* Abnormal, specimen, specified
    cerebrospinal — *see* Abnormal, cerebrospinal fluid
    peritoneal — *see* Abnormal, specimen, digestive organs
    pleural — *see* Abnormal, specimen, respiratory organs
    synovial — *see* Abnormal, specimen, specified
    thorax (bronchial washings) (pleural fluid) — *see* Abnormal, specimen, respiratory organs
    vaginal — *see* Abnormal, specimen, female genital organs

Abnormal, abnormality, abnormalities — *continued*
form
  teeth K00.2
  uterus — *see* Anomaly, uterus
function studies
  auditory R94.120
  bladder R94.8
  brain R94.09
  cardiovascular R94.30
  ear R94.128
  endocrine NEC R94.7
  eye NEC R94.118
  kidney R94.4
  liver R94.5
  nervous system
    central NEC R94.09
    peripheral NEC R94.138
  pancreas R94.8
  placenta R94.8
  pulmonary R94.2
  special senses NEC R94.128
  spleen R94.8
  thyroid R94.6
  vestibular R94.121
gait — *see* Gait
  hysterical F44.4
gastrin secretion E16.4
globulin R77.1
  cortisol-binding E27.8
  thyroid-binding E07.89
glomerular, minor — *see also* N00-N07 with fourth
  character .0 N05.0
glucagon secretion E16.3
glucose tolerance (test) (non-fasting) R73.09
gravitational (G) forces or states (effect of) T75.81 ☑
hair (color) (shaft) L67.9
  specified NEC L67.8
hard tissue formation in pulp (dental) K04.3
head movement R25.0
heart
  rate R00.9
    specified NEC R00.8
  shadow R93.1
  sounds NEC R01.2
hemoglobin (disease) — *see also* Disease, hemoglobin
  D58.2
  trait — *see* Trait, hemoglobin, abnormal
histology NEC R89.7
immunological findings R89.4
  in serum R76.9
    specified NEC R76.8
increase in appetite R63.2
involuntary movement — *see* Abnormal, movement,
  involuntary
jaw closure M26.51
karyotype R89.8
kidney function test R94.4
knee jerk R29.2
leukocyte (cell) (differential) NEC D72.9
liver function test — *see also* Elevated, liver function,
  test R79.89
loss of
  height R29.890
  weight R63.4
mammogram NEC R92.8
  calcification (calculus) R92.1
  microcalcification R92.0
Mantoux test R76.11
movement (disorder) — *see also* Disorder, movement
  head R25.0
  involuntary R25.9
    fasciculation R25.3
    of head R25.0
    spasm R25.2
    specified type NEC R25.8
    tremor R25.1
myoglobin (Aberdeen) (Annapolis) R89.7
neonatal screening P09.9
  for
    congenital adrenal hyperplasia P09.2
    congenital endocrine disease P09.2
    congenital hematologic disorders P09.3
    critical congenital heart disease P09.5
    cystic fibrosis P09.4
    hemoglobinothies P09.3
    hypothyroidism P09.2
    inborn errors of metabolism P09.1

Abnormal, abnormality, abnormalities — *continued*
neonatal screening — *continued*
  for — *continued*
    neonatal hearing loss P09.6
    red cell membrane defects P09.3
    sickle cell P09.3
    specified NEC P09.8
oculomotor study R94.113
palmar creases Q82.8
Papanicolaou (smear)
  anus R85.619
    atypical squamous cells cannot exclude high
      grade squamous intraepithelial lesion
      (ASC-H) R85.611
    atypical squamous cells of undetermined signif-
      icance (ASC-US) R85.610
    cytologic evidence of malignancy R85.614
    high grade squamous intraepithelial lesion
      (HGSIL) R85.613
    human papillomavirus (HPV) DNA test
      high risk positive R85.81
      low risk postive R85.82
    inadequate smear R85.615
    low grade squamous intraepithelial lesion (LGSIL)
      R85.612
    satisfactory anal smear but lacking transforma-
      tion zone R85.616
    specified NEC R85.618
    unsatisfactory smear R85.615
  bronchial washings R84.6
  cerebrospinal fluid R83.6
  cervix R87.629
    atypical squamous cells cannot exclude high
      grade squamous intraepithelial lesion
      (ASC-H) R87.611
    atypical squamous cells of undetermined signif-
      icance (ASC-US) R87.610
    cytologic evidence of malignancy R87.614
    high grade squamous intraepithelial lesion
      (HGSIL) R87.613
    inadequate smear R87.615
    low grade squamous intraepithelial lesion (LGSIL)
      R87.612
    non-atypical endometrial cells R87.618
    satisfactory cervical smear but lacking transfor-
      mation zone R87.616
    specified NEC R87.618
    thin preparaton R87.619
    unsatisfactory smear R87.615
  nasal secretions R84.6
  nipple discharge R89.6
  peritoneal fluid R85.69
  pleural fluid R84.6
  prostatic secretions R86.6
  saliva R85.69
  seminal fluid R86.6
  sites NEC R89.6
  sputum R84.6
  synovial fluid R89.6
  throat scrapings R84.6
  vagina R87.629
    atypical squamous cells cannot exclude high
      grade squamous intraepithelial lesion
      (ASC-H) R87.621
    atypical squamous cells of undetermined signif-
      icance (ASC-US) R87.620
    cytologic evidence of malignancy R87.624
    high grade squamous intraepithelial lesion
      (HGSIL) R87.623
    inadequate smear R87.625
    low grade squamous intraepithelial lesion (LGSIL)
      R87.622
    specified NEC R87.628
    thin preparation R87.629
    unsatisfactory smear R87.625
  vulva R87.69
  wound secretions R89.6
partial thromboplastin time (PTT) R79.1
pelvis (bony) — *see* Deformity, pelvis
percussion, chest (tympany) R09.89
periods (grossly) — *see* Menstruation
phonocardiogram R94.39
plantar reflex R29.2
plasma
  protein R77.9
    specified NEC R77.8
  viscosity R70.1
pleural (folds) Q34.0

Abnormal, abnormality, abnormalities — *continued*
posture R29.3
product of conception O02.9
  specified type NEC O02.89
prothrombin time (PT) R79.1
pulmonary
  artery, congenital Q25.79
  function, newborn P28.89
  test results R94.2
pulsations in neck R00.2
pupillary H21.56- ☑
  function (reaction) (reflex) — *see* Anomaly, pupil,
    function
radiological examination — *see* Abnormal, diagnostic
  imaging
red blood cell(s) (morphology) (volume) R71.8
reflex — *see* Reflex
renal function test R94.4
response to nerve stimulation R94.130
retinal correspondence H53.31
retinal function study R94.111
rhythm, heart — *see also* Arrhythmia
saliva — *see* Abnormal, specimen, digestive organs
scan
  kidney R94.4
  liver R93.2
  thyroid R94.6
secretion
  gastrin E16.4
  glucagon E16.3
semen, seminal fluid — *see* Abnormal, specimen, male
  genital organs
serum level (of)
  acid phosphatase R74.8
  alkaline phosphatase R74.8
  amylase R74.8
  enzymes R74.9
    specified NEC R74.8
  lipase R74.8
  triacylglycerol lipase R74.8
shape
  gravid uterus — *see* Anomaly, uterus
sinus venosus Q21.16
size, tooth, teeth K00.2
spacing, tooth, teeth, fully erupted M26.30
specimen
  digestive organs (peritoneal fluid) (saliva) R85.9
    cytology R85.69
    drug level R85.2
    enzyme level R85.0
    histology R85.7
    hormones R85.1
    immunology R85.4
    microbiology R85.5
    nonmedicinal level R85.3
    specified type NEC R85.89
  female genital organs (secretions) (smears) R87.9
    cytology R87.69
      cervix R87.619
        human papillomavirus (HPV) DNA test
          high risk positive R87.810
          low risk positive R87.820
        inadequate (unsatisfactory) smear
          R87.615
        non-atypical endometrial cells R87.618
        specified NEC R87.618
      vagina R87.629
        human papillomavirus (HPV) DNA test
          high risk positive R87.811
          low risk positive R87.821
        inadequate (unsatisfactory) smear
          R87.625
      vulva R87.69
    drug level R87.2
    enzyme level R87.0
    histological R87.7
    hormones R87.1
    immunology R87.4
    microbiology R87.5
    nonmedicinal level R87.3
    specified type NEC R87.89
  male genital organs (prostatic secretions) (semen)
    R86.9
    cytology R86.6
    drug level R86.2
    enzyme level R86.0
    histological R86.7

Abnormal, abnormality, abnormalities — *continued*
  specimen — *continued*
    male genital organs — *continued*
      hormones R86.1
      immunology R86.4
      microbiology R86.5
      nonmedicinal level R86.3
      specified type NEC R86.8
    nipple discharge — *see* Abnormal, specimen, specified
    respiratory organs (bronchial washings) (nasal secretions) (pleural fluid) (sputum) R84.9
      cytology R84.6
      drug level R84.2
      enzyme level R84.0
      histology R84.7
      hormones R84.1
      immunology R84.4
      microbiology R84.5
      nonmedicinal level R84.3
      specified type NEC R84.8
    specified organ, system and tissue NOS R89.9
      cytology R89.6
      drug level R89.2
      enzyme level R89.0
      histology R89.7
      hormones R89.1
      immunology R89.4
      microbiology R89.5
      nonmedicinal level R89.3
      specified type NEC R89.8
    synovial fluid — *see* Abnormal, specimen, specified
    thorax (bronchial washings) (pleural fluids) — *see* Abnormal, specimen, respiratory organs
    vagina (secretion) (smear) R87.629
    vulva (secretion) (smear) R87.69
    wound secretion — *see* Abnormal, specimen, specified
   spermatozoa — *see* Abnormal, specimen, male genital organs
  sputum (amount) (color) (odor) R09.3
  stool (color) (contents) (mucus) R19.5
   bloody K92.1
   guaiac positive R19.5
  synchondrosis Q78.8
  thermography — *see also* Abnormal, diagnostic imaging R93.89
  thyroid-binding globulin E07.89
  tooth, teeth (form) (size) K00.2
  toxicology (findings) R78.9
  transport protein E88.09
  tumor marker NEC R97.8
  ultrasound results — *see* Abnormal, diagnostic imaging
  umbilical cord complicating delivery O69.9 ☑
  urination NEC R39.198
  urine (constituents) R82.90
   bile R82.2
   cytological examination R82.89
   drugs R82.5
   fat R82.0
   glucose R81
   heavy metals R82.6
   hemoglobin R82.3
   histological examination R82.89
   ketones R82.4
   microbiological examination (culture) R82.79
   myoglobin R82.1
   positive culture R82.79
   protein — *see* Proteinuria
   specified substance NEC R82.998
    chromoabnormality NEC R82.91
   substances nonmedical R82.6
  uterine hemorrhage — *see* Hemorrhage, uterus
  vectorcardiogram R94.39
  visually evoked potential (VEP) R94.112
  white blood cells D72.9
   specified NEC D72.89
  X-ray examination — *see* Abnormal, diagnostic imaging
Abnormity (any organ or part) — *see* Anomaly
Abocclusion M26.29
  hemolytic disease (newborn) P55.1
  incompatibility reaction ABO — *see* Complication(s), transfusion, incompatibility reaction, ABO
Abolition, language R48.8
Aborter, habitual or recurrent — *see* Loss (of), pregnancy, recurrent
Abortion (complete) (spontaneous) O03.9

Abortion — *continued*
  with
   retained products of conception — *see* Abortion, incomplete
  attempted (elective) (failed) O07.4
   complicated by O07.30
    afibrinogenemia O07.1
    cardiac arrest O07.36
    chemical damage of pelvic organ(s) O07.34
    circulatory collapse O07.31
    cystitis O07.38
    defibrination syndrome O07.1
    electrolyte imbalance O07.33
    embolism (air) (amniotic fluid) (blood clot) (fat) (pulmonary) (septic) (soap) O07.2
    endometritis O07.0
    genital tract and pelvic infection O07.0
    hemolysis O07.1
    hemorrhage (delayed) (excessive) O07.1
    infection
     genital tract or pelvic O07.0
     urinary tract tract O07.38
    intravascular coagulation O07.1
    laceration of pelvic organ(s) O07.34
    metabolic disorder O07.33
    oliguria O07.32
    oophoritis O07.0
    parametritis O07.0
    pelvic peritonitis O07.0
    perforation of pelvic organ(s) O07.34
    renal failure or shutdown O07.32
    salpingitis or salpingo-oophoritis O07.0
    sepsis O07.37
    shock O07.31
    specified condition NEC O07.39
    tubular necrosis (renal) O07.32
    uremia O07.32
    urinary tract infection O07.38
    venous complication NEC O07.35
     embolism (air) (amniotic fluid) (blood clot) (fat) (pulmonary) (septic) (soap) O07.2
  complicated (by) (following) O03.80
   afibrinogenemia O03.6
   cardiac arrest O03.86
   chemical damage of pelvic organ(s) O03.84
   circulatory collapse O03.81
   cystitis O03.88
   defibrination syndrome O03.6
   electrolyte imbalance O03.83
   embolism (air) (amniotic fluid) (blood clot) (fat) (pulmonary) (septic) (soap) O03.7
   endometritis O03.5
   genital tract and pelvic infection O03.5
   hemolysis O03.6
   hemorrhage (delayed) (excessive) O03.6
   infection
    genital tract or pelvic O03.5
    urinary tract O03.88
   intravascular coagulation O03.6
   laceration of pelvic organ(s) O03.84
   metabolic disorder O03.83
   oliguria O03.82
   oophoritis O03.5
   parametritis O03.5
   pelvic peritonitis O03.5
   perforation of pelvic organ(s) O03.84
   renal failure or shutdown O03.82
   salpingitis or salpingo-oophoritis O03.5
   sepsis O03.87
   shock O03.81
   specified condition NEC O03.89
   tubular necrosis (renal) O03.82
   uremia O03.82
   urinary tract infection O03.88
   venous complication NEC O03.85
    embolism (air) (amniotic fluid) (blood clot) (fat) (pulmonary) (septic) (soap) O03.7
  failed — *see* Abortion, attempted
  habitual or recurrent N96
   with current abortion — *see* categories O03-O04
   without current pregnancy N96
   care in current pregnancy O26.2- ☑
  incomplete (spontaneous) O03.4
   complicated (by) (following) O03.30
    afibrinogenemia O03.1
    cardiac arrest O03.36
    chemical damage of pelvic organ(s) O03.34
    circulatory collapse O03.31
    cystitis O03.38

Abortion — *continued*
  incomplete — *continued*
   complicated — *continued*
    defibrination syndrome O03.1
    electrolyte imbalance O03.33
    embolism (air) (amniotic fluid) (blood clot) (fat) (pulmonary) (septic) (soap) O03.2
    endometritis O03.0
    genital tract and pelvic infection O03.0
    hemolysis O03.1
    hemorrhage (delayed) (excessive) O03.1
    infection
     genital tract or pelvic O03.0
     urinary tract O03.38
    intravascular coagulation O03.1
    laceration of pelvic organ(s) O03.34
    metabolic disorder O03.33
    oliguria O03.32
    oophoritis O03.0
    parametritis O03.0
    pelvic peritonitis O03.0
    perforation of pelvic organ(s) O03.34
    renal failure or shutdown O03.32
    salpingitis or salpingo-oophoritis O03.0
    sepsis O03.37
    shock O03.31
    specified condition NEC O03.39
    tubular necrosis (renal) O03.32
    uremia O03.32
    urinary infection O03.38
    venous complication NEC O03.35
     embolism (air) (amniotic fluid) (blood clot) (fat) (pulmonary) (septic) (soap) O03.2
  induced (encounter for) Z33.2
   complicated by O04.80
    afibrinogenemia O04.6
    cardiac arrest O04.86
    chemical damage of pelvic organ(s) O04.84
    circulatory collapse O04.81
    cystitis O04.88
    defibrination syndrome O04.6
    electrolyte imbalance O04.83
    embolism (air) (amniotic fluid) (blood clot) (fat) (pulmonary) (septic) (soap) O04.7
    endometritis O04.5
    genital tract and pelvic infection O04.5
    hemolysis O04.6
    hemorrhage (delayed) (excessive) O04.6
    infection
     genital tract or pelvic O04.5
     urinary tract O04.88
    intravascular coagulation O04.6
    laceration of pelvic organ(s) O04.84
    metabolic disorder O04.83
    oliguria O04.82
    oophoritis O04.5
    parametritis O04.5
    pelvic peritonitis O04.5
    perforation of pelvic organ(s) O04.84
    renal failure or shutdown O04.82
    salpingitis or salpingo-oophoritis O04.5
    sepsis O04.87
    shock O04.81
    specified condition NEC O04.89
    tubular necrosis (renal) O04.82
    uremia O04.82
    urinary tract infection O04.88
    venous complication NEC O04.85
     embolism (air) (amniotic fluid) (blood clot) (fat) (pulmonary) (septic) (soap) O04.7
  inevitable O03.4
  missed O02.1
  spontaneous — *see* Abortion (complete) (spontaneous)
   threatened O20.0
  threatened (spontaneous) O20.0
  tubal O00.10-
   with intrauterine pregnancy O00.11- ☑
Abortus fever A23.1
Aboulomania F60.7
Abrami's disease D59.8
Abramov-Fiedler myocarditis (acute isolated myocarditis) I40.1
Abrasion T14.8 ☑
  abdomen, abdominal (wall) S30.811 ☑
  alveolar process S00.512 ☑
  ankle S90.51- ☑
  antecubital space — *see* Abrasion, elbow
  anus S30.817 ☑

Abrasion — continued
 arm (upper) S40.81- ☑
 auditory canal — see Abrasion, ear
 auricle — see Abrasion, ear
 axilla — see Abrasion, arm
 back, lower S30.810 ☑
 breast S20.11- ☑
 brow S00.81 ☑
 buttock S30.810 ☑
 calf — see Abrasion, leg
 canthus — see Abrasion, eyelid
 cheek S00.81 ☑
  internal S00.512 ☑
 chest wall — see Abrasion, thorax
 chin S00.81 ☑
 clitoris S30.814 ☑
 cornea S05.0- ☑
 costal region — see Abrasion, thorax
 dental K03.1
 digit(s)
  foot — see Abrasion, toe
  hand — see Abrasion, finger
 ear S00.41- ☑
 elbow S50.31- ☑
 epididymis S30.813 ☑
 epigastric region S30.811 ☑
 epiglottis S10.11 ☑
 esophagus (thoracic) S27.818 ☑
  cervical S10.11 ☑
 eyebrow — see Abrasion, eyelid
 eyelid S00.21- ☑
 face S00.81 ☑
 finger(s) S60.41- ☑
  index S60.41- ☑
  little S60.41- ☑
  middle S60.41- ☑
  ring S60.41- ☑
 flank S30.811 ☑
 foot (except toe(s) alone) S90.81- ☑
  toe — see Abrasion, toe
 forearm S50.81- ☑
  elbow only — see Abrasion, elbow
 forehead S00.81 ☑
 genital organs, external
  female S30.816 ☑
  male S30.815 ☑
 groin S30.811 ☑
 gum S00.512 ☑
 hand S60.51- ☑
 head S00.91 ☑
  ear — see Abrasion, ear
  eyelid — see Abrasion, eyelid
  lip S00.511 ☑
  nose S00.31 ☑
  oral cavity S00.512 ☑
  scalp S00.01 ☑
  specified site NEC S00.81 ☑
 heel — see Abrasion, foot
 hip S70.21- ☑
 inguinal region S30.811 ☑
 interscapular region S20.419 ☑
 jaw S00.81 ☑
 knee S80.21- ☑
 labium (majus) (minus) S30.814 ☑
 larynx S10.11 ☑
 leg (lower) S80.81- ☑
  knee — see Abrasion, knee
  upper — see Abrasion, thigh
 lip S00.511 ☑
 lower back S30.810 ☑
 lumbar region S30.810 ☑
 malar region S00.81 ☑
 mammary — see Abrasion, breast
 mastoid region S00.81 ☑
 mouth S00.512 ☑
 nail
  finger — see Abrasion, finger
  toe — see Abrasion, toe
 nape S10.81 ☑
 nasal S00.31 ☑
 neck S10.91 ☑
  specified site NEC S10.81 ☑
  throat S10.11 ☑
 nose S00.31 ☑
 occipital region S00.01 ☑
 oral cavity S00.512 ☑

Abrasion — continued
 orbital region — see Abrasion, eyelid
 palate S00.512 ☑
 palm — see Abrasion, hand
 parietal region S00.01 ☑
 pelvis S30.810 ☑
 penis S30.812 ☑
 perineum
  female S30.814 ☑
  male S30.810 ☑
 periocular area — see Abrasion, eyelid
 phalanges
  finger — see Abrasion, finger
  toe — see Abrasion, toe
 pharynx S10.11 ☑
 pinna — see Abrasion, ear
 popliteal space — see Abrasion, knee
 prepuce S30.812 ☑
 pubic region S30.810 ☑
 pudendum
  female S30.816 ☑
  male S30.815 ☑
 sacral region S30.810 ☑
 scalp S00.01 ☑
 scapular region — see Abrasion, shoulder
 scrotum S30.813 ☑
 shin — see Abrasion, leg
 shoulder S40.21- ☑
 skin NEC T14.8 ☑
 sternal region S20.319 ☑
 submaxillary region S00.81 ☑
 submental region S00.81 ☑
 subungual
  finger(s) — see Abrasion, finger
  toe(s) — see Abrasion, toe
 supraclavicular fossa S10.81 ☑
 supraorbital S00.81 ☑
 temple S00.81 ☑
 temporal region S00.81 ☑
 testis S30.813 ☑
 thigh S70.31- ☑
 thorax, thoracic (wall) S20.91 ☑
  back S20.41- ☑
  front S20.31- ☑
 throat S10.11 ☑
 thumb S60.31- ☑
 toe(s) (lesser) S90.416 ☑
  great S90.41- ☑
 tongue S00.512 ☑
 tooth, teeth (dentifrice) (habitual) (hard tissues) (occupational) (ritual) (traditional) K03.1
 trachea S10.11 ☑
 tunica vaginalis S30.813 ☑
 tympanum, tympanic membrane — see Abrasion, ear
 uvula S00.512 ☑
 vagina S30.814 ☑
 vocal cords S10.11 ☑
 vulva S30.814 ☑
 wrist S60.81- ☑
Abrism — see Poisoning, food, noxious, plant
Abruptio placentae O45.9- ☑
 with
  afibrinogenemia O45.01- ☑
  coagulation defect O45.00- ☑
   specified NEC O45.09- ☑
  disseminated intravascular coagulation O45.02- ☑
  hypofibrinogenemia O45.01- ☑
 specified NEC O45.8- ☑

Abruption, placenta — see Abruptio placentae
Abscess (connective tissue) (embolic) (fistulous) (infective) (metastatic) (multiple) (pernicious) (pyogenic) (septic) L02.91
 with
  diverticular disease (intestine) K57.80
   with bleeding K57.81
   large intestine K57.20
    with
     bleeding K57.21
     small intestine K57.40
      with bleeding K57.41
   small intestine K57.00
    with
     bleeding K57.01
     large intestine K57.40
      with bleeding K57.41

Abscess — continued
 with — continued
  lymphangitis — code by site under Abscess
 abdomen, abdominal
  cavity K65.1
  wall L02.211
 abdominopelvic K65.1
 accessory sinus — see Sinusitis
 adrenal (capsule) (gland) E27.8
 alveolar K04.7
  with sinus K04.6
 amebic A06.4
  brain (and liver or lung abscess) A06.6
  genitourinary tract A06.82
  liver (without mention of brain or lung abscess) A06.4
  lung (and liver) (without mention of brain abscess) A06.5
  specified site NEC A06.89
  spleen A06.89
 anerobic A48.0
 ankle — see Abscess, lower limb
 anorectal K61.2
 antecubital space — see Abscess, upper limb
 antrum (chronic) (Highmore) — see Sinusitis, maxillary
 anus K61.0
 apical (tooth) K04.7
  with sinus (alveolar) K04.6
 appendix K35.33
 areola (acute) (chronic) (nonpuerperal) N61.1
  puerperal, postpartum or gestational — see Infection, nipple
 arm (any part) — see Abscess, upper limb
 artery (wall) I77.89
 atheromatous I77.2
 auricle, ear — see Abscess, ear, external
 axilla (region) L02.41- ☑
  lymph gland or node L04.2
 back (any part, except buttock) L02.212
 Bartholin's gland N75.1
  with
   abortion — see Abortion, by type complicated by, sepsis
   ectopic or molar pregnancy O08.0
  following ectopic or molar pregnancy O08.0
 Bezold's — see Mastoiditis, acute
 bilharziasis B65.1
 bladder (wall) — see Cystitis, specified type NEC
 bone (subperiosteal) — see also Osteomyelitis, specified type NEC
  accessory sinus (chronic) — see Sinusitis
  chronic or old — see Osteomyelitis, chronic
  jaw (lower) (upper) M27.2
  mastoid — see Mastoiditis, acute, subperiosteal
  petrous — see Petrositis
  spinal (tuberculous) A18.01
   nontuberculous — see Osteomyelitis, vertebra
 bowel K63.0
 brain (any part) (cystic) (otogenic) G06.0
  amebic (with abscess of any other site) A06.6
  gonococcal A54.82
  pheomycotic (chromomycotic) B43.1
  tuberculous A17.81
 breast (acute) (chronic) (nonpuerperal) N61.1
  newborn P39.0
  puerperal, postpartum, gestational — see Mastitis, obstetric, purulent
 broad ligament N73.2
  acute N73.0
  chronic N73.1
 Brodie's (localized) (chronic) M86.8X- ☑
 bronchi J98.09
 buccal cavity K12.2
 bulbourethral gland N34.0
 bursa M71.00
  ankle M71.07- ☑
  elbow M71.02- ☑
  foot M71.07- ☑
  hand M71.04- ☑
  hip M71.05- ☑
  knee M71.06- ☑
  multiple sites M71.09
  pharyngeal J39.1
  shoulder M71.01- ☑
  specified site NEC M71.08
  wrist M71.03- ☑
 buttock L02.31
 canthus — see Blepharoconjunctivitis

Abscess — *continued*

cartilage — *see* Disorder, cartilage, specified type NEC
cecum K35.33
cerebellum, cerebellar G06.0
  sequelae G09
cerebral (embolic) G06.0
  sequelae G09
cervical (meaning neck) L02.11
  lymph gland or node L04.0
cervix (stump) (uteri) — *see* Cervicitis
cheek (external) L02.01
  inner K12.2
chest J86.9
  with fistula J86.0
  wall L02.213
chin L02.01
choroid — *see* Inflammation, chorioretinal
circumtonsillar J36
cold (lung) (tuberculous) — *see also* Tuberculosis, abscess, lung
  articular — *see* Tuberculosis, joint
colon (wall) K63.0
colostomy K94.02
conjunctiva — *see* Conjunctivitis, acute
cornea H16.31- ☑
corpus
  cavernosum N48.21
  luteum — *see* Oophoritis
Cowper's gland N34.0
cranium G06.0
cul-de-sac (Douglas') (posterior) — *see* Peritonitis, pelvic, female
cutaneous — *see* Abscess, by site
dental K04.7
  with sinus (alveolar) K04.6
dentoalveolar K04.7
  with sinus K04.6
diaphragm, diaphragmatic K65.1
Douglas' cul-de-sac or pouch — *see* Peritonitis, pelvic, female
Dubois A50.59
ear (middle) — *see also* Otitis, media, suppurative
  acute — *see* Otitis, media, suppurative, acute
  external H60.0- ☑
entamebic — *see* Abscess, amebic
enterostomy K94.12
epididymis N45.4
epidural G06.2
  brain G06.0
  spinal cord G06.1
epiglottis J38.7
epiploon, epiploic K65.1
erysipelatous — *see* Erysipelas
esophagus K20.80
ethmoid (bone) (chronic) (sinus) J32.2
external auditory canal — *see* Abscess, ear, external
extradural G06.2
  brain G06.0
    sequelae G09
  spinal cord G06.1
extraperitoneal K68.19
eye — *see* Endophthalmitis, purulent
eyelid H00.03- ☑
face (any part, except ear, eye and nose) L02.01
fallopian tube — *see* Salpingitis
fascia M72.8
fauces J39.1
fecal K63.0
femoral (region) — *see* Abscess, lower limb
filaria, filarial — *see* Infestation, filarial
finger (any) — *see also* Abscess, hand
  nail — *see* Cellulitis, finger
foot L02.61- ☑
forehead L02.01
frontal sinus (chronic) J32.1
gallbladder K81.0
genital organ or tract
  female (external) N76.4
  male N49.9
    multiple sites N49.8
    specified NEC N49.8
gestational mammary O91.11- ☑
gestational subareolar O91.11- ☑
gingival
  aggressive K05.20
    generalized K05.229
      moderate K05.222
      severe K05.223

Abscess — *continued*

gingival — *continued*
  aggressive — *continued*
    generalized — *continued*
      slight K05.221
    localized K05.219
      moderate K05.212
      severe K05.213
      slight K05.211
gland, glandular (lymph) (acute) — *see* Lymphadenitis, acute
gluteal (region) L02.31
gonococcal — *see* Gonococcus
groin L02.214
gum
  aggressive K05.20
    generalized K05.229
      moderate K05.222
      severe K05.223
      slight K05.221
    localized K05.219
      moderate K05.212
      severe K05.213
      slight K05.211
hand L02.51- ☑
head NEC L02.811
  face (any part, except ear, eye and nose) L02.01
heart — *see* Carditis
heel — *see* Abscess, foot
helminthic — *see* Infestation, helminth
hepatic (cholangitic) (hematogenic) (lymphogenic) (pylephlebitic) K75.0
  amebic A06.4
hip (region) — *see* Abscess, lower limb
horseshoe K61.31
ileocecal K35.33
ileostomy (bud) K94.12
iliac (region) L02.214
  fossa K35.33
infraclavicular (fossa) — *see* Abscess, upper limb
inguinal (region) L02.214
  lymph gland or node L04.1
intersphincteric K61.4
intestine, intestinal NEC K63.0
  rectal K61.1
intra-abdominal — *see also* Abscess, peritoneum K65.1
  following procedure T81.43 ☑
    obstetrical O86.03
  postprocedural T81.43 ☑
    retroperitoneal K68.11
intracranial G06.0
intramammary — *see* Abscess, breast
intramuscular, following procedure T81.42 ☑
  obstetrical O86.02
intraorbital — *see* Abscess, orbit
intraperitoneal K65.1
intrasphincteric (anus) K61.4
intraspinal G06.1
intratonsillar J36
ischiorectal (fossa) (specified NEC) K61.39
jaw (bone) (lower) (upper) M27.2
joint — *see* Arthritis, pyogenic or pyemic
  spine (tuberculous) A18.01
    nontuberculous — *see* Spondylopathy, infective
kidney N15.1
  with calculus N20.0
    with hydronephrosis N13.6
  puerperal (postpartum) O86.21
knee — *see also* Abscess, lower limb
  joint M00.9
labium (majus) (minus) N76.4
lacrimal
  caruncle — *see* Inflammation, lacrimal, passages, acute
  gland — *see* Dacryoadenitis
  passages (duct) (sac) — *see* Inflammation, lacrimal, passages, acute
lacunar N34.0
larynx J38.7
lateral (alveolar) K04.7
  with sinus K04.6
leg (any part) — *see* Abscess, lower limb
lens H27.8
lingual K14.0
  tonsil J36
lip K13.0
Littre's gland N34.0

Abscess — *continued*

liver (cholangitic) (hematogenic) (lymphogenic) (pylephlebitic) (pyogenic) K75.0
  amebic (due to Entamoeba histolytica) (dysenteric) (tropical) A06.4
    with
      brain abscess (and liver or lung abscess) A06.6
      lung abscess A06.5
loin (region) L02.211
lower limb L02.41- ☑
lumbar (tuberculous) A18.01
  nontuberculous L02.212
lung (miliary) (putrid) J85.2
  with pneumonia J85.1
    due to specified organism (see Pneumonia, in (due to))
  amebic (with liver abscess) A06.5
    with
      brain abscess A06.6
      pneumonia A06.5
lymph, lymphatic, gland or node (acute) — *see also* Lymphadenitis, acute
  mesentery I88.0
malar M27.2
mammary gland — *see* Abscess, breast
marginal, anus K61.0
mastoid — *see* Mastoiditis, acute
maxilla, maxillary M27.2
  molar (tooth) K04.7
    with sinus K04.6
  premolar K04.7
  sinus (chronic) J32.0
mediastinum J85.3
meibomian gland — *see* Hordeolum
meninges G06.2
mesentery, mesenteric K65.1
mesosalpinx — *see* Salpingitis
mons pubis L02.215
mouth (floor) K12.2
muscle — *see* Myositis, infective
myocardium I40.0
nabothian (follicle) — *see* Cervicitis
nasal J34.9
nasopharyngeal J39.1
navel L02.216
  newborn P38.9
    with mild hemorrhage P38.1
    without hemorrhage P38.9
neck (region) L02.11
  lymph gland or node L04.0
nephritic — *see* Abscess, kidney
nipple N61.1
  associated with
    lactation — *see* Pregnancy, complicated by
    pregnancy — *see* Pregnancy, complicated by
nose (external) (fossa) (septum) J34.0
  sinus (chronic) — *see* Sinusitis
omentum K65.1
operative wound T81.49 ☑
orbit, orbital — *see* Cellulitis, orbit
otogenic G06.0
ovary, ovarian (corpus luteum) — *see* Oophoritis
oviduct — *see* Oophoritis
palate (soft) K12.2
  hard M27.2
palmar (space) — *see* Abscess, hand
pancreas (duct) — *see* Pancreatitis, acute
parafrenal N48.21
parametric, parametrium N73.2
  acute N73.0
  chronic N73.1
paranephric N15.1
parapancreatic — *see* Pancreatitis, acute
parapharyngeal J39.0
pararectal K61.1
parasinus — *see* Sinusitis
parauterine — *see also* Disease, pelvis, inflammatory N73.2
paravaginal — *see* Vaginitis
parietal region (scalp) L02.811
parodontal — *see* Periodontitis, aggressive, localized
parotid (duct) (gland) K11.3
  region K12.2
pectoral (region) L02.213
pelvis, pelvic
  female — *see* Disease, pelvis, inflammatory
  male, peritoneal K65.1
penis N48.21

Abscess — *continued*
  penis — *continued*
    gonococcal (accessory gland) (periurethral) A54.1
  perianal K61.0
  periapical K04.7
    with sinus (alveolar) K04.6
  periappendicular K35.33
  pericardial I30.1
  pericecal K35.33
  pericemental — *see* Periodontitis, aggressive, localized
  pericholecystic — *see* Cholecystitis, acute
  pericoronal — *see* Periodontitis, aggressive, localized
  peridental — *see* Periodontitis, aggressive, localized
  perimetric — *see also* Disease, pelvis, inflammatory N73.2
  perinephric, perinephritic — *see* Abscess, kidney
  perineum, perineal (superficial) L02.215
    urethra N34.0
  periodontal (parietal) — *see* Periodontitis, aggressive, localized
    apical K04.7
  periosteum, periosteal — *see also* Osteomyelitis, specified type NEC
    with osteomyelitis — *see also* Osteomyelitis, specified type NEC
      acute — *see* Osteomyelitis, acute
      chronic — *see* Osteomyelitis, chronic
  peripharyngeal J39.0
  peripleuritic J86.9
    with fistula J86.0
  periprostatic N41.2
  perirectal K61.1
  perirenal (tissue) — *see* Abscess, kidney
  perisinuous (nose) — *see* Sinusitis
  peritoneum, peritoneal (perforated) (ruptured) K65.1
    with appendicitis — *see also* Appendicitis K35.33
    pelvic
      female — *see* Peritonitis, pelvic, female
      male K65.1
    postoperative T81.43 ☑
    puerperal, postpartum, childbirth O85
    tuberculous A18.31
  peritonsillar J36
  perityphlic K35.33
  periureteral N28.89
  periurethral N34.0
    gonococcal (accessory gland) (periurethral) A54.1
  periuterine — *see also* Disease, pelvis, inflammatory N73.2
  perivesical — *see* Cystitis, specified type NEC
  petrous bone — *see* Petrositis
  phagedenic NOS L02.91
    chancroid A57
  pharynx, pharyngeal (lateral) J39.1
  pilonidal L05.01
  pituitary (gland) E23.6
  pleura J86.9
    with fistula J86.0
  popliteal — *see* Abscess, lower limb
  postcecal K35.33
  postlaryngeal J38.7
  postnasal J34.0
  postoperative (any site) — *see also* Infection, postoperative wound T81.49 ☑
    retroperitoneal K68.11
  postpharyngeal J39.0
  posttonsillar J36
  post-typhoid A01.09
  pouch of Douglas — *see* Peritonitis, pelvic, female
  premammary — *see* Abscess, breast
  prepatellar — *see* Abscess, lower limb
  presacral K68.19
  prostate N41.2
    gonococcal (acute) (chronic) A54.22
  psoas muscle K68.12
  puerperal — *code by* site under Puerperal, abscess
  pulmonary — *see* Abscess, lung
  pulp, pulpal (dental) K04.01
    irreversible K04.02
    reversible K04.01
  rectovaginal septum K63.0
  rectovesical — *see* Cystitis, specified type NEC
  rectum K61.1
  renal — *see* Abscess, kidney
  retina — *see* Inflammation, chorioretinal
  retrobulbar — *see* Abscess, orbit
  retrocecal K65.1
  retrolaryngeal J38.7

Abscess — *continued*
  retromammary — *see* Abscess, breast
  retroperitoneal NEC K68.19
    postprocedural K68.11
  retropharyngeal J39.0
  retrouterine — *see* Peritonitis, pelvic, female
  retrovesical — *see* Cystitis, specified type NEC
  root, tooth K04.7
    with sinus (alveolar) K04.6
  round ligament — *see also* Disease, pelvis, inflammatory N73.2
  rupture (spontaneous) NOS L02.91
  sacrum (tuberculous) A18.01
    nontuberculous M46.28
  salivary (duct) (gland) K11.3
  scalp (any part) L02.811
  scapular — *see* Osteomyelitis, specified type NEC
  sclera — *see* Scleritis
  scrofulous (tuberculous) A18.2
  scrotum N49.2
  seminal vesicle N49.0
  septal, dental K04.7
    with sinus (alveolar) K04.6
  serous — *see* Periostitis
  shoulder (region) — *see* Abscess, upper limb
  sigmoid K63.0
  sinus (accessory) (chronic) (nasal) — *see also* Sinusitis
    intracranial venous (any) G06.0
  Skene's duct or gland N34.0
  skin — *see* Abscess, by site
  specified site NEC L02.818
  spermatic cord N49.1
  sphenoidal (sinus) (chronic) J32.3
  spinal cord (any part) (staphylococcal) G06.1
    tuberculous A17.81
  spine (column) (tuberculous) A18.01
    epidural G06.1
    nontuberculous — *see* Osteomyelitis, vertebra
  spleen D73.3
    amebic A06.89
  stitch T81.41 ☑
    following an obstetrical procedure O86.01
  subarachnoid G06.2
    brain G06.0
    spinal cord G06.1
  subareolar — *see* Abscess, breast
  subcecal K35.33
  subcutaneous — *see also* Abscess, by site
    following procedure T81.41 ☑
      obstetrical O86.01
    pheomycotic (chromomycotic) B43.2
  subdiaphragmatic K65.1
  subdural G06.2
    brain G06.0
      sequelae G09
    spinal cord G06.1
  sub-fascial, following an obstetrical procedure O86.02
  subgaleal L02.811
  subhepatic K65.1
  sublingual K12.2
    gland K11.3
  submammary — *see* Abscess, breast
  submandibular (region) (space) (triangle) K12.2
    gland K11.3
  submaxillary (region) L02.01
    gland K11.3
  submental L02.01
    gland K11.3
  subperiosteal — *see* Osteomyelitis, specified type NEC
  subphrenic K65.1
    following an obstetrical procedure O86.03
    postoperative T81.43 ☑
  suburethral N34.0
  sudoriparous L75.8
  supraclavicular (fossa) — *see* Abscess, upper limb
  supralevator K61.5
  suprapelvic, acute N73.0
  suprarenal (capsule) (gland) E27.8
  sweat gland L74.8
  tear duct — *see* Inflammation, lacrimal, passages, acute
  temple L02.01
  temporal region L02.01
  temporosphenoidal G06.0
  tendon (sheath) M65.00
    ankle M65.07- ☑
    foot M65.07- ☑
    forearm M65.03- ☑
    hand M65.04- ☑

Abscess — *continued*
  tendon — *continued*
    lower leg M65.06- ☑
    pelvic region M65.05- ☑
    shoulder region M65.01- ☑
    specified site NEC M65.08
    thigh M65.05- ☑
    upper arm M65.02- ☑
  testis N45.4
  thigh — *see* Abscess, lower limb
  thorax J86.9
    with fistula J86.0
  throat J39.1
  thumb — *see also* Abscess, hand
    nail — *see* Cellulitis, finger
  thymus (gland) E32.1
  thyroid (gland) E06.0
  toe (any) — *see also* Abscess, foot
    nail — *see* Cellulitis, toe
  tongue (staphylococcal) K14.0
  tonsil(s) (lingual) J36
  tonsillopharyngeal J36
  tooth, teeth (root) K04.7
    with sinus (alveolar) K04.6
    supporting structures NEC — *see* Periodontitis, aggressive, localized
  trachea J39.8
  trunk L02.219
    abdominal wall L02.211
    back L02.212
    chest wall L02.213
    groin L02.214
    perineum L02.215
    umbilicus L02.216
  tubal — *see* Salpingitis
  tuberculous — *see* Tuberculosis, abscess
  tubo-ovarian — *see* Salpingo-oophoritis
  tunica vaginalis N49.1
  umbilicus L02.216
  upper
    limb L02.41- ☑
    respiratory J39.8
  urethral (gland) N34.0
  urinary N34.0
  uterus, uterine (wall) — *see also* Endometritis
    ligament — *see also* Disease, pelvis, inflammatory N73.2
    neck — *see* Cervicitis
  uvula K12.2
  vagina (wall) — *see* Vaginitis
  vaginorectal — *see* Vaginitis
  vas deferens N49.1
  vermiform appendix K35.33
  vertebra (column) (tuberculous) A18.01
    nontuberculous — *see* Osteomyelitis, vertebra
  vesical — *see* Cystitis, specified type NEC
  vesico-uterine pouch — *see* Peritonitis, pelvic, female
  vitreous (humor) — *see* Endophthalmitis, purulent
  vocal cord J38.3
  von Bezold's — *see* Mastoiditis, acute
  vulva N76.4
  vulvovaginal gland N75.1
  web space — *see* Abscess, hand
  wound T81.49 ☑
  wrist — *see* Abscess, upper limb
Absence (of) (organ or part) (complete or partial)
  adrenal (gland) (congenital) Q89.1
    acquired E89.6
  albumin in blood E88.09
  alimentary tract (congenital) Q45.8
    upper Q40.8
  alveolar process (acquired) — *see* Anomaly, alveolar
  ankle (acquired) Z89.44- ☑
  anus (congenital) Q42.3
    with fistula Q42.2
  aorta (congenital) Q25.41
  appendix, congenital Q42.8
  arm (acquired) Z89.20- ☑
    above elbow Z89.22- ☑
      congenital (with hand present) — *see* Agenesis, arm, with hand present
      and hand — *see* Agenesis, forearm, and hand
    below elbow Z89.21- ☑
      congenital (with hand present) — *see* Agenesis, arm, with hand present
      and hand — *see* Agenesis, forearm, and hand
    congenital — *see* Defect, reduction, upper limb

Absence — *continued*
  arm — *continued*
    shoulder (following explantation of shoulder joint prosthesis) (joint) (with or without presence of antibiotic-impregnated cement spacer) Z89.23- ☑
      congenital (with hand present) — *see* Agenesis, arm, with hand present
  artery (congenital) (peripheral) Q27.8
    brain Q28.3
    coronary Q24.5
    pulmonary Q25.79
    specified NEC Q27.8
    umbilical Q27.0
  atrial septum (congenital) Q21.19
  auditory canal (congenital) (external) Q16.1
  auricle (ear), congenital Q16.0
  bile, biliary duct, congenital Q44.5
  bladder (acquired) Z90.6
    congenital Q64.5
  bowel sounds R19.11
  brain Q00.0
    part of Q04.3
  breast(s) (and nipple(s)) (acquired) Z90.1- ☑
    congenital Q83.8
  broad ligament Q50.6
  bronchus (congenital) Q32.4
  canaliculus lacrimalis, congenital Q10.4
  cerebellum (vermis) Q04.3
  cervix (acquired) (with uterus) Z90.710
    with remaining uterus Z90.712
    congenital Q51.5
  chin, congenital Q18.8
  cilia (congenital) Q10.3
    acquired — *see* Madarosis
  clitoris (congenital) Q52.6
  coccyx, congenital Q76.49
  cold sense R20.8
  congenital
    lumen — *see* Atresia
    organ or site NEC — *see* Agenesis
    septum — *see* Imperfect, closure
  corpus callosum Q04.0
  cricoid cartilage, congenital Q31.8
  diaphragm (with hernia), congenital Q79.1
  digestive organ(s) or tract, congenital Q45.8
    acquired NEC Z90.49
    upper Q40.8
  ductus arteriosus Q28.8
  duodenum (acquired) Z90.49
    congenital Q41.0
  ear, congenital Q16.9
    acquired H93.8- ☑
    auricle Q16.0
    external Q16.0
    inner Q16.5
    lobe, lobule Q17.8
    middle, except ossicles Q16.4
      ossicles Q16.3
    ossicles Q16.3
  ejaculatory duct (congenital) Q55.4
  endocrine gland (congenital) NEC Q89.2
    acquired E89.89
  epididymis (congenital) Q55.4
    acquired Z90.79
  epiglottis, congenital Q31.8
  esophagus (congenital) Q39.8
    acquired (partial) Z90.49
  eustachian tube (congenital) Q16.2
  extremity (acquired) Z89.9
    congenital Q73.0
    knee (following explantation of knee joint prosthesis) (joint) (with or without presence of antibiotic-impregnated cement spacer) Z89.52- ☑
    lower (above knee) Z89.619
      below knee Z89.51- ☑
    upper — *see* Absence, arm
  eye (acquired) Z90.01
    congenital Q11.1
    muscle (congenital) Q10.3
  eyeball (acquired) Z90.01
  eyelid (fold) (congenital) Q10.3
    acquired Z90.01
  face, specified part NEC Q18.8
  fallopian tube(s) (acquired) Z90.79
    congenital Q50.6
  family member (causing problem in home) NEC — *see also* Disruption, family Z63.32

Absence — *continued*
  femur, congenital — *see* Defect, reduction, lower limb, longitudinal, femur
  fibrinogen (congenital) D68.2
    acquired D65
  finger(s) (acquired) Z89.02- ☑
    congenital — *see* Agenesis, hand
  foot (acquired) Z89.43- ☑
    congenital — *see* Agenesis, foot
  forearm (acquired) — *see* Absence, arm, below elbow
  gallbladder (acquired) Z90.49
    congenital Q44.0
  gamma globulin in blood D80.1
    hereditary D80.0
  genital organs
    acquired (female) (male) Z90.79
    female, congenital Q52.8
      external Q52.71
      internal NEC Q52.8
    male, congenital Q55.8
  genitourinary organs, congenital NEC
    female Q52.8
    male Q55.8
  globe (acquired) Z90.01
    congenital Q11.1
  glottis, congenital Q31.8
  hand and wrist (acquired) Z89.11- ☑
    congenital — *see* Agenesis, hand
  head, part (acquired) NEC Z90.09
  heat sense R20.8
  hip (following explantation of hip joint prosthesis) (joint) (with or without presence of antibiotic-impregnated cement spacer) Z89.62- ☑
  hymen (congenital) Q52.4
  ileum (acquired) Z90.49
    congenital Q41.2
  immunoglobulin, isolated NEC D80.3
    IgA D80.2
    IgG D80.3
    IgM D80.4
  incus (acquired) — *see* Loss, ossicles, ear
    congenital Q16.3
  inner ear, congenital Q16.5
  intestine (acquired) (small) Z90.49
    congenital Q41.9
      specified NEC Q41.8
    large Z90.49
      congenital Q42.9
        specified NEC Q42.8
  iris, congenital Q13.1
  jejunum (acquired) Z90.49
    congenital Q41.1
  joint
    acquired
      hip (following explantation of hip joint prosthesis) (with or without presence of antibiotic-impregnated cement spacer) Z89.62- ☑
      knee (following explantation of knee joint prosthesis) (with or without presence of antibiotic-impregnated cement spacer) Z89.52- ☑
      shoulder (following explantation of shoulder joint prosthesis) (with or without presence of antibiotic-impregnated cement spacer) Z89.23- ☑
    congenital NEC Q74.8
  kidney(s) (acquired) Z90.5
    congenital Q60.2
      bilateral Q60.1
      unilateral Q60.0
  knee (following explantation of knee joint prosthesis) (joint) (with or without presence of antibiotic-impregnated cement spacer) Z89.52- ☑
  labyrinth, membranous Q16.5
  larynx (congenital) Q31.8
    acquired Z90.02
  leg (acquired) (above knee) Z89.61- ☑
    below knee (acquired) Z89.51- ☑
    congenital — *see* Defect, reduction, lower limb
  lens (acquired) — *see also* Aphakia
    congenital Q12.3
    post cataract extraction Z98.4- ☑
  limb (acquired) — *see* Absence, extremity
  lip Q38.6
  liver (congenital) Q44.7
  lung (fissure) (lobe) (bilateral) (unilateral) (congenital) Q33.3
    acquired (any part) Z90.2

Absence — *continued*
  menstruation — *see* Amenorrhea
  muscle (congenital) (pectoral) Q79.8
    ocular Q10.3
  neck, part Q18.8
  neutrophil — *see* Agranulocytosis
  nipple(s) (with breast(s)) (acquired) Z90.1- ☑
    congenital Q83.2
  nose (congenital) Q30.1
    acquired Z90.09
  organ
    of Corti, congenital Q16.5
    or site, congenital NEC Q89.8
      acquired NEC Z90.89
  osseous meatus (ear) Q16.4
  ovary (acquired)
    bilateral Z90.722
    congenital
      bilateral Q50.02
      unilateral Q50.01
    unilateral Z90.721
  oviduct (acquired)
    bilateral Z90.722
    congenital Q50.6
    unilateral Z90.721
  pancreas (congenital) Q45.0
    acquired Z90.410
      complete Z90.410
      partial Z90.411
      total Z90.410
  parathyroid gland (acquired) E89.2
    congenital Q89.2
  patella, congenital Q74.1
  penis (congenital) Q55.5
    acquired Z90.79
  pericardium (congenital) Q24.8
  pituitary gland (congenital) Q89.2
    acquired E89.3
  prostate (acquired) Z90.79
    congenital Q55.4
  pulmonary valve Q22.0
  punctum lacrimale (congenital) Q10.4
  radius, congenital — *see* Defect, reduction, upper limb, longitudinal, radius
  rectum (congenital) Q42.1
    with fistula Q42.0
    acquired Z90.49
  respiratory organ NOS Q34.9
  rib (acquired) Z90.89
    congenital Q76.6
  sacrum, congenital Q76.49
  salivary gland(s), congenital Q38.4
  scrotum, congenital Q55.29
  seminal vesicles (congenital) Q55.4
    acquired Z90.79
  septum
    atrial (congenital) Q21.19
    between aorta and pulmonary artery Q21.4
    ventricular (congenital) Q20.4
  sex chromosome
    female phenotype Q97.8
    male phenotype Q98.8
  skull bone (congenital) Q75.8
    with
      anencephaly Q00.0
      encephalocele — *see* Encephalocele
      hydrocephalus Q03.9
        with spina bifida — *see* Spina bifida, by site, with hydrocephalus
      microcephaly Q02
  spermatic cord, congenital Q55.4
  spine, congenital Q76.49
  spleen (congenital) Q89.01
    acquired Z90.81
  sternum, congenital Q76.7
  stomach (acquired) (partial) Z90.3
    congenital Q40.2
  superior vena cava, congenital Q26.8
  teeth, tooth (congenital) K00.0
    acquired (complete) K08.109
      class I K08.101
      class II K08.102
      class III K08.103
      class IV K08.104
      due to
        caries K08.139
          class I K08.131
          class II K08.132
          class III K08.133

Absence — *continued*
  teeth, tooth — *continued*
    acquired — *continued*
      due to — *continued*
        caries — *continued*
          class IV K08.134
          periodontal disease K08.129
            class I K08.121
            class II K08.122
            class III K08.123
            class IV K08.124
          specified NEC K08.199
            class I K08.191
            class II K08.192
            class III K08.193
            class IV K08.194
          trauma K08.119
            class I K08.111
            class II K08.112
            class III K08.113
            class IV K08.114
        partial K08.409
          class I K08.401
          class II K08.402
          class III K08.403
          class IV K08.404
          due to
            caries K08.439
              class I K08.431
              class II K08.432
              class III K08.433
              class IV K08.434
            periodontal disease K08.429
              class I K08.421
              class II K08.422
              class III K08.423
              class IV K08.424
            specified NEC K08.499
              class I K08.491
              class II K08.492
              class III K08.493
              class IV K08.494
            trauma K08.419
              class I K08.411
              class II K08.412
              class III K08.413
              class IV K08.414
  tendon (congenital) Q79.8
  testis (congenital) Q55.0
    acquired Z90.79
  thumb (acquired) Z89.01- ☑
    congenital — *see* Agenesis, hand
  thymus gland Q89.2
  thyroid (gland) (acquired) E89.0
    cartilage, congenital Q31.8
    congenital E03.1
  toe(s) (acquired) Z89.42- ☑
    with foot — *see* Absence, foot and ankle
    congenital — *see* Agenesis, foot
    great Z89.41- ☑
  tongue, congenital Q38.3
  trachea (cartilage), congenital Q32.1
  transverse aortic arch, congenital Q25.49
  tricuspid valve Q22.4
  umbilical artery, congenital Q27.0
  upper arm and forearm with hand present, congenital
    — *see* Agenesis, arm, with hand present
  ureter (congenital) Q62.4
    acquired Z90.6
  urethra, congenital Q64.5
  uterus (acquired) Z90.710
    with cervix Z90.710
    with remaining cervical stump Z90.711
    congenital Q51.0
  uvula, congenital Q38.5
  vagina, congenital Q52.0
  vas deferens (congenital) Q55.4
    acquired Z90.79
  vein (peripheral) congenital NEC Q27.8
    cerebral Q28.3
    digestive system Q27.8
    great Q26.8
    lower limb Q27.8
    portal Q26.5
    precerebral Q28.1
    specified site NEC Q27.8
    upper limb Q27.8
  vena cava (inferior) (superior), congenital Q26.8

Absence — *continued*
  ventricular septum Q20.4
  vertebra, congenital Q76.49
  von Willebrand factor, complete (near) — *see also*
    Disease, von Willebrand D68.03
  vulva, congenital Q52.71
  wrist (acquired) Z89.12- ☑
Absorbent system disease I87.8
Absorption
  carbohydrate, disturbance K90.49
  chemical — *see* Table of Drugs and Chemicals
    through placenta (newborn) P04.9
      environmental substance P04.6
      nutritional substance P04.5
      obstetric anesthetic or analgesic drug P04.0
  drug NEC — *see* Table of Drugs and Chemicals
    addictive
      through placenta (newborn) — *see also* New-
        born, affected by, maternal, use of P04.40
        cocaine P04.41
        hallucinogens P04.42
        specified drug NEC P04.49
    medicinal
      through placenta (newborn) P04.19
    through placenta (newborn) P04.19
    obstetric anesthetic or analgesic drug P04.0
  fat, disturbance K90.49
    pancreatic K90.3
  noxious substance — *see* Table of Drugs and Chemicals
  protein, disturbance K90.49
  starch, disturbance K90.49
  toxic substance — *see* Table of Drugs and Chemicals
  uremic — *see* Uremia
Abstinence symptoms, syndrome
  alcohol F10.239
    with delirium F10.231
  cocaine F14.23
  neonatal P96.1
  nicotine — *see* Dependence, drug, nicotine, with,
    withdrawal
  opioid F11.93
    with dependence F11.23
  psychoactive NEC F19.939
    with
      delirium F19.931
      dependence F19.239
        with
          delirium F19.231
          perceptual disturbance F19.232
        uncomplicated F19.230
      perceptual disturbance F19.932
    uncomplicated F19.930
  sedative F13.939
    with
      delirium F13.931
      dependence F13.239
        with
          delirium F13.231
          perceptual disturbance F13.232
        uncomplicated F13.230
      perceptual disturbance F13.932
    uncomplicated F13.930
  stimulant NEC F15.93
    with dependence F15.23
Abulia R68.89
Abulomania F60.7
Abuse
  adult — *see* Maltreatment, adult
    as reason for
      couple seeking advice (including offender) Z63.0
  alcohol (non-dependent) F10.10
    with
      anxiety disorder F10.180
      intoxication F10.129
        with delirium F10.121
        uncomplicated F10.120
      mood disorder F10.14
      other specified disorder F10.188
      psychosis F10.159
        delusions F10.150
        hallucinations F10.151
      sexual dysfunction F10.181
      sleep disorder F10.182
      unspecified disorder F10.19
      withdrawal F10.139
        with
          perceptual disturbance F10.132
        delirium F10.131

Abuse — *continued*
  alcohol — *continued*
    with — *continued*
      withdrawal — *continued*
        uncomplicated F10.130
    counseling and surveillance Z71.41
    in remission (early) (sustained) F10.11
  amphetamine (or related substance) — *see also* Abuse,
    drug, stimulant NEC
    stimulant NEC F15.10
      with
        anxiety disorder F15.180
        intoxication F15.129
          with
            delirium F15.121
            perceptual disturbance F15.122
        withdrawal F15.13
  analgesics (non-prescribed) (over the counter) F55.8
  antacids F55.0
  antidepressants — *see* Abuse, drug, psychoactive NEC
  anxiolytic — *see* Abuse, drug, sedative
  barbiturates — *see* Abuse, drug, sedative
  caffeine — *see* Abuse, drug, stimulant NEC
  cannabis, cannabinoids — *see* Abuse, drug, cannabis
  child — *see* Maltreatment, child
  cocaine — *see* Abuse, drug, cocaine
  drug NEC (non-dependent) F19.10
    with sleep disorder F19.182
    amphetamine type — *see* Abuse, drug, stimulant
      NEC
    analgesics (non-prescribed) (over the counter) F55.8
    antacids F55.0
    antidepressants — *see* Abuse, drug, psychoactive
      NEC
    anxiolytics — *see* Abuse, drug, sedative
    barbiturates — *see* Abuse, drug, sedative
    caffeine — *see* Abuse, drug, stimulant NEC
    cannabis F12.10
      with
        anxiety disorder F12.180
        intoxication F12.129
          with
            delirium F12.121
            perceptual disturbance F12.122
          uncomplicated F12.120
        other specified disorder F12.188
        psychosis F12.159
          delusions F12.150
          hallucinations F12.151
        unspecified disorder F12.19
        withdrawal F12.13
      in remission (early) (sustained) F12.11
    cocaine F14.10
      with
        anxiety disorder F14.180
        intoxication F14.129
          with
            delirium F14.121
            perceptual disturbance F14.122
          uncomplicated F14.120
        mood disorder F14.14
        other specified disorder F14.188
        psychosis F14.159
          delusions F14.150
          hallucinations F14.151
        sexual dysfunction F14.181
        sleep disorder F14.182
        unspecified disorder F14.19
        withdrawal F14.13
      in remission (early) (sustained) F14.11
    counseling and surveillance Z71.51
    hallucinogen F16.10
      with
        anxiety disorder F16.180
        flashbacks F16.183
        intoxication F16.129
          with
            delirium F16.121
            perceptual disturbance F16.122
          uncomplicated F16.120
        mood disorder F16.14
        other specified disorder F16.188
        perception disorder, persisting F16.183
        psychosis F16.159
          delusions F16.150
          hallucinations F16.151
        unspecified disorder F16.19
      in remission (early) (sustained) F16.11

☑ **Additional Character Required** — **Refer to the Tabular List for Character Selection**

Abuse — *continued*
  drug — *continued*
    hashish — *see* Abuse, drug, cannabis
    herbal or folk remedies F55.1
    hormones F55.3
    hypnotics — *see* Abuse, drug, sedative
    in remission (early) (sustained) F19.11
    inhalant F18.10
      with
        anxiety disorder F18.180
        dementia, persisting F18.17
        intoxication F18.129
          with delirium F18.121
          uncomplicated F18.120
        mood disorder F18.14
        other specified disorder F18.188
        psychosis F18.159
          delusions F18.150
          hallucinations F18.151
        unspecified disorder F18.19
    in remission (early) (sustained) F18.11
    laxatives F55.2
    LSD — *see* Abuse, drug, hallucinogen
    marihuana — *see* Abuse, drug, cannabis
    morphine type (opioids) — *see* Abuse, drug, opioid
    opioid F11.10
      with
        intoxication F11.129
          with
            delirium F11.121
            perceptual disturbance F11.122
          uncomplicated F11.120
        mood disorder F11.14
        other specified disorder F11.188
        psychosis F11.159
          delusions F11.150
          hallucinations F11.151
        sexual dysfunction F11.181
        sleep disorder F11.182
        unspecified disorder F11.19
        withdrawal F11.13
    in remission (early) (sustained) F11.11
    PCP (phencyclidine) (or related substance) — *see* Abuse, drug, hallucinogen
    psychoactive NEC F19.10
      with
        amnestic disorder F19.16
        anxiety disorder F19.180
        dementia F19.17
        intoxication F19.129
          with
            delirium F19.121
            perceptual disturbance F19.122
          uncomplicated F19.120
        mood disorder F19.14
        other specified disorder F19.188
        psychosis F19.159
          delusions F19.150
          hallucinations F19.151
        sexual dysfunction F19.181
        sleep disorder F19.182
        unspecified disorder F19.19
        withdrawal F19.139
          with
            perceptual disturbance F19.132
          delirium F19.131
          uncomplicated F19.130
    sedative, hypnotic or anxiolytic F13.10
      with
        anxiety disorder F13.180
        intoxication F13.129
          with delirium F13.121
          uncomplicated F13.120
        mood disorder F13.14
        other specified disorder F13.188
        psychosis F13.159
          delusions F13.150
          hallucinations F13.151
        sexual dysfunction F13.181
        sleep disorder F13.182
        unspecified disorder F13.19
        withdrawal F13.139
          with
            perceptual disturbance F13.132
          delirium F13.131
          uncomplicated F13.130
    in remission (early) (sustained) F13.11
    solvent — *see* Abuse, drug, inhalant

Abuse — *continued*
  drug — *continued*
    steroids F55.3
    stimulant NEC F15.10
      with
        anxiety disorder F15.180
        intoxication F15.129
          with
            delirium F15.121
            perceptual disturbance F15.122
          uncomplicated F15.120
        mood disorder F15.14
        other specified disorder F15.188
        psychosis F15.159
          delusions F15.150
          hallucinations F15.151
        sexual dysfunction F15.181
        sleep disorder F15.182
        unspecified disorder F15.19
        withdrawal F15.13
    in remission (early) (sustained) F15.11
    tranquilizers — *see* Abuse, drug, sedative
    vitamins F55.4
  hallucinogens — *see* Abuse, drug, hallucinogen
  hashish — *see* Abuse, drug, cannabis
  herbal or folk remedies F55.1
  hormones F55.3
  hypnotic — *see* Abuse, drug, sedative
  inhalant — *see* Abuse, drug, inhalant
  laxatives F55.2
  LSD — *see* Abuse, drug, hallucinogen
  marihuana — *see* Abuse, drug, cannabis
  morphine type (opioids) — *see* Abuse, drug, opioid
  non-psychoactive substance NEC F55.8
    antacids F55.0
    folk remedies F55.1
    herbal remedies F55.1
    hormones F55.3
    laxatives F55.2
    steroids F55.3
    vitamins F55.4
  opioids — *see* Abuse, drug, opioid
  PCP (phencyclidine) (or related substance) — *see* Abuse, drug, hallucinogen
  physical (adult) (child) — *see* Maltreatment
  psychoactive substance — *see* Abuse, drug, psychoactive NEC
  psychological (adult) (child) — *see* Maltreatment
  sedative — *see* Abuse, drug, sedative
  sexual — *see* Maltreatment
  solvent — *see* Abuse, drug, inhalant
  steroids F55.3
  vitamins F55.4
Acalculia R48.8
  developmental F81.2
Acanthamebiasis (with) B60.10
  conjunctiva B60.12
  keratoconjunctivitis B60.13
  meningoencephalitis B60.11
  other specified B60.19
Acanthocephaliasis B83.8
Acanthocheilonemiasis B74.4
Acanthocytosis E78.6
Acantholysis L11.9
Acanthosis (acquired) (nigricans) L83
  benign Q82.8
  congenital Q82.8
  seborrheic L82.1
    inflamed L82.0
  tongue K14.3
Acapnia E87.3
Acarbia E87.29
Acardia, acardius Q89.8
Acardiacus amorphus Q89.8
Acardiotrophia I51.4
Acariasis B88.0
  scabies B86
Acarodermatitis (urticarioides) B88.0
Acarophobia F40.218
Acatalasemia, acatalasia E80.3
Acathisia (drug induced) G25.71
Accelerated atrioventricular conduction I45.6
Accentuation of personality traits (type A) Z73.1
Accessory (congenital)
  adrenal gland Q89.1
  anus Q43.4
  appendix Q43.4
  atrioventricular conduction I45.6

Accessory — *continued*
  auditory ossicles Q16.3
  auricle (ear) Q17.0
  biliary duct or passage Q44.5
  bladder Q64.79
  blood vessels NEC Q27.9
    coronary Q24.5
  bone NEC Q79.8
  breast tissue, axilla Q83.1
  carpal bones Q74.0
  cecum Q43.4
  chromosome(s) NEC (nonsex) Q92.9
    with complex rearrangements NEC Q92.5
      seen only at prometaphase Q92.8
    13 — *see* Trisomy, 13
    18 — *see* Trisomy, 18
    21 — *see* Trisomy, 21
    partial Q92.9
    sex
      female phenotype Q97.8
  coronary artery Q24.5
  cusp(s), heart valve NEC Q24.8
    pulmonary Q22.3
  cystic duct Q44.5
  digit(s) Q69.9
  ear (auricle) (lobe) Q17.0
  endocrine gland NEC Q89.2
  eye muscle Q10.3
  eyelid Q10.3
  face bone(s) Q75.8
  fallopian tube (fimbria) (ostium) Q50.6
  finger(s) Q69.0
  foreskin N47.8
  frontonasal process Q75.8
  gallbladder Q44.1
  genital organ(s)
    female Q52.8
      external Q52.79
      internal NEC Q52.8
    male Q55.8
  genitourinary organs NEC Q89.8
    female Q52.8
    male Q55.8
  hallux Q69.2
  heart Q24.8
    valve NEC Q24.8
      pulmonary Q22.3
  hepatic ducts Q44.5
  hymen Q52.4
  intestine (large) (small) Q43.4
  kidney Q63.0
  lacrimal canal Q10.6
  leaflet, heart valve NEC Q24.8
  ligament, broad Q50.6
  liver Q44.7
    duct Q44.5
  lobule (ear) Q17.0
  lung (lobe) Q33.1
  muscle Q79.8
  navicular of carpus Q74.0
  nervous system, part NEC Q07.8
  nipple Q83.3
  nose Q30.8
  organ or site not listed — *see* Anomaly, by site
  ovary Q50.31
  oviduct Q50.6
  pancreas Q45.3
  parathyroid gland Q89.2
  parotid gland (and duct) Q38.4
  pituitary gland Q89.2
  preauricular appendage Q17.0
  prepuce N47.8
  renal arteries (multiple) Q27.2
  rib Q76.6
    cervical Q76.5
  roots (teeth) K00.2
  salivary gland Q38.4
  sesamoid bones Q74.8
    foot Q74.2
    hand Q74.0
  skin tags Q82.8
  spleen Q89.09
  sternum Q76.7
  submaxillary gland Q38.4
  tarsal bones Q74.2
  teeth, tooth K00.1
  tendon Q79.8
  thumb Q69.1
  thymus gland Q89.2

Accessory — *continued*
  thyroid gland Q89.2
  toes Q69.2
  tongue Q38.3
  tooth, teeth K00.1
  tragus Q17.0
  ureter Q62.5
  urethra Q64.79
  urinary organ or tract NEC Q64.8
  uterus Q51.28
  vagina Q52.10
  valve, heart NEC Q24.8
    pulmonary Q22.3
  vertebra Q76.49
  vocal cords Q31.8
  vulva Q52.79
Accident
  birth — *see* Birth, injury
  cardiac — *see* Infarct, myocardium
  cerebral I63.9
  cerebrovascular (embolic) (ischemic) (thrombotic) I63.9
    aborted I63.9
    hemorrhagic — *see* Hemorrhage, intracranial, intrac-erebral
    old (without sequelae) Z86.73
      with sequelae (of) — *see* Sequelae, infarction, cerebral
  coronary — *see* Infarct, myocardium
  craniovascular I63.9
  vascular, brain I63.9
Accidental — *see* condition
Accommodation (disorder) — *see also* condition
  hysterical paralysis of F44.89
  insufficiency of H52.4
  paresis — *see* Paresis, of accommodation
  spasm — *see* Spasm, of accommodation
Accouchement — *see* Delivery
Accreta placenta O43.21- ☑
Accretio cordis (nonrheumatic) I31.0
Accretions, tooth, teeth K03.6
Acculturation difficulty Z60.3
Accumulation secretion, prostate N42.89
Acephalia, acephalism, acephalus, acephaly Q00.0
Acephalobrachia monster Q89.8
Acephalochirus monster Q89.8
Acephalogaster Q89.8
Acephalostomus monster Q89.8
Acephalothorax Q89.8
Acerophobia F40.298
Acetonemia R79.89
  in Type 1 diabetes E10.10
    with coma E10.11
Acetonuria R82.4
Achalasia (cardia) (esophagus) K22.0
  congenital Q39.5
  pylorus Q40.0
  sphincteral NEC K59.89
Ache(s) — *see* Pain
Acheilia Q38.6
Achillobursitis — *see* Tendinitis, Achilles
Achillodynia — *see* Tendinitis, Achilles
Achlorhydria, achlorhydric (neurogenic) K31.83
  anemia D50.8
  diarrhea K31.83
  psychogenic F45.8
  secondary to vagotomy K91.1
Achluophobia F40.228
Acholia K82.8
Acholuric jaundice (familial) (splenomegalic) — *see also* Spherocytosis
  acquired D59.8
Achondrogenesis Q77.0
Achondroplasia (osteosclerosis congenita) Q77.4
Achroma, cutis L80
Achromat (ism), achromatopsia (acquired) (congenital) H53.51
Achromia, congenital — *see* Albinism
Achromia parasitica B36.0
Achylia gastrica K31.89
  psychogenic F45.8
Acid
  burn — *see* Corrosion
  deficiency
    amide nicotinic E52
    ascorbic E54
    folic E53.8
    nicotinic E52

Acid — *continued*
  deficiency — *continued*
    pantothenic E53.8
  intoxication — *see also* Acidosis E87.29
  peptic disease K30
  phosphatase deficiency E83.39
  stomach K30
    psychogenic F45.8
Acidemia — *see also* Acidosis E87.20
  argininosuccinic E72.22
  isovaleric E71.110
  metabolic (newborn) P19.9
    first noted before onset of labor P19.0
    first noted during labor P19.1
    noted at birth P19.2
  methylmalonic E71.120
  pipecolic E72.3
  propionic E71.121
Acidity, gastric (high) K30
  psychogenic F45.8
Acidocytopenia — *see* Agranulocytosis
Acidocytosis D72.10
Acidopenia — *see* Agranulocytosis
Acidosis (lactic) E87.20
  in Type 1 diabetes E10.10
    with coma E10.11
  kidney, tubular N25.89
  lactic E87.20
    acute E87.21
    chronic E87.22
  metabolic NEC E87.20
    with respiratory acidosis E87.4
    acute E87.21
    chronic E87.22
    hyperchloremic, of newborn P74.421
    late, of newborn P74.0
  mixed metabolic and respiratory, newborn P84
  newborn P84
  renal (hyperchloremic) (tubular) N25.89
  respiratory E87.29
    acute J96.02
    chronic J96.12
    complicated by
      metabolic
        acidosis E87.4
        alkalosis E87.4
  specified NEC E87.29
Aciduria
  4-hydroxybutyric E72.81
  argininosuccinic E72.22
  gamma-hydroxybutyric E72.81
  glutaric (type I) E72.3
    type II E71.313
    type III E71.5- ☑
  orotic (congenital) (hereditary) (pyrimidine deficiency) E79.8
    anemia D53.0
Acladiosis (skin) B36.0
Aclasis, diaphyseal Q78.6
Acleistocardia Q21.19
Aclusion — *see* Anomaly, dentofacial, malocclusion
Acne L70.9
  artificialis L70.8
  atrophica L70.2
  cachecticorum (Hebra) L70.8
  conglobata L70.1
  cystic L70.0
  decalvans L66.2
  excoriée (des jeunes filles) L70.5
  frontalis L70.2
  indurata L70.0
  infantile L70.4
  keloid L73.0
  lupoid L70.2
  necrotic, necrotica (miliaris) L70.2
  neonatal L70.4
  nodular L70.0
  occupational L70.8
  picker's L70.5
  pustular L70.0
  rodens L70.2
  rosacea L71.9
  specified NEC L70.8
  tropica L70.3
  varioliformis L70.2
  vulgaris L70.0
Acnitis (primary) A18.4
Acosta's disease T70.29 ☑

Acoustic — *see* condition
Acousticophobia F40.298
ACPO (acute colonic pseudo-obstruction) K59.81
Acquired — *see also* condition
  immunodeficiency syndrome (AIDS) B20
Acrania Q00.0
Acroangiodermatitis I78.9
Acroasphyxia, chronic I73.89
Acrobystitis N47.7
Acrocephalopolysyndactyly Q87.0
Acrocephalosyndactyly Q87.0
Acrocephaly Q75.0
Acrochondrohyperplasia — *see* Syndrome, Marfan's
Acrocyanosis I73.89
  newborn P28.2
    meaning transient blue hands and feet — *omit code*
Acrodermatitis L30.8
  atrophicans (chronica) L90.4
  continua (Hallopeau) L40.2
  enteropathica (hereditary) E83.2
  Hallopeau's L40.2
  infantile papular L44.4
  perstans L40.2
  pustulosa continua L40.2
  recalcitrant pustular L40.2
Acrodynia — *see* Poisoning, mercury
Acromegaly, acromegalia E22.0
Acromelalgia I73.81
Acromicria, acromikria Q79.8
Acronyx L60.0
Acropachy, thyroid — *see* Thyrotoxicosis
Acroparesthesia (simple) (vasomotor) I73.89
Acropathy, thyroid — *see* Thyrotoxicosis
Acrophobia F40.241
Acroposthitis N47.7
Acroscleriasis, acroscleroderma, acrosclerosis — *see* Sclerosis, systemic
Acrosphacelus I96
Acrospiroma, eccrine — *see* Neoplasm, skin, benign
Acrostealgia — *see* Osteochondropathy
Acrotrophodynia — *see* Immersion
ACTH ectopic syndrome E24.3
Actinic — *see* condition
Actinobacillosis, actinobacillus A28.8
  mallei A24.0
  muris A25.1
Actinomyces israelii (infection) — *see* Actinomycosis
Actinomycetoma (foot) B47.1
Actinomycosis, actinomycotic A42.9
  with pneumonia A42.0
  abdominal A42.1
  cervicofacial A42.2
  cutaneous A42.89
  gastrointestinal A42.1
  pulmonary A42.0
  sepsis A42.7
  specified site NEC A42.89
Actinoneuritis G62.82
Action, heart
  disorder I49.9
  irregular I49.9
    psychogenic F45.8
Activated protein C resistance D68.51
Activation
  mast cell (disorder) (syndrome) D89.40
    idiopathic D89.42
    monoclonal D89.41
    secondary D89.43
    specified type NEC D89.49
Active — *see* condition
Acute — *see also* condition
  abdomen R10.0
  gallbladder — *see* Cholecystitis, acute
Acyanotic heart disease (congenital) Q24.9
Acystia Q64.5
Adair-Dighton syndrome (brittle bones and blue sclera, deafness) Q78.0
Adamantinoblastoma — *see* Ameloblastoma
Adamantinoma — *see also* Cyst, calcifying odontogenic
  long bones C40.90
    lower limb C40.2- ☑
    upper limb C40.0- ☑
  malignant C41.1
    jaw (bone) (lower) C41.1
      upper C41.0
  tibial C40.2- ☑
Adamantoblastoma — *see* Ameloblastoma

Adams-Stokes (-Morgagni) disease or syndrome I45.9
Adaption reaction — *see* Disorder, adjustment
Addiction — *see also* Dependence F19.20
  alcohol, alcoholic (ethyl) (methyl) (wood) (without remission) F10.20
    with remission F10.21
  drug — *see* Dependence, drug
  ethyl alcohol (without remission) F10.20
    with remission F10.21
  heroin — *see* Dependence, drug, opioid
  methyl alcohol (without remission) F10.20
    with remission F10.21
  methylated spirit (without remission) F10.20
    with remission F10.21
  morphine (-like substances) — *see* Dependence, drug, opioid
  nicotine — *see* Dependence, drug, nicotine
  opium and opioids — *see* Dependence, drug, opioid
  tobacco — *see* Dependence, drug, nicotine
Addison-Biermer anemia (pernicious) D51.0
Addisonian crisis E27.2
Addison's
  anemia (pernicious) D51.0
  disease (bronze) or syndrome E27.1
    tuberculous A18.7
  keloid L94.0
Addison-Schilder complex E71.528
Additional — *see also* Accessory
  chromosome(s) Q99.8
    21 — *see* Trisomy, 21
    sex — *see* Abnormal, chromosome, sex
Adduction contracture, hip or other joint — *see* Contraction, joint
Adenitis — *see also* Lymphadenitis
  acute, unspecified site L04.9
  axillary I88.9
    acute L04.2
    chronic or subacute I88.1
  Bartholin's gland N75.8
  bulbourethral gland — *see* Urethritis
  cervical I88.9
    acute L04.0
    chronic or subacute I88.1
  chancroid (Hemophilus ducreyi) A57
  chronic, unspecified site I88.1
  Cowper's gland — *see* Urethritis
  due to Pasteurella multocida (P. septica) A28.0
  epidemic, acute B27.09
  gangrenous L04.9
  gonorrheal NEC A54.89
  groin I88.9
    acute L04.1
    chronic or subacute I88.1
  infectious (acute) (epidemic) B27.09
  inguinal I88.9
    acute L04.1
    chronic or subacute I88.1
  lymph gland or node, except mesenteric I88.9
    acute — *see* Lymphadenitis, acute
    chronic or subacute I88.1
  mesenteric (acute) (chronic) (nonspecific) (subacute) I88.0
  parotid gland (suppurative) — *see* Sialoadenitis
  salivary gland (any) (suppurative) — *see* Sialoadenitis
  scrofulous (tuberculous) A18.2
  Skene's duct or gland — *see* Urethritis
  strumous, tuberculous A18.2
  subacute, unspecified site I88.1
  sublingual gland (suppurative) — *see* Sialoadenitis
  submandibular gland (suppurative) — *see* Sialoadenitis
  submaxillary gland (suppurative) — *see* Sialoadenitis
  tuberculous — *see* Tuberculosis, lymph gland
  urethral gland — *see* Urethritis
  Wharton's duct (suppurative) — *see* Sialoadenitis
Adenoacanthoma — *see* Neoplasm, malignant, by site
Adenoameloblastoma — *see* Cyst, calcifying odontogenic
Adenocarcinoid (tumor) — *see* Neoplasm, malignant, by site
Adenocarcinoma — *see also* Neoplasm, malignant, by site
  acidophil
    specified site — *see* Neoplasm, malignant, by site
    unspecified site C75.1
  adrenal cortical C74.0- ☑
  alveolar — *see* Neoplasm, lung, malignant
  apocrine
    breast — *see* Neoplasm, breast, malignant

Adenocarcinoma — *continued*
  apocrine — *continued*
    in situ
      breast D05.8- ☑
      specified site NEC — *see* Neoplasm, skin, in situ
      unspecified site D04.9
    specified site NEC — *see* Neoplasm, skin, malignant
    unspecified site C44.99
  basal cell
    specified site — *see* Neoplasm, skin, malignant
    unspecified site C08.9
  basophil
    specified site — *see* Neoplasm, malignant, by site
    unspecified site C75.1
  bile duct type C22.1
    liver C22.1
    specified site NEC — *see* Neoplasm, malignant, by site
    unspecified site C22.1
  bronchiolar — *see* Neoplasm, lung, malignant
  bronchioloalveolar — *see* Neoplasm, lung, malignant
  ceruminous C44.29- ☑
  cervix, in situ — *see also* Carcinoma, cervix uteri, in situ D06.9
  chromophobe
    specified site — *see* Neoplasm, malignant, by site
    unspecified site C75.1
  diffuse type
    specified site — *see* Neoplasm, malignant, by site
    unspecified site C16.9
  duct
    infiltrating
      with Paget's disease — *see* Neoplasm, breast, malignant
      specified site — *see* Neoplasm, malignant, by site
      unspecified site (female) C50.91- ☑
        male C50.92- ☑
    specified site — *see* Neoplasm, malignant, by site
    unspecified site
      female C56.9
      male C61
  eosinophil
    specified site — *see* Neoplasm, malignant, by site
    unspecified site C75.1
  follicular
    with papillary C73
    moderately differentiated C73
    specified site — *see* Neoplasm, malignant, by site
    trabecular C73
    unspecified site C73
    well differentiated C73
  Hurthle cell C73
  in
    adenomatous
      polyposis coli C18.9
  infiltrating duct
    with Paget's disease — *see* Neoplasm, breast, malignant
    specified site — *see* Neoplasm, by site, malignant
    unspecified site (female) C50.91- ☑
      male C50.92- ☑
  inflammatory
    specified site — *see* Neoplasm, by site, malignant
    unspecified site (female) C50.91- ☑
      male C50.92- ☑
  intestinal type
    specified site — *see* Neoplasm, by site, malignant
    unspecified site C16.9
  intracystic papillary
  intraductal
    breast D05.1- ☑
    noninfiltrating
      breast D05.1- ☑
      papillary
        with invasion
          specified site — *see* Neoplasm, by site, malignant
          unspecified site (female) C50.91- ☑
            male C50.92- ☑
        breast D05.1- ☑
        specified site NEC — *see* Neoplasm, in situ, by site
        unspecified site D05.1- ☑
      specified site NEC — *see* Neoplasm, in situ, by site
      unspecified site D05.1- ☑

Adenocarcinoma — *continued*
  intraductal — *continued*
    papillary
      with invasion
        specified site — *see* Neoplasm, malignant, by site
        unspecified site (female) C50.91- ☑
          male C50.92- ☑
      breast D05.1- ☑
      specified site — *see* Neoplasm, in situ, by site
      unspecified site D05.1- ☑
    specified site NEC — *see* Neoplasm, in situ, by site
    unspecified site D05.1- ☑
  islet cell
    with exocrine, mixed
      specified site — *see* Neoplasm, malignant, by site
      unspecified site C25.9
    pancreas C25.4
    specified site NEC — *see* Neoplasm, malignant, by site
    unspecified site C25.4
  lobular
    in situ
      breast D05.0- ☑
      specified site NEC — *see* Neoplasm, in situ, by site
      unspecified site D05.0- ☑
    specified site — *see* Neoplasm, malignant, by site
    unspecified site (female) C50.91- ☑
      male C50.92- ☑
  mucoid — *see also* Neoplasm, malignant, by site
    cell
      specified site — *see* Neoplasm, malignant, by site
      unspecified site C75.1
  nonencapsulated sclerosing C73
  papillary
    with follicular C73
    follicular variant C73
    intraductal (noninfiltrating)
      with invasion
        specified site — *see* Neoplasm, malignant, by site
        unspecified site (female) C50.91- ☑
          male C50.92- ☑
      breast D05.1- ☑
      specified site NEC — *see* Neoplasm, in situ, by site
      unspecified site D05.1- ☑
    serous
      specified site — *see* Neoplasm, malignant, by site
      unspecified site C56.9
  papillocystic
    specified site — *see* Neoplasm, malignant, by site
    unspecified site C56.9
  pseudomucinous
    specified site — *see* Neoplasm, malignant, by site
    unspecified site C56.9
  renal cell C64- ☑
  sebaceous — *see* Neoplasm, skin, malignant
  serous — *see also* Neoplasm, malignant, by site
    papillary
      specified site — *see* Neoplasm, malignant, by site
      unspecified site C56.9
  sweat gland — *see* Neoplasm, skin, malignant
  water-clear cell C75.0
Adenocarcinoma-in-situ — *see also* Neoplasm, in situ, by site
  breast D05.9- ☑
Adenofibroma
  clear cell — *see* Neoplasm, benign, by site
  endometrioid D27.9
    borderline malignancy D39.10
    malignant C56- ☑
  mucinous
    specified site — *see* Neoplasm, benign, by site
    unspecified site D27.9
  papillary
    specified site — *see* Neoplasm, benign, by site
    unspecified site D27.9
  prostate — *see* Enlargement, enlarged, prostate
  serous
    specified site — *see* Neoplasm, benign, by site
    unspecified site D27.9

Adenofibroma — *continued*
   specified site — *see* Neoplasm, benign, by site
   unspecified site D27.9
Adenofibrosis
   breast — *see* Fibroadenosis, breast
   endometrioid N80.00
Adenoiditis (chronic) J35.02
   with tonsillitis J35.03
   acute J03.90
      recurrent J03.91
      specified organism NEC J03.80
         recurrent J03.81
      staphylococcal J03.80
         recurrent J03.81
      streptococcal J03.00
         recurrent J03.01
Adenoids — *see* condition
Adenolipoma — *see* Neoplasm, benign, by site
Adenolipomatosis, Launois-Bensaude E88.89
Adenolymphoma
   specified site — *see* Neoplasm, benign, by site
   unspecified site D11.9
Adenoma — *see also* Neoplasm, benign, by site
   acidophil
      specified site — *see* Neoplasm, benign, by site
      unspecified site D35.2
   acidophil-basophil, mixed
      specified site — *see* Neoplasm, benign, by site
      unspecified site D35.2
   adrenal (cortical) D35.00
      clear cell D35.00
      compact cell D35.00
      glomerulosa cell D35.00
      heavily pigmented variant D35.00
      mixed cell D35.00
   alpha-cell
      pancreas D13.7
      specified site NEC — *see* Neoplasm, benign, by site
      unspecified site D13.7
   alveolar D14.30
   apocrine
      breast D24- ☑
      specified site NEC — *see* Neoplasm, skin, benign, by site
      unspecified site D23.9
   basal cell D11.9
   basophil
      specified site — *see* Neoplasm, benign, by site
      unspecified site D35.2
   basophil-acidophil, mixed
      specified site — *see* Neoplasm, benign, by site
      unspecified site D35.2
   beta-cell
      pancreas D13.7
      specified site NEC — *see* Neoplasm, benign, by site
      unspecified site D13.7
   bile duct D13.4
      common D13.5
      extrahepatic D13.5
      intrahepatic D13.4
      specified site NEC — *see* Neoplasm, benign, by site
      unspecified site D13.4
   black D35.00
   bronchial D38.1
      cylindroid type — *see* Neoplasm, lung, malignant
   ceruminous D23.2- ☑
   chief cell D35.1
   chromophobe
      specified site — *see* Neoplasm, benign, by site
      unspecified site D35.2
   colloid
      specified site — *see* Neoplasm, benign, by site
      unspecified site D34
   eccrine, papillary — *see* Neoplasm, skin, benign
   endocrine, multiple
      single specified site — *see* Neoplasm, uncertain behavior, by site
      two or more specified sites D44- ☑
      unspecified site D44.9
   endometrioid — *see also* Neoplasm, benign
      borderline malignancy — *see* Neoplasm, uncertain behavior, by site
   eosinophil
      specified site — *see* Neoplasm, benign, by site
      unspecified site D35.2
   fetal
      specified site — *see* Neoplasm, benign, by site
      unspecified site D34

Adenoma — *continued*
   follicular
      specified site — *see* Neoplasm, benign, by site
      unspecified site D34
   hepatocellular D13.4
   Hurthle cell D34
   islet cell
      pancreas D13.7
      specified site NEC — *see* Neoplasm, benign, by site
      unspecified site D13.7
   liver cell D13.4
   macrofollicular
      specified site — *see* Neoplasm, benign, by site
      unspecified site D34
   malignant, malignum — *see* Neoplasm, malignant, by site
   microcystic
      pancreas D13.6
      specified site NEC — *see* Neoplasm, benign, by site
      unspecified site D13.6
   microfollicular
      specified site — *see* Neoplasm, benign, by site
      unspecified site D34
   mucoid cell
      specified site — *see* Neoplasm, benign, by site
      unspecified site D35.2
   multiple endocrine
      single specified site — *see* Neoplasm, uncertain behavior, by site
      two or more specified sites D44- ☑
      unspecified site D44.9
   nipple D24- ☑
   papillary — *see also* Neoplasm, benign, by site
      eccrine — *see* Neoplasm, skin, benign, by site
   Pick's tubular
      specified site — *see* Neoplasm, benign, by site
      unspecified site
         female D27.9
         male D29.20
   pleomorphic
      carcinoma in — *see* Neoplasm, salivary gland, malignant
      specified site — *see* Neoplasm, malignant, by site
      unspecified site C08.9
   polypoid — *see also* Neoplasm, benign
      adenocarcinoma in — *see* Neoplasm, malignant, by site
      adenocarcinoma in situ — *see* Neoplasm, in situ, by site
   prostate — *see* Neoplasm, benign, prostate
   rete cell D29.20
   sebaceous — *see* Neoplasm, skin, benign
   Sertoli cell
      specified site — *see* Neoplasm, benign, by site
      unspecified site
         female D27.9
         male D29.20
   skin appendage — *see* Neoplasm, skin, benign
   sudoriferous gland — *see* Neoplasm, skin, benign
   sweat gland — *see* Neoplasm, skin, benign
   testicular
      specified site — *see* Neoplasm, benign, by site
      unspecified site
         female D27.9
         male D29.20
   tubular — *see also* Neoplasm, benign, by site
      adenocarcinoma in — *see* Neoplasm, malignant, by site
      adenocarcinoma in situ — *see* Neoplasm, in situ, by site
      Pick's
         specified site — *see* Neoplasm, benign, by site
         unspecified site
            female D27.9
            male D29.20
   tubulovillous — *see also* Neoplasm, benign, by site
      adenocarcinoma in — *see* Neoplasm, malignant, by site
      adenocarcinoma in situ — *see* Neoplasm, in situ, by site
   villous — *see* Neoplasm, uncertain behavior, by site
      adenocarcinoma in — *see* Neoplasm, malignant, by site
      adenocarcinoma in situ — *see* Neoplasm, in situ, by site
   water-clear cell D35.1

Adenomatosis
   endocrine (multiple) E31.20
      single specified site — *see* Neoplasm, uncertain behavior, by site
   erosive of nipple D24- ☑
   pluriendocrine — *see* Adenomatosis, endocrine
   pulmonary D38.1
      malignant — *see* Neoplasm, lung, malignant
   specified site — *see* Neoplasm, benign, by site
   unspecified site D12.6
Adenomatous
   goiter (nontoxic) E04.9
      with hyperthyroidism — *see* Hyperthyroidism, with, goiter, nodular
      toxic — *see* Hyperthyroidism, with, goiter, nodular
Adenomyoma — *see also* Neoplasm, benign, by site
   prostate — *see* Enlarged, prostate
Adenomyometritis N80.00
Adenomyosis (uterus) N80.03
Adenopathy (lymph gland) R59.9
   generalized R59.1
   inguinal R59.0
   localized R59.0
   mediastinal R59.0
   mesentery R59.0
   syphilitic (secondary) A51.49
   tracheobronchial R59.0
      tuberculous A15.4
         primary (progressive) A15.7
   tuberculous — *see also* Tuberculosis, lymph gland
      tracheobronchial A15.4
         primary (progressive) A15.7
Adenosalpingitis — *see* Salpingitis
Adenosarcoma — *see* Neoplasm, malignant, by site
Adenosclerosis I88.8
Adenosis (sclerosing) breast — *see* Fibroadenosis, breast
Adenovirus, as cause of disease classified elsewhere B97.0
Adentia (complete) (partial) — *see* Absence, teeth
Adherent — *see also* Adhesions
   labia (minora) N90.89
   pericardium (nonrheumatic) I31.0
      rheumatic I09.2
   placenta (with hemorrhage) O72.0
      without hemorrhage O73.0
   prepuce, newborn N47.0
   scar (skin) L90.5
   tendon in scar L90.5
Adhesions, adhesive (postinfective) K66.0
   with intestinal obstruction K56.50
      complete K56.52
      incomplete K56.51
      partial K56.51
   abdominal (wall) — *see* Adhesions, peritoneum
   appendix K38.8
   bile duct (common) (hepatic) K83.8
   bladder (sphincter) N32.89
   bowel — *see* Adhesions, peritoneum
   cardiac I31.0
      rheumatic I09.2
   cecum — *see* Adhesions, peritoneum
   cervicovaginal N88.1
      congenital Q52.8
      postpartal O90.89
         old N88.1
   cervix N88.1
   ciliary body NEC — *see* Adhesions, iris
   clitoris N90.89
   colon — *see* Adhesions, peritoneum
   common duct K83.8
   congenital — *see also* Anomaly, by site
      fingers — *see* Syndactylism, complex, fingers
      omental, anomalous Q43.3
      peritoneal Q43.3
      tongue (to gum or roof of mouth) Q38.3
   conjunctiva (acquired) H11.21- ☑
      congenital Q15.8
   cystic duct K82.8
   diaphragm — *see* Adhesions, peritoneum
   due to foreign body — *see* Foreign body
   duodenum — *see* Adhesions, peritoneum
   ear
      middle H74.1- ☑
   epididymis N50.89
   epidural — *see* Adhesions, meninges
   epiglottis J38.7
   eyelid H02.59
   female pelvis N73.6

Adhesions, adhesive — *continued*
  gallbladder K82.8
  globe H44.89
  heart I31.Ø
    rheumatic IØ9.2
  ileocecal (coil) — *see* Adhesions, peritoneum
  ileum — *see* Adhesions, peritoneum
  intestine — *see also* Adhesions, peritoneum
    with obstruction K56.5Ø
      complete K56.52
      incomplete K56.51
      partial K56.51
  intra-abdominal — *see* Adhesions, peritoneum
  iris H21.5Ø- ☑
    anterior H21.51- ☑
    goniosynechiae H21.52- ☑
    posterior H21.54- ☑
    to corneal graft T85.898 ☑
  joint — *see* Ankylosis
    knee M23.8X ☑
    temporomandibular M26.61- ☑
  labium (majus) (minus), congenital Q52.5
  liver — *see* Adhesions, peritoneum
  lung J98.4
  mediastinum J98.59
  meninges (cerebral) (spinal) G96.12
    congenital QØ7.8
    tuberculous (cerebral) (spinal) A17.Ø
  mesenteric — *see* Adhesions, peritoneum
  nasal (septum) (to turbinates) J34.89
  ocular muscle — *see* Strabismus, mechanical
  omentum — *see* Adhesions, peritoneum
  ovary N73.6
    congenital (to cecum, kidney or omentum) Q5Ø.39
  paraovarian N73.6
  pelvic (peritoneal)
    female N73.6
      postprocedural N99.4
    male — *see* Adhesions, peritoneum
    postpartal (old) N73.6
    tuberculous A18.17
  penis to scrotum (congenital) Q55.8
  periappendiceal — *see also* Adhesions, peritoneum
  pericardium (nonrheumatic) I31.Ø
    focal I31.8
    rheumatic IØ9.2
    tuberculous A18.84
  pericholecystic K82.8
  perigastric — *see* Adhesions, peritoneum
  periovarian N73.6
  periprostatic N42.89
  perirectal — *see* Adhesions, peritoneum
  perirenal N28.89
  peritoneum, peritoneal (postinfective) K66.Ø
    with obstruction (intestinal) K56.5Ø
      complete K56.52
      incomplete K56.51
      partial K56.51
    congenital Q43.3
    pelvic, female N73.6
      postprocedural N99.4
    postpartal, pelvic N73.6
    postprocedural K66.Ø
    to uterus N73.6
  peritubal N73.6
  periureteral N28.89
  periuterine N73.6
  perivesical N32.89
  perivesicular (seminal vesicle) N5Ø.89
  pleura, pleuritic J94.8
    tuberculous NEC A15.6
  pleuropericardial J94.8
  postoperative (gastrointestinal tract) K66.Ø
    with obstruction — *see also* Obstruction, intestine, postoperative K91.3Ø
    due to foreign body accidentally left in wound — *see* Foreign body, accidentally left during a procedure
    pelvic peritoneal N99.4
    urethra — *see* Stricture, urethra, postprocedural
    vagina N99.2
  postpartal, old (vulva or perineum) N9Ø.89
  preputial, prepuce N47.5
  pulmonary J98.4
  pylorus — *see* Adhesions, peritoneum
  sciatic nerve — *see* Lesion, nerve, sciatic
  seminal vesicle N5Ø.89
  shoulder (joint) — *see* Capsulitis, adhesive

Adhesions, adhesive — *continued*
  sigmoid flexure — *see* Adhesions, peritoneum
  spermatic cord (acquired) N5Ø.89
    congenital Q55.4
  spinal canal G96.12
  stomach — *see* Adhesions, peritoneum
  subscapular — *see* Capsulitis, adhesive
  temporomandibular M26.61- ☑
  tendinitis (*see also* Tenosynovitis, specified type NEC)
    shoulder — *see* Capsulitis, adhesive
  testis N44.8
  tongue, congenital (to gum or roof of mouth) Q38.3
    acquired K14.8
  trachea J39.8
  tubo-ovarian N73.6
  tunica vaginalis N44.8
  uterus N73.6
    internal N85.6
    to abdominal wall N73.6
  vagina (chronic) N89.5
    postoperative N99.2
  vitreomacular H43.82- ☑
  vitreous H43.89
  vulva N9Ø.89
Adiaspiromycosis B48.8
Adie (-Holmes) **pupil or syndrome** — *see* Anomaly, pupil, function, tonic pupil
Adiponecrosis neonatorum P83.88
Adiposis — *see also* Obesity
  cerebralis E23.6
  dolorosa E88.2
Adiposity — *see also* Obesity
  heart — *see* Degeneration, myocardial
  localized E65
Adiposogenital dystrophy E23.6
Adjustment
  disorder — *see* Disorder, adjustment
  implanted device — *see* Encounter (for), adjustment (of)
  prosthesis, external — *see* Fitting
  reaction — *see* Disorder, adjustment
Administration of tPA (rtPA) in a different facility within the last 24 hours prior to admission to current facility Z92.82
Admission (for) — *see also* Encounter (for)
  adjustment (of)
    artificial
      arm Z44.ØØ- ☑
        complete Z44.Ø1- ☑
        partial Z44.Ø2- ☑
      eye Z44.2 ☑
      leg Z44.1Ø- ☑
        complete Z44.11- ☑
        partial Z44.12- ☑
    brain neuropacemaker Z46.2
      implanted Z45.42
    breast
      implant Z45.81 ☑
      prosthesis (external) Z44.3 ☑
    colostomy belt Z46.89
    contact lenses Z46.Ø
    cystostomy device Z46.6
    dental prosthesis Z46.3
    device NEC
      abdominal Z46.89
      implanted Z45.89
        cardiac Z45.Ø9
          defibrillator (with synchronous cardiac pacemaker) Z45.Ø2
          pacemaker (cardiac resynchronization therapy (CRT-P)) Z45.Ø18
            pulse generator Z45.Ø1Ø
          resynchronization therapy defibrillator (CRT-D) Z45.Ø2
        hearing device Z45.328
          bone conduction Z45.32Ø
          cochlear Z45.321
        infusion pump Z45.1
        nervous system Z45.49
          CSF drainage Z45.41
          hearing device — *see* Admission, adjustment, device, implanted, hearing device
          neuropacemaker Z45.42
          visual substitution Z45.31
        specified NEC Z45.89
        vascular access Z45.2
        visual substitution Z45.31

Admission — *continued*
  adjustment — *continued*
    device — *continued*
      nervous system Z46.2
        implanted — *see* Admission, adjustment, device, implanted, nervous system
      orthodontic Z46.4
      prosthetic Z44.9
        arm — *see* Admission, adjustment, artificial, arm
        breast Z44.3 ☑
        dental Z46.3
        eye Z44.2 ☑
        leg — *see* Admission, adjustment, artificial, leg
        specified type NEC Z44.8
      substitution
        auditory Z46.2
          implanted — *see* Admission, adjustment, device, implanted, hearing device
        nervous system Z46.2
          implanted — *see* Admission, adjustment, device, implanted, nervous system
        visual Z46.2
          implanted Z45.31
      urinary Z46.6
    hearing aid Z46.1
      implanted — *see* Admission, adjustment, device, implanted, hearing device
    ileostomy device Z46.89
    intestinal appliance or device NEC Z46.89
    neuropacemaker (brain) (peripheral nerve) (spinal cord) Z46.2
      implanted Z45.42
    orthodontic device Z46.4
    orthopedic (brace) (cast) (device) (shoes) Z46.89
    pacemaker (cardiac resynchronization therapy (CRT-P))
      cardiac Z45.Ø18
        pulse generator Z45.Ø1Ø
      nervous system Z46.2
        implanted Z45.42
    portacath (port-a-cath) Z45.2
    prosthesis Z44.9
      arm — *see* Admission, adjustment, artificial, arm
      breast Z44.3 ☑
      dental Z46.3
      eye Z44.2 ☑
      leg — *see* Admission, adjustment, artificial, leg
      specified NEC Z44.8
    spectacles Z46.Ø
  aftercare — *see also* Aftercare Z51.89
    postpartum
      immediately after delivery Z39.Ø
      routine follow-up Z39.2
    radiation therapy (antineoplastic) Z51.Ø
  attention to artificial opening (of) Z43.9
    artificial vagina Z43.7
    colostomy Z43.3
    cystostomy Z43.5
    enterostomy Z43.4
    gastrostomy Z43.1
    ileostomy Z43.2
    jejunostomy Z43.4
    nephrostomy Z43.6
    specified site NEC Z43.8
      intestinal tract Z43.4
      urinary tract Z43.6
    tracheostomy Z43.Ø
    ureterostomy Z43.6
    urethrostomy Z43.6
  breast augmentation or reduction Z41.1
  breast reconstruction following mastectomy Z42.1
  change of
    dressing (nonsurgical) Z48.ØØ
    neuropacemaker device (brain) (peripheral nerve) (spinal cord) Z46.2
      implanted Z45.42
    surgical dressing Z48.Ø1
  circumcision, ritual or routine (in absence of diagnosis) Z41.2
  clinical research investigation (control) (normal comparison) (participant) ZØØ.6
  contraceptive management Z3Ø.9
  cosmetic surgery NEC Z41.1
  counseling — *see also* Counseling
    dietary Z71.3
    gestational carrier Z31.7

Admission — *continued*
  counseling — *see also* Counseling — *continued*
    HIV Z71.7
    human immunodeficiency virus Z71.7
    nonattending third party Z71.0
    procreative management NEC Z31.69
  delivery, full-term, uncomplicated O80
    cesarean, without indication O82
  desensitization to allergens Z51.6
  dietary surveillance and counseling Z71.3
  ear piercing Z41.3
  examination at health care facility (adult) — *see also* Examination Z00.00
    with abnormal findings Z00.01
    clinical research investigation (control) (normal comparison) (participant) Z00.6
    dental Z01.20
      with abnormal findings Z01.21
    donor (potential) Z00.5
    ear Z01.10
      with abnormal findings NEC Z01.118
    eye Z01.00
      with abnormal findings Z01.01
      following failed vision screening Z01.020
        with abnormal findings Z01.021
    general, specified reason NEC Z00.8
    hearing Z01.10
      with abnormal findings NEC Z01.118
      infant or child (over 28 days old) Z00.129
        with abnormal findings Z00.121
    postpartum checkup Z39.2
    psychiatric (general) Z00.8
      requested by authority Z04.6
    vision Z01.00
      with abnormal findings Z01.01
      following failed vision screening Z01.020
        with abnormal findings Z01.021
      infant or child (over 28 days old) Z00.129
        with abnormal findings Z00.121
  fitting (of)
    artificial
      arm — *see* Admission, adjustment, artificial, arm
      eye Z44.2 ☑
      leg — *see* Admission, adjustment, artificial, leg
    brain neuropacemaker Z46.2
      implanted Z45.42
    breast prosthesis (external) Z44.3 ☑
    colostomy belt Z46.89
    contact lenses Z46.0
    cystostomy device Z46.6
    dental prosthesis Z46.3
    dentures Z46.3
    device NEC
      abdominal Z46.89
      nervous system Z46.2
        implanted — *see* Admission, adjustment, device, implanted, nervous system
      orthodontic Z46.4
      prosthetic Z44.9
        breast Z44.3 ☑
        dental Z46.3
        eye Z44.2 ☑
      substitution
        auditory Z46.2
          implanted — *see* Admission, adjustment, device, implanted, hearing device
        nervous system Z46.2
          implanted — *see* Admission, adjustment, device, implanted, nervous system
        visual Z46.2
          implanted Z45.31
    hearing aid Z46.1
    ileostomy device Z46.89
    intestinal appliance or device NEC Z46.89
    neuropacemaker (brain) (peripheral nerve) (spinal cord) Z46.2
      implanted Z45.42
    orthodontic device Z46.4
    orthopedic device (brace) (cast) (shoes) Z46.89
    prosthesis Z44.9
      arm — *see* Admission, adjustment, artificial, arm
      breast Z44.3 ☑
      dental Z46.3
      eye Z44.2 ☑
      leg — *see* Admission, adjustment, artificial, leg
      specified type NEC Z44.8
    spectacles Z46.0
  follow-up examination Z09

Admission — *continued*
  intrauterine device management Z30.431
    initial prescription Z30.014
  mental health evaluation Z00.8
    requested by authority Z04.6
  observation — *see* Observation
  Papanicolaou smear, cervix Z12.4
    for suspected malignant neoplasm Z12.4
  plastic and reconstructive surgery following medical procedure or healed injury NEC Z42.8
  plastic surgery, cosmetic NEC Z41.1
  postpartum observation
    immediately after delivery Z39.0
    routine follow-up Z39.2
  poststerilization (for restoration) Z31.0
    aftercare Z31.42
  procreative management Z31.9
  prophylactic (measure) — *see also* Encounter, prophylactic measures
    organ removal Z40.00
      breast Z40.01
      fallopian tube(s) Z40.03
        with ovary(s) Z40.02
      ovary(s) Z40.02
      specified organ NEC Z40.09
      testes Z40.09
      vaccination Z23
  psychiatric examination (general) Z00.8
    requested by authority Z04.6
  radiation therapy (antineoplastic) Z51.0
  reconstructive surgery following medical procedure or healed injury NEC Z42.8
  removal of
    cystostomy catheter Z43.5
    drains Z48.03
    dressing (nonsurgical) Z48.00
    implantable subdermal contraceptive Z30.46
    intrauterine contraceptive device Z30.432
    neuropacemaker (brain) (peripheral nerve) (spinal cord) Z46.2
      implanted Z45.42
    staples Z48.02
    surgical dressing Z48.01
    sutures Z48.02
    ureteral stent Z46.6
  respirator [ventilator] use during power failure Z99.12
  restoration of organ continuity (poststerilization) Z31.0
    aftercare Z31.42
  sensitivity test — *see also* Test, skin
    allergy NEC Z01.82
    Mantoux Z11.1
  tuboplasty following previous sterilization Z31.0
    aftercare Z31.42
  vasoplasty following previous sterilization Z31.0
    aftercare Z31.42
  vision examination Z01.00
    with abnormal findings Z01.01
    following failed vision screening Z01.020
      with abnormal findings Z01.021
    infant or child (over 28 days old) Z00.129
      with abnormal findings Z00.121
  waiting period for admission to other facility Z75.1
Adnexitis (suppurative) — *see* Salpingo-oophoritis
Adolescent X-linked adrenoleukodystrophy E71.521
Adrenal (gland) — *see* condition
Adrenalism, tuberculous A18.7
Adrenalitis, adrenitis E27.8
  autoimmune E27.1
  meningococcal, hemorrhagic A39.1
Adrenarche, premature E27.0
Adrenocortical syndrome — *see* Cushing's, syndrome
Adrenogenital syndrome E25.9
  acquired E25.8
  congenital E25.0
  salt loss E25.0
Adrenogenitalism, congenital E25.0
Adrenoleukodystrophy E71.529
  neonatal E71.511
  X-linked E71.529
    Addison only phenotype E71.528
    Addison-Schilder E71.528
    adolescent E71.521
    adrenomyeloneuropathy E71.522
    childhood cerebral E71.520
    other specified E71.528
Adrenomyeloneuropathy E71.522
Adventitious bursa — *see* Bursopathy, specified type NEC

Adverse effect — *see* Table of Drugs and Chemicals, categories T36-T50, with 6th character 5
Advice — *see* Counseling
Adynamia (episodica) (hereditary) (periodic) G72.3
Aeration lung imperfect, newborn — *see* Atelectasis
Aerobullosis T70.3 ☑
Aerocele — *see* Embolism, air
Aerodermectasia
  subcutaneous (traumatic) T79.7 ☑
Aerodontalgia T70.29 ☑
Aeroembolism T70.3 ☑
Aerogenes capsulatus infection A48.0
Aero-otitis media T70.0 ☑
Aerophagy, aerophagia (psychogenic) F45.8
Aerophobia F40.228
Aerosinusitis T70.1 ☑
Aerotitis T70.0 ☑
Affection — *see* Disease
Afibrinogenemia — *see also* Defect, coagulation D68.8
  acquired D65
  congenital D68.2
  following ectopic or molar pregnancy O08.1
  in abortion — *see* Abortion, by type, complicated by, afibrinogenemia
  puerperal O72.3
African
  sleeping sickness B56.9
  tick fever A68.1
  trypanosomiasis B56.9
    gambian B56.0
    rhodesian B56.1
Aftercare — *see also* Care Z51.89
  following surgery (for) (on)
    amputation Z47.81
    attention to
      drains Z48.03
      dressings (nonsurgical) Z48.00
        surgical Z48.01
      sutures Z48.02
    circulatory system Z48.812
    delayed (planned) wound closure Z48.1
    digestive system Z48.815
    explantation of joint prosthesis (staged procedure)
      hip Z47.32
      knee Z47.33
      shoulder Z47.31
    genitourinary system Z48.816
    joint replacement Z47.1
    neoplasm Z48.3
    nervous system Z48.811
    oral cavity Z48.814
    organ transplant
      bone marrow Z48.290
      heart Z48.21
      heart-lung Z48.280
      kidney Z48.22
      liver Z48.23
      lung Z48.24
      multiple organs NEC Z48.288
      specified NEC Z48.298
    orthopedic NEC Z47.89
    planned wound closure Z48.1
    removal of internal fixation device Z47.2
    respiratory system Z48.813
    scoliosis Z47.82
    sense organs Z48.810
    skin and subcutaneous tissue Z48.817
    specified body system
      circulatory Z48.812
      digestive Z48.815
      genitourinary Z48.816
      nervous Z48.811
      oral cavity Z48.814
      respiratory Z48.813
      sense organs Z48.810
      skin and subcutaneous tissue Z48.817
      teeth Z48.814
    specified NEC Z48.89
    spinal Z47.89
    teeth Z48.814
  fracture — *code to* fracture with seventh character D
  involving
    removal of
      drains Z48.03
      dressings (nonsurgical) Z48.00
      staples Z48.02
      surgical dressings Z48.01
      sutures Z48.02

Aftercare — *continued*
- neuropacemaker (brain) (peripheral nerve) (spinal cord) Z46.2
  - implanted Z45.42
- orthopedic NEC Z47.89
- postprocedural — *see* Aftercare, following surgery

After-cataract — *see* Cataract, secondary

Agalactia (primary) O92.3
- elective, secondary or therapeutic O92.5

Agammaglobulinemia (acquired (secondary) (nonfamilial) D80.1
- with
  - immunoglobulin-bearing B-lymphocytes D80.1
  - lymphopenia D81.9
- autosomal recessive (Swiss type) D80.0
- Bruton's X-linked D80.0
- common variable (CVAgamma) D80.1
- congenital sex-linked D80.0
- hereditary D80.0
- lymphopenic D81.9
- Swiss type (autosomal recessive) D80.0
- X-linked (with growth hormone deficiency) (Bruton) D80.0

Aganglionosis (bowel) (colon) Q43.1

Age (old) — *see* Senility

Agenesis
- adrenal (gland) Q89.1
- alimentary tract (complete) (partial) NEC Q45.8
  - upper Q40.8
- anus, anal (canal) Q42.3
  - with fistula Q42.2
- aorta Q25.41
- appendix Q42.8
- arm (complete) Q71.0- ☑
  - with hand present Q71.1- ☑
- artery (peripheral) Q27.9
  - brain Q28.3
  - coronary Q24.5
  - pulmonary Q25.79
  - specified NEC Q27.8
  - umbilical Q27.0
- auditory (canal) (external) Q16.1
- auricle (ear) Q16.0
- bile duct or passage Q44.5
- bladder Q64.5
- bone Q79.9
- brain Q00.0
  - part of Q04.3
- breast (with nipple present) Q83.8
  - with absent nipple Q83.0
- bronchus Q32.4
- canaliculus lacrimalis Q10.4
- carpus — *see* Agenesis, hand
- cartilage Q79.9
- cecum Q42.8
- cerebellum Q04.3
- cervix Q51.5
- chin Q18.8
- cilia Q10.3
- circulatory system, part NOS Q28.9
- clavicle Q74.0
- clitoris Q52.6
- coccyx Q76.49
- colon Q42.9
  - specified NEC Q42.8
- corpus callosum Q04.0
- cricoid cartilage Q31.8
- diaphragm (with hernia) Q79.1
- digestive organ(s) or tract (complete) (partial) NEC Q45.8
  - upper Q40.8
- ductus arteriosus Q28.8
- duodenum Q41.0
- ear Q16.9
  - auricle Q16.0
  - lobe Q17.8
- ejaculatory duct Q55.4
- endocrine (gland) NEC Q89.2
- epiglottis Q31.8
- esophagus Q39.8
- eustachian tube Q16.2
- eye Q11.1
  - adnexa Q15.8
- eyelid (fold) Q10.3
- face
  - bones NEC Q75.8
  - specified part NEC Q18.8
- fallopian tube Q50.6

Agenesis — *continued*
- femur — *see* Defect, reduction, lower limb, longitudinal, femur
- fibula — *see* Defect, reduction, lower limb, longitudinal, fibula
- finger (complete) (partial) — *see* Agenesis, hand
- foot (and toes) (complete) (partial) Q72.3- ☑
- forearm (with hand present) — *see* Agenesis, arm, with hand present
  - and hand Q71.2- ☑
- gallbladder Q44.0
- gastric Q40.2
- genitalia, genital (organ(s))
  - female Q52.8
    - external Q52.71
    - internal NEC Q52.8
  - male Q55.8
- glottis Q31.8
- hair Q84.0
- hand (and fingers) (complete) (partial) Q71.3- ☑
- heart Q24.8
  - valve NEC Q24.8
    - pulmonary Q22.0
- hepatic Q44.7
- humerus — *see* Defect, reduction, upper limb
- hymen Q52.4
- ileum Q41.2
- incus Q16.3
- intestine (small) Q41.9
  - large Q42.9
    - specified NEC Q42.8
- iris (dilator fibers) Q13.1
- jaw M26.09
- jejunum Q41.1
- kidney(s) (partial) Q60.2
  - bilateral Q60.1
  - unilateral Q60.0
- labium (majus) (minus) Q52.71
- labyrinth, membranous Q16.5
- lacrimal apparatus Q10.4
- larynx Q31.8
- leg (complete) Q72.0- ☑
  - with foot present Q72.1- ☑
  - lower leg (with foot present) — *see* Agenesis, leg, with foot present
  - and foot Q72.2- ☑
- lens Q12.3
- limb (complete) Q73.0
  - lower — *see* Agenesis, leg
  - upper — *see* Agenesis, arm
- lip Q38.0
- liver Q44.7
- lung (fissure) (lobe) (bilateral) (unilateral) Q33.3
- mandible, maxilla M26.09
- metacarpus — *see* Agenesis, hand
- metatarsus — *see* Agenesis, foot
- muscle Q79.8
  - eyelid Q10.3
  - ocular Q15.8
- musculoskeletal system NEC Q79.8
- nail(s) Q84.3
- neck, part Q18.8
- nerve Q07.8
- nervous system, part NEC Q07.8
- nipple Q83.2
- nose Q30.1
- nuclear Q07.8
- organ
  - of Corti Q16.5
  - or site not listed — *see* Anomaly, by site
- osseous meatus (ear) Q16.1
- ovary
  - bilateral Q50.02
  - unilateral Q50.01
- oviduct Q50.6
- pancreas Q45.0
- parathyroid (gland) Q89.2
- parotid gland(s) Q38.4
- patella Q74.1
- pelvic girdle (complete) (partial) Q74.2
- penis Q55.5
- pericardium Q24.8
- pituitary (gland) Q89.2
- prostate Q55.4
- punctum lacrimale Q10.4
- radioulnar — *see* Defect, reduction, upper limb
- radius — *see* Defect, reduction, upper limb, longitudinal, radius

Agenesis — *continued*
- rectum Q42.1
  - with fistula Q42.0
- renal Q60.2
  - bilateral Q60.1
  - unilateral Q60.0
- respiratory organ NEC Q34.8
- rib Q76.6
- roof of orbit Q75.8
- round ligament Q52.8
- sacrum Q76.49
- salivary gland Q38.4
- scapula Q74.0
- scrotum Q55.29
- seminal vesicles Q55.4
- septum
  - atrial Q21.19
  - between aorta and pulmonary artery Q21.4
  - ventricular Q20.4
- shoulder girdle (complete) (partial) Q74.0
- skull (bone) Q75.8
  - with
    - anencephaly Q00.0
    - encephalocele — *see* Encephalocele
    - hydrocephalus Q03.9
      - with spina bifida — *see* Spina bifida, by site, with hydrocephalus
    - microcephaly Q02
- spermatic cord Q55.4
- spinal cord Q06.0
- spine Q76.49
- spleen Q89.01
- sternum Q76.7
- stomach Q40.2
- submaxillary gland(s) (congenital) Q38.4
- tarsus — *see* Agenesis, foot
- tendon Q79.8
- testicle Q55.0
- thymus (gland) Q89.2
- thyroid (gland) E03.1
  - cartilage Q31.8
- tibia — *see* Defect, reduction, lower limb, longitudinal, tibia
- tibiofibular — *see* Defect, reduction, lower limb, specified type NEC
- toe (and foot) (complete) (partial) — *see* Agenesis, foot
- tongue Q38.3
- trachea (cartilage) Q32.1
- ulna — *see* Defect, reduction, upper limb, longitudinal, ulna
- upper limb — *see* Agenesis, arm
- ureter Q62.4
- urethra Q64.5
- urinary tract NEC Q64.8
- uterus Q51.0
- uvula Q38.5
- vagina Q52.0
- vas deferens Q55.4
- vein(s) (peripheral) Q27.9
  - brain Q28.3
  - great NEC Q26.8
  - portal Q26.5
- vena cava (inferior) (superior) Q26.8
- vermis of cerebellum Q04.3
- vertebra Q76.49
- vulva Q52.71

Ageusia R43.2

Agitated — *see* condition

Agitation R45.1

Aglossia (congenital) Q38.3

Aglossia-adactylia syndrome Q87.0

Aglycogenosis E74.00

Agnosia (body image) (other senses) (tactile) R48.1
- developmental F88
- verbal R48.1
  - auditory R48.1
    - developmental F80.2
  - developmental F80.2
- visual (object) R48.3

Agoraphobia F40.00
- with panic disorder F40.01
- without panic disorder F40.02

Agrammatism R48.8

Agranulocytopenia — *see* Agranulocytosis

Agranulocytosis (chronic) (cyclical) (genetic) (infantile) (periodic) (pernicious) — *see also* Neutropenia D70.9
- congenital D70.0

Agranulocytosis — continued
cytoreductive cancer chemotherapy sequela D70.1
drug-induced D70.2
  due to cytoreductive cancer chemotherapy D70.1
due to infection D70.3
secondary D70.4
  drug-induced D70.2
    due to cytoreductive cancer chemotherapy D70.1
Agraphia (absolute) R48.8
with alexia R48.0
developmental F81.81
Ague (dumb) — see Malaria
Agyria Q04.3
Ahumada-del Castillo syndrome E23.0
Aichomophobia F40.298
AIDS (related complex) B20
Ailment heart — see Disease, heart
Ailurophobia F40.218
AIN — see Neoplasia, intraepithelial, anal
Ainhum (disease) L94.6
AIPHI (acute idiopathic pulmonary hemorrhage in infants (over 28 days old)) R04.81
Air
anterior mediastinum J98.2
compressed, disease T70.3 ☑
conditioner lung or pneumonitis J67.7
embolism (artery) (cerebral) (any site) T79.0 ☑
  with ectopic or molar pregnancy O08.2
  due to implanted device NEC — see Complications, by site and type, specified NEC
  following
    abortion — see Abortion by type, complicated by, embolism
    ectopic or molar pregnancy O08.2
    infusion, therapeutic injection or transfusion T80.0 ☑
  in pregnancy, childbirth or puerperium — see Embolism, obstetric
  traumatic T79.0 ☑
hunger, psychogenic F45.8
rarefied, effects of — see Effect, adverse, high altitude
sickness T75.3 ☑
Airplane sickness T75.3 ☑
Akathisia (drug-induced) (treatment-induced) G25.71
neuroleptic induced (acute) G25.71
tardive G25.71
Akinesia R29.898
Akinetic mutism R41.89
Akureyri's disease G93.39
Alactasia, congenital E73.0
Alagille's syndrome Q44.7
Alastrim B03
Albers-Schönberg syndrome Q78.2
Albert's syndrome — see Tendinitis, Achilles
Albinism, albino E70.30
with hematologic abnormality E70.339
  Chédiak-Higashi syndrome E70.330
  Hermansky-Pudlak syndrome E70.331
  other specified E70.338
  I E70.320
  II E70.321
ocular E70.319
  autosomal recessive E70.311
  other specified E70.318
  X-linked E70.310
oculocutaneous E70.329
  other specified E70.328
  tyrosinase (ty) negative E70.320
  tyrosinase (ty) positive E70.321
other specified E70.39
Albinismus E70.30
Albright (-McCune)(-Sternberg) syndrome Q78.1
Albuminous — see condition
Albuminuria, albuminuric (acute) (chronic) (subacute) — see also Proteinuria R80.9
complicating pregnancy — see Proteinuria, gestational
  with
    gestational hypertension — see Pre-eclampsia
    pre-existing hypertension — see Hypertension, complicating pregnancy, pre-existing, with, pre-eclampsia
gestational — see Proteinuria, gestational
  with
    gestational hypertension — see Pre-eclampsia
    pre-existing hypertension — see Hypertension, complicating pregnancy, pre-existing, with, pre-eclampsia

Albuminuria, albuminuric — continued
orthostatic R80.2
postural R80.2
pre-eclamptic — see Pre-eclampsia
scarlatinal A38.8
Albuminurophobia F40.298
Alcaptonuria E70.29
Alcohol, alcoholic, alcohol-induced
addiction (without remission) F10.20
  with remission F10.21
amnestic disorder, persisting F10.96
  with dependence F10.26
anxiety disorder F10.980
bipolar and related disorder F10.94
brain syndrome, chronic F10.97
  with dependence F10.27
cardiopathy I42.6
counseling and surveillance Z71.41
  family member Z71.42
delirium (acute) (tremens) (withdrawal) F10.921
  with intoxication F10.921
  in
    abuse F10.121
    dependence F10.221
  dependence (acute) (tremens) (withdrawal) F10.231
dementia F10.97
  with dependence F10.27
depressive disorder F10.94
deterioration F10.97
  with dependence F10.27
hallucinosis (acute) F10.951
  in
    abuse F10.151
    dependence F10.251
insanity F10.959
intoxication (acute) (without dependence) F10.129
  with
    delirium F10.121
    dependence F10.229
      with delirium F10.221
      uncomplicated F10.220
    uncomplicated F10.120
jealousy F10.988
Korsakoff's, Korsakov's, Korsakow's F10.26
liver K70.9
  acute — see Disease, liver, alcoholic, hepatitis
major neurocognitive disorder, amnestic-confabulatory type F10.96
major neurocognitive disorder, nonamnestic-confabulatory type F10.97
mania (acute) (chronic) F10.959
mild neurocognitive disorder F10.988
paranoia, paranoid (type) psychosis F10.950
pellagra E52
poisoning, accidental (acute) NEC — see Table of Drugs and Chemicals, alcohol, poisoning
psychosis — see Psychosis, alcoholic
psychotic disorder F10.959
sexual dysfunction F10.981
sleep disorder F10.982
withdrawal (without convulsions) F10.239
  with delirium F10.231
Alcoholism (chronic) (without remission) F10.20
with
  psychosis — see Psychosis, alcoholic
  remission F10.21
Korsakov's F10.96
  with dependence F10.26
Alder (-Reilly) **anomaly or syndrome** (leukocyte granulation) D72.0
Aldosteronism E26.9
familial (type I) E26.02
glucocorticoid-remediable E26.02
primary (due to (bilateral) adrenal hyperplasia) E26.09
primary NEC E26.09
secondary E26.1
specified NEC E26.89
Aldosteronoma D44.10
Aldrich (-Wiskott) **syndrome** (eczema-thrombocytopenia) D82.0
Alektorophobia F40.218
Aleppo boil B55.1
Aleukemic — see condition
Aleukia
congenital D70.0
hemorrhagica D61.9
  congenital D61.09
splenica D73.1

Alexia R48.0
developmental F81.0
secondary to organic lesion R48.0
Algoneurodystrophy M89.00
ankle M89.07- ☑
foot M89.07- ☑
forearm M89.03- ☑
hand M89.04- ☑
lower leg M89.06- ☑
multiple sites M89.0- ☑
shoulder M89.01- ☑
specified site NEC M89.08
thigh M89.05- ☑
upper arm M89.02- ☑
Algophobia F40.298
Alienation, mental — see Psychosis
Alkalemia E87.3
Alkalosis E87.3
metabolic E87.3
  with respiratory acidosis E87.4
  of newborn P74.41
respiratory E87.3
Alkaptonuria E70.29
Allen-Masters syndrome N83.8
Allergy, allergic (reaction) (to) T78.40 ☑
air-borne substance NEC (rhinitis) J30.89
alveolitis (extrinsic) J67.9
  due to
    Aspergillus clavatus J67.4
    Cryptostroma corticale J67.6
    organisms (fungal, thermophilic actinomycete) growing in ventilation (air conditioning) systems J67.7
    specified type NEC J67.8
anaphylactic reaction or shock T78.2 ☑
angioneurotic edema T78.3 ☑
animal (dander) (epidermal) (hair) (rhinitis) J30.81
bee sting (anaphylactic shock) — see Toxicity, venom, arthropod, bee
biological — see Allergy, drug
colitis — see also Colitis, allergic K52.29
dander (animal) (rhinitis) J30.81
dandruff (rhinitis) J30.81
dental restorative material (existing) K08.55
dermatitis — see Dermatitis, contact, allergic
diathesis — see History, allergy
drug, medicament & biological (any) (external) (internal) T78.40 ☑
  correct substance properly administered — see Table of Drugs and Chemicals, by drug, adverse effect
  wrong substance given or taken NEC (by accident) — see Table of Drugs and Chemicals, by drug, poisoning
due to pollen J30.1
dust (house) (stock) (rhinitis) J30.89
  with asthma — see Asthma, allergic extrinsic
eczema — see Dermatitis, contact, allergic
epidermal (animal) (rhinitis) J30.81
feathers (rhinitis) J30.89
food (any) (ingested) NEC T78.1 ☑
  anaphylactic shock — see Shock, anaphylactic, due to food
  dermatitis — see Dermatitis, due to, food
  dietary counseling and surveillance Z71.3
  in contact with skin L23.6
  rhinitis J30.5
  status (without reaction) Z91.018
    beef Z91.014
    eggs Z91.012
    lamb Z91.014
    mammalian meats Z91.014
    milk products Z91.011
    peanuts Z91.010
    pork Z91.014
    red meats Z91.014
    seafood Z91.013
    specified NEC Z91.018
  gastrointestinal — see also specific type of allergic reaction
    meaning colitis — see also Colitis, allergic K52.29
    meaning gastroenteritis — see also Gastroenteritis, allergic K52.29
    meaning other adverse food reaction not elsewhere classified T78.1 ☑
grain J30.1
grass (hay fever) (pollen) J30.1

Allergy, allergic — *continued*
  grass — *continued*
    asthma — *see* Asthma, allergic extrinsic
  hair (animal) (rhinitis) J30.81
  history (of) — *see* History, allergy
  horse serum — *see* Allergy, serum
  inhalant (rhinitis) J30.89
    pollen J30.1
  kapok (rhinitis) J30.89
  medicine — *see* Allergy, drug
  milk protein — *see also* Allergy, food Z91.011
    anaphylactic reaction T78.07 ☑
    dermatitis L27.2
    enterocolitis syndrome K52.21
    enteropathy K52.22
    gastroenteritis K52.29
    gastroesophageal reflux — *see also* Reaction, adverse, food K21.9
      with esophagitis (without bleeding) K21.00
        with bleeding K21.01
    proctocolitis K52.29
  nasal, seasonal due to pollen J30.1
  pneumonia J82.89
  pollen (any) (hay fever) J30.1
    asthma — *see* Asthma, allergic extrinsic
  primrose J30.1
  primula J30.1
  proctocolitis K52.29
  purpura D69.0
  ragweed (hay fever) (pollen) J30.1
    asthma — *see* Asthma, allergic extrinsic
  rose (pollen) J30.1
  seasonal NEC J30.2
  Senecio jacobae (pollen) J30.1
  serum — *see also* Reaction, serum T80.69 ☑
    anaphylactic shock T80.59 ☑
  shock (anaphylactic) T78.2 ☑
    due to
      administration of blood and blood products T80.51 ☑
      adverse effect of correct medicinal substance properly administered T88.6 ☑
      immunization T80.52 ☑
      serum NEC T80.59 ☑
      vaccination T80.52 ☑
  specific NEC T78.49 ☑
  tree (any) (hay fever) (pollen) J30.1
    asthma — *see* Asthma, allergic extrinsic
  upper respiratory J30.9
  urticaria L50.0
  vaccine — *see* Allergy, serum
  wheat — *see* Allergy, food
Allescheriasis B48.2
Alligator skin disease Q80.9
Allocheiria, allochiria R20.8
Almeida's disease — *see* Paracoccidioidomycosis
Alopecia (hereditaria) (seborrheica) L65.9
  androgenic L64.9
    drug-induced L64.0
    specified NEC L64.8
  areata L63.9
    ophiasis L63.2
    specified NEC L63.8
    totalis L63.0
    universalis L63.1
  cicatricial L66.9
    specified NEC L66.8
  circumscripta L63.9
  congenital, congenitalis Q84.0
  due to cytotoxic drugs NEC L65.8
  mucinosa L65.2
  postinfective NEC L65.8
  postpartum L65.0
  premature L64.8
  specific (syphilitic) A51.32
  specified NEC L65.8
  syphilitic (secondary) A51.32
  totalis (capitis) L63.0
  universalis (entire body) L63.1
  X-ray L58.1
Alpers' disease G31.81
Alpine sickness T70.29 ☑
Alport syndrome Q87.81
ALTE (apparent life threatening event) **in newborn and infant** R68.13
Alteration (of), **Altered**
  awareness
    transient R40.4

Alteration (of), **Altered** — *continued*
  awareness — *continued*
    unintended under general anesthesia, during procedure T88.53 ☑
  mental status R41.82
  pattern of family relationships affecting child Z62.898
  sensation
    following
      cerebrovascular disease I69.998
        cerebral infarction I69.398
        intracerebral hemorrhage I69.198
        nontraumatic intracranial hemorrhage NEC I69.298
        specified disease NEC I69.898
        subarachnoid hemorrhage I69.098
Alternating — *see* condition
Altitude, high (effects) — *see* Effect, adverse, high altitude
Aluminosis (of lung) J63.0
Alveolitis
  allergic (extrinsic) — *see* Pneumonitis, hypersensitivity
  due to
    Aspergillus clavatus J67.4
    Cryptostroma corticale J67.6
  fibrosing (cryptogenic) (idiopathic) J84.112
  jaw M27.3
  sicca dolorosa M27.3
Alveolus, alveolar — *see* condition
Alymphocytosis D72.810
  thymic (with immunodeficiency) D82.1
Alymphoplasia, thymic D82.1
Alzheimer's disease or sclerosis — *see* Disease, Alzheimer's
Amastia (with nipple present) Q83.8
  with absent nipple Q83.0
Amathophobia F40.228
Amaurosis (acquired) (congenital) — *see also* Blindness
  fugax G45.3
  hysterical F44.6
  Leber's congenital H35.50
  uremic — *see* Uremia
Amaurotic idiocy (infantile) (juvenile) (late) E75.4
Amaxophobia F40.248
Ambiguous genitalia Q56.4
Amblyopia (congenital) (ex anopsia) (partial) (suppression) H53.00- ☑
  anisometropic — *see* Amblyopia, refractive
  deprivation H53.01- ☑
  hysterical F44.6
  nocturnal — *see also* Blindness, night
    vitamin A deficiency E50.5
  refractive H53.02- ☑
  strabismic H53.03- ☑
  suspect H53.04- ☑
  tobacco H53.8
  toxic NEC H53.8
  uremic — *see* Uremia
Ameba, amebic (histolytica) — *see also* Amebiasis
  abscess (liver) A06.4
Amebiasis A06.9
  with abscess — *see* Abscess, amebic
  acute A06.0
  chronic (intestine) A06.1
    with abscess — *see* Abscess, amebic
  cutaneous A06.7
  cutis A06.7
  cystitis A06.81
  genitourinary tract NEC A06.82
  hepatic — *see* Abscess, liver, amebic
  intestine A06.0
  nondysenteric colitis A06.2
  skin A06.7
  specified site NEC A06.89
Ameboma (of intestine) A06.3
Amelia Q73.0
  lower limb — *see* Agenesis, leg
  upper limb — *see* Agenesis, arm
Ameloblastoma — *see also* Cyst, calcifying odontogenic
  long bones C40.9- ☑
    lower limb C40.2- ☑
    upper limb C40.0- ☑
  malignant C41.1
    jaw (bone) (lower) C41.1
      upper C41.0
  tibial C40.2- ☑
Amelogenesis imperfecta K00.5
  nonhereditaria (segmentalis) K00.4

Amenorrhea N91.2
  hyperhormonal E28.8
  primary N91.0
  secondary N91.1
Amentia — *see* Disability, intellectual
  Meynert's (nonalcoholic) F04
American
  leishmaniasis B55.2
  mountain tick fever A93.2
Ametropia — *see* Disorder, refraction
AMH (asymptomatic microscopic hematuria) R31.21
Amianthosis J61
Amimia R48.8
Amino-acid disorder E72.9
  anemia D53.0
Aminoacidopathy E72.9
Aminoaciduria E72.9
Amnesia R41.3
  anterograde R41.1
  auditory R48.8
  dissociative F44.0
    with dissociative fugue F44.1
  hysterical F44.0
  postictal in epilepsy — *see* Epilepsy
  psychogenic F44.0
  retrograde R41.2
  transient global G45.4
Amnes(t)ic syndrome (post-traumatic) F04
  induced by
    alcohol F10.96
      with dependence F10.26
    psychoactive NEC F19.96
      with
        abuse F19.16
        dependence F19.26
    sedative F13.96
      with dependence F13.26
Amnion, amniotic — *see* condition
Amnionitis — *see* Pregnancy, complicated by
Amok F68.8
Amoral traits F60.89
Amphetamine (or other stimulant) **-induced**
  anxiety disorder F15.980
  bipolar and related disorder F15.94
  delirium F15.921
  depressive disorder F15.94
  obsessive-compulsive and related disorder F15.988
  psychotic disorder F15.959
  sexual dysfunction F15.981
  sleep disorder F15.982
  stimulant withdrawal F15.23
Ampulla
  lower esophagus K22.89
  phrenic K22.89
Amputation — *see also* Absence, by site, acquired
  neuroma (postoperative) (traumatic) — *see* Complications, amputation stump, neuroma
  stump (surgical)
    abnormal, painful, or with complication (late) — *see* Complications, amputation stump
    healed or old NOS Z89.9
  traumatic (complete) (partial)
    arm (upper) (complete) S48.91- ☑
      at
        elbow S58.01- ☑
          partial S58.02- ☑
        shoulder joint (complete) S48.01- ☑
          partial S48.02- ☑
      between
        elbow and wrist (complete) S58.11- ☑
          partial S58.12- ☑
        shoulder and elbow (complete) S48.11- ☑
          partial S48.12- ☑
      partial S48.92- ☑
    breast (complete) S28.21- ☑
      partial S28.22- ☑
    clitoris (complete) S38.211 ☑
      partial S38.212
    ear (complete) S08.11- ☑
      partial S08.12- ☑
    finger (complete) (metacarpophalangeal) S68.11- ☑
      index S68.11- ☑
      little S68.11- ☑
      middle S68.11- ☑
      partial S68.12- ☑
        index S68.12- ☑
        little S68.12- ☑

Amputation — *continued*
  traumatic — *continued*
    finger — *continued*
      partial — *continued*
        middle S68.12- ☑
        ring S68.12- ☑
      ring S68.11- ☑
      thumb — *see* Amputation, traumatic, thumb
      transphalangeal (complete) S68.61- ☑
        index S68.61- ☑
        little S68.61- ☑
        middle S68.61- ☑
        partial S68.62- ☑
          index S68.62- ☑
          little S68.62- ☑
          middle S68.62- ☑
          ring S68.62- ☑
        ring S68.61- ☑
    foot (complete) S98.91- ☑
      at ankle level S98.01- ☑
        partial S98.02- ☑
      midfoot S98.31- ☑
        partial S98.32- ☑
      partial S98.92- ☑
    forearm (complete) S58.91- ☑
      at elbow level (complete) S58.01- ☑
        partial S58.02- ☑
      between elbow and wrist (complete) S58.11- ☑
        partial S58.12- ☑
      partial S58.92- ☑
    genital organ(s) (external)
      female (complete) S38.211 ☑
        partial S38.212 ☑
      male
        penis (complete) S38.221 ☑
          partial S38.222 ☑
        scrotum (complete) S38.231 ☑
          partial S38.232 ☑
        testes (complete) S38.231 ☑
          partial S38.232 ☑
    hand (complete) (wrist level) S68.41- ☑
      finger(s) alone — *see* Amputation, traumatic, finger
      partial S68.42- ☑
      thumb alone — *see* Amputation, traumatic, thumb
      transmetacarpal (complete) S68.71- ☑
        partial S68.72- ☑
    head
      ear — *see* Amputation, traumatic, ear
      nose (partial) S08.812 ☑
        complete S08.811 ☑
      part S08.89 ☑
        scalp S08.0 ☑
    hip (and thigh) (complete) S78.91- ☑
      at hip joint (complete) S78.01- ☑
        partial S78.02- ☑
      between hip and knee (complete) S78.11- ☑
        partial S78.12- ☑
      partial S78.92- ☑
    labium (majus) (minus) (complete) S38.21- ☑
      partial S38.21- ☑
    leg (lower) S88.91- ☑
      at knee level S88.01- ☑
        partial S88.02- ☑
      between knee and ankle S88.11- ☑
        partial S88.12- ☑
      partial S88.92- ☑
    nose (partial) S08.812 ☑
      complete S08.811 ☑
    penis (complete) S38.221 ☑
      partial S38.222 ☑
    scrotum (complete) S38.231 ☑
      partial S38.232 ☑
    shoulder — *see* Amputation, traumatic, arm
      at shoulder joint — *see* Amputation, traumatic, arm, at shoulder joint
    testes (complete) S38.231 ☑
      partial S38.232 ☑
    thigh — *see* Amputation, traumatic, hip
    thorax, part of S28.1 ☑
      breast — *see* Amputation, traumatic, breast
    thumb (complete) (metacarpophalangeal)
      S68.01- ☑
      partial S68.02- ☑
      transphalangeal (complete) S68.51- ☑

Amputation — *continued*
  traumatic — *continued*
    thumb — *continued*
      transphalangeal — *continued*
        partial S68.52- ☑
    toe (lesser) S98.13- ☑
      great S98.11- ☑
        partial S98.12- ☑
      more than one S98.21- ☑
        partial S98.22- ☑
      partial S98.14- ☑
    vulva (complete) S38.211 ☑
      partial S38.212 ☑
Amputee (bilateral) (old) Z89.9
Amsterdam dwarfism Q87.19
Amusia R48.8
  developmental F80.89
Amyelencephalus, amyelencephaly Q00.0
Amyelia Q06.0
Amygdalitis — *see* Tonsillitis
Amygdalolith J35.8
Amyloid heart (disease) E85.4 *[I43]*
Amyloidosis (generalized) (primary) E85.9
  with lung involvement E85.4 *[J99]*
  familial E85.2
  genetic E85.2
  heart E85.4 *[I43]*
  hemodialysis-associated E85.3
  light chain (AL) E85.81
  liver E85.4 *[K77]*
  localized E85.4
  neuropathic heredofamilial E85.1
  non-neuropathic heredofamilial E85.0
  organ limited E85.4
  Portuguese E85.1
  pulmonary E85.4 *[J99]*
  secondary systemic E85.3
  senile systemic (SSA) E85.82
  skin (lichen) (macular) E85.4 *[L99]*
  specified NEC E85.89
  subglottic E85.4 *[J99]*
  wild-type transthyretin-related (ATTR) E85.82
Amylopectinosis (brancher enzyme deficiency) E74.03
Amylophagia — *see* Pica
Amyoplasia congenita Q79.8
Amyotonia M62.89
  congenita G70.2
Amyotrophia, amyotrophy, amyotrophic G71.8
  congenita Q79.8
  diabetic — *see* Diabetes, amyotrophy
  lateral sclerosis G12.21
  neuralgic G54.5
  spinal progressive G12.25
Anacidity, gastric K31.83
  psychogenic F45.8
Anaerosis of newborn P28.89
Analbuminemia E88.09
Analgesia — *see* Anesthesia
Analphalipoproteinemia E78.6
Anaphylactic
  purpura D69.0
  shock or reaction — *see* Shock, anaphylactic
Anaphylactoid shock or reaction — *see* Shock, anaphylactic
Anaphylactoid syndrome of pregnancy O88.01- ☑
Anaphylaxis — *see* Shock, anaphylactic
Anaplasia cervix — *see also* Dysplasia, cervix N87.9
Anaplasmosis [A. phagocytophilum] (transfusion transmitted) A79.82
  human A77.49
Anarthria R47.1
Anasarca R60.1
  cardiac — *see* Failure, heart, congestive
  lung J18.2
  newborn P83.2
  nutritional E43
  pulmonary J18.2
  renal N04.9
Anastomosis
  aneurysmal — *see* Aneurysm
  arteriovenous ruptured brain I60.8
    intracerebral I61.8
    intraparenchymal I61.8
    intraventricular I61.5
    subarachnoid I60.8
  intestinal K63.89
    complicated NEC K91.89

Anastomosis — *continued*
  intestinal — *continued*
    complicated — *continued*
      involving urinary tract N99.89
  retinal and choroidal vessels (congenital) Q14.8
Anatomical narrow angle H40.03- ☑
Ancylostoma, ancylostomiasis (braziliense) (caninum) (ceylanicum) (duodenale) B76.0
  Necator americanus B76.1
Andersen's disease (glycogen storage) E74.09
Anderson-Fabry disease E75.21
Andes disease T70.29 ☑
Andrews' disease (bacterid) L08.89
Androblastoma
  benign
    specified site — *see* Neoplasm, benign, by site
    unspecified site
      female D27.9
      male D29.20
  malignant
    specified site — *see* Neoplasm, malignant, by site
    unspecified site
      female C56.9
      male C62.90
  specified site — *see* Neoplasm, uncertain behavior, by site
  tubular
    with lipid storage
      specified site — *see* Neoplasm, benign, by site
      unspecified site
        female D27.9
        male D29.20
    specified site — *see* Neoplasm, benign, by site
    unspecified site
      female D27.9
      male D29.20
  unspecified site
    female D39.10
    male D40.10
Androgen insensitivity syndrome — *see also* Syndrome, androgen insensitivity E34.50
Androgen resistance syndrome — *see also* Syndrome, androgen insensitivity E34.50
Android pelvis Q74.2
  with disproportion (fetopelvic) O33.3 ☑
    causing obstructed labor O65.3
Androphobia F40.290
Anectasis, pulmonary (newborn) — *see* Atelectasis
Anemia (essential) (general) (hemoglobin deficiency) (infantile) (primary) (profound) D64.9
  with (due to) (in)
    disorder of
      anaerobic glycolysis D55.29
      pentose phosphate pathway D55.1
    koilonychia D50.9
  achlorhydric D50.8
  achrestic D53.1
  Addison (-Biermer) (pernicious) D51.0
  agranulocytic — *see* Agranulocytosis
  amino-acid-deficiency D53.0
  aplastic D61.9
    congenital D61.09
    drug-induced D61.1
    due to
      drugs D61.1
      external agents NEC D61.2
      infection D61.2
      radiation D61.2
    idiopathic D61.3
    red cell (pure) D60.9
      chronic D60.0
      congenital D61.01
      specified type NEC D60.8
      transient D60.1
    specified type NEC D61.89
    toxic D61.2
  aregenerative
    congenital D61.09
  asiderotic D50.9
  atypical (primary) D64.9
  Baghdad spring D55.0
  Balantidium coli A07.0
  Biermer's (pernicious) D51.0
  blood loss (chronic) D50.0
    acute D62
  bothriocephalus B70.0 *[D63.8]*
  brickmaker's B76.9 *[D63.8]*
  cerebral I67.89

Anemia — *continued*
  childhood D58.9
  chlorotic D50.8
  chronic
    blood loss D50.0
    hemolytic D58.9
      idiopathic D59.9
    simple D53.9
  chronica congenita aregenerativa D61.09
  combined system disease NEC D51.0 *[G32.0]*
    due to dietary vitamin B12 deficiency D51.3 *[G32.0]*
  complicating pregnancy, childbirth or puerperium —
    see Pregnancy, complicated by (management
    affected by), anemia
  congenital P61.4
    aplastic D61.09
    due to isoimmunization NOS P55.9
    dyserythropoietic, dyshematopoietic D64.4
    following fetal blood loss P61.3
    Heinz body D58.2
    hereditary hemolytic NOS D58.9
    pernicious D51.0
    spherocytic D58.0
  Cooley's (erythroblastic) D56.1
  cytogenic D51.0
  deficiency D53.9
    2, 3 diphosphoglycurate mutase D55.29
    2, 3 PG D55.29
    6 phosphogluconate dehydrogenase D55.1
    6-PGD D55.1
    amino-acid D53.0
    combined B12 and folate D53.1
    enzyme D55.9
      drug-induced (hemolytic) D59.2
      glucose-6-phosphate dehydrogenase (G6PD)
        D55.0
      glycolytic D55.29
      nucleotide metabolism D55.3
      related to hexose monophosphate (HMP) shunt
        pathway NEC D55.1
      specified type NEC D55.8
    erythrocytic glutathione D55.1
    folate D52.9
      dietary D52.0
      drug-induced D52.1
    folic acid D52.9
      dietary D52.0
      drug-induced D52.1
    G SH D55.1
    G6PD D55.0
    GGS-R D55.1
    glucose-6-phosphate dehydrogenase D55.0
    glutathione reductase D55.1
    glyceraldehyde phosphate dehydrogenase D55.29
    hexokinase D55.29
    iron D50.9
      secondary to blood loss (chronic) D50.0
    nutritional D53.9
      with
        poor iron absorption D50.8
        specified deficiency NEC D53.8
    phosphofructo-aldolase D55.29
    phosphoglycerate kinase D55.29
    PK D55.21
    protein D53.0
    pyruvate kinase D55.21
    transcobalamin II D51.2
    triose-phosphate isomerase D55.29
    vitamin B12 NOS D51.9
      dietary D51.3
      due to
        intrinsic factor deficiency D51.0
        selective vitamin B12 malabsorption with
          proteinuria D51.1
      pernicious D51.0
      specified type NEC D51.8
  Diamond-Blackfan (congenital hypoplastic) D61.01
  dibothriocephalus B70.0 *[D63.8]*
  dimorphic D53.1
  diphasic D53.1
  Diphyllobothrium (Dibothriocephalus) B70.0 *[D63.8]*
  due to (in) (with)
    antineoplastic chemotherapy D64.81
    blood loss (chronic) D50.0
      acute D62
    chemotherapy, antineoplastic D64.81
    chronic disease classified elsewhere NEC D63.8
    chronic kidney disease D63.1

Anemia — *continued*
  due to — *continued*
    deficiency
      amino-acid D53.0
      copper D53.8
      folate (folic acid) D52.9
        dietary D52.0
        drug-induced D52.1
      molybdenum D53.8
      protein D53.0
      zinc D53.8
    dietary vitamin B12 deficiency D51.3
    disorder of
      glutathione metabolism D55.1
      nucleotide metabolism D55.3
    drug — *see* Anemia, by type — *see also* Table of
      Drugs and Chemicals
    end stage renal disease D63.1
    enzyme disorder D55.9
    fetal blood loss P61.3
    fish tapeworm (D.latum) infestation B70.0 *[D63.8]*
    hemorrhage (chronic) D50.0
      acute D62
    impaired absorption D50.9
    loss of blood (chronic) D50.0
      acute D62
    myxedema E03.9 *[D63.8]*
    Necator americanus B76.1 *[D63.8]*
    prematurity P61.2
    selective vitamin B12 malabsorption with protein-
      uria D51.1
    transcobalamin II deficiency D51.2
  Dyke-Young type (secondary) (symptomatic) D59.19
  dyserythropoietic (congenital) D64.4
  dyshematopoietic (congenital) D64.4
  Egyptian B76.9 *[D63.8]*
  elliptocytosis — *see* Elliptocytosis
  enzyme-deficiency, drug-induced D59.2
  epidemic — *see also* Ancylostomiasis B76.9 *[D63.8]*
  erythroblastic
    familial D56.1
    newborn — *see also* Disease, hemolytic P55.9
    of childhood D56.1
  erythrocytic glutathione deficiency D55.1
  erythropoietin-resistant anemia (EPO resistant anemia)
    D63.1
  Faber's (achlorhydric anemia) D50.9
  factitious (self-induced blood letting) D50.0
  familial erythroblastic D56.1
  Fanconi's (congenital pancytopenia) D61.09
  favism D55.0
  fish tapeworm (D. latum) infestation B70.0 *[D63.8]*
  folate (folic acid) deficiency D52.9
  glucose-6-phosphate dehydrogenase (G6PD) deficiency
    D55.0
  glutathione-reductase deficiency D55.1
  goat's milk D52.0
  granulocytic — *see* Agranulocytosis
  Heinz body, congenital D58.2
  hemolytic D58.9
    acquired D59.9
      with hemoglobinuria NEC D59.6
      autoimmune NEC D59.19
      infectious D59.4
      specified type NEC D59.8
      toxic D59.4
    acute D59.9
      due to enzyme deficiency specified type NEC
        D55.8
      Lederer's D59.19
    autoimmune D59.10
      cold D59.12
      drug-induced D59.0
      mixed D59.13
      warm D59.11
    chronic D58.9
      idiopathic D59.9
    cold type (primary) (secondary) (symptomatic)
      D59.12
    congenital (spherocytic) — *see* Spherocytosis
    due to
      cardiac conditions D59.4
      drugs (nonautoimmune) D59.2
        autoimmune D59.0
      enzyme disorder D55.9
        drug-induced D59.2
      presence of shunt or other internal prosthetic
        device D59.4

Anemia — *continued*
  hemolytic — *continued*
    familial D58.9
    hereditary D58.9
      due to enzyme disorder D55.9
        specified type NEC D55.8
      specified type NEC D58.8
    idiopathic (chronic) D59.9
    mechanical D59.4
    microangiopathic D59.4
    mixed type (primary) (secondary) (symptomatic)
      D59.13
    nonautoimmune D59.4
      drug-induced D59.2
    nonspherocytic
      congenital or hereditary NEC D55.8
        glucose-6-phosphate dehydrogenase deficien-
          cy D55.0
        pyruvate kinase deficiency D55.21
        type
          I D55.1
          II D55.29
      type
        I D55.1
        II D55.29
    primary
      autoimmune
        cold type D59.12
        mixed type D59.13
        warm type D59.11
    secondary D59.4
      autoimmune
        cold type D59.12
        mixed type D59.13
        warm type D59.11
    specified (hereditary) type NEC D58.8
    Stransky-Regala type — *see also* Hemoglobinopathy
      D58.8
    symptomatic D59.4
      autoimmune
        cold type D59.12
        mixed type D59.13
        warm type D59.11
    toxic D59.4
    warm type (primary) (secondary) (symptomatic)
      D59.11
  hemorrhagic (chronic) D50.0
    acute D62
  Herrick's D57.1
  hexokinase deficiency D55.29
  hookworm B76.9 *[D63.8]*
  hypochromic (idiopathic) (microcytic) (normoblastic)
    D50.9
    due to blood loss (chronic) D50.0
      acute D62
    familial sex-linked D64.0
    pyridoxine-responsive D64.3
    sideroblastic, sex-linked D64.0
  hypoplasia, red blood cells D61.9
    congenital or familial D61.01
  hypoplastic (idiopathic) D61.9
    congenital or familial (of childhood) D61.01
  hypoproliferative (refractive) D61.9
  idiopathic D64.9
    aplastic D61.3
    hemolytic, chronic D59.9
  in (due to) (with)
    chronic kidney disease D63.1
    end stage renal disease D63.1
    failure, kidney (renal) D63.1
    neoplastic disease — *see also* Neoplasm D63.0
  intertropical — *see also* Ancylostomiasis D63.8
  iron deficiency D50.9
    secondary to blood loss (chronic) D50.0
      acute D62
    specified type NEC D50.8
  Joseph-Diamond-Blackfan (congenital hypoplastic)
    D61.01
  Lederer's (hemolytic) D59.19
  leukoerythroblastic D61.82
  macrocytic D53.9
    nutritional D52.0
    tropical D52.8
  malarial — *see also* Malaria B54 *[D63.8]*
  malignant (progressive) D51.0
  malnutrition D53.9
  marsh — *see also* Malaria B54 *[D63.8]*
  Mediterranean (with other hemoglobinopathy) D56.9
  megaloblastic D53.1

Anemia — *continued*
 megaloblastic — *continued*
  combined B12 and folate deficiency D53.1
  hereditary D51.1
  nutritional D52.0
  orotic aciduria D53.0
  refractory D53.1
  specified type NEC D53.1
 megalocytic D53.1
 microcytic (hypochromic) D50.9
  due to blood loss (chronic) D50.0
   acute D62
  familial D56.8
 microdrepanocytosis D57.40
 microelliptopoikilocytic (Rietti-Greppi- Micheli) D56.9
 miner's B76.9 *[D63.8]*
 myelodysplastic D46.9
 myelofibrosis D75.81
 myelogenous D64.89
 myelopathic D64.89
 myelophthisic D61.82
 myeloproliferative D47.Z9 (*following* D47.4)
 newborn P61.4
  due to
   ABO (antibodies, isoimmunization, maternal/fetal incompatibility) P55.1
   Rh (antibodies, isoimmunization, maternal/fetal incompatibility) P55.0
  following fetal blood loss P61.3
  posthemorrhagic (fetal) P61.3
 nonspherocytic hemolytic — *see* Anemia, hemolytic, nonspherocytic
 normocytic (infectional) D64.9
  due to blood loss (chronic) D50.0
   acute D62
  myelophthisic D61.82
 nutritional (deficiency) D53.9
  with
   poor iron absorption D50.8
   specified deficiency NEC D53.8
  megaloblastic D52.0
 of prematurity P61.2
 orotaciduric (congenital) (hereditary) D53.0
 osteosclerotic D64.89
 ovalocytosis (hereditary) — *see* Elliptocytosis
 paludal — *see also* Malaria B54 *[D63.8]*
 pernicious (congenital) (malignant) (progressive) D51.0
 pleochromic D64.89
  of sprue D52.8
 posthemorrhagic (chronic) D50.0
  acute D62
  newborn P61.3
 postoperative (postprocedural)
  due to (acute) blood loss D62
   chronic blood loss D50.0
  specified NEC D64.89
 postpartum O90.81
 pressure D64.89
 progressive D64.9
  malignant D51.0
  pernicious D51.0
 protein-deficiency D53.0
 pseudoleukemica infantum D64.89
 pure red cell D60.9
  congenital D61.01
 pyridoxine-responsive D64.3
 pyruvate kinase deficiency D55.21
 refractory D46.4
  with
   excess of blasts D46.20
    1 (RAEB 1) D46.21
    2 (RAEB 2) D46.22
    in transformation (RAEB T) — *see* Leukemia, acute myeloblastic
   hemochromatosis D46.1
   sideroblasts (ring) (RARS) D46.1
  megaloblastic D53.1
  sideroblastic D46.1
  sideropenic D50.9
  without ring sideroblasts, so stated D46.0
  without sideroblasts without excess of blasts D46.0
 Rietti-Greppi-Micheli D56.9
 scorbutic D53.2
 secondary to
  blood loss (chronic) D50.0
   acute D62
  hemorrhage (chronic) D50.0
   acute D62
 semiplastic D61.89

Anemia — *continued*
 sickle-cell — *see* Disease, sickle-cell
 sideroblastic D64.3
  hereditary D64.0
  hypochromic, sex-linked D64.0
  pyridoxine-responsive NEC D64.3
  refractory D46.1
  secondary (due to)
   disease D64.1
   drugs and toxins D64.2
  specified type NEC D64.3
 sideropenic (refractory) D50.9
  due to blood loss (chronic) D50.0
   acute D62
 simple chronic D53.9
 specified type NEC D64.89
 spherocytic (hereditary) — *see* Spherocytosis
 splenic D64.89
 splenomegalic D64.89
 stomatocytosis D58.8
 syphilitic (acquired) (late) A52.79 *[D63.8]*
 target cell D64.89
 thalassemia D56.9
 thrombocytopenic — *see* Thrombocytopenia
 toxic D61.2
 tropical B76.9 *[D63.8]*
  macrocytic D52.8
 tuberculous A18.89 *[D63.8]*
 vegan D51.3
 vitamin
  B12 deficiency (dietary) pernicious D51.0
  B6-responsive D64.3
 von Jaksch's D64.89
 Witts' (achlorhydric anemia) D50.8
Anemophobia F40.228
Anencephalus, anencephaly Q00.0
Anergasia — *see* Psychosis, organic
Anesthesia, anesthetic R20.0
 complication or reaction NEC — *see also* Complications, anesthesia T88.59 ☑
  due to
   correct substance properly administered — *see* Table of Drugs and Chemicals, by drug, adverse effect
   overdose or wrong substance given — *see* Table of Drugs and Chemicals, by drug, poisoning
  unintended awareness under general anesthesia
   during procedure T88.53 ☑
   personal history of Z92.84
 cornea H18.81- ☑
 dissociative F44.6
 functional (hysterical) F44.6
 hyperesthetic, thalamic G89.0
 hysterical F44.6
 local skin lesion R20.0
 sexual (psychogenic) F52.1
 shock (due to) T88.2 ☑
 skin R20.0
 testicular N50.9
Anetoderma (maculosum) (of) L90.8
 Jadassohn-Pellizzari L90.2
 Schweninger-Buzzi L90.1
Aneurin deficiency E51.9
Aneurysm (anastomotic) (artery) (cirsoid) (diffuse) (false) (fusiform) (multiple) (saccular) I72.9
 abdominal (aorta) I71.40
  infrarenal I71.43
   ruptured I71.33
  juxtarenal I71.42
   ruptured I71.32
  pararenal I71.41
   ruptured I71.31
  ruptured I71.30
  syphilitic A52.01
 aorta, aortic (nonsyphilitic) I71.9
  abdominal I71.40
   dissecting — *see* Dissection, aorta, abdominal
   ruptured I71.30
  arch I71.22
   ruptured I71.12
  arteriosclerotic I71.9
   ruptured I71.8
  ascending I71.21
   ruptured I71.11
  congenital Q25.43
  descending I71.9
   abdominal I71.40

Aneurysm — *continued*
 aorta, aortic — *continued*
  descending — *continued*
   abdominal — *continued*
    ruptured I71.30
   ruptured I71.8
   thoracic I71.23
    ruptured I71.13
  dissecting — *see* Dissection, aorta
  root Q25.43
  ruptured I71.8
  sinus, congenital Q25.43
  syphilitic A52.01
  thoracic I71.20
   ruptured I71.10
  thoracoabdominal I71.60
   paravisceral I71.62
    ruptured I71.52
   ruptured I71.50
   supraceliac I71.61
    ruptured I71.51
  thorax, thoracic I71.20
   arch I71.22
    ruptured I71.12
   ascending I71.21
    ruptured I71.11
   descending I71.23
    ruptured I71.13
   ruptured I71.10
   arch I71.12
   ascending I71.11
   descending I71.13
  transverse I71.22
   ruptured I71.12
  valve (heart) — *see also* Endocarditis, aortic I35.8
 arteriosclerotic I72.9
  cerebral I67.1
   ruptured — *see* Hemorrhage, intracranial, subarachnoid
 arteriovenous (congenital) — *see also* Malformation, arteriovenous
  acquired I77.0
   brain I67.1
    ruptured — *see* Aneurysm, arteriovenous, brain, ruptured
   coronary I25.41
   pulmonary I28.0
  brain Q28.2
   ruptured I60.8
    intracerebral I61.8
    intraparenchymal I61.8
    intraventricular I61.5
    subarachnoid I60.8
  peripheral — *see* Malformation, arteriovenous, peripheral
  precerebral vessels Q28.0
  specified site NEC — *see also* Malformation, arteriovenous
   acquired I77.0
 basal — *see* Aneurysm, brain
 basilar (trunk) I72.5
 berry (congenital) (nonruptured) I67.1
  ruptured I60.7
 brain I67.1
  arteriosclerotic I67.1
   ruptured — *see* Hemorrhage, intracranial, subarachnoid
  arteriovenous (congenital) (nonruptured) Q28.2
   acquired I67.1
    ruptured — *see* Aneurysm, arteriovenous, brain, ruptured I60.8-
   ruptured — *see* Aneurysm, arteriovenous, brain, ruptured I60.8-
  berry (congenital) (nonruptured) I67.1
   ruptured — *see also* Hemorrhage, intracranial, subarachnoid I60.7
  congenital Q28.3
   ruptured I60.7
  meninges I67.1
   ruptured I60.8
  miliary (congenital) (nonruptured) I67.1
   ruptured — *see also* Hemorrhage, intracranial, subarachnoid I60.7
  mycotic I33.0
   ruptured — *see* Aneurysm, arteriovenous, brain, ruptured I60.8
  syphilitic (hemorrhage) A52.05
 cardiac (false) — *see also* Aneurysm, heart I25.3

☑ Additional Character Required — Refer to the Tabular List for Character Selection

Aneurysm — *continued*
  carotid artery (common) (external) I72.0
    internal (intracranial) I67.1
      extracranial portion I72.0
      ruptured into brain I60.0- ☑
    syphilitic A52.09
      intracranial A52.05
  cavernous sinus I67.1
    arteriovenous (congenital) (nonruptured) Q28.3
      ruptured I60.8
  celiac I72.8
  central nervous system, syphilitic A52.05
  cerebral — *see* Aneurysm, brain
  chest — *see* Aneurysm, thorax
  circle of Willis I67.1
    congenital Q28.3
      ruptured I60.6
    ruptured I60.6
  common iliac artery I72.3
  congenital (peripheral) Q27.8
    aorta (root) (sinus) Q25.43
    brain Q28.3
      ruptured I60.7
    coronary Q24.5
    digestive system Q27.8
    lower limb Q27.8
    pulmonary Q25.79
    retina Q14.1
    specified site NEC Q27.8
    upper limb Q27.8
  conjunctiva — *see* Abnormality, conjunctiva, vascular
  conus arteriosus — *see* Aneurysm, heart
  coronary (arteriosclerotic) (artery) I25.41
    arteriovenous, congenital Q24.5
    congenital Q24.5
    ruptured — *see* Infarct, myocardium
    syphilitic A52.06
    vein I25.89
  cylindroid (aorta) I71.9
    ruptured I71.8
    syphilitic A52.01
  ductus arteriosus Q25.0
  endocardial, infective (any valve) I33.0
  femoral (artery) (ruptured) I72.4
  gastroduodenal I72.8
  gastroepiploic I72.8
  heart (wall) (chronic or with a stated duration of over
      4 weeks) I25.3
    valve — *see* Endocarditis
  hepatic I72.8
  iliac (common) (artery) (ruptured) I72.3
  infective I72.9
    endocardial (any valve) I33.0
  innominate (nonsyphilitic) I72.8
    syphilitic A52.09
  interauricular septum — *see* Aneurysm, heart
  interventricular septum — *see* Aneurysm, heart
  intrathoracic (nonsyphilitic) — *see also* Aneurysm,
      aorta, thorax I71.20
    ruptured — *see also* Aneurysm, aorta, thorax, rup-
        tured I71.10
    syphilitic A52.01
  lower limb I72.4
  lung (pulmonary artery) I28.1
  mediastinal (nonsyphilitic) I72.8
    syphilitic A52.09
  miliary (congenital) I67.1
    ruptured — *see* Hemorrhage, intracerebral, sub-
        arachnoid, intracranial
  mitral (heart) (valve) I34.89
  mural — *see* Aneurysm, heart
  mycotic I72.9
    endocardial (any valve) I33.0
    ruptured, brain — *see* Hemorrhage, intracerebral,
        subarachnoid
  myocardium — *see* Aneurysm, heart
  neck I72.0
  pancreaticoduodenal I72.8
  patent ductus arteriosus Q25.0
  peripheral NEC I72.8
    congenital Q27.8
      digestive system Q27.8
      lower limb Q27.8
      specified site NEC Q27.8
      upper limb Q27.8
  popliteal (artery) (ruptured) I72.4
  precerebral
    congenital (nonruptured) Q28.1

Aneurysm — *continued*
  precerebral — *continued*
    specified site, NEC I72.5
  pulmonary I28.1
    arteriovenous Q25.72
      acquired I28.0
    syphilitic A52.09
    valve (heart) — *see* Endocarditis, pulmonary
  racemose (peripheral) I72.9
    congenital — *see* Aneurysm, congenital
  radial I72.1
  Rasmussen NEC A15.0
  renal (artery) I72.2
  retina — *see also* Disorder, retina, microaneurysms
    congenital Q14.1
    diabetic — *see* E08-E13 with .3-
  sinus of Valsalva Q25.49
  specified NEC I72.8
  spinal (cord) I72.8
    syphilitic (hemorrhage) A52.09
  splenic I72.8
  subclavian (artery) (ruptured) I72.8
    syphilitic A52.09
  superior mesenteric I72.8
  syphilitic (aorta) A52.01
    central nervous system A52.05
    congenital (late) A50.54 [I79.0]
    spine, spinal A52.09
  thoracoabdominal (aorta) I71.60
    ruptured I71.50
    syphilitic A52.01
  thorax, thoracic (aorta) (arch) (nonsyphilitic) — *see*
      Aneurysm, aorta, thorax
    ruptured — *see* Aneurysm, aorta, thorax, ruptured
    syphilitic A52.01
  traumatic (complication) (early), specified site — *see*
      Injury, blood vessel
  tricuspid (heart) (valve) I07.8
  ulnar I72.1
  upper limb (ruptured) I72.1
  valve, valvular — *see* Endocarditis
  venous — *see also* Varix I86.8
    congenital Q27.8
      digestive system Q27.8
      lower limb Q27.8
      specified site NEC Q27.8
      upper limb Q27.8
  ventricle — *see* Aneurysm, heart
  vertebral artery I72.6
  visceral NEC I72.8
Angelman syndrome Q93.51
Anger R45.4
Angiectasis, angiectopia I99.8
Angiitis I77.6
  allergic granulomatous M30.1
  hypersensitivity M31.0
  necrotizing M31.9
    specified NEC M31.8
  nervous system, granulomatous I67.7
Angina (attack) (cardiac) (chest) (heart) (pectoris) (syn-
    drome) (vasomotor) I20.9
  with
    atherosclerotic heart disease — *see* Arteriosclerosis,
        coronary (artery),
    documented spasm I20.1
  abdominal K55.1
  accelerated — *see* Angina, unstable
  agranulocytic — *see* Agranulocytosis
  angiospastic — *see* Angina, with documented spasm
  aphthous B08.5
  crescendo — *see* Angina, unstable
  croupous J05.0
  cruris I73.9
  de novo effort — *see* Angina, unstable
  diphtheritic, membranous A36.0
  equivalent I20.8
  exudative, chronic J37.0
  following acute myocardial infarction I23.7
  gangrenous diphtheritic A36.0
  intestinal K55.1
  Ludovici K12.2
  Ludwig's K12.2
  malignant diphtheritic A36.0
  membranous J05.0
    diphtheritic A36.0
    Vincent's A69.1
  mesenteric K55.1
  monocytic — *see* Mononucleosis, infectious

Angina — *continued*
  of effort — *see* Angina, specified NEC
  phlegmonous J36
    diphtheritic A36.0
  post-infarctional I23.7
  pre-infarctional — *see* Angina, unstable
  Prinzmetal — *see* Angina, with documented spasm
  progressive — *see* Angina, unstable
  pseudomembranous A69.1
  pultaceous, diphtheritic A36.0
  refractory I20.2
  spasm-induced — *see* Angina, with documented spasm
  specified NEC I20.8
  stable I20.8
  stenocardia — *see* Angina, specified NEC
  stridulous, diphtheritic A36.2
  tonsil J36
  trachealis J05.0
  unstable I20.0
  variant — *see* Angina, with documented spasm
  Vincent's A69.1
  worsening effort — *see* Angina, unstable
Angioblastoma — *see* Neoplasm, connective tissue,
    uncertain behavior
Angiocholecystitis — *see* Cholecystitis, acute
Angiocholitis — *see also* Cholecystitis, acute K83.09
Angiodysgenesis spinalis G95.19
Angiodysplasia (cecum) (colon) K55.20
  with bleeding K55.21
  duodenum (and stomach) K31.819
    with bleeding K31.811
  stomach (and duodenum) K31.819
    with bleeding K31.811
Angioedema (allergic) (any site) (with urticaria) T78.3 ☑
  episodic, with eosinophilia D72.118
  hereditary D84.1
Angioendothelioma — *see* Neoplasm, uncertain behav-
    ior, by site
  benign D18.00
    intra-abdominal D18.03
    intracranial D18.02
    skin D18.01
    specified site NEC D18.09
  bone — *see* Neoplasm, bone, malignant
  Ewing's — *see* Neoplasm, bone, malignant
Angioendotheliomatosis C85.8- ☑
Angiofibroma — *see also* Neoplasm, benign, by site
  juvenile
    specified site — *see* Neoplasm, benign, by site
    unspecified site D10.6
Angiohemophilia (A) (B) — *see* Disease, von Willebrand
Angioid streaks (choroid) (macula) (retina) H35.33
Angiokeratoma — *see* Neoplasm, skin, benign
  corporis diffusum E75.21
Angioleiomyoma — *see* Neoplasm, connective tissue,
    benign
Angiolipoma — *see also* Lipoma
  infiltrating — *see* Lipoma
Angioma — *see also* Hemangioma, by site
  capillary I78.1
  hemorrhagicum hereditaria I78.0
  intra-abdominal D18.03
  intracranial D18.02
  malignant — *see* Neoplasm, connective tissue, malig-
    nant
  plexiform D18.00
    intra-abdominal D18.03
    intracranial D18.02
    skin D18.01
    specified site NEC D18.09
  senile I78.1
  serpiginosum L81.7
  skin D18.01
  specified site NEC D18.09
  spider I78.1
  stellate I78.1
  venous Q28.3
Angiomatosis Q82.8
  bacillary A79.89
  encephalotrigeminal Q85.89
  hemorrhagic familial I78.0
  hereditary familial I78.0
  liver K76.4
Angiomyolipoma — *see* Lipoma
Angiomyoliposarcoma — *see* Neoplasm, connective
    tissue, malignant
Angiomyoma — *see* Neoplasm, connective tissue, benign

Index

Angiomyosarcoma — Anomaly, anomalous

Angiomyosarcoma — *see* Neoplasm, connective tissue, malignant
Angiomyxoma — *see* Neoplasm, connective tissue, uncertain behavior
Angioneurosis F45.8
Angioneurotic edema (allergic) (any site) (with urticaria) T78.3 ☑
  hereditary D84.1
Angiopathia, angiopathy I99.9
  cerebral I67.9
    amyloid E85.4 *[I68.0]*
  diabetic (peripheral) — *see* Diabetes, angiopathy
  peripheral I73.9
    diabetic — *see* Diabetes, angiopathy
    specified type NEC I73.89
  retinae syphilitica A52.05
  retinalis (juvenilis)
    diabetic — *see* Diabetes, retinopathy
    proliferative — *see* Retinopathy, proliferative
Angiosarcoma — *see also* Neoplasm, connective tissue, malignant
  liver C22.3
Angiosclerosis — *see* Arteriosclerosis
Angiospasm (peripheral) (traumatic) (vessel) I73.9
  brachial plexus G54.0
  cerebral G45.9
  cervical plexus G54.2
  nerve
    arm — *see* Mononeuropathy, upper limb
      axillary G54.0
      median — *see* Lesion, nerve, median
      ulnar — *see* Lesion, nerve, ulnar
    axillary G54.0
    leg — *see* Mononeuropathy, lower limb
    median — *see* Lesion, nerve, median
    plantar — *see* Lesion, nerve, plantar
    ulnar — *see* Lesion, nerve, ulnar
Angiospastic disease or edema I73.9
Angiostrongyliasis
  due to
    Parastrongylus
      cantonensis B83.2
      costaricensis B81.3
    intestinal B81.3
Anguillulosis — *see* Strongyloidiasis
Angulation
  cecum — *see* Obstruction, intestine
  coccyx (acquired) — *see also* subcategory M43.8 ☑
    congenital NEC Q76.49
  femur (acquired) — *see also* Deformity, limb, specified type NEC, thigh
    congenital Q74.2
  intestine (large) (small) — *see* Obstruction, intestine
  sacrum (acquired) — *see also* subcategory M43.8 ☑
    congenital NEC Q76.49
  sigmoid (flexure) — *see* Obstruction, intestine
  spine — *see* Dorsopathy, deforming, specified NEC
  tibia (acquired) — *see also* Deformity, limb, specified type NEC, lower leg
    congenital Q74.2
  ureter N13.5
    with infection N13.6
  wrist (acquired) — *see also* Deformity, limb, specified type NEC, forearm
    congenital Q74.0
Angulus infectiosus (lips) K13.0
Anhedonia R45.84
  sexual F52.0
Anhidrosis L74.4
Anhydration E86.0
Anhydremia E86.0
Anidrosis L74.4
Aniridia (congenital) Q13.1
Anisakiasis (infection) (infestation) B81.0
Anisakis larvae infestation B81.0
Aniseikonia H52.32
Anisocoria (pupil) H57.02
  congenital Q13.2
Anisocytosis R71.8
Anisometropia (congenital) H52.31
Ankle — *see* condition
Ankyloblepharon (eyelid) (acquired) — *see also* Blepharophimosis
  filiforme (adnatum) (congenital) Q10.3
  total Q10.3
Ankyloglossia Q38.1
Ankylosis (fibrous) (osseous) (joint) M24.60

Ankylosis — *continued*
  ankle M24.67- ☑
  arthrodesis status Z98.1
  cricoarytenoid (cartilage) (joint) (larynx) J38.7
  dental K03.5
  ear ossicles H74.31- ☑
  elbow M24.62- ☑
  foot M24.67- ☑
  hand M24.64- ☑
  hip M24.65- ☑
  incostapedial joint (infectional) — *see* Ankylosis, ear ossicles
  jaw (temporomandibular) M26.61- ☑
  knee M24.66- ☑
  lumbosacral (joint) M43.27
  postoperative (status) Z98.1
  produced by surgical fusion, status Z98.1
  sacro-iliac (joint) M43.28
  shoulder M24.61- ☑
  specified site NEC M24.69
  spine (joint) — *see also* Fusion, spine
    spondylitic — *see* Spondylitis, ankylosing
  surgical Z98.1
  temporomandibular M26.61- ☑
  tooth, teeth (hard tissues) K03.5
  wrist M24.63- ☑
Ankylostoma — *see* Ancylostoma
Ankylostomiasis — *see* Ancylostomiasis
Ankylurethria — *see* Stricture, urethra
Annular — *see also* condition
  detachment, cervix N88.8
  organ or site, congenital NEC — *see* Distortion
  pancreas (congenital) Q45.1
Anoctaminopathy G71.035
Anodontia (complete) (partial) (vera) K00.0
  acquired K08.10 ☑
Anomaly, anomalous (congenital) (unspecified type) Q89.9
  abdominal wall NEC Q79.59
  acoustic nerve Q07.8
  adrenal (gland) Q89.1
  Alder (-Reilly) (leukocyte granulation) D72.0
  alimentary tract Q45.9
    upper Q40.9
  alveolar M26.70
    hyperplasia M26.79
      mandibular M26.72
      maxillary M26.71
    hypoplasia M26.79
      mandibular M26.74
      maxillary M26.73
    ridge (process) M26.79
    specified NEC M26.79
  ankle (joint) Q74.2
  anus Q43.9
  aorta (arch) NEC Q25.40
    coarctation (preductal) (postductal) Q25.1
  aortic cusp or valve Q23.9
  appendix Q43.8
  apple peel syndrome Q41.1
  aqueduct of Sylvius Q03.0
    with spina bifida — *see* Spina bifida, with hydrocephalus
  arm Q74.0
  arteriovenous NEC
    coronary Q24.5
    gastrointestinal Q27.33
      acquired — *see* Angiodysplasia
  artery (peripheral) Q27.9
    basilar NEC Q28.1
    cerebral Q28.3
    coronary Q24.5
    digestive system Q27.8
    eye Q15.8
    great Q25.9
      specified NEC Q25.8
    lower limb Q27.8
    peripheral Q27.9
      specified NEC Q27.8
    pulmonary NEC Q25.79
    renal Q27.2
    retina Q14.1
    specified site NEC Q27.8
    subclavian Q27.8
      origin Q25.48
    umbilical Q27.0
    upper limb Q27.8
    vertebral NEC Q28.1

Anomaly, anomalous — *continued*
  aryteno-epiglottic folds Q31.8
  atrial
    bands or folds Q20.8
    septa Q21.10
  atrioventricular
    excitation I45.6
    septum Q21.0
  auditory canal Q17.8
  auricle
    ear Q17.8
      causing impairment of hearing Q16.9
    heart Q20.8
  Axenfeld's Q15.0
  back Q89.9
  band
    atrial Q20.8
    heart Q24.8
    ventricular Q24.8
  Bartholin's duct Q38.4
  biliary duct or passage Q44.5
  bladder Q64.70
    absence Q64.5
    diverticulum Q64.6
    exstrophy Q64.10
      cloacal Q64.12
      extroversion Q64.19
      specified type NEC Q64.19
      supravesical fissure Q64.11
    neck obstruction Q64.31
    specified type NEC Q64.79
  bone Q79.9
    arm Q74.0
    face Q75.9
    leg Q74.2
    pelvic girdle Q74.2
    shoulder girdle Q74.0
    skull Q75.9
      with
        anencephaly Q00.0
        encephalocele — *see* Encephalocele
        hydrocephalus Q03.9
          with spina bifida — *see* Spina bifida, by site, with hydrocephalus
        microcephaly Q02
  brain (multiple) Q04.9
    vessel Q28.3
  breast Q83.9
  broad ligament Q50.6
  bronchus Q32.4
  bulbus cordis Q21.9
  bursa Q79.9
  canal of Nuck Q52.4
  canthus Q10.3
  capillary Q27.9
  cardiac Q24.9
    chambers Q20.9
      specified NEC Q20.8
    septal closure Q21.9
      specified NEC Q21.8
    valve NEC Q24.8
      pulmonary Q22.3
  cardiovascular system Q28.8
  carpus Q74.0
  caruncle, lacrimal Q10.6
  cascade stomach Q40.2
  cauda equina Q06.3
  cecum Q43.9
  cerebral Q04.9
    vessels Q28.3
  cervix Q51.9
  Chédiak-Higashi (-Steinbrinck) (congenital gigantism of peroxidase granules) E70.330
  cheek Q18.9
  chest wall Q67.8
    bones Q76.9
  chin Q18.9
  chordae tendineae Q24.8
  choroid Q14.3
    plexus Q07.8
  chromosomes, chromosomal Q99.9
    D (1) — *see* condition, chromosome 13
    E (3) — *see* condition, chromosome 18
    G — *see* condition, chromosome 21
    sex
      female phenotype Q97.8
      gonadal dysgenesis (pure) Q99.1
      Klinefelter's Q98.4
      male phenotype Q98.9

Anomaly, anomalous — *continued*
  chromosomes, chromosomal — *continued*
    sex — *continued*
      Turner's Q96.9
      specified NEC Q99.8
  cilia Q10.3
  circulatory system Q28.9
  clavicle Q74.0
  clitoris Q52.6
  coccyx Q76.49
  colon Q43.9
  common duct Q44.5
  communication
    coronary artery Q24.5
    left ventricle with right atrium Q21.0
  concha (ear) Q17.3
  connection
    portal vein Q26.5
    pulmonary venous Q26.4
      partial Q26.3
      total Q26.2
    renal artery with kidney Q27.2
  cornea (shape) Q13.4
  coronary artery or vein Q24.5
  cranium — *see* Anomaly, skull
  cricoid cartilage Q31.8
  cystic duct Q44.5
  dental
    alveolar — *see* Anomaly, alveolar
    arch relationship M26.20
      specified NEC M26.29
  dentofacial M26.9
    alveolar — *see* Anomaly, alveolar
    dental arch relationship M26.20
      specified NEC M26.29
    functional M26.50
      specified NEC M26.59
    jaw size M26.00
      macrogenia M26.05
      mandibular
        hyperplasia M26.03
        hypoplasia M26.04
      maxillary
        hyperplasia M26.01
        hypoplasia M26.02
      microgenia M26.06
      specified type NEC M26.09
    jaw-cranial base relationship M26.10
      asymmetry M26.12
        maxillary M26.11
      specified type NEC M26.19
    malocclusion M26.4
      dental arch relationship NEC M26.29
      jaw size — *see* Anomaly, dentofacial, jaw size
      jaw-cranial base relationship — *see* Anomaly,
        dentofacial, jaw-cranial base relationship
    specified type NEC M26.89
    temporomandibular joint M26.60- ☑
      adhesions M26.61- ☑
      ankylosis M26.61- ☑
      arthralgia M26.62- ☑
      articular disc M26.63- ☑
      specified type NEC M26.69
    tooth position, fully erupted M26.30
      specified NEC M26.39
  dermatoglyphic Q82.8
  diaphragm (apertures) NEC Q79.1
  digestive organ(s) or tract Q45.9
    lower Q43.9
    upper Q40.9
  distance, interarch (excessive) (inadequate) M26.25
  distribution, coronary artery Q24.5
  ductus
    arteriosus Q25.0
    botalli Q25.0
  duodenum Q43.9
  dura (brain) Q04.9
    spinal cord Q06.9
  ear (external) Q17.9
    causing impairment of hearing Q16.9
    inner Q16.5
    middle (causing impairment of hearing) Q16.4
    ossicles Q16.3
  Ebstein's (heart) (tricuspid valve) Q22.5
  ectodermal Q82.9
  Eisenmenger's (ventricular septal defect) Q21.8
  ejaculatory duct Q55.4
  elbow Q74.0

Anomaly, anomalous — *continued*
  endocrine gland NEC Q89.2
  epididymis Q55.4
  epiglottis Q31.8
  esophagus Q39.9
  eustachian tube Q17.8
  eye Q15.9
    anterior segment Q13.9
      specified NEC Q13.89
    posterior segment Q14.9
      specified NEC Q14.8
    ptosis (eyelid) Q10.0
    specified NEC Q15.8
  eyebrow Q18.8
  eyelid Q10.3
    ptosis Q10.0
  face Q18.9
    bone(s) Q75.9
  fallopian tube Q50.6
  fascia Q79.9
  femur NEC Q74.2
  fibula NEC Q74.2
  finger Q74.0
  fixation, intestine Q43.3
  flexion (joint) NOS Q74.9
    hip or thigh Q65.89
  foot NEC Q74.2
    varus (congenital) Q66.3- ☑
  foramen
    Botalli Q21.12
    ovale Q21.12
  forearm Q74.0
  forehead Q75.8
  form, teeth K00.2
  fovea centralis Q14.1
  frontal bone — *see* Anomaly, skull
  gallbladder (position) (shape) (size) Q44.1
  Gartner's duct Q52.4
  gastrointestinal tract Q45.9
  genitalia, genital organ(s) or system
    female Q52.9
      external Q52.70
      internal NOS Q52.9
    male Q55.9
      hydrocele P83.5
      specified NEC Q55.8
  genitourinary NEC
    female Q52.9
    male Q55.9
  Gerbode Q21.0
  glottis Q31.8
  granulation or granulocyte, genetic (constitutional)
    (leukocyte) D72.0
  gum Q38.6
  gyri Q07.9
  hair Q84.2
  hand Q74.0
  hard tissue formation in pulp K04.3
  head — *see* Anomaly, skull
  heart Q24.9
    auricle Q20.8
    bands or folds Q24.8
    fibroelastosis cordis I42.4
    obstructive NEC Q22.6
    patent ductus arteriosus (Botalli) Q25.0
    septum Q21.9
      auricular Q21.19
      interatrial Q21.19
      interventricular Q21.0
        with pulmonary stenosis or atresia, dextrapo-
          sition of aorta and hypertrophy of right
          ventricle Q21.3
      specified NEC Q21.8
      ventricular Q21.0
        with pulmonary stenosis or atresia, dextrapo-
          sition of aorta and hypertrophy of right
          ventricle Q21.3
    tetralogy of Fallot Q21.3
    valve NEC Q24.8
      aortic
        bicuspid valve Q23.1
        insufficiency Q23.1
        stenosis Q23.0
          subaortic Q24.4
      mitral
        insufficiency Q23.3
        stenosis Q23.2
      pulmonary Q22.3
        atresia Q22.0

Anomaly, anomalous — *continued*
  heart — *continued*
    valve — *continued*
      pulmonary — *continued*
        insufficiency Q22.2
        stenosis Q22.1
          infundibular Q24.3
          subvalvular Q24.3
      tricuspid
        atresia Q22.4
        stenosis Q22.4
    ventricle Q20.8
  heel NEC Q74.2
  Hegglin's D72.0
  hemianencephaly Q00.0
  hemicephaly Q00.0
  hemicrania Q00.0
  hepatic duct Q44.5
  hip NEC Q74.2
  hourglass stomach Q40.2
  humerus Q74.2
  hydatid of Morgagni
    female Q50.5
    male (epididymal) Q55.4
      testicular Q55.29
  hymen Q52.4
  hypersegmentation of neutrophils, hereditary D72.0
  hypophyseal Q89.2
  ileocecal (coil) (valve) Q43.9
  ileum Q43.9
  ilium NEC Q74.2
  integument Q84.9
    specified NEC Q84.8
  interarch distance (excessive) (inadequate) M26.25
  intervertebral cartilage or disc Q76.49
  intestine (large) (small) Q43.9
    with anomalous adhesions, fixation or malrotation
      Q43.3
  iris Q13.2
  ischium NEC Q74.2
  jaw — *see* Anomaly, dentofacial
    alveolar — *see* Anomaly, alveolar
  jaw-cranial base relationship — *see* Anomaly, dentofa-
    cial, jaw-cranial base relationship
  jejunum Q43.8
  joint Q74.9
    specified NEC Q74.8
  Jordan's D72.0
  kidney(s) (calyx) (pelvis) Q63.9
    artery Q27.2
    specified NEC Q63.8
  Klippel-Feil (brevicollis) Q76.1
  knee Q74.1
  labium (majus) (minus) Q52.70
  labyrinth, membranous Q16.5
  lacrimal apparatus or duct Q10.6
  larynx, laryngeal (muscle) Q31.9
    web (bed) Q31.0
  lens Q12.9
  leukocytes, genetic D72.0
    granulation (constitutional) D72.0
  lid (fold) Q10.3
  ligament Q79.9
    broad Q50.6
    round Q52.8
  limb Q74.9
    lower NEC Q74.2
      reduction deformity — *see* Defect, reduction,
        lower limb
    upper Q74.0
  lip Q38.0
  liver Q44.7
    duct Q44.5
  lower limb NEC Q74.2
  lumbosacral (joint) (region) Q76.49
    kyphosis — *see* Kyphosis, congenital
    lordosis — *see* Lordosis, congenital
  lung (fissure) (lobe) Q33.9
  mandible — *see* Anomaly, dentofacial
  maxilla — *see* Anomaly, dentofacial
  May (-Hegglin) D72.0
  meatus urinarius NEC Q64.79
  meningeal bands or folds Q07.9
    constriction of Q07.8
    spinal Q06.9
  meninges Q07.9
    cerebral Q04.8
    spinal Q06.9

Anomaly, anomalous — *continued*
  meningocele Q05.9
  mesentery Q45.9
  metacarpus Q74.0
  metatarsus NEC Q74.2
  middle ear Q16.4
    ossicles Q16.3
  mitral (leaflets) (valve) Q23.9
    insufficiency Q23.3
    specified NEC Q23.8
    stenosis Q23.2
  mouth Q38.6
  Müllerian — *see also* Anomaly, by site
    uterus NEC Q51.818
  multiple NEC Q89.7
  muscle Q79.9
    eyelid Q10.3
  musculoskeletal system, except limbs Q79.9
  myocardium Q24.8
  nail Q84.6
  narrowness, eyelid Q10.3
  nasal sinus (wall) Q30.8
  neck (any part) Q18.9
  nerve Q07.9
    acoustic Q07.8
    optic Q07.8
  nervous system (central) Q07.9
  nipple Q83.9
  nose, nasal (bones) (cartilage) (septum) (sinus) Q30.9
    specified NEC Q30.8
  ocular muscle Q15.8
  omphalomesenteric duct Q43.0
  opening, pulmonary veins Q26.4
  optic
    disc Q14.2
    nerve Q07.8
  opticociliary vessels Q13.2
  orbit (eye) Q10.7
  organ Q89.9
    of Corti Q16.5
  origin
    artery
      innominate Q25.8
      pulmonary Q25.79
      renal Q27.2
      subclavian Q25.48
  osseous meatus (ear) Q16.1
  ovary Q50.39
  oviduct Q50.6
  palate (hard) (soft) NEC Q38.5
  pancreas or pancreatic duct Q45.3
  papillary muscles Q24.8
  parathyroid gland Q89.2
  paraurethral ducts Q64.79
  parotid (gland) Q38.4
  patella Q74.1
  Pelger-Huët (hereditary hyposegmentation) D72.0
  pelvic girdle NEC Q74.2
  pelvis (bony) NEC Q74.2
    rachitic E64.3
  penis (glans) Q55.69
  pericardium Q24.8
  peripheral vascular system Q27.9
  Peter's Q13.4
  pharynx Q38.8
  pigmentation L81.9
    congenital Q82.8
  pituitary (gland) Q89.2
  pleural (folds) Q34.0
  portal vein Q26.5
    connection Q26.5
  position, tooth, teeth, fully erupted M26.30
    specified NEC M26.39
  precerebral vessel Q28.1
  prepuce Q55.69
  prostate Q55.4
  pulmonary Q33.9
    artery NEC Q25.79
    valve Q22.3
      atresia Q22.0
      insufficiency Q22.2
      specified type NEC Q22.3
      stenosis Q22.1
        infundibular Q24.3
        subvalvular Q24.3
    venous connection Q26.4
      partial Q26.3
      total Q26.2
  pupil Q13.2

Anomaly, anomalous — *continued*
  pupil — *continued*
    function H57.00
      anisocoria H57.02
      Argyll Robertson pupil H57.01
      miosis H57.03
      mydriasis H57.04
      specified type NEC H57.09
      tonic pupil H57.05- ☑
  pylorus Q40.3
  radius Q74.0
  rectum Q43.9
  reduction (extremity) (limb)
    femur (longitudinal) — *see* Defect, reduction, lower limb, longitudinal, femur
    fibula (longitudinal) — *see* Defect, reduction, lower limb, longitudinal, fibula
    lower limb — *see* Defect, reduction, lower limb
    radius (longitudinal) — *see* Defect, reduction, upper limb, longitudinal, radius
    tibia (longitudinal) — *see* Defect, reduction, lower limb, longitudinal, tibia
    ulna (longitudinal) — *see* Defect, reduction, upper limb, longitudinal, ulna
    upper limb — *see* Defect, reduction, upper limb
  refraction — *see* Disorder, refraction
  renal Q63.9
    artery Q27.2
    pelvis Q63.9
    specified NEC Q63.8
  respiratory system Q34.9
    specified NEC Q34.8
  retina Q14.1
  rib Q76.6
    cervical Q76.5
  Rieger's Q13.81
  rotation — *see* Malrotation
    hip or thigh Q65.89
  round ligament Q52.8
  sacroiliac (joint) NEC Q74.2
  sacrum NEC Q76.49
    kyphosis — *see* Kyphosis, congenital
    lordosis — *see* Lordosis, congenital
  saddle nose, syphilitic A50.57
  salivary duct or gland Q38.4
  scapula Q74.0
  scrotum — *see* Malformation, testis and scrotum
  sebaceous gland Q82.9
  seminal vesicles Q55.4
  sense organs NEC Q07.8
  sex chromosomes NEC — *see also* Anomaly, chromosomes
    female phenotype Q97.8
    male phenotype Q98.9
  shoulder (girdle) (joint) Q74.0
  sigmoid (flexure) Q43.9
  simian crease Q82.8
  sinus of Valsalva Q25.49
  skeleton generalized Q78.9
  skin (appendage) Q82.9
  skull Q75.9
    with
      anencephaly Q00.0
      encephalocele — *see* Encephalocele
      hydrocephalus Q03.9
        with spina bifida — *see* Spina bifida, by site, with hydrocephalus
      microcephaly Q02
  specified organ or site NEC Q89.8
  spermatic cord Q55.4
  spine, spinal NEC Q76.49
    column NEC Q76.49
      kyphosis — *see* Kyphosis, congenital
      lordosis — *see* Lordosis, congenital
    cord Q06.9
    nerve root Q07.8
  spleen Q89.09
    agenesis Q89.01
  stenonian duct Q38.4
  sternum NEC Q76.7
  stomach Q40.3
  submaxillary gland Q38.4
  tarsus NEC Q74.2
  tendon Q79.9
  testis — *see* Malformation, testis and scrotum
  thigh NEC Q74.2
  thorax (wall) Q67.8
    bony Q76.9

Anomaly, anomalous — *continued*
  throat Q38.8
  thumb Q74.0
  thymus gland Q89.2
  thyroid (gland) Q89.2
    cartilage Q31.8
  tibia NEC Q74.2
    saber A50.56
  toe Q74.2
  tongue Q38.3
  tooth, teeth K00.9
    eruption K00.6
    position, fully erupted M26.30
    spacing, fully erupted M26.30
  trachea (cartilage) Q32.1
  tragus Q17.9
  tricuspid (leaflet) (valve) Q22.9
    atresia or stenosis Q22.4
    Ebstein's Q22.5
  Uhl's (hypoplasia of myocardium, right ventricle) Q24.8
  ulna Q74.0
  umbilical artery Q27.0
  union
    cricoid cartilage and thyroid cartilage Q31.8
    thyroid cartilage and hyoid bone Q31.8
    trachea with larynx Q31.8
  upper limb Q74.0
  urachus Q64.4
  ureter Q62.8
    obstructive NEC Q62.39
      cecoureterocele Q62.32
      orthotopic ureterocele Q62.31
  urethra Q64.70
    absence Q64.5
    double Q64.74
    fistula to rectum Q64.73
    obstructive Q64.39
      stricture Q64.32
    prolapse Q64.71
    specified type NEC Q64.79
  urinary tract Q64.9
  uterus Q51.9
    with only one functioning horn Q51.4
  uvula Q38.5
  vagina Q52.4
  valleculae Q31.8
  valve (heart) NEC Q24.8
    coronary sinus Q24.5
    inferior vena cava Q24.8
    pulmonary Q22.3
    sinus coronario Q24.5
    venae cavae inferioris Q24.8
  vas deferens Q55.4
  vascular Q27.9
    brain Q28.3
    ring Q25.45
  vein(s) (peripheral) Q27.9
    brain Q28.3
    cerebral Q28.3
    coronary Q24.5
    developmental Q28.3
    great Q26.9
      specified NEC Q26.8
  vena cava (inferior) (superior) Q26.9
  venous — *see* Anomaly, vein(s)
  venous return Q26.8
  ventricular
    bands or folds Q24.8
    septa Q21.0
  vertebra Q76.49
    kyphosis — *see* Kyphosis, congenital
    lordosis — *see* Lordosis, congenital
  vesicourethral orifice Q64.79
  vessel(s) Q27.9
    optic papilla Q14.2
    precerebral Q28.1
  vitelline duct Q43.0
  vitreous body or humor Q14.0
  vulva Q52.70
  wrist (joint) Q74.0
Anomia R48.8
Anonychia (congenital) Q84.3
  acquired L60.8
Anophthalmos, anophthalmus (congenital) (globe) Q11.1
  acquired Z90.01
Anopia, anopsia H53.46- ☑
  quadrant H53.46- ☑

Anorchia, anorchism, anorchidism Q55.0
Anorexia R63.0
  hysterical F44.89
  nervosa F50.00
    atypical F50.9
    binge-eating type F50.2
      with purging F50.02
    restricting type F50.01
Anorgasmy, psychogenic (female) F52.31
  male F52.32
Anosmia R43.0
  hysterical F44.6
  postinfectional J39.8
Anosognosia R41.89
Anosteoplasia Q78.9
Anovulatory cycle N97.0
Anoxemia R09.02
  newborn P84
Anoxia (pathological) R09.02
  altitude T70.29 ☑
  cerebral G93.1
    complicating
      anesthesia (general) (local) or other sedation
        T88.59 ☑
        in labor and delivery O74.3
        in pregnancy O29.21- ☑
        postpartum, puerperal O89.2
      delivery (cesarean) (instrumental) O75.4
    during a procedure G97.81
    newborn P84
    resulting from a procedure G97.82
  due to
    drowning T75.1 ☑
    high altitude T70.29 ☑
  heart — see Insufficiency, coronary
  intrauterine P84
  myocardial — see Insufficiency, coronary
  newborn P84
  spinal cord G95.11
  systemic (by suffocation) (low content in atmosphere)
    — see Asphyxia, traumatic
Anteflexion — see Anteversion
Antenatal
  care (normal pregnancy) Z34.90
  screening (encounter for) of mother — see also En-
    counter, antenatal screening Z36.9
Antepartum — see condition
Anterior — see condition
Antero-occlusion M26.220
Anteversion
  cervix — see Anteversion, uterus
  femur (neck), congenital Q65.89
  uterus, uterine (cervix) (postinfectional) (postpartal,
    old) N85.4
    congenital Q51.818
    in pregnancy or childbirth — see Pregnancy, com-
      plicated by
Anthophobia F40.228
Anthracosilicosis J60
Anthracosis (lung) (occupational) J60
  lingua K14.3
Anthrax A22.9
  with pneumonia A22.1
  cerebral A22.8
  colitis A22.2
  cutaneous A22.0
  gastrointestinal A22.2
  inhalation A22.1
  intestinal A22.2
  meningitis A22.8
  pulmonary A22.1
  respiratory A22.1
  sepsis A22.7
  specified manifestation NEC A22.8
Anthropoid pelvis Q74.2
  with disproportion (fetopelvic) O33.0
Anthropophobia F40.10
  generalized F40.11
Antibodies, maternal (blood group) — see Isoimmunization, affecting management of pregnancy
  anti-D — see Isoimmunization, affecting management
    of pregnancy, Rh
  newborn P55.0
Antibody
  anticardiolipin R76.0
    with
      hemorrhagic disorder D68.312
      hypercoagulable state D68.61

Antibody — continued
  antiphosphatidylglycerol R76.0
    with
      hemorrhagic disorder D68.312
      hypercoagulable state D68.61
  antiphosphatidylinositol R76.0
    with
      hemorrhagic disorder D68.312
      hypercoagulable state D68.61
  antiphosphatidylserine R76.0
    with
      hemorrhagic disorder D68.312
      hypercoagulable state D68.61
  antiphospholipid R76.0
    with
      hemorrhagic disorder D68.312
      hypercoagulable state D68.61
Anticardiolipin syndrome D68.61
Anticoagulant, circulating (intrinsic) — see also Disor-
  der, hemorrhagic D68.318
  drug-induced (extrinsic) — see also Disorder, hemor-
    rhagic D68.32
  iatrogenic D68.32
Antidiuretic hormone syndrome E22.2
Antimonial cholera — see Poisoning, antimony
Antiphospholipid
  antibody
    with hemorrhagic disorder D68.312
    syndrome D68.61
Antisocial personality F60.2
Antithrombinemia — see Circulating anticoagulants
Antithromboplastinemia D68.318
Antithromboplastinogenemia D68.318
Antitoxin complication or reaction — see Complications, vaccination
Antlophobia F40.228
Antritis J32.0
  maxilla J32.0
    acute J01.00
      recurrent J01.01
  stomach K29.50
    with bleeding K29.51
Antrum, antral — see condition
Anuria R34
  calculous (impacted) (recurrent) — see also Calculus,
    urinary N20.9
  following
    abortion — see Abortion by type complicated by,
      renal failure
    ectopic or molar pregnancy O08.4
  newborn P96.0
  postprocedural N99.0
  postrenal N13.8
  traumatic (following crushing) T79.5 ☑
Anus, anal — see condition
Anusitis K62.89
Anxiety F41.9
  depression F41.8
  episodic paroxysmal F41.0
  generalized F41.1
  hysteria F41.8
  neurosis F41.1
  panic type F41.0
  reaction F41.1
  separation, abnormal (of childhood) F93.0
  specified NEC F41.8
  state F41.1
Aorta, aortic — see condition
Aortectasia — see Ectasia, aorta
  with aneurysm — see Aneurysm, aorta
Aortitis (nonsyphilitic) (calcific) I77.6
  arteriosclerotic I70.0
  Doehle-Heller A52.02
  luetic A52.02
  rheumatic — see Endocarditis, acute, rheumatic
  specific (syphilitic) A52.02
  syphilitic A52.02
    congenital A50.54 [I79.1]
Apathetic thyroid storm — see Thyrotoxicosis
Apathy R45.3
Apeirophobia F40.228
Apepsia K30
  psychogenic F45.8
Aperistalsis, esophagus K22.0
Apertognathia M26.29
Apert's syndrome Q87.0
Aphagia R13.0
  psychogenic F50.9

Aphakia (acquired) (postoperative) H27.0- ☑
  congenital Q12.3
Aphasia (amnestic) (global) (nominal) (semantic) (syntac-
  tic) R47.01
  acquired, with epilepsy (Landau-Kleffner syndrome)
    — see Epilepsy, specified NEC
  auditory (developmental) F80.2
  developmental (receptive type) F80.2
    expressive type F80.1
    Wernicke's F80.2
  following
    cerebrovascular disease I69.920
      cerebral infarction I69.320
      intracerebral hemorrhage I69.120
      nontraumatic intracranial hemorrhage NEC
        I69.220
      specified disease NEC I69.820
      subarachnoid hemorrhage I69.020
  primary progressive — see also Dementia, in, diseases
    specified elsewhere G31.01 [F02.80]
    with behavioral disturbance — see also Dementia,
      in, diseases specified elsewhere
      G31.01 [F02.81-] ☑
  progressive isolated — see also Dementia, in, diseases
    specified elsewhere G31.01 [F02.80]
    with behavioral disturbance — see also Dementia,
      in, diseases specified elsewhere
      G31.01 [F02.81-] ☑
  sensory F80.2
  syphilis, tertiary A52.19
  Wernicke's (developmental) F80.2
Aphonia (organic) R49.1
  hysterical F44.4
  psychogenic F44.4
Aphthae, aphthous — see also condition
  Bednar's K12.0
  cachectic K14.0
  epizootic B08.8
  fever B08.8
  oral (recurrent) K12.0
  stomatitis (major) (minor) K12.0
  thrush B37.0
  ulcer (oral) (recurrent) K12.0
    genital organ(s) NEC
      female N76.6
      male N50.89
    larynx J38.7
Apical — see condition
Apiphobia F40.218
Aplasia — see also Agenesis
  abdominal muscle syndrome Q79.4
  alveolar process (acquired) — see Anomaly, alveolar
    congenital Q38.6
  aorta (congenital) Q25.41
  axialis extracorticalis (congenita) E75.29
  bone marrow (myeloid) D61.9
    congenital D61.01
  brain Q00.0
    part of Q04.3
  bronchus Q32.4
  cementum K00.4
  cerebellum Q04.3
  cervix (congenital) Q51.5
  congenital pure red cell D61.01
  corpus callosum Q04.0
  cutis congenita Q84.8
  erythrocyte congenital D61.01
  extracortical axial E75.29
  eye Q11.1
  fovea centralis (congenital) Q14.1
  gallbladder, congenital Q44.0
  iris Q13.1
  labyrinth, membranous Q16.5
  limb (congenital) Q73.8
    lower — see Defect, reduction, lower limb
    upper — see Agenesis, arm
  lung, congenital (bilateral) (unilateral) Q33.3
  pancreas Q45.0
  parathyroid-thymic D82.1
  Pelizaeus-Merzbacher E75.29
  penis Q55.5
  prostate Q55.4
  red cell (with thymoma) D60.9
    acquired D60.9
      due to drugs D60.9
    adult D60.9
    chronic D60.0
    congenital D61.01

Aplasia — *continued*
  red cell — *continued*
    constitutional D61.01
    due to drugs D60.9
    hereditary D61.01
    of infants D61.01
    primary D61.01
    pure D61.01
      due to drugs D60.9
    specified type NEC D60.8
    transient D60.1
  round ligament Q52.8
  skin Q84.8
  spermatic cord Q55.4
  spleen Q89.01
  testicle Q55.0
  thymic, with immunodeficiency D82.1
  thyroid (congenital) (with myxedema) E03.1
  uterus Q51.0
  ventral horn cell Q06.1
Apnea, apneic (of) (spells) R06.81
  newborn P28.40
    central P28.41
    mixed P28.43
    obstructive P28.42
    sleep
      primary P28.30
        central P28.31
        mixed P28.33
        obstructive P28.32
        specified NEC P28.39
    specified NEC P28.49
  prematurity P28.49
  sleep G47.30
    central (primary) G47.31
      idiopathic G47.31
      in conditions classified elsewhere G47.37
    obstructive (adult) (pediatric) G47.33
      hypopnea G47.33
    primary central G47.31
    specified NEC G47.39
Apneumatosis, newborn P28.0
Apocrine metaplasia (breast) — *see* Dysplasia, mammary, specified type NEC
Apophysitis (bone) — *see also* Osteochondropathy
  calcaneus M92.8
  juvenile M92.9
Apoplectiform convulsions (cerebral ischemia) I67.82
Apoplexia, apoplexy, apoplectic
  adrenal A39.1
  heart (auricle) (ventricle) — *see* Infarct, myocardium
  heat T67.01 ☑
  hemorrhagic (stroke) — *see* Hemorrhage, intracranial
  meninges, hemorrhagic — *see* Hemorrhage, intracranial, subarachnoid
  uremic N18.9 *[I68.8]*
Appearance
  bizarre R46.1
  specified NEC R46.89
  very low level of personal hygiene R46.0
Appendage
  epididymal (organ of Morgagni) Q55.4
  intestine (epiploic) Q43.8
  preauricular Q17.0
  testicular (organ of Morgagni) Q55.29
Appendicitis (pneumococcal) (retrocecal) K37
  with
    gangrene K35.891
      with localized peritonitis K35.31
    perforation NOS K35.32
    peritoneal abscess K35.33
    peritonitis NEC K35.33
      generalized (with perforation or rupture) K35.20
        with abscess K35.21
      localized K35.30
        with
          gangrene K35.31
          perforation K35.32
            and abscess K35.33
    rupture (with localized peritonitis) K35.32
  acute (catarrhal) (fulminating) (obstructive) (retrocecal) (suppurative) K35.80
    with
      gangrene K35.891
      peritoneal abscess K35.33
      peritonitis NEC K35.33
        generalized (with perforation or rupture) K35.20
          with abscess K35.21
        localized K35.30
          with
            gangrene K35.31
            perforation K35.32
              and abscess K35.33
      specified NEC K35.890
        with gangrene K35.891
          with localized peritonitis K35.31
  amebic A06.89
  chronic (recurrent) K36
  exacerbation — *see* Appendicitis, with, gangrene
  gangrenous — *see* Appendicitis, acute
  healed (obliterative) K36
  interval K36
  neurogenic K36
  obstructive K36
  recurrent K36
  relapsing K36
  ruptured NOS (with localized peritonitis) K35.32
  subacute (adhesive) K36
  subsiding K36
  suppurative — *see* Appendicitis, acute
  tuberculous A18.32
Appendicopathia oxyurica B80
Appendix, appendicular — *see also* condition
  epididymis Q55.4
  Morgagni
    female Q50.5
    male (epididymal) Q55.4
      testicular Q55.29
  testis Q55.29
Appetite
  depraved — *see* Pica
  excessive R63.2
  lack or loss — *see also* Anorexia R63.0
    nonorganic origin F50.89
    psychogenic F50.89
  perverted (hysterical) — *see* Pica
Apple peel syndrome Q41.1
Apprehension state F41.1
Apprehensiveness, abnormal F41.9
Approximal wear K03.0
Apraxia (classic) (ideational) (ideokinetic) (ideomotor) (motor) (verbal) R48.2
  following
    cerebrovascular disease I69.990
      cerebral infarction I69.390
      intracerebral hemorrhage I69.190
      nontraumatic intracranial hemorrhage NEC I69.290
      specified disease NEC I69.890
      subarachnoid hemorrhage I69.090
  oculomotor, congenital H51.8
Aptyalism K11.7
Apudoma — *see* Neoplasm, uncertain behavior, by site
Aqueous misdirection H40.83- ☑
Arabicum elephantiasis — *see* Infestation, filarial
Arachnitis — *see* Meningitis
Arachnodactyly — *see* Syndrome, Marfan's
Arachnoiditis (acute) (adhesive) (basal) (brain) (cerebrospinal) — *see* Meningitis
Arachnophobia F40.210
Arboencephalitis, Australian A83.4
Arborization block (heart) I45.5
ARC (AIDS-related complex) B20
Arch
  aortic Q25.49
  bovine Q25.49
Arches — *see* condition
Arcuate uterus Q51.810
Arcuatus uterus Q51.810
Arcus (cornea) senilis — *see* Degeneration, cornea, senile
Arc-welder's lung J63.4
Areflexia R29.2
Areola — *see* condition
Argentaffinoma — *see also* Neoplasm, uncertain behavior, by site
  malignant — *see* Neoplasm, malignant, by site
  syndrome E34.0
Argininemia E72.21
Arginosuccinic aciduria E72.22

Argyll Robertson phenomenon, pupil or syndrome (syphilitic) A52.19
  atypical H57.09
  nonsyphilitic H57.09
Argyria, argyriasis
  conjunctival H11.13- ☑
  from drug or medicament — *see* Table of Drugs and Chemicals, by substance
Argyrosis, conjunctival H11.13- ☑
Arhinencephaly Q04.1
Ariboflavinosis E53.0
Arm — *see* condition
Arnold-Chiari disease, obstruction or syndrome (type II) Q07.00
  with
    hydrocephalus Q07.02
      with spina bifida Q07.03
    spina bifida Q07.01
      with hydrocephalus Q07.03
  type III — *see* Encephalocele
  type IV Q04.8
Aromatic amino-acid metabolism disorder E70.9
  specified NEC E70.89
Arousals, confusional G47.51
Arrest, arrested
  cardiac I46.9
    complicating
      abortion — *see* Abortion, by type, complicated by, cardiac arrest
      anesthesia (general) (local) or other sedation — *see* Table of Drugs and Chemicals, by drug
        in labor and delivery O74.2
        in pregnancy O29.11- ☑
        postpartum, puerperal O89.1
      delivery (cesarean) (instrumental) O75.4
    due to
      cardiac condition I46.2
      specified condition NEC I46.8
    intraoperative I97.71- ☑
    newborn P29.81
    personal history, successfully resuscitated Z86.74
    postprocedural I97.12- ☑
      obstetric procedure O75.4
  cardiorespiratory — *see* Arrest, cardiac
  circulatory — *see* Arrest, cardiac
  deep transverse O64.0 ☑
  development or growth
    bone — *see* Disorder, bone, development or growth
    child R62.50
    tracheal rings Q32.1
  epiphyseal
    complete
      femur M89.15- ☑
      humerus M89.12- ☑
      tibia M89.16- ☑
      ulna M89.13- ☑
      forearm M89.13- ☑
        specified NEC M89.13- ☑
        ulna — *see* Arrest, epiphyseal, by type, ulna
      lower leg M89.16- ☑
        specified NEC M89.168
        tibia — *see* Arrest, epiphyseal, by type, tibia
    partial
      femur M89.15- ☑
      humerus M89.12- ☑
      tibia M89.16- ☑
      ulna M89.13- ☑
      specified NEC M89.18
  granulopoiesis — *see* Agranulocytosis
  growth plate — *see* Arrest, epiphyseal
  heart — *see* Arrest, cardiac
  legal, anxiety concerning Z65.3
  physeal — *see* Arrest, epiphyseal
  respiratory R09.2
    newborn P28.81
  sinus I45.5
  spermatogenesis (complete) — *see* Azoospermia
    incomplete — *see* Oligospermia
  transverse (deep) O64.0 ☑
Arrhenoblastoma
  benign
    specified site — *see* Neoplasm, benign, by site
    unspecified site
      female D27.9
      male D29.20
  malignant
    specified site — *see* Neoplasm, malignant, by site

Arrhenoblastoma — *continued*
   malignant — *continued*
      unspecified site
         female C56.9
         male C62.90
   specified site — *see* Neoplasm, uncertain behavior, by
      site
   unspecified site
      female D39.10
      male D40.10
Arrhythmia (auricle) (cardiac) (juvenile) (nodal) (reflex)
   (supraventricular) (transitory) (ventricle) I49.9
   block I45.9
   extrasystolic I49.49
   newborn
      bradycardia P29.12
      occurring before birth P03.819
         before onset of labor P03.810
         during labor P03.811
      tachycardia P29.11
   psychogenic F45.8
   sinus I49.8
   specified NEC I49.8
   vagal R55
   ventricular re-entry I47.0
Arrillaga-Ayerza syndrome (pulmonary sclerosis with
   pulmonary hypertension) I27.0
Arsenical pigmentation L81.8
   from drug or medicament — *see* Table of Drugs and
      Chemicals
Arsenism — *see* Poisoning, arsenic
Arterial — *see* condition
Arteriofibrosis — *see* Arteriosclerosis
Arteriolar sclerosis — *see* Arteriosclerosis
Arteriolith — *see* Arteriosclerosis
Arteriolitis I77.6
   necrotizing, kidney I77.5
   renal — *see* Hypertension, kidney
Arteriolosclerosis — *see* Arteriosclerosis
Arterionephrosclerosis — *see* Hypertension, kidney
Arteriopathy I77.9
   cerebral autosomal dominant, with subcortical infarcts
      and leukoencephalopathy (CADASIL) I67.850
Arteriosclerosis, arteriosclerotic (diffuse) (obliterans)
   (of) (senile) (with calcification) I70.90
   with
      chronic limb-threatening ischemia — *see* Arteriosclerosis, with critical limb ischemia
      critical limb ischemia
         bypass graft I70.329
            autologous vein graft I70.429
               leg I70.429
                  with
                     gangrene (and intermittent claudication, rest pain, and ulcer)
                        I70.469
                     rest pain (and intermittent claudication) I70.429
                bilateral I70.423
                  with
                     gangrene (and intermittent claudication, rest pain, and ulcer) I70.463
                     rest pain (and intermittent claudication) I70.423
                left I70.422
                  with
                     gangrene (and intermittent claudication, rest pain, and ulcer) I70.462
                     rest pain (and intermittent claudication) I70.422
                     ulceration (and intermittent claudication and rest pain) I70.449
                       ankle I70.443
                       calf I70.442
                       foot site NEC I70.445
                       heel I70.444
                       lower leg NEC I70.448
                       mid foot I70.444
                       thigh I70.441
                right I70.421
                  with
                     gangrene (and intermittent claudication, rest pain, and ulcer) I70.461

Arteriosclerosis, arteriosclerotic — *continued*
   with — *continued*
      critical limb ischemia — *continued*
         bypass graft — *continued*
            autologous vein graft — *continued*
               leg — *continued*
                  right — *continued*
                    with — *continued*
                     rest pain (and intermittent claudication) I70.421
                     ulceration (and intermittent claudication and rest pain) I70.439
                       ankle I70.433
                       calf I70.432
                       foot site NEC I70.435
                       heel I70.434
                       lower leg NEC I70.438
                       midfoot I70.434
                       thigh I70.431
            leg I70.329
               with
                  gangrene (and intermittent claudication, rest pain, and ulcer) I70.369
                  rest pain (and intermittent claudication) I70.329
               bilateral I70.323
                 with
                  gangrene (and intermittent claudication, rest pain, and ulcer) I70.363
                  rest pain (and intermittent claudication) I70.323
               left I70.322
                 with
                  gangrene (and intermittent claudication, rest pain, and ulcer) I70.362
                  rest pain (and intermittent claudication) I70.322
                  ulceration (and intermittent claudication and rest pain) I70.349
                   ankle I70.343
                   calf I70.342
                   foot site NEC I70.345
                   heel I70.344
                   lower leg NEC I70.348
                   midfoot I70.344
                   thigh I70.341
              right I70.321
                with
                 gangrene (and intermittent claudication, rest pain, and ulcer) I70.361
                 rest pain (and intermittent claudication) I70.321
                 ulceration (and intermittent claudication and rest pain) I70.339
                  ankle I70.333
                  calf I70.332
                  foot site NEC I70.335
                  heel I70.334
                  lower leg NEC I70.338
                  midfoot I70.334
                  thigh I70.331
            nonautologous biological graft I70.529
               leg I70.529
                 with
                  gangrene (and intermittent claudication, rest pain, and ulcer) I70.569
                  rest pain (and intermittent claudication) I70.529
               bilateral I70.523
                 with
                  gangrene (and intermittent claudication, rest pain, and ulcer) I70.563
                  rest pain (and intermittent claudication) I70.523
               left I70.522
                 with
                  gangrene (and intermittent claudication, rest pain, and ulcer) I70.562
                  rest pain (and intermittent claudication) I70.522

Arteriosclerosis, arteriosclerotic — *continued*
   with — *continued*
      critical limb ischemia — *continued*
         bypass graft — *continued*
            nonautologous biological graft — *continued*
               leg — *continued*
                  left — *continued*
                    with — *continued*
                     ulceration (and intermittent claudication and rest pain) I70.549
                       ankle I70.543
                       calf I70.542
                       foot site NEC I70.545
                       heel I70.544
                       lower leg NEC I70.548
                       midfoot I70.544
                       thigh I70.541
                right I70.521
                  with
                     gangrene (and intermittent claudication, rest pain, and ulcer) I70.561
                     rest pain (and intermittent claudication) I70.521
                     ulceration (and intermittent claudication and rest pain) I70.539
                       ankle I70.533
                       calf I70.532
                       foot site NEC I70.535
                       heel I70.534
                       lower leg NEC I70.538
                       midfoot I70.534
                       thigh I70.531
            nonbiological graft I70.629
               leg I70.629
                 with
                  gangrene (and intermittent claudication, rest pain, and ulcer) I70.669
                  rest pain (and intermittent claudication) I70.629
               bilateral I70.623
                 with
                  gangrene (and intermittent claudication, rest pain, and ulcer) I70.663
                  rest pain (intermittent claudication) I70.623
               left I70.622
                 with
                  gangrene (and intermittent claudication, rest pain, and ulcer) I70.662
                  rest pain (and intermittent claudication) I70.622
                  ulceration (and intermittent claudication and rest pain) I70.649
                   ankle I70.643
                   calf I70.642
                   foot site NEC I70.645
                   heel I70.644
                   lower leg NEC I70.648
                   midfoot I70.644
                   thigh I70.641
              right I70.621
                with
                  gangrene (and intermittent claudication, rest pain, and ulcer) I70.661
                  rest pain (and intermittent claudication) I70.621
                  ulceration (and intermittent claudication and rest pain) I70.639
                   ankle I70.633
                   calf I70.632
                   foot site NEC I70.635
                   heel I70.634
                   lower leg NEC I70.638
                   midfoot I70.634
                   thigh I70.631
            specified graft NEC I70.729
               leg I70.729

Arteriosclerosis, arteriosclerotic — *continued*
  with — *continued*
    critical limb ischemia — *continued*
      bypass graft — *continued*
        specified graft — *continued*
          leg — *continued*
            with
              gangrene (and intermittent claudication, rest pain, and ulcer) I70.769
              rest pain (and intermittent claudication) I70.729
            bilateral I70.723
              with
                gangrene (and intermittent claudication, rest pain, and ulcer) I70.763
                rest pain (and intermittent claudication) I70.723
            left I70.722
              with
                gangrene (and intermittent claudication, rest pain, and ulcer) I70.762
                rest pain (and intermittent claudication) I70.722
                ulceration (and intermittent claudication and rest pain) I70.749
                  ankle I70.743
                  calf I70.742
                  foot site NEC I70.745
                  heel I70.744
                  lower leg NEC I70.748
                  midfoot I70.744
                  thigh I70.741
            right I70.721
              with
                gangrene (and intermittent claudication, rest pain, and ulcer) I70.761
                rest pain (and intermittent claudication) I70.721
                ulceration (and intermittent claudication and rest pain) I70.739
                  ankle I70.733
                  calf I70.732
                  foot site NEC I70.735
                  heel I70.734
                  lower leg NEC I70.738
                  midfoot I70.734
                  thigh I70.731
      leg I70.229
        with
          gangrene (and intermittent claudication, rest pain, and ulcer) I70.269
          rest pain (and intermittent claudication) I70.229
        bilateral I70.223
          with
            gangrene (and intermittent claudication, rest pain, and ulcer) I70.263
            rest pain (and intermittent claudication) I70.223
        left I70.222
          with
            gangrene (and intermittent claudication, rest pain, and ulcer) I70.262
            rest pain (and intermittent claudication) I70.222
            ulceration (and intermittent claudication and rest pain) I70.249
              ankle I70.243
              calf I70.242
              foot site NEC I70.245
              heel I70.244
              lower leg NEC I70.248
              midfoot I70.244
              thigh I70.241
        right I70.221
          with
            gangrene (and intermittent claudication, rest pain, and ulcer) I70.261
            rest pain (and intermittent claudication) I70.221

Arteriosclerosis, arteriosclerotic — *continued*
  with — *continued*
    critical limb ischemia — *continued*
      leg — *continued*
        right — *continued*
          with — *continued*
            ulceration (and intermittent claudication and rest pain) I70.239
              ankle I70.233
              calf I70.232
              foot site NEC I70.235
              heel I70.234
              lower leg NEC I70.238
              midfoot I70.234
              thigh I70.231
  aorta I70.0
  arteries of extremities — *see* Arteriosclerosis, extremities
    with
      chronic limb-threatening ischemia — *see* Arteriosclerosis, with critical limb ischemia
      critical limb ischemia — *see* Arteriosclerosis, with critical limb ischemia
  brain I67.2
  bypass graft
    with
      chronic limb-threatening ischemia — *see* Arteriosclerosis, with critical limb ischemia
      critical limb ischemia — *see* Arteriosclerosis, with critical limb ischemia
      coronary — *see* Arteriosclerosis, coronary, bypass graft
      extremities — *see* Arteriosclerosis, extremities, bypass graft
  cardiac — *see* Disease, heart, ischemic, atherosclerotic
  cardiopathy — *see* Disease, heart, ischemic, atherosclerotic
  cardiorenal — *see* Hypertension, cardiorenal
  cardiovascular — *see* Disease, heart, ischemic, atherosclerotic
  carotid — *see also* Occlusion, artery, carotid I65.2- ☑
  central nervous system I67.2
  cerebral I67.2
  cerebrovascular I67.2
  coronary (artery) I25.10
    due to
      calcified coronary lesion (severely) I25.84
      lipid rich plaque I25.83
    bypass graft I25.810
      with
        angina pectoris I25.709
          with documented spasm I25.701
          refractory I25.702
          specified type NEC I25.708
          unstable I25.700
        ischemic chest pain I25.709
      autologous artery I25.810
        with
          angina pectoris I25.729
            with documented spasm I25.721
            refractory I25.722
            specified type I25.728
            unstable I25.720
          ischemic chest pain I25.729
      autologous vein I25.810
        with
          angina pectoris I25.719
            with documented spasm I25.711
            refractory I25.712
            specified type I25.718
            unstable I25.710
          ischemic chest pain I25.719
      nonautologous biological I25.810
        with
          angina pectoris I25.739
            with documented spasm I25.731
            refractory I25.732
            specified type I25.738
            unstable I25.730
          ischemic chest pain I25.739
      specified type NEC I25.810
        with
          angina pectoris I25.799
            with documented spasm I25.791
            refractory I25.792
            specified type I25.798
            unstable I25.790
          ischemic chest pain I25.799

Arteriosclerosis, arteriosclerotic — *continued*
  coronary — *continued*
    native vessel
      with
        angina pectoris I25.119
          with documented spasm I25.111
          refractory I25.112
          specified type NEC I25.118
          unstable I25.110
        ischemic chest pain I25.119
    transplanted heart I25.811
      bypass graft I25.812
        with
          angina pectoris I25.769
            with documented spasm I25.761
            refractory I25.762
            specified type I25.768
            unstable I25.760
          ischemic chest pain I25.769
      native coronary artery I25.811
        with
          angina pectoris I25.759
            with documented spasm I25.751
            refractory I25.752
            specified type I25.758
            unstable I25.750
          ischemic chest pain I25.759
  extremities (native arteries) I70.209
    with
      chronic limb-threatening ischemia — *see* Arteriosclerosis, with critical limb ischemia
      critical limb ischemia — *see* Arteriosclerosis, with critical limb ischemia
    bypass graft I70.309
      with
        chronic limb-threatening ischemia — *see* Arteriosclerosis, with critical limb ischemia
        critical limb ischemia — *see* Arteriosclerosis, with critical limb ischemia
      autologous vein graft I70.409
        leg I70.409
          with
            gangrene (and intermittent claudication, rest pain and ulcer) I70.469
            intermittent claudication I70.419
            rest pain (and intermittent claudication) I70.429
          bilateral I70.403
            with
              gangrene (and intermittent claudication, rest pain and ulcer) I70.463
              intermittent claudication I70.463
              rest pain (and intermittent claudication) I70.423
            specified type NEC I70.493
          left I70.402
            with
              gangrene (and intermittent claudication, rest pain and ulcer) I70.462
              intermittent claudication I70.412
              rest pain (and intermittent claudication) I70.422
              ulceration (and intermittent claudication and rest pain) I70.449
                ankle I70.443
                calf I70.442
                foot site NEC I70.445
                heel I70.444
                lower leg NEC I70.448
                midfoot I70.444
                thigh I70.441
            specified type NEC I70.492
          right I70.401
            with
              gangrene (and intermittent claudication, rest pain and ulcer) I70.461
              intermittent claudication I70.411
              rest pain (and intermittent claudication) I70.421
              ulceration (and intermittent claudication and rest pain) I70.439
                ankle I70.433
                calf I70.432
                foot site NEC I70.435
                heel I70.434
                lower leg NEC I70.438

Arteriosclerosis, arteriosclerotic — *continued*
  extremities — *continued*
    bypass graft — *continued*
      autologous vein graft — *continued*
        leg — *continued*
          right — *continued*
            with — *continued*
              ulceration — *continued*
                midfoot I70.434
                thigh I70.431
            specified type NEC I70.491
          specified type NEC I70.499
        specified type NEC I70.408
          with
            gangrene (and intermittent claudication, rest pain and ulcer) I70.468
            intermittent claudication I70.418
            rest pain (and intermittent claudication) I70.428
            ulceration (and intermittent claudication and rest pain) I70.45
        specified type NEC I70.498
      leg I70.309
        with
          gangrene (and intermittent claudication, rest pain and ulcer) I70.369
          intermittent claudication I70.319
          rest pain (and intermittent claudication) I70.329
        bilateral I70.303
          with
            gangrene (and intermittent claudication, rest pain and ulcer) I70.363
            intermittent claudication I70.313
            rest pain (and intermittent claudication) I70.323
          specified type NEC I70.393
        left I70.302
          with
            gangrene (and intermittent claudication, rest pain and ulcer) I70.362
            intermittent claudication I70.312
            rest pain (and intermittent claudication) I70.322
            ulceration (and intermittent claudication and rest pain) I70.349
              ankle I70.343
              calf I70.342
              foot site NEC I70.345
              heel I70.344
              lower leg NEC I70.348
              midfoot I70.344
              thigh I70.341
          specified type NEC I70.392
        right I70.301
          with
            gangrene (and intermittent claudication, rest pain and ulcer) I70.361
            intermittent claudication I70.311
            rest pain (and intermittent claudication) I70.321
            ulceration (and intermittent claudication and rest pain I70.339
              ankle I70.333
              calf I70.332
              foot site NEC I70.335
              heel I70.334
              lower leg NEC I70.338
              midfoot I70.334
              thigh I70.331
          specified type NEC I70.391
        specified type NEC I70.399
      nonautologous biological graft I70.509
        leg I70.509
          with
            gangrene (and intermittent claudication, rest pain and ulcer) I70.569
            intermittent claudication I70.519
            rest pain (and intermittent claudication) I70.529
        bilateral I70.503
          with
            gangrene (and intermittent claudication, rest pain and ulcer) I70.563
            intermittent claudication I70.513
            rest pain (and intermittent claudication) I70.523
          specified type NEC I70.593

Arteriosclerosis, arteriosclerotic — *continued*
  extremities — *continued*
    bypass graft — *continued*
      nonautologous biological graft — *continued*
        leg — *continued*
          left I70.502
            with
              gangrene (and intermittent claudication, rest pain and ulcer) I70.562
              intermittent claudication I70.512
              rest pain (and intermittent claudication) I70.522
              ulceration (and intermittent claudication and rest pain) I70.549
                ankle I70.543
                calf I70.542
                foot site NEC I70.545
                heel I70.544
                lower leg NEC I70.548
                midfoot I70.544
                thigh I70.541
          specified type NEC I70.592
          right I70.501
            with
              gangrene (and intermittent claudication, rest pain and ulcer) I70.561
              intermittent claudication I70.511
              rest pain (and intermittent claudication) I70.521
              ulceration (and intermittent claudication and rest pain) I70.539
                ankle I70.533
                calf I70.532
                foot site NEC I70.535
                heel I70.534
                lower leg NEC I70.538
                midfoot I70.534
                thigh I70.531
          specified type NEC I70.591
        specified type NEC I70.599
        specified NEC I70.508
          with
            gangrene (and intermittent claudication, rest pain and ulcer) I70.568
            intermittent claudication I70.518
            rest pain (and intermittent claudication) I70.528
            ulceration (and intermittent claudication and rest pain) I70.55
        specified type NEC I70.598
      nonbiological graft I70.609
        leg I70.609
          with
            gangrene (and intermittent claudication, rest pain and ulcer) I70.669
            intermittent claudication I70.619
            rest pain (and intermittent claudication) I70.629
        bilateral I70.603
          with
            gangrene (and intermittent claudication, rest pain and ulcer) I70.663
            intermittent claudication I70.613
            rest pain (and intermittent claudication) I70.623
          specified type NEC I70.693
        left I70.602
          with
            gangrene (and intermittent claudication, rest pain and ulcer) I70.662
            intermittent claudication I70.612
            rest pain (and intermittent claudication) I70.622
            ulceration (and intermittent claudication and rest pain) I70.649
              ankle I70.643
              calf I70.642
              foot site NEC I70.645
              heel I70.644
              lower leg NEC I70.648
              midfoot I70.644
              thigh I70.641
          specified type NEC I70.692
        right I70.601

Arteriosclerosis, arteriosclerotic — *continued*
  extremities — *continued*
    bypass graft — *continued*
      nonbiological graft — *continued*
        leg — *continued*
          right — *continued*
            with
              gangrene (and intermittent claudication, rest pain and ulcer) I70.661
              intermittent claudication I70.611
              rest pain (and intermittent claudication) I70.621
              ulceration (and intermittent claudication and rest pain) I70.639
                ankle I70.633
                calf I70.632
                foot site NEC I70.635
                heel I70.634
                lower leg NEC I70.638
                midfoot I70.634
                thigh I70.631
          specified type NEC I70.691
        specified type NEC I70.699
        specified NEC I70.608
          with
            gangrene (and intermittent claudication, rest pain and ulcer) I70.668
            intermittent claudication I70.618
            rest pain (and intermittent claudication) I70.628
            ulceration (and intermittent claudication and rest pain) I70.65
        specified type NEC I70.698
      specified graft NEC I70.709
        leg I70.709
          with
            gangrene (and intermittent claudication, rest pain and ulcer) I70.769
            intermittent claudication I70.719
            rest pain (and intermittent claudication) I70.729
        bilateral I70.703
          with
            gangrene (and intermittent claudication, rest pain and ulcer) I70.763
            intermittent claudication I70.713
            rest pain (and intermittent claudication) I70.723
          specified type NEC I70.793
        left I70.702
          with
            gangrene (and intermittent claudication, rest pain and ulcer) I70.762
            intermittent claudication I70.712
            rest pain (and intermittent claudication) I70.722
            ulceration (and intermittent claudication and rest pain) I70.749
              ankle I70.743
              calf I70.742
              foot site NEC I70.745
              heel I70.744
              lower leg NEC I70.748
              midfoot I70.744
              thigh I70.741
          specified type NEC I70.792
        right I70.701
          with
            gangrene (and intermittent claudication, rest pain and ulcer) I70.761
            intermittent claudication I70.711
            rest pain (and intermittent claudication) I70.721
            ulceration (and intermittent claudication and rest pain) I70.739
              ankle I70.733
              calf I70.732
              foot site NEC I70.735
              heel I70.734
              lower leg NEC I70.738
              midfoot I70.734
              thigh I70.731
          specified type NEC I70.791
        specified type NEC I70.799
        specified NEC I70.708

Arteriosclerosis, arteriosclerotic — *continued*
  extremities — *continued*
    bypass graft — *continued*
      specified graft — *continued*
        specified — *continued*
          with
            gangrene (and intermittent claudication, rest pain and ulcer) I70.768
            intermittent claudication I70.718
            rest pain (and intermittent claudication) I70.728
            ulceration (and intermittent claudication and rest pain) I70.75
          specified type NEC I70.798
      specified NEC I70.308
        with
          gangrene (and intermittent claudication, rest pain and ulcer) I70.368
          intermittent claudication I70.318
          rest pain (and intermittent claudication) I70.328
          ulceration (and intermittent claudication and rest pain) I70.35
        specifiec type NEC I70.398
    leg I70.209
      with
        gangrene (and intermittent claudication, rest pain and ulcer) I70.269
        intermittent claudication I70.219
        rest pain (and intermittent claudication) I70.229
      bilateral I70.203
        with
          gangrene (and intermittent claudication, rest pain and ulcer) I70.263
          intermittent claudication I70.213
          rest pain (and intermittent claudication) I70.223
        specified type NEC I70.293
      left I70.202
        with
          gangrene (and intermittent claudication, rest pain and ulcer) I70.262
          intermittent claudication I70.212
          rest pain (and intermittent claudication) I70.222
          ulceration (and intermittent claudication and rest pain) I70.249
            ankle I70.243
            calf I70.242
            foot site NEC I70.245
            heel I70.244
            lower leg NEC I70.248
            midfoot I70.244
            thigh I70.241
        specified type NEC I70.292
      right I70.201
        with
          gangrene (and intermittent claudication, rest pain and ulcer) I70.261
          intermittent claudication I70.211
          rest pain (and intermittent claudication) I70.221
          ulceration (and intermittent claudication and rest pain) I70.239
            ankle I70.233
            calf I70.232
            foot site NEC I70.235
            heel I70.234
            lower leg NEC I70.238
            midfoot I70.234
            thigh I70.231
        specified type NEC I70.291
      specified type NEC I70.299
    specified site NEC I70.208
      with
        gangrene (and intermittent claudication, rest pain and ulcer) I70.268
        intermittent claudication I70.218
        rest pain (and intermittent claudication) I70.228
        ulceration (and intermittent claudication and rest pain) I70.25
      specified type NEC I70.298
  generalized I70.91
  heart (disease) — *see* Arteriosclerosis, coronary (artery), kidney — *see* Hypertension, kidney
  medial — *see* Arteriosclerosis, extremities
  mesenteric (artery) K55.1

Arteriosclerosis, arteriosclerotic — *continued*
  Mönckeberg's — *see* Arteriosclerosis, extremities
  myocarditis I51.4
  peripheral (of extremities) — *see* Arteriosclerosis, extremities
  pulmonary (idiopathic) I27.0
  renal (arterioles) — *see also* Hypertension, kidney
    artery I70.1
  retina (vascular) I70.8 *[H35.0-]* ☑
  specified artery NEC I70.8
  spinal (cord) G95.19
  vertebral (artery) I67.2
Arteriospasm I73.9
Arteriovenous — *see* condition
Arteritis I77.6
  allergic M31.0
  aorta (nonsyphilitic) I77.6
    syphilitic A52.02
  aortic arch M31.4
  brachiocephalic M31.4
  brain I67.7
    syphilitic A52.04
  cerebral I67.7
    in systemic lupus erythematosus M32.19
    listerial A32.89
    syphilitic A52.04
    tuberculous A18.89
  coronary (artery) I25.89
    rheumatic I01.8
      chronic I09.89
    syphilitic A52.06
  cranial (left) (right), giant cell M31.6
  deformans — *see* Arteriosclerosis
  giant cell NEC M31.6
    with polymyalgia rheumatica M31.5
  necrosing or necrotizing M31.9
    specified NEC M31.8
  nodosa M30.0
  obliterans — *see* Arteriosclerosis
  pulmonary I28.8
  rheumatic — *see* Fever, rheumatic
  senile — *see* Arteriosclerosis
  suppurative I77.2
  syphilitic (general) A52.09
    brain A52.04
    coronary A52.06
    spinal A52.09
  temporal, giant cell M31.6
  young female aortic arch syndrome M31.4
Artery, arterial — *see also* condition
  abscess I77.89
  single umbilical Q27.0
Arthralgia (allergic) — *see also* Pain, joint
  in caisson disease T70.3 ☑
  temporomandibular M26.62- ☑
Arthritis, arthritic (acute) (chronic) (nonpyogenic) (subacute) M19.90
  allergic — *see* Arthritis, specified form NEC
  ankylosing (crippling) (spine) — *see also* Spondylitis, ankylosing
    sites other than spine — *see* Arthritis, specified form NEC
  atrophic — *see* Osteoarthritis
    spine — *see* Spondylitis, ankylosing
  back — *see* Spondylopathy, inflammatory
  blennorrhagic (gonococcal) A54.42
  Charcot's — *see* Arthropathy, neuropathic
    diabetic — *see* Diabetes, arthropathy, neuropathic
    syringomyelic G95.0
  chylous (filarial) — *see also* category M01 B74.9
  climacteric (any site) NEC — *see* Arthritis, specified form NEC
  crystal (-induced) — *see* Arthritis, in, crystals
  deformans — *see* Osteoarthritis
  degenerative — *see* Osteoarthritis
  due to or associated with
    acromegaly E22.0
    brucellosis — *see* Brucellosis
    caisson disease T70.3 ☑
    diabetes — *see* Diabetes, arthropathy
    dracontiasis — *see also* category M01 B72
    enteritis NEC
      regional — *see* Enteritis, regional
    erysipelas — *see also* category M01 A46
    erythema
      epidemic A25.1
      nodosum L52
    filariasis NOS B74.9

Arthritis, arthritic — *continued*
  due to or associated with — *continued*
    glanders A24.0
    helminthiasis — *see also* category M01 B83.9
    hemophilia D66 *[M36.2]*
    Henoch- (Schönlein) purpura D69.0 *[M36.4]*
    human parvovirus — *see also* category M01 B97.6
    infectious disease NEC M01 ☑
    leprosy (see also category M01) — *see also* Leprosy A30.9
    Lyme disease A69.23
    mycobacteria — *see also* category M01 A31.8
    parasitic disease NEC — *see also* category M01 B89
    paratyphoid fever (see also category M01) — *see also* Fever, paratyphoid A01.4
    rat bite fever — *see also* category M01 A25.1
    regional enteritis — *see* Enteritis, regional
    respiratory disorder NOS J98.9
    serum sickness — *see also* Reaction, serum T80.69 ☑
    syringomyelia G95.0
    typhoid fever A01.04
  epidemic erythema A25.1
  facet joint — *see also* Spondylosis M47.819
  febrile — *see* Fever, rheumatic
  gonococcal A54.42
  gouty (acute) — *see* Gout
  in (due to)
    acromegaly — *see also* subcategory M14.8- E22.0
    amyloidosis — *see also* subcategory M14.8- E85.4
    bacterial disease — *see also* subcategory M01 A49.9
    Behçet's syndrome M35.2
    caisson disease — *see also* subcategory M14.8- T70.3 ☑
    coliform bacilli (Escherichia coli) — *see* Arthritis, in, pyogenic organism NEC
    crystals M11.9
      dicalcium phosphate — *see* Arthritis, in, crystals, specified type NEC
      hydroxyapatite M11.0- ☑
      pyrophosphate — *see* Arthritis, in, crystals, specified type NEC
      specified type NEC M11.80
        ankle M11.87- ☑
        elbow M11.82- ☑
        foot joint M11.87- ☑
        hand joint M11.84- ☑
        hip M11.85- ☑
        knee M11.86- ☑
        multiple sites M11.8- ☑
        shoulder M11.81- ☑
        vertebrae M11.88
        wrist M11.83- ☑
    dermatoarthritis, lipoid E78.81
    dracontiasis (dracunculiasis) — *see also* category M01 B72
    endocrine disorder NEC — *see also* subcategory M14.8- E34.9
    enteritis, infectious NEC — *see also* category M01 A09
      specified organism NEC — *see also* category M01 A08.8
    erythema
      multiforme — *see also* subcategory M14.8- L51.9
      nodosum — *see also* subcategory M14.8- L52
    gout — *see* Gout
    helminthiasis NEC — *see also* category M01 B83.9
    hemochromatosis — *see also* subcategory M14.8- E83.118
    hemoglobinopathy NEC D58.2 *[M36.3]*
    hemophilia NEC D66 *[M36.2]*
    Hemophilus influenzae M00.8- ☑ *[B96.3]*
    Henoch (-Schönlein) purpura D69.0 *[M36.4]*
    hyperparathyroidism NEC — *see also* subcategory M14.8- E21.3
    hypersensitivity reaction NEC T78.49 ☑ *[M36.4]*
    hypogammaglobulinemia — *see also* subcategory M14.8- D80.1
    hypothyroidism NEC — *see also* subcategory M14.8- E03.9
    infection — *see* Arthritis, pyogenic or pyemic
      spine — *see* Spondylopathy, infective
    infectious disease NEC M01 ☑
    leprosy — *see also* category M01 A30.9
    leukemia NEC C95.9- ☑ *[M36.1]*
    lipoid dermatoarthritis E78.81
    Lyme disease A69.23

Arthritis, arthritic — *continued*
　in — *continued*
　　Mediterranean fever, familial — *see also* subcategory M14.8- M04.1
　　Meningococcus A39.83
　　metabolic disorder NEC — *see also* subcategory M14.8- E88.9
　　multiple myelomatosis C90.0- ☑ *[M36.1]*
　　mumps B26.85
　　mycosis NEC — *see also* category M01 B49
　　myelomatosis (multiple) C90.0- ☑ *[M36.1]*
　　neurological disorder NEC G98.0
　　ochronosis — *see also* subcategory M14.8- E70.29
　　O'nyong-nyong — *see also* category M01 A92.1
　　parasitic disease NEC — *see also* category M01 B89
　　paratyphoid fever — *see also* category M01 A01.4
　　Pseudomonas — *see* Arthritis, pyogenic, bacterial NEC
　　psoriasis L40.50
　　pyogenic organism NEC — *see* Arthritis, pyogenic, bacterial NEC
　　Reiter's disease — *see* Reiter's disease
　　respiratory disorder NEC — *see also* subcategory M14.8- J98.9
　　reticulosis, malignant — *see also* subcategory M14.8- C86.0
　　rubella B06.82
　　Salmonella (arizonae) (cholerae-suis) (enteritidis) (typhimurium) A02.23
　　sarcoidosis D86.86
　　specified bacteria NEC — *see* Arthritis, pyogenic, bacterial NEC
　　sporotrichosis B42.82
　　syringomyelia G95.0
　　thalassemia NEC D56.9 *[M36.3]*
　　tuberculosis — *see* Tuberculosis, arthritis
　　typhoid fever A01.04
　　urethritis, Reiter's — *see* Reiter's disease
　　viral disease NEC — *see also* category M01 B34.9
　infectious or infective — *see also* Arthritis, pyogenic or pyemic
　　spine — *see* Spondylopathy, infective
　juvenile M08.90
　　with systemic onset — *see* Still's disease
　　ankle M08.97- ☑
　　elbow M08.92- ☑
　　foot joint M08.97- ☑
　　hand joint M08.94- ☑
　　hip M08.95- ☑
　　knee M08.96- ☑
　　multiple site M08.99
　　pauciarticular M08.40
　　　ankle M08.47- ☑
　　　elbow M08.42- ☑
　　　foot joint M08.47- ☑
　　　hand joint M08.44- ☑
　　　hip M08.45- ☑
　　　knee M08.46- ☑
　　　shoulder M08.41- ☑
　　　specified site NEC M08.4A
　　　vertebrae M08.48
　　　wrist M08.43- ☑
　　psoriatic L40.54
　　rheumatoid — *see* Arthritis, rheumatoid, juvenile
　　shoulder M08.91- ☑
　　specified site NEC M08.9A
　　specified type NEC M08.80
　　　ankle M08.87- ☑
　　　elbow M08.82- ☑
　　　foot joint M08.87- ☑
　　　hand joint M08.84- ☑
　　　hip M08.85- ☑
　　　knee M08.86- ☑
　　　multiple site M08.89
　　　shoulder M08.81- ☑
　　　specified joint NEC M08.88
　　　vertebrae M08.88
　　　wrist M08.83- ☑
　　wrist M08.93- ☑
　meaning osteoarthritis — *see* Osteoarthritis
　meningococcal A39.83
　menopausal (any site) NEC — *see* Arthritis, specified form NEC
　mutilans (psoriatic) L40.52
　mycotic NEC — *see also* category M01 B49
　neuropathic (Charcot) — *see* Arthropathy, neuropathic
　　diabetic — *see* Diabetes, arthropathy, neuropathic

Arthritis, arthritic — *continued*
　neuropathic — *see* Arthropathy, neuropathic — *continued*
　　nonsyphilitic NEC G98.0
　　syringomyelic G95.0
　ochronotic — *see also* subcategory M14.8- E70.29
　palindromic (any site) — *see* Rheumatism, palindromic
　pneumococcal M00.10
　　ankle M00.17- ☑
　　elbow M00.12- ☑
　　foot joint — *see* Arthritis, pneumococcal, ankle
　　hand joint M00.14- ☑
　　hip M00.15- ☑
　　knee M00.16- ☑
　　multiple site M00.19
　　shoulder M00.11- ☑
　　vertebra M00.18
　　wrist M00.13- ☑
　postdysenteric — *see* Arthropathy, postdysenteric
　postmeningococcal A39.84
　postrheumatic, chronic — *see* Arthropathy, postrheumatic, chronic
　primary progressive — *see also* Arthritis, specified form NEC
　　spine — *see* Spondylitis, ankylosing
　psoriatic L40.50
　purulent (any site except spine) — *see* Arthritis, pyogenic or pyemic
　　spine — *see* Spondylopathy, infective
　pyogenic or pyemic (any site except spine) M00.9
　　bacterial NEC M00.80
　　　ankle M00.87- ☑
　　　elbow M00.82- ☑
　　　foot joint — *see* Arthritis, pyogenic, bacterial NEC, ankle
　　　hand joint M00.84- ☑
　　　hip M00.85- ☑
　　　knee M00.86- ☑
　　　multiple site M00.89
　　　shoulder M00.81- ☑
　　　vertebra M00.88
　　　wrist M00.83- ☑
　　pneumococcal — *see* Arthritis, pneumococcal
　　spine — *see* Spondylopathy, infective
　　staphylococcal — *see* Arthritis, staphylococcal
　　streptococcal — *see* Arthritis, streptococcal NEC
　　　pneumococcal — *see* Arthritis, pneumococcal
　reactive — *see* Reiter's disease
　rheumatic — *see also* Arthritis, rheumatoid
　　acute or subacute — *see* Fever, rheumatic
　rheumatoid M06.9
　　with
　　　carditis — *see* Rheumatoid, carditis
　　　endocarditis — *see* Rheumatoid, carditis
　　　heart involvement NEC — *see* Rheumatoid, carditis
　　　lung involvement — *see* Rheumatoid, lung
　　　myocarditis — *see* Rheumatoid, carditis
　　　myopathy — *see* Rheumatoid, myopathy
　　　pericarditis — *see* Rheumatoid, carditis
　　　polyneuropathy — *see* Rheumatoid, polyneuropathy
　　　rheumatoid factor — *see* Arthritis, rheumatoid, seropositive
　　　splenoadenomegaly and leukopenia — *see* Felty's syndrome
　　　vasculitis — *see* Rheumatoid, vasculitis
　　　visceral involvement NEC — *see* Rheumatoid, arthritis, with involvement of organs NEC
　　juvenile (with or without rheumatoid factor) M08.00
　　　with systemic onset — *see* Still's disease
　　　ankle M08.07- ☑
　　　elbow M08.02- ☑
　　　foot joint M08.07- ☑
　　　hand joint M08.04- ☑
　　　hip M08.05- ☑
　　　knee M08.06- ☑
　　　multiple site M08.09
　　　shoulder M08.01- ☑
　　　specified site NEC M08.0A
　　　vertebra M08.08
　　　wrist M08.03- ☑
　　seronegative M06.00
　　　ankle M06.07- ☑
　　　elbow M06.02- ☑
　　　foot joint M06.07- ☑
　　　hand joint M06.04- ☑

Arthritis, arthritic — *continued*
　rheumatoid — *continued*
　　seronegative — *continued*
　　　hip M06.05- ☑
　　　knee M06.06- ☑
　　　multiple site M06.09
　　　shoulder M06.01- ☑
　　　specified site NEC M06.0A
　　　vertebra M06.08
　　　wrist M06.03- ☑
　　seropositive M05.9
　　　specified NEC M05.80
　　　　ankle M05.87- ☑
　　　　elbow M05.82- ☑
　　　　foot joint M05.87- ☑
　　　　hand joint M05.84- ☑
　　　　hip M05.85- ☑
　　　　knee M05.86- ☑
　　　　multiple sites M05.89
　　　　shoulder M05.81- ☑
　　　　specified site NEC M05.8A
　　　　vertebra — *see* Spondylitis, ankylosing
　　　　wrist M05.83- ☑
　　　without organ involvement M05.70
　　　　ankle M05.77- ☑
　　　　elbow M05.72- ☑
　　　　foot joint M05.77- ☑
　　　　hand joint M05.74- ☑
　　　　hip M05.75- ☑
　　　　knee M05.76- ☑
　　　　multiple sites M05.79
　　　　shoulder M05.71- ☑
　　　　specified site NEC M05.7A
　　　　vertebra — *see* Spondylitis, ankylosing
　　　　wrist M05.73- ☑
　　specified type NEC M06.80
　　　ankle M06.87- ☑
　　　elbow M06.82- ☑
　　　foot joint M06.87- ☑
　　　hand joint M06.84- ☑
　　　hip M06.85- ☑
　　　knee M06.86- ☑
　　　multiple site M06.89
　　　shoulder M06.81- ☑
　　　specified site NEC M06.8A
　　　vertebra M06.88
　　　wrist M06.83- ☑
　　spine — *see* Spondylitis, ankylosing
　rubella B06.82
　scorbutic — *see also* subcategory M14.8- E54
　senile or senescent — *see* Osteoarthritis
　septic (any site except spine) — *see* Arthritis, pyogenic or pyemic
　　spine — *see* Spondylopathy, infective
　serum (nontherapeutic) (therapeutic) — *see* Arthropathy, postimmunization
　specified form NEC M13.80
　　ankle M13.87- ☑
　　elbow M13.82- ☑
　　foot joint M13.87- ☑
　　hand joint M13.84- ☑
　　hip M13.85- ☑
　　knee M13.86- ☑
　　multiple site M13.89
　　shoulder M13.81- ☑
　　specified joint NEC M13.88
　　wrist M13.83- ☑
　spine — *see also* Spondylosis
　　infectious or infective NEC — *see* Spondylopathy, infective
　　Marie-Strümpell — *see* Spondylitis, ankylosing
　　pyogenic — *see* Spondylopathy, infective
　　rheumatoid — *see* Spondylitis, ankylosing
　　traumatic (old) — *see* Spondylopathy, traumatic
　　tuberculous A18.01
　staphylococcal M00.00
　　ankle M00.07- ☑
　　elbow M00.02- ☑
　　foot joint — *see* Arthritis, staphylococcal, ankle
　　hand joint M00.04- ☑
　　hip M00.05- ☑
　　knee M00.06- ☑
　　multiple site M00.09
　　shoulder M00.01- ☑
　　vertebra M00.08
　　wrist M00.03- ☑
　streptococcal NEC M00.20

Arthritis, arthritic — *continued*
  streptococcal — *continued*
    ankle M00.27- ☑
    elbow M00.22- ☑
    foot joint — *see* Arthritis, streptococcal, ankle
    hand joint M00.24- ☑
    hip M00.25- ☑
    knee M00.26- ☑
    multiple site M00.29
    shoulder M00.21- ☑
    vertebra M00.28
    wrist M00.23- ☑
  suppurative — *see* Arthritis, pyogenic or pyemic
  syphilitic (late) A52.16
    congenital A50.55 [M12.80]
  syphilitica deformans (Charcot) A52.16
  temporomandibular joint M26.64- ☑
  toxic of menopause (any site) — *see* Arthritis, specified
    form NEC
  transient — *see* Arthropathy, specified form NEC
  traumatic (chronic) — *see* Arthropathy, traumatic
  tuberculous A18.02
    spine A18.01
  uratic — *see* Gout
  urethritica (Reiter's) — *see* Reiter's disease
  vertebral — *see* Spondylopathy, inflammatory
  villous (any site) — *see* Arthropathy, specified form
    NEC
Arthrocele — *see* Effusion, joint
Arthrodesis status Z98.1
Arthrodynia — *see also* Pain, joint
Arthrodysplasia Q74.9
Arthrofibrosis, joint — *see* Ankylosis
Arthrogryposis (congenital) Q68.8
  multiplex congenita Q74.3
Arthrokatadysis M24.7
Arthropathy — *see also* Arthritis M12.9
  Charcot's — *see* Arthropathy, neuropathic
    diabetic — *see* Diabetes, arthropathy, neuropathic
    syringomyelic G95.0
  cricoarytenoid J38.7
  crystal (-induced) — *see* Arthritis, in, crystals
  diabetic NEC — *see* Diabetes, arthropathy
  distal interphalangeal, psoriatic L40.51
  enteropathic M07.60
    ankle M07.67- ☑
    elbow M07.62- ☑
    foot joint M07.67- ☑
    hand joint M07.64- ☑
    hip M07.65- ☑
    knee M07.66- ☑
    multiple site M07.69
    shoulder M07.61- ☑
    vertebra M07.68
    wrist M07.63- ☑
  facet joint — *see also* Spondylosis M47.819
  following intestinal bypass M02.00
    ankle M02.07- ☑
    elbow M02.02- ☑
    foot joint M02.07- ☑
    hand joint M02.04- ☑
    hip M02.05- ☑
    knee M02.06- ☑
    multiple site M02.09
    shoulder M02.01- ☑
    vertebra M02.08
    wrist M02.03- ☑
  gouty — *see also* Gout
    in (due to)
      Lesch-Nyhan syndrome E79.1 [M14.8-] ☑
      sickle-cell disorders D57- ☑ [M14.8-] ☑
  hemophilic NEC D66 [M36.2]
    in (due to)
      hyperparathyroidism NEC E21.3 [M14.8-] ☑
      metabolic disease NOS E88.9 [M14.8-] ☑
  in (due to)
    acromegaly E22.0 [M14.8-] ☑
    amyloidosis E85.4 [M14.8-] ☑
    blood disorder NOS D75.9 [M36.3]
    diabetes — *see* Diabetes, arthropathy
    endocrine disease NOS E34.9 [M14.8-] ☑
    erythema
      multiforme L51.9 [M14.8-] ☑
      nodosum L52 [M14.8-] ☑
    hemochromatosis E83.118 [M14.8-] ☑
    hemoglobinopathy NEC D58.2 [M36.3]

Arthropathy — *continued*
  in — *continued*
    hemophilia NEC D66 [M36.2]
    Henoch-Schönlein purpura D69.0 [M36.4]
    hyperthyroidism E05.90 [M14.8-] ☑
    hypothyroidism E03.9 [M14.8-] ☑
    infective endocarditis I33.0 [M12.80]
    leukemia NEC C95.9- ☑ [M36.1]
    malignant histiocytosis C96.A [M36.1]
    metabolic disease NOS E88.9 [M14.8-] ☑
    multiple myeloma C90.0- ☑ [M36.1]
    neoplastic disease NOS (*see also* Neoplasm)
      D49.9 [M36.1]
    nutritional deficiency — *see also* subcategory
      M14.8- E63.9
    psoriasis NOS L40.50
    sarcoidosis D86.86
    syphilis (late) A52.77
      congenital A50.55 [M12.80]
    thyrotoxicosis — *see also* subcategory M14.8-
      E05.90
    ulcerative colitis K51.90 [M07.60]
    viral hepatitis (postinfectious) NEC B19.9 [M12.80]
    Whipple's disease — *see also* subcategory M14.8-
      K90.81
  Jaccoud — *see* Arthropathy, postrheumatic, chronic
  juvenile — *see* Arthritis, juvenile
    psoriatic L40.54
  mutilans (psoriatic) L40.52
  neuropathic (Charcot) M14.60
    ankle M14.67- ☑
    diabetic — *see* Diabetes, arthropathy, neuropathic
    elbow M14.62- ☑
    foot joint M14.67- ☑
    hand joint M14.64- ☑
    hip M14.65- ☑
    knee M14.66- ☑
    multiple site M14.69
    nonsyphilitic NEC G98.0
    shoulder M14.61- ☑
    syringomyelic G95.0
    vertebra M14.68
    wrist M14.63- ☑
  osteopulmonary — *see* Osteoarthropathy, hyper-
    trophic, specified NEC
  postdysenteric M02.10
    ankle M02.17- ☑
    elbow M02.12- ☑
    foot joint M02.17- ☑
    hand joint M02.14- ☑
    hip M02.15- ☑
    knee M02.16- ☑
    multiple site M02.19
    shoulder M02.11- ☑
    vertebra M02.18
    wrist M02.13- ☑
  postimmunization M02.20
    ankle M02.27- ☑
    elbow M02.22- ☑
    foot joint M02.27- ☑
    hand joint M02.24- ☑
    hip M02.25- ☑
    knee M02.26- ☑
    multiple site M02.29
    shoulder M02.21- ☑
    vertebra M02.28
    wrist M02.23- ☑
  postinfectious NEC B99 ☑ [M12.80]
    in (due to)
      enteritis due to Yersinia enterocolitica
        A04.6 [M12.80]
      syphilis A52.77
      viral hepatitis NEC B19.9 [M12.80]
  postrheumatic, chronic (Jaccoud) M12.00
    ankle M12.07- ☑
    elbow M12.02- ☑
    foot joint M12.07- ☑
    hand joint M12.04- ☑
    hip M12.05- ☑
    knee M12.06- ☑
    multiple site M12.09
    shoulder M12.01- ☑
    specified joint NEC M12.08
    vertebrae M12.08
    wrist M12.03- ☑
  psoriatic NEC L40.59
    interphalangeal, distal L40.51

Arthropathy — *continued*
  reactive M02.9
    in (due to)
      infective endocarditis I33.0 [M02.9]
    specified type NEC M02.80
      ankle M02.87- ☑
      elbow M02.82- ☑
      foot joint M02.87- ☑
      hand joint M02.84- ☑
      hip M02.85- ☑
      knee M02.86- ☑
      multiple site M02.89
      shoulder M02.81- ☑
      vertebra M02.88
      wrist M02.83- ☑
  specified form NEC M12.80
    ankle M12.87- ☑
    elbow M12.82- ☑
    foot joint M12.87- ☑
    hand joint M12.84- ☑
    hip M12.85- ☑
    knee M12.86- ☑
    multiple site M12.89
    shoulder M12.81- ☑
    specified joint NEC M12.88
    vertebrae M12.88
    wrist M12.83- ☑
  syringomyelic G95.0
  tabes dorsalis A52.16
  tabetic A52.16
  temporomandibular joint M26.65- ☑
  transient — *see* Arthropathy, specified form NEC
  traumatic M12.50
    ankle M12.57- ☑
    elbow M12.52- ☑
    foot joint M12.57- ☑
    hand joint M12.54- ☑
    hip M12.55- ☑
    knee M12.56- ☑
    multiple site M12.59
    shoulder M12.51- ☑
    specified joint NEC M12.58
    vertebrae M12.58
    wrist M12.53- ☑
Arthropyosis — *see* Arthritis, pyogenic or pyemic
Arthrosis (deformans) (degenerative) (localized) — *see
  also* Osteoarthritis M19.90
  spine — *see* Spondylosis
Arthus' phenomenon or reaction T78.41 ☑
  due to
    drug — *see* Table of Drugs and Chemicals, by drug
Articular — *see* condition
Articulation, reverse (teeth) M26.24
Artificial
  insemination complication — *see* Complications, arti-
    ficial, fertilization
  opening status (functioning) (without complication)
    Z93.9
    anus (colostomy) Z93.3
    colostomy Z93.3
    cystostomy Z93.50
      appendico-vesicostomy Z93.52
      cutaneous Z93.51
      specified NEC Z93.59
    enterostomy Z93.4
    gastrostomy Z93.1
    ileostomy Z93.2
    intestinal tract NEC Z93.4
    jejunostomy Z93.4
    nephrostomy Z93.6
    specified site NEC Z93.8
    tracheostomy Z93.0
    ureterostomy Z93.6
    urethrostomy Z93.6
    urinary tract NEC Z93.6
    vagina Z93.8
  vagina status Z93.8
Arytenoid — *see* condition
Asbestosis (occupational) J61
Ascariasis B77.9
  with
    complications NEC B77.89
    intestinal complications B77.0
    pneumonia, pneumonitis B77.81
Ascaridosis, ascaridiasis — *see* Ascariasis
Ascaris (infection) (infestation) (lumbricoides) — *see* As-
  cariasis

Ascending — *see* condition
ASC-H (atypical squamous cells cannot exclude high grade squamous intraepithelial lesion on cytologic smear)
　anus R85.611
　cervix R87.611
　vagina R87.621
Aschoff's bodies — *see* Myocarditis, rheumatic
Ascites (abdominal) R18.8
　cardiac — *see also* Failure, heart, right I50.810
　chylous (nonfilarial) I89.8
　　filarial — *see* Infestation, filarial
　due to
　　cirrhosis, alcoholic K70.31
　　hepatitis
　　　alcoholic K70.11
　　　chronic active K71.51
　　　S. japonicum B65.2
　heart — *see also* Failure, heart, right I50.810
　malignant R18.0
　pseudochylous R18.8
　syphilitic A52.74
　tuberculous A18.31
ASC-US (atypical squamous cells of undetermined significance on cytologic smear)
　anus R85.610
　cervix R87.610
　vagina R87.620
Aseptic — *see* condition
Asherman's syndrome N85.6
Asialia K11.7
Asiatic cholera — *see* Cholera
Asimultagnosia (simultanagnosia) R48.3
Askin's tumor — *see* Neoplasm, connective tissue, malignant
Asocial personality F60.2
Asomatognosia R41.4
Aspartylglucosaminuria E77.1
Asperger's disease or syndrome F84.5
Aspergilloma — *see* Aspergillosis
Aspergillosis (with pneumonia) B44.9
　bronchopulmonary, allergic B44.81
　disseminated B44.7
　generalized B44.7
　pulmonary NEC B44.1
　　allergic B44.81
　　invasive B44.0
　specified NEC B44.89
　tonsillar B44.2
Aspergillus (flavus) (fumigatus) (infection) (terreus) — *see* Aspergillosis
Aspermatogenesis — *see* Azoospermia
Aspermia (testis) — *see* Azoospermia
Asphyxia, asphyxiation (by) R09.01
　antenatal P84
　birth P84
　bunny bag — *see* Asphyxia, due to, mechanical threat to breathing, trapped in bed clothes
　crushing S28.0 ☑
　drowning T75.1 ☑
　gas, fumes, or vapor — *see* Table of Drugs and Chemicals
　inhalation — *see* Inhalation
　intrauterine P84
　local I73.00
　　with gangrene I73.01
　mucus — *see also* Foreign body, respiratory tract, causing asphyxia
　newborn P84
　pathological R09.01
　postnatal P84
　　mechanical — *see* Asphyxia, due to, mechanical threat to breathing
　prenatal P84
　reticularis R23.1
　strangulation — *see* Asphyxia, due to, mechanical threat to breathing
　submersion T75.1 ☑
　traumatic T71.9 ☑
　　due to
　　　crushed chest S28.0 ☑
　　　foreign body (in) — *see* Foreign body, respiratory tract, causing asphyxia
　　　low oxygen content of ambient air T71.20 ☑
　　　　due to
　　　　　being trapped in
　　　　　　low oxygen environment T71.29 ☑
　　　　　　　in car trunk T71.221 ☑

Asphyxia, asphyxiation — *continued*
　traumatic — *continued*
　　due to — *continued*
　　　low oxygen content of ambient air — *continued*
　　　　due to — *continued*
　　　　　being trapped in — *continued*
　　　　　　low oxygen environment — *continued*
　　　　　　　in car trunk — *continued*
　　　　　　　　circumstances undetermined T71.224 ☑
　　　　　　　　done with intent to harm by
　　　　　　　　　another person T71.223 ☑
　　　　　　　　　self T71.222 ☑
　　　　　　　in refrigerator T71.231 ☑
　　　　　　　　circumstances undetermined T71.234 ☑
　　　　　　　　done with intent to harm by
　　　　　　　　　another person T71.233 ☑
　　　　　　　　　self T71.232 ☑
　　　cave-in T71.21 ☑
　　mechanical threat to breathing (accidental) T71.191 ☑
　　　circumstances undetermined T71.194 ☑
　　　done with intent to harm by
　　　　another person T71.193 ☑
　　　　self T71.192 ☑
　　　hanging T71.161 ☑
　　　　circumstances undetermined T71.164 ☑
　　　　done with intent to harm by
　　　　　another person T71.163 ☑
　　　　　self T71.162 ☑
　　　plastic bag T71.121 ☑
　　　　circumstances undetermined T71.124 ☑
　　　　done with intent to harm by
　　　　　another person T71.123 ☑
　　　　　self T71.122 ☑
　　　smothering
　　　　in furniture T71.151 ☑
　　　　　circumstances undetermined T71.154 ☑
　　　　　done with intent to harm by
　　　　　　another person T71.153 ☑
　　　　　　self T71.152 ☑
　　　　under
　　　　　another person's body T71.141 ☑
　　　　　　circumstances undetermined T71.144 ☑
　　　　　　done with intent to harm T71.143 ☑
　　　　　pillow T71.111 ☑
　　　　　　circumstances undetermined T71.114 ☑
　　　　　　done with intent to harm by
　　　　　　　another person T71.113 ☑
　　　　　　　self T71.112 ☑
　　　trapped in bed clothes T71.131 ☑
　　　　circumstances undetermined T71.134 ☑
　　　　done with intent to harm by
　　　　　another person T71.133 ☑
　　　　　self T71.132 ☑
　vomiting, vomitus — *see* Foreign body, respiratory tract, causing asphyxia
Aspiration
　amniotic (clear) fluid (newborn) P24.10
　　with
　　　pneumonia (pneumonitis) P24.11
　　　respiratory symptoms P24.11
　blood
　　newborn (without respiratory symptoms) P24.20
　　　with
　　　　pneumonia (pneumonitis) P24.21
　　　　respiratory symptoms P24.21
　　specified age NEC — *see* Foreign body, respiratory tract
　bronchitis J69.0
　food or foreign body — *see* Foreign body, by site
　liquor (amnii) (newborn) P24.10
　　with
　　　pneumonia (pneumonitis) P24.11
　　　respiratory symptoms P24.11
　meconium (newborn) (without respiratory symptoms) P24.00
　　with
　　　pneumonitis (pneumonitis) P24.01
　　　respiratory symptoms P24.01
　milk (newborn) (without respiratory symptoms) P24.30

Aspiration — *continued*
　milk — *continued*
　　with
　　　pneumonia (pneumonitis) P24.31
　　　respiratory symptoms P24.31
　　specified age NEC — *see* Foreign body, respiratory tract
　mucus — *see also* Foreign body, by site, causing asphyxia
　　newborn P24.10
　　　with
　　　　pneumonia (pneumonitis) P24.11
　　　　respiratory symptoms P24.11
　　neonatal P24.9
　　　specific NEC (without respiratory symptoms) P24.80
　　　　with
　　　　　pneumonia (pneumonitis) P24.81
　　　　　respiratory symptoms P24.81
　　newborn P24.9
　　　specific NEC (without respiratory symptoms) P24.80
　　　　with
　　　　　pneumonia (pneumonitis) P24.81
　　　　　respiratory symptoms P24.81
　pneumonia J69.0
　pneumonitis J69.0
　syndrome of newborn — *see* Aspiration, by substance, with pneumonia
　vernix caseosa (newborn) P24.80
　　with
　　　pneumonia (pneumonitis) P24.81
　　　respiratory symptoms P24.81
　vomitus — *see also* Foreign body, respiratory tract
　　newborn (without respiratory symptoms) P24.30
　　　with
　　　　pneumonia (pneumonitis) P24.31
　　　　respiratory symptoms P24.31
Asplenia (congenital) Q89.01
　postsurgical Z90.81
Assam fever B55.0
Assault, sexual — *see* Maltreatment
Assmann's focus NEC A15.0
Astasia (-abasia) (hysterical) F44.4
Asteatosis cutis L85.3
Astereognosia, astereognosis R48.1
Asterixis R27.8
　in liver disease K71.3
Asteroid hyalitis — *see* Deposit, crystalline
Asthenia, asthenic R53.1
　cardiac — *see also* Failure, heart I50.9
　　psychogenic F45.8
　cardiovascular — *see also* Failure, heart I50.9
　　psychogenic F45.8
　heart — *see also* Failure, heart I50.9
　　psychogenic F45.8
　hysterical F44.4
　myocardial — *see also* Failure, heart I50.9
　　psychogenic F45.8
　nervous F48.8
　neurocirculatory F45.8
　neurotic F48.8
　psychogenic F48.8
　psychoneurotic F48.8
　psychophysiologic F48.8
　reaction (psychophysiologic) F48.8
　senile R54
Asthenopia — *see also* Discomfort, visual
　hysterical F44.6
　psychogenic F44.6
Asthenospermia — *see* Abnormal, specimen, male genital organs
Asthma, asthmatic (bronchial) (catarrh) (spasmodic) J45.909
　with
　　chronic obstructive bronchitis J44.9
　　　with
　　　　acute lower respiratory infection J44.0
　　　　exacerbation (acute) J44.1
　　chronic obstructive pulmonary disease J44.9
　　　with
　　　　acute lower respiratory infection J44.0
　　　　exacerbation (acute) J44.1
　　exacerbation (acute) J45.901
　　hay fever — *see* Asthma, allergic extrinsic
　　rhinitis, allergic — *see* Asthma, allergic extrinsic
　　status asthmaticus J45.902
　allergic extrinsic J45.909
　　with
　　　exacerbation (acute) J45.901

Asthma, asthmatic — *continued*
  allergic extrinsic — *continued*
    with — *continued*
      status asthmaticus J45.902
  atopic — *see* Asthma, allergic extrinsic
  cardiac — *see* Failure, ventricular, left
  cardiobronchial I50.1
  childhood J45.909
    with
      exacerbation (acute) J45.901
      status asthmaticus J45.902
  chronic obstructive J44.9
    with
      acute lower respiratory infection J44.0
      exacerbation (acute) J44.1
  collier's J60
  cough variant J45.991
  detergent J69.8
  due to
    detergent J69.8
    inhalation of fumes J68.3
  eosinophilic J82.83
  extrinsic, allergic — *see* Asthma, allergic extrinsic
  grinder's J62.8
  hay — *see* Asthma, allergic extrinsic
  heart I50.1
  idiosyncratic — *see* Asthma, nonallergic
  intermittent (mild) J45.20
    with
      exacerbation (acute) J45.21
      status asthmaticus J45.22
  intrinsic, nonallergic — *see* Asthma, nonallergic
  Kopp's E32.8
  late-onset J45.909
    with
      exacerbation (acute) J45.901
      status asthmaticus J45.902
  mild intermittent J45.20
    with
      exacerbation (acute) J45.21
      status asthmaticus J45.22
  mild persistent J45.30
    with
      exacerbation (acute) J45.31
      status asthmaticus J45.32
  Millar's (laryngismus stridulus) J38.5
  miner's J60
  mixed J45.909
    with
      exacerbation (acute) J45.901
      status asthmaticus J45.902
  moderate persistent J45.40
    with
      exacerbation (acute) J45.41
      status asthmaticus J45.42
  nervous — *see* Asthma, nonallergic
  nonallergic (intrinsic) J45.909
    with
      exacerbation (acute) J45.901
      status asthmaticus J45.902
  persistent
    mild J45.30
      with
        exacerbation (acute) J45.31
        status asthmaticus J45.32
    moderate J45.40
      with
        exacerbation (acute) J45.41
        status asthmaticus J45.42
    severe J45.50
      with
        exacerbation (acute) J45.51
        status asthmaticus J45.52
  platinum J45.998
  pneumoconiotic NEC J64
  potter's J62.8
  predominantly allergic J45.909
  psychogenic F54
  pulmonary eosinophilic J82.83
  red cedar J67.8
  Rostan's I50.1
  sandblaster's J62.8
  sequoiosis J67.8
  severe persistent J45.50
    with
      exacerbation (acute) J45.51
      status asthmaticus J45.52
  specified NEC J45.998

Asthma, asthmatic — *continued*
  stonemason's J62.8
  thymic E32.8
  tuberculous — *see* Tuberculosis, pulmonary
  Wichmann's (laryngismus stridulus) J38.5
  wood J67.8

Astigmatism (compound) (congenital) H52.20- ☑
  irregular H52.21- ☑
  regular H52.22- ☑

Astraphobia F40.220

Astroblastoma
  specified site — *see* Neoplasm, malignant, by site
  unspecified site C71.9

Astrocytoma (cystic)
  anaplastic
    specified site — *see* Neoplasm, malignant, by site
    unspecified site C71.9
  fibrillary
    specified site — *see* Neoplasm, malignant, by site
    unspecified site C71.9
  fibrous
    specified site — *see* Neoplasm, malignant, by site
    unspecified site C71.9
  gemistocytic
    specified site — *see* Neoplasm, malignant, by site
    unspecified site C71.9
  juvenile
    specified site — *see* Neoplasm, malignant, by site
    unspecified site C71.9
  pilocytic
    specified site — *see* Neoplasm, malignant, by site
    unspecified site C71.9
  piloid
    specified site — *see* Neoplasm, malignant, by site
    unspecified site C71.9
  protoplasmic
    specified site — *see* Neoplasm, malignant, by site
    unspecified site C71.9
  specified site NEC — *see* Neoplasm, malignant, by site
  subependymal D43.2
    giant cell
      specified site — *see* Neoplasm, uncertain behavior, by site
      unspecified site D43.2
    specified site — *see* Neoplasm, uncertain behavior, by site
    unspecified site D43.2
  unspecified site C71.9

Astroglioma
  specified site — *see* Neoplasm, malignant, by site
  unspecified site C71.9

Asymbolia R48.8

Asymmetry — *see also* Distortion
  between native and reconstructed breast N65.1
  face Q67.0
  jaw (lower) — *see* Anomaly, dentofacial, jaw-cranial base relationship, asymmetry

Asynergia, asynergy R27.8
  ventricular I51.89

Asystole (heart) — *see* Arrest, cardiac

At risk
  for
    dental caries Z91.849
      high Z91.843
      low Z91.841
      moderate Z91.842
    falling Z91.81

Ataxia, ataxy, ataxic R27.0
  acute R27.8
  autosomal recessive Friedreich G11.11
  brain (hereditary) G11.9
  cerebellar (hereditary) G11.9
    with defective DNA repair G11.3
      alcoholic G31.2
    early-onset G11.10
      with
        essential tremor G11.19
        myoclonus [Hunt's ataxia] G11.19
        retained tendon reflexes G11.19
      in
        alcoholism G31.2
        myxedema E03.9 *[G13.2]*
        neoplastic disease — *see also* Neoplasm D49.9 *[G32.81]*
        specified disease NEC G32.81
    late-onset (Marie's) G11.2
  cerebral (hereditary) G11.9
  congenital nonprogressive G11.0

Ataxia, ataxy, ataxic — *continued*
  family, familial — *see* Ataxia, hereditary
  following
    cerebrovascular disease I69.993
      cerebral infarction I69.393
      intracerebral hemorrhage I69.193
      nontraumatic intracranial hemorrhage NEC I69.293
      specified disease NEC I69.893
      subarachnoid hemorrhage I69.093
  Friedreich's (heredofamilial) (cerebellar) (spinal) (with retained reflexes) G11.11
  gait R26.0
    hysterical F44.4
  general R27.8
  gluten M35.9 *[G32.81]*
    with celiac disease K90.0 *[G32.81]*
  hereditary G11.9
    with neuropathy G60.2
    cerebellar — *see* Ataxia, cerebellar
    spastic G11.4
    specified NEC G11.8
    spinal (Friedreich's) G11.11
  heredofamilial — *see* Ataxia, hereditary
  Hunt's G11.19
  hysterical F44.4
  locomotor (progressive) (syphilitic) (partial) (spastic) A52.11
    diabetic — *see* Diabetes, ataxia
  Marie's (cerebellar) (heredofamilial) (late- onset) G11.2
  nonorganic origin F44.4
  nonprogressive, congenital G11.0
  psychogenic F44.4
  Roussy-Lévy G60.0
  Sanger-Brown's (hereditary) G11.2
  spastic hereditary G11.4
  spinal
    hereditary (Friedreich's) G11.11
    progressive (syphilitic) A52.11
  spinocerebellar, X-linked recessive G11.19
  telangiectasia (Louis-Bar) G11.3

Ataxia-telangiectasia (Louis-Bar) G11.3

Atelectasis (massive) (partial) (pressure) (pulmonary) J98.11
  newborn P28.10
    due to resorption P28.11
    partial P28.19
    primary P28.0
    secondary P28.19
  primary (newborn) P28.0
  tuberculous — *see* Tuberculosis, pulmonary

Atelocardia Q24.9

Atelomyelia Q06.1

Atheroembolism
  of
    extremities
      lower I75.02- ☑
      upper I75.01- ☑
    kidney I75.81
    specified NEC I75.89

Atheroma, atheromatous — *see also* Arteriosclerosis I70.90
  aorta, aortic I70.0
    valve — *see also* Endocarditis, aortic I35.8
  aorto-iliac I70.0
  artery — *see* Arteriosclerosis
  basilar (artery) I67.2
  carotid (artery) (common) (internal) I67.2
  cerebral (arteries) I67.2
  coronary (artery) I25.10
    with angina pectoris — *see* Arteriosclerosis, coronary (artery),
  degeneration — *see* Arteriosclerosis
  heart, cardiac — *see* Disease, heart, ischemic, atherosclerotic
  mitral (valve) I34.89
  myocardium, myocardial — *see* Disease, heart, is-chemic, atherosclerotic
  pulmonary valve (heart) — *see also* Endocarditis, pulmonary I37.8
  tricuspid (heart) (valve) I36.8
  valve, valvular — *see* Endocarditis
  vertebral (artery) I67.2

Atheromatosis — *see* Arteriosclerosis

Atherosclerosis — *see also* Arteriosclerosis
  coronary
    artery I25.10

Atherosclerosis — *continued*
  coronary — *continued*
    artery — *continued*
      with angina pectoris — *see* Arteriosclerosis,
        coronary (artery),
      due to
        calcified coronary lesion (severely) I25.84
        lipid rich plaque I25.83
    transplanted heart I25.811
      bypass graft I25.812
        with angina pectoris — *see* Arteriosclerosis,
          coronary (artery),
      native coronary artery I25.811
        with angina pectoris — *see* Arteriosclerosis,
          coronary (artery),
Athetosis (acquired) R25.8
  bilateral (congenital) G80.3
  congenital (bilateral) (double) G80.3
  double (congenital) G80.3
  unilateral R25.8
Athlete's
  foot B35.3
  heart I51.7
Athrepsia E41
Athyrea (acquired) — *see also* Hypothyroidism
  congenital E03.1
Atonia, atony, atonic
  bladder (sphincter) (neurogenic) N31.2
  capillary I78.8
  cecum K59.89
    psychogenic F45.8
  colon — *see* Atony, intestine
  congenital P94.2
  esophagus K22.89
  intestine K59.89
    psychogenic F45.8
  stomach K31.89
    neurotic or psychogenic F45.8
  uterus (during labor) O62.2
    with hemorrhage (postpartum) O72.1
    postpartum (with hemorrhage) O72.1
      without hemorrhage O75.89
Atopy — *see* History, allergy
Atransferrinemia, congenital E88.09
Atresia, atretic
  alimentary organ or tract NEC Q45.8
    upper Q40.8
  ani, anus, anal (canal) Q42.3
    with fistula Q42.2
  aorta (ring) Q25.29
  aortic (orifice) (valve) Q23.0
    arch Q25.21
    congenital with hypoplasia of ascending aorta and
      defective development of left ventricle (with
      mitral stenosis) Q23.4
    in hypoplastic left heart syndrome Q23.4
  aqueduct of Sylvius Q03.0
    with spina bifida — *see* Spina bifida, with hydro-
      cephalus
  artery NEC Q27.8
    cerebral Q28.3
    coronary Q24.5
    digestive system Q27.8
    eye Q15.8
    lower limb Q27.8
    pulmonary Q25.5
    specified site NEC Q27.8
    umbilical Q27.0
    upper limb Q27.8
  auditory canal (external) Q16.1
  bile duct (common) (congenital) (hepatic) Q44.2
    acquired — *see* Obstruction, bile duct
  bladder (neck) Q64.39
    obstruction Q64.31
  bronchus Q32.4
  cecum Q42.8
  cervix (acquired) N88.2
    congenital Q51.828
    in pregnancy or childbirth — *see* Anomaly, cervix,
      in pregnancy or childbirth
      causing obstructed labor O65.5
  choana Q30.0
  colon Q42.9
    specified NEC Q42.8
  common duct Q44.2
  cricoid cartilage Q31.8
  cystic duct Q44.2
    acquired K82.8

Atresia, atretic — *continued*
  cystic duct — *continued*
    acquired — *continued*
      with obstruction K82.0
  digestive organs NEC Q45.8
  duodenum Q41.0
  ear canal Q16.1
  ejaculatory duct Q55.4
  epiglottis Q31.8
  esophagus Q39.0
    with tracheoesophageal fistula Q39.1
  eustachian tube Q17.8
  fallopian tube (congenital) Q50.6
    acquired N97.1
  follicular cyst N83.0- ☑
  foramen of
    Luschka Q03.1
      with spina bifida — *see* Spina bifida, with hydro-
        cephalus
    Magendie Q03.1
      with spina bifida — *see* Spina bifida, with hydro-
        cephalus
  gallbladder Q44.1
  genital organ
    external
      female Q52.79
      male Q55.8
    internal
      female Q52.8
      male Q55.8
  glottis Q31.8
  gullet Q39.0
    with tracheoesophageal fistula Q39.1
  heart valve NEC Q24.8
    pulmonary Q22.0
    tricuspid Q22.4
  hymen Q52.3
    acquired (postinfective) N89.6
  ileum Q41.2
  intestine (small) Q41.9
    large Q42.9
      specified NEC Q42.8
  iris, filtration angle Q15.0
  jejunum Q41.1
  lacrimal apparatus Q10.4
  larynx Q31.8
  meatus urinarius Q64.33
  mitral valve Q23.2
    in hypoplastic left heart syndrome Q23.4
  nares (anterior) (posterior) Q30.0
  nasopharynx Q34.8
  nose, nostril Q30.0
    acquired J34.89
  organ or site NEC Q89.8
  osseous meatus (ear) Q16.1
  oviduct (congenital) Q50.6
    acquired N97.1
  parotid duct Q38.4
    acquired K11.8
  pulmonary (artery) Q25.5
    valve Q22.0
  pulmonic Q22.0
  pupil Q13.2
  rectum Q42.1
    with fistula Q42.0
  salivary duct Q38.4
    acquired K11.8
  sublingual duct Q38.4
    acquired K11.8
  submandibular duct Q38.4
    acquired K11.8
  submaxillary duct Q38.4
    acquired K11.8
  thyroid cartilage Q31.8
  trachea Q32.1
  tricuspid valve Q22.4
  ureter Q62.10
    pelvic junction Q62.11
    vesical orifice Q62.12
  ureteropelvic junction Q62.11
  ureterovesical orifice Q62.12
  urethra (valvular) Q64.39
    stricture Q64.32
  urinary tract NEC Q64.8
  uterus Q51.818
    acquired N85.8
  vagina (congenital) Q52.4
    acquired (postinfectional) (senile) N89.5
  vas deferens Q55.3

Atresia, atretic — *continued*
  vascular NEC Q27.8
    cerebral Q28.3
    digestive system Q27.8
    lower limb Q27.8
    specified site NEC Q27.8
    upper limb Q27.8
  vein NEC Q27.8
    digestive system Q27.8
    great Q26.8
    lower limb Q27.8
    portal Q26.5
    pulmonary Q26.4
      partial Q26.3
      total Q26.2
    specified site NEC Q27.8
    upper limb Q27.8
  vena cava (inferior) (superior) Q26.8
  vesicourethral orifice Q64.31
  vulva Q52.79
    acquired N90.5
Atrichia, atrichosis — *see* Alopecia
Atrophia — *see also* Atrophy
  cutis senilis L90.8
    due to radiation L57.8
  gyrata of choroid and retina H31.23
  senilis R54
    dermatological L90.8
      due to radiation (nonionizing) (solar) L57.8
  unguium L60.3
    congenita Q84.6
Atrophie blanche (en plaque) (de Milian) L95.0
Atrophoderma, atrophodermia (of) L90.9
  diffusum (idiopathic) L90.4
  maculatum L90.8
    et striatum L90.8
      due to syphilis A52.79
    syphilitic A51.39
  neuriticum L90.8
  Pasini and Pierini L90.3
  pigmentosum Q82.1
  reticulatum symmetricum faciei L66.4
  senile L90.8
    due to radiation (nonionizing) (solar) L57.8
  vermiculata (cheeks) L66.4
Atrophy, atrophic (of)
  adrenal (capsule) (gland) E27.49
    primary (autoimmune) E27.1
  alveolar process or ridge (edentulous) K08.20
  anal sphincter (disuse) N81.84
  appendix K38.8
  arteriosclerotic — *see* Arteriosclerosis
  bile duct (common) (hepatic) K83.8
  bladder N32.89
    neurogenic N31.8
  blanche (en plaque) (of Milian) L95.0
  bone (senile) NEC — *see also* Disorder, bone, specified
    type NEC
    due to
      tabes dorsalis (neurogenic) A52.11
  brain (cortex) (progressive) G31.9
    frontotemporal circumscribed — *see also* Dementia,
      in, diseases specified elsewhere
      G31.01 *[F02.80]*
      with behavioral disturbance — *see also* Demen-
        tia, in, diseases specified elsewhere
        G31.01 *[F02.81-]* ☑
    senile NEC G31.1
  breast N64.2
    obstetric — *see* Disorder, breast, specified type NEC
  buccal cavity K13.79
  cardiac — *see* Degeneration, myocardial
  cartilage (infectional) (joint) — *see* Disorder, cartilage,
    specified NEC
  cerebellar — *see* Atrophy, brain
  cerebral — *see* Atrophy, brain
  cervix (mucosa) (senile) (uteri) N88.8
    menopausal N95.8
  Charcot-Marie-Tooth G60.0
  choroid (central) (macular) (myopic) (retina) H31.10- ☑
    diffuse secondary H31.12- ☑
    gyrate H31.23
    senile H31.11- ☑
  ciliary body — *see* Atrophy, iris
  conjunctiva (senile) H11.89
  corpus cavernosum N48.89
  cortical — *see* Atrophy, brain
  cystic duct K82.8

Atrophy, atrophic — *continued*
Déjérine-Thomas G23.8
disuse NEC — *see* Atrophy, muscle
Duchenne-Aran G12.21
ear H93.8- ☑
edentulous alveolar ridge K08.20
endometrium (senile) N85.8
   cervix N88.8
enteric K63.89
epididymis N50.89
eyeball — *see* Disorder, globe, degenerated condition,
   atrophy
eyelid (senile) — *see* Disorder, eyelid, degenerative
facial (skin) L90.9
fallopian tube (senile) N83.32- ☑
   with ovary N83.33- ☑
fascioscapulohumeral (Landouzy- Déjérine) G71.02
fatty, thymus (gland) E32.8
gallbladder K82.8
gastric K29.40
   with bleeding K29.41
gastrointestinal K63.89
glandular I89.8
globe H44.52- ☑
gum — *see* Recession, gingival
hair L67.8
heart (brown) — *see* Degeneration, myocardial
hemifacial Q67.4
   Romberg G51.8
infantile E41
   paralysis, acute — *see* Poliomyelitis, paralytic
intestine K63.89
iris (essential) (progressive) H21.26- ☑
   specified NEC H21.29
kidney (senile) (terminal) — *see also* Sclerosis, renal
   N26.1
   congenital or infantile Q60.5
     bilateral Q60.4
     unilateral Q60.3
   hydronephrotic — *see* Hydronephrosis
lacrimal gland (primary) H04.14- ☑
   secondary H04.15- ☑
Landouzy-Déjérine G71.02
laryngitis, infective J37.0
larynx J38.7
Leber's optic (hereditary) H47.22
lip K13.0
liver (yellow) K72.90
   with coma K72.91
   acute, subacute K72.00
     with coma K72.01
   chronic K72.10
     with coma K72.11
lung (senile) J98.4
macular (dermatological) L90.8
   syphilitic, skin A51.39
     striated A52.79
mandible (edentulous) K08.20
   minimal K08.21
   moderate K08.22
   severe K08.23
maxilla K08.20
   minimal K08.24
   moderate K08.25
   severe K08.26
muscle, muscular (diffuse) (general) (idiopathic) (primary) M62.50
   ankle M62.57- ☑
   back M62.5A9
     cervical M62.5A0
     lumbosacral M62.5A2
     thoracic M62.5A1
   Duchenne-Aran G12.21
   foot M62.57- ☑
   forearm M62.53- ☑
   hand M62.54- ☑
   infantile spinal G12.0
   lower leg M62.56- ☑
   multiple sites M62.59
   myelopathic — *see* Atrophy, muscle, spinal
   myotonic G71.11
   neuritic G58.9
   neuropathic (peroneal) (progressive) G60.0
   pelvic (disuse) N81.84
   peroneal G60.0
   progressive (bulbar) G12.21
     adult G12.1
     infantile (spinal) G12.0

Atrophy, atrophic — *continued*
muscle, muscular — *continued*
   progressive — *continued*
     spinal G12.25
       adult G12.1
       infantile G12.0
   pseudohypertrophic G71.02
   shoulder region M62.51- ☑
   specified site NEC M62.58
   spinal G12.9
     adult form G12.1
     Aran-Duchenne G12.21
     childhood form, type II G12.1
     distal G12.1
     hereditary NEC G12.1
     infantile, type I (Werdnig-Hoffmann) G12.0
     juvenile form, type III (Kugelberg- Welander)
       G12.1
     progressive G12.25
     scapuloperoneal form G12.1
     specified NEC G12.8
   syphilitic A52.78
   thigh M62.55- ☑
   upper arm M62.52- ☑
myocardium — *see* Degeneration, myocardial
myometrium (senile) N85.8
   cervix N88.8
myopathic NEC — *see* Atrophy, muscle
myotonia G71.11
nail L60.3
nasopharynx J31.1
nerve — *see also* Disorder, nerve
   abducens — *see* Strabismus, paralytic, sixth nerve
   accessory G52.8
   acoustic or auditory H93.3 ☑
   cranial G52.9
     eighth (auditory) H93.3 ☑
     eleventh (accessory) G52.8
     fifth (trigeminal) G50.8
     first (olfactory) G52.0
     fourth (trochlear) — *see* Strabismus, paralytic,
       fourth nerve
     second (optic) H47.20
     sixth (abducens) — *see* Strabismus, paralytic,
       sixth nerve
     tenth (pneumogastric) (vagus) G52.2
     third (oculomotor) — *see* Strabismus, paralytic,
       third nerve
     twelfth (hypoglossal) G52.3
   hypoglossal G52.3
   oculomotor — *see* Strabismus, paralytic, third nerve
   olfactory G52.0
   optic (papillomacular bundle)
     syphilitic (late) A52.15
       congenital A50.44
   pneumogastric G52.2
   trigeminal G50.8
   trochlear — *see* Strabismus, paralytic, fourth nerve
   vagus (pneumogastric) G52.2
neurogenic, bone, tabetic A52.11
nutritional E43
   with marasmus E41
old age R54
olivopontocerebellar G23.8
optic (nerve) H47.20
   glaucomatous H47.23- ☑
   hereditary H47.22
   primary H47.21- ☑
   specified type NEC H47.29- ☑
   syphilitic (late) A52.15
     congenital A50.44
orbit H05.31- ☑
ovary (senile) N83.31- ☑
   with fallopian tube N83.33- ☑
oviduct (senile) — *see* Atrophy, fallopian tube
palsy, diffuse (progressive) G12.22
pancreas (duct) (senile) K86.89
parotid gland K11.0
pelvic muscle N81.84
penis N48.89
pharynx J39.2
pluriglandular E31.8
   autoimmune E31.0
polyarthritis M15.9
prostate N42.89
pseudohypertrophic (muscle) G71.02
renal — *see also* Sclerosis, renal N26.1
retina, retinal (postinfectional) H35.89

Atrophy, atrophic — *continued*
rhinitis J31.0
salivary gland K11.0
scar L90.5
sclerosis, lobar (of brain) — *see also* Dementia, in, diseases specified elsewhere G31.09 *[F02.80]*
   with behavioral disturbance — *see also* Dementia,
     in, diseases specified elsewhere
     G31.09 *[F02.81-]* ☑
scrotum N50.89
seminal vesicle N50.89
senile R54
   due to radiation (nonionizing) (solar) L57.8
skin (patches) (spots) L90.9
   degenerative (senile) L90.8
   due to radiation (nonionizing) (solar) L57.8
   senile L90.8
spermatic cord N50.89
spinal (acute) (cord) G95.89
   muscular — *see* Atrophy, muscle, spinal
   paralysis G12.20
     acute — *see* Poliomyelitis, paralytic
     meaning progressive muscular atrophy G12.25
spine (column) — *see* Spondylopathy, specified NEC
spleen (senile) D73.0
stomach K29.40
   with bleeding K29.41
striate (skin) L90.6
   syphilitic A52.79
subcutaneous L90.9
sublingual gland K11.0
submandibular gland K11.0
submaxillary gland K11.0
Sudeck's — *see* Algoneurodystrophy
suprarenal (capsule) (gland) E27.49
   primary E27.1
systemic affecting central nervous system
   in
     myxedema E03.9 *[G13.2]*
     neoplastic disease — *see also* Neoplasm
       D49.9 *[G13.1]*
     specified disease NEC G13.8
tarso-orbital fascia, congenital Q10.3
testis N50.0
thenar, partial — *see* Syndrome, carpal tunnel
thymus (fatty) E32.8
thyroid (gland) (acquired) E03.4
   with cretinism E03.1
   congenital (with myxedema) E03.1
tongue (senile) K14.8
   papillae K14.4
trachea J39.8
tunica vaginalis N50.89
turbinate J34.89
tympanic membrane (nonflaccid) H73.82- ☑
   flaccid H73.81- ☑
upper respiratory tract J39.8
uterus, uterine (senile) N85.8
   cervix N88.8
   due to radiation (intended effect) N85.8
     adverse effect or misadventure N99.89
vagina (senile) N95.2
vas deferens N50.89
vascular I99.8
vertebra (senile) — *see* Spondylopathy, specified NEC
vulva (senile) N90.5
Werdnig-Hoffmann G12.0
yellow — *see* Failure, hepatic
Attack, attacks
with alteration of consciousness (with automatisms)
   — *see* Epilepsy, localization-related, symptomatic, with complex partial seizures
Adams-Stokes I45.9
akinetic — *see* Epilepsy, generalized, specified NEC
angina — *see* Angina
atonic — *see* Epilepsy, generalized, specified NEC
benign shuddering G25.83
cataleptic — *see* Catalepsy
coronary — *see* Infarct, myocardium
cyanotic, newborn P28.2
drop NEC R55
epileptic — *see* Epilepsy
heart — *see* infarct, myocardium
hysterical F44.9
jacksonian — *see* Epilepsy, localization-related, symptomatic, with simple partial seizures
myocardium, myocardial — *see* Infarct, myocardium
myoclonic — *see* Epilepsy, generalized, specified NEC

Attack, attacks — *continued*
　panic F41.Ø
　psychomotor — *see* Epilepsy, localization-related, symptomatic, with complex partial seizures
　salaam — *see* Epilepsy, spasms
　schizophreniform, brief F23
　shuddering, benign G25.83
　Stokes-Adams I45.9
　syncope R55
　transient ischemic (TIA) G45.9
　　specified NEC G45.8
　unconsciousness R55
　　hysterical F44.89
　vasomotor R55
　vasovagal (paroxysmal) (idiopathic) R55
　without alteration of consciousness — *see* Epilepsy, localization-related, symptomatic, with simple partial seizures
Attention (to)
　artificial
　　opening (of) Z43.9
　　　digestive tract NEC Z43.4
　　　　colon Z43.3
　　　　ilium Z43.2
　　　　stomach Z43.1
　　　specified NEC Z43.8
　　　trachea Z43.Ø
　　　urinary tract NEC Z43.6
　　　　cystostomy Z43.5
　　　　nephrostomy Z43.6
　　　　ureterostomy Z43.6
　　　　urethrostomy Z43.6
　　　vagina Z43.7
　colostomy Z43.3
　cystostomy Z43.5
　deficit disorder or syndrome F98.8
　　with hyperactivity — *see* Disorder, attention-deficit hyperactivity
　gastrostomy Z43.1
　ileostomy Z43.2
　jejunostomy Z43.4
　nephrostomy Z43.6
　surgical dressings Z48.Ø1
　sutures Z48.Ø2
　tracheostomy Z43.Ø
　ureterostomy Z43.6
　urethrostomy Z43.6
Attrition
　gum — *see* Recession, gingival
　tooth, teeth (excessive) (hard tissues) KØ3.Ø
Atypical, atypism — *see also* condition
　cells (on cytolgocial smear) (endocervical) (endometrial) (glandular)
　　cervix R87.619
　　vagina R87.629
　cervical N87.9
　endometrium N85.9
　　hyperplasia N85.ØØ
　parenting situation Z62.9
Auditory — *see* condition
Aujeszky's disease B33.8
Aurantiasis, cutis E67.1
Auricle, auricular — *see also* condition
　cervical Q18.2
Auriculotemporal syndrome G5Ø.8
Austin Flint murmur (aortic insufficiency) I35.1
Australian
　Q fever A78
　X disease A83.4
Autism, autistic (childhood) (infantile) F84.Ø
　atypical F84.9
　spectrum disorder F84.Ø
Autodigestion R68.89
Autoerythrocyte sensitization (syndrome) D69.2
Autographism L5Ø.3
Autoimmune
　disease (systemic) M35.9
　inhibitors to clotting factors D68.311
　lymphoproliferative syndrome [ALPS] D89.82
　thyroiditis EØ6.3
Autointoxication R68.89
Automatism G93.89
　with temporal sclerosis G93.81
　epileptic — *see* Epilepsy, localization-related, symptomatic, with complex partial seizures
　paroxysmal, idiopathic — *see* Epilepsy, localization-related, symptomatic, with complex partial seizures

Autonomic, autonomous
　bladder (neurogenic) N31.2
　hysteria seizure F44.5
Autosensitivity, erythrocyte D69.2
Autosensitization, cutaneous L3Ø.2
Autosome — *see* condition by chromosome involved
Autotopagnosia R48.1
Autotoxemia R68.89
Autumn — *see* condition
Avellis' syndrome G46.8
Aversion
　oral R63.39
　　newborn P92.- ☑
　　nonorganic origin F98.2 ☑
　sexual F52.1
Aviator's
　disease or sickness — *see* Effect, adverse, high altitude
　ear T7Ø.Ø ☑
Avitaminosis (multiple) — *see also* Deficiency, vitamin
　E56.9
　B E53.9
　　with
　　　beriberi E51.11
　　　pellagra E52
　B2 E53.Ø
　B6 E53.1
　B12 E53.8
　D E55.9
　　with rickets E55.Ø
　G E53.Ø
　K E56.1
　nicotinic acid E52
AVNRT (atrioventricular nodal re-entrant tachycardia) I47.1
AVRT (atrioventricular nodal re-entrant tachycardia) I47.1
Avulsion (traumatic)
　blood vessel — *see* Injury, blood vessel
　bone — *see* Fracture, by site
　cartilage — *see also* Dislocation, by site
　　symphyseal (inner), complicating delivery O71.6
　external site other than limb — *see* Wound, open, by site
　eye SØ5.7- ☑
　head (intracranial)
　　external site NEC SØ8.89 ☑
　　scalp SØ8.Ø ☑
　internal organ or site — *see* Injury, by site
　joint — *see also* Dislocation, by site
　　capsule — *see* Sprain, by site
　kidney S37.Ø6- ☑
　ligament — *see* Sprain, by site
　limb — *see also* Amputation, traumatic, by site
　　skin and subcutaneous tissue — *see* Wound, open, by site
　muscle — *see* Injury, muscle
　nerve (root) — *see* Injury, nerve
　scalp SØ8.Ø ☑
　skin and subcutaneous tissue — *see* Wound, open, by site
　spleen S36.Ø32 ☑
　symphyseal cartilage (inner), complicating delivery O71.6
　tendon — *see* Injury, muscle
　tooth SØ3.2 ☑
Awareness of heart beat RØØ.2
Axenfeld's
　anomaly or syndrome Q15.Ø
　degeneration (calcareous) Q13.4
Axilla, axillary — *see also* condition
　breast Q83.1
Axonotmesis — *see* Injury, nerve
Ayerza's disease or syndrome (pulmonary artery sclerosis with pulmonary hypertension) I27.Ø
Azoospermia (organic) N46.Ø1
　due to
　　drug therapy N46.Ø21
　　efferent duct obstruction N46.Ø23
　　infection N46.Ø22
　　radiation N46.Ø24
　　specified cause NEC N46.Ø29
　　systemic disease N46.Ø25
Azotemia R79.89
　meaning uremia N19
Aztec ear Q17.3
Azygos
　continuation inferior vena cava Q26.8
　lobe (lung) Q33.1

B

Baastrup's disease — *see* Kissing spine
Babesiosis B6Ø.ØØ
　due to
　　Babesia
　　　divergens B6Ø.Ø3
　　　duncani B6Ø.Ø2
　　　KO-1 B6Ø.Ø9
　　　microti B6Ø.Ø1
　　　MO-1 B6Ø.Ø3
　　　species
　　　　unspecified B6Ø.ØØ
　　　venatorum B6Ø.Ø9
　　specified NEC B6Ø.Ø9
Babington's disease (familial hemorrhagic telangiectasia) I78.Ø
Babinski's syndrome A52.79
Baby
　crying constantly R68.11
　floppy (syndrome) P94.2
Bacillary — *see* condition
Bacilluria R82.71
Bacillus — *see also* Infection, bacillus
　abortus infection A23.1
　anthracis infection A22.9
　coli infection — *see also* Escherichia coli B96.2Ø
　Flexner's AØ3.1
　mallei infection A24.Ø
　Shiga's AØ3.Ø
　suipestifer infection — *see* Infection, salmonella
Back — *see* condition
Backache (postural) M54.9
　sacroiliac M53.3
　specified NEC M54.89
Backflow — *see* Reflux
Backward reading (dyslexia) F81.Ø
Bacteremia R78.81
　with sepsis — *see* Sepsis
Bactericholia — *see* Cholecystitis, acute
Bacterid, bacteride (pustular) L4Ø.3
Bacterium, bacteria, bacterial
　agent NEC, as cause of disease classified elsewhere B96.89
　in blood — *see* Bacteremia
　in urine — *see* Bacteriuria
Bacteriuria, bacteruria R82.71
　asymptomatic R82.71
Bacteroides
　fragilis, as cause of disease classified elsewhere B96.6
Bad
　heart — *see* Disease, heart
　trip
　　due to drug abuse — *see* Abuse, drug, hallucinogen
　　due to drug dependence — *see* Dependence, drug, hallucinogen
Baelz's disease (cheilitis glandularis apostematosa) K13.Ø
Baerensprung's disease (eczema marginatum) B35.6
Bagasse disease or pneumonitis J67.1
Bagassosis J67.1
Baker's cyst — *see* Cyst, Baker's
Bakwin-Krida syndrome (metaphyseal dysplasia) Q78.5
Balancing side interference M26.56
Balanitis (circinata) (erosiva) (gangrenosa) (phagedenic) (vulgaris) N48.1
　amebic AØ6.82
　candidal B37.42
　due to Haemophilus ducreyi A57
　gonococcal (acute) (chronic) A54.23
　xerotica obliterans N48.Ø
Balanoposthitis N47.6
　gonococcal (acute) (chronic) A54.23
　ulcerative (specific) A63.8
Balanorrhagia — *see* Balanitis
Balantidiasis, balantidiosis AØ7.Ø
Bald tongue K14.4
Baldness — *see also* Alopecia
　male-pattern — *see* Alopecia, androgenic
Balkan grippe A78
Balloon disease — *see* Effect, adverse, high altitude
Balo's disease (concentric sclerosis) G37.5
Bamberger-Marie disease — *see* Osteoarthropathy, hypertrophic, specified type NEC
Bancroft's filariasis B74.Ø
Band(s)
　adhesive — *see* Adhesions, peritoneum

Band(s) — *continued*
  anomalous or congenital — *see also* Anomaly, by site
    heart (atrial) (ventricular) Q24.8
    intestine Q43.3
    omentum Q43.3
  cervix N88.1
  constricting, congenital Q79.8
  gallbladder (congenital) Q44.1
  intestinal (adhesive) — *see* Adhesions, peritoneum
  obstructive
    intestine K56.50
      complete K56.52
      incomplete K56.51
      partial K56.51
    peritoneum K56.50
      complete K56.52
      incomplete K56.51
      partial K56.51
  periappendiceal, congenital Q43.3
  peritoneal (adhesive) — *see* Adhesions, peritoneum
  uterus N73.6
    internal N85.6
  vagina N89.5
Bandemia D72.825
Bandl's ring (contraction), complicating delivery O62.4
Bangkok hemorrhagic fever A91
Bang's disease (brucella abortus) A23.1
Bankruptcy (anxiety concerning) Z59.86
Bannister's disease T78.3 ☑
  hereditary D84.1
Banti's disease or syndrome (with cirrhosis) (with portal hypertension) K76.6
Bar, median, prostate — *see* Enlargement, enlarged, prostate
Barcoo disease or rot — *see* Ulcer, skin
Barlow's disease E54
Barodontalgia T70.29 ☑
Baron Münchausen syndrome — *see* Disorder, factitious
Barosinusitis T70.1 ☑
Barotitis T70.0 ☑
Barotrauma T70.29 ☑
  odontalgia T70.29 ☑
  otitic T70.0 ☑
  sinus T70.1 ☑
Barraquer (-Simons) **disease or syndrome** (progressive lipodystrophy) E88.1
Barré-Guillain disease or syndrome G61.0
Barrel chest M95.4
Barré-Liéou syndrome (posterior cervical sympathetic) M53.0
Barrett's
  disease — *see* Barrett's, esophagus
  esophagus K22.70
    with dysplasia K22.719
      high grade K22.711
      low grade K22.710
    without dysplasia K22.70
  syndrome — *see* Barrett's, esophagus
  ulcer K22.10
    with bleeding K22.11
    without bleeding K22.10
Bársony (-Polgár) (-Teschendorf) **syndrome** (corkscrew esophagus) K22.4
Barth syndrome E78.71
Bartholinitis (suppurating) N75.8
  gonococcal (acute) (chronic) (with abscess) A54.1
Bartonellosis A44.9
  cutaneous A44.1
  mucocutaneous A44.1
  specified NEC A44.8
  systemic A44.0
Barton's fracture S52.56- ☑
Bartter's syndrome E26.81
Basal — *see* condition
Basan's (hidrotic) ectodermal dysplasia Q82.4
Baseball finger — *see* Dislocation, finger
Basedow's disease (exophthalmic goiter) — *see* Hyperthyroidism, with, goiter
Basic — *see* condition
Basilar — *see* condition
Bason's (hidrotic) ectodermal dysplasia Q82.4
Basopenia — *see* Agranulocytosis
Basophilia D72.824
Basophilism (cortico-adrenal) (Cushing's) (pituitary) E24.0
Bassen-Kornzweig disease or syndrome E78.6
Bat ear Q17.5

Bateman's
  disease B08.1
  purpura (senile) D69.2
Bathing cramp T75.1 ☑
Bathophobia F40.248
Batten (-Mayou) **disease** E75.4
  retina E75.4 *[H36]*
Batten-Steinert syndrome G71.11
Battered — *see* Maltreatment
Battey Mycobacterium infection A31.0
Battle exhaustion F43.0
Battledore placenta O43.19- ☑
Baumgarten-Cruveilhier cirrhosis, disease or syndrome K74.69
Bauxite fibrosis (of lung) J63.1
Bayle's disease (general paresis) A52.17
Bazin's disease (primary) (tuberculous) A18.4
Beach ear — *see* Swimmer's, ear
Beaded hair (congenital) Q84.1
Béal conjunctivitis or syndrome B30.2
Beard's disease (neurasthenia) F48.8
Beat(s)
  atrial, premature I49.1
  ectopic I49.49
  elbow — *see* Bursitis, elbow
  escaped, heart I49.49
  hand — *see* Bursitis, hand
  knee — *see* Bursitis, knee
  premature I49.40
    atrial I49.1
    auricular I49.1
    supraventricular I49.1
Beau's
  disease or syndrome — *see* Degeneration, myocardial
  lines (transverse furrows on fingernails) L60.4
Bechterev's syndrome — *see* Spondylitis, ankylosing
Becker's
  cardiomyopathy I42.8
  disease
    idiopathic mural endomyocardial disease I42.3
    myotonia congenita, recessive form G71.12
  dystrophy G71.01
  pigmented hairy nevus D22.5
Beck's syndrome (anterior spinal artery occlusion) I65.8
Beckwith-Wiedemann syndrome Q87.3
Bed confinement status Z74.01
Bed sore — *see* Ulcer, pressure, by site
Bedbug bite(s) — *see* Bite(s), by site, superficial, insect
Bedclothes, asphyxiation or suffocation by — *see* Asphyxia, traumatic, due to, mechanical, trapped
Bednar's
  aphthae K12.0
  tumor — *see* Neoplasm, malignant, by site
Bedridden Z74.01
Bed-sharing, infant Z72.823
Bedsore — *see* Ulcer, pressure, by site
Bedwetting — *see* Enuresis
Bee sting (with allergic or anaphylactic shock) — *see* Toxicity, venom, arthropod, bee
Beer drinker's heart (disease) I42.6
Begbie's disease (exophthalmic goiter) — *see* Hyperthyroidism, with, goiter
Behavior
  antisocial
    adult Z72.811
    child or adolescent Z72.810
  disorder, disturbance — *see* Disorder, conduct
  disruptive — *see* Disorder, conduct
  drug seeking Z76.5
  inexplicable R46.2
  marked evasiveness R46.5
  obsessive-compulsive R46.81
  overactivity R46.3
  poor responsiveness R46.4
  self-damaging (life-style) Z72.89
  sleep-incompatible Z72.821
  slowness R46.4
  specified NEC R46.89
  strange (and inexplicable) R46.2
  suspiciousness R46.5
  type A pattern Z73.1
  undue concern or preoccupation with stressful events R46.6
  verbosity and circumstantial detail obscuring reason for contact R46.7
Behçet's disease or syndrome M35.2
Behr's disease — *see* Degeneration, macula

Beigel's disease or morbus (white piedra) B36.2
Bejel A65
Bekhterev's syndrome — *see* Spondylitis, ankylosing
Belching — *see* Eructation
Bell's
  mania F30.8
  palsy, paralysis G51.0
    infant or newborn P11.3
  spasm G51.3- ☑
Bence Jones albuminuria or proteinuria NEC R80.3
Bends T70.3 ☑
Benedikt's paralysis or syndrome G46.3
Benign — *see also* condition
  prostatic hyperplasia — *see* Hyperplasia, prostate
Bennett's fracture (displaced) S62.21- ☑
Benson's disease — *see* Deposit, crystalline
Bent
  back (hysterical) F44.4
  nose M95.0
    congenital Q67.4
Bereavement (uncomplicated) Z63.4
Bergeron's disease (hysterical chorea) F44.4
Berger's disease — *see* Nephropathy, IgA
Beriberi (dry) E51.11
  heart (disease) E51.12
  polyneuropathy E51.11
  wet E51.12
    involving circulatory system E51.11
Berlin's disease or edema (traumatic) S05.8X- ☑
Berlock (berloque) **dermatitis** L56.2
Bernard-Horner syndrome G90.2
Bernard-Soulier disease or thrombopathia D69.1
Bernhardt (-Roth) **disease** — *see* Mononeuropathy, lower limb, meralgia paresthetica
Bernheim's syndrome — *see* Failure, heart, right
Bertielliasis B71.8
Berylliosis (lung) J63.2
Besnier-Boeck (-Schaumann) **disease** — *see* Sarcoidosis
Besnier's
  lupus pernio D86.3
  prurigo L20.0
Bestiality F65.89
Best's disease H35.50
Betalipoproteinemia, broad or floating E78.2
Beta-mercaptolactate-cysteine disulfiduria E72.09
Betting and gambling Z72.6
  pathological (compulsive) F63.0
Bezoar T18.9 ☑
  intestine T18.3 ☑
  stomach T18.2 ☑
Bezold's abscess — *see* Mastoiditis, acute
Bianchi's syndrome R48.8
Bicornate or bicornis uterus Q51.3
  in pregnancy or childbirth O34.00
    causing obstructed labor O65.5
Bicuspid aortic valve Q23.1
Biedl-Bardet syndrome Q87.89
Bielschowsky (-Jansky) disease E75.4
Biermer's (pernicious) anemia or disease D51.0
Biett's disease L93.0
Bifid (congenital)
  apex, heart Q24.8
  clitoris Q52.6
  kidney Q63.8
  nose Q30.2
  patella Q74.1
  scrotum Q55.29
  toe NEC Q74.2
  tongue Q38.3
  ureter Q62.8
  uterus Q51.3
  uvula Q35.7
Biforis uterus (suprasimplex) Q51.3
Bifurcation (congenital)
  gallbladder Q44.1
  kidney pelvis Q63.8
  renal pelvis Q63.8
  rib Q76.6
  tongue, congenital Q38.3
  trachea Q32.1
  ureter Q62.8
  urethra Q64.74
  vertebra Q76.49
Big spleen syndrome D73.1
Bigeminal pulse R00.8
Bilateral — *see* condition

Bite(s) — *continued*
- genital organs, external
  - female S31.552 ☑
    - superficial NEC S30.876 ☑
      - insect S30.866 ☑
    - vagina and vulva — *see* Bite, vulva
  - male S31.551 ☑
    - penis — *see* Bite, penis
    - scrotum — *see* Bite, scrotum
    - superficial NEC S30.875 ☑
      - insect S30.865 ☑
    - testes — *see* Bite, testis
- groin — *see* Bite, abdomen, wall
- gum — *see* Bite, oral cavity
- hand S61.45- ☑
  - finger — *see* Bite, finger
  - superficial NEC S60.57- ☑
    - insect S60.56- ☑
  - thumb — *see* Bite, thumb
- head S01.95 ☑
  - cheek — *see* Bite, cheek
  - ear — *see* Bite, ear
  - eyelid — *see* Bite, eyelid
  - lip — *see* Bite, lip
  - nose — *see* Bite, nose
  - oral cavity — *see* Bite, oral cavity
  - scalp — *see* Bite, scalp
  - specified site NEC S01.85 ☑
    - superficial NEC S00.87 ☑
      - insect S00.86 ☑
  - superficial NEC S00.97 ☑
    - insect S00.96 ☑
  - temporomandibular area — *see* Bite, cheek
- heel — *see* Bite, foot
- hip S71.05- ☑
  - superficial NEC S70.27- ☑
    - insect S70.26- ☑
- hymen S31.45 ☑
- hypochondrium — *see* Bite, abdomen, wall
- hypogastric region — *see* Bite, abdomen, wall
- inguinal region — *see* Bite, abdomen, wall
- insect — *see* Bite, by site, superficial, insect
- instep — *see* Bite, foot
- interscapular region — *see* Bite, thorax, back
- jaw — *see* Bite, head, specified site NEC
- knee S81.05- ☑
  - superficial NEC S80.27- ☑
    - insect S80.26- ☑
- labium (majus) (minus) — *see* Bite, vulva
- lacrimal duct — *see* Bite, eyelid
- larynx S11.015 ☑
  - superficial NEC S10.17 ☑
    - insect S10.16 ☑
- leg (lower) S81.85- ☑
  - ankle — *see* Bite, ankle
  - foot — *see* Bite, foot
  - knee — *see* Bite, knee
  - superficial NEC S80.87- ☑
    - insect S80.86- ☑
  - toe — *see* Bite, toe
  - upper — *see* Bite, thigh
- lip S01.551 ☑
  - superficial NEC S00.571 ☑
    - insect S00.561 ☑
- lizard (venomous) — *see* Venom, bite, reptile
- loin — *see* Bite, abdomen, wall
- lower back — *see* Bite, back, lower
- lumbar region — *see* Bite, back, lower
- malar region — *see* Bite, head, specified site NEC
- mammary — *see* Bite, breast
- marine animals (venomous) — *see* Toxicity, venom, marine animal
- mastoid region — *see* Bite, head, specified site NEC
- mouth — *see* Bite, oral cavity
- nail
  - finger — *see* Bite, finger
  - toe — *see* Bite, toe
- nape — *see* Bite, neck, specified site NEC
- nasal (septum) (sinus) — *see* Bite, nose
- nasopharynx — *see* Bite, head, specified site NEC
- neck S11.95 ☑
  - involving
    - cervical esophagus — *see* Bite, esophagus, cervical
    - larynx — *see* Bite, larynx
    - pharynx — *see* Bite, pharynx

Bite(s) — *continued*
- neck — *continued*
  - involving — *continued*
    - thyroid gland S11.15 ☑
    - trachea — *see* Bite, trachea
  - specified site NEC S11.85 ☑
    - superficial NEC S10.87 ☑
      - insect S10.86 ☑
  - superficial NEC S10.97 ☑
    - insect S10.96 ☑
  - throat S11.85 ☑
    - superficial NEC S10.17 ☑
      - insect S10.16 ☑
- nose (septum) (sinus) S01.25 ☑
  - superficial NEC S00.37 ☑
    - insect S00.36 ☑
- occipital region — *see* Bite, scalp
- oral cavity S01.552 ☑
  - superficial NEC S00.572 ☑
    - insect S00.562 ☑
- orbital region — *see* Bite, eyelid
- palate — *see* Bite, oral cavity
- palm — *see* Bite, hand
- parietal region — *see* Bite, scalp
- pelvis S31.050 ☑
  - with penetration into retroperitoneal space S31.051 ☑
  - superficial NEC S30.870 ☑
    - insect S30.860 ☑
- penis S31.25 ☑
  - superficial NEC S30.872 ☑
    - insect S30.862 ☑
- perineum
  - female — *see* Bite, vulva
  - male — *see* Bite, pelvis
- periocular area (with or without lacrimal passages) — *see* Bite, eyelid
- phalanges
  - finger — *see* Bite, finger
  - toe — *see* Bite, toe
- pharynx S11.25 ☑
  - superficial NEC S10.17 ☑
    - insect S10.16 ☑
- pinna — *see* Bite, ear
- poisonous — *see* Venom
- popliteal space — *see* Bite, knee
- prepuce — *see* Bite, penis
- pubic region — *see* Bite, abdomen, wall
- rectovaginal septum — *see* Bite, vulva
- red bug B88.0
- reptile NEC — *see also* Venom, bite, reptile
  - nonvenomous — *see* Bite, by site
  - snake — *see* Venom, bite, snake
- sacral region — *see* Bite, back, lower
- sacroiliac region — *see* Bite, back, lower
- salivary gland — *see* Bite, oral cavity
- scalp S01.05 ☑
  - superficial NEC S00.07 ☑
    - insect S00.06 ☑
- scapular region — *see* Bite, shoulder
- scrotum S31.35 ☑
  - superficial NEC S30.873 ☑
    - insect S30.863 ☑
- sea-snake (venomous) — *see* Toxicity, venom, snake, sea snake
- shin — *see* Bite, leg
- shoulder S41.05- ☑
  - superficial NEC S40.27- ☑
    - insect S40.26- ☑
- snake — *see also* Venom, bite, snake
  - nonvenomous — *see* Bite, by site
- spermatic cord — *see* Bite, testis
- spider (venomous) — *see* Toxicity, venom, spider
  - nonvenomous — *see* Bite, by site, superficial, insect
- sternal region — *see* Bite, thorax, front
- submaxillary region — *see* Bite, head, specified site NEC
- submental region — *see* Bite, head, specified site NEC
- subungual
  - finger(s) — *see* Bite, finger
  - toe — *see* Bite, toe
- superficial — *see* Bite, by site, superficial
- supraclavicular fossa S11.85 ☑
- supraorbital — *see* Bite, head, specified site NEC
- temple, temporal region — *see* Bite, head, specified site NEC

Bite(s) — *continued*
- temporomandibular area — *see* Bite, cheek
- testis S31.35 ☑
  - superficial NEC S30.873 ☑
    - insect S30.863 ☑
- thigh S71.15- ☑
  - superficial NEC S70.37- ☑
    - insect S70.36- ☑
- thorax, thoracic (wall) S21.95 ☑
  - back S21.25- ☑
    - with penetration into thoracic cavity S21.45- ☑
  - breast — *see* Bite, breast
  - front S21.15- ☑
    - with penetration into thoracic cavity S21.35- ☑
  - superficial NEC S20.97 ☑
    - back S20.47- ☑
    - front S20.37- ☑
    - insect S20.96 ☑
      - back S20.46- ☑
      - front S20.36- ☑
- throat — *see* Bite, neck, throat
- thumb S61.05- ☑
  - with
    - damage to nail S61.15- ☑
  - superficial NEC S60.37- ☑
    - insect S60.36- ☑
- thyroid S11.15 ☑
  - superficial NEC S10.87 ☑
    - insect S10.86 ☑
- toe(s) S91.15- ☑
  - with
    - damage to nail S91.25- ☑
  - great S91.15- ☑
    - with
      - damage to nail S91.25- ☑
  - lesser S91.15- ☑
    - with
      - damage to nail S91.25- ☑
  - superficial NEC S90.47- ☑
    - great S90.47- ☑
    - insect S90.46- ☑
      - great S90.46- ☑
- tongue S01.552 ☑
- trachea S11.025 ☑
  - superficial NEC S10.17 ☑
    - insect S10.16 ☑
- tunica vaginalis — *see* Bite, testis
- tympanum, tympanic membrane — *see* Bite, ear
- umbilical region S31.155 ☑
- uvula — *see* Bite, oral cavity
- vagina — *see* Bite, vulva
- venomous — *see* Venom
- vocal cords S11.035 ☑
  - superficial NEC S10.17 ☑
    - insect S10.16 ☑
- vulva S31.45 ☑
  - superficial NEC S30.874 ☑
    - insect S30.864 ☑
- wrist S61.55- ☑
  - superficial NEC S60.87- ☑
    - insect S60.86- ☑

Biting, cheek or lip K13.1
Biventricular failure (heart) I50.82
Björck (-Thorson) **syndrome** (malignant carcinoid) E34.0
Black
- death A20.9
- eye S00.1- ☑
- hairy tongue K14.3
- heel (foot) S90.3- ☑
- lung (disease) J60
- palm (hand) S60.22- ☑

Blackfan-Diamond anemia or syndrome (congenital hypoplastic anemia) D61.01
Blackhead L70.0
Blackout R55
Bladder — *see* condition
Blast (air) (hydraulic) (immersion) (underwater)
- blindness S05.8X- ☑
- injury
  - abdomen or thorax — *see* Injury, by site
  - ear (acoustic nerve trauma) — *see* Injury, nerve, acoustic, specified type NEC
  - syndrome NEC T70.8
Blastoma — *see* Neoplasm, malignant, by site
- pulmonary — *see* Neoplasm, lung, malignant
Blastomycosis, blastomycotic B40.9

Blastomycosis, blastomycotic — *continued*
- Brazilian — *see* Paracoccidioidomycosis
- cutaneous B40.3
- disseminated B40.7
- European — *see* Cryptococcosis
- generalized B40.7
- keloidal B48.0
- North American B40.9
- primary pulmonary B40.0
- pulmonary B40.2
  - acute B40.0
  - chronic B40.1
- skin B40.3
- South American — *see* Paracoccidioidomycosis
- specified NEC B40.89

Bleb(s) R23.8
- emphysematous (lung) (solitary) J43.9
- endophthalmitis H59.43
- filtering (vitreous), after glaucoma surgery Z98.83
- inflamed (infected), postprocedural H59.40
  - stage 1 H59.41
  - stage 2 H59.42
  - stage 3 H59.43
- lung (ruptured) J43.9
  - congenital — *see* Atelectasis
  - newborn P25.8
- subpleural (emphysematous) J43.9

Blebitis, postprocedural H59.40
- stage 1 H59.41
- stage 2 H59.42
- stage 3 H59.43

Bleeder (familial) (hereditary) — *see* Hemophilia

Bleeding — *see also* Hemorrhage
- anal K62.5
- anovulatory N97.0
- atonic, following delivery O72.1
- capillary I78.8
  - puerperal O72.2
- contact (postcoital) N93.0
- due to uterine subinvolution N85.3
- ear — *see* Otorrhagia
- excessive, associated with menopausal onset N92.4
- familial — *see* Defect, coagulation
- following intercourse N93.0
- gastrointestinal K92.2
- hemorrhoids — *see* Hemorrhoids
- intermenstrual (regular) N92.3
  - irregular N92.1
- intraoperative — *see* Complication, intraoperative, hemorrhage
- irregular N92.6
- menopausal N92.4
- newborn, intraventricular — *see* Newborn, affected by, hemorrhage, intraventricular
- nipple N64.59
- nose R04.0
- ovulation N92.3
- perimenopausal N92.4
- postclimacteric N95.0
- postcoital N93.0
- postmenopausal N95.0
- postoperative — *see* Complication, postprocedural, hemorrhage
- preclimacteric N92.4
- pre-pubertal vaginal N93.1
- puberty (excessive, with onset of menstrual periods) N92.2
- rectum, rectal K62.5
  - newborn P54.2
- tendencies — *see* Defect, coagulation
- throat R04.1
- tooth socket (post-extraction) K91.840
- umbilical stump P51.9
- uterus, uterine NEC N93.9
  - climacteric N92.4
  - dysfunctional or functional N93.8
  - menopausal N92.4
  - preclimacteric or premenopausal N92.4
  - unrelated to menstrual cycle N93.9
- vagina, vaginal (abnormal) N93.9
  - dysfunctional or functional N93.8
  - newborn P54.6
  - pre-pubertal N93.1
- vicarious N94.89

Blennorrhagia, blennorrhagic — *see* Gonorrhea

Blennorrhea (acute) (chronic) — *see also* Gonorrhea
- inclusion (neonatal) (newborn) P39.1
- lower genitourinary tract (gonococcal) A54.00

Blennorrhea — *continued*
- neonatorum (gonococcal ophthalmia) A54.31

Blepharelosis — *see* Entropion

Blepharitis (angularis) (ciliaris) (eyelid) (marginal) (nonulcerative) H01.009
- herpes zoster B02.39
- left H01.006
  - lower H01.005
  - upper H01.004
  - upper and lower H01.00B
- right H01.003
  - lower H01.002
  - upper H01.001
  - upper and lower H01.00A
- squamous H01.029
  - left H01.026
    - lower H01.025
    - upper H01.024
    - upper and lower H01.02B
  - right H01.023
    - lower H01.022
    - upper H01.021
    - upper and lower H01.02A
- ulcerative H01.019
  - left H01.016
    - lower H01.015
    - upper H01.014
    - upper and lower H01.01B
  - right H01.013
    - lower H01.012
    - upper H01.011
    - upper and lower H01.01A

Blepharochalasis H02.30
- congenital Q10.0
- left H02.36
  - lower H02.35
  - upper H02.34
- right H02.33
  - lower H02.32
  - upper H02.31

Blepharoclonus H02.59

Blepharoconjunctivitis H10.50- ☑
- angular H10.52- ☑
- contact H10.53- ☑
- ligneous H10.51- ☑

Blepharophimosis (eyelid) H02.529
- congenital Q10.3
- left H02.526
  - lower H02.525
  - upper H02.524
- right H02.523
  - lower H02.522
  - upper H02.521

Blepharoptosis H02.40- ☑
- congenital Q10.0
- mechanical H02.41- ☑
- myogenic H02.42- ☑
- neurogenic H02.43- ☑
- paralytic H02.43- ☑

Blepharopyorrhea, gonococcal A54.39

Blepharospasm G24.5
- drug induced G24.01

Blighted ovum O02.0

Blind — *see also* Blindness
- bronchus (congenital) Q32.4
- loop syndrome K90.2
  - congenital Q43.8
- sac, fallopian tube (congenital) Q50.6
- spot, enlarged — *see* Defect, visual field, localized, scotoma, blind spot area
- tract or tube, congenital NEC — *see* Atresia, by site

Blindness (acquired) (congenital) (both eyes) H54.0X- ☑
- blast S05.8X- ☑
- color — *see* Deficiency, color vision
- concussion S05.8X- ☑
- cortical H47.619
  - left brain H47.612
  - right brain H47.611
- day H53.11
- due to injury (current episode) S05.9- ☑
  - sequelae — *code to* injury with seventh character S
- eclipse (total) — *see* Retinopathy, solar
- emotional (hysterical) F44.6
- face H53.16
- hysterical F44.6
- legal (both eyes) (USA definition) H54.8
- mind R48.8

Blindness — *continued*
- night H53.60
  - abnormal dark adaptation curve H53.61
  - acquired H53.62
  - congenital H53.63
  - specified type NEC H53.69
  - vitamin A deficiency E50.5
- one eye (other eye normal) H54.40
  - left (normal vision on right) H54.4- ☑
    - low vision on right H54.12- ☑
  - low vision, other eye H54.10
  - right (normal vision on left) H54.41- ☑
    - low vision on left H54.11- ☑
- psychic R48.8
- river B73.01
- snow — *see* Photokeratitis
- sun, solar — *see* Retinopathy, solar
- transient — *see* Disturbance, vision, subjective, loss, transient
- traumatic (current episode) S05.9- ☑
- word (developmental) F81.0
  - acquired R48.0
  - secondary to organic lesion R48.0

Blister (nonthermal)
- abdominal wall S30.821 ☑
- alveolar process S00.522 ☑
- ankle S90.52- ☑
- antecubital space — *see* Blister, elbow
- anus S30.827 ☑
- arm (upper) S40.82- ☑
- auditory canal — *see* Blister, ear
- auricle — *see* Blister, ear
- axilla — *see* Blister, arm
- back, lower S30.820 ☑
- beetle dermatitis L24.89
- breast S20.12- ☑
- brow S00.82 ☑
- calf — *see* Blister, leg
- canthus — *see* Blister, eyelid
- cheek S00.82 ☑
  - internal S00.522 ☑
- chest wall — *see* Blister, thorax
- chin S00.82 ☑
- costal region — *see* Blister, thorax
- digit(s)
  - foot — *see* Blister, toe
  - hand — *see* Blister, finger
- due to burn — *see* Burn, by site, second degree
- ear S00.42- ☑
- elbow S50.32- ☑
- epiglottis S10.12 ☑
- esophagus, cervical S10.12 ☑
- eyebrow — *see* Blister, eyelid
- eyelid S00.22- ☑
- face S00.82 ☑
- fever B00.1
- finger(s) S60.429 ☑
  - index S60.42- ☑
  - little S60.42- ☑
  - middle S60.42- ☑
  - ring S60.42- ☑
- foot (except toe(s) alone) S90.82- ☑
  - toe — *see* Blister, toe
- forearm S50.82- ☑
  - elbow only — *see* Blister, elbow
- forehead S00.82 ☑
- fracture — *omit code*
- genital organ
  - female S30.826 ☑
  - male S30.825 ☑
- gum S00.522 ☑
- hand S60.52- ☑
- head S00.92 ☑
  - ear — *see* Blister, ear
  - eyelid — *see* Blister, eyelid
  - lip S00.521 ☑
  - nose S00.32 ☑
  - oral cavity S00.522 ☑
  - scalp S00.02 ☑
  - specified site NEC S00.82 ☑
- heel — *see* Blister, foot
- hip S70.22- ☑
- interscapular region S20.429 ☑
- jaw S00.82 ☑
- knee S80.22- ☑
- larynx S10.12 ☑

Blister — *continued*
leg (lower) S80.82- ☑
  knee — *see* Blister, knee
  upper — *see* Blister, thigh
lip S00.521 ☑
malar region S00.82 ☑
mammary — *see* Blister, breast
mastoid region S00.82 ☑
mouth S00.522 ☑
multiple, skin, nontraumatic R23.8
nail
  finger — *see* Blister, finger
  toe — *see* Blister, toe
nasal S00.32 ☑
neck S10.92 ☑
  specified site NEC S10.82 ☑
  throat S10.12 ☑
nose S00.32 ☑
occipital region S00.02 ☑
oral cavity S00.522 ☑
orbital region — *see* Blister, eyelid
palate S00.522 ☑
palm — *see* Blister, hand
parietal region S00.02 ☑
pelvis S30.820 ☑
penis S30.822 ☑
periocular area — *see* Blister, eyelid
phalanges
  finger — *see* Blister, finger
  toe — *see* Blister, toe
pharynx S10.12 ☑
pinna — *see* Blister, ear
popliteal space — *see* Blister, knee
scalp S00.02 ☑
scapular region — *see* Blister, shoulder
scrotum S30.823 ☑
shin — *see* Blister, leg
shoulder S40.22- ☑
sternal region S20.329 ☑
submaxillary region S00.82 ☑
submental region S00.82 ☑
subungual
  finger(s) — *see* Blister, finger
  toe(s) — *see* Blister, toe
supraclavicular fossa S10.82 ☑
supraorbital S00.82 ☑
temple S00.82 ☑
temporal region S00.82 ☑
testis S30.823 ☑
thermal — *see* Burn, second degree, by site
thigh S70.32- ☑
thorax, thoracic (wall) S20.92 ☑
  back S20.42- ☑
  front S20.32- ☑
throat S10.12 ☑
thumb S60.32- ☑
toe(s) S90.42- ☑
  great S90.42- ☑
tongue S00.522 ☑
trachea S10.12 ☑
tympanum, tympanic membrane — *see* Blister, ear
upper arm — *see* Blister, arm (upper)
uvula S00.522 ☑
vagina S30.824 ☑
vocal cords S10.12 ☑
vulva S30.824 ☑
wrist S60.82- ☑
Bloating R14.0
Bloch-Sulzberger disease or syndrome Q82.3
Block, blocked
alveolocapillary J84.10
arborization (heart) I45.5
arrhythmic I45.9
atrioventricular (incomplete) (partial) I44.30
  with atrioventricular dissociation I44.2
  complete I44.2
    congenital Q24.6
  congenital Q24.6
  first degree I44.0
  second degree (types I and II) I44.1
  specified NEC I44.39
  third degree I44.2
  types I and II I44.1
auriculoventricular — *see* Block, atrioventricular
bifascicular (cardiac) I45.2
bundle-branch (complete) (false) (incomplete) I44.4

Block, blocked — *continued*
bundle-branch — *continued*
  bilateral I45.2
  left I44.7
    with right bundle branch block I45.2
    hemiblock I44.60
      anterior I44.4
      posterior I44.5
    incomplete I44.7
      with right bundle branch block I45.2
  right I45.10
    with
      left bundle branch block I45.2
      left fascicular block I45.2
    specified NEC I45.19
  Wilson's type I45.19
cardiac I45.9
conduction I45.9
  complete I44.2
fascicular (left) I44.60
  anterior I44.4
  posterior I44.5
  right I45.0
  specified NEC I44.69
foramen Magendie (acquired) G91.1
  congenital Q03.1
    with spina bifida — *see* Spina bifida, by site, with hydrocephalus
heart I45.9
  bundle branch I45.4
    bilateral I45.2
  complete (atrioventricular) I44.2
  congenital Q24.6
  first degree (atrioventricular) I44.0
  second degree (atrioventricular) I44.1
  specified type NEC I45.5
  third degree (atrioventricular) I44.2
hepatic vein I82.0
intraventricular (nonspecific) I45.4
  bundle branch
    bilateral I45.2
kidney N28.9
  postcystoscopic or postprocedural N99.0
Mobitz (types I and II) I44.1
myocardial — *see* Block, heart
nodal I45.5
organ or site, congenital NEC — *see* Atresia, by site
portal (vein) I81
second degree (types I and II) I44.1
sinoatrial I45.5
sinoauricular I45.5
third degree I44.2
trifascicular I45.3
tubal N97.1
vein NOS I82.90
Wenckebach (types I and II) I44.1
Blockage — *see* Obstruction
Blocq's disease F44.4
Blood
constituents, abnormal R78.9
disease D75.9
donor — *see* Donor, blood
dyscrasia D75.9
  with
    abortion — *see* Abortion, by type, complicated by, hemorrhage
    ectopic pregnancy O08.1
    molar pregnancy O08.1
  following ectopic or molar pregnancy O08.1
  newborn P61.9
  puerperal, postpartum O72.3
flukes NEC — *see* Schistosomiasis
in
  feces K92.1
    occult R19.5
  urine — *see* Hematuria
mole O02.0
occult in feces R19.5
pressure
  decreased, due to shock following injury T79.4 ☑
  examination only Z01.30
  fluctuating I99.8
  high — *see* Hypertension
    borderline R03.0
    incidental reading, without diagnosis of hypertension R03.0
  low — *see also* Hypotension

Blood — *continued*
pressure — *continued*
  low — *see also* Hypotension — *continued*
    incidental reading, without diagnosis of hypotension R03.1
spitting — *see* Hemoptysis
staining cornea — *see* Pigmentation, cornea, stromal
transfusion
  reaction or complication — *see* Complications, transfusion
type
  A (Rh positive) Z67.10
    Rh negative Z67.11
  AB (Rh positive) Z67.30
    Rh negative Z67.31
  B (Rh positive) Z67.20
    Rh negative Z67.21
  O (Rh positive) Z67.40
    Rh negative Z67.41
  Rh (positive) Z67.90
    negative Z67.91
vessel rupture — *see* Hemorrhage
vomiting — *see* Hematemesis
Blood-forming organs, disease D75.9
Bloodgood's disease — *see* Mastopathy, cystic
Bloom (-Machacek)(-Torre) **syndrome** Q82.8
Blount disease or osteochondrosis M92.51- ☑
Blue
baby Q24.9
diaper syndrome E72.09
dome cyst (breast) — *see* Cyst, breast
dot cataract Q12.0
nevus D22.9
sclera Q13.5
  with fragility of bone and deafness Q78.0
toe syndrome I75.02- ☑
Blueness — *see* Cyanosis
Blues, postpartal O90.6
  baby O90.6
Blurring, visual H53.8
Blushing (abnormal) (excessive) R23.2
BMI — *see* Body, mass index
Boarder, hospital NEC Z76.4
accompanying sick person Z76.3
healthy infant or child Z76.2
  foundling Z76.1
Bockhart's impetigo L01.02
Bodechtel-Guttman disease (subacute sclerosing panencephalitis) A81.1
Boder-Sedgwick syndrome (ataxia-telangiectasia) G11.3
Body, bodies
Aschoff's — *see* Myocarditis, rheumatic
asteroid, vitreous — *see* Deposit, crystalline
cytoid (retina) — *see* Occlusion, artery, retina
drusen (degenerative) (macula) (retinal) — *see also* Degeneration, macula, drusen
  optic disc — *see* Drusen, optic disc
foreign — *see* Foreign body
loose
  joint, except knee — *see* Loose, body, joint
    knee M23.4- ☑
  sheath, tendon — *see* Disorder, tendon, specified type NEC
mass index (BMI)
  adult
    19.9 or less Z68.1
    20.0-20.9 Z68.20
    21.0-21.9 Z68.21
    22.0-22.9 Z68.22
    23.0-23.9 Z68.23
    24.0-24.9 Z68.24
    25.0-25.9 Z68.25
    26.0-26.9 Z68.26
    27.0-27.9 Z68.27
    28.0-28.9 Z68.28
    29.0-29.9 Z68.29
    30.0-30.9 Z68.30
    31.0-31.9 Z68.31
    32.0-32.9 Z68.32
    33.0-33.9 Z68.33
    34.0-34.9 Z68.34
    35.0-35.9 Z68.35
    36.0-36.9 Z68.36
    37.0-37.9 Z68.37
    38.0-38.9 Z68.38
    39.0-39.9 Z68.39
    40.0-44.9 Z68.41
    45.0-49.9 Z68.42

☑ **Additional Character Required** — **Refer to the Tabular List for Character Selection**

Body, bodies — *continued*
　mass index — *continued*
　　adult — *continued*
　　　50.0-59.9 Z68.43
　　　60.0-69.9 Z68.44
　　　70 and over Z68.45
　　pediatric
　　　5th percentile to less than 85th percentile for
　　　　age Z68.52
　　　85th percentile to less than 95th percentile for
　　　　age Z68.53
　　　greater than or equal to ninety-fifth percentile
　　　　for age Z68.54
　　　less than fifth percentile for age Z68.51
　　Mooser's A75.2
　　rice — *see also* Loose, body, joint
　　　knee M23.4- ☑
　　rocking F98.4
Boeck's
　disease or sarcoid — *see* Sarcoidosis
　lupoid (miliary) D86.3
Boerhaave's syndrome (spontaneous esophageal rupture) K22.3
Boggy
　cervix N88.8
　uterus N85.8
Boil — *see also* Furuncle, by site
　Aleppo B55.1
　Baghdad B55.1
　Delhi B55.1
　lacrimal
　　gland — *see* Dacryoadenitis
　　passages (duct) (sac) — *see* Inflammation, lacrimal,
　　　passages, acute
　Natal B55.1
　orbit, orbital — *see* Abscess, orbit
　tropical B55.1
Bold hives — *see* Urticaria
Bombé, iris — *see* Membrane, pupillary
Bone — *see* condition
Bonnevie-Ullrich syndrome — *see also* Turner's syndrome Q87.19
Bonnier's syndrome H81.8 ☑
Bonvale dam fever T73.3 ☑
Bony block of joint — *see* Ankylosis
BOOP (bronchiolitis obliterans organized pneumonia)
　J84.89
Borderline
　diabetes mellitus R73.03
　hypertension R03.0
　osteopenia M85.8- ☑
　pelvis, with obstruction during labor O65.1
　personality F60.3
Borna disease A83.9
Bornholm disease B33.0
Boston exanthem A88.0
Botalli, ductus (patent) (persistent) Q25.0
Bothriocephalus latus infestation B70.0
Botulism (foodborne intoxication) A05.1
　infant A48.51
　non-foodborne A48.52
　wound A48.52
Bouba — *see* Yaws
Bouchard's nodes (with arthropathy) M15.2
Bouffée délirante F23
Bouillaud's disease or syndrome (rheumatic heart
　disease) I01.9
Bourneville's disease Q85.1
Boutonniere deformity (finger) — *see* Deformity, finger,
　boutonniere
Bouveret (-Hoffmann) **syndrome** (paroxysmal tachycardia) I47.9
Bovine heart — *see* Hypertrophy, cardiac
Bowel — *see* condition
Bowen's
　dermatosis (precancerous) — *see* Neoplasm, skin, in
　　situ
　disease — *see* Neoplasm, skin, in situ
　epithelioma — *see* Neoplasm, skin, in situ
　type
　　epidermoid carcinoma-in-situ — *see* Neoplasm,
　　　skin, in situ
　　intraepidermal squamous cell carcinoma — *see*
　　　Neoplasm, skin, in situ
Bowing
　femur — *see also* Deformity, limb, specified type NEC,
　　thigh

Bowing — *continued*
　femur — *see also* Deformity, limb, specified type, thigh
　　— *continued*
　　congenital Q68.3
　fibula — *see also* Deformity, limb, specified type NEC,
　　lower leg
　　congenital Q68.4
　forearm — *see also* Deformity, limb, specified type NEC,
　　forearm
　leg(s), long bones, congenital Q68.5
　radius — *see* Deformity, limb, specified type NEC,
　　forearm
　tibia — *see also* Deformity, limb, specified type NEC,
　　lower leg
　　congenital Q68.4
Bowleg(s) (acquired) M21.16- ☑
　congenital Q68.5
　rachitic E64.3
Boyd's dysentery A03.2
Brachial — *see* condition
Brachycardia R00.1
Brachycephaly Q75.0
Bradley's disease A08.19
Bradyarrhythmia, cardiac I49.8
Bradycardia (sinoatrial) (sinus) (vagal) R00.1
　neonatal P29.12
　reflex G90.09
　tachycardia syndrome I49.5
Bradykinesia R25.8
Bradypnea R06.89
Bradytachycardia I49.5
Brailsford's disease or osteochondrosis — *see* Osteochondrosis, juvenile, radius
Brain — *see also* condition
　death G93.82
　syndrome — *see* Syndrome, brain
Branched-chain amino-acid disorder E71.2
Branchial — *see* condition
　cartilage, congenital Q18.2
Branchiogenic remnant (in neck) Q18.0
Brandt's syndrome (acrodermatitis enteropathica) E83.2
Brash (water) R12
Bravais-jacksonian epilepsy — *see* Epilepsy, localization-related, symptomatic, with simple partial
　seizures
Braxton Hicks contractions — *see* False, labor
Brazilian leishmaniasis B55.2
BRBPR K62.5
Break, retina (without detachment) H33.30- ☑
　with retinal detachment — *see* Detachment, retina
　horseshoe tear H33.31- ☑
　multiple H33.33- ☑
　round hole H33.32- ☑
Breakdown
　device, graft or implant — *see also* Complications, by
　　site and type, mechanical T85.618 ☑
　　arterial graft NEC — *see* Complication, cardiovascular device, mechanical, vascular
　　breast (implant) T85.41 ☑
　　catheter NEC T85.618 ☑
　　　cystostomy T83.010 ☑
　　　dialysis (renal) T82.41 ☑
　　　　intraperitoneal T85.611 ☑
　　　Hopkins T83.018 ☑
　　　ileostomy T83.018 ☑
　　　infusion NEC T82.514 ☑
　　　　cranial T85.610- ☑
　　　　epidural T85.610 ☑
　　　　intrathecal T85.610 ☑
　　　　spinal T85.610 ☑
　　　　subarachnoid T85.610 ☑
　　　　subdural T85.610 ☑
　　　nephrostomy T83.012 ☑
　　　urethral indwelling T83.011 ☑
　　　urinary NEC T83.018 ☑
　　　urostomy T83.018 ☑
　　electronic (electrode) (pulse generator) (stimulator)
　　　bone T84.310 ☑
　　　cardiac T82.119 ☑
　　　　electrode T82.110 ☑
　　　　pulse generator T82.111 ☑
　　　　specified type NEC T82.118 ☑
　　　nervous system — *see* Complication, prosthetic
　　　　device, mechanical, electronic nervous
　　　　system stimulator
　　　urinary — *see* Complication, genitourinary, device, urinary, mechanical

Breakdown — *continued*
　device, graft or implant — *see also* Complications, by
　　site and type, mechanical — *continued*
　　fixation, internal (orthopedic) NEC — *see* Complication, fixation device, mechanical
　　gastrointestinal — *see* Complications, prosthetic
　　　device, mechanical, gastrointestinal device
　　genital NEC T83.418 ☑
　　　intrauterine contraceptive device T83.31 ☑
　　　penile prosthesis (cylinder) (implanted) (pump)
　　　　(resevoir) T83.410 ☑
　　　testicular prosthesis T83.411 ☑
　　heart NEC — *see* Complication, cardiovascular device, mechanical
　　intrathecal infusion pump T85.615 ☑
　　joint prosthesis — *see* Complications, joint prosthesis, internal, mechanical, by site
　　nervous system, specified device NEC T85.615 ☑
　　ocular NEC — *see* Complications, prosthetic device,
　　　mechanical, ocular device
　　orthopedic NEC — *see* Complication, orthopedic,
　　　device, mechanical
　　specified NEC T85.618 ☑
　　subcutaneous device pocket
　　　nervous system prosthetic device, implant, or
　　　　graft T85.890 ☑
　　　other internal prosthetic device, implant, or graft
　　　　T85.898 ☑
　　sutures, permanent T85.612 ☑
　　　used in bone repair — *see* Complications, fixation
　　　　device, internal (orthopedic), mechanical
　　urinary NEC T83.118 ☑
　　　graft T83.21 ☑
　　　sphincter, implanted T83.111 ☑
　　　stent (ileal conduit) (nephroureteral) T83.113 ☑
　　　　ureteral indwelling T83.112 ☑
　　vascular NEC — *see* Complication, cardiovascular
　　　device, mechanical
　　ventricular intracranial shunt T85.01 ☑
　nervous F48.8
　perineum O90.1
　respirator J95.850
　　specified NEC J95.859
　ventilator J95.850
　　specified NEC J95.859
Breast — *see also* condition
　buds E30.1
　　in newborn P96.89
　dense R92.2
　nodule — *see also* Lump, breast N63.0
Breath
　foul R19.6
　holder, child R06.89
　holding spell R06.89
　shortness R06.02
Breathing
　labored — *see* Hyperventilation
　mouth R06.5
　　causing malocclusion M26.5 ☑
　periodic R06.3
　　high altitude G47.32
Breathlessness R06.81
Breda's disease — *see* Yaws
Breech presentation (mother) O32.1 ☑
　causing obstructed labor O64.1 ☑
　footling O32.8 ☑
　　causing obstructed labor O64.8 ☑
　incomplete O32.8 ☑
　　causing obstructed labor O64.8 ☑
Breisky's disease N90.4
Brennemann's syndrome I88.0
Brenner
　tumor (benign) D27.9
　　borderline malignancy D39.1- ☑
　　malignant C56 ☑
　　proliferating D39.1- ☑
Bretonneau's disease or angina A36.0
Breus' mole O02.0
Brevicollis Q76.49
Brickmakers' anemia B76.9 *[D63.8]*
Bridge, myocardial Q24.5
Bright red blood per rectum (BRBPR) K62.5
Bright's disease — *see also* Nephritis
　arteriosclerotic — *see* Hypertension, kidney
Brill (-Zinsser) **disease** (recrudescent typhus) A75.1
Brill-Symmers' disease C82.90
Brion-Kayser disease — *see* Fever, parathyroid

Briquet's disorder or syndrome F45.0
Brissaud's
  infantilism or dwarfism E23.0
  motor-verbal tic F95.2
Brittle
  bones disease Q78.0
  nails L60.3
    congenital Q84.6
Broad — *see also* condition
  beta disease E78.2
  ligament laceration syndrome N83.8
Broad- or floating-betalipoproteinemia E78.2
Brock's syndrome (atelectasis due to enlarged lymph
  nodes) J98.19
Brocq-Duhring disease (dermatitis herpetiformis) L13.0
Brodie's abscess or disease M86.8X- ☑
Broken
  arches — *see also* Deformity, limb, flat foot
  arm (meaning upper limb) — *see* Fracture, arm
  back — *see* Fracture, vertebra
  bone — *see* Fracture
  implant or internal device — *see* Complications, by site
    and type, mechanical
  leg (meaning lower limb) — *see* Fracture, leg
  nose S02.2 ☑
  tooth, teeth — *see* Fracture, tooth
Bromhidrosis, bromidrosis L75.0
Bromidism, bromism G92.8
  due to
    correct substance properly administered — *see* Ta-
      ble of Drugs and Chemicals, by drug, adverse
      effect
    overdose or wrong substance given or taken — *see*
      Table of Drugs and Chemicals, by drug, poi-
      soning
  chronic (dependence) F13.20
Bromidrosiphobia F40.298
Bronchi, bronchial — *see* condition
Bronchiectasis (cylindrical) (diffuse) (fusiform) (localized)
  (saccular) J47.9
  with
    acute
      bronchitis J47.0
      lower respiratory infection J47.0
    exacerbation (acute) J47.1
  congenital Q33.4
  tuberculous NEC — *see* Tuberculosis, pulmonary
Bronchiolectasis — *see* Bronchiectasis
Bronchiolitis (acute) (infective) (subacute) J21.9
  with
    bronchospasm or obstruction J21.9
    influenza, flu or grippe — *see* Influenza, with, respi-
      ratory manifestations NEC
  chemical (chronic) J68.4
    acute J68.0
  chronic (fibrosing) (obliterative) J44.9
  due to
    external agent — *see* Bronchitis, acute, due to
    human metapneumovirus J21.1
    respiratory syncytial virus (RSV) J21.0
    specified organism NEC J21.8
  fibrosa obliterans J44.9
  influenzal — *see* Influenza, with, respiratory manifesta-
    tions NEC
  obliterans J42
    with organizing pneumonia (BOOP) J84.89
  obliterative (chronic) (subacute) J44.9
    due to fumes or vapors J68.4
    due to chemicals, gases, fumes or vapors (inhalation)
      J68.4
  respiratory, interstitial lung disease J84.115
Bronchitis (diffuse) (fibrinous) (hypostatic) (infective)
  (membranous) J40
  with
    influenza, flu or grippe — *see* Influenza, with, respi-
      ratory manifestations NEC
    obstruction (airway) (lung) J44.9
    tracheitis (15 years of age and above) J40
      acute or subacute J20.9
      chronic J42
      under 15 years of age J20.9
  acute or subacute (with bronchospasm or obstruction)
    J20.9
    with
      bronchiectasis J47.0
      chronic obstructive pulmonary disease J44.0
    chemical (due to gases, fumes or vapors) J68.0

Bronchitis — *continued*
  acute or subacute — *continued*
    due to
      fumes or vapors J68.0
      Haemophilus influenzae J20.1
      Mycoplasma pneumoniae J20.0
      radiation J70.0
      specified organism NEC J20.8
      Streptococcus J20.2
      virus
        coxsackie J20.3
        echovirus J20.7
        parainfluenzae J20.4
        respiratory syncytial (RSV) J20.5
        rhinovirus J20.6
    viral NEC J20.8
  allergic (acute) J45.909
    with
      exacerbation (acute) J45.901
      status asthmaticus J45.902
  arachidic T17.528 ☑
  aspiration (due to food and vomit) J69.0
  asthmatic J45.9 ☑
    chronic J44.9
      with
        acute lower respiratory infection J44.0
        exacerbation (acute) J44.1
  capillary — *see* Pneumonia, broncho
  caseous (tuberculous) A15.5
  Castellani's A69.8
  catarrhal (15 years of age and above) J40
    acute — *see* Bronchitis, acute
    chronic J41.0
    under 15 years of age J20.9
  chemical (acute) (subacute) J68.0
    chronic J68.4
    due to fumes or vapors J68.0
      chronic J68.4
  chronic J42
    with
      airways obstruction J44.9
      tracheitis (chronic) J42
    asthmatic (obstructive) J44.9
    catarrhal J41.0
    chemical (due to fumes or vapors) J68.4
    due to
      chemicals, gases, fumes or vapors (inhalation)
        J68.4
      radiation J70.1
      tobacco smoking J41.0
    emphysematous J44.9
    mucopurulent J41.1
    non-obstructive J41.0
    obliterans J44.9
    obstructive J44.9
    purulent J41.1
    simple J41.0
  croupous — *see* Bronchitis, acute
  due to gases, fumes or vapors (chemical) J68.0
  emphysematous (obstructive) J44.9
  exudative — *see* Bronchitis, acute
  fetid J41.1
  grippal — *see* Influenza, with, respiratory manifesta-
    tions NEC
  in those under 15 years age — *see* Bronchitis, acute
    chronic — *see* Bronchitis, chronic
  influenzal — *see* Influenza, with, respiratory manifesta-
    tions NEC
  mixed simple and mucopurulent J41.8
  moulder's J62.8
  mucopurulent (chronic) (recurrent) J41.1
    acute or subacute J20.9
    simple (mixed) J41.8
  obliterans (chronic) J44.9
  obstructive (chronic) (diffuse) J44.9
  pituitous J41.1
  pneumococcal, acute or subacute J20.2
  pseudomembranous, acute or subacute — *see* Bronchi-
    tis, acute
  purulent (chronic) (recurrent) J41.1
    acute or subacute — *see* Bronchitis, acute
  putrid J41.1
  senile (chronic) J42
  simple and mucopurulent (mixed) J41.8
  smokers' J41.0
  spirochetal NEC A69.8
  subacute — *see* Bronchitis, acute
  suppurative (chronic) J41.1

Bronchitis — *continued*
  suppurative — *continued*
    acute or subacute — *see* Bronchitis, acute
    tuberculous A15.5
  under 15 years of age — *see* Bronchitis, acute
    chronic — *see* Bronchitis, chronic
  viral NEC, acute or subacute — *see also* Bronchitis,
    acute J20.8
Bronchoalveolitis J18.0
Bronchoaspergillosis B44.1
Bronchocele meaning goiter E04.0
Broncholithiasis J98.09
  tuberculous NEC A15.5
Bronchomalacia J98.09
  congenital Q32.2
Bronchomycosis NOS B49 *[J99]*
  candidal B37.1
Bronchopleuropneumonia — *see* Pneumonia, broncho
Bronchopneumonia — *see* Pneumonia, broncho
Bronchopneumonitis — *see* Pneumonia, broncho
Bronchopulmonary — *see* condition
Bronchopulmonitis — *see* Pneumonia, broncho
Bronchorrhagia (see Hemoptysis)
Bronchorrhea J98.09
  acute J20.9
  chronic (infective) (purulent) J42
Bronchospasm (acute) J98.01
  with
    bronchiolitis, acute J21.9
    bronchitis, acute (conditions in J20) — *see* Bronchi-
      tis, acute
  due to external agent — *see* condition, respiratory,
    acute, due to
  exercise induced J45.990
Bronchospirochetosis A69.8
  Castellani A69.8
Bronchostenosis J98.09
Bronchus — *see* condition
Brontophobia F40.220
Bronze baby syndrome P83.88
Brooke's tumor — *see* Neoplasm, skin, benign
Brown enamel of teeth (hereditary) K00.5
Brown's sheath syndrome H50.61- ☑
Brown-Séquard disease, paralysis or syndrome
  G83.81
Bruce sepsis A23.0
Brucellosis (infection) A23.9
  abortus A23.1
  canis A23.3
  dermatitis A23.9
  melitensis A23.0
  mixed A23.8
  sepsis A23.9
    melitensis A23.0
    specified NEC A23.8
  suis A23.2
Bruck-de Lange disease Q87.19
Bruck's disease — *see* Deformity, limb
BRUE (brief resolved unexplained event) R68.13
Brugsch's syndrome Q82.8
Bruise (skin surface intact) — *see also* Contusion
  with
    open wound — *see* Wound, open
  internal organ — *see* Injury, by site
  newborn P54.5
  scalp, due to birth injury, newborn P12.3
  umbilical cord O69.5 ☑
Bruit (arterial) R09.89
  cardiac R01.1
Brush burn — *see* Abrasion, by site
Bruton's X-linked agammaglobulinemia D80.0
Bruxism
  psychogenic F45.8
  sleep related G47.63
Bubbly lung syndrome P27.0
Bubo I88.8
  blennorrhagic (gonococcal) A54.89
  chancroidal A57
  climatic A55
  due to Haemophilus ducreyi A57
  gonococcal A54.89
  indolent (nonspecific) I88.8
  inguinal (nonspecific) I88.8
    chancroidal A57
    climatic A55
    due to H. ducreyi A57
    infective I88.8

Bubo — *continued*
　scrofulous (tuberculous) A18.2
　soft chancre A57
　suppurating — *see* Lymphadenitis, acute
　syphilitic (primary) A51.0
　　congenital A50.07
　tropical A55
　virulent (chancroidal) A57
Bubonic plague A20.0
Bubonocele — *see* Hernia, inguinal
Buccal — *see* condition
Buchanan's disease or osteochondrosis M91.0
Buchem's syndrome (hyperostosis corticalis) M85.2
Bucket-handle fracture or tear (semilunar cartilage)
　　 — *see* Tear, meniscus
Budd-Chiari syndrome (hepatic vein thrombosis) I82.0
Budgerigar fancier's disease or lung J67.2
Buds
　breast E30.1
　　in newborn P96.89
Buerger's disease (thromboangiitis obliterans) I73.1
Bulbar — *see* condition
Bulbus cordis (left ventricle) (persistent) Q21.8
Bulimia (nervosa) F50.2
　atypical F50.9
　normal weight F50.9
Bulky
　stools R19.5
　uterus N85.2
Bulla (e) R23.8
　lung (emphysematous) (solitary) J43.9
　　newborn P25.8
Bullet wound — *see also* Puncture
　fracture — *code as* Fracture, by site
　internal organ — *see* Injury, by site
Bundle
　branch block (complete) (false) (incomplete) — *see*
　　Block, bundle-branch
　of His — *see* condition
Bunion M21.61- ☑
　tailor's M21.62- ☑
Bunionette M21.62- ☑
Buphthalmia, buphthalmos (congenital) Q15.0
Burdwan fever B55.0
Bürger-Grütz disease or syndrome E78.3
Buried
　penis (congenital) Q55.64
　　acquired N48.83
　roots K08.3
Burke's syndrome K86.89
Burkitt
　cell leukemia C91.0- ☑
　lymphoma (malignant) C83.7- ☑
　　small noncleaved, diffuse C83.7- ☑
　　spleen C83.77
　undifferentiated C83.7- ☑
　tumor C83.7- ☑
　type
　　acute lymphoblastic leukemia C91.0- ☑
　　undifferentiated C83.7- ☑
Burn (electricity) (flame) (hot gas, liquid or hot object)
　　(radiation) (steam) (thermal) T30.0
　abdomen, abdominal (muscle) (wall) T21.02 ☑
　　first degree T21.12 ☑
　　second degree T21.22 ☑
　　third degree T21.32 ☑
　above elbow T22.039 ☑
　　first degree T22.139 ☑
　　left T22.032 ☑
　　　first degree T22.132 ☑
　　　second degree T22.232 ☑
　　　third degree T22.332 ☑
　　right T22.031 ☑
　　　first degree T22.131 ☑
　　　second degree T22.231 ☑
　　　third degree T22.331 ☑
　　second degree T22.239 ☑
　　third degree T22.339 ☑
　acid (caustic) (external) (internal) — *see* Corrosion, by
　　site
　alimentary tract NEC T28.2 ☑
　　esophagus T28.1 ☑
　　mouth T28.0 ☑
　　pharynx T28.0 ☑
　alkaline (caustic) (external) (internal) — *see* Corrosion,
　　by site

Burn — *continued*
　ankle T25.019 ☑
　　first degree T25.119 ☑
　　left T25.012 ☑
　　　first degree T25.112 ☑
　　　second degree T25.212 ☑
　　　third degree T25.312 ☑
　　multiple with foot — *see* Burn, lower, limb, multiple,
　　　ankle and foot
　　right T25.011 ☑
　　　first degree T25.111 ☑
　　　second degree T25.211 ☑
　　　third degree T25.311 ☑
　　second degree T25.219 ☑
　　third degree T25.319 ☑
　anus — *see* Burn, buttock
　arm (lower) (upper) — *see* Burn, upper, limb
　axilla T22.049 ☑
　　first degree T22.149 ☑
　　left T22.042 ☑
　　　first degree T22.142 ☑
　　　second degree T22.242 ☑
　　　third degree T22.342 ☑
　　right T22.041 ☑
　　　first degree T22.141 ☑
　　　second degree T22.241 ☑
　　　third degree T22.341 ☑
　　second degree T22.249 ☑
　　third degree T22.349 ☑
　back (lower) T21.04 ☑
　　first degree T21.14 ☑
　　second degree T21.24 ☑
　　third degree T21.34 ☑
　　upper T21.03 ☑
　　　first degree T21.13 ☑
　　　second degree T21.23 ☑
　　　third degree T21.33 ☑
　blisters — *code as* Burn, second degree, by site
　breast(s) — *see* Burn, chest wall
　buttock(s) T21.05 ☑
　　first degree T21.15 ☑
　　second degree T21.25 ☑
　　third degree T21.35 ☑
　calf T24.039 ☑
　　first degree T24.139 ☑
　　left T24.032 ☑
　　　first degree T24.132 ☑
　　　second degree T24.232 ☑
　　　third degree T24.332 ☑
　　right T24.031 ☑
　　　first degree T24.131 ☑
　　　second degree T24.231 ☑
　　　third degree T24.331 ☑
　　second degree T24.239 ☑
　　third degree T24.339 ☑
　canthus (eye) — *see* Burn, eyelid
　caustic acid or alkaline — *see* Corrosion, by site
　cervix T28.3 ☑
　cheek T20.06 ☑
　　first degree T20.16 ☑
　　second degree T20.26 ☑
　　third degree T20.36 ☑
　chemical (acids) (alkalines) (caustics) (external) (inter-
　　nal) — *see* Corrosion, by site
　chest wall T21.01 ☑
　　first degree T21.11 ☑
　　second degree T21.21 ☑
　　third degree T21.31 ☑
　chin T20.03 ☑
　　first degree T20.13 ☑
　　second degree T20.23 ☑
　　third degree T20.33 ☑
　colon T28.2 ☑
　conjunctiva (and cornea) — *see* Burn, cornea
　cornea (and conjunctiva) T26.1- ☑
　　chemical — *see* Corrosion, cornea
　corrosion (external) (internal) — *see* Corrosion, by site
　deep necrosis of underlying tissue — *code as* Burn,
　　third degree, by site
　dorsum of hand T23.069 ☑
　　first degree T23.169 ☑
　　left T23.062 ☑
　　　first degree T23.162 ☑
　　　second degree T23.262 ☑
　　　third degree T23.362 ☑
　　right T23.061 ☑

Burn — *continued*
　dorsum of hand — *continued*
　　right — *continued*
　　　first degree T23.161 ☑
　　　second degree T23.261 ☑
　　　third degree T23.361 ☑
　　second degree T23.269 ☑
　　third degree T23.369 ☑
　due to ingested chemical agent — *see* Corrosion, by
　　site
　ear (auricle) (external) (canal) T20.01 ☑
　　first degree T20.11 ☑
　　second degree T20.21 ☑
　　third degree T20.31 ☑
　elbow T22.029 ☑
　　first degree T22.129 ☑
　　left T22.022 ☑
　　　first degree T22.122 ☑
　　　second degree T22.222 ☑
　　　third degree T22.322 ☑
　　right T22.021 ☑
　　　first degree T22.121 ☑
　　　second degree T22.221 ☑
　　　third degree T22.321 ☑
　　second degree T22.229 ☑
　　third degree T22.329 ☑
　epidermal loss — *code as* Burn, second degree, by site
　erythema, erythematous — *code as* Burn, first degree,
　　by site
　esophagus T28.1 ☑
　extent (percentage of body surface)
　　less than 10 percent T31.0
　　10-19 percent T31.10
　　　with 0-9 percent third degree burns T31.10
　　　with 10-19 percent third degree burns T31.11
　　20-29 percent T31.20
　　　with 0-9 percent third degree burns T31.20
　　　with 10-19 percent third degree burns T31.21
　　　with 20-29 percent third degree burns T31.22
　　30-39 percent T31.30
　　　with 0-9 percent third degree burns T31.30
　　　with 10-19 percent third degree burns T31.31
　　　with 20-29 percent third degree burns T31.32
　　　with 30-39 percent third degree burns T31.33
　　40-49 percent T31.40
　　　with 0-9 percent third degree burns T31.40
　　　with 10-19 percent third degree burns T31.41
　　　with 20-29 percent third degree burns T31.42
　　　with 30-39 percent third degree burns T31.43
　　　with 40-49 percent third degree burns T31.44
　　50-59 percent T31.50
　　　with 0-9 percent third degree burns T31.50
　　　with 10-19 percent third degree burns T31.51
　　　with 20-29 percent third degree burns T31.52
　　　with 30-39 percent third degree burns T31.53
　　　with 40-49 percent third degree burns T31.54
　　　with 50-59 percent third degree burns T31.55
　　60-69 percent T31.60
　　　with 0-9 percent third degree burns T31.60
　　　with 10-19 percent third degree burns T31.61
　　　with 20-29 percent third degree burns T31.62
　　　with 30-39 percent third degree burns T31.63
　　　with 40-49 percent third degree burns T31.64
　　　with 50-59 percent third degree burns T31.65
　　　with 60-69 percent third degree burns T31.66
　　70-79 percent T31.70
　　　with 0-9 percent third degree burns T31.70
　　　with 10-19 percent third degree burns T31.71
　　　with 20-29 percent third degree burns T31.72
　　　with 30-39 percent third degree burns T31.73
　　　with 40-49 percent third degree burns T31.74
　　　with 50-59 percent third degree burns T31.75
　　　with 60-69 percent third degree burns T31.76
　　　with 70-79 percent third degree burns T31.77
　　80-89 percent T31.80
　　　with 0-9 percent third degree burns T31.80
　　　with 10-19 percent third degree burns T31.81
　　　with 20-29 percent third degree burns T31.82
　　　with 30-39 percent third degree burns T31.83
　　　with 40-49 percent third degree burns T31.84
　　　with 50-59 percent third degree burns T31.85
　　　with 60-69 percent third degree burns T31.86
　　　with 70-79 percent third degree burns T31.87
　　　with 80-89 percent third degree burns T31.88
　　90 percent or more T31.90
　　　with 0-9 percent third degree burns T31.90
　　　with 10-19 percent third degree burns T31.91
　　　with 20-29 percent third degree burns T31.92

Burn — *continued*
  extent — *continued*
    90 percent or more — *continued*
      with 30-39 percent third degree burns T31.93
      with 40-49 percent third degree burns T31.94
      with 50-59 percent third degree burns T31.95
      with 60-69 percent third degree burns T31.96
      with 70-79 percent third degree burns T31.97
      with 80-89 percent third degree burns T31.98
      with 90 percent or more third degree burns T31.99
  extremity — *see* Burn, limb
  eye(s) and adnexa T26.4- ☑
    with resulting rupture and destruction of eyeball T26.2- ☑
    conjunctival sac — *see* Burn, cornea
    cornea — *see* Burn, cornea
    lid — *see* Burn, eyelid
    periocular area — *see* Burn, eyelid
    specified site NEC T26.3- ☑
  eyeball — *see* Burn, eye
  eyelid(s) T26.0- ☑
    chemical — *see* Corrosion, eyelid
  face — *see* Burn, head
  finger T23.029 ☑
    first degree T23.129 ☑
    left T23.022 ☑
      first degree T23.122 ☑
      second degree T23.222 ☑
      third degree T23.322 ☑
    multiple sites (without thumb) T23.039 ☑
      with thumb T23.049 ☑
        first degree T23.149 ☑
        left T23.042 ☑
          first degree T23.142 ☑
          second degree T23.242 ☑
          third degree T23.342 ☑
        right T23.041 ☑
          first degree T23.141 ☑
          second degree T23.241 ☑
          third degree T23.341 ☑
        second degree T23.249 ☑
        third degree T23.349 ☑
      first degree T23.139 ☑
      left T23.032 ☑
        first degree T23.132 ☑
        second degree T23.232 ☑
        third degree T23.332 ☑
      right T23.031 ☑
        first degree T23.131 ☑
        second degree T23.231 ☑
        third degree T23.331 ☑
      second degree T23.239 ☑
      third degree T23.339 ☑
    right T23.021 ☑
      first degree T23.121 ☑
      second degree T23.221 ☑
      third degree T23.321 ☑
    second degree T23.229 ☑
    third degree T23.329 ☑
  flank — *see* Burn, abdominal wall
  foot T25.029 ☑
    first degree T25.129 ☑
    left T25.022 ☑
      first degree T25.122 ☑
      second degree T25.222 ☑
      third degree T25.322 ☑
    multiple with ankle — *see* Burn, lower, limb, multiple, ankle and foot
    right T25.021 ☑
      first degree T25.121 ☑
      second degree T25.221 ☑
      third degree T25.321 ☑
    second degree T25.229 ☑
    third degree T25.329 ☑
  forearm T22.019 ☑
    first degree T22.119 ☑
    left T22.012 ☑
      first degree T22.112 ☑
      second degree T22.212 ☑
      third degree T22.312 ☑
    right T22.011 ☑
      first degree T22.111 ☑
      second degree T22.211 ☑
      third degree T22.311 ☑
    second degree T22.219 ☑

Burn — *continued*
  forearm — *continued*
    third degree T22.319 ☑
  forehead T20.06 ☑
    first degree T20.16 ☑
    second degree T20.26 ☑
    third degree T20.36 ☑
  fourth degree — *code as* Burn, third degree, by site
  friction — *see* Burn, by site
  from swallowing caustic or corrosive substance NEC — *see* Corrosion, by site
  full thickness skin loss — *code as* Burn, third degree, by site
  gastrointestinal tract NEC T28.2 ☑
    from swallowing caustic or corrosive substance T28.7 ☑
  genital organs
    external
      female T21.07 ☑
        first degree T21.17 ☑
        second degree T21.27 ☑
        third degree T21.37 ☑
      male T21.06 ☑
        first degree T21.16 ☑
        second degree T21.26 ☑
        third degree T21.36 ☑
    internal T28.3 ☑
      from caustic or corrosive substance T28.8 ☑
  groin — *see* Burn, abdominal wall
  hand(s) T23.009 ☑
    back — *see* Burn, dorsum of hand
    finger — *see* Burn, finger
    first degree T23.109 ☑
    left T23.002 ☑
      first degree T23.102 ☑
      second degree T23.202 ☑
      third degree T23.302 ☑
    multiple sites with wrist T23.099 ☑
      first degree T23.199 ☑
      left T23.092 ☑
        first degree T23.192 ☑
        second degree T23.292 ☑
        third degree T23.392 ☑
      right T23.091 ☑
        first degree T23.191 ☑
        second degree T23.291 ☑
        third degree T23.391 ☑
      second degree T23.299 ☑
      third degree T23.399 ☑
    palm — *see* Burn, palm
    right T23.001 ☑
      first degree T23.101 ☑
      second degree T23.201 ☑
      third degree T23.301 ☑
    second degree T23.209 ☑
    third degree T23.309 ☑
    thumb — *see* Burn, thumb
  head (and face) (and neck) T20.00 ☑
    cheek — *see* Burn, cheek
    chin — *see* Burn, chin
    ear — *see* Burn, ear
    eye(s) only — *see* Burn, eye
    first degree T20.10 ☑
    forehead — *see* Burn, forehead
    lip — *see* Burn, lip
    multiple sites T20.09 ☑
      first degree T20.19 ☑
      second degree T20.29 ☑
      third degree T20.39 ☑
    neck — *see* Burn, neck
    nose — *see* Burn, nose
    scalp — *see* Burn, scalp
    second degree T20.20 ☑
    third degree T20.30 ☑
  hip(s) — *see* Burn, thigh
  inhalation — *see* Burn, respiratory tract
    caustic or corrosive substance (fumes) — *see* Corrosion, respiratory tract
  internal organ(s) T28.40 ☑
    alimentary tract T28.2 ☑
      esophagus T28.1 ☑
    eardrum T28.41 ☑
    esophagus T28.1 ☑
    from caustic or corrosive substance (swallowing) NEC — *see* Corrosion, by site
    genitourinary T28.3 ☑

Burn — *continued*
  internal organ(s) — *continued*
    mouth T28.0 ☑
    pharynx T28.0 ☑
    respiratory tract — *see* Burn, respiratory tract
    specified organ NEC T28.49 ☑
  interscapular region — *see* Burn, back, upper
  intestine (large) (small) T28.2 ☑
  knee T24.029 ☑
    first degree T24.129 ☑
    left T24.022 ☑
      first degree T24.122 ☑
      second degree T24.222 ☑
      third degree T24.322 ☑
    right T24.021 ☑
      first degree T24.121 ☑
      second degree T24.221 ☑
      third degree T24.321 ☑
    second degree T24.229 ☑
    third degree T24.329 ☑
  labium (majus) (minus) — *see* Burn, genital organs, external, female
  lacrimal apparatus, duct, gland or sac — *see* Burn, eye, specified site NEC
  larynx T27.0 ☑
    with lung T27.1 ☑
  leg(s) (lower) (upper) — *see* Burn, lower, limb
  lightning — *see* Burn, by site
  limb(s)
    lower (except ankle or foot alone) — *see* Burn, lower, limb
    upper — *see* Burn, upper limb
  lip(s) T20.02 ☑
    first degree T20.12 ☑
    second degree T20.22 ☑
    third degree T20.32 ☑
  lower
    back — *see* Burn, back
    limb T24.009 ☑
      ankle — *see* Burn, ankle
      calf — *see* Burn, calf
      first degree T24.109 ☑
      foot — *see* Burn, foot
      hip — *see* Burn, thigh
      knee — *see* Burn, knee
      left T24.002 ☑
        first degree T24.102 ☑
        second degree T24.202 ☑
        third degree T24.302 ☑
      multiple sites, except ankle and foot T24.099 ☑
        ankle and foot T25.099 ☑
          first degree T25.199 ☑
          left T25.092 ☑
            first degree T25.192 ☑
            second degree T25.292 ☑
            third degree T25.392 ☑
          right T25.091 ☑
            first degree T25.191 ☑
            second degree T25.291 ☑
            third degree T25.391 ☑
          second degree T25.299 ☑
          third degree T25.399 ☑
        first degree T24.199 ☑
        left T24.092 ☑
          first degree T24.192 ☑
          second degree T24.292 ☑
          third degree T24.392 ☑
        right T24.091 ☑
          first degree T24.191 ☑
          second degree T24.291 ☑
          third degree T24.391 ☑
        second degree T24.299 ☑
        third degree T24.399 ☑
      right T24.001 ☑
        first degree T24.101 ☑
        second degree T24.201 ☑
        third degree T24.301 ☑
      second degree T24.209 ☑
      thigh — *see* Burn, thigh
      third degree T24.309 ☑
      toe — *see* Burn, toe
  lung (with larynx and trachea) T27.1 ☑
  mouth T28.0 ☑
  neck T20.07 ☑
    first degree T20.17 ☑
    second degree T20.27 ☑

Burn — *continued*
neck — *continued*
    third degree T20.37 ✓
nose (septum) T20.04 ✓
  first degree T20.14 ✓
  second degree T20.24 ✓
  third degree T20.34 ✓
ocular adnexa — *see* Burn, eye
orbit region — *see* Burn, eyelid
palm T23.059 ✓
  first degree T23.159 ✓
  left T23.052 ✓
    first degree T23.152 ✓
    second degree T23.252 ✓
    third degree T23.352 ✓
  right T23.051 ✓
    first degree T23.151 ✓
    second degree T23.251 ✓
    third degree T23.351 ✓
  second degree T23.259 ✓
  third degree T23.359 ✓
partial thickness — *code as* Burn, by site, second degree
pelvis — *see* Burn, trunk
penis — *see* Burn, genital organs, external, male
perineum
  female — *see* Burn, genital organs, external, female
  male — *see* Burn, genital organs, external, male
periocular area — *see* Burn, eyelid
pharynx T28.0 ✓
rectum T28.2 ✓
respiratory tract T27.3 ✓
  larynx — *see* Burn, larynx
  specified part NEC T27.2 ✓
  trachea — *see* Burn, trachea
sac, lacrimal — *see* Burn, eye, specified site NEC
scalp T20.05 ✓
  first degree T20.15 ✓
  second degree T20.25 ✓
  third degree T20.35 ✓
scapular region T22.069 ✓
  first degree T22.169 ✓
  left T22.062 ✓
    first degree T22.162 ✓
    second degree T22.262 ✓
    third degree T22.362 ✓
  right T22.061 ✓
    first degree T22.161 ✓
    second degree T22.261 ✓
    third degree T22.361 ✓
  second degree T22.269 ✓
  third degree T22.369 ✓
sclera — *see* Burn, eye, specified site NEC
scrotum — *see* Burn, genital organs, external, male
shoulder T22.059 ✓
  first degree T22.159 ✓
  left T22.052 ✓
    first degree T22.152 ✓
    second degree T22.252 ✓
    third degree T22.352 ✓
  right T22.051 ✓
    first degree T22.151 ✓
    second degree T22.251 ✓
    third degree T22.351 ✓
  second degree T22.259 ✓
  third degree T22.359 ✓
stomach T28.2 ✓
temple — *see* Burn, head
testis — *see* Burn, genital organs, external, male
thigh T24.019 ✓
  first degree T24.119 ✓
  left T24.012 ✓
    first degree T24.112 ✓
    second degree T24.212 ✓
    third degree T24.312 ✓
  right T24.011 ✓
    first degree T24.111 ✓
    second degree T24.211 ✓
    third degree T24.311 ✓
  second degree T24.219 ✓
  third degree T24.319 ✓
thorax (external) — *see* Burn, trunk
throat (meaning pharynx) T28.0 ✓
thumb(s) T23.019 ✓
  first degree T23.119 ✓
  left T23.012 ✓
    first degree T23.112 ✓

Burn — *continued*
thumb(s) — *continued*
  left — *continued*
    second degree T23.212 ✓
    third degree T23.312 ✓
  multiple sites with fingers T23.049 ✓
    first degree T23.149 ✓
    left T23.042 ✓
      first degree T23.142 ✓
      second degree T23.242 ✓
      third degree T23.342 ✓
    right T23.041 ✓
      first degree T23.141 ✓
      second degree T23.241 ✓
      third degree T23.341 ✓
    second degree T23.249 ✓
    third degree T23.349 ✓
  right T23.011 ✓
    first degree T23.111 ✓
    second degree T23.211 ✓
    third degree T23.311 ✓
  second degree T23.219 ✓
  third degree T23.319 ✓
toe T25.039 ✓
  first degree T25.139 ✓
  left T25.032 ✓
    first degree T25.132 ✓
    second degree T25.232 ✓
    third degree T25.332 ✓
  right T25.031 ✓
    first degree T25.131 ✓
    second degree T25.231 ✓
    third degree T25.331 ✓
  second degree T25.239 ✓
  third degree T25.339 ✓
tongue T28.0 ✓
tonsil(s) T28.0 ✓
trachea T27.0 ✓
  with lung T27.1 ✓
trunk T21.00 ✓
  abdominal wall — *see* Burn, abdominal wall
  anus — *see* Burn, buttock
  axilla — *see* Burn, upper limb
  back — *see* Burn, back
  breast — *see* Burn, chest wall
  buttock — *see* Burn, buttock
  chest wall — *see* Burn, chest wall
  first degree T21.10 ✓
  flank — *see* Burn, abdominal wall
  genital
    female — *see* Burn, genital organs, external, female
    male — *see* Burn, genital organs, external, male
  groin — *see* Burn, abdominal wall
  interscapular region — *see* Burn, back, upper
  labia — *see* Burn, genital organs, external, female
  lower back — *see* Burn, back
  penis — *see* Burn, genital organs, external, male
  perineum
    female — *see* Burn, genital organs, external, female
    male — *see* Burn, genital organs, external, male
  scapula region — *see* Burn, scapular region
  scrotum — *see* Burn, genital organs, external, male
  second degree T21.20 ✓
  specified site NEC T21.09 ✓
    first degree T21.19 ✓
    second degree T21.29 ✓
    third degree T21.39 ✓
  testes — *see* Burn, genital organs, external, male
  third degree T21.30 ✓
  upper back — *see* Burn, back, upper
  vulva — *see* Burn, genital organs, external, female
unspecified site with extent of body surface involved
  specified
    less than 10 percent T31.0
    10-19 percent (0-9 percent third degree) T31.10
      with 10-19 percent third degree T31.11
    20-29 percent (0-9 percent third degree) T31.20
      with
        10-19 percent third degree T31.21
        20-29 percent third degree T31.22
    30-39 percent (0-9 percent third degree) T31.30
      with
        10-19 percent third degree T31.31
        20-29 percent third degree T31.32

Burn — *continued*
unspecified site with extent of body surface involved
  specified — *continued*
    30-39 percent — *continued*
      with — *continued*
        30-39 percent third degree T31.33
    40-49 percent (0-9 percent third degree) T31.40
      with
        10-19 percent third degree T31.41
        20-29 percent third degree T31.42
        30-39 percent third degree T31.43
        40-49 percent third degree T31.44
    50-59 percent (0-9 percent third degree) T31.50
      with
        10-19 percent third degree T31.51
        20-29 percent third degree T31.52
        30-39 percent third degree T31.53
        40-49 percent third degree T31.54
        50-59 percent third degree T31.55
    60-69 percent (0-9 percent third degree) T31.60
      with
        10-19 percent third degree T31.61
        20-29 percent third degree T31.62
        30-39 percent third degree T31.63
        40-49 percent third degree T31.64
        50-59 percent third degree T31.65
        60-69 percent third degree T31.66
    70-79 percent (0-9 percent third degree) T31.70
      with
        10-19 percent third degree T31.71
        20-29 percent third degree T31.72
        30-39 percent third degree T31.73
        40-49 percent third degree T31.74
        50-59 percent third degree T31.75
        60-69 percent third degree T31.76
        70-79 percent third degree T31.77
    80-89 percent (0-9 percent third degree) T31.80
      with
        10-19 percent third degree T31.81
        20-29 percent third degree T31.82
        30-39 percent third degree T31.83
        40-49 percent third degree T31.84
        50-59 percent third degree T31.85
        60-69 percent third degree T31.86
        70-79 percent third degree T31.87
        80-89 percent third degree T31.88
    90 percent or more (0-9 percent third degree) T31.90
      with
        10-19 percent third degree T31.91
        20-29 percent third degree T31.92
        30-39 percent third degree T31.93
        40-49 percent third degree T31.94
        50-59 percent third degree T31.95
        60-69 percent third degree T31.96
        70-79 percent third degree T31.97
        80-89 percent third degree T31.98
        90-99 percent third degree T31.99
upper limb T22.00 ✓
  above elbow — *see* Burn, above elbow
  axilla — *see* Burn, axilla
  elbow — *see* Burn, elbow
  first degree T22.10 ✓
  forearm — *see* Burn, forearm
  hand — *see* Burn, hand
  interscapular region — *see* Burn, back, upper
  multiple sites T22.099 ✓
    first degree T22.199 ✓
    left T22.092 ✓
      first degree T22.192 ✓
      second degree T22.292 ✓
      third degree T22.392 ✓
    right T22.091 ✓
      first degree T22.191 ✓
      second degree T22.291 ✓
      third degree T22.391 ✓
    second degree T22.299 ✓
    third degree T22.399 ✓
  scapular region — *see* Burn, scapular region
  second degree T22.20 ✓
  shoulder — *see* Burn, shoulder
  third degree T22.30 ✓
  wrist — *see* Burn, wrist
uterus T28.3 ✓
vagina T28.3 ✓
vulva — *see* Burn, genital organs, external, female
wrist T23.079 ✓
  first degree T23.179 ✓
  left T23.072 ✓

Burn — continued
  wrist — continued
    left — continued
      first degree T23.172 ☑
      second degree T23.272 ☑
      third degree T23.372 ☑
      multiple sites with hand T23.099 ☑
        first degree T23.199 ☑
        left T23.092 ☑
          first degree T23.192 ☑
          second degree T23.292 ☑
          third degree T23.392 ☑
        right T23.091 ☑
          first degree T23.191 ☑
          second degree T23.291 ☑
          third degree T23.391 ☑
        second degree T23.299 ☑
        third degree T23.399 ☑
      right T23.071 ☑
        first degree T23.171 ☑
        second degree T23.271 ☑
        third degree T23.371 ☑
      second degree T23.279 ☑
      third degree T23.379 ☑
Burnett's syndrome E83.52
Burning
  feet syndrome E53.9
  sensation R20.8
  tongue K14.6
Burn-out (state) Z73.0
Burns' disease or osteochondrosis — see Osteochondrosis, juvenile, ulna
Bursa — see condition
Bursitis M71.9
  Achilles — see Tendinitis, Achilles
  adhesive — see Bursitis, specified NEC
  ankle — see Enthesopathy, lower limb, ankle, specified type NEC
  calcaneal — see Enthesopathy, foot, specified type NEC
  collateral ligament, tibial — see Bursitis, tibial collateral
  due to use, overuse, pressure — see also Disorder, soft tissue, due to use, specified type NEC
    specified NEC — see Disorder, soft tissue, due to use, specified NEC
  Duplay's M75.0
  elbow NEC M70.3- ☑
    olecranon M70.2- ☑
  finger — see Disorder, soft tissue, due to use, specified type NEC, hand
  foot — see Enthesopathy, foot, specified type NEC
  gonococcal A54.49
  gouty — see Gout
  hand M70.1- ☑
  hip NEC M70.7- ☑
    trochanteric M70.6- ☑
  infective NEC M71.10
    abscess — see Abscess, bursa
    ankle M71.17- ☑
    elbow M71.12- ☑
    foot M71.17- ☑
    hand M71.14- ☑
    hip M71.15- ☑
    knee M71.16- ☑
    multiple sites M71.19
    shoulder M71.11- ☑
    specified site NEC M71.18
    wrist M71.13- ☑
  ischial — see Bursitis, hip
  knee NEC M70.5- ☑
    prepatellar M70.4- ☑
  occupational NEC — see also Disorder, soft tissue, due to, use
  olecranon — see Bursitis, elbow, olecranon
  pharyngeal J39.1
  popliteal — see Bursitis, knee
  prepatellar M70.4- ☑
  radiohumeral M70.3- ☑
  rheumatoid M06.20
    ankle M06.27- ☑
    elbow M06.22- ☑
    foot joint M06.27- ☑
    hand joint M06.24- ☑
    hip M06.25- ☑
    knee M06.26- ☑
    multiple site M06.29
    shoulder M06.21- ☑

Bursitis — continued
  rheumatoid — continued
    vertebra M06.28
    wrist M06.23- ☑
  scapulohumeral — see Bursitis, shoulder
  semimembranous muscle (knee) — see Bursitis, knee
  shoulder M75.5- ☑
    adhesive — see Capsulitis, adhesive
  specified NEC M71.50
    ankle M71.57- ☑
    due to use, overuse or pressure — see Disorder, soft tissue, due to, use
    elbow M71.52- ☑
    foot M71.57- ☑
    hand M71.54- ☑
    hip M71.55- ☑
    knee M71.56- ☑
    shoulder — see Bursitis, shoulder
    specified site NEC M71.58
    tibial collateral M76.4- ☑
    wrist M71.53- ☑
  subacromial — see Bursitis, shoulder
  subcoracoid — see Bursitis, shoulder
  subdeltoid — see Bursitis, shoulder
  syphilitic A52.78
  Thornwaldt, Tornwaldt J39.2
  tibial collateral M76.4- ☑
  toe — see Enthesopathy, foot, specified type NEC
  trochanteric (area) — see Bursitis, hip, trochanteric
  wrist — see Bursitis, hand
Bursopathy M71.9
  specified type NEC M71.80
    ankle M71.87- ☑
    elbow M71.82- ☑
    foot M71.87- ☑
    hand M71.84- ☑
    hip M71.85- ☑
    knee M71.86- ☑
    multiple sites M71.89
    shoulder M71.81- ☑
    specified site NEC M71.88
    wrist M71.83- ☑
Burst stitches or sutures (complication of surgery) T81.31 ☑
  external operation wound T81.31 ☑
  internal operation wound T81.32 ☑
Buruli ulcer A31.1
Bury's disease L95.1
Buschke's
  disease — see Cryptococcosis by site
  scleredema — see Sclerosis, systemic
Busse-Buschke disease — see Cryptococcosis by site
Buttock — see condition
Button
  Biskra B55.1
  Delhi B55.1
  oriental B55.1
Buttonhole deformity (finger) — see Deformity, finger, boutonniere
Bwamba fever A92.8
Byssinosis J66.0
Bywaters' syndrome T79.5 ☑

C

Cachexia R64
  cancerous R64
  cardiac — see Disease, heart
  dehydration E86.0
  due to malnutrition R64
  exophthalmic — see Hyperthyroidism
  heart — see Disease, heart
  hypophyseal E23.0
  hypopituitary E23.0
  lead — see Poisoning, lead
  malignant R64
  marsh — see Malaria
  nervous F48.8
  old age R54
  paludal — see Malaria
  pituitary E23.0
  pulmonary R64
  renal N28.9
  saturnine — see Poisoning, lead
  senile R54
  Simmonds' E23.0
  splenica D73.0

Cachexia — continued
  strumipriva E03.4
  tuberculous NEC — see Tuberculosis
CADASIL (cerebral autosomal dominant arteriopathy with subcortical infarcts and leukoencephalopathy) I67.850
Café, au lait spots L81.3
Caffeine-induced
  anxiety disorder F15.980
  sleep disorder F15.982
Caffey's syndrome Q78.8
Caisson disease T70.3 ☑
Cake kidney Q63.1
Caked breast (puerperal, postpartum) O92.79
Calabar swelling B74.3
Calcaneal spur — see Spur, bone, calcaneal
Calcaneo-apophysitis M92.8
Calcareous — see condition
Calcicosis J62.8
Calciferol (vitamin D) deficiency E55.9
  with rickets E55.0
Calcification
  adrenal (capsule) (gland) E27.49
    tuberculous B90.8 [E35]
  aorta I70.0
  artery (annular) — see Arteriosclerosis
  auricle (ear) — see Disorder, pinna, specified type NEC
  basal ganglia G23.8
  bladder N32.89
    due to Schistosoma hematobium B65.0
  brain (cortex) — see Calcification, cerebral
  bronchus J98.09
  bursa M71.40
    ankle M71.47- ☑
    elbow M71.42- ☑
    foot M71.47- ☑
    hand M71.44- ☑
    hip M71.45- ☑
    knee M71.46- ☑
    multiple sites M71.49
    shoulder M75.3- ☑
    specified site NEC M71.48
    wrist M71.43- ☑
  cardiac — see Degeneration, myocardial
  cerebral (cortex) G93.89
    artery I67.2
  cervix (uteri) N88.8
  choroid plexus G93.89
  conjunctiva — see Concretion, conjunctiva
  corpora cavernosa (penis) N48.89
  cortex (brain) — see Calcification, cerebral
  dental pulp (nodular) K04.2
  dentinal papilla K00.4
  fallopian tube N83.8
  falx cerebri G96.198
  gallbladder K82.8
  general E83.59
  heart — see also Degeneration, myocardial
    valve — see also Endocarditis
      mitral — see Calcification, mitral
  idiopathic infantile arterial (IIAC) Q28.8
  intervertebral cartilage or disc (postinfective) — see Disorder, disc, specified NEC
  intracranial — see Calcification, cerebral
  joint — see Disorder, joint, specified type NEC
  kidney N28.89
    tuberculous N29 [B90.1]
  larynx (senile) J38.7
  lens — see Cataract, specified NEC
  lung (active) (postinfectional) J98.4
    tuberculous B90.9
  lymph gland or node (postinfectional) I89.8
    tuberculous — see also Tuberculosis, lymph gland B90.8
  mammographic R92.1
  massive (paraplegic) — see Myositis, ossificans, in, quadriplegia
  medial — see Arteriosclerosis, extremities
  meninges (cerebral) (spinal) G96.198
  metastatic E83.59
  mitral (valve)
    annular I34.81
      nonrheumatic I34.81
      rheumatic I05.8
    annulus I34.81
      nonrheumatic I34.81
      rheumatic I05.8

Calcification — continued
　Mönckeberg's — see Arteriosclerosis, extremities
　muscle M61.9
　　due to burns — see Myositis, ossificans, in, burns
　　paralytic — see Myositis, ossificans, in, quadriplegia
　　specified type NEC M61.40
　　　ankle M61.47- ☑
　　　foot M61.47- ☑
　　　forearm M61.43- ☑
　　　hand M61.44- ☑
　　　lower leg M61.46- ☑
　　　multiple sites M61.49
　　　pelvic region M61.45- ☑
　　　shoulder region M61.41- ☑
　　　specified site NEC M61.48
　　　thigh M61.45- ☑
　　　upper arm M61.42- ☑
　myocardium, myocardial — see Degeneration, myocardial
　ovary N83.8
　pancreas K86.89
　penis N48.89
　periarticular — see Disorder, joint, specified type NEC
　pericardium — see also Pericarditis I31.1
　pineal gland E34.8
　pleura J94.8
　　postinfectional J94.8
　　tuberculous NEC B90.9
　pulpal (dental) (nodular) K04.2
　sclera H15.89
　spleen D73.89
　subcutaneous L94.2
　suprarenal (capsule) (gland) E27.49
　tendon (sheath) — see also Tenosynovitis, specified type NEC
　　with bursitis, synovitis or tenosynovitis — see Tendinitis, calcific
　trachea J39.8
　ureter N28.89
　uterus N85.8
　vitreous — see Deposit, crystalline
Calcified — see Calcification
Calcinosis (interstitial) (tumoral) (universalis) E83.59
　with Raynaud's phenomenon, esophageal dysfunction, sclerodactyly, telangiectasia (CREST syndrome) M34.1
　circumscripta (skin) L94.2
　cutis L94.2
Calciphylaxis — see also Calcification, by site E83.59
Calcium
　deposits — see Calcification, by site
　metabolism disorder E83.50
　salts or soaps in vitreous — see Deposit, crystalline
Calciuria R82.994
Calculi — see Calculus
Calculosis, intrahepatic — see Calculus, bile duct
Calculus, calculi, calculous
　ampulla of Vater — see Calculus, bile duct
　anuria (impacted) (recurrent) — see also Calculus, urinary N20.9
　appendix K38.1
　bile duct (common) (hepatic) K80.50
　　with
　　　calculus of gallbladder — see Calculus, gallbladder and bile duct
　　　cholangitis K80.30
　　　　with
　　　　　cholecystitis — see Calculus, bile duct, with cholecystitis
　　　　　obstruction K80.31
　　　　acute K80.32
　　　　　with
　　　　　　chronic cholangitis K80.36
　　　　　　　with obstruction K80.37
　　　　　　obstruction K80.33
　　　　chronic K80.34
　　　　　with
　　　　　　acute cholangitis K80.36
　　　　　　　with obstruction K80.37
　　　　　　obstruction K80.35
　　　　cholecystitis (with cholangitis) K80.40
　　　　　with obstruction K80.41
　　　　　acute K80.42
　　　　　　with
　　　　　　　chronic cholecystitis K80.46
　　　　　　　　with obstruction K80.47
　　　　　　　obstruction K80.43
　　　　　chronic K80.44

Calculus, calculi, calculous — continued
　bile duct — continued
　　with — continued
　　　cholecystitis — continued
　　　　chronic — continued
　　　　　with
　　　　　　acute cholecystitis K80.46
　　　　　　　with obstruction K80.47
　　　　　　obstruction K80.45
　biliary — see also Calculus, gallbladder
　　specified NEC K80.80
　　　with obstruction K80.81
　bilirubin, multiple — see Calculus, gallbladder
　bladder (encysted) (impacted) (urinary) (diverticulum) N21.0
　bronchus J98.09
　calyx (kidney) (renal) — see Calculus, kidney
　cholesterol (pure) (solitary) — see Calculus, gallbladder
　common duct (bile) — see Calculus, bile duct
　conjunctiva — see Concretion, conjunctiva
　cystic N21.0
　　duct — see Calculus, gallbladder
　dental (subgingival) (supragingival) K03.6
　diverticulum
　　bladder N21.0
　　kidney N20.0
　epididymis N50.89
　gallbladder K80.20
　　with
　　　bile duct calculus — see Calculus, gallbladder and bile duct
　　　cholecystitis K80.10
　　　　with obstruction K80.11
　　　　acute K80.00
　　　　　with
　　　　　　chronic cholecystitis K80.12
　　　　　　　with obstruction K80.13
　　　　　　obstruction K80.01
　　　　chronic K80.10
　　　　　with
　　　　　　acute cholecystitis K80.12
　　　　　　　with obstruction K80.13
　　　　　　obstruction K80.11
　　　　specified NEC K80.18
　　　　　with obstruction K80.19
　　　obstruction K80.21
　gallbladder and bile duct K80.70
　　with
　　　cholecystitis K80.60
　　　　with obstruction K80.61
　　　　acute K80.62
　　　　　with
　　　　　　chronic cholecystitis K80.66
　　　　　　　with obstruction K80.67
　　　　　　obstruction K80.63
　　　　chronic K80.64
　　　　　with
　　　　　　acute cholecystitis K80.66
　　　　　　　with obstruction K80.67
　　　　　　obstruction K80.65
　　　obstruction K80.71
　hepatic (duct) — see Calculus, bile duct
　ileal conduit N21.8
　intestinal (impaction) (obstruction) K56.49
　kidney (impacted) (multiple) (pelvis) (recurrent) (staghorn) N20.0
　　with calculus, ureter N20.2
　　congenital Q63.8
　lacrimal passages — see Dacryolith
　liver (impacted) — see Calculus, bile duct
　lung J98.4
　mammographic R92.1
　nephritic (impacted) (recurrent) — see Calculus, kidney
　nose J34.89
　pancreas (duct) K86.89
　parotid duct or gland K11.5
　pelvis, encysted — see Calculus, kidney
　prostate N42.0
　pulmonary J98.4
　pyelitis (impacted) (recurrent) N20.0
　　with hydronephrosis N13.6
　pyelonephritis (impacted) (recurrent) — see category N20 ☑
　　with hydronephrosis N13.6
　renal (impacted) (recurrent) — see Calculus, kidney
　salivary (duct) (gland) K11.5
　seminal vesicle N50.89
　staghorn — see Calculus, kidney

Calculus, calculi, calculous — continued
　Stensen's duct K11.5
　stomach K31.89
　sublingual duct or gland K11.5
　　congenital Q38.4
　submandibular duct, gland or region K11.5
　submaxillary duct, gland or region K11.5
　suburethral N21.8
　tonsil J35.8
　tooth, teeth (subgingival) (supragingival) K03.6
　tunica vaginalis N50.89
　ureter (impacted) (recurrent) N20.1
　　with calculus, kidney N20.2
　　　with hydronephrosis N13.2
　　　　with infection N13.6
　ureteropelvic junction N20.1
　urethra (impacted) N21.1
　urinary (duct) (impacted) (passage) (tract) N20.9
　　with hydronephrosis N13.2
　　　with infection N13.6
　　in (due to)
　　lower N21.9
　　　specified NEC N21.8
　vagina N89.8
　vesical (impacted) N21.0
　Wharton's duct K11.5
　xanthine E79.8 [N22]
Calicectasis N28.89
Caliectasis N28.89
California
　disease B38.9
　encephalitis A83.5
Caligo cornea — see Opacity, cornea, central
Callositas, callosity (infected) L84
Callus (infected) L84
　bone — see Osteophyte
　　excessive, following fracture — code as Sequelae of fracture
CALME (childhood asymmetric labium majus enlargement) N90.61
Calorie deficiency or malnutrition — see also Malnutrition E46
Calpainopathy (primary) G71.032
　autosomal dominant G71.031
　autosomal recessive G71.032
Calvé-Perthes disease — see Legg-Calvé-Perthes disease
Calvé's disease — see Osteochondrosis, juvenile, spine
Calvities — see Alopecia, androgenic
Cameroon fever — see Malaria
Camptocormia (hysterical) F44.4
Camurati-Engelmann syndrome Q78.3
Canal — see also condition
　atrioventricular Q21.20
　　common Q21.23
　　incomplete Q21.21
　　intermediate Q21.22
　　partial Q21.21
　　transitional Q21.22
Canaliculitis (lacrimal) (acute) (subacute) H04.33- ☑
　Actinomyces A42.89
　chronic H04.42- ☑
Canavan's disease E75.29
Canceled procedure (surgical) Z53.9
　because of
　　contraindication Z53.09
　　　smoking Z53.01
　　left against medical advice (AMA) Z53.29
　　patient's decision Z53.20
　　　for reasons of belief or group pressure Z53.1
　　　specified reason NEC Z53.29
　　specified reason NEC Z53.8
Cancer — see also Neoplasm, by site, malignant
　bile duct type liver C22.1
　blood — see Leukemia
　breast — see also Neoplasm, breast, malignant C50.91- ☑
　hepatocellular C22.0
　lung — see also Neoplasm, lung, malignant C34.90
　ovarian — see also Neoplasm ovary, malignant C56.9
　unspecified site (primary) C80.1
Cancer (o) phobia F45.29
Cancerous — see Neoplasm, malignant, by site
Cancrum oris A69.0
Candidiasis, candidal B37.9
　balanitis B37.42
　bronchitis B37.1
　cheilitis B37.83

Candidiasis, candidal — *continued*
  congenital P37.5
  cystitis B37.41
  disseminated B37.7
  endocarditis B37.6
  enteritis B37.82
  esophagitis B37.81
  intertrigo B37.2
  lung B37.1
  meningitis B37.5
  mouth B37.0
  nails B37.2
  neonatal P37.5
  onychia B37.2
  oral B37.0
  osteomyelitis B37.89
  otitis externa B37.84
  paronychia B37.2
  perionyxis B37.2
  pneumonia B37.1
  proctitis B37.82
  pulmonary B37.1
  pyelonephritis B37.49
  sepsis B37.7
  skin B37.2
  specified site NEC B37.89
  stomatitis B37.0
  systemic B37.7
  urethritis B37.41
  urogenital site NEC B37.49
  vagina (acute) B37.31
    chronic (recurrent) B37.32
  vulva (acute) B37.31
    chronic (recurrent) B37.32
  vulvovaginitis (acute) B37.31
    chronic (recurrent) B37.32
Candidid L30.2
Candidosis — *see* Candidiasis
Candiru infection or infestation B88.8
Canities (premature) L67.1
  congenital Q84.2
Canker (mouth) (sore) K12.0
  rash A38.9
Cannabinosis J66.2
Cannabis induced
  anxiety disorder F12.980
  psychotic disorder F12.959
  sleep disorder F12.988
Canton fever A75.9
Cantrell's syndrome Q87.89
Capillariasis (intestinal) B81.1
  hepatic B83.8
Capillary — *see* condition
Caplan's syndrome — *see* Rheumatoid, lung
Capsule — *see* condition
Capsulitis (joint) — *see also* Enthesopathy
  adhesive (shoulder) M75.0- ☑
  hepatic K65.8
  labyrinthine — *see* Otosclerosis, specified NEC
  thyroid E06.9
Caput
  crepitus Q75.8
  medusae I86.8
  succedaneum P12.81
Car sickness T75.3 ☑
Carapata (disease) A68.0
Carate — *see* Pinta
Carbon lung J60
Carbuncle L02.93
  abdominal wall L02.231
  anus K61.0
  auditory canal, external — *see* Abscess, ear, external
  auricle ear — *see* Abscess, ear, external
  axilla L02.43- ☑
  back (any part) L02.232
  breast N61.1
  buttock L02.33
  cheek (external) L02.03
  chest wall L02.233
  chin L02.03
  corpus cavernosum N48.21
  ear (any part) (external) (middle) — *see* Abscess, ear, external
  external auditory canal — *see* Abscess, ear, external
  eyelid — *see* Abscess, eyelid
  face NEC L02.03
  femoral (region) — *see* Carbuncle, lower limb
  finger — *see* Carbuncle, hand

Carbuncle — *continued*
  flank L02.231
  foot L02.63- ☑
  forehead L02.03
  genital — *see* Abscess, genital
  gluteal (region) L02.33
  groin L02.234
  hand L02.53- ☑
  head NEC L02.831
  heel — *see* Carbuncle, foot
  hip — *see* Carbuncle, lower limb
  kidney — *see* Abscess, kidney
  knee — *see* Carbuncle, lower limb
  labium (majus) (minus) N76.4
  lacrimal
    gland — *see* Dacryoadenitis
    passages (duct) (sac) — *see* Inflammation, lacrimal, passages, acute
  leg — *see* Carbuncle, lower limb
  lower limb L02.43- ☑
  malignant A22.0
  navel L02.236
  neck L02.13
  nose (external) (septum) J34.0
  orbit, orbital — *see* Abscess, orbit
  palmar (space) — *see* Carbuncle, hand
  partes posteriores L02.33
  pectoral region L02.233
  penis N48.21
  perineum L02.235
  pinna — *see* Abscess, ear, external
  popliteal — *see* Carbuncle, lower limb
  scalp L02.831
  seminal vesicle N49.0
  shoulder — *see* Carbuncle, upper limb
  specified site NEC L02.838
  temple (region) L02.03
  thumb — *see* Carbuncle, hand
  toe — *see* Carbuncle, foot
  trunk L02.239
    abdominal wall L02.231
    back L02.232
    chest wall L02.233
    groin L02.234
    perineum L02.235
    umbilicus L02.236
  umbilicus L02.236
  upper limb L02.43- ☑
  urethra N34.0
  vulva N76.4
Carbunculus — *see* Carbuncle
Carcinoid (tumor) — *see* Tumor, carcinoid
Carcinoidosis E34.0
Carcinoma (malignant) — *see also* Neoplasm, by site, malignant
  acidophil
    specified site — *see* Neoplasm, malignant, by site
    unspecified site C75.1
  acidophil-basophil, mixed
    specified site — *see* Neoplasm, malignant, by site
    unspecified site C75.1
  adnexal (skin) — *see* Neoplasm, skin, malignant
  adrenal cortical C74.0- ☑
  alveolar — *see* Neoplasm, lung, malignant
    cell — *see* Neoplasm, lung, malignant
  ameloblastic C41.1
    upper jaw (bone) C41.0
  apocrine
    breast — *see* Neoplasm, breast, malignant
    specified site NEC — *see* Neoplasm, skin, malignant
    unspecified site C44.99
  basal cell (pigmented) (*see also* Neoplasm, skin, malignant) C44.91
    fibro-epithelial — *see* Neoplasm, skin, malignant
    morphea — *see* Neoplasm, skin, malignant
    multicentric — *see* Neoplasm, skin, malignant
  basaloid
  basal-squamous cell, mixed — *see* Neoplasm, skin, malignant
  basophil
    specified site — *see* Neoplasm, malignant, by site
    unspecified site C75.1
  basophil-acidophil, mixed
    specified site — *see* Neoplasm, malignant, by site
    unspecified site C75.1
  basosquamous — *see* Neoplasm, skin, malignant

Carcinoma — *continued*
  bile duct
    with hepatocellular, mixed C22.0
    liver C22.1
    specified site NEC — *see* Neoplasm, malignant, by site
    unspecified site C22.1
  branchial or branchiogenic C10.4
  bronchial or bronchogenic — *see* Neoplasm, lung, malignant
  bronchiolar — *see* Neoplasm, lung, malignant
  bronchioloalveolar — *see* Neoplasm, lung, malignant
  C cell
    specified site — *see* Neoplasm, malignant, by site
    unspecified site C73
  ceruminous C44.29- ☑
  cervix uteri
    in situ D06.9
      endocervix D06.0
      exocervix D06.1
      specified site NEC D06.7
  chorionic
    specified site — *see* Neoplasm, malignant, by site
    unspecified site
      female C58
      male C62.90
  chromophobe
    specified site — *see* Neoplasm, malignant, by site
    unspecified site C75.1
  cloacogenic
    specified site — *see* Neoplasm, malignant, by site
    unspecified site C21.2
  diffuse type
    specified site — *see* Neoplasm, malignant, by site
    unspecified site C16.9
  duct (cell)
    with Paget's disease — *see* Neoplasm, breast, malignant
    infiltrating
      with lobular carcinoma (in situ)
        specified site — *see* Neoplasm, malignant, by site
        unspecified site (female) C50.91- ☑
          male C50.92- ☑
      specified site — *see* Neoplasm, malignant, by site
      unspecified site (female) C50.91- ☑
        male C50.92- ☑
  ductal
    with lobular
      specified site — *see* Neoplasm, malignant, by site
      unspecified site (female) C50.91- ☑
        male C50.92- ☑
  ductular, infiltrating
    specified site — *see* Neoplasm, malignant, by site
    unspecified site (female) C50.91- ☑
      male C50.92- ☑
  embryonal
    liver C22.7
  endometrioid
    specified site — *see* Neoplasm, malignant, by site
    unspecified site
      female C56.9
      male C61
  eosinophil
    specified site — *see* Neoplasm, malignant, by site
    unspecified site C75.1
  epidermoid — *see also* Neoplasm, skin, malignant
    in situ, Bowen's type — *see* Neoplasm, skin, in situ
  fibroepithelial, basal cell — *see* Neoplasm, skin, malignant
  follicular
    with papillary (mixed) C73
    moderately differentiated C73
    pure follicle C73
    specified site — *see* Neoplasm, malignant, by site
    trabecular C73
    unspecified site C73
    well differentiated C73
  generalized, with unspecified primary site C80.0
  glycogen-rich — *see* Neoplasm, breast, malignant
  granulosa cell C56- ☑
  hepatic cell C22.0
  hepatocellular C22.0
    with bile duct, mixed C22.0
    fibrolamellar C22.0
  hepatocholangiolitic C22.0

Carcinoma — *continued*
  Hurthle cell C73
  in
    adenomatous
      polyposis coli C18.9
    pleomorphic adenoma — *see* Neoplasm, salivary
      glands, malignant
    situ — *see* Carcinoma-in-situ
  infiltrating
    duct
      with lobular
        specified site — *see* Neoplasm, malignant, by
          site
        unspecified site (female) C50.91- ☑
          male C50.92- ☑
      with Paget's disease — *see* Neoplasm, breast,
        malignant
      specified site — *see* Neoplasm, malignant
      unspecified site (female) C50.91- ☑
        male C50.92- ☑
    ductular
      specified site — *see* Neoplasm, malignant
      unspecified site (female) C50.91- ☑
        male C50.92- ☑
    lobular
      specified site — *see* Neoplasm, malignant
      unspecified site (female) C50.91- ☑
        male C50.92- ☑
  inflammatory
    specified site — *see* Neoplasm, malignant
    unspecified site (female) C50.91- ☑
      male C50.92- ☑
  intestinal type
    specified site — *see* Neoplasm, malignant, by site
    unspecified site C16.9
  intracystic
    noninfiltrating — *see* Neoplasm, in situ, by site
  intraductal (noninfiltrating)
    with Paget's disease — *see* Neoplasm, breast, ma-
      lignant
    breast D05.1- ☑
    papillary
      with invasion
        specified site — *see* Neoplasm, malignant, by
          site
        unspecified site (female) C50.91- ☑
          male C50.92- ☑
      breast D05.1- ☑
      specified site NEC — *see* Neoplasm, in situ, by
        site
      unspecified site (female) D05.1- ☑
    specified site NEC — *see* Neoplasm, in situ, by site
    unspecified site (female) D05.1- ☑
  intraepidermal — *see* Neoplasm, in situ
    squamous cell, Bowen's type — *see* Neoplasm, skin,
      in situ
  intraepithelial — *see* Neoplasm, in situ, by site
    squamous cell — *see* Neoplasm, in situ, by site
  intraosseous C41.1
    upper jaw (bone) C41.0
  islet cell
    with exocrine, mixed
      specified site — *see* Neoplasm, malignant, by
        site
      unspecified site C25.9
    pancreas C25.4
    specified site NEC — *see* Neoplasm, malignant, by
      site
    unspecified site C25.4
  juvenile, breast — *see* Neoplasm, breast, malignant
  large cell
    small cell
      specified site — *see* Neoplasm, malignant, by
        site
      unspecified site C34.90
  Leydig cell (testis)
    specified site — *see* Neoplasm, malignant, by site
    unspecified site
      female C56.9
      male C62.90
  lipid-rich (female) C50.91- ☑
    male C50.92- ☑
  liver cell C22.0
  liver NEC C22.7

Carcinoma — *continued*
  lobular (infiltrating)
    with intraductal
      specified site — *see* Neoplasm, malignant, by
        site
      unspecified site (female) C50.91- ☑
        male C50.92- ☑
    noninfiltrating
      breast D05.0- ☑
      specified site NEC — *see* Neoplasm, in situ, by
        site
      unspecified site D05.0- ☑
    specified site — *see* Neoplasm, malignant, by site
    unspecified site (female) C50.91- ☑
      male C50.92- ☑
  medullary
    with
      amyloid stroma
        specified site — *see* Neoplasm, malignant, by
          site
        unspecified site C73
      lymphoid stroma
        specified site — *see* Neoplasm, malignant, by
          site
        unspecified site (female) C50.91- ☑
          male C50.92- ☑
  Merkel cell C4A.9 (*following* C43)
    anal margin C4A.51 (*following* C43)
    anal skin C4A.51 (*following* C43)
    canthus C4A.1- ☑ (*following* C43)
    ear and external auricular canal C4A.2- ☑ (*following*
      C43)
    external auricular canal C4A.2- ☑ (*following* C43)
    eyelid, including canthus C4A.1- ☑ (*following* C43)
    face C4A.30 (*following* C43)
      specified NEC C4A.39 (*following* C43)
    hip C4A.7- ☑ (*following* C43)
    lip C4A.0 (*following* C43)
    lower limb, including hip C4A.7- ☑ (*following* C43)
    neck C4A.4 (*following* C43)
    nodal presentation C7B.1 (*following* C75)
    nose C4A.31 (*following* C43)
    overlapping sites C4A.8 (*following* C43)
    perianal skin C4A.51 (*following* C43)
    scalp C4A.4 (*following* C43)
    secondary C7B.1 (*following* C75)
    shoulder C4A.6- ☑ (*following* C43)
    skin of breast C4A.52 (*following* C43)
    trunk NEC C4A.59 (*following* C43)
    upper limb, including shoulder C4A.6- ☑ (*following*
      C43)
    visceral metastatic C7B.1 (*following* C75)
  metastatic — *see* Neoplasm, secondary, by site
  metatypical — *see* Neoplasm, skin, malignant
  morphea, basal cell — *see* Neoplasm, skin, malignant
  mucoid
    cell
      specified site — *see* Neoplasm, malignant, by
        site
      unspecified site C75.1
  neuroendocrine — *see also* Tumor, neuroendocrine
    high grade, any site C7A.1 (*following* C75)
    poorly differentiated, any site C7A.1 (*following* C75)
  nonencapsulated sclerosing C73
  noninfiltrating
    intracystic — *see* Neoplasm, in situ, by site
    intraductal
      breast D05.1- ☑
      papillary
        breast D05.1- ☑
        specified site NEC — *see* Neoplasm, in situ,
          by site
        unspecified site D05.1- ☑
      specified site — *see* Neoplasm, in situ, by site
      unspecified site D05.1- ☑
    lobular
      breast D05.0- ☑
      specified site NEC — *see* Neoplasm, in situ, by
        site
      unspecified site (female) D05.0- ☑
  oat cell
    specified site — *see* Neoplasm, malignant, by site
    unspecified site C34.90
  odontogenic C41.1
    upper jaw (bone) C41.0
  papillary
    with follicular (mixed) C73

Carcinoma — *continued*
  papillary — *continued*
    follicular variant C73
    intraductal (noninfiltrating)
      with invasion
        specified site — *see* Neoplasm, malignant, by
          site
        unspecified site (female) C50.91- ☑
          male C50.92- ☑
      breast D05.1- ☑
      specified site NEC — *see* Neoplasm, in situ, by
        site
      unspecified site D05.1- ☑
    serous
      specified site — *see* Neoplasm, malignant, by
        site
      surface
        specified site — *see* Neoplasm, malignant, by
          site
        unspecified site C56.9
      unspecified site C56.9
  papillocystic
    specified site — *see* Neoplasm, malignant, by site
    unspecified site C56.9
  parafollicular cell
    specified site — *see* Neoplasm, malignant, by site
    unspecified site C73
  pilomatrix — *see* Neoplasm, skin, malignant
  pseudomucinous
    specified site — *see* Neoplasm, malignant, by site
    unspecified site C56.9
  renal cell C64- ☑
  Schmincke — *see* Neoplasm, nasopharynx, malignant
  Schneiderian
    specified site — *see* Neoplasm, malignant, by site
    unspecified site C30.0
  sebaceous — *see* Neoplasm, skin, malignant
  secondary — *see also* Neoplasm, secondary, by site
    Merkel cell C7B.1 (*following* C75)
  secretory, breast — *see* Neoplasm, breast, malignant
  serous
    papillary
      specified site — *see* Neoplasm, malignant, by
        site
      unspecified site C56.9
    surface, papillary
      specified site — *see* Neoplasm, malignant, by
        site
      unspecified site C56.9
  Sertoli cell
    specified site — *see* Neoplasm, malignant, by site
    unspecified site C62.90
      female C56.9
      male C62.90
  skin appendage — *see* Neoplasm, skin, malignant
  small cell
    fusiform cell
      specified site — *see* Neoplasm, malignant, by
        site
      unspecified site C34.90
    intermediate cell
      specified site — *see* Neoplasm, malignant, by
        site
      unspecified site C34.90
    large cell
      specified site — *see* Neoplasm, malignant, by
        site
      unspecified site C34.90
  solid
    with amyloid stroma
      specified site — *see* Neoplasm, malignant, by
        site
      unspecified site C73
    microinvasive
      specified site — *see* Neoplasm, malignant, by
        site
      unspecified site C53.9
  sweat gland — *see* Neoplasm, skin, malignant
  theca cell C56.- ☑
  thymic C37
  unspecified site (primary) C80.1
  water-clear cell C75.0
Carcinoma-in-situ — *see also* Neoplasm, in situ, by site
  breast NOS D05.9- ☑
    specified type NEC D05.8- ☑
  epidermoid — *see also* Neoplasm, in situ, by site
    with questionable stromal invasion
      cervix D06.9

Carcinoma-in-situ — *continued*
  epidermoid — *see also* Neoplasm, in situ, by site — *continued*
    with questionable stromal invasion — *continued*
      specified site NEC — *see* Neoplasm, in situ, by site
      unspecified site D06.9
  Bowen's type — *see* Neoplasm, skin, in situ
  intraductal
    breast D05.1- ☑
    specified site NEC — *see* Neoplasm, in situ, by site
    unspecified site D05.1- ☑
  lobular
    with
      infiltrating duct
        breast (female) C50.91- ☑
          male C50.92- ☑
        specified site NEC — *see* Neoplasm, malignant, by site
        unspecified site (female) C50.91- ☑
          male C50.92- ☑
      intraductal
        breast D05.8- ☑
        specified site NEC — *see* Neoplasm, in situ, by site
        unspecified site (female) D05.8- ☑
    breast D05.0- ☑
    specified site NEC — *see* Neoplasm, in situ, by site
    unspecified site D05.0- ☑
  squamous cell — *see also* Neoplasm, in situ, by site
    with questionable stromal invasion
      cervix D06.9
      specified site NEC — *see* Neoplasm, in situ, by site
      unspecified site D06.9
Carcinomaphobia F45.29
Carcinomatosis C80.0
  peritonei C78.6
  unspecified site (primary) (secondary) C80.0
Carcinosarcoma — *see* Neoplasm, malignant, by site
  embryonal — *see* Neoplasm, malignant, by site
Cardia, cardial — *see* condition
Cardiac — *see also* condition
  death, sudden — *see* Arrest, cardiac
  pacemaker
    in situ Z95.0
    management or adjustment Z45.018
  tamponade I31.4
Cardialgia — *see* Pain, precordial
Cardiectasis — *see* Hypertrophy, cardiac
Cardiochalasia K21.9
Cardiomalacia I51.5
Cardiomegalia glycogenica diffusa E74.02 *[I43]*
Cardiomegaly — *see also* Hypertrophy, cardiac
  congenital Q24.8
  glycogen E74.02 *[I43]*
  idiopathic I51.7
Cardiomyoliposis I51.5
Cardiomyopathy (familial) (idiopathic) I42.9
  alcoholic I42.6
  amyloid E85.4 *[I43]*
    transthyretin-related (ATTR) familial E85.4 *[I43]*
  arteriosclerotic — *see* Disease, heart, ischemic, atherosclerotic
  beriberi E51.12
  cobalt-beer I42.6
  congenital I42.4
  congestive I42.0
  constrictive NOS I42.5
  dilated I42.0
  due to
    alcohol I42.6
    beriberi E51.12
    cardiac glycogenosis E74.02 *[I43]*
    drugs I42.7
    external agents NEC I42.7
    Friedreich's ataxia G11.11
    myotonia atrophica G71.11 *[I43]*
    progressive muscular dystrophy — *see also* Dystrophy, muscular, by type G71.09 *[I43]*
  glycogen storage E74.02 *[I43]*
  hypertensive — *see* Hypertension, heart
  hypertrophic (nonobstructive) I42.2
    obstructive I42.1
      congenital Q24.8
  in
    Chagas' disease (chronic) B57.2
      acute B57.0

Cardiomyopathy — *continued*
  in — *continued*
    sarcoidosis D86.85
  ischemic I25.5
  metabolic E88.9 *[I43]*
    thyrotoxic E05.90 *[I43]*
      with thyroid storm E05.91 *[I43]*
  newborn I42.8
    congenital I42.4
  non-ischemic — *see also* by cause I42.8
  nutritional E63.9 *[I43]*
    beriberi E51.12
  obscure of Africa I42.8
  peripartum O90.3
  postpartum O90.3
  restrictive NEC I42.5
  rheumatic I09.0
  secondary I42.9
  specified NEC I42.8
  stress induced I51.81
  takotsubo I51.81
  thyrotoxic E05.90 *[I43]*
    with thyroid storm E05.91 *[I43]*
  toxic NEC I42.7
  transthyretin-related (ATTR) familial amyloid E85.4
  tuberculous A18.84
  viral B33.24
Cardionephritis — *see* Hypertension, cardiorenal
Cardionephropathy — *see* Hypertension, cardiorenal
Cardionephrosis — *see* Hypertension, cardiorenal
Cardiopathia nigra I27.0
Cardiopathy — *see also* Disease, heart I51.9
  idiopathic I42.9
  mucopolysaccharidosis E76.3 *[I52]*
Cardiopericarditis — *see* Pericarditis
Cardiophobia F45.29
Cardiorenal — *see* condition
Cardiorrhexis — *see* Infarct, myocardium
Cardiosclerosis — *see* Disease, heart, ischemic, atherosclerotic
Cardiosis — *see* Disease, heart
Cardiospasm (esophagus) (reflex) (stomach) K22.0
  congenital Q39.5
    with megaesophagus Q39.5
Cardiostenosis — *see* Disease, heart
Cardiosymphysis I31.0
Cardiovascular — *see* condition
Carditis (acute) (bacterial) (chronic) (subacute) I51.89
  meningococcal A39.50
  rheumatic — *see* Disease, heart, rheumatic
  rheumatoid — *see* Rheumatoid, carditis
  viral B33.20
Care (of) (for) (following)
  child (routine) Z76.2
  family member (handicapped) (sick)
    creating problem for family Z63.6
    provided away from home for holiday relief Z75.5
    unavailable, due to
      absence (person rendering care) (sufferer) Z74.2
      inability (any reason) of person rendering care Z74.2
  foundling Z76.1
  holiday relief Z75.5
  improper — *see* Maltreatment
  lack of (at or after birth) (infant) — *see* Maltreatment, child, neglect
  lactating mother Z39.1
  palliative Z51.5
  postpartum
    immediately after delivery Z39.0
    routine follow-up Z39.2
  respite Z75.5
  unavailable, due to
    absence of person rendering care Z74.2
    inability (any reason) of person rendering care Z74.2
  well-baby Z76.2
Caries
  bone NEC A18.03
  dental (dentino enamel junction) (early childhood) (of dentine) (pre-eruptive) (recurrent) (to the pulp) K02.9
    arrested (coronal) (root) K02.3
    chewing surface
      limited to enamel K02.51
      penetrating into dentin K02.52
      penetrating into pulp K02.53

Caries — *continued*
  dental — *continued*
    coronal surface
      chewing surface
        limited to enamel K02.51
        penetrating into dentin K02.52
        penetrating into pulp K02.53
      pit and fissure surface
        limited to enamel K02.51
        penetrating into dentin K02.52
        penetrating into pulp K02.53
      smooth surface
        limited to enamel K02.61
        penetrating into dentin K02.62
        penetrating into pulp K02.63
    pit and fissure surface
      limited to enamel K02.51
      penetrating into dentin K02.52
      penetrating into pulp K02.53
    primary, cervical origin K02.52
    root K02.7
    smooth surface
      limited to enamel K02.61
      penetrating into dentin K02.62
      penetrating into pulp K02.63
  external meatus — *see* Disorder, ear, external, specified type NEC
  hip (tuberculous) A18.02
  initial (tooth)
    chewing surface K02.51
    pit and fissure surface K02.51
    smooth surface K02.61
  knee (tuberculous) A18.02
  labyrinth H83.8 ☑
  limb NEC (tuberculous) A18.03
  mastoid process (chronic) — *see* Mastoiditis, chronic
    tuberculous A18.03
  middle ear H74.8 ☑
  nose (tuberculous) A18.03
  orbit (tuberculous) A18.03
  ossicles, ear — *see* Abnormal, ear ossicles
  petrous bone — *see* Petrositis
  root (dental) (tooth) K02.7
  sacrum (tuberculous) A18.01
  spine, spinal (column) (tuberculous) A18.01
  syphilitic A52.77
    congenital (early) A50.02 *[M90.80]*
  tooth, teeth — *see* Caries, dental
  tuberculous A18.03
  vertebra (column) (tuberculous) A18.01
Carious teeth — *see* Caries, dental
Carneous mole O02.0
Carnitine insufficiency E71.40
Carotenemia (dietary) E67.1
Carotenosis (cutis) (skin) E67.1
Carotid body or sinus syndrome G90.01
Carotidynia G90.01
Carpal tunnel syndrome — *see* Syndrome, carpal tunnel
Carpenter's syndrome Q87.0
Carpopedal spasm — *see* Tetany
Carr-Barr-Plunkett syndrome Q97.1
Carrier (suspected) of
  amebiasis Z22.1
  bacterial disease NEC Z22.39
    diphtheria Z22.2
    intestinal infectious NEC Z22.1
      typhoid Z22.0
    meningococcal Z22.31
    sexually transmitted Z22.4
    specified NEC Z22.39
    staphylococcal (Methicillin susceptible) Z22.321
      Methicillin resistant Z22.322
    streptococcal Z22.338
      group B Z22.330
        complicating pregnancy or delivery O99.82- ☑
    typhoid Z22.0
  cholera Z22.1
  diphtheria Z22.2
  gastrointestinal pathogens NEC Z22.1
  genetic Z14.8
    cystic fibrosis Z14.1
    hemophilia A (asymptomatic) Z14.01
      symptomatic Z14.02
  gestational, pregnant Z33.1
  gonorrhea Z22.4
  HAA (hepatitis Australian-antigen) B18.8
  HB (c)(s)-AG B18.1

Carcinoma-in-situ — Carrier

Carrier of — *continued*
  hepatitis (viral) B18.9
    Australia-antigen (HAA) B18.8
    B surface antigen (HBsAg) B18.1
      with acute delta- (super)infection B17.0
    C B18.2
    specified NEC B18.8
  human T-cell lymphotropic virus type-1 (HTLV-1) infection Z22.6
  infectious organism Z22.9
    specified NEC Z22.8
  meningococci Z22.31
  Salmonella typhosa Z22.0
  serum hepatitis — *see* Carrier, hepatitis
  staphylococci (Methicillin susceptible) Z22.321
    Methicillin resistant Z22.322
  streptococci Z22.338
    group B Z22.330
      complicating pregnancy or delivery O99.82- ☑
  syphilis Z22.4
  typhoid Z22.0
  venereal disease NEC Z22.4
Carrion's disease A44.0
Carter's relapsing fever (Asiatic) A68.1
Cartilage — *see* condition
Caruncle (inflamed)
  conjunctiva (acute) — *see* Conjunctivitis, acute
  labium (majus) (minus) N90.89
  lacrimal — *see* Inflammation, lacrimal, passages
  myrtiform N89.8
  urethral (benign) N36.2
Cascade stomach K31.2
Caseation lymphatic gland (tuberculous) A18.2
Cassidy (-Scholte) syndrome (malignant carcinoid) E34.0
Castellani's disease A69.8
Castration, traumatic, male S38.231 ☑
Casts in urine R82.998
Cat
  cry syndrome Q93.4
  ear Q17.3
  eye syndrome Q92.8
Catabolism, senile R54
Catalepsy (hysterical) F44.2
  schizophrenic F20.2
Cataplexy (idiopathic) — *see* Narcolepsy
Cataract (cortical) (immature) (incipient) H26.9
  with
    neovascularization — *see* Cataract, complicated
  age-related — *see* Cataract, senile
  anterior
    and posterior axial embryonal Q12.0
    pyramidal Q12.0
  associated with
    galactosemia E74.21 *[H28]*
    myotonic disorders G71.19 *[H28]*
  blue Q12.0
  central Q12.0
  cerulean Q12.0
  complicated H26.20
    with
      neovascularization H26.21- ☑
      ocular disorder H26.22- ☑
    glaucomatous flecks H26.23- ☑
  congenital Q12.0
  coraliform Q12.0
  coronary Q12.0
  crystalline Q12.0
  diabetic — *see* Diabetes, cataract
  drug-induced H26.3- ☑
  due to
    ocular disorder — *see* Cataract, complicated
    radiation H26.8
  electric H26.8
  extraction status Z98.4- ☑
  glass-blower's H26.8
  heat ray H26.8
  heterochromic — *see* Cataract, complicated
  hypermature — *see* Cataract, senile, morgagnian type
  in (due to)
    chronic iridocyclitis — *see* Cataract, complicated
    diabetes — *see* Diabetes, cataract
    endocrine disease E34.9 *[H28]*
    eye disease — *see* Cataract, complicated
    hypoparathyroidism E20.9 *[H28]*
    malnutrition-dehydration E46 *[H28]*
    metabolic disease E88.9 *[H28]*
    myotonic disorders G71.19 *[H28]*

Cataract — *continued*
  in — *continued*
    nutritional disease E63.9 *[H28]*
  infantile — *see* Cataract, presenile
  irradiational — *see* Cataract, specified NEC
  juvenile — *see* Cataract, presenile
  malnutrition-dehydration E46 *[H28]*
  morgagnian — *see* Cataract, senile, morgagnian type
  myotonic G71.19 *[H28]*
  myxedema E03.9 *[H28]*
  nuclear
    embryonal Q12.0
    sclerosis — *see* Cataract, senile, nuclear
  presenile H26.00- ☑
    combined forms H26.06- ☑
    cortical H26.01- ☑
    lamellar — *see* Cataract, presenile, cortical
    nuclear H26.03- ☑
    specified NEC H26.09
    subcapsular polar (anterior) H26.04- ☑
      posterior H26.05- ☑
    zonular — *see* Cataract, presenile, cortical
  secondary H26.40
    Soemmering's ring H26.41- ☑
    specified NEC H26.49- ☑
    to eye disease — *see* Cataract, complicated
  senile H25.9
    brunescens — *see* Cataract, senile, nuclear
    combined forms H25.81- ☑
    coronary — *see* Cataract, senile, incipient
    cortical H25.01- ☑
    hypermature — *see* Cataract, senile, morgagnian type
    incipient (mature) (total) H25.09- ☑
      cortical — *see* Cataract, senile, cortical
      subcapsular — *see* Cataract, senile, subcapsular
    morgagnian type (hypermature) H25.2- ☑
    nuclear (sclerosis) H25.1- ☑
    polar subcapsular (anterior) (posterior) — *see* Cataract, senile, incipient
    punctate — *see* Cataract, senile, incipient
    specified NEC H25.89
    subcapsular polar (anterior) H25.03- ☑
      posterior H25.04- ☑
  snowflake — *see* Diabetes, cataract
  specified NEC H26.8
  toxic — *see* Cataract, drug-induced
  traumatic H26.10- ☑
    localized H26.11- ☑
    partially resolved H26.12- ☑
    total H26.13- ☑
  zonular (perinuclear) Q12.0
Cataracta — *see also* Cataract
  brunescens — *see* Cataract, senile, nuclear
  centralis pulverulenta Q12.0
  cerulea Q12.0
  complicata — *see* Cataract, complicated
  congenita Q12.0
  coralliformis Q12.0
  coronaria Q12.0
  diabetic — *see* Diabetes, cataract
  membranacea
    accreta — *see* Cataract, secondary
    congenita Q12.0
  nigra — *see* Cataract, senile, nuclear
  sunflower — *see* Cataract, complicated
Catarrh, catarrhal (acute) (febrile) (infectious) (inflammation) — *see also* condition J00
  bronchial — *see* Bronchitis
  chest — *see* Bronchitis
  chronic J31.0
  due to congenital syphilis A50.03
  enteric — *see* Enteritis
  eustachian H68.009
  fauces — *see* Pharyngitis
  gastrointestinal — *see* Enteritis
  gingivitis K05.00
    nonplaque induced K05.01
    plaque induced K05.00
  hay — *see* Fever, hay
  intestinal — *see* Enteritis
  larynx, chronic J37.0
  liver B15.9
    with hepatic coma B15.0
  lung — *see* Bronchitis
  middle ear, chronic — *see* Otitis, media, nonsuppurative, chronic, serous

Catarrh, catarrhal — *continued*
  mouth K12.1
  nasal (chronic) — *see* Rhinitis
  nasobronchial J31.1
  nasopharyngeal (chronic) J31.1
    acute J00
  pulmonary — *see* Bronchitis
  spring (eye) (vernal) — *see* Conjunctivitis, acute, atopic
  summer (hay) — *see* Fever, hay
  throat J31.2
  tubotympanal — *see also* Otitis, media, nonsuppurative
    chronic — *see* Otitis, media, nonsuppurative, chronic, serous
Catatonia (schizophrenic) F20.2
Catatonic
  disorder due to known physiologic condition F06.1
  schizophrenia F20.2
  stupor R40.1
Cat-scratch — *see also* Abrasion
  disease or fever A28.1
Cauda equina — *see* condition
Cauliflower ear M95.1- ☑
Causalgia (upper limb) G56.4- ☑
  lower limb G57.7- ☑
Cause
  external, general effects T75.89 ☑
Caustic burn — *see* Corrosion, by site
Cavare's disease (familial periodic paralysis) G72.3
Cave-in, injury
  crushing (severe) — *see* Crush
  suffocation — *see* Asphyxia, traumatic, due to low oxygen, due to cave-in
Cavernitis (penis) N48.29
Cavernositis N48.29
Cavernous — *see* condition
Cavitation of lung — *see also* Tuberculosis, pulmonary
  nontuberculous J98.4
Cavities, dental — *see* Caries, dental
Cavity
  lung — *see* Cavitation of lung
  optic papilla Q14.2
  pulmonary — *see* Cavitation of lung
Cavovarus foot, congenital Q66.1- ☑
Cavus foot (congenital) Q66.7- ☑
  acquired — *see* Deformity, limb, foot, specified NEC
Cazenave's disease L10.2
CDKL5 (Cyclin-Dependent Kinase-Like 5 Deficiency Disorder) G40.42
Cecitis K52.9
  with perforation, peritonitis, or rupture K65.8
Cecoureterocele Q62.32
Cecum — *see* condition
Celiac
  artery compression syndrome I77.4
  disease (with steatorrhea) K90.0
  infantilism K90.0
Cell(s), **cellular** — *see also* condition
  in urine R82.998
Cellulitis (diffuse) (phlegmonous) (septic) (suppurative) L03.90
  abdominal wall L03.311
  anaerobic A48.0
  ankle — *see* Cellulitis, lower limb
  anus K61.0
  arm — *see* Cellulitis, upper limb
  auricle (ear) — *see* Cellulitis, ear
  axilla L03.11- ☑
  back (any part) L03.312
  breast (acute) (nonpuerperal) (subacute) N61.0
    nipple N61.0
  broad ligament
    acute N73.0
  buttock L03.317
  cervical (meaning neck) L03.221
  cervix (uteri) — *see* Cervicitis
  cheek (external) L03.211
    internal K12.2
  chest wall L03.313
  chronic L03.90
  clostridial A48.0
  corpus cavernosum N48.22
  digit
    finger — *see* Cellulitis, finger
    toe — *see* Cellulitis, toe
  Douglas' cul-de-sac or pouch
    acute N73.0
  drainage site (following operation) T81.49 ☑

Cellulitis — *continued*
ear (external) H60.1- ☑
eosinophilic (granulomatous) L98.3
erysipelatous — *see* Erysipelas
external auditory canal — *see* Cellulitis, ear
eyelid — *see* Abscess, eyelid
face NEC L03.211
finger (intrathecal) (periosteal) (subcutaneous) (subcuticular) L03.01- ☑
foot — *see* Cellulitis, lower limb
gangrenous — *see* Gangrene
genital organ NEC
female (external) N76.4
male N49.9
multiple sites N49.8
specified NEC N49.8
gluteal (region) L03.317
gonococcal A54.89
groin L03.314
hand — *see* Cellulitis, upper limb
head NEC L03.811
face (any part, except ear, eye and nose) L03.211
heel — *see* Cellulitis, lower limb
hip — *see* Cellulitis, lower limb
jaw (region) L03.211
knee — *see* Cellulitis, lower limb
labium (majus) (minus) — *see* Vulvitis
lacrimal passages — *see* Inflammation, lacrimal, passages
larynx J38.7
leg — *see* Cellulitis, lower limb
lip K13.0
lower limb L03.11- ☑
toe — *see* Cellulitis, toe
mouth (floor) K12.2
multiple sites, so stated L03.90
nasopharynx J39.1
navel L03.316
newborn P38.9
with mild hemorrhage P38.1
without hemorrhage P38.9
neck (region) L03.221
nipple (acute) (nonpuerperal) (subacute) N61.0
nose (septum) (external) J34.0
orbit, orbital H05.01- ☑
palate (soft) K12.2
pectoral (region) L03.313
pelvis, pelvic (chronic)
female — *see also* Disease, pelvis, inflammatory N73.2
acute N73.0
following ectopic or molar pregnancy O08.0
male K65.0
penis N48.22
perineal, perineum L03.315
periorbital L03.213
perirectal K61.1
peritonsillar J36
periurethral N34.0
periuterine — *see also* Disease, pelvis, inflammatory N73.2
acute N73.0
pharynx J39.1
preseptal L03.213
rectum K61.1
retroperitoneal K68.9
round ligament
acute N73.0
scalp (any part) L03.811
scrotum N49.2
seminal vesicle N49.0
shoulder — *see* Cellulitis, upper limb
specified site NEC L03.818
submandibular (region) (space) (triangle) K12.2
gland K11.3
submaxillary (region) K12.2
gland K11.3
thigh — *see* Cellulitis, lower limb
thumb (intrathecal) (periosteal) (subcutaneous) (subcuticular) — *see* Cellulitis, finger
toe (intrathecal) (periosteal) (subcutaneous) (subcuticular) L03.03- ☑
tonsil J36
trunk L03.319
abdominal wall L03.311
back (any part) L03.312
buttock L03.317
chest wall L03.313

Cellulitis — *continued*
trunk — *continued*
groin L03.314
perineal, perineum L03.315
umbilicus L03.316
tuberculous (primary) A18.4
umbilicus L03.316
upper limb L03.11- ☑
axilla — *see* Cellulitis, axilla
finger — *see* Cellulitis, finger
thumb — *see* Cellulitis, finger
vaccinal T88.0 ☑
vocal cord J38.3
vulva — *see* Vulvitis
wrist — *see* Cellulitis, upper limb
Cementoblastoma, benign — *see* Cyst, calcifying odontogenic
Cementoma — *see* Cyst, calcifying odontogenic
Cementoperiostitis — *see* Periodontitis
Cementosis K03.4
Central auditory processing disorder H93.25
Central pain syndrome G89.0
Cephalematocele, cephal (o)hematocele
newborn P52.8
birth injury P10.8
traumatic — *see* Hematoma, brain
Cephalematoma, cephalhematoma (calcified)
newborn (birth injury) P12.0
traumatic — *see* Hematoma, brain
Cephalgia, cephalalgia — *see also* Headache
histamine G44.009
intractable G44.001
not intractable G44.009
trigeminal autonomic (TAC) NEC G44.099
intractable G44.091
not intractable G44.099
Cephalic — *see* condition
Cephalitis — *see* Encephalitis
Cephalocele — *see* Encephalocele
Cephalomenia N94.89
Cephalopelvic — *see* condition
Cerclage (with cervical incompetence) in pregnancy — *see* Incompetence, cervix, in pregnancy
Cerebellitis — *see* Encephalitis
Cerebellum, cerebellar — *see* condition
Cerebral — *see* condition
Cerebritis — *see* Encephalitis
Cerebro-hepato-renal syndrome Q87.89
Cerebromalacia — *see* Softening, brain
sequelae of cerebrovascular disease I69.398
Cerebroside lipidosis E75.22
Cerebrospasticity (congenital) G80.1
Cerebrospinal — *see* condition
Cerebrum — *see* condition
Ceroid-lipofuscinosis, neuronal E75.4
Cerumen (accumulation) (impacted) H61.2- ☑
Cervical — *see also* condition
auricle Q18.2
dysplasia in pregnancy — *see* Abnormal, cervix, in pregnancy or childbirth
erosion in pregnancy — *see* Abnormal, cervix, in pregnancy or childbirth
fibrosis in pregnancy — *see* Abnormal, cervix, in pregnancy or childbirth
fusion syndrome Q76.1
rib Q76.5
shortening (complicating pregnancy) O26.87- ☑
Cervicalgia M54.2
Cervicitis (acute) (atrophic) (chronic) (nonvenereal) (senile) (subacute) (with ulceration) N72
with
abortion — *see* Abortion, by type complicated by genital tract and pelvic infection
ectopic pregnancy O08.0
molar pregnancy O08.0
chlamydial A56.09
gonococcal A54.03
herpesviral A60.03
puerperal (postpartum) O86.11
syphilitic A52.76
trichomonal A59.09
tuberculous A18.16
Cervicocolpitis (emphysematosa) — *see also* Cervicitis N72
Cervix — *see* condition
Cesarean delivery, previous, affecting management of pregnancy O34.219

Cesarean delivery, previous, affecting management of pregnancy — *continued*
classical (vertical) scar O34.212
isthmocele (non-pregnant state) N85.A
maternal care for O34.22
low transverse scar O34.211
mid-transverse T incision O34.218
scar
defect (non-pregnant state) N85.A
maternal care for O34.22
specified type NEC O34.218
Céstan (-Chenais) paralysis or syndrome G46.3
Céstan-Raymond syndrome I65.8
Cestode infestation B71.9
specified type NEC B71.8
Cestodiasis B71.9
Chabert's disease A22.9
Chacaleh E53.8
Chafing L30.4
Chagas' (-Mazza) disease (chronic) B57.2
with
cardiovascular involvement NEC B57.2
digestive system involvement B57.30
megacolon B57.32
megaesophagus B57.31
other specified B57.39
megacolon B57.32
megaesophagus B57.31
myocarditis B57.2
nervous system involvement B57.40
meningitis B57.41
meningoencephalitis B57.42
other specified B57.49
specified organ involvement NEC B57.5
acute (with) B57.1
cardiovascular NEC B57.0
myocarditis B57.0
Chagres fever B50.9
Chairridden Z74.09
Chalasia (cardiac sphincter) K21.9
Chalazion H00.19
left H00.16
lower H00.15
upper H00.14
right H00.13
lower H00.12
upper H00.11
Chalcosis — *see also* Disorder, globe, degenerative, chalcosis
cornea — *see* Deposit, cornea
crystalline lens — *see* Cataract, complicated
retina H35.89
Chalicosis (pulmonum) J62.8
Chancre (any genital site) (hard) (hunterian) (mixed) (primary) (seronegative) (seropositive) (syphilitic) A51.0
congenital A50.07
conjunctiva NEC A51.2
Ducrey's A57
extragenital A51.2
eyelid A51.2
lip A51.2
nipple A51.2
Nisbet's A57
of
carate A67.0
pinta A67.0
yaws A66.0
palate, soft A51.2
phagedenic A57
simple A57
soft A57
bubo A57
palate A51.2
urethra A51.0
yaws A66.0
Chancroid (anus) (genital) (penis) (perineum) (rectum) (urethra) (vulva) A57
Chandler's disease (osteochondritis dissecans, hip) — *see* Osteochondritis, dissecans, hip
Change(s) (in) (of) — *see also* Removal
arteriosclerotic — *see* Arteriosclerosis
bone — *see also* Disorder, bone
diabetic — *see* Diabetes, bone change
bowel habit R19.4
cardiorenal (vascular) — *see* Hypertension, cardiorenal
cardiovascular — *see* Disease, cardiovascular
circulatory I99.9

Change(s) — *continued*
  cognitive (mild) (organic) R41.89
  color, tooth, teeth
    during formation K00.8
    posteruptive K03.7
  contraceptive device Z30.433
  corneal membrane H18.30
    Bowman's membrane fold or rupture H18.31- ☑
    Descemet's membrane
      fold H18.32- ☑
      rupture H18.33- ☑
  coronary — *see* Disease, heart, ischemic
  degenerative, spine or vertebra — *see* Spondylosis
  dental pulp, regressive K04.2
  dressing (nonsurgical) Z48.00
    surgical Z48.01
  heart — *see* Disease, heart
  hip joint — *see* Derangement, joint, hip
  hyperplastic larynx J38.7
  hypertrophic
    nasal sinus J34.89
    turbinate, nasal J34.3
    upper respiratory tract J39.8
  indwelling catheter Z46.6
  inflammatory — *see also* Inflammation
    sacroiliac M46.1
  job, anxiety concerning Z56.1
  joint — *see* Derangement, joint
  life — *see* Menopause
  mental status R41.82
  minimal (glomerular) — *see also* N00-N07 with fourth
    character .0 N05.0
  myocardium, myocardial — *see* Degeneration, myocardial
  of life — *see* Menopause
  pacemaker Z45.018
    pulse generator Z45.010
  personality (enduring) F68.8
    due to (secondary to)
      general medical condition F07.0
      secondary (nonspecific) F60.89
  regressive, dental pulp K04.2
  renal — *see* Disease, renal
  retina H35.9
    myopic — *see also* Myopia, degenerative H44.2- ☑
  sacroiliac joint M53.3
  senile — *see also* condition R54
  sensory R20.8
  skin R23.9
    acute, due to ultraviolet radiation L56.9
      specified NEC L56.8
    chronic, due to nonionizing radiation L57.9
      specified NEC L57.8
    cyanosis R23.0
    flushing R23.2
    pallor R23.1
    petechiae R23.3
    specified change NEC R23.8
    swelling — *see* Mass, localized
    texture R23.4
  trophic
    arm — *see* Mononeuropathy, upper limb
    leg — *see* Mononeuropathy, lower limb
  vascular I99.9
  vasomotor I73.9
  voice R49.9
    psychogenic F44.4
    specified NEC R49.8
Changing sleep-work schedule, affecting sleep G47.26
Changuinola fever A93.1
Chapping skin T69.8 ☑
Charcot-Marie-Tooth disease, paralysis or syndrome G60.0
Charcot's
  arthropathy — *see* Arthropathy, neuropathic
  cirrhosis K74.3
  disease (tabetic arthropathy) A52.16
  joint (disease) (tabetic) A52.16
    diabetic — *see* Diabetes, with, arthropathy
    syringomyelic G95.0
  syndrome (intermittent claudication) I73.9
CHARGE association Q89.8
Charley-horse (quadriceps) M62.831
  traumatic (quadriceps) S76.11- ☑
Charlouis' disease — *see* Yaws
Cheadle's disease E54

Checking (of)
  cardiac pacemaker (battery) (electrode(s)) Z45.018
    pulse generator Z45.010
  implantable subdermal contraceptive Z30.46
  intrauterine contraceptive device Z30.431
  wound Z48.0- ☑
    due to injury — code to Injury, by site, using appropriate seventh character for subsequent encounter
Check-up — *see* Examination
Chédiak-Higashi (-Steinbrinck) **syndrome** (congenital gigantism of peroxidase granules) E70.330
Cheek — *see* condition
Cheese itch B88.0
Cheese-washer's lung J67.8
Cheese-worker's lung J67.8
Cheilitis (acute) (angular) (catarrhal) (chronic) (exfoliative) (gangrenous) (glandular) (infectional) (suppurative) (ulcerative) (vesicular) K13.0
  actinic (due to sun) L56.8
    other than from sun L59.8
  candidal B37.83
Cheilodynia K13.0
Cheiloschisis — *see* Cleft, lip
Cheilosis (angular) K13.0
  with pellagra E52
  due to
    vitamin B2 (riboflavin) deficiency E53.0
Cheiromegaly M79.89
Cheiropompholyx L30.1
Cheloid — *see* Keloid
Chemical burn — *see* Corrosion, by site
Chemodectoma — *see* Paraganglioma, nonchromaffin
Chemosis, conjunctiva — *see* Edema, conjunctiva
Chemotherapy (session) (for)
  cancer Z51.11
  neoplasm Z51.11
Cherubism M27.8
Chest — *see* condition
Cheyne-Stokes breathing (respiration) R06.3
Chiari's
  disease or syndrome (hepatic vein thrombosis) I82.0
  malformation
    type I G93.5
    type II — *see* Spina bifida
  net Q24.8
Chicago disease B40.9
Chickenpox — *see* Varicella
Chiclero ulcer or sore B55.1
Chigger (infestation) B88.0
Chignon (disease) B36.8
  newborn (from vacuum extraction) (birth injury) P12.1
Chilaiditi's syndrome (subphrenic displacement, colon) Q43.3
Chilblain(s) (lupus) T69.1 ☑
Child
  custody dispute Z65.3
Childbirth — *see* Delivery
Childhood
  cerebral X-linked adrenoleukodystrophy E71.520
  period of rapid growth Z00.2
Chill(s) R68.83
  with fever R50.9
  congestive in malarial regions B54
  without fever R68.83
Chilomastigiasis A07.8
Chimera 46,XX/46,XY Q99.0
Chin — *see* condition
Chinese dysentery A03.9
Chionophobia F40.228
Chitral fever A93.1
Chlamydia, chlamydial A74.9
  cervicitis A56.09
  conjunctivitis A74.0
  cystitis A56.01
  endometritis A56.11
  epididymitis A56.19
  female
    pelvic inflammatory disease A56.11
    pelviperitonitis A56.11
  orchitis A56.19
  peritonitis A74.81
  pharyngitis A56.4
  proctitis A56.3
  psittaci (infection) A70
  salpingitis A56.11
  sexually-transmitted infection NEC A56.8

Chlamydia, chlamydial — *continued*
  specified NEC A74.89
  urethritis A56.01
  vulvovaginitis A56.02
Chlamydiosis — *see* Chlamydia
Chloasma (skin) (idiopathic) (symptomatic) L81.1
  eyelid H02.719
    hyperthyroid E05.90 [H02.719]
      with thyroid storm E05.91 [H02.719]
    left H02.716
      lower H02.715
      upper H02.714
    right H02.713
      lower H02.712
      upper H02.711
Chloroma C92.3- ☑
Chlorosis D50.9
  Egyptian B76.9 [D63.8]
  miner's B76.9 [D63.8]
Chlorotic anemia D50.8
Chocolate cyst (ovary) N80.10- ☑
Choked
  disc or disk — *see* Papilledema
  on food, phlegm, or vomitus NOS — *see* Foreign body, by site
  while vomiting NOS — *see* Foreign body, by site
Chokes (resulting from bends) T70.3 ☑
Choking sensation R09.89
Cholangiectasis K83.8
Cholangiocarcinoma
  with hepatocellular carcinoma, combined C22.0
  liver C22.1
  specified site NEC — *see* Neoplasm, malignant, by site
  unspecified site C22.1
Cholangiohepatitis K83.8
  due to fluke infestation B66.1
Cholangiohepatoma C22.0
Cholangiolitis (acute) (chronic) (extrahepatic) (gangrenous) (intrahepatic) K83.09
  paratyphoidal — *see* Fever, paratyphoid
  typhoidal A01.09
Cholangioma D13.4
  malignant — *see* Cholangiocarcinoma
Cholangitis (ascending) (recurrent) (secondary) (stenosing) (suppurative) K83.09
  with calculus, bile duct — *see* Calculus, bile duct, with cholangitis
  chronic nonsuppurative destructive K74.3
  primary K83.09
    sclerosing K83.01
  sclerosing K83.09
Cholecystectasia K82.8
Cholecystitis K81.9
  with
    calculus, stones in
      bile duct (common) (hepatic) — *see* Calculus, bile duct, with cholecystitis
      cystic duct — *see* Calculus, gallbladder, with cholecystitis
      gallbladder — *see* Calculus, gallbladder, with cholecystitis
      choledocholithiasis — *see* Calculus, bile duct, with cholecystitis
      cholelithiasis — *see* Calculus, gallbladder, with cholecystitis
    gangrene of gallbladder K82.A1
    perforation of gallbladder K82.A2
  acute (emphysematous) (gangrenous) (suppurative) K81.0
    with
      calculus, stones in
        cystic duct — *see* Calculus, gallbladder, with cholecystitis, acute
        gallbladder — *see* Calculus, gallbladder, with cholecystitis, acute
        choledocholithiasis — *see* Calculus, bile duct, with cholecystitis, acute
        cholelithiasis — *see* Calculus, gallbladder, with cholecystitis, acute
    chronic cholecystitis K81.2
      with gallbladder calculus K80.12
        with obstruction K80.13
  chronic K81.1
    with acute cholecystitis K81.2
      with gallbladder calculus K80.12
        with obstruction K80.13
  emphysematous (acute) — *see* Cholecystitis, acute

Index

Cholecystitis — Chromomycosis

Cholecystitis — *continued*
  gangrenous — *see* Cholecystitis, acute
  paratyphoidal, current A01.4
  suppurative — *see* Cholecystitis, acute
  typhoidal A01.09
Cholecystolithiasis — *see* Calculus, gallbladder
Choledochitis (suppurative) K83.09
Choledocholith — *see* Calculus, bile duct
Choledocholithiasis (common duct) (hepatic duct) —
    see Calculus, bile duct
  cystic — *see* Calculus, gallbladder
  typhoidal A01.09
Cholelithiasis (cystic duct) (gallbladder) (impacted)
    (multiple) — *see* Calculus, gallbladder
  bile duct (common) (hepatic) — *see* Calculus, bile duct
  hepatic duct — *see* Calculus, bile duct
  specified NEC K80.80
    with obstruction K80.81
Cholemia — *see also* Jaundice
  familial (simple) (congenital) E80.4
  Gilbert's E80.4
Choleperitoneum, choleperitonitis K65.3
Cholera (Asiatic) (epidemic) (malignant) A00.9
  antimonial — *see* Poisoning, antimony
  classical A00.0
  due to Vibrio cholerae 01 A00.9
    biovar cholerae A00.0
    biovar eltor A00.1
    el tor A00.1
  el tor A00.1
Cholerine — *see* Cholera
Cholestasis NEC K83.1
  with hepatocyte injury K71.0
  due to total parenteral nutrition (TPN) K76.89
  pure K71.0
Cholesteatoma (ear) (middle) (with reaction) H71.9- ☑
  attic H71.0- ☑
  external ear (canal) H60.4- ☑
  mastoid H71.2- ☑
  postmastoidectomy cavity (recurrent) — *see* Complications, postmastoidectomy, recurrent cholesteatoma
  recurrent (postmastoidectomy) — *see* Complications, postmastoidectomy, recurrent cholesteatoma
  tympanum H71.1- ☑
Cholesteatosis, diffuse H71.3- ☑
Cholesteremia E78.00
Cholesterin in vitreous — *see* Deposit, crystalline
Cholesterol
  deposit
    retina H35.89
    vitreous — *see* Deposit, crystalline
  elevated (high) E78.00
    with elevated (high) triglycerides E78.2
    screening for Z13.220
  imbibition of gallbladder K82.4
Cholesterolemia (essential) (pure) E78.00
  familial E78.01
  hereditary E78.01
Cholesterolosis, cholesterosis (gallbladder) K82.4
  cerebrotendinous E75.5
Cholocolic fistula K82.3
Choluria R82.2
Chondritis M94.8X9
  auricular H61.03- ☑
  costal (Tietze's) M94.0
  external ear H61.03- ☑
  patella, posttraumatic — *see* Chondromalacia, patella
  pinna H61.03- ☑
  purulent M94.8X- ☑
  tuberculous NEC A18.02
    intervertebral A18.01
Chondroblastoma — *see also* Neoplasm, bone, benign
  malignant — *see* Neoplasm, bone, malignant
Chondrocalcinosis M11.20
  ankle M11.27- ☑
  elbow M11.22- ☑
  familial M11.10
    ankle M11.17- ☑
    elbow M11.12- ☑
    foot joint M11.17- ☑
    hand joint M11.14- ☑
    hip M11.15- ☑
    knee M11.16- ☑
    multiple site M11.19
    shoulder M11.11- ☑
    vertebrae M11.18

Chondrocalcinosis — *continued*
  familial — *continued*
    wrist M11.13- ☑
  foot joint M11.27- ☑
  hand joint M11.24- ☑
  hip M11.25- ☑
  knee M11.26- ☑
  multiple site M11.29
  shoulder M11.21- ☑
  specified type NEC M11.20
    ankle M11.27- ☑
    elbow M11.22- ☑
    foot joint M11.27- ☑
    hand joint M11.24- ☑
    hip M11.25- ☑
    knee M11.26- ☑
    multiple site M11.29
    shoulder M11.21- ☑
    vertebrae M11.28
    wrist M11.23- ☑
  vertebrae M11.28
  wrist M11.23- ☑
Chondrodermatitis nodularis helicis or anthelicis —
    see Perichondritis, ear
Chondrodysplasia Q78.9
  with hemangioma Q78.4
  calcificans congenita Q77.3
  fetalis Q77.4
  metaphyseal (Jansen's) (McKusick's) (Schmid's) Q78.8
  punctata Q77.3
Chondrodystrophy, chondrodystrophia (familial) (fetalis) (hypoplastic) Q78.9
  calcificans congenita Q77.3
  myotonic (congenital) G71.13
  punctata Q77.3
Chondroectodermal dysplasia Q77.6
Chondrogenesis imperfecta Q77.4
Chondrolysis M94.35- ☑
Chondroma — *see also* Neoplasm, cartilage, benign
  juxtacortical — *see* Neoplasm, bone, benign
  periosteal — *see* Neoplasm, bone, benign
Chondromalacia (systemic) M94.20
  acromioclavicular joint M94.21- ☑
  ankle M94.27- ☑
  elbow M94.22- ☑
  foot joint M94.27- ☑
  glenohumeral joint M94.21- ☑
  hand joint M94.24- ☑
  hip M94.25- ☑
  knee M94.26- ☑
    patella M22.4- ☑
  multiple sites M94.29
  patella M22.4- ☑
  rib M94.28
  sacroiliac joint M94.259
  shoulder M94.21- ☑
  sternoclavicular joint M94.21- ☑
  vertebral joint M94.28
  wrist M94.23- ☑
Chondromatosis — *see also* Neoplasm, cartilage, uncertain behavior
  internal Q78.4
Chondromyxosarcoma — *see* Neoplasm, cartilage, malignant
Chondro-osteodysplasia (Morquio-Brailsford type) E76.219
Chondro-osteodystrophy E76.29
Chondro-osteoma — *see* Neoplasm, bone, benign
Chondropathia tuberosa M94.0
Chondrosarcoma — *see* Neoplasm, cartilage, malignant
  juxtacortical — *see* Neoplasm, bone, malignant
  mesenchymal — *see* Neoplasm, connective tissue, malignant
  myxoid — *see* Neoplasm, cartilage, malignant
Chordee (nonvenereal) N48.89
  congenital Q54.4
  gonococcal A54.09
Chorditis (fibrinous) (nodosa) (tuberosa) J38.2
Chordoma — *see* Neoplasm, vertebral (column), malignant
Chorea (chronic) (gravis) (posthemiplegic) (senile) (spasmodic) G25.5
  with
    heart involvement I02.0
      active or acute (conditions in I01-) I02.0
      rheumatic I02.9
        with valvular disorder I02.0

Chorea — *continued*
  with — *continued*
    rheumatic heart disease (chronic) (inactive) (quiescent) — *code to* rheumatic heart condition involved
  drug-induced G25.4
  habit F95.8
  hereditary G10
  Huntington's G10
  hysterical F44.4
  minor I02.9
    with heart involvement I02.0
  progressive G25.5
    hereditary G10
  rheumatic (chronic) I02.9
    with heart involvement I02.0
  Sydenham's I02.9
    with heart involvement — *see* Chorea, with rheumatic heart disease
  nonrheumatic G25.5
Choreoathetosis (paroxysmal) G25.5
Chorioadenoma (destruens) D39.2
Chorioamnionitis O41.12- ☑
Chorioangioma D26.7
Choriocarcinoma — *see* Neoplasm, malignant, by site
  combined with
    embryonal carcinoma — *see* Neoplasm, malignant, by site
    other germ cell elements — *see* Neoplasm, malignant, by site
    teratoma — *see* Neoplasm, malignant, by site
  specified site — *see* Neoplasm, malignant, by site
  unspecified site
    female C58
    male C62.90
Chorioencephalitis (acute) (lymphocytic) (serous) A87.2
Chorioepithelioma — *see* Choriocarcinoma
Choriomeningitis (acute) (lymphocytic) (serous) A87.2
Chorionepithelioma — *see* Choriocarcinoma
Chorioretinitis — *see also* Inflammation, chorioretinal,
  disseminated — *see also* Inflammation, chorioretinal, disseminated
    in neurosyphilis A52.19
  Egyptian B76.9 *[D63.8]*
  focal — *see also* Inflammation, chorioretinal, focal
  histoplasmic B39.9 *[H32]*
  in (due to)
    histoplasmosis B39.9 *[H32]*
    syphilis (secondary) A51.43
      late A52.71
    toxoplasmosis (acquired) B58.01
      congenital (active) P37.1 *[H32]*
    tuberculosis A18.53
  juxtapapillary, juxtapapillaris — *see* Inflammation, chorioretinal, focal, juxtapapillary
  leprous A30.9 *[H32]*
  miner's B76.9 *[D63.8]*
  progressive myopia (degeneration) — *see also* Myopia, degenerative H44.2- ☑
  syphilitic (secondary) A51.43
    congenital (early) A50.01 *[H32]*
    late A50.32
    late A52.71
  tuberculous A18.53
Chorioretinopathy, central serous H35.71- ☑
Choroid — *see* condition
Choroideremia H31.21
Choroiditis — *see* Chorioretinitis
Choroidopathy — *see* Disorder, choroid
Choroidoretinitis — *see* Chorioretinitis
Choroidoretinopathy, central serous — *see* Chorioretinopathy, central serous
Christian-Weber disease M35.6
Christmas disease D67
Chromaffinoma — *see also* Neoplasm, benign, by site
  malignant — *see* Neoplasm, malignant, by site
Chromatopsia — *see* Deficiency, color vision
Chromhidrosis, chromidrosis L75.1
Chromoblastomycosis — *see* Chromomycosis
Chromoconversion R82.91
Chromomycosis B43.9
  brain abscess B43.1
  cerebral B43.1
  cutaneous B43.0
  skin B43.0
  specified NEC B43.8
  subcutaneous abscess or cyst B43.2

☑ **Additional Character Required** — **Refer to the Tabular List for Character Selection**

Chromophytosis B36.0
Chromosome — *see* Anomaly, by chromosome involved
   D (1) — *see* Anomaly, chromosome 13
   E (3) — *see* Anomaly, chromosome 18
   G — *see* Anomaly, chromosome 21
Chromotrichomycosis B36.8
Chronic — *see* condition
   fracture — *see* Fracture, pathological
Churg-Strauss syndrome M30.1
Chyle cyst, mesentery I89.8
Chylocele (nonfilarial) I89.8
   filarial — *see also* Infestation, filarial B74.9 [N51]
   tunica vaginalis N50.89
     filarial — *see also* Infestation, filarial B74.9 [N51]
Chylomicronemia (fasting) (with hyperprebetalipopro-
   teinemia) E78.3
Chylopericardium I31.39
   acute I30.9
Chylothorax (nonfilarial) J94.0
   filarial — *see also* Infestation, filarial B74.9 [J91.8]
Chylous — *see* condition
Chyluria (nonfilarial) R82.0
   due to
     bilharziasis B65.0
     Brugia (malayi) B74.1
       timori B74.2
     schistosomiasis (bilharziasis) B65.0
     Wuchereria (bancrofti) B74.0
   filarial — *see* Infestation, filarial
Cicatricial (deformity) — *see* Cicatrix
Cicatrix (adherent) (contracted) (painful) (vicious) — *see also* Scar L90.5
   adenoid (and tonsil) J35.8
   alveolar process M26.79
   anus K62.89
   auricle — *see* Disorder, pinna, specified type NEC
   bile duct (common) (hepatic) K83.8
   bladder N32.89
   bone — *see* Disorder, bone, specified type NEC
   brain G93.89
   cervix (postoperative) (postpartal) N88.1
   common duct K83.8
   cornea H17.9
     tuberculous A18.59
   duodenum (bulb), obstructive K31.5
   esophagus K22.2
   eyelid — *see* Disorder, eyelid function
   hypopharynx J39.2
   lacrimal passages — *see* Obstruction, lacrimal
   larynx J38.7
   lung J98.4
   middle ear H74.8 ☑
   mouth K13.79
   muscle M62.89
     with contracture — *see* Contraction, muscle NEC
   nasopharynx J39.2
   palate (soft) K13.79
   penis N48.89
   pharynx J39.2
   prostate N42.89
   rectum K62.89
   retina — *see* Scar, chorioretinal
   semilunar cartilage — *see* Derangement, meniscus
   seminal vesicle N50.89
   skin L90.5
     infected L08.89
     postinfective L90.5
     tuberculous B90.8
   specified site NEC L90.5
   throat J39.2
   tongue K14.8
   tonsil (and adenoid) J35.8
   trachea J39.8
   tuberculous NEC B90.9
   urethra N36.8
   uterus N85.8
   vagina N89.8
     postoperative N99.2
   vocal cord J38.3
   wrist, constricting (annular) L90.5
CIDP (chronic inflammatory demyelinating polyneuropathy) G61.81
CIN — *see* Neoplasia, intraepithelial, cervix
CINCA (chronic infantile neurological, cutaneous and articular syndrome) M04.2
Cinchonism — *see* Deafness, ototoxic
   correct substance properly administered — *see* Table of Drugs and Chemicals, by drug, adverse effect

Cinchonism — *continued*
   overdose or wrong substance given or taken — *see* Table of Drugs and Chemicals, by drug, poisoning
Circle of Willis — *see* condition
Circular — *see* condition
Circulating anticoagulants — *see also* Disorder, hemorrhagic D68.318
   due to drugs — *see also* Disorder, hemorrhagic D68.32
   following childbirth O72.3
Circulation
   collateral, any site I99.8
   defective (lower extremity) I99.9
     congenital Q28.9
   embryonic Q28.9
   failure (peripheral) R57.9
     newborn P29.89
   fetal, persistent P29.38
   heart, incomplete Q28.9
Circulatory system — *see* condition
Circulus senilis (cornea) — *see* Degeneration, cornea, senile
Circumcision (in absence of medical indication) (ritual) (routine) Z41.2
Circumscribed — *see* condition
Circumvallate placenta O43.11- ☑
Cirrhosis, cirrhotic (hepatic) (liver) K74.60
   alcoholic K70.30
     with ascites K70.31
   atrophic — *see* Cirrhosis, liver
   Baumgarten-Cruveilhier K74.69
   biliary (cholangiolitic) (cholangitic) (hypertrophic) (obstructive) (pericholangiolitic) K74.5
     due to
       Clonorchiasis B66.1
       flukes B66.3
     primary K74.3
     secondary K74.4
   cardiac (of liver) K76.1
   Charcot's K74.3
   cholangiolitic, cholangitic, cholostatic (primary) K74.3
   congestive K76.1
   Cruveilhier-Baumgarten K74.69
   cryptogenic (liver) K74.69
   due to
     hepatolenticular degeneration E83.01
     Wilson's disease E83.01
     xanthomatosis E78.2
   fatty K76.0
     alcoholic K70.0
   Hanot's (hypertrophic) K74.3
   hepatic — *see* Cirrhosis, liver
   hypertrophic K74.3
   Indian childhood K74.69
   kidney — *see* Sclerosis, renal
   Laennec's K70.30
     with ascites K70.31
     alcoholic K70.30
       with ascites K70.31
     nonalcoholic K74.69
   liver K74.60
     alcoholic K70.30
       with ascites K70.31
       fatty K70.0
     congenital P78.81
     syphilitic A52.74
   lung (chronic) J84.10
   macronodular K74.69
     alcoholic K70.30
       with ascites K70.31
   micronodular K74.69
     alcoholic K70.30
       with ascites K70.31
   mixed type K74.69
   monolobular K74.3
   nephritis — *see* Sclerosis, renal
   nutritional K74.69
     alcoholic K70.30
       with ascites K70.31
   obstructive — *see* Cirrhosis, biliary
   ovarian N83.8
   pancreas (duct) K86.89
   pigmentary E83.110
   portal K74.69
     alcoholic K70.30
       with ascites K70.31
   postnecrotic K74.69
     alcoholic K70.30
       with ascites K70.31

Cirrhosis, cirrhotic — *continued*
   pulmonary J84.10
   renal — *see* Sclerosis, renal
   spleen D73.2
   stasis K76.1
   Todd's K74.3
   unilobar K74.3
   xanthomatous (biliary) K74.5
     due to xanthomatosis (familial) (metabolic) (prima-
     ry) E78.2
Cistern, subarachnoid R93.0
Citrullinemia E72.23
Citrullinuria E72.23
Civatte's disease or poikiloderma L57.3
Clam digger's itch B65.3
Clammy skin R23.1
Clap — *see* Gonorrhea
Clarke-Hadfield syndrome (pancreatic infantilism) K86.89
Clark's paralysis G80.9
Clastothrix L67.8
Claude Bernard-Horner syndrome G90.2
   traumatic — *see* Injury, nerve, cervical sympathetic
Claude's disease or syndrome G46.3
Claudicatio venosa intermittens I87.8
Claudication (intermittent) I73.9
   cerebral (artery) G45.9
   spinal cord (arteriosclerotic) G95.19
     syphilitic A52.09
   venous (axillary) I87.8
Claustrophobia F40.240
Clavus (infected) L84
Clawfoot (congenital) Q66.89
   acquired — *see* Deformity, limb, clawfoot
Clawhand (acquired) — *see also* Deformity, limb, clawhand
   congenital Q68.1
Clawtoe (congenital) Q66.89
   acquired — *see* Deformity, toe, specified NEC
Clay eating — *see* Pica
Cleansing of artificial opening — *see* Attention to, artificial, opening
Cleft (congenital) — *see also* Imperfect, closure
   alveolar process M26.79
   branchial (persistent) Q18.2
     cyst Q18.0
       fistula Q18.0
       sinus Q18.0
   cricoid cartilage, posterior Q31.8
   cyst Q18.0
     fistula Q18.0
     sinus Q18.0
   foot Q72.7 ☑
   hand Q71.6 ☑
   lip (unilateral) Q36.9
     with cleft palate Q37.9
       hard Q37.1
         with soft Q37.5
       soft Q37.3
         with hard Q37.5
     bilateral Q36.0
       with cleft palate Q37.8
         hard Q37.0
           with soft Q37.4
         soft Q37.2
           with hard Q37.4
     median Q36.1
   nose Q30.2
   palate Q35.9
     with cleft lip (unilateral) Q37.9
       bilateral Q37.8
     hard Q35.1
       with
         cleft lip (unilateral) Q37.1
           bilateral Q37.0
         soft Q35.5
           with cleft lip (unilateral) Q37.5
             bilateral Q37.4
     medial Q35.5
     soft Q35.3
       with
         cleft lip (unilateral) Q37.3
           bilateral Q37.2
         hard Q35.5
           with cleft lip (unilateral) Q37.5
             bilateral Q37.4
   penis Q55.69
   scrotum Q55.29

Cleft — *continued*
- thyroid cartilage Q31.8
- uvula Q35.7

Cleidocranial dysostosis Q74.0

Cleptomania F63.2

Clicking hip (newborn) R29.4

Climacteric (female) — *see also* Menopause
- arthritis (any site) NEC — *see* Arthritis, specified form NEC
- depression (single episode) F32.89
  - recurrent episode F33.8
- male (symptoms) (syndrome) NEC N50.89
- melancholia (single episode) F32.89
  - recurrent episode F33.8
- paranoid state F22
- polyarthritis NEC — *see* Arthritis, specified form NEC
- symptoms (female) N95.1

Clinical research investigation (clinical trial) (control subject) (normal comparison) (participant) Z00.6

Clitoris — *see* condition

Cloaca (persistent) Q43.7

Clonorchiasis, clonorchis infection (liver) B66.1

Clonus R25.8

Closed bite M26.29

Clostridium (C.) **perfringens, as cause of disease classified elsewhere** B96.7

Closure
- congenital, nose Q30.0
- cranial sutures, premature Q75.0
- defective or imperfect NEC — *see* Imperfect, closure
- fistula, delayed — *see* Fistula
- foramen ovale, imperfect Q21.12
- hymen N89.6
- interauricular septum, defective Q21.19
- interventricular septum, defective Q21.0
- lacrimal duct — *see also* Stenosis, lacrimal, duct
  - congenital Q10.5
- nose (congenital) Q30.0
  - acquired M95.0
- of artificial opening — *see* Attention to, artificial, opening
- vagina N89.5
- valve — *see* Endocarditis
- vulva N90.5

Clot (blood) — *see also* Embolism
- artery (obstruction) (occlusion) — *see* Embolism
- bladder N32.89
- brain (intradural or extradural) — *see* Occlusion, artery, cerebral
- circulation I74.9
- heart — *see also* Infarct, myocardium
  - not resulting in infarction I51.3
- vein — *see* Thrombosis

Clouded state R40.1
- epileptic — *see* Epilepsy, specified NEC
- paroxysmal — *see* Epilepsy, specified NEC

Cloudy antrum, antra J32.0

Clouston's (hidrotic) **ectodermal dysplasia** Q82.4

Clubbed nail pachydermoperiostosis M89.40 *[L62]*

Clubbing of finger(s) (nails) R68.3

Clubfinger R68.3
- congenital Q68.1

Clubfoot (congenital) Q66.89
- acquired — *see* Deformity, limb, clubfoot
- equinovarus Q66.0- ☑
- paralytic — *see* Deformity, limb, clubfoot

Clubhand (congenital) (radial) Q71.4- ☑
- acquired — *see* Deformity, limb, clubhand

Clubnail R68.3
- congenital Q84.6

Clump, kidney Q63.1

Clumsiness, clumsy child syndrome F82

Cluttering F80.81

Clutton's joints A50.51 *[M12.80]*

Coagulation, intravascular (diffuse) (disseminated) — *see also* Defibrination syndrome
- complicating abortion — *see* Abortion, by type, complicated by, intravascular coagulation
- following ectopic or molar pregnancy O08.1

Coagulopathy — *see also* Defect, coagulation
- consumption D65
- intravascular D65
  - newborn P60

Coalition
- calcaneo-scaphoid Q66.89
- tarsal Q66.89

Coalminer's
- elbow — *see* Bursitis, elbow, olecranon
- lung or pneumoconiosis J60

Coalworker's lung or pneumoconiosis J60

Coarctation
- aorta (preductal) (postductal) Q25.1
- pulmonary artery Q25.71

Coated tongue K14.3

Coats' disease (exudative retinopathy) — *see* Retinopathy, exudative

Cocaine-induced
- anxiety disorder F14.980
- bipolar and related disorder F14.94
- depressive disorder F14.94
- obsessive-compulsive and related disorder F14.988
- psychotic disorder F14.959
- sexual dysfunction F14.981
- sleep disorder F14.982

Cocainism — *see* Disorder, cocaine use

Coccidioidomycosis B38.9
- cutaneous B38.3
- disseminated B38.7
- generalized B38.7
- meninges B38.4
- prostate B38.81
- pulmonary B38.2
  - acute B38.0
  - chronic B38.1
- skin B38.3
- specified NEC B38.89

Coccidioidosis — *see* Coccidioidomycosis

Coccidiosis (intestinal) A07.3

Coccyx — *see* condition

Cochin-China diarrhea K90.1

Cockayne's syndrome Q87.19

Cocked up toe — *see* Deformity, toe, specified NEC

Cock's peculiar tumor L72.3

Codman's tumor — *see* Neoplasm, bone, benign

Coenurosis B71.8

Coffee-worker's lung J67.8

Cogan's syndrome H16.32- ☑
- oculomotor apraxia H51.8

Coitus, painful (female) N94.10
- male N53.12
- psychogenic F52.6

Cold J00
- with influenza, flu, or grippe — *see* Influenza, with, respiratory manifestations NEC
- agglutinin disease or hemoglobinuria (chronic) D59.12
- bronchial — *see* Bronchitis
- chest — *see* Bronchitis
- common (head) J00
- effects of T69.9 ☑
  - specified effect NEC T69.8 ☑
- excessive, effects of T69.9 ☑
  - specified effect NEC T69.8 ☑
- exhaustion from T69.8 ☑
- exposure to T69.9 ☑
  - specified effect NEC T69.8 ☑
- head J00
- injury syndrome (newborn) P80.0
- on lung — *see* Bronchitis
- rose J30.1
- sensitivity, auto-immune D59.12
- symptoms J00
- virus J00

Coldsore B00.1

Colibacillosis A49.8
- as the cause of other disease — *see also* Escherichia coli B96.20
- generalized A41.50

Colic (bilious) (infantile) (intestinal) (recurrent) (spasmodic) R10.83
- abdomen R10.83
  - psychogenic F45.8
- appendix, appendicular K38.8
- bile duct — *see* Calculus, bile duct
- biliary — *see* Calculus, bile duct
- common duct — *see* Calculus, bile duct
- cystic duct — *see* Calculus, gallbladder
- Devonshire NEC — *see* Poisoning, lead
- gallbladder — *see* Calculus, gallbladder
- gallstone — *see* Calculus, gallbladder
  - gallbladder or cystic duct — *see* Calculus, gallbladder
- hepatic (duct) — *see* Calculus, bile duct

Colic — *continued*
- hysterical F45.8
- kidney N23
- lead NEC — *see* Poisoning, lead
- mucous K58.9
  - with diarrhea K58.0
  - psychogenic F54
- nephritic N23
- painter's NEC — *see* Poisoning, lead
- pancreas K86.89
- psychogenic F45.8
- renal N23
- saturnine NEC — *see* Poisoning, lead
- ureter N23
- urethral N36.8
  - due to calculus N21.1
- uterus NEC N94.89
  - menstrual — *see* Dysmenorrhea
- worm NOS B83.9

Colicystitis — *see* Cystitis

Colitis (acute) (catarrhal) (chronic) (noninfective) (hemorrhagic) — *see also* Enteritis K52.9
- allergic K52.29
  - with
    - food protein-induced enterocolitis syndrome K52.21
    - proctocolitis K52.29
- amebic (acute) — *see also* Amebiasis A06.0
  - nondysenteric A06.2
- anthrax A22.2
- bacillary — *see* Infection, Shigella
- balantidial A07.0
- Clostridium difficile
  - not specified as recurrent A04.72
  - recurrent A04.71
- coccidial A07.3
- collagenous K52.831
- cystica superficialis K52.89
- dietary counseling and surveillance (for) Z71.3
- dietetic — *see also* Colitis, allergic K52.29
- drug-induced K52.1
- due to radiation K52.0
- eosinophilic K52.82
- food hypersensitivity — *see also* Colitis, allergic K52.29
- giardial A07.1
- granulomatous — *see* Enteritis, regional, large intestine
- indeterminate, so stated K52.3
- infectious — *see* Enteritis, infectious
- ischemic K55.9
  - acute (subacute) — *see also* Ischemia, intestine, acute K55.039
  - chronic K55.1
  - due to mesenteric artery insufficiency K55.1
  - fulminant (acute) — *see also* Ischemia, intestine, acute K55.039
- left sided K51.50
  - with
    - abscess K51.514
    - complication K51.519
      - specified NEC K51.518
    - fistula K51.513
    - obstruction K51.512
    - rectal bleeding K51.511
- lymphocytic K52.832
- membranous
  - psychogenic F54
- microscopic K52.839
  - specified NEC K52.838
- mucous — *see* Syndrome, irritable, bowel
  - psychogenic F54
- noninfective K52.9
  - specified NEC K52.89
- polyposa — *see* Polyp, colon, inflammatory
- protozoal A07.9
- pseudomembranous
  - not specified as recurrent A04.72
  - recurrent A04.71
- pseudomucinous — *see* Syndrome, irritable, bowel
- regional — *see* Enteritis, regional, large intestine
  - infectious A09
- segmental — *see* Enteritis, regional, large intestine
- septic — *see* Enteritis, infectious
- spastic K58.9
  - with diarrhea K58.0
  - psychogenic F54
- staphylococcal A04.8
  - foodborne A05.0

Cleft — Colitis

Colitis — *continued*
  subacute ischemic — *see also* Ischemia, intestine, acute
    K55.039
  thromboulcerative — *see also* Ischemia, intestine, acute
    K55.039
  toxic NEC K52.1
    due to Clostridium difficile
      not specified as recurrent A04.72
      recurrent A04.71
  transmural — *see* Enteritis, regional, large intestine
  trichomonal A07.8
  tuberculous (ulcerative) A18.32
  ulcerative (chronic) K51.90
    with
      complication K51.919
        abscess K51.914
        fistula K51.913
        obstruction K51.912
        rectal bleeding K51.911
        specified complication NEC K51.918
    enterocolitis — *see* Enterocolitis, ulcerative
    ileocolitis — *see* Ileocolitis, ulcerative
    mucosal proctocolitis — *see* Proctocolitis, mucosal
    proctitis — *see* Proctitis, ulcerative
    pseudopolyposis —*see* Polyp, colon, inflammatory
    psychogenic F54
    rectosigmoiditis — *see* Rectosigmoiditis, ulcerative
    specified type NEC K51.80
      with
        complication K51.819
          abscess K51.814
          fistula K51.813
          obstruction K51.812
          rectal bleeding K51.811
          specified complication NEC K51.818
Collagenosis, collagen disease (nonvascular) (vascular)
  M35.9
  cardiovascular I42.8
  reactive perforating L87.1
  specified NEC M35.89
Collapse R55
  adrenal E27.2
  cardiorespiratory R57.0
  cardiovascular R57.0
    newborn P29.89
  circulatory (peripheral) R57.9
    during or after labor and delivery O75.1
    following ectopic or molar pregnancy O08.3
    newborn P29.89
  during or
    after labor and delivery O75.1
    resulting from a procedure, not elsewhere classified
      T81.10 ☑
  external ear canal — *see* Stenosis, external ear canal
  general R55
  heart — *see* Disease, heart
  heat T67.1 ☑
  hysterical F44.89
  labyrinth, membranous (congenital) Q16.5
  lung (massive) — *see also* Atelectasis J98.19
    pressure due to anesthesia (general) (local) or other
      sedation T88.2 ☑
      during labor and delivery O74.1
      in pregnancy O29.02- ☑
      postpartum, puerperal O89.09
  myocardial — *see* Disease, heart
  nervous F48.8
  neurocirculatory F45.8
  nose M95.0
  postoperative T81.10 ☑
  pulmonary — *see also* Atelectasis J98.19
    newborn — *see* Atelectasis
  trachea J39.8
  tracheobronchial J98.09
  valvular — *see* Endocarditis
  vascular (peripheral) R57.9
    during or after labor and delivery O75.1
    following ectopic or molar pregnancy O08.3
    newborn P29.89
  vertebra M48.50- ☑
    cervical region M48.52- ☑
    cervicothoracic region M48.53- ☑
    in (due to)
      neoplasm (metastasis) M84.58- ☑
      osteoporosis — *see also* Osteoporosis M80.88 ☑
        cervical region M80.88 ☑
        cervicothoracic region M80.88 ☑
        lumbar region M80.88 ☑

Collapse — *continued*
  vertebra — *continued*
    in — *continued*
      osteoporosis — *see also* Osteoporosis — *continued*
        lumbosacral region M80.88 ☑
        multiple sites M80.88 ☑
        occipito-atlanto-axial region M80.88 ☑
        sacrococcygeal region M80.88 ☑
        thoracic region M80.88 ☑
        thoracolumbar region M80.88 ☑
      specified disease NEC M48.50- ☑
        cervical region M48.52- ☑
        cervicothoracic region M48.53- ☑
        lumbar region M48.56- ☑
        lumbosacral region M48.57- ☑
        occipito-atlanto-axial region M48.51- ☑
        sacrococcygeal region M48.58- ☑
        thoracic region M48.54- ☑
        thoracolumbar region M48.55- ☑
    lumbar region M48.56- ☑
    lumbosacral region M48.57- ☑
    occipito-atlanto-axial region M48.51- ☑
    sacrococcygeal region M48.58- ☑
    thoracic region M48.54- ☑
    thoracolumbar region M48.55- ☑
Collateral — *see also* condition
  circulation (venous) I87.8
  dilation, veins I87.8
Colles' fracture S52.53- ☑
Collet (-Sicard) syndrome G52.7
Collier's asthma or lung J60
Collodion baby Q80.2
Colloid nodule (of thyroid) (cystic) E04.1
Coloboma (iris) Q13.0
  eyelid Q10.3
  fundus Q14.8
  lens Q12.2
  optic disc (congenital) Q14.2
    acquired H47.31- ☑
Coloenteritis — *see* Enteritis
Colon — *see* condition
Colonization
  MRSA (Methicillin resistant Staphylococcus aureus)
    Z22.322
  MSSA (Methicillin susceptible Staphylococcus aureus)
    Z22.321
  status — *see* Carrier (suspected) of
Coloptosis K63.4
Color blindness — *see* Deficiency, color vision
Colostomy
  attention to Z43.3
  fitting or adjustment Z46.89
  malfunctioning K94.03
  status Z93.3
Colpitis (acute) — *see* Vaginitis
Colpocele N81.5
Colpocystitis — *see* Vaginitis
Colpospasm N94.2
Column, spinal, vertebral — *see* condition
Coma R40.20
  with
    motor response (none) R40.231 ☑
      abnormal extensor posturing to pain or noxious
        stimuli (< 2 years of age) R40.232 ☑
      abnormal flexure posturing to pain or noxious
        stimuli (0-5 years of age) R40.233 ☑
      extensor posturing to pain or noxious stimuli (2-
        5 years of age) R40.232 ☑
      flexion/decorticate posturing (< 2 years of age)
        R40.233 ☑
      localizes pain (2-5 years of age) R40.235 ☑
      normal or spontaneous movement (< 2 years of
        age) R40.236 ☑
      obeys commands (2-5 years of age) R40.236 ☑
      score of
        1 R40.231 ☑
        2 R40.232 ☑
        3 R40.233 ☑
        4 R40.234 ☑
        5 R40.235 ☑
        6 R40.236 ☑
      withdraws from pain or noxious stimuli (0-5 years
        of age) R40.234 ☑
      withdraws to touch (< 2 years of age) R40.235 ☑
    opening of eyes (never) R40.211 ☑

Coma — *continued*
  with — *continued*
    opening of eyes — *continued*
      in response to
        pain R40.212 ☑
        sound R40.213 ☑
      score of
        1 R40.211 ☑
        2 R40.212 ☑
        3 R40.213 ☑
        4 R40.214 ☑
      spontaneous R40.214 ☑
    verbal response (none) R40.221 ☑
      confused conversation R40.224 ☑
      cooing or babbling or crying appropriately (<2
        years of age) R40.225 ☑
      inappropriate crying or screaming (< 2 years of
        age) R40.223 ☑
      inappropriate words (2-5 years of age)
        R40.224 ☑
      inappropriate words R40.223 ☑
      incomprehensible sounds (2-5 years of age)
        R40.222 ☑
      incomprehensible words R40.222 ☑
      irritable cries (< 2 years of age) R40.224 ☑
      moans/grunts to pain; restless (< 2 years old)
        R40.222 ☑
      oriented R40.225 ☑
      score of
        1 R40.221 ☑
        2 R40.222 ☑
        3 R40.223 ☑
        4 R40.224 ☑
        5 R40.225 ☑
      screaming (2-5 years of age) R40.223 ☑
      uses appropriate words (2-5 years of age)
        R40.225 ☑
  eclamptic — *see* Eclampsia
  epileptic — *see* Epilepsy
  Glasgow, scale score — *see* Glasgow coma scale
  hepatic — *see* Failure, hepatic, by type, with coma
  hyperglycemic (diabetic) — *see* Diabetes, by type, with
    hyperosmolarity, with coma
  hyperosmolar (diabetic) — *see* Diabetes, by type, with
    hyperosmolarity, with coma
  hypoglycemic (diabetic) — *see* Diabetes, by type, with
    hypoglycemia, with coma
    nondiabetic E15
  in diabetes — *see* Diabetes, coma
  insulin-induced — *see* Coma, hypoglycemic
  ketoacidotic (diabetic) — *see* Diabetes, by type, with
    ketoacidosis, with coma
  myxedematous E03.5
  newborn P91.5
  persistent vegetative state R40.3
  specified NEC, without documented Glasgow coma
    scale score, or with partial Glasgow coma scale
    score reported R40.244 ☑
Comatose — *see* Coma
Combat fatigue F43.0
Combined — *see* condition
Comedo, comedones (giant) L70.0
Comedocarcinoma — *see also* Neoplasm, breast, malignant
  noninfiltrating
    breast D05.8- ☑
    specified site — *see* Neoplasm, in situ, by site
    unspecified site D05.8- ☑
Comedomastitis — *see* Ectasia, mammary duct
Comminuted fracture — *code as* Fracture, closed
Common
  arterial trunk Q20.0
  atrioventricular canal Q21.23
  atrium Q21.19
  cold (head) J00
  truncus (arteriosus) Q20.0
  variable immunodeficiency — *see* Immunodeficiency,
    common variable
  ventricle Q20.4
Commotio, commotion (current)
  brain — *see* Injury, intracranial, concussion
  cerebri — *see* Injury, intracranial, concussion
  retinae S05.8X- ☑
  spinal cord — *see* Injury, spinal cord, by region
  spinalis — *see* Injury, spinal cord, by region

Index

Colitis — Commotio, commotion

Communication

between
- base of aorta and pulmonary artery Q21.4
- left ventricle and right atrium Q20.5
- pericardial sac and pleural sac Q34.8
- pulmonary artery and pulmonary vein, congenital Q25.72
- congenital between uterus and digestive or urinary tract Q51.7

Compartment syndrome (deep) (posterior) (traumatic) T79.A0 ☑ (*following* T79.7)
- abdomen T79.A3 ☑ (*following* T79.7)
- lower extremity (hip, buttock, thigh, leg, foot, toes) T79.A2 ☑ (*following* T79.7)
- nontraumatic
  - abdomen M79.A3 (*following* M79.7)
  - lower extremity (hip, buttock, thigh, leg, foot, toes) M79.A2- ☑ (*following* M79.7)
  - specified site NEC M79.A9 (*following* M79.7)
  - upper extremity (shoulder, arm, forearm, wrist, hand, fingers) M79.A1- ☑ (*following* M79.7)
- specified site NEC T79.A9 ☑ (*following* T79.7)
- upper extremity (shoulder, arm, forearm, wrist, hand, fingers) T79.A1- ☑ (*following* T79.7)

Compensation
- failure — *see* Disease, heart
- neurosis, psychoneurosis — *see* Disorder, factitious

Complaint — *see also* Disease
- bowel, functional K59.9
  - psychogenic F45.8
- intestine, functional K59.9
  - psychogenic F45.8
- kidney — *see* Disease, renal
- miners' J60

Complete — *see* condition

Complex
- Addison-Schilder E71.528
- cardiorenal — *see* Hypertension, cardiorenal
- Costen's M26.69
- disseminated mycobacterium avium- intracellulare (DMAC) A31.2
- Eisenmenger's (ventricular septal defect) I27.83
- hypersexual F52.8
- jumped process, spine — *see* Dislocation, vertebra
- primary, tuberculous A15.7
- Schilder-Addison E71.528
- subluxation (vertebral) M99.19
  - abdomen M99.19
  - acromioclavicular M99.17
  - cervical region M99.11
  - cervicothoracic M99.11
  - costochondral M99.18
  - costovertebral M99.18
  - head region M99.10
  - hip M99.15
  - lower extremity M99.16
  - lumbar region M99.13
  - lumbosacral M99.13
  - occipitocervical M99.10
  - pelvic region M99.15
  - pubic M99.15
  - rib cage M99.18
  - sacral region M99.14
  - sacrococcygeal M99.14
  - sacroiliac M99.14
  - specified NEC M99.19
  - sternochondral M99.18
  - sternoclavicular M99.17
  - thoracic region M99.12
  - thoracolumbar M99.12
  - upper extremity M99.17
- Taussig-Bing (transposition, aorta and overriding pulmonary artery) Q20.1

Complication(s) (from) (of)
- accidental puncture or laceration during a procedure (of) — *see* Complications, intraoperative (intraprocedural), puncture or laceration
- amputation stump (surgical) (late) NEC T87.9
  - dehiscence T87.81
  - infection or inflammation T87.40
    - lower limb T87.4- ☑
    - upper limb T87.4- ☑
  - necrosis T87.50
    - lower limb T87.5- ☑
    - upper limb T87.5- ☑
  - neuroma T87.30
    - lower limb T87.3- ☑
    - upper limb T87.3- ☑

Complication(s) — *continued*
- amputation stump — *continued*
  - specified type NEC T87.89
- anastomosis (and bypass) — *see also* Complications, prosthetic device or implant
  - intestinal (internal) NEC K91.89
    - involving urinary tract N99.89
  - urinary tract (involving intestinal tract) N99.89
  - vascular — *see* Complications, cardiovascular device or implant
- anesthesia, anesthetic — *see also* Anesthesia, complication T88.59 ☑
  - brain, postpartum, puerperal O89.2
  - cardiac
    - in
      - labor and delivery O74.2
      - pregnancy O29.19-
    - postpartum, puerperal O89.1
  - central nervous system
    - in
      - labor and delivery O74.3
      - pregnancy O29.29-
    - postpartum, puerperal O89.2
  - difficult or failed intubation T88.4 ☑
    - in pregnancy O29.6-
  - failed sedation (conscious) (moderate) during procedure T88.52 ☑
  - general, unintended awareness during procedure T88.53 ☑
  - hyperthermia, malignant T88.3 ☑
  - hypothermia T88.51 ☑
  - intubation failure T88.4 ☑
  - malignant hyperthermia T88.3 ☑
  - pulmonary
    - in
      - labor and delivery O74.1
      - pregnancy NEC O29.09-
    - postpartum, puerperal O89.09
  - shock T88.2 ☑
  - spinal and epidural
    - in
      - labor and delivery NEC O74.6
        - headache O74.5
      - pregnancy NEC O29.5X- ☑
    - postpartum, puerperal NEC O89.5
      - headache O89.4
  - unintended awareness under general anesthesia during procedure T88.53 ☑
- anti-reflux device — *see* Complications, esophageal anti-reflux device
- aortic (bifurcation) graft — *see* Complications, graft, vascular
- aortocoronary (bypass) graft — *see* Complications, coronary artery (bypass) graft
- aortofemoral (bypass) graft — *see* Complications, extremity artery (bypass) graft
- arteriovenous
  - fistula, surgically created T82.9 ☑
    - embolism T82.818 ☑
    - fibrosis T82.828 ☑
    - hemorrhage T82.838 ☑
    - infection or inflammation T82.7 ☑
    - mechanical
      - breakdown T82.510 ☑
      - displacement T82.520 ☑
      - leakage T82.530 ☑
      - malposition T82.520 ☑
      - obstruction T82.590 ☑
      - perforation T82.590 ☑
      - protrusion T82.590 ☑
    - pain T82.848 ☑
    - specified type NEC T82.898 ☑
    - stenosis T82.858 ☑
    - thrombosis T82.868 ☑
  - shunt, surgically created T82.9 ☑
    - embolism T82.818 ☑
    - fibrosis T82.828 ☑
    - hemorrhage T82.838 ☑
    - infection or inflammation T82.7 ☑
    - mechanical
      - breakdown T82.511 ☑
      - displacement T82.521 ☑
      - leakage T82.531 ☑
      - malposition T82.521 ☑
      - obstruction T82.591 ☑
      - perforation T82.591 ☑
      - protrusion T82.591 ☑

Complication(s) — *continued*
- arteriovenous — *continued*
  - shunt, surgically created — *continued*
    - pain T82.848 ☑
    - specified type NEC T82.898 ☑
    - stenosis T82.858 ☑
    - thrombosis T82.868 ☑
  - arthroplasty — *see* Complications, joint prosthesis
  - artificial
    - fertilization or insemination N98.9
      - attempted introduction (of)
        - embryo in embryo transfer N98.3
        - ovum following in vitro fertilization N98.2
      - hyperstimulation of ovaries N98.1
      - infection N98.0
      - specified NEC N98.8
    - heart T82.9 ☑
      - embolism T82.817 ☑
      - fibrosis T82.827 ☑
      - hemorrhage T82.837 ☑
      - infection or inflammation T82.7 ☑
      - mechanical
        - breakdown T82.512 ☑
        - displacement T82.522 ☑
        - leakage T82.532 ☑
        - malposition T82.522 ☑
        - obstruction T82.592 ☑
        - perforation T82.592 ☑
        - protrusion T82.592 ☑
      - pain T82.847 ☑
      - specified type NEC T82.897 ☑
      - stenosis T82.857 ☑
      - thrombosis T82.867 ☑
    - opening
      - cecostomy — *see* Complications, colostomy
      - colostomy — *see* Complications, colostomy
      - cystostomy — *see* Complications, cystostomy
      - enterostomy — *see* Complications, enterostomy
      - gastrostomy — *see* Complications, gastrostomy
      - ileostomy — *see* Complications, enterostomy
      - jejunostomy — *see* Complications, enterostomy
      - nephrostomy — *see* Complications, stoma, urinary tract
      - tracheostomy — *see* Complications, tracheostomy
      - ureterostomy — *see* Complications, stoma, urinary tract
      - urethrostomy — *see* Complications, stoma, urinary tract
- balloon implant or device
  - gastrointestinal T85.9 ☑
    - embolism T85.818 ☑
    - fibrosis T85.828 ☑
    - hemorrhage T85.838 ☑
    - infection and inflammation T85.79 ☑
    - pain T85.848 ☑
    - specified type NEC T85.898 ☑
    - stenosis T85.858 ☑
    - thrombosis T85.868 ☑
  - vascular (counterpulsation) T82.9 ☑
    - embolism T82.818 ☑
    - fibrosis T82.828 ☑
    - hemorrhage T82.838 ☑
    - infection or inflammation T82.7 ☑
    - mechanical
      - breakdown T82.513 ☑
      - displacement T82.523 ☑
      - leakage T82.533 ☑
      - malposition T82.523 ☑
      - obstruction T82.593 ☑
      - perforation T82.593 ☑
      - protrusion T82.593 ☑
    - pain T82.848 ☑
    - specified type NEC T82.898 ☑
    - stenosis T82.858 ☑
    - thrombosis T82.868 ☑
- bariatric procedure
  - gastric band procedure K95.09
    - infection K95.01
  - specified procedure NEC K95.89
    - infection K95.81
- bile duct implant (prosthetic) T85.9 ☑
  - embolism T85.818 ☑
  - fibrosis T85.828 ☑
  - hemorrhage T85.838 ☑
  - infection and inflammation T85.79 ☑

Complication(s) — *continued*
- bile duct implant — *continued*
  - mechanical
    - breakdown T85.510 ☑
    - displacement T85.520 ☑
    - malfunction T85.510 ☑
    - malposition T85.520 ☑
    - obstruction T85.590 ☑
    - perforation T85.590 ☑
    - protrusion T85.590 ☑
    - specified NEC T85.590 ☑
  - pain T85.848 ☑
  - specified type NEC T85.898 ☑
  - stenosis T85.858 ☑
  - thrombosis T85.868 ☑
- bladder device (auxiliary) — *see* Complications, genitourinary, device or implant, urinary system
- bleeding (postoperative) — *see* Complication, postoperative, hemorrhage
  - intraoperative — *see* Complication, intraoperative, hemorrhage
- blood vessel graft — *see* Complications, graft, vascular
- bone
  - device NEC T84.9 ☑
    - embolism T84.81 ☑
    - fibrosis T84.82 ☑
    - hemorrhage T84.83 ☑
    - infection or inflammation T84.7 ☑
    - mechanical
      - breakdown T84.318 ☑
      - displacement T84.328 ☑
      - malposition T84.328 ☑
      - obstruction T84.398 ☑
      - perforation T84.398 ☑
      - protrusion T84.398 ☑
    - pain T84.84 ☑
    - specified type NEC T84.89 ☑
    - stenosis T84.85 ☑
    - thrombosis T84.86 ☑
  - graft — *see* Complications, graft, bone
  - growth stimulator (electrode) — *see* Complications, electronic stimulator device, bone
  - marrow transplant — *see* Complications, transplant, bone, marrow
- brain neurostimulator (electrode) — *see* Complications, electronic stimulator device, brain
- breast implant (prosthetic) T85.9 ☑
  - capsular contracture T85.44 ☑
  - embolism T85.818 ☑
  - fibrosis T85.828 ☑
  - hemorrhage T85.838 ☑
  - infection and inflammation T85.79 ☑
  - mechanical
    - breakdown T85.41 ☑
    - displacement T85.42 ☑
    - leakage T85.43 ☑
    - malposition T85.42 ☑
    - obstruction T85.49 ☑
    - perforation T85.49 ☑
    - protrusion T85.49 ☑
    - specified NEC T85.49 ☑
  - pain T85.848 ☑
  - specified type NEC T85.898 ☑
  - stenosis T85.858 ☑
  - thrombosis T85.868 ☑
- bypass — *see also* Complications, prosthetic device or implant
  - aortocoronary — *see* Complications, coronary artery (bypass) graft
  - arterial — *see also* Complications, graft, vascular
    - extremity — *see* Complications, extremity artery (bypass) graft
- cardiac — *see also* Disease, heart
  - device, implant or graft T82.9 ☑
    - embolism T82.817 ☑
    - fibrosis T82.827 ☑
    - hemorrhage T82.837 ☑
    - infection or inflammation T82.7 ☑
      - valve prosthesis T82.6 ☑
    - mechanical
      - breakdown T82.519 ☑
        - specified device NEC T82.518 ☑
      - displacement T82.529 ☑
        - specified device NEC T82.528 ☑
      - leakage T82.539 ☑
        - specified device NEC T82.538 ☑

Complication(s) — *continued*
- cardiac — *see also* Disease, heart — *continued*
  - device, implant or graft — *continued*
    - mechanical — *continued*
      - malposition T82.529 ☑
        - specified device NEC T82.528 ☑
      - obstruction T82.599 ☑
        - specified device NEC T82.598 ☑
      - perforation T82.599 ☑
        - specified device NEC T82.598 ☑
      - protrusion T82.599 ☑
        - specified device NEC T82.598 ☑
    - pain T82.847 ☑
    - specified type NEC T82.897 ☑
    - stenosis T82.857 ☑
    - thrombosis T82.867 ☑
- cardiovascular device, graft or implant T82.9 ☑
  - aortic graft — *see* Complications, graft, vascular
  - arteriovenous
    - fistula, artificial — *see* Complication, arteriovenous, fistula, surgically created
    - shunt — *see* Complication, arteriovenous, shunt, surgically created
  - artificial heart — *see* Complication, artificial, heart
  - balloon (counterpulsation) device — *see* Complication, balloon implant, vascular
  - carotid artery graft — *see* Complications, graft, vascular
  - coronary bypass graft — *see* Complication, coronary artery (bypass) graft
  - dialysis catheter (vascular) — *see* Complication, catheter, dialysis
  - electronic T82.9 ☑
    - electrode T82.9 ☑
      - embolism T82.817 ☑
      - fibrosis T82.827 ☑
      - hemorrhage T82.837 ☑
      - infection T82.7 ☑
      - mechanical
        - breakdown T82.110 ☑
        - displacement T82.120 ☑
        - leakage T82.190 ☑
        - obstruction T82.190 ☑
        - perforation T82.190 ☑
        - protrusion T82.190 ☑
        - specified type NEC T82.190 ☑
      - pain T82.847 ☑
      - specified NEC T82.897 ☑
      - stenosis T82.857 ☑
      - thrombosis T82.867 ☑
    - embolism T82.817 ☑
    - fibrosis T82.827 ☑
    - hemorrhage T82.837 ☑
    - infection T82.7 ☑
    - mechanical
      - breakdown T82.119 ☑
      - displacement T82.129 ☑
      - leakage T82.199 ☑
      - obstruction T82.199 ☑
      - perforation T82.199 ☑
      - protrusion T82.199 ☑
      - specified type NEC T82.199 ☑
    - pain T82.847 ☑
    - pulse generator T82.9 ☑
      - embolism T82.817 ☑
      - fibrosis T82.827 ☑
      - hemorrhage T82.837 ☑
      - infection T82.7 ☑
      - mechanical
        - breakdown T82.111 ☑
        - displacement T82.121 ☑
        - leakage T82.191 ☑
        - obstruction T82.191 ☑
        - perforation T82.191 ☑
        - protrusion T82.191 ☑
        - specified type NEC T82.191 ☑
      - pain T82.847 ☑
      - specified NEC T82.897 ☑
      - stenosis T82.857 ☑
      - thrombosis T82.867 ☑
    - specified condition NEC T82.897 ☑
    - specified device NEC T82.9 ☑
      - embolism T82.817 ☑
      - fibrosis T82.827 ☑
      - hemorrhage T82.837 ☑
      - infection T82.7 ☑

Complication(s) — *continued*
- cardiovascular device, graft or implant — *continued*
  - electronic — *continued*
    - specified device — *continued*
      - mechanical
        - breakdown T82.118 ☑
        - displacement T82.128 ☑
        - leakage T82.198 ☑
        - obstruction T82.198 ☑
        - perforation T82.198 ☑
        - protrusion T82.198 ☑
        - specified type NEC T82.198 ☑
      - pain T82.847 ☑
      - specified NEC T82.897 ☑
      - stenosis T82.857 ☑
      - thrombosis T82.867 ☑
    - stenosis T82.857 ☑
    - thrombosis T82.867 ☑
  - extremity artery graft — *see* Complication, extremity artery (bypass) graft
  - femoral artery graft — *see* Complication, extremity artery (bypass) graft
  - heart
    - transplant — *see* Complication, transplant, heart
    - valve — *see* Complication, prosthetic device, heart valve
      - graft — *see* Complication, heart, valve, graft
  - heart-lung transplant — *see* Complication, transplant, heart, with lung
  - infection or inflammation T82.7 ☑
  - umbrella device — *see* Complication, umbrella device, vascular
  - vascular graft (or anastomosis) — *see* Complication, graft, vascular
- carotid artery (bypass) graft — *see* Complications, graft, vascular
- catheter (device) NEC — *see also* Complications, prosthetic device or implant
  - cranial infusion
    - infection and inflammation T85.735 ☑
    - mechanical
      - breakdown T85.610 ☑
      - displacement T85.620 ☑
      - leakage T85.630 ☑
      - malfunction T85.690 ☑
      - malposition T85.620 ☑
      - obstruction T85.690 ☑
      - perforation T85.690 ☑
      - protrusion T85.690 ☑
      - specified NEC T85.690 ☑
  - cystostomy T83.9 ☑
    - embolism T83.81 ☑
    - fibrosis T83.82 ☑
    - hemorrhage T83.83 ☑
    - infection and inflammation T83.510 ☑
    - mechanical
      - breakdown T83.010 ☑
      - displacement T83.020 ☑
      - leakage T83.030 ☑
      - malposition T83.020 ☑
      - obstruction T83.090 ☑
      - perforation T83.090 ☑
      - protrusion T83.090 ☑
      - specified NEC T83.090 ☑
    - pain T83.84 ☑
    - specified type NEC T83.89 ☑
    - stenosis T83.85 ☑
    - thrombosis T83.86 ☑
  - dialysis (vascular) T82.9 ☑
    - embolism T82.818 ☑
    - fibrosis T82.828 ☑
    - hemorrhage T82.838 ☑
    - infection and inflammation T82.7 ☑
    - intraperitoneal — *see* Complications, catheter, intraperitoneal
    - mechanical
      - breakdown T82.41 ☑
      - displacement T82.42 ☑
      - leakage T82.43 ☑
      - malposition T82.42 ☑
      - obstruction T82.49 ☑
      - perforation T82.49 ☑
      - protrusion T82.49 ☑
    - pain T82.848 ☑
    - specified type NEC T82.898 ☑
    - stenosis T82.858 ☑

Complication(s) — *continued*
catheter — *see also* Complications, prosthetic device or implant — *continued*
  dialysis — *continued*
    thrombosis T82.868 ☑
  epidural infusion T85.9 ☑
    embolism T85.810 ☑
    fibrosis T85.820 ☑
    hemorrhage T85.830 ☑
    infection and inflammation T85.735 ☑
    mechanical
      breakdown T85.610 ☑
      displacement T85.620 ☑
      leakage T85.630 ☑
      malfunction T85.610 ☑
      malposition T85.620 ☑
      obstruction T85.690 ☑
      perforation T85.690 ☑
      protrusion T85.690 ☑
      specified NEC T85.690 ☑
    pain T85.840 ☑
    specified type NEC T85.890 ☑
    stenosis T85.850 ☑
    thrombosis T85.860 ☑
  intraperitoneal dialysis T85.9 ☑
    embolism T85.818 ☑
    fibrosis T85.828 ☑
    hemorrhage T85.838 ☑
    infection and inflammation T85.71 ☑
    mechanical
      breakdown T85.611 ☑
      displacement T85.621 ☑
      leakage T85.631 ☑
      malfunction T85.611 ☑
      malposition T85.621 ☑
      obstruction T85.691 ☑
      perforation T85.691 ☑
      protrusion T85.691 ☑
      specified NEC T85.691 ☑
    pain T85.848 ☑
    specified type NEC T85.898 ☑
    stenosis T85.858 ☑
    thrombosis T85.868 ☑
  intrathecal infusion
    infection and inflammation T85.735 ☑
    mechanical
      breakdown T85.610 ☑
      displacement T85.620 ☑
      leakage T85.630 ☑
      malfunction T85.690 ☑
      malposition T85.620 ☑
      obstruction T85.690 ☑
      perforation T85.690 ☑
      protrusion T85.690 ☑
      specified NEC T85.690 ☑
  intravenous infusion T82.9 ☑
    embolism T82.818 ☑
    fibrosis T82.828 ☑
    hemorrhage T82.838 ☑
    infection or inflammation T82.7 ☑
    mechanical
      breakdown T82.514 ☑
      displacement T82.524 ☑
      leakage T82.534 ☑
      malposition T82.524 ☑
      obstruction T82.594 ☑
      perforation T82.594 ☑
      protrusion T82.594 ☑
    pain T82.848 ☑
    specified type NEC T82.898 ☑
    stenosis T82.858 ☑
    thrombosis T82.868 ☑
  spinal infusion
    infection and inflammation T85.735 ☑
    mechanical
      breakdown T85.610 ☑
      displacement T85.620 ☑
      leakage T85.630 ☑
      malfunction T85.690 ☑
      malposition T85.620 ☑
      obstruction T85.690 ☑
      perforation T85.690 ☑
      protrusion T85.690 ☑
      specified NEC T85.690 ☑
  subarachnoid infusion
    infection and inflammation T85.735 ☑

Complication(s) — *continued*
catheter — *see also* Complications, prosthetic device or implant — *continued*
  subarachnoid infusion — *continued*
    mechanical
      breakdown T85.610 ☑
      displacement T85.620 ☑
      leakage T85.630 ☑
      malfunction T85.690 ☑
      malposition T85.620 ☑
      obstruction T85.690 ☑
      perforation T85.690 ☑
      protrusion T85.690 ☑
      specified NEC T85.690 ☑
  subdural infusion T85.9 ☑
    embolism T85.810 ☑
    fibrosis T85.820 ☑
    hemorrhage T85.830 ☑
    infection and inflammation T85.735 ☑
    mechanical
      breakdown T85.610 ☑
      displacement T85.620 ☑
      leakage T85.630 ☑
      malfunction T85.610 ☑
      malposition T85.620 ☑
      obstruction T85.690 ☑
      perforation T85.690 ☑
      protrusion T85.690 ☑
      specified NEC T85.690 ☑
    pain T85.840 ☑
    specified type NEC T85.890 ☑
    stenosis T85.850 ☑
    thrombosis T85.860 ☑
  urethral T83.9 ☑
    displacement T83.028 ☑
    embolism T83.81 ☑
    fibrosis T83.82 ☑
    hemorrhage T83.83 ☑
    indwelling
      breakdown T83.011 ☑
      displacement T83.021 ☑
      infection and inflammation T83.511 ☑
      leakage T83.031 ☑
      specified complication NEC T83.091 ☑
    infection and inflammation T83.511 ☑
    leakage T83.038 ☑
    malposition T83.028 ☑
    mechanical
      breakdown T83.011 ☑
    obstruction (mechanical) T83.091 ☑
    pain T83.84 ☑
    perforation T83.091 ☑
    protrusion T83.091 ☑
    specified type NEC T83.091 ☑
    stenosis T83.85 ☑
    thrombosis T83.86 ☑
  urinary NEC
    breakdown T83.018 ☑
    displacement T83.028 ☑
    infection and inflammation T83.518 ☑
    leakage T83.038 ☑
    specified complication NEC T83.098 ☑
cecostomy (stoma) — *see* Complications, colostomy
cesarean delivery wound NEC O90.89
  disruption O90.0
  hematoma O90.2
  infection (following delivery) O86.00
chemotherapy (antineoplastic) NEC T88.7 ☑
chimeric antigen receptor (CAR-T) cell therapy T80.82 ☑
chin implant (prosthetic) — *see* Complication, prosthetic device or implant, specified NEC
circulatory system I99.8
  intraoperative I97.88
  postprocedural I97.89
    following cardiac surgery — *see also* Infarct, myocardium, associated with revascularization procedure I97.19-
      postcardiotomy syndrome I97.0
    hypertension I97.3
    lymphedema after mastectomy I97.2
    postcardiotomy syndrome I97.0
    specified NEC I97.89
colostomy (stoma) K94.00
  hemorrhage K94.01
  infection K94.02

Complication(s) — *continued*
colostomy — *continued*
  malfunction K94.03
  mechanical K94.03
  specified complication NEC K94.09
contraceptive device, intrauterine — *see* Complications, intrauterine, contraceptive device
cord (umbilical) — *see* Complications, umbilical cord
corneal graft — *see* Complications, graft, cornea
coronary artery (bypass) graft T82.9 ☑
  atherosclerosis — *see* Arteriosclerosis, coronary (artery)
  embolism T82.817 ☑
  fibrosis T82.827 ☑
  hemorrhage T82.837 ☑
  infection and inflammation T82.7 ☑
  mechanical
    breakdown T82.211 ☑
    displacement T82.212 ☑
    leakage T82.213 ☑
    malposition T82.212 ☑
    obstruction T82.218 ☑
    perforation T82.218 ☑
    protrusion T82.218 ☑
    specified NEC T82.218 ☑
  pain T82.847 ☑
  specified type NEC T82.898 ☑
  stenosis T82.857 ☑
  thrombosis T82.867 ☑
counterpulsation device (balloon), intra- aortic — *see* Complications, balloon implant, vascular
cystostomy (stoma) N99.518
  catheter — *see* Complications, catheter, cystostomy
  hemorrhage N99.510
  infection N99.511
  malfunction N99.512
  specified type NEC N99.518
delivery — *see also* Complications, obstetric O75.9
  procedure (instrumental) (manual) (surgical) O75.4
  specified NEC O75.89
dialysis (peritoneal) (renal) — *see also* Complications, infusion
  catheter (vascular) — *see* Complication, catheter, dialysis
    peritoneal, intraperitoneal — *see* Complications, catheter, intraperitoneal
dorsal column (spinal) neurostimulator — *see* Complications, electronic stimulator device, spinal cord
drug NEC T88.7 ☑
ear procedure — *see also* Disorder, ear
  intraoperative H95.88
    hematoma — *see* Complications, intraoperative, hemorrhage (hematoma) of, ear
    hemorrhage — *see* Complications, intraoperative, hemorrhage (hematoma) (of), ear
    laceration — *see* Complications, intraoperative, puncture or laceration, ear
    specified NEC H95.88
  postoperative H95.89
    external ear canal stenosis H95.81- ☑
    hematoma — *see* Complications, postprocedural, hematoma (of), ear
    hemorrhage — *see* Complications, postprocedural, hemorrhage (of), ear
    postmastoidectomy — *see* Complications, postmastoidectomy
    seroma — *see* Complications, postprocedural, seroma (of), mastoid process
    specified NEC H95.89
ectopic pregnancy O08.9
  damage to pelvic organs O08.6
  embolism O08.2
  genital infection O08.0
  hemorrhage (delayed) (excessive) O08.1
  metabolic disorder O08.5
  renal failure O08.4
  shock O08.3
  specified type NEC O08.0
  venous complication NEC O08.7
electronic stimulator device
  bladder (urinary) — *see* Complications, electronic stimulator device, urinary
  bone T84.9 ☑
    breakdown T84.310 ☑
    displacement T84.320 ☑
    embolism T84.81 ☑
    fibrosis T84.82 ☑

Complication(s) — *continued*
  electronic stimulator device — *continued*
    bone — *continued*
      hemorrhage T84.83 ☑
      infection or inflammation T84.7 ☑
      malfunction T84.310 ☑
      malposition T84.320 ☑
      mechanical NEC T84.390 ☑
      obstruction T84.390 ☑
      pain T84.84 ☑
      perforation T84.390 ☑
      protrusion T84.390 ☑
      specified type NEC T84.89 ☑
      stenosis T84.85 ☑
      thrombosis T84.86 ☑
    brain T85.9 ☑
      embolism T85.810 ☑
      fibrosis T85.820 ☑
      hemorrhage T85.830 ☑
      infection and inflammation T85.731 ☑
      mechanical
        breakdown T85.110 ☑
        displacement T85.120 ☑
        leakage T85.190 ☑
        malposition T85.120 ☑
        obstruction T85.190 ☑
        perforation T85.190 ☑
        protrusion T85.190 ☑
        specified NEC T85.190 ☑
      pain T85.840 ☑
      specified type NEC T85.890 ☑
      stenosis T85.850 ☑
      thrombosis T85.860 ☑
    cardiac (defibrillator) (pacemaker) — *see* Complications, cardiovascular device or implant, electronic
    generator (brain) (gastric) (peripheral) (sacral) (spinal)
      breakdown T85.113 ☑
      displacement T85.123 ☑
      leakage T85.193 ☑
      malposition T85.123 ☑
      obstruction T85.193 ☑
      perforation T85.193 ☑
      protrusion T85.193 ☑
      specified type NEC T85.193 ☑
    muscle T84.9 ☑
      breakdown T84.418 ☑
      displacement T84.428 ☑
      embolism T84.81 ☑
      fibrosis T84.82 ☑
      hemorrhage T84.83 ☑
      infection or inflammation T84.7 ☑
      mechanical NEC T84.498 ☑
      pain T84.84 ☑
      specified type NEC T84.89 ☑
      stenosis T84.85 ☑
      thrombosis T84.86 ☑
    nervous system T85.9 ☑
      brain — *see* Complications, electronic stimulator device, brain
      cranial nerve — *see* Complications, electronic stimulator device, peripheral nerve
      embolism T85.810 ☑
      fibrosis T85.820 ☑
      gastric nerve — *see* Complications, electronic stimulator device, peripheral nerve
      hemorrhage T85.830 ☑
      infection and inflammation T85.738 ☑
      mechanical
        breakdown T85.118 ☑
        displacement T85.128 ☑
        leakage T85.199 ☑
        malposition T85.128 ☑
        obstruction T85.199 ☑
        perforation T85.199 ☑
        protrusion T85.199 ☑
        specified NEC T85.199 ☑
      pain T85.840 ☑
      peripheral nerve — *see* Complications, electronic stimulator device, peripheral nerve
      sacral nerve — *see* Complications, electronic stimulator device, peripheral nerve
      specified type NEC T85.890 ☑
      spinal cord — *see* Complications, electronic stimulator device, spinal cord

Complication(s) — *continued*
  electronic stimulator device — *continued*
    nervous system — *continued*
      stenosis T85.850 ☑
      thrombosis T85.860 ☑
      vagal nerve — *see* Complications, electronic stimulator device, peripheral nerve
    peripheral nerve T85.9 ☑
      embolism T85.810 ☑
      fibrosis T85.820 ☑
      hemorrhage T85.830 ☑
      infection and inflammation T85.732 ☑
      mechanical
        breakdown T85.111 ☑
        displacement T85.121 ☑
        leakage T85.191 ☑
        malposition T85.121 ☑
        obstruction T85.191 ☑
        perforation T85.191 ☑
        protrusion T85.191 ☑
        specified NEC T85.191 ☑
      pain T85.840 ☑
      specified type NEC T85.890 ☑
      stenosis T85.850 ☑
      thrombosis T85.860 ☑
    spinal cord T85.9 ☑
      embolism T85.810 ☑
      fibrosis T85.820 ☑
      hemorrhage T85.830 ☑
      infection and inflammation T85.733 ☑
      mechanical
        breakdown T85.112 ☑
        displacement T85.122 ☑
        leakage T85.192 ☑
        malposition T85.122 ☑
        obstruction T85.192 ☑
        perforation T85.192 ☑
        protrusion T85.192 ☑
        specified NEC T85.192 ☑
      pain T85.840 ☑
      specified type NEC T85.890 ☑
      stenosis T85.850 ☑
      thrombosis T85.860 ☑
    urinary T83.9 ☑
      embolism T83.81 ☑
      fibrosis T83.82 ☑
      hemorrhage T83.83 ☑
      infection and inflammation T83.598 ☑
      mechanical
        breakdown T83.110 ☑
        displacement T83.120 ☑
        malposition T83.120 ☑
        perforation T83.190 ☑
        protrusion T83.190 ☑
        specified NEC T83.190 ☑
      pain T83.84 ☑
      specified type NEC T83.89 ☑
      stenosis T83.85 ☑
      thrombosis T83.86 ☑
  electroshock therapy T88.9 ☑
    specified NEC T88.8 ☑
  endocrine E34.9
    postprocedural
      adrenal hypofunction E89.6
      hypoinsulinemia E89.1
      hypoparathyroidism E89.2
      hypopituitarism E89.3
      hypothyroidism E89.0
      ovarian failure E89.40
        asymptomatic E89.40
        symptomatic E89.41
      specified NEC E89.89
      testicular hypofunction E89.5
  endodontic treatment NEC M27.59
  enterostomy (stoma) K94.10
    hemorrhage K94.11
    infection K94.12
    malfunction K94.13
    mechanical K94.13
    specified complication NEC K94.19
  episiotomy, disruption O90.1
  esophageal anti-reflux device T85.9 ☑
    embolism T85.818 ☑
    fibrosis T85.828 ☑
    hemorrhage T85.838 ☑
    infection and inflammation T85.79 ☑

Complication(s) — *continued*
  esophageal anti-reflux device — *continued*
    mechanical
      breakdown T85.511 ☑
      displacement T85.521 ☑
      malfunction T85.511 ☑
      malposition T85.521 ☑
      obstruction T85.591 ☑
      perforation T85.591 ☑
      protrusion T85.591 ☑
      specified NEC T85.591 ☑
    pain T85.848 ☑
    specified type NEC T85.898 ☑
    stenosis T85.858 ☑
    thrombosis T85.868 ☑
  esophagostomy K94.30
    hemorrhage K94.31
    infection K94.32
    malfunction K94.33
    mechanical K94.33
    specified complication NEC K94.39
  extracorporeal circulation T80.90 ☑
  extremity artery (bypass) graft T82.9 ☑
    arteriosclerosis — *see* Arteriosclerosis, extremities, bypass graft
    embolism T82.818 ☑
    fibrosis T82.828 ☑
    hemorrhage T82.838 ☑
    infection and inflammation T82.7 ☑
    mechanical
      breakdown T82.318 ☑
        femoral artery T82.312 ☑
      displacement T82.328 ☑
        femoral artery T82.322 ☑
      leakage T82.338 ☑
        femoral artery T82.332 ☑
      malposition T82.328 ☑
        femoral artery T82.322 ☑
      obstruction T82.398 ☑
        femoral artery T82.392 ☑
      perforation T82.398 ☑
        femoral artery T82.392 ☑
      protrusion T82.398 ☑
        femoral artery T82.392 ☑
    pain T82.848 ☑
    specified type NEC T82.898 ☑
    stenosis T82.858 ☑
    thrombosis T82.868 ☑
  eye H57.9
    corneal graft — *see* Complications, graft, cornea
    implant (prosthetic) T85.9 ☑
      embolism T85.818 ☑
      fibrosis T85.828 ☑
      hemorrhage T85.838 ☑
      infection and inflammation T85.79 ☑
      mechanical
        breakdown T85.318 ☑
        displacement T85.328 ☑
        leakage T85.398 ☑
        malposition T85.328 ☑
        obstruction T85.398 ☑
        perforation T85.398 ☑
        protrusion T85.398 ☑
        specified NEC T85.398 ☑
      pain T85.848 ☑
      specified type NEC T85.898 ☑
      stenosis T85.858 ☑
      thrombosis T85.868 ☑
    intraocular lens — *see* Complications, intraocular lens
    orbital prosthesis — *see* Complications, orbital prosthesis
  female genital N94.9
    device, implant or graft NEC — *see* Complications, genitourinary, device or implant, genital tract
  femoral artery (bypass) graft — *see* Complication, extremity artery (bypass) graft
  fixation device, internal (orthopedic) T84.9 ☑
    infection and inflammation T84.60 ☑
      arm T84.61- ☑
        humerus T84.61- ☑
        radius T84.61- ☑
        ulna T84.61- ☑
      leg T84.629 ☑
        femur T84.62- ☑
        fibula T84.62- ☑

Complication(s) — *continued*
  fixation device, internal — *continued*
    infection and inflammation — *continued*
      leg — *continued*
        tibia T84.62- ☑
      specified site NEC T84.89 ☑
      spine T84.63 ☑
    mechanical
      breakdown
        limb T84.119 ☑
          carpal T84.210 ☑
          femur T84.11- ☑
          fibula T84.11- ☑
          humerus T84.11- ☑
          metacarpal T84.210 ☑
          metatarsal T84.213 ☑
          phalanx
            foot T84.213 ☑
            hand T84.210 ☑
          radius T84.11- ☑
          tarsal T84.213 ☑
          tibia T84.11- ☑
          ulna T84.11- ☑
        specified bone NEC T84.218 ☑
        spine T84.216 ☑
      displacement
        limb T84.129 ☑
          carpal T84.220 ☑
          femur T84.12- ☑
          fibula T84.12- ☑
          humerus T84.12- ☑
          metacarpal T84.220 ☑
          metatarsal T84.223 ☑
          phalanx
            foot T84.223 ☑
            hand T84.220 ☑
          radius T84.12- ☑
          tarsal T84.223 ☑
          tibia T84.12- ☑
          ulna T84.12- ☑
        specified bone NEC T84.228 ☑
        spine T84.226 ☑
      malposition — *see* Complications, fixation device, internal, mechanical, displacement
      obstruction — *see* Complications, fixation device, internal, mechanical, specified type NEC
      perforation — *see* Complications, fixation device, internal, mechanical, specified type NEC
      protrusion — *see* Complications, fixation device, internal, mechanical, specified type NEC
      specified type NEC
        limb T84.199 ☑
          carpal T84.290 ☑
          femur T84.19- ☑
          fibula T84.19- ☑
          humerus T84.19- ☑
          metacarpal T84.290 ☑
          metatarsal T84.293 ☑
          phalanx
            foot T84.293 ☑
            hand T84.290 ☑
          radius T84.19- ☑
          tarsal T84.293 ☑
          tibia T84.19- ☑
          ulna T84.19- ☑
        specified bone NEC T84.298 ☑
        vertebra T84.296 ☑
    specified type NEC T84.89 ☑
      embolism T84.81 ☑
      fibrosis T84.82 ☑
      hemorrhage T84.83 ☑
      pain T84.84 ☑
      specified complication NEC T84.89 ☑
      stenosis T84.85 ☑
      thrombosis T84.86 ☑
  following
    acute myocardial infarction NEC I23.8
      aneurysm (false) (of cardiac wall) (of heart wall) (ruptured) I23.3
      angina I23.7
      atrial
        septal defect I23.1
        thrombosis I23.6
      cardiac wall rupture I23.3
      chordae tendinae rupture I23.4

Complication(s) — *continued*
  following — *continued*
    acute myocardial infarction — *continued*
      defect
        septal
          atrial (heart) I23.1
          ventricular (heart) I23.2
      hemopericardium I23.0
      papillary muscle rupture I23.5
      rupture
        cardiac wall I23.3
          with hemopericardium I23.0
        chordae tendineae I23.4
        papillary muscle I23.5
      specified NEC I23.8
      thrombosis
        atrium I23.6
        auricular appendage I23.6
        ventricle (heart) I23.6
      ventricular
        septal defect I23.2
        thrombosis I23.6
    ectopic or molar pregnancy O08.9
      cardiac arrest O08.81
      sepsis O08.82
      specified type NEC O08.89
      urinary tract infection O08.83
    termination of pregnancy — *see* Abortion
  gastrointestinal K92.9
    bile duct prosthesis — *see* Complications, bile duct implant
    esophageal anti-reflux device — *see* Complications, esophageal anti-reflux device
    postoperative
      colostomy — *see* Complications, colostomy
      dumping syndrome K91.1
      enterostomy — *see* Complications, enterostomy
      gastrostomy — *see* Complications, gastrostomy
      malabsorption NEC K91.2
      obstruction — *see also* Obstruction, intestine, postoperative K91.30
      postcholecystectomy syndrome K91.5
      specified NEC K91.89
      vomiting after GI surgery K91.0
    prosthetic device or implant
      bile duct prosthesis — *see* Complications, bile duct implant
      esophageal anti-reflux device — *see* Complications, esophageal anti-reflux device
      specified type NEC
        embolism T85.818 ☑
        fibrosis T85.828 ☑
        hemorrhage T85.838 ☑
        mechanical
          breakdown T85.518 ☑
          displacement T85.528 ☑
          malfunction T85.518 ☑
          malposition T85.528 ☑
          obstruction T85.598 ☑
          perforation T85.598 ☑
          protrusion T85.598 ☑
          specified NEC T85.598 ☑
        pain T85.848 ☑
        specified complication NEC T85.898 ☑
        stenosis T85.858 ☑
        thrombosis T85.868 ☑
  gastrostomy (stoma) K94.20
    hemorrhage K94.21
    infection K94.22
    malfunction K94.23
    mechanical K94.23
    specified complication NEC K94.29
  genitourinary
    device or implant T83.9 ☑
      genital tract T83.9 ☑
        infection or inflammation T83.69 ☑
        intrauterine contraceptive device — *see* Complications, intrauterine, contraceptive device
        mechanical — *see* Complications, by device, mechanical
        mesh — *see* Complications, prosthetic device or implant, mesh
        penile prosthesis — *see* Complications, prosthetic device, penile
        specified type NEC T83.89 ☑
          embolism T83.81 ☑

Complication(s) — *continued*
  genitourinary — *continued*
    device or implant — *continued*
      genital tract — *continued*
        specified type — *continued*
          fibrosis T83.82 ☑
          hemorrhage T83.83 ☑
          pain T83.84 ☑
          specified complication NEC T83.89 ☑
          stenosis T83.85 ☑
          thrombosis T83.86 ☑
        vaginal mesh — *see* Complications, prosthetic device or implant, mesh
      urinary system T83.9 ☑
        cystostomy catheter — *see* Complication, catheter, cystostomy
        electronic stimulator — *see* Complications, electronic stimulator device, urinary
        indwelling urethral catheter — *see* Complications, catheter, urethral, indwelling
        infection or inflammation T83.598 ☑
          indwelling urethral catheter T83.511 ☑
        kidney transplant — *see* Complication, transplant, kidney
        organ graft — *see* Complication, graft, urinary organ
        specified type NEC T83.89 ☑
          embolism T83.81 ☑
          fibrosis T83.82 ☑
          hemorrhage T83.83 ☑
          mechanical T83.198 ☑
            breakdown T83.118 ☑
            displacement T83.128 ☑
            malfunction T83.118 ☑
            malposition T83.128 ☑
            obstruction T83.198 ☑
            perforation T83.198 ☑
            protrusion T83.198 ☑
            specified NEC T83.198 ☑
          sphincter implant — *see* Complications, implant, urinary sphincter
          sphincter, implanted T83.191 ☑
          stent (ileal conduit) (nephroureteral) T83.193 ☑
          pain T83.84 ☑
          specified complication NEC T83.89 ☑
          stenosis T83.85 ☑
          thrombosis T83.86 ☑
          ureteral indwelling T83.192 ☑
    postprocedural
      pelvic peritoneal adhesions N99.4
      renal failure N99.0
      specified NEC N99.89
      stoma — *see* Complications, stoma, urinary tract
      urethral stricture — *see* Stricture, urethra, postprocedural
      vaginal
        adhesions N99.2
        vault prolapse N99.3
  graft (bypass) (patch) — *see also* Complications, prosthetic device or implant
    aorta — *see* Complications, graft, vascular
    arterial — *see* Complication, graft, vascular
    bone T86.839
      failure T86.831
      infection T86.832
      mechanical T84.318 ☑
        breakdown T84.318 ☑
        displacement T84.328 ☑
        protrusion T84.398 ☑
        specified type NEC T84.398 ☑
      rejection T86.830
      specified type NEC T86.838
    carotid artery — *see* Complications, graft, vascular
    cornea T86.849- ☑
      failure T86.841- ☑
      infection T86.842- ☑
      mechanical T85.398 ☑
        breakdown T85.318 ☑
        displacement T85.328 ☑
        protrusion T85.398 ☑
        specified type NEC T85.398 ☑
      rejection T86.840- ☑
      retroprosthetic membrane T85.398 ☑
      specified type NEC T86.848- ☑
    femoral artery (bypass) — *see* Complication, extremity artery (bypass) graft

Complication(s) — *continued*
  graft — *see also* Complications, prosthetic device or
    implant — *continued*
    genital organ or tract — *see* Complications, geni-
      tourinary, device or implant, genital tract
    muscle T84.9 ☑
      breakdown T84.410 ☑
      displacement T84.420 ☑
      embolism T84.81 ☑
      fibrosis T84.82 ☑
      hemorrhage T84.83 ☑
      infection and inflammation T84.7 ☑
      mechanical NEC T84.490 ☑
      pain T84.84 ☑
      specified type NEC T84.89 ☑
      stenosis T84.85 ☑
      thrombosis T84.86 ☑
    nerve — *see* Complication, prosthetic device or im-
      plant, specified NEC
    skin — *see* Complications, prosthetic device or im-
      plant, skin graft
    tendon T84.9 ☑
      breakdown T84.410 ☑
      displacement T84.420 ☑
      embolism T84.81 ☑
      fibrosis T84.82 ☑
      hemorrhage T84.83 ☑
      infection and inflammation T84.7 ☑
      mechanical NEC T84.490 ☑
      pain T84.84 ☑
      specified type NEC T84.89 ☑
      stenosis T84.85 ☑
      thrombosis T84.86 ☑
    urinary organ T83.9 ☑
      embolism T83.81 ☑
      fibrosis T83.82 ☑
      hemorrhage T83.83 ☑
      infection and inflammation T83.598 ☑
        indwelling urethral catheter T83.511 ☑
      mechanical
        breakdown T83.21 ☑
        displacement T83.22 ☑
        erosion T83.24 ☑
        exposure T83.25 ☑
        leakage T83.23 ☑
        malposition T83.22 ☑
        obstruction T83.29 ☑
        perforation T83.29 ☑
        protrusion T83.29 ☑
        specified NEC T83.29 ☑
      pain T83.84 ☑
      specified type NEC T83.89 ☑
      stenosis T83.85 ☑
      thrombosis T83.86 ☑
    vascular T82.9 ☑
      embolism T82.818 ☑
      femoral artery — *see* Complication, extremity
        artery (bypass) graft
      fibrosis T82.828 ☑
      hemorrhage T82.838 ☑
      mechanical
        breakdown T82.319 ☑
          aorta (bifurcation) T82.310 ☑
          carotid artery T82.311 ☑
          specified vessel NEC T82.318 ☑
        displacement T82.329 ☑
          aorta (bifurcation) T82.320 ☑
          carotid artery T82.321 ☑
          specified vessel NEC T82.328 ☑
        leakage T82.339 ☑
          aorta (bifurcation) T82.330 ☑
          carotid artery T82.331 ☑
          specified vessel NEC T82.338 ☑
        malposition T82.329 ☑
          aorta (bifurcation) T82.320 ☑
          carotid artery T82.321 ☑
          specified vessel NEC T82.328 ☑
        obstruction T82.399 ☑
          aorta (bifurcation) T82.390 ☑
          carotid artery T82.391 ☑
          specified vessel NEC T82.398 ☑
        perforation T82.399 ☑
          aorta (bifurcation) T82.390 ☑
          carotid artery T82.391 ☑
          specified vessel NEC T82.398 ☑
        protrusion T82.399 ☑

Complication(s) — *continued*
  graft — *see also* Complications, prosthetic device or
    implant — *continued*
    vascular — *continued*
      mechanical — *continued*
        protrusion — *continued*
          aorta (bifurcation) T82.390 ☑
          carotid artery T82.391 ☑
          specified vessel NEC T82.398 ☑
        pain T82.848 ☑
        specified complication NEC T82.898 ☑
        stenosis T82.858 ☑
        thrombosis T82.868 ☑
  heart I51.9
    assist device
      infection and inflammation T82.7 ☑
    following acute myocardial infarction — *see* Com-
      plications, following, acute myocardial infarc-
      tion
    postoperative — *see* Complications, circulatory
      system
    transplant — *see* Complication, transplant, heart
      and lung(s) — *see* Complications, transplant,
      heart, with lung
    valve
      graft (biological) T82.9 ☑
        embolism T82.817 ☑
        fibrosis T82.827 ☑
        hemorrhage T82.837 ☑
        infection and inflammation T82.7 ☑
        mechanical T82.228 ☑
          breakdown T82.221 ☑
          displacement T82.222 ☑
          leakage T82.223 ☑
          malposition T82.222 ☑
          obstruction T82.228 ☑
          perforation T82.228 ☑
          protrusion T82.228 ☑
        pain T82.847 ☑
        specified type NEC T82.897 ☑
        stenosis T82.857 ☑
        thrombosis T82.867 ☑
      prosthesis T82.9 ☑
        embolism T82.817 ☑
        fibrosis T82.827 ☑
        hemorrhage T82.837 ☑
        infection or inflammation T82.6 ☑
        mechanical T82.09 ☑
          breakdown T82.01 ☑
          displacement T82.02 ☑
          leakage T82.03 ☑
          malposition T82.02 ☑
          obstruction T82.09 ☑
          perforation T82.09 ☑
          protrusion T82.09 ☑
        pain T82.847 ☑
        specified type NEC T82.897 ☑
          mechanical T82.09 ☑
        stenosis T82.857 ☑
        thrombosis T82.867 ☑
  hematoma
    intraoperative — *see* Complication, intraoperative,
      hemorrhage
    postprocedural — *see* Complication, postprocedu-
      ral, hematoma
  hemodialysis — *see* Complications, dialysis
  hemorrhage
    intraoperative — *see* Complication, intraoperative,
      hemorrhage
    postprocedural — *see* Complication, postprocedu-
      ral, hemorrhage
  IEC (immune effector cellular) therapy T80.82 ☑
  ileostomy (stoma) — *see* Complications, enterostomy
  immune effector cellular (IEC) therapy T80.82 ☑
  immunization (procedure) — *see* Complications, vacci-
    nation
  implant — *see also* Complications, by site and type
    urinary sphincter T83.9 ☑
      embolism T83.81 ☑
      fibrosis T83.82 ☑
      hemorrhage T83.83 ☑
      infection and inflammation T83.591 ☑
      mechanical
        breakdown T83.111 ☑
        displacement T83.121 ☑
        leakage T83.191 ☑

Complication(s) — *continued*
  implant — *see also* Complications, by site and type —
    continued
    urinary sphincter — *continued*
      mechanical — *continued*
        malposition T83.121 ☑
        obstruction T83.191 ☑
        perforation T83.191 ☑
        protrusion T83.191 ☑
        specified NEC T83.191 ☑
      pain T83.84 ☑
      specified type NEC T83.89 ☑
      stenosis T83.85 ☑
      thrombosis T83.86 ☑
  infusion (procedure) T80.90 ☑
    air embolism T80.0 ☑
    blood — *see* Complications, transfusion
    catheter — *see* Complications, catheter
    infection T80.29 ☑
    pump — *see* Complications, cardiovascular, device
      or implant
    sepsis T80.29 ☑
    serum reaction — *see also* Reaction, serum
      T80.69 ☑
      anaphylactic shock — *see also* Shock, anaphylac-
        tic T80.59 ☑
    specified type NEC T80.89 ☑
  inhalation therapy NEC T81.81 ☑
  injection (procedure) T80.90 ☑
    drug reaction — *see* Reaction, drug
    infection T80.29 ☑
    sepsis T80.29 ☑
    serum (prophylactic) (therapeutic) — *see* Complica-
      tions, vaccination
    specified type NEC T80.89 ☑
    vaccine (any) — *see* Complications, vaccination
  inoculation (any) — *see* Complications, vaccination
  insulin pump
    infection and inflammation T85.72 ☑
    mechanical
      breakdown T85.614 ☑
      displacement T85.624 ☑
      leakage T85.633 ☑
      malposition T85.624 ☑
      obstruction T85.694 ☑
      perforation T85.694 ☑
      protrusion T85.694 ☑
      specified NEC T85.694 ☑
  intestinal pouch NEC K91.858
  intraocular lens (prosthetic) T85.9 ☑
    embolism T85.818 ☑
    fibrosis T85.828 ☑
    hemorrhage T85.838 ☑
    infection and inflammation T85.79 ☑
    mechanical
      breakdown T85.21 ☑
      displacement T85.22 ☑
      malposition T85.22 ☑
      obstruction T85.29 ☑
      perforation T85.29 ☑
      protrusion T85.29 ☑
      specified NEC T85.29 ☑
    pain T85.848 ☑
    specified type NEC T85.898 ☑
    stenosis T85.858 ☑
    thrombosis T85.868 ☑
  intraoperative (intraprocedural)
    cardiac arrest — *see also* Infarct, myocardium, asso-
      ciated with revascularization procedure
      during cardiac surgery I97.710
      during other surgery I97.711
    cardiac functional disturbance NEC — *see also* In-
      farct, myocardium, associated with revascular-
      ization procedure
      during cardiac surgery I97.790
      during other surgery I97.791
    hemorrhage (hematoma) (of)
      circulatory system organ or structure
        during cardiac bypass I97.411
        during cardiac catheterization I97.410
        during other circulatory system procedure
          I97.418
        during other procedure I97.42
      digestive system organ
        during procedure on digestive system K91.61
        during procedure on other organ K91.62

Complication(s) — *continued*
intraoperative — *continued*
  hemorrhage — *continued*
    ear
      during procedure on ear and mastoid process H95.21
      during procedure on other organ H95.22
    endocrine system organ or structure
      during procedure on endocrine system organ or structure E36.01
      during procedure on other organ E36.02
    eye and adnexa
      during ophthalmic procedure H59.11- ☑
      during other procedure H59.12- ☑
    genitourinary organ or structure
      during procedure on genitourinary organ or structure N99.61
      during procedure on other organ N99.62
    mastoid process
      during procedure on ear and mastoid process H95.21
      during procedure on other organ H95.22
    musculoskeletal structure
      during musculoskeletal surgery M96.810
      during non-orthopedic surgery M96.811
      during orthopedic surgery M96.810
    nervous system
      during a nervous system procedure G97.31
      during other procedure G97.32
    respiratory system
      during other procedure J95.62
      during procedure on respiratory system organ or structure J95.61
    skin and subcutaneous tissue
      during a dermatologic procedure L76.01
      during a procedure on other organ L76.02
    spleen
      during a procedure on other organ D78.02
      during a procedure on the spleen D78.01
  puncture or laceration (accidental) (unintentional) (of)
    brain
      during a nervous system procedure G97.48
      during other procedure G97.49
    circulatory system organ or structure
      during circulatory system procedure I97.51
      during other procedure I97.52
    digestive system
      during procedure on digestive system K91.71
      during procedure on other organ K91.72
    ear
      during procedure on ear and mastoid process H95.31
      during procedure on other organ H95.32
    endocrine system organ or structure
      during procedure on endocrine system organ or structure E36.11
      during procedure on other organ E36.12
    eye and adnexa
      during ophthalmic procedure H59.21- ☑
      during other procedure H59.22- ☑
    genitourinary organ or structure
      during procedure on genitourinary organ or structure N99.71
      during procedure on other organ N99.72
    mastoid process
      during procedure on ear and mastoid process H95.31
      during procedure on other organ H95.32
    musculoskeletal structure
      during musculoskeletal surgery M96.820
      during non-orthopedic surgery M96.821
      during orthopedic surgery M96.820
    nervous system
      during a nervous system procedure G97.48
      during other procedure G97.49
    respiratory system
      during other procedure J95.72
      during procedure on respiratory system organ or structure J95.71
    skin and subcutaneous tissue
      during a dermatologic procedure L76.11
      during a procedure on other organ L76.12
    spleen
      during a procedure on other organ D78.12
      during a procedure on the spleen D78.11
  specified NEC
    circulatory system I97.88
    digestive system K91.81

Complication(s) — *continued*
intraoperative — *continued*
  specified — *continued*
    ear H95.88
    endocrine system E36.8
    eye and adnexa H59.88
    genitourinary system N99.81
    mastoid process H95.88
    musculoskeletal structure M96.89
    nervous system G97.81
    respiratory system J95.88
    skin and subcutaneous tissue L76.81
    spleen D78.81
intraperitoneal catheter (dialysis) (infusion) — *see* Complication(s), catheter, intraperitoneal dialysis
intrathecal infusion pump
  infection and inflammation T85.738 ☑
  mechanical
    breakdown T85.615 ☑
    displacement T85.625 ☑
    leakage T85.635 ☑
    malfunction T85.695 ☑
    malposition T85.625 ☑
    obstruction T85.695 ☑
    perforation T85.695 ☑
    protrusion T85.695 ☑
    specified NEC T85.695 ☑
intrauterine
  contraceptive device
    embolism T83.81 ☑
    fibrosis T83.82 ☑
    hemorrhage T83.83 ☑
    infection and inflammation T83.69 ☑
    mechanical
      breakdown T83.31 ☑
      displacement T83.32 ☑
      malposition T83.32 ☑
      obstruction T83.39 ☑
      perforation T83.39 ☑
      protrusion T83.39 ☑
      specified NEC T83.39 ☑
    pain T83.84 ☑
    specified type NEC T83.89 ☑
    stenosis T83.85 ☑
    thrombosis T83.86 ☑
  procedure (fetal), to newborn P96.5
jejunostomy (stoma) — *see* Complications, enterostomy
joint prosthesis, internal T84.9 ☑
  breakage (fracture) T84.01- ☑
  dislocation T84.02- ☑
  fracture T84.01- ☑
  infection or inflammation T84.50 ☑
    hip T84.5- ☑
    knee T84.5- ☑
    specified joint NEC T84.59 ☑
  instability T84.02- ☑
  malposition — *see* Complications, joint prosthesis, mechanical, displacement
  mechanical
    breakage, broken T84.01- ☑
    dislocation T84.02- ☑
    fracture T84.01- ☑
    instability T84.02- ☑
    leakage — *see* Complications, joint prosthesis, mechanical, specified NEC
    loosening T84.039 ☑
      hip T84.03- ☑
      knee T84.03- ☑
      specified joint NEC T84.038 ☑
    obstruction — *see* Complications, joint prosthesis, mechanical, specified NEC
    perforation — *see* Complications, joint prosthesis, mechanical, specified NEC
    osteolysis T84.059 ☑
      hip T84.05- ☑
      knee T84.05- ☑
      other specified joint T84.058 ☑
    periprosthetic osteolysis, by site T84.05- ☑
    protrusion — *see* Complications, joint prosthesis, mechanical, specified NEC
    specified complication NEC T84.099 ☑
      hip T84.09- ☑
      knee T84.09- ☑
      other specified joint T84.098 ☑
    subluxation T84.02- ☑

Complication(s) — *continued*
joint prosthesis, internal — *continued*
  mechanical — *continued*
    wear of articular bearing surface T84.069 ☑
      hip T84.06- ☑
      knee T84.06- ☑
      other specified joint T84.068 ☑
    specified joint NEC T84.89 ☑
      embolism T84.81 ☑
      fibrosis T84.82 ☑
      hemorrhage T84.83 ☑
      pain T84.84 ☑
      specified complication NEC T84.89 ☑
      stenosis T84.85 ☑
      thrombosis T84.86 ☑
    subluxation T84.02- ☑
kidney transplant — *see* Complications, transplant, kidney
labor O75.9
  specified NEC O75.89
liver transplant (immune or nonimmune) — *see* Complications, transplant, liver
lumbar puncture G97.1
  cerebrospinal fluid leak G97.0
  headache or reaction G97.1
lung transplant — *see* Complications, transplant, lung and heart — *see* Complications, transplant, lung, with heart
male genital N50.9
  device, implant or graft — *see* Complications, genitourinary, device or implant, genital tract
  postprocedural or postoperative — *see* Complications, genitourinary, postprocedural
  specified NEC N99.89
mastoid (process) procedure
  intraoperative H95.88
    hematoma — *see* Complications, intraoperative, hemorrhage (hematoma) (of), mastoid process
    hemorrhage — *see* Complications, intraoperative, hemorrhage (hematoma) (of), mastoid process
    laceration — *see* Complications, intraoperative, puncture or laceration, mastoid process
    specified NEC H95.88
  postmastoidectomy — *see* Complications, postmastoidectomy
  postoperative H95.89
    external ear canal stenosis H95.81 ☑
    hematoma — *see* Complications, postprocedural, hematoma (of), mastoid process
    hemorrhage — *see* Complications, postprocedural, hemorrhage (of), mastoid process
    postmastoidectomy — *see* Complications, postmastoidectomy
    seroma — *see* Complications, postprocedural, seroma (of), mastoid process
    specified NEC H95.89
mastoidectomy cavity — *see* Complications, postmastoidectomy
mechanical — *see* Complications, by site and type, mechanical
medical procedures — *see also* Complication(s), intraoperative T88.9 ☑
metabolic E88.9
  postoperative E89.89
    specified NEC E89.89
molar pregnancy NOS O08.9
  damage to pelvic organs O08.6
  embolism O08.2
  genital infection O08.0
  hemorrhage (delayed) (excessive) O08.1
  metabolic disorder O08.5
  renal failure O08.4
  shock O08.3
  specified type NEC O08.0
  venous complication NEC O08.7
musculoskeletal system — *see also* Complication, intraoperative (intraprocedural), by site
  device, implant or graft NEC — *see* Complications, orthopedic, device or implant
  internal fixation (nail) (plate) (rod) — *see* Complications, fixation device, internal
  joint prosthesis — *see* Complications, joint prosthesis
  post radiation M96.89
    kyphosis M96.2

☑ Additional Character Required — Refer to the Tabular List for Character Selection

Complication(s) — *continued*
  musculoskeletal system — *see also* Complication, intra-
      operative, by site — *continued*
    post radiation — *continued*
      scoliosis M96.5
      specified complication NEC M96.89
    postoperative (postprocedural) M96.89
      with osteoporosis — *see* Osteoporosis
      fracture following insertion of device — *see*
          Fracture, following insertion of orthopedic
          implant, joint prosthesis or bone plate
      joint instability after prosthesis removal M96.89
      lordosis M96.4
      postlaminectomy syndrome NEC M96.1
          kyphosis M96.3
      pseudarthrosis M96.0
      specified complication NEC M96.89
  nephrostomy (stoma) — *see* Complications, stoma,
      urinary tract, external NEC
  nervous system G98.8
    central G96.9
      device, implant or graft — *see also* Complication,
          prosthetic device or implant, specified NEC
      electronic stimulator (electrode(s)) — *see* Com-
          plications, electronic stimulator device
      specified NEC
          infection and inflammation T85.738 ☑
          mechanical T85.695 ☑
              breakdown T85.615 ☑
              displacement T85.625 ☑
              leakage T85.635 ☑
              malfunction T85.695 ☑
              malposition T85.625 ☑
              obstruction T85.695 ☑
              perforation T85.695 ☑
              protrusion T85.695 ☑
              specified NEC T85.695 ☑
      ventricular shunt — *see* Complications, ventricu-
          lar shunt
    electronic stimulator (electrode(s)) — *see* Complica-
        tions, electronic stimulator device
    postprocedural G97.82
        intracranial hypotension G97.2
        specified NEC G97.82
        spinal fluid leak G97.0
  newborn, due to intrauterine (fetal) procedure P96.5
  nonabsorbable (permanent) sutures — *see* Complica-
      tion, sutures, permanent
  obstetric O75.9
    procedure (instrumental) (manual) (surgical) speci-
        fied NEC O75.4
    specified NEC O75.89
    surgical wound NEC O90.89
        hematoma O90.2
        infection O86.00
  ocular lens implant — *see* Complications, intraocular
      lens
  ophthalmologic
    postprocedural bleb — *see* Blebitis
  orbital prosthesis T85.9 ☑
    embolism T85.818 ☑
    fibrosis T85.828 ☑
    hemorrhage T85.838 ☑
    infection and inflammation T85.79 ☑
    mechanical
        breakdown T85.31- ☑
        displacement T85.32- ☑
        malposition T85.32- ☑
        obstruction T85.39- ☑
        perforation T85.39- ☑
        protrusion T85.39- ☑
        specified NEC T85.39- ☑
    pain T85.848 ☑
    specified type NEC T85.898 ☑
    stenosis T85.858 ☑
    thrombosis T85.868 ☑
  organ or tissue transplant (partial) (total) — *see* Com-
      plications, transplant
  orthopedic — *see also* Disorder, soft tissue
    device or implant T84.9 ☑
        bone
            device or implant — *see* Complication, bone,
                device NEC
            graft — *see* Complication, graft, bone
            breakdown T84.418 ☑
            displacement T84.428 ☑

Complication(s) — *continued*
  orthopedic — *see also* Disorder, soft tissue — *contin-
      ued*
    device or implant — *continued*
        electronic bone stimulator — *see* Complications,
            electronic stimulator device, bone
        embolism T84.81 ☑
        fibrosis T84.82 ☑
        fixation device — *see* Complication, fixation de-
            vice, internal
        hemorrhage T84.83 ☑
        infection or inflammation T84.7 ☑
        joint prosthesis — *see* Complication, joint pros-
            thesis, internal
        malfunction T84.418 ☑
        malposition T84.428 ☑
        mechanical NEC T84.498 ☑
        muscle graft — *see* Complications, graft, muscle
        obstruction T84.498 ☑
        pain T84.84 ☑
        perforation T84.498 ☑
        protrusion T84.498 ☑
        specified complication NEC T84.89 ☑
        stenosis T84.85 ☑
        tendon graft — *see* Complications, graft, tendon
        thrombosis T84.86 ☑
    fracture (following insertion of device) — *see* Frac-
        ture, following insertion of orthopedic im-
        plant, joint prosthesis or bone plate
    postprocedural M96.89
        fracture — *see* Fracture, following insertion of
            orthopedic implant, joint prosthesis or
            bone plate
        postlaminectomy syndrome NEC M96.1
            kyphosis M96.3
            lordosis M96.4
        postradiation
            kyphosis M96.2
            scoliosis M96.5
        pseudarthrosis post-fusion M96.0
        specified type NEC M96.89
  pacemaker (cardiac) — *see* Complications, cardiovas-
      cular device or implant, electronic
  pancreas transplant — *see* Complications, transplant,
      pancreas
  penile prosthesis (implant) — *see* Complications,
      prosthetic device, penile
  perfusion NEC T80.90 ☑
  perineal repair (obstetrical) NEC O90.89
    disruption O90.1
    hematoma O90.2
    infection (following delivery) O86.09
  phototherapy T88.9 ☑
    specified NEC T88.8 ☑
  postmastoidectomy NEC H95.19- ☑
    cyst, mucosal H95.13- ☑
    granulation H95.12- ☑
    inflammation, chronic H95.11- ☑
    recurrent cholesteatoma H95.0- ☑
  postoperative — *see* Complications, postprocedural
    circulatory — *see* Complications, circulatory system
    ear — *see* Complications, ear
    endocrine — *see* Complications, endocrine
    eye — *see* Complications, eye
    lumbar puncture G97.1
        cerebrospinal fluid leak G97.0
    nervous system (central) (peripheral) — *see* Compli-
        cations, nervous system
    respiratory system — *see* Complications, respiratory
        system
  postprocedural — *see also* Complications, surgical
      procedure
    cardiac arrest — *see also* Infarct, myocardium, asso-
        ciated with revascularization procedure
        following cardiac surgery I97.120
        following other surgery I97.121
    cardiac functional disturbance NEC — *see also* In-
        farct, myocardium, associated with revascular-
        ization procedure
        following cardiac surgery I97.190
        following other surgery I97.191
    cardiac insufficiency
        following cardiac surgery I97.110
        following other surgery I97.111
    chorioretinal scars following retinal surgery
        H59.81- ☑

Complication(s) — *continued*
  postprocedural — *see also* Complications, surgical
      procedure — *continued*
    following cataract surgery
        cataract (lens) fragments H59.02- ☑
        cystoid macular edema H59.03- ☑
        specified NEC H59.09- ☑
        vitreous (touch) syndrome H59.01- ☑
    heart failure
        following cardiac surgery I97.130
        following other surgery I97.131
    hematoma (of)
        circulatory system organ or structure
            following cardiac bypass I97.631
            following cardiac catheterization I97.630
            following other circulatory system procedure
                I97.638
            following other procedure I97.621
        digestive system
            following procedure on digestive system
                K91.870
            following procedure on other organ K91.871
        ear
            following other procedure H95.52
            following procedure on ear and mastoid pro-
                cess H95.51
        endocrine system
            following endocrine system procedure
                E89.820
            following other procedure E89.821
        eye and adnexa
            following ophthalmic procedure H59.33- ☑
            following other procedure H59.34- ☑
        genitourinary organ or structure
            following procedure on genitourinary organ
                or structure N99.840
            following procedure on other organ N99.841
        mastoid process
            following other procedure H95.52
            following procedure on ear and mastoid pro-
                cess H95.51
        musculoskeletal structure
            following musculoskeletal surgery M96.840
            following non-orthopedic surgery M96.841
            following orthopedic surgery M96.840
        nervous system
            following nervous system procedure G97.61
            following other procedure G97.62
        respiratory system
            following other procedure J95.861
            following procedure on respiratory system
                organ or structure J95.860
        skin and subcutaneous tissue
            following dermatologic procedure L76.31
            following procedure on other organ L76.32
        spleen
            following procedure on other organ D78.32
            following procedure on the spleen D78.31
    hemorrhage (of)
        circulatory system organ or structure
            following cardiac bypass I97.611
            following cardiac catheterization I97.610
            following other circulatory system procedure
                I97.618
            following other procedure I97.620
        digestive system
            following procedure on digestive system
                K91.840
            following procedure on other organ K91.841
        ear
            following other procedure H95.42
            following procedure on ear and mastoid pro-
                cess H95.41
        endocrine system
            following endocrine system procedure
                E89.810
            following other procedure E89.811
        eye and adnexa
            following ophthalmic procedure H59.31- ☑
            following other procedure H59.32- ☑
        genitourinary organ or structure
            following procedure on genitourinary organ
                or structure N99.820
            following procedure on other organ N99.821
        mastoid process
            following other procedure H95.42
            following procedure on ear and mastoid pro-
                cess H95.41

Complication(s) — *continued*
- postprocedural — *see also* Complications, surgical procedure — *continued*
  - hemorrhage — *continued*
    - musculoskeletal structure
      - following musculoskeletal surgery M96.830
      - following non-orthopedic surgery M96.831
      - following orthopedic surgery M96.830
    - nervous system
      - following nervous system procedure G97.51
      - following other procedure G97.52
    - respiratory system
      - following a respiratory system procedure J95.830
      - following other procedure J95.831
    - skin and subcutaneous tissue
      - following a procedure on other organ L76.22
      - following dermatologic procedure L76.21
    - spleen
      - following procedure on other organ D78.22
      - following procedure on the spleen D78.21
  - seroma (of)
    - circulatory system organ or structure
      - following cardiac bypass I97.641
      - following cardiac catheterization I97.640
      - following other circulatory system procedure I97.648
      - following other procedure I97.622
    - digestive system
      - following procedure on digestive system K91.872
      - following procedure on other organ K91.873
    - ear
      - following other procedure H95.54
      - following procedure on ear and mastoid process H95.53
    - endocrine system
      - following endocrine system procedure E89.822
      - following other procedure E89.823
    - eye and adnexa
      - following ophthalmic procedure H59.35-
      - following other procedure H59.36-
    - genitourinary organ or structure
      - following procedure on genitourinary organ or structure N99.842
      - following procedure on other organ N99.843
    - mastoid process
      - following other procedure H95.54
      - following procedure on ear and mastoid process H95.53
    - musculoskeletal structure
      - following musculoskeletal surgery M96.842
      - following non-orthopedic surgery M96.843
      - following orthopedic surgery M96.842
    - nervous system
      - following nervous system procedure G97.63
      - following other procedure G97.64
    - respiratory system
      - following other procedure J95.863
      - following procedure on respiratory system organ or structure J95.862
    - skin and subcutaneous tissue
      - following dermatologic procedure L76.33
      - following procedure on other organ L76.34
    - spleen
      - following procedure on other organ D78.34
      - following procedure on the spleen D78.33
  - specified NEC
    - circulatory system I97.89
    - digestive K91.89
    - ear H95.89
    - endocrine E89.89
    - eye and adnexa H59.89
    - genitourinary N99.89
    - mastoid process H95.89
    - metabolic E89.89
    - musculoskeletal structure M96.89
    - nervous system G97.82
    - respiratory system J95.89
    - skin and subcutaneous tissue L76.82
    - spleen D78.89
- pregnancy NEC — *see* Pregnancy, complicated by
- prosthetic device or implant T85.9
  - bile duct — *see* Complications, bile duct implant
  - breast — *see* Complications, breast implant

Complication(s) — *continued*
- prosthetic device or implant — *continued*
  - bulking agent
    - ureteral
      - erosion T83.714
      - exposure T83.724
    - urethral
      - erosion T83.713
      - exposure T83.723
  - cardiac and vascular NEC — *see* Complications, cardiovascular device or implant
  - corneal transplant — *see* Complications, graft, cornea
  - electronic nervous system stimulator — *see* Complications, electronic stimulator device
  - epidural infusion catheter — *see* Complications, catheter, epidural
  - esophageal anti-reflux device — *see* Complications, esophageal anti-reflux device
  - genital organ or tract — *see* Complications, genitourinary, device or implant, genital tract
    - specified NEC T83.79-
  - heart valve — *see* Complications, heart, valve, prosthesis
  - infection or inflammation T85.79
    - intestine transplant T86.852
    - liver transplant T86.43
    - lung transplant T86.812
    - pancreas transplant T86.892
    - skin graft T86.822
  - intraocular lens — *see* Complications, intraocular lens
  - intraperitoneal (dialysis) catheter — *see* Complication(s), catheter, intraperitoneal dialysis
  - joint — *see* Complications, joint prosthesis, internal
  - mechanical NEC T85.698
    - dialysis catheter (vascular) — *see also* Complication, catheter, dialysis, mechanical
      - peritoneal — *see* Complication(s), catheter, intraperitoneal dialysis
    - gastrointestinal device T85.598
    - ocular device T85.398
    - subdural (infusion) catheter T85.690
    - suture, permanent T85.692
      - that for bone repair — *see* Complications, fixation device, internal (orthopedic), mechanical
    - ventricular shunt
      - breakdown T85.01
      - displacement T85.02
      - leakage T85.03
      - malposition T85.02
      - obstruction T85.09
      - perforation T85.09
      - protrusion T85.09
      - specified NEC T85.09
    - mesh
      - erosion (to surrounding organ or tissue) T83.718
        - urethral (into pelvic floor muscles) T83.712
        - vaginal (into pelvic floor muscles) T83.711
      - exposure (into surrounding organ or tissue) T83.728
        - urethral (through urethral wall) T83.722
        - vaginal (into vagina) (through vaginal wall) T83.721
    - orbital — *see* Complications, orbital prosthesis
    - penile T83.9
      - embolism T83.81
      - fibrosis T83.82
      - hemorrhage T83.83
      - infection and inflammation T83.61
      - mechanical
        - breakdown T83.410
        - displacement T83.420
        - leakage T83.490
        - malposition T83.420
        - obstruction T83.490
        - perforation T83.490
        - protrusion T83.490
        - specified NEC T83.490
      - pain T83.84
      - specified type NEC T83.89
      - stenosis T83.85
      - thrombosis T83.86

Complication(s) — *continued*
- prosthetic device or implant — *continued*
  - prosthetic materials NEC
    - erosion (to surrounding organ or tissue) T83.718
    - exposure (into surrounding organ or tissue) T83.728
  - skin graft T86.829
    - artificial skin or decellularized allodermis
      - embolism T85.818
      - fibrosis T85.828
      - hemorrhage T85.838
      - infection and inflammation T85.79
      - mechanical
        - breakdown T85.613
        - displacement T85.623
        - malfunction T85.613
        - malposition T85.623
        - obstruction T85.693
        - perforation T85.693
        - protrusion T85.693
        - specified NEC T85.693
      - pain T85.848
      - specified type NEC T85.898
      - stenosis T85.858
      - thrombosis T85.868
    - failure T86.821
    - infection T86.822
    - rejection T86.820
    - specified NEC T86.828
  - sling
    - urethral (female) (male)
      - erosion T83.712
      - exposure T83.722
  - specified NEC T85.9
    - embolism T85.818
    - fibrosis T85.828
    - hemorrhage T85.838
    - infection and inflammation T85.79
    - mechanical
      - breakdown T85.618
      - displacement T85.628
      - leakage T85.638
      - malfunction T85.618
      - malposition T85.628
      - obstruction T85.698
      - perforation T85.698
      - protrusion T85.698
      - specified NEC T85.698
    - pain T85.848
    - specified type NEC T85.898
    - stenosis T85.858
    - thrombosis T85.868
  - subdural infusion catheter — *see* Complications, catheter, subdural
  - sutures — *see* Complications, sutures
  - urinary organ or tract NEC — *see* Complications, genitourinary, device or implant, urinary system
  - vascular — *see* Complications, cardiovascular device or implant
  - ventricular shunt — *see* Complications, ventricular shunt (device)
- puerperium — *see* Puerperal
- puncture, spinal G97.1
  - cerebrospinal fluid leak G97.0
  - headache or reaction G97.1
- pyelogram N99.89
- radiation
  - kyphosis M96.2
  - scoliosis M96.5
- reattached
  - extremity (infection) (rejection)
    - lower T87.1X-
    - upper T87.0X-
  - specified body part NEC T87.2
- reconstructed breast
  - asymmetry between native and reconstructed breast N65.1
  - deformity N65.0
  - disproportion between native and reconstructed breast N65.1
  - excess tissue N65.0
  - misshapen N65.0
- reimplant NEC — *see also* Complications, prosthetic device or implant

☑ Additional Character Required — Refer to the Tabular List for Character Selection

Complication(s) — *continued*
  reimplant — *see also* Complications, prosthetic device
      or implant — *continued*
    limb (infection) (rejection) — *see* Complications,
        reattached, extremity
    organ (partial) (total) — *see* Complications, trans-
        plant
    prosthetic device NEC — *see* Complications, pros-
        thetic device
  renal N28.9
    allograft — *see* Complications, transplant, kidney
    dialysis — *see* Complications, dialysis
  respirator
    mechancial J95.850
      specified NEC J95.859
  respiratory system J98.9
    device, implant or graft — *see* Complication, pros-
        thetic device or implant, specified NEC
    lung transplant — *see* Complications, prosthetic
        device or implant, lung transplant
    postoperative J95.89
      air leak J95.812
      Mendelson's syndrome (chemical pneumonitis)
          J95.4
      pneumothorax J95.811
      pulmonary insufficiency (acute) (after nontho-
          racic surgery) J95.2
        chronic J95.3
        following thoracic surgery J95.1
      respiratory failure (acute) J95.821
        acute and chronic J95.822
      specified NEC J95.89
      subglottic stenosis J95.5
      tracheostomy complication — *see* Complica-
          tions, tracheostomy
    therapy T81.89 ☑
  sedation during labor and delivery O74.9
    cardiac O74.2
    central nervous system O74.3
    pulmonary NEC O74.1
  shunt — *see also* Complications, prosthetic device or
      implant
    arteriovenous — *see* Complications, arteriovenous,
        shunt
    ventricular (communicating) — *see* Complications,
        ventricular shunt
  skin
    graft T86.829
      failure T86.821
      infection T86.822
      rejection T86.820
      specified type NEC T86.828
  spinal
    anesthesia — *see* Complications, anesthesia, spinal
    catheter (epidural) (subdural) — *see* Complications,
        catheter
    puncture or tap G97.1
      cerebrospinal fluid leak G97.0
      headache or reaction G97.1
  stent
    bile duct — *see* Complications, bile duct prosthesis
    ureteral indwelling
      breakdown T83.112 ☑
      displacement T83.122 ☑
      leakage T83.192 ☑
      malposition T83.122 ☑
      obstruction T83.192 ☑
      perforation T83.192 ☑
      protrusion T83.192 ☑
      specified NEC T83.192 ☑
    urinary NEC (ileal conduit) (nephroureteral)
        T83.193 ☑
      embolism T83.81 ☑
      fibrosis T83.82 ☑
      hemorrhage T83.83 ☑
      infection and inflammation T83.593 ☑
      mechanical
        breakdown T83.113 ☑
        displacement T83.123 ☑
        leakage T83.193 ☑
        malposition T83.123 ☑
        obstruction T83.193 ☑
        perforation T83.193 ☑
        protrusion T83.193 ☑
        specified NEC T83.193 ☑
      pain T83.84 ☑
      specified type NEC T83.89 ☑

Complication(s) — *continued*
  stent — *continued*
    urinary — *continued*
      stenosis T83.85 ☑
      thrombosis T83.86 ☑
    vascular
      end stent stenosis — *see* Restenosis, stent
      in stent stenosis — *see* Restenosis, stent
  stoma
    digestive tract
      colostomy — *see* Complications, colostomy
      enterostomy — *see* Complications, enterostomy
      esophagostomy — *see* Complications,
          esophagostomy
      gastrostomy — *see* Complications, gastrostomy
    urinary tract N99.528
      continent N99.538
        hemorrhage N99.530
        herniation N99.533
        infection N99.531
        malfunction N99.532
        specified type NEC N99.538
        stenosis N99.534
      cystostomy — *see* Complications, cystostomy
      external NOS N99.528
      hemorrhage N99.520
      herniation N99.523
      incontinent N99.528
        hemorrhage N99.520
        herniation N99.523
        infection N99.521
        malfunction N99.522
        specified type NEC N99.528
        stenosis N99.524
      infection N99.521
      malfunction N99.522
      specified type NEC N99.528
      stenosis N99.524
  stomach banding — *see* Complication(s), bariatric
      procedure
  stomach stapling — *see* Complication(s), bariatric
      procedure
  surgical material, nonabsorbable — *see* Complication,
      suture, permanent
  surgical procedure (on) T81.9 ☑
    amputation stump (late) — *see* Complications,
        amputation stump
    cardiac — *see* Complications, circulatory system
    cholesteatoma, recurrent — *see* Complications,
        postmastoidectomy, recurrent cholesteatoma
    circulatory (early) — *see* Complications, circulatory
        system
    digestive system — *see* Complications, gastrointesti-
        nal
    dumping syndrome (postgastrectomy) K91.1
    ear — *see* Complications, ear
    elephantiasis or lymphedema I97.89
      postmastectomy I97.2
    emphysema (surgical) T81.82 ☑
    endocrine — *see* Complications, endocrine
    eye — *see* Complications, eye
    fistula (persistent postoperative) T81.83 ☑
    foreign body inadvertently left in wound (sponge)
        (suture) (swab) — *see* Foreign body, acciden-
        tally left during a procedure
    gastrointestinal — *see* Complications, gastrointesti-
        nal
    genitourinary NEC N99.89
    hematoma
      intraoperative — *see* Complication, intraopera-
          tive, hemorrhage
      postprocedural — *see* Complication, postproce-
          dural, hematoma
    hemorrhage
      intraoperative — *see* Complication, intraopera-
          tive, hemorrhage
      postprocedural — *see* Complication, postproce-
          dural, hemorrhage
    hepatic failure K91.82
    hyperglycemia (postpancreatectomy) E89.1
    hypoinsulinemia (postpancreatectomy) E89.1
    hypoparathyroidism (postparathyroidectomy) E89.2
    hypopituitarism (posthypophysectomy) E89.3
    hypothyroidism (post-thyroidectomy) E89.0
    intestinal obstruction — *see also* Obstruction, intes-
        tine, postoperative K91.30
    intracranial hypotension following ventricular
        shunting (ventriculostomy) G97.2

Complication(s) — *continued*
  surgical procedure — *continued*
    lymphedema I97.89
      postmastectomy I97.2
    malabsorption (postsurgical) NEC K91.2
      osteoporosis — *see* Osteoporosis, postsurgical
          malabsorption
    mastoidectomy cavity NEC — *see* Complications,
        postmastoidectomy
    metabolic E89.89
      specified NEC E89.89
    musculoskeletal — *see* Complications, musculoskele-
        tal system
    nervous system (central) (peripheral) — *see* Compli-
        cations, nervous system
    ovarian failure E89.40
      asymptomatic E89.40
      symptomatic E89.41
    peripheral vascular — *see* Complications, surgical
        procedure, vascular
    postcardiotomy syndrome I97.0
    postcholecystectomy syndrome K91.5
    postcommissurotomy syndrome I97.0
    postgastrectomy dumping syndrome K91.1
    postlaminectomy syndrome NEC M96.1
      kyphosis M96.3
    postmastectomy lymphedema syndrome I97.2
    postmastoidectomy cholesteatoma — *see* Compli-
        cations, postmastoidectomy, recurrent
        cholesteatoma
    postvagotomy syndrome K91.1
    postvalvulotomy syndrome I97.0
    pulmonary insufficiency (acute) J95.2
      chronic J95.3
      following thoracic surgery J95.1
    reattached body part — *see* Complications, reat-
        tached
    respiratory — *see* Complications, respiratory system
    shock (hypovolemic) T81.19 ☑
    spleen (postoperative) D78.89
      intraoperative D78.81
    stitch abscess T81.41 ☑
    subglottic stenosis (postsurgical) J95.5
    testicular hypofunction E89.5
    transplant — *see* Complications, organ or tissue
        transplant
    urinary NEC N99.89
    vaginal vault prolapse (posthysterectomy) N99.3
    vascular (peripheral)
      artery T81.719 ☑
        mesenteric T81.710 ☑
        renal T81.711 ☑
        specified NEC T81.718 ☑
      vein T81.72 ☑
    wound infection T81.49 ☑
  suture, permanent (wire) NEC T85.9 ☑
    with repair of bone — *see* Complications, fixation
        device, internal
    embolism T85.818 ☑
    fibrosis T85.828 ☑
    hemorrhage T85.838 ☑
    infection and inflammation T85.79 ☑
    mechanical
      breakdown T85.612 ☑
      displacement T85.622 ☑
      malfunction T85.612 ☑
      malposition T85.622 ☑
      obstruction T85.692 ☑
      perforation T85.692 ☑
      protrusion T85.692 ☑
      specified NEC T85.692 ☑
    pain T85.848 ☑
    specified type NEC T85.898 ☑
    stenosis T85.858 ☑
    thrombosis T85.868 ☑
  tracheostomy J95.00
    granuloma J95.09
    hemorrhage J95.01
    infection J95.02
    malfunction J95.03
    mechanical J95.03
    obstruction J95.03
    specified type NEC J95.09
    tracheo-esophageal fistula J95.04
  transfusion (blood) (lymphocytes) (plasma) T80.92 ☑
    air emblism T80.0 ☑
    circulatory overload E87.71

Complication(s) — *continued*
 transfusion — *continued*
  febrile nonhemolytic transfusion reaction R50.84
  hemochromatosis E83.111
  hemolysis T80.89 ☑
  hemolytic reaction (antigen unspecified) T80.919 ☑
  incompatibility reaction (antigen unspecified)
    T80.919 ☑
    ABO T80.30 ☑
     delayed serologic (DSTR) T80.39 ☑
     hemolytic transfusion reaction (HTR) (unspec-
       ified time after transfusion) T80.319 ☑
      acute (AHTR) (less than 24 hours after
        transfusion) T80.310 ☑
      delayed (DHTR) (24 hours or more after
        transfusion) T80.311 ☑
     specified NEC T80.39 ☑
    acute (antigen unspecified) T80.910 ☑
    delayed (antigen unspecified) T80.911 ☑
    delayed serologic (DSTR) T80.89 ☑
    non-ABO (minor antigens (Duffy) (K) (Kell) (Kidd)
      (Lewis) (M) (N) (P) (S)) T80.A0 ☑ (*following*
      T80.4)
     delayed serologic (DSTR) T80.A9 ☑ (*following*
       T80.4)
     hemolytic transfusion reaction (HTR) (unspec-
       ified time after transfusion) T80.A19 ☑
       (*following* T80.4)
      acute (AHTR) (less than 24 hours after
        transfusion) T80.A10 ☑ (*following*
        T80.4)
      delayed (DHTR) (24 hours or more after
        transfusion) T80.A11 ☑ (*following*
        T80.4)
     specified NEC T80.A9 ☑ (*following* T80.4)
    Rh (antigens (C) (c) (D) (E) (e)) (factor) T80.40 ☑
     delayed serologic (DSTR) T80.49 ☑
     hemolytic transfusion reaction (HTR) (unspec-
       ified time after transfusion) T80.419 ☑
      acute (AHTR) (less than 24 hours after
        transfusion) T80.410 ☑
      delayed (DHTR) (24 hours or more after
        transfusion) T80.411 ☑
     specified NEC T80.49 ☑
  infection T80.29 ☑
    acute T80.22- ☑
  reaction NEC T80.89 ☑
  sepsis T80.29 ☑
  shock T80.89 ☑
 transplant T86.90
  bone T86.839
   failure T86.831
   infection T86.832
   rejection T86.830
   specified type NEC T86.838
  bone marrow T86.00
   failure T86.02
   infection T86.03
   rejection T86.01
   specified type NEC T86.09
  cornea T86.849- ☑
   failure T86.841- ☑
   infection T86.842- ☑
   rejection T86.840- ☑
   specified type NEC T86.848- ☑
  failure T86.92
  heart T86.20
   with lung T86.30
   cardiac allograft vasculopathy T86.290
    failure T86.32
    infection T86.33
    rejection T86.31
    specified type NEC T86.39
   failure T86.22
   infection T86.23
   rejection T86.21
   specified type NEC T86.298
  infection T86.93
  intestine T86.859
   failure T86.851
   infection T86.852
   rejection T86.850
   specified type NEC T86.858
  kidney T86.10
   failure T86.12
   infection T86.13
   rejection T86.11

Complication(s) — *continued*
 transplant — *continued*
  kidney — *continued*
   specified type NEC T86.19
  liver T86.40
   failure T86.42
   infection T86.43
   rejection T86.41
   specified type NEC T86.49
  lung T86.819
   with heart T86.30
    failure T86.32
    infection T86.33
    rejection T86.31
    specified type NEC T86.39
   failure T86.811
   infection T86.812
   rejection T86.810
   specified type NEC T86.818
  malignant neoplasm C80.2
  pancreas T86.899
   failure T86.891
   infection T86.892
   rejection T86.890
   specified type NEC T86.898
  peripheral blood stem cells T86.5
  post-transplant lymphoproliferative disorder (PTLD)
    D47.Z1 (*following* D47.4)
  rejection T86.91
  skin T86.829
   failure T86.821
   infection T86.822
   rejection T86.820
   specified type NEC T86.828
  specified
   tissue T86.899
    failure T86.891
    infection T86.892
    rejection T86.890
    specified type NEC T86.898
   type NEC T86.99
  stem cell (from peripheral blood) (from umbilical
    cord) T86.5
  umbilical cord stem cells T86.5
 trauma (early) T79.9 ☑
  specified NEC T79.8 ☑
 ultrasound therapy NEC T88.9 ☑
 umbilical cord NEC
  complicating delivery O69.9 ☑
   specified NEC O69.89 ☑
 umbrella device, vascular T82.9 ☑
  embolism T82.818 ☑
  fibrosis T82.828 ☑
  hemorrhage T82.838 ☑
  infection or inflammation T82.7 ☑
  mechanical
   breakdown T82.515 ☑
   displacement T82.525 ☑
   leakage T82.535 ☑
   malposition T82.525 ☑
   obstruction T82.595 ☑
   perforation T82.595 ☑
   protrusion T82.595 ☑
  pain T82.848 ☑
  specified type NEC T82.898 ☑
  stenosis T82.858 ☑
  thrombosis T82.868 ☑
 urethral catheter — *see* Complications, catheter, urethral, indwelling
 vaccination T88.1 ☑
  anaphylaxis NEC T80.52 ☑
  arthropathy — *see* Arthropathy, postimmunization
  cellulitis T88.0 ☑
  encephalitis or encephalomyelitis G04.02
  infection (general) (local) NEC T88.0 ☑
  meningitis G03.8
  myelitis G04.02
  protein sickness T80.62 ☑
  rash T88.1 ☑
  reaction (allergic) T88.1 ☑
   serum T80.62 ☑
  sepsis T88.0 ☑
  serum intoxication, sickness, rash, or other serum
    reaction NEC T80.62 ☑
   anaphylactic shock T80.52 ☑
  shock (allergic) (anaphylactic) T80.52 ☑
  vaccinia (generalized) (localized) T88.1 ☑

Complication(s) — *continued*
 vas deferens device or implant — *see* Complications,
   genitourinary, device or implant, genital tract
 vascular I99.9
  device or implant T82.9 ☑
   embolism T82.818 ☑
   fibrosis T82.828 ☑
   hemorrhage T82.838 ☑
   infection or inflammation T82.7 ☑
   mechanical
    breakdown T82.519 ☑
     specified device NEC T82.518 ☑
    displacement T82.529 ☑
     specified device NEC T82.528 ☑
    leakage T82.539 ☑
     specified device NEC T82.538 ☑
    malposition T82.529 ☑
     specified device NEC T82.528 ☑
    obstruction T82.599 ☑
     specified device NEC T82.598 ☑
    perforation T82.599 ☑
     specified device NEC T82.598 ☑
    protrusion T82.599 ☑
     specified device NEC T82.598 ☑
   pain T82.848 ☑
   specified type NEC T82.898 ☑
   stenosis T82.858 ☑
   thrombosis T82.868 ☑
  dialysis catheter — *see* Complication, catheter,
    dialysis
  following infusion, therapeutic injection or transfu-
    sion T80.1 ☑
  graft T82.9 ☑
   embolism T82.818 ☑
   fibrosis T82.828 ☑
   hemorrhage T82.838 ☑
   mechanical
    breakdown T82.319 ☑
     aorta (bifurcation) T82.310 ☑
     carotid artery T82.311 ☑
     specified vessel NEC T82.318 ☑
    displacement T82.329 ☑
     aorta (bifurcation) T82.320 ☑
     carotid artery T82.321 ☑
     specified vessel NEC T82.328 ☑
    leakage T82.339 ☑
     aorta (bifurcation) T82.330 ☑
     carotid artery T82.331 ☑
     femoral artery T82.332 ☑
     specified vessel NEC T82.338 ☑
    malposition T82.329 ☑
     aorta (bifurcation) T82.320 ☑
     carotid artery T82.321 ☑
     specified vessel NEC T82.328 ☑
    obstruction T82.399 ☑
     aorta (bifurcation) T82.390 ☑
     carotid artery T82.391 ☑
     specified vessel NEC T82.398 ☑
    perforation T82.399 ☑
     aorta (bifurcation) T82.390 ☑
     carotid artery T82.391 ☑
     specified vessel NEC T82.398 ☑
    protrusion T82.399 ☑
     aorta (bifurcation) T82.390 ☑
     carotid artery T82.391 ☑
     specified vessel NEC T82.398 ☑
   pain T82.848 ☑
   specified complication NEC T82.898 ☑
   stenosis T82.858 ☑
   thrombosis T82.868 ☑
  postoperative — *see* Complications, postoperative,
    circulatory
 vena cava device (filter) (sieve) (umbrella) — *see*
   Complications, umbrella device, vascular
 ventilation therapy NEC T81.81 ☑
 ventilator
  mechanical J95.850
   specified NEC J95.859
 ventricular (communicating) shunt (device) T85.9 ☑
  embolism T85.810 ☑
  fibrosis T85.820 ☑
  hemorrhage T85.830 ☑
  infection and inflammation T85.730 ☑
  mechanical
   breakdown T85.01 ☑
   displacement T85.02 ☑

☑ Additional Character Required — Refer to the Tabular List for Character Selection

Complication(s) — *continued*
  ventricular shunt — *continued*
    mechanical — *continued*
      leakage T85.03 ☑
      malposition T85.02 ☑
      obstruction T85.09 ☑
      perforation T85.09 ☑
      protrusion T85.09 ☑
      specified NEC T85.09 ☑
    pain T85.840 ☑
    specified type NEC T85.890 ☑
    stenosis T85.850 ☑
    thrombosis T85.860 ☑
  wire suture, permanent (implanted) — *see* Complications, suture, permanent
Compressed air disease T70.3 ☑
Compression
  with injury — code by Nature of injury
  artery I77.1
    celiac, syndrome I77.4
  brachial plexus G54.0
  brain (stem) G93.5
    due to
      contusion (diffuse) — *see also* Injury, intracranial, diffuse S06.A0 ☑
        with herniation S06.A1 ☑
        focal — *see also* Injury, intracranial, focal S06.A0 ☑
          with herniation S06.A1 ☑
      injury NEC — *see also* Injury, intracranial, diffuse S06.A0 ☑
      nontraumatic G93.5
      traumatic — *see also* Injury, intracranial, diffuse S06.A0 ☑
        with herniation S06.A1 ☑
  bronchus J98.09
  cauda equina G83.4
  celiac (artery) (axis) I77.4
  cerebral — *see* Compression, brain
  cervical plexus G54.2
  cord
    spinal — *see* Compression, spinal
    umbilical — *see* Compression, umbilical cord
  cranial nerve G52.9
    eighth H93.3 ☑
    eleventh G52.8
    fifth G50.8
    first G52.0
    fourth — *see* Strabismus, paralytic, fourth nerve
    ninth G52.1
    second — *see* Disorder, nerve, optic
    seventh G51.8
    sixth — *see* Strabismus, paralytic, sixth nerve
    tenth G52.2
    third — *see* Strabismus, paralytic, third nerve
    twelfth G52.3
  diver's squeeze T70.3 ☑
  during birth (newborn) P15.9
  esophagus K22.2
  eustachian tube — *see* Obstruction, eustachian tube, cartilaginous
  facies Q67.1
  fracture
    nontraumatic NOS — *see* Collapse, vertebra
    pathological — *see* Fracture, pathological
    traumatic — *see* Fracture, traumatic
  heart — *see* Disease, heart
  intestine — *see* Obstruction, intestine
  laryngeal nerve, recurrent G52.2
    with paralysis of vocal cords and larynx J38.00
      bilateral J38.02
      unilateral J38.01
  lumbosacral plexus G54.1
  lung J98.4
  lymphatic vessel I89.0
  medulla — *see* Compression, brain
  nerve — *see also* Disorder, nerve G58.9
    arm NEC — *see* Mononeuropathy, upper limb
    axillary G54.0
    cranial — *see* Compression, cranial nerve
    leg NEC — *see* Mononeuropathy, lower limb
    median (in carpal tunnel) — *see* Syndrome, carpal tunnel
    optic — *see* Disorder, nerve, optic
    plantar — *see* Lesion, nerve, plantar
    posterior tibial (in tarsal tunnel) — *see* Syndrome, tarsal tunnel

Compression — *continued*
  nerve — *see also* Disorder, nerve — *continued*
    root or plexus NOS (in) G54.9
      intervertebral disc disorder NEC — *see* Disorder, disc, with, radiculopathy
        with myelopathy — *see* Disorder, disc, with, myelopathy
      neoplastic disease — *see also* Neoplasm D49.9 *[G55]*
      spondylosis — *see* Spondylosis, with radiculopathy
    sciatic (acute) — *see* Lesion, nerve, sciatic
    sympathetic G90.8
    traumatic — *see* Injury, nerve
    ulnar — *see* Lesion, nerve, ulnar
    upper extremity NEC — *see* Mononeuropathy, upper limb
  spinal (cord) G95.20
    by displacement of intervertebral disc NEC — *see also* Disorder, disc, with, myelopathy
    nerve root NOS G54.9
      due to displacement of intervertebral disc NEC — *see* Disorder, disc, with, radiculopathy
      with myelopathy — *see* Disorder, disc, with, myelopathy
    specified NEC G95.29
    spondylogenic (cervical) (lumbar, lumbosacral) (thoracic) — *see* Spondylosis, with myelopathy NEC
    anterior — *see* Syndrome, anterior, spinal artery, compression
    traumatic — *see* Injury, spinal cord, by region
  subcostal nerve (syndrome) — *see* Mononeuropathy, upper limb, specified NEC
  sympathetic nerve NEC G90.8
  syndrome T79.5 ☑
  trachea J39.8
  ulnar nerve (by scar tissue) — *see* Lesion, nerve, ulnar
  umbilical cord
    complicating delivery O69.2 ☑
      cord around neck O69.1 ☑
      prolapse O69.0 ☑
      specified NEC O69.2 ☑
  ureter N13.5
  vein I87.1
  vena cava (inferior) (superior) I87.1
Compulsion, compulsive
  gambling F63.0
  neurosis F42.8
  personality F60.5
  states F42.8
  swearing F42.8
    in Gilles de la Tourette's syndrome F95.2
  tics and spasms F95.9
Concato's disease (pericardial polyserositis) A19.9
  nontubercular I31.1
  pleural — *see* Pleurisy, with effusion
Concavity chest wall M95.4
Concealed penis Q55.64
Concern (normal) **about sick person in family** Z63.6
Concrescence (teeth) K00.2
Concretio cordis I31.1
  rheumatic I09.2
Concretion — *see also* Calculus
  appendicular K38.1
  canaliculus — *see* Dacryolith
  clitoris N90.89
  conjunctiva H11.12- ☑
  eyelid — *see* Disorder, eyelid, specified type NEC
  lacrimal passages — *see* Dacryolith
  prepuce (male) N47.8
  salivary gland (any) K11.5
  seminal vesicle N50.89
  tonsil J35.8
Concussion (brain) (cerebral) (current) S06.0X9 ☑
  with
    loss of consciousness
      30 minutes or less S06.0X1 ☑
      brief S06.0X1 ☑
      status unknown S06.0XA ☑
      unspecified S06.0X9 ☑
    no loss of consciousness S06.0X0 ☑
  blast (air) (hydraulic) (immersion) (underwater)
    abdomen or thorax — *see* Injury, blast, by site
    ear with acoustic nerve injury — *see* Injury, nerve, acoustic, specified type NEC
  cauda equina S34.3 ☑

Concussion — *continued*
  conus medullaris S34.02 ☑
  ocular S05.8X- ☑
  spinal (cord)
    cervical S14.0 ☑
    lumbar S34.01 ☑
    sacral S34.02 ☑
    thoracic S24.0 ☑
  syndrome F07.81
  without loss of consciousness S06.0X0 ☑
Condition — *see also* Disease
  post COVID-19 U09.9
Conditions arising in the perinatal period — *see* Newborn, affected by
Conduct disorder — *see* Disorder, conduct
Condyloma A63.0
  acuminatum A63.0
  gonorrheal A54.09
  latum A51.31
  syphilitic A51.31
    congenital A50.07
  venereal, syphilitic A51.31
Conflagration — *see also* Burn
  asphyxia (by inhalation of gases, fumes or vapors) — *see also* Table of Drugs and Chemicals T59.9- ☑
Conflict (with) — *see also* Discord
  family Z73.9
  marital Z63.0
    involving divorce or estrangement Z63.5
  parent-child Z62.820
    parent-adopted child Z62.821
    parent-biological child Z62.820
    parent-foster child Z62.822
  social role NEC Z73.5
Confluent — *see* condition
Confusion, confused R41.0
  epileptic F05
  mental state (psychogenic) F44.89
  psychogenic F44.89
  reactive (from emotional stress, psychological trauma) F44.89
Confusional arousals G47.51
Congelation T69.9 ☑
Congenital — *see also* condition
  aortic septum Q25.49
  intrinsic factor deficiency D51.0
  malformation — *see* Anomaly
Congestion, congestive
  bladder N32.89
  bowel K63.89
  brain G93.89
  breast N64.59
  bronchial J98.09
  catarrhal J31.0
  chest R09.89
  chill, malarial — *see* Malaria
  circulatory NEC I99.8
  duodenum K31.89
  eye — *see* Hyperemia, conjunctiva
  facial, due to birth injury P15.4
  general R68.89
  glottis J37.0
  heart — *see* Failure, heart, congestive
  hepatic K76.1
  hypostatic (lung) — *see* Edema, lung
  intestine K63.89
  kidney N28.89
  labyrinth H83.8 ☑
  larynx J37.0
  liver K76.1
  lung R09.89
    active or acute — *see* Pneumonia
  malaria, malarial — *see* Malaria
  nasal R09.81
  nose R09.81
  orbit, orbital — *see also* Exophthalmos
    inflammatory (chronic) — *see* Inflammation, orbit
  ovary N83.8
  pancreas K86.89
  pelvic, female N94.89
  pleural J94.8
  prostate (active) N42.1
  pulmonary — *see* Congestion, lung
  renal N28.89
  retina H35.81
  seminal vesicle N50.1
  spinal cord G95.19
  spleen (chronic) D73.2

Congestion, congestive — *continued*
  stomach K31.89
  trachea — *see* Tracheitis
  urethra N36.8
  uterus N85.8
    with subinvolution N85.3
  venous (passive) I87.8
  viscera R68.89
Congestive — *see* Congestion
Conical
  cervix (hypertrophic elongation) N88.4
  cornea — *see* Keratoconus
  teeth K00.2
Conjoined twins Q89.4
Conjugal maladjustment Z63.0
  involving divorce or estrangement Z63.5
Conjunctiva — *see* condition
Conjunctivitis (staphylococcal) (streptococcal) NOS H10.9
  Acanthamoeba B60.12
  acute H10.3- ☑
    atopic H10.1- ☑
    chemical — *see also* Corrosion, cornea H10.21- ☑
    mucopurulent H10.02- ☑
      follicular H10.01- ☑
    pseudomembranous H10.22- ☑
    serous except viral H10.23- ☑
      viral — *see* Conjunctivitis, viral
    toxic H10.21- ☑
  adenoviral (acute) (follicular) B30.1
  allergic (acute) — *see* Conjunctivitis, acute, atopic
    chronic H10.45
      vernal H10.44
  anaphylactic — *see* Conjunctivitis, acute, atopic
  Apollo B30.3
  atopic (acute) — *see* Conjunctivitis, acute, atopic
  Béal's B30.2
  blennorrhagic (gonococcal) (neonatorum) A54.31
  chemical (acute) — *see also* Corrosion, cornea
    H10.21- ☑
  chlamydial A74.0
    due to trachoma A71.1
    neonatal P39.1
  chronic (nodosa) (petrificans) (phlyctenular) H10.40- ☑
    allergic H10.45
      vernal H10.44
    follicular H10.43- ☑
    giant papillary H10.41- ☑
    simple H10.42- ☑
    vernal H10.44
  coxsackievirus 24 B30.3
  diphtheritic A36.86
  due to
    dust — *see* Conjunctivitis, acute, atopic
    filariasis B74.9
    mucocutaneous leishmaniasis B55.2
  enterovirus type 70 (hemorrhagic) B30.3
  epidemic (viral) B30.9
    hemorrhagic B30.3
  gonococcal (neonatorum) A54.31
  granular (trachomatous) A71.1
    sequelae (late effect) B94.0
  hemorrhagic (acute) (epidemic) B30.3
  herpes zoster B02.31
  in (due to)
    Acanthamoeba B60.12
    adenovirus (acute) (follicular) B30.1
    Chlamydia A74.0
    coxsackievirus 24 B30.3
    diphtheria A36.86
    enterovirus type 70 (hemorrhagic) B30.3
    filariasis B74.9
    gonococci A54.31
    herpes (simplex) virus B00.53
      zoster B02.31
    infectious disease NEC B99 ☑
    meningococci A39.89
    mucocutaneous leishmaniasis B55.2
    rosacea H10.82- ☑
    syphilis (late) A52.71
    zoster B02.31
  inclusion A74.0
  infantile P39.1
    gonococcal A54.31
  Koch-Weeks' — *see* Conjunctivitis, acute, mucopurulent
  light — *see* Conjunctivitis, acute, atopic
  ligneous — *see* Blepharoconjunctivitis, ligneous
  meningococcal A39.89

Conjunctivitis — *continued*
  mucopurulent — *see* Conjunctivitis, acute, mucopurulent
  neonatal P39.1
    gonococcal A54.31
  Newcastle B30.8
  of Béal B30.2
  parasitic
    filariasis B74.9
    mucocutaneous leishmaniasis B55.2
  Parinaud's H10.89
  petrificans H10.89
  rosacea H10.82- ☑
  specified NEC H10.89
  swimming-pool B30.1
  trachomatous A71.1
    acute A71.0
    sequelae (late effect) B94.0
  traumatic NEC H10.89
  tuberculous A18.59
  tularemic A21.1
  tularensis A21.1
  viral B30.9
    due to
      adenovirus B30.1
      enterovirus B30.3
    specified NEC B30.8
Conjunctivochalasis H11.82- ☑
Connective tissue — *see* condition
Conn's syndrome E26.01
Conradi (-Hunermann) **disease** Q77.3
Consanguinity Z84.3
  counseling Z71.89
Conscious simulation (of illness) Z76.5
Consecutive — *see* condition
Consolidation lung (base) — *see* Pneumonia, lobar
Constipation (atonic) (neurogenic) (simple) (spastic)
    K59.00
  chronic K59.09
    idiopathic K59.04
  drug-induced K59.03
  functional K59.04
  outlet dysfunction K59.02
  psychogenic F45.8
  slow transit K59.01
  specified NEC K59.09
Constitutional — *see also* condition
  substandard F60.7
Constitutionally substandard F60.7
Constriction — *see also* Stricture
  auditory canal — *see* Stenosis, external ear canal
  bronchial J98.09
  duodenum K31.5
  esophagus K22.2
  external
    abdomen, abdominal (wall) S30.841 ☑
    alveolar process S00.542 ☑
    ankle S90.54- ☑
    antecubital space — *see* Constriction, external, forearm
    arm (upper) S40.84- ☑
    auricle — *see* Constriction, external, ear
    axilla — *see* Constriction, external, arm
    back, lower S30.840 ☑
    breast S20.14- ☑
    brow S00.84 ☑
    buttock S30.840 ☑
    calf — *see* Constriction, external, leg
    canthus — *see* Constriction, external, eyelid
    cheek S00.84 ☑
      internal S00.542 ☑
    chest wall — *see* Constriction, external, thorax
    chin S00.84 ☑
    clitoris S30.844 ☑
    costal region — *see* Constriction, external, thorax
    digit(s)
      foot — *see* Constriction, external, toe
      hand — *see* Constriction, external, finger
    ear S00.44- ☑
    elbow S50.34- ☑
    epididymis S30.843 ☑
    epigastric region S30.841 ☑
    esophagus, cervical S10.14 ☑
    eyebrow — *see* Constriction, external, eyelid
    eyelid S00.24- ☑
    face S00.84 ☑
    finger(s) S60.44- ☑

Constriction — *continued*
  external — *continued*
    finger(s) — *continued*
      index S60.44- ☑
      little S60.44- ☑
      middle S60.44- ☑
      ring S60.44- ☑
    flank S30.841 ☑
    foot (except toe(s) alone) S90.84- ☑
      toe — *see* Constriction, external, toe
    forearm S50.84- ☑
      elbow only — *see* Constriction, external, elbow
    forehead S00.84 ☑
    genital organs, external
      female S30.846 ☑
      male S30.845 ☑
    groin S30.841 ☑
    gum S00.542 ☑
    hand S60.54- ☑
    head S00.94 ☑
      ear — *see* Constriction, external, ear
      eyelid — *see* Constriction, external, eyelid
      lip S00.541 ☑
      nose S00.34 ☑
      oral cavity S00.542 ☑
      scalp S00.04 ☑
      specified site NEC S00.84 ☑
    heel — *see* Constriction, external, foot
    hip S70.24- ☑
    inguinal region S30.841 ☑
    interscapular region S20.449 ☑
    jaw S00.84 ☑
    knee S80.24- ☑
    labium (majus) (minus) S30.844 ☑
    larynx S10.14 ☑
    leg (lower) S80.84- ☑
      knee — *see* Constriction, external, knee
      upper — *see* Constriction, external, thigh
    lip S00.541 ☑
    lower back S30.840 ☑
    lumbar region S30.840 ☑
    malar region S00.84 ☑
    mammary — *see* Constriction, external, breast
    mastoid region S00.84 ☑
    mouth S00.542 ☑
    nail
      finger — *see* Constriction, external, finger
      toe — *see* Constriction, external, toe
    nasal S00.34 ☑
    neck S10.94 ☑
      specified site NEC S10.84 ☑
      throat S10.14 ☑
    nose S00.34 ☑
    occipital region S00.04 ☑
    oral cavity S00.542 ☑
    orbital region — *see* Constriction, external, eyelid
    palate S00.542 ☑
    palm — *see* Constriction, external, hand
    parietal region S00.04 ☑
    pelvis S30.840 ☑
    penis S30.842 ☑
    perineum
      female S30.844 ☑
      male S30.840 ☑
    periocular area — *see* Constriction, external, eyelid
    phalanges
      finger — *see* Constriction, external, finger
      toe — *see* Constriction, external, toe
    pharynx S10.14 ☑
    pinna — *see* Constriction, external, ear
    popliteal space — *see* Constriction, external, knee
    prepuce S30.842 ☑
    pubic region S30.840 ☑
    pudendum
      female S30.846 ☑
      male S30.845 ☑
    sacral region S30.840 ☑
    scalp S00.04 ☑
    scapular region — *see* Constriction, external, shoulder
    scrotum S30.843 ☑
    shin — *see* Constriction, external, leg
    shoulder S40.24- ☑
    sternal region S20.349 ☑
    submaxillary region S00.84 ☑
    submental region S00.84 ☑

Constriction — *continued*
  external — *continued*
    subungual
      finger(s) — *see* Constriction, external, finger
      toe(s) — *see* Constriction, external, toe
    supraclavicular fossa S10.84 ☑
    supraorbital S00.84 ☑
    temple S00.84 ☑
    temporal region S00.84 ☑
    testis S30.843 ☑
    thigh S70.34- ☑
    thorax, thoracic (wall) S20.94 ☑
      back S20.44- ☑
      front S20.34- ☑
    throat S10.14 ☑
    thumb S60.34- ☑
    toe(s) (lesser) S90.44- ☑
      great S90.44- ☑
    tongue S00.542 ☑
    trachea S10.14 ☑
    tunica vaginalis S30.843 ☑
    uvula S00.542 ☑
    vagina S30.844 ☑
    vulva S30.844 ☑
    wrist S60.84- ☑
  gallbladder — *see* Obstruction, gallbladder
  intestine — *see* Obstruction, intestine
  larynx J38.6
    congenital Q31.8
      specified NEC Q31.8
      subglottic Q31.1
  organ or site, congenital NEC — *see* Atresia, by site
  prepuce (acquired) (congenital) N47.1
  pylorus (adult hypertrophic) K31.1
    congenital or infantile Q40.0
    newborn Q40.0
  ring dystocia (uterus) O62.4
  spastic — *see also* Spasm
    ureter N13.5
  ureter N13.5
    with infection N13.6
  urethra — *see* Stricture, urethra
  visual field (peripheral) (functional) — *see* Defect, visual field

Constrictive — *see* condition
Consultation
  medical — *see* Counseling, medical
  religious Z71.81
  specified reason NEC Z71.89
  spiritual Z71.81
  without complaint or sickness Z71.9
    feared complaint unfounded Z71.1
    specified reason NEC Z71.89
Consumption — *see* Tuberculosis
Contact (with) — *see also* Exposure (to)
  acariasis Z20.7
  AIDS virus Z20.6
  air pollution Z77.110
  algae and algae toxins Z77.121
  algae bloom Z77.121
  anthrax Z20.810
  aromatic amines Z77.020
  aromatic (hazardous) compounds NEC Z77.028
  aromatic dyes NOS Z77.028
  arsenic Z77.010
  asbestos Z77.090
  bacterial disease NEC Z20.818
  benzene Z77.021
  blue-green algae bloom Z77.121
  body fluids (potentially hazardous) Z77.21
  brown tide Z77.121
  chemicals (chiefly nonmedicinal) (hazardous) NEC Z77.098
  cholera Z20.09
  chromium compounds Z77.018
  communicable disease Z20.9
    bacterial NEC Z20.818
    specified NEC Z20.89
    viral NEC Z20.828
    Zika virus Z20.821
  coronavirus (disease) (novel) 2019 Z20.822
  COVID-19 Z20.822
  cyanobacteria bloom Z77.121
  dyes Z77.098
  Escherichia coli (E. coli) Z20.01
  fiberglass — *see* Table of Drugs and Chemicals, fiberglass
  German measles Z20.4

Contact — *continued*
  gonorrhea Z20.2
  hazardous metals NEC Z77.018
  hazardous substances NEC Z77.29
  hazards in the physical environment NEC Z77.128
  hazards to health NEC Z77.9
  HIV Z20.6
  HTLV-III/LAV Z20.6
  human immunodeficiency virus (HIV) Z20.6
  infection Z20.9
    specified NEC Z20.89
  infestation (parasitic) NEC Z20.7
  intestinal infectious disease NEC Z20.09
    Escherichia coli (E. coli) Z20.01
  lead Z77.011
  meningococcus Z20.811
  mold (toxic) Z77.120
  nickel dust Z77.018
  noise Z77.122
  parasitic disease Z20.7
  pediculosis Z20.7
  pfiesteria piscicida Z77.121
  poliomyelitis Z20.89
  pollution
    air Z77.110
    environmental NEC Z77.118
    soil Z77.112
    water Z77.111
  polycyclic aromatic hydrocarbons Z77.028
  positive maternal group B streptococcus P00.82
  rabies Z20.3
  radiation, naturally occurring NEC Z77.123
  radon Z77.123
  red tide (Florida) Z77.121
  rubella Z20.4
  SARS-CoV-2 Z20.822
  sexually-transmitted disease Z20.2
  smallpox (laboratory) Z20.89
  syphilis Z20.2
  tuberculosis Z20.1
  uranium Z77.012
  varicella Z20.820
  venereal disease Z20.2
  viral disease NEC Z20.828
  viral hepatitis Z20.5
  water pollution Z77.111
  Zika virus Z20.821
Contamination, food — *see* Intoxication, foodborne
Contraception, contraceptive
  advice Z30.09
  counseling Z30.09
  device (intrauterine) (in situ) Z97.5
    causing menorrhagia T83.83 ☑
    checking Z30.431
    complications — *see* Complications, intrauterine, contraceptive device
    in place Z97.5
    initial prescription Z30.014
    reinsertion Z30.433
    removal Z30.432
    replacement Z30.433
  emergency (postcoital) Z30.012
  initial prescription Z30.019
    barrier Z30.018
    diaphragm Z30.018
    injectable Z30.013
    intrauterine device Z30.014
    pills Z30.011
    postcoital (emergency) Z30.012
    specified type NEC Z30.018
    subdermal implantable Z30.017
    transdermal patch hormonal Z30.016
    vaginal ring hormonal Z30.015
  maintenance Z30.40
    barrier Z30.49
    diaphragm Z30.49
    examination Z30.8
    injectable Z30.42
    intrauterine device Z30.431
    pills Z30.41
    specified type NEC Z30.49
    subdermal implantable Z30.46
    transdermal patch hormonal Z30.45
    vaginal ring hormonal Z30.44
  management Z30.9
    specified NEC Z30.8
  postcoital (emergency) Z30.012
  prescription Z30.019
    repeat Z30.40

Contraception, contraceptive — *continued*
  sterilization Z30.2
  surveillance (drug) — *see* Contraception, maintenance
Contraction(s), contracture, contracted
  Achilles tendon — *see also* Short, tendon, Achilles
    congenital Q66.89
  amputation stump (surgical) (flexion) (late) (next proximal joint) T87.89
  anus K59.89
  bile duct (common) (hepatic) K83.8
  bladder N32.89
    neck or sphincter N32.0
  bowel, cecum, colon or intestine, any part — *see* Obstruction, intestine
  Braxton Hicks — *see* False, labor
  breast implant, capsular T85.44 ☑
  bronchial J98.09
  burn (old) — *see* Cicatrix
  cervix — *see* Stricture, cervix
  cicatricial — *see* Cicatrix
  conjunctiva, trachomatous, active A71.1
    sequelae (late effect) B94.0
  Dupuytren's M72.0
  eyelid — *see* Disorder, eyelid function
  fascia (lata) (postural) M72.8
    Dupuytren's M72.0
    palmar M72.0
    plantar M72.2
  finger NEC — *see also* Deformity, finger
    congenital Q68.1
    joint — *see* Contraction, joint, hand
  flaccid — *see* Contraction, paralytic
  gallbladder K82.0
  heart valve — *see* Endocarditis
  hip — *see* Contraction, joint, hip
  hourglass
    bladder N32.89
      congenital Q64.79
    gallbladder K82.0
      congenital Q44.1
    stomach K31.89
      congenital Q40.2
      psychogenic F45.8
    uterus (complicating delivery) O62.4
  hysterical F44.4
  internal os — *see* Stricture, cervix
  joint (abduction) (acquired) (adduction) (flexion) (rotation) M24.50
    ankle M24.57- ☑
    congenital NEC Q68.8
      hip Q65.89
    elbow M24.52- ☑
    foot joint M24.57- ☑
    hand joint M24.54- ☑
    hip M24.55- ☑
      congenital Q65.89
    hysterical F44.4
    knee M24.56- ☑
    shoulder M24.51- ☑
    specified site NEC M24.59
    wrist M24.53- ☑
  kidney (granular) (secondary) N26.9
    congenital Q63.8
    hydronephritic — *see* Hydronephrosis
    Page N26.2
    pyelonephritic — *see* Pyelitis, chronic
    tuberculous A18.11
  ligament — *see also* Disorder, ligament
    congenital Q79.8
  muscle (postinfective) (postural) NEC M62.40
    with contracture of joint — *see* Contraction, joint
    ankle M62.47- ☑
    congenital Q79.8
      sternocleidomastoid Q68.0
    extraocular — *see* Strabismus
    eye (extrinsic) — *see* Strabismus
    foot M62.47- ☑
    forearm M62.43- ☑
    hand M62.44- ☑
    hysterical F44.4
    ischemic (Volkmann's) T79.6 ☑
    lower leg M62.46- ☑
    multiple sites M62.49
    pelvic region M62.45- ☑
    posttraumatic — *see* Strabismus, paralytic
    psychogenic F45.8
      conversion reaction F44.4

Contraction(s), contracture, contracted — *continued*
- muscle — *continued*
  - shoulder region M62.41- ☑
  - specified site NEC M62.48
  - thigh M62.45- ☑
  - upper arm M62.42- ☑
- neck — *see* Torticollis
- ocular muscle — *see* Strabismus
- organ or site, congenital NEC — *see* Atresia, by site
- outlet (pelvis) — *see* Contraction, pelvis
- palmar fascia M72.0
- paralytic
  - joint — *see* Contraction, joint
  - muscle — *see also* Contraction, muscle NEC
    - ocular — *see* Strabismus, paralytic
- pelvis (acquired) (general) M95.5
  - with disproportion (fetopelvic) O33.1
    - causing obstructed labor O65.1
    - inlet O33.2
    - mid-cavity O33.3 ☑
    - outlet O33.3 ☑
- plantar fascia M72.2
- premature
  - atrium I49.1
  - auriculoventricular I49.49
  - heart I49.49
  - junctional I49.2
  - supraventricular I49.1
  - ventricular I49.3
- prostate N42.89
- pylorus NEC — *see also* Pylorospasm
  - psychogenic F45.8
- rectum, rectal (sphincter) K59.89
- ring (Bandl's) (complicating delivery) O62.4
- scar — *see* Cicatrix
- spine — *see* Dorsopathy, deforming
- sternocleidomastoid (muscle), congenital Q68.0
- stomach K31.89
  - hourglass K31.89
    - congenital Q40.2
    - psychogenic F45.8
  - psychogenic F45.8
- tendon (sheath) M62.40
  - with contracture of joint — *see* Contraction, joint
  - Achilles — *see* Short, tendon, Achilles
  - ankle M62.47- ☑
    - Achilles — *see* Short, tendon, Achilles
  - foot M62.47- ☑
  - forearm M62.43- ☑
  - hand M62.44- ☑
  - lower leg M62.46- ☑
  - multiple sites M62.49
  - neck M62.48
  - pelvic region M62.45- ☑
  - shoulder region M62.41- ☑
  - specified site NEC M62.48
  - thigh M62.45- ☑
  - thorax M62.48
  - trunk M62.48
  - upper arm M62.42- ☑
- toe — *see* Deformity, toe, specified NEC
- ureterovesical orifice (postinfectional) N13.5
  - with infection N13.6
- urethra — *see also* Stricture, urethra
  - orifice N32.0
- uterus N85.8
  - abnormal NEC O62.9
  - clonic (complicating delivery) O62.4
  - dyscoordinate (complicating delivery) O62.4
  - hourglass (complicating delivery) O62.4
  - hypertonic O62.4
  - hypotonic NEC O62.2
  - inadequate
    - primary O62.0
    - secondary O62.1
  - incoordinate (complicating delivery) O62.4
  - poor O62.2
  - tetanic (complicating delivery) O62.4
- vagina (outlet) N89.5
- vesical N32.89
  - neck or urethral orifice N32.0
- visual field — *see* Defect, visual field, generalized
- Volkmann's (ischemic) T79.6
Contusion (skin surface intact) T14.8 ☑
- abdomen, abdominal (muscle) (wall) S30.1 ☑
- adnexa, eye NEC S05.8X- ☑

Contusion — *continued*
- adrenal gland S37.812 ☑
- alveolar process S00.532 ☑
- ankle S90.0- ☑
- antecubital space — *see* Contusion, forearm
- anus S30.3 ☑
- arm (upper) S40.02- ☑
  - lower (with elbow) — *see* Contusion, forearm
- auditory canal — *see* Contusion, ear
- auricle — *see* Contusion, ear
- axilla — *see* Contusion, arm, upper
- back — *see also* Contusion, thorax, back
  - lower S30.0 ☑
- bile duct S36.13 ☑
- bladder S37.22 ☑
- bone NEC T14.8 ☑
- brain (diffuse) — *see* Injury, intracranial, diffuse
  - focal — *see* Injury, intracranial, focal
- brainstem S06.38- ☑
- breast S20.0- ☑
- broad ligament S37.892 ☑
- brow S00.83 ☑
- buttock S30.0 ☑
- canthus, eye S00.1- ☑
- cauda equina S34.3 ☑
- cerebellar, traumatic S06.37- ☑
- cerebral S06.33- ☑
  - left side S06.32- ☑
  - right side S06.31- ☑
- cheek S00.83 ☑
  - internal S00.532 ☑
- chest (wall) — *see* Contusion, thorax
- chin S00.83 ☑
- clitoris S30.23 ☑
- colon — *see* Injury, intestine, large, contusion
- common bile duct S36.13 ☑
- conjunctiva S05.1- ☑
  - with foreign body (in conjunctival sac) — *see* Foreign body, conjunctival sac
- conus medullaris (spine) S34.139 ☑
- cornea — *see* Contusion, eyeball
  - with foreign body — *see* Foreign body, cornea
- corpus cavernosum S30.21 ☑
- cortex (brain) (cerebral) — *see* Injury, intracranial, diffuse
  - focal — *see* Injury, intracranial, focal
- costal region — *see* Contusion, thorax
- cystic duct S36.13 ☑
- diaphragm S27.802 ☑
- duodenum S36.420 ☑
- ear S00.43- ☑
- elbow S50.0- ☑
  - with forearm — *see* Contusion, forearm
- epididymis S30.22 ☑
- epigastric region S30.1 ☑
- epiglottis S10.0 ☑
- esophagus (thoracic) S27.812 ☑
  - cervical S10.0 ☑
- eyeball S05.1- ☑
- eyebrow S00.1- ☑
- eyelid (and periocular area) S00.1- ☑
- face NEC S00.83 ☑
- fallopian tube S37.529 ☑
  - bilateral S37.522 ☑
  - unilateral S37.521 ☑
- femoral triangle S30.1 ☑
- finger(s) S60.00 ☑
  - with damage to nail (matrix) S60.10 ☑
  - index S60.02- ☑
    - with damage to nail S60.12- ☑
  - little S60.05- ☑
    - with damage to nail S60.15- ☑
  - middle S60.03- ☑
    - with damage to nail S60.13- ☑
  - ring S60.04- ☑
    - with damage to nail S60.14- ☑
  - thumb — *see* Contusion, thumb
- flank S30.1 ☑
- foot (except toe(s) alone) S90.3- ☑
  - toe — *see* Contusion, toe
- forearm S50.1- ☑
  - elbow only — *see* Contusion, elbow
- forehead S00.83 ☑
- gallbladder S36.122 ☑
- genital organs, external
  - female S30.202 ☑

Contusion — *continued*
- genital organs, external — *continued*
  - male S30.201 ☑
- globe (eye) — *see* Contusion, eyeball
- groin S30.1 ☑
- gum S00.532 ☑
- hand S60.22- ☑
  - finger(s) — *see* Contusion, finger
  - wrist — *see* Contusion, wrist
- head S00.93 ☑
  - ear — *see* Contusion, ear
  - eyelid — *see* Contusion, eyelid
  - lip S00.531 ☑
  - nose S00.33 ☑
  - oral cavity S00.532 ☑
  - scalp S00.03 ☑
  - specified part NEC S00.83 ☑
- heart — *see also* Injury, heart S26.91 ☑
- heel — *see* Contusion, foot
- hepatic duct S36.13 ☑
- hip S70.0- ☑
- ileum S36.428 ☑
- iliac region S30.1 ☑
- inguinal region S30.1 ☑
- interscapular region S20.229 ☑
- intra-abdominal organ S36.92 ☑
  - colon — *see* Injury, intestine, large, contusion
  - liver S36.112 ☑
  - pancreas — *see* Contusion, pancreas
  - rectum S36.62 ☑
  - small intestine — *see* Injury, intestine, small, contusion
  - specified organ NEC S36.892 ☑
  - spleen — *see* Contusion, spleen
  - stomach S36.32 ☑
- iris (eye) — *see* Contusion, eyeball
- jaw S00.83 ☑
- jejunum S36.428 ☑
- kidney S37.01- ☑
  - major (greater than 2 cm) S37.02- ☑
  - minor (less than 2 cm) S37.01- ☑
- knee S80.0- ☑
- labium (majus) (minus) S30.23 ☑
- lacrimal apparatus, gland or sac S05.8X- ☑
- larynx S10.0 ☑
- leg (lower) S80.1- ☑
  - knee — *see* Contusion, knee
- lens — *see* Contusion, eyeball
- lip S00.531 ☑
- liver S36.112 ☑
- lower back S30.0 ☑
- lumbar region S30.0 ☑
- lung S27.329 ☑
  - bilateral S27.322 ☑
  - unilateral S27.321 ☑
- malar region S00.83 ☑
- mastoid region S00.83 ☑
- membrane, brain — *see* Injury, intracranial, diffuse
  - focal — *see* Injury, intracranial, focal
- mesentery S36.892 ☑
- mesosalpinx S37.892 ☑
- mouth S00.532 ☑
- muscle — *see* Contusion, by site
- nail
  - finger — *see* Contusion, finger, with damage to nail
  - toe — *see* Contusion, toe, with damage to nail
- nasal S00.33 ☑
- neck S10.93 ☑
  - specified site NEC S10.83 ☑
  - throat S10.0 ☑
- nerve — *see* Injury, nerve
- newborn P54.5
- nose S00.33 ☑
- occipital
  - lobe (brain) — *see* Injury, intracranial, diffuse
    - focal — *see* Injury, intracranial, focal
  - region (scalp) S00.03 ☑
- orbit (region) (tissues) S05.1- ☑
- ovary S37.429 ☑
  - bilateral S37.422 ☑
  - unilateral S37.421 ☑
- palate S00.532 ☑
- pancreas S36.229 ☑
  - body S36.221 ☑
  - head S36.220 ☑
  - tail S36.222 ☑

☑ **Additional Character Required — Refer to the Tabular List for Character Selection**

Contusion — *continued*
 parietal
  lobe (brain) — *see* Injury, intracranial, diffuse
   focal — *see* Injury, intracranial, focal
  region (scalp) S00.03 ☑
 pelvic organ S37.92 ☑
  adrenal gland S37.812 ☑
  bladder S37.22 ☑
  fallopian tube — *see* Contusion, fallopian tube
  kidney — *see* Contusion, kidney
  ovary — *see* Contusion, ovary
  prostate S37.822 ☑
  specified organ NEC S37.892 ☑
  ureter S37.12 ☑
  urethra S37.32 ☑
  uterus S37.62 ☑
 pelvis S30.0 ☑
 penis S30.21 ☑
 perineum
  female S30.23 ☑
  male S30.0 ☑
 periocular area S00.1- ☑
 peritoneum S36.81 ☑
 periurethral tissue — *see* Contusion, urethra
 pharynx S10.0 ☑
 pinna — *see* Contusion, ear
 popliteal space — *see* Contusion, knee
 prepuce S30.21 ☑
 prostate S37.822 ☑
 pubic region S30.1 ☑
 pudendum
  female S30.202 ☑
  male S30.201 ☑
 quadriceps femoris — *see* Contusion, thigh
 rectum S36.62 ☑
 retroperitoneum S36.892 ☑
 round ligament S37.892 ☑
 sacral region S30.0 ☑
 scalp S00.03 ☑
  due to birth injury P12.3
 scapular region — *see* Contusion, shoulder
 sclera — *see* Contusion, eyeball
 scrotum S30.22 ☑
 seminal vesicle S37.892 ☑
 shoulder S40.01- ☑
 skin NEC T14.8 ☑
 small intestine — *see* Injury, intestine, small, contusion
 spermatic cord S30.22 ☑
 spinal cord — *see* Injury, spinal cord, by region
  cauda equina S34.3 ☑
  conus medullaris S34.139 ☑
 spleen S36.029 ☑
  major S36.021 ☑
  minor S36.020 ☑
 sternal region S20.219 ☑
 stomach S36.32 ☑
 subconjunctival S05.1- ☑
 subcutaneous NEC T14.8 ☑
 submaxillary region S00.83 ☑
 submental region S00.83 ☑
 subperiosteal NEC T14.8 ☑
 subungual
  finger — *see* Contusion, finger, with damage to nail
  toe — *see* Contusion, toe, with damage to nail
 supraclavicular fossa S10.83 ☑
 supraorbital S00.83 ☑
 suprarenal gland S37.812 ☑
 temple (region) S00.83 ☑
 temporal
  lobe (brain) — *see* Injury, intracranial, diffuse
   focal — *see* Injury, intracranial, focal
  region S00.83 ☑
 testis S30.22 ☑
 thigh S70.1- ☑
 thorax (wall) S20.20 ☑
  back S20.22- ☑
  front S20.21- ☑
 throat S10.0 ☑
 thumb S60.01- ☑
  with damage to nail S60.11- ☑
 toe(s) (lesser) S90.12- ☑
  with damage to nail S90.22- ☑
  great S90.11- ☑
   with damage to nail S90.21- ☑
 tongue S00.532 ☑
 trachea (cervical) S10.0 ☑

Contusion — *continued*
 trachea — *continued*
  thoracic S27.52 ☑
  tunica vaginalis S30.22 ☑
 tympanum, tympanic membrane — *see* Contusion, ear
 ureter S37.12 ☑
 urethra S37.32 ☑
 urinary organ NEC S37.892 ☑
 uterus S37.62 ☑
 uvula S00.532 ☑
 vagina S30.23 ☑
 vas deferens S37.892 ☑
 vesical S37.22 ☑
 vocal cord(s) S10.0 ☑
 vulva S30.23 ☑
 wrist S60.21- ☑
Conus (congenital) (any type) Q14.8
 cornea — *see* Keratoconus
 medullaris syndrome G95.81
Conversion hysteria, neurosis or reaction F44.9
Converter, tuberculosis (test reaction) R76.11
Conviction (legal), anxiety concerning Z65.0
 with imprisonment Z65.1
Convulsions (idiopathic) — *see also* Seizure(s) R56.9
 apoplectiform (cerebral ischemia) I67.82
 dissociative F44.5
 epileptic — *see* Epilepsy
 epileptiform, epileptoid — *see* Seizure, epileptiform
 ether (anesthetic) — *see* Table of Drugs and Chemicals, by drug
 febrile R56.00
  with status epilepticus G40.901
  complex R56.01
   with status epilepticus G40.901
  simple R56.00
 hysterical F44.5
 infantile P90
  epilepsy — *see* Epilepsy
 jacksonian — *see* Epilepsy, localization-related, symptomatic, with simple partial seizures
 myoclonic G25.3
 newborn P90
 obstetrical (nephritic) (uremic) — *see* Eclampsia
 paretic A52.17
 post traumatic R56.1
 psychomotor — *see* Epilepsy, localization-related, symptomatic, with complex partial seizures
 recurrent R56.9
 reflex R25.8
 scarlatinal A38.8
 tetanus, tetanic — *see* Tetanus
 thymic E32.8
Convulsive — *see also* Convulsions
Cooley's anemia D56.1
Coolie itch B76.9
Cooper's
 disease — *see* Mastopathy, cystic
 hernia — *see* Hernia, abdomen, specified site NEC
Copra itch B88.0
Coprophagy F50.89
Coprophobia F40.298
Coproporphyria, hereditary E80.29
Cor
 biloculare Q20.8
 bovis, bovinum — *see* Hypertrophy, cardiac
 pulmonale (chronic) I27.81
  acute I26.09
 triatriatum, triatrium Q24.2
 triloculare Q20.8
  biatrium Q20.4
  biventriculare Q21.19
Corbus' disease (gangrenous balanitis) N48.1
Cord — *see also* condition
 around neck
  complicating delivery O69.81 ☑
   with compression O69.1 ☑
 bladder G95.89
  tabetic A52.19
Cordis ectopia Q24.8
Corditis (spermatic) N49.1
Corectopia Q13.2
Cori's disease (glycogen storage) E74.03
Corkhandler's disease or lung J67.3
Corkscrew esophagus K22.4
Corkworker's disease or lung J67.3
Corn (infected) L84

Cornea — *see also* condition
 donor Z52.5
 plana Q13.4
Cornelia de Lange syndrome Q87.19
Cornu cutaneum L85.8
Cornual gestation or pregnancy O00.80
 with intrauterine pregnancy O00.81
Coronary (artery) — *see* condition
Coronavirus (infection)
 2019 — *see also* COVID-19 U07.1
 as cause of diseases classified elsewhere B97.29
 coronavirus-19 — *see also* COVID-19 U07.1
 COVID-19 — *see also* COVID-19 U07.1
 SARS-associated B97.21
Corpora — *see also* condition
 amylacea, prostate N42.89
 cavernosa — *see* condition
Corpulence — *see* Obesity
Corpus — *see* condition
Corrected transposition Q20.5
Corrosion (injury) (acid) (caustic) (chemical) (lime) (external) (internal) T30.4
 abdomen, abdominal (muscle) (wall) T21.42 ☑
  first degree T21.52 ☑
  second degree T21.62 ☑
  third degree T21.72 ☑
 above elbow T22.439 ☑
  first degree T22.539 ☑
  left T22.432 ☑
   first degree T22.532 ☑
   second degree T22.632 ☑
   third degree T22.732 ☑
  right T22.431 ☑
   first degree T22.531 ☑
   second degree T22.631 ☑
   third degree T22.731 ☑
  second degree T22.639 ☑
  third degree T22.739 ☑
 alimentary tract NEC T28.7 ☑
 ankle T25.419 ☑
  first degree T25.519 ☑
  left T25.412 ☑
   first degree T25.512 ☑
   second degree T25.612 ☑
   third degree T25.712 ☑
  multiple with foot — *see* Corrosion, lower, limb, multiple, ankle and foot
  right T25.411 ☑
   first degree T25.511 ☑
   second degree T25.611 ☑
   third degree T25.711 ☑
  second degree T25.619 ☑
  third degree T25.719 ☑
 anus — *see* Corrosion, buttock
 arm(s) (meaning upper limb(s)) — *see* Corrosion, upper limb
 axilla T22.449 ☑
  first degree T22.549 ☑
  left T22.442 ☑
   first degree T22.542 ☑
   second degree T22.642 ☑
   third degree T22.742 ☑
  right T22.441 ☑
   first degree T22.541 ☑
   second degree T22.641 ☑
   third degree T22.741 ☑
  second degree T22.649 ☑
  third degree T22.749 ☑
 back (lower) T21.44 ☑
  first degree T21.54 ☑
  second degree T21.64 ☑
  third degree T21.74 ☑
  upper T21.43 ☑
   first degree T21.53 ☑
   second degree T21.63 ☑
   third degree T21.73 ☑
 blisters — *code as* Corrosion, second degree, by site
 breast(s) — *see* Corrosion, chest wall
 buttock(s) T21.45 ☑
  first degree T21.55 ☑
  second degree T21.65 ☑
  third degree T21.75 ☑
 calf T24.439 ☑
  first degree T24.539 ☑
  left T24.432 ☑
   first degree T24.532 ☑

Corrosion — *continued*
  calf — *continued*
    left — *continued*
      second degree T24.632 ☑
      third degree T24.732 ☑
      right T24.431 ☑
        first degree T24.531 ☑
        second degree T24.631 ☑
        third degree T24.731 ☑
      second degree T24.639 ☑
      third degree T24.739 ☑
  canthus (eye) — *see* Corrosion, eyelid
  cervix T28.8 ☑
  cheek T20.46 ☑
    first degree T20.56 ☑
    second degree T20.66 ☑
    third degree T20.76 ☑
  chest wall T21.41 ☑
    first degree T21.51 ☑
    second degree T21.61 ☑
    third degree T21.71 ☑
  chin T20.43 ☑
    first degree T20.53 ☑
    second degree T20.63 ☑
    third degree T20.73 ☑
  colon T28.7 ☑
  conjunctiva (and cornea) — *see* Corrosion, cornea
  cornea (and conjunctiva) T26.6- ☑
  deep necrosis of underlying tissue — *code as* Corrosion, third degree, by site
  dorsum of hand T23.469 ☑
    first degree T23.569 ☑
    left T23.462 ☑
      first degree T23.562 ☑
      second degree T23.662 ☑
      third degree T23.762 ☑
    right T23.461 ☑
      first degree T23.561 ☑
      second degree T23.661 ☑
      third degree T23.761 ☑
    second degree T23.669 ☑
    third degree T23.769 ☑
  ear (auricle) (external) (canal) T20.41 ☑
    drum T28.91 ☑
    first degree T20.51 ☑
    second degree T20.61 ☑
    third degree T20.71 ☑
  elbow T22.429 ☑
    first degree T22.529 ☑
    left T22.422 ☑
      first degree T22.522 ☑
      second degree T22.622 ☑
      third degree T22.722 ☑
    right T22.421 ☑
      first degree T22.521 ☑
      second degree T22.621 ☑
      third degree T22.721 ☑
    second degree T22.629 ☑
    third degree T22.729 ☑
  entire body — *see* Corrosion, multiple body regions
  epidermal loss — *code as* Corrosion, second degree, by site
  epiglottis T27.4 ☑
  erythema, erythematous — *code as* Corrosion, first degree, by site
  esophagus T28.6 ☑
  extent (percentage of body surface)
    less than 10 percent T32.0
    10-19 percent (0-9 percent third degree) T32.10
      with 10-19 percent third degree T32.11
    20-29 percent (0-9 percent third degree) T32.20
      with
        10-19 percent third degree T32.21
        20-29 percent third degree T32.22
    30-39 percent (0-9 percent third degree) T32.30
      with
        10-19 percent third degree T32.31
        20-29 percent third degree T32.32
        30-39 percent third degree T32.33
    40-49 percent (0-9 percent third degree) T32.40
      with
        10-19 percent third degree T32.41
        20-29 percent third degree T32.42
        30-39 percent third degree T32.43
        40-49 percent third degree T32.44
    50-59 percent (0-9 percent third degree) T32.50

Corrosion — *continued*
  extent — *continued*
    50-59 percent — *continued*
      with
        10-19 percent third degree T32.51
        20-29 percent third degree T32.52
        30-39 percent third degree T32.53
        40-49 percent third degree T32.54
        50-59 percent third degree T32.55
    60-69 percent (0-9 percent third degree) T32.60
      with
        10-19 percent third degree T32.61
        20-29 percent third degree T32.62
        30-39 percent third degree T32.63
        40-49 percent third degree T32.64
        50-59 percent third degree T32.65
        60-69 percent third degree T32.66
    70-79 percent (0-9 percent third degree) T32.70
      with
        10-19 percent third degree T32.71
        20-29 percent third degree T32.72
        30-39 percent third degree T32.73
        40-49 percent third degree T32.74
        50-59 percent third degree T32.75
        60-69 percent third degree T32.76
        70-79 percent third degree T32.77
    80-89 percent (0-9 percent third degree) T32.80
      with
        10-19 percent third degree T32.81
        20-29 percent third degree T32.82
        30-39 percent third degree T32.83
        40-49 percent third degree T32.84
        50-59 percent third degree T32.85
        60-69 percent third degree T32.86
        70-79 percent third degree T32.87
        80-89 percent third degree T32.88
    90 percent or more (0-9 percent third degree) T32.90
      with
        10-19 percent third degree T32.91
        20-29 percent third degree T32.92
        30-39 percent third degree T32.93
        40-49 percent third degree T32.94
        50-59 percent third degree T32.95
        60-69 percent third degree T32.96
        70-79 percent third degree T32.97
        80-89 percent third degree T32.98
        90-99 percent third degree T32.99
  extremity — *see* Corrosion, limb
  eye(s) and adnexa T26.9- ☑
    with resulting rupture and destruction of eyeball T26.7- ☑
    conjunctival sac — *see* Corrosion, cornea
    cornea — *see* Corrosion, cornea
    lid — *see* Corrosion, eyelid
    periocular area — *see* Corrosion eyelid
    specified site NEC T26.8- ☑
  eyeball — *see* Corrosion, eye
  eyelid(s) T26.5- ☑
  face — *see* Corrosion, head
  finger T23.429 ☑
    first degree T23.529 ☑
    left T23.422 ☑
      first degree T23.522 ☑
      second degree T23.622 ☑
      third degree T23.722 ☑
    multiple sites (without thumb) T23.439 ☑
      with thumb T23.449 ☑
        first degree T23.549 ☑
        left T23.442 ☑
          first degree T23.542 ☑
          second degree T23.642 ☑
          third degree T23.742 ☑
        right T23.441 ☑
          first degree T23.541 ☑
          second degree T23.641 ☑
          third degree T23.741 ☑
        second degree T23.649 ☑
        third degree T23.749 ☑
      first degree T23.539 ☑
      left T23.432 ☑
        first degree T23.532 ☑
        second degree T23.632 ☑
        third degree T23.732 ☑
      right T23.431 ☑
        first degree T23.531 ☑
        second degree T23.631 ☑
        third degree T23.731 ☑

Corrosion — *continued*
  finger — *continued*
    multiple sites — *continued*
      second degree T23.639 ☑
      third degree T23.739 ☑
      right T23.421 ☑
        first degree T23.521 ☑
        second degree T23.621 ☑
        third degree T23.721 ☑
      second degree T23.629 ☑
      third degree T23.729 ☑
  flank — *see* Corrosion, abdomen
  foot T25.429 ☑
    first degree T25.529 ☑
    left T25.422 ☑
      first degree T25.522 ☑
      second degree T25.622 ☑
      third degree T25.722 ☑
    multiple with ankle — *see* Corrosion, lower, limb, multiple, ankle and foot
    right T25.421 ☑
      first degree T25.521 ☑
      second degree T25.621 ☑
      third degree T25.721 ☑
    second degree T25.629 ☑
    third degree T25.729 ☑
  forearm T22.419 ☑
    first degree T22.519 ☑
    left T22.412 ☑
      first degree T22.512 ☑
      second degree T22.612 ☑
      third degree T22.712 ☑
    right T22.411 ☑
      first degree T22.511 ☑
      second degree T22.611 ☑
      third degree T22.711 ☑
    second degree T22.619 ☑
    third degree T22.719 ☑
  forehead T20.46 ☑
    first degree T20.56 ☑
    second degree T20.66 ☑
    third degree T20.76 ☑
  fourth degree — *code as* Corrosion, third degree, by site
  full thickness skin loss — *code as* Corrosion, third degree, by site
  gastrointestinal tract NEC T28.7 ☑
  genital organs
    external
      female T21.47 ☑
        first degree T21.57 ☑
        second degree T21.67 ☑
        third degree T21.77 ☑
      male T21.46 ☑
        first degree T21.56 ☑
        second degree T21.66 ☑
        third degree T21.76 ☑
    internal T28.8 ☑
  groin — *see* Corrosion, abdominal wall
  hand(s) T23.409 ☑
    back — *see* Corrosion, dorsum of hand
    finger — *see* Corrosion, finger
    first degree T23.509 ☑
    left T23.402 ☑
      first degree T23.502 ☑
      second degree T23.602 ☑
      third degree T23.702 ☑
    multiple sites with wrist T23.499 ☑
      first degree T23.599 ☑
      left T23.492 ☑
        first degree T23.592 ☑
        second degree T23.692 ☑
        third degree T23.792 ☑
      right T23.491 ☑
        first degree T23.591 ☑
        second degree T23.691 ☑
        third degree T23.791 ☑
      second degree T23.699 ☑
      third degree T23.799 ☑
    palm — *see* Corrosion, palm
    right T23.401 ☑
      first degree T23.501 ☑
      second degree T23.601 ☑
      third degree T23.701 ☑
    second degree T23.609 ☑
    third degree T23.709 ☑

Corrosion — *continued*
  hand(s) — *continued*
    thumb — *see* Corrosion, thumb
  head (and face) (and neck) T20.40 ☑
    cheek — *see* Corrosion, cheek
    chin — *see* Corrosion, chin
    ear — *see* Corrosion, ear
    eye(s) only — *see* Corrosion, eye
    first degree T20.50 ☑
    forehead — *see* Corrosion, forehead
    lip — *see* Corrosion, lip
    multiple sites T20.49 ☑
      first degree T20.59 ☑
      second degree T20.69 ☑
      third degree T20.79 ☑
    neck — *see* Corrosion, neck
    nose — *see* Corrosion, nose
    scalp — *see* Corrosion, scalp
    second degree T20.60 ☑
    third degree T20.70 ☑
  hip(s) — *see* Corrosion, lower, limb
  inhalation — *see* Corrosion, respiratory tract
  internal organ(s) — *see also* Corrosion, by site
    T28.90 ☑
    alimentary tract T28.7 ☑
      esophagus T28.6 ☑
    esophagus T28.6 ☑
    genitourinary T28.8 ☑
    mouth T28.5 ☑
    pharynx T28.5 ☑
    specified organ NEC T28.99 ☑
  interscapular region — *see* Corrosion, back, upper
  intestine (large) (small) T28.7 ☑
  knee T24.429 ☑
    first degree T24.529 ☑
    left T24.422 ☑
      first degree T24.522 ☑
      second degree T24.622 ☑
      third degree T24.722 ☑
    right T24.421 ☑
      first degree T24.521 ☑
      second degree T24.621 ☑
      third degree T24.721 ☑
    second degree T24.629 ☑
    third degree T24.729 ☑
  labium (majus) (minus) — *see* Corrosion, genital organs, external, female
  lacrimal apparatus, duct, gland or sac — *see* Corrosion, eye, specified site NEC
  larynx T27.4 ☑
    with lung T27.5 ☑
  leg(s) (meaning lower limb(s)) — *see* Corrosion, lower, limb
  limb(s)
    lower — *see* Corrosion, lower, limb
    upper — *see* Corrosion, upper limb
  lip(s) T20.42 ☑
    first degree T20.52 ☑
    second degree T20.62 ☑
    third degree T20.72 ☑
  lower
    back — *see* Corrosion, back
    limb T24.409 ☑
      ankle — *see* Corrosion, ankle
      calf — *see* Corrosion, calf
      first degree T24.509 ☑
      foot — *see* Corrosion, foot
      knee — *see* Corrosion, knee
      left T24.402 ☑
        first degree T24.502 ☑
        second degree T24.602 ☑
        third degree T24.702 ☑
      multiple sites, except ankle and foot T24.499 ☑
        ankle and foot T25.499 ☑
          first degree T25.599 ☑
          left T25.492 ☑
            first degree T25.592 ☑
            second degree T25.692 ☑
            third degree T25.792 ☑
          right T25.491 ☑
            first degree T25.591 ☑
            second degree T25.691 ☑
            third degree T25.791 ☑
          second degree T25.699 ☑
          third degree T25.799 ☑
        first degree T24.599 ☑

Corrosion — *continued*
  lower — *continued*
    limb — *continued*
      multiple sites, except ankle and foot — *continued*
        left T24.492 ☑
          first degree T24.592 ☑
          second degree T24.692 ☑
          third degree T24.792 ☑
        right T24.491 ☑
          first degree T24.591 ☑
          second degree T24.691 ☑
          third degree T24.791 ☑
        second degree T24.699 ☑
        third degree T24.799 ☑
      right T24.401 ☑
        first degree T24.501 ☑
        second degree T24.601 ☑
        third degree T24.701 ☑
      second degree T24.609 ☑
      thigh — *see* Corrosion, thigh
      third degree T24.709 ☑
  lung (with larynx and trachea) T27.5 ☑
  mouth T28.5 ☑
  neck T20.47 ☑
    first degree T20.57 ☑
    second degree T20.67 ☑
    third degree T20.77 ☑
  nose (septum) T20.44 ☑
    first degree T20.54 ☑
    second degree T20.64 ☑
    third degree T20.74 ☑
  ocular adnexa — *see* Corrosion, eye
  orbit region — *see* Corrosion, eyelid
  palm T23.459 ☑
    first degree T23.559 ☑
    left T23.452 ☑
      first degree T23.552 ☑
      second degree T23.652 ☑
      third degree T23.752 ☑
    right T23.451 ☑
      first degree T23.551 ☑
      second degree T23.651 ☑
      third degree T23.751 ☑
    second degree T23.659 ☑
    third degree T23.759 ☑
  partial thickness — *code as* Corrosion, unspecified degree, by site
  pelvis — *see* Corrosion, trunk
  penis — *see* Corrosion, genital organs, external, male
  perineum
    female — *see* Corrosion, genital organs, external, female
    male — *see* Corrosion, genital organs, external, male
  periocular area — *see* Corrosion, eyelid
  pharynx T28.5 ☑
  rectum T28.7 ☑
  respiratory tract T27.7 ☑
    larynx — *see* Corrosion, larynx
    specified part NEC T27.6 ☑
    trachea — *see* Corrosion, larynx
  sac, lacrimal — *see* Corrosion, eye, specified site NEC
  scalp T20.45 ☑
    first degree T20.55 ☑
    second degree T20.65 ☑
    third degree T20.75 ☑
  scapular region T22.469 ☑
    first degree T22.569 ☑
    left T22.462 ☑
      first degree T22.562 ☑
      second degree T22.662 ☑
      third degree T22.762 ☑
    right T22.461 ☑
      first degree T22.561 ☑
      second degree T22.661 ☑
      third degree T22.761 ☑
    second degree T22.669 ☑
    third degree T22.769 ☑
  sclera — *see* Corrosion, eye, specified site NEC
  scrotum — *see* Corrosion, genital organs, external, male
  shoulder T22.459 ☑
    first degree T22.559 ☑
    left T22.452 ☑
      first degree T22.552 ☑
      second degree T22.652 ☑

Corrosion — *continued*
  shoulder — *continued*
    left — *continued*
      third degree T22.752 ☑
    right T22.451 ☑
      first degree T22.551 ☑
      second degree T22.651 ☑
      third degree T22.751 ☑
    second degree T22.659 ☑
    third degree T22.759 ☑
  stomach T28.7 ☑
  temple — *see* Corrosion, head
  testis — *see* Corrosion, genital organs, external, male
  thigh T24.419 ☑
    first degree T24.519 ☑
    left T24.412 ☑
      first degree T24.512 ☑
      second degree T24.612 ☑
      third degree T24.712 ☑
    right T24.411 ☑
      first degree T24.511 ☑
      second degree T24.611 ☑
      third degree T24.711 ☑
    second degree T24.619 ☑
    third degree T24.719 ☑
  thorax (external) — *see* Corrosion, trunk
  throat (meaning pharynx) T28.5 ☑
  thumb(s) T23.419 ☑
    first degree T23.519 ☑
    left T23.412 ☑
      first degree T23.512 ☑
      second degree T23.612 ☑
      third degree T23.712 ☑
    multiple sites with fingers T23.449 ☑
      first degree T23.549 ☑
      left T23.442 ☑
        first degree T23.542 ☑
        second degree T23.642 ☑
        third degree T23.742 ☑
      right T23.441 ☑
        first degree T23.541 ☑
        second degree T23.641 ☑
        third degree T23.741 ☑
      second degree T23.649 ☑
      third degree T23.749 ☑
    right T23.411 ☑
      first degree T23.511 ☑
      second degree T23.611 ☑
      third degree T23.711 ☑
    second degree T23.619 ☑
    third degree T23.719 ☑
  toe T25.439 ☑
    first degree T25.539 ☑
    left T25.432 ☑
      first degree T25.532 ☑
      second degree T25.632 ☑
      third degree T25.732 ☑
    right T25.431 ☑
      first degree T25.531 ☑
      second degree T25.631 ☑
      third degree T25.731 ☑
    second degree T25.639 ☑
    third degree T25.739 ☑
  tongue T28.5 ☑
  tonsil(s) T28.5 ☑
  total body — *see* Corrosion, multiple body regions
  trachea T27.4 ☑
    with lung T27.5 ☑
  trunk T21.40 ☑
    abdominal wall — *see* Corrosion, abdominal wall
    anus — *see* Corrosion, buttock
    axilla — *see* Corrosion, upper limb
    back — *see* Corrosion, back
    breast — *see* Corrosion, chest wall
    buttock — *see* Corrosion, buttock
    chest wall — *see* Corrosion, chest wall
    first degree T21.50 ☑
    flank — *see* Corrosion, abdominal wall
    genital
      female — *see* Corrosion, genital organs, external, female
      male — *see* Corrosion, genital organs, external, male
    groin — *see* Corrosion, abdominal wall
    interscapular region — *see* Corrosion, back, upper

Corrosion — *continued*
- trunk — *continued*
  - labia — *see* Corrosion, genital organs, external, female
  - lower back — *see* Corrosion, back
  - penis — *see* Corrosion, genital organs, external, male
  - perineum
    - female — *see* Corrosion, genital organs, external, female
    - male — *see* Corrosion, genital organs, external, male
  - scapular region — *see* Corrosion, upper limb
  - scrotum — *see* Corrosion, genital organs, external, male
  - second degree T21.60 ☑
  - shoulder — *see* Corrosion, upper limb
  - specified site NEC T21.49 ☑
    - first degree T21.59 ☑
    - second degree T21.69 ☑
    - third degree T21.79 ☑
  - testes — *see* Corrosion, genital organs, external, male
  - third degree T21.70 ☑
  - upper back — *see* Corrosion, back, upper
  - vagina T28.8 ☑
  - vulva — *see* Corrosion, genital organs, external, female
- unspecified site with extent of body surface involved
  - specified
    - less than 10 percent T32.0
    - 10-19 percent (0-9 percent third degree) T32.10
      - with 10-19 percent third degree T32.11
    - 20-29 percent (0-9 percent third degree) T32.20
      - with
        - 10-19 percent third degree T32.21
        - 20-29 percent third degree T32.22
    - 30-39 percent (0-9 percent third degree) T32.30
      - with
        - 10-19 percent third degree T32.31
        - 20-29 percent third degree T32.32
        - 30-39 percent third degree T32.33
    - 40-49 percent (0-9 percent third degree) T32.40
      - with
        - 10-19 percent third degree T32.41
        - 20-29 percent third degree T32.42
        - 30-39 percent third degree T32.43
        - 40-49 percent third degree T32.44
    - 50-59 percent (0-9 percent third degree) T32.50
      - with
        - 10-19 percent third degree T32.51
        - 20-29 percent third degree T32.52
        - 30-39 percent third degree T32.53
        - 40-49 percent third degree T32.54
        - 50-59 percent third degree T32.55
    - 60-69 percent (0-9 percent third degree) T32.60
      - with
        - 10-19 percent third degree T32.61
        - 20-29 percent third degree T32.62
        - 30-39 percent third degree T32.63
        - 40-49 percent third degree T32.64
        - 50-59 percent third degree T32.65
        - 60-69 percent third degree T32.66
    - 70-79 percent (0-9 percent third degree) T32.70
      - with
        - 10-19 percent third degree T32.71
        - 20-29 percent third degree T32.72
        - 30-39 percent third degree T32.73
        - 40-49 percent third degree T32.74
        - 50-59 percent third degree T32.75
        - 60-69 percent third degree T32.76
        - 70-79 percent third degree T32.77
    - 80-89 percent (0-9 percent third degree) T32.80
      - with
        - 10-19 percent third degree T32.81
        - 20-29 percent third degree T32.82
        - 30-39 percent third degree T32.83
        - 40-49 percent third degree T32.84
        - 50-59 percent third degree T32.85
        - 60-69 percent third degree T32.86
        - 70-79 percent third degree T32.87
        - 80-89 percent third degree T32.88
    - 90 percent or more (0-9 percent third degree) T32.90
      - with
        - 10-19 percent third degree T32.91
        - 20-29 percent third degree T32.92
        - 30-39 percent third degree T32.93
        - 40-49 percent third degree T32.94

Corrosion — *continued*
- unspecified site with extent of body surface involved
  - specified — *continued*
    - 90 percent or more — *continued*
      - with — *continued*
        - 50-59 percent third degree T32.95
        - 60-69 percent third degree T32.96
        - 70-79 percent third degree T32.97
        - 80-89 percent third degree T32.98
        - 90-99 percent third degree T32.99
- upper limb (axilla) (scapular region) T22.40 ☑
  - above elbow — *see* Corrosion, above elbow
  - axilla — *see* Corrosion, axilla
  - elbow — *see* Corrosion, elbow
  - first degree T22.50 ☑
  - forearm — *see* Corrosion, forearm
  - hand — *see* Corrosion, hand
  - interscapular region — *see* Corrosion, back, upper
  - multiple sites T22.499 ☑
    - first degree T22.599 ☑
    - left T22.492 ☑
      - first degree T22.592 ☑
      - second degree T22.692 ☑
      - third degree T22.792 ☑
    - right T22.491 ☑
      - first degree T22.591 ☑
      - second degree T22.691 ☑
      - third degree T22.791 ☑
    - second degree T22.699 ☑
    - third degree T22.799 ☑
  - scapular region — *see* Corrosion, scapular region
  - second degree T22.60 ☑
  - shoulder — *see* Corrosion, shoulder
  - third degree T22.70 ☑
  - wrist — *see* Corrosion, hand
- uterus T28.8 ☑
- vagina T28.8 ☑
- vulva — *see* Corrosion, genital organs, external, female
- wrist T23.479 ☑
  - first degree T23.579 ☑
  - left T23.472 ☑
    - first degree T23.572 ☑
    - second degree T23.672 ☑
    - third degree T23.772 ☑
  - multiple sites with hand T23.499 ☑
    - first degree T23.599 ☑
    - left T23.492 ☑
      - first degree T23.592 ☑
      - second degree T23.692 ☑
      - third degree T23.792 ☑
    - right T23.491 ☑
      - first degree T23.591 ☑
      - second degree T23.691 ☑
      - third degree T23.791 ☑
    - second degree T23.699 ☑
    - third degree T23.799 ☑
  - right T23.471 ☑
    - first degree T23.571 ☑
    - second degree T23.671 ☑
    - third degree T23.771 ☑
  - second degree T23.679 ☑
  - third degree T23.779 ☑

Corrosive burn — *see* Corrosion
Corsican fever — *see* Malaria
Cortical — *see* condition
Cortico-adrenal — *see* condition
Coryza (acute) J00
- with grippe or influenza — *see* Influenza, with, respiratory manifestations NEC
- syphilitic
  - congenital (chronic) A50.05
Co-sleeping, child-caregiver Z72.823
Costen's syndrome or complex M26.69
Costiveness — *see* Constipation
Costochondritis M94.0
Cot death R99
Cotard's syndrome F22
Cotia virus B08.8
Cotton wool spots (retinal) H35.81
Cotungo's disease — *see* Sciatica
Cough (affected) (epidemic) (nervous) R05.9
- with hemorrhage — *see* Hemoptysis
- acute R05.1
- bronchial R05.8
  - with grippe or influenza — *see* Influenza, with, respiratory manifestations NEC

Cough — *continued*
- chronic R05.3
- functional F45.8
- hysterical F45.8
- laryngeal, spasmodic R05.8
- paroxysmal, due to Bordetella pertussis (without pneumonia) A37.00
  - with pneumonia A37.01
- persistent R05.3
- psychogenic F45.8
- refractory R05.3
- smokers' J41.0
- specified NEC R05.8
- subacute R05.2
- syncope R05.4
- tea taster's B49
- unexplained R05.3
Counseling (for) Z71.9
- abuse NEC
  - perpetrator Z69.82
  - victim Z69.81
- alcohol abuser Z71.41
  - family Z71.42
- child abuse
  - nonparental
    - perpetrator Z69.021
    - victim Z69.020
  - parental
    - perpetrator Z69.011
    - victim Z69.010
- consanguinity Z71.89
- contraceptive Z30.09
- dietary Z71.3
- drug abuser Z71.51
  - family member Z71.52
- exercise Z71.82
- family Z71.89
- fertility preservation (prior to cancer therapy) (prior to removal of gonads) Z31.62
- for non-attending third party Z71.0
  - related to sexual behavior or orientation Z70.2
- genetic
  - nonprocreative Z71.83
  - procreative NEC Z31.5
- gestational carrier Z31.7
- health (advice) (education) (instruction) — *see* Counseling, medical
  - risk for travel (international) Z71.84
- human immunodeficiency virus (HIV) Z71.7
- immunization safety Z71.85
- impotence Z70.1
- insulin pump use Z46.81
- medical (for) Z71.9
  - boarding school resident Z59.3
  - consanguinity Z71.89
  - feared complaint and no disease found Z71.1
  - human immunodeficiency virus (HIV) Z71.7
  - institutional resident Z59.3
  - on behalf of another Z71.0
    - related to sexual behavior or orientation Z70.2
  - person living alone Z60.2
  - specified reason NEC Z71.89
- natural family planning
  - procreative Z31.61
  - to avoid pregnancy Z30.02
- pediatric-to-adult transition Z71.87
- perpetrator (of)
  - abuse NEC Z69.82
  - child abuse
    - non-parental Z69.021
    - parental Z69.011
  - rape NEC Z69.82
  - spousal abuse Z69.12
- procreative NEC Z31.69
  - fertility preservation (prior to cancer therapy) (prior to removal of gonads) Z31.62
  - using natural family planning Z31.61
- promiscuity Z70.1
- rape victim Z69.81
- religious Z71.81
- safety for travel (international) Z71.84
- sex, sexual (related to) Z70.9
  - attitude(s) Z70.0
  - behavior or orientation Z70.1
  - combined concerns Z70.3
  - non-responsiveness Z70.1
  - on behalf of third party Z70.2
  - specified reason NEC Z70.8
- socioeconomic factors Z71.88

Crush, crushed, crushing — *continued*
 finger(s) — *continued*
  thumb — *see* Crush, thumb
 foot S97.8- ☑
  toe — *see* Crush, toe
 forearm S57.8- ☑
 genitalia, external
  female S38.002 ☑
   vagina S38.03 ☑
   vulva S38.03 ☑
  male S38.001 ☑
   penis S38.01 ☑
   scrotum S38.02 ☑
   testis S38.02 ☑
 hand (except fingers alone) S67.2- ☑
  with wrist S67.4- ☑
 head S07.9
  specified NEC S07.8 ☑
 heel — *see* Crush, foot
 hip S77.0- ☑
  with thigh S77.2- ☑
 internal organ (abdomen, chest, or pelvis) NEC T14.8 ☑
 knee S87.0- ☑
 labium (majus) (minus) S38.03 ☑
 larynx S17.0 ☑
 leg (lower) S87.8- ☑
  knee — *see* Crush, knee
 lip S07.0 ☑
 lower
  back S38.1 ☑
  leg — *see* Crush, leg
 neck S17.9 ☑
 nerve — *see* Injury, nerve
 nose S07.0 ☑
 pelvis S38.1 ☑
 penis S38.01 ☑
 scalp S07.8 ☑
 scapular region — *see* Crush, arm
 scrotum S38.02 ☑
 severe, unspecified site T14.8 ☑
 shoulder (and upper arm) — *see* Crush, arm
 skull S07.1 ☑
 syndrome (complication of trauma) T79.5 ☑
 testis S38.02 ☑
 thigh S77.1- ☑
  with hip S77.2- ☑
 throat S17.8 ☑
 thumb S67.0- ☑
  with hand (and wrist) — *see* Crush, hand, specified
   site NEC
 toe(s) S97.10- ☑
  great S97.11- ☑
  lesser S97.12- ☑
 trachea S17.0 ☑
 vagina S38.03 ☑
 vulva S38.03 ☑
 wrist S67.3- ☑
  with hand S67.4- ☑
Crusta lactea L21.0
Crusts R23.4
Crutch paralysis — *see* Injury, brachial plexus
Cruveilhier-Baumgarten cirrhosis, disease or syndrome K74.69
Cruveilhier's atrophy or disease G12.8
Crying (constant) (continuous) (excessive)
 child, adolescent, or adult R45.83
 infant (baby) (newborn) R68.11
Cryofibrinogenemia D89.2
Cryoglobulinemia (essential) (idiopathic) (mixed) (primary) (purpura) (secondary) (vasculitis) D89.1
 with lung involvement D89.1 *[J99]*
Cryptitis (anal) (rectal) K62.89
Cryptococcosis, cryptococcus (infection) (neoformans) B45.9
 bone B45.3
 cerebral B45.1
 cutaneous B45.2
 disseminated B45.7
 generalized B45.7
 meningitis B45.1
 meningocerebralis B45.1
 osseous B45.3
 pulmonary B45.0
 skin B45.2
 specified NEC B45.8
Cryptopapillitis (anus) K62.89

Cryptophthalmos Q11.2
 syndrome Q87.0
Cryptorchid, cryptorchism, cryptorchidism Q53.9
 bilateral Q53.20
  abdominal Q53.211
  perineal Q53.22
 unilateral Q53.10
  abdominal Q53.111
  perineal Q53.12
Cryptosporidiosis A07.2
 hepatobiliary B88.8
 respiratory B88.8
Cryptostromosis J67.6
Crystalluria R82.998
Cubitus
 congenital Q68.8
 valgus (acquired) M21.0- ☑
  congenital Q68.8
  sequelae (late effect) of rickets E64.3
 varus (acquired) M21.1- ☑
  congenital Q68.8
  sequelae (late effect) of rickets E64.3
Cultural deprivation or shock Z60.3
Curling esophagus K22.4
Curling's ulcer — *see* Ulcer, peptic, acute
Curschmann (-Batten) (-Steinert) **disease or syndrome** G71.11
Curse, Ondine's — *see* Apnea, sleep
Curvature
 organ or site, congenital NEC — *see* Distortion
 penis (lateral) Q55.61
 Pott's (spinal) A18.01
 radius, idiopathic, progressive (congenital) Q74.0
 spine (acquired) (angular) (idiopathic) (incorrect) (postural) — *see* Dorsopathy, deforming
  congenital Q67.5
  due to or associated with
   Charcot-Marie-Tooth disease — *see also* subcategory M49.8 G60.0
   osteitis
    deformans M88.88
    fibrosa cystica — *see also* subcategory M49.8 E21.0
   tuberculosis (Pott's curvature) A18.01
  sequelae (late effect) of rickets E64.3
  tuberculous A18.01
Cushingoid due to steroid therapy E24.2
 correct substance properly administered — *see* Table of Drugs and Chemicals, by drug, adverse effect
 overdose or wrong substance given or taken — *see* Table of Drugs and Chemicals, by drug, poisoning
Cushing's
 syndrome or disease E24.9
  drug-induced E24.2
  iatrogenic E24.2
  pituitary-dependent E24.0
  specified NEC E24.8
 ulcer — *see* Ulcer, peptic, acute
Cusp, Carabelli — *omit code*
Cut (external) — *see also* Laceration
 muscle — *see* Injury, muscle
Cutaneous — *see also* condition
 hemorrhage R23.3
 larva migrans B76.9
Cutis — *see also* condition
 hyperelastica Q82.8
  acquired L57.4
 laxa (hyperelastica) — *see* Dermatolysis
 marmorata R23.8
 osteosis L94.2
 pendula — *see* Dermatolysis
 rhomboidalis nuchae L57.2
 verticis gyrata Q82.8
  acquired L91.8
Cyanosis R23.0
 due to
  patent foramen botalli Q21.12
  persistent foramen ovale Q21.12
 enterogenous D74.8
 paroxysmal digital — *see* Raynaud's disease
  with gangrene I73.01
 retina, retinal H35.89
Cyanotic heart disease I24.9
 congenital Q24.9
Cycle
 anovulatory N97.0
 menstrual, irregular N92.6
Cyclencephaly Q04.9

Cyclical vomiting, in migraine — *see also* Vomiting, cyclical G43.A0 (*following* G43.7)
 psychogenic F50.89
Cyclitis — *see also* Iridocyclitis H20.9
 chronic — *see* Iridocyclitis, chronic
 Fuchs' heterochromic H20.81- ☑
 granulomatous — *see* Iridocyclitis, chronic
 lens-induced — *see* Iridocyclitis, lens-induced
 posterior H30.2- ☑
Cycloid personality F34.0
Cyclophoria H50.54
Cyclopia, cyclops Q87.0
Cyclopism Q87.0
Cyclosporiasis A07.4
Cyclothymia F34.0
Cyclothymic personality F34.0
Cyclotropia H50.41- ☑
Cylindroma — *see also* Neoplasm, malignant, by site
 eccrine dermal — *see* Neoplasm, skin, benign
 skin — *see* Neoplasm, skin, benign
Cylindruria R82.998
Cynanche
 diphtheritic A36.2
 tonsillaris J36
Cynophobia F40.218
Cynorexia R63.2
Cyphosis — *see* Kyphosis
Cyprus fever — *see* Brucellosis
Cyst (colloid) (mucous) (simple) (retention)
 adenoid (infected) J35.8
 adrenal gland E27.8
  congenital Q89.1
 air, lung J98.4
 allantoic Q64.4
 alveolar process (jaw bone) M27.40
 amnion, amniotic O41.8X- ☑
 aneurysmal M27.49
 anterior
  chamber (eye) — *see* Cyst, iris
  nasopalatine K09.1
 antrum J34.1
 anus K62.89
 apical (tooth) (periodontal) K04.8
 appendix K38.8
 arachnoid, brain (acquired) G93.0
  congenital Q04.6
 arytenoid J38.7
 Baker's M71.2- ☑
  ruptured M66.0
  tuberculous A18.02
 Bartholin's gland N75.0
 bile duct (common) (hepatic) K83.5
 bladder (multiple) (trigone) N32.89
 blue dome (breast) — *see* Cyst, breast
 bone (local) NEC M85.60
  aneurysmal M85.50
   ankle M85.57- ☑
   foot M85.57- ☑
   forearm M85.53- ☑
   hand M85.54- ☑
   jaw M27.49
   lower leg M85.56- ☑
   multiple site M85.59
   neck M85.58
   rib M85.58
   shoulder M85.51- ☑
   skull M85.58
   specified site NEC M85.58
   thigh M85.55- ☑
   toe M85.57- ☑
   upper arm M85.52- ☑
   vertebra M85.58
  solitary M85.40
   ankle M85.47- ☑
   fibula M85.46- ☑
   foot M85.47- ☑
   hand M85.44- ☑
   humerus M85.42- ☑
   jaw M27.49
   neck M85.48
   pelvis M85.45- ☑
   radius M85.43- ☑
   rib M85.48
   shoulder M85.41- ☑
   skull M85.48
   specified site NEC M85.48
   tibia M85.46- ☑

Cyst — *continued*
  bone — *continued*
    solitary — *continued*
      toe M85.47- ☑
      ulna M85.43- ☑
      vertebra M85.48
    specified type NEC M85.60
      ankle M85.67- ☑
      foot M85.67- ☑
      forearm M85.63- ☑
      hand M85.64- ☑
      jaw M27.40
        developmental (nonodontogenic) K09.1
          odontogenic K09.0
        latent M27.0
      lower leg M85.66- ☑
      multiple site M85.69
      neck M85.68
      rib M85.68
      shoulder M85.61- ☑
      skull M85.68
      specified site NEC M85.68
      thigh M85.65- ☑
      toe M85.67- ☑
      upper arm M85.62- ☑
      vertebra M85.68
  brain (acquired) G93.0
    congenital Q04.6
    hydatid B67.99 [G94]
    third ventricle (colloid), congenital Q04.6
  branchial (cleft) Q18.0
  branchiogenic Q18.0
  breast (benign) (blue dome) (pedunculated) (solitary) N60.0- ☑
    involution — *see* Dysplasia, mammary, specified type NEC
    sebaceous — *see* Dysplasia, mammary, specified type NEC
  broad ligament (benign) N83.8
  bronchogenic (mediastinal) (sequestration) J98.4
    congenital Q33.0
  buccal K09.8
  bulbourethral gland N36.8
  bursa, bursal NEC M71.30
    with rupture — *see* Rupture, synovium
    ankle M71.37- ☑
    elbow M71.32- ☑
    foot M71.37- ☑
    hand M71.34- ☑
    hip M71.35- ☑
    multiple sites M71.39
    pharyngeal J39.2
    popliteal space — *see* Cyst, Baker's
    shoulder M71.31- ☑
    specified site NEC M71.38
    wrist M71.33- ☑
  calcifying odontogenic D16.5
    upper jaw (bone) (maxilla) D16.4
  canal of Nuck (female) N94.89
    congenital Q52.4
  canthus — *see* Cyst, conjunctiva
  carcinomatous — *see* Neoplasm, malignant, by site
  cauda equina G95.89
  cavum septi pellucidi — *see* Cyst, brain
  celomic (pericardium) Q24.8
  cerebellopontine (angle) — *see* Cyst, brain
  cerebellum — *see* Cyst, brain
  cerebral — *see* Cyst, brain
  cervical lateral Q18.0
  cervix NEC N88.8
    embryonic Q51.6
    nabothian N88.8
  chiasmal optic NEC — *see* Disorder, optic, chiasm
  chocolate (ovary) N80.10- ☑
  choledochus, congenital Q44.4
  chorion O41.8X- ☑
  choroid plexus G93.0
    congenital Q04.6
  ciliary body — *see* Cyst, iris
  clitoris N90.7
  colon K63.89
  common (bile) duct K83.5
  congenital NEC Q89.8
    adrenal gland Q89.1
    epiglottis Q31.8
    esophagus Q39.8
    fallopian tube Q50.4

Cyst — *continued*
  congenital — *continued*
    kidney Q61.00
      more than one (multiple) Q61.02
        specified as polycystic Q61.3
          adult type Q61.2
          infantile type NEC Q61.19
            collecting duct dilation Q61.11
      solitary Q61.01
    larynx Q31.8
    liver Q44.6
    lung Q33.0
    mediastinum Q34.1
    ovary Q50.1
    oviduct Q50.4
    periurethral (tissue) Q64.79
    prepuce Q55.69
    salivary gland (any) Q38.4
    sublingual Q38.6
    submaxillary gland Q38.6
    thymus (gland) Q89.2
    tongue Q38.3
    ureterovesical orifice Q62.8
    vulva Q52.79
  conjunctiva H11.44- ☑
  cornea H18.89- ☑
  corpora quadrigemina G93.0
  corpus
    albicans N83.29- ☑
    luteum (hemorrhagic) (ruptured) N83.1- ☑
  Cowper's gland (benign) (infected) N36.8
  cranial meninges G93.0
  craniobuccal pouch E23.6
  craniopharyngeal pouch E23.6
  cystic duct K82.8
  Cysticercus — *see* Cysticercosis
  Dandy-Walker Q03.1
    with spina bifida — *see* Spina bifida
  dental (root) K04.8
    developmental K09.0
    eruption K09.0
    primordial K09.0
  dentigerous (mandible) (maxilla) K09.0
  dermoid — *see* Neoplasm, benign, by site
    with malignant transformation C56.- ☑
    implantation
      external area or site (skin) NEC L72.0
      iris — *see* Cyst, iris, implantation
      vagina N89.8
      vulva N90.7
    mouth K09.8
    oral soft tissue K09.8
    sacrococcygeal — *see* Cyst, pilonidal
  developmental K09.1
    odontogenic K09.0
    oral region (nonodontogenic) K09.1
    ovary, ovarian Q50.1
  dura (cerebral) G93.0
    spinal G96.198
  ear (external) Q18.1
  echinococcal — *see* Echinococcus
  embryonic
    cervix uteri Q51.6
    fallopian tube Q50.4
    vagina Q52.4
  endometrium, endometrial (uterus) N85.8
    ectopic — *see* Endometriosis
  enterogenous Q43.8
  epidermal, epidermoid (inclusion) (*see also* Cyst, skin) L72.0
    mouth K09.8
    oral soft tissue K09.8
  epididymis N50.3
  epiglottis J38.7
  epiphysis cerebri E34.8
  epithelial (inclusion) L72.0
  epoophoron Q50.5
  eruption K09.0
  esophagus K22.89
  ethmoid sinus J34.1
  external female genital organs NEC N90.7
  eyelid (sebaceous) H02.829
    infected — *see* Hordeolum
    left H02.826
      lower H02.825
      upper H02.824
    right H02.823
      lower H02.822

Cyst — *continued*
  eyelid — *continued*
    right — *continued*
      upper H02.821
  eye NEC H57.89
    congenital Q15.8
  fallopian tube N83.8
    congenital Q50.4
  fimbrial (twisted) Q50.4
  fissural (oral region) K09.1
  follicle (graafian) (hemorrhagic) N83.0- ☑
    nabothian N88.8
  follicular (atretic) (hemorrhagic) (ovarian) N83.0- ☑
    dentigerous K09.0
    odontogenic K09.0
    skin L72.9
      specified NEC L72.8
  frontal sinus J34.1
  gallbladder K82.8
  ganglion — *see* Ganglion
  Gartner's duct Q52.4
  gingiva K09.0
  gland of Moll — *see* Cyst, eyelid
  globulomaxillary K09.1
  graafian follicle (hemorrhagic) N83.0- ☑
  granulosal lutein (hemorrhagic) N83.1- ☑
  hemangiomatous D18.00
    intra-abdominal D18.03
    intracranial D18.02
    skin D18.01
    specified site NEC D18.09
  hemorrhagic M27.49
  hydatid — *see also* Echinococcus B67.90
    brain B67.99 [G94]
    liver — *see also* Cyst, liver, hydatid B67.8
    lung NEC B67.99 [J99]
    Morgagni
      female Q50.5
      male (epididymal) Q55.4
        testicular Q55.29
    specified site NEC B67.99
  hymen N89.8
    embryonic Q52.4
  hypopharynx J39.2
  hypophysis, hypophyseal (duct) (recurrent) E23.6
    cerebri E23.6
  implantation (dermoid)
    external area or site (skin) NEC L72.0
    iris — *see* Cyst, iris, implantation
    vagina N89.8
    vulva N90.7
  incisive canal K09.1
  inclusion (epidermal) (epithelial) (epidermoid) (squamous) L72.0
    not of skin — *code under* Cyst, by site
  intestine (large) (small) K63.89
  intracranial — *see* Cyst, brain
  intraligamentous — *see also* Disorder, ligament
    knee — *see* Derangement, knee
  intrasellar E23.6
  iris H21.309
    exudative H21.31- ☑
    idiopathic H21.30- ☑
    implantation H21.32- ☑
    parasitic H21.33- ☑
    pars plana (primary) H21.34- ☑
      exudative H21.35- ☑
  jaw (bone) M27.40
    aneurysmal M27.49
    developmental (odontogenic) K09.0
    fissural K09.1
    hemorrhagic M27.49
    traumatic M27.49
  joint NEC — *see* Disorder, joint, specified type NEC
  kidney N28.1
    acquired N28.1
    calyceal — *see* Hydronephrosis
    congenital Q61.00
    more than one (multiple) Q61.02
      specified as polycystic Q61.3
        adult type (autosomal dominant) Q61.2
        infantile type (autosomal recessive) NEC Q61.19
          collecting duct dilation Q61.11
    pyelogenic — *see* Hydronephrosis
    simple N28.1
    solitary (single) N28.1
      acquired N28.1

Cyst — *continued*
  kidney — *continued*
    solitary — *continued*
      congenital Q61.01
  labium (majus) (minus) N90.7
    sebaceous N90.7
  lacrimal — *see also* Disorder, lacrimal system, specified NEC
    gland H04.13- ☑
    passages or sac — *see* Disorder, lacrimal system, specified NEC
  larynx J38.7
  lateral periodontal K09.0
  lens H27.8
    congenital Q12.8
  lip (gland) K13.0
  liver (idiopathic) (simple) K76.89
    congenital Q44.6
    hydatid B67.8
      granulosus B67.0
      multilocularis B67.5
  lung J98.4
    congenital Q33.0
    giant bullous J43.9
  lutein N83.1- ☑
  lymphangiomatous D18.1
  lymphoepithelial, oral soft tissue K09.8
  macula — *see* Degeneration, macula, hole
  malignant — *see* Neoplasm, malignant, by site
  mammary gland — *see* Cyst, breast
  mandible M27.40
    dentigerous K09.0
    radicular K04.8
  maxilla M27.40
    dentigerous K09.0
    radicular K04.8
  medial, face and neck Q18.8
  median
    anterior maxillary K09.1
    palatal K09.1
  mediastinum, congenital Q34.1
  meibomian (gland) — *see* Chalazion
    infected — *see* Hordeolum
  membrane, brain G93.0
  meninges (cerebral) G93.0
    spinal G96.198
  meniscus, knee — *see* Derangement, knee, meniscus, cystic
  mesentery, mesenteric K66.8
    chyle I89.8
  mesonephric duct
    female Q50.5
    male Q55.4
  milk N64.89
  Morgagni (hydatid)
    female Q50.5
    male (epididymal) Q55.4
      testicular Q55.29
  mouth K09.8
  Müllerian duct Q50.4
    appendix testis Q55.29
    cervix Q51.6
    fallopian tube Q50.4
    female Q50.4
    male Q55.29
    prostatic utricle Q55.4
    vagina (embryonal) Q52.4
  multilocular (ovary) D39.10
    benign — *see* Neoplasm, benign, by site
  myometrium N85.8
  nabothian (follicle) (ruptured) N88.8
  nasoalveolar K09.1
  nasolabial K09.1
  nasopalatine (anterior) (duct) K09.1
  nasopharynx J39.2
  neoplastic — *see* Neoplasm, uncertain behavior, by site
    benign — *see* Neoplasm, benign, by site
  nerve root
    cervical G96.191
    lumbar G96.191
    sacral G96.191
    thoracic G96.191
  nervous system NEC G96.89
  neuroenteric (congenital) Q06.8
  nipple — *see* Cyst, breast
  nose (turbinates) J34.1
    sinus J34.1

Cyst — *continued*
  odontogenic, developmental K09.0
  omentum (lesser) K66.8
    congenital Q45.8
  ora serrata — *see* Cyst, retina, ora serrata
  oral
    region K09.9
      developmental (nonodontogenic) K09.1
      specified NEC K09.8
    soft tissue K09.9
      specified NEC K09.8
  orbit H05.81- ☑
  ovary, ovarian (twisted) N83.20- ☑
    adherent N83.20- ☑
    chocolate N80.10- ☑
    corpus
      albicans N83.29- ☑
      luteum (hemorrhagic) N83.1- ☑
    dermoid D27.9
    developmental Q50.1
    due to failure of involution NEC N83.20- ☑
    endometrial N80.10- ☑
    follicular (graafian) (hemorrhagic) N83.0- ☑
    hemorrhagic N83.20- ☑
    in pregnancy or childbirth O34.8- ☑
      with obstructed labor O65.5
    multilocular D39.10
    pseudomucinous D27.9
    retention N83.29- ☑
    serous N83.20- ☑
    specified NEC N83.29- ☑
    theca lutein (hemorrhagic) N83.1- ☑
    tuberculous A18.18
  oviduct N83.8
  palate (median) (fissural) K09.1
  palatine papilla (jaw) K09.1
  pancreas, pancreatic (hemorrhagic) (true) K86.2
    congenital Q45.2
    false K86.3
  paralabral
    hip M24.85- ☑
    shoulder S43.43- ☑
  paramesonephric duct Q50.4
    female Q50.4
    male Q55.29
  paranephric N28.1
  paraphysis, cerebri, congenital Q04.6
  parasitic B89
  parathyroid (gland) E21.4
  paratubal N83.8
  paraurethral duct N36.8
  paroophoron Q50.5
  parotid gland K11.6
  parovarian Q50.5
  pelvis, female N94.89
    in pregnancy or childbirth O34.8- ☑
      causing obstructed labor O65.5
  penis (sebaceous) N48.89
  periapical K04.8
  pericardial (congenital) Q24.8
    acquired (secondary) I31.8
  pericoronal K09.0
  perineural G96.191
  periodontal K04.8
    lateral K09.0
  peripelvic (lymphatic) N28.1
  peritoneum K66.8
    chylous I89.8
  periventricular, acquired, newborn P91.1
  pharynx (wall) J39.2
  pilar L72.11
  pilonidal (infected) (rectum) L05.91
    with abscess L05.01
    malignant C44.59- ☑
  pituitary (duct) (gland) E23.6
  placenta O43.19- ☑
  pleura J94.8
  popliteal — *see* Cyst, Baker's
  porencephalic Q04.6
    acquired G93.0
  postanal (infected) — *see* Cyst, pilonidal
  postmastoidectomy cavity (mucosal) — *see* Complications, postmastoidectomy, cyst
  preauricular Q18.1
  prepuce N47.4
    congenital Q55.69
  primordial (jaw) K09.0
  prostate N42.83

Cyst — *continued*
  pseudomucinous (ovary) D27.9
  pupillary, miotic H21.27- ☑
  radicular (residual) K04.8
  radiculodental K04.8
  ranular K11.8
  Rathke's pouch E23.6
  rectum (epithelium) (mucous) K62.89
  renal — *see* Cyst, kidney
  residual (radicular) K04.8
  retention (ovary) N83.29- ☑
    salivary gland K11.6
  retina H33.19- ☑
    ora serrata H33.11- ☑
    parasitic H33.12- ☑
  retroperitoneal K68.9
  sacrococcygeal (dermoid) — *see* Cyst, pilonidal
  salivary gland or duct (mucous extravasation or retention) K11.6
  Sampson's N80.10- ☑
  sclera H15.89
  scrotum L72.9
    sebaceous L72.3
  sebaceous (duct) (gland) L72.3
    breast — *see* Dysplasia, mammary, specified type NEC
    eyelid — *see* Cyst, eyelid
    genital organ NEC
      female N94.89
      male N50.89
    scrotum L72.3
  semilunar cartilage (knee) (multiple) — *see* Derangement, knee, meniscus, cystic
  seminal vesicle N50.89
  serous (ovary) N83.20- ☑
  sinus (accessory) (nasal) J34.1
  Skene's gland N36.8
  skin L72.9
    breast — *see* Dysplasia, mammary, specified type NEC
    epidermal, epidermoid L72.0
    epithelial L72.0
    eyelid — *see* Cyst, eyelid
    genital organ NEC
      female N90.7
      male N50.89
    inclusion L72.0
    scrotum L72.9
    sebaceous L72.3
    sweat gland or duct L74.8
  solitary
    bone — *see* Cyst, bone, solitary
    jaw M27.40
    kidney N28.1
  spermatic cord N50.89
  sphenoid sinus J34.1
  spinal meninges G96.198
  spleen NEC D73.4
    congenital Q89.09
    hydatid — *see also* Echinococcus B67.99 *[D77]*
  Stafne's M27.0
  subarachnoid intrasellar R93.0
  subcutaneous, pheomycotic (chromomycotic) B43.2
  subdural (cerebral) G93.0
    spinal cord G96.198
  sublingual gland K11.6
  submandibular gland K11.6
  submaxillary gland K11.6
  suburethral N36.8
  suprarenal gland E27.8
  suprasellar — *see* Cyst, brain
  sweat gland or duct L74.8
  synovial — *see also* Cyst, bursa
    ruptured — *see* Rupture, synovium
  Tarlov G96.191
  tarsal — *see* Chalazion
  tendon (sheath) — *see* Disorder, tendon, specified type NEC
  testis N44.2
    tunica albuginea N44.1
  theca lutein (ovary) N83.1- ☑
  Thornwaldt's J39.2
  thymus (gland) E32.8
  thyroglossal duct (infected) (persistent) Q89.2
  thyroid (gland) E04.1
  thyrolingual duct (infected) (persistent) Q89.2
  tongue K14.8
  tonsil J35.8

Cyst — *continued*
tooth — *see* Cyst, dental
Tornwaldt's J39.2
trichilemmal (proliferating) L72.12
trichodermal L72.12
tubal (fallopian) N83.8
inflammatory — *see* Salpingitis, chronic
tubo-ovarian N83.8
inflammatory N70.13
tunica
albuginea testis N44.1
vaginalis N50.89
turbinate (nose) J34.1
Tyson's gland N48.89
urachus, congenital Q64.4
ureter N28.89
ureterovesical orifice N28.89
urethra, urethral (gland) N36.8
uterine ligament N83.8
uterus (body) (corpus) (recurrent) N85.8
embryonic Q51.818
cervix Q51.6
vagina, vaginal (implantation) (inclusion) (squamous cell) (wall) N89.8
embryonic Q52.4
vallecula, vallecular (epiglottis) J38.7
vesical (orifice) N32.89
vitreous body H43.89
vulva (implantation) (inclusion) N90.7
congenital Q52.79
sebaceous gland N90.7
vulvovaginal gland N90.7
wolffian
female Q50.5
male Q55.4
Cystadenocarcinoma — *see* Neoplasm, malignant, by site
bile duct C22.1
endometrioid — *see* Neoplasm, malignant, by site
specified site — *see* Neoplasm, malignant, by site
unspecified site
female C56.9
male C61
mucinous
papillary
specified site — *see* Neoplasm, malignant, by site
unspecified site C56.9
specified site — *see* Neoplasm, malignant, by site
unspecified site C56.9
papillary
mucinous
specified site — *see* Neoplasm, malignant, by site
unspecified site C56.9
pseudomucinous
specified site — *see* Neoplasm, malignant, by site
unspecified site C56.9
serous
specified site — *see* Neoplasm, malignant, by site
unspecified site C56.9
specified site — *see* Neoplasm, malignant, by site
unspecified site C56.9
pseudomucinous
papillary
specified site — *see* Neoplasm, malignant, by site
unspecified site C56.9
specified site — *see* Neoplasm, malignant, by site
unspecified site C56.9
serous
papillary
specified site — *see* Neoplasm, malignant, by site
unspecified site C56.9
specified site — *see* Neoplasm, malignant, by site
unspecified site C56.9
Cystadenofibroma
clear cell — *see* Neoplasm, benign, by site
endometrioid D27.9
borderline malignancy D39.1- ☑
malignant C56.- ☑
mucinous
specified site — *see* Neoplasm, benign, by site
unspecified site D27.9

Cystadenofibroma — *continued*
serous
specified site — *see* Neoplasm, benign, by site
unspecified site D27.9
specified site — *see* Neoplasm, benign, by site
unspecified site D27.9
Cystadenoma — *see also* Neoplasm, benign, by site
bile duct D13.4
endometrioid — *see* Neoplasm, benign, by site
borderline malignancy — *see* Neoplasm, uncertain behavior, by site
malignant — *see* Neoplasm, malignant, by site
mucinous
borderline malignancy
ovary C56.- ☑
specified site NEC — *see* Neoplasm, uncertain behavior, by site
unspecified site C56.9
papillary
borderline malignancy
ovary C56.- ☑
specified site NEC — *see* Neoplasm, uncertain behavior, by site
specified site — *see* Neoplasm, benign, by site
unspecified site D27.9
specified site — *see* Neoplasm, benign, by site
unspecified site D27.9
papillary
borderline malignancy
ovary C56.- ☑
specified site NEC — *see* Neoplasm, uncertain behavior, by site
unspecified site C56.9
lymphomatosum
specified site — *see* Neoplasm, benign, by site
unspecified site D11.9
mucinous
borderline malignancy
ovary C56.- ☑
specified site NEC — *see* Neoplasm, uncertain behavior, by site
unspecified site C56.9
specified site — *see* Neoplasm, benign, by site
unspecified site D27.9
pseudomucinous
borderline malignancy
ovary C56.- ☑
specified site NEC — *see* Neoplasm, uncertain behavior, by site
unspecified site C56.9
specified site — *see* Neoplasm, benign, by site
unspecified site D27.9
serous
borderline malignancy
ovary C56.- ☑
specified site NEC — *see* Neoplasm, uncertain behavior, by site
unspecified site C56.9
specified site — *see* Neoplasm, benign, by site
unspecified site D27.9
specified site — *see* Neoplasm, benign, by site
unspecified site D27.9
pseudomucinous
borderline malignancy
ovary C56.- ☑
specified site NEC — *see* Neoplasm, uncertain behavior, by site
unspecified site C56.9
papillary
borderline malignancy
ovary C56.- ☑
specified site NEC — *see* Neoplasm, uncertain behavior, by site
unspecified site C56.9
specified site — *see* Neoplasm, benign, by site
unspecified site D27.9
specified site — *see* Neoplasm, benign, by site
unspecified site D27.9
serous
borderline malignancy
ovary C56.- ☑
specified site NEC — *see* Neoplasm, uncertain behavior, by site
unspecified site C56.9
papillary
borderline malignancy
ovary C56.- ☑

Cystadenoma — *continued*
serous — *continued*
papillary — *continued*
borderline malignancy — *continued*
specified site NEC — *see* Neoplasm, uncertain behavior, by site
unspecified site C56.9
specified site — *see* Neoplasm, benign, by site
unspecified site D27.9
specified site — *see* Neoplasm, benign, by site
unspecified site D27.9
Cystathionine synthase deficiency E72.11
Cystathioninemia E72.19
Cystathioninuria E72.19
Cystic — *see also* condition
breast (chronic) — *see* Mastopathy, cystic
corpora lutea (hemorrhagic) N83.1- ☑
duct — *see* condition
eyeball (congenital) Q11.0
fibrosis — *see* Fibrosis, cystic
kidney (congenital) Q61.9
adult type Q61.2
infantile type NEC Q61.19
collecting duct dilatation Q61.11
medullary Q61.5
liver, congenital Q44.6
lung disease J98.4
congenital Q33.0
mastitis, chronic — *see* Mastopathy, cystic
medullary, kidney Q61.5
meniscus — *see* Derangement, knee, meniscus, cystic
ovary N83.20- ☑
Cysticercosis, cysticerciasis B69.9
with
epileptiform fits B69.0
myositis B69.81
brain B69.0
central nervous system B69.0
cerebral B69.0
ocular B69.1
specified NEC B69.89
Cysticercus cellulose infestation — *see* Cysticercosis
Cystinosis (malignant) E72.04
Cystinuria E72.01
Cystitis (exudative) (hemorrhagic) (septic) (suppurative) N30.90
with
fibrosis — *see* Cystitis, chronic, interstitial
hematuria N30.91
leukoplakia — *see* Cystitis, chronic, interstitial
malakoplakia — *see* Cystitis, chronic, interstitial
metaplasia — *see* Cystitis, chronic, interstitial
prostatitis N41.3
acute N30.00
with hematuria N30.01
of trigone N30.30
with hematuria N30.31
allergic — *see* Cystitis, specified type NEC
amebic A06.81
bilharzial B65.9 *[N33]*
blennorrhagic (gonococcal) A54.01
bullous — *see* Cystitis, specified type NEC
calculous N21.0
chlamydial A56.01
chronic N30.20
with hematuria N30.21
interstitial N30.10
with hematuria N30.11
of trigone N30.30
with hematuria N30.31
specified NEC N30.20
with hematuria N30.21
cystic (a) — *see* Cystitis, specified type NEC
diphtheritic A36.85
echinococcal
granulosus B67.39
multilocularis B67.69
emphysematous — *see* Cystitis, specified type NEC
encysted — *see* Cystitis, specified type NEC
eosinophilic — *see* Cystitis, specified type NEC
follicular — *see* Cystitis, of trigone
gangrenous — *see* Cystitis, specified type NEC
glandularis — *see* Cystitis, specified type NEC
gonococcal A54.01
incrusted — *see* Cystitis, specified type NEC
interstitial (chronic) — *see* Cystitis, chronic, interstitial
irradiation N30.40
with hematuria N30.41

Cystitis — *continued*
   irritation — *see* Cystitis, specified type NEC
   malignant — *see* Cystitis, specified type NEC
   of trigone N3Ø.3Ø
      with hematuria N3Ø.31
   panmural — *see* Cystitis, chronic, interstitial
   polyposa — *see* Cystitis, specified type NEC
   prostatic N41.3
   puerperal (postpartum) O86.22
   radiation — *see* Cystitis, irradiation
   specified type NEC N3Ø.8Ø
      with hematuria N3Ø.81
   subacute — *see* Cystitis, chronic
   submucous — *see* Cystitis, chronic, interstitial
   syphilitic (late) A52.76
   trichomonal A59.Ø3
   tuberculous A18.12
   ulcerative — *see* Cystitis, chronic, interstitial
Cystocele (-urethrocele)
   female N81.1Ø
      with prolapse of uterus — *see* Prolapse, uterus
      lateral N81.12
      midline N81.11
      paravaginal N81.12

Cystocele — *continued*
   in pregnancy or childbirth O34.8- ☑
      causing obstructed labor O65.5
   male N32.89
Cystolithiasis N21.Ø
Cystoma — *see also* Neoplasm, benign, by site
   endometrial, ovary N8Ø.1Ø- ☑
   mucinous
      specified site — *see* Neoplasm, benign, by site
      unspecified site D27.9
   serous
      specified site — *see* Neoplasm, benign, by site
      unspecified site D27.9
   simple (ovary) N83.29- ☑
Cystoplegia N31.2
Cystoptosis N32.89
Cystopyelitis — *see* Pyelonephritis
Cystorrhagia N32.89
Cystosarcoma phyllodes D48.6- ☑
   benign D24- ☑
   malignant — *see* Neoplasm, breast, malignant
Cystostomy
   attention to Z43.5
   complication — *see* Complications, cystostomy

Cystostomy — *continued*
   status Z93.5Ø
      appendico-vesicostomy Z93.52
      cutaneous Z93.51
      specified NEC Z93.59
Cystourethritis — *see* Urethritis
Cystourethrocele — *see also* Cystocele
   female N81.1Ø
      with uterine prolapse — *see* Prolapse, uterus
      lateral N81.12
      midline N81.11
      paravaginal N81.12
   male N32.89
Cytomegalic inclusion disease
   congenital P35.1
Cytomegalovirus infection B25.9
Cytomycosis (reticuloendothelial) B39.4
Cytopenia D75.9
   refractory
      with multilineage dysplasia D46.A (*following* D46.2)
         and ring sideroblasts (RCMD RS) D46.B (*following* D46.2)
Czerny's disease (periodic hydrarthrosis of the knee) —
      see Effusion, joint, knee

D

Da Costa's syndrome F45.8
Daae (-Finsen) **disease** (epidemic pleurodynia) B33.0
Dabney's grip B33.0
Dacryoadenitis, dacryadenitis H04.00- ☑
  acute H04.01- ☑
  chronic H04.02- ☑
Dacryocystitis H04.30- ☑
  acute H04.32- ☑
  chronic H04.41- ☑
  neonatal P39.1
  phlegmonous H04.31- ☑
  syphilitic A52.71
    congenital (early) A50.01
  trachomatous, active A71.1
    sequelae (late effect) B94.0
Dacryocystoblenorrhea — *see* Inflammation, lacrimal, passages, chronic
Dacryocystocele — *see* Disorder, lacrimal system, changes
Dacryolith, dacryolithiasis H04.51- ☑
Dacryoma — *see* Disorder, lacrimal system, changes
Dacryopericystitis — *see* Dacryocystitis
Dacryops H04.11- ☑
Dacryostenosis — *see also* Stenosis, lacrimal
  congenital Q10.5
Dactylitis
  bone — *see* Osteomyelitis
  sickle-cell D57.00
    Hb C D57.219
    Hb SS D57.00
    specified NEC D57.819
  skin L08.9
  syphilitic A52.77
  tuberculous A18.03
Dactylolysis spontanea (ainhum) L94.6
Dactylosymphysis Q70.9
  fingers — *see* Syndactylism, complex, fingers
  toes — *see* Syndactylism, complex, toes
Damage
  arteriosclerotic — *see* Arteriosclerosis
  brain (nontraumatic) G93.9
    anoxic, hypoxic G93.1
      resulting from a procedure G97.82
    child NEC G80.9
      due to birth injury P11.2
  cardiorenal (vascular) — *see* Hypertension, cardiorenal
  cerebral NEC — *see* Damage, brain
  coccyx, complicating delivery O71.6
  coronary — *see* Disease, heart, ischemic
  deep tissue, pressure-induced — *see also* L89 with final character .6
  eye, birth injury P15.3
  liver (nontraumatic) K76.9
    alcoholic K70.9
    due to drugs — *see* Disease, liver, toxic
    toxic — *see* Disease, liver, toxic
  lung
    dabbing (related) U07.0
    electronic cigarette (related) U07.0
    vaping (associated) (device) (product) (use) U07.0
  medication T88.7 ☑
  organ
    dabbing (related) U07.0
    electronic cigarette (related) U07.0
    vaping (associated) (device) (product) (use) U07.0
  pelvic
    joint or ligament, during delivery O71.6
    organ NEC
      during delivery O71.5
      following ectopic or molar pregnancy O08.6
  renal — *see* Disease, renal
  subendocardium, subendocardial — *see* Degeneration, myocardial
  vascular I99.9
Dana-Putnam syndrome (subacute combined sclerosis with pernicious anemia) — *see* Degeneration, combined
Danbolt (-Cross) **syndrome** (acrodermatitis enteropathica) E83.2
Dandruff L21.0
Dandy-Walker syndrome Q03.1
  with spina bifida — *see* Spina bifida
Danlos' syndrome — *see also* Syndrome, Ehlers-Danlos Q79.60

Darier (-White) **disease** (congenital) Q82.8
  meaning erythema annulare centrifugum L53.1
Darier-Roussy sarcoid D86.3
Darling's disease or histoplasmosis B39.4
Darwin's tubercle Q17.8
Dawson's (inclusion body) **encephalitis** A81.1
De Beurmann (-Gougerot) **disease** B42.1
De la Tourette's syndrome F95.2
De Lange's syndrome Q87.19
De Morgan's spots (senile angiomas) I78.1
De Quervain's
  disease (tendon sheath) M65.4
  syndrome E34.51
  thyroiditis (subacute granulomatous thyroiditis) E06.1
De Toni-Fanconi (-Debré) **syndrome** E72.09
  with cystinosis E72.04
Dead
  fetus, retained (mother) O36.4 ☑
    early pregnancy O02.1
  labyrinth H83.2 ☑
  ovum, retained O02.0
Deaf nonspeaking NEC H91.3
Deafmutism (acquired) (congenital) NEC H91.3
  hysterical F44.6
  syphilitic, congenital — *see also* subcategory H94.8 A50.09
Deafness (acquired) (complete) (hereditary) (partial) H91.9- ☑
  with blue sclera and fragility of bone Q78.0
  auditory fatigue — *see* Deafness, specified type NEC
  aviation T70.0 ☑
    nerve injury — *see* Injury, nerve, acoustic, specified type NEC
  boilermaker's H83.3 ☑
  central — *see* Deafness, sensorineural
  conductive H90.2
    and sensorineural
      mixed H90.8
        bilateral H90.6
    bilateral H90.0
    unilateral H90.1- ☑
      with restricted hearing on the contralateral side H90.A- ☑
  congenital H90.5
    with blue sclera and fragility of bone Q78.0
  due to toxic agents — *see* Deafness, ototoxic
  emotional (hysterical) F44.6
  functional (hysterical) F44.6
  high frequency H91.9- ☑
  hysterical F44.6
  low frequency H91.9- ☑
  mental R48.8
  mixed conductive and sensorineural H90.8
    bilateral H90.6
    unilateral H90.7- ☑
  nerve — *see* Deafness, sensorineural
  neural — *see* Deafness, sensorineural
  noise-induced — *see also* subcategory H83.3 ☑
    nerve injury — *see* Injury, nerve, acoustic, specified type NEC
  nonspeaking H91.3
  ototoxic H91.0 ☑
  perceptive — *see* Deafness, sensorineural
  psychogenic (hysterical) F44.6
  sensorineural H90.5
    and conductive
      bilateral H90.6
      mixed H90.8
        bilateral H90.6
    bilateral H90.3
    unilateral H90.4- ☑
      with restricted hearing on the contralateral side H90.A- ☑
  sensory — *see* Deafness, sensorineural
  specified type NEC H91.8 ☑
  sudden (idiopathic) H91.2- ☑
  syphilitic A52.15
  transient ischemic H93.01- ☑
  traumatic — *see* Injury, nerve, acoustic, specified type NEC
  word (developmental) H93.25
Death (cause unknown) (of) (unexplained) (unspecified cause) R99
  brain G93.82
  cardiac (sudden) (with successful resuscitation) — *see* Arrest, cardiac
    family history of Z82.41

Death — *continued*
  cardiac — *see* Arrest, cardiac — *continued*
    personal history of Z86.74
  family member (assumed) Z63.4
Debility (chronic) (general) (nervous) R53.81
  congenital or neonatal NOS P96.9
  nervous R53.81
  old age R54
  senile R54
Débove's disease (splenomegaly) R16.1
Debt, burdensome Z59.86
Decalcification
  bone — *see* Osteoporosis
  teeth K03.89
Decapsulation, kidney N28.89
Decay
  dental — *see* Caries, dental
  senile R54
  tooth, teeth — *see* Caries, dental
Deciduitis (acute)
  following ectopic or molar pregnancy O08.0
Decline (general) — *see* Debility
  cognitive, age-associated R41.81
Decompensation
  cardiac (acute) (chronic) — *see* Disease, heart
  cardiovascular — *see* Disease, cardiovascular
  heart — *see* Disease, heart
  hepatic — *see* Failure, hepatic
  myocardial (acute) (chronic) — *see* Disease, heart
  respiratory J98.8
Decompression sickness T70.3 ☑
Decrease (d)
  absolute neutrophil count — *see* Neutropenia
  blood
    platelets — *see* Thrombocytopenia
    pressure R03.1
      due to shock following
        injury T79.4 ☑
        operation T81.19 ☑
  estrogen E28.39
    postablative E89.40
      asymptomatic E89.40
      symptomatic E89.41
  fragility of erythrocytes D58.8
  function
    lipase (pancreatic) K90.3
    ovary in hypopituitarism E23.0
    parenchyma of pancreas K86.89
    pituitary (gland) (anterior) (lobe) E23.0
      posterior (lobe) E23.0
  functional activity R68.89
  glucose R73.09
  hematocrit R71.0
  hemoglobin R71.0
  leukocytes D72.819
    specified NEC D72.818
  libido R68.82
  lymphocytes D72.810
  platelets D69.6
  respiration, due to shock following injury T79.4 ☑
  sexual desire R68.82
  tear secretion NEC — *see* Syndrome, dry eye
  tolerance
    fat K90.49
    glucose R73.09
    pancreatic K90.3
    salt and water E87.8
  vision NEC H54.7
  white blood cell count D72.819
    specified NEC D72.818
Decubitus (ulcer) — *see* Ulcer, pressure, by site
  cervix N86
Deepening acetabulum — *see* Derangement, joint, specified type NEC, hip
Defect, defective Q89.9
  3-beta-hydroxysteroid dehydrogenase E25.0
  11-hydroxylase E25.0
  21-hydroxylase E25.0
  abdominal wall, congenital Q79.59
  antibody immunodeficiency D80.9
  aorticopulmonary septum Q21.4
  atrial septal Q21.10
    coronary sinus Q21.13
    following acute myocardial infarction (current complication) I23.1
    ostium primum type (type I) Q21.20

Defect, defective — *continued*
  atrial septal — *continued*
    ostium primum type — *continued*
      with
        common atrioventricular valves and moderate or larger inlet VSD Q21.23
        separate atrioventricular valves and small or restrictive inlet VSD Q21.22
    ostium secundum type (patent persistent) (type II) Q21.11
    sinus venosus Q21.16
      inferior Q21.15
      superior Q21.14
    specified NEC Q21.19
    vena cava type
      inferior Q21.15
      superior Q21.14
  atrioventricular
    canal Q21.20
    septal
      common Q21.23
      complete Q21.23
      incomplete Q21.21
      intermediate Q21.22
      partial Q21.21
      transitional Q21.22
      unspecified as to partial or complete Q21.20
    septum Q21.20
  auricular septal Q21.10
  bilirubin excretion NEC E80.6
  biosynthesis, androgen (testicular) E29.1
  bulbar septum Q21.0
  catalase E80.3
  cell membrane receptor complex (CR3) D71
  circulation I99.9
    congenital Q28.9
    newborn Q28.9
  coagulation (factor) — *see also* Deficiency, factor D68.9
    with
      ectopic pregnancy O08.1
      molar pregnancy O08.1
    acquired D68.4
    antepartum with hemorrhage — *see* Hemorrhage, antepartum, with coagulation defect
    due to
      liver disease D68.4
      vitamin K deficiency D68.4
    hereditary NEC D68.2
    intrapartum O67.0
    newborn, transient P61.6
    postpartum O99.13
      with hemorrhage O72.3
    specified type NEC D68.8
  complement system D84.1
  conduction (heart) I45.9
    bone — *see* Deafness, conductive
  congenital, organ or site not listed — *see* Anomaly, by site
  coronary sinus Q21.13
  cushion, endocardial Q21.20
    common Q21.23
    incomplete Q21.21
    intermediate Q21.22
    transitional Q21.22
  degradation, glycoprotein E77.1
  dental bridge, crown, fillings — *see* Defect, dental restoration
  dental restoration K08.50
    specified NEC K08.59
  dentin (hereditary) K00.5
  Descemet's membrane, congenital Q13.89
  developmental — *see also* Anomaly
    cauda equina Q06.3
  diaphragm
    with elevation, eventration or hernia — *see* Hernia, diaphragm
    congenital Q79.1
      with hernia Q79.0
      gross (with hernia) Q79.0
  ectodermal, congenital Q82.9
  Eisenmenger's Q21.8
  enzyme
    catalase E80.3
    peroxidase E80.3
  esophagus, congenital Q39.9
  extensor retinaculum M62.89
  fibrin polymerization D68.2

Defect, defective — *continued*
  filling
    bladder R93.41
    kidney R93.42- ☑
    renal pelvis R93.41
    stomach R93.3
    ureter R93.41
    urinary organs, specified NEC R93.49
  GABA (gamma aminobutyric acid) metabolic E72.81
  Gerbode Q21.0
  glucose transport, blood-brain barrier E74.810
  glycoprotein degradation E77.1
  Hageman (factor) D68.2
  hearing — *see* Deafness
  high grade F70
  interatrial septal Q21.19
  interauricular septal Q21.19
  interventricular septal Q21.0
    with dextroposition of aorta, pulmonary stenosis and hypertrophy of right ventricle Q21.3
    in tetralogy of Fallot Q21.3
  intervertebral annular fibrosis — *see also* Disease, intervertebral disc, by site M51.9
    lumbar M51.A0
      large M51.A2
      small M51.A1
    lumbosacral M51.A3
      large M51.A5
      small M51.A4
  learning (specific) — *see* Disorder, learning
  lymphocyte function antigen-1 (LFA-1) D84.0
  lysosomal enzyme, post-translational modification E77.0
  major osseous M89.70
    ankle M89.77- ☑
    carpus M89.74- ☑
    clavicle M89.71- ☑
    femur M89.75- ☑
    fibula M89.76- ☑
    fingers M89.74- ☑
    foot M89.77- ☑
    forearm M89.73- ☑
    hand M89.74- ☑
    humerus M89.72- ☑
    lower leg M89.76- ☑
    metacarpus M89.74- ☑
    metatarsus M89.77- ☑
    multiple sites M89.79
    pelvic region M89.75- ☑
    pelvis M89.75- ☑
    radius M89.73- ☑
    scapula M89.71- ☑
    shoulder region M89.71- ☑
    specified NEC M89.78
    tarsus M89.77- ☑
    thigh M89.75- ☑
    tibia M89.76- ☑
    toes M89.77- ☑
    ulna M89.73- ☑
  mental — *see* Disability, intellectual
  modification, lysosomal enzymes, post-translational E77.0
  obstructive, congenital
    renal pelvis Q62.39
    ureter Q62.39
      atresia — *see* Atresia, ureter
      cecoureterocele Q62.32
      megaureter Q62.2
      orthotopic ureterocele Q62.31
  osseous, major M89.70
    ankle M89.77- ☑
    carpus M89.74- ☑
    clavicle M89.71- ☑
    femur M89.75- ☑
    fibula M89.76- ☑
    fingers M89.74- ☑
    foot M89.77- ☑
    forearm M89.73- ☑
    hand M89.74- ☑
    humerus M89.72- ☑
    lower leg M89.76- ☑
    metacarpus M89.74- ☑
    metatarsus M89.77- ☑
    multiple sites M89.9
    pelvic region M89.75- ☑
    pelvis M89.75- ☑
    radius M89.73- ☑

Defect, defective — *continued*
  osseous, major — *continued*
    scapula M89.71- ☑
    shoulder region M89.71- ☑
    specified NEC M89.78
    tarsus M89.77- ☑
    thigh M89.75- ☑
    tibia M89.76- ☑
    toes M89.77- ☑
    ulna M89.73- ☑
  osteochondral NEC — *see also* Deformity M95.8
  ostium
    primum Q21.20
    secundum Q21.11
  peroxidase E80.3
  placental blood supply — *see* Insufficiency, placental
  platelets, qualitative D69.1
    constitutional — *see* Disease, von Willebrand
  postural NEC, spine — *see* Dorsopathy, deforming
  qualitative, of von Willebrand factor
    with
      decreased platelet adhesion and selective deficiency of high-molecular-weight multimers — *see also* Disease, von Willebrand D68.020
      defective platelet adhesion with a normal size distribution of von Willebrand factor multimers — *see also* Disease, von Willebrand D68.022
      defective von Willebrand factor to factor VIII binding — *see also* Disease, von Willebrand D68.023
      high-molecular-weight von Willebrand factor loss — *see also* Disease, von Willebrand D68.021
      hyper-adhesive forms — *see also* Disease, von Willebrand D68.021
      increased affinity for platelet glycoprotein Ib — *see also* Disease, von Willebrand D68.021
      markedly decreased affinity for factor VIII — *see also* Disease, von Willebrand D68.023
    in von Willebrand factor function, with no further subtyping — *see also* Disease, von Willebrand D68.029
  reduction
    limb Q73.8
      lower Q72.9- ☑
        absence — *see* Agenesis, leg
          foot — *see* Agenesis, foot
        longitudinal
          femur Q72.4- ☑
          fibula Q72.6- ☑
          tibia Q72.5- ☑
        specified type NEC Q72.89- ☑
        split foot Q72.7- ☑
      specified type NEC Q73.8
      upper Q71.9- ☑
        absence — *see* Agenesis, arm
          forearm — *see* Agenesis, forearm
          hand — *see* Agenesis, hand
        lobster-claw hand Q71.6- ☑
        longitudinal
          radius Q71.4- ☑
          ulna Q71.5- ☑
        specified type NEC Q71.89- ☑
  renal pelvis Q63.8
    obstructive Q62.39
  respiratory system, congenital Q34.9
  restoration, dental K08.50
    specified NEC K08.59
  retinal nerve bundle fibers H35.89
  septal (heart) NOS Q21.9
    acquired (atrial) (auricular) (ventricular) (old) I51.0
    atrial — *see also* Defect, atrial septal Q21.10
      concurrent with acute myocardial infarction — *see* Infarct, myocardium
      following acute myocardial infarction (current complication) I23.1
    ventricular — *see also* Defect, ventricular septal Q21.0
  sinus venosus — *see also* Defect, atrial septal, sinus venosus Q21.16
  speech — *see* Disorder, speech
    developmental F80.9
    specified NEC R47.89
  Taussig-Bing (aortic transposition and overriding pulmonary artery) Q20.1

☑ **Additional Character Required** — Refer to the Tabular List for Character Selection

Defect, defective — *continued*
　teeth, wedge K03.1
　vascular (local) I99.9
　　congenital Q27.9
　ventricular septal Q21.0
　　concurrent with acute myocardial infarction — *see*
　　　Infarct, myocardium
　　following acute myocardial infarction (current
　　　complication) I23.2
　　in tetralogy of Fallot Q21.3
　vision NEC H54.7
　visual field H53.40
　　bilateral
　　　heteronymous H53.47
　　　homonymous H53.46- ☑
　　generalized contraction H53.48- ☑
　　localized
　　　arcuate H53.43- ☑
　　　scotoma (central area) H53.41- ☑
　　　　blind spot area H53.42- ☑
　　　sector H53.43- ☑
　　　specified type NEC H53.45- ☑
　voice R49.9
　　specified NEC R49.8
　wedge, tooth, teeth (abrasion) K03.1
Deferentitis N49.1
　gonorrheal (acute) (chronic) A54.23
Defibrination (syndrome) D65
　antepartum — *see* Hemorrhage, antepartum, with
　　coagulation defect, disseminated intravascular
　　coagulation
　following ectopic or molar pregnancy O08.1
　intrapartum O67.0
　newborn P60
　postpartum O72.3
Deficiency, deficient
　3-beta hydroxysteroid dehydrogenase E25.0
　5-alpha reductase (with male pseudohermaphroditism)
　　E29.1
　11-hydroxylase E25.0
　21-hydroxylase E25.0
　AADC (aromatic L-amino acid decarboxylase) E70.81
　abdominal muscle syndrome Q79.4
　AC globulin (congenital) (hereditary) D68.2
　　acquired D68.4
　accelerator globulin (Ac G) (blood) D68.2
　acid phosphatase E83.39
　acid sphingomyelinase (ASMD) E75.249
　　type
　　　A E75.240
　　　A/B E75.244
　　　B E75.241
　activating factor (blood) D68.2
　ADA2 (adenosine deaminase 2) D81.32
　adenosine deaminase (ADA) D81.30
　　with severe combined immunodeficiency (SCID)
　　　D81.31
　　partial (type 1) D81.39
　　specified NEC D81.39
　　type 1 (without SCID) (without severe combined
　　　immunodeficiency) D81.39
　　type 2 D81.32
　aldolase (hereditary) E74.19
　alpha-1-antitrypsin E88.01
　amino-acids E72.9
　aneurin E51.9
　antibody with
　　hyperimmunoglobulinemia D80.6
　　near-normal immunoglobins D80.6
　antidiuretic hormone E23.2
　anti-hemophilic
　　factor (A) D66
　　　B D67
　　　C D68.1
　　globulin (AHG) NEC D66
　antithrombin (antithrombin III) D68.59
　aromatic L-amino acid decarboxylase (AADC) E70.81
　ascorbic acid E54
　attention (disorder) (syndrome) F98.8
　　with hyperactivity — *see* Disorder, attention-deficit
　　　hyperactivity
　autoprothrombin
　　I D68.2
　　II D67
　　C D68.2
　beta-glucuronidase E76.29
　biotin E53.8

Deficiency, deficient — *continued*
　biotin-dependent carboxylase D81.819
　biotinidase D81.810
　brancher enzyme (amylopectinosis) E74.03
　C1 esterase inhibitor (C1-INH) D84.1
　calciferol E55.9
　　with
　　　adult osteomalacia M83.8
　　　rickets — *see* Rickets
　calcium (dietary) E58
　calorie, severe E43
　　with marasmus E41
　　　and kwashiorkor E42
　cardiac — *see* Insufficiency, myocardial
　carnitine E71.40
　　due to
　　　hemodialysis E71.43
　　　inborn errors of metabolism E71.42
　　　Valproic acid therapy E71.43
　　iatrogenic E71.43
　　muscle palmityltransferase E71.314
　　primary E71.41
　　secondary E71.448
　carotene E50.9
　central nervous system G96.89
　ceruloplasmin (Wilson) E83.01
　choline E53.8
　Christmas factor D67
　chromium E61.4
　chronic neurovisceral acid sphingomyelinase E75.244
　chronic visceral acid sphingomyelinase E75.241
　clotting (blood) — *see also* Deficiency, coagulation
　　factor D68.9
　clotting factor NEC (hereditary) — *see also* Deficiency,
　　factor D68.2
　coagulation NOS D68.9
　　with
　　　ectopic pregnancy O08.1
　　　molar pregnancy O08.1
　　acquired (any) D68.4
　　antepartum hemorrhage — *see* Hemorrhage, an-
　　　tepartum, with coagulation defect
　　clotting factor NEC — *see also* Deficiency, factor
　　　D68.2
　　due to
　　　hyperprothrombinemia D68.4
　　　liver disease D68.4
　　　vitamin K deficiency D68.4
　　newborn, transient P61.6
　　postpartum O72.3
　　specified NEC D68.8
　cognitive F09
　color vision H53.50
　　achromatopsia H53.51
　　acquired H53.52
　　deuteranomaly H53.53
　　protanomaly H53.54
　　specified type NEC H53.59
　　tritanomaly H53.55
　combined glucocorticoid and mineralocorticoid E27.49
　contact factor D68.2
　copper (nutritional) E61.0
　corticoadrenal E27.40
　　primary E27.1
　craniofacial axis Q75.0
　cyanocobalamin E53.8
　debrancher enzyme (limit dextrinosis) E74.03
　dehydrogenase
　　long chain/very long chain acyl CoA E71.310
　　　medium chain acyl CoA E71.311
　　　short chain acyl CoA E71.312
　diet E63.9
　dihydropyrimidine dehydrogenase (DPD) E88.89
　disaccharidase E73.9
　edema — *see* Malnutrition, severe
　endocrine E34.9
　energy-supply — *see* Malnutrition
　enzymes, circulating NEC E88.09
　ergosterol E55.9
　　with
　　　adult osteomalacia M83.8
　　　rickets — *see* Rickets
　essential fatty acid (EFA) E63.0
　eye movements
　　saccadic H55.81
　　smooth pursuit H55.82
　factor — *see also* Deficiency, coagulation
　　Hageman D68.2

Deficiency, deficient — *continued*
　factor — *see also* Deficiency, coagulation — *contin-*
　　ued
　　I (congenital) (hereditary) D68.2
　　II (congenital) (hereditary) D68.2
　　IX (congenital) (functional) (hereditary) (with func-
　　　tional defect) D67
　　multiple (congenital) D68.8
　　　acquired D68.4
　　V (congenital) (hereditary) D68.2
　　VII (congenital) (hereditary) D68.2
　　VIII (congenital) (functional) (hereditary) (with
　　　functional defect) D66
　　　with vascular defect — *see* Disease, von Wille-
　　　　brand
　　X (congenital) (hereditary) D68.2
　　XI (congenital) (hereditary) D68.1
　　XII (congenital) (hereditary) D68.2
　　XIII (congenital) (hereditary) D68.2
　femoral, proximal focal (congenital) — *see* Defect, re-
　　duction, lower limb, longitudinal, femur
　fibrinase D68.2
　fibrinogen (congenital) (hereditary) D68.2
　　acquired D65
　fibrin-stabilizing factor (congenital) (hereditary) D68.2
　　acquired D68.4
　folate E53.8
　folic acid E53.8
　foreskin N47.3
　fructokinase E74.11
　fructose 1,6-diphosphatase E74.19
　fructose-1-phosphate aldolase E74.19
　GABA (gamma aminobutyric acid) transaminase E72.81
　GABA-T (gamma aminobutyric acid transaminase)
　　E72.81
　galactokinase E74.29
　galactose-1-phosphate uridyl transferase E74.29
　gammaglobulin in blood D80.1
　　hereditary D80.0
　glass factor D68.2
　glucocorticoid E27.49
　　mineralocorticoid E27.49
　glucose transporter protein type 1 E74.810
　glucose-6-phosphatase E74.01
　glucose-6-phosphate dehydrogenase
　　anemia D55.0
　　without anemia D75.A
　glucuronyl transferase E80.5
　Glut1 E74.810
　glycogen synthetase E74.09
　gonadotropin (isolated) E23.0
　growth hormone (idiopathic) (isolated) E23.0
　Hageman factor D68.2
　hemoglobin D64.9
　hepatophosphorylase E74.09
　homogentisate 1,2-dioxygenase E70.29
　hormone
　　anterior pituitary (partial) NEC E23.0
　　　growth E23.0
　　growth (isolated) E23.0
　　pituitary E23.0
　　testicular E29.1
　hypoxanthine- (guanine)-phosphoribosyltransferase
　　(HG- PRT) (total H-PRT) E79.1
　immunity D84.9
　　cell-mediated D84.89
　　　with thrombocytopenia and eczema D82.0
　　combined D81.9
　　humoral D80.9
　　IgA (secretory) D80.2
　　IgG D80.3
　　IgM D80.4
　immuno — *see* Immunodeficiency
　immunoglobulin, selective
　　A (IgA) D80.2
　　G (IgG) (subclasses) D80.3
　　M (IgM) D80.4
　infantile neurovisceral acid sphingomyelinase E75.240
　inositol (B complex) E53.8
　intrinsic
　　factor (congenital) D51.0
　　sphincter N36.42
　　　with urethral hypermobility N36.43
　iodine E61.8
　　congenital syndrome — *see* Syndrome, iodine-defi-
　　　ciency, congenital
　iron E61.1
　　anemia D50.9
　kalium E87.6

Deficiency, deficient — *continued*
  kappa-light chain D80.8
  labile factor (congenital) (hereditary) D68.2
    acquired D68.4
  lacrimal fluid (acquired) — *see also* Syndrome, dry eye
    congenital Q10.6
  lactase
    congenital E73.0
    secondary E73.1
  Laki-Lorand factor D68.2
  lecithin cholesterol acyltransferase E78.6
  lipocaic K86.89
  lipoprotein (familial) (high density) E78.6
  liver phosphorylase E74.09
  lysosomal alpha-1, 4 glucosidase E74.02
  magnesium E61.2
  major histocompatibility complex
    class I D81.6
    class II D81.7
  manganese E61.3
  menadione (vitamin K) E56.1
    newborn P53
  mental (familial) (hereditary) — *see* Disability, intellectual
  methylenetetrahydrofolate reductase (MTHFR) E72.12
  mevalonate kinase M04.1
  mineralocorticoid E27.49
    with glucocorticoid E27.49
  mineral NEC E61.8
  molybdenum (nutritional) E61.5
  moral F60.2
  multiple nutrient elements E61.7
  multiple sulfatase (MSD) E75.26
  muscle
    carnitine (palmityltransferase) E71.314
    phosphofructokinase E74.09
  myoadenylate deaminase E79.2
  myocardial — *see* Insufficiency, myocardial
  myophosphorylase E74.04
  NADH diaphorase or reductase (congenital) D74.0
  NADH-methemoglobin reductase (congenital) D74.0
  natrium E87.1
  niacin (amide) (-tryptophan) E52
  nicotinamide E52
  nicotinic acid E52
  number of teeth — *see* Anodontia
  nutrient element E61.9
    multiple E61.7
    specified NEC E61.8
  nutrition, nutritional — *see also* Nutrition deficient E63.9
    sequelae — *see* Sequelae, nutritional deficiency
    specified NEC E63.8
  of interleukin 1 receptor antagonist [DIRA] M04.8
  ornithine transcarbamylase E72.4
  ovarian E28.39
  oxygen — *see* Anoxia
  pantothenic acid E53.8
  parathyroid (gland) E20.9
  perineum (female) N81.89
  phenylalanine hydroxylase E70.1
  phosphoenolpyruvate carboxykinase E74.4
  phosphofructokinase E74.19
  phosphomannomutase E74.818
  phosphomannose isomerase E74.818
  phosphomannosyl mutase E74.818
  phosphorylase kinase, liver E74.09
  pituitary hormone (isolated) E23.0
  plasma thromboplastin
    antecedent (PTA) D68.1
    component (PTC) D67
  plasminogen (type 1) (type 2) E88.02
  platelet NEC D69.1
    constitutional — *see* Disease, von Willebrand
  polyglandular E31.8
    autoimmune E31.0
  potassium (K) E87.6
  prepuce N47.3
  proaccelerin (congenital) (hereditary) D68.2
    acquired D68.4
  proconvertin factor (congenital) (hereditary) D68.2
    acquired D68.4
  protein — *see also* Malnutrition E46
    anemia D53.0
    C D68.59
    S D68.59
  prothrombin (congenital) (hereditary) D68.2
    acquired D68.4

Deficiency, deficient — *continued*
  Prower factor D68.2
  pseudocholinesterase E88.09
  PTA (plasma thromboplastin antecedent) D68.1
  PTC (plasma thromboplastin component) D67
  purine nucleoside phosphorylase (PNP) D81.5
  pyracin (alpha) (beta) E53.1
  pyridoxal E53.1
  pyridoxamine E53.1
  pyridoxine (derivatives) E53.1
  pyruvate
    carboxylase E74.4
    dehydrogenase E74.4
  riboflavin (vitamin B2) E53.0
  salt E87.1
  secretion
    ovary E28.39
    salivary gland (any) K11.7
    urine R34
  selenium (dietary) E59
  serum antitrypsin, familial E88.01
  short stature homeobox gene (SHOX)
    with
      dyschondrosteosis Q78.8
      short stature (idiopathic) E34.328
      Turner's syndrome Q96.9
  sodium (Na) E87.1
  SPCA (factor VII) D68.2
  sphincter, intrinsic N36.42
    with urethral hypermobility N36.43
  stable factor (congenital) (hereditary) D68.2
    acquired D68.4
  Stuart-Prower (factor X) D68.2
  succinic semialdehyde dehydrogenase E72.81
  sucrase E74.39
  sulfatase E75.26
  sulfite oxidase E72.19
  thiamin, thiaminic (chloride) E51.9
    beriberi (dry) E51.11
    wet E51.12
  thrombokinase D68.2
    newborn P53
  thyroid (gland) — *see* Hypothyroidism
  tocopherol E56.0
  tooth bud K00.0
  transcobalamine II (anemia) D51.2
  vanadium E61.6
  vascular I99.9
  vasopressin E23.2
  vertical ridge K06.8
  viosterol — *see* Deficiency, calciferol
  vitamin (multiple) NOS E56.9
    A E50.9
      with
        Bitot's spot (corneal) E50.1
        follicular keratosis E50.8
        keratomalacia E50.4
        manifestations NEC E50.8
        night blindness E50.5
        scar of cornea, xerophthalmic E50.6
        xeroderma E50.8
        xerophthalmia E50.7
        xerosis
          conjunctival E50.0
            and Bitot's spot E50.1
          cornea E50.2
            and ulceration E50.3
      sequelae E64.1
    B (complex) NOS E53.9
      with
        beriberi (dry) E51.11
          wet E51.12
        pellagra E52
    B1 NOS E51.9
      beriberi (dry) E51.11
        with circulatory system manifestations E51.11
        wet E51.12
    B12 E53.8
    B2 (riboflavin) E53.0
    B6 E53.1
    C E54
      sequelae E64.2
    D E55.9
      with
        adult osteomalacia M83.8
        rickets — *see* Rickets
      25-hydroxylase E83.32
    E E56.0
    folic acid E53.8

Deficiency, deficient — *continued*
  vitamin — *continued*
    G E53.0
    group B E53.9
      specified NEC E53.8
    H (biotin) E53.8
    K E56.1
      of newborn P53
    nicotinic E52
    P E56.8
    PP (pellagra-preventing) E52
    specified NEC E56.8
    thiamin E51.9
      beriberi — *see* Beriberi
  von Willebrand factor
    partial quantitative — *see also* Disease, von Willebrand D68.01
    total quantitative — *see also* Disease, von Willebrand D68.03
  zinc, dietary E60
Deficit — *see also* Deficiency
  attention and concentration R41.840
    disorder — *see* Attention, deficit
    following
      cerebral infarction I69.310
      cerebrovascular disease I69.910
        specified disease NEC I69.810
      nontraumatic
        intracerebral hemorrhage I69.110
        specified intracranial hemorrhage NEC I69.210
        subarachnoid hemorrhage I69.010
  cognitive
    communication R41.841
    emotional
      following
        cerebral infarction I69.315
        cerebrovascular disease I69.915
          specified disease NEC I69.815
        nontraumatic
          intracerebral hemorrhage I69.115
          specified intracranial hemorrhage NEC I69.215
          subarachnoid hemorrhage I69.015
    following
      cerebral infarction I69.319
      cerebrovascular disease I69.919
        specified disease NEC I69.819
      nontraumatic
        intracerebral hemorrhage I69.119
        specified intracranial hemorrhage NEC I69.219
        subarachnoid hemorrhage I69.019
    social
      following
        cerebral infarction I69.315
        cerebrovascular disease I69.915
          specified disease NEC I69.815
        nontraumatic
          intracerebral hemorrhage I69.115
          specified intracranial hemorrhage NEC I69.215
          subarachnoid hemorrhage I69.015
  cognitive NEC R41.89
    following
      cerebral infarction I69.318
      cerebrovascular disease I69.918
        specified disease NEC I69.818
      nontraumatic
        intracerebral hemorrhage I69.118
        specified intracranial hemorrhage NEC I69.218
        subarachnoid hemorrhage I69.018
  concentration R41.840
  executive function R41.844
    following
      cerebral infarction I69.314
      cerebrovascular disease I69.914
        specified disease NEC I69.814
      nontraumatic
        intracerebral hemorrhage I69.114
        specified intracranial hemorrhage NEC I69.214
        subarachnoid hemorrhage I69.014
  frontal lobe R41.844
    following
      cerebral infarction I69.314
      cerebrovascular disease I69.914
        specified disease NEC I69.814
      nontraumatic
        intracerebral hemorrhage I69.114
        specified intracranial hemorrhage NEC I69.214
        subarachnoid hemorrhage I69.014

Deficit — *continued*
- memory
  - following
    - cerebral infarction I69.311
    - cerebrovascular disease I69.911
      - specified disease NEC I69.811
    - nontraumatic
      - intracerebral hemorrhage I69.111
      - specified intracranial hemorrhage NEC I69.211
      - subarachnoid hemorrhage I69.011
- neurologic NEC R29.818
  - ischemic
    - reversible (RIND) I63.9
      - prolonged (PRIND) I63.9
- oxygen R09.02
- prolonged reversible ischemic neurologic (PRIND) I63.9
- psychomotor R41.843
  - following
    - cerebral infarction I69.313
    - cerebrovascular disease I69.913
      - specified disease NEC I69.813
    - nontraumatic
      - intracerebral hemorrhage I69.113
      - specified intracranial hemorrhage NEC I69.213
      - subarachnoid hemorrhage I69.013
- visuospatial R41.842
  - following
    - cerebral infarction I69.312
    - cerebrovascular disease I69.912
      - specified disease NEC I69.812
    - nontraumatic
      - intracerebral hemorrhage I69.112
      - specified intracranial hemorrhage NEC I69.212
      - subarachnoid hemorrhage I69.012

Deflection
- radius — *see* Deformity, limb, specified type NEC, forearm
- septum (acquired) (nasal) (nose) J34.2
- spine — *see* Curvature, spine
- turbinate (nose) J34.2

Defluvium
- capillorum — *see* Alopecia
- ciliorum — *see* Madarosis
- unguium L60.8

Deformity Q89.9
- abdomen, congenital Q89.9
- abdominal wall
  - acquired M95.8
  - congenital Q79.59
- acquired (unspecified site) M95.9
- adrenal gland Q89.1
- alimentary tract, congenital Q45.9
  - upper Q40.9
- ankle (joint) (acquired) — *see also* Deformity, limb, lower leg
  - abduction — *see* Contraction, joint, ankle
  - congenital Q68.8
  - contraction — *see* Contraction, joint, ankle
  - specified type NEC — *see* Deformity, limb, foot, specified NEC
- anus (acquired) K62.89
  - congenital Q43.9
- aorta (arch) (congenital) Q25.40
  - acquired I77.89
- aortic
  - arch, acquired I77.89
  - cusp or valve (congenital) Q23.8
    - acquired — *see also* Endocarditis, aortic I35.8
- arm (acquired) (upper) — *see* Deformity, limb, upper arm
  - congenital Q68.8
  - forearm — *see* Deformity, limb, forearm
- artery (congenital) (peripheral) NOS Q27.9
  - acquired I77.89
  - coronary (acquired) I25.9
    - congenital Q24.5
  - umbilical Q27.0
- atrial septal — *see also* Defect, atrial septal Q21.10
- auditory canal (external) (congenital) — *see also* Malformation, ear, external
  - acquired — *see* Disorder, ear, external, specified type NEC
- auricle
  - ear (congenital) — *see also* Malformation, ear, external
    - acquired — *see* Disorder, pinna, deformity
- back — *see* Dorsopathy, deforming
- bile duct (common) (congenital) (hepatic) Q44.5

Deformity — *continued*
- bile duct — *continued*
  - acquired K83.8
- biliary duct or passage (congenital) Q44.5
  - acquired K83.8
- bladder (neck) (trigone) (sphincter) (acquired) N32.89
  - congenital Q64.79
- bone (acquired) NOS M95.9
  - congenital Q79.9
  - turbinate M95.0
- brain (congenital) Q04.9
  - acquired G93.89
  - reduction Q04.3
- breast (acquired) N64.89
  - congenital Q83.9
  - reconstructed N65.0
- bronchus (congenital) Q32.4
  - acquired NEC J98.09
- bursa, congenital Q79.9
- canaliculi (lacrimalis) (acquired) — *see also* Disorder, lacrimal system, changes
  - congenital Q10.6
- canthus, acquired — *see* Disorder, eyelid, specified type NEC
- capillary (acquired) I78.8
- cardiovascular system, congenital Q28.9
- caruncle, lacrimal (acquired) — *see also* Disorder, lacrimal system, changes
  - congenital Q10.6
- cascade, stomach K31.2
- cecum (congenital) Q43.9
  - acquired K63.89
- cerebral, acquired G93.89
  - congenital Q04.9
- cervix (uterus) (acquired) NEC N88.8
  - congenital Q51.9
- cheek (acquired) M95.2
  - congenital Q18.9
- chest (acquired) (wall) M95.4
  - congenital Q67.8
  - sequelae (late effect) of rickets E64.3
- chin (acquired) M95.2
  - congenital Q18.9
- choroid (congenital) Q14.3
  - acquired H31.8
  - plexus Q07.8
    - acquired G96.198
- cicatricial — *see* Cicatrix
- cilia, acquired — *see* Disorder, eyelid, specified type NEC
- clavicle (acquired) M95.8
  - congenital Q68.8
- clitoris (congenital) Q52.6
  - acquired N90.89
- clubfoot — *see* Clubfoot
- coccyx (acquired) — *see* subcategory M43.8 ☑
- colon (congenital) Q43.9
  - acquired K63.89
- concha (ear), congenital — *see also* Malformation, ear, external
  - acquired — *see* Disorder, pinna, deformity
- cornea (acquired) H18.70
  - congenital Q13.4
  - descemetocele — *see* Descemetocele
  - ectasia — *see* Ectasia, cornea
  - specified NEC H18.79- ☑
  - staphyloma — *see* Staphyloma, cornea
- coronary artery (acquired) I25.9
  - congenital Q24.5
- cranium (acquired) — *see* Deformity, skull
- cricoid cartilage (congenital) Q31.8
  - acquired J38.7
- cystic duct (congenital) Q44.5
  - acquired K82.8
- Dandy-Walker Q03.1
  - with spina bifida — *see* Spina bifida
- diaphragm (congenital) Q79.1
  - acquired J98.6
- digestive organ NOS Q45.9
- ductus arteriosus Q25.0
- duodenal bulb K31.89
- duodenum (congenital) Q43.9
  - acquired K31.89
- dura — *see* Deformity, meninges
- ear (acquired) — *see also* Disorder, pinna, deformity
  - congenital (external) Q17.9
    - internal Q16.5
    - middle Q16.4

Deformity — *continued*
- ear — *see also* Disorder, pinna, deformity — *continued*
  - congenital — *continued*
    - middle — *continued*
      - ossicles Q16.3
    - ossicles Q16.3
- ectodermal (congenital) NEC Q84.9
- ejaculatory duct (congenital) Q55.4
  - acquired N50.89
- elbow (joint) (acquired) — *see also* Deformity, limb, upper arm
  - congenital Q68.8
  - contraction — *see* Contraction, joint, elbow
- endocrine gland NEC Q89.2
- epididymis (congenital) Q55.4
  - acquired N50.89
- epiglottis (congenital) Q31.8
  - acquired J38.7
- esophagus (congenital) Q39.9
  - acquired K22.89
- eustachian tube (congenital) NEC Q17.8
- eye, congenital Q15.9
- eyebrow (congenital) Q18.8
- eyelid (acquired) — *see also* Disorder, eyelid, specified type NEC
  - congenital Q10.3
- face (acquired) M95.2
  - congenital Q18.9
- fallopian tube, acquired N83.8
- femur (acquired) — *see* Deformity, limb, specified type NEC, thigh
- fetal
  - with fetopelvic disproportion O33.7 ☑
  - causing obstructed labor O66.3
- finger (acquired) M20.00- ☑
  - boutonniere M20.02- ☑
  - congenital Q68.1
  - flexion contracture — *see* Contraction, joint, hand
  - mallet finger M20.01- ☑
  - specified NEC M20.09- ☑
  - swan-neck M20.03- ☑
- flexion (joint) (acquired) — *see also* Deformity, limb, flexion M21.20
  - congenital NOS Q74.9
  - hip Q65.89
- foot (acquired) — *see also* Deformity, limb, lower leg
  - cavovarus (congenital) Q66.1- ☑
  - congenital NOS Q66.9- ☑
    - specified type NEC Q66.89
  - specified type NEC — *see* Deformity, limb, foot, specified NEC
  - valgus (congenital) Q66.6
    - acquired — *see* Deformity, valgus, ankle
  - varus (congenital) NEC Q66.3- ☑
    - acquired — *see* Deformity, varus, ankle
- forearm (acquired) — *see also* Deformity, limb, forearm
  - congenital Q68.8
- forehead (acquired) M95.2
  - congenital Q75.8
- frontal bone (acquired) M95.2
  - congenital Q75.8
- gallbladder (congenital) Q44.1
  - acquired K82.8
- gastrointestinal tract (congenital) NOS Q45.9
  - acquired K63.89
- genitalia, genital organ(s) or system NEC
  - female (congenital) Q52.9
    - acquired N94.89
    - external Q52.70
  - male (congenital) Q55.9
    - acquired N50.89
- globe (eye) (congenital) Q15.8
  - acquired H44.89
- gum, acquired NEC K06.8
- hand (acquired) — *see* Deformity, limb, hand
  - congenital Q68.1
- head (acquired) M95.2
  - congenital Q75.8
- heart (congenital) Q24.9
  - septum Q21.9
    - auricular — *see also* Defect, atrial septal Q21.10
    - ventricular Q21.0
  - valve (congenital) NEC Q24.8
    - acquired — *see* Endocarditis
- heel (acquired) — *see* Deformity, foot
- hepatic duct (congenital) Q44.5
  - acquired K83.8

Deformity — *continued*
  hip (joint) (acquired) (*see also* Deformity, limb, thigh)
    congenital Q65.9
    due to (previous) juvenile osteochondrosis — *see* Coxa, plana
    flexion — *see* Contraction, joint, hip
  hourglass — *see* Contraction, hourglass
  humerus (acquired) M21.82- ☑
    congenital Q74.0
  hypophyseal (congenital) Q89.2
  ileocecal (coil) (valve) (acquired) K63.89
    congenital Q43.9
  ileum (congenital) Q43.9
    acquired K63.89
  ilium (acquired) M95.5
    congenital Q74.2
  integument (congenital) Q84.9
  intervertebral cartilage or disc (acquired) — *see* Disorder, disc, specified NEC
  intestine (large) (small) (congenital) NOS Q43.9
    acquired K63.89
  intrinsic minus or plus (hand) — *see* Deformity, limb, specified type NEC, forearm
  iris (acquired) H21.89
    congenital Q13.2
  ischium (acquired) M95.5
    congenital Q74.2
  jaw (acquired) (congenital) M26.9
  joint (acquired) NEC M21.90
    congenital Q68.8
    elbow M21.92- ☑
    hand M21.94- ☑
    hip M21.95- ☑
    knee M21.96- ☑
    shoulder M21.92- ☑
    wrist M21.93- ☑
  kidney(s) (calyx) (pelvis) (congenital) Q63.9
    acquired N28.89
    artery (congenital) Q27.2
      acquired I77.89
  Klippel-Feil (brevicollis) Q76.1
  knee (acquired) NEC — *see also* Deformity, limb, lower leg
    congenital Q68.2
  labium (majus) (minus) (congenital) Q52.79
    acquired N90.89
  lacrimal passages or duct (congenital) NEC Q10.6
    acquired — *see* Disorder, lacrimal system, changes
  larynx (muscle) (congenital) Q31.8
    acquired J38.7
    web (glottic) Q31.0
  leg (upper) (acquired) NEC — *see also* Deformity, limb, thigh
    congenital Q68.8
    lower leg — *see* Deformity, limb, lower leg
  lens (acquired) H27.8
    congenital Q12.9
  lid (fold) (acquired) — *see also* Disorder, eyelid, specified type NEC
    congenital Q10.3
  ligament (acquired) — *see* Disorder, ligament
    congenital Q79.9
  limb (acquired) M21.90
    clawfoot M21.53- ☑
    clawhand M21.51- ☑
      congenital Q68.1
    clubfoot M21.54- ☑
    clubhand M21.52- ☑
    congenital, except reduction deformity Q74.9
    flat foot M21.4- ☑
    flexion M21.20
      ankle M21.27- ☑
      elbow M21.22- ☑
      finger M21.24- ☑
      hip M21.25- ☑
      knee M21.26- ☑
      shoulder M21.21- ☑
      toe M21.27- ☑
      wrist M21.23- ☑
    foot
      claw — *see* Deformity, limb, clawfoot
      club — *see* Deformity, limb, clubfoot
      drop M21.37- ☑
      flat — *see* Deformity, limb, flat foot
      specified NEC M21.6X- ☑
    forearm M21.93- ☑
    hand M21.94- ☑

Deformity — *continued*
  limb — *continued*
    lower leg M21.96- ☑
    specified type NEC M21.80
      forearm M21.83- ☑
      lower leg M21.86- ☑
      thigh M21.85- ☑
      upper arm M21.82- ☑
    thigh M21.95- ☑
    unequal length M21.70
      short site is
        femur M21.75- ☑
        fibula M21.76- ☑
        humerus M21.72- ☑
        radius M21.73- ☑
        tibia M21.76- ☑
        ulna M21.73- ☑
    upper arm M21.92- ☑
    valgus — *see* Deformity, valgus
    varus — *see* Deformity, varus
    wrist drop M21.33- ☑
  lip (acquired) NEC K13.0
    congenital Q38.0
  liver (congenital) Q44.7
    acquired K76.89
  lumbosacral (congenital) (joint) (region) Q76.49
    acquired — *see* subcategory M43.8 ☑
    kyphosis — *see* Kyphosis, congenital
    lordosis — *see* Lordosis, congenital
  lung (congenital) Q33.9
    acquired J98.4
  lymphatic system, congenital Q89.9
  Madelung's (radius) Q74.0
  mandible (acquired) (congenital) M26.9
  maxilla (acquired) (congenital) M26.9
  meninges or membrane (congenital) Q07.9
    cerebral Q04.8
      acquired G96.198
    spinal cord (congenital) Q06.- ☑
      acquired G96.198
  metacarpus (acquired) — *see* Deformity, limb, forearm
    congenital Q74.0
  metatarsus (acquired) — *see* Deformity, foot
    congenital Q66.9- ☑
  middle ear (congenital) Q16.4
    ossicles Q16.3
  mitral (leaflets) (valve) I05.8
    parachute Q23.2
    stenosis, congenital Q23.2
  mouth (acquired) K13.79
    congenital Q38.6
  multiple, congenital NEC Q89.7
  muscle (acquired) M62.89
    congenital Q79.9
      sternocleidomastoid Q68.0
  musculoskeletal system (acquired) M95.9
    congenital Q79.9
    specified NEC M95.8
  nail (acquired) L60.8
    congenital Q84.6
  nasal — *see* Deformity, nose
  neck (acquired) M95.3
    congenital Q18.9
      sternocleidomastoid Q68.0
  nervous system (congenital) Q07.9
  nipple (congenital) Q83.9
    acquired N64.89
  nose (acquired) (cartilage) M95.0
    bone (turbinate) M95.0
    congenital Q30.9
      bent or squashed Q67.4
    saddle M95.0
      syphilitic A50.57
    septum (acquired) J34.2
      congenital Q30.8
    sinus (wall) (congenital) Q30.8
      acquired M95.0
    syphilitic (congenital) A50.57
      late A52.73
  ocular muscle (congenital) Q10.3
    acquired — *see* Strabismus, mechanical
  opticociliary vessels (congenital) Q13.2
  orbit (eye) (acquired) H05.30
    atrophy — *see* Atrophy, orbit
    congenital Q10.7
    due to
      bone disease NEC H05.32- ☑
      trauma or surgery H05.33- ☑

Deformity — *continued*
  orbit — *continued*
    enlargement — *see* Enlargement, orbit
    exostosis — *see* Exostosis, orbit
  organ of Corti (congenital) Q16.5
  ovary (congenital) Q50.39
    acquired N83.8
  oviduct, acquired N83.8
  palate (congenital) Q38.5
    acquired M27.8
    cleft (congenital) — *see* Cleft, palate
  pancreas (congenital) Q45.3
    acquired K86.89
  parathyroid (gland) Q89.2
  parotid (gland) (congenital) Q38.4
    acquired K11.8
  patella (acquired) — *see* Disorder, patella, specified NEC
  pelvis, pelvic (acquired) (bony) M95.5
    with disproportion (fetopelvic) O33.0
      causing obstructed labor O65.0
    congenital Q74.2
    rachitic sequelae (late effect) E64.3
  penis (glans) (congenital) Q55.69
    acquired N48.89
  pericardium (congenital) Q24.8
    acquired — *see* Pericarditis
  pharynx (congenital) Q38.8
    acquired J39.2
  pinna, acquired — *see also* Disorder, pinna, deformity
    congenital Q17.9
  pituitary (congenital) Q89.2
  posture — *see* Dorsopathy, deforming
  prepuce (congenital) Q55.69
    acquired N47.8
  prostate (congenital) Q55.4
    acquired N42.89
  pupil (congenital) Q13.2
    acquired — *see* Abnormality, pupillary
  pylorus (congenital) Q40.3
    acquired K31.89
  rachitic (acquired), old or healed E64.3
  radius (acquired) — *see also* Deformity, limb, forearm
    congenital Q68.8
  rectum (congenital) Q43.9
    acquired K62.89
  reduction (extremity) (limb), congenital — *see also* condition and site Q73.8
    brain Q04.3
    lower — *see* Defect, reduction, lower limb
    upper — *see* Defect, reduction, upper limb
  renal — *see* Deformity, kidney
  respiratory system (congenital) Q34.9
  rib (acquired) M95.4
    congenital Q76.6
      cervical Q76.5
  rotation (joint) (acquired) — *see* Deformity, limb, specified site NEC
    congenital Q74.9
    hip — *see* Deformity, limb, specified type NEC, thigh
      congenital Q65.89
  sacroiliac joint (congenital) — *see* subcategory Q74.2
    acquired — *see* subcategory M43.8 ☑
  sacrum (acquired) — *see* subcategory M43.8 ☑
  saddle
    back — *see* Lordosis
    nose M95.0
      syphilitic A50.57
  salivary gland or duct (congenital) Q38.4
    acquired K11.8
  scapula (acquired) M95.8
    congenital Q68.8
  scrotum (congenital) — *see also* Malformation, testis and scrotum
    acquired N50.89
  seminal vesicles (congenital) Q55.4
    acquired N50.89
  septum, nasal (acquired) J34.2
  shoulder (joint) (acquired) — *see* Deformity, limb, upper arm
    congenital Q74.0
    contraction — *see* Contraction, joint, shoulder
  sigmoid (flexure) (congenital) Q43.9
    acquired K63.89
  skin (congenital) Q82.9
  skull (acquired) M95.2
    congenital Q75.8

Deformity — *continued*
 skull — *continued*
  congenital — *continued*
   with
    anencephaly Q00.0
    encephalocele — *see* Encephalocele
    hydrocephalus Q03.9
     with spina bifida — *see* Spina bifida, by site, with hydrocephalus
    microcephaly Q02
 soft parts, organs or tissues (of pelvis)
  in pregnancy or childbirth NEC O34.8- ☑
   causing obstructed labor O65.5
 spermatic cord (congenital) Q55.4
  acquired N50.89
   torsion — *see* Torsion, spermatic cord
 spinal — *see* Dorsopathy, deforming
  column (acquired) — *see* Dorsopathy, deforming
  congenital Q67.5
  cord (congenital) Q06.9
   acquired G95.89
  nerve root (congenital) Q07.9
 spine (acquired) — *see also* Dorsopathy, deforming
  congenital Q67.5
  rachitic E64.3
  specified NEC — *see* Dorsopathy, deforming, specified NEC
 spleen
  acquired D73.89
  congenital Q89.09
 Sprengel's (congenital) Q74.0
 sternocleidomastoid (muscle), congenital Q68.0
 sternum (acquired) M95.4
  congenital NEC Q76.7
 stomach (congenital) Q40.3
  acquired K31.89
 submandibular gland (congenital) Q38.4
 submaxillary gland (congenital) Q38.4
  acquired K11.8
 talipes — *see* Talipes
 testis (congenital) — *see also* Malformation, testis and scrotum
  acquired N44.8
   torsion — *see* Torsion, testis
 thigh (acquired) — *see also* Deformity, limb, thigh
  congenital NEC Q68.8
 thorax (acquired) (wall) M95.4
  congenital Q67.8
  sequelae of rickets E64.3
 thumb (acquired) — *see also* Deformity, finger
  congenital NEC Q68.1
 thymus (tissue) (congenital) Q89.2
 thyroid (gland) (congenital) Q89.2
  cartilage Q31.8
   acquired J38.7
 tibia (acquired) — *see also* Deformity, limb, specified type NEC, lower leg
  congenital NEC Q68.8
  saber (syphilitic) A50.56
 toe (acquired) M20.6- ☑
  congenital Q66.9- ☑
  hallux rigidus M20.2- ☑
  hallux valgus M20.1- ☑
  hallux varus M20.3- ☑
  hammer toe M20.4- ☑
  specified NEC M20.5X- ☑
 tongue (congenital) Q38.3
  acquired K14.8
 tooth, teeth K00.2
 trachea (rings) (congenital) Q32.1
  acquired J39.8
 transverse aortic arch (congenital) Q25.49
 tricuspid (leaflets) (valve) I07.8
  atresia or stenosis Q22.4
  Ebstein's Q22.5
 trunk (acquired) M95.8
  congenital Q89.9
 ulna (acquired) — *see also* Deformity, limb, forearm
  congenital NEC Q68.8
 urachus, congenital Q64.4
 ureter (opening) (congenital) Q62.8
  acquired N28.89
 urethra (congenital) Q64.79
  acquired N36.8
 urinary tract (congenital) Q64.9
  urachus Q64.4
 uterus (congenital) Q51.9
  acquired N85.8

Deformity — *continued*
 uvula (congenital) Q38.5
 vagina (acquired) N89.8
  congenital Q52.4
 valgus NEC M21.00
  ankle M21.07- ☑
  elbow M21.02- ☑
  hip M21.05- ☑
  knee M21.06- ☑
 valve, valvular (congenital) (heart) Q24.8
  acquired — *see* Endocarditis
 varus NEC M21.10
  ankle M21.17- ☑
  elbow M21.12- ☑
  hip M21.15 ☑
  knee M21.16- ☑
  tibia — *see* Osteochondrosis, juvenile, tibia
 vas deferens (congenital) Q55.4
  acquired N50.89
 vein (congenital) Q27.9
  great Q26.9
 vertebra — *see* Dorsopathy, deforming
 vertical talus (congenital) Q66.80
  left foot Q66.82
  right foot Q66.81
 vesicourethral orifice (acquired) N32.89
  congenital NEC Q64.79
 vessels of optic papilla (congenital) Q14.2
 visual field (contraction) — *see* Defect, visual field
 vitreous body, acquired H43.89
 vulva (congenital) Q52.79
  acquired N90.89
 wrist (joint) (acquired) — *see also* Deformity, limb, forearm
  congenital Q68.8
  contraction — *see* Contraction, joint, wrist

Degeneration, degenerative
 adrenal (capsule) (fatty) (gland) (hyaline) (infectional) E27.8
 amyloid — *see also* Amyloidosis E85.9
 anterior cornua, spinal cord G12.29
 anterior labral S43.49- ☑
 aorta, aortic I70.0
  fatty I77.89
 aortic valve (heart) — *see* Endocarditis, aortic
 arteriovascular — *see* Arteriosclerosis
 artery, arterial (atheromatous) (calcareous) — *see also* Arteriosclerosis
  cerebral, amyloid E85.4 [I68.0]
  medial — *see* Arteriosclerosis, extremities
 articular cartilage NEC — *see* Derangement, joint, articular cartilage, by site
 atheromatous — *see* Arteriosclerosis
 basal nuclei or ganglia G23.9
  specified NEC G23.8
 bone NEC — *see* Disorder, bone, specified type NEC
 brachial plexus G54.0
 brain (cortical) (progressive) G31.9
  alcoholic G31.2
  arteriosclerotic I67.2
  childhood G31.9
   specified NEC G31.89
  cystic G31.89
   congenital Q04.6
  in
   alcoholism G31.2
   beriberi E51.2
   cerebrovascular disease I67.9
   congenital hydrocephalus Q03.9
    with spina bifida — *see also* Spina bifida
   Fabry-Anderson disease E75.21
   Gaucher's disease E75.22
   Hunter's syndrome E76.1
   lipidosis
    cerebral E75.4
    generalized E75.6
   mucopolysaccharidosis — *see* Mucopolysaccharidosis
   myxedema E03.9 [G32.89]
   neoplastic disease — *see also* Neoplasm D49.6 [G32.89]
   Niemann-Pick disease E75.249 [G32.89]
   sphingolipidosis E75.3 [G32.89]
   vitamin B12 deficiency E53.8 [G32.89]
  senile NEC G31.1
 breast N64.89
 Bruch's membrane — *see* Degeneration, choroid
 capillaries (fatty) I78.8

Degeneration, degenerative — *continued*
 capillaries — *continued*
  amyloid E85.89 [I79.8]
 cardiac — *see also* Degeneration, myocardial
  valve, valvular — *see* Endocarditis
 cardiorenal — *see* Hypertension, cardiorenal
 cardiovascular — *see also* Disease, cardiovascular
  renal — *see* Hypertension, cardiorenal
 cerebellar NOS G31.9
  alcoholic G31.2
  primary (hereditary) (sporadic) G11.9
 cerebral — *see* Degeneration, brain
 cerebrovascular I67.9
  due to hypertension I67.4
 cervical plexus G54.2
 cervix N88.8
  due to radiation (intended effect) N88.8
   adverse effect or misadventure N99.89
 chamber angle H21.21- ☑
 changes, spine or vertebra — *see* Spondylosis
 chorioretinal — *see also* Degeneration, choroid
  hereditary H31.20
 choroid (colloid) (drusen) H31.10- ☑
  atrophy — *see* Atrophy, choroidal
  hereditary — *see* Dystrophy, choroidal, hereditary
 ciliary body H21.22- ☑
 cochlear — *see* subcategory H83.8 ☑
 combined (spinal cord) (subacute) E53.8 [G32.0]
  with anemia (pernicious) D51.0 [G32.0]
   due to dietary vitamin B12 deficiency D51.3 [G32.0]
  in (due to)
   vitamin B12 deficiency E53.8 [G32.0]
    anemia D51.9 [G32.0]
 conjunctiva H11.10
  concretions — *see* Concretion, conjunctiva
  deposits — *see* Deposit, conjunctiva
  pigmentations — *see* Pigmentation, conjunctiva
  pinguecula — *see* Pinguecula
  xerosis — *see* Xerosis, conjunctiva
 cornea H18.40
  calcerous H18.43
   band keratopathy H18.42- ☑
  familial, hereditary — *see* Dystrophy, cornea
  hyaline (of old scars) H18.49
  keratomalacia — *see* Keratomalacia
  nodular H18.45- ☑
  peripheral H18.46- ☑
  senile H18.41- ☑
  specified type NEC H18.49
 cortical (cerebellar) (parenchymatous) G31.89
  alcoholic G31.2
  diffuse, due to arteriopathy I67.2
 corticobasal G31.85
 cutis L98.8
  amyloid E85.4 [L99]
 dental pulp K04.2
 disc disease — *see* Degeneration, intervertebral disc, by site
 dorsolateral (spinal cord) — *see* Degeneration, combined
 extrapyramidal G25.9
 eye, macular — *see also* Degeneration, macula
  congenital or hereditary — *see* Dystrophy, retina
 facet joints — *see* Spondylosis
 fatty
  liver NEC K76.0
   alcoholic K70.0
 grey matter (brain) (Alpers') G31.81
 heart — *see also* Degeneration, myocardial
  amyloid E85.4 [I43]
  atheromatous — *see* Disease, heart, ischemic, atherosclerotic
  ischemic — *see* Disease, heart, ischemic
 hepatolenticular (Wilson's) E83.01
 hepatorenal K76.7
 hyaline (diffuse) (generalized)
  localized — *see* Degeneration, by site
 infrapatellar fat pad M79.4
 intervertebral disc NOS
  with
   myelopathy — *see* Disorder, disc, with, myelopathy
   radiculitis or radiculopathy — *see* Disorder, disc, with, radiculopathy
   cervical, cervicothoracic — *see* Disorder, disc, cervical, degeneration

Degeneration, degenerative — *continued*
  intervertebral disc — *continued*
    cervical, cervicothoracic — *see* Disorder, disc, cervical, degeneration — *continued*
      with
        myelopathy — *see* Disorder, disc, cervical, with myelopathy
        neuritis, radiculitis or radiculopathy — *see* Disorder, disc, cervical, with neuritis
    lumbar region M51.36
      with
        myelopathy M51.06
        neuritis, radiculitis, radiculopathy or sciatica M51.16
    lumbosacral region M51.37
      with
        neuritis, radiculitis, radiculopathy or sciatica M51.17
    sacrococcygeal region M53.3
    thoracic region M51.34
      with
        myelopathy M51.04
        neuritis, radiculitis, radiculopathy M51.14
    thoracolumbar region M51.35
      with
        myelopathy M51.05
        neuritis, radiculitis, radiculopathy M51.15
  intestine, amyloid E85.4
  iris (pigmentary) H21.23- ☑
  ischemic — *see* Ischemia
  joint disease — *see* Osteoarthritis
  kidney N28.89
    amyloid E85.4 [N29]
    cystic, congenital Q61.9
    fatty N28.89
    polycystic Q61.3
      adult type (autosomal dominant) Q61.2
      infantile type (autosomal recessive) NEC Q61.19
        collecting duct dilatation Q61.11
    Kuhnt-Junius — *see also* Degeneration, macula
      H35.32- ☑
  lens — *see* Cataract
  lenticular (familial) (progressive) (Wilson's) (with cirrhosis of liver) E83.01
  liver (diffuse) NEC K76.89
    amyloid E85.4 [K77]
    cystic K76.89
      congenital Q44.6
    fatty NEC K76.0
      alcoholic K70.0
    hypertrophic K76.89
    parenchymatous, acute or subacute K72.00
      with coma K72.01
    pigmentary K76.89
    toxic (acute) K71.9
  lung J98.4
  lymph gland I89.8
    hyaline I89.8
  macula, macular (acquired) (age-related) (senile) H35.30
    angioid streaks H35.33
    atrophic age-related H35.31- ☑
    congenital or hereditary — *see* Dystrophy, retina
    cystoid H35.35- ☑
    drusen H35.36- ☑
    dry age-related H35.31- ☑
    exudative H35.32- ☑
    hole H35.34- ☑
    nonexudative H35.31- ☑
    puckering H35.37- ☑
    toxic H35.38- ☑
    wet age-related H35.32- ☑
  membranous labyrinth, congenital (causing impairment of hearing) Q16.5
  meniscus — *see* Derangement, meniscus
  mitral — *see* Insufficiency, mitral
  Mönckeberg's — *see* Arteriosclerosis, extremities
  motor centers, senile G31.1
  multi-system G90.3
  mural — *see* Degeneration, myocardial
  muscle (fatty) (fibrous) (hyaline) (progressive) M62.89
    heart — *see* Degeneration, myocardial
  myelin, central nervous system G37.9
  myocardial, myocardium (fatty) (hyaline) (senile) I51.5
    with rheumatic fever (conditions in I00) I09.0
      active, acute or subacute I01.2
        with chorea I02.0
      inactive or quiescent (with chorea) I09.0

Degeneration, degenerative — *continued*
  myocardial, myocardium — *continued*
    hypertensive — *see* Hypertension, heart
    rheumatic — *see* Degeneration, myocardial, with rheumatic fever
    syphilitic A52.06
  nasal sinus (mucosa) J32.9
    frontal J32.1
    maxillary J32.0
  nerve — *see* Disorder, nerve
  nervous system G31.9
    alcoholic G31.2
    amyloid E85.4 [G99.8]
    autonomic G90.9
    fatty G31.89
    specified NEC G31.89
  nipple N64.89
  olivopontocerebellar (hereditary) (familial) G23.8
  osseous labyrinth — *see* subcategory H83.8 ☑
  ovary N83.8
    cystic N83.20- ☑
    microcystic N83.20- ☑
  pallidal pigmentary (progressive) G23.0
  pancreas K86.89
    tuberculous A18.83
  penis N48.89
  pigmentary (diffuse) (general)
    localized — *see* Degeneration, by site
    pallidal (progressive) G23.0
  pineal gland E34.8
  pituitary (gland) E23.6
  popliteal fat pad M79.4
  posterolateral (spinal cord) — *see* Degeneration, combined
  pulmonary valve (heart) I37.8
  pulp (tooth) K04.2
  pupillary margin H21.24- ☑
  renal — *see* Degeneration, kidney
  retina H35.9
    hereditary (cerebroretinal) (congenital) (juvenile) (macula) (peripheral) (pigmentary) — *see* Dystrophy, retina
    Kuhnt-Junius — *see also* Degeneration, macula
      H35.32- ☑
    macula (cystic) (exudative) (hole) (nonexudative) (pseudohole) (senile) (toxic) — *see* Degeneration, macula
    peripheral H35.40
      lattice H35.41- ☑
      microcystoid H35.42- ☑
      paving stone H35.43- ☑
      secondary
        pigmentary H35.45- ☑
        vitreoretinal H35.46- ☑
      senile reticular H35.44- ☑
    pigmentary (primary) — *see also* Dystrophy, retina
      secondary — *see* Degeneration, retina, peripheral, secondary
    posterior pole — *see* Degeneration, macula
  saccule, congenital (causing impairment of hearing) Q16.5
  senile R54
    brain G31.1
    cardiac, heart or myocardium — *see* Degeneration, myocardial
    motor centers G31.1
    vascular — *see* Arteriosclerosis
  sinus (cystic) — *see also* Sinusitis
    polypoid J33.1
  skin L98.8
    amyloid E85.4 [L99]
    colloid L98.8
  spinal (cord) G31.89
    amyloid E85.4 [G32.89]
    combined (subacute) — *see* Degeneration, combined
    dorsolateral — *see* Degeneration, combined
    familial NEC G31.89
    fatty G31.89
    funicular — *see* Degeneration, combined
    posterolateral — *see* Degeneration, combined
    subacute combined — *see* Degeneration, combined
    tuberculous A17.81
  spleen D73.0
    amyloid E85.4 [D77]
  stomach K31.89
  striatonigral G23.2
  suprarenal (capsule) (gland) E27.8

Degeneration, degenerative — *continued*
  synovial membrane (pulpy) — *see* Disorder, synovium, specified type NEC
  tapetoretinal — *see* Dystrophy, retina
  thymus (gland) E32.8
    fatty E32.8
  thyroid (gland) E07.89
  tricuspid (heart) (valve) I07.9
  tuberculous NEC — *see* Tuberculosis
  turbinate J34.89
  uterus (cystic) N85.8
  vascular (senile) — *see* Arteriosclerosis
    hypertensive — *see* Hypertension
  vitreoretinal, secondary — *see* Degeneration, retina, peripheral, secondary, vitreoretinal
  vitreous (body) H43.81- ☑
  Wallerian — *see* Disorder, nerve
  Wilson's hepatolenticular E83.01
Deglutition
  paralysis R13.0
    hysterical F44.4
  pneumonia J69.0
Degos' disease I77.89
Dehiscence (of)
  amputation stump T87.81
  cesarean wound O90.0
  closure of
    cornea T81.31 ☑
    craniotomy T81.32 ☑
    fascia (muscular) (superficial) T81.32 ☑
    internal organ or tissue T81.32 ☑
    laceration (external) (internal) T81.33 ☑
    ligament T81.32 ☑
    mucosa T81.31 ☑
    muscle or muscle flap T81.32 ☑
    ribs or rib cage T81.32 ☑
    skin and subcutaneous tissue (full-thickness) (superficial) T81.31 ☑
    skull T81.32 ☑
    sternum (sternotomy) T81.32 ☑
    tendon T81.32 ☑
    traumatic laceration (external) (internal) T81.33 ☑
  episiotomy O90.1
  operation wound NEC T81.31 ☑
    external operation wound (superficial) T81.31 ☑
    internal operation wound (deep) T81.32 ☑
  perineal wound (postpartum) O90.1
  traumatic injury wound repair T81.33 ☑
  wound T81.30 ☑
    traumatic repair T81.33 ☑
Dehydration E86.0
  newborn P74.1
Déjérine-Roussy syndrome G89.0
Déjérine-Sottas disease or neuropathy (hypertrophic) G60.0
Déjérine-Thomas atrophy G23.8
Delay, delayed
  any plane in pelvis
    complicating delivery O66.9
  birth or delivery NOS O63.9
  closure, ductus arteriosus (Botalli) P29.38
  coagulation — *see* Defect, coagulation
  conduction (cardiac) (ventricular) I45.9
  delivery, second twin, triplet, etc O63.2
  development R62.50
    global F88
    intellectual (specific) F81.9
    language F80.9
      due to hearing loss F80.4
    learning F81.9
    milestone R62.0
    pervasive F84.9
    physiological R62.50
      specified stage NEC R62.0
    reading F81.0
    sexual E30.0
    speech F80.9
      due to hearing loss F80.4
    spelling F81.81
  ejaculation F52.32
  gastric emptying K30
  menarche E30.0
  menstruation (cause unknown) N91.0
  milestone R62.0
  passage of meconium (newborn) P76.0
  primary respiration P28.9
  puberty (constitutional) E30.0

Delay, delayed — *continued*
 separation of umbilical cord P96.82
 sexual maturation, female E30.0
 sleep phase syndrome G47.21
 union, fracture — *see* Fracture, by site
 vaccination Z28.9
Deletion(s)
 autosome Q93.9
  identified by fluorescence in situ hybridization (FISH) Q93.89
  identified by in situ hybridization (ISH) Q93.89
 chromosome
  with complex rearrangements NEC Q93.7
  part of NEC Q93.59
  seen only at prometaphase Q93.89
  short arm
   22q11.2 Q93.81
   4 Q93.3
   5p Q93.4
  specified NEC Q93.89
 long arm chromosome 18 or 21 Q93.89
  with complex rearrangements NEC Q93.7
 microdeletions NEC Q93.88
Delhi boil or button B55.1
Delinquency (juvenile) (neurotic) F91.8
 group Z72.810
Delinquent immunization status Z28.39
 COVID-19 Z28.31- ☑
Delirium, delirious (acute or subacute) (not alcohol- or drug-induced) (with dementia) R41.0
 alcoholic (acute) (tremens) (withdrawal) F10.921
  with intoxication F10.921
   in
    abuse F10.121
    dependence F10.221
 due to (secondary to)
  alcohol
   intoxication F10.921
    in
     abuse F10.121
     dependence F10.221
   withdrawal F10.231
  amphetamine intoxication F15.921
   in
    abuse F15.121
    dependence F15.221
  anxiolytic
   intoxication F13.921
    in
     abuse F13.121
     dependence F13.221
   withdrawal F13.231
  cannabis intoxication (acute) F12.921
   in
    abuse F12.121
    dependence F12.221
  cocaine intoxication (acute) F14.921
   in
    abuse F14.121
    dependence F14.221
  general medical condition F05
  hallucinogen intoxication F16.921
   in
    abuse F16.121
    dependence F16.221
  hypnotic
   intoxication F13.921
    in
     abuse F13.121
     dependence F13.221
   withdrawal F13.231
  inhalant intoxication (acute) F18.921
   in
    abuse F18.121
    dependence F18.221
  multiple etiologies F05
  opioid intoxication (acute) F11.921
   in
    abuse F11.121
    dependence F11.221
  other (or unknown) substance F19.921
  phencyclidine intoxication (acute) F16.921
   in
    abuse F16.121
    dependence F16.221
  psychoactive substance NEC intoxication (acute) F19.921

Delirium, delirious — *continued*
 due to — *continued*
  psychoactive substance intoxication — *continued*
   in
    abuse F19.121
    dependence F19.221
  sedative
   intoxication F13.921
    in
     abuse F13.121
     dependence F13.221
   withdrawal F13.231
  unknown etiology R41.0
 exhaustion F43.0
 hysterical F44.89
 postprocedural (postoperative) F05
 puerperal F05
 thyroid — *see* Thyrotoxicosis with thyroid storm
 traumatic — *see* Injury, intracranial
 tremens (alcohol-induced) F10.231
  sedative-induced F13.231
Delivery (childbirth) (labor)
 arrested active phase O62.1
 cesarean (for)
  abnormal
   pelvis (bony) (deformity) (major) NEC with disproportion (fetopelvic) O33.0
    with obstructed labor O65.0
   presentation or position O32.9 ☑
  abruptio placentae — *see also* Abruptio placentae O45.9- ☑
  acromion presentation O32.2 ☑
  atony, uterus O62.2
  breech presentation O32.1 ☑
   incomplete O32.8 ☑
  brow presentation O32.3 ☑
  cephalopelvic disproportion O33.9
  cerclage O34.3- ☑
  chin presentation O32.3 ☑
  cicatrix of cervix O34.4- ☑
  contracted pelvis (general)
   inlet O33.2
   outlet O33.3 ☑
  cord presentation or prolapse O69.0 ☑
  cystocele O34.8- ☑
  deformity (acquired) (congenital)
   pelvic organs or tissues NEC O34.8- ☑
   pelvis (bony) NEC O33.0
  disproportion NOS O33.9
  eclampsia — *see* Eclampsia
  face presentation O32.3 ☑
  failed
   forceps O66.5
   induction of labor O61.9
    instrumental O61.1
    mechanical O61.1
    medical O61.0
    specified NEC O61.8
    surgical O61.1
   trial of labor NOS O66.40
    following previous cesarean delivery O66.41
   vacuum extraction O66.5
   ventouse O66.5
  fetal-maternal hemorrhage O43.01- ☑
  hemorrhage (intrapartum) O67.9
   with coagulation defect O67.0
   specified cause NEC O67.8
  high head at term O32.4 ☑
  hydrocephalic fetus O33.6 ☑
  incarceration of uterus O34.51- ☑
  incoordinate uterine action O62.4
  increased size, fetus O33.5 ☑
  inertia, uterus O62.2
   primary O62.0
   secondary O62.1
  isthmocele O34.22
  lateroversion, uterus O34.59- ☑
  mal lie O32.9 ☑
  malposition
   fetus O32.9 ☑
   pelvic organs or tissues NEC O34.8- ☑
   uterus NEC O34.59- ☑
  malpresentation NOS O32.9 ☑
  oblique presentation O32.2 ☑
  occurring after 37 completed weeks of gestation but before 39 completed weeks gestation due to (spontaneous) onset of labor O75.82

Delivery — *continued*
 cesarean — *continued*
  oversize fetus O33.5 ☑
  pelvic tumor NEC O34.8- ☑
  placenta previa O44.0- ☑
   complete O44.0- ☑
    with hemorrhage O44.1- ☑
  placental insufficiency O36.51- ☑
  planned, occurring after 37 completed weeks of gestation but before 39 completed weeks gestation due to (spontaneous) onset of labor O75.82
  polyp, cervix O34.4- ☑
   causing obstructed labor O65.5
  poor dilatation, cervix O62.0
  pre-eclampsia O14.94
   mild O14.04
   moderate O14.04
   severe O14.14
    with hemolysis, elevated liver enzymes and low platelet count (HELLP) O14.24
  previous
   cesarean delivery O34.219
    classical (vertical) scar O34.212
    isthmocele O34.22
    low transverse scar O34.211
    mid-transverse T incision O34.218
    scar
     defect (isthmocele) O34.22
     specified type NEC O34.218
   surgery (to)
    cervix O34.4- ☑
    gynecological NEC O34.8- ☑
    rectum O34.7- ☑
    uterus O34.29
    vagina O34.6- ☑
  prolapse
   arm or hand O32.2 ☑
   uterus O34.52- ☑
  prolonged labor NOS O63.9
  rectocele O34.8- ☑
  retroversion
   uterus O34.53- ☑
  rigid
   cervix O34.4- ☑
   pelvic floor O34.8- ☑
   perineum O34.7- ☑
   vagina O34.6- ☑
   vulva O34.7- ☑
  sacculation, pregnant uterus O34.59- ☑
  scar(s)
   cervix O34.4- ☑
   cesarean delivery O34.219
    classical (vertical) O34.212
    isthmocele O34.22
    low transverse O34.211
    mid-transverse T incision O34.218
    scar
     defect (isthmocele) O34.22
     specified type NEC O34.218
   defect (isthmocele) O34.22
   transmural uterine O34.29
   uterus O34.29
  Shirodkar suture in situ O34.3- ☑
  shoulder presentation O32.2 ☑
  stenosis or stricture, cervix O34.4- ☑
  streptococcus group B (GBS) carrier state O99.824
  transmural uterine scar O34.29
  transverse presentation or lie O32.2 ☑
  tumor, pelvic organs or tissues NEC O34.8- ☑
   cervix O34.4- ☑
  umbilical cord presentation or prolapse O69.0 ☑
  without indication O82
 completely normal case O80
 complicated O75.9
  by
   abnormal, abnormality (of)
    forces of labor O62.9
     specified type NEC O62.8
    glucose O99.814
    uterine contractions NOS O62.9
   abruptio placentae — *see also* Abruptio placentae O45.9- ☑
   abuse
    physical O9A.32 (*following* O99)
    psychological O9A.52 (*following* O99)
    sexual O9A.42 (*following* O99)

Delivery — *continued*
  complicated — *continued*
    by — *continued*
      adherent placenta O72.0
        without hemorrhage O73.0
      alcohol use O99.314
      anemia (pre-existing) O99.02
      anesthetic death O74.8
      annular detachment of cervix O71.3
      atony, uterus O62.2
      attempted vacuum extraction and forceps O66.5
      Bandl's ring O62.4
      bariatric surgery status O99.844
      biliary tract disorder O26.62
      bleeding — *see* Delivery, complicated by, hemorrhage
      blood disorder NEC O99.12
      cervical dystocia (hypotonic) O62.2
        primary O62.0
        secondary O62.1
      circulatory system disorder O99.42
      compression of cord (umbilical) NEC O69.2 ☑
      condition NEC O99.892
      contraction, contracted ring O62.4
      cord (umbilical)
        around neck
          with compression O69.1 ☑
          without compression O69.81 ☑
        bruising O69.5 ☑
        complication O69.9 ☑
          specified NEC O69.89 ☑
        compression NEC O69.2 ☑
        entanglement O69.2 ☑
          without compression O69.82 ☑
        hematoma O69.5 ☑
        presentation O69.0 ☑
        prolapse O69.0 ☑
        short O69.3 ☑
        thrombosis (vessels) O69.5 ☑
        vascular lesion O69.5 ☑
      Couvelaire uterus O45.8X- ☑
      damage to (injury to) NEC
        perineum O71.82
        periurethral tissue O71.82
        vulva O71.82
      delay following rupture of membranes (spontaneous) — *see* Pregnancy, complicated by, premature rupture of membranes
      depressed fetal heart tones O76
      diabetes O24.92
        gestational O24.429
          diet controlled O24.420
          insulin controlled O24.424
          oral drug controlled (antidiabetic) (hypoglycemic) O24.425
        pre-existing O24.32
          specified NEC O24.82
          type 1 O24.02
          type 2 O24.12
      diastasis recti (abdominis) O71.89
      dilatation
        bladder O66.8
        cervix incomplete, poor or slow O62.0
      disease NEC O99.892
      disruptio uteri — *see* Delivery, complicated by, rupture, uterus
      drug use O99.324
      dysfunction, uterus NOS O62.9
        hypertonic O62.4
        hypotonic O62.2
          primary O62.0
          secondary O62.1
        incoordinate O62.4
      eclampsia O15.1
      embolism (pulmonary) — *see* Embolism, obstetric
      endocrine, nutritional or metabolic disease NEC O99.284
      failed
        attempted vaginal birth after previous cesarean delivery O66.41
        induction of labor O61.9
          instrumental O61.1
          mechanical O61.1
          medical O61.0
          specified NEC O61.8
          surgical O61.1
        trial of labor O66.40

Delivery — *continued*
  complicated — *continued*
    by — *continued*
      female genital mutilation O65.5
      fetal
        abnormal acid-base balance O68
        acidemia O68
        acidosis O68
        alkalosis O68
        death, early O02.1
        deformity O66.3
        heart rate or rhythm (abnormal) (non-reassuring) O76
        hypoxia O77.8
        stress O77.9
          due to drug administration O77.1
          electrocardiographic evidence of O77.8
          specified NEC O77.8
          ultrasound evidence of O77.8
      fever during labor O75.2
      gastric banding status O99.844
      gastric bypass status O99.844
      gastrointestinal disease NEC O99.62
      gestational
        diabetes O24.429
          diet controlled O24.420
          insulin (and diet) controlled O24.424
          oral drug controlled (antidiabetic) (hypoglycemic) O24.425
        edema O12.04
          with proteinuria O12.24
        proteinuria O12.14
      gonorrhea O98.22
      hematoma O71.7
        ischial spine O71.7
        pelvic O71.7
        vagina O71.7
        vulva or perineum O71.7
      hemorrhage (uterine) O67.9
        associated with
          afibrinogenemia O67.0
          coagulation defect O67.0
          hyperfibrinolysis O67.0
          hypofibrinogenemia O67.0
        due to
          low implantation of placenta O44.5- ☑
          low-lying placenta O44.5- ☑
          placenta previa O44.1- ☑
            marginal O44.3- ☑
            partial O44.3- ☑
          premature separation of placenta (normally implanted) — *see also* Abruptio placentae O45.9- ☑
        retained placenta O72.0
        uterine leiomyoma O67.8
        placenta NEC O67.8
        postpartum NEC (atonic) (immediate) O72.1
          with retained or trapped placenta O72.0
          delayed O72.2
          secondary O72.2
          third stage O72.0
      hourglass contraction, uterus O62.4
      hypertension, hypertensive (pre-existing) — *see* Hypertension, complicated by, childbirth (labor)
      hypotension O26.5- ☑
      incomplete dilatation (cervix) O62.0
      incoordinate uterus contractions O62.4
      inertia, uterus O62.2
        during latent phase of labor O62.0
        primary O62.0
        secondary O62.1
      infection (maternal) O98.92
        carrier state NEC O99.834
        gonorrhea O98.22
        human immunodeficiency virus (HIV) O98.72
        sexually transmitted NEC O98.32
        specified NEC O98.82
        syphilis O98.12
        tuberculosis O98.02
        viral hepatitis O98.42
        viral NEC O98.52
      injury (to mother) — *see also* Delivery, complicated by, damage to O71.9
      nonobstetric O9A.22 (*following* O99)
        caused by abuse — *see* Delivery, complicated by, abuse
      intrauterine fetal death, early O02.1

Delivery — *continued*
  complicated — *continued*
    by — *continued*
      inversion, uterus O71.2
      laceration (perineal) O70.9
        anus (sphincter) O70.4
          with third degree laceration — *see also* Delivery, complicated, by, laceration, perineum, third degree O70.20
            with mucosa O70.3
          without third degree laceration O70.2 ☑
        bladder (urinary) O71.5
        bowel O71.5
        cervix (uteri) O71.3
        fourchette O70.0
        hymen O70.0
        labia O70.0
        pelvic
          floor O70.1
          organ NEC O71.5
        perineum, perineal O70.9
          first degree O70.0
          fourth degree O70.3
          muscles O70.1
          second degree O70.1
          skin O70.0
          slight O70.0
          third degree O70.20
            with
              both external anal sphincter (EAS) and internal anal sphincter (IAS) torn (IIIc) O70.23
              less than 50% of external anal sphincter (EAS) thickness torn (IIIa) O70.21
              more than 50% external anal sphincter (EAS) thickness torn (IIIb) O70.22
            IIIa O70.21
            IIIb O70.22
            IIIc O70.23
        peritoneum (pelvic) O71.5
        rectovaginal (septum) (without perineal laceration) O71.4
          with perineum — *see also* Delivery, complicated, by, laceration, perineum, third degree O70.20
          with anal or rectal mucosa O70.3
        specified NEC O71.89
        sphincter ani — *see* Delivery, complicated, by, laceration, anus (sphincter)
        urethra O71.5
        uterus O71.81
          before labor O71.81
        vagina, vaginal (deep) (high) (without perineal laceration) O71.4
          with perineum O70.0
          muscles, with perineum O70.1
        vulva O70.0
      liver disorder O26.62
      malignancy O9A.12 (*following* O99)
      malnutrition O25.2
      malposition, malpresentation
        uterus or cervix O65.5
        placenta O44.0- ☑
          with hemorrhage O44.1- ☑
        without obstruction — *see also* Delivery, complicated by, obstruction O32.9 ☑
          breech O32.1 ☑
          compound O32.6 ☑
          face (brow) (chin) O32.3 ☑
          footling O32.8 ☑
          high head O32.4 ☑
          oblique O32.2 ☑
          specified NEC O32.8 ☑
          transverse O32.2 ☑
          unstable lie O32.0 ☑
      meconium in amniotic fluid O77.0
      mental disorder NEC O99.344
      metrorrhexis — *see* Delivery, complicated by, rupture, uterus
      nervous system disorder O99.354
      obesity (pre-existing) O99.214
      obesity surgery status O99.844
      obstetric trauma O71.9
        specified NEC O71.89

Delivery — *continued*
- complicated — *continued*
  - by — *continued*
    - obstructed labor
      - due to
        - breech (complete) (frank) presentation O64.1 ☑
          - incomplete O64.8 ☑
        - brow presentation O64.3 ☑
        - buttock presentation O64.1 ☑
        - chin presentation O64.2 ☑
        - compound presentation O64.5 ☑
        - contracted pelvis O65.1
        - deep transverse arrest O64.0 ☑
        - deformed pelvis O65.0
        - dystocia (fetal) O66.9
          - due to
            - conjoined twins O66.3
            - fetal
              - abnormality NEC O66.3
              - ascites O66.3
              - hydrops O66.3
              - meningomyelocele O66.3
              - sacral teratoma O66.3
              - tumor O66.3
            - hydrocephalic fetus O66.3
            - shoulder O66.0
        - face presentation O64.2 ☑
        - fetopelvic disproportion O65.4
        - footling presentation O64.8 ☑
        - impacted shoulders O66.0
        - incomplete rotation of fetal head O64.0 ☑
        - large fetus O66.2
        - locked twins O66.1
        - malposition O64.9 ☑
          - specified NEC O64.8 ☑
        - malpresentation O64.9 ☑
          - specified NEC O64.8 ☑
        - multiple fetuses NEC O66.6
        - pelvic
          - abnormality (maternal) O65.9
            - organ O65.5
              - specified NEC O65.8
          - contraction
            - inlet O65.2
            - mid-cavity O65.3
            - outlet O65.3
        - persistent (position)
          - occipitoiliac O64.0 ☑
          - occipitoposterior O64.0 ☑
          - occipitosacral O64.0 ☑
          - occipitotransverse O64.0 ☑
        - prolapsed arm O64.4 ☑
        - shoulder presentation O64.4 ☑
      - specified NEC O66.8
    - pathological retraction ring, uterus O62.4
    - penetration, pregnant uterus by instrument O71.1
    - perforation — *see* Delivery, complicated by, laceration
    - placenta, placental
      - ablatio — *see also* Abruptio placentae O45.9- ☑
      - abnormality O43.9- ☑
        - specified NEC O43.89- ☑
      - abruptio — *see also* Abruptio placentae O45.9- ☑
      - accreta O43.21- ☑
      - adherent (with hemorrhage) O72.0
        - without hemorrhage O73.0
      - detachment (premature) — *see also* Abruptio placentae O45.9- ☑
      - disorder O43.9- ☑
        - specified NEC O43.89- ☑
      - hemorrhage NEC O67.8
      - increta O43.22- ☑
      - low (implantation) (lying) O44.4- ☑
        - with hemorrhage O44.5- ☑
      - malformation O43.10- ☑
      - malposition O44.0- ☑
        - without hemorrhage O44.1- ☑
      - percreta O43.23- ☑
      - previa (central) (complete) (lateral) (total) O44.0- ☑
        - with hemorrhage O44.1- ☑
          - marginal O44.2- ☑

Delivery — *continued*
- complicated — *continued*
  - by — *continued*
    - placenta, placental — *continued*
      - previa — *continued*
        - marginal — *continued*
          - with hemorrhage O44.3- ☑
          - partial O44.2- ☑
            - with hemorrhage O44.3- ☑
      - retained (with hemorrhage) O72.0
        - without hemorrhage O73.0
      - separation (premature) O45.9- ☑
        - specified NEC O45.8X- ☑
      - vicious insertion O44.1- ☑
    - precipitate labor O62.3
    - premature rupture, membranes — *see also* Pregnancy, complicated by, premature rupture of membranes O42.90
    - prolapse
      - arm or hand O32.2 ☑
      - cord (umbilical) O69.0 ☑
      - foot or leg O32.8 ☑
      - uterus O34.52- ☑
    - prolonged labor O63.9
      - first stage O63.0
      - second stage O63.1
    - protozoal disease (maternal) O98.62
    - respiratory disease NEC O99.52
    - retained membranes or portions of placenta O72.2
      - without hemorrhage O73.1
    - retarded birth O63.9
    - retention of secundines (with hemorrhage) O72.0
      - without hemorrhage O73.0
      - partial O72.2
        - without hemorrhage O73.1
    - rupture
      - bladder (urinary) O71.5
      - cervix O71.3
      - pelvic organ NEC O71.5
      - urethra O71.5
      - uterus (during or after labor) O71.1
        - before labor O71.0- ☑
    - separation, pubic bone (symphysis pubis) O71.6
    - shock O75.1
    - shoulder presentation O64.4 ☑
    - skin disorder NEC O99.72
    - spasm, cervix O62.4
    - stenosis or stricture, cervix O65.5
    - streptococcus group B (GBS) carrier state O99.824
    - subluxation of symphysis (pubis) O26.72
    - syphilis (maternal) O98.12
    - tear — *see* Delivery, complicated by, laceration
    - tetanic uterus O62.4
    - trauma (obstetrical) — *see also* Delivery, complicated, by, damage to O71.9
      - non-obstetric O9A.22 (*following* O99)
      - periurethral O71.82
      - specified NEC O71.89
    - tuberculosis (maternal) O98.02
    - tumor, pelvic organs or tissues NEC O65.5
    - umbilical cord around neck
      - with compression O69.1 ☑
      - without compression O69.81 ☑
    - uterine inertia O62.2
      - during latent phase of labor O62.0
      - primary O62.0
      - secondary O62.1
    - vasa previa O69.4 ☑
    - velamentous insertion of cord O43.12- ☑
  - specified complication NEC O75.89
- delayed NOS O63.9
  - following rupture of membranes
    - artificial O75.5
  - second twin, triplet, etc. O63.2
- forceps, low following failed vacuum extraction O66.5
- missed (at or near term) O36.4 ☑
- normal O80
- obstructed — *see* Delivery, complicated by, obstructed labor
- precipitate O62.3
- preterm — *see also* Pregnancy, complicated by, preterm labor O60.10 ☑
- spontaneous O80
- term pregnancy NOS O80
- uncomplicated O80
- vaginal, following previous cesarean delivery O34.219
  - classical (vertical) scar O34.212

Delivery — *continued*
- vaginal, following previous cesarean delivery — *continued*
  - low transverse scar O34.211
  - mid-transverse T incision O34.218
  - scar
    - defect (isthmocele) O34.22
    - specified type NEC O34.218

Delusions (paranoid) — *see* Disorder, delusional

Dementia (degenerative (primary)) (old age) (persisting) (unspecified severity) (without behavioral disturbance, psychotic disturbance, mood disturbance, and anxiety) F03.90
- with
  - aberrant motor behavior (exit-seeking) (pacing) (restlessness) (rocking) F03.911
  - agitation F03.911
  - anxiety F03.94
  - behavioral disturbances (sexual disinhibition) (sleep disturbance) (social disinhibition) F03.918
    - specified NEC F03.918
  - Lewy bodies — *see also* Dementia, in, diseases specified elsewhere G31.83 *[F02.80]*
    - with behavioral disturbance — *see also* Dementia, in, diseases specified elsewhere G31.83 *[F02.81-]* ☑
  - mood disturbance (anhedonia) (apathy) (depression) F03.93
  - Parkinsonism — *see also* Dementia, in, diseases specified elsewhere G20 *[F02.80]*
    - with behavioral disturbance — *see also* Dementia, in, diseases specified elsewhere G20 *[F02.81-]* ☑
  - Parkinson's disease — *see also* Dementia, in, diseases specified elsewhere G20 *[F02.80]*
    - with behavioral disturbance — *see also* Dementia, in, diseases specified elsewhere G20 *[F02.81-]* ☑
  - psychotic disturbance (delusional state) (hallucinations) (paranoia) (suspiciousness) F03.92
  - verbal or physical behaviors (anger) (aggression) (combativeness) (profanity) (shouting) (threatening) (violence) F03.911
- alcoholic F10.97
  - with dependence F10.27
- Alzheimer's type — *see* Disease, Alzheimer's
- arteriosclerotic — *see* Dementia, vascular
- atypical, Alzheimer's type — *see* Disease, Alzheimer's, specified NEC
- congenital — *see* Disability, intellectual
- frontal (lobe) — *see also* Dementia, in, diseases specified elsewhere G31.09 *[F02.80]*
  - with behavioral disturbance — *see also* Dementia, in, diseases specified elsewhere G31.09 *[F02.81-]* ☑
- frontotemporal G31.09 *[F02.80]*
  - with behavioral disturbance G31.09 *[F02.81]* ☑
  - specified NEC — *see also* Dementia, in, diseases specified elsewhere G31.09 *[F02.80]*
    - with behavioral disturbance — *see also* Dementia, in, diseases specified elsewhere G31.09 *[F02.81-]* ☑
- in (due to)
  - alcohol F10.97
    - with dependence F10.27
  - Alzheimer's disease — *see* Disease, Alzheimer's
  - arteriosclerotic brain disease — *see* Dementia, vascular
  - cerebral lipidoses — *see also* Dementia, in, diseases specified elsewhere E75.- ☑ *[F02.80]*
    - with behavioral disturbance — *see also* Dementia, in, diseases specified elsewhere E75.- ☑ *[F02.81-]* ☑
  - Creutzfeldt-Jakob disease — *see also* Creutzfeldt-Jakob disease or syndrome (with dementia) A81.00
  - diseases specified elsewhere (unspecified severity) (without behavioral disturbance, psychotic disturbance, mood disturbance, and anxiety) F02.80
    - with
      - aberrant motor behavior (exit-seeking) (pacing) (restlessness) (rocking) F02.811
      - agitation F02.811
      - anxiety F02.84

Dementia — *continued*
  in — *continued*
    diseases specified elsewhere — *continued*
      with — *continued*
        behavioral disturbances (sexual disinhibition) (sleep disturbance) (social disinhibition) F02.818
          specified NEC F02.818
        mood disturbance (anhedonia) (apathy) (depression) F02.83
        psychotic disturbance (delusional state) (hallucinations) (paranoia) (suspiciousness) F02.82
        verbal or physical behaviors (anger) (aggression) (combativeness) (profanity) (shouting) (threatening) (violence) F02.811
    mild F02.A0
      with
        aberrant motor behavior (exit-seeking) (pacing) (restlessness) (rocking) F02.A11
        agitation F02.A11
        anxiety F02.A4
        behavioral disturbances (sexual disinhibition) (sleep disturbance) (social disinhibition) F02.A18
          specified NEC F02.A18
        mood disturbance (anhedonia) (apathy) (depression) F02.A3
        psychotic disturbance (delusional state) (hallucinations) (paranoia) (suspiciousness) F02.A2
        verbal or physical behaviors (anger) (aggression) (combativeness) (profanity) (shouting) (threatening) (violence) F02.A11
    moderate F02.B0
      with
        aberrant motor behavior (exit-seeking) (pacing) (restlessness) (rocking) F02.B11
        agitation F02.B11
        anxiety F02.B4
        behavioral disturbances (sexual disinhibition) (sleep disturbance) (social disinhibition) F02.B18
          specified NEC F02.B18
        mood disturbance (anhedonia) (apathy) (depression) F02.B3
        psychotic disturbance (delusional state) (hallucinations) (paranoia) (suspiciousness) F02.B2
        verbal or physical behaviors (anger) (aggression) (combativeness) (profanity) (shouting) (threatening) (violence) F02.B11
    severe F02.C0
      with
        aberrant motor behavior (exit-seeking) (pacing) (restlessness) (rocking) F02.C11
        agitation F02.C11
        anxiety F02.C4
        behavioral disturbances (sexual disinhibition) (sleep disturbance) (social disinhibition) F02.C18
          specified NEC F02.C18
        mood disturbance (anhedonia) (apathy) (depression) F02.C3
        psychotic disturbance (delusional state) (hallucinations) (paranoia) (suspiciousness) F02.C2
        verbal or physical behaviors (anger) (aggression) (combativeness) (profanity) (shouting) (threatening) (violence) F02.C11
    epilepsy — *see also* Dementia, in, diseases specified elsewhere G40.- *[F02.80]*
      with behavioral disturbance — *see also* Dementia, in, diseases specified elsewhere G40.- ☑ *[F02.81-]* ☑
    hepatolenticular degeneration — *see also* Dementia, in, diseases specified elsewhere E83.01 *[F02.80]*
      with behavioral disturbance — *see also* Dementia, in, diseases specified elsewhere E83.01 *[F02.81-]* ☑

    human immunodeficiency virus (HIV) disease — *see also* Dementia, in, diseases specified elsewhere B20 *[F02.80]*
      with behavioral disturbance — *see also* Dementia, in, diseases specified elsewhere B20 *[F02.81-]* ☑
    Huntington's disease or chorea — *see also* Dementia, in, diseases specified elsewhere G10 *[F02.80]*
      with behavioral disturbance — *see also* Dementia, in, diseases specified elsewhere G10 *[F02.81-]* ☑
    hypercalcemia — *see also* Dementia, in, diseases specified elsewhere E83.52 *[F02.80]*
      with behavioral disturbance — *see also* Dementia, in, diseases specified elsewhere E83.52 *[F02.81-]* ☑
    hypothyroidism, acquired — *see also* Dementia, in, diseases specified elsewhere E03.9 *[F02.80]*
      with behavioral disturbance — *see also* Dementia, in, diseases specified elsewhere E03.9 *[F02.81-]* ☑
      due to iodine deficiency — *see also* Dementia, in, diseases specified elsewhere E01.8 *[F02.80]*
        with behavioral disturbance — *see also* Dementia, in, diseases specified elsewhere E01.8 *[F02.81-]* ☑
    inhalants F18.97
      with dependence F18.27
    multiple
      etiologies F03 ☑
      sclerosis — *see also* Dementia, in, diseases specified elsewhere G35 *[F02.80]*
        with behavioral disturbance — *see also* Dementia, in, diseases specified elsewhere G35 *[F02.81-]* ☑
    neurosyphilis — *see also* Dementia, in, diseases specified elsewhere A52.17 *[F02.80]*
      with behavioral disturbance — *see also* Dementia, in, diseases specified elsewhere A52.17 *[F02.81-]* ☑
      juvenile — *see also* Dementia, in, diseases specified elsewhere A50.49 *[F02.80]*
        with behavioral disturbance — *see also* Dementia, in, diseases specified elsewhere A50.49 *[F02.81-]* ☑
    niacin deficiency — *see also* Dementia, in, diseases specified elsewhere E52 *[F02.80]*
      with behavioral disturbance — *see also* Dementia, in, diseases specified elsewhere E52 *[F02.81-]* ☑
    paralysis agitans — *see also* Dementia, in, diseases specified elsewhere G20 *[F02.80]*
      with behavioral disturbance — *see also* Dementia, in, diseases specified elsewhere G20 *[F02.81-]* ☑
    Parkinson's disease — *see also* Dementia, in, diseases specified elsewhere G20 *[F02.80]*
    pellagra — *see also* Dementia, in, diseases specified elsewhere E52 *[F02.80]*
      with behavioral disturbance — *see also* Dementia, in, diseases specified elsewhere E52 *[F02.81-]* ☑
    Pick's — *see also* Dementia, in, diseases specified elsewhere G31.01 *[F02.80]*
      with behavioral disturbance — *see also* Dementia, in, diseases specified elsewhere G31.01 *[F02.81-]* ☑
    polyarteritis nodosa — *see also* Dementia, in, diseases specified elsewhere M30.0 *[F02.80]*
      with behavioral disturbance — *see also* Dementia, in, diseases specified elsewhere M30.0 *[F02.81-]* ☑
    psychoactive drug F19.97
      with dependence F19.27
      inhalants F18.97
        with dependence F18.27
      sedatives, hypnotics or anxiolytics F13.97
        with dependence F13.27
    sedatives, hypnotics or anxiolytics F13.97
      with dependence F13.27
    systemic lupus erythematosus — *see also* Dementia, in, diseases specified elsewhere M32.- ☑ *[F02.80]*

    systemic lupus erythematosus — *see also* Dementia, in, diseases specified elsewhere — *continued*
      with behavioral disturbance — *see also* Dementia, in, diseases specified elsewhere M32.- *[F02.81-]* ☑
    trypanosomiasis
      African — *see also* Dementia, in, diseases specified elsewhere B56.9 *[F02.80]*
        with behavioral disturbance — *see also* Dementia, in, diseases specified elsewhere B56.9 *[F02.81-]* ☑
    unknown etiology F03.- ☑
    vitamin B12 deficiency — *see also* Dementia, in, diseases specified elsewhere E53.8 *[F02.80]*
      with behavioral disturbance — *see also* Dementia, in, diseases specified elsewhere E53.8 *[F02.81-]* ☑
    volatile solvents F18.97
      with dependence F18.27
  infantile, infantilis F84.3
  Lewy body — *see also* Dementia, in, diseases specified elsewhere G31.83 *[F02.80]*
    with behavioral disturbance — *see also* Dementia, in, diseases specified elsewhere G31.83 *[F02.81-]* ☑
  mild F03.A0
    with
      aberrant motor behavior (exit-seeking) (pacing) (restlessness) (rocking) F03.A11
      agitation F03.A11
      anxiety F03.A4
      behavioral disturbances (sexual disinhibition) (sleep disturbance) (social disinhibition) F03.A18
        specified NEC F03.A18
      mood disturbance (anhedonia) (apathy) (depression) F03.A3
      psychotic disturbance (delusional state) (hallucinations) (paranoia) (suspiciousness) F03.A2
      verbal or physical behaviors (anger) (aggression) (combativeness) (profanity) (shouting) (threatening) (violence) F03.A11
  moderate F03.B0
    with
      aberrant motor behavior (exit-seeking) (pacing) (restlessness) (rocking) F03.B11
      agitation F03.B11
      anxiety F03.B4
      behavioral disturbances (sexual disinhibition) (sleep disturbance) (social disinhibition) F03.B18
        specified NEC F03.B18
      mood disturbance (anhedonia) (apathy) (depression) F03.B3
      psychotic disturbance (delusional state) (hallucinations) (paranoia) (suspiciousness) F03.B2
      verbal or physical behaviors (anger) (aggression) (combativeness) (profanity) (shouting) (threatening) (violence) F03.B11
  multi-infarct — *see* Dementia, vascular
  paralytica, paralytic (syphilitic) — *see also* Dementia, in, diseases specified elsewhere A52.17 *[F02.80]*
    with behavioral disturbance — *see also* Dementia, in, diseases specified elsewhere A52.17 *[F02.81-]* ☑
    juvenilis A50.45
  paretic A52.17
  praecox — *see* Schizophrenia
  presenile F03 ☑
    Alzheimer's type — *see* Disease, Alzheimer's, early onset
  primary degenerative F03 ☑
  progressive, syphilitic A52.17
  senile F03 ☑
    with acute confusional state F05
    Alzheimer's type — *see* Disease, Alzheimer's, late onset
    depressed or paranoid type F03 ☑
  severe F03.C0
    with
      aberrant motor behavior (exit-seeking) (pacing) (restlessness) (rocking) F03.C11
      agitation F03.C11
      anxiety F03.C4

Dementia — *continued*
- severe — *continued*
  - with — *continued*
    - behavioral disturbances (sexual disinhibition) (sleep disturbance) (social disinhibition) F03.C18
      - specified NEC F03.C18
    - mood disturbance (anhedonia) (apathy) (depression) F03.C3
    - psychotic disturbance (delusional state) (hallucinations) (paranoia) (suspiciousness) F03.C2
    - verbal or physical behaviors (anger) (aggression) (combativeness) (profanity) (shouting) (threatening) (violence) F03.C11
- vascular (acute onset) (mixed) (multi-infarct) (subcortical) (unspecified severity) (without behavioral disturbance, psychotic disturbance, mood disturbance, and anxiety) F01.50
  - with
    - aberrant motor behavior (exit-seeking) (pacing) (restlessness) (rocking) F01.511
    - agitation F01.511
    - anxiety F01.54
    - behavioral disturbances (sleep disturbance) (sexual disinhibition) (social disinhibition) F01.518
      - specified NEC F01.518
    - mood disturbance (anhedonia) (apathy) (depression) F01.53
    - psychotic disturbance (delusional state) (hallucinations) (paranoia) (suspiciousness) F01.52
    - verbal or physical behaviors (anger) (aggression) (combativeness) (profanity) (shouting) (threatening) (violence) F01.511
  - mild F01.A0
    - with
      - aberrant motor behavior (exit-seeking) (pacing) (restlessness) (rocking) F01.A11
      - agitation F01.A11
      - anxiety F01.A4
      - behavioral disturbances (sleep disturbance) (sexual disinhibition) (social disinhibition) F01.A18
        - specified NEC F01.A18
      - mood disturbance (anhedonia) (apathy) (depression) F01.A3
      - psychotic disturbance (delusional state) (hallucinations) (paranoia) (suspiciousness) F01.A2
      - verbal or physical behaviors (anger) (aggression) (combativeness) (profanity) (shouting) (threatening) (violence) F01.A11
  - moderate F01.B0
    - with
      - aberrant motor behavior (exit-seeking) (pacing) (restlessness) (rocking) F01.B11
      - agitation F01.B11
      - anxiety F01.B4
      - behavioral disturbances (sleep disturbance) (sexual disinhibition) (social disinhibition) F01.B18
        - specified NEC F01.B18
      - mood disturbance (anhedonia) (apathy) (depression) F01.B3
      - psychotic disturbance (delusional state) (hallucinations) (paranoia) (suspiciousness) F01.B2
      - verbal or physical behaviors (anger) (aggression) (combativeness) (profanity) (shouting) (threatening) (violence) F01.B11
  - severe F01.C0
    - with
      - aberrant motor behavior (exit-seeking) (pacing) (restlessness) (rocking) F01.C11
      - agitation F01.C11
      - anxiety F01.C4
      - behavioral disturbances (sleep disturbance) (sexual disinhibition) (social disinhibition) F01.C18
        - specified NEC F01.C18
      - mood disturbance (anhedonia) (apathy) (depression) F01.C3
      - psychotic disturbance (delusional state) (hallucinations) (paranoia) (suspiciousness) F01.C2

Dementia — *continued*
- vascular — *continued*
  - severe — *continued*
    - with — *continued*
      - verbal or physical behaviors (anger) (aggression) (combativeness) (profanity) (shouting) (threatening) (violence) F01.C11
Demineralization, bone — *see* Osteoporosis
Demodex folliculorum (infestation) B88.0
Demophobia F40.248
Demoralization R45.3
Demyelination, demyelinization
- central nervous system G37.9
  - specified NEC G37.8
- corpus callosum (central) G37.1
- disseminated, acute G36.9
  - specified NEC G36.8
- global G35
- in optic neuritis G36.0
Dengue (classical) (fever) A90
- hemorrhagic A91
- sandfly A93.1
Dennie-Marfan syphilitic syndrome A50.45
Dens evaginatus, in dente or invaginatus K00.2
Dense breasts R92.2
Density
- increased, bone (disseminated) (generalized) (spotted) — *see* Disorder, bone, density and structure, specified type NEC
- lung (nodular) J98.4
Dental — *see also* condition
- examination Z01.20
  - with abnormal findings Z01.21
- restoration
  - aesthetically inadequate or displeasing K08.56
  - defective K08.50
    - specified NEC K08.59
  - failure of marginal integrity K08.51
  - failure of periodontal anatomical integrity K08.54
Dentia praecox K00.6
Denticles (pulp) K04.2
Dentigerous cyst K09.0
Dentin
- irregular (in pulp) K04.3
- opalescent K00.5
- secondary (in pulp) K04.3
- sensitive K03.89
Dentinogenesis imperfecta K00.5
Dentinoma — *see* Cyst, calcifying odontogenic
Dentition (syndrome) K00.7
- delayed K00.6
- difficult K00.7
- precocious K00.6
- premature K00.6
- retarded K00.6
Dependence (on) (syndrome) F19.20
- with remission F19.21
- alcohol (ethyl) (methyl) (without remission) F10.20
  - with
    - amnestic disorder, persisting F10.26
    - anxiety disorder F10.280
    - dementia, persisting F10.27
    - intoxication F10.229
      - with delirium F10.221
      - uncomplicated F10.220
    - mood disorder F10.24
    - psychotic disorder F10.259
      - with
        - delusions F10.250
        - hallucinations F10.251
    - remission F10.21
    - sexual dysfunction F10.281
    - sleep disorder F10.282
    - specified disorder NEC F10.288
    - withdrawal F10.239
      - with
        - delirium F10.231
        - perceptual disturbance F10.232
      - uncomplicated F10.230
  - counseling and surveillance Z71.41
  - in remission F10.21
- amobarbital — *see* Dependence, drug, sedative
- amphetamine(s) (type) — *see* Dependence, drug, stimulant NEC
- amytal (sodium) — *see* Dependence, drug, sedative
- analgesic NEC F55.8

Dependence — *continued*
- anesthetic (agent) (gas) (general) (local) NEC — *see* Dependence, drug, psychoactive NEC
- anxiolytic NEC — *see* Dependence, drug, sedative
- barbital(s) — *see* Dependence, drug, sedative
- barbiturate(s) (compounds) (drugs classifiable to T42) — *see* Dependence, drug, sedative
- benzedrine — *see* Dependence, drug, stimulant NEC
- bhang — *see* Dependence, drug, cannabis
- bromide(s) NEC — *see* Dependence, drug, sedative
- caffeine — *see* Dependence, drug, stimulant NEC
- cannabis (sativa) (indica) (resin) (derivatives) (type) — *see* Dependence, drug, cannabis
- chloral (betaine) (hydrate) — *see* Dependence, drug, sedative
- chlordiazepoxide — *see* Dependence, drug, sedative
- coca (leaf) (derivatives) — *see* Dependence, drug, cocaine
- cocaine — *see* Dependence, drug, cocaine
- codeine — *see* Dependence, drug, opioid
- combinations of drugs F19.20
- dagga — *see* Dependence, drug, cannabis
- demerol — *see* Dependence, drug, opioid
- dexamphetamine — *see* Dependence, drug, stimulant NEC
- dexedrine — *see* Dependence, drug, stimulant NEC
- dextromethorphan — *see* Dependence, drug, opioid
- dextromoramide — *see* Dependence, drug, opioid
- dextro-nor-pseudo-ephedrine — *see* Dependence, drug, stimulant NEC
- dextrorphan — *see* Dependence, drug, opioid
- diazepam — *see* Dependence, drug, sedative
- dilaudid — *see* Dependence, drug, opioid
- D-lysergic acid diethylamide — *see* Dependence, drug, hallucinogen
- drug NEC F19.20
  - with sleep disorder F19.282
  - cannabis F12.20
    - with
      - anxiety disorder F12.280
      - intoxication F12.229
        - with
          - delirium F12.221
          - perceptual disturbance F12.222
        - uncomplicated F12.220
      - other specified disorder F12.288
      - psychosis F12.259
        - delusions F12.250
        - hallucinations F12.251
      - unspecified disorder F12.29
      - withdrawal F12.23
    - in remission F12.21
  - cocaine F14.20
    - with
      - anxiety disorder F14.280
      - intoxication F14.229
        - with
          - delirium F14.221
          - perceptual disturbance F14.222
        - uncomplicated F14.220
      - mood disorder F14.24
      - other specified disorder F14.288
      - psychosis F14.259
        - delusions F14.250
        - hallucinations F14.251
      - sexual dysfunction F14.281
      - sleep disorder F14.282
      - unspecified disorder F14.29
      - withdrawal F14.23
    - in remission F14.21
    - withdrawal symptoms in newborn P96.1
  - counseling and surveillance Z71.51
  - hallucinogen F16.20
    - with
      - anxiety disorder F16.280
      - flashbacks F16.283
      - intoxication F16.229
        - with delirium F16.221
        - uncomplicated F16.220
      - mood disorder F16.24
      - other specified disorder F16.288
      - perception disorder, persisting F16.283
      - psychosis F16.259
        - delusions F16.250
        - hallucinations F16.251
      - unspecified disorder F16.29
    - in remission F16.21
  - in remission F19.21

Dependence — continued
  drug — continued
    inhalant F18.20
      with
        anxiety disorder F18.280
        dementia, persisting F18.27
        intoxication F18.229
          with delirium F18.221
          uncomplicated F18.220
        mood disorder F18.24
        other specified disorder F18.288
        psychosis F18.259
          delusions F18.250
          hallucinations F18.251
        unspecified disorder F18.29
      in remission F18.21
    nicotine F17.200
      with disorder F17.209
        in remission F17.201
        specified disorder NEC F17.208
        withdrawal F17.203
      chewing tobacco F17.220
        with disorder F17.229
          in remission F17.221
          specified disorder NEC F17.228
          withdrawal F17.223
      cigarettes F17.210
        with disorder F17.219
          in remission F17.211
          specified disorder NEC F17.218
          withdrawal F17.213
      specified product NEC F17.290
        with disorder F17.299
          remission F17.291
          specified disorder NEC F17.298
          withdrawal F17.293
    opioid F11.20
      with
        intoxication F11.229
          with
            delirium F11.221
            perceptual disturbance F11.222
          uncomplicated F11.220
        mood disorder F11.24
        other specified disorder F11.288
        psychosis F11.259
          delusions F11.250
          hallucinations F11.251
        sexual dysfunction F11.281
        sleep disorder F11.282
        unspecified disorder F11.29
        withdrawal F11.23
      in remission F11.21
    psychoactive NEC F19.20
      with
        amnestic disorder F19.26
        anxiety disorder F19.280
        dementia F19.27
        intoxication F19.229
          with
            delirium F19.221
            perceptual disturbance F19.222
          uncomplicated F19.220
        mood disorder F19.24
        other specified disorder F19.288
        psychosis F19.259
          delusions F19.250
          hallucinations F19.251
        sexual dysfunction F19.281
        sleep disorder F19.282
        unspecified disorder F19.29
        withdrawal F19.239
          with
            delirium F19.231
            perceptual disturbance F19.232
          uncomplicated F19.230
    sedative, hypnotic or anxiolytic F13.20
      with
        amnestic disorder F13.26
        anxiety disorder F13.280
        dementia, persisting F13.27
        intoxication F13.229
          with delirium F13.221
          uncomplicated F13.220
        mood disorder F13.24
        other specified disorder F13.288
        psychosis F13.259
          delusions F13.250
          hallucinations F13.251

Dependence — continued
  drug — continued
    sedative, hypnotic or anxiolytic — continued
      with — continued
        sexual dysfunction F13.281
        sleep disorder F13.282
        unspecified disorder F13.29
        withdrawal F13.239
          with
            delirium F13.231
            perceptual disturbance F13.232
          uncomplicated F13.230
      in remission F13.21
    stimulant NEC F15.20
      with
        anxiety disorder F15.280
        intoxication F15.229
          with
            delirium F15.221
            perceptual disturbance F15.222
          uncomplicated F15.220
        mood disorder F15.24
        other specified disorder F15.288
        psychosis F15.259
          delusions F15.250
          hallucinations F15.251
        sexual dysfunction F15.281
        sleep disorder F15.282
        unspecified disorder F15.29
        withdrawal F15.23
      in remission F15.21
    ethyl
      alcohol (without remission) F10.20
        with remission F10.21
      bromide — see Dependence, drug, sedative
      carbamate F19.20
      chloride F19.20
      morphine — see Dependence, drug, opioid
    ganja — see Dependence, drug, cannabis
    glue (airplane) (sniffing) — see Dependence, drug, inhalant
    glutethimide — see Dependence, drug, sedative
    hallucinogenics — see Dependence, drug, hallucinogen
    hashish — see Dependence, drug, cannabis
    hemp — see Dependence, drug, cannabis
    heroin (salt) (any) — see Dependence, drug, opioid
    hypnotic NEC — see Dependence, drug, sedative
    Indian hemp — see Dependence, drug, cannabis
    inhalants — see Dependence, drug, inhalant
    khat — see Dependence, drug, stimulant NEC
    laudanum — see Dependence, drug, opioid
    LSD (-25) (derivatives) — see Dependence, drug, hallucinogen
    luminal — see Dependence, drug, sedative
    lysergic acid — see Dependence, drug, hallucinogen
    maconha — see Dependence, drug, cannabis
    marihuana — see Dependence, drug, cannabis
    meprobamate — see Dependence, drug, sedative
    mescaline — see Dependence, drug, hallucinogen
    methadone — see Dependence, drug, opioid
    methamphetamine(s) — see Dependence, drug, stimulant NEC
    methaqualone — see Dependence, drug, sedative
    methyl
      alcohol (without remission) F10.20
        with remission F10.21
      bromide — see Dependence, drug, sedative
      morphine — see Dependence, drug, opioid
    phenidate — see Dependence, drug, stimulant NEC
    sulfonal — see Dependence, drug, sedative
    morphine (sulfate) (sulfite) (type) — see Dependence, drug, opioid
    narcotic (drug) NEC — see Dependence, drug, opioid
    nembutal — see Dependence, drug, sedative
    neraval — see Dependence, drug, sedative
    neravan — see Dependence, drug, sedative
    neurobarb — see Dependence, drug, sedative
    nicotine — see Dependence, drug, nicotine
    nitrous oxide F19.20
    nonbarbiturate sedatives and tranquilizers with similar effect — see Dependence, drug, sedative
  on
    artificial heart (fully implantable) (mechanical) Z95.812
    aspirator Z99.0
    care provider (because of) Z74.9
      impaired mobility Z74.09

Dependence — continued
  on — continued
    care provider — continued
      need for
        assistance with personal care Z74.1
        continuous supervision Z74.3
      no other household member able to render care Z74.2
      specified reason NEC Z74.8
    machine Z99.89
      enabling NEC Z99.89
      specified type NEC Z99.89
    renal dialysis (hemodialysis) (peritoneal) Z99.2
    respirator Z99.11
    ventilator Z99.11
    wheelchair Z99.3
  opiate — see Dependence, drug, opioid
  opioids — see Dependence, drug, opioid
  opium (alkaloids) (derivatives) (tincture) — see Dependence, drug, opioid
  oxygen (long-term) (supplemental) Z99.81
  paraldehyde — see Dependence, drug, sedative
  paregoric — see Dependence, drug, opioid
  PCP (phencyclidine) (or related substance) — see Dependence, drug, hallucinogen
  pentobarbital — see Dependence, drug, sedative
  pentobarbitone (sodium) — see Dependence, drug, sedative
  pentothal — see Dependence, drug, sedative
  peyote — see Dependence, drug, hallucinogen
  phencyclidine (PCP) (or related substance) — see Dependence, drug, hallucinogen
  phenmetrazine — see Dependence, drug, stimulant NEC
  phenobarbital — see Dependence, drug, sedative
  polysubstance F19.20
  psilocibin, psilocin, psilocyn, psilocyline — see Dependence, drug, hallucinogen
  psychostimulant NEC — see Dependence, drug, stimulant NEC
  secobarbital — see Dependence, drug, sedative
  seconal — see Dependence, drug, sedative
  sedative NEC — see Dependence, drug, sedative
  specified drug NEC — see Dependence, drug
  stimulant NEC — see Dependence, drug, stimulant NEC
  substance NEC — see Dependence, drug
  supplemental oxygen Z99.81
  tobacco — see Dependence, drug, nicotine
    counseling and surveillance Z71.6
  tranquilizer NEC — see Dependence, drug, sedative
  vitamin B6 E53.1
  volatile solvents — see Dependence, drug, inhalant
Dependency
  care-provider Z74.9
  passive F60.7
  reactions (persistent) F60.7
Depersonalization (in neurotic state) (neurotic) (syndrome) F48.1
Depletion
  extracellular fluid E86.9
  plasma E86.1
  potassium E87.6
    nephropathy N25.89
  salt or sodium E87.1
    causing heat exhaustion or prostration T67.4 ☑
    nephropathy N28.9
  volume NOS E86.9
Deployment (current) (military) status Z56.82
  in theater or in support of military war, peacekeeping and humanitarian operations Z56.82
  personal history of Z91.82
    military war, peacekeeping and humanitarian deployment (current or past conflict) Z91.82
  returned from Z91.82
Depolarization, premature I49.40
  atrial I49.1
  junctional I49.2
  specified NEC I49.49
  ventricular I49.3
Deposit
  bone in Boeck's sarcoid D86.89
  calcareous, calcium — see Calcification
  cholesterol
    retina H35.89
    vitreous (body) (humor) — see Deposit, crystalline
  conjunctiva H11.11- ☑
  cornea H18.00- ☑
    argentous H18.02- ☑

Deposit — *continued*
- cornea — *continued*
  - due to metabolic disorder H18.03- ☑
  - Kayser-Fleischer ring H18.04- ☑
  - pigmentation — *see* Pigmentation, cornea
- crystalline, vitreous (body) (humor) H43.2- ☑
- hemosiderin in old scars of cornea — *see* Pigmentation, cornea, stromal
- metallic in lens — *see* Cataract, specified NEC
- skin R23.8
- tooth, teeth (betel) (black) (green) (materia alba) (orange) (tobacco) K03.6
- urate, kidney — *see* Calculus, kidney

Depraved appetite — *see* Pica

Depressed
- HDL cholesterol E78.6

Depression (acute) (mental) F32.A
- agitated (single episode) F32.2
- anaclitic — *see* Disorder, adjustment
- anxiety F41.8
  - persistent F34.1
- arches — *see also* Deformity, limb, flat foot
- atypical (single episode) F32.89
  - recurrent episode F33.8
- basal metabolic rate R94.8
- bone marrow D75.89
- central nervous system R09.2
- cerebral R29.818
  - newborn P91.4
- cerebrovascular I67.9
- chest wall M95.4
- climacteric (single episode) F32.89
  - recurrent episode F33.8
- endogenous (without psychotic symptoms) F33.2
  - with psychotic symptoms F33.3
- functional activity R68.89
- hysterical F44.89
- involutional (single episode) F32.89
  - recurrent episode F33.8
- major F32.9
  - with psychotic symptoms F32.3
  - recurrent — *see* Disorder, depressive, recurrent
- manic-depressive — *see* Disorder, depressive, recurrent
- masked (single episode) F32.89
- medullary G93.89
- menopausal (single episode) F32.89
  - recurrent episode F33.8
- metatarsus — *see* Depression, arches
- monopolar F33.9
- nervous F34.1
- neurotic F34.1
- nose M95.0
- postnatal (NOS) F53.0
- postpartum (NOS) F53.0
- post-psychotic of schizophrenia F32.89
- post-schizophrenic F32.89
- psychogenic (reactive) (single episode) F32.9
- psychoneurotic F34.1
- psychotic (single episode) F32.3
  - recurrent F33.3
- reactive (psychogenic) (single episode) F32.9
  - psychotic (single episode) F32.3
- recurrent — *see* Disorder, depressive, recurrent
- respiratory center G93.89
- seasonal — *see* Disorder, depressive, recurrent
- senile F03 ☑
- severe, single episode F32.2
- situational F43.21
- skull Q67.4
- specified NEC (single episode) F32.89
- sternum M95.4
- visual field — *see* Defect, visual field
- vital (recurrent) (without psychotic symptoms) F33.2
  - with psychotic symptoms F33.3
  - single episode F32.2

Deprivation
- cultural Z60.3
- effects NOS T73.9 ☑
  - specified NEC T73.8 ☑
- emotional NEC Z65.8
  - affecting infant or child — *see* Maltreatment, child, psychological
- food T73.0 ☑
- material Z59.87
- protein — *see* Malnutrition
- sleep Z72.820
- social Z60.4

Deprivation — *continued*
- social — *continued*
  - affecting infant or child — *see* Maltreatment, child, psychological
- specified NEC T73.8 ☑
- vitamins — *see* Deficiency, vitamin
- water T73.1 ☑

Derangement
- ankle (internal) — *see* Derangement, joint, articular cartilage, ankle
- cartilage (articular) NEC — *see* Derangement, joint, articular cartilage, by site
  - recurrent — *see* Dislocation, recurrent
- cruciate ligament, anterior, current injury — *see* Sprain, knee, cruciate, anterior
- elbow (internal) — *see* Derangement, joint, articular cartilage, elbow
- hip (joint) (internal) (old) — *see* Derangement, joint, articular cartilage, hip
- joint (internal) M24.9
  - ankylosis — *see* Ankylosis
  - articular cartilage M24.10
    - ankle M24.17- ☑
    - elbow M24.12- ☑
    - foot M24.17- ☑
    - hand M24.14- ☑
    - hip M24.15- ☑
    - knee NEC M23.9- ☑
    - loose body — *see* Loose, body
    - shoulder M24.11- ☑
    - specified site NEC M24.19
    - wrist M24.13- ☑
  - contracture — *see* Contraction, joint
  - current injury — *see also* Dislocation
    - knee, meniscus or cartilage — *see* Tear, meniscus
  - dislocation
    - pathological — *see* Dislocation, pathological
    - recurrent — *see* Dislocation, recurrent
  - knee — *see* Derangement, knee
  - ligament — *see* Disorder, ligament
  - loose body — *see* Loose, body
  - recurrent — *see* Dislocation, recurrent
  - specified type NEC M24.80
    - ankle M24.87- ☑
    - elbow M24.82- ☑
    - foot joint M24.87- ☑
    - hand joint M24.84- ☑
    - hip M24.85- ☑
    - shoulder M24.81- ☑
    - specified site NEC M24.89
    - wrist M24.83- ☑
  - temporomandibular M26.69
- knee (recurrent) M23.9- ☑
  - ligament disruption, spontaneous M23.60- ☑
    - anterior cruciate M23.61- ☑
    - capsular M23.67- ☑
    - instability, chronic M23.5- ☑
    - lateral collateral M23.64- ☑
    - medial collateral M23.63- ☑
    - posterior cruciate M23.62- ☑
  - loose body M23.4- ☑
  - meniscus M23.30- ☑
    - cystic M23.00- ☑
      - lateral M23.002
        - anterior horn M23.04- ☑
        - posterior horn M23.05- ☑
        - specified NEC M23.06- ☑
      - medial M23.005
        - anterior horn M23.01- ☑
        - posterior horn M23.02- ☑
        - specified NEC M23.03- ☑
    - degenerate — *see* Derangement, knee, meniscus, specified NEC
    - detached — *see* Derangement, knee, meniscus, specified NEC
    - due to old tear or injury M23.20- ☑
      - lateral M23.20- ☑
        - anterior horn M23.24- ☑
        - posterior horn M23.25- ☑
        - specified NEC M23.26- ☑
      - medial M23.20- ☑
        - anterior horn M23.21- ☑
        - posterior horn M23.22- ☑
        - specified NEC M23.23- ☑
    - retained — *see* Derangement, knee, meniscus, specified NEC

Derangement — *continued*
- knee — *continued*
  - meniscus — *continued*
    - specified NEC M23.30- ☑
      - lateral M23.30- ☑
        - anterior horn M23.34- ☑
        - posterior horn M23.35- ☑
        - specified NEC M23.36- ☑
      - medial M23.30- ☑
        - anterior horn M23.31- ☑
        - posterior horn M23.32- ☑
        - specified NEC M23.33- ☑
    - old M23.8X- ☑
    - specified NEC — *see* subcategory M23.8 ☑
  - low back NEC — *see* Dorsopathy, specified NEC
  - meniscus — *see* Derangement, knee, meniscus
  - mental — *see* Psychosis
  - patella, specified NEC — *see* Disorder, patella, derangement NEC
  - semilunar cartilage (knee) — *see* Derangement, knee, meniscus, specified NEC
  - shoulder (internal) — *see* Derangement, joint, shoulder

Dercum's disease E88.2

Derealization (neurotic) F48.1

Dermal — *see* condition

Dermaphytid — *see* Dermatophytosis

Dermatitis (eczematous) L30.9
- ab igne L59.0
- acarine B88.0
- actinic (due to sun) L57.8
  - other than from sun L59.8
- allergic — *see* Dermatitis, contact, allergic
- ambustionis, due to burn or scald — *see* Burn
- amebic A06.7
- ammonia L22
- arsenical (ingested) L27.8
- artefacta L98.1
  - psychogenic F54
- atopic L20.9
  - psychogenic F54
  - specified NEC L20.89
- autoimmune progesterone L30.8
- berlock, berloque L56.2
- blastomycotic B40.3
- blister beetle L24.89
- bullous, bullosa L13.9
  - mucosynechial, atrophic L12.1
  - seasonal L30.8
  - specified NEC L13.8
- calorica L59.0
  - due to burn or scald — *see* Burn
- caterpillar L24.89
- cercarial B65.3
- combustionis L59.0
  - due to burn or scald — *see* Burn
- congelationis T69.1 ☑
- contact (occupational) L25.9
  - allergic L23.9
    - due to
      - adhesives L23.1
      - cement L23.5
      - chemical products NEC L23.5
      - chromium L23.0
      - cosmetics L23.2
      - dander (cat) (dog) L23.81
      - drugs in contact with skin L23.3
      - dyes L23.4
      - food in contact with skin L23.6
      - hair (cat) (dog) L23.81
      - insecticide L23.5
      - metals L23.0
      - nickel L23.0
      - plants, non-food L23.7
      - plastic L23.5
      - rubber L23.5
      - specified agent NEC L23.89
    - due to
      - cement L25.3
      - chemical products NEC L25.3
      - cosmetics L25.0
      - dander (cat) (dog) L23.81
      - drugs in contact with skin L25.1
      - dyes L25.2
      - food in contact with skin L25.4
      - hair (cat) (dog) L23.81
      - plants, non-food L25.5
      - specified agent NEC L25.8
    - irritant L24.9

Dermatitis — *continued*
　contact — *continued*
　　irritant — *continued*
　　　due to
　　　　body fluids L24.A0
　　　　　incontinence (dual) (fecal) (urinary)
　　　　　　L24.A2
　　　　　saliva L24.A1
　　　　　specified NEC L24.A9
　　　　cement L24.5
　　　　chemical products NEC L24.5
　　　　cosmetics L24.3
　　　　detergents L24.0
　　　　drugs in contact with skin L24.4
　　　　food in contact with skin L24.6
　　　　oils and greases L24.1
　　　　plants, non-food L24.7
　　　　solvents L24.2
　　　　specified agent NEC L24.89
　　　related to
　　　　colostomy L24.B3
　　　　endotracheal tube L24.A9
　　　　enterocutaneous fistula L24.B3
　　　　gastrostomy L24.B1
　　　　ileostomy L24.B3
　　　　jejunostomy L24.B1
　　　　saliva or spit fistula L24.B1
　　　　stoma or fistula L24.B0
　　　　　digestive L24.B1
　　　　　fecal or urinary L24.B3
　　　　　respiratory L24.B2
　　　　tracheostomy L24.B2
　contusiformis L52
　desquamative L30.8
　diabetic — *see* E08-E13 with .620
　diaper L22
　diphtheritica A36.3
　dry skin L85.3
　due to
　　acetone (contact) (irritant) L24.2
　　acids (contact) (irritant) L24.5
　　adhesive(s) (allergic) (contact) (plaster) L23.1
　　　irritant L24.5
　　alcohol (irritant) (skin contact) (substances in cate-
　　　gory T51) L24.2
　　　taken internally L27.8
　　alkalis (contact) (irritant) L24.5
　　arsenic (ingested) L27.8
　　carbon disulfide (contact) (irritant) L24.2
　　caustics (contact) (irritant) L24.5
　　cement (contact) L25.3
　　cereal (ingested) L27.2
　　chemical(s) NEC L25.3
　　　taken internally L27.8
　　chlorocompounds L24.2
　　chromium (contact) (irritant) L24.81
　　coffee (ingested) L27.2
　　cold weather L30.8
　　cosmetics (contact) L25.0
　　　allergic L23.2
　　　irritant L24.3
　　cyclohexanes L24.2
　　dander (cat) (dog) L23.81
　　Demodex species B88.0
　　Dermanyssus gallinae B88.0
　　detergents (contact) (irritant) L24.0
　　dichromate L24.81
　　drugs and medicaments (generalized) (internal use)
　　　L27.0
　　　external — *see* Dermatitis, due to, drugs, in
　　　　contact with skin
　　　in contact with skin L25.1
　　　　allergic L23.3
　　　　irritant L24.4
　　　localized skin eruption L27.1
　　　specified substance — *see* Table of Drugs and
　　　　Chemicals
　　dyes (contact) L25.2
　　　allergic L23.4
　　　irritant L24.89
　　epidermophytosis — *see* Dermatophytosis
　　esters L24.2
　　external irritant NEC L24.9
　　fish (ingested) L27.2
　　flour (ingested) L27.2
　　food (ingested) L27.2
　　　in contact with skin L25.4
　　fruit (ingested) L27.2
　　furs (allergic) (contact) L23.81

Dermatitis — *continued*
　due to — *continued*
　　glues — *see* Dermatitis, due to, adhesives
　　glycols L24.2
　　greases NEC (contact) (irritant) L24.1
　　hair (cat) (dog) L23.81
　　hot
　　　objects and materials — *see* Burn
　　　weather or places L59.0
　　hydrocarbons L24.2
　　infrared rays L59.8
　　ingestion, ingested substance L27.9
　　　chemical NEC L27.8
　　　drugs and medicaments — *see* Dermatitis, due
　　　　to, drugs
　　　food L27.2
　　　specified NEC L27.8
　　insecticide in contact with skin L24.5
　　internal agent L27.9
　　　drugs and medicaments (generalized) — *see*
　　　　Dermatitis, due to, drugs
　　　food L27.2
　　irradiation — *see* Dermatitis, due to, radioactive
　　　substance
　　ketones L24.2
　　lacquer tree (allergic) (contact) L23.7
　　light (sun) NEC L57.8
　　　acute L56.8
　　　other L59.8
　　Liponyssoides sanguineus B88.0
　　low temperature L30.8
　　meat (ingested) L27.2
　　metals, metal salts (contact) (irritant) L24.81
　　milk (ingested) L27.2
　　nickel (contact) (irritant) L24.81
　　nylon (contact) (irritant) L24.5
　　oils NEC (contact) (irritant) L24.1
　　paint solvent (contact) (irritant) L24.2
　　petroleum products (contact) (irritant) (substances
　　　in T52.0) L24.2
　　plants NEC (contact) L25.5
　　　allergic L23.7
　　　irritant L24.7
　　plasters (adhesive) (any) (allergic) (contact) L23.1
　　　irritant L24.5
　　plastic (contact) L25.3
　　preservatives (contact) — *see* Dermatitis, due to,
　　　chemical, in contact with skin
　　primrose (allergic) (contact) L23.7
　　primula (allergic) (contact) L23.7
　　radiation L59.8
　　　nonionizing (chronic exposure) L57.8
　　　sun NEC L57.8
　　　　acute L56.8
　　radioactive substance L58.9
　　　acute L58.0
　　　chronic L58.1
　　radium L58.9
　　　acute L58.0
　　　chronic L58.1
　　ragweed (allergic) (contact) L23.7
　　Rhus (allergic) (contact) (diversiloba) (radicans)
　　　(toxicodendron) (venenata) (verniciflua) L23.7
　　rubber (contact) L24.5
　　Senecio jacobaea (allergic) (contact) L23.7
　　solvents (contact) (irritant) (substances in category
　　　T52) L24.2
　　specified agent NEC (contact) L25.8
　　　allergic L23.89
　　　irritant L24.89
　　sunshine NEC L57.8
　　　acute L56.8
　　tetrachlorethylene (contact) (irritant) L24.2
　　toluene (contact) (irritant) L24.2
　　turpentine (contact) L24.2
　　ultraviolet rays (sun NEC) (chronic exposure) L57.8
　　　acute L56.8
　　vaccine or vaccination L27.0
　　　specified substance — *see* Table of Drugs and
　　　　Chemicals
　　varicose veins — *see* Varix, leg, with, inflammation
　　X-rays L58.9
　　　acute L58.0
　　　chronic L58.1
　dyshydrotic L30.1
　dysmenorrheica N94.6
　escharotica — *see* Burn
　exfoliative, exfoliativa (generalized) L26

Dermatitis — *continued*
　exfoliative, exfoliativa — *continued*
　　neonatorum L00
　　eyelid — *see also* Dermatosis, eyelid H01.9
　　　allergic H01.119
　　　　left H01.116
　　　　　lower H01.115
　　　　　upper H01.114
　　　　right H01.113
　　　　　lower H01.112
　　　　　upper H01.111
　　　contact — *see* Dermatitis, eyelid, allergic
　　　due to
　　　　Demodex species B88.0
　　　　herpes (zoster) B02.39
　　　　　simplex B00.59
　　　eczematous H01.139
　　　　left H01.136
　　　　　lower H01.135
　　　　　upper H01.134
　　　　right H01.133
　　　　　lower H01.132
　　　　　upper H01.131
　　　specified NEC H01.8
　facta, factitia, factitial L98.1
　　psychogenic F54
　flexural NEC L20.82
　friction L30.4
　fungus B36.9
　　specified type NEC B36.8
　gangrenosa, gangrenous infantum L08.0
　harvest mite B88.0
　heat L59.0
　herpesviral, vesicular (ear) (lip) B00.1
　herpetiformis (bullous) (erythematous) (pustular)
　　(vesicular) L13.0
　　juvenile L12.2
　　senile L12.0
　hiemalis L30.8
　hypostatic, hypostatica — *see* Varix, leg, with, inflam-
　　mation
　infectious eczematoid L30.3
　infective L30.3
　irritant — *see* Dermatitis, contact, irritant
　Jacquet's (diaper dermatitis) L22
　Leptus B88.0
　lichenified NEC L28.0
　medicamentosa (generalized) (internal use) — *see*
　　Dermatitis, due to drugs
　mite B88.0
　multiformis L13.0
　　juvenile L12.2
　napkin L22
　neurotica L13.0
　nummular L30.0
　papillaris capillitii L73.0
　pellagrous E52
　perioral L71.0
　photocontact L56.2
　polymorpha dolorosa L13.0
　pruriginosa L13.0
　pruritic NEC L30.8
　psychogenic F54
　purulent L08.0
　pustular
　　contagious B08.02
　　subcorneal L13.1
　pyococcal L08.0
　pyogenica L08.0
　repens L40.2
　Ritter's (exfoliativa) L00
　Schamberg's L81.7
　schistosome B65.3
　seasonal bullous L30.8
　seborrheic L21.9
　　infantile L21.1
　　specified NEC L21.8
　sensitization NOS L23.9
　septic L08.0
　solare L57.8
　specified NEC L30.8
　stasis I87.2
　　with
　　　varicose ulcer — *see* Varix, leg, with ulcer, with
　　　　inflammation
　　　varicose veins — *see* Varix, leg, with, inflamma-
　　　　tion

Dermatitis — *continued*
  stasis — *continued*
      due to postthrombotic syndrome — *see* Syndrome, postthrombotic
    suppurative L08.0
    traumatic NEC L30.4
    trophoneurotica L13.0
    ultraviolet (sun) (chronic exposure) L57.8
      acute L56.8
    varicose — *see* Varix, leg, with, inflammation
    vegetans L10.1
    verrucosa B43.0
    vesicular, herpesviral B00.1
Dermatoarthritis, lipoid E78.81
Dermatochalasis, eyelid H02.839
  left H02.836
    lower H02.835
    upper H02.834
  right H02.833
    lower H02.832
    upper H02.831
Dermatofibroma (lenticulare) — *see* Neoplasm, skin, benign
  protuberans — *see* Neoplasm, skin, uncertain behavior
Dermatofibrosarcoma (pigmented) (protuberans) — *see* Neoplasm, skin, malignant
Dermatographia L50.3
Dermatolysis (exfoliativa) (congenital) Q82.8
  acquired L57.4
  eyelids — *see* Blepharochalasis
  palpebrarum — *see* Blepharochalasis
  senile L57.4
Dermatomegaly NEC Q82.8
Dermatomucosomyositis — *see also* Dermatomyositis M33.10
  with
    myopathy M33.12
    respiratory involvement M33.11
    specified organ involvement NEC M33.19
Dermatomycosis B36.9
  furfuracea B36.0
  specified type NEC B36.8
Dermatomyositis (acute) (chronic) — *see also* Dermatopolymyositis
  adult — *see also* Dermatomyositis, specified NEC M33.10
  in (due to) neoplastic disease — *see also* Neoplasm D49.9 *[M36.0]*
  juvenile M33.00
    with
      myopathy M33.02
      respiratory involvement M33.01
      specified organ involvement NEC M33.09
    amyopathic M33.03
    without myopathy M33.03
  specified NEC M33.10
    with
      myopathy M33.12
      respiratory involvement M33.11
      specified organ involvement NEC M33.19
    amyopathic M33.13
    without myopathy M33.13
Dermatoneuritis of children — *see* Poisoning, mercury
Dermatophilosis A48.8
Dermatophytid L30.2
Dermatophytide — *see* Dermatophytosis
Dermatophytosis (epidermophyton) (infection) (Microsporum) (tinea) (Trichophyton) B35.9
  beard B35.0
  body B35.4
  capitis B35.0
  corporis B35.4
  deep-seated B35.8
  disseminated B35.8
  foot B35.3
  granulomatous B35.8
  groin B35.6
  hand B35.2
  nail B35.1
  perianal (area) B35.6
  scalp B35.0
  specified NEC B35.8
Dermatopolymyositis M33.90
  with
    myopathy M33.92
    respiratory involvement M33.91
    specified organ involvement NEC M33.99
  amyopathic M33.93

Dermatopolymyositis — *continued*
  in neoplastic disease — *see also* Neoplasm D49.9 *[M36.0]*
  juvenile M33.00
    with
      myopathy M33.02
      respiratory involvement M33.01
      specified organ involvement NEC M33.09
    amyopathic M33.03
    without myopathy M33.03
  specified NEC M33.10
    amyopathic M33.13
    myopathy M33.12
    respiratory involvement M33.11
    specified organ involvement NEC M33.19
    without myopathy M33.13
  without myopathy M33.93
Dermatopolyneuritis — *see* Poisoning, mercury
Dermatorrhexis — *see also* Syndrome, Ehlers-Danlos Q79.60
  acquired L57.4
Dermatosclerosis — *see also* Scleroderma
  localized L94.0
Dermatosis L98.9
  Andrews' L08.89
  Bowen's — *see* Neoplasm, skin, in situ
  bullous L13.9
    specified NEC L13.8
  exfoliativa L26
  eyelid (noninfectious) — *see also* Dermatitis, eyelid H01.9
    discoid lupus erythematosus — *see* Lupus, erythematosus, eyelid
    xeroderma — *see* Xeroderma, acquired, eyelid
  factitial L98.1
  febrile neutrophilic L98.2
  gonococcal A54.89
  herpetiformis L13.0
    juvenile L12.2
  linear IgA L13.8
  menstrual NEC L98.8
  neutrophilic, febrile L98.2
  occupational — *see* Dermatitis, contact
  papulosa nigra L82.1
  pigmentary L81.9
    progressive L81.7
    Schamberg's L81.7
  psychogenic F54
  purpuric, pigmented L81.7
  pustular, subcorneal L13.1
  transient acantholytic L11.1
Dermographia, dermographism L50.3
Dermoid (cyst) — *see also* Neoplasm, benign, by site
  with malignant transformation C56- ☑
  due to radiation (nonionizing) L57.8
Dermopathy
  infiltrative with thyrotoxicosis — *see* Thyrotoxicosis
  nephrogenic fibrosing L90.8
Dermophytosis — *see* Dermatophytosis
Descemetocele H18.73- ☑
Descemet's membrane — *see* condition
Descending — *see* condition
Descensus uteri — *see* Prolapse, uterus
Desert
  rheumatism B38.0
  sore — *see* Ulcer, skin
Desertion (newborn) — *see* Maltreatment
Desmoid (extra-abdominal) (tumor) — *see* Neoplasm, connective tissue, uncertain behavior
  abdominal D48.1
Despondency F32.A
Desquamation, skin R23.4
Destruction, destructive — *see also* Damage
  articular facet — *see also* Derangement, joint, specified type NEC
    knee M23.8X- ☑
    vertebra — *see* Spondylosis
  bone — *see also* Disorder, bone, specified type NEC
    syphilitic A52.77
  joint — *see also* Derangement, joint, specified type NEC
    sacroiliac M53.3
  rectal sphincter K62.89
  septum (nasal) J34.89
  tuberculous NEC — *see* Tuberculosis
  tympanum, tympanic membrane (nontraumatic) — *see* Disorder, tympanic membrane, specified NEC
  vertebral disc — *see* Degeneration, intervertebral disc

Destructiveness — *see also* Disorder, conduct
  adjustment reaction — *see* Disorder, adjustment
Desultory labor O62.2
Detachment
  cartilage — *see* Sprain
  cervix, annular N88.8
    complicating delivery O71.3
  choroid (old) (postinfectional) (simple) (spontaneous) H31.40- ☑
    hemorrhagic H31.41- ☑
    serous H31.42- ☑
  ligament — *see* Sprain
  meniscus (knee) — *see also* Derangement, knee, meniscus, specified NEC
    current injury — *see* Tear, meniscus
    due to old tear or injury — *see* Derangement, knee, meniscus, due to old tear
  retina (without retinal break) (serous) H33.2- ☑
    with retinal:
      break H33.00- ☑
        giant H33.03- ☑
        multiple H33.02- ☑
        single H33.01- ☑
      dialysis H33.04- ☑
    pigment epithelium — *see* Degeneration, retina, separation of layers, pigment epithelium detachment
    rhegmatogenous — *see* Detachment, retina, with retinal, break
    specified NEC H33.8
    total H33.05- ☑
    traction H33.4- ☑
  vitreous (body) H43.81 ☑
Detergent asthma J69.8
Deterioration
  epileptic F06.8
  general physical R53.81
  heart, cardiac — *see* Degeneration, myocardial
  mental — *see* Psychosis
  myocardial, myocardium — *see* Degeneration, myocardial
  senile (simple) R54
Deuteranomaly (anomalous trichromat) H53.53
Deuteranopia (complete) (incomplete) H53.53
Development
  abnormal, bone Q79.9
  arrested R62.50
    bone — *see* Arrest, development or growth, bone
    child R62.50
    due to malnutrition E45
  defective, congenital — *see also* Anomaly, by site
    cauda equina Q06.3
    left ventricle Q24.8
      in hypoplastic left heart syndrome Q23.4
    valve Q24.8
      pulmonary Q22.3
  delayed — *see also* Delay, development R62.50
    arithmetical skills F81.2
    language (skills) (expressive) F80.1
    learning skill F81.9
    mixed skills F88
    motor coordination F82
    reading F81.0
    specified learning skill NEC F81.89
    speech F80.9
    spelling F81.81
    written expression F81.81
  imperfect, congenital — *see also* Anomaly, by site
    heart Q24.9
    lungs Q33.6
  incomplete
    bronchial tree Q32.4
    organ or site not listed — *see* Hypoplasia, by site
    respiratory system Q34.9
  sexual, precocious NEC E30.1
  tardy, mental — *see also* Disability, intellectual F79
Developmental — *see* condition
  testing, infant or child — *see* Examination, child
Devergie's disease (pityriasis rubra pilaris) L44.0
Deviation (in)
  conjugate palsy (eye) (spastic) H51.0
  esophagus (acquired) K22.89
  eye, skew H51.8
  midline (jaw) (teeth) (dental arch) M26.29
    specified site NEC — *see* Malposition
  nasal septum J34.2
    congenital Q67.4

☑ **Additional Character Required** — **Refer to the Tabular List for Character Selection**

Deviation — *continued*
opening and closing of the mandible M26.53
organ or site, congenital NEC — *see* Malposition, congenital
septum (nasal) (acquired) J34.2
congenital Q67.4
sexual F65.9
bestiality F65.89
erotomania F52.8
exhibitionism F65.2
fetishism, fetishistic F65.0
transvestism F65.1
frotteurism F65.81
masochism F65.51
multiple F65.89
necrophilia F65.89
nymphomania F52.8
pederosis F65.4
pedophilia F65.4
sadism, sadomasochism F65.52
satyriasis F52.8
specified type NEC F65.89
transvestism F64.1
voyeurism F65.3
teeth, midline M26.29
trachea J39.8
ureter, congenital Q62.61
Device
cerebral ventricle (communicating) in situ Z98.2
contraceptive — *see* Contraceptive, device
drainage, cerebrospinal fluid, in situ Z98.2
Devic's disease G36.0
Devil's
grip B33.0
pinches (purpura simplex) D69.2
Devitalized tooth K04.99
Devonshire colic — *see* Poisoning, lead
Dextraposition, aorta Q20.3
in tetralogy of Fallot Q21.3
Dextrinosis, limit (debrancher enzyme deficiency) E74.03
Dextrocardia (true) Q24.0
with
complete transposition of viscera Q89.3
situs inversus Q89.3
Dextrotransposition, aorta Q20.3
d-glyceric acidemia E72.59
Dhat syndrome F48.8
Dhobi itch B35.6
Di George's syndrome D82.1
Di Guglielmo's disease C94.0- ☑
Diabetes, diabetic (mellitus) (sugar) E11.9
with
amyotrophy E11.44
arthropathy NEC E11.618
autonomic (poly)neuropathy E11.43
cataract E11.36
Charcot's joints E11.610
chronic kidney disease E11.22
circulatory complication NEC E11.59
coma due to
hyperosmolarity E11.01
hypoglycemia E11.641
ketoacidosis E11.11
complication E11.8
specified NEC E11.69
dermatitis E11.620
foot ulcer E11.621
gangrene E11.52
gastroparalysis E11.43
gastroparesis E11.43
glomerulonephrosis, intracapillary E11.21
glomerulosclerosis, intercapillary E11.21
hyperglycemia E11.65
hyperosmolarity E11.00
with coma E11.01
hypoglycemia E11.649
with coma E11.641
ketoacidosis E11.10
with coma E11.11
kidney complications NEC E11.29
Kimmelstiel-Wilson disease E11.21
loss of protective sensation (LOPS) — *see* Diabetes, by type, with neuropathy
mononeuropathy E11.41
myasthenia E11.44
necrobiosis lipoidica E11.620
nephropathy E11.21
neuralgia E11.42

Diabetes, diabetic — *continued*
with — *continued*
neurologic complication NEC E11.49
neuropathic arthropathy E11.610
neuropathy E11.40
ophthalmic complication NEC E11.39
oral complication NEC E11.638
osteomyelitis E11.69
periodontal disease E11.630
peripheral angiopathy E11.51
with gangrene E11.52
polyneuropathy E11.42
renal complication NEC E11.29
renal tubular degeneration E11.29
retinopathy E11.319
with macular edema E11.311
resolved following treatment E11.37- ☑
nonproliferative E11.329 ☑
with macular edema E11.321 ☑
mild E11.329 ☑
with macular edema E11.321 ☑
moderate E11.339 ☑
with macular edema E11.331 ☑
severe E11.349 ☑
with macular edema E11.341 ☑
proliferative E11.359 ☑
with
combined traction retinal detachment and rhegmatogenous retinal detachment E11.354 ☑
macular edema E11.351 ☑
stable proliferative diabetic retinopathy E11.355 ☑
traction retinal detachment involving the macula E11.352 ☑
traction retinal detachment not involving the macula E11.353 ☑
skin complication NEC E11.628
skin ulcer NEC E11.622
brittle — *see* Diabetes, type 1
bronzed E83.110
complicating pregnancy — *see* Pregnancy, complicated by, diabetes
dietary counseling and surveillance Z71.3
due to
autoimmune process — *see* Diabetes, type 1
immune mediated pancreatic islet beta-cell destruction — *see* Diabetes, type 1
due to drug or chemical E09.9
with
amyotrophy E09.44
arthropathy NEC E09.618
autonomic (poly)neuropathy E09.43
cataract E09.36
Charcot's joints E09.610
chronic kidney disease E09.22
circulatory complication NEC E09.59
complication E09.8
specified NEC E09.69
dermatitis E09.620
foot ulcer E09.621
gangrene E09.52
gastroparalysis E09.43
gastroparesis E09.43
glomerulonephrosis, intracapillary E09.21
glomerulosclerosis, intercapillary E09.21
hyperglycemia E09.65
hyperosmolarity E09.00
with coma E09.01
hypoglycemia E09.649
with coma E09.641
ketoacidosis E09.10
with coma E09.11
kidney complications NEC E09.29
Kimmelstiel-Wilson disease E09.21
mononeuropathy E09.41
myasthenia E09.44
necrobiosis lipoidica E09.620
nephropathy E09.21
neuralgia E09.42
neurologic complication NEC E09.49
neuropathic arthropathy E09.610
neuropathy E09.40
ophthalmic complication NEC E09.39
oral complication NEC E09.638
periodontal disease E09.630
peripheral angiopathy E09.51
with gangrene E09.52

Diabetes, diabetic — *continued*
due to drug or chemical — *continued*
with — *continued*
polyneuropathy E09.42
renal complication NEC E09.29
renal tubular degeneration E09.29
retinopathy E09.319
with macular edema E09.311
resolved following treatment E09.37 ☑
nonproliferative E09.329 ☑
with macular edema E09.321 ☑
mild E09.329 ☑
with macular edema E09.321 ☑
moderate E09.339 ☑
with macular edema E09.331 ☑
severe E09.349 ☑
with macular edema E09.341 ☑
proliferative E09.359 ☑
with
combined traction retinal detachment and rhegmatogenous retinal detachment E09.354 ☑
macular edema E09.351 ☑
stable proliferative diabetic retinopathy E09.355 ☑
traction retinal detachment involving the macula E09.352 ☑
traction retinal detachment not involving the macula E09.353 ☑
skin complication NEC E09.628
skin ulcer NEC E09.622
due to underlying condition E08.9
with
amyotrophy E08.44
arthropathy NEC E08.618
autonomic (poly)neuropathy E08.43
cataract E08.36
Charcot's joints E08.610
chronic kidney disease E08.22
circulatory complication NEC E08.59
complication E08.8
specified NEC E08.69
dermatitis E08.620
foot ulcer E08.621
gangrene E08.52
gastroparalysis E08.43
gastroparesis E08.43
glomerulonephrosis, intracapillary E08.21
glomerulosclerosis, intercapillary E08.21
hyperglycemia E08.65
hyperosmolarity E08.00
with coma E08.01
hypoglycemia E08.649
with coma E08.641
ketoacidosis E08.10
with coma E08.11
kidney complications NEC E08.29
Kimmelstiel-Wilson disease E08.21
mononeuropathy E08.41
myasthenia E08.44
necrobiosis lipoidica E08.620
nephropathy E08.21
neuralgia E08.42
neurologic complication NEC E08.49
neuropathic arthropathy E08.610
neuropathy E08.40
ophthalmic complication NEC E08.39
oral complication NEC E08.638
periodontal disease E08.630
peripheral angiopathy E08.51
with gangrene E08.52
polyneuropathy E08.42
renal complication NEC E08.29
renal tubular degeneration E08.29
retinopathy E08.319
with macular edema E08.311
resolved following treatment E08.37 ☑
nonproliferative E08.329 ☑
with macular edema E08.321 ☑
mild E08.329 ☑
with macular edema E08.321 ☑
moderate E08.339 ☑
with macular edema E08.331 ☑
severe E08.349 ☑
with macular edema E08.341 ☑
proliferative E08.359 ☑

Diabetes, diabetic — *continued*
  due to underlying condition — *continued*
    with — *continued*
      retinopathy — *continued*
        proliferative — *continued*
          with
            combined traction retinal detachment and rhegmatogenous retinal detachment E08.354 ☑
            macular edema E08.351 ☑
            stable proliferative diabetic retinopathy E08.355 ☑
            traction retinal detachment involving the macula E08.352 ☑
            traction retinal detachment not involving the macula E08.353 ☑
      skin complication NEC E08.628
      skin ulcer NEC E08.622
  gestational (in pregnancy) O24.419
    affecting newborn P70.0
    diet controlled O24.410
    in childbirth O24.429
      diet controlled O24.420
      insulin (and diet) controlled O24.424
      oral drug controlled (antidiabetic) (hypoglycemic) O24.425
    insulin (and diet) controlled O24.414
    oral drug controlled (antidiabetic) (hypoglycemic) O24.415
    puerperal O24.439
      diet controlled O24.430
      insulin (and diet) controlled O24.434
      oral drug controlled (antidiabetic) (hypoglycemic) O24.435
  hepatogenous E13.9
  idiopathic — *see* Diabetes, type 1
  inadequately controlled — *see* Diabetes, by type, with hyperglycemia
  insipidus E23.2
    nephrogenic N25.1
    pituitary E23.2
    vasopressin resistant N25.1
  insulin dependent — *code to* type of diabetes
  juvenile-onset — *see* Diabetes, type 1
  ketosis-prone — *see* Diabetes, type 1
  latent R73.03
  neonatal (transient) P70.2
  non-insulin dependent — *code to* type of diabetes
  out of control — *see* Diabetes, by type, with hyperglycemia
  phosphate E83.39
  poorly controlled — *see* Diabetes, by type, with hyperglycemia
  postpancreatectomy — *see* Diabetes, specified type NEC
  postprocedural — *see* Diabetes, specified type NEC
  retina, hemorrhage E13.39
  secondary diabetes mellitus NEC — *see* Diabetes, specified type NEC
  specified type NEC E13.9
    with
      amyotrophy E13.44
      arthropathy NEC E13.618
      autonomic (poly)neuropathy E13.43
      cataract E13.36
      Charcot's joints E13.610
      chronic kidney disease E13.22
      circulatory complication NEC E13.59
      complication E13.8
        specified NEC E13.69
      dermatitis E13.620
      foot ulcer E13.621
      gangrene E13.52
      gastroparalysis E13.43
      gastroparesis E13.43
      glomerulonephrosis, intracapillary E13.21
      glomerulosclerosis, intercapillary E13.21
      hyperglycemia E13.65
      hyperosmolarity E13.00
        with coma E13.01
      hypoglycemia E13.649
        with coma E13.641
      ketoacidosis E13.10
        with coma E13.11
      kidney complications NEC E13.29
      Kimmelstiel-Wilson disease E13.21
      mononeuropathy E13.41
      myasthenia E13.44

Diabetes, diabetic — *continued*
  specified type — *continued*
    with — *continued*
      necrobiosis lipoidica E13.620
      nephropathy E13.21
      neuralgia E13.42
      neurologic complication NEC E13.49
      neuropathic arthropathy E13.610
      neuropathy E13.40
      ophthalmic complication NEC E13.39
      oral complication NEC E13.638
      periodontal disease E13.630
      peripheral angiopathy E13.51
        with gangrene E13.52
      polyneuropathy E13.42
      renal complication NEC E13.29
      renal tubular degeneration E13.29
      retinopathy E13.319
        with macular edema E13.311
        resolved following treatment E13.37 ☑
        nonproliferative E13.329 ☑
          with macular edema E13.321 ☑
          mild E13.329 ☑
            with macular edema E13.321 ☑
          moderate E13.339 ☑
            with macular edema E13.331 ☑
          severe E13.349 ☑
            with macular edema E13.341 ☑
        proliferative E13.359 ☑
          with
            combined traction retinal detachment and rhegmatogenous retinal detachment E13.354 ☑
            macular edema E13.351 ☑
            stable proliferative diabetic retinopathy E13.355 ☑
            traction retinal detachment involving the macula E13.352 ☑
            traction retinal detachment not involving the macula E13.353 ☑
      skin complication NEC E13.628
      skin ulcer NEC E13.622
  steroid-induced — *see* Diabetes, due to, drug or chemical
  type 1 E10.9
    with
      amyotrophy E10.44
      arthropathy NEC E10.618
      autonomic (poly)neuropathy E10.43
      cataract E10.36
      Charcot's joints E10.610
      chronic kidney disease E10.22
      circulatory complication NEC E10.59
      coma due to
        hyperosmolarity E11.01
        hypoglycemia E11.641
        ketoacidosis E10.11
      complication E10.8
        specified NEC E10.69
      dermatitis E10.620
      foot ulcer E10.621
      gangrene E10.52
      gastroparalysis E10.43
      gastroparesis E10.43
      glomerulonephrosis, intracapillary E10.21
      glomerulosclerosis, intercapillary E10.21
      hyperglycemia E10.65
      hypoglycemia E10.649
        with coma E10.641
      ketoacidosis E10.10
        with coma E10.11
      kidney complications NEC E10.29
      Kimmelstiel-Wilson disease E10.21
      mononeuropathy E10.41
      myasthenia E10.44
      necrobiosis lipoidica E10.620
      nephropathy E10.21
      neuralgia E10.42
      neurologic complication NEC E10.49
      neuropathic arthropathy E10.610
      neuropathy E10.40
      ophthalmic complication NEC E10.39
      oral complication NEC E10.638
      osteomyelitis E10.69
      periodontal disease E10.630
      peripheral angiopathy E10.51
        with gangrene E10.52
      polyneuropathy E10.42

Diabetes, diabetic — *continued*
  type 1 — *continued*
    with — *continued*
      renal complication NEC E10.29
      renal tubular degeneration E10.29
      retinopathy E10.319
        with macular edema E10.311
        resolved following treatment E10.37 ☑
        nonproliferative E10.329 ☑
          with macular edema E10.321 ☑
          mild E10.329 ☑
            with macular edema E10.321 ☑
          moderate E10.339 ☑
            with macular edema E10.331 ☑
          severe E10.349 ☑
            with macular edema E10.341 ☑
        proliferative E10.359 ☑
          with
            combined traction retinal detachment and rhegmatogenous retinal detachment E10.354 ☑
            macular edema E10.351 ☑
            stable proliferative diabetic retinopathy E10.355 ☑
            traction retinal detachment involving the macula E10.352 ☑
            traction retinal detachment not involving the macula E10.353 ☑
      skin complication NEC E10.628
      skin ulcer NEC E10.622
  type 2 E11.9
    with
      amyotrophy E11.44
      arthropathy NEC E11.618
      autonomic (poly)neuropathy E11.43
      cataract E11.36
      Charcot's joints E11.610
      chronic kidney disease E11.22
      circulatory complication NEC E11.59
      coma due to
        hyperosmolarity E11.01
        hypoglycemia E11.641
        ketoacidosis E11.1- ☑
      complication E11.8
        specified NEC E11.69
      dermatitis E11.620
      foot ulcer E11.621
      gangrene E11.52
      gastroparalysis E11.43
      gastroparesis E11.43
      glomerulonephrosis, intracapillary E11.21
      glomerulosclerosis, intercapillary E11.21
      hyperglycemia E11.65
      hyperosmolarity E11.00
        with coma E11.01
      hypoglycemia E11.649
        with coma E11.641
      ketoacidosis E11.10
        with coma E11.11
      kidney complications NEC E11.29
      Kimmelstiel-Wilson disease E11.21
      mononeuropathy E11.41
      myasthenia E11.44
      necrobiosis lipoidica E11.620
      nephropathy E11.21
      neuralgia E11.42
      neurologic complication NEC E11.49
      neuropathic arthropathy E11.610
      neuropathy E11.40
      ophthalmic complication NEC E11.39
      oral complication NEC E11.638
      osteomyelitis E11.69
      periodontal disease E11.630
      peripheral angiopathy E11.51
        with gangrene E11.52
      polyneuropathy E11.42
      renal complication NEC E11.29
      renal tubular degeneration E11.29
      retinopathy E11.319
        with macular edema E11.311
        resolved following treatment E11.37 ☑
        nonproliferative E11.329 ☑
          with macular edema E11.321 ☑
          mild E11.329 ☑
            with macular edema E11.321 ☑
          moderate E11.339 ☑
            with macular edema E11.331 ☑
          severe E11.349 ☑

Diabetes, diabetic — *continued*
  type 2 — *continued*
    with — *continued*
      retinopathy — *continued*
        nonproliferative — *continued*
          severe — *continued*
            with macular edema E11.341 ☑
          proliferative E11.359 ☑
            with
              combined traction retinal detachment and rhegmatogenous retinal detachment E11.354 ☑
              macular edema E11.351 ☑
              stable proliferative diabetic retinopathy E11.355 ☑
              traction retinal detachment involving the macula E11.352 ☑
              traction retinal detachment not involving the macula E11.353 ☑
          skin complication NEC E11.628
          skin ulcer NEC E11.622
    uncontrolled
      meaning
        hyperglycemia — *see* Diabetes, by type, with, hyperglycemia
        hypoglycemia — *see* Diabetes, by type, with, hypoglycemia
Diacyclothrombopathia D69.1
Diagnosis deferred R69
Dialysis (intermittent) (treatment)
  noncompliance (with) Z91.15
  renal (hemodialysis) (peritoneal), status Z99.2
  retina, retinal — *see* Detachment, retina, with retinal, dialysis
Diamond-Blackfan anemia (congenital hypoplastic) D61.01
Diamond-Gardener syndrome (autoerythrocyte sensitization) D69.2
Diaper rash L22
Diaphoresis (excessive) R61
Diaphragm — *see* condition
Diaphragmalgia R07.1
Diaphragmatitis, diaphragmitis J98.6
Diaphysial aclasis Q78.6
Diaphysitis — *see* Osteomyelitis, specified type NEC
Diarrhea, diarrheal (disease) (infantile) (inflammatory) R19.7
  achlorhydric K31.83
  allergic K52.29
    due to
      colitis — *see* Colitis, allergic
      enteritis — *see* Enteritis, allergic
  amebic — *see also* Amebiasis A06.0
    with abscess — *see* Abscess, amebic
    acute A06.0
    chronic A06.1
    nondysenteric A06.2
  bacillary — *see* Dysentery, bacillary
  balantidial A07.0
  cachectic NEC K52.89
  Chilomastix A07.8
  choleriformis A00.1
  chronic (noninfectious) K52.9
  coccidial A07.3
  Cochin-China K90.1
    strongyloidiasis B78.0
  Dientamoeba A07.8
  dietetic — *see also* Diarrhea, allergic K52.29
  drug-induced K52.1
  due to
    bacteria A04.9
      specified NEC A04.8
    Campylobacter A04.5
    Capillaria philippinensis B81.1
    Clostridium difficile
      not specified as recurrent A04.72
      recurrent A04.71
    Clostridium perfringens (C) (F) A04.8
    Cryptosporidium A07.2
    drugs K52.1
    Escherichia coli A04.4
      enteroaggregative A04.4
      enterohemorrhagic A04.3
      enteroinvasive A04.2
      enteropathogenic A04.0
      enterotoxigenic A04.1
      specified NEC A04.4

Diarrhea, diarrheal — *continued*
  due to — *continued*
    food hypersensitivity — *see also* Diarrhea, allergic K52.29
    Necator americanus B76.1
    S. japonicum B65.2
    specified organism NEC A08.8
      bacterial A04.8
      viral A08.39
    Staphylococcus A04.8
    Trichuris trichiuria B79
    virus — *see* Enteritis, viral
    Yersinia enterocolitica A04.6
  dysenteric A09
  endemic A09
  epidemic A09
  flagellate A07.9
  Flexner's (ulcerative) A03.1
  functional K59.1
    following gastrointestinal surgery K91.89
    psychogenic F45.8
  Giardia lamblia A07.1
  giardial A07.1
  hill K90.1
  infectious A09
  malarial — *see* Malaria
  mite B88.0
  mycotic NEC B49
  neonatal (noninfectious) P78.3
  nervous F45.8
  neurogenic K59.1
  noninfectious K52.9
  postgastrectomy K91.1
  postvagotomy K91.1
  protozoal A07.9
    specified NEC A07.8
  psychogenic F45.8
  specified
    bacterium NEC A04.8
    virus NEC A08.39
  strongyloidiasis B78.0
  toxic K52.1
  trichomonal A07.8
  tropical K90.1
  tuberculous A18.32
  viral — *see* Enteritis, viral
Diastasis
  cranial bones M84.88
    congenital NEC Q75.8
  joint (traumatic) — *see* Dislocation
  muscle M62.00
    ankle M62.07- ☑
    congenital Q79.8
    foot M62.07- ☑
    forearm M62.03- ☑
    hand M62.04- ☑
    lower leg M62.06- ☑
    pelvic region M62.05- ☑
    shoulder region M62.01- ☑
    specified site NEC M62.08
    thigh M62.05- ☑
    upper arm M62.02- ☑
  recti (abdomen)
    complicating delivery O71.89
    congenital Q79.59
Diastema, tooth, teeth, fully erupted M26.32
Diastematomyelia Q06.2
Diataxia, cerebral G80.4
Diathesis
  allergic — *see* History, allergy
  bleeding (familial) D69.9
  cystine (familial) E72.00
  gouty — *see* Gout
  hemorrhagic (familial) D69.9
    newborn NEC P53
  spasmophilic R29.0
Diaz's disease or osteochondrosis (juvenile) (talus) — *see* Osteochondrosis, juvenile, tarsus
Dibothriocephalus, dibothriocephaliasis (latus) (infection) (infestation) B70.0
  larval B70.1
Dicephalus, dicephaly Q89.4
Dichotomy, teeth K00.2
Dichromat, dichromatopsia (congenital) — *see* Deficiency, color vision
Dichuchwa A65
Dicroceliasis B66.2
Didelphia, didelphys — *see* Double uterus

Didymytis N45.1
  with orchitis N45.3
Dietary
  inadequacy or deficiency E63.9
  surveillance and counseling Z71.3
Dietl's crisis N13.8
Dieulafoy lesion (hemorrhagic)
  duodenum K31.82
  esophagus K22.89
  intestine (colon) K63.81
  stomach K31.82
Difficult, difficulty (in)
  acculturation Z60.3
  feeding R63.30
    newborn P92.9
      breast P92.5
      specified NEC P92.8
    nonorganic (infant or child) F98.29
    specified NEC R63.39
  intubation, in anesthesia T88.4 ☑
  mechanical, gastroduodenal stoma K91.89
    causing obstruction — *see also* Obstruction, intestine, postoperative K91.30
  micturition
    need to immediately re-void R39.191
    position dependent R39.192
    specified NEC R39.198
  reading (developmental) F81.0
    secondary to emotional disorders F93.9
  spelling (specific) F81.81
    with reading disorder F81.89
    due to inadequate teaching Z55.8
  swallowing — *see* Dysphagia
  walking R26.2
  work
    conditions NEC Z56.5
    schedule Z56.3
Diffuse — *see* condition
Digestive — *see* condition
Dihydropyrimidine dehydrogenase disease (DPD) E88.89
Diktyoma — *see* Neoplasm, malignant, by site
Dilaceration, tooth K00.4
Dilatation
  anus K59.89
    venule — *see* Hemorrhoids
  aorta (focal) (general) — *see* Ectasia, aorta
    with aneuysm — *see* Aneurysm, aorta
    congenital Q25.44
  artery — *see* Aneurysm
  bladder (sphincter) N32.89
    congenital Q64.79
  blood vessel I99.8
  bronchial J47.9
    with
      exacerbation (acute) J47.1
      lower respiratory infection J47.0
  calyx N28.89
    due to obstruction — *see* Hydronephrosis
  capillaries I78.8
  cardiac (acute) (chronic) — *see also* Hypertrophy, cardiac
    congenital Q24.8
      valve NEC Q24.8
        pulmonary Q22.3
    valve — *see* Endocarditis
  cavum septi pellucidi Q06.8
  cervix (uteri) — *see also* Incompetency, cervix
    incomplete, poor, slow complicating delivery O62.0
  colon K59.39
    congenital Q43.1
    psychogenic F45.8
    toxic K59.31
  common duct (acquired) K83.8
    congenital Q44.5
  cystic duct (acquired) K82.8
    congenital Q44.5
  duct, mammary — *see* Ectasia, mammary duct
  duodenum K59.89
  esophagus K22.89
    congenital Q39.5
    due to achalasia K22.0
  eustachian tube, congenital Q17.8
  gallbladder K82.8
  gastric — *see* Dilatation, stomach
  heart (acute) (chronic) — *see also* Hypertrophy, cardiac
    congenital Q24.8
    valve — *see* Endocarditis

☑ Additional Character Required — Refer to the Tabular List for Character Selection

Dilatation — continued
  Ileum K59.89
    psychogenic F45.8
  jejunum K59.89
    psychogenic F45.8
  kidney (calyx) (collecting structures) (cystic)
      (parenchyma) (pelvis) (idiopathic) N28.89
    due to obstruction — see Hydronephrosis
  lacrimal passages or duct — see Disorder, lacrimal
      system, changes
  lymphatic vessel I89.0
  mammary duct — see Ectasia, mammary duct
  Meckel's diverticulum (congenital) Q43.0
    malignant — see Table of Neoplasms, small intes-
        tine, malignant
  myocardium (acute) (chronic) — see Hypertrophy,
      cardiac
  organ or site, congenital NEC — see Distortion
  pancreatic duct K86.89
  pericardium — see Pericarditis
  pharynx J39.2
  prostate N42.89
  pulmonary
    artery (idiopathic) I28.8
    valve, congenital Q22.3
  pupil H57.04
  rectum K59.39
  saccule, congenital Q16.5
  salivary gland (duct) K11.8
  sphincter ani K62.89
  stomach K31.89
    acute K31.0
    psychogenic F45.8
  submaxillary duct K11.8
  trachea, congenital Q32.1
  ureter (idiopathic) N28.82
    congenital Q62.2
    due to obstruction N13.4
  urethra (acquired) N36.8
  vasomotor I73.9
  vein I86.8
  ventricular, ventricle (acute) (chronic) — see also Hy-
      pertrophy, cardiac
    cerebral, congenital Q04.8
  venule NEC I86.8
  vesical orifice N32.89
Dilated, dilation — see Dilatation
Diminished, diminution
  hearing (acuity) — see Deafness
  sense or sensation (cold) (heat) (tactile) (vibratory)
      R20.8
  vision NEC H54.7
  vital capacity R94.2
Diminuta taenia B71.0
Dimitri-Sturge-Weber disease Q85.89
Dimple
  congenital sacral Q82.6
  parasacral Q82.6
  pilonidal or postanal — see Cyst, pilonidal
Dioctophyme renalis (infection) (infestation) B83.8
Dipetalonemiasis B74.4
Diphallus Q55.69
Diphtheria, diphtheritic (gangrenous) (hemorrhagic)
      A36.9
  carrier (suspected) Z22.2
  cutaneous A36.3
  faucial A36.0
  infection of wound A36.3
  laryngeal A36.2
  myocarditis A36.81
  nasal, anterior A36.89
  nasopharyngeal A36.1
  neurological complication A36.89
  pharyngeal A36.0
  specified site NEC A36.89
  tonsillar A36.0
Diphyllobothriasis (intestine) B70.0
  larval B70.1
Diplacusis H93.22- ☑
Diplegia (upper limbs) G83.0
  congenital (cerebral) G80.8
  facial G51.0
  lower limbs G82.20
  spastic G80.1
Diplococcus, diplococcal — see condition
Diplopia H53.2
Dipsomania F10.20

Dipsomania — continued
  with
    psychosis — see Psychosis, alcoholic
    remission F10.21
Dipylidiasis B71.1
DIRA (deficiency of interleukin 1 receptor antagonist)
      M04.8
Direction, teeth, abnormal, fully erupted M26.30
Dirofilariasis B74.8
Dirt-eating child F98.3
Disability, disabilities
  heart — see Disease, heart
  intellectual F79
    with
      autistic features F84.9
      pathogenic CHAMP1 (genetic) (variant) F78.A9
      pathogenic HNRNPH2 (genetic) (variant) F78.A9
      pathogenic SATB2 (genetic) (variant) F78.A9
      pathogenic SETBP1 (genetic) (variant) F78.A9
      pathogenic STXBP1 (genetic) (variant) F78.A9
      pathogenic SYNGAP1 (genetic) (variant) F78.A1
    autosomal dominant F78.A9
    autosomal recessive F78.A9
    genetic related F78.A9
      with
        pathogenic CHAMP1 (variant) F78.A9
        pathogenic HNRNPH2 (variant) F78.A9
        pathogenic SATB2 (variant) F78.A9
        pathogenic SETBP1 (variant) F78.A9
        pathogenic STXBP1 (variant) F78.A9
        pathogenic SYNGAP1 (variant) F78.A1
      specified NEC F78.A9
      SYNGAP1-related F78.A1
    in
      autosomal dominant mental retardation F78.A9
      autosomal recessive mental retardation F78.A9
      SATB2-associated syndrome F78.A9
      SETBP1 disorder F78.A9
      STXBP1 encephalopathy with epilepsy — see
          also Encephalopathy; and — see also
          Epilepsy
      X-linked mental retardation (syndromic) (Bain
          type) F78.A9
    mild (I.Q. 50-69) F70
    moderate (I.Q. 35-49) F71
    profound (I.Q. under 20) F73
    severe (I.Q. 20-34) F72
    specified level NEC F78.A9
    SYNGAP1-related F78.A1
    X-linked (syndromic) (Bain type) F78.A9
  knowledge acquisition F81.9
  learning F81.9
  limiting activities Z73.6
  spelling, specific F81.81
Disappearance of family member Z63.4
Disarticulation — see Amputation
  meaning traumatic amputation — see Amputation,
      traumatic
Discharge (from)
  abnormal finding in — see Abnormal, specimen
  breast (female) (male) N64.52
  diencephalic autonomic idiopathic — see Epilepsy,
      specified NEC
  ear — see also Otorrhea
    blood — see Otorrhagia
  excessive urine R35.89
  nipple N64.52
  penile R36.9
  postnasal R09.82
  prison, anxiety concerning Z65.2
  urethral R36.9
    without blood R36.0
      hematospermia R36.1
  vaginal N89.8
Discitis, diskitis M46.40
  cervical region M46.42
  cervicothoracic region M46.43
  lumbar region M46.46
  lumbosacral region M46.47
  multiple sites M46.49
  occipito-atlanto-axial region M46.41
  pyogenic — see Infection, intervertebral disc, pyogenic
  sacrococcygeal region M46.48
  thoracic region M46.44
  thoracolumbar region M46.45
Discoid
  meniscus (congenital) Q68.6

Discoid — continued
  semilunar cartilage (congenital) — see Derangement,
      knee, meniscus, specified NEC
Discoloration
  nails L60.8
  teeth (posteruptive) K03.7
    during formation K00.8
Discomfort
  chest R07.89
  visual H53.14- ☑
Discontinuity, ossicles, ear H74.2- ☑
Discord (with)
  boss Z56.4
  classmates Z55.4
  counselor Z64.4
  employer Z56.4
  family Z63.8
  fellow employees Z56.4
  in-laws Z63.1
  landlord Z59.2
  lodgers Z59.2
  neighbors Z59.2
  probation officer Z64.4
  social worker Z64.4
  teachers Z55.4
  workmates Z56.4
Discordant connection
  atrioventricular (congenital) Q20.5
  ventriculoarterial Q20.3
Discrepancy
  centric occlusion maximum intercuspation M26.55
  leg length (acquired) — see Deformity, limb, unequal
      length
    congenital — see Defect, reduction, lower limb
  uterine size date O26.84- ☑
Discrimination
  ethnic Z60.5
  political Z60.5
  racial Z60.5
  religious Z60.5
  sex Z60.5
Disease, diseased — see also Syndrome
  absorbent system I87.8
  acid-peptic K30
  Acosta's T70.29 ☑
  Adams-Stokes (-Morgagni) (syncope with heart block)
      I45.9
  Addison's anemia (pernicious) D51.0
  adenoids (and tonsils) J35.9
  adrenal (capsule) (cortex) (gland) (medullary) E27.9
    hyperfunction E27.0
    specified NEC E27.8
  ainhum L94.6
  airway
    obstructive, chronic J44.9
      due to
        cotton dust J66.0
        specific organic dusts NEC J66.8
    reactive — see Asthma
  akamushi (scrub typhus) A75.3
  Albers-Schönberg (marble bones) Q78.2
  Albert's — see Tendinitis, Achilles
  alimentary canal K63.9
  alligator-skin Q80.9
    acquired L85.0
  alpha heavy chain C88.3
  alpine T70.29 ☑
  altitude T70.20 ☑
  alveolar ridge
    edentulous K06.9
      specified NEC K06.8
  alveoli, teeth K08.9
  Alzheimer's — see also Dementia, in, diseases specified
      elsewhere G30.9 [F02.80]
    with behavioral disturbance — see also Dementia,
        in, diseases specified elsewhere
        G30.9 [F02.81-] ☑
    early onset — see also Dementia, in, diseases spec-
        ified elsewhere G30.0 [F02.80]
      with behavioral disturbance — see also Demen-
          tia, in, diseases specified elsewhere
          G30.0 [F02.81-] ☑
    late onset — see also Dementia, in, diseases speci-
        fied elsewhere G30.1 [F02.80]
      with behavioral disturbance — see also Demen-
          tia, in, diseases specified elsewhere
          G30.1 [F02.81-] ☑

Disease, diseased — *continued*
  Alzheimer's — *see also* Dementia, in, diseases specified elsewhere — *continued*
    specified NEC — *see also* Dementia, in, diseases specified elsewhere G30.8 *[F02.80]*
      with behavioral disturbance — *see also* Dementia, in, diseases specified elsewhere G30.8 *[F02.81]* ☑
  amyloid — *see* Amyloidosis
  Andersen's (glycogenosis IV) E74.09
  Andes T70.29 ☑
  Andrews' (bacterid) L08.89
  angiospastic I73.9
    cerebral G45.9
    vein I87.8
  anterior
    chamber H21.9
    horn cell G12.29
  antiglomerular basement membrane (anti- GBM) antibody M31.0
    tubulo-interstitial nephritis N12
  antral — *see* Sinusitis, maxillary
  anus K62.9
    specified NEC K62.89
  aorta (nonsyphilitic) I77.9
    syphilitic NEC A52.02
  aortic (heart) (valve) I35.9
    rheumatic I06.9
  Apollo B30.3
  aponeuroses — *see* Enthesopathy
  appendix K38.9
    specified NEC K38.8
  aqueous (chamber) H21.9
  Arnold-Chiari — *see* Arnold-Chiari disease
  arterial I77.9
    occlusive — *see* Occlusion, by site
      due to stricture or stenosis I77.1
    peripheral I73.9
  arteriocardiorenal — *see* Hypertension, cardiorenal
  arteriolar (generalized) (obliterative) I77.9
  arteriorenal — *see* Hypertension, kidney
  arteriosclerotic — *see also* Arteriosclerosis
    cardiovascular — *see* Disease, heart, ischemic, atherosclerotic
    coronary (artery) — *see* Disease, heart, ischemic, atherosclerotic
    heart — *see* Disease, heart, ischemic, atherosclerotic
  artery I77.9
    cerebral I67.9
    coronary I25.10
      with angina pectoris — *see* Arteriosclerosis, coronary (artery)
    peripheral I73.9
  arthropod-borne NOS (viral) A94
    specified type NEC A93.8
  atticoantral, chronic H66.20
    left H66.22
      with right H66.23
    right H66.21
      with left H66.23
  auditory canal — *see* Disorder, ear, external
  auricle, ear NEC — *see* Disorder, pinna
  Australian X A83.4
  autoimmune (systemic) NOS M35.9
    hemolytic D59.10
      cold type (primary) (secondary) (symptomatic) D59.12
      drug-induced D59.0
      mixed type (primary) (secondary) (symptomatic) D59.13
      warm type (primary) (secondary) (symptomatic) D59.11
    thyroid E06.3
  autoinflammatory M04.9
    NOD2-associated M04.8
    specified type NEC M04.8
  aviator's — *see* Effect, adverse, high altitude
  Ayerza's (pulmonary artery sclerosis with pulmonary hypertension) I27.0
  Babington's (familial hemorrhagic telangiectasia) I78.0
  bacterial A49.9
    specified NEC A48.8
    zoonotic A28.9
      specified type NEC A28.8
  Baelz's (cheilitis glandularis apostematosa) K13.0
  bagasse J67.1
  balloon — *see* Effect, adverse, high altitude
  Bang's (brucella abortus) A23.1

Disease, diseased — *continued*
  Bannister's T78.3 ☑
  barometer makers' — *see* Poisoning, mercury
  Barraquer (-Simons') (progressive lipodystrophy) E88.1
  Barrett's — *see* Barrett's, esophagus
  Bartholin's gland N75.9
  basal ganglia G25.9
    degenerative G23.9
      specified NEC G23.8
    specified NEC G25.89
  Basedow's (exophthalmic goiter) — *see* Hyperthyroidism, with, goiter (diffuse)
  Bateman's B08.1
  Batten-Steinert G71.11
  Battey A31.0
  Beard's (neurasthenia) F48.8
  Becker
    idiopathic mural endomyocardial I42.3
    myotonia congenita G71.12
  Begbie's (exophthalmic goiter) — *see* Hyperthyroidism, with, goiter (diffuse)
  behavioral, organic F07.9
  Beigel's (white piedra) B36.2
  Benson's — *see* Deposit, crystalline
  Bernard-Soulier (thrombopathy) D69.1
  Bernhardt (-Roth) — *see* Mononeuropathy, lower limb, meralgia paresthetica
  Biermer's (pernicious anemia) D51.0
  bile duct (common) (hepatic) K83.9
    with calculus, stones — *see* Calculus, bile duct
    specified NEC K83.8
  biliary (tract) K83.9
    specified NEC K83.8
  Billroth's — *see* Spina bifida
  bird fancier's J67.2
  black lung J60
  bladder N32.9
    in (due to)
      schistosomiasis (bilharziasis) B65.0 *[N33]*
    specified NEC N32.89
  bleeder's D66
  blood D75.9
    forming organs D75.9
    vessel I99.9
  Bloodgood's — *see* Mastopathy, cystic
  Blount M92.51- ☑
  Bodechtel-Guttmann (subacute sclerosing panencephalitis) A81.1
  bone — *see also* Disorder, bone
    aluminum M83.4
    fibrocystic NEC
      jaw M27.49
  bone-marrow D75.9
  Borna A83.9
  Bornholm (epidemic pleurodynia) B33.0
  Bouchard's (myopathic dilatation of the stomach) K31.0
  Bouillaud's (rheumatic heart disease) I01.9
  Bourneville (-Brissaud) (tuberous sclerosis) Q85.1
  Bouveret (-Hoffmann) (paroxysmal tachycardia) I47.9
  bowel K63.9
    functional K59.9
      psychogenic F45.8
  brain — *see also* Dementia, in, diseases specified elsewhere G93.9
    arterial, artery I67.9
    arteriosclerotic I67.2
    congenital Q04.9
    degenerative — *see* Degeneration, brain
    inflammatory — *see* Encephalitis
    organic G93.9
      arteriosclerotic I67.2
    parasitic B71.9 *[G94]*
    senile NEC G31.1
    specified NEC G93.89
  breast — *see also* Disorder, breast N64.9
    cystic (chronic) — *see* Mastopathy, cystic
    fibrocystic — *see* Mastopathy, cystic
    Paget's
      female, unspecified side C50.91- ☑
      male, unspecified side C50.92- ☑
    specified NEC N64.89
  Breda's — *see* Yaws
  Bretonneau's (diphtheritic malignant angina) A36.0
  Bright's — *see* Nephritis
    arteriosclerotic — *see* Hypertension, kidney
  Brill's (recrudescent typhus) A75.1
  Brill-Zinsser (recrudescent typhus) A75.1
  Brion-Kayser — *see* Fever, paratyphoid

Disease, diseased — *continued*
  broad
    beta E78.2
    ligament (noninflammatory) N83.9
      inflammatory — *see* Disease, pelvis, inflammatory
      specified NEC N83.8
  Brocq-Duhring (dermatitis herpetiformis) L13.0
  Brocq's
    meaning
      dermatitis herpetiformis L13.0
      prurigo L28.2
  bronchopulmonary J98.4
  bronchus NEC J98.09
  bronze Addison's E27.1
    tuberculous A18.7
  budgerigar fancier's J67.2
  Buerger's (thromboangiitis obliterans) I73.1
  bullous L13.9
    chronic of childhood L12.2
    specified NEC L13.8
  Bürger-Grütz (essential familial hyperlipemia) E78.3
  bursa — *see* Bursopathy
  caisson T70.3 ☑
  California — *see* Coccidioidomycosis
  capillaries I78.9
    specified NEC I78.8
  Carapata A68.0
  cardiac — *see* Disease, heart
  cardiopulmonary, chronic I27.9
  cardiorenal (hepatic) (hypertensive) (vascular) — *see* Hypertension, cardiorenal
  cardiovascular (atherosclerotic) I25.10
    with angina pectoris — *see* Arteriosclerosis, coronary (artery),
    congenital Q28.9
    hypertensive — *see* Hypertension, heart
    newborn P29.9
      specified NEC P29.89
    renal (hypertensive) — *see* Hypertension, cardiorenal
    syphilitic (asymptomatic) A52.00
  cartilage — *see* Disorder, cartilage
  Castellani's A69.8
  Castleman (unicentric) (multicentric) D47.Z2
    HHV-8-associated — *see also* Herpesvirus, human, 8 D47.Z2
  cat-scratch A28.1
  Cavare's (familial periodic paralysis) G72.3
  cecum K63.9
  celiac (adult) (infantile) (with steatorrhea) K90.0
  cellular tissue L98.9
  central core G71.29
  cerebellar, cerebellum — *see* Disease, brain
  cerebral — *see also* Disease, brain
    degenerative — *see* Degeneration, brain
  cerebrospinal G96.9
  cerebrovascular I67.9
    acute I67.89
      embolic I63.4- ☑
      thrombotic I63.3- ☑
    arteriosclerotic I67.2
    hereditary NEC I67.858
    specified NEC I67.89
  cervix (uteri) (noninflammatory) N88.9
    inflammatory — *see* Cervicitis
    specified NEC N88.8
  Chabert's A22.9
  Chandler's (osteochondritis dissecans, hip) — *see* Osteochondritis, dissecans, hip
  Charlouis — *see* Yaws
  Chédiak-Steinbrinck (-Higashi) (congenital gigantism of peroxidase granules) E70.330
  chest J98.9
  Chiari's (hepatic vein thrombosis) I82.0
  Chicago B40.9
  Chignon B36.8
  chigo, chigoe B88.1
  childhood granulomatous D71
  Chinese liver fluke B66.1
  chlamydial A74.9
    specified NEC A74.89
  cholecystic K82.9
  choroid H31.9
    specified NEC H31.8
  Christmas D67
  chronic bullous of childhood L12.2
  chylomicron retention E78.3

Disease, diseased — *continued*
- ciliary body H21.9
  - specified NEC H21.89
- circulatory (system) NEC I99.8
  - newborn P29.9
  - syphilitic A52.00
    - congenital A50.54
- coagulation factor deficiency (congenital) — *see* Defect, coagulation
- coccidioidal — *see* Coccidioidomycosis
- cold
  - agglutinin or hemoglobinuria D59.12
    - paroxysmal D59.6
  - hemagglutinin (chronic) D59.12
- collagen NOS (nonvascular) (vascular) M35.9
  - specified NEC M35.89
- colon K63.9
  - functional K59.9
    - congenital Q43.2
  - ischemic — *see also* Ischemia, intestine, acute K55.039
- colonic inflammatory bowel, unclassified (IBDU) K52.3
- combined system — *see* Degeneration, combined
- compressed air T70.3 ☑
- Concato's (pericardial polyserositis) A19.9
  - nontubercular I31.1
  - pleural — *see* Pleurisy, with effusion
- conjunctiva H11.9
  - chlamydial A74.0
  - specified NEC H11.89
  - viral B30.9
    - specified NEC B30.8
- connective tissue, systemic (diffuse) M35.9
  - in (due to)
    - hypogammaglobulinemia D80.1 *[M36.8]*
    - ochronosis E70.29 *[M36.8]*
  - specified NEC M35.89
- Conor and Bruch's (boutonneuse fever) A77.1
- Cooper's — *see* Mastopathy, cystic
- Cori's (glycogenosis III) E74.03
- corkhandler's or corkworker's J67.3
- cornea H18.9
  - specified NEC H18.89- ☑
- coronary (artery) — *see* Disease, heart, ischemic, atherosclerotic
  - congenital Q24.5
  - ostial, syphilitic (aortic) (mitral) (pulmonary) A52.03
- corpus cavernosum N48.9
  - specified NEC N48.89
- Cotugno's — *see* Sciatica
- COVID-19 U07.1
- coxsackie (virus) NEC B34.1
- cranial nerve NOS G52.9
- Creutzfeldt-Jakob — *see* Creutzfeldt-Jakob disease or syndrome
- Crocq's (acrocyanosis) I73.89
- Crohn's — *see* Enteritis, regional
- Curschmann G71.11
- cystic
  - breast (chronic) — *see* Mastopathy, cystic
  - kidney, congenital Q61.9
  - liver, congenital Q44.6
  - lung J98.4
    - congenital Q33.0
- cytomegalic inclusion (generalized) B25.9
  - with pneumonia B25.0
  - congenital P35.1
- cytomegaloviral B25.9
  - specified NEC B25.8
- Czerny's (periodic hydrarthrosis of the knee) — *see* Effusion, joint, knee
- Daae (-Finsen) (epidemic pleurodynia) B33.0
- Darling's — *see* Histoplasmosis capsulati
- de Quervain's (tendon sheath) M65.4
  - thyroid (subacute granulomatous thyroiditis) E06.1
- Débove's (splenomegaly) R16.1
- deer fly — *see* Tularemia
- Degos' I77.89
- demyelinating, demyelinizating (nervous system) G37.9
  - multiple sclerosis G35
  - specified NEC G37.8
- dense deposit — *see also* N00-N07 with fourth character .6 N05.6
- deposition, hydroxyapatite — *see* Disease, hydroxyapatite deposition
- Devergie's (pityriasis rubra pilaris) L44.0
- Devic's G36.0
- diaphorase deficiency D74.0

Disease, diseased — *continued*
- diaphragm J98.6
- diarrheal, infectious NEC A09
- digestive system K92.9
  - specified NEC K92.89
- disc, degenerative — *see* Degeneration, intervertebral disc
- discogenic — *see also* Displacement, intervertebral disc NEC
  - with myelopathy — *see* Disorder, disc, with, myelopathy
- diverticular — *see* Diverticula
- Dubois (thymus) A50.59 *[E35]*
- Duchenne-Griesinger G71.01
- Duchenne's
  - muscular dystrophy G71.01
  - pseudohypertrophy, muscles G71.01
- ductless glands E34.9
- Duhring's (dermatitis herpetiformis) L13.0
- duodenum K31.9
  - specified NEC K31.89
- Dupré's (meningism) R29.1
- Dupuytren's (muscle contracture) M72.0
- Durand-Nicholas-Favre (climatic bubo) A55
- Duroziez's (congenital mitral stenosis) Q23.2
- ear — *see* Disorder, ear
- Eberth's — *see* Fever, typhoid
- Ebola (virus) A98.4
- Ebstein's heart Q22.5
- Echinococcus — *see* Echinococcus
- echovirus NEC B34.1
- Eddowes' (brittle bones and blue sclera) Q78.0
- edentulous (alveolar) ridge K06.9
  - specified NEC K06.8
- Edsall's T67.2 ☑
- Eichstedt's (pityriasis versicolor) B36.0
- Eisenmenger's (irreversible) I27.83
- Ellis-van Creveld (chondroectodermal dysplasia) Q77.6
- end stage renal (ESRD) N18.6
  - due to hypertension I12.0
- endocrine glands or system NEC E34.9
- endomyocardial (eosinophilic) I42.3
- English (rickets) E55.0
- enteroviral, enterovirus NEC B34.1
  - central nervous system NEC A88.8
- epidemic B99.9
  - specified NEC B99.8
- epididymis N50.9
- Erb (-Landouzy) G71.02
- Erdheim-Chester (ECD) E88.89
- esophagus K22.9
  - functional K22.4
    - psychogenic F45.8
  - specified NEC K22.89
- Eulenburg's (congenital paramyotonia) G71.19
- eustachian tube — *see* Disorder, eustachian tube
- external
  - auditory canal — *see* Disorder, ear, external
  - ear — *see* Disorder, ear, external
- extrapyramidal G25.9
  - specified NEC G25.89
- eye H57.9
  - anterior chamber H21.9
  - inflammatory NEC H57.89
  - muscle (external) — *see* Strabismus
  - specified NEC H57.89
  - syphilitic — *see* Oculopathy, syphilitic
- eyeball H44.9
  - specified NEC H44.89
- eyelid — *see* Disorder, eyelid
  - specified NEC — *see* Disorder, eyelid, specified type NEC
- eyeworm of Africa B74.3
- facial nerve (seventh) G51.9
  - newborn (birth injury) P11.3
- Fahr (of brain) G23.8
- Fahr Volhard (of kidney) I12.- ☑
- fallopian tube (noninflammatory) N83.9
  - inflammatory — *see* Salpingo-oophoritis
  - specified NEC N83.8
- familial periodic paralysis G72.3
- Fanconi's (congenital pancytopenia) D61.09
- fascia NEC — *see also* Disorder, muscle
  - inflammatory — *see* Myositis
  - specified NEC M62.89
- Fauchard's (periodontitis) — *see* Periodontitis
- Favre-Durand-Nicolas (climatic bubo) A55
- Fede's K14.0

Disease, diseased — *continued*
- Feer's — *see* Poisoning, mercury
- female pelvic inflammatory — *see also* Disease, pelvis, inflammatory N73.9
  - syphilitic (secondary) A51.42
  - tuberculous A18.17
- Fernels' (aortic aneurysm) I71.9
- fibrocaseous of lung — *see* Tuberculosis, pulmonary
- fibrocystic — *see* Fibrocystic disease
- Fiedler's (leptospiral jaundice) A27.0
- fifth B08.3
- file-cutter's — *see* Poisoning, lead
- fish-skin Q80.9
  - acquired L85.0
- Flajani (-Basedow) (exophthalmic goiter) — *see* Hyper-thyroidism, with, goiter (diffuse)
- flax-dresser's J66.1
- fluke — *see* Infestation, fluke
- foot and mouth B08.8
- foot process N04.9
- Forbes' (glycogenosis III) E74.03
- Fordyce-Fox (apocrine miliaria) L75.2
- Fordyce's (ectopic sebaceous glands) (mouth) Q38.6
- Forestier's (rhizomelic pseudopolyarthritis) M35.3
  - meaning ankylosing hyperostosis — *see* Hyperosto-sis, ankylosing
- Fothergill's
  - neuralgia — *see* Neuralgia, trigeminal
  - scarlatina anginosa A38.9
- Fournier (gangrene) N49.3
  - female N76.82
  - vagina and vulva N76.82
- fourth B08.8
- Fox (-Fordyce) (apocrine miliaria) L75.2
- Francis' — *see* Tularemia
- Franklin C88.2
- Frei's (climatic bubo) A55
- Friedreich's
  - combined systemic or ataxia G11.11
  - myoclonia G25.3
- frontal sinus — *see* Sinusitis, frontal
- fungus NEC B49
- Gaisböck's (polycythemia hypertonica) D75.1
- gallbladder K82.9
  - calculus — *see* Calculus, gallbladder
  - cholecystitis — *see* Cholecystitis
  - cholesterolosis K82.4
  - fistula — *see* Fistula, gallbladder
  - hydrops K82.1
  - obstruction — *see* Obstruction, gallbladder
  - perforation K82.2
  - specified NEC K82.8
- gamma heavy chain C88.2
- Gamna's (siderotic splenomegaly) D73.2
- Gamstorp's (adynamia episodica hereditaria) G72.3
- Gandy-Nanta (siderotic splenomegaly) D73.2
- ganister J62.8
- gastric — *see* Disease, stomach
- gastroesophageal reflux (GERD) K21.9
  - with esophagitis (without bleeding) K21.00
    - with bleeding K21.01
- gastrointestinal (tract) K92.9
  - amyloid E85.4
  - functional K59.9
    - psychogenic F45.8
  - specified NEC K92.89
- Gee (-Herter) (-Heubner) (-Thaysen) (nontropical sprue) K90.0
- genital organs
  - female N94.9
  - male N50.9
- Gerhardt's (erythromelalgia) I73.81
- Gibert's (pityriasis rosea) L42
- Gierke's (glycogenosis I) E74.01
- Gilles de la Tourette's (motor-verbal tic) F95.2
- gingiva K06.9
  - plaque induced K05.00
  - specified NEC K06.8
- gland (lymph) I89.9
- Glanzmann's (hereditary hemorrhagic thrombasthenia) D69.1
- glass-blower's (cataract) — *see* Cataract, specified NEC
  - salivary gland hypertrophy K11.1
- Glisson's — *see* Rickets
- globe H44.9
  - specified NEC H44.89
- glomerular — *see also* Glomerulonephritis
  - with edema — *see* Nephrosis

Disease, diseased — *continued*
  glomerular — *see also* Glomerulonephritis — *continued*
    acute — *see* Nephritis, acute
    chronic — *see* Nephritis, chronic
    minimal change N05.0
    rapidly progressive N01.9
  glycogen storage E74.00
    Andersen's E74.09
    Cori's E74.03
    Forbes' E74.03
    generalized E74.00
    glucose-6-phosphatase deficiency E74.01
    heart E74.02 *[I43]*
    hepatorenal E74.09
    Hers' E74.09
    liver and kidney E74.09
    McArdle's E74.04
    muscle phosphofructokinase E74.09
    myocardium E74.02 *[I43]*
    Pompe's E74.02
    Tauri's E74.09
    type 0 E74.09
    type I E74.01
    type II E74.02
    type III E74.03
    type IV E74.09
    type V E74.04
    type VI-XI E74.09
    Von Gierke's E74.01
  Goldstein's (familial hemorrhagic telangiectasia) I78.0
  gonococcal NOS A54.9
  graft-versus-host (GVH) D89.813
    acute D89.810
    acute on chronic D89.812
    chronic D89.811
  grainhandler's J67.8
  granulomatous (childhood) (chronic) D71
  Graves' (exophthalmic goiter) — *see* Hyperthyroidism, with, goiter (diffuse)
  Griesinger's — *see* Ancylostomiasis
  Grisel's M43.6
  Gruby's (tinea tonsurans) B35.0
  Guillain-Barré G61.0
  Guinon's (motor-verbal tic) F95.2
  gum K06.9
  gynecological N94.9
  H (Hartnup's) E72.02
  Haff — *see* Poisoning, mercury
  Hageman (congenital factor XII deficiency) D68.2
  hair (color) (shaft) L67.9
    follicles L73.9
      specified NEC L73.8
  Hamman's (spontaneous mediastinal emphysema) J98.2
  hand, foot and mouth B08.4
  Hansen's — *see* Leprosy
  Hantavirus, with pulmonary manifestations B33.4
    with renal manifestations A98.5
  Harada's H30.81- ☑
  Hartnup (pellagra-cerebellar ataxia-renal aminoaciduria) E72.02
  Hart's (pellagra-cerebellar ataxia-renal aminoaciduria) E72.02
  Hashimoto's (struma lymphomatosa) E06.3
  Hb — *see* Disease, hemoglobin
  heart (organic) I51.9
    with
      pulmonary edema (acute) — *see also* Failure, ventricular, left I50.1
      rheumatic fever (conditions in I00)
        active I01.9
          with chorea I02.0
          specified NEC I01.8
        inactive or quiescent (with chorea) I09.9
          specified NEC I09.89
    amyloid E85.4 *[I43]*
    aortic (valve) I35.9
    arteriosclerotic or sclerotic (senile) — *see* Disease, heart, ischemic, atherosclerotic
    artery, arterial — *see* Disease, heart, ischemic, atherosclerotic
    beer drinkers' I42.6
    beriberi (wet) E51.12
    black I27.0
    congenital Q24.9
      cyanotic Q24.9
      specified NEC Q24.8

Disease, diseased — *continued*
  heart — *continued*
    coronary — *see* Disease, heart, ischemic
    cryptogenic I51.9
    fibroid — *see* Myocarditis
    functional I51.89
      psychogenic F45.8
    glycogen storage E74.02 *[I43]*
    gonococcal A54.83
    hypertensive — *see* Hypertension, heart
    hyperthyroid — *see also* Hyperthyroidism E05.90 *[I43]*
      with thyroid storm E05.91 *[I43]*
    ischemic (chronic or with a stated duration of over 4 weeks) I25.9
      atherosclerotic (of) I25.10
        with angina pectoris — *see* Arteriosclerosis, coronary (artery)
        coronary artery bypass graft — *see* Arteriosclerosis, coronary (artery),
      cardiomyopathy I25.5
      diagnosed on ECG or other special investigation, but currently presenting no symptoms I25.6
      silent I25.6
      specified form NEC I25.89
    kyphoscoliotic I27.1
    meningococcal A39.50
      endocarditis A39.51
      myocarditis A39.52
      pericarditis A39.53
    mitral I05.9
      specified NEC I05.8
    muscular — *see* Degeneration, myocardial
    psychogenic (functional) F45.8
    pulmonary (chronic) I27.9
      in schistosomiasis B65.9 *[I52]*
      specified NEC I27.89
    rheumatic (chronic) (inactive) (old) (quiescent) (with chorea) I09.9
      active or acute I01.9
        with chorea (acute) (rheumatic) (Sydenham's) I02.0
      specified NEC I09.89
    senile — *see* Myocarditis
    syphilitic A52.06
      aortic A52.03
        aneurysm A52.01
      congenital A50.54 *[I52]*
    thyrotoxic — *see also* Thyrotoxicosis E05.90 *[I43]*
      with thyroid storm E05.91 *[I43]*
    valve, valvular (obstructive) (regurgitant) — *see also* Endocarditis
      congenital NEC Q24.8
      pulmonary Q22.3
    vascular — *see* Disease, cardiovascular
  heavy chain NEC C88.2
    alpha C88.3
    gamma C88.2
    mu C88.2
  Hebra's
    pityriasis
      maculata et circinata L42
      rubra pilaris L44.0
    prurigo L28.2
  hematopoietic organs D75.9
  hemoglobin or Hb
    abnormal (mixed) NEC D58.2
      with thalassemia D56.9
    AS genotype D57.3
    Bart's D56.0
    C (Hb-C) D58.2
      with other abnormal hemoglobin NEC D58.2
      elliptocytosis D58.1
      Hb-S D57.2- ☑
      sickle-cell D57.2- ☑
      thalassemia D56.8
    Constant Spring D58.2
    D (Hb-D) D58.2
    E (Hb-E) D58.2
    E-beta thalassemia D56.5
    elliptocytosis D58.1
    H (Hb-H) (thalassemia) D56.0
      with other abnormal hemoglobin NEC D56.9
      Constant Spring D56.0
    I thalassemia D56.9
    M D74.0
    S or SS D57.1

Disease, diseased — *continued*
  hemoglobin or Hb — *continued*
    S or SS — *continued*
      with
        acute chest syndrome D57.01
        cerebral vascular involvement D57.03
        crisis (painful) D57.00
          with complication specified NEC D57.09
        splenic sequestration D57.02
        vasoocclusive pain D57.00
      beta plus D57.44
        with
          acute chest syndrome D57.451
          cerebral vascular involvement D57.453
          crisis D57.459
            with specified complication NEC D57.458
          splenic sequestration D57.452
          vasoocclusive pain D57.459
        without crisis D57.44
      beta zero D57.42
        with
          acute chest syndrome D57.431
          cerebral vascular involvement D57.433
          crisis D57.439
            with specified complication NEC D57.438
          splenic sequestration D57.432
          vasoocclusive pain
        without crisis D57.42
    SC D57.2- ☑
    SD D57.8- ☑
    SE D57.8- ☑
    spherocytosis D58.0
    unstable, hemolytic D58.2
  hemolytic (newborn) P55.9
    autoimmune D59.10
      cold type (primary) (secondary) (symptomatic) D59.12
      mixed type (primary) (secondary) (symptomatic) D59.13
      warm type (primary) (secondary) (symptomatic) D59.11
    drug-induced D59.0
    due to or with
      incompatibility
        ABO (blood group) P55.1
        blood (group) (Duffy) (K) (Kell) (Kidd) (Lewis) (M) (S) NEC P55.8
        Rh (blood group) (factor) P55.0
      Rh negative mother P55.0
    specified type NEC P55.8
    unstable hemoglobin D58.2
  hemorrhagic D69.9
    newborn P53
  Henoch (-Schönlein) (purpura nervosa) D69.0
  hepatic — *see* Disease, liver
  hepatolenticular E83.01
  heredodegenerative NEC
    spinal cord G95.89
  herpesviral, disseminated B00.7
  Hers' (glycogenosis VI) E74.09
  Herter (-Gee) (-Heubner) (nontropical sprue) K90.0
  Heubner-Herter (nontropical sprue) K90.0
  high fetal gene or hemoglobin thalassemia D56.9
  Hildenbrand's — *see* Typhus
  hip (joint) M25.9
    congenital Q65.89
    suppurative M00.9
    tuberculous A18.02
  His (-Werner) (trench fever) A79.0
  Hodgson's — *see also* Aneurysm, aorta, thorax I71.20
    ruptured — *see also* Aneurysm, aorta, thorax, ruptured I71.10
  Holla — *see* Spherocytosis
  hookworm B76.9
    specified NEC B76.8
  host-versus-graft D89.813
    acute D89.810
    acute on chronic D89.812
    chronic D89.811
  human immunodeficiency virus (HIV) B20
  Huntington's G10
    with dementia — *see also* Dementia, in, diseases specified elsewhere G10 *[F02.80]*
  Hutchinson's (cheiropompholyx) — *see* Hutchinson's disease
  hyaline (diffuse) (generalized)

Disease, diseased — *continued*
  hyaline — *continued*
    membrane (lung) (newborn) P22.0
      adult J80
  hydatid — *see* Echinococcus
  hydroxyapatite deposition M11.00
    ankle M11.07- ☑
    elbow M11.02- ☑
    foot joint M11.07- ☑
    hand joint M11.04- ☑
    hip M11.05- ☑
    knee M11.06- ☑
    multiple site M11.09
    shoulder M11.01- ☑
    vertebra M11.08
    wrist M11.03- ☑
  hyperkinetic — *see* Hyperkinesia
  hypertensive — *see* Hypertension
  hypophysis E23.7
  Iceland G93.39
  I-cell E77.0
  immune D89.9
  immunoproliferative (malignant) C88.9
    small intestinal C88.3
    specified NEC C88.8
  inclusion B25.9
    salivary gland B25.9
  infectious, infective B99.9
    congenital P37.9
      specified NEC P37.8
      viral P35.9
        specified type NEC P35.8
    specified NEC B99.8
  inflammatory
    penis N48.29
      abscess N48.21
      cellulitis N48.22
    prepuce N47.7
      balanoposthitis N47.6
    tubo-ovarian — *see* Salpingo-oophoritis
  intervertebral disc — *see also* Disorder, disc
    with myelopathy — *see* Disorder, disc, with, myelopathy
    cervical, cervicothoracic — *see* Disorder, disc, cervical
    with
      myelopathy — *see* Disorder, disc, cervical, with myelopathy
      neuritis, radiculitis or radiculopathy — *see* Disorder, disc, cervical, with neuritis
      specified NEC — *see* Disorder, disc, cervical, specified type NEC
    lumbar (with)
      myelopathy M51.06
      neuritis, radiculitis, radiculopathy or sciatica M51.16
      specified NEC M51.86
    lumbosacral (with)
      neuritis, radiculitis, radiculopathy or sciatica M51.17
      specified NEC M51.87
    specified NEC — *see* Disorder, disc, specified NEC
    thoracic (with)
      myelopathy M51.04
      neuritis, radiculitis or radiculopathy M51.14
      specified NEC M51.84
    thoracolumbar (with)
      myelopathy M51.05
      neuritis, radiculitis or radiculopathy M51.15
      specified NEC M51.85
  intestine K63.9
    functional K59.9
      psychogenic F45.8
      specified NEC K59.89
    organic K63.9
    protozoal A07.9
    specified NEC K63.89
  iris H21.9
    specified NEC H21.89
  iron metabolism or storage E83.10
  island (scrub typhus) A75.3
  itai-itai — *see* Poisoning, cadmium
  Jakob-Creutzfeldt — *see* Creutzfeldt-Jakob disease or syndrome
  jaw M27.9
    fibrocystic M27.49
    specified NEC M27.8
  jigger B88.1

Disease, diseased — *continued*
  joint — *see also* Disorder, joint
    Charcot's — *see* Arthropathy, neuropathic (Charcot)
    degenerative — *see* Osteoarthritis
      multiple M15.9
      spine — *see* Spondylosis
    facet joint — *see also* Spondylosis M47.819
    hypertrophic — *see* Osteoarthritis
    sacroiliac M53.3
    specified NEC — *see* Disorder, joint, specified type NEC
    spine NEC — *see* Dorsopathy
    suppurative — *see* Arthritis, pyogenic or pyemic
  Jourdain's (acute gingivitis) K05.00
    nonplaque induced K05.01
    plaque induced K05.00
  Kaschin-Beck (endemic polyarthritis) M12.10
    ankle M12.17- ☑
    elbow M12.12- ☑
    foot joint M12.17- ☑
    hand joint M12.14- ☑
    hip M12.15- ☑
    knee M12.16- ☑
    multiple site M12.19
    shoulder M12.11- ☑
    vertebra M12.18
    wrist M12.13- ☑
  Katayama B65.2
  Kedani (scrub typhus) A75.3
  Keshan E59
  kidney (functional) (pelvis) N28.9
    chronic N18.9
      hypertensive — *see* Hypertension, kidney
      stage 1 N18.1
      stage 2 (mild) N18.2
      stage 3 (moderate) N18.30
      stage 3a N18.31
      stage 3b N18.32
      stage 4 (severe) N18.4
      stage 5 N18.5
    complicating pregnancy — *see* Pregnancy, complicated by, renal disease
    cystic (congenital) Q61.9
    fibrocystic (congenital) Q61.8
    hypertensive — *see* Hypertension, kidney
    in (due to)
      schistosomiasis (bilharziasis) B65.9 *[N29]*
    multicystic Q61.4
    polycystic Q61.3
      adult type Q61.2
      childhood type NEC Q61.19
        collecting duct dilatation Q61.11
  Kimmelstiel (-Wilson) (intercapillary polycystic (congenital) glomerulosclerosis) — *see* E08-E13 with .21
  Kinnier Wilson's (hepatolenticular degeneration) E83.01
  kissing — *see* Mononucleosis, infectious
  Klebs' — *see also* Glomerulonephritis N05- ☑
  Klippel-Feil (brevicollis) Q76.1
  Köhler-Pellegrini-Stieda (calcification, knee joint) — *see* Bursitis, tibial collateral
  Kok Q89.8
  König's (osteochondritis dissecans) — *see* Osteochondritis, dissecans
  Korsakoff's (nonalcoholic) F04
    alcoholic F10.96
      with dependence F10.26
  Kostmann's (infantile genetic agranulocytosis) D70.0
  kuru A81.81
  Kyasanur Forest A98.2
  labyrinth, ear — *see* Disorder, ear, inner
  lacrimal system — *see* Disorder, lacrimal system
  Lafora's — *see* Epilepsy, generalized, idiopathic
  Lancereaux-Mathieu (leptospiral jaundice) A27.0
  Landry's G61.0
  Larrey-Weil (leptospiral jaundice) A27.0
  larynx J38.7
  legionnaires' A48.1
    nonpneumonic A48.2
  Lenegre's I44.2
  lens H27.9
    specified NEC H27.8
  Lev's (acquired complete heart block) I44.2
  Lewy body (dementia) — *see also* Dementia, in, diseases specified elsewhere G31.83 *[F02.80]*
    with behavioral disturbance — *see also* Dementia, in, diseases specified elsewhere G31.83 *[F02.81-]* ☑

Disease, diseased — *continued*
  Lichtheim's (subacute combined sclerosis with pernicious anemia) D51.0
  Lightwood's (renal tubular acidosis) N25.89
  Lignac's (cystinosis) E72.04
  lip K13.0
  lipid-storage E75.6
    specified NEC E75.5
  Lipschütz's N76.6
  liver (chronic) (organic) K76.9
    alcoholic (chronic) K70.9
      acute — *see* Disease, liver, alcoholic, hepatitis
      cirrhosis K70.30
        with ascites K70.31
      failure K70.40
        with coma K70.41
      fatty liver K70.0
      fibrosis K70.2
      hepatitis K70.10
        with ascites K70.11
      sclerosis K70.2
    cystic, congenital Q44.6
    drug-induced (idiosyncratic) (toxic) (predictable) (unpredictable) — *see* Disease, liver, toxic
    end stage K72.1- ☑
      due to hepatitis — *see* Hepatitis
      with coma K72.11
    fatty, nonalcoholic (NAFLD) K76.0
      alcoholic K70.0
    fibrocystic (congenital) Q44.6
    fluke
      Chinese B66.1
      oriental B66.1
      sheep B66.3
    gestational alloimmune (GALD) P78.84
    glycogen storage E74.09 *[K77]*
    in (due to)
      schistosomiasis (bilharziasis) B65.9 *[K77]*
    inflammatory K75.9
      alcoholic K70.1 ☑
      specified NEC K75.89
    polycystic (congenital) Q44.6
    toxic K71.9
      with
        cholestasis K71.0
        cirrhosis (liver) K71.7
        fibrosis (liver) K71.7
        focal nodular hyperplasia K71.8
        hepatic granuloma K71.8
        hepatic necrosis K71.10
          with coma K71.11
        hepatitis NEC K71.6
          acute K71.2
          chronic
            active K71.50
              with ascites K71.51
            lobular K71.4
            persistent K71.3
        lupoid K71.50
          with ascites K71.51
        peliosis hepatis K71.8
        veno-occlusive disease (VOD) of liver K71.8
    veno-occlusive K76.5
  Lobo's (keloid blastomycosis) B48.0
  Lobstein's (brittle bones and blue sclera) Q78.0
  Ludwig's (submaxillary cellulitis) K12.2
  lumbosacral region M53.87
  lung J98.4
    black J60
    congenital Q33.9
    cystic J98.4
      congenital Q33.0
    dabbing (related) U07.0
    electronic cigarette (related) U07.0
    fibroid (chronic) — *see* Fibrosis, lung
    fluke B66.4
      oriental B66.4
    in
      amyloidosis E85.4 *[J99]*
      sarcoidosis D86.0
      Sjögren's syndrome M35.02
      systemic
        lupus erythematosus M32.13
        sclerosis M34.81
    interstitial J84.9
      of childhood, specified NEC J84.848
      respiratory bronchiolitis J84.115
      specified NEC J84.89

Disease, diseased — *continued*
- lung — *continued*
  - interstitial — *continued*
    - with progressive fibrotic phenotype, in diseases classified elsewhere J84.170
    - obstructive (chronic) J44.9
      - with
        - acute
          - bronchitis J44.0
          - exacerbation NEC J44.1
          - lower respiratory infection J44.0
        - alveolitis, allergic J67.9
        - asthma J44.9
        - bronchiectasis J47.9
          - with
            - exacerbation (acute) J47.1
            - lower respiratory infection J47.0
        - bronchitis J44.9
          - with
            - exacerbation (acute) J44.1
            - lower respiratory infection J44.0
        - emphysema J43.9
        - hypersensitivity pneumonitis J67.9
      - decompensated J44.1
        - with
          - exacerbation (acute) J44.1
    - polycystic J98.4
      - congenital Q33.0
    - rheumatoid (diffuse) (interstitial) — *see* Rheumatoid, lung
    - vaping (associated) (device) (product) (use) U07.0
- Lutembacher's (atrial septal defect with mitral stenosis) Q21.19
- Lyme A69.20
- lymphatic (gland) (system) (channel) (vessel) I89.9
- lymphoproliferative D47.9
  - specified NEC D47.Z9 (*following* D47.4)
  - T-gamma D47.Z9 (*following* D47.4)
  - X-linked D82.3
- Magitot's M27.2
- malarial — *see* Malaria
- malignant — *see also* Neoplasm, malignant, by site
- Manson's B65.1
- maple bark J67.6
- maple-syrup-urine E71.0
- Marburg (virus) A98.3
- Marion's (bladder neck obstruction) N32.0
- Marsh's (exophthalmic goiter) — *see* Hyperthyroidism, with, goiter (diffuse)
- mastoid (process) — *see* Disorder, ear, middle
- Mathieu's (leptospiral jaundice) A27.0
- Maxcy's A75.2
- McArdle (-Schmid-Pearson) (glycogenosis V) E74.04
- mediastinum J98.59
- medullary center (idiopathic) (respiratory) G93.89
- Meige's (chronic hereditary edema) Q82.0
- meningococcal — *see* Infection, meningococcal
- mental F99
  - organic F09
- mesenchymal M35.9
- mesenteric embolic — *see also* Ischemia, intestine, acute K55.039
- metabolic, metabolism E88.9
  - bilirubin E80.7
- metal-polisher's J62.8
- metastatic — *see also* Neoplasm, secondary, by site C79.9
- microvascular - code to condition
- microvillus
  - atrophy Q43.8
  - inclusion (MVD) Q43.8
- middle ear — *see* Disorder, ear, middle
- Mikulicz' (dryness of mouth, absent or decreased lacrimation) K11.8
- Milroy's (chronic hereditary edema) Q82.0
- Minamata — *see* Poisoning, mercury
- minicore G71.29
- Minor's G95.19
- Minot's (hemorrhagic disease, newborn) P53
- Minot-von Willebrand-Jürgens (angiohemophilia) — *see* Disease, von Willebrand
- Mitchell's (erythromelalgia) I73.81
- mitral (valve) I05.9
  - nonrheumatic I34.9
- mixed connective tissue M35.1
- moldy hay J67.0
- Monge's T70.29 ☑

Disease, diseased — *continued*
- Morgagni-Adams-Stokes (syncope with heart block) I45.9
- Morgagni's (syndrome) (hyperostosis frontalis interna) M85.2
- Morton's (with metatarsalgia) — *see* Lesion, nerve, plantar
- Morvan's G60.8
- motor neuron (bulbar) (mixed type) (spinal) G12.20
  - amyotrophic lateral sclerosis G12.21
  - familial G12.24
  - progressive bulbar palsy G12.22
  - specified NEC G12.29
- moyamoya I67.5
- mu heavy chain disease C88.2
- multicore G71.29
- multiminicore G71.29
- muscle — *see also* Disorder, muscle
  - inflammatory — *see* Myositis
  - ocular (external) — *see* Strabismus
- musculoskeletal system, soft tissue — *see also* Disorder, soft tissue
  - specified NEC — *see* Disorder, soft tissue, specified type NEC
- mushroom workers' J67.5
- mycotic B49
- myelodysplastic — *see also* Syndrome, myelodysplasia C94.6
- myelodysplastic/myeloproliferative neoplasm, unclassifiable C94.6
- myeloproliferative D47.1
  - chronic D47.1
  - not classified C94.6
  - specified NEC C94.6
  - unclassifiable C94.6
- myocardium, myocardial — *see also* Degeneration, myocardial I51.5
  - primary (idiopathic) I42.9
- myoneural G70.9
- Naegeli's D69.1
- nails L60.9
  - specified NEC L60.8
- Nairobi (sheep virus) A93.8
- nasal J34.9
- nemaline body G71.21
- nerve — *see* Disorder, nerve
- nervous system G98.8
  - autonomic G90.9
  - central G96.9
    - specified NEC G96.89
  - congenital Q07.9
  - parasympathetic G90.9
  - specified NEC G98.8
  - sympathetic G90.9
  - vegetative G90.9
- neuromuscular system G70.9
- Newcastle B30.8
- Nicolas (-Durand)-Favre (climatic bubo) A55
- nipple N64.9
  - Paget's C50.01- ☑
    - female C50.01- ☑
    - male C50.02- ☑
- Nishimoto (-Takeuchi) I67.5
- nonarthropod-borne NOS (viral) B34.9
  - enterovirus NEC B34.1
- nonautoimmune hemolytic D59.4
  - drug-induced D59.2
- Nonne-Milroy-Meige (chronic hereditary edema) Q82.0
- nose J34.9
- nucleus pulposus — *see* Disorder, disc
- nutritional E63.9
- oast-house-urine E72.19
  - ocular
    - herpesviral B00.50
    - zoster B02.30
- obliterative vascular I77.1
- Ohara's — *see* Tularemia
- Opitz's (congestive splenomegaly) D73.2
- Oppenheim-Urbach (necrobiosis lipoidica diabeticorum) — *see* E08-E13 with .620
- optic nerve NEC — *see* Disorder, nerve, optic
- orbit — *see* Disorder, orbit
- organ
  - dabbing (related) U07.0
  - electronic cigarette (related) U07.0
  - vaping (associated) (device) (product) (use) U07.0
- Oriental liver fluke B66.1
- Oriental lung fluke B66.4

Disease, diseased — *continued*
- Ormond's N13.5
- Oropouche virus A93.0
- Osler-Rendu (familial hemorrhagic telangiectasia) I78.0
- osteofibrocystic E21.0
- Otto's M24.7
- outer ear — *see* Disorder, ear, external
- ovary (noninflammatory) N83.9
  - cystic N83.20- ☑
  - inflammatory — *see* Salpingo-oophoritis
  - polycystic E28.2
  - specified NEC N83.8
- Owren's (congenital) — *see* Defect, coagulation
- p110d-activating mutation causing senescent T cells, lymphadenopathy, and immunodeficiency [PASLI] D81.82
- pancreas K86.9
  - cystic K86.2
  - fibrocystic E84.9
  - specified NEC K86.89
- panvalvular I08.9
  - specified NEC I08.8
- parametrium (noninflammatory) N83.9
- parasitic B89
  - cerebral NEC B71.9 *[G94]*
  - intestinal NOS B82.9
  - mouth B37.0
  - skin NOS B88.9
  - specified type — *see* Infestation
  - tongue B37.0
- parathyroid (gland) E21.5
  - specified NEC E21.4
- Parkinson's G20
- parodontal K05.6
- Parrot's (syphilitic osteochondritis) A50.02
- Parry's (exophthalmic goiter) — *see* Hyperthyroidism, with, goiter (diffuse)
- Parson's (exophthalmic goiter) — *see* Hyperthyroidism, with, goiter (diffuse)
- Paxton's (white piedra) B36.2
- pearl-worker's — *see* Osteomyelitis, specified type NEC
- Pellegrini-Stieda (calcification, knee joint) — *see* Bursitis, tibial collateral
- pelvis, pelvic
  - female NOS N94.9
    - specified NEC N94.89
  - gonococcal (acute) (chronic) A54.24
  - inflammatory (female) N73.9
    - acute N73.0
    - chlamydial A56.11
    - chronic N73.1
    - specified NEC N73.8
    - syphilitic (secondary) A51.42
      - late A52.76
    - tuberculous A18.17
  - organ, female N94.9
  - peritoneum, female NEC N94.89
- penis N48.9
  - inflammatory N48.29
    - abscess N48.21
    - cellulitis N48.22
  - specified NEC N48.89
- periapical tissues NOS K04.90
- periodontal K05.6
  - specified NEC K05.5
- periosteum — *see* Disorder, bone, specified type NEC
- peripheral
  - arterial I73.9
  - autonomic nervous system G90.9
  - nerves — *see* Polyneuropathy
  - vascular NOS I73.9
- peritoneum K66.9
  - pelvic, female NEC N94.89
  - specified NEC K66.8
- persistent mucosal (middle ear) H66.20
  - left H66.22
    - with right H66.23
  - right H66.21
    - with left H66.23
- Petit's — *see* Hernia, abdomen, specified site NEC
- pharynx J39.2
  - specified NEC J39.2
- Phocas' — *see* Mastopathy, cystic
- photochromogenic (acid-fast bacilli) (pulmonary) A31.0
  - nonpulmonary A31.9
- Pick's — *see also* Dementia, in, diseases specified elsewhere G31.01 *[F02.80]*

☑ Additional Character Required — Refer to the Tabular List for Character Selection

Disease, diseased — *continued*
  Pick's — *see also* Dementia, in, diseases specified
    elsewhere — *continued*
    with behavioral disturbance — *see also* Dementia,
      in, diseases specified elsewhere
      G31.01 *[F02.81-]* ☑
    brain G31.01 *[F02.80]*
      with behavioral disturbance — *see also* Demen-
        tia, in, diseases specified elsewhere
        G31.01 *[F02.81-]* ☑
    of pericardium (pericardial pseudocirrhosis of liver)
      I31.1
  pigeon fancier's J67.2
  pineal gland E34.8
  pink — *see* Poisoning, mercury
  Pinkus' (lichen nitidus) L44.1
  pinworm B80
  Piry virus A93.8
  pituitary (gland) E23.7
  pituitary-snuff-taker's J67.8
  pleura (cavity) J94.9
    specified NEC J94.8
  pneumatic drill (hammer) T75.21 ☑
  Pollitzer's (hidradenitis suppurativa) L73.2
  polycystic
    kidney or renal Q61.3
      adult type Q61.2
      childhood type NEC Q61.19
        collecting duct dilatation Q61.11
    liver or hepatic Q44.6
    lung or pulmonary J98.4
      congenital Q33.0
    ovary, ovaries E28.2
    spleen Q89.09
  polyethylene T84.05- ☑
  Pompe's (glycogenosis II) E74.02
  Posadas-Wernicke B38.9
  Potain's (pulmonary edema) — *see* Edema, lung
  prepuce N47.8
    inflammatory N47.7
      balanoposthitis N47.6
  Pringle's (tuberous sclerosis) Q85.1
  prion, central nervous system A81.9
    specified NEC A81.89
  prostate N42.9
    specified NEC N42.89
  protozoal B64
    acanthamebiasis — *see* Acanthamebiasis
    African trypanosomiasis — *see* African trypanosomi-
      asis
    babesiosis — *see also* Babesiosis B60.00
    Chagas disease — *see* Chagas disease
    intestine, intestinal A07.9
    leishmaniasis — *see* Leishmaniasis
    malaria — *see* Malaria
    naegleriasis B60.2
    pneumocystosis B59
    specified organism NEC B60.8
    toxoplasmosis — *see* Toxoplasmosis
  pseudo-Hurler's E77.0
  psychiatric F99
  psychotic — *see* Psychosis
  Puente's (simple glandular cheilitis) K13.0
  puerperal — *see also* Puerperal O90.89
  pulmonary — *see also* Disease, lung
    artery I28.9
    chronic obstructive J44.9
      with
        acute bronchitis J44.0
        exacerbation (acute) J44.1
        lower respiratory infection (acute) J44.0
      decompensated J44.1
        with
          exacerbation (acute) J44.1
    heart I27.9
      specified NEC I27.89
    hypertensive (vascular) — *see also* Hypertension,
      pulmonary I27.20
      NEC I27.2 ☑
      primary (idiopathic) I27.0
    valve I37.9
      rheumatic I09.89
  pulp (dental) NOS K04.90
  pulseless M31.4
  Putnam's (subacute combined sclerosis with pernicious
    anemia) D51.0
  Pyle (-Cohn) (metaphyseal dysplasia) Q78.5
  ragpicker's or ragsorter's A22.1

Disease, diseased — *continued*
  Raynaud's — *see* Raynaud's disease
  reactive airway — *see* Asthma
  Reclus' (cystic) — *see* Mastopathy, cystic
  rectum K62.9
    specified NEC K62.89
  Refsum's (heredopathia atactica polyneuritiformis)
    G60.1
  renal (functional) (pelvis) — *see also* Disease, kidney
    N28.9
    with
      edema — *see* Nephrosis
      glomerular lesion — *see* Glomerulonephritis
        with edema — *see* Nephrosis
      interstitial nephritis N12
    acute N28.9
    chronic — *see also* Disease, kidney, chronic N18.9
    cystic, congenital Q61.9
    diabetic — *see* E08-E13 with .22
    end-stage (failure) N18.6
      due to hypertension I12.0
    fibrocystic (congenital) Q61.8
    hypertensive — *see* Hypertension, kidney
    lupus M32.14
    phosphate-losing (tubular) N25.0
    polycystic (congenital) Q61.3
      adult type Q61.2
      childhood type NEC Q61.19
        collecting duct dilatation Q61.11
    rapidly progressive N01.9
    subacute N01.9
  Rendu-Osler-Weber (familial hemorrhagic telangiecta-
    sia) I78.0
  renovascular (arteriosclerotic) — *see* Hypertension,
    kidney
  respiratory (tract) J98.9
    acute or subacute NOS J06.9
      due to
        chemicals, gases, fumes or vapors (inhalation)
          J68.3
        external agent J70.9
          specified NEC J70.8
        radiation J70.0
        smoke inhalation J70.5
      noninfectious J39.8
    chronic NOS J98.9
      due to
        chemicals, gases, fumes or vapors J68.4
        external agent J70.9
          specified NEC J70.8
        radiation J70.1
      newborn P27.9
        specified NEC P27.8
    due to
      chemicals, gases, fumes or vapors J68.9
        acute or subacute NEC J68.3
        chronic J68.4
      external agent J70.9
        specified NEC J70.8
      newborn P28.9
        specified type NEC P28.89
    upper J39.9
      acute or subacute J06.9
      noninfectious NEC J39.8
      specified NEC J39.8
      streptococcal J06.9
  retina, retinal H35.9
    Batten's or Batten-Mayou E75.4 *[H36]*
    specified NEC H35.89
  rheumatoid — *see* Arthritis, rheumatoid
  rickettsial NOS A79.9
    specified type NEC A79.89
  Riga (-Fede) (cachectic aphthae) K14.0
  Riggs' (compound periodontitis) — *see* Periodontitis
  Ritter's L00
  Rivalta's (cervicofacial actinomycosis) A42.2
  Robles' (onchocerciasis) B73.01
  rod body G71.21
  Roger's (congenital interventricular septal defect) Q21.0
  Rosenthal's (factor XI deficiency) D68.1
  Ross River B33.1
  Rossbach's (hyperchlorhydria) K31.89
    psychogenic F45.8
  Rotes Quérol — *see* Hyperostosis, ankylosing
  Roth (-Bernhardt) — *see* Mononeuropathy, lower limb,
    meralgia paresthetica
  Runeberg's (progressive pernicious anemia) D51.0
  sacroiliac NEC M53.3

Disease, diseased — *continued*
  salivary gland or duct K11.9
    inclusion B25.9
    specified NEC K11.8
    virus B25.9
  sandworm B76.9
  Schimmelbusch's — *see* Mastopathy, cystic
  Schmorl's — *see* Schmorl's disease or nodes
  Schönlein (-Henoch) (purpura rheumatica) D69.0
  Schottmüller's — *see* Fever, paratyphoid
  Schultz's (agranulocytosis) — *see* Agranulocytosis
  Schwalbe-Ziehen-Oppenheim G24.1
  Schwartz-Jampel G71.13
  sclera H15.9
    specified NEC H15.89
  scrofulous (tuberculous) A18.2
  scrotum N50.9
  sebaceous glands L73.9
  semilunar cartilage, cystic — *see also* Derangement,
    knee, meniscus, cystic
  seminal vesicle N50.9
  serum NEC — *see also* Reaction, serum T80.69 ☑
  sexually transmitted A64
    anogenital
      herpesviral infection — *see* Herpes, anogenital
      warts A63.0
    chancroid A57
    chlamydial infection — *see* Chlamydia
    gonorrhea — *see* Gonorrhea
    granuloma inguinale A58
    specified organism NEC A63.8
    syphilis — *see* Syphilis
    trichomoniasis — *see* Trichomoniasis
  Sézary C84.1- ☑
  shimamushi (scrub typhus) A75.3
  shipyard B30.0
  sickle-cell D57.1
    with
      acute chest syndrome D57.01
      cerebral vascular involvement D57.03
      crisis (painful) D57.00
        with complication specified NEC D57.09
      splenic sequestration D57.02
      vasoocclusive pain D57.00
    elliptocytosis D57.8- ☑
    Hb-C D57.20
      with
        acute chest syndrome D57.211
        cerebral vascular involvement D57.213
        crisis D57.219
          with specified complication NEC D57.218
        splenic sequestration D57.212
        vasoocclusive pain D57.219
      without crisis D57.20
    Hb-SD D57.80
      with
        acute chest syndrome D57.811
        cerebral vascular involvement D57.813
        crisis D57.819
          with complication specified NEC D57.818
        splenic sequestration D57.812
        vasoocclusive pain D57.819
      without crisis D57.80
    Hb-SE D57.80
      with
        acute chest syndrome D57.811
        cerebral vascular involvement D57.813
        crisis D57.819
          with complication specified NEC D57.818
        splenic sequestration D57.812
        vasoocclusive pain D57.819
      without crisis D57.80
    specified NEC D57.80
      with
        acute chest syndrome D57.811
        cerebral vascular involvement D57.813
        crisis D57.819
          with complication specified NEC D57.818
        splenic sequestration D57.812
        vasoocclusive pain D57.819
      without crisis D57.80
    spherocytosis D57.80
      with
        acute chest syndrome D57.811
        cerebral vascular involvement D57.813
        crisis D57.819
          with complication specified NEC D57.818
        splenic sequestration D57.812

Disease, diseased — *continued*
- sickle-cell — *continued*
  - spherocytosis — *continued*
    - with — *continued*
      - vasoocclusive pain D57.819
      - without crisis D57.80
    - thalassemia D57.40
      - with
        - acute chest syndrome D57.411
        - cerebral vascular involvement D57.413
        - crisis (painful) D57.419
          - with specified complication NEC D57.418
        - splenic sequestration D57.412
        - vasoocclusive pain D57.419
      - beta plus D57.44
        - with
          - acute chest syndrome D57.451
          - cerebral vascular involvement D57.453
          - crisis D57.459
            - with specified complication NEC D57.458
          - splenic sequestration D57.452
          - vasoocclusive pain D57.459
        - without crisis D57.44
      - beta zero D57.42
        - with
          - acute chest syndrome D57.431
          - cerebral vascular involvement D57.433
          - crisis D57.439
            - with specified complication NEC D57.438
          - splenic sequestration D57.432
          - vasoocclusive pain D57.439
        - without crisis D57.42
- silo-filler's J68.8
  - bronchitis J68.0
  - pneumonitis J68.0
  - pulmonary edema J68.1
- simian B B00.4
- Simons' (progressive lipodystrophy) E88.1
- sin nombre virus B33.4
- sinus — *see* Sinusitis
- Sirkari's B55.0
- sixth B08.20
  - due to human herpesvirus 6 B08.21
  - due to human herpesvirus 7 B08.22
- skin L98.9
  - due to metabolic disorder NEC E88.9 [L99]
  - specified NEC L98.8
- slim (HIV) B20
- small vessel I73.9
- Sneddon-Wilkinson (subcorneal pustular dermatosis) L13.1
- South African creeping B88.0
- spinal (cord) G95.9
  - congenital Q06.9
  - specified NEC G95.89
- spine — *see also* Spondylopathy
  - joint — *see* Dorsopathy
  - tuberculous A18.01
- spinocerebellar (hereditary) G11.9
  - specified NEC G11.8
- spleen D73.9
  - amyloid E85.4 [D77]
  - organic D73.9
  - polycystic Q89.09
  - postinfectional D73.89
- sponge-diver's — *see* Toxicity, venom, marine animal, sea anemone
- Startle Q89.8
- Steinert's G71.11
- Sticker's (erythema infectiosum) B08.3
- Stieda's (calcification, knee joint) — *see* Bursitis, tibial collateral
- Stokes' (exophthalmic goiter) — *see* Hyperthyroidism, with, goiter (diffuse)
- Stokes-Adams (syncope with heart block) I45.9
- stomach K31.9
  - functional, psychogenic F45.8
  - specified NEC K31.89
- stonemason's J62.8
- storage
  - glycogen — *see* Disease, glycogen storage
  - mucopolysaccharide — *see* Mucopolysaccharidosis
- striatopallidal system NEC G25.89
- Stuart-Prower (congenital factor X deficiency) D68.2
- Stuart's (congenital factor X deficiency) D68.2
- subcutaneous tissue — *see* Disease, skin

Disease, diseased — *continued*
- supporting structures of teeth K08.9
  - specified NEC K08.89
- suprarenal (capsule) (gland) E27.9
  - hyperfunction E27.0
  - specified NEC E27.8
- sweat glands L74.9
  - specified NEC L74.8
- Sweeley-Klionsky E75.21
- Swift (-Feer) — *see* Poisoning, mercury
- swimming-pool granuloma A31.1
- Sylvest's (epidemic pleurodynia) B33.0
- sympathetic nervous system G90.9
- synovium — *see* Disorder, synovium
- syphilitic — *see* Syphilis
- systemic tissue mast cell D47.02
- tanapox (virus) B08.71
- Tangier E78.6
- Tarral-Besnier (pityriasis rubra pilaris) L44.0
- Tauri's E74.09
- tear duct — *see* Disorder, lacrimal system
- tendon, tendinous — *see also* Disorder, tendon
  - nodular — *see* Trigger finger
- terminal vessel I73.9
- testis N50.9
- thalassemia Hb-S — *see* Disease, sickle-cell, thalassemia
- Thaysen-Gee (nontropical sprue) K90.0
- Thomsen G71.12
- throat J39.2
  - septic J02.0
- thromboembolic — *see* Embolism
- thymus (gland) E32.9
  - specified NEC E32.8
- thyroid (gland) E07.9
  - heart — *see also* Hyperthyroidism E05.90 [I43]
    - with thyroid storm E05.91 [I43]
  - specified NEC E07.89
- Tietze's M94.0
- tongue K14.9
  - specified NEC K14.8
- tonsils, tonsillar (and adenoids) J35.9
- tooth, teeth K08.9
  - hard tissues K03.9
    - specified NEC K03.89
  - pulp NEC K04.99
  - specified NEC K08.89
- Tourette's F95.2
- trachea NEC J39.8
- tricuspid I07.9
  - nonrheumatic I36.9
- triglyceride-storage E75.5
- trophoblastic — *see* Mole, hydatidiform
- tsutsugamushi A75.3
- tube (fallopian) (noninflammatory) N83.9
  - inflammatory — *see* Salpingitis
  - specified NEC N83.8
- tuberculous NEC — *see* Tuberculosis
- tubo-ovarian (noninflammatory) N83.9
  - inflammatory — *see* Salpingo-oophoritis
  - specified NEC N83.8
- tubotympanic, chronic — *see* Otitis, media, suppurative, chronic, tubotympanic
- tubulo-interstitial N15.9
  - specified NEC N15.8
- tympanum — *see* Disorder, tympanic membrane
- Uhl's Q24.8
- Underwood's (sclerema neonatorum) P83.0
- Unverricht (-Lundborg) — *see* Epilepsy, generalized, idiopathic
- Urbach-Oppenheim (necrobiosis lipoidica diabeticorum) — *see* E08-E13 with .620
- ureter N28.9
  - in (due to)
    - schistosomiasis (bilharziasis) B65.0 [N29]
- urethra N36.9
  - specified NEC N36.8
- urinary (tract) N39.9
  - bladder N32.9
    - specified NEC N32.89
  - specified NEC N39.8
- uterus (noninflammatory) N85.9
  - infective — *see* Endometritis
  - inflammatory — *see* Endometritis
  - specified NEC N85.8
- uveal tract (anterior) H21.9
  - posterior H31.9
- vagabond's B85.1
- vagina, vaginal (noninflammatory) N89.9

Disease, diseased — *continued*
- vagina, vaginal — *continued*
  - inflammatory NEC N76.89
  - specified NEC N89.8
- valve, valvular I38
  - multiple I08.9
    - specified NEC I08.8
- van Creveld-von Gierke (glycogenosis I) E74.01
- vas deferens N50.9
- vascular I99.9
  - arteriosclerotic — *see* Arteriosclerosis
  - ciliary body NEC — *see* Disorder, iris, vascular
  - hypertensive — *see* Hypertension
  - iris NEC — *see* Disorder, iris, vascular
  - obliterative I77.1
    - peripheral I73.9
  - occlusive I99.8
  - peripheral (occlusive) I73.9
    - in diabetes mellitus — *see* E08-E13 with .51
- vasomotor I73.9
- vasospastic I73.9
- vein I87.9
- venereal — *see also* Disease, sexually transmitted A64
  - chlamydial NEC A56.8
    - anus A56.3
    - genitourinary NOS A56.2
    - pharynx A56.4
    - rectum A56.3
  - fifth A55
  - sixth A55
  - specified nature or type NEC A63.8
- vertebra, vertebral — *see also* Spondylopathy
  - disc — *see* Disorder, disc
- vibration — *see* Vibration, adverse effects
- viral, virus — *see also* Disease, by type of virus B34.9
  - arbovirus NOS A94
  - arthropod-borne NOS A94
  - congenital P35.9
    - specified NEC P35.8
  - Hanta (with renal manifestations) (Dobrava) (Puumala) (Seoul) A98.5
    - with pulmonary manifestations (Andes) (Bayou) (Bermejo) (Black Creek Canal) (Choclo) (Juquitiba) (Laguna negra) (Lechiguanas) (New York) (Oran) (Sin nombre) B33.4
  - Hantaan (Korean hemorrhagic fever) A98.5
  - human immunodeficiency (HIV) B20
  - Kunjin A83.4
  - nonarthropod-borne NOS B34.9
  - Powassan A84.81
  - Rocio (encephalitis) A83.6
  - Sin nombre (Hantavirus) (cardio)-pulmonary syndrome B33.4
  - Tahyna B33.8
  - vesicular stomatitis A93.8
- vitreous H43.9
  - specified NEC H43.89
- vocal cord J38.3
- Volkmann's, acquired T79.6 ☑
- von Eulenburg's (congenital paramyotonia) G71.19
- von Gierke's (glycogenosis I) E74.01
- von Graefe's — *see* Strabismus, paralytic, ophthalmoplegia, progressive
- von Willebrand (-Jürgens) (angiohemophilia) D68.00
  - acquired D68.04
  - platelet-type D68.09
  - pseudo D68.09
  - specified NEC D68.09
  - type 1 D68.01
  - type 1C D68.01
  - type 2 D68.029
    - type 2A D68.020
    - type 2B D68.021
    - type 2M D68.022
    - type 2N D68.023
  - type 3 D68.03
- Vrolik's (osteogenesis imperfecta) Q78.0
- vulva (noninflammatory) N90.9
  - inflammatory NEC N76.89
  - specified NEC N90.89
- Wallgren's (obstruction of splenic vein with collateral circulation) I87.8
- Wassilieff's (leptospiral jaundice) A27.0
- wasting NEC R64
  - due to malnutrition E43
    - with marasmus E41
- Waterhouse-Friderichsen A39.1
- Wegner's (syphilitic osteochondritis) A50.02

Disease, diseased — *continued*
- Weil's (leptospiral jaundice of lung) A27.Ø
- Weir Mitchell's (erythromelalgia) I73.81
- Werdnig-Hoffmann G12.Ø
- Wermer's E31.21
- Werner-His (trench fever) A79.Ø
- Werner-Schultz (neutropenic splenomegaly) D73.81
- Wernicke-Posadas B38.9
- whipworm B79
- white blood cells D72.9
  - specified NEC D72.89
- white matter R9Ø.82
- white-spot, meaning lichen sclerosus et atrophicus L9Ø.Ø
  - penis N48.Ø
  - vulva N9Ø.4
- Wilkie's K55.1
- Wilkinson-Sneddon (subcorneal pustular dermatosis) L13.1
- Willis' — *see* Diabetes
- Wilson's (hepatolenticular degeneration) E83.Ø1
- woolsorter's A22.1
- yaba monkey tumor BØ8.72
- yaba pox (virus) BØ8.72
- Zika virus A92.5
  - congenital P35.4
- zoonotic, bacterial A28.9
  - specified type NEC A28.8

Disfigurement (due to scar) L9Ø.5
Disgerminoma — *see* Dysgerminoma
DISH (diffuse idiopathic skeletal hyperostosis) — *see* Hyperostosis, ankylosing
Disinsertion, retina — *see* Detachment, retina
Dislocatable hip, congenital Q65.6
Dislocation (articular)
- with fracture — *see* Fracture
- acromioclavicular (joint) S43.1Ø-☑
  - with displacement
    - 1ØØ%-2ØØ% S43.12-☑
    - more than 2ØØ% S43.13-☑
  - inferior S43.14-☑
  - posterior S43.15-☑
- ankle S93.Ø-☑
- astragalus — *see* Dislocation, ankle
- atlantoaxial S13.121 ☑
- atlantooccipital S13.111 ☑
- atloidooccipital S13.111 ☑
- breast bone S23.29 ☑
- capsule, joint — *code by* site under Dislocation
- carpal (bone) — *see* Dislocation, wrist
- carpometacarpal (joint) NEC S63.Ø5-☑
  - thumb S63.Ø4-☑
- cartilage (joint) — *code by* site under Dislocation
- cervical spine (vertebra) — *see* Dislocation, vertebra, cervical
- chronic — *see* Dislocation, recurrent
- clavicle — *see* Dislocation, acromioclavicular joint
- coccyx S33.2
- congenital NEC Q68.8
- coracoid — *see* Dislocation, shoulder
- costal cartilage S23.29 ☑
- costochondral S23.29 ☑
- cricoarytenoid articulation S13.29 ☑
- cricothyroid articulation S13.29 ☑
- dorsal vertebra — *see* Dislocation, vertebra, thoracic
- ear ossicle — *see* Discontinuity, ossicles, ear
- elbow S53.1Ø-☑
  - congenital Q68.8
  - pathological — *see* Dislocation, pathological NEC, elbow
  - radial head alone — *see* Dislocation, radial head
  - recurrent — *see* Dislocation, recurrent, elbow
  - traumatic S53.1Ø-☑
    - anterior S53.11-☑
    - lateral S53.14-☑
    - medial S53.13-☑
    - posterior S53.12-☑
    - specified type NEC S53.19-☑
- eye, nontraumatic — *see* Luxation, globe
- eyeball, nontraumatic — *see* Luxation, globe
- femur
  - distal end — *see* Dislocation, knee
  - proximal end — *see* Dislocation, hip
- fibula
  - distal end — *see* Dislocation, ankle
  - proximal end — *see* Dislocation, knee
- finger S63.25-☑

Dislocation — *continued*
- finger — *continued*
  - index S63.25-☑
  - interphalangeal S63.27-☑
    - distal S63.29-☑
      - index S63.29-☑
      - little S63.29-☑
      - middle S63.29-☑
      - ring S63.29-☑
    - index S63.27-☑
    - little S63.27-☑
    - middle S63.27-☑
    - proximal S63.28-☑
      - index S63.28-☑
      - little S63.28-☑
      - middle S63.28-☑
      - ring S63.28-☑
    - ring S63.27-☑
  - little S63.25-☑
  - metacarpophalangeal S63.26-☑
    - index S63.26-☑
    - little S63.26-☑
    - middle S63.26-☑
    - ring S63.26-☑
  - middle S63.25-☑
  - recurrent — *see* Dislocation, recurrent, finger
  - ring S63.25-☑
  - thumb — *see* Dislocation, thumb
- foot S93.3Ø-☑
  - recurrent — *see* Dislocation, recurrent, foot
  - specified site NEC S93.33-☑
  - tarsal joint S93.31-☑
  - tarsometatarsal joint S93.32-☑
  - toe — *see* Dislocation, toe
- fracture — *see* Fracture
- glenohumeral (joint) — *see* Dislocation, shoulder
- glenoid — *see* Dislocation, shoulder
- habitual — *see* Dislocation, recurrent
- hip S73.ØØ-☑
  - anterior S73.Ø3-☑
    - obturator S73.Ø2-☑
  - central S73.Ø4-☑
  - congenital (total) Q65.2
    - bilateral Q65.1
    - partial Q65.5
      - bilateral Q65.4
      - unilateral Q65.3-☑
    - unilateral Q65.Ø-☑
  - developmental M24.85-☑
  - pathological — *see* Dislocation, pathological NEC, hip
  - posterior S73.Ø1-☑
  - recurrent — *see* Dislocation, recurrent, hip
- humerus, proximal end — *see* Dislocation, shoulder
- incomplete — *see* Subluxation, by site
- incus — *see* Discontinuity, ossicles, ear
- infracoracoid — *see* Dislocation, shoulder
- innominate (pubic junction) (sacral junction) S33.39 ☑
  - acetabulum — *see* Dislocation, hip
- interphalangeal (joint(s))
  - finger S63.279 ☑
    - distal S63.29-☑
      - index S63.29-☑
      - little S63.29-☑
      - middle S63.29-☑
      - ring S63.29-☑
    - index S63.27-☑
    - little S63.27-☑
    - middle S63.27-☑
    - proximal S63.28-☑
      - index S63.28-☑
      - little S63.28-☑
      - middle S63.28-☑
      - ring S63.28-☑
    - ring S63.27-☑
  - foot or toe — *see* Dislocation, toe
  - thumb S63.12-☑
- jaw (cartilage) (meniscus) SØ3.Ø-☑
- joint prosthesis — *see* Complications, joint prosthesis, mechanical, displacement, by site
- knee S83.1Ø6 ☑
  - cap — *see* Dislocation, patella
  - congenital Q68.2
  - old M23.8X-☑
  - patella — *see* Dislocation, patella

Dislocation — *continued*
- knee — *continued*
  - pathological — *see* Dislocation, pathological NEC, knee
  - proximal tibia
    - anteriorly S83.11-☑
    - laterally S83.14-☑
    - medially S83.13-☑
    - posteriorly S83.12-☑
  - recurrent — *see also* Derangement, knee, specified NEC
  - specified type NEC S83.19-☑
- lacrimal gland HØ4.16-☑
- lens (complete) H27.1Ø
  - anterior H27.12-☑
  - congenital Q12.1
  - ocular implant — *see* Complications, intraocular lens
  - partial H27.11-☑
  - posterior H27.13-☑
  - traumatic SØ5.8X-☑
- ligament — *code by* site under Dislocation
- lumbar (vertebra) — *see* Dislocation, vertebra, lumbar
- lumbosacral (vertebra) — *see also* Dislocation, vertebra, lumbar
  - congenital Q76.49
- mandible SØ3.Ø-☑
- meniscus (knee) — *see* Tear, meniscus
  - other sites - code by site under Dislocation
- metacarpal (bone)
  - distal end — *see* Dislocation, finger
  - proximal end S63.Ø6-☑
- metacarpophalangeal (joint)
  - finger S63.26-☑
    - index S63.26-☑
    - little S63.26-☑
    - middle S63.26-☑
    - ring S63.26-☑
  - thumb S63.11-☑
- metatarsal (bone) — *see* Dislocation, foot
- metatarsophalangeal (joint(s)) — *see* Dislocation, toe
- midcarpal (joint) S63.Ø3-☑
- midtarsal (joint) — *see* Dislocation, foot
- neck S13.2Ø ☑
  - specified site NEC S13.29 ☑
  - vertebra — *see* Dislocation, vertebra, cervical
- nose (septal cartilage) SØ3.1 ☑
- occipitoatloid S13.111 ☑
- old — *see* Derangement, joint, specified type NEC
- ossicles, ear — *see* Discontinuity, ossicles, ear
- partial — *see* Subluxation, by site
- patella S83.ØØ6 ☑
  - congenital Q74.1
  - lateral S83.Ø1-☑
  - recurrent (nontraumatic) M22.Ø-☑
    - incomplete M22.1-☑
  - specified type NEC S83.Ø9-☑
- pathological NEC M24.3Ø
  - ankle M24.37-☑
  - elbow M24.32-☑
  - foot joint M24.37-☑
  - hand joint M24.34-☑
  - hip M24.35-☑
  - knee M24.36-☑
  - lumbosacral joint — *see* subcategory M53.2 ☑
  - pelvic region — *see* Dislocation, pathological, hip
  - sacroiliac — *see* subcategory M53.2 ☑
  - shoulder M24.31-☑
  - specified site NEC M24.39
  - wrist M24.33-☑
- pelvis NEC S33.3Ø ☑
  - specified NEC S33.39 ☑
- phalanx
  - finger or hand — *see* Dislocation, finger
  - foot or toe — *see* Dislocation, toe
- prosthesis, internal — *see* Complications, prosthetic device, by site, mechanical
- radial head S53.ØØ6 ☑
  - anterior S53.Ø1-☑
  - posterior S53.Ø2-☑
  - specified type NEC S53.Ø9-☑
- radiocarpal (joint) S63.Ø2-☑
- radiohumeral (joint) — *see* Dislocation, radial head
- radioulnar (joint)
  - distal S63.Ø1-☑
  - proximal — *see* Dislocation, elbow

Dislocation — *continued*
 radius
  distal end — *see* Dislocation, wrist
  proximal end — *see* Dislocation, radial head
 recurrent M24.40
  ankle M24.47- ✓
  elbow M24.42- ✓
  finger M24.44- ✓
  foot joint M24.47- ✓
  hand joint M24.44- ✓
  hip M24.45- ✓
  knee M24.46- ✓
   patella — *see* Dislocation, patella, recurrent
  patella — *see* Dislocation, patella, recurrent
  sacroiliac — *see* subcategory M53.2 ✓
  shoulder M24.41- ✓
  specified site NEC M24.49
  toe M24.47- ✓
  vertebra — *see also* subcategory M43.5 ✓
   atlantoaxial M43.4
    with myelopathy M43.3
  wrist M24.43- ✓
 rib (cartilage) S23.29 ✓
 sacrococcygeal S33.2 ✓
 sacroiliac (joint) (ligament) S33.2 ✓
  congenital Q74.2
  recurrent — *see* subcategory M53.2 ✓
 sacrum S33.2 ✓
 scaphoid (bone) (hand) (wrist) — *see* Dislocation, wrist
  foot — *see* Dislocation, foot
 scapula — *see* Dislocation, shoulder, girdle, scapula
 semilunar cartilage, knee — *see* Tear, meniscus
 septal cartilage (nose) S03.1 ✓
 septum (nasal) (old) J34.2
 sesamoid bone — *code by* site under Dislocation
 shoulder (blade) (ligament) (joint) (traumatic)
   S43.006 ✓
  acromioclavicular — *see* Dislocation, acromioclavicular
  chronic — *see* Dislocation, recurrent, shoulder
  congenital Q68.8
  girdle S43.30- ✓
   scapula S43.31- ✓
   specified site NEC S43.39- ✓
  humerus S43.00- ✓
   anterior S43.01- ✓
   inferior S43.03- ✓
   posterior S43.02- ✓
  pathological — *see* Dislocation, pathological NEC, shoulder
  recurrent — *see* Dislocation, recurrent, shoulder
  specified type NEC S43.08- ✓
 spine
  cervical — *see* Dislocation, vertebra, cervical
  congenital Q76.49
  due to birth trauma P11.5
  lumbar — *see* Dislocation, vertebra, lumbar
  thoracic — *see* Dislocation, vertebra, thoracic
 spontaneous — *see* Dislocation, pathological
 sternoclavicular (joint) S43.206 ✓
  anterior S43.21- ✓
  posterior S43.22- ✓
 sternum S23.29 ✓
 subglenoid — *see* Dislocation, shoulder
 symphysis pubis S33.4 ✓
 talus — *see* Dislocation, ankle
 tarsal (bone(s)) (joint(s)) — *see* Dislocation, foot
 tarsometatarsal (joint(s)) — *see* Dislocation, foot
 temporomandibular (joint) S03.0- ✓
 thigh, proximal end — *see* Dislocation, hip
 thorax S23.20 ✓
  specified site NEC S23.29 ✓
  vertebra — *see* Dislocation, vertebra
 thumb S63.10- ✓
  interphalangeal joint — *see* Dislocation, interphalangeal (joint), thumb
  metacarpophalangeal joint — *see* Dislocation, metacarpophalangeal (joint), thumb
 thyroid cartilage S13.29 ✓
 tibia
  distal end — *see* Dislocation, ankle
  proximal end — *see* Dislocation, knee
 tibiofibular (joint)
  distal — *see* Dislocation, ankle
  superior — *see* Dislocation, knee
 toe(s) S93.106 ✓

Dislocation — *continued*
 toe(s) — *continued*
  great S93.10- ✓
   interphalangeal joint S93.11- ✓
   metatarsophalangeal joint S93.12- ✓
  interphalangeal joint S93.119 ✓
  lesser S93.106 ✓
   interphalangeal joint S93.11- ✓
   metatarsophalangeal joint S93.12- ✓
  metatarsophalangeal joint S93.12- ✓
 tooth S03.2 ✓
 trachea S23.29 ✓
 ulna
  distal end S63.07- ✓
  proximal end — *see* Dislocation, elbow
 ulnohumeral (joint) — *see* Dislocation, elbow
 vertebra (articular process) (body) (traumatic)
  cervical S13.101 ✓
   atlantoaxial joint S13.121 ✓
   atlantooccipital joint S13.111 ✓
   atloidooccipital joint S13.111 ✓
   joint between
    C0 and C1 S13.111 ✓
    C1 and C2 S13.121 ✓
    C2 and C3 S13.131 ✓
    C3 and C4 S13.141 ✓
    C4 and C5 S13.151 ✓
    C5 and C6 S13.161 ✓
    C6 and C7 S13.171 ✓
    C7 and T1 S13.181 ✓
   occipitoatloid joint S13.111 ✓
  congenital Q76.49
  lumbar S33.101 ✓
   joint between
    L1 and L2 S33.111 ✓
    L2 and L3 S33.121 ✓
    L3 and L4 S33.131 ✓
    L4 and L5 S33.141 ✓
  nontraumatic — *see* Displacement, intervertebral disc
  partial — *see* Subluxation, by site
  recurrent NEC — *see* subcategory M43.5 ✓
  thoracic S23.101 ✓
   joint between
    T1 and T2 S23.111 ✓
    T2 and T3 S23.121 ✓
    T3 and T4 S23.123 ✓
    T4 and T5 S23.131 ✓
    T5 and T6 S23.133 ✓
    T6 and T7 S23.141 ✓
    T7 and T8 S23.143 ✓
    T8 and T9 S23.151 ✓
    T9 and T10 S23.153 ✓
    T10 and T11 S23.161 ✓
    T11 and T12 S23.163 ✓
    T12 and L1 S23.171 ✓
 wrist (carpal bone) S63.006 ✓
  carpometacarpal joint — *see* Dislocation, carpometacarpal (joint)
  distal radioulnar joint — *see* Dislocation, radioulnar (joint), distal
  metacarpal bone, proximal — *see* Dislocation, metacarpal (bone), proximal end
  midcarpal — *see* Dislocation, midcarpal (joint)
  radiocarpal joint — *see* Dislocation, radiocarpal (joint)
  recurrent — *see* Dislocation, recurrent, wrist
  specified site NEC S63.09- ✓
  ulna — *see* Dislocation, ulna, distal end
 xiphoid cartilage S23.29 ✓
Disorder (of) — *see also* Disease
 acantholytic L11.9
  specified NEC L11.8
 acute
  psychotic — *see* Psychosis, acute
  stress F43.0
 adjustment (grief) F43.20
  with
   anxiety F43.22
    with depressed mood F43.23
   conduct disturbance F43.24
    with emotional disturbance F43.25
   depressed mood F43.21
    with anxiety F43.23
   other specified symptom F43.29
 adrenal (capsule) (gland) (medullary) E27.9

Disorder — *continued*
 adrenal — *continued*
  specified NEC E27.8
 adrenogenital — *see also* Adrenogenital syndrome E25.9
  drug-induced E25.8
  iatrogenic E25.8
  idiopathic E25.8
 adult personality (and behavior) F69
  specified NEC F68.8
 affective (mood) — *see* Disorder, mood
 aggressive, unsocialized F91.1
 alcohol use
  mild F10.10
   with
    alcohol intoxication F10.129
     delirium F10.121
    alcohol-induced
     anxiety disorder F10.180
     bipolar and related disorder F10.14
     depressive disorder F10.14
     psychotic disorder F10.159
     sexual dysfunction F10.181
     sleep disorder F10.182
   in remission (early) (sustained) F10.11
  moderate or severe F10.20
   with
    alcohol intoxication F10.229
     delirium F10.221
    alcohol-induced
     anxiety disorder F10.280
     bipolar and related disorder F10.24
     depressive disorder F10.24
     major neurocognitive disorder, amnestic-confabulatory type F10.26
     major neurocognitive disorder, non-amnestic-confabulatory type F10.27
     mild neurocognitive disorder F10.288
     psychotic disorder F10.259
     sexual dysfunction F10.281
     sleep disorder F10.282
   in remission (early) (sustained) F10.21
 alcohol-related F10.99
  with
   amnestic disorder, persisting F10.96
   anxiety disorder F10.980
   dementia, persisting F10.97
   intoxication F10.929
    with delirium F10.921
    uncomplicated F10.920
   mood disorder F10.94
   other specified F10.988
   psychotic disorder F10.959
    with
     delusions F10.950
     hallucinations F10.951
   sexual dysfunction F10.981
   sleep disorder F10.982
 allergic — *see* Allergy
 alveolar NEC J84.09
 amino-acid
  cystathioninuria E72.19
  cystinosis E72.04
  cystinuria E72.01
  glycinuria E72.09
  homocystinuria E72.11
  metabolism — *see* Disturbance, metabolism, amino-acid
   specified NEC E72.89
  neonatal, transitory P74.8
  renal transport NEC E72.09
  transport NEC E72.09
 amnesic, amnestic
  alcohol-induced F10.96
   with dependence F10.26
  due to (secondary to) general medical condition F04
  psychoactive NEC-induced F19.96
   with
    abuse F19.16
    dependence F19.26
  sedative, hypnotic or anxiolytic-induced F13.96
   with dependence F13.26
 amphetamine (or other stimulant) use
  mild
   with
    amphetamine, cocaine, or other stimulant intoxication
     with perceptual disturbances F15.122

Disorder — *continued*
  amphetamine use — *continued*
    mild — *continued*
      with — *continued*
        amphetamine, cocaine, or other stimulant
            intoxication — *continued*
          without perceptual disturbances F15.129
        amphetamine (or other stimulant) -induced
          anxiety disorder F15.180
          bipolar and related disorder F15.14
          depressive disorder F15.14
          obsessive-compulsive and related disor-
              der F15.188
          psychotic disorder F15.159
          sexual dysfunction F15.181
        intoxication delirium F15.121
    moderate or severe
      with
        amphetamine, cocaine, or other stimulant
            intoxication
          with perceptual disturbances F15.222
          without perceptual disturbances F15.229
        amphetamine (or other stimulant) -induced
          anxiety disorder F15.280
          bipolar and related disorder F15.24
          depressive disorder F15.24
          obsessive-compulsive and related disor-
              der F15.288
          psychotic disorder F15.259
          sexual dysfunction F15.281
        intoxication delirium F15.221
  amphetamine-type substance use
    mild F15.10
      in remission (early) (sustained) F15.11
    moderate F15.20
      in remission (early) (sustained) F15.21
    severe F15.20
      in remission (early) (sustained) F15.21
  anaerobic glycolysis with anemia D55.29
  anxiety F41.9
    due to (secondary to)
      alcohol F10.980
        in
          abuse F10.180
          dependence F10.280
      amphetamine F15.980
        in
          abuse F15.180
          dependence F15.280
      anxiolytic F13.980
        in
          abuse F13.180
          dependence F13.280
      caffeine F15.980
        in
          abuse F15.180
          dependence F15.280
      cannabis F12.980
        in
          abuse F12.180
          dependence F12.280
      cocaine F14.980
        in
          abuse F14.180
          dependence F14.180
      general medical condition F06.4
      hallucinogen F16.980
        in
          abuse F16.180
          dependence F16.280
      hypnotic F13.980
        in
          abuse F13.180
          dependence F13.280
      inhalant F18.980
        in
          abuse F18.180
          dependence F18.280
      phencyclidine F16.980
        in
          abuse F16.180
          dependence F16.280
      psychoactive substance NEC F19.980
        in
          abuse F19.180
          dependence F19.280
      sedative F13.980
        in
          abuse F13.180

Disorder — *continued*
  anxiety — *continued*
    due to — *continued*
      sedative — *continued*
        in — *continued*
          dependence F13.280
      volatile solvents F18.980
        in
          abuse F18.180
          dependence F18.280
    generalized F41.1
    illness F45.21
    mixed
      with depression (mild) F41.8
      specified NEC F41.3
    organic F06.4
    phobic F40.9
      of childhood F40.8
    specified NEC F41.8
  aortic valve — *see* Endocarditis, aortic
  aromatic amino-acid metabolism E70.9
    specified NEC E70.89
  arteriole NEC I77.89
  artery NEC I77.89
  articulation — *see* Disorder, joint
  attachment (childhood)
    disinhibited F94.2
    reactive F94.1
  attention-deficit hyperactivity (adolescent) (adult)
      (child) F90.9
    combined
      presentation F90.2
      type F90.2
    hyperactive
      impulsive presentation F90.1
      type F90.1
    inattentive
      presentation F90.0
      type F90.0
    specified type NEC F90.8
  attention-deficit without hyperactivity (adolescent)
      (adult) (child) F98.8
  auditory processing (central) H93.25
  autism spectrum F84.0
  autistic F84.0
  autoimmune D89.89
  autonomic nervous system G90.9
    specified NEC G90.8
  avoidant
    child or adolescent F40.10
    restrictive food intake F50.82
  balance
    acid-base E87.8
      mixed E87.4
    electrolyte E87.8
    fluid NEC E87.8
  behavioral (disruptive) — *see* Disorder, conduct
  bereavement, persistent complex F43.81
  beta-amino-acid metabolism E72.89
  bile acid and cholesterol metabolism E78.70
    Barth syndrome E78.71
    other specified E78.79
    Smith-Lemli-Opitz syndrome E78.72
  bilirubin excretion E80.6
  binge eating F50.81
  binocular
    movement H51.9
      convergence
        excess H51.12
        insufficiency H51.11
      internuclear ophthalmoplegia — *see* Ophthalmo-
          plegia, internuclear
      palsy of conjugate gaze H51.0
      specified type NEC H51.8
    vision NEC — *see* Disorder, vision, binocular
  bipolar (I) seasonal) (type I) F31.9
    and related due to a known physiological condition
      with
        manic features F06.33
        manic- or hypomanic-like episodes F06.33
        mixed features F06.34
    current (or most recent) episode
      depressed F31.9
        with psychotic features F31.5
        without psychotic features F31.30
          mild F31.31
          moderate F31.32
          severe (without psychotic features) F31.4
            with psychotic features F31.5

Disorder — *continued*
  bipolar seasonal — *continued*
    current episode — *continued*
      hypomanic F31.0
      manic F31.9
        with psychotic features F31.2
        without psychotic features F31.10
          mild F31.11
          moderate F31.12
          severe (without psychotic features)
              F31.13
            with psychotic features F31.2
      mixed F31.60
        mild F31.61
        moderate F31.62
        severe (without psychotic features) F31.63
          with psychotic features F31.64
      severe depression (without psychotic features)
          F31.4
        with psychotic features F31.5
    II (type 2) F31.81
    in remission (currently) F31.70
      in full remission
        most recent episode
          depressed F31.76
          hypomanic F31.72
          manic F31.74
          mixed F31.78
      in partial remission
        most recent episode
          depressed F31.75
          hypomanic F31.71
          manic F31.73
          mixed F31.77
    organic F06.30
    single manic episode F30.9
      mild F30.11
      moderate F30.12
      severe (without psychotic symptoms) F30.13
        with psychotic symptoms F30.2
    specified NEC F31.89
  bladder N32.9
    functional NEC N31.9
    in schistosomiasis B65.0 *[N33]*
    specified NEC N32.89
  bleeding D68.9
  blood D75.9
    in congenital early syphilis A50.09 *[D77]*
  body dysmorphic F45.22
  bone M89.9
    continuity M84.9
      specified type NEC M84.80
        ankle M84.87- ☑
        fibula M84.86- ☑
        foot M84.87- ☑
        hand M84.84- ☑
        humerus M84.82- ☑
        neck M84.88
        pelvis M84.859
        radius M84.83- ☑
        rib M84.88
        shoulder M84.81- ☑
        skull M84.88
        thigh M84.85- ☑
        tibia M84.86- ☑
        ulna M84.83- ☑
        vertebra M84.88
    density and structure M85.9
    cyst — *see also* Cyst, bone, specified type NEC
      aneurysmal — *see* Cyst, bone, aneurysmal
      solitary — *see* Cyst, bone, solitary
    diffuse idiopathic skeletal hyperostosis — *see*
        Hyperostosis, ankylosing
    fibrous dysplasia (monostotic) — *see* Dysplasia,
        fibrous, bone
    fluorosis — *see* Fluorosis, skeletal
    hyperostosis of skull M85.2
    osteitis condensans — *see* Osteitis, condensans
    specified type NEC M85.8- ☑
      ankle M85.87- ☑
      foot M85.87- ☑
      forearm M85.83- ☑
      hand M85.84- ☑
      lower leg M85.86- ☑
      multiple sites M85.89
      neck M85.88
      rib M85.88
      shoulder M85.81- ☑

Disorder — *continued*
  bone — *continued*
    density and structure — *continued*
      specified type — *continued*
        skull M85.88
        thigh M85.85- ☑
        upper arm M85.82- ☑
        vertebra M85.88
    development and growth NEC M89.20
      carpus M89.24- ☑
      clavicle M89.21- ☑
      femur M89.25- ☑
      fibula M89.26- ☑
      finger M89.24- ☑
      humerus M89.22- ☑
      ilium M89.259
      ischium M89.259
      metacarpus M89.24- ☑
      metatarsus M89.27- ☑
      multiple sites M89.29
      neck M89.28
      radius M89.23- ☑
      rib M89.28
      scapula M89.21- ☑
      skull M89.28
      tarsus M89.27- ☑
      tibia M89.26- ☑
      toe M89.27- ☑
      ulna M89.23- ☑
      vertebra M89.28
      specified type NEC M89.8X- ☑
  brachial plexus G54.0
  branched-chain amino-acid metabolism E71.2
    specified NEC E71.19
  breast N64.9
    agalactia — *see* Agalactia
    associated with
      lactation O92.70
        specified NEC O92.79
      pregnancy O92.20
        specified NEC O92.29
      puerperium O92.20
        specified NEC O92.29
    cracked nipple — *see* Cracked nipple
    galactorrhea — *see* Galactorrhea
    hypogalactia O92.4
    lactation disorder NEC O92.79
    mastitis — *see* Mastitis
    nipple infection — *see* Infection, nipple
    retracted nipple — *see* Retraction, nipple
    specified type NEC N64.89
  Briquet's F45.0
  bullous, in diseases classified elsewhere L14
  caffeine use
    mild
      with
        caffeine-induced
          anxiety disorder F15.180
          sleep disorder F15.182
    moderate or severe
      with
        caffeine-induced
          anxiety disorder F15.280
          sleep disorder F15.282
  cannabis use
    mild F12.10
      with
        cannabis intoxication delirium F12.121
          with perceptual disturbances F12.122
          without perceptual disturbances F12.129
        cannabis-induced
          anxiety disorder F12.180
          psychotic disorder F12.159
          sleep disorder F12.188
      in remission (early) (sustained) F12.11
    moderate or severe F12.20
      with
        cannabis intoxication
          with perceptual disturbances F12.222
          without perceptual disturbances F12.229
        cannabis-induced
          anxiety disorder F12.280
          psychotic disorder F12.259
          sleep disorder F12.288
        delirium F12.221
      in remission (early) (sustained) F12.21
  carbohydrate
    absorption, intestinal NEC E74.39

Disorder — *continued*
  carbohydrate — *continued*
    metabolism (congenital) E74.9
      specified NEC E74.89
  cardiac, functional I51.89
  carnitine metabolism E71.40
  cartilage M94.9
    articular NEC — *see* Derangement, joint, articular
      cartilage
    chondrocalcinosis — *see* Chondrocalcinosis
    specified type NEC M94.8X- ☑
      articular — *see* Derangement, joint, articular
        cartilage
      multiple sites M94.8X0
  catatonia (due to known physiological condition) (with another mental disorder) F06.1
  catatonic
    due to (secondary to) known physiological condition F06.1
    organic F06.1
  central auditory processing H93.25
  cervical
    region NEC M53.82
    root (nerve) NEC G54.2
  character NOS F60.9
  childhood disintegrative NEC F84.3
  cholesterol and bile acid metabolism E78.70
    Barth syndrome E78.71
    other specified E78.79
    Smith-Lemli-Opitz syndrome E78.72
  choroid H31.9
    atrophy — *see* Atrophy, choroid
    degeneration — *see* Degeneration, choroid
    detachment — *see* Detachment, choroid
    dystrophy — *see* Dystrophy, choroid
    hemorrhage — *see* Hemorrhage, choroid
    rupture — *see* Rupture, choroid
    scar — *see* Scar, chorioretinal
    solar retinopathy — *see* Retinopathy, solar
    specified type NEC H31.8
  ciliary body — *see* Disorder, iris
    degeneration — *see* Degeneration, ciliary body
  coagulation (factor) — *see also* Defect, coagulation D68.9
    newborn, transient P61.6
  cocaine use
    mild F14.10
      with
        amphetamine, cocaine, or other stimulant intoxication
          with perceptual disturbances F14.122
          without perceptual disturbances F14.129
        cocaine intoxication delirium F14.121
        cocaine-induced
          anxiety disorder F14.180
          bipolar and related disorder F14.14
          depressive disorder F14.14
          obsessive-compulsive and related disorder F14.188
          psychotic disorder F14.159
          sexual dysfunction F14.181
          sleep disorder F14.182
      in remission (early) (sustained) F14.11
    moderate or severe F14.20
      with
        amphetamine, cocaine, or other stimulant intoxication
          with perceptual disturbances F14.222
          without perceptual disturbances F14.229
        cocaine intoxication delirium F14.221
        cocaine-induced
          anxiety disorder F14.280
          bipolar and related disorder F14.24
          depressive disorder F14.24
          obsessive-compulsive and related disorder F14.288
          psychotic disorder F14.259
          sexual dysfunction F14.281
          sleep disorder F14.282
      in remission (early) (sustained) F14.21
  coccyx NEC M53.3
  cognitive F09
    due to (secondary to) general medical condition F09
    persisting R41.89
      due to
        alcohol F10.97
          with dependence F10.27
        anxiolytics F13.97

Disorder — *continued*
  cognitive — *continued*
    persisting — *continued*
      due to — *continued*
        anxiolytics — *continued*
          with dependence F13.27
        hypnotics F13.97
          with dependence F13.27
        sedatives F13.97
          with dependence F13.27
        specified substance NEC F19.97
          with
            abuse F19.17
            dependence F19.27
  communication F80.9
    social pragmatic F80.82
  conduct (childhood) F91.9
    adjustment reaction — *see* Disorder, adjustment
    adolescent onset type F91.2
    childhood onset type F91.1
    compulsive F63.9
    confined to family context F91.0
    depressive F91.8
    group type F91.2
    hyperkinetic — *see* Disorder, attention-deficit hyperactivity
    oppositional defiance F91.3
    socialized F91.2
    solitary aggressive type F91.1
    specified NEC F91.8
    unsocialized (aggressive) F91.1
  conduction, heart I45.9
  congenital glycosylation (CDG) E74.89
  conjunctiva H11.9
    infection — *see* Conjunctivitis
  connective tissue, localized L94.9
    specified NEC L94.8
  conversion (functional neurological symptom disorder)
    with
      abnormal movement F44.4
      anesthesia or sensory loss F44.6
      attacks or seizures F44.5
      mixed symptoms F44.7
      special sensory symptoms F44.6
      speech symptoms F44.4
      swallowing symptoms F44.4
      weakness or paralysis F44.4
  convulsive (secondary) — *see* Convulsions
  cornea H18.9
    deformity — *see* Deformity, cornea
    degeneration — *see* Degeneration, cornea
    deposits — *see* Deposit, cornea
    due to contact lens H18.82- ☑
      specified as edema — *see* Edema, cornea
    edema — *see* Edema, cornea
    keratitis — *see* Keratitis
    keratoconjunctivitis — *see* Keratoconjunctivitis
    membrane change — *see* Change, corneal membrane
    neovascularization — *see* Neovascularization, cornea
    scar — *see* Opacity, cornea
    specified type NEC H18.89- ☑
    ulcer — *see* Ulcer, cornea
  corpus cavernosum N48.9
  cranial nerve — *see* Disorder, nerve, cranial
  Cyclin-Dependent Kinase-Like 5 Deficiency (CDKL5) G40.42
  cyclothymic F34.0
  defiant oppositional F91.3
  delusional (persistent) (systematized) F22
    induced F24
  depersonalization F48.1
  depressive F32.A
    due to known physiological condition
      with
        depressive features F06.31
        major depressive-like episode F06.32
        mixed features F06.34
    major F32.9
      with psychotic symptoms F32.3
      in remission (full) F32.5
        partial F32.4
      recurrent F33.9
        with psychotic features F33.3
      single episode F32.9
        mild F32.0
        moderate F32.1

☑ Additional Character Required — Refer to the Tabular List for Character Selection

Disorder — *continued*
  depressive — *continued*
    major — *continued*
      single episode — *continued*
        severe (without psychotic symptoms) F32.2
          with psychotic symptoms F32.3
    organic F06.31
    persistent F34.1
    recurrent F33.9
      current episode
        mild F33.0
        moderate F33.1
        severe (without psychotic symptoms) F33.2
          with psychotic symptoms F33.3
      in remission F33.40
        full F33.42
        partial F33.41
      specified NEC F33.8
    single episode — *see* Episode, depressive
    specified NEC F32.89
  developmental F89
    arithmetical skills F81.2
    coordination (motor) F82
    expressive writing F81.81
    language F80.9
      expressive F80.1
      mixed receptive and expressive F80.2
      receptive type F80.2
      specified NEC F80.89
    learning F81.9
      arithmetical F81.2
      reading F81.0
    mixed F88
    motor coordination or function F82
    pervasive F84.9
      specified NEC F84.8
    phonological F80.0
    reading F81.0
    scholastic skills — *see also* Disorder, learning
      mixed F81.89
    specified NEC F88
    speech F80.9
      articulation F80.0
      specified NEC F80.89
    written expression F81.81
  diaphragm J98.6
  digestive (system) K92.9
    newborn P78.9
      specified NEC P78.89
    postprocedural — *see* Complication, gastrointestinal
    psychogenic F45.8
  disc (intervertebral) M51.9
    with
      myelopathy
        cervical region M50.00
        cervicothoracic region M50.03
        high cervical region M50.01
        lumbar region M51.06
        mid-cervical region M50.020
        sacrococcygeal region M53.3
        thoracic region M51.04
        thoracolumbar region M51.05
      radiculopathy
        cervical region M50.10
        cervicothoracic region M50.13
        high cervical region M50.11
        lumbar region M51.16
        lumbosacral region M51.17
        mid-cervical region M50.120
        sacrococcygeal region M53.3
        thoracic region M51.14
        thoracolumbar region M51.15
    cervical M50.90
      with
        myelopathy M50.00
          C2-C3 M50.01
          C3-C4 M50.01
          C4-C5 M50.021
          C5-C6 M50.022
          C6-C7 M50.023
          C7-T1 M50.03
          cervicothoracic region M50.03
          high cervical region M50.01
          mid-cervical region M50.020
        neuritis, radiculitis or radiculopathy M50.10
          C2-C3 M50.11
          C3-C4 M50.11
          C4-C5 M50.121
          C5-C6 M50.122

Disorder — *continued*
  disc — *continued*
    cervical — *continued*
      with — *continued*
        neuritis, radiculitis or radiculopathy — *continued*
          C6-C7 M50.123
          C7-T1 M50.13
          cervicothoracic region M50.13
          high cervical region M50.11
          mid-cervical region M50.120
        C2-C3 M50.91
        C3-C4 M50.91
        C4-C5 M50.921
        C5-C6 M50.922
        C6-C7 M50.923
        C7-T1 M50.93
        cervicothoracic region M50.93
        degeneration M50.30
          C2-C3 M50.31
          C3-C4 M50.31
          C4-C5 M50.321
          C5-C6 M50.322
          C6-C7 M50.323
          C7-T1 M50.33
          cervicothoracic region M50.33
          high cervical region M50.31
          mid-cervical region M50.320
        displacement M50.20
          C2-C3 M50.21
          C3-C4 M50.21
          C4-C5 M50.221
          C5-C6 M50.222
          C6-C7 M50.223
          C7-T1 M50.23
          cervicothoracic region M50.23
          high cervical region M50.21
          mid-cervical region M50.220
        high cervical region M50.91
        mid-cervical region M50.920
        specified type NEC M50.80
          C2-C3 M50.81
          C3-C4 M50.81
          C4-C5 M50.821
          C5-C6 M50.822
          C6-C7 M50.823
          C7-T1 M50.83
          cervicothoracic region M50.83
          high cervical region M50.81
          mid-cervical region M50.820
    specified NEC
      lumbar region M51.86
      lumbosacral region M51.87
      sacrococcygeal region M53.3
      thoracic region M51.84
      thoracolumbar region M51.85
  disinhibited attachment (childhood) F94.2
  disintegrative, childhood NEC F84.3
  disruptive F91.9
    mood dysregulation F34.81
    specified NEC F91.8
  disruptive behavior — *see* Disorder, conduct
  dissocial personality F60.2
  dissociative F44.9
    affecting
      motor function F44.4
        and sensation F44.7
      sensation F44.6
        and motor function F44.7
    brief reactive F43.0
    due to (secondary to) general medical condition
      F06.8
    mixed F44.7
    organic F06.8
    other specified NEC F44.89
  double heterozygous sickling — *see* Disease, sickle-cell
  dream anxiety F51.5
  drug induced hemorrhagic D68.32
  drug related F19.99
    abuse — *see* Abuse, drug
    dependence — *see* Dependence, drug
  dysmorphic body F45.22
  dysthymic F34.1
  ear H93.9- ☑
    bleeding — *see* Otorrhagia
    deafness — *see* Deafness
    degenerative H93.09- ☑
    discharge — *see* Otorrhea

Disorder — *continued*
  ear — *continued*
    external H61.9- ☑
      auditory canal stenosis — *see* Stenosis, external
        ear canal
      exostosis — *see* Exostosis, external ear canal
      impacted cerumen — *see* Impaction, cerumen
      otitis — *see* Otitis, externa
      perichondritis — *see* Perichondritis, ear
      pinna — *see* Disorder, pinna
      specified type NEC H61.89- ☑
    inner H83.9- ☑
      vestibular dysfunction — *see* Disorder, vestibular
        function
    middle H74.9- ☑
      adhesive H74.1- ☑
      ossicle — *see* Abnormal, ear ossicles
      polyp — *see* Polyp, ear (middle)
      specified NEC, in diseases classified elsewhere
        H75.8- ☑
    postprocedural — *see* Complications, ear, procedure
    specified NEC, in diseases classified elsewhere
      H94.8- ☑
  eating (adult) (psychogenic) F50.9
    anorexia — *see* Anorexia
    binge F50.81
    bulimia F50.2
    child F98.29
      pica F98.3
      rumination disorder F98.21
    pica F50.89
      childhood F98.3
  electrolyte (balance) NEC E87.8
    with
      abortion — *see* Abortion by type complicated
        by specified condition NEC
      ectopic pregnancy O08.5
      molar pregnancy O08.5
    acidosis (lactic) (metabolic) E87.20
      acute E87.21
      chronic E87.22
      respiratory E87.29
      specified NEC E87.29
    alkalosis (metabolic) (respiratory) E87.3
  elimination, transepidermal L87.9
    specified NEC L87.8
  emotional (persistent) F34.9
    of childhood F93.9
      specified NEC F93.8
  endocrine E34.9
    postprocedural E89.89
      specified NEC E89.89
  erectile (male) (organic) — *see also* Dysfunction, sexual,
    male, erectile N52.9
    nonorganic F52.21
  erythematous — *see* Erythema
  esophagus K22.9
    functional K22.4
    psychogenic F45.8
  eustachian tube H69.9- ☑
    infection — *see* Salpingitis, eustachian
    obstruction — *see* Obstruction, eustachian tube
    patulous — *see* Patulous, eustachian tube
    specified NEC H69.8- ☑
  exhibitionistic F65.2
  extrapyramidal G25.9
    in deseases classified elsewhere — *see* category
      G26
    specified type NEC G25.89
  eye H57.9
    postprocedural — *see* Complication, postprocedu-
      ral, eye
  eyelid H02.9
    cyst — *see* Cyst, eyelid
    degenerative H02.70
      chloasma — *see* Chloasma, eyelid
      madarosis — *see* Madarosis
      specified type NEC H02.79
      vitiligo — *see* Vitiligo, eyelid
      xanthelasma — *see* Xanthelasma
    dermatochalasis — *see* Dermatochalasis
    edema — *see* Edema, eyelid
    elephantiasis — *see* Elephantiasis, eyelid
    foreign body, retained — *see* Foreign body, re-
      tained, eyelid
    function H02.59

Index

Disorder — Disorder

Disorder — *continued*
  eyelid — *continued*
    function — *continued*
      abnormal innervation syndrome — *see* Syndrome, abnormal innervation
      blepharochalasis — *see* Blepharochalasis
      blepharoclonus — *see* Blepharoclonus
      blepharophimosis — *see* Blepharophimosis
      blepharoptosis — *see* Blepharoptosis
      lagophthalmos — *see* Lagophthalmos
      lid retraction — *see* Retraction, lid
    hypertrichosis — *see* Hypertrichosis, eyelid
    specified type NEC H02.89
    vascular H02.879
      left H02.876
        lower H02.875
        upper H02.874
      right H02.873
        lower H02.872
        upper H02.871
  factitious
    by proxy F68.A
    imposed on another F68.A
    imposed on self F68.10
      with predominantly
        psychological symptoms F68.11
          with physical symptoms F68.13
        physical symptoms F68.12
          with psychological symptoms F68.13
  factor, coagulation — *see* Defect, coagulation
  fatty acid
    metabolism E71.30
      specified NEC E71.39
    oxidation
      LCAD E71.310
      MCAD E71.311
      SCAD E71.312
      specified deficiency NEC E71.318
  feeding (infant or child) — *see also* Disorder, eating R63.30
    or eating disorder F50.9
    pediatric
      acute R63.31
      chronic R63.32
      specified NEC F50.9
  feigned (with obvious motivation) Z76.5
    without obvious motivation — *see* Disorder, factitious
  female
    hypoactive sexual desire F52.0
    orgasmic F52.31
    sexual interest/arousal F52.22
  fetishistic F65.0
  fibroblastic M72.9
    specified NEC M72.8
  fluency
    adult onset F98.5
    childhood onset F80.81
    following
      cerebral infarction I69.323
      cerebrovascular disease I69.923
        specified disease NEC I69.823
      intracerebral hemorrhage I69.123
      nontraumatic intracranial hemorrhage NEC I69.223
      subarachnoid hemorrhage I69.023
    in conditions classified elsewhere R47.82
  fluid balance E87.8
  follicular (skin) L73.9
    specified NEC L73.8
  frotteuristic F65.81
  fructose metabolism E74.10
    essential fructosuria E74.11
    fructokinase deficiency E74.11
    fructose-1, 6-diphosphatase deficiency E74.19
    hereditary fructose intolerance E74.12
    other specified E74.19
  functional polymorphonuclear neutrophils D71
  gallbladder, biliary tract and pancreas in diseases classified elsewhere K87
  gambling F63.0
  gamma aminobutyric acid (GABA) metabolism E72.81
  gamma-glutamyl cycle E72.89
  gastric (functional) K31.9
    motility K30
    psychogenic F45.8
    secretion K30
  gastrointestinal (functional) NOS K92.9

Disorder — *continued*
  gastrointestinal — *continued*
    newborn P78.9
    psychogenic F45.8
  gender-identity or -role F64.9
    childhood F64.2
    effect on relationship F66
    of adolescence or adulthood F64.0
      nontranssexual F64.8
    specified NEC F64.8
    uncertainty F66
  genito-pelvic pain penetration F52.6
  genitourinary system
    female N94.9
    male N50.9
    psychogenic F45.8
  globe H44.9
    degenerated condition H44.50
      absolute glaucoma H44.51- ☑
      atrophy H44.52- ☑
      leucocoria H44.53- ☑
    degenerative H44.30
      chalcosis H44.31- ☑
      myopia — *see also* Myopia, degenerative H44.2- ☑
      siderosis H44.32- ☑
      specified type NEC H44.39- ☑
    endophthalmitis — *see* Endophthalmitis
    foreign body, retained — *see* Foreign body, intraocular, old, retained
    hemophthalmos — *see* Hemophthalmos
    hypotony H44.40
      due to
        ocular fistula H44.42- ☑
        specified disorder NEC H44.43- ☑
      flat anterior chamber H44.41- ☑
      primary H44.44- ☑
    luxation — *see* Luxation, globe
    specified type NEC H44.89
  glomerular (in) N05.9
    amyloidosis E85.4 *[N08]*
    cryoglobulinemia D89.1 *[N08]*
    disseminated intravascular coagulation D65 *[N08]*
    Fabry's disease E75.21 *[N08]*
    familial lecithin cholesterol acyltransferase deficiency E78.6 *[N08]*
    Goodpasture's syndrome M31.0
    hemolytic-uremic syndrome — *see* Syndrome, hemolytic-uremic
    Henoch (-Schönlein) purpura D69.0 *[N08]*
    malariae malaria B52.0
    microscopic polyangiitis M31.7 *[N08]*
    multiple myeloma C90.0- ☑ *[N08]*
    mumps B26.83
    schistosomiasis B65.9 *[N08]*
    sepsis NEC A41.- ☑ *[N08]*
      streptococcal A40.- ☑ *[N08]*
    sickle-cell disorders D57.- ☑ *[N08]*
    strongyloidiasis B78.9 *[N08]*
    subacute bacterial endocarditis I33.0 *[N08]*
    syphilis A52.75
    systemic lupus erythematosus M32.14
    thrombotic thrombocytopenic purpura M31.19 *[N08]*
    Waldenström macroglobulinemia C88.0 *[N08]*
    Wegener's granulomatosis M31.31
  gluconeogenesis E74.4
  glucosaminoglycan metabolism — *see* Disorder, metabolism, glucosaminoglycan
  glucose transport E74.819
    specified NEC E74.818
  glycine metabolism E72.50
    d-glycericacidemia E72.59
    hyperhydroxyprolinemia E72.59
    hyperoxaluria R82.992
      primary E72.53
    hyperprolinemia E72.59
    non-ketotic hyperglycinemia E72.51
    oxalosis E72.53
    oxaluria E72.53
    sarcosinemia E72.59
    trimethylaminuria E72.52
  glycoprotein metabolism E77.9
    specified NEC E77.8
  grief
    complicated F43.81
    prolonged F43.81
  habit (and impulse) F63.9

Disorder — *continued*
  habit — *continued*
    involving sexual behavior NEC F65.9
    specified NEC F63.89
  hallucinogen use
    mild F16.10
      with
        hallucinogen intoxication delirium F16.121
        hallucinogen-induced
          anxiety disorder F16.180
          bipolar and related disorder F16.14
          depressive disorder F16.14
          psychotic disorder F16.159
        other hallucinogen intoxication F16.129
      in remission (early) (sustained) F16.11
    moderate or severe F16.20
      with
        hallucinogen intoxication delirium F16.221
        hallucinogen-induced
          anxiety disorder F16.280
          bipolar and related disorder F16.24
          depressive disorder F16.24
          psychotic disorder F16.259
        other hallucinogen intoxication F16.229
      in remission (early) (sustained) F16.21
  heart action I49.9
  hematological D75.9
    newborn (transient) P61.9
      specified NEC P61.8
  hematopoietic organs D75.9
  hemorrhagic NEC D69.9
    drug-induced D68.32
    due to
      extrinsic circulating anticoagulants D68.32
      increase in
        anti-IIa D68.32
        anti-Xa D68.32
      intrinsic
        circulating anticoagulants D68.318
        increase in
          anti-IXa D68.318
          antithrombin D68.318
          anti-VIIIa D68.318
          anti-XIa D68.318
    following childbirth O72.3
  hemostasis — *see* Defect, coagulation
  histidine metabolism E70.40
    histidinemia E70.41
    other specified E70.49
  hoarding F42.3
  hyperkinetic — *see* Disorder, attention-deficit hyperactivity
  hyperleucine-isoleucinemia E71.19
  hypervalinemia E71.19
  hypoactive sexual desire F52.0
  hypochondriacal F45.20
    body dysmorphic F45.22
    neurosis F45.21
    other specified F45.29
  identity
    dissociative F44.81
    illness anxiety F45.21
    of childhood F93.8
  immune mechanism (immunity) D89.9
    specified type NEC D89.89
  impaired renal tubular function N25.9
    specified NEC N25.89
  impulse (control) F63.9
  inflammatory
    pelvic, in diseases classified elsewhere — *see* category N74
    penis N48.29
      abscess N48.21
      cellulitis N48.22
  inhalant use
    mild F18.10
      with
        inhalant intoxication F18.129
        inhalant intoxication delirium F18.121
        inhalant-induced
          anxiety disorder F18.180
          depressive disorder F18.14
          major neurocognitive disorder F18.17
          mild neurocognitive disorder F18.188
          psychotic disorder F18.159
      in remission (early) (sustained) F18.11
    moderate or severe F18.20
      with
        inhalant intoxication F18.229

☑ Additional Character Required — Refer to the Tabular List for Character Selection

Disorder — *continued*
  inhalant use — *continued*
    moderate or severe — *continued*
      with — *continued*
        inhalant intoxication delirium F18.221
        inhalant-induced
          anxiety disorder F18.280
          depressive disorder F18.24
          major neurocognitive disorder F18.27
          mild neurocognitive disorder F18.288
          psychotic disorder F18.259
      in remission (early) (sustained) F18.21
  integument, newborn P83.9
    specified NEC P83.88
  intermittent explosive F63.81
  internal secretion pancreas — *see* Increased, secretion,
    pancreas, endocrine
  intestine, intestinal
    carbohydrate absorption NEC E74.39
      postoperative K91.2
    functional NEC K59.9
      postoperative K91.89
    psychogenic F45.8
    vascular K55.9
      chronic K55.1
      specified NEC K55.8
  intraoperative (intraprocedural) — *see* Complications,
    intraoperative
  involuntary emotional expression (IEED) F07.89
  iris H21.9
    adhesions — *see* Adhesions, iris
    atrophy — *see* Atrophy, iris
    chamber angle recession — *see* Recession, chamber
      angle
    cyst — *see* Cyst, iris
    degeneration — *see* Degeneration, iris
    in diseases classified elsewhere H22
    iridodialysis — *see* Iridodialysis
    iridoschisis — *see* Iridoschisis
    miotic pupillary cyst — *see* Cyst, pupillary
    pupillary
      abnormality — *see* Abnormality, pupillary
      membrane — *see* Membrane, pupillary
    specified type NEC H21.89
    vascular NEC H21.1X- ☑
  iron metabolism E83.10
    specified NEC E83.19
  isovaleric acidemia E71.110
  jaw, developmental M27.0
    temporomandibular — *see also* Anomaly, dentofa-
      cial, temporomandibular joint M26.60- ☑
  joint M25.9
    derangement — *see* Derangement, joint
    effusion — *see* Effusion, joint
    fistula — *see* Fistula, joint
    hemarthrosis — *see* Hemarthrosis
    instability — *see* Instability, joint
    osteophyte — *see* Osteophyte
    pain — *see* Pain, joint
    psychogenic F45.8
    specified type NEC M25.80
      ankle M25.87- ☑
      elbow M25.82- ☑
      foot joint M25.87- ☑
      hand joint M25.84- ☑
      hip M25.85- ☑
      knee M25.86- ☑
      shoulder M25.81- ☑
      wrist M25.83- ☑
    stiffness — *see* Stiffness, joint
  ketone metabolism E71.32
  kidney N28.9
    functional (tubular) N25.9
    in
      schistosomiasis B65.9 [N29]
    tubular function N25.9
      specified NEC N25.89
  lacrimal system H04.9
    changes H04.69
      fistula — *see* Fistula, lacrimal
    gland H04.19
      atrophy — *see* Atrophy, lacrimal gland
      cyst — *see* Cyst, lacrimal, gland
      dacryops — *see* Dacryops
      dislocation — *see* Dislocation, lacrimal gland
      dry eye syndrome — *see* Syndrome, dry eye
      infection — *see* Dacryoadenitis

Disorder — *continued*
  lacrimal system — *continued*
    granuloma — *see* Granuloma, lacrimal
    inflammation — *see* Inflammation, lacrimal
    obstruction — *see* Obstruction, lacrimal
    specified NEC H04.89
  lactation NEC O92.79
  language (developmental) F80.9
    expressive F80.1
    mixed receptive and expressive F80.2
    receptive F80.2
  late luteal phase dysphoric N94.89
  learning (specific) F81.9
    acalculia R48.8
    alexia R48.0
    mathematics F81.2
    reading F81.0
    specified
      with impairment in
        mathematics F81.2
        reading F81.0
        written expression F81.81
    specified NEC F81.89
    spelling F81.81
    written expression F81.81
  lens H27.9
    aphakia — *see* Aphakia
    cataract — *see* Cataract
    dislocation — *see* Dislocation, lens
    specified type NEC H27.8
  ligament M24.20
    ankle M24.27- ☑
    attachment, spine — *see* Enthesopathy, spinal
    elbow M24.22- ☑
    foot joint M24.27- ☑
    hand joint M24.24- ☑
    hip M24.25- ☑
    knee — *see* Derangement, knee, specified NEC
    shoulder M24.21- ☑
    specified site NEC M24.29
    vertebra M24.28
    wrist M24.23- ☑
  ligamentous attachments — *see also* Enthesopathy
    spine — *see* Enthesopathy, spinal
  lipid
    metabolism, congenital E78.9
    storage E75.6
      specified NEC E75.5
  lipoprotein
    deficiency (familial) E78.6
    metabolism E78.9
      specified NEC E78.89
  liver K76.9
    malarial B54 [K77]
  low back — *see also* Dorsopathy, specified NEC
  lumbosacral
    plexus G54.1
    root (nerve) NEC G54.4
  lung, interstitial, drug-induced J70.4
    acute J70.2
    chronic J70.3
    dabbing (related) U07.0
    e-cigarette (related) U07.0
    electronic cigarette (related) U07.0
    vaping (associated) (device) (product) (related) (use)
      U07.0
  lymphoproliferative, post-transplant (PTLD) D47.Z1
    (*following* D47.4)
  lysine and hydroxylysine metabolism E72.3
  major neurocognitive — *see also* Dementia, in (due to)
    F03- ☑
  male
    erectile (organic) — *see also* Dysfunction, sexual,
      male, erectile N52.9
      nonorganic F52.21
    hypoactive sexual desire F52.0
    orgasmic F52.32
  manic F30.9
    organic F06.33
  mast cell activation — *see* Activation, mast cell
  mastoid — *see also* Disorder, ear, middle
    postprocedural — *see* Complications, ear, procedure
  meninges, specified type NEC G96.198
  meniscus — *see* Derangement, knee, meniscus
  menopausal N95.9
    specified NEC N95.8
  menstrual N92.6
    psychogenic F45.8

Disorder — *continued*
  menstrual — *continued*
    specified NEC N92.5
  mental (or behavioral) (nonpsychotic) F99
    due to (secondary to)
      amphetamine
        due to drug abuse — *see* Abuse, drug, stimu-
          lant
        due to drug dependence — *see* Dependence,
          drug, stimulant
      brain disease, damage and dysfunction F09
      caffeine use
        due to drug abuse — *see* Abuse, drug, stimu-
          lant
        due to drug dependence — *see* Dependence,
          drug, stimulant
      cannabis use
        due to drug abuse — *see* Abuse, drug,
          cannabis
        due to drug dependence — *see* Dependence,
          drug, cannabis
      general medical condition F09
      sedative or hypnotic use
        due to drug abuse — *see* Abuse, drug, seda-
          tive
        due to drug dependence — *see* Dependence,
          drug, sedative
      tobacco (nicotine) use — *see* Dependence, drug,
        nicotine
    following organic brain damage F07.9
      frontal lobe syndrome F07.0
      personality change F07.0
      postconcussional syndrome F07.81
      specified NEC F07.89
    infancy, childhood or adolescence F98.9
    neurotic — *see* Neurosis
    organic or symptomatic F09
    presenile, psychotic F03 ☑
    problem NEC
    psychoneurotic — *see* Neurosis
    psychotic — *see* Psychosis
    puerperal F53.0
    senile, psychotic NEC F03 ☑
  metabolic, amino acid, transitory, newborn P74.8
  metabolism NOS E88.9
    amino-acid E72.9
      aromatic E70.9
        albinism — *see* Albinism
        histidine E70.40
          histidinemia E70.41
          other specified E70.49
        hyperphenylalaninemia E70.1
          classical phenylketonuria E70.0
        other specified E70.89
        tryptophan E70.5
        tyrosine E70.20
          hypertyrosinemia E70.21
          other specified E70.29
      branched chain E71.2
        3-methylglutaconic aciduria E71.111
        hyperleucine-isoleucinemia E71.19
        hypervalinemia E71.19
        isovaleric acidemia E71.110
        maple syrup urine disease E71.0
        methylmalonic acidemia E71.120
        organic aciduria NEC E71.118
        other specified E71.19
        proprionate NEC E71.128
        proprionic acidemia E71.121
      glycine E72.50
        d-glycericacidemia E72.59
        hyperhydroxyprolinemia E72.59
        hyperoxaluria R82.992
          primary E72.53
        hyperprolinemia E72.59
        non-ketotic hyperglycinemia E72.51
        other specified E72.59
        sarcosinemia E72.59
        trimethylaminuria E72.52
      hydroxylysine E72.3
      lysine E72.3
      ornithine E72.4
      other specified E72.89
        beta-amino acid E72.89
        gamma-glutamyl cycle E72.89
      straight-chain E72.89
      sulfur-bearing E72.10
        homocystinuria E72.11

Disorder — continued
- metabolism — continued
  - amino-acid — continued
    - sulfur-bearing — continued
      - methylenetetrahydrofolate reductase deficiency E72.12
      - other specified E72.19
  - bile acid and cholesterol metabolism E78.70
  - bilirubin E80.7
    - specified NEC E80.6
  - calcium E83.50
    - hypercalcemia E83.52
    - hypocalcemia E83.51
    - other specified E83.59
  - carbohydrate E74.9
    - specified NEC E74.89
  - cholesterol and bile acid metabolism E78.70
  - congenital E88.9
  - copper E83.00
    - specified type NEC E83.09
    - Wilson's disease E83.01
  - cystinuria E72.01
  - fructose E74.10
  - galactose E74.20
  - glucosaminoglycan E76.9
    - mucopolysaccharidosis — see Mucopolysaccharidosis
    - specified NEC E76.8
  - glutamine E72.89
  - glycine E72.50
  - glycogen storage (hepatorenal) E74.09
  - glycoprotein E77.9
    - specified NEC E77.8
  - glycosaminoglycan E76.9
    - specified NEC E76.8
  - in labor and delivery O75.89
  - iron E83.10
  - isoleucine E71.19
  - leucine E71.19
  - lipoid E78.9
  - lipoprotein E78.9
    - specified NEC E78.89
  - magnesium E83.40
    - hypermagnesemia E83.41
    - hypomagnesemia E83.42
    - other specified E83.49
  - mineral E83.9
    - specified NEC E83.89
  - mitochondrial E88.40
    - MELAS syndrome E88.41
    - MERRF syndrome (myoclonic epilepsy associated with ragged-red fibers) E88.42
    - other specified E88.49
  - ornithine E72.4
  - phosphatases E83.30
  - phosphorus E83.30
    - acid phosphatase deficiency E83.39
    - hypophosphatasia E83.39
    - hypophosphatemia E83.39
      - familial E83.31
    - other specified E83.39
    - pseudovitamin D deficiency E83.32
  - plasma protein NEC E88.09
  - porphyrin — see Porphyria
  - postprocedural E89.89
    - specified NEC E89.89
  - purine E79.9
    - specified NEC E79.8
  - pyrimidine E79.9
    - specified NEC E79.8
  - pyruvate E74.4
  - serine E72.89
  - sodium E87.8
  - specified NEC E88.89
  - threonine E72.89
  - valine E71.19
  - zinc E83.2
- methylmalonic acidemia E71.120
- micturition NEC — see also Difficulty, micturition R39.198
  - feeling of incomplete emptying R39.14
  - hesitancy R39.11
  - poor stream R39.12
  - psychogenic F45.8
  - split stream R39.13
  - straining R39.16
  - urgency R39.15
- mild neurocognitive G31.84

Disorder — continued
- mild neurocognitive — continued
  - due to known physiological condition (without behavioral disturbance) F06.70
  - with behavioral disturbance F06.71
- mitochondrial metabolism E88.40
- mitral (valve) — see Endocarditis, mitral
- mixed
  - anxiety and depressive F41.8
  - of scholastic skills (developmental) F81.89
  - receptive expressive language F80.2
- mood F39
  - bipolar — see Disorder, bipolar
  - depressive — see Disorder, depressive
  - due to (secondary to)
    - alcohol F10.94
    - amphetamine F15.94
      - in
        - abuse F15.14
        - dependence F15.24
    - anxiolytic F13.94
      - in
        - abuse F13.14
        - dependence F13.24
    - cocaine F14.94
      - in
        - abuse F14.14
        - dependence F14.24
    - general medical condition F06.30
    - hallucinogen F16.94
      - in
        - abuse F16.14
        - dependence F16.24
    - hypnotic F13.94
      - in
        - abuse F13.14
        - dependence F13.24
    - inhalant F18.94
      - in
        - abuse F18.14
        - dependence F18.24
    - opioid F11.94
      - in
        - abuse F11.14
        - dependence F11.24
    - phencyclidine (PCP) F16.94
      - in
        - abuse F16.14
        - dependence F16.24
    - physiological condition F06.30
      - with
        - depressive features F06.31
        - major depressive-like episode F06.32
        - manic features F06.33
        - mixed features F06.34
    - psychoactive substance NEC F19.94
      - in
        - abuse F19.14
        - dependence F19.24
    - sedative F13.94
      - in
        - abuse F13.14
        - dependence F13.24
    - volatile solvents F18.94
      - in
        - abuse F18.14
        - dependence F18.24
  - manic episode F30.9
    - with psychotic symptoms F30.2
    - in remission (full) F30.4
      - partial F30.3
    - specified type NEC F30.8
    - without psychotic symptoms F30.10
      - mild F30.11
      - moderate F30.12
      - severe F30.13
  - organic F06.30
    - right hemisphere F07.89
  - persistent F34.9
    - cyclothymia F34.0
    - dysthymia F34.1
    - specified type NEC F34.89
  - recurrent F39
  - right hemisphere organic F07.89
- movement G25.9
  - drug-induced G25.70
    - akathisia G25.71
    - specified NEC G25.79
  - hysterical F44.4

Disorder — continued
- movement — continued
  - in diseases classified elsewhere — see category G26
  - periodic limb G47.61
    - sleep related G47.61
  - sleep related NEC G47.69
  - specified NEC G25.89
  - stereotyped F98.4
  - treatment-induced G25.9
- multiple personality F44.81
- muscle M62.9
  - attachment, spine — see Enthesopathy, spinal
  - in trichinellosis — see Trichinellosis, with muscle disorder
  - psychogenic F45.8
  - specified type NEC M62.89
  - tone, newborn P94.9
    - specified NEC P94.8
- muscular
  - attachments — see also Enthesopathy
    - spine — see Enthesopathy, spinal
  - urethra N36.44
- musculoskeletal system, soft tissue — see Disorder, soft tissue
  - postprocedural M96.89
  - psychogenic F45.8
- myoneural G70.9
  - due to lead G70.1
  - specified NEC G70.89
  - toxic G70.1
- myotonic NEC G71.19
- nail, in diseases classified elsewhere L62
- neck region NEC — see Dorsopathy, specified NEC
- neonatal onset multisystemic inflammatory (NOMID) M04.2
- nerve G58.9
  - abducent NEC — see Strabismus, paralytic, sixth nerve
  - accessory G52.8
  - acoustic — see subcategory H93.3 ☑
  - auditory — see subcategory H93.3 ☑
  - auriculotemporal G50.8
  - axillary G54.0
  - cerebral — see Disorder, nerve, cranial
  - cranial G52.9
    - eighth — see subcategory H93.3 ☑
    - eleventh G52.8
    - fifth G50.9
    - first G52.0
    - fourth NEC — see Strabismus, paralytic, fourth nerve
    - multiple G52.7
    - ninth G52.1
    - second NEC — see Disorder, nerve, optic
    - seventh NEC G51.8
    - sixth NEC — see Strabismus, paralytic, sixth nerve
    - specified NEC G52.8
    - tenth G52.2
    - third NEC — see Strabismus, paralytic, third nerve
    - twelfth G52.3
  - entrapment — see Neuropathy, entrapment
  - facial G51.9
    - specified NEC G51.8
  - femoral — see Lesion, nerve, femoral
  - glossopharyngeal NEC G52.1
  - hypoglossal G52.3
  - intercostal G58.0
  - lateral
    - cutaneous of thigh — see Mononeuropathy, lower limb, meralgia paresthetica
    - popliteal — see Lesion, nerve, popliteal
  - lower limb — see Mononeuropathy, lower limb
  - medial popliteal — see Lesion, nerve, popliteal, medial
  - median NEC — see Lesion, nerve, median
  - multiple G58.7
  - oculomotor NEC — see Strabismus, paralytic, third nerve
  - olfactory G52.0
  - optic NEC H47.09- ☑
    - hemorrhage into sheath — see Hemorrhage, optic nerve
    - ischemic H47.01- ☑
  - peroneal — see Lesion, nerve, popliteal
  - phrenic G58.8
  - plantar — see Lesion, nerve, plantar
  - pneumogastric G52.2
  - posterior tibial — see Syndrome, tarsal tunnel

Disorder — *continued*
nerve — *continued*
  radial — *see* Lesion, nerve, radial
  recurrent laryngeal G52.2
  root G54.9
    cervical G54.2
    lumbosacral G54.1
    specified NEC G54.8
    thoracic G54.3
  sciatic NEC — *see* Lesion, nerve, sciatic
  specified NEC G58.8
    lower limb — *see* Mononeuropathy, lower limb, specified NEC
    upper limb — *see* Mononeuropathy, upper limb, specified NEC
  sympathetic G90.9
  tibial — *see* Lesion, nerve, popliteal, medial
  trigeminal G50.9
    specified NEC G50.8
  trochlear NEC — *see* Strabismus, paralytic, fourth nerve
  ulnar — *see* Lesion, nerve, ulnar
  upper limb — *see* Mononeuropathy, upper limb
  vagus G52.2
nervous system G98.8
  autonomic (peripheral) G90.9
    specified NEC G90.8
  central G96.9
    specified NEC G96.89
  parasympathetic G90.9
  specified NEC G98.8
  sympathetic G90.9
  vegetative G90.9
neurocognitive R41.9
  with Lewy bodies — *see also* Dementia, in, diseases specified elsewhere G31.83 *[F02.-]* ☑
  frontotemporal, specified NEC — *see also* Dementia, in, diseases specified elsewhere G31.09 *[F02.-]* ☑
  major — *see also* Dementia F03.- ☑
    due to vascular disease — *see* Dementia, vascular
    mild — *see* Dementia, vascular, mild
    moderate — *see* Dementia, vascular, moderate
    severe — *see* Dementia, vascular, severe
    in (due to) (other diseases classified elsewhere) — *see also* Dementia, in (due to) F02.80
      with
        aggressive behavior — *see also* Dementia, in (due to) F02.81- ☑
        combative behavior — *see also* Dementia, in (due to) F02.81- ☑
        violent behavior — *see also* Dementia, in (due to) F02.81- ☑
  mild (of uncertain or unknown etiology) — *see also* Disorder, mild neurocognitive G31.84
neurodevelopmental F89
  specified NEC F88
neurohypophysis NEC E23.3
neurological NEC R29.818
neuromuscular G70.9
  hereditary NEC G71.9
  specified NEC G70.89
  toxic G70.1
neurotic F48.9
  specified NEC F48.8
neutrophil, polymorphonuclear D71
nicotine use — *see* Dependence, drug, nicotine
nightmare F51.5
non-rapid eye movement sleep arousal
  sleep terror type F51.4
  sleepwalking type F51.3
nose J34.9
  specified NEC J34.89
obsessive-compulsive F42.9
  and related disorder due to a known physiological condition F06.8
odontogenesis NOS K00.9
opioid use
  with
    opioid-induced psychotic disorder F11.959
      with
        delusions F11.950
        hallucinations F11.951
  due to drug abuse — *see* Abuse, drug, opioid
  due to drug dependence — *see* Dependence, drug, opioid
  mild F11.10

Disorder — *continued*
opioid use — *continued*
  mild — *continued*
    with
      opioid-induced
        anxiety disorder F11.188
        depressive disorder F11.14
        sexual dysfunction F11.181
      opioid intoxication
        with perceptual disturbances F11.122
        delirium F11.121
        without perceptual disturbances F11.129
    in remission (early) (sustained) F11.11
  moderate or severe F11.20
    with
      opioid-induced
        anxiety disorder F11.288
        anxiety disorder F11.988
        depressive disorder F11.24
        depressive disorder F11.94
        sexual dysfunction F11.281
        sexual dysfunction F11.981
      opioid intoxication
        with perceptual disturbances F11.222
        delirium F11.221
        without perceptual disturbances F11.229
    in remission (early) (sustained) F11.21
oppositional defiant F91.3
optic
  chiasm H47.49
    due to
      inflammatory disorder H47.41
      neoplasm H47.42
      vascular disorder H47.43
  disc H47.39- ☑
    coloboma — *see* Coloboma, optic disc
    drusen — *see* Drusen, optic disc
    pseudopapilledema — *see* Pseudopapilledema
  radiations — *see* Disorder, visual, pathway
  tracts — *see* Disorder, visual, pathway
orbit H05.9
  cyst — *see* Cyst, orbit
  deformity — *see* Deformity, orbit
  edema — *see* Edema, orbit
  enophthalmos — *see* Enophthalmos
  exophthalmos — *see* Exophthalmos
  hemorrhage — *see* Hemorrhage, orbit
  inflammation — *see* Inflammation, orbit
  myopathy — *see* Myopathy, extraocular muscles
  retained foreign body — *see* Foreign body, orbit, old
  specified type NEC H05.89
organic
  anxiety F06.4
  catatonic F06.1
  delusional F06.2
  dissociative F06.8
  emotionally labile (asthenic) F06.8
  mood (affective) F06.30
  schizophrenia-like F06.2
orgasmic (female) F52.31
  male F52.32
ornithine metabolism E72.4
overanxious F41.1
  of childhood F93.8
pain
  with related psychological factors F45.42
  exclusively related to psychological factors F45.41
  genito-pelvic penetration disorder F52.6
pancreatic internal secretion E16.9
  specified NEC E16.8
panic F41.0
  with agoraphobia F40.01
papulosquamous L44.9
  in diseases classified elsewhere L45
  specified NEC L44.8
paranoid F22
  induced F24
  shared F24
paraphilic F65.9
  specified NEC F65.89
parathyroid (gland) E21.5
  specified NEC E21.4
parietoalveolar NEC J84.09
paroxysmal, mixed R56.9
patella M22.9- ☑
  chondromalacia — *see* Chondromalacia, patella
  derangement NEC M22.3X- ☑

Disorder — *continued*
patella — *continued*
  recurrent
    dislocation — *see* Dislocation, patella, recurrent
    subluxation — *see* Dislocation, patella, recurrent, incomplete
  specified NEC M22.8X- ☑
patellofemoral M22.2X- ☑
pedophilic F65.4
pentose phosphate pathway with anemia D55.1
perception, due to hallucinogens F16.983
  in
    abuse F16.183
    dependence F16.283
peripheral nervous system NEC G64
peroxisomal E71.50
  biogenesis
    neonatal adrenoleukodystrophy E71.511
    specified disorder NEC E71.518
    Zellweger syndrome E71.510
  rhizomelic chondrodysplasia punctata E71.540
  specified form NEC E71.548
    group 1 E71.518
    group 2 E71.53
    group 3 E71.542
  X-linked adrenoleukodystrophy E71.529
    adolescent E71.521
    adrenomyeloneuropathy E71.522
    childhood E71.520
    specified form NEC E71.528
  Zellweger-like syndrome E71.541
persistent
  (somatoform) pain F45.41
  affective (mood) F34.9
personality — *see also* Personality F60.9
  affective F34.0
  aggressive F60.3
  amoral F60.2
  anankastic F60.5
  antisocial F60.2
  anxious F60.6
  asocial F60.2
  asthenic F60.7
  avoidant F60.6
  borderline F60.3
  change (secondary) due to general medical condition F07.0
  compulsive F60.5
  cyclothymic F34.0
  dependent (passive) F60.7
  depressive F34.1
  dissocial F60.2
  emotional instability F60.3
  expansive paranoid F60.0
  explosive F60.3
  following organic brain damage F07.9
  histrionic F60.4
  hyperthymic F34.0
  hypothymic F34.1
  hysterical F60.4
  immature F60.89
  inadequate F60.7
  labile F60.3
  mixed (nonspecific) F60.89
  moral deficiency F60.2
  narcissistic F60.81
  negativistic F60.89
  obsessional F60.5
  obsessive (-compulsive) F60.5
  organic F07.9
  overconscientious F60.5
  paranoid F60.0
  passive (-dependent) F60.7
  passive-aggressive F60.89
  pathological NEC F60.9
  pseudosocial F60.2
  psychopathic F60.2
  schizoid F60.1
  schizotypal F21
  self-defeating F60.7
  specified NEC F60.89
  type A F60.5
  unstable (emotional) F60.3
pervasive, developmental F84.9
phencyclidine use
  mild F16.10
    with
      phencyclidine intoxication F16.129
      phencyclidine intoxication delirium F16.121

Disorder — *continued*
  phencyclidine use — *continued*
    mild — *continued*
      with — *continued*
        phencyclidine-induced
          anxiety disorder F16.180
          bipolar and related disorder F16.14
          depressive disorder F16.14
          psychotic disorder F16.159
        in remission (early) (sustained) F16.11
    moderate or severe F16.20
      with
        phencyclidine intoxication F16.229
        phencyclidine intoxication delirium F16.221
        phencyclidine-induced
          anxiety disorder F16.280
          bipolar and related disorder F16.14
          depressive disorder F16.24
          psychotic disorder F16.259
        in remission (early) (sustained) F16.21
  phobic anxiety, childhood F40.8
  phosphate-losing tubular N25.0
  pigmentation L81.9
    choroid, congenital Q14.3
    diminished melanin formation L81.6
    iron L81.8
    specified NEC L81.8
  pinna (noninfective) H61.10- ☑
    deformity, acquired H61.11- ☑
    hematoma H61.12- ☑
    perichondritis — *see* Perichondritis, ear
    specified type NEC H61.19- ☑
  pituitary gland E23.7
    iatrogenic (postprocedural) E89.3
    specified NEC E23.6
  platelet-activating anti-PF4, specified NEC D75.84
  platelets D69.1
  plexus G54.9
    specified NEC G54.8
  polymorphonuclear neutrophils D71
  porphyrin metabolism — *see* Porphyria
  postconcussional F07.81
  posthallucinogen perception F16.983
    in
      abuse F16.183
      dependence F16.283
  postmenopausal N95.9
    specified NEC N95.8
  postprocedural (postoperative) — *see* Complications, postprocedural
  post-transplant lymphoproliferative D47.Z1 (*following* D47.4)
  post-traumatic stress (PTSD) F43.10
    acute F43.11
    chronic F43.12
  premenstrual dysphoric (PMDD) F32.81
  prepuce N47.8
  propionic acidemia E71.121
  prostate N42.9
    specified NEC N42.89
  psychogenic NOS — *see also* condition F45.9
    anxiety F41.8
    appetite F50.9
    asthenic F48.8
    cardiovascular (system) F45.8
    compulsive F42.8
    cutaneous F54
    depressive F32.9
    digestive (system) F45.8
    dysmenorrheic F45.8
    dyspneic F45.8
    endocrine (system) F54
    eye NEC F45.8
    feeding — *see* Disorder, eating
    functional NEC F45.8
    gastric F45.8
    gastrointestinal (system) F45.8
    genitourinary (system) F45.8
    heart (function) (rhythm) F45.8
    hyperventilatory F45.8
    hypochondriacal — *see* Disorder, hypochondriacal
    intestinal F45.8
    joint F45.8
    learning F81.9
    limb F45.8
    lymphatic (system) F45.8
    menstrual F45.8
    micturition F45.8

Disorder — *continued*
  psychogenic — *see also* condition — *continued*
    monoplegic NEC F44.4
    motor F44.4
    muscle F45.8
    musculoskeletal F45.8
    neurocirculatory F45.8
    obsessive F42.8
    occupational F48.8
    organ or part of body NEC F45.8
    paralytic NEC F44.4
    phobic F40.9
    physical NEC F45.8
    rectal F45.8
    respiratory (system) F45.8
    rheumatic F45.8
    sexual (function) F52.9
    skin (allergic) (eczematous) F54
    sleep F51.9
    specified part of body NEC F45.8
    stomach F45.8
  psychological F99
    associated with
      disease classified elsewhere F54
      sexual
        development F66
        relationship F66
        uncertainty about gender identity F64.9
  psychomotor NEC F44.4
    hysterical F44.4
  psychoneurotic — *see also* Neurosis
    mixed NEC F48.8
  psychophysiologic — *see* Disorder, somatoform
  psychosexual F65.9
    development F66
    identity of childhood F64.2
  psychosomatic NOS — *see* Disorder, somatoform
    multiple F45.0
    undifferentiated F45.1
  psychotic — *see* Psychosis
    transient (acute) F23
  puberty E30.9
    specified NEC E30.8
  pulmonary (valve) — *see* Endocarditis, pulmonary
  purine metabolism E79.9
  pyrimidine metabolism E79.9
  pyruvate metabolism E74.4
  reactive attachment (childhood) F94.1
  reading R48.0
    developmental (specific) F81.0
  receptive language F80.2
  receptor, hormonal, peripheral — *see also* Syndrome, androgen insensitivity E34.50
  recurrent brief depressive F33.8
  reflex R29.2
  refraction H52.7
    aniseikonia H52.32
    anisometropia H52.31
    astigmatism — *see* Astigmatism
    hypermetropia — *see* Hypermetropia
    myopia — *see* Myopia
    presbyopia H52.4
    specified NEC H52.6
  relationship F68.8
    due to sexual orientation F66
  REM sleep behavior G47.52
  renal function, impaired (tubular) N25.9
  resonance R49.9
    specified NEC R49.8
  respiratory function, impaired — *see also* Failure, respiration
    postprocedural — *see* Complication, postoperative, respiratory system
    psychogenic F45.8
  retina H35.9
    angioid streaks H35.33
    changes in vascular appearance H35.01- ☑
    degeneration — *see* Degeneration, retina
    dystrophy (hereditary) — *see* Dystrophy, retina
    edema H35.81
    hemorrhage — *see* Hemorrhage, retina
    ischemia H35.82
    macular degeneration — *see* Degeneration, macula
    microaneurysms H35.04- ☑
    microvascular abnormality NEC H35.09
    neovascularization — *see* Neovascularization, retina
    retinopathy — *see* Retinopathy
    separation of layers H35.70

Disorder — *continued*
  retina — *continued*
    separation of layers — *continued*
      central serous chorioretinopathy H35.71- ☑
      pigment epithelium detachment (serous) H35.72- ☑
        hemorrhagic H35.73- ☑
      specified type NEC H35.89
    telangiectasis — *see* Telangiectasis, retina
    vasculitis — *see* Vasculitis, retina
  retroperitoneal K68.9
  right hemisphere organic affective F07.89
  rumination (infant or child) F98.21
  sacrum, sacrococcygeal NEC M53.3
  schizoaffective F25.9
    bipolar type F25.0
    depressive type F25.1
    manic type F25.0
    mixed type F25.0
    specified NEC F25.8
  schizoid of childhood F84.5
  schizophrenia spectrum and other psychotic disorder F29
    specified NEC F28
  schizophreniform F20.81
    brief F23
  schizotypal (personality) F21
  seasonal affective, recurrent episodes F33.- ☑
  secretion, thyrocalcitonin E07.0
  sedative, hypnotic, or anxiolytic use
    mild F13.10
      with
        sedative, hypnotic, or anxiolytic intoxication F13.129
        sedative, hypnotic, or anxiolytic intoxication delirium F13.121
        sedative, hypnotic, or anxiolytic-induced
          anxiety disorder F13.180
          bipolar and related disorder F13.14
          depressive disorder F13.14
          psychotic disorder F13.159
          sexual dysfunction F13.181
        in remission (early) (sustained) F13.11
    moderate or severe F13.20
      with
        sedative, hypnotic, or anxiolytic intoxication F13.229
        sedative, hypnotic, or anxiolytic intoxication delirium F13.221
        sedative, hypnotic, or anxiolytic-induced
          anxiety disorder F13.280
          bipolar and related disorder F13.24
          depressive disorder F13.24
          major neurocognitive disorder F13.27
          mild neurocognitive disorder F13.288
          psychotic disorder F13.259
          sexual dysfunction F13.281
        in remission (early) (sustained) F13.21
  seizure — *see also* Epilepsy G40.909
    intractable G40.919
      with status epilepticus G40.911
  semantic pragmatic F80.89
    with autism F84.0
  sense of smell R43.1
    psychogenic F45.8
  separation anxiety, of childhood F93.0
  sexual
    aversion F52.1
    function, psychogenic F52.9
    interest/arousal, female F52.22
    masochism F65.51
    maturation F66
    nonorganic F52.9
    preference — *see also* Deviation, sexual F65.9
      fetishistic transvestism F65.1
    relationship F66
    sadism F65.52
  shyness, of childhood and adolescence F40.10
  sibling rivalry F93.8
  sickle-cell (sickling) (homozygous) — *see* Disease, sickle-cell
    heterozygous D57.3
    specified type NEC D57.8- ☑
    trait D57.3
  sinus (nasal) J34.9
    specified NEC J34.89
  skin L98.9
    atrophic L90.9

Disorder — Disorder

Disorder — *continued*
  skin — *continued*
    atrophic — *continued*
      specified NEC L90.8
    granulomatous L92.9
      specified NEC L92.8
    hypertrophic L91.9
      specified NEC L91.8
    infiltrative NEC L98.6
    newborn P83.9
      specified NEC P83.88
    picking F42.4
    psychogenic (allergic) (eczematous) F54
  sleep G47.9
    breathing-related — *see* Apnea, sleep
    circadian rhythm G47.20
      advance sleep phase type G47.22
      delayed sleep phase type G47.21
      due to
        alcohol
          abuse F10.182
          dependence F10.282
          use F10.982
        amphetamines
          abuse F15.182
          dependence F15.282
          use F15.982
        caffeine
          abuse F15.182
          dependence F15.282
          use F15.982
        cocaine
          abuse F14.182
          dependence F14.282
          use F14.982
        drug NEC
          abuse F19.182
          dependence F19.282
          use F19.982
        opioid
          abuse F11.182
          dependence F11.282
          use F11.982
        psychoactive substance NEC
          abuse F19.182
          dependence F19.282
          use F19.982
        sedative, hypnotic, or anxiolytic
          abuse F13.182
          dependence F13.282
          use F13.982
        stimulant NEC
          abuse F15.182
          dependence F15.282
          use F15.982
      free running type G47.24
      in conditions classified elsewhere G47.27
      irregular sleep wake type G47.23
      jet lag type G47.25
      non-24-hour sleep-wake type G47.24
      shift work type G47.26
      specified NEC G47.29
    due to
      alcohol
        abuse F10.182
        dependence F10.282
        use F10.982
      amphetamine
        abuse F15.182
        dependence F15.282
        use F15.982
      anxiolytic
        abuse F13.182
        dependence F13.282
        use F13.982
      caffeine
        abuse F15.182
        dependence F15.282
        use F15.982
      cocaine
        abuse F14.182
        dependence F14.282
        use F14.982
      drug NEC
        abuse F19.182
        dependence F19.282
        use F19.982
      hypnotic
        abuse F13.182

Disorder — *continued*
  sleep — *continued*
    due to
      hypnotic — *continued*
        dependence F13.282
        use F13.982
      opioid
        abuse F11.182
        dependence F11.282
        use F11.982
      psychoactive substance NEC
        abuse F19.182
        dependence F19.282
        use F19.982
      sedative
        abuse F13.182
        dependence F13.282
        use F13.982
      stimulant NEC
        abuse F15.182
        dependence F15.282
        use F15.982
    emotional F51.9
    excessive somnolence — *see* Hypersomnia
    hypersomnia type — *see* Hypersomnia
    initiating or maintaining — *see* Insomnia
    nightmares F51.5
    nonorganic F51.9
      specified NEC F51.8
    parasomnia type G47.50
    specified NEC G47.8
    terrors F51.4
    walking F51.3
  sleep-wake pattern or schedule — *see also* Disorder, sleep, circadian rhythm G47.9
    specified NEC G47.8
  social
    anxiety (of childhood) F40.10
      generalized F40.11
    functioning in childhood F94.9
      specified NEC F94.8
    pragmatic F80.82
  soft tissue M79.9
    ankle M79.9
    due to use, overuse and pressure M70.90
      ankle M70.97- ☑
      bursitis — *see* Bursitis
      foot M70.97- ☑
      forearm M70.93- ☑
      hand M70.94- ☑
      lower leg M70.96- ☑
      multiple sites M70.99
      pelvic region M70.95- ☑
      shoulder region M70.91- ☑
      specified site NEC M70.98
      specified type NEC M70.80
        ankle M70.87- ☑
        foot M70.87- ☑
        forearm M70.83- ☑
        hand M70.84- ☑
        lower leg M70.86- ☑
        multiple sites M70.89
        pelvic region M70.85- ☑
        shoulder region M70.81- ☑
        specified site NEC M70.88
        thigh M70.85- ☑
        upper arm M70.82- ☑
      thigh M70.95- ☑
      upper arm M70.92- ☑
    foot M79.9
    forearm M79.9
    hand M79.9
    lower leg M79.9
    multiple sites M79.9
    occupational — *see* Disorder, soft tissue, due to use, overuse and pressure
    pelvic region M79.9
    shoulder region M79.9
    specified type NEC M79.89
    thigh M79.9
    upper arm M79.9
  somatic symptom F45.1
  somatization F45.0
  somatoform F45.9
    pain (persistent) F45.41
    somatization (multiple) (long-lasting) F45.0
    specified NEC F45.8
    undifferentiated F45.1

Disorder — *continued*
  somnolence, excessive — *see* Hypersomnia
  specific
    arithmetical F81.2
    developmental, of motor F82
    reading F81.0
    speech and language F80.9
    spelling F81.81
    written expression F81.81
  speech R47.9
    articulation (functional) (specific) F80.0
    developmental F80.9
    specified NEC R47.89
  speech-sound F80.0
  spelling (specific) F81.81
  spine — *see also* Dorsopathy
    ligamentous or muscular attachments, peripheral — *see* Enthesopathy, spinal
    specified NEC — *see* Dorsopathy, specified NEC
  stereotyped, habit or movement F98.4
  stimulant use (other) (unspecified)
    mild F15.10
      in remission (early) (sustained) F15.11
    moderate or severe F15.20
      in remission (early) (sustained) F15.21
  stomach (functional) — *see* Disorder, gastric
  stress F43.9
    acute F43.0
    post-traumatic F43.10
      acute F43.11
      chronic F43.12
  substance use (other) (unknown)
    mild F19.10
      with substance-induced
        anxiety disorder F19.180
        bipolar and related disorder F19.14
        depressive disorder F19.14
        major neurocognitive disorder F19.17
        mild neurocognitive disorder F19.188
        obsessive-compulsive and related disorder F19.188
        sexual dysfunction F19.181
      substance intoxication F19.129
      substance intoxication delirium F19.121
    moderate or severe F19.20
      with substance-induced
        anxiety disorder F19.280
        bipolar and related disorder F19.24
        depressive disorder F19.24
        major neurocognitive disorder F19.27
        mild neurocognitive disorder F19.288
        obsessive-compulsive and related disorder F19.288
        sexual dysfunction F19.281
      in remission (early) (sustained) F19.21
      substance intoxication F19.229
      substance intoxication delirium F19.221
  sulfur-bearing amino-acid metabolism E72.10
  sweat gland (eccrine) L74.9
    apocrine L75.9
      specified NEC L75.8
    specified NEC L74.8
  synovium M67.90
    acromioclavicular M67.91- ☑
    ankle M67.97- ☑
    elbow M67.92- ☑
    foot M67.97- ☑
    forearm M67.93- ☑
    hand M67.94- ☑
    hip M67.95- ☑
    knee M67.96- ☑
    multiple sites M67.99
    rupture — *see* Rupture, synovium
    shoulder M67.91- ☑
    specified type NEC M67.80
      acromioclavicular M67.81- ☑
      ankle M67.87- ☑
      elbow M67.82- ☑
      foot M67.87- ☑
      hand M67.84- ☑
      hip M67.85- ☑
      knee M67.86- ☑
      multiple sites M67.89
      wrist M67.83- ☑
    synovitis — *see* Synovitis
    upper arm M67.92- ☑
    wrist M67.93- ☑
  temperature regulation, newborn P81.9

Disorder — *continued*
  temperature regulation, newborn — *continued*
    specified NEC P81.8
  temporomandibular joint M26.60- ☑
  tendon M67.90
    acromioclavicular M67.91- ☑
    ankle M67.97- ☑
    contracture — *see* Contracture, tendon
    elbow M67.92- ☑
    foot M67.97- ☑
    forearm M67.93- ☑
    hand M67.94- ☑
    hip M67.95- ☑
    knee M67.96- ☑
    multiple sites M67.99
    rupture — *see* Rupture, tendon
    shoulder M67.91- ☑
    specified type NEC M67.80
      acromioclavicular M67.81- ☑
      ankle M67.87- ☑
      elbow M67.82- ☑
      foot M67.87- ☑
      hand M67.84- ☑
      hip M67.85- ☑
      knee M67.86- ☑
      multiple sites M67.89
      trunk M67.88
      wrist M67.83- ☑
    synovitis — *see* Synovitis
    tendinitis — *see* Tendinitis
    tenosynovitis — *see* Tenosynovitis
    trunk M67.98
    upper arm M67.92- ☑
    wrist M67.93- ☑
  thoracic root (nerve) NEC G54.3
  thyrocalcitonin hypersecretion E07.0
  thyroid (gland) E07.9
    function NEC, neonatal, transitory P72.2
    iodine-deficiency related E01.8
    specified NEC E07.89
  tic — *see* Tic
  tobacco use
    chewing tobacco (mild) (moderate) (severe) F17.221
      in remission (early) (sustained) F17.221
    cigarettes (mild) (moderate) (severe)
      in remission (early) (sustained) F17.211
    mild F17.200
      in remission (early) (sustained) F17.201
    moderate F17.200
      in remission (early) (sustained) F17.201
    severe F17.200
      in remission (early) (sustained) F17.201
    specified product NEC (mild) (moderate) (severe)
      in remission (early) (sustained) F17.291
  tooth K08.9
    development K00.9
      specified NEC K00.8
    eruption K00.6
  Tourette's F95.2
  trance and possession F44.89
  transvestic F65.1
  trauma and stressor-related NOS F43.9
    other specified F43.89
    unspecified F43.9
  tricuspid (valve) — *see* Endocarditis, tricuspid
  tryptophan metabolism E70.5
  tubular, phosphate-losing N25.0
  tubulo-interstitial (in)
    brucellosis A23.9 *[N16]*
    cystinosis E72.04
    diphtheria A36.84
    glycogen storage disease E74.00 *[N16]*
    leukemia NEC C95.9- ☑ *[N16]*
    lymphoma NEC C85.9- ☑ *[N16]*
    mixed cryoglobulinemia D89.1 *[N16]*
    multiple myeloma C90.0- ☑ *[N16]*
    Salmonella infection A02.25
    sarcoidosis D86.84
    sepsis A41.9 *[N16]*
      streptococcal A40.9 *[N16]*
    systemic lupus erythematosus M32.15
    toxoplasmosis B58.83
    transplant rejection T86.91 *[N16]*
    Wilson's disease E83.01 *[N16]*
  tubulo-renal function, impaired N25.9
    specified NEC N25.89
  tympanic membrane H73.9- ☑

Disorder — *continued*
  tympanic membrane — *continued*
    atrophy — *see* Atrophy, tympanic membrane
    infection — *see* Myringitis
    perforation — *see* Perforation, tympanum
    specified NEC H73.89- ☑
  unsocialized aggressive F91.1
  urea cycle metabolism E72.20
    argininemia E72.21
    arginosuccinic aciduria E72.22
    citrullinemia E72.23
    ornithine transcarbamylase deficiency E72.4
    other specified E72.29
  ureter (in) N28.9
    schistosomiasis B65.0 *[N29]*
    tuberculosis A18.11
  urethra N36.9
    specified NEC N36.8
  urinary system N39.9
    specified NEC N39.8
  valve, heart
    aortic — *see* Endocarditis, aortic
    mitral — *see* Endocarditis, mitral
    pulmonary — *see* Endocarditis, pulmonary
    rheumatic
      aortic — *see* Endocarditis, aortic, rheumatic
      mitral — *see* Endocarditis, mitral
      pulmonary — *see* Endocarditis, pulmonary, rheumatic
      tricuspid — *see* Endocarditis, tricuspid
    tricuspid — *see* Endocarditis, tricuspid
  vestibular function H81.9- ☑
    specified NEC — *see* subcategory H81.8 ☑
    in diseases classified elsewhere H82.- ☑
    vertigo — *see* Vertigo
  vision, binocular H53.30
    abnormal retinal correspondence H53.31
    diplopia H53.2
    fusion with defective stereopsis H53.32
    simultaneous perception H53.33
    suppression H53.34
  visual
    cortex
      blindness H47.619
        left brain H47.612
        right brain H47.611
      due to
        inflammatory disorder H47.629
          left brain H47.622
          right brain H47.621
        neoplasm H47.639
          left brain H47.632
          right brain H47.631
        vascular disorder H47.649
          left brain H47.642
          right brain H47.641
    pathway H47.9
      due to
        inflammatory disorder H47.51- ☑
        neoplasm H47.52- ☑
        vascular disorder H47.53- ☑
    optic chiasm — *see* Disorder, optic, chiasm
  vitreous body H43.9
    crystalline deposits — *see* Deposit, crystalline
    degeneration — *see* Degeneration, vitreous
    hemorrhage — *see* Hemorrhage, vitreous
    opacities — *see* Opacity, vitreous
    prolapse — *see* Prolapse, vitreous
    specified type NEC H43.89
  voice R49.9
    specified type NEC R49.8
  volatile solvent use
    due to drug abuse — *see* Abuse, drug, inhalant
    due to drug dependence — *see* Dependence, drug, inhalant
  voyeuristic F65.3
  white blood cells D72.9
    specified NEC D72.89
  withdrawing, child or adolescent F40.10
Disorientation R41.0
Displacement, displaced
  acquired traumatic of bone, cartilage, joint, tendon NEC — *see* Dislocation
  adrenal gland (congenital) Q89.1
  appendix, retrocecal (congenital) Q43.8
  auricle (congenital) Q17.4
  bladder (acquired) N32.89
    congenital Q64.19

Displacement, displaced — *continued*
  brachial plexus (congenital) Q07.8
  brain stem, caudal (congenital) Q04.8
  canaliculus (lacrimalis), congenital Q10.6
  cardia through esophageal hiatus (congenital) Q40.1
  cerebellum, caudal (congenital) Q04.8
  cervix — *see* Malposition, uterus
  colon (congenital) Q43.3
  device, implant or graft — *see also* Complications, by site and type, mechanical T85.628 ☑
    arterial graft NEC — *see* Complication, cardiovascular device, mechanical, vascular
    breast (implant) T85.42 ☑
    catheter NEC T85.628 ☑
      dialysis (renal) T82.42 ☑
        intraperitoneal T85.621 ☑
      infusion NEC T82.524 ☑
        spinal (epidural) (subdural) T85.620 ☑
      urinary
        cystostomy T83.020 ☑
        Hopkins T83.028 ☑
        ileostomy T83.028 ☑
        indwelling T83.021 ☑
        nephrostomy T83.022 ☑
        specified NEC T83.028 ☑
        urostomy T83.028 ☑
    electronic (electrode) (pulse generator) (stimulator) — *see* Complication, electronic stimulator
    fixation, internal (orthopedic) NEC — *see* Complication, fixation device, mechanical
    gastrointestinal — *see* Complications, prosthetic device, mechanical, gastrointestinal device
    genital NEC T83.428 ☑
      intrauterine contraceptive device (string) T83.32 ☑
      penile prosthesis (cylinder) (implanted) (pump) (reservoir) T83.420 ☑
      testicular prosthesis T83.421 ☑
    heart NEC — *see* Complication, cardiovascular device, mechanical
    joint prosthesis — *see* Complications, joint prosthesis, mechanical
    ocular — *see* Complications, prosthetic device, mechanical, ocular device
    orthopedic NEC — *see* Complication, orthopedic, device or graft, mechanical
    specified NEC T85.628 ☑
    urinary NEC T83.128 ☑
      graft T83.22 ☑
      sphincter, implanted T83.121 ☑
      stent (ileal conduit) (nephroureteral) T83.123 ☑
      ureteral indwelling T83.122 ☑
    vascular NEC — *see* Complication, cardiovascular device, mechanical
    ventricular intracranial shunt T85.02 ☑
  electronic stimulator
    bone T84.320 ☑
    cardiac — *see* Complications, cardiac device, electronic
    nervous system — *see* Complication, prosthetic device, mechanical, electronic nervous system stimulator
    urinary — *see* Complications, electronic stimulator, urinary
  esophageal mucosa into cardia of stomach, congenital Q39.8
  esophagus (acquired) K22.89
    congenital Q39.8
  eyeball (acquired) (lateral) (old) — *see* Displacement, globe
    congenital Q15.8
    current — *see* Avulsion, eye
  fallopian tube (acquired) N83.4- ☑
    congenital Q50.6
    opening (congenital) Q50.6
  gallbladder (congenital) Q44.1
  gastric mucosa (congenital) Q40.2
  globe (acquired) (old) (lateral) H05.21- ☑
    current — *see* Avulsion, eye
  heart (congenital) Q24.8
    acquired I51.89
  hymen (upward) (congenital) Q52.4
  intervertebral disc NEC
    with myelopathy — *see* Disorder, disc, with, myelopathy
    cervical, cervicothoracic (with) M50.20

Displacement, displaced — *continued*
  intervertebral disc — *continued*
    cervical, cervicothoracic — *continued*
      myelopathy — *see* Disorder, disc, cervical, with myelopathy
      neuritis, radiculitis or radiculopathy — *see* Disorder, disc, cervical, with neuritis
      due to trauma — *see* Dislocation, vertebra
    lumbar region M51.26
      with
        myelopathy M51.06
        neuritis, radiculitis, radiculopathy or sciatica M51.16
    lumbosacral region M51.27
      with
        neuritis, radiculitis, radiculopathy or sciatica M51.17
    sacrococcygeal region M53.3
    thoracic region M51.24
      with
        myelopathy M51.04
        neuritis, radiculitis, radiculopathy M51.14
    thoracolumbar region M51.25
      with
        myelopathy M51.05
        neuritis, radiculitis, radiculopathy M51.15
  intrauterine device (string) T83.32 ☑
  kidney (acquired) N28.83
    congenital Q63.2
  lachrymal, lacrimal apparatus or duct (congenital) Q10.6
  lens, congenital Q12.1
  macula (congenital) Q14.1
  Meckel's diverticulum Q43.0
    malignant — *see* Table of Neoplasms, small intestine, malignant
  nail (congenital) Q84.6
    acquired L60.8
  opening of Wharton's duct in mouth Q38.4
  organ or site, congenital NEC — *see* Malposition, congenital
  ovary (acquired) N83.4- ☑
    congenital Q50.39
    free in peritoneal cavity (congenital) Q50.39
    into hernial sac N83.4- ☑
  oviduct (acquired) N83.4- ☑
    congenital Q50.6
  parathyroid (gland) E21.4
  parotid gland (congenital) Q38.4
  punctum lacrimale (congenital) Q10.6
  sacro-iliac (joint) (congenital) Q74.2
    current injury S33.2 ☑
    old — *see* subcategory M53.2 ☑
  salivary gland (any) (congenital) Q38.4
  spleen (congenital) Q89.09
  stomach, congenital Q40.2
  sublingual duct Q38.4
  tongue (downward) (congenital) Q38.3
  tooth, teeth, fully erupted M26.30
    horizontal M26.33
    vertical M26.34
  trachea (congenital) Q32.1
  ureter or ureteric opening or orifice (congenital) Q62.62
  uterine opening of oviducts or fallopian tubes Q50.6
  uterus, uterine — *see* Malposition, uterus
  ventricular septum Q21.0
    with rudimentary ventricle Q20.4
Disproportion
  between native and reconstructed breast N65.1
  fiber-type G71.20
    congenital G71.29
Disruptio uteri — *see* Rupture, uterus
Disruption (of)
  ciliary body NEC H21.89
  closure of
    cornea T81.31 ☑
    craniotomy T81.32 ☑
    fascia (muscular) (superficial) T81.32 ☑
    internal organ or tissue T81.32 ☑
    laceration (external) (internal) T81.33 ☑
    ligament T81.32 ☑
    mucosa T81.31 ☑
    muscle or muscle flap T81.32 ☑
    ribs or rib cage T81.32 ☑
    skin and subcutaneous tissue (full-thickness) (superficial) T81.31 ☑
    skull T81.32 ☑
    sternum (sternotomy) T81.32 ☑
    tendon T81.32 ☑

Disruption — *continued*
  closure of — *continued*
    traumatic laceration (external) (internal) T81.33 ☑
  family Z63.8
    due to
      absence of family member due to military deployment Z63.31
      absence of family member NEC Z63.32
      alcoholism and drug addiction in family Z63.72
      bereavement Z63.4
      death (assumed) or disappearance of family member Z63.4
      divorce or separation Z63.5
      drug addiction in family Z63.72
      return of family member from military deployment (current or past conflict) Z63.71
      stressful life events NEC Z63.79
  iris NEC H21.89
  ligament(s) — *see also* Sprain
    knee
      current injury — *see* Dislocation, knee
      old (chronic) — *see* Derangement, knee, instability
      spontaneous NEC — *see* Derangement, knee, disruption ligament
  ossicular chain — *see* Discontinuity, ossicles, ear
  pelvic ring (stable) S32.810 ☑
    unstable S32.811 ☑
  traumatic injury wound repair T81.33 ☑
  wound T81.30 ☑
    episiotomy O90.1
    operation T81.31 ☑
      cesarean O90.0
      external operation wound (superficial) T81.31 ☑
      internal operation wound (deep) T81.32 ☑
    perineal (obstetric) O90.1
    traumatic injury repair T81.33 ☑
Dissatisfaction with
  employment Z56.9
  school environment Z55.4
Dissecting — *see* condition
Dissection
  aorta I71.00
    abdominal I71.02
    thoracic I71.019
      aortic arch I71.011
      ascending aorta I71.010
      descending thoracic aorta I71.012
    thoracoabdominal I71.03
  artery I77.70
    basilar (trunk) I77.75
    carotid I77.71
    cerebral (nonruptured) I67.0
      ruptured — *see* Hemorrhage, intracranial, subarachnoid
    coronary I25.42
    extremity
      lower I77.77
      upper I77.76
    iliac I77.72
    precerebral
      congenital (nonruptured) Q28.1
      specified site NEC I77.75
    renal I77.73
    specified NEC I77.79
    vertebral I77.74
  precerebral artery, congenital (nonruptured) Q28.1
  Heartland A93.8
  traumatic — *see* Wound, open, by site
  vascular I99.8
  wound — *see* Wound, open
Disseminated — *see* condition
Dissociation
  auriculoventricular or atrioventricular (AV) (any degree) (isorhythmic) I45.89
    with heart block I44.2
  interference I45.89
Dissociative reaction, state F44.9
Dissolution, vertebra — *see* Osteoporosis
Distension, distention
  abdomen R14.0
  bladder N32.89
  cecum K63.89
  colon K63.89
  gallbladder K82.8
  intestine K63.89
  kidney N28.89
  liver K76.89

Distension, distention — *continued*
  seminal vesicle N50.89
  stomach K31.89
    acute K31.0
    psychogenic F45.8
  ureter — *see* Dilatation, ureter
  uterus N85.8
Distoma hepaticum infestation B66.3
Distomiasis B66.9
  bile passages B66.3
  hemic B65.9
  hepatic B66.3
    due to Clonorchis sinensis B66.1
  intestinal B66.5
  liver B66.3
    due to Clonorchis sinensis B66.1
  lung B66.4
  pulmonary B66.4
Distomolar (fourth molar) K00.1
Disto-occlusion (Division I) (Division II) M26.212
Distortion(s) (congenital)
  adrenal (gland) Q89.1
  arm NEC Q68.8
  bile duct or passage Q44.5
  bladder Q64.79
  brain Q04.9
  cervix (uteri) Q51.9
  chest (wall) Q67.8
    bones Q76.8
  clavicle Q74.0
  clitoris Q52.6
  coccyx Q76.49
  common duct Q44.5
  coronary Q24.5
  cystic duct Q44.5
  ear (auricle) (external) Q17.3
    inner Q16.5
    middle Q16.4
      ossicles Q16.3
  endocrine NEC Q89.2
  eustachian tube Q17.8
  eye (adnexa) Q15.8
  face bone(s) NEC Q75.8
  fallopian tube Q50.6
  femur NEC Q68.8
  fibula NEC Q68.8
  finger(s) Q68.1
  foot Q66.9- ☑
  genitalia, genital organ(s)
    female Q52.8
      external Q52.79
      internal NEC Q52.8
  gyri Q04.8
  hand bone(s) Q68.1
  heart (auricle) (ventricle) Q24.8
    valve (cusp) Q24.8
  hepatic duct Q44.5
  humerus NEC Q68.8
  hymen Q52.4
  intrafamilial communications Z63.8
  jaw NEC M26.89
  labium (majus) (minus) Q52.79
  leg NEC Q68.8
  lens Q12.8
  liver Q44.7
  lumbar spine Q76.49
    with disproportion O33.8
      causing obstructed labor O65.0
  lumbosacral (joint) (region) Q76.49
    kyphosis — *see* Kyphosis, congenital
    lordosis — *see* Lordosis, congenital
  nerve Q07.8
  nose Q30.8
  organ
    of Corti Q16.5
    or site not listed — *see* Anomaly, by site
  ossicles, ear Q16.3
  oviduct Q50.6
  pancreas Q45.3
  parathyroid (gland) Q89.2
  pituitary (gland) Q89.2
  radius NEC Q68.8
  sacroiliac joint Q74.2
  sacrum Q76.49
  scapula Q74.0
  shoulder girdle Q74.0
  skull bone(s) NEC Q75.8

Distortion(s) — *continued*
  skull bone(s) — *continued*
    with
      anencephalus Q00.0
      encephalocele — *see* Encephalocele
      hydrocephalus Q03.9
        with spina bifida — *see* Spina bifida, with hydrocephalus
      microcephaly Q02
  spinal cord Q06.8
  spine Q76.49
    kyphosis — *see* Kyphosis, congenital
    lordosis — *see* Lordosis, congenital
  spleen Q89.09
  sternum NEC Q76.7
  thorax (wall) Q67.8
    bony Q76.8
  thymus (gland) Q89.2
  thyroid (gland) Q89.2
  tibia NEC Q68.8 ☑
  toe(s) Q66.9- ☑
  tongue Q38.3
  trachea (cartilage) Q32.1
  ulna NEC Q68.8
  ureter Q62.8
  urethra Q64.79
    causing obstruction Q64.39
  uterus Q51.9
  vagina Q52.4
  vertebra Q76.49
    kyphosis — *see* Kyphosis, congenital
    lordosis — *see* Lordosis, congenital
  visual — *see also* Disturbance, vision
    shape and size H53.15
  vulva Q52.79
  wrist (bones) (joint) Q68.8
Distress
  abdomen — *see* Pain, abdominal
  acute respiratory R06.03
    syndrome (adult) (child) J80
  epigastric R10.13
  fetal P84
    complicating pregnancy — *see* Stress, fetal
  gastrointestinal (functional) K30
    psychogenic F45.8
  intestinal (functional) NOS K59.9
    psychogenic F45.8
  maternal, during labor and delivery O75.0
  relationship, with spouse or intimate partner Z63.0
  respiratory (adult) (child) R06.03
    newborn P22.9
      specified NEC P22.8
    orthopnea R06.01
    psychogenic F45.8
    shortness of breath R06.02
    specified type NEC R06.09
Distribution vessel, atypical Q27.9
  coronary artery Q24.5
  precerebral Q28.1
Distichiasis L68.8
Disturbance(s) — *see also* Disease
  absorption K90.9
    calcium E58
    carbohydrate K90.49
    fat K90.49
      pancreatic K90.3
    protein K90.49
    starch K90.49
    vitamin — *see* Deficiency, vitamin
  acid-base equilibrium E87.8
    mixed E87.4
  activity and attention (with hyperkinesis) — *see* Disorder, attention-deficit hyperactivity
  amino acid transport E72.00
  assimilation, food K90.9
  auditory nerve, except deafness — *see* subcategory H93.3 ☑
  behavior — *see* Disorder, conduct
  blood clotting (mechanism) — *see also* Defect, coagulation D68.9
  cerebral
    nerve — *see* Disorder, nerve, cranial
    status, newborn P91.9
      specified NEC P91.88
  circulatory I99.9
  conduct — *see also* Disorder, conduct F91.9
    adjustment reaction — *see* Disorder, adjustment
    compulsive F63.9

Disturbance(s) — *continued*
  conduct — *see also* Disorder, conduct — *continued*
    disruptive F91.9
    hyperkinetic — *see* Disorder, attention-deficit hyperactivity
    socialized F91.2
    specified NEC F91.8
    unsocialized F91.1
  coordination R27.8
  cranial nerve — *see* Disorder, nerve, cranial
  deep sensibility — *see* Disturbance, sensation
  digestive K30
    psychogenic F45.8
  electrolyte — *see also* Imbalance, electrolyte
    newborn, transitory P74.49
      hyperammonemia P74.6
      hyperchloremia P74.421
      hyperchloremic metabolic acidosis P74.421
      hypochloremia P74.422
      potassium balance
        hyperkalemia P74.31
        hypokalemia P74.32
      sodium balance
        hypernatremia P74.21
        hyponatremia P74.22
      specified type NEC P74.49
  emotions specific to childhood and adolescence F93.9
    with
      anxiety and fearfulness NEC F93.8
      elective mutism F94.0
      oppositional disorder F91.3
      sensitivity (withdrawal) F40.10
      shyness F40.10
      social withdrawal F40.10
    involving relationship problems F93.8
    mixed F93.8
    specified NEC F93.8
  endocrine (gland) E34.9
    neonatal, transitory P72.9
      specified NEC P72.8
  equilibrium R42
  fructose metabolism E74.10
  gait — *see* Gait
    hysterical F44.4
    psychogenic F44.4
  gastrointestinal (functional) K30
    psychogenic F45.8
  habit, child F98.9
  hearing, except deafness and tinnitus — *see* Abnormal, auditory perception
  heart, functional (conditions in I44-I50)
    due to presence of (cardiac) prosthesis I97.19- ☑
    postoperative I97.89
      cardiac surgery — *see also* Infarct, myocardium, associated with revascularization procedure I97.19- ☑
  hormones E34.9
  innervation uterus (parasympathetic) (sympathetic) N85.8
  keratinization NEC
    gingiva K05.10
      nonplaque induced K05.11
      plaque induced K05.10
    lip K13.0
    oral (mucosa) (soft tissue) K13.29
    tongue K13.29
  learning (specific) — *see* Disorder, learning
  memory — *see* Amnesia
    mild, following organic brain damage F06.8
  mental F99
    associated with diseases classified elsewhere F54
  metabolism E88.9
    with
      abortion — *see* Abortion, by type with other specified complication
      ectopic pregnancy O08.5
      molar pregnancy O08.5
    amino-acid E72.9
      aromatic E70.9
      branched-chain E71.2
      straight-chain E72.89
      sulfur-bearing E72.10
    ammonia E72.20
    arginine E72.21
    arginosuccinic acid E72.22
    carbohydrate E74.9
    cholesterol E78.9
    citrulline E72.23

Disturbance(s) — *continued*
  metabolism — *continued*
    cystathionine E72.19
    general E88.9
    glutamine E72.89
    histidine E70.40
    homocystine E72.19
    hydroxylysine E72.3
    in labor or delivery O75.89
    iron E83.10
    lipoid E78.9
    lysine E72.3
    methionine E72.19
    neonatal, transitory P74.9
      calcium and magnesium P71.9
        specified type NEC P71.8
      carbohydrate metabolism P70.9
        specified type NEC P70.8
      specified NEC P74.8
    ornithine E72.4
    phosphate E83.39
    sodium NEC E87.8
    threonine E72.89
    tryptophan E70.5
    tyrosine E70.20
    urea cycle E72.20
  motor R29.2
  nervous, functional R45.0
  neuromuscular mechanism (eye), due to syphilis A52.15
  nutritional E63.9
    nail L60.3
  ocular motion H51.9
    psychogenic F45.8
  oculogyric H51.8
    psychogenic F45.8
  oculomotor H51.9
    psychogenic F45.8
  olfactory nerve R43.1
  optic nerve NEC — *see* Disorder, nerve, optic
  oral epithelium, including tongue NEC K13.29
  perceptual due to
    alcohol withdrawal F10.232
    amphetamine intoxication F15.922
      in
        abuse F15.122
        dependence F15.222
    anxiolytic withdrawal F13.232
    cannabis intoxication (acute) F12.922
      in
        abuse F12.122
        dependence F12.222
    cocaine intoxication (acute) F14.922
      in
        abuse F14.122
        dependence F14.222
    hypnotic withdrawal F13.232
    opioid intoxication (acute) F11.922
      in
        abuse F11.122
        dependence F11.222
    phencyclidine intoxication (acute) F16.122
    sedative withdrawal F13.232
  personality (pattern) (trait) — *see also* Disorder, personality F60.9
    following organic brain damage F07.9
  polyglandular E31.9
    specified NEC E31.8
  potassium balance, newborn
    hyperkalemia P74.31
    hypokalemia P74.32
  psychogenic F45.9
  psychomotor F44.4
  psychophysical visual H53.16
  pupillary — *see* Anomaly, pupil, function
  reflex R29.2
  rhythm, heart I49.9
  salivary secretion K11.7
  sensation (cold) (heat) (localization) (tactile discrimination) (texture) (vibratory) NEC R20.9
    hysterical F44.6
    skin R20.9
      anesthesia R20.0
      hyperesthesia R20.3
      hypoesthesia R20.1
      paresthesia R20.2
      specified type NEC R20.8
    smell R43.9
      and taste (mixed) R43.8
      anosmia R43.0

Disturbance(s) — *continued*
  sensation — *continued*
    smell — *continued*
      parosmia R43.1
      specified NEC R43.8
    taste R43.9
      and smell (mixed) R43.8
      parageusia R43.2
      specified NEC R43.8
  sensory — *see* Disturbance, sensation
  situational (transient) — *see also* Disorder, adjustment
    acute F43.0
  sleep G47.9
    nonorganic origin F51.9
  smell — *see* Disturbance, sensation, smell
  sociopathic F60.2
  sodium balance, newborn
    hypernatremia P74.21
    hyponatremia P74.22
  speech R47.9
    developmental F80.9
    specified NEC R47.89
  stomach (functional) K31.9
  sympathetic (nerve) G90.9
  taste — *see* Disturbance, sensation, taste
  temperature
    regulation, newborn P81.9
      specified NEC P81.8
    sense R20.8
      hysterical F44.6
  tooth
    eruption K00.6
    formation K00.4
    structure, hereditary NEC K00.5
  touch — *see* Disturbance, sensation
  vascular I99.9
    arteriosclerotic — *see* Arteriosclerosis
  vasomotor I73.9
  vasospastic I73.9
  vision, visual H53.9
    following
      cerebral infarction I69.398
      cerebrovascular disease I69.998
        specified NEC I69.898
      intracerebral hemorrhage I69.198
      nontraumatic intracranial hemorrhage NEC I69.298
      specified disease NEC I69.898
      subarachnoid hemorrhage I69.098
    psychophysical H53.16
    specified NEC H53.8
    subjective H53.10
      day blindness H53.11
      discomfort H53.14- ☑
      distortions of shape and size H53.15
      loss
        sudden H53.13- ☑
        transient H53.12- ☑
      specified type NEC H53.19
  voice R49.9
    psychogenic F44.4
    specified NEC R49.8
Diuresis R35.89
Diver's palsy, paralysis or squeeze T70.3 ☑
Diverticulitis (acute) K57.92
  bladder — *see* Cystitis
  ileum — *see* Diverticulitis, intestine, small
  intestine K57.92
    with
      abscess, perforation K57.80
        with bleeding K57.81
      bleeding K57.93
    congenital Q43.8
    large K57.32
      with
        abscess, perforation K57.20
          with bleeding K57.21
        bleeding K57.33
        small intestine K57.52
          with
            abscess, perforation K57.40
              with bleeding K57.41
            bleeding K57.53
    small K57.12
      with
        abscess, perforation K57.00
          with bleeding K57.01
        bleeding K57.13

Diverticulitis — *continued*
  intestine — *continued*
    small — *continued*
      with — *continued*
        large intestine K57.52
          with
            abscess, perforation K57.40
              with bleeding K57.41
            bleeding K57.53
Diverticulosis K57.90
  with bleeding K57.91
  large intestine K57.30
    with
      bleeding K57.31
      small intestine K57.50
        with bleeding K57.51
  small intestine K57.10
    with
      bleeding K57.11
      large intestine K57.50
        with bleeding K57.51
Diverticulum, diverticula (multiple) K57.90
  appendix (noninflammatory) K38.2
  bladder (sphincter) N32.3
    congenital Q64.6
  bronchus (congenital) Q32.4
    acquired J98.09
  calyx, calyceal (kidney) N28.89
  cardia (stomach) K31.4
  cecum — *see* Diverticulosis, intestine, large
    congenital Q43.8
  colon — *see* Diverticulosis, intestine, large
    congenital Q43.8
  duodenum — *see* Diverticulosis, intestine, small
    congenital Q43.8
  epiphrenic (esophagus) K22.5
  esophagus (congenital) Q39.6
    acquired (epiphrenic) (pulsion) (traction) K22.5
  eustachian tube — *see* Disorder, eustachian tube, specified NEC
  fallopian tube N83.8
  gastric K31.4
  heart (congenital) Q24.8
  ileum — *see* Diverticulosis, intestine, small
  jejunum — *see* Diverticulosis, intestine, small
  kidney (pelvis) (calyces) N28.89
    with calculus — *see* Calculus, kidney
  Meckel's (displaced) (hypertrophic) Q43.0
    malignant — *see* Table of Neoplasms, small intestine, malignant
  midthoracic K22.5
  organ or site, congenital NEC — *see* Distortion
  pericardium (congenital) (cyst) Q24.8
    acquired I31.8
  pharyngoesophageal (congenital) Q39.6
    acquired K22.5
  pharynx (congenital) Q38.7
  rectosigmoid — *see* Diverticulosis, intestine, large
    congenital Q43.8
  rectum — *see* Diverticulosis, intestine, large
  Rokitansky's K22.5
  seminal vesicle N50.89
  sigmoid — *see* Diverticulosis, intestine, large
    congenital Q43.8
  stomach (acquired) K31.4
    congenital Q40.2
  trachea (acquired) J39.8
  ureter (acquired) N28.89
    congenital Q62.8
  ureterovesical orifice N28.89
  urethra (acquired) N36.1
    congenital Q64.79
  ventricle, left (congenital) Q24.8
  vesical N32.3
    congenital Q64.6
  Zenker's (esophagus) K22.5
Division
  cervix uteri (acquired) N88.8
  glans penis Q55.69
  labia minora (congenital) Q52.79
  ligament (partial or complete) (current) — *see also* Sprain
    with open wound — *see* Wound, open
  muscle (partial or complete) (current) — *see also* Injury, muscle
    with open wound — *see* Wound, open
  nerve (traumatic) — *see* Injury, nerve
  spinal cord — *see* Injury, spinal cord, by region

Division — *continued*
  vein I87.8
Divorce, causing family disruption Z63.5
Dix-Hallpike neurolabyrinthitis — *see* Neuronitis, vestibular
Dizziness R42
  hysterical F44.89
  psychogenic F45.8
DMAC (disseminated mycobacterium avium- intracellulare complex) A31.2
DNR (do not resuscitate) Z66
Doan-Wiseman syndrome (primary splenic neutropenia) — *see* Agranulocytosis
Doehle-Heller aortitis A52.02
Dog bite — *see* Bite
Dohle body panmyelopathic syndrome D72.0
Dolichocephaly Q67.2
Dolichocolon Q43.8
Dolichostenomelia — *see* Syndrome, Marfan's
Donohue's syndrome E34.8
Donor (organ or tissue) Z52.9
  blood (whole) Z52.000
    autologous Z52.010
    specified component (lymphocytes) (platelets) NEC Z52.008
      autologous Z52.018
      specified donor NEC Z52.098
      specified donor NEC Z52.090
    stem cells Z52.001
      autologous Z52.011
      specified donor NEC Z52.091
  bone Z52.20
    autologous Z52.21
    marrow Z52.3
    specified type NEC Z52.29
  cornea Z52.5
  egg (Oocyte) Z52.819
    age 35 and over Z52.812
      anonymous recipient Z52.812
      designated recipient Z52.813
    under age 35 Z52.810
      anonymous recipient Z52.810
      designated recipient Z52.811
  kidney Z52.4
  liver Z52.6
  lung Z52.89
  lymphocyte — *see* Donor, blood, specified components NEC
  Oocyte — *see* Donor, egg
  platelets Z52.008
  potential, examination of Z00.5
  semen Z52.89
  skin Z52.10
    autologous Z52.11
    specified type NEC Z52.19
  specified organ or tissue NEC Z52.89
  sperm Z52.89
Donovanosis A58
Dorsalgia M54.9
  psychogenic F45.41
  specified NEC M54.89
Dorsopathy M53.9
  deforming M43.9
    specified NEC — *see* subcategory M43.8 ☑
  specified NEC M53.80
    cervical region M53.82
    cervicothoracic region M53.83
    lumbar region M53.86
    lumbosacral region M53.87
    occipito-atlanto-axial region M53.81
    sacrococcygeal region M53.88
    thoracic region M53.84
    thoracolumbar region M53.85
Double
  albumin E88.09
  aortic arch Q25.45
  auditory canal Q17.8
  auricle (heart) Q20.8
  bladder Q64.79
  cervix Q51.820
    with doubling of uterus (and vagina) Q51.10
      with obstruction Q51.11
  inlet ventricle Q20.4
  kidney with double pelvis (renal) Q63.0
  meatus urinarius Q64.75
  monster Q89.4
  outlet
    left ventricle Q20.2

Double — continued
   outlet — continued
      right ventricle Q20.1
   pelvis (renal) with double ureter Q62.5
   tongue Q38.3
   ureter (one or both sides) Q62.5
      with double pelvis (renal) Q62.5
   urethra Q64.74
   urinary meatus Q64.75
   uterus Q51.28
      with
         doubling of cervix (and vagina) Q51.10
            with obstruction Q51.11
         complete Q51.21
         in pregnancy or childbirth O34.0- ☑
            causing obstructed labor O65.5
         partial Q51.22
         specified NEC Q51.28
   vagina Q52.10
      with doubling of uterus (and cervix) Q51.10
         with obstruction Q51.11
   vision H53.2
   vulva Q52.79
Doubled up Z59.01
Douglas' pouch, cul-de-sac — see condition
Down syndrome Q90.9
   meiotic nondisjunction Q90.0
   mitotic nondisjunction Q90.1
   mosaicism Q90.1
   translocation Q90.2
DPD (dihydropyrimidine dehydrogenase deficiency) E88.89
Dracontiasis B72
Dracunculiasis, dracunculosis B72
Dream state, hysterical F44.89
Drepanocytic anemia — see Disease, sickle-cell
Dresbach's syndrome (elliptocytosis) D58.1
Dreschlera (hawaiiensis) (infection) B43.8
Dressler's syndrome I24.1
Drift, ulnar — see Deformity, limb, specified type NEC, forearm
Drinking (alcohol)
   excessive, to excess NEC (without dependence) F10.10
      habitual (continual) (without remission) F10.20
         with remission F10.21
Drip, postnasal (chronic) R09.82
   due to
      allergic rhinitis — see Rhinitis, allergic
      common cold J00
      gastroesophageal reflux — see Reflux, gastroesophageal
      nasopharyngitis — see Nasopharyngitis
      other known condition — code to condition
      sinusitis — see Sinusitis
Droop
   facial R29.810
      cerebrovascular disease I69.992
         cerebral infarction I69.392
         intracerebral hemorrhage I69.192
         nontraumatic intracranial hemorrhage NEC I69.292
         specified disease NEC I69.892
         subarachnoid hemorrhage I69.092
Drop (in)
   attack NEC R55
   finger — see Deformity, finger
   foot — see Deformity, limb, foot, drop
   hematocrit (precipitous) R71.0
   hemoglobin R71.0
   toe — see Deformity, toe, specified NEC
   wrist — see Deformity, limb, wrist drop
Dropped heart beats I45.9
Dropsy, dropsical — see also Hydrops
   abdomen R18.8
   brain — see Hydrocephalus
   cardiac, heart — see Failure, heart, congestive
   gangrenous — see Gangrene
   heart — see Failure, heart, congestive
   kidney — see Nephrosis
   lung — see Edema, lung
   newborn due to isoimmunization P56.0
   pericardium — see Pericarditis
Drowned, drowning (near) T75.1 ☑
Drowsiness R40.0
Drug
   abuse counseling and surveillance Z71.51
   addiction — see Dependence

Drug — continued
   dependence — see Dependence
   habit — see Dependence
   harmful use — see Abuse, drug
   induced fever R50.2
   overdose — see Table of Drugs and Chemicals, by drug, poisoning
   poisoning — see Table of Drugs and Chemicals, by drug, poisoning
   resistant organism infection — see also Resistant, organism, to, drug Z16.30
   therapy
      long term (current) (prophylactic) — see Therapy, drug long-term (current) (prophylactic)
      short term — omit code
   wrong substance given or taken in error — see Table of Drugs and Chemicals, by drug, poisoning
Drunkenness (without dependence) F10.129
   acute in alcoholism F10.229
   chronic (without remission) F10.20
      with remission F10.21
   pathological (without dependence) F10.129
      with dependence F10.229
   sleep F51.9
Drusen
   macula (degenerative) (retina) — see Degeneration, macula, drusen
   optic disc H47.32- ☑
Dry, dryness — see also condition
   larynx J38.7
   mouth R68.2
      due to dehydration E86.0
   nose J34.89
   socket (teeth) M27.3
   throat J39.2
DSAP L56.5
Duane's syndrome H50.81- ☑
Dubin-Johnson disease or syndrome E80.6
Dubois' disease (thymus gland) A50.59 [E35]
Dubowitz' syndrome Q87.19
Duchenne-Aran muscular atrophy G12.21
Duchenne-Griesinger disease G71.01
Duchenne's
   disease or syndrome
      motor neuron disease G12.22
      muscular dystrophy G71.01
      locomotor ataxia (syphilitic) A52.11
   paralysis
      birth injury P14.0
      due to or associated with
         motor neuron disease G12.22
         muscular dystrophy G71.01
Ducrey's chancre A57
Duct, ductus — see condition
Duhring's disease (dermatitis herpetiformis) L13.0
Dullness, cardiac (decreased) (increased) R01.2
Dumb ague — see Malaria
Dumbness — see Aphasia
Dumdum fever B55.0
Dumping syndrome (postgastrectomy) K91.1
Duodenitis (nonspecific) (peptic) K29.80
   with bleeding K29.81
Duodenocholangitis — see Cholangitis
Duodenum, duodenal — see condition
Duplay's bursitis or periarthritis M75.0 ☑
Duplication, duplex — see also Accessory
   alimentary tract Q45.8
   anus Q43.4
   appendix (and cecum) Q43.4
   biliary duct (any) Q44.5
   bladder Q64.79
   cecum (and appendix) Q43.4
   cervix Q51.820
   chromosome NEC
      with complex rearrangements NEC Q92.5
      seen only at prometaphase Q92.8
   cystic duct Q44.5
   digestive organs Q45.8
   esophagus Q39.8
   frontonasal process Q75.8
   intestine (large) (small) Q43.4
   kidney Q63.0
   liver Q44.7
   pancreas Q45.3
   penis Q55.69
   respiratory organs NEC Q34.8
   salivary duct Q38.4
   spinal cord (incomplete) Q06.2

Duplication, duplex — continued
   stomach Q40.2
Dupré's disease (meningism) R29.1
Dupuytren's contraction or disease M72.0
Durand-Nicolas-Favre disease A55
Durotomy (inadvertent) (incidental) G97.41
Duroziez's disease (congenital mitral stenosis) Q23.2
Dutton's relapsing fever (West African) A68.1
Dwarfism — see also Stature, short E34.328
   achondroplastic Q77.4
   congenital — see also Stature, short E34.328
   constitutional E34.31
   hypochondroplastic Q77.4
   hypophyseal E23.0
   infantile — see also Stature, short E34.328
   Laron-type — see also Stature, short E34.321
   Lorain (-Levi) type E23.0
   metatropic Q77.8
   nephrotic-glycosuric (with hypophosphatemic rickets) E72.09
   nutritional E45
   pancreatic K86.89
   pituitary E23.0
   renal N25.0
   thanatophoric Q77.1
Dyke-Young anemia (secondary) (symptomatic) D59.19
Dysacusis — see Abnormal, auditory perception
Dysadrenocortism E27.9
   hyperfunction E27.0
Dysarthria R47.1
   following
      cerebral infarction I69.322
      cerebrovascular disease I69.922
         specified disease NEC I69.822
      intracerebral hemorrhage I69.122
      nontraumatic intracranial hemorrhage NEC I69.222
      subarachnoid hemorrhage I69.022
Dysautonomia (familial) G90.1
Dysbarism T70.3 ☑
Dysbasia R26.2
   angiosclerotica intermittens I73.9
   hysterical F44.4
   lordotica (progressiva) G24.1
   nonorganic origin F44.4
   psychogenic F44.4
Dysbetalipoproteinemia (familial) E78.2
Dyscalculia R48.8
   developmental F81.2
Dyschezia K59.00
Dyschondroplasia (with hemangiomata) Q78.4
Dyschromia (skin) L81.9
Dyscollagenosis M35.9
Dyscranio-pygo-phalangy Q87.0
Dyscrasia
   blood (with) D75.9
      antepartum hemorrhage — see Hemorrhage, antepartum, with coagulation defect
      intrapartum hemorrhage O67.0
      newborn P61.9
         specified type NEC P61.8
      puerperal, postpartum O72.3
   polyglandular, pluriglandular E31.9
Dysendocrinism E34.9
Dysentery, dysenteric (catarrhal) (diarrhea) (epidemic) (hemorrhagic) (infectious) (sporadic) (tropical) A09
   abscess, liver A06.4
   amebic — see also Amebiasis A06.0
      with abscess — see Abscess, amebic
      acute A06.0
      chronic A06.1
   arthritis — see also category M01 A09
      bacillary (see also category M01) A03.9
   bacillary A03.9
      arthritis — see also category M01 A03.9
      Boyd A03.2
      Flexner A03.1
      Schmitz (-Stutzer) A03.0
      Shiga (-Kruse) A03.0
      Shigella A03.9
         boydii A03.2
         dysenteriae A03.0
         flexneri A03.1
         group A A03.0
         group B A03.1
         group C A03.2
         group D A03.3
         sonnei A03.3
         specified type NEC A03.8

Dysentery, dysenteric — *continued*
   bacillary — *continued*
      Sonne A03.3
      specified type NEC A03.8
   balantidial A07.0
   Balantidium coli A07.0
   Boyd's A03.2
   candidal B37.82
   Chilomastix A07.8
   Chinese A03.9
   coccidial A07.3
   Dientamoeba (fragilis) A07.8
   Embadomonas A07.8
   Entamoeba, entamebic — *see* Dysentery, amebic
   Flexner-Boyd A03.2
   Flexner's A03.1
   Giardia lamblia A07.1
   Hiss-Russell A03.1
   Lamblia A07.1
   leishmanial B55.0
   malarial — *see* Malaria
   metazoal B82.0
   monilial B37.82
   protozoal A07.9
   Salmonella A02.0
   schistosomal B65.1
   Schmitz (-Stutzer) A03.0
   Shiga (-Kruse) A03.0
   Shigella NOS — *see* Dysentery, bacillary
   Sonne A03.3
   strongyloidiasis B78.0
   trichomonal A07.8
   viral — *see also* Enteritis, viral A08.4
Dysequilibrium R42
Dysesthesia R20.8
   hysterical F44.6
Dysferlinopathy G71.033
Dysfibrinogenemia (congenital) D68.2
Dysfunction
   adrenal E27.9
      hyperfunction E27.0
   autonomic
      due to alcohol G31.2
      somatoform F45.8
   bladder N31.9
      neurogenic NOS — *see* Dysfunction, bladder, neuromuscular
      neuromuscular NOS N31.9
         atonic (motor) (sensory) N31.2
         autonomous N31.2
         flaccid N31.2
         nonreflex N31.2
         reflex N31.1
         specified NEC N31.8
         uninhibited N31.0
   bleeding, uterus N93.8
   cerebral G93.89
   colon K59.9
      psychogenic F45.8
   colostomy K94.03
   cystic duct K82.8
   cystostomy (stoma) — *see* Complications, cystostomy
   ejaculatory N53.19
      anejaculatory orgasm N53.13
      painful N53.12
      premature F52.4
      retarded N53.11
   endocrine NOS E34.9
   endometrium N85.8
   enterostomy K94.13
   erectile — *see* Dysfunction, sexual, male, erectile
   feeding, pediatric
      acute R63.31
      chronic R63.32
   gallbladder K82.8
   gastrostomy (stoma) K94.23
   gland, glandular NOS E34.9
      meibomian, of eyelid — *see* Dysfunction, meibomian gland
   heart I51.89
   hemoglobin D75.89
   hepatic K76.89
   hypophysis E23.7
   hypothalamic NEC E23.3
   ileostomy (stoma) K94.13
   jejunostomy (stoma) K94.13
   kidney — *see* Disease, renal
   labyrinthine — *see* subcategory H83.2 ☑

Dysfunction — *continued*
   left ventricular, following sudden emotional stress I51.81
   liver K76.89
   male — *see* Dysfunction, sexual, male
   meibomian gland, of eyelid H02.889
      left H02.886
         lower H02.885
         upper H02.884
         upper and lower eyelids H02.88B
      right H02.883
         lower H02.882
         upper H02.881
         upper and lower eyelids H02.88A
   orgasmic (female) F52.31
      male F52.32
   ovary E28.9
      specified NEC E28.8
   papillary muscle I51.89
   parathyroid E21.4
   physiological NEC R68.89
      psychogenic F59
   pineal gland E34.8
   pituitary (gland) E23.3
   platelets D69.1
   polyglandular E31.9
      specified NEC E31.8
   psychophysiologic F59
   psychosexual F52.9
      with
         dyspareunia F52.6
         premature ejaculation F52.4
         vaginismus F52.5
   pylorus K31.9
   rectum K59.9
      psychogenic F45.8
   reflex (sympathetic) — *see* Syndrome, pain, complex regional I
   segmental — *see* Dysfunction, somatic
   senile R54
   sexual (due to) R37
      alcohol F10.981
      amphetamine F15.981
         in
            abuse F15.181
            dependence F15.281
      anxiolytic F13.981
         in
            abuse F13.181
            dependence F13.281
      cocaine F14.981
         in
            abuse F14.181
            dependence F14.281
      excessive sexual drive F52.8
      failure of genital response (male) F52.21
         female F52.22
      female N94.9
         aversion F52.1
         dyspareunia N94.10
            psychogenic F52.6
         frigidity F52.22
         nymphomania F52.8
         orgasmic F52.31
         psychogenic F52.9
            aversion F52.1
            dyspareunia F52.6
            frigidity F52.22
            nymphomania F52.8
            orgasmic F52.31
            vaginismus F52.5
         vaginismus N94.2
            psychogenic F52.5
      hypnotic F13.981
         in
            abuse F13.181
            dependence F13.281
      inhibited orgasm (female) F52.31
         male F52.32
      lack
         of sexual enjoyment F52.1
         or loss of sexual desire F52.0
      male N53.9
         anejaculatory orgasm N53.13
         ejaculatory N53.19
            painful N53.12
            premature F52.4
            retarded N53.11
         erectile N52.9

Dysfunction — *continued*
   sexual — *continued*
      male — *continued*
         erectile — *continued*
            drug induced N52.2
            due to
               disease classified elsewhere N52.1
               drug N52.2
            postoperative (postprocedural) N52.39
               following
                  cryotherapy N52.37
                  interstitial seed therapy N52.36
                  prostate ablative therapy N52.37
                  prostatectomy N52.34
                     radical N52.31
                  radiation therapy N52.35
                  radical cystectomy N52.32
                  ultrasound ablative therapy N52.37
                  urethral surgery N52.33
            psychogenic F52.21
            specified cause NEC N52.8
            vasculogenic
               arterial insufficiency N52.01
                  with corporo-venous occlusive N52.03
               corporo-venous occlusive N52.02
                  with arterial insufficiency N52.03
         impotence — *see* Dysfunction, sexual, male, erectile
         psychogenic F52.9
            aversion F52.1
            erectile F52.21
            orgasmic F52.32
            premature ejaculation F52.4
            satyriasis F52.8
            specified type NEC F52.8
         specified type NEC N53.8
      nonorganic F52.9
         specified NEC F52.8
      opioid F11.981
         in
            abuse F11.181
            dependence F11.281
      orgasmic dysfunction (female) F52.31
         male F52.32
      premature ejaculation F52.4
      psychoactive substances NEC F19.981
         in
            abuse F19.181
            dependence F19.281
      psychogenic F52.9
      sedative F13.981
         in
            abuse F13.181
            dependence F13.281
      sexual aversion F52.1
      vaginismus (nonorganic) (psychogenic) F52.5
   sinoatrial node I49.5
   somatic M99.09
      abdomen M99.09
      acromioclavicular M99.07
      cervical region M99.01
      cervicothoracic M99.01
      costochondral M99.08
      costovertebral M99.08
      head region M99.00
      hip M99.05
      lower extremity M99.06
      lumbar region M99.03
      lumbosacral M99.03
      occipitocervical M99.00
      pelvic region M99.05
      pubic M99.05
      rib cage M99.08
      sacral region M99.04
      sacrococcygeal M99.04
      sacroiliac M99.04
      specified NEC M99.09
      sternochondral M99.08
      sternoclavicular M99.07
      thoracic region M99.02
      thoracolumbar M99.02
      upper extremity M99.07
   somatoform autonomic F45.8
   stomach K31.89
      psychogenic F45.8
   suprarenal E27.9
      hyperfunction E27.0
   symbolic R48.9
      specified type NEC R48.8

Dysfunction — *continued*
  temporomandibular (joint) M26.69
    joint-pain syndrome M26.62- ☑
  testicular (endocrine) E29.9
    specified NEC E29.8
  thymus E32.9
  thyroid E07.9
  ureterostomy (stoma) — *see* Complications, stoma, urinary tract
  urethrostomy (stoma) — *see* Complications, stoma, urinary tract
  uterus, complicating delivery O62.9
    hypertonic O62.4
    hypotonic O62.2
      primary O62.0
      secondary O62.1
  ventricular I51.9
    with congestive heart failure — *see also* Failure, heart I50.9
    left, reversible, following sudden emotional stress I51.81
Dysgenesis
  gonadal (due to chromosomal anomaly) Q96.9
    pure Q99.1
  renal Q60.5
    bilateral Q60.4
    unilateral Q60.3
  reticular D72.0
  tidal platelet D69.3
Dysgerminoma
  specified site — *see* Neoplasm, malignant, by site
  unspecified site
    female C56.9
    male C62.90
Dysgeusia R43.2
Dysgraphia R27.8
Dyshidrosis, dysidrosis L30.1
Dyskaryotic cervical smear R87.619
Dyskeratosis L85.8
  cervix — *see* Dysplasia, cervix
  congenital Q82.8
  uterus NEC N85.8
Dyskinesia G24.9
  biliary (cystic duct or gallbladder) K82.8
  drug induced
    orofacial G24.01
  esophagus K22.4
  hysterical F44.4
  intestinal K59.89
  nonorganic origin F44.4
  orofacial (idiopathic) G24.4
    drug induced G24.01
  psychogenic F44.4
  subacute, drug induced G24.01
  tardive G24.01
    neuroleptic induced G24.01
  trachea J39.8
  tracheobronchial J98.09
Dyslalia (developmental) F80.0
Dyslexia R48.0
  developmental F81.0
Dyslipidemia E78.5
  depressed HDL cholesterol E78.6
  elevated fasting triglycerides E78.1
Dysmaturity — *see also* Light for dates
  pulmonary (newborn) (Wilson-Mikity) P27.0
Dysmenorrhea (essential) (exfoliative) N94.6
  congestive (syndrome) N94.6
  primary N94.4
  psychogenic F45.8
  secondary N94.5
Dysmetabolic syndrome X E88.81
Dysmetria R27.8
Dysmorphism (due to)
  alcohol Q86.0
  exogenous cause NEC Q86.8
  hydantoin Q86.1
  warfarin Q86.2
Dysmorphophobia (nondelusional) F45.22
  delusional F22
Dysnomia R47.01
Dysorexia R63.0
  psychogenic F50.89
Dysostosis
  cleidocranial, cleidocranialis Q74.0
  craniofacial Q75.1
  Fairbank's (idiopathic familial generalized osteophytosis) Q78.9

Dysostosis — *continued*
  mandibulofacial (incomplete) Q75.4
  multiplex E76.01
  oculomandibular Q75.5
Dyspareunia (female) N94.10
  deep N94.12
  male N53.12
  nonorganic F52.6
  psychogenic F52.6
  secondary N94.19
  specified NEC N94.19
  superficial (introital) N94.11
Dyspepsia R10.13
  atonic K30
  functional (allergic) (congenital) (gastrointestinal) (occupational) (reflex) K30
  intestinal K59.89
  nervous F45.8
  neurotic F45.8
  psychogenic F45.8
Dysphagia R13.10
  cervical R13.19
  following
    cerebral infarction I69.391
    cerebrovascular disease I69.991
      specified NEC I69.891
    intracerebral hemorrhage I69.191
    nontraumatic intracranial hemorrhage NEC I69.291
    specified disease NEC I69.891
    subarachnoid hemorrhage I69.091
  functional (hysterical) F45.8
  hysterical F45.8
  nervous (hysterical) F45.8
  neurogenic R13.19
  oral phase R13.11
  oropharyngeal phase R13.12
  pharyngeal phase R13.13
  pharyngoesophageal phase R13.14
  psychogenic F45.8
  sideropenic D50.1
  spastica K22.4
  specified NEC R13.19
Dysphagocytosis, congenital D71
Dysphasia R47.02
  developmental
    expressive type F80.1
    receptive type F80.2
  following
    cerebrovascular disease I69.921
      cerebral infarction I69.321
      intracerebral hemorrhage I69.121
      nontraumatic intracranial hemorrhage NEC I69.221
      specified disease NEC I69.821
      subarachnoid hemorrhage I69.021
Dysphonia R49.0
  functional F44.4
  hysterical F44.4
  psychogenic F44.4
  spastica J38.3
Dysphoria
  gender F64.9
    in
      adolescence and adulthood F64.0
      children F64.2
    specified NEC F64.8
  postpartal O90.6
Dyspituitarism E23.3
Dysplasia — *see also* Anomaly *[handwritten: vulva intraepithelial Neoplasia (VIN)]*
  acetabular, congenital Q65.89
  alveolar capillary, with vein misalignment J84.843
  anus (histologically confirmed) (mild) (moderate) K62.82
    severe D01.3
  arrhythmogenic right ventricular I42.8
  arterial, fibromuscular I77.3
  asphyxiating thoracic (congenital) Q77.2
  brain Q07.9
  bronchopulmonary, perinatal P27.1
  cervix (uteri) N87.9 *[handwritten: metaplasia]*
    mild N87.0
    moderate N87.1
    severe D06.9 *[handwritten: CIS]*
  chondroectodermal Q77.6
  colon D12.6
  craniometaphyseal Q78.8
  dentinal K00.5
  diaphyseal, progressive Q78.3

Dysplasia — *continued*
  dystrophic Q77.5
  ectodermal (anhidrotic) (congenital) (hereditary) Q82.4
    hydrotic Q82.8
  epithelial, uterine cervix — *see* Dysplasia, cervix
  eye (congenital) Q11.2
  fibrous
    bone NEC (monostotic) M85.00
      ankle M85.07- ☑
      foot M85.07- ☑
      forearm M85.03- ☑
      hand M85.04- ☑
      lower leg M85.06- ☑
      multiple site M85.09
      neck M85.08
      rib M85.08
      shoulder M85.01- ☑
      skull M85.08
      specified site NEC M85.08
      thigh M85.05- ☑
      toe M85.07- ☑
      upper arm M85.02- ☑
      vertebra M85.08
    diaphyseal, progressive Q78.3
    jaw M27.8
    polyostotic Q78.1
  florid osseous — *see also* Cyst, calcifying odontogenic
  high grade, focal D12.6
  hip, congenital Q65.89
  joint, congenital Q74.8
  kidney Q61.4
    multicystic Q61.4
  leg Q74.2
  lung, congenital (not associated with short gestation) Q33.6
  mammary (gland) (benign) N60.9- ☑
    cyst (solitary) — *see* Cyst, breast
    cystic — *see* Mastopathy, cystic
    duct ectasia — *see* Ectasia, mammary duct
    fibroadenosis — *see* Fibroadenosis, breast
    fibrosclerosis — *see* Fibrosclerosis, breast
    specified type NEC N60.8- ☑
  metaphyseal Q78.5
  muscle Q79.8
  oculodentodigital Q87.0
  periapical (cemental) (cemento-osseous) — *see* Cyst, calcifying odontogenic
  periosteum — *see* Disorder, bone, specified type NEC
  polyostotic fibrous Q78.1
  prostate — *see also* Neoplasia, intraepithelial, prostate N42.30
    severe D07.5
    specified NEC N42.39
  renal Q61.4
    multicystic Q61.4
  retinal, congenital Q14.1
  right ventricular, arrhythmogenic I42.8
  septo-optic Q04.4
  skin L98.8
  spinal cord Q06.1
  spondyloepiphyseal Q77.7
  thymic, with immunodeficiency D82.1
  vagina N89.3
    mild N89.0
    moderate N89.1
    severe NEC D07.2
  vulva N90.3
    mild N90.0
    moderate N90.1
    severe NEC D07.1 *[handwritten: VIN III (CIS)]*
Dysplasminogenemia E88.02
Dyspnea (nocturnal) (paroxysmal) R06.00
  asthmatic (bronchial) J45.909
    with
      bronchitis J45.909
        with
          exacerbation (acute) J45.901
          status asthmaticus J45.902
        chronic J44.9
        exacerbation (acute) J45.901
        status asthmaticus J45.902
      cardiac — *see* Failure, ventricular, left
  cardiac — *see* Failure, ventricular, left
  functional F45.8
  hyperventilation R06.4
  hysterical F45.8
  newborn P28.89
  orthopnea R06.01

☑ **Additional Character Required** — Refer to the Tabular List for Character Selection

Dyspnea — *continued*
- psychogenic F45.8
- shortness of breath R06.02
- specified type NEC R06.09
- transfusion-associated [TAD] J95.87

Dyspraxia R27.8
- developmental (syndrome) F82

Dysproteinemia E88.09

Dysreflexia, autonomic G90.4

Dysrhythmia
- cardiac I49.9
  - newborn
    - bradycardia P29.12
      - occurring before birth P03.819
        - before onset of labor P03.810
          - during labor P03.811
    - tachycardia P29.11
  - postoperative I97.89
- cerebral or cortical — *see* Epilepsy

Dyssomnia — *see* Disorder, sleep

Dyssynergia
- biliary K83.8
- bladder sphincter N36.44
- cerebellaris myoclonica (Hunt's ataxia) G11.19

Dysthymia F34.1

Dysthyroidism E07.9

Dystocia O66.9
- affecting newborn P03.1
- cervical (hypotonic) O62.2
  - affecting newborn P03.6
  - primary O62.0
  - secondary O62.1
- contraction ring O62.4
- fetal O66.9
  - abnormality NEC O66.3
  - conjoined twins O66.3
  - oversize O66.2
- maternal O66.9
- positional O64.9 ☑
- shoulder (girdle) O66.0
  - causing obstructed labor O66.0
- uterine NEC O62.4

Dystonia G24.9
- cervical G24.3
- deformans progressiva G24.1
- drug induced NEC G24.09
  - acute G24.02
  - specified NEC G24.09
- familial G24.1
- idiopathic G24.1
  - familial G24.1
  - nonfamilial G24.2
  - orofacial G24.4
- lenticularis G24.8
- musculorum deformans G24.1
- neuroleptic induced (acute) G24.02
- orofacial (idiopathic) G24.4
- oromandibular G24.4
  - due to drug G24.01
- specified NEC G24.8
- torsion (familial) (idiopathic) G24.1
  - acquired G24.8
  - genetic G24.1
  - symptomatic (nonfamilial) G24.2

Dystonic movements R25.8

Dystrophy, dystrophia
- adiposogenital E23.6
- autosomal recessive, childhood type, muscular dystrophy resembling Duchenne or Becker G71.01
- Becker's type G71.01
- cervical sympathetic G90.2
- choroid (hereditary) H31.20
  - central areolar H31.22
  - choroideremia H31.21
  - gyrate atrophy H31.23
  - specified type NEC H31.29
- cornea (hereditary) H18.50- ☑
  - endothelial H18.51- ☑
  - epithelial H18.52- ☑
  - granular H18.53- ☑
  - lattice H18.54- ☑
  - macular H18.55- ☑
  - specified type NEC H18.59- ☑
- Duchenne's type G71.01
- due to malnutrition E45
- Erb's G71.02
- Fuchs' H18.51- ☑
- Gower's muscular G71.01

Dystrophy, dystrophia — *continued*
- hair L67.8
- infantile neuroaxonal G31.89
- Landouzy-Déjérine G71.02
- Leyden-Möbius — *see also* Dystrophy, muscular, limb-girdle, by type G71.039
  - meaning Limb girdle muscular dystrophy NOS G71.039
  - meaning Limb girdle muscular dystrophy, other specified type — *see* by type
  - meaning Limb girdle muscular dystrophy, specified type NEC G71.038
  - meaning Limb girdle muscular dystrophy type 2A (autosomal recessive) G71.032
- muscular G71.00
  - autosomal recessive, childhood type, muscular dystrophy resembling Duchenne or Becker G71.01
  - benign (Becker type) G71.01
    - scapuloperoneal with early contractures [Emery-Dreifuss] G71.09
  - congenital (hereditary) (progressive) (with specific morphological abnormalities of the muscle fiber) G71.09
    - myotonic G71.11
  - distal G71.09
  - Duchenne type G71.01
  - Emery-Dreifuss G71.09
  - Erb type G71.02
  - facioscapulohumeral G71.02
  - Gower's G71.01
  - hereditary (progressive) — *see also* Dystrophy, muscular, by type G71.09
  - Landouzy-Déjérine type G71.02
  - limb-girdle G71.039
    - alpha-sarcoglycan-relate G71.0341
    - anoctamin-5-related autosomal recessive (R12) G71.035
    - autosomal recessive NEC G71.038
    - beta-sarcoglycan-related G71.0342
    - calpain-3-related G71.032
      - autosomal dominant G71.031
      - autosomal recessive G71.032
    - collagen VI related
      - autosomal dominant G71.031
      - autosomal recessive G71.038
    - D1 (autosomal dominant) G71.031
    - D2 (autosomal dominant) G71.031
    - D3 (autosomal dominant) G71.031
    - D4 (autosomal dominant) G71.031
    - D5 (autosomal dominant) G71.031
    - delta-sarcoglycan-related G71.0349
    - due to
      - alpha sarcoglycan dysfunction G71.0341
      - anoctamin-5 dysfunction G71.035
      - beta sarcoglycan dysfunction G71.0342
      - fukutin related protein dysfunction G71.038
      - sarcoglycan dysfunction, specified NEC G71.0349
    - FKRP-related autosomal recessive G71.038
    - gamma-sarcoglycan-related G71.0349
    - R1 (autosomal recessive) G71.032
    - R2 (autosomal recessive) G71.033
    - R3 (autosomal recessive) G71.0341
    - R4 (autosomal recessive) G71.0342
    - R5 (autosomal recessive) G71.0349
    - R6 (autosomal recessive) G71.0349
    - R7 (autosomal recessive) G71.038
    - R8 (autosomal recessive) G71.038
    - R9 (autosomal recessive) G71.038
    - R10 (autosomal recessive) G71.038
    - R11 (autosomal recessive) G71.038
    - R12 (autosomal recessive) G71.035
    - R13 (autosomal recessive) G71.038
    - R14 (autosomal recessive) G71.038
    - R15 (autosomal recessive) G71.038
    - R16 (autosomal recessive) G71.038
    - R17 (autosomal recessive) G71.038
    - R18 (autosomal recessive) G71.038
    - R19 (autosomal recessive) G71.038
    - R20 (autosomal recessive) G71.038
    - R21 (autosomal recessive) G71.038
    - R22 (autosomal recessive) G71.038
    - R23 (autosomal recessive) G71.038
    - R24 (autosomal recessive) G71.038
    - type 1 (autosomal dominant) G71.031
    - type 1A (autosomal dominant) G71.031
    - type 1B (autosomal dominant) G71.031
    - type 1C (autosomal dominant) G71.031

Dystrophy, dystrophia — *continued*
- muscular — *continued*
  - limb-girdle — *continued*
    - type 1E (autosomal dominant) G71.031
    - type 1H (autosomal dominant) G71.031
    - type 1I (autosomal dominant) G71.031
    - type 2 (autosomal recessive) G71.038
      - specified NEC G71.038
    - type 2A (autosomal recessive) G71.032
    - type 2B (autosomal recessive) G71.033
    - type 2C (autosomal recessive) G71.0349
    - type 2D (autosomal recessive) G71.0341
    - type 2E (autosomal recessive) G71.0342
    - type 2F (autosomal recessive) G71.0349
    - type 2I (autosomal recessive) G71.038
    - type 2L (autosomal recessive) G71.035
  - myotonic G71.11
  - progressive (hereditary) — *see also* Dystrophy, muscular, by type G71.09
    - Charcot-Marie (-Tooth) type G60.0
  - pseudohypertrophic (infantile) G71.01
  - scapulohumeral G71.02
  - scapuloperoneal G71.09
  - severe (Duchenne type) G71.01
  - specified type NEC G71.09
- myocardium, myocardial — *see* Degeneration, myocardial
- nail L60.3
  - congenital Q84.6
- nutritional E45
- ocular G71.09
- oculocerebrorenal E72.03
- oculopharyngeal G71.09
- ovarian N83.8
- polyglandular E31.8
- reflex (neuromuscular) (sympathetic) — *see* Syndrome, pain, complex regional I
- retinal (hereditary) H35.50
  - in
    - lipid storage disorders E75.6 *[H36]*
    - systemic lipidoses E75.6 *[H36]*
  - involving
    - pigment epithelium H35.54
    - sensory area H35.53
  - pigmentary H35.52
  - vitreoretinal H35.51
- Salzmann's nodular — *see* Degeneration, cornea, nodular
- scapuloperoneal G71.09
- skin NEC L98.8
- sympathetic (reflex) — *see* Syndrome, pain, complex regional I
  - cervical G90.2
- tapetoretinal H35.54
- thoracic, asphyxiating Q77.2
- unguium L60.3
  - congenital Q84.6
- vitreoretinal H35.51
- vulva N90.4
- yellow (liver) — *see* Failure, hepatic

Dysuria R30.0
- psychogenic F45.8

E

Eales' disease H35.06- ☑

Ear — *see also* condition
- piercing Z41.3
- tropical NEC B36.9 *[H62.40]*
  - in
    - aspergillosis B44.89
    - candidiasis B37.84
    - moniliasis B37.84
- wax (impacted) H61.20
  - left H61.22
    - with right H61.23
  - right H61.21
    - with left H61.23

Earache — *see* subcategory H92.0 ☑

Early satiety R68.81

Eaton-Lambert syndrome — *see* Syndrome, Lambert-Eaton

Eberth's disease (typhoid fever) A01.00

Ebola virus disease A98.4

Ebstein's anomaly or syndrome (heart) Q22.5

Eccentro-osteochondrodysplasia E76.29

Ecchondroma — *see* Neoplasm, bone, benign

Ecchondrosis D48.0

Ecchymosis R58
- conjunctiva — *see* Hemorrhage, conjunctiva
- eye (traumatic) — *see* Contusion, eyeball
- eyelid (traumatic) — *see* Contusion, eyelid
- newborn P54.5
- spontaneous R23.3
- traumatic — *see* Contusion

Echinocicciasis — *see* Echinococcus
Echinococcosis — *see* Echinococcus
Echinococcus (infection) B67.90
- granulosus B67.4
  - bone B67.2
  - liver B67.0
  - lung B67.1
  - multiple sites B67.32
  - specified site NEC B67.39
  - thyroid B67.31
- liver NOS B67.8
  - granulosus B67.0
  - multilocularis B67.5
- lung NEC B67.99
  - granulosus B67.1
  - multilocularis B67.69
- multilocularis B67.7
  - liver B67.5
  - multiple sites B67.61
  - specified site NEC B67.69
- specified site NEC B67.99
  - granulosus B67.39
  - multilocularis B67.69
- thyroid NEC B67.99
  - granulosus B67.31
  - multilocularis B67.69 *[E35]*

Echinorhynchiasis B83.8
Echinostomiasis B66.8
Echolalia R48.8
Echovirus, as cause of disease classified elsewhere B97.12
Eclampsia, eclamptic (coma) (convulsions) (delirium) (with hypertension) NEC O15.9
- complicating
  - labor and delivery O15.1
  - postpartum O15.2
  - pregnancy O15.0- ☑
  - puerperium O15.2

Economic circumstances affecting care Z59.9
Economo's disease A85.8
Ectasia, ectasis
- annuloaortic I35.8
- aorta I77.819
  - with aneurysm — *see* Aneurysm, aorta
  - abdominal I77.811
  - thoracic I77.810
  - thoracoabdominal I77.812
- breast — *see* Ectasia, mammary duct
- capillary I78.8
- cornea H18.71- ☑
- gastric antral vascular (GAVE) K31.819
  - with hemorrhage K31.811
  - without hemorrhage K31.819
- mammary duct N60.4- ☑
- salivary gland (duct) K11.8
- sclera — *see* Sclerectasia

Ecthyma L08.0
- contagiosum B08.02
- gangrenosum L08.0
- infectiosum B08.02

Ectocardia Q24.8
Ectodermal dysplasia (anhidrotic) Q82.4
Ectodermosis erosiva pluriorificialis L51.1
Ectopic, ectopia (congenital)
- abdominal viscera Q45.8
  - due to defect in anterior abdominal wall Q79.59
- ACTH syndrome E24.3
- adrenal gland Q89.1
- anus Q43.5
- atrial beats I49.1
- beats I49.49
  - atrial I49.1
  - ventricular I49.3
- bladder Q64.10
- bone and cartilage in lung Q33.5
- brain Q04.8
- breast tissue Q83.8
- cardiac Q24.8
- cerebral Q04.8
- cordis Q24.8
- endometrium — *see* Endometriosis

Ectopic, ectopia — *continued*
- gastric mucosa Q40.2
- gestation — *see* Pregnancy, by site
- heart Q24.8
- hormone secretion NEC E34.2
- kidney (crossed) (pelvis) Q63.2
- lens, lentis Q12.1
- mole — *see* Pregnancy, by site
- organ or site NEC — *see* Malposition, congenital
- pancreas Q45.3
- pregnancy — *see* Pregnancy, ectopic
- pupil — *see* Abnormality, pupillary
- renal Q63.2
- sebaceous glands of mouth Q38.6
- spleen Q89.09
- testis Q53.00
  - bilateral Q53.02
  - unilateral Q53.01
- thyroid Q89.2
- tissue in lung Q33.5
- ureter Q62.63
- ventricular beats I49.3
- vesicae Q64.10

Ectromelia Q73.8
- lower limb — *see* Defect, reduction, limb, lower, specified type NEC
- upper limb — *see* Defect, reduction, limb, upper, specified type NEC

Ectropion H02.109
- cervix N86
  - with cervicitis N72
- congenital Q10.1
- eyelid H02.109
  - cicatricial H02.119
    - left H02.116
      - lower H02.115
      - upper H02.114
    - right H02.113
      - lower H02.112
      - upper H02.111
  - congenital Q10.1
  - left H02.106
    - lower H02.105
    - upper H02.104
  - mechanical H02.129
    - left H02.126
      - lower H02.125
      - upper H02.124
    - right H02.123
      - lower H02.122
      - upper H02.121
  - paralytic H02.159
    - left H02.156
      - lower H02.155
      - upper H02.154
    - right H02.153
      - lower H02.152
      - upper H02.151
  - right H02.103
    - lower H02.102
    - upper H02.101
  - senile H02.139
    - left H02.136
      - lower H02.135
      - upper H02.134
    - right H02.133
      - lower H02.132
      - upper H02.131
  - spastic H02.149
    - left H02.146
      - lower H02.145
      - upper H02.144
    - right H02.143
      - lower H02.142
      - upper H02.141
- iris H21.89
- lip (acquired) K13.0
  - congenital Q38.0
- urethra N36.8
- uvea H21.89

Eczema (acute) (chronic) (erythematous) (fissum) (rubrum) (squamous) — *see also* Dermatitis L30.9
- contact — *see* Dermatitis, contact
- dyshidrotic L30.1
- external ear — *see* Otitis, externa, acute, eczematoid
- flexural L20.82
- herpeticum B00.0
- hypertrophicum L28.0

Eczema — *continued*
- hypostatic — *see* Varix, leg, with, inflammation
- impetiginous L01.1
- infantile (due to any substance) L20.83
  - intertriginous L21.1
  - seborrheic L21.1
- intertriginous NEC L30.4
  - infantile L21.1
- intrinsic (allergic) L20.84
- lichenified NEC L28.0
- marginatum (hebrae) B35.6
- pustular L30.3
- stasis I87.2
  - with varicose veins — *see* Varix, leg, with, inflammation
- vaccination, vaccinatum T88.1 ☑
- varicose — *see* Varix, leg, with, inflammation

Eczematid L30.2
Eddowes (-Spurway) **syndrome** Q78.0
Edema, edematous (infectious) (pitting) (toxic) R60.9
- with nephritis — *see* Nephrosis
- allergic T78.3 ☑
- amputation stump (surgical) (sequelae) (late effect)) T87.89
- angioneurotic (allergic) (any site) (with urticaria) T78.3 ☑
  - hereditary D84.1
- angiospastic I73.9
- Berlin's (traumatic) S05.8X- ☑
- brain (cytotoxic) (vasogenic) G93.6
  - due to birth injury P11.0
  - newborn (anoxia or hypoxia) P52.4
    - birth injury P11.0
  - traumatic — *see* Injury, intracranial, cerebral edema
- cardiac — *see* Failure, heart, congestive
- cardiovascular — *see* Failure, heart, congestive
- cerebral — *see* Edema, brain
- cerebrospinal — *see* Edema, brain
- cervix (uteri) (acute) N88.8
  - puerperal, postpartum O90.89
- chronic hereditary Q82.0
- circumscribed, acute T78.3 ☑
  - hereditary D84.1
- conjunctiva H11.42- ☑
- cornea H18.2- ☑
  - idiopathic H18.22- ☑
  - secondary H18.23- ☑
    - due to contact lens H18.21- ☑
- due to
  - lymphatic obstruction I89.0
  - salt retention E87.0
- epiglottis — *see* Edema, glottis
- essential, acute T78.3 ☑
  - hereditary D84.1
- extremities, lower — *see* Edema, legs
- eyelid NEC H02.849
  - left H02.846
    - lower H02.845
    - upper H02.844
  - right H02.843
    - lower H02.842
    - upper H02.841
- familial, hereditary Q82.0
- famine — *see* Malnutrition, severe
- generalized R60.1
- glottis, glottic, glottidis (obstructive) (passive) J38.4
  - allergic T78.3 ☑
    - hereditary D84.1
- heart — *see* Failure, heart, congestive
- heat T67.7 ☑
- hereditary Q82.0
- inanition — *see* Malnutrition, severe
- intracranial G93.6
- iris H21.89
- joint — *see* Effusion, joint
- larynx — *see* Edema, glottis
- legs R60.0
  - due to venous obstruction I87.1
  - hereditary Q82.0
- localized R60.0
  - due to venous obstruction I87.1
- lower limbs — *see* Edema, legs
- lung J81.1
  - with heart condition or failure — *see* Failure, ventricular, left
  - acute J81.0
  - chemical (acute) J68.1
    - chronic J68.1

Edema, edematous — *continued*
  lung — *continued*
    chronic J81.1
      due to
        chemicals, gases, fumes or vapors (inhalation)
          J68.1
        external agent J70.9
          specified NEC J70.8
        radiation J70.1
    due to
      chemicals, fumes or vapors (inhalation) J68.1
      external agent J70.9
        specified NEC J70.8
      high altitude T70.29 ☑
      near drowning T75.1 ☑
      radiation J70.0
    meaning failure, left ventricle I50.1
  lymphatic I89.0
    due to mastectomy I97.2
  macula H35.81
    cystoid, following cataract surgery — *see* Complications, postprocedural, following cataract surgery
    diabetic — *see* Diabetes, by type, with, retinopathy, with macular edema
  malignant — *see* Gangrene, gas
  Milroy's Q82.0
  nasopharynx J39.2
  newborn P83.30
    hydrops fetalis — *see* Hydrops, fetalis
    specified NEC P83.39
  nutritional — *see also* Malnutrition, severe
    with dyspigmentation, skin and hair E40
  optic disc or nerve — *see* Papilledema
  orbit H05.22- ☑
  pancreas K86.89
  papilla, optic — *see* Papilledema
  penis N48.89
  periodic T78.3 ☑
    hereditary D84.1
  pharynx J39.2
  pulmonary — *see* Edema, lung
  Quincke's T78.3 ☑
    hereditary D84.1
  renal — *see* Nephrosis
  retina H35.81
    diabetic — *see* Diabetes, by type, with, retinopathy, with macular edema
  salt E87.0
  scrotum N50.89
  seminal vesicle N50.89
  spermatic cord N50.89
  spinal (cord) (vascular) (nontraumatic) G95.19
  starvation — *see* Malnutrition, severe
  stasis — *see* Hypertension, venous, (chronic)
  subglottic — *see* Edema, glottis
  supraglottic — *see* Edema, glottis
  testis N44.8
  tunica vaginalis N50.89
  vas deferens N50.89
  vulva (acute) N90.89
Edentulism — *see* Absence, teeth, acquired
Edsall's disease T67.2 ☑
Educational handicap Z55.9
  less than a high school diploma Z55.5
  no general equivalence degree (GED) Z55.5
  specified NEC Z55.8
Edward's syndrome — *see* Trisomy, 18
Effect(s) (of) (from) — *see* Effect, adverse NEC
Effect, adverse
  abnormal gravitational (G) forces or states T75.81 ☑
  abuse — *see* Maltreatment
  air pressure T70.9 ☑
    specified NEC T70.8 ☑
  altitude (high) — *see* Effect, adverse, high altitude
  anesthesia — *see also* Anesthesia T88.59 ☑
    in labor and delivery O74.9
    local, toxic
      in labor and delivery O74.4
      in pregnancy NEC O29.3- ☑
      postpartum, puerperal O89.3
    postpartum, puerperal O89.9
    specified NEC T88.59 ☑
      in labor and delivery O74.8
      postpartum, puerperal O89.8
    spinal and epidural T88.59 ☑
      headache T88.59 ☑

Effect, adverse — *continued*
  anesthesia — *see also* Anesthesia — *continued*
    spinal and epidural — *continued*
      headache — *continued*
        in labor and delivery O74.5
        postpartum, puerperal O89.4
      specified NEC
        in labor and delivery O74.6
        postpartum, puerperal O89.5
  antitoxin — *see* Complications, vaccination
  atmospheric pressure T70.9 ☑
    due to explosion T70.8 ☑
    high T70.3 ☑
    low — *see* Effect, adverse, high altitude
    specified NEC T70.8 ☑
  biological, correct substance properly administered — *see* Effect, adverse, drug
  blood (derivatives) (serum) (transfusion) — *see* Complications, transfusion
  chemical substance — *see* Table of Drugs and Chemicals
  cold (temperature) (weather) T69.9 ☑
    chilblains T69.1 ☑
    frostbite — *see* Frostbite
    specified effect NEC T69.8 ☑
  drugs and medicaments T88.7 ☑
    specified drug — *see* Table of Drugs and Chemicals, by drug, adverse effect
    specified effect — *code to* condition
  electric current, electricity (shock) T75.4 ☑
    burn — *see* Burn
  exertion (excessive) T73.3 ☑
  exposure — *see* Exposure
  external cause NEC T75.89 ☑
  foodstuffs T78.1 ☑
    allergic reaction — *see* Allergy, food
      causing anaphylaxis — *see* Shock, anaphylactic, due to food
    noxious — *see* Poisoning, food, noxious
  gases, fumes, or vapors T59.9- ☑
    specified agent — *see* Table of Drugs and Chemicals
  glue (airplane) sniffing
    due to drug abuse — *see* Abuse, drug, inhalant
    due to drug dependence — *see* Dependence, drug, inhalant
  heat — *see* Heat
  high altitude NEC T70.29 ☑
    anoxia T70.29 ☑
    on
      ears T70.0 ☑
      sinuses T70.1 ☑
    polycythemia D75.1
  high pressure fluids T70.4 ☑
  hot weather — *see* Heat
  hunger T73.0 ☑
  immersion, foot — *see* Immersion
  immunization — *see* Complications, vaccination
  immunological agents — *see* Complications, vaccination
  infrared (radiation) (rays) NOS T66 ☑
    dermatitis or eczema L59.8
  infusion — *see* Complications, infusion
  lack of care of infants — *see* Maltreatment, child
  lightning — *see* Lightning
  medical care T88.9 ☑
    specified NEC T88.8 ☑
  medicinal substance, correct, properly administered — *see* Effect, adverse, drug
  motion T75.3 ☑
  noise, on inner ear — *see* subcategory H83.3 ☑
  overheated places — *see* Heat
  psychosocial, of work environment Z56.5
  radiation (diagnostic) (infrared) (natural source) (therapeutic) (ultraviolet) (X-ray) NOS T66 ☑
    dermatitis or eczema — *see* Dermatitis, due to, radiation
    fibrosis of lung J70.1
    pneumonitis J70.0
    pulmonary manifestations
      acute J70.0
      chronic J70.1
    skin L59.9
  radioactive substance NOS
    dermatitis or eczema — *see* Radiodermatitis
  reduced temperature T69.9 ☑
    immersion foot or hand — *see* Immersion
    specified effect NEC T69.8 ☑

Effect, adverse — *continued*
  serum NEC — *see also* Reaction, serum T80.69 ☑
  specified NEC T78.8 ☑
    external cause NEC T75.89 ☑
  strangulation — *see* Asphyxia, traumatic
  submersion T75.1 ☑
  thirst T73.1 ☑
  toxic — *see* Toxicity
  transfusion — *see* Complications, transfusion
  ultraviolet (radiation) (rays) NOS T66 ☑
    burn — *see* Burn
    dermatitis or eczema — *see* Dermatitis, due to, ultraviolet rays
      acute L56.8
  vaccine (any) — *see* Complications, vaccination
  vibration — *see* Vibration, adverse effects
  water pressure NEC T70.9 ☑
    specified NEC T70.8 ☑
  weightlessness T75.82 ☑
  whole blood — *see* Complications, transfusion
  work environment Z56.5
Effects, late — *see* Sequelae
Effluvium
  anagen L65.1
  telogen L65.0
Effort syndrome (psychogenic) F45.8
Effusion
  amniotic fluid — *see* Pregnancy, complicated by, premature rupture of membranes
  brain (serous) G93.6
  bronchial — *see* Bronchitis
  cerebral G93.6
  cerebrospinal — *see also* Meningitis
    vessel G93.6
  chest — *see* Effusion, pleura
  chylous, chyliform (pleura) J94.0
  intracranial G93.6
  joint M25.40
    ankle M25.47- ☑
    elbow M25.42- ☑
    foot joint M25.47- ☑
    hand joint M25.44- ☑
    hip M25.45- ☑
    knee M25.46- ☑
    shoulder M25.41- ☑
    specified joint NEC M25.48
    wrist M25.43- ☑
  malignant pleural J91.0
  meninges — *see* Meningitis
  pericardium, pericardial (noninflammatory) I31.39
    acute — *see* Pericarditis, acute
    malignant, in disease classified elsewhere I31.31
    specified type, NEC I31.39
  peritoneal (chronic) R18.8
  pleura, pleurisy, pleuritic, pleuropericardial J90
    chylous, chyliform J94.0
    due to systemic lupus erythematosis M32.13
    in conditions classified elsewhere J91.8
    influenzal — *see* Influenza, with, respiratory manifestations NEC
    malignant J91.0
    newborn P28.89
    tuberculous NEC A15.6
      primary (progressive) A15.7
  spinal — *see* Meningitis
  thorax, thoracic — *see* Effusion, pleura
Egg shell nails L60.3
  congenital Q84.6
EGPA (eosinophilic granulomatosis with polyangiitis) M30.1
Egyptian splenomegaly B65.1
Ehlers-Danlos syndrome — *see also* Syndrome, Ehlers-Danlos Q79.60
Ehrlichiosis A77.40
  due to
    E. chafeensis A77.41
    E. ewingii A77.49
    E. muris euclairensis A77.49
    E. sennetsu A79.81
    specified organism NEC A77.49
Eichstedt's disease B36.0
Eisenmenger's
  complex or syndrome I27.83
  defect Q21.8
Ejaculation
  delayed F52.32
  painful N53.12

Ejaculation — *continued*
premature F52.4
retarded N53.11
retrograde N53.14
semen, painful N53.12
psychogenic F52.6
Ekbom's syndrome (restless legs) G25.81
Ekman's syndrome (brittle bones and blue sclera) Q78.0
Elastic skin Q82.8
acquired L57.4
Elastofibroma — *see* Neoplasm, connective tissue, benign
Elastoma (juvenile) Q82.8
Miescher's L87.2
Elastomyofibrosis I42.4
Elastosis
actinic, solar L57.8
atrophicans (senile) L57.4
perforans serpiginosa L87.2
senilis L57.4
Elbow — *see* condition
Electric current, electricity, effects (concussion) (fatal) (nonfatal) (shock) T75.4 ☑
burn — *see* Burn
Electric feet syndrome E53.8
Electrocution T75.4 ☑
from electroshock gun (taser) T75.4 ☑
Electrolyte imbalance E87.8
with
abortion — *see* Abortion by type, complicated by, electrolyte imbalance
ectopic pregnancy O08.5
molar pregnancy O08.5
Elephantiasis (nonfilarial) I89.0
arabicum — *see* Infestation, filarial
bancroftian B74.0
congenital (any site) (hereditary) Q82.0
due to
Brugia (malayi) B74.1
timori B74.2
mastectomy I97.2
Wuchereria (bancrofti) B74.0
eyelid H02.859
left H02.856
lower H02.855
upper H02.854
right H02.853
lower H02.852
upper H02.851
filarial, filariensis — *see* Infestation, filarial
glandular I89.0
graecorum A30.9
lymphangiectatic I89.0
lymphatic vessel I89.0
due to mastectomy I97.2
scrotum (nonfilarial) I89.0
streptococcal I89.0
surgical I97.89
postmastectomy I97.2
telangiectodes I89.0
vulva (nonfilarial) N90.89
Elevated, elevation
alanine transaminase (ALT) R74.01
ALT (alanine transaminase) R74.01
antibody titer R76.0
aspartate transaminase (AST) R74.01
AST (aspartate transaminase) R74.01
basal metabolic rate R94.8
blood pressure — *see also* Hypertension
reading (incidental) (isolated) (nonspecific), no diagnosis of hypertension R03.0
blood sugar R73.9
body temperature (of unknown origin) R50.9
cancer antigen 125 [CA 125] R97.1
carcinoembryonic antigen [CEA] R97.0
cholesterol E78.00
with high triglycerides E78.2
conjugate, eye H51.0
C-reactive protein (CRP) R79.82
diaphragm, congenital Q79.1
erythrocyte sedimentation rate R70.0
fasting glucose R73.01
fasting triglycerides E78.1
finding on laboratory examination — *see* Findings, abnormal, inconclusive, without diagnosis, by type of exam

Elevated, elevation — *continued*
GFR (glomerular filtration rate) — *see* Findings, abnormal, inconclusive, without diagnosis, by type of exam
glucose tolerance (oral) R73.02
immunoglobulin level R76.8
indoleacetic acid R82.5
lactic acid dehydrogenase (LDH) level R74.02
leukocytes D72.829
lipoprotein a (Lp(a)) level E78.41
liver function
study R94.5
test R79.89
alkaline phosphatase R74.8
aminotransferase R74.01
bilirubin R17
hepatic enzyme R74.8
lactate dehydrogenase R74.02
Lp(a) (lipoprotein(a)) E78.41
lymphocytes D72.820
prostate specific antigen [PSA] R97.20
Rh titer — *see* Complication(s), transfusion, incompatibility reaction, Rh (factor)
scapula, congenital Q74.0
sedimentation rate R70.0
SGOT R74.01
SGPT R74.01
transaminase level R74.01
triglycerides E78.1
with high cholesterol E78.2
troponin R77.8
tumor associated antigens [TAA] NEC R97.8
tumor specific antigens [TSA] NEC R97.8
urine level of
17-ketosteroids R82.5
catecholamine R82.5
indoleacetic acid R82.5
steroids R82.5
vanillylmandelic acid (VMA) R82.5
venous pressure I87.8
white blood cell count D72.829
specified NEC D72.828
Elliptocytosis (congenital) (hereditary) D58.1
Hb C (disease) D58.1
hemoglobin disease D58.1
sickle-cell (disease) D57.8- ☑
trait D57.3
Ellison-Zollinger syndrome E16.4
Ellis-van Creveld syndrome (chondroectodermal dysplasia) Q77.6
Elongated, elongation (congenital) — *see also* Distortion
bone Q79.9
cervix (uteri) Q51.828
acquired N88.4
hypertrophic N88.4
colon Q43.8
common bile duct Q44.5
cystic duct Q44.5
frenulum, penis Q55.69
labia minora (acquired) N90.69
ligamentum patellae Q74.1
petiolus (epiglottidis) Q31.8
tooth, teeth K00.2
uvula Q38.6
Eltor cholera A00.1
Emaciation R64
due to malnutrition E43
Embadomoniasis A07.8
Embedded tooth, teeth K01.0
root only K08.3
Embolic — *see* condition
Embolism (multiple) (paradoxical) I74.9
air (any site) (traumatic) T79.0 ☑
following
abortion — *see* Abortion by type complicated by embolism
ectopic pregnancy O08.2
infusion, therapeutic injection or transfusion T80.0 ☑
molar pregnancy O08.2
procedure NEC ☑
artery T81.719 ☑
mesenteric T81.710 ☑
renal T81.711 ☑
specified NEC T81.718 ☑
vein T81.72 ☑

Embolism — *continued*
air — *continued*
in pregnancy, childbirth or puerperium — *see* Embolism, obstetric
amniotic fluid (pulmonary) — *see also* Embolism, obstetric
following
abortion — *see* Abortion by type complicated by embolism
ectopic pregnancy O08.2
molar pregnancy O08.2
aorta, aortic I74.10
abdominal I74.09
saddle I74.01
bifurcation I74.09
saddle I74.01
thoracic I74.11
artery I74.9
auditory, internal I65.8
basilar — *see* Occlusion, artery, basilar
carotid (common) (internal) — *see* Occlusion, artery, carotid
cerebellar (anterior inferior) (posterior inferior) (superior) I66.3
cerebral — *see* Occlusion, artery, cerebral
choroidal (anterior) I65.8
communicating posterior I65.8
coronary — *see also* Infarct, myocardium
not resulting in infarction I24.0
extremity I74.4
lower I74.3
upper I74.2
hypophyseal I65.8
iliac I74.5
limb I74.4
lower I74.3
upper I74.2
mesenteric (with gangrene) — *see also* Ischemia, intestine, acute K55.059
ophthalmic — *see* Occlusion, artery, retina
peripheral I74.4
pontine I65.8
precerebral — *see* Occlusion, artery, precerebral
pulmonary — *see* Embolism, pulmonary
renal N28.0
retinal — *see* Occlusion, artery, retina
septic I76
specified NEC I74.8
vertebral — *see* Occlusion, artery, vertebral
basilar (artery) I65.1
blood clot
following
abortion — *see* Abortion by type complicated by embolism
ectopic or molar pregnancy O08.2
in pregnancy, childbirth or puerperium — *see* Embolism, obstetric
brain — *see also* Occlusion, artery, cerebral
following
abortion — *see* Abortion by type complicated by embolism
ectopic or molar pregnancy O08.2
puerperal, postpartum, childbirth — *see* Embolism, obstetric
capillary I78.8
cardiac — *see also* Infarct, myocardium
not resulting in infarction I51.3
carotid (artery) (common) (internal) — *see* Occlusion, artery, carotid
cavernous sinus (venous) — *see* Embolism, intracranial venous sinus
cerebral — *see* Occlusion, artery, cerebral
cholesterol — *see* Atheroembolism
coronary (artery or vein) (systemic) — *see* Occlusion, coronary
due to device, implant or graft — *see also* Complications, by site and type, specified NEC
arterial graft NEC T82.818 ☑
breast (implant) T85.818 ☑
catheter NEC T85.818 ☑
dialysis (renal) T82.818 ☑
intraperitoneal T85.818 ☑
infusion NEC T82.818 ☑
spinal (epidural) (subdural) T85.810 ☑
urinary (indwelling) T83.81 ☑
electronic (electrode) (pulse generator) (stimulator)
bone T84.81 ☑
cardiac T82.817 ☑

Embolism — *continued*
  due to device, implant or graft — *see also* Complications, by site and type, specified — *continued*
    electronic — *continued*
      nervous system (brain) (peripheral nerve) (spinal) T85.810 ☑
      urinary T83.81 ☑
    fixation, internal (orthopedic) NEC T84.81 ☑
    gastrointestinal (bile duct) (esophagus) T85.818 ☑
    genital NEC T83.81 ☑
    heart (graft) (valve) T82.817 ☑
    joint prosthesis T84.81 ☑
    ocular (corneal graft) (orbital implant) T85.818 ☑
    orthopedic (bone graft) NEC T86.838
    specified NEC T85.818 ☑
    urinary (graft) NEC T83.81 ☑
    vascular NEC T82.818 ☑
    ventricular intracranial shunt T85.810 ☑
  extremities
    lower — *see* Embolism, vein, lower extremity
      arterial I74.3
    upper I74.2
  eye H34.9
  fat (cerebral) (pulmonary) (systemic) T79.1 ☑
    complicating delivery — *see* Embolism, obstetric
    following
      abortion — *see* Abortion by type complicated by embolism
      ectopic or molar pregnancy O08.2
  following
    abortion — *see* Abortion by type complicated by embolism
    ectopic or molar pregnancy O08.2
    infusion, therapeutic injection or transfusion
      air T80.0 ☑
  heart (fatty) — *see also* Infarct, myocardium
    not resulting in infarction I51.3
  hepatic (vein) I82.0
  in pregnancy, childbirth or puerperium — *see* Embolism, obstetric
  intestine (artery) (vein) (with gangrene) — *see also* Ischemia, intestine, acute K55.039
  intracranial — *see also* Occlusion, artery, cerebral
    venous sinus (any) G08
      nonpyogenic I67.6
  intraspinal venous sinuses or veins G08
    nonpyogenic G95.19
  kidney (artery) N28.0
  lateral sinus (venous) — *see* Embolism, intracranial, venous sinus
  leg — *see* Embolism, vein, lower extremity
    arterial I74.3
  longitudinal sinus (venous) — *see* Embolism, intracranial, venous sinus
  lung (massive) — *see* Embolism, pulmonary
  meninges I66.8
  mesenteric (artery) (vein) (with gangrene) — *see also* Ischemia, intestine, acute K55.059
  obstetric (in) (pulmonary)
    childbirth O88.22
      air O88.02
      amniotic fluid O88.12
      blood clot O88.22
      fat O88.82
      pyemic O88.32
      septic O88.32
      specified type NEC O88.82
    pregnancy O88.21- ☑
      air O88.01- ☑
      amniotic fluid O88.11- ☑
      blood clot O88.21- ☑
      fat O88.81- ☑
      pyemic O88.31- ☑
      septic O88.31- ☑
      specified type NEC O88.81- ☑
    puerperal O88.23
      air O88.03
      amniotic fluid O88.13
      blood clot O88.23
      fat O88.83
      pyemic O88.33
      septic O88.33
      specified type NEC O88.83
  ophthalmic — *see* Occlusion, artery, retina
  penis N48.81
  peripheral artery NOS I74.4
  pituitary E23.6

Embolism — *continued*
  popliteal (artery) I74.3
  portal (vein) I81
  postoperative, postprocedural
    artery T81.719 ☑
      mesenteric T81.710 ☑
      renal T81.711 ☑
      specified NEC T81.718 ☑
    vein T81.72 ☑
  precerebral artery — *see* Occlusion, artery, precerebral
  puerperal — *see* Embolism, obstetric
  pulmonary (acute) (artery) (vein) I26.99
    with acute cor pulmonale I26.09
    chronic I27.82
    following
      abortion — *see* Abortion by type complicated by embolism
      ectopic or molar pregnancy O08.2
    healed or old Z86.711
    in pregnancy, childbirth or puerperium — *see* Embolism, obstetric
    multiple subsegmental without acute cor pulmonale I26.94
    personal history of Z86.711
    saddle I26.92
      with acute cor pulmonale I26.02
    septic I26.90
      with acute cor pulmonale I26.01
    single subsegmental without acute cor pulmonale I26.93
    subsegmental NOS I26.93
  pyemic (multiple) I76
    following
      abortion — *see* Abortion by type complicated by embolism
      ectopic or molar pregnancy O08.2
    Hemophilus influenzae A41.3
    pneumococcal A40.3
      with pneumonia J13
    puerperal, postpartum, childbirth (any organism) — *see* Embolism, obstetric
    specified organism NEC A41.89
    staphylococcal A41.2
    streptococcal A40.9
  renal (artery) N28.0
    vein I82.3
  retina, retinal — *see* Occlusion, artery, retina
  saddle
    abdominal aorta I74.01
    pulmonary artery I26.92
      with acute cor pulmonale I26.02
  septic (arterial) I76
    complicating abortion — *see* Abortion, by type, complicated by, embolism
  sinus — *see* Embolism, intracranial, venous sinus
  soap complicating abortion — *see* Abortion, by type, complicated by, embolism
  spinal cord G95.19
    pyogenic origin G06.1
  spleen, splenic (artery) I74.8
  upper extremity I74.2
  vein (acute) I82.90
    antecubital I82.61- ☑
      chronic I82.71- ☑
    axillary I82.A1- ☑ (*following* I82.7)
      chronic I82.A2- ☑ (*following* I82.7)
    basilic I82.61- ☑
      chronic I82.71- ☑
    brachial I82.62- ☑
      chronic I82.72- ☑
    brachiocephalic (innominate) I82.290
      chronic I82.291
    calf, muscle I82.46- ☑
      chronic I82.56- ☑
    cephalic I82.61- ☑
      chronic I82.71- ☑
    chronic I82.91
    deep (DVT) I82.40- ☑
      calf I82.4Z- ☑
        chronic I82.5Z- ☑
      lower leg I82.4Z- ☑
        chronic I82.5Z- ☑
      thigh I82.4Y- ☑
        chronic I82.5Y- ☑
      upper leg I82.4Y
        chronic I82.5Y-
    femoral I82.41- ☑

Embolism — *continued*
  vein — *continued*
    femoral — *continued*
      chronic I82.51- ☑
      gastrocnemial I82.46- ☑
        chronic I82.56- ☑
      iliac (iliofemoral) I82.42- ☑
        chronic I82.52- ☑
      innominate I82.290
        chronic I82.291
      internal jugular I82.C1- ☑ (*following* I82.7)
        chronic I82.C2- ☑ (*following* I82.7)
      lower extremity
        deep I82.40- ☑
          chronic I82.50- ☑
          specified NEC I82.49- ☑
            chronic NEC I82.59- ☑
        distal
          deep I82.4Z- ☑
        proximal
          deep I82.4Y- ☑
            chronic I82.5Y- ☑
        superficial I82.81- ☑
      peroneal I82.45- ☑
        chronic I82.55- ☑
      popliteal I82.43- ☑
        chronic I82.53- ☑
      radial I82.62- ☑
        chronic I82.72- ☑
      renal I82.3
      saphenous (greater) (lesser) I82.81- ☑
      soleal I82.46- ☑
        chronic I82.56- ☑
      specified NEC I82.890
        chronic NEC I82.891
      subclavian I82.B1- ☑ (*following* I82.7)
        chronic I82.B2- ☑ (*following* I82.7)
      thoracic NEC I82.290
        chronic I82.291
      tibial I82.44- ☑
        chronic I82.54- ☑
      ulnar I82.62- ☑
        chronic I82.72- ☑
      upper extremity I82.60- ☑
        chronic I82.70- ☑
        deep I82.62- ☑
          chronic I82.72- ☑
        superficial I82.61- ☑
          chronic I82.71- ☑
    vena cava
      inferior (acute) I82.220
        chronic I82.221
      superior (acute) I82.210
        chronic I82.211
    venous sinus G08
  vessels of brain — *see* Occlusion, artery, cerebral
Embolus — *see* Embolism
Embryoma — *see also* Neoplasm, uncertain behavior, by site
  benign — *see* Neoplasm, benign, by site
  kidney C64.- ☑
  liver C22.0
  malignant — *see also* Neoplasm, malignant, by site
    kidney C64.- ☑
    liver C22.0
    testis C62.9- ☑
      descended (scrotal) C62.1- ☑
      undescended C62.0- ☑
  testis C62.9- ☑
    descended (scrotal) C62.1- ☑
    undescended C62.0- ☑
Embryonic
  circulation Q28.9
  heart Q28.9
  vas deferens Q55.4
Embryopathia NOS Q89.9
Embryotoxon Q13.4
Emesis — *see* Vomiting
Emotional lability R45.86
Emotionality, pathological F60.3
Emotogenic disease — *see* Disorder, psychogenic
Emphysema (atrophic) (bullous) (chronic) (interlobular) (lung) (obstructive) (pulmonary) (senile) (vesicular) J43.9
  cellular tissue (traumatic) T79.7 ☑
    surgical T81.82 ☑

Emphysema — continued
- centrilobular J43.2
- compensatory J98.3
- congenital (interstitial) P25.0
- conjunctiva H11.89
- connective tissue (traumatic) T79.7 ☑
  - surgical T81.82 ☑
- due to chemicals, gases, fumes or vapors J68.4
- eyelid(s) — see Disorder, eyelid, specified type NEC
  - surgical T81.82 ☑
  - traumatic T79.7 ☑
- interstitial J98.2
  - congenital P25.0
  - perinatal period P25.0
- laminated tissue T79.7 ☑
  - surgical T81.82 ☑
- mediastinal J98.2
  - newborn P25.2
- orbit, orbital — see Disorder, orbit, specified type NEC
- panacinar J43.1
- panlobular J43.1
- specified NEC J43.8
- subcutaneous (traumatic) T79.7 ☑
  - nontraumatic J98.2
  - postprocedural T81.82 ☑
  - surgical T81.82 ☑
- surgical T81.82 ☑
- thymus (gland) (congenital) E32.8
- traumatic (subcutaneous) T79.7 ☑
- unilateral J43.0

Empty nest syndrome Z60.0

Empyema (acute) (chest) (double) (pleura) (supradiaphragmatic) (thorax) J86.9
- with fistula J86.0
- accessory sinus (chronic) — see Sinusitis
- antrum (chronic) — see Sinusitis, maxillary
- brain (any part) — see Abscess, brain
- ethmoidal (chronic) (sinus) — see Sinusitis, ethmoidal
- extradural — see Abscess, extradural
- frontal (chronic) (sinus) — see Sinusitis, frontal
- gallbladder K81.0
- mastoid (process) (acute) — see Mastoiditis, acute
- maxilla, maxillary M27.2
  - sinus (chronic) — see Sinusitis, maxillary
- nasal sinus (chronic) — see Sinusitis
- sinus (accessory) (chronic) (nasal) — see Sinusitis
- sphenoidal (sinus) (chronic) — see Sinusitis, sphenoidal
- subarachnoid — see Abscess, extradural
- subdural — see Abscess, subdural
- tuberculous A15.6
- ureter — see Ureteritis
- ventricular — see Abscess, brain

En coup de sabre lesion L94.1

Enamel pearls K00.2

Enameloma K00.2

Enanthema, viral B09

Encephalitis (chronic) (hemorrhagic) (idiopathic) (nonepidemic) (spurious) (subacute) G04.90
- acute — see also Encephalitis, viral A86
  - disseminated G04.00
    - infectious G04.01
    - noninfectious G04.81
    - postimmunization (postvaccination) G04.02
    - postinfectious G04.01
  - inclusion body A85.8
  - necrotizing hemorrhagic G04.30
    - postimmunization G04.32
    - postinfectious G04.31
    - specified NEC G04.39
- arboviral, arbovirus NEC A85.2
- arthropod-borne NEC (viral) A85.2
- Australian A83.4
- California (virus) A83.5
- Central European (tick-borne) A84.1
- Czechoslovakian A84.1
- Dawson's (inclusion body) A81.1
- diffuse sclerosing A81.1
- disseminated, acute G04.00
- due to
  - cat scratch disease A28.1
  - human immunodeficiency virus (HIV) disease B20 [G05.3]
  - malaria — see Malaria
  - rickettsiosis — see Rickettsiosis
  - smallpox inoculation G04.02
  - typhus — see Typhus
- Eastern equine A83.2

Encephalitis — continued
- endemic (viral) A86
- epidemic NEC (viral) A86
- equine (acute) (infectious) (viral) A83.9
  - Eastern A83.2
  - Venezuelan A92.2
  - Western A83.1
- Far Eastern (tick-borne) A84.0
- following vaccination or other immunization procedure G04.02
- herpes zoster B02.0
- herpesviral B00.4
  - due to herpesvirus 6 B10.01
  - due to herpesvirus 7 B10.09
  - specified NEC B10.09
- Ilheus (virus) A83.8
- in (due to)
  - actinomycosis A42.82
  - adenovirus A85.1
  - African trypanosomiasis B56.9 [G05.3]
  - Chagas' disease (chronic) B57.42
  - cytomegalovirus B25.8
  - enterovirus A85.0
  - herpes (simplex) virus B00.4
    - due to herpesvirus 6 B10.01
    - due to herpesvirus 7 B10.09
    - specified NEC B10.09
  - infectious disease NEC B99 ☑ [G05.3]
  - influenza — see Influenza, with, encephalopathy
  - listeriosis A32.12
  - measles B05.0
  - mumps B26.2
  - naegleriasis B60.2
  - parasitic disease NEC B89 [G05.3]
  - poliovirus A80.9 [G05.3]
  - rubella B06.01
  - syphilis
    - congenital A50.42
    - late A52.14
  - systemic lupus erythematosus M32.19
  - toxoplasmosis (acquired) B58.2
    - congenital P37.1
  - tuberculosis A17.82
  - zoster B02.0
- inclusion body A81.1
- infectious (acute) (virus) NEC A86
- Japanese (B type) A83.0
- La Crosse A83.5
- lead — see Poisoning, lead
- lethargica (acute) (infectious) A85.8
- louping ill A84.89
- lupus erythematosus, systemic M32.19
- lymphatica A87.2
- Mengo A85.8
- meningococcal A39.81
- Murray Valley A83.4
- otitic NEC H66.40 [G05.3]
- parasitic NOS B71.9
- periaxial G37.0
- periaxialis (concentrica) (diffuse) G37.5
- postchickenpox B01.11
- postexanthematous NEC B09
- postimmunization G04.02
- postinfectious NEC G04.01
- postmeasles B05.0
- postvaccinal G04.02
- postvaricella B01.11
- postviral NEC A86
- Powassan A84.81
- Rasmussen G04.81
- Rio Bravo A85.8
- Russian
  - autumnal A83.0
  - spring-summer (taiga) A84.0
- saturnine — see Poisoning, lead
- specified NEC G04.81
- St. Louis A83.3
- subacute sclerosing A81.1
- summer A83.0
- suppurative G04.81
- tick-borne A84.9
- Torula, torular (cryptococcal) B45.1
- toxic NEC G92.8
- trichinosis B75 [G05.3]
- type
  - B A83.0
  - C A83.3
- van Bogaert's A81.1

Encephalitis — continued
- Venezuelan equine A92.2
- Vienna A85.8
- viral, virus A86
  - arthropod-borne NEC A85.2
    - mosquito-borne A83.9
      - Australian X disease A83.4
      - California virus A83.5
      - Eastern equine A83.2
      - Japanese (B type) A83.0
      - Murray Valley A83.4
      - specified NEC A83.8
      - St. Louis A83.3
      - type B A83.0
      - type C A83.3
      - Western equine A83.1
    - tick-borne A84.9
      - biundulant A84.1
      - central European A84.1
      - Czechoslovakian A84.1
      - diphasic meningoencephalitis A84.1
      - Far Eastern A84.0
      - Russian spring-summer (taiga) A84.0
      - specified NEC A84.89
  - specified type NEC A85.8
  - tick-borne, specified NEC A84.89
- Western equine A83.1

Encephalocele Q01.9
- frontal Q01.0
- nasofrontal Q01.1
- occipital Q01.2
- specified NEC Q01.8

Encephalocystocele — see Encephalocele

Encephaloduroarteriomyosynangiosis (EDAMS) I67.5

Encephalomalacia (brain) (cerebellar) (cerebral) — see Softening, brain

Encephalomeningitis — see Meningoencephalitis

Encephalomeningocele — see Encephalocele

Encephalomeningomyelitis — see Meningoencephalitis

Encephalomyelitis — see also Encephalitis G04.90
- acute disseminated G04.00
  - infectious G04.01
  - noninfectious G04.81
  - postimmunization G04.02
  - postinfectious G04.01
- acute necrotizing hemorrhagic G04.30
  - postimmunization G04.32
  - postinfectious G04.31
  - specified NEC G04.39
- equine A83.9
  - Eastern A83.2
  - Venezuelan A92.2
  - Western A83.1
- in diseases classified elsewhere G05.3
- myalgic G93.32
  - chronic fatigue syndrome [ME/CFS] G93.32
- postchickenpox B01.11
- postinfectious NEC G04.01
- postmeasles B05.0
- postvaccinal G04.02
- postvaricella B01.11
- rubella B06.01
- specified NEC G04.81
- Venezuelan equine A92.2

Encephalomyelocele — see Encephalocele

Encephalomyelomeningitis — see Meningoencephalitis

Encephalomyelopathy G96.9

Encephalomyeloradiculitis (acute) G61.0

Encephalomyeloradiculoneuritis (acute) (Guillain-Barré) G61.0

Encephalomyeloradiculopathy G96.9

Encephalopathia hyperbilirubinemica, newborn P57.9
- due to isoimmunization (conditions in P55) P57.0

Encephalopathy (acute) G93.40
- acute necrotizing hemorrhagic G04.30
  - postimmunization G04.32
  - postinfectious G04.31
  - specified NEC G04.39
- alcoholic G31.2
- anoxic — see Damage, brain, anoxic
- arteriosclerotic I67.2
- centrolobar progressive (Schilder) G37.0
- congenital Q07.9
- degenerative, in specified disease NEC G32.89
- demyelinating callosal G37.1

Encephalopathy — continued
- due to
  - drugs — see also Table of Drugs and Chemicals G92.8
  - hepatic (without coma) K76.82
  - hyperbilirubinemic, newborn P57.9
    - due to isoimmunization (conditions in P55) P57.0
  - hypertensive I67.4
  - hypoglycemic E16.2
  - hypoxic — see Damage, brain, anoxic
  - hypoxic ischemic P91.60
    - mild P91.61
    - moderate P91.62
    - severe P91.63
- in (due to) (with)
  - birth injury P11.1
  - hyperinsulinism E16.1 [G94]
  - influenza — see Influenza, with, encephalopathy
  - lack of vitamin — see also Deficiency, vitamin E56.9 [G32.89]
  - neoplastic disease — see also Neoplasm D49.9 [G13.1]
  - serum — see also Reaction, serum T80.69 ☑
  - syphilis A52.17
  - trauma (postconcussional) F07.81
    - current injury — see Injury, intracranial
  - vaccination G04.02
- lead — see Poisoning, lead
- metabolic G93.41
  - drug induced G92.8
  - toxic G92.8
- myoclonic, early, symptomatic — see Epilepsy, generalized, specified NEC
- necrotizing, subacute (Leigh) G31.82
- neonatal P91.819
  - in diseases classified elsewhere P91.811
- pellagrous E52 [G32.89]
- portal-systemic K76.82
- postcontusional F07.81
  - current injury — see Injury, intracranial, diffuse
- posthypoglycemic (coma) E16.1 [G94]
- postradiation G93.89
- saturnine — see Poisoning, lead
- septic G93.41
- specified NEC G93.49
- spongiform, subacute (viral) A81.09
- toxic G92.9
  - metabolic G92.8
- traumatic (postconcussional) F07.81
  - current injury — see Injury, intracranial
- vitamin B deficiency NEC E53.9 [G32.89]
  - vitamin B1 E51.2
- Wernicke's E51.2

Encephalorrhagia — see Hemorrhage, intracranial, intracerebral

Encephalosis, posttraumatic F07.81

Enchondroma — see also Neoplasm, bone, benign

Enchondromatosis (cartilaginous) (multiple) Q78.4

Encopresis R15.9
- functional F98.1
- nonorganic origin F98.1
- psychogenic F98.1

Encounter (with health service) (for) Z76.89
- adjustment and management (of)
  - breast implant Z45.81 ☑
  - implanted device NEC Z45.89
  - myringotomy device (stent) (tube) Z45.82
  - neurostimulator (brain) (gastric) (peripheral nerve) (sacral nerve) (spinal cord) (vagus nerve) Z45.42
- administrative purpose only Z02.9
  - examination for
    - adoption Z02.82
    - armed forces Z02.3
    - disability determination Z02.71
    - driving license Z02.4
    - employment Z02.1
    - insurance Z02.6
    - medical certificate NEC Z02.79
    - paternity testing Z02.81
    - residential institution admission Z02.2
    - school admission Z02.0
    - sports Z02.5
  - specified reason NEC Z02.89
- aftercare — see Aftercare
- antenatal screening Z36.9
  - cervical length Z36.86
  - chromosomal anomalies Z36.0

Encounter — continued
- antenatal screening — continued
  - congenital cardiac abnormalities Z36.83
  - elevated maternal serum alphafetoprotein Z36.1
  - fetal growth retardation Z36.4
  - fetal lung maturity Z36.84
  - fetal macrosomia Z36.88
  - hydrops fetalis Z36.81
  - intrauterine growth restriction (IUGR) /small-for-dates Z36.4
  - isoimmunization Z36.5
  - large-for-dates Z36.88
  - malformations Z36.3
  - non-visualized anatomy on a previous scan Z36.2
  - nuchal translucency Z36.82
  - raised alphafetoprotein level Z36.1
  - risk of pre-term labor Z36.86
  - specified follow-up NEC Z36.2
  - specified genetic defects NEC Z36.8A
  - specified type NEC Z36.89
  - Streptococcus B Z36.85
  - suspected anomaly Z36.3
  - uncertain dates Z36.87
- assisted reproductive fertility procedure cycle Z31.83
- blood typing Z01.83
  - Rh typing Z01.83
- breast augmentation or reduction Z41.1
- breast implant exchange (different material) (different size) Z45.81 ☑
- breast reconstruction following mastectomy Z42.1
- check-up — see Examination
- chemotherapy for neoplasm Z51.11
- colonoscopy, screening Z12.11
- counseling — see Counseling
- delivery, full-term, uncomplicated O80
  - cesarean, without indication O82
- desensitization to allergens Z51.6
- ear piercing Z41.3
- examination — see Examination
- expectant parent(s) (adoptive) pre-birth pediatrician visit Z76.81
- fertility preservation procedure (prior to cancer therapy) (prior to removal of gonads) Z31.84
- fitting (of) — see Fitting (and adjustment) (of)
- genetic
  - counseling
    - nonprocreative Z71.83
    - procreative Z31.5
  - testing — see Test, genetic
- hearing conservation and treatment Z01.12
- immunotherapy for neoplasm Z51.12
- in vitro fertilization cycle Z31.83
- instruction (in)
  - child care (postpartal) (prenatal) Z32.3
  - childbirth Z32.2
  - natural family planning
    - procreative Z31.61
    - to avoid pregnancy Z30.02
- insulin pump titration Z46.81
- joint prosthesis insertion following prior explantation of joint prosthesis (staged procedure)
  - hip Z47.32
  - knee Z47.33
  - shoulder Z47.31
- laboratory (as part of a general medical examination) Z00.00
  - with abnormal findings Z00.01
- mental health services (for)
  - abuse NEC
    - perpetrator Z69.82
    - victim Z69.81
  - child abuse
    - nonparental
      - perpetrator Z69.021
      - victim Z69.020
    - parental
      - perpetrator Z69.011
      - victim Z69.010
  - child neglect
    - nonparental
      - perpetrator Z69.021
      - victim Z69.020
    - parental
      - perpetrator Z69.011
      - victim Z69.010
  - child psychological abuse
    - nonparental
      - perpetrator Z69.021
      - victim Z69.020

Encounter — continued
- mental health services — continued
  - child psychological abuse — continued
    - parental
      - perpetrator Z69.011
      - victim Z69.010
  - child sexual abuse
    - nonparental
      - perpetrator Z69.021
      - victim Z69.020
    - parental
      - perpetrator Z69.011
      - victim Z69.010
  - non-spousal adult abuse
    - perpetrator Z69.82
    - victim Z69.81
  - spousal or partner
    - abuse
      - perpetrator Z69.12
      - victim Z69.11
    - neglect
      - perpetrator Z69.12
      - victim Z69.11
    - psychological abuse
      - perpetrator Z69.12
      - victim Z69.11
    - violence
      - perpetrator (physical) (sexual) Z69.12
      - victim (physical) Z69.11
        - sexual Z69.81
- observation (for) (ruled out)
  - alarm, without findings
    - apnea Z03.83
    - bradycardia Z03.83
    - oximeter Z03.83
  - condition suspected related to home physiologic monitoring device Z03.83
  - exposure to (suspected)
    - anthrax Z03.810
    - biological agent NEC Z03.818
  - malfunction of home cardiorespiratory monitor Z03.83
  - non-specific findings home physiologic monitoring device Z03.83
- pediatrician visit, by expectant parent(s) (adoptive) Z76.81
- placental sample (taken vaginally) — see also Encounter, antenatal screening Z36.9
- plastic and reconstructive surgery following medical procedure or healed injury NEC Z42.8
- pregnancy
  - supervision of — see Pregnancy, supervision of
  - test Z32.00
    - result negative Z32.02
    - result positive Z32.01
- procreative management and counseling for gestational carrier Z31.7
- prophylactic measures Z29.9
  - antivenin Z29.12
  - fluoride administration Z29.3
  - immunotherapy for respiratory syncytial virus (RSV) Z29.11
  - rabies immune globin Z29.14
  - Rho (D) immune globulin Z29.13
  - specified NEC Z29.8
- radiation therapy (antineoplastic) Z51.0
- radiological (as part of a general medical examination) Z00.00
  - with abnormal findings Z00.01
- reconstructive surgery following medical procedure or healed injury NEC Z42.8
- removal (of) — see also Removal
  - artificial
    - arm Z44.00- ☑
      - complete Z44.01- ☑
      - partial Z44.02- ☑
    - eye Z44.2- ☑
    - leg Z44.10- ☑
      - complete Z44.11- ☑
      - partial Z44.12- ☑
  - breast implant Z45.81 ☑
    - tissue expander (with or without synchronous insertion of permanent implant) Z45.81 ☑
  - device Z46.9
    - specified NEC Z46.89

Encounter — *continued*
  removal — *see also* Removal — *continued*
    external
      fixation device — *code to* fracture with seventh character D
      prosthesis, prosthetic device Z44.9
        breast Z44.3- ☑
        specified NEC Z44.8
    implanted device NEC Z45.89
    insulin pump Z46.81
    internal fixation device Z47.2
    myringotomy device (stent) (tube) Z45.82
    nervous system device NEC Z46.2
      brain neuropacemaker Z46.2
      visual substitution device Z46.2
        implanted Z45.31
    non-vascular catheter Z46.82
    orthodontic device Z46.4
    stent
      ureteral Z46.6
    urinary device Z46.6
  repeat cervical smear to confirm findings of recent normal smear following initial abnormal smear Z01.42
  respirator [ventilator] use during power failure Z99.12
  Rh typing Z01.83
  screening — *see* Screening
  specified NEC Z76.89
  sterilization Z30.2 *tubal ligation*
  suspected condition, ruled out
    amniotic cavity and membrane Z03.71
    cervical shortening Z03.75
    fetal anomaly Z03.73
    fetal growth Z03.74
    maternal and fetal conditions NEC Z03.79
    oligohydramnios Z03.71
    placental problem Z03.72
    polyhydramnios Z03.71
  suspected exposure (to), ruled out
    anthrax Z03.810
    biological agents NEC Z03.818
  termination of pregnancy, elective Z33.2
  testing — *see* Test
  therapeutic drug level monitoring Z51.81
  titration, insulin pump Z46.81
  to determine fetal viability of pregnancy O36.80 ☑
  training
    insulin pump Z46.81
  X-ray of chest (as part of a general medical examination) Z00.00
    with abnormal findings Z00.01
Encystment — *see* Cyst
Endarteritis (bacterial, subacute) (infective) I77.6
  brain I67.7
  cerebral or cerebrospinal I67.7
  deformans — *see* Arteriosclerosis
  embolic — *see* Embolism
  obliterans — *see also* Arteriosclerosis
    pulmonary I28.8
  pulmonary I28.8
  retina — *see* Vasculitis, retina
  senile — *see* Arteriosclerosis
  syphilitic A52.09
    brain or cerebral A52.04
    congenital A50.54 [I79.8]
  tuberculous A18.89
Endemic — *see* condition
Endocarditis (chronic) (marantic) (nonbacterial) (thrombotic) (valvular) I38
  with rheumatic fever (conditions in I00)
    active — *see* Endocarditis, acute, rheumatic
    inactive or quiescent (with chorea) I09.1
  acute or subacute I33.9
    infective I33.0
    rheumatic (aortic) (mitral) (pulmonary) (tricuspid) I01.1
      with chorea (acute) (rheumatic) (Sydenham's) I02.0
  aortic (heart) (nonrheumatic) (valve) I35.8
    with
      mitral disease I08.0
        with tricuspid (valve) disease I08.3
          active or acute I01.1
            with chorea (acute) (rheumatic) (Sydenham's) I02.0
        rheumatic fever (conditions in I00)
          active — *see* Endocarditis, acute, rheumatic
          inactive or quiescent (with chorea) I06.9

Endocarditis — *continued*
  aortic — *continued*
    with — *continued*
      tricuspid (valve) disease I08.2
        with mitral (valve) disease I08.3
    acute or subacute I33.9
    arteriosclerotic I35.8
    rheumatic I06.9
      with mitral disease I08.0
        with tricuspid (valve) disease I08.3
          active or acute I01.1
            with chorea (acute) (rheumatic) (Sydenham's) I02.0
      active or acute I01.1
        with chorea (acute) (rheumatic) (Sydenham's) I02.0
      specified NEC I06.8
    specified cause NEC I35.8
    syphilitic A52.03
  arteriosclerotic I38
  atypical verrucous (Libman-Sacks) M32.11
  bacterial (acute) (any valve) (subacute) I33.0
  candidal B37.6
  congenital Q24.8
  constrictive I33.0
  Coxiella burnetii A78 [I39]
  Coxsackie B33.21
  due to
    prosthetic cardiac valve T82.6 ☑
    Q fever A78 [I39]
    Serratia marcescens I33.0
    typhoid (fever) A01.02
  gonococcal A54.83
  infectious or infective (acute) (any valve) (subacute) I33.0
  lenta (acute) (any valve) (subacute) I33.0
  Libman-Sacks M32.11
  listerial A32.82
  Löffler's I42.3
  malignant (acute) (any valve) (subacute) I33.0
  meningococcal A39.51
  mitral (chronic) (double) (fibroid) (heart) (inactive) (valve) (with chorea) I05.9
    with
      aortic (valve) disease I08.0
        with tricuspid (valve) disease I08.3
          active or acute I01.1
            with chorea (acute) (rheumatic) (Sydenham's) I02.0
      rheumatic fever (conditions in I00)
        active — *see* Endocarditis, acute, rheumatic
        inactive or quiescent (with chorea) I05.9
      tricuspid (valve) disease I08.1
        with aortic (valve) disease I08.3
    active or acute I01.1
      with chorea (acute) (rheumatic) (Sydenham's) I02.0
    bacterial I33.0
    arteriosclerotic I34.89
    nonrheumatic I34.89
      acute or subacute I33.9
    specified NEC I05.8
  monilial B37.6
  multiple valves I08.9
    specified disorders I08.8
  mycotic (acute) (any valve) (subacute) I33.0
  pneumococcal (acute) (any valve) (subacute) I33.0
  pulmonary (chronic) (heart) (valve) I37.8
    with rheumatic fever (conditions in I00)
      active — *see* Endocarditis, acute, rheumatic
      inactive or quiescent (with chorea) I09.89
        with aortic, mitral or tricuspid disease I08.8
    acute or subacute I33.9
      rheumatic I01.1
        with chorea (acute) (rheumatic) (Sydenham's) I02.0
    arteriosclerotic I37.8
    congenital Q22.2
    rheumatic (chronic) (inactive) (with chorea) I09.89
      active or acute I01.1
        with chorea (acute) (rheumatic) (Sydenham's) I02.0
    syphilitic A52.03
  purulent (acute) (any valve) (subacute) I33.0
  Q fever A78 [I39]
  rheumatic (chronic) (inactive) (with chorea) I09.1
    active or acute (aortic) (mitral) (pulmonary) (tricuspid) I01.1

Endocarditis — *continued*
  rheumatic — *continued*
    active or acute — *continued*
      with chorea (acute) (rheumatic) (Sydenham's) I02.0
  rheumatoid — *see* Rheumatoid, carditis
  septic (acute) (any valve) (subacute) I33.0
  streptococcal (acute) (any valve) (subacute) I33.0
  subacute — *see* Endocarditis, acute
  suppurative (acute) (any valve) (subacute) I33.0
  syphilitic A52.03
  toxic I33.9
  tricuspid (chronic) (heart) (inactive) (rheumatic) (valve) (with chorea) I07.9
    with
      aortic (valve) disease I08.2
        mitral (valve) disease I08.3
      mitral (valve) disease I08.1
        aortic (valve) disease I08.3
      rheumatic fever (conditions in I00)
        active — *see* Endocarditis, acute, rheumatic
        inactive or quiescent (with chorea) I07.8
    active or acute I01.1
      with chorea (acute) (rheumatic) (Sydenham's) I02.0
    arteriosclerotic I36.8
    nonrheumatic I36.8
      acute or subacute I33.9
    specified cause, except rheumatic I36.8
  tuberculous — *see* Tuberculosis, endocarditis
  typhoid A01.02
  ulcerative (acute) (any valve) (subacute) I33.0
  vegetative (acute) (any valve) (subacute) I33.0
  verrucous (atypical) (nonbacterial) (nonrheumatic) M32.11
Endocardium, endocardial — *see also* condition
  cushion defect Q21.20
Endocervicitis — *see also* Cervicitis
  due to intrauterine (contraceptive) device T83.69 ☑
  hyperplastic N72
Endocrine — *see* condition
Endocrinopathy, pluriglandular E31.9
Endodontic
  overfill M27.52
  underfill M27.53
Endodontitis K04.01
  irreversible K04.02
  reversible K04.01
Endomastoiditis — *see* Mastoiditis
Endometrioma N80.12- ☑
Endometriosis N80.9
  abdomen, abdominal N80.C0
    specified site, NEC N80.C9
      wall N80.C19
        fascia and muscular layers N80.C11
        subcutaneous tissue N80.C10
        unspecified depth N80.C19
  appendix N80.549
    deep N80.542
    superficial N80.541
  bladder (unspecified depth) N80.A0
    deep N80.A2
    superficial N80.A1
  bowel N80.50
  broad ligament N80.3C ☑
  cardiothoracic space N80.B6
  cecum N80.539
    deep N80.532
    superficial N80.531
  cervix N80.0- ☑
  colon N80.559
    descending N80.559
      deep N80.552
      superficial N80.551
    sigmoid N80.529
      deep N80.522
      superficial N80.521
    transverse N80.559
      deep N80.552
      superficial N80.551
  cul-de-sac (Douglas')
    anterior (unspecified depth) N80.319
      deep N80.312
      superficial N80.311
    posterior (unspecified depth) N80.329
      deep N80.322
      superficial N80.321

Endometriosis — *continued*
deep
involving muscular wall of fallopian tube N80.22 ☑
retrocervical N80.02
diaphragm N80.B39
deep N80.B32
superficial N80.B31
unspecified depth N80.B39
exocervix N80.01
extra-pelvic abdominal peritoneum N80.C4
fallopian tube (unspecified depth) N80.20- ☑
deep N80.22- ☑
superficial N80.21- ☑
female genital organ NEC N80.8
gallbladder N80.8
in scar of skin N80.6
inguinal canal N80.C3
internal N80.02
intestine N80.50
lung N80.B2
mediastinal space N80.B5
myometrium N80.03
nerve
femoral N80.D6
obturator N80.D3
pelvic N80.D0
splanchnic N80.D1
pudendal N80.D5
retroperitoneum, NEC N80.D9
sacral splanchnic N80.D1
sciatic N80.D4
specified, NEC N80.D9
ovary (unspecified depth) N80.10- ☑
deep N80.12- ☑
superficial N80.11- ☑
parametrium N80.399
pelvic
brim N80.38- ☑
deep N80.37- ☑
superficial N80.36- ☑
peritoneum N80.30
specified sites, NEC N80.399
deep N80.392
superficial N80.391
sidewall N80.35- ☑
deep N80.34- ☑
superficial N80.33- ☑
pericardial space N80.B4
peritoneal (pelvic) N80.30
pleura N80.B1
rectovaginal septum N80.40
with involvement of vagina N80.42
without involvement of vagina N80.41
rectum N80.519
deep (multifocal) N80.512
superficial N80.511
retroperitoneum N80.30
round ligament N80.3C9
sacral nerve roots N80.D2
skin (scar) N80.6
small N80.569
deep (multifocal) N80.562
superficial N80.561
specified site NEC N80.8
stromal D39.0
thorax N80.B- ☑
umbilicus N80.C2
ureter N80.A69
deep N80.A5- ☑
extrinsic N80.A4- ☑
intrinsic N80.A5- ☑
superficial N80.A4- ☑
unspecified depth N80.A6- ☑
uterosacral ligament(s) N80.3C- ☑
deep N80.3B- ☑
superficial N80.3A- ☑
uterus N80.00
deep N80.02
internal N80.02
superficial N80.01
vagina N80.42
vulva N80.8
Endometritis (decidual) (nonspecific) (purulent) (senile)
(atrophic) (suppurative) N71.9
with ectopic pregnancy O08.0
acute N71.0
blenorrhagic (gonococcal) (acute) (chronic) A54.24

Endometritis — *continued*
cervix, cervical (with erosion or ectropion) — *see also*
Cervicitis
hyperplastic N72
chlamydial A56.11
chronic N71.1
following
abortion — *see* Abortion by type complicated by
genital infection
ectopic or molar pregnancy O08.0
gonococcal, gonorrheal (acute) (chronic) A54.24
hyperplastic — *see also* Hyperplasia, endometrial
N85.00
cervix N72
puerperal, postpartum, childbirth O86.12
subacute N71.0
tuberculous A18.17
Endometrium — *see* condition
Endomyocardiopathy, South African I42.3
Endomyocarditis — *see* Endocarditis
Endomyofibrosis I42.3
Endomyometritis — *see* Endometritis
Endopericarditis — *see* Endocarditis
Endoperineuritis — *see* Disorder, nerve
Endophlebitis — *see* Phlebitis
Endophthalmia — *see* Endophthalmitis, purulent
Endophthalmitis (acute) (infective) (metastatic) (subacute) H44.009
bleb associated — *see also* Bleb, inflamed (infected),
postprocedural H59.4 ☑
gonorrheal A54.39
in (due to)
cysticercosis B69.1
onchocerciasis B73.01
toxocariasis B83.0
panuveitis — *see* Panuveitis
parasitic H44.12- ☑
purulent H44.00- ☑
panophthalmitis — *see* Panophthalmitis
vitreous abscess H44.02- ☑
specified NEC H44.19
sympathetic — *see* Uveitis, sympathetic
Endosalpingioma D28.2
Endosalpingiosis N94.89
Endosteitis — *see* Osteomyelitis
Endothelioma, bone — *see* Neoplasm, bone, malignant
Endotheliosis (hemorrhagic infectional) D69.8
Endotoxemia — code to condition
Endotrachelitis — *see* Cervicitis
Engelmann (-Camurati) **syndrome** Q78.3
English disease — *see* Rickets
Engman's disease L30.3
Engorgement
breast N64.59
newborn P83.4
puerperal, postpartum O92.79
lung (passive) — *see* Edema, lung
pulmonary (passive) — *see* Edema, lung
stomach K31.89
venous, retina — *see* Occlusion, retina, vein, engorgement
Enlargement, enlarged — *see also* Hypertrophy
adenoids J35.2
with tonsils J35.3
alveolar ridge K08.89
congenital — *see* Anomaly, alveolar
apertures of diaphragm (congenital) Q79.1
gingival K06.1
heart, cardiac — *see* Hypertrophy, cardiac
labium majus, childhood asymmetric (CALME) N90.61
lacrimal gland, chronic H04.03- ☑
liver — *see* Hypertrophy, liver
lymph gland or node R59.9
generalized R59.1
localized R59.0
orbit H05.34- ☑
organ or site, congenital NEC — *see* Anomaly, by site
parathyroid (gland) E21.0
pituitary fossa R93.0
prostate N40.0
with lower urinary tract symptoms (LUTS) N40.1
without lower urinary tract symptoms (LUTS) N40.0
sella turcica R93.0
spleen — *see* Splenomegaly
thymus (gland) (congenital) E32.0
thyroid (gland) — *see* Goiter
tongue K14.8

Enlargement, enlarged — *continued*
tonsils J35.1
with adenoids J35.3
uterus N85.2
vestibular aqueduct Q16.5
Enophthalmos H05.40- ☑
due to
orbital tissue atrophy H05.41- ☑
trauma or surgery H05.42- ☑
Enostosis M27.8
Entamebic, entamebiasis — *see* Amebiasis
Entanglement
umbilical cord(s) O69.82 ☑
with compression O69.2 ☑
around neck (with compression) O69.81 ☑
with compression O69.1 ☑
without compression O69.81 ☑
of twins in monoamniotic sac O69.2 ☑
without compression O69.82 ☑
Enteralgia — *see* Pain, abdominal
Enteric — *see* condition
Enteritis (acute) (diarrheal) (hemorrhagic) (noninfective)
K52.9
adenovirus A08.2
aertrycke infection A02.0
allergic K52.29
with
eosinophilic gastritis or gastroenteritis K52.81
food protein-induced enterocolitis syndrome
K52.21
food protein-induced enteropathy K52.22
FPIES K52.21
amebic (acute) A06.0
with abscess — *see* Abscess, amebic
chronic A06.1
with abscess — *see* Abscess, amebic
nondysenteric A06.2
nondysenteric A06.2
astrovirus A08.32
bacillary NOS A03.9
bacterial A04.9
specified NEC A04.8
calicivirus A08.31
candidal B37.82
Chilomastix A07.8
choleriformis A00.1
chronic (noninfectious) K52.9
ulcerative — *see* Colitis, ulcerative
cicatrizing (chronic) — *see* Enteritis, regional, small intestine
Clostridium
botulinum (food poisoning) A05.1
difficile
not specified as recurrent A04.72
recurrent A04.71
coccidial A07.3
coxsackie virus A08.39
dietetic — *see also* Enteritis, allergic K52.29
drug-induced K52.1
due to
astrovirus A08.32
calicivirus A08.31
coxsackie virus A08.39
drugs K52.1
echovirus A08.39
enterovirus NEC A08.39
food hypersensitivity — *see also* Enteritis, allergic
K52.29
infectious organism (bacterial) (viral) — *see* Enteritis,
infectious
torovirus A08.39
Yersinia enterocolitica A04.6
echovirus A08.39
eltor A00.1
enterovirus NEC A08.39
eosinophilic K52.81
epidemic (infectious) A09
fulminant — *see also* Ischemia, intestine, acute K55.019
gangrenous — *see* Enteritis, infectious
giardial A07.1
infectious NOS A09
due to
adenovirus A08.2
Aerobacter aerogenes A04.8
Arizona (bacillus) A02.0
bacteria NOS A04.9
specified NEC A04.8
Campylobacter A04.5

Enteritis — *continued*
- infectious — *continued*
  - due to — *continued*
    - Clostridium difficile
      - not specified as recurrent A04.72
      - recurrent A04.71
    - Clostridium perfringens A04.8
    - Enterobacter aerogenes A04.8
    - enterovirus A08.39
    - Escherichia coli A04.4
      - enteroaggregative A04.4
      - enterohemorrhagic A04.3
      - enteroinvasive A04.2
      - enteropathogenic A04.0
      - enterotoxigenic A04.1
      - specified NEC A04.4
    - specified
      - bacteria NEC A04.8
      - virus NEC A08.39
    - Staphylococcus A04.8
    - virus NEC A08.4
      - specified type NEC A08.39
    - Yersinia enterocolitica A04.6
  - specified organism NEC A08.8
- influenzal — *see* Influenza, with, digestive manifestations
- ischemic K55.9
  - acute — *see also* Ischemia, intestine, acute K55.019
  - chronic K55.1
- microsporidial A07.8
- mucomembranous, myxomembranous — *see* Syndrome, irritable bowel
- mucous — *see* Syndrome, irritable bowel
- necroticans A05.2
- necrotizing of newborn — *see* Enterocolitis, necrotizing, in newborn
- neurogenic — *see* Syndrome, irritable bowel
- newborn necrotizing — *see* Enterocolitis, necrotizing, in newborn
- noninfectious K52.9
- norovirus A08.11
- parasitic NEC B82.9
- paratyphoid (fever) — *see* Fever, paratyphoid
- protozoal A07.9
  - specified NEC A07.8
- radiation K52.0
- regional (of) K50.90
  - with
    - complication K50.919
      - abscess K50.914
      - fistula K50.913
      - intestinal obstruction K50.912
      - rectal bleeding K50.911
      - specified complication NEC K50.918
  - colon — *see* Enteritis, regional, large intestine
  - duodenum — *see* Enteritis, regional, small intestine
  - ileum — *see* Enteritis, regional, small intestine
  - jejunum — *see* Enteritis, regional, small intestine
  - large bowel — *see* Enteritis, regional, large intestine
  - large intestine (colon) (rectum) K50.10
    - with
      - complication K50.119
        - abscess K50.114
        - fistula K50.113
        - intestinal obstruction K50.112
        - rectal bleeding K50.111
        - small intestine (duodenum) (ileum) (jejunum) involvement K50.80
          - with
            - complication K50.819
              - abscess K50.814
              - fistula K50.813
              - intestinal obstruction K50.812
              - rectal bleeding K50.811
              - specified complication NEC K50.818
        - specified complication NEC K50.118
  - rectum — *see* Enteritis, regional, large intestine
  - small intestine (duodenum) (ileum) (jejunum) K50.00
    - with
      - complication K50.019
        - abscess K50.014
        - fistula K50.013
        - intestinal obstruction K50.012
        - large intestine (colon) (rectum) involvement K50.80

Enteritis — *continued*
- regional — *continued*
  - small intestine — *continued*
    - with — *continued*
      - complication — *continued*
        - large intestine involvement — *continued*
          - with
            - complication K50.819
              - abscess K50.814
              - fistula K50.813
              - intestinal obstruction K50.812
              - rectal bleeding K50.811
              - specified complication NEC K50.818
        - rectal bleeding K50.011
        - specified complication NEC K50.018
- rotaviral A08.0
- Salmonella, salmonellosis (arizonae) (cholerae-suis) (enteritidis) (typhimurium) A02.0
- segmental — *see* Enteritis, regional
- septic A09
- Shigella — *see* Infection, Shigella
- small round structured NEC A08.19
- spasmodic, spastic — *see* Syndrome, irritable bowel
- staphylococcal A04.8
  - due to food A05.0
- torovirus A08.39
- toxic NEC K52.1
  - due to Clostridium difficile
    - not specified as recurrent A04.72
    - recurrent A04.71
- trichomonal A07.8
- tuberculous A18.32
- typhosa A01.00
- ulcerative (chronic) — *see* Colitis, ulcerative
- viral A08.4
  - adenovirus A08.2
  - enterovirus A08.39
  - Rotavirus A08.0
  - small round structured NEC A08.19
  - specified NEC A08.39
  - virus specified NEC A08.39

Enterobiasis B80
Enterobius vermicularis (infection) (infestation) B80
Enterocele — *see also* Hernia, abdomen
- pelvic, pelvis (acquired) (congenital) N81.5
- vagina, vaginal (acquired) (congenital) NEC N81.5

Enterocolitis — *see also* Enteritis K52.9
- due to Clostridium difficile
  - not specified as recurrent A04.72
  - recurrent A04.71
- fulminant ischemic — *see also* Ischemia, intestine, acute K55.059
- granulomatous — *see* Enteritis, regional
- hemorrhagic (acute) — *see also* Ischemia, intestine, acute K55.059
- chronic K55.1
- infectious NEC A09
- ischemic K55.9
- necrotizing K55.30
  - with
    - perforation K55.33
    - pneumatosis K55.32
      - and perforation K55.33
  - due to Clostridium difficile
    - not specified as recurrent A04.72
    - recurrent A04.71
  - in non-newborn K55.30
    - stage 1 (without pneumatosis, without perforation) K55.31
    - stage 2 (with pneumatosis, without perforation) K55.32
    - stage 3 (with pneumatosis, with perforation) K55.33
  - in newborn P77.9
    - stage 1 (without pneumatosis, without perforation) P77.1
    - stage 2 (with pneumatosis, without perforation) P77.2
    - stage 3 (with pneumatosis, with perforation) P77.3
  - without pneumatosis or perforation K55.31
- noninfectious K52.9
  - newborn — *see* Enterocolitis, necrotizing, in newborn
- pseudomembranous (newborn)
  - not specified as recurrent A04.72

Enterocolitis — *continued*
- pseudomembranous — *continued*
  - recurrent A04.71
- radiation K52.0
  - newborn — *see* Enterocolitis, necrotizing, in newborn
- ulcerative (chronic) — *see* Pancolitis, ulcerative (chronic)
Enterogastritis — *see* Enteritis
Enteropathy K63.9
- celiac-gluten-sensitive K90.0
  - non-celiac K90.41
- food protein-induced K52.22
- hemorrhagic, terminal — *see also* Ischemia, intestine, acute K55.059
- protein-losing K90.49
Enteroperitonitis — *see* Peritonitis
Enteroptosis K63.4
Enterorrhagia K92.2
Enterospasm — *see also* Syndrome, irritable, bowel
- psychogenic F45.8
Enterostenosis — *see also* Obstruction, intestine, specified NEC K56.699
Enterostomy
- complication — *see* Complication, enterostomy
- status Z93.4
Enterovirus, as cause of disease classified elsewhere B97.10
- coxsackievirus B97.11
- echovirus B97.12
- other specified B97.19
Enthesopathy (peripheral) M77.9
- Achilles tendinitis — *see* Tendinitis, Achilles
- ankle and tarsus M77.5- ☑
  - specified type NEC — *see* Enthesopathy, foot, specified type NEC
- anterior tibial syndrome M76.81- ☑
- calcaneal spur — *see* Spur, bone, calcaneal
- elbow region M77.8
  - lateral epicondylitis — *see* Epicondylitis, lateral
  - medial epicondylitis — *see* Epicondylitis, medial
- foot NEC M77.8
  - metatarsalgia — *see* Metatarsalgia
  - specified type NEC M77.5- ☑
- forearm M77.8
- gluteal tendinitis — *see* Tendinitis, gluteal
- hand M77.8
- hip — *see* Enthesopathy, lower limb, specified type NEC
- iliac crest spur — *see* Spur, bone, iliac crest
- iliotibial band syndrome — *see* Syndrome, iliotibial band
- knee — *see* Enthesopathy, lower limb, lower leg, specified type NEC
- lateral epicondylitis — *see* Epicondylitis, lateral
- lower limb (excluding foot) M76.9
  - Achilles tendinitis — *see* Tendinitis, Achilles
  - ankle and tarsus M77.5- ☑
    - specified type NEC — *see* Enthesopathy, foot, specified type NEC
  - anterior tibial syndrome M76.81- ☑
  - gluteal tendinitis — *see* Tendinitis, gluteal
  - iliac crest spur — *see* Spur, bone, iliac crest
  - iliotibial band syndrome — *see* Syndrome, iliotibial band
  - patellar tendinitis — *see* Tendinitis, patellar
  - pelvic region — *see* Enthesopathy, lower limb, specified type NEC
  - peroneal tendinitis — *see* Tendinitis, peroneal
  - posterior tibial syndrome M76.82- ☑
  - psoas tendinitis — *see* Tendinitis, psoas
  - specified type NEC M76.89- ☑
  - tibial collateral bursitis — *see* Bursitis, tibial collateral
- medial epicondylitis — *see* Epicondylitis, medial
- metatarsalgia — *see* Metatarsalgia
- multiple sites M77.8
- patellar tendinitis — *see* Tendinitis, patellar
- pelvis M77.8
- periarthritis of wrist — *see* Periarthritis, wrist
- peroneal tendinitis — *see* Tendinitis, peroneal
- posterior tibial syndrome M76.82- ☑
- psoas tendinitis — *see* Tendinitis, psoas
- shoulder M77.8
- shoulder region — *see* Lesion, shoulder
- specified type NEC M77.8
- spinal M46.00

Enthesopathy — *continued*
  spinal — *continued*
    cervical region M46.02
    cervicothoracic region M46.03
    lumbar region M46.06
    lumbosacral region M46.07
    multiple sites M46.09
    occipito-atlanto-axial region M46.01
    sacrococcygeal region M46.08
    thoracic region M46.04
    thoracolumbar region M46.05
  tibial collateral bursitis — *see* Bursitis, tibial collateral
  upper arm M77.8
  wrist and carpus NEC M77.8
    calcaneal spur — *see* Spur, bone, calcaneal
    periarthritis of wrist — *see* Periarthritis, wrist
Entomophobia F40.218
Entomophthoromycosis B46.8
Entrance, air into vein — *see* Embolism, air
Entrapment, nerve — *see* Neuropathy, entrapment
Entropion (eyelid) (paralytic) H02.009
  cicatricial H02.019
    left H02.016
      lower H02.015
      upper H02.014
    right H02.013
      lower H02.012
      upper H02.011
  congenital Q10.2
  left H02.006
    lower H02.005
    upper H02.004
  mechanical H02.029
    left H02.026
      lower H02.025
      upper H02.024
    right H02.023
      lower H02.022
      upper H02.021
  right H02.003
    lower H02.002
    upper H02.001
  senile H02.039
    left H02.036
      lower H02.035
      upper H02.034
    right H02.033
      lower H02.032
      upper H02.031
  spastic H02.049
    left H02.046
      lower H02.045
      upper H02.044
    right H02.043
      lower H02.042
      upper H02.041
Enucleated eye (traumatic, current) S05.7- ☑
Enuresis R32
  functional F98.0
  habit disturbance F98.0
  nocturnal N39.44
    psychogenic F98.0
  nonorganic origin F98.0
  psychogenic F98.0
Eosinopenia — *see* Agranulocytosis
Eosinophilia (allergic) (idiopathic) (secondary) D72.10
  with
    angiolymphoid hyperplasia (ALHE) D18.01
  familial D72.19
  hereditary D72.19
  in disease classified elsewhere D72.18
  infiltrative — *see* Eosinophilia, pulmonary
  Löffler's J82.89
  peritoneal — *see* Peritonitis, eosinophilic
  pulmonary NEC J82.89
    acute J82.82
    asthmatic J82.83
    chronic J82.81
  specified NEC D72.19
  tropical (pulmonary) J82.89
Eosinophilia-myalgia syndrome M35.89
Ependymitis (acute) (cerebral) (chronic) (granular) — *see* Encephalomyelitis
Ependymoblastoma
  specified site — *see* Neoplasm, malignant, by site
  unspecified site C71.9

Ependymoma (epithelial) (malignant)
  anaplastic
    specified site — *see* Neoplasm, malignant, by site
    unspecified site C71.9
  benign
    specified site — *see* Neoplasm, benign, by site
    unspecified site D33.2
  myxopapillary D43.2
    specified site — *see* Neoplasm, uncertain behavior, by site
    unspecified site D43.2
  papillary D43.2
    specified site — *see* Neoplasm, uncertain behavior, by site
    unspecified site D43.2
  specified site — *see* Neoplasm, malignant, by site
  unspecified site C71.9
Ependymopathy G93.89
Ephelis, ephelides L81.2
Epiblepharon (congenital) Q10.3
Epicanthus, epicanthic fold (eyelid) (congenital) Q10.3
Epicondylitis (elbow)
  lateral M77.1- ☑
  medial M77.0- ☑
Epicystitis — *see* Cystitis
Epidemic — *see* condition
Epidermidalization, cervix — *see* Dysplasia, cervix
Epidermis, epidermal — *see* condition
Epidermodysplasia verruciformis B07.8
Epidermolysis
  bullosa (congenital) Q81.9
    acquired L12.30
      drug-induced L12.31
      specified cause NEC L12.35
    dystrophica Q81.2
    letalis Q81.1
    simplex Q81.0
    specified NEC Q81.8
  necroticans combustiformis L51.2
    due to drug — *see* Table of Drugs and Chemicals, by drug
Epidermophytid — *see* Dermatophytosis
Epidermophytosis (infected) — *see* Dermatophytosis
Epididymis — *see* condition
Epididymitis (acute) (nonvenereal) (recurrent) (residual) N45.1
  with orchitis N45.3
  blennorrhagic (gonococcal) A54.23
  caseous (tuberculous) A18.15
  chlamydial A56.19
  filarial — *see also* Infestation, filarial B74.9 *[N51]*
  gonococcal A54.23
  syphilitic A52.76
  tuberculous A18.15
Epididymo-orchitis — *see also* Epididymitis N45.3
Epidural — *see* condition
Epigastrium, epigastric — *see* condition
Epigastrocele — *see* Hernia, ventral
Epiglottis — *see* condition
Epiglottitis, epiglottiditis (acute) J05.10
  with obstruction J05.11
  chronic J37.0
Epignathus Q89.4
Epilepsia partialis continua — *see also* Kozhevnikof's epilepsy G40.1- ☑
Epilepsy, epileptic, epilepsia (attack) (cerebral) (convulsion) (fit) (seizure) G40.909

> *Note: the following terms are to be considered equivalent to intractable: pharmacoresistant (pharmacologically resistant), treatment resistant, refractory (medically) and poorly controlled*

  with
    complex partial seizures — *see* Epilepsy, localization-related, symptomatic, with complex partial seizures
    grand mal seizures on awakening — *see* Epilepsy, generalized, specified NEC
    myoclonic absences — *see* Epilepsy, generalized, specified NEC
    myoclonic-astatic seizures — *see* Epilepsy, generalized, specified NEC
    simple partial seizures — *see* Epilepsy, localization-related, symptomatic, with simple partial seizures
  akinetic — *see* Epilepsy, generalized, specified NEC

Epilepsy, epileptic, epilepsia — *continued*
  benign childhood with centrotemporal EEG spikes — *see* Epilepsy, localization-related, idiopathic
  benign myoclonic in infancy G40.80- ☑
  Bravais-jacksonian — *see* Epilepsy, localization-related, symptomatic, with simple partial seizures
  childhood
    with occipital EEG paroxysms — *see* Epilepsy, localization-related, idiopathic
    absence G40.A09 (*following* G40.3)
      intractable G40.A19 (*following* G40.3)
        with status epilepticus G40.A11 (*following* G40.3)
        without status epilepticus G40.A19 (*following* G40.3)
      not intractable G40.A09 (*following* G40.3)
        with status epilepticus G40.A01 (*following* G40.3)
        without status epilepticus G40.A09 (*following* G40.3)
  climacteric — *see* Epilepsy, specified NEC
  cysticercosis B69.0
  deterioration (mental) F06.8
  due to syphilis A52.19
  focal — *see* Epilepsy, localization-related, symptomatic, with simple partial seizures
  generalized
    idiopathic G40.309
      intractable G40.319
        with status epilepticus G40.311
        without status epilepticus G40.319
      not intractable G40.309
        with status epilepticus G40.301
        without status epilepticus G40.309
    specified NEC G40.409
      intractable G40.419
        with status epilepticus G40.411
        without status epilepticus G40.419
      not intractable G40.409
        with status epilepticus G40.401
        without status epilepticus G40.409
  impulsive petit mal — *see* Epilepsy, juvenile myoclonic
  intractable G40.919
    with status epilepticus G40.911
    without status epilepticus G40.919
  juvenile absence G40.A09 (*following* G40.3)
    intractable G40.A19 (*following* G40.3)
      with status epilepticus G40.A11 (*following* G40.3)
      without status epilepticus G40.A19 (*following* G40.3)
    not intractable G40.A09 (*following* G40.3)
      with status epilepticus G40.A01 (*following* G40.3)
      without status epilepticus G40.A09 (*following* G40.3)
  juvenile myoclonic G40.B09 (*following* G40.3)
    intractable G40.B19 (*following* G40.3)
      with status epilepticus G40.B11 (*following* G40.3)
      without status epilepticus G40.B19 (*following* G40.3)
    not intractable G40.B09 (*following* G40.3)
      with status epilepticus G40.B01 (*following* G40.3)
      without status epilepticus G40.B09 (*following* G40.3)
  localization-related (focal) (partial)
    idiopathic G40.009
      with seizures of localized onset G40.009
        intractable G40.019
          with status epilepticus G40.011
          without status epilepticus G40.019
        not intractable G40.009
          with status epilepticus G40.001
          without status epilepticus G40.009
    symptomatic
      with complex partial seizures G40.209
        intractable G40.219
          with status epilepticus G40.211
          without status epilepticus G40.219
        not intractable G40.209
          with status epilepticus G40.201
          without status epilepticus G40.209
      with simple partial seizures G40.109
        intractable G40.119
          with status epilepticus G40.111
          without status epilepticus G40.119
        not intractable G40.109
          with status epilepticus G40.101
          without status epilepticus G40.109

Epilepsy, epileptic, epilepsia — *continued*
  myoclonus, myoclonic — *see also* Epilepsy, generalized, specified NEC
    progressive — *see* Epilepsy, generalized, idiopathic
    severe, in infancy (SMEI) G40.83- ☑
    not intractable G40.909
      with status epilepticus G40.901
      without status epilepticus G40.909
    on awakening — *see* Epilepsy, generalized, specified NEC
  parasitic NOS B71.9 *[G94]*
  partialis continua — *see also* Kozhevnikof's epilepsy G40.1- ☑
  peripheral — *see* Epilepsy, specified NEC
  polymorphic, in infancy (PMEI) G40.83- ☑
  procursiva — *see* Epilepsy, localization-related, symptomatic, with simple partial seizures
  progressive (familial) myoclonic — *see* Epilepsy, generalized, idiopathic
  reflex — *see* Epilepsy, specified NEC
  related to
    alcohol G40.509
      not intractable G40.509
        with status epilepticus G40.501
        without status epliepticus G40.509
    drugs G40.509
      not intractable G40.509
        with status epilepticus G40.501
        without status epliepticus G40.509
    external causes G40.509
      not intractable G40.509
        with status epilepticus G40.501
        without status epliepticus G40.509
    hormonal changes G40.509
      not intractable G40.509
        with status epilepticus G40.501
        without status epliepticus G40.509
    sleep deprivation G40.509
      not intractable G40.509
        with status epilepticus G40.501
        without status epliepticus G40.509
    stress G40.509
      not intractable G40.509
        with status epilepticus G40.501
        without status epliepticus G40.509
  somatomotor — *see* Epilepsy, localization-related, symptomatic, with simple partial seizures
  somatosensory — *see* Epilepsy, localization-related, symptomatic, with simple partial seizures
  spasms G40.822
    intractable G40.824
      with status epilepticus G40.823
      without status epilepticus G40.824
    not intractable G40.822
      with status epilepticus G40.821
      without status epilepticus G40.822
    specified NEC G40.802
      intractable G40.804
        with status epilepticus G40.803
        without status epilepticus G40.804
      not intractable G40.802
        with status epilepticus G40.801
        without status epilepticus G40.802
  syndromes
    generalized
      idiopathic G40.309
        intractable G40.319
          with status epilepticus G40.311
          without status epilepticus G40.319
        not intractable G40.309
          with status epilepticus G40.301
          without status epilepticus G40.309
      specified NEC G40.409
        intractable G40.419
          with status epilepticus G40.411
          without status epilepticus G40.419
        not intractable G40.409
          with status epilepticus G40.401
          without status epilepticus G40.409
    localization-related (focal) (partial)
      idiopathic G40.009
        with seizures of localized onset G40.009
          intractable G40.019
            with status epilepticus G40.011
            without status epilepticus G40.019
          not intractable G40.009
            with status epilepticus G40.001
            without status epilepticus G40.009

Epilepsy, epileptic, epilepsia — *continued*
  syndromes — *continued*
    localization-related — *continued*
      symptomatic
        with complex partial seizures G40.209
          intractable G40.219
            with status epilepticus G40.211
            without status epilepticus G40.219
          not intractable G40.209
            with status epilepticus G40.201
            without status epilepticus G40.209
        with simple partial seizures G40.109
          intractable G40.119
            with status epilepticus G40.111
            without status epilepticus G40.119
          not intractable G40.109
            with status epilepticus G40.101
            without status epilepticus G40.109
      specified NEC G40.802
        intractable G40.804
          with status epilepticus G40.803
          without status epilepticus G40.804
        not intractable G40.802
          with status epilepticus G40.801
          without status epilepticus G40.802
    tonic (-clonic) — *see* Epilepsy, generalized, specified NEC
    twilight F05
    uncinate (gyrus) — *see* Epilepsy, localization-related, symptomatic, with complex partial seizures
    Unverricht (-Lundborg) (familial myoclonic) — *see* Epilepsy, generalized, idiopathic
    visceral — *see* Epilepsy, specified NEC
    visual — *see* Epilepsy, specified NEC
Epiloia Q85.1
Epimenorrhea N92.0
Epipharyngitis — *see* Nasopharyngitis
Epiphora H04.20- ☑
  due to
    excess lacrimation H04.21- ☑
    insufficient drainage H04.22- ☑
Epiphyseal arrest — *see* Arrest, epiphyseal
Epiphyseolysis, epiphysiolysis — *see* Osteochondropathy
Epiphysitis — *see also* Osteochondropathy
  juvenile M92.9
  syphilitic (congenital) A50.02
Epiplocele — *see* Hernia, abdomen
Epiploitis — *see* Peritonitis
Epiplosarcomphalocele — *see* Hernia, umbilicus
Episcleritis (suppurative) H15.10- ☑
  in (due to)
    syphilis A52.71
    tuberculosis A18.51
  nodular H15.12- ☑
  periodica fugax H15.11- ☑
    angioneurotic — *see* Edema, angioneurotic
  syphilitic (late) A52.71
  tuberculous A18.51
Episode
  affective, mixed F39
  depersonalization (in neurotic state) F48.1
  depressive F32.A
    major F32.9
      mild F32.0
      moderate F32.1
      severe (without psychotic symptoms) F32.2
        with psychotic symptoms F32.3
    recurrent F33.9
      brief F33.8
    specified NEC F32.89
  hypomanic F30.8
  manic F30.9
    with
      psychotic symptoms F30.2
      remission (full) F30.4
        partial F30.3
    other specified F30.8
    recurrent F31.89
    without psychotic symptoms F30.10
      mild F30.11
      moderate F30.12
      severe (without psychotic symptoms) F30.13
        with psychotic symptoms F30.2
  psychotic F23
    organic F06.8
  schizophrenic (acute) NEC, brief F23
Epispadias (female) (male) Q64.0

Episplenitis D73.89
Epistaxis (multiple) R04.0
  hereditary I78.0
  vicarious menstruation N94.89
Epithelioma (malignant) — *see also* Neoplasm, malignant, by site
  adenoides cysticum — *see* Neoplasm, skin, benign
  basal cell — *see* Neoplasm, skin, malignant
  benign — *see* Neoplasm, benign, by site
  Bowen's — *see* Neoplasm, skin, in situ
  calcifying, of Malherbe — *see* Neoplasm, skin, benign
  external site — *see* Neoplasm, skin, malignant
  intraepidermal, Jadassohn — *see* Neoplasm, skin, benign
  squamous cell — *see* Neoplasm, malignant, by site
Epitheliomatosis pigmented Q82.1
Epitheliopathy, multifocal placoid pigment H30.14- ☑
Epithelium, epithelial — *see* condition
Epituberculosis (with atelectasis) (allergic) A15.7
Eponychia Q84.6
Epstein's
  nephrosis or syndrome — *see* Nephrosis
  pearl K09.8
Epulis (gingiva) (fibrous) (giant cell) K06.8
Equinia A24.0
Equinovarus (congenital) (talipes) Q66.0- ☑
  acquired — *see* Deformity, limb, clubfoot
Equivalent
  convulsive (abdominal) — *see* Epilepsy, specified NEC
  epileptic (psychic) — *see* Epilepsy, localization-related, symptomatic, with complex partial seizures
Erb (-Duchenne) **paralysis** (birth injury) (newborn) P14.0
Erb-Goldflam disease or syndrome G70.00
  with exacerbation (acute) G70.01
  in crisis G70.01
Erb's
  disease G71.02
  palsy, paralysis (brachial) (birth) (newborn) P14.0
    spinal (spastic) syphilitic A52.17
  pseudohypertrophic muscular dystrophy G71.02
Erdheim's syndrome (acromegalic macrospondylitis) E22.0
Erection, painful (persistent) — *see* Priapism
Ergosterol deficiency (vitamin D) E55.9
  with
    adult osteomalacia M83.8
    rickets — *see* Rickets
Ergotism — *see also* Poisoning, food, noxious, plant
  from ergot used as drug (migraine therapy) — *see* Table of Drugs and Chemicals
Erosio interdigitalis blastomycetica B37.2
Erosion
  artery I77.2
    without rupture I77.89
  bone — *see* Disorder, bone, density and structure, specified NEC
  bronchus J98.09
  cartilage (joint) — *see* Disorder, cartilage, specified type NEC
  cervix (uteri) (acquired) (chronic) (congenital) N86
    with cervicitis N72
  cornea (nontraumatic) — *see* Ulcer, cornea
    recurrent H18.83- ☑
    traumatic — *see* Abrasion, cornea
  dental (idiopathic) (occupational) (due to diet, drugs or vomiting) K03.2
  duodenum, postpyloric — *see* Ulcer, duodenum
  esophagus K22.10
    with bleeding K22.11
  gastric — *see* Ulcer, stomach
  gastrojejunal — *see* Ulcer, gastrojejunal
  implanted mesh — *see* Complications, prosthetic device or implant, mesh
  intestine K63.3
  lymphatic vessel I89.8
  pylorus, pyloric (ulcer) — *see* Ulcer, stomach
  spine, aneurysmal A52.09
  stomach — *see* Ulcer, stomach
  subcutaneous device pocket
    nervous system prosthetic device, implant, or graft T85.890 ☑
    other internal prosthetic device, implant, or graft T85.898 ☑
  teeth (idiopathic) (occupational) (due to diet, drugs or vomiting) K03.2
  urethra N36.8

Erosion — *continued*
  uterus N85.8
Erotomania F52.8
Error
  metabolism, inborn — *see* Disorder, metabolism
  refractive — *see* Disorder, refraction
Eructation R14.2
  nervous or psychogenic F45.8
Eruption
  creeping B76.9
  drug (generalized) (taken internally) L27.0
    fixed L27.1
    in contact with skin — *see* Dermatitis, due to drugs
    localized L27.1
  Hutchinson, summer L56.4
  Kaposi's varicelliform B00.0
  napkin L22
  polymorphous light (sun) L56.4
  recalcitrant pustular L13.8
  ringed R23.8
  skin (nonspecific) R21
    creeping (meaning hookworm) B76.9
    due to inoculation/vaccination (generalized) — *see also* Dermatitis, due to, vaccine L27.0
      localized L27.1
    erysipeloid A26.0
    feigned L98.1
    Kaposi's varicelliform B00.0
    lichenoid L28.0
    meaning dermatitis — *see* Dermatitis
    toxic NEC L53.0
  tooth, teeth, abnormal (incomplete) (late) (premature) (sequence) K00.6
  vesicular R23.8
Erysipelas (gangrenous) (infantile) (newborn) (phlegmonous) (suppurative) A46
  external ear A46 *[H62.40]*
  puerperal, postpartum O86.89
Erysipeloid A26.9
  cutaneous (Rosenbach's) A26.0
  disseminated A26.8
  sepsis A26.7
  specified NEC A26.8
Erythema, erythematous (infectional) (inflammation) L53.9
  ab igne L59.0
  annulare (centrifugum) (rheumaticum) L53.1
  arthriticum epidemicum A25.1
  brucellum — *see* Brucellosis
  chronic figurate NEC L53.3
  chronicum migrans (Borrelia burgdorferi) A69.20
  diaper L22
  due to
    chemical NEC L53.0
      in contact with skin L24.5
    drug (internal use) — *see* Dermatitis, due to, drugs
  elevatum diutinum L95.1
  endemic E52
  epidemic, arthritic A25.1
  figuratum perstans L53.3
  gluteal L22
  heat — *code by site under* Burn, first degree
  ichthyosiforme congenitum bullous Q80.3
  in diseases classified elsewhere L54
  induratum (nontuberculous) L52
    tuberculous A18.4
  infectiosum B08.3
  intertrigo L30.4
  iris L51.9
  marginatum L53.2
    in (due to) acute rheumatic fever I00
  medicamentosum — *see* Dermatitis, due to, drugs
  migrans A26.0
    chronicum A69.20
    tongue K14.1
  multiforme (major) (minor) L51.9
    bullous, bullosum L51.1
    conjunctiva L51.1
    nonbullous L51.0
    pemphigoides L12.0
    specified NEC L51.8
  napkin L22
  neonatorum P83.88
    toxic P83.1
  nodosum L52
    tuberculous A18.4
  palmar L53.8
  pernio T69.1 ☑

Erythema, erythematous — *continued*
  rash, newborn P83.88
  scarlatiniform (recurrent) (exfoliative) L53.8
  solare L55.0
  specified NEC L53.8
  toxic, toxicum NEC L53.0
    newborn P83.1
  tuberculous (primary) A18.4
Erythematous, erythematosus — *see* condition
Erythralgia (primary) I73.81
Erythralgia I73.81
Erythrasma L08.1
Erythredema (polyneuropathy) — *see* Poisoning, mercury
Erythremia (acute) C94.0- ☑
  chronic D45
  secondary D75.1
Erythroblastopenia — *see also* Aplasia, red cell D60.9
  congenital D61.01
Erythroblastophthisis D61.09
Erythroblastosis (fetalis) (newborn) P55.9
  due to
    ABO (antibodies) (incompatibility) (isoimmunization) P55.1
    Rh (antibodies) (incompatibility) (isoimmunization) P55.0
Erythrocyanosis (crurum) I73.89
Erythrocythemia — *see* Erythremia
Erythrocytosis (megalosplenic) (secondary) D75.1
  familial D75.0
  oval, hereditary — *see* Elliptocytosis
  secondary D75.1
  stress D75.1
Erythroderma (secondary) — *see also* Erythema L53.9
  bullous ichthyosiform, congenital Q80.3
  desquamativum L21.1
  ichthyosiform, congenital (bullous) Q80.3
  neonatorum P83.88
  psoriaticum L40.8
Erythrodysesthesia, palmar plantar (PPE) L27.1
Erythrogenesis imperfecta D61.09
Erythroleukemia C94.0- ☑
Erythromelalgia I73.81
Erythrophagocytosis D75.89
Erythrophobia F40.298
Erythroplakia, oral epithelium, and tongue K13.29
Erythroplasia (Queyrat) D07.4
  specified site — *see* Neoplasm, skin, in situ
  unspecified site D07.4
Escherichia coli (E. coli), **as cause of disease classified elsewhere** B96.20
  non-O157 Shiga toxin-producing (with known O group) B96.22
  non-Shiga toxin-producing B96.29
  O157 B96.21
  O157 with confirmation of Shiga toxin when H antigen is unknown, or is not H7 B96.21
  O157:H- (nonmotile) with confirmation of Shiga toxin B96.21
  O157:H7 with or without confirmation of Shiga toxin-production B96.21
    specified NEC B96.22
  Shiga toxin-producing (with unspecified O group) (STEC) B96.23
  specified NEC B96.29
Esophagismus K22.4
Esophagitis (acute) (alkaline) (chemical) (chronic) (infectional) (necrotic) (peptic) (postoperative) (without bleeding) K20.90
  with bleeding K20.91
  candidal B37.81
  due to gastrointestinal reflux disease (without bleeding) K21.00
    with bleeding K21.01
  eosinophilic K20.0
  reflux K21.00
  specified NEC (without bleeding) K20.80
    with bleeding K20.81
  tuberculous A18.83
  ulcerative K22.10
    with bleeding K22.11
Esophagocele K22.5
Esophagomalacia K22.89
Esophagospasm K22.4
Esophagostenosis K22.2
Esophagostomiasis B81.8
Esophagotracheal — *see* condition
Esophagus — *see* condition

Esophoria H50.51
  convergence, excess H51.12
  divergence, insufficiency H51.8
Esotropia — *see* Strabismus, convergent concomitant
Espundia B55.2
Essential — *see* condition
Esthesioneuroblastoma C30.0
Esthesioneurocytoma C30.0
Esthesioneuroepithelioma C30.0
Esthiomene A55
Estrangement (marital) Z63.5
  parent-child NEC Z62.890
Estriasis — *see* Myiasis
Estivo-autumnal malaria (fever) B50.9
Ethanolism — *see* Alcoholism
Etherism — *see* Dependence, drug, inhalant
Ethmoid, ethmoidal — *see* condition
Ethmoiditis (chronic) (nonpurulent) (purulent) — *see also* Sinusitis, ethmoidal
  influenzal — *see* Influenza, with, respiratory manifestations NEC
  Woakes' J33.1
Ethylism — *see* Alcoholism
Eulenburg's disease (congenital paramyotonia) G71.19
Eumycetoma B47.0
Eunuchoidism E29.1
  hypogonadotropic E23.0
European blastomycosis — *see* Cryptococcosis
Eustachian — *see* condition
Evaluation (for) (of)
  development state
    adolescent Z00.3
    period of
      delayed growth in childhood Z00.70
        with abnormal findings Z00.71
      rapid growth in childhood Z00.2
    puberty Z00.3
  growth and developmental state (period of rapid growth) Z00.2
    delayed growth Z00.70
      with abnormal findings Z00.71
  mental health (status) Z00.8
    requested by authority Z04.6
  period of
    delayed growth in childhood Z00.70
      with abnormal findings Z00.71
    rapid growth in childhood Z00.2
  suspected condition — *see* Observation
Evans syndrome D69.41
Event
  apparent life threatening in newborn and infant (ALTE) R68.13
  brief resolved unexplained event (BRUE) R68.13
Eventration — *see also* Hernia, ventral
  colon into chest — *see* Hernia, diaphragm
  diaphragm (congenital) Q79.1
Eversion
  bladder N32.89
  cervix (uteri) N86
    with cervicitis N72
  foot NEC — *see also* Deformity, valgus, ankle
    congenital Q66.6
  punctum lacrimale (postinfectional) (senile) H04.52- ☑
  ureter (meatus) N28.89
  urethra (meatus) N36.8
  uterus N81.4
Evidence
  cytologic
    of malignancy on anal smear R85.614
    of malignancy on cervical smear R87.614
    of malignancy on vaginal smear R87.624
Evisceration
  birth injury P15.8
  traumatic NEC
    eye — *see* Enucleated eye
Evulsion — *see* Avulsion
Ewing's sarcoma or tumor — *see* Neoplasm, bone, malignant
Examination (for) (following) (general) (of) (routine) Z00.00
  with abnormal findings Z00.01
  abuse, physical (alleged), ruled out
    adult Z04.71
    child Z04.72
  adolescent (development state) Z00.3
  alleged rape or sexual assault (victim), ruled out
    adult Z04.41
    child Z04.42

Examination — *continued*
allergy Z01.82
annual (adult) (periodic) (physical) Z00.00
　with abnormal findings Z00.01
　gynecological Z01.419
　　with abnormal findings Z01.411
antibody response Z01.84
blood — *see* Examination, laboratory
blood pressure Z01.30
　with abnormal findings Z01.31
cancer staging — *see* Neoplasm, malignant, by site
cervical Papanicolaou smear Z12.4
　as part of routine gynecological examination Z01.419
　　with abnormal findings Z01.411
child (over 28 days old) Z00.129
　with abnormal findings Z00.121
　under 28 days old — *see* Newborn, examination
clinical research control or normal comparison (control) (participant) Z00.6
contraceptive (drug) maintenance (routine) Z30.8
　device (intrauterine) Z30.431
dental Z01.20
　with abnormal findings Z01.21
developmental — *see* Examination, child
donor (potential) Z00.5
ear Z01.10
　with abnormal findings NEC Z01.118
eye Z01.00
　with abnormal findings Z01.01
　following failed vision screening Z01.020
　　with abnormal findings Z01.021
follow-up (routine) (following) Z09
　chemotherapy NEC Z09
　　malignant neoplasm Z08
　fracture Z09
　malignant neoplasm Z08
　postpartum Z39.2
　psychotherapy Z09
　radiotherapy NEC Z09
　　malignant neoplasm Z08
　surgery NEC Z09
　　malignant neoplasm Z08
following
　accident NEC Z04.3
　　transport Z04.1
　　work Z04.2
　assault, alleged, ruled out
　　adult Z04.71
　　child Z04.72
　motor vehicle accident Z04.1
　treatment (for) Z09
　　combined NEC Z09
　　　fracture Z09
　　　malignant neoplasm Z08
　　malignant neoplasm Z08
　　mental disorder Z09
　　specified condition NEC Z09
forced sexual exploitation Z04.81
forced labor exploitation Z04.82
gynecological Z01.419
　with abnormal findings Z01.411
　for contraceptive maintenance Z30.8
health — *see* Examination, medical
hearing Z01.10
　with abnormal findings NEC Z01.118
　following failed hearing screening Z01.110
　infant or child (over 28 days old) Z00.129
　　with abnormal findings Z00.121
immunity status testing Z01.84
laboratory (as part of a general medical examination) Z00.00
　with abnormal findings Z00.01
　preprocedural Z01.812
lactating mother Z39.1
medical (adult) (for) (of) Z00.00
　with abnormal findings Z00.01
　administrative purpose only Z02.9
　　specified NEC Z02.89
　admission to
　　armed forces Z02.3
　　old age home Z02.2
　　prison Z02.89
　　residential institution Z02.2
　　school Z02.0
　　　following illness or medical treatment Z02.0
　　summer camp Z02.89
　adoption Z02.82
　blood alcohol or drug level Z02.83

Examination — *continued*
medical — *continued*
　camp (summer) Z02.89
　clinical research, normal subject (control) (participant) Z00.6
　control subject in clinical research (normal comparison) (participant) Z00.6
　donor (potential) Z00.5
　driving license Z02.4
　general (adult) Z00.00
　　with abnormal findings Z00.01
　immigration Z02.89
　insurance purposes Z02.6
　marriage Z02.89
　medicolegal reasons NEC Z04.89
　naturalization Z02.89
　participation in sport Z02.5
　paternity testing Z02.81
　population survey Z00.8
　pre-employment Z02.1
　pre-operative — *see* Examination, pre-procedural
　pre-procedural
　　cardiovascular Z01.810
　　respiratory Z01.811
　　specified NEC Z01.818
　preschool children
　　for admission to school Z02.0
　prisoners
　　for entrance into prison Z02.89
　recruitment for armed forces Z02.3
　specified NEC Z00.8
　sport competition Z02.5
medicolegal reason NEC Z04.89
　following
　　forced sexual exploitation Z04.81
　　forced labor exploitation Z04.82
newborn — *see* Newborn, examination
pelvic (annual) (periodic) Z01.419
　with abnormal findings Z01.411
period of rapid growth in childhood Z00.2
periodic (adult) (annual) (routine) Z00.00
　with abnormal findings Z00.01
physical (adult) — *see also* Examination, medical Z00.00
　sports Z02.5
postpartum
　immediately after delivery Z39.0
　routine follow-up Z39.2
pre-chemotherapy (antineoplastic) Z01.818
prenatal (normal pregnancy) — *see also* Pregnancy, normal Z34.9- ☑
pre-procedural (pre-operative)
　cardiovascular Z01.810
　laboratory Z01.812
　respiratory Z01.811
　specified NEC Z01.818
prior to chemotherapy (antineoplastic) Z01.818
psychiatric NEC Z00.8
　follow-up not needing further care Z09
　requested by authority Z04.6
radiological (as part of a general medical examination) Z00.00
　with abnormal findings Z00.01
repeat cervical smear to confirm findings of recent normal smear following initial abnormal smear Z01.42
skin (hypersensitivity) Z01.82
special — *see also* Examination, by type Z01.89
　specified type NEC Z01.89
specified type or reason NEC Z04.89
teeth Z01.20
　with abnormal findings Z01.21
urine — *see* Examination, laboratory
vision Z01.00
　with abnormal findings Z01.01
　following failed vision screening Z01.020
　　with abnormal findings Z01.021
　infant or child (over 28 days old) Z00.129
　　with abnormal findings Z00.121

Exanthem, exanthema — *see also* Rash
with enteroviral vesicular stomatitis B08.4
Boston A88.0
epidemic with meningitis A88.0 *[G02]*
subitum B08.20
　due to human herpesvirus 6 B08.21
　due to human herpesvirus 7 B08.22
viral, virus B09
　specified type NEC B08.8

Excess, excessive, excessively
alcohol level in blood R78.0
androgen (ovarian) E28.1
attrition, tooth, teeth K03.0
carotene, carotin (dietary) E67.1
cold, effects of T69.9 ☑
　specified effect NEC T69.8 ☑
convergence H51.12
crying
　in child, adolescent, or adult R45.83
　in infant R68.11
development, breast N62
divergence H51.8
drinking (alcohol) NEC (without dependence) F10.10
　habitual (continual) (without remission) F10.20
eating R63.2
estrogen E28.0
fat — *see also* Obesity
　in heart — *see* Degeneration, myocardial
　localized E65
foreskin N47.8
gas R14.0
glucagon E16.3
heat — *see* Heat
intermaxillary vertical dimension of fully erupted teeth M26.37
interocclusal distance of fully erupted teeth M26.37
kalium E87.5
large
　colon K59.39
　　congenital Q43.8
　infant P08.0
　organ or site, congenital NEC — *see* Anomaly, by site
long
　organ or site, congenital NEC — *see* Anomaly, by site
menstruation (with regular cycle) N92.0
　with irregular cycle N92.1
napping Z72.821
natrium E87.0
number of teeth K00.1
nutrient (dietary) NEC R63.2
potassium (K) E87.5
salivation K11.7
secretion — *see also* Hypersecretion
　milk O92.6
　sputum R09.3
　sweat R61
sexual drive F52.8
short
　organ or site, congenital NEC — *see* Anomaly, by site
　umbilical cord in labor or delivery O69.3 ☑
skin L98.7
　and subcutaneous tissue L98.7
　eyelid (acquired) — *see* Blepharochalasis
　　congenital Q10.3
sodium (Na) E87.0
spacing of fully erupted teeth M26.32
sputum R09.3
sweating R61
thirst R63.1
　due to deprivation of water T73.1 ☑
transportation time Z59.82
tuberosity of jaw M26.07
vitamin
　A (dietary) E67.0
　　administered as drug (prolonged intake) — *see* Table of Drugs and Chemicals, vitamins, adverse effect
　　overdose or wrong substance given or taken — *see* Table of Drugs and Chemicals, vitamins, poisoning
　D (dietary) E67.3
　　administered as drug (prolonged intake) — *see* Table of Drugs and Chemicals, vitamins, adverse effect
　　overdose or wrong substance given or taken — *see* Table of Drugs and Chemicals, vitamins, poisoning
weight
　gain R63.5
　loss R63.4
Excitability, abnormal, under minor stress (personality disorder) F60.3
Excitation
anomalous atrioventricular I45.6

Excitation — *continued*
  psychogenic F3Ø.8
  reactive (from emotional stress, psychological trauma) F3Ø.8
Excitement
  hypomanic F3Ø.8
  manic F3Ø.9
  mental, reactive (from emotional stress, psychological trauma) F3Ø.8
  state, reactive (from emotional stress, psychological trauma) F3Ø.8
Excoriation (traumatic) — *see also* Abrasion
  neurotic L98.1
  skin picking disorder F42.4
Exfoliation
  due to erythematous conditions according to extent of body surface involved L49.Ø
    1Ø-19 percent of body surface L49.1
    2Ø-29 percent of body surface L49.2
    3Ø-39 percent of body surface L49.3
    4Ø-49 percent of body surface L49.4
    5Ø-59 percent of body surface L49.5
    6Ø-69 percent of body surface L49.6
    7Ø-79 percent of body surface L49.7
    8Ø-89 percent of body surface L49.8
    9Ø-99 percent of body surface L49.9
    less than 1Ø percent of body surface L49.Ø
  teeth, due to systemic causes KØ8.Ø
Exfoliative — *see* condition
Exhaustion, exhaustive (physical NEC) R53.83
  battle F43.Ø
  cardiac — *see* Failure, heart
  delirium F43.Ø
  due to
    cold T69.8 ☑
    excessive exertion T73.3 ☑
    exposure T73.2 ☑
    neurasthenia F48.8
  heart — *see* Failure, heart
  heat — *see also* Heat, exhaustion T67.5 ☑
    due to
      salt depletion T67.4 ☑
      water depletion T67.3 ☑
  maternal, complicating delivery O75.81
  mental F48.8
  myocardium, myocardial — *see* Failure, heart
  nervous F48.8
  old age R54
  psychogenic F48.8
  psychosis F43.Ø
  senile R54
  vital NEC Z73.Ø
Exhibitionism F65.2
Exocervicitis — *see* Cervicitis
Exomphalos Q79.2
  meaning hernia — *see* Hernia, umbilicus
Exophoria H5Ø.52
  convergence, insufficiency H51.11
  divergence, excess H51.8
Exophthalmos HØ5.2- ☑
  congenital Q15.8
  constant NEC HØ5.24- ☑
  displacement, globe — *see* Displacement, globe
  due to thyrotoxicosis (hyperthyroidism) — *see* Hyperthyroidism, with, goiter (diffuse)
  dysthyroid — *see* Hyperthyroidism, with, goiter (diffuse)
  goiter — *see* Hyperthyroidism, with, goiter (diffuse)
  intermittent NEC HØ5.25- ☑
  malignant — *see* Hyperthyroidism, with, goiter (diffuse)
  orbital
    edema — *see* Edema, orbit
    hemorrhage — *see* Hemorrhage, orbit
  pulsating NEC HØ5.26- ☑
  thyrotoxic, thyrotropic — *see* Hyperthyroidism, with, goiter (diffuse)
Exostosis — *see also* Disorder, bone
  cartilaginous — *see* Neoplasm, bone, benign
  congenital (multiple) Q78.6
  external ear canal H61.81- ☑
  gonococcal A54.49
  jaw (bone) M27.8
  multiple, congenital Q78.6
  orbit HØ5.35- ☑
  osteocartilaginous — *see* Neoplasm, bone, benign
  syphilitic A52.77
Exotropia — *see* Strabismus, divergent concomitant

Explanation of
  investigation finding Z71.2
  medication Z71.89
Exploitation
  labor
    confirmed
      adult forced T74.61 ☑
      child forced T74.62 ☑
    suspected
      adult forced T76.61 ☑
      child forced T76.62 ☑
  sexual
    confirmed
      adult forced T74.51 ☑
      child T74.52 ☑
    suspected
      adult forced T76.51 ☑
      child T76.52 ☑
Exposure (to) — *see also* Contact, with T75.89 ☑
  acariasis Z2Ø.7
  AIDS virus Z2Ø.6
  air pollution Z77.11Ø
  algae and algae toxins Z77.121
  algae bloom Z77.121
  anthrax Z2Ø.81Ø
  aromatic amines Z77.Ø2Ø
  aromatic (hazardous) compounds NEC Z77.Ø28
  aromatic dyes NOS Z77.Ø28
  arsenic Z77.Ø1Ø
  asbestos Z77.Ø9Ø
  bacterial disease NEC Z2Ø.818
  benzene Z77.Ø21
  blue-green algae bloom Z77.121
  body fluids (potentially hazardous) Z77.21
  brown tide Z77.121
  chemicals (chiefly nonmedicinal) (hazardous) NEC Z77.Ø98
  cholera Z2Ø.Ø9
  chromium compounds Z77.Ø18
  cold, effects of T69.9 ☑
    specified effect NEC T69.8 ☑
  communicable disease Z2Ø.9
    bacterial NEC Z2Ø.818
    specified NEC Z2Ø.89
    viral NEC Z2Ø.828
    Zika virus Z2Ø.821
  coronavirus (disease) (novel) 2Ø19 Z2Ø.822
  COVID-19 Z2Ø.822
  cyanobacteria bloom Z77.121
  disaster Z65.5
  discrimination Z6Ø.5
  dyes Z77.Ø98
  effects of T73.9 ☑
  environmental tobacco smoke (acute) (chronic) Z77.22
  Escherichia coli (E. coli) Z2Ø.Ø1
  exhaustion due to T73.2 ☑
  fiberglass — *see* Table of Drugs and Chemicals, fiberglass
  German measles Z2Ø.4
  gonorrhea Z2Ø.2
  hazardous metals NEC Z77.Ø18
  hazardous substances NEC Z77.29
  hazards in the physical environment NEC Z77.128
  hazards to health NEC Z77.9
  human immunodeficiency virus (HIV) Z2Ø.6
  human T-lymphotropic virus type-1 (HTLV-1) Z2Ø.89
  implanted
    mesh — *see* Complications, prosthetic device or implant, mesh
    prosthetic materials NEC — *see* Complications, prosthetic materials NEC
  infestation (parasitic) NEC Z2Ø.7
  intestinal infectious disease NEC Z2Ø.Ø9
    Escherichia coli (E. coli) Z2Ø.Ø1
  lead Z77.Ø11
  meningococcus Z2Ø.811
  mold (toxic) Z77.12Ø
  nickel dust Z77.Ø18
  noise Z77.122
  occupational
    air contaminants NEC Z57.39
    dust Z57.2
    environmental tobacco smoke Z57.31
    extreme temperature Z57.6
    noise Z57.Ø
    radiation Z57.1
    risk factors Z57.9
      specified NEC Z57.8

Exposure — *continued*
  occupational — *continued*
    toxic agents (gases) (liquids) (solids) (vapors) in agriculture Z57.4
    toxic agents (gases) (liquids) (solids) (vapors) in industry NEC Z57.5
    vibration Z57.7
  parasitic disease NEC Z2Ø.7
  pediculosis Z2Ø.7
  persecution Z6Ø.5
  pfiesteria piscicida Z77.121
  poliomyelitis Z2Ø.89
  pollution
    air Z77.11Ø
    environmental NEC Z77.118
    soil Z77.112
    water Z77.111
  polycyclic aromatic hydrocarbons Z77.Ø28
  prenatal (drugs) (toxic chemicals) — *see* Newborn, affected by, noxious substances transmitted via placenta or breast milk
  rabies Z2Ø.3
  radiation, naturally occurring NEC Z77.123
  radon Z77.123
  red tide (Florida) Z77.121
  rubella Z2Ø.4
  SARS-CoV-2 Z2Ø.822
  second hand tobacco smoke (acute) (chronic) Z77.22
    in the perinatal period P96.81
  sexually-transmitted disease Z2Ø.2
  smallpox (laboratory) Z2Ø.89
  syphilis Z2Ø.2
  terrorism Z65.4
  torture Z65.4
  tuberculosis Z2Ø.1
  uranium Z77.Ø12
  varicella Z2Ø.82Ø
  venereal disease Z2Ø.2
  viral disease NEC Z2Ø.828
  war Z65.5
  water pollution Z77.111
  Zika virus Z2Ø.821
Exsanguination — *see* Hemorrhage
Exstrophy
  abdominal contents Q45.8
  bladder Q64.1Ø
    cloacal Q64.12
    specified type NEC Q64.19
    supravesical fissure Q64.11
Extensive — *see* condition
Extra — *see also* Accessory
  marker chromosomes (normal individual) Q92.61
    in abnormal individual Q92.62
  rib Q76.6
    cervical Q76.5
Extrasystoles (supraventricular) I49.49
  atrial I49.1
  auricular I49.1
  junctional I49.2
  ventricular I49.3
Extrauterine gestation or pregnancy — *see* Pregnancy, by site
Extravasation
  blood R58
  chyle into mesentery I89.8
  pelvicalyceal N13.8
  pyelosinus N13.8
  urine (from ureter) R39.Ø
  vesicant agent
    antineoplastic chemotherapy T8Ø.81Ø ☑
    other agent NEC T8Ø.818 ☑
Extremity — *see* condition, limb
Extrophy — *see* Exstrophy
Extroversion
  bladder Q64.19
  uterus N81.4
    complicating delivery O71.2
    postpartal (old) N81.4
Extruded tooth (teeth) M26.34
Extrusion
  breast implant (prosthetic) T85.42 ☑
  eye implant (globe) (ball) T85.328 ☑
  intervertebral disc — *see* Displacement, intervertebral disc
  ocular lens implant (prosthetic) — *see* Complications, intraocular lens
  vitreous — *see* Prolapse, vitreous

Exudate
Exudate
- pleural — *see* Effusion, pleura
- retina H35.89
- wound fluids L24.A9

Exudative — *see* condition
Eye, eyeball, eyelid — *see* condition
Eyestrain — *see* Disturbance, vision, subjective
Eyeworm disease of Africa B74.3

F

Faber's syndrome (achlorhydric anemia) D50.9
Fabry (-Anderson) **disease** E75.21
Facet syndrome M47.89- ☑
Faciocephalalgia, autonomic — *see also* Neuropathy, peripheral, autonomic G90.09
Factor(s)
- psychic, associated with diseases classified elsewhere F54
- psychological
  - affecting physical conditions F54
  - or behavioral
    - affecting general medical condition F54
    - associated with disorders or diseases classified elsewhere F54

Fahr disease (of brain) G23.8
Fahr Volhard disease (of kidney) I12.- ☑
Failure, failed
- abortion — *see* Abortion, attempted
- aortic (valve) I35.8
  - rheumatic I06.8
- attempted abortion — *see* Abortion, attempted
- biventricular I50.82
  - due to left heart failure I50.814
- bone marrow — *see* Anemia, aplastic
- cardiac — *see* Failure, heart
- cardiorenal (chronic) — *see also* Failure, renal, and Failure, heart I50.9
  - hypertensive I13.2
- cardiorespiratory — *see also* Failure, heart R09.2
- cardiovascular (chronic) — *see* Failure, heart
- cerebrovascular I67.9
- cervical dilatation in labor O62.0
- circulation, circulatory (peripheral) R57.9
  - newborn P29.89
- compensation — *see* Disease, heart
- compliance with medical treatment or regimen — *see* Noncompliance
- congestive — *see* Failure, heart, congestive
- dental implant (endosseous) M27.69
  - due to
    - failure of dental prosthesis M27.63
    - lack of attached gingiva M27.62
    - occlusal trauma (poor prosthetic design) M27.62
    - parafunctional habits M27.62
    - periodontal infection (peri-implantitis) M27.62
    - poor oral hygiene M27.62
    - osseointegration M27.61
      - due to
        - complications of systemic disease M27.61
        - poor bone quality M27.61
      - iatrogenic M27.61
    - post-osseointegration
      - biological M27.62
      - due to complications of systemic disease M27.62
      - iatrogenic M27.62
      - mechanical M27.63
    - pre-integration M27.61
    - pre-osseointegration M27.61
    - specified NEC M27.69
- descent of head (at term) of pregnancy (mother) O32.4 ☑
- endosseous dental implant — *see* Failure, dental implant
- engagement of head (term of pregnancy) (mother) O32.4 ☑
- erection (penile) — *see also* Dysfunction, sexual, male, erectile N52.9
  - nonorganic F52.21
- examination(s), anxiety concerning Z55.2
- expansion terminal respiratory units (newborn) (primary) P28.0
- forceps NOS (with subsequent cesarean delivery) O66.5
- gain weight (child over 28 days old) R62.51
  - adult R62.7
  - newborn P92.6
- genital response (male) F52.21
  - female F52.22

Failure, failed — *continued*
- heart (acute) (senile) (sudden) I50.9
  - with
    - acute pulmonary edema — *see* Failure, ventricular, left
    - decompensation I50.9
      - with
        - normal ejection fraction I50.33
        - preserved ejection fraction I50.33
        - reduced ejection fraction I50.23
          - with diastolic dysfunction I50.43
      - combined systolic and diastolic I50.43
      - diastolic I50.33
      - right I50.813
      - systolic I50.23
    - dilatation — *see* Disease, heart
    - hypertension — *see* Hypertension, heart
    - normal ejection fraction — *see* Failure, heart, diastolic
    - preserved ejection fraction — *see* Failure, heart, diastolic
    - reduced ejection fraction — *see* Failure, heart, systolic
  - arteriosclerotic I70.90
  - biventricular I50.82
    - due to left heart failure I50.814
  - combined left-right sided I50.82
    - due to left heart failure I50.814
  - compensated — *see also* Failure, heart, by type as diastolic or systolic, chronic I50.9
  - complicating
    - anesthesia (general) (local) or other sedation
      - in labor and delivery O74.2
      - in pregnancy O29.12- ☑
      - postpartum, puerperal O89.1
    - delivery (cesarean) (instrumental) O75.4
  - congestive I50.9
    - with rheumatic fever (conditions in I00)
      - active I01.8
      - inactive or quiescent (with chorea) I09.81
    - newborn P29.0
    - rheumatic (chronic) (inactive) (with chorea) I09.81
      - active or acute I01.8
        - with chorea I02.0
  - decompensated — *see also* Failure, heart, by type as diastolic or systolic, acute and chronic I50.9
  - degenerative — *see* Degeneration, myocardial
  - diastolic (congestive) (left ventricular) I50.30
    - acute (congestive) I50.31
      - and (on) chronic (congestive) I50.33
    - chronic (congestive) I50.32
      - and (on) acute (congestive) I50.33
    - combined with systolic (congestive) I50.40
      - acute (congestive) I50.41
        - and (on) chronic (congestive) I50.43
      - chronic (congestive) I50.42
        - and (on) acute (congestive) I50.43
  - due to presence of cardiac prosthesis I97.13- ☑
  - end stage — *see also* Failure, heart, by type as diastolic or systolic, chronic I50.84
  - following cardiac surgery I97.13- ☑
  - high output NOS I50.83
  - hypertensive — *see* Hypertension, heart
  - left (ventricular) — *see also* Failure, ventricular, left
    - combined diastolic and systolic — *see* Failure, heart, diastolic, combined with systolic
    - diastolic — *see* Failure, heart, diastolic
    - systolic — *see* Failure, heart, systolic
  - low output (syndrome) NOS I50.9
  - newborn P29.0
  - organic — *see* Disease, heart
  - peripartum O90.3
  - postprocedural I97.13- ☑
  - rheumatic (chronic) (inactive) I09.9
  - right (isolated) (ventricular) I50.810
    - acute I50.811
      - and (on) chronic I50.813
    - chronic I50.812
      - and acute I50.813
    - secondary to left heart failure I50.814
  - specified NEC I50.89

Note: heart failure stages A, B, C, and D are based on the American College of Cardiology and American Heart Association stages of heart failure, which complement and should not be confused with the New York Heart Association Classification of Heart Failure, into Class I, Class II, Class III, and Class IV

Failure, failed — *continued*
- heart — *continued*
  - stage A Z91.89
  - stage B — *see also* Failure, heart, by type as diastolic or systolic I50.9
  - stage C — *see also* Failure, heart, by type as diastolic or systolic I50.9
  - stage D — *see also* Failure, heart, by type as diastolic or systolic, chronic I50.84
  - systolic (congestive) (left ventricular) I50.20
    - acute (congestive) I50.21
      - and (on) chronic (congestive) I50.23
    - chronic (congestive) I50.22
      - and (on) acute (congestive) I50.23
    - combined with diastolic (congestive) I50.40
      - acute (congestive) I50.41
        - and (on) chronic (congestive) I50.43
      - chronic (congestive) I50.42
        - and (on) acute (congestive) I50.43
  - thyrotoxic — *see also* Thyrotoxicosis E05.90 *[I43]*
    - with
      - high output — *see also* Thyrotoxicosis I50.83
      - thyroid storm E05.91 *[I43]*
        - high output — *see also* Thyrotoxicosis I50.83
  - valvular — *see* Endocarditis
- hepatic K72.90
  - with coma K72.91
  - acute or subacute K72.00
    - with coma K72.01
    - due to drugs K71.10
      - with coma K71.11
  - alcoholic (acute) (chronic) (subacute) K70.40
    - with coma K70.41
  - chronic K72.10
    - with coma K72.11
    - due to drugs (acute) (subacute) (chronic) K71.10
      - with coma K71.11
  - due to drugs (acute) (subacute) (chronic) K71.10
    - with coma K71.11
  - postprocedural K91.82
- hepatorenal K76.7
- induction (of labor) O61.9
  - abortion — *see* Abortion, attempted
  - by
    - oxytocic drugs O61.0
    - prostaglandins O61.0
  - instrumental O61.1
  - mechanical O61.1
  - medical O61.0
  - specified NEC O61.8
  - surgical O61.1
- intubation during anesthesia T88.4 ☑
  - in pregnancy O29.6- ☑
  - labor and delivery O74.7
  - postpartum, puerperal O89.6
- involution, thymus (gland) E32.0
- kidney — *see also* Disease, kidney, chronic N19
  - acute — *see also* Failure, renal, acute N17.9
- lactation (complete) O92.3
  - partial O92.4
- Leydig's cell, adult E29.1
- liver — *see* Failure, hepatic
- menstruation at puberty N91.0
- mitral I05.8
- myocardial, myocardium — *see also* Failure, heart I50.9
  - chronic — *see also* Failure, heart, congestive I50.9
  - congestive — *see also* Failure, heart, congestive I50.9
- newborn screening — *see* Abnormal, neonatal screening
- neonatal congenital heart disease P09.5
- orgasm (female) (psychogenic) F52.31
  - male F52.32
- ovarian (primary) E28.39
  - iatrogenic E89.40
    - asymptomatic E89.40
    - symptomatic E89.41
  - postprocedural (postablative) (postirradiation) (postsurgical) E89.40
    - asymptomatic E89.40
    - symptomatic E89.41
- ovulation causing infertility N97.0
- polyglandular, autoimmune E31.0
- prosthetic joint implant — *see* Complications, joint prosthesis, mechanical, breakdown, by site
- renal N19

☑ **Additional Character Required — Refer to the Tabular List for Character Selection**

Failure, failed — *continued*
  renal — *continued*
    with
      tubular necrosis (acute) N17.0
    acute N17.9
      with
        cortical necrosis N17.1
        medullary necrosis N17.2
        tubular necrosis N17.0
      specified NEC N17.8
    chronic N18.9
      hypertensive — *see* Hypertension, kidney
    congenital P96.0
    end stage (chronic) N18.6
      due to hypertension I12.0
    following
      abortion — *see* Abortion by type complicated
        by specified condition NEC
      crushing T79.5 ☑
      ectopic or molar pregnancy O08.4
      labor and delivery (acute) O90.4
    hypertensive — *see* Hypertension, kidney
    postprocedural N99.0
  respiration, respiratory J96.90
    with
      hypercapnia J96.92
      hypercarbia J96.92
      hypoxia J96.91
    acute J96.00
      with
        hypercapnia J96.02
        hypercarbia J96.02
        hypoxia J96.01
    center G93.89
    acute and (on) chronic J96.20
      with
        hypercapnia J96.22
        hypercarbia J96.22
        hypoxia J96.21
    chronic J96.10
      with
        hypercapnia J96.12
        hypercarbia J96.12
        hypoxia J96.11
    newborn P28.5
    postprocedural (acute) J95.821
      acute and chronic J95.822
  rotation
    cecum Q43.3
    colon Q43.3
    intestine Q43.3
    kidney Q63.2
  sedation (conscious) (moderate) during procedure
    T88.52 ☑
    history of Z92.83
  segmentation — *see also* Fusion
    fingers — *see* Syndactylism, complex, fingers
    vertebra Q76.49
      with scoliosis Q76.3
  seminiferous tubule, adult E29.1
  senile (general) R54
  sexual arousal (male) F52.21
    female F52.22
  testicular endocrine function E29.1
  to thrive (child over 28 days old) R62.51
    adult R62.7
    newborn P92.6
  transplant T86.92
    bone T86.831
      marrow T86.02
    cornea T86.841- ☑
    heart T86.22
      with lung(s) T86.32
    intestine T86.851
    kidney T86.12
    liver T86.42
    lung(s) T86.811
      with heart T86.32
    pancreas T86.891
    skin (allograft) (autograft) T86.821
    specified organ or tissue NEC T86.891
    stem cell (peripheral blood) (umbilical cord) T86.5
  trial of labor (with subsequent cesarean delivery)
    O66.40
    following previous cesarean delivery O66.41
  tubal ligation N99.89
  urinary — *see* Disease, kidney, chronic

Failure, failed — *continued*
  vacuum extraction NOS (with subsequent cesarean
    delivery) O66.5
  vasectomy N99.89
  ventouse NOS (with subsequent cesarean delivery)
    O66.5
  ventricular — *see also* Failure, heart I50.9
    left — *see also* Failure, heart, left I50.1
      with rheumatic fever (conditions in I00)
        active I01.8
          with chorea I02.0
        inactive or quiescent (with chorea) I09.81
        rheumatic (chronic) (inactive) (with chorea)
          I09.81
          active or acute I01.8
            with chorea I02.0
    right — *see* Failure, heart, right
  vital centers, newborn P91.88
Fainting (fit) R55
Fallen arches — *see* Deformity, limb, flat foot
Falling, falls (repeated) R29.6
  any organ or part — *see* Prolapse
Fallopian
  insufflation Z31.41
  tube — *see* condition
Fallot's
  pentalogy Q21.8
  tetrad or tetralogy Q21.3
  triad or trilogy Q22.3
False — *see also* condition
  croup J38.5
  joint — *see* Nonunion, fracture
  labor (pains) O47.9
    at or after 37 completed weeks of gestation O47.1
    before 37 completed weeks of gestation O47.0- ☑
  passage, urethra (prostatic) N36.5
  pregnancy F45.8
Family, familial — *see also* condition
  disruption Z63.8
    involving divorce or separation Z63.5
  Li-Fraumeni (syndrome) Z15.01
  planning advice Z30.09
  problem Z63.9
    specified NEC Z63.8
  retinoblastoma C69.2- ☑
Famine (effects of) T73.0 ☑
  edema — *see* Malnutrition, severe
Fanconi (-de Toni)(-Debré) **syndrome** E72.09
  with cystinosis E72.04
Fanconi's anemia (congenital pancytopenia) D61.09
Farber's disease or syndrome E75.29
Farcy A24.0
Farmer's
  lung J67.0
  skin L57.8
Farsightedness — *see* Hypermetropia
Fascia — *see* condition
Fasciculation R25.3
Fasciitis M72.9
  diffuse (eosinophilic) M35.4
  infective M72.8
    necrotizing M72.6
  necrotizing M72.6
  nodular M72.4
  perirenal (with ureteral obstruction) N13.5
    with infection N13.6
  plantar M72.2
  specified NEC M72.8
  traumatic (old) M72.8
    current — *code by* site under Sprain
Fascioliasis B66.3
Fasciolopsis, fasciolopsiasis (intestinal) B66.5
Fascioscapulohumeral myopathy G71.02
Fast pulse R00.0
Fat
  embolism — *see* Embolism, fat
  excessive — *see also* Obesity
    in heart — *see* Degeneration, myocardial
  in stool R19.5
  localized (pad) E65
    heart — *see* Degeneration, myocardial
    knee M79.4
    retropatellar M79.4
  necrosis
    breast N64.1
    mesentery K65.4
    omentum K65.4
  pad E65

Fat — *continued*
  pad — *continued*
    knee M79.4
Fatigue R53.83
  auditory deafness — *see* Deafness
  chronic R53.82
  combat F43.0
  general R53.83
    psychogenic F48.8
  heat (transient) T67.6 ☑
  muscle M62.89
  myocardium — *see* Failure, heart
  neoplasm-related R53.0
  nervous, neurosis F48.8
  operational F48.8
  psychogenic (general) F48.8
  senile R54
  voice R49.8
Fatness — *see* Obesity
Fatty — *see also* condition
  apron E65
  degeneration — *see* Degeneration, fatty
  heart (enlarged) — *see* Degeneration, myocardial
  liver NEC K76.0
    alcoholic K70.0
    nonalcoholic K76.0
  necrosis — *see* Degeneration, fatty
Fauces — *see* condition
Fauchard's disease (periodontitis) — *see* Periodontitis
Faucitis J02.9
Favism (anemia) D55.0
Favus — *see* Dermatophytosis
Fazio-Londe disease or syndrome G12.1
Fear complex or reaction F40.9
Fear of — *see* Phobia
Feared complaint unfounded Z71.1
Febris, febrile — *see also* Fever
  flava — *see also* Fever, yellow A95.9
  melitensis A23.0
  pestis — *see* Plague
  recurrens — *see* Fever, relapsing
  rubra A38.9
Fecal
  incontinence R15.9
  smearing R15.1
  soiling R15.1
  urgency R15.2
Fecalith (impaction) K56.41
  appendix K38.1
  congenital P76.8
Fede's disease K14.0
Feeble rapid pulse due to shock following injury
  T79.4 ☑
Feeble-minded F70
Feeding
  difficulties R63.30
  problem (elderly) (infant) R63.39
    newborn P92.9
      specified NEC P92.8
    nonorganic (adult) — *see* Disorder, eating
Feeling (of)
  foreign body in throat R09.89
Feer's disease — *see* Poisoning, mercury
Feet — *see* condition
Feigned illness Z76.5
Feil-Klippel syndrome (brevicollis) Q76.1
Feinmesser's (hidrotic) **ectodermal dysplasia** Q82.4
Felinophobia F40.218
Felon — *see also* Cellulitis, digit
  with lymphangitis — *see* Lymphangitis, acute, digit
Felty's syndrome M05.00
  ankle M05.07- ☑
  elbow M05.02- ☑
  foot joint M05.07- ☑
  hand joint M05.04- ☑
  hip M05.05- ☑
  knee M05.06- ☑
  multiple site M05.09
  shoulder M05.01- ☑
  vertebra — *see* Spondylitis, ankylosing
  wrist M05.03- ☑
Female genital cutting status — *see* Female genital
  mutilation status (FGM)
Female genital mutilation status (FGM) N90.810
  specified NEC N90.818
  type I (clitorectomy status) N90.811

Female genital mutilation status — *continued*
  type II (clitorectomy with excision of labia minora status) N90.812
  type III (infibulation status) N90.813
  type IV N90.818
Femur, femoral — *see* condition
Fenestration, fenestrated — *see also* Imperfect, closure
  aortico-pulmonary Q21.4
  atrial septum Q21.11
  cusps, heart valve NEC Q24.8
    pulmonary Q22.3
  pulmonic cusps Q22.3
Fernell's disease (aortic aneurysm) I71.9
Fertile eunuch syndrome E23.0
Fetid
  breath R19.6
  sweat L75.0
Fetishism F65.0
  transvestic F65.1
Fetus, fetal — *see also* condition
  alcohol syndrome (dysmorphic) Q86.0
  compressus O31.0- ☑
  hydantoin syndrome Q86.1
  lung tissue P28.0
  papyraceous O31.0- ☑
Fever (inanition) (of unknown origin) (persistent) (with chills) (with rigor) R50.9
  abortus A23.1
  Aden (dengue) A90
  African tick bite A77.8
  African tick-borne A68.1
  American
    mountain (tick) A93.2
      spotted A77.0
  aphthous B08.8
  arbovirus, arboviral A94
    hemorrhagic A94
    specified NEC A93.8
  Argentinian hemorrhagic A96.0
  Assam B55.0
  Australian Q A78
  Bangkok hemorrhagic A91
  Barmah forest A92.8
  Bartonella A44.0
  bilious, hemoglobinuric B50.8
  blackwater B50.8
  blister B00.1
  Bolivian hemorrhagic A96.1
  Bonvale dam T73.3 ☑
  boutonneuse A77.1
  brain — *see* Encephalitis
  Brazilian purpuric A48.4
  breakbone A90
  Bullis A77.0
  Bunyamwera A92.8
  Burdwan B55.0
  Bwamba A92.8
  Cameroon — *see* Malaria
  Canton A75.9
  catarrhal (acute) J00
    chronic J31.0
  cat-scratch A28.1
  Central Asian hemorrhagic A98.0
  cerebral — *see* Encephalitis
  cerebrospinal meningococcal A39.0
  Chagres B50.9
  Chandipura A92.8
  Changuinola A93.1
  Charcot's (biliary) (hepatic) (intermittent) — *see* Calculus, bile duct
  Chikungunya (viral) (hemorrhagic) A92.0
  Chitral A93.1
  Colombo — *see* Fever, paratyphoid
  Colorado tick (virus) A93.2
  congestive (remittent) — *see* Malaria
  Congo virus A98.0
  continued malarial B50.9
  Corsican — *see* Malaria
  Crimean-Congo hemorrhagic A98.0
  Cyprus — *see* Brucellosis
  dandy A90
  deer fly — *see* Tularemia
  dengue (virus) A90
    hemorrhagic A91
    sandfly A93.1
  desert B38.0
  drug induced R50.2

Fever — *continued*
  due to
    conditions classified elsewhere R50.81
    heat T67.01 ☑
  enteric A01.00
  enteroviral exanthematous (Boston exanthem) A88.0
  ephemeral (of unknown origin) R50.9
  epidemic hemorrhagic A98.5
  erysipelatous — *see* Erysipelas
  estivo-autumnal (malarial) B50.9
  famine A75.0
  five day A79.0
  following delivery O86.4
  Fort Bragg A27.89
  gastroenteric A01.00
  gastromalarial — *see* Malaria
  Gibraltar — *see* Brucellosis
  glandular — *see* Mononucleosis, infectious
  Guama (viral) A92.8
  Haverhill A25.1
  hay (allergic) J30.1
    with asthma (bronchial) J45.909
      with
        exacerbation (acute) J45.901
        status asthmaticus J45.902
    due to
      allergen other than pollen J30.89
      pollen, any plant or tree J30.1
  heat (effects) T67.01 ☑
  hematuric, bilious B50.8
  hemoglobinuric (malarial) (bilious) B50.8
  hemorrhagic (arthropod-borne) NOS A94
    with renal syndrome A98.5
    arenaviral A96.9
      specified NEC A96.8
    Argentinian A96.0
    Bangkok A91
    Bolivian A96.1
    Central Asian A98.0
    Chikungunya A92.0
    Crimean-Congo A98.0
    dengue (virus) A91
    epidemic A98.5
    Junin (virus) A96.0
    Korean A98.5
    Kyasanur forest A98.2
    Machupo (virus) A96.1
    mite-borne A93.8
    mosquito-borne A92.8
    Omsk A98.1
    Philippine A91
    Russian A98.5
    Singapore A91
    Southeast Asia A91
    Thailand A91
    tick-borne NEC A93.8
    viral A99
      specified NEC A98.8
  hepatic — *see* Cholecystitis
  herpetic — *see* Herpes
  icterohemorrhagic A27.0
  Indiana A93.8
  infective B99.9
    specified NEC B99.8
  intermittent (bilious) — *see also* Malaria
    of unknown origin R50.9
    pernicious B50.9
  iodide R50.2
  Japanese river A75.3
  jungle — *see also* Malaria
    yellow A95.0
  Junin (virus) hemorrhagic A96.0
  Katayama B65.2
  kedani A75.3
  Kenya (tick) A77.1
  Kew Garden A79.1
  Korean hemorrhagic A98.5
  Lassa A96.2
  Lone Star A77.0
  Machupo (virus) hemorrhagic A96.1
  malaria, malarial — *see* Malaria
  Malta A23.9
  Marseilles A77.1
  marsh — *see* Malaria
  Mayaro A92.8
  Mediterranean — *see also* Brucellosis A23.9
    familial M04.1
    tick A77.1

Fever — *continued*
  meningeal — *see* Meningitis
  Meuse A79.0
  Mexican A75.2
  mianeh A68.1
  miasmatic — *see* Malaria
  mosquito-borne (viral) A92.9
    hemorrhagic A92.8
  mountain — *see also* Brucellosis
    meaning Rocky Mountain spotted fever A77.0
    tick (American) (Colorado) (viral) A93.2
  Mucambo (viral) A92.8
  mud A27.9
  Neapolitan — *see* Brucellosis
  neutropenic D70.9
  newborn P81.9
    environmental P81.0
  Nine-Mile A78
  non-exanthematous tick A93.2
  North Asian tick-borne A77.2
  Omsk hemorrhagic A98.1
  O'nyong-nyong (viral) A92.1
  Oropouche (viral) A93.0
  Oroya A44.0
  pacific coast tick A77.8
  paludal — *see* Malaria
  Panama (malarial) B50.9
  Pappataci A93.1
  paratyphoid A01.4
    A A01.1
    B A01.2
    C A01.3
  parrot A70
  periodic (Mediterranean) M04.1
  persistent (of unknown origin) R50.9
  petechial A39.0
  pharyngoconjunctival B30.2
  Philippine hemorrhagic A91
  phlebotomus A93.1
  Piry (virus) A93.8
  Pixuna (viral) A92.8
  Plasmodium ovale B53.0
  polioviral (nonparalytic) A80.4
  Pontiac A48.2
  postimmunization R50.83
  postoperative R50.82
    due to infection T81.40 ☑
  posttransfusion R50.84
  postvaccination R50.83
  presenting with conditions classified elsewhere R50.81
  pretibial A27.89
  puerperal O86.4
  Q A78
  quadrilateral A78
  quartan (malaria) B52.9
  Queensland (coastal) (tick) A77.3
  quintan A79.0
  rabbit — *see* Tularemia
  rat-bite A25.9
    due to
      Spirillum A25.0
      Streptobacillus moniliformis A25.1
  recurrent — *see* Fever, relapsing
  relapsing (Borrelia) A68.9
    Carter's (Asiatic) A68.1
    Dutton's (West African) A68.1
    Koch's A68.9
    louse-borne A68.0
    Novy's
      louse-borne A68.0
      tick-borne A68.1
    Obermeyer's (European) A68.0
    tick-borne A68.1
  remittent (bilious) (congestive) (gastric) — *see* Malaria
  rheumatic (active) (acute) (chronic) (subacute) I00
    with central nervous system involvement I02.9
    active with heart involvement — *see* category I01 ☑
    inactive or quiescent with
      cardiac hypertrophy I09.89
      carditis I09.9
      endocarditis I09.1
        aortic (valve) I06.9
          with mitral (valve) disease I08.0
        mitral (valve) I05.9
          with aortic (valve) disease I08.0
        pulmonary (valve) I09.89
        tricuspid (valve) I07.8
      heart disease NEC I09.89

Fever — *continued*
  rheumatic — *continued*
    inactive or quiescent with — *continued*
      heart failure (congestive) (conditions in category
        I50.) I09.81
      left ventricular failure (conditions in I50.1-I50.4-)
        I09.81
      myocarditis, myocardial degeneration (condi-
        tions in I51.4) I09.0
      pancarditis I09.9
      pericarditis I09.2
  Rift Valley (viral) A92.4
  Rocky Mountain spotted A77.0
  rose J30.1
  Ross River B33.1
  Russian hemorrhagic A98.5
  San Joaquin (Valley) B38.0
  sandfly A93.1
  Sao Paulo A77.0
  scarlet A38.9
  seven day (leptospirosis) (autumnal) (Japanese) A27.89
    dengue A90
  shin-bone A79.0
  Singapore hemorrhagic A91
  solar A90
  Songo A98.5
  sore B00.1
  South African tick-bite A68.1
  Southeast Asia hemorrhagic A91
  spinal — *see* Meningitis
  spirillary A25.0
  splenic — *see* Anthrax
  spotted A77.9
    American A77.0
    Brazilian A77.0
    cerebrospinal meningitis A39.0
    Colombian A77.0
    due to Rickettsia
      africae (African tick bite fever) A77.8
      australis A77.3
      conorii A77.1
      parkeri A77.8
      rickettsii A77.0
      sibirica A77.2
      specified type NEC A77.8
    Ehrlichiosis A77.40
      due to
        E. chafeensis A77.41
        specified organism NEC A77.49
    Rocky Mountain A77.0
  steroid R50.2
  streptobacillary A25.1
  subtertian B50.9
  Sumatran mite A75.3
  sun A90
  swamp A27.9
  swine A02.8
  sylvatic, yellow A95.0
  Tahyna B33.8
  tertian — *see* Malaria, tertian
  Thailand hemorrhagic A91
  thermic T67.01 ☑
  three-day A93.1
  tick
    American mountain A93.2
    Colorado A93.2
    Kemerovo A93.8
    Mediterranean A77.1
    mountain A93.2
    nonexanthematous A93.2
    Quaranfil A93.8
  tick-bite NEC A93.8
  tick-borne (hemorrhagic) NEC A93.8
  trench A79.0
  tsutsugamushi A75.3
  typhogastric A01.00
  typhoid (abortive) (hemorrhagic) (intermittent) (malig-
    nant) A01.00
    complicated by
      arthritis A01.04
      heart involvement A01.02
      meningitis A01.01
      osteomyelitis A01.05
      pneumonia A01.03
      specified NEC A01.09
  typhomalarial — *see* Malaria
  typhus — *see* Typhus (fever)
  undulant — *see* Brucellosis

Fever — *continued*
  unknown origin R50.9
  uveoparotid D86.89
  valley B38.0
  Venezuelan equine A92.2
  vesicular stomatitis A93.8
  viral hemorrhagic — *see* Fever, hemorrhagic, by type
    of virus
  Volhynian A79.0
  Wesselsbron (viral) A92.8
  West
    African B50.8
    Nile (viral) A92.30
      with
        complications NEC A92.39
        cranial nerve disorders A92.32
        encephalitis A92.31
        encephalomyelitis A92.31
        neurologic manifestation NEC A92.32
        optic neuritis A92.32
        polyradiculitis A92.32
  Whitmore's — *see* Melioidosis
  Wolhynian A79.0
  worm B83.9
  yellow A95.9
    jungle A95.0
    sylvatic A95.0
    urban A95.1
  Zika virus A92.5
Fibrillation
  atrial or auricular (established) I48.91
    chronic I48.20
      persistent I48.19
    paroxysmal I48.0
    permanent I48.21
    persistent (chronic) (NOS) (other) I48.19
      longstanding I48.11
  cardiac I49.8
  heart I49.8
  muscular M62.89
  ventricular I49.01
Fibrin
  ball or bodies, pleural (sac) J94.1
  chamber, anterior (eye) (gelatinous exudate) — *see*
    Iridocyclitis, acute
Fibrinogenolysis — *see* Fibrinolysis
Fibrinogenopenia D68.8
  acquired D65
  congenital D68.2
Fibrinolysis (hemorrhagic) (acquired) D65
  antepartum hemorrhage — *see* Hemorrhage, antepar-
    tum, with coagulation defect
  following
    abortion — *see* Abortion by type complicated by
      hemorrhage
    ectopic or molar pregnancy O08.1
  intrapartum O67.0
  newborn, transient P60
  postpartum O72.3
Fibrinopenia (hereditary) D68.2
  acquired D68.4
Fibrinopurulent — *see* condition
Fibrinous — *see* condition
Fibroadenoma
  cellular intracanalicular D24- ☑
  giant D24- ☑
  intracanalicular
    cellular D24- ☑
    giant D24- ☑
    specified site — *see* Neoplasm, benign, by site
    unspecified site D24- ☑
  juvenile D24- ☑
  pericanalicular
    specified site — *see* Neoplasm, benign, by site
    unspecified site D24- ☑
  phyllodes D24- ☑
  prostate D29.1
  specified site NEC — *see* Neoplasm, benign, by site
  unspecified site D24- ☑
Fibroadenosis, breast (chronic) (cystic) (diffuse) (periodic) (segmental) N60.2- ☑
Fibroangioma — *see also* Neoplasm, benign, by site
  juvenile
    specified site — *see* Neoplasm, benign, by site
    unspecified site D10.6
Fibrochondrosarcoma — *see* Neoplasm, cartilage, malignant

Fibrocystic
  disease — *see also* Fibrosis, cystic
    breast — *see* Mastopathy, cystic
    jaw M27.49
    kidney (congenital) Q61.8
    liver Q44.6
    pancreas E84.9
  kidney (congenital) Q61.8
Fibrodysplasia ossificans progressiva — *see* Myositis,
  ossificans, progressiva
Fibroelastosis (cordis) (endocardial) (endomyocardial)
  I42.4
Fibroid (tumor) — *see also* Neoplasm, connective tissue,
  benign
  disease, lung (chronic) — *see* Fibrosis, lung
  heart (disease) — *see* Myocarditis
  in pregnancy or childbirth O34.1- ☑
    causing obstructed labor O65.5
  induration, lung (chronic) — *see* Fibrosis, lung
  lung — *see* Fibrosis, lung
  pneumonia (chronic) — *see* Fibrosis, lung
  uterus — *see also* Leiomyoma, uterus D25.9
Fibrolipoma — *see* Lipoma
Fibroliposarcoma — *see* Neoplasm, connective tissue,
  malignant
Fibroma — *see also* Neoplasm, connective tissue, benign
  ameloblastic — *see* Cyst, calcifying odontogenic
  bone (nonossifying) — *see* Disorder, bone, specified
    type NEC
    ossifying — *see* Neoplasm, bone, benign
  cementifying — *see* Neoplasm, bone, benign
  chondromyxoid — *see* Neoplasm, bone, benign
  desmoplastic — *see* Neoplasm, connective tissue, un-
    certain behavior
  durum — *see* Neoplasm, connective tissue, benign
  fascial — *see* Neoplasm, connective tissue, benign
  invasive — *see* Neoplasm, connective tissue, uncertain
    behavior
  molle — *see* Lipoma
  myxoid — *see* Neoplasm, connective tissue, benign
  nasopharynx, nasopharyngeal (juvenile) D10.6
  nonosteogenic (nonossifying) — *see* Dysplasia, fibrous
  odontogenic (central) — *see* Cyst, calcifying odonto-
    genic
  ossifying — *see* Neoplasm, bone, benign
  periosteal — *see* Neoplasm, bone, benign
  soft — *see* Lipoma
Fibromatosis M72.9
  abdominal — *see* Neoplasm, connective tissue, uncer-
    tain behavior
  aggressive — *see* Neoplasm, connective tissue, uncer-
    tain behavior
  congenital generalized — *see* Neoplasm, connective
    tissue, uncertain behavior
  Dupuytren's M72.0
  gingival K06.1
  palmar (fascial) M72.0
  plantar (fascial) M72.2
  pseudosarcomatous (proliferative) (subcutaneous)
    M72.4
  retroperitoneal D48.3
  specified NEC M72.8
Fibromyalgia M79.7
Fibromyoma — *see also* Neoplasm, connective tissue,
  benign
  uterus (corpus) — *see also* Leiomyoma, uterus
    in pregnancy or childbirth — *see* Fibroid, in preg-
      nancy or childbirth
    causing obstructed labor O65.5
Fibromyositis M79.7
Fibromyxolipoma D17.9
Fibromyxoma — *see* Neoplasm, connective tissue, benign
Fibromyxosarcoma — *see* Neoplasm, connective tissue,
  malignant
Fibro-odontoma, ameloblastic — *see* Cyst, calcifying
  odontogenic
Fibro-osteoma — *see* Neoplasm, bone, benign
Fibroplasia, retrolental H35.17- ☑
Fibropurulent — *see* condition
Fibrosarcoma — *see also* Neoplasm, connective tissue,
  malignant
  ameloblastic C41.1
    upper jaw (bone) C41.0
  congenital — *see* Neoplasm, connective tissue, malig-
    nant
  fascial — *see* Neoplasm, connective tissue, malignant

Fibrosarcoma — *continued*
infantile — *see* Neoplasm, connective tissue, malignant
odontogenic C41.1
upper jaw (bone) C41.0
periosteal — *see* Neoplasm, bone, malignant
Fibrosclerosis
breast N60.3- ☑
multifocal M35.5
penis (corpora cavernosa) N48.6
Fibrosis, fibrotic
adrenal (gland) E27.8
amnion O41.8X- ☑
anal papillae K62.89
arteriocapillary — *see* Arteriosclerosis
bladder N32.89
interstitial — *see* Cystitis, chronic, interstitial
localized submucosal — *see* Cystitis, chronic, interstitial
panmural — *see* Cystitis, chronic, interstitial
breast — *see* Fibrosclerosis, breast
capillary — *see also* Arteriosclerosis I70.90
lung (chronic) — *see* Fibrosis, lung
cardiac — *see* Myocarditis
cervix N88.8
chorion O41.8X- ☑
corpus cavernosum (sclerosing) N48.6
cystic (of pancreas) E84.9
with
distal intestinal obstruction syndrome E84.19
fecal impaction E84.19
intestinal manifestations NEC E84.19
pulmonary manifestations E84.0
specified manifestations NEC E84.8
due to device, implant or graft — *see also* Complications, by site and type, specified NEC T85.828 ☑
arterial graft NEC T82.828 ☑
breast (implant) T85.828 ☑
catheter NEC T85.828 ☑
dialysis (renal) T82.828 ☑
intraperitoneal T85.828 ☑
infusion NEC T82.828 ☑
spinal (epidural) (subdural) T85.820 ☑
urinary (indwelling) T83.82 ☑
electronic (electrode) (pulse generator) (stimulator)
bone T84.82 ☑
cardiac T82.827 ☑
nervous system (brain) (peripheral nerve) (spinal) T85.820 ☑
urinary T83.82 ☑
fixation, internal (orthopedic) NEC T84.82 ☑
gastrointestinal (bile duct) (esophagus) T85.828 ☑
genital NEC T83.82 ☑
heart NEC T82.827 ☑
joint prosthesis T84.82 ☑
ocular (corneal graft) (orbital implant) NEC T85.828 ☑
orthopedic NEC T84.82 ☑
specified NEC T85.828 ☑
urinary NEC T83.82 ☑
vascular NEC T82.828 ☑
ventricular intracranial shunt T85.820 ☑
ejaculatory duct N50.89
endocardium — *see* Endocarditis
endomyocardial (tropical) I42.3
epididymis N50.89
eye muscle — *see* Strabismus, mechanical
heart — *see* Myocarditis
hepatic — *see* Fibrosis, liver
hepatolienal (portal hypertension) K76.6
hepatosplenic (portal hypertension) K76.6
infrapatellar fat pad M79.4
intrascrotal N50.89
kidney N26.9
liver K74.00
with sclerosis K74.2
advanced K74.02
alcoholic K70.2
early K74.01
stage
F1 or F2 K74.01
F3 K74.02
lung (atrophic) (chronic) (confluent) (massive) (perialveolar) (peribronchial) J84.10
with
anthracosilicosis J60
anthracosis J60
asbestosis J61

Fibrosis, fibrotic — *continued*
lung — *continued*
with — *continued*
bagassosis J67.1
bauxite J63.1
berylliosis J63.2
byssinosis J66.0
calcicosis J62.8
chalicosis J62.8
dust reticulation J64
farmer's lung J67.0
ganister disease J62.8
graphite J63.3
pneumoconiosis NOS J64
siderosis J63.4
silicosis J62.8
capillary J84.10
congenital P27.8
diffuse (idiopathic) J84.10
chemicals, gases, fumes or vapors (inhalation) J68.4
interstitial J84.10
acute J84.114
talc J62.0
following radiation J70.1
idiopathic J84.112
postinflammatory J84.10
silicotic J62.8
tuberculous — *see* Tuberculosis, pulmonary
lymphatic gland I89.8
median bar — *see* Hyperplasia, prostate
mediastinum (idiopathic) J98.59
meninges G96.198
myocardium, myocardial — *see* Myocarditis
ovary N83.8
oviduct N83.8
pancreas K86.89
penis NEC N48.6
pericardium I31.0
perineum, in pregnancy or childbirth O34.7- ☑
causing obstructed labor O65.5
pleura J94.1
popliteal fat pad M79.4
prostate (chronic) — *see* Hyperplasia, prostate
pulmonary — *see also* Fibrosis, lung J84.10
congenital P27.8
idiopathic J84.112
rectal sphincter K62.89
retroperitoneal, idiopathic (with ureteral obstruction) N13.5
with infection N13.6
sclerosing mesenteric (idiopathic) K65.4
scrotum N50.89
seminal vesicle N50.89
senile R54
skin L90.5
spermatic cord N50.89
spleen D73.89
in schistosomiasis (bilharziasis) B65.9 *[D77]*
subepidermal nodular — *see* Neoplasm, skin, benign
submucous (oral) (tongue) K13.5
testis N44.8
chronic, due to syphilis A52.76
thymus (gland) E32.8
tongue, submucous K13.5
tunica vaginalis N50.89
uterus (non-neoplastic) N85.8
vagina N89.8
valve, heart — *see* Endocarditis
vas deferens N50.89
vein I87.8
Fibrositis (periarticular) M79.7
nodular, chronic (Jaccoud's) (rheumatoid) — *see* Arthropathy, postrheumatic, chronic
Fibrothorax J94.1
Fibrotic — *see* Fibrosis
Fibrous — *see* condition
Fibroxanthoma — *see also* Neoplasm, connective tissue, benign
atypical — *see* Neoplasm, connective tissue, uncertain behavior
malignant — *see* Neoplasm, connective tissue, malignant
Fibroxanthosarcoma — *see* Neoplasm, connective tissue, malignant
Fiedler's
disease (icterohemorrhagic leptospirosis) A27.0
myocarditis (acute) I40.1

Fifth disease B08.3
venereal A55
Filaria, filarial, filariasis — *see* Infestation, filarial
Filatov's disease — *see* Mononucleosis, infectious
File-cutter's disease — *see* Poisoning, lead
Filling defect
biliary tract R93.2
bladder R93.41
duodenum R93.3
gallbladder R93.2
gastrointestinal tract R93.3
intestine R93.3
kidney R93.42- ☑
stomach R93.3
ureter R93.41
urinary organs, specified NEC R93.49
Fimbrial cyst Q50.4
Financial problem affecting care NOS Z59.9
bankruptcy Z59.89
foreclosure on loan Z59.89
home loan Z59.81- ☑
strain Z59.86
Findings, abnormal, inconclusive, without diagnosis
— *see also* Abnormal
17-ketosteroids, elevated R82.5
acetonuria R82.4
alcohol in blood R78.0
anisocytosis R71.8
antenatal screening of mother O28.9
biochemical O28.1
chromosomal O28.5
cytological O28.2
genetic O28.5
hematological O28.0
radiological O28.4
specified NEC O28.8
ultrasonic O28.3
antibody titer, elevated R76.0
anticardiolipin antibody R76.0
antiphosphatidylglycerol antibody R76.0
antiphosphatidylinositol antibody R76.0
antiphosphatidylserine antibody R76.0
antiphospholipid antibody R76.0
bacteriuria R82.71
bicarbonate E87.8
bile in urine R82.2
blood sugar R73.09
high R73.9
low (transient) E16.2
body fluid or substance, specified NEC R88.8
casts, urine R82.998
catecholamines R82.5
cells, urine R82.998
chloride E87.8
cholesterol E78.9
high E78.00
with high triglycerides E78.2
chyluria R82.0
cloudy
dialysis effluent R88.0
urine R82.90
creatinine clearance R94.4
crystals, urine R82.998
culture
blood R78.81
positive — *see* Positive, culture
echocardiogram R93.1
electrolyte level, urinary R82.998
function study NEC R94.8
bladder R94.8
endocrine NEC R94.7
thyroid R94.6
kidney R94.4
liver R94.5
pancreas R94.8
placenta R94.8
pulmonary R94.2
spleen R94.8
gallbladder, nonvisualization R93.2
glucose (tolerance test) (non-fasting) R73.09
glycosuria R81
heart
shadow R93.1
sounds R01.2
hematinuria R82.3
hematocrit drop (precipitous) R71.0
hemoglobinuria R82.3

Findings, abnormal, inconclusive, without diagnosis
— *continued*
  human papillomavirus (HPV) DNA test positive
    cervix
      high risk R87.810
      low risk R87.820
    vagina
      high risk R87.811
      low risk R87.821
  in blood (of substance not normally found in blood)
    R78.9
    addictive drug NEC R78.4
    alcohol (excessive level) R78.0
    cocaine R78.2
    hallucinogen R78.3
    heavy metals (abnormal level) R78.79
    lead R78.71
    lithium (abnormal level) R78.89
    opiate drug R78.1
    psychotropic drug R78.5
    specified substance NEC R78.89
    steroid agent R78.6
  indoleacetic acid, elevated R82.5
  ketonuria R82.4
  lactic acid dehydrogenase (LDH) R74.02
  liver function test — *see also* Elevated, liver function,
    test R79.89
  mammogram NEC R92.8
    calcification (calculus) R92.1
    inconclusive result (due to dense breasts) R92.2
    microcalcification R92.0
  mediastinal shift R93.89
  melanin, urine R82.998
  myoglobinuria R82.1
  neonatal screening — *see* Abnormal, neonatal
    screening
  newborn screens, state mandated — *see* Abnormal,
    neonatal screening
  nonvisualization of gallbladder R93.2
  odor of urine NOS R82.90
  Papanicolaou cervix R87.619
    non-atypical endometrial cells R87.618
  pneumoencephalogram R93.0
  poikilocytosis R71.8
  potassium (deficiency) E87.6
    excess E87.5
  PPD R76.11
  radiologic (X-ray) R93.89
    abdomen R93.5
    biliary tract R93.2
    breast R92.8
    gastrointestinal tract R93.3
    genitourinary organs R93.89
    head R93.0
    inconclusive due to excess body fat of patient R93.9
    intrathoracic organs NEC R93.1
    musculoskeletal
      limbs R93.6
      other than limb R93.7
    placenta R93.89
    retroperitoneum R93.5
    skin R93.89
    skull R93.0
    subcutaneous tissue R93.89
    testis R93.81- ☑
  red blood cell (count) (morphology) (sickling) (volume)
    R71.8
  scan NEC R94.8
    bladder R94.8
    bone R94.8
    kidney R94.4
    liver R93.2
    lung R94.2
    pancreas R94.8
    placental R94.8
    spleen R94.8
    thyroid R94.6
  sedimentation rate, elevated R70.0
  SGOT R74.01
  SGPT R74.01
  sodium (deficiency) E87.1
    excess E87.0
  specified body fluid NEC R88.8
  stress test R94.39
  testis R93.81- ☑
  thyroid (function) (metabolic rate) (scan) (uptake) R94.6
  transaminase (level) R74.01
  triglycerides E78.9
    high E78.1

Findings, abnormal, inconclusive, without diagnosis
— *continued*
  triglycerides — *continued*
    high — *continued*
      with high cholesterol E78.2
  tuberculin skin test (without active tuberculosis) R76.11
  urine R82.90
    acetone R82.4
    bacteria R82.71
    bile R82.2
    casts or cells R82.998
    chyle R82.0
    culture positive R82.79
    glucose R81
    hemoglobin R82.3
    ketone R82.4
    sugar R81
  vanillylmandelic acid (VMA), elevated R82.5
  vectorcardiogram (VCG) R94.39
  ventriculogram R93.0
  white blood cell (count) (differential) (morphology)
    D72.9
  xerography R92.8
Finger — *see* condition
Fire, Saint Anthony's — *see* Erysipelas
Fire-setting
  pathological (compulsive) F63.1
Fish hook stomach K31.89
Fishmeal-worker's lung J67.8
Fissure, fissured
  anus, anal K60.2
    acute K60.0
    chronic K60.1
    congenital Q43.8
  ear, lobule, congenital Q17.8
  epiglottis (congenital) Q31.8
  larynx J38.7
    congenital Q31.8
  lip K13.0
    congenital — *see* Cleft, lip
  nipple N64.0
    associated with
      lactation O92.13
      pregnancy O92.11- ☑
      puerperium O92.12
  nose Q30.2
  palate (congenital) — *see* Cleft, palate
  skin R23.4
  spine (congenital) — *see also* Spina bifida
    with hydrocephalus — *see* Spina bifida, by site, with
      hydrocephalus
  tongue (acquired) K14.5
    congenital Q38.3
Fistula (cutaneous) L98.8
  abdomen (wall) K63.2
    bladder N32.2
    intestine NEC K63.2
    ureter N28.89
    uterus N82.5
  abdominorectal K63.2
  abdominosigmoidal K63.2
  abdominothoracic J86.0
  abdominouterine N82.5
    congenital Q51.7
  abdominovesical N32.2
  accessory sinuses — *see* Sinusitis
  actinomycotic — *see* Actinomycosis
  alveolar antrum — *see* Sinusitis, maxillary
  alveolar process K04.6
  anorectal K60.5
  antrobuccal — *see* Sinusitis, maxillary
  antrum — *see* Sinusitis, maxillary
  anus, anal (recurrent) (infectional) K60.3
    congenital Q43.6
      with absence, atresia and stenosis Q42.2
    tuberculous A18.32
  aorta-duodenal I77.2
  appendix, appendicular K38.3
  arteriovenous (acquired) (nonruptured) I77.0
    brain I67.1
      congenital Q28.2
        ruptured — *see* Fistula, arteriovenous, brain,
          ruptured
      ruptured I60.8
        intracerebral I61.8
        intraparenchymal I61.8
        intraventricular I61.5
        subarachnoid I60.8

Fistula — *continued*
  arteriovenous — *continued*
    cerebral — *see* Fistula, arteriovenous, brain
    congenital (peripheral) — *see also* Malformation,
      arteriovenous
      brain Q28.2
        ruptured — *see* Fistula, arteriovenous, brain,
          ruptured
      coronary Q24.5
      pulmonary Q25.72
    coronary I25.41
      congenital Q24.5
    pulmonary I28.0
      congenital Q25.72
    surgically created (for dialysis) Z99.2
      complication — *see* Complication, arteriovenous,
        fistula, surgically created
    traumatic — *see* Injury, blood vessel
  artery I77.2
  aural (mastoid) — *see* Mastoiditis, chronic
  auricle — *see also* Disorder, pinna, specified type NEC
    congenital Q18.1
  Bartholin's gland N82.8
  bile duct (common) (hepatic) K83.3
    with calculus, stones — *see also* Calculus, bile duct
      K83.3
  biliary (tract) — *see* Fistula, bile duct
  bladder (sphincter) NEC — *see* Fistula, vesico-
    N32.2
    into seminal vesicle N32.2
  bone — *see also* Disorder, bone, specified type NEC
    with osteomyelitis, chronic — *see* Osteomyelitis,
      chronic, with draining sinus
  brain G93.89
    arteriovenous (acquired) — *see also* Fistula, arteri-
      ovenous, brain I67.1
    congenital Q28.2
  branchial (cleft) Q18.0
  branchiogenous Q18.0
  breast N61.0
    puerperal, postpartum or gestational, due to mastitis
      (purulent) — *see* Mastitis, obstetric, purulent
  bronchial J86.0
  bronchocutaneous, bronchomediastinal, bronchopleu-
    ral, bronchopleuromediastinal (infective) J86.0
    tuberculous NEC A15.5
  bronchoesophageal J86.0
    congenital Q39.2
      with atresia of esophagus Q39.1
  bronchovisceral J86.0
  buccal cavity (infective) K12.2
  cecosigmoidal K63.2
  cecum K63.2
  cerebrospinal (fluid) G96.08
  cervical, lateral Q18.1
  cervicoaural Q18.1
  cervicosigmoidal N82.4
  cervicovesical N82.1
  cervix N82.8
  chest (wall) J86.0
  cholecystenteric — *see* Fistula, gallbladder
  cholecystocolic — *see* Fistula, gallbladder
  cholecystocolonic — *see* Fistula, gallbladder
  cholecystoduodenal — *see* Fistula, gallbladder
  cholecystogastric — *see* Fistula, gallbladder
  cholecystointestinal — *see* Fistula, gallbladder
  choledochoduodenal — *see* Fistula, bile duct
  cholocolic K82.3
  coccyx — *see* Sinus, pilonidal
  colon K63.2
  colostomy K94.09
  colovesical N32.1
  common duct — *see* Fistula, bile duct
  congenital, site not listed — *see* Anomaly, by site
  coronary, arteriovenous I25.41
    congenital Q24.5
  costal region J86.0
  cul-de-sac, Douglas' N82.8
  cystic duct — *see also* Fistula, gallbladder
    congenital Q44.5
  dental K04.6
  diaphragm J86.0
  duodenum K31.6
  ear (external) (canal) — *see* Disorder, ear, external,
    specified type NEC
  enterocolic K63.2
  enterocutaneous K63.2
  enterouterine N82.4

Fistula — continued

enterouterine — continued
   congenital Q51.7
enterovaginal N82.4
   congenital Q52.2
   large intestine N82.3
   small intestine N82.2
enterovesical N32.1
epididymis N50.89
   tuberculous A18.15
esophagobronchial J86.0
   congenital Q39.2
     with atresia of esophagus Q39.1
esophagocutaneous K22.89
esophagopleural-cutaneous J86.0
esophagotracheal J86.0
   congenital Q39.2
     with atresia of esophagus Q39.1
esophagus K22.89
   congenital Q39.2
     with atresia of esophagus Q39.1
ethmoid — see Sinusitis, ethmoidal
eyeball (cornea) (sclera) — see Disorder, globe, hypotony
eyelid H01.8
fallopian tube, external N82.5
fecal K63.2
   congenital Q43.6
from periapical abscess K04.6
frontal sinus — see Sinusitis, frontal
gallbladder K82.3
   with calculus, cholelithiasis, stones — see Calculus, gallbladder
gastric K31.6
gastrocolic K31.6
   congenital Q40.2
   tuberculous A18.32
gastroenterocolic K31.6
gastroesophageal K31.6
gastrojejunal K31.6
gastrojejunocolic K31.6
genital tract (female) N82.9
   specified NEC N82.8
   to intestine NEC N82.4
   to skin N82.5
hepatic artery-portal vein, congenital Q26.6
hepatopleural J86.0
hepatopulmonary J86.0
ileorectal or ileosigmoidal K63.2
ileovaginal N82.2
ileovesical N32.1
ileum K63.2
in ano K60.3
   tuberculous A18.32
inner ear (labyrinth) — see subcategory H83.1 ☑
intestine NEC K63.2
intestinocolonic (abdominal) K63.2
intestinoureteral N28.89
intestinouterine N82.4
intestinovaginal N82.4
   large intestine N82.3
   small intestine N82.2
intestinovesical N32.1
ischiorectal (fossa) K61.39
jejunum K63.2
joint M25.10
   ankle M25.17- ☑
   elbow M25.12- ☑
   foot joint M25.17- ☑
   hand joint M25.14- ☑
   hip M25.15- ☑
   knee M25.16- ☑
   shoulder M25.11- ☑
   specified joint NEC M25.18
   tuberculous — see Tuberculosis, joint
   vertebrae M25.18
   wrist M25.13- ☑
kidney N28.89
labium (majus) (minus) N82.8
labyrinth — see subcategory H83.1 ☑
lacrimal (gland) (sac) H04.61- ☑
lacrimonasal duct — see Fistula, lacrimal
laryngotracheal, congenital Q34.8
larynx J38.7
lip K13.0
   congenital Q38.0
lumbar, tuberculous A18.01
lung J86.0

Fistula — continued

lymphatic I89.8
mammary (gland) N61.0
mastoid (process) (region) — see Mastoiditis, chronic
maxillary J32.0
medial, face and neck Q18.8
mediastinal J86.0
mediastinobronchial J86.0
mediastinocutaneous J86.0
middle ear — see subcategory H74.8 ☑
mouth K12.2
nasal J34.89
   sinus — see Sinusitis
nasopharynx J39.2
nipple N64.0
nose J34.89
oral (cutaneous) K12.2
   maxillary J32.0
   nasal (with cleft palate) — see Cleft, palate
orbit, orbital — see Disorder, orbit, specified type NEC
oroantral J32.0
oviduct, external N82.5
palate (hard) M27.8
pancreatic K86.89
pancreaticoduodenal K86.89
parotid (gland) K11.4
   region K12.2
penis N48.89
perianal K60.3
pericardium (pleura) (sac) — see Pericarditis
pericecal K63.2
perineorectal K60.4
perineosigmoidal K63.2
perineum, perineal (with urethral involvement) NEC N36.0
   tuberculous A18.13
   ureter N28.89
perirectal K60.4
   tuberculous A18.32
peritoneum K65.9
pharyngoesophageal J39.2
pharynx J39.2
   branchial cleft (congenital) Q18.0
pilonidal (infected) (rectum) — see Sinus, pilonidal
pleura, pleural, pleurocutaneous, pleuroperitoneal J86.0
   tuberculous NEC A15.6
pleuropericardial I31.8
portal vein-hepatic artery, congenital Q26.6
postauricular H70.81- ☑
postoperative, persistent T81.83 ☑
   specified site — see Fistula, by site
preauricular (congenital) Q18.1
prostate N42.89
pulmonary J86.0
   arteriovenous I28.0
     congenital Q25.72
   tuberculous — see Tuberculosis, pulmonary
pulmonoperitoneal J86.0
rectolabial N82.4
rectosigmoid (intercommunicating) K63.2
rectoureteral N28.89
rectourethral N36.0
   congenital Q64.73
rectouterine N82.4
   congenital Q51.7
rectovaginal N82.3
   congenital Q52.2
   tuberculous A18.18
rectovesical N32.1
   congenital Q64.79
rectovesicovaginal N82.3
rectovulval N82.4
   congenital Q52.79
rectum (to skin) K60.4
   congenital Q43.6
     with absence, atresia and stenosis Q42.0
   tuberculous A18.32
renal N28.89
retroauricular — see Fistula, postauricular
salivary duct or gland (any) K11.4
   congenital Q38.4
scrotum (urinary) N50.89
   tuberculous A18.15
semicircular canals — see subcategory H83.1 ☑
sigmoid K63.2
   to bladder N32.1
sinus — see Sinusitis

Fistula — continued

skin L98.8
   to genital tract (female) N82.5
splenocolic D73.89
stercoral K63.3
stomach K31.6
sublingual gland K11.4
submandibular gland K11.4
submaxillary (gland) K11.4
   region K12.2
thoracic J86.0
   duct I89.8
thoracoabdominal J86.0
thoracogastric J86.0
thoracointestinal J86.0
thorax J86.0
thyroglossal duct Q89.2
thyroid E07.89
trachea, congenital (external) (internal) Q32.1
tracheoesophageal J86.0
   congenital Q39.2
     with atresia of esophagus Q39.1
   following tracheostomy J95.04
traumatic arteriovenous — see Injury, blood vessel, by site
tuberculous — code by site under Tuberculosis
typhoid A01.09
umbilicourinary Q64.8
urachus, congenital Q64.4
ureter (persistent) N28.89
ureteroabdominal N28.89
ureterorectal N28.89
ureterosigmoido-abdominal N28.89
ureterovaginal N82.1
ureterovesical N32.2
urethra N36.0
   congenital Q64.79
   tuberculous A18.13
urethroperineal N36.0
urethroperineovesical N32.2
urethrorectal N36.0
   congenital Q64.73
urethroscrotal N50.89
urethrovaginal N82.1
urethrovesical N32.2
urinary (tract) (persistent) (recurrent) N36.0
uteroabdominal N82.5
   congenital Q51.7
uteroenteric, uterointestinal N82.4
   congenital Q51.7
uterorectal N82.4
   congenital Q51.7
uteroureteric N82.1
uterourethral Q51.7
uterovaginal N82.8
uterovesical N82.1
   congenital Q51.7
uterus N82.8
vagina (postpartal) (wall) N82.8
vaginocutaneous (postpartal) N82.5
vaginointestinal NEC N82.4
   large intestine N82.3
   small intestine N82.2
vaginoperineal N82.5
vasocutaneous, congenital Q55.7
vesical NEC N32.2
vesicoabdominal N32.2
vesicocervicovaginal N82.1
vesicocolic N32.1
vesicocutaneous N32.2
vesicoenteric N32.1
vesicointestinal N32.1
vesicometrorectal N82.4
vesicoperineal N32.2
vesicorectal N32.1
   congenital Q64.79
vesicosigmoidal N32.1
vesicosigmoidovaginal N82.3
vesicoureteral N32.2
vesicoureterovaginal N82.1
vesicourethral N32.2
vesicourethrorectal N32.1
vesicouterine N82.1
   congenital Q51.7
vesicovaginal N82.0
vulvorectal N82.4
   congenital Q52.79

Fit R56.9
   epileptic — see Epilepsy

☑ Additional Character Required — Refer to the Tabular List for Character Selection

Fit — *continued*
  fainting R55
  hysterical F44.5
  newborn P90
Fitting (and adjustment) (of)
  artificial
    arm — *see* Admission, adjustment, artificial, arm
    breast Z44.3 ☑
    eye Z44.2 ☑
    leg — *see* Admission, adjustment, artificial, leg
  automatic implantable cardiac defibrillator (with synchronous cardiac pacemaker) Z45.02
  brain neuropacemaker Z46.2
    implanted Z45.42
  cardiac defibrillator — *see* Fitting (and adjustment) (of), automatic implantable cardiac defibrillator
  catheter, non-vascular Z46.82
  colostomy belt Z46.89
  contact lenses Z46.0
  CRT-D (resynchronization therapy defibrillator) Z45.02
  CRT-P (cardiac resynchronization therapy pacemaker) Z45.018
    pulse generator Z45.010
  cystostomy device Z46.6
  defibrillator, cardiac — *see* Fitting (and adjustment) (of), automatic implantable cardiac defibrillator
  dentures Z46.3
  device NOS Z46.9
    abdominal Z46.89
    gastrointestinal NEC Z46.59
    implanted NEC Z45.89
    nervous system Z46.2
      implanted — *see* Admission, adjustment, device, implanted, nervous system
    orthodontic Z46.4
    orthoptic Z46.0
    orthotic Z46.89
    prosthetic (external) Z44.9
      breast Z44.3 ☑
      dental Z46.3
      eye Z44.2 ☑
      specified NEC Z44.8
    specified NEC Z46.89
    substitution
      auditory Z46.2
        implanted — *see* Admission, adjustment, device, implanted, hearing device
      nervous system Z46.2
        implanted — *see* Admission, adjustment, device, implanted, nervous system
      visual Z46.2
        implanted Z45.31
    urinary Z46.6
  gastric lap band Z46.51
  gastrointestinal appliance NEC Z46.59
  glasses (reading) Z46.0
  hearing aid Z46.1
  ileostomy device Z46.89
  insulin pump Z46.81
  intestinal appliance NEC Z46.89
  myringotomy device (stent) (tube) Z45.82
  neuropacemaker Z46.2
    implanted Z45.42
  non-vascular catheter Z46.82
  orthodontic device Z46.4
  orthopedic device (brace) (cast) (corset) (shoes) Z46.89
  pacemaker (cardiac) (cardiac resynchronization therapy (CRT-P)) Z45.018
    nervous system (brain) (peripheral nerve) (spinal cord) Z46.2
      implanted Z45.42
    pulse generator Z45.010
  portacath (port-a-cath) Z45.2
  prosthesis (external) Z44.9
    arm — *see* Admission, adjustment, artificial, arm
    breast Z44.3 ☑
    dental Z46.3
    eye Z44.2 ☑
    leg — *see* Admission, adjustment, artificial, leg
    specified NEC Z44.8
  spectacles Z46.0
  wheelchair Z46.89
Fitzhugh-Curtis syndrome
  due to
    Chlamydia trachomatis A74.81
    Neisseria gonorrhorea (gonococcal peritonitis) A54.85

Fitz's syndrome (acute hemorrhagic pancreatitis) — *see also* Pancreatitis, acute K85.80
Fixation
  joint — *see* Ankylosis
  larynx J38.7
  stapes — *see* Ankylosis, ear ossicles
    deafness — *see* Deafness, conductive
  uterus (acquired) — *see* Malposition, uterus
  vocal cord J38.3
Flabby ridge K06.8
Flaccid — *see also* condition
  palate, congenital Q38.5
Flail
  chest S22.5 ☑
    associated with chest compression and cardiopulmonary resuscitation M96.A4
    newborn (birth injury) P13.8
  joint (paralytic) M25.20
    ankle M25.27- ☑
    elbow M25.22- ☑
    foot joint M25.27- ☑
    hand joint M25.24- ☑
    hip M25.25- ☑
    knee M25.26- ☑
    shoulder M25.21- ☑
    specified joint NEC M25.28
    wrist M25.23- ☑
Flajani's disease — *see* Hyperthyroidism, with, goiter (diffuse)
Flap, liver K71.3
Flashbacks (residual to hallucinogen use) F16.283
Flat
  chamber (eye) — *see* Disorder, globe, hypotony, flat anterior chamber
  chest, congenital Q67.8
  foot (acquired) (fixed type) (painful) (postural) — *see also* Deformity, limb, flat foot
    congenital (rigid) (spastic) (everted) Q66.5- ☑
    rachitic sequelae (late effect) E64.3
  organ or site, congenital NEC — *see* Anomaly, by site
  pelvis M95.5
    with disproportion (fetopelvic) O33.0
      causing obstructed labor O65.0
    congenital Q74.2
Flatau-Schilder disease G37.0
Flatback syndrome M40.30
  lumbar region M40.36
  lumbosacral region M40.37
  thoracolumbar region M40.35
Flattening
  head, femur M89.8X5
  hip — *see* Coxa, plana
  lip (congenital) Q18.8
  nose (congenital) Q67.4
    acquired M95.0
Flatulence R14.3
  psychogenic F45.8
Flatus R14.3
  vaginalis N89.8
Flax-dresser's disease J66.1
Flea bite — *see* Injury, bite, by site, superficial, insect
Flecks, glaucomatous (subcapsular) — *see* Cataract, complicated
Fleischer (-Kayser) **ring** (cornea) H18.04- ☑
Fleshy mole O02.0
Flexibilitas cerea — *see* Catalepsy
Flexion
  amputation stump (surgical) T87.89
  cervix — *see* Malposition, uterus
  contracture, joint — *see* Contraction, joint
  deformity, joint — *see also* Deformity, limb, flexion M21.20
    hip, congenital Q65.89
  uterus — *see also* Malposition, uterus
    lateral — *see* Lateroversion, uterus
Flexner-Boyd dysentery A03.2
Flexner's dysentery A03.1
Flexure — *see* Flexion
Flint murmur (aortic insufficiency) I35.1
Floater, vitreous — *see* Opacity, vitreous
Floating
  cartilage (joint) — *see also* Loose, body, joint
    knee — *see* Derangement, knee, loose body
  gallbladder, congenital Q44.1
  kidney N28.89
    congenital Q63.8
  spleen D73.89

Flooding N92.0
Floor — *see* condition
Floppy
  baby syndrome (nonspecific) P94.2
  iris syndrome (intraoperative) (IFIS) H21.81
  nonrheumatic mitral valve syndrome I34.1
Flu — *see also* Influenza
  avian — *see also* Influenza, due to, identified novel influenza A virus J09.X2
  bird — *see also* Influenza, due to, identified novel influenza A virus J09.X2
  intestinal NEC A08.4
  swine (viruses that normally cause infections in pigs) — *see also* Influenza, due to, identified novel influenza A virus J09.X2
Fluctuating blood pressure I99.8
Fluid
  abdomen R18.8
  chest J94.8
  heart — *see* Failure, heart, congestive
  joint — *see* Effusion, joint
  loss (acute) E86.9
  lung — *see* Edema, lung
  overload E87.70
    specified NEC E87.79
  peritoneal cavity R18.8
  pleural cavity J94.8
  retention R60.9
Flukes NEC — *see also* Infestation, fluke
  blood NEC — *see* Schistosomiasis
  liver B66.3
Fluor (vaginalis) N89.8
  trichomonal or due to Trichomonas (vaginalis) A59.00
Fluorosis
  dental K00.3
  skeletal M85.10
    ankle M85.17- ☑
    foot M85.17- ☑
    forearm M85.13- ☑
    hand M85.14- ☑
    lower leg M85.16- ☑
    multiple site M85.19
    neck M85.18
    rib M85.18
    shoulder M85.11- ☑
    skull M85.18
    specified site NEC M85.18
    thigh M85.15- ☑
    toe M85.17- ☑
    upper arm M85.12- ☑
    vertebra M85.18
Flush syndrome E34.0
Flushing R23.2
  menopausal N95.1
Flutter
  atrial or auricular I48.92
    atypical I48.4
      type I I48.3
      type II I48.4
    typical I48.3
  heart I49.8
    atrial or auricular I48.92
      atypical I48.4
        type I I48.3
        type II I48.4
      typical I48.3
    ventricular I49.02
  ventricular I49.02
FNHTR (febrile nonhemolytic transfusion reaction) R50.84
Fochier's abscess — *code by* site under Abscess
Focus, Assmann's — *see* Tuberculosis, pulmonary
Fogo selvagem L10.3
Foix-Alajouanine syndrome G95.19
Fold, folds (anomalous) — *see* Anomaly, by site
  Descemet's membrane — *see* Change, corneal membrane, Descemet's, fold
  epicanthic Q10.3
  heart Q24.8
Folie à deux F24
Follicle
  cervix (nabothian) (ruptured) N88.8
  graafian, ruptured, with hemorrhage N83.0- ☑
  nabothian N88.8
Follicular — *see* condition
Folliculitis (superficial) L73.9
  abscedens et suffodiens L66.3
  cyst N83.0- ☑

Folliculitis — *continued*
  decalvans L66.2
  deep — *see* Furuncle, by site
  gonococcal (acute) (chronic) A54.01
  keloid, keloidalis L73.0
  pustular L01.02
  ulerythematosa reticulata L66.4
Folliculome lipidique
  specified site — *see* Neoplasm, benign, by site
  unspecified site
    female D27.9
    male D29.20
Følling's disease E70.0
Follow-up — *see* Examination, follow-up
Fong's syndrome (hereditary osteo-onychodysplasia) Q87.2
Food
  allergy L27.2
  asphyxia (from aspiration or inhalation) — *see* Foreign body, by site
  choked on — *see* Foreign body, by site
  deprivation T73.0
    specified kind of food NEC E63.8
  insecurity Z59.41
  intoxication — *see* Poisoning, food
  lack of T73.0
  poisoning — *see* Poisoning, food
  rejection NEC — *see* Disorder, eating
  strangulation or suffocation — *see* Foreign body, by site
  toxemia — *see* Poisoning, food
Foot — *see* condition
Foramen ovale (nonclosure) (patent) (persistent) Q21.12
Forbes' glycogen storage disease E74.03
Fordyce-Fox disease L75.2
Fordyce's disease (mouth) Q38.6
Forearm — *see* condition
Foreclosure on loan Z59.89
Foreign body
  with
    laceration — *see* Laceration, by site, with foreign body
    puncture wound — *see* Puncture, by site, with foreign body
  accidentally left following a procedure T81.509 ☑
    aspiration T81.506 ☑
      resulting in
        adhesions T81.516 ☑
        obstruction T81.526 ☑
        perforation T81.536 ☑
        specified complication NEC T81.596 ☑
    cardiac catheterization T81.505 ☑
      resulting in
        acute reaction T81.60 ☑
          aseptic peritonitis T81.61 ☑
          specified NEC T81.69 ☑
        adhesions T81.515 ☑
        obstruction T81.525 ☑
        perforation T81.535 ☑
        specified complication NEC T81.595 ☑
    causing
      acute reaction T81.60 ☑
        aseptic peritonitis T81.61 ☑
        specified complication NEC T81.69 ☑
      adhesions T81.519 ☑
      aseptic peritonitis T81.61 ☑
      obstruction T81.529 ☑
      perforation T81.539 ☑
      specified complication NEC T81.599 ☑
    endoscopy T81.504 ☑
      resulting in
        adhesions T81.514 ☑
        obstruction T81.524 ☑
        perforation T81.534 ☑
        specified complication NEC T81.594 ☑
    immunization T81.503 ☑
      resulting in
        adhesions T81.513 ☑
        obstruction T81.523 ☑
        perforation T81.533 ☑
        specified complication NEC T81.593 ☑
    infusion T81.501 ☑
      resulting in
        adhesions T81.511 ☑
        obstruction T81.521 ☑
        perforation T81.531 ☑

Foreign body — *continued*
  accidentally left following a procedure — *continued*
    infusion — *continued*
      resulting in — *continued*
        specified complication NEC T81.591 ☑
    injection T81.503 ☑
      resulting in
        adhesions T81.513 ☑
        obstruction T81.523 ☑
        perforation T81.533 ☑
        specified complication NEC T81.593 ☑
    kidney dialysis T81.502 ☑
      resulting in
        adhesions T81.512 ☑
        obstruction T81.522 ☑
        perforation T81.532 ☑
        specified complication NEC T81.592 ☑
    packing removal T81.507 ☑
      resulting in
        acute reaction T81.60 ☑
          aseptic peritonitis T81.61 ☑
          specified NEC T81.69 ☑
        adhesions T81.517 ☑
        obstruction T81.527 ☑
        perforation T81.537 ☑
        specified complication NEC T81.597 ☑
    puncture T81.506 ☑
      resulting in
        adhesions T81.516 ☑
        obstruction T81.526 ☑
        perforation T81.536 ☑
        specified complication NEC T81.596 ☑
    specified procedure NEC T81.508 ☑
      resulting in
        acute reaction T81.60 ☑
          aseptic peritonitis T81.61 ☑
          specified NEC T81.69 ☑
        adhesions T81.518 ☑
        obstruction T81.528 ☑
        perforation T81.538 ☑
        specified complication NEC T81.598 ☑
    surgical operation T81.500 ☑
      resulting in
        acute reaction T81.60 ☑
          aseptic peritonitis T81.61 ☑
          specified NEC T81.69 ☑
        adhesions T81.510 ☑
        obstruction T81.520 ☑
        perforation T81.530 ☑
        specified complication NEC T81.590 ☑
    transfusion T81.501 ☑
      resulting in
        adhesions T81.511 ☑
        obstruction T81.521 ☑
        perforation T81.531 ☑
        specified complication NEC T81.591 ☑
  alimentary tract T18.9 ☑
    anus T18.5 ☑
    colon T18.4 ☑
    esophagus — *see* Foreign body, esophagus
    mouth T18.0 ☑
    multiple sites T18.8 ☑
    rectosigmoid (junction) T18.5 ☑
    rectum T18.5 ☑
    small intestine T18.3 ☑
    specified site NEC T18.8 ☑
    stomach T18.2 ☑
  anterior chamber (eye) S05.5-
  auditory canal — *see* Foreign body, entering through orifice, ear
  bronchus T17.508 ☑
    causing
      asphyxiation T17.500 ☑
        food (bone) (seed) T17.520 ☑
        gastric contents (vomitus) T17.510 ☑
        specified type NEC T17.590 ☑
      injury NEC T17.508 ☑
        food (bone) (seed) T17.528 ☑
        gastric contents (vomitus) T17.518 ☑
        specified type NEC T17.598 ☑
  canthus — *see* Foreign body, conjunctival sac
  ciliary body (eye) S05.5- ☑
  conjunctival sac T15.1- ☑
  cornea T15.0- ☑
  entering through orifice
    accessory sinus T17.0 ☑

Foreign body — *continued*
  entering through orifice — *continued*
    alimentary canal T18.9 ☑
      multiple parts T18.8 ☑
      specified part NEC T18.8 ☑
    alveolar process T18.0 ☑
    antrum (Highmore's) T17.0 ☑
    anus T18.5 ☑
    appendix T18.4 ☑
    auditory canal — *see* Foreign body, entering through orifice, ear
    auricle — *see* Foreign body, entering through orifice, ear
    bladder T19.1 ☑
    bronchioles — *see* Foreign body, respiratory tract, specified site NEC
    bronchus (main) — *see* Foreign body, bronchus
    buccal cavity T18.0 ☑
    canthus (inner) — *see* Foreign body, conjunctival sac
    cecum T18.4 ☑
    cervix (canal) (uteri) T19.3 ☑
    colon T18.4 ☑
    conjunctival sac — *see* Foreign body, conjunctival sac
    cornea — *see* Foreign body, cornea
    digestive organ or tract NOS T18.9 ☑
      multiple parts T18.8 ☑
      specified part NEC T18.8 ☑
    duodenum T18.3 ☑
    ear (external) T16.-
    esophagus — *see* Foreign body, esophagus
    eye (external) NOS T15.9-
      conjunctival sac — *see* Foreign body, conjunctival sac
      cornea — *see* Foreign body, cornea
      specified part NEC T15.8-
    eyeball — *see also* Foreign body, entering through orifice, eye, specified part NEC
      with penetrating wound — *see* Puncture, eyeball
    eyelid — *see also* Foreign body, conjunctival sac
      with
        laceration — *see* Laceration, eyelid, with foreign body
        puncture — *see* Puncture, eyelid, with foreign body
        superficial injury — *see* Foreign body, superficial, eyelid
    gastrointestinal tract T18.9 ☑
      multiple parts T18.8 ☑
      specified part NEC T18.8 ☑
    genitourinary tract T19.9 ☑
      multiple parts T19.8 ☑
      specified part NEC T19.8 ☑
    globe — *see* Foreign body, entering through orifice, eyeball
    gum T18.0 ☑
    Highmore's antrum T17.0 ☑
    hypopharynx — *see* Foreign body, pharynx
    ileum T18.3 ☑
    intestine (small) T18.3 ☑
      large T18.4 ☑
    lacrimal apparatus (punctum) — *see* Foreign body, entering through orifice, eye, specified part NEC
    large intestine T18.4 ☑
    larynx — *see* Foreign body, larynx
    lung — *see* Foreign body, respiratory tract, specified site NEC
    maxillary sinus T17.0 ☑
    mouth T18.0 ☑
    nasal sinus T17.0 ☑
    nasopharynx — *see* Foreign body, pharynx
    nose (passage) T17.1 ☑
    nostril T17.1 ☑
    oral cavity T18.0 ☑
    palate T18.0 ☑
    penis T19.4 ☑
    pharynx — *see* Foreign body, pharynx
    piriform sinus — *see* Foreign body, pharynx
    rectosigmoid (junction) T18.5 ☑
    rectum T18.5 ☑
    respiratory tract — *see* Foreign body, respiratory tract
    sinus (accessory) (frontal) (maxillary) (nasal) T17.0 ☑
      piriform — *see* Foreign body, pharynx

Foreign body — *continued*

  entering through orifice — *continued*

    small intestine T18.3 ☑

    stomach T18.2 ☑

    suffocation by — *see* Foreign body, by site

    tear ducts or glands — *see* Foreign body, entering through orifice, eye, specified part NEC

    throat — *see* Foreign body, pharynx

    tongue T18.0 ☑

    tonsil, tonsillar (fossa) — *see* Foreign body, pharynx

    trachea — *see* Foreign body, trachea

    ureter T19.8 ☑

    urethra T19.0 ☑

    uterus (any part) T19.3 ☑

    vagina T19.2 ☑

    vulva T19.2 ☑

  esophagus T18.108 ☑

    causing

      injury NEC T18.108 ☑

        food (bone) (seed) T18.128 ☑

        gastric contents (vomitus) T18.118 ☑

        specified type NEC T18.198 ☑

      tracheal compression T18.100 ☑

        food (bone) (seed) T18.120 ☑

        gastric contents (vomitus) T18.110 ☑

        specified type NEC T18.190 ☑

  feeling of, in throat R09.89

  fragment — *see* Retained, foreign body fragments (type of)

  genitourinary tract T19.9 ☑

    bladder T19.1 ☑

    multiple parts T19.8 ☑

    penis T19.4 ☑

    specified site NEC T19.8 ☑

    urethra T19.0 ☑

    uterus T19.3 ☑

      IUD Z97.5

    vagina T19.2 ☑

      contraceptive device Z97.5

    vulva T19.2 ☑

  granuloma (old) (soft tissue) — *see also* Granuloma, foreign body

    skin L92.3

  in

    laceration — *see* Laceration, by site, with foreign body

    puncture wound — *see* Puncture, by site, with foreign body

    soft tissue (residual) M79.5

  inadvertently left in operation wound — *see* Foreign body, accidentally left during a procedure

  ingestion, ingested NOS T18.9 ☑

  inhalation or inspiration — *see* Foreign body, by site

  internal organ, not entering through a natural orifice — code as specific injury with foreign body

  intraocular S05.5- ☑

    old, retained (nonmagnetic) H44.70- ☑

      anterior chamber H44.71- ☑

      ciliary body H44.72- ☑

      iris H44.72- ☑

      lens H44.73- ☑

      magnetic H44.60- ☑

        anterior chamber H44.61- ☑

        ciliary body H44.62- ☑

        iris H44.62- ☑

        lens H44.63- ☑

        posterior wall H44.64- ☑

        specified site NEC H44.69- ☑

        vitreous body H44.65- ☑

      posterior wall H44.74- ☑

      specified site NEC H44.79- ☑

      vitreous body H44.75- ☑

  iris — *see* Foreign body, intraocular

  lacrimal punctum — *see* Foreign body, entering through orifice, eye, specified part NEC

  larynx T17.308 ☑

    causing

      asphyxiation T17.300 ☑

        food (bone) (seed) T17.320 ☑

        gastric contents (vomitus) T17.310 ☑

        specified type NEC T17.390 ☑

      injury NEC T17.308 ☑

        food (bone) (seed) T17.328 ☑

        gastric contents (vomitus) T17.318 ☑

        specified type NEC T17.398 ☑

  lens — *see* Foreign body, intraocular

Foreign body — *continued*

  ocular muscle S05.4- ☑

    old, retained — *see* Foreign body, orbit, old

  old or residual

    soft tissue (residual) M79.5

  operation wound, left accidentally — *see* Foreign body, accidentally left during a procedure

  orbit S05.4- ☑

    old, retained H05.5- ☑

  pharynx T17.208 ☑

    causing

      asphyxiation T17.200 ☑

        food (bone) (seed) T17.220 ☑

        gastric contents (vomitus) T17.210 ☑

        specified type NEC T17.290 ☑

      injury NEC T17.208 ☑

        food (bone) (seed) T17.228 ☑

        gastric contents (vomitus) T17.218 ☑

        specified type NEC T17.298 ☑

  respiratory tract T17.908 ☑

    bronchioles — *see* Foreign body, respiratory tract, specified site NEC

    bronchus — *see* Foreign body, bronchus

    causing

      asphyxiation T17.900 ☑

        food (bone) (seed) T17.920 ☑

        gastric contents (vomitus) T17.910 ☑

        specified type NEC T17.990 ☑

      injury NEC T17.908 ☑

        food (bone) (seed) T17.928 ☑

        gastric contents (vomitus) T17.918 ☑

        specified type NEC T17.998 ☑

    larynx — *see* Foreign body, larynx

    lung — *see* Foreign body, respiratory tract, specified site NEC

    multiple parts — *see* Foreign body, respiratory tract, specified site NEC

    nasal sinus T17.0 ☑

    nasopharynx — *see* Foreign body, pharynx

    nose T17.1 ☑

    nostril T17.1 ☑

    pharynx — *see* Foreign body, pharynx

    specified site NEC T17.808 ☑

      causing

        asphyxiation T17.800 ☑

          food (bone) (seed) T17.820 ☑

          gastric contents (vomitus) T17.810 ☑

          specified type NEC T17.890 ☑

        injury NEC T17.808 ☑

          food (bone) (seed) T17.828 ☑

          gastric contents (vomitus) T17.818 ☑

          specified type NEC T17.898 ☑

    throat — *see* Foreign body, pharynx

    trachea — *see* Foreign body, trachea

  retained (old) (nonmagnetic) (in)

    anterior chamber (eye) — *see* Foreign body, intraocular, old, retained, anterior chamber

      magnetic — *see* Foreign body, intraocular, old, retained, magnetic, anterior chamber

    ciliary body — *see* Foreign body, intraocular, old, retained, ciliary body

      magnetic — *see* Foreign body, intraocular, old, retained, magnetic, ciliary body

    eyelid H02.819

      left H02.816

        lower H02.815

        upper H02.814

      right H02.813

        lower H02.812

        upper H02.811

    fragments — *see* Retained, foreign body fragments (type of)

    globe — *see* Foreign body, intraocular, old, retained

      magnetic — *see* Foreign body, intraocular, old, retained, magnetic

    intraocular — *see* Foreign body, intraocular, old, retained

      magnetic — *see* Foreign body, intraocular, old, retained, magnetic

    iris — *see* Foreign body, intraocular, old, retained, iris

      magnetic — *see* Foreign body, intraocular, old, retained, magnetic, iris

    lens — *see* Foreign body, intraocular, old, retained, lens

      magnetic — *see* Foreign body, intraocular, old, retained, magnetic, lens

Foreign body — *continued*

  retained — *continued*

    muscle — *see* Foreign body, retained, soft tissue

    orbit — *see* Foreign body, orbit, old

    posterior wall of globe — *see* Foreign body, intraocular, old, retained, posterior wall

      magnetic — *see* Foreign body, intraocular, old, retained, magnetic, posterior wall

    retrobulbar — *see* Foreign body, orbit, old, retrobulbar

    soft tissue M79.5

    vitreous — *see* Foreign body, intraocular, old, retained, vitreous body

      magnetic — *see* Foreign body, intraocular, old, retained, magnetic, vitreous body

  retina S05.5- ☑

  superficial, without open wound

    abdomen, abdominal (wall) S30.851 ☑

    alveolar process S00.552 ☑

    ankle S90.55- ☑

    antecubital space — *see* Foreign body, superficial, forearm

    anus S30.857 ☑

    arm (upper) S40.85- ☑

    auditory canal — *see* Foreign body, superficial, ear

    auricle — *see* Foreign body, superficial, ear

    axilla — *see* Foreign body, superficial, arm

    back, lower S30.850 ☑

    breast S20.15- ☑

    brow S00.85 ☑

    buttock S30.850 ☑

    calf — *see* Foreign body, superficial, leg

    canthus — *see* Foreign body, superficial, eyelid

    cheek S00.85 ☑

      internal S00.552 ☑

    chest wall — *see* Foreign body, superficial, thorax

    chin S00.85 ☑

    clitoris S30.854 ☑

    costal region — *see* Foreign body, superficial, thorax

    digit(s)

      foot — *see* Foreign body, superficial, toe

      hand — *see* Foreign body, superficial, finger

    ear S00.45- ☑

    elbow S50.35- ☑

    epididymis S30.853 ☑

    epigastric region S30.851 ☑

    epiglottis S10.15 ☑

    esophagus, cervical S10.15 ☑

    eyebrow — *see* Foreign body, superficial, eyelid

    eyelid S00.25- ☑

    face S00.85 ☑

    finger(s) S60.459 ☑

      index S60.45- ☑

      little S60.45- ☑

      middle S60.45- ☑

      ring S60.45- ☑

    flank S30.851 ☑

    foot (except toe(s) alone) S90.85- ☑

      toe — *see* Foreign body, superficial, toe

    forearm S50.85- ☑

      elbow only — *see* Foreign body, superficial, elbow

    forehead S00.85 ☑

    genital organs, external

      female S30.856 ☑

      male S30.855 ☑

    groin S30.851 ☑

    gum S00.552 ☑

    hand S60.55- ☑

    head S00.95 ☑

      ear — *see* Foreign body, superficial, ear

      eyelid — *see* Foreign body, superficial, eyelid

      lip S00.551 ☑

      nose S00.35 ☑

      oral cavity S00.552 ☑

      scalp S00.05 ☑

      specified site NEC S00.85 ☑

    heel — *see* Foreign body, superficial, foot

    hip S70.25- ☑

    inguinal region S30.851 ☑

    interscapular region S20.459 ☑

    jaw S00.85 ☑

    knee S80.25- ☑

    labium (majus) (minus) S30.854 ☑

    larynx S10.15 ☑

    leg (lower) S80.85- ☑

Foreign body — *continued*
  superficial, without open wound — *continued*
    leg — *continued*
      knee — *see* Foreign body, superficial, knee
      upper — *see* Foreign body, superficial, thigh
    lip S00.551 ☑
    lower back S30.850 ☑
    lumbar region S30.850 ☑
    malar region S00.85 ☑
    mammary — *see* Foreign body, superficial, breast
    mastoid region S00.85 ☑
    mouth S00.552 ☑
    nail
      finger — *see* Foreign body, superficial, finger
      toe — *see* Foreign body, superficial, toe
    nape S10.85 ☑
    nasal S00.35 ☑
    neck S10.95 ☑
      specified site NEC S10.85 ☑
      throat S10.15 ☑
    nose S00.35 ☑
    occipital region S00.05 ☑
    oral cavity S00.552 ☑
    orbital region — *see* Foreign body, superficial, eyelid
    palate S00.552 ☑
    palm — *see* Foreign body, superficial, hand
    parietal region S00.05 ☑
    pelvis S30.850 ☑
    penis S30.852 ☑
    perineum
      female S30.854 ☑
      male S30.850 ☑
    periocular area — *see* Foreign body, superficial, eyelid
    phalanges
      finger — *see* Foreign body, superficial, finger
      toe — *see* Foreign body, superficial, toe
    pharynx S10.15 ☑
    pinna — *see* Foreign body, superficial, ear
    popliteal space — *see* Foreign body, superficial, knee
    prepuce S30.852 ☑
    pubic region S30.850 ☑
    pudendum
      female S30.856 ☑
      male S30.855 ☑
    sacral region S30.850 ☑
    scalp S00.05 ☑
    scapular region — *see* Foreign body, superficial, shoulder
    scrotum S30.853 ☑
    shin — *see* Foreign body, superficial, leg
    shoulder S40.25- ☑
    sternal region S20.359 ☑
    submaxillary region S00.85 ☑
    submental region S00.85 ☑
    subungual
      finger(s) — *see* Foreign body, superficial, finger
      toe(s) — *see* Foreign body, superficial, toe
    supraclavicular fossa S10.85 ☑
    supraorbital S00.85 ☑
    temple S00.85 ☑
    temporal region S00.85 ☑
    testis S30.853 ☑
    thigh S70.35- ☑
    thorax, thoracic (wall) S20.95 ☑
      back S20.45- ☑
      front S20.35- ☑
    throat S10.15 ☑
    thumb S60.35- ☑
    toe(s) (lesser) S90.456 ☑
      great S90.45- ☑
    tongue S00.552 ☑
    trachea S10.15 ☑
    tunica vaginalis S30.853 ☑
    tympanum, tympanic membrane — *see* Foreign body, superficial, ear
    uvula S00.552 ☑
    vagina S30.854 ☑
    vocal cords S10.15 ☑
    vulva S30.854 ☑
    wrist S60.85- ☑
  swallowed T18.9 ☑
  trachea T17.408 ☑
    causing
      asphyxiation T17.400 ☑

Foreign body — *continued*
  trachea — *continued*
    causing — *continued*
      asphyxiation — *continued*
        food (bone) (seed) T17.420 ☑
        gastric contents (vomitus) T17.410 ☑
        specified type NEC T17.490 ☑
      injury NEC T17.408 ☑
        food (bone) (seed) T17.428 ☑
        gastric contents (vomitus) T17.418 ☑
        specified type NEC T17.498 ☑
    type of fragment — *see* Retained, foreign body fragments (type of)
  vitreous (humor) S05.5- ☑
Forestier's disease (rhizomelic pseudopolyarthritis) M35.3
  meaning ankylosing hyperostosis — *see* Hyperostosis, ankylosing
Formation
  hyalin in cornea — *see* Degeneration, cornea
  sequestrum in bone (due to infection) — *see* Osteomyelitis, chronic
  valve
    colon, congenital Q43.8
    ureter (congenital) Q62.39
Formication R20.2
Fort Bragg fever A27.89
Fossa — *see also* condition
  pyriform — *see* condition
Foster-Kennedy syndrome H47.14- ☑
Fothergill's
  disease (trigeminal neuralgia) — *see also* Neuralgia, trigeminal
    scarlatina anginosa A38.9
Foul breath R19.6
Foundling Z76.1
Fournier disease or gangrene N49.3
  female N76.82
  vagina and vulva N76.82
Fourth
  cranial nerve — *see* condition
  molar K00.1
Foville's (peduncular) **disease or syndrome** G46.3
Fox (-Fordyce) disease (apocrine miliaria) L75.2
FPIES (food protein-induced enterocolitis syndrome) K52.21
Fracture, burst — *see* Fracture, traumatic, by site
Fracture, chronic — *see* Fracture, pathological, by site
Fracture, insufficiency — *see* Fracture, pathological, by site
Fracture, nontraumatic, NEC
  atypical
    femur M84.750- ☑
      complete
        oblique M84.759 ☑
          left side M84.758 ☑
          right side M84.757 ☑
        transverse M84.756 ☑
          left side M84.755 ☑
          right side M84.754 ☑
      incomplete M84.753 ☑
        left side M84.752 ☑
        right side M84.751 ☑
Fracture, pathological (pathologic) — *see also* Fracture, traumatic M84.40 ☑
  ankle M84.47- ☑
  carpus M84.44- ☑
  clavicle M84.41- ☑
  compression (not due to trauma) — *see also* Collapse, vertebra M48.50- ☑
  dental implant M27.63
  dental restorative material K08.539
    with loss of material K08.531
    without loss of material K08.530
  due to
    neoplastic disease NEC — *see also* Neoplasm M84.50 ☑
      ankle M84.57- ☑
      carpus M84.54- ☑
      clavicle M84.51- ☑
      femur M84.55- ☑
      fibula M84.56- ☑
      finger M84.54- ☑
      hip M84.559 ☑
      humerus M84.52- ☑
      ilium M84.550 ☑

Fracture, pathological — *continued*
  due to — *continued*
    neoplastic disease — *see also* Neoplasm — *continued*
      ischium M84.550 ☑
      metacarpus M84.54- ☑
      metatarsus M84.57- ☑
      neck M84.58 ☑
      pelvis M84.550 ☑
      radius M84.53- ☑
      rib M84.58 ☑
      scapula M84.51- ☑
      skull M84.58 ☑
      specified site NEC M84.58 ☑
      tarsus M84.57- ☑
      tibia M84.56- ☑
      toe M84.57- ☑
      ulna M84.53- ☑
      vertebra M84.58 ☑
    osteoporosis M80.00 ☑
      disuse — *see* Osteoporosis, specified type NEC, with pathological fracture
      drug-induced — *see* Osteoporosis, drug induced, with pathological fracture
      idiopathic — *see* Osteoporosis, specified type NEC, with pathological fracture
      postmenopausal — *see* Osteoporosis, postmenopausal, with pathological fracture
      postoophorectomy — *see* Osteoporosis, postoophorectomy, with pathological fracture
      postsurgical malabsorption — *see* Osteoporosis, specified type NEC, with pathological fracture
      specified cause NEC — *see* Osteoporosis, specified type NEC, with pathological fracture
    specified disease NEC M84.60 ☑
      ankle M84.67- ☑
      carpus M84.64- ☑
      clavicle M84.61- ☑
      femur M84.65- ☑
      fibula M84.66- ☑
      finger M84.64- ☑
      hip M84.65- ☑
      humerus M84.62- ☑
      ilium M84.650 ☑
      ischium M84.650 ☑
      metacarpus M84.64- ☑
      metatarsus M84.67- ☑
      neck M84.68 ☑
      radius M84.63- ☑
      rib M84.68 ☑
      scapula M84.61- ☑
      skull M84.68 ☑
      tarsus M84.67- ☑
      tibia M84.66- ☑
      toe M84.67- ☑
      ulna M84.63- ☑
      vertebra M84.68 ☑
  femur M84.45- ☑
  fibula M84.46- ☑
  finger M84.44- ☑
  hip M84.459 ☑
  humerus M84.42- ☑
  ilium M84.454 ☑
  ischium M84.454 ☑
  joint prosthesis — *see* Complications, joint prosthesis, mechanical, breakdown, by site
    periprosthetic — *see* Fracture, pathological, periprosthetic
  metacarpus M84.44- ☑
  metatarsus M84.47- ☑
  neck M84.48 ☑
  pelvis M84.454 ☑
  periprosthetic M97.9 ☑
    ankle M97.2- ☑
    elbow M97.4- ☑
    finger M97.8 ☑
    hip M97.0- ☑
    knee M97.1- ☑
    other specified joint M97.8 ☑
    shoulder M97.3- ☑
    spinal joint M97.8 ☑
    toe joint M97.8 ☑
    wrist joint M97.8 ☑
  radius M84.43- ☑
  restorative material (dental) K08.539

☑ **Additional Character Required** — **Refer to the Tabular List for Character Selection**

Fracture, pathological — *continued*
  restorative material — *continued*
    with loss of material K08.531
    without loss of material K08.530
  rib M84.48 ☑
  scapula M84.41- ☑
  skull M84.48 ☑
  tarsus M84.47- ☑
  tibia M84.46- ☑
  toe M84.47- ☑
  ulna M84.43- ☑
  vertebra M84.48 ☑
Fracture, traumatic (abduction) (adduction) (separation)
  — *see also* Fracture, pathological T14.8 ☑
  acetabulum S32.40- ☑
    column
      anterior (displaced) (iliopubic) S32.43- ☑
        nondisplaced S32.436
      posterior (displaced) (ilioischial) S32.443 ☑
        nondisplaced S32.44- ☑
    dome (displaced) S32.48- ☑
      nondisplaced S32.48 ☑
    specified NEC S32.49- ☑
    transverse (displaced) S32.45- ☑
      with associated posterior wall fracture (displaced)
        S32.46- ☑
        nondisplaced S32.46- ☑
      nondisplaced S32.45- ☑
    wall
      anterior (displaced) S32.41- ☑
        nondisplaced S32.41- ☑
      medial (displaced) S32.47- ☑
        nondisplaced S32.47- ☑
      posterior (displaced) S32.42- ☑
        with associated transverse fracture (displaced)
          S32.46- ☑
          nondisplaced S32.46- ☑
        nondisplaced S32.42- ☑
  acromion — *see* Fracture, scapula, acromial process
  ankle S82.899 ☑
    bimalleolar (displaced) S82.84- ☑
      nondisplaced S82.84- ☑
    lateral malleolus only (displaced) S82.6- ☑
      nondisplaced S82.6- ☑
    medial malleolus (displaced) S82.5- ☑
      associated with Maisonneuve's fracture — *see*
        Fracture, Maisonneuve's
      nondisplaced S82.5- ☑
    talus — *see* Fracture, tarsal, talus
    trimalleolar (displaced) S82.85- ☑
      nondisplaced S82.85- ☑
  arm (upper) — *see also* Fracture, humerus, shaft
    humerus — *see* Fracture, humerus
    radius — *see* Fracture, radius
    ulna — *see* Fracture, ulna
  associated with chest compression and cardiopul-
    monary resuscitation M96.A9
  astragalus — *see* Fracture, tarsal, talus
  atlas — *see* Fracture, neck, cervical vertebra, first
  axis — *see* Fracture, neck, cervical vertebra, second
  back — *see* Fracture, vertebra
  Barton's — *see* Barton's fracture
  base of skull — *see* Fracture, skull, base
  basicervical (basal) (femoral) S72.0 ☑
  Bennett's — *see* Bennett's fracture
  bimalleolar — *see* Fracture, ankle, bimalleolar
  blow-out S02.3- ☑
  bone NEC T14.8 ☑
    birth injury P13.9
    following insertion of orthopedic implant, joint
      prosthesis or bone plate — *see* Fracture, fol-
      lowing insertion of orthopedic implant, joint
      prosthesis or bone plate
    in (due to) neoplastic disease NEC — *see* Fracture,
      pathological, due to, neoplastic disease
    pathological (cause unknown) — *see* Fracture,
      pathological
  breast bone — *see* Fracture, sternum
  bucket handle (semilunar cartilage) — *see* Tear,
    meniscus
  buckle — *see* Fracture, by site, torus
  burst — *see* Fracture, traumatic, by site
  calcaneus — *see* Fracture, tarsal, calcaneus
  carpal bone(s) S62.10- ☑
    capitate (displaced) S62.13- ☑
      nondisplaced S62.13- ☑

Fracture, traumatic — *continued*
  carpal bone(s) — *continued*
    cuneiform — *see* Fracture, carpal bone, triquetrum
    hamate (body) (displaced) S62.143 ☑
      hook process (displaced) S62.15- ☑
        nondisplaced S62.15- ☑
      nondisplaced S62.14- ☑
    larger multangular — *see* Fracture, carpal bones,
      trapezium
    lunate (displaced) S62.12- ☑
      nondisplaced S62.12- ☑
    navicular S62.00- ☑
      distal pole (displaced) S62.01- ☑
        nondisplaced S62.01- ☑
      middle third (displaced) S62.02- ☑
        nondisplaced S62.02- ☑
      proximal third (displaced) S62.03- ☑
        nondisplaced S62.03- ☑
      volar tuberosity — *see* Fracture, carpal bones,
        navicular, distal pole
    os magnum — *see* Fracture, carpal bones, capitate
    pisiform (displaced) S62.16- ☑
      nondisplaced S62.16- ☑
    semilunar — *see* Fracture, carpal bones, lunate
    smaller multangular — *see* Fracture, carpal bones,
      trapezoid
    trapezium (displaced) S62.17- ☑
      nondisplaced S62.17- ☑
    trapezoid (displaced) S62.18- ☑
      nondisplaced S62.18- ☑
    triquetrum (displaced) S62.11- ☑
      nondisplaced S62.11- ☑
    unciform — *see* Fracture, carpal bones, hamate
  cervical — *see* Fracture, vertebra, cervical
  clavicle S42.00- ☑
    acromial end (displaced) S42.03- ☑
      nondisplaced S42.03- ☑
    birth injury P13.4
    lateral end — *see* Fracture, clavicle, acromial end
    shaft (displaced) S42.02- ☑
      nondisplaced S42.02- ☑
    sternal end (anterior) (displaced) S42.01- ☑
      nondisplaced S42.01- ☑
      posterior S42.01- ☑
  coccyx S32.2 ☑
  collapsed — *see* Collapse, vertebra
  collar bone — *see* Fracture, clavicle
  Colles' — *see* Colles' fracture
  coronoid process — *see* Fracture, ulna, upper end,
    coronoid process
  corpus cavernosum penis S39.840 ☑
  costochondral cartilage S23.41 ☑
  costochondral, costosternal junction — *see* Fracture,
    rib
  cranium — *see* Fracture, skull
  cricoid cartilage S12.8 ☑
  cuboid (ankle) — *see* Fracture, tarsal, cuboid
  cuneiform
    foot — *see* Fracture, tarsal, cuneiform
    wrist — *see* Fracture, carpal, triquetrum
  delayed union — *see* Delay, union, fracture
  dental restorative material K08.539
    with loss of material K08.531
    without loss of material K08.530
  due to
    birth injury — *see* Birth, injury, fracture
    osteoporosis — *see* Osteoporosis, with fracture
  Dupuytren's — *see* Fracture, ankle, lateral malleolus
  elbow S42.40- ☑
  ethmoid (bone) (sinus) — *see* Fracture, skull, base
  face bone S02.92 ☑
  fatigue — *see also* Fracture, stress
    vertebra M48.40 ☑
      cervical region M48.42 ☑
      cervicothoracic region M48.43 ☑
      lumbar region M48.46 ☑
      lumbosacral region M48.47 ☑
      occipito-atlanto-axial region M48.41 ☑
      sacrococcygeal region M48.48 ☑
      thoracic region M48.44 ☑
      thoracolumbar region M48.45 ☑
  femur, femoral S72.9- ☑
    basicervical (basal) S72.0 ☑
    birth injury P13.2
    capital epiphyseal S79.01- ☑

Fracture, traumatic — *continued*
  femur, femoral — *continued*
    condyles, epicondyles — *see* Fracture, femur, lower
      end
    distal end — *see* Fracture, femur, lower end
    epiphysis
      head — *see* Fracture, femur, upper end, epiphysis
      lower — *see* Fracture, femur, lower end, epiph-
        ysis
      upper — *see* Fracture, femur, upper end, epiph-
        ysis
    following insertion of implant, prosthesis or plate
      M96.66- ☑
    head — *see* Fracture, femur, upper end, head
    intertrochanteric — *see* Fracture, femur,
      trochanteric
    intratrochanteric — *see* Fracture, femur,
      trochanteric
    lower end S72.40- ☑
      condyle (displaced) S72.41- ☑
        lateral (displaced) S72.42- ☑
          nondisplaced S72.42- ☑
        medial (displaced) S72.43- ☑
          nondisplaced S72.43- ☑
        nondisplaced S72.41- ☑
      epiphysis (displaced) S72.44- ☑
        nondisplaced S72.44- ☑
      physeal S79.10- ☑
        Salter-Harris
          Type I S79.11- ☑
          Type II S79.12- ☑
          Type III S79.13- ☑
          Type IV S79.14- ☑
        specified NEC S79.19- ☑
      specified NEC S72.49- ☑
      supracondylar (displaced) S72.45- ☑
        with intracondylar extension (displaced)
          S72.46- ☑
          nondisplaced S72.46- ☑
        nondisplaced S72.45- ☑
      torus S72.47- ☑
    neck — *see* Fracture, femur, upper end, neck
    pertrochanteric — *see* Fracture, femur, trochanteric
    shaft (lower third) (middle third) (upper third)
      S72.30- ☑
      comminuted (displaced) S72.35- ☑
        nondisplaced S72.35- ☑
      oblique (displaced) S72.33- ☑
        nondisplaced S72.33- ☑
      segmental (displaced) S72.36- ☑
        nondisplaced S72.36- ☑
      specified NEC S72.39- ☑
      spiral (displaced) S72.34- ☑
        nondisplaced S72.34- ☑
      transverse (displaced) S72.32- ☑
        nondisplaced S72.32- ☑
    specified site NEC — *see* subcategory S72.8 ☑
    subcapital (displaced) S72.01- ☑
    subtrochanteric (region) (section) (displaced)
      S72.2- ☑
      nondisplaced S72.2- ☑
    transcervical — *see* Fracture, femur, midcervical
    transtrochanteric — *see* Fracture, femur,
      trochanteric
    trochanteric S72.10- ☑
      apophyseal (displaced) S72.13- ☑
        nondisplaced S72.13- ☑
      greater trochanter (displaced) S72.11- ☑
        nondisplaced S72.11- ☑
      intertrochanteric (displaced) S72.14- ☑
        nondisplaced S72.14- ☑
      lesser trochanter (displaced) S72.12- ☑
        nondisplaced S72.12- ☑
    upper end S72.00- ☑
      apophyseal (displaced) S72.13- ☑
        nondisplaced S72.13- ☑
      cervicotrochanteric — *see* Fracture, femur, upper
        end, neck, base
      epiphysis (displaced) S72.02- ☑
        nondisplaced S72.02- ☑
      head S72.05- ☑
        articular (displaced) S72.06- ☑
          nondisplaced S72.06- ☑
        specified NEC S72.09- ☑
      intertrochanteric (displaced) S72.14- ☑
        nondisplaced S72.14- ☑

Fracture, traumatic — *continued*
femur, femoral — *continued*
upper end — *continued*
intracapsular S72.01- ☑
midcervical (displaced) S72.03- ☑
nondisplaced S72.03- ☑
neck S72.00- ☑
base (displaced) S72.04- ☑
nondisplaced S72.04- ☑
specified NEC S72.09- ☑
pertrochanteric — *see* Fracture, femur, upper end, trochanteric
physeal S79.00- ☑
Salter-Harris type I S79.01- ☑
specified NEC S79.09- ☑
subcapital (displaced) S72.01- ☑
subtrochanteric (displaced) S72.2- ☑
nondisplaced S72.2- ☑
transcervical — *see* Fracture, femur, upper end, midcervical
trochanteric S72.10- ☑
greater (displaced) S72.11- ☑
nondisplaced S72.11- ☑
lesser (displaced) S72.12- ☑
nondisplaced S72.12- ☑
fibula (shaft) (styloid) S82.40- ☑
comminuted (displaced) S82.45- ☑
nondisplaced S82.45- ☑
following insertion of implant, prosthesis or plate M96.67- ☑
involving ankle or malleolus — *see* Fracture, fibula, lateral malleolus
lateral malleolus (displaced) S82.6- ☑
nondisplaced S82.6- ☑
lower end
physeal S89.30- ☑
Salter-Harris
Type I S89.31- ☑
Type II S89.32- ☑
specified NEC S89.39- ☑
specified NEC S82.83- ☑
torus S82.82- ☑
oblique (displaced) S82.43- ☑
nondisplaced S82.43- ☑
segmental (displaced) S82.46- ☑
nondisplaced S82.46- ☑
specified NEC S82.49- ☑
spiral (displaced) S82.44- ☑
nondisplaced S82.44- ☑
transverse (displaced) S82.42- ☑
nondisplaced S82.42- ☑
upper end
physeal S89.20- ☑
Salter-Harris
Type I S89.21- ☑
Type II S89.22- ☑
specified NEC S89.29- ☑
specified NEC S82.83- ☑
torus S82.81- ☑
finger (except thumb) S62.60- ☑
distal phalanx (displaced) S62.63- ☑
nondisplaced S62.66- ☑
index S62.60- ☑
distal phalanx (displaced) S62.63- ☑
nondisplaced S62.66- ☑
middle phalanx (displaced) S62.62- ☑
nondisplaced S62.65- ☑
proximal phalanx (displaced) S62.61- ☑
nondisplaced S62.64- ☑
little S62.60- ☑
distal phalanx (displaced) S62.63- ☑
nondisplaced S62.66- ☑
middle phalanx (displaced) S62.62- ☑
nondisplaced S62.65- ☑
proximal phalanx (displaced) S62.61- ☑
nondisplaced S62.64- ☑
middle S62.60- ☑
distal phalanx (displaced) S62.63- ☑
nondisplaced S62.66- ☑
middle phalanx (displaced) S62.62- ☑
nondisplaced S62.65- ☑
proximal phalanx (displaced) S62.61- ☑
nondisplaced S62.64- ☑
middle phalanx (displaced) S62.62- ☑
nondisplaced S62.65- ☑
proximal phalanx (displaced) S62.61- ☑

Fracture, traumatic — *continued*
finger — *continued*
proximal phalanx — *continued*
nondisplaced S62.64- ☑
ring S62.60- ☑
distal phalanx (displaced) S62.63- ☑
nondisplaced S62.66- ☑
middle phalanx (displaced) S62.62- ☑
nondisplaced S62.65- ☑
proximal phalanx (displaced) S62.61- ☑
nondisplaced S62.64- ☑
thumb — *see* Fracture, thumb
following insertion (intraoperative) (postoperative) of orthopedic implant, joint prosthesis or bone plate M96.69
femur M96.66- ☑
fibula M96.67- ☑
humerus M96.62- ☑
pelvis M96.65
radius M96.63- ☑
specified bone NEC M96.69
tibia M96.67- ☑
ulna M96.63- ☑
foot S92.90- ☑
astragalus — *see* Fracture, tarsal, talus
calcaneus — *see* Fracture, tarsal, calcaneus
cuboid — *see* Fracture, tarsal, cuboid
cuneiform — *see* Fracture, tarsal, cuneiform
metatarsal — *see* Fracture, metatarsal
navicular — *see* Fracture, tarsal, navicular
sesamoid S92.81- ☑
specified NEC S92.81- ☑
talus — *see* Fracture, tarsal, talus
tarsal — *see* Fracture, tarsal
toe — *see* Fracture, toe
forearm S52.9- ☑
radius — *see* Fracture, radius
ulna — *see* Fracture, ulna
fossa (anterior) (middle) (posterior) S02.19 ☑
fragility — *see* Fracture, pathological, due to osteoporosis
frontal (bone) (skull) S02.0 ☑
sinus S02.19 ☑
glenoid (cavity) (scapula) — *see* Fracture, scapula, glenoid cavity
greenstick — *see* Fracture, by site
hallux — *see* Fracture, toe, great
hand S62.9- ☑
carpal — *see* Fracture, carpal bone
finger (except thumb) — *see* Fracture, finger
metacarpal — *see* Fracture, metacarpal
navicular (scaphoid) (hand) — *see* Fracture, carpal bone, navicular
thumb — *see* Fracture, thumb
healed or old
with complications — *code by* Nature of the complication
heel bone — *see* Fracture, tarsal, calcaneus
Hill-Sachs S42.29- ☑
hip — *see* Fracture, femur, neck
humerus S42.30- ☑
anatomical neck — *see* Fracture, humerus, upper end
articular process — *see* Fracture, humerus, lower end
capitellum — *see* Fracture, humerus, lower end, condyle, lateral
distal end — *see* Fracture, humerus, lower end
epiphysis
lower — *see* Fracture, humerus, lower end, physeal
upper — *see* Fracture, humerus, upper end, physeal
external condyle — *see* Fracture, humerus, lower end, condyle, lateral
following insertion of implant, prosthesis or plate M96.62- ☑
great tuberosity — *see* Fracture, humerus, upper end, greater tuberosity
intercondylar — *see* Fracture, humerus, lower end
internal epicondyle — *see* Fracture, humerus, lower end, epicondyle, medial
lesser tuberosity — *see* Fracture, humerus, upper end, lesser tuberosity
lower end S42.40- ☑
condyle
lateral (displaced) S42.45- ☑

Fracture, traumatic — *continued*
humerus — *continued*
lower end — *continued*
condyle — *continued*
lateral — *continued*
nondisplaced S42.45- ☑
medial (displaced) S42.46- ☑
nondisplaced S42.46- ☑
epicondyle
lateral (displaced) S42.43- ☑
nondisplaced S42.43- ☑
medial (displaced) S42.44- ☑
incarcerated S42.44- ☑
nondisplaced S42.44- ☑
physeal S49.10- ☑
Salter-Harris
Type I S49.11- ☑
Type II S49.12- ☑
Type III S49.13- ☑
Type IV S49.14- ☑
specified NEC S49.19- ☑
specified NEC (displaced) S42.49- ☑
nondisplaced S42.49- ☑
supracondylar (simple) (displaced) S42.41- ☑
with intercondylar fracture — *see* Fracture, humerus, lower end
comminuted (displaced) S42.42- ☑
nondisplaced S42.42- ☑
nondisplaced S42.41- ☑
torus S42.48- ☑
transcondylar (displaced) S42.47- ☑
nondisplaced S42.47- ☑
proximal end — *see* Fracture, humerus, upper end
shaft S42.30- ☑
comminuted (displaced) S42.35- ☑
nondisplaced S42.35- ☑
greenstick S42.31- ☑
oblique (displaced) S42.33- ☑
nondisplaced S42.33- ☑
segmental (displaced) S42.36- ☑
nondisplaced S42.36- ☑
specified NEC S42.39- ☑
spiral (displaced) S42.34- ☑
nondisplaced S42.34- ☑
transverse (displaced) S42.32- ☑
nondisplaced S42.32- ☑
supracondylar — *see* Fracture, humerus, lower end
surgical neck — *see* Fracture, humerus, upper end, surgical neck
trochlea — *see* Fracture, humerus, lower end, condyle, medial
tuberosity — *see* Fracture, humerus, upper end
upper end S42.20- ☑
anatomical neck — *see* Fracture, humerus, upper end, specified NEC
articular head — *see* Fracture, humerus, upper end, specified NEC
epiphysis — *see* Fracture, humerus, upper end, physeal
greater tuberosity (displaced) S42.25- ☑
nondisplaced S42.25- ☑
lesser tuberosity (displaced) S42.26- ☑
nondisplaced S42.26- ☑
physeal S49.00- ☑
Salter-Harris
Type I S49.01- ☑
Type II S49.02- ☑
Type III S49.03- ☑
Type IV S49.04- ☑
specified NEC S49.09- ☑
specified NEC (displaced) S42.29- ☑
nondisplaced S42.29- ☑
surgical neck (displaced) S42.21- ☑
four-part S42.24- ☑
nondisplaced S42.21- ☑
three-part S42.23- ☑
two-part (displaced) S42.22- ☑
nondisplaced S42.22- ☑
torus S42.27- ☑
transepiphyseal — *see* Fracture, humerus, upper end, physeal
hyoid bone S12.8 ☑
ilium S32.30- ☑
with disruption of pelvic ring — *see* Disruption, pelvic ring
avulsion (displaced) S32.31- ☑

☑ Additional Character Required — Refer to the Tabular List for Character Selection

Fracture, traumatic — *continued*
  ilium — *continued*
    avulsion — *continued*
      nondisplaced S32.31- ☑
      specified NEC S32.39- ☑
    impaction, impacted — *code as* Fracture, by site
    innominate bone — *see* Fracture, ilium
  instep — *see* Fracture, foot
  ischium S32.60- ☑
    with disruption of pelvic ring — *see* Disruption, pelvic ring
    avulsion (displaced) S32.61- ☑
      nondisplaced S32.61- ☑
    specified NEC S32.69- ☑
  jaw (bone) (lower) — *see* Fracture, mandible
    upper — *see* Fracture, maxilla
  joint prosthesis — *see* Complications, joint prosthesis, mechanical, breakdown, by site
    periprosthetic — *see* Fracture, traumatic, periprosthetic
  knee cap — *see* Fracture, patella
  larynx S12.8 ☑
  late effects — *see* Sequelae, fracture
  leg (lower) S82.9- ☑
    ankle — *see* Fracture, ankle
    femur — *see* Fracture, femur
    fibula — *see* Fracture, fibula
    malleolus — *see* Fracture, ankle
    patella — *see* Fracture, patella
    specified site NEC S82.89- ☑
    tibia — *see* Fracture, tibia
  lumbar spine — *see* Fracture, vertebra, lumbar
  lumbosacral spine S32.9 ☑
  Maisonneuve's (displaced) S82.86- ☑
    nondisplaced S82.86- ☑
  malar bone — *see also* Fracture, maxilla S02.400 ☑
    left side S02.40B ☑
    right side S02.40A ☑
  malleolus — *see* Fracture, ankle
  malunion — *see* Fracture, by site
  mandible (lower jaw (bone)) S02.609 ☑
    alveolus S02.67- ☑
    angle (of jaw) S02.65- ☑
    body, unspecified S02.600 ☑
      left side S02.602 ☑
      right side S02.601 ☑
    condylar process S02.61- ☑
    coronoid process S02.63- ☑
    ramus, unspecified S02.64- ☑
    specified site NEC S02.69 ☑
    subcondylar process S02.62- ☑
    symphysis S02.66 ☑
  manubrium (sterni) S22.21 ☑
    dissociation from sternum S22.23 ☑
  march — *see* Fracture, traumatic, stress, by site
  maxilla, maxillary (bone) (sinus) (superior) (upper jaw) S02.401 ☑
    alveolus S02.42 ☑
    inferior — *see* Fracture, mandible
    LeFort I S02.411 ☑
    LeFort II S02.412 ☑
    LeFort III S02.413 ☑
    left side S02.40D ☑
    right side S02.40C ☑
  metacarpal S62.309 ☑
    base (displaced) S62.319 ☑
      nondisplaced S62.349 ☑
    fifth S62.30- ☑
      base (displaced) S62.31- ☑
        nondisplaced S62.34- ☑
      neck (displaced) S62.33- ☑
        nondisplaced S62.36- ☑
      shaft (displaced) S62.32- ☑
        nondisplaced S62.35- ☑
      specified NEC S62.398 ☑
    first S62.20- ☑
      base NEC (displaced) S62.23- ☑
        nondisplaced S62.23- ☑
      Bennett's — *see* Bennett's fracture
      neck (displaced) S62.25- ☑
        nondisplaced S62.25- ☑
      shaft (displaced) S62.24- ☑
        nondisplaced S62.24- ☑
      specified NEC S62.29- ☑
    fourth S62.30- ☑
      base (displaced) S62.31- ☑

Fracture, traumatic — *continued*
  metacarpal — *continued*
    fourth — *continued*
      base — *continued*
        nondisplaced S62.34- ☑
      neck (displaced) S62.33- ☑
        nondisplaced S62.36- ☑
      shaft (displaced) S62.32- ☑
        nondisplaced S62.35- ☑
      specified NEC S62.39- ☑
    neck (displaced) S62.33- ☑
      nondisplaced S62.36- ☑
    Rolando's — *see* Rolando's fracture
    second S62.30- ☑
      base (displaced) S62.31- ☑
        nondisplaced S62.34- ☑
      neck (displaced) S62.33- ☑
        nondisplaced S62.36- ☑
      shaft (displaced) S62.32- ☑
        nondisplaced S62.35- ☑
      specified NEC S62.39- ☑
    shaft (displaced) S62.32- ☑
      nondisplaced S62.35- ☑
    specified NEC S62.399 ☑
    third S62.30- ☑
      base (displaced) S62.31- ☑
        nondisplaced S62.34- ☑
      neck (displaced) S62.33- ☑
        nondisplaced S62.36- ☑
      shaft (displaced) S62.32- ☑
        nondisplaced S62.35- ☑
      specified NEC S62.39- ☑
  metaphyseal — *see* Fracture, traumatic, by site, shaft
  metastatic — *see* Fracture, pathological, due to, neoplastic disease — *see also* Neoplasm
  metatarsal bone S92.30- ☑
    fifth (displaced) S92.35- ☑
      nondisplaced S92.35- ☑
    first (displaced) S92.31- ☑
      nondisplaced S92.31- ☑
    fourth (displaced) S92.34- ☑
      nondisplaced S92.34- ☑
    physeal S99.10- ☑
      Salter-Harris
        Type I S99.11- ☑
        Type II S99.12- ☑
        Type III S99.13- ☑
        Type IV S99.14- ☑
      specified NEC S99.19- ☑
    second (displaced) S92.32- ☑
      nondisplaced S92.32- ☑
    third (displaced) S92.33- ☑
      nondisplaced S92.33- ☑
  Monteggia's — *see* Monteggia's fracture
  multiple
    hand (and wrist) NEC — *see* Fracture, by site
    ribs — *see* Fracture, rib, multiple
  nasal (bone(s)) S02.2 ☑
  navicular (scaphoid) (foot) — *see also* Fracture, tarsal, navicular
    hand — *see* Fracture, carpal, navicular
  neck S12.9 ☑
    cervical vertebra S12.9 ☑
      fifth (displaced) S12.400 ☑
        nondisplaced S12.401 ☑
        specified type NEC (displaced) S12.490 ☑
          nondisplaced S12.491 ☑
      first (displaced) S12.000 ☑
        burst (stable) S12.01 ☑
          unstable S12.02 ☑
        lateral mass (displaced) S12.040 ☑
          nondisplaced S12.041 ☑
        nondisplaced S12.001 ☑
        posterior arch (displaced) S12.030 ☑
          nondisplaced S12.031 ☑
        specified type NEC (displaced) S12.090 ☑
          nondisplaced S12.091 ☑
      fourth (displaced) S12.300 ☑
        nondisplaced S12.301 ☑
        specified type NEC (displaced) S12.390 ☑
          nondisplaced S12.391 ☑
      second (displaced) S12.100 ☑
        dens (anterior) (displaced) (type II) S12.110 ☑
          nondisplaced S12.112 ☑
          posterior S12.111 ☑
          specified type NEC (displaced) S12.120 ☑

Fracture, traumatic — *continued*
  neck — *continued*
    cervical vertebra — *continued*
      second — *continued*
        dens — *continued*
          specified type — *continued*
            nondisplaced S12.121 ☑
        nondisplaced S12.101 ☑
        specified type NEC (displaced) S12.190 ☑
          nondisplaced S12.191 ☑
      seventh (displaced) S12.600 ☑
        nondisplaced S12.601 ☑
        specified type NEC (displaced) S12.690 ☑
          nondisplaced S12.691 ☑
      sixth (displaced) S12.500 ☑
        nondisplaced S12.501 ☑
        specified type NEC (displaced) S12.590 ☑
          nondisplaced S12.591 ☑
      third (displaced) S12.200 ☑
        nondisplaced S12.201 ☑
        specified type NEC (displaced) S12.290 ☑
          nondisplaced S12.291 ☑
    hyoid bone S12.8 ☑
    larynx S12.8 ☑
    specified site NEC S12.8 ☑
    thyroid cartilage S12.8 ☑
    trachea S12.8 ☑
  neoplastic NEC — *see* Fracture, pathological, due to, neoplastic disease
  neural arch — *see* Fracture, vertebra
  newborn — *see* Birth, injury, fracture
  nontraumatic — *see* Fracture, pathological
  nonunion — *see* Nonunion, fracture
  nose, nasal (bone) (septum) S02.2 ☑
  occiput — *see* Fracture, skull, base, occiput
  odontoid process — *see* Fracture, neck, cervical vertebra, second
  olecranon (process) (ulna) — *see* Fracture, ulna, upper end, olecranon process
  orbit, orbital (bone) (region) S02.85 ☑
    floor (blow-out) S02.3- ☑
    roof S02.12- ☑
    wall S02.85 ☑
      lateral S02.84- ☑
      medial S02.83- ☑
  os
    calcis — *see* Fracture, tarsal, calcaneus
    magnum — *see* Fracture, carpal, capitate
    pubis — *see* Fracture, pubis
  palate S02.8- ☑
  parietal bone (skull) S02.0 ☑
  patella S82.00- ☑
    comminuted (displaced) S82.04- ☑
      nondisplaced S82.04- ☑
    longitudinal (displaced) S82.02- ☑
      nondisplaced S82.02- ☑
    osteochondral (displaced) S82.01- ☑
      nondisplaced S82.01- ☑
    specified NEC S82.09- ☑
    transverse (displaced) S82.03- ☑
      nondisplaced S82.03- ☑
  pedicle (of vertebral arch) — *see* Fracture, vertebra
  pelvis, pelvic (bone) S32.9 ☑
    acetabulum — *see* Fracture, acetabulum
    circle — *see* Disruption, pelvic ring
    following insertion of implant, prosthesis or plate M96.65
    ilium — *see* Fracture, ilium
    ischium — *see* Fracture, ischium
    multiple
      with disruption of pelvic ring (circle) — *see* Disruption, pelvic ring
      without disruption of pelvic ring (circle) S32.82 ☑
    pubis — *see* Fracture, pubis
    sacrum — *see* Fracture, sacrum
    specified site NEC S32.89 ☑
  periprosthetic, around internal prosthetic joint M97.9 ☑
    ankle M97.2- ☑
    elbow M97.4- ☑
    finger M97.8 ☑
    hip M97.0- ☑
    knee M97.1- ☑
    shoulder M97.3- ☑
    specified joint NEC M97.8 ☑

☑ **Additional Character Required — Refer to the Tabular List for Character Selection**

Fracture, traumatic — *continued*
- periprosthetic, around internal prosthetic joint — *continued*
  - spine M97.8 ☑
  - toe M97.8 ☑
  - wrist M97.8 ☑
- phalanx
  - foot — *see* Fracture, toe
  - hand — *see* Fracture, finger
- pisiform — *see* Fracture, carpal, pisiform
- pond — *see* Fracture, skull
- prosthetic device, internal — *see* Complications, prosthetic device, by site, mechanical
- pubis S32.50- ☑
  - with disruption of pelvic ring — *see* Disruption, pelvic ring
  - specified site NEC S32.59- ☑
  - superior rim S32.51- ☑
- radius S52.9- ☑
  - distal end — *see* Fracture, radius, lower end
  - following insertion of implant, prosthesis or plate M96.63- ☑
  - head — *see* Fracture, radius, upper end, head
  - lower end S52.50- ☑
    - Barton's — *see* Barton's fracture
    - Colles' — *see* Colles' fracture
    - extraarticular NEC S52.55- ☑
    - intraarticular NEC S52.57- ☑
    - physeal S59.20- ☑
      - Salter-Harris
        - Type I S59.21- ☑
        - Type II S59.22- ☑
        - Type III S59.23- ☑
        - Type IV S59.24- ☑
        - specified NEC S59.29- ☑
    - Smith's — *see* Smith's fracture
    - specified NEC S52.59- ☑
    - styloid process (displaced) S52.51- ☑
      - nondisplaced S52.51- ☑
    - torus S52.52- ☑
  - neck — *see* Fracture, radius, upper end
  - proximal end — *see* Fracture, radius, upper end
  - shaft S52.30- ☑
    - bent bone S52.38- ☑
    - comminuted (displaced) S52.35- ☑
      - nondisplaced S52.35- ☑
    - Galeazzi's — *see* Galeazzi's fracture
    - greenstick S52.31- ☑
    - oblique (displaced) S52.33- ☑
      - nondisplaced S52.33- ☑
    - segmental (displaced) S52.36- ☑
      - nondisplaced S52.36- ☑
    - specified NEC S52.39- ☑
    - spiral (displaced) S52.34- ☑
      - nondisplaced S52.34- ☑
    - transverse (displaced) S52.32- ☑
      - nondisplaced S52.32- ☑
  - upper end S52.10- ☑
    - head (displaced) S52.12- ☑
      - nondisplaced S52.12- ☑
    - neck (displaced) S52.13- ☑
      - nondisplaced S52.13- ☑
    - physeal S59.10- ☑
      - Salter-Harris
        - Type I S59.11- ☑
        - Type II S59.12- ☑
        - Type III S59.13- ☑
        - Type IV S59.14- ☑
        - specified NEC S59.19- ☑
    - specified NEC S52.18- ☑
    - torus S52.11- ☑
- ramus
  - inferior or superior, pubis — *see* Fracture, pubis
  - mandible — *see* Fracture, mandible
- restorative material (dental) K08.539
  - with loss of material K08.531
  - without loss of material K08.530
- rib S22.3- ☑
  - with flail chest — *see* Flail, chest
  - associated with chest compression and cardiopulmonary resuscitation M96.A2
  - multiple S22.4- ☑
    - with flail chest — *see* Flail, chest
    - associated with chest compression and cardiopulmonary resuscitation M96.A3
- root, tooth — *see* Fracture, tooth

Fracture, traumatic — *continued*
- sacrum S32.10 ☑
  - specified NEC S32.19 ☑
  - Type
    - 1 S32.14 ☑
    - 2 S32.15 ☑
    - 3 S32.16 ☑
    - 4 S32.17 ☑
  - Zone
    - I S32.119 ☑
      - displaced (minimally) S32.111 ☑
        - severely S32.112 ☑
      - nondisplaced S32.110 ☑
    - II S32.129 ☑
      - displaced (minimally) S32.121 ☑
        - severely S32.122 ☑
      - nondisplaced S32.120 ☑
    - III S32.139 ☑
      - displaced (minimally) S32.131 ☑
        - severely S32.132 ☑
      - nondisplaced S32.130 ☑
- scaphoid (hand) — *see also* Fracture, carpal, navicular
  - foot — *see* Fracture, tarsal, navicular
- scapula S42.10- ☑
  - acromial process (displaced) S42.12- ☑
    - nondisplaced S42.12- ☑
  - body (displaced) S42.11- ☑
    - nondisplaced S42.11- ☑
  - coracoid process (displaced) S42.13- ☑
    - nondisplaced S42.13- ☑
  - glenoid cavity (displaced) S42.14- ☑
    - nondisplaced S42.14- ☑
  - neck (displaced) S42.15- ☑
    - nondisplaced S42.15- ☑
  - specified NEC S42.19- ☑
- semilunar bone, wrist — *see* Fracture, carpal, lunate
- sequelae — *see* Sequelae, fracture
- sesamoid bone
  - foot S92.81- ☑
  - hand — *see* Fracture, carpal
  - other — *see* Fracture, traumatic, by site
- shepherd's — *see* Fracture, tarsal, talus
- shoulder (girdle) S42.9- ☑
  - blade — *see* Fracture, scapula
- sinus (ethmoid) (frontal) S02.19 ☑
- skull S02.91 ☑
  - base S02.10- ☑
    - occiput S02.119 ☑
      - condyle S02.113 ☑
        - specified NEC S02.118 ☑
          - left side S02.11H ☑
          - right side S02.11G ☑
        - type I S02.110 ☑
          - left side S02.11B ☑
          - right side S02.11A ☑
        - type II S02.111 ☑
          - left side S02.11D ☑
          - right side S02.11C ☑
        - type III S02.112 ☑
          - left side S02.11F ☑
          - right side S02.11E ☑
    - specified NEC S02.19 ☑
  - birth injury P13.0
  - frontal bone S02.0 ☑
  - parietal bone S02.0 ☑
  - specified site NEC S02.8- ☑
  - temporal bone S02.19 ☑
  - vault S02.0 ☑
- Smith's — *see* Smith's fracture
- sphenoid (bone) (sinus) S02.19 ☑
- spine — *see* Fracture, vertebra
- spinous process — *see* Fracture, vertebra
- spontaneous (cause unknown) — *see* Fracture, pathological
- stave (of thumb) — *see* Fracture, metacarpal, first
- sternum S22.20 ☑
  - with flail chest — *see* Flail, chest
  - associated with chest compression and cardiopulmonary resuscitation M96.A1
  - body S22.22 ☑
  - manubrium S22.21 ☑
  - xiphoid (process) S22.24 ☑
    - associated with chest compression and cardiopulmonary resuscitation M96.A1
- stress M84.30 ☑
  - ankle M84.37- ☑

Fracture, traumatic — *continued*
- stress — *continued*
  - carpus M84.34- ☑
  - clavicle M84.31- ☑
  - femoral neck M84.359 ☑
  - femur M84.35- ☑
  - fibula M84.36- ☑
  - finger M84.34- ☑
  - hip M84.359 ☑
  - humerus M84.32- ☑
  - ilium M84.350 ☑
  - ischium M84.350 ☑
  - metacarpus M84.34- ☑
  - metatarsus M84.37- ☑
  - neck — *see* Fracture, fatigue, vertebra
  - pelvis M84.350 ☑
  - radius M84.33- ☑
  - rib M84.38 ☑
  - scapula M84.31- ☑
  - skull M84.38 ☑
  - tarsus M84.37- ☑
  - tibia M84.36- ☑
  - toe M84.37- ☑
  - ulna M84.33- ☑
  - vertebra — *see* Fracture, fatigue, vertebra
- supracondylar, elbow — *see* Fracture, humerus, lower end, supracondylar
- symphysis pubis — *see* Fracture, pubis
- talus (ankle bone) — *see* Fracture, tarsal, talus
- tarsal bone(s) S92.20- ☑
  - astragalus — *see* Fracture, tarsal, talus
  - calcaneus S92.00- ☑
    - anterior process (displaced) S92.02- ☑
      - nondisplaced S92.02- ☑
    - body (displaced) S92.01- ☑
      - nondisplaced S92.01- ☑
    - extraarticular NEC (displaced) S92.05- ☑
      - nondisplaced S92.05- ☑
    - intraarticular (displaced) S92.06- ☑
      - nondisplaced S92.06- ☑
    - physeal S99.00- ☑
      - Salter-Harris
        - Type I S99.01- ☑
        - Type II S99.02- ☑
        - Type III S99.03- ☑
        - Type IV S99.04- ☑
        - specified NEC S99.09- ☑
    - tuberosity (displaced) S92.04- ☑
      - avulsion (displaced) S92.03- ☑
        - nondisplaced S92.03- ☑
      - nondisplaced S92.04- ☑
  - cuboid (displaced) S92.21- ☑
    - nondisplaced S92.21- ☑
  - cuneiform
    - intermediate (displaced) S92.23- ☑
      - nondisplaced S92.23- ☑
    - lateral (displaced) S92.22- ☑
      - nondisplaced S92.22- ☑
    - medial (displaced) S92.24- ☑
      - nondisplaced S92.24- ☑
  - navicular (displaced) S92.25- ☑
    - nondisplaced S92.25- ☑
  - scaphoid — *see* Fracture, tarsal, navicular
  - talus S92.10- ☑
    - avulsion (displaced) S92.15- ☑
      - nondisplaced S92.15- ☑
    - body (displaced) S92.12- ☑
      - nondisplaced S92.12- ☑
    - dome (displaced) S92.14- ☑
      - nondisplaced S92.14- ☑
    - head (displaced) S92.12- ☑
      - nondisplaced S92.12- ☑
    - lateral process (displaced) S92.14- ☑
      - nondisplaced S92.14- ☑
    - neck (displaced) S92.11- ☑
      - nondisplaced S92.11- ☑
    - posterior process (displaced) S92.13- ☑
      - nondisplaced S92.13- ☑
    - specified NEC S92.19- ☑
  - temporal bone (styloid) S02.19 ☑
- thorax (bony) S22.9 ☑
  - with flail chest — *see* Flail, chest
  - rib S22.3- ☑
    - multiple S22.4- ☑
      - with flail chest — *see* Flail, chest
  - sternum S22.20 ☑

☑ **Additional Character Required** — Refer to the Tabular List for Character Selection

Fracture, traumatic — *continued*
  thorax — *continued*
    sternum — *continued*
      body S22.22
      manubrium S22.21 ☑
      xiphoid process S22.24 ☑
        associated with chest compression and cardiopulmonary resuscitation M96.A1
    vertebra (displaced) S22.009 ☑
      burst (stable) S22.001 ☑
        unstable S22.002 ☑
      eighth S22.069 ☑
        burst (stable) S22.061 ☑
          unstable S22.062 ☑
        specified type NEC S22.068 ☑
        wedge compression S22.060 ☑
      eleventh S22.089 ☑
        burst (stable) S22.081 ☑
          unstable S22.082 ☑
        specified type NEC S22.088 ☑
        wedge compression S22.080 ☑
      fifth S22.059 ☑
        burst (stable) S22.051 ☑
          unstable S22.052 ☑
        specified type NEC S22.058 ☑
        wedge compression S22.050 ☑
      first S22.019 ☑
        burst (stable) S22.011 ☑
          unstable S22.012 ☑
        specified type NEC S22.018 ☑
        wedge compression S22.010 ☑
      fourth S22.049 ☑
        burst (stable) S22.041 ☑
          unstable S22.042 ☑
        specified type NEC S22.048 ☑
        wedge compression S22.040 ☑
      ninth S22.079 ☑
        burst (stable) S22.071 ☑
          unstable S22.072 ☑
        specified type NEC S22.078 ☑
        wedge compression S22.070 ☑
      nondisplaced S22.001 ☑
      second S22.029 ☑
        burst (stable) S22.021 ☑
          unstable S22.022 ☑
        specified type NEC S22.028 ☑
        wedge compression S22.020 ☑
      seventh S22.069 ☑
        burst (stable) S22.061 ☑
          unstable S22.062 ☑
        specified type NEC S22.068 ☑
        wedge compression S22.060 ☑
      sixth S22.059 ☑
        burst (stable) S22.051 ☑
          unstable S22.052 ☑
        specified type NEC S22.058 ☑
        wedge compression S22.050 ☑
      specified type NEC S22.008 ☑
      tenth S22.079 ☑
        burst (stable) S22.071 ☑
          unstable S22.072 ☑
        specified type NEC S22.078 ☑
        wedge compression S22.070 ☑
      third S22.039 ☑
        burst (stable) S22.031 ☑
          unstable S22.032 ☑
        specified type NEC S22.038 ☑
        wedge compression S22.030 ☑
      twelfth S22.089 ☑
        burst (stable) S22.081 ☑
          unstable S22.082 ☑
        specified type NEC S22.088 ☑
        wedge compression S22.080 ☑
      wedge compression S22.000 ☑
  thumb S62.50- ☑
    distal phalanx (displaced) S62.52- ☑
    nondisplaced S62.52- ☑
    proximal phalanx (displaced) S62.51- ☑
    nondisplaced S62.51- ☑
  thyroid cartilage S12.8
  tibia (shaft) S82.20- ☑
    comminuted (displaced) S82.25- ☑
    nondisplaced S82.25- ☑
    condyles — *see* Fracture, tibia, upper end
    distal end — *see* Fracture, tibia, lower end

Fracture, traumatic — *continued*
  tibia — *continued*
    epiphysis
      lower — *see* Fracture, tibia, lower end
      upper — *see* Fracture, tibia, upper end
    following insertion of implant, prosthesis or plate M96.67- ☑
    head (involving knee joint) — *see* Fracture, tibia, upper end
    intercondyloid eminence — *see* Fracture, tibia, upper end
    involving ankle or malleolus — *see* Fracture, ankle, medial malleolus
    lower end S82.30- ☑
      physeal S89.10- ☑
        Salter-Harris
          Type I S89.11- ☑
          Type II S89.12- ☑
          Type III S89.13- ☑
          Type IV S89.14- ☑
        specified NEC S89.19- ☑
      pilon (displaced) S82.87- ☑
        nondisplaced S82.87- ☑
      specified NEC S82.39- ☑
      torus S82.31- ☑
    malleolus — *see* Fracture, ankle, medial malleolus
    oblique (displaced) S82.23- ☑
      nondisplaced S82.23- ☑
    pilon — *see* Fracture, tibia, lower end, pilon
    proximal end — *see* Fracture, tibia, upper end
    segmental (displaced) S82.26- ☑
      nondisplaced S82.26- ☑
    specified NEC S82.29- ☑
    spine — *see* Fracture, tibia, upper end, spine
    spiral (displaced) S82.24- ☑
      nondisplaced S82.24- ☑
    transverse (displaced) S82.22- ☑
      nondisplaced S82.22- ☑
    tuberosity — *see* Fracture, tibia, upper end, tuberosity
    upper end S82.10- ☑
      bicondylar (displaced) S82.14- ☑
        nondisplaced S82.14- ☑
      lateral condyle (displaced) S82.12- ☑
        nondisplaced S82.12- ☑
      medial condyle (displaced) S82.13- ☑
        nondisplaced S82.13- ☑
      physeal S89.00- ☑
        Salter-Harris
          Type I S89.01- ☑
          Type II S89.02- ☑
          Type III S89.03- ☑
          Type IV S89.04- ☑
        specified NEC S89.09- ☑
      plateau — *see* Fracture, tibia, upper end, bicondylar
      specified NEC S82.19- ☑
      spine (displaced) S82.11- ☑
        nondisplaced S82.11- ☑
      torus S82.16- ☑
      tuberosity (displaced) S82.15- ☑
        nondisplaced S82.15- ☑
  toe S92.91- ☑
    great (displaced) S92.40- ☑
      distal phalanx (displaced) S92.42- ☑
        nondisplaced S92.42- ☑
      nondisplaced S92.40- ☑
      proximal phalanx (displaced) S92.41- ☑
        nondisplaced S92.41- ☑
      specified NEC S92.49- ☑
    lesser (displaced) S92.50- ☑
      distal phalanx (displaced) S92.53- ☑
        nondisplaced S92.53- ☑
      middle phalanx (displaced) S92.52- ☑
        nondisplaced S92.52- ☑
      nondisplaced S92.50- ☑
      proximal phalanx (displaced) S92.51- ☑
        nondisplaced S92.51- ☑
      specified NEC S92.59- ☑
    physeal
      phalanx S99.20- ☑
        Salter-Harris
          Type I S99.21- ☑
          Type II S99.22- ☑
          Type III S99.23- ☑
          Type IV S99.24- ☑

Fracture, traumatic — *continued*
  toe — *continued*
    physeal — *continued*
      phalanx — *continued*
        specified NEC S99.29- ☑
  tooth (root) S02.5 ☑
  trachea (cartilage) S12.8 ☑
  transverse process — *see* Fracture, vertebra
  trapezium or trapezoid bone — *see* Fracture, carpal
  trimalleolar — *see* Fracture, ankle, trimalleolar
  triquetrum (cuneiform of carpus) — *see* Fracture, carpal, triquetrum
  trochanter — *see* Fracture, femur, trochanteric
  tuberosity (external) — *see* Fracture, traumatic, by site
  ulna (shaft) S52.20- ☑
    bent bone S52.28- ☑
    coronoid process — *see* Fracture, ulna, upper end, coronoid process
    distal end — *see* Fracture, ulna, lower end
    following insertion of implant, prosthesis or plate M96.63- ☑
    head S52.60- ☑
    lower end S52.60- ☑
      physeal S59.00- ☑
        Salter-Harris
          Type I S59.01- ☑
          Type II S59.02- ☑
          Type III S59.03- ☑
          Type IV S59.04- ☑
        specified NEC S59.09- ☑
      specified NEC S52.69- ☑
      styloid process (displaced) S52.61- ☑
        nondisplaced S52.61- ☑
      torus S52.62- ☑
    proximal end — *see* Fracture, ulna, upper end
    shaft S52.20- ☑
      comminuted (displaced) S52.25- ☑
        nondisplaced S52.25- ☑
      greenstick S52.21- ☑
      Monteggia's — *see* Monteggia's fracture
      oblique (displaced) S52.23- ☑
        nondisplaced S52.23- ☑
      segmental (displaced) S52.26- ☑
        nondisplaced S52.26- ☑
      specified NEC S52.29- ☑
      spiral (displaced) S52.24- ☑
        nondisplaced S52.24- ☑
      transverse (displaced) S52.22- ☑
        nondisplaced S52.22- ☑
    upper end S52.00- ☑
      coronoid process (displaced) S52.04- ☑
        nondisplaced S52.04- ☑
      olecranon process (displaced) S52.02- ☑
        with intraarticular extension S52.03- ☑
        nondisplaced S52.02- ☑
          with intraarticular extension S52.03- ☑
      specified NEC S52.09- ☑
      torus S52.01- ☑
  unciform — *see* Fracture, carpal, hamate
  vault of skull S02.0 ☑
  vertebra, vertebral (arch) (body) (column) (neural arch) (pedicle) (spinous process) (transverse process)
    atlas — *see* Fracture, neck, cervical vertebra, first
    axis — *see* Fracture, neck, cervical vertebra, second
    cervical (teardrop) S12.9
      axis — *see* Fracture, neck, cervical vertebra, second
      first (atlas) — *see* Fracture, neck, cervical vertebra, first
      second (axis) — *see* Fracture, neck, cervical vertebra, second
    chronic M84.48 ☑
    coccyx S32.2 ☑
    dorsal — *see* Fracture, thorax, vertebra
    lumbar S32.009 ☑
      burst (stable) S32.001 ☑
        unstable S32.002 ☑
      fifth S32.059 ☑
        burst (stable) S32.051 ☑
          unstable S32.052 ☑
        specified type NEC S32.058 ☑
        wedge compression S32.050 ☑
      first S32.019 ☑
        burst (stable) S32.011 ☑
          unstable S32.012 ☑
        specified type NEC S32.018 ☑

Fracture, traumatic — continued
  vertebra, vertebral — continued
    lumbar — continued
      first — continued
        wedge compression S32.010 ☑
        fourth S32.049 ☑
          burst (stable) S32.041 ☑
            unstable S32.042 ☑
          specified type NEC S32.048 ☑
          wedge compression S32.040 ☑
        second S32.029 ☑
          burst (stable) S32.021 ☑
            unstable S32.022 ☑
          specified type NEC S32.028 ☑
          wedge compression S32.020 ☑
        specified type NEC S32.008 ☑
        third S32.039 ☑
          burst (stable) S32.031 ☑
            unstable S32.032 ☑
          specified type NEC S32.038 ☑
          wedge compression S32.030 ☑
        wedge compression S32.000 ☑
      metastatic — see Collapse, vertebra, in, specified
          disease NEC — see also Neoplasm
      newborn (birth injury) P11.5
      sacrum S32.10 ☑
        specified NEC S32.19 ☑
        Type
          1 S32.14 ☑
          2 S32.15 ☑
          3 S32.16 ☑
          4 S32.17 ☑
        Zone
          I S32.119 ☑
            displaced (minimally) S32.111 ☑
              severely S32.112 ☑
            nondisplaced S32.110 ☑
          II S32.129 ☑
            displaced (minimally) S32.121 ☑
              severely S32.122 ☑
            nondisplaced S32.120 ☑
          III S32.139 ☑
            displaced (minimally) S32.131 ☑
              severely S32.132 ☑
            nondisplaced S32.130 ☑
      thoracic — see Fracture, thorax, vertebra
    vertex S02.0 ☑
    vomer (bone) S02.2 ☑
    wrist S62.10- ☑
      carpal — see Fracture, carpal bone
      navicular (scaphoid) (hand) — see Fracture, carpal,
          navicular
    xiphisternum, xiphoid (process) S22.24 ☑
      associated with chest compression and cardiopul-
          monary resuscitation M96.A1
    zygoma S02.402 ☑
      left side S02.40F ☑
      right side S02.40E ☑
Fragile, fragility
  autosomal site Q95.5
  bone, congenital (with blue sclera) Q78.0
  capillary (hereditary) D69.8
  hair L67.8
  nails L60.3
  non-sex chromosome site Q95.5
  X chromosome Q99.2
Fragilitas
  crinium L67.8
  ossium (with blue sclerae) (hereditary) Q78.0
  unguium L60.3
    congenital Q84.6
Fragments, cataract (lens), **following cataract surgery**
    H59.02- ☑
  retained foreign body — see Retained, foreign body
      fragments (type of)
Frailty (frail) R54
  mental R41.81
Frambesia, frambesial (tropica) — see also Yaws
  initial lesion or ulcer A66.0
  primary A66.0
Frambeside
  gummatous A66.4
  of early yaws A66.2
Frambesioma A66.1
Franceschetti-Klein (-Wildervanck) **disease or syn-**
    drome Q75.4
Francis' disease — see Tularemia

Franklin disease C88.2
Frank's essential thrombocytopenia D69.3
Fraser's syndrome Q87.0
Freckle(s) L81.2
  malignant melanoma in — see Melanoma
  melanotic (Hutchinson's) — see Melanoma, in situ
  retinal D49.81
Frederickson's hyperlipoproteinemia, type
  I and V E78.3
  IIA E78.00
  IIB and III E78.2
  IV E78.1
Freeman Sheldon syndrome Q87.0
Freezing — see also Effect, adverse, cold T69.9 ☑
Freiberg's disease (infraction of metatarsal head or os-
    teochondrosis) — see Osteochondrosis, juvenile,
    metatarsus
Frei's disease A55
Fremitus, friction, cardiac R01.2
Frenum, frenulum
  external os Q51.828
  tongue (shortening) (congenital) Q38.1
Frequency micturition (nocturnal) R35.0
  psychogenic F45.8
Frey's syndrome
  auriculotemporal G50.8
  hyperhidrosis L74.52
Friction
  burn — see Burn, by site
  fremitus, cardiac R01.2
  precordial R01.2
  sounds, chest R09.89
Friderichsen-Waterhouse syndrome or disease A39.1
Friedländer's B (bacillus) **NEC** — see also condition A49.8
Friedreich's
  ataxia G11.11
  combined systemic disease G11.11
  facial hemihypertrophy Q67.4
  sclerosis (cerebellum) (spinal cord) G11.11
Frigidity F52.22
Fröhlich's syndrome E23.6
Frontal — see also condition
  lobe syndrome F07.0
Frostbite (superficial) T33.90 ☑
  with
    partial thickness skin loss — see Frostbite (superfi-
        cial), by site
    tissue necrosis T34.90 ☑
  abdominal wall T33.3 ☑
    with tissue necrosis T34.3 ☑
  ankle T33.81- ☑
    with tissue necrosis T34.81- ☑
  arm T33.4- ☑
    with tissue necrosis T34.4- ☑
    finger(s) — see Frostbite, finger
    hand — see Frostbite, hand
    wrist — see Frostbite, wrist
  ear T33.01- ☑
    with tissue necrosis T34.01- ☑
  face T33.09 ☑
    with tissue necrosis T34.09 ☑
  finger T33.53- ☑
    with tissue necrosis T34.53- ☑
  foot T33.82- ☑
    with tissue necrosis T34.82- ☑
  hand T33.52- ☑
    with tissue necrosis T34.52- ☑
  head T33.09 ☑
    with tissue necrosis T34.09 ☑
    ear — see Frostbite, ear
    nose — see Frostbite, nose
  hip (and thigh) T33.6- ☑
    with tissue necrosis T34.6- ☑
  knee T33.7- ☑
    with tissue necrosis T34.7- ☑
  leg T33.9- ☑
    with tissue necrosis T34.9- ☑
    ankle — see Frostbite, ankle
    foot — see Frostbite, foot
    knee — see Frostbite, knee
    lower T33.7- ☑
      with tissue necrosis T34.7- ☑
    thigh — see Frostbite, hip
    toe — see Frostbite, toe
  limb
    lower T33.99 ☑

Frostbite — continued
  limb — continued
    lower — continued
      with tissue necrosis T34.99 ☑
    upper — see Frostbite, arm
  neck T33.1 ☑
    with tissue necrosis T34.1 ☑
  nose T33.02 ☑
    with tissue necrosis T34.02 ☑
  pelvis T33.3 ☑
    with tissue necrosis T34.3 ☑
  specified site NEC T33.99 ☑
    with tissue necrosis T34.99 ☑
  thigh — see Frostbite, hip
  thorax T33.2 ☑
    with tissue necrosis T34.2 ☑
  toes T33.83- ☑
    with tissue necrosis T34.83- ☑
  trunk T33.99 ☑
    with tissue necrosis T34.99 ☑
  wrist T33.51- ☑
    with tissue necrosis T34.51- ☑
Frotteurism F65.81
Frozen — see also Effect, adverse, cold T69.9 ☑
  pelvis (female) N94.89
    male K66.8
  shoulder — see Capsulitis, adhesive
Fructokinase deficiency E74.11
Fructose 1,6 diphosphatase deficiency E74.19
Fructosemia (benign) (essential) E74.12
Fructosuria (benign) (essential) E74.11
Fuchs'
  black spot (myopic) — see also Myopia, degenerative
      H44.2- ☑
  dystrophy (corneal endothelium) H18.51- ☑
  heterochromic cyclitis — see Cyclitis, Fuchs' hete-
      rochromic
Fucosidosis E77.1
Fugue R68.89
  dissociative F44.1
  hysterical (dissociative) F44.1
  postictal in epilepsy — see Epilepsy
  reaction to exceptional stress (transient) F43.0
Fulminant, fulminating — see condition
Functional — see also condition
  bleeding (uterus) N93.8
Functioning, intellectual, borderline R41.83
Fundus — see condition
Fungemia NOS B49
Fungus, fungous
  cerebral G93.89
  disease NOS B49
  infection — see Infection, fungus
Funiculitis (acute) (chronic) (endemic) N49.1
  gonococcal (acute) (chronic) A54.23
  tuberculous A18.15
Funnel
  breast (acquired) M95.4
    congenital Q67.6
    sequelae (late effect) of rickets E64.3
  chest (acquired) M95.4
    congenital Q67.6
    sequelae (late effect) of rickets E64.3
  pelvis (acquired) M95.5
    with disproportion (fetopelvic) O33.3 ☑
      causing obstructed labor O65.3
    congenital Q74.2
FUO (fever of unknown origin) R50.9
Furfur L21.0
  microsporon B36.0
Furrier's lung J67.8
Furrowed K14.5
  nail(s) (transverse) L60.4
    congenital Q84.6
  tongue K14.5
    congenital Q38.3
Furuncle L02.92
  abdominal wall L02.221
  ankle — see Furuncle, lower limb
  antecubital space — see Furuncle, upper limb
  anus K61.0
  arm — see Furuncle, upper limb
  auditory canal, external — see Abscess, ear, external
  auricle (ear) — see Abscess, ear, external
  axilla (region) L02.42- ☑
  back (any part) L02.222
  breast N61.1

Furuncle — *continued*
- buttock LØ2.32
- cheek (external) LØ2.Ø2
- chest wall LØ2.223
- chin LØ2.Ø2
- corpus cavernosum N48.21
- ear, external — *see* Abscess, ear, external
- external auditory canal — *see* Abscess, ear, external
- eyelid — *see* Abscess, eyelid
- face LØ2.Ø2
- femoral (region) — *see* Furuncle, lower limb
- finger — *see* Furuncle, hand
- flank LØ2.221
- foot LØ2.62- ☑
- forehead LØ2.Ø2
- gluteal (region) LØ2.32
- groin LØ2.224
- hand LØ2.52- ☑
- head LØ2.821
  - face LØ2.Ø2
- hip — *see* Furuncle, lower limb
- kidney — *see* Abscess, kidney
- knee — *see* Furuncle, lower limb
- labium (majus) (minus) N76.4
- lacrimal
  - gland — *see* Dacryoadenitis
  - passages (duct) (sac) — *see* Inflammation, lacrimal, passages, acute
- leg (any part) — *see* Furuncle, lower limb
- lower limb LØ2.42- ☑
- malignant A22.Ø
- mouth K12.2
- navel LØ2.226
- neck LØ2.12
- nose J34.Ø
- orbit, orbital — *see* Abscess, orbit
- palmar (space) — *see* Furuncle, hand
- partes posteriores LØ2.32
- pectoral region LØ2.223
- penis N48.21
- perineum LØ2.225
- pinna — *see* Abscess, ear, external
- popliteal — *see* Furuncle, lower limb

Furuncle — *continued*
- prepatellar — *see* Furuncle, lower limb
- scalp LØ2.821
- seminal vesicle N49.Ø
- shoulder — *see* Furuncle, upper limb
- specified site NEC LØ2.828
- submandibular K12.2
- temple (region) LØ2.Ø2
- thumb — *see* Furuncle, hand
- toe — *see* Furuncle, foot
- trunk LØ2.229
  - abdominal wall LØ2.221
  - back LØ2.222
  - chest wall LØ2.223
  - groin LØ2.224
  - perineum LØ2.225
  - umbilicus LØ2.226
- umbilicus LØ2.226
- upper limb LØ2.42- ☑
- vulva N76.4

Furunculosis — *see* Furuncle

Fused — *see* Fusion, fused

Fusion, fused (congenital)
- astragaloscaphoid Q74.2
- atria Q21.19
- auditory canal Q16.1
- auricles, heart Q21.19
- binocular with defective stereopsis H53.32
- bone Q79.8
- cervical spine M43.22
- choanal Q3Ø.Ø
- commissure, mitral valve Q23.2
- cusps, heart valve NEC Q24.8
  - mitral Q23.2
  - pulmonary Q22.1
  - tricuspid Q22.4
- ear ossicles Q16.3
- fingers Q7Ø.Ø ☑
- hymen Q52.3
- joint (acquired) — *see also* Ankylosis
  - congenital Q74.8
- kidneys (incomplete) Q63.1
- labium (majus) (minus) Q52.5
- larynx and trachea Q34.8

Fusion, fused — *continued*
- limb, congenital Q74.8
  - lower Q74.2
  - upper Q74.Ø
- lobes, lung Q33.8
- lumbosacral (acquired) M43.27
  - arthrodesis status Z98.1
  - congenital Q76.49
  - postprocedural status Z98.1
- nares, nose, nasal, nostril(s) Q3Ø.Ø
- organ or site not listed — *see* Anomaly, by site
- ossicles Q79.9
  - auditory Q16.3
- pulmonic cusps Q22.1
- ribs Q76.6
- sacroiliac (joint) (acquired) M43.28
  - arthrodesis status Z98.1
  - congenital Q74.2
  - postprocedural status Z98.1
- spine (acquired) NEC M43.2Ø
  - arthrodesis status Z98.1
  - cervical region M43.22
  - cervicothoracic region M43.23
  - congenital Q76.49
  - lumbar M43.26
  - lumbosacral region M43.27
  - occipito-atlanto-axial region M43.21
  - postoperative status Z98.1
  - sacrococcygeal region M43.28
  - thoracic region M43.24
  - thoracolumbar region M43.25
- sublingual duct with submaxillary duct at opening in mouth Q38.4
- testes Q55.1
- toes Q7Ø.2- ☑
- tooth, teeth KØØ.2
- trachea and esophagus Q39.8
- twins Q89.4
- vagina Q52.4
- ventricles, heart Q21.Ø
- vertebra (arch) — *see* Fusion, spine
- vulva Q52.5

Fusospirillosis (mouth) (tongue) (tonsil) A69.1
Fussy baby R68.12

G

Gain in weight (abnormal) (excessive) — *see also* Weight, gain
Gaisböck's disease (polycythemia hypertonica) D75.1
Gait abnormality R26.9
  ataxic R26.0
  falling R29.6
  hysterical (ataxic) (staggering) F44.4
  paralytic R26.1
  spastic R26.1
  specified type NEC R26.89
  staggering R26.0
  unsteadiness R26.81
  walking difficulty NEC R26.2
Galactocele (breast) N64.89
  puerperal, postpartum O92.79
Galactokinase deficiency E74.29
Galactophoritis N61.0
  gestational, puerperal, postpartum O91.2- ☑
Galactorrhea O92.6
  not associated with childbirth N64.3
Galactosemia (classic) (congenital) E74.21
Galactosuria E74.29
Galacturia R82.0
  schistosomiasis (bilharziasis) B65.0
GALD (gestational alloimmune liver disease) P78.84
Galeazzi's fracture S52.37- ☑
Galen's vein — *see* condition
Galeophobia F40.218
Gall duct — *see* condition
Gallbladder — *see also* condition
  acute K81.0
Gallop rhythm R00.8
Gallstone (colic) (cystic duct) (gallbladder) (impacted) (multiple) — *see also* Calculus, gallbladder
  with
    cholecystitis — *see* Calculus, gallbladder, with cholecystitis
  bile duct (common) (hepatic) — *see* Calculus, bile duct
  causing intestinal obstruction K56.3
  specified NEC K80.80
    with obstruction K80.81
Gambling Z72.6
  pathological (compulsive) F63.0
Gammopathy (of undetermined significance [MGUS]) D47.2
  associated with lymphoplasmacytic dyscrasia D47.2
  monoclonal D47.2
  polyclonal D89.0
Gamna's disease (siderotic splenomegaly) D73.1
Gamophobia F40.298
Gampsodactylia (congenital) Q66.7- ☑
Gamstorp's disease (adynamia episodica hereditaria) G72.3
Gandy-Nanta disease (siderotic splenomegaly) D73.1
Gang
  membership offenses Z72.810
Gangliocytoma D36.10
Ganglioglioma — *see* Neoplasm, uncertain behavior, by site
Ganglion (compound) (diffuse) (joint) (tendon (sheath)) M67.40
  ankle M67.47- ☑
  foot M67.47- ☑
  forearm M67.43- ☑
  hand M67.44- ☑
  lower leg M67.46- ☑
  multiple sites M67.49
  of yaws (early) (late) A66.6
  pelvic region M67.45- ☑
  periosteal — *see* Periostitis
  shoulder region M67.41- ☑
  specified site NEC M67.48
  thigh region M67.45- ☑
  tuberculous A18.09
  upper arm M67.42- ☑
  wrist M67.43- ☑
Ganglioneuroblastoma — *see* Neoplasm, nerve, malignant
Ganglioneuroma D36.10
  malignant — *see* Neoplasm, nerve, malignant
Ganglioneuromatosis D36.10
Ganglionitis
  fifth nerve — *see* Neuralgia, trigeminal
  gasserian (postherpetic) (postzoster) B02.21

Ganglionitis — *continued*
  geniculate G51.1
    newborn (birth injury) P11.3
    postherpetic, postzoster B02.21
  herpes zoster B02.21
  postherpetic geniculate B02.21
Gangliosidosis E75.10
  GM1 E75.19
  GM2 E75.00
    other specified E75.09
    Sandhoff disease E75.01
    Tay-Sachs disease E75.02
  GM3 E75.19
  mucolipidosis IV E75.11
Gangosa A66.5
Gangrene, gangrenous (connective tissue) (dropsical) (dry) (moist) (skin) (ulcer) — *see also* Necrosis I96
  with diabetes (mellitus) — *see* Diabetes, with, gangrene
  abdomen (wall) I96
  alveolar M27.3
  appendix K35.80
    with
      peritonitis, localized — *see also* Appendicitis K35.31
  arteriosclerotic (general) (senile) — *see* Arteriosclerosis, extremities, with, gangrene
  auricle I96
  Bacillus welchii A48.0
  bladder (infectious) — *see* Cystitis, specified type NEC
  bowel, cecum, or colon — *see* Gangrene, intestine
  Clostridium perfringens or welchii A48.0
  cornea H18.89- ☑
  corpora cavernosa N48.29
    noninfective N48.89
  cutaneous, spreading I96
  decubital — *see* Ulcer, pressure, by site
  diabetic (any site) — *see* Diabetes, with, gangrene
  emphysematous — *see* Gangrene, gas
  epidemic — *see* Poisoning, food, noxious, plant
  epididymis (infectional) N45.1
  erysipelas — *see* Erysipelas
  extremity (lower) (upper) I96
  Fournier N49.3
    female N76.82
    vagina and vulva N76.82
  fusospirochetal A69.0
  gallbladder — *see* Cholecystitis, acute
  gas (bacillus) A48.0
    following
      abortion — *see* Abortion by type complicated by infection
      ectopic or molar pregnancy O08.0
  glossitis K14.0
  hernia — *see* Hernia, by site, with gangrene
  intestine, intestinal (hemorrhagic) (massive) — *see also* Infarct, intestine K55.069
    with
      mesenteric embolism — *see also* Infarct, intestine K55.069
      obstruction — *see* Obstruction, intestine
  laryngitis J04.0
  limb (lower) (upper) I96
  lung J85.0
    spirochetal A69.8
  lymphangitis I89.1
  Meleney's (synergistic) — *see* Ulcer, skin
  mesentery — *see also* Infarct, intestine K55.069
    with
      embolism — *see also* Infarct, intestine K55.069
      intestinal obstruction — *see* Obstruction, intestine
  mouth A69.0
  ovary — *see* Oophoritis
  pancreas — *see* Pancreatitis, acute
  penis N48.29
    noninfective N48.89
  perineum I96
  pharynx — *see also* Pharyngitis
    Vincent's A69.1
  presenile I73.1
  progressive synergistic — *see* Ulcer, skin
  pulmonary J85.0
  pulpal (dental) K04.1
  quinsy J36
  Raynaud's (symmetric gangrene) I73.01
  retropharyngeal J39.2
  scrotum N49.3
    noninfective N50.89

Gangrene, gangrenous — *continued*
  senile (atherosclerotic) — *see* Arteriosclerosis, extremities, with, gangrene
  spermatic cord N49.1
    noninfective N50.89
  spine I96
  spirochetal NEC A69.8
  spreading cutaneous I96
  stomatitis A69.0
  symmetrical I73.01
  testis (infectional) N45.2
    noninfective N44.8
  throat — *see also* Pharyngitis
    diphtheritic A36.0
    Vincent's A69.1
  thyroid (gland) E07.89
  tooth (pulp) K04.1
  tuberculous NEC — *see* Tuberculosis
  tunica vaginalis N49.1
    noninfective N50.89
  umbilicus I96
  uterus — *see* Endometritis
  uvulitis K12.2
  vas deferens N49.1
    noninfective N50.89
  vulva N76.82
Ganister disease J62.8
Ganser's syndrome (hysterical) F44.89
Gardner-Diamond syndrome (autoerythrocyte sensitization) D69.2
Gargoylism E76.01
Garré's disease, osteitis (sclerosing), osteomyelitis — *see* Osteomyelitis, specified type NEC
Garrod's pad, knuckle M72.1
Gartner's duct
  cyst Q52.4
  persistent Q50.6
Gas R14.3
  asphyxiation, inhalation, poisoning, suffocation NEC — *see* Table of Drugs and Chemicals
  excessive R14.0
  gangrene A48.0
    following
      abortion — *see* Abortion by type complicated by infection
      ectopic or molar pregnancy O08.0
  on stomach R14.0
  pains R14.1
Gastralgia — *see also* Pain, abdominal
Gastrectasis K31.0
  psychogenic F45.8
Gastric — *see* condition
Gastrinoma
  malignant
    pancreas C25.4
    specified site NEC — *see* Neoplasm, malignant, by site
    unspecified site C25.4
  specified site — *see* Neoplasm, uncertain behavior
  unspecified site D37.9
Gastritis (simple) K29.70
  with bleeding K29.71
  acute (erosive) K29.00
    with bleeding K29.01
  alcoholic K29.20
    with bleeding K29.21
  allergic K29.60
    with bleeding K29.61
  atrophic (chronic) K29.40
    with bleeding K29.41
  chronic (antral) (fundal) K29.50
    with bleeding K29.51
    atrophic K29.40
      with bleeding K29.41
    superficial K29.30
      with bleeding K29.31
  dietary counseling and surveillance Z71.3
  due to diet deficiency E63.9
  eosinophilic K52.81
  giant hypertrophic K29.60
    with bleeding K29.61
  granulomatous K29.60
    with bleeding K29.61
  hypertrophic (mucosa) K29.60
    with bleeding K29.61
  nervous F54
  spastic K29.60
    with bleeding K29.61

Gastritis — continued
  specified NEC K29.60
    with bleeding K29.61
  superficial chronic K29.30
    with bleeding K29.31
  tuberculous A18.83
  viral NEC A08.4
Gastrocarcinoma — see Neoplasm, malignant, stomach
Gastrocolic — see condition
Gastrodisciasis, gastrodiscoidiasis B66.8
Gastroduodenitis K29.90
  with bleeding K29.91
  virus, viral A08.4
    specified type NEC A08.39
Gastrodynia — see Pain, abdominal
Gastroenteritis (acute) (chronic) (noninfectious) — see
  also Enteritis K52.9
  allergic K52.29
    with
      eosinophilic gastritis or gastroenteritis K52.81
      food protein-induced enterocolitis syndrome
        K52.21
      food protein-induced enteropathy K52.22
  dietetic — see also Gastroenteritis, allergic K52.29
  drug-induced K52.1
  due to
    Cryptosporidium A07.2
    drugs K52.1
    food poisoning — see Intoxication, foodborne
    radiation K52.0
  eosinophilic K52.81
  epidemic (infectious) A09
  food hypersensitivity — see also Gastroenteritis, allergic
    K52.29
  infectious — see Enteritis, infectious
  influenzal — see Influenza, with gastroenteritis
  noninfectious K52.9
    specified NEC K52.89
  rotaviral A08.0
  Salmonella A02.0
  toxic K52.1
  viral NEC A08.4
    acute infectious A08.39
      type Norwalk A08.11
    infantile (acute) A08.39
    Norwalk agent A08.11
    rotaviral A08.0
    severe of infants A08.39
    specified type NEC A08.39
Gastroenteropathy — see also Gastroenteritis K52.9
  acute, due to Norovirus A08.11
  acute, due to Norwalk agent A08.11
  infectious A09
Gastroenteroptosis K63.4
**Gastroesophageal laceration- hemorrhage syn-
  drome** K22.6
Gastrointestinal — see condition
Gastrojejunal — see condition
Gastrojejunitis — see also Enteritis K52.9
Gastrojejunocolic — see condition
Gastroliths K31.89
Gastromalacia K31.89
Gastroparalysis K31.84
  diabetic — see Diabetes, gastroparalysis
Gastroparesis K31.84
  diabetic — see Diabetes, by type, with gastroparesis
Gastropathy K31.9
  congestive portal — see also Hypertension, portal
    K31.89
  erythematous K29.70
  exudative K90.89
  portal hypertensive — see also Hypertension, portal
    K31.89
Gastroptosis K31.89
Gastrorrhagia K92.2
  psychogenic F45.8
Gastroschisis (congenital) Q79.3
Gastrospasm (neurogenic) (reflex) K31.89
  neurotic F45.8
  psychogenic F45.8
Gastrostaxis — see Gastritis, with bleeding
Gastrostenosis K31.89
Gastrostomy
  attention to Z43.1
  status Z93.1
Gastrosuccorrhea (continuous) (intermittent) K31.89
  neurotic F45.8
  psychogenic F45.8

Gatophobia F40.218
Gaucher's disease or splenomegaly (adult) (infantile)
  E75.22
Gee (-Herter)(-Thaysen) **disease** (nontropical sprue) K90.0
Gélineau's syndrome G47.419
  with cataplexy G47.411
Gemination, tooth, teeth K00.2
Gemistocytoma
  specified site — see Neoplasm, malignant, by site
  unspecified site C71.9
General, generalized — see condition
Genetic
  carrier (status)
    cystic fibrosis Z14.1
    hemophilia A (asymptomatic) Z14.01
      symptomatic Z14.02
    specified NEC Z14.8
  susceptibility to disease NEC Z15.89
    malignant neoplasm Z15.09
      breast Z15.01
      endometrium Z15.04
      ovary Z15.02
      prostate Z15.03
      specified NEC Z15.09
    multiple endocrine neoplasia Z15.81
Genital — see condition
Genito-anorectal syndrome A55
Genitourinary system — see condition
Genu
  congenital Q74.1
  extrorsum (acquired) — see also Deformity, varus, knee
    congenital Q74.1
    sequelae (late effect) of rickets E64.3
  introrsum (acquired) — see also Deformity, valgus,
    knee
    congenital Q74.1
    sequelae (late effect) of rickets E64.3
  rachitic (old) E64.3
  recurvatum (acquired) — see also Deformity, limb,
    specified type NEC, lower leg
    congenital Q68.2
    sequelae (late effect) of rickets E64.3
  valgum (acquired) (knock-knee) M21.06- ☑
    congenital Q74.1
    sequelae (late effect) of rickets E64.3
  varum (acquired) (bowleg) M21.16- ☑
    congenital Q74.1
    sequelae (late effect) of rickets E64.3
Geographic tongue K14.1
Geophagia — see Pica
Geotrichosis B48.3
  stomatitis B48.3
Gephyrophobia F40.242
Gerbode defect Q21.0
GERD (gastroesophageal reflux disease) K21.9
Gerhardt's
  disease (erythromelalgia) I73.81
  syndrome (vocal cord paralysis) J38.00
    bilateral J38.02
    unilateral J38.01
German measles — see also Rubella
  exposure to Z20.4
Germinoblastoma (diffuse) C85.9- ☑
  follicular C82.9- ☑
Germinoma — see Neoplasm, malignant, by site
Gerontoxon — see Degeneration, cornea, senile
Gerstmann's syndrome R48.8
  developmental F81.2
Gerstmann-Sträussler-Scheinker syndrome (GSS)
  A81.82
Gestation (period) — see also Pregnancy
  ectopic — see Pregnancy, by site
  multiple O30.9- ☑
    greater than quadruplets — see Pregnancy, multiple
      (gestation), specified NEC
    specified NEC — see Pregnancy, multiple (gesta-
      tion), specified NEC
Gestational
  mammary abscess O91.11- ☑
  purulent mastitis O91.11- ☑
  subareolar abscess O91.11- ☑
Ghon tubercle, primary infection A15.7
Ghost
  teeth K00.4
  vessels (cornea) H16.41- ☑
Ghoul hand A66.3
Gianotti-Crosti disease L44.4

Giant
  cell
    epulis K06.8
    peripheral granuloma K06.8
  esophagus, congenital Q39.5
  kidney, congenital Q63.3
  urticaria T78.3 ☑
    hereditary D84.1
Giardiasis A07.1
Gibert's disease or pityriasis L42
Giddiness R42
  hysterical F44.89
  psychogenic F45.8
Gierke's disease (glycogenosis I) E74.01
Gigantism (cerebral) (hypophyseal) (pituitary) E22.0
  constitutional E34.4
Gilbert's disease or syndrome E80.4
Gilchrist's disease B40.9
Gilford-Hutchinson disease E34.8
Gilles de la Tourette's disease or syndrome (motor-
  verbal tic) F95.2
Gingivitis K05.10
  acute (catarrhal) K05.00
    necrotizing A69.1
    nonplaque induced K05.01
    plaque induced K05.00
  chronic (desquamative) (hyperplastic) (simple marginal)
    (pregnancy associated) (ulcerative) K05.10
    nonplaque induced K05.11
    plaque induced K05.10
  expulsiva — see Periodontitis
  necrotizing ulcerative (acute) A69.1
  pellagrous E52
    acute necrotizing A69.1
  Vincent's A69.1
Gingivoglossitis K14.0
Gingivopericementitis — see Periodontitis
Gingivosis — see Gingivitis, chronic
Gingivostomatitis K05.10
  herpesviral B00.2
  necrotizing ulcerative (acute) A69.1
Gland, glandular — see condition
Glanders A24.0
Glanzmann (-Naegeli) **disease or thrombasthenia**
  D69.1
Glasgow coma scale
  total score
    3-8 R40.243 ☑
    9-12 R40.242 ☑
    13-15 R40.241 ☑
Glass-blower's disease (cataract) — see Cataract, spec-
  ified NEC
Glaucoma H40.9
  with
    increased episcleral venous pressure H40.81- ☑
    pseudoexfoliation of lens — see Glaucoma, open
      angle, primary, capsular
  absolute H44.51- ☑
  angle-closure (primary) H40.20- ☑
    acute (attack) (crisis) H40.21- ☑
    chronic H40.22- ☑
    intermittent H40.23- ☑
    residual stage H40.24- ☑
  borderline H40.00- ☑
  capsular (with pseudoexfoliation of lens) — see Glau-
    coma, open angle, primary, capsular
  childhood Q15.0
  closed angle — see Glaucoma, angle-closure
  congenital Q15.0
  corticosteroid-induced — see Glaucoma, secondary,
    drugs
  hypersecretion H40.82- ☑
  in (due to)
    amyloidosis E85.4 [H42]
    aniridia Q13.1 [H42]
    concussion of globe — see Glaucoma, secondary,
      trauma
    dislocation of lens — see Glaucoma, secondary
    disorder of lens NEC — see Glaucoma, secondary
    drugs — see Glaucoma, secondary, drugs
    endocrine disease NOS E34.9 [H42]
    eye
      inflammation — see Glaucoma, secondary, in-
        flammation
      trauma — see Glaucoma, secondary, trauma
    hypermature cataract — see Glaucoma, secondary

Glaucoma — *continued*
 in — *continued*
  iridocyclitis — *see* Glaucoma, secondary, inflammation
  lens disorder — *see* Glaucoma, secondary
  Lowe's syndrome E72.03 *[H42]*
  metabolic disease NOS E88.9 *[H42]*
  ocular disorders NEC — *see* Glaucoma, secondary
  onchocerciasis B73.02
  pupillary block — *see* Glaucoma, secondary
  retinal vein occlusion — *see* Glaucoma, secondary
  Rieger's anomaly Q13.81 *[H42]*
  rubeosis of iris — *see* Glaucoma, secondary
  tumor of globe — *see* Glaucoma, secondary
 infantile Q15.0
 low tension — *see* Glaucoma, open angle, primary, low-tension
 malignant H40.83- ☑
 narrow angle — *see* Glaucoma, angle-closure
 newborn Q15.0
 noncongestive (chronic) — *see* Glaucoma, open angle
 nonobstructive — *see* Glaucoma, open angle
 obstructive — *see also* Glaucoma, angle-closure
  due to lens changes — *see* Glaucoma, secondary
 open angle H40.10- ☑
  primary H40.11- ☑
   capsular (with pseudoexfoliation of lens) H40.14-
   low-tension H40.12- ☑
   pigmentary H40.13- ☑
   residual stage H40.15- ☑
 phacolytic — *see* Glaucoma, secondary
 pigmentary — *see* Glaucoma, open angle, primary, pigmentary
 postinfectious — *see* Glaucoma, secondary, inflammation
 secondary (to) H40.5- ☑
  drugs H40.6- ☑
  inflammation H40.4- ☑
  trauma H40.3- ☑
 simple (chronic) H40.11- ☑
 simplex H40.11- ☑
 specified type NEC H40.89
 suspect H40.00- ☑
 syphilitic A52.71
 traumatic — *see also* Glaucoma, secondary, trauma
  newborn (birth injury) P15.3
 tuberculous A18.59
Glaucomatous flecks (subcapsular) — *see* Cataract, complicated
Glazed tongue K14.4
Gleet (gonococcal) A54.01
Glénard's disease K63.4
Glioblastoma (multiforme)
 with sarcomatous component
  specified site — *see* Neoplasm, malignant, by site
  unspecified site C71.9
 giant cell
  specified site — *see* Neoplasm, malignant, by site
  unspecified site C71.9
 specified site — *see* Neoplasm, malignant, by site
 unspecified site C71.9
Glioma (malignant)
 astrocytic
  specified site — *see* Neoplasm, malignant, by site
  unspecified site C71.9
 mixed
  specified site — *see* Neoplasm, malignant, by site
  unspecified site C71.9
 nose Q30.8
 specified site NEC — *see* Neoplasm, malignant, by site
 subependymal D43.2
  specified site — *see* Neoplasm, uncertain behavior, by site
  unspecified site D43.2
 unspecified site C71.9
Gliomatosis cerebri C71.0
Glioneuroma — *see* Neoplasm, uncertain behavior, by site
Gliosarcoma
 specified site — *see* Neoplasm, malignant, by site
 unspecified site C71.9
Gliosis (cerebral) G93.89
 spinal G95.89
Glisson's disease — *see* Rickets
Globinuria R82.3
Globus (hystericus) F45.8

Glomangioma D18.00
 intra-abdominal D18.03
 intracranial D18.02
 skin D18.01
 specified site NEC D18.09
Glomangiomyoma D18.00
 intra-abdominal D18.03
 intracranial D18.02
 skin D18.01
 specified site NEC D18.09
Glomangiosarcoma — *see* Neoplasm, connective tissue, malignant
Glomerular
 disease in syphilis A52.75
 nephritis — *see* Glomerulonephritis
Glomerulitis — *see* Glomerulonephritis
Glomerulonephritis — *see also* Nephritis N05.9
 with
  C3
   glomerulonephritis N05.A
   glomerulopathy N05.A
    with dense deposit disease N05.6
  edema — *see* Nephrosis
  minimal change N05.0
  minor glomerular abnormality N05.0
 acute N00.9
 chronic N03.9
 crescentic (diffuse) NEC — *see also* N00-N07 with fourth character .7 N05.7
 dense deposit — *see also* N00-N07 with fourth character .6 N05.6
 diffuse
  crescentic — *see also* N00-N07 with fourth character .7 N05.7
  endocapillary proliferative — *see also* N00-N07 with fourth character .4 N05.4
  membranous — *see also* N00-N07 with fourth character .2 N05.2
  mesangial proliferative — *see also* N00-N07 with fourth character .3 N05.3
  mesangiocapillary — *see also* N00-N07 with fourth character .5 N05.5
  sclerosing N18.9
 endocapillary proliferative (diffuse) NEC — *see also* N00-N07 with fourth character .4 N05.4
 extracapillary NEC — *see also* N00-N07 with fourth character .7 N05.7
 focal (and segmental) NEC — *see also* N00-N07 with fourth character .1 N05.1
 hypocomplementemic — *see* Glomerulonephritis, membranoproliferative
 IgA — *see* Nephropathy, IgA
 immune complex (circulating) NEC N05.8
 in (due to)
  amyloidosis E85.4 *[N08]*
  bilharziasis B65.9 *[N08]*
  cryoglobulinemia D89.1 *[N08]*
  defibrination syndrome D65 *[N08]*
  diabetes mellitus — *see* Diabetes, glomerulosclerosis
  disseminated intravascular coagulation D65 *[N08]*
  Fabry (-Anderson) disease E75.21 *[N08]*
  Goodpasture's syndrome M31.0
  hemolytic-uremic syndrome — *see* Syndrome, hemolytic-uremic
  Henoch (-Schönlein) purpura D69.0 *[N08]*
  lecithin cholesterol acyltransferase deficiency E78.6 *[N08]*
  microscopic polyangiitis M31.7 *[N08]*
  multiple myeloma C90.0- ☑ *[N08]*
  Plasmodium malariae B52.0
  schistosomiasis B65.9 *[N08]*
  sepsis A41.9 *[N08]*
   streptococcal A40- ☑ *[N08]*
  sickle-cell disorders D57.- *[N08]*
  strongyloidiasis B78.9 *[N08]*
  subacute bacterial endocarditis I33.0 *[N08]*
  syphilis (late) congenital A50.59 *[N08]*
  systemic lupus erythematosus M32.14
  thrombotic thrombocytopenic purpura M31.19 *[N08]*
  typhoid fever A01.09
  Waldenström macroglobulinemia C88.0 *[N08]*
  Wegener's granulomatosis M31.31
 latent or quiescent N03.9
 lobular, lobulonodular — *see* Glomerulonephritis, membranoproliferative

Glomerulonephritis — *continued*
 membranoproliferative (diffuse)(type 1 or 3) — *see also* N00-N07 with fourth character .5 N05.5
  dense deposit (type 2) NEC — *see also* N00-N07 with fourth character .6 N05.6
 membranous (diffuse) NEC — *see also* N00-N07 with fourth character .2 N05.2
 mesangial
  IgA/IgG — *see* Nephropathy, IgA
  proliferative (diffuse) NEC — *see also* N00-N07 with fourth character .3 N05.3
 mesangiocapillary (diffuse) NEC — *see also* N00-N07 with fourth character .5 N05.5
 necrotic, necrotizing NEC — *see also* N00-N07 with fourth character .8 N05.8
 nodular — *see* Glomerulonephritis, membranoproliferative
 poststreptococcal NEC N05.9
  acute N00.9
  chronic N03.9
  rapidly progressive N01.9
 proliferative NEC — *see also* N00-N07 with fourth character .8 N05.8
  diffuse (lupus) M32.14
 rapidly progressive N01.9
 sclerosing, diffuse N18.9
 specified pathology NEC — *see also* N00-N07 with fourth character .8 N05.8
 subacute N01.9
Glomerulopathy — *see* Glomerulonephritis
Glomerulosclerosis — *see also* Sclerosis, renal
 intercapillary (nodular) (with diabetes) — *see* Diabetes, glomerulosclerosis
 intracapillary — *see* Diabetes, glomerulosclerosis
Glossagra K14.6
Glossalgia K14.6
Glossitis (chronic superficial) (gangrenous) (Moeller's) K14.0
 areata exfoliativa K14.1
 atrophic K14.4
 benign migratory K14.1
 cortical superficial, sclerotic K14.0
 Hunter's D51.0
 interstitial, sclerous K14.0
 median rhomboid K14.2
 pellagrous E52
 superficial, chronic K14.0
Glossocele K14.8
Glossodynia K14.6
 exfoliativa K14.4
Glossoncus K14.8
Glossopathy K14.9
Glossophytia K14.3
Glossoplegia K14.8
Glossoptosis K14.8
Glossopyrosis K14.6
Glossotrichia K14.3
Glossy skin L90.8
Glottis — *see* condition
Glottitis — *see also* Laryngitis J04.0
Glucagonoma
 pancreas
  benign D13.7
  malignant C25.4
  uncertain behavior D37.8
 specified site NEC
  benign — *see* Neoplasm, benign, by site
  malignant — *see* Neoplasm, malignant, by site
  uncertain behavior — *see* Neoplasm, uncertain behavior, by site
 unspecified site
  benign D13.7
  malignant C25.4
  uncertain behavior D37.8
Glucoglycinuria E72.51
Glucose-galactose malabsorption E74.39
Glue
 ear — *see* Otitis, media, nonsuppurative, chronic, mucoid
 sniffing (airplane) — *see* Abuse, drug, inhalant
  dependence — *see* Dependence, drug, inhalant
GLUT1 deficiency syndrome 1, infantile onset E74.810
GLUT1 deficiency syndrome 2, childhood onset E74.810
Glutaric aciduria E72.3
Glycinemia E72.51
Glycinuria (renal) (with ketosis) E72.09

Glycogen
infiltration — *see* Disease, glycogen storage
storage disease — *see* Disease, glycogen storage
Glycogenosis (diffuse) (generalized) — *see also* Disease, glycogen storage
cardiac E74.02 *[I43]*
diabetic, secondary — *see* Diabetes, glycogenosis, secondary
pulmonary interstitial J84.842
Glycopenia E16.2
Glycosuria R81
renal E74.818
Gnathostoma spinigerum (infection) (infestation), **gnathostomiasis** (wandering swelling) B83.1
Goiter (plunging) (substernal) E04.9
with
hyperthyroidism (recurrent) — *see* Hyperthyroidism, with, goiter
thyrotoxicosis — *see* Hyperthyroidism, with, goiter
adenomatous — *see* Goiter, nodular
cancerous C73
congenital (nontoxic) E03.0
diffuse E03.0
parenchymatous E03.0
transitory, with normal functioning P72.0
cystic E04.2
due to iodine-deficiency E01.1
due to
enzyme defect in synthesis of thyroid hormone E07.1
iodine-deficiency (endemic) E01.2
dyshormonogenetic (familial) E07.1
endemic (iodine-deficiency) E01.2
diffuse E01.0
multinodular E01.1
exophthalmic — *see* Hyperthyroidism, with, goiter
iodine-deficiency (endemic) E01.2
diffuse E01.0
multinodular E01.1
nodular E01.1
lingual Q89.2
lymphadenoid E06.3
malignant C73
multinodular (cystic) (nontoxic) E04.2
toxic or with hyperthyroidism E05.20
with thyroid storm E05.21
neonatal NEC P72.0
nodular (nontoxic) (due to) E04.9
with
hyperthyroidism E05.20
with thyroid storm E05.21
thyrotoxicosis E05.20
with thyroid storm E05.21
endemic E01.1
iodine-deficiency E01.1
sporadic E04.9
toxic E05.20
with thyroid storm E05.21
nontoxic E04.9
diffuse (colloid) E04.0
multinodular E04.2
simple E04.0
specified NEC E04.8
uninodular E04.1
simple E04.0
toxic — *see* Hyperthyroidism, with, goiter
uninodular (nontoxic) E04.1
toxic or with hyperthyroidism E05.10
with thyroid storm E05.11
Goiter-deafness syndrome E07.1
Goldberg syndrome Q89.8
Goldberg-Maxwell syndrome E34.51
Goldblatt's hypertension or kidney I70.1
Goldenhar (-Gorlin) **syndrome** Q87.0
Goldflam-Erb disease or syndrome G70.00
with exacerbation (acute) G70.01
in crisis G70.01
Goldscheider's disease Q81.8
Goldstein's disease (familial hemorrhagic telangiectasia) I78.0
Golfer's elbow — *see* Epicondylitis, medial
Gonadoblastoma
specified site — *see* Neoplasm, uncertain behavior, by site
unspecified site
female D39.10
male D40.10
Gonecystitis — *see* Vesiculitis

Gongylonemiasis B83.8
Goniosynechiae — *see* Adhesions, iris, goniosynechiae
Gonococcemia A54.86
Gonococcus, gonococcal (disease) (infection) — *see also* condition A54.9
anus A54.6
bursa, bursitis A54.49
conjunctiva, conjunctivitis (neonatorum) A54.31
endocardium A54.83
eye A54.30
conjunctivitis A54.31
iridocyclitis A54.32
keratitis A54.33
newborn A54.31
other specified A54.39
fallopian tubes (acute) (chronic) A54.24
genitourinary (organ) (system) (tract) (acute)
lower A54.00
with abscess (accessory gland) (periurethral) A54.1
upper — *see also* condition A54.29
heart A54.83
iridocyclitis A54.32
joint A54.42
lymphatic (gland) (node) A54.89
meninges, meningitis A54.81
musculoskeletal A54.40
arthritis A54.42
osteomyelitis A54.43
other specified A54.49
spondylopathy A54.41
pelviperitonitis A54.24
pelvis (acute) (chronic) A54.24
pharynx A54.5
proctitis A54.6
pyosalpinx (acute) (chronic) A54.24
rectum A54.6
skin A54.89
specified site NEC A54.89
tendon sheath A54.49
throat A54.5
urethra (acute) (chronic) A54.01
with abscess (accessory gland) (periurethral) A54.1
vulva (acute) (chronic) A54.02
Gonocytoma
specified site — *see* Neoplasm, uncertain behavior, by site
unspecified site
female D39.10
male D40.10
Gonorrhea (acute) (chronic) A54.9
Bartholin's gland (acute) (chronic) (purulent) A54.02
with abscess (accessory gland) (periurethral) A54.1
bladder A54.01
cervix A54.03
conjunctiva, conjunctivitis (neonatorum) A54.31
contact Z20.2
Cowper's gland (with abscess) A54.1
exposure to Z20.2
fallopian tube (acute) (chronic) A54.24
kidney (acute) (chronic) A54.21
lower genitourinary tract A54.00
with abscess (accessory gland) (periurethral) A54.1
ovary (acute) (chronic) A54.24
pelvis (acute) (chronic) A54.24
female pelvic inflammatory disease A54.24
penis A54.09
prostate (acute) (chronic) A54.22
seminal vesicle (acute) (chronic) A54.23
specified site not listed — *see also* Gonococcus A54.89
spermatic cord (acute) (chronic) A54.23
urethra A54.01
with abscess (accessory gland) (periurethral) A54.1
vagina A54.02
vas deferens (acute) (chronic) A54.23
vulva A54.02
Goodall's disease A08.19
Goodpasture's syndrome M31.0
Gopalan's syndrome (burning feet) E53.0
Gorlin-Chaudry-Moss syndrome Q87.0
Gottron's papules L94.4
Gougerot-Blum syndrome (pigmented purpuric lichenoid dermatitis) L81.7
Gougerot-Carteaud disease or syndrome (confluent reticulate papillomatosis) L83
Gougerot's syndrome (trisymptomatic) L81.7
Gouley's syndrome (constrictive pericarditis) I31.1
Goundou A66.6

Gout, chronic — *see also* Gout, gouty M1A.9 ☑ *(following M08)*
drug-induced M1A.20 ☑ *(following M08)*
ankle M1A.27- ☑ *(following M08)*
elbow M1A.22- ☑ *(following M08)*
foot joint M1A.27- ☑ *(following M08)*
hand joint M1A.24- ☑ *(following M08)*
hip M1A.25- ☑ *(following M08)*
knee M1A.26- ☑ *(following M08)*
multiple site M1A.29- ☑ *(following M08)*
shoulder M1A.21- ☑ *(following M08)*
vertebrae M1A.28 ☑ *(following M08)*
wrist M1A.23- ☑ *(following M08)*
idiopathic M1A.00 ☑ *(following M08)*
ankle M1A.07- ☑ *(following M08)*
elbow M1A.02- ☑ *(following M08)*
foot joint M1A.07- ☑ *(following M08)*
hand joint M1A.04- ☑ *(following M08)*
hip M1A.05- ☑ *(following M08)*
knee M1A.06- ☑ *(following M08)*
multiple site M1A.09 ☑ *(following M08)*
shoulder M1A.01- ☑ *(following M08)*
vertebrae M1A.08 ☑ *(following M08)*
wrist M1A.03- ☑ *(following M08)*
in (due to) renal impairment M1A.30 ☑ *(following M08)*
ankle M1A.37- ☑ *(following M08)*
elbow M1A.32- ☑ *(following M08)*
foot joint M1A.37- ☑ *(following M08)*
hand joint M1A.34- ☑ *(following M08)*
hip M1A.35- ☑ *(following M08)*
knee M1A.36- ☑ *(following M08)*
multiple site M1A.39 ☑ *(following M08)*
shoulder M1A.31- ☑ *(following M08)*
vertebrae M1A.38 ☑ *(following M08)*
wrist M1A.33- ☑ *(following M08)*
lead-induced M1A.10 ☑ *(following M08)*
ankle M1A.17- ☑ *(following M08)*
elbow M1A.12- ☑ *(following M08)*
foot joint M1A.17- ☑ *(following M08)*
hand joint M1A.14- ☑ *(following M08)*
hip M1A.15- ☑ *(following M08)*
knee M1A.16- ☑ *(following M08)*
multiple site M1A.19 ☑ *(following M08)*
shoulder M1A.11- ☑ *(following M08)*
vertebrae M1A.18 ☑ *(following M08)*
wrist M1A.13- ☑ *(following M08)*
primary — *see* Gout, chronic, idiopathic
saturnine — *see* Gout, chronic, lead-induced
secondary NEC M1A.40 ☑ *(following M08)*
ankle M1A.47- ☑ *(following M08)*
elbow M1A.42- ☑ *(following M08)*
foot joint M1A.47- ☑ *(following M08)*
hand joint M1A.44- ☑ *(following M08)*
hip M1A.45- ☑ *(following M08)*
knee M1A.46- ☑ *(following M08)*
multiple site M1A.49 ☑ *(following M08)*
shoulder M1A.41- ☑ *(following M08)*
vertebrae M1A.48 ☑ *(following M08)*
wrist M1A.43- ☑ *(following M08)*
syphilitic — *see also* subcategory M14.8- A52.77
tophi M1A.9 ☑ *(following M08)*
Gout, gouty (acute) (attack) (flare) — *see also* Gout, chronic M10.9
drug-induced M10.20
ankle M10.27- ☑
elbow M10.22- ☑
foot joint M10.27- ☑
hand joint M10.24- ☑
hip M10.25- ☑
knee M10.26- ☑
multiple site M10.29
shoulder M10.21- ☑
vertebrae M10.28
wrist M10.23- ☑
idiopathic M10.00
ankle M10.07- ☑
elbow M10.02- ☑
foot joint M10.07- ☑
hand joint M10.04- ☑
hip M10.05- ☑
knee M10.06- ☑
multiple site M10.09
shoulder M10.01- ☑
vertebrae M10.08
wrist M10.03- ☑
in (due to) renal impairment M10.30

Gout, gouty — *continued*
  in renal impairment — *continued*
    ankle M10.37- ☑
    elbow M10.32- ☑
    foot joint M10.37- ☑
    hand joint M10.34- ☑
    hip M10.35- ☑
    knee M10.36- ☑
    multiple site M10.39
    shoulder M10.31- ☑
    vertebrae M10.38
    wrist M10.33- ☑
  lead-induced M10.10
    ankle M10.17- ☑
    elbow M10.12- ☑
    foot joint M10.17- ☑
    hand joint M10.14- ☑
    hip M10.15- ☑
    knee M10.16- ☑
    multiple site M10.19
    shoulder M10.11- ☑
    vertebrae M10.18
    wrist M10.13- ☑
  primary — *see* Gout, idiopathic
  saturnine — *see* Gout, lead-induced
  secondary NEC M10.40
    ankle M10.47- ☑
    elbow M10.42- ☑
    foot joint M10.47- ☑
    hand joint M10.44- ☑
    hip M10.45- ☑
    knee M10.46- ☑
    multiple site M10.49
    shoulder M10.41- ☑
    vertebrae M10.48
    wrist M10.43- ☑
  syphilitic — *see also* subcategory M14.8- A52.77
  tophi — *see* Gout, chronic
Gower's
  muscular dystrophy G71.01
  syndrome (vasovagal attack) R55
Gradenigo's syndrome — *see* Otitis, media, suppurative, acute
Graefe's disease — *see* Strabismus, paralytic, ophthalmoplegia, progressive
Graft-versus-host disease D89.813
  acute D89.810
  acute on chronic D89.812
  chronic D89.811
Grain mite (itch) B88.0
Grainhandler's disease or lung J67.8
Grand mal — *see* Epilepsy, generalized, specified NEC
Grand multipara status only (not pregnant) Z64.1
  pregnant — *see* Pregnancy, complicated by, grand multiparity
Granite worker's lung J62.8
Granular — *see also* condition
  inflammation, pharynx J31.2
  kidney (contracting) — *see* Sclerosis, renal
  liver K74.69
Granulation tissue (abnormal) (excessive) L92.9
  postmastoidectomy cavity — *see* Complications, postmastoidectomy, granulation
Granulocytopenia (primary) (malignant) — *see* Agranulocytosis
Granuloma L92.9
  abdomen K66.8
    from residual foreign body L92.3
    pyogenicum L98.0
  actinic L57.5
  annulare (perforating) L92.0
  apical K04.5
  aural — *see* Otitis, externa, specified NEC
  beryllium (skin) L92.3
  bone
    eosinophilic C96.6
    from residual foreign body — *see* Osteomyelitis, specified type NEC
    lung C96.6
  brain (any site) G06.0
    schistosomiasis B65.9 *[G07]*
  canaliculus lacrimalis — *see* Granuloma, lacrimal
  candidal (cutaneous) B37.2
  cerebral (any site) G06.0
  coccidioidal (primary) (progressive) B38.7
    lung B38.1
    meninges B38.4

Granuloma — *continued*
  colon K63.89
  conjunctiva H11.22- ☑
  dental K04.5
  ear, middle — *see* Cholesteatoma
  eosinophilic C96.6
    bone C96.6
    lung C96.6
    oral mucosa K13.4
    skin L92.2
  eyelid H01.8
  facial (e) L92.2
  foreign body (in soft tissue) NEC M60.20
    ankle M60.27- ☑
    foot M60.27- ☑
    forearm M60.23- ☑
    hand M60.24- ☑
    in operation wound — *see* Foreign body, accidentally left during a procedure
    lower leg M60.26- ☑
    pelvic region M60.25- ☑
    shoulder region M60.21- ☑
    skin L92.3
    specified site NEC M60.28
    subcutaneous tissue L92.3
    thigh M60.25- ☑
    upper arm M60.22- ☑
  gangraenescens M31.2
  genito-inguinale A58
  giant cell (central) (reparative) (jaw) M27.1
    gingiva (peripheral) K06.8
  gland (lymph) I88.8
  hepatic NEC K75.3
    in (due to)
      berylliosis J63.2 *[K77]*
      sarcoidosis D86.89
  Hodgkin C81.9 ☑
  ileum K63.89
  infectious B99.9
    specified NEC B99.8
  inguinale (Donovan) (venereal) A58
  intestine NEC K63.89
  intracranial (any site) G06.0
  intraspinal (any part) G06.1
  iridocyclitis — *see* Iridocyclitis, chronic
  jaw (bone) (central) M27.1
    reparative giant cell M27.1
  kidney — *see also* Infection, kidney N15.8
  lacrimal H04.81- ☑
  larynx J38.7
  lethal midline (faciale(e)) M31.2
  liver NEC — *see* Granuloma, hepatic
  lung (infectious) — *see also* Fibrosis, lung
    coccidioidal B38.1
    eosinophilic C96.6
  Majocchi's B35.8
  malignant (facial(e)) M31.2
  mandible (central) M27.1
  midline (lethal) M31.2
  monilial (cutaneous) B37.2
  nasal sinus — *see* Sinusitis
  operation wound T81.89 ☑
    foreign body — *see* Foreign body, accidentally left during a procedure
    stitch T81.89 ☑
    talc — *see* Foreign body, accidentally left during a procedure
  oral mucosa K13.4
  orbit, orbital H05.11- ☑
  paracoccidioidal B41.8
  penis, venereal A58
  periapical K04.5
  peritoneum K66.8
    due to ova of helminths NOS — *see also* Helminthiasis B83.9 *[K67]*
  postmastoidectomy cavity — *see* Complications, postmastoidectomy, recurrent cholesteatoma
  prostate N42.89
  pudendi (ulcerating) A58
  pulp, internal (tooth) K03.3
  pyogenic, pyogenicum (of) (skin) L98.0
    gingiva K06.8
    maxillary alveolar ridge K04.5
    oral mucosa K13.4
  rectum K62.89
  reticulohistiocytic D76.3
  rubrum nasi L74.8
  Schistosoma — *see* Schistosomiasis

Granuloma — *continued*
  septic (skin) L98.0
  silica (skin) L92.3
  sinus (accessory) (infective) (nasal) — *see* Sinusitis
  skin L92.9
    from residual foreign body L92.3
    pyogenicum L98.0
  spine
    syphilitic (epidural) A52.19
    tuberculous A18.01
  stitch (postoperative) T81.89 ☑
  suppurative (skin) L98.0
  swimming pool A31.1
  talc — *see also* Granuloma, foreign body
    in operation wound — *see* Foreign body, accidentally left during a procedure
  telangiectaticum (skin) L98.0
  tracheostomy J95.09
  trichophyticum B35.8
  tropicum A66.4
  umbilical P83.81
  umbilicus P83.81
  urethra N36.8
  uveitis — *see* Iridocyclitis, chronic
  vagina A58
  venereum A58
  vocal cord J38.3
Granulomatosis L92.9
  with polyangiitis M31.3- ☑
  eosinophilic, with polyangiitis [EGPA] M30.1
  lymphoid C83.8- ☑
  miliary (listerial) A32.89
  necrotizing, respiratory M31.30
  progressive septic D71
  specified NEC L92.8
  Wegener's M31.30
    with renal involvement M31.31
Granulomatous tissue (abnormal) (excessive) L92.9
Granulosis rubra nasi L74.8
Graphite fibrosis (of lung) J63.3
Graphospasm F48.8
  organic G25.89
Grating scapula M89.8X1
Gravel (urinary) — *see* Calculus, urinary
Graves' disease — *see* Hyperthyroidism, with, goiter
Gravis — *see* condition
Grawitz tumor C64.- ☑
Gray syndrome (newborn) P93.0
Grayness, hair (premature) L67.1
  congenital Q84.2
Green sickness D50.8
Greenfield's disease
  meaning
    concentric sclerosis (encephalitis periaxialis concentrica) G37.5
    metachromatic leukodystrophy E75.25
Greenstick fracture — *code as* Fracture, by site
Grey syndrome (newborn) P93.0
Grief F43.21
  complicated F34.81
  prolonged F43.29
  reaction — *see also* Disorder, adjustment F43.20
Griesinger's disease B76.0
Grinder's lung or pneumoconiosis J62.8
Grinding, teeth
  psychogenic F45.8
  sleep related G47.63
Grip
  Dabney's B33.0
  devil's B33.0
Grippe, grippal — *see also* Influenza
  Balkan A78
  summer, of Italy A93.1
Grisel's disease M43.6
Groin — *see* condition
Grooved tongue K14.5
Ground itch B76.9
Grover's disease or syndrome L11.1
Growing pains, children R29.898
Growth (fungoid) (neoplastic) (new) — *see also* Neoplasm
  adenoid (vegetative) J35.8
  benign — *see* Neoplasm, benign, by site
  malignant — *see* Neoplasm, malignant, by site
  rapid, childhood Z00.2
  secondary — *see* Neoplasm, secondary, by site
Gruby's disease B35.0
Gubler-Millard paralysis or syndrome G46.3

Guerin-Stern syndrome Q74.3
Guidance, insufficient anterior (occlusal) M26.54
Guillain-Barré disease or syndrome G61.0
　　sequelae G65.0
Guinea worms (infection) (infestation) B72
Guinon's disease (motor-verbal tic) F95.2
Gull's disease E03.4
Gum — see condition
Gumboil K04.7
　　with sinus K04.6
Gumma (syphilitic) A52.79
　　artery A52.09
　　　　cerebral A52.04
　　bone A52.77
　　　　of yaws (late) A66.6
　　brain A52.19
　　cauda equina A52.19
　　central nervous system A52.3
　　ciliary body A52.71
　　congenital A50.59
　　eyelid A52.71
　　heart A52.06
　　intracranial A52.19
　　iris A52.71
　　kidney A52.75
　　larynx A52.73
　　leptomeninges A52.19
　　liver A52.74
　　meninges A52.19
　　myocardium A52.06
　　nasopharynx A52.73
　　neurosyphilitic A52.3
　　nose A52.73
　　orbit A52.71
　　palate (soft) A52.79
　　penis A52.76
　　pericardium A52.06
　　pharynx A52.73
　　pituitary A52.79
　　scrofulous (tuberculous) A18.4
　　skin A52.79
　　specified site NEC A52.79
　　spinal cord A52.19
　　tongue A52.79
　　tonsil A52.73
　　trachea A52.73
　　tuberculous A18.4
　　ulcerative due to yaws A66.4
　　ureter A52.75
　　yaws A66.4
　　　　bone A66.6
Gunn's syndrome Q07.8
Gunshot wound — see also Puncture, open
　　fracture — code as Fracture, by site
　　internal organs — see Injury, by site
Gynandrism Q56.0
Gynandroblastoma
　　specified site — see Neoplasm, uncertain behavior, by
　　　　site
　　unspecified site
　　　　female D39.10
　　　　male D40.10
Gynecological examination (periodic) (routine) Z01.419
　　with abnormal findings Z01.411
Gynecomastia N62
Gynephobia F40.291
Gyrate scalp Q82.8

H

H (Hartnup's) **disease** E72.02
Haas' disease or osteochondrosis (juvenile) (head of
　　humerus) — see Osteochondrosis, juvenile, humerus
Habit, habituation
　　bad sleep Z72.821
　　chorea F95.8
　　disturbance, child F98.9
　　drug — see Dependence, drug
　　irregular sleep Z72.821
　　laxative F55.2
　　spasm — see Tic
　　tic — see Tic
Haemophilus (H.) **influenzae, as cause of disease
　　classified elsewhere** B96.3
Haff disease — see Poisoning, mercury
Hageman's factor defect, deficiency or disease D68.2

Haglund's disease or osteochondrosis (juvenile) (os
　　tibiale externum) — see Osteochondrosis, juvenile,
　　tarsus
Hailey-Hailey disease Q82.8
Hair — see also condition
　　plucking F63.3
　　　　in stereotyped movement disorder F98.4
　　tourniquet syndrome — see also Constriction, external,
　　　　by site
　　　　finger S60.44- ☑
　　　　penis S30.842 ☑
　　　　thumb S60.34- ☑
　　　　toe S90.44- ☑
Hairball in stomach T18.2 ☑
Hair-pulling, pathological (compulsive) F63.3
Hairy black tongue K14.3
Half vertebra Q76.49
Halitosis R19.6
Hallerman-Streiff syndrome Q87.0
Hallervorden-Spatz disease G23.0
Hallopeau's acrodermatitis or disease L40.2
Hallucination R44.3
　　auditory R44.0
　　gustatory R44.2
　　olfactory R44.2
　　specified NEC R44.2
　　tactile R44.2
　　visual R44.1
Hallucinosis (chronic) F28
　　alcoholic (acute) F10.951
　　　　in
　　　　　　abuse F10.151
　　　　　　dependence F10.251
　　drug-induced F19.951
　　　　cannabis F12.951
　　　　cocaine F14.951
　　　　hallucinogen F16.151
　　　　in
　　　　　　abuse F19.151
　　　　　　　　cannabis F12.151
　　　　　　　　cocaine F14.151
　　　　　　　　hallucinogen F16.151
　　　　　　　　inhalant F18.151
　　　　　　　　opioid F11.151
　　　　　　　　sedative, anxiolytic or hypnotic F13.151
　　　　　　　　stimulant NEC F15.151
　　　　　　dependence F19.251
　　　　　　　　cannabis F12.251
　　　　　　　　cocaine F14.251
　　　　　　　　hallucinogen F16.251
　　　　　　　　inhalant F18.251
　　　　　　　　opioid F11.251
　　　　　　　　sedative, anxiolytic or hypnotic F13.251
　　　　　　　　stimulant NEC F15.251
　　　　inhalant F18.951
　　　　opioid F11.951
　　　　sedative, anxiolytic or hypnotic F13.951
　　　　stimulant NEC F15.951
　　organic F06.0
Hallux
　　deformity (acquired) NEC M20.5X- ☑
　　limitus M20.5X- ☑
　　malleus (acquired) NEC M20.3- ☑
　　rigidus (acquired) M20.2- ☑
　　　　congenital Q74.2
　　　　sequelae (late effect) of rickets E64.3
　　valgus (acquired) M20.1- ☑
　　　　congenital Q66.6
　　varus (acquired) M20.3- ☑
　　　　congenital Q66.3- ☑
Halo, visual H53.19
Hamartoma, hamartoblastoma Q85.9
　　epithelial (gingival), odontogenic, central or peripheral
　　　　— see Cyst, calcifying odontogenic
Hamartosis Q85.9
Hamman-Rich syndrome J84.114
Hammer toe (acquired) NEC — see also Deformity, toe,
　　hammer toe
　　congenital Q66.89
　　sequelae (late effect) of rickets E64.3
Hand — see condition
Hand-foot syndrome L27.1
Handicap, handicapped
　　educational Z55.9
　　　　specified NEC Z55.8
Hand-Schüller-Christian disease or syndrome C96.5

Hanging (asphyxia) (strangulation) (suffocation) — see
　　Asphyxia, traumatic, due to mechanical threat
Hangnail — see also Cellulitis, digit
　　with lymphangitis — see Lymphangitis, acute, digit
Hangover (alcohol) F10.129
Hanhart's syndrome Q87.0
Hanot-Chauffard (-Troisier) **syndrome** E83.19
Hanot's cirrhosis or disease K74.3
Hansen's disease — see Leprosy
Hantaan virus disease (Korean hemorrhagic fever) A98.5
Hantavirus disease (with renal manifestations) (Dobrava)
　　(Puumala) (Seoul) A98.5
　　with pulmonary manifestations (Andes) (Bayou)
　　　　(Bermejo) (Black Creek Canal) (Choclo) (Juquitiba)
　　　　(Laguna negra) (Lechiguanas) (New York) (Oran)
　　　　(Sin nombre) B33.4
Happy puppet syndrome Q93.51
Harada's disease or syndrome H30.81- ☑
Hardening
　　artery — see Arteriosclerosis
　　brain G93.89
Hardship, material Z59.87
Harelip (complete) (incomplete) — see Cleft, lip
Harlequin (newborn) Q80.4
Harley's disease D59.6
Harmful use (of)
　　alcohol F10.10
　　anxiolytics — see Abuse, drug, sedative
　　cannabinoids — see Abuse, drug, cannabis
　　cocaine — see Abuse, drug, cocaine
　　drug — see Abuse, drug
　　hallucinogens — see Abuse, drug, hallucinogen
　　hypnotics — see Abuse, drug, sedative
　　opioids — see Abuse, drug, opioid
　　PCP (phencyclidine) — see Abuse, drug, hallucinogen
　　sedatives — see Abuse, drug, sedative
　　stimulants NEC — see Abuse, drug, stimulant
Harris' lines — see Arrest, epiphyseal
Hartnup's disease E72.02
Harvester's lung J67.0
Harvesting ovum for in vitro fertilization Z31.83
Hashimoto's disease or thyroiditis E06.3
Hashitoxicosis (transient) E06.3
Hassal-Henle bodies or warts (cornea) H18.49
Haut mal — see Epilepsy, generalized, specified NEC
Haverhill fever A25.1
Hay fever — see also Fever, hay J30.1
Hayem-Widal syndrome D59.8
Haygarth's nodes M15.8
Haymaker's lung J67.0
Hb (abnormal)
　　Bart's disease D56.0
　　disease — see Disease, hemoglobin
　　trait — see Trait
Head — see condition
Headache R51.9
　　with
　　　　orthostatic component NEC R51.0
　　　　positional component NEC R51.0
　　allergic NEC G44.89
　　associated with sexual activity G44.82
　　cervicogenic G44.86
　　chronic daily R51.9
　　cluster G44.009
　　　　chronic G44.029
　　　　　　intractable G44.021
　　　　　　not intractable G44.029
　　　　episodic G44.019
　　　　　　intractable G44.011
　　　　　　not intractable G44.019
　　　　intractable G44.001
　　　　not intractable G44.009
　　cough (primary) G44.83
　　daily chronic R51.9
　　drug-induced NEC G44.40
　　　　intractable G44.41
　　　　not intractable G44.40
　　exertional (primary) G44.84
　　histamine G44.009
　　　　intractable G44.001
　　　　not intractable G44.009
　　hypnic G44.81
　　lumbar puncture G97.1
　　medication overuse G44.40
　　　　intractable G44.41
　　　　not intractable G44.40
　　menstrual — see Migraine, menstrual

Headache — *continued*
  migraine (type) — *see also* Migraine G43.909
  nasal septum R51.9
  neuralgiform, short lasting unilateral, with conjunctival injection and tearing (SUNCT) G44.059
    intractable G44.051
    not intractable G44.059
  new daily persistent (NDPH) G44.52
  orgasmic G44.82
  periodic syndromes in adults and children G43.C0 (*following* G43.7)
    with refractory migraine G43.C1 (*following* G43.7)
    intractable G43.C1 (*following* G43.7)
    not intractable G43.C0 (*following* G43.7)
    without refractory migraine G43.C0 (*following* G43.7)
  postspinal puncture G97.1
  post-traumatic G44.309
    acute G44.319
      intractable G44.311
      not intractable G44.319
    chronic G44.329
      intractable G44.321
      not intractable G44.329
    intractable G44.301
    not intractable G44.309
  pre-menstrual — *see* Migraine, menstrual
  preorgasmic G44.82
  primary
    cough G44.83
    exertional G44.84
    stabbing G44.85
    thunderclap G44.53
  rebound G44.40
    intractable G44.41
    not intractable G44.40
  short lasting unilateral neuralgiform, with conjunctival injection and tearing (SUNCT) G44.059
    intractable G44.051
    not intractable G44.059
  specified syndrome NEC G44.89
  spinal and epidural anesthesia - induced T88.59 ☑
    in labor and delivery O74.5
    in pregnancy O29.4- ☑
    postpartum, puerperal O89.4
  spinal fluid loss (from puncture) G97.1
  stabbing (primary) G44.85
  tension (-type) G44.209
    chronic G44.229
      intractable G44.221
      not intractable G44.229
    episodic G44.219
      intractable G44.211
      not intractable G44.219
    intractable G44.201
    not intractable G44.209
  thunderclap (primary) G44.53
  vascular NEC G44.1
Healthy
  infant
    accompanying sick mother Z76.3
    receiving care Z76.2
  person accompanying sick person Z76.3
Hearing examination Z01.10
  with abnormal findings NEC Z01.118
  following failed hearing screening Z01.110
  for hearing conservation and treatment Z01.12
  infant or child (over 28 days old) Z00.129
    with abnormal findings Z00.121
Heart — *see* condition
Heart beat
  abnormality R00.9
    specified NEC R00.8
  awareness R00.2
  rapid R00.0
  slow R00.1
Heartburn R12
  psychogenic F45.8
Heartland virus disease A93.8
Heat (effects) T67.9 ☑
  apoplexy T67.01 ☑
  burn — *see also* Burn L55.9
  collapse T67.1 ☑
  cramps T67.2 ☑
  dermatitis or eczema L59.0
  edema T67.7 ☑
  erythema — *code by site under* Burn, first degree
  excessive T67.9 ☑
    specified effect NEC T67.8 ☑

Heat — *continued*
  exhaustion T67.5 ☑
    anhydrotic T67.3 ☑
    due to
      salt (and water) depletion T67.4 ☑
      water depletion T67.3 ☑
        with salt depletion T67.4 ☑
  fatigue (transient) T67.6 ☑
  fever T67.01 ☑
  hyperpyrexia T67.01 ☑
  prickly L74.0
  prostration — *see* Heat, exhaustion
  pyrexia T67.01 ☑
  rash L74.0
  specified effect NEC T67.8 ☑
  stroke T67.01 ☑
    exertional T67.02 ☑
    specified NEC T67.09 ☑
  sunburn — *see* Sunburn
  syncope T67.1 ☑
Heavy-for-dates NEC (infant) (4000g to 4499g) P08.1
  exceptionally (4500g or more) P08.0
Hebephrenia, hebephrenic (schizophrenia) F20.1
Heberden's disease or nodes (with arthropathy) M15.1
Hebra's
  pityriasis L26
  prurigo L28.2
Heel — *see* condition
Heerfordt's disease D86.89
Hegglin's anomaly or syndrome D72.0
Heilmeyer-Schoner disease D45
Heine-Medin disease A80.9
Heinz body anemia, congenital D58.2
Heliophobia F40.228
Heller's disease or syndrome F84.3
HELLP syndrome (hemolysis, elevated liver enzymes and low platelet count) O14.2- ☑
  complicating
    childbirth O14.24
    puerperium O14.25
Helminthiasis — *see also* Infestation, helminth
  Ancylostoma B76.0
  intestinal B82.0
    mixed types (types classifiable to more than one of the titles B65.0-B81.3 and B81.8) B81.4
    specified type NEC B81.8
  mixed types (intestinal) (types classifiable to more than one of the titles B65.0-B81.3 and B81.8) B81.4
  Necator (americanus) B76.1
  specified type NEC B83.8
Heloma L84
Hemangioblastoma — *see* Neoplasm, connective tissue, uncertain behavior
  malignant — *see* Neoplasm, connective tissue, malignant
Hemangioendothelioma — *see also* Neoplasm, uncertain behavior, by site
  benign D18.00
    intra-abdominal D18.03
    intracranial D18.02
    skin D18.01
    specified site NEC D18.09
  bone (diffuse) — *see* Neoplasm, bone, malignant
  epithelioid — *see also* Neoplasm, uncertain behavior, by site
    malignant — *see* Neoplasm, malignant, by site
  malignant — *see* Neoplasm, connective tissue, malignant
Hemangiofibroma — *see* Neoplasm, benign, by site
Hemangiolipoma — *see* Lipoma
Hemangioma D18.00
  arteriovenous D18.00
    intra-abdominal D18.03
    intracranial D18.02
    skin D18.01
    specified site NEC D18.09
  capillary I78.1
    intra-abdominal D18.03
    intracranial D18.02
    skin D18.01
    specified site NEC D18.09
  cavernous D18.00
    intra-abdominal D18.03
    intracranial D18.02
    skin D18.01
    specified site NEC D18.09
  epithelioid D18.00

Hemangioma — *continued*
  epithelioid — *continued*
    intra-abdominal D18.03
    intracranial D18.02
    skin D18.01
    specified site NEC D18.09
  histiocytoid D18.00
    intra-abdominal D18.03
    intracranial D18.02
    skin D18.01
    specified site NEC D18.09
  infantile D18.00
    intra-abdominal D18.03
    intracranial D18.02
    skin D18.01
    specified site NEC D18.09
  intra-abdominal D18.03
  intracranial D18.02
  intramuscular D18.00
    intra-abdominal D18.03
    intracranial D18.02
    skin D18.01
    specified site NEC D18.09
  intrathoracic structures D18.09
  juvenile D18.00
  malignant — *see* Neoplasm, connective tissue, malignant
  plexiform D18.00
    intra-abdominal D18.03
    intracranial D18.02
    skin D18.01
    specified site NEC D18.09
  racemose D18.00
    intra-abdominal D18.03
    intracranial D18.02
    skin D18.01
    specified site NEC D18.09
  sclerosing — *see* Neoplasm, skin, benign
  simplex D18.00
    intra-abdominal D18.03
    intracranial D18.02
    skin D18.01
    specified site NEC D18.09
  skin D18.01
  specified site NEC D18.09
  venous D18.00
    intra-abdominal D18.03
    intracranial D18.02
    skin D18.01
    specified site NEC D18.09
  verrucous keratotic D18.00
    intra-abdominal D18.03
    intracranial D18.02
    skin D18.01
    specified site NEC D18.09
Hemangiomatosis (systemic) I78.8
  involving single site — *see* Hemangioma
Hemangiopericytoma — *see also* Neoplasm, connective tissue, uncertain behavior
  benign — *see* Neoplasm, connective tissue, benign
  malignant — *see* Neoplasm, connective tissue, malignant
Hemangiosarcoma — *see* Neoplasm, connective tissue, malignant
Hemarthrosis (nontraumatic) M25.00
  ankle M25.07- ☑
  elbow M25.02- ☑
  foot joint M25.07- ☑
  hand joint M25.04- ☑
  hip M25.05- ☑
  in hemophilic arthropathy — *see* Arthropathy, hemophilic
  knee M25.06- ☑
  shoulder M25.01- ☑
  specified joint NEC M25.08
  traumatic — *see* Sprain, by site
  vertebrae M25.08
  wrist M25.03- ☑
Hematemesis K92.0
  with ulcer — *code by site under* Ulcer, with hemorrhage K27.4
  newborn, neonatal P54.0
    due to swallowed maternal blood P78.2
Hematidrosis L74.8
Hematinuria — *see also* Hemoglobinuria
  malarial B50.8
Hematobilia K83.8

Hematocele
  female NEC N94.89
    with ectopic pregnancy O00.90
      with intrauterine pregnancy O00.91
      ovary N83.8
  male N50.1
Hematochezia — see also Melena K92.1
Hematochyluria — see also Infestation, filarial
    schistosomiasis (bilharziasis) B65.0
Hematocolpos (with hematometra or hematosalpinx)
    N89.7
Hematocornea — see Pigmentation, cornea, stromal
Hematogenous — see condition
Hematoma (traumatic) (skin surface intact) — see also
    Contusion
  with
    injury of internal organs — see Injury, by site
    open wound — see Wound, open
  amputation stump (surgical) (late) T87.89
  aorta, dissecting I71.00
    abdominal I71.02
    thoracic — see also Dissection, aorta, thoracic
      I71.019
    thoracoabdominal I71.03
  aortic intramural — see Dissection, aorta
  arterial (complicating trauma) — see Injury, blood
      vessel, by site
  auricle — see Contusion, ear
    nontraumatic — see Disorder, pinna, hematoma
  birth injury NEC P15.8
  brain (traumatic)
    with
      cerebral laceration or contusion (diffuse) — see
        Injury, intracranial, diffuse
      focal — see Injury, intracranial, focal
    cerebellar, traumatic S06.37- ☑
    intracerebral, traumatic — see Injury, intracranial,
      intracerebral hemorrhage
    newborn NEC P52.4
      birth injury P10.1
    nontraumatic — see Hemorrhage, intracranial
    subarachnoid, arachnoid, traumatic — see Injury,
      intracranial, subarachnoid hemorrhage
    subdural, traumatic — see Injury, intracranial, sub-
      dural hemorrhage
  breast (nontraumatic) N64.89
  broad ligament (nontraumatic) N83.7
    traumatic S37.892 ☑
  cerebellar, traumatic S06.37- ☑
  cerebral — see Hematoma, brain
  cerebrum S06.36- ☑
    left S06.35- ☑
    right S06.34- ☑
  cesarean delivery wound O90.2
  complicating delivery (perineal) (pelvic) (vagina) (vulva)
      O71.7
  corpus cavernosum (nontraumatic) N48.89
  epididymis (nontraumatic) N50.1
  epidural (traumatic) — see Injury, intracranial, epidural
      hemorrhage
    spinal — see Injury, spinal cord, by region
  episiotomy O90.2
  face, birth injury P15.4
  genital organ NEC (nontraumatic)
    female (nonobstetric) N94.89
      traumatic S30.202 ☑
    male N50.1
      traumatic S30.201 ☑
  internal organs — see Injury, by site
  intracerebral, traumatic — see Injury, intracranial, in-
      tracerebral hemorrhage
  intraoperative — see Complications, intraoperative,
      hemorrhage
  labia (nontraumatic) (nonobstetric) N90.89
  liver (subcapsular) (nontraumatic) K76.89
    birth injury P15.0
  mediastinum — see Injury, intrathoracic
  mesosalpinx (nontraumatic) N83.7
    traumatic S37.898 ☑
  muscle — code by site under Contusion
  nontraumatic
    muscle M79.81
    soft tissue M79.81
  obstetrical surgical wound O90.2
  orbit, orbital (nontraumatic) — see also Hemorrhage,
      orbit
    traumatic — see Contusion, orbit

Hematoma — continued
  pelvis (female) (nontraumatic) (nonobstetric) N94.89
    obstetric O71.7
    traumatic — see Injury, by site
  penis (nontraumatic) N48.89
    birth injury P15.5
  perianal (nontraumatic) K64.5
  perineal S30.23 ☑
    complicating delivery O71.7
  perirenal — see Injury, kidney
  pinna — see Contusion, ear
    nontraumatic — see Disorder, pinna, hematoma
  placenta O43.89- ☑
  postoperative (postprocedural) — see Complication,
      postprocedural, hematoma
  retroperitoneal (nontraumatic) K66.1
    traumatic S36.892 ☑
  scrotum, superficial S30.22 ☑
    birth injury P15.5
  seminal vesicle (nontraumatic) N50.1
    traumatic S37.892 ☑
  spermatic cord (traumatic) S37.892 ☑
    nontraumatic N50.1
  spinal (cord) (meninges) — see also Injury, spinal cord,
      by region
    newborn (birth injury) P11.5
  spleen D73.5
    intraoperative — see Complications, intraoperative,
      hemorrhage, spleen
    postprocedural (postoperative) — see Complica-
      tions, postprocedural, hemorrhage, spleen
  sternocleidomastoid, birth injury P15.2
  sternomastoid, birth injury P15.2
  subarachnoid (traumatic) — see Injury, intracranial,
      subarachnoid hemorrhage
    newborn (nontraumatic) P52.5
      due to birth injury P10.3
    nontraumatic — see Hemorrhage, intracranial,
      subarachnoid
  subdural (traumatic) — see Injury, intracranial, subdural
      hemorrhage
    newborn (localized) P52.8
      birth injury P10.0
    nontraumatic — see Hemorrhage, intracranial,
      subdural
  superficial, newborn P54.5
  testis (nontraumatic) N50.1
    birth injury P15.5
  tunica vaginalis (nontraumatic) N50.1
  umbilical cord, complicating delivery O69.5 ☑
  uterine ligament (broad) (nontraumatic) N83.7
    traumatic S37.892 ☑
  vagina (ruptured) (nontraumatic) N89.8
    complicating delivery O71.7
  vas deferens (nontraumatic) N50.1
    traumatic S37.892 ☑
  vitreous — see Hemorrhage, vitreous
  vulva (nontraumatic) (nonobstetric) N90.89
    complicating delivery O71.7
    newborn (birth injury) P15.5
Hematometra N85.7
  with hematocolpos N89.7
Hematomyelia (central) G95.19
  newborn (birth injury) P11.5
  traumatic T14.8 ☑
Hematomyelitis G04.90
Hematoperitoneum — see Hemoperitoneum
Hematophobia F40.230
Hematopneumothorax (see Hemothorax)
Hematopoiesis, cyclic D70.4
Hematoporphyria — see Porphyria
Hematorachis, hematorrhachis G95.19
  newborn (birth injury) P11.5
Hematosalpinx N83.6
  with
    hematocolpos N89.7
    hematometra N85.7
      with hematocolpos N89.7
  infectional — see Salpingitis
Hematospermia R36.1
Hematothorax (see Hemothorax)
Hematuria R31.9
  benign (familial) (of childhood) — see also Hematuria,
      idiopathic
    essential microscopic R31.1
  due to sulphonamide, sulfonamide — see Table of
      Drugs and Chemicals, by drug

Hematuria — continued
  endemic — see also Schistosomiasis B65.0
  gross R31.0
  idiopathic N02.9
    with glomerular lesion
      C3
        glomerulonephritis N02.A
        glomerulopathy N02.A
          with dense deposit disease N02.6
      crescentic (diffuse) glomerulonephritis N02.7
      dense deposit disease N02.6
      endocapillary proliferative glomerulonephritis
        N02.4
      focal and segmental hyalinosis or sclerosis N02.1
      membranoproliferative (diffuse) N02.5
      membranous (diffuse) N02.2
      mesangial proliferative (diffuse) N02.3
      mesangiocapillary (diffuse) N02.5
      minor abnormality N02.0
      proliferative NEC N02.8
      specified pathology NEC N02.8
  intermittent — see Hematuria, idiopathic
  malarial B50.8
  microscopic NEC (with symptoms) R31.29
    asymptomatic R31.21
    benign essential R31.1
  paroxysmal — see also Hematuria, idiopathic
    nocturnal D59.5
  persistent — see Hematuria, idiopathic
  recurrent — see Hematuria, idiopathic
  tropical — see also Schistosomiasis B65.0
  tuberculous A18.13
Hemeralopia (day blindness) H53.11
  vitamin A deficiency E50.5
Hemi-akinesia R41.4
Hemialgesia R20.0
Hemianencephaly Q00.0
Hemianesthesia R20.0
Hemianopia, hemianopsia (heteronymous) H53.47
  homonymous H53.46- ☑
  syphilitic A52.71
Hemiathetosis R25.8
Hemiatrophy R68.89
  cerebellar G31.9
  face, facial, progressive (Romberg) G51.8
  tongue K14.8
Hemiballism (us) G25.5
Hemicardia Q24.8
Hemicephalus, hemicephaly Q00.0
Hemichorea G25.5
Hemicolitis, left — see Colitis, left sided
Hemicrania
  congenital malformation Q00.0
  continua G44.51
  meaning migraine — see also Migraine G43.909
  paroxysmal G44.039
    chronic G44.049
      intractable G44.041
      not intractable G44.049
    episodic G44.039
      intractable G44.031
      not intractable G44.039
    intractable G44.031
    not intractable G44.039
Hemidystrophy — see Hemiatrophy
Hemiectromelia Q73.8
Hemihypalgesia R20.8
Hemihypesthesia R20.1
Hemi-inattention R41.4
Hemimelia Q73.8
  lower limb — see Defect, reduction, lower limb, speci-
      fied type NEC
  upper limb — see Defect, reduction, upper limb, spec-
      ified type NEC
Hemiparalysis — see Hemiplegia
Hemiparesis — see Hemiplegia
Hemiparesthesia R20.2
Hemiparkinsonism G20
Hemiplegia G81.9- ☑
  alternans facialis G83.89
  ascending NEC G81.90
    spinal G95.89
  congenital (cerebral) G80.8
    spastic G80.2
  embolic (current episode) I63.4- ☑
  flaccid G81.0- ☑
  following
    cerebrovascular disease I69.959

Hemiplegia — *continued*
  following — *continued*
    cerebrovascular disease — *continued*
      cerebral infarction I69.35- ☑
      intracerebral hemorrhage I69.15- ☑
      nontraumatic intracranial hemorrhage NEC
        I69.25- ☑
      specified disease NEC I69.85- ☑
      stroke NOS I69.35- ☑
      subarachnoid hemorrhage I69.05- ☑
  hysterical F44.4
  newborn NEC P91.88
    birth injury P11.9
  spastic G81.1- ☑
    congenital G80.2
  thrombotic (current episode) I63.3- ☑
Hemisection, spinal cord — *see* Injury, spinal cord, by
  region
Hemispasm (facial) R25.2
Hemisporosis B48.8
Hemitremor R25.1
Hemivertebra Q76.49
  failure of segmentation with scoliosis Q76.3
  fusion with scoliosis Q76.3
Hemochromatosis E83.119
  with refractory anemia D46.1
  due to repeated red blood cell transfusion E83.111
  hereditary (primary) E83.110
  neonatal P78.84
  primary E83.110
  specified NEC E83.118
Hemoglobin — *see also* condition
  abnormal (disease) — *see* Disease, hemoglobin
  AS genotype D57.3
  Constant Spring D58.2
  E-beta thalassemia D56.5
  fetal, hereditary persistence (HPFH) D56.4
  H Constant Spring D56.0
  low NOS D64.9
  S (Hb S), heterozygous D57.3
Hemoglobinemia D59.9
  due to blood transfusion T80.89 ☑
  paroxysmal D59.6
  nocturnal D59.5
Hemoglobinopathy (mixed) D58.2
  with thalassemia D56.8
  sickle-cell D57.1
    with thalassemia D57.40
      with
        acute chest syndrome D57.411
        cerebral vascular involvement D57.413
        crisis (painful) D57.419
          with specified complication NEC D57.418
        splenic sequestration D57.412
        vasoocclusive pain D57.419
      without crisis D57.40
Hemoglobinuria R82.3
  with anemia, hemolytic, acquired (chronic) NEC D59.6
  cold (paroxysmal) (with Raynaud's syndrome) D59.6
    agglutinin D59.12
  due to exertion or hemolysis NEC D59.6
  intermittent D59.6
  malarial B50.8
  march D59.6
  nocturnal (paroxysmal) D59.5
  paroxysmal (cold) D59.6
    nocturnal D59.5
Hemolymphangioma D18.1
Hemolysis
  intravascular
    with
      abortion — *see* Abortion, by type, complicated
        by, hemorrhage
      ectopic or molar pregnancy O08.1
      hemorrhage
        antepartum — *see* Hemorrhage, antepartum,
          with coagulation defect
        intrapartum — *see also* Hemorrhage, compli-
          cating, delivery O67.0
      postpartum O72.3
  neonatal (excessive) P58.9
    specified NEC P58.8
Hemolytic — *see* condition
Hemopericardium I31.2
  following acute myocardial infarction (current compli-
    cation) I23.0
  newborn P54.8
  traumatic — *see* Injury, heart, with hemopericardium

Hemoperitoneum K66.1
  infectional K65.9
  traumatic S36.899 ☑
    with open wound — *see* Wound, open, with pene-
      tration into peritoneal cavity
Hemophilia (classical) (familial) (hereditary) D66
  A D66
  acquired D68.311
  autoimmune D68.311
  B D67
  C D68.1
  calcipriva — *see also* Defect, coagulation D68.4
  nonfamilial — *see also* Defect, coagulation D68.4
  secondary D68.311
  vascular — *see* Disease, von Willebrand
Hemophthalmos H44.81- ☑
Hemopneumothorax — *see also* Hemothorax
  traumatic S27.2 ☑
Hemoptysis R04.2
  newborn P26.9
  tuberculous — *see* Tuberculosis, pulmonary
Hemorrhage, hemorrhagic (concealed) R58
  abdomen R58
  accidental antepartum — *see* Hemorrhage, antepartum
  acute idiopathic pulmonary, in infants R04.81
  adenoid J35.8
  adrenal (capsule) (gland) E27.49
    medulla E27.8
    newborn P54.4
  after delivery — *see* Hemorrhage, postpartum
  alveolar
    lung, newborn P26.8
    process K08.89
  alveolus K08.89
  amputation stump (surgical) T87.89
  anemia (chronic) D50.0
    acute D62
  antepartum (with) O46.90
    with coagulation defect O46.00- ☑
      afibrinogenemia O46.01- ☑
      disseminated intravascular coagulation
        O46.02- ☑
      hypofibrinogenemia O46.01- ☑
      specified defect NEC O46.09- ☑
    before 20 weeks gestation O20.9
      specified type NEC O20.8
      threatened abortion O20.0
    due to
      abruptio placenta — *see also* Abruptio placentae
        O45.9- ☑
      leiomyoma, uterus — *see* Hemorrhage, antepar-
        tum, specified cause NEC
      placenta previa O44.1- ☑
    specified cause NEC — *see* subcategory O46.8X- ☑
  anus (sphincter) K62.5
  apoplexy (stroke) — *see* Hemorrhage, intracranial, in-
    tracerebral
  arachnoid — *see* Hemorrhage, intracranial, subarach-
    noid
  artery R58
    brain — *see* Hemorrhage, intracranial, intracerebral
  basilar (ganglion) I61.0
  bladder N32.89
  bowel K92.2
    newborn P54.3
  brain (miliary) (nontraumatic) — *see* Hemorrhage, in-
    tracranial, intracerebral
    due to
      birth injury P10.1
      syphilis A52.05
    epidural or extradural (traumatic) — *see* Injury, in-
      tracranial, epidural hemorrhage
    newborn P52.4
      birth injury P10.1
    subarachnoid — *see* Hemorrhage, intracranial,
      subarachnoid
    subdural — *see* Hemorrhage, intracranial, subdural
  brainstem (nontraumatic) I61.3
    traumatic S06.38- ☑
  breast N64.59
  bronchial tube — *see* Hemorrhage, lung
  bronchopulmonary — *see* Hemorrhage, lung
  bronchus — *see* Hemorrhage, lung
  bulbar I61.5
  capillary I78.8
    primary D69.8
  cecum K92.2

Hemorrhage, hemorrhagic — *continued*
  cerebellar, cerebellum (nontraumatic) I61.4
    newborn P52.6
    traumatic S06.37- ☑
  cerebral, cerebrum — *see also* Hemorrhage, intracra-
    nial, intracerebral
    lobe I61.1
    newborn (anoxic) P52.4
      birth injury P10.1
  cerebromeningeal I61.8
  cerebrospinal — *see* Hemorrhage, intracranial, intrac-
    erebral
  cervix (uteri) (stump) NEC N88.8
  chamber, anterior (eye) — *see* Hyphema
  childbirth — *see* Hemorrhage, complicating, delivery
  choroid H31.30- ☑
    expulsive H31.31- ☑
  ciliary body — *see* Hyphema
  cochlea — *see* subcategory H83.8 ☑
  colon K92.2
  complicating
    abortion — *see* Abortion, by type, complicated by,
      hemorrhage
    delivery O67.9
      associated with coagulation defect (afibrinogen-
        emia) (DIC) (hyperfibrinolysis) O67.0
      specified cause NEC O67.8
      surgical procedure — *see* Hemorrhage, intraopera-
        tive
  conjunctiva H11.3- ☑
    newborn P54.8
  cord, newborn (stump) P51.9
  corpus luteum (ruptured) cyst N83.1- ☑
  cortical (brain) I61.1
  cranial — *see* Hemorrhage, intracranial
  cutaneous R23.3
    due to autosensitivity, erythrocyte D69.2
    newborn P54.5
  delayed
    following ectopic or molar pregnancy O08.1
    postpartum O72.2
  diathesis (familial) D69.9
  disease D69.9
    newborn P53
    specified type NEC D69.8
  due to or associated with
    afibrinogenemia or other coagulation defect (condi-
      tions in categories D65- D69)
      antepartum — *see* Hemorrhage, antepartum,
        with coagulation defect
      intrapartum O67.0
    dental implant M27.61
    device, implant or graft — *see also* Complications,
      by site and type, specified NEC T85.838 ☑
      arterial graft NEC T82.838 ☑
      breast T85.838 ☑
      catheter NEC T85.838 ☑
        dialysis (renal) T82.838 ☑
          intraperitoneal T85.838 ☑
        infusion NEC T82.838 ☑
          spinal (epidural) (subdural) T85.830 ☑
        urinary (indwelling) T83.83 ☑
      electronic (electrode) (pulse generator) (stimula-
        tor)
        bone T84.83 ☑
        cardiac T82.837 ☑
        nervous system (brain) (peripheral nerve)
          (spinal) T85.830 ☑
        urinary T83.83 ☑
      fixation, internal (orthopedic) NEC T84.83 ☑
      gastrointestinal (bile duct) (esophagus)
        T85.838 ☑
      genital NEC T83.83 ☑
      heart NEC T82.837 ☑
      joint prosthesis T84.83 ☑
      ocular (corneal graft) (orbital implant) NEC
        T85.838 ☑
      orthopedic NEC T84.83 ☑
        bone graft T86.838 ☑
      specified NEC T85.838 ☑
      urinary NEC T83.83 ☑
      vascular NEC T82.838 ☑
      ventricular intracranial shunt T85.830 ☑
  duodenum, duodenal K92.2
    ulcer — *see* Ulcer, duodenum, with hemorrhage
  dura mater — *see* Hemorrhage, intracranial, subdural
  endotracheal — *see* Hemorrhage, lung

Hemorrhage, hemorrhagic — *continued*
  epicranial subaponeurotic (massive), birth injury P12.2
  epidural (traumatic) — *see also* Injury, intracranial,
      epidural hemorrhage
    nontraumatic I62.1
  esophagus K22.89
    varix I85.01
      secondary I85.11
  excessive, following ectopic gestation (subsequent
      episode) O08.1
  extradural (traumatic) — *see* Injury, intracranial,
      epidural hemorrhage
    birth injury P10.8
    newborn (anoxic) (nontraumatic) P52.8
    nontraumatic I62.1
  eye NEC H57.89
    fundus — *see* Hemorrhage, retina
    lid — *see* Disorder, eyelid, specified type NEC
  fallopian tube N83.6
  fibrinogenolysis — *see* Fibrinolysis
  fibrinolytic (acquired) — *see* Fibrinolysis
  from
    ear (nontraumatic) — *see* Otorrhagia
    tracheostomy stoma J95.01
  fundus, eye — *see* Hemorrhage, retina
  funis — *see* Hemorrhage, umbilicus, cord
  gastric — *see* Hemorrhage, stomach
  gastroenteric K92.2
    newborn P54.3
  gastrointestinal (tract) K92.2
    newborn P54.3
  genital organ, male N50.1
  genitourinary (tract) NOS R31.9
  gingiva K06.8
  globe (eye) — *see* Hemophthalmos
  graafian follicle cyst (ruptured) N83.0- ☑
  gum K06.8
  heart I51.89
  hypopharyngeal (throat) R04.1
  intermenstrual (regular) N92.3
    irregular N92.1
  internal (organs) NEC R58
    capsule I61.0
    ear — *see* subcategory H83.8 ☑
    newborn P54.8
  intestine K92.2
    newborn P54.3
  intra-abdominal R58
  intra-alveolar (lung), newborn P26.8
  intracerebral (nontraumatic) — *see* Hemorrhage, in-
      tracranial, intracerebral
  intracranial (nontraumatic) I62.9
    birth injury P10.9
    epidural, nontraumatic I62.1
    extradural, nontraumatic I62.1
    intracerebral (nontraumatic) (in) I61.9
      brain stem I61.3
      cerebellum I61.4
      hemisphere I61.2
        cortical (superficial) I61.1
        subcortical (deep) I61.0
      intraoperative
        during a nervous system procedure G97.31
        during other procedure G97.32
      intraventricular I61.5
      multiple localized I61.6
      newborn P52.4
        birth injury P10.1
      postprocedural
        following a nervous system procedure G97.51
        following other procedure G97.52
      specified NEC I61.8
      superficial I61.1
      traumatic (diffuse) — *see* Injury, intracranial,
        diffuse
      focal — *see* Injury, intracranial, focal
    newborn P52.9
      specified NEC P52.8
    subarachnoid (nontraumatic) (from) I60.9
      intracranial (cerebral) artery I60.7
        anterior communicating I60.2
        basilar I60.4
        carotid siphon and bifurcation I60.0- ☑
        communicating I60.7
          anterior I60.2
          posterior I60.3- ☑
        middle cerebral I60.1- ☑
        posterior communicating I60.3- ☑

Hemorrhage, hemorrhagic — *continued*
  intracranial — *continued*
    subarachnoid — *continued*
      intracranial artery — *continued*
        specified artery NEC I60.6
        vertebral I60.5- ☑
      newborn P52.5
        birth injury P10.3
      specified NEC I60.8
      traumatic S06.6X- ☑
    subdural (nontraumatic) I62.00
      acute I62.01
      birth injury P10.0
      chronic I62.03
      newborn (anoxic) (hypoxic) P52.8
        birth injury P10.0
      spinal G95.19
      subacute I62.02
      traumatic — *see* Injury, intracranial, subdural
        hemorrhage
    traumatic — *see* Injury, intracranial, focal brain in-
      jury
  intramedullary NEC G95.19
  intraocular — *see* Hemophthalmos
  intraoperative, intraprocedural — *see* Complication,
      hemorrhage (hematoma), intraoperative (in-
      traprocedural), by site
  intrapartum — *see* Hemorrhage, complicating, delivery
  intrapelvic
    female N94.89
    male K66.1
  intraperitoneal K66.1
  intrapontine I61.3
  intraprocedural — *see* Complication, hemorrhage
      (hematoma), intraoperative (intraprocedural),
      by site
  intrauterine N85.7
    complicating delivery — *see also* Hemorrhage,
      complicating, delivery O67.9
    postpartum — *see* Hemorrhage, postpartum
  intraventricular I61.5
    newborn (nontraumatic) — *see also* Newborn, af-
      fected by, hemorrhage P52.3
      due to birth injury P10.2
      grade
        1 P52.0
        2 P52.1
        3 P52.21
        4 P52.22
  intravesical N32.89
  iris (postinfectional) (postinflammatory) (toxic) — *see*
      Hyphema
  joint (nontraumatic) — *see* Hemarthrosis
  kidney N28.89
  knee (joint) (nontraumatic) — *see* Hemarthrosis, knee
  labyrinth — *see* subcategory H83.8 ☑
  lenticular striate artery I61.0
  ligature, vessel — *see* Hemorrhage, postoperative
  liver K76.89
  lung R04.89
    newborn P26.9
      massive P26.1
      specified NEC P26.8
    tuberculous — *see* Tuberculosis, pulmonary
  massive umbilical, newborn P51.0
  mediastinum — *see* Hemorrhage, lung
  medulla I61.3
  membrane (brain) I60.8
    spinal cord — *see* Hemorrhage, spinal cord
  meninges, meningeal (brain) (middle) I60.8
    spinal cord — *see* Hemorrhage, spinal cord
  mesentery K66.1
  metritis — *see* Endometritis
  mouth K13.79
  mucous membrane NEC R58
    newborn P54.8
  muscle M62.89
  nail (subungual) L60.8
  nasal turbinate R04.0
    newborn P54.8
  navel, newborn P51.9
  newborn P54.9
    specified NEC P54.8
  nipple N64.59
  nose R04.0
    newborn P54.8
  omentum K66.1
  optic nerve (sheath) H47.02- ☑

Hemorrhage, hemorrhagic — *continued*
  orbit, orbital H05.23- ☑
  ovary NEC N83.8
  oviduct N83.6
  pancreas K86.89
  parathyroid (gland) (spontaneous) E21.4
  parturition — *see* Hemorrhage, complicating, delivery
  penis N48.89
  pericardium, pericarditis I31.2
  peritoneum, peritoneal K66.1
  peritonsillar tissue J35.8
    due to infection J36
  petechial R23.3
    due to autosensitivity, erythrocyte D69.2
  pituitary (gland) E23.6
  pleura — *see* Hemorrhage, lung
  polioencephalitis, superior E51.2
  polymyositis — *see* Polymyositis
  pons, pontine I61.3
  posterior fossa (nontraumatic) I61.8
    newborn P52.6
  postmenopausal N95.0
  postnasal R04.0
  postoperative — *see* Complications, postprocedural,
      hemorrhage, by site
  postpartum NEC (following delivery of placenta) O72.1
    delayed or secondary O72.2
    retained placenta O72.0
    third stage O72.0
  pregnancy — *see* Hemorrhage, antepartum
  preretinal — *see* Hemorrhage, retina
  prostate N42.1
  puerperal — *see* Hemorrhage, postpartum
    delayed or secondary O72.2
  pulmonary R04.89
    newborn P26.9
      massive P26.1
      specified NEC P26.8
    tuberculous — *see* Tuberculosis, pulmonary
  purpura (primary) D69.3
  rectum (sphincter) K62.5
    newborn P54.2
  recurring, following initial hemorrhage at time of injury
      T79.2 ☑
  renal N28.89
  respiratory passage or tract R04.9
    specified NEC R04.89
  retina, retinal (vessels) H35.6- ☑
    diabetic — *see* Microaneurysm, retinal, diabetic
  retroperitoneal R58
  scalp R58
  scrotum N50.1
  secondary (nontraumatic) R58
    following initial hemorrhage at time of injury
      T79.2 ☑
  seminal vesicle N50.1
  skin R23.3
    newborn P54.5
  slipped umbilical ligature P51.8
  spermatic cord N50.1
  spinal (cord) G95.19
    newborn (birth injury) P11.5
  spleen D73.5
    intraoperative — *see* Complications, intraoperative,
      hemorrhage, spleen
    postprocedural — *see* Complications, postprocedu-
      ral, hemorrhage, spleen
  stomach K92.2
    newborn P54.3
    ulcer — *see* Ulcer, stomach, with hemorrhage
  subarachnoid (nontraumatic) — *see* Hemorrhage, in-
      tracranial, subarachnoid
  subconjunctival — *see also* Hemorrhage, conjunctiva
    birth injury P15.3
  subcortical (brain) I61.0
  subcutaneous R23.3
  subdiaphragmatic R58
  subdural (acute) (nontraumatic) — *see* Hemorrhage,
      intracranial, subdural
  subependymal
    newborn P52.0
      with intraventricular extension P52.1
        and intracerebral extension P52.22
  subgaleal P12.2
  subhyaloid — *see* Hemorrhage, retina
  subperiosteal — *see* Disorder, bone, specified type NEC
  subretinal — *see* Hemorrhage, retina
  subtentorial — *see* Hemorrhage, intracranial, subdural

Hemorrhage, hemorrhagic — *continued*
- subungual L60.8
- suprarenal (capsule) (gland) E27.49
    - newborn P54.4
- tentorium (traumatic) NEC — *see* Hemorrhage, brain
    - newborn (birth injury) P10.4
- testis N50.1
- third stage (postpartum) O72.0
- thorax — *see* Hemorrhage, lung
- throat R04.1
- thymus (gland) E32.8
- thyroid (cyst) (gland) E07.89
- tongue K14.8
- tonsil J35.8
- trachea — *see* Hemorrhage, lung
- tracheobronchial R04.89
    - newborn P26.0
- traumatic — *code to* specific injury
    - cerebellar — *see* Hemorrhage, brain
    - intracranial — *see* Hemorrhage, brain
    - recurring or secondary (following initial hemorrhage at time of injury) T79.2 ☑
- tuberculous NEC — *see also* Tuberculosis, pulmonary A15.0
- tunica vaginalis N50.1
- ulcer — *code by* site under Ulcer, with hemorrhage K27.4
- umbilicus, umbilical
    - cord
        - after birth, newborn P51.9
        - complicating delivery O69.5 ☑
    - newborn P51.9
        - massive P51.0
        - slipped ligature P51.8
    - stump P51.9
- urethra (idiopathic) N36.8
- uterus, uterine (abnormal) N93.9
    - climacteric N92.4
    - complicating delivery — *see* Hemorrhage, complicating, delivery
    - dysfunctional or functional N93.8
    - intermenstrual (regular) N92.3
        - irregular N92.1
    - postmenopausal N95.0
    - postpartum — *see* Hemorrhage, postpartum
    - preclimacteric or premenopausal N92.4
    - prepubertal N93.8
    - pubertal N92.2
- vagina (abnormal) N93.9
    - newborn P54.6
- vas deferens N50.1
- vasa previa O69.4 ☑
- ventricular I61.5
- vesical N32.89
- viscera NEC R58
    - newborn P54.8
- vitreous (humor) (intraocular) H43.1- ☑
- vulva N90.89

Hemorrhoids (bleeding) (without mention of degree) K64.9
- 1st degree (grade/stage I) (without prolapse outside of anal canal) K64.0
- 2nd degree (grade/stage II) (that prolapse with straining but retract spontaneously) K64.1
- 3rd degree (grade/stage III) (that prolapse with straining and require manual replacement back inside anal canal) K64.2
- 4th degree (grade/stage IV) (with prolapsed tissue that cannot be manually replaced) K64.3
- complicating
    - pregnancy O22.4 ☑
    - puerperium O87.2
- external K64.4
    - with
        - thrombosis K64.5
- internal (without mention of degree) K64.8
- prolapsed K64.8
- skin tags
    - anus K64.4
    - residual K64.4
- specified NEC K64.8
- strangulated — *see also* Hemorrhoids, by degree K64.8
- thrombosed — *see also* Hemorrhoids, by degree K64.5
- ulcerated — *see also* Hemorrhoids, by degree K64.8

Hemosalpinx N83.6
- with
    - hematocolpos N89.7
    - hematometra N85.7

Hemosalpinx — *continued*
- with — *continued*
    - hematometra — *continued*
        - with hematocolpos N89.7

Hemosiderosis (dietary) E83.19
- pulmonary, idiopathic E83.1- ☑ [J84.03]
- transfusion T80.89 ☑

Hemothorax (bacterial) (nontuberculous) J94.2
- newborn P54.8
- traumatic S27.1 ☑
    - with pneumothorax S27.2 ☑
- tuberculous NEC A15.6

Henoch (-Schönlein) **disease or syndrome** (purpura) D69.0

Henpue, henpuye A66.6

Hepar lobatum (syphilitic) A52.74

Hepatalgia K76.89

Hepatitis K75.9
- acute B17.9
    - with coma K72.01
    - with hepatic failure — *see* Failure, hepatic
    - alcoholic — *see* Hepatitis, alcoholic
    - infectious B17.9
    - non-viral K72.0 ☑
    - viral B17.9
- alcoholic (acute) (chronic) K70.10
    - with ascites K70.11
- amebic — *see* Abscess, liver, amebic
- anicteric, (viral) — *see* Hepatitis, viral
- antigen-associated (HAA) — *see* Hepatitis, B
- Australia-antigen (positive) — *see* Hepatitis, B
- autoimmune K75.4
- B B19.10
    - with hepatic coma B19.11
    - acute B16.9
        - with
            - delta-agent (coinfection) (without hepatic coma) B16.1
                - with hepatic coma B16.0
            - hepatic coma (without delta-agent coinfection) B16.2
    - chronic B18.1
        - with delta-agent B18.0
- bacterial NEC K75.89
- C (viral) B19.20
    - with hepatic coma B19.21
    - acute B17.10
        - with hepatic coma B17.11
    - chronic B18.2
- catarrhal (acute) B15.9
    - with hepatic coma B15.0
- cholangiolitic K75.89
- cholestatic K75.89
- chronic K73.9
    - active NEC K73.2
    - lobular NEC K73.1
    - persistent NEC K73.0
    - specified NEC K73.8
- cytomegaloviral B25.1
- due to ethanol (acute) (chronic) — *see* Hepatitis, alcoholic
- epidemic B15.9
    - with hepatic coma B15.0
- fulminant NEC (viral) — *see* Hepatitis, viral
- granulomatous NEC K75.3
- herpesviral B00.81
- history of
    - B Z86.19
    - C Z86.19
- homologous serum — *see* Hepatitis, viral, type B
- in (due to)
    - mumps B26.81
    - toxoplasmosis (acquired) B58.1
        - congenital (active) P37.1 [K77]
- infectious, infective B15.9
    - acute (subacute) B17.9
    - chronic B18.9
- inoculation — *see* Hepatitis, viral, type B
- interstitial (chronic) K74.69
- ischemia, ischemic K72.00
- lupoid NEC K75.4
- malignant NEC (with hepatic failure) K72.90
    - with coma K72.91
- neonatal (idiopathic) (toxic) P59.29
- neonatal giant cell P59.29
- newborn P59.29
- non-viral K72.0 ☑
- postimmunization — *see* Hepatitis, viral, type B

Hepatitis — *continued*
- post-transfusion — *see* Hepatitis, viral, type B
- reactive, nonspecific K75.2
- serum — *see* Hepatitis, viral, type B
- shock K72.00
- specified type NEC
    - with hepatic failure — *see* Failure, hepatic
- syphilitic (late) A52.74
    - congenital (early) A50.08 [K77]
        - late A50.59 [K77]
    - secondary A51.45
- toxic — *see also* Disease, liver, toxic K71.6
- tuberculous A18.83
- viral, virus B19.9
    - with hepatic coma B19.0
    - acute B17.9
    - chronic B18.9
        - specified NEC B18.8
        - type
            - B B18.1
                - with delta-agent B18.0
            - C B18.2
    - congenital P35.3
    - coxsackie B33.8 [K77]
    - cytomegalic inclusion B25.1
    - in remission, any type — *code to* Hepatitis, chronic, by type
    - non-A, non-B B17.8
    - specified type NEC (with or without coma) B17.8
    - type
        - A B15.9
            - with hepatic coma B15.0
        - B B19.10
            - with hepatic coma B19.11
            - acute B16.9
                - with
                    - delta-agent (coinfection) (without hepatic coma) B16.1
                        - with hepatic coma B16.0
                    - hepatic coma (without delta-agent coinfection) B16.2
            - chronic B18.1
                - with delta-agent B18.0
        - C B19.20
            - with hepatic coma B19.21
            - acute B17.10
                - with hepatic coma B17.11
            - chronic B18.2
        - E B17.2
        - non-A, non-B B17.8

Hepatization lung (acute) — *see* Pneumonia, lobar

Hepatoblastoma C22.2

Hepatocarcinoma C22.0

Hepatocholangiocarcinoma C22.0

Hepatocholangioma, benign D13.4

Hepatocholangitis K75.89

Hepatolenticular degeneration E83.01

Hepatoma (malignant) C22.0
- benign D13.4
- embryonal C22.0

Hepatomegaly — *see also* Hypertrophy, liver
- with splenomegaly R16.2
- congenital Q44.7
- in mononucleosis
    - gammaherpesviral B27.09
    - infectious specified NEC B27.89

Hepatoptosis K76.89

Hepatorenal syndrome following labor and delivery O90.4

Hepatosis K76.89

Hepatosplenomegaly R16.2
- hyperlipemic (Bürger-Grütz type) E78.3 [K77]

Hereditary — *see* condition

Hereditary alpha tryptasemia (syndrome) D89.44

Heredodegeneration, macular — *see* Dystrophy, retina

Heredopathia atactica polyneuritiformis G60.1

Heredosyphilis — *see* Syphilis, congenital

Herlitz' syndrome Q81.1

Hermansky-Pudlak syndrome E70.331

Hermaphrodite, hermaphroditism (true) Q56.0
- 46,XX with streak gonads Q99.1
- 46,XX/46,XY Q99.0
- 46,XY with streak gonads Q99.1
- chimera 46,XX/46,XY Q99.0

Hernia, hernial (acquired) (recurrent) K46.9
- with
    - gangrene — *see* Hernia, by site, with, gangrene
    - incarceration — *see* Hernia, by site, with, obstruction

☑ **Additional Character Required** — **Refer to the Tabular List for Character Selection**

Hernia, hernial — *continued*
  with — *continued*
    irreducible — *see* Hernia, by site, with, obstruction
    obstruction — *see* Hernia, by site, with, obstruction
    strangulation — *see* Hernia, by site, with, obstruction
  abdomen, abdominal K46.9
    with
      gangrene (and obstruction) K46.1
      obstruction K46.0
    femoral — *see* Hernia, femoral
    incisional — *see* Hernia, incisional
    inguinal — *see* Hernia, inguinal
    specified site NEC K45.8
      with
        gangrene (and obstruction) K45.1
        obstruction K45.0
    umbilical — *see* Hernia, umbilical
    wall — *see* Hernia, ventral
  appendix — *see* Hernia, abdomen
  bladder (mucosa) (sphincter)
    congenital (female) (male) Q79.51
    female — *see* Cystocele
    male N32.89
  brain, congenital — *see* Encephalocele
  cartilage, vertebra — *see* Displacement, intervertebral disc
  cerebral, congenital — *see also* Encephalocele
    endaural Q01.8
  ciliary body (traumatic) S05.2- ☑
  colon — *see* Hernia, abdomen
  Cooper's — *see* Hernia, abdomen, specified site NEC
  crural — *see* Hernia, femoral
  diaphragm, diaphragmatic K44.9
    with
      gangrene (and obstruction) K44.1
      obstruction K44.0
    congenital Q79.0
  direct (inguinal) — *see* Hernia, inguinal
  diverticulum, intestine — *see* Hernia, abdomen
  double (inguinal) — *see* Hernia, inguinal, bilateral
  due to adhesions (with obstruction) K56.50
  epigastric — *see also* Hernia, ventral K43.9
  esophageal hiatus — *see* Hernia, hiatal
  external (inguinal) — *see* Hernia, inguinal
  fallopian tube N83.4- ☑
  fascia M62.89
  femoral K41.90
    with
      gangrene (and obstruction) K41.40
        not specified as recurrent K41.40
        recurrent K41.41
      obstruction K41.30
        not specified as recurrent K41.30
        recurrent K41.31
    not specified as recurrent K41.90
    recurrent K41.91
    bilateral K41.20
      with
        gangrene (and obstruction) K41.10
          not specified as recurrent K41.10
          recurrent K41.11
        obstruction K41.00
          not specified as recurrent K41.00
          recurrent K41.01
      not specified as recurrent K41.20
      recurrent K41.21
    unilateral K41.90
      with
        gangrene (and obstruction) K41.40
          not specified as recurrent K41.40
          recurrent K41.41
        obstruction K41.30
          not specified as recurrent K41.30
          recurrent K41.31
      not specified as recurrent K41.90
      recurrent K41.91
  foramen magnum G93.5
    congenital Q01.8
  funicular (umbilical) — *see also* Hernia, umbilicus
    spermatic (cord) — *see* Hernia, inguinal
  gastrointestinal tract — *see* Hernia, abdomen
  Hesselbach's — *see* Hernia, femoral, specified site NEC
  hiatal (esophageal) (sliding) K44.9
    with
      gangrene (and obstruction) K44.1
      obstruction K44.0
    congenital Q40.1

Hernia, hernial — *continued*
  hypogastric — *see* Hernia, ventral
  incarcerated — *see also* Hernia, by site, with obstruction
    with gangrene — *see* Hernia, by site, with gangrene
  incisional K43.2
    with
      gangrene (and obstruction) K43.1
      obstruction K43.0
  indirect (inguinal) — *see* Hernia, inguinal
  inguinal (direct) (external) (funicular) (indirect) (internal) (oblique) (scrotal) (sliding) K40.90
    with
      gangrene (and obstruction) K40.40
        not specified as recurrent K40.40
        recurrent K40.41
      obstruction K40.30
        not specified as recurrent K40.30
        recurrent K40.31
    not specified as recurrent K40.90
    recurrent K40.91
    bilateral K40.20
      with
        gangrene (and obstruction) K40.10
          not specified as recurrent K40.10
          recurrent K40.11
        obstruction K40.00
          not specified as recurrent K40.00
          recurrent K40.01
      not specified as recurrent K40.20
      recurrent K40.21
    unilateral K40.90
      with
        gangrene (and obstruction) K40.40
          not specified as recurrent K40.40
          recurrent K40.41
        obstruction K40.30
          not specified as recurrent K40.30
          recurrent K40.31
      not specified as recurrent K40.90
      recurrent K40.91
  internal — *see also* Hernia, abdomen
    inguinal — *see* Hernia, inguinal
  interstitial — *see* Hernia, abdomen
  intervertebral cartilage or disc — *see* Displacement, intervertebral disc
  intestine, intestinal — *see* Hernia, by site
  intra-abdominal — *see* Hernia, abdomen
  iris (traumatic) S05.2- ☑
  irreducible — *see also* Hernia, by site, with obstruction
    with gangrene — *see* Hernia, by site, with gangrene
  ischiatic — *see* Hernia, abdomen, specified site NEC
  ischiorectal — *see* Hernia, abdomen, specified site NEC
  lens (traumatic) S05.2- ☑
  linea (alba) (semilunaris) — *see* Hernia, ventral
  Littre's — *see* Hernia, abdomen
  lumbar — *see* Hernia, abdomen, specified site NEC
  lung (subcutaneous) J98.4
  mediastinum J98.59
  mesenteric (internal) — *see* Hernia, abdomen
  midline — *see* Hernia, ventral
  muscle (sheath) M62.89
  nucleus pulposus — *see* Displacement, intervertebral disc
  oblique (inguinal) — *see* Hernia, inguinal
  obstructive — *see also* Hernia, by site, with obstruction
    with gangrene — *see* Hernia, by site, with gangrene
  obturator — *see* Hernia, abdomen, specified site NEC
  omental — *see* Hernia, abdomen
  ovary N83.4- ☑
  oviduct N83.4- ☑
  paraesophageal — *see also* Hernia, diaphragm
    congenital Q40.1
  parastomal K43.5
    with
      gangrene (and obstruction) K43.4
      obstruction K43.3
  paraumbilical — *see* Hernia, umbilicus
  perineal — *see* Hernia, abdomen, specified site NEC
  Petit's — *see* Hernia, abdomen, specified site NEC
  postoperative — *see* Hernia, incisional
  pregnant uterus — *see* Abnormal, uterus in pregnancy or childbirth
  prevesical N32.89
  properitoneal — *see* Hernia, abdomen, specified site NEC
  pudendal — *see* Hernia, abdomen, specified site NEC
  rectovaginal N81.6

Hernia, hernial — *continued*
  retroperitoneal — *see* Hernia, abdomen, specified site NEC
  Richter's — *see* Hernia, abdomen, with obstruction
  Rieux's, Riex's — *see* Hernia, abdomen, specified site NEC
  sac condition (adhesion) (dropsy) (inflammation) (laceration) (suppuration) — *code by site under Hernia*
  sciatic — *see* Hernia, abdomen, specified site NEC
  scrotum, scrotal — *see* Hernia, inguinal
  sliding (inguinal) — *see also* Hernia, inguinal
    hiatus — *see* Hernia, hiatal
  spigelian — *see* Hernia, ventral
  spinal — *see* Spina bifida
  strangulated — *see also* Hernia, by site, with obstruction
    with gangrene — *see* Hernia, by site, with gangrene
  subxiphoid — *see* Hernia, ventral
  supra-umbilicus — *see* Hernia, ventral
  tendon — *see* Disorder, tendon, specified type NEC
  Treitz's (fossa) — *see* Hernia, abdomen, specified site NEC
  tunica vaginalis Q55.29
  umbilicus, umbilical K42.9
    with
      gangrene (and obstruction) K42.1
      obstruction K42.0
  ureter N28.89
  urethra, congenital Q64.79
  urinary meatus, congenital Q64.79
  uterus N81.4
    pregnant — *see* Abnormal, uterus in pregnancy or childbirth
  vaginal (anterior) (wall) — *see* Cystocele
  Velpeau's — *see* Hernia, femoral
  ventral K43.9
    with
      gangrene (and obstruction) K43.7
      obstruction K43.6
    incisional K43.2
      with
        gangrene (and obstruction) K43.1
        obstruction K43.0
    recurrent — *see* Hernia, incisional
    specified NEC K43.9
      with
        gangrene (and obstruction) K43.7
        obstruction K43.6
  vesical
    congenital (female) (male) Q79.51
    female — *see* Cystocele
    male N32.89
  vitreous (into wound) S05.2- ☑
    into anterior chamber — *see* Prolapse, vitreous
Herniation — *see also* Hernia
  brain (stem) G93.5
    nontraumatic G93.5
    traumatic S06.A1 ☑
      cerebellar S06.A1 ☑
      subfalcine (cingulate) S06.A1 ☑
      tonsillar S06.A1 ☑
      transtentorial (central) (upward cerebellar) S06.A1 ☑
      uncal S06.A1 ☑
  cerebral G93.5
    nontraumatic G93.5
    traumatic S06.A1 ☑
  mediastinum J98.59
  nucleus pulposus — *see* Displacement, intervertebral disc
Herpangina B08.5
Herpes, herpesvirus, herpetic B00.9
  anogenital A60.9
    perianal skin A60.1
    rectum A60.1
    urogenital tract A60.00
      cervix A60.03
      male genital organ NEC A60.02
      penis A60.01
      specified site NEC A60.09
      vagina A60.04
      vulva A60.04
  blepharitis (zoster) B02.39
    simplex B00.59
  circinatus B35.4
    bullosus L12.0
  conjunctivitis (simplex) B00.53

Herpes, herpesvirus, herpetic — *continued*
conjunctivitis — *continued*
zoster B02.31
cornea B02.33
encephalitis B00.4
due to herpesvirus 6 B10.01
due to herpesvirus 7 B10.09
specified NEC B10.09
eye (zoster) B02.30
simplex B00.50
eyelid (zoster) B02.39
simplex B00.59
facialis B00.1
febrilis B00.1
geniculate ganglionitis B02.21
genital, genitalis A60.00
female A60.09
male A60.02
gestational, gestationis O26.4- ☑
gingivostomatitis B00.2
human B00.9
1 — *see* Herpes, simplex
2 — *see* Herpes, simplex
3 — *see* Varicella
4 — *see* Mononucleosis, Epstein-Barr (virus)
5 — *see* Disease, cytomegalic inclusion (generalized)
6
encephalitis B10.01
specified NEC B10.81
7
encephalitis B10.09
specified NEC B10.82
8 B10.89
infection NEC B10.89
Kaposi's sarcoma associated B10.89
iridocyclitis (simplex) B00.51
zoster B02.32
iris (vesicular erythema multiforme) L51.9
iritis (simplex) B00.51
Kaposi's sarcoma associated B10.89
keratitis (simplex) (dendritic) (disciform) (interstitial) B00.52
zoster (interstitial) B02.33
keratoconjunctivitis (simplex) B00.52
zoster B02.33
labialis B00.1
lip B00.1
meningitis (simplex) B00.3
zoster B02.1
ophthalmicus (zoster) NEC B02.30
simplex B00.50
penis A60.01
perianal skin A60.1
pharyngitis, pharyngotonsillitis B00.2
rectum A60.1
scrotum A60.02
sepsis B00.7
simplex B00.9
complicated NEC B00.89
congenital P35.2
conjunctivitis B00.53
external ear B00.1
eyelid B00.59
hepatitis B00.81
keratitis (interstitial) B00.52
myelitis B00.82
specified complication NEC B00.89
visceral B00.89
stomatitis B00.2
tonsurans B35.0
visceral B00.89
vulva A60.04
whitlow B00.89
zoster — *see also* condition B02.9
auricularis B02.21
complicated NEC B02.8
conjunctivitis B02.31
disseminated B02.7
encephalitis B02.0
eye (lid) B02.39
geniculate ganglionitis B02.21
keratitis (interstitial) B02.33
meningitis B02.1
myelitis B02.24
neuritis, neuralgia B02.29
ophthalmicus NEC B02.30
oticus B02.21
polyneuropathy B02.23

Herpes, herpesvirus, herpetic — *continued*
zoster — *see also* condition — *continued*
specified complication NEC B02.8
trigeminal neuralgia B02.22
Herpesvirus (human) — *see* Herpes
Herpetophobia F40.218
Herrick's anemia — *see* Disease, sickle-cell
Hers' disease E74.09
Herter-Gee syndrome K90.0
Herxheimer's reaction R68.89
Hesitancy
of micturition R39.11
urinary R39.11
Hesselbach's hernia — *see* Hernia, femoral, specified site NEC
Heterochromia (congenital) Q13.2
cataract — *see* Cataract, complicated
cyclitis (Fuchs) — *see* Cyclitis, Fuchs' heterochromic hair L67.1
iritis — *see* Cyclitis, Fuchs' heterochromic
retained metallic foreign body (nonmagnetic) — *see* Foreign body, intraocular, old, retained
magnetic — *see* Foreign body, intraocular, old, retained, magnetic
uveitis — *see* Cyclitis, Fuchs' heterochromic
Heterophoria — *see* Strabismus, heterophoria
Heterophyes, heterophyiasis (small intestine) B66.8
Heterotopia, heterotopic — *see also* Malposition, congenital
cerebralis Q04.8
Heterotropia — *see* Strabismus
Heubner-Herter disease K90.0
Hexadactylism Q69.9
HGSIL (cytology finding) (high grade squamous intraepithelial lesion on cytologic smear) (Pap smear finding)
anus R85.613
cervix R87.613
biopsy (histology) finding — *see* Neoplasia, intraepithelial, cervix, grade II or grade III
vagina R87.623
biopsy (histology) finding — *see* Neoplasia, intraepithelial, cervix, grade II or grade III
Hibernoma — *see* Lipoma
Hiccup, hiccough R06.6
epidemic B33.0
psychogenic F45.8
Hidden penis (congenital) Q55.64
acquired N48.83
Hidradenitis (axillaris) (suppurative) L73.2
Hidradenoma (nodular) — *see also* Neoplasm, skin, benign
clear cell — *see* Neoplasm, skin, benign
papillary — *see* Neoplasm, skin, benign
Hidrocystoma — *see* Neoplasm, skin, benign
High
altitude effects T70.20 ☑
anoxia T70.29 ☑
on
ears T70.0 ☑
sinuses T70.1 ☑
polycythemia D75.1
arch
foot Q66.7- ☑
palate, congenital Q38.5
arterial tension — *see* Hypertension
basal metabolic rate R94.8
blood pressure — *see also* Hypertension
borderline R03.0
reading (incidental) (isolated) (nonspecific), without diagnosis of hypertension R03.0
cholesterol E78.00
with high triglycerides E78.2
diaphragm (congenital) Q79.1
expressed emotional level within family Z63.8
head at term O32.4 ☑
palate, congenital Q38.5
risk
infant NEC Z76.2
sexual behavior (heterosexual) Z72.51
bisexual Z72.53
homosexual Z72.52
scrotal testis, testes
bilateral Q53.23
unilateral Q53.13
temperature (of unknown origin) R50.9
thoracic rib Q76.6

High — *continued*
triglycerides E78.1
with high cholesterol E78.2
Hildenbrand's disease A75.0
Hilum — *see* condition
Hip — *see* condition
Hippel's disease Q85.83
Hippophobia F40.218
Hippus H57.09
Hirschsprung's disease or megacolon Q43.1
Hirsutism, hirsuties L68.0
Hirudiniasis
external B88.3
internal B83.4
Hiss-Russell dysentery A03.1
Histidinemia, histidinuria E70.41
Histiocytoma — *see also* Neoplasm, skin, benign
fibrous — *see also* Neoplasm, skin, benign
atypical — *see* Neoplasm, connective tissue, uncertain behavior
malignant — *see* Neoplasm, connective tissue, malignant
Histiocytosis D76.3
acute differentiated progressive C96.0
Langerhans' cell NEC C96.6
multifocal X
multisystemic (disseminated) C96.0
unisystemic C96.5
pulmonary, adult (adult PLCH) J84.82
unifocal (X) C96.6
lipid, lipoid D76.3
essential E75.29
malignant C96.A (*following* C96.6)
mononuclear phagocytes NEC D76.1
Langerhans' cells C96.6
non-Langerhans cell D76.3
polyostotic sclerosing D76.3
sinus, with massive lymphadenopathy D76.3
syndrome NEC D76.3
X NEC C96.6
acute (progressive) C96.0
chronic C96.6
multifocal C96.5
multisystemic C96.0
unifocal C96.6
Histoplasmosis B39.9
with pneumonia NEC B39.2
African B39.5
American — *see* Histoplasmosis, capsulati
capsulati B39.4
disseminated B39.3
generalized B39.3
pulmonary B39.2
acute B39.0
chronic B39.1
Darling's B39.4
duboisii B39.5
lung NEC B39.2
History
family (of) — *see also* History, personal (of)
alcohol abuse Z81.1
allergy NEC Z84.89
anemia Z83.2
arthritis Z82.61
asthma Z82.5
blindness Z82.1
cardiac death (sudden) Z82.41
carrier of genetic disease Z84.81
chromosomal anomaly Z82.79
chronic
disabling disease NEC Z82.8
lower respiratory disease Z82.5
colonic polyps Z83.71
congenital malformations and deformations Z82.79
polycystic kidney Z82.71
consanguinity Z84.3
deafness Z82.2
diabetes mellitus Z83.3
disability NEC Z82.8
disease or disorder (of)
allergic NEC Z84.89
behavioral NEC Z81.8
blood and blood-forming organs Z83.2
cardiovascular NEC Z82.49
chronic disabling NEC Z82.8
digestive Z83.79
ear NEC Z83.52
elevated lipoprotein (a) (Lp(a)) Z83.430

History — *continued*
  family — *see also* History, personal — *continued*
    disease or disorder — *continued*
      endocrine NEC Z83.49
      eye NEC Z83.518
        glaucoma Z83.511
      familial hypercholesterolemia Z83.42
      genitourinary NEC Z84.2
      glaucoma Z83.511
      hematological Z83.2
      immune mechanism Z83.2
      infectious NEC Z83.1
      ischemic heart Z82.49
      kidney Z84.1
      lipoprotein metabolism Z83.438
      mental NEC Z81.8
      metabolic Z83.49
      musculoskeletal NEC Z82.69
      neurological NEC Z82.0
      nutritional Z83.49
      parasitic NEC Z83.1
      psychiatric NEC Z81.8
      respiratory NEC Z83.6
      skin and subcutaneous tissue NEC Z84.0
      specified NEC Z84.89
    drug abuse NEC Z81.3
    elevated lipoprotein (a) (Lp(a)) Z83.430
    epilepsy Z82.0
    familial hypercholesterolemia Z83.42
    genetic disease carrier Z84.81
    glaucoma Z83.511
    hearing loss Z82.2
    human immunodeficiency virus (HIV) infection Z83.0
    Huntington's chorea Z82.0
    hyperlipidemia, familial combined Z83.438
    intellectual disability Z81.0
    leukemia Z80.6
    lipidemia NEC Z83.438
    malignant neoplasm (of) NOS Z80.9
      bladder Z80.52
      breast Z80.3
      bronchus Z80.1
      digestive organ Z80.0
      gastrointestinal tract Z80.0
      genital organ Z80.49
        ovary Z80.41
        prostate Z80.42
        specified organ NEC Z80.49
        testis Z80.43
      hematopoietic NEC Z80.7
      intrathoracic organ NEC Z80.2
      kidney Z80.51
      lung Z80.1
      lymphatic NEC Z80.7
      ovary Z80.41
      prostate Z80.42
      respiratory organ NEC Z80.2
      specified site NEC Z80.8
      testis Z80.43
      trachea Z80.1
      urinary organ or tract Z80.59
        bladder Z80.52
        kidney Z80.51
    mental
      disorder NEC Z81.8
    multiple endocrine neoplasia (MEN) syndrome Z83.41
    osteoporosis Z82.62
    polycystic kidney Z82.71
    polyps (colon) Z83.71
    psychiatric disorder Z81.8
    psychoactive substance abuse NEC Z81.3
    respiratory condition NEC Z83.6
      asthma and other lower respiratory conditions Z82.5
    self-harmful behavior Z81.8
    SIDS (sudden infant death syndrome) Z84.82
    skin condition Z84.0
    specified condition NEC Z84.89
    stroke (cerebrovascular) Z82.3
    substance abuse NEC Z81.4
      alcohol Z81.1
      drug NEC Z81.3
      psychoactive NEC Z81.3
      tobacco Z81.2
    sudden
      cardiac death Z82.41
      infant death syndrome (SIDS) Z84.82
    tobacco abuse Z81.2

History — *continued*
  family — *see also* History, personal — *continued*
    violence, violent behavior Z81.8
    visual loss Z82.1
  personal (of) — *see also* History, family (of)
    abuse
      adult Z91.419
        forced labor or sexual exploitation Z91.42
        physical and sexual Z91.410
        psychological Z91.411
      childhood Z62.819
        forced labor or sexual exploitation in childhood Z62.813
        physical Z62.810
        psychological Z62.811
        sexual Z62.810
    alcohol dependence F10.21
    allergy (to) Z88.9
      analgesic agent NEC Z88.6
      anesthetic Z88.4
      antibiotic agent NEC Z88.1
      anti-infective agent NEC Z88.3
      contrast media Z91.041
      drugs, medicaments and biological substances Z88.9
        specified NEC Z88.8
      food Z91.018
        additives Z91.02
        beef Z91.014
        eggs Z91.012
        lamb Z91.014
        mammalian meats Z91.014
        milk products Z91.011
        peanuts Z91.010
        pork Z91.014
        red meats Z91.014
        seafood Z91.013
        specified food NEC Z91.018
      insect Z91.038
        bee Z91.030
      latex Z91.040
      medicinal agents Z88.9
        specified NEC Z88.8
      narcotic agent NEC Z88.5
      nonmedicinal agents Z91.048
      penicillin Z88.0
      serum Z88.7
      specified NEC Z91.09
      sulfonamides Z88.2
      vaccine Z88.7
    anaphylactic shock Z87.892
    anaphylaxis Z87.892
    behavioral disorders Z86.59
    benign carcinoid tumor Z86.012
    benign neoplasm Z86.018
      brain Z86.011
      carcinoid Z86.012
      colonic polyps Z86.010
    brain injury (traumatic) Z87.820
    breast implant removal Z98.86
    calculi, renal Z87.442
    cancer — *see* History, personal (of), malignant neoplasm (of)
    cardiac arrest (death), successfully resuscitated Z86.74
    CAR-T (Chimeric Antigen Receptor T-cell) therapy Z92.850
    cellular therapy Z92.859
      specified NEC Z92.858
    cerebral infarction without residual deficit Z86.73
    certain (corrected) conditions arising in the perinatal period, specified NEC Z87.68
    cervical dysplasia Z87.410
    chemotherapy for neoplastic condition Z92.21
    childhood abuse — *see* History, personal (of), abuse
    Chimeric Antigen Receptor T-cell (CAR-T) therapy Z92.850
    cleft lip (corrected) Z87.730
    cleft palate (corrected) Z87.730
    cloaca, persistent Z87.732
    cloacal malformations Z87.732
    collapsed vertebra (healed) Z87.311
      due to osteoporosis Z87.310
    combat and operational stress reaction Z86.51
    congenital malformation (corrected) Z87.798
      circulatory system (corrected) Z87.74
      diaphragmatic hernia Z87.760
      digestive system (corrected) NEC Z87.738
      ear (corrected) Z87.721

History — *continued*
  personal — *see also* History, family — *continued*
    congenital malformation — *continued*
      eye (corrected) Z87.720
      face and neck (corrected) Z87.790
      gastroschisis Z87.761
      genitourinary system (corrected) NEC Z87.718
      heart (corrected) Z87.74
      integument (corrected) Z87.768
      limb(s) (corrected) Z87.768
      malformations
        abdominal wall Z87.763
        diaphragm NEC Z87.760
        integument Z87.768
        limbs Z87.768
        musculoskeletal system Z87.768
        prune belly Z87.762
      musculoskeletal system (corrected) Z87.768
      neck (corrected) Z87.790
      nervous system (corrected) NEC Z87.728
      respiratory system (corrected) Z87.75
      sense organs (corrected) NEC Z87.728
      specified NEC Z87.798
    contraception Z92.0
    coronavirus (disease) (novel) 2019 Z86.16
    COVID-19 Z86.16
    deployment (military) Z91.82
    diabetic foot ulcer Z86.31
    disease or disorder (of) Z87.898
      anaphylaxis Z87.892
      blood and blood-forming organs Z86.2
      circulatory system Z86.79
        specified condition NEC Z86.79
      connective tissue Z87.39
      digestive system Z87.19
        colonic polyp Z86.010
        peptic ulcer disease Z87.11
        specified condition NEC Z87.19
      ear Z86.69
      endocrine Z86.39
        diabetic foot ulcer Z86.31
        gestational diabetes Z86.32
        specified type NEC Z86.39
      eye Z86.69
      genital (track) system NEC
        female Z87.42
        male Z87.438
      hematological Z86.2
      Hodgkin Z85.71
      immune mechanism Z86.2
      infectious Z86.19
        coronavirus (disease) (novel) 2019 Z86.16
        COVID-19 Z86.16
        malaria Z86.13
        Methicillin resistant Staphylococcus aureus (MRSA) Z86.14
        poliomyelitis Z86.12
        SARS-CoV-2 Z86.16
        specified NEC Z86.19
        tuberculosis Z86.11
      mental NEC Z86.59
      metabolic Z86.39
        diabetic foot ulcer Z86.31
        gestational diabetes Z86.32
        specified type NEC Z86.39
      musculoskeletal NEC Z87.39
      nervous system Z86.69
      nutritional Z86.39
      parasitic Z86.19
      respiratory system NEC Z87.09
      sense organs Z86.69
      skin Z87.2
      specified site or type NEC Z87.898
      subcutaneous tissue Z87.2
      trophoblastic Z87.59
      urinary system NEC Z87.448
    drug dependence — *see* Dependence, drug, by type, in remission
    drug therapy
      antineoplastic chemotherapy Z92.21
      estrogen Z92.23
      immunosuppression Z92.25
      inhaled steroids Z92.240
      monoclonal drug Z92.22
      specified NEC Z92.29
      steroid Z92.241
      systemic steroids Z92.241
    dysplasia
      cervical (mild) (moderate) Z87.410

History — *continued*
personal — *see also* History, family — *continued*
  dysplasia — *continued*
    cervical — *continued*
      severe (grade III) Z86.001
    prostatic Z87.430
    vaginal (mild) (moderate) Z87.411
      severe (grade III) Z86.002
    vulvar (mild) (moderate) Z87.412
      severe (grade III) Z86.002
  embolism (venous) Z86.718
    pulmonary Z86.711
  encephalitis Z86.61
  estrogen therapy Z92.23
  extracorporeal membrane oxygenation (ECMO) Z92.81
  failed conscious sedation Z92.83
  failed moderate sedation Z92.83
  fall, falling Z91.81
  forced labor or sexual exploitation Z91.42
    in childhood Z62.813
  fracture (healed)
    fatigue Z87.312
    fragility Z87.310
    osteoporosis Z87.310
    pathological NEC Z87.311
    stress Z87.312
    traumatic Z87.81
  gene therapy Z92.86
  gestational diabetes Z86.32
  hepatitis
    B Z86.19
    C Z86.19
  Hodgkin disease Z85.71
  hyperthermia, malignant Z88.4
  hypospadias (corrected) Z87.710
  hysterectomy Z90.710
  immunosuppression therapy Z92.25
  in situ neoplasm
    breast Z86.000
    cervix uteri Z86.001
    digestive organs, specified NEC Z86.004
    esophagus Z86.003
    genital organs, specified NEC Z86.002
    melanoma Z86.006
    middle ear Z86.005
    oral cavity Z86.003
    respiratory system Z86.005
    skin Z86.007
    specified NEC Z86.008
    stomach Z86.003
  in utero procedure during pregnancy Z98.870
  in utero procedure while a fetus Z98.871
  infection NEC Z86.19
    central nervous system Z86.61
    coronavirus (disease) (novel) 2019 Z86.16
    COVID-19 Z86.16
    latent tuberculosis Z86.15
    Methicillin resistant Staphylococcus aureus (MRSA) Z86.14
    SARS-CoV-2 Z86.16
    urinary (recurrent) (tract) Z87.440
  injury NEC Z87.828
  irradiation Z92.3
  kidney stones Z87.442
  latent tuberculosis infection Z86.15
  leukemia Z85.6
  lymphoma (non-Hodgkin) Z85.72
  malignant melanoma (skin) Z85.820
  malignant neoplasm (of) Z85.9
    accessory sinuses Z85.22
    anus NEC Z85.048
      carcinoid Z85.040
    bladder Z85.51
    bone Z85.830
    brain Z85.841
    breast Z85.3
    bronchus NEC Z85.118
      carcinoid Z85.110
    carcinoid — *see* History, personal (of), malignant neoplasm, by site, carcinioid
    cervix Z85.41
    colon NEC Z85.038
      carcinoid Z85.030
    digestive organ Z85.00
      specified NEC Z85.09
    endocrine gland NEC Z85.858
    epididymis Z85.48
    esophagus Z85.01

History — *continued*
personal — *see also* History, family — *continued*
  malignant neoplasm — *continued*
    eye Z85.840
    gastrointestinal tract — *see* History, malignant neoplasm, digestive organ
    genital organ
      female Z85.40
        specified NEC Z85.44
      male Z85.45
        specified NEC Z85.49
    hematopoietic Z85.79
    intrathoracic organ Z85.20
    kidney NEC Z85.528
      carcinoid Z85.520
    large intestine NEC Z85.038
      carcinoid Z85.030
    larynx Z85.21
    liver Z85.05
    lung NEC Z85.118
      carcinoid Z85.110
    mediastinum Z85.29
    Merkel cell Z85.821
    middle ear Z85.22
    nasal cavities Z85.22
    nervous system NEC Z85.848
    oral cavity Z85.819
      specified site NEC Z85.818
    ovary Z85.43
    pancreas Z85.07
    pelvis Z85.53
    pharynx Z85.819
      specified site NEC Z85.818
    pleura Z85.29
    prostate Z85.46
    rectosigmoid junction NEC Z85.048
      carcinoid Z85.040
    rectum NEC Z85.048
      carcinoid Z85.040
    respiratory organ Z85.20
    sinuses, accessory Z85.22
    skin NEC Z85.828
      melanoma Z85.820
      Merkel cell Z85.821
    small intestine NEC Z85.068
      carcinoid Z85.060
    soft tissue Z85.831
    specified site NEC Z85.89
    stomach NEC Z85.028
      carcinoid Z85.020
    testis Z85.47
    thymus NEC Z85.238
      carcinoid Z85.230
    thyroid Z85.850
    tongue Z85.810
    trachea Z85.12
    urinary organ or tract Z85.50
      specified NEC Z85.59
    uterus Z85.42
  maltreatment Z91.89
  medical treatment NEC Z92.89
  melanoma Z85.820
    in situ Z86.006
    malignant (skin) Z85.820
  meningitis Z86.61
  mental disorder Z86.59
  Merkel cell carcinoma (skin) Z85.821
  Methicillin resistant Staphylococcus aureus (MRSA) Z86.14
  military deployment Z91.82
  military war, peacekeeping and humanitarian deployment (current or past conflict) Z91.82
  myocardial infarction (old) I25.2
  necrotizing enterocolitis of newborn (corrected) Z87.61
  neglect (in)
    adult Z91.412
    childhood Z62.812
  neoplasia
    anal intraepithelial, III [AIN III] Z86.004
    high-grade prostatic intraepithelial, III [HGPIN III] Z86.002
    vaginal intraepithelial, III [VAIN III] Z86.002
    vulvar intraepithelial, III [VIN III] Z86.002
  neoplasm
    benign Z86.018
      brain Z86.011
      colon polyp Z86.010

History — *continued*
personal — *see also* History, family — *continued*
  neoplasm — *continued*
    in situ
      breast Z86.000
      cervix uteri Z86.001
      digestive organs, specified NEC Z86.004
      esophagus Z86.003
      genital organs, specified NEC Z86.002
      melanoma Z86.006
      middle ear Z86.005
      oral cavity Z86.003
      respiratory system Z86.005
      skin Z86.007
      specified NEC Z86.008
      stomach Z86.003
    malignant — *see* History of, malignant neoplasm
    uncertain behavior Z86.03
  nephrotic syndrome Z87.441
  nicotine dependence Z87.891
  noncompliance with medical treatment or regimen — *see* Noncompliance
  nutritional deficiency Z86.39
  obstetric complications Z87.59 *Cesarean*
    childbirth Z87.59
    pregnancy Z87.59
    pre-term labor Z87.51
    puerperium Z87.59
  osteoporosis fractures Z87.31 ☑
  parasuicide (attempt) Z91.51
  physical trauma NEC Z87.828
    self-harm or suicide attempt Z91.51
  pneumonia (recurrent) Z87.01
  poisoning NEC Z91.89
    self-harm or suicide attempt Z91.51
  poor personal hygiene Z91.89
  preterm labor Z87.51
  procedure during pregnancy Z98.870
  procedure while a fetus Z98.871
  prolonged reversible ischemic neurologic deficit (PRIND) Z86.73
  prostatic dysplasia Z87.430
  psychological
    abuse
      adult Z91.411
      child Z62.811
    trauma, specified NEC Z91.49
  radiation therapy Z92.3
  removal
    implant
      breast Z98.86
  renal calculi Z87.442
  respiratory condition NEC Z87.09
  retained foreign body fully removed Z87.821
  risk factors NEC Z91.89
  SARS-CoV-2 infection Z86.16
  self-harm
    nonsuicidal Z91.52
    suicidal Z91.51
  self-inflicted injury without suicidal intent Z91.52
  self-injury
    nonsuicidal Z91.52
  self-mutilation Z91.52
  self-poisoning attempt Z91.51
  sex reassignment Z87.890
  sleep-wake cycle problem Z72.821
  specified NEC Z87.898
  steroid therapy (systemic) Z92.241
    inhaled Z92.240
  stroke without residual deficits Z86.73
  substance abuse NEC F10-F19
  sudden cardiac arrest Z86.74
  sudden cardiac death successfully resuscitated Z86.74
  suicidal behavior Z91.51
  suicide attempt Z91.51
  surgery NEC Z98.890
    with uterine scar Z98.891
    sex reassignment Z87.890
    transplant — *see* Transplant
  thrombophlebitis Z86.72
  thrombosis (venous) Z86.718
    pulmonary Z86.711
  tobacco dependence Z87.891
  tracheoesophageal
    atresia Z87.731
    fistula Z87.731
  transient ischemic attack (TIA) without residual deficits Z86.73

☑ Additional Character Required — Refer to the Tabular List for Character Selection

History — History

History — *continued*
  personal — *see also* History, family — *continued*
    trauma (physical) NEC Z87.828
      psychological NEC Z91.49
      self-harm Z91.51
    traumatic brain injury Z87.820
    tuberculosis, latent infection Z86.15
    unhealthy sleep-wake cycle Z72.821
    unintended awareness under general anesthesia Z92.84
    urinary calculi Z87.442
    urinary (recurrent) (tract) infection(s) Z87.440
    uterine scar from previous surgery Z98.891
    vaginal dysplasia Z87.411
    venous thrombosis or embolism Z86.718
      pulmonary Z86.711
    vulvar dysplasia Z87.412
His-Werner disease A79.0
HIV — *see also* Human, immunodeficiency virus B20
  laboratory evidence (nonconclusive) R75
  nonconclusive test (in infants) R75
  positive, seropositive Z21
Hives (bold) — *see* Urticaria
Hoarseness R49.0
Hobo Z59.00
Hodgkin disease — *see* Lymphoma, Hodgkin
Hodgson's — *see also* Aneurysm, aorta, thorax I71.20
  ruptured — *see also* Aneurysm, aorta, thorax, ruptured I71.10
Hoffa-Kastert disease E88.89
Hoffa's disease E88.89
Hoffmann-Bouveret syndrome I47.9
Hoffmann's syndrome E03.9 *[G73.7]*
Hole (round)
  macula H35.34- ☑
  retina (without detachment) — *see* Break, retina, round hole
    with detachment — *see* Detachment, retina, with retinal, break
Holiday relief care Z75.5
Hollenhorst's plaque — *see* Occlusion, artery, retina
Hollow foot (congenital) Q66.7- ☑
  acquired — *see* Deformity, limb, foot, specified NEC
Holoprosencephaly Q04.2
Holt-Oram syndrome Q87.2
Homelessness Z59.00
  sheltered Z59.01
  unsheltered Z59.02
Homesickness — *see* Disorder, adjustment
Homocysteinemia R79.83
Homocystinemia, homocystinuria E72.11
Homogentisate 1,2-dioxygenase deficiency E70.29
Homologous serum hepatitis (prophylactic) (therapeutic) — *see* Hepatitis, viral, type B
Honeycomb lung J98.4
  congenital Q33.0
Hooded
  clitoris Q52.6
  penis Q55.69
Hookworm (disease) (infection) (infestation) B76.9
  with anemia B76.9 *[D63.8]*
  specified NEC B76.8
Hordeolum (eyelid) (externum) (recurrent) H00.019
  internum H00.029
    left H00.026
      lower H00.025
      upper H00.024
    right H00.023
      lower H00.022
      upper H00.021
  left H00.016
    lower H00.015
    upper H00.014
  right H00.013
    lower H00.012
    upper H00.011
Horn
  cutaneous L85.8
  nail L60.2
    congenital Q84.6
Horner (-Claude Bernard) **syndrome** G90.2
  traumatic — *see* Injury, nerve, cervical sympathetic
Horseshoe kidney (congenital) Q63.1
Horton's headache or neuralgia G44.099
  intractable G44.091
  not intractable G44.099
Hospital hopper syndrome — *see* Disorder, factitious

Hospitalism in children — *see* Disorder, adjustment
Hostility R45.5
  towards child Z62.3
Hot flashes
  menopausal N95.1
Hourglass (contracture) — *see also* Contraction, hourglass
  stomach K31.89
    congenital Q40.2
    stricture K31.2
Household, housing circumstance affecting care Z59.9
  specified NEC Z59.89
Housemaid's knee — *see* Bursitis, prepatellar
HSCT-TMA (hematopoietic stem cell transplantation-associated thrombotic microangiopathy) M31.11
Hudson (-Ståhli) **line** (cornea) — *see* Pigmentation, cornea, anterior
Human
  bite (open wound) — *see also* Bite
    intact skin surface — *see* Bite, superficial
  herpesvirus — *see* Herpes
  immunodeficiency virus (HIV) disease (infection) B20
    asymptomatic status Z21
    contact Z20.6
    counseling Z71.7
    dementia — *see also* Dementia, in, diseases specified elsewhere B20 *[F02.80]*
      with behavioral disturbance — *see also* Dementia, in, diseases specified elsewhere B20 *[F02.81-]* ☑
    exposure to Z20.6
    laboratory evidence R75
    type-2 (HIV 2) as cause of disease classified elsewhere B97.35
  papillomavirus (HPV)
    DNA test positive

[handwritten: high risk.]

      high risk
        cervix R87.810
        vagina R87.811
      low risk
        cervix R87.820
        vagina R87.821
    screening for Z11.51
  T-cell lymphotropic virus
    type-1 (HTLV-I) infection B33.3
      as cause of disease classified elsewhere B97.33
      carrier Z22.6
    type-2 (HTLV-II) as cause of disease classified elsewhere B97.34
Humidifier lung or pneumonitis J67.7
Humiliation (experience) **in childhood** Z62.898
Humpback (acquired) — *see* Kyphosis
Hunchback (acquired) — *see* Kyphosis
Hunger T73.0 ☑
  air, psychogenic F45.8
Hungry bone syndrome E83.81
Hunner's ulcer — *see* Cystitis, chronic, interstitial
Hunter's
  glossitis D51.0
  syndrome E76.1
Huntington's disease or chorea G10
  with dementia — *see also* Dementia, in, diseases specified elsewhere G10 *[F02.80]*
    with behavioral disturbance — *see also* Dementia, in, diseases specified elsewhere G10 *[F02.81-]* ☑
Hunt's
  disease or syndrome (herpetic geniculate ganglionitis) B02.21
    dyssynergia cerebellaris myoclonica G11.19
  neuralgia B02.21
Hurler (-Scheie) **disease or syndrome** E76.02
Hurst's disease G36.1
Hurthle cell
  adenocarcinoma C73
  adenoma D34
  carcinoma C73
  tumor D34
Hutchinson-Boeck disease or syndrome — *see* Sarcoidosis
Hutchinson-Gilford disease or syndrome E34.8
Hutchinson's
  disease, meaning
    angioma serpiginosum L81.7
    pompholyx (cheiropompholyx) L30.1
    prurigo estivalis L56.4
    summer eruption or summer prurigo L56.4

Hutchinson's — *continued*
  melanotic freckle — *see* Melanoma, in situ
    malignant melanoma in — *see* Melanoma
  teeth or incisors (congenital syphilis) A50.52
  triad (congenital syphilis) A50.53
Hyalin plaque, sclera, senile H15.89
Hyaline membrane (disease) (lung) (pulmonary) (newborn) P22.0
Hyalinosis
  cutis (et mucosae) E78.89
  focal and segmental (glomerular) — *see also* N00-N07 with fourth character .1 N05.1
Hyalitis, hyalosis, asteroid — *see also* Deposit, crystalline
  syphilitic (late) A52.71
Hydatid
  cyst or tumor — *see* Echinococcus
  mole — *see* Hydatidiform mole
  Morgagni
    female Q50.5
    male (epididymal) Q55.4
      testicular Q55.29
Hydatidiform mole (benign) (complicating pregnancy) (delivered) (undelivered) O01.9
  classical O01.0
  complete O01.0
  incomplete O01.1
  invasive D39.2
  malignant D39.2
  partial O01.1
Hydatidosis — *see* Echinococcus
Hydradenitis (axillaris) (suppurative) L73.2
Hydradenoma — *see* Hidradenoma
Hydramnios O40.- ☑
Hydrancephaly, hydranencephaly Q04.3
  with spina bifida — *see* Spina bifida, with hydrocephalus
Hydrargyrism NEC — *see* Poisoning, mercury
Hydrarthrosis — *see also* Effusion, joint
  gonococcal A54.42
  intermittent M12.40
    ankle M12.47- ☑
    elbow M12.42- ☑
    foot joint M12.47- ☑
    hand joint M12.44- ☑
    hip M12.45- ☑
    knee M12.46- ☑
    multiple site M12.49
    shoulder M12.41- ☑
    specified joint NEC M12.48
    wrist M12.43- ☑
  of yaws (early) (late) — *see also* subcategory M14.8-A66.6
  syphilitic (late) A52.77
    congenital A50.55 *[M12.80]*
Hydremia D64.89
Hydrencephalocele (congenital) — *see* Encephalocele
Hydrencephalomeningocele (congenital) — *see* Encephalocele
Hydroa R23.8
  aestivale L56.4
  vacciniforme L56.4
Hydroadenitis (axillaris) (suppurative) L73.2
Hydrocalycosis — *see* Hydronephrosis
Hydrocele (spermatic cord) (testis) (tunica vaginalis) N43.3
  canal of Nuck N94.89
  communicating N43.2
    congenital P83.5
  congenital P83.5
  encysted N43.0
  female NEC N94.89
  infected N43.1
  newborn P83.5
  round ligament N94.89
  specified NEC N43.2
  spinalis — *see* Spina bifida
  vulva N90.89
Hydrocephalus (acquired) (external) (internal) (malignant) (recurrent) G91.9
  aqueduct Sylvius stricture Q03.0
  causing disproportion O33.6 ☑
    with obstructed labor O66.3
  communicating G91.0
  congenital (external) (internal) Q03.9
    with spina bifida Q05.4
      cervical Q05.0

Index — side tab

Hydrocephalus — *continued*
  congenital — *continued*
    with spina bifida — *continued*
      dorsal Q05.1
      lumbar Q05.2
      lumbosacral Q05.2
      sacral Q05.3
      thoracic Q05.1
      thoracolumbar Q05.1
      specified NEC Q03.8
  due to toxoplasmosis (congenital) P37.1
  foramen Magendie block (acquired) G91.1
    congenital — *see also* Hydrocephalus, congenital Q03.1
  in (due to)
    infectious disease NEC B89 *[G91.4]*
    neoplastic disease NEC — *see also* Neoplasm G91.4
    parasitic disease B89 *[G91.4]*
  newborn Q03.9
    with spina bifida — *see* Spina bifida, with hydrocephalus
  noncommunicating G91.1
  normal pressure G91.2
    secondary G91.0
  obstructive G91.1
  otitic G93.2
  post-traumatic NEC G91.3
  secondary G91.4
    post-traumatic G91.3
  specified NEC G91.8
  syphilitic, congenital A50.49
Hydrocolpos (congenital) N89.8
Hydrocystoma — *see* Neoplasm, skin, benign
Hydroencephalocele (congenital) — *see* Encephalocele
Hydroencephalomeningocele (congenital) — *see* Encephalocele
Hydrohematopneumothorax — *see* Hemothorax
Hydromeningitis — *see* Meningitis
Hydromeningocele (spinal) — *see also* Spina bifida
  cranial — *see* Encephalocele
Hydrometra N85.8
Hydrometrocolpos N89.8
Hydromicrocephaly Q02
Hydromphalos (since birth) Q45.8
Hydromyelia Q06.4
Hydromyelocele — *see* Spina bifida
Hydronephrosis (atrophic) (early) (functionless) (intermittent) (primary) (secondary) NEC N13.30
  with
    infection N13.6
    obstruction (by) (of)
      renal calculus N13.2
        with infection N13.6
      ureteral NEC N13.1
        with infection N13.6
        calculus N13.2
          with infection N13.6
      ureteropelvic junction (congenital) Q62.11
        acquired N13.0
          with infection N13.6
      ureteral stricture NEC N13.1
        with infection N13.6
  congenital Q62.0
    due to acquired occlusion of ureteropelvic junction N13.0
  specified type NEC N13.39
  tuberculous A18.11
Hydropericarditis — *see* Pericarditis
Hydropericardium — *see* Pericarditis
Hydroperitoneum R18.8
Hydrophobia — *see* Rabies
Hydrophthalmos Q15.0
Hydropneumohemothorax — *see* Hemothorax
Hydropneumopericarditis — *see* Pericarditis
Hydropneumopericardium — *see* Pericarditis
Hydropneumothorax J94.8
  traumatic — *see* Injury, intrathoracic, lung
  tuberculous NEC A15.6
Hydrops R60.9
  abdominis R18.8
  articulorum intermittens — *see* Hydrarthrosis, intermittent
  cardiac — *see* Failure, heart, congestive
  causing obstructed labor (mother) O66.3
  endolymphatic H81.0- ☑
  fetal — *see* Pregnancy, complicated by, hydrops, fetalis
  fetalis P83.2

Hydrops — *continued*
  fetalis — *continued*
    due to
      ABO isoimmunization P56.0
      alpha thalassemia D56.0
      hemolytic disease P56.90
        specified NEC P56.99
      isoimmunization (ABO) (Rh) P56.0
      other specified nonhemolytic disease NEC P83.2
      Rh incompatibility P56.0
    during pregnancy — *see* Pregnancy, complicated by, hydrops, fetalis
  gallbladder K82.1
  joint — *see* Effusion, joint
  labyrinth H81.0- ☑
  newborn (idiopathic) P83.2
    due to
      ABO isoimmunization P56.0
      alpha thalassemia D56.0
      hemolytic disease P56.90
        specified NEC P56.99
      isoimmunization (ABO) (Rh) P56.0
      Rh incompatibility P56.0
  nutritional — *see* Malnutrition, severe
  pericardium — *see* Pericarditis
  pleura — *see* Hydrothorax
  spermatic cord — *see* Hydrocele
Hydropyonephrosis N13.6
Hydrorachis Q06.4
Hydrorrhea (nasal) J34.89
  pregnancy — *see* Rupture, membranes, premature
Hydrosadenitis (axillaris) (suppurative) L73.2
Hydrosalpinx (fallopian tube) (follicularis) N70.11
Hydrothorax (double) (pleura) J94.8
  chylous (nonfilarial) I89.8
    filarial — *see also* Infestation, filarial B74.9 *[J91.8]*
  traumatic — *see* Injury, intrathoracic
  tuberculous NEC (non primary) A15.6
Hydroureter — *see also* Hydronephrosis N13.4
  with infection N13.6
  congenital Q62.39
Hydroureteronephrosis — *see* Hydronephrosis
Hydrourethra N36.8
Hydroxykynureninuria E70.89
Hydroxylysinemia E72.3
Hydroxyprolinemia E72.59
Hygiene, sleep
  abuse Z72.821
  inadequate Z72.821
  poor Z72.821
Hygroma (congenital) (cystic) D18.1
  praepatellare, prepatellar — *see* Bursitis, prepatellar
Hymen — *see* condition
Hymenolepis, hymenolepiasis (diminuta) (infection) (infestation) (nana) B71.0
Hypalgesia R20.8
Hyperacidity (gastric) K31.89
  psychogenic F45.8
Hyperactive, hyperactivity F90.9
  basal cell, uterine cervix — *see* Dysplasia, cervix
  bowel sounds R19.12
  cervix epithelial (basal) — *see* Dysplasia, cervix
  child F90.9
    attention deficit — *see* Disorder, attention-deficit hyperactivity
  detrusor muscle N32.81
  gastrointestinal K31.89
    psychogenic F45.8
  nasal mucous membrane J34.3
  stomach K31.89
  thyroid (gland) — *see* Hyperthyroidism
Hyperacusis H93.23- ☑
Hyperadrenalism E27.5
Hyperadrenocorticism E24.9
  congenital E25.0
  iatrogenic E24.2
    correct substance properly administered — *see* Table of Drugs and Chemicals, by drug, adverse effect
    overdose or wrong substance given or taken — *see* Table of Drugs and Chemicals, by drug, poisoning
  not associated with Cushing's syndrome E27.0
  pituitary-dependent E24.0
Hyperaldosteronism E26.9
  familial (type I) E26.02
  glucocorticoid-remediable E26.02

Hyperaldosteronism — *continued*
  primary (due to (bilateral) adrenal hyperplasia) E26.09
  primary NEC E26.09
  secondary E26.1
  specified NEC E26.89
Hyperalgesia R20.8
Hyperalimentation R63.2
  carotene, carotin E67.1
  specified NEC E67.8
  vitamin
    A E67.0
    D E67.3
Hyperaminoaciduria
  arginine E72.21
  cystine E72.01
  lysine E72.3
  ornithine E72.4
Hyperammonemia (congenital) E72.20
Hyperazotemia — *see* Uremia
Hyperbetalipoproteinemia (familial) E78.00
  with prebetalipoproteinemia E78.2
Hyperbicarbonatemia P74.41
Hyperbilirubinemia
  constitutional E80.6
  familial conjugated E80.6
  neonatal (transient) — *see* Jaundice, newborn
Hypercalcemia, hypocalciuric, familial E83.52
Hypercalciuria, idiopathic R82.994
Hypercapnia R06.89
  newborn P84
Hypercarotenemia (dietary) E67.1
Hypercementosis K03.4
Hyperchloremia E87.8
Hyperchlorhydria K31.89
  neurotic F45.8
  psychogenic F45.8
Hypercholesterinemia — *see* Hypercholesterolemia
Hypercholesterolemia (essential) (primary) (pure) E78.00
  with hyperglyceridemia, endogenous E78.2
  dietary counseling and surveillance Z71.3
  familial E78.01
  hereditary E78.01
Hyperchylia gastrica, psychogenic F45.8
Hyperchylomicronemia (familial) (primary) E78.3
  with hyperbetalipoproteinemia E78.3
Hypercoagulable (state) D68.59
  activated protein C resistance D68.51
  antithrombin (III) deficiency D68.59
  factor V Leiden mutation D68.51
  primary NEC D68.59
  protein C deficiency D68.59
  protein S deficiency D68.59
  prothrombin gene mutation D68.52
  secondary D68.69
  specified NEC D68.69
Hypercoagulation (state) D68.59
Hypercorticalism, pituitary-dependent E24.0
Hypercorticosolism — *see* Cushing's, syndrome
Hypercorticosteronism E24.2
  correct substance properly administered — *see* Table of Drugs and Chemicals, by drug, adverse effect
  overdose or wrong substance given or taken — *see* Table of Drugs and Chemicals, by drug, poisoning
Hypercortisonism E24.2
  correct substance properly administered — *see* Table of Drugs and Chemicals, by drug, adverse effect
  overdose or wrong substance given or taken — *see* Table of Drugs and Chemicals, by drug, poisoning
Hyperekplexia Q89.8
Hyperelectrolytemia E87.8
Hyperemesis R11.10
  with nausea R11.2
  gravidarum (mild) O21.0
    with
      carbohydrate depletion O21.1
      dehydration O21.1
      electrolyte imbalance O21.1
      metabolic disturbance O21.1
    severe (with metabolic disturbance) O21.1
  projectile R11.12
  psychogenic F45.8
Hyperemia (acute) (passive) R68.89
  anal mucosa K62.89
  bladder N32.89
  cerebral I67.89
  conjunctiva H11.43- ☑
  ear internal, acute — *see* subcategory H83.0 ☑
  enteric K59.89

Hyperemia — *continued*
  eye — *see* Hyperemia, conjunctiva
  eyelid (active) (passive) — *see* Disorder, eyelid, specified type NEC
  intestine K59.89
  iris — *see* Disorder, iris, vascular
  kidney N28.89
  labyrinth — *see* subcategory H83.0 ☑
  liver (active) K76.89
  lung (passive) — *see* Edema, lung
  pulmonary (passive) — *see* Edema, lung
  renal N28.89
  retina H35.89
  stomach K31.89
Hyperesthesia (body surface) R20.3
  larynx (reflex) J38.7
    hysterical F44.89
  pharynx (reflex) J39.2
    hysterical F44.89
Hyperestrogenism (drug-induced) (iatrogenic) E28.0
Hyperexplexia Q89.8
Hyperfibrinolysis — *see* Fibrinolysis
Hyperfructosemia E74.19
Hyperfunction
  adrenal cortex, not associated with Cushing's syndrome E27.0
    medulla E27.5
      adrenomedullary E27.5
    virilism E25.9
      congenital E25.0
  ovarian E28.8
  pancreas K86.89
  parathyroid (gland) E21.3
  pituitary (gland) (anterior) E22.9
    specified NEC E22.8
  polyglandular E31.1
  testicular E29.0
Hypergammaglobulinemia D89.2
  polyclonal D89.0
  Waldenström D89.0
Hypergastrinemia E16.4
Hyperglobulinemia R77.1
Hyperglycemia, hyperglycemic (transient) R73.9
  coma — *see* Diabetes, by type, with coma
  postpancreatectomy E89.1
Hyperglyceridemia (endogenous) (essential) (familial) (hereditary) (pure) E78.1
  mixed E78.3
Hyperglycinemia (non-ketotic) E72.51
Hypergonadism
  ovarian E28.8
  testicular (primary) (infantile) E29.0
Hyperheparinemia D68.32
Hyperhidrosis, hyperidrosis R61
  focal
    primary L74.519
      axilla L74.510
      face L74.511
      palms L74.512
      soles L74.513
    secondary L74.52
  generalized R61
  localized
    primary L74.519
      axilla L74.510
      face L74.511
      palms L74.512
      soles L74.513
    secondary L74.52
  psychogenic F45.8
  secondary R61
    focal L74.52
Hyperhistidinemia E70.41
Hyperhomocysteinemia E72.11
Hyperhydroxyprolinemia E72.59
Hyperinsulinism (functional) E16.1
  with
    coma (hypoglycemic) E15
    encephalopathy E16.1 *[G94]*
  ectopic E16.1
  therapeutic misadventure (from administration of insulin) — *see* subcategory T38.3 ☑
Hyperkalemia E87.5
Hyperkeratosis — *see also* Keratosis L85.9
  cervix N88.0
  due to yaws (early) (late) (palmar or plantar) A66.3
  follicularis Q82.8
    penetrans (in cutem) L87.0

Hyperkeratosis — *continued*
  palmoplantaris climacterica L85.1
  pinta A67.1
  senile (with pruritus) L57.0
  universalis congenita Q80.8
  vocal cord J38.3
  vulva N90.4
Hyperkinesia, hyperkinetic (disease) (reaction) (syndrome) (childhood) (adolescence) — *see also* Disorder, attention-deficit hyperactivity
  heart I51.89
Hyperleucine-isoleucinemia E71.19
Hyperlipemia, hyperlipidemia E78.5
  combined E78.2
    familial E78.49
  group
    A E78.00
    B E78.1
    C E78.2
    D E78.3
  mixed E78.2
  specified NEC E78.49
Hyperlipidosis E75.6
  hereditary NEC E75.5
Hyperlipoproteinemia E78.5
  Fredrickson's type
    I E78.3
    IIa E78.00
    IIb E78.2
    III E78.2
    IV E78.1
    V E78.3
  low-density-lipoprotein-type (LDL) E78.00
  very-low-density-lipoprotein-type (VLDL) E78.1
Hyperlucent lung, unilateral J43.0
Hyperlysinemia E72.3
Hypermagnesemia E83.41
  neonatal P71.8
Hypermenorrhea N92.0
Hypermethioninemia E72.19
Hypermetropia (congenital) H52.0- ☑
Hypermobility, hypermotility
  cecum — *see* Syndrome, irritable bowel
  coccyx — *see* subcategory M53.2 ☑
  colon — *see* Syndrome, irritable bowel
    psychogenic F45.8
  ileum K58.9
  intestine — *see also* Syndrome, irritable bowel K58.9
    psychogenic F45.8
  meniscus (knee) — *see* Derangement, knee, meniscus
  scapula — *see* Instability, joint, shoulder
  stomach K31.89
    psychogenic F45.8
  syndrome M35.7
  urethra N36.41
    with intrinsic sphincter deficiency N36.43
Hypernasality R49.21
Hypernatremia E87.0
Hypernephroma C64.- ☑
Hyperopia — *see* Hypermetropia
Hyperorexia nervosa F50.2
Hyperornithinemia E72.4
Hyperosmia R43.1
Hyperosmolality E87.0
Hyperostosis (monomelic) — *see also* Disorder, bone, density and structure, specified NEC
  ankylosing (spine) M48.10
    cervical region M48.12
    cervicothoracic region M48.13
    lumbar region M48.16
    lumbosacral region M48.17
    multiple sites M48.19
    occipito-atlanto-axial region M48.11
    sacrococcygeal region M48.18
    thoracic region M48.14
    thoracolumbar region M48.15
  cortical (skull) M85.2
    infantile M89.8X- ☑
  frontal, internal of skull M85.2
  interna frontalis M85.2
  skeletal, diffuse idiopathic — *see* Hyperostosis, ankylosing
  skull M85.2
    congenital Q75.8
  vertebral, ankylosing — *see* Hyperostosis, ankylosing
Hyperovarism E28.8
Hyperoxaluria R82.992
  primary E72.53

Hyperparathyroidism E21.3
  primary E21.0
  secondary (renal) N25.81
    non-renal E21.1
  specified NEC E21.2
  tertiary E21.2
Hyperpathia R20.8
Hyperperistalsis R19.2
  psychogenic F45.8
Hyperpermeability, capillary I78.8
Hyperphagia R63.2
Hyperphenylalaninemia NEC E70.1
Hyperphoria (alternating) H50.53
Hyperphosphatemia E83.39
Hyperpiesis, hyperpiesia — *see* Hypertension
Hyperpigmentation — *see also* Pigmentation
  melanin NEC L81.4
  postinflammatory L81.0
Hyperpinealism E34.8
Hyperpituitarism E22.9
Hyperplasia, hyperplastic
  adenoids J35.2
  adrenal (capsule) (cortex) (gland) E27.8
    with
      sexual precocity (male) E25.9
        congenital E25.0
      virilism, adrenal E25.9
        congenital E25.0
      virilization (female) E25.9
        congenital E25.0
    congenital E25.0
    salt-losing E25.0
  adrenomedullary E27.5
  angiolymphoid, eosinophilia (ALHE) D18.01
  appendix (lymphoid) K38.0
  artery, fibromuscular I77.3
  bone — *see also* Hypertrophy, bone
    marrow D75.89
  breast — *see also* Hypertrophy, breast
    atypical, atypia N60.9- ☑
      ductal N60.9- ☑
      lobular N60.9- ☑
  C-cell, thyroid E07.0
  cementation (tooth) (teeth) K03.4
  cervical gland R59.0
  cervix (uteri) (basal cell) (endometrium) (polypoid) — *see also* Dysplasia, cervix
    congenital Q51.828
  clitoris, congenital Q52.6
  denture K06.2
  endocervicitis N72
  endometrium, endometrial (adenomatous) (cystic) (glandular) (glandular-cystic) (polypoid) N85.00
    with atypia N85.02
    benign N85.01
    cervix — *see* Dysplasia, cervix
    complex (without atypia) N85.01
    simple (without atypia) N85.01
  epithelial L85.9
    focal, oral, including tongue K13.29
    nipple N62
    skin L85.9
    tongue K13.29
    vaginal wall N89.3
  erythroid D75.89
  fibromuscular of artery (carotid) (renal) I77.3
  genital
    female NEC N94.89
    male N50.89
  gingiva K06.1
  glandularis cystica uteri (interstitialis) — *see also* Hyperplasia, endometrial N85.00
  gum K06.1
  hymen, congenital Q52.4
  irritative, edentulous (alveolar) K06.2
  jaw M26.09
    alveolar M26.79
      lower M26.03
        alveolar M26.72
      upper M26.01
        alveolar M26.71
  kidney (congenital) Q63.3
  labia N90.69
    epithelial N90.3
  liver (congenital) Q44.7
    nodular, focal K76.89
  lymph gland or node R59.9
  mandible, mandibular M26.03

Hyperplasia, hyperplastic — *continued*
  mandible, mandibular — *continued*
    alveolar M26.72
    unilateral condylar M27.8
   maxilla, maxillary M26.01
    alveolar M26.71
  myometrium, myometrial N85.2
  neuroendocrine cell, of infancy J84.841
  nose
   lymphoid J34.89
   polypoid J33.9
  oral mucosa (irritative) K13.6
  organ or site, congenital NEC — *see* Anomaly, by site
  ovary N83.8
  palate, papillary (irritative) K13.6
  pancreatic islet cells E16.9
   alpha E16.8
    with excess
     gastrin E16.4
     glucagon E16.3
   beta E16.1
  parathyroid (gland) E21.0
  pharynx (lymphoid) J39.2
  prostate (adenofibromatous) (nodular) N40.0
   with lower urinary tract symptoms (LUTS) N40.1
   without lower urinary tract symtpoms (LUTS) N40.0
  renal artery I77.89
  reticulo-endothelial (cell) D75.89
  salivary gland (any) K11.1
  Schimmelbusch's — *see* Mastopathy, cystic
  suprarenal capsule (gland) E27.8
  thymus (gland) (persistent) E32.0
  thyroid (gland) — *see* Goiter
  tonsils (faucial) (infective) (lingual) (lymphoid) J35.1
   with adenoids J35.3
  unilateral condylar M27.8
  uterus, uterine N85.2
   endometrium (glandular) — *see also* Hyperplasia, endometrial N85.00
  vulva N90.69
   epithelial N90.3
Hyperpnea — *see* Hyperventilation
Hyperpotassemia E87.5
Hyperprebetalipoproteinemia (familial) E78.1
Hyperprolactinemia E22.1
Hyperprolinemia (type I) (type II) E72.59
Hyperproteinemia E88.09
Hyperprothrombinemia, causing coagulation factor deficiency D68.4
Hyperpyrexia R50.9
  heat (effects) T67.01 ☑
  malignant, due to anesthetic T88.3 ☑
  rheumatic — *see* Fever, rheumatic
  unknown origin R50.9
Hyper-reflexia R29.2
Hypersalivation K11.7
Hypersecretion
  ACTH (not associated with Cushing's syndrome) E27.0
   pituitary E24.0
  adrenaline E27.5
  adrenomedullary E27.5
  androgen (testicular) E29.0
   ovarian (drug-induced) (iatrogenic) E28.1
  calcitonin E07.0
  catecholamine E27.5
  corticoadrenal E24.9
  cortisol E24.9
  epinephrine E27.5
  estrogen E28.0
  gastric K31.89
   psychogenic F45.8
  gastrin E16.4
  glucagon E16.3
  hormone(s)
   ACTH (not associated with Cushing's syndrome) E27.0
    pituitary E24.0
   antidiuretic E22.2
   growth E22.0
   intestinal NEC E34.1
   ovarian androgen E28.1
   pituitary E22.9
   testicular E29.0
   thyroid stimulating E05.80
    with thyroid storm E05.81
  insulin — *see* Hyperinsulinism
  lacrimal glands — *see* Epiphora
  medulloadrenal E27.5

Hypersecretion — *continued*
  milk O92.6
  ovarian androgens E28.1
  salivary gland (any) K11.7
  thyrocalcitonin E07.0
  upper respiratory J39.8
Hypersegmentation, leukocytic, hereditary D72.0
Hypersensitive, hypersensitiveness, hypersensitivity — *see also* Allergy
  carotid sinus G90.01
  colon — *see* Irritable, colon
  drug T88.7 ☑
  gastrointestinal K52.29
   immediate K52.29
   psychogenic F45.8
  labyrinth — *see* subcategory H83.2 ☑
  pain R20.8
  pneumonitis — *see* Pneumonitis, allergic
  reaction T78.40 ☑
   upper respiratory tract NEC J39.3
Hypersomnia (organic) G47.10
  due to
   alcohol
    abuse F10.182
    dependence F10.282
    use F10.982
   amphetamines
    abuse F15.182
    dependence F15.282
    use F15.982
   caffeine
    abuse F15.182
    dependence F15.282
    use F15.982
   cocaine
    abuse F14.182
    dependence F14.282
    use F14.982
   drug NEC
    abuse F19.182
    dependence F19.282
    use F19.982
   medical condition G47.14
   mental disorder F51.13
   opioid
    abuse F11.182
    dependence F11.282
    use F11.982
   psychoactive substance NEC
    abuse F19.182
    dependence F19.282
    use F19.982
   sedative, hypnotic, or anxiolytic
    abuse F13.182
    dependence F13.282
    use F13.982
   stimulant NEC
    abuse F15.182
    dependence F15.282
    use F15.982
  idiopathic G47.11
   with long sleep time G47.11
   without long sleep time G47.12
  menstrual related G47.13
  nonorganic origin F51.11
   specified NEC F51.19
  not due to a substance or known physiological condition F51.11
   specified NEC F51.19
  primary F51.11
  recurrent G47.13
  specified NEC G47.19
Hypersplenia, hypersplenism D73.1
Hyperstimulation, ovaries (associated with induced ovulation) N98.1
Hypersusceptibility — *see* Allergy
Hypertelorism (ocular) (orbital) Q75.2
Hypertension, hypertensive (accelerated) (benign) (essential) (idiopathic) (malignant) (systemic) I10
  with
   heart failure (congestive) I11.0
   heart involvement (conditions in I50.- or I51.4-I51.7, I51.89, I51.9, due to hypertension) — *see* Hypertension, heart
   kidney involvement — *see* Hypertension, kidney
  benign, intracranial G93.2
  borderline R03.0
  cardiorenal (disease) I13.10

Hypertension, hypertensive — *continued*
  cardiorenal — *continued*
   with heart failure I13.0
    with stage 1 through stage 4 chronic kidney disease I13.0
    with stage 5 or end stage renal disease I13.2
   without heart failure I13.10
    with stage 1 through stage 4 chronic kidney disease I13.10
    with stage 5 or end stage renal disease I13.11
  cardiovascular
   disease (arteriosclerotic) (sclerotic) — *see* Hypertension, heart
   renal (disease) — *see* Hypertension, cardiorenal
  chronic venous — *see* Hypertension, venous (chronic)
  complicating
   childbirth (labor) O16.4
    pre-existing O10.92
     with
      heart disease O10.12
       with renal disease O10.32
      pre-eclampsia O11.4
      renal disease O10.22
       with heart disease O10.32
     essential O10.02
     secondary O10.42
   pregnancy O16.- ☑
    with edema — *see also* Pre-eclampsia O14.9- ☑
    gestational (pregnancy induced) (without proteinuria) O13.- ☑
     with proteinuria O14.9- ☑
      mild pre-eclampsia O14.0- ☑
      moderate pre-eclampsia O14.0- ☑
      severe pre-eclampsia O14.1- ☑
       with hemolysis, elevated liver enzymes and low platelet count (HELLP) O14.2- ☑
    pre-existing O10.91- ☑
     with
      heart disease O10.11- ☑
       with renal disease O10.31- ☑
      pre-eclampsia — *see* category O11
      renal disease O10.21- ☑
       with heart disease O10.31- ☑
     essential O10.01- ☑
     secondary O10.41- ☑
    transient O13- ☑
   puerperium, pre-existing O16.5
    pre-existing
     with
      heart disease O10.13
       with renal disease O10.33
      pre-eclampsia O11.5
      renal disease O10.23
       with heart disease O10.33
     essential O10.03
    pregnancy-induced O13.9
    secondary O10.43
  crisis I16.9
  due to
   endocrine disorders I15.2
   pheochromocytoma I15.2
   renal disorders NEC I15.1
    arterial I15.0
   renovascular disorders I15.0
   specified disease NEC I15.8
  emergency I16.1
  encephalopathy I67.4
  gestational (without significant proteinuria) (pregnancy-induced) (transient) O13.- ☑
   with significant proteinuria — *see* Pre-eclampsia
   complicating
    delivery O13.4
    puerperium O13.5
  Goldblatt's I70.1
  heart (disease) (conditions in I51.4-I51.9 due to hypertension) I11.9
   with
    heart failure (congestive) I11.0
    kidney disease (chronic) — *see* Hypertension, cardiorenal
  intracranial, benign G93.2
  kidney I12.9
   with
    heart disease — *see* Hypertension, cardiorenal
    stage 1 through stage 4 chronic kidney disease I12.9

☑ **Additional Character Required** — Refer to the Tabular List for Character Selection

Hypertension, hypertensive — continued
kidney — continued
  with — continued
    stage 5 chronic kidney disease (CKD) or end stage
      renal disease (ESRD) I12.0
lesser circulation I27.0
maternal O16- ☑
newborn P29.2
  pulmonary (persistent) P29.30
ocular H40.05- ☑
pancreatic duct — code to underlying condition
  with chronic pancreatitis K86.1
portal (due to chronic liver disease) (idiopathic) K76.6
  gastropathy K31.89
  in (due to) schistosomiasis (bilharziasis) B65.9 [K77]
postoperative I97.3
psychogenic F45.8
pulmonary I27.20
  with
    cor pulmonale (chronic) I27.29
      acute I26.09
    right heart ventricular strain/failure I27.29
      acute I26.09
    right to left shunt related to congenital heart
      disease I27.83
    unclear multifactorial mechanisms I27.29
  arterial (associated) (drug-induced) (toxin-induced)
    I27.21
  chronic thromboembolic I27.24
  due to
    hematologic disorders I27.29
    kyphoscoliotic heart disease I27.1
    left heart disease I27.22
    lung diseases and hypoxia I27.23
    metabolic disorders I27.29
    specified systemic disorders I27.29
  group 1 (associated) (drug-induced) (toxin-induced)
    I27.21
  group 2 I27.22
  group 3 I27.23
  group 4 I27.24
  group 5 I27.29
  of newborn (persistent) P29.30
  primary (idiopathic) I27.0
  secondary
    arterial I27.21
    specified NEC I27.29
renal — see Hypertension, kidney
renovascular I15.0
secondary NEC I15.9
  due to
    endocrine disorders I15.2
    pheochromocytoma I15.2
    renal disorders NEC I15.1
      arterial I15.0
    renovascular disorders I15.0
  specified NEC I15.8
transient R03.0
  of pregnancy O13.- ☑
urgency I16.0
venous (chronic)
  due to
    deep vein thrombosis — see Syndrome, post-
      thrombotic
  idiopathic I87.309
    with
      inflammation I87.32- ☑
        with ulcer I87.33- ☑
      specified complication NEC I87.39- ☑
      ulcer I87.31- ☑
        with inflammation I87.33- ☑
      asymptomatic I87.30- ☑
Hypertensive urgency — see Hypertension
Hyperthecosis ovary E28.8
Hyperthermia (of unknown origin) — see also Hyperpyrexia
  malignant, due to anesthesia T88.3 ☑
  newborn P81.9
    environmental P81.0
Hyperthyroid (recurrent) — see Hyperthyroidism
Hyperthyroidism (latent) (pre-adult) (recurrent) E05.90
  with
    goiter (diffuse) E05.00
      with thyroid storm E05.01
    nodular (multinodular) E05.20
      with thyroid storm E05.21
      uninodular E05.10
        with thyroid storm E05.11

Hyperthyroidism — continued
  with — continued
    storm E05.91
  due to ectopic thyroid tissue E05.30
    with thyroid storm E05.31
  neonatal, transitory P72.1
  specified NEC E05.80
    with thyroid storm E05.81
Hypertony, hypertonia, hypertonicity
  bladder N31.8
  congenital P94.1
  stomach K31.89
    psychogenic F45.8
  uterus, uterine (contractions) (complicating delivery)
    O62.4
Hypertrichosis L68.9
  congenital Q84.2
  eyelid H02.869
    left H02.866
      lower H02.865
      upper H02.864
    right H02.863
      lower H02.862
      upper H02.861
  lanuginosa Q84.2
    acquired L68.1
  localized L68.2
  specified NEC L68.8
Hypertriglyceridemia, essential E78.1
Hypertrophy, hypertrophic
  adenofibromatous, prostate — see Enlargement, en-
    larged, prostate
  adenoids (infective) J35.2
    with tonsils J35.3
  adrenal cortex E27.8
  alveolar process or ridge — see Anomaly, alveolar
  anal papillae K62.89
  artery I77.89
    congenital NEC Q27.8
      digestive system Q27.8
      lower limb Q27.8
      specified site NEC Q27.8
      upper limb Q27.8
  auricular — see Hypertrophy, cardiac
  Bartholin's gland N75.8
  bile duct (common) (hepatic) K83.8
  bladder (sphincter) (trigone) N32.89
  bone M89.30
    carpus M89.34- ☑
    clavicle M89.31- ☑
    femur M89.35- ☑
    fibula M89.36- ☑
    finger M89.34- ☑
    humerus M89.32- ☑
    ilium M89.359
    ischium M89.359
    metacarpus M89.34- ☑
    metatarsus M89.37- ☑
    multiple sites M89.39
    neck M89.38
    radius M89.33- ☑
    rib M89.38
    scapula M89.31- ☑
    skull M89.38
    tarsus M89.37- ☑
    tibia M89.36- ☑
    toe M89.37- ☑
    ulna M89.33- ☑
    vertebra M89.38
  brain G93.89
  breast N62
    cystic — see Mastopathy, cystic
    newborn P83.4
    pubertal, massive N62
    puerperal, postpartum — see Disorder, breast,
      specified type NEC
    senile (parenchymatous) N62
  cardiac (chronic) (idiopathic) I51.7
    with rheumatic fever (conditions in I00)
      active I01.8
      inactive or quiescent (with chorea) I09.89
    congenital NEC Q24.8
    fatty — see Degeneration, myocardial
    hypertensive — see Hypertension, heart
    rheumatic (with chorea) I09.89
      active or acute I01.8
        with chorea I02.0
    valve — see Endocarditis

Hypertrophy, hypertrophic — continued
  cartilage — see Disorder, cartilage, specified type NEC
  cecum — see Megacolon
  cervix (uteri) N88.8
    congenital Q51.828
    elongation N88.4
  clitoris (cirrhotic) N90.89
    congenital Q52.6
  colon — see also Megacolon
    congenital Q43.2
  conjunctiva, lymphoid H11.89
  corpora cavernosa N48.89
  cystic duct K82.8
  duodenum K31.89
  endometrium (glandular) — see also Hyperplasia, en-
    dometrial N85.00
    cervix N88.8
  epididymis N50.89
  esophageal hiatus (congenital) Q79.1
    with hernia — see Hernia, hiatal
  eyelid — see Disorder, eyelid, specified type NEC
  facet joint — see also Spondylosis M47.819
  fat pad E65
    knee (infrapatellar) (popliteal) (prepatellar)
      (retropatellar) M79.4
  foot (congenital) Q74.2
  frenulum, frenum (tongue) K14.8
    lip K13.0
  gallbladder K82.8
  gastric mucosa K29.60
    with bleeding K29.61
  gland, glandular R59.9
    generalized R59.1
    localized R59.0
  gum (mucous membrane) K06.1
  heart (idiopathic) — see also Hypertrophy, cardiac
    valve — see also Endocarditis I38
  hemifacial Q67.4
  hepatic — see Hypertrophy, liver
  hiatus (esophageal) Q79.1
  hilus gland R59.0
  hymen, congenital Q52.4
  ileum K63.89
  intestine NEC K63.89
  jejunum K63.89
  kidney (compensatory) N28.81
    congenital Q63.3
  labium (majus) (minus) N90.60
  ligament — see Disorder, ligament
  lingual tonsil (infective) J35.1
    with adenoids J35.3
  lip K13.0
    congenital Q18.6
  liver R16.0
    acute K76.89
    cirrhotic — see Cirrhosis, liver
    congenital Q44.7
    fatty — see Fatty, liver
  lymph, lymphatic gland R59.9
    generalized R59.1
    localized R59.0
    tuberculous — see Tuberculosis, lymph gland
  mammary gland — see Hypertrophy, breast
  Meckel's diverticulum (congenital) Q43.0
    malignant — see Table of Neoplasms, small intes-
      tine, malignant
  median bar — see Hyperplasia, prostate
  meibomian gland — see Chalazion
  meniscus, knee, congenital Q74.1
  metatarsal head — see Hypertrophy, bone, metatarsus
  metatarsus — see Hypertrophy, bone, metatarsus
  mucous membrane
    alveolar ridge K06.2
    gum K06.1
    nose (turbinate) J34.3
  muscle M62.89
  muscular coat, artery I77.89
  myocardium — see also Hypertrophy, cardiac
    idiopathic I42.2
  myometrium N85.2
  nail L60.2
    congenital Q84.5
  nasal J34.89
    alae J34.89
    bone J34.89
    cartilage J34.89
    mucous membrane (septum) J34.3
    sinus J34.89

Hypertrophy, hypertrophic — *continued*
- nasal — *continued*
  - turbinate J34.3
- nasopharynx, lymphoid (infectional) (tissue) (wall) J35.2
- nipple N62
- organ or site, congenital NEC — *see* Anomaly, by site
- ovary N83.8
- palate (hard) M27.8
  - soft K13.79
- pancreas, congenital Q45.3
- parathyroid (gland) E21.0
- parotid gland K11.1
- penis N48.89
- pharyngeal tonsil J35.2
- pharynx J39.2
  - lymphoid (infectional) (tissue) (wall) J35.2
- pituitary (anterior) (fossa) (gland) E23.6
- prepuce (congenital) N47.8
  - female N90.89
- prostate — *see* Enlargement, enlarged, prostate
  - congenital Q55.4
- pseudomuscular — *see also* Dystrophy, muscular, by type, if applicable G71.09
- pylorus (adult) (muscle) (sphincter) K31.1
  - congenital or infantile Q40.0
- rectal, rectum (sphincter) K62.89
- rhinitis (turbinate) J31.0
- salivary gland (any) K11.1
  - congenital Q38.4
- scaphoid (tarsal) — *see* Hypertrophy, bone, tarsus
- scar L91.0
- scrotum N50.89
- seminal vesicle N50.89
- sigmoid — *see* Megacolon
- skin L91.9
  - specified NEC L91.8
- spermatic cord N50.89
- spleen — *see* Splenomegaly
- spondylitis — *see* Spondylosis
- stomach K31.89
- sublingual gland K11.1
- submandibular gland K11.1
- suprarenal cortex (gland) E27.8
- synovial NEC M67.20
  - acromioclavicular M67.21- ☑
  - ankle M67.27- ☑
  - elbow M67.22- ☑
  - foot M67.27- ☑
  - hand M67.24- ☑
  - hip M67.25- ☑
  - knee M67.26- ☑
  - multiple sites M67.29
  - specified site NEC M67.28
  - wrist M67.23- ☑
- tendon — *see* Disorder, tendon, specified type NEC
- testis N44.8
  - congenital Q55.29
- thymic, thymus (gland) (congenital) E32.0
- thyroid (gland) — *see* Goiter
- toe (congenital) Q74.2
  - acquired — *see also* Deformity, toe, specified NEC
- tongue K14.8
  - congenital Q38.2
  - papillae (foliate) K14.3
- tonsils (faucial) (infective) (lingual) (lymphoid) J35.1
  - with adenoids J35.3
- tunica vaginalis N50.89
- ureter N28.89
- urethra N36.8
- uterus N85.2
  - neck (with elongation) N88.4
  - puerperal O90.89
- uvula K13.79
- vagina N89.8
- vas deferens N50.89
- vein I87.8
- ventricle, ventricular (heart) — *see also* Hypertrophy, cardiac
  - congenital Q24.8
  - in tetralogy of Fallot Q21.3
- verumontanum N36.8
- vocal cord J38.3
- vulva N90.60
  - stasis (nonfilarial) N90.69

Hypertropia H50.2- ☑
Hypertyrosinemia E70.21
Hyperuricemia (asymptomatic) E79.0
Hyperuricosuria R82.993

Hypervalinemia E71.19
Hyperventilation (tetany) R06.4
- hysterical F45.8
- psychogenic F45.8
- syndrome F45.8

Hypervitaminosis (dietary) NEC E67.8
- A E67.0
  - administered as drug (prolonged intake) — *see* Table of Drugs and Chemicals, vitamins, adverse effect
  - overdose or wrong substance given or taken — *see* Table of Drugs and Chemicals, vitamins, poisoning
- B6 E67.2
- D E67.3
  - administered as drug (prolonged intake) — *see* Table of Drugs and Chemicals, vitamins, adverse effect
  - overdose or wrong substance given or taken — *see* Table of Drugs and Chemicals, vitamins, poisoning
- K E67.8
  - administered as drug (prolonged intake) — *see* Table of Drugs and Chemicals, vitamins, adverse effect
  - overdose or wrong substance given or taken — *see* Table of Drugs and Chemicals, vitamins, poisoning

Hypervolemia E87.70
- specified NEC E87.79

Hypesthesia R20.1
- cornea — *see* Anesthesia, cornea

Hyphema H21.0- ☑
- traumatic S05.1- ☑

Hypoacidity, gastric K31.89
- psychogenic F45.8

Hypoadrenalism, hypoadrenia E27.40
- primary E27.1
- tuberculous A18.7

Hypoadrenocorticism E27.40
- pituitary E23.0
- primary E27.1

Hypoalbuminemia E88.09
Hypoaldosteronism E27.40
Hypoalphalipoproteinemia E78.6
Hypobarism T70.29 ☑
Hypobaropathy T70.29 ☑
Hypobetalipoproteinemia (familial) E78.6
Hypocalcemia E83.51
- dietary E58
- neonatal P71.1
  - due to cow's milk P71.0
- phosphate-loading (newborn) P71.1

Hypochloremia E87.8
Hypochlorhydria K31.89
- neurotic F45.8
- psychogenic F45.8

Hypochondria, hypochondriac, hypochondriasis (reaction) F45.21
- sleep F51.03

Hypochondrogenesis Q77.0
Hypochondroplasia Q77.4
Hypochromasia, blood cells D50.8
Hypocitraturia R82.991
Hypodontia — *see* Anodontia
Hypoeosinophilia D72.89
Hypoesthesia R20.1
Hypofibrinogenemia D68.8
- acquired D65
- congenital (hereditary) D68.2

Hypofunction
- adrenocortical E27.40
  - drug-induced E27.3
  - postprocedural E89.6
  - primary E27.1
- adrenomedullary, postprocedural E89.6
- cerebral R29.818
- corticoadrenal NEC E27.40
- intestinal K59.89
- labyrinth — *see* subcategory H83.2 ☑
- ovary E28.39
- pituitary (gland) (anterior) E23.0
- testicular E29.1
  - postprocedural (postsurgical) (postirradiation) (iatrogenic) E89.5

Hypogalactia O92.4

Hypogammaglobulinemia — *see also* Agammaglobulinemia D80.1
- hereditary D80.0
- nonfamilial D80.1
- transient, of infancy D80.7

Hypogenitalism (congenital) — *see* Hypogonadism
Hypoglossia Q38.3
Hypoglycemia (spontaneous) E16.2
- coma E15
  - diabetic — *see* Diabetes, by type, with hypoglycemia, with coma
- diabetic — *see* Diabetes, hypoglycemia
- dietary counseling and surveillance Z71.3
- drug-induced E16.0
  - with coma (nondiabetic) E15
- due to insulin E16.0
  - with coma (nondiabetic) E15
  - therapeutic misadventure — *see* subcategory T38.3 ☑
- functional, nonhyperinsulinemic E16.1
- iatrogenic E16.0
  - with coma (nondiabetic) E15
- in infant of diabetic mother P70.1
  - gestational diabetes P70.0
- infantile E16.1
- leucine-induced E71.19
- neonatal (transitory) P70.4
  - iatrogenic P70.3
- reactive (not drug-induced) E16.1
- transitory neonatal P70.4

Hypogonadism
- female E28.39
- hypogonadotropic E23.0
- male E29.1
- ovarian (primary) E28.39
- pituitary E23.0
- testicular (primary) E29.1

Hypohidrosis, hypoidrosis L74.4
Hypoinsulinemia, postprocedural E89.1
Hypokalemia E87.6
Hypoleukocytosis — *see* Agranulocytosis
Hypolipoproteinemia (alpha) (beta) E78.6
Hypomagnesemia E83.42
- neonatal P71.2

Hypomania, hypomanic reaction F30.8
Hypomenorrhea — *see* Oligomenorrhea
Hypometabolism R63.8
Hypomotility
- gastrointestinal (tract) K31.89
  - psychogenic F45.8
- intestine K59.89
  - psychogenic F45.8
- stomach K31.89
  - psychogenic F45.8

Hyponasality R49.22
Hyponatremia E87.1
Hypo-osmolality E87.1
Hypo-ovarianism, hypo-ovarism E28.39
Hypoparathyroidism E20.9
- familial E20.8
- idiopathic E20.0
- neonatal, transitory P71.4
- postprocedural E89.2
- specified NEC E20.8

Hypoperfusion (in)
- newborn P96.89

Hypopharyngitis — *see* Laryngopharyngitis
Hypophoria H50.53
Hypophosphatemia, hypophosphatasia (acquired) (congenital) (renal) E83.39
- familial E83.31

Hypophyseal, hypophysis — *see also* condition
- dwarfism E23.0
- gigantism E22.0

Hypopiesis — *see* Hypotension
Hypopinealism E34.8
Hypopituitarism (juvenile) E23.0
- drug-induced E23.1
- due to
  - hypophysectomy E89.3
  - radiotherapy E89.3
- iatrogenic NEC E23.1
- postirradiation E89.3
- postpartum O99.285
- postprocedural E89.3

Hypoplasia, hypoplastic
- adrenal (gland), congenital Q89.1
- alimentary tract, congenital Q45.8

Hypoplasia, hypoplastic — *continued*

alimentary tract, congenital — *continued*
  upper Q40.8
anus, anal (canal) Q42.3
  with fistula Q42.2
aorta, aortic Q25.42
  ascending, in hypoplastic left heart syndrome Q23.4
  valve Q23.1
    in hypoplastic left heart syndrome Q23.4
areola, congenital Q83.8
arm (congenital) — *see* Defect, reduction, upper limb
artery (peripheral) Q27.8
  brain (congenital) Q28.3
  coronary Q24.5
  digestive system Q27.8
  lower limb Q27.8
  pulmonary Q25.79
    functional, unilateral J43.0
  retinal (congenital) Q14.1
  specified site NEC Q27.8
  umbilical Q27.0
  upper limb Q27.8
auditory canal Q17.8
  causing impairment of hearing Q16.9
biliary duct or passage Q44.5
bone NOS Q79.9
  face Q75.8
  marrow D61.9
    megakaryocytic D69.49
  skull — *see* Hypoplasia, skull
brain Q02
  gyri Q04.3
  part of Q04.3
breast (areola) N64.82
bronchus Q32.4
cardiac Q24.8
carpus — *see* Defect, reduction, upper limb, specified type NEC
cartilage hair Q78.8
cecum Q42.8
cementum K00.4
cephalic Q02
cerebellum Q04.3
cervix (uteri), congenital Q51.821
clavicle (congenital) Q74.0
coccyx Q76.49
colon Q42.9
  specified NEC Q42.8
corpus callosum Q04.0
cricoid cartilage Q31.2
digestive organ(s) or tract NEC Q45.8
  upper (congenital) Q40.8
ear (auricle) (lobe) Q17.2
  middle Q16.4
enamel of teeth (neonatal) (postnatal) (prenatal) K00.4
endocrine (gland) NEC Q89.2
endometrium N85.8
epididymis (congenital) Q55.4
epiglottis Q31.2
erythroid, congenital D61.01
esophagus (congenital) Q39.8
eustachian tube Q17.8
eye Q11.2
eyelid (congenital) Q10.3
face Q18.8
  bone(s) Q75.8
femur (congenital) — *see* Defect, reduction, lower limb, specified type NEC
fibula (congenital) — *see* Defect, reduction, lower limb, specified type NEC
finger (congenital) — *see* Defect, reduction, upper limb, specified type NEC
focal dermal Q82.8
foot — *see* Defect, reduction, lower limb, specified type NEC
gallbladder Q44.0
genitalia, genital organ(s)
  female, congenital Q52.8
    external Q52.79
    internal NEC Q52.8
    in adiposogenital dystrophy E23.6
  glottis Q31.2
hair Q84.2
hand (congenital) — *see* Defect, reduction, upper limb, specified type NEC
heart Q24.8
humerus (congenital) — *see* Defect, reduction, upper limb, specified type NEC

Hypoplasia, hypoplastic — *continued*

intestine (small) Q41.9
  large Q42.9
    specified NEC Q42.8
jaw M26.09
  alveolar M26.79
  lower M26.04
    alveolar M26.74
  upper M26.02
    alveolar M26.73
kidney(s) Q60.5
  bilateral Q60.4
  unilateral Q60.3
labium (majus) (minus), congenital Q52.79
larynx Q31.2
left heart syndrome Q23.4
leg (congenital) — *see* Defect, reduction, lower limb
limb Q73.8
  lower (congenital) — *see* Defect, reduction, lower limb
  upper (congenital) — *see* Defect, reduction, upper limb
liver Q44.7
lung (lobe) (not associated with short gestation) Q33.6
  associated with immaturity, low birth weight, prematurity, or short gestation P28.0
mammary (areola), congenital Q83.8
mandible, mandibular M26.04
  alveolar M26.74
  unilateral condylar M27.8
maxillary M26.02
  alveolar M26.73
medullary D61.9
megakaryocytic D69.49
metacarpus — *see* Defect, reduction, upper limb, specified type NEC
metatarsus — *see* Defect, reduction, lower limb, specified type NEC
muscle Q79.8
nail(s) Q84.6
nose, nasal Q30.1
optic nerve H47.03- ☑
osseous meatus (ear) Q17.8
ovary, congenital Q50.39
pancreas Q45.0
parathyroid (gland) Q89.2
parotid gland Q38.4
patella Q74.1
pelvis, pelvic girdle Q74.2
penis (congenital) Q55.62
peripheral vascular system Q27.8
  digestive system Q27.8
  lower limb Q27.8
  specified site NEC Q27.8
  upper limb Q27.8
pituitary (gland) (congenital) Q89.2
pulmonary (not associated with short gestation) Q33.6
  artery, functional J43.0
  associated with short gestation P28.0
radioulnar — *see* Defect, reduction, upper limb, specified type NEC
radius — *see* Defect, reduction, upper limb
rectum Q42.1
  with fistula Q42.0
respiratory system NEC Q34.8
rib Q76.6
right heart syndrome Q22.6
sacrum Q76.49
scapula Q74.0
scrotum Q55.1
shoulder girdle Q74.0
skin Q82.8
skull (bone) Q75.8
  with
    anencephaly Q00.0
    encephalocele — *see* Encephalocele
    hydrocephalus Q03.9
      with spina bifida — *see* Spina bifida, by site, with hydrocephalus
    microcephaly Q02
spinal (cord) (ventral horn cell) Q06.1
spine Q76.49
sternum Q76.7
tarsus — *see* Defect, reduction, lower limb, specified type NEC
testis Q55.1
thymic, with immunodeficiency D82.1
thymus (gland) Q89.2

Hypoplasia, hypoplastic — *continued*

thymus — *continued*
  with immunodeficiency D82.1
thyroid (gland) E03.1
  cartilage Q31.2
tibiofibular (congenital) — *see* Defect, reduction, lower limb, specified type NEC
toe — *see* Defect, reduction, lower limb, specified type NEC
tongue Q38.3
Turner's K00.4
ulna (congenital) — *see* Defect, reduction, upper limb
umbilical artery Q27.0
unilateral condylar M27.8
ureter Q62.8
uterus, congenital Q51.811
vagina Q52.4
vascular NEC peripheral Q27.8
  brain Q28.3
  digestive system Q27.8
  lower limb Q27.8
  specified site NEC Q27.8
  upper limb Q27.8
vein(s) (peripheral) Q27.8
  brain Q28.3
  digestive system Q27.8
  great Q26.8
  lower limb Q27.8
  specified site NEC Q27.8
  upper limb Q27.8
vena cava (inferior) (superior) Q26.8
vertebra Q76.49
vulva, congenital Q52.79
zonule (ciliary) Q12.8
Hypoplasminogenemia E88.02
Hypopnea, obstructive sleep apnea G47.33
Hypopotassemia E87.6
Hypoproconvertinemia, congenital (hereditary) D68.2
Hypoproteinemia E77.8
Hypoprothrombinemia (congenital) (hereditary) (idiopathic) D68.2
  acquired D68.4
  newborn, transient P61.6
Hypoptyalism K11.7
Hypopyon (eye) (anterior chamber) — *see* Iridocyclitis, acute, hypopyon
Hypopyrexia R68.0
Hyporeflexia R29.2
Hyposecretion
  ACTH E23.0
  antidiuretic hormone E23.2
  ovary E28.39
  salivary gland (any) K11.7
  vasopressin E23.2
Hyposegmentation, leukocytic, hereditary D72.0
Hyposiderinemia D50.9
Hypospadias Q54.9
  balanic Q54.0
  coronal Q54.0
  glandular Q54.0
  penile Q54.1
  penoscrotal Q54.2
  perineal Q54.3
  specified NEC Q54.8
Hypospermatogenesis — *see* Oligospermia
Hyposplenism D73.0
Hypostasis pulmonary, passive — *see* Edema, lung
Hypostatic — *see* condition
Hyposthenuria N28.89
Hypotension (arterial) (constitutional) I95.9
  chronic I95.89
  due to (of) hemodialysis I95.3
  drug-induced I95.2
  iatrogenic I95.89
  idiopathic (permanent) I95.0
  intracranial G96.810
    following
      lumbar cerebrospinal fluid shunting G97.83
      specified procedure NEC G97.84
      ventricular shunting (ventriculostomy) G97.2
    specified NEC G96.819
    spontaneous G96.811
  intra-dialytic I95.3
  maternal, syndrome (following labor and delivery) O26.5- ☑
  neurogenic, orthostatic G90.3
  orthostatic (chronic) I95.1
    due to drugs I95.2

Hypotension — *continued*
  orthostatic — *continued*
    neurogenic G90.3
  postoperative I95.81
  postural I95.1
  specified NEC I95.89
Hypothermia (accidental) T68 ☑
  due to anesthesia, anesthetic T88.51 ☑
  low environmental temperature T68 ☑
  neonatal P80.9
    environmental (mild) NEC P80.8
    mild P80.8
    severe (chronic) (cold injury syndrome) P80.0
    specified NEC P80.8
  not associated with low environmental temperature R68.0
Hypothyroidism (acquired) E03.9
  autoimmune — *see* Thyroiditis, autoimmune
  congenital (without goiter) E03.1
    with goiter (diffuse) E03.0
  due to
    exogenous substance NEC E03.2
    iodine-deficiency, acquired E01.8
      subclinical E02
    irradiation therapy E89.0
    medicament NEC E03.2
    P-aminosalicylic acid (PAS) E03.2
    phenylbutazone E03.2
    resorcinol E03.2
    sulfonamide E03.2
    surgery E89.0
    thiourea group drugs E03.2
  iatrogenic NEC E03.2
  iodine-deficiency (acquired) E01.8
    congenital — *see* Syndrome, iodine- deficiency, congenital
    subclinical E02
  neonatal, transitory P72.2
  postinfectious E03.3
  postirradiation E89.0
  postprocedural E89.0
  postsurgical E89.0
  specified NEC E03.8
  subclinical, iodine-deficiency related E02
Hypotonia, hypotonicity, hypotony
  bladder N31.2
  congenital (benign) P94.2
  eye — *see* Disorder, globe, hypotony
Hypotrichosis — *see* Alopecia
Hypotropia H50.2- ☑
Hypoventilation R06.89
  congenital central alveolar G47.35
  sleep related
    idiopathic nonobstructive alveolar G47.34
    in conditions classified elsewhere G47.36
Hypovitaminosis — *see* Deficiency, vitamin
Hypovolemia E86.1
  surgical shock T81.19 ☑
  traumatic (shock) T79.4 ☑
Hypoxemia R09.02
  newborn P84
  sleep related, in conditions classified elsewhere G47.36
Hypoxia — *see also* Anoxia R09.02
  cerebral, during a procedure NEC G97.81
    postprocedural NEC G97.82
  intrauterine P84
  myocardial — *see* Insufficiency, coronary
  newborn P84
  sleep-related G47.34
Hypsarrhythmia — *see* Epilepsy, generalized, specified NEC
Hysteralgia, pregnant uterus O26.89- ☑
Hysteria, hysterical (conversion) (dissociative state) F44.9
  anxiety F41.8
  convulsions F44.5
  psychosis, acute F44.9
Hysteroepilepsy F44.5

I

IBDU (colonic inflammatory bowel dissease unclassified) K52.3
ICANS (immune effector cell-associated neurotoxicity syndrome) — *see* Syndrome, immune effector cell-associated neurotoxicity
Ichthyoparasitism due to Vandellia cirrhosa B88.8
Ichthyosis (congenital) Q80.9

Ichthyosis — *continued*
  acquired L85.0
  fetalis Q80.4
  hystrix Q80.8
  lamellar Q80.2
  lingual K13.29
  palmaris and plantaris Q82.8
  simplex Q80.0
  vera Q80.8
  vulgaris Q80.0
  X-linked Q80.1
Ichthyotoxism — *see* Poisoning, fish
  bacterial — *see* Intoxication, foodborne
Icteroanemia, hemolytic (acquired) D59.9
  congenital — *see* Spherocytosis
Icterus — *see also* Jaundice
  conjunctiva R17
  gravis, newborn P55.0
  hematogenous (acquired) D59.9
  hemolytic (acquired) D59.9
    congenital — *see* Spherocytosis
  hemorrhagic (acute) (leptospiral) (spirochetal) A27.0
    newborn P53
  infectious B15.9
    with hepatic coma B15.0
    leptospiral A27.0
    spirochetal A27.0
  neonatorum — *see* Jaundice, newborn
  newborn P59.9
  spirochetal A27.0
Ictus solaris, solis T67.01 ☑
Id reaction (due to bacteria) L30.2
Ideation
  homicidal R45.850
  suicidal R45.851
Identity disorder (child) F64.9
  gender role F64.2
  psychosexual F64.2
Idioglossia F80.0
Idiopathic — *see* condition
Idiot, idiocy (congenital) F73
  amaurotic (Bielschowsky(-Jansky)) (family) (infantile (late)) (juvenile (late)) (Vogt-Spielmeyer) E75.4
  microcephalic Q02
IgE asthma J45.909
IIAC (idiopathic infantile arterial calcification) Q28.8
Ileitis (chronic) (noninfectious) — *see also* Enteritis K52.9
  backwash — *see* Pancolitis, ulcerative (chronic)
  infectious A09
  regional (ulcerative) — *see* Enteritis, regional, small intestine
  segmental — *see* Enteritis, regional
  terminal (ulcerative) — *see* Enteritis, regional, small intestine
Ileocolitis — *see also* Enteritis K52.9
  infectious A09
  regional — *see* Enteritis, regional
  ulcerative K51.0- ☑
Ileostomy
  attention to Z43.2
  malfunctioning K94.13
  status Z93.2
    with complication — *see* Complications, enterostomy
Ileotyphus — *see* Typhoid
Ileum — *see* condition
Ileus (bowel) (colon) (inhibitory) (intestine) K56.7
  adynamic K56.0
  due to gallstone (in intestine) K56.3
  duodenal (chronic) K31.5
  gallstone K56.3
  mechanical NEC — *see also* Obstruction, intestine, specified NEC K56.699
  meconium P76.0
    in cystic fibrosis E84.11
    meaning meconium plug (without cystic fibrosis) P76.0
  myxedema K59.89
  neurogenic K56.0
    Hirschsprung's disease or megacolon Q43.1
  newborn
    due to meconium P76.0
      in cystic fibrosis E84.11
      meaning meconium plug (without cystic fibrosis) P76.0
    transitory P76.1
  obstructive — *see also* Obstruction, intestine, specified NEC K56.699

Ileus — *continued*
  paralytic K56.0
  postoperative K91.89
Iliac — *see* condition
Iliotibial band syndrome M76.3- ☑
Illiteracy Z55.0
Illness — *see also* Disease R69
  manic-depressive — *see* Disorder, bipolar
Imbalance R26.89
  autonomic G90.8
  constituents of food intake E63.1
  electrolyte E87.8
    with
      abortion — *see* Abortion by type, complicated by, electrolyte imbalance
      molar pregnancy O08.5
    due to hyperemesis gravidarum O21.1
    following ectopic or molar pregnancy O08.5
    neonatal, transitory NEC P74.49
      potassium
        hyperkalemia P74.31
        hypokalemia P74.32
      sodium
        hypernatremia P74.21
        hyponatremia P74.22
  endocrine E34.9
  eye muscle NOS H50.9
  hormone E34.9
  hysterical F44.4
  labyrinth — *see* subcategory H83.2 ☑
  posture R29.3
  protein-energy — *see* Malnutrition
  sympathetic G90.8
Imbecile, imbecility (I.Q. 35-49) F71
Imbedding, intrauterine device T83.39 ☑
Imbibition, cholesterol (gallbladder) K82.4
Imbrication, teeth,, fully erupted M26.30
Imerslund (-Gräsbeck) **syndrome** D51.1
Immature — *see also* Immaturity
  birth (less than 37 completed weeks) — *see* Preterm, newborn
    extremely (less than 28 completed weeks) — *see* Immaturity, extreme
  personality F60.89
Immaturity (less than 37 completed weeks) — *see also* Preterm, newborn
  extreme of newborn (less than 28 completed weeks of gestation) (less than 196 completed days of gestation) (unspecified weeks of gestation) P07.20
    gestational age
      23 completed weeks (23 weeks, 0 days through 23 weeks, 6 days) P07.22
      24 completed weeks (24 weeks, 0 days through 24 weeks, 6 days) P07.23
      25 completed weeks (25 weeks, 0 days through 25 weeks, 6 days) P07.24
      26 completed weeks (26 weeks, 0 days through 26 weeks, 6 days) P07.25
      27 completed weeks (27 weeks, 0 days through 27 weeks, 6 days) P07.26
      less than 23 completed weeks P07.21
  fetus or infant light-for-dates — *see* Light-for-dates
  lung, newborn P28.0
  organ or site NEC — *see* Hypoplasia
  pulmonary, newborn P28.0
  reaction F60.89
  sexual (female) (male), after puberty E30.0
Immersion T75.1 ☑
  foot T69.02- ☑
  hand T69.01- ☑
Immobile, immobility
  complete, due to severe physical disability or frailty R53.2
  intestine K59.89
  syndrome (paraplegic) M62.3
Immune reconstitution (inflammatory) syndrome [IRIS] D89.3
Immunization — *see also* Vaccination
  ABO — *see* Incompatibility, ABO
    in newborn P55.1
  appropriate for age
    child (over 28 days old) Z00.129
      with abnormal findings Z00.121
  complication — *see* Complications, vaccination
  encounter for Z23
  not done (not carried out) — *see also* Underimmunization status Z28.9

☑ **Additional Character Required — Refer to the Tabular List for Character Selection**

Immunization — *continued*
  not done — *see also* Underimmunization status — *continued*
    because (of)
      acute illness of patient Z28.01
      allergy to vaccine (or component) Z28.04
      caregiver refusal Z28.82
      chronic illness of patient Z28.02
      contraindication NEC Z28.09
      delay in delivery of vaccine Z28.83
      group pressure Z28.1
      guardian refusal Z28.82
      immune compromised state of patient Z28.03
      lack of availability of vaccine Z28.83
      manufacturer delay of vaccine Z28.83
      parent refusal Z28.82
      patient had disease being vaccinated against Z28.81
      patient refusal Z28.21
      patient's belief Z28.1
      religious beliefs of patient Z28.1
      specified reason NEC Z28.89
        of patient Z28.29
      unavailability of vaccine Z28.83
      unspecified patient reason Z28.20
  partial — *see also* Underimmunization status
    for COVID-19 Z28.311
  Rh factor
    affecting management of pregnancy NEC O36.09- ☑
      anti-D antibody O36.01- ☑
    from transfusion — *see* Complication(s), transfusion, incompatibility reaction, Rh (factor)
Immunocompromised NOS D84.9
Immunocytoma C83.0- ☑
Immunodeficiency D84.9
  with
    adenosine-deaminase deficiency — *see also* Deficiency, adenosine deaminase D81.30
    antibody defects D80.9
      specified type NEC D80.8
    hyperimmunoglobulinemia D80.6
    increased immunoglobulin M (IgM) D80.5
    major defect D82.9
      specified type NEC D82.8
    partial albinism D82.8
    short-limbed stature D82.2
    thrombocytopenia and eczema D82.0
  antibody with
    hyperimmunoglobulinemia D80.6
    near-normal immunoglobulins D80.6
  autosomal recessive, Swiss type D80.0
  combined D81.9
    biotin-dependent carboxylase D81.819
      biotinidase D81.810
      holocarboxylase synthetase D81.818
      specified type NEC D81.818
    severe (SCID) D81.9
      with
        low or normal B-cell numbers D81.2
        low T- and B-cell numbers D81.1
        reticular dysgenesis D81.0
    specified type NEC D81.89
  common variable D83.9
    with
      abnormalities of B-cell numbers and function D83.0
      autoantibodies to B- or T-cells D83.2
      immunoregulatory T-cell disorders D83.1
    specified type NEC D83.8
  due to
    conditions classified elsewhere D84.81
    drugs D84.821
    external causes D84.822
    medication (current or past) D84.821
  following hereditary defective response to Epstein-Barr virus (EBV) D82.3
  selective, immunoglobulin
    A (IgA) D80.2
    G (IgG) (subclasses) D80.3
    M (IgM) D80.4
  severe combined (SCID) D81.9
    due to adenosine deaminase deficiency D81.31
  specified type NEC D84.89
  X-linked, with increased IgM D80.5
Immunodeficient NOS D84.9
Immunosuppressed NOS D84.9
Immunotherapy (encounter for)
  antineoplastic Z51.12

Impaction, impacted
  bowel, colon, rectum — *see also* Impaction, fecal K56.49
    by gallstone K56.3
  calculus — *see* Calculus
  cerumen (ear) (external) H61.2- ☑
  cuspid — *see* Impaction, tooth
  dental (same or adjacent tooth) K01.1
  fecal, feces K56.41
  fracture — *see* Fracture, by site
  gallbladder — *see* Calculus, gallbladder
  gallstone(s) — *see* Calculus, gallbladder
    bile duct (common) (hepatic) — *see* Calculus, bile duct
    cystic duct — *see* Calculus, gallbladder
    in intestine, with obstruction (any part) K56.3
  intestine (calculous) NEC — *see also* Impaction, fecal K56.49
    gallstone, with ileus K56.3
  intrauterine device (IUD) T83.39 ☑
  molar — *see* Impaction, tooth
  shoulder, causing obstructed labor O66.0
  tooth, teeth K01.1
  turbinate J34.89
Impaired, impairment (function)
  auditory discrimination — *see* Abnormal, auditory perception
  cognitive, mild, of uncertain or unknown etiology G31.84
  dual sensory Z73.82
  fasting glucose R73.01
  glucose tolerance (oral) R73.02
  hearing — *see* Deafness
  heart — *see* Disease, heart
  kidney N28.9
    disorder resulting from N25.9
      specified NEC N25.89
  liver K72.90
    with coma K72.91
  mastication K08.89
  mild cognitive G31.84
    of uncertain or unknown etiology G31.84
  mild neurocognitive
    due to known physiological condition (without behavioral disturbance) F06.70
      with behavioral disturbance F06.71
  mobility
    ear ossicles — *see* Ankylosis, ear ossicles
    requiring care provider Z74.09
  myocardium, myocardial — *see* Insufficiency, myocardial
  rectal sphincter R19.8
  renal (acute) (chronic) N28.9
    disorder resulting from N25.9
      specified NEC N25.89
  vision NEC H54.7
    both eyes H54.3
Impediment, speech — *see also* Disorder, speech R47.9
  psychogenic (childhood) F98.8
  slurring R47.81
  specified NEC R47.89
Impending
  coronary syndrome I20.0
  delirium tremens F10.239
  myocardial infarction I20.0
Imperception auditory (acquired) — *see also* Deafness
  congenital H93.25
Imperfect
  aeration, lung (newborn) NEC — *see* Atelectasis
  closure (congenital)
    alimentary tract NEC Q45.8
      lower Q43.8
      upper Q40.8
    atrioventricular ostium Q21.20
    atrium (secundum) Q21.11
    branchial cleft NOS Q18.2
      cyst Q18.0
      fistula Q18.0
      sinus Q18.0
    choroid Q14.3
    cricoid cartilage Q31.8
    cusps, heart valve NEC Q24.8
      pulmonary Q22.3
    ductus
      arteriosus Q25.0
      Botalli Q25.0
    ear drum (causing impairment of hearing) Q16.4

Imperfect — *continued*
  closure — *continued*
    esophagus with communication to bronchus or trachea Q39.1
    eyelid Q10.3
    foramen
      botalli Q21.12
      ovale Q21.12
    genitalia, genital organ(s) or system
      female Q52.8
        external Q52.79
        internal NEC Q52.8
      male Q55.8
    glottis Q31.8
    interatrial ostium or septum Q21.19
    interauricular ostium or septum Q21.19
    interventricular ostium or septum Q21.0
    larynx Q31.8
    lip — *see* Cleft, lip
    nasal septum Q30.3
    nose Q30.2
    omphalomesenteric duct Q43.0
    optic nerve entry Q14.2
    organ or site not listed — *see* Anomaly, by site
    ostium
      interatrial Q21.19
      interauricular Q21.19
      interventricular Q21.0
    palate — *see* Cleft, palate
    preauricular sinus Q18.1
    retina Q14.1
    roof of orbit Q75.8
    sclera Q13.5
    septum
      aorticopulmonary Q21.4
      atrial (secundum) Q21.19
      between aorta and pulmonary artery Q21.4
      heart Q21.9
      interatrial (secundum) Q21.19
      interauricular (secundum) Q21.19
      interventricular Q21.0
        in tetralogy of Fallot Q21.3
      nasal Q30.3
      ventricular Q21.0
        with pulmonary stenosis or atresia, dextraposition of aorta, and hypertrophy of right ventricle Q21.3
        in tetralogy of Fallot Q21.3
    skull Q75.0
      with
        anencephaly Q00.0
        encephalocele — *see* Encephalocele
        hydrocephalus Q03.9
          with spina bifida — *see* Spina bifida, by site, with hydrocephalus
        microcephaly Q02
    spine (with meningocele) — *see* Spina bifida
    trachea Q32.1
    tympanic membrane (causing impairment of hearing) Q16.4
    uterus Q51.818
    vitelline duct Q43.0
  erection — *see* Dysfunction, sexual, male, erectile
  fusion — *see* Imperfect, closure
  inflation, lung (newborn) — *see* Atelectasis
  posture R29.3
  rotation, intestine Q43.3
  septum, ventricular Q21.0
Imperfectly descended testis — *see* Cryptorchid
Imperforate (congenital) — *see also* Atresia
  anus Q42.3
    with fistula Q42.2
  cervix (uteri) Q51.828
  esophagus Q39.0
    with tracheoesophageal fistula Q39.1
  hymen Q52.3
  jejunum Q41.1
  pharynx Q38.8
  rectum Q42.1
    with fistula Q42.0
  urethra Q64.39
  vagina Q52.4
Impervious (congenital) — *see also* Atresia
  anus Q42.3
    with fistula Q42.2
  bile duct Q44.2
  esophagus Q39.0
    with tracheoesophageal fistula Q39.1

Impervious — *continued*
- intestine (small) Q41.9
  - large Q42.9
    - specified NEC Q42.8
  - rectum Q42.1
    - with fistula Q42.0
  - ureter — *see* Atresia, ureter
  - urethra Q64.39

Impetiginization of dermatoses L01.1
Impetigo (any organism) (any site) (circinate) (contagiosa) (simplex) (vulgaris) L01.00
- Bockhart's L01.02
- bullous, bullosa L01.03
- external ear L01.00 [H62.40]
- follicularis L01.02
- furfuracea L30.5
- herpetiformis L40.1
  - nonobstetrical L40.1
- neonatorum L01.03
- nonbullous L01.01
- specified type NEC L01.09
- ulcerative L01.09

Impingement (on teeth)
- joint — *see* Disorder, joint, specified type NEC
- soft tissue
  - anterior M26.81
  - posterior M26.82

Implant, endometrial N80.9
Implantation
- anomalous — *see* Anomaly, by site
  - ureter Q62.63
- cyst
  - external area or site (skin) NEC L72.0
  - iris — *see* Cyst, iris, implantation
  - vagina N89.8
  - vulva N90.7
- dermoid (cyst) — *see* Implantation, cyst

Impotence (sexual) N52.9
- counseling Z70.1
- organic origin — *see also* Dysfunction, sexual, male, erectile N52.9
- psychogenic F52.21

Impression, basilar Q75.8
Imprisonment, anxiety concerning Z65.1
Improper care (child) (newborn) — *see* Maltreatment
Improperly tied umbilical cord (causing hemorrhage) P51.8
Impulsiveness (impulsive) R45.87
Inability to swallow — *see* Aphagia
- comply with dietary regimen Z91.118
- swallow — *see* Aphagia

Inaccessible, inaccessibility
- health care NEC Z75.3
  - due to
    - waiting period Z75.2
      - for admission to facility elsewhere Z75.1
  - other helping agencies Z75.4
  - transportation Z59.82

Inactive — *see* condition
Inadequate, inadequacy
- aesthetics of dental restoration K08.56
- biologic, constitutional, functional, or social F60.7
- development
  - child R62.50
  - genitalia
    - after puberty NEC E30.0
    - congenital
      - female Q52.8
        - external Q52.79
        - internal Q52.8
      - male Q55.8
  - lungs Q33.6
    - associated with short gestation P28.0
  - organ or site not listed — *see* Anomaly, by site
- diet (causing nutritional deficiency) E63.9
- drinking-water supply Z58.6
- eating habits Z72.4
- environment, household Z59.1
- family support Z63.8
- food (supply) NEC Z59.48
  - hunger effects T73.0 ☑
- functional F60.7
- household care, due to
  - family member
    - handicapped or ill Z74.2
    - on vacation Z75.5
    - temporarily away from home Z74.2
  - technical defects in home Z59.1

Inadequate, inadequacy — *continued*
- household care, due to — *continued*
  - temporary absence from home of person rendering care Z74.2
- housing (heating) (space) Z59.1
- income (financial) Z59.6
- intrafamilial communication Z63.8
- material resources Z59.87
- mental — *see* Disability, intellectual
- parental supervision or control of child Z62.0
- personality F60.7
- pulmonary
  - function R06.89
    - newborn P28.5
  - ventilation, newborn P28.5
- sample of cytologic smear
  - anus R85.615
  - cervix R87.615
  - vagina R87.625
- social F60.7
  - insurance Z59.7
  - skills NEC Z73.4
- supervision of child by parent Z62.0
- teaching affecting education Z55.8
- transportation Z59.82
- welfare support Z59.7

Inanition R64
- with edema — *see* Malnutrition, severe
- due to
  - deprivation of food T73.0 ☑
  - malnutrition — *see* Malnutrition
- fever R50.9

Inappropriate
- change in quantitative human chorionic gonadotropin (hCG) in early pregnancy O02.81
- diet or eating habits Z72.4
- level of quantitative human chorionic gonadotropin (hCG) for gestational age in early pregnancy O02.81
- secretion
  - antidiuretic hormone (ADH) (excessive) E22.2
    - deficiency E23.2
  - pituitary (posterior) E22.2

Inattention at or after birth — *see* Neglect
Incarceration, incarcerated
- enterocele K46.0
  - gangrenous K46.1
- epiplocele K46.0
  - gangrenous K46.1
- exomphalos K42.0
  - gangrenous K42.1
- hernia — *see also* Hernia, by site, with obstruction
  - with gangrene — *see* Hernia, by site, with gangrene
- iris, in wound — *see* Injury, eye, laceration, with prolapse
- lens, in wound — *see* Injury, eye, laceration, with prolapse
- omphalocele K42.0
- prison, anxiety concerning Z65.1
- rupture — *see* Hernia, by site
- sarcoepiplocele K46.0
  - gangrenous K46.1
- sarcoepiplomphalocele K42.0
  - with gangrene K42.1
- uterus N85.8
  - gravid O34.51- ☑
    - causing obstructed labor O65.5

Incised wound
- external — *see* Laceration
- internal organs — *see* Injury, by site

Incision, incisional
- hernia K43.2
  - with
    - gangrene (and obstruction) K43.1
    - obstruction K43.0
  - surgical, complication — *see* Complications, surgical procedure
- traumatic
  - external — *see* Laceration
  - internal organs — *see* Injury, by site

Inclusion
- azurophilic leukocytic D72.0
- blennorrhea (neonatal) (newborn) P39.1
- gallbladder in liver (congenital) Q44.1

Incompatibility
- ABO
  - affecting management of pregnancy O36.11- ☑
    - anti-A sensitization O36.11- ☑

Incompatibility — *continued*
- ABO — *continued*
  - affecting management of pregnancy — *continued*
    - anti-B sensitization O36.19- ☑
    - specified NEC O36.19- ☑
  - infusion or transfusion reaction — *see* Complication(s), transfusion, incompatibility reaction, ABO
  - newborn P55.1
- blood (group) (Duffy) (K) (Kell) (Kidd) (Lewis) (M) (S) NEC
  - affecting management of pregnancy O36.11- ☑
    - anti-A sensitization O36.11- ☑
    - anti-B sensitization O36.19- ☑
  - infusion or transfusion reaction T80.89 ☑
  - newborn P55.8
- divorce or estrangement Z63.5
- Rh (blood group) (factor) Z31.82
  - affecting management of pregnancy NEC O36.09- ☑
    - anti-D antibody O36.01- ☑
  - infusion or transfusion reaction — *see* Complication(s), transfusion, incompatibility reaction, Rh (factor)
  - newborn P55.0
- rhesus — *see* Incompatibility, Rh

Incompetency, incompetent, incompetence
- annular
  - aortic (valve) — *see* Insufficiency, aortic
  - mitral (valve) I34.0
  - pulmonary valve (heart) I37.1
- aortic (valve) — *see* Insufficiency, aortic
- cardiac valve — *see* Endocarditis
- cervix, cervical (os) N88.3
  - in pregnancy O34.3- ☑
- chronotropic I45.89
  - with
    - autonomic dysfunction G90.8
    - ischemic heart disease I25.89
    - left ventricular dysfunction I51.89
    - sinus node dysfunction I49.8
- esophagogastric (junction) (sphincter) K22.0
- mitral (valve) — *see* Insufficiency, mitral
- pelvic fundus N81.89
- pubocervical tissue N81.82
- pulmonary valve (heart) I37.1
  - congenital Q22.3
- rectovaginal tissue N81.83
- tricuspid (annular) (valve) — *see* Insufficiency, tricuspid
- valvular — *see* Endocarditis
  - congenital Q24.8
- vein, venous (saphenous) (varicose) — *see* Varix, leg

Incomplete — *see also* condition
- atrioventricular
  - canal Q21.21
  - septal defect Q21.21
- bladder, emptying R33.9
- defecation R15.0
- endocardial cushion defect Q21.21
- expansion lungs (newborn) NEC — *see* Atelectasis
- rotation, intestine Q43.3

Inconclusive
- diagnostic imaging due to excess body fat of patient R93.9
- findings on diagnostic imaging of breast NEC R92.8
- mammogram (due to dense breasts) R92.2

Incontinence R32
- anal sphincter R15.9
- coital N39.491
- feces R15.9
  - nonorganic origin F98.1
- insensible (urinary) N39.42
- overflow N39.490
- postural (urinary) N39.492
- psychogenic F45.8
- rectal R15.9
- reflex N39.498
- stress (female) (male) N39.3
  - and urge N39.46
- urethral sphincter R32
- urge N39.41
  - and stress (female) (male) N39.46
- urine (urinary) R32
  - continuous N39.45
  - due to cognitive impairment, or severe physical disability or immobility R39.81
  - functional R39.81
  - insensible N39.42

☑ Additional Character Required — Refer to the Tabular List for Character Selection

Incontinence — *continued*
  urine — *continued*
    mixed (stress and urge) N39.46
    nocturnal N39.44
    nonorganic origin F98.0
    overflow N39.490
    post dribbling N39.43
    postural N39.492
    reflex N39.498
    specified NEC N39.498
    stress (female) (male) N39.3
      and urge N39.46
    total N39.498
    unaware N39.42
    urge N39.41
      and stress (female) (male) N39.46
Incontinentia pigmenti Q82.3
Incoordinate, incoordination
  esophageal-pharyngeal (newborn) — *see* Dysphagia
  muscular R27.8
  uterus (action) (contractions) (complicating delivery) O62.4
Increase, increased
  abnormal, in development R63.8
  androgens (ovarian) E28.1
  anticoagulants (antithrombin) (anti-VIIIa) (anti-IXa) (anti-Xa) (anti-XIa) — *see* Circulating anticoagulants
  cold sense R20.8
  estrogen E28.0
  function
    adrenal
      cortex — *see* Cushing's, syndrome
      medulla E27.5
    pituitary (gland) (anterior) (lobe) E22.9
      posterior E22.2
  heat sense R20.8
  intracranial pressure (benign) G93.2
  permeability, capillaries I78.8
  pressure, intracranial G93.2
  secretion
    gastrin E16.4
    glucagon E16.3
    pancreas, endocrine E16.9
      growth hormone-releasing hormone E16.8
      pancreatic polypeptide E16.8
      somatostatin E16.8
      vasoactive-intestinal polypeptide E16.8
  sphericity, lens Q12.4
  splenic activity D73.1
  venous pressure I87.8
    portal K76.6
Increta placenta O43.22- ☑
Incrustation, cornea, foreign body (lead)(zinc) — *see* Foreign body, cornea
Incyclophoria H50.54
Incyclotropia — *see* Cyclotropia
Indeterminate sex Q56.4
India rubber skin Q82.8
Indigestion (acid) (bilious) (functional) K30
  catarrhal K31.89
  due to decomposed food NOS A05.9
  nervous F45.8
  psychogenic F45.8
Indirect — *see* condition
Induratio penis plastica N48.6
Induration, indurated
  brain G93.89
  breast (fibrous) N64.51
    puerperal, postpartum O92.29
  broad ligament N83.8
  chancre
    anus A51.1
    congenital A50.07
    extragenital NEC A51.2
  corpora cavernosa (penis) (plastic) N48.6
  liver (chronic) K76.89
  lung (black) (chronic) (fibroid) — *see also* Fibrosis, lung J84.10
    essential brown J84.03
  penile (plastic) N48.6
  phlebitic — *see* Phlebitis
  skin R23.4
Inebriety (without dependence) — *see* Alcohol, intoxication
Inefficiency, kidney N28.9
Inelasticity, skin R23.4

Inequality, leg (length) (acquired) — *see also* Deformity, limb, unequal length
  congenital — *see* Defect, reduction, lower limb
  lower leg — *see* Deformity, limb, unequal length
Inertia
  bladder (neurogenic) N31.2
  stomach K31.89
    psychogenic F45.8
  uterus, uterine during labor O62.2
    during latent phase of labor O62.0
    primary O62.0
    secondary O62.1
  vesical (neurogenic) N31.2
Infancy, infantile, infantilism — *see also* condition
  celiac K90.0
  genitalia, genitals (after puberty) E30.0
  Herter's (nontropical sprue) K90.0
  intestinal K90.0
  Lorain E23.0
  pancreatic K86.89
  pelvis M95.5
    with disproportion (fetopelvic) O33.1
      causing obstructed labor O65.1
  pituitary E23.0
  renal N25.0
  uterus — *see* Infantile, genitalia
Infant(s) — *see also* Infancy
  excessive crying R68.11
  irritable child R68.12
  lack of care — *see* Neglect
  liveborn (singleton) Z38.2
    born in hospital Z38.00
      by cesarean Z38.01
    born outside hospital Z38.1
    multiple NEC Z38.8
      born in hospital Z38.68
        by cesarean Z38.69
      born outside hospital Z38.7
    quadruplet Z38.8
      born in hospital Z38.63
        by cesarean Z38.64
      born outside hospital Z38.7
    quintuplet Z38.8
      born in hospital Z38.65
        by cesarean Z38.66
      born outside hospital Z38.7
    triplet Z38.8
      born in hospital Z38.61
        by cesarean Z38.62
      born outside hospital Z38.7
    twin Z38.5
      born in hospital Z38.30
        by cesarean Z38.31
      born outside hospital Z38.4
  of diabetic mother (syndrome of) P70.1
    gestational diabetes P70.0
Infantile — *see also* condition
  genitalia, genitals E30.0
  os, uterine E30.0
  penis E30.0
  testis E29.1
  uterus E30.0
Infantilism — *see* Infancy
Infarct, infarction
  adrenal (capsule) (gland) E27.49
  appendices epiploicae — *see also* Infarct, intestine K55.069
  bowel — *see also* Infarct, intestine K55.069
  brain (stem) — *see* Infarct, cerebral
  breast N64.89
  brewer's (kidney) N28.0
  cardiac — *see* Infarct, myocardium
  cerebellar — *see* Infarct, cerebral
  cerebral (acute) (chronic) — *see also* Occlusion, artery cerebral or precerebral, with infarction I63.9-
    aborted I63.9
    cortical I63.9
    due to
      cerebral venous thrombosis, nonpyogenic I63.6
      embolism
        cerebral arteries I63.4- ☑
        precerebral arteries I63.1- ☑
      occlusion NEC
        cerebral arteries I63.5- ☑
        precerebral arteries I63.2- ☑
        small artery I63.81
      stenosis NEC
        cerebral arteries I63.5- ☑

Infarct, infarction — *continued*
  cerebral — *see also* Occlusion, artery cerebral or precerebral, with infarction — *continued*
    due to — *continued*
      stenosis — *continued*
        precerebral arteries I63.2- ☑
        small artery I63.81
      thrombosis
        cerebral artery I63.3- ☑
        precerebral artery I63.0- ☑
    intraoperative
      during cardiac surgery I97.810
      during other surgery I97.811
    neonatal P91.82- ☑
    perinatal (arterial ischemic) P91.82- ☑
    postprocedural
      following cardiac surgery I97.820
      following other surgery I97.821
    specified NEC I63.89
  colon (acute) (agnogenic) (embolic) (hemorrhagic) (nonocclusive) (nonthrombotic) (occlusive) (segmental) (thrombotic) (with gangrene) — *see also* Infarct, intestine K55.049
  coronary artery — *see* Infarct, myocardium
  embolic — *see* Embolism
  fallopian tube N83.8
  gallbladder K82.8
  heart — *see* Infarct, myocardium
  hepatic K76.3
  hypophysis (anterior lobe) E23.6
  impending (myocardium) I20.0
  intestine (acute) (agnogenic) (embolic) (hemorrhagic) (nonocclusive) (nonthrombotic) (occlusive) (thrombotic) (with gangrene) K55.069
    diffuse K55.062
    focal K55.061
    large K55.049
      diffuse K55.042
      focal K55.041
    small K55.029
      diffuse K55.022
      focal K55.021
  kidney N28.0
  lacunar I63.81
  liver K76.3
  lung (embolic) (thrombotic) — *see* Embolism, pulmonary
  lymph node I89.8
  mesentery, mesenteric (embolic) (thrombotic) (with gangrene) — *see also* Infarct, intestine K55.069
  muscle (ischemic) M62.20
    ankle M62.27- ☑
    foot M62.27- ☑
    forearm M62.23- ☑
    hand M62.24- ☑
    lower leg M62.26- ☑
    pelvic region M62.25- ☑
    shoulder region M62.21- ☑
    specified site NEC M62.28
    thigh M62.25- ☑
    upper arm M62.22- ☑
  myocardium, myocardial (acute) (with stated duration of 4 weeks or less) I21.9
    associated with revascularization procedure I21.A9
    diagnosed on ECG, but presenting no symptoms I25.2
    due to
      demand ischemia I21.A1
      ischemic imbalance I21.A1
    healed or old I25.2
    intraoperative — *see also* Infarct, myocardium, associated with revascularization procedure
      during cardiac surgery I97.790
      during other surgery I97.791
    non-Q wave I21.4
    non-ST elevation (NSTEMI) I21.4
      subsequent I22.2
    nontransmural I21.4
    past (diagnosed on ECG or other investigation, but currently presenting no symptoms) I25.2
    postprocedural — *see also* Infarct, myocardium, associated with revascularization procedure
      following cardiac surgery — *see also* Infarct, myocardium, type 4 or type 5 I97.190
      following other surgery I97.191
    Q wave (*see also* Infarct, myocardium, by site) I21.3
    secondary to
      demand ischemia I21.A1

Infarct, infarction — continued
  myocardium, myocardial — continued
    secondary to — continued
      ischemic imbalance I21.A1
    ST elevation (STEMI) I21.3
      anterior (anteroapical) (anterolateral) (anteroseptal) (Q wave) (wall) I21.09
        subsequent I22.0
      inferior (diaphragmatic) (inferolateral) (inferoposterior) (wall) NEC I21.19
        subsequent I22.1
      inferoposterior transmural (Q wave) I21.11
      involving
        coronary artery of anterior wall NEC I21.09
        coronary artery of inferior wall NEC I21.19
        diagonal coronary artery I21.02
        left anterior descending coronary artery I21.02
        left circumflex coronary artery I21.21
        left main coronary artery I21.01
        oblique marginal coronary artery I21.21
        right coronary artery I21.11
      lateral (apical-lateral) (basal-lateral) (high) I21.29
        subsequent I22.8
      posterior (posterobasal) (posterolateral) (posteroseptal) (true) I21.29
        subsequent I22.8
      septal I21.29
        subsequent I22.8
      specified NEC I21.29
        subsequent I22.8
      subsequent I22.9
    subsequent (recurrent) (reinfarction) I22.9
      anterior (anteroapical) (anterolateral) (anteroseptal) (wall) I22.0
      diaphragmatic (wall) I22.1
      inferior (diaphragmatic) (inferolateral) (inferoposterior) (wall) I22.1
      lateral (apical-lateral) (basal-lateral) (high) I22.8
      non-ST elevation (NSTEMI) I22.2
      posterior (posterobasal) (posterolateral) (posteroseptal) (true) I22.8
      septal I22.8
      specified NEC I22.8
      ST elevation I22.9
        anterior (anteroapical) (anterolateral) (anteroseptal) (wall) I22.0
        inferior (diaphragmatic) (inferolateral) (inferoposterior) (wall) I22.1
        specified NEC I22.8
      subendocardial I22.2
      transmural I22.9
        anterior (anteroapical) (anterolateral) (anteroseptal) (wall) I22.0
        diaphragmatic (wall) I22.1
        inferior (diaphragmatic) (inferolateral) (inferoposterior) (wall) I22.1
        lateral (apical-lateral) (basal-lateral) (high) I22.8
        posterior (posterobasal) (posterolateral) (posteroseptal) (true) I22.8
        specified NEC I22.8
      type 1 — see also Infarction, myocardial, subsequent, by site, or by ST elevation or non-ST elevation I22.9
      type 2 I21.A1
      type 3 I21.A9
      type 4 I21.A9
      type 5 I21.A9
    syphilitic A52.06
    transmural I21.9
      anterior (anteroapical) (anterolateral) (anteroseptal) (Q wave) (wall) NEC I21.09
      inferior (diaphragmatic) (inferolateral) (inferoposterior) (Q wave) (wall) NEC I21.19
      inferoposterior (Q wave) I21.11
      lateral (apical-lateral) (basal-lateral) (high) NEC I21.29
      posterior (posterobasal) (posterolateral) (posteroseptal) (true) NEC I21.29
      septal NEC I21.29
      specified NEC I21.29
    type 1 — see also Infarction, myocardial, by site, or by ST elevation or non-ST elevation I21.9
    type 2 I21.A1
    type 3 I21.A9
    type 4 (a) (b) (c) I21.A9
    type 5 I21.A9
  nontransmural I21.4
  omentum — see also Infarct, intestine K55.069

Infarct, infarction — continued
  ovary N83.8
  pancreas K86.89
  papillary muscle — see Infarct, myocardium
  parathyroid gland E21.4
  pituitary (gland) E23.6
  placenta O43.81- ☑
  prostate N42.89
  pulmonary (artery) (vein) (hemorrhagic) — see Embolism, pulmonary
  renal (embolic) (thrombotic) N28.0
  retina, retinal (artery) — see Occlusion, artery, retina
  spinal (cord) (acute) (embolic) (nonembolic) G95.11
  spleen D73.5
    embolic or thrombotic I74.8
  subendocardial (acute) (nontransmural) I21.4
  suprarenal (capsule) (gland) E27.49
  testis N50.1
  thrombotic — see also Thrombosis
    artery, arterial — see Embolism
  thyroid (gland) E07.89
  ventricle (heart) — see Infarct, myocardium
Infecting — see condition
Infection, infected, infective (opportunistic) B99.9
  with
    drug resistant organism — see Resistance (to), drug — see also specific organism
    lymphangitis — see Lymphangitis
    organ dysfunction (acute) R65.20
      with septic shock R65.21
  abscess (skin) — code by site under Abscess
  Absidia — see Mucormycosis
  Acanthamoeba — see Acanthamebiasis
  Acanthocheilonema (perstans) (streptocerca) B74.4
  accessory sinus (chronic) — see Sinusitis
  achorion — see Dermatophytosis
  Acremonium falciforme B47.0
  acromioclavicular M00.9
  Actinobacillus (actinomycetem-comitans) A28.8
    mallei A24.0
    muris A25.1
  Actinomadura B47.1
  Actinomyces (israelii) — see also Actinomycosis A42.9
  Actinomycetales — see Actinomycosis
  actinomycotic NOS — see Actinomycosis
  adenoid (and tonsil) J03.90
    chronic J35.02
  adenovirus NEC
    as cause of disease classified elsewhere B97.0
    unspecified nature or site B34.0
  aerogenes capsulatus A48.0
  aertrycke — see Infection, salmonella
  alimentary canal NOS — see Enteritis, infectious
  Allescheria boydii B48.2
  Alternaria B48.8
  alveolus, alveolar (process) K04.7
  Ameba, amebic (histolytica) — see Amebiasis
  amniotic fluid, sac or cavity O41.10- ☑
    chorioamnionitis O41.12- ☑
    placentitis O41.14- ☑
  amputation stump (surgical) — see Complication, amputation stump, infection
  Ancylostoma (duodenalis) B76.0
  Anisakiasis, Anisakis larvae B81.0
  anthrax — see Anthrax
  antrum (chronic) — see Sinusitis, maxillary
  anus, anal (papillae) (sphincter) K62.89
  arbovirus (arbor virus) A94
    specified type NEC A93.8
  artificial insemination N98.0
  Ascaris lumbricoides — see Ascariasis
  Ascomycetes B47.0
  Aspergillus (flavus) (fumigatus) (terreus) — see Aspergillosis
  atypical
    acid-fast (bacilli) — see Mycobacterium, atypical
    mycobacteria — see Mycobacterium, atypical
    virus A81.9
      specified type NEC A81.89
  auditory meatus (external) — see Otitis, externa, infective
  auricle (ear) — see Otitis, externa, infective
  axillary gland (lymph) L04.2
  Bacillus A49.9
    abortus A23.1
    anthracis — see Anthrax
    Ducrey's (any location) A57
    Flexner's A03.1

Infection, infected, infective — continued
  Bacillus — continued
    Friedländer's NEC A49.8
    gas (gangrene) A48.0
    mallei A24.0
    melitensis A23.0
    paratyphoid, paratyphosus A01.4
      A A01.1
      B A01.2
      C A01.3
    Shiga (-Kruse) A03.0
    suipestifer — see Infection, salmonella
    swimming pool A31.1
    typhosa A01.00
    welchii — see Gangrene, gas
  bacterial NOS A49.9
    as cause of disease classified elsewhere B96.89
      Bacteroides fragilis [B. fragilis] B96.6
      Clostridium perfringens [C. perfringens] B96.7
      Enterobacter sakazakii B96.89
      Enterococcus B95.2
      Escherichia coli [E. coli] — see also Escherichia coli B96.20
      Helicobacter pylori [H.pylori] B96.81
      Hemophilus influenzae [H. influenzae] B96.3
      Klebsiella pneumoniae [K. pneumoniae] B96.1
      Mycoplasma pneumoniae [M. pneumoniae] B96.0
      Proteus (mirabilis) (morganii) B96.4
      Pseudomonas (aeruginosa) (mallei) (pseudomallei) B96.5
      Staphylococcus B95.8
        aureus (methicillin susceptible) (MSSA) B95.61
        methicillin resistant (MRSA) B95.62
        specified NEC B95.7
      Streptococcus B95.5
        group A B95.0
        group B B95.1
        pneumoniae B95.3
        specified NEC B95.4
      Vibrio vulnificus B96.82
    specified NEC A48.8
  Bacterium
    paratyphosum A01.4
      A A01.1
      B A01.2
      C A01.3
    typhosum A01.00
  Bacteroides NEC A49.8
    fragilis, as cause of disease classified elsewhere B96.6
  Balantidium coli A07.0
  Bartholin's gland N75.8
  Basidiobolus B46.8
  bile duct (common) (hepatic) — see Cholangitis
  bladder — see Cystitis
  Blastomyces, blastomycotic — see also Blastomycosis
    brasiliensis — see Paracoccidioidomycosis
    dermatitidis — see Blastomycosis
    European — see Cryptococcosis
    Loboi B48.0
    North American B40.9
    South American — see Paracoccidioidomycosis
  bleb, postprocedure — see Blebitis
  bone — see Osteomyelitis
  Bordetella — see Whooping cough
  Borrelia bergdorfi A69.20
  brain — see also Encephalitis G04.90
    membranes — see Meningitis
    septic G06.0
      meninges — see Meningitis, bacterial
  branchial cyst Q18.0
  breast — see Mastitis
  bronchus — see Bronchitis
  Brucella A23.9
    abortus A23.1
    canis A23.3
    melitensis A23.0
    mixed A23.8
    specified NEC A23.8
    suis A23.2
  Brugia (malayi) B74.1
    timori B74.2
  bursa — see Bursitis, infective
  buttocks (skin) L08.9
  Campylobacter, intestinal A04.5
    as cause of disease classified elsewhere B96.81
  Candida (albicans) (tropicalis) — see Candidiasis

☑ Additional Character Required — Refer to the Tabular List for Character Selection

Infection, infected, infective — *continued*
- candiru B88.8
- Capillaria (intestinal) B81.1
  - hepatica B83.8
  - philippinensis B81.1
- cartilage — *see* Disorder, cartilage, specified type NEC
- cat liver fluke B66.0
- catheter-related bloodstream (CRBSI) T80.211 ☑
- cellulitis — *code by* site under Cellulitis
- central line-associated T80.219 ☑
  - bloodstream (CLABSI) T80.211 ☑
  - specified NEC T80.218 ☑
- Cephalosporium falciforme B47.0
- cerebrospinal — *see* Meningitis
- cervical gland (lymph) L04.0
- cervix — *see* Cervicitis
- cesarean delivery wound (puerperal) O86.00
- cestodes — *see* Infestation, cestodes
- chest J22
- Chilomastix (intestinal) A07.8
- Chlamydia, chlamydial A74.9
  - anus A56.3
  - genitourinary tract A56.2
    - lower A56.00
    - specified NEC A56.19
  - lymphogranuloma A55
  - pharynx A56.4
  - psittaci A70
  - rectum A56.3
  - sexually transmitted NEC A56.8
- cholera — *see* Cholera
- Cladosporium
  - bantianum (brain abscess) B43.1
  - carrionii B43.0
  - castellanii B36.1
  - trichoides (brain abscess) B43.1
  - werneckii B36.1
- Clonorchis (sinensis) (liver) B66.1
- Clostridium NEC
  - bifermentans A48.0
  - botulinum (food poisoning) A05.1
    - infant A48.51
    - wound A48.52
  - difficile
    - as cause of disease classified elsewhere B96.89
    - foodborne (disease)
      - not specified as recurrent A04.72
      - recurrent A04.71
    - gas gangrene A48.0
    - necrotizing enterocolitis
      - not specified as recurrent A04.72
      - recurrent A04.71
    - sepsis A41.4
  - gas-forming NEC A48.0
  - histolyticum A48.0
  - novyi, causing gas gangrene A48.0
  - oedematiens A48.0
  - perfringens
    - as cause of disease classified elsewhere B96.7
    - due to food A05.2
    - foodborne (disease) A05.2
    - gas gangrene A48.0
    - sepsis A41.4
  - septicum, causing gas gangrene A48.0
  - sordellii, causing gas gangrene A48.0
  - welchii
    - as cause of disease classified elsewhere B96.7
    - foodborne (disease) A05.2
    - gas gangrene A48.0
    - necrotizing enteritis A05.2
    - sepsis A41.4
- Coccidioides (immitis) — *see* Coccidioidomycosis
- colon — *see* Enteritis, infectious
- colostomy K94.02
- common duct — *see* Cholangitis
- congenital P39.9
  - Candida (albicans) P37.5
  - cytomegalovirus P35.1
  - hepatitis, viral P35.3
  - herpes simplex P35.2
  - infectious or parasitic disease P37.9
    - specified NEC P37.8
  - listeriosis (disseminated) P37.2
  - malaria NEC P37.4
    - falciparum P37.3
  - Plasmodium falciparum P37.3
  - poliomyelitis P35.8
  - rubella P35.0

Infection, infected, infective — *continued*
- congenital — *continued*
  - skin P39.4
  - toxoplasmosis (acute) (subacute) (chronic) P37.1
  - tuberculosis P37.0
  - urinary (tract) P39.3
  - vaccinia P35.8
  - virus P35.9
    - specified type NEC P35.8
- Conidiobolus B46.8
- coronavirus-2019 U07.1
- coronavirus NEC B34.2
  - as cause of disease classified elsewhere B97.29
  - severe acute respiratory syndrome (SARS associated) B97.21
- corpus luteum — *see* Salpingo-oophoritis
- Corynebacterium diphtheriae — *see* Diphtheria
- cotia virus B08.8
- Coxiella burnetii A78
- coxsackie — *see* Coxsackie
- Cryptococcus neoformans — *see* Cryptococcosis
- Cryptosporidium A07.2
- Cunninghamella — *see* Mucormycosis
- cyst — *see* Cyst
- cystic duct — *see also* Cholecystitis K81.9
- Cysticercus cellulosae — *see* Cysticercosis
- cytomegalovirus, cytomegaloviral B25.9
  - congenital P35.1
  - maternal, maternal care for (suspected) damage to fetus O35.3 ☑
  - mononucleosis B27.10
    - with
      - complication NEC B27.19
      - meningitis B27.12
      - polyneuropathy B27.11
- delta-agent (acute), in hepatitis B carrier B17.0
- dental (pulpal origin) K04.7
- Deuteromycetes B47.0
- Dicrocoelium dendriticum B66.2
- Dipetalonema (perstans) (streptocerca) B74.4
- diphtherial — *see* Diphtheria
- Diphyllobothrium (adult) (latum) (pacificum) B70.0
  - larval B70.1
- Diplogonoporus (grandis) B71.8
- Dipylidium caninum B67.4
- Dirofilaria B74.8
- Dracunculus medinensis B72
- Drechslera (hawaiiensis) B43.8
- Ducrey Haemophilus (any location) A57
- due to or resulting from
  - artificial insemination N98.0
  - Babesia
    - divergens (-like) strain B60.03
    - duncani (-type) species B60.02
    - microti B60.01
    - species
      - specified NEC B60.09
  - central venous catheter T80.219 ☑
    - bloodstream T80.211 ☑
    - exit or insertion site T80.212 ☑
    - localized T80.212 ☑
    - port or reservoir T80.212 ☑
    - specified NEC T80.218 ☑
    - tunnel T80.212 ☑
  - device, implant or graft — *see also* Complications, by site and type, infection or inflammation T85.79 ☑
    - arterial graft NEC T82.7 ☑
    - breast (implant) T85.79 ☑
    - catheter NEC T85.79 ☑
      - dialysis (renal) T82.7 ☑
        - central line T80.211 ☑
        - intraperitoneal T85.71 ☑
      - infusion NEC T82.7 ☑
        - cranial T85.735 ☑
        - intrathecal T85.735 ☑
        - spinal (epidural) (subdural) T85.735 ☑
        - subarachnoid T85.735 ☑
      - urinary T83.518 ☑
        - cystostomy T83.510 ☑
        - Hopkins T83.518 ☑
        - ileostomy T83.518 ☑
        - nephrostomy T83.512 ☑
        - specified NEC T83.518 ☑
        - urethral indwelling T83.511 ☑
        - urostomy T83.518 ☑

Infection, infected, infective — *continued*
- due to or resulting from — *continued*
  - device, implant or graft — *see also* Complications, by site and type, infection or inflammation — *continued*
    - electronic (electrode) (pulse generator) (stimulator)
      - bone T84.7 ☑
      - cardiac T82.7 ☑
      - nervous system T85.738 ☑
        - brain T85.731 ☑
        - cranial nerve T85.732 ☑
        - gastric nerve T85.732 ☑
        - generator pocket T85.734 ☑
        - neurostimulator generator T85.734 ☑
        - peripheral nerve T85.732 ☑
        - sacral nerve T85.732 ☑
        - spinal cord T85.733 ☑
        - vagal nerve T85.732 ☑
      - urinary (indwelling) T83.51 ☑
    - fixation, internal (orthopedic) NEC — *see* Complication, fixation device, infection
    - gastrointestinal (bile duct) (esophagus) T85.79 ☑
      - neurostimulator electrode (lead) T85.732 ☑
    - genital NEC T83.69 ☑
    - heart NEC T82.7 ☑
      - valve (prosthesis) T82.6 ☑
        - graft T82.7 ☑
    - joint prosthesis — *see* Complication, joint prosthesis, infection
    - ocular (corneal graft) (orbital implant) NEC T85.79 ☑
    - orthopedic NEC T84.7 ☑
    - penile (cylinder) (pump) (resevoir) T83.61 ☑
    - specified NEC T85.79 ☑
    - testicular T83.62 ☑
    - urinary NEC T83.598 ☑
      - ileal conduit stent T83.593 ☑
      - implanted neurostimulation T83.590 ☑
      - implanted sphincter T83.591 ☑
      - indwelling ureteral stent T83.592 ☑
      - nephroureteral stent T83.593 ☑
      - specified stent NEC T83.593 ☑
    - vascular NEC T82.7 ☑
    - ventricular intracranial (communicating) shunt T85.730 ☑
  - Hickman catheter T80.219 ☑
    - bloodstream T80.211 ☑
    - localized T80.212 ☑
    - specified NEC T80.218 ☑
  - immunization or vaccination T88.0 ☑
  - infusion, injection or transfusion NEC T80.29 ☑
  - injury NEC — *code by* site under Wound, open
  - peripherally inserted central catheter (PICC) T80.219 ☑
    - bloodstream T80.211 ☑
    - localized T80.212 ☑
    - specified NEC T80.218 ☑
  - portacath (port-a-cath) T80.219 ☑
    - bloodstream T80.211 ☑
    - localized T80.212 ☑
    - specified NEC T80.218 ☑
  - protozoa of the order Piroplasmida NEC B60.09
  - pulmonary artery catheter — *see* Infection, due to or resulting from, central venous catheter
  - surgery T81.40 ☑
  - Swan Ganz catheter — *see* Infection, due to or resulting from, central venous catheter
  - triple lumen catheter T80.219 ☑
    - bloodstream T80.211 ☑
    - localized T80.212 ☑
    - specified NEC T80.218 ☑
  - umbilical venous catheter T80.219 ☑
    - bloodstream T80.211 ☑
    - localized T80.212 ☑
    - specified NEC T80.218 ☑
- during labor NEC O75.3
- ear (middle) — *see also* Otitis media
  - external — *see* Otitis, externa, infective
  - inner — *see* subcategory H83.0 ☑
- Eberthella typhosa A01.00
- Echinococcus — *see* Echinococcus
- echovirus
  - as cause of disease classified elsewhere B97.12
  - unspecified nature or site B34.1
- endocardium I33.0

Infection, infected, infective — *continued*
- endocervix — *see* Cervicitis
- Entamoeba — *see* Amebiasis
- enteric — *see* Enteritis, infectious
- Enterobacter sakazakii B96.89
- Enterobius vermicularis B80
- enterostomy K94.12
- enterovirus B34.1
  - as cause of disease classified elsewhere B97.10
    - coxsackievirus B97.11
    - echovirus B97.12
    - specified NEC B97.19
- Entomophthora B46.8
- Epidermophyton — *see* Dermatophytosis
- epididymis — *see* Epididymitis
- episiotomy (puerperal) O86.09
- Erysipelothrix (insidiosa) (rhusiopathiae) — *see* Erysipeloid
- erythema infectiosum B08.3
- Escherichia (E.) coli NEC A49.8
  - as cause of disease classified elsewhere — *see also* Escherichia coli B96.20
  - congenital P39.8
    - sepsis P36.4
  - generalized A41.51
  - intestinal — *see* Enteritis, infectious, due to, Escherichia coli
- ethmoidal (chronic) (sinus) — *see* Sinusitis, ethmoidal
- eustachian tube (ear) — *see* Salpingitis, eustachian
- external auditory canal (meatus) NEC — *see* Otitis, externa, infective
- eye (purulent) — *see* Endophthalmitis, purulent
- eyelid — *see* Inflammation, eyelid
- fallopian tube — *see* Salpingo-oophoritis
- Fasciola (gigantica) (hepatica) (indica) B66.3
- Fasciolopsis (buski) B66.5
- filarial — *see* Infestation, filarial
- finger (skin) L08.9
  - nail L03.01- ☑
    - fungus B35.1
- fish tapeworm B70.0
  - larval B70.1
- flagellate, intestinal A07.9
- fluke — *see* Infestation, fluke
- focal
  - teeth (pulpal origin) K04.7
  - tonsils J35.01
- Fonsecaea (compactum) (pedrosoi) B43.0
- food — *see* Intoxication, foodborne
- foot (skin) L08.9
  - dermatophytic fungus B35.3
- Francisella tularensis — *see* Tularemia
- frontal (sinus) (chronic) — *see* Sinusitis, frontal
- fungus NOS B49
  - beard B35.0
  - dermatophytic — *see* Dermatophytosis
  - foot B35.3
  - groin B35.6
  - hand B35.2
  - nail B35.1
  - pathogenic to compromised host only B48.8
  - perianal (area) B35.6
  - scalp B35.0
  - skin B36.9
    - foot B35.3
    - hand B35.2
    - toenails B35.1
- Fusarium B48.8
- gallbladder — *see* Cholecystitis
- gas bacillus — *see* Gangrene, gas
- gastrointestinal — *see* Enteritis, infectious
- generalized NEC — *see* Sepsis
- generator pocket, implanted electronic neurostimulator T85.734 ☑
- genital organ or tract
  - female — *see* Disease, pelvis, inflammatory
  - male N49.9
    - multiple sites N49.8
    - specified NEC N49.8
- Ghon tubercle, primary A15.7
- Giardia lamblia A07.1
- gingiva (chronic) K05.10
  - acute K05.00
    - nonplaque induced K05.01
    - plaque induced K05.00
  - nonplaque induced K05.11
  - plaque induced K05.10
- glanders A24.0

Infection, infected, infective — *continued*
- glenosporopsis B48.0
- Gnathostoma (spinigerum) B83.1
- Gongylonema B83.8
- gonococcal — *see* Gonococcus
- gram-negative bacilli NOS A49.9
- guinea worm B72
- gum (chronic) K05.10
  - acute K05.00
    - nonplaque induced K05.01
    - plaque induced K05.00
  - nonplaque induced K05.11
  - plaque induced K05.10
- Haemophilus — *see* Infection, Hemophilus
- heart — *see* Carditis
- Helicobacter pylori A04.8
  - as cause of disease classified elsewhere B96.81
- helminths B83.9
  - intestinal B82.0
    - mixed (types classifiable to more than one of the titles B65.0-B81.3 and B81.8) B81.4
    - specified type NEC B81.8
  - specified type NEC B83.8
- Hemophilus
  - aegyptius, systemic A48.4
  - ducrey (any location) A57
  - generalized A41.3
  - influenzae NEC A49.2
    - as cause of disease classified elsewhere B96.3
- herpes (simplex) — *see also* Herpes
  - congenital P35.2
  - disseminated B00.7
  - zoster B02.9
- herpesvirus, herpesviral — *see* Herpes
- Heterophyes (heterophyes) B66.8
- hip (joint) NEC M00.9
  - due to internal joint prosthesis
    - left T84.52 ☑
    - right T84.51 ☑
  - skin NEC L08.9
- Histoplasma — *see* Histoplasmosis
  - American B39.4
  - capsulatum B39.4
- hookworm B76.9
- human
  - papilloma virus A63.0
  - T-cell lymphotropic virus type-1 (HTLV-1) B33.3
- hydrocele N43.0
- Hymenolepis B71.0
- hypopharynx — *see* Pharyngitis
- inguinal (lymph) glands L04.1
  - due to soft chancre A57
- intervertebral disc, pyogenic M46.30
  - cervical region M46.32
  - cervicothoracic region M46.33
  - lumbar region M46.36
  - lumbosacral region M46.37
  - multiple sites M46.39
  - occipito-atlanto-axial region M46.31
  - sacrococcygeal region M46.38
  - thoracic region M46.34
  - thoracolumbar region M46.35
- intestine, intestinal — *see* Enteritis, infectious
  - specified NEC A08.8
- intra-amniotic affecting newborn NEC P39.2
- intrauterine inflammation O41.12- ☑
- Isospora belli or hominis A07.3
- Japanese B encephalitis A83.0
- jaw (bone) (lower) (upper) M27.2
- joint NEC M00.9
  - due to internal joint prosthesis T84.50 ☑
- kidney (cortex) (hematogenous) N15.9
  - with calculus N20.0
    - with hydronephrosis N13.6
  - following ectopic gestation O08.83
  - pelvis and ureter (cystic) N28.85
  - puerperal (postpartum) O86.21
  - specified NEC N15.8
- Klebsiella (K.) pneumoniae NEC A49.8
  - as cause of disease classified elsewhere B96.1
- knee (joint) NEC M00.9
  - joint M00.9
  - due to internal joint prosthesis
    - left T84.54 ☑
    - right T84.53 ☑
  - skin L08.9
- Koch's — *see* Tuberculosis
- labia (majora) (minora) (acute) — *see* Vulvitis

Infection, infected, infective — *continued*
- lacrimal
  - gland — *see* Dacryoadenitis
  - passages (duct) (sac) — *see* Inflammation, lacrimal, passages
- lancet fluke B66.2
- larynx NEC J38.7
- leg (skin) NOS L08.9
- Legionella pneumophila A48.1
  - nonpneumonic A48.2
- Leishmania — *see also* Leishmaniasis
  - aethiopica B55.1
  - braziliensis B55.2
  - chagasi B55.0
  - donovani B55.0
  - infantum B55.0
  - major B55.1
  - mexicana B55.1
  - tropica B55.1
- lentivirus, as cause of disease classified elsewhere B97.31
- Leptosphaeria senegalensis B47.0
- Leptospira interrogans A27.9
  - autumnalis A27.89
  - canicola A27.89
  - hebdomadis A27.89
  - icterohaemorrhagiae A27.0
  - pomona A27.89
  - specified type NEC A27.89
- leptospirochetal NEC — *see* Leptospirosis
- Listeria monocytogenes — *see also* Listeriosis
  - congenital P37.2
- Loa loa B74.3
  - with conjunctival infestation B74.3
  - eyelid B74.3
- Loboa loboi B48.0
- local, skin (staphylococcal) (streptococcal) L08.9
  - abscess — *code by* site under Abscess
  - cellulitis — *code by* site under Cellulitis
  - specified NEC L08.89
  - ulcer — *see* Ulcer, skin
- Loefflerella mallei A24.0
- lung — *see also* Pneumonia J18.9
  - atypical Mycobacterium A31.0
  - spirochetal A69.8
  - tuberculous — *see* Tuberculosis, pulmonary
  - virus — *see* Pneumonia, viral
- lymph gland — *see also* Lymphadenitis, acute
  - mesenteric I88.0
- lymphoid tissue, base of tongue or posterior pharynx, NEC (chronic) J35.03
- Madurella (grisea) (mycetomii) B47.0
- major
  - following ectopic or molar pregnancy O08.0
  - puerperal, postpartum, childbirth O85
- Malassezia furfur B36.0
- Malleomyces
  - mallei A24.0
  - pseudomallei (whitmori) — *see* Melioidosis
- mammary gland N61.0
- Mansonella (ozzardi) (perstans) (streptocerca) B74.4
- mastoid — *see* Mastoiditis
- maxilla, maxillary M27.2
  - sinus (chronic) — *see* Sinusitis, maxillary
- mediastinum J98.51
- Medina (worm) B72
- meibomian cyst or gland — *see* Hordeolum
- meninges — *see* Meningitis, bacterial
- meningococcal — *see also* condition A39.9
  - adrenals A39.1
  - brain A39.81
  - cerebrospinal A39.0
  - conjunctiva A39.89
  - endocardium A39.51
  - heart A39.50
    - endocardium A39.51
    - myocardium A39.52
    - pericardium A39.53
  - joint A39.83
  - meninges A39.0
  - meningococcemia A39.4
    - acute A39.2
    - chronic A39.3
  - myocardium A39.52
  - pericardium A39.53
  - retrobulbar neuritis A39.82
  - specified site NEC A39.89
- mesenteric lymph nodes or glands NEC I88.0

Infection, infected, infective — *continued*
Metagonimus B66.8
metatarsophalangeal M00.9
methicillin
resistant Staphylococcus aureus (MRSA) A49.02
susceptible Staphylococcus aureus (MSSA) A49.01
Microsporum, microsporic — *see* Dermatophytosis
mixed flora (bacterial) NEC A49.8
Monilia — *see* Candidiasis
Monosporium apiospermum B48.2
mouth, parasitic B37.0
Mucor — *see* Mucormycosis
muscle NEC — *see* Myositis, infective
mycelium NOS B49
mycetoma B47.9
actinomycotic NEC B47.1
mycotic NEC B47.0
Mycobacterium, mycobacterial — *see* Mycobacterium
Mycoplasma NEC A49.3
pneumoniae, as cause of disease classified elsewhere B96.0
mycotic NOS B49
pathogenic to compromised host only B48.8
skin NOS B36.9
myocardium NEC I40.0
nail (chronic)
with lymphangitis — *see* Lymphangitis, acute, digit
finger L03.01- ☑
fungus B35.1
ingrowing L60.0
toe L03.03- ☑
fungus B35.1
nasal sinus (chronic) — *see* Sinusitis
nasopharynx — *see* Nasopharyngitis
navel L08.82
Necator americanus B76.1
Neisseria — *see* Gonococcus
Neotestudina rosatii B47.0
newborn P39.9
intra-amniotic NEC P39.2
skin P39.4
specified type NEC P39.8
nipple N61.0
associated with
lactation O91.03
pregnancy O91.01- ☑
puerperium O91.02
Nocardia — *see* Nocardiosis
obstetrical surgical wound (puerperal) O86.00
incisional site
deep O86.02
superficial O86.01
organ and space site O86.03
surgical site specified NEC O86.09
Oesophagostomum (apiostomum) B81.8
Oestrus ovis — *see* Myiasis
Oidium albicans B37.9
Onchocerca (volvulus) — *see* Onchocerciasis
oncovirus, as cause of disease classified elsewhere
B97.32
operation wound T81.49 ☑
Opisthorchis (felineus) (viverrini) B66.0
orbit, orbital — *see* Inflammation, orbit
orthopoxvirus NEC B08.09
ovary — *see* Salpingo-oophoritis
Oxyuris vermicularis B80
pancreas (acute) — *see* Pancreatitis, acute
abscess — *see* Pancreatitis, acute
specified NEC — *see also* Pancreatitis, acute K85.80
papillomavirus, as cause of disease classified elsewhere
B97.7
papovavirus NEC B34.4
Paracoccidioides brasiliensis — *see* Paracoccidioidomycosis
Paragonimus (westermani) B66.4
parainfluenza virus B34.8
parameningococcus NOS A39.9
parapoxvirus B08.60
specified NEC B08.69
parasitic B89
Parastrongylus
cantonensis B83.2
costaricensis B81.3
paratyphoid A01.4
Type A A01.1
Type B A01.2
Type C A01.3
paraurethral ducts N34.2

Infection, infected, infective — *continued*
parotid gland — *see* Sialoadenitis
parvovirus NEC B34.3
as cause of disease classified elsewhere B97.6
Pasteurella NEC A28.9
multocida A28.0
pestis — *see* Plague
pseudotuberculosis A28.0
septica (cat bite) (dog bite) A28.0
tularensis — *see* Tularemia
pelvic, female — *see* Disease, pelvis, inflammatory
Penicillium (marneffei) B48.4
penis (glans) (retention) NEC N48.29
periapical K04.5
peridental, periodontal K05.20
generalized — *see* Periodontitis, aggressive, generalized
localized — *see* Periodontitis, aggressive, localized
perinatal period P39.9
specified type NEC P39.8
perineal repair (puerperal) O86.09
periorbital — *see* Inflammation, orbit
perirectal K62.89
perirenal — *see* Infection, kidney
peritoneal — *see* Peritonitis
periureteral N28.89
Petriellidium boydii B48.2
pharynx — *see also* Pharyngitis
coxsackievirus B08.5
posterior, lymphoid (chronic) J35.03
Phialophora
gougerotii (subcutaneous abscess or cyst) B43.2
jeanselmei (subcutaneous abscess or cyst) B43.2
verrucosa (skin) B43.0
Piedraia hortae B36.3
pinta A67.9
intermediate A67.1
late A67.2
mixed A67.3
primary A67.0
pinworm B80
pityrosporum furfur B36.0
pleuro-pneumonia-like organism (PPLO) NEC A49.3
as cause of disease classified elsewhere B96.0
pneumococcus, pneumococcal NEC A49.1
as cause of disease classified elsewhere B95.3
generalized (purulent) A40.3
with pneumonia J13
Pneumocystis carinii (pneumonia) B59
Pneumocystis jiroveci (pneumonia) B59
port or reservoir T80.212 ☑
postoperative T81.40 ☑
postoperative wound T81.49 ☑
surgical site
deep incisional T81.42 ☑
organ and space T81.43 ☑
specified NEC T81.49 ☑
superficial incisional T81.41 ☑
postprocedural T81.40 ☑
postvaccinal T88.0 ☑
prepuce NEC N47.7
with penile inflammation N47.6
prion — *see* Disease, prion, central nervous system
prostate (capsule) — *see* Prostatitis
Proteus (mirabilis) (morganii) (vulgaris) NEC A49.8
as cause of disease classified elsewhere B96.4
protozoal NEC B64
intestinal A07.9
specified NEC A07.8
specified NEC B60.8
Pseudoallescheria boydii B48.2
Pseudomonas NEC A49.8
as cause of disease classified elsewhere B96.5
mallei A24.0
pneumonia J15.1
pseudomallei — *see* Melioidosis
puerperal O86.4
genitourinary tract NEC O86.89
major or generalized O85
minor O86.4
specified NEC O86.89
pulmonary — *see* Infection, lung
purulent — *see* Abscess
Pyrenochaeta romeroi B47.0
Q fever A78
rectum (sphincter) K62.89
renal — *see also* Infection, kidney
pelvis and ureter (cystic) N28.85

Infection, infected, infective — *continued*
reovirus, as cause of disease classified elsewhere B97.5
respiratory (tract) NEC J98.8
acute J22
chronic J98.8
influenzal (upper) (acute) — *see* Influenza, with,
respiratory manifestations NEC
lower (acute) J22
chronic — *see* Bronchitis, chronic
rhinovirus J00
syncytial virus (RSV) — *see* Infection, virus, respiratory syncytial (RSV)
upper (acute) NOS J06.9
chronic J39.8
streptococcal J06.9
viral NOS J06.9
due to respiratory syncytial virus (RSV)
J06.9 *[B97.4]*
resulting from
presence of internal prosthesis, implant, graft —
see Complications, by site and type, infection
retortamoniasis A07.8
retroperitoneal NEC K68.9
retrovirus B33.3
as cause of disease classified elsewhere B97.30
human
immunodeficiency, type 2 (HIV 2) B97.35
T-cell lymphotropic
type I (HTLV-I) B97.33
type II (HTLV-II) B97.34
lentivirus B97.31
oncovirus B97.32
specified NEC B97.39
Rhinosporidium (seeberi) B48.1
rhinovirus
as cause of disease classified elsewhere B97.89
unspecified nature or site B34.8
Rhizopus — *see* Mucormycosis
rickettsial NOS A79.9
roundworm (large) NEC B82.0
Ascariasis — *see also* Ascariasis B77.9
rubella — *see* Rubella
Saccharomyces — *see* Candidiasis
salivary duct or gland (any) — *see* Sialoadenitis
Salmonella (aertrycke) (arizonae) (callinarum) (cholerae-
suis) (enteritidis) (suipestifer) (typhimurium)
A02.9
with
(gastro)enteritis A02.0
sepsis A02.1
specified manifestation NEC A02.8
due to food (poisoning) A02.9
hirschfeldii A01.3
localized A02.20
arthritis A02.23
meningitis A02.21
osteomyelitis A02.24
pneumonia A02.22
pyelonephritis A02.25
specified NEC A02.29
paratyphi A01.4
A A01.1
B A01.2
C A01.3
schottmuelleri A01.2
typhi, typhosa — *see* Typhoid
Sarcocystis A07.8
SARS-CoV-2 — *see* Infection, COVID-19
scabies B86
Schistosoma — *see* Infestation, Schistosoma
scrotum (acute) NEC N49.2
seminal vesicle — *see* Vesiculitis
septic
localized, skin — *see* Abscess
sheep liver fluke B66.3
Shigella A03.9
boydii A03.2
dysenteriae A03.0
flexneri A03.1
group
A A03.0
B A03.1
C A03.2
D A03.3
Schmitz (-Stutzer) A03.0
schmitzii A03.0
shigae A03.0
sonnei A03.3

Infection, infected, infective — *continued*
  Shigella — *continued*
    specified NEC A03.8
  shoulder (joint) NEC M00.9
    due to internal joint prosthesis T84.59 ☑
    skin NEC L08.9
  sinus (accessory) (chronic) (nasal) — *see also* Sinusitis
    pilonidal — *see* Sinus, pilonidal
    skin NEC L08.89
  Skene's duct or gland — *see* Urethritis
  skin (local) (staphylococcal) (streptococcal) L08.9
    abscess — *code by* site under Abscess
    cellulitis — *code by* site under Cellulitis
    due to fungus B36.9
      specified type NEC B36.8
    mycotic B36.9
      specified type NEC B36.8
    newborn P39.4
    ulcer — *see* Ulcer, skin
  slow virus A81.9
    specified NEC A81.89
  Sparganum (mansoni) (proliferum) (baxteri) B70.1
  specific — *see also* Syphilis
    to perinatal period — *see* Infection, congenital
  specified NEC B99.8
  spermatic cord NEC N49.1
  sphenoidal (sinus) — *see* Sinusitis, sphenoidal
  spinal cord NOS — *see also* Myelitis G04.91
    abscess G06.1
    meninges — *see* Meningitis
    streptococcal G04.89
  Spirillum A25.0
  spirochetal NOS A69.9
    lung A69.8
    specified NEC A69.8
  Spirometra larvae B70.1
  spleen D73.89
  Sporotrichum, Sporothrix (schenckii) — *see* Sporotrichosis
  staphylococcal, unspecified site
    as cause of disease classified elsewhere B95.8
      aureus (methicillin susceptible) (MSSA) B95.61
        methicillin resistant (MRSA) B95.62
        specified NEC B95.7
      aureus (methicillin susceptible) (MSSA) A49.01
        methicillin resistant (MRSA) A49.02
    food poisoning A05.0
    generalized (purulent) A41.2
    pneumonia — *see* Pneumonia, staphylococcal
  Stellantchasmus falcatus B66.8
  streptobacillus moniliformis A25.1
  streptococcal NEC A49.1
    as cause of disease classified elsewhere B95.5
    B genitourinary complicating
      childbirth O98.82
      pregnancy O98.81- ☑
      puerperium O98.83
    congenital
      sepsis P36.10
        group B P36.0
        specified NEC P36.19
    generalized (purulent) A40.9
  Streptomyces B47.1
  Strongyloides (stercoralis) — *see* Strongyloidiasis
  stump (amputation) (surgical) — *see* Complication, amputation stump, infection
  subcutaneous tissue, local L08.9
  suipestifer — *see* Infection, salmonella
  swimming pool bacillus A31.1
  Taenia — *see* Infestation, Taenia
  Taeniarhynchus saginatus B68.1
  tapeworm — *see* Infestation, tapeworm
  tendon (sheath) — *see* Tenosynovitis, infective NEC
  Ternidens diminutus B81.8
  testis — *see* Orchitis
  threadworm B80
  throat — *see* Pharyngitis
  thyroglossal duct K14.8
  toe (skin) L08.9
    cellulitis L03.03- ☑
      fungus B35.1
    nail L03.03- ☑
      fungus B35.1
  tongue NEC K14.0
    parasitic B37.0
  tonsil (and adenoid) (faucial) (lingual) (pharyngeal) — *see* Tonsillitis
  tooth, teeth K04.7

Infection, infected, infective — *continued*
  tooth, teeth — *continued*
    periapical K04.7
    peridental, periodontal K05.20
      generalized — *see* Periodontitis, aggressive, generalized
      localized — *see* Periodontitis, aggressive, localized
    pulp K04.01
      irreversible K04.02
      reversible K04.01
    socket M27.3
  TORCH — *see* Infection, congenital
    without active infection P00.2
  Torula histolytica — *see* Cryptococcosis
  Toxocara (canis) (cati) (felis) B83.0
  Toxoplasma gondii — *see* Toxoplasma
  trachea, chronic J42
  trematode NEC — *see* Infestation, fluke
  trench fever A79.0
  Treponema pallidum — *see* Syphilis
  Trichinella (spiralis) B75
  Trichomonas A59.9
    cervix A59.09
    intestine A07.8
    prostate A59.02
    specified site NEC A59.8
    urethra A59.03
    urogenitalis A59.00
    vagina A59.01
    vulva A59.01
  Trichophyton, trichophytic — *see* Dermatophytosis
  Trichosporon (beigelii) cutaneum B36.2
  Trichostrongylus B81.2
  Trichuris (trichiura) B79
  Trombicula (irritans) B88.0
  Trypanosoma
    brucei
      gambiense B56.0
      rhodesiense B56.1
    cruzi — *see* Chagas' disease
  tubal — *see* Salpingo-oophoritis
  tuberculous
    latent (LTBI) Z22.7
    NEC — *see* Tuberculosis
  tubo-ovarian — *see* Salpingo-oophoritis
  tunica vaginalis N49.1
  tunnel T80.212 ☑
  tympanic membrane NEC — *see* Myringitis
  typhoid (abortive) (ambulant) (bacillus) — *see* Typhoid
  typhus A75.9
    flea-borne A75.2
    mite-borne A75.3
    recrudescent A75.1
    tick-borne A77.9
      African A77.1
      North Asian A77.2
  umbilicus L08.82
  ureter — *see* Ureteritis
  urethra — *see* Urethritis
  urinary (tract) N39.0
    bladder — *see* Cystitis
    complicating
      pregnancy O23.4- ☑
        specified type NEC O23.3- ☑
    kidney — *see* Infection, kidney
    newborn P39.3
    puerperal (postpartum) O86.20
    tuberculous A18.13
    urethra — *see* Urethritis
  uterus, uterine — *see* Endometritis
  vaccination T88.0 ☑
  vaccinia not from vaccination B08.011
  vagina (acute) — *see* Vaginitis
  varicella B01.9
  varicose veins — *see* Varix
  vas deferens NEC N49.1
  vesical — *see* Cystitis
  Vibrio
    cholerae A00.0
      El Tor A00.1
    parahaemolyticus (food poisoning) A05.3
    vulnificus
      as cause of disease classified elsewhere B96.82
      foodborne intoxication A05.5
  Vincent's (gum) (mouth) (tonsil) A69.1
  virus, viral NOS B34.9

Infection, infected, infective — *continued*
  virus, viral — *continued*
    adenovirus
      as cause of disease classified elsewhere B97.0
      unspecified nature or site B34.0
    arbovirus, arbovirus arthropod-borne A94
    as cause of disease classified elsewhere B97.89
      adenovirus B97.0
      coronavirus B97.29
        SARS-associated B97.21
      coxsackievirus B97.11
      echovirus B97.12
      enterovirus B97.10
        coxsackievirus B97.11
        echovirus B97.12
        specified NEC B97.19
      human
        immunodeficiency, type 2 (HIV 2) B97.35
        metapneumovirus B97.81
        T-cell lymphotropic,
          type I (HTLV-I) B97.33
          type II (HTLV-II) B97.34
      papillomavirus B97.7
      parvovirus B97.6
      reovirus B97.5
      respiratory syncytial (RSV) — *see* Infection, virus, respiratory syncytial (RSV)
      retrovirus B97.30
        human
          immunodeficiency, type 2 (HIV 2) B97.35
          T-cell lymphotropic,
            type I (HTLV-I) B97.33
            type II (HTLV-II) B97.34
        lentivirus B97.31
        oncovirus B97.32
        specified NEC B97.39
      specified NEC B97.89
    central nervous system A89
      atypical A81.9
        specified NEC A81.89
      enterovirus NEC A88.8
        meningitis A87.0
      slow virus A81.9
        specified NEC A81.89
      specified NEC A88.8
    chest J98.8
    cotia B08.8
    COVID-19 U07.1
    coxsackie — *see also* Infection, coxsackie B34.1
      as cause of disease classified elsewhere B97.11
    ECHO
      as cause of disease classified elsewhere B97.12
      unspecified nature or site B34.1
    encephalitis, tick-borne A84.9
    enterovirus, as cause of disease classified elsewhere B97.10
      coxsackievirus B97.11
      echovirus B97.12
      specified NEC B97.19
    exanthem NOS B09
    human metapneumovirus as cause of disease classified elsewhere B97.81
    human papilloma as cause of disease classified elsewhere B97.7
    intestine — *see* Enteritis, viral
    respiratory syncytial (RSV)
      as cause of disease classified elsewhere B97.4
      bronchiolitis J21.0
      bronchitis J20.5
      bronchopneumonia J12.1
      otitis media H65- ☑ *[B97.4]*
      pneumonia J12.1
      upper respiratory infection J06.9 *[B97.4]*
    rhinovirus
      as cause of disease classified elsewhere B97.89
      unspecified nature or site B34.8
    slow A81.9
      specified NEC A81.89
    specified type NEC B33.8
      as cause of disease classified elsewhere B97.89
      unspecified nature or site B34.8
    unspecified nature or site B34.9
    West Nile — *see* Virus, West Nile
  vulva (acute) — *see* Vulvitis
  West Nile — *see* Virus, West Nile
  whipworm B79
  worms B83.9
    specified type NEC B83.8

☑ **Additional Character Required — Refer to the Tabular List for Character Selection**

Infection, infected, infective — *continued*
  Wuchereria (bancrofti) B74.0
    malayi B74.1
  yatapoxvirus B08.70
    specified NEC B08.79
  yeast — *see also* Candidiasis B37.9
  yellow fever — *see* Fever, yellow
  Yersinia
    enterocolitica (intestinal) A04.6
    pestis — *see* Plague
    pseudotuberculosis A28.2
  Zeis' gland — *see* Hordeolum
  Zika virus A92.5
    congenital P35.4
  zoonotic bacterial NOS A28.9
  Zopfia senegalensis B47.0
Infective, infectious — *see* condition
Infertility
  female N97.9
    age-related N97.8
    associated with
      anovulation N97.0
      cervical (mucus) disease or anomaly N88.3
      congenital anomaly
        cervix N88.3
        fallopian tube N97.1
        uterus N97.2
        vagina N97.8
      dysmucorrhea N88.3
      fallopian tube disease or anomaly N97.1
      pituitary-hypothalamic origin E23.0
      specified origin NEC N97.8
      Stein-Leventhal syndrome E28.2
      uterine disease or anomaly N97.2
      vaginal disease or anomaly N97.8
    due to
      cervical anomaly N88.3
      fallopian tube anomaly N97.1
      ovarian failure E28.39
      Stein-Leventhal syndrome E28.2
      uterine anomaly N97.2
      vaginal anomaly N97.8
    nonimplantation N97.2
    origin
      cervical N88.3
      tubal (block) (occlusion) (stenosis) N97.1
      uterine N97.2
      vaginal N97.8
  male N46.9
    azoospermia N46.01
      extratesticular cause N46.029
        drug therapy N46.021
        efferent duct obstruction N46.023
        infection N46.022
        radiation N46.024
        specified cause NEC N46.029
        systemic disease N46.025
    oligospermia N46.11
      extratesticular cause N46.129
        drug therapy N46.121
        efferent duct obstruction N46.123
        infection N46.122
        radiation N46.124
        specified cause NEC N46.129
        systemic disease N46.125
    specified type NEC N46.8
Infestation B88.9
  Acanthocheilonema (perstans) (streptocerca) B74.4
  Acariasis B88.0
    demodex folliculorum B88.0
    sarcoptes scabiei B86
    trombiculae B88.0
  Agamofilaria streptocerca B74.4
  Ancylostoma, ankylostoma (braziliense) (caninum) (ceylanicum) (duodenale) B76.0
    americanum B76.1
    new world B76.1
  Anisakis larvae, anisakiasis B81.0
  arthropod NEC B88.2
  Ascaris lumbricoides — *see* Ascariasis
  Balantidium coli A07.0
  beef tapeworm B68.1
  Bothriocephalus (latus) B70.0
    larval B70.1
  broad tapeworm B70.0
    larval B70.1
  Brugia (malayi) B74.1
    timori B74.2

Infestation — *continued*
  candiru B88.8
  Capillaria
    hepatica B83.8
    philippinensis B81.1
  cat liver fluke B66.0
  cestodes B71.9
    diphyllobothrium — *see* Infestation, diphyllobothrium
    dipylidiasis B71.1
    hymenolepiasis B71.0
    specified type NEC B71.8
  chigger B88.0
  chigo, chigoe B88.1
  Clonorchis (sinensis) (liver) B66.1
  coccidial A07.3
  crab-lice B85.3
  Cysticercus cellulosae — *see* Cysticercosis
  Demodex (folliculorum) B88.0
  Dermanyssus gallinae B88.0
  Dermatobia (hominis) — *see* Myiasis
  Dibothriocephalus (latus) B70.0
    larval B70.1
  Dicrocoelium dendriticum B66.2
  Diphyllobothrium (adult) (latum) (intestinal) (pacificum) B70.0
    larval B70.1
  Diplogonoporus (grandis) B71.8
  Dipylidium caninum B67.4
  Distoma hepaticum B66.3
  dog tapeworm B67.4
  Dracunculus medinensis B72
  dragon worm B72
  dwarf tapeworm B71.0
  Echinococcus — *see* Echinococcus
  Echinostomum ilocanum B66.8
  Entamoeba (histolytica) — *see* Infection, Ameba
  Enterobius vermicularis B80
  eyelid
    in (due to)
      leishmaniasis B55.1
      loiasis B74.3
      onchocerciasis B73.09
      phthiriasis B85.3
    parasitic NOS B89
  eyeworm B74.3
  Fasciola (gigantica) (hepatica) (indica) B66.3
  Fasciolopsis (buski) (intestine) B66.5
  filarial B74.9
    bancroftian B74.0
    conjunctiva B74.9
    due to
      Acanthocheilonema (perstans) (streptocerca) B74.4
      Brugia (malayi) B74.1
        timori B74.2
      Dracunculus medinensis B72
      guinea worm B72
      loa loa B74.3
      Mansonella (ozzardi) (perstans) (streptocerca) B74.4
      Onchocerca volvulus B73.00
        eye B73.00
        eyelid B73.09
      Wuchereria (bancrofti) B74.0
    Malayan B74.1
    ozzardi B74.4
    specified type NEC B74.8
  fish tapeworm B70.0
    larval B70.1
  fluke B66.9
    blood NOS — *see* Schistosomiasis
    cat liver B66.0
    intestinal B66.5
    lancet B66.2
    liver (sheep) B66.3
      cat B66.0
      Chinese B66.1
      due to clonorchiasis B66.1
      oriental B66.1
    lung (oriental) B66.4
    sheep liver B66.3
    specified type NEC B66.8
  fly larvae — *see* Myiasis
  Gasterophilus (intestinalis) — *see* Myiasis
  Gastrodiscoides hominis B66.8
  Giardia lamblia A07.1
  Gnathostoma (spinigerum) B83.1

Infestation — *continued*
  Gongylonema B83.8
  guinea worm B72
  helminth B83.9
    angiostrongyliasis B83.2
      intestinal B81.3
    gnathostomiasis B83.1
    hirudiniasis, internal B83.4
    intestinal B82.0
      angiostrongyliasis B81.3
      anisakiasis B81.0
      ascariasis — *see* Ascariasis
      capillariasis B81.1
      cysticercosis — *see* Cysticercosis
      diphyllobothriasis — *see* Infestation, diphyllobothriasis
      dracunculiasis B72
      echinococcus — *see* Echinococcosis
      enterobiasis B80
      filariasis — *see* Infestation, filarial
      fluke — *see* Infestation, fluke
      hookworm — *see* Infestation, hookworm
      mixed (types classifiable to more than one of the titles B65.0-B81.3 and B81.8) B81.4
      onchocerciasis — *see* Onchocerciasis
      schistosomiasis — *see* Infestation, schistosoma
      specified
        cestode NEC — *see* Infestation, cestode
        type NEC B81.8
      strongyloidiasis — *see* Strongyloidiasis
      taenia — *see* Infestation, taenia
      trichinellosis B75
      trichostrongyliasis B81.2
      trichuriasis B79
    specified type NEC B83.8
    syngamiasis B83.3
    visceral larva migrans B83.0
  Heterophyes (heterophyes) B66.8
  hookworm B76.9
    ancylostomiasis B76.0
    necatoriasis B76.1
    specified type NEC B76.8
  Hymenolepis (diminuta) (nana) B71.0
  intestinal NEC B82.9
  leeches (aquatic) (land) — *see* Hirudiniasis
  Leishmania — *see* Leishmaniasis
  lice, louse — *see* Infestation, Pediculus
  Linguatula B88.8
  Liponyssoides sanguineus B88.0
  Loa loa B74.3
    conjunctival B74.3
    eyelid B74.3
  louse — *see* Infestation, Pediculus
  maggots — *see* Myiasis
  Mansonella (ozzardi) (perstans) (streptocerca) B74.4
  Medina (worm) B72
  Metagonimus (yokogawai) B66.8
  microfilaria streptocerca — *see* Onchocerciasis
    eye B73.00
    eyelid B73.09
  mites B88.9
    scabic B86
  Monilia (albicans) — *see* Candidiasis
  mouth B37.0
  Necator americanus B76.1
  nematode NEC (intestinal) B82.0
    Ancylostoma B76.0
    conjunctiva NEC B83.9
    Enterobius vermicularis B80
    Gnathostoma spinigerum B83.1
    physaloptera B80
    specified NEC B81.8
    trichostrongylus B81.2
    trichuris (trichuria) B79
  Oesophagostomum (apiostomum) B81.8
  Oestrus ovis — *see also* Myiasis B87.9
  Onchocerca (volvulus) — *see* Onchocerciasis
  Opisthorchis (felineus) (viverrini) B66.0
  orbit, parasitic NOS B89
  Oxyuris vermicularis B80
  Paragonimus (westermani) B66.4
  parasite, parasitic B89
    eyelid B89
    intestinal NOS B82.9
    mouth B37.0
    skin B88.9
    tongue B37.0

Infestation — *continued*
  Parastrongylus
    cantonensis B83.2
    costaricensis B81.3
  Pediculus B85.2
    body B85.1
    capitis (humanus) (any site) B85.Ø
    corporis (humanus) (any site) B85.1
    head B85.Ø
    mixed (classifiable to more than one of the titles B85.Ø - B85.3) B85.4
    pubis (any site) B85.3
  Pentastoma B88.8
  Phthirus (pubis) (any site) B85.3
    with any infestation classifiable to B85.Ø - B85.2 B85.4
  pinworm B8Ø
  pork tapeworm (adult) B68.Ø
  protozoal NEC B64
    intestinal AØ7.9
      specified NEC AØ7.8
    specified NEC B6Ø.8
  pubic, louse B85.3
  rat tapeworm B71.Ø
  red bug B88.Ø
  roundworm (large) NEC B82.Ø
    Ascariasis — *see also* Ascariasis B77.9
  sandflea B88.1
  Sarcoptes scabiei B86
  scabies B86
  Schistosoma B65.9
    bovis B65.8
    cercariae B65.3
    haematobium B65.Ø
    intercalatum B65.8
    japonicum B65.2
    mansoni B65.1
    mattheei B65.8
    mekongi B65.8
    specified type NEC B65.8
    spindale B65.8
  screw worms — *see* Myiasis
  skin NOS B88.9
  Sparganum (mansoni) (proliferum) (baxteri) B7Ø.1
    larval B7Ø.1
  specified type NEC B88.8
  Spirometra larvae B7Ø.1
  Stellantchasmus falcatus B66.8
  Strongyloides stercoralis — *see* Strongyloidiasis
  Taenia B68.9
    diminuta B71.Ø
    echinococcus — *see* Echinococcus
    mediocanellata B68.1
    nana B71.Ø
    saginata B68.1
    solium (intestinal form) B68.Ø
      larval form — *see* Cysticercosis
  Taeniarhynchus saginatus B68.1
  tapeworm B71.9
    beef B68.1
    broad B7Ø.Ø
      larval B7Ø.1
    dog B67.4
    dwarf B71.Ø
    fish B7Ø.Ø
      larval B7Ø.1
    pork B68.Ø
    rat B71.Ø
  Ternidens diminutus B81.8
  Tetranychus molestissimus B88.Ø
  threadworm B8Ø
  tongue B37.Ø
  Toxocara (canis) (cati) (felis) B83.Ø
  trematode(s) NEC — *see* Infestation, fluke
  Trichinella (spiralis) B75
  Trichocephalus B79
  Trichomonas — *see* Trichomoniasis
  Trichostrongylus B81.2
  Trichuris (trichiura) B79
  Trombicula (irritans) B88.Ø
  Tunga penetrans B88.1
  Uncinaria americana B76.1
  Vandellia cirrhosa B88.8
  whipworm B79
  worms B83.9
    intestinal B82.Ø
  Wuchereria (bancrofti) B74.Ø

Infiltrate, infiltration
  amyloid (generalized) (localized) — *see* Amyloidosis
  calcareous NEC R89.7
    localized — *see* Degeneration, by site
  calcium salt R89.7
  cardiac
    fatty — *see* Degeneration, myocardial
    glycogenic E74.Ø2 *[I43]*
  corneal — *see* Edema, cornea
  eyelid — *see* Inflammation, eyelid
  glycogen, glycogenic — *see* Disease, glycogen storage
  heart, cardiac
    fatty — *see* Degeneration, myocardial
    glycogenic E74.Ø2 *[I43]*
  inflammatory in vitreous H43.89
  kidney N28.89
  leukemic — *see* Leukemia
  liver K76.89
    fatty — *see* Fatty, liver NEC
    glycogen — *see also* Disease, glycogen storage E74.Ø3 *[K77]*
  lung R91.8
    eosinophilic — *see* Eosinophilia, pulmonary
  lymphatic — *see also* Leukemia, lymphatic C91.9- ☑
    gland I88.9
  muscle, fatty M62.89
  myocardium, myocardial
    fatty — *see* Degeneration, myocardial
    glycogenic E74.Ø2 *[I43]*
  on chest x-ray R91.8
  pulmonary R91.8
    with eosinophilia — *see* Eosinophilia, pulmonary
  skin (lymphocytic) L98.6
  thymus (gland) (fatty) E32.8
  urine R39.Ø
  vesicant agent
    antineoplastic chemotherapy T8Ø.81Ø ☑
    other agent NEC T8Ø.818 ☑
  vitreous body H43.89

Infirmity R68.89
  senile R54

Inflammation, inflamed, inflammatory (with exudation)
  abducent (nerve) — *see* Strabismus, paralytic, sixth nerve
  accessory sinus (chronic) — *see* Sinusitis
  adrenal (gland) E27.8
  alveoli, teeth M27.3
    scorbutic E54
  anal canal, anus K62.89
  antrum (chronic) — *see* Sinusitis, maxillary
  appendix — *see* Appendicitis
  arachnoid — *see* Meningitis
  areola N61.Ø
    puerperal, postpartum or gestational — *see* Infection, nipple
  areolar tissue NOS LØ8.9
  artery — *see* Arteritis
  auditory meatus (external) — *see* Otitis, externa
  Bartholin's gland N75.8
  bile duct (common) (hepatic) or passage — *see* Cholangitis
  bladder — *see* Cystitis
  bone — *see* Osteomyelitis
  brain — *see also* Encephalitis
    membrane — *see* Meningitis
  breast N61.Ø
    puerperal, postpartum, gestational — *see* Mastitis, obstetric
  broad ligament — *see* Disease, pelvis, inflammatory
  bronchi — *see* Bronchitis
  catarrhal JØØ
  cecum — *see* Appendicitis
  cerebral — *see also* Encephalitis
    membrane — *see* Meningitis
  cerebrospinal
    meningococcal A39.Ø
  cervix (uteri) — *see* Cervicitis
  chest J98.8
  chorioretinal H3Ø.9- ☑
    cyclitis — *see* Cyclitis
    disseminated H3Ø.1Ø- ☑
      generalized H3Ø.13- ☑
      peripheral H3Ø.12- ☑
      posterior pole H3Ø.11- ☑
    epitheliopathy — *see* Epitheliopathy
    focal H3Ø.ØØ- ☑

Inflammation, inflamed, inflammatory — *continued*
  chorioretinal — *continued*
    focal — *continued*
      juxtapapillary H3Ø.Ø1- ☑
      macular H3Ø.Ø4- ☑
      paramacular — *see* Inflammation, chorioretinal, focal, macular
      peripheral H3Ø.Ø3- ☑
      posterior pole H3Ø.Ø2- ☑
    specified type NEC H3Ø.89- ☑
  choroid — *see* Inflammation, chorioretinal
  chronic, postmastoidectomy cavity — *see* Complications, postmastoidectomy, inflammation
  colon — *see* Enteritis
  connective tissue (diffuse) NEC — *see* Disorder, soft tissue, specified type NEC
  cornea — *see* Keratitis
  corpora cavernosa N48.29
  cranial nerve — *see* Disorder, nerve, cranial
  Douglas' cul-de-sac or pouch (chronic) N73.Ø
  due to device, implant or graft — *see also* Complications, by site and type, infection or inflammation
    arterial graft T82.7 ☑
    breast (implant) T85.79 ☑
    catheter T85.79 ☑
      dialysis (renal) T82.7 ☑
        intraperitoneal T85.71 ☑
      infusion T82.7 ☑
        cranial T85.735 ☑
        intrathecal T85.735 ☑
        spinal (epidural) (subdural) T85.735 ☑
        subarachnoid T85.735 ☑
      urinary T83.518 ☑
        cystostomy T83.51Ø ☑
        Hopkins T83.518 ☑
        ileostomy T83.518 ☑
        nephrostomy T83.512 ☑
        specified NEC T83.518 ☑
        urethral indwelling T83.511 ☑
        urostomy T83.518 ☑
    electronic (electrode) (pulse generator) (stimulator)
      bone T84.7 ☑
      cardiac T82.7 ☑
      nervous system T85.738 ☑
        brain T85.731 ☑
        cranial nerve T85.732 ☑
        gastric nerve T85.732 ☑
        neurostimulator generator T85.734 ☑
        peripheral nerve T85.732 ☑
        sacral nerve T85.732 ☑
        spinal cord T85.733 ☑
        vagal nerve T85.732 ☑
      urinary T83.59Ø ☑
    fixation, internal (orthopedic) NEC — *see* Complication, fixation device, infection
    gastrointestinal (bile duct) (esophagus) T85.79 ☑
      neurostimulator electrode (lead) T85.732 ☑
    genital NEC T83.69 ☑
    heart NEC T82.7 ☑
      valve (prosthesis) T82.6 ☑
        graft T82.7 ☑
    joint prosthesis — *see* Complication, joint prosthesis, infection
    ocular (corneal graft) (orbital implant) NEC T85.79 ☑
    orthopedic NEC T84.7 ☑
    penile (cylinder) (pump) (resevoir) T83.61 ☑
    specified NEC T85.79 ☑
    testicular T83.62 ☑
    urinary NEC T83.598 ☑
      ileal conduit stent T83.593 ☑
      implanted neurostimulation T83.59Ø ☑
      implanted sphincter T83.591 ☑
      indwelling ureteral stent T83.592 ☑
      nephroureteral stent T83.593 ☑
      specified stent NEC T83.593 ☑
    vascular NEC T82.7 ☑
    ventricular intracranial (communicating) shunt T85.73Ø ☑
  duodenum K29.8Ø
    with bleeding K29.81
  dura mater — *see* Meningitis
  ear (middle) — *see also* Otitis, media
    external — *see* Otitis, externa
    inner — *see* subcategory H83.Ø ☑
  epididymis — *see* Epididymitis

☑ Additional Character Required — Refer to the Tabular List for Character Selection

Inflammation, inflamed, inflammatory — *continued*
- esophagus — *see* Esophagitis
- ethmoidal (sinus) (chronic) — *see* Sinusitis, ethmoidal
- eustachian tube (catarrhal) — *see* Salpingitis, eustachian
- eyelid H01.9
  - abscess — *see* Abscess, eyelid
  - blepharitis — *see* Blepharitis
  - chalazion — *see* Chalazion
  - dermatosis (noninfectious) — *see* Dermatosis, eyelid
  - hordeolum — *see* Hordeolum
  - specified NEC H01.8
- fallopian tube — *see* Salpingo-oophoritis
- fascia — *see* Myositis
- follicular, pharynx J31.2
- frontal (sinus) (chronic) — *see* Sinusitis, frontal
- gallbladder — *see* Cholecystitis
- gastric — *see* Gastritis
- gastrointestinal — *see* Enteritis
- genital organ (internal) (diffuse)
  - female — *see* Disease, pelvis, inflammatory
  - male N49.9
    - multiple sites N49.8
    - specified NEC N49.8
- gland (lymph) — *see* Lymphadenitis
- glottis — *see* Laryngitis
- granular, pharynx J31.2
- gum K05.10
  - nonplaque induced K05.11
  - plaque induced K05.10
- heart — *see* Carditis
- hepatic duct — *see* Cholangitis
- ileoanal (internal) pouch K91.850
- ileum — *see also* Enteritis
  - regional or terminal — *see* Enteritis, regional
- intestinal pouch K91.850
- intestine (any part) — *see* Enteritis
- jaw (acute) (bone) (chronic) (lower) (suppurative) (upper) M27.2
- joint NEC — *see* Arthritis
  - sacroiliac M46.1
- kidney — *see* Nephritis
- knee (joint) M13.169
  - tuberculous A18.02
- labium (majus) (minus) — *see* Vulvitis
- lacrimal
  - gland — *see* Dacryoadenitis
  - passages (duct) (sac) — *see also* Dacryocystitis
    - canaliculitis — *see* Canaliculitis, lacrimal
- larynx — *see* Laryngitis
- leg NOS L08.9
- lip K13.0
- liver (capsule) — *see also* Hepatitis
  - chronic K73.9
  - suppurative K75.0
- lung (acute) — *see also* Pneumonia
  - chronic J98.4
- lymph gland or node — *see* Lymphadenitis
- lymphatic vessel — *see* Lymphangitis
- maxilla, maxillary M27.2
  - sinus (chronic) — *see* Sinusitis, maxillary
- membranes of brain or spinal cord — *see* Meningitis
- meninges — *see* Meningitis
- mouth K12.1
- muscle — *see* Myositis
- myocardium — *see* Myocarditis
- nasal sinus (chronic) — *see* Sinusitis
- nasopharynx — *see* Nasopharyngitis
- navel L08.82
- nerve NEC — *see* Neuritis
- nipple N61.0
  - puerperal, postpartum or gestational — *see* Infection, nipple
- nose — *see* Rhinitis
- oculomotor (nerve) — *see* Strabismus, paralytic, third nerve
- optic nerve — *see* Neuritis, optic
- orbit (chronic) H05.10
  - acute H05.00
    - abscess — *see* Abscess, orbit
    - cellulitis — *see* Cellulitis, orbit
    - osteomyelitis — *see* Osteomyelitis, orbit
    - periostitis — *see* Periostitis, orbital
    - tenonitis — *see* Tenonitis, eye
  - granuloma — *see* Granuloma, orbit
  - myositis — *see* Myositis, orbital

Inflammation, inflamed, inflammatory — *continued*
- ovary — *see* Salpingo-oophoritis
- oviduct — *see* Salpingo-oophoritis
- pancreas (acute) — *see* Pancreatitis
- parametrium N73.0
- parotid region L08.9
- pelvis, female — *see* Disease, pelvis, inflammatory
- penis (corpora cavernosa) N48.29
- perianal K62.89
- pericardium — *see* Pericarditis
- perineum (female) (male) L08.9
- perirectal K62.89
- peritoneum — *see* Peritonitis
- periuterine — *see* Disease, pelvis, inflammatory
- perivesical — *see* Cystitis
- petrous bone (acute) (chronic) — *see* Petrositis
- pharynx (acute) — *see* Pharyngitis
- pia mater — *see* Meningitis
- pleura — *see* Pleurisy
- polyp, colon — *see also* Polyp, colon, inflammatory K51.40
- prostate — *see also* Prostatitis
  - specified type NEC N41.8
- rectosigmoid — *see* Rectosigmoiditis
- rectum — *see also* Proctitis K62.89
- respiratory, upper — *see also* Infection, respiratory, upper J06.9
  - acute, due to radiation J70.0
  - chronic, due to external agent — *see* condition, respiratory, chronic, due to
  - due to
    - chemicals, gases, fumes or vapors (inhalation) J68.2
    - radiation J70.1
- retina — *see* Chorioretinitis
- retrocecal — *see* Appendicitis
- retroperitoneal — *see* Peritonitis
- salivary duct or gland (any) (suppurative) — *see* Sialoadenitis
- scorbutic, alveoli, teeth E54
- scrotum N49.2
- seminal vesicle — *see* Vesiculitis
- sigmoid — *see* Enteritis
- sinus — *see* Sinusitis
- Skene's duct or gland — *see* Urethritis
- skin L08.9
- spermatic cord N49.1
- sphenoidal (sinus) — *see* Sinusitis, sphenoidal
- spinal
  - cord — *see* Encephalitis
  - membrane — *see* Meningitis
  - nerve — *see* Disorder, nerve
- spine — *see* Spondylopathy, inflammatory
- spleen (capsule) D73.89
- stomach — *see* Gastritis
- subcutaneous tissue L08.9
- suprarenal (gland) E27.8
- synovial — *see* Tenosynovitis
- tendon (sheath) NEC — *see* Tenosynovitis
- testis — *see* Orchitis
- throat (acute) — *see* Pharyngitis
- thymus (gland) E32.8
- thyroid (gland) — *see* Thyroiditis
- tongue K14.0
- tonsil — *see* Tonsillitis
- trachea — *see* Tracheitis
- trochlear (nerve) — *see* Strabismus, paralytic, fourth nerve
- tubal — *see* Salpingo-oophoritis
- tuberculous NEC — *see* Tuberculosis
- tubo-ovarian — *see* Salpingo-oophoritis
- tunica vaginalis N49.1
- tympanic membrane — *see* Tympanitis
- umbilicus, umbilical L08.82
- uterine ligament — *see* Disease, pelvis, inflammatory
- uterus (catarrhal) — *see* Endometritis
- uveal tract (anterior) NOS — *see also* Iridocyclitis
  - posterior — *see* Chorioretinitis
- vagina — *see* Vaginitis
- vas deferens N49.1
- vein — *see also* Phlebitis
  - intracranial or intraspinal (septic) G08
  - thrombotic I80.9
    - leg — *see* Phlebitis, leg
    - lower extremity — *see* Phlebitis, leg
- vocal cord J38.3

Inflammation, inflamed, inflammatory — *continued*
- vulva — *see* Vulvitis
- Wharton's duct (suppurative) — *see* Sialoadenitis
Inflation, lung, imperfect (newborn) — *see* Atelectasis
Influenza (bronchial) (epidemic) (respiratory (upper)) (unidentified influenza virus) J11.1
- with
  - digestive manifestations J11.2
  - encephalopathy J11.81
  - enteritis J11.2
  - gastroenteritis J11.2
  - gastrointestinal manifestations J11.2
  - laryngitis J11.1
  - myocarditis J11.82
  - otitis media J11.83
  - pharyngitis J11.1
  - pneumonia J11.00
    - specified type J11.08
  - respiratory manifestations NEC J11.1
  - specified manifestation NEC J11.89
- A (non-novel) J10- ☑
- A/H5N1 — *see also* Influenza, due to, identified novel influenza A virus J09.X2
- avian — *see also* Influenza, due to, identified novel influenza A virus J09.X2
- B J10- ☑
- bird — *see also* Influenza, due to, identified novel influenza A virus J09.X2
- C J10- ☑
- due to
  - avian — *see also* Influenza, due to, identified novel influenza A virus J09.X2
  - identified influenza virus NEC J10.1
    - with
      - digestive manifestations J10.2
      - encephalopathy J10.81
      - enteritis J10.2
      - gastroenteritis J10.2
      - gastrointestinal manifestations J10.2
      - laryngitis J10.1
      - myocarditis J10.82
      - otitis media J10.83
      - pharyngitis J10.1
      - pneumonia (unspecified type) J10.00
        - with same identified influenza virus J10.01
        - specified type NEC J10.08
      - respiratory manifestations NEC J10.1
      - specified manifestation NEC J10.89
  - identified novel influenza A virus J09.X2
    - with
      - digestive manifestations J09.X3
      - encephalopathy J09.X9
      - enteritis J09.X3
      - gastroenteritis J09.X3
      - gastrointestinal manifestations J09.X3
      - laryngitis J09.X2
      - myocarditis J09.X9
      - otitis media J09.X9
      - pharyngitis J09.X2
      - pneumonia J09.X1
      - respiratory manifestations NEC J09.X2
      - specified manifestation NEC J09.X9
      - upper respiratory symptoms J09.X2
  - novel (2009) H1N1 influenza — *see also* Influenza, due to, identified influenza virus NEC J10.1
  - novel influenza A/H1N1 — *see also* Influenza, due to, identified influenza virus NEC J10.1
  - of other animal origin, not bird or swine — *see also* Influenza, due to, identified novel influenza A virus J09.X2
  - swine (viruses that normally cause infections in pigs) — *see also* Influenza, due to, identified novel influenza A virus J09.X2
Influenzal — *see* Influenza
Influenza-like disease — *see* Influenza
Infraction, Freiberg's (metatarsal head) — *see* Osteochondrosis, juvenile, metatarsus
Infraeruption of tooth (teeth) M26.34
Infusion complication, misadventure, or reaction — *see* Complications, infusion
Ingestion
- chemical — *see* Table of Drugs and Chemicals, by substance, poisoning

Ingestion — *continued*
  drug or medicament
    correct substance properly administered — *see* Table of Drugs and Chemicals, by drug, adverse effect
    overdose or wrong substance given or taken — *see* Table of Drugs and Chemicals, by drug, poisoning
  foreign body — *see* Foreign body, alimentary tract
  multiple drug — *see* Table of Drugs and Chemicals, multiple
  tularemia A21.3
Ingrowing
  hair (beard) L73.1
  nail (finger) (toe) L60.0
Inguinal — *see also* condition
  testicle Q53.9
    bilateral Q53.212
    unilateral Q53.112
Inhalant-induced
  anxiety disorder F18.980
  depressive disorder F18.94
  major neurocognitive disorder F18.97
  mild neurocognitive disorder F18.988
  psychotic disorder F18.959
Inhalation
  anthrax A22.1
  flame T27.3 ☑
  food or foreign body — *see* Foreign body, by site
  gases, fumes, or vapors T59.9- ☑
    specified agent NEC — *see* Table of Drugs and Chemicals, by substance T59.89- ☑
  liquid or vomitus — *see* Asphyxia
  meconium (newborn) P24.00
    with
      with respiratory symptoms P24.01
      pneumonia (pneumonitis) P24.01
  mucus — *see* Asphyxia, mucus
  oil or gasoline (causing suffocation) — *see* Foreign body, by site
  smoke T59.81- ☑
    with respiratory conditions J70.5
    due to chemicals, gases, fumes and vapors J68.9
  steam — *see also* Burn, respiratory tract T59.9- ☑
  stomach contents or secretions — *see* Foreign body, by site
    due to anesthesia (general) (local) or other sedation T88.59 ☑
    in labor and delivery O74.0
    in pregnancy O29.01- ☑
    postpartum, puerperal O89.01
Inhibition, orgasm
  female F52.31
  male F52.32
Inhibitor, systemic lupus erythematosus (presence of) D68.62
Iniencephalus, iniencephaly Q00.2
Injection, traumatic jet (air) (industrial) (water) (paint or dye) T70.4 ☑
Injury — *see also* specified injury type T14.90 ☑
  abdomen, abdominal S39.91 ☑
    blood vessel — *see* Injury, blood vessel, abdomen
    cavity — *see* Injury, intra-abdominal
    contusion S30.1 ☑
    internal — *see* Injury, intra-abdominal
    intra-abdominal organ — *see* Injury, intra-abdominal
    nerve — *see* Injury, nerve, abdomen
    open — *see* Wound, open, abdomen
    specified NEC S39.81 ☑
    superficial — *see* Injury, superficial, abdomen
  Achilles tendon S86.00- ☑
    laceration S86.02- ☑
    specified type NEC S86.09- ☑
    strain S86.01- ☑
  acoustic, resulting in deafness — *see* Injury, nerve, acoustic
  adrenal (gland) S37.819 ☑
    contusion S37.812 ☑
    laceration S37.813 ☑
    specified type NEC S37.818 ☑
  alveolar (process) S09.93 ☑
  ankle S99.91- ☑
    contusion — *see* Contusion, ankle
    dislocation — *see* Dislocation, ankle
    fracture — *see* Fracture, ankle
    nerve — *see* Injury, nerve, ankle

Injury — *continued*
  ankle — *continued*
    open — *see* Wound, open, ankle
    specified type NEC S99.81- ☑
    sprain — *see* Sprain, ankle
    superficial — *see* Injury, superficial, ankle
  anterior chamber, eye — *see* Injury, eye, specified site NEC
  anus — *see* Injury, abdomen
  aorta (thoracic) S25.00 ☑
    abdominal S35.00 ☑
      laceration (minor) (superficial) S35.01 ☑
        major S35.02 ☑
      specified type NEC S35.09 ☑
    laceration (minor) (superficial) S25.01 ☑
      major S25.02 ☑
    specified type NEC S25.09 ☑
  arm (upper) S49.9- ☑
    blood vessel — *see* Injury, blood vessel, arm
    contusion — *see* Contusion, arm, upper
    fracture — *see* Fracture, humerus
    lower — *see* Injury, forearm
    muscle — *see* Injury, muscle, shoulder
    nerve — *see* Injury, nerve, arm
    open — *see* Wound, open, arm
    specified type NEC S49.8- ☑
    superficial — *see* Injury, superficial, arm
  artery (complicating trauma) — *see also* Injury, blood vessel, by site
    cerebral or meningeal — *see* Injury, intracranial
  auditory canal (external) (meatus) S09.91 ☑
  auricle, auris, ear S09.91 ☑
  axilla — *see* Injury, shoulder
  back — *see* Injury, back, lower
  bile duct S36.13 ☑
  birth — *see also* Birth, injury P15.9
  bladder (sphincter) S37.20 ☑
    at delivery O71.5
    contusion S37.22 ☑
    laceration S37.23 ☑
    obstetrical trauma O71.5
    specified type NEC S37.29 ☑
  blast (air) (hydraulic) (immersion) (underwater) NEC T14.8 ☑
    acoustic nerve trauma — *see* Injury, nerve, acoustic
    bladder — *see* Injury, bladder
    brain — *see* Concussion
      primary, specified NEC S06.8A- ☑
    colon — *see* Injury, intestine, large
    ear (primary) S09.31- ☑
      secondary S09.39- ☑
    generalized T70.8 ☑
    lung — *see* Injury, intrathoracic, lung
    multiple body organs T70.8 ☑
    peritoneum S36.81 ☑
    rectum S36.61 ☑
    retroperitoneum S36.898 ☑
    small intestine S36.419 ☑
      duodenum S36.410 ☑
      specified site NEC S36.418 ☑
    specified
      intra-abdominal organ NEC S36.898 ☑
      pelvic organ NEC S37.899 ☑
  blood vessel NEC T14.8 ☑
    abdomen S35.9 ☑
      aorta — *see* Injury, aorta, abdominal
      celiac artery — *see* Injury, blood vessel, celiac artery
      iliac vessel — *see* Injury, blood vessel, iliac
      laceration S35.91 ☑
      mesenteric vessel — *see* Injury, mesenteric
      portal vein — *see* Injury, blood vessel, portal vein
      renal vessel — *see* Injury, blood vessel, renal
      specified vessel NEC S35.8X- ☑
      splenic vessel — *see* Injury, blood vessel, splenic
      vena cava — *see* Injury, vena cava, inferior
    ankle — *see* Injury, blood vessel, foot
    aorta (abdominal) (thoracic) — *see* Injury, aorta
    arm (upper) NEC S45.90- ☑
      forearm — *see* Injury, blood vessel, forearm
      laceration S45.91- ☑
      specified
        site NEC S45.80- ☑
          laceration S45.81- ☑
          specified type NEC S45.89- ☑
        type NEC S45.99- ☑

Injury — *continued*
  blood vessel — *continued*
    arm — *continued*
      superficial vein S45.30- ☑
        laceration S45.31- ☑
        specified type NEC S45.39- ☑
      axillary
        artery S45.00- ☑
          laceration S45.01- ☑
          specified type NEC S45.09- ☑
        vein S45.20- ☑
          laceration S45.21- ☑
          specified type NEC S45.29- ☑
      azygos vein — *see* Injury, blood vessel, thoracic, specified site NEC
      brachial
        artery S45.10- ☑
          laceration S45.11- ☑
          specified type NEC S45.19- ☑
        vein S45.20- ☑
          laceration S45.219 ☑
          specified type NEC S45.29- ☑
      carotid artery (common) (external) (internal, extracranial) S15.00- ☑
        internal, intracranial S06.8- ☑
        laceration (minor) (superficial) S15.01- ☑
          major S15.02- ☑
        specified type NEC S15.09- ☑
      celiac artery S35.219 ☑
        branch S35.299 ☑
          laceration (minor) (superficial) S35.291 ☑
            major S35.292 ☑
          specified NEC S35.298 ☑
        laceration (minor) (superficial) S35.211 ☑
          major S35.212 ☑
        specified type NEC S35.218 ☑
      cerebral — *see* Injury, intracranial
      deep plantar — *see* Injury, blood vessel, plantar artery
      digital (hand) — *see* Injury, blood vessel, finger
      dorsal
        artery (foot) S95.00- ☑
          laceration S95.01- ☑
          specified type NEC S95.09- ☑
        vein (foot) S95.20- ☑
          laceration S95.21- ☑
          specified type NEC S95.29- ☑
      due to accidental laceration during procedure — *see* Laceration, accidental complicating surgery
      extremity — *see* Injury, blood vessel, limb
      femoral
        artery (common) (superficial) S75.00- ☑
          laceration (minor) (superficial) S75.01- ☑
            major S75.02- ☑
          specified type NEC S75.09- ☑
        vein (hip level) (thigh level) S75.10- ☑
          laceration (minor) (superficial) S75.11- ☑
            major S75.12- ☑
          specified type NEC S75.19- ☑
      finger S65.50- ☑
        index S65.50- ☑
          laceration S65.51- ☑
          specified type NEC S65.59- ☑
        laceration S65.51- ☑
        little S65.50- ☑
          laceration S65.51- ☑
          specified type NEC S65.59- ☑
        middle S65.50- ☑
          laceration S65.51- ☑
          specified type NEC S65.59- ☑
        specified type NEC S65.59- ☑
        thumb — *see* Injury, blood vessel, thumb
      foot S95.90- ☑
        dorsal
          artery — *see* Injury, blood vessel, dorsal, artery
          vein — *see* Injury, blood vessel, dorsal, vein
        laceration S95.91- ☑
        plantar artery — *see* Injury, blood vessel, plantar artery
        specified
          site NEC S95.80- ☑
            laceration S95.81- ☑
            specified type NEC S95.89- ☑
          specified type NEC S95.99- ☑

☑ Additional Character Required — Refer to the Tabular List for Character Selection

Injury — *continued*
  blood vessel — *continued*
    forearm S55.90- ☑
      laceration S55.91- ☑
      radial artery — *see* Injury, blood vessel, radial artery
      specified
        site NEC S55.80- ☑
          laceration S55.81- ☑
          specified type NEC S55.89- ☑
        type NEC S55.99- ☑
      ulnar artery — *see* Injury, blood vessel, ulnar artery
      vein S55.20- ☑
        laceration S55.21- ☑
        specified type NEC S55.29- ☑
    gastric
      artery — *see* Injury, mesenteric, artery, branch
      vein — *see* Injury, blood vessel, abdomen
    gastroduodenal artery — *see* Injury, mesenteric, artery, branch
    greater saphenous vein (lower leg level) S85.30- ☑
      hip (and thigh) level S75.20- ☑
        laceration (minor) (superficial) S75.21- ☑
          major S75.22- ☑
        specified type NEC S75.29- ☑
      laceration S85.31- ☑
      specified type NEC S85.39- ☑
    hand (level) S65.90- ☑
      finger — *see* Injury, blood vessel, finger
      laceration S65.91- ☑
      palmar arch — *see* Injury, blood vessel, palmar arch
      radial artery — *see* Injury, blood vessel, radial artery, hand
      specified
        site NEC S65.80- ☑
          laceration S65.81- ☑
          specified type NEC S65.89- ☑
        type NEC S65.99- ☑
      thumb — *see* Injury, blood vessel, thumb
      ulnar artery — *see* Injury, blood vessel, ulnar artery, hand
    head S09.0 ☑
      intracranial — *see* Injury, intracranial
      multiple S09.0 ☑
    hepatic
      artery — *see* Injury, mesenteric, artery
      vein — *see* Injury, vena cava, inferior
    hip S75.90- ☑
      femoral artery — *see* Injury, blood vessel, femoral, artery
      femoral vein — *see* Injury, blood vessel, femoral, vein
      greater saphenous vein — *see* Injury, blood vessel, greater saphenous, hip level
      laceration S75.91- ☑
      specified
        site NEC S75.80- ☑
          laceration S75.81- ☑
          specified type NEC S75.89- ☑
        type NEC S75.99- ☑
    hypogastric (artery) (vein) — *see* Injury, blood vessel, iliac
    iliac S35.5- ☑
      artery S35.51- ☑
      specified vessel NEC S35.5- ☑
      uterine vessel — *see* Injury, blood vessel, uterine
      vein S35.51- ☑
    innominate — *see* Injury, blood vessel, thoracic, innominate
    intercostal (artery) (vein) — *see* Injury, blood vessel, thoracic, intercostal
    jugular vein (external) S15.20- ☑
      internal S15.30- ☑
        laceration (minor) (superficial) S15.31- ☑
          major S15.32- ☑
        specified type NEC S15.39- ☑
      laceration (minor) (superficial) S15.21- ☑
        major S15.22- ☑
      specified type NEC S15.29- ☑
    leg (level) (lower) S85.90- ☑
      greater saphenous — *see* Injury, blood vessel, greater saphenous
      laceration S85.91- ☑

Injury — *continued*
  blood vessel — *continued*
    leg — *continued*
      lesser saphenous — *see* Injury, blood vessel, lesser saphenous
      peroneal artery — *see* Injury, blood vessel, peroneal artery
      popliteal
        artery — *see* Injury, blood vessel, popliteal, artery
        vein — *see* Injury, blood vessel, popliteal, vein
      specified
        site NEC S85.80- ☑
          laceration S85.81- ☑
          specified type NEC S85.89- ☑
        type NEC S85.99- ☑
      thigh — *see* Injury, blood vessel, hip
      tibial artery — *see* Injury, blood vessel, tibial artery
    lesser saphenous vein (lower leg level) S85.40- ☑
      laceration S85.41- ☑
      specified type NEC S85.49- ☑
    limb
      lower — *see* Injury, blood vessel, leg
      upper — *see* Injury, blood vessel, arm
    lower back — *see* Injury, blood vessel, abdomen
    specified NEC — *see* Injury, blood vessel, abdomen, specified, site NEC
    mammary (artery) (vein) — *see* Injury, blood vessel, thoracic, specified site NEC
    mesenteric (inferior) (superior)
      artery — *see* Injury, mesenteric, artery
      vein — *see* Injury, blood vessel, mesenteric, vein
    neck S15.9 ☑
      specified site NEC S15.8 ☑
    ovarian (artery) (vein) — *see* subcategory S35.8 ☑
    palmar arch (superficial) S65.20- ☑
      deep S65.30- ☑
        laceration S65.31- ☑
        specified type NEC S65.39- ☑
      laceration S65.21- ☑
      specified type NEC S65.29- ☑
    pelvis — *see* Injury, blood vessel, abdomen
    specified NEC — *see* Injury, blood vessel, abdomen, specified, site NEC
    peroneal artery S85.20- ☑
      laceration S85.21- ☑
      specified type NEC S85.29- ☑
    plantar artery (deep) (foot) S95.10- ☑
      laceration S95.11- ☑
      specified type NEC S95.19- ☑
    popliteal
      artery S85.00- ☑
        laceration S85.01- ☑
        specified type NEC S85.09- ☑
      vein S85.50- ☑
        laceration S85.51- ☑
        specified type NEC S85.59- ☑
    portal vein S35.319 ☑
      laceration S35.311 ☑
      specified type NEC S35.318 ☑
    precerebral — *see* Injury, blood vessel, neck
    pulmonary (artery) (vein) — *see* Injury, blood vessel, thoracic, pulmonary
    radial artery (forearm level) S55.10- ☑
      hand and wrist (level) S65.10- ☑
        laceration S65.11- ☑
        specified type NEC S65.19- ☑
      laceration S55.01- ☑
      specified type NEC S55.19- ☑
    renal
      artery S35.40- ☑
        laceration S35.41- ☑
        specified NEC S35.49- ☑
      vein S35.40- ☑
        laceration S35.41- ☑
        specified NEC S35.49- ☑
    saphenous vein (greater) (lower leg level) — *see* Injury, blood vessel, greater saphenous
      hip and thigh level — *see* Injury, blood vessel, greater saphenous, hip level
      lesser — *see* Injury, blood vessel, lesser saphenous
    shoulder
      specified NEC — *see* Injury, blood vessel, arm, specified site NEC

Injury — *continued*
  blood vessel — *continued*
    shoulder — *continued*
      superficial vein — *see* Injury, blood vessel, arm, superficial vein
    specified NEC T14.8 ☑
    splenic
      artery — *see* Injury, blood vessel, celiac artery, branch
      vein S35.329 ☑
        laceration S35.321 ☑
        specified NEC S35.328 ☑
    subclavian — *see* Injury, blood vessel, thoracic, innominate
    thigh — *see* Injury, blood vessel, hip
    thoracic S25.90 ☑
      aorta S25.00 ☑
        laceration (minor) (superficial) S25.01 ☑
          major S25.02 ☑
        specified type NEC S25.09 ☑
      azygos vein — *see* Injury, blood vessel, thoracic, specified, site NEC
      innominate
        artery S25.10- ☑
          laceration (minor) (superficial) S25.11- ☑
            major S25.12- ☑
          specified type NEC S25.19- ☑
        vein S25.30- ☑
          laceration (minor) (superficial) S25.31- ☑
            major S25.32- ☑
          specified type NEC S25.39- ☑
      intercostal S25.50- ☑
        laceration S25.51- ☑
        specified type NEC S25.59- ☑
      laceration S25.91 ☑
      mammary vessel — *see* Injury, blood vessel, thoracic, specified, site NEC
      pulmonary S25.40- ☑
        laceration (minor) (superficial) S25.41- ☑
          major S25.42- ☑
        specified type NEC S25.49- ☑
      specified
        site NEC S25.80- ☑
          laceration S25.81 ☑
          specified type NEC S25.89 ☑
        type NEC S25.99 ☑
      subclavian — *see* Injury, blood vessel, thoracic, innominate
      vena cava (superior) S25.20 ☑
        laceration (minor) (superficial) S25.21 ☑
          major S25.22 ☑
        specified type NEC S25.29 ☑
    thumb S65.40- ☑
      laceration S65.41- ☑
      specified type NEC S65.49- ☑
    tibial artery S85.10- ☑
      anterior S85.13- ☑
        laceration S85.14- ☑
        specified injury NEC S85.15- ☑
      laceration S85.11- ☑
      posterior S85.16- ☑
        laceration S85.17- ☑
        specified injury NEC S85.18- ☑
      specified injury NEC S85.12- ☑
    ulnar artery (forearm level) S55.00- ☑
      hand and wrist (level) S65.00- ☑
        laceration S65.01- ☑
        specified type NEC S65.09- ☑
      laceration S55.01- ☑
      specified type NEC S55.09- ☑
    upper arm (level) — *see* Injury, blood vessel, arm
      superficial vein — *see* Injury, blood vessel, arm, superficial vein
    uterine S35.5- ☑
      artery S35.53- ☑
      vein S35.53- ☑
    vena cava — *see* Injury, vena cava
    vertebral artery S15.10- ☑
      laceration (minor) (superficial) S15.11- ☑
        major S15.12- ☑
      specified type NEC S15.19- ☑
    wrist (level) — *see* Injury, blood vessel, hand
  brachial plexus S14.3 ☑
    newborn P14.3
  brain (traumatic) S06.9- ☑
    diffuse (axonal) S06.2X- ☑

Injury — *continued*
  brain — *continued*
    focal S06.30- ☑
    brainstem S06.38- ☑
  breast NOS S29.9 ☑
  broad ligament — *see* Injury, pelvic organ, specified site NEC
  bronchus, bronchi — *see* Injury, intrathoracic, bronchus
  brow S09.90 ☑
  buttock S39.92 ☑
  canthus, eye S05.90 ☑
  cardiac plexus — *see* Injury, nerve, thorax, sympathetic
  cauda equina S34.3 ☑
  cavernous sinus — *see* Injury, intracranial
  cecum — *see* Injury, colon
  celiac ganglion or plexus — *see* Injury, nerve, lumbosacral, sympathetic
  cerebellum — *see* Injury, intracranial
  cerebral — *see* Injury, intracranial
  cervix (uteri) — *see* Injury, uterus
  cheek (wall) S09.93 ☑
  chest — *see* Injury, thorax
  childbirth (newborn) — *see also* Birth, injury
    maternal NEC O71.9
  chin S09.93 ☑
  choroid (eye) — *see* Injury, eye, specified site NEC
  clitoris S39.94 ☑
  coccyx — *see also* Injury, back, lower
    complicating delivery O71.6
  colon — *see* Injury, intestine, large
  common bile duct — *see* Injury, liver
  conjunctiva (superficial) — *see* Injury, eye, conjunctiva
  conus medullaris — *see* Injury, spinal, sacral
  cord
    spermatic (pelvic region) S37.898 ☑
      scrotal region S39.848 ☑
    spinal — *see* Injury, spinal cord, by region
  cornea — *see* Injury, eye, specified site NEC
    abrasion — *see* Injury, eye, cornea, abrasion
  cortex (cerebral) — *see also* Injury, intracranial
    visual — *see* Injury, nerve, optic
  costal region NEC S29.9 ☑
  costochondral NEC S29.9 ☑
  cranial
    cavity — *see* Injury, intracranial
    nerve — *see* Injury, nerve, cranial
  crushing — *see* Crush
  cutaneous sensory nerve
  cystic duct — *see* Injury, liver
  deep tissue — *see* Contusion, by site
    meaning pressure ulcer — *see* Ulcer, pressure L89 with final character .6
  delivery (newborn) P15.9
    maternal NEC O71.9
  Descemet's membrane — *see* Injury, eyeball, penetrating
  diaphragm — *see* Injury, intrathoracic, diaphragm
  duodenum — *see* Injury, intestine, small, duodenum
  ear (auricle) (external) (canal) S09.91 ☑
    abrasion — *see* Abrasion, ear
    bite — *see* Bite, ear
    blister — *see* Blister, ear
    bruise — *see* Contusion, ear
    contusion — *see* Contusion, ear
    external constriction — *see* Constriction, external, ear
    hematoma — *see* Hematoma, ear
    inner — *see* Injury, ear, middle
    laceration — *see* Laceration, ear
    middle S09.30- ☑
      blast — *see* Injury, blast, ear
      specified NEC S09.39- ☑
    puncture — *see* Puncture, ear
    superficial — *see* Injury, superficial, ear
  eighth cranial nerve (acoustic or auditory) — *see* Injury, nerve, acoustic
  elbow S59.90- ☑
    contusion — *see* Contusion, elbow
    dislocation — *see* Dislocation, elbow
    fracture — *see* Fracture, ulna, upper end
    open — *see* Wound, open, elbow
    specified NEC S59.80- ☑
    sprain — *see* Sprain, elbow
    superficial — *see* Injury, superficial, elbow
  eleventh cranial nerve (accessory) — *see* Injury, nerve, accessory

Injury — *continued*
  epididymis S39.94 ☑
  epigastric region S39.91 ☑
  epiglottis NEC S19.89 ☑
  esophageal plexus — *see* Injury, nerve, thorax, sympathetic
  esophagus (thoracic part) — *see also* Injury, intrathoracic, esophagus
    cervical NEC S19.85 ☑
  eustachian tube S09.30 ☑
  eye S05.9- ☑
    avulsion S05.7- ☑
    ball — *see* Injury, eyeball
    conjunctiva S05.0- ☑
    cornea
      abrasion S05.0- ☑
      laceration S05.3- ☑
        with prolapse S05.2- ☑
    lacrimal apparatus S05.8X- ☑
    orbit penetration S05.4- ☑
    specified site NEC S05.8X- ☑
  eyeball S05.8X- ☑
    contusion S05.1- ☑
    penetrating S05.6- ☑
      with
        foreign body S05.5- ☑
        prolapse or loss of intraocular tissue S05.2- ☑
      without prolapse or loss of intraocular tissue S05.3- ☑
    specified type NEC S05.8- ☑
  eyebrow S09.93 ☑
  eyelid S09.93 ☑
    abrasion — *see* Abrasion, eyelid
    contusion — *see* Contusion, eyelid
    open — *see* Wound, open, eyelid
  face S09.93 ☑
  fallopian tube S37.509 ☑
    bilateral S37.502 ☑
      blast injury S37.512 ☑
      contusion S37.522 ☑
      laceration S37.532 ☑
      specified type NEC S37.592 ☑
    blast injury (primary) S37.519 ☑
      bilateral S37.512 ☑
      secondary — *see* Injury, fallopian tube, specified type NEC
      unilateral S37.511 ☑
    contusion S37.529 ☑
      bilateral S37.522 ☑
      unilateral S37.521 ☑
    laceration S37.539 ☑
      bilateral S37.532 ☑
      unilateral S37.531 ☑
    specified type NEC S37.599 ☑
      bilateral S37.592 ☑
      unilateral S37.591 ☑
    unilateral S37.501 ☑
      blast injury S37.511 ☑
      contusion S37.521 ☑
      laceration S37.531 ☑
      specified type NEC S37.591 ☑
  fascia — *see* Injury, muscle
  fifth cranial nerve (trigeminal) — *see* Injury, nerve, trigeminal
  finger (nail) S69.9- ☑
    blood vessel — *see* Injury, blood vessel, finger
    contusion — *see* Contusion, finger
    dislocation — *see* Dislocation, finger
    fracture — *see* Fracture, finger
    muscle — *see* Injury, muscle, finger
    nerve — *see* Injury, nerve, digital, finger
    open — *see* Wound, open, finger
    specified NEC S69.8- ☑
    sprain — *see* Sprain, finger
    superficial — *see* Injury, superficial, finger
  first cranial nerve (olfactory) — *see* Injury, nerve, olfactory
  flank — *see* Injury, abdomen
  foot S99.92- ☑
    blood vessel — *see* Injury, blood vessel, foot
    contusion — *see* Contusion, foot
    dislocation — *see* Dislocation, foot
    fracture — *see* Fracture, foot
    muscle — *see* Injury, muscle, foot
    open — *see* Wound, open, foot
    specified type NEC S99.82- ☑

Injury — *continued*
  foot — *continued*
    sprain — *see* Sprain, foot
    superficial — *see* Injury, superficial, foot
  forceps NOS P15.9
  forearm S59.91- ☑
    blood vessel — *see* Injury, blood vessel, forearm
    contusion — *see* Contusion, forearm
    fracture — *see* Fracture, forearm
    muscle — *see* Injury, muscle, forearm
    nerve — *see* Injury, nerve, forearm
    open — *see* Wound, open, forearm
    specified NEC S59.81- ☑
    superficial — *see* Injury, superficial, forearm
  forehead S09.90 ☑
  fourth cranial nerve (trochlear) — *see* Injury, nerve, trochlear
  gallbladder S36.129 ☑
    contusion S36.122 ☑
    laceration S36.123 ☑
    specified NEC S36.128 ☑
  ganglion
    celiac, coeliac — *see* Injury, nerve, lumbosacral, sympathetic
    gasserian — *see* Injury, nerve, trigeminal
    stellate — *see* Injury, nerve, thorax, sympathetic
    thoracic sympathetic — *see* Injury, nerve, thorax, sympathetic
  gasserian ganglion — *see* Injury, nerve, trigeminal
  gastric artery — *see* Injury, blood vessel, celiac artery, branch
  gastroduodenal artery — *see* Injury, blood vessel, celiac artery, branch
  gastrointestinal tract — *see* Injury, intra-abdominal
    with open wound into abdominal cavity — *see* Wound, open, with penetration into peritoneal cavity
    colon — *see* Injury, intestine, large
    rectum — *see* Injury, intestine, large, rectum
      with open wound into abdominal cavity S36.61
    small intestine — *see* Injury, intestine, small
    specified site NEC — *see* Injury, intra-abdominal, specified, site NEC
    stomach — *see* Injury, stomach
  genital organ(s)
    external S39.94 ☑
      specified NEC S39.848 ☑
    internal S37.90 ☑
      fallopian tube — *see* Injury, fallopian tube
      ovary — *see* Injury, ovary
      prostate — *see* Injury, prostate
      seminal vesicle — *see* Injury, pelvis, organ, specified site NEC
      uterus — *see* Injury, uterus
      vas deferens — *see* Injury, pelvis, organ, specified site NEC
    obstetrical trauma O71.9
  gland
    lacrimal laceration — *see* Injury, eye, specified site NEC
    salivary S09.93 ☑
    thyroid NEC S19.84 ☑
  globe (eye) S05.90 ☑
    specified NEC S05.8X- ☑
  groin — *see* Injury, abdomen
  gum S09.90 ☑
  hand S69.9- ☑
    blood vessel — *see* Injury, blood vessel, hand
    contusion — *see* Contusion, hand
    fracture — *see* Fracture, hand
    muscle — *see* Injury, muscle, hand
    nerve — *see* Injury, nerve, hand
    open — *see* Wound, open, hand
    specified NEC S69.8- ☑
    sprain — *see* Sprain, hand
    superficial — *see* Injury, superficial, hand
  head S09.90 ☑
    with loss of consciousness S06.9- ☑
    specified NEC S09.8 ☑
  heart (traumatic) S26.90 ☑
    with hemopericardium S26.00 ☑
      contusion S26.01 ☑
      laceration (mild) S26.020 ☑
        major S26.022 ☑
        moderate S26.021 ☑

Injury — continued
  heart — continued
    with hemopericardium — continued
      specified type NEC S26.09 ☑
    contusion S26.91 ☑
    laceration S26.92 ☑
    non-traumatic (acute) (chronic) (non-ischemic) I5A
    specified type NEC S26.99 ☑
    without hemopericardium S26.10 ☑
      contusion S26.11 ☑
      laceration S26.12 ☑
      specified type NEC S26.19 ☑
  heel — see Injury, foot
  hepatic
    artery — see Injury, blood vessel, celiac artery,
      branch
    duct — see Injury, liver
    vein — see Injury, vena cava, inferior
  hip S79.91- ☑
    blood vessel — see Injury, blood vessel, hip
    contusion — see Contusion, hip
    dislocation — see Dislocation, hip
    fracture — see Fracture, femur, neck
    muscle — see Injury, muscle, hip
    nerve — see Injury, nerve, hip
    open — see Wound, open, hip
    specified NEC S79.81- ☑
    sprain — see Sprain, hip
    superficial — see Injury, superficial, hip
  hymen S39.94 ☑
  hypogastric
    blood vessel — see Injury, blood vessel, iliac
    plexus — see Injury, nerve, lumbosacral, sympathet-
      ic
  ileum — see Injury, intestine, small
  iliac region S39.91 ☑
  instrumental (during surgery) — see Laceration, acci-
    dental complicating surgery
    birth injury — see Birth, injury
    nonsurgical — see Injury, by site
    obstetrical O71.9
      bladder O71.5
      cervix O71.3
      high vaginal O71.4
      perineal NOS O70.9
      urethra O71.5
      uterus O71.5
        with rupture or perforation O71.1
  internal T14.8 ☑
    aorta — see Injury, aorta
    bladder (sphincter) — see Injury, bladder
      with
        ectopic or molar pregnancy O08.6
        following ectopic or molar pregnancy O08.6
        obstetrical trauma O71.5
    bronchus, bronchi — see Injury, intrathoracic,
      bronchus
    cecum — see Injury, intestine, large
    cervix (uteri) — see also Injury, uterus
      with ectopic or molar pregnancy O08.6
      following ectopic or molar pregnancy O08.6
      obstetrical trauma O71.3
    chest — see Injury, intrathoracic
    gastrointestinal tract — see Injury, intra-abdominal
    heart — see Injury, heart
    intestine NEC — see Injury, intestine
    intrauterine — see Injury, uterus
    mesentery — see Injury, intra-abdominal, specified,
      site NEC
    pelvis, pelvic (organ) S37.90 ☑
      following ectopic or molar pregnancy (subse-
        quent episode) O08.6
      obstetrical trauma NEC O71.5
        rupture or perforation O71.1
      specified NEC S39.83 ☑
    rectum — see Injury, intestine, large, rectum
    stomach — see Injury, stomach
    ureter — see Injury, ureter
    urethra (sphincter) following ectopic or molar
      pregnancy O08.6
    uterus — see Injury, uterus
  interscapular area — see Injury, thorax
  intestine
    large S36.509 ☑
      ascending (right) S36.500 ☑
        blast injury (primary) S36.510 ☑
          secondary S36.590 ☑

Injury — continued
  intestine — continued
    large — continued
      ascending — continued
        contusion S36.520 ☑
        laceration S36.530 ☑
        specified type NEC S36.590 ☑
      blast injury (primary) S36.519 ☑
        ascending (right) S36.510 ☑
        descending (left) S36.512 ☑
        rectum S36.61 ☑
        sigmoid S36.513 ☑
        specified site NEC S36.518 ☑
        transverse S36.511 ☑
      contusion S36.529 ☑
        ascending (right) S36.520 ☑
        descending (left) S36.522 ☑
        rectum S36.62 ☑
        sigmoid S36.523 ☑
        specified site NEC S36.528 ☑
        transverse S36.521 ☑
      descending (left) S36.502 ☑
        blast injury (primary) S36.512 ☑
          secondary S36.592 ☑
        contusion S36.522 ☑
        laceration S36.532 ☑
        specified type NEC S36.592 ☑
      laceration S36.539 ☑
        ascending (right) S36.530 ☑
        descending (left) S36.532 ☑
        rectum S36.63 ☑
        sigmoid S36.533 ☑
        specified site NEC S36.538 ☑
        transverse S36.531 ☑
      rectum S36.60 ☑
        blast injury (primary) S36.61 ☑
          secondary S36.69 ☑
        contusion S36.62 ☑
        laceration S36.63 ☑
        specified type NEC S36.69 ☑
      sigmoid S36.503 ☑
        blast injury (primary) S36.513 ☑
          secondary S36.593 ☑
        contusion S36.523 ☑
        laceration S36.533 ☑
        specified type NEC S36.593 ☑
      specified
        site NEC S36.508 ☑
          blast injury (primary) S36.518 ☑
            secondary S36.598 ☑
          contusion S36.528 ☑
          laceration S36.538 ☑
          specified type NEC S36.598 ☑
        type NEC S36.599 ☑
          ascending (right) S36.590 ☑
          descending (left) S36.592 ☑
          rectum S36.69 ☑
          sigmoid S36.593 ☑
          specified site NEC S36.598 ☑
          transverse S36.591 ☑
      transverse S36.501 ☑
        blast injury (primary) S36.511 ☑
          secondary S36.591 ☑
        contusion S36.521 ☑
        laceration S36.531 ☑
        specified type NEC S36.591 ☑
    small S36.409 ☑
      blast injury (primary) S36.419 ☑
        duodenum S36.410 ☑
        secondary S36.499 ☑
          duodenum S36.490 ☑
          specified site NEC S36.498 ☑
        specified site NEC S36.418 ☑
      contusion S36.429 ☑
        duodenum S36.420 ☑
        specified site NEC S36.428 ☑
      duodenum S36.400 ☑
        blast injury (primary) S36.410 ☑
          secondary S36.490 ☑
        contusion S36.420 ☑
        laceration S36.430 ☑
        specified NEC S36.490 ☑
      laceration S36.439 ☑
        duodenum S36.430 ☑
        specified site NEC S36.438 ☑

Injury — continued
  intestine — continued
    small — continued
      specified
        site NEC S36.408 ☑
        type NEC S36.499 ☑
          duodenum S36.490 ☑
          specified site NEC S36.498 ☑
  intra-abdominal S36.90 ☑
    adrenal gland — see Injury, adrenal gland
    bladder — see Injury, bladder
    colon — see Injury, intestine, large
    contusion S36.92 ☑
    fallopian tube — see Injury, fallopian tube
    gallbladder — see Injury, gallbladder
    intestine — see Injury, intestine
    kidney — see Injury, kidney
    laceration S36.93 ☑
    liver — see Injury, liver
    ovary — see Injury, ovary
    pancreas — see Injury, pancreas
    pelvic NOS S37.90 ☑
    peritoneum — see Injury, intra-abdominal, specified,
      site NEC
    prostate — see Injury, prostate
    rectum — see Injury, intestine, large, rectum
    retroperitoneum — see Injury, intra-abdominal,
      specified, site NEC
    seminal vesicle — see Injury, pelvis, organ, specified
      site NEC
    small intestine — see Injury, intestine, small
    specified
      pelvic S37.90 ☑
        specified
          site NEC S37.899 ☑
            specified type NEC S37.898 ☑
          type NEC S37.99 ☑
      site NEC S36.899 ☑
        contusion S36.892 ☑
        laceration S36.893 ☑
        specified type NEC S36.898 ☑
      type NEC S36.99 ☑
    spleen — see Injury, spleen
    stomach — see Injury, stomach
    ureter — see Injury, ureter
    urethra — see Injury, urethra
    uterus — see Injury, uterus
    vas deferens — see Injury, pelvis, organ, specified
      site NEC
  intracranial (traumatic) — see also if applicable, Com-
    pression, brain, traumatic S06.9- ☑
    cerebellar hemorrhage, traumatic — see Injury, in-
      tracranial, focal
    cerebral edema, traumatic S06.1X- ☑
      diffuse S06.1X- ☑
      focal S06.1X- ☑
    diffuse (axonal) S06.2X- ☑
    epidural hemorrhage (traumatic) S06.4X- ☑
    focal brain injury S06.30- ☑
      contusion — see Contusion, cerebral
      laceration — see Laceration, cerebral
      intracerebral hemorrhage, traumatic S06.36- ☑
        left side S06.35- ☑
        right side S06.34- ☑
      specified NEC S06.89- ☑
    subarachnoid hemorrhage, traumatic S06.6X- ☑
    subdural hemorrhage, traumatic S06.5X- ☑
  intraocular — see Injury, eyeball, penetrating
  intrathoracic S27.9 ☑
    bronchus S27.409 ☑
      bilateral S27.402 ☑
      blast injury (primary) S27.419 ☑
        bilateral S27.412 ☑
        secondary — see Injury, intrathoracic,
          bronchus, specified type NEC
        unilateral S27.411 ☑
      contusion S27.429 ☑
        bilateral S27.422 ☑
        unilateral S27.421 ☑
      laceration S27.439 ☑
        bilateral S27.432 ☑
        unilateral S27.431 ☑
      specified type NEC S27.499 ☑
        bilateral S27.492 ☑
        unilateral S27.491 ☑
      unilateral S27.401 ☑

☑ Additional Character Required — Refer to the Tabular List for Character Selection

Injury — *continued*
  intrathoracic — *continued*
    diaphragm S27.809 ☑
      contusion S27.802 ☑
      laceration S27.803 ☑
      specified type NEC S27.808 ☑
    esophagus (thoracic) S27.819 ☑
      contusion S27.812 ☑
      laceration S27.813 ☑
      specified type NEC S27.818 ☑
    heart — *see* Injury, heart
    hemopneumothorax S27.2 ☑
    hemothorax S27.1 ☑
    lung S27.309 ☑
      aspiration J69.0
      bilateral S27.302 ☑
      blast injury (primary) S27.319 ☑
        bilateral S27.312 ☑
        secondary — *see* Injury, intrathoracic, lung, specified type NEC
        unilateral S27.311 ☑
      contusion S27.329 ☑
        bilateral S27.322 ☑
        unilateral S27.321 ☑
      laceration S27.339 ☑
        bilateral S27.332 ☑
        unilateral S27.331 ☑
      specified type NEC S27.399 ☑
        bilateral S27.392 ☑
        unilateral S27.391 ☑
      unilateral S27.301 ☑
    pleura S27.60 ☑
      laceration S27.63 ☑
      specified type NEC S27.69 ☑
    pneumothorax S27.0 ☑
    specified organ NEC S27.899 ☑
      contusion S27.892 ☑
      laceration S27.893 ☑
      specified type NEC S27.898 ☑
    thoracic duct — *see* Injury, intrathoracic, specified organ NEC
    thymus gland — *see* Injury, intrathoracic, specified organ NEC
    trachea, thoracic S27.50 ☑
      blast (primary) S27.51 ☑
      contusion S27.52 ☑
      laceration S27.53 ☑
      specified type NEC S27.59 ☑
  iris — *see* Injury, eye, specified site NEC
    penetrating — *see* Injury, eyeball, penetrating
  jaw S09.93 ☑
  jejunum — *see* Injury, intestine, small
  joint NOS T14.8 ☑
    old or residual — *see* Disorder, joint, specified type NEC
  kidney S37.00- ☑
    acute (nontraumatic) N17.9
    contusion — *see* Contusion, kidney
    laceration — *see* Laceration, kidney
    specified NEC S37.09- ☑
  knee S89.9- ☑
    contusion — *see* Contusion, knee
    dislocation — *see* Dislocation, knee
    meniscus (lateral) (medial) — *see* Sprain, knee, specified site NEC
      old injury or tear — *see* Derangement, knee, meniscus, due to old injury
    open — *see* Wound, open, knee
    specified NEC S89.8- ☑
    sprain — *see* Sprain, knee
    superficial — *see* Injury, superficial, knee
  labium (majus) (minus) S39.94 ☑
  labyrinth, ear S09.30- ☑
  lacrimal apparatus, duct, gland, or sac — *see* Injury, eye, specified site NEC
  larynx NEC S19.81 ☑
  leg (lower) S89.9- ☑
    blood vessel — *see* Injury, blood vessel, leg
    contusion — *see* Contusion, leg
    fracture — *see* Fracture, leg
    muscle — *see* Injury, muscle, leg
    nerve — *see* Injury, nerve, leg
    open — *see* Wound, open, leg
    specified NEC S89.8- ☑
    superficial — *see* Injury, superficial, leg
  lens, eye — *see* Injury, eye, specified site NEC

Injury — *continued*
  lens, eye — *see* Injury, eye, specified site — *continued*
    penetrating — *see* Injury, eyeball, penetrating
  limb NEC T14.8 ☑
  lip S09.93 ☑
  liver S36.119 ☑
    contusion S36.112 ☑
    laceration S36.113 ☑
      major (stellate) S36.116 ☑
      minor S36.114 ☑
      moderate S36.115 ☑
    specified NEC S36.118 ☑
  lower back S39.92 ☑
    specified NEC S39.82 ☑
  lumbar, lumbosacral (region) S39.92 ☑
    plexus — *see* Injury, lumbosacral plexus
  lumbosacral plexus S34.4 ☑
  lung — *see also* Injury, intrathoracic, lung
    aspiration J69.0
    dabbing (related) U07.0
    electronic cigarette (related) U07.0
    EVALI - [e-cigarette, or vaping, product use associated] U07.0
    transfusion-related (TRALI) J95.84
    vaping (associated) (device) (product) (use) U07.0
  lymphatic thoracic duct — *see* Injury, intrathoracic, specified organ NEC
  malar region S09.93 ☑
  mastoid region S09.90 ☑
  maxilla S09.93 ☑
  mediastinum — *see* Injury, intrathoracic, specified organ NEC
  membrane, brain — *see* Injury, intracranial
  meningeal artery — *see* Injury, intracranial, subdural hemorrhage
  meninges (cerebral) — *see* Injury, intracranial
  mesenteric
    artery
      branch S35.299 ☑
        laceration (minor) (superficial) S35.291 ☑
          major S35.292 ☑
        specified NEC S35.298 ☑
      inferior S35.239 ☑
        laceration (minor) (superficial) S35.231 ☑
          major S35.232 ☑
        specified NEC S35.238 ☑
      superior S35.229 ☑
        laceration (minor) (superficial) S35.221 ☑
          major S35.222 ☑
        specified NEC S35.228 ☑
      plexus (inferior) (superior) — *see* Injury, nerve, lumbosacral, sympathetic
    vein
      inferior S35.349 ☑
        laceration S35.341 ☑
        specified NEC S35.348 ☑
      superior S35.339 ☑
        laceration S35.331 ☑
        specified NEC S35.338 ☑
  mesentery — *see* Injury, intra-abdominal, specified site NEC
  mesosalpinx — *see* Injury, pelvic organ, specified site NEC
  middle ear S09.30- ☑
  midthoracic region NOS S29.9 ☑
  mouth S09.93 ☑
  multiple NOS T07 ☑
  muscle (and fascia) (and tendon)
    abdomen S39.001 ☑
      laceration S39.021 ☑
      specified type NEC S39.091 ☑
      strain S39.011 ☑
    abductor
      thumb, forearm level — *see* Injury, muscle, thumb, abductor
    adductor
      thigh S76.20- ☑
        laceration S76.22- ☑
        specified type NEC S76.29- ☑
        strain S76.21- ☑
    ankle — *see* Injury, muscle, foot
    anterior muscle group, at leg level (lower) S86.20- ☑
      laceration S86.22- ☑
      specified type NEC S86.29- ☑
      strain S86.21- ☑

Injury — *continued*
  muscle — *continued*
    arm (upper) — *see* Injury, muscle, shoulder
    biceps (parts NEC) S46.20- ☑
      laceration S46.22- ☑
      long head S46.10- ☑
        laceration S46.12- ☑
        specified type NEC S46.19- ☑
        strain S46.11- ☑
      specified type NEC S46.29- ☑
      strain S46.21- ☑
    extensor
      finger(s) (other than thumb) — *see* Injury, muscle, finger by site, extensor
      forearm level, specified NEC — *see* Injury, muscle, forearm, extensor
      thumb — *see* Injury, muscle, thumb, extensor
      toe (large) (ankle level) (foot level) — *see* Injury, muscle, toe, extensor
    finger
      extensor (forearm level) S56.40- ☑
        hand level S66.309 ☑
          laceration S66.329 ☑
          specified type NEC S66.399 ☑
          strain S66.319 ☑
        laceration S56.429 ☑
        specified type NEC S56.499 ☑
        strain S56.419 ☑
      flexor (forearm level) S56.10- ☑
        hand level S66.109 ☑
          laceration S66.129 ☑
          specified type NEC S66.199 ☑
          strain S66.119 ☑
        laceration S56.129 ☑
        specified type NEC S56.199 ☑
        strain S56.119 ☑
    index
      extensor (forearm level)
        hand level S66.308 ☑
          laceration S66.32- ☑
          specified type NEC S66.39- ☑
          strain S66.31- ☑
        specified type NEC S56.492- ☑
      flexor (forearm level)
        hand level S66.108 ☑
          laceration S66.12- ☑
          specified type NEC S66.19- ☑
          strain S66.11- ☑
        specified type NEC S56.19- ☑
        strain S56.11- ☑
      intrinsic S66.50- ☑
        laceration S66.52- ☑
        specified type NEC S66.59- ☑
        strain S66.51- ☑
      intrinsic S66.509 ☑
        laceration S66.529 ☑
        specified type NEC S66.599 ☑
        strain S66.519 ☑
    little
      extensor (forearm level)
        hand level S66.30- ☑
          laceration S66.32- ☑
          specified type NEC S66.39- ☑
          strain S66.31- ☑
        laceration S56.42- ☑
        specified type NEC S56.49- ☑
        strain S56.41- ☑
      flexor (forearm level)
        hand level S66.10- ☑
          laceration S66.12- ☑
          specified type NEC S66.19- ☑
          strain S66.11- ☑
        laceration S56.12- ☑
        specified type NEC S56.19- ☑
        strain S56.11- ☑
      intrinsic S66.50- ☑
        laceration S66.52- ☑
        specified type NEC S66.59- ☑
        strain S66.51- ☑
    middle
      extensor (forearm level)
        hand level S66.30- ☑
          laceration S66.32- ☑
          specified type NEC S66.39- ☑
          strain S66.31- ☑
        laceration S56.42- ☑

Injury — continued
  muscle — continued
    finger — continued
      middle — continued
        extensor — continued
          specified type NEC S56.49- ☑
          strain S56.41- ☑
        flexor (forearm level)
          hand level S66.10- ☑
            laceration S66.12- ☑
            specified type NEC S66.19- ☑
            strain S66.11- ☑
          laceration S56.12- ☑
          specified type NEC S56.19- ☑
          strain S56.11- ☑
        intrinsic S66.50- ☑
          laceration S66.52- ☑
          specified type NEC S66.59- ☑
          strain S66.51- ☑
      ring
        extensor (forearm level)
          hand level S66.30- ☑
            laceration S66.32- ☑
            specified type NEC S66.39- ☑
            strain S66.31- ☑
          laceration S56.42- ☑
          specified type NEC S56.49- ☑
          strain S56.41- ☑
        flexor (forearm level)
          hand level S66.10- ☑
            laceration S66.12- ☑
            specified type NEC S66.19- ☑
            strain S66.11- ☑
          laceration S56.12- ☑
          specified type NEC S56.19- ☑
          strain S56.11- ☑
        intrinsic S66.50- ☑
          laceration S66.52- ☑
          specified type NEC S66.59- ☑
          strain S66.51- ☑
  flexor
    finger(s) (other than thumb) — see Injury, muscle, finger
    forearm level, specified NEC — see Injury, muscle, forearm, flexor
    thumb — see Injury, muscle, thumb, flexor
    toe (long) (ankle level) (foot level) — see Injury, muscle, toe, flexor
  foot S96.90- ☑
    intrinsic S96.20- ☑
      laceration S96.22- ☑
      specified type NEC S96.29- ☑
      strain S96.21- ☑
    laceration S96.92- ☑
    long extensor, toe — see Injury, muscle, toe, extensor
    long flexor, toe — see Injury, muscle, toe, flexor
    specified
      site NEC S96.80- ☑
        laceration S96.82- ☑
        specified type NEC S96.89- ☑
        strain S96.81- ☑
      type S96.99- ☑
    strain S96.91- ☑
  forearm (level) S56.90- ☑
    extensor S56.50- ☑
      laceration S56.52- ☑
      specified type NEC S56.59- ☑
      strain S56.51- ☑
    flexor S56.20- ☑
      laceration S56.22- ☑
      specified type NEC S56.29- ☑
      strain S56.21- ☑
    laceration S56.92- ☑
    specified S56.99- ☑
      site NEC S56.80- ☑
        laceration S56.82- ☑
        strain S56.81- ☑
        type NEC S56.89- ☑
    strain S56.91- ☑
  hand (level) S66.90- ☑
    laceration S66.92- ☑
    specified
      site NEC S66.80- ☑
        laceration S66.82- ☑
        specified type NEC S66.89- ☑

Injury — continued
  muscle — continued
    hand — continued
      specified — continued
        site — continued
          strain S66.81- ☑
          type NEC S66.99- ☑
      strain S66.91- ☑
    head S09.10 ☑
      laceration S09.12 ☑
      specified type NEC S09.19 ☑
      strain S09.11 ☑
    hip NEC S76.00- ☑
      laceration S76.02- ☑
      specified type NEC S76.09- ☑
      strain S76.01- ☑
    intrinsic
      ankle and foot level — see Injury, muscle, foot, intrinsic
      finger (other than thumb) — see Injury, muscle, finger by site, intrinsic
      foot (level) — see Injury, muscle, foot, intrinsic
      thumb — see Injury, muscle, thumb, intrinsic
    leg (level) (lower) S86.90- ☑
      Achilles tendon — see Injury, Achilles tendon
      anterior muscle group — see Injury, muscle, anterior muscle group
      laceration S86.92- ☑
      peroneal muscle group — see Injury, muscle, peroneal muscle group
      posterior muscle group — see Injury, muscle, posterior muscle group, leg level
      specified
        site NEC S86.80- ☑
          laceration S86.82- ☑
          specified type NEC S86.89- ☑
          strain S86.81- ☑
        type NEC S86.99- ☑
      strain S86.91- ☑
    long
      extensor toe, at ankle and foot level — see Injury, muscle, toe, extensor
      flexor, toe, at ankle and foot level — see Injury, muscle, toe, flexor
      head, biceps — see Injury, muscle, biceps, long head
    lower back S39.002 ☑
      laceration S39.022 ☑
      specified type NEC S39.092 ☑
      strain S39.012 ☑
    neck (level) S16.9 ☑
      laceration S16.2 ☑
      specified type NEC S16.8 ☑
      strain S16.1 ☑
    pelvis S39.003 ☑
      laceration S39.023 ☑
      specified type NEC S39.093 ☑
      strain S39.013 ☑
    peroneal muscle group, at leg level (lower) S86.30- ☑
      laceration S86.32- ☑
      specified type NEC S86.39- ☑
      strain S86.31- ☑
    posterior muscle (group)
      leg level (lower) S86.10- ☑
        laceration S86.12- ☑
        specified type NEC S86.19- ☑
        strain S86.11- ☑
      thigh level S76.30- ☑
        laceration S76.32- ☑
        specified type NEC S76.39- ☑
        strain S76.31- ☑
    quadriceps (thigh) S76.10- ☑
      laceration S76.12- ☑
      specified type NEC S76.19- ☑
      strain S76.11- ☑
    shoulder S46.90- ☑
      laceration S46.92- ☑
      rotator cuff — see Injury, rotator cuff
      specified site NEC S46.80- ☑
        laceration S46.82- ☑
        specified type NEC S46.89- ☑
        strain S46.81- ☑
      specified type NEC S46.99- ☑
      strain S46.91- ☑
    thigh NEC (level) S76.90- ☑

Injury — continued
  muscle — continued
    thigh — continued
      adductor — see Injury, muscle, adductor, thigh
      laceration S76.92- ☑
      posterior muscle (group) — see Injury, muscle, posterior muscle, thigh level
      quadriceps — see Injury, muscle, quadriceps
      specified
        site NEC S76.80- ☑
          laceration S76.82- ☑
          specified type NEC S76.89- ☑
          strain S76.81- ☑
        type NEC S76.99- ☑
      strain S76.91- ☑
    thorax (level) S29.009 ☑
      back wall S29.002 ☑
      front wall S29.001 ☑
      laceration S29.029 ☑
        back wall S29.022 ☑
        front wall S29.021 ☑
      specified type NEC S29.099 ☑
        back wall S29.092 ☑
        front wall S29.091 ☑
      strain S29.019 ☑
        back wall S29.012 ☑
        front wall S29.011 ☑
    thumb
      abductor (forearm level) S56.30- ☑
        laceration S56.32- ☑
        specified type NEC S56.39- ☑
        strain S56.31- ☑
      extensor (forearm level) S56.30- ☑
        hand level S66.20- ☑
          laceration S66.22- ☑
          specified type NEC S66.29- ☑
          strain S66.21- ☑
        laceration S56.32- ☑
        specified type NEC S56.39- ☑
        strain S56.31- ☑
      flexor (forearm level) S56.00- ☑
        hand level S66.00- ☑
          laceration S66.02- ☑
          specified type NEC S66.09- ☑
          strain S66.01- ☑
        laceration S56.02- ☑
        specified type NEC S56.09- ☑
        strain S56.01- ☑
        wrist level — see Injury, muscle, thumb, flexor, hand level
      intrinsic S66.40- ☑
        laceration S66.42- ☑
        specified type NEC S66.49- ☑
        strain S66.41- ☑
      toe — see also Injury, muscle, foot
      extensor, long S96.10- ☑
        laceration S96.12- ☑
        specified type NEC S96.19- ☑
        strain S96.11- ☑
      flexor, long S96.00- ☑
        laceration S96.02- ☑
        specified type NEC S96.09- ☑
        strain S96.01- ☑
    triceps S46.30- ☑
      laceration S46.32- ☑
      specified type NEC S46.39- ☑
      strain S46.31- ☑
    wrist (and hand) level — see Injury, muscle, hand
  musculocutaneous nerve — see Injury, nerve, musculocutaneous
  myocardial (acute) (chronic) (non-ischemic) (non-traumatic) I5A
    traumatic — see Injury, heart
  myocardium — see also Injury, heart
    non-traumatic — see Injury, myocardial
  nape — see Injury, neck
  nasal (septum) (sinus) S09.92 ☑
  nasopharynx S09.92 ☑
  neck S19.9 ☑
    specified NEC S19.80 ☑
      specified site NEC S19.89 ☑
  nerve NEC T14.8 ☑
    abdomen S34.9 ☑
      peripheral S34.6 ☑
        specified site NEC S34.8 ☑
    abducens S04.4- ☑

Injury — *continued*
  nerve — *continued*
    abducens — *continued*
      contusion S04.4- ☑
      laceration S04.4- ☑
      specified type NEC S04.4- ☑
    abducent — *see* Injury, nerve, abducens
    accessory S04.7- ☑
      contusion S04.7- ☑
      laceration S04.7- ☑
      specified type NEC S04.7- ☑
    acoustic S04.6- ☑
      contusion S04.6- ☑
      laceration S04.6- ☑
      specified type NEC S04.6- ☑
    ankle S94.9- ☑
      cutaneous sensory S94.3- ☑
      specified site NEC — *see* subcategory S94.8 ☑
    anterior crural, femoral — *see* Injury, nerve, femoral
    arm (upper) S44.9- ☑
      axillary — *see* Injury, nerve, axillary
      cutaneous — *see* Injury, nerve, cutaneous, arm
      median — *see* Injury, nerve, median, upper arm
      musculocutaneous — *see* Injury, nerve, musculocutaneous
      radial — *see* Injury, nerve, radial, upper arm
      specified site NEC — *see* subcategory S44.8 ☑
      ulnar — *see* Injury, nerve, ulnar, arm
    auditory — *see* Injury, nerve, acoustic
    axillary S44.3- ☑
    brachial plexus — *see* Injury, brachial plexus
    cervical sympathetic S14.5 ☑
    cranial S04.9 ☑
      contusion S04.9 ☑
      eighth (acoustic or auditory) — *see* Injury, nerve, acoustic
      eleventh (accessory) — *see* Injury, nerve, accessory
      fifth (trigeminal) — *see* Injury, nerve, trigeminal
      first (olfactory) — *see* Injury, nerve, olfactory
      fourth (trochlear) — *see* Injury, nerve, trochlear
      laceration S04.9 ☑
      ninth (glossopharyngeal) — *see* Injury, nerve, glossopharyngeal
      second (optic) — *see* Injury, nerve, optic
      seventh (facial) — *see* Injury, nerve, facial
      sixth (abducent) — *see* Injury, nerve, abducens
      specified
        nerve NEC S04.89- ☑
          contusion S04.89- ☑
          laceration S04.89- ☑
          specified type NEC S04.89- ☑
        type NEC S04.9 ☑
      tenth (pneumogastric or vagus) — *see* Injury, nerve, vagus
      third (oculomotor) — *see* Injury, nerve, oculomotor
      twelfth (hypoglossal) — *see* Injury, nerve, hypoglossal
    cutaneous sensory
      ankle (level) S94.3- ☑
      arm (upper) (level) S44.5- ☑
      foot (level) — *see* Injury, nerve, cutaneous sensory, ankle
      forearm (level) S54.3- ☑
      hip (level) S74.2- ☑
      leg (lower level) S84.2- ☑
      shoulder (level) — *see* Injury, nerve, cutaneous sensory, arm
      thigh (level) — *see* Injury, nerve, cutaneous sensory, hip
    deep peroneal — *see* Injury, nerve, peroneal, foot
    digital
      finger S64.4- ☑
        index S64.49- ☑
        little S64.49- ☑
        middle S64.49- ☑
        ring S64.49- ☑
      thumb S64.3- ☑
      toe — *see* Injury, nerve, ankle, specified site NEC
    eighth cranial (acoustic or auditory) — *see* Injury, nerve, acoustic
    eleventh cranial (accessory) — *see* Injury, nerve, accessory
    facial S04.5- ☑
      contusion S04.5- ☑

Injury — *continued*
  nerve — *continued*
    facial — *continued*
      laceration S04.5- ☑
      newborn P11.3
      specified type NEC S04.5- ☑
    femoral (hip level) (thigh level) S74.1- ☑
    fifth cranial (trigeminal) — *see* Injury, nerve, trigeminal
    finger (digital) — *see* Injury, nerve, digital, finger
    first cranial (olfactory) — *see* Injury, nerve, olfactory
    foot S94.9- ☑
      cutaneous sensory S94.3- ☑
      deep peroneal S94.2- ☑
      lateral plantar S94.0- ☑
      medial plantar S94.1- ☑
      specified site NEC — *see* subcategory S94.8 ☑
    forearm (level) S54.9- ☑
      cutaneous sensory — *see* Injury, nerve, cutaneous sensory, forearm
      median — *see* Injury, nerve, median
      radial — *see* Injury, nerve, radial
      specified site NEC — *see* subcategory S54.8 ☑
      ulnar — *see* Injury, nerve, ulnar
    fourth cranial (trochlear) — *see* Injury, nerve, trochlear
    glossopharyngeal S04.89- ☑
      specified type NEC S04.89- ☑
    hand S64.9- ☑
      median — *see* Injury, nerve, median, hand
      radial — *see* Injury, nerve, radial, hand
      specified NEC — *see* subcategory S64.8 ☑
      ulnar — *see* Injury, nerve, ulnar, hand
    hip (level) S74.9- ☑
      cutaneous sensory — *see* Injury, nerve, cutaneous sensory, hip
      femoral — *see* Injury, nerve, femoral
      sciatic — *see* Injury, nerve, sciatic
      specified site NEC — *see* subcategory S74.8 ☑
    hypoglossal S04.89- ☑
      specified type NEC S04.89- ☑
    lateral plantar S94.0- ☑
    leg (lower) S84.9- ☑
      cutaneous sensory — *see* Injury, nerve, cutaneous sensory, leg
      peroneal — *see* Injury, nerve, peroneal
      specified site NEC — *see* subcategory S84.8 ☑
      tibial — *see* Injury, nerve, tibial
      upper — *see* Injury, nerve, thigh
    lower
      back — *see* Injury, nerve, abdomen, specified site NEC
        peripheral — *see* Injury, nerve, abdomen, peripheral
      limb — *see* Injury, nerve, leg
    lumbar plexus — *see* Injury, nerve, lumbosacral, sympathetic
    lumbar spinal — *see* Injury, spinal, lumbar
      peripheral S34.6 ☑
      root S34.21 ☑
      sympathetic S34.5 ☑
    lumbosacral
      plexus — *see* Injury, nerve, lumbosacral, sympathetic
      sympathetic S34.5 ☑
    medial plantar S94.1- ☑
    median (forearm level) S54.1- ☑
      hand (level) S64.1- ☑
      upper arm (level) S44.1- ☑
      wrist (level) — *see* Injury, nerve, median, hand
    musculocutaneous S44.4- ☑
    musculospiral (upper arm level) — *see* Injury, nerve, radial, upper arm
    neck S14.9 ☑
      peripheral S14.4 ☑
      specified site NEC S14.8 ☑
      sympathetic S14.5 ☑
    ninth cranial (glossopharyngeal) — *see* Injury, nerve, glossopharyngeal
    oculomotor S04.1- ☑
      contusion S04.1- ☑
      laceration S04.1- ☑
      specified type NEC S04.1- ☑
    olfactory S04.81- ☑
      specified type NEC S04.81- ☑
    optic S04.01- ☑

Injury — *continued*
  nerve — *continued*
    optic — *continued*
      contusion S04.01- ☑
      laceration S04.01- ☑
      specified type NEC S04.01- ☑
    pelvic girdle — *see* Injury, nerve, hip
    pelvis — *see* Injury, nerve, abdomen, specified site NEC
      peripheral — *see* Injury, nerve, abdomen, peripheral
    peripheral NEC T14.8 ☑
      abdomen — *see* Injury, nerve, abdomen, peripheral
      lower back — *see* Injury, nerve, abdomen, peripheral
      neck — *see* Injury, nerve, neck, peripheral
      pelvis — *see* Injury, nerve, abdomen, peripheral
      specified NEC T14.8 ☑
    peroneal (lower leg level) S84.1- ☑
      foot S94.2- ☑
    plexus
      brachial — *see* Injury, brachial plexus
      celiac, coeliac — *see* Injury, nerve, lumbosacral, sympathetic
      mesenteric, inferior — *see* Injury, nerve, lumbosacral, sympathetic
      sacral — *see* Injury, lumbosacral plexus
      spinal
        brachial — *see* Injury, brachial plexus
        lumbosacral — *see* Injury, lumbosacral plexus
    pneumogastric — *see* Injury, nerve, vagus
    radial (forearm level) S54.2- ☑
      hand (level) S64.2- ☑
      upper arm (level) S44.2- ☑
      wrist (level) — *see* Injury, nerve, radial, hand
    root — *see* Injury, nerve, spinal, root
    sacral plexus — *see* Injury, lumbosacral plexus
    sacral spinal — *see* Injury, spinal, sacral
      peripheral S34.6 ☑
      root S34.22 ☑
      sympathetic S34.5 ☑
    sciatic (hip level) (thigh level) S74.0- ☑
    second cranial (optic) — *see* Injury, nerve, optic
    seventh cranial (facial) — *see* Injury, nerve, facial
    shoulder — *see* Injury, nerve, arm
    sixth cranial (abducent) — *see* Injury, nerve, abducens
    spinal
      plexus — *see* Injury, nerve, plexus, spinal
      root
        cervical S14.2 ☑
        dorsal S24.2 ☑
        lumbar S34.21 ☑
        sacral S34.22 ☑
        thoracic — *see* Injury, nerve, spinal, root, dorsal
    splanchnic — *see* Injury, nerve, lumbosacral, sympathetic
    sympathetic NEC — *see* Injury, nerve, lumbosacral, sympathetic
      cervical — *see* Injury, nerve, cervical sympathetic
    tenth cranial (pneumogastric or vagus) — *see* Injury, nerve, vagus
    thigh (level) — *see* Injury, nerve, hip
      cutaneous sensory — *see* Injury, nerve, cutaneous sensory, hip
      femoral — *see* Injury, nerve, femoral
      sciatic — *see* Injury, nerve, sciatic
      specified NEC — *see* Injury, nerve, hip
    third cranial (oculomotor) — *see* Injury, nerve, oculomotor
    thorax S24.9 ☑
      peripheral S24.3 ☑
      specified site NEC S24.8 ☑
      sympathetic S24.4 ☑
    thumb, digital — *see* Injury, nerve, digital, thumb
    tibial (lower leg level) (posterior) S84.0- ☑
    toe — *see* Injury, nerve, ankle
    trigeminal S04.3- ☑
      contusion S04.3- ☑
      laceration S04.3- ☑
      specified type NEC S04.3- ☑
    trochlear S04.2- ☑
      contusion S04.2- ☑
      laceration S04.2- ☑

Injury — *continued*
  nerve — *continued*
    trochlear — *continued*
      specified type NEC S04.2- ☑
    twelfth cranial (hypoglossal) — *see* Injury, nerve, hypoglossal
    ulnar (forearm level) S54.0- ☑
      arm (upper) (level) S44.0- ☑
      hand (level) S64.0- ☑
      wrist (level) — *see* Injury, nerve, ulnar, hand
    vagus S04.89- ☑
      specified type NEC S04.89- ☑
    wrist (level) — *see* Injury, nerve, hand
    ninth cranial nerve (glossopharyngeal) — *see* Injury, nerve, glossopharyngeal
  nose (septum) S09.92 ☑
  obstetrical O71.9
    specified NEC O71.89
  occipital (region) (scalp) S09.90 ☑
    lobe — *see* Injury, intracranial
  optic chiasm S04.02 ☑
  optic radiation S04.03- ☑
  optic tract and pathways S04.03- ☑
  orbit, orbital (region) — *see* Injury, eye
    penetrating (with foreign body) — *see* Injury, eye, orbit, penetrating
    specified NEC — *see* Injury, eye, specified site NEC
  ovary, ovarian S37.409 ☑
    bilateral S37.402 ☑
      contusion S37.422 ☑
      laceration S37.432 ☑
      specified type NEC S37.492 ☑
    blood vessel — *see* Injury, blood vessel, ovarian
    contusion S37.429 ☑
      bilateral S37.422 ☑
      unilateral S37.421 ☑
    laceration S37.439 ☑
      bilateral S37.432 ☑
      unilateral S37.431 ☑
    specified type NEC S37.499 ☑
      bilateral S37.492 ☑
      unilateral S37.491 ☑
    unilateral S37.401 ☑
      contusion S37.421 ☑
      laceration S37.431 ☑
      specified type NEC S37.491 ☑
  palate (hard) (soft) S09.93 ☑
  pancreas S36.209 ☑
    body S36.201 ☑
      contusion S36.221 ☑
      laceration S36.231 ☑
        major S36.261 ☑
        minor S36.241 ☑
        moderate S36.251 ☑
      specified type NEC S36.291 ☑
    contusion S36.229 ☑
    head S36.200 ☑
      contusion S36.220 ☑
      laceration S36.230 ☑
        major S36.260 ☑
        minor S36.240 ☑
        moderate S36.250 ☑
      specified type NEC S36.290 ☑
    laceration S36.239 ☑
      major S36.269 ☑
      minor S36.249 ☑
      moderate S36.259 ☑
    specified type NEC S36.299 ☑
    tail S36.202 ☑
      contusion S36.222 ☑
      laceration S36.232 ☑
        major S36.262 ☑
        minor S36.242 ☑
        moderate S36.252 ☑
      specified type NEC S36.292 ☑
  parietal (region) (scalp) S09.90 ☑
    lobe — *see* Injury, intracranial
  patellar ligament (tendon) S76.10- ☑
    laceration S76.12- ☑
    specified NEC S76.19- ☑
    strain S76.11- ☑
  pelvis, pelvic (floor) S39.93 ☑
    complicating delivery O70.1
    joint or ligament, complicating delivery O71.6
    organ S37.90 ☑
      with ectopic or molar pregnancy O08.6

Injury — *continued*
  pelvis, pelvic — *continued*
    organ — *continued*
      complication of abortion — *see* Abortion
      contusion S37.92 ☑
      following ectopic or molar pregnancy O08.6
      laceration S37.93 ☑
      obstetrical trauma NEC O71.5
      specified
        site NEC S37.899 ☑
          contusion S37.892 ☑
          laceration S37.893 ☑
          specified type NEC S37.898 ☑
        type NEC S37.99 ☑
      specified NEC S39.83 ☑
  penis S39.94 ☑
  perineum S39.94 ☑
  peritoneum S36.81 ☑
    laceration S36.893 ☑
  periurethral tissue — *see* Injury, urethra
    complicating delivery O71.82
  phalanges
    foot — *see* Injury, foot
    hand — *see* Injury, hand
  pharynx NEC S19.85 ☑
  pleura — *see* Injury, intrathoracic, pleura
  plexus
    brachial — *see* Injury, brachial plexus
    cardiac — *see* Injury, nerve, thorax, sympathetic
    celiac, coeliac — *see* Injury, nerve, lumbosacral, sympathetic
    esophageal — *see* Injury, nerve, thorax, sympathetic
    hypogastric — *see* Injury, nerve, lumbosacral, sympathetic
    lumbar, lumbosacral — *see* Injury, lumbosacral plexus
    mesenteric — *see* Injury, nerve, lumbosacral, sympathetic
    pulmonary — *see* Injury, nerve, thorax, sympathetic
  postcardiac surgery (syndrome) I97.0
  prepuce S39.94 ☑
  pressure
    injury — *see* Ulcer, pressure, by site
  prostate S37.829 ☑
    contusion S37.822 ☑
    laceration S37.823 ☑
    specified type NEC S37.828 ☑
  pubic region S39.94 ☑
  pudendum S39.94 ☑
  pulmonary plexus — *see* Injury, nerve, thorax, sympathetic
  rectovaginal septum NEC S39.83 ☑
  rectum — *see* Injury, intestine, large, rectum
  retina — *see* Injury, eye, specified site NEC
    penetrating — *see* Injury, eyeball, penetrating
  retroperitoneal — *see* Injury, intra-abdominal, specified site NEC
  rotator cuff (muscle(s)) (tendon(s)) S46.00- ☑
    laceration S46.02- ☑
    specified type NEC S46.09- ☑
    strain S46.01- ☑
  round ligament — *see* Injury, pelvic organ, specified site NEC
  sacral plexus — *see* Injury, lumbosacral plexus
  salivary duct or gland S09.93 ☑
  scalp S09.90 ☑
    newborn (birth injury) P12.9
      due to monitoring (electrode) (sampling incision) P12.4
      specified NEC P12.89
        caput succedaneum P12.81
  scapular region — *see* Injury, shoulder
  sclera — *see* Injury, eye, specified site NEC
    penetrating — *see* Injury, eyeball, penetrating
  scrotum S39.94 ☑
  second cranial nerve (optic) — *see* Injury, nerve, optic
  self-inflicted, without suicidal intent R45.88
  seminal vesicle — *see* Injury, pelvic organ, specified site NEC
  seventh cranial nerve (facial) — *see* Injury, nerve, facial
  shoulder S49.9- ☑
    blood vessel — *see* Injury, blood vessel, arm
    contusion — *see* Contusion, shoulder
    dislocation — *see* Dislocation, shoulder
    fracture — *see* Fracture, shoulder
    muscle — *see* Injury, muscle, shoulder
    nerve — *see* Injury, nerve, shoulder

Injury — *continued*
  shoulder — *continued*
    open — *see* Wound, open, shoulder
    specified type NEC S49.8- ☑
    sprain — *see* Sprain, shoulder girdle
    superficial — *see* Injury, superficial, shoulder
  sinus
    cavernous — *see* Injury, intracranial
    nasal S09.92 ☑
  sixth cranial nerve (abducent) — *see* Injury, nerve, abducens
  skeleton, birth injury P13.9
    specified part NEC P13.8
  skin NEC T14.8 ☑
    surface intact — *see* Injury, superficial
  skull NEC S09.90 ☑
  specified NEC T14.8 ☑
  spermatic cord (pelvic region) S37.898 ☑
    scrotal region S39.848 ☑
  spinal (cord)
    cervical (neck) S14.109 ☑
      anterior cord syndrome S14.139 ☑
        C1 level S14.131 ☑
        C2 level S14.132 ☑
        C3 level S14.133 ☑
        C4 level S14.134 ☑
        C5 level S14.135 ☑
        C6 level S14.136 ☑
        C7 level S14.137 ☑
        C8 level S14.138 ☑
      Brown-Séquard syndrome S14.149 ☑
        C1 level S14.141 ☑
        C2 level S14.142 ☑
        C3 level S14.143 ☑
        C4 level S14.144 ☑
        C5 level S14.145 ☑
        C6 level S14.146 ☑
        C7 level S14.147 ☑
        C8 level S14.148 ☑
      C1 level S14.101 ☑
      C2 level S14.102 ☑
      C3 level S14.103 ☑
      C4 level S14.104 ☑
      C5 level S14.105 ☑
      C6 level S14.106 ☑
      C7 level S14.107 ☑
      C8 level S14.108 ☑
      central cord syndrome S14.129 ☑
        C1 level S14.121 ☑
        C2 level S14.122 ☑
        C3 level S14.123 ☑
        C4 level S14.124 ☑
        C5 level S14.125 ☑
        C6 level S14.126 ☑
        C7 level S14.127 ☑
        C8 level S14.128 ☑
      complete lesion S14.119 ☑
        C1 level S14.111 ☑
        C2 level S14.112 ☑
        C3 level S14.113 ☑
        C4 level S14.114 ☑
        C5 level S14.115 ☑
        C6 level S14.116 ☑
        C7 level S14.117 ☑
        C8 level S14.118 ☑
      concussion S14.0 ☑
      edema S14.0 ☑
      incomplete lesion specified NEC S14.159 ☑
        C1 level S14.151 ☑
        C2 level S14.152 ☑
        C3 level S14.153 ☑
        C4 level S14.154 ☑
        C5 level S14.155 ☑
        C6 level S14.156 ☑
        C7 level S14.157 ☑
        C8 level S14.158 ☑
      posterior cord syndrome S14.159 ☑
        C1 level S14.151 ☑
        C2 level S14.152 ☑
        C3 level S14.153 ☑
        C4 level S14.154 ☑
        C5 level S14.155 ☑
        C6 level S14.156 ☑
        C7 level S14.157 ☑
        C8 level S14.158 ☑
    dorsal — *see* Injury, spinal, thoracic

Injury — *continued*
- spinal — *continued*
  - lumbar S34.109 ☑
    - complete lesion S34.119 ☑
      - L1 level S34.111 ☑
      - L2 level S34.112 ☑
      - L3 level S34.113 ☑
      - L4 level S34.114 ☑
      - L5 level S34.115 ☑
    - concussion S34.01 ☑
    - edema S34.01 ☑
    - incomplete lesion S34.129 ☑
      - L1 level S34.121 ☑
      - L2 level S34.122 ☑
      - L3 level S34.123 ☑
      - L4 level S34.124 ☑
      - L5 level S34.125 ☑
    - L1 level S34.101 ☑
    - L2 level S34.102 ☑
    - L3 level S34.103 ☑
    - L4 level S34.104 ☑
    - L5 level S34.105 ☑
  - nerve root NEC
    - cervical — *see* Injury, nerve, spinal, root, cervical
    - dorsal — *see* Injury, nerve, spinal, root, dorsal
    - lumbar S34.21
    - sacral S34.22 ☑
    - thoracic — *see* Injury, nerve, spinal, root, dorsal
  - plexus
    - brachial — *see* Injury, brachial plexus
    - lumbosacral — *see* Injury, lumbosacral plexus
  - sacral S34.139 ☑
    - complete lesion S34.131 ☑
    - incomplete lesion S34.132 ☑
  - thoracic S24.109 ☑
    - anterior cord syndrome S24.139 ☑
      - T1 level S24.131 ☑
      - T2-T6 level S24.132 ☑
      - T7-T10 level S24.133 ☑
      - T11-T12 level S24.134 ☑
    - Brown-Séquard syndrome S24.149 ☑
      - T1 level S24.141 ☑
      - T2-T6 level S24.142 ☑
      - T7-T10 level S24.143 ☑
      - T11-T12 level S24.144 ☑
    - complete lesion S24.119 ☑
      - T1 level S24.111 ☑
      - T2-T6 level S24.112 ☑
      - T7-T10 level S24.113 ☑
      - T11-T12 level S24.114 ☑
    - concussion S24.0 ☑
    - edema S24.0 ☑
    - incomplete lesion specified NEC S24.159 ☑
      - T1 level S24.151 ☑
      - T2-T6 level S24.152 ☑
      - T7-T10 level S24.153 ☑
      - T11-T12 level S24.154 ☑
    - posterior cord syndrome S24.159 ☑
      - T1 level S24.151 ☑
      - T2-T6 level S24.152 ☑
      - T7-T10 level S24.153 ☑
      - T11-T12 level S24.154 ☑
    - T1 level S24.101 ☑
    - T2-T6 level S24.102 ☑
    - T7-T10 level S24.103 ☑
    - T11-T12 level S24.104 ☑
  - splanchnic nerve — *see* Injury, nerve, lumbosacral, sympathetic
  - spleen S36.00 ☑
    - contusion S36.029 ☑
      - major S36.021 ☑
      - minor S36.020 ☑
    - laceration S36.039 ☑
      - major (massive) (stellate) S36.032 ☑
      - moderate S36.031 ☑
      - superficial (capsular) (minor) S36.030 ☑
    - specified type NEC S36.09 ☑
  - splenic artery — *see* Injury, blood vessel, celiac artery, branch
  - stellate ganglion — *see* Injury, nerve, thorax, sympathetic
  - sternal region S29.9 ☑
  - stomach S36.30 ☑
    - contusion S36.32 ☑
    - laceration S36.33 ☑
    - specified type NEC S36.39 ☑

Injury — *continued*
- subconjunctival — *see* Injury, eye, conjunctiva
- subcutaneous NEC T14.8 ☑
- submaxillary region S09.93 ☑
- submental region S09.93 ☑
- subungual
  - fingers — *see* Injury, hand
  - toes — *see* Injury, foot
- superficial NEC T14.8 ☑
  - abdomen, abdominal (wall) S30.92 ☑
    - abrasion S30.811 ☑
    - bite S30.871 ☑
      - insect S30.861 ☑
    - contusion S30.1 ☑
    - external constriction S30.841 ☑
    - foreign body S30.851 ☑
  - abrasion — *see* Abrasion, by site
  - adnexa, eye NEC — *see* Injury, eye, specified site NEC
  - alveolar process — *see* Injury, superficial, oral cavity
  - ankle S90.91- ☑
    - abrasion — *see* Abrasion, ankle
    - bite — *see* Bite, ankle
    - blister — *see* Blister, ankle
    - contusion — *see* Contusion, ankle
    - external constriction — *see* Constriction, external, ankle
    - foreign body — *see* Foreign body, superficial, ankle
  - anus S30.98 ☑
  - arm (upper) S40.92- ☑
    - abrasion — *see* Abrasion, arm
    - bite — *see* Bite, superficial, arm
    - blister — *see* Blister, arm (upper)
    - contusion — *see* Contusion, arm
    - external constriction — *see* Constriction, external, arm
    - foreign body — *see* Foreign body, superficial, arm
  - auditory canal (external) (meatus) — *see* Injury, superficial, ear
  - auricle — *see* Injury, superficial, ear
  - axilla — *see* Injury, superficial, arm
  - back — *see also* Injury, superficial, thorax, back
    - lower S30.91 ☑
      - abrasion S30.810 ☑
      - contusion S30.0 ☑
      - external constriction S30.840 ☑
      - superficial
        - bite NEC S30.870 ☑
          - insect S30.860 ☑
        - foreign body S30.850 ☑
  - bite NEC — *see* Bite, superficial NEC, by site
  - blister — *see* Blister, by site
  - breast S20.10- ☑
    - abrasion — *see* Abrasion, breast
    - bite — *see* Bite, superficial, breast
    - contusion — *see* Contusion, breast
    - external constriction — *see* Constriction, external, breast
    - foreign body — *see* Foreign body, superficial, breast
  - brow — *see* Injury, superficial, head, specified NEC
  - buttock S30.91 ☑
  - calf — *see* Injury, superficial, leg
  - canthus, eye — *see* Injury, superficial, periocular area
  - cheek (external) — *see* Injury, superficial, head, specified NEC
    - internal — *see* Injury, superficial, oral cavity
  - chest wall — *see* Injury, superficial, thorax
  - chin — *see* Injury, superficial, head NEC
  - clitoris S30.95 ☑
  - conjunctiva — *see* Injury, eye, conjunctiva
    - with foreign body (in conjunctival sac) — *see* Foreign body, conjunctival sac
  - contusion — *see* Contusion, by site
  - costal region — *see* Injury, superficial, thorax
  - digit(s)
    - hand — *see* Injury, superficial, finger
  - ear (auricle) (canal) (external) S00.40- ☑
    - abrasion — *see* Abrasion, ear
    - bite — *see* Bite, superficial, ear
    - contusion — *see* Contusion, ear
    - external constriction — *see* Constriction, external, ear

Injury — *continued*
- superficial — *continued*
  - ear — *continued*
    - foreign body — *see* Foreign body, superficial, ear
  - elbow S50.90- ☑
    - abrasion — *see* Abrasion, elbow
    - bite — *see* Bite, superficial, elbow
    - blister — *see* Blister, elbow
    - contusion — *see* Contusion, elbow
    - external constriction — *see* Constriction, external, elbow
    - foreign body — *see* Foreign body, superficial, elbow
  - epididymis S30.94 ☑
  - epigastric region S30.92 ☑
  - epiglottis — *see* Injury, superficial, throat
  - esophagus
    - cervical — *see* Injury, superficial, throat
  - external constriction — *see* Constriction, external, by site
  - extremity NEC T14.8 ☑
  - eyeball NEC — *see* Injury, eye, specified site NEC
  - eyebrow — *see* Injury, superficial, periocular area
  - eyelid S00.20- ☑
    - abrasion — *see* Abrasion, eyelid
    - bite — *see* Bite, superficial, eyelid
    - contusion — *see* Contusion, eyelid
    - external constriction — *see* Constriction, external, eyelid
    - foreign body — *see* Foreign body, superficial, eyelid
  - face NEC — *see* Injury, superficial, head, specified NEC
  - finger(s) S60.949 ☑
    - abrasion — *see* Abrasion, finger
    - bite — *see* Bite, superficial, finger
    - blister — *see* Blister, finger
    - contusion — *see* Contusion, finger
    - external constriction — *see* Constriction, external, finger
    - foreign body — *see* Foreign body, superficial, finger
    - index S60.94- ☑
    - insect bite — *see* Bite, by site, superficial, insect
    - little S60.94- ☑
    - middle S60.94- ☑
    - ring S60.94- ☑
  - flank S30.92 ☑
  - foot S90.92- ☑
    - abrasion — *see* Abrasion, foot
    - bite — *see* Bite, foot
    - blister — *see* Blister, foot
    - contusion — *see* Contusion, foot
    - external constriction — *see* Constriction, external, foot
    - foreign body — *see* Foreign body, superficial, foot
  - forearm S50.91- ☑
    - abrasion — *see* Abrasion, forearm
    - bite — *see* Bite, forearm, superficial
    - blister — *see* Blister, forearm
    - contusion — *see* Contusion, forearm
    - elbow only — *see* Injury, superficial, elbow
    - external constriction — *see* Constriction, external, forearm
    - foreign body — *see* Foreign body, superficial, forearm
  - forehead — *see* Injury, superficial, head NEC
  - foreign body — *see* Foreign body, superficial
  - genital organs, external
    - female S30.97 ☑
    - male S30.96 ☑
  - globe (eye) — *see* Injury, eye, specified site NEC
  - groin S30.92 ☑
  - gum — *see* Injury, superficial, oral cavity
  - hand S60.92- ☑
    - abrasion — *see* Abrasion, hand
    - bite — *see* Bite, superficial, hand
    - contusion — *see* Contusion, hand
    - external constriction — *see* Constriction, external, hand
    - foreign body — *see* Foreign body, superficial, hand
  - head S00.90 ☑
    - ear — *see* Injury, superficial, ear

☑ **Additional Character Required** — **Refer to the Tabular List for Character Selection**

Injury — *continued*
  superficial — *continued*
    head — *continued*
      eyelid — *see* Injury, superficial, eyelid
      nose S00.30 ☑
      oral cavity S00.502 ☑
      scalp S00.00 ☑
      specified site NEC S00.80 ☑
    heel — *see* Injury, superficial, foot
    hip S70.91- ☑
      abrasion — *see* Abrasion, hip
      bite — *see* Bite, superficial, hip
      blister — *see* Blister, hip
      contusion — *see* Contusion, hip
      external constriction — *see* Constriction, external, hip
      foreign body — *see* Foreign body, superficial, hip
    iliac region — *see* Injury, superficial, abdomen
    inguinal region — *see* Injury, superficial, abdomen
    insect bite — *see* Bite, by site, superficial, insect
    interscapular region — *see* Injury, superficial, thorax, back
    jaw — *see* Injury, superficial, head, specified NEC
    knee S80.91- ☑
      abrasion — *see* Abrasion, knee
      bite — *see* Bite, superficial, knee
      blister — *see* Blister, knee
      contusion — *see* Contusion, knee
      external constriction — *see* Constriction, external, knee
      foreign body — *see* Foreign body, superficial, knee
    labium (majus) (minus) S30.95 ☑
    lacrimal (apparatus) (gland) (sac) — *see* Injury, eye, specified site NEC
    larynx — *see* Injury, superficial, throat
    leg (lower) S80.92- ☑
      abrasion — *see* Abrasion, leg
      bite — *see* Bite, superficial, leg
      contusion — *see* Contusion, leg
      external constriction — *see* Constriction, external, leg
      foreign body — *see* Foreign body, superficial, leg
      knee — *see* Injury, superficial, knee
    limb NEC T14.8 ☑
    lip S00.501 ☑
    lower back S30.91 ☑
    lumbar region S30.91 ☑
    malar region — *see* Injury, superficial, head, specified NEC
    mammary — *see* Injury, superficial, breast
    mastoid region — *see* Injury, superficial, head, specified NEC
    mouth — *see* Injury, superficial, oral cavity
    muscle NEC T14.8 ☑
    nail NEC T14.8 ☑
      finger — *see* Injury, superficial, finger
      toe — *see* Injury, superficial, toe
    nasal (septum) — *see* Injury, superficial, nose
    neck S10.90 ☑
      specified site NEC S10.80 ☑
    nose (septum) S00.30 ☑
    occipital region — *see* Injury, superficial, scalp
    oral cavity S00.502 ☑
    orbital region — *see* Injury, superficial, periocular area
    palate — *see* Injury, superficial, oral cavity
    palm — *see* Injury, superficial, hand
    parietal region — *see* Injury, superficial, scalp
    pelvis S30.91 ☑
      girdle — *see* Injury, superficial, hip
    penis S30.93 ☑
    perineum
      female S30.95 ☑
      male S30.91 ☑
    periocular area S00.20- ☑
      abrasion — *see* Abrasion, eyelid
      bite — *see* Bite, superficial, eyelid
      contusion — *see* Contusion, eyelid
      external constriction — *see* Constriction, external, eyelid
      foreign body — *see* Foreign body, superficial, eyelid

Injury — *continued*
  superficial — *continued*
    phalanges
      finger — *see* Injury, superficial, finger
      toe — *see* Injury, superficial, toe
    pharynx — *see* Injury, superficial, throat
    pinna — *see* Injury, superficial, ear
    popliteal space — *see* Injury, superficial, knee
    prepuce S30.93 ☑
    pubic region S30.91 ☑
    pudendum
      female S30.97 ☑
      male S30.96 ☑
    sacral region S30.91 ☑
    scalp S00.00 ☑
    scapular region — *see* Injury, superficial, shoulder
    sclera — *see* Injury, eye, specified site NEC
    scrotum S30.94 ☑
    shin — *see* Injury, superficial, leg
    shoulder S40.91- ☑
      abrasion — *see* Abrasion, shoulder
      bite — *see* Bite, superficial, shoulder
      blister — *see* Blister, shoulder
      contusion — *see* Contusion, shoulder
      external constriction — *see* Constriction, external, shoulder
      foreign body — *see* Foreign body, superficial, shoulder
    skin NEC T14.8 ☑
    sternal region — *see* Injury, superficial, thorax, front
    subconjunctival — *see* Injury, eye, specified site NEC
    subcutaneous NEC T14.8 ☑
    submaxillary region — *see* Injury, superficial, head, specified NEC
    submental region — *see* Injury, superficial, head, specified NEC
    subungual
      finger(s) — *see* Injury, superficial, finger
      toe(s) — *see* Injury, superficial, toe
    supraclavicular fossa — *see* Injury, superficial, neck
    supraorbital — *see* Injury, superficial, head, specified NEC
    temple — *see* Injury, superficial, head, specified NEC
    temporal region — *see* Injury, superficial, head, specified NEC
    testis S30.94 ☑
    thigh S70.92- ☑
      abrasion — *see* Abrasion, thigh
      bite — *see* Bite, superficial, thigh
      blister — *see* Blister, thigh
      contusion — *see* Contusion, thigh
      external constriction — *see* Constriction, external, thigh
      foreign body — *see* Foreign body, superficial, thigh
    thorax, thoracic (wall) S20.90 ☑
      abrasion — *see* Abrasion, thorax
      back S20.40- ☑
      bite — *see* Bite, thorax, superficial
      blister — *see* Blister, thorax
      contusion — *see* Contusion, thorax
      external constriction — *see* Constriction, external, thorax
      foreign body — *see* Foreign body, superficial, thorax
      front S20.30- ☑
    throat S10.10 ☑
      abrasion S10.11 ☑
      bite S10.17 ☑
        insect S10.16 ☑
      blister S10.12 ☑
      contusion S10.0 ☑
      external constriction S10.14 ☑
      foreign body S10.15 ☑
    thumb S60.93- ☑
      abrasion — *see* Abrasion, thumb
      bite — *see* Bite, superficial, thumb
      blister — *see* Blister, thumb
      contusion — *see* Contusion, thumb
      external constriction — *see* Constriction, external, thumb
      foreign body — *see* Foreign body, superficial, thumb
      insect bite — *see* Bite, by site, superficial, insect
      specified type NEC S60.39 ☑
    toe(s) S90.93- ☑

Injury — *continued*
  superficial — *continued*
    toe(s) — *continued*
      abrasion — *see* Abrasion, toe
      bite — *see* Bite, toe
      blister — *see* Blister, toe
      contusion — *see* Contusion, toe
      external constriction — *see* Constriction, external, toe
      foreign body — *see* Foreign body, superficial, toe
      great S90.93- ☑
    tongue — *see* Injury, superficial, oral cavity
    tooth, teeth — *see* Injury, superficial, oral cavity
    trachea S10.10 ☑
    tunica vaginalis S30.94 ☑
    tympanum, tympanic membrane — *see* Injury, superficial, ear
    uvula — *see* Injury, superficial, oral cavity
    vagina S30.95 ☑
    vocal cords — *see* Injury, superficial, throat
    vulva S30.95 ☑
    wrist S60.91- ☑
  supraclavicular region — *see* Injury, neck
  supraorbital S09.93 ☑
  suprarenal gland (multiple) — *see* Injury, adrenal
  surgical complication (external or internal site) — *see* Laceration, accidental complicating surgery
  temple S09.90 ☑
  temporal region S09.90 ☑
  tendon — *see also* Injury, muscle, by site
    abdomen — *see* Injury, muscle, abdomen
    Achilles — *see* Injury, Achilles tendon
    lower back — *see* Injury, muscle, lower back
    pelvic organs — *see* Injury, muscle, pelvis
  tenth cranial nerve (pneumogastric or vagus) — *see* Injury, nerve, vagus
  testis S39.94 ☑
  thigh S79.92- ☑
    blood vessel — *see* Injury, blood vessel, hip
    contusion — *see* Contusion, thigh
    fracture — *see* Fracture, femur
    muscle — *see* Injury, muscle, thigh
    nerve — *see* Injury, nerve, thigh
    open — *see* Wound, open, thigh
    specified NEC S79.82- ☑
    superficial — *see* Injury, superficial, thigh
  third cranial nerve (oculomotor) — *see* Injury, nerve, oculomotor
  thorax, thoracic S29.9 ☑
    blood vessel — *see* Injury, blood vessel, thorax
    cavity — *see* Injury, intrathoracic
    dislocation — *see* Dislocation, thorax
    external (wall) S29.9 ☑
      contusion — *see* Contusion, thorax
      nerve — *see* Injury, nerve, thorax
      open — *see* Wound, open, thorax
      specified NEC S29.8 ☑
      sprain — *see* Sprain, thorax
      superficial — *see* Injury, superficial, thorax
    fracture — *see* Fracture, thorax
    internal — *see* Injury, intrathoracic
    intrathoracic organ — *see* Injury, intrathoracic
    sympathetic ganglion — *see* Injury, nerve, thorax, sympathetic
  throat — *see also* Injury, neck S19.9 ☑
  thumb S69.9- ☑
    blood vessel — *see* Injury, blood vessel, thumb
    contusion — *see* Contusion, thumb
    dislocation — *see* Dislocation, thumb
    fracture — *see* Fracture, thumb
    muscle — *see* Injury, muscle, thumb
    nerve — *see* Injury, nerve, digital, thumb
    open — *see* Wound, open, thumb
    specified NEC S69.8- ☑
    sprain — *see* Sprain, thumb
    superficial — *see* Injury, superficial, thumb
  thymus (gland) — *see* Injury, intrathoracic, specified organ NEC
  thyroid (gland) NEC S19.84 ☑
  toe S99.92- ☑
    contusion — *see* Contusion, toe
    dislocation — *see* Dislocation, toe
    fracture — *see* Fracture, toe
    muscle — *see* Injury, muscle, toe
    open — *see* Wound, open, toe

Injury — *continued*
  toe — *continued*
    specified type NEC S99.82- ☑
    sprain — *see* Sprain, toe
    superficial — *see* Injury, superficial, toe
  tongue S09.93 ☑
  tonsil S09.93 ☑
  tooth S09.93 ☑
  trachea (cervical) NEC S19.82 ☑
    thoracic — *see* Injury, intrathoracic, trachea, thoracic
  transfusion-related acute lung (TRALI) J95.84
  tunica vaginalis S39.94 ☑
  twelfth cranial nerve (hypoglossal) — *see* Injury, nerve, hypoglossal
  ureter S37.10 ☑
    contusion S37.12 ☑
    laceration S37.13 ☑
    specified type NEC S37.19 ☑
  urethra (sphincter) S37.30 ☑
    at delivery O71.5
    contusion S37.32 ☑
    laceration S37.33 ☑
    specified type NEC S37.39 ☑
  urinary organ S37.90 ☑
    contusion S37.92 ☑
    laceration S37.93 ☑
    specified
      site NEC S37.899 ☑
        contusion S37.892 ☑
        laceration S37.893 ☑
        specified type NEC S37.898 ☑
      type NEC S37.99 ☑
  uterus, uterine S37.60 ☑
    with ectopic or molar pregnancy O08.6
    blood vessel — *see* Injury, blood vessel, iliac
    contusion S37.62 ☑
    laceration S37.63 ☑
      cervix at delivery O71.3
    rupture associated with obstetrics — *see* Rupture, uterus
    specified type NEC S37.69 ☑
  uvula S09.93 ☑
  vagina S39.93 ☑
    abrasion S30.814 ☑
    bite S31.45 ☑
      insect S30.864 ☑
      superficial NEC S30.874 ☑
    contusion S30.23 ☑
    crush S38.03 ☑
    during delivery — *see* Laceration, vagina, during delivery
    external constriction S30.844 ☑
    insect bite S30.864 ☑
    laceration S31.41 ☑
      with foreign body S31.42 ☑
    open wound S31.40 ☑
    puncture S31.43 ☑
      with foreign body S31.44 ☑
    superficial S30.95 ☑
      foreign body S30.854 ☑
  vas deferens — *see* Injury, pelvic organ, specified site NEC
  vascular NEC T14.8 ☑
  vein — *see* Injury, blood vessel
  vena cava (superior) S25.20 ☑
    inferior S35.10 ☑
      laceration (minor) (superficial) S35.11 ☑
        major S35.12 ☑
      specified type NEC S35.19 ☑
    laceration (minor) (superficial) S25.21 ☑
      major S25.22 ☑
    specified type NEC S25.29 ☑
  vesical (sphincter) — *see* Injury, bladder
  visual cortex S04.04- ☑
  vitreous (humor) S05.90 ☑
    specified NEC S05.8X- ☑
  vocal cord NEC S19.83 ☑
  vulva S39.94 ☑
    abrasion S30.814 ☑
    bite S31.45 ☑
      insect S30.864 ☑
      superficial NEC S30.874 ☑
    contusion S30.23 ☑
    crush S38.03 ☑
    during delivery — *see* Laceration, perineum, female, during delivery

Injury — *continued*
  vulva — *continued*
    external constriction S30.844 ☑
    insect bite S30.864 ☑
    laceration S31.41 ☑
      with foreign body S31.42 ☑
    open wound S31.40 ☑
    puncture S31.43 ☑
      with foreign body S31.44 ☑
    superficial S30.95 ☑
      foreign body S30.854 ☑
  whiplash (cervical spine) S13.4 ☑
  wrist S69.9- ☑
    blood vessel — *see* Injury, blood vessel, hand
    contusion — *see* Contusion, wrist
    dislocation — *see* Dislocation, wrist
    fracture — *see* Fracture, wrist
    muscle — *see* Injury, muscle, hand
    nerve — *see* Injury, nerve, hand
    open — *see* Wound, open, wrist
    specified NEC S69.8- ☑
    sprain — *see* Sprain, wrist
    superficial — *see* Injury, superficial, wrist
Inoculation — *see also* Vaccination
  complication or reaction — *see* Complications, vaccination
Insanity, insane — *see also* Psychosis
  adolescent — *see* Schizophrenia
  confusional F28
    acute or subacute F05
  delusional F22
  senile F03 ☑
Insect
  bite — *see* Bite, by site, superficial, insect
  venomous, poisoning NEC (by) — *see* Venom, arthropod
Insecurity
  financial Z59.86
  food Z59.41
  transportation Z59.82
Insensitivity
  adrenocorticotropin hormone (ACTH) E27.49
  androgen E34.50
    complete E34.51
    partial E34.52
Insertion
  cord (umbilical) lateral or velamentous O43.12- ☑
  intrauterine contraceptive device (encounter for) — *see* Intrauterine contraceptive device
Insolation (sunstroke) T67.01 ☑
Insomnia (organic) G47.00
  adjustment F51.02
  adjustment disorder F51.02
  behavioral, of childhood Z73.819
    combined type Z73.812
    limit setting type Z73.811
    sleep-onset association type Z73.810
  childhood Z73.819
  chronic F51.04
    somatized tension F51.04
  conditioned F51.04
  due to
    alcohol
      abuse F10.182
      dependence F10.282
      use F10.982
    amphetamines
      abuse F15.182
      dependence F15.282
      use F15.982
    anxiety disorder F51.05
    caffeine
      abuse F15.182
      dependence F15.282
      use F15.982
    cocaine
      abuse F14.182
      dependence F14.282
      use F14.982
    depression F51.05
    drug NEC
      abuse F19.182
      dependence F19.282
      use F19.982
    medical condition G47.01
    mental disorder NEC F51.05

Insomnia — *continued*
  due to — *continued*
    opioid
      abuse F11.182
      dependence F11.282
      use F11.982
    psychoactive substance NEC
      abuse F19.182
      dependence F19.182
      use F19.982
    sedative, hypnotic, or anxiolytic
      abuse F13.182
      dependence F13.282
      use F13.982
    stimulant NEC
      abuse F15.182
      dependence F15.282
      use F15.982
  fatal familial (FFI) A81.83
  idiopathic F51.01
  learned F51.3
  nonorganic origin F51.01
  not due to a substance or known physiological condition F51.01
    specified NEC F51.09
  paradoxical F51.03
  primary F51.01
  psychiatric F51.05
  psychophysiologic F51.04
  related to psychopathology F51.05
  short-term F51.02
  specified NEC G47.09
  stress-related F51.02
  transient F51.02
  without objective findings F51.02
Inspiration
  food or foreign body — *see* Foreign body, by site
  mucus — *see* Asphyxia, mucus
Inspissated bile syndrome (newborn) P59.1
Instability
  emotional (excessive) F60.3
  housing
    housed Z59.819
      with risk of homelessness Z59.811
      homelessness in past 12 months Z59.812
  joint (post-traumatic) M25.30
    ankle M25.37- ☑
    due to old ligament injury — *see* Disorder, ligament
    elbow M25.32- ☑
    flail — *see* Flail, joint
    foot M25.37- ☑
    hand M25.34- ☑
    hip M25.35- ☑
    knee M25.36- ☑
    lumbosacral — *see* subcategory M53.2 ☑
    prosthesis — *see* Complications, joint prosthesis, mechanical, displacement, by site
    sacroiliac — *see* subcategory M53.2 ☑
    secondary to
      old ligament injury — *see* Disorder, ligament
      removal of joint prosthesis M96.89
    shoulder (region) M25.31- ☑
    specified site NEC M25.39
    spine — *see* subcategory M53.2 ☑
    wrist M25.33- ☑
  knee (chronic) M23.5- ☑
  lumbosacral — *see* subcategory M53.2 ☑
  nervous F48.8
  personality (emotional) F60.3
  spine — *see* Instability, joint, spine
  vasomotor R55
Institutional syndrome (childhood) F94.2
Institutionalization, affecting child Z62.22
  disinhibited attachment F94.2
Insufficiency, insufficient
  accommodation, old age H52.4
  adrenal (gland) E27.40
    primary E27.1
  adrenocortical E27.40
    drug-induced E27.3
    iatrogenic E27.3
    primary E27.1
  anatomic crown height K08.89
  anterior (occlusal) guidance M26.54
  anus K62.89
  aortic (valve) I35.1
    with
      mitral (valve) disease I08.0

Insufficiency, insufficient — *continued*
  aortic — *continued*
    with — *continued*
      mitral disease — *continued*
        with tricuspid (valve) disease I08.3
        stenosis I35.2
        tricuspid (valve) disease I08.2
          with mitral (valve) disease I08.3
      congenital Q23.1
      rheumatic I06.1
        with
          mitral (valve) disease I08.0
            with tricuspid (valve) disease I08.3
            stenosis I06.2
              with mitral (valve) disease I08.0
                with tricuspid (valve) disease I08.3
            tricuspid (valve) disease I08.2
              with mitral (valve) disease I08.3
    specified cause NEC I35.1
    syphilitic A52.03
  arterial I77.1
    basilar G45.0
    carotid (hemispheric) G45.1
    cerebral I67.81
    coronary (acute or subacute) I24.8
    mesenteric K55.1
    peripheral I73.9
    precerebral (multiple) (bilateral) G45.2
    vertebral G45.0
  arteriovenous I99.8
  biliary K83.8
  cardiac — *see also* Insufficiency, myocardial
    due to presence of (cardiac) prosthesis I97.11- ☑
    postprocedural I97.11- ☑
  cardiorenal, hypertensive I13.2
  cardiovascular — *see* Disease, cardiovascular
  cerebrovascular (acute) I67.81
    with transient focal neurological signs and symp-
      toms G45.8
  circulatory NEC I99.8
    newborn P29.89
  clinical crown length K08.89
  convergence H51.11
  coronary (acute or subacute) I24.8
    chronic or with a stated duration of over 4 weeks
      I25.89
  corticoadrenal E27.40
    primary E27.1
  dietary E63.9
  divergence H51.8
  food T73.0 ☑
  gastroesophageal K22.89
  gonadal
    ovary E28.39
    testis E29.1
  heart — *see also* Insufficiency, myocardial
    newborn P29.0
    valve — *see* Endocarditis
  hepatic — *see* Failure, hepatic
  idiopathic autonomic G90.09
  interocclusal distance of fully erupted teeth (ridge)
    M26.36
  kidney N28.9
    acute N28.9
    chronic N18.9
  lacrimal (secretion) H04.12- ☑
    passages — *see* Stenosis, lacrimal
  liver — *see* Failure, hepatic
  lung — *see* Insufficiency, pulmonary
  mental (congenital) — *see* Disability, intellectual
  mesenteric K55.1
  mitral (valve) I34.0
    with
      aortic valve disease I08.0
        with tricuspid (valve) disease I08.3
      obstruction or stenosis I05.2
        with aortic valve disease I08.0
      tricuspid (valve) disease I08.1
        with aortic (valve) disease I08.3
    congenital Q23.3
    rheumatic I05.1
      with
        aortic valve disease I08.0
          with tricuspid (valve) disease I08.3
        obstruction or stenosis I05.2
          with aortic valve disease I08.0
            with tricuspid (valve) disease I08.3
        tricuspid (valve) disease I08.1

Insufficiency, insufficient — *continued*
  mitral — *continued*
    rheumatic — *continued*
      with — *continued*
        tricuspid disease — *continued*
          with aortic (valve) disease I08.3
      active or acute I01.1
        with chorea, rheumatic (Sydenham's) I02.0
    specified cause, except rheumatic I34.0
  muscle — *see also* Disease, muscle
    heart — *see* Insufficiency, myocardial
    ocular NEC H50.9
  myocardial, myocardium (with arteriosclerosis) — *see*
    also Failure, heart I50.9
    with
      rheumatic fever (conditions in I00) I09.0
        active, acute or subacute I01.2
          with chorea I02.0
        inactive or quiescent (with chorea) I09.0
    congenital Q24.8
    hypertensive — *see* Hypertension, heart
    newborn P29.0
    rheumatic I09.0
      active, acute, or subacute I01.2
    syphilitic A52.06
  nourishment — *see also* Nutrition deficient T73.0 ☑
  pancreatic K86.89
    exocrine K86.81
  parathyroid (gland) E20.9
  peripheral vascular (arterial) I73.9
  pituitary E23.0
  placental (mother) O36.51- ☑
  platelets D69.6
  prenatal care affecting management of pregnancy
    O09.3- ☑
  progressive pluriglandular E31.0
  pulmonary J98.4
    acute, following surgery (nonthoracic) J95.2
      thoracic J95.1
    chronic, following surgery J95.3
    following
      shock J98.4
      trauma J98.4
    newborn P28.89
    valve I37.1
      with stenosis I37.2
      congenital Q22.2
      rheumatic I09.89
        with aortic, mitral or tricuspid (valve) disease
          I08.8
  pyloric K31.89
  renal (acute) N28.9
    chronic N18.9
  respiratory R06.89
    newborn P28.5
  rotation — *see* Malrotation
  sleep syndrome F51.12
  social insurance Z59.7
  suprarenal E27.40
    primary E27.1
  tarso-orbital fascia, congenital Q10.3
  testis E29.1
  thyroid (gland) (acquired) E03.9
    congenital E03.1
  tricuspid (valve) (rheumatic) I07.1
    with
      aortic (valve) disease I08.2
        with mitral (valve) disease I08.3
      mitral (valve) disease I08.1
        with aortic (valve) disease I08.3
      obstruction or stenosis I07.2
        with aortic (valve) disease I08.2
          with mitral (valve) disease I08.3
    congenital Q22.8
    nonrheumatic I36.1
      with stenosis I36.2
  urethral sphincter R32
  valve, valvular (heart) I38
    aortic — *see* Insufficiency, aortic (valve)
    congenital Q24.8
    mitral — *see* Insufficiency, mitral (valve)
    pulmonary — *see* Insufficiency, pulmonary, valve
    tricuspid — *see* Insufficiency, tricuspid (valve)
  vascular I99.8
    intestine K55.9
      acute — *see also* Ischemia, intestine, acute
        K55.059
    mesenteric K55.1

Insufficiency, insufficient — *continued*
  vascular — *continued*
    peripheral I73.9
    renal — *see* Hypertension, kidney
  velopharyngeal
    acquired K13.79
    congenital Q38.8
  venous (chronic) (peripheral) I87.2
  ventricular — *see* Insufficiency, myocardial
  welfare support Z59.7
Insufflation, fallopian Z31.41
Insular — *see* condition
Insulinoma
  pancreas
    benign D13.7
    malignant C25.4
    uncertain behavior D37.8
  specified site
    benign — *see* Neoplasm, by site, benign
    malignant — *see* Neoplasm, by site, malignant
    uncertain behavior — *see* Neoplasm, by site, uncer-
      tain behavior
  unspecified site
    benign D13.7
    malignant C25.4
    uncertain behavior D37.8
Insuloma — *see* Insulinoma
Interference
  balancing side M26.56
  non-working side M26.56
Intermenstrual — *see* condition
Intermittent — *see* condition
Internal — *see* condition
Interrogation
  cardiac defibrillator (automatic) (implantable) Z45.02
  cardiac pacemaker Z45.018
  cardiac (event) (loop) recorder Z45.09
  infusion pump (implanted) (intrathecal) Z45.1
  neurostimulator Z46.2
Interruption
  aortic arch Q25.21
  bundle of His I44.30
  phase-shift, sleep cycle — *see* Disorder, sleep, circadian
    rhythm
  sleep phase-shift, or 24 hour sleep-wake cycle — *see*
    Disorder, sleep, circadian rhythm
Interstitial — *see* condition
Intertrigo L30.4
  labialis K13.0
Intervertebral disc — *see* condition
Intestine, intestinal — *see* condition
Intolerance
  carbohydrate K90.49
  disaccharide, hereditary E73.0
  fat NEC K90.49
    pancreatic K90.3
  food K90.49
    dietary counseling and surveillance Z71.3
  fructose E74.10
    hereditary E74.12
  glucose (-galactose) E74.39
  gluten K90.41
  lactose E73.9
    specified NEC E73.8
  lysine E72.3
  milk NEC K90.49
    lactose E73.9
  orthostatic, chronic G90.A
  protein K90.49
  starch NEC K90.49
  sucrose (-isomaltose) E74.31
Intoxicated NEC (without dependence) — *see* Alcohol,
  intoxication
Intoxication
  acid — *see also* Acidosis E87.29
  alcoholic (acute) (without dependence) — *see* Alcohol,
    intoxication
  alimentary canal K52.1
  amphetamine (without dependence) — *see also* Abuse,
    drug, stimulant, with intoxication
    with dependence — *see* Dependence, drug, stimu-
      lant, with intoxication
    stimulant NEC F15.10
      with
        anxiety disorder F15.180
        intoxication F15.129
          with
            delirium F15.121

Intoxication — *continued*
amphetamine — *see also* Abuse, drug, stimulant, with intoxication — *continued*
  stimulant — *continued*
    with — *continued*
      intoxication — *continued*
        with — *continued*
          perceptual disturbance F15.122
anxiolytic (acute) (without dependence) — *see* Abuse, drug, sedative, with intoxication
  with dependence — *see* Dependence, drug, sedative, with intoxication
caffeine F15.929
  with dependence — *see* Dependence, drug, stimulant, with intoxication
cannabinoids (acute) (without dependence) — *see* Use, cannabis, with intoxication
  with
    abuse — *see* Abuse, drug, cannabis, with intoxication
    dependence — *see* Dependence, drug, cannabis, with intoxication
chemical — *see* Table of Drugs and Chemicals
  via placenta or breast milk — *see* - Absorption, chemical, through placenta
cocaine (acute) (without dependence) — *see* Abuse, drug, cocaine, with intoxication
  with dependence — *see* Dependence, drug, cocaine, with intoxication
drug
  acute (without dependence) — *see* Abuse, drug, by type with intoxication
    with dependence — *see* Dependence, drug, by type with intoxication
  addictive
    via placenta or breast milk — *see* Absorption, drug, addictive, through placenta
  newborn P93.8
    gray baby syndrome P93.0
  overdose or wrong substance given or taken — *see* Table of Drugs and Chemicals, by drug, poisoning
enteric K52.1
foodborne A05.9
  bacterial A05.9
  classical (Clostridium botulinum) A05.1
  due to
    Bacillus cereus A05.4
    bacterium A05.9
      specified NEC A05.8
    Clostridium
      botulinum A05.1
      perfringens A05.2
      welchii A05.2
    Salmonella A02.9
      with
        (gastro)enteritis A02.0
        localized infection(s) A02.20
          arthritis A02.23
          meningitis A02.21
          osteomyelitis A02.24
          pneumonia A02.22
          pyelonephritis A02.25
          specified NEC A02.29
        sepsis A02.1
        specified manifestation NEC A02.8
    Staphylococcus A05.0
    Vibrio
      parahaemolyticus A05.3
      vulnificus A05.5
  enterotoxin, staphylococcal A05.0
  noxious — *see* Poisoning, food, noxious
gastrointestinal K52.1
hallucinogenic (without dependence) — *see* Abuse, drug, hallucinogen, with intoxication
  with dependence — *see* Dependence, drug, hallucinogen, with intoxication
hepatocerebral intoxication K76.82
hypnotic (acute) (without dependence) — *see* Abuse, drug, sedative, with intoxication
  with dependence — *see* Dependence, drug, sedative, with intoxication
inhalant (acute) (without dependence) — *see* Abuse, drug, inhalant, with intoxication
  with dependence — *see* Dependence, drug, inhalant, with intoxication
meaning
  inebriation — *see* category F10 ☑

Intoxication — *continued*
meaning — *continued*
  poisoning — *see* Table of Drugs and Chemicals
  methyl alcohol (acute) (without dependence) — *see* Alcohol, intoxication
  opioid (acute) (without dependence) — *see* Abuse, drug, opioid, with intoxication
    with dependence — *see* Dependence, drug, opioid, with intoxication
  pathologic NEC (without dependence) — *see* Alcohol, intoxication
  phencyclidine (without dependence) — *see* Abuse, drug, hallucinogen, with intoxication
    with dependence — *see* Dependence, drug, hallucinogen, with intoxication
  potassium (K) E87.5
  psychoactive substance NEC (without dependence) — *see* Abuse, drug, psychoactive NEC, with intoxication
    with dependence — *see* Dependence, drug, psychoactive NEC, with intoxication
  sedative (acute) (without dependence) — *see* Abuse, drug, sedative, with intoxication
    with dependence — *see* Dependence, drug, sedative, with intoxication
  serum — *see also* Reaction, serum T80.69 ☑
  uremic — *see* Uremia
  volatile solvents (acute) (without dependence) — *see* Abuse, drug, inhalant, with intoxication
    with dependence — *see* Dependence, drug, inhalant, with intoxication
  water E87.79
Intraabdominal testis, testes
bilateral Q53.211
unilateral Q53.111
Intracranial — *see* condition
Intrahepatic gallbladder Q44.1
Intraligamentous — *see* condition
Intrathoracic — *see also* condition
kidney Q63.2
Intrauterine contraceptive device
checking Z30.431
in situ Z97.5
insertion Z30.430
  immediately following removal Z30.433
management Z30.431
reinsertion Z30.433
removal Z30.432
replacement Z30.433
retention in pregnancy O26.3- ☑
Intraventricular — *see* condition
Intrinsic deformity — *see* Deformity
Intubation, difficult or failed T88.4 ☑
Intumescence, lens (eye) (cataract) — *see* Cataract
Intussusception (bowel) (colon) (enteric) (ileocecal) (ileocolic) (intestine) (rectum) K56.1
appendix K38.8
congenital Q43.8
ureter (with obstruction) N13.5
Invagination (bowel, colon, intestine or rectum) K56.1
Inversion
albumin-globulin (A-G) ratio E88.09
bladder N32.89
cecum — *see* Intussusception
cervix N88.8
chromosome in normal individual Q95.1
circadian rhythm — *see* Disorder, sleep, circadian rhythm
nipple N64.59
  congenital Q83.8
  gestational — *see* Retraction, nipple
  puerperal, postpartum — *see* Retraction, nipple
nyctohemeral rhythm — *see* Disorder, sleep, circadian rhythm
optic papilla Q14.2
organ or site, congenital NEC — *see* Anomaly, by site
sleep rhythm — *see* Disorder, sleep, circadian rhythm
testis (congenital) Q55.29
uterus (chronic) (postinfectional) (postpartal, old) N85.5
  postpartum O71.2
vagina (posthysterectomy) N99.3
ventricular Q20.5
Investigation — *see also* Examination Z04.9
clinical research subject (control) (normal comparison) (participant) Z00.6
Involuntary movement, abnormal R25.9
Involution, involutional — *see also* condition

Involution, involutional — *continued*
breast, cystic — *see* Dysplasia, mammary, specified type NEC
depression (single episode) F32.89
  recurrent episode F33.9
melancholia (single episode) F32.89
  recurrent episode F33.8
ovary, senile — *see* Atrophy, ovary
thymus failure E32.8
I.Q.
20-34 F72
35-49 F71
50-69 F70
under 20 F73
IRDS (type I) P22.0
type II P22.1
Irideremia Q13.1
Iridis rubeosis — *see* Disorder, iris, vascular
Iridochoroiditis (panuveitis) — *see* Panuveitis
Iridocyclitis H20.9
acute H20.0- ☑
  hypopyon H20.05- ☑
  primary H20.01- ☑
  recurrent H20.02- ☑
  secondary (noninfectious) H20.04- ☑
    infectious H20.03- ☑
chronic H20.1- ☑
due to allergy — *see* Iridocyclitis, acute, secondary
endogenous — *see* Iridocyclitis, acute, primary
Fuchs' — *see* Cyclitis, Fuchs' heterochromic
gonococcal A54.32
granulomatous — *see* Iridocyclitis, chronic
herpes, herpetic (simplex) B00.51
  zoster B02.32
hypopyon — *see* Iridocyclitis, acute, hypopyon
in (due to)
  ankylosing spondylitis M45.9
  gonococcal infection A54.32
  herpes (simplex) virus B00.51
    zoster B02.32
  infectious disease NOS B99 ☑
  parasitic disease NOS B89 *[H22]*
  sarcoidosis D86.83
  syphilis A51.43
  tuberculosis A18.54
  zoster B02.32
lens-induced H20.2- ☑
nongranulomatous — *see* Iridocyclitis, acute
recurrent — *see* Iridocyclitis, acute, recurrent
rheumatic — *see* Iridocyclitis, chronic
subacute — *see* Iridocyclitis, acute
sympathetic — *see* Uveitis, sympathetic
syphilitic (secondary) A51.43
tuberculous (chronic) A18.54
Vogt-Koyanagi H20.82- ☑
Iridocyclochoroiditis (panuveitis) — *see* Panuveitis
Iridodialysis H21.53- ☑
Iridodonesis H21.89
Iridoplegia (complete) (partial) (reflex) H57.09
Iridoschisis H21.25- ☑
Iris — *see also* condition
bombé — *see* Membrane, pupillary
Iritis — *see also* Iridocyclitis
chronic — *see* Iridocyclitis, chronic
diabetic — *see* E08-E13 with .39
due to
  herpes simplex B00.51
  leprosy A30.9 *[H22]*
gonococcal A54.32
gouty — *see also* Gout, by type M10.9 *[H22]*
granulomatous — *see* Iridocyclitis, chronic
lens induced — *see* Iridocyclitis, lens-induced
papulosa (syphilitic) A52.71
rheumatic — *see* Iridocyclitis, chronic
syphilitic (secondary) A51.43
  congenital (early) A50.01
  late A52.71
tuberculous A18.54
Iron — *see* condition
Iron-miner's lung J63.4
Irradiated enamel (tooth, teeth) K03.89
Irradiation effects, adverse T66 ☑
Irreducible, irreducibility — *see* condition
Irregular, irregularity
action, heart I49.9
alveolar process K08.89
bleeding N92.6

Irregular, irregularity — *continued*
  breathing R06.89
  contour of cornea (acquired) — *see* Deformity, cornea
    congenital Q13.4
  contour, reconstructed breast N65.0
  dentin (in pulp) K04.3
  eye movements H55.89
    deficient
      saccadic H55.81
      smooth H55.82
    nystagmus — *see* Nystagmus
  labor O62.2
  menstruation (cause unknown) N92.6
  periods N92.6
  prostate N42.9
  pupil — *see* Abnormality, pupillary
  reconstructed breast N65.0
  respiratory R06.89
  septum (nasal) J34.2
  shape, organ or site, congenital NEC — *see* Distortion
  sleep-wake pattern (rhythm) G47.23
Irritable, irritability R45.4
  bladder N32.89
  bowel (syndrome) K58.9
    with
      constipation K58.1
      diarrhea K58.0
    mixed K58.2
    psychogenic F45.8
    specified NEC K58.8
  bronchial — *see* Bronchitis
  cerebral, in newborn P91.3
  colon — *see also* Irritable, bowel K58.9
    with diarrhea K58.0
    psychogenic F45.8
  duodenum K59.89
  heart (psychogenic) F45.8
  hip — *see* Derangement, joint, specified type NEC, hip
  ileum K59.89
  infant R68.12
  jejunum K59.89
  rectum K59.89
  stomach K31.89
    psychogenic F45.8
  sympathetic G90.8
  urethra N36.8
Irritation
  anus K62.89
  axillary nerve G54.0
  bladder N32.89
  brachial plexus G54.0
  bronchial — *see* Bronchitis
  cervical plexus G54.2
  cervix — *see* Cervicitis
  choroid, sympathetic — *see* Endophthalmitis
  cranial nerve — *see* Disorder, nerve, cranial
  gastric K31.89
    psychogenic F45.8
  globe, sympathetic — *see* Uveitis, sympathetic
  labyrinth — *see* subcategory H83.2 ☑
  lumbosacral plexus G54.1
  meninges (traumatic) — *see* Injury, intracranial
    nontraumatic — *see* Meningismus
  nerve — *see* Disorder, nerve
  nervous R45.0
  penis N48.89
  perineum NEC L29.3
  peripheral autonomic nervous system G90.8
  peritoneum — *see* Peritonitis
  pharynx J39.2
  plantar nerve — *see* Lesion, nerve, plantar
  spinal (cord) (traumatic) — *see also* Injury, spinal cord, by region
    nerve G58.9
      root NEC — *see* Radiculopathy
    nontraumatic — *see* Myelopathy
  stomach K31.89
    psychogenic F45.8
  sympathetic nerve NEC G90.8
  ulnar nerve — *see* Lesion, nerve, ulnar
  vagina N89.8
Ischemia, ischemic I99.8
  bowel (transient)
    acute — *see also* Ischemia, intestine, acute K55.059
    chronic K55.1
    due to mesenteric artery insufficiency K55.1
  brain — *see* Ischemia, cerebral
  cardiac (see Disease, heart, ischemic)

Ischemia, ischemic — *continued*
  cardiomyopathy I25.5
  cerebral (chronic) (generalized) I67.82
    arteriosclerotic I67.2
    intermittent G45.9
    newborn P91.0
    recurrent focal G45.8
    transient G45.9
  colon chronic (due to mesenteric artery insufficiency) K55.1
  coronary — *see* Disease, heart, ischemic
  demand (coronary) — *see also* Angina I24.8
    with myocardial infarction I21.A1
    resulting in myocardial infarction I21.A1
  heart (chronic or with a stated duration of over 4 weeks) I25.9
    acute or with a stated duration of 4 weeks or less I24.9
    subacute I24.9
  infarction, muscle — *see* Infarct, muscle
  intestine (large) (small) (transient) K55.9
    acute K55.059
      diffuse K55.052
      focal K55.051
      large K55.039
        diffuse K55.032
        focal K55.031
      small K55.019
        diffuse K55.012
        focal K55.011
    chronic K55.1
    due to mesenteric artery insufficiency K55.1
  kidney N28.0
  limb, critical — *see* Arteriosclerosis, with critical limb ischemia
  limb-threatening, chronic — *see* Arteriosclerosis, with critical limb ischemia
  mesenteric, acute — *see also* Ischemia, intestine, acute K55.059
  muscle, traumatic T79.6 ☑
  myocardium, myocardial (chronic or with a stated duration of over 4 weeks) I25.9
    acute, without myocardial infarction I51.3
    silent (asymptomatic) I25.6
    transient of newborn P29.4
  renal N28.0
  retina, retinal — *see* Occlusion, artery, retina
  small bowel
    acute K55.019
      diffuse K55.012
      focal K55.011
    chronic K55.1
    due to mesenteric artery insufficiency K55.1
  spinal cord G95.11
  subendocardial — *see* Insufficiency, coronary
  supply (coronary) — *see also* Angina I25.9
    due to vasospasm I20.1
Ischial spine — *see* condition
Ischialgia — *see* Sciatica
Ischiopagus Q89.4
Ischium, ischial — *see* condition
Ischuria R34
Iselin's disease or osteochondrosis — *see* Osteochondrosis, juvenile, metatarsus
Islands of
  parotid tissue in
    lymph nodes Q38.6
    neck structures Q38.6
  submaxillary glands in
    fascia Q38.6
    lymph nodes Q38.6
    neck muscles Q38.6
Islet cell tumor, pancreas D13.7
Isoimmunization NEC — *see also* Incompatibility
  affecting management of pregnancy (ABO) (with hydrops fetalis) O36.11- ☑
    anti-A sensitization O36.11- ☑
    anti-B sensitization O36.19- ☑
    anti-c sensitization O36.09- ☑
    anti-C sensitization O36.09- ☑
    anti-e sensitization O36.09- ☑
    anti-E sensitization O36.09- ☑
    Rh NEC O36.09- ☑
      anti-D antibody O36.01- ☑
    specified NEC O36.19- ☑
  newborn P55.9
    with
      hydrops fetalis P56.0

Isoimmunization — *continued*
  newborn — *continued*
    with — *continued*
      kernicterus P57.0
    ABO (blood groups) P55.1
    Rhesus (Rh) factor P55.0
    specified type NEC P55.8
Isolation, isolated
  dwelling Z59.89
  family Z63.79
  social Z60.4
Isoleucinosis E71.19
Isomerism atrial appendages (with asplenia or polysplenia) Q20.6
Isosporiasis, isosporosis A07.3
Isovaleric acidemia E71.110
Issue of
  medical certificate Z02.79
    for disability determination Z02.71
  repeat prescription (appliance) (glasses) (medicinal substance, medicament, medicine) Z76.0
    contraception — *see* Contraception
Itch, itching — *see also* Pruritus
  baker's L23.6
  barber's B35.0
  bricklayer's L24.5
  cheese B88.0
  clam digger's B65.3
  coolie B76.9
  copra B88.0
  dew B76.9
  dhobi B35.6
  filarial — *see* Infestation, filarial
  grain B88.0
  grocer's B88.0
  ground B76.9
  harvest B88.0
  jock B35.6
  Malabar B35.5
    beard B35.0
    foot B35.3
    scalp B35.0
  meaning scabies B86
  Norwegian B86
  perianal L29.0
  poultrymen's B88.0
  sarcoptic B86
  scabies B86
  scrub B88.0
  straw B88.0
  swimmer's B65.3
  water B76.9
  winter L29.8
Ivemark's syndrome (asplenia with congenital heart disease) Q89.01
Ivory bones Q78.2
Ixodiasis NEC B88.8

J

Jaccoud's syndrome — *see* Arthropathy, postrheumatic, chronic
Jackson's
  membrane Q43.3
  paralysis or syndrome G83.89
  veil Q43.3
Jacquet's dermatitis (diaper dermatitis) L22
Jadassohn-Pellizari's disease or anetoderma L90.2
Jadassohn's
  blue nevus — *see* Nevus
  intraepidermal epithelioma — *see* Neoplasm, skin, benign
Jaffe-Lichtenstein (-Uehlinger) **syndrome** — *see* Dysplasia, fibrous, bone NEC
Jakob-Creutzfeldt disease or syndrome — *see* Creutzfeldt-Jakob disease or syndrome
Jaksch-Luzet disease D64.89
Jamaican
  neuropathy G92.8
  paraplegic tropical ataxic-spastic syndrome G92.8
Janet's disease F48.8
Janiceps Q89.4
Jansky-Bielschowsky amaurotic idiocy E75.4
Japanese
  B-type encephalitis A83.0
  river fever A75.3
Jaundice (yellow) R17

Jaundice — *continued*
- acholuric (familial) (splenomegalic) — *see also* Spherocytosis
  - acquired D59.8
- breast-milk (inhibitor) P59.3
- catarrhal (acute) B15.9
  - with hepatic coma B15.0
- cholestatic (benign) R17
- due to or associated with
  - delayed conjugation P59.8
    - associated with (due to) preterm delivery P59.0
  - preterm delivery P59.0
- epidemic (catarrhal) B15.9
  - with hepatic coma B15.0
  - leptospiral A27.0
  - spirochetal A27.0
- familial nonhemolytic (congenital) (Gilbert) E80.4
  - Crigler-Najjar E80.5
- febrile (acute) B15.9
  - with hepatic coma B15.0
  - leptospiral A27.0
  - spirochetal A27.0
- hematogenous D59.9
- hemolytic (acquired) D59.9
  - congenital — *see* Spherocytosis
- hemorrhagic (acute) (leptospiral) (spirochetal) A27.0
- infectious (acute) (subacute) B15.9
  - with hepatic coma B15.0
  - leptospiral A27.0
  - spirochetal A27.0
- leptospiral (hemorrhagic) A27.0
- malignant (without coma) K72.90
  - with coma K72.91
- neonatal — *see* Jaundice, newborn
- newborn P59.9
  - due to or associated with
    - ABO
      - antibodies P55.1
      - incompatibility, maternal/fetal P55.1
      - isoimmunization P55.1
    - absence or deficiency of enzyme system for bilirubin conjugation (congenital) P59.8
    - bleeding P58.1
    - breast milk inhibitors to conjugation P59.3
      - associated with preterm delivery P59.0
    - bruising P58.0
    - Crigler-Najjar syndrome E80.5
    - delayed conjugation P59.8
      - associated with preterm delivery P59.0
    - drugs or toxins
      - given to newborn P58.42
      - transmitted from mother P58.41
    - excessive hemolysis P58.9
      - due to
        - bleeding P58.1
        - bruising P58.0
        - drugs or toxins
          - given to newborn P58.42
          - transmitted from mother P58.41
        - infection P58.2
        - polycythemia P58.3
        - swallowed maternal blood P58.5
      - specified type NEC P58.8
    - galactosemia E74.21
    - Gilbert syndrome E80.4
    - hemolytic disease P55.9
      - ABO isoimmunization P55.1
      - Rh isoimmunization P55.0
      - specified NEC P55.8
    - hepatocellular damage P59.20
      - specified NEC P59.29
    - hereditary hemolytic anemia P58.8
    - hypothyroidism, congenital E03.1
    - incompatibility, maternal/fetal NOS P55.9
    - infection P58.2
    - inspissated bile syndrome P59.1
    - isoimmunization NOS P55.9
    - mucoviscidosis E84.9
    - polycythemia P58.3
    - preterm delivery P59.0
    - Rh
      - antibodies P55.0
      - incompatibility, maternal/fetal P55.0
      - isoimmunization P55.0
    - specified cause NEC P59.8
    - swallowed maternal blood P58.5
  - spherocytosis (congenital) D58.0
- nonhemolytic congenital familial (Gilbert) E80.4

Jaundice — *continued*
- nuclear, newborn — *see also* Kernicterus of newborn P57.9
- obstructive — *see also* Obstruction, bile duct K83.1
- post-immunization — *see* Hepatitis, viral, type, B
- post-transfusion — *see* Hepatitis, viral, type, B
- regurgitation — *see also* Obstruction, bile duct K83.1
- serum (homologous) (prophylactic) (therapeutic) — *see* Hepatitis, viral, type, B
- spirochetal (hemorrhagic) A27.0
- symptomatic R17
  - newborn P59.9
Jaw — *see* condition
Jaw-winking phenomenon or syndrome Q07.8
Jealousy
- alcoholic F10.988
- childhood F93.8
- sibling F93.8
Jejunitis — *see* Enteritis
Jejunostomy status Z93.4
Jejunum, jejunal — *see* condition
Jensen's disease — *see* Inflammation, chorioretinal, focal, juxtapapillary
Jerks, myoclonic G25.3
Jervell-Lange-Nielsen syndrome I45.81
Jeune's disease Q77.2
Jigger disease B88.1
Job's syndrome (chronic granulomatous disease) D71
Joint — *see also* condition
- mice — *see* Loose, body, joint
  - knee M23.4- ☑
Jordan's anomaly or syndrome D72.0
Joseph-Diamond-Blackfan anemia (congenital hypoplastic) D61.01
Jungle yellow fever A95.0
Jüngling's disease — *see* Sarcoidosis
Juvenile — *see* condition

K

Kahler's disease C90.0- ☑
Kakke E51.11
Kala-azar B55.0
Kallmann's syndrome E23.0
Kanner's syndrome (autism) — *see* Psychosis, childhood
Kaposi's
- dermatosis (xeroderma pigmentosum) Q82.1
- lichen ruber L44.0
  - acuminatus L44.0
- sarcoma
  - colon C46.4
  - connective tissue C46.1
  - gastrointestinal organ C46.4
  - lung C46.5- ☑
  - lymph node (multiple) C46.3
  - palate (hard) (soft) C46.2
  - rectum C46.4
  - skin (multiple sites) C46.0
  - specified site NEC C46.7
  - stomach C46.4
  - unspecified site C46.9
- varicelliform eruption B00.0
  - vaccinia T88.1 ☑
Kartagener's syndrome or triad (sinusitis, bronchiectasis, situs inversus) Q89.3
Karyotype
- with abnormality except iso (Xq) Q96.2
- 45,X Q96.0
- 46,X
  - iso (Xq) Q96.1
- 46,XX Q98.3
  - with streak gonads Q50.32
  - hermaphrodite (true) Q99.1
  - male Q98.3
- 46,XY
  - with streak gonads Q56.1
  - female Q97.3
  - hermaphrodite (true) Q99.1
- 47,XXX Q97.0
- 47,XXY Q98.0
- 47,XYY Q98.5
Kaschin-Beck disease — *see* Disease, Kaschin-Beck
Katayama's disease or fever B65.2
Kawasaki's syndrome M30.3
Kayser-Fleischer ring (cornea) (pseudosclerosis)
- H18.04- ☑

Kaznelson's syndrome (congenital hypoplastic anemia) D61.01
Kearns-Sayre syndrome H49.81- ☑
Kedani fever A75.3
Kelis L91.0
Kelly (-Patterson) **syndrome** (sideropenic dysphagia) D50.1
Keloid, cheloid L91.0
- acne L73.0
- Addison's L94.0
- cornea — *see* Opacity, cornea
- Hawkin's L91.0
- scar L91.0
Keloma L91.0
Kenya fever A77.1
Keratectasia — *see also* Ectasia, cornea
- congenital Q13.4
Keratinization of alveolar ridge mucosa
- excessive K13.23
- minimal K13.22
Keratinized residual ridge mucosa
- excessive K13.23
- minimal K13.22
Keratitis (nodular) (nonulcerative) (simple) (zonular) H16.9
- with ulceration (central) (marginal) (perforated) (ring) — *see* Ulcer, cornea
- actinic — *see* Photokeratitis
- arborescens (herpes simplex) B00.52
- areolar H16.11- ☑
- bullosa H16.8
- deep H16.309
  - specified type NEC H16.399
- dendritic (a) (herpes simplex) B00.52
- disciform (is) (herpes simplex) B00.52
  - varicella B01.81
- filamentary H16.12- ☑
- gonococcal (congenital or prenatal) A54.33
- herpes, herpetic (simplex) B00.52
  - zoster B02.33
- in (due to)
  - acanthamebiasis B60.13
  - adenovirus B30.0
  - exanthema — *see also* Exanthem B09
  - herpes (simplex) virus B00.52
  - measles B05.81
  - syphilis A50.31
  - tuberculosis A18.52
  - zoster B02.33
- interstitial (nonsyphilitic) H16.30- ☑
  - diffuse H16.32- ☑
  - herpes, herpetic (simplex) B00.52
    - zoster B02.33
  - sclerosing H16.33- ☑
  - specified type NEC H16.39- ☑
  - syphilitic (congenital) (late) A50.31
  - tuberculous A18.52
- macular H16.11- ☑
- nummular H16.11- ☑
- oyster shuckers' H16.8
- parenchymatous — *see* Keratitis, interstitial
- petrificans H16.8
- postmeasles B05.81
- punctata
  - leprosa A30.9 *[H16.14-]* ☑
  - syphilitic (profunda) A50.31
- punctate H16.14- ☑
- purulent H16.8
- rosacea L71.8
- sclerosing H16.33- ☑
- specified type NEC H16.8
- stellate H16.11- ☑
- striate H16.11- ☑
- superficial H16.10- ☑
  - with conjunctivitis — *see* Keratoconjunctivitis
  - due to light — *see* Photokeratitis
- suppurative H16.8
- syphilitic (congenital) (prenatal) A50.31
- trachomatous A71.1
  - sequelae B94.0
- tuberculous A18.52
- vesicular H16.8
- xerotic — *see also* Keratomalacia H16.8
  - vitamin A deficiency E50.4
Keratoacanthoma L85.8
Keratocele — *see* Descemetocele
Keratoconjunctivitis H16.20- ☑

Keratoconjunctivitis — *continued*
- Acanthamoeba B6Ø.13
- adenoviral B3Ø.Ø
- epidemic B3Ø.Ø
- exposure H16.21- ☑
- herpes, herpetic (simplex) BØØ.52
  - zoster BØ2.33
- in exanthema — *see also* Exanthem BØ9
- infectious B3Ø.Ø
- lagophthalmic — *see* Keratoconjunctivitis, specified type NEC
- neurotrophic H16.23- ☑
- phlyctenular H16.25- ☑
- postmeasles BØ5.81
- shipyard B3Ø.Ø
- sicca (Sjogren's) M35.Ø- ☑
  - not Sjogren's H16.22- ☑
- specified type NEC H16.29- ☑
- tuberculous (phlyctenular) A18.52
- vernal H16.26- ☑

Keratoconus H18.6Ø- ☑
- congenital Q13.4
- stable H18.61- ☑
- unstable H18.62- ☑

Keratocyst (dental) (odontogenic) — *see* Cyst, calcifying odontogenic

Keratoderma, keratodermia (congenital) (palmaris et plantaris) (symmetrical) Q82.8
- acquired L85.1
  - in diseases classified elsewhere L86
- climactericum L85.1
- gonococcal A54.89
- gonorrheal A54.89
- punctata L85.2
- Reiter's — *see* Reiter's disease

Keratodermatocele — *see* Descemetocele

Keratohemia — *see* Pigmentation, cornea, stromal

Keratoiritis — *see also* Iridocyclitis
- syphilitic A5Ø.39
- tuberculous A18.54

Keratoma L57.Ø
- palmaris and plantaris hereditarium Q82.8
- senile L57.Ø

Keratomalacia H18.44- ☑
- vitamin A deficiency E5Ø.4

Keratomegaly Q13.4

Keratomycosis B49
- nigrans, nigricans (palmaris) B36.1

Keratopathy H18.9
- band H18.42- ☑
- bullous (aphakic), following cataract surgery H59.Ø1- ☑
- bullous H18.1- ☑

Keratoscleritis, tuberculous A18.52

Keratosis L57.Ø
- actinic L57.Ø
- arsenical L85.8
- congenital, specified NEC Q8Ø.8
- female genital NEC N94.89
- follicularis Q82.8
  - acquired L11.Ø
  - congenita Q82.8
  - et parafollicularis in cutem penetrans L87.Ø
  - spinulosa (decalvans) Q82.8
  - vitamin A deficiency E5Ø.8
- gonococcal A54.89
- male genital (external) N5Ø.89
- nigricans L83
- obturans, external ear (canal) — *see* Cholesteatoma, external ear
- palmaris et plantaris (inherited) (symmetrical) Q82.8
  - acquired L85.1
- penile N48.89
- pharynx J39.2
- pilaris, acquired L85.8
- punctata (palmaris et plantaris) L85.2
- scrotal N5Ø.89
- seborrheic L82.1
  - inflamed L82.Ø
- senile L57.Ø
- solar L57.Ø
- tonsillaris J35.8
- vagina N89.4
- vegetans Q82.8
- vitamin A deficiency E5Ø.8
- vocal cord J38.3

Kerato-uveitis — *see* Iridocyclitis

Kerion (celsi) B35.Ø

Kernicterus of newborn (not due to isoimmunization) P57.9
- due to isoimmunization (conditions in P55.Ø-P55.9) P57.Ø
- specified type NEC P57.8

Kerunoparalysis T75.Ø9 ☑

Keshan disease E59

Ketoacidosis E87.29
- diabetic — *see* Diabetes, by type, with ketoacidosis

Ketonuria R82.4

Ketosis NEC E88.89
- diabetic — *see* Diabetes, by type, with ketoacidosis

Kew Garden fever A79.1

Kidney — *see* condition

Kienböck's disease — *see also* Osteochondrosis, juvenile, hand, carpal lunate
- adult M93.1

Kimmelstiel (-Wilson) disease — *see* Diabetes, Kimmelstiel (-Wilson) disease

Kink, kinking
- artery I77.1
- hair (acquired) L67.8
- ileum or intestine — *see* Obstruction, intestine
- Lane's — *see* Obstruction, intestine
- organ or site, congenital NEC — *see* Anomaly, by site
- ureter (pelvic junction) N13.5
  - with
    - hydronephrosis N13.1
      - with infection N13.6
    - pyelonephritis (chronic) N11.1
  - congenital Q62.39
- vein(s) I87.8
  - caval I87.1
  - peripheral I87.1

Kinnier Wilson's disease (hepatolenticular degeneration) E83.Ø1

Kissing spine M48.2Ø
- cervical region M48.22
- cervicothoracic region M48.23
- lumbar region M48.26
- lumbosacral region M48.27
- occipito-atlanto-axial region M48.21
- thoracic region M48.24
- thoracolumbar region M48.25

Klatskin's tumor C22.1

Klauder's disease A26.8

Klebs' disease — *see also* Glomerulonephritis NØ5- ☑

Klebsiella (K.) pneumoniae, as cause of disease classified elsewhere B96.1

Klein (e)-**Levin syndrome** G47.13

Kleptomania F63.2

Klinefelter's syndrome Q98.4
- karyotype 47,XXY Q98.Ø
- male with more than two X chromosomes Q98.1

Klippel-Feil deficiency, disease, or syndrome (brevicollis) Q76.1

Klippel's disease I67.2

Klippel-Trenaunay (-Weber) syndrome Q87.2

Klumpke (-Déjerine) palsy, paralysis (birth) (newborn) P14.1

Knee — *see* condition

Knock knee (acquired) M21.Ø6- ☑
- congenital Q74.1

Knot(s)
- intestinal, syndrome (volvulus) K56.2
- surfer S89.8- ☑
- umbilical cord (true) O69.2 ☑

Knotting (of)
- hair L67.8
- intestine K56.2

Knuckle pad (Garrod's) M72.1

Koch's
- infection — *see* Tuberculosis
- relapsing fever A68.9

Koch-Weeks' conjunctivitis — *see* Conjunctivitis, acute, mucopurulent

Köebner's syndrome Q81.8

Köenig's disease (osteochondritis dissecans) — *see* Osteochondritis, dissecans

Köhler-Pellegrini-Steida disease or syndrome (calcification, knee joint) — *see* Bursitis, tibial collateral

Köhler's disease
- patellar — *see* Osteochondrosis, juvenile, patella
- tarsal navicular — *see* Osteochondrosis, juvenile, tarsus

Koilonychia L6Ø.3

Koilonychia — *continued*
- congenital Q84.6

Kojevnikov's, epilepsy — *see* Kozhevnikof's epilepsy

Koplik's spots BØ5.9

Kopp's asthma E32.8

Korsakoff's (Wernicke) disease, psychosis or syndrome (alcoholic) F1Ø.96
- with dependence F1Ø.26
- drug-induced
  - due to drug abuse — *see* Abuse, drug, by type, with amnestic disorder
  - due to drug dependence — *see* Dependence, drug, by type, with amnestic disorder
- nonalcoholic FØ4

Korsakov's disease, psychosis or syndrome — *see* Korsakoff's disease

Korsakow's disease, psychosis or syndrome — *see* Korsakoff's disease

Kostmann's disease or syndrome (infantile genetic agranulocytosis) — *see* Agranulocytosis

Kozhevnikof's epilepsy G4Ø.1Ø9
- intractable G4Ø.119
  - with status epilepticus G4Ø.111
  - without status epilepticus G4Ø.119
- not intractable G4Ø.1Ø9
  - with status epilepticus G4Ø.1Ø1
  - without status epilepticus G4Ø.1Ø9

Krabbe's
- disease E75.23
- syndrome, congenital muscle hypoplasia Q79.8

Kraepelin-Morel disease — *see* Schizophrenia

Kraft-Weber-Dimitri disease Q85.89

Kraurosis
- ani K62.89
- penis N48.Ø
- vagina N89.8
- vulva N9Ø.4

Kreotoxism AØ5.9

Krukenberg's
- spindle — *see* Pigmentation, cornea, posterior
- tumor C79.6- ☑

Kufs' disease E75.4

Kugelberg-Welander disease G12.1

Kuhnt-Junius degeneration — *see also* Degeneration, macula H35.32- ☑

Kümmell's disease or spondylitis — *see* Spondylopathy, traumatic

Kupffer cell sarcoma C22.3

Kuru A81.81

Kussmaul's
- disease M3Ø.Ø
- respiration E87.29
  - in diabetic acidosis — *see* Diabetes, by type, with ketoacidosis

Kwashiorkor E4Ø
- marasmic, marasmus type E42

Kyasanur Forest disease A98.2

Kyphoscoliosis, kyphoscoliotic (acquired) — *see also* Scoliosis M41.9
- congenital Q67.5
- heart (disease) I27.1
- sequelae of rickets E64.3
- tuberculous A18.Ø1

Kyphosis, kyphotic (acquired) M4Ø.2Ø9
- cervical region M4Ø.2Ø2
- cervicothoracic region M4Ø.2Ø3
- congenital Q76.419
  - cervical region Q76.412
  - cervicothoracic region Q76.413
  - occipito-atlanto-axial region Q76.411
  - thoracic region Q76.414
  - thoracolumbar region Q76.415
- Morquio-Brailsford type (spinal) — *see also* subcategory M49.8 E76.219
- postlaminectomy M96.3
- postradiation therapy M96.2
- postural (adolescent) M4Ø.ØØ
  - cervicothoracic region M4Ø.Ø3
  - thoracic region M4Ø.Ø4
  - thoracolumbar region M4Ø.Ø5
- secondary NEC M4Ø.1Ø
  - cervical region M4Ø.12
  - cervicothoracic region M4Ø.13
  - thoracic region M4Ø.14
  - thoracolumbar region M4Ø.15
- sequelae of rickets E64.3
- specified type NEC M4Ø.299
  - cervical region M4Ø.292

Kyphosis, kyphotic — *continued*
  specified type — *continued*
    cervicothoracic region M40.293
    thoracic region M40.294
    thoracolumbar region M40.295
  syphilitic, congenital A50.56
  thoracic region M40.204
  thoracolumbar region M40.205
  tuberculous A18.01
Kyrle disease L87.0

L

Labia, labium — *see* condition
Labile
  blood pressure R09.89
  vasomotor system I73.9
Labioglossal paralysis G12.29
Labium leporinum — *see* Cleft, lip
Labor — *see* Delivery
Labored breathing — *see* Hyperventilation
Labyrinthitis (circumscribed) (destructive) (diffuse) (inner
  ear) (latent) (purulent) (suppurative) — *see also*
  subcategory H83.0 ☑
  syphilitic A52.79
Laceration
  with abortion — *see* Abortion, by type, complicated
    by laceration of pelvic organs
  abdomen, abdominal
    wall S31.119 ☑
      with
        foreign body S31.129 ☑
        penetration into peritoneal cavity S31.619 ☑
          with foreign body S31.629 ☑
      epigastric region S31.112 ☑
        with
          foreign body S31.122 ☑
          penetration into peritoneal cavity
            S31.612 ☑
              with foreign body S31.622 ☑
      left
        lower quadrant S31.114 ☑
          with
            foreign body S31.124 ☑
            penetration into peritoneal cavity
              S31.614 ☑
                with foreign body S31.624 ☑
        upper quadrant S31.111 ☑
          with
            foreign body S31.121 ☑
            penetration into peritoneal cavity
              S31.611 ☑
                with foreign body S31.621 ☑
      periumbilic region S31.115 ☑
        with
          foreign body S31.125 ☑
          penetration into peritoneal cavity
             S31.615 ☑
              with foreign body S31.625 ☑
      right
        lower quadrant S31.113 ☑
          with
            foreign body S31.123 ☑
            penetration into peritoneal cavity
              S31.613 ☑
                with foreign body S31.623 ☑
        upper quadrant S31.110 ☑
          with
            foreign body S31.120 ☑
            penetration into peritoneal cavity
              S31.610 ☑
                with foreign body S31.620 ☑
  accidental, complicating surgery — *see* Complications,
    surgical, accidental puncture or laceration
  Achilles tendon S86.02- ☑
  adrenal gland S37.813 ☑
  alveolar (process) — *see* Laceration, oral cavity
  ankle S91.01- ☑
    with
      foreign body S91.02- ☑
  antecubital space — *see* Laceration, elbow
  anus (sphincter) S31.831 ☑
    with
      ectopic or molar pregnancy O08.6
      foreign body S31.832 ☑
    complicating delivery — *see* Delivery, complicated,
      by, laceration, anus (sphincter)

Laceration — *continued*
  anus — *continued*
    following ectopic or molar pregnancy O08.6
    nontraumatic, nonpuerperal — *see* Fissure, anus
  arm (upper) S41.11- ☑
    with foreign body S41.12- ☑
    lower — *see* Laceration, forearm
  auditory canal (external) (meatus) — *see* Laceration,
    ear
  auricle, ear — *see* Laceration, ear
  axilla — *see* Laceration, arm
  back — *see also* Laceration, thorax, back
    lower S31.010 ☑
      with
        foreign body S31.020 ☑
          with penetration into retroperitoneal
            space S31.021 ☑
        penetration into retroperitoneal space
          S31.011 ☑
  bile duct S36.13 ☑
  bladder S37.23 ☑
    with ectopic or molar pregnancy O08.6
    following ectopic or molar pregnancy O08.6
    obstetrical trauma O71.5
  blood vessel — *see* Injury, blood vessel
  bowel — *see also* Laceration, intestine
    with ectopic or molar pregnancy O08.6
    complicating abortion — *see* Abortion, by type,
      complicated by, specified condition NEC
    following ectopic or molar pregnancy O08.6
    obstetrical trauma O71.5
  brain (any part) (cortex) (diffuse) (membrane) — *see
    also* Injury, intracranial, diffuse
    during birth P10.8
      with hemorrhage P10.1
    focal — *see* Injury, intracranial, focal brain injury
  brainstem S06.38- ☑
  breast S21.01- ☑
    with foreign body S21.02- ☑
  broad ligament S37.893 ☑
    with ectopic or molar pregnancy O08.6
    following ectopic or molar pregnancy O08.6
    laceration syndrome N83.8
    obstetrical trauma O71.6
    syndrome (laceration) N83.8
  buttock S31.801 ☑
    with foreign body S31.802 ☑
    left S31.821 ☑
      with foreign body S31.822 ☑
    right S31.811 ☑
      with foreign body S31.812 ☑
  calf — *see* Laceration, leg
  canaliculus lacrimalis — *see* Laceration, eyelid
  canthus, eye — *see* Laceration, eyelid
  capsule, joint — *see* Sprain
  causing eversion of cervix uteri (old) N86
  central (perineal), complicating delivery O70.9
  cerebellum, traumatic S06.37- ☑
  cerebral S06.33- ☑
    during birth P10.8
      with hemorrhage P10.1
    left side S06.32- ☑
    right side S06.31- ☑
  cervix (uteri)
    with ectopic or molar pregnancy O08.6
    following ectopic or molar pregnancy O08.6
    nonpuerperal, nontraumatic N88.1
    obstetrical trauma (current) O71.3
    old (postpartal) N88.1
    traumatic S37.63 ☑
  cheek (external) S01.41- ☑
    with foreign body S01.42- ☑
    internal — *see* Laceration, oral cavity
  chest wall — *see* Laceration, thorax
  chin — *see* Laceration, head, specified site NEC
  chordae tendinae NEC I51.1
    concurrent with acute myocardial infarction — *see*
      Infarct, myocardium
    following acute myocardial infarction (current
      complication) I23.4
  clitoris — *see* Laceration, vulva
  colon — *see* Laceration, intestine, large, colon
  common bile duct S36.13 ☑
  cortex (cerebral) — *see* Injury, intracranial, diffuse
  costal region — *see* Laceration, thorax
  cystic duct S36.13 ☑
  diaphragm S27.803 ☑

Laceration — *continued*
  digit(s)
    foot — *see* Laceration, toe
    hand — *see* Laceration, finger
  duodenum S36.430 ☑
  ear (canal) (external) S01.31- ☑
    with foreign body S01.32- ☑
    drum S09.2- ☑
  elbow S51.01- ☑
    with
      foreign body S51.02- ☑
  epididymis — *see* Laceration, testis
  epigastric region — *see* Laceration, abdomen, wall,
    epigastric region
  esophagus K22.89
    traumatic
      cervical S11.21 ☑
        with foreign body S11.22 ☑
      thoracic S27.813 ☑
  eye (ball) S05.3- ☑
    with prolapse or loss of intraocular tissue S05.2- ☑
    penetrating S05.6- ☑
  eyebrow — *see* Laceration, eyelid
  eyelid S01.11- ☑
    with foreign body S01.12- ☑
  face NEC — *see* Laceration, head, specified site NEC
  fallopian tube S37.539 ☑
    bilateral S37.532 ☑
    unilateral S37.531 ☑
  finger(s) S61.219 ☑
    with
      damage to nail S61.319 ☑
        with
          foreign body S61.329 ☑
      foreign body S61.229 ☑
    index S61.218 ☑
      with
        damage to nail S61.318 ☑
          with
            foreign body S61.328 ☑
        foreign body S61.228 ☑
      left S61.211 ☑
        with
          damage to nail S61.311 ☑
            with
              foreign body S61.321 ☑
          foreign body S61.221 ☑
      right S61.210 ☑
        with
          damage to nail S61.310 ☑
            with
              foreign body S61.320 ☑
          foreign body S61.220 ☑
    little S61.218 ☑
      with
        damage to nail S61.318 ☑
          with
            foreign body S61.328 ☑
        foreign body S61.228 ☑
      left S61.217 ☑
        with
          damage to nail S61.317 ☑
            with
              foreign body S61.327 ☑
          foreign body S61.227 ☑
      right S61.216 ☑
        with
          damage to nail S61.316 ☑
            with
              foreign body S61.326 ☑
          foreign body S61.226 ☑
    middle S61.218 ☑
      with
        damage to nail S61.318 ☑
          with
            foreign body S61.328 ☑
        foreign body S61.228 ☑
      left S61.213 ☑
        with
          damage to nail S61.313 ☑
            with
              foreign body S61.323 ☑
          foreign body S61.223 ☑
      right S61.212 ☑
        with
          damage to nail S61.312 ☑

Laceration — *continued*
  finger(s) — *continued*
    middle — *continued*
      right — *continued*
        with — *continued*
          damage to nail — *continued*
            with
              foreign body S61.322 ☑
          foreign body S61.222 ☑
    ring S61.218 ☑
      with
        damage to nail S61.318 ☑
          with
            foreign body S61.328 ☑
        foreign body S61.228 ☑
      left S61.215 ☑
        with
          damage to nail S61.315 ☑
            with
              foreign body S61.325 ☑
          foreign body S61.225 ☑
      right S61.214 ☑
        with
          damage to nail S61.314 ☑
            with
              foreign body S61.324 ☑
          foreign body S61.224 ☑
  flank S31.119 ☑
    with foreign body S31.129 ☑
  foot (except toe(s) alone) S91.319 ☑
    with foreign body S91.329 ☑
    left S91.312 ☑
      with foreign body S91.322 ☑
    right S91.311 ☑
      with foreign body S91.321 ☑
    toe — *see* Laceration, toe
  forearm S51.819 ☑
    with
      foreign body S51.829 ☑
    elbow only — *see* Laceration, elbow
    left S51.812 ☑
      with
        foreign body S51.822 ☑
    right S51.811 ☑
      with
        foreign body S51.821 ☑
  forehead S01.81 ☑
    with foreign body S01.82 ☑
  fourchette O70.0
    with ectopic or molar pregnancy O08.6
    complicating delivery O70.0
    following ectopic or molar pregnancy O08.6
  gallbladder S36.123 ☑
  genital organs, external
    female S31.512 ☑
      with foreign body S31.522 ☑
      vagina — *see* Laceration, vagina
      vulva — *see* Laceration, vulva
    male S31.511 ☑
      with foreign body S31.521 ☑
      penis — *see* Laceration, penis
      scrotum — *see* Laceration, scrotum
      testis — *see* Laceration, testis
  groin — *see* Laceration, abdomen, wall
  gum — *see* Laceration, oral cavity
  hand S61.419 ☑
    with
      foreign body S61.429 ☑
    finger — *see* Laceration, finger
    left S61.412 ☑
      with
        foreign body S61.422 ☑
    right S61.411 ☑
      with
        foreign body S61.421 ☑
    thumb — *see* Laceration, thumb
  head S01.91 ☑
    with foreign body S01.92 ☑
    cheek — *see* Laceration, cheek
    ear — *see* Laceration, ear
    eyelid — *see* Laceration — eyelid
    lip — *see* Laceration, lip
    nose — *see* Laceration, nose
    oral cavity — *see* Laceration, oral cavity
    scalp S01.01 ☑
      with foreign body S01.02 ☑

Laceration — *continued*
  head — *continued*
    specified site NEC S01.81 ☑
      with foreign body S01.82 ☑
    temporomandibular area — *see* Laceration, cheek
  heart — *see* Injury, heart, laceration
  heel — *see* Laceration, foot
  hepatic duct S36.13 ☑
  hip S71.019 ☑
    with foreign body S71.029 ☑
    left S71.012 ☑
      with foreign body S71.022 ☑
    right S71.011 ☑
      with foreign body S71.021 ☑
  hymen — *see* Laceration, vagina
  hypochondrium — *see* Laceration, abdomen, wall
  hypogastric region — *see* Laceration, abdomen, wall
  ileum S36.438 ☑
  inguinal region — *see* Laceration, abdomen, wall
  instep — *see* Laceration, foot
  internal organ — *see* Injury, by site
  interscapular region — *see* Laceration, thorax, back
  intestine
    large
      colon S36.539 ☑
        ascending S36.530 ☑
        descending S36.532 ☑
        sigmoid S36.533 ☑
        specified site NEC S36.538 ☑
      rectum S36.63 ☑
      transverse S36.531 ☑
    small S36.439 ☑
      duodenum S36.430 ☑
      specified site NEC S36.438 ☑
  intra-abdominal organ S36.93 ☑
    intestine — *see* Laceration, intestine
    liver — *see* Laceration, liver
    pancreas — *see* Laceration, pancreas
    peritoneum S36.81 ☑
    specified site NEC S36.893 ☑
    spleen — *see* Laceration, spleen
    stomach — *see* Laceration, stomach
  intracranial NEC — *see also* Injury, intracranial, diffuse
    birth injury P10.9
  jaw — *see* Laceration, head, specified site NEC
  jejunum S36.438 ☑
  joint capsule — *see* Sprain, by site
  kidney S37.03- ☑
    major (greater than 3 cm) (massive) (stellate)
      S37.06- ☑
    minor (less than 1 cm) S37.04- ☑
    moderate (1 to 3 cm) S37.05- ☑
      multiple S37.06- ☑
  knee S81.01- ☑
    with foreign body S81.02- ☑
  labium (majus) (minus) — *see* Laceration, vulva
  lacrimal duct — *see* Laceration, eyelid
  large intestine — *see* Laceration, intestine, large
  larynx S11.011 ☑
    with foreign body S11.012 ☑
  leg (lower) S81.819 ☑
    with foreign body S81.829 ☑
    foot — *see* Laceration, foot
    knee — *see* Laceration, knee
    left S81.812 ☑
      with foreign body S81.822 ☑
    right S81.811 ☑
      with foreign body S81.821 ☑
    upper — *see* Laceration, thigh
  ligament — *see* Sprain
  lip S01.511 ☑
    with foreign body S01.521 ☑
  liver S36.113 ☑
    major (stellate) S36.116 ☑
    minor S36.114 ☑
    moderate S36.115 ☑
  loin — *see* Laceration, abdomen, wall
  lower back — *see* Laceration, back, lower
  lumbar region — *see* Laceration, back, lower
  lung S27.339 ☑
    bilateral S27.332 ☑
    unilateral S27.331 ☑
  malar region — *see* Laceration, head, specified site NEC
  mammary — *see* Laceration, breast
  mastoid region — *see* Laceration, head, specified site NEC

Laceration — *continued*
  meninges — *see* Injury, intracranial, diffuse
  meniscus — *see* Tear, meniscus
  mesentery S36.893 ☑
  mesosalpinx S37.893 ☑
  mouth — *see* Laceration, oral cavity
  muscle — *see* Injury, muscle, by site, laceration
  nail
    finger — *see* Laceration, finger, with damage to nail
    toe — *see* Laceration, toe, with damage to nail
  nasal (septum) (sinus) — *see* Laceration, nose
  nasopharynx — *see* Laceration, head, specified site NEC
  neck S11.91 ☑
    with foreign body S11.92 ☑
    involving
      cervical esophagus S11.21 ☑
        with foreign body S11.22 ☑
      larynx — *see* Laceration, larynx
      pharynx — *see* Laceration, pharynx
      thyroid gland — *see* Laceration, thyroid gland
      trachea — *see* Laceration, trachea
    specified site NEC S11.81 ☑
      with foreign body S11.82 ☑
  nerve — *see* Injury, nerve
  nose (septum) (sinus) S01.21 ☑
    with foreign body S01.22 ☑
  ocular NOS S05.3- ☑
    adnexa NOS S01.11- ☑
  oral cavity S01.512 ☑
    with foreign body S01.522 ☑
  orbit (eye) — *see* Wound, open, ocular, orbit
  ovary S37.439 ☑
    bilateral S37.432 ☑
    unilateral S37.431 ☑
  palate — *see* Laceration, oral cavity
  palm — *see* Laceration, hand
  pancreas S36.239 ☑
  pelvic S31.010 ☑
    with
      foreign body S31.020 ☑
        penetration into retroperitoneal cavity S31.021 ☑
      penetration into retroperitoneal cavity S31.011 ☑
    floor — *see also* Laceration, back, lower
      with ectopic or molar pregnancy O08.6
      complicating delivery O70.1
      following ectopic or molar pregnancy O08.6
      old (postpartal) N81.89
    organ S37.93 ☑
  penis S31.21 ☑
    with foreign body S31.22 ☑
  perineum
    female S31.41 ☑
      with
        ectopic or molar pregnancy O08.6
        foreign body S31.42 ☑
      during delivery O70.9
        first degree O70.0
        fourth degree O70.3
        second degree O70.1
        third degree — *see also* Delivery, complicated, by, laceration, perineum, third degree O70.20
      old (postpartal) N81.89
      postpartal N81.89
      secondary (postpartal) O90.1
    male S31.119 ☑
      with foreign body S31.129 ☑
  periocular area (with or without lacrimal passages) — *see* Laceration, eyelid
  peritoneum S36.893 ☑
  periumbilic region — *see* Laceration, abdomen, wall, periumbilic
  periurethral tissue — *see* Laceration, urethra
  phalanges
    finger — *see* Laceration, finger
    toe — *see* Laceration, toe
  pharynx S11.21 ☑
    with foreign body S11.22 ☑
  pinna — *see* Laceration, ear
  popliteal space — *see* Laceration, knee
  prepuce — *see* Laceration, penis
  prostate S37.823 ☑
  pubic region S31.119 ☑
    with foreign body S31.129 ☑

Laceration — *continued*
pudendum — *see* Laceration, genital organs, external
rectovaginal septum — *see* Laceration, vagina
rectum S36.63 ☑
retroperitoneum S36.893 ☑
round ligament S37.893 ☑
sacral region — *see* Laceration, back, lower
sacroiliac region — *see* Laceration, back, lower
salivary gland — *see* Laceration, oral cavity
scalp S01.01 ☑
　with foreign body S01.02 ☑
scapular region — *see* Laceration, shoulder
scrotum S31.31 ☑
　with foreign body S31.32 ☑
seminal vesicle S37.893 ☑
shin — *see* Laceration, leg
shoulder S41.019 ☑
　with foreign body S41.029 ☑
　left S41.012 ☑
　　with foreign body S41.022 ☑
　right S41.011 ☑
　　with foreign body S41.021 ☑
small intestine — *see* Laceration, intestine, small
spermatic cord — *see* Laceration, testis
spinal cord (meninges) — *see also* Injury, spinal cord, by region
　due to injury at birth P11.5
　newborn (birth injury) P11.5
spleen S36.039 ☑
　major (massive) (stellate) S36.032 ☑
　moderate S36.031 ☑
　superficial (minor) S36.030 ☑
sternal region — *see* Laceration, thorax, front
stomach S36.33 ☑
submaxillary region — *see* Laceration, head, specified site NEC
submental region — *see* Laceration, head, specified site NEC
subungual
　finger(s) — *see* Laceration, finger, with damage to nail
　toe(s) — *see* Laceration, toe, with damage to nail
suprarenal gland — *see* Laceration, adrenal gland
temple, temporal region — *see* Laceration, head, specified site NEC
temporomandibular area — *see* Laceration, cheek
tendon — *see* Injury, muscle, by site, laceration
　Achilles S86.02- ☑
tentorium cerebelli — *see* Injury, intracranial, diffuse
testis S31.31 ☑
　with foreign body S31.32 ☑
thigh S71.11- ☑
　with foreign body S71.12- ☑
thorax, thoracic (wall) S21.91 ☑
　with foreign body S21.92 ☑
　　back S21.22- ☑
　　　with penetration into thoracic cavity S21.42- ☑
　　front S21.12- ☑
　　　with penetration into thoracic cavity S21.32- ☑
　　back S21.21- ☑
　　　with
　　　　foreign body S21.22- ☑
　　　　　with penetration into thoracic cavity S21.42- ☑
　　　　penetration into thoracic cavity S21.41- ☑
　　breast — *see* Laceration, breast
　　front S21.11- ☑
　　　with
　　　　foreign body S21.12- ☑
　　　　　with penetration into thoracic cavity S21.32- ☑
　　　　penetration into thoracic cavity S21.31- ☑
thumb S61.019 ☑
　with
　　damage to nail S61.119 ☑
　　　with
　　　　foreign body S61.129 ☑
　　foreign body S61.029 ☑
　left S61.012 ☑
　　with
　　　damage to nail S61.112 ☑
　　　　with
　　　　　foreign body S61.122 ☑
　　　foreign body S61.022 ☑

Laceration — *continued*
thumb — *continued*
　right S61.011 ☑
　　with
　　　damage to nail S61.111 ☑
　　　　with
　　　　　foreign body S61.121 ☑
　　　foreign body S61.021 ☑
thyroid gland S11.11 ☑
　with foreign body S11.12 ☑
toe(s) S91.119 ☑
　with
　　damage to nail S91.219 ☑
　　　with
　　　　foreign body S91.229 ☑
　　foreign body S91.129 ☑
　great S91.113 ☑
　　with
　　　damage to nail S91.213 ☑
　　　　with
　　　　　foreign body S91.223 ☑
　　　foreign body S91.123 ☑
　　left S91.112 ☑
　　　with
　　　　damage to nail S91.212 ☑
　　　　　with
　　　　　　foreign body S91.222 ☑
　　　　foreign body S91.122 ☑
　　right S91.111 ☑
　　　with
　　　　damage to nail S91.211 ☑
　　　　　with
　　　　　　foreign body S91.221 ☑
　　　　foreign body S91.121 ☑
　lesser S91.116 ☑
　　with
　　　damage to nail S91.216 ☑
　　　　with
　　　　　foreign body S91.226 ☑
　　foreign body S91.126 ☑
　　left S91.115 ☑
　　　with
　　　　damage to nail S91.215 ☑
　　　　　with
　　　　　　foreign body S91.225 ☑
　　　　foreign body S91.125 ☑
　　right S91.114 ☑
　　　with
　　　　damage to nail S91.214 ☑
　　　　　with
　　　　　　foreign body S91.224 ☑
　　　　foreign body S91.124 ☑
tongue — *see* Laceration, oral cavity
trachea S11.021 ☑
　with foreign body S11.022 ☑
tunica vaginalis — *see* Laceration, testis
tympanum, tympanic membrane — *see* Laceration, ear, drum
umbilical region S31.115 ☑
　with foreign body S31.125 ☑
ureter S37.13 ☑
urethra S37.33 ☑
　with or following ectopic or molar pregnancy O08.6
　obstetrical trauma O71.5
urinary organ NEC S37.893 ☑
uterus S37.63 ☑
　with ectopic or molar pregnancy O08.6
　following ectopic or molar pregnancy O08.6
　nonpuerperal, nontraumatic N85.8
　obstetrical trauma NEC O71.81
　old (postpartal) N85.8
uvula — *see* Laceration, oral cavity
vagina S31.41 ☑
　with
　　ectopic or molar pregnancy O08.6
　　foreign body S31.42 ☑
　during delivery O71.4
　　with perineal laceration — *see* Laceration, perineum, female, during delivery
　following ectopic or molar pregnancy O08.6
　nonpuerperal, nontraumatic N89.8
　old (postpartal) N89.8
vas deferens S37.893 ☑
vesical — *see* Laceration, bladder
vocal cords S11.031 ☑
　with foreign body S11.032 ☑
vulva S31.41 ☑

Laceration — *continued*
vulva — *continued*
　with
　　ectopic or molar pregnancy O08.6
　　foreign body S31.42 ☑
　complicating delivery O70.0
　following ectopic or molar pregnancy O08.6
　nonpuerperal, nontraumatic N90.89
　old (postpartal) N90.89
wrist S61.519 ☑
　with
　　foreign body S61.529 ☑
　left S61.512 ☑
　　with
　　　foreign body S61.522 ☑
　right S61.511 ☑
　　with
　　　foreign body S61.521 ☑
Lack of
achievement in school Z55.3
adequate
　food Z59.48
　intermaxillary vertical dimension of fully erupted teeth M26.36
　sleep Z72.820
appetite (see Anorexia) R63.0
awareness R41.9
care
　in home Z74.2
　of infant (at or after birth) T76.02 ☑
　　confirmed T74.02 ☑
cognitive functions R41.9
coordination R27.9
　ataxia R27.0
　specified type NEC R27.8
development (physiological) R62.50
　failure to thrive (child over 28 days old) R62.51
　　adult R62.7
　　newborn P92.6
　short stature R62.52
　specified type NEC R62.59
energy R53.83
financial resources Z59.6
food Z59.48
growth R62.52
heating Z59.1
housing (permanent) (temporary) Z59.00
　adequate Z59.1
learning experiences in childhood Z62.898
leisure time (affecting life-style) Z73.2
material resources Z59.87
memory — *see also* Amnesia
　mild, following organic brain damage F06.8
ovulation N97.0
parental supervision or control of child Z62.0
person able to render necessary care Z74.2
physical exercise Z72.3
play experience in childhood Z62.898
posterior occlusal support M26.57
relaxation (affecting life-style) Z73.2
safe drinking water Z58.6
sexual
　desire F52.0
　enjoyment F52.1
shelter Z59.02
sleep (adequate) Z72.820
supervision of child by parent Z62.0
support, posterior occlusal M26.57
transportation Z59.82
water T73.1 ☑
　safe drinking Z58.6
Lacrimal — *see* condition
Lacrimation, abnormal — *see* Epiphora
Lacrimonasal duct — *see* condition
Lactation, lactating (breast) (puerperal, postpartum)
associated
　cracked nipple O92.13
　retracted nipple O92.03
defective O92.4
disorder NEC O92.79
excessive O92.6
failed (complete) O92.3
　partial O92.4
mastitis NEC — *see* Mastitis, obstetric
mother (care and/or examination) Z39.1
nonpuerperal N64.3
Lacticemia, excessive — *see also* Acidosis E87.20
Lacunar skull Q75.8

☑ Additional Character Required — Refer to the Tabular List for Character Selection

Laennec's cirrhosis K70.30
  with ascites K70.31
  nonalcoholic K74.69
Lafora's disease — *see* Epilepsy, generalized, idiopathic
Lag, lid (nervous) — *see* Retraction, lid
Lagophthalmos (eyelid) (nervous) H02.209
  bilateral, upper and lower eyelids H02.20C
  cicatricial H02.219
    bilateral, upper and lower eyelids H02.21C
    left H02.216
      lower H02.215
      upper H02.214
      upper and lower eyelids H02.21B
    right H02.213
      lower H02.212
      upper H02.211
      upper and lower eyelids H02.21A
  keratoconjunctivitis — *see* Keratoconjunctivitis
  left H02.206
    lower H02.205
    upper H02.204
    upper and lower eyelids H02.20B
  mechanical H02.229
    bilateral, upper and lower eyelids H02.22C
    left H02.226
      lower H02.225
      upper H02.224
      upper and lower eyelids H02.22B
    right H02.223
      lower H02.222
      upper H02.221
      upper and lower eyelids H02.22A
  paralytic H02.239
    bilateral, upper and lower eyelids H02.23C
    left H02.236
      lower H02.235
      upper H02.234
      upper and lower eyelids H02.23B
    right H02.233
      lower H02.232
      upper H02.231
      upper and lower eyelids H02.23A
  right H02.203
    lower H02.202
    upper H02.201
    upper and lower eyelids H02.20A
Laki-Lorand factor deficiency — *see* Defect, coagulation, specified type NEC
Lalling F80.0
Lambert-Eaton syndrome — *see* Syndrome, Lambert-Eaton
Lambliasis, lambliosis A07.1
Landau-Kleffner syndrome — *see* Epilepsy, specified NEC
Landouzy-Déjérine dystrophy or facioscapulohumeral atrophy G71.02
Landouzy's disease (icterohemorrhagic leptospirosis) A27.0
Landry-Guillain-Barré, syndrome or paralysis G61.0
Landry's disease or paralysis G61.0
Lane's
  band Q43.3
  kink — *see* Obstruction, intestine
  syndrome K90.2
Langdon Down syndrome — *see* Trisomy, 21
Lapsed immunization schedule status Z28.39
Large
  baby (regardless of gestational age) (4000g to 4499g) P08.1
  ear, congenital Q17.1
  physiological cup Q14.2
  stature R68.89
Large-for-dates NEC (infant) (4000g to 4499g) P08.1
  affecting management of pregnancy O36.6- ☑
  exceptionally (4500g or more) P08.0
Larsen-Johansson disease orosteochondrosis — *see* Osteochondrosis, juvenile, patella
Larsen's syndrome (flattened facies and multiple congenital dislocations) Q74.8
Larva migrans
  cutaneous B76.9
    Ancylostoma B76.0
  visceral B83.0
Laryngeal — *see* condition
Laryngismus (stridulus) J38.5
  congenital P28.89
  diphtheritic A36.2

Laryngitis (acute) (edematous) (fibrinous) (infective) (infiltrative) (malignant) (membranous) (phlegmonous) (pneumococcal) (pseudomembranous) (septic) (subglottic) (suppurative) (ulcerative) J04.0
  with
    influenza, flu, or grippe — *see* Influenza, with, laryngitis
    tracheitis (acute) — *see* Laryngotracheitis
  atrophic J37.0
  catarrhal J37.0
  chronic J37.0
    with tracheitis (chronic) J37.1
  diphtheritic A36.2
  due to external agent — *see* Inflammation, respiratory, upper, due to
  H. influenzae J04.0
  Hemophilus influenzae J04.0
  hypertrophic J37.0
  influenzal — *see* Influenza, with, respiratory manifestations NEC
  obstructive J05.0
  sicca J37.0
  spasmodic J05.0
    acute J04.0
  streptococcal J04.0
  stridulous J05.0
  syphilitic (late) A52.73
    congenital A50.59 *[J99]*
      early A50.03 *[J99]*
  tuberculous A15.5
  Vincent's A69.1
Laryngocele (congenital) (ventricular) Q31.3
Laryngofissure J38.7
  congenital Q31.8
Laryngomalacia (congenital) Q31.5
Laryngopharyngitis (acute) J06.0
  chronic J37.0
  due to external agent — *see* Inflammation, respiratory, upper, due to
Laryngoplegia J38.00
  bilateral J38.02
  unilateral J38.01
Laryngoptosis J38.7
Laryngospasm J38.5
Laryngostenosis J38.6
Laryngotracheitis (acute) (Infectional) (infective) (viral) J04.2
  atrophic J37.1
  catarrhal J37.1
  chronic J37.1
  diphtheritic A36.2
  due to external agent — *see* Inflammation, respiratory, upper, due to
  Hemophilus influenzae J04.2
  hypertrophic J37.1
  influenzal — *see* Influenza, with, respiratory manifestations NEC
  pachydermic J38.7
  sicca J37.1
  spasmodic J38.5
    acute J05.0
  streptococcal J04.2
  stridulous J38.5
  syphilitic (late) A52.73
    congenital A50.59 *[J99]*
      early A50.03 *[J99]*
  tuberculous A15.5
  Vincent's A69.1
Laryngotracheobronchitis — *see* Bronchitis
Larynx, laryngeal — *see* condition
Lassa fever A96.2
Lassitude — *see* Weakness
Late
  talker R62.0
  walker R62.0
Late effect(s) — *see* Sequelae
Latent — *see* condition
Laterocession — *see* Lateroversion
Lateroflexion — *see* Lateroversion
Lateroversion
  cervix — *see* Lateroversion, uterus
  uterus, uterine (cervix) (postinfectional) (postpartal, old) N85.4
    congenital Q51.818
    in pregnancy or childbirth O34.59- ☑
Lathyrism — *see* Poisoning, food, noxious, plant
Launois' syndrome (pituitary gigantism) E22.0
Launois-Bensaude adenolipomatosis E88.89

Laurence-Moon (-Bardet)-**Biedl syndrome** Q87.89
Lax, laxity — *see also* Relaxation
  ligament (ous) — *see also* Disorder, ligament
    familial M35.7
    knee — *see* Derangement, knee
  skin (acquired) L57.4
    congenital Q82.8
Laxative habit F55.2
Lazy leukocyte syndrome D70.8
Lead miner's lung J63.6
Leak, leakage
  air NEC J93.82
    postprocedural J95.812
  amniotic fluid — *see* Rupture, membranes, premature
  blood (microscopic), fetal, into maternal circulation affecting management of pregnancy — *see* Pregnancy, complicated by
  cerebrospinal fluid G96.00
    cranial
      postoperative G96.08
      specified NEC G96.08
      spontaneous G96.01
      traumatic G96.08
    from spinal (lumbar) puncture G97.0
    spinal
      postoperative G96.09
      post-traumatic G96.09
      specified NEC G96.09
      spontaneous G96.02
    spontaneous
      from
        skull base G96.01
        spine G96.02
  CSF — *see* Leak, cerebrospinal fluid
  device, implant or graft — *see also* Complications, by site and type, mechanical
    arterial graft NEC — *see* Complication vascular, graft, mechanical, leakage T82.838 ☑
    breast (implant) T85.43 ☑
    catheter NEC T85.638 ☑
      dialysis (renal) T82.43 ☑
        intraperitoneal T85.631 ☑
      infusion NEC T82.534 ☑
        spinal (epidural) (subdural) T85.630 ☑
      urinary T83.038 ☑
        cystostomy T83.030 ☑
        Hopkins T83.038 ☑
        ileostomy T83.038 ☑
        indwelling T83.031 ☑
        nephrostomy T83.032 ☑
        specified T83.038 ☑
        urostomy T83.038 ☑
    gastrointestinal — *see* Complications, prosthetic device, mechanical, gastrointestinal device
    genital NEC T83.498 ☑
      penile prosthesis (cylinder) (implanted) (pump) (reservoir) T83.490 ☑
      testicular prosthesis T83.491 ☑
    heart NEC — *see* Complication, cardiovascular device, mechanical
    joint prosthesis — *see* Complications, joint prosthesis, mechanical, specified NEC, by site
    ocular NEC — *see* Complications, prosthetic device, mechanical, ocular device
    orthopedic NEC — *see* Complication, orthopedic, device, mechanical
    persistent air J93.82
    specified NEC T85.638 ☑
    urinary NEC — *see also* Complication, genitourinary, device, urinary, mechanical
      graft T83.23 ☑
    vascular NEC — *see* Complication, cardiovascular device, mechanical
    ventricular intracranial shunt T85.03 ☑
  urine — *see* Incontinence
Leaky heart — *see* Endocarditis
Learning defect (specific) F81.9
Leather bottle stomach C16.9
Leber's
  congenital amaurosis H35.50
  optic atrophy (hereditary) H47.22
Lederer's anemia D59.19
Leeches (external) — *see* Hirudiniasis
Leg — *see* condition
Legg (-Calvé)-**Perthes disease, syndrome or osteochondrosis** M91.1- ☑
Legionellosis A48.1

Legionellosis — *continued*
  nonpneumonic A48.2
Legionnaires'
  disease A48.1
    nonpneumonic A48.2
  pneumonia A48.1
Leigh's disease G31.82
Leiner's disease L21.1
Leiofibromyoma — *see* Leiomyoma
Leiomyoblastoma — *see* Neoplasm, connective tissue, benign
Leiomyofibroma — *see also* Neoplasm, connective tissue, benign
  uterus (cervix) (corpus) D25.9
Leiomyoma — *see also* Neoplasm, connective tissue, benign
  bizarre — *see* Neoplasm, connective tissue, benign
  cellular — *see* Neoplasm, connective tissue, benign
  epithelioid — *see* Neoplasm, connective tissue, benign
  uterus (cervix) (corpus) D25.9
    intramural D25.1
    submucous D25.0
    subserosal D25.2
  vascular — *see* Neoplasm, connective tissue, benign
Leiomyoma, leiomyomatosis (intravascular) — *see* Neoplasm, connective tissue, uncertain behavior
Leiomyosarcoma — *see also* Neoplasm, connective tissue, malignant
  epithelioid — *see* Neoplasm, connective tissue, malignant
  myxoid — *see* Neoplasm, connective tissue, malignant
Leishmaniasis B55.9
  American (mucocutaneous) B55.2
    cutaneous B55.1
  Asian Desert B55.1
  Brazilian B55.2
  cutaneous (any type) B55.1
  dermal — *see also* Leishmaniasis, cutaneous
    post-kala-azar B55.0
  eyelid B55.1
  infantile B55.0
  Mediterranean B55.0
  mucocutaneous (American) (New World) B55.2
  naso-oral B55.2
  nasopharyngeal B55.2
  old world B55.1
  tegumentaria diffusa B55.1
  visceral B55.0
Leishmanoid, dermal — *see also* Leishmaniasis, cutaneous
  post-kala-azar B55.0
Lenegre's disease I44.2
Lengthening, leg — *see* Deformity, limb, unequal length
Lennert's lymphoma — *see* Lymphoma, Lennert's
Lennox-Gastaut syndrome G40.812
  intractable G40.814
    with status epilepticus G40.813
    without status epilepticus G40.814
  not intractable G40.812
    with status epilepticus G40.811
    without status epilepticus G40.812
Lens — *see* condition
Lenticonus (anterior) (posterior) (congenital) Q12.8
Lenticular degeneration, progressive E83.01
Lentiglobus (posterior) (congenital) Q12.8
Lentigo (congenital) L81.4
  maligna — *see also* Melanoma, in situ
    melanoma — *see* Melanoma
Lentivirus, as cause of disease classified elsewhere B97.31
Leontiasis
  ossium M85.2
  syphilitic (late) A52.78
    congenital A50.59
Lepothrix A48.8
Lepra — *see* Leprosy
Leprechaunism E34.8
Leprosy A30.- ☑
  with muscle disorder A30.9 [M63.80]
    ankle A30.9 [M63.87-] ☑
    foot A30.9 [M63.87-] ☑
    forearm A30.9 [M63.83-] ☑
    hand A30.9 [M63.84-] ☑
    lower leg A30.9 [M63.86-] ☑
    multiple sites A30.9 [M63.89]
    pelvic region A30.9 [M63.85-] ☑
    shoulder region A30.9 [M63.81-] ☑

Leprosy — *continued*
  with muscle disorder — *continued*
    specified site NEC A30.9 [M63.88]
      thigh A30.9 [M63.85-] ☑
      upper arm A30.9 [M63.82-] ☑
  anesthetic A30.9
  BB A30.3
  BL A30.4
  borderline (infiltrated) (neuritic) A30.3
    lepromatous A30.4
    tuberculoid A30.2
  BT A30.2
  dimorphous (infiltrated) (neuritic) A30.3
  I A30.0
  indeterminate (macular) (neuritic) A30.0
  lepromatous (diffuse) (infiltrated) (macular) (neuritic) (nodular) A30.5
  LL A30.5
  macular (early) (neuritic) (simple) A30.9
  maculoanesthetic A30.9
  mixed A30.3
  neural A30.9
  nodular A30.5
  primary neuritic A30.3
  specified type NEC A30.8
  TT A30.1
  tuberculoid (major) (minor) A30.1
Leptocytosis, hereditary D56.9
Leptomeningitis (chronic) (circumscribed) (hemorrhagic) (nonsuppurative) — *see* Meningitis
Leptomeningopathy G96.198
Leptospiral — *see* condition
Leptospirochetal — *see* condition
Leptospirosis A27.9
  canicola A27.89
  due to Leptospira interrogans serovar icterohaemorrhagiae A27.0
  icterohemorrhagica A27.0
  pomona A27.89
  Weil's disease A27.0
Leptus dermatitis B88.0
Leriche's syndrome (aortic bifurcation occlusion) I74.09
Leri's pleonosteosis Q78.8
Leri-Weill syndrome Q77.8
Lermoyez' syndrome — *see* Vertigo, peripheral NEC
Lesch-Nyhan syndrome E79.1
Leser-Trélat disease L82.1
  inflamed L82.0
Lesion(s) (nontraumatic)
  abducens nerve — *see* Strabismus, paralytic, sixth nerve
  alveolar process K08.9
  angiocentric immunoproliferative D47.Z9 (*following* D47.4)
  anorectal K62.9
  aortic (valve) I35.9
  auditory nerve — *see* subcategory H93.3 ☑
  basal ganglion G25.9
  bile duct — *see* Disease, bile duct
  biomechanical M99.9
    specified type NEC M99.89
      abdomen M99.89
      acromioclavicular M99.87
      cervical region M99.81
      cervicothoracic M99.81
      costochondral M99.88
      costovertebral M99.88
      head region M99.80
      hip M99.85
      lower extremity M99.86
      lumbar region M99.83
      lumbosacral M99.83
      occipitocervical M99.80
      pelvic region M99.85
      pubic M99.85
      rib cage M99.88
      sacral region M99.84
      sacrococcygeal M99.84
      sacroiliac M99.84
      specified NEC M99.89
      sternochondral M99.88
      sternoclavicular M99.87
      thoracic region M99.82
      thoracolumbar M99.82
      upper extremity M99.87
  bladder N32.9
  bone — *see* Disorder, bone
  brachial plexus G54.0
  brain G93.9

Lesion(s) — *continued*
  brain — *continued*
    congenital Q04.9
    vascular I67.9
      degenerative I67.9
      hypertensive I67.4
  buccal cavity K13.79
  calcified — *see* Calcification
  canthus — *see* Disorder, eyelid
  carate — *see* Pinta, lesions
  cardia K31.9
  cardiac — *see also* Disease, heart I51.9
    congenital Q24.9
    valvular — *see* Endocarditis
  cauda equina G83.4
  cecum K63.9
  cerebral — *see* Lesion, brain
  cerebrovascular I67.9
    degenerative I67.9
    hypertensive I67.4
  cervical (nerve) root NEC G54.2
  chiasmal — *see* Disorder, optic, chiasm
  chorda tympani G51.8
  coin, lung R91.1
  colon K63.9
  combined periodontic - endodontic K05.5
  congenital — *see* Anomaly, by site
  conjunctiva H11.9
  conus medullaris — *see* Injury, conus medullaris
  coronary artery — *see* Ischemia, heart
  cranial nerve G52.9
    eighth — *see* Disorder, ear
    eleventh G52.9
    fifth G50.9
    first G52.0
    fourth — *see* Strabismus, paralytic, fourth nerve
    seventh G51.9
    sixth — *see* Strabismus, paralytic, sixth nerve
    tenth G52.2
    twelfth G52.3
  cystic — *see* Cyst
  degenerative — *see* Degeneration
  duodenum K31.9
  edentulous (alveolar) ridge, associated with trauma, due to traumatic occlusion K06.2
  en coup de sabre L94.1
  eyelid — *see* Disorder, eyelid
  gasserian ganglion G50.8
  gastric K31.9
  gastroduodenal K31.9
  gastrointestinal K63.9
  gingiva, associated with trauma K06.2
  glomerular
    focal and segmental — *see also* N00-N07 with fourth character .1 N05.1
    minimal change — *see also* N00-N07 with fourth character .0 N05.0
  heart (organic) — *see* Disease, heart
  hyperchromic, due to pinta (carate) A67.1
  hyperkeratotic — *see* Hyperkeratosis
  hypothalamic E23.7
  ileocecal K63.9
  ileum K63.9
  iliohypogastric nerve G57.8- ☑
  inflammatory — *see* Inflammation
  intestine K63.9
  intracerebral — *see* Lesion, brain
  intrachiasmal (optic) — *see* Disorder, optic, chiasm
  intracranial, space-occupying R90.0
  joint — *see* Disorder, joint
    sacroiliac (old) M53.3
  keratotic — *see* Keratosis
  kidney — *see* Disease, renal
  laryngeal nerve (recurrent) G52.2
  lip K13.0
  liver K76.9
  lumbosacral
    plexus G54.1
    root (nerve) NEC G54.4
  lung (coin) R91.1
  maxillary sinus J32.0
  mitral I05.9
  Morel-Lavallée — *see* Hematoma, by site
  motor cortex NEC G93.89
  mouth K13.79
  nerve G58.9
    femoral G57.2- ☑
    median G56.1- ☑

Lesion(s) — *continued*
 nerve — *continued*
  median — *continued*
   carpal tunnel syndrome — *see* Syndrome, carpal tunnel
  plantar G57.6- ☑
  popliteal (lateral) G57.3- ☑
   medial G57.4- ☑
  radial G56.3- ☑
  sciatic G57.0- ☑
  spinal — *see* Injury, nerve, spinal
  ulnar G56.2- ☑
 nervous system, congenital Q07.9
 nonallopathic — *see* Lesion, biomechanical
 nose (internal) J34.89
 obstructive — *see* Obstruction
 obturator nerve G57.8- ☑
 oral mucosa K13.70
 organ or site NEC — *see* Disease, by site
 osteolytic — *see* Osteolysis
 peptic K27.9
 periodontal, due to traumatic occlusion K05.5
 pharynx J39.2
 pigment, pigmented (skin) L81.9
 pinta — *see* Pinta, lesions
 polypoid — *see* Polyp
 prechiasmal (optic) — *see* Disorder, optic, chiasm
 primary — *see also* Syphilis, primary A51.0
  carate A67.0
  pinta A67.0
  yaws A66.0
 pulmonary J98.4
  valve I37.9
 pylorus K31.9
 rectosigmoid K63.9
 retina, retinal H35.9
 sacroiliac (joint) (old) M53.3
 salivary gland K11.9
  benign lymphoepithelial K11.8
 saphenous nerve G57.8- ☑
 sciatic nerve G57.0- ☑
 secondary — *see* Syphilis, secondary
 shoulder (region) M75.9- ☑
  specified NEC M75.8- ☑
 sigmoid K63.9
 sinus (accessory) (nasal) J34.89
 skin L98.9
  suppurative L08.0
 SLAP S43.43- ☑
 spinal cord G95.9
  congenital Q06.9
 spleen D73.89
 stomach K31.9
 superior glenoid labrum S43.43- ☑
 syphilitic — *see* Syphilis
 tertiary — *see* Syphilis, tertiary
 thoracic root (nerve) NEC G54.3
 tonsillar fossa J35.9
 tooth, teeth K08.9
  white spot
   chewing surface K02.51
   pit and fissure surface K02.51
   smooth surface K02.61
 traumatic — *see* specific type of injury by site
 tricuspid (valve) I07.9
  nonrheumatic I36.9
 trigeminal nerve G50.9
 ulcerated or ulcerative — *see* Ulcer, skin
 uterus N85.9
 vagina N89.8
 vagus nerve G52.2
 valvular — *see* Endocarditis
 vascular I99.9
  affecting central nervous system I67.9
  following trauma NEC T14.8 ☑
  umbilical cord, complicating delivery O69.5 ☑
 vulva N90.89
 warty — *see* Verruca
 white spot (tooth)
  chewing surface K02.51
  pit and fissure surface K02.51
  smooth surface K02.61
Less than a high school diploma Z55.5
Lethargic — *see* condition
Lethargy R53.83
Letterer-Siwe's disease C96.0
Leukemia, leukemic C95.9- ☑

Leukemia, leukemic — *continued*
 acute basophilic C94.8- ☑
 acute bilineal C95.0- ☑
 acute erythroid C94.0- ☑
 acute lymphoblastic C91.0- ☑
 acute megakaryoblastic C94.2- ☑
 acute megakaryocytic C94.2- ☑
 acute mixed lineage C95.0- ☑
 acute monoblastic (monoblastic/monocytic) C93.0- ☑
 acute monocytic (monoblastic/monocytic) C93.0- ☑
 acute myeloblastic (minimal differentiation) (with maturation) C92.0- ☑
 acute myeloid, NOS C92.0- ☑
  with
   11q23-abnormality C92.6- ☑
   dysplasia of remaining hematopoesis and/or myelodysplastic disease in its history C92.A- ☑ (*following* C92.6)
   multilineage dysplasia C92.A- ☑ (*following* C92.6)
   variation of MLL-gene C92.6- ☑
  M6 (a)(b) C94.0- ☑
  M7 C94.2- ☑
 acute myelomonocytic C92.5- ☑
 acute promyelocytic C92.4- ☑
 adult T-cell (HTLV-1-associated) (acute variant) (chronic variant) (lymphomatoid variant) (smouldering variant) C91.5- ☑
 aggressive NK-cell C94.8- ☑
 AML (1/ETO) (M0) (M1) (M2) (without a FAB classification) C92.0- ☑
 AML M3 C92.4- ☑
 AML M4 (Eo with inv(16) or t(16;16)) C92.5- ☑
 AML M5 C93.0- ☑
 AML M5a C93.0- ☑
 AML M5b C93.0- ☑
 AML Me with t (15;17) and variants C92.4- ☑
 atypical chronic myeloid, BCR/ABL-negative C92.2- ☑
 biphenotypic acute C95.0- ☑
 blast cell C95.0- ☑
 Burkitt-type, mature B-cell C91.A- ☑ (*following* C91.6)
 chronic eosinophilic — *see also* Syndrome, hypereosinophilic, myeloid C94.8- ☑
 chronic lymphocytic, of B-cell type C91.1- ☑
 chronic monocytic C93.1- ☑
 chronic myelogenous (Philadelphia chromosome (Ph1) positive) (t(9;22)) (q34;q11) (with crisis of blast cells) C92.1- ☑
 chronic myeloid, BCR/ABL-positive C92.1- ☑
  atypical, BCR/ABL-negative C92.2- ☑
 chronic myelomonocytic C93.1- ☑
 chronic neutrophilic D47.1
 CMML (-1) (-2) (with eosinophilia) C93.1- ☑
 granulocytic — *see also* Category C92 C92.9- ☑
 hairy cell C91.4- ☑
 juvenile myelomonocytic C93.3- ☑
 lymphoid C91.9- ☑
  specified NEC C91.Z- ☑ (*following* C91.6)
 mast cell C94.3- ☑
 mature B-cell, Burkitt-type C91.A- ☑ (*following* C91.6)
 monocytic (subacute) C93.9- ☑
  specified NEC C93.Z- ☑ (*following* C93.3)
 myelogenous — *see also* Category C92 C92.9- ☑
 myeloid C92.9- ☑
  specified NEC C92.Z- ☑ (*following* C92.6)
 plasma cell C90.1- ☑
 plasmacytic C90.1- ☑
 prolymphocytic
  of B-cell type C91.3- ☑
  of T-cell type C91.6- ☑
 specified NEC C94.8- ☑
 stem cell, of unclear lineage C95.0- ☑
 subacute lymphocytic C91.9- ☑
 T-cell large granular lymphocytic C91.Z- ☑ (*following* C91.6)
 unspecified cell type C95.9- ☑
  acute C95.0- ☑
  chronic C95.1- ☑
Leukemoid reaction — *see also* Reaction, leukemoid D72.823
Leukoaraiosis (hypertensive) I67.81
Leukoariosis — *see* Leukoaraiosis
Leukocoria — *see* Disorder, globe, degenerated condition, leucocoria
Leukocytopenia D72.819
Leukocytosis D72.829

Leukocytosis — *continued*
 eosinophilic D72.19
Leukoderma, leukodermia NEC L81.5
 syphilitic A51.39
  late A52.79
Leukodystrophy E75.29
Leukoedema, oral epithelium K13.29
Leukoencephalitis G04.81
 acute (subacute) hemorrhagic G36.1
  postimmunization or postvaccinal G04.02
 postinfectious G04.01
 subacute sclerosing A81.1
 van Bogaert's (sclerosing) A81.1
Leukoencephalopathy — *see also* Encephalopathy G93.49
 Binswanger's I67.3
 heroin vapor G92.8
 metachromatic E75.25
 multifocal (progressive) A81.2
 postimmunization and postvaccinal G04.02
 progressive multifocal A81.2
 reversible, posterior G93.6
 van Bogaert's (sclerosing) A81.1
 vascular, progressive I67.3
Leukoerythroblastosis D75.9
Leukokeratosis — *see also* Leukoplakia
 mouth K13.21
 nicotina palati K13.24
 oral mucosa K13.21
 tongue K13.21
 vocal cord J38.3
Leukokraurosis vulva (e) N90.4
Leukoma (cornea) — *see also* Opacity, cornea
 adherent H17.0- ☑
 interfering with central vision — *see* Opacity, cornea, central
Leukomalacia, cerebral, newborn P91.2
 periventricular P91.2
Leukomelanopathy, hereditary D72.0
Leukonychia (punctata) (striata) L60.8
 congenital Q84.4
Leukopathia unguium L60.8
 congenital Q84.4
Leukopenia D72.819
 basophilic D72.818
 chemotherapy (cancer) induced D70.1
 congenital D70.0
 cyclic D70.0
 drug induced NEC D70.2
  due to cytoreductive cancer chemotherapy D70.1
 eosinophilic D72.818
 familial D70.0
 infantile genetic D70.0
 malignant D70.9
 periodic D70.0
 transitory neonatal P61.5
Leukopenic — *see* condition
Leukoplakia
 anus K62.89
 bladder (postinfectional) N32.89
 buccal K13.21
 cervix (uteri) N88.0
 esophagus K22.89
 gingiva K13.21
 hairy (oral mucosa) (tongue) K13.3
 kidney (pelvis) N28.89
 larynx J38.7
 lip K13.21
 mouth K13.21
 oral epithelium, including tongue (mucosa) K13.21
 palate K13.21
 pelvis (kidney) N28.89
 penis (infectional) N48.0
 rectum K62.89
 syphilitic (late) A52.79
 tongue K13.21
 ureter (postinfectional) N28.89
 urethra (postinfectional) N36.8
 uterus N85.8
 vagina N89.4
 vocal cord J38.3
 vulva N90.4
Leukorrhea N89.8
 due to Trichomonas (vaginalis) A59.00
 trichomonal A59.00
Leukosarcoma C85.9- ☑
Levocardia (isolated) Q24.1
 with situs inversus Q89.3

Levotransposition Q20.5
Lev's disease or syndrome (acquired complete heart block) I44.2
Levulosuria — *see* Fructosuria
Levurid L30.2
Lewy body (ies) (disease) G31.83
Leyden-Möbius dystrophy — *see* Dystrophy, Leyden-Möbius
Leydig cell
 carcinoma
  specified site — *see* Neoplasm, malignant, by site
  unspecified site
   female C56.9
   male C62.9- ☑
 tumor
  benign
   specified site — *see* Neoplasm, benign, by site
   unspecified site
    female D27.- ☑
    male D29.2- ☑
  malignant
   specified site — *see* Neoplasm, malignant, by site
   unspecified site
    female C56.- ☑
    male C62.9- ☑
  specified site — *see* Neoplasm, uncertain behavior, by site
  unspecified site
   female D39.1- ☑
   male D40.1- ☑
Leydig-Sertoli cell tumor
 specified site — *see* Neoplasm, benign, by site
 unspecified site
  female D27.- ☑
  male D29.2- ☑
LGMD — *see* Dystrophy, muscular, limb-girdle
LGSIL (Low grade squamous intraepithelial lesion on cytologic smear of)
 anus R85.612
 cervix R87.612
 vagina R87.622
Liar, pathologic F60.2
Libido
 decreased R68.82
Libman-Sacks disease M32.11
Lice (infestation) B85.2
 body (Pediculus corporis) B85.1
 crab B85.3
 head (Pediculus capitis) B85.0
 mixed (classifiable to more than one of the titles B85.0-B85.3) B85.4
 pubic (Phthirus pubis) B85.3
Lichen L28.0
 albus L90.0
  penis N48.0
  vulva N90.4
 amyloidosis E85.4 *[L99]*
 atrophicus L90.0
  penis N48.0
  vulva N90.4
 congenital Q82.8
 myxedematosus L98.5
 nitidus L44.1
 pilaris Q82.8
  acquired L85.8
 planopilaris L66.1
 planus (chronicus) L43.9
  annularis L43.8
  bullous L43.1
  follicular L66.1
  hypertrophic L43.0
  moniliformis L44.3
  of Wilson L43.9
  specified NEC L43.8
  subacute (active) L43.3
  tropicus L43.3
 ruber
  acuminatus L44.0
  moniliformis L44.3
  planus L43.9
 sclerosus (et atrophicus) L90.0
  penis N48.0
  vulva N90.4
 scrofulosus (primary) (tuberculous) A18.4
 simplex (chronicus) (circumscriptus) L28.0
 striatus L44.2
 urticatus L28.2

Lichenification L28.0
Lichenoides tuberculosis (primary) A18.4
Lichtheim's disease or syndrome D51.0
Lien migrans D73.89
Ligament — *see* condition
Light
 for gestational age — *see* Light for dates
 headedness R42
Light-for-dates (infant) P05.00
 with weight of
  499 grams or less P05.01
  500-749 grams P05.02
  750-999 grams P05.03
  1000-1249 grams P05.04
  1250-1499 grams P05.05
  1500-1749 grams P05.06
  1750-1999 grams P05.07
  2000-2499 grams P05.08
  2500 grams and over P05.09
 affecting management of pregnancy O36.59- ☑
 and small-for-dates — *see* Small for dates
 specified NEC P05.09
Lightning (effects) (stroke) (struck by) T75.00 ☑
 burn — *see* Burn
 foot E53.8
 shock T75.01 ☑
 specified effect NEC T75.09 ☑
Lightwood-Albright syndrome N25.89
Lightwood's disease or syndrome (renal tubular acidosis) N25.89
Lignac (-de Toni) (-Fanconi) (-Debré) **disease or syndrome** E72.09
 with cystinosis E72.04
Ligneous thyroiditis E06.5
Likoff's syndrome I20.8
Limb — *see* condition
Limbic epilepsy personality syndrome F07.0
Limitation, limited
 activities due to disability Z73.6
 cardiac reserve — *see* Disease, heart
 eye muscle duction, traumatic — *see* Strabismus, mechanical
 mandibular range of motion M26.52
Lindau (-von Hippel) **disease** Q85.83
Line(s)
 Beau's L60.4
 Harris' — *see* Arrest, epiphyseal
 Hudson's (cornea) — *see* Pigmentation, cornea, anterior
 Stähli's (cornea) — *see* Pigmentation, cornea, anterior
Linea corneae senilis — *see* Change, cornea, senile
Lingua
 geographica K14.1
 nigra (villosa) K14.3
 plicata K14.5
 tylosis K13.29
Lingual — *see* condition
Linguatulosis B88.8
Linitis (gastric) **plastica** C16.9
Lip — *see* condition
Lipedema — *see* Edema
Lipemia — *see also* Hyperlipidemia
 retina, retinalis E78.3
Lipidosis E75.6
 cerebral (infantile) (juvenile) (late) E75.4
 cerebroretinal E75.4
 cerebroside E75.22
 cholesterol (cerebral) E75.5
 glycolipid E75.21
 hepatosplenomegalic E78.3
 sphingomyelin — *see* Niemann-Pick disease or syndrome
 sulfatide E75.29
Lipoadenoma — *see* Neoplasm, benign, by site
Lipoblastoma — *see* Lipoma
Lipoblastomatosis — *see* Lipoma
Lipochondrodystrophy E76.01
Lipochrome histiocytosis (familial) D71
Lipodermatosclerosis — *see* Varix, leg, with, inflammation
 ulcerated — *see* Varix, leg, with, ulcer, with inflammation by site
Lipodystrophia progressiva E88.1
Lipodystrophy (progressive) E88.1
 insulin E88.1
 intestinal K90.81
 mesenteric K65.4
Lipofibroma — *see* Lipoma

Lipofuscinosis, neuronal (with ceroidosis) E75.4
Lipogranuloma, sclerosing L92.8
Lipogranulomatosis E78.89
Lipoid — *see also* condition
 histiocytosis D76.3
  essential E75.29
 nephrosis N04.9
 proteinosis of Urbach E78.89
Lipoidemia — *see* Hyperlipidemia
Lipoidosis — *see* Lipidosis
Lipoma D17.9
 fetal D17.9
  fat cell D17.9
 infiltrating D17.9
 intramuscular D17.9
 pleomorphic D17.9
 site classification
  arms (skin) (subcutaneous) D17.2- ☑
  connective tissue D17.30
   intra-abdominal D17.5
   intrathoracic D17.4
   peritoneum D17.79
   retroperitoneum D17.79
   specified site NEC D17.39
   spermatic cord D17.6
  face (skin) (subcutaneous) D17.0
  genitourinary organ NEC D17.72
  head (skin) (subcutaneous) D17.0
  intra-abdominal D17.5
  intrathoracic D17.4
  kidney D17.71
  legs (skin) (subcutaneous) D17.2- ☑
  neck (skin) (subcutaneous) D17.0
  peritoneum D17.79
  retroperitoneum D17.79
  skin D17.30
   specified site NEC D17.39
  specified site NEC D17.79
  spermatic cord D17.6
  subcutaneous D17.30
   specified site NEC D17.39
  trunk (skin) (subcutaneous) D17.1
  unspecified D17.9
 spindle cell D17.9
Lipomatosis E88.2
 dolorosa (Dercum) E88.2
 fetal — *see* Lipoma
 Launois-Bensaude E88.89
Lipomyoma — *see* Lipoma
Lipomyxoma — *see* Lipoma
Lipomyxosarcoma — *see* Neoplasm, connective tissue, malignant
Lipoprotein metabolism disorder E78.9
Lipoproteinemia E78.5
 broad-beta E78.2
 floating-beta E78.2
 hyper-pre-beta E78.1
Liposarcoma — *see also* Neoplasm, connective tissue, malignant
 dedifferentiated — *see* Neoplasm, connective tissue, malignant
 differentiated type — *see* Neoplasm, connective tissue, malignant
 embryonal — *see* Neoplasm, connective tissue, malignant
 mixed type — *see* Neoplasm, connective tissue, malignant
 myxoid — *see* Neoplasm, connective tissue, malignant
 pleomorphic — *see* Neoplasm, connective tissue, malignant
 round cell — *see* Neoplasm, connective tissue, malignant
 well differentiated type — *see* Neoplasm, connective tissue, malignant
Liposynovitis prepatellaris E88.89
Lipping, cervix N86
Lipschütz disease or ulcer N76.6
Lipuria R82.0
 schistosomiasis (bilharziasis) B65.0
Lisping F80.0
Lissauer's paralysis A52.17
Lissencephalia, lissencephaly Q04.3
Listeriosis, listerellosis A32.9
 congenital (disseminated) P37.2
 cutaneous A32.0
 neonatal, newborn (disseminated) P37.2
 oculoglandular A32.81
 specified NEC A32.89

Lithemia E79.0
Lithiasis — *see* Calculus
Lithosis J62.8
Lithuria R82.998
Litigation, anxiety concerning Z65.3
Little leaguer's elbow — *see* Epicondylitis, medial
Little's disease G80.9
Littre's
   gland — *see* condition
   hernia — *see* Hernia, abdomen
Littritis — *see* Urethritis
Livedo (annularis) (racemosa) (reticularis) R23.1
Liver — *see* condition
Living alone (problems with) Z60.2
   with handicapped person Z74.2
Living in a shelter (motel) (scattered site housing)
   (temporary or transitional living situation) Z59.01
Lloyd's syndrome — *see* Adenomatosis, endocrine
Loa loa, loaiasis, loasis B74.3
Lobar — *see* condition
Lobomycosis B48.0
Lobo's disease B48.0
Lobotomy syndrome F07.0
Lobstein (-Ekman) **disease or syndrome** Q78.0
Lobster-claw hand Q71.6- ☑
Lobulation (congenital) — *see also* Anomaly, by site
   kidney, Q63.1
   liver, abnormal Q44.7
   spleen Q89.09
Lobule, lobular — *see* condition
Local, localized — *see* condition
Locked twins causing obstructed labor O66.1
Locked-in state G83.5
Locking
   joint — *see* Derangement, joint, specified type NEC
      knee — *see* Derangement, knee
Lockjaw — *see* Tetanus
Löffler's
   endocarditis I42.3
   eosinophilia J82.89
   pneumonia J82.89
   syndrome (eosinophilic pneumonitis) J82.89
Loiasis (with conjunctival infestation) (eyelid) B74.3
Lone Star fever A77.0
Long
   COVID (-19) — *see also* COVID-19 U09.9
   labor O63.9
      first stage O63.0
      second stage O63.1
   QT syndrome I45.81
Longitudinal stripes or grooves, nails L60.8
   congenital Q84.6
Long-term (current) (prophylactic) **drug therapy** (use
   of)
   5-fluorouracil Z79.631
   6-mercaptopurine Z79.631
   adalimumab Z79.620
   agents affecting estrogen receptors and estrogen levels
      NEC Z79.818
   alkylating agent Z79.630
   anastrozole (Arimidex) Z79.811
   antibiotics Z79.2
      short-term use — *omit code*
   anticoagulants Z79.01
   antidiabetic drugs, injectable, non-insulin Z79.85
   anti-inflammatory, non-steroidal (NSAID) Z79.1
   antimetabolite agent Z79.631
   antiplatelet Z79.02
   antithrombotics Z79.02
   antitumor antibiotic Z79.632
   apremilast Z79.61
   aromatase inhibitors Z79.811
   aspirin Z79.82
   azathioprine Z79.624
   birth control pill or patch Z79.3
   bisphosphonates Z79.83
   bleomycin Z79.632
   calcineurin inhibitor Z79.621
   chlorambucil Z79.630
   cisplatin Z79.630
   contraceptive, oral Z79.3
   cyclophosphamide Z79.630
   cyclosporine Z79.621
   cytarabine Z79.631
   doxorubicin Z79.632
   drug, specified NEC Z79.899
   estrogen receptor downregulators Z79.818

Long-term (current) (prophylactic) **drug therapy** —
   continued
   etanercept Z79.620
   etoposide Z79.634
   Evista Z79.810
   exemestane (Aromasin) Z79.811
   Fareston Z79.810
   fulvestrant (Faslodex) Z79.818
   gonadotropin-releasing hormone (GnRH) agonist
      Z79.818
   goserelin acetate (Zoladex) Z79.818
   hormone replacement Z79.890
   hydroxyurea Z79.64
   immunomodulators, unspecified Z79.60
      specified NEC Z79.69
   immunomodulatory imide drug Z79.61
   immunosuppressants, unspecified Z79.60
      specified NEC Z79.69
   immunosuppressive biologic Z79.620
   infliximab Z79.620
   inhibitors of nucleotide synthesis Z79.624
   insulin Z79.4
   irinotecan Z79.634
   Janus kinase inhibitor Z79.622
   lenalidomide Z79.61
   letrozole (Femara) Z79.811
   leuprolide acetate (leuprorelin) (Lupron) Z79.818
   mammalian target of rapamycin (mTOR) inhibitor
      Z79.623
   megestrol acetate (Megace) Z79.818
   methadone for pain management Z79.891
   mitomycin C Z79.632
   mitotic inhibitor Z79.633
   monoclonal antibodies Z79.620
   myelosuppressive agent Z79.64
   Nolvadex Z79.810
   non-insulin antidiabetic drug, injectable Z79.899
   non-steroidal anti-inflammatories (NSAID) Z79.1
   omycophenolate Z79.624
   opiate analgesic Z79.891
   oral
      antidiabetic Z79.84
      contraceptive Z79.3
      hypoglycemic Z79.84
   paclitaxel Z79.633
   plant alkaloids Z79.633
   pomalidomide Z79.61
   purine synthesis (IMDH) inhibitors Z79.624
   raloxifene (Evista) Z79.810
   selective estrogen receptor modulators (SERMs)
      Z79.810
   sirolimus Z79.623
   steroids
      inhaled Z79.51
      systemic Z79.52
   tacrolimus Z79.621
   tamoxifen (Nolvadex) Z79.810
   tofacitinib Z79.622
   topoisomerase inhibitor Z79.634
   topotecan Z79.634
   toremifene (Fareston) Z79.810
   vinblastine Z79.633
   vincristine Z79.633
Loop
   intestine — *see* Volvulus
   vascular on papilla (optic) Q14.2
Loose — *see also* condition
   body
      joint M24.00
         ankle M24.07- ☑
         elbow M24.02- ☑
         hand M24.04- ☑
         hip M24.05- ☑
         knee M23.4- ☑
         shoulder (region) M24.01- ☑
         specified site NEC M24.08
         toe M24.07- ☑
         vertebra M24.08
         wrist M24.03- ☑
      knee M23.4- ☑
      sheath, tendon — *see* Disorder, tendon, specified
        type NEC
   cartilage — *see* Loose, body, joint
   skin and subcutaneous tissue (following bariatric
      surgery weight loss) (following dietary weight
      loss) L98.7
   tooth, teeth K08.89

Loosening
   aseptic
      joint prosthesis — *see* Complications, joint prosthe-
        sis, mechanical, loosening, by site
   epiphysis — *see* Osteochondropathy
   mechanical
      joint prosthesis — *see* Complications, joint prosthe-
        sis, mechanical, loosening, by site
Looser-Milkman (-Debray) **syndrome** M83.8
Lop ear (deformity) Q17.3
Lorain (-Levi) **short stature syndrome** E23.0
Lordosis M40.50
   acquired — *see* Lordosis, specified type NEC
   congenital Q76.429
      lumbar region Q76.426
      lumbosacral region Q76.427
      sacral region Q76.428
      sacrococcygeal region Q76.428
      thoracolumbar region Q76.425
   lumbar region M40.56
   lumbosacral region M40.57
   postsurgical M96.4
   postural — *see* Lordosis, specified type NEC
   rachitic (late effect) (sequelae) E64.3
   sequelae of rickets E64.3
   specified type NEC M40.40
      lumbar region M40.46
      lumbosacral region M40.47
      thoracolumbar region M40.45
   thoracolumbar region M40.55
   tuberculous A18.01
Loss (of)
   appetite — *see also* Anorexia R63.0
      hysterical F50.89
      nonorganic origin F50.89
      psychogenic F50.89
   blood — *see* Hemorrhage
   bone —*see* Loss, substance of, bone
   consciousness, transient R55
      traumatic — *see* Injury, intracranial
   control, sphincter, rectum R15.9
      nonorganic origin F98.1
   elasticity, skin R23.4
   family (member) in childhood Z62.898
   fluid (acute) E86.9
   function of labyrinth — *see* subcategory H83.2 ☑
   hair, nonscarring — *see* Alopecia
   hearing — *see also* Deafness
      central NOS H90.5
      conductive H90.2
        bilateral H90.0
        unilateral
          with
            restricted hearing on the contralateral
              side H90.A1- ☑
            unrestricted hearing on the contralateral
              side H90.1- ☑
      mixed conductive and sensorineural hearing loss
        H90.8
        bilateral H90.6
        unilateral
          with
            restricted hearing on the contralateral
              side H90.A3- ☑
            unrestricted hearing on the contralateral
              side H90.7- ☑
      neural NOS H90.5
      perceptive NOS H90.5
      sensorineural NOS H90.5
        bilateral H90.3
        unilateral
          with
            restricted hearing onthe contralateral
              side H90.A2- ☑
            unrestricted hearing on the contralateral
              side H90.4- ☑
      sensory NOS H90.5
   height R29.890
   limb or member, traumatic, current — *see* Amputation,
      traumatic
   love relationship in childhood Z62.898
   memory — *see also* Amnesia
      mild, following organic brain damage F06.8
   mind — *see* Psychosis
   occlusal vertical dimension of fully erupted teeth
      M26.37
   organ or part — *see* Absence, by site, acquired
   ossicles, ear (partial) H74.32- ☑

Loss — *continued*
  parent in childhood Z63.4
  pregnancy, recurrent N96
    care in current pregnancy O26.2- ☑
    without current pregnancy N96
  recurrent pregnancy — *see* Loss, pregnancy, recurrent
  self-esteem, in childhood Z62.898
  sense of
    smell — *see* Disturbance, sensation, smell
    taste — *see* Disturbance, sensation, taste
    touch R20.8
  sensory R44.9
    dissociative F44.6
  sexual desire F52.0
  sight (acquired) (complete) (congenital) — *see* Blindness
  substance of
    bone — *see* Disorder, bone, density and structure, specified NEC
      horizontal alveolar K06.3
    cartilage — *see* Disorder, cartilage, specified type NEC
      auricle (ear) — *see* Disorder, pinna, specified type NEC
    vitreous (humor) H15.89
  tooth, teeth — *see* Absence, teeth, acquired
  vision, visual H54.7
    both eyes H54.3
    one eye H54.60
      left (normal vision on right) H54.62
      right (normal vision on left) H54.61
    specified as blindness — *see* Blindness
    subjective
      sudden H53.13- ☑
      transient H53.12- ☑
  vitreous — *see* Prolapse, vitreous
  voice — *see* Aphonia
  weight (abnormal) (cause unknown) R63.4
Louis-Bar syndrome (ataxia-telangiectasia) G11.3
Louping ill (encephalitis) A84.89
Louse, lousiness — *see* Lice
Low
  achiever, school Z55.3
  back syndrome M54.50
  basal metabolic rate R94.8
  birthweight (2499 grams or less) P07.10
    with weight of
      1000-1249 grams P07.14
      1250-1499 grams P07.15
      1500-1749 grams P07.16
      1750-1999 grams P07.17
      2000-2499 grams P07.18
    extreme (999 grams or less) P07.00
      with weight of
        499 grams or less P07.01
        500-749 grams P07.02
        750-999 grams P07.03
    for gestational age — *see* Light for dates
  blood pressure — *see also* Hypotension
    reading (incidental) (isolated) (nonspecific) R03.1
  cardiac reserve — *see* Disease, heart
  function — *see also* Hypofunction
    kidney N28.9
  hematocrit D64.9
  hemoglobin D64.9
  income Z59.6
  level of literacy Z55.0
  lying
    kidney N28.89
    organ or site, congenital — *see* Malposition, congenital
  output syndrome (cardiac) — *see* Failure, heart
  platelets (blood) — *see* Thrombocytopenia
  reserve, kidney N28.89
  salt syndrome E87.1
  self esteem R45.81
  set ears Q17.4
  vision H54.2X- ☑
    one eye (other eye normal) H54.50
      left (normal vision on right) H54.52A- ☑
      other eye blind — *see* Blindness
      right (normal vision on left) H54.511- ☑
  von Willebrand factor R79.1
Low-density-lipoprotein-type (LDL) **hyperlipoproteinemia** E78.00
Lowe's syndrome E72.03
Lown-Ganong-Levine syndrome I45.6
LSD reaction (acute) (without dependence) F16.90

LSD reaction — *continued*
  with dependence F16.20
L-shaped kidney Q63.8
LTBI (latent tuberculosis infection) Z22.7
Ludwig's angina or disease K12.2
Lues (venerea), **luetic** — *see* Syphilis
Luetscher's syndrome (dehydration) E86.0
Lumbago, lumbalgia M54.50
  with sciatica M54.4- ☑
    due to intervertebral disc disorder M51.17
  due to displacement, intervertebral disc M51.27
    with sciatica M51.17
Lumbar — *see* condition
Lumbarization, vertebra, congenital Q76.49
Lumbermen's itch B88.0
Lump — *see also* Mass
  breast N63.0
    axillary tail
      left N63.32
      right N63.31
    left
      lower inner quadrant N63.24
      lower outer quadrant N63.23
      overlapping quadrants N63.25
      unspecified quadrant N63.20
      upper inner quadrant N63.22
      upper outer quadrant N63.21
    right
      lower inner quadrant N63.14
      lower outer quadrant N63.13
      overlapping quadrants N63.15
      unspecified quadrant N63.10
      upper inner quadrant N63.12
      upper outer quadrant N63.11
    subareolar
      left N63.42
      right N63.41
Lunacy — *see* Psychosis
Lung — *see* condition
Lupoid (miliary) **of Boeck** D86.3
Lupus
  anticoagulant D68.62
    with
      hemorrhagic disorder D68.312
      hypercoagulable state D68.62
    finding without diagnosis R76.0
  discoid (local) L93.0
  erythematosus (discoid) (local) L93.0
    disseminated — *see* Lupus, erythematosus, systemic
    eyelid H01.129
      left H01.126
        lower H01.125
        upper H01.124
      right H01.123
        lower H01.122
        upper H01.121
    profundus L93.2
    specified NEC L93.2
    subacute cutaneous L93.1
    systemic M32.9
      with organ or system involvement M32.10
        endocarditis M32.11
        lung M32.13
        pericarditis M32.12
        renal (glomerular) M32.14
          tubulo-interstitial M32.15
        specified organ or system NEC M32.19
      drug-induced M32.0
    inhibitor (presence of) D68.62
      with
        hemorrhagic disorder D68.312
        hypercoagulable state D68.62
      finding without diagnosis R76.0
    specified NEC M32.8
  exedens A18.4
  hydralazine M32.0
    correct substance properly administered — *see* Table of Drugs and Chemicals, by drug, adverse effect
    overdose or wrong substance given or taken — *see* Table of Drugs and Chemicals, by drug, poisoning
  nephritis (chronic) M32.14
  nontuberculous, not disseminated L93.0
  panniculitis L93.2
  pernio (Besnier) D86.3
  systemic — *see* Lupus, erythematosus, systemic
  tuberculous A18.4

Lupus — *continued*
  tuberculous — *continued*
    eyelid A18.4
    vulgaris A18.4
      eyelid A18.4
Luteinoma D27.- ☑
Lutembacher's disease or syndrome (atrial septal defect with mitral stenosis) Q21.19
Luteoma D27.- ☑
Lutz (-Splendore-de Almeida) **disease** — *see* Paracoccidioidomycosis
Luxation — *see also* Dislocation
  eyeball (nontraumatic) — *see* Luxation, globe
    birth injury P15.3
  globe, nontraumatic H44.82- ☑
  lacrimal gland — *see* Dislocation, lacrimal gland
  lens (old) (partial) (spontaneous)
    congenital Q12.1
    syphilitic A50.39
Lycanthropy F22
Lyell's syndrome L51.2
  due to drug L51.2
    correct substance properly administered — *see* Table of Drugs and Chemicals, by drug, adverse effect
    overdose or wrong substance given or taken — *see* Table of Drugs and Chemicals, by drug, poisoning
Lyme disease A69.20
Lymph
  gland or node — *see* condition
  scrotum — *see* Infestation, filarial
Lymphadenitis I88.9
  with ectopic or molar pregnancy O08.0
  acute L04.9
    axilla L04.2
    face L04.0
    head L04.0
    hip L04.3
    limb
      lower L04.3
      upper L04.2
    neck L04.0
    shoulder L04.2
    specified site NEC L04.8
    trunk L04.1
  anthracosis (occupational) J60
  any site, except mesenteric I88.9
    chronic I88.1
    subacute I88.1
  breast
    gestational — *see* Mastitis, obstetric
    puerperal, postpartum (nonpurulent) O91.22
  chancroidal (congenital) A57
  chronic I88.1
    mesenteric I88.0
  due to
    Brugia (malayi) B74.1
      timori B74.2
    chlamydial lymphogranuloma A55
    diphtheria (toxin) A36.89
    lymphogranuloma venereum A55
    Wuchereria bancrofti B74.0
  following ectopic or molar pregnancy O08.0
  gonorrheal A54.89
  infective — *see* Lymphadenitis, acute
  mesenteric (acute) (chronic) (nonspecific) (subacute) I88.0
    due to Salmonella typhi A01.09
    tuberculous A18.39
  mycobacterial A31.8
  purulent — *see* Lymphadenitis, acute
  pyogenic — *see* Lymphadenitis, acute
  regional, nonbacterial I88.8
  septic — *see* Lymphadenitis, acute
  subacute, unspecified site I88.1
  suppurative — *see* Lymphadenitis, acute
  syphilitic (early) (secondary) A51.49
    late A52.79
  tuberculous — *see* Tuberculosis, lymph gland
  venereal (chlamydial) A55
Lymphadenoid goiter E06.3
Lymphadenopathy (generalized) R59.1
  angioimmunoblastic, with dysproteinemia (AILD) C86.5
  due to toxoplasmosis (acquired) B58.89
    congenital (acute) (subacute) (chronic) P37.1
  localized R59.0
  syphilitic (early) (secondary) A51.49

Lymphadenosis R59.1
Lymphangiectasis I89.0
 conjunctiva H11.89
 postinfectional I89.0
 scrotum I89.0
Lymphangiectatic elephantiasis, nonfilarial I89.0
Lymphangioendothelioma D18.1
 malignant — *see* Neoplasm, connective tissue, malignant
Lymphangioleiomyomatosis J84.81
Lymphangioma D18.1
 capillary D18.1
 cavernous D18.1
 cystic D18.1
 malignant — *see* Neoplasm, connective tissue, malignant
Lymphangiomyoma D18.1
Lymphangiomyomatosis J84.81
Lymphangiosarcoma — *see* Neoplasm, connective tissue, malignant
Lymphangitis I89.1
 with
  abscess — *code by* site under Abscess
  cellulitis — *code by* site under Cellulitis
  ectopic or molar pregnancy O08.0
 acute L03.91
  abdominal wall L03.321
  ankle — *see* Lymphangitis, acute, lower limb
  arm — *see* Lymphangitis, acute, upper limb
  auricle (ear) — *see* Lymphangitis, acute, ear
  axilla L03.12-
  back (any part) L03.322
  buttock L03.327
  cervical (meaning neck) L03.222
  cheek (external) L03.212
  chest wall L03.323
  digit
   finger — *see* Lymphangitis, acute, finger
   toe — *see* Lymphangitis, acute, toe
  ear (external) H60.1-
  external auditory canal — *see* Lymphangitis, acute, ear
  eyelid — *see* Abscess, eyelid
  face NEC L03.212
  finger (intrathecal) (periosteal) (subcutaneous) (subcuticular) L03.02-
  foot — *see* Lymphangitis, acute, lower limb
  gluteal (region) L03.327
  groin L03.324
  hand — *see* Lymphangitis, acute, upper limb
  head NEC L03.891
   face (any part, except ear, eye and nose) L03.212
  heel — *see* Lymphangitis, acute, lower limb
  hip — *see* Lymphangitis, acute, lower limb
  jaw (region) L03.212
  knee — *see* Lymphangitis, acute, lower limb
  leg — *see* Lymphangitis, acute, lower limb
  lower limb L03.12-
   toe — *see* Lymphangitis, acute, toe
  navel L03.326
  neck (region) L03.222
  orbit, orbital — *see* Cellulitis, orbit
  pectoral (region) L03.323
  perineal, perineum L03.325
  scalp (any part) L03.891
  shoulder — *see* Lymphangitis, acute, upper limb
  specified site NEC L03.898
  thigh — *see* Lymphangitis, acute, lower limb
  thumb (intrathecal) (periosteal) (subcutaneous) (subcuticular) — *see* Lymphangitis, acute, finger
  toe (intrathecal) (periosteal) (subcutaneous) (subcuticular) L03.04-
  trunk L03.329
   abdominal wall L03.321
   back (any part) L03.322
   buttock L03.327
   chest wall L03.323
   groin L03.324
   perineal, perineum L03.325
   umbilicus L03.326
  umbilicus L03.326
  upper limb L03.12-
   axilla — *see* Lymphangitis, acute, axilla
   finger — *see* Lymphangitis, acute, finger
   thumb — *see* Lymphangitis, acute, finger
   wrist — *see* Lymphangitis, acute, upper limb

Lymphangitis — *continued*
 breast
  gestational — *see* Mastitis, obstetric
 chancroidal A57
 chronic (any site) I89.1
 due to
  Brugia (malayi) B74.1
   timori B74.2
  Wuchereria bancrofti B74.0
 following ectopic or molar pregnancy O08.89
 penis
  acute N48.29
   gonococcal (acute) (chronic) A54.09
 puerperal, postpartum, childbirth O86.89
 strumous, tuberculous A18.2
 subacute (any site) I89.1
 tuberculous — *see* Tuberculosis, lymph gland
Lymphatic (vessel) — *see* condition
Lymphatism E32.8
Lymphectasia I89.0
Lymphedema (acquired) — *see also* Elephantiasis
 congenital Q82.0
 hereditary (chronic) (idiopathic) Q82.0
 postmastectomy I97.2
 praecox I89.0
 secondary I89.0
 surgical NEC I97.89
  postmastectomy (syndrome) I97.2
Lymphoblastic — *see* condition
Lymphoblastoma (diffuse) — *see* Lymphoma, lymphoblastic (diffuse)
 giant follicular — *see* Lymphoma, lymphoblastic (diffuse)
 macrofollicular — *see* Lymphoma, lymphoblastic (diffuse)
Lymphocele I89.8
Lymphocytic
 chorioencephalitis (acute) (serous) A87.2
 choriomeningitis (acute) (serous) A87.2
 meningoencephalitis A87.2
Lymphocytoma, benign cutis L98.8
Lymphocytopenia D72.810
Lymphocytosis (symptomatic) D72.820
 infectious (acute) B33.8
Lymphoepithelioma — *see* Neoplasm, malignant, by site
Lymphogranuloma (malignant) — *see also* Lymphoma, Hodgkin
 chlamydial A55
 inguinale A55
 venereum (any site) (chlamydial) (with stricture of rectum) A55
Lymphogranulomatosis (malignant) — *see also* Lymphoma, Hodgkin
 benign (Boeck's sarcoid) (Schaumann's) D86.1
Lymphohistiocytosis, hemophagocytic (familial) D76.1
Lymphoid — *see* condition
Lymphoma (of) (malignant) C85.90
 adult T-cell (HTLV-1-associated) (acute variant) (chronic variant) (lymphomatoid variant) (smouldering variant) C91.5-
 anaplastic large cell
  ALK-negative C84.7-
  ALK-positive C84.6-
  breast implant associated (BIA-ALCL) C84.7A
  CD30-positive C84.6-
  primary cutaneous C86.6
 angioimmunoblastic T-cell C86.5
 BALT C88.4
 B-cell C85.1-
 blastic NK-cell C86.4
 blastic plasmacytoid dendritic cell neoplasm (BPDCN) C86.4
 B-precursor C83.5-
 bronchial-associated lymphoid tissue [BALT-lymphoma] C88.4
 Burkitt (atypical) C83.7-
 Burkitt-like C83.7-
 centrocytic C83.1-
 cutaneous follicle center C82.6-
 cutaneous T-cell C84.A- (*following* C84.7)
 diffuse follicle center C82.5-
 diffuse large cell C83.3-
  anaplastic C83.3-
  B-cell C83.3-
  CD30-positive C83.3-
  centroblastic C83.3-

Lymphoma — *continued*
 diffuse large cell — *continued*
  immunoblastic C83.3-
  plasmablastic C83.3-
  subtype not specified C83.3-
  T-cell rich C83.3-
 enteropathy-type (associated) (intestinal) T-cell C86.2
 extranodal marginal zone B-cell lymphoma of mucosa-associated lymphoid tissue [MALT-lymphoma] C88.4
 extranodal NK/T-cell, nasal type C86.0
 follicular C82.9-
  grade
   I C82.0-
   II C82.1-
   III C82.2-
   IIIa C82.3-
   IIIb C82.4-
  specified NEC C82.8-
 hepatosplenic T-cell (alpha-beta) (gamma-delta) C86.1
 histiocytic C85.9-
  true C96.A (*following* C96.6)
 Hodgkin C81.9
  lymphocyte depleted (classical) C81.3-
  lymphocyte-rich (classical) C81.4-
  mixed cellularity (classical) C81.2-
  nodular
   lymphocyte predominant C81.0-
   sclerosis (classical) C81.1-
  nodular sclerosis (classical) C81.1-
  specified NEC (classical) C81.7-
 intravascular large B-cell C83.8-
 Lennert's C84.4-
 lymphoblastic (diffuse) C83.5-
 lymphoblastic B-cell C83.5-
 lymphoblastic T-cell C83.5-
 lymphoepithelioid C84.4-
 lymphoplasmacytic C83.0-
  with IgM-production C88.0
 MALT C88.4
 mantle cell C83.1-
 mature T-cell NEC C84.4-
 mature T/NK-cell C84.9-
  specified NEC C84.Z- (*following* C84.7)
 mediastinal (thymic) large B-cell C85.2-
 Mediterranean C88.3
 mucosa-associated lymphoid tissue [MALT-lymphoma] C88.4
 NK/T cell C84.9-
 nodal marginal zone C83.0-
 non-follicular (diffuse) C83.9-
  specified NEC C83.8-
 non-Hodgkin — *see also* Lymphoma, by type C85.9-
  specified NEC C85.8-
 non-leukemic variant of B-CLL C83.0-
 peripheral T-cell NEC C84.4-
 primary cutaneous
  anaplastic large cell C86.6
  CD30-positive large T-cell C86.6
 primary effusion B-cell C83.8-
 SALT C88.4
 skin-associated lymphoid tissue [SALT-lymphoma] C88.4
 small cell B-cell C83.0-
 splenic marginal zone C83.0-
 subcutaneous panniculitis-like T-cell C86.3
 T-precursor C83.5-
 true histiocytic C96.A (*following* C96.6)
Lymphomatosis — *see* Lymphoma
Lymphopathia venereum, veneris A55
Lymphopenia D72.810
Lymphoplasmacytic leukemia — *see* Leukemia, chronic lymphocytic, B-cell type
Lymphoproliferation, X-linked disease D82.3
Lymphoreticulosis, benign (of inoculation) A28.1
Lymphorrhea I89.8
Lymphosarcoma (diffuse) — *see also* Lymphoma C85.9-
Lymphostasis I89.8
Lypemania — *see* Melancholia
Lysine and hydroxylysine metabolism disorder E72.3
Lyssa — *see* Rabies

M

Macacus ear Q17.3

Maceration, wet feet, tropical (syndrome) T69.02- ☑
MacLeod's syndrome J43.0
Macrocephalia, macrocephaly Q75.3
Macrocheilia, macrochilia (congenital) Q18.6
Macrocolon — *see also* Megacolon Q43.1
Macrocornea Q15.8
    with glaucoma Q15.0
Macrocytic — *see* condition
Macrocytosis D75.89
Macrodactylia, macrodactylism (fingers) (thumbs)
        Q74.0
    toes Q74.2
Macrodontia K00.2
Macrogenia M26.05
Macrogenitosomia (adrenal) (male) (praecox) E25.9
    congenital E25.0
Macroglobulinemia (idiopathic) (primary) C88.0
    monoclonal (essential) D47.2
    Waldenström C88.0
Macroglossia (congenital) Q38.2
    acquired K14.8
Macrognathia, macrognathism (congenital)
        (mandibular) (maxillary) M26.09
Macrogyria (congenital) Q04.8
Macrohydrocephalus — *see* Hydrocephalus
Macromastia — *see* Hypertrophy, breast
Macrophthalmos Q11.3
    in congenital glaucoma Q15.0
Macropsia H53.15
Macrosigmoid K59.39
    congenital Q43.2
Macrospondylitis , acromegalic E22.0
Macrostomia (congenital) Q18.4
Macrotia (external ear) (congenital) Q17.1
Macula
    cornea, corneal — *see* Opacity, cornea
    degeneration (atrophic) (exudative) (senile) — *see also*
        Degeneration, macula
    hereditary — *see* Dystrophy, retina
Maculae ceruleae B85.1
Maculopathy, toxic — *see* Degeneration, macula, toxic
Madarosis (eyelid) H02.729
    left H02.726
        lower H02.725
        upper H02.724
    right H02.723
        lower H02.722
        upper H02.721
Madelung's
    deformity (radius) Q74.0
    disease
        radial deformity Q74.0
        symmetrical lipomas, neck E88.89
Madness — *see* Psychosis
Madura
    foot B47.9
        actinomycotic B47.1
        mycotic B47.0
Maduromycosis B47.0
Maffucci's syndrome Q78.4
Magnesium metabolism disorder — *see* Disorder,
        metabolism, magnesium
Main en griffe (acquired) — *see also* Deformity, limb,
        clawhand
    congenital Q68.1
Maintenance (encounter for)
    antineoplastic chemotherapy Z51.11
    antineoplastic radiation therapy Z51.0
    methadone F11.20
Majocchi's
    disease L81.7
    granuloma B35.8
Major — *see* condition
Mal de los pintos — *see* Pinta
Mal de mer T75.3 ☑
Malabar itch (any site) B35.5
Malabsorption K90.9
    calcium K90.89
    carbohydrate K90.49
    disaccharide E73.9
    fat K90.49
    galactose E74.20
    glucose (-galactose) E74.39
    intestinal K90.9
        specified NEC K90.89
    isomaltose E74.31
    lactose E73.9

Malabsorption — *continued*
    methionine E72.19
    monosaccharide E74.39
    postgastrectomy K91.2
    postsurgical K91.2
    protein K90.49
    starch K90.49
    sucrose E74.39
    syndrome K90.9
        postsurgical K91.2
Malacia, bone (adult) M83.9
    juvenile — *see* Rickets
Malacoplakia
    bladder N32.89
    pelvis (kidney) N28.89
    ureter N28.89
    urethra N36.8
Malacosteon, juvenile — *see* Rickets
Maladaptation — *see* Maladjustment
Maladie de Roger Q21.0
Maladjustment
    conjugal Z63.0
        involving divorce or estrangement Z63.5
    educational Z55.4
    family Z63.9
    marital Z63.0
        involving divorce or estrangement Z63.5
    occupational NEC Z56.89
    simple, adult — *see* Disorder, adjustment
    situational — *see* Disorder, adjustment
    social Z60.9
        due to
            acculturation difficulty Z60.3
            discrimination and persecution (perceived) Z60.5
            exclusion and isolation Z60.4
            life-cycle (phase of life) transition Z60.0
            rejection Z60.4
            specified reason NEC Z60.8
Malaise R53.81
Malakoplakia — *see* Malacoplakia
Malaria, malarial (fever) B54
    with
        blackwater fever B50.8
            hemoglobinuric (bilious) B50.8
        hemoglobinuria B50.8
    accidentally induced (therapeutically) — *code by* type
        under Malaria
    algid B50.9
    cerebral B50.0 *[G94]*
    clinically diagnosed (without parasitological confirma-
        tion) B54
    congenital NEC P37.4
        falciparum P37.3
    congestion, congestive B54
    continued (fever) B50.9
    estivo-autumnal B50.9
    falciparum B50.9
        with complications NEC B50.8
            cerebral B50.0 *[G94]*
        severe B50.8
    hemorrhagic B54
    malariae B52.9
        with
            complications NEC B52.8
            glomerular disorder B52.0
    malignant (tertian) — *see* Malaria, falciparum
    mixed infections — *code to* first listed type in B50-B53
    ovale B53.0
    parasitologically confirmed NEC B53.8
    pernicious, acute — *see* Malaria, falciparum
    Plasmodium (P.)
        falciparum NEC — *see* Malaria, falciparum
        malariae NEC B52.9
            with Plasmodium
                falciparum (and or vivax) — *see* Malaria, falci-
                    parum
                vivax — *see also* Malaria, vivax
                    and falciparum — *see* Malaria, falciparum
        ovale B53.0
            with Plasmodium malariae — *see also* Malaria,
                malariae
            and vivax — *see also* Malaria, vivax
                and falciparum — *see* Malaria, falciparum
        simian B53.1
            with Plasmodium malariae — *see also* Malaria,
                malariae
            and vivax — *see also* Malaria, vivax
                and falciparum — *see* Malaria, falciparum

Malaria, malarial — *continued*
    Plasmodium — *continued*
        vivax NEC B51.9
            with Plasmodium falciparum — *see* Malaria, fal-
                ciparum
        quartan — *see* Malaria, malariae
        quotidian — *see* Malaria, falciparum
        recurrent B54
        remittent B54
        specified type NEC (parasitologically confirmed) B53.8
        spleen B54
        subtertian (fever) — *see* Malaria, falciparum
        tertian (benign) — *see also* Malaria, vivax
            malignant B50.9
        tropical B50.9
        typhoid B54
        vivax B51.9
            with
                complications NEC B51.8
                ruptured spleen B51.0
Malassez's disease (cystic) N50.89
Malassimilation K90.9
Maldescent, testis Q53.9
    bilateral Q53.20
        abdominal Q53.211
        perineal Q53.22
    unilateral Q53.10
        abdominal Q53.111
        perineal Q53.12
Maldevelopment — *see also* Anomaly
    brain Q07.9
    colon Q43.9
    hip Q74.2
        congenital dislocation Q65.2
            bilateral Q65.1
            unilateral Q65.0- ☑
    mastoid process Q75.8
    middle ear Q16.4
        except ossicles Q16.4
        ossicles Q16.3
    ossicles Q16.3
    spine Q76.49
    toe Q74.2
Male type pelvis Q74.2
    with disproportion (fetopelvic) O33.3 ☑
        causing obstructed labor O65.3
Malformation (congenital) — *see also* Anomaly
    adrenal gland Q89.1
    affecting multiple systems with skeletal changes NEC
        Q87.5
    alimentary tract Q45.9
        specified type NEC Q45.8
        upper Q40.9
            specified type NEC Q40.8
    aorta Q25.40
        absence Q25.41
        aneurysm, congenital Q25.43
        aplasia Q25.41
        atresia Q25.29
            aortic arch Q25.21
        coarctation (preductal) (postductal) Q25.1
        dilatation, congenital Q25.44
        hypoplasia Q25.42
        patent ductus arteriosus Q25.0
        specified type NEC Q25.49
        stenosis Q25.1
            supravalvular Q25.3
    aortic valve Q23.9
        specified NEC Q23.8
    arteriovenous, aneurysmatic (congenital) Q27.30
        brain Q28.2
            ruptured I60.8
                intracerebral I61.8
                intraparenchymal I61.8
                intraventricular I61.5
                subarachnoid I60.8
        cerebral — *see also* Malformation, arteriovenous,
            brain Q28.2
        peripheral Q27.30
            digestive system — *see* Angiodysplasia
                congenital Q27.33
            lower limb Q27.32
            other specified site Q27.39
            renal vessel Q27.34
            upper limb Q27.31
        precerebral vessels (nonruptured) Q28.0
    auricle
        ear (congenital) Q17.3

Malformation — *continued*
  auricle — *continued*
    ear — *continued*
      acquired H61.119
        left H61.112
          with right H61.113
        right H61.111
          with left H61.113
  bile duct Q44.5
  bladder Q64.79
    aplasia Q64.5
    diverticulum Q64.6
    exstrophy — *see* Exstrophy, bladder
    neck obstruction Q64.31
  bone Q79.9
    face Q75.9
      specified type NEC Q75.8
    skull Q75.9
      specified type NEC Q75.8
  brain (multiple) Q04.9
    arteriovenous Q28.2
    specified type NEC Q04.8
  branchial cleft Q18.2
  breast Q83.9
    specified type NEC Q83.8
  broad ligament Q50.6
  bronchus Q32.4
  bursa Q79.9
  cardiac
    chambers Q20.9
      specified type NEC Q20.8
    septum Q21.9
      specified type NEC Q21.8
  cerebral Q04.9
    vessels Q28.3
  cervix uteri Q51.9
    specified type NEC Q51.828
  Chiari
    Type I G93.5
    Type II Q07.01
  choroid (congenital) Q14.3
    plexus Q07.8
  circulatory system Q28.9
  cochlea Q16.5
  cornea Q13.4
  coronary vessels Q24.5
  corpus callosum (congenital) Q04.0
  diaphragm Q79.1
  digestive system NEC, specified type NEC Q45.8
  dura Q07.9
    brain Q04.9
    spinal Q06.9
  ear Q17.9
    causing impairment of hearing Q16.9
    external Q17.9
      accessory auricle Q17.0
      causing impairment of hearing Q16.9
        absence of
          auditory canal Q16.1
          auricle Q16.0
      macrotia Q17.1
      microtia Q17.2
      misplacement Q17.4
      misshapen NEC Q17.3
      prominence Q17.5
      specified type NEC Q17.8
    inner Q16.5
    middle Q16.4
      absence of eustachian tube Q16.2
      ossicles (fusion) Q16.3
    ossicles Q16.3
    specified type NEC Q17.8
  epididymis Q55.4
  esophagus Q39.9
    specified type NEC Q39.8
  eye Q15.9
    lid Q10.3
    specified NEC Q15.8
  fallopian tube Q50.6
  genital organ — *see* Anomaly, genitalia
  great
    artery Q25.9
      aorta — *see* Malformation, aorta
      pulmonary artery — *see* Malformation, pulmonary, artery
      specified type NEC Q25.8
    vein Q26.9
      anomalous
        portal venous connection Q26.5

Malformation — *continued*
  great — *continued*
    vein — *continued*
      anomalous — *continued*
        pulmonary venous connection Q26.4
          partial Q26.3
          total Q26.2
      persistent left superior vena cava Q26.1
      portal vein-hepatic artery fistula Q26.6
      specified type NEC Q26.8
      vena cava stenosis, congenital Q26.0
  gum Q38.6
  hair Q84.2
  heart Q24.9
    specified type NEC Q24.8
  integument Q84.9
    specified type NEC Q84.8
  internal ear Q16.5
  intestine Q43.9
    specified type NEC Q43.8
  iris Q13.2
  joint Q74.9
    ankle Q74.2
    lumbosacral Q76.49
    sacroiliac Q74.2
    specified type NEC Q74.8
  kidney Q63.9
    accessory Q63.0
    giant Q63.3
    horseshoe Q63.1
    hydronephrosis Q62.0
    malposition Q63.2
    specified type NEC Q63.8
  lacrimal apparatus Q10.6
  lingual Q38.3
  lip Q38.0
  liver Q44.7
  lung Q33.9
  meninges or membrane (congenital) Q07.9
    cerebral Q04.8
    spinal (cord) Q06.9
  middle ear Q16.4
    ossicles Q16.3
  mitral valve Q23.9
    specified NEC Q23.8
  Mondini's (congenital) (malformation, cochlea) Q16.5
  mouth (congenital) Q38.6
  multiple types NEC Q89.7
  musculoskeletal system Q79.9
  myocardium Q24.8
  nail Q84.6
  nervous system (central) Q07.9
  nose Q30.9
    specified type NEC Q30.8
  optic disc Q14.2
  orbit Q10.7
  ovary Q50.39
  palate Q38.5
  parathyroid gland Q89.2
  pelvic organs or tissues NEC
    in pregnancy or childbirth O34.8- ☑
      causing obstructed labor O65.5
  penis Q55.69
    aplasia Q55.5
    curvature (lateral) Q55.61
    hypoplasia Q55.62
  pericardium Q24.8
  peripheral vascular system Q27.9
    specified type NEC Q27.8
  pharynx Q38.8
  precerebral vessels Q28.1
  prostate Q55.4
  pulmonary
    arteriovenous Q25.72
    artery Q25.9
      atresia Q25.5
      specified type NEC Q25.79
      stenosis Q25.6
    valve Q22.3
  renal artery Q27.2
  respiratory system Q34.9
  retina Q14.1
  scrotum — *see* Malformation, testis and scrotum
  seminal vesicles Q55.4
  sense organs NEC Q07.9
  skin Q82.9
  specified NEC Q89.8
  spinal
    cord Q06.9

Malformation — *continued*
  spinal — *continued*
    nerve root Q07.8
  spine Q76.49
    kyphosis — *see* Kyphosis, congenital
    lordosis — *see* Lordosis, congenital
  spleen Q89.09
  stomach Q40.3
    specified type NEC Q40.2
  teeth, tooth K00.9
  tendon Q79.9
  testis and scrotum Q55.20
    aplasia Q55.0
    hypoplasia Q55.1
    polyorchism Q55.21
    retractile testis Q55.22
    scrotal transposition Q55.23
    specified NEC Q55.29
  thorax, bony Q76.9
  throat Q38.8
  thyroid gland Q89.2
  tongue (congenital) Q38.3
    hypertrophy Q38.2
    tie Q38.1
  trachea Q32.1
  tricuspid valve Q22.9
    specified type NEC Q22.8
  umbilical cord NEC (complicating delivery) O69.89 ☑
  umbilicus Q89.9
  ureter Q62.8
    agenesis Q62.4
    duplication Q62.5
    malposition — *see* Malposition, congenital, ureter
    obstructive defect — *see* Defect, obstructive, ureter
    vesico-uretero-renal reflux Q62.7
  urethra Q64.79
    aplasia Q64.5
    duplication Q64.74
    posterior valves Q64.2
    prolapse Q64.71
    stricture Q64.32
  urinary system Q64.9
  uterus Q51.9
    specified type NEC Q51.818
  vagina Q52.4
  vas deferens Q55.4
    atresia Q55.3
  vascular system, peripheral Q27.9
  venous — *see* Anomaly, vein(s)
  vulva Q52.70
Malfunction — *see also* Dysfunction
  cardiac electronic device T82.119 ☑
    electrode T82.110 ☑
    pulse generator T82.111 ☑
    specified type NEC T82.118 ☑
  catheter device NEC T85.618 ☑
    cystostomy T83.010 ☑
    dialysis (renal) (vascular) T82.41 ☑
      intraperitoneal T85.611 ☑
    infusion NEC T82.514 ☑
      cranial T85.610 ☑
      epidural T85.610 ☑
      intrathecal T85.610 ☑
      spinal T85.610 ☑
      subarachnoid T85.610 ☑
      subdural T85.610 ☑
    urinary — *see also* Breakdown, device, catheter T83.018 ☑
  colostomy K94.03
    valve K94.03
  cystostomy (stoma) N99.512
    catheter T83.010 ☑
  enteric stoma K94.13
  enterostomy K94.13
  esophagostomy K94.33
  gastroenteric K31.89
  gastrostomy K94.23
  ileostomy K94.13
    valve K94.13
  intrathecal infusion pump T85.615 ☑
  jejunostomy K94.13
  nervous system device, implant or graft, specified NEC T85.615 ☑
  pacemaker — *see* Malfunction, cardiac electronic device
  prosthetic device, internal — *see* Complications, prosthetic device, by site, mechanical
  tracheostomy J95.03

Malfunction — *continued*
  urinary device NEC — *see* Complication, genitourinary, device, urinary, mechanical
  valve
    colostomy K94.03
    heart T82.09 ☑
    ileostomy K94.13
  vascular graft or shunt NEC — *see* Complication, cardiovascular device, mechanical, vascular
  ventricular (communicating shunt) T85.01 ☑
Malherbe's tumor — *see* Neoplasm, skin, benign
Malibu disease L98.8
Malignancy — *see also* Neoplasm, malignant, by site
  unspecified site (primary) C80.1
Malignant — *see* condition
Malingerer, malingering Z76.5
Mallet finger (acquired) — *see* Deformity, finger, mallet finger
  congenital Q74.0
  sequelae of rickets E64.3
Malleus A24.0
Mallory's bodies R89.7
Mallory-Weiss syndrome K22.6
Malnutrition E46
  degree
    first E44.1
    mild (protein) E44.1
    moderate (protein) E44.0
    second E44.0
    severe (protein-energy) E43
      intermediate form E42
        with
          kwashiorkor E42
          marasmus E41
    third E43
  following gastrointestinal surgery K91.2
  intrauterine
    light-for-dates — *see* Light for dates
    small-for-dates — *see* Small for dates
  lack of care, or neglect (child) (infant) T76.02 ☑
    confirmed T74.02 ☑
  malignant E40
  protein E46
    calorie E46
      mild E44.1
      moderate E44.0
      severe E43
        intermediate form E42
          with
            kwashiorkor (and marasmus) E42
            marasmus E41
    energy E46
      mild E44.1
      moderate E44.0
      severe E43
        intermediate form E42
          with
            kwashiorkor (and marasmus) E42
            marasmus E41
  severe (protein-energy) E43
    with
      kwashiorkor (and marasmus) E42
      marasmus E41
Malocclusion (teeth) M26.4
  Angle's M26.219
    class I M26.211
    class II M26.212
    class III M26.213
  due to
    abnormal swallowing M26.59
    mouth breathing M26.59
    tongue, lip or finger habits M26.59
  temporomandibular (joint) M26.69
Malposition
  cervix — *see* Malposition, uterus
  congenital
    adrenal (gland) Q89.1
    alimentary tract Q45.8
      lower Q43.8
      upper Q40.8
    aorta Q25.49
    appendix Q43.8
    arterial trunk Q20.0
    artery (peripheral) Q27.8
      coronary Q24.5
      digestive system Q27.8
      lower limb Q27.8
      pulmonary Q25.79

Malposition — *continued*
  congenital — *continued*
    artery — *continued*
      specified site NEC Q27.8
      upper limb Q27.8
    auditory canal Q17.8
      causing impairment of hearing Q16.9
    auricle (ear) Q17.4
      causing impairment of hearing Q16.9
      cervical Q18.2
    biliary duct or passage Q44.5
    bladder (mucosa) — *see* Exstrophy, bladder
    brachial plexus Q07.8
    brain tissue Q04.8
    breast Q83.8
    bronchus Q32.4
    cecum Q43.8
    clavicle Q74.0
    colon Q43.8
    digestive organ or tract NEC Q45.8
      lower Q43.8
      upper Q40.8
    ear (auricle) (external) Q17.4
      ossicles Q16.3
    endocrine (gland) NEC Q89.2
    epiglottis Q31.8
    eustachian tube Q17.8
    eye Q15.8
    facial features Q18.8
    fallopian tube Q50.6
    finger(s) Q68.1
      supernumerary Q69.0
    foot Q66.9- ☑
    gallbladder Q44.1
    gastrointestinal tract Q45.8
    genitalia, genital organ(s) or tract
      female Q52.8
        external Q52.79
        internal NEC Q52.8
      male Q55.8
    glottis Q31.8
    hand Q68.1
    heart Q24.8
      dextrocardia Q24.0
        with complete transposition of viscera Q89.3
    hepatic duct Q44.5
    hip (joint) Q65.89
    intestine (large) (small) Q43.8
      with anomalous adhesions, fixation or malrotation Q43.3
    joint NEC Q68.8
    kidney Q63.2
    larynx Q31.8
    limb Q68.8
      lower Q68.8
      upper Q68.8
    liver Q44.7
    lung (lobe) Q33.8
    nail(s) Q84.6
    nerve Q07.8
    nervous system NEC Q07.8
    nose, nasal (septum) Q30.8
    organ or site not listed — *see* Anomaly, by site
    ovary Q50.39
    pancreas Q45.3
    parathyroid (gland) Q89.2
    patella Q74.1
    peripheral vascular system Q27.8
    pituitary (gland) Q89.2
    respiratory organ or system NEC Q34.8
    rib (cage) Q76.6
      supernumerary in cervical region Q76.5
    scapula Q74.0
    shoulder Q74.0
    spinal cord Q06.8
    spleen Q89.09
    sternum NEC Q76.7
    stomach Q40.2
    symphysis pubis Q74.2
    thymus (gland) Q89.2
    thyroid (gland) (tissue) Q89.2
      cartilage Q31.8
    toe(s) Q66.9- ☑
      supernumerary Q69.2
    tongue Q38.3
    trachea Q32.1
    ureter Q62.60
      deviation Q62.61
      displacement Q62.62

Malposition — *continued*
  congenital — *continued*
    ureter — *continued*
      ectopia Q62.63
      specified type NEC Q62.69
    uterus Q51.818
    vein(s) (peripheral) Q27.8
      great Q26.8
    vena cava (inferior) (superior) Q26.8
  device, implant or graft — *see also* Complications, by site and type, mechanical T85.628 ☑
    arterial graft NEC — *see* Complication, cardiovascular device, mechanical, vascular
    breast (implant) T85.42 ☑
    catheter NEC T85.628 ☑
      cystostomy T83.020 ☑
      dialysis (renal) T82.42 ☑
        intraperitoneal T85.621 ☑
      infusion NEC T82.524 ☑
        spinal (epidural) (subdural) T85.620 ☑
      urinary — *see also* Displacement, device, catheter, urinary T83.028 ☑
    electronic (electrode) (pulse generator) (stimulator)
      bone T84.320 ☑
      cardiac T82.129 ☑
        electrode T82.120 ☑
        pulse generator T82.121 ☑
        specified type NEC T82.128 ☑
      nervous system — *see* Complication, prosthetic device, mechanical, electronic nervous system stimulator
      urinary — *see* Complication, genitourinary, device, urinary, mechanical
    fixation, internal (orthopedic) NEC — *see* Complication, fixation device, mechanical
    gastrointestinal — *see* Complications, prosthetic device, mechanical, gastrointestinal device
    genital NEC T83.428 ☑
      intrauterine contraceptive device (string) T83.32 ☑
      penile prosthesis (cylinder) (implanted) (pump) (reservoir) T83.420 ☑
      testicular prosthesis T83.421 ☑
    heart NEC — *see* Complication, cardiovascular device, mechanical
    joint prosthesis — *see* Complication, joint prosthesis, mechanical
    ocular NEC — *see* Complications, prosthetic device, mechanical, ocular device
    orthopedic NEC — *see* Complication, orthopedic, device, mechanical
    specified NEC T85.628 ☑
    urinary NEC — *see also* Complication, genitourinary, device, urinary, mechanical
      graft T83.22 ☑
    vascular NEC — *see* Complication, cardiovascular device, mechanical
    ventricular intracranial shunt T85.02 ☑
  fetus — *see* Pregnancy, complicated by (management affected by), presentation, fetal
  gallbladder K82.8
  gastrointestinal tract, congenital Q45.8
  heart, congenital NEC Q24.8
  joint prosthesis — *see* Complications, joint prosthesis, mechanical, displacement, by site
  stomach K31.89
    congenital Q40.2
  tooth, teeth, fully erupted M26.30
  uterus (acute) (acquired) (adherent) (asymptomatic) (postinfectional) (postpartal, old) N85.4
    anteflexion or anteversion N85.4
      congenital Q51.818
    flexion N85.4
      lateral — *see* Lateroversion, uterus
    inversion N85.5
    lateral (flexion) (version) — *see* Lateroversion, uterus
      in pregnancy or childbirth — *see* subcategory O34.5 ☑
    retroflexion or retroversion — *see* Retroversion, uterus
Malposture R29.3
Malrotation
  cecum Q43.3
  colon Q43.3
  intestine Q43.3
  kidney Q63.2
Malta fever — *see* Brucellosis

☑ Additional Character Required — Refer to the Tabular List for Character Selection

Maltreatment
  adult
    abandonment
      confirmed T74.01 ☑
      suspected T76.01 ☑
    bullying
      confirmed T74.31 ☑
      suspected T76.31 ☑
    confirmed T74.91 ☑
    history of Z91.419
    intimidation (through social media)
      confirmed T74.31 ☑
      suspected T76.31 ☑
    neglect
      confirmed T74.01 ☑
      suspected T76.01 ☑
    physical abuse
      confirmed T74.11 ☑
      suspected T76.11 ☑
    psychological abuse
      confirmed T74.31 ☑
      history of Z91.411
      suspected T76.31 ☑
    sexual abuse
      confirmed T74.21 ☑
      suspected T76.21 ☑
    suspected T76.91 ☑
  child
    abandonment
      confirmed T74.02 ☑
      suspected T76.02 ☑
    bullying
      confirmed T74.32 ☑
      suspected T76.32 ☑
    confirmed T74.92 ☑
    history of — see History, personal (of), abuse
    intimidation (through social media)
      confirmed T74.32 ☑
      suspected T76.32 ☑
    neglect
      confirmed T74.02 ☑
      history of — see History, personal (of), abuse
      suspected T76.02 ☑
    physical abuse
      confirmed T74.12 ☑
      history of — see History, personal (of), abuse
      suspected T76.12 ☑
    psychological abuse
      confirmed T74.32 ☑
      history of — see History, personal (of), abuse
      suspected T76.32 ☑
    sexual abuse
      confirmed T74.22 ☑
      history of — see History, personal (of), abuse
      suspected T76.22 ☑
    suspected T76.92 ☑
  personal history of Z91.89
Maltworker's lung J67.4
Malunion, fracture — see Fracture, by site
Mammillitis N61.0
  puerperal, postpartum O91.02
Mammitis — see Mastitis
Mammogram (examination) Z12.39
  routine Z12.31
Mammoplasia N62
Management (of)
  bone conduction hearing device (implanted) Z45.320
  cardiac pacemaker NEC Z45.018
  cerebrospinal fluid drainage device Z45.41
  cochlear device (implanted) Z45.321
  contraceptive Z30.9
    specified NEC Z30.8
  implanted device Z45.9
    specified NEC Z45.89
  infusion pump Z45.1
  procreative Z31.9
    male factor infertility in female Z31.81
    specified NEC Z31.89
  prosthesis (external) — see also Fitting Z44.9
    implanted Z45.9
      specified NEC Z45.89
  renal dialysis catheter Z49.01
  vascular access device Z45.2
Mangled — see specified injury by site
Mania (monopolar) — see also Disorder, mood, manic episode
  with psychotic symptoms F30.2

Mania — continued
  without psychotic symptoms F30.10
    mild F30.11
    moderate F30.12
    severe F30.13
  Bell's F30.8
  chronic (recurrent) F31.89
  hysterical F44.89
  puerperal F30.8
  recurrent F31.89
Manic depression F31.9
Manic-depressive insanity, psychosis, or syndrome — see Disorder, bipolar
Mannosidosis E77.1
Mansonelliasis, mansonellosis B74.4
Manson's
  disease B65.1
  schistosomiasis B65.1
Manual — see condition
Maple-bark-stripper's lung (disease) J67.6
Maple-syrup-urine disease E71.0
Marable's syndrome (celiac artery compression) I77.4
Marasmus E41
  due to malnutrition E41
  intestinal E41
  nutritional E41
  senile R54
  tuberculous NEC — see Tuberculosis
Marble
  bones Q78.2
  skin R23.8
Marburg virus disease A98.3
March
  fracture — see Fracture, traumatic, stress, by site
  hemoglobinuria D59.6
Marchesani (-Weill) **syndrome** Q87.0
Marchiafava (-Bignami) **syndrome or disease** G37.1
Marchiafava-Micheli syndrome D59.5
Marcus Gunn's syndrome Q07.8
Marfan's syndrome — see Syndrome, Marfan's
Marie-Bamberger disease — see Osteoarthropathy, hypertrophic, specified NEC
Marie-Charcot-Tooth neuropathic muscular atrophy G60.0
Marie's
  cerebellar ataxia (late-onset) G11.2
  disease or syndrome (acromegaly) E22.0
Marie-Strümpell arthritis, disease or spondylitis — see Spondylitis, ankylosing
Marion's disease (bladder neck obstruction) N32.0
Marital conflict Z63.0
Mark
  port wine Q82.5
  raspberry Q82.5
  strawberry Q82.5
  stretch L90.6
  tattoo L81.8
Marker heterochromatin — see Extra, marker chromosomes
Maroteaux-Lamy syndrome (mild) (severe) E76.29
Marrow (bone)
  arrest D61.9
  poor function D75.89
Marseilles fever A77.1
Marsh fever — see Malaria
Marshall's (hidrotic) **ectodermal dysplasia** Q82.4
Marsh's disease (exophthalmic goiter) E05.00
  with storm E05.01
Masculinization (female) **with adrenal hyperplasia** E25.9
  congenital E25.0
Masculinovoblastoma D27.- ☑
Masochism (sexual) F65.51
Mason's lung J62.8
Mass
  abdominal R19.00
    epigastric R19.06
    generalized R19.07
    left lower quadrant R19.04
    left upper quadrant R19.02
    periumbilic R19.05
    right lower quadrant R19.03
    right upper quadrant R19.01
    specified site NEC R19.09
  breast — see also Lump, breast N63.0
  chest R22.2
  cystic — see Cyst

Mass — continued
  ear H93.8- ☑
  head R22.0
  intra-abdominal (diffuse) (generalized) — see Mass, abdominal
  kidney N28.89
  liver R16.0
  localized (skin) R22.9
    chest R22.2
    head R22.0
    limb
      lower R22.4- ☑
      upper R22.3- ☑
    neck R22.1
    trunk R22.2
  lung R91.8
  malignant — see Neoplasm, malignant, by site
  neck R22.1
  pelvic (diffuse) (generalized) — see Mass, abdominal
  specified organ NEC — see Disease, by site
  splenic R16.1
  substernal thyroid — see Goiter
  superficial (localized) R22.9
  umbilical (diffuse) (generalized) R19.09
Massive — see condition
Mast cell
  disease, systemic tissue D47.02
  leukemia C94.3- ☑
  neoplasm
    malignant C96.20
      specified type NEC C96.29
    of uncertain behavior NEC D47.09
  sarcoma C96.22
  tumor D47.09
Mastalgia N64.4
Masters-Allen syndrome N83.8
Mastitis (acute) (diffuse) (nonpuerperal) (subacute) N61.0
  with abscess N61.1
  chronic (cystic) — see Mastopathy, cystic
  cystic (Schimmelbusch's type) — see Mastopathy, cystic
  fibrocystic — see Mastopathy, cystic
  granulomatous N61.2- ☑
  infective N61.0
    newborn P39.0
  interstitial, gestational or puerperal — see Mastitis, obstetric
  neonatal (noninfective) P83.4
    infective P39.0
  obstetric (interstitial) (nonpurulent)
    associated with
      lactation O91.23
      pregnancy O91.21- ☑
      puerperium O91.22
    purulent
      associated with
        lactation O91.13
        pregnancy O91.11- ☑
        puerperium O91.12
  periductal — see Ectasia, mammary duct
  phlegmonous — see Mastopathy, cystic
  plasma cell — see Ectasia, mammary duct
  without abscess N61.0
Mastocytoma (extracutaneous) D47.09
  malignant C96.29
  solitary D47.01
Mastocytosis D47.09
  aggressive systemic C96.21
  cutaneous (diffuse) (maculopapular) D47.01
    congenital Q82.2
    of neonatal onset Q82.2
    of newborn onset Q82.2
  indolent systemic D47.02
  isolated bone marrow D47.02
  malignant C96.29
  systemic (indolent) (smoldering)
    with an associated hematological non-mast cell lineage disease (SM-AHNMD) D47.02
Mastodynia N64.4
Mastoid — see condition
Mastoidalgia — see subcategory H92.0 ☑
Mastoiditis (coalescent) (hemorrhagic) (suppurative) H70.9- ☑
  acute, subacute H70.00- ☑
    complicated NEC H70.09- ☑
    subperiosteal H70.01- ☑
  chronic (necrotic) (recurrent) H70.1- ☑

Mastoiditis — *continued*
in (due to)
infectious disease NEC B99 ☑ *[H75.0-]* ☑
parasitic disease NEC B89 *[H75.0-]* ☑
tuberculosis A18.03
petrositis — *see* Petrositis
postauricular fistula — *see* Fistula, postauricular
specified NEC H70.89- ☑
tuberculous A18.03
Mastopathy, mastopathia N64.9
chronica cystica — *see* Mastopathy, cystic
cystic (chronic) (diffuse) N60.1- ☑
with epithelial proliferation N60.3- ☑
diffuse cystic — *see* Mastopathy, cystic
estrogenic, oestrogenica N64.89
ovarian origin N64.89
Mastoplasia, mastoplastia N62
Masturbation (excessive) F98.8
Maternal care (for) — *see* Pregnancy (complicated by)
(management affected by)
Matheiu's disease (leptospiral jaundice) A27.0
Mauclaire's disease or osteochondrosis — *see* Osteochondrosis, juvenile, hand, metacarpal
Maxcy's disease A75.2
Maxilla, maxillary — *see* condition
May (-Hegglin) **anomaly or syndrome** D72.0
McArdle (-Schmid)(-Pearson) **disease** (glycogen storage)
E74.04
McCune-Albright syndrome Q78.1
McQuarrie's syndrome (idiopathic familial hypo-
glycemia) E16.2
Meadow's syndrome Q86.1
Measles (black) (hemorrhagic) (suppressed) B05.9
with
complications NEC B05.89
encephalitis B05.0
intestinal complications B05.4
keratitis (keratoconjunctivitis) B05.81
meningitis B05.1
otitis media B05.3
pneumonia B05.2
French — *see* Rubella
German — *see* Rubella
Liberty — *see* Rubella
Meatitis, urethral — *see* Urethritis
Meatus, meatal — *see* condition
Meat-wrappers' asthma J68.9
ME/CFS (myalgic encephalomyelitis/chronic fatigue syndrome) G93.32
Meckel-Gruber syndrome Q61.9
Meckel's diverticulitis, diverticulum (displaced) (hypertrophic) Q43.0
malignant — *see* Table of Neoplasms, small intestine,
malignant
Meconium
ileus, newborn P76.0
in cystic fibrosis E84.11
meaning meconium plug (without cystic fibrosis)
P76.0
obstruction, newborn P76.0
due to fecaliths P76.0
in mucoviscidosis E84.11
peritonitis P78.0
plug syndrome (newborn) NEC P76.0
Median — *see also* condition
arcuate ligament syndrome I77.4
bar (prostate) (vesical orifice) — *see* Hyperplasia,
prostate
rhomboid glossitis K14.2
Mediastinal shift R93.89
Mediastinitis (acute) (chronic) J98.51
syphilitic A52.73
tuberculous A15.8
Mediastinopericarditis — *see also* Pericarditis
acute I30.9
adhesive I31.0
chronic I31.8
rheumatic I09.2
Mediastinum, mediastinal — *see* condition
Medicine poisoning — *see* Table of Drugs and Chemicals, by drug, poisoning
Mediterranean
fever — *see* Brucellosis
familial M04.1
tick A77.1
kala-azar B55.0
leishmaniasis B55.0

Mediterranean — *continued*
tick fever A77.1
Medulla — *see* condition
Medullary cystic kidney Q61.5
Medullated fibers
optic (nerve) Q14.8
retina Q14.1
Medulloblastoma
desmoplastic C71.6
specified site — *see* Neoplasm, malignant, by site
unspecified site C71.6
Medulloepithelioma — *see also* Neoplasm, malignant,
by site
teratoid — *see* Neoplasm, malignant, by site
Medullomyoblastoma
specified site — *see* Neoplasm, malignant, by site
unspecified site C71.6
Meekeren-Ehlers-Danlos syndrome — *see also* Syndrome, Ehlers-Danlos Q79.69
Megacolon (acquired) (functional) (not Hirschsprung's
disease) (in) K59.39
Chagas' disease B57.32
congenital, congenitum (aganglionic) Q43.1
Hirschsprung's (disease) Q43.1
toxic NEC K59.31
due to Clostridium difficile
not specified as recurrent A04.72
recurrent A04.71
Megaesophagus (functional) K22.0
congenital Q39.5
in (due to) Chagas' disease B57.31
Megalencephaly Q04.5
Megalerythema (epidemic) B08.3
Megaloappendix Q43.8
Megalocephalus, megalocephaly NEC Q75.3
Megalocornea Q15.8
with glaucoma Q15.0
Megalocytic anemia D53.1
Megalodactylia (fingers) (thumbs) (congenital) Q74.0
toes Q74.2
Megaloduodenum Q43.8
Megaloesophagus (functional) K22.0
congenital Q39.5
Megalogastria (acquired) K31.89
congenital Q40.2
Megalophthalmos Q11.3
Megalopsia H53.15
Megalosplenia — *see* Splenomegaly
Megaloureter N28.82
congenital Q62.2
Megarectum K62.89
Megasigmoid K59.39
congenital Q43.2
Megaureter N28.82
congenital Q62.2
Megavitamin-B6 syndrome E67.2
Megrim — *see* Migraine
Meibomian
cyst, infected — *see* Hordeolum
gland — *see* condition
sty, stye — *see* Hordeolum
Meibomitis — *see* Hordeolum
Meige-Milroy disease (chronic hereditary edema) Q82.0
Meige's syndrome Q82.0
Melalgia, nutritional E53.8
Melancholia F32.A
climacteric (single episode) F32.89
recurrent episode F33.8
hypochondriac F45.29
intermittent (single episode) F32.89
recurrent episode F33.8
involutional (single episode) F32.89
recurrent episode F33.8
menopausal (single episode) F32.89
recurrent episode F33.8
puerperal F32.89
reactive (emotional stress or trauma) F32.3
recurrent F33.9
senile F03 ☑
stuporous (single episode) F32.89
recurrent episode F33.8
Melanemia R79.89
Melanoameloblastoma — *see* Neoplasm, bone, benign
Melanoblastoma — *see* Melanoma
Melanocarcinoma — *see* Melanoma
Melanocytoma, eyeball D31.9- ☑
Melanocytosis, neurocutaneous Q82.8

Melanoderma, melanodermia L81.4
Melanodontia, infantile K03.89
Melanodontoclasia K03.89
Melanoepithelioma — *see* Melanoma
Melanoma (malignant) C43.9
acral lentiginous, malignant — *see* Melanoma, skin, by
site
amelanotic — *see* Melanoma, skin, by site
balloon cell — *see* Melanoma, skin, by site
benign — *see* Nevus
desmoplastic, malignant — *see* Melanoma, skin, by
site
epithelioid cell — *see* Melanoma, skin, by site
with spindle cell, mixed — *see* Melanoma, skin, by
site
in
giant pigmented nevus — *see* Melanoma, skin, by
site
Hutchinson's melanotic freckle — *see* Melanoma,
skin, by site
junctional nevus — *see* Melanoma, skin, by site
precancerous melanosis — *see* Melanoma, skin, by
site
in situ D03.9
abdominal wall D03.59
ala nasi D03.39
ankle D03.7- ☑
anus, anal (margin) (skin) D03.51
arm D03.6- ☑
auditory canal D03.2- ☑
auricle (ear) D03.2- ☑
auricular canal (external) D03.2- ☑
axilla, axillary fold D03.59
back D03.59
breast D03.52
brow D03.39
buttock D03.59
canthus (eye) D03.1- ☑
cheek (external) D03.39
chest wall D03.59
chin D03.39
choroid D03.8
conjunctiva D03.8
ear (external) D03.2- ☑
external meatus (ear) D03.2- ☑
eye D03.8
eyebrow D03.39
eyelid (lower) (upper) D03.1- ☑
face D03.30
specified NEC D03.39
female genital organ (external) NEC D03.8
finger D03.6- ☑
flank D03.59
foot D03.7- ☑
forearm D03.6- ☑
forehead D03.39
foreskin D03.8
gluteal region D03.59
groin D03.59
hand D03.6- ☑
heel D03.7- ☑
helix D03.2- ☑
hip D03.7- ☑
interscapular region D03.59
iris D03.8
jaw D03.39
knee D03.7- ☑
labium (majus) (minus) D03.8
lacrimal gland D03.8
leg D03.7- ☑
lip (lower) (upper) D03.0
lower limb NEC D03.7- ☑
male genital organ (external) NEC D03.8
nail D03.9
finger D03.6- ☑
toe D03.7- ☑
neck D03.4
nose (external) D03.39
orbit D03.8
penis D03.8
perianal skin D03.51
perineum D03.51
pinna D03.2- ☑
popliteal fossa or space D03.7- ☑
prepuce D03.8
pudendum D03.8
retina D03.8

☑ **Additional Character Required** — **Refer to the Tabular List for Character Selection**

Melanoma — *continued*
  in situ — *continued*
    retrobulbar D03.8
    scalp D03.4
    scrotum D03.8
    shoulder D03.6- ☑
    specified site NEC D03.8
    submammary fold D03.52
    temple D03.39
    thigh D03.7- ☑
    toe D03.7- ☑
    trunk NEC D03.59
    umbilicus D03.59
    upper limb NEC D03.6- ☑
    vulva D03.8
  juvenile — *see* Nevus
  malignant, of soft parts except skin — *see* Neoplasm, connective tissue, malignant
  metastatic
    breast C79.81
    genital organ C79.82
    specified site NEC C79.89
  neurotropic, malignant — *see* Melanoma, skin, by site
  nodular — *see* Melanoma, skin, by site
  regressing, malignant — *see* Melanoma, skin, by site
  skin C43.9
    abdominal wall C43.59
    ala nasi C43.31
    ankle C43.7- ☑
    anus, anal (skin) C43.51
    arm C43.6- ☑
    auditory canal (external) C43.2- ☑
    auricle (ear) C43.2- ☑
    auricular canal (external) C43.2- ☑
    axilla, axillary fold C43.59
    back C43.59
    breast (female) (male) C43.52
    brow C43.39
    buttock C43.59
    canthus (eye) C43.1- ☑
    cheek (external) C43.39
    chest wall C43.59
    chin C43.39
    ear (external) C43.2- ☑
    elbow C43.6- ☑
    external meatus (ear) C43.2- ☑
    eyebrow C43.39
    eyelid (lower) (upper) C43.1- ☑
    face C43.30
      specified NEC C43.39
    female genital organ (external) NEC C51.9
    finger C43.6- ☑
    flank C43.59
    foot C43.7- ☑
    forearm C43.6- ☑
    forehead C43.39
    foreskin C60.0
    glabella C43.39
    gluteal region C43.59
    groin C43.59
    hand C43.6- ☑
    heel C43.7- ☑
    helix C43.2- ☑
    hip C43.7- ☑
    interscapular region C43.59
    jaw (external) C43.39
    knee C43.7- ☑
    labium C51.9
      majus C51.0
      minus C51.1
    leg C43.7- ☑
    lip (lower) (upper) C43.0
    lower limb NEC C43.7- ☑
    male genital organ (external) NEC C63.9
    nail
      finger C43.6- ☑
      toe C43.7- ☑
    nasolabial groove C43.39
    nates C43.59
    neck C43.4
    nose (external) C43.31
    overlapping site C43.8
    palpebra C43.1- ☑
    penis C60.9
    perianal skin C43.51
    perineum C43.51
    pinna C43.2- ☑

Melanoma — *continued*
  skin — *continued*
    popliteal fossa or space C43.7- ☑
    prepuce C60.0
    pudendum C51.9
    scalp C43.4
    scrotum C63.2
    shoulder C43.6- ☑
    skin NEC C43.9
    submammary fold C43.52
    temple C43.39
    thigh C43.7- ☑
    toe C43.7- ☑
    trunk NEC C43.59
    umbilicus C43.59
    upper limb NEC C43.6- ☑
    vulva C51.9
      overlapping sites C51.8
  spindle cell
    with epithelioid, mixed — *see* Melanoma, skin, by site
    type A C69.4- ☑
    type B C69.4- ☑
  superficial spreading — *see* Melanoma, skin, by site
Melanosarcoma — *see also* Melanoma
  epithelioid cell — *see* Melanoma
Melanosis L81.4
  addisonian E27.1
    tuberculous A18.7
  adrenal E27.1
  colon K63.89
  conjunctiva — *see* Pigmentation, conjunctiva
    congenital Q13.89
  cornea (presenile) (senile) — *see also* Pigmentation, cornea
    congenital Q13.4
  eye NEC H57.89
    congenital Q15.8
  lenticularis progressiva Q82.1
  liver K76.89
  precancerous — *see also* Melanoma, in situ
    malignant melanoma in — *see* Melanoma
  Riehl's L81.4
  sclera H15.89
    congenital Q13.89
  suprarenal E27.1
  tar L81.4
  toxic L81.4
Melanuria R82.998
MELAS syndrome E88.41
Melasma L81.1
  adrenal (gland) E27.1
  suprarenal (gland) E27.1
Melena K92.1
  with ulcer — *code by* site under Ulcer, with hemorrhage K27.4
  due to swallowed maternal blood P78.2
  newborn, neonatal P54.1
    due to swallowed maternal blood P78.2
Meleney's
  gangrene (cutaneous) — *see* Ulcer, skin
  ulcer (chronic undermining) — *see* Ulcer, skin
Melioidosis A24.9
  acute A24.1
  chronic A24.2
  fulminating A24.1
  pneumonia A24.1
  pulmonary (chronic) A24.2
    acute A24.1
    subacute A24.2
  sepsis A24.1
  specified NEC A24.3
  subacute A24.2
Melitensis, febris A23.0
Melkersson (-Rosenthal) **syndrome** G51.2
Mellitus, diabetes — *see* Diabetes
Melorheostosis (bone) — *see* Disorder, bone, density and structure, specified NEC
Meloschisis Q18.4
Melotia Q17.4
Membrana
  capsularis lentis posterior Q13.89
  epipapillaris Q14.2
Membranacea placenta O43.19- ☑
Membranaceous uterus N85.8
Membrane(s), membranous — *see also* condition
  cyclitic — *see* Membrane, pupillary

Membrane(s), membranous — *continued*
  folds, congenital — *see* Web
  Jackson's Q43.3
  over face of newborn P28.9
  premature rupture — *see* Rupture, membranes, premature
  pupillary H21.4- ☑
    persistent Q13.89
  retained (with hemorrhage) (complicating delivery) O72.2
    without hemorrhage O73.1
  secondary cataract — *see* Cataract, secondary
  unruptured (causing asphyxia) — *see* Asphyxia, newborn
  vitreous — *see* Opacity, vitreous, membranes and strands
Membranitis — *see* Chorioamnionitis
Memory disturbance, lack or loss — *see also* Amnesia
  mild, following organic brain damage F06.8
Menadione deficiency E56.1
Menarche
  delayed E30.0
  precocious E30.1
Mendacity, pathologic F60.2
Mendelson's syndrome (due to anesthesia) J95.4
  in labor and delivery O74.0
  in pregnancy O29.01- ☑
  obstetric O74.0
  postpartum, puerperal O89.01
Ménétrier's disease or syndrome K29.60
  with bleeding K29.61
Ménière's disease, syndrome or vertigo H81.0- ☑
Meninges, meningeal — *see* condition
Meningioma — *see also* Neoplasm, meninges, benign
  angioblastic — *see* Neoplasm, meninges, benign
  angiomatous — *see* Neoplasm, meninges, benign
  atypical — *see* Neoplasm, meninges, uncertain behavior
  endotheliomatous — *see* Neoplasm, meninges, benign
  fibroblastic — *see* Neoplasm, meninges, benign
  fibrous — *see* Neoplasm, meninges, benign
  hemangioblastic — *see* Neoplasm, meninges, benign
  hemangiopericytic — *see* Neoplasm, meninges, benign
  malignant — *see* Neoplasm, meninges, malignant
  meningiothelial — *see* Neoplasm, meninges, benign
  meningotheliomatous — *see* Neoplasm, meninges, benign
  mixed — *see* Neoplasm, meninges, benign
  multiple — *see* Neoplasm, meninges, uncertain behavior
  papillary — *see* Neoplasm, meninges, uncertain behavior
  psammomatous — *see* Neoplasm, meninges, benign
  syncytial — *see* Neoplasm, meninges, benign
  transitional — *see* Neoplasm, meninges, benign
Meningiomatosis (diffuse) — *see* Neoplasm, meninges, uncertain behavior
Meningism — *see* Meningismus
Meningismus (infectional) (pneumococcal) R29.1
  due to serum or vaccine R29.1
  influenzal — *see* Influenza, with, manifestations NEC
Meningitis (basal) (basic) (brain) (cerebral) (cervical) (congestive) (diffuse) (hemorrhagic) (infantile) (membranous) (metastatic) (nonspecific) (pontine) (progressive) (simple) (spinal) (subacute) (sympathetic) (toxic) G03.9
  abacterial G03.0
  actinomycotic A42.81
  adenoviral A87.1
  arbovirus A87.8
  aseptic (acute) G03.0
  bacterial G00.9
    Escherichia coli (E. coli) G00.8
    Friedländer (bacillus) G00.8
    gram-negative G00.9
    H. influenzae G00.0
    Klebsiella G00.8
    pneumococcal G00.1
    specified organism NEC G00.8
    staphylococcal G00.3
    streptococcal (acute) G00.2
  benign recurrent (Mollaret) G03.2
  candidal B37.5
  caseous (tuberculous) A17.0
  cerebrospinal A39.0
  chronic NEC G03.1
  clear cerebrospinal fluid NEC G03.0

Meningitis — *continued*
- coxsackievirus A87.0
- cryptococcal B45.1
- diplococcal (gram positive) A39.0
- echovirus A87.0
- enteroviral A87.0
- eosinophilic B83.2
- epidemic NEC A39.0
- Escherichia coli (E. coli) G00.8
- fibrinopurulent G00.9
  - specified organism NEC G00.8
- Friedländer (bacillus) G00.8
- gonococcal A54.81
- gram-negative cocci G00.9
- gram-positive cocci G00.9
- H. influenzae G00.0
- Haemophilus (influenzae) G00.0
- in (due to)
  - adenovirus A87.1
  - African trypanosomiasis B56.9 *[G02]*
  - anthrax A22.8
  - bacterial disease NEC A48.8 *[G01]*
  - Chagas' disease (chronic) B57.41
  - chickenpox B01.0
  - coccidioidomycosis B38.4
  - Diplococcus pneumoniae G00.1
  - enterovirus A87.0
  - herpes (simplex) virus B00.3
    - zoster B02.1
  - infectious mononucleosis B27.92
  - leptospirosis A27.81
  - Listeria monocytogenes A32.11
  - Lyme disease A69.21
  - measles B05.1
  - mumps (virus) B26.1
  - neurosyphilis (late) A52.13
  - parasitic disease NEC B89 *[G02]*
  - poliovirus A80.9 *[G02]*
  - preventive immunization, inoculation or vaccination G03.8
  - rubella B06.02
  - Salmonella infection A02.21
  - specified cause NEC G03.8
  - Streptococcal pneumoniae G00.1
  - typhoid fever A01.01
  - varicella B01.0
  - viral disease NEC A87.8
  - whooping cough A37.90
  - zoster B02.1
- infectious G00.9
- influenzal (H. influenzae) G00.0
- Klebsiella G00.8
- leptospiral (aseptic) A27.81
- lymphocytic (acute) (benign) (serous) A87.2
- meningococcal A39.0
- Mima polymorpha G00.8
- Mollaret (benign recurrent) G03.2
- monilial B37.5
- mycotic NEC B49 *[G02]*
- Neisseria A39.0
- nonbacterial G03.0
- nonpyogenic NEC G03.0
- ossificans G96.198
- pneumococcal streptococcus pneumoniae G00.1
- poliovirus A80.9 *[G02]*
- postmeasles B05.1
- purulent G00.9
  - specified organism NEC G00.8
- pyogenic G00.9
  - specified organism NEC G00.8
- Salmonella (arizonae) (Cholerae-Suis) (enteritidis) (typhimurium) A02.21
- septic G00.9
  - specified organism NEC G00.8
- serosa circumscripta NEC G03.0
- serous NEC G93.2
- specified organism NEC G00.8
- sporotrichosis B42.81
- staphylococcal G00.3
- sterile G03.0
- Streptococcal (acute) G00.2
  - pneumoniae G00.1
- suppurative G00.9
  - specified organism NEC G00.8
- syphilitic (late) (tertiary) A52.13
  - acute A51.41
  - congenital A50.41
  - secondary A51.41
- Torula histolytica (cryptococcal) B45.1

Meningitis — *continued*
- traumatic (complication of injury) T79.8 ☑
- tuberculous A17.0
- typhoid A01.01
- viral NEC A87.9
- Yersinia pestis A20.3

Meningocele (spinal) — *see also* Spina bifida
- with hydrocephalus — *see* Spina bifida, by site, with hydrocephalus
- acquired (traumatic) G96.198
- cerebral — *see* Encephalocele

Meningocerebritis — *see* Meningoencephalitis

Meningococcemia A39.4
- acute A39.2
- chronic A39.3

Meningococcus, meningococcal — *see also* condition A39.9
- adrenalitis, hemorrhagic A39.1
- carrier (suspected) of Z22.31
- meningitis (cerebrospinal) A39.0

Meningoencephalitis — *see also* Encephalitis G04.90
- acute NEC — *see also* Encephalitis, viral A86
- bacterial NEC G04.2
- California A83.5
- diphasic A84.1
- eosinophilic B83.2
- epidemic A39.81
- herpesviral, herpetic B00.4
  - due to herpesvirus 6 B10.01
  - due to herpesvirus 7 B10.09
  - specified NEC B10.09
- in (due to)
  - blastomycosis NEC B40.81
  - diseases classified elsewhere G05.3
  - free-living amebae B60.2
  - H. influenzae G00.0
  - Hemophilus influenzae (H .influenzae) G00.0
  - herpes B00.4
    - due to herpesvirus 6 B10.01
    - due to herpesvirus 7 B10.09
    - specified NEC B10.09
  - Lyme disease A69.22
  - mercury — *see* subcategory T56.1 ☑
  - mumps B26.2
  - Naegleria (amebae) (organisms) (fowleri) B60.2
  - Parastrongylus cantonensis B83.2
  - toxoplasmosis (acquired) B58.2
    - congenital P37.1
- infectious (acute) (viral) A86
- influenzal (H. influenzae) G00.0
- Listeria monocytogenes A32.12
- lymphocytic (serous) A87.2
- mumps B26.2
- parasitic NEC B89 *[G05.3]*
- pneumococcal G04.2
- primary ambic B60.2
- specific (syphilitic) A52.14
- specified organism NEC G04.81
- staphylococcal G04.2
- streptococcal G04.2
- syphilitic A52.14
- toxic NEC G92.8
  - due to mercury — *see* subcategory T56.1 ☑
- tuberculous A17.82
- virus NEC A86

Meningoencephalocele — *see also* Encephalocele
- syphilitic A52.19
  - congenital A50.49

Meningoencephalomyelitis — *see also* Meningoencephalitis
- acute NEC (viral) A86
  - disseminated G04.00
    - postimmunization or postvaccination G04.02
    - postinfectious G04.01
  - due to
    - actinomycosis A42.82
    - Torula B45.1
    - Toxoplasma or toxoplasmosis (acquired) B58.2
      - congenital P37.1
  - postimmunization or postvaccination G04.02

Meningoencephalomyelopathy G96.9

Meningoencephalopathy G96.9

Meningomyelitis — *see also* Meningoencephalitis
- bacterial NEC G04.2
- blastomycotic NEC B40.81
- cryptococcal B45.1
- in diseases classified elsewhere G05.4
- meningococcal A39.81

Meningomyelitis — *continued*
- syphilitic A52.14
- tuberculous A17.82

Meningomyelocele — *see also* Spina bifida
- syphilitic A52.19

Meningomyeloneuritis — *see* Meningoencephalitis

Meningoradiculitis — *see* Meningitis

Meningovascular — *see* condition

Menkes' disease or syndrome E83.09
- meaning maple-syrup-urine disease E71.0

Menometrorrhagia N92.1

Menopause, menopausal (asymptomatic) (state) Z78.0
- arthritis (any site) NEC — *see* Arthritis, specified form NEC
- bleeding N92.4
- depression (single episode) F32.89
  - agitated (single episode) F32.2
    - recurrent episode F33.9
  - psychotic (single episode) F32.89
    - recurrent episode F33.9
  - recurrent episode F33.8
- melancholia (single episode) F32.89
  - recurrent episode F33.8
- paranoid state F22
- postirradiation (postprocedural)
  - asymptomatic E89.40
  - symptomatic E89.41
- premature E28.319
  - asymptomatic E28.319
    - postirradiation E89.40
    - postsurgical E89.40
  - symptomatic E28.310
    - postirradiation E89.41
    - postsurgical E89.41
- psychosis NEC F28
- symptomatic N95.1
- toxic polyarthritis NEC — *see* Arthritis, specified form NEC

Menorrhagia (primary) N92.0
- climacteric N92.4
  - menopausal N92.4
- menopausal N92.4
- perimenopausal N92.4
- postclimacteric N95.0
- postmenopausal N95.0
- preclimacteric or premenopausal N92.4
- pubertal (menses retained) N92.2

Menostaxis N92.0

Menses, retention N94.89

Menstrual — *see* Menstruation

Menstruation
- absent — *see* Amenorrhea
- anovulatory N97.0
- cycle, irregular N92.6
- delayed N91.0
- disorder N93.9
  - psychogenic F45.8
- during pregnancy O20.8
- excessive (with regular cycle) N92.0
  - with irregular cycle N92.1
  - at puberty N92.2
- frequent N92.0
- infrequent — *see* Oligomenorrhea
- irregular N92.6
  - specified NEC N92.5
- latent N92.5
- membranous N92.5
- painful — *see also* Dysmenorrhea N94.6
  - primary N94.4
  - psychogenic F45.8
  - secondary N94.5
- passage of clots N92.0
- precocious E30.1
- protracted N92.5
- rare — *see* Oligomenorrhea
- retained N94.89
- retrograde N92.5
- scanty — *see* Oligomenorrhea
- suppression N94.89
- vicarious (nasal) N94.89

Mental — *see also* condition
- deficiency — *see* Disability, intellectual
- deterioration — *see* Psychosis
- disorder — *see* Disorder, mental
- exhaustion F48.8
- insufficiency (congenital) — *see* Disability, intellectual
- observation without need for further medical care Z03.89

☑ **Additional Character Required** — Refer to the Tabular List for Character Selection

Mental — *continued*
  retardation — *see* Disability, intellectual
  subnormality — *see* Disability, intellectuall
  upset — *see* Disorder, mental
Meralgia paresthetica G57.1- ☑
Mercurial — *see* condition
Mercurialism — *see* subcategory T56.1 ☑
Merkel cell tumor — *see* Carcinoma, Merkel cell
Merocele — *see* Hernia, femoral
Meromelia
  lower limb — *see* Defect, reduction, lower limb
    intercalary
      femur — *see* Defect, reduction, lower limb,
        specified type NEC
        tibiofibular (complete) (incomplete) — *see*
          Defect, reduction, lower limb
    upper limb — *see* Defect, reduction, upper limb
      intercalary, humeral, radioulnar — *see* Agenesis,
        arm, with hand present
MERRF syndrome (myoclonic epilepsy associated with
  ragged-red fiber) E88.42
Merzbacher-Pelizaeus disease E75.29
Mesaortitis — *see* Aortitis
Mesarteritis — *see* Arteritis
Mesencephalitis — *see* Encephalitis
Mesenchymoma — *see also* Neoplasm, connective tis-
  sue, uncertain behavior
  benign — *see* Neoplasm, connective tissue, benign
  malignant — *see* Neoplasm, connective tissue, malig-
    nant
Mesenteritis
  retractile K65.4
  sclerosing K65.4
Mesentery, mesenteric — *see* condition
Mesiodens, mesiodentes K00.1
Mesio-occlusion M26.213
Mesocolon — *see* condition
Mesonephroma (malignant) — *see* Neoplasm, malig-
  nant, by site
  benign — *see* Neoplasm, benign, by site
Mesophlebitis — *see* Phlebitis
Mesostromal dysgenesia Q13.89
Mesothelioma (malignant) C45.9
  benign
    mesentery D19.1
    mesocolon D19.1
    omentum D19.1
    peritoneum D19.1
    pleura D19.0
    specified site NEC D19.7
    unspecified site D19.9
  biphasic C45.9
    benign
      mesentery D19.1
      mesocolon D19.1
      omentum D19.1
      peritoneum D19.1
      pleura D19.0
      specified site NEC D19.7
      unspecified site D19.9
  cystic D48.4
  epithelioid C45.9
    benign
      mesentery D19.1
      mesocolon D19.1
      omentum D19.1
      peritoneum D19.1
      pleura D19.0
      specified site NEC D19.7
      unspecified site D19.9
  fibrous C45.9
    benign
      mesentery D19.1
      mesocolon D19.1
      omentum D19.1
      peritoneum D19.1
      pleura D19.0
      specified site NEC D19.7
      unspecified site D19.9
  site classification
    liver C45.7
    lung C45.7
    mediastinum C45.7
    mesentery C45.1
    mesocolon C45.1
    omentum C45.1
    pericardium C45.2
    peritoneum C45.1

Mesothelioma — *continued*
  site classification — *continued*
    pleura C45.0
      parietal C45.0
    retroperitoneum C45.7
    specified site NEC C45.7
    unspecified C45.9
Metabolic syndrome E88.81
Metagonimiasis B66.8
Metagonimus infestation (intestine) B66.8
Metal
  pigmentation L81.8
  polisher's disease J62.8
Metamorphopsia H53.15
Metaplasia
  apocrine (breast) — *see* Dysplasia, mammary, specified
    type NEC
  cervix (squamous) — *see* Dysplasia, cervix
  endometrium (squamous) (uterus) N85.8
  esophagus K22.7- ☑
  gastric intestinal K31.A0
    with dysplasia K31.A29
      high grade K31.A22
      low grade K31.A21
    indefinite for dysplasia K31.A0
    without dysplasia K31.A19
      involving
        antrum K31.A11
        body (corpus) K31.A12
        cardia K31.A14
        fundus K31.A13
        multiple sites K31.A15
  kidney (pelvis) (squamous) N28.89
  myelogenous D73.1
  myeloid (agnogenic) (megakaryocytic) D73.1
  spleen D73.1
  squamous cell, bladder N32.89
Metastasis, metastatic
  abscess — *see* Abscess
  calcification E83.59
  cancer
    from specified site — *see* Neoplasm, malignant, by
      site
    to specified site — *see* Neoplasm, secondary, by site
  deposits (in) — *see* Neoplasm, secondary, by site
  disease — *see also* Neoplasm, secondary, by site C79.9
  spread (to) — *see* Neoplasm, secondary, by site
Metastrongyliasis B83.8
Metatarsalgia M77.4- ☑
  anterior G57.6- ☑
  Morton's G57.6- ☑
Metatarsus, metatarsal — *see also* condition
  adductus, congenital Q66.22- ☑
  valgus (abductus), congenital Q66.6
  varus (congenital) Q66.22- ☑
    primus Q66.21- ☑
Methadone use — *see* Use, opioid
Methemoglobinemia D74.9
  acquired (with sulfhemoglobinemia) D74.8
  congenital D74.0
  enzymatic (congenital) D74.0
  Hb M disease D74.0
  hereditary D74.0
  toxic D74.8
Methemoglobinuria — *see* Hemoglobinuria
Methioninemia E72.19
Methylmalonic acidemia E71.120
Metritis (catarrhal) (hemorrhagic) (septic) (suppurative)
    — *see also* Endometritis
  cervical — *see* Cervicitis
Metropathia hemorrhagica N93.8
Metroperitonitis — *see* Peritonitis, pelvic, female
Metrorrhagia N92.1
  climacteric N92.4
  menopausal N92.4
  perimenopausal N92.4
  postpartum NEC (atonic) (following delivery of placen-
    ta) O72.1
    delayed or secondary O72.2
  preclimacteric or premenopausal N92.4
  psychogenic F45.8
Metrorrhexis — *see* Rupture, uterus
Metrosalpingitis N70.91
Metrostaxis N93.8
Metrovaginitis — *see* Endometritis
Meyer-Schwickerath and Weyers syndrome Q87.0
Meynert's amentia (nonalcoholic) F04

Meynert's amentia — *continued*
  alcoholic F10.96
    with dependence F10.26
Mibelli's disease (porokeratosis) Q82.8
Mice, joint — *see* Loose, body, joint
  knee M23.4- ☑
Micrencephalon, micrencephaly Q02
Microalbuminuria R80.9
Microaneurysm, retinal — *see also* Disorder, retina,
    microaneurysms
  diabetic — *see* E08-E13 with .31
Microangiopathy (peripheral) I73.9
  thrombotic M31.10
    hematopoietic stem cell transplantation-associated
      [HSCT-TMA] M31.10
Microcalcifications, breast R92.0
Microcephalus, microcephalic, microcephaly Q02
  due to toxoplasmosis (congenital) P37.1
Microcheilia Q18.7
Microcolon (congenital) Q43.8
Microcornea (congenital) Q13.4
Microcytic — *see* condition
Microdeletions NEC Q93.88
Microdontia K00.2
Microdrepanocytosis D57.40
  with
    acute chest syndrome D57.411
    cerebral vascular involvement D57.413
    crisis (painful) D57.419
      with specified complication NEC D57.418
    splenic sequestration D57.412
    vasoocclusive pain D57.419
Microembolism
  atherothrombotic — *see* Atheroembolism
  retinal — *see* Occlusion, artery, retina
Microencephalon Q02
Microfilaria streptocerca infestation — *see* Onchocer-
    ciasis
Microgastria (congenital) Q40.2
Microgenia M26.06
Microgenitalia, congenital
  female Q52.8
  male Q55.8
Microglioma — *see* Lymphoma, non-Hodgkin, specified
    NEC
Microglossia (congenital) Q38.3
Micrognathia, micrognathism (congenital) (mandibu-
    lar) (maxillary) M26.09
Microgyria (congenital) Q04.3
Microinfarct of heart — *see* Insufficiency, coronary
Microlentia (congenital) Q12.8
Microlithiasis, alveolar, pulmonary J84.02
Micromastia N64.82
Micromyelia (congenital) Q06.8
Micropenis Q55.62
Microphakia (congenital) Q12.8
Microphthalmos, microphthalmia (congenital) Q11.2
  due to toxoplasmosis P37.1
Micropsia H53.15
Microscopic polyangiitis (polyarteritis) M31.7
Microsporidiosis B60.8
  intestinal A07.8
Microsporon furfur infestation B36.0
Microsporosis — *see also* Dermatophytosis
  nigra B36.1
Microstomia (congenital) Q18.5
Microtia (congenital) (external ear) Q17.2
Microtropia H50.40
Microvillus inclusion disease (MVD) (MVID) Q43.8
Micturition
  disorder NEC — *see also* Difficulty, micturition R39.198
    psychogenic F45.8
  frequency R35.0
    psychogenic F45.8
  hesitancy R39.11
  incomplete emptying R39.14
  nocturnal R35.1
  painful R30.9
    dysuria R30.0
    psychogenic F45.8
    tenesmus R30.1
  poor stream R39.12
  position dependent R39.192
  split stream R39.13
  straining R39.16
  urgency R39.15
Mid plane — *see* condition

Middle
ear — *see* condition
lobe (right) syndrome J98.19
Miescher's elastoma L87.2
Mietens' syndrome Q87.2
Migraine (idiopathic) G43.909
with refractory migraine G43.919
with status migrainosus G43.911
without status migrainosus G43.919
with aura (acute-onset) (prolonged) (typical) (without headache) G43.109
with refractory migraine G43.119
with status migrainosus G43.111
without status migrainosus G43.119
intractable G43.119
with status migrainosus G43.111
without status migrainosus G43.119
not intractable G43.109
with status migrainosus G43.101
without status migrainosus G43.109
persistent G43.509
with cerebral infarction G43.609
with refractory migraine G43.619
with status migrainosus G43.611
without status migrainosus G43.619
intractable G43.619
with status migrainosus G43.611
without status migrainosus G43.619
not intractable G43.609
with status migrainosus G43.601
without status migrainosus G43.609
without refractory migraine G43.609
with status migrainosus G43.601
without status migrainosus H43.609
without cerebral infarction G43.509
with refractory migraine G43.519
with status migrainosus G43.511
without status migrainosus G43.519
intractable G43.519
with status migrainosus G43.511
without status migrainosus G43.519
not intractable G43.509
with status migrainosus G43.501
without status migrainosus G43.509
without refractory migraine G43.509
with status migrainosus G43.501
without status migrainosus G43.509
without mention of refractory migraine G43.109
with status migrainosus G43.101
without status migrainosus G43.109
abdominal G43.D0 (*following* G43.7)
with refractory migraine G43.D1 (*following* G43.7)
intractable G43.D1 (*following* G43.7)
not intractable G43.D0 (*following* G43.7)
without refractory migraine G43.D0 (*following* G43.7)
basilar — *see* Migraine, with aura
classical — *see* Migraine, with aura
common — *see* Migraine, without aura
complicated G43.109
equivalents — *see* Migraine, with aura
familiar — *see* Migraine, hemiplegic
hemiplegic G43.409
with refractory migraine G43.419
with status migrainosus G43.411
without status migrainosus G43.419
intractable G43.419
with status migrainosus G43.411
without status migrainosus G43.419
not intractable G43.409
with status migrainosus G43.401
without status migrainosus G43.409
without refractory migraine G43.409
with status migrainosus G43.401
without status migrainosus G43.409
intractable G43.919
with status migrainosus G43.911
without status migrainosus G43.919
menstrual G43.829
with refractory migraine G43.839
with status migrainosus G43.831
without status migrainosus G43.839
intractable G43.839
with status migrainosus G43.831
without status migrainosus G43.839
not intractable G43.829
with status migrainosus G43.821
without status migrainosus G43.829
without refractory migraine G43.829

Migraine — *continued*
menstrual — *continued*
without refractory migraine — *continued*
with status migrainosus G43.821
without status migrainosus G43.829
menstrually related — *see* Migraine, menstrual
not intractable G43.909
with status migrainosus G43.901
without status migrainosus G43.919
ophthalmoplegic G43.B0 (*following* G43.7)
with refractory migraine G43.B1 (*following* G43.7)
intractable G43.B1 (*following* G43.7)
not intractable G43.B0 (*following* G43.7)
without refractory migraine G43.B0 (*following* G43.7)
persistent aura (with, without) cerebral infarction — *see* Migraine, with aura
preceded or accompanied by transient focal neurological phenomena — *see* Migraine, with aura
pre-menstrual — *see* Migraine, menstrual
pure menstrual — *see* Migraine, menstrual
retinal — *see* Migraine, with aura
specified NEC G43.809
intractable G43.819
with status migrainosus G43.811
without status migrainosus G43.819
not intractable G43.809
with status migrainosus G43.801
without status migrainosus G43.809
sporadic — *see* Migraine, hemiplegic
transformed — *see* Migraine, without aura, chronic
triggered seizures — *see* Migraine, with aura
without aura G43.009
with refractory migraine G43.019
with status migrainosus G43.011
without status migrainosus G43.019
chronic G43.709
with refractory migraine G43.719
with status migrainosus G43.711
without status migrainosus G43.719
intractable
with status migrainosus G43.711
without status migrainosus G43.719
not intractable
with status migrainosus G43.701
without status migrainosus G43.709
without refractory migraine G43.709
with status migrainosus G43.701
without status migrainosus G43.709
intractable
with status migrainosus G43.011
without status migrainosus G43.019
not intractable
with status migrainosus G43.001
without status migrainosus G43.009
without mention of refractory migraine G43.009
with status migrainosus G43.001
without status migrainosus G43.009
without refractory migraine G43.909
with status migrainosus G43.901
without status migrainosus G43.909
Migrant, social Z59.00
Migration, anxiety concerning Z60.3
Migratory, migrating — *see also* condition
person Z59.00
testis Q55.29
Mikity-Wilson disease or syndrome P27.0
Mikulicz' disease or syndrome K11.8
Miliaria L74.3
alba L74.1
apocrine L75.2
crystallina L74.1
profunda L74.2
rubra L74.0
tropicalis L74.2
Miliary — *see* condition
Milium L72.0
colloid L57.8
Milk
crust L21.0
excessive secretion O92.6
poisoning — *see* Poisoning, food, noxious
retention O92.79
sickness — *see* Poisoning, food, noxious
spots I31.0
Milk-alkali disease or syndrome E83.52
Milk-leg (deep vessels) (nonpuerperal) — *see* Embolism, vein, lower extremity
complicating pregnancy O22.3- ☑

Milk-leg — *continued*
puerperal, postpartum, childbirth O87.1
Milkman's disease or syndrome M83.8
Milky urine — *see* Chyluria
Millard-Gubler (-Foville) **paralysis or syndrome** G46.3
Millar's asthma J38.5
Miller Fisher syndrome G61.0
Mills' disease — *see* Hemiplegia
Millstone maker's pneumoconiosis J62.8
Milroy's disease (chronic hereditary edema) Q82.0
Minamata disease T56.1 ☑
Miners' asthma or lung J60
Minkowski-Chauffard syndrome — *see* Spherocytosis
Minor — *see* condition
Minor's disease (hematomyelia) G95.19
Minot's disease (hemorrhagic disease), newborn P53
Minot-von Willebrand-Jurgens disease or syndrome (angiohemophilia) — *see* Disease, von Willebrand
Minus (and plus) **hand** (intrinsic) — *see* Deformity, limb, specified type NEC, forearm
Miosis (pupil) H57.03
Mirizzi's syndrome (hepatic duct stenosis) K83.1
Mirror writing F81.0
MIS-A M35.81
Misadventure (of) (prophylactic) (therapeutic) — *see also* Complications T88.9 ☑
administration of insulin (by accident) — *see* subcategory T38.3 ☑
infusion — *see* Complications, infusion
local applications (of fomentations, plasters, etc.) T88.9 ☑
burn or scald — *see* Burn
specified NEC T88.8 ☑
medical care (early) (late) T88.9 ☑
adverse effect of drugs or chemicals — *see* Table of Drugs and Chemicals
burn or scald — *see* Burn
specified NEC T88.8 ☑
specified NEC T88.8 ☑
surgical procedure (early) (late) — *see* Complications, surgical procedure
transfusion — *see* Complications, transfusion
vaccination or other immunological procedure — *see* Complications, vaccination
MIS-C M35.81
Miscarriage O03.9
Misdirection, aqueous H40.83- ☑
Misperception, sleep state F51.02
Misplaced, misplacement
ear Q17.4
kidney (acquired) N28.89
congenital Q63.2
organ or site, congenital NEC — *see* Malposition, congenital
Missed
abortion O02.1
delivery O36.4 ☑
Missing — *see also* Absence
string of intrauterine contraceptive device T83.32- ☑
Misuse of drugs F19.99
Mitchell's disease (erythromelalgia) I73.81
Mite(s) (infestation) B88.9
diarrhea B88.0
grain (itch) B88.0
hair follicle (itch) B88.0
in sputum B88.0
Mitral — *see* condition
Mittelschmerz N94.0
Mixed — *see* condition
MMN (multifocal motor neuropathy) G61.82
MNGIE (Mitochondrial Neurogastrointestinal Encephalopathy) **syndrome** E88.49
Mobile, mobility
cecum Q43.3
excessive — *see* Hypermobility
gallbladder, congenital Q44.1
kidney N28.89
organ or site, congenital NEC — *see* Malposition, congenital
Mobitz heart block (atrioventricular) I44.1
Moebius, Möbius
disease (ophthalmoplegic migraine) — *see* Migraine, ophthalmoplegic
syndrome Q87.0
congenital oculofacial paralysis (with other anomalies) Q87.0

☑ Additional Character Required — Refer to the Tabular List for Character Selection

Moebius, Möbius — *continued*
  syndrome — *continued*
    ophthalmoplegic migraine — *see* Migraine, ophthalmoplegic
Moeller's glossitis K14.0
Mohr's syndrome (Types I and II) Q87.0
Mola destruens D39.2
Molar pregnancy O02.0
Molarization of premolars K00.2
Molding, head (during birth) — *omit code*
Mole (pigmented) — *see also* Nevus
  blood O02.0
  Breus' O02.0
  cancerous — *see* Melanoma
  carneous O02.0
  destructive D39.2
  fleshy O02.0
  hydatid, hydatidiform (benign) (complicating pregnancy) (delivered) (undelivered) O01.9
    classical O01.0
    complete O01.0
    incomplete O01.1
    invasive D39.2
    malignant D39.2
    partial O01.1
  intrauterine O02.0
  invasive (hydatidiform) D39.2
  malignant
    meaning
      malignant hydatidiform mole D39.2
      melanoma — *see* Melanoma
  nonhydatidiform O02.0
  nonpigmented — *see* Nevus
  pregnancy NEC O02.0
  skin — *see* Nevus
  tubal O00.10- ☑
    with intrauterine pregnancy O00.11- ☑
  vesicular — *see* Mole, hydatidiform
Molimen, molimina (menstrual) N94.3
Molluscum contagiosum (epitheliale) B08.1
Mönckeberg's arteriosclerosis, disease, or sclerosis
  — *see* Arteriosclerosis, extremities
Mondini's malformation (cochlea) Q16.5
Mondor's disease I80.8
Monge's disease T70.29 ☑
Monilethrix (congenital) Q84.1
Moniliasis — *see also* Candidiasis B37.9
  neonatal P37.5
Monitoring (encounter for)
  therapeutic drug level Z51.81
Monkey malaria B53.1
Monkeypox B04
Monoarthritis M13.10
  ankle M13.17- ☑
  elbow M13.12- ☑
  foot joint M13.17- ☑
  hand joint M13.14- ☑
  hip M13.15- ☑
  knee M13.16- ☑
  shoulder M13.11- ☑
  wrist M13.13- ☑
Monoblastic — *see* condition
Monochromat (ism), monochromatopsia (acquired) (congenital) H53.51
Monocytic — *see* condition
Monocytopenia D72.818
Monocytosis (symptomatic) D72.821
Monomania — *see* Psychosis
Mononeuritis G58.9
  cranial nerve — *see* Disorder, nerve, cranial
  femoral nerve G57.2- ☑
  lateral
    cutaneous nerve of thigh G57.1- ☑
    popliteal nerve G57.3- ☑
  lower limb G57.9- ☑
    specified nerve NEC G57.8- ☑
  medial popliteal nerve G57.4- ☑
  median nerve G56.1- ☑
  multiplex G58.7
  plantar nerve G57.6- ☑
  posterior tibial nerve G57.5- ☑
  radial nerve G56.3- ☑
  sciatic nerve G57.0- ☑
  specified NEC G58.8
  tibial nerve G57.4- ☑
  ulnar nerve G56.2- ☑
  upper limb G56.9- ☑

Mononeuritis — *continued*
  upper limb — *continued*
    specified nerve NEC G56.8- ☑
  vestibular — *see* subcategory H93.3 ☑
Mononeuropathy G58.9
  carpal tunnel syndrome — *see* Syndrome, carpal tunnel
  diabetic NEC — *see* E08-E13 with .41
  femoral nerve — *see* Lesion, nerve, femoral
  ilioinguinal nerve G57.8- ☑
  in diseases classified elsewhere — *see* category G59
  intercostal G58.0
  lower limb G57.9- ☑
    causalgia — *see* Causalgia, lower limb
    femoral nerve — *see* Lesion, nerve, femoral
    meralgia paresthetica G57.1- ☑
    plantar nerve — *see* Lesion, nerve, plantar
    popliteal nerve — *see* Lesion, nerve, popliteal
    sciatic nerve — *see* Lesion, nerve, sciatic
    specified NEC G57.8- ☑
    tarsal tunnel syndrome — *see* Syndrome, tarsal tunnel
  median nerve — *see* Lesion, nerve, median
  multiplex G58.7
  obturator nerve G57.8- ☑
  popliteal nerve — *see* Lesion, nerve, popliteal
  radial nerve — *see* Lesion, nerve, radial
  saphenous nerve G57.8- ☑
  specified NEC G58.8
  tarsal tunnel syndrome — *see* Syndrome, tarsal tunnel
  tuberculous A17.83
  ulnar nerve — *see* Lesion, nerve, ulnar
  upper limb G56.9- ☑
    carpal tunnel syndrome — *see* Syndrome, carpal tunnel
    causalgia — *see* Causalgia
    median nerve — *see* Lesion, nerve, median
    radial nerve — *see* Lesion, nerve, radial
    specified site NEC G56.8- ☑
    ulnar nerve — *see* Lesion, nerve, ulnar
Mononucleosis, infectious B27.90
  with
    complication NEC B27.99
    meningitis B27.92
    polyneuropathy B27.91
  cytomegaloviral B27.10
    with
      complication NEC B27.19
      meningitis B27.12
      polyneuropathy B27.11
  Epstein-Barr (virus) B27.00
    with
      complication NEC B27.09
      meningitis B27.02
      polyneuropathy B27.01
  gammaherpesviral B27.00
    with
      complication NEC B27.09
      meningitis B27.02
      polyneuropathy B27.01
  specified NEC B27.80
    with
      complication NEC B27.89
      meningitis B27.82
      polyneuropathy B27.81
Monoplegia G83.3- ☑
  congenital (cerebral) G80.8
    spastic G80.1
  embolic (current episode) I63.4- ☑
  following
    cerebrovascular disease
      cerebral infarction
        lower limb I69.34- ☑
        upper limb I69.33- ☑
      intracerebral hemorrhage
        lower limb I69.14- ☑
        upper limb I69.13- ☑
      lower limb I69.94- ☑
      nontraumatic intracranial hemorrhage NEC
        lower limb I69.24- ☑
        upper limb I69.23- ☑
      specified disease NEC
        lower limb I69.84- ☑
        upper limb I69.83- ☑
      stroke NOS
        lower limb I69.34- ☑
        upper limb I69.33- ☑

Monoplegia — *continued*
  following — *continued*
    cerebrovascular disease — *continued*
      subarachnoid hemorrhage
        lower limb I69.04- ☑
        upper limb I69.03- ☑
      upper limb I69.93- ☑
  hysterical (transient) F44.4
  lower limb G83.1- ☑
  psychogenic (conversion reaction) F44.4
  thrombotic (current episode) I63.3- ☑
  transient R29.818
  upper limb G83.2- ☑
Monorchism, monorchidism Q55.0
Monosomy — *see also* Deletion, chromosome Q93.9
  specified NEC Q93.89
  whole chromosome
    meiotic nondisjunction Q93.0
    mitotic nondisjunction Q93.1
    mosaicism Q93.1
  X Q96.9
Monster, monstrosity (single) Q89.7
  acephalic Q00.0
  twin Q89.4
Monteggia's fracture (-dislocation) S52.27- ☑
Mooren's ulcer (cornea) — *see* Ulcer, cornea, Mooren's
Moore's syndrome — *see* Epilepsy, specified NEC
Mooser-Neill reaction A75.2
Mooser's bodies A75.2
Morbidity not stated or unknown R69
Morbilli — *see* Measles
Morbus — *see also* Disease
  angelicus, anglorum E55.0
  Beigel B36.2
  caducus — *see* Epilepsy
  celiacus K90.0
  comitialis — *see* Epilepsy
  cordis — *see also* Disease, heart I51.9
    valvulorum — *see* Endocarditis
  coxae senilis M16.9
    tuberculous A18.02
  hemorrhagicus neonatorum P53
  maculosus neonatorum P54.5
Morel (-Stewart)(-Morgagni) **syndrome** M85.2
Morel-Kraepelin disease — *see* Schizophrenia
Morel-Moore syndrome M85.2
Morgagni's
  cyst, organ, hydatid, or appendage
    female Q50.5
    male (epididymal) Q55.4
      testicular Q55.29
  syndrome M85.2
Morgagni-Stewart-Morel syndrome M85.2
Morgagni-Stokes-Adams syndrome I45.9
Morgagni-Turner (-Albright) **syndrome** Q96.9
Moria F07.0
Moron (I.Q. 50-69) F70
Morphea L94.0
Morphinism (without remission) F11.20
  with remission F11.21
Morphinomania (without remission) F11.20
  with remission F11.21
Morquio (-Ullrich)(-Brailsford) **disease or syndrome** — *see* Mucopolysaccharidosis
Mortification (dry) (moist) — *see* Gangrene
Morton's metatarsalgia (neuralgia) (neuroma) (syndrome) G57.6- ☑
Morvan's disease or syndrome G60.8
Mosaicism, mosaic (autosomal) (chromosomal)
  45,X/46,XX Q96.3
  45,X/other cell lines NEC with abnormal sex chromosome Q96.4
  sex chromosome
    female Q97.8
    lines with various numbers of X chromosomes Q97.2
    male Q98.7
  XY Q96.3
Moschowitz' disease M31.19
Mother yaw A66.0
Motion sickness (from travel, any vehicle) (from roundabouts or swings) T75.3 ☑
Mottled, mottling, teeth (enamel) (endemic) (nonendemic) K00.3
Mounier-Kuhn syndrome Q32.4
  with bronchiectasis J47.9
    exacerbation (acute) J47.1
    lower respiratory infection J47.0

Mounier-Kuhn syndrome — *continued*
　acquired J98.09
　　with bronchiectasis J47.9
　　　with
　　　　exacerbation (acute) J47.1
　　　　lower respiratory infection J47.0
Mountain
　sickness T70.29 ☑
　　with polycythemia , acquired (acute) D75.1
　tick fever A93.2
Mouse, joint — *see* Loose, body, joint
　knee M23.4- ☑
Mouth — *see* condition
Movable
　coccyx — *see* subcategory M53.2 ☑
　kidney N28.89
　　congenital Q63.8
　spleen D73.89
Movements, dystonic R25.8
Moyamoya disease I67.5
MRSA (Methicillin resistant Staphylococcus aureus)
　infection A49.02
　　as the cause of diseases classified elsewhere B95.62
　sepsis A41.02
MSD (multiple sulfatase deficiency) E75.26
MSSA (Methicillin susceptible Staphylococcus aureus)
　infection A49.01
　　as the cause of diseases classified elsewhere B95.61
　sepsis A41.01
Mucha-Habermann disease L41.0
Mucinosis (cutaneous) (focal) (papular) (skin) L98.5
　oral K13.79
Mucocele
　appendix K38.8
　buccal cavity K13.79
　gallbladder K82.1
　lacrimal sac, chronic H04.43- ☑
　nasal sinus J34.1
　nose J34.1
　salivary gland (any) K11.6
　sinus (accessory) (nasal) J34.1
　turbinate (bone) (middle) (nasal) J34.1
　uterus N85.8
Mucolipidosis
　I E77.1
　II, III E77.0
　IV E75.11
Mucopolysaccharidosis E76.3
　beta-gluduronidase deficiency E76.29
　cardiopathy E76.3 *[I52]*
　Hunter's syndrome E76.1
　Hurler's syndrome E76.01
　Hurler-Scheie syndrome E76.02
　Maroteaux-Lamy syndrome E76.29
　Morquio syndrome E76.219
　　A E76.210
　　B E76.211
　　classic E76.210
　Sanfilippo syndrome E76.22
　Scheie's syndrome E76.03
　specified NEC E76.29
　type
　　I
　　　Hurler's syndrome E76.01
　　　Hurler-Scheie syndrome E76.02
　　　Scheie's syndrome E76.03
　　II E76.1
　　III E76.22
　　IV E76.219
　　IVA E76.210
　　IVB E76.211
　　VI E76.29
　　VII E76.29
Mucormycosis B46.5
　cutaneous B46.3
　disseminated B46.4
　gastrointestinal B46.2
　generalized B46.4
　pulmonary B46.0
　rhinocerebral B46.1
　skin B46.3
　subcutaneous B46.3
Mucositis (ulcerative) K12.30
　due to drugs NEC K12.32
　gastrointestinal K92.81
　mouth (oral) (oropharyngeal) K12.30
　　due to antineoplastic therapy K12.31
　　due to drugs NEC K12.32

Mucositis — *continued*
　mouth — *continued*
　　due to radiation K12.33
　　specified NEC K12.39
　　viral K12.39
　nasal J34.81
　oral cavity — *see* Mucositis, mouth
　oral soft tissues — *see* Mucositis, mouth
　vagina and vulva N76.81
Mucositis necroticans agranulocytica — *see* Agranu-
　locytosis
Mucous — *see also* condition
　patches (syphilitic) A51.39
　　congenital A50.07
Mucoviscidosis E84.9
　with meconium obstruction E84.11
Mucus
　asphyxia or suffocation — *see* Asphyxia, mucus
　in stool R19.5
　plug — *see* Asphyxia, mucus
Muguet B37.0
Mulberry molars (congenital syphilis) A50.52
Müllerian mixed tumor
　specified site — *see* Neoplasm, malignant, by site
　unspecified site C54.9
Multicystic kidney (development) Q61.4
Multiparity (grand) Z64.1
　affecting management of pregnancy, labor and delivery
　　(supervision only) O09.4- ☑
　requiring contraceptive management — *see* Contra-
　　ception
Multipartita placenta O43.19- ☑
Multiple, multiplex — *see also* condition
　digits (congenital) Q69.9
　endocrine neoplasia — *see* Neoplasia, endocrine,
　　multiple (MEN)
　personality F44.81
Multisystem inflammatory syndrome (in adult) (in
　children) M35.81
Mumps B26.9
　arthritis B26.85
　complication NEC B26.89
　encephalitis B26.2
　hepatitis B26.81
　meningitis (aseptic) B26.1
　meningoencephalitis B26.2
　myocarditis B26.82
　oophoritis B26.89
　orchitis B26.0
　pancreatitis B26.3
　polyneuropathy B26.84
Mumu — *see also* Infestation, filarial B74.9 *[N51]*
Münchhausen's syndrome — *see* Disorder, factitious
Münchmeyer's syndrome — *see* Myositis, ossificans,
　progressiva
Mural — *see* condition
Murmur (cardiac) (heart) (organic) R01.1
　abdominal R19.15
　aortic (valve) — *see* Endocarditis, aortic
　benign R01.0
　diastolic — *see* Endocarditis
　Flint I35.1
　functional R01.0
　Graham Steell I37.1
　innocent R01.0
　mitral (valve) — *see* Insufficiency, mitral
　nonorganic R01.0
　presystolic, mitral — *see* Insufficiency, mitral
　pulmonic (valve) I37.8
　systolic R01.1
　tricuspid (valve) I07.9
　valvular — *see* Endocarditis
Murri's disease (intermittent hemoglobinuria) D59.6
Muscle, muscular — *see also* condition
　carnitine (palmityltransferase) deficiency E71.314
Musculoneuralgia — *see* Neuralgia
Mushrooming hip — *see* Derangement, joint, specified
　NEC, hip
Mushroom-workers' (pickers') **disease or lung** J67.5
Mutation(s)
　factor V Leiden D68.51
　prothrombin gene D68.52
　surfactant, of lung J84.83
Mutism — *see also* Aphasia
　deaf (acquired) (congenital) NEC H91.3
　elective (adjustment reaction) (childhood) F94.0
　hysterical F44.4

Mutism — *continued*
　selective (childhood) F94.0
MVD (microvillus inclusion disease) Q43.8
MVID (microvillus inclusion disease) Q43.8
Myalgia M79.10
　auxiliary muscles, head and neck M79.12
　epidemic (cervical) B33.0
　mastication muscle M79.11
　site specified NEC M79.18
　traumatic NEC T14.8 ☑
Myasthenia G70.9
　congenital G70.2
　cordis — *see* Failure, heart
　developmental G70.2
　gravis G70.00
　　with exacerbation (acute) G70.01
　　in crisis G70.01
　　neonatal, transient P94.0
　　pseudoparalytica G70.00
　　　with exacerbation (acute) G70.01
　　　in crisis G70.01
　stomach, psychogenic F45.8
　syndrome
　　in
　　　diabetes mellitus — *see* E08-E13 with .44
　　　neoplastic disease — *see also* Neoplasm
　　　　D49.9 *[G73.3]*
　　　pernicious anemia D51.0 *[G73.3]*
　　　thyrotoxicosis E05.90 *[G73.3]*
　　　　with thyroid storm E05.91 *[G73.3]*
Myasthenic M62.81
Mycelium infection B49
Mycetismus — *see* Poisoning, food, noxious, mushroom
Mycetoma B47.9
　actinomycotic B47.1
　bone (mycotic) B47.9 *[M90.80]*
　eumycotic B47.0
　foot B47.9
　　actinomycotic B47.1
　　mycotic B47.0
　madurae NEC B47.9
　　mycotic B47.0
　maduromycotic B47.0
　mycotic B47.0
　nocardial B47.1
Mycobacteriosis — *see* Mycobacterium
Mycobacterium, mycobacterial (infection) A31.9
　anonymous A31.9
　atypical A31.9
　　cutaneous A31.1
　　pulmonary A31.0
　　　tuberculous — *see* Tuberculosis, pulmonary
　　specified site NEC A31.8
　avium (intracellulare complex) A31.0
　balnei A31.1
　Battey A31.0
　chelonei A31.8
　cutaneous A31.1
　extrapulmonary systemic A31.8
　fortuitum A31.8
　intracellulare (Battey bacillus) A31.0
　kakaferifu A31.8
　kansasii (yellow bacillus) A31.0
　kasongo A31.8
　leprae — *see also* Leprosy A30.9
　luciflavum A31.1
　marinum (M. balnei) A31.1
　nonspecific — *see* Mycobacterium, atypical
　pulmonary (atypical) A31.0
　　tuberculous — *see* Tuberculosis, pulmonary
　scrofulaceum A31.8
　simiae A31.8
　systemic, extrapulmonary A31.8
　szulgai A31.8
　terrae A31.8
　triviale A31.8
　tuberculosis (human, bovine) — *see* Tuberculosis
　ulcerans A31.1
　xenopi A31.8
Mycoplasma (M.) **pneumoniae, as cause of disease
　classified elsewhere** B96.0
Mycosis, mycotic B49
　cutaneous NEC B36.9
　ear B36.9
　　in
　　　aspergillosis B44.89
　　　candidiasis B37.84
　　　moniliasis B37.84

Mycosis, mycotic — *continued*
 fungoides (extranodal) (solid organ) C84.0- ☑
 mouth B37.0
 nails B35.1
 opportunistic B48.8
 skin NEC B36.9
 specified NEC B48.8
 stomatitis B37.0
 vagina, vaginitis (candidal) (acute) B37.31
  chronic (recurrent) B37.32
Mydriasis (pupil) H57.04
Myelatelia Q06.1
Myelinolysis, pontine, central G37.2
Myelitis (acute) (ascending) (childhood) (chronic) (descending) (diffuse) (disseminated) (idiopathic) (pressure) (progressive) (spinal cord) (subacute) — *see also* Encephalitis G04.91
 flaccid G04.82
 herpes simplex B00.82
 herpes zoster B02.24
 in diseases classified elsewhere G05.4
 necrotizing, subacute G37.4
 optic neuritis in G36.0
 postchickenpox B01.12
 postherpetic B02.24
 postimmunization G04.02
 postinfectious NEC G04.89
 postvaccinal G04.02
 specified NEC G04.89
 syphilitic (transverse) A52.14
 toxic G92.9
 transverse (in demyelinating diseases of central nervous system) G37.3
 tuberculous A17.82
 varicella B01.12
Myeloblastic — *see* condition
Myeloblastoma
 granular cell — *see also* Neoplasm, connective tissue
  malignant — *see* Neoplasm, connective tissue, malignant
  tongue D10.1
Myelocele — *see* Spina bifida
Myelocystocele — *see* Spina bifida
Myelocytic — *see* condition
Myelodysplasia D46.9
 specified NEC D46.Z (*following* D46.4)
 spinal cord (congenital) Q06.1
Myelodysplastic syndrome — *see also* Syndrome, myelodysplastic D46.9
 with
  5q deletion D46.C (*following* D46.2)
  isolated del (5q) chromosomal abnormality D46.C (*following* D46.2)
 specified NEC D46.Z (*following* D46.4)
Myeloencephalitis — *see* Encephalitis
Myelofibrosis D75.81
 with myeloid metaplasia D47.4
 acute C94.4- ☑
 idiopathic (chronic) D47.4
 primary D47.1
 secondary D75.81
  in myeloproliferative disease D47.4
Myelogenous — *see* condition
Myeloid — *see* condition
Myelokathexis D70.9
Myeloleukodystrophy E75.29
Myelolipoma — *see* Lipoma
Myeloma (multiple) C90.0- ☑
 monostotic C90.3 ☑
  plasma cell C90.0- ☑
 plasma cell C90.0- ☑
 solitary — *see also* Plasmacytoma, solitary C90.3- ☑
Myelomalacia G95.89
Myelomatosis C90.0- ☑
Myelomeningitis — *see* Meningoencephalitis
Myelomeningocele (spinal cord) — *see* Spina bifida
Myelo-osteo-musculodysplasia hereditaria Q79.8
Myelopathic
 anemia D64.89
 muscle atrophy — *see* Atrophy, muscle, spinal
 pain syndrome G89.0
Myelopathy (spinal cord) G95.9
 drug-induced G95.89
 in (due to)
  degeneration or displacement, intervertebral disc NEC — *see* Disorder, disc, with, myelopathy
  infection — *see* Encephalitis

Myelopathy — *continued*
 in — *continued*
  intervertebral disc disorder — *see also* Disorder, disc, with, myelopathy
  mercury — *see* subcategory T56.1 ☑
  neoplastic disease — *see also* Neoplasm D49.9 [G99.2]
  pernicious anemia D51.0 [G99.2]
  spondylosis — *see* Spondylosis, with myelopathy NEC
 necrotic (subacute) (vascular) G95.19
 radiation-induced G95.89
 spondylogenic NEC — *see* Spondylosis, with myelopathy NEC
 toxic G95.89
 transverse, acute G37.3
 vascular G95.19
 vitamin B12 E53.8 [G32.0]
Myelophthisis D61.82
Myeloradiculitis G04.91
Myeloradiculodysplasia (spinal) Q06.1
Myelosarcoma C92.3- ☑
Myelosclerosis D75.89
 with myeloid metaplasia D47.4
 disseminated, of nervous system G35
 megakaryocytic D47.4
  with myeloid metaplasia D47.4
Myelosis
 acute C92.0- ☑
 aleukemic C92.9- ☑
 chronic D47.1
 erythremic (acute) C94.0- ☑
 megakaryocytic C94.2- ☑
 nonleukemic D72.828
 subacute C92.9- ☑
Myiasis (cavernous) B87.9
 aural B87.4
 creeping B87.0
 cutaneous B87.0
 dermal B87.0
 ear (external) (middle) B87.4
 eye B87.2
 genitourinary B87.81
 intestinal B87.82
 laryngeal B87.3
 nasopharyngeal B87.3
 ocular B87.2
 orbit B87.2
 skin B87.0
 specified site NEC B87.89
 traumatic B87.1
 wound B87.1
Myoadenoma, prostate — *see* Hyperplasia, prostate
Myoblastoma
 granular cell — *see also* Neoplasm, connective tissue, benign
  malignant — *see* Neoplasm, connective tissue, malignant
  tongue D10.1
Myocardial — *see* condition
Myocardiopathy (congestive) (constrictive) (familial) (hypertrophic nonobstructive) (idiopathic) (infiltrative) (obstructive) (primary) (restrictive) (sporadic) — *see also* Cardiomyopathy I42.9
 alcoholic I42.6
 cobalt-beer I42.6
 glycogen storage E74.02 [I43]
 hypertrophic obstructive I42.1
 in (due to)
  beriberi E51.12
  cardiac glycogenosis E74.02 [I43]
  Friedreich's ataxia G11.11 [I43]
  myotonia atrophica G71.11 [I43]
  progressive muscular dystrophy — *see also* Dystrophy, muscular, by type G71.09 [I43]
 obscure (African) I42.8
 secondary I42.9
 thyrotoxic E05.90 [I43]
  with storm E05.91 [I43]
 toxic NEC I42.7
Myocarditis (with arteriosclerosis) (chronic) (fibroid) (interstitial) (old) (progressive) (senile) I51.4
 with
  rheumatic fever (conditions in I00) I09.0
   active — *see* Myocarditis, acute, rheumatic
   inactive or quiescent (with chorea) I09.0
 active I40.9

Myocarditis — *continued*
 active — *continued*
  rheumatic I01.2
   with chorea (acute) (rheumatic) (Sydenham's) I02.0
 acute or subacute (interstitial) I40.9
  due to
   streptococcus (beta-hemolytic) I01.2
   idiopathic I40.1
   rheumatic I01.2
    with chorea (acute) (rheumatic) (Sydenham's) I02.0
   specified NEC I40.8
 aseptic of newborn B33.22
 bacterial (acute) I40.0
 Coxsackie (virus) B33.22
 diphtheritic A36.81
 eosinophilic I40.1
 epidemic of newborn (Coxsackie) B33.22
 Fiedler's (acute) (isolated) I40.1
 giant cell (acute) (subacute) I40.1
 gonococcal A54.83
 granulomatous (idiopathic) (isolated) (nonspecific) I40.1
 hypertensive — *see* Hypertension, heart
 idiopathic (granulomatous) I40.1
 in (due to)
  diphtheria A36.81
  epidemic louse-borne typhus A75.0 [I41]
  Lyme disease A69.29
  sarcoidosis D86.85
  scarlet fever A38.1
  toxoplasmosis (acquired) B58.81
  typhoid A01.02
  typhus NEC A75.9 [I41]
 infective I40.0
 influenzal — *see* Influenza, with, myocarditis
 isolated (acute) I40.1
 meningococcal A39.52
 mumps B26.82
 nonrheumatic, active I40.9
 parenchymatous I40.9
 pneumococcal I40.0
 rheumatic (chronic) (inactive) (with chorea) I09.0
  active or acute I01.2
   with chorea (acute) (rheumatic) (Sydenham's) I02.0
 rheumatoid — *see* Rheumatoid, carditis
 septic I40.0
 staphylococcal I40.0
 suppurative I40.0
 syphilitic (chronic) A52.06
 toxic I40.8
  rheumatic — *see* Myocarditis, acute, rheumatic
 tuberculous A18.84
 typhoid A01.02
 valvular — *see* Endocarditis
 virus, viral I40.0
  of newborn (Coxsackie) B33.22
Myocardium, myocardial — *see* condition
Myocardosis — *see* Cardiomyopathy
Myoclonus, myoclonic, myoclonia (familial) (essential) (multifocal) (simplex) G25.3
 drug-induced G25.3
 epilepsy — *see also* Epilepsy, generalized, specified NEC G40.4- ☑
  familial (progressive) G25.3
 epileptica G40.409
  with status epilepticus G40.401
 facial G51.3- ☑
 familial progressive G25.3
 Friedreich's G25.3
 jerks G25.3
 massive G25.3
 palatal G25.3
 pharyngeal G25.3
Myocytolysis I51.5
Myodiastasis — *see* Diastasis, muscle
Myoendocarditis — *see* Endocarditis
Myoepithelioma — *see* Neoplasm, benign, by site
Myofasciitis (acute) — *see* Myositis
Myofibroma — *see also* Neoplasm, connective tissue, benign
 uterus (cervix) (corpus) — *see* Leiomyoma
Myofibromatosis D48.1
 infantile Q89.8
Myofibrosis M62.89
 heart — *see* Myocarditis
 scapulohumeral — *see* Lesion, shoulder, specified NEC

Myofibrositis M79.7
  scapulohumeral — *see* Lesion, shoulder, specified NEC
Myoglobulinuria, myoglobinuria (primary) R82.1
Myokymia, facial G51.4
Myolipoma — *see* Lipoma
Myoma — *see also* Neoplasm, connective tissue, benign
  malignant — *see* Neoplasm, connective tissue, malig-
    nant
  prostate D29.1
  uterus (cervix) (corpus) — *see* Leiomyoma
Myomalacia M62.89
Myometritis — *see* Endometritis
Myometrium — *see* condition
Myonecrosis, clostridial A48.0
Myopathy G72.9
  acute
    necrotizing G72.81
      quadriplegic G72.81
  alcoholic G72.1
  benign congenital G71.20
  central core G71.29
  centronuclear G71.228
    autosomal (dominant) (recessive) G71.228
    other specified NEC G71.228
  congenital (benign) G71.20
  critical illness G72.81
  distal G71.09
  drug-induced G72.0
  endocrine NEC E34.9 [G73.7]
  extraocular muscles H05.82- ☑
  facioscapulohumeral G71.02
  hereditary G71.9
    specified NEC G71.8
  hyaline body G71.29
  immune NEC G72.49
  in (due to)
    Addison's disease E27.1 [G73.7]
    alcohol G72.1
    amyloidosis E85.0 [G73.7]
    cretinism E00.9 [G73.7]
    Cushing's syndrome E24.9 [G73.7]
    drugs G72.0
    endocrine disease NEC E34.9 [G73.7]
    giant cell arteritis M31.6 [G73.7]
    glycogen storage disease E74.00 [G73.7]
    hyperadrenocorticism E24.9 [G73.7]
    hyperparathyroidism NEC E21.3 [G73.7]
    hypoparathyroidism E20.9 [G73.7]
    hypopituitarism E23.0 [G73.7]
    hypothyroidism E03.9 [G73.7]
    infectious disease NEC B99 ☑ [G73.7]
    lipid storage disease E75.6 [G73.7]
    metabolic disease NEC E88.9 [G73.7]
    myxedema E03.9 [G73.7]
    parasitic disease NEC B89 [G73.7]
    polyarteritis nodosa M30.0 [G73.7]
    rheumatoid arthritis — *see* Rheumatoid, myopathy
    sarcoidosis D86.87
    scleroderma M34.82
    sicca syndrome M35.03
    Sjögren's syndrome M35.03
    systemic lupus erythematosus M32.19
    thyrotoxicosis (hyperthyroidism) E05.90 [G73.7]
      with thyroid storm E05.91 [G73.7]
    toxic agent NEC G72.2
  inflammatory NEC G72.49
  intensive care (ICU) G72.81
  limb-girdle — *see* Dystrophy, muscular, limb-girdle
  mitochondrial NEC
  Miyoshi, type 3 G71.035
  myosin storage G71.29
  myotubular (centronuclear) G71.220
    X-linked G71.220
  mytonic, proximal (PROMM) G71.11
  nemaline G71.21
  ocular G71.09
  oculopharyngeal G71.09
  of critical illness G72.81
  primary G71.9
    specified NEC G71.8
  progressive NEC G72.89
  proximal myotonic (PROMM) G71.11
  rod (body) G71.21
  scapulohumeral G71.02
  specified NEC G72.89
  toxic G72.2
Myopericarditis — *see also* Pericarditis
  chronic rheumatic I09.2

Myopia (axial) (congenital) H52.1- ☑
  degenerative (malignant) H44.20
    with
      choroidal neovascularization H44.2A- ☑
      foveoschisis H44.2D- ☑
      macular hole H44.2B- ☑
      retinal detachment H44.2C- ☑
      specified maculopathy NEC H44.2E- ☑
    bilateral H44.23
    left eye H44.22
    right eye H44.21
  malignant — *see also* Myopia, degenerative H44.2- ☑
  pernicious — *see also* Myopia, degenerative H44.2- ☑
  progressive high (degenerative) — *see also* Myopia,
    degenerative H44.2- ☑
Myosarcoma — *see* Neoplasm, connective tissue, malignant
Myosis (pupil) H57.03
  stromal (endolymphatic) D39.0
Myositis M60.9
  clostridial A48.0
  due to posture — *see* Myositis, specified type NEC
  epidemic B33.0
  fibrosa or fibrous (chronic), Volkmann's T79.6 ☑
  foreign body granuloma — *see* Granuloma, foreign
    body
  in (due to)
    bilharziasis B65.9 [M63.8-] ☑
    cysticercosis B69.81
    leprosy A30.9 [M63.8-] ☑
    mycosis B49 [M63.8-] ☑
    sarcoidosis D86.87
    schistosomiasis B65.9 [M63.8-] ☑
    syphilis
      late A52.78
      secondary A51.49
    toxoplasmosis (acquired) B58.82
    trichinellosis B75 [M63.8-] ☑
    tuberculosis A18.09
  inclusion body [IBM] G72.41
  infective M60.009
    arm M60.002
      left M60.001
      right M60.000
    leg M60.005
      left M60.004
      right M60.003
    lower limb M60.005
      ankle M60.07- ☑
      foot M60.07- ☑
      lower leg M60.06- ☑
      thigh M60.05- ☑
      toe M60.07- ☑
    multiple sites M60.09
    specified site NEC M60.08
    upper limb M60.002
      finger M60.04- ☑
      forearm M60.03- ☑
      hand M60.04- ☑
      shoulder region M60.01- ☑
      upper arm M60.02- ☑
  interstitial M60.10
    ankle M60.17- ☑
    foot M60.17- ☑
    forearm M60.13- ☑
    hand M60.14- ☑
    lower leg M60.16- ☑
    multiple sites M60.19
    shoulder region M60.11- ☑
    specified site NEC M60.18
    thigh M60.15- ☑
    upper arm M60.12- ☑
  mycotic B49 [M63.8-] ☑
  orbital, chronic H05.12- ☑
  ossificans or ossifying (circumscripta) — *see also* Ossi-
    fication, muscle, specified NEC
    in (due to)
      burns M61.30
        ankle M61.37- ☑
        foot M61.37- ☑
        forearm M61.33- ☑
        hand M61.34- ☑
        lower leg M61.36- ☑
        multiple sites M61.39
        pelvic region M61.35- ☑
        shoulder region M61.31- ☑
        specified site NEC M61.38

Myositis — *continued*
  ossificans or ossifying — *see also* Ossification, muscle,
    specified — *continued*
    in — *continued*
      burns — *continued*
        thigh M61.35- ☑
        upper arm M61.32- ☑
      quadriplegia or paraplegia M61.20
        ankle M61.27- ☑
        foot M61.27- ☑
        forearm M61.23- ☑
        hand M61.24- ☑
        lower leg M61.26- ☑
        multiple sites M61.29
        pelvic region M61.25- ☑
        shoulder region M61.21- ☑
        specified site NEC M61.28
        thigh M61.25- ☑
        upper arm M61.22- ☑
    progressiva M61.10
      ankle M61.17- ☑
      finger M61.14- ☑
      foot M61.17- ☑
      forearm M61.13- ☑
      hand M61.14- ☑
      lower leg M61.16- ☑
      multiple sites M61.19
      pelvic region M61.15- ☑
      shoulder region M61.11- ☑
      specified site NEC M61.18
      thigh M61.15- ☑
      toe M61.17- ☑
      upper arm M61.12- ☑
    traumatica M61.00
      ankle M61.07- ☑
      foot M61.07- ☑
      forearm M61.03- ☑
      hand M61.04- ☑
      lower leg M61.06- ☑
      multiple sites M61.09
      pelvic region M61.05- ☑
      shoulder region M61.01- ☑
      specified site NEC M61.08
      thigh M61.05- ☑
      upper arm M61.02- ☑
  purulent — *see* Myositis, infective
  specified type NEC M60.80
    ankle M60.87- ☑
    foot M60.87- ☑
    forearm M60.83- ☑
    hand M60.84- ☑
    lower leg M60.86- ☑
    multiple sites M60.89
    pelvic region M60.85- ☑
    shoulder region M60.81- ☑
    specified site NEC M60.88
    thigh M60.85- ☑
    upper arm M60.82- ☑
  suppurative — *see* Myositis, infective
  traumatic (old) — *see* Myositis, specified type NEC
Myospasia impulsiva F95.2
Myotonia (acquisita) (intermittens) M62.89
  atrophica G71.11
  chondrodystrophic G71.13
  congenita (acetazolamide responsive) (dominant) (re-
    cessive) G71.12
  drug-induced G71.14
  dystrophica G71.11
  fluctuans G71.19
  levior G71.12
  permanens G71.19
  symptomatic G71.19
Myotonic pupil — *see* Anomaly, pupil, function, tonic
  pupil
Myriapodiasis B88.2
Myringitis H73.2- ☑
  with otitis media — *see* Otitis, media
  acute H73.00- ☑
    bullous H73.01- ☑
    specified NEC H73.09- ☑
  bullous — *see* Myringitis, acute, bullous
  chronic H73.1- ☑
Mysophobia F40.228
Mytilotoxism — *see* Poisoning, fish
Myxadenitis labialis K13.0

☑ **Additional Character Required** — Refer to the Tabular List for Character Selection

Myxedema (adult) (idiocy) (infantile) (juvenile) — see
    also Hypothyroidism E03.9
    circumscribed E05.90
        with storm E05.91
    coma E03.5
    congenital E00.1
    cutis L98.5
    localized (pretibial) E05.90
        with storm E05.91

Myxedema — *continued*
    papular L98.5
Myxochondrosarcoma — *see* Neoplasm, cartilage, malignant
Myxofibroma — *see* Neoplasm, connective tissue, benign
    odontogenic — *see* Cyst, calcifying odontogenic
Myxofibrosarcoma — *see* Neoplasm, connective tissue, malignant

Myxolipoma D17.9
Myxoliposarcoma — *see* Neoplasm, connective tissue, malignant
Myxoma — *see also* Neoplasm, connective tissue, benign
    nerve sheath — *see* Neoplasm, nerve, benign
    odontogenic — *see* Cyst, calcifying odontogenic
Myxosarcoma — *see* Neoplasm, connective tissue, malignant

N

Naegeli's
disease Q82.8
leukemia, monocytic C93.1- ☑
Naegleriasis (with meningoencephalitis) B60.2
Naffziger's syndrome G54.0
Naga sore — *see* Ulcer, skin
Nägele's pelvis M95.5
with disproportion (fetopelvic) O33.0
causing obstructed labor O65.0
Nail — *see also* condition
biting F98.8
patella syndrome Q87.2
Nanism, nanosomia — *see* Dwarfism
Nanophyetiasis B66.8
Nanukayami A27.89
Napkin rash L22
Narcolepsy G47.419
with cataplexy G47.411
in conditions classified elsewhere G47.429
with cataplexy G47.421
Narcosis R06.89
Narcotism — *see* Dependence
NARP (Neuropathy, Ataxia and Retinitis pigmentosa)
syndrome E88.49
Narrow
anterior chamber angle H40.03- ☑
gingival width (of periodontal soft tissue) K05.5
pelvis — *see* Contraction, pelvis
Narrowing — *see also* Stenosis
artery I77.1
auditory, internal I65.8
basilar — *see* Occlusion, artery, basilar
carotid — *see* Occlusion, artery, carotid
cerebellar — *see* Occlusion, artery, cerebellar
cerebral — *see* Occlusion artery, cerebral
choroidal — *see* Occlusion, artery, precerebral,
specified NEC
communicating posterior — *see* Occlusion, artery,
precerebral, specified NEC
coronary — *see also* Disease, heart, ischemic,
atherosclerotic
congenital Q24.5
syphilitic A50.54 *[I52]*
due to syphilis NEC A52.06
hypophyseal — *see* Occlusion, artery, precerebral,
specified NEC
pontine — *see* Occlusion, artery, precerebral, specified NEC
precerebral — *see* Occlusion, artery, precerebral
vertebral — *see* Occlusion, artery, vertebral
auditory canal (external) — *see* Stenosis, external ear
canal
eustachian tube — *see* Obstruction, eustachian tube
eyelid — *see* Disorder, eyelid function
larynx J38.6
mesenteric artery — *see also* Ischemia, intestine, acute
K55.059
palate M26.89
palpebral fissure — *see* Disorder, eyelid function
ureter N13.5
with infection N13.6
urethra — *see* Stricture, urethra
Narrowness, abnormal, eyelid Q10.3
Nasal — *see* condition
Nasolachrymal, nasolacrimal — *see* condition
Nasopharyngeal — *see also* condition
pituitary gland Q89.2
torticollis M43.6
Nasopharyngitis (acute) (infective) (streptococcal)
(subacute) J00
chronic (suppurative) (ulcerative) J31.1
Nasopharynx, nasopharyngeal — *see* condition
Natal tooth, teeth K00.6
Nausea (without vomiting) R11.0
with vomiting R11.2
gravidarum — *see* Hyperemesis, gravidarum
marina T75.3 ☑
navalis T75.3 ☑
Navel — *see* condition
Neapolitan fever — *see* Brucellosis
Near drowning T75.1 ☑
Nearsightedness — *see* Myopia
Near-syncope R55
Nebula, cornea — *see* Opacity, cornea

Necator americanus infestation B76.1
Necatoriasis B76.1
Neck — *see* condition
Necrobiosis R68.89
lipoidica NEC L92.1
with diabetes — *see* E08-E13 with .620
Necrolysis, toxic epidermal L51.2
due to drug
correct substance properly administered — *see* Table of Drugs and Chemicals, by drug, adverse
effect
overdose or wrong substance given or taken — *see*
Table of Drugs and Chemicals, by drug, poisoning
Necrophilia F65.89
Necrosis, necrotic (ischemic) — *see also* Gangrene
adrenal (capsule) (gland) E27.49
amputation stump (surgical) (late) T87.50
arm T87.5- ☑
leg T87.5- ☑
antrum J32.0
aorta (hyaline) — *see also* Aneurysm, aorta
cystic medial — *see* Dissection, aorta
artery I77.5
bladder (aseptic) (sphincter) N32.89
bone — *see also* Osteonecrosis M87.9
aseptic or avascular — *see* Osteonecrosis
idiopathic M87.00
ethmoid J32.2
jaw M27.2
tuberculous — *see* Tuberculosis, bone
brain I67.89
breast (aseptic) (fat) (segmental) N64.1
bronchus J98.09
central nervous system NEC I67.89
cerebellar I67.89
cerebral I67.89
colon — *see also* Infarct, intestine K55.049
cornea H18.89- ☑
cortical (acute) (renal) N17.1
cystic medial (aorta) — *see* Dissection, aorta
dental pulp K04.1
esophagus K22.89
ethmoid (bone) J32.2
eyelid — *see* Disorder, eyelid, degenerative
fat, fatty (generalized) — *see also* Disorder, soft tissue,
specified type NEC
abdominal wall K65.4
breast (aseptic) (segmental) N64.1
localized — *see* Degeneration, by site, fatty
mesentery K65.4
omentum K65.4
pancreas K86.89
peritoneum K65.4
skin (subcutaneous) P83.0
subcutaneous, due to birth injury P15.6
gallbladder — *see* Cholecystitis, acute
heart — *see* Infarct, myocardium
hip, aseptic or avascular — *see* Osteonecrosis, by type,
femur
intestine (acute) (hemorrhagic) (massive) — *see also*
Infarct, intestine K55.069
jaw M27.2
kidney (bilateral) N28.0
acute N17.9
cortical (acute) (bilateral) N17.1
with ectopic or molar pregnancy O08.4
medullary (bilateral) (in acute renal failure) (papillary) N17.2
papillary (bilateral) (in acute renal failure) N17.2
tubular N17.0
with ectopic or molar pregnancy O08.4
complicating
abortion — *see* Abortion, by type, complicated by, tubular necrosis
ectopic or molar pregnancy O08.4
pregnancy — *see* Pregnancy, complicated by,
diseases of, specified type or system
NEC
following ectopic or molar pregnancy O08.4
traumatic T79.5 ☑
larynx J38.7
liver (with hepatic failure) (cell) — *see* Failure, hepatic
hemorrhagic, central K76.2
lung J85.0
lymphatic gland — *see* Lymphadenitis, acute
mammary gland (fat) (segmental) N64.1
mastoid (chronic) — *see* Mastoiditis, chronic

Necrosis, necrotic — *continued*
medullary (acute) (renal) N17.2
mesentery — *see also* Infarct, intestine K55.069
fat K65.4
mitral valve — *see* Insufficiency, mitral
myocardium, myocardial — *see* Infarct, myocardium
nose J34.0
omentum (with mesenteric infarction) — *see also* Infarct, intestine K55.069
fat K65.4
orbit, orbital — *see* Osteomyelitis, orbit
ossicles, ear — *see* Abnormal, ear ossicles
ovary N70.92
pancreas (aseptic) (duct) (fat) K86.89
acute (infective) — *see* Pancreatitis, acute
infective — *see* Pancreatitis, acute
papillary (acute) (renal) N17.2
perineum N90.89
peritoneum (with mesenteric infarction) — *see also*
Infarct, intestine K55.069
fat K65.4
pharynx J02.9
in granulocytopenia — *see* Neutropenia
Vincent's A69.1
phosphorus — *see* subcategory T54.2 ☑
pituitary (gland) E23.0
postpartum O99.285
Sheehan O99.285
pressure — *see* Ulcer, pressure, by site
pulmonary J85.0
pulp (dental) K04.1
radiation — *see* Necrosis, by site
radium — *see* Necrosis, by site
renal — *see* Necrosis, kidney
sclera H15.89
scrotum N50.89
skin or subcutaneous tissue NEC I96
spine, spinal (column) — *see also* Osteonecrosis, by
type, vertebra
cord G95.19
spleen D73.5
stomach K31.89
stomatitis (ulcerative) A69.0
subcutaneous fat, newborn P83.88
subendocardial (acute) I21.4
chronic I25.89
suprarenal (capsule) (gland) E27.49
testis N50.89
thymus (gland) E32.8
tonsil J35.8
trachea J39.8
tuberculous NEC — *see* Tuberculosis
tubular (acute) (anoxic) (renal) (toxic) N17.0
postprocedural N99.0
vagina N89.8
vertebra — *see also* Osteonecrosis, by type, vertebra
tuberculous A18.01
vulva N90.89
X-ray — *see* Necrosis, by site
Necrospermia — *see* Infertility, male
Need (for)
care provider because (of)
assistance with personal care Z74.1
continuous supervision required Z74.3
impaired mobility Z74.09
no other household member able to render care
Z74.2
specified reason NEC Z74.8
immunization — *see* Vaccination
vaccination — *see* Vaccination
Neglect
adult
confirmed T74.01 ☑
history of Z91.412
suspected T76.01 ☑
child (childhood)
confirmed T74.02 ☑
history of Z62.812
suspected T76.02 ☑
emotional, in childhood Z62.898
hemispatial R41.4
left-sided R41.4
sensory R41.4
visuospatial R41.4
Neisserian infection NEC — *see* Gonococcus
Nelaton's syndrome G60.8
Nelson's syndrome E24.1
Nematodiasis (intestinal) B82.0

☑ **Additional Character Required — Refer to the Tabular List for Character Selection**

Nematodiasis — *continued*
  Ancylostoma B76.Ø
Neonatal — *see also* Newborn
  acne L7Ø.4
  bradycardia P29.12
  screening, abnormal findings on — *see* Abnormal,
    neonatal screening
  tachycardia P29.11
  tooth, teeth KØØ.6
Neonatorum — *see* condition
Neoplasia
  endocrine, multiple (MEN) E31.2Ø
    type I E31.21
    type IIA E31.22
    type IIB E31.23
  intraepithelial (histologically confirmed)
    anal (AIN) (histologically confirmed) K62.82
      grade I K62.82
      grade II K62.82
      severe DØ1.3
    cervical glandular (histologically confirmed) DØ6.9
    cervix (uteri) (CIN) (histologically confirmed) N87.9
      glandular DØ6.9
      grade I N87.Ø
      grade II N87.1
      grade III (severe dysplasia) — *see also* Carcinoma,
        cervix uteri, in situ DØ6.9
    prostate (histologically confirmed) (PIN) N42.31
      grade I N42.31
      grade II N42.31
      grade III (severe dysplasia) DØ7.5
    vagina (histologically confirmed) (VAIN) N89.3
      grade I N89.Ø
      grade II N89.1
      grade III (severe dysplasia) DØ7.2
    vulva (histologically confirmed) (VIN) N9Ø.3
      grade I N9Ø.Ø
      grade II N9Ø.1
      grade III (severe dysplasia) DØ7.1
Neoplasm, neoplastic — *see also* Table of Neoplasms
  lipomatous, benign — *see* Lipoma
  malignant mast cell C96.2Ø
    specified type NEC C96.29
  mast cell, of uncertain behavior NEC D47.Ø9
  myelodysplastic/myeloproliferative, unclassifiable
    C94.6
Neovascularization
  ciliary body — *see* Disorder, iris, vascular
  cornea H16.4Ø- ☑
    deep H16.44- ☑
    ghost vessels — *see* Ghost, vessels
    localized H16.43- ☑
    pannus — *see* Pannus
  iris — *see* Disorder, iris, vascular
  retina H35.Ø5- ☑
Nephralgia N23
Nephritis, nephritic (albuminuric) (azotemic) (congenital) (disseminated) (epithelial) (familial) (focal) (granulomatous) (hemorrhagic) (infantile) (nonsuppurative, excretory) (uremic) NØ5.9
  with
    C3
      glomerulonephritis NØ5.A
      glomerulopathy NØ5.A
        with dense deposit disease NØ5.6
      dense deposit disease NØ5.6
      diffuse
        crescentic glomerulonephritis NØ5.7
        endocapillary proliferative glomerulonephritis
          NØ5.4
        membranous glomerulonephritis NØ5.2
        mesangial proliferative glomerulonephritis NØ5.3
        mesangiocapillary glomerulonephritis NØ5.5
      edema — *see* Nephrosis
      focal and segmental glomerular lesions NØ5.1
      foot process disease NØ4.9
      glomerular lesion
        diffuse sclerosing NØ5.8
        hypocomplementemic — *see* Nephritis, membranoproliferative
        IgA — *see* Nephropathy, IgA
        lobular, lobulonodular — *see* Nephritis, membranoproliferative
        nodular — *see* Nephritis, membranoproliferative
      lesion of
        glomerulonephritis, proliferative NØ5.8
        renal necrosis NØ5.9
      minor glomerular abnormality NØ5.Ø

Nephritis, nephritic — *continued*
  with — *continued*
    specified morphological changes NEC NØ5.8
  acute NØØ.9
    with
      C3
        glomerulonephritis NØØ.A
        glomerulopathy NØØ.A
          with dense deposit disease NØØ.6
        dense deposit disease NØØ.6
        diffuse
          crescentic glomerulonephritis NØØ.7
          endocapillary proliferative glomerulonephritis
            NØØ.4
          membranous glomerulonephritis NØØ.2
          mesangial proliferative glomerulonephritis
            NØØ.3
          mesangiocapillary glomerulonephritis NØØ.5
        focal and segmental glomerular lesions NØØ.1
        minor glomerular abnormality NØØ.Ø
        specified morphological changes NEC NØØ.8
  amyloid E85.4 *[NØ8]*
  antiglomerular basement membrane (anti-GBM) antibody NEC
    in Goodpasture's syndrome M31.Ø
  antitubular basement membrane (tubulo-interstitial)
    NEC N12
    toxic — *see* Nephropathy, toxic
  arteriolar — *see* Hypertension, kidney
  arteriosclerotic — *see* Hypertension, kidney
  ascending — *see* Nephritis, tubulo-interstitial
  atrophic NØ3.9
  Balkan (endemic) N15.Ø
  calculous, calculus — *see* Calculus, kidney
  cardiac — *see* Hypertension, kidney
  cardiovascular — *see* Hypertension, kidney
  chronic NØ3.9
    with
      C3
        glomerulonephritis NØ3.A
        glomerulopathy NØ3.A
          with dense deposit disease NØ3.6
        dense deposit disease NØ3.6
        diffuse
          crescentic glomerulonephritis NØ3.7
          endocapillary proliferative glomerulonephritis
            NØ3.4
          membranous glomerulonephritis NØ3.2
          mesangial proliferative glomerulonephritis
            NØ3.3
          mesangiocapillary glomerulonephritis NØ3.5
        focal and segmental glomerular lesions NØ3.1
        minor glomerular abnormality NØ3.Ø
        specified morphological changes NEC NØ3.8
    arteriosclerotic — *see* Hypertension, kidney
  cirrhotic N26.9
  complicating pregnancy O26.83- ☑
  croupous NØØ.9
  degenerative — *see* Nephrosis
  diffuse sclerosing NØ5.8
  due to
    diabetes mellitus — *see* EØ8-E13 with .21
    subacute bacterial endocarditis I33.Ø
    systemic lupus erythematosus (chronic) M32.14
    typhoid fever AØ1.Ø9
  gonococcal (acute) (chronic) A54.21
  hypocomplementemic — *see* Nephritis, membranoproliferative
  IgA — *see* Nephropathy, IgA
  immune complex (circulating) NEC NØ5.8
  infective — *see* Nephritis, tubulo-interstitial
  interstitial — *see* Nephritis, tubulo-interstitial
  lead N14.3
  membranoproliferative (diffuse) (type 1 or 3) — *see
    also* NØØ-NØ7 with fourth character .5 NØ5.5
    type 2 — *see also* NØØ-NØ7 with fourth character .6
      NØ5.6
  minimal change NØ5.Ø
  necrotic, necrotizing NEC — *see also* NØØ-NØ7 with
    fourth character .8 NØ5.8
  nephrotic — *see* Nephrosis
  nodular — *see* Nephritis, membranoproliferative
  polycystic Q61.3
    adult type Q61.2
    autosomal
      dominant Q61.2
      recessive NEC Q61.19
    childhood type NEC Q61.19

Nephritis, nephritic — *continued*
  polycystic — *continued*
    infantile type NEC Q61.19
  poststreptococcal NØ5.9
    acute NØØ.9
    chronic NØ3.9
    rapidly progressive NØ1.9
  proliferative NEC — *see also* NØØ-NØ7 with fourth
    character .8 NØ5.8
  purulent — *see* Nephritis, tubulo-interstitial
  rapidly progressive NØ1.9
    with
      C3
        glomerulonephritis NØ1.A
        glomerulopathy NØ1.A
          with dense deposit disease NØ1.6
        dense deposit disease NØ1.6
        diffuse
          crescentic glomerulonephritis NØ1.7
          endocapillary proliferative glomerulonephritis
            NØ1.4
          membranous glomerulonephritis NØ1.2
          mesangial proliferative glomerulonephritis
            NØ1.3
          mesangiocapillary glomerulonephritis NØ1.5
        focal and segmental glomerular lesions NØ1.1
        minor glomerular abnormality NØ1.Ø
        specified morphological changes NEC NØ1.8
  salt losing or wasting NEC N28.89
  saturnine N14.3
  sclerosing, diffuse NØ5.8
  septic — *see* Nephritis, tubulo-interstitial
  specified pathology NEC — *see also* NØØ-NØ7 with
    fourth character .8 NØ5.8
  subacute NØ1.9
  suppurative — *see* Nephritis, tubulo-interstitial
  syphilitic (late) A52.75
    congenital A5Ø.59 *[NØ8]*
    early (secondary) A51.44
  toxic — *see* Nephropathy, toxic
  tubal, tubular — *see* Nephritis, tubulo-interstitial
  tuberculous A18.11
  tubulo-interstitial (in) N12
    acute (infectious) N1Ø
    chronic (infectious) N11.9
      nonobstructive N11.8
        reflux-associated N11.Ø
      obstructive N11.1
      specified NEC N11.8
    due to
      brucellosis A23.9 *[N16]*
      cryoglobulinemia D89.1 *[N16]*
      glycogen storage disease E74.ØØ *[N16]*
      Sjögren's syndrome M35.Ø4
  vascular — *see* Hypertension, kidney
  war NØØ.9
Nephroblastoma (epithelial) (mesenchymal) C64- ☑
Nephrocalcinosis E83.59 *[N29]*
Nephrocystitis, pustular — *see* Nephritis, tubulo-interstitial
Nephrolithiasis (congenital) (pelvis) (recurrent) — *see
  also* Calculus, kidney
Nephroma C64- ☑
  mesoblastic D41.Ø- ☑
Nephronephritis — *see* Nephrosis
Nephronophthisis Q61.5
Nephropathia epidemica A98.5
Nephropathy — *see also* Nephritis N28.9
  with
    edema — *see* Nephrosis
    glomerular lesion — *see* Glomerulonephritis
  amyloid, hereditary E85.Ø
  analgesic N14.Ø
    with medullary necrosis, acute N17.2
  Balkan (endemic) N15.Ø
  chemical — *see* Nephropathy, toxic
  contrast medium, radiography N14.11
  contrast-induced N14.11
  diabetic — *see* EØ8-E13 with .21
  drug-induced N14.2
    contrast-induced N14.11
    specified NEC N14.19
  focal and segmental hyalinosis or sclerosis NØ2.1
  heavy metal-induced N14.3
  hereditary NEC NØ7.9
    with
      C3
        glomerulonephritis NØ7.A

Nephropathy — *continued*
  hereditary — *continued*
    with — *continued*
      C3 — *continued*
        glomerulopathy N07.A
          with dense deposit disease N07.6
        dense deposit disease N07.6
        diffuse
          crescentic glomerulonephritis N07.7
          endocapillary proliferative glomerulonephritis N07.4
          membranous glomerulonephritis N07.2
          mesangial proliferative glomerulonephritis N07.3
          mesangiocapillary glomerulonephritis N07.5
        focal and segmental glomerular lesions N07.1
        minor glomerular abnormality N07.0
        specified morphological changes NEC N07.8
  hypercalcemic N25.89
  hypertensive — *see* Hypertension, kidney
  hypokalemic (vacuolar) N25.89
  IgA N02.8
    with glomerular lesion N02.9
      focal and segmental hyalinosis or sclerosis N02.1
      membranoproliferative (diffuse) N02.5
      membranous (diffuse) N02.2
      mesangial proliferative (diffuse) N02.3
      mesangiocapillary (diffuse) N02.5
      proliferative NEC N02.8
      specified pathology NEC N02.8
  lead N14.3
  membranoproliferative (diffuse) N02.5
  membranous (diffuse) N02.2
  mesangial (IgA/IgG) — *see* Nephropathy, IgA
    proliferative (diffuse) N02.3
  mesangiocapillary (diffuse) N02.5
  obstructive N13.8
  phenacetin N17.2
  phosphate-losing N25.0
  potassium depletion N25.89
  pregnancy-related O26.83- ☑
  proliferative NEC — *see also* N00-N07 with fourth character .8 N05.8
  protein-losing N25.89
  saturnine N14.3
  sickle-cell D57.- ☑ *[N08]*
  toxic NEC N14.4
    due to
      drugs N14.2
        analgesic N14.0
        specified NEC N14.19
      heavy metals N14.3
  vasomotor N17.0
  water-losing N25.89
Nephroptosis N28.83
Nephropyosis — *see* Abscess, kidney
Nephrorrhagia N28.89
Nephrosclerosis (arteriolar) (arteriosclerotic) (chronic) (hyaline) — *see also* Hypertension, kidney
  hyperplastic — *see* Hypertension, kidney
  senile N26.9
Nephrosis, nephrotic (Epstein's) (syndrome) (congenital) N04.9
  with
    foot process disease N04.9
    glomerular lesion N04.1
    hypocomplementemic N04.5
  acute N04.9
  anoxic — *see* Nephrosis, tubular
  chemical — *see* Nephrosis, tubular
  cholemic K76.7
  diabetic — *see* E08-E13 with .21
  Finnish type (congenital) Q89.8
  hemoglobin N10
  hemoglobinuric — *see* Nephrosis, tubular
  in
    amyloidosis E85.4 *[N08]*
    diabetes mellitus — *see* E08-E13 with .21
    epidemic hemorrhagic fever A98.5
    malaria (malariae) B52.0
  ischemic — *see* Nephrosis, tubular
  lipoid N04.9
  lower nephron — *see* Nephrosis, tubular
  malarial (malariae) B52.0
  minimal change N04.0
  myoglobin N10
  necrotizing — *see* Nephrosis, tubular
  osmotic (sucrose) N25.89

Nephrosis, nephrotic — *continued*
  radiation N04.9
  syphilitic (late) A52.75
  toxic — *see* Nephrosis, tubular
  tubular (acute) N17.0
    postprocedural N99.0
    radiation N04.9
Nephrosonephritis, hemorrhagic (endemic) A98.5
Nephrostomy
  attention to Z43.6
  status Z93.6
Nerve — *see also* condition
  injury — *see* Injury, nerve, by body site
Nerves R45.0
Nervous — *see also* condition R45.0
  heart F45.8
  stomach F45.8
  tension R45.0
Nervousness R45.0
Nesidioblastoma
  pancreas D13.7
  specified site NEC — *see* Neoplasm, benign, by site
  unspecified site D13.7
Nettleship's syndrome — *see* Urticaria pigmentosa
Neumann's disease or syndrome L10.1
Neuralgia, neuralgic (acute) M79.2
  accessory (nerve) G52.8
  acoustic (nerve) — *see* subcategory H93.3 ☑
  auditory (nerve) — *see* subcategory H93.3 ☑
  ciliary G44.009
    intractable G44.001
    not intractable G44.009
  cranial
    nerve — *see also* Disorder, nerve, cranial
      fifth or trigeminal — *see* Neuralgia, trigeminal
      postherpetic, postzoster B02.29
  ear — *see* subcategory H92.0 ☑
  facialis vera G51.1
  Fothergill's — *see* Neuralgia, trigeminal
  glossopharyngeal (nerve) G52.1
  Horton's G44.009
    intractable G44.091
    not intractable G44.099
  Hunt's B02.21
  hypoglossal (nerve) G52.3
  infraorbital — *see* Neuralgia, trigeminal
  malarial — *see* Malaria
  migrainous G44.009
    intractable G44.001
    not intractable G44.009
  Morton's G57.6- ☑
  nerve, cranial — *see* Disorder, nerve, cranial
  nose G52.0
  occipital M54.81
  olfactory G52.0
  penis N48.9
  perineum R10.2
  postherpetic NEC B02.29
    trigeminal B02.22
  pubic region R10.2
  scrotum R10.2
  Sluder's G44.89
  specified nerve NEC G58.8
  spermatic cord R10.2
  sphenopalatine (ganglion) G90.09
  trifacial — *see* Neuralgia, trigeminal
  trigeminal G50.0
    postherpetic, postzoster B02.22
  vagus (nerve) G52.2
  writer's F48.8
    organic G25.89
Neurapraxia — *see* Injury, nerve
Neurasthenia F48.8
  cardiac F45.8
  gastric F45.8
  heart F45.8
Neurilemmoma — *see also* Neoplasm, nerve, benign
  acoustic (nerve) D33.3
  malignant — *see also* Neoplasm, nerve, malignant
    acoustic (nerve) C72.4- ☑
Neurilemmosarcoma — *see* Neoplasm, nerve, malignant
Neurinoma — *see* Neoplasm, nerve, benign
Neurinomatosis — *see* Neoplasm, nerve, uncertain behavior
Neuritis (rheumatoid) M79.2
  abducens (nerve) — *see* Strabismus, paralytic, sixth nerve
  accessory (nerve) G52.8

Neuritis — *continued*
  acoustic (nerve) — *see also* subcategory H93.3 ☑
    in (due to)
      infectious disease NEC B99 ☑ *[H94.0-]* ☑
      parasitic disease NEC B89 *[H94.0-]* ☑
    syphilitic A52.15
  alcoholic G62.1
    with psychosis — *see* Psychosis, alcoholic
  amyloid, any site E85.4 *[G63]*
  auditory (nerve) — *see* subcategory H93.3 ☑
  brachial — *see* Radiculopathy
    due to displacement, intervertebral disc — *see* Disorder, disc, cervical, with neuritis
  cranial
    due to Lyme disease A69.22
    eighth or acoustic or auditory — *see* subcategory H93.3 ☑
    eleventh or accessory G52.8
    fifth or trigeminal G50.- ☑
    first or olfactory G52.0
    fourth or trochlear — *see* Strabismus, paralytic, fourth nerve
    second or optic — *see* Neuritis, optic
    seventh or facial G51.8
      newborn (birth injury) P11.3
    sixth or abducent — *see* Strabismus, paralytic, sixth nerve
    tenth or vagus G52.2
    third or oculomotor — *see* Strabismus, paralytic, third nerve
    twelfth or hypoglossal G52.3
  Déjérine-Sottas G60.0
  diabetic (mononeuropathy) — *see* E08-E13 with .41
    polyneuropathy — *see* E08-E13 with .42
  due to
    beriberi E51.11
    displacement, prolapse or rupture, intervertebral disc — *see* Disorder, disc, with, radiculopathy
    herniation, nucleus pulposus M51.9 *[G55]*
  endemic E51.11
  facial G51.8
    newborn (birth injury) P11.3
  general — *see* Polyneuropathy
  geniculate ganglion G51.1
    due to herpes (zoster) B02.21
  gouty — *see also* Gout, by type M10.9 *[G63]*
  hypoglossal (nerve) G52.3
  ilioinguinal (nerve) NEC G57.9- ☑
  infectious (multiple) NEC G61.0
  interstitial hypertrophic progressive G60.0
  lumbar M54.16
  lumbosacral M54.17
  multiple — *see also* Polyneuropathy
    endemic E51.11
    infective, acute G61.0
  multiplex endemica E51.11
  nerve root — *see* Radiculopathy
  oculomotor (nerve) — *see* Strabismus, paralytic, third nerve
  olfactory nerve G52.0
  optic (nerve) (hereditary) (sympathetic) H46.9
    with demyelination G36.0
    in myelitis G36.0
    nutritional H46.2
    papillitis — *see* Papillitis, optic
    retrobulbar H46.1- ☑
    specified type NEC H46.8
    toxic H46.3
  peripheral (nerve) G62.9
    multiple — *see* Polyneuropathy
    single — *see* Mononeuritis
  pneumogastric (nerve) G52.2
  postherpetic, postzoster B02.29
  progressive hypertrophic interstitial G60.0
  retrobulbar — *see also* Neuritis, optic, retrobulbar
    in (due to)
      late syphilis A52.15
      meningococcal infection A39.82
    meningococcal A39.82
    syphilitic A52.15
  sciatic (nerve) — *see also* Sciatica
    due to displacement of intervertebral disc — *see* Disorder, disc, with, radiculopathy
  serum — *see also* Reaction, serum T80.69 ☑
  shoulder-girdle G54.5
  specified nerve NEC G58.8
  spinal (nerve) root — *see* Radiculopathy
  syphilitic A52.15

Neuritis — *continued*
   thenar (median) G56.1- ☑
   thoracic M54.14
   toxic NEC G62.2
   trochlear (nerve) — *see* Strabismus, paralytic, fourth
      nerve
   vagus (nerve) G52.2
Neuroastrocytoma — *see* Neoplasm, uncertain behavior,
      by site
Neuroavitaminosis E56.9 *[G99.8]*
Neuroblastoma
   olfactory C30.0
   specified site — *see* Neoplasm, malignant, by site
   unspecified site C74.90
Neurochorioretinitis — *see* Chorioretinitis
Neurocirculatory asthenia F45.8
Neurocysticercosis B69.0
Neurocytoma — *see* Neoplasm, benign, by site
Neurodermatitis (circumscribed) (circumscripta) (local)
      L28.0
   atopic L20.81
   diffuse (Brocq) L20.81
   disseminated L20.81
Neuroencephalomyelopathy, optic G36.0
Neuroepithelioma — *see also* Neoplasm, malignant, by
      site
   olfactory C30.0
Neurofibroma — *see also* Neoplasm, nerve, benign
   melanotic — *see* Neoplasm, nerve, benign
   multiple — *see* Neurofibromatosis
   plexiform — *see* Neoplasm, nerve, benign
Neurofibromatosis (multiple) (nonmalignant) Q85.00
   acoustic Q85.02
   malignant — *see* Neoplasm, nerve, malignant
   specified NEC Q85.09
   type 1 (von Recklinghausen) Q85.01
   type 2 Q85.02
Neurofibrosarcoma — *see* Neoplasm, nerve, malignant
Neurogenic — *see also* condition
   bladder — *see also* Dysfunction, bladder, neuromuscu-
      lar N31.9
      cauda equina syndrome G83.4
   bowel NEC K59.2
   heart F45.8
Neuroglioma — *see* Neoplasm, uncertain behavior, by
      site
Neurolabyrinthitis (of Dix and Hallpike) — *see* Neuroni-
      tis, vestibular
Neurolathyrism — *see* Poisoning, food, noxious, plant
Neuroleprosy A30.9
Neuroma — *see also* Neoplasm, nerve, benign
   acoustic (nerve) D33.3
   amputation (stump) (traumatic) (surgical complication)
      (late) T87.3- ☑
      arm T87.3- ☑
      leg T87.3- ☑
   digital (toe) G57.6- ☑
   interdigital G58.8
      lower limb (toe) G57.8- ☑
      upper limb G56.8- ☑
   intermetatarsal G57.8- ☑
   Morton's G57.6- ☑
   nonneoplastic
      arm G56.9- ☑
      leg G57.9- ☑
      lower extremity G57.9- ☑
      upper extremity G56.9- ☑
   optic (nerve) D33.3
   plantar G57.6- ☑
   plexiform — *see* Neoplasm, nerve, benign
   surgical (nonneoplastic)
      arm G56.9- ☑
      leg G57.9- ☑
      lower extremity G57.9- ☑
      upper extremity G56.9- ☑
Neuromyalgia — *see* Neuralgia
Neuromyasthenia (epidemic) (postinfectious) G93.39
Neuromyelitis G36.9
   ascending G61.0
   optica G36.0
Neuromyopathy G70.9
   paraneoplastic D49.9 *[G13.0]*
Neuromyotonia (Isaacs) G71.19
Neuronevus — *see* Nevus
Neuronitis G58.9
   ascending (acute) G57.2- ☑
   vestibular H81.2- ☑

Neuroparalytic — *see* condition
Neuropathy, neuropathic G62.9
   acute motor G62.81
   alcoholic G62.1
      with psychosis — *see* Psychosis, alcoholic
   arm G56.9- ☑
   autonomic, peripheral — *see* Neuropathy, peripheral,
      autonomic
   axillary G56.9- ☑
   bladder N31.9
      atonic (motor) (sensory) N31.2
      autonomous N31.2
      flaccid N31.2
      nonreflex N31.2
      reflex N31.1
      uninhibited N31.0
   brachial plexus G54.0
   cervical plexus G54.2
   chronic
      progressive segmentally demyelinating G62.89
      relapsing demyelinating G62.89
   Déjérine-Sottas G60.0
   diabetic — *see* E08-E13 with .40
      mononeuropathy — *see* E08-E13 with .41
      polyneuropathy — *see* E08-E13 with .42
   entrapment G58.9
      iliohypogastric nerve G57.8- ☑
      ilioinguinal nerve G57.8- ☑
      lateral cutaneous nerve of thigh G57.1- ☑
      median nerve G56.0- ☑
      obturator nerve G57.8- ☑
      peroneal nerve G57.3- ☑
      posterior tibial nerve G57.5- ☑
      saphenous nerve G57.8- ☑
      ulnar nerve G56.2- ☑
   facial nerve G51.9
   hereditary G60.9
      motor and sensory (types I-IV) G60.0
      sensory G60.8
      specified NEC G60.8
   hypertrophic G60.0
      Charcot-Marie-Tooth G60.0
      Déjérine-Sottas G60.0
      interstitial progressive G60.0
      of infancy G60.0
      Refsum G60.1
   idiopathic G60.9
      progressive G60.3
      specified NEC G60.8
   in association with hereditary ataxia G60.2
   intercostal G58.0
   ischemic — *see* Disorder, nerve
   Jamaica (ginger) G62.2
   leg NEC G57.9- ☑
   lower extremity G57.9- ☑
   lumbar plexus G54.1
   median nerve G56.1- ☑
   motor and sensory — *see also* Polyneuropathy
      hereditary (types I-IV) G60.0
   multifocal motor (MMN) G61.82
   multiple (acute) (chronic) — *see* Polyneuropathy
   optic (nerve) — *see also* Neuritis, optic
      ischemic H47.01- ☑
   paraneoplastic (sensorial) (Denny Brown) D49.9 *[G13.0]*
   peripheral (nerve) — *see also* Polyneuropathy G62.9
      autonomic G90.9
         idiopathic G90.09
         in (due to)
            amyloidosis E85.4 *[G99.0]*
            diabetes mellitus — *see* E08-E13 with .43
            endocrine disease NEC E34.9 *[G99.0]*
            gout M10.00 *[G99.0]*
            hyperthyroidism E05.90 *[G99.0]*
               with thyroid storm E05.91 *[G99.0]*
            metabolic disease NEC E88.9 *[G99.0]*
      idiopathic G60.9
         progressive G60.3
      in (due to)
         antitetanus serum G62.0
         arsenic G62.2
         drugs NEC G62.0
         lead G62.2
         organophosphate compounds G62.2
         toxic agent NEC G62.2
   plantar nerves G57.6- ☑
   progressive
      hypertrophic interstitial G60.0

Neuropathy, neuropathic — *continued*
   progressive — *continued*
      inflammatory G62.81
   radicular NEC — *see* Radiculopathy
   sacral plexus G54.1
   sciatic G57.0- ☑
   serum G61.1
   toxic NEC G62.2
   trigeminal sensory G50.8
   ulnar nerve G56.2- ☑
   uremic N18.9 *[G63]*
   vitamin B12 E53.8 *[G63]*
      with anemia (pernicious) D51.0 *[G63]*
         due to dietary deficiency D51.3 *[G63]*
Neurophthisis — *see also* Disorder, nerve
   peripheral, diabetic — *see* E08-E13 with .42
Neuroretinitis — *see* Chorioretinitis
Neuroretinopathy, hereditary optic H47.22
Neurosarcoma — *see* Neoplasm, nerve, malignant
Neurosclerosis — *see* Disorder, nerve
Neurosis, neurotic F48.9
   anankastic F42.8
   anxiety (state) F41.1
      panic type F41.0
   asthenic F48.8
   bladder F45.8
   cardiac (reflex) F45.8
   cardiovascular F45.8
   character F60.9
   colon F45.8
   compensation F68.10
   compulsive, compulsion F42.8
   conversion F44.9
   craft F48.8
   cutaneous F45.8
   depersonalization F48.1
   depressive (reaction) (type) F34.1
   environmental F48.8
   excoriation L98.1
   fatigue F48.8
   functional — *see* Disorder, somatoform
   gastric F45.8
   gastrointestinal F45.8
   heart F45.8
   hypochondriacal F45.21
   hysterical F44.9
   incoordination F45.8
      larynx F45.8
      vocal cord F45.8
   intestine F45.8
   larynx (sensory) F45.8
      hysterical F44.4
   mixed NEC F48.8
   musculoskeletal F45.8
   obsessional F42.8
   obsessive-compulsive F42.8
   occupational F48.8
   ocular NEC F45.8
   organ — *see* Disorder, somatoform
   pharynx F45.8
   phobic F40.9
   posttraumatic (situational) F43.10
      acute F43.11
      chronic F43.12
   psychasthenic (type) F48.8
   railroad F48.8
   rectum F45.8
   respiratory F45.8
   rumination F45.8
   sexual F65.9
   situational F48.8
   social F40.10
      generalized F40.11
   specified type NEC F48.8
   state F48.9
      with depersonalization episode F48.1
   stomach F45.8
   traumatic F43.10
      acute F43.11
      chronic F43.12
   vasomotor F45.8
   visceral F45.8
   war F48.8
Neurospongioblastosis diffusa Q85.1
Neurosyphilis (arrested) (early) (gumma) (late) (latent)
      (recurrent) (relapse) A52.3
   with ataxia (cerebellar) (locomotor) (spastic) (spinal)
      A52.19

Neurosyphilis — continued

Neurosyphilis — continued
- aneurysm (cerebral) A52.05
- arachnoid (adhesive) A52.13
- arteritis (any artery) (cerebral) A52.04
- asymptomatic A52.2
- congenital A50.40
- dura (mater) A52.13
- general paresis A52.17
- hemorrhagic A52.05
- juvenile (asymptomatic) (meningeal) A50.40
- leptomeninges (aseptic) A52.13
- meningeal, meninges (adhesive) A52.13
- meningitis A52.13
- meningovascular (diffuse) A52.13
- optic atrophy A52.15
- parenchymatous (degenerative) A52.19
- paresis, paretic A52.17
  - juvenile A50.45
- remission in (sustained) A52.3
- serological (without symptoms) A52.2
- specified nature or site NEC A52.19
- tabes, tabetic (dorsalis) A52.11
  - juvenile A50.45
- taboparesis A52.17
  - juvenile A50.45
- thrombosis (cerebral) A52.05
- vascular (cerebral) NEC A52.05

Neurothekeoma — see Neoplasm, nerve, benign

Neurotic — see Neurosis

Neurotoxemia — see Toxemia

Neutroclusion M26.211

Neutropenia, neutropenic (chronic) (genetic) (idiopathic) (immune) (infantile) (malignant) (pernicious) (splenic) D70.9
- congenital (primary) D70.0
- cyclic D70.4
- cytoreductive cancer chemotherapy sequela D70.1
- drug-induced D70.2
  - due to cytoreductive cancer chemotherapy D70.1
- due to infection D70.3
- fever D70.9
- neonatal, transitory (isoimmune) (maternal transfer) P61.5
- periodic D70.4
- secondary (cyclic) (periodic) (splenic) D70.4
  - drug-induced D70.2
    - due to cytoreductive cancer chemotherapy D70.1
- toxic D70.8

Neutrophilia, hereditary giant D72.0

Nevocarcinoma — see Melanoma

Nevus D22.9
- achromic — see Neoplasm, skin, benign
- amelanotic — see Neoplasm, skin, benign
- angiomatous D18.00
  - intra-abdominal D18.03
  - intracranial D18.02
  - skin D18.01
  - specified site NEC D18.09
- araneus I78.1
- balloon cell — see Neoplasm, skin, benign
- bathing trunk D48.5
- blue — see Neoplasm, skin, benign
  - cellular — see Neoplasm, skin, benign
  - giant — see Neoplasm, skin, benign
  - Jadassohn's — see Neoplasm, skin, benign
  - malignant — see Melanoma
- capillary D18.00
  - intra-abdominal D18.03
  - intracranial D18.02
  - skin D18.01
  - specified site NEC D18.09
- cavernous D18.00
  - intra-abdominal D18.03
  - intracranial D18.02
  - skin D18.01
  - specified site NEC D18.09
- cellular — see Neoplasm, skin, benign
  - blue — see Neoplasm, skin, benign
- choroid D31.3- ☑
- comedonicus Q82.5
- conjunctiva D31.0- ☑
- dermal — see Neoplasm, skin, benign
  - with epidermal nevus — see Neoplasm, skin, benign
- dysplastic — see Neoplasm, skin, benign
- eye D31.9- ☑
- flammeus Q82.5
- hemangiomatous D18.00
  - intra-abdominal D18.03

Nevus — continued

Nevus — continued
- hemangiomatous — continued
  - intracranial D18.02
  - skin D18.01
  - specified site NEC D18.09
- iris D31.4- ☑
- lacrimal gland D31.5- ☑
- lymphatic D18.1
- magnocellular
  - specified site — see Neoplasm, benign, by site
  - unspecified site D31.40
- malignant — see Melanoma
- meaning hemangioma D18.00
  - intra-abdominal D18.03
  - intracranial D18.02
  - skin D18.01
  - specified site NEC D18.09
- mouth (mucosa) D10.30
  - specified site NEC D10.39
  - white sponge Q38.6
- multiplex Q85.1
- non-neoplastic I78.1
- oral mucosa D10.30
  - specified site NEC D10.39
  - white sponge Q38.6
- orbit D31.6- ☑
- pigmented
  - giant — see also Neoplasm, skin, uncertain behavior D48.5
    - malignant melanoma in — see Melanoma
- portwine Q82.5
- retina D31.2- ☑
- retrobulbar D31.6- ☑
- sanguineous Q82.5
- senile I78.1
- skin D22.9
  - abdominal wall D22.5
  - ala nasi D22.39
  - ankle D22.7- ☑
  - anus, anal D22.5
  - arm D22.6- ☑
  - auditory canal (external) D22.2- ☑
  - auricle (ear) D22.2- ☑
  - auricular canal (external) D22.2- ☑
  - axilla, axillary fold D22.5
  - back D22.5
  - breast D22.5
  - brow D22.39
  - buttock D22.5
  - canthus (eye) D22.1- ☑
  - cheek (external) D22.39
  - chest wall D22.5
  - chin D22.39
  - ear (external) D22.2- ☑
  - external meatus (ear) D22.2- ☑
  - eyebrow D22.39
  - eyelid (lower) (upper) D22.1- ☑
  - face D22.30
    - specified NEC D22.39
  - female genital organ (external) NEC D28.0
  - finger D22.6- ☑
  - flank D22.5
  - foot D22.7- ☑
  - forearm D22.6- ☑
  - forehead D22.39
  - foreskin D29.0
  - genital organ (external) NEC
    - female D28.0
    - male D29.9
  - gluteal region D22.5
  - groin D22.5
  - hand D22.6- ☑
  - heel D22.7- ☑
  - helix D22.2- ☑
  - hip D22.7- ☑
  - interscapular region D22.5
  - jaw D22.39
  - knee D22.7- ☑
  - labium (majus) (minus) D28.0
  - leg D22.7- ☑
  - lip (lower) (upper) D22.0
  - lower limb D22.7- ☑
  - male genital organ (external) D29.9
  - nail D22.9
    - finger D22.6- ☑
    - toe D22.7- ☑
  - nasolabial groove D22.39
  - nates D22.5

Nevus — continued

Nevus — continued
- skin — continued
  - neck D22.4
  - nose (external) D22.39
  - palpebra D22.1- ☑
  - penis D29.0
  - perianal skin D22.5
  - perineum D22.5
  - pinna D22.2- ☑
  - popliteal fossa or space D22.7- ☑
  - prepuce D29.0
  - pudendum D28.0
  - scalp D22.4
  - scrotum D29.4
  - shoulder D22.6- ☑
  - submammary fold D22.5
  - temple D22.39
  - thigh D22.7- ☑
  - toe D22.7- ☑
  - trunk NEC D22.5
  - umbilicus D22.5
  - upper limb D22.6- ☑
  - vulva D28.0
- specified site NEC — see Neoplasm, by site, benign
- spider I78.1
- stellar I78.1
- strawberry Q82.5
- Sutton's benign D22.9
- unius lateris Q82.5
- Unna's Q82.5
- vascular Q82.5
- verrucous Q82.5

Newborn (infant) (liveborn) (singleton) Z38.2
- abstinence syndrome P96.1
- acne L70.4
- affected by
  - abnormalities of membranes P02.9
    - specified NEC P02.8
  - abruptio placenta P02.1
  - amino-acid metabolic disorder, transitory P74.8
  - amniocentesis (while in utero) P00.6
  - amnionitis P02.78
  - apparent life threatening event (ALTE) R68.13
  - bleeding (into)
    - cerebral cortex P52.22
    - germinal matrix P52.0
    - ventricles P52.1
  - breech delivery P03.0
  - cardiac arrest P29.81
  - cardiomyopathy I42.8
    - congenital I42.4
  - cerebral ischemia P91.0
  - Cesarean delivery P03.4
  - chemotherapy agents P04.11
  - chorioamnionitis P02.78
  - cocaine (crack) P04.41
  - complications of labor and delivery P03.9
    - specified NEC P03.89
  - compression of umbilical cord NEC P02.5
  - contracted pelvis P03.1
  - cyanosis P28.2
  - delivery P03.9
    - Cesarean P03.4
    - forceps P03.2
    - vacuum extractor P03.3
  - drugs of addiction P04.40
    - cocaine P04.41
    - hallucinogens P04.42
    - specified drug NEC P04.49
  - entanglement (knot) in umbilical cord P02.5
  - environmental chemicals P04.6
  - fetal (intrauterine)
    - growth retardation P05.9
    - inflammatory response syndrome (FIRS) P02.70
    - malnutrition not light or small for gestational age P05.2
  - FIRS (fetal inflammatory response syndrome) P02.70
  - forceps delivery P03.2
  - heart rate abnormalities
    - bradycardia P29.12
    - intrauterine P03.819
      - before onset of labor P03.810
      - during labor P03.811
    - tachycardia P29.11
  - hemorrhage (antepartum) P02.1
    - cerebellar (nontraumatic) P52.6
    - intracerebral (nontraumatic) P52.4
    - intracranial (nontraumatic) P52.9

☑ **Additional Character Required** — Refer to the Tabular List for Character Selection

Newborn — *continued*
  affected by — *continued*
    hemorrhage — *continued*
      intracranial — *continued*
        specified NEC P52.8
        intraventricular (nontraumatic) P52.3
          grade 1 P52.0
          grade 2 P52.1
          grade 3 P52.21
          grade 4 P52.22
        posterior fossa (nontraumatic) P52.6
        subarachnoid (nontraumatic) P52.5
        subependymal P52.0
          with intracerebral extension P52.22
          with intraventricular extension P52.1
            with enlargment of ventricles P52.21
          without intraventricular extension P52.0
    hypoxic ischemic encephalopathy [HIE] P91.60
      mild P91.61
      moderate P91.62
      severe P91.63
    induction of labor P03.89
    intestinal perforation P78.0
    intrauterine (fetal) blood loss P50.9
      due to (from)
        cut end of co-twin cord P50.5
        hemorrhage into
          co-twin P50.3
            maternal circulation P50.4
        placenta P50.2
        ruptured cord blood P50.1
        vasa previa P50.0
      specified NEC P50.8
    intrauterine (fetal) hemorrhage P50.9
    intrauterine (in utero) procedure P96.5
    malpresentation (malposition) NEC P03.1
    maternal (complication of) (use of)
      alcohol P04.3
      amphetamines P04.16
      analgesia (maternal) P04.0
      anesthesia (maternal) P04.0
      anticonvulsants P04.13
      antidepressants P04.15
      antineoplastic chemotherapy P04.11
      anxiolytics P04.1A
      blood loss P02.1
      cannabis P04.81
      circulatory disease P00.3
      condition P00.9
        specified NEC P00.89
      cytotoxic drugs P04.12
      delivery P03.9
        Cesarean P03.4
        forceps P03.2
        vacuum extractor P03.3
      diabetes mellitus (pre-existing) P70.1
      disorder P00.9
        specified NEC P00.89
      drugs (addictive) (illegal) NEC P04.49
      ectopic pregnancy P01.4
      gestational diabetes P70.0
      group B streptococcus (GBS) colonization (positive) P00.82
      hemorrhage P02.1
      hypertensive disorder P00.0
      incompetent cervix P01.0
      infectious disease P00.2
      injury P00.5
      labor and delivery P03.9
      malpresentation before labor P01.7
      maternal death P01.6
      medical procedure P00.7
      medication P04.19
        specified type NEC P04.18
      multiple pregnancy P01.5
      nutritional disorder P00.4
      oligohydramnios P01.2
      opiates P04.14
        administered for procedures during pregnancy or labor and delivery P04.0
      parasitic disease P00.2
      periodontal disease P00.81
      placenta previa P02.0
      polyhydramnios P01.3
      precipitate delivery P03.5
      pregnancy P01.9
        specified P01.8
      premature rupture of membranes P01.1
      renal disease P00.1

Newborn — *continued*
  affected by — *continued*
    maternal — *continued*
      respiratory disease P00.3
      sedative-hypnotics P04.17
      surgical procedure P00.6
      tranquilizers administered for procedures during pregnancy or labor and delivery P04.0
      urinary tract disease P00.1
      uterine contraction (abnormal) P03.6
    meconium peritonitis P78.0
    medication (legal) (maternal use) (prescribed) P04.19
    membrane abnormalities P02.9
      specified NEC P02.8
    membranitis P02.78
    methamphetamine(s) P04.49
    mixed metabolic and respiratory acidosis P84
    neonatal abstinence syndrome P96.1
    noxious substances transmitted via placenta or breast milk P04.9
      cannabis P04.81
      specified NEC P04.89
    nutritional supplements P04.5
    placenta previa P02.0
    placental
      abnormality (functional) (morphological) P02.20
        specified NEC P02.29
      dysfunction P02.29
      infarction P02.29
      insufficiency P02.29
      separation NEC P02.1
      transfusion syndromes P02.3
    placentitis P02.78
    precipitate delivery P03.5
    prolapsed cord P02.4
    respiratory arrest P28.81
    slow intrauterine growth P05.9
    tobacco P04.2
    twin to twin transplacental transfusion P02.3
    umbilical cord (tightly) around neck P02.5
    umbilical cord condition P02.60
      short cord P02.69
      specified NEC P02.69
    uterine contractions (abnormal) P03.6
    vasa previa P02.69
      from intrauterine blood loss P50.0
  apnea — *see also* Apnea, newborn P28.40
    obstructive P28.42
    primary — *see also* Apnea, newborn, sleep, primary P28.30
    sleep (central) (obstructive) (primary) — *see also* Apnea, newborn, sleep, primary P28.30
  born in hospital Z38.00
    by cesarean Z38.01
  born outside hospital Z38.1
  breast buds P96.89
  breast engorgement P83.4
  check-up — *see* Newborn, examination
  convulsion P90
  dehydration P74.1
  examination
    8 to 28 days old Z00.111
    under 8 days old Z00.110
  fever P81.9
    environmentally-induced P81.0
  hyperbilirubinemia P59.9
    of prematurity P59.0
  hypernatremia P74.21
  hyponatremia P74.22
  infection P39.9
    candidal P37.5
    specified NEC P39.8
    urinary tract P39.3
  jaundice P59.9
    due to
      breast milk inhibitor P59.3
      hepatocellular damage P59.20
        specified NEC P59.29
      preterm delivery P59.0
    of prematurity P59.0
    specified NEC P59.8
  late metabolic acidosis P74.0
  mastitis P39.0
    infective P39.0
    noninfective P83.4
  multiple born NEC Z38.8
    born in hospital Z38.68
      by cesarean Z38.69

Newborn — *continued*
  multiple born — *continued*
    born outside hospital Z38.7
  omphalitis P38.9
    with mild hemorrhage P38.1
    without hemorrhage P38.9
  post-term P08.21
  prolonged gestation (over 42 completed weeks) P08.22
  quadruplet Z38.8
    born in hospital Z38.63
      by cesarean Z38.64
    born outside hospital Z38.7
  quintuplet Z38.8
    born in hospital Z38.65
      by cesarean Z38.66
    born outside hospital Z38.7
  seizure P90
  sepsis (congenital) P36.9
    due to
      anaerobes NEC P36.5
      Escherichia coli P36.4
      Staphylococcus P36.30
        aureus P36.2
        specified NEC P36.39
      Streptococcus P36.10
        group B P36.0
        specified NEC P36.19
      specified NEC P36.8
  triplet Z38.8
    born in hospital Z38.61
      by cesarean Z38.62
    born outside hospital Z38.7
  twin Z38.5
    born in hospital Z38.30
      by cesarean Z38.31
    born outside hospital Z38.4
  vomiting P92.09
    bilious P92.01
  weight check Z00.111
Newcastle conjunctivitis or disease B30.8
Nezelof's syndrome (pure alymphocytosis) D81.4
Niacin (amide) **deficiency** E52
Nicolas (-Durand)-**Favre disease** A55
Nicotine — *see* Tobacco
Nicotinic acid deficiency E52
Niemann-Pick disease or syndrome E75.249
  specified NEC E75.248
  type
    A E75.240
    A/B E75.244
    B E75.241
    C E75.242
    D E75.243
Night
  blindness — *see* Blindness, night
  sweats R61
  terrors (child) F51.4
Nightmares (REM sleep type) F51.5
NIHSS (National Institutes of Health Stroke Scale) **score** R29.7- ☑
Nipple — *see* condition
Nisbet's chancre A57
Nishimoto (-Takeuchi) **disease** I67.5
Nitritoid crisis or reaction — *see* Crisis, nitritoid
Nitrosohemoglobinemia D74.8
Njovera A65
No general equivalence degree (GED) Z55.5
Nocardiosis, nocardiasis A43.9
  cutaneous A43.1
  lung A43.0
  pneumonia A43.0
  pulmonary A43.0
  specified site NEC A43.8
Nocturia R35.1
  psychogenic F45.8
Nocturnal — *see* condition
Nodal rhythm I49.8
Node(s) — *see also* Nodule
  Bouchard's (with arthropathy) M15.2
  Haygarth's M15.8
  Heberden's (with arthropathy) M15.1
  larynx J38.7
  lymph — *see* condition
  milker's B08.03
  Osler's I33.0
  Schmorl's — *see* Schmorl's disease
  singer's J38.2
  teacher's J38.2

Node(s) — *continued*
tuberculous — *see* Tuberculosis, lymph gland
vocal cord J38.2
Nodule(s), **nodular**
actinomycotic — *see* Actinomycosis
breast NEC — *see also* Lump, breast N63.0
colloid (cystic), thyroid E04.1
cutaneous — *see* Swelling, localized
endometrial (stromal) D26.1
Haygarth's M15.8
inflammatory — *see* Inflammation
juxta-articular
syphilitic A52.77
yaws A66.7
larynx J38.7
lung, solitary (subsegmental branch of the bronchial
tree) R91.1
multiple R91.8
milker's B08.03
prostate N40.2
with lower urinary tract symptoms (LUTS) N40.3
without lower urinary tract symtpoms (LUTS) N40.2
pulmonary, solitary (subsegmental branch of the
bronchial tree) R91.1
retrocardiac R09.89
rheumatoid M06.30
ankle M06.37- ☑
elbow M06.32- ☑
foot joint M06.37- ☑
hand joint M06.34- ☑
hip M06.35- ☑
knee M06.36- ☑
multiple site M06.39
shoulder M06.31- ☑
vertebra M06.38
wrist M06.33- ☑
scrotum (inflammatory) N49.2
singer's J38.2
solitary, lung (subsegmental branch of the bronchial
tree) R91.1
multiple R91.8
subcutaneous — *see* Swelling, localized
teacher's J38.2
thyroid (cold) (gland) (nontoxic) E04.1
with thyrotoxicosis E05.20
with thyroid storm E05.21
toxic or with hyperthyroidism E05.20
with thyroid storm E05.21
vocal cord J38.2
Noma (gangrenous) (hospital) (infective) A69.0
auricle I96
mouth A69.0
pudendi N76.89
vulvae N76.89
Nomad, nomadism Z59.00
NOMID (neonatal onset multisystemic inflammatory disorder) M04.2
Nonadherence to medical treatment, specified NEC
Z91.199
due to
financial hardship Z91.190
specified reason NEC Z91.198
Nonautoimmune hemolytic anemia D59.4
drug-induced D59.2
Nonclosure — *see also* Imperfect, closure
ductus arteriosus (Botallo's) Q25.0
foramen
botalli Q21.12
ovale Q21.12
Noncompliance Z91.199
with
dialysis Z91.15
dietary regimen Z91.119
due to
financial hardship Z91.110
specified reason NEC Z91.118
medical treatment, specified NEC Z91.199
due to
financial hardship Z91.190
specified reason NEC Z91.198
medication regimen NEC Z91.14
underdosing — *see also* Table of Drugs and
Chemicals, categories T36-T50, with final
character 6 Z91.14
intentional NEC Z91.128
by caregiver Z91.A4
due to
financial hardship Z91.A20

Noncompliance — *continued*
with — *continued*
medication regimen — *continued*
underdosing — *see also* Table of Drugs and
Chemicals, categories T36-T50, with final
character 6 — *continued*
intentional — *continued*
by caregiver — *continued*
due to — *continued*
specified reason NEC Z91.A28
due to financial hardship of patient
Z91.120
unintentional NEC Z91.138
by caregiver Z91.A3
due to patient's age related debility
Z91.130
renal dialysis Z91.15
caregiver
with patient's
dietary regimen
due to
financial hardship Z91.A10
specified reason NEC Z91.A18
medical treatment and regimen Z91.A9
medication regimen, specified NEC Z91.A4
renal dialysis Z91.A5
Nondescent (congenital) — *see also* Malposition, congenital
cecum Q43.3
colon Q43.3
testicle Q53.9
bilateral Q53.20
abdominal Q53.211
perineal Q53.22
unilateral Q53.10
abdominal Q53.111
perineal Q53.12
Nondevelopment
brain Q02
part of Q04.3
heart Q24.8
organ or site, congenital NEC — *see* Hypoplasia
Nonengagement
head NEC O32.4 ☑
in labor, causing obstructed labor O64.8 ☑
Nonexanthematous tick fever A93.2
Nonexpansion, lung (newborn) P28.0
Nonfunctioning
cystic duct — *see also* Disease, gallbladder K82.8
gallbladder — *see also* Disease, gallbladder K82.8
kidney N28.9
labyrinth — *see* subcategory H83.2 ☑
Non-Hodgkin lymphoma NEC — *see* Lymphoma, non-Hodgkin
Nonimplantation, ovum N97.2
Noninsufflation, fallopian tube N97.1
Non-ketotic hyperglycinemia E72.51
Nonne-Milroy syndrome Q82.0
Nonovulation N97.0
Non-palpable testicle(s)
bilateral R39.84
unilateral R39.83
Nonpatent fallopian tube N97.1
Nonpneumatization, lung NEC P28.0
Nonrotation — *see* Malrotation
Nonsecretion, urine — *see* Anuria
Nonunion
fracture — *see* Fracture, by site
joint, following fusion or arthrodesis M96.0
organ or site, congenital NEC — *see* Imperfect, closure
symphysis pubis, congenital Q74.2
Nonvisualization, gallbladder R93.2
Nonvital, nonvitalized tooth K04.99
Non-working side interference M26.56
Noonan's syndrome Q87.19
Normocytic anemia (infectional) due to blood loss
(chronic) D50.0
acute D62
Norrie's disease (congenital) Q15.8
North American blastomycosis B40.9
Norwegian itch B86
Nose, nasal — *see* condition
Nosebleed R04.0
Nose-picking F98.8
Nosomania F45.21
Nosophobia F45.22
Nostalgia F43.20

Notch of iris Q13.2
Notching nose, congenital (tip) Q30.2
Nothnagel's
syndrome — *see* Strabismus, paralytic, third nerve
vasomotor acroparesthesia I73.89
Novy's relapsing fever A68.9
louse-borne A68.0
tick-borne A68.1
Noxious
foodstuffs, poisoning by — *see* Poisoning, food, noxious, plant
substances transmitted through placenta or breast milk
P04.9
Nucleus pulposus — *see* condition
Numbness R20.0
Nuns' knee — *see* Bursitis, prepatellar
Nursemaid's elbow S53.03- ☑
Nutcracker esophagus K22.4
Nutmeg liver K76.1
Nutrient element deficiency E61.9
specified NEC E61.8
Nutrition deficient or insufficient — *see also* Malnutrition E63.9
due to
insufficient food T73.0 ☑
lack of
care (child) T76.02 ☑
adult T76.01 ☑
food T73.0 ☑
specific element deficiency — *see* Nutrient element
deficiency, or by element
sequelae — *see* Sequelae, nutritional deficiency
specified NEC E63.8
Nutritional stunting E45
Nyctalopia (night blindness) — *see* Blindness, night
Nycturia R35.1
psychogenic F45.8
Nymphomania F52.8
Nystagmus H55.00
benign paroxysmal — *see* Vertigo, benign paroxysmal
central positional H81.4
congenital H55.01
dissociated H55.04
latent H55.02
miners' H55.09
positional
benign paroxysmal H81.4
central H81.4
specified form NEC H55.09
visual deprivation H55.03

O

Obermeyer's relapsing fever (European) A68.0
Obesity E66.9
with alveolar hypoventilation E66.2
adrenal E27.8
complicating
childbirth O99.214
pregnancy O99.21- ☑
puerperium O99.215
constitutional E66.8
dietary counseling and surveillance Z71.3
drug-induced E66.1
due to
drug E66.1
excess calories E66.09
morbid E66.01
severe E66.01
endocrine E66.8
endogenous E66.8
exogenous E66.09
familial E66.8
glandular E66.8
hypothyroid — *see* Hypothyroidism
hypoventilation syndrome (OHS) E66.2
morbid E66.01
with
alveolar hypoventilation E66.2
obesity hypoventilation syndrome (OHS) E66.2
due to excess calories E66.01
nutritional E66.09
pituitary E23.6
severe E66.01
specified type NEC E66.8
Oblique — *see* condition

Obliteration
  appendix (lumen) K38.8
  artery I77.1
  bile duct (noncalculous) K83.1
  common duct (noncalculous) K83.1
  cystic duct — see Obstruction, gallbladder
  disease, arteriolar I77.1
  endometrium N85.8
  eye, anterior chamber — see Disorder, globe, hypotony
  fallopian tube N97.1
  lymphatic vessel I89.0
    due to mastectomy I97.2
  organ or site, congenital NEC — see Atresia, by site
  ureter N13.5
    with infection N13.6
  urethra — see Stricture, urethra
  vein I87.8
  vestibule (oral) K08.89
Observation (following) (for) (without need for further
    medical care) Z04.9
  accident NEC Z04.3
    at work Z04.2
    transport Z04.1
  adverse effect of drug Z03.6
  alleged rape or sexual assault (victim), ruled out
    adult Z04.41
    child Z04.42
  criminal assault Z04.89
  development state
    adolescent Z00.3
    period of rapid growth in childhood Z00.2
    puberty Z00.3
  disease, specified NEC Z03.89
  following work accident Z04.2
  forced sexual exploitation Z04.81
  forced labor exploitation Z04.82
  growth and development state — see Observation,
    development state
  injuries (accidental) NEC — see also Observation, acci-
    dent
  newborn (for)
    suspected condition, related to exposure from the
        mother or birth process — see Newborn, af-
        fected by, maternal
    ruled out Z05.9
        cardiac Z05.0
        connective tissue Z05.73
        gastrointestinal Z05.5
        genetic Z05.41
        genitourinary Z05.6
        immunologic Z05.43
        infectious Z05.1
        metabolic Z05.42
        musculoskeletal Z05.72
        neurological Z05.2
        respiratory Z05.3
        skin and subcutaneous tissue Z05.71
        specified condition NEC Z05.8
  postpartum
    immediately after delivery Z39.0
    routine follow-up Z39.2
  pregnancy (normal) (without complication) Z34.9- ☑
    high risk O09.9- ☑
  suicide attempt, alleged NEC Z03.89
    self-poisoning Z03.6
  suspected, ruled out — see also Suspected condition,
    ruled out
    abuse, physical
        adult Z04.71
        child Z04.72
    accident at work Z04.2
    adult battering victim Z04.71
    child battering victim Z04.72
    condition NEC Z03.89
        newborn — see also Observation, newborn (for),
            suspected condition, ruled out Z05.9
    drug poisoning or adverse effect Z03.6
    exposure (to)
        anthrax Z03.810
        biological agent NEC Z03.818
    foreign body
        aspirated (inhaled) Z03.822
        ingested Z03.821
        inserted (injected), in (eye) (orifice) (skin) Z03.823
    inflicted injury NEC Z04.89
    suicide attempt, alleged Z03.89
        self-poisoning Z03.6

Observation — continued
  suspected, ruled out — see also Suspected condition,
    ruled out — continued
    toxic effects from ingested substance (drug) (poison)
        Z03.6
  toxic effects from ingested substance (drug) (poison)
    Z03.6
Obsession, obsessional state F42.8
  mixed thoughts and acts F42.2
Obsessive-compulsive neurosis or reaction F42.8
Obstetric embolism, septic — see Embolism, obstetric,
    septic
Obstetrical trauma (complicating delivery) O71.9
  with or following ectopic or molar pregnancy O08.6
  specified type NEC O71.89
Obstipation — see Constipation
Obstruction, obstructed, obstructive
  airway J98.8
    with
        allergic alveolitis J67.9
        asthma J45.909
            with
                exacerbation (acute) J45.901
                status asthmaticus J45.902
        bronchiectasis J47.9
            with
                exacerbation (acute) J47.1
                lower respiratory infection J47.0
        bronchitis (chronic) J44.9
        emphysema J43.9
    chronic J44.9
        with
            allergic alveolitis — see Pneumonitis, hyper-
                sensitivity
            bronchiectasis J47.9
                with
                    exacerbation (acute) J47.1
                    lower respiratory infection J47.0
    due to
        foreign body — see Foreign body, by site, caus-
            ing asphyxia
        inhalation of fumes or vapors J68.9
        laryngospasm J38.5
  ampulla of Vater K83.1
  aortic (heart) (valve) — see Stenosis, aortic
  aortoiliac I74.09
  aqueduct of Sylvius G91.1
    congenital Q03.0
        with spina bifida — see Spina bifida, by site, with
            hydrocephalus
  Arnold-Chiari — see Arnold-Chiari disease
  artery — see also Atherosclerosis, artery I70.9 ☑
    basilar (complete) (partial) — see Occlusion, artery,
        basilar
    carotid (complete) (partial) — see Occlusion, artery,
        carotid
    cerebellar — see Occlusion, artery, cerebellar
    cerebral (anterior) (middle) (posterior) — see Occlu-
        sion, artery, cerebral
    precerebral — see Occlusion, artery, precerebral
    renal N28.0
    retinal NEC — see Occlusion, artery, retina
    stent — see Restenosis, stent
    vertebral (complete) (partial) — see Occlusion,
        artery, vertebral
  band (intestinal) — see also Obstruction, intestine,
    specified NEC K56.699
  bile duct or passage (common) (hepatic) (noncalculous)
    K83.1
    with calculus K80.51
    congenital (causing jaundice) Q44.3
  biliary (duct) (tract) K83.1
    gallbladder K82.0
  bladder-neck (acquired) N32.0
    congenital Q64.31
    due to hyperplasia (hypertrophy) of prostate — see
        Hyperplasia, prostate
  bowel — see Obstruction, intestine
  bronchus J98.09
  canal, ear — see Stenosis, external ear canal
  cardia K22.2
  caval veins (inferior) (superior) I87.1
  cecum — see Obstruction, intestine
  circulatory I99.8
  colon — see Obstruction, intestine
  common duct (noncalculous) K83.1
  coronary (artery) — see Occlusion, coronary
  cystic duct — see also Obstruction, gallbladder

Obstruction, obstructed, obstructive — continued
  cystic duct — see also Obstruction, gallbladder —
    continued
    with calculus K80.21
  device, implant or graft — see also Complications, by
    site and type, mechanical T85.698 ☑
    arterial graft NEC — see Complication, cardiovascu-
        lar device, mechanical, vascular
    catheter NEC T85.628 ☑
        cystostomy T83.090 ☑
        dialysis (renal) T82.49 ☑
            intraperitoneal T85.691 ☑
        Hopkins T83.098 ☑
        ileostomy T83.098 ☑
        infusion NEC T82.594 ☑
            spinal (epidural) (subdural) T85.690 ☑
        nephrostomy T83.092 ☑
        urethral indwelling T83.091 ☑
        urinary T83.098 ☑
        urostomy T83.098 ☑
    due to infection T85.79 ☑
    gastrointestinal — see Complications, prosthetic
        device, mechanical, gastrointestinal device
    genital NEC T83.498 ☑
        intrauterine contraceptive device T83.39 ☑
        penile prosthesis (cylinder) (implanted) (pump)
            (resevoir) T83.490 ☑
        testicular prosthesis T83.491 ☑
    heart NEC — see Complication, cardiovascular de-
        vice, mechanical
    joint prosthesis — see Complications, joint prosthe-
        sis, mechanical, specified NEC, by site
    orthopedic NEC — see Complication, orthopedic,
        device, mechanical
    specified NEC T85.628 ☑
    urinary NEC — see also Complication, genitourinary,
        device, urinary, mechanical
        graft T83.29 ☑
    vascular NEC — see Complication, cardiovascular
        device, mechanical
    ventricular intracranial shunt T85.09 ☑
  due to foreign body accidentally left in operative
    wound T81.529 ☑
  duodenum K31.5
  ejaculatory duct N50.89
  esophagus K22.2
  eustachian tube (complete) (partial) H68.10- ☑
    cartilagenous (extrinsic) H68.13- ☑
        intrinsic H68.12- ☑
    osseous H68.11- ☑
  fallopian tube (bilateral) N97.1
  fecal K56.41
    with hernia — see Hernia, by site, with obstruction
  foramen of Monro (congenital) Q03.8
    with spina bifida — see Spina bifida, by site, with
        hydrocephalus
  foreign body — see Foreign body
  gallbladder K82.0
    with calculus, stones K80.21
    congenital Q44.1
  gastric outlet K31.1
  gastrointestinal — see Obstruction, intestine
  hepatic K76.89
    duct (noncalculous) K83.1
  ileum — see Obstruction, intestine
  iliofemoral (artery) I74.5
  intestine K56.609
    with
        adhesions (intestinal) (peritoneal) K56.50
            complete K56.52
            incomplete K56.51
            partial K56.51
    adynamic K56.0
    by gallstone K56.3
    complete K56.601
    congenital (small) Q41.9
        large Q42.9
            specified part NEC Q42.8
    incomplete K56.600
    neurogenic K56.0
        Hirschsprung's disease or megacolon Q43.1
    newborn P76.9
        due to
            fecaliths P76.8
            inspissated milk P76.2
            meconium (plug) P76.0
                in mucoviscidosis E84.11

Obstruction, obstructed, obstructive — *continued*
  intestine — *continued*
    newborn — *continued*
      specified NEC P76.8
    partial K56.600
    postoperative K91.30
      complete K91.32
      incomplete K91.31
      partial K91.31
    reflex K56.0
    specified NEC K56.699
      complete K56.691
      incomplete K56.690
      partial K56.690
    volvulus K56.2
  intracardiac ball valve prosthesis T82.09 ☑
  jejunum — *see* Obstruction, intestine
  joint prosthesis — *see* Complications, joint prosthesis, mechanical, specified NEC, by site
  kidney (calices) — *see also* Hydronephrosis N28.89
  labor — *see* Delivery
  lacrimal (passages) (duct)
    by
      dacryolith — *see* Dacryolith
      stenosis — *see* Stenosis, lacrimal
    congenital Q10.5
    neonatal H04.53- ☑
  lacrimonasal duct — *see* Obstruction, lacrimal
  lacteal, with steatorrhea K90.2
  laryngitis — *see* Laryngitis
  larynx NEC J38.6
    congenital Q31.8
  lung J98.4
    disease, chronic J44.9
  lymphatic I89.0
  meconium (plug)
    newborn P76.0
      due to fecaliths P76.0
      in mucoviscidosis E84.11
  mitral — *see* Stenosis, mitral
  nasal J34.89
  nasolacrimal duct — *see also* Obstruction, lacrimal
    congenital Q10.5
  nasopharynx J39.2
  nose J34.89
  organ or site, congenital NEC — *see* Atresia, by site
  pancreatic duct K86.89
  parotid duct or gland K11.8
  pelviureteral junction N13.5
    with hydronephrosis N13.0
    congenital Q62.39
  pharynx J39.2
  portal (circulation) (vein) I81
  prostate — *see also* Hyperplasia, prostate
    valve (urinary) N32.0
  pulmonary valve (heart) I37.0
  pyelonephritis (chronic) N11.1
  pylorus
    adult K31.1
    congenital or infantile Q40.0
  rectosigmoid — *see* Obstruction, intestine
  rectum K62.4
  renal — *see also* Hydronephrosis N28.89
    outflow N13.8
    pelvis, congenital Q62.39
  respiratory J98.8
    chronic J44.9
  retinal (vessels) H34.9
  salivary duct (any) K11.8
    with calculus K11.5
  sigmoid — *see* Obstruction, intestine
  sinus (accessory) (nasal) J34.89
  Stensen's duct K11.8
  stomach NEC K31.89
    acute K31.0
    congenital Q40.2
    due to pylorospasm K31.3
  submandibular duct K11.8
  submaxillary gland K11.8
    with calculus K11.5
  thoracic duct I89.0
  thrombotic — *see* Thrombosis
  trachea J39.8
  tracheostomy airway J95.03
  tricuspid (valve) — *see* Stenosis, tricuspid
  upper respiratory, congenital Q34.8
  ureter (functional) (pelvic junction) NEC N13.5

Obstruction, obstructed, obstructive — *continued*
  ureter — *continued*
    with
      hydronephrosis N13.1
        with infection N13.6
        congenital Q62.39
      pyelonephritis (chronic) N11.1
    congenital Q62.39
    due to calculus — *see* Calculus, ureter
  urethra NEC N36.8
    congenital Q64.39
  urinary (moderate) N13.9
    due to hyperplasia (hypertrophy) of prostate — *see* Hyperplasia, prostate
    organ or tract (lower) N13.9
    prostatic valve N32.0
    specified NEC N13.8
  uropathy N13.9
  uterus N85.8
  vagina N89.5
  valvular — *see* Endocarditis
  vein, venous I87.1
    caval (inferior) (superior) I87.1
    thrombotic — *see* Thrombosis
  vena cava (inferior) (superior) I87.1
  vesical NEC N32.0
  vesicourethral orifice N32.0
    congenital Q64.31
  vessel NEC I99.8
    stent — *see* Restenosis, stent

Obturator — *see* condition
Occlusal wear, teeth K03.0
Occlusio pupillae — *see* Membrane, pupillary
Occlusion, occluded
  anus K62.4
    congenital Q42.3
      with fistula Q42.2
  aortoiliac (chronic) I74.09
  aqueduct of Sylvius G91.1
    congenital Q03.0
      with spina bifida — *see* Spina bifida, by site, with hydrocephalus
  artery — *see also* Atherosclerosis, artery I70.9 ☑
    auditory, internal I65.8
    basilar I65.1
      with
        infarction I63.22
          due to
            embolism I63.12
            thrombosis I63.02
    brain or cerebral I66.9
      with infarction (due to) I63.5- ☑
        embolism I63.4- ☑
        thrombosis I63.3- ☑
    carotid I65.2- ☑
      with
        infarction I63.23- ☑
          due to
            embolism I63.13- ☑
            thrombosis I63.03- ☑
    cerebellar (anterior inferior) (posterior inferior) (superior) I66.3
      with infarction I63.54- ☑
        due to
          embolism I63.44- ☑
          thrombosis I63.34- ☑
    cerebral I66.9
      with infarction I63.50
        due to
          embolism I63.40
            specified NEC I63.49
          thrombosis I63.30
            specified NEC I63.39
      anterior I66.1-
        with infarction I63.52- ☑
          due to
            embolism I63.42- ☑
            thrombosis I63.32- ☑
      middle I66.0- ☑
        with infarction I63.51- ☑
          due to
            embolism I63.41- ☑
            thrombosis I63.31- ☑
      posterior I66.2- ☑
        with infarction I63.53- ☑
          due to
            embolism I63.43- ☑

Occlusion, occluded — *continued*
  artery — *see also* Atherosclerosis, artery — *continued*
    cerebral — *continued*
      posterior — *continued*
        with infarction — *continued*
          due to — *continued*
            thrombosis I63.33- ☑
        specified NEC I66.8
          with infarction I63.59
            due to
              embolism I63.4- ☑
              thrombosis I63.3- ☑
    choroidal (anterior) — *see* Occlusion, artery, precerebral, specified NEC
    communicating posterior — *see* Occlusion, artery, precerebral, specified NEC
    complete
      coronary I25.82
      extremities I70.92
    coronary (acute) (thrombotic) (without myocardial infarction) I24.0
      with myocardial infarction — *see* Infarction, myocardium
      chronic total I25.82
      complete I25.82
      healed or old I25.2
      total (chronic) I25.82
    hypophyseal — *see* Occlusion, artery, precerebral, specified NEC
    iliac I74.5
    lower extremities due to stenosis or stricture I77.1
    mesenteric (embolic) (thrombotic) — *see also* Infarct, intestine K55.069
    perforating — *see* Occlusion, artery, cerebral, specified NEC
    peripheral I77.9
      thrombotic or embolic I74.4
    pontine — *see* Occlusion, artery, precerebral, specified NEC
    precerebral I65.9
      with infarction I63.20
        specified NEC I63.29
          due to
            embolism I63.10
              specified NEC I63.19
            thrombosis I63.00
              specified NEC I63.09
      basilar — *see* Occlusion, artery, basilar
      carotid — *see* Occlusion, artery, carotid
      puerperal O88.23
      specified NEC I65.8
        with infarction I63.29
          due to
            embolism I63.19
            thrombosis I63.09
      vertebral — *see* Occlusion, artery, vertebral
    renal N28.0
    retinal
      branch H34.23- ☑
      central H34.1- ☑
      partial H34.21- ☑
      transient H34.0- ☑
    spinal — *see* Occlusion, artery, precerebral, vertebral
    total (chronic)
      coronary I25.82
      extremities I70.92
    vertebral I65.0- ☑
      with
        infarction I63.21- ☑
          due to
            embolism I63.11- ☑
            thrombosis I63.01- ☑
  basilar artery — *see* Occlusion, artery, basilar
  bile duct (common) (hepatic) (noncalculous) K83.1
  bowel — *see* Obstruction, intestine
  carotid (artery) (common) (internal) — *see* Occlusion, artery, carotid
  centric (of teeth) M26.59
    maximum intercuspation discrepancy M26.55
  cerebellar (artery) — *see* Occlusion, artery, cerebellar
  cerebral (artery) — *see* Occlusion, artery, cerebral
  cerebrovascular — *see also* Occlusion, artery, cerebral
    with infarction I63.5- ☑
  cervical canal — *see* Stricture, cervix
  cervix (uteri) — *see* Stricture, cervix
  choanal Q30.0

☑ **Additional Character Required — Refer to the Tabular List for Character Selection**

Occlusion, occluded — *continued*
  choroidal (artery) — *see* Occlusion, artery, precerebral,
    specified NEC
  colon — *see* Obstruction, intestine
  communicating posterior artery — *see* Occlusion,
    artery, precerebral, specified NEC
  coronary (artery) (vein) (thrombotic) — *see also* Infarct,
    myocardium
    chronic total I25.82
    healed or old I25.2
    not resulting in infarction I24.0
    total (chronic) I25.82
  cystic duct — *see* Obstruction, gallbladder
  embolic — *see* Embolism
  fallopian tube N97.1
    congenital Q50.6
  gallbladder — *see also* Obstruction, gallbladder
    congenital (causing jaundice) Q44.1
  gingiva, traumatic K06.2
  hymen N89.6
    congenital Q52.3
  hypophyseal (artery) — *see* Occlusion, artery, precere-
    bral, specified NEC
  iliac artery I74.5
  intestine — *see* Obstruction, intestine
  lacrimal passages — *see* Obstruction, lacrimal
  lung J98.4
  lymph or lymphatic channel I89.0
  mammary duct N64.89
  mesenteric artery (embolic) (thrombotic) — *see also*
    Infarct, intestine K55.069
  nose J34.89
    congenital Q30.0
  organ or site, congenital NEC — *see* Atresia, by site
  oviduct N97.1
    congenital Q50.6
  peripheral arteries
    due to stricture or stenosis I77.1
    upper extremity I74.2
  pontine (artery) — *see* Occlusion, artery, precerebral,
    specified NEC
  posterior lingual, of mandibular teeth M26.29
  precerebral artery — *see* Occlusion, artery, precerebral
  punctum lacrimale — *see* Obstruction, lacrimal
  pupil — *see* Membrane, pupillary
  pylorus, adult — *see also* Stricture, pylorus K31.1
  renal artery N28.0
  retina, retinal
    artery — *see* Occlusion, artery, retinal
    vein (central) H34.81- ☑
      engorgement H34.82- ☑
      tributary H34.83- ☑
      vessels H34.9
  spinal artery — *see* Occlusion, artery, precerebral, ver-
    tebral
  teeth (mandibular) (posterior lingual) M26.29
  thoracic duct I89.0
  thrombotic — *see* Thrombosis, artery
  traumatic
    edentulous (alveolar) ridge K06.2
    gingiva K06.2
    periodontal K05.5
  tubal N97.1
  ureter (complete) (partial) N13.5
    congenital Q62.10
  ureteropelvic junction N13.5
    congenital Q62.11
  ureterovesical orifice N13.5
    congenital Q62.12
  urethra — *see* Stricture, urethra
  uterus N85.8
  vagina N89.5
  vascular NEC I99.8
  vein — *see* Thrombosis
    retinal — *see* Occlusion, retinal, vein
  vena cava (inferior) (superior) — *see* Embolism, vena
    cava
  ventricle (brain) NEC G91.1
  vertebral (artery) — *see* Occlusion, artery, vertebral
  vessel (blood) I99.8
  vulva N90.5
Occult
  blood in feces (stools) R19.5
Occupational
  problems NEC Z56.89
Ochlophobia — *see* Agoraphobia
Ochronosis (endogenous) E70.29
Ocular muscle — *see* condition

Oculogyric crisis or disturbance H51.8
  psychogenic F45.8
Oculomotor syndrome H51.9
Oculopathy
  syphilitic NEC A52.71
    congenital
      early A50.01
      late A50.30
    early (secondary) A51.43
    late A52.71
Oddi's sphincter spasm K83.4
Odontalgia K08.89
Odontoameloblastoma — *see* Cyst, calcifying odonto-
  genic
Odontoclasia K03.89
Odontodysplasia, regional K00.4
Odontogenesis imperfecta K00.5
Odontoma (ameloblastic) (complex) (compound) (fi-
  broameloblastic) — *see* Cyst, calcifying odontogenic
Odontomyelitis (closed) (open) K04.01
  irreversible K04.02
  reversible K04.01
Odontorrhagia K08.89
Odontosarcoma, ameloblastic C41.1
  upper jaw (bone) C41.0
Oestriasis — *see* Myiasis
Oguchi's disease H53.63
Ohara's disease — *see* Tularemia
OHS (obesity hypoventilation syndrome) E66.2
Oidiomycosis — *see* Candidiasis
Oidium albicans infection — *see* Candidiasis
Old age (without mention of debility) R54
  dementia F03 ☑
Old (previous) **myocardial infarction** I25.2
Olfactory — *see* condition
Oligemia — *see* Anemia
Oligoastrocytoma
  specified site — *see* Neoplasm, malignant, by site
  unspecified site C71.9
Oligocythemia D64.9
Oligodendroblastoma
  specified site — *see* Neoplasm, malignant
  unspecified site C71.9
Oligodendroglioma
  anaplastic type
    specified site — *see* Neoplasm, malignant, by site
    unspecified site C71.9
  specified site — *see* Neoplasm, malignant, by site
  unspecified site C71.9
Oligodontia — *see* Anodontia
Oligoencephalon Q02
Oligohidrosis L74.4
Oligohydramnios O41.0- ☑
Oligohydrosis L74.4
Oligomenorrhea N91.5
  primary N91.3
  secondary N91.4
Oligophrenia — *see also* Disability, intellectual
  phenylpyruvic E70.0
Oligospermia N46.11
  due to
    drug therapy N46.121
    efferent duct obstruction N46.123
    infection N46.122
    radiation N46.124
    specified cause NEC N46.129
    systemic disease N46.125
Oligotrichia — *see* Alopecia
Oliguria R34
  with, complicating or following ectopic or molar preg-
    nancy O08.4
  postprocedural N99.0
Ollier's disease Q78.4
Omenotocele — *see* Hernia, abdomen, specified site NEC
Omentitis — *see* Peritonitis
Omentum, omental — *see* condition
Omphalitis (congenital) (newborn) P38.9
  with mild hemorrhage P38.1
  without hemorrhage P38.9
  not of newborn L08.82
  tetanus A33
Omphalocele Q79.2
Omphalomesenteric duct, persistent Q43.0
Omphalorrhagia, newborn P51.9
Omsk hemorrhagic fever A98.1
Onanism (excessive) F98.8
Onchocerciasis, onchocercosis B73.1

Onchocerciasis, onchocercosis — *continued*
  with
    eye disease B73.00
      endophthalmitis B73.01
      eyelid B73.09
      glaucoma B73.02
      specified NEC B73.09
    eyelid B73.09
    eye NEC B73.00
Oncocytoma — *see* Neoplasm, benign, by site
Oncovirus, as cause of disease classified elsewhere
  B97.32
Ondine's curse — *see* Apnea, sleep
Oneirophrenia F23
Onychauxis L60.2
  congenital Q84.5
Onychia — *see also* Cellulitis, digit
  with lymphangitis — *see* Lymphangitis, acute, digit
  candidal B37.2
  dermatophytic B35.1
Onychitis — *see also* Cellulitis, digit
  with lymphangitis — *see* Lymphangitis, acute, digit
Onychocryptosis L60.0
Onychodystrophy L60.3
  congenital Q84.6
Onychogryphosis, onychogryposis L60.2
Onycholysis L60.1
Onychomadesis L60.8
Onychomalacia L60.3
Onychomycosis (finger) (toe) B35.1
Onycho-osteodysplasia Q87.2
Onychophagia F98.8
Onychophosis L60.8
Onychoptosis L60.8
Onychorrhexis L60.3
  congenital Q84.6
Onychoschizia L60.3
Onyxis (finger) (toe) L60.0
Onyxitis — *see also* Cellulitis, digit
  with lymphangitis — *see* Lymphangitis, acute, digit
Oophoritis (cystic) (infectional) (interstitial) N70.92
  with salpingitis N70.93
  acute N70.02
    with salpingitis N70.03
  chronic N70.12
    with salpingitis N70.13
  complicating abortion — *see* Abortion, by type, com-
    plicated by, oophoritis
Oophorocele N83.4- ☑
Opacity, opacities
  cornea H17.- ☑
    central H17.1- ☑
    congenital Q13.3
    degenerative — *see* Degeneration, cornea
    hereditary — *see* Dystrophy, cornea
    inflammatory — *see* Keratitis
    minor H17.81- ☑
    peripheral H17.82- ☑
    sequelae of trachoma (healed) B94.0
    specified NEC H17.89
  enamel (teeth) (fluoride) (nonfluoride) K00.3
  lens — *see* Cataract
  snowball — *see* Deposit, crystalline
  vitreous (humor) NEC H43.39- ☑
    congenital Q14.0
    membranes and strands H43.31- ☑
Opalescent dentin (hereditary) K00.5
Open, opening
  abnormal, organ or site, congenital — *see* Imperfect,
    closure
  angle with
    borderline
      findings
        high risk H40.02- ☑
        low risk H40.01- ☑
      intraocular pressure H40.00- ☑
    cupping of discs H40.01- ☑
    glaucoma (primary) — *see* Glaucoma, open angle
  bite
    anterior M26.220
    posterior M26.221
  false — *see* Imperfect, closure
  margin on tooth restoration K08.51
  restoration margins of tooth K08.51
  wound — *see* Wound, open
Operational fatigue F48.8
Operative — *see* condition

Operculitis — see Periodontitis
Operculum — see Break, retina
Ophiasis L63.2
Ophthalmia — see also Conjunctivitis H10.9
  actinic rays — see Photokeratitis
  allergic (acute) — see Conjunctivitis, acute, atopic
  blennorrhagic (gonococcal) (neonatorum) A54.31
  diphtheritic A36.86
  Egyptian A71.1
  electrica — see Photokeratitis
  gonococcal (neonatorum) A54.31
  metastatic — see Endophthalmitis, purulent
  migraine — see Migraine, ophthalmoplegic
  neonatorum, newborn P39.1
    gonococcal A54.31
  nodosa H16.24- ☑
  purulent — see Conjunctivitis, acute, mucopurulent
  spring — see Conjunctivitis, acute, atopic
  sympathetic — see Uveitis, sympathetic
Ophthalmitis — see Ophthalmia
Ophthalmocele (congenital) Q15.8
Ophthalmoneuromyelitis G36.0
Ophthalmoplegia — see also Strabismus, paralytic
  anterior internuclear — see Ophthalmoplegia, internuclear
  ataxia-areflexia G61.0
  diabetic — see E08-E13 with .39
  exophthalmic E05.00
    with thyroid storm E05.01
  external H49.88- ☑
    progressive H49.4- ☑
      with pigmentary retinopathy — see Kearns-Sayre syndrome
    total H49.3- ☑
  internal (complete) (total) H52.51- ☑
  internuclear H51.2- ☑
  migraine — see Migraine, ophthalmoplegic
  Parinaud's H49.88- ☑
  progressive external — see Ophthalmoplegia, external, progressive
  supranuclear, progressive G23.1
  total (external) — see Ophthalmoplegia, external, total
Opioid(s)
  abuse — see Abuse, drug, opioids
  dependence — see Dependence, drug, opioids
  induced, without use disorder
    anxiety disorder F11.988
    delirium F11.921
    depressive disorder F11.94
    sexual dysfunction F11.981
    sleep disorder F11.982
Opisthognathism M26.09
Opisthorchiasis (felineus) (viverrini) B66.0
Opitz' disease D73.2
Opiumism — see Dependence, drug, opioid
Oppenheim's disease G70.2
Oppenheim-Urbach disease (necrobiosis lipoidica diabeticorum) — see E08-E13 with .620
Optic nerve — see condition
Orbit — see condition
Orchioblastoma C62.9- ☑
Orchitis (gangrenous) (nonspecific) (septic) (suppurative) N45.2
  blennorrhagic (gonococcal) (acute) (chronic) A54.23
  chlamydial A56.19
  filarial — see also Infestation, filarial B74.9 [N51]
  gonococcal (acute) (chronic) A54.23
  mumps B26.0
  syphilitic A52.76
  tuberculous A18.15
Orf (virus disease) B08.02
Organic — see also condition
  brain syndrome F09
  heart — see Disease, heart
  mental disorder F09
  psychosis F09
Orgasm
  anejaculatory N53.13
Oriental
  bilharziasis B65.2
  schistosomiasis B65.2
Orifice — see condition
Origin of both great vessels from right ventricle Q20.1
Ormond's disease (with ureteral obstruction) N13.5
  with infection N13.6
Ornithine metabolism disorder E72.4

Ornithinemia (Type I) (Type II) E72.4
Ornithosis A70
Orotacidosis, oroticaciduria (congenital) (hereditary) (pyrimidine deficiency) E79.8
  anemia D53.0
Orthodontics
  adjustment Z46.4
  fitting Z46.4
Orthopnea R06.01
Orthopoxvirus B08.09
Os, uterus — see condition
Osgood-Schlatter disease or osteochondrosis M92.52- ☑
Osler (-Weber)-**Rendu disease** I78.0
Osler's nodes I33.0
Osmidrosis L75.0
Osseous — see condition
Ossification
  artery — see Arteriosclerosis
  auricle (ear) — see Disorder, pinna, specified type NEC
  bronchial J98.09
  cardiac — see Degeneration, myocardial
  cartilage (senile) — see Disorder, cartilage, specified type NEC
  coronary (artery) — see Disease, heart, ischemic, atherosclerotic
  diaphragm J98.6
  ear, middle — see Otosclerosis
  falx cerebri G96.198
  fontanel, premature Q75.0
  heart — see also Degeneration, myocardial
    valve — see Endocarditis
  larynx J38.7
  ligament — see Disorder, tendon, specified type NEC
    posterior longitudinal — see Spondylopathy, specified NEC
  meninges (cerebral) (spinal) G96.198
  multiple, eccentric centers — see Disorder, bone, development or growth
  muscle — see also Calcification, muscle
    due to burns — see Myositis, ossificans, in, burns
    paralytic — see Myositis, ossificans, in, quadriplegia
    progressive — see Myositis, ossificans, progressiva
    specified NEC M61.50
      ankle M61.57- ☑
      foot M61.57- ☑
      forearm M61.53- ☑
      hand M61.54- ☑
      lower leg M61.56- ☑
      multiple sites M61.59
      pelvic region M61.55- ☑
      shoulder region M61.51- ☑
      specified site NEC M61.58
      thigh M61.55- ☑
      upper arm M61.52- ☑
    traumatic — see Myositis, ossificans, traumatica
  myocardium, myocardial — see Degeneration, myocardial
  penis N48.89
  periarticular — see Disorder, joint, specified type NEC
  pinna — see Disorder, pinna, specified type NEC
  rider's bone — see Ossification, muscle, specified NEC
  sclera H15.89
  subperiosteal, post-traumatic M89.8X- ☑
  tendon — see Disorder, tendon, specified type NEC
  trachea J39.8
  tympanic membrane — see Disorder, tympanic membrane, specified NEC
  vitreous (humor) — see Deposit, crystalline
Osteitis — see also Osteomyelitis
  alveolar M27.3
  condensans M85.30
    ankle M85.37- ☑
    foot M85.37- ☑
    forearm M85.33- ☑
    hand M85.34- ☑
    lower leg M85.36- ☑
    multiple site M85.39
    neck M85.38
    rib M85.38
    shoulder M85.31- ☑
    skull M85.38
    specified site NEC M85.38
    thigh M85.35- ☑
    toe M85.37- ☑
    upper arm M85.32- ☑
    vertebra M85.38

Osteitis — continued
  deformans M88.9
    in (due to)
      malignant neoplasm of bone C41.9 [M90.60]
      neoplastic disease — see also Neoplasm D49.9 [M90.60]
        carpus D49.9 [M90.64-] ☑
        clavicle D49.9 [M90.61-] ☑
        femur D49.9 [M90.65-] ☑
        fibula D49.9 [M90.66-] ☑
        finger D49.9 [M90.64-] ☑
        humerus D49.9 [M90.62-] ☑
        ilium D49.9 [M90.65-] ☑
        ischium D49.9 [M90.65-] ☑
        metacarpus D49.9 [M90.64-] ☑
        metatarsus D49.9 [M90.67-] ☑
        multiple sites D49.9 [M90.69]
        neck D49.9 [M90.68]
        radius D49.9 [M90.63-] ☑
        rib D49.9 [M90.68]
        scapula D49.9 [M90.61-] ☑
        skull D49.9 [M90.68]
        tarsus D49.9 [M90.67-] ☑
        tibia D49.9 [M90.66-] ☑
        toe D49.9 [M90.67-] ☑
        ulna D49.9 [M90.63-] ☑
        vertebra D49.9 [M90.68]
    skull M88.0
    specified NEC — see Paget's disease, bone, by site
    vertebra M88.1
  due to yaws A66.6
  fibrosa NEC — see Cyst, bone, by site
    circumscripta — see Dysplasia, fibrous, bone NEC
    cystica (generalisata) E21.0
    disseminata Q78.1
    osteoplastica E21.0
  fragilitans Q78.0
  Garr's (sclerosing) — see Osteomyelitis, specified type NEC
  jaw (acute) (chronic) (lower) (suppurative) (upper) M27.2
  parathyroid E21.0
  petrous bone (acute) (chronic) — see Petrositis
  sclerotic, nonsuppurative — see Osteomyelitis, specified type NEC
  tuberculosa A18.09
    cystica D86.89
    multiplex cystoides D86.89
Osteoarthritis M19.90
  ankle M19.07- ☑
    post-traumatic M19.17- ☑
    primary M19.07- ☑
    secondary M19.27- ☑
  elbow M19.02- ☑
    post-traumatic M19.12- ☑
    primary M19.02- ☑
    secondary M19.22- ☑
  foot joint M19.07- ☑
    post-traumatic M19.17- ☑
    primary M19.07- ☑
    secondary M19.27- ☑
  generalized (multiple joints) M15.9
    erosive M15.4
    primary M15.0
    specified NEC M15.8
  hand joint M19.04- ☑
    first carpometacarpal joint M18.9
      post-traumatic — see Osteoarthritis, post-traumatic NEC, hand joint, first carpometacarpal joint
      primary — see Osteoarthritis, primary, hand joint, first carpometacarpal joint
      secondary — see Osteoarthritis, secondary, hand joint, first carpometacarpal joint
    post-traumatic M19.14- ☑
    primary M19.04- ☑
    secondary M19.24- ☑
  hip M16.9
    bilateral M16.0
      due to hip dysplasia M16.2
      post-traumatic M16.4
      secondary M16.6
    due to hip dysplasia (unilateral) M16.3- ☑
      bilateral M16.2
    post-traumatic — see Osteoarthritis, post-traumatic, hip
    primary M16.1- ☑

☑ Additional Character Required — Refer to the Tabular List for Character Selection

Osteoarthritis — *continued*
  hip — *continued*
    secondary — *see* Osteoarthritis, secondary, hip
    unilateral M16.1- ☑
      due to hip dysplasia M16.3- ☑
      post-traumatic M16.5- ☑
      primary M16.1- ☑
      secondary NEC M16.7
  interphalangeal
    distal (Heberden) M15.1
    proximal (Bouchard) M15.2
  knee M17.9
    bilateral M17.0
      post-traumatic M17.2
      secondary M17.4
    post-traumatic — *see* Osteoarthritis, post-traumatic,
      knee
    primary M17.1- ☑
      bilateral M17.0
    secondary — *see* Osteoarthritis, secondary, knee
    unilateral M17.1- ☑
      post-traumatic M17.3- ☑
      primary M17.1- ☑
      secondary NEC M17.5
  post-traumatic NEC M19.92
    ankle M19.17- ☑
    elbow M19.12- ☑
    foot joint M19.17- ☑
    hand joint M19.14- ☑
      first carpometacarpal joint M18.3- ☑
        bilateral M18.2
    hip M16.5- ☑
      bilateral M16.4
    knee M17.3- ☑
      bilateral M17.2
    shoulder M19.11- ☑
    specified site NEC M19.19
    wrist M19.13- ☑
  primary M19.91
    ankle M19.07- ☑
    elbow M19.02- ☑
    foot joint M19.07- ☑
    hand joint M19.04- ☑
      first carpometacarpal joint M18.1- ☑
        bilateral M18.0
    hip M16.1- ☑
      bilateral M16.0
    knee M17.1- ☑
      bilateral M17.0
    multiple sites M15.9
    shoulder M19.01- ☑
    specified site NEC M19.09
    spine — *see* Spondylosis
    wrist M19.03- ☑
  secondary M19.93
    ankle M19.27- ☑
    elbow M19.22- ☑
    foot joint M19.27- ☑
    hand joint M19.24- ☑
      first carpometacarpal joint M18.5- ☑
        bilateral M18.4
    hip M16.7-
      bilateral M16.6
    knee M17.5-
      bilateral M17.4
    multiple M15.3
    shoulder M19.21- ☑
    specified site NEC M19.29
    spine — *see* Spondylosis
    wrist M19.23- ☑
  shoulder M19.01- ☑
    post-traumatic M19.11- ☑
    primary M19.01- ☑
    secondary M19.21- ☑
  specified site NEC M19.09
  spine — *see* Spondylosis
  wrist M19.03- ☑
    first carpometacarpal joint — *see* Osteoarthritis,
      hand joint, first carpometacarpal joint
    post-traumatic M19.13- ☑
    primary M19.03- ☑
    secondary M19.23 ☑
Osteoarthropathy (hypertrophic) M19.90
  ankle — *see* Osteoarthritis, primary, ankle
  elbow — *see* Osteoarthritis, primary, elbow
  foot joint — *see* Osteoarthritis, primary, foot
  hand joint — *see* Osteoarthritis, primary, hand joint

Osteoarthropathy — *continued*
  knee joint — *see* Osteoarthritis, primary, knee
  multiple site — *see* Osteoarthritis, primary, multiple
    joint
  pulmonary — *see also* Osteoarthropathy, specified
    type NEC
    hypertrophic — *see* Osteoarthropathy, hypertrophic,
      specified type NEC
  secondary — *see* Osteoarthropathy, specified type NEC
  secondary hypertrophic — *see* Osteoarthropathy,
    specified type NEC
  shoulder — *see* Osteoarthritis, primary, shoulder
  specified joint NEC — *see* Osteoarthritis, primary,
    specified joint NEC
  specified type NEC M89.40
    carpus M89.44- ☑
    clavicle M89.41- ☑
    femur M89.45- ☑
    fibula M89.46- ☑
    finger M89.44- ☑
    humerus M89.42- ☑
    ilium M89.459
    ischium M89.459
    metacarpus M89.44- ☑
    metatarsus M89.47- ☑
    multiple sites M89.49
    neck M89.48
    radius M89.43- ☑
    rib M89.48
    scapula M89.41- ☑
    skull M89.48
    tarsus M89.47- ☑
    tibia M89.46- ☑
    toe M89.47- ☑
    ulna M89.43- ☑
    vertebra M89.48
  spine — *see* Spondylosis
  wrist — *see* Osteoarthritis, primary, wrist
Osteoarthrosis (degenerative) (hypertrophic) (joint) —
  see also Osteoarthritis
  deformans alkaptonurica E70.29 *[M36.8]*
  erosive M15.4
  generalized M15.9
    primary M15.0
  polyarticular M15.9
  spine — *see* Spondylosis
Osteoblastoma — *see* Neoplasm, bone, benign
  aggressive — *see* Neoplasm, bone, uncertain behavior
Osteochondritis — *see also* Osteochondropathy, by site
  Brailsford's — *see* Osteochondrosis, juvenile, radius
  dissecans M93.20
    ankle M93.27- ☑
    elbow M93.22- ☑
    foot M93.27- ☑
    hand M93.24- ☑
    hip M93.25- ☑
    knee M93.26- ☑
    multiple sites M93.29
    shoulder joint M93.21- ☑
    specified site NEC M93.28
    wrist M93.23- ☑
  juvenile M92.9
    patellar — *see* Osteochondrosis, juvenile, patella
  syphilitic (congenital) (early) A50.02 *[M90.80]*
    ankle A50.02 *[M90.87-]* ☑
    elbow A50.02 *[M90.82-]* ☑
    foot A50.02 *[M90.87-]* ☑
    forearm A50.02 *[M90.83-]* ☑
    hand A50.02 *[M90.84-]* ☑
    hip A50.02 *[M90.85-]* ☑
    knee A50.02 *[M90.86-]* ☑
    multiple sites A50.02 *[M90.89]*
    shoulder joint A50.02 *[M90.81-]* ☑
    specified site NEC A50.02 *[M90.88]*
Osteochondroarthrosis deformans endemica — *see*
  Disease, Kaschin-Beck
Osteochondrodysplasia Q78.9
  with defects of growth of tubular bones and spine
    Q77.9
    specified NEC Q77.8
  specified NEC Q78.8
Osteochondrodystrophy E78.9
Osteochondrolysis — *see* Osteochondritis, dissecans
Osteochondroma — *see* Neoplasm, bone, benign
Osteochondromatosis D16.9
  syndrome Q78.4

Osteochondromyxosarcoma — *see* Neoplasm, bone,
  malignant
Osteochondropathy M93.90
  ankle M93.97- ☑
  elbow M93.92- ☑
  foot M93.97- ☑
  hand M93.94- ☑
  hip M93.95- ☑
  Kienböck's disease of adults M93.1
  knee M93.96- ☑
  multiple joints M93.99
  osteochondritis dissecans — *see* Osteochondritis, dis-
    secans
  osteochondrosis — *see* Osteochondrosis
  shoulder region M93.91- ☑
  slipped upper femoral epiphysis — *see* Slipped, epiph-
    ysis, upper femoral
  specified joint NEC M93.98
  specified type NEC M93.80
    ankle M93.87- ☑
    elbow M93.82- ☑
    foot M93.87- ☑
    hand M93.84- ☑
    hip M93.85- ☑
    knee M93.86- ☑
    multiple joints M93.89
    shoulder region M93.81- ☑
    specified joint NEC M93.88
    wrist M93.83- ☑
  syphilitic, congenital
    early A50.02 *[M90.80]*
    late A50.56 *[M90.80]*
  wrist M93.93- ☑
Osteochondrosarcoma — *see* Neoplasm, bone, malignant
Osteochondrosis — *see also* Osteochondropathy, by
  site
  acetabulum (juvenile) M91.0
  adult — *see* Osteochondropathy, specified type NEC,
    by site
  astragalus (juvenile) — *see* Osteochondrosis, juvenile,
    tarsus
  Blount M92.51- ☑
  Buchanan's M91.0
  Burns' — *see* Osteochondrosis, juvenile, ulna
  calcaneus (juvenile) — *see* Osteochondrosis, juvenile,
    tarsus
  capitular epiphysis (femur) (juvenile) — *see* Legg-Calvé-
    Perthes disease
  carpal (juvenile) (lunate) (scaphoid) — *see* Osteochon-
    drosis, juvenile, hand, carpal lunate
    adult M93.1
  coxae juvenilis — *see* Legg-Calvé-Perthes disease
  deformans juvenilis, coxae — *see* Legg-Calvé-Perthes
    disease
  Diaz's — *see* Osteochondrosis, juvenile, tarsus
  dissecans (knee) (shoulder) — *see* Osteochondritis,
    dissecans
  femoral capital epiphysis (juvenile) — *see* Legg-Calvé-
    Perthes disease
  femur (head), juvenile — *see* Legg-Calvé-Perthes dis-
    ease
  fibula (juvenile) — *see* Osteochondrosis, juvenile,
    fibula
  foot NEC (juvenile) M92.8
  Freiberg's — *see* Osteochondrosis, juvenile, metatarsus
  Haas' (juvenile) — *see* Osteochondrosis, juvenile,
    humerus
  Haglund's — *see* Osteochondrosis, juvenile, tarsus
  hip (juvenile) — *see* Legg-Calvé-Perthes disease
  humerus (capitulum) (head) (juvenile) — *see* Osteo-
    chondrosis, juvenile, humerus
  ilium, iliac crest (juvenile) M91.0
  ischiopubic synchondrosis M91.0
  Iselin's — *see* Osteochondrosis, juvenile, metatarsus
  juvenile, juvenilis M92.9
    after congenital dislocation of hip reduction — *see*
      Osteochondrosis, juvenile, hip, specified NEC
    arm — *see* Osteochondrosis, juvenile, upper limb
      NEC
    capitular epiphysis (femur) — *see* Legg-Calvé-
      Perthes disease
    clavicle, sternal epiphysis — *see* Osteochondrosis,
      juvenile, upper limb NEC
    coxae — *see* Legg-Calvé-Perthes disease
    deformans M92.9
    fibula M92.50- ☑

Osteochondrosis — continued
  juvenile, juvenilis — continued
    foot NEC M92.8
    hand M92.20- ☑
      carpal lunate M92.21- ☑
      metacarpal head M92.22- ☑
      specified site NEC M92.29- ☑
    head of femur — see Legg-Calvé-Perthes disease
    hip and pelvis M91.9- ☑
      coxa plana — see Coxa, plana
      femoral head — see Legg-Calvé-Perthes disease
      pelvis M91.0
      pseudocoxalgia — see Pseudocoxalgia
      specified NEC M91.8- ☑
    humerus M92.0- ☑
    limb
      lower NEC M92.8
      upper NEC — see Osteochondrosis, juvenile, upper limb NEC
    medial cuneiform bone — see Osteochondrosis, juvenile, tarsus
    metatarsus M92.7- ☑
    patella M92.4- ☑
    radius M92.1- ☑
    specified
      site NEC M92.8
      type NEC M92.8
        tibia and fibula M92.59- ☑
    spine M42.00
      cervical region M42.02
      cervicothoracic region M42.03
      lumbar region M42.06
      lumbosacral region M42.07
      multiple sites M42.09
      occipito-atlanto-axial region M42.01
      sacrococcygeal region M42.08
      thoracic region M42.04
      thoracolumbar region M42.05
    tarsus M92.6- ☑
    tibia M92.50- ☑
      proximal M92.51- ☑
      tubercle M92.52- ☑
    ulna M92.1- ☑
    upper limb NEC M92.3- ☑
    vertebra (body) (epiphyseal plates) (Calvé's) (Scheuermann's) — see Osteochondrosis, juvenile, spine
  Kienböck's — see Osteochondrosis, juvenile, hand, carpal lunate
    adult M93.1
  Köhler's
    patellar — see Osteochondrosis, juvenile, patella
    tarsal navicular — see Osteochondrosis, juvenile, tarsus
  Legg-Perthes (-Calvé) (-Waldenström) — see Legg-Calvé-Perthes disease
  limb
    lower NEC (juvenile) M92.8
      tibia and fibula M92.59- ☑
    upper NEC (juvenile) — see Osteochondrosis, juvenile, upper limb NEC
  lunate bone (carpal) (juvenile) — see also Osteochondrosis, juvenile, hand, carpal lunate
    adult M93.1
  Mauclaire's — see Osteochondrosis, juvenile, hand, metacarpal
  metacarpal (head) (juvenile) — see Osteochondrosis, juvenile, hand, metacarpal
  metatarsus (fifth) (head) (juvenile) (second) — see Osteochondrosis, juvenile, metatarsus
  navicular (juvenile) — see Osteochondrosis, juvenile, tarsus
  os
    calcis (juvenile) — see Osteochondrosis, juvenile, tarsus
    tibiale externum (juvenile) — see Osteochondrosis, juvenile, tarsus
  Osgood-Schlatter M92.52- ☑
  Panner's — see Osteochondrosis, juvenile, humerus
  patellar center (juvenile) (primary) (secondary) — see Osteochondrosis, juvenile, patella
  pelvis (juvenile) M91.0
  Pierson's M91.0
  radius (head) (juvenile) — see Osteochondrosis, juvenile, radius
  Scheuermann's — see Osteochondrosis, juvenile, spine
  Sever's — see Osteochondrosis, juvenile, tarsus

Osteochondrosis — continued
  Sinding-Larsen — see Osteochondrosis, juvenile, patella
  spine M42.9
    adult M42.10
      cervical region M42.12
      cervicothoracic region M42.13
      lumbar region M42.16
      lumbosacral region M42.17
      multiple sites M42.19
      occipito-atlanto-axial region M42.11
      sacrococcygeal region M42.18
      thoracic region M42.14
      thoracolumbar region M42.15
    juvenile — see Osteochondrosis, juvenile, spine
  symphysis pubis (juvenile) M91.0
  syphilitic (congenital) A50.02
  talus (juvenile) — see Osteochondrosis, juvenile, tarsus
  tarsus (navicular) (juvenile) — see Osteochondrosis, juvenile, tarsus
  tibia (proximal) (tubercle) (juvenile) — see Osteochondrosis, juvenile, tibia
  tuberculous — see Tuberculosis, bone
  ulna (lower) (juvenile) — see Osteochondrosis, juvenile, ulna
  van Neck's M91.0
  vertebral — see Osteochondrosis, spine
Osteoclastoma D48.0
  malignant — see Neoplasm, bone, malignant
Osteodynia — see Disorder, bone, specified type NEC
Osteodystrophy Q78.9
  azotemic N25.0
  congenital Q78.9
  parathyroid, secondary E21.1
  renal N25.0
Osteofibroma — see Neoplasm, bone, benign
Osteofibrosarcoma — see Neoplasm, bone, malignant
Osteogenesis imperfecta Q78.0
Osteogenic — see condition
Osteolysis M89.50
  carpus M89.54- ☑
  clavicle M89.51- ☑
  femur M89.55- ☑
  fibula M89.56- ☑
  finger M89.54- ☑
  humerus M89.52- ☑
  ilium M89.559
  ischium M89.559
  joint prosthesis (periprosthetic) — see Complications, joint prosthesis, mechanical, periprosthetic, osteolysis, by site
  metacarpus M89.54- ☑
  metatarsus M89.57- ☑
  multiple sites M89.59
  neck M89.58
  periprosthetic — see Complications, joint prosthesis, mechanical, periprosthetic, osteolysis, by site
  radius M89.53- ☑
  rib M89.58
  scapula M89.51- ☑
  skull M89.58
  tarsus M89.57- ☑
  tibia M89.56- ☑
  toe M89.57- ☑
  ulna M89.53- ☑
  vertebra M89.58
Osteoma — see also Neoplasm, bone, benign
  osteoid — see also Neoplasm, bone, benign
    giant — see Neoplasm, bone, benign
Osteomalacia M83.9
  adult M83.9
    drug-induced NEC M83.5
    due to
      malabsorption (postsurgical) M83.2
      malnutrition M83.3
    specified NEC M83.8
  aluminium-induced M83.4
  infantile — see Rickets
  juvenile — see Rickets
  oncogenic E83.89
  pelvis M83.8
  puerperal M83.0
  senile M83.1
  vitamin-D-resistant in adults E83.31 [M90.8-] ☑
    carpus E83.31 [M90.84-] ☑
    clavicle E83.31 [M90.81-] ☑
    femur E83.31 [M90.85-] ☑

Osteomalacia — continued
  vitamin-D-resistant in adults — continued
    fibula E83.31 [M90.86-] ☑
    finger E83.31 [M90.84-] ☑
    humerus E83.31 [M90.82-] ☑
    ilium E83.31 [M90.859]
    ischium E83.31 [M90.859]
    metacarpus E83.31 [M90.84-] ☑
    metatarsus E83.31 [M90.87-] ☑
    multiple sites E83.31 [M90.89]
    neck E83.31 [M90.88]
    radius E83.31 [M90.83-] ☑
    rib E83.31 [M90.88]
    scapula E83.31 [M90.819]
    skull E83.31 [M90.88]
    tarsus E83.31 [M90.879]
    tibia E83.31 [M90.869]
    toe E83.31 [M90.879]
    ulna E83.31 [M90.839]
    vertebra E83.31 [M90.88]
Osteomyelitis (general) (infective) (localized) (neonatal) (purulent) (septic) (staphylococcal) (streptococcal) (suppurative) (with periostitis) M86.9
  acute M86.10
    carpus M86.14- ☑
    clavicle M86.11- ☑
    femur M86.15- ☑
    fibula M86.16- ☑
    finger M86.14- ☑
    hematogenous M86.00
      carpus M86.04- ☑
      clavicle M86.01- ☑
      femur M86.05- ☑
      fibula M86.06- ☑
      finger M86.04- ☑
      humerus M86.02- ☑
      ilium M86.08
      ischium M86.08
      mandible M27.2
      metacarpus M86.04- ☑
      metatarsus M86.07- ☑
      multiple sites M86.09
      neck M86.08
      orbit H05.02- ☑
      petrous bone — see Petrositis
      radius M86.03- ☑
      rib M86.08
      scapula M86.01- ☑
      skull M86.08
      tarsus M86.07- ☑
      tibia M86.06- ☑
      toe M86.07- ☑
      ulna M86.03- ☑
      vertebra — see Osteomyelitis, vertebra
    humerus M86.12- ☑
    ilium M86.18
    ischium M86.18
    mandible M27.2
    metacarpus M86.14- ☑
    metatarsus M86.17- ☑
    multiple sites M86.19
    neck M86.18
    orbit H05.02- ☑
    petrous bone — see Petrositis
    radius M86.13- ☑
    rib M86.18
    scapula M86.11- ☑
    skull M86.18
    tarsus M86.17- ☑
    tibia M86.16- ☑
    toe M86.17- ☑
    ulna M86.13- ☑
    vertebra — see Osteomyelitis, vertebra
  chronic (or old) M86.60
    with draining sinus M86.40
      carpus M86.44- ☑
      clavicle M86.41- ☑
      femur M86.45- ☑
      fibula M86.46- ☑
      finger M86.44- ☑
      humerus M86.42- ☑
      ilium M86.459
      ischium M86.459
      mandible M27.2
      metacarpus M86.44- ☑
      metatarsus M86.47- ☑

Osteomyelitis — *continued*
  chronic — *continued*
    with draining sinus — *continued*
      multiple sites M86.49
      neck M86.48
      orbit H05.02- ☑
      petrous bone — *see* Petrositis
      radius M86.43- ☑
      rib M86.48
      scapula M86.41- ☑
      skull M86.48
      tarsus M86.47- ☑
      tibia M86.46- ☑
      toe M86.47- ☑
      ulna M86.43- ☑
      vertebra — *see* Osteomyelitis, vertebra
    carpus M86.64- ☑
    clavicle M86.61- ☑
    femur M86.65- ☑
    fibula M86.66- ☑
    finger M86.64- ☑
    hematogenous NEC M86.50
      carpus M86.54- ☑
      clavicle M86.51- ☑
      femur M86.55- ☑
      fibula M86.56- ☑
      finger M86.54- ☑
      humerus M86.52- ☑
      ilium M86.559
      ischium M86.559
      mandible M27.2
      metacarpus M86.54- ☑
      metatarsus M86.57- ☑
      multifocal M86.30
        carpus M86.34- ☑
        clavicle M86.31- ☑
        femur M86.35- ☑
        fibula M86.36- ☑
        finger M86.34- ☑
        humerus M86.32- ☑
        ilium M86.359
        ischium M86.359
        metacarpus M86.34- ☑
        metatarsus M86.37- ☑
        multiple sites M86.39
        neck M86.38
        radius M86.33- ☑
        rib M86.38
        scapula M86.31- ☑
        skull M86.38
        tarsus M86.37- ☑
        tibia M86.36- ☑
        toe M86.37- ☑
        ulna M86.33- ☑
        vertebra — *see* Osteomyelitis, vertebra
      multiple sites M86.59
      neck M86.58
      orbit H05.02- ☑
      petrous bone — *see* Petrositis
      radius M86.53- ☑
      rib M86.58
      scapula M86.51- ☑
      skull M86.58
      tarsus M86.57- ☑
      tibia M86.56- ☑
      toe M86.57- ☑
      ulna M86.53- ☑
      vertebra — *see* Osteomyelitis, vertebra
    humerus M86.62- ☑
    ilium M86.659
    ischium M86.659
    mandible M27.2
    metacarpus M86.64- ☑
    metatarsus M86.67- ☑
    multifocal — *see* Osteomyelitis, chronic,
      hematogenous, multifocal
    multiple sites M86.69
    neck M86.68
    orbit H05.02- ☑
    petrous bone — *see* Petrositis
    radius M86.63- ☑
    rib M86.68
    scapula M86.61- ☑
    skull M86.68
    tarsus M86.67- ☑
    tibia M86.66- ☑
    toe M86.67- ☑

Osteomyelitis — *continued*
  chronic — *continued*
    ulna M86.63- ☑
    vertebra — *see* Osteomyelitis, vertebra
  echinococcal B67.2
  Garr's — *see* Osteomyelitis, specified type NEC
  in diabetes mellitus — *see* E08-E13 with .69
  jaw (acute) (chronic) (lower) (neonatal) (suppurative)
    (upper) M27.2
  nonsuppurating — *see* Osteomyelitis, specified type
    NEC
  orbit H05.02- ☑
  petrous bone — *see* Petrositis
  Salmonella (arizonae) (cholerae-suis) (enteritidis) (ty-
    phimurium) A02.24
  sclerosing, nonsuppurative — *see* Osteomyelitis,
    specified type NEC
  specified type NEC — *see also* subcategory M86.8X- ☑
    mandible M27.2
    orbit H05.02- ☑
    petrous bone — *see* Petrositis
    vertebra — *see* Osteomyelitis, vertebra
  subacute M86.20
    carpus M86.24- ☑
    clavicle M86.21- ☑
    femur M86.25- ☑
    fibula M86.26- ☑
    finger M86.24- ☑
    humerus M86.22- ☑
    mandible M27.2
    metacarpus M86.24- ☑
    metatarsus M86.27- ☑
    multiple sites M86.29
    neck M86.28
    orbit H05.02- ☑
    petrous bone — *see* Petrositis
    radius M86.23- ☑
    rib M86.28
    scapula M86.21- ☑
    skull M86.28
    tarsus M86.27- ☑
    tibia M86.26- ☑
    toe M86.27- ☑
    ulna M86.23- ☑
    vertebra — *see* Osteomyelitis, vertebra
  syphilitic A52.77
    congenital (early) A50.02 [M90.80]
  tuberculous — *see* Tuberculosis, bone
  typhoid A01.05
  vertebra M46.20
    cervical region M46.22
    cervicothoracic region M46.23
    lumbar region M46.26
    lumbosacral region M46.27
    occipito-atlanto-axial region M46.21
    sacrococcygeal region M46.28
    thoracic region M46.24
    thoracolumbar region M46.25
Osteomyelofibrosis D47.4
Osteomyelosclerosis D75.89
Osteonecrosis M87.9
  due to
    drugs — *see* Osteonecrosis, secondary, due to, drugs
    trauma — *see* Osteonecrosis, secondary, due to,
      trauma
  idiopathic aseptic M87.00
    ankle M87.07- ☑
    carpus M87.03- ☑
    clavicle M87.01- ☑
    femur M87.05- ☑
    fibula M87.06- ☑
    finger M87.04- ☑
    humerus M87.02- ☑
    ilium M87.050
    ischium M87.050
    metacarpus M87.04- ☑
    metatarsus M87.07- ☑
    multiple sites M87.09
    neck M87.08
    pelvis M87.050
    radius M87.03- ☑
    rib M87.08
    scapula M87.01- ☑
    skull M87.08
    tarsus M87.07- ☑
    tibia M87.06- ☑
    toe M87.07- ☑

Osteonecrosis — *continued*
  idiopathic aseptic — *continued*
    ulna M87.03- ☑
    vertebra M87.08
  secondary NEC M87.30
    carpus M87.33- ☑
    clavicle M87.31- ☑
    due to
      drugs M87.10
        carpus M87.13- ☑
        clavicle M87.11- ☑
        femur M87.15- ☑
        fibula M87.16- ☑
        finger M87.14- ☑
        humerus M87.12- ☑
        ilium M87.159
        ischium M87.159
        jaw M87.180
        metacarpus M87.14- ☑
        metatarsus M87.17- ☑
        multiple sites M87.19
        neck M87.18
        radius M87.13- ☑
        rib M87.18
        scapula M87.11- ☑
        skull M87.18
        tarsus M87.17- ☑
        tibia M87.16- ☑
        toe M87.17- ☑
        ulna M87.13- ☑
        vertebra M87.18
      hemoglobinopathy NEC D58.2 [M90.50]
        carpus D58.2 [M90.54-] ☑
        clavicle D58.2 [M90.51-] ☑
        femur D58.2 [M90.55-] ☑
        fibula D58.2 [M90.56-] ☑
        finger D58.2 [M90.54-] ☑
        humerus D58.2 [M90.52-] ☑
        ilium D58.2 [M90.55-] ☑
        ischium D58.2 [M90.55-] ☑
        metacarpus D58.2 [M90.54-] ☑
        metatarsus D58.2 [M90.57-] ☑
        multiple sites D58.2 [M90.58]
        neck D58.2 [M90.58]
        radius D58.2 [M90.53-] ☑
        rib D58.2 [M90.58]
        scapula D58.2 [M90.51-] ☑
        skull D58.2 [M90.58]
        tarsus D58.2 [M90.57-] ☑
        tibia D58.2 [M90.56-] ☑
        toe D58.2 [M90.57-] ☑
        ulna D58.2 [M90.53-] ☑
        vertebra D58.2 [M90.58]
      trauma (previous) M87.20
        carpus M87.23- ☑
        clavicle M87.21- ☑
        femur M87.25- ☑
        fibula M87.26- ☑
        finger M87.24- ☑
        humerus M87.22- ☑
        ilium M87.25- ☑
        ischium M87.25- ☑
        metacarpus M87.24- ☑
        metatarsus M87.27- ☑
        multiple sites M87.29
        neck M87.28
        radius M87.23- ☑
        rib M87.28
        scapula M87.21- ☑
        skull M87.28
        tarsus M87.27- ☑
        tibia M87.26- ☑
        toe M87.27- ☑
        ulna M87.23- ☑
        vertebra M87.28
    femur M87.35- ☑
    fibula M87.36- ☑
    finger M87.34- ☑
    humerus M87.32- ☑
    ilium M87.350
    in
      caisson disease T70.3 ☑ [M90.50]
        carpus T70.3 ☑ [M90.54-]
        clavicle T70.3 ☑ [M90.51-]
        femur T70.3 ☑ [M90.55-] ☑
        fibula T70.3 ☑ [M90.56-]

Osteonecrosis — continued
  secondary — continued
    in — continued
      caisson disease — continued
        finger T70.3 ✓ [M90.54-] ✓
        humerus T70.3 ✓ [M90.52-] ✓
        ilium T70.3 ✓ [M90.55-] ✓
        ischium T70.3 ✓ [M90.55-] ✓
        metacarpus T70.3 ✓ [M90.54-] ✓
        metatarsus T70.3 ✓ [M90.57-] ✓
        multiple sites T70.3 ✓ [M90.59]
        neck T70.3 ✓ [M90.58]
        radius T70.3 ✓ [M90.53-] ✓
        rib T70.3 ✓ [M90.58]
        scapula T70.3 ✓ [M90.51-] ✓
        skull T70.3 ✓ [M90.58]
        tarsus T70.3 ✓ [M90.57-] ✓
        tibia T70.3 ✓ [M90.56-] ✓
        toe T70.3 ✓ [M90.57-] ✓
        ulna T70.3 ✓ [M90.53-] ✓
        vertebra T70.3 ✓ [M90.58]
    ischium M87.350
    metacarpus M87.34- ✓
    metatarsus M87.37- ✓
    multiple site M87.39
    neck M87.38
    radius M87.33- ✓
    rib M87.38
    scapula M87.319
    skull M87.38
    tarsus M87.379
    tibia M87.366
    toe M87.379
    ulna M87.33- ✓
    vertebra M87.38
  specified type NEC M87.80
    carpus M87.83- ✓
    clavicle M87.81- ✓
    femur M87.85- ✓
    fibula M87.86- ✓
    finger M87.84- ✓
    humerus M87.82- ✓
    ilium M87.85- ✓
    ischium M87.85- ✓
    metacarpus M87.84- ✓
    metatarsus M87.87- ✓
    multiple sites M87.89
    neck M87.88
    radius M87.83- ✓
    rib M87.88
    scapula M87.81- ✓
    skull M87.88
    tarsus M87.87- ✓
    tibia M87.86- ✓
    toe M87.87- ✓
    ulna M87.83- ✓
    vertebra M87.88
Osteo-onycho-arthro-dysplasia Q87.2
Osteo-onychodysplasia, hereditary Q87.2
Osteopathia condensans disseminata Q78.8
Osteopathy — see also Osteomyelitis, Osteonecrosis,
    Osteoporosis
  after poliomyelitis M89.60
    carpus M89.64- ✓
    clavicle M89.61- ✓
    femur M89.65- ✓
    fibula M89.66- ✓
    finger M89.64- ✓
    humerus M89.62- ✓
    ilium M89.659
    ischium M89.659
    metacarpus M89.64- ✓
    metatarsus M89.67- ✓
    multiple sites M89.69
    neck M89.68
    radius M89.63- ✓
    rib M89.68
    scapula M89.61- ✓
    skull M89.68
    tarsus M89.67- ✓
    tibia M89.66- ✓
    toe M89.67- ✓
    ulna M89.63- ✓
    vertebra M89.68
  in (due to)
    renal osteodystrophy N25.0

Osteopathy — continued
  in — continued
    specified diseases classified elsewhere — see sub-
        category M90.8 ✓
Osteopenia M85.8- ✓
  borderline M85.8- ✓
Osteoperiostitis — see Osteomyelitis, specified type
    NEC
Osteopetrosis (familial) Q78.2
Osteophyte M25.70
  ankle M25.77- ✓
  elbow M25.72- ✓
  foot joint M25.77- ✓
  hand joint M25.74- ✓
  hip M25.75- ✓
  knee M25.76- ✓
  shoulder M25.71- ✓
  spine M25.78
  vertebrae M25.78
  wrist M25.73- ✓
Osteopoikilosis Q78.8
Osteoporosis (female) (male) M81.0
  with current pathological fracture M80.00 ✓
  age-related M81.0
    with current pathologic fracture M80.00 ✓
      carpus M80.04- ✓
      clavicle M80.01- ✓
      fibula M80.06- ✓
      finger M80.04- ✓
      humerus M80.02- ✓
      ilium M80.05- ✓
      ischium M80.05- ✓
      metacarpus M80.04- ✓
      metatarsus M80.07- ✓
      pelvis M80.05- ✓
      radius M80.03- ✓
      rib(s) — see Osteoporosis, specified site NEC
      scapula M80.01- ✓
      site specified NEC M80.0A ✓
      specified site NEC M80.0A ✓
      tarsus M80.07- ✓
      tibia M80.06- ✓
      toe M80.07- ✓
      ulna M80.03- ✓
      vertebra M80.08 ✓
  disuse M81.8
    with current pathological fracture M80.80 ✓
      carpus M80.84- ✓
      clavicle M80.81- ✓
      fibula M80.86- ✓
      finger M80.84- ✓
      humerus M80.82- ✓
      ilium M80.85- ✓
      ischium M80.85- ✓
      metacarpus M80.84- ✓
      metatarsus M80.87- ✓
      pelvis M80.85- ✓
      radius M80.83- ✓
      scapula M80.81- ✓
      site specified NEC M80.8A ✓
      tarsus M80.87- ✓
      tibia M80.86- ✓
      toe M80.87- ✓
      ulna M80.83- ✓
      vertebra M80.88 ✓
  drug-induced — see Osteoporosis, specified type NEC
  idiopathic — see Osteoporosis, specified type NEC
  involutional — see Osteoporosis, age-related
  Lequesne M81.6
  localized M81.6
  postmenopausal M81.0
    with pathological fracture M80.00 ✓
      carpus M80.04- ✓
      clavicle M80.01- ✓
      fibula M80.06- ✓
      finger M80.04- ✓
      humerus M80.02- ✓
      ilium M80.05- ✓
      ischium M80.05- ✓
      metacarpus M80.04- ✓
      metatarsus M80.07- ✓
      pelvis M80.05- ✓
      radius M80.03- ✓
      scapula M80.01- ✓
      site specified NEC M80.0A ✓
      tarsus M80.07- ✓

Osteoporosis — continued
  postmenopausal — continued
    with pathological fracture — continued
      tibia M80.06- ✓
      toe M80.07- ✓
      ulna M80.03- ✓
      vertebra M80.08 ✓
  postoophorectomy — see Osteoporosis, specified type
    NEC
  postsurgical malabsorption — see Osteoporosis,
    specified type NEC
  post-traumatic — see Osteoporosis, specified type NEC
  senile — see Osteoporosis, age-related
  specified type NEC M81.8
    with pathological fracture M80.80 ✓
      carpus M80.84- ✓
      clavicle M80.81- ✓
      fibula M80.86- ✓
      finger M80.84- ✓
      humerus M80.82- ✓
      ilium M80.85- ✓
      ischium M80.85- ✓
      metacarpus M80.84- ✓
      metatarsus M80.87- ✓
      pelvis M80.85- ✓
      radius M80.83- ✓
      scapula M80.81- ✓
      site specified NEC M80.8A ✓
      tarsus M80.87- ✓
      tibia M80.86- ✓
      toe M80.87- ✓
      ulna M80.83- ✓
      vertebra M80.88 ✓
Osteopsathyrosis (idiopathica) Q78.0
Osteoradionecrosis, jaw (acute) (chronic) (lower) (sup-
    purative) (upper) M27.2
Osteosarcoma (any form) — see Neoplasm, bone, malig-
    nant
Osteosclerosis Q78.2
  acquired M85.8- ✓
  congenita Q77.4
  fragilitas (generalisata) Q78.2
  myelofibrosis D75.81
Osteosclerotic anemia D64.89
Osteosis
  cutis L94.2
  renal fibrocystic N25.0
Österreicher-Turner syndrome Q87.2
Ostium
  atrioventriculare commune Q21.23
  primum (arteriosum) (defect) (persistent) Q21.20
  secundum (arteriosum) (defect) (patent) (persistent)
    Q21.11
Ostrum-Furst syndrome Q75.8
Otalgia H92.0
Otitis (acute) H66.90
  with effusion — see also Otitis, media, nonsuppurative
    purulent — see Otitis, media, suppurative
  adhesive — see subcategory H74.1 ✓
  chronic — see also Otitis, media, chronic
    with effusion — see also Otitis, media, nonsuppura-
      tive, chronic
  externa H60.9- ✓
    abscess — see Abscess, ear, external
    acute (noninfective) H60.50- ✓
      actinic H60.51- ✓
      chemical H60.52- ✓
      contact H60.53- ✓
      eczematoid H60.54- ✓
      infective — see Otitis, externa, infective
      reactive H60.55- ✓
      specified NEC H60.59- ✓
    cellulitis — see Cellulitis, ear
    chronic H60.6- ✓
    diffuse — see Otitis, externa, infective, diffuse
    hemorrhagic — see Otitis, externa, infective, hem-
      orrhagic
    in (due to)
      aspergillosis B44.89
      candidiasis B37.84
      erysipelas A46 [H62.40]
      herpes (simplex) virus infection B00.1
        zoster B02.8
      impetigo L01.00 [H62.40]
      infectious disease NEC B99 ✓ [H62.4-] ✓
      mycosis NEC B36.9 [H62.40]

Otitis — *continued*
externa — *continued*
in — *continued*
parasitic disease NEC B89 *[H62.40]*
viral disease NEC B34.9 *[H62.40]*
zoster B02.8
infective NEC H60.39- ☑
abscess — *see* Abscess, ear, external
cellulitis — *see* Cellulitis, ear
diffuse H60.31- ☑
hemorrhagic H60.32- ☑
swimmer's ear — *see* Swimmer's, ear
malignant H60.2- ☑
mycotic NEC B36.9 *[H62.40]*
in
aspergillosis B44.89
candidiasis B37.84
moniliasis B37.84
necrotizing — *see* Otitis, externa, malignant
Pseudomonas aeruginosa — *see* Otitis, externa, malignant
reactive — *see* Otitis, externa, acute, reactive
specified NEC — *see* subcategory H60.8 ☑
tropical NEC B36.9 *[H62.40]*
in
aspergillosis B44.89
candidiasis B37.84
moniliasis B37.84
insidiosa — *see* Otosclerosis
interna H83.0 ☑
media (hemorrhagic) (staphylococcal) (streptococcal) H66.9- ☑
with effusion (nonpurulent) — *see* Otitis, media, nonsuppurative
acute, subacute H66.90
allergic — *see* Otitis, media, nonsuppurative, acute, allergic
exudative — *see* Otitis, media, suppurative, acute
mucoid — *see* Otitis, media, nonsuppurative, acute
necrotizing — *see also* Otitis, media, suppurative, acute
in
measles B05.3
scarlet fever A38.0
nonsuppurative NEC — *see* Otitis, media, nonsuppurative, acute
purulent — *see* Otitis, media, suppurative, acute
sanguinous — *see* Otitis, media, nonsuppurative, acute
secretory — *see* Otitis, media, nonsuppurative, acute, serous
seromucinous — *see* Otitis, media, nonsuppurative, acute
serous — *see* Otitis, media, nonsuppurative, acute, serous
suppurative — *see* Otitis, media, suppurative, acute
allergic — *see* Otitis, media, nonsuppurative
catarrhal — *see* Otitis, media, nonsuppurative
chronic H66.90
with effusion (nonpurulent) — *see* Otitis, media, nonsuppurative, chronic
allergic — *see* Otitis, media, nonsuppurative, chronic, allergic
benign suppurative — *see* Otitis, media, suppurative, chronic, tubotympanic
catarrhal — *see* Otitis, media, nonsuppurative, chronic, serous
exudative — *see* Otitis, media, nonsuppurative, chronic
mucinous — *see* Otitis, media, nonsuppurative, chronic, mucoid
mucoid — *see* Otitis, media, nonsuppurative, chronic, mucoid
nonsuppurative NEC — *see* Otitis, media, nonsuppurative, chronic
purulent — *see* Otitis, media, suppurative, chronic
secretory — *see* Otitis, media, nonsuppurative, chronic, mucoid
seromucinous — *see* Otitis, media, nonsuppurative, chronic
serous — *see* Otitis, media, nonsuppurative, chronic, serous
suppurative — *see* Otitis, media, suppurative, chronic

Otitis — *continued*
media — *continued*
chronic — *continued*
transudative — *see* Otitis, media, nonsuppurative, chronic, mucoid
exudative — *see* Otitis, media, suppurative
in (due to) (with)
influenza — *see* Influenza, with, otitis media
measles B05.3
scarlet fever A38.0
tuberculosis A18.6
viral disease NEC B34.- ☑ *[H67.-]*
mucoid — *see* Otitis, media, nonsuppurative
nonsuppurative H65.9- ☑
acute or subacute NEC H65.19- ☑
allergic H65.11- ☑
recurrent H65.11- ☑
recurrent H65.19- ☑
secretory — *see* Otitis, media, nonsuppurative, serous
serous H65.0- ☑
recurrent H65.0- ☑
chronic H65.49- ☑
allergic H65.41- ☑
mucoid H65.3- ☑
serous H65.2- ☑
postmeasles B05.3
purulent — *see* Otitis, media, suppurative
secretory — *see* Otitis, media, nonsuppurative
seromucinous — *see* Otitis, media, nonsuppurative
serous — *see* Otitis, media, nonsuppurative
suppurative H66.4- ☑
acute H66.00- ☑
with rupture of ear drum H66.01- ☑
recurrent H66.00- ☑
with rupture of ear drum H66.01- ☑
chronic — *see also* subcategory H66.3 ☑
atticoantral H66.2- ☑
benign — *see* Otitis, media, suppurative, chronic, tubotympanic
tubotympanic H66.1- ☑
transudative — *see* Otitis, media, nonsuppurative
tuberculous A18.6
Otocephaly Q18.2
Otolith syndrome — *see* subcategory H81.8 ☑
Otomycosis (diffuse) **NEC** B36.9 *[H62.40]*
in
aspergillosis B44.89
candidiasis B37.84
moniliasis B37.84
Otoporosis — *see* Otosclerosis
Otorrhagia (nontraumatic) H92.2- ☑
traumatic — *code by* Type of injury
Otorrhea H92.1- ☑
cerebrospinal (fluid) G96.01
postoperative G96.08
specified NEC G96.08
spontaneous G96.01
traumatic G96.08
Otosclerosis (general) H80.9- ☑
cochlear (endosteal) H80.2- ☑
involving
otic capsule — *see* Otosclerosis, cochlear
oval window
nonobliterative H80.0- ☑
obliterative H80.1- ☑
round window — *see* Otosclerosis, cochlear
nonobliterative — *see* Otosclerosis, involving, oval window, nonobliterative
obliterative — *see* Otosclerosis, involving, oval window, obliterative
specified NEC H80.8- ☑
Otospongiosis — *see* Otosclerosis
Otto's disease or pelvis M24.7
Outcome of delivery Z37.9
multiple births Z37.9
all liveborn Z37.50
quadruplets Z37.52
quintuplets Z37.53
sextuplets Z37.54
specified number NEC Z37.59
triplets Z37.51
all stillborn Z37.7
some liveborn Z37.60
quadruplets Z37.62
quintuplets Z37.63
sextuplets Z37.64

Outcome of delivery — *continued*
multiple births — *continued*
some liveborn — *continued*
specified number NEC Z37.69
triplets Z37.61
single NEC Z37.9
liveborn Z37.0
stillborn Z37.1
twins NEC Z37.9
both liveborn Z37.2
both stillborn Z37.4
one liveborn, one stillborn Z37.3
Outlet — *see* condition
Ovalocytosis (congenital) (hereditary) — *see* Elliptocytosis
Ovarian — *see* Condition
Ovariocele N83.4- ☑
Ovaritis (cystic) — *see* Oophoritis
Ovary, ovarian — *see also* condition
resistant syndrome E28.39
vein syndrome N13.8
Overactive — *see also* Hyperfunction
adrenal cortex NEC E27.0
bladder N32.81
hypothalamus E23.3
thyroid — *see* Hyperthyroidism
Overactivity R46.3
child — *see* Disorder, attention-deficit hyperactivity
Overbite (deep) (excessive) (horizontal) (vertical) M26.29
Overbreathing — *see* Hyperventilation
Overconscientious personality F60.5
Overdevelopment — *see* Hypertrophy
Overdistension — *see* Distension
Overdose, overdosage (drug) — *see* Table of Drugs and Chemicals, by drug, poisoning
Overeating R63.2
nonorganic origin F50.89
psychogenic F50.89
Overexertion (effects) (exhaustion) T73.3 ☑
Overexposure (effects) T73.9 ☑
exhaustion T73.2 ☑
Overfeeding — *see* Overeating
newborn P92.4
Overfill, endodontic M27.52
Overgrowth, bone — *see* Hypertrophy, bone
Overhanging of dental restorative material (unrepairable) K08.52
Overheated (places) (effects) — *see* Heat
Overjet (excessive horizontal) M26.23
Overlaid, overlying (suffocation) — *see* Asphyxia, traumatic, due to mechanical threat
Overlap, excessive horizontal (teeth) M26.23
Overlapping toe (acquired) — *see also* Deformity, toe, specified NEC
congenital (fifth toe) Q66.89
Overload
circulatory, due to transfusion (blood) (blood components) (TACO) E87.71
fluid E87.70
due to transfusion (blood) (blood components) E87.71
specified NEC E87.79
iron, due to repeated red blood cell transfusions E83.111
potassium (K) E87.5
sodium (Na) E87.0
Overnutrition — *see* Hyperalimentation
Overproduction — *see also* Hypersecretion
ACTH E27.0
catecholamine E27.5
growth hormone E22.0
Overprotection, child by parent Z62.1
Overriding
aorta Q25.49
finger (acquired) — *see* Deformity, finger
congenital Q68.1
toe (acquired) — *see also* Deformity, toe, specified NEC
congenital Q66.89
Overstrained R53.83
heart — *see* Hypertrophy, cardiac
Overuse, muscle NEC M70.8- ☑
Overweight E66.3
Overworked R53.83
Oviduct — *see* condition
Ovotestis Q56.0
Ovulation (cycle)
failure or lack of N97.0

☑ **Additional Character Required** — Refer to the Tabular List for Character Selection

Ovulation — *continued*
  pain N94.0
Ovum — *see* condition
Owren's disease or syndrome (parahemophilia) D68.2
Ox heart — *see* Hypertrophy, cardiac
Oxalosis E72.53
Oxaluria E72.53
Oxycephaly, oxycephalic Q75.0
  syphilitic, congenital A50.02
Oxyuriasis B80
Oxyuris vermicularis (infestation) B80
Ozena J31.0

P

Pachyderma, pachydermia L85.9
  larynx (verrucosa) J38.7
Pachydermatocele (congenital) Q82.8
Pachydermoperiostosis — *see also* Osteoarthropathy, hypertrophic, specified type NEC
  clubbed nail M89.40 *[L62]*
Pachygyria Q04.3
Pachymeningitis (adhesive) (basal) (brain) (cervical) (chronic) (circumscribed) (external) (fibrous) (hemorrhagic) (hypertrophic) (internal) (purulent) (spinal) (suppurative) — *see* Meningitis
Pachyonychia (congenital) Q84.5
Pacinian tumor — *see* Neoplasm, skin, benign
Pad, knuckle or Garrod's M72.1
Paget's disease
  with infiltrating duct carcinoma — *see* Neoplasm, breast, malignant
  bone M88.9
    carpus M88.84- ☑
    clavicle M88.81- ☑
    femur M88.85- ☑
    fibula M88.86- ☑
    finger M88.84- ☑
    humerus M88.82- ☑
    ilium M88.85- ☑
    in neoplastic disease — *see* Osteitis, deformans, in neoplastic disease
    ischium M88.85- ☑
    metacarpus M88.84- ☑
    metatarsus M88.87- ☑
    multiple sites M88.89
    neck M88.88
    radius M88.83- ☑
    rib M88.88
    scapula M88.81- ☑
    skull M88.0
    specified NEC M88.88
    tarsus M88.87- ☑
    tibia M88.86- ☑
    toe M88.87- ☑
    ulna M88.83- ☑
    vertebra M88.1
  breast (female) C50.01- ☑
    male C50.02- ☑
  extramammary — *see also* Neoplasm, skin, malignant
    anus C21.0
      margin C44.590
      skin C44.590
  intraductal carcinoma — *see* Neoplasm, breast, malignant
  malignant — *see* Neoplasm, skin, malignant
    breast (female) C50.01- ☑
      male C50.02- ☑
    unspecified site (female) C50.01- ☑
      male C50.02- ☑
  mammary — *see* Paget's disease, breast
  nipple — *see* Paget's disease, breast
  osteitis deformans — *see* Paget's disease, bone
Paget-Schroetter syndrome I82.890
Pain(s) — *see also* Painful R52
  abdominal R10.9
    colic R10.83
    generalized R10.84
      with acute abdomen R10.0
    lower R10.30
      left quadrant R10.32
      pelvic or perineal R10.2
      periumbilical R10.33
      right quadrant R10.31
    rebound — *see* Tenderness, abdominal, rebound
    severe with abdominal rigidity R10.0
    tenderness — *see* Tenderness, abdominal

Pain(s) — *continued*
  abdominal — *continued*
    upper R10.10
      epigastric R10.13
      left quadrant R10.12
      right quadrant R10.11
  acute R52
    due to trauma G89.11
    neoplasm related G89.3
    postprocedural NEC G89.18
    post-thoracotomy G89.12
    specified by site — *code to* Pain, by site
  adnexa (uteri) R10.2
  anginoid — *see* Pain, precordial
  anus K62.89
  arm — *see* Pain, limb, upper
  axillary (axilla) M79.62- ☑
  back (postural) M54.9
  bladder R39.89
    associated with micturition — *see* Micturition, painful
    chronic R39.82
  bone — *see* Disorder, bone, specified type NEC
  breast N64.4
  broad ligament R10.2
  cancer associated (acute) (chronic) G89.3
  cecum — *see* Pain, abdominal
  cervicobrachial M53.1
  chest (central) R07.9
    anterior wall R07.89
    atypical R07.89
    ischemic I20.9
    musculoskeletal R07.89
    non-cardiac R07.89
    on breathing R07.1
    pleurodynia R07.81
    precordial R07.2
    wall (anterior) R07.89
  chronic G89.29
    associated with significant psychosocial dysfunction G89.4
    due to trauma G89.21
    neoplasm related G89.3
    postoperative NEC G89.28
    postprocedural NEC G89.28
    post-thoracotomy G89.22
    specified NEC G89.29
  coccyx M53.3
  colon — *see* Pain, abdominal
  coronary — *see* Angina
  costochondral R07.1
  diaphragm R07.1
  due to cancer G89.3
  due to device, implant or graft — *see also* Complications, by site and type, specified NEC T85.848 ☑
    arterial graft NEC T82.848 ☑
    breast (implant) T85.848 ☑
    catheter NEC T85.848 ☑
      dialysis (renal) T82.848 ☑
        intraperitoneal T85.848 ☑
      infusion NEC T82.848 ☑
        spinal (epidural) (subdural) T85.840 ☑
      urinary (indwelling) T83.84 ☑
    electronic (electrode) (pulse generator) (stimulator)
      bone T85.840 ☑
      cardiac T82.847 ☑
      nervous system (brain) (peripheral nerve) (spinal) T85.84 ☑
      urinary T83.84 ☑
    fixation, internal (orthopedic) NEC T84.84 ☑
    gastrointestinal (bile duct) (esophagus) T85.848 ☑
    genital NEC T83.84 ☑
    heart NEC T82.847 ☑
      infusion NEC T85.848 ☑
    joint prosthesis T84.84 ☑
    ocular (corneal graft) (orbital implant) NEC T85.848 ☑
    orthopedic NEC T84.84 ☑
    specified NEC T85.848 ☑
    urinary NEC T83.84 ☑
    vascular NEC T82.848 ☑
    ventricular intracranial shunt T85.840 ☑
  due to malignancy (primary) (secondary) G89.3
  ear — *see* subcategory H92.0 ☑
  epigastric, epigastrium R10.13
  eye — *see* Pain, ocular
  face, facial R51.9

Pain(s) — *continued*
  face, facial — *continued*
    atypical G50.1
  female genital organs NEC N94.89
  finger — *see* Pain, limb, upper
  flank — *see* Pain, abdominal
  foot — *see* Pain, limb, lower
  gallbladder K82.9
  gas (intestinal) R14.1
  gastric — *see* Pain, abdominal
  generalized NOS R52
  genital organ
    female N94.89
    male N50.89
  groin — *see* Pain, abdominal, lower
  hand — *see* Pain, limb, upper
  head — *see* Headache
  heart — *see* Pain, precordial
  infra-orbital — *see* Neuralgia, trigeminal
  intercostal R07.82
  intermenstrual N94.0
  jaw R68.84
  joint M25.50
    ankle M25.57- ☑
    elbow M25.52- ☑
    finger M25.54- ☑
    foot M25.57- ☑
    hand M25.54- ☑
    hip M25.55- ☑
    knee M25.56- ☑
    shoulder M25.51- ☑
    specified site NEC M25.59
    toe M25.57- ☑
    wrist M25.53- ☑
  kidney N23
  laryngeal R07.0
  leg — *see* Pain, limb, lower
  limb M79.609
    lower M79.60- ☑
      foot M79.67- ☑
      lower leg M79.66- ☑
      thigh M79.65- ☑
      toe M79.67- ☑
    upper M79.60- ☑
      axilla M79.62- ☑
      finger M79.64- ☑
      forearm M79.63- ☑
      hand M79.64- ☑
      upper arm M79.62- ☑
  loin M54.50
  low back M54.50
    specified NEC M54.59
    vertebral end plate M54.51
    vertebrogenic M54.51
  lumbar region M54.50
    vertebral end plate M54.51
    vertebrogenic M54.51
  mandibular R68.84
  mastoid — *see* subcategory H92.0 ☑
  maxilla R68.84
  menstrual — *see also* Dysmenorrhea N94.6
  metacarpophalangeal (joint) — *see* Pain, joint, hand
  metatarsophalangeal (joint) — *see* Pain, joint, foot
  mouth K13.79
  muscle — *see* Myalgia
  musculoskeletal — *see also* Pain, by site M79.18
  myofascial M79.18
  nasal J34.89
  nasopharynx J39.2
  neck NEC M54.2
  nerve NEC — *see* Neuralgia
  neuromuscular — *see* Neuralgia
  nose J34.89
  ocular H57.1- ☑
  ophthalmic — *see* Pain, ocular
  orbital region — *see* Pain, ocular
  ovary N94.89
  over heart — *see* Pain, precordial
  ovulation N94.0
  pelvic (female) R10.2
  penis N48.89
  pericardial — *see* Pain, precordial
  perineal, perineum R10.2
  pharynx J39.2
  pleura, pleural, pleuritic R07.81
  postoperative NOS G89.18
  postprocedural NOS G89.18

☑ **Additional Character Required** — **Refer to the Tabular List for Character Selection**

Pain(s) — *continued*
  post-thoracotomy G89.12
  precordial (region) R07.2
  premenstrual N94.3
  psychogenic (persistent) (any site) F45.41
  radicular (spinal) — *see* Radiculopathy
  rectum K62.89
  respiration R07.1
  retrosternal R07.2
  rheumatoid, muscular — *see* Myalgia
  rib R07.81
  root (spinal) — *see* Radiculopathy
  round ligament (stretch) R10.2
  sacroiliac M53.3
  sciatic — *see* Sciatica
  scrotum N50.82
  seminal vesicle N50.89
  shoulder M25.51- ☑
  spermatic cord N50.89
  spinal root — *see* Radiculopathy
  spine M54.9
    cervical M54.2
    low back M54.50
      with sciatica M54.4- ☑
    thoracic M54.6
  stomach — *see* Pain, abdominal
  substernal R07.2
  temporomandibular (joint) M26.62- ☑
  testis N50.81- ☑
  thoracic spine M54.6
    with radicular and visceral pain M54.14
  throat R07.0
  tibia — *see* Pain, limb, lower
  toe — *see* Pain, limb, lower
  tongue K14.6
  tooth K08.89
  trigeminal — *see* Neuralgia, trigeminal
  tumor associated G89.3
  ureter N23
  urinary (organ) (system) N23
  uterus NEC N94.89
  vagina R10.2
  vertebral end plate — *see* Pain, vertebrogenic
  vertebrogenic M54.89
    low back M54.51
    lumbar M54.51
    syndrome M54.89
  vesical R39.89
    associated with micturition — *see* Micturition,
      painful
  vulva R10.2
Painful — *see also* Pain
  coitus
    female N94.10
    male N53.12
    psychogenic F52.6
  ejaculation (semen) N53.12
    psychogenic F52.6
  erection — *see* Priapism
  feet syndrome E53.8
  joint replacement (hip) (knee) T84.84 ☑
  menstruation — *see* Dysmenorrhea
    psychogenic F45.8
  micturition — *see* Micturition, painful
  respiration R07.1
  scar NEC L90.5
  wire sutures T81.89 ☑
Painter's colic — *see* subcategory T56.0 ☑
Palate — *see* condition
Palatoplegia K13.79
Palatoschisis — *see* Cleft, palate
Palilalia R48.8
Palliative care Z51.5
Pallor R23.1
  optic disc, temporal — *see* Atrophy, optic
Palmar — *see also* condition
  fascia — *see* condition
Palpable
  cecum K63.89
  kidney N28.89
  ovary N83.8
  prostate N42.9
  spleen — *see* Splenomegaly
Palpitations (heart) R00.2
  psychogenic F45.8
Palsy — *see also* Paralysis G83.9
  atrophic diffuse (progressive) G12.22
  Bell's — *see also* Palsy, facial

Palsy — *continued*
  Bell's — *see also* Palsy, facial — *continued*
    newborn P11.3
  brachial plexus NEC G54.0
    newborn (birth injury) P14.3
  brain — *see* Palsy, cerebral
  bulbar (progressive) (chronic) G12.22
    of childhood (Fazio-Londe) G12.1
    pseudo NEC G12.29
    supranuclear (progressive) G23.1
  cerebral (congenital) G80.9
    ataxic G80.4
    athetoid G80.3
    choreathetoid G80.3
    diplegic G80.8
      spastic G80.1
    dyskinetic G80.3
      athetoid G80.3
      choreathetoid G80.3
      distonic G80.3
    dystonic G80.3
    hemiplegic G80.8
      spastic G80.2
    mixed G80.8
    monoplegic G80.8
      spastic G80.1
    paraplegic G80.8
      spastic G80.1
    quadriplegic G80.8
      spastic G80.0
    spastic G80.1
      diplegic G80.1
      hemiplegic G80.2
      monoplegic G80.1
      quadriplegic G80.0
      specified NEC G80.1
      tetrapelgic G80.0
    specified NEC G80.8
    syphilitic A52.12
      congenital A50.49
    tetraplegic G80.8
      spastic G80.0
  cranial nerve — *see also* Disorder, nerve, cranial
    multiple G52.7
      in
        infectious disease B99 ☑ *[G53]*
        neoplastic disease — *see also* Neoplasm
          D49.9 *[G53]*
        parasitic disease B89 *[G53]*
        sarcoidosis D86.82
  creeping G12.22
  diver's T70.3 ☑
  Erb's P14.0
  facial G51.0
    newborn (birth injury) P11.3
  glossopharyngeal G52.1
  Klumpke (-Déjérine) P14.1
  lead — *see* subcategory T56.0 ☑
  median nerve (tardy) G56.1- ☑
  nerve G58.9
    specified NEC G58.8
  peroneal nerve (acute) (tardy) G57.3- ☑
  progressive supranuclear G23.1
  pseudobulbar NEC G12.29
  radial nerve (acute) G56.3- ☑
  seventh nerve — *see also* Palsy, facial
    newborn P11.3
  shaking — *see* Parkinsonism
  spastic (cerebral) (spinal) G80.1
  ulnar nerve (tardy) G56.2- ☑
  wasting G12.29
Paludism — *see* Malaria
Panangiitis M30.0
Panaris, panaritium — *see also* Cellulitis, digit
  with lymphangitis — *see* Lymphangitis, acute, digit
Panarteritis nodosa M30.0
  brain or cerebral I67.7
Pancake heart R93.1
  with cor pulmonale (chronic) I27.81
Pancarditis (acute) (chronic) I51.89
  rheumatic I09.89
    active or acute I01.8
Pancoast's syndrome or tumor C34.1- ☑
Pancolitis, ulcerative (chronic) K51.00
  with
    abscess K51.014
    complication K51.019
    fistula K51.013

Pancolitis, ulcerative — *continued*
  with — *continued*
    obstruction K51.012
    rectal bleeding K51.011
    specified complication NEC K51.018
Pancreas, pancreatic — *see* condition
Pancreatitis (annular) (apoplectic) (calcareous) (edematous) (hemorrhagic) (malignant) (subacute) (suppurative) K85.90
  with necrosis (uninfected) K85.91
    infected K85.92
  acute (without necrosis or infection) K85.90
    with necrosis (uninfected) K85.91
      infected K85.92
    alcohol induced (without necrosis or infection)
      K85.20
      with necrosis (uninfected) K85.21
        infected K85.22
    biliary (without necrosis or infection) K85.10
      with necrosis (uninfected) K85.11
        infected K85.12
    drug induced (without necrosis or infection) K85.30
      with necrosis (uninfected) K85.31
        infected K85.32
    gallstone (without necrosis or infection) K85.10
      with necrosis (uninfected) K85.11
        infected K85.12
    idiopathic (without necrosis or infection) K85.00
      with necrosis (uninfected) K85.01
        infected K85.02
    specified NEC (without necrosis or infection) K85.80
      with necrosis (uninfected) K85.81
        infected K85.82
  chronic (infectious) K86.1
    alcohol-induced K86.0
    recurrent K86.1
    relapsing K86.1
  cystic (chronic) K86.1
  cytomegaloviral B25.2
  fibrous (chronic) K86.1
  gallstone (without necrosis or infection) K85.10
    with necrosis (uninfected) K85.11
      infected K85.12
  gangrenous — *see* Pancreatitis, acute
  interstitial (chronic) K86.1
    acute — *see also* Pancreatitis, acute K85.80
  mumps B26.3
  recurrent
    acute — *see* Pancreatitis, acute by type
    chronic K86.1
  relapsing, chronic K86.1
  syphilitic A52.74
Pancreatoblastoma — *see* Neoplasm, pancreas, malignant
Pancreolithiasis K86.89
Pancytolysis D75.89
Pancytopenia (acquired) D61.818
  with
    malformations D61.09
    myelodysplastic syndrome — *see* Syndrome,
      myelodysplastic
  antineoplastic chemotherapy induced D61.810
  congenital D61.09
  drug-induced NEC D61.811
PANDAS (pediatric autoimmune neuropsychiatric disorders associated with streptococcal infections syndrome) D89.89
Panencephalitis, subacute, sclerosing A81.1
Panhematopenia D61.9
  congenital D61.09
  constitutional D61.09
  splenic, primary D73.1
Panhemocytopenia D61.9
  congenital D61.09
  constitutional D61.09
Panhypogonadism E29.1
Panhypopituitarism E23.0
  prepubertal E23.0
Panic (attack) (state) F41.0
  reaction to exceptional stress (transient) F43.0
Panmyelopathy, familial, constitutional D61.09
Panmyelophthisis D61.82
  congenital D61.09
Panmyelosis (acute) (with myelofibrosis) C94.4- ☑
Panner's disease — *see* Osteochondrosis, juvenile,
  humerus
Panneuritis endemica E51.11
Panniculitis (nodular) (nonsuppurative) M79.3

Panniculitis — *continued*
  back M54.00
    cervical region M54.02
    cervicothoracic region M54.03
    lumbar region M54.06
    lumbosacral region M54.07
    multiple sites M54.09
    occipito-atlanto-axial region M54.01
    sacrococcygeal region M54.08
    thoracic region M54.04
    thoracolumbar region M54.05
  lupus L93.2
  mesenteric K65.4
  neck M54.02
    cervicothoracic region M54.03
    occipito-atlanto-axial region M54.01
  relapsing M35.6
Panniculus adiposus (abdominal) E65
Pannus (allergic) (cornea) (degenerativus) (keratic) H16.42- ☑
  abdominal (symptomatic) E65
  trachomatosus, trachomatous (active) A71.1
Panophthalmitis H44.01- ☑
Pansinusitis (chronic) (hyperplastic) (nonpurulent) (purulent) J32.4
  acute J01.40
    recurrent J01.41
  tuberculous A15.8
Panuveitis (sympathetic) H44.11- ☑
Panvalvular disease I08.9
  specified NEC I08.8
PAPA (pyogenic arthritis, pyoderma gangrenosum, and acne syndrome) M04.8
Papanicolaou smear, cervix Z12.4
  as part of routine gynecological examination Z01.419
    with abnormal findings Z01.411
  for suspected neoplasm Z12.4
  nonspecific abnormal finding R87.619
  routine Z01.419
    with abnormal findings Z01.411
Papilledema (choked disc) H47.10
  associated with
    decreased ocular pressure H47.12
    increased intracranial pressure H47.11
    retinal disorder H47.13
  Foster-Kennedy syndrome H47.14- ☑
Papillitis H46.00
  anus K62.89
  chronic lingual K14.4
  necrotizing, kidney N17.2
  optic H46.0- ☑
  rectum K62.89
  renal, necrotizing N17.2
  tongue K14.0
Papilloma — *see also* Neoplasm, benign, by site
  acuminatum (female) (male) (anogenital) A63.0
  basal cell L82.1
    inflamed L82.0
  benign pinta (primary) A67.0
  bladder (urinary) (transitional cell) D41.4
  choroid plexus (lateral ventricle) (third ventricle) D33.0
    anaplastic C71.5
    fourth ventricle D33.1
    malignant C71.5
  renal pelvis (transitional cell) D41.1- ☑
    benign D30.1- ☑
  Schneiderian
    specified site — *see* Neoplasm, benign, by site
    unspecified site D14.0
  serous surface
    borderline malignancy
      specified site — *see* Neoplasm, uncertain behavior, by site
      unspecified site D39.10
    specified site — *see* Neoplasm, benign, by site
    unspecified site D27.9
  transitional (cell)
    bladder (urinary) D41.4
    inverted type — *see* Neoplasm, uncertain behavior, by site
    renal pelvis D41.1- ☑
    ureter D41.2- ☑
  ureter (transitional cell) D41.2- ☑
    benign D30.2- ☑
  urothelial — *see* Neoplasm, uncertain behavior, by site
  villous — *see* Neoplasm, uncertain behavior, by site
    adenocarcinoma in — *see* Neoplasm, malignant, by site

Papilloma — *continued*
  villous — *see* Neoplasm, uncertain behavior, by site — *continued*
    adenocarcinoma in — *see* Neoplasm, malignant, by site — *continued*
      in situ — *see* Neoplasm, in situ
  yaws, plantar or palmar A66.1
Papillomata, multiple, of yaws A66.1
Papillomatosis — *see also* Neoplasm, benign, by site
  confluent and reticulated L83
  cystic, breast — *see* Mastopathy, cystic
  ductal, breast — *see* Mastopathy, cystic
  intraductal (diffuse) — *see* Neoplasm, benign, by site
  subareolar duct D24- ☑
Papillomavirus, as cause of disease classified elsewhere B97.7
Papillon-Léage and Psaume syndrome Q87.0
Papule(s) R23.8
  carate (primary) A67.0
  fibrous, of nose D22.39
  Gottron's L94.4
  pinta (primary) A67.0
Papulosis
  lymphomatoid C86.6
  malignant I77.89
Papyraceous fetus O31.0- ☑
Para-albuminemia E88.09
Paracephalus Q89.7
Parachute mitral valve Q23.2
Paracoccidioidomycosis B41.9
  disseminated B41.7
  generalized B41.7
  mucocutaneous-lymphangitic B41.8
  pulmonary B41.0
  specified NEC B41.8
  visceral B41.8
Paradentosis K05.4
Paraffinoma T88.8 ☑
Paraganglioma D44.7
  adrenal D35.0- ☑
    malignant C74.1- ☑
  aortic body D44.7
    malignant C75.5
  carotid body D44.6
    malignant C75.4
  chromaffin — *see also* Neoplasm, benign, by site
    malignant — *see* Neoplasm, malignant, by site
  extra-adrenal D44.7
    malignant C75.5
      specified site — *see* Neoplasm, malignant, by site
      unspecified site C75.5
    specified site — *see* Neoplasm, uncertain behavior, by site
    unspecified site D44.7
  gangliocytic D13.2
    specified site — *see* Neoplasm, benign, by site
    unspecified site D13.2
  glomus jugulare D44.7
    malignant C75.5
  jugular D44.7
  malignant C75.5
    specified site — *see* Neoplasm, malignant, by site
    unspecified site C75.5
  nonchromaffin D44.7
    malignant C75.5
      specified site — *see* Neoplasm, malignant, by site
      unspecified site C75.5
    specified site — *see* Neoplasm, uncertain behavior, by site
    unspecified site D44.7
  parasympathetic D44.7
    specified site — *see* Neoplasm, uncertain behavior, by site
    unspecified site D44.7
  specified site — *see* Neoplasm, uncertain behavior, by site
  sympathetic D44.7
    specified site — *see* Neoplasm, uncertain behavior, by site
    unspecified site D44.7
  unspecified site D44.7
Parageusia R43.2
  psychogenic F45.8
Paragonimiasis B66.4

Paragranuloma, Hodgkin — *see* Lymphoma, Hodgkin, specified NEC
Parahemophilia — *see also* Defect, coagulation D68.2
Parakeratosis R23.4
  variegata L41.0
Paralysis, paralytic (complete) (incomplete) G83.9
  with
    syphilis A52.17
  abducens, abducent (nerve) — *see* Strabismus, paralytic, sixth nerve
  abductor, lower extremity G57.9- ☑
  accessory nerve G52.8
  accommodation — *see also* Paresis, of accommodation
    hysterical F44.89
  acoustic nerve (except Deafness) H93.3 ☑
  agitans — *see also* Parkinsonism G20
    arteriosclerotic G21.4
  alternating (oculomotor) G83.89
  amyotrophic G12.21
  ankle G57.9- ☑
  anus (sphincter) K62.89
  arm — *see* Monoplegia, upper limb
  ascending (spinal), acute G61.0
  association G12.29
  asthenic bulbar G70.00
    with exacerbation (acute) G70.01
    in crisis G70.01
  ataxic (hereditary) G11.9
    general (syphilitic) A52.17
  atrophic G58.9
    infantile, acute — *see* Poliomyelitis, paralytic
    progressive G12.22
    spinal (acute) — *see* Poliomyelitis, paralytic
  axillary G54.0
  Babinski-Nageotte's G83.89
  Bell's G51.0
    newborn P11.3
  Benedikt's G46.3
  birth injury P14.9
    spinal cord P11.5
  bladder (neurogenic) (sphincter) N31.2
  bowel, colon or intestine K56.0
  brachial plexus G54.0
    birth injury P14.3
    newborn (birth injury) P14.3
  brain G83.9
    diplegia G83.0
    triplegia G83.89
  bronchial J98.09
  Brown-Séquard G83.81
  bulbar (chronic) (progressive) G12.22
    infantile — *see* Poliomyelitis, paralytic
    poliomyelitic — *see* Poliomyelitis, paralytic
    pseudo G12.29
  bulbospinal G70.00
    with exacerbation (acute) G70.01
    in crisis G70.01
  cardiac — *see also* Failure, heart I50.9
  cerebrocerebellar, diplegic G80.1
  cervical
    plexus G54.2
    sympathetic G90.09
  Céstan-Chenais G46.3
  Charcot-Marie-Tooth type G60.0
  Clark's G80.9
  colon K56.0
  compressed air T70.3 ☑
  compression
    arm G56.9- ☑
    leg G57.9- ☑
    lower extremity G57.9- ☑
    upper extremity G56.9- ☑
  congenital (cerebral) — *see* Palsy, cerebral
  conjugate movement (gaze) (of eye) H51.0
    cortical (nuclear) (supranuclear) H51.0
  cordis — *see* Failure, heart
  cranial or cerebral nerve G52.9
  creeping G12.22
  crossed leg G83.89
  crutch — *see* Injury, brachial plexus
  deglutition R13.0
    hysterical F44.4
  dementia A52.17
  descending (spinal) NEC G12.29
  diaphragm (flaccid) J98.6
    due to accidental dissection of phrenic nerve during procedure — *see* Puncture, accidental complicating surgery

Paralysis, paralytic — *continued*
digestive organs NEC K59.89
diplegic — *see* Diplegia
divergence (nuclear) H51.8
diver's T70.3 ☑
Duchenne's
 birth injury P14.0
 due to or associated with
 motor neuron disease G12.22
 muscular dystrophy G71.01
due to intracranial or spinal birth injury — *see* Palsy,
 cerebral
embolic (current episode) I63.4- ☑
Erb (-Duchenne) (birth) (newborn) P14.0
Erb's syphilitic spastic spinal A52.17
esophagus K22.89
eye muscle (extrinsic) H49.9
 intrinsic — *see also* Paresis, of accommodation
facial (nerve) G51.0
 birth injury P11.3
 congenital P11.3
 following operation NEC — *see* Puncture, accidental
 complicating surgery
 newborn (birth injury) P11.3
familial (recurrent) (periodic) G72.3
 spastic G11.4
fauces J39.2
finger G56.9- ☑
gait R26.1
gastric nerve (nondiabetic) G52.2
gaze, conjugate H51.0
general (progressive) (syphilitic) A52.17
 juvenile A50.45
glottis J38.00
 bilateral J38.02
 unilateral J38.01
gluteal G54.1
Gubler (-Millard) G46.3
hand — *see* Monoplegia, upper limb
heart — *see* Arrest, cardiac
hemiplegic — *see* Hemiplegia
hyperkalemic periodic (familial) G72.3
hypoglossal (nerve) G52.3
hypokalemic periodic G72.3
hysterical F44.4
ileus K56.0
infantile — *see also* Poliomyelitis, paralytic A80.30
 bulbar — *see* Poliomyelitis, paralytic
 cerebral — *see* Palsy, cerebral
 spastic — *see* Palsy, cerebral, spastic
infective — *see* Poliomyelitis, paralytic
inferior nuclear G83.9
internuclear — *see* Ophthalmoplegia, internuclear
intestine K56.0
iris H57.09
 due to diphtheria (toxin) A36.89
ischemic, Volkmann's (complicating trauma) T79.6 ☑
Jackson's G83.89
jake — *see* Poisoning, food, noxious, plant
Jamaica ginger (jake) G62.2
juvenile general A50.45
Klumpke (-Déjérine) (birth) (newborn) P14.1
labioglossal (laryngeal) (pharyngeal) G12.29
Landry's G61.0
laryngeal nerve (recurrent) (superior) (unilateral) J38.00
 bilateral J38.02
 unilateral J38.01
larynx J38.00
 bilateral J38.02
 due to diphtheria (toxin) A36.2
 unilateral J38.01
lateral G12.23
lead T56.0 ☑
left side — *see* Hemiplegia
leg G83.1- ☑
 both — *see* Paraplegia
 crossed G83.89
 hysterical F44.4
 psychogenic F44.4
 transient or transitory R29.818
 traumatic NEC — *see* Injury, nerve, leg
levator palpebrae superioris — *see* Blepharoptosis,
 paralytic
limb — *see* Monoplegia
lip K13.0
Lissauer's A52.17
lower limb — *see* Monoplegia, lower limb
 both — *see* Paraplegia

Paralysis, paralytic — *continued*
lung J98.4
median nerve G56.1- ☑
medullary (tegmental) G83.89
mesencephalic NEC G83.89
 tegmental G83.89
middle alternating G83.89
Millard-Gubler-Foville G46.3
monoplegic — *see* Monoplegia
motor G83.9
muscle, muscular NEC G72.89
 due to nerve lesion G58.9
 eye (extrinsic) H49.9
 intrinsic — *see* Paresis, of accommodation
 oblique — *see* Strabismus, paralytic, fourth nerve
 iris sphincter H21.9
 ischemic (Volkmann's) (complicating trauma)
 T79.6 ☑
 progressive G12.21
 progressive, spinal G12.25
 pseudohypertrophic G71.02
 spinal progressive G12.25
musculocutaneous nerve G56.9- ☑
musculospiral G56.9- ☑
nerve — *see also* Disorder, nerve
 abducent — *see* Strabismus, paralytic, sixth nerve
 accessory G52.8
 auditory (except Deafness) H93.3 ☑
 birth injury P14.9
 cranial or cerebral G52.9
 facial G51.0
 birth injury P11.3
 congenital P11.3
 newborn (birth injury) P11.3
 fourth or trochlear — *see* Strabismus, paralytic,
 fourth nerve
 newborn (birth injury) P14.9
 oculomotor — *see* Strabismus, paralytic, third nerve
 phrenic (birth injury) P14.2
 radial G56.3- ☑
 seventh or facial G51.0
 newborn (birth injury) P11.3
 sixth or abducent — *see* Strabismus, paralytic, sixth
 nerve
 syphilitic A52.15
 third or oculomotor — *see* Strabismus, paralytic,
 third nerve
 trigeminal G50.9
 trochlear — *see* Strabismus, paralytic, fourth nerve
 ulnar G56.2- ☑
normokalemic periodic G72.3
ocular H49.9
 alternating G83.89
oculofacial, congenital (Moebius) Q87.0
oculomotor (external bilateral) (nerve) — *see* Strabismus, paralytic, third nerve
palate (soft) K13.79
paratrigeminal G50.9
periodic (familial) (hyperkalemic) (hypokalemic) (myotonic) (normokalemic) (potassium sensitive)
 (secondary) G72.3
peripheral autonomic nervous system — *see* Neuropathy, peripheral, autonomic
peroneal (nerve) G57.3- ☑
pharynx J39.2
phrenic nerve G56.8- ☑
plantar nerve(s) G57.6- ☑
pneumogastric nerve G52.2
poliomyelitis (current) — *see* Poliomyelitis, paralytic
popliteal nerve G57.3- ☑
postepileptic transitory G83.84
progressive (atrophic) (bulbar) (spinal) G12.22
 general A52.17
 infantile acute — *see* Poliomyelitis, paralytic
 supranuclear G23.1
pseudobulbar G12.29
pseudohypertrophic (muscle) — *see also* Dystrophy,
 muscular, by type, if applicable G71.09
psychogenic F44.4
quadriceps G57.9- ☑
quadriplegic — *see* Tetraplegia
radial nerve G56.3- ☑
rectus muscle (eye) H49.9
recurrent isolated sleep G47.53
respiratory (muscle) (system) (tract) R06.81
 center NEC G93.89
 congenital P28.89
 newborn P28.89

Paralysis, paralytic — *continued*
right side — *see* Hemiplegia
saturnine T56.0 ☑
sciatic nerve G57.0- ☑
senile G83.9
shaking — *see* Parkinsonism
shoulder G56.9- ☑
sleep, recurrent isolated G47.53
spastic G83.9
 cerebral — *see* Palsy, cerebral, spastic
 congenital (cerebral) — *see* Palsy, cerebral, spastic
 familial G11.4
 hereditary G11.4
 quadriplegic G80.0
 syphilitic (spinal) A52.17
sphincter, bladder — *see* Paralysis, bladder
spinal (cord) G83.9
 accessory nerve G52.8
 acute — *see* Poliomyelitis, paralytic
 ascending acute G61.0
 atrophic (acute) — *see also* Poliomyelitis, paralytic
 spastic, syphilitic A52.17
 congenital NEC — *see* Palsy, cerebral
 hereditary G95.89
 infantile — *see* Poliomyelitis, paralytic
 progressive G12.21
 muscle G12.25
 sequelae NEC G83.89
sternomastoid G52.8
stomach K31.84
 diabetic — *see* Diabetes, by type, with gastroparesis
 nerve G52.2
 diabetic — *see* Diabetes, by type, with gastroparesis
stroke — *see* Infarct, brain
subcapsularis G56.8- ☑
supranuclear (progressive) G23.1
sympathetic G90.8
 cervical G90.09
 nervous system — *see* Neuropathy, peripheral, autonomic
syndrome G83.9
 specified NEC G83.89
syphilitic spastic spinal (Erb's) A52.17
thigh G57.9- ☑
throat J39.2
 diphtheritic A36.0
 muscle J39.2
thrombotic (current episode) I63.3- ☑
thumb G56.9- ☑
tick — *see* Toxicity, venom, arthropod, specified NEC
Todd's (postepileptic transitory paralysis) G83.84
toe G57.6- ☑
tongue K14.8
transient R29.5
 arm or leg NEC R29.818
 traumatic NEC — *see* Injury, nerve
trapezius G52.8
traumatic, transient NEC — *see* Injury, nerve
trembling — *see* Parkinsonism
triceps brachii G56.9- ☑
trigeminal nerve G50.9
trochlear (nerve) — *see* Strabismus, paralytic, fourth
 nerve
ulnar nerve G56.2- ☑
upper limb — *see* Monoplegia, upper limb
uremic N18.9 *[G99.8]*
uveoparotitic D86.89
uvula K13.79
 postdiphtheritic A36.0
vagus nerve G52.2
vasomotor NEC G90.8
velum palati K13.79
vesical — *see* Paralysis, bladder
vestibular nerve (except Vertigo) H93.3 ☑
vocal cords J38.00
 bilateral J38.02
 unilateral J38.01
Volkmann's (complicating trauma) T79.6 ☑
wasting G12.29
Weber's G46.3
wrist G56.9- ☑
Paramedial urethrovesical orifice Q64.79
Paramenia N92.6
Parametritis — *see also* Disease, pelvis, inflammatory
 N73.2
 acute N73.0

Parametritis — *continued*
  complicating abortion — *see* Abortion, by type, complicated by, parametritis
Parametrium, parametric — *see* condition
Paramnesia — *see* Amnesia
Paramolar K00.1
Paramyloidosis E85.89
Paramyoclonus multiplex G25.3
Paramyotonia (congenita) G71.19
Parangi — *see* Yaws
Paranoia (querulans) F22
  senile F03 ☑
Paranoid
  dementia (senile) F03 ☑
    praecox — *see* Schizophrenia
  personality F60.0
  psychosis (climacteric) (involutional) (menopausal) F22
    psychogenic (acute) F23
      senile F03 ☑
  reaction (acute) F23
    chronic F22
  schizophrenia F20.0
  state (climacteric) (involutional) (menopausal) (simple) F22
    senile F03 ☑
  tendencies F60.0
  traits F60.0
  trends F60.0
  type, psychopathic personality F60.0
Paraparesis — *see* Paraplegia
Paraphasia R47.02
Paraphilia F65.9
Paraphimosis (congenital) N47.2
  chancroidal A57
Paraphrenia, paraphrenic (late) F22
  schizophrenia F20.0
Paraplegia (lower) G82.20
  ataxic — *see* Degeneration, combined, spinal cord
  complete G82.21
  congenital (cerebral) G80.8
    spastic G80.1
  familial spastic G11.4
  functional (hysterical) F44.4
  hereditary, spastic G11.4
  hysterical F44.4
  incomplete G82.22
  Pott's A18.01
  psychogenic F44.4
  spastic
    Erb's spinal, syphilitic A52.17
    hereditary G11.4
    tropical G04.1
  syphilitic (spastic) A52.17
  traumatic
    current injury — code to injury with seventh character A
    sequela of previous injury — code to injury with seventh character S
  tropical spastic G04.1
Parapoxvirus B08.60
  specified NEC B08.69
Paraproteinemia D89.2
  benign (familial) D89.2
  monoclonal D47.2
  secondary to malignant disease D47.2
Parapsoriasis L41.9
  en plaques L41.4
  guttata L41.1
  large plaque L41.4
  retiform, retiformis L41.5
  small plaque L41.3
  specified NEC L41.8
  varioliformis (acuta) L41.0
Parasitic — *see also* condition
  disease NEC B89
  stomatitis B37.0
  sycosis (beard) (scalp) B35.0
  twin Q89.4
Parasitism B89
  intestinal B82.9
  skin B88.9
  specified — *see* Infestation
Parasitophobia F40.218
Parasomnia G47.50
  due to
    alcohol
      abuse F10.182
      dependence F10.282

Parasomnia — *continued*
  due to — *continued*
    alcohol — *continued*
      use F10.982
    amphetamines
      abuse F15.182
      dependence F15.282
      use F15.982
    caffeine
      abuse F15.182
      dependence F15.282
      use F15.982
    cocaine
      abuse F14.182
      dependence F14.282
      use F14.982
    drug NEC
      abuse F19.182
      dependence F19.282
      use F19.982
    opioid
      abuse F11.182
      dependence F11.282
      use F11.982
    psychoactive substance NEC
      abuse F19.182
      dependence F19.282
      use F19.982
    sedative, hypnotic, or anxiolytic
      abuse F13.182
      dependence F13.282
      use F13.982
    stimulant NEC
      abuse F15.182
      dependence F15.282
      use F15.982
  in conditions classified elsewhere G47.54
  nonorganic origin F51.8
  organic G47.50
  specified NEC G47.59
Paraspadias Q54.9
Paraspasmus facialis G51.8
Parasuicide (attempt)
  history of (personal) Z91.51
    in family Z81.8
Parathyroid gland — *see* condition
Parathyroid tetany E20.9
Paratrachoma A74.0
Paratyphilitis — *see* Appendicitis
Paratyphoid (fever) — *see* Fever, paratyphoid
Paratyphus — *see* Fever, paratyphoid
Paraurethral duct Q64.79
Paraurethritis — *see also* Urethritis
  gonococcal (acute) (chronic) (with abscess) A54.1
Paravaccinia NEC B08.04
Paravaginitis — *see* Vaginitis
Parencephalitis — *see also* Encephalitis
  sequelae G09
Parent-child conflict — *see* Conflict, parent-child
  estrangement NEC Z62.890
Paresis — *see also* Paralysis
  accommodation — *see* Paresis, of accommodation
  Bernhardt's G57.1- ☑
  bladder (sphincter) — *see also* Paralysis, bladder
    tabetic A52.17
  bowel, colon or intestine K56.0
  extrinsic muscle, eye H49.9
  general (progressive) (syphilitic) A52.17
    juvenile A50.45
  heart — *see* Failure, heart
  insane (syphilitic) A52.17
  juvenile (general) A50.45
  of accommodation H52.52- ☑
  peripheral progressive (idiopathic) G60.3
  pseudohypertrophic — *see also* Dystrophy, muscular, by type, if applicable G71.09
  senile G83.9
  syphilitic (general) A52.17
    congenital A50.45
  vesical NEC N31.2
Paresthesia — *see also* Disturbance, sensation, skin R20.2
  Bernhardt G57.1- ☑
Paretic — *see* condition
Parinaud's
  conjunctivitis H10.89
  oculoglandular syndrome H10.89
  ophthalmoplegia H49.88- ☑
Parkinsonism (idiopathic) (primary) G20

Parkinsonism — *continued*
  with neurogenic orthostatic hypotension (symptomatic) G90.3
  arteriosclerotic G21.4
  dementia — *see also* Dementia, in, diseases specified elsewhere G20 [F02.80]
    with behavioral disturbance — *see also* Dementia, in, diseases specified elsewhere G20 [F02.81-] ☑
  due to
    drugs NEC G21.19
      neuroleptic G21.11
    medication-induced NEC G21.19
    neuroleptic induced G21.11
    postencephalitic G21.3
    secondary G21.9
      due to
        arteriosclerosis G21.4
        drugs NEC G21.19
          neuroleptic G21.11
        encephalitis G21.3
        external agents NEC G21.2
        syphilis A52.19
      specified NEC G21.8
    syphilitic A52.19
    treatment-induced NEC G21.19
    vascular G21.4
Parkinson's disease, syndrome or tremor — *see* Parkinsonism
Parodontitis — *see* Periodontitis
Parodontosis K05.4
Paronychia — *see also* Cellulitis, digit
  with lymphangitis — *see* Lymphangitis, acute, digit
  candidal (chronic) B37.2
  tuberculous (primary) A18.4
Parorexia (psychogenic) F50.89
Parosmia R43.1
  psychogenic F45.8
Parotid gland — *see* condition
Parotitis, parotiditis (allergic) (nonspecific toxic) (purulent) (septic) (suppurative) — *see also* Sialoadenitis
  epidemic — *see* Mumps
  infectious — *see* Mumps
  postoperative K91.89
  surgical K91.89
Parrot fever A70
Parrot's disease (early congenital syphilitic pseudoparalysis) A50.02
Parry-Romberg syndrome G51.8
Parry's disease or syndrome E05.00
  with thyroid storm E05.01
Pars planitis — *see* Cyclitis
Parsonage (-Aldren)-**Turner syndrome** G54.5
Parson's disease (exophthalmic goiter) E05.00
  with thyroid storm E05.01
Particolored infant Q82.8
Parturition — *see* Delivery
Parulis K04.7
  with sinus K04.6
Parvovirus, as cause of disease classified elsewhere B97.6
Pasini and Pierini's atrophoderma L90.3
Passage
  false, urethra N36.5
  meconium (newborn) during delivery P03.82
  of sounds or bougies — *see* Attention to, artificial, opening
Passive — *see* condition
  smoking Z77.22
Past due on rent or mortgage Z59.81- ☑
Pasteurella septica A28.0
Pasteurellosis — *see* Infection, Pasteurella
PAT (paroxysmal atrial tachycardia) I47.1
Patau's syndrome — *see* Trisomy, 13
Patches
  mucous (syphilitic) A51.39
    congenital A50.07
  smokers' (mouth) K13.24
Patellar — *see* condition
Patent — *see also* Imperfect, closure
  canal of Nuck Q52.4
  cervix N88.3
  ductus arteriosus or Botallo's Q25.0
  foramen
    botalli Q21.12
    ovale Q21.12
  interauricular septum Q21.19

☑ **Additional Character Required — Refer to the Tabular List for Character Selection**

Patent — *continued*
  interventricular septum Q21.0
  omphalomesenteric duct Q43.0
  os (uteri) — *see* Patent, cervix
  ostium secundum (type II) Q21.11
  urachus Q64.4
  vitelline duct Q43.0
Paterson (-Brown) (-Kelly) **syndrome or web** D50.1
Pathologic, pathological — *see also* condition
  asphyxia R09.01
  fire-setting F63.1
  gambling F63.0
  ovum O02.0
  resorption, tooth K03.3
  stealing F63.2
Pathology (of) — *see* Disease
  periradicular, associated with previous endodontic
    treatment NEC M27.59
Pattern, sleep-wake, irregular G47.23
Patulous — *see also* Imperfect, closure (congenital)
  alimentary tract Q45.8
    lower Q43.8
    upper Q40.8
  eustachian tube H69.0- ☑
Pause, sinoatrial I49.5
Paxton's disease B36.2
Pearl(s)
  enamel K00.2
  Epstein's K09.8
Pearl-worker's disease — *see* Osteomyelitis, specified
  type NEC
Pectenosis K62.4
Pectoral — *see* condition
Pectus
  carinatum (congenital) Q67.7
    acquired M95.4
    rachitic sequelae (late effect) E64.3
  excavatum (congenital) Q67.6
    acquired M95.4
    rachitic sequelae (late effect) E64.3
  recurvatum (congenital) Q67.6
Pedatrophia E41
Pederosis F65.4
Pediatric inflammatory multisystem syndrome
  M35.81
Pediculosis (infestation) B85.2
  capitis (head-louse) (any site) B85.0
  corporis (body-louse) (any site) B85.1
  eyelid B85.0
  mixed (classifiable to more than one of the titles B85.0-
    B85.3) B85.4
  pubis (pubic louse) (any site) B85.3
  vestimenti B85.1
  vulvae B85.3
Pediculus (infestation) — *see* Pediculosis
Pedophilia F65.4
Peg-shaped teeth K00.2
Pelade — *see* Alopecia, areata
Pelger-Huët anomaly or syndrome D72.0
Peliosis (rheumatica) D69.0
  hepatis K76.4
    with toxic liver disease K71.8
Pelizaeus-Merzbacher disease E75.29
Pellagra (alcoholic) (with polyneuropathy) E52
Pellagra-cerebellar-ataxia-renal aminoaciduria
  syndrome E72.02
Pellegrini (-Stieda) **disease or syndrome** — *see* Bursitis,
  tibial collateral
Pellizzi's syndrome E34.8
Pel's crisis A52.11
Pelvic — *see also* condition
  examination (periodic) (routine) Z01.419
    with abnormal findings Z01.411
  kidney, congenital Q63.2
Pelviolithiasis — *see* Calculus, kidney
Pelviperitonitis — *see also* Peritonitis, pelvic
  gonococcal A54.24
  puerperal O85
Pelvis — *see* condition or type
Pemphigoid L12.9
  benign, mucous membrane L12.1
  bullous L12.0
  cicatricial L12.1
  juvenile L12.2
  ocular L12.1
  specified NEC L12.8
Pemphigus L10.9
  benign familial (chronic) Q82.8

Pemphigus — *continued*
  Brazilian L10.3
  circinatus L13.0
  conjunctiva L12.1
  drug-induced L10.5
  erythematosus L10.4
  foliaceous L10.2
  gangrenous — *see* Gangrene
  neonatorum L01.03
  ocular L12.1
  paraneoplastic L10.81
  specified NEC L10.89
  syphilitic (congenital) A50.06
  vegetans L10.1
  vulgaris L10.0
  wildfire L10.3
Pendred's syndrome E07.1
Pendulous
  abdomen, in pregnancy — *see* Pregnancy, complicated
    by, abnormal, pelvic organs or tissues NEC
  breast N64.89
Penetrating wound — *see also* Puncture
  with internal injury — *see* Injury, by site
  eyeball — *see* Puncture, eyeball
  orbit (with or without foreign body) — *see* Puncture,
    orbit
  uterus by instrument with or following ectopic or molar
    pregnancy O08.6
Penicillosis B48.4
Penis — *see* condition
Penitis N48.29
Pentalogy of Fallot Q21.8
Pentasomy X syndrome Q97.1
Pentosuria (essential) E74.89
Percreta placenta - O43.23 ☑
Peregrinating patient — *see* Disorder, factitious
Perforation, perforated (nontraumatic) (of)
  accidental during procedure (blood vessel) (nerve)
    (organ) — *see* Complication, accidental puncture
    or laceration
  antrum — *see* Sinusitis, maxillary
  appendix K35.32
    with localized peritonitis K35.32
  atrial septum, multiple Q21.19
  attic, ear — *see* Perforation, tympanum, attic
  bile duct (common) (hepatic) K83.2
    cystic K82.2
  bladder (urinary)
    with or following ectopic or molar pregnancy O08.6
    obstetrical trauma O71.5
    traumatic S37.29 ☑
      at delivery O71.5
  bowel K63.1
    with or following ectopic or molar pregnancy O08.6
    newborn P78.0
    obstetrical trauma O71.5
    traumatic — *see* Laceration, intestine
  broad ligament N83.8
    with or following ectopic or molar pregnancy O08.6
    obstetrical trauma O71.6
  by
    device, implant or graft — *see also* Complications,
      by site and type, mechanical T85.628 ☑
      arterial graft NEC — *see* Complication, cardiovas-
        cular device, mechanical, vascular
      breast (implant) T85.49 ☑
      catheter NEC T85.698 ☑
        cystostomy T83.090 ☑
        dialysis (renal) T82.49 ☑
          intraperitoneal T85.691 ☑
        infusion NEC T82.594 ☑
          spinal (epidural) (subdural) T85.690 ☑
        urinary — *see also* Complications, catheter,
          urinary T83.098 ☑
      electronic (electrode) (pulse generator) (stimula-
        tor)
        bone T84.390 ☑
        cardiac T82.199 ☑
          electrode T82.190 ☑
          pulse generator T82.191 ☑
          specified type NEC T82.198 ☑
        nervous system — *see* Complication, prosthet-
          ic device, mechanical, electronic ner-
          vous system stimulator
        urinary — *see* Complication, genitourinary,
          device, urinary, mechanical

Perforation, perforated — *continued*
  by — *continued*
    device, implant or graft — *see also* Complications,
      by site and type, mechanical — *continued*
      fixation, internal (orthopedic) NEC — *see* Compli-
        cation, fixation device, mechanical
      gastrointestinal — *see* Complications, prosthetic
        device, mechanical, gastrointestinal device
      genital NEC T83.498 ☑
        intrauterine contraceptive device T83.39 ☑
        penile prosthesis T83.490 ☑
      heart NEC — *see* Complication, cardiovascular
        device, mechanical
      joint prosthesis — *see* Complications, joint
        prosthesis, mechanical, specified NEC, by
        site
      ocular NEC — *see* Complications, prosthetic de-
        vice, mechanical, ocular device
      orthopedic NEC — *see* Complication, orthopedic,
        device, mechanical
      specified NEC T85.628 ☑
      urinary NEC — *see also* Complication, genitouri-
        nary, device, urinary, mechanical
        graft T83.29 ☑
      vascular NEC — *see* Complication, cardiovascular
        device, mechanical
      ventricular intracranial shunt T85.09 ☑
    foreign body left accidentally in operative wound
      T81.539 ☑
    instrument (any) during a procedure, accidental —
      see Puncture, accidental complicating surgery
  cecum K35.32
    with localized peritonitis K35.32
  cervix (uteri) N88.8
    with or following ectopic or molar pregnancy O08.6
    obstetrical trauma O71.3
  colon K63.1
    newborn P78.0
    obstetrical trauma O71.5
    traumatic — *see* Laceration, intestine, large
  common duct (bile) K83.2
  cornea (due to ulceration) — *see* Ulcer, cornea, perfo-
    rated
  cystic duct K82.2
  diverticulum (intestine) K57.80
    with bleeding K57.81
    large intestine K57.20
      with
        bleeding K57.21
        small intestine K57.40
          with bleeding K57.41
    small intestine K57.00
      with
        bleeding K57.01
        large intestine K57.40
          with bleeding K57.41
  ear drum — *see* Perforation, tympanum
  esophagus K22.3
  ethmoidal sinus — *see* Sinusitis, ethmoidal
  frontal sinus — *see* Sinusitis, frontal
  gallbladder K82.2
  heart valve — *see* Endocarditis
  ileum K63.1
    newborn P78.0
    obstetrical trauma O71.5
    traumatic — *see* Laceration, intestine, small
  instrumental, surgical (accidental) (blood vessel) (nerve)
    (organ) — *see* Puncture, accidental complicating
    surgery
  intestine NEC K63.1
    with ectopic or molar pregnancy O08.6
    newborn P78.0
    obstetrical trauma O71.5
    traumatic — *see* Laceration, intestine
    ulcerative NEC K63.1
      newborn P78.0
  jejunum, jejunal K63.1
    obstetrical trauma O71.5
    traumatic — *see* Laceration, intestine, small
    ulcer — *see* Ulcer, gastrojejunal, with perforation
  joint prosthesis — *see* Complications, joint prosthesis,
    mechanical, specified NEC, by site
  mastoid (antrum) (cell) — *see* Disorder, mastoid,
    specified NEC
  maxillary sinus — *see* Sinusitis, maxillary
  membrana tympani — *see* Perforation, tympanum
  nasal
    septum J34.89

Perforation, perforated — continued
nasal — continued
   septum — continued
     congenital Q30.3
     syphilitic A52.73
   sinus J34.89
     congenital Q30.8
     due to sinusitis — see Sinusitis
palate — see also Cleft, palate Q35.9
   syphilitic A52.79
palatine vault — see also Cleft, palate, hard Q35.1
   syphilitic A52.79
   congenital A50.59
pars flaccida (ear drum) — see Perforation, tympanum, attic
pelvic
   floor S31.030 ☑
     with
       ectopic or molar pregnancy O08.6
       penetration into retroperitoneal space S31.031 ☑
       retained foreign body S31.040 ☑
         with penetration into retroperitoneal space S31.041 ☑
     following ectopic or molar pregnancy O08.6
     obstetrical trauma O70.1
   organ S37.99 ☑
     adrenal gland S37.818 ☑
     bladder — see Perforation, bladder
     fallopian tube S37.599 ☑
       bilateral S37.592 ☑
       unilateral S37.591 ☑
     kidney S37.09- ☑
     obstetrical trauma O71.5
     ovary S37.499 ☑
       bilateral S37.492 ☑
       unilateral S37.491 ☑
     prostate S37.828 ☑
     specified organ NEC S37.898 ☑
     ureter — see Perforation, ureter
     urethra — see Perforation, urethra
     uterus — see Perforation, uterus
perineum — see Laceration, perineum
pharynx J39.2
rectum K63.1
   newborn P78.0
   obstetrical trauma O71.5
   traumatic S36.63 ☑
root canal space due to endodontic treatment M27.51
sigmoid K63.1
   newborn P78.0
   obstetrical trauma O71.5
   traumatic S36.533 ☑
sinus (accessory) (chronic) (nasal) J34.89
sphenoidal sinus — see Sinusitis, sphenoidal
surgical (accidental) (by instrument) (blood vessel) (nerve) (organ) — see Puncture, accidental
   complicating surgery
traumatic
   external — see Puncture
   eye — see Puncture, eyeball
   internal organ — see Injury, by site
tympanum, tympanic (membrane) (persistent post-traumatic) (postinflammatory) H72.9- ☑
   attic H72.1- ☑
     multiple — see Perforation, tympanum, multiple
     total — see Perforation, tympanum, total
   central H72.0- ☑
     multiple — see Perforation, tympanum, multiple
     total — see Perforation, tympanum, total
   marginal NEC — see subcategory H72.2 ☑
   multiple H72.81- ☑
   pars flaccida — see Perforation, tympanum, attic
   total H72.82- ☑
   traumatic, current episode S09.2- ☑
typhoid, gastrointestinal — see Typhoid
ulcer — see Ulcer, by site, with perforation
ureter N28.89
   traumatic S37.19 ☑
urethra N36.8
   with ectopic or molar pregnancy O08.6
   following ectopic or molar pregnancy O08.6
   obstetrical trauma O71.5
   traumatic S37.39 ☑
     at delivery O71.5
uterus
   with ectopic or molar pregnancy O08.6

Perforation, perforated — continued
uterus — continued
   by intrauterine contraceptive device T83.39 ☑
   following ectopic or molar pregnancy O08.6
   obstetrical trauma O71.1
   traumatic S37.69 ☑
     obstetric O71.1
uvula K13.79
   syphilitic A52.79
vagina O71.4
   obstetrical trauma O71.4
   other trauma — see Puncture, vagina
Periadenitis mucosa necrotica recurrens K12.0
Periappendicitis (acute) — see Appendicitis
Periarteritis nodosa (disseminated) (infectious) (necrotizing) M30.0
Periarthritis (joint) — see also Enthesopathy
   Duplay's M75.0- ☑
   gonococcal A54.42
   humeroscapularis — see Capsulitis, adhesive
   scapulohumeral — see Capsulitis, adhesive
   shoulder — see Capsulitis, adhesive
   wrist M77.2- ☑
Periarthrosis (angioneural) — see Enthesopathy
Pericapsulitis, adhesive (shoulder) — see Capsulitis, adhesive
Pericarditis (with decompensation) (with effusion) I31.9
   with rheumatic fever (conditions in I00)
     active — see Pericarditis, rheumatic
     inactive or quiescent I09.2
   acute (hemorrhagic) (nonrheumatic) (Sicca) I30.9
     with chorea (acute) (rheumatic) (Sydenham's) I02.0
     benign I30.8
     nonspecific I30.0
     rheumatic I01.0
       with chorea (acute) (Sydenham's) I02.0
   adhesive or adherent (chronic) (external) (internal) I31.0
     acute — see Pericarditis, acute
     rheumatic I09.2
   bacterial (acute) (subacute) (with serous or seropurulent effusion) I30.1
   calcareous I31.1
   cholesterol (chronic) I31.8
     acute I30.9
   chronic (nonrheumatic) I31.9
     rheumatic I09.2
   constrictive (chronic) I31.1
   coxsackie B33.23
   fibrinocaseous (tuberculous) A18.84
   fibrinopurulent I30.1
   fibrinous I30.8
   fibrous I31.0
   gonococcal A54.83
   idiopathic I30.0
   in systemic lupus erythematosus M32.12
   infective I30.1
   meningococcal A39.53
   neoplastic (chronic) I31.8
     acute I30.9
   obliterans, obliterating I31.0
   plastic I31.0
   pneumococcal I30.1
   postinfarction I24.1
   purulent I30.1
   rheumatic (active) (acute) (with effusion) (with pneumonia) I01.0
     with chorea (acute) (rheumatic) (Sydenham's) I02.0
     chronic or inactive (with chorea) I09.2
   rheumatoid — see Rheumatoid, carditis
   septic I30.1
   serofibrinous I30.8
   staphylococcal I30.1
   streptococcal I30.1
   suppurative I30.1
   syphilitic A52.06
   tuberculous A18.84
   uremic N18.9 [I32]
   viral I30.1
Pericardium, pericardial — see condition
Pericellulitis — see Cellulitis
Pericementitis (chronic) (suppurative) — see also Periodontitis
   acute K05.20
     generalized — see Periodontitis, aggressive, generalized
     localized — see Periodontitis, aggressive, localized
Perichondritis
   auricle — see Perichondritis, ear

Perichondritis — continued
   bronchus J98.09
   ear (external) H61.00- ☑
     acute H61.01- ☑
     chronic H61.02- ☑
   external auditory canal — see Perichondritis, ear
   larynx J38.7
     syphilitic A52.73
     typhoid A01.09
   nose J34.89
   pinna — see Perichondritis, ear
   trachea J39.8
Periclasia K05.4
Pericoronitis — see Periodontitis
Pericystitis N30.90
   with hematuria N30.91
Peridiverticulitis (intestine) K57.92
   cecum — see Diverticulitis, intestine, large
   colon — see Diverticulitis, intestine, large
   duodenum — see Diverticulitis, intestine, small
   intestine — see Diverticulitis, intestine
   jejunum — see Diverticulitis, intestine, small
   rectosigmoid — see Diverticulitis, intestine, large
   rectum — see Diverticulitis, intestine, large
   sigmoid — see Diverticulitis, intestine, large
Periendocarditis — see Endocarditis
Periepididymitis N45.1
Perifolliculitis L01.02
   abscedens, caput, scalp L66.3
   capitis, abscedens (et suffodiens) L66.3
   superficial pustular L01.02
Perihepatitis K65.8
Perilabyrinthitis (acute) — see subcategory H83.0 ☑
Perimeningitis — see Meningitis
Perimetritis — see Endometritis
Perimetrosalpingitis — see Salpingo-oophoritis
Perineocele N81.81
Perinephric, perinephritic — see condition
Perinephritis — see also Infection, kidney
   purulent — see Abscess, kidney
Perineum, perineal — see condition
Perineuritis NEC — see Neuralgia
Periodic — see condition
Periodontitis (chronic) (complex) (compound) (local) (simplex) K05.30
   acute K05.20
     generalized K05.229
       moderate K05.222
       severe K05.223
       slight K05.221
     localized K05.219
       moderate K05.212
       severe K05.213
       slight K05.211
   aggressive K05.20
     generalized K05.229
       moderate K05.222
       severe K05.223
       slight K05.221
     localized K05.219
       moderate K05.212
       severe K05.213
       slight K05.211
   apical K04.5
     acute (pulpal origin) K04.4
   generalized K05.329
     moderate K05.322
     severe K05.323
     slight K05.321
   localized K05.319
     moderate K05.312
     severe K05.313
     slight K05.311
Periodontoclasia K05.4
Periodontosis (juvenile) K05.4
Periods — see also Menstruation
   heavy N92.0
   irregular N92.6
   shortened intervals (irregular) N92.1
Perionychia — see also Cellulitis, digit
   with lymphangitis — see Lymphangitis, acute, digit
Perioophoritis — see Salpingo-oophoritis
Periorchitis N45.2
Periosteum, periosteal — see condition
Periostitis (albuminosa) (circumscribed) (diffuse) (infective) (monomelic) — see also Osteomyelitis
   alveolar M27.3

Periostitis — *continued*
  alveolodental M27.3
  dental M27.3
  gonorrheal A54.43
  jaw (lower) (upper) M27.2
  orbit H05.03- ☑
  syphilitic A52.77
    congenital (early) A50.02 *[M90.80]*
    secondary A51.46
  tuberculous — *see* Tuberculosis, bone
  yaws (hypertrophic) (early) (late) A66.6 *[M90.80]*
Periostosis (hyperplastic) — *see also* Disorder, bone,
    specified type NEC
  with osteomyelitis — *see* Osteomyelitis, specified type
    NEC
Peripartum
  cardiomyopathy O90.3
Periphlebitis — *see* Phlebitis
Periproctitis K62.89
Periprostatitis — *see* Prostatitis
Perirectal — *see* condition
Perirenal — *see* condition
Perisalpingitis — *see* Salpingo-oophoritis
Perisplenitis (infectional) D73.89
Peristalsis, visible or reversed R19.2
Peritendinitis — *see* Enthesopathy
Peritoneum, peritoneal — *see* condition
Peritonitis (adhesive) (bacterial) (fibrinous) (hemorrhagic)
    (idiopathic) (localized) (perforative) (primary) (with
    adhesions) (with effusion) K65.9
  with or following
    abscess K65.1
    appendicitis
      with perforation or rupture K35.32
      generalized — *see also* Appendicitis K35.20
      localized — *see also* Appendicitis K35.30
    diverticular disease (intestine) K57.80
      with bleeding K57.81
      ectopic or molar pregnancy O08.0
      large intestine K57.20
        with
          bleeding K57.21
          small intestine K57.40
            with bleeding K57.41
        small intestine K57.00
          with
            bleeding K57.01
            large intestine K57.40
              with bleeding K57.41
  acute (generalized) K65.0
  aseptic T81.61 ☑
  bile, biliary K65.3
  chemical T81.61 ☑
  chlamydial A74.81
  chronic proliferative K65.8
  complicating abortion — *see* Abortion, by type, com-
    plicated by, pelvic peritonitis
  congenital P78.1
  diaphragmatic K65.0
  diffuse K65.0
  diphtheritic A36.89
  disseminated K65.0
  due to
    bile K65.3
    foreign
      body or object accidentally left during a proce-
        dure (instrument) (sponge) (swab)
        T81.599 ☑
      substance accidentally left during a procedure
        (chemical) (powder) (talc) T81.61 ☑
    talc T81.61 ☑
    urine K65.8
  eosinophilic K65.8
    acute K65.0
  fibrocaseous (tuberculous) A18.31
  fibropurulent K65.0
  following ectopic or molar pregnancy O08.0
  general (ized) K65.0
  gonococcal A54.85
  meconium (newborn) P78.0
  neonatal P78.1
    meconium P78.0
  pancreatic K65.0
  paroxysmal, familial E85.0
    benign E85.0
  pelvic
    female N73.5
      acute N73.3

Peritonitis — *continued*
  pelvic — *continued*
    female — *continued*
      chronic N73.4
        with adhesions N73.6
    male K65.0
  periodic, familial E85.0
  proliferative, chronic K65.8
  puerperal, postpartum, childbirth O85
  purulent K65.0
  septic K65.0
  specified NEC K65.8
  spontaneous bacterial K65.2
  subdiaphragmatic K65.0
  subphrenic K65.0
  suppurative K65.0
  syphilitic A52.74
    congenital (early) A50.08 *[K67]*
  talc T81.61 ☑
  tuberculous A18.31
  urine K65.8
Peritonsillar — *see* condition
Peritonsillitis J36
Perityphlitis — *see also* Cecitis K37
Periureteritis N28.89
Periurethral — *see* condition
Periurethritis (gangrenous) — *see* Urethritis
Periuterine — *see* condition
Perivaginitis — *see* Vaginitis
Perivasculitis, retinal H35.06- ☑
Perivasitis (chronic) N49.1
Perivesiculitis (seminal) — *see* Vesiculitis
Perlèche NEC K13.0
  due to
    candidiasis B37.83
    moniliasis B37.83
    riboflavin deficiency E53.0
    vitamin B2 (riboflavin) deficiency E53.0
Pernicious — *see* condition
Pernio, perniosis T69.1 ☑
Perpetrator (of abuse) — *see* Index to External Causes
    of Injury, Perpetrator
Persecution
  delusion F22
  social Z60.5
Perseveration (tonic) R48.8
Persistence, persistent (congenital)
  anal membrane Q42.3
    with fistula Q42.2
  arteria stapedia Q16.3
  atrioventricular canal Q21.20
  branchial cleft NOS Q18.2
    cyst Q18.0
    fistula Q18.0
    sinus Q18.0
  bulbus cordis in left ventricle Q21.8
  canal of Cloquet Q14.0
  capsule (opaque) Q12.8
  cilioretinal artery or vein Q14.8
  cloaca Q43.7
  communication — *see* Fistula, congenital
  convolutions
    aortic arch Q25.46
    fallopian tube Q50.6
    oviduct Q50.6
    uterine tube Q50.6
  double aortic arch Q25.45
  ductus arteriosus (Botalli) Q25.0
  fetal
    circulation P29.38
    form of cervix (uteri) Q51.828
    hemoglobin, hereditary (HPFH) D56.4
  foramen
    Botalli Q21.12
    ovale Q21.12
  Gartner's duct Q52.4
  hemoglobin, fetal (hereditary) (HPFH) D56.4
  hyaloid
    artery (generally incomplete) Q14.0
    system Q14.8
  hymen, in pregnancy or childbirth — *see* Pregnancy,
    complicated by, abnormal, vulva
  lanugo Q84.2
  left
    posterior cardinal vein Q26.8
    root with right arch of aorta Q25.49
    superior vena cava Q26.1
  Meckel's diverticulum Q43.0

Persistence, persistent — *continued*
  Meckel's diverticulum — *continued*
    malignant — *see* Table of Neoplasms, small intes-
      tine, malignant
  mucosal disease (middle ear) — *see* Otitis, media,
    suppurative, chronic, tubotympanic
  nail(s), anomalous Q84.6
  omphalomesenteric duct Q43.0
  organ or site not listed — *see* Anomaly, by site
  ostium
    atrioventriculare commune Q21.23
    primum Q21.20
    secundum Q21.11
  ovarian rests in fallopian tube Q50.6
  pancreatic tissue in intestinal tract Q43.8
  primary (deciduous)
    teeth K00.6
    vitreous hyperplasia Q14.0
  pupillary membrane Q13.89
  rhesus (Rh) titer — *see* Complication(s), transfusion,
    incompatibility reaction, Rh (factor)
  right aortic arch Q25.47
  sinus
    urogenitalis
      female Q52.8
      male Q55.8
    venosus with imperfect incorporation in right auricle
      Q26.8
  thymus (gland) (hyperplasia) E32.0
  thyroglossal duct Q89.2
  thyrolingual duct Q89.2
  truncus arteriosus or communis Q20.0
  tunica vasculosa lentis Q12.2
  umbilical sinus Q64.4
  urachus Q64.4
  vitelline duct Q43.0
Person (with)
  admitted for clinical research, as a control subject
    (normal comparison) (participant) Z00.6
  awaiting admission to adequate facility elsewhere
    Z75.1
  concern (normal) about sick person in family Z63.6
  consulting on behalf of another Z71.0
  feigning illness Z76.5
  living (in)
    alone Z60.2
    boarding school Z59.3
    residential institution Z59.3
    without
      adequate housing (heating) (space) Z59.1
      housing (permanent) (temporary) Z59.00
      person able to render necessary care Z74.2
      shelter Z59.02
  on waiting list Z75.1
  sick or handicapped in family Z63.6
Personality (disorder) F60.9
  accentuation of traits (type A pattern) Z73.1
  affective F34.0
  aggressive F60.3
  amoral F60.2
  anacastic, anankastic F60.5
  antisocial F60.2
  anxious F60.6
  asocial F60.2
  asthenic F60.7
  avoidant F60.6
  borderline F60.3
  change due to organic condition (enduring) F07.0
  compulsive F60.5
  cycloid F34.0
  cyclothymic F34.0
  dependent F60.7
  depressive F34.1
  dissocial F60.2
  dual F44.81
  eccentric F60.89
  emotionally unstable F60.3
  expansive paranoid F60.0
  explosive F60.3
  fanatic F60.0
  haltlose type F60.89
  histrionic F60.4
  hyperthymic F34.0
  hypothymic F34.1
  hysterical F60.4
  immature F60.89
  inadequate F60.7
  labile (emotional) F60.3
  mixed (nonspecific) F60.89

Personality — Phobia, phobic

Index

Personality — *continued*
  morally defective F60.2
  multiple F44.81
  narcissistic F60.81
  obsessional F60.5
  obsessive (-compulsive) F60.5
  organic F07.0
  overconscientious F60.5
  paranoid F60.0
  passive (-dependent) F60.7
  passive-aggressive F60.89
  pathologic F60.9
  pattern defect or disturbance F60.9
  pseudopsychopathic (organic) F07.0
  pseudoretarded (organic) F07.0
  psychoinfantile F60.4
  psychoneurotic NEC F60.89
  psychopathic F60.2
  querulant F60.0
  sadistic F60.89
  schizoid F60.1
  self-defeating F60.89
  sensitive paranoid F60.0
  sociopathic (amoral) (antisocial) (asocial) (dissocial)
      F60.2
  specified NEC F60.89
  type A Z73.1
  unstable (emotional) F60.3
Perthes' disease — *see* Legg-Calvé-Perthes disease
Pertussis — *see also* Whooping cough A37.90
Perversion, perverted
  appetite F50.89
      psychogenic F50.89
  function
      pituitary gland E23.2
          posterior lobe E22.2
  sense of smell and taste R43.8
      psychogenic F45.8
  sexual — *see* Deviation, sexual
Pervious, congenital — *see also* Imperfect, closure
  ductus arteriosus Q25.0
Pes (congenital) — *see also* Talipes
  acquired — *see also* Deformity, limb, foot, specified
      NEC
      planus — *see* Deformity, limb, flat foot
  adductus Q66.89
  cavus Q66.7- ☑
  deformity NEC, acquired — *see* Deformity, limb, foot,
      specified NEC
  planus (acquired) (any degree) — *see also* Deformity,
      limb, flat foot
      rachitic sequelae (late effect) E64.3
  valgus Q66.6
Pest, pestis — *see* Plague
Petechia, petechiae R23.3
  newborn P54.5
Petechial typhus A75.9
Peter's anomaly Q13.4
Petit mal seizure — *see* Epilepsy, childhood, absence
Petit's hernia — *see* Hernia, abdomen, specified site NEC
Petrellidosis B48.2
Petrositis H70.20- ☑
  acute H70.21- ☑
  chronic H70.22- ☑
Peutz-Jeghers disease or syndrome Q85.89
Peyronie's disease N48.6
PFAPA (periodic fever, aphthous stomatitis, pharyngitis,
      and adenopathy syndrome) M04.8
Pfeiffer's disease — *see* Mononucleosis, infectious
Phagedena (dry) (moist) (sloughing) — *see also* Gan-
      grene
  geometric L88
  penis N48.29
  tropical — *see* Ulcer, skin
  vulva N76.6
Phagedenic — *see* condition
Phakoma H35.89
Phakomatosis — *see also* specific eponymous syndromes
      Q85.9
  Bourneville's Q85.1
  specified NEC Q85.89
Phantom limb syndrome (without pain) G54.7
  with pain G54.6
Pharyngeal pouch syndrome D82.1
Pharyngitis (acute) (catarrhal) (gangrenous) (infective)
      (malignant) (membranous) (phlegmonous) (pseu-
      domembranous) (simple) (subacute) (suppurative)
      (ulcerative) (viral) J02.9

Pharyngitis — *continued*
  with influenza, flu, or grippe — *see* Influenza, with,
      pharyngitis
  aphthous B08.5
  atrophic J31.2
  chlamydial A56.4
  chronic (atrophic) (granular) (hypertrophic) J31.2
  coxsackievirus B08.5
  diphtheritic A36.0
  enteroviral vesicular B08.5
  follicular (chronic) J31.2
  fusospirochetal A69.1
  gonococcal A54.5
  granular (chronic) J31.2
  herpesviral B00.2
  hypertrophic J31.2
  infectional, chronic J31.2
  influenzal — *see* Influenza, with, respiratory manifesta-
      tions NEC
  lymphonodular, acute (enteroviral) B08.8
  pneumococcal J02.8
  purulent J02.9
  putrid J02.9
  septic J02.0
  sicca J31.2
  specified organism NEC J02.8
  staphylococcal J02.8
  streptococcal J02.0
  syphilitic, congenital (early) A50.03
  tuberculous A15.8
  vesicular, enteroviral B08.5
  viral NEC J02.8
Pharyngoconjunctivitis, viral B30.2
Pharyngolaryngitis (acute) J06.0
  chronic J37.0
Pharyngoplegia J39.2
Pharyngotonsillitis, herpesviral B00.2
Pharyngotracheitis, chronic J42
Pharynx, pharyngeal — *see* condition
Phencyclidine-induced
  anxiety disorder F16.980
  bipolar and related disorder F16.94
  depressive disorder F16.94
  psychotic disorder F16.959
Phenomenon
  Arthus' — *see* Arthus' phenomenon
  jaw-winking Q07.8
  lupus erythematosus (LE) cell M32.9
  Raynaud's (secondary) I73.00
      with gangrene I73.01
  vasomotor R55
  vasospastic I73.9
  vasovagal R55
  Wenckebach's I44.1
Phenylketonuria E70.1
  classical E70.0
  maternal E70.1
Pheochromoblastoma
  specified site — *see* Neoplasm, malignant, by site
  unspecified site C74.10
Pheochromocytoma
  malignant
      specified site — *see* Neoplasm, malignant, by site
      unspecified site C74.10
  specified site — *see* Neoplasm, benign, by site
  unspecified site D35.00
Pheohyphomycosis — *see* Chromomycosis
Pheomycosis — *see* Chromomycosis
Phimosis (congenital) (due to infection) N47.1
  chancroidal A57
Phlebectasia — *see also* Varix
  congenital Q27.4
Phlebitis (infective) (pyemic) (septic) (suppurative) I80.9
  antepartum — *see* Thrombophlebitis, antepartum
  blue — *see* Phlebitis, leg, deep
  breast, superficial I80.8
  calf muscular vein (NOS) I80.25- ☑
  cavernous (venous) sinus — *see* Phlebitis, intracranial
      (venous) sinus
  cerebral (venous) sinus — *see* Phlebitis, intracranial
      (venous) sinus
  chest wall, superficial I80.8
  cranial (venous) sinus — *see* Phlebitis, intracranial
      (venous) sinus
  deep (vessels) — *see* Phlebitis, leg, deep
  due to implanted device — *see* Complications, by site
      and type, specified NEC
  during or resulting from a procedure T81.72 ☑

Phlebitis — *continued*
  femoral vein (superficial) I80.1- ☑
  femoropopliteal vein I80.0- ☑
  gastrocnemial vein I80.25- ☑
  gestational — *see* Phlebopathy, gestational
  hepatic veins I80.8
  iliac vein (common) (external) (internal) I80.21- ☑
  iliofemoral — *see* Phlebitis, femoral vein
  intracranial (venous) sinus (any) G08
      nonpyogenic I67.6
  intraspinal venous sinuses and veins G08
      nonpyogenic G95.19
  lateral (venous) sinus — *see* Phlebitis, intracranial (ve-
      nous) sinus
  leg I80.3
      antepartum — *see* Thrombophlebitis, antepartum
      deep (vessels) NEC I80.20- ☑
          iliac I80.21- ☑
          popliteal vein I80.22- ☑
          specified vessel NEC I80.29- ☑
          tibial vein (anterior) (posterior) I80.23- ☑
      femoral vein (superficial) I80.1- ☑
      superficial (vessels) I80.0- ☑
  longitudinal sinus — *see* Phlebitis, intracranial (venous)
      sinus
  lower limb — *see* Phlebitis, leg
  migrans, migrating (superficial) I82.1
  pelvic
      with ectopic or molar pregnancy O08.0
      following ectopic or molar pregnancy O08.0
      puerperal, postpartum O87.1
  peroneal vein I80.24- ☑
  popliteal vein — *see* Phlebitis, leg, deep, popliteal
  portal (vein) K75.1
  postoperative T81.72 ☑
  pregnancy — *see* Thrombophlebitis, antepartum
  puerperal, postpartum, childbirth O87.0
      deep O87.1
      pelvic O87.1
      superficial O87.0
  retina — *see* Vasculitis, retina
  saphenous (accessory) (great) (long) (small) — *see*
      Phlebitis, leg, superficial
  sinus (meninges) — *see* Phlebitis, intracranial (venous)
      sinus
  soleal vein I80.25- ☑
  specified site NEC I80.8
  syphilitic A52.09
  tibial vein — *see* Phlebitis, leg, deep, tibial
  ulcerative I80.9
      leg — *see* Phlebitis, leg
  umbilicus I80.8
  uterus (septic) — *see* Endometritis
  varicose (leg) (lower limb) — *see* Varix, leg, with, inflam-
      mation
Phlebofibrosis I87.8
Phleboliths I87.8
Phlebopathy,
  gestational O22.9- ☑
  puerperal O87.9
Phlebosclerosis I87.8
Phlebothrombosis — *see also* Thrombosis
  antepartum — *see* Thrombophlebitis, antepartum
  pregnancy — *see* Thrombophlebitis, antepartum
  puerperal — *see* Thrombophlebitis, puerperal
Phlebotomus fever A93.1
Phlegmasia
  alba dolens O87.1
      nonpuerperal — *see* Phlebitis, femoral vein
  cerulea dolens — *see* Phlebitis, leg, deep
Phlegmon — *see* Abscess
Phlegmonous — *see* condition
Phlyctenulosis (allergic) (keratoconjunctivitis) (nontuber-
      culous) — *see also* Keratoconjunctivitis
  cornea — *see* Keratoconjunctivitis
  tuberculous A18.52
Phobia, phobic F40.9
  animal F40.218
      spiders F40.210
  examination F40.298
  reaction F40.9
  simple F40.298
  social F40.10
      generalized F40.11
  specific (isolated) F40.298
      animal F40.218
          spiders F40.210

Phobia, phobic — *continued*
  specific — *continued*
    blood F40.230
    injection F40.231
    injury F40.233
    men F40.290
    natural environment F40.228
      thunderstorms F40.220
    situational F40.248
      bridges F40.242
      closed in spaces F40.240
      flying F40.243
      heights F40.241
    specified focus NEC F40.298
    transfusion F40.231
    women F40.291
  specified NEC F40.8
    medical care NEC F40.232
  state F40.9
Phocas' disease — *see* Mastopathy, cystic
Phocomelia Q73.1
  lower limb — *see* Agenesis, leg, with foot present
  upper limb — *see* Agenesis, arm, with hand present
Phoria H50.50
Phosphate-losing tubular disorder N25.0
Phosphatemia E83.39
Phosphaturia E83.39
Photodermatitis (sun) L56.8
  chronic L57.8
  due to drug L56.8
  light other than sun L59.8
Photokeratitis H16.13- ☑
Photophobia H53.14- ☑
Photophthalmia — *see* Photokeratitis
Photopsia H53.19
Photoretinitis — *see* Retinopathy, solar
Photosensitivity, photosensitization (sun) skin L56.8
  light other than sun L59.8
Phrenitis — *see* Encephalitis
Phrynoderma (vitamin A deficiency) E50.8
Phthiriasis (pubis) B85.3
  with any infestation classifiable to B85.0-B85.2 B85.4
Phthirus infestation — *see* Phthiriasis
Phthisis — *see also* Tuberculosis
  bulbi (infectional) — *see* Disorder, globe, degenerated condition, atrophy
  eyeball (due to infection) — *see* Disorder, globe, degenerated condition, atrophy
PHTS Q85.81
Phycomycosis — *see* Zygomycosis
Physalopteriasis B81.8
Physical restraint status Z78.1
Phytobezoar T18.9 ☑
  intestine T18.3 ☑
  stomach T18.2 ☑
Pian — *see* Yaws
Pianoma A66.1
Pica F50.89
  in adults F50.89
  infant or child F98.3
Picking, nose F98.8
Pick-Niemann disease — *see* Niemann-Pick disease or syndrome
Pick's
  cerebral atrophy — *see also* Dementia, in, diseases specified elsewhere G31.01 *[F02.80]*
    with behavioral disturbance — *see also* Dementia, in, diseases specified elsewhere G31.01 *[F02.81-]* ☑
  disease or syndrome (brain) — *see also* Dementia, in, diseases specified elsewhere G31.01 *[F02.80]*
    with behavioral disturbance — *see also* Dementia, in, diseases specified elsewhere G31.01 *[F02.81-]* ☑
  brain — *see also* Dementia, in, diseases specified elsewhere G31.01 *[F02.80]*
    with behavioral disturbance — *see also* Dementia, in, diseases specified elsewhere G31.01 *[F02.81-]* ☑
  pericardium (pericardial pseudocirrhosis of liver) I31.1
  syndrome
    brain — *see also* Dementia, in, diseases specified elsewhere G31.01 *[F02.80]*
      with behavioral disturbance — *see also* Dementia, in, diseases specified elsewhere G31.01 *[F02.81-]* ☑

Pick's — *continued*
  syndrome — *continued*
    of heart (pericardial pseudocirrhosis of liver) I31.1
Pickwickian syndrome E66.2
Piebaldism E70.39
Piedra (beard) (scalp) B36.8
  black B36.3
  white B36.2
Pierre Robin deformity or syndrome Q87.0
Pierson's disease or osteochondrosis M91.0
Pig-bel A05.2
Pigeon
  breast or chest (acquired) M95.4
    congenital Q67.7
      rachitic sequelae (late effect) E64.3
  breeder's disease or lung J67.2
  fancier's disease or lung J67.2
  toe — *see* Deformity, toe, specified NEC
Pigmentation (abnormal) (anomaly) L81.9
  conjunctiva H11.13- ☑
  cornea (anterior) H18.01- ☑
    posterior H18.05- ☑
    stromal H18.06- ☑
  diminished melanin formation NEC L81.6
  iron L81.8
  lids, congenital Q82.8
  limbus corneae — *see* Pigmentation, cornea
  metals L81.8
  optic papilla, congenital Q14.2
  retina, congenital (grouped) (nevoid) Q14.1
  scrotum, congenital Q82.8
  tattoo L81.8
Piles — *see also* Hemorrhoids K64.9
Pili
  annulati or torti (congenital) Q84.1
  incarnati L73.1
Pill roller hand (intrinsic) — *see* Parkinsonism
Pilomatrixoma — *see* Neoplasm, skin, benign
  malignant — *see* Neoplasm, skin, malignant
Pilonidal — *see* condition
Pimple R23.8
PIMS M35.81
PIN — *see* Neoplasia, intraepithelial, prostate
Pinched nerve — *see* Neuropathy, entrapment
Pindborg tumor — *see* Cyst, calcifying odontogenic
Pineal body or gland — *see* condition
Pinealoblastoma C75.3
Pinealoma D44.5
  malignant C75.3
Pineoblastoma C75.3
Pineocytoma D44.5
Pinguecula H11.15- ☑
Pingueculitis H10.81- ☑
Pinhole meatus — *see also* Stricture, urethra N35.919
Pink
  disease — *see* subcategory T56.1 ☑
  eye — *see* Conjunctivitis, acute, mucopurulent
Pinkus' disease (lichen nitidus) L44.1
Pinpoint
  meatus — *see* Stricture, urethra
  os (uteri) — *see* Stricture, cervix
Pins and needles R20.2
Pinta A67.9
  cardiovascular lesions A67.2
  chancre (primary) A67.0
  erythematous plaques A67.1
  hyperchromic lesions A67.1
  hyperkeratosis A67.1
  lesions A67.9
    cardiovascular A67.2
    hyperchromic A67.1
    intermediate A67.1
    late A67.2
    mixed A67.3
    primary A67.0
    skin (achromic) (cicatricial) (dyschromic) A67.2
      hyperchromic A67.1
      mixed (achromic and hyperchromic) A67.3
  papule (primary) A67.0
  skin lesions (achromic) (cicatricial) (dyschromic) A67.2
    hyperchromic A67.1
    mixed (achromic and hyperchromic) A67.3
  vitiligo A67.2
Pintids A67.1
Pinworm (disease) (infection) (infestation) B80
Piroplasmosis — *see also* Babesiosis B60.00
  specified NEC B60.09

Pistol wound — *see* Gunshot wound
Pitchers' elbow — *see* Derangement, joint, specified type NEC, elbow
Pithecoid pelvis Q74.2
  with disproportion (fetopelvic) O33.0
    causing obstructed labor O65.0
Pithiatism F48.8
Pitted — *see* Pitting
Pitting — *see also* Edema R60.9
  lip R60.0
  nail L60.8
  teeth K00.4
Pituitary gland — *see* condition
Pituitary-snuff-taker's disease J67.8
Pityriasis (capitis) L21.0
  alba L30.5
  circinata (et maculata) L42
  furfuracea L21.0
  Hebra's L26
  lichenoides L41.0
    chronica L41.1
    et varioliformis (acuta) L41.0
  maculata (et circinata) L30.5
  nigra B36.1
  pilaris, Hebra's L44.0
  rosea L42
  rotunda L44.8
  rubra (Hebra) pilaris L44.0
  simplex L30.5
  specified type NEC L30.5
  streptogenes L30.5
  versicolor (scrotal) B36.0
Placenta, placental — *see* Pregnancy, complicated by (care of) (management affected by), specified condition
Placentitis O41.14- ☑
Plagiocephaly Q67.3
Plague A20.9
  abortive A20.8
  ambulatory A20.8
  asymptomatic A20.8
  bubonic A20.0
  cellulocutaneous A20.1
  cutaneobubonic A20.1
  lymphatic gland A20.0
  meningitis A20.3
  pharyngeal A20.8
  pneumonic (primary) (secondary) A20.2
  pulmonary, pulmonic A20.2
  septicemic A20.7
  tonsillar A20.8
    septicemic A20.7
Planning, family
  contraception Z30.9
  procreation Z31.69
Plaque(s)
  artery, arterial — *see* Arteriosclerosis
  calcareous — *see* Calcification
  coronary, lipid rich I25.83
  epicardial I31.8
  erythematous, of pinta A67.1
  Hollenhorst's — *see* Occlusion, artery, retina
  lipid rich, coronary I25.83
  pleural (without asbestos) J92.9
    with asbestos J92.0
  tongue K13.29
Plasmacytoma C90.3- ☑
  extramedullary C90.2- ☑
  medullary C90.0- ☑
  solitary C90.3- ☑
Plasmacytopenia D72.818
Plasmacytosis D72.822
Plaster ulcer — *see* Ulcer, pressure, by site
Plateau iris syndrome (post-iridectomy) (postprocedural) (without glaucoma) H21.82
  with glaucoma H40.22- ☑
Platybasia Q75.8
Platyonychia (congenital) Q84.6
  acquired L60.8
Platypelloid pelvis M95.5
  with disproportion (fetopelvic) O33.0
    causing obstructed labor O65.0
  congenital Q74.2
Platyspondylisis Q76.49
Plaut (-Vincent) **disease** — *see also* Vincent's A69.1
Plethora R23.2
  newborn P61.1
Pleura, pleural — *see* condition

Pleuralgia R07.81
Pleurisy (acute) (adhesive) (chronic) (costal) (diaphragmatic) (double) (dry) (fibrinous) (fibrous) (interlobar) (latent) (plastic) (primary) (residual) (sicca) (sterile) (subacute) (unresolved) R09.1
  with
    adherent pleura J86.0
    effusion J90
      chylous, chyliform J94.0
      tuberculous (non primary) A15.6
        primary (progressive) A15.7
      tuberculosis — see Pleurisy, tuberculous (non primary)
  encysted — see Pleurisy, with effusion
  exudative — see Pleurisy, with effusion
  fibrinopurulent, fibropurulent — see Pyothorax
  hemorrhagic — see Hemothorax
  pneumococcal J90
  purulent — see Pyothorax
  septic — see Pyothorax
  serofibrinous — see Pleurisy, with effusion
  seropurulent — see Pyothorax
  serous — see Pleurisy, with effusion
  staphylococcal J86.9
  streptococcal J90
  suppurative — see Pyothorax
  traumatic (post) (current) — see Injury, intrathoracic, pleura
  tuberculous (with effusion) (non primary) A15.6
    primary (progressive) A15.7
Pleuritis sicca — see Pleurisy
Pleurobronchopneumonia — see Pneumonia, broncho-
Pleurodynia R07.81
  epidemic B33.0
  viral B33.0
Pleuropericarditis — see also Pericarditis
  acute I30.9
Pleuropneumonia (acute) (bilateral) (double) (septic) — see also Pneumonia J18.8
  chronic — see Fibrosis, lung
Pleuro-pneumonia-like-organism (PPLO), as cause of disease classified elsewhere B96.0
Pleurorrhea — see Pleurisy, with effusion
Plexitis, brachial G54.0
Plica
  polonica B85.0
  syndrome, knee M67.5- ☑
  tonsil J35.8
Plicated tongue K14.5
Plug
  bronchus NEC J98.09
  meconium (newborn) NEC syndrome P76.0
  mucus — see Asphyxia, mucus
Plumbism — see subcategory T56.0 ☑
Plummer's disease E05.20
  with thyroid storm E05.21
Plummer-Vinson syndrome D50.1
Pluricarential syndrome of infancy E40
Plus (and minus) **hand** (intrinsic) — see Deformity, limb, specified type NEC, forearm
PMEI (polymorphic epilepsy in infancy) G40.83- ☑
Pneumathemia — see Air, embolism
Pneumatic hammer (drill) syndrome T75.21 ☑
Pneumatocele (lung) J98.4
  intracranial G93.89
  tension J44.9
Pneumatosis
  cystoides intestinalis K63.89
  intestinalis K63.89
  peritonei K66.8
Pneumaturia R39.89
Pneumoblastoma — see Neoplasm, lung, malignant
Pneumocephalus G93.89
Pneumococcemia A40.3
Pneumococcus, pneumococcal — see condition
Pneumoconiosis (due to) (inhalation of) J64
  with tuberculosis (any type in A15) J65
  aluminum J63.0
  asbestos J61
  bagasse, bagassosis J67.1
  bauxite J63.1
  beryllium J63.2
  coal miners' (simple) J60
  coalworkers' (simple) J60
  collier's J60
  cotton dust J66.0
  diatomite (diatomaceous earth) J62.8

Pneumoconiosis — continued
  dust
    inorganic NEC J63.6
    lime J62.8
    marble J62.8
    organic NEC J66.8
  fumes or vapors (from silo) J68.9
  graphite J63.3
  grinder's J62.8
  kaolin J62.8
  mica J62.8
  millstone maker's J62.8
  mineral fibers NEC J61
  miner's J60
  moldy hay J67.0
  potter's J62.8
  rheumatoid — see Rheumatoid, lung
  sandblaster's J62.8
  silica, silicate NEC J62.8
    with carbon J60
  stonemason's J62.8
  talc (dust) J62.0
Pneumocystis carinii pneumonia B59
Pneumocystis jiroveci (pneumonia) B59
Pneumocystosis (with pneumonia) B59
Pneumohemopericardium I31.2
Pneumohemothorax J94.2
  traumatic S27.2 ☑
Pneumohydropericardium — see Pericarditis
Pneumohydrothorax — see Hydrothorax
Pneumomediastinum J98.2
  congenital or perinatal P25.2
Pneumomycosis B49 [J99]
Pneumonia (acute) (double) (migratory) (purulent) (septic) (unresolved) J18.9
  with
    influenza — see Influenza, with, pneumonia
    lung abscess J85.1
      due to specified organism — see Pneumonia, in (due to)
  2019 (novel) coronavirus J12.82
  adenoviral J12.0
  adynamic J18.2
  alba A50.04
  allergic — see also Pneumonitis, hypersensitivity J82.89
  alveolar — see Pneumonia, lobar
  anaerobes J15.8
  anthrax A22.1
  apex, apical — see Pneumonia, lobar
  Ascaris B77.81
  aspiration J69.0
    due to
      aspiration of microorganisms
        bacterial J15.9
        viral J12.9
      food (regurgitated) J69.0
      gastric secretions J69.0
      milk (regurgitated) J69.0
      oils, essences J69.1
      solids, liquids NEC J69.8
      vomitus J69.0
    newborn P24.81
      amniotic fluid (clear) P24.11
      blood P24.21
      food (regurgitated) P24.31
      liquor (amnii) P24.11
      meconium P24.01
      milk P24.31
      mucus P24.11
      specified NEC P24.81
      stomach contents P24.31
    postprocedural J95.4
  atypical NEC J18.9
  bacillus J15.9
    specified NEC J15.8
  bacterial J15.9
    specified NEC J15.8
  Bacteroides (fragilis) (oralis) (melaninogenicus) J15.8
  basal, basic, basilar — see Pneumonia, by type
  bronchiolitis obliterans organized (BOOP) J84.89
  broncho-, bronchial (confluent) (croupous) (diffuse) (disseminated) (hemorrhagic) (involving lobes) (lobar) (terminal) J18.0
    allergic — see also Pneumonitis, hypersensitivity J82.89
    aspiration — see Pneumonia, aspiration
    bacterial J15.9
      specified NEC J15.8

Pneumonia — continued
  broncho-, bronchial — continued
    chronic — see Fibrosis, lung
    diplococcal J13
    Eaton's agent J15.7
    Escherichia coli (E. coli) J15.5
    Friedländer's bacillus J15.0
    Hemophilus influenzae J14
    hypostatic J18.2
    inhalation — see also Pneumonia, aspiration
      due to fumes or vapors (chemical) J68.0
      of oils or essences J69.1
    Klebsiella (pneumoniae) J15.0
    lipid, lipoid J69.1
      endogenous J84.89
    Mycoplasma (pneumoniae) J15.7
    pleuro-pneumonia-like-organisms (PPLO) J15.7
    pneumococcal J13
    Proteus J15.6
    Pseudomonas J15.1
    Serratia marcescens J15.6
    specified organism NEC J16.8
    staphylococcal — see Pneumonia, staphylococcal
    streptococcal NEC J15.4
      group B J15.3
      pneumoniae J13
    viral, virus — see Pneumonia, viral
  Butyrivibrio (fibriosolvens) J15.8
  Candida B37.1
  caseous — see Tuberculosis, pulmonary
  catarrhal — see Pneumonia, broncho
  chlamydial J16.0
    congenital P23.1
  cholesterol J84.89
  cirrhotic (chronic) — see Fibrosis, lung
  Clostridium (haemolyticum) (novyi) J15.8
  confluent — see Pneumonia, broncho
  congenital (infective) P23.9
    due to
      bacterium NEC P23.6
      Chlamydia P23.1
      Escherichia coli P23.4
      Haemophilus influenzae P23.6
      infective organism NEC P23.8
      Klebsiella pneumoniae P23.6
      Mycoplasma P23.6
      Pseudomonas P23.5
      Staphylococcus P23.2
      Streptococcus (except group B) P23.6
        group B P23.3
      viral agent P23.0
    specified NEC P23.8
  coronavirus (novel) (disease) 2019 J12.82
  COVID-19 J12.82
  croupous — see Pneumonia, lobar
  cryptogenic organizing J84.116
  cytomegalic inclusion B25.0
  cytomegaloviral B25.0
  deglutition — see Pneumonia, aspiration
  desquamative interstitial J84.117
  diffuse — see Pneumonia, broncho
  diplococcal, diplococcus (broncho-) (lobar) J13
  disseminated (focal) — see Pneumonia, broncho
  Eaton's agent J15.7
  embolic, embolism — see Embolism, pulmonary
  Enterobacter J15.6
  eosinophilic J82.81
    acute J82.82
    chronic J82.81
  Escherichia coli (E. coli) J15.5
  Eubacterium J15.8
  fibrinous — see Pneumonia, lobar
  fibroid, fibrous (chronic) — see Fibrosis, lung
  Friedländer's bacillus J15.0
  Fusobacterium (nucleatum) J15.8
  gangrenous J85.0
  giant cell (measles) B05.2
  gonococcal A54.84
  gram-negative bacteria NEC J15.6
    anaerobic J15.8
  Hemophilus influenzae (broncho) (lobar) J14
  human metapneumovirus J12.3
  hypostatic (broncho) (lobar) J18.2
  in (due to)
    actinomycosis A42.0
    adenovirus J12.0
    anthrax A22.1
    ascariasis B77.81

Pneumonia — *continued*
  in — *continued*
    aspergillosis B44.9
    Bacillus anthracis A22.1
    Bacterium anitratum J15.6
    candidiasis B37.1
    chickenpox B01.2
    Chlamydia J16.0
      neonatal P23.1
    coccidioidomycosis B38.2
      acute B38.0
      chronic B38.1
    cytomegalovirus disease B25.0
    Diplococcus (pneumoniae) J13
    Eaton's agent J15.7
    Enterobacter J15.6
    Escherichia coli (E. coli) J15.5
    Friedländer's bacillus J15.0
    fumes and vapors (chemical) (inhalation) J68.0
    gonorrhea A54.84
    Hemophilus influenzae (H. influenzae) J14
    Herellea J15.6
    histoplasmosis B39.2
      acute B39.0
      chronic B39.1
    human metapneumovirus J12.3
    Klebsiella (pneumoniae) J15.0
    measles B05.2
    Mycoplasma (pneumoniae) J15.7
    nocardiosis, nocardiasis A43.0
    ornithosis A70
    parainfluenza virus J12.2
    pleuro-pneumonia-like-organism (PPLO) J15.7
    pneumococcus J13
    pneumocystosis (Pneumocystis carinii) (Pneumocystis jiroveci) B59
    Proteus J15.6
    Pseudomonas NEC J15.1
      pseudomallei A24.1
    psittacosis A70
    Q fever A78
    respiratory syncytial virus (RSV) J12.1
    rheumatic fever I00 *[J17]*
    rubella B06.81
    Salmonella (infection) A02.22
      typhi A01.03
    schistosomiasis B65.9 *[J17]*
    Serratia marcescens J15.6
    specified
      bacterium NEC J15.8
      organism NEC J16.8
    spirochetal NEC A69.8
    Staphylococcus J15.20
      aureus (methicillin susceptible) (MSSA) J15.211
        methicillin resistant (MRSA) J15.212
      specified NEC J15.29
    Streptococcus J15.4
      group B J15.3
      pneumoniae J13
      specified NEC J15.4
    toxoplasmosis B58.3
    tularemia A21.2
    typhoid (fever) A01.03
    varicella B01.2
    virus — *see* Pneumonia, viral
    whooping cough A37.91
      due to
        Bordetella parapertussis A37.11
        Bordetella pertussis A37.01
        specified NEC A37.81
    Yersinia pestis A20.2
  inhalation of food or vomit — *see* Pneumonia, aspiration
  interstitial J84.9
    chronic J84.111
    desquamative J84.117
    due to
      collagen vascular disease J84.178
      known underlying cause J84.178
    idiopathic NOS J84.111
    in disease classified elsewhere J84.178
    lymphocytic (due to collagen vascular disease) (in diseases classified elsewhere) J84.178
    lymphoid J84.2
    non-specific J84.89
      due to
        collagen vascular disease J84.178
        known underlying cause J84.178
        idiopathic J84.113

Pneumonia — *continued*
  interstitial — *continued*
    non-specific — *continued*
      in diseases classified elsewhere J84.178
      plasma cell B59
      pseudomonas J15.1
      usual J84.112
        due to collagen vascular disease J84.178
        idiopathic J84.112
        in diseases classified elsewhere J84.178
    Klebsiella (pneumoniae) J15.0
    lipid, lipoid (exogenous) J69.1
      endogenous J84.89
    lobar (disseminated) (double) (interstitial) J18.1
      bacterial J15.9
        specified NEC J15.8
      chronic — *see* Fibrosis, lung
      Escherichia coli (E. coli) J15.5
      Friedländer's bacillus J15.0
      Hemophilus influenzae J14
      hypostatic J18.2
      Klebsiella (pneumoniae) J15.0
      pneumococcal J13
      Proteus J15.6
      Pseudomonas J15.1
      specified organism NEC J16.8
      staphylococcal — *see* Pneumonia, staphylococcal
      streptococcal NEC J15.4
      Streptococcus pneumoniae J13
      viral, virus — *see* Pneumonia, viral
    lobular — *see* Pneumonia, broncho
    Löffler's J82.89
    lymphoid interstitial J84.2
    massive — *see* Pneumonia, lobar
    meconium P24.01
    MRSA (methicillin resistant Staphylococcus aureus) J15.212
    MSSA (methicillin susceptible Staphylococcus aureus) J15.211
    multilobar — *see* Pneumonia, by type
    Mycoplasma (pneumoniae) J15.7
    necrotic J85.0
    neonatal P23.9
      aspiration — *see* Aspiration, by substance, with pneumonia
    nitrogen dioxide J68.0
    organizing J84.89
      due to
        collagen vascular disease J84.178
        known underlying cause J84.178
      in diseases classified elsewhere J84.178
    orthostatic J18.2
    parainfluenza virus J12.2
    parenchymatous — *see* Fibrosis, lung
    passive J18.2
    patchy — *see* Pneumonia, broncho
    Peptococcus J15.8
    Peptostreptococcus J15.8
    plasma cell (of infants) B59
    pleurolobar — *see* Pneumonia, lobar
    pleuro-pneumonia-like organism (PPLO) J15.7
    pneumococcal (broncho) (lobar) J13
    Pneumocystis (carinii) (jiroveci) B59
    postinfectional NEC B99 ☑ *[J17]*
    postmeasles B05.2
    Proteus J15.6
    Pseudomonas J15.1
    psittacosis A70
    radiation J70.0
    respiratory syncytial virus (RSV) J12.1
    resulting from a procedure J95.89
    rheumatic I00 *[J17]*
    Salmonella (arizonae) (cholerae-suis) (enteritidis) (typhimurium) A02.22
      typhi A01.03
      typhoid fever A01.03
    SARS-associated coronavirus J12.81
    SARS-CoV-2 J12.82
    segmented, segmental — *see* Pneumonia, broncho-
    Serratia marcescens J15.6
    specified NEC J18.8
      bacterium NEC J15.8
      organism NEC J16.8
      virus NEC J12.89
    spirochetal NEC A69.8
    staphylococcal (broncho) (lobar) J15.20
      aureus (methicillin susceptible) (MSSA) J15.211
        methicillin resistant (MRSA) J15.212

Pneumonia — *continued*
  staphylococcal — *continued*
    specified NEC J15.29
  static, stasis J18.2
  streptococcal NEC (broncho) (lobar) J15.4
    group
      A J15.4
      B J15.3
    specified NEC J15.4
  Streptococcus pneumoniae J13
  syphilitic, congenital (early) A50.04
  traumatic (complication) (early) (secondary) T79.8 ☑
  tuberculous (any) — *see* Tuberculosis, pulmonary
  tularemic A21.2
  varicella B01.2
  Veillonella J15.8
  ventilator associated J95.851
  viral, virus (broncho) (interstitial) (lobar) J12.9
    adenoviral J12.0
    congenital P23.0
    human metapneumovirus J12.3
    parainfluenza J12.2
    respiratory syncytial (RSV) J12.1
    SARS-associated coronavirus J12.81
    specified NEC J12.89
  white (congenital) A50.04
Pneumonic — *see* condition
Pneumonitis (acute) (primary) — *see also* Pneumonia
  air-conditioner J67.7
  allergic (due to) J67.9
    organic dust NEC J67.8
    red cedar dust J67.8
    sequoiosis J67.8
    wood dust J67.8
  aspiration J69.0
    due to
      anesthesia J95.4
        during
          labor and delivery O74.0
          pregnancy O29.01- ☑
          puerperium O89.01
      fumes or gases J68.0
    obstetric O74.0
  chemical (due to gases, fumes or vapors) (inhalation) J68.0
    due to anesthesia J95.4
  cholesterol J84.89
  chronic — *see* Fibrosis, lung
  congenital rubella P35.0
  crack (cocaine) J68.0
  due to
    beryllium J68.0
    cadmium J68.0
    crack (cocaine) J68.0
    detergent J69.8
    fluorocarbon-polymer J68.0
    food, vomit (aspiration) J69.0
    fumes or vapors J68.0
    gases, fumes or vapors (inhalation) J68.0
    inhalation
      blood J69.8
      essences J69.1
      food (regurgitated), milk, vomit J69.0
      oils, essences J69.1
      saliva J69.0
      solids, liquids NEC J69.8
    manganese J68.0
    nitrogen dioxide J68.0
    oils, essences J69.1
    solids, liquids NEC J69.8
    toxoplasmosis (acquired) B58.3
      congenital P37.1
    vanadium J68.0
    ventilator J95.851
  eosinophilic J82.81
    acute J82.82
    chronic J82.81
  hypersensitivity J67.9
    air conditioner lung J67.7
    bagassosis J67.1
    bird fancier's lung J67.2
    farmer's lung J67.0
    maltworker's lung J67.4
    maple bark-stripper's lung J67.6
    mushroom worker's lung J67.5
    specified organic dust NEC J67.8
    suberosis J67.3
  interstitial (chronic) J84.89

Pneumonitis — *continued*
- interstitial — *continued*
  - acute J84.114
  - lymphoid J84.2
  - non-specific J84.89
    - idiopathic J84.113
- lymphoid, interstitial J84.2
- meconium P24.01
- postanesthetic J95.4
  - correct substance properly administered — *see* Table of Drugs and Chemicals, by drug, adverse effect
  - in labor and delivery O74.0
  - in pregnancy O29.01- ☑
  - obstetric O74.0
  - overdose or wrong substance given or taken (by accident) — *see* Table of Drugs and Chemicals, by drug, poisoning
  - postpartum, puerperal O89.01
- postoperative J95.4
  - obstetric O74.0
- radiation J70.0
- rubella, congenital P35.0
- ventilation (air-conditioning) J67.7
- ventilator associated J95.851
- wood-dust J67.8

Pneumoconiosis — *see* Pneumoconiosis
Pneumoparotid K11.8
Pneumopathy NEC J98.4
- alveolar J84.09
- due to organic dust NEC J66.8
- parietoalveolar J84.09

Pneumopericarditis — *see also* Pericarditis
- acute I30.9
Pneumopericardium — *see also* Pericarditis
- congenital P25.3
- newborn P25.3
- traumatic (post) — *see* Injury, heart
Pneumophagia (psychogenic) F45.8
Pneumopleurisy, pneumopleuritis — *see also* Pneumonia J18.8
Pneumopyopericardium I30.1
Pneumopyothorax — *see* Pyopneumothorax
- with fistula J86.0
Pneumorrhagia — *see also* Hemorrhage, lung
- tuberculous — *see* Tuberculosis, pulmonary
Pneumothorax NOS J93.9
- acute J93.83
- chronic J93.81
- congenital P25.1
- perinatal period P25.1
- postprocedural J95.811
- specified NEC J93.83
- spontaneous NOS J93.83
  - newborn P25.1
  - primary J93.11
  - secondary J93.12
  - tension J93.0
- tense valvular, infectional J93.0
- tension (spontaneous) J93.0
- traumatic S27.0 ☑
  - with hemothorax S27.2 ☑
- tuberculous — *see* Tuberculosis, pulmonary
Podagra — *see also* Gout M10.9
Podencephalus Q01.9
Poikilocytosis R71.8
Poikiloderma L81.6
- Civatte's L57.3
- congenital Q82.8
- vasculare atrophicans L94.5
Poikilodermatomyositis M33.10
- with
  - myopathy M33.12
  - respiratory involvement M33.11
  - specified organ involvement NEC M33.19
- amyopathic M33.13
- without myopathy M33.13
Pointed ear (congenital) Q17.3
Poison ivy, oak, sumac or other plant dermatitis (allergic) (contact) L23.7
Poisoning (acute) — *see also* Table of Drugs and Chemicals
- algae and toxins T65.82- ☑
- Bacillus B (aertrycke) (cholerae (suis)) (paratyphosus) (suipestifer) A02.9
  - botulinus A05.1
- bacterial toxins A05.9
- berries, noxious — *see* Poisoning, food, noxious, berries

Poisoning — *continued*
- botulism A05.1
- ciguatera fish T61.0- ☑
- Clostridium botulinum A05.1
- death-cap (Amanita phalloides) (Amanita verna) — *see* Poisoning, food, noxious, mushrooms
- drug — *see* Table of Drugs and Chemicals, by drug, poisoning
- epidemic, fish (noxious) — *see* Poisoning, seafood
  - bacterial A05.9
- fava bean D55.0
- fish (noxious) T61.9- ☑
  - bacterial — *see* Intoxication, foodborne, by agent
  - ciguatera fish — *see* Poisoning, ciguatera fish
  - scombroid fish — *see* Poisoning, scombroid fish
  - specified type NEC T61.77- ☑
- food NEC A05.9
  - bacterial — *see* Intoxication, foodborne, by agent
  - due to
    - Bacillus (aertrycke) (choleraesuis) (paratyphosus) (suipestifer) A02.9
      - botulinus A05.1
    - Clostridium (perfringens) (Welchii) A05.2
    - salmonella (aertrycke) (callinarum) (choleraesuis) (enteritidis) (paratyphi) (suipestifer) A02.9
      - with
        - gastroenteritis A02.0
        - sepsis A02.1
    - staphylococcus A05.0
    - Vibrio
      - parahaemolyticus A05.3
      - vulnificus A05.5
  - noxious or naturally toxic T62.9- ☑
    - berries — *see* subcategory T62.1 ☑
    - fish — *see* Poisoning, seafood
    - mushrooms — *see* subcategory T62.0X ☑
    - plants NEC — *see* subcategory T62.2X ☑
    - seafood — *see* Poisoning, seafood
    - specified NEC — *see* subcategory T62.8X ☑
- ichthyotoxism — *see* Poisoning, seafood
- kreotoxism, food A05.9
- latex T65.81- ☑
- lead T56.0- ☑
- mushroom — *see* Poisoning, food, noxious, mushroom
- mussels — *see also* Poisoning, shellfish
  - bacterial — *see* Intoxication, foodborne, by agent
- nicotine (tobacco) T65.2- ☑
- noxious foodstuffs — *see* Poisoning, food, noxious
- plants, noxious — *see* Poisoning, food, noxious, plants NEC
- ptomaine — *see* Poisoning, food
- radiation J70.0
- Salmonella (arizonae) (cholerae-suis) (enteritidis) (typhimurium) A02.9
- scombroid fish T61.1- ☑
- seafood (noxious) T61.9- ☑
  - bacterial — *see* Intoxication, foodborne, by agent
  - fish — *see* Poisoning, fish
  - shellfish — *see* Poisoning, shellfish
  - specified NEC — *see* subcategory T61.8X ☑
- shellfish (amnesic) (azaspiracid) (diarrheic) (neurotoxic) (noxious) (paralytic) T61.78- ☑
  - bacterial — *see* Intoxication, foodborne, by agent
  - ciguatera mollusk — *see* Poisoning, ciguatera fish
- specified substance NEC T65.891 ☑
- Staphylococcus, food A05.0
- tobacco (nicotine) T65.2- ☑
- water E87.79
Poker spine — *see* Spondylitis, ankylosing
Poland syndrome Q79.8
Polioencephalitis (acute) (bulbar) A80.9
- inferior G12.22
- influenzal — *see* Influenza, with, encephalopathy
- superior hemorrhagic (acute) (Wernicke's) E51.2
- Wernicke's E51.2
Polioencephalomyelitis (acute) (anterior) A80.9
- with beriberi E51.2
Polioencephalopathy, superior hemorrhagic E51.2
- with
  - beriberi E51.11
  - pellagra E52
Poliomeningoencephalitis — *see* Meningoencephalitis
Poliomyelitis (acute) (anterior) (epidemic) A80.9
- with paralysis (bulbar) — *see* Poliomyelitis, paralytic
- abortive A80.4
- ascending (progressive) — *see* Poliomyelitis, paralytic
- bulbar (paralytic) — *see* Poliomyelitis, paralytic

Poliomyelitis — *continued*
- congenital P35.8
- nonepidemic A80.9
- nonparalytic A80.4
- paralytic A80.30
  - specified NEC A80.39
  - vaccine-associated A80.0
  - wild virus
    - imported A80.1
    - indigenous A80.2
- spinal, acute A80.9
Poliosis (eyebrow) (eyelashes) L67.1
- circumscripta, acquired L67.1
Pollakiuria R35.0
- psychogenic F45.8
Pollinosis J30.1
Pollitzer's disease L73.2
Polyadenitis — *see also* Lymphadenitis
- malignant A20.0
Polyalgia M79.89
Polyangiitis M30.0
- microscopic M31.7
- overlap syndrome M30.8
Polyarteritis
- microscopic M31.7
- nodosa M30.0
  - with lung involvement M30.1
  - juvenile M30.2
  - related condition NEC M30.8
Polyarthralgia — *see* Pain, joint
Polyarthritis, polyarthropathy — *see also* Arthritis M13.0
- due to or associated with other specified conditions — *see* Arthritis
- epidemic (Australian) (with exanthema) B33.1
- infective — *see* Arthritis, pyogenic or pyemic
- inflammatory M06.4
- juvenile (chronic) (seronegative) M08.3
- migratory M13.8- ☑
- rheumatic, acute — *see* Fever, rheumatic
Polyarthrosis M15.9
- post-traumatic M15.3
- primary M15.0
- specified NEC M15.8
Polycarential syndrome of infancy E40
Polychondritis (atrophic) (chronic) — *see also* Disorder, cartilage, specified type NEC
- relapsing M94.1
Polycoria Q13.2
Polycystic (disease)
- degeneration, kidney Q61.3
  - autosomal dominant (adult type) Q61.2
  - autosomal recessive (infantile type) NEC Q61.19
- kidney Q61.3
  - autosomal
    - dominant Q61.2
    - recessive NEC Q61.19
  - autosomal dominant (adult type) Q61.2
  - autosomal recessive (childhood type) NEC Q61.19
  - infantile type NEC Q61.19
- liver Q44.6
- lung J98.4
  - congenital Q33.0
- ovary, ovaries E28.2
- spleen Q89.09
Polycythemia (secondary) D75.1
- acquired D75.1
- benign (familial) D75.0
- due to
  - donor twin P61.1
  - erythropoietin D75.1
  - fall in plasma volume D75.1
  - high altitude D75.1
  - maternal-fetal transfusion P61.1
  - stress D75.1
- emotional D75.1
- erythropoietin D75.1
- familial (benign) D75.0
- Gaisböck's (hypertonica) D75.1
- high altitude D75.1
- hypertonica D75.1
- hypoxemic D75.1
- neonatorum P61.1
- nephrogenous D75.1
- relative D75.1
- secondary D75.1
- spurious D75.1
- stress D75.1

☑ Additional Character Required — Refer to the Tabular List for Character Selection

Polycythemia — *continued*
  vera D45
Polycytosis cryptogenica D75.1
Polydactylism, polydactyly Q69.9
  toes Q69.2
Polydipsia R63.1
Polydystrophy, pseudo-Hurler E77.Ø
Polyembryoma — *see* Neoplasm, malignant, by site
Polyglandular
  deficiency E31.Ø
  dyscrasia E31.9
  dysfunction E31.9
  syndrome E31.8
Polyhydramnios O4Ø.- ☑
Polymastia Q83.1
Polymenorrhea N92.Ø
Polymyalgia M35.3
  arteritica, giant cell M31.5
  rheumatica M35.3
    with giant cell arteritis M31.5
Polymyositis (acute) (chronic) (hemorrhagic) M33.2Ø
  with
    myopathy M33.22
    respiratory involvement M33.21
    skin involvement — *see* Dermatopolymyositis
    specified organ involvement NEC M33.29
  ossificans (generalisata) (progressiva) — *see* Myositis,
    ossificans, progressiva
Polyneuritis, polyneuritic — *see also* Polyneuropathy
  acute (post-)infective G61.Ø
  alcoholic G62.1
  cranialis G52.7
  demyelinating, chronic inflammatory (CIDP) G61.81
  diabetic — *see* Diabetes, polyneuropathy
  diphtheritic A36.83
  due to lack of vitamin NEC E56.9 *[G63]*
  endemic E51.11
  erythredema — *see* subcategory T56.1 ☑
  febrile, acute G61.Ø
  hereditary ataxic G6Ø.1
  idiopathic, acute G61.Ø
  infective (acute) G61.Ø
  inflammatory, chronic demyelinating (CIDP) G61.81
  nutritional E63.9 *[G63]*
  postinfective (acute) G61.Ø
  specified NEC G62.89
Polyneuropathy (peripheral) G62.9
  alcoholic G62.1
  amyloid (Portuguese) E85.1 *[G63]*
    transthyretin-related (ATTR) familial E85.1 *[G63]*
  arsenical G62.2
  critical illness G62.81
  demyelinating, chronic inflammatory (CIDP) G61.81
  diabetic — *see* Diabetes, polyneuropathy
  drug-induced G62.Ø
  hereditary G6Ø.9
    specified NEC G6Ø.8
  idiopathic G6Ø.9
    progressive G6Ø.3
  in (due to)
    alcohol G62.1
      sequelae G65.2
    amyloidosis, familial (Portuguese) E85.1 *[G63]*
    antitetanus serum G61.1
    arsenic G62.2
      sequelae G65.2
    avitaminosis NEC E56.9 *[G63]*
    beriberi E51.11
    collagen vascular disease NEC M35.9 *[G63]*
    deficiency (of)
      B (-complex) vitamins E53.9 *[G63]*
      vitamin B6 E53.1 *[G63]*
    diabetes — *see* Diabetes, polyneuropathy
    diphtheria A36.83
    drug or medicament G62.Ø
      correct substance properly administered — *see*
        Table of Drugs and Chemicals, by drug,
        adverse effect
      overdose or wrong substance given or taken —
        see Table of Drugs and Chemicals, by drug,
        poisoning
    endocrine disease NEC E34.9 *[G63]*
    herpes zoster B02.23
    hypoglycemia E16.2 *[G63]*
    infectious
      disease NEC B99 ☑ *[G63]*
      mononucleosis B27.91
    lack of vitamin NEC E56.9 *[G63]*

Polyneuropathy — *continued*
  in — *continued*
    lead G62.2
      sequelae G65.2
    leprosy A3Ø.9 *[G63]*
    Lyme disease A69.22
    metabolic disease NEC E88.9 *[G63]*
    microscopic polyangiitis M31.7 *[G63]*
    mumps B26.84
    neoplastic disease — *see also* Neoplasm D49.9 *[G63]*
    nutritional deficiency NEC E63.9 *[G63]*
    organophosphate compounds G62.2
      sequelae G65.2
    parasitic disease NEC B89 *[G63]*
    pellagra E52 *[G63]*
    polyarteritis nodosa M3Ø.Ø
    porphyria E8Ø.2Ø *[G63]*
    radiation G62.82
    rheumatoid arthritis — *see* Rheumatoid, polyneu-
      ropathy
    sarcoidosis D86.89
    serum G61.1
    syphilis (late) A52.15
      congenital A5Ø.43
    systemic
      connective tissue disorder M35.9 *[G63]*
      lupus erythematosus M32.19
    toxic agent NEC G62.2
      sequelae G65.2
    transthyretin-related (ATTR) familial amyloid E85.1
    triorthocresyl phosphate G62.2
      sequelae G65.2
    tuberculosis A17.89
    uremia N18.9 *[G63]*
    vitamin B12 deficiency E53.8 *[G63]*
      with anemia (pernicious) D51.Ø *[G63]*
        due to dietary deficiency D51.3, G63
    zoster B02.23
  inflammatory G61.9
    chronic demyelinating (CIDP) G61.81
    sequelae G65.1
    specified NEC G61.89
  lead G62.2
    sequelae G65.2
  nutritional NEC E63.9 *[G63]*
  postherpetic (zoster) B02.23
  progressive G6Ø.3
  radiation-induced G62.82
  sensory (hereditary) (idiopathic) G6Ø.8
  specified NEC G62.89
  syphilitic (late) A52.15
    congenital A5Ø.43
Polyopia H53.8
Polyorchism, polyorchidism Q55.21
Polyosteoarthritis — *see also* Osteoarthritis, generalized
  M15.9
  post-traumatic M15.3
  specified NEC M15.8
Polyostotic fibrous dysplasia Q78.1
Polyotia Q17.Ø
Polyp, polypus
  accessory sinus J33.8
  adenocarcinoma in — *see* Neoplasm, malignant, by
    site
  adenocarcinoma in situ in — *see* Neoplasm, in situ, by
    site
  adenoid tissue J33.Ø
  adenomatous — *see also* Neoplasm, benign, by site
    adenocarcinoma in — *see* Neoplasm, malignant, by
      site
    adenocarcinoma in situ in — *see* Neoplasm, in situ,
      by site
    carcinoma in — *see* Neoplasm, malignant, by site
    carcinoma in situ in — *see* Neoplasm, in situ, by site
    multiple — *see* Neoplasm, benign
      adenocarcinoma in — *see* Neoplasm, malignant,
        by site
      adenocarcinoma in situ in — *see* Neoplasm, in
        situ, by site
  antrum J33.8
  anus, anal (canal) K62.Ø
  Bartholin's gland N84.3
  bladder D41.4
  carcinoma in — *see* Neoplasm, malignant, by site
  carcinoma in situ in — *see* Neoplasm, in situ, by site
  cecum D12.Ø
  cervix (uteri) N84.1

Polyp, polypus — *continued*
  cervix — *continued*
    in pregnancy or childbirth — *see* Pregnancy, com-
      plicated by, abnormal, cervix
    mucous N84.1
    nonneoplastic N84.1
  choanal J33.Ø
  cholesterol K82.4
  clitoris N84.3
  colon K63.5
    adenomatous D12.6
      ascending D12.2
      cecum D12.Ø
      descending D12.4
      sigmoid D12.5
      transverse D12.3
    ascending K63.5
    cecum K63.5
    descending K63.5
    hyperplastic, (any site) K63.5
    inflammatory K51.4Ø
      with
        abscess K51.414
        complication K51.419
          specified NEC K51.418
        fistula K51.413
        intestinal obstruction K51.412
        rectal bleeding K51.411
    sigmoid K63.5
    transverse K63.5
  corpus uteri N84.Ø
  dental KØ4.Ø1
    irreversible KØ4.Ø2
    reversible KØ4.Ø1
  duodenum K31.7
  ear (middle) H74.4- ☑
  endometrium N84.Ø
  esophageal K22.81
  esophagogastric junction K22.82
  ethmoidal (sinus) J33.8
  fallopian tube N84.8
  female genital tract N84.9
    specified NEC N84.8
  frontal (sinus) J33.8
  gallbladder K82.4
  gingiva, gum KØ6.8
  labia, labium (majus) (minus) N84.3
  larynx (mucous) J38.1
    adenomatous D14.1
  malignant — *see* Neoplasm, malignant, by site
  maxillary (sinus) J33.8
  middle ear — *see* Polyp, ear (middle)
  myometrium N84.Ø
  nares
    anterior J33.9
    posterior J33.Ø
  nasal (mucous) J33.9
    cavity J33.Ø
    septum J33.Ø
  nasopharyngeal J33.Ø
  nose (mucous) J33.9
  oviduct N84.8
  pharynx J39.2
  placenta O9Ø.89
  prostate — *see* Enlargement, enlarged, prostate
  pudenda, pudendum N84.3
  pulpal (dental) KØ4.Ø1
    irreversible KØ4.Ø2
    reversible KØ4.Ø1
  rectum (nonadenomatous) K62.1
    adenomatous — *see* Polyp, adenomatous
  septum (nasal) J33.Ø
  sinus (accessory) (ethmoidal) (frontal) (maxillary)
    (sphenoidal) J33.8
  sphenoidal (sinus) J33.8
  stomach K31.7
    adenomatous D13.1
  tube, fallopian N84.8
  turbinate, mucous membrane J33.8
  umbilical, newborn P83.6
  ureter N28.89
  urethra N36.2
  uterus (body) (corpus) (mucous) N84.Ø
    cervix N84.1
    in pregnancy or childbirth — *see* Pregnancy, com-
      plicated by, tumor, uterus
  vagina N84.2
  vocal cord (mucous) J38.1

Polyp, polypus — *continued*
  vulva N84.3
Polyphagia R63.2
Polyploidy Q92.7
Polypoid — *see* condition
Polyposis — *see also* Polyp
  coli (adenomatous) D12.6
    adenocarcinoma in C18.9
    adenocarcinoma in situ in — *see* Neoplasm, in situ,
      by site
    carcinoma in C18.9
  colon (adenomatous) D12.6
  familial D12.6
    adenocarcinoma in situ in — *see* Neoplasm, in situ,
      by site
  intestinal (adenomatous) D12.6
  malignant lymphomatous C83.1- ☑
  multiple, adenomatous — *see also* Neoplasm, benign
    D36.9
Polyradiculitis — *see* Polyneuropathy
Polyradiculoneuropathy (acute) (postinfective) (seg-
  mentally demyelinating) G61.0
Polyserositis
  due to pericarditis I31.1
  pericardial I31.1
  periodic, familial E85.0
  tuberculous A19.9
    acute A19.1
    chronic A19.8
Polysplenia syndrome Q89.09
Polysyndactyly — *see also* Syndactylism, syndactyly
  Q70.4
Polytrichia L68.3
Polyunguia Q84.6
Polyuria R35.89
  nocturnal R35.81
  psychogenic F45.8
  specified NEC R35.89
Pompe's disease (glycogen storage) E74.02
Pompholyx L30.1
Poncet's disease (tuberculous rheumatism) A18.09
Pond fracture — *see* Fracture, skull
Ponos B55.0
Pons, pontine — *see* condition
Poor
  aesthetic of existing restoration of tooth K08.56
  contractions, labor O62.2
  gingival margin to tooth restoration K08.51
  personal hygiene R46.0
  prenatal care, affecting management of pregnancy —
    see Pregnancy, complicated by, insufficient,
    prenatal care
  sucking reflex (newborn) R29.2
  urinary stream R39.12
  vision NEC H54.7
Poradenitis, nostras inguinalis or venerea A55
Porencephaly (congenital) (developmental) (true) Q04.6
  acquired G93.0
  nondevelopmental G93.0
  traumatic (post) F07.89
Porocephaliasis B88.8
Porokeratosis Q82.8
Poroma, eccrine — *see* Neoplasm, skin, benign
Porphyria (South African) E80.20
  acquired E80.20
  acute intermittent (hepatic) (Swedish) E80.21
  cutanea tarda (hereditary) (symptomatic) E80.1
  due to drugs E80.20
    correct substance properly administered — *see* Ta-
      ble of Drugs and Chemicals, by drug, adverse
      effect
    overdose or wrong substance given or taken — *see*
      Table of Drugs and Chemicals, by drug, poi-
      soning
  erythropoietic (congenital) (hereditary) E80.0
  hepatocutaneous type E80.1
  secondary E80.20
  toxic NEC E80.20
  variegata E80.20
Porphyrinuria — *see* Porphyria
Porphyruria — *see* Porphyria
Port wine nevus, mark, or stain Q82.5
Portal — *see* condition
Posadas-Wernicke disease B38.9
Positive
  culture (nonspecific)
    blood R78.81
    bronchial washings R84.5

Positive — *continued*
  culture — *continued*
    cerebrospinal fluid R83.5
    cervix uteri R87.5
    nasal secretions R84.5
    nipple discharge R89.5
    nose R84.5
      staphylococcus (Methicillin susceptible) Z22.321
        Methicillin resistant Z22.322
    peritoneal fluid R85.5
    pleural fluid R84.5
    prostatic secretions R86.5
    saliva R85.5
    seminal fluid R86.5
    sputum R84.5
    synovial fluid R89.5
    throat scrapings R84.5
    urine R82.79
    vagina R87.5
    vulva R87.5
    wound secretions R89.5
  PPD (skin test) R76.11
  serology for syphilis A53.0
    false R76.8
    with signs or symptoms — *code as* Syphilis, by site
      and stage
  skin test, tuberculin (without active tuberculosis) R76.11
  test, human immunodeficiency virus (HIV) R75
  VDRL A53.0
    with signs or symptoms — *code by* site and stage
      under Syphilis A53.9
  Wassermann reaction A53.0
Post COVID-19 condition, unspecified U09.9
Postcardiotomy syndrome I97.0
Postcaval ureter Q62.62
Postcholecystectomy syndrome K91.5
Postclimacteric bleeding N95.0
Postcommissurotomy syndrome I97.0
Postconcussional syndrome F07.81
Postcontusional syndrome F07.81
Postcricoid region — *see* condition
Post-dates (40-42 weeks) (pregnancy) (mother) O48.0
  more than 42 weeks gestation O48.1
Postencephalitic syndrome F07.89
Posterior — *see* condition
Posterolateral sclerosis (spinal cord) — *see* Degenera-
  tion, combined
Postexanthematous — *see* condition
Postfebrile — *see* condition
Postgastrectomy dumping syndrome K91.1
Posthemiplegic chorea — *see* Monoplegia
Posthemorrhagic anemia (chronic) D50.0
  acute D62
  newborn P61.3
Postherpetic neuralgia (zoster) B02.29
  trigeminal B02.22
Posthitis N47.7
Postimmunization complication or reaction — *see*
  Complications, vaccination
Postinfectious — *see* condition
Postlaminectomy syndrome NEC M96.1
Postleukotomy syndrome F07.0
Postmastectomy lymphedema (syndrome) I97.2
Postmaturity, postmature (over 42 weeks)
  maternal (over 42 weeks gestation) O48.1
  newborn P08.22
Postmeasles complication NEC — *see also* condition
  B05.89
Postmenopausal
  endometrium (atrophic) N95.8
    suppurative — *see also* Endometritis N71.9
  osteoporosis — *see* Osteoporosis, postmenopausal
Postnasal drip R09.82
  due to
    allergic rhinitis — *see* Rhinitis, allergic
    common cold J00
    gastroesophageal reflux — *see* Reflux, gastroe-
      sophageal
    nasopharyngitis — *see* Nasopharyngitis
    other known condition — *code to* condition
    sinusitis — *see* Sinusitis
Postnatal — *see* condition
Postoperative (postprocedural) — *see* Complication,
  postoperative
  pneumothorax, therapeutic Z98.3
  state NEC Z98.890
Postpancreatectomy hyperglycemia E89.1

Postpartum — *see* Puerperal
Postphlebitic syndrome — *see* Syndrome, postthrom-
  botic
Postpolio (myelitic) **syndrome** G14
Postpoliomyelitic — *see also* condition
  osteopathy — *see* Osteopathy, after poliomyelitis
Postprocedural — *see also* Postoperative
  hypoinsulinemia E89.1
Postschizophrenic depression F32.89
Postsurgery status — *see also* Status (post)
  pneumothorax, therapeutic Z98.3
Post-term (40-42 weeks) (pregnancy) (mother) O48.0
  infant P08.21
  more than 42 weeks gestation (mother) O48.1
Post-traumatic brain syndrome, nonpsychotic F07.81
Post-typhoid abscess A01.09
Postures, hysterical F44.2
Postvaccinal reaction or complication — *see* Complications, vaccination
Postvalvulotomy syndrome I97.0
Potain's
  disease (pulmonary edema) — *see* Edema, lung
  syndrome (gastrectasis with dyspepsia) K31.0
POTS (postural orthostatic tachycardia syndrome) G90.A
Potter's
  asthma J62.8
  facies Q60.6
  lung J62.8
  syndrome (with renal agenesis) Q60.6
Pott's
  curvature (spinal) A18.01
  disease or paraplegia A18.01
  spinal curvature A18.01
  tumor, puffy — *see* Osteomyelitis, specified type NEC
Pouch
  bronchus Q32.4
  Douglas' — *see* condition
  esophagus, esophageal, congenital Q39.6
    acquired K22.5
  gastric K31.4
  Hartmann's K82.8
  pharynx, pharyngeal (congenital) Q38.7
Pouchitis K91.850
Poultrymen's itch B88.0
Poverty NEC Z59.6
  extreme Z59.5
Poxvirus NEC B08.8
Prader-Willi syndrome Q87.11
Prader-Willi-like syndrome Q87.19
Preauricular appendage or tag Q17.0
Prebetalipoproteinemia (acquired) (essential) (familial)
  (hereditary) (primary) (secondary) E78.1
  with chylomicronemia E78.3
Precipitate labor or delivery O62.3
Preclimacteric bleeding (menorrhagia) N92.4
Precocious
  adrenarche E30.1
  menarche E30.1
  menstruation E30.1
  pubarche E30.1
  puberty E30.1
    central E22.8
  sexual development NEC E30.1
  thelarche E30.8
Precocity, sexual (constitutional) (cryptogenic) (female)
  (idiopathic) (male) E30.1
  with adrenal hyperplasia E25.9
    congenital E25.0
Precordial pain R07.2
Predeciduous teeth K00.2
Prediabetes, prediabetic R73.03
  complicating
    pregnancy — *see* Pregnancy, complicated by, dis-
      eases of, specified type or system NEC
    puerperium O99.893
Predislocation status of hip at birth Q65.6
Pre-eclampsia O14.9- ☑
  with pre-existing hypertension — *see* Hypertension,
    complicating pregnancy, pre-existing, with, pre-
    eclampsia
  complicating
    childbirth O14.94
    puerperium O14.95
  mild O14.0- ☑
    complicating
      childbirth O14.04
      puerperium O14.05

Pre-eclampsia — *continued*
  moderate O14.0- ☑
    complicating
      childbirth O14.04
      puerperium O14.05
  severe O14.1- ☑
    with hemolysis, elevated liver enzymes and low
        platelet count (HELLP) O14.2- ☑
    complicating
      childbirth O14.24
      puerperium O14.25
    complicating
      childbirth O14.14
      puerperium O14.15
Pre-eruptive color change, teeth, tooth K00.8
Pre-excitation atrioventricular conduction I45.6
Preglaucoma H40.00- ☑
Pregnancy (single) (uterine) — *see also* Delivery and
    Puerperal Z33.1

> *Note: The Tabular must be reviewed for assignment of appropriate seventh character for multiple gestation codes in Chapter 15*

> *Note: The Tabular must be reviewed for assignment of the appropriate character indicating the trimester of the pregnancy*

  abdominal (ectopic) O00.00
    with intrauterine pregnancy O00.01
    with viable fetus O36.7- ☑
  ampullar O00.10- ☑
    with intrauterine pregnancy O00.11- ☑
  biochemical O02.81
  broad ligament O00.80
    with intrauterine pregnancy O00.81
  cervical O00.8
    with intrauterine pregnancy O00.81
  chemical O02.81
  complicated by (care of) (management affected by)
    abnormal, abnormality
      cervix O34.4- ☑
        causing obstructed labor O65.5
      cord (umbilical) O69.9
      fetal heart rate or rhythm O36.83- ☑
      findings on antenatal screening of mother O28.9
        biochemical O28.1
        chromosomal O28.5
        cytological O28.2
        genetic O28.5
        hematological O28.0
        radiological O28.4
        specified NEC O28.8
        ultrasonic O28.3
      glucose (tolerance) NEC O99.810
      pelvic organs O34.9- ☑
        specified NEC O34.8- ☑
          causing obstructed labor O65.5
      pelvis (bony) (major) NEC O33.0
      perineum O34.7- ☑
      position
        placenta O44.0- ☑
          with hemorrhage O44.1- ☑
        uterus O34.59- ☑
      uterus O34.59- ☑
        causing obstructed labor O65.5
        congenital O34.0- ☑
      vagina O34.6- ☑
        causing obstructed labor O65.5
      vulva O34.7- ☑
        causing obstructed labor O65.5
    abruptio placentae — *see* Abruptio placentae
    abscess or cellulitis
      bladder O23.1- ☑
      breast O91.11- ☑
      genital organ or tract O23.9- ☑
    abuse
      physical O9A.31 ☑ (*following* O99)
      psychological O9A.51 ☑ (*following* O99)
      sexual O9A.41 ☑ (*following* O99)
    adverse effect anesthesia O29.9- ☑
      aspiration pneumonitis O29.01- ☑
      cardiac arrest O29.11- ☑
      cardiac complication NEC O29.19- ☑
      cardiac failure O29.12- ☑
      central nervous system complication NEC
        O29.29- ☑
      cerebral anoxia O29.21- ☑

Pregnancy — *continued*
  complicated by — *continued*
    adverse effect anesthesia — *continued*
      failed or difficult intubation O29.6- ☑
      inhalation of stomach contents or secretions NOS
        O29.01- ☑
      local, toxic reaction O29.3X
      Mendelson's syndrome O29.01- ☑
      pressure collapse of lung O29.02- ☑
      pulmonary complications NEC O29.09- ☑
      specified NEC O29.8X- ☑
      spinal and epidural type NEC O29.5X ☑
        induced headache O29.4- ☑
    albuminuria — *see also* Proteinuria, gestational
      O12.1- ☑
    alcohol use O99.31- ☑
    amnionitis O41.12- ☑
    anaphylactoid syndrome of pregnancy O88.01- ☑
    anemia (conditions in D50-D64) (pre-existing)
      O99.01- ☑
      complicating the puerperium O99.03
    antepartum hemorrhage O46.9-
      with coagulation defect — *see* Hemorrhage,
        antepartum, with coagulation defect
      specified NEC O46.8X- ☑
    appendicitis O99.61- ☑
    atrophy (yellow) (acute) liver (subacute) O26.61- ☑
    bariatric surgery status O99.84- ☑
    bicornis or bicornuate uterus O34.0- ☑
    biliary tract problems O26.61- ☑
    breech presentation O32.1
    cardiovascular diseases (conditions in I00-I09, I20-
      I52, I70-I99) O99.41- ☑
    cerebrovascular disorders (conditions in I60-I69)
      O99.41- ☑
    cervical shortening O26.87- ☑
    cervicitis O23.51- ☑
    cesarean scar defect (isthmocele) O34.22
    chloasma (gravidarum) O26.89- ☑
    cholecystitis O99.61- ☑
    cholestasis (intrahepatic) O26.61- ☑
    chorioamnionitis O41.12- ☑
    circulatory system disorder (conditions in I00-I09,
      I20-I99, O99.41-)
    compound presentation O32.6 ☑
    conjoined twins O30.02- ☑
    connective system disorders (conditions in M00-
      M99) O99.891
    contracted pelvis (general) O33.1
      inlet O33.2
      outlet O33.3 ☑
    convulsions (eclamptic) (uremic) — *see also*
      Eclampsia O15.9
    cracked nipple O92.11- ☑
    cystitis O23.1- ☑
    cystocele O34.8- ☑
    death of fetus (near term) O36.4 ☑
      early pregnancy O02.1
      of one fetus or more in multiple gestation
        O31.2- ☑
    deciduitis O41.14- ☑
    decreased fetal movement O36.81- ☑
    dental problems O99.61- ☑
    diabetes (mellitus) O24.91- ☑
      gestational (pregnancy induced) — *see* Diabetes,
        gestational
      pre-existing O24.31- ☑
        specified NEC O24.81- ☑
        type 1 O24.01- ☑
        type 2 O24.11- ☑
    digestive system disorders (conditions in K00-K93)
      O99.61- ☑
    diseases of — *see* Pregnancy, complicated by,
      specified body system disease
      biliary tract O26.61- ☑
      blood NEC (conditions in D65-D77) O99.11- ☑
      liver O26.61- ☑
      specified NEC O99.891
    disorders of — *see* Pregnancy, complicated by,
      specified body system disorder
      amniotic fluid and membranes O41.9- ☑
        specified NEC O41.8X- ☑
      biliary tract O26.61- ☑
      ear and mastoid process (conditions in H60-H95)
        O99.891
      eye and adnexa (conditions in H00-H59) O99.891

Pregnancy — *continued*
  complicated by — *continued*
    disorders of — *see* Pregnancy, complicated by,
      specified body system disorder — *continued*
      liver O26.61- ☑
      skin (conditions in L00-L99) O99.71- ☑
      specified NEC O99.891
    displacement, uterus NEC O34.59- ☑
      causing obstructed labor O65.5
    disproportion (due to) O33.9
      fetal (ascites) (hydrops) (meningomyelocele)
        (sacral teratoma) (tumor) deformities NEC
        O33.7
      generally contracted pelvis O33.1
      hydrocephalic fetus O33.6 ☑
      inlet contraction of pelvis O33.2
      mixed maternal and fetal origin O33.4 ☑
      specified NEC O33.8
    double uterus O34.0- ☑
      causing obstructed labor O65.5
    drug use (conditions in F11-F19) O99.32- ☑
    eclampsia, eclamptic (coma) (convulsions) (delirium)
      (nephritis) (uremia) — *see also* Eclampsia
      O15.- ☑
    ectopic pregnancy — *see* Pregnancy, ectopic
    edema O12.0- ☑
      with
        gestational hypertension, mild — *see also*
          Pre-eclampsia O14.0- ☑
        proteinuria O12.2- ☑
    effusion, amniotic fluid — *see* Pregnancy, complicated by, premature rupture of membranes
    elderly
      multigravida O09.52- ☑
      primigravida O09.51- ☑
    embolism — *see also* Embolism, obstetric, pregnancy O88.- ☑
    endocrine diseases NEC O99.28- ☑
    endometritis O86.12
    excessive weight gain O26.0- ☑
    exhaustion O26.81- ☑
      during labor and delivery O75.81
    face presentation O32.3
    failed induction of labor O61.9
      instrumental O61.1
      mechanical O61.1
      medical O61.0
      specified NEC O61.8
      surgical O61.1
    failed or difficult intubation for anesthesia O29.6- ☑
    false labor (pains) O47.9
      at or after 37 completed weeks of pregnancy
        O47.1
      before 37 completed weeks of pregnancy
        O47.0- ☑
    fatigue O26.81- ☑
      during labor and delivery O75.81
    fatty metamorphosis of liver O26.61- ☑
    female genital mutilation O34.8- ☑ *[N90.81-]* ☑
    fetal (maternal care for)
      abnormality or damage O35.9 ☑
        acid-base balance O68
        specified type NEC O35.8 ☑
      acidemia O68
      acidosis O68
      agenesis of corpus callosum O35.01 ☑
      alkalosis O68
      anemia and thrombocytopenia O36.82- ☑
      anencephaly O35.02 ☑
      bradycardia O36.83- ☑
      cardiac anomalies O35.B ☑
      central nervous system malformation or damage
        O35.00 ☑
        specified type NEC O35.09 ☑
      choroid plexus cysts O35.03 ☑
      chromosomal abnormality (conditions in Q90-
        Q99) O35.10 ☑
        sex chromosome O35.15 ☑
        specified NEC O35.19 ☑
        Trisomy 13 O35.11 ☑
        Trisomy 18 O35.12 ☑
        Trisomy 21 O35.13 ☑
        Turner Syndrome O35.14 ☑
      conjoined twins O30.02- ☑
      damage from
        amniocentesis O35.7 ☑

Pregnancy — *continued*
  complicated by — *continued*
    fetal — *continued*
      damage from — *continued*
        biopsy procedures O35.7 ☑
        drug addiction O35.5 ☑
        hematological investigation O35.7 ☑
        intrauterine contraceptive device O35.7 ☑
        maternal
          alcohol addiction O35.4 ☑
          cytomegalovirus infection O35.3 ☑
          disease NEC O35.8 ☑
          drug addiction O35.5 ☑
          listeriosis O35.8 ☑
          rubella O35.3 ☑
          toxoplasmosis O35.8 ☑
          viral infection O35.3 ☑
        medical procedure NEC O35.7 ☑
        radiation O35.6 ☑
      death (near term) O36.4 ☑
        early pregnancy O02.1
      decreased movement O36.81- ☑
      depressed heart rate tones O36.83- ☑
      disproportion due to deformity (fetal) O33.7 ☑
      encephalocele O35.04 ☑
      excessive growth (large for dates) O36.6- ☑
      facial anomalies O35.A ☑
      gastrointestinal anomalies O35.D ☑
      genitourinary anomalies O35.E ☑
      growth retardation O36.59- ☑
        light for dates O36.59- ☑
        small for dates O36.59- ☑
      heart rate irregularity (abnormal variability)
          (bradycardia) (decelerations) (tachycardia)
          O36.83- ☑
      hereditary disease O35.2 ☑
      holoprosencephaly O35.05 ☑
      hydrocephalus O35.06 ☑
      hydrocephaly O35.06 ☑
      intrauterine death O36.4 ☑
      microcephaly O35.07 ☑
      musculoskeletal anomalies
        lower extremities O35.H ☑
        trunk O35.F ☑
        upper extremities O35.G ☑
      non-reassuring heart rate or rhythm O36.83- ☑
      poor growth O36.59- ☑
        light for dates O36.59- ☑
        small for dates O36.59- ☑
      problem O36.9- ☑
        specified NEC O36.89- ☑
      pulmonary anomalies O35.C ☑
      reduction (elective) O31.3- ☑
      selective termination O31.3- ☑
      spina bifida O35.08 ☑
      thrombocytopenia O36.82- ☑
    fibroid (tumor) (uterus) O34.1- ☑
    fissure of nipple O92.11- ☑
    gallstones O99.61- ☑
    gastric banding status O99.84- ☑
    gastric bypass status O99.84- ☑
    genital herpes (asymptomatic) (history of) (inactive)
        O98.3- ☑
    genital tract infection O23.9- ☑
    glomerular diseases (conditions in N00-N07)
        O26.83- ☑
      with hypertension, pre-existing — *see* Hyperten-
          sion, complicating, pregnancy, pre-exist-
          ing, with, renal disease
    gonorrhea O98.21- ☑
    grand multiparity O09.4 ☑
    habitual aborter — *see* Pregnancy, complicated by,
        recurrent pregnancy loss
    HELLP syndrome (hemolysis, elevated liver enzymes
        and low platelet count) O14.2- ☑
    hemorrhage
      antepartum — *see* Hemorrhage, antepartum
      before 20 completed weeks gestation O20.9
        specified NEC O20.8
      due to premature separation, placenta — *see*
          also Abruptio placentae O45.9- ☑
      early O20.9
        specified NEC O20.8
      threatened abortion O20.0
    hemorrhoids O22.4- ☑
    hepatitis (viral) O98.41- ☑

Pregnancy — *continued*
  complicated by — *continued*
    herniation of uterus O34.59- ☑
    high
      head at term O32.4 ☑
      risk — *see* Supervision (of) (for), high-risk
    history of in utero procedure during previous preg-
        nancy O09.82- ☑
    HIV O98.71- ☑
    human immunodeficiency virus (HIV) disease
        O98.71- ☑
    hydatidiform mole — *see also* Mole, hydatidiform
        O01.9
    hydramnios O40.- ☑
    hydrocephalic fetus (disproportion) O33.6 ☑
    hydrops
      amnii O40.- ☑
      fetalis O36.2- ☑
        associated with isoimmunization — *see also*
            Pregnancy, complicated by, isoimmu-
            nization O36.11- ☑
    hydrorrhea O42.90
    hyperemesis (gravidarum) (mild) — *see also* Hyper-
        emesis, gravidarum O21.0
    hypertension — *see* Hypertension, complicating
        pregnancy
    hypertensive
      heart and renal disease, pre-existing — *see* Hy-
          pertension, complicating, pregnancy, pre-
          existing, with, heart disease, with renal
          disease
      heart disease, pre-existing — *see* Hypertension,
          complicating, pregnancy, pre-existing,
          with, heart disease
      renal disease, pre-existing — *see* Hypertension,
          complicating, pregnancy, pre-existing,
          with, renal disease
    hypotension O26.5- ☑
    immune disorders NEC (conditions in D80-D89)
        O99.11- ☑
    incarceration, uterus O34.51- ☑
    incompetent cervix O34.3- ☑
    inconclusive fetal viability O36.80 ☑
    infection(s) O98.91- ☑
      amniotic fluid or sac O41.10- ☑
      bladder O23.1- ☑
      carrier state NEC O99.830
        streptococcus B O99.820
      genital organ or tract O23.9- ☑
        specified NEC O23.59- ☑
      genitourinary tract O23.9- ☑
      gonorrhea O98.21- ☑
      hepatitis (viral) O98.41- ☑
      HIV O98.71- ☑
      human immunodeficiency virus (HIV) O98.71- ☑
      intrauterine O41.12 ☑
      kidney O23.0- ☑
      nipple O91.01- ☑
      parasitic disease O98.91- ☑
        specified NEC O98.81- ☑
      protozoal disease O98.61- ☑
      sexually transmitted NEC O98.31- ☑
      specified type NEC O98.81- ☑
      syphilis O98.11- ☑
      tuberculosis O98.01- ☑
      urethra O23.2- ☑
      urinary (tract) O23.4- ☑
        specified NEC O23.3- ☑
      viral disease O98.51- ☑
    inflammation
      intrauterine O41.12 ☑
    injury or poisoning (conditions in S00-T88)
        O9A.21- ☑ (*following* O99)
      due to abuse
        physical O9A.31- ☑ (*following* O99)
        psychological O9A.51- ☑ (*following* O99)
        sexual O9A.41- ☑ (*following* O99)
    insufficient
      prenatal care O09.3- ☑
      weight gain O26.1- ☑
    insulin resistance O26.89 ☑
    intrauterine fetal death (near term) O36.4 ☑
      early pregnancy O02.1
      multiple gestation (one fetus or more) O31.2- ☑
    isoimmunization O36.11- ☑
      anti-A sensitization O36.11- ☑

Pregnancy — *continued*
  complicated by — *continued*
    isoimmunization — *continued*
      anti-B sensitization O36.19- ☑
      Rh O36.09- ☑
        anti-D antibody O36.01- ☑
      specified NEC O36.19- ☑
    laceration of uterus NEC O71.81
    malformation
      central nervous system O35.00 ☑
        specified type NEC O35.09 ☑
      placenta, placental (vessel) O43.10- ☑
        specified NEC O43.19- ☑
      uterus (congenital) O34.0- ☑
    malnutrition (conditions in E40-E46) O25.1- ☑
    maternal hypotension syndrome O26.5- ☑
    mental disorders (conditions in F01-F09, F20-F52
        and F54-F99) O99.34- ☑
      alcohol use O99.31- ☑
      drug use O99.32- ☑
      smoking O99.33- ☑
    mentum presentation O32.3 ☑
    metabolic disorders O99.28- ☑
    missed
      abortion O02.1
      delivery O36.4 ☑
    multiple gestations O30.9- ☑
      conjoined twins O30.02- ☑
      quadruplet — *see* Pregnancy, quadruplet
      specified complication NEC O31.8X- ☑
      specified number of multiples NEC — *see* Preg-
          nancy, multiple (gestation), specified NEC
      triplet — *see* Pregnancy, triplet
      twin — *see* Pregnancy, twin
    musculoskeletal condition (conditions is M00-M99)
        O99.891
    necrosis, liver (conditions in K72) O26.61- ☑
    neoplasm
      benign
        cervix O34.4- ☑
        corpus uteri O34.1- ☑
        uterus O34.1- ☑
      malignant O9A.11- ☑ (*following* O99)
    nephropathy NEC O26.83- ☑
    nervous system condition (conditions in G00-G99)
        O99.35- ☑
    nutritional diseases NEC O99.28- ☑
    obesity (pre-existing) O99.21- ☑
    obesity surgery status O99.84- ☑
    oblique lie or presentation O32.2 ☑
    older mother — *see* Pregnancy, complicated by,
        elderly
    oligohydramnios O41.0- ☑
      with premature rupture of membranes — *see*
          also Pregnancy, complicated by, prema-
          ture rupture of membranes O42.- ☑
    onset (spontaneous) of labor after 37 completed
        weeks of gestation but before 39 completed
        weeks gestation, with delivery by (planned)
        cesarean section O75.82
    oophoritis O23.52- ☑
    overdose, drug — *see also* Table of Drugs and
        Chemicals, by drug, poisoning O9A.21- ☑
        (*following* O99)
    oversize fetus O33.5 ☑
    papyraceous fetus O31.0- ☑
    pelvic inflammatory disease O99.891
    periodontal disease O99.61- ☑
    peripheral neuritis O26.82- ☑
    peritoneal (pelvic) adhesions O99.891
    phlebitis O22.9- ☑
    phlebopathy O22.9- ☑
    phlebothrombosis (superficial) O22.2- ☑
      deep O22.3- ☑
    placenta accreta O43.21- ☑
    placenta increta O43.22- ☑
    placenta percreta O43.23- ☑
    placenta previa O44.0- ☑
      complete O44.0- ☑
        with hemorrhage O44.1- ☑
      marginal O44.2- ☑
        with hemorrhage O44.3- ☑
      partial O44.2- ☑
        with hemorrhage O44.3- ☑
    placental disorder O43.9- ☑
      specified NEC O43.89- ☑

Pregnancy — *continued*
  complicated by — *continued*
    placental dysfunction O43.89- ☑
    placental infarction O43.81- ☑
    placental insufficiency O36.51- ☑
    placental transfusion syndromes
      fetomaternal O43.01- ☑
      fetus to fetus O43.02- ☑
      maternofetal O43.01- ☑
    placentitis O41.14- ☑
    pneumonia O99.51- ☑
    poisoning — *see also* Table of Drugs and Chemicals
      O9A.21 ☑ (*following* O99)
    polyhydramnios O40- ☑
    polymorphic eruption of pregnancy O26.86
    poor obstetric history NEC O09.29- ☑
    postmaturity (post-term) (40 to 42 weeks) O48.0
      more than 42 completed weeks gestation (prolonged) O48.1
    pre-eclampsia O14.9- ☑
      mild O14.0- ☑
      moderate O14.0- ☑
      severe O14.1- ☑
        with hemolysis, elevated liver enzymes and
          low platelet count (HELLP) O14.2- ☑
    premature labor — *see* Pregnancy, complicated by,
      preterm labor
    premature rupture of membranes O42.90
      with onset of labor
        within 24 hours O42.00
          at or after 37 weeks gestation, onset of
            labor within 24 hours of rupture
            O42.02
          pre-term (before 37 completed weeks of
            gestation) O42.01- ☑
        after 24 hours O42.10
          at or after 37 weeks gestation, onset of
            labor more than 24 hours following
            rupture O42.12
          pre-term (before 37 completed weeks of
            gestation) O42.11- ☑
        at or after 37 weeks gestation, unspecified as to
          length of time between rupture and onset
          of labor O42.92
        full-term, unspecified as to length of time between rupture and onset of labor O42.92
        pre-term (before 37 completed weeks of gestation) O42.91- ☑
    premature separation of placenta — *see also*
      Abruptio placentae O45.9- ☑
    presentation, fetal — *see* Delivery, complicated by,
      malposition
    preterm delivery O60.10 ☑
    preterm labor
      with delivery O60.10 ☑
        preterm O60.10 ☑
        term O60.20 ☑
      second trimester
        with term delivery O60.22 ☑
        without delivery O60.02
        with preterm delivery
          second trimester O60.12 ☑
          third trimester O60.13 ☑
      third trimester
        with term delivery O60.23 ☑
        without delivery O60.03
        with third trimester preterm delivery
          O60.14 ☑
      without delivery O60.00
        second trimester O60.02
        third trimester O60.03
    previous history of — *see* Pregnancy, supervision
      of, high-risk
    prolapse, uterus O34.52- ☑
    proteinuria (gestational) — *see also* Proteinuria,
      gestational O12.1- ☑
      with edema O12.2- ☑
    pruritic urticarial papules and plaques of pregnancy
      (PUPPP) O26.86
    pruritus (neurogenic) O26.89- ☑
    psychosis or psychoneurosis (puerperal) F53.1
    ptyalism O26.89- ☑
    PUPPP (pruritic urticarial papules and plaques of
      pregnancy) O26.86
    pyelitis O23.0- ☑
    recurrent pregnancy loss O26.2- ☑
    renal disease or failure NEC O26.83- ☑

Pregnancy — *continued*
  complicated by — *continued*
    renal disease or failure — *continued*
      with secondary hypertension, pre-existing —
        see Hypertension, complicating, pregnancy, pre-existing, secondary
      hypertensive, pre-existing — *see* Hypertension,
        complicating, pregnancy, pre-existing,
        with, renal disease
    respiratory condition (conditions in J00-J99)
      O99.51- ☑
    retained, retention
      dead ovum O02.0
      intrauterine contraceptive device O26.3- ☑
    retroversion, uterus O34.53- ☑
    Rh immunization, incompatibility or sensitization
      NEC O36.09- ☑
      anti-D antibody O36.01- ☑
    rupture
      amnion (premature) — *see also* Pregnancy,
        complicated by, premature rupture of
        membranes O42-
      membranes (premature) — *see also* Pregnancy,
        complicated by, premature rupture of
        membranes O42-
      uterus (during labor) O71.1
        before onset of labor O71.0- ☑
    salivation (excessive) O26.89- ☑
    salpingitis O23.52- ☑
    salpingo-oophoritis O23.52- ☑
    sepsis (conditions in A40, A41) O98.81- ☑
    size date discrepancy (uterine) O26.84- ☑
    skin condition (conditions in L00-L99) O99.71- ☑
    smoking (tobacco) O99.33- ☑
    social problem O09.7- ☑
    specified condition NEC O26.89- ☑
    spotting O26.85- ☑
    streptococcus group B (GBS) carrier state O99.820
    subluxation of symphysis (pubis) O26.71- ☑
    syphilis (conditions in A50-A53) O98.11- ☑
    threatened
      abortion O20.0
      labor O47.9
        at or after 37 completed weeks of gestation
          O47.1
        before 37 completed weeks of gestation
          O47.0- ☑
    thrombophlebitis (superficial) O22.2- ☑
    thrombosis O22.9- ☑
      cerebral venous O22.5- ☑
      cerebrovenous sinus O22.5- ☑
      deep O22.3- ☑
    tobacco use disorder (smoking) O99.33- ☑
    torsion of uterus O34.59- ☑
    toxemia O14.9- ☑
    transverse lie or presentation O32.2 ☑
    tuberculosis (conditions in A15-A19) O98.01- ☑
    tumor (benign)
      cervix O34.4- ☑
      malignant O9A.11- ☑ (*following* O99)
      uterus O34.1- ☑
    unstable lie O32.0 ☑
    upper respiratory infection O99.51- ☑
    urethritis O23.2- ☑
    uterine size date discrepancy O26.84- ☑
    vaginitis or vulvitis O23.59- ☑
    varicose veins (lower extremities) O22.0- ☑
      genitals O22.1- ☑
      legs O22.0- ☑
      perineal O22.1- ☑
      vaginal or vulval O22.1- ☑
    venereal disease NEC (conditions in A63.8)
      O98.31- ☑
    venous disorders O22.9- ☑
      specified NEC O22.8X- ☑
    very young mother — *see* Pregnancy, complicated
      by, young mother
    viral diseases (conditions in A80-B09, B25-B34)
      O98.51- ☑
    vomiting O21.9
      due to diseases classified elsewhere O21.8
      hyperemesis gravidarum (mild) — *see also* Hyperemesis, gravidarum O21.0
      late (occurring after 20 weeks of gestation) O21.2
    young mother
      multigravida O09.62- ☑
      primigravida O09.61- ☑

Pregnancy — *continued*
  complicated NOS O26.9- ☑
  concealed O09.3- ☑
  continuing following
    elective fetal reduction of one or more fetus
      O31.3- ☑
    intrauterine death of one or more fetus O31.2- ☑
    spontaneous abortion of one or more fetus
      O31.1- ☑
  cornual O00.80
    with intrauterine pregnancy O00.81
  ectopic (ruptured) O00.90
    with intrauterine pregnancy O00.91
    abdominal O00.00
      with
        intrauterine pregnancy O00.01
          viable fetus O36.7- ☑
    cervical O00.80
      with intrauterine pregnancy O00.81
    complicated (by) O08.9
      afibrinogenemia O08.1
      cardiac arrest O08.81
      chemical damage of pelvic organ(s) O08.6
      circulatory collapse O08.3
      defibrination syndrome O08.1
      electrolyte imbalance O08.5
      embolism (amniotic fluid) (blood clot) (pulmonary) (septic) O08.2
      endometritis O08.0
      genital tract and pelvic infection O08.0
      hemorrhage (delayed) (excessive) O08.1
      infection
        genital tract or pelvic O08.0
        kidney O08.83
        urinary tract O08.83
      intravascular coagulation O08.1
      laceration of pelvic organ(s) O08.6
      metabolic disorder O08.5
      oliguria O08.4
      oophoritis O08.0
      parametritis O08.0
      pelvic peritonitis O08.0
      perforation of pelvic organ(s) O08.6
      renal failure or shutdown O08.4
      salpingitis or salpingo-oophoritis O08.0
      sepsis O08.82
      shock O08.83
        septic O08.82
      specified condition NEC O08.89
      tubular necrosis (renal) O08.4
      uremia O08.4
      urinary infection O08.83
      venous complication NEC O08.7
        embolism O08.2
    cornual O00.80
      with intrauterine pregnancy O00.81
    intraligamentous O00.80
      with intrauterine pregnancy O00.81
    mural O00.80
      with intrauterine pregnancy O00.81
    ovarian O00.20- ☑
      with intrauterine pregnancy O00.21- ☑
    specified site NEC O00.80
      with intrauterine pregnancy O00.81
    tubal (ruptured) O00.10- ☑
      with intrauterine pregnancy O00.11- ☑
  examination (normal) Z34.9- ☑
    first Z34.0- ☑
    high-risk — *see* Pregnancy, supervision of, high-risk
    specified Z34.8- ☑
  extrauterine — *see* Pregnancy, ectopic
  fallopian O00.10- ☑
    with intrauterine pregnancy O00.11- ☑
  false F45.8
  gestational carrier Z33.3
  heptachorionic, hepta-amniotic (septuplets) O30.83- ☑
  hexachorionic, hexa-amniotic (sextuplets) O30.83- ☑
  hidden O09.3- ☑
  high-risk — *see* Pregnancy, supervision of, high-risk
  incidental finding Z33.1
  interstitial O00.80
    with intrauterine pregnancy O00.81
  intraligamentous O00.80
    with intrauterine pregnancy O00.81
  intramural O00.80
    with intrauterine pregnancy O00.81
  intraperitoneal O00.00
    with intrauterine pregnancy O00.01

Pregnancy — *continued*
  isthmian O00.10- ☑
    with intrauterine pregnancy O00.11- ☑
  mesometric (mural) O00.80
    with intrauterine pregnancy O00.81
  molar NEC O02.0
    complicated (by) O08.9
      afibrinogenemia O08.1
      cardiac arrest O08.81
      chemical damage of pelvic organ(s) O08.6
      circulatory collapse O08.3
      defibrination syndrome O08.1
      electrolyte imbalance O08.5
      embolism (amniotic fluid) (blood clot) (pulmonary) (septic) O08.2
      endometritis O08.0
      genital tract and pelvic infection O08.0
      hemorrhage (delayed) (excessive) O08.1
      infection
        genital tract or pelvic O08.0
        kidney O08.83
        urinary tract O08.83
      intravascular coagulation O08.1
      laceration of pelvic organ(s) O08.6
      metabolic disorder O08.5
      oliguria O08.4
      oophoritis O08.0
      parametritis O08.0
      pelvic peritonitis O08.0
      perforation of pelvic organ(s) O08.6
      renal failure or shutdown O08.4
      salpingitis or salpingo-oophoritis O08.0
      sepsis O08.82
      shock O08.3
        septic O08.82
      specified condition NEC O08.89
      tubular necrosis (renal) O08.4
      uremia O08.4
      urinary infection O08.83
      venous complication NEC O08.7
        embolism O08.2
  hydatidiform — *see also* Mole, hydatidiform O01.9
  multiple (gestation) O30.9- ☑
    greater than quadruplets — *see* Pregnancy, multiple (gestation), specified NEC
    specified NEC O30.80- ☑
      with
        two or more monoamniotic fetuses O30.82- ☑
        two or more monochorionic fetuses O30.81- ☑
        number of chorions and amnions are both equal to the number of fetuses O30.83- ☑
        two or more monoamniotic fetuses O30.82- ☑
        two or more monochorionic fetuses O30.81- ☑
        unable to determine number of placenta and number of amniotic sacs O30.89- ☑
        unspecified number of placenta and unspecified number of amniotic sacs O30.80- ☑
  mural O00.80
    with intrauterine pregnancy O00.81
  normal (supervision of) Z34.9- ☑
    first Z34.0- ☑
    high-risk — *see* Pregnancy, supervision of, high-risk
    specified Z34.8- ☑
  ovarian O00.20- ☑
    with intrauterine pregnancy O00.21- ☑
  pentachorionic, penta-amniotic (quintuplets) O30.83- ☑
  postmature (40 to 42 weeks) O48.0
    more than 42 weeks gestation O48.1
  post-term (40 to 42 weeks) O48.0
  prenatal care only Z34.9- ☑
    first Z34.0- ☑
    high-risk — *see* Pregnancy, supervision of, high-risk
    specified Z34.8- ☑
  prolonged (more than 42 weeks gestation) O48.1
  quadruplet O30.20- ☑
    with
      two or more monoamniotic fetuses O30.22- ☑
      two or more monochorionic fetuses O30.21- ☑
    quadrachorionic/quadra-amniotic O30.23- ☑
    two or more monoamniotic fetuses O30.22- ☑
    two or more monochorionic fetuses O30.21- ☑
    unable to determine number of placenta and number of amniotic sacs O30.29- ☑
    unspecified number of placenta and unspecified number of amniotic sacs O30.20- ☑

Pregnancy — *continued*
  quintuplet — *see* Pregnancy, multiple (gestation), specified NEC
  sextuplet — *see* Pregnancy, multiple (gestation), specified NEC
  supervision of
    concealed pregnancy O09.3- ☑
    elderly mother
      multigravida O09.52- ☑
      primigravida O09.51- ☑
    hidden pregnancy O09.3- ☑
    high-risk O09.9- ☑
      due to (history of)
        ectopic pregnancy O09.1- ☑
        elderly — *see* Pregnancy, supervision, elderly mother
        grand multiparity O09.4 ☑
        in utero procedure during previous pregnancy O09.82- ☑
        in vitro fertilization O09.81- ☑
        infertility O09.0- ☑
        insufficient prenatal care O09.3- ☑
        molar pregnancy O09.A- ☑
        multiple previous pregnancies O09.4- ☑
        older mother — *see* Pregnancy, supervision of, elderly mother
        poor reproductive or obstetric history NEC O09.29- ☑ *stillbirth*
        pre-term labor O09.21- ☑
        previous
          neonatal death O09.29- ☑
        social problems O09.7- ☑
        specified NEC O09.89- ☑
        very young mother — *see* Pregnancy, supervision, young mother
      resulting from in vitro fertilization O09.81- ☑
    normal Z34.9- ☑
      first Z34.0- ☑
      specified NEC Z34.8- ☑
    young mother
      multigravida O09.62- ☑
      primigravida O09.61- ☑
  triplet O30.10- ☑
    with
      two or more monoamniotic fetuses O30.12- ☑
      two or more monochorionic fetuses O30.11- ☑
    trichorionic/triamniotic O30.13- ☑
    two or more monoamniotic fetuses O30.12- ☑
    two or more monochorionic fetuses O30.11- ☑
    unable to determine number of placenta and number of amniotic sacs O30.19- ☑
    unspecified number of placenta and unspecified number of amniotic sacs O30.10- ☑
  tubal (with abortion) (with rupture) O00.10- ☑
    with intrauterine pregnancy O00.11- ☑
  twin O30.00- ☑
    conjoined O30.02- ☑
    dichorionic/diamniotic (two placenta, two amniotic sacs) O30.04- ☑
    monochorionic/diamniotic (one placenta, two amniotic sacs) O30.03- ☑
    monochorionic/monoamniotic (one placenta, one amniotic sac) O30.01- ☑
    unable to determine number of placenta and number of amniotic sacs O30.09- ☑
    unspecified number of placenta and unspecified number of amniotic sacs O30.00- ☑
  unwanted Z64.0
  weeks of gestation
    8 weeks Z3A.08 (*following* Z36)
    9 weeks Z3A.09 (*following* Z36)
    10 weeks Z3A.10 (*following* Z36)
    11 weeks Z3A.11 (*following* Z36)
    12 weeks Z3A.12 (*following* Z36)
    13 weeks Z3A.13 (*following* Z36)
    14 weeks Z3A.14 (*following* Z36)
    15 weeks Z3A.15 (*following* Z36)
    16 weeks Z3A.16 (*following* Z36)
    17 weeks Z3A.17 (*following* Z36)
    18 weeks Z3A.18 (*following* Z36)
    19 weeks Z3A.19 (*following* Z36)
    20 weeks Z3A.20 (*following* Z36)
    21 weeks Z3A.21 (*following* Z36)
    22 weeks Z3A.22 (*following* Z36)
    23 weeks Z3A.23 (*following* Z36)
    24 weeks Z3A.24 (*following* Z36)
    25 weeks Z3A.25 (*following* Z36)

Pregnancy — *continued*
  weeks of gestation — *continued*
    26 weeks Z3A.26 (*following* Z36)
    27 weeks Z3A.27 (*following* Z36)
    28 weeks Z3A.28 (*following* Z36)
    29 weeks Z3A.29 (*following* Z36)
    30 weeks Z3A.30 (*following* Z36)
    31 weeks Z3A.31 (*following* Z36)
    32 weeks Z3A.32 (*following* Z36)
    33 weeks Z3A.33 (*following* Z36)
    34 weeks Z3A.34 (*following* Z36)
    35 weeks Z3A.35 (*following* Z36)
    36 weeks Z3A.36 (*following* Z36)
    37 weeks Z3A.37 (*following* Z36)
    38 weeks Z3A.38 (*following* Z36)
    39 weeks Z3A.39 (*following* Z36)
    40 weeks Z3A.40 (*following* Z36)
    41 weeks Z3A.41 (*following* Z36)
    42 weeks Z3A.42 (*following* Z36)
    greater than 42 weeks Z3A.49 (*following* Z36)
    less than 8 weeks Z3A.01 (*following* Z36)
    not specified Z3A.00 (*following* Z36)
Preiser's disease — *see* Osteonecrosis, secondary, due to, trauma, metacarpus
Pre-kwashiorkor — *see* Malnutrition, severe
Preleukemia (syndrome) D46.9
Preluxation, hip, congenital Q65.6
Premature — *see also* condition
  adrenarche E27.0
  aging E34.8
  beats I49.40
    atrial I49.1
    auricular I49.1
    supraventricular I49.1
  birth NEC — *see* Preterm, newborn
  closure, foramen ovale Q21.8
  contraction
    atrial I49.1
    atrioventricular I49.2
    auricular I49.1
    auriculoventricular I49.49
    heart (extrasystole) I49.49
    junctional I49.2
    ventricular I49.3
  delivery — *see also* Pregnancy, complicated by, preterm labor O60.10 ☑
  ejaculation F52.4
  infant NEC — *see* Preterm, newborn
    light-for-dates — *see* Light for dates
  labor — *see* Pregnancy, complicated by, preterm labor
  lungs P28.0
  menopause E28.319
    asymptomatic E28.319
    symptomatic E28.310
  newborn
    extreme (less than 28 completed weeks) — *see* Immaturity, extreme
    less than 37 completed weeks — *see* Preterm, newborn
  puberty E30.1
  rupture membranes or amnion — *see* Pregnancy, complicated by, premature rupture of membranes
  senility E34.8
  thelarche E30.8
  ventricular systole I49.3
Prematurity NEC (less than 37 completed weeks) — *see* Preterm, newborn
  extreme (less than 28 completed weeks) — *see* Immaturity, extreme
Premenstrual
  dysphoric disorder (PMDD) F32.81
  tension (syndrome) N94.3
Premolarization, cuspids K00.2
Prenatal
  care, normal pregnancy — *see* Pregnancy, normal
  screening of mother — *see also* Encounter, antenatal screening Z36.9
  teeth K00.6
Preparatory care for subsequent treatment NEC
  for dialysis Z49.01
    peritoneal Z49.02
Prepartum — *see* condition
Preponderance, left or right ventricular I51.7
Prepuce — *see* condition
PRES (posterior reversible encephalopathy syndrome) I67.83
Presbycardia R54

☑ **Additional Character Required** — Refer to the Tabular List for Character Selection

Presbycusis, presbyacusia H91.1- ☑
Presbyesophagus K22.89
Presbyophrenia F03 ☑
Presbyopia H52.4
Prescription of contraceptives (initial) Z30.019
  barrier Z30.018
  diaphragm Z30.018
  emergency (postcoital) Z30.012
  implantable subdermal Z30.017
  injectable Z30.013
  intrauterine contraceptive device Z30.014
  pills Z30.011
  postcoital (emergency) Z30.012
  repeat Z30.40
    barrier Z30.49
    diaphragm Z30.49
    implantable subdermal Z30.46
    injectable Z30.42
    pills Z30.41
    specified type NEC Z30.49
    transdermal patch hormonal Z30.45
    vaginal ring hormonal Z30.44
  specified type NEC Z30.018
    transdermal patch hormonal Z30.016
    vaginal ring hormonal Z30.015
Presence (of)
  ankle-joint implant (functional) (prosthesis) Z96.66- ☑
  aortocoronary (bypass) graft Z95.1
  arterial-venous shunt (dialysis) Z99.2
  artificial
    eye (globe) Z97.0
    heart (fully implantable) (mechanical) Z95.812
      valve Z95.2
    larynx Z96.3
    lens (intraocular) Z96.1
    limb (complete) (partial) Z97.1- ☑
      arm Z97.1- ☑
        bilateral Z97.15
      leg Z97.1- ☑
        bilateral Z97.16
  audiological implant (functional) Z96.29
  bladder implant (functional) Z96.0
  bone
    conduction hearing device Z96.29
    implant (functional) NEC Z96.7
    joint (prosthesis) — see Presence, joint implant
  cardiac
    defibrillator (functional) (with synchronous cardiac
      pacemaker) Z95.810
    implant or graft Z95.9
      specified type NEC Z95.818
    pacemaker Z95.0
    resynchronization therapy
      defibrillator Z95.810
      pacemaker Z95.0
  cardioverter-defibrillator (ICD) Z95.810
  cerebrospinal fluid drainage device Z98.2
  cochlear implant (functional) Z96.21
  contact lens (es) Z97.3
  coronary artery graft or prosthesis Z95.5
  CRT-D (cardiac resynchronization therapy defibrillator)
    Z95.810
  CRT-P (cardiac resynchronization therapy pacemaker)
    Z95.0
  CSF shunt Z98.2
  dental prosthesis device Z97.2
  dentures Z97.2
  device (external) NEC Z97.8
    cardiac NEC Z95.818
    heart assist Z95.811
    implanted (functional) Z96.9
      specified NEC Z96.89
    prosthetic Z97.8
  ear implant Z96.20
    cochlear implant Z96.21
    myringotomy tube Z96.22
    specified type NEC Z96.29
  elbow-joint implant (functional) (prosthesis) Z96.62- ☑
  endocrine implant (functional) NEC Z96.49
  eustachian tube stent or device (functional) Z96.29
  external hearing-aid or device Z97.4
  finger-joint implant (functional) (prosthetic) Z96.69- ☑
  functional implant Z96.9
    specified NEC Z96.89
  graft
    cardiac NEC Z95.818
    vascular NEC Z95.828
  hearing-aid or device (external) Z97.4

Presence — continued
  hearing-aid or device — continued
    implant (bone) (cochlear) (functional) Z96.21
  heart assist device Z95.811
  heart valve implant (functional) Z95.2
    prosthetic Z95.2
    specified type NEC Z95.4
    xenogenic Z95.3
  hip-joint implant (functional) (prosthesis) Z96.64- ☑
  ICD (cardioverter-defibrillator) Z95.810
  implanted device (artificial) (functional) (prosthetic)
    Z96.9
    automatic cardiac defibrillator (with synchronous
      cardiac pacemaker) Z95.810
    cardiac pacemaker Z95.0
    cochlear Z96.21
    dental Z96.5
    heart Z95.812
    heart valve Z95.2
      prosthetic Z95.2
      specified NEC Z95.4
      xenogenic Z95.3
    insulin pump Z96.41
    intraocular lens Z96.1
    joint Z96.60
      ankle Z96.66- ☑
      elbow Z96.62- ☑
      finger Z96.69- ☑
      hip Z96.64- ☑
      knee Z96.65- ☑
      shoulder Z96.61- ☑
      specified NEC Z96.698
      wrist Z96.63- ☑
    larynx Z96.3
    myringotomy tube Z96.22
    otological Z96.20
      cochlear Z96.21
      eustachian stent Z96.29
      myringotomy Z96.22
      specified NEC Z96.29
      stapes Z96.29
    skin Z96.81
    skull plate Z96.7
    specified NEC Z96.89
    urogenital Z96.0
  insulin pump (functional) Z96.41
  intestinal bypass or anastomosis Z98.0
  intraocular lens (functional) Z96.1
  intrauterine contraceptive device (IUD) Z97.5
  intravascular implant (functional) (prosthetic) NEC
    Z95.9
    coronary artery Z95.5
    defibrillator (with synchronous cardiac pacemaker)
      Z95.810
    peripheral vessel (with angioplasty) Z95.820
  joint implant (prosthetic) (any) Z96.60
    ankle — see Presence, ankle joint implant
    elbow — see Presence, elbow joint implant
    finger — see Presence, finger joint implant
    hip — see Presence, hip joint implant
    knee — see Presence, knee joint implant
    shoulder — see Presence, shoulder joint implant
    specified joint NEC Z96.698
    wrist — see Presence, wrist joint implant
  knee-joint implant (functional) (prosthesis) Z96.65- ☑
  laryngeal implant (functional) Z96.3
  mandibular implant (dental) Z96.5
  myringotomy tube(s) Z96.22
  neurostimulator (brain) (gastric) (peripheral nerve)
    (sacral nerve) (spinal cord) (vagus nerve) Z96.82
  orthopedic-joint implant (prosthetic) (any) — see
    Presence, joint implant
  otological implant (functional) Z96.29
  shoulder-joint implant (functional) (prosthesis)
    Z96.61- ☑
  skull-plate implant Z96.7
  spectacles Z97.3
  stapes implant (functional) Z96.29
  systemic lupus erythematosus [SLE] inhibitor D68.62
  tendon implant (functional) (graft) Z96.7
  tooth root(s) implant Z96.5
  ureteral stent Z96.0
  urethral stent Z96.0
  urogenital implant (functional) Z96.0
  vascular implant or device Z95.9
    access port device Z95.828
    specified type NEC Z95.828
  wrist-joint implant (functional) (prosthesis) Z96.63- ☑

Presenile — see also condition
  dementia F03 ☑
  premature aging E34.8
Presentation, fetal — see Delivery, complicated by,
  malposition
Prespondylolisthesis (congenital) Q76.2
Pressure
  area, skin — see Ulcer, pressure, by site
  brachial plexus G54.0
  brain G93.5
    injury at birth NEC P11.1
  cerebral — see Pressure, brain
  chest R07.89
  cone, tentorial G93.5
  hyposystolic — see also Hypotension
    incidental reading, without diagnosis of hypoten-
      sion R03.1
  increased
    intracranial benign G93.2
      injury at birth P11.0
    intraocular H40.05- ☑
  injury — see Ulcer, pressure, by site
  lumbosacral plexus G54.1
  mediastinum J98.59
  necrosis (chronic) — see Ulcer, pressure, by site
  parental, inappropriate (excessive) Z62.6
  sore (chronic) — see Ulcer, pressure, by site
  spinal cord G95.20
  ulcer (chronic) — see Ulcer, pressure, by site
  venous, increased I87.8
Pre-syncope R55
Preterm
  delivery — see also Pregnancy, complicated by,
    preterm labor O60.10 ☑
  labor — see Pregnancy, complicated by, preterm labor
  newborn (infant) P07.30
    gestational age
      28 completed weeks (28 weeks, 0 days through
        28 weeks, 6 days) P07.31
      29 completed weeks (29 weeks, 0 days through
        29 weeks, 6 days) P07.32
      30 completed weeks (30 weeks, 0 days through
        30 weeks, 6 days) P07.33
      31 completed weeks (31 weeks, 0 days through
        31 weeks, 6 days) P07.34
      32 completed weeks (32 weeks, 0 days through
        32 weeks, 6 days) P07.35
      33 completed weeks (33 weeks, 0 days through
        33 weeks, 6 days) P07.36
      34 completed weeks (34 weeks, 0 days through
        34 weeks, 6 days) P07.37
      35 completed weeks (35 weeks, 0 days through
        35 weeks, 6 days) P07.38
      36 completed weeks (36 weeks, 0 days through
        36 weeks, 6 days) P07.39
Previa
  placenta (total) (without hemorrhage) O44.0- ☑
    with hemorrhage O44.1- ☑
    complete O44.0- ☑
      with hemorrhage O44.1- ☑
    low — see also Delivery, complicated, by, placenta,
      low O44.4- ☑
      with hemorrhage O44.5- ☑
    marginal O44.2- ☑
      with hemorrhage O44.3- ☑
    partial O44.2- ☑
      with hemorrhage O44.3- ☑
  vasa O69.4 ☑
Priapism N48.30
  due to
    disease classified elsewhere N48.32
    drug N48.33
    specified cause NEC N48.39
    trauma N48.31
Prickling sensation (skin) R20.2
Prickly heat L74.0
Primary — see condition
Primigravida
  elderly, affecting management of pregnancy, labor and
    delivery (supervision only) — see Pregnancy,
    complicated by, elderly, primigravida
  older, affecting management of pregnancy, labor and
    delivery (supervision only) — see Pregnancy,
    complicated by, elderly, primigravida
  very young, affecting management of pregnancy, labor
    and delivery (supervision only) — see Pregnancy,
    complicated by, young mother, primigravida

Primipara
  elderly, affecting management of pregnancy, labor and delivery (supervision only) — *see* Pregnancy, complicated by, elderly, primigravida
  older, affecting management of pregnancy, labor and delivery (supervision only) — *see* Pregnancy, complicated by, elderly, primigravida
  very young, affecting management of pregnancy, labor and delivery (supervision only) — *see* Pregnancy, complicated by, young mother, primigravida
Primus varus Q66.21- ☑
PRIND (Prolonged reversible ischemic neurologic deficit) I63.9
Pringle's disease (tuberous sclerosis) Q85.1
Prinzmetal angina I20.1
Prizefighter ear — *see* Cauliflower ear
Problem (with) (related to)
  academic Z55.8
  acculturation Z60.3
  adjustment (to)
    change of job Z56.1
    life-cycle transition Z60.0
    pension Z60.0
    retirement Z60.0
  adopted child Z62.821
  alcoholism in family Z63.72
  atypical parenting situation Z62.9
  bankruptcy Z59.89
  behavioral (adult) F69
    drug seeking Z76.5
  birth of sibling affecting child Z62.898
  care (of)
    provider dependency Z74.9
      specified NEC Z74.8
    sick or handicapped person in family or household Z63.6
  child
    abuse (affecting the child) — *see* Maltreatment, child
    custody or support proceedings Z65.3
    in care of non-parental family member Z62.21
    in foster care Z62.21
    in welfare custody Z62.21
    living in orphanage or group home Z62.22
  child-rearing Z62.9
    specified NEC Z62.898
  communication (developmental) F80.9
  conflict or discord (with)
    boss Z56.4
    classmates Z55.4
    counselor Z64.4
    employer Z56.4
    family Z63.9
      specified NEC Z63.8
    probation officer Z64.4
    social worker Z64.4
    teachers Z55.4
    workmates Z56.4
  conviction in legal proceedings Z65.0
    with imprisonment Z65.1
  counselor Z64.4
  creditors Z59.89
  digestive K92.9
  drug addict in family Z63.72
  ear — *see* Disorder, ear
  economic Z59.9
    affecting care Z59.9
    specified NEC Z59.89
    strain Z59.86
  education Z55.9
    specified NEC Z55.8
  employment Z56.9
    change of job Z56.1
    discord Z56.4
    environment Z56.5
    sexual harassment Z56.81
    specified NEC Z56.89
    stressful schedule Z56.3
    stress NEC Z56.6
    threat of job loss Z56.2
    unemployment Z56.0
  enuresis, child F98.0
  eye H57.9
  failed examinations (school) Z55.2
  falling Z91.81
  family — *see also* Disruption, family Z63.9
    specified NEC Z63.8
  feeding (elderly) (infant) R63.39

Problem — *continued*
  feeding — *continued*
    newborn P92.9
      breast P92.5
      overfeeding P92.4
      slow P92.2
      specified NEC P92.8
      underfeeding P92.3
    nonorganic F50.89
  finance Z59.9
    specified NEC Z59.89
  foreclosure on loan Z59.89
  foster child Z62.822
  frightening experience(s) in childhood Z62.898
  genital NEC
    female N94.9
    male N50.9
  health care Z75.9
    specified NEC Z75.8
  hearing — *see* Deafness
  homelessness Z59.00
  housing Z59.9
    inadequate Z59.1
    isolated Z59.89
    specified NEC Z59.89
  identity (of childhood) F93.8
  illegitimate pregnancy (unwanted) Z64.0
  illiteracy Z55.0
  impaired mobility Z74.09
  imprisonment or incarceration Z65.1
  inadequate teaching affecting education Z55.8
  inappropriate (excessive) parental pressure Z62.6
  influencing health status NEC Z78.9
  in-law Z63.1
  institutionalization, affecting child Z62.22
  intrafamilial communication Z63.8
  jealousy, child F93.8
  landlord Z59.2
  language (developmental) F80.9
  learning (developmental) F81.9
  legal Z65.3
    conviction without imprisonment Z65.0
    imprisonment Z65.1
    release from prison Z65.2
  life-management Z73.9
    specified NEC Z73.89
  life-style Z72.9
    gambling Z72.6
    high-risk sexual behavior (heterosexual) Z72.51
      bisexual Z72.53
      homosexual Z72.52
    inappropriate eating habits Z72.4
    self-damaging behavior NEC Z72.89
    specified NEC Z72.89
    tobacco use Z72.0
  literacy Z55.9
    low level Z55.0
    specified NEC Z55.8
  living alone Z60.2
  lodgers Z59.2
  loss of love relationship in childhood Z62.898
  marital Z63.0
    involving
      divorce Z63.5
      estrangement Z63.5
      gender identity F66
  mastication K08.89
  medical
    care, within family Z63.6
    facilities Z75.9
      specified NEC Z75.8
  mental F48.9
  money Z59.86
  multiparity Z64.1
  negative life events in childhood Z62.9
    altered pattern of family relationships Z62.898
    frightening experience Z62.898
    loss of
      love relationship Z62.898
      self-esteem Z62.898
    physical abuse (alleged) — *see* Maltreatment, child
    removal from home Z62.29
    specified event NEC Z62.898
  neighbor Z59.9
  neurological NEC R29.818
  new step-parent affecting child Z62.898
  none (feared complaint unfounded) Z71.1
  occupational NEC Z56.89
  parent-child — *see* Conflict, parent-child

Problem — *continued*
  personal hygiene Z91.89
  personality F69
  phase-of-life transition, adjustment Z60.0
  presence of sick or disabled person in family or household Z63.79
    needing care Z63.6
  primary support group (family) Z63.9
    specified NEC Z63.8
  probation officer Z64.4
  psychiatric F99
  psychosexual (development) F66
  psychosocial Z65.9
    religious or spiritual Z65.8
    specified NEC Z65.8
  relationship Z63.9
    childhood F93.8
  release from prison Z65.2
    religious or spiritual Z65.8
  removal from home affecting child Z62.29
  seeking and accepting known hazardous and harmful
    behavioral or psychological interventions Z65.8
    chemical, nutritional or physical interventions Z65.8
  sexual function (nonorganic) F52.9
  sight H54.7
  sleep disorder, child F51.9
  smell — *see* Disturbance, sensation, smell
  social
    environment Z60.9
      specified NEC Z60.8
    exclusion and rejection Z60.4
    worker Z64.4
  speech R47.9
    developmental F80.9
    specified NEC R47.89
  swallowing — *see* Dysphagia
  taste — *see* Disturbance, sensation, taste
  tic, child F95.0
  underachievement in school Z55.3
  unemployment Z56.0
    threatened Z56.2
  unwanted pregnancy Z64.0
  upbringing Z62.9
    specified NEC Z62.898
  urinary N39.9
  voice production R47.89
  work schedule (stressful) Z56.3
Procedure (surgical)
  converted
    arthroscopic to open Z53.33
    laparoscopic to open Z53.31
    specified procedure NEC to open Z53.39
    thoracoscopic to open Z53.32
  for purpose other than remedying health state Z41.9
    specified NEC Z41.8
  not done Z53.9
    because of
      administrative reasons Z53.8
      contraindication Z53.09
        smoking Z53.01
      patient's decision Z53.20
        for reasons of belief or group pressure Z53.1
        left against medical advice (AMA) Z53.29
        left without being seen Z53.21
        specified reason NEC Z53.29
      specified reason NEC Z53.8
Procidentia (uteri) N81.3
Proctalgia K62.89
  fugax K59.4
  spasmodic K59.4
Proctitis K62.89
  amebic (acute) A06.0
  chlamydial A56.3
  gonococcal A54.6
  granulomatous — *see* Enteritis, regional, large intestine
  herpetic A60.1
  radiation K62.7
  tuberculous A18.32
  ulcerative (chronic) K51.20
    with
      complication K51.219
        abscess K51.214
        fistula K51.213
        obstruction K51.212
        rectal bleeding K51.211
        specified NEC K51.218
Proctocele
  female (without uterine prolapse) N81.6

☑ **Additional Character Required — Refer to the Tabular List for Character Selection**

Proctocele — *continued*
  female — *continued*
    with uterine prolapse N81.2
      complete N81.3
  male K62.3
Proctocolitis
  allergic K52.29
  food protein-induced K52.29
  food-induced eosinophilic K52.29
  milk protein-induced K52.29
  mucosal — *see* Rectosigmoiditis, ulcerative
Proctoptosis K62.3
Proctorrhagia K62.5
Proctosigmoiditis K63.89
  ulcerative (chronic) — *see* Rectosigmoiditis, ulcerative
Proctospasm K59.4
  psychogenic F45.8
Profichet's disease — *see* Disorder, soft tissue, specified type NEC
Progeria E34.8
Prognathism (mandibular) (maxillary) M26.19
Progonoma (melanotic) — *see* Neoplasm, benign, by site
Progressive — *see* condition
Prolactinoma
  specified site — *see* Neoplasm, benign, by site
  unspecified site D35.2
Prolapse, prolapsed
  anus, anal (canal) (sphincter) K62.2
  arm or hand O32.2 ☑
    causing obstructed labor O64.4 ☑
  bladder (mucosa) (sphincter) (acquired)
    congenital Q79.4
    female — *see* Cystocele
    male N32.89
  breast implant (prosthetic) T85.49 ☑
  cecostomy K94.09
  cecum K63.4
  cervix, cervical (hypertrophied) N81.2
    anterior lip, obstructing labor O65.5
    congenital Q51.828
    postpartal, old N81.2
    stump N81.85
  ciliary body (traumatic) — *see* Laceration, eye(ball), with prolapse or loss of interocular tissue
  colon (pedunculated) K63.4
  colostomy K94.09
  disc (intervertebral) — *see* Displacement, intervertebral disc
  eye implant (orbital) T85.398 ☑
    lens (ocular) — *see* Complications, intraocular lens
  fallopian tube N83.4- ☑
  gastric (mucosa) K31.89
  genital, female N81.9
    specified NEC N81.89
  globe, nontraumatic — *see* Luxation, globe
  ileostomy bud K94.19
  intervertebral disc — *see* Displacement, intervertebral disc
  intestine (small) K63.4
  iris (traumatic) — *see* Laceration, eye(ball), with prolapse or loss of interocular tissue
    nontraumatic H21.89
  kidney N28.83
    congenital Q63.2
  laryngeal muscles or ventricle J38.7
  liver K76.89
  meatus urinarius N36.8
  mitral (valve) I34.1
  ocular lens implant — *see* Complications, intraocular lens
  organ or site, congenital NEC — *see* Malposition, congenital
  ovary N83.4- ☑
  pelvic floor, female N81.89
  perineum, female N81.89
  rectum (mucosa) (sphincter) K62.3
    due to trichuris trichuria B79
  spleen D73.89
  stomach K31.89
  umbilical cord
    complicating delivery O69.0 ☑
  urachus, congenital Q64.4
  ureter N28.89
    with obstruction N13.5
      with infection N13.6
  ureterovesical orifice N28.89
  urethra (acquired) (infected) (mucosa) N36.8

Prolapse, prolapsed — *continued*
  urethra — *continued*
    congenital Q64.71
    urinary meatus N36.8
    congenital Q64.72
  uterovaginal N81.4
    complete N81.3
    incomplete N81.2
  uterus (with prolapse of vagina) N81.4   *w Cystocele*
    complete N81.3
    congenital Q51.818
    first degree N81.2
    in pregnancy or childbirth — *see* Pregnancy, complicated by, abnormal, uterus
    incomplete N81.2
    postpartal (old) N81.4
    second degree N81.2
    third degree N81.3
  uveal (traumatic) — *see* Laceration, eye(ball), with prolapse or loss of interocular tissue
  vagina (anterior) (wall) — *see* Cystocele
    with prolapse of uterus N81.4
      complete N81.3
      incomplete N81.2
    posterior wall N81.6
    posthysterectomy N99.3
  vitreous (humor) H43.0- ☑
    in wound — *see* Laceration, eye(ball), with prolapse or loss of interocular tissue
  womb — *see* Prolapse, uterus
Prolapsus, female N81.9
  specified NEC N81.89
Proliferation(s)
  primary cutaneous CD30-positive large T-cell C86.6
  prostate, atypical small acinar N42.32
Proliferative — *see* condition
Prolonged, prolongation (of)
  bleeding (time) (idiopathic) R79.1
  coagulation (time) R79.1
  gestation (over 42 completed weeks)
    mother O48.1
    newborn P08.22
  interval I44.0
  labor O63.9
    first stage O63.0
    second stage O63.1
  partial thromboplastin time (PTT) R79.1
  pregnancy (more than 42 weeks gestation) O48.1
  prothrombin time R79.1
  QT interval R94.31
  uterine contractions in labor O62.4
Prominence, prominent
  auricle (congenital) (ear) Q17.5
  ischial spine or sacral promontory with disproportion (fetopelvic) O33.0
    causing obstructed labor O65.0
  nose (congenital) acquired M95.0
Promiscuity — *see* High, risk, sexual behavior
Pronation
  ankle — *see* Deformity, limb, foot, specified NEC
  foot — *see also* Deformity, limb, foot, specified NEC
    congenital Q74.2
Prophylactic
  administration of
    antibiotics, long-term Z79.2
      short-term use — *omit code*
    drug — *see also* Long-term (current) drug therapy (use of) Z79.899
  medication Z79.899
  organ removal (for neoplasia management) Z40.00
    breast Z40.01
    fallopian tube(s) Z40.03
      with ovary(s) Z40.02
    ovary(s) Z40.02
    specified site NEC Z40.09
  surgery Z40.9
    for risk factors related to malignant neoplasm — *see* Prophylactic, organ removal
    specified NEC Z40.8
  vaccination Z23
Propionic acidemia E71.121
Proptosis (ocular) — *see also* Exophthalmos
  thyroid — *see* Hyperthyroidism, with goiter
Prosection, anxiety concerning Z65.3
Prosopagnosia R48.3
Prostadynia N42.81
Prostate, prostatic — *see* condition
Prostatism — *see* Hyperplasia, prostate

Prostatitis (congestive) (suppurative) (with cystitis) N41.9
  acute N41.0
  cavitary N41.8
  chronic N41.1
  diverticular N41.8
  due to Trichomonas (vaginalis) A59.02
  fibrous N41.8
  gonococcal (acute) (chronic) A54.22
  granulomatous N41.4
  hypertrophic N41.1
  subacute N41.1
  trichomonal A59.02
  tuberculous A18.14
Prostatocystitis N41.3
Prostatorrhea N42.89
Prostatosis N42.82
Prostration R53.83
  heat — *see also* Heat, exhaustion
    anhydrotic T67.3 ☑
    due to
      salt (and water) depletion T67.4 ☑
      water depletion T67.3 ☑
  nervous F48.8
  senile R54
Protanomaly (anomalous trichromat) H53.54
Protanopia (complete) (incomplete) H53.54
Protection (against) (from) — *see* Prophylactic
Protein
  deficiency NEC — *see* Malnutrition
  malnutrition — *see* Malnutrition
  sickness — *see also* Reaction, serum T80.69 ☑
Proteinemia R77.9
Proteinosis
  alveolar (pulmonary) J84.01
  lipid or lipoid (of Urbach) E78.89
Proteinuria R80.9
  Bence Jones R80.3
  complicating pregnancy — *see* Proteinuria, gestational
  gestational
    complicating
      childbirth O12.14
      pregnancy O12.1- ☑
        with edema O12.2- ☑
      puerperium O12.15
  idiopathic R80.0
  isolated R80.0
    with glomerular lesion N06.9
      C3
        glomerulonephritis N06.A
        glomerulopathy N06.A
          with dense deposit disease N06.6
        dense deposit disease N06.6
        diffuse
          crescentic glomerulonephritis N06.7
          endocapillary proliferative glomerulonephritis N06.4
          mesangiocapillary glomerulonephritis N06.5
        focal and segmental hyalinosis or sclerosis N06.1
        membranous (diffuse) N06.2
        mesangial proliferative (diffuse) N06.3
        minimal change N06.0
        specified pathology NEC N06.8
  orthostatic R80.2
    with glomerular lesion — *see* Proteinuria, isolated, with glomerular lesion
  persistent R80.1
    with glomerular lesion — *see* Proteinuria, isolated, with glomerular lesion
  postural R80.2
    with glomerular lesion — *see* Proteinuria, isolated, with glomerular lesion
  pre-eclamptic — *see* Pre-eclampsia
  puerperal O12.15
  specified type NEC R80.8
Proteolysis, pathologic D65
Proteus (mirabilis) (morganii), **as cause of disease classified elsewhere** B96.4
Prothrombin gene mutation D68.52
Protoporphyria, erythropoietic E80.0
Protozoal — *see also* condition
  disease B64
  specified NEC B60.8
Protrusion, protrusio
  acetabuli M24.7
  acetabulum (into pelvis) M24.7
  device, implant or graft — *see also* Complications, by site and type, mechanical T85.698 ☑

Index

Protrusion, protrusio — Psychosis, psychotic

Protrusion, protrusio — *continued*
  device, implant or graft — *see also* Complications, by
    site and type, mechanical — *continued*
    arterial graft NEC — *see* Complication, cardiovascular device, mechanical, vascular
    breast (implant) T85.49 ☑
    catheter NEC T85.698 ☑
      cystostomy T83.090 ☑
      dialysis (renal) T82.49 ☑
        intraperitoneal T85.691 ☑
      infusion NEC T82.594 ☑
        spinal (epidural) (subdural) T85.690 ☑
      urinary — *see also* Complications, catheter, urinary T83.098 ☑
    electronic (electrode) (pulse generator) (stimulator)
      bone T84.390 ☑
      nervous system — *see* Complication, prosthetic device, mechanical, electronic nervous system stimulator
    fixation, internal (orthopedic) NEC — *see* Complication, fixation device, mechanical
    gastrointestinal — *see* Complications, prosthetic device, mechanical, gastrointestinal device
    genital NEC T83.498 ☑
      intrauterine contraceptive device T83.39 ☑
      penile prosthesis (cylinder) (implanted) (pump) (resevoir) T83.490 ☑
      testicular prosthesis T83.491 ☑
    heart NEC — *see* Complication, cardiovascular device, mechanical
    joint prosthesis — *see* Complications, joint prosthesis, mechanical, specified NEC, by site
    ocular NEC — *see* Complications, prosthetic device, mechanical, ocular device
    orthopedic NEC — *see* Complication, orthopedic, device, mechanical
    specified NEC T85.628 ☑
    urinary NEC — *see also* Complication, genitourinary, device, urinary, mechanical
      graft T83.29 ☑
    vascular NEC — *see* Complication, cardiovascular device, mechanical
    ventricular intracranial shunt T85.09 ☑
  intervertebral disc — *see* Displacement, intervertebral disc
  joint prosthesis — *see* Complications, joint prosthesis, mechanical, specified NEC, by site
  nucleus pulposus — *see* Displacement, intervertebral disc
Prune belly (syndrome) Q79.4
Prurigo (ferox) (gravis) (Hebrae) (Hebra's) (mitis) (simplex) L28.2
  Besnier's L20.0
  estivalis L56.4
  nodularis L28.1
  psychogenic F45.8
Pruritus, pruritic (essential) L29.9
  ani, anus L29.0
    psychogenic F45.8
  anogenital L29.3
    psychogenic F45.8
  due to onchocerca volvulus B73.1
  gravidarum — *see* Pregnancy, complicated by, specified pregnancy-related condition NEC
  hiemalis L29.8
  neurogenic (any site) F45.8
  perianal L29.0
  psychogenic (any site) F45.8
  scroti, scrotum L29.1
    psychogenic F45.8
  senile, senilis L29.8
  specified NEC L29.8
    psychogenic F45.8
  Trichomonas A59.9
  vulva, vulvae L29.2
    psychogenic F45.8
Pseudarthrosis, pseudoarthrosis (bone) — *see* Nonunion, fracture
  clavicle, congenital Q74.0
  joint, following fusion or arthrodesis M96.0
Pseudoaneurysm — *see* Aneurysm
Pseudoangina (pectoris) — *see* Angina
Pseudoangioma I81
Pseudoarteriosus Q28.8
Pseudoarthrosis — *see* Pseudarthrosis
Pseudobulbar affect (PBA) F48.2
Pseudochromhidrosis L67.8

Pseudocirrhosis, liver, pericardial I31.1
Pseudocowpox B08.03
Pseudocoxalgia M91.3- ☑
Pseudocroup J38.5
Pseudo-Cushing's syndrome, alcohol-induced E24.4
Pseudocyesis F45.8
Pseudocyst
  lung J98.4
  pancreas K86.3
  retina — *see* Cyst, retina
Pseudoelephantiasis neuroarthritica Q82.0
Pseudoexfoliation, capsule (lens) — *see* Cataract, specified NEC
Pseudofolliculitis barbae L73.1
Pseudoglioma H44.89
Pseudohemophilia (Bernuth's) (hereditary) (type B) — *see* Disease, von Willebrand
  Type A D69.8
  vascular D69.8
Pseudohermaphroditism Q56.3
  adrenal E25.8
  female — *see also* Disorder, adrenogenital Q56.2
    with adrenocortical disorder E25.8
    without adrenocortical disorder Q56.2
    adrenal (congenital) E25.0
  male — *see also* Disorder, adrenogenital Q56.1
    with
      5-alpha-reductase deficiency E29.1
      adrenocortical disorder E25.8
      androgen resistance E34.51
      cleft scrotum Q56.1
      feminizing testis E34.51
    without gonadal disorder Q56.1
  adrenal E25.8
Pseudo-Hurler's polydystrophy E77.0
Pseudohydrocephalus G93.2
Pseudohypertrophic muscular dystrophy (Erb's) G71.02
Pseudohypertrophy, muscle — *see also* Dystrophy, muscular, by type, if applicable G71.09
Pseudohypoparathyroidism E20.1
Pseudoinsomnia F51.03
Pseudoleukemia, infantile D64.89
Pseudomembranous — *see* condition
Pseudomeningocele (cerebral) (infective) (post-traumatic) G96.198
  postprocedural (spinal) G97.82
Pseudomenses (newborn) P54.6
Pseudomenstruation (newborn) P54.6
Pseudomonas
  aeruginosa, as cause of disease classified elsewhere B96.5
  mallei infection A24.0
    as cause of disease classified elsewhere B96.5
  pseudomallei, as cause of disease classified elsewhere B96.5
Pseudomyotonia G71.19
Pseudomyxoma peritonei C78.6
Pseudoneuritis, optic (nerve) (disc) (papilla), **congenital** Q14.2
Pseudo-obstruction intestine (acute) (chronic) (idiopathic) (intermittent secondary) (primary) K59.89
  colonic K59.81
Pseudopapilledema H47.33- ☑
  congenital Q14.2
Pseudoparalysis
  arm or leg R29.818
  atonic, congenital P94.2
Pseudopelade L66.0
Pseudophakia Z96.1
Pseudopolyarthritis, rhizomelic M35.3
Pseudopolycythemia D75.1
Pseudopseudohypoparathyroidism E20.1
Pseudopterygium H11.81- ☑
Pseudoptosis (eyelid) — *see* Blepharochalasis
Pseudopuberty, precocious
  female heterosexual E25.8
  male isosexual E25.8
Pseudorickets (renal) N25.0
Pseudorubella B08.20
Pseudosclerema, newborn P83.88
Pseudosclerosis (brain)
  Jakob's — *see* Creutzfeldt-Jakob disease or syndrome of Westphal (Strümpell) E83.01
  spastic — *see* Creutzfeldt-Jakob disease or syndrome
Pseudotetanus — *see* Convulsions
Pseudotetany R29.0

Pseudotetany — *continued*
  hysterical F44.5
Pseudotruncus arteriosus Q25.49
Pseudotuberculosis A28.2
  enterocolitis A04.8
  pasteurella (infection) A28.0
Pseudotumor G93.2
  cerebri G93.2
  orbital H05.11 ☑
Pseudoxanthoma elasticum Q82.8
Psilosis (sprue) (tropical) K90.1
  nontropical K90.0
Psittacosis A70
Psoitis M60.88
Psoriasis L40.9
  arthropathic L40.50
    arthritis mutilans L40.52
    distal interphalangeal L40.51
    juvenile L40.54
    other specified L40.59
    spondylitis L40.53
  buccal K13.29
  flexural L40.8
  guttate L40.4
  mouth K13.29
  nummular L40.0
  plaque L40.0
  psychogenic F54
  pustular (generalized) L40.1
    palmaris et plantaris L40.3
  specified NEC L40.8
  vulgaris L40.0
Psychasthenia F48.8
Psychiatric disorder or problem F99
Psychogenic — *see also* condition
  factors associated with physical conditions F54
Psychological and behavioral factors affecting medical condition F59
Psychoneurosis, psychoneurotic — *see also* Neurosis
  anxiety (state) F41.1
  depersonalization F48.1
  hypochondriacal F45.21
  hysteria F44.9
  neurasthenic F48.8
  personality NEC F60.89
Psychopathy, psychopathic
  affectionless F94.2
  autistic F84.5
  constitution, post-traumatic F07.81
  personality — *see* Disorder, personality
  sexual — *see* Deviation, sexual
  state F60.2
Psychosexual identity disorder of childhood F64.2
Psychosis, psychotic F29
  acute (transient) F23
    hysterical F44.9
  affective — *see* Disorder, mood
  alcoholic F10.959
    with
      abuse F10.159
      anxiety disorder F10.980
        with
          abuse F10.180
          dependence F10.280
      delirium tremens F10.231
      delusions F10.950
        with
          abuse F10.150
          dependence F10.250
      dementia F10.97
        with dependence F10.27
      dependence F10.259
      hallucinosis F10.951
        with
          abuse F10.151
          dependence F10.251
      mood disorder F10.94
        with
          abuse F10.14
          dependence F10.24
      paranoia F10.950
        with
          abuse F10.150
          dependence F10.250
      persisting amnesia F10.96
        with dependence F10.26
    amnestic confabulatory F10.96
      with dependence F10.26

Psychosis, psychotic — *continued*
  alcoholic — *continued*
    delirium tremens F10.231
    Korsakoff's, Korsakov's, Korsakow's F10.26
    paranoid type F10.950
      with
        abuse F10.150
        dependence F10.250
  anergastic — *see* Psychosis, organic
  arteriosclerotic (simple type) (uncomplicated) — *see also* Dementia, vascular F01.50
    with behavioral disturbance — *see* Dementia, vascular
  childhood F84.0
    atypical F84.8
  climacteric — *see* Psychosis, involutional
  confusional F29
    acute or subacute F05
    reactive F23
  cycloid F23
  depressive — *see* Disorder, depressive
  disintegrative (childhood) F84.3
  drug-induced — *see* F11-F19 with .X59
    paranoid and hallucinatory states — *see* F11-F19 with .X50 or .X51
  due to or associated with
    addiction, drug — *see* F11-F19 with .X59
    dependence
      alcohol F10.259
      drug — *see* F11-F19 with .X59
    epilepsy F06.8
    Huntington's chorea F06.8
    ischemia, cerebrovascular (generalized) F06.8
    multiple sclerosis F06.8
    physical disease F06.8
    presenile dementia F03 ☑
    senile dementia F03 ☑
    vascular disease (arteriosclerotic) (cerebral) — *see also* Dementia, vascular F01.50
      with behavioral disturbance — *see* Dementia, vascular
  epileptic F06.8
  episode F23
    due to or associated with physical condition F06.8
  exhaustive F43.0
  hallucinatory, chronic F28
  hypomanic F30.8
  hysterical (acute) F44.9
  induced F24
  infantile F84.0
    atypical F84.8
  infective (acute) (subacute) F05
  involutional F28
    depressive — *see* Disorder, depressive
    melancholic — *see* Disorder, depressive
    paranoid (state) F22
  Korsakoff's, Korsakov's, Korsakow's (nonalcoholic) F04
    alcoholic F10.96
      in dependence F10.26
    induced by other psychoactive substance — *see* categories F11-F19 with .X5X
  mania, manic (single episode) F30.2
    recurrent type F31.89
  manic-depressive — *see* Disorder, bipolar
  menopausal — *see* Psychosis, involutional
  mixed schizophrenic and affective F25.8
  multi-infarct (cerebrovascular) — *see also* Dementia, vascular F01.50
    with behavioral disturbance — *see* Dementia, vascular
  nonorganic F29
    specified NEC F28
  organic F09
    due to or associated with
      arteriosclerosis (cerebral) — *see* Psychosis, arteriosclerotic
      cerebrovascular disease, arteriosclerotic — *see* Psychosis, arteriosclerotic
      childbirth — *see* Psychosis, puerperal
      Creutzfeldt-Jakob disease or syndrome — *see* Creutzfeldt-Jakob disease or syndrome
      dependence, alcohol F10.259
      disease
        alcoholic liver F10.259
        brain, arteriosclerotic — *see* Psychosis, arteriosclerotic
        cerebrovascular — *see also* Dementia, vascular F01.50

Psychosis, psychotic — *continued*
  organic — *continued*
    due to or associated with — *continued*
      disease — *continued*
        cerebrovascular — *see also* Dementia, vascular — *continued*
          with behavioral disturbance — *see* Dementia, vascular
        Creutzfeldt-Jakob — *see* Creutzfeldt-Jakob disease or syndrome
        endocrine or metabolic F06.8
          acute or subacute F05
        liver, alcoholic F10.259
      epilepsy transient (acute) F05
      infection
        brain (intracranial) F06.8
          acute or subacute F05
      intoxication
        alcoholic (acute) F10.259
        drug F11-F19 with .x59
      ischemia, cerebrovascular (generalized) — *see* Psychosis, arteriosclerotic
      puerperium — *see* Psychosis, puerperal
      trauma, brain (birth) (from electric current) (surgical) F06.8
        acute or subacute F05
    infective F06.8
      acute or subacute F05
    post-traumatic F06.8
      acute or subacute F05
  paranoiac F22
  paranoid (climacteric) (involutional) (menopausal) F22
    psychogenic (acute) F23
    schizophrenic F20.0
    senile F03 ☑
  postpartum (NOS) F53.1
  presbyophrenic (type) F03 ☑
  presenile F03 ☑
  psychogenic (paranoid) F23
    depressive F32.3
  puerperal (NOS) F53.1
    specified type — *see* Psychosis, by type
  reactive (brief) (transient) (emotional stress) (psychological trauma) F23
    depressive F32.3
      recurrent F33.3
    excitative type F30.8
  schizoaffective F25.9
    depressive type F25.1
    manic type F25.0
  schizophrenia, schizophrenic — *see* Schizophrenia
  schizophrenia-like, in epilepsy F06.2
  schizophreniform F20.81
    affective type F25.9
    brief F23
    confusional type F23
    mixed type F25.0
  senile NEC F03 ☑
    depressed or paranoid type F03 ☑
    simple deterioration F03 ☑
    specified type — *code to* condition
  shared F24
  situational (reactive) F23
  symbiotic (childhood) F84.3
  symptomatic F09
Psychosomatic — *see* Disorder, psychosomatic
Psychosyndrome, organic F07.9
Psychotic episode due to or associated with physical condition F06.8
Pterygium (eye) H11.00- ☑
  amyloid H11.01- ☑
  central H11.02- ☑
  colli Q18.3
  double H11.03- ☑
  peripheral
    progressive H11.05- ☑
    stationary H11.04- ☑
  recurrent H11.06- ☑
Ptilosis (eyelid) — *see* Madarosis
Ptomaine (poisoning) — *see* Poisoning, food
Ptosis — *see also* Blepharoptosis
  adiposa (false) — *see* Blepharoptosis
  breast N64.81-
  brow H57.81- ☑
  cecum K63.4
  colon K63.4
  congenital (eyelid) Q10.0
    specified site NEC — *see* Anomaly, by site

Ptosis — *continued*
  eyebrow H57.81- ☑
  eyelid — *see* Blepharoptosis
    congenital Q10.0
  gastric K31.89
  intestine K63.4
  kidney N28.83
  liver K76.89
  renal N28.83
  splanchnic K63.4
  spleen D73.89
  stomach K31.89
  viscera K63.4
PTP D69.51
Ptyalism (periodic) K11.7
  hysterical F45.8
  pregnancy — *see* Pregnancy, complicated by, specified pregnancy-related condition NEC
  psychogenic F45.8
Ptyalolithiasis K11.5
Pubarche, precocious E30.1
Pubertas praecox E30.1
Puberty (development state) Z00.3
  bleeding (excessive) N92.2
  delayed E30.0
  precocious (constitutional) (cryptogenic) (idiopathic) E30.1
    central E22.8
    due to
      ovarian hyperfunction E28.1
        estrogen E28.0
      testicular hyperfunction E29.0
  premature E30.1
    due to
      adrenal cortical hyperfunction E25.8
      pineal tumor E34.8
      pituitary (anterior) hyperfunction E22.8
Puckering, macula — *see* Degeneration, macula, puckering
Pudenda, pudendum — *see* condition
Puente's disease (simple glandular cheilitis) K13.0
Puerperal, puerperium (complicated by, complications)
  abnormal glucose (tolerance test) O99.815
  abscess
    areola O91.02
      associated with lactation O91.03
    Bartholin's gland O86.19
    breast O91.12
      associated with lactation O91.13
    cervix (uteri) O86.11
    genital organ NEC O86.19
    kidney O86.21
    mammary O91.12
      associated with lactation O91.13
    nipple O91.02
      associated with lactation O91.03
    peritoneum O85
    subareolar O91.12
      associated with lactation O91.13
    urinary tract — *see* Puerperal, infection, urinary
    uterus O86.12
    vagina (wall) O86.13
    vaginorectal O86.13
    vulvovaginal gland O86.13
  adnexitis O86.19
  afibrinogenemia, or other coagulation defect O72.3
  albuminuria (acute) (subacute) — *see* Proteinuria, gestational
  alcohol use O99.315
  anemia O90.81
    pre-existing (pre-pregnancy) O99.03
  anesthetic death O89.8
  apoplexy O99.43
  bariatric surgery status O99.845
  blood disorder NEC O99.13
  blood dyscrasia O72.3
  cardiomyopathy O90.3
  cerebrovascular disorder (conditions in I60-I69) O99.43
  cervicitis O86.11
  circulatory system disorder O99.43
  coagulopathy (any) O99.13
    with hemorrhage O72.3
  complications O90.9
    specified NEC O90.89
  convulsions — *see* Eclampsia
  cystitis O86.22
  cystopyelitis O86.29
  delirium NEC F05

☑ **Additional Character Required** — **Refer to the Tabular List for Character Selection**

Puncture — *continued*
  abdomen, abdominal — *continued*
    wall — *continued*
      epigastric region — *continued*
        with
          foreign body S31.142 ☑
          penetration into peritoneal cavity S31.632 ☑
            with foreign body S31.642 ☑
      left
        lower quadrant S31.134 ☑
          with
            foreign body S31.144 ☑
            penetration into peritoneal cavity S31.634 ☑
              with foreign body S31.644 ☑
        upper quadrant S31.131 ☑
          with
            foreign body S31.141 ☑
            penetration into peritoneal cavity S31.631 ☑
              with foreign body S31.641 ☑
      periumbilic region S31.135 ☑
        with
          foreign body S31.145 ☑
          penetration into peritoneal cavity S31.635 ☑
            with foreign body S31.645 ☑
      right
        lower quadrant S31.133 ☑
          with
            foreign body S31.143 ☑
            penetration into peritoneal cavity S31.633 ☑
              with foreign body S31.643 ☑
        upper quadrant S31.130 ☑
          with
            foreign body S31.140 ☑
            penetration into peritoneal cavity S31.630 ☑
              with foreign body S31.640 ☑
  accidental, complicating surgery — *see* Complication, accidental puncture or laceration
  alveolar (process) — *see* Puncture, oral cavity
  ankle S91.039 ☑
    with
      foreign body S91.049 ☑
    left S91.032 ☑
      with
        foreign body S91.042 ☑
    right S91.031 ☑
      with
        foreign body S91.041 ☑
  anus S31.833 ☑
    with foreign body S31.834 ☑
  arm (upper) S41.139 ☑
    with foreign body S41.149 ☑
    left S41.132 ☑
      with foreign body S41.142 ☑
    lower — *see* Puncture, forearm
    right S41.131 ☑
      with foreign body S41.141 ☑
  auditory canal (external) (meatus) — *see* Puncture, ear
  auricle, ear — *see* Puncture, ear
  axilla — *see* Puncture, arm
  back — *see also* Puncture, thorax, back
    lower S31.030 ☑
      with
        foreign body S31.040 ☑
          with penetration into retroperitoneal space S31.041 ☑
        penetration into retroperitoneal space S31.031 ☑
  bladder (traumatic) S37.29 ☑
    nontraumatic N32.89
  breast S21.039 ☑
    with foreign body S21.049 ☑
    left S21.032 ☑
      with foreign body S21.042 ☑
    right S21.031 ☑
      with foreign body S21.041 ☑
  buttock S31.803 ☑
    with foreign body S31.804 ☑
    left S31.823 ☑
      with foreign body S31.824 ☑
    right S31.813 ☑

Puncture — *continued*
  buttock — *continued*
    right — *continued*
      with foreign body S31.814 ☑
  by
    device, implant or graft — *see* Complications, by site and type, mechanical
    foreign body left accidentally in operative wound T81.539 ☑
    instrument (any) during a procedure, accidental — *see* Puncture, accidental complicating surgery
  calf — *see* Puncture, leg
  canaliculus lacrimalis — *see* Puncture, eyelid
  canthus, eye — *see* Puncture, eyelid
  cervical esophagus S11.23 ☑
    with foreign body S11.24 ☑
  cheek (external) S01.439 ☑
    with foreign body S01.449 ☑
    internal — *see* Puncture, oral cavity
    left S01.432 ☑
      with foreign body S01.442 ☑
    right S01.431 ☑
      with foreign body S01.441 ☑
  chest wall — *see* Puncture, thorax
  chin — *see* Puncture, head, specified site NEC
  clitoris — *see* Puncture, vulva
  costal region — *see* Puncture, thorax
  digit(s)
    foot — *see* Puncture, toe
    hand — *see* Puncture, finger
  ear (canal) (external) S01.339 ☑
    with foreign body S01.349 ☑
    drum S09.2- ☑
    left S01.332 ☑
      with foreign body S01.342 ☑
    right S01.331 ☑
      with foreign body S01.341 ☑
  elbow S51.039 ☑
    with
      foreign body S51.049 ☑
    left S51.032 ☑
      with
        foreign body S51.042 ☑
    right S51.031 ☑
      with
        foreign body S51.041 ☑
  epididymis — *see* Puncture, testis
  epigastric region — *see* Puncture, abdomen, wall, epigastric
  epiglottis S11.83 ☑
    with foreign body S11.84 ☑
  esophagus
    cervical S11.23 ☑
      with foreign body S11.24 ☑
    thoracic S27.818 ☑
  eyeball S05.6- ☑
    with foreign body S05.5- ☑
  eyebrow — *see* Puncture, eyelid
  eyelid S01.13- ☑
    with foreign body S01.14- ☑
    left S01.132 ☑
      with foreign body S01.142 ☑
    right S01.131 ☑
      with foreign body S01.141 ☑
  face NEC — *see* Puncture, head, specified site NEC
  finger(s) S61.239 ☑
    with
      damage to nail S61.339 ☑
        with
          foreign body S61.349 ☑
      foreign body S61.249 ☑
    index S61.238 ☑
      with
        damage to nail S61.338 ☑
          with
            foreign body S61.348 ☑
        foreign body S61.248 ☑
      left S61.231 ☑
        with
          damage to nail S61.331 ☑
            with
              foreign body S61.341 ☑
          foreign body S61.241 ☑
      right S61.230 ☑
        with
          damage to nail S61.330 ☑

Puncture — *continued*
  finger(s) — *continued*
    index — *continued*
      right — *continued*
        with — *continued*
          damage to nail — *continued*
            with
              foreign body S61.340 ☑
          foreign body S61.240 ☑
    little S61.238 ☑
      with
        damage to nail S61.338 ☑
          with
            foreign body S61.348 ☑
        foreign body S61.248 ☑
      left S61.237 ☑
        with
          damage to nail S61.337 ☑
            with
              foreign body S61.347 ☑
          foreign body S61.247 ☑
      right S61.236 ☑
        with
          damage to nail S61.336 ☑
            with
              foreign body S61.346 ☑
          foreign body S61.246 ☑
    middle S61.238 ☑
      with
        damage to nail S61.338 ☑
          with
            foreign body S61.348 ☑
        foreign body S61.248 ☑
      left S61.233 ☑
        with
          damage to nail S61.333 ☑
            with
              foreign body S61.343 ☑
          foreign body S61.243 ☑
      right S61.232 ☑
        with
          damage to nail S61.332 ☑
            with
              foreign body S61.342 ☑
          foreign body S61.242 ☑
    ring S61.238 ☑
      with
        damage to nail S61.338 ☑
          with
            foreign body S61.348 ☑
        foreign body S61.248 ☑
      left S61.235 ☑
        with
          damage to nail S61.335 ☑
            with
              foreign body S61.345 ☑
          foreign body S61.245 ☑
      right S61.234 ☑
        with
          damage to nail S61.334 ☑
            with
              foreign body S61.344 ☑
          foreign body S61.244 ☑
  flank S31.139 ☑
    with foreign body S31.149 ☑
  foot (except toe(s) alone) S91.339 ☑
    with foreign body S91.349 ☑
    left S91.332 ☑
      with foreign body S91.342 ☑
    right S91.331 ☑
      with foreign body S91.341 ☑
    toe — *see* Puncture, toe
  forearm S51.839 ☑
    with
      foreign body S51.849 ☑
    elbow only — *see* Puncture, elbow
    left S51.832 ☑
      with
        foreign body S51.842 ☑
    right S51.831 ☑
      with
        foreign body S51.841 ☑
  forehead — *see* Puncture, head, specified site NEC
  genital organs, external
    female S31.532 ☑
      with foreign body S31.542 ☑

Puncture — *continued*

  genital organs, external — *continued*
    female — *continued*
      vagina — *see* Puncture, vagina
      vulva — *see* Puncture, vulva
    male S31.531 ☑
      with foreign body S31.541 ☑
      penis — *see* Puncture, penis
      scrotum — *see* Puncture, scrotum
      testis — *see* Puncture, testis
  groin — *see* Puncture, abdomen, wall
  gum — *see* Puncture, oral cavity
  hand S61.439 ☑
    with
      foreign body S61.449 ☑
    finger — *see* Puncture, finger
    left S61.432 ☑
      with
        foreign body S61.442 ☑
    right S61.431 ☑
      with
        foreign body S61.441 ☑
    thumb — *see* Puncture, thumb
  head S01.93 ☑
    with foreign body S01.94 ☑
    cheek — *see* Puncture, cheek
    ear — *see* Puncture, ear
    eyelid — *see* Puncture, eyelid
    lip — *see* Puncture, oral cavity
    nose — *see* Puncture, nose
    oral cavity — *see* Puncture, oral cavity
    scalp S01.03 ☑
      with foreign body S01.04 ☑
    specified site NEC S01.83 ☑
      with foreign body S01.84 ☑
    temporomandibular area — *see* Puncture, cheek
  heart S26.99 ☑
    with hemopericardium S26.09 ☑
    without hemopericardium S26.19 ☑
  heel — *see* Puncture, foot
  hip S71.039 ☑
    with foreign body S71.049 ☑
    left S71.032 ☑
      with foreign body S71.042 ☑
    right S71.031 ☑
      with foreign body S71.041 ☑
  hymen — *see* Puncture, vagina
  hypochondrium — *see* Puncture, abdomen, wall
  hypogastric region — *see* Puncture, abdomen, wall
  inguinal region — *see* Puncture, abdomen, wall
  instep — *see* Puncture, foot
  internal organs — *see* Injury, by site
  interscapular region — *see* Puncture, thorax, back
  intestine
    large
      colon S36.599 ☑
        ascending S36.590 ☑
        descending S36.592 ☑
        sigmoid S36.593 ☑
        specified site NEC S36.598 ☑
        transverse S36.591 ☑
      rectum S36.69 ☑
    small S36.499 ☑
      duodenum S36.490 ☑
      specified site NEC S36.498 ☑
  intra-abdominal organ S36.99 ☑
    gallbladder S36.128 ☑
    intestine — *see* Puncture, intestine
    liver S36.118 ☑
    pancreas — *see* Puncture, pancreas
    peritoneum S36.81 ☑
    specified site NEC S36.898 ☑
    spleen S36.09 ☑
    stomach S36.39 ☑
  jaw — *see* Puncture, head, specified site NEC
  knee S81.039 ☑
    with foreign body S81.049 ☑
    left S81.032 ☑
      with foreign body S81.042 ☑
    right S81.031 ☑
      with foreign body S81.041 ☑
  labium (majus) (minus) — *see* Puncture, vulva
  lacrimal duct — *see* Puncture, eyelid
  larynx S11.013 ☑
    with foreign body S11.014 ☑
  leg (lower) S81.839 ☑

Puncture — *continued*

  leg — *continued*
    with foreign body S81.849 ☑
    foot — *see* Puncture, foot
    knee — *see* Puncture, knee
    left S81.832 ☑
      with foreign body S81.842 ☑
    right S81.831 ☑
      with foreign body S81.841 ☑
    upper — *see* Puncture, thigh
  lip S01.531 ☑
    with foreign body S01.541 ☑
  loin — *see* Puncture, abdomen, wall
  lower back — *see* Puncture, back, lower
  lumbar region — *see* Puncture, back, lower
  malar region — *see* Puncture, head, specified site NEC
  mammary — *see* Puncture, breast
  mastoid region — *see* Puncture, head, specified site NEC
  mouth — *see* Puncture, oral cavity
  nail
    finger — *see* Puncture, finger, with damage to nail
    toe — *see* Puncture, toe, with damage to nail
  nasal (septum) (sinus) — *see* Puncture, nose
  nasopharynx — *see* Puncture, head, specified site NEC
  neck S11.93 ☑
    with foreign body S11.94 ☑
    involving
      cervical esophagus — *see* Puncture, cervical esophagus
      larynx — *see* Puncture, larynx
      pharynx — *see* Puncture, pharynx
      thyroid gland — *see* Puncture, thyroid gland
      trachea — *see* Puncture, trachea
    specified site NEC S11.83 ☑
      with foreign body S11.84 ☑
  nose (septum) (sinus) S01.23 ☑
    with foreign body S01.24 ☑
  ocular — *see* Puncture, eyeball
  oral cavity S01.532 ☑
    with foreign body S01.542 ☑
  orbit S05.4- ☑
  palate — *see* Puncture, oral cavity
  palm — *see* Puncture, hand
  pancreas S36.299 ☑
    body S36.291 ☑
    head S36.290 ☑
    tail S36.292 ☑
  pelvis — *see* Puncture, back, lower
  penis S31.23 ☑
    with foreign body S31.24 ☑
  perineum
    female S31.43 ☑
      with foreign body S31.44 ☑
    male S31.139 ☑
      with foreign body S31.149 ☑
  periocular area (with or without lacrimal passages) — *see* Puncture, eyelid
  phalanges
    finger — *see* Puncture, finger
    toe — *see* Puncture, toe
  pharynx S11.23 ☑
    with foreign body S11.24 ☑
  pinna — *see* Puncture, ear
  popliteal space — *see* Puncture, knee
  prepuce — *see* Puncture, penis
  pubic region S31.139 ☑
    with foreign body S31.149 ☑
  pudendum — *see* Puncture, genital organs, external
  rectovaginal septum — *see* Puncture, vagina
  sacral region — *see* Puncture, back, lower
  sacroiliac region — *see* Puncture, back, lower
  salivary gland — *see* Puncture, oral cavity
  scalp S01.03 ☑
    with foreign body S01.04 ☑
  scapular region — *see* Puncture, shoulder
  scrotum S31.33 ☑
    with foreign body S31.34 ☑
  shin — *see* Puncture, leg
  shoulder S41.039 ☑
    with foreign body S41.049 ☑
    left S41.032 ☑
      with foreign body S41.042 ☑
    right S41.031 ☑
      with foreign body S41.041 ☑
  spermatic cord — *see* Puncture, testis

Puncture — *continued*

  sternal region — *see* Puncture, thorax, front
  submaxillary region — *see* Puncture, head, specified site NEC
  submental region — *see* Puncture, head, specified site NEC
  subungual
    finger(s) — *see* Puncture, finger, with damage to nail
    toe — *see* Puncture, toe, with damage to nail
  supraclavicular fossa — *see* Puncture, neck, specified site NEC
  temple, temporal region — *see* Puncture, head, specified site NEC
  temporomandibular area — *see* Puncture, cheek
  testis S31.33 ☑
    with foreign body S31.34 ☑
  thigh S71.139 ☑
    with foreign body S71.149 ☑
    left S71.132 ☑
      with foreign body S71.142 ☑
    right S71.131 ☑
      with foreign body S71.141 ☑
  thorax, thoracic (wall) S21.93 ☑
    with foreign body S21.94 ☑
    back S21.23- ☑
      with
        foreign body S21.24- ☑
          with penetration S21.44 ☑
        penetration S21.43 ☑
    breast — *see* Puncture, breast
    front S21.13- ☑
      with
        foreign body S21.14- ☑
          with penetration S21.34 ☑
        penetration S21.33 ☑
  throat — *see* Puncture, neck
  thumb S61.039 ☑
    with
      damage to nail S61.139 ☑
        with
          foreign body S61.149 ☑
      foreign body S61.049 ☑
    left S61.032 ☑
      with
        damage to nail S61.132 ☑
          with
            foreign body S61.142 ☑
        foreign body S61.042 ☑
    right S61.031 ☑
      with
        damage to nail S61.131 ☑
          with
            foreign body S61.141 ☑
        foreign body S61.041 ☑
  thyroid gland S11.13 ☑
    with foreign body S11.14 ☑
  toe(s) S91.139 ☑
    with
      damage to nail S91.239 ☑
        with
          foreign body S91.249 ☑
      foreign body S91.149 ☑
    great S91.133 ☑
      with
        damage to nail S91.233 ☑
          with
            foreign body S91.243 ☑
        foreign body S91.143 ☑
      left S91.132 ☑
        with
          damage to nail S91.232 ☑
            with
              foreign body S91.242 ☑
          foreign body S91.142 ☑
      right S91.131 ☑
        with
          damage to nail S91.231 ☑
            with
              foreign body S91.241 ☑
          foreign body S91.141 ☑
    lesser S91.136 ☑
      with
        damage to nail S91.236 ☑
          with
            foreign body S91.246 ☑

☑ **Additional Character Required** — **Refer to the Tabular List for Character Selection**

Puncture — *continued*
 toe(s) — *continued*
  lesser — *continued*
   with — *continued*
    foreign body S91.146 ☑
    left S91.135 ☑
     with
      damage to nail S91.235 ☑
       with
        foreign body S91.245 ☑
      foreign body S91.145 ☑
    right S91.134 ☑
     with
      damage to nail S91.234 ☑
       with
        foreign body S91.244 ☑
      foreign body S91.144 ☑
 tongue — *see* Puncture, oral cavity
 trachea S11.023 ☑
  with foreign body S11.024 ☑
 tunica vaginalis — *see* Puncture, testis
 tympanum, tympanic membrane S09.2- ☑
 umbilical region S31.135 ☑
  with foreign body S31.145 ☑
 uvula — *see* Puncture, oral cavity
 vagina S31.43 ☑
  with foreign body S31.44 ☑
 vocal cords S11.033 ☑
  with foreign body S11.034 ☑
 vulva S31.43 ☑
  with foreign body S31.44 ☑
 wrist S61.539 ☑
  with
   foreign body S61.549 ☑
  left S61.532 ☑
   with
    foreign body S61.542 ☑
  right S61.531 ☑
   with
    foreign body S61.541 ☑
PUO (pyrexia of unknown origin) R50.9
Pupillary membrane (persistent) Q13.89
Pupillotonia — *see* Anomaly, pupil, function, tonic pupil
Purpura D69.2
 abdominal D69.0
 allergic D69.0
 anaphylactoid D69.0
 annularis telangiectodes L81.7
 arthritic D69.0
 autoerythrocyte sensitization D69.2
 autoimmune D69.0
 bacterial D69.0
 Bateman's (senile) D69.2
 capillary fragility (hereditary) (idiopathic) D69.8
 cryoglobulinemic D89.1
 Devil's pinches D69.2
 fibrinolytic — *see* Fibrinolysis
 fulminans, fulminous D65
 gangrenous D65
 hemorrhagic, hemorrhagica D69.3
  not due to thrombocytopenia D69.0
 Henoch (-Schönlein) (allergic) D69.0
 hypergammaglobulinemic (benign) (Waldenström) D89.0
 idiopathic (thrombocytopenic) D69.3
  nonthrombocytopenic D69.0
 immune thrombocytopenic D69.3
 infectious D69.0
 malignant D69.0
 neonatorum P54.5
 nervosa D69.0
 newborn P54.5
 nonthrombocytopenic D69.2
  hemorrhagic D69.0
  idiopathic D69.0
 nonthrombopenic D69.2
 peliosis rheumatica D69.0
 posttransfusion (post-transfusion) (from (fresh) whole blood or blood products) D69.51
 primary D69.49
 red cell membrane sensitivity D69.2
 rheumatica D69.0
 Schönlein (-Henoch) (allergic) D69.0
 scorbutic E54 *[D77]*
 senile D69.2
 simplex D69.2
 symptomatica D69.0

Purpura — *continued*
 telangiectasia annularis L81.7
 thrombocytopenic D69.49
  congenital D69.42
  hemorrhagic D69.3
  hereditary D69.42
  idiopathic D69.3
  immune D69.3
  neonatal, transitory P61.0
  thrombotic M31.19
 thrombohemolytic — *see* Fibrinolysis
 thrombolytic — *see* Fibrinolysis
 thrombopenic D69.49
 thrombotic, thrombocytopenic M31.19
 toxic D69.0
 vascular D69.0
 visceral symptoms D69.0
Purpuric spots R23.3
Purulent — *see* condition
Pus
 in
  stool R19.5
  urine N39.0
 tube (rupture) — *see* Salpingo-oophoritis
Pustular rash L08.0
Pustule (nonmalignant) L08.9
 malignant A22.0
Pustulosis palmaris et plantaris L40.3
Putnam (-Dana) **disease or syndrome** — *see* Degeneration, combined
Putrescent pulp (dental) K04.1
Pyarthritis, pyarthrosis — *see* Arthritis, pyogenic or pyemic
 tuberculous — *see* Tuberculosis, joint
Pyelectasis — *see* Hydronephrosis
Pyelitis (congenital) (uremic) — *see also* Pyelonephritis
 with
  calculus — *see* category N20 ☑
   with hydronephrosis N13.6
  contracted kidney N11.9
 acute N10
 chronic N11.9
  with calculus — *see* category N20 ☑
   with hydronephrosis N13.6
 cystica N28.84
 puerperal (postpartum) O86.21
 tuberculous A18.11
Pyelocystitis — *see* Pyelonephritis
Pyelonephritis — *see also* Nephritis, tubulo-interstitial
 with
  calculus — *see* category N20 ☑
   with hydronephrosis N13.6
  contracted kidney N11.9
 acute N10
 calculous — *see* category N20 ☑
  with hydronephrosis N13.6
 chronic N11.9
  with calculus — *see* category N20 ☑
   with hydronephrosis N13.6
  associated with ureteral obstruction or stricture N11.1
  nonobstructive N11.8
   with reflux (vesicoureteral) N11.0
  obstructive N11.1
  specified NEC N11.8
 in (due to)
  brucellosis A23.9 *[N16]*
  cryoglobulinemia (mixed) D89.1 *[N16]*
  cystinosis E72.04
  diphtheria A36.84
  glycogen storage disease E74.09 *[N16]*
  leukemia NEC C95.9- ☑ *[N16]*
  lymphoma NEC C85.90 *[N16]*
  multiple myeloma C90.0- ☑ *[N16]*
  obstruction N11.1
  Salmonella infection A02.25
  sarcoidosis D86.84
  sepsis A41.9 *[N16]*
  Sjögren's disease M35.04
  toxoplasmosis B58.83
  transplant rejection T86.91 *[N16]*
  Wilson's disease E83.01 *[N16]*
 nonobstructive N12
  with reflux (vesicoureteral) N11.0
  chronic N11.8
 syphilitic A52.75
Pyelonephrosis (obstructive) N11.1
 chronic N11.9

Pyelophlebitis I80.8
Pyeloureteritis cystica N28.85
Pyemia, pyemic (fever) (infection) (purulent) — *see also* Sepsis
 joint — *see* Arthritis, pyogenic or pyemic
 liver K75.1
 pneumococcal A40.3
 portal K75.1
 postvaccinal T88.0 ☑
 puerperal, postpartum, childbirth O85
 specified organism NEC A41.89
 tuberculous — *see* Tuberculosis, miliary
Pygopagus Q89.4
Pyknoepilepsy (idiopathic) — *see* Pyknolepsy
Pyknolepsy G40.A09 (*following* G40.3)
 intractable G40.A19 (*following* G40.3)
  with status epilepticus G40.A11 (*following* G40.3)
  without status epilepticus G40.A19 (*following* G40.3)
 not intractable G40.A09 (*following* G40.3)
  with status epilepticus G40.A01 (*following* G40.3)
  without status epilepticus G40.A09 (*following* G40.3)
Pylephlebitis K75.1
Pyle's syndrome Q78.5
Pylethrombophlebitis K75.1
Pylethrombosis K75.1
Pyloritis K29.90
 with bleeding K29.91
Pylorospasm (reflex) **NEC** K31.3
 congenital or infantile Q40.0
 neurotic F45.8
 newborn Q40.0
 psychogenic F45.8
Pylorus, pyloric — *see* condition
Pyoarthrosis — *see* Arthritis, pyogenic or pyemic
Pyocele
 mastoid — *see* Mastoiditis, acute
 sinus (accessory) — *see* Sinusitis
 turbinate (bone) J32.9
 urethra — *see also* Urethritis N34.0
Pyocolpos — *see* Vaginitis
Pyocystitis N30.80
 with hematuria N30.81
Pyoderma, pyodermia L08.0
 gangrenosum L88
 newborn P39.4
 phagedenic L88
 vegetans L08.81
Pyodermatitis L08.0
 vegetans L08.81
Pyogenic — *see* condition
Pyohydronephrosis N13.6
Pyometra, pyometrium, pyometritis — *see* Endometritis
Pyomyositis (tropical) — *see* Myositis, infective
Pyonephritis N12
Pyonephrosis N13.6
 tuberculous A18.11
Pyo-oophoritis — *see* Salpingo-oophoritis
Pyo-ovarium — *see* Salpingo-oophoritis
Pyopericarditis, pyopericardium I30.1
Pyophlebitis — *see* Phlebitis
Pyopneumopericardium I30.1
Pyopneumothorax (infective) J86.9
 with fistula J86.0
 tuberculous NEC A15.6
Pyosalpinx, pyosalpingitis — *see also* Salpingo-oophoritis
Pyothorax J86.9
 with fistula J86.0
 tuberculous NEC A15.6
Pyoureter N28.89
 tuberculous A18.11
Pyramidopallidonigral syndrome G20
Pyrexia (of unknown origin) R50.9
 atmospheric T67.01 ☑
 during labor NEC O75.2
 heat T67.01 ☑
 newborn P81.9
  environmentally-induced P81.0
 persistent R50.9
 puerperal O86.4
Pyroglobulinemia NEC E88.09
Pyromania F63.1
Pyrosis R12
Pyuria (bacterial) (sterile) R82.81

Q

Q fever A78
  with pneumonia A78
Quadricuspid aortic valve Q23.8
Quadrilateral fever A78
Quadriparesis — *see* Quadriplegia
  meaning muscle weakness M62.81
Quadriplegia G82.50
  complete
    C1-C4 level G82.51
    C5-C7 level G82.53
  congenital (cerebral) (spinal) G80.8
    spastic G80.0
  embolic (current episode) I63.4- ☑
  functional R53.2
  incomplete
    C1-C4 level G82.52
    C5-C7 level G82.54
  thrombotic (current episode) I63.3- ☑
  traumatic — *code to* injury with seventh character S
    current episode — *see* Injury, spinal (cord), cervical
Quadruplet, pregnancy — *see* Pregnancy, quadruplet
Quarrelsomeness F60.3
Queensland fever A77.3
Quervain's disease M65.4
  thyroid E06.1
Queyrat's erythroplasia D07.4
  penis D07.4
  specified site — *see* Neoplasm, skin, in situ
  unspecified site D07.4
Quincke's disease or edema T78.3 ☑
  hereditary D84.1
Quinsy (gangrenous) J36
Quintan fever A79.0
Quintuplet, pregnancy — *see* Pregnancy, quintuplet

R

Rabbit fever — *see* Tularemia
Rabies A82.9
  contact Z20.3
  exposure to Z20.3
  inoculation reaction — *see* Complications, vaccination
  sylvatic A82.0
  urban A82.1
Rachischisis — *see* Spina bifida
Rachitic — *see also* condition
  deformities of spine (late effect) (sequelae) E64.3
  pelvis (late effect) (sequelae) E64.3
    with disproportion (fetopelvic) O33.0
      causing obstructed labor O65.0
Rachitis, rachitism (acute) (tarda) — *see also* Rickets
  renalis N25.0
  sequelae E64.3
Radial nerve — *see* condition
Radiation
  burn — *see* Burn
  effects NOS T66 ☑
  sickness NOS T66 ☑
  therapy, encounter for Z51.0
Radiculitis (pressure) (vertebrogenic) — *see* Radiculopathy
Radiculomyelitis — *see also* Encephalitis
  toxic, due to
    Clostridium tetani A35
    Corynebacterium diphtheriae A36.82
Radiculopathy M54.10
  cervical region M54.12
  cervicothoracic region M54.13
  due to
    disc disorder
      C3 M50.11
      C4 M50.11
      C5 M50.121
      C6 M50.122
      C7 M50.123
    displacement of intervertebral disc — *see* Disorder, disc, with, radiculopathy
  leg M54.1- ☑
  lumbar region M54.16
  lumbosacral region M54.17
  occipito-atlanto-axial region M54.11
  postherpetic B02.29
  sacrococcygeal region M54.18
  syphilitic A52.11

Radiculopathy — *continued*
  thoracic region (with visceral pain) M54.14
  thoracolumbar region M54.15
Radiodermal burns (acute, chronic, or occupational) — *see* Burn
Radiodermatitis L58.9
  acute L58.0
  chronic L58.1
Radiotherapy session Z51.0
RAEB (refractory anemia with excess blasts) D46.2- ☑
Rage, meaning rabies — *see* Rabies
Ragpicker's disease A22.1
Ragsorter's disease A22.1
Raillietiniasis B71.8
Railroad neurosis F48.8
Railway spine F48.8
Raised — *see also* Elevated
  antibody titer R76.0
Rake teeth, tooth M26.39
Rales R09.89
Ramifying renal pelvis Q63.8
Ramsay-Hunt disease or syndrome — *see also* Hunt's disease B02.21
  meaning dyssynergia cerebellaris myoclonica G11.19
Ranula K11.6
  congenital Q38.4
Rape
  adult
    confirmed T74.21 ☑
    suspected T76.21 ☑
  alleged, observation or examination, ruled out
    adult Z04.41
    child Z04.42
  child
    confirmed T74.22 ☑
    suspected T76.22 ☑
Rapid
  feeble pulse, due to shock, following injury T79.4 ☑
  heart (beat) R00.0
    psychogenic F45.8
  second stage (delivery) O62.3
  time-zone change syndrome G47.25
Rarefaction, bone — *see* Disorder, bone, density and structure, specified NEC
Rash (toxic) R21
  canker A38.9
  diaper L22
  drug (internal use) L27.0
    contact — *see also* Dermatitis, due to, drugs, external L25.1
  following immunization T88.1 ☑
  food — *see* Dermatitis, due to, food
  heat L74.0
  napkin (psoriasiform) L22
  nettle — *see* Urticaria
  pustular L08.0
  rose R21
    epidemic B06.9
  scarlet A38.9
  serum — *see also* Reaction, serum T80.69 ☑
  wandering tongue K14.1
Rasmussen aneurysm — *see* Tuberculosis, pulmonary
Rasmussen encephalitis G04.81
Rat-bite fever A25.9
  due to Streptobacillus moniliformis A25.1
  spirochetal (morsus muris) A25.0
Rathke's pouch tumor D44.3
Raymond (-Céstan) **syndrome** I65.8
Raynaud's disease, phenomenon or syndrome (secondary) I73.00
  with gangrene (symmetric) I73.01
RDS (newborn) (type I) P22.0
  type II P22.1
Reaction — *see also* Disorder
  withdrawing, child or adolescent F93.8
  adaptation — *see* Disorder, adjustment
  adjustment (anxiety) (conduct disorder) (depressiveness) (distress) — *see* Disorder, adjustment
    with
      mutism, elective (child) (adolescent) F94.0
  adverse
    food (any) (ingested) NEC T78.1 ☑
      anaphylactic — *see* Shock, anaphylactic, due to food
  affective — *see* Disorder, mood
  allergic — *see* Allergy
  anaphylactic — *see* Shock, anaphylactic

Reaction — *continued*
  anaphylactoid — *see* Shock, anaphylactic
  anesthesia — *see* Anesthesia, complication
  antitoxin (prophylactic) (therapeutic) — *see* Complications, vaccination
  anxiety F41.1
  Arthus — *see* Arthus' phenomenon
  asthenic F48.8
  combat and operational stress F43.0
  compulsive F42.8
  conversion F44.9
  crisis, acute F43.0
  deoxyribonuclease (DNA) (DNase) hypersensitivity D69.2
  depressive (single episode) F32.9
    affective (single episode) F31.4
      recurrent episode F33.9
    neurotic F34.1
    psychoneurotic F34.1
    psychotic F32.3
    recurrent — *see* Disorder, depressive, recurrent
  dissociative F44.9
  drug NEC T88.7 ☑
    addictive — *see* Dependence, drug
      transmitted via placenta or breast milk — *see* Absorption, drug, addictive, through placenta
    allergic — *see* Allergy, drug
    lichenoid L43.2
    newborn P93.8
      gray baby syndrome P93.0
    overdose or poisoning (by accident) — *see* Table of Drugs and Chemicals, by drug, poisoning
    photoallergic L56.1
    phototoxic L56.0
    withdrawal — *see* Dependence, by drug, with, withdrawal
      infant of dependent mother P96.1
      newborn P96.1
    wrong substance given or taken (by accident) — *see* Table of Drugs and Chemicals, by drug, poisoning
  fear F40.9
    child (abnormal) F93.8
  febrile nonhemolytic transfusion (FNHTR) R50.84
  fluid loss, cerebrospinal G97.1
  foreign
    body NEC — *see* Granuloma, foreign body
      in operative wound (inadvertently left) — *see* Foreign body, accidentally left during a procedure
    substance accidentally left during a procedure (chemical) (powder) (talc) T81.60 ☑
      aseptic peritonitis T81.61 ☑
      body or object (instrument) (sponge) (swab) — *see* Foreign body, accidentally left during a procedure
      specified reaction NEC T81.69 ☑
  grief — *see* Disorder, adjustment
  Herxheimer's R68.89
  hyperkinetic — *see* Hyperkinesia
  hypochondriacal F45.20
  hypoglycemic, due to insulin E16.0
    with coma (diabetic) — *see* Diabetes, coma
      nondiabetic E15
    therapeutic misadventure — *see* subcategory T38.3 ☑
  hypomanic F30.8
  hysterical F44.9
  immunization — *see* Complications, vaccination
  incompatibility
    ABO blood group (infusion) (transfusion) — *see* Complication(s), transfusion, incompatibility reaction, ABO
      delayed serologic T80.39 ☑
      minor blood group (Duffy) (E) (K) (Kell) (Kidd) (Lewis) (M) (N) (P) (S) T80.89 ☑
      Rh (factor) (infusion) (transfusion) — *see* Complication(s), transfusion, incompatibility reaction, Rh (factor)
  inflammatory — *see* Infection
  infusion — *see* Complications, infusion
  inoculation (immune serum) — *see* Complications, vaccination
  insulin T38.3- ☑
  involutional psychotic — *see* Disorder, depressive
  leukemoid D72.823
    basophilic D72.823

☑ **Additional Character Required** — Refer to the Tabular List for Character Selection

Reaction — *continued*
  leukemoid — *continued*
    lymphocytic D72.823
    monocytic D72.823
    myelocytic D72.823
    neutrophilic D72.823
  LSD (acute)
    due to drug abuse — *see* Abuse, drug, hallucinogen
    due to drug dependence — *see* Dependence, drug, hallucinogen
  lumbar puncture G97.1
  manic-depressive — *see* Disorder, bipolar
  neurasthenic F48.8
  neurogenic — *see* Neurosis
  neurotic F48.9
  neurotic-depressive F34.1
  nitritoid — *see* Crisis, nitritoid
  nonspecific
    to
      cell mediated immunity measurement of gamma interferon antigen response without active tuberculosis R76.12
      QuantiFERON-TB test (QFT) without active tuberculosis R76.12
      tuberculin test — *see also* Reaction, tuberculin skin test R76.11
  obsessive-compulsive F42.8
  organic, acute or subacute — *see* Delirium
  paranoid (acute) F23
    chronic F22
    senile F03 ☑
  passive dependency F60.7
  phobic F40.9
  post-traumatic stress, uncomplicated Z73.3
  psychogenic F99
  psychoneurotic — *see also* Neurosis
    compulsive F42.8
    depersonalization F48.1
    depressive F34.1
    hypochondriacal F45.20
    neurasthenic F48.8
    obsessive F42.8
  psychophysiologic — *see* Disorder, somatoform
  psychosomatic — *see* Disorder, somatoform
  psychotic — *see* Psychosis
  scarlet fever toxin — *see* Complications, vaccination
  schizophrenic F23
    acute (brief) (undifferentiated) F23
    latent F21
    undifferentiated (acute) (brief) F23
  serological for syphilis — *see* Serology for syphilis
  serum T80.69 ☑
    anaphylactic (immediate) — *see also* Shock, anaphylactic T80.59 ☑
    specified reaction NEC
      due to
        administration of blood and blood products T80.61 ☑
        immunization T80.62 ☑
        serum specified NEC T80.69 ☑
        vaccination T80.62 ☑
  situational — *see* Disorder, adjustment
  somatization — *see* Disorder, somatoform
  spinal puncture G97.1
    dural G97.1
  stress (severe) F43.9
    acute (agitation) ("daze") (disorientation) (disturbance of consciousness) (flight reaction) (fugue) F43.0
    specified NEC F43.89
  surgical procedure — *see* Complications, surgical procedure
  tetanus antitoxin — *see* Complications, vaccination
  toxic, to local anesthesia T88.59 ☑
    in labor and delivery O74.4
    in pregnancy O29.3X- ☑
    postpartum, puerperal O89.3
  toxin-antitoxin — *see* Complications, vaccination
  transfusion (blood) (bone marrow) (lymphocytes) (allergic) — *see* Complications, transfusion
  tuberculin skin test, abnormal R76.11
  vaccination (any) — *see* Complications, vaccination
Reactive airway disease — *see* Asthma
Reactive depression — *see* Reaction, depressive
Rearrangement
  chromosomal
    balanced (in) Q95.9
      abnormal individual (autosomal) Q95.2

Rearrangement — *continued*
  chromosomal — *continued*
    balanced — *continued*
      abnormal individual — *continued*
        non-sex (autosomal) chromosomes Q95.2
        sex/non-sex chromosomes Q95.3
      specified NEC Q95.8
Recalcitrant patient — *see* Noncompliance
Recanalization, thrombus — *see* Thrombosis
Recession, receding
  chamber angle (eye) H21.55- ☑
  chin M26.09
  gingival (postinfective) (postoperative)
    generalized K06.020
      minimal K06.021
      moderate K06.022
      severe K06.023
    localized K06.010
      minimal K06.011
      moderate K06.012
      severe K06.013
Recklinghausen disease Q85.01
  bones E21.0
Reclus' disease (cystic) — *see* Mastopathy, cystic
Recrudescent typhus (fever) A75.1
Recruitment, auditory H93.21- ☑
Rectalgia K62.89
Rectitis K62.89
Rectocele
  female (without uterine prolapse) N81.6
    with uterine prolapse N81.4
      incomplete N81.2
  in pregnancy — *see* Pregnancy, complicated by, abnormal, pelvic organs or tissues NEC
  male K62.3
Rectosigmoid junction — *see* condition
Rectosigmoiditis K63.89
  ulcerative (chronic) K51.30
    with
      complication K51.319
        abscess K51.314
        fistula K51.313
        obstruction K51.312
        rectal bleeding K51.311
        specified NEC K51.318
Rectourethral — *see* condition
Rectovaginal — *see* condition
Rectovesical — *see* condition
Rectum, rectal — *see* condition
Recurrent — *see* condition
  pregnancy loss — *see* Loss (of), pregnancy, recurrent
Red bugs B88.0
Red tide — *see also* Table of Drugs and Chemicals T65.82- ☑
Red-cedar lung or pneumonitis J67.8
Reduced
  mobility Z74.09
  ventilatory or vital capacity R94.2
Redundant, redundancy
  anus (congenital) Q43.8
  clitoris N90.89
  colon (congenital) Q43.8
  foreskin (congenital) N47.8
  intestine (congenital) Q43.8
  labia N90.69
  organ or site, congenital NEC — *see* Accessory
  panniculus (abdominal) E65
  prepuce (congenital) N47.8
  pylorus K31.89
  rectum (congenital) Q43.8
  scrotum N50.89
  sigmoid (congenital) Q43.8
  skin L98.7
    and subcutaneous tissue L98.7
    of face L57.4
    eyelids — *see* Blepharochalasis
  stomach K31.89
Reduplication — *see* Duplication
Reflex R29.2
  hyperactive gag J39.2
  pupillary, abnormal — *see* Anomaly, pupil, function
  vasoconstriction I73.9
  vasovagal R55
Reflux K21.9
  acid K21.9
  esophageal K21.9
    with esophagitis (without bleeding) K21.00
      with bleeding K21.01

Reflux — *continued*
  esophageal — *continued*
    newborn P78.83
  gastroesophageal K21.9
    with esophagitis (without bleeding) K21.00
      with bleeding K21.01
  mitral — *see* Insufficiency, mitral
  ureteral — *see* Reflux, vesicoureteral
  vesicoureteral (with scarring) N13.70
    with
      nephropathy N13.729
        with hydroureter N13.739
          bilateral N13.732
          unilateral N13.731
        bilateral N13.722
        unilateral N13.721
        without hydroureter N13.729
          bilateral N13.722
          unilateral N13.721
      pyelonephritis (chronic) N11.0
    congenital Q62.7
    without nephropathy N13.71
Reforming, artificial openings — *see* Attention to, artificial, opening
Refractive error — *see* Disorder, refraction
Refsum's disease or syndrome G60.1
Refusal of
  food, psychogenic F50.89
  treatment (because of) Z53.20
    left against medical advice (AMA) Z53.29
    left without being seen Z53.21
    patient's decision NEC Z53.29
    reasons of belief or group pressure Z53.1
Regional — *see* condition
Regurgitation R11.10
  aortic (valve) — *see* Insufficiency, aortic
  food — *see also* Vomiting
    with reswallowing — *see* Rumination
    newborn P92.1
  gastric contents — *see* Vomiting
  heart — *see* Endocarditis
  mitral (valve) — *see* Insufficiency, mitral
    congenital Q23.3
  myocardial — *see* Endocarditis
  pulmonary (valve) (heart) I37.1
    congenital Q22.2
    syphilitic A52.03
  tricuspid — *see* Insufficiency, tricuspid
  valve, valvular — *see* Endocarditis
    congenital Q24.8
  vesicoureteral — *see* Reflux, vesicoureteral
Reichmann's disease or syndrome K31.89
Reifenstein syndrome E34.52
Reinsertion
  implantable subdermal contraceptive Z30.46
  intrauterine contraceptive device Z30.433
Reiter's disease, syndrome, or urethritis M02.30
  ankle M02.37- ☑
  elbow M02.32- ☑
  foot joint M02.37- ☑
  hand joint M02.34- ☑
  hip M02.35- ☑
  knee M02.36- ☑
  multiple site M02.39
  shoulder M02.31- ☑
  vertebra M02.38
  wrist M02.33- ☑
Rejection
  food, psychogenic F50.89
  transplant T86.91
    bone T86.830
      marrow T86.01
    cornea T86.840- ☑
    heart T86.21
      with lung(s) T86.31
    intestine T86.850
    kidney T86.11
    liver T86.41
    lung(s) T86.810
      with heart T86.31
    organ (immune or nonimmune cause) T86.91
    pancreas T86.890
    skin (allograft) (autograft) T86.820
    specified NEC T86.890
    stem cell (peripheral blood) (umbilical cord) T86.5
Relapsing fever A68.9
  Carter's (Asiatic) A68.1
  Dutton's (West African) A68.1

Relapsing fever — *continued*
  Koch's A68.9
  louse-borne (epidemic) A68.0
  Novy's (American) A68.1
  Obermeyers's (European) A68.0
  Spirillum A68.9
  tick-borne (endemic) A68.1
Relationship
  occlusal
    open anterior M26.220
    open posterior M26.221
Relaxation
  anus (sphincter) K62.89
    psychogenic F45.8
  arch (foot) — *see also* Deformity, limb, flat foot
  back ligaments — *see* Instability, joint, spine
  bladder (sphincter) N31.2
  cardioesophageal K21.9
  cervix — *see* Incompetency, cervix
  diaphragm J98.6
  joint (capsule) (ligament) (paralytic) — *see* Flail, joint
    congenital NEC Q74.8
  lumbosacral (joint) — *see* subcategory M53.2 ☑
  pelvic floor N81.89
  perineum N81.89
  posture R29.3
  rectum (sphincter) K62.89
  sacroiliac (joint) — *see* subcategory M53.2 ☑
  scrotum N50.89
  urethra (sphincter) N36.44
  vesical N31.2
Release from prison, anxiety concerning Z65.2
Remains
  canal of Cloquet Q14.0
  capsule (opaque) Q14.8
Remittent fever (malarial) B54
Remnant
  canal of Cloquet Q14.0
  capsule (opaque) Q14.8
  cervix, cervical stump (acquired) (postoperative) N88.8
  cystic duct, postcholecystectomy K91.5
  fingernail L60.8
    congenital Q84.6
  meniscus, knee — *see* Derangement, knee, meniscus,
    specified NEC
  thyroglossal duct Q89.2
  tonsil J35.8
    infected (chronic) J35.01
  urachus Q64.4
Removal (from) (of)
  artificial
    arm Z44.00- ☑
      complete Z44.01- ☑
      partial Z44.02- ☑
    eye Z44.2- ☑
    leg Z44.10- ☑
      complete Z44.11- ☑
      partial Z44.12- ☑
  breast implant Z45.81 ☑
  cardiac pulse generator (battery) (end-of-life) Z45.010
  catheter (urinary) (indwelling) Z46.6
    from artificial opening — *see* Attention to, artificial,
      opening
    non-vascular Z46.82
    vascular NEC Z45.2
  device Z46.9
    contraceptive Z30.432
      implantable subdermal Z30.46
    implanted NEC Z45.89
    specified NEC Z46.89
  drains Z48.03
  dressing (nonsurgical) Z48.00
    surgical Z48.01
  external
    fixation device — *code to* fracture with seventh
      character D
    prosthesis, prosthetic device Z44.9
      breast Z44.3- ☑
      specified NEC Z44.8
  home in childhood (to foster home or institution)
    Z62.29
  ileostomy Z43.2
  insulin pump Z46.81
  myringotomy device (stent) (tube) Z45.82
  nervous system device NEC Z46.2
    brain neuropacemaker Z46.2
    visual substitution device Z46.2
      implanted Z45.31

Removal — *continued*
  non-vascular catheter Z46.82
  organ, prophylactic (for neoplasia management) —
    see Prophylactic, organ removal
  orthodontic device Z46.4
  staples Z48.02
  stent
    ureteral Z46.6
  suture Z48.02
  urinary device Z46.6
  vascular access device or catheter Z45.2
Ren
  arcuatus Q63.1
  mobile, mobilis N28.89
    congenital Q63.8
  unguliformis Q63.1
Renal — *see* condition
Rendu-Osler-Weber disease or syndrome I78.0
Reninoma D41.0- ☑
Renon-Delille syndrome E23.3
Reovirus, as cause of disease classified elsewhere
  B97.5
Repeated falls NEC R29.6
Replaced chromosome by dicentric ring Q93.2
**Replacement by artificial or mechanical device or
  prosthesis of**
  bladder Z96.0
  blood vessel NEC Z95.828
  bone NEC Z96.7
  cochlea Z96.21
  coronary artery Z95.5
  eustachian tube Z96.29
  eye globe Z97.0
  heart Z95.812
    valve Z95.2
      prosthetic Z95.2
      specified NEC Z95.4
      xenogenic Z95.3
  intestine Z96.89
  joint Z96.60
    hip — *see* Presence, hip joint implant
    knee — *see* Presence, knee joint implant
    specified site NEC Z96.698
  larynx Z96.3
  lens Z96.1
  limb(s) — *see* Presence, artificial, limb
  mandible NEC (for tooth root implant(s)) Z96.5
  organ NEC Z96.89
  peripheral vessel NEC Z95.828
  stapes Z96.29
  teeth Z97.2
  tendon Z96.7
  tissue NEC Z96.89
  tooth root(s) Z96.5
  vessel NEC Z95.828
    coronary (artery) Z95.5
Request for expert evidence Z04.89
Reserve, decreased or low
  cardiac — *see* Disease, heart
  kidney N28.89
Residing
  in place not meant for human habitation (abandoned
    building) (car) (park) (sidewalk) Z59.02
  on the street Z59.02
Residual — *see also* condition
  ovary syndrome N99.83
  state, schizophrenic F20.5
  urine R39.198
Resistance, resistant (to)
  activated protein C D68.51
  complicating pregnancy O26.89 ☑
  insulin E88.81
  organism(s)
    to
      drug Z16.30
        aminoglycosides Z16.29
        amoxicillin Z16.11
        ampicillin Z16.11
        antibiotic(s) Z16.20
          multiple Z16.24
          specified NEC Z16.29
        antifungal Z16.32
        antimicrobial (single) Z16.30
          multiple Z16.35
          specified NEC Z16.39
        antimycobacterial (single) Z16.341
          multiple Z16.342
        antiparasitic Z16.31

Resistance, resistant — *continued*
  organism(s) — *continued*
    to — *continued*
      drug — *continued*
        antiviral Z16.33
        beta lactam antibiotics Z16.10
          specified NEC Z16.19
        cephalosporins Z16.19
        extended beta lactamase (ESBL) Z16.12
        fluoroquinolones Z16.23
        macrolides Z16.29
        methicillin — *see* MRSA
        multiple drugs (MDRO)
          antibiotics Z16.24
          antimicrobial Z16.35
          antimycobacterials Z16.342
        penicillins Z16.11
        quinine (and related compounds) Z16.31
        quinolones Z16.23
        sulfonamides Z16.29
        tetracyclines Z16.29
        tuberculostatics (single) Z16.341
          multiple Z16.342
        vancomycin Z16.21
          related antibiotics Z16.22
  thyroid hormone E07.89
Resorption
  dental (roots) K03.3
    alveoli M26.79
  teeth (external) (internal) (pathological) (roots) K03.3
Respiration
  Cheyne-Stokes R06.3
  decreased due to shock, following injury T79.4 ☑
  disorder of, psychogenic F45.8
  insufficient, or poor R06.89
    newborn P28.5
  painful R07.1
  sighing, psychogenic F45.8
Respiratory — *see also* condition
  distress syndrome (newborn) (type I) P22.0
    type II P22.1
  syncytial virus, as cause of disease classified elsewhere
    — *see also* Virus, respiratory syncytial (RSV) B97.4
Respite care Z75.5
Response (drug)
  photoallergic L56.1
  phototoxic L56.0
Restenosis
  stent
    vascular
      end stent
        adjacent to stent — *see* Arteriosclerosis
        within the stent
          coronary T82.855 ☑
          peripheral T82.856 ☑
      in stent
        coronary vessel T82.855 ☑
        peripheral vessel T82.856 ☑
Restless legs (syndrome) G25.81
Restlessness R45.1
Restoration (of)
  dental
    aesthetically inadequate or displeasing K08.56
    defective K08.50
      specified NEC K08.59
    failure of marginal integrity K08.51
    failure of periodontal anatomical intergrity K08.54
    organ continuity from previous sterilization (tuboplas-
      ty) (vasoplasty) Z31.0
      aftercare Z31.42
    tooth (existing)
      contours biologically incompatible with oral health
        K08.54
      open margins K08.51
      overhanging K08.52
      poor aesthetic K08.56
      poor gingival margins K08.51
    unsatisfactory, of tooth K08.50
      specified NEC K08.59
Restorative material (dental)
  allergy to K08.55
  fractured K08.539
    with loss of material K08.531
    without loss of material K08.530
  unrepairable overhanging of K08.52
Restriction of housing space Z59.1
Rests, ovarian, in fallopian tube Q50.6
Restzustand (schizophrenic) F20.5

Index

Retained — see also Retention
  cholelithiasis following cholecystectomy K91.86
  foreign body fragments (type of) Z18.9
    acrylics Z18.2
    animal quill(s) or spines Z18.31
    cement Z18.83
    concrete Z18.83
    crystalline Z18.83
    depleted isotope Z18.09
    depleted uranium Z18.01
    diethylhexyl phthalates Z18.2
    glass Z18.81
    isocyanate Z18.2
    magnetic metal Z18.11
    metal Z18.10
    nonmagnectic metal Z18.12
    nontherapeutic radioactive Z18.09
    organic NEC Z18.39
    plastic Z18.2
    quill(s) (animal) Z18.31
    radioactive (nontherapeutic) NEC Z18.09
    specified NEC Z18.89
    spine(s) (animal) Z18.31
    stone Z18.83
    tooth (teeth) Z18.32
    wood Z18.33
  fragments (type of) Z18.9
    acrylics Z18.2
    animal quill(s) or spines Z18.31
    cement Z18.83
    concrete Z18.83
    crystalline Z18.83
    depleted isotope Z18.09
    depleted uranium Z18.01
    diethylhexyl phthalates Z18.2
    glass Z18.81
    isocyanate Z18.2
    magnetic metal Z18.11
    metal Z18.10
    nonmagnectic metal Z18.12
    nontherapeutic radioactive Z18.09
    organic NEC Z18.39
    plastic Z18.2
    quill(s) (animal) Z18.31
    radioactive (nontherapeutic) NEC Z18.09
    specified NEC Z18.89
    spine(s) (animal) Z18.31
    stone Z18.83
    tooth (teeth) Z18.32
    wood Z18.33
  gallstones, following cholecystectomy K91.86
Retardation
  development, developmental, specific — see Disorder,
    developmental
  endochondral bone growth — see Disorder, bone, de-
    velopment or growth
  growth R62.50
    due to malnutrition E45
  mental — see Disability, intellectual
  motor function, specific F82
  physical (child) R62.52
    due to malnutrition E45
  reading (specific) F81.0
  spelling (specific) (without reading disorder) F81.81
Retching — see Vomiting
Retention — see also Retained
  bladder — see Retention, urine
  carbon dioxide E87.29
  cholelithiasis following cholecystectomy K91.86
  cyst — see Cyst
  dead
    fetus (at or near term) (mother) O36.4 ☑
      early fetal death O02.1
      ovum O02.0
  decidua (fragments) (following delivery) (with hemor-
    rhage) O72.2
    without hemorrhage O73.1
  deciduous tooth K00.6
  dental root K08.3
  fecal — see Constipation
  fetus
    dead O36.4 ☑
      early O02.1
  fluid R60.9
  foreign body — see also Foreign body, retained
    current trauma — code as Foreign body, by site or
      type
  gallstones, following cholecystectomy K91.86

Retention — continued
  gastric K31.89
  intrauterine contraceptive device, in pregnancy — see
    Pregnancy, complicated by, retention, intrauter-
    ine device
  membranes (complicating delivery) (with hemorrhage)
    O72.2
    with abortion — see Abortion, by type
    without hemorrhage O73.1
  meniscus — see Derangement, meniscus
  menses N94.89
  milk (puerperal, postpartum) O92.79
  nitrogen, extrarenal R39.2
  ovary syndrome N99.83
  placenta (total) (with hemorrhage) O72.0
    without hemorrhage O73.0
    portions or fragments (with hemorrhage) O72.2
      without hemorrhage O73.1
  products of conception
    early pregnancy (dead fetus) O02.1
    following
      delivery (with hemorrhage) O72.2
        without hemorrhage O73.1
  secundines (following delivery) (with hemorrhage)
    O72.0
    without hemorrhage O73.0
    complicating puerperium (delayed hemorrhage)
      O72.2
    partial O72.2
      without hemorrhage O73.1
  smegma, clitoris N90.89
  urine R33.9
    due to hyperplasia (hypertrophy) of prostate — see
      Hyperplasia, prostate
    drug-induced R33.0
    organic R33.8
      drug-induced R33.0
    psychogenic F45.8
    specified NEC R33.8
  water (in tissues) — see Edema
Reticulation, dust — see Pneumoconiosis
Reticulocytosis R70.1
Reticuloendotheliosis
  acute infantile C96.0
  leukemic C91.4- ☑
  nonlipid C96.0
Reticulohistiocytoma (giant-cell) D76.3
Reticuloid, actinic L57.1
Reticulosis (skin)
  acute of infancy C96.0
  hemophagocytic, familial D76.1
  histiocytic medullary C96.A (following C96.6)
  lipomelanotic I89.8
  malignant (midline) C86.0
  polymorphic C83.8- ☑
  Sézary — see Sézary disease
Retina, retinal — see also condition
  dark area D49.81
Retinitis — see also Inflammation, chorioretinal
  albuminurica N18.9 [H32]
  diabetic — see Diabetes, retinitis
  disciformis — see Degeneration, macula
  focal — see Inflammation, chorioretinal, focal
  gravidarum — see Pregnancy, complicated by, speci-
    fied pregnancy-related condition NEC
  juxtapapillaris — see Inflammation, chorioretinal, focal,
    juxtapapillary
  luetic — see Retinitis, syphilitic
  pigmentosa H35.52
  proliferans — see Disorder, globe, degenerative, spec-
    ified type NEC
  proliferating — see Disorder, globe, degenerative,
    specified type NEC
  renal N18.9 [H32]
  syphilitic (early) (secondary) A51.43
    central, recurrent A52.71
    congenital (early) A50.01 [H32]
    late A52.71
  tuberculous A18.53
Retinoblastoma C69.2- ☑
  differentiated C69.2- ☑
  undifferentiated C69.2- ☑
Retinochoroiditis — see also Inflammation, chorioretinal
  disseminated — see Inflammation, chorioretinal, dis-
    seminated
    syphilitic A52.71
  focal — see Inflammation, chorioretinal

Retinochoroiditis — continued
  juxtapapillaris — see Inflammation, chorioretinal, focal,
    juxtapapillary
Retinopathy (background) H35.00
  arteriosclerotic I70.8 [H35.0-] ☑
  atherosclerotic I70.8 [H35.0-] ☑
  central serous — see Chorioretinopathy, central serous
  Coats H35.02- ☑
  diabetic — see Diabetes, retinopathy
  exudative H35.02- ☑
  hypertensive H35.03- ☑
  in (due to)
    diabetes — see Diabetes, retinopathy
    sickle-cell disorders D57.- ☑ [H36]
  of prematurity H35.10- ☑
    stage 0 H35.11- ☑
    stage 1 H35.12- ☑
    stage 2 H35.13- ☑
    stage 3 H35.14- ☑
    stage 4 H35.15- ☑
    stage 5 H35.16- ☑
  pigmentary, congenital — see Dystrophy, retina
  proliferative NEC H35.2- ☑
    diabetic — see Diabetes, retinopathy, proliferative
    sickle-cell D57.- ☑ [H36]
  solar H31.02- ☑
Retinoschisis H33.10- ☑
  congenital Q14.1
  specified type NEC H33.19- ☑
Retortamoniasis A07.8
Retractile testis Q55.22
Retraction
  cervix — see Retroversion, uterus
  drum (membrane) — see Disorder, tympanic mem-
    brane, specified NEC
  finger — see Deformity, finger
  lid H02.539
    left H02.536
      lower H02.535
      upper H02.534
    right H02.533
      lower H02.532
      upper H02.531
  lung J98.4
  mediastinum J98.59
  nipple N64.53
    associated with
      lactation O92.03
      pregnancy O92.01- ☑
      puerperium O92.02
    congenital Q83.8
  palmar fascia M72.0
  pleura — see Pleurisy
  ring, uterus (Bandl's) (pathological) O62.4
  sternum (congenital) Q76.7
    acquired M95.4
  uterus — see Retroversion, uterus
  valve (heart) — see Endocarditis
Retrobulbar — see condition
Retrocecal — see condition
Retrocession — see Retroversion
Retrodisplacement — see Retroversion
Retroflection, retroflexion — see Retroversion
Retrognathia, retrognathism (mandibular) (maxillary)
  M26.19
Retrograde menstruation N92.5
Retroperineal — see condition
Retroperitoneal — see condition
Retroperitonitis K68.9
Retropharyngeal — see condition
Retroplacental — see condition
Retroposition — see Retroversion
Retroprosthetic membrane T85.398 ☑
Retrosternal thyroid (congenital) Q89.2
Retroversion, retroverted
  cervix — see Retroversion, uterus
  female NEC — see Retroversion, uterus
  iris H21.89
  testis (congenital) Q55.29
  uterus (acquired) (acute) (any degree) (asymptomatic)
    (cervix) (postinfectional) (postpartal, old) N85.4
    congenital Q51.818
    in pregnancy O34.53- ☑
Retrovirus, as cause of disease classified elsewhere
  B97.30
  human
    immunodeficiency, type 2 (HIV 2) B97.35

Retained — Retrovirus, as cause of disease classified elsewhere

Retrovirus, as cause of disease classified elsewhere
— *continued*
  human — *continued*
    T-cell lymphotropic
      type I (HTLV-I) B97.33
      type II (HTLV-II) B97.34
  lentivirus B97.31
  oncovirus B97.32
  specified NEC B97.39
Retrusion, premaxilla (developmental) M26.09
Rett's disease or syndrome F84.2
Reverse peristalsis R19.2
Reye's syndrome G93.7
Rh (factor)
  hemolytic disease (newborn) P55.0
  incompatibility, immunization or sensitization
    affecting management of pregnancy NEC O36.09- ☑
      anti-D antibody O36.01- ☑
    newborn P55.0
    transfusion reaction — *see* Complication(s), transfusion, incompatibility reaction, Rh (factor)
  negative mother affecting newborn P55.0
  titer elevated — *see* Complication(s), transfusion, incompatibility reaction, Rh (factor)
  transfusion reaction — *see* Complication(s), transfusion, incompatibility reaction, Rh (factor)
Rhabdomyolysis (idiopathic) NEC M62.82
  traumatic T79.6 ☑
Rhabdomyoma — *see also* Neoplasm, connective tissue, benign
  adult — *see* Neoplasm, connective tissue, benign
  fetal — *see* Neoplasm, connective tissue, benign
  glycogenic — *see* Neoplasm, connective tissue, benign
Rhabdomyosarcoma (any type) — *see* Neoplasm, connective tissue, malignant
Rhabdosarcoma — *see* Rhabdomyosarcoma
Rhesus (factor) **incompatibility** — *see* Rh, incompatibility
Rheumatic (acute) (subacute)
  adherent pericardium I09.2
  chronic I09.89
  coronary arteritis I01.8
  degeneration, myocardium I09.0
  fever (acute) — *see* Fever, rheumatic
  heart — *see* Disease, heart, rheumatic
  myocardial degeneration — *see* Degeneration, myocardium
  myocarditis (chronic) (inactive) (with chorea) I09.0
    active or acute I01.2
      with chorea (acute) (rheumatic) (Sydenham's) I02.0
  pancarditis, acute I01.8
    with chorea (acute) (rheumatic) Sydenham's) I02.0
  pericarditis (active) (acute) (with effusion) (with pneumonia) I01.0
    with chorea (acute) (rheumatic) (Sydenham's) I02.0
    chronic or inactive I09.2
  pneumonia I00 [J17]
  torticollis M43.6
  typhoid fever A01.09
Rheumatism (articular) (neuralgic) (nonarticular) M79.0
  gout — *see* Arthritis, rheumatoid
  intercostal, meaning Tietze's disease M94.0
  palindromic (any site) M12.30
    ankle M12.37- ☑
    elbow M12.32- ☑
    foot joint M12.37- ☑
    hand joint M12.34- ☑
    hip M12.35- ☑
    knee M12.36- ☑
    multiple site M12.39
    shoulder M12.31- ☑
    specified joint NEC M12.38
    vertebrae M12.38
    wrist M12.33- ☑
  sciatic M54.4- ☑
Rheumatoid — *see also* condition
  arthritis — *see also* Arthritis, rheumatoid
    with involvement of organs NEC M05.60
      ankle M05.67- ☑
      elbow M05.62- ☑
      foot joint M05.67- ☑
      hand joint M05.64- ☑
      hip M05.65- ☑
      knee M05.66- ☑
      multiple site M05.69
      shoulder M05.61- ☑
      vertebra — *see* Spondylitis, ankylosing

Rheumatoid — *continued*
  arthritis — *see also* Arthritis, rheumatoid — *continued*
    with involvement of organs — *continued*
      wrist M05.63- ☑
    seronegative — *see* Arthritis, rheumatoid, seronegative
    seropositive — *see* Arthritis, rheumatoid, seropositive
  carditis M05.30
    ankle M05.37- ☑
    elbow M05.32- ☑
    foot joint M05.37- ☑
    hand joint M05.34- ☑
    hip M05.35- ☑
    knee M05.36- ☑
    multiple site M05.39
    shoulder M05.31- ☑
    vertebra — *see* Spondylitis, ankylosing
    wrist M05.33- ☑
  endocarditis — *see* Rheumatoid, carditis
  lung (disease) M05.10
    ankle M05.17- ☑
    elbow M05.12- ☑
    foot joint M05.17- ☑
    hand joint M05.14- ☑
    hip M05.15- ☑
    knee M05.16- ☑
    multiple site M05.19
    shoulder M05.11- ☑
    vertebra — *see* Spondylitis, ankylosing
    wrist M05.13- ☑
  myocarditis — *see* Rheumatoid, carditis
  myopathy M05.40
    ankle M05.47- ☑
    elbow M05.42- ☑
    foot joint M05.47- ☑
    hand joint M05.44- ☑
    hip M05.45- ☑
    knee M05.46- ☑
    multiple site M05.49
    shoulder M05.41- ☑
    vertebra — *see* Spondylitis, ankylosing
    wrist M05.43- ☑
  pericarditis — *see* Rheumatoid, carditis
  polyarthritis — *see* Arthritis, rheumatoid
  polyneuropathy M05.50
    ankle M05.57- ☑
    elbow M05.52- ☑
    foot joint M05.57- ☑
    hand joint M05.54- ☑
    hip M05.55- ☑
    knee M05.56- ☑
    multiple site M05.59
    shoulder M05.51- ☑
    vertebra — *see* Spondylitis, ankylosing
    wrist M05.53- ☑
  vasculitis M05.20
    ankle M05.27- ☑
    elbow M05.22- ☑
    foot joint M05.27- ☑
    hand joint M05.24- ☑
    hip M05.25- ☑
    knee M05.26- ☑
    multiple site M05.29
    shoulder M05.21- ☑
    vertebra — *see* Spondylitis, ankylosing
    wrist M05.23- ☑
Rhinitis (atrophic) (catarrhal) (chronic) (croupous) (fibrinous) (granulomatous) (hyperplastic) (hypertrophic) (membranous) (obstructive) (purulent) (suppurative) (ulcerative) J31.0
  with
    sore throat — *see* Nasopharyngitis
  acute J00
  allergic J30.9
    with asthma J45.909
      with
        exacerbation (acute) J45.901
        status asthmaticus J45.902
    due to
      food J30.5
      pollen J30.1
    nonseasonal J30.89
    perennial J30.89
    seasonal NEC J30.2
    specified NEC J30.89

Rhinitis — *continued*
  infective J00
  pneumococcal J00
  syphilitic A52.73
    congenital A50.05 [J99]
  tuberculous A15.8
  vasomotor J30.0
Rhinoantritis (chronic) — *see* Sinusitis, maxillary
Rhinodacryolith — *see* Dacryolith
Rhinolith (nasal sinus) J34.89
Rhinomegaly J34.89
Rhinopharyngitis (acute) (subacute) — *see also* Nasopharyngitis
  chronic J31.1
  destructive ulcerating A66.5
  mutilans A66.5
Rhinophyma L71.1
Rhinorrhea J34.89
  cerebrospinal (fluid) G96.01
    postoperative G96.08
    specified NEC G96.08
    spontaneous G96.01
    traumatic G96.08
  paroxysmal — *see* Rhinitis, allergic
  spasmodic — *see* Rhinitis, allergic
Rhinosalpingitis — *see* Salpingitis, eustachian
Rhinoscleroma A48.8
Rhinosporidiosis B48.1
Rhinovirus infection NEC B34.8
Rhizomelic chondrodysplasia punctata E71.540
Rhythm
  atrioventricular nodal I49.8
  disorder I49.9
    coronary sinus I49.8
    ectopic I49.8
    nodal I49.8
  escape I49.9
  heart, abnormal I49.9
  idioventricular I44.2
  nodal I49.8
  sleep, inversion G47.2- ☑
    nonorganic origin — *see* Disorder, sleep, circadian rhythm, psychogenic
Rhytidosis facialis L98.8
Rib — *see also* condition
  cervical Q76.5
Riboflavin deficiency E53.0
Rice bodies — *see also* Loose, body, joint
  knee M23.4- ☑
Richter syndrome — *see* Leukemia, chronic lymphocytic, B-cell type
Richter's hernia — *see* Hernia, abdomen, with obstruction
Ricinism — *see* Poisoning, food, noxious, plant
Rickets (active) (acute) (adolescent) (chest wall) (congenital) (current) (infantile) (intestinal) E55.0
  adult — *see* Osteomalacia
  celiac K90.0
  hypophosphatemic with nephrotic-glycosuric dwarfism E72.09
  inactive E64.3
  kidney N25.0
  renal N25.0
  sequelae, any E64.3
  vitamin-D-resistant E83.31 [M90.80]
Rickettsia 364D/R. philipii (Pacific Coast tick fever) A77.8
Rickettsial disease A79.9
  specified type NEC A79.89
Rickettsialpox (Rickettsia akari) A79.1
Rickettsiosis A79.9
  due to
    Ehrlichia sennetsu A79.81
    Neorickettsia sennetsu A79.81
    Rickettsia akari (rickettsialpox) A79.1
  specified type NEC A79.89
  tick-borne A77.9
  vesicular A79.1
Rider's bone — *see* Ossification, muscle, specified NEC
Ridge, alveolus — *see also* condition
  flabby K06.8
Ridged ear, congenital Q17.3
Riedel's
  lobe, liver Q44.7
  struma, thyroiditis or disease E06.5
Rieger's anomaly or syndrome Q13.81
Riehl's melanosis L81.4

Rietti-Greppi-Micheli anemia D56.9
Rieux's hernia — *see* Hernia, abdomen, specified site NEC
Riga (-Fede) **disease** K14.0
Riggs' disease — *see* Periodontitis
Right aortic arch Q25.47
Right middle lobe syndrome J98.11
Rigid, rigidity — *see also* condition
　abdominal R19.30
　　with severe abdominal pain R10.0
　　epigastric R19.36
　　generalized R19.37
　　left lower quadrant R19.34
　　left upper quadrant R19.32
　　periumbilic R19.35
　　right lower quadrant R19.33
　　right upper quadrant R19.31
　articular, multiple, congenital Q68.8
　cervix (uteri) in pregnancy — *see* Pregnancy, complicated by, abnormal, cervix
　hymen (acquired) (congenital) N89.6
　nuchal R29.1
　pelvic floor in pregnancy — *see* Pregnancy, complicated by, abnormal, pelvic organs or tissues NEC
　perineum or vulva in pregnancy — *see* Pregnancy, complicated by, abnormal, vulva
　spine — *see* Dorsopathy, specified NEC
　vagina in pregnancy — *see* Pregnancy, complicated by, abnormal, vagina
Rigors R68.89
　with fever R50.9
Riley-Day syndrome G90.1
RIND (reversible ischemic neurologic deficit) I63.9
Ring(s)
　aorta (vascular) Q25.45
　Bandl's O62.4
　contraction, complicating delivery O62.4
　esophageal, lower (muscular) K22.2
　Fleischer's (cornea) H18.04- ☑
　hymenal, tight (acquired) (congenital) N89.6
　Kayser-Fleischer (cornea) H18.04- ☑
　retraction, uterus, pathological O62.4
　Schatzki's (esophagus) (lower) K22.2
　　congenital Q39.3
　Soemmerring's — *see* Cataract, secondary
　vascular (congenital) Q25.8
　　aorta Q25.45
Ringed hair (congenital) Q84.1
Ringworm B35.9
　beard B35.0
　black dot B35.0
　body B35.4
　Burmese B35.5
　corporeal B35.4
　foot B35.3
　groin B35.6
　hand B35.2
　honeycomb B35.0
　nails B35.1
　perianal (area) B35.6
　scalp B35.0
　specified NEC B35.8
　Tokelau B35.5
Rise, venous pressure I87.8
Rising, PSA following treatment for malignant neoplasm of prostate R97.21
Risk
　for
　　dental caries Z91.849
　　　high Z91.843
　　　low Z91.841
　　　moderate Z91.842
　　homelessness, imminent Z59.811
　　suffocation (smothering) under another while sleeping Z72.823
　suicidal
　　meaning personal history of attempted suicide Z91.51
　　meaning suicidal ideation — *see* Ideation, suicidal
Ritter's disease L00
Rivalry, sibling Z62.891
Rivalta's disease A42.2
River blindness B73.01
Robert's pelvis Q74.2
　with disproportion (fetopelvic) O33.0
　　causing obstructed labor O65.0
Robin (-Pierre) **syndrome** Q87.0
Robinow-Silvermann-Smith syndrome Q87.19

Robinson's (hidrotic) **ectodermal dysplasia or syndrome** Q82.4
Robles' disease B73.01
Rocky Mountain (spotted) **fever** A77.0
Roetheln — *see* Rubella
Roger's disease Q21.0
Rokitansky-Aschoff sinuses (gallbladder) K82.8
Rolando's fracture (displaced) S62.22- ☑
　nondisplaced S62.22-
Romano-Ward (prolonged QT interval) **syndrome** I45.81
Romberg's disease or syndrome G51.8
Roof, mouth — *see* condition
Rosacea L71.9
　acne L71.9
　keratitis L71.8
　specified NEC L71.8
Rosary, rachitic E55.0
Rose
　cold J30.1
　fever J30.1
　rash R21
　　epidemic B06.9
Rosenbach's erysipeloid A26.0
Rosenthal's disease or syndrome D68.1
Roseola B09
　infantum B08.20
　　due to human herpesvirus 6 B08.21
　　due to human herpesvirus 7 B08.22
Ross River disease or fever B33.1
Rossbach's disease K31.89
　psychogenic F45.8
Rostan's asthma (cardiac) — *see* Failure, ventricular, left
Rotation
　anomalous, incomplete or insufficient, intestine Q43.3
　cecum (congenital) Q43.3
　colon (congenital) Q43.3
　spine, incomplete or insufficient — *see* Dorsopathy, deforming, specified NEC
　tooth, teeth, fully erupted M26.35
　vertebra, incomplete or insufficient — *see* Dorsopathy, deforming, specified NEC
Rotes Quérol disease or syndrome — *see* Hyperostosis, ankylosing
Roth (-Bernhardt) **disease or syndrome** — *see* Meralgia paraesthetica
Rothmund (-Thomson) **syndrome** Q82.8
Rotor's disease or syndrome E80.6
Round
　back (with wedging of vertebrae) — *see* Kyphosis
　　sequelae (late effect) of rickets E64.3
　worms (large) (infestation) NEC B82.0
　　Ascariasis — *see also* Ascariasis B77.9
Roussy-Lévy syndrome G60.0
Rubella (German measles) B06.9
　complication NEC B06.09
　　neurological B06.00
　congenital P35.0
　contact Z20.4
　exposure to Z20.4
　maternal
　　care for (suspected) damage to fetus O35.3 ☑
　　manifest rubella in infant P35.0
　　suspected damage to fetus affecting management of pregnancy O35.3 ☑
　specified complications NEC B06.89
Rubeola (meaning measles) — *see* Measles
　meaning rubella — *see* Rubella
Rubeosis, iris — *see* Disorder, iris, vascular
Rubinstein-Taybi syndrome Q87.2
Rudimentary (congenital) — *see also* Agenesis
　arm — *see* Defect, reduction, upper limb
　bone Q79.9
　cervix uteri Q51.828
　eye Q11.2
　lobule of ear Q17.3
　patella Q74.1
　respiratory organs in thoracopagus Q89.4
　tracheal bronchus Q32.4
　uterus Q51.818
　　in male Q56.1
　vagina Q52.0
Ruled out condition — *see* Observation, suspected
Rumination R11.10
　with nausea R11.2
　disorder of infancy F98.21
　neurotic F42.8
　newborn P92.1

Rumination — *continued*
　obsessional F42.8
　psychogenic F42.8
Runeberg's disease D51.0
Running out of money Z59.86
Runny nose R09.89
Rupia (syphilitic) A51.39
　congenital A50.06
　tertiary A52.79
Rupture, ruptured
　abscess (spontaneous) — *code by* site under Abscess
　aneurysm — *see* Aneurysm
　anus (sphincter) — *see* Laceration, anus
　aorta, aortic I71.8
　　abdominal I71.30
　　　infrarenal I71.33
　　　juxtarenal I71.32
　　　pararenal I71.31
　　arch I71.12
　　ascending I71.11
　　descending I71.8
　　　abdominal I71.30
　　　thoracic I71.13
　　syphilitic A52.01
　　thoracoabdominal I71.50
　　　paravisceral I71.52
　　　supraceliac I71.51
　　thorax, thoracic I71.10
　　transverse I71.12
　　traumatic — *see* Injury, aorta, laceration, major
　　valve or cusp — *see also* Endocarditis, aortic I35.8
　appendix (with peritonitis) — *see also* Appendicitis K35.32
　　with localized peritonitis — *see also* Appendicitis K35.32
　arteriovenous fistula, brain — *see* Fistula, arteriovenous, brain, ruptured
　artery I77.2
　　brain — *see* Hemorrhage, intracranial, intracerebral
　　coronary — *see* Infarct, myocardium
　　heart — *see* Infarct, myocardium
　　pulmonary I28.8
　　traumatic (complication) — *see* Injury, blood vessel
　bile duct (common) (hepatic) K83.2
　　cystic K82.2
　bladder (sphincter) (nontraumatic) (spontaneous) N32.89
　　following ectopic or molar pregnancy O08.6
　　obstetrical trauma O71.5
　　traumatic S37.29 ☑
　blood vessel — *see also* Hemorrhage
　　brain — *see* Hemorrhage, intracranial, intracerebral
　　heart — *see* Infarct, myocardium
　　traumatic (complication) — *see* Injury, blood vessel, laceration, major, by site
　bone — *see* Fracture
　bowel (nontraumatic) K63.1
　brain
　　aneurysm (congenital) — *see also* Hemorrhage, intracranial, subarachnoid
　　　syphilitic A52.05
　　hemorrhagic — *see* Hemorrhage, intracranial, intracerebral
　capillaries I78.8
　cardiac (auricle) (ventricle) (wall) I23.3
　　with hemopericardium I23.0
　　infectional I40.9
　　traumatic — *see* Injury, heart
　cartilage (articular) (current) — *see also* Sprain
　　knee S83.3- ☑
　　semilunar — *see* Tear, meniscus
　cecum (with peritonitis) K65.0
　　with peritoneal abscess K35.33
　　traumatic S36.598 ☑
　celiac artery, traumatic — *see* Injury, blood vessel, celiac artery, laceration, major
　cerebral aneurysm (congenital) (see Hemorrhage, intracranial, subarachnoid)
　cervix (uteri)
　　with ectopic or molar pregnancy O08.6
　　following ectopic or molar pregnancy O08.6
　　obstetrical trauma O71.3
　　traumatic S37.69 ☑
　chordae tendineae NEC I51.1
　　concurrent with acute myocardial infarction — *see* Infarct, myocardium
　　following acute myocardial infarction (current complication) I23.4

Rupture, ruptured — *continued*
  choroid (direct) (indirect) (traumatic) H31.32- ☑
  circle of Willis I60.6
  colon (nontraumatic) K63.1
    traumatic — *see* Injury, intestine, large
  cornea (traumatic) — *see* Injury, eye, laceration
  coronary (artery) (thrombotic) — *see* Infarct, myocardium
  corpus luteum (infected) (ovary) N83.1- ☑
  cyst — *see* Cyst
  cystic duct K82.2
  Descemet's membrane — *see* Change, corneal membrane, Descemet's, rupture
    traumatic — *see* Injury, eye, laceration
  diaphragm, traumatic — *see* Injury, intrathoracic, diaphragm
  disc — *see* Rupture, intervertebral disc
  diverticulum (intestine) K57.80
    with bleeding K57.81
    bladder N32.3
    large intestine K57.20
      with
        bleeding K57.21
        small intestine K57.40
          with bleeding K57.41
      small intestine K57.00
        with
          bleeding K57.01
          large intestine K57.40
            with bleeding K57.41
  duodenal stump K31.89
  ear drum (nontraumatic) — *see also* Perforation, tympanum
    traumatic S09.2- ☑
      due to blast injury — *see* Injury, blast, ear
  esophagus K22.3
  eye (without prolapse or loss of intraocular tissue) — *see* Injury, eye, laceration
  fallopian tube NEC (nonobstetric) (nontraumatic) N83.8
    due to pregnancy O00.10- ☑
      with intrauterine pregnancy O00.11- ☑
  fontanel P13.1
  gallbladder K82.2
    traumatic S36.128 ☑
  gastric — *see also* Rupture, stomach
    vessel K92.2
  globe (eye) (traumatic) — *see* Injury, eye, laceration
  graafian follicle (hematoma) N83.0- ☑
  heart — *see* Rupture, cardiac
  hymen (nontraumatic) (nonintentional) N89.8
  internal organ, traumatic — *see* Injury, by site
  intervertebral disc — *see* Displacement, intervertebral disc
    traumatic — *see* Rupture, traumatic, intervertebral disc
  intestine NEC (nontraumatic) K63.1
    traumatic — *see* Injury, intestine
  iris — *see also* Abnormality, pupillary
    traumatic — *see* Injury, eye, laceration
  joint capsule, traumatic — *see* Sprain
  kidney (traumatic) S37.06- ☑
    birth injury P15.8
    nontraumatic N28.89
  lacrimal duct (traumatic) — *see* Injury, eye, specified site NEC
  lens (cataract) (traumatic) — *see* Cataract, traumatic
  ligament, traumatic — *see* Rupture, traumatic, ligament, by site
  liver S36.116 ☑
    birth injury P15.0
  lymphatic vessel I89.8
  marginal sinus (placental) (with hemorrhage) — *see* Hemorrhage, antepartum, specified cause NEC
  membrana tympani (nontraumatic) — *see* Perforation, tympanum
  membranes (spontaneous)
    artificial
      delayed delivery following O75.5
      delayed delivery following — *see* Pregnancy, complicated by, premature rupture of membranes
  meningeal artery I60.8
  meniscus (knee) — *see also* Tear, meniscus
    old — *see* Derangement, meniscus
    site other than knee — *code as* Sprain
  mesenteric artery, traumatic — *see* Injury, mesenteric, artery, laceration, major
  mesentery (nontraumatic) K66.8

Rupture, ruptured — *continued*
  mesentery — *continued*
    traumatic — *see* Injury, intra-abdominal, specified, site NEC
  mitral (valve) I34.89
  muscle (traumatic) — *see also* Strain
    diastasis — *see* Diastasis, muscle
    nontraumatic M62.10
      ankle M62.17- ☑
      foot M62.17- ☑
      forearm M62.13- ☑
      hand M62.14- ☑
      lower leg M62.16- ☑
      pelvic region M62.15- ☑
      shoulder region M62.11- ☑
      specified site NEC M62.18
      thigh M62.15- ☑
      upper arm M62.12- ☑
    traumatic — *see* Strain, by site
  musculotendinous junction NEC, nontraumatic — *see* Rupture, tendon, spontaneous
  mycotic aneurysm causing cerebral hemorrhage — *see* Hemorrhage, intracranial, subarachnoid
  myocardium, myocardial — *see* Rupture, cardiac
    traumatic — *see* Injury, heart
  nontraumatic, meaning hernia — *see* Hernia
  obstructed — *see* Hernia, by site, obstructed
  operation wound — *see* Disruption, wound, operation
  ovary, ovarian N83.8
    corpus luteum cyst N83.1- ☑
    follicle (graafian) N83.0- ☑
  oviduct (nonobstetric) (nontraumatic) N83.8
    due to pregnancy O00.10- ☑
      with intrauterine pregnancy O00.11- ☑
  pancreas (nontraumatic) K86.89
    traumatic S36.299 ☑
  papillary muscle NEC I51.2
    following acute myocardial infarction (current complication) I23.5
  pelvic
    floor, complicating delivery O70.1
    organ NEC, obstetrical trauma O71.5
  perineum (nonobstetric) (nontraumatic) N90.89
    complicating delivery — *see* Delivery, complicated, by, laceration, anus (sphincter)
  postoperative wound — *see* Disruption, wound, operation
  prostate (traumatic) S37.828 ☑
  pulmonary
    artery I28.8
    valve (heart) I37.8
    vein I28.8
    vessel I28.8
  pus tube — *see* Salpingitis
  pyosalpinx — *see* Salpingitis
  rectum (nontraumatic) K63.1
    traumatic S36.69 ☑
  retina, retinal (traumatic) (without detachment) — *see also* Break, retina
    with detachment — *see* Detachment, retina, with retinal, break
  rotator cuff (nontraumatic) M75.10- ☑
    complete M75.12- ☑
    incomplete M75.11- ☑
  sclera — *see* Injury, eye, laceration
  sigmoid (nontraumatic) K63.1
    traumatic S36.593 ☑
  spinal cord — *see also* Injury, spinal cord, by region
    due to injury at birth P11.5
    newborn (birth injury) P11.5
  spleen (traumatic) S36.09 ☑
    birth injury P15.1
    congenital (birth injury) P15.1
    due to P. vivax malaria B51.0
    nontraumatic D73.5
    spontaneous D73.5
  splenic vein R58
    traumatic — *see* Injury, blood vessel, splenic vein
  stomach (nontraumatic) (spontaneous) K31.89
    traumatic S36.39 ☑
  supraspinatus (complete) (incomplete) (nontraumatic) — *see* Tear, rotator cuff
  symphysis pubis
    obstetric O71.6
    traumatic S33.4 ☑
  synovium (cyst) M66.10
    ankle M66.17- ☑

Rupture, ruptured — *continued*
  synovium — *continued*
    elbow M66.12- ☑
    finger M66.14- ☑
    foot M66.17- ☑
    forearm M66.13- ☑
    hand M66.14- ☑
    pelvic region M66.15- ☑
    shoulder region M66.11- ☑
    specified site NEC M66.18
    thigh M66.15- ☑
    toe M66.17- ☑
    upper arm M66.12- ☑
    wrist M66.13- ☑
  tendon (traumatic) — *see* Strain
    nontraumatic (spontaneous) M66.9
      ankle M66.87- ☑
      extensor M66.20
        ankle M66.27- ☑
        foot M66.27- ☑
        forearm M66.23- ☑
        hand M66.24- ☑
        lower leg M66.26- ☑
        multiple sites M66.29
        pelvic region M66.25- ☑
        shoulder region M66.21- ☑
        specified site NEC M66.28
        thigh M66.25- ☑
        upper arm M66.22- ☑
      flexor M66.30
        ankle M66.37- ☑
        foot M66.37- ☑
        forearm M66.33- ☑
        hand M66.34- ☑
        lower leg M66.36- ☑
        multiple sites M66.39
        pelvic region M66.35- ☑
        shoulder region M66.31- ☑
        specified site NEC M66.38
        thigh M66.35- ☑
        upper arm M66.32- ☑
      foot M66.87- ☑
      forearm M66.83- ☑
      hand M66.84- ☑
      lower leg M66.86- ☑
      multiple sites M66.89
      pelvic region M66.85- ☑
      shoulder region M66.81- ☑
      specified
        site NEC M66.88
        tendon M66.80
      thigh M66.85- ☑
      upper arm M66.82- ☑
  thoracic duct I89.8
  tonsil J35.8
  traumatic
    aorta — *see* Injury, aorta, laceration, major
    diaphragm — *see* Injury, intrathoracic, diaphragm
    external site — *see* Wound, open, by site
    eye — *see* Injury, eye, laceration
    internal organ — *see* Injury, by site
    intervertebral disc
      cervical S13.0 ☑
      lumbar S33.0 ☑
      thoracic S23.0 ☑
    kidney S37.06- ☑
    ligament — *see also* Sprain
      ankle — *see* Sprain, ankle
      carpus — *see* Rupture, traumatic, ligament, wrist
      collateral (hand) — *see* Rupture, traumatic, ligament, finger, collateral
      finger (metacarpophalangeal) (interphalangeal) S63.40- ☑
        collateral S63.41- ☑
          index S63.41- ☑
          little S63.41- ☑
          middle S63.41- ☑
          ring S63.41- ☑
        index S63.40- ☑
        little S63.40- ☑
        middle S63.40- ☑
        palmar S63.42- ☑
          index S63.42- ☑
          little S63.42- ☑
          middle S63.42- ☑
          ring S63.42- ☑

Rupture, ruptured — continued
  traumatic — continued
    ligament — see also Sprain — continued
      finger — continued
        ring S63.40- ☑
        specified site NEC S63.499 ☑
          index S63.49- ☑
          little S63.49- ☑
          middle S63.49- ☑
          ring S63.49- ☑
        volar plate S63.43- ☑
          index S63.43- ☑
          little S63.43- ☑
          middle S63.43- ☑
          ring S63.43- ☑
      foot — see Sprain, foot
      radial collateral S53.2- ☑
      radiocarpal — see Rupture, traumatic, ligament,
        wrist, radiocarpal
      ulnar collateral S53.3- ☑
      ulnocarpal — see Rupture, traumatic, ligament,
        wrist, ulnocarpal
      wrist S63.30- ☑
        collateral S63.31- ☑
        radiocarpal S63.32- ☑
        specified site NEC S63.39- ☑
        ulnocarpal (palmar) S63.33- ☑
    liver S36.116 ☑
    membrana tympani — see Rupture, ear drum,
      traumatic
    muscle or tendon — see Strain
    myocardium — see Injury, heart
    pancreas S36.299 ☑
    rectum S36.69 ☑
    sigmoid S36.593 ☑
    spleen S36.09 ☑
    stomach S36.39 ☑
    symphysis pubis S33.4 ☑
    tympanum, tympanic (membrane) — see Rupture,
      ear drum, traumatic
    ureter S37.19 ☑
    uterus S37.69 ☑
    vagina — see Injury, vagina
    vena cava — see Injury, vena cava, laceration, major
  tricuspid (heart) (valve) I07.8
  tube, tubal (nonobstetric) (nontraumatic) N83.8
    abscess — see Salpingitis
    due to pregnancy O00.10- ☑
      with intrauterine pregnancy O00.11- ☑
  tympanum, tympanic (membrane) (nontraumatic) —
    see also Perforation, tympanic membrane
    H72.9- ☑
    traumatic — see Rupture, ear drum, traumatic
  umbilical cord, complicating delivery O69.89 ☑
  ureter (traumatic) S37.19 ☑
    nontraumatic N28.89
  urethra (nontraumatic) N36.8
    with ectopic or molar pregnancy O08.6
    following ectopic or molar pregnancy O08.6
    obstetrical trauma O71.5
    traumatic S37.39 ☑
  uterosacral ligament (nonobstetric) (nontraumatic)
    N83.8
  uterus (traumatic) S37.69 ☑
    before labor O71.0- ☑
    during or after labor O71.1
    nonpuerperal, nontraumatic N85.8
    pregnant (during labor) O71.1
      before labor O71.0- ☑
  vagina — see Injury, vagina
  valve, valvular (heart) — see Endocarditis
  varicose vein — see Varix
  varix — see Varix
  vena cava R58
    traumatic — see Injury, vena cava, laceration, major
  vesical (urinary) N32.89
  vessel (blood) R58
    pulmonary I28.8
    traumatic — see Injury, blood vessel
  viscus R19.8
  vulva complicating delivery O70.0
Russell-Silver syndrome Q87.19
Russian spring-summer type encephalitis A84.0
Rust's disease (tuberculous cervical spondylitis) A18.01
Ruvalcaba-Myhre-Smith syndrome E71.440
Rytand-Lipsitch syndrome I44.2

S

Saber, sabre shin or tibia (syphilitic) A50.56 [M90.8-] ☑
Sac lacrimal — see condition
Saccharomyces infection B37.9
Saccharopinuria E72.3
Saccular — see condition
Sacculation
  aorta (nonsyphilitic) — see Aneurysm, aorta
  bladder N32.3
  intralaryngeal (congenital) (ventricular) Q31.3
  larynx (congenital) (ventricular) Q31.3
  organ or site, congenital — see Distortion
  pregnant uterus — see Pregnancy, complicated by,
    abnormal, uterus
  ureter N28.89
  urethra N36.1
  vesical N32.3
Sachs' amaurotic familial idiocy or disease E75.02
Sachs-Tay disease E75.02
Sacks-Libman disease M32.11
Sacralgia M53.3
Sacralization Q76.49
Sacrodynia M53.3
Sacroiliac joint — see condition
Sacroiliitis NEC M46.1
Sacrum — see condition
Saddle
  back — see Lordosis
  embolus
    abdominal aorta I74.01
    pulmonary artery I26.92
      with acute cor pulmonale I26.02
  injury — code to condition
  nose M95.0
    due to syphilis A50.57
Sadism (sexual) F65.52
Sadness, postpartal O90.6
Sadomasochism F65.50
Saemisch's ulcer (cornea) — see Ulcer, cornea, central
Sagging
  skin and subcutaneous tissue (following bariatric
    surgery weight loss) (following dietary weight
    loss) L98.7
Sahib disease B55.0
Sailors' skin L57.8
Saint
  Anthony's fire — see Erysipelas
  triad — see Hernia, diaphragm
  Vitus' dance — see Chorea, Sydenham's
Salaam
  attack(s) — see Epilepsy, spasms
  tic R25.8
Salicylism
  abuse F55.8
  overdose or wrong substance given — see Table of
    Drugs and Chemicals, by drug, poisoning
Salivary duct or gland — see condition
Salivation, excessive K11.7
Salmonella — see Infection, Salmonella
Salmonellosis A02.0
Salpingitis (catarrhal) (fallopian tube) (nodular) (pseud-
  ofollicular) (purulent) (septic) N70.91
  with oophoritis N70.93
  acute N70.01
    with oophoritis N70.03
  chlamydial A56.11
  chronic N70.11
    with oophoritis N70.13
  complicating abortion — see Abortion, by type, com-
    plicated by, salpingitis
  ear — see Salpingitis, eustachian
  eustachian (tube) H68.00- ☑
    acute H68.01- ☑
    chronic H68.02- ☑
  follicularis N70.11
    with oophoritis N70.13
  gonococcal (acute) (chronic) A54.24
  interstitial, chronic N70.11
    with oophoritis N70.13
  isthmica nodosa N70.11
    with oophoritis N70.13
  specific (gonococcal) (acute) (chronic) A54.24
  tuberculous (acute) (chronic) A18.17
  venereal (gonococcal) (acute) (chronic) A54.24
Salpingocele N83.4- ☑

Salpingo-oophoritis (catarrhal) (purulent) (ruptured)
  (septic) (suppurative) N70.93
  acute N70.03
    with ectopic or molar pregnancy O08.0
    following ectopic or molar pregnancy O08.0
    gonococcal A54.24
  chronic N70.13
  following ectopic or molar pregnancy O08.0
  gonococcal (acute) (chronic) A54.24
  puerperal O86.19
  specific (gonococcal) (acute) (chronic) A54.24
  subacute N70.03
  tuberculous (acute) (chronic) A18.17
  venereal (gonococcal) (acute) (chronic) A54.24
Salpingo-ovaritis — see Salpingo-oophoritis
Salpingoperitonitis — see Salpingo-oophoritis
Salzmann's nodular dystrophy — see Degeneration,
  cornea, nodular
Sampson's cyst or tumor N80.10- ☑
San Joaquin (Valley) **fever** B38.0
Sandblaster's asthma, lung or pneumoconiosis J62.8
Sander's disease (paranoia) F22
Sandfly fever A93.1
Sandhoff's disease E75.01
Sanfilippo (Type B) (Type C) (Type D) **syndrome** E76.22
Sanger-Brown ataxia G11.2
Sao Paulo fever or typhus A77.0
Saponification, mesenteric K65.8
Sarcocele (benign)
  syphilitic A52.76
    congenital A50.59
Sarcocystosis A07.8
Sarcoepiplocele — see Hernia
Sarcoepiplomphalocele Q79.2
Sarcoglycanopathy G71.0340
  alpha G71.0341
  beta G71.0342
  delta G71.0349
  gamma G71.0349
Sarcoid — see also Sarcoidosis
  arthropathy D86.86
  Boeck's D86.9
  Darier-Roussy D86.3
  iridocyclitis D86.83
  meningitis D86.81
  myocarditis D86.85
  myositis D86.87
  pyelonephritis D86.84
  Spiegler-Fendt L08.89
Sarcoidosis D86.9
  with
    cranial nerve palsies D86.82
    hepatic granuloma D86.89
    polyarthritis D86.86
    tubulo-interstitial nephropathy D86.84
  combined sites NEC D86.89
  lung D86.0
    and lymph nodes D86.2
  lymph nodes D86.1
    and lung D86.2
  meninges D86.81
  skin D86.3
  specified type NEC D86.89
Sarcoma (of) — see also Neoplasm, connective tissue,
  malignant
  alveolar soft part — see Neoplasm, connective tissue,
    malignant
  ameloblastic C41.1
    upper jaw (bone) C41.0
  botryoid — see Neoplasm, connective tissue, malignant
  botryoides — see Neoplasm, connective tissue, malig-
    nant
  cerebellar C71.6
    circumscribed (arachnoidal) C71.6
  circumscribed (arachnoidal) cerebellar C71.6
  clear cell — see also Neoplasm, connective tissue, ma-
    lignant
    kidney C64.- ☑
  dendritic cells (accessory cells) C96.4
  embryonal — see Neoplasm, connective tissue, malig-
    nant
  endometrial (stromal) C54.1
    isthmus C54.0
  epithelioid (cell) — see Neoplasm, connective tissue,
    malignant
  Ewing's — see Neoplasm, bone, malignant
  follicular dendritic cell C96.4

Index

Sarcoma — Schmidt's syndrome

Sarcoma — *continued*
- germinoblastic (diffuse) — *see* Lymphoma, diffuse large cell
  - follicular — *see* Lymphoma, follicular, specified NEC
- giant cell (except of bone) — *see also* Neoplasm, connective tissue, malignant
  - bone — *see* Neoplasm, bone, malignant
- glomoid — *see* Neoplasm, connective tissue, malignant
- granulocytic C92.3- ☑
- hemangioendothelial — *see* Neoplasm, connective tissue, malignant
- hemorrhagic, multiple — *see* Sarcoma, Kaposi's
- histiocytic C96.A *(following C96.6)*
- Hodgkin — *see* Lymphoma, Hodgkin
- immunoblastic (diffuse) — *see* Lymphoma, diffuse large cell
- interdigitating dendritic cell C96.4
- Kaposi's
  - colon C46.4
  - connective tissue C46.1
  - gastrointestinal organ C46.4
  - lung C46.5- ☑
  - lymph node(s) C46.3
  - palate (hard) (soft) C46.2
  - rectum C46.4
  - skin C46.0
  - specified site NEC C46.7
  - stomach C46.4
  - unspecified site C46.9
- Kupffer cell C22.3
- Langerhans cell C96.4
- leptomeningeal — *see* Neoplasm, meninges, malignant
- liver NEC C22.4
- lymphangioendothelial — *see* Neoplasm, connective tissue, malignant
- lymphoblastic — *see* Lymphoma, lymphoblastic (diffuse)
- lymphocytic — *see* Lymphoma, small cell B-cell
- mast cell C96.22
- melanotic — *see* Melanoma
- meningeal — *see* Neoplasm, meninges, malignant
- meningothelial — *see* Neoplasm, meninges, malignant
- mesenchymal — *see also* Neoplasm, connective tissue, malignant
  - mixed — *see* Neoplasm, connective tissue, malignant
- mesothelial — *see* Mesothelioma
- monstrocellular
  - specified site — *see* Neoplasm, malignant, by site
  - unspecified site C71.9
- myeloid C92.3- ☑
- neurogenic — *see* Neoplasm, nerve, malignant
- odontogenic C41.1
  - upper jaw (bone) C41.0
- osteoblastic — *see* Neoplasm, bone, malignant
- osteogenic — *see also* Neoplasm, bone, malignant
  - juxtacortical — *see* Neoplasm, bone, malignant
  - periosteal — *see* Neoplasm, bone, malignant
- periosteal — *see also* Neoplasm, bone, malignant
  - osteogenic — *see* Neoplasm, bone, malignant
- pleomorphic cell — *see* Neoplasm, connective tissue, malignant
- reticulum cell (diffuse) — *see* Lymphoma, diffuse large cell
  - nodular — *see* Lymphoma, follicular
  - pleomorphic cell type — *see* Lymphoma, diffuse large cell
- rhabdoid — *see* Neoplasm, malignant, by site
- round cell — *see* Neoplasm, connective tissue, malignant
- small cell — *see* Neoplasm, connective tissue, malignant
- soft tissue — *see* Neoplasm, connective tissue, malignant
- spindle cell — *see* Neoplasm, connective tissue, malignant
- stromal (endometrial) C54.1
  - isthmus C54.0
- synovial — *see also* Neoplasm, connective tissue, malignant
  - biphasic — *see* Neoplasm, connective tissue, malignant
  - epithelioid cell — *see* Neoplasm, connective tissue, malignant
  - spindle cell — *see* Neoplasm, connective tissue, malignant

Sarcomatosis
- meningeal — *see* Neoplasm, meninges, malignant
- specified site NEC — *see* Neoplasm, connective tissue, malignant
- unspecified site C80.1

Sarcopenia (age-related) M62.84
Sarcosinemia E72.59
Sarcosporidiosis (intestinal) A07.8
SARS-CoV-2 — *see also* COVID-19
- sequelae (post acute) U09.9
Satiety, early R68.81
Saturnine — *see* condition
Saturnism
- overdose or wrong substance given or taken — *see* Table of Drugs and Chemicals, by drug, poisoning
Satyriasis F52.8
Sauriasis — *see* Ichthyosis
SBE (subacute bacterial endocarditis) I33.0
Scabies (any site) B86
Scabs R23.4
Scaglietti-Dagnini syndrome E22.0
Scald — *see* Burn
Scalenus anticus (anterior) **syndrome** G54.0
Scales R23.4
Scaling, skin R23.4
Scalp — *see* condition
Scapegoating affecting child Z62.3
Scaphocephaly Q75.0
Scapulalgia M89.8X1
Scapulohumeral myopathy G71.02
Scar, scarring — *see also* Cicatrix L90.5
- adherent L90.5
- atrophic L90.5
- cervix
  - in pregnancy or childbirth — *see* Pregnancy, complicated by, abnormal cervix
- cheloid L91.0
- chorioretinal H31.00- ☑
  - posterior pole macula H31.01- ☑
  - postsurgical H59.81- ☑
  - solar retinopathy H31.02- ☑
  - specified type NEC H31.09- ☑
- choroid — *see* Scar, chorioretinal
- conjunctiva H11.24- ☑
- cornea H17.9
  - xerophthalmic — *see also* Opacity, cornea
    - vitamin A deficiency E50.6
- defect (isthmocele) O34.22
- duodenum, obstructive K31.5
- hypertrophic L91.0
- keloid L91.0
- labia N90.89
- lung (base) J98.4
- macula — *see* Scar, chorioretinal, posterior pole
- muscle M62.89
- myocardium, myocardial I25.2
- painful L90.5
- posterior pole (eye) — *see* Scar, chorioretinal, posterior pole
- retina — *see* Scar, chorioretinal
- trachea J39.8
- transmural uterine, in pregnancy O34.29
- uterus N85.8
  - in pregnancy O34.29
- vagina N89.8
  - postoperative N99.2
- vulva N90.89
Scarabiasis B88.2
Scarlatina (anginosa) (maligna) A38.9
- myocarditis (acute) A38.1
  - old — *see* Myocarditis
- otitis media A38.0
- ulcerosa A38.8
Scarlet fever (albuminuria) (angina) A38.9
Schamberg's disease (progressive pigmentary dermatosis) L81.7
Schatzki's ring (acquired) (esophagus) (lower) K22.2
- congenital Q39.3
Schaufenster krankheit I20.8
Schaumann's
- benign lymphogranulomatosis D86.1
- disease or syndrome — *see* Sarcoidosis
Scheie's syndrome E76.03
Schenck's disease B42.1
Scheuermann's disease or osteochondrosis — *see* Osteochondrosis, juvenile, spine
Schilder (-Flatau) **disease** G37.0

Schilling-type monocytic leukemia C93.0- ☑
Schimmelbusch's disease, cystic mastitis, or hyperplasia — *see* Mastopathy, cystic
Schistosoma infestation — *see* Infestation, Schistosoma
Schistosomiasis B65.9
- with muscle disorder B65.9 *[M63.80]*
  - ankle B65.9 *[M63.87-]* ☑
  - foot B65.9 *[M63.87-]* ☑
  - forearm B65.9 *[M63.83-]* ☑
  - hand B65.9 *[M63.84-]* ☑
  - lower leg B65.9 *[M63.86-]* ☑
  - multiple sites B65.9 *[M63.89]*
  - pelvic region B65.9 *[M63.85-]* ☑
  - shoulder region B65.9 *[M63.81-]* ☑
  - specified site NEC B65.9 *[M63.88]*
  - thigh B65.9 *[M63.85-]* ☑
  - upper arm B65.9 *[M63.82-]* ☑
- Asiatic B65.2
- bladder B65.0
- chestermani B65.8
- colon B65.1
- cutaneous B65.3
- due to
  - S. haematobium B65.0
  - S. japonicum B65.2
  - S. mansoni B65.1
  - S. mattheii B65.8
- Eastern B65.2
- genitourinary tract B65.0
- intestinal B65.1
- lung NEC B65.9 *[J99]*
  - pneumonia B65.9 *[J17]*
- Manson's (intestinal) B65.1
- oriental B65.2
- pulmonary NEC B65.9 *[J99]*
  - pneumonia B65.9
- Schistosoma
  - haematobium B65.0
  - japonicum B65.2
  - mansoni B65.1
- specified type NEC B65.8
- urinary B65.0
- vesical B65.0
Schizencephaly Q04.6
Schizoaffective psychosis F25.9
Schizodontia K00.2
Schizoid personality F60.1
Schizophrenia, schizophrenic F20.9
- acute (brief) (undifferentiated) F23
- atypical (form) F20.3
- borderline F21
- catalepsy F20.2
- catatonic (type) (excited) (withdrawn) F20.2
- cenesthopathic, cenesthesiopathic F20.89
- childhood type F84.5
- chronic undifferentiated F20.9
- cyclic F25.0
- disorganized (type) F20.1
- flexibilitas cerea F20.2
- hebephrenic (type) F20.1
- incipient F21
- latent F21
- negative type F20.5
- paranoid (type) F20.0
- paraphrenic F20.0
- post-psychotic depression F32.89
- prepsychotic F21
- prodromal F21
- pseudoneurotic F21
- pseudopsychopathic F21
- reaction F23
- residual (state) (type) F20.5
- restzustand F20.5
- schizoaffective (type) — *see* Psychosis, schizoaffective
- simple (type) F20.89
- simplex F20.89
- specified type NEC F20.89
- spectrum and other psychotic disorder F29
  - specified NEC F28
- stupor F20.2
- syndrome of childhood F84.5
- undifferentiated (type) F20.3
  - chronic F20.9
Schizothymia (persistent) F60.1
Schlatter-Osgood disease or osteochondrosis M92.52- ☑
Schlatter's tibia — *see* Osteochondrosis, juvenile, tibia
Schmidt's syndrome (polyglandular, autoimmune) E31.0

Schmincke's carcinoma or tumor — *see* Neoplasm, nasopharynx, malignant
Schmitz (-Stutzer) dysentery A03.0
Schmorl's disease or nodes
  lumbar region M51.46
  lumbosacral region M51.47
  sacrococcygeal region M53.3
  thoracic region M51.44
  thoracolumbar region M51.45
Schneiderian
  papilloma — *see* Neoplasm, nasopharynx, benign
    specified site — *see* Neoplasm, benign, by site
    unspecified site D14.0
  specified site — *see* Neoplasm, malignant, by site
    unspecified site C30.0
Scholte's syndrome (malignant carcinoid) E34.0
Scholz (-Bielchowsky-Henneberg) disease or syndrome E75.25
Schönlein (-Henoch) disease or purpura (primary) (rheumatic) D69.0
Schottmuller's disease A01.4
Schroeder's syndrome (endocrine hypertensive) E27.0
Schüller-Christian disease or syndrome C96.5
Schultze's type acroparesthesia, simple I73.89
Schultz's disease or syndrome — *see* Agranulocytosis
Schwalbe-Ziehen-Oppenheim disease G24.1
Schwannoma — *see also* Neoplasm, nerve, benign
  malignant — *see also* Neoplasm, nerve, malignant
    with rhabdomyoblastic differentiation — *see* Neoplasm, nerve, malignant
  melanocytic — *see* Neoplasm, nerve, benign
  pigmented — *see* Neoplasm, nerve, benign
Schwannomatosis Q85.03
Schwartz (-Jampel) syndrome G71.13
Schwartz-Bartter syndrome E22.2
Schweniger-Buzzi anetoderma L90.1
Sciatic — *see* condition
Sciatica (infective) M54.3 ☑
  with lumbago M54.4- ☑
    due to intervertebral disc disorder — *see* Disorder, disc, with, radiculopathy
  due to displacement of intervertebral disc (with lumbago) — *see* Disorder, disc, with, radiculopathy
  wallet M54.3- ☑
Scimitar syndrome Q26.8
Sclera — *see* condition
Sclerectasia H15.84- ☑
Scleredema
  adultorum — *see* Sclerosis, systemic
  Buschke's — *see* Sclerosis, systemic
  newborn P83.0
Sclerema (adiposum) (edematosum) (neonatorum) (newborn) P83.0
  adultorum — *see* Sclerosis, systemic
Scleriasis — *see* Scleroderma
Scleritis H15.00- ☑
  with corneal involvement H15.04- ☑
  anterior H15.01- ☑
  brawny H15.02- ☑
  in (due to) zoster B02.34
  posterior H15.03- ☑
  specified type NEC H15.09- ☑
  syphilitic A52.71
  tuberculous (nodular) A18.51
Sclerochoroiditis H31.8
Scleroconjunctivitis — *see* Scleritis
Sclerocystic ovary syndrome E28.2
Sclerodactyly, sclerodactylia L94.3
Scleroderma, sclerodermia (acrosclerotic) (diffuse) (generalized) (progressive) (pulmonary) — *see also* Sclerosis, systemic M34.9
  circumscribed L94.0
  linear L94.1
  localized L94.0
  newborn P83.88
  systemic M34.9
Sclerokeratitis H16.8
  tuberculous A18.52
Scleroma nasi A48.8
Scleromalacia (perforans) H15.05- ☑
Scleromyxedema L98.5
Sclérose en plaques G35
Sclerosis, sclerotic
  adrenal (gland) E27.8
  Alzheimer's — *see* Disease, Alzheimer's
  amyotrophic (lateral) G12.21
  aorta, aortic I70.0

Sclerosis, sclerotic — *continued*
  aorta, aortic — *continued*
    valve — *see* Endocarditis, aortic
  artery, arterial, arteriolar, arteriovascular — *see* Arteriosclerosis
  ascending multiple G35
  brain (generalized) (lobular) G37.9
    artery, arterial I67.2
    diffuse G37.0
    disseminated G35
    insular G35
    Krabbe's E75.23
    miliary G35
    multiple G35
    presenile (Alzheimer's) — *see* Disease, Alzheimer's, early onset
    senile (arteriosclerotic) I67.2
    stem, multiple G35
    tuberous Q85.1
  bulbar, multiple G35
  bundle of His I44.39
  cardiac — *see* Disease, heart, ischemic, atherosclerotic
  cardiorenal — *see* Hypertension, cardiorenal
  cardiovascular — *see also* Disease, cardiovascular
    renal — *see* Hypertension, cardiorenal
  cerebellar — *see* Sclerosis, brain
  cerebral — *see* Sclerosis, brain
  cerebrospinal (disseminated) (multiple) G35
  cerebrovascular I67.2
  choroid — *see* Degeneration, choroid
  combined (spinal cord) — *see also* Degeneration, combined
    multiple G35
  concentric (Balo) G37.5
  cornea — *see* Opacity, cornea
  coronary (artery) I25.10
    with angina pectoris — *see* Arteriosclerosis, coronary (artery),
  corpus cavernosum
    female N90.89
    male N48.6
  diffuse (brain) (spinal cord) G37.0
  disseminated G35
  dorsal G35
  dorsolateral (spinal cord) — *see* Degeneration, combined
  endometrium N85.5
  extrapyramidal G25.9
  eye, nuclear (senile) — *see* Cataract, senile, nuclear
  focal and segmental (glomerular) — *see also* N00-N07
    with fourth character .1 N05.1
  Friedreich's (spinal cord) G11.11
  funicular (spermatic cord) N50.89
  general (vascular) — *see* Arteriosclerosis
  gland (lymphatic) I89.8
  hepatic K74.1
    alcoholic K70.2
  hereditary
    cerebellar G11.9
    spinal (Friedreich's ataxia) G11.11
  hippocampal G93.81
  insular G35
  kidney — *see* Sclerosis, renal
  larynx J38.7
  lateral (amyotrophic) (descending) (spinal) G12.21
    primary G12.23
  lens, senile nuclear — *see* Cataract, senile, nuclear
  liver K74.1
    with fibrosis K74.2
      alcoholic K70.2
    alcoholic K70.2
    cardiac K76.1
  lung — *see* Fibrosis, lung
  mastoid — *see* Mastoiditis, chronic
  mesial temporal G93.81
  mitral I05.8
  Mönckeberg's (medial) — *see* Arteriosclerosis, extremities
  multiple (brain stem) (cerebral) (generalized) (spinal cord) G35
  myocardium, myocardial — *see* Disease, heart, ischemic, atherosclerotic
  nuclear (senile), eye — *see* Cataract, senile, nuclear
  ovary N83.8
  pancreas K86.89
  penis N48.6
  peripheral arteries — *see* Arteriosclerosis, extremities
  plaques G35

Sclerosis, sclerotic — *continued*
  pluriglandular E31.8
  polyglandular E31.8
  posterolateral (spinal cord) — *see* Degeneration, combined
  presenile (Alzheimer's) — *see* Disease, Alzheimer's, early onset
  primary, lateral G12.23
  progressive, systemic M34.0
  pulmonary — *see* Fibrosis, lung
    artery I27.0
    valve (heart) — *see* Endocarditis, pulmonary
  renal N26.9
    with
      cystine storage disease E72.09
      hypertensive heart disease (conditions in I11) — *see* Hypertension, cardiorenal
    arteriolar (hyaline) (hyperplastic) — *see* Hypertension, kidney
  retina (senile) (vascular) H35.00
  senile (vascular) — *see* Arteriosclerosis
  spinal (cord) (progressive) G95.89
    ascending G61.0
    combined — *see also* Degeneration, combined
      multiple G35
      syphilitic A52.11
    disseminated G35
    dorsolateral — *see* Degeneration, combined
    hereditary (Friedreich's) (mixed form) G11.11
    lateral (amyotrophic) G12.21
      progressive G12.23
    multiple G35
    posterior (syphilitic) A52.11
  stomach K31.89
  subendocardial, congenital I42.4
  systemic M34.9
    with
      lung involvement M34.81
      myopathy M34.82
      polyneuropathy M34.83
    drug-induced M34.2
    due to chemicals NEC M34.2
    progressive M34.0
    specified NEC M34.89
  temporal (mesial) G93.81
  tricuspid (heart) (valve) I07.8
  tuberous (brain) Q85.1
  tympanic membrane — *see* Disorder, tympanic membrane, specified NEC
  valve, valvular (heart) — *see* Endocarditis
  vascular — *see* Arteriosclerosis
  vein I87.8
Scoliosis (acquired) (postural) M41.9
  adolescent (idiopathic) — *see* Scoliosis, idiopathic, adolescent
  congenital Q67.5
    due to bony malformation Q76.3
    failure of segmentation (hemivertebra) Q76.3
    hemivertebra fusion Q76.3
    postural Q67.5
  degenerative M41.5- ☑
  idiopathic M41.20
    adolescent M41.129
      cervical region M41.122
      cervicothoracic region M41.123
      lumbar region M41.126
      lumbosacral region M41.127
      thoracic region M41.124
      thoracolumbar region M41.125
    cervical region M41.22
    cervicothoracic region M41.23
    infantile M41.00
      cervical region M41.02
      cervicothoracic region M41.03
      lumbar region M41.06
      lumbosacral region M41.07
      sacrococcygeal region M41.08
      thoracic region M41.04
      thoracolumbar region M41.05
    juvenile M41.119
      cervical region M41.112
      cervicothoracic region M41.113
      lumbar region M41.116
      lumbosacral region M41.117
      thoracic region M41.114
      thoracolumbar region M41.115
    lumbar region M41.26
    lumbosacral region M41.27

Scoliosis — *continued*
  idiopathic — *continued*
    thoracic region M41.24
    thoracolumbar region M41.25
  infantile — *see* Scoliosis, idiopathic, infantile
  neuromuscular M41.40
    cervical region M41.42
    cervicothoracic region M41.43
    lumbar region M41.46
    lumbosacral region M41.47
    occipito-atlanto-axial region M41.41
    thoracic region M41.44
    thoracolumbar region M41.45
  paralytic — *see* Scoliosis, neuromuscular
  postradiation therapy M96.5
  rachitic (late effect or sequelae) E64.3 *[M49.80]*
    cervical region E64.3 *[M49.82]*
    cervicothoracic region E64.3 *[M49.83]*
    lumbar region E64.3 *[M49.86]*
    lumbosacral region E64.3 *[M49.87]*
    multiple sites E64.3 *[M49.89]*
    occipito-atlanto-axial region E64.3 *[M49.81]*
    sacrococcygeal region E64.3 *[M49.88]*
    thoracic region E64.3 *[M49.84]*
    thoracolumbar region E64.3 *[M49.85]*
  sciatic M54.4- ☑
  secondary (to) NEC M41.50
    cerebral palsy, Friedreich's ataxia, poliomyelitis, neuromuscular disorders — *see* Scoliosis, neuromuscular
    cervical region M41.52
    cervicothoracic region M41.53
    lumbar region M41.56
    lumbosacral region M41.57
    thoracic region M41.54
    thoracolumbar region M41.55
  specified form NEC M41.80
    cervical region M41.82
    cervicothoracic region M41.83
    lumbar region M41.86
    lumbosacral region M41.87
    thoracic region M41.84
    thoracolumbar region M41.85
  thoracogenic M41.30
    thoracic region M41.34
    thoracolumbar region M41.35
  tuberculous A18.01
Scoliotic pelvis
  with disproportion (fetopelvic) O33.0
    causing obstructed labor O65.0
Scorbutus, scorbutic — *see also* Scurvy
  anemia D53.2
Score, NIHSS (National Institutes of Health Stroke Scale) R29.7- ☑
Scotoma (arcuate) (Bjerrum) (central) (ring) — *see also* Defect, visual field, localized, scotoma
  scintillating H53.12- ☑
Scratch — *see* Abrasion
Scratchy throat R09.89
Screening (for) Z13.9
  alcoholism Z13.39
  anemia Z13.0
  anomaly, congenital Z13.89
  antenatal, of mother — *see also* Encounter, antenatal screening Z36.9
  arterial hypertension Z13.6
  arthropod-borne viral disease NEC Z11.59
  autism Z13.41
  bacteriuria, asymptomatic Z13.89
  behavioral disorder Z13.30
    specified NEC Z13.39
  brain injury, traumatic Z13.850
  bronchitis, chronic Z13.83
  brucellosis Z11.2
  cardiovascular disorder Z13.6
  cataract Z13.5
  chlamydial diseases Z11.8
  cholera Z11.0
  chromosomal abnormalities (nonprocreative) NEC Z13.79
  colonoscopy Z12.11
  congenital
    dislocation of hip Z13.89
    eye disorder Z13.5
    malformation or deformation Z13.89
  contamination NEC Z13.88
  coronavirus (disease) (novel) 2019 Z11.52
  COVID-19 Z11.52

Screening — *continued*
  cystic fibrosis Z13.228
  dengue fever Z11.59
  dental disorder Z13.84
  depression (adult) (adolescent) (child) Z13.31
    maternal Z13.32
    perinatal Z13.32
  developmental
    delays Z13.40
      global (milestones) Z13.42
      specified NEC Z13.49
    handicap Z13.42
      in early childhood Z13.42
  diabetes mellitus Z13.1
  diphtheria Z11.2
  disability, intellectual Z13.39
  disease or disorder Z13.9
    bacterial NEC Z11.2
      intestinal infectious Z11.0
      respiratory tuberculosis Z11.1
    behavioral Z13.30
      specified NEC Z13.39
    blood or blood-forming organ Z13.0
    cardiovascular Z13.6
    Chagas' Z11.6
    chlamydial Z11.8
    coronavirus (novel) 2019 Z11.52
    COVID-19 Z11.52
    dental Z13.89
    developmental delays Z13.40
      global (milestones) Z13.42
      specified NEC Z13.49
    digestive tract NEC Z13.818
      lower GI Z13.811
      upper GI Z13.810
    ear Z13.5
    endocrine Z13.29
    eye Z13.5
    genitourinary Z13.89
    heart Z13.6
    human immunodeficiency virus (HIV) infection Z11.4
    immunity Z13.0
    infection
      intestinal Z11.0
        specified NEC Z11.6
    infectious Z11.9
    mental health and behavioral Z13.30
      specified NEC Z13.39
    metabolic Z13.228
    neurological Z13.89
    nutritional Z13.21
      metabolic Z13.228
        lipoid disorders Z13.220
    protozoal Z11.6
      intestinal Z11.0
    respiratory Z13.83
    rheumatic Z13.828
    rickettsial Z11.8
    sexually-transmitted NEC Z11.3
      human immunodeficiency virus (HIV) Z11.4
    sickle-cell (trait) Z13.0
    skin Z13.89
    specified NEC Z13.89
    spirochetal Z11.8
    thyroid Z13.29
    vascular Z13.6
    venereal Z11.3
    viral NEC Z11.59
      coronavirus (novel) 2019 Z11.52
      COVID-19 Z11.52
      human immunodeficiency virus (HIV) Z11.4
      intestinal Z11.0
      SARS-CoV-2 Z11.52
  elevated titer Z13.89
  emphysema Z13.83
  encephalitis, viral (mosquito- or tick-borne) Z11.59
  exposure to contaminants (toxic) Z13.88
  fever
    dengue Z11.59
    hemorrhagic Z11.59
    yellow Z11.59
  filariasis Z11.6
  galactosemia Z13.228
  gastrointestinal condition Z13.818
  genetic (nonprocreative) - for procreative management — *see* Testing, genetic, for procreative management
    disease carrier status (nonprocreative) Z13.71
    specified NEC (nonprocreative) Z13.79

Screening — *continued*
  genitourinary condition Z13.89
  glaucoma Z13.5
  gonorrhea Z11.3
  gout Z13.89
  helminthiasis (intestinal) Z11.6
  hematopoietic malignancy Z12.89
  hemoglobinopathies NEC Z13.0
  hemorrhagic fever Z11.59
  Hodgkin disease Z12.89
  human immunodeficiency virus (HIV) Z11.4
  human papillomavirus Z11.51
  hypertension Z13.6
  immunity disorders Z13.0
  infant or child (over 28 days old) Z00.129
    with abnormal findings Z00.121
  infection
    mycotic Z11.8
    parasitic Z11.8
  ingestion of radioactive substance Z13.88
  intellectual disability Z13.39
  intestinal
    helminthiasis Z11.6
    infectious disease Z11.0
  leishmaniasis Z11.6
  leprosy Z11.2
  leptospirosis Z11.8
  leukemia Z12.89
  lymphoma Z12.89
  malaria Z11.6
  malnutrition Z13.29
    metabolic Z13.228
    nutritional Z13.21
  measles Z11.59
  mental health disorder Z13.30
    specified NEC Z13.39
  metabolic errors, inborn Z13.228
  multiphasic Z13.89
  musculoskeletal disorder Z13.828
    osteoporosis Z13.820
  mycoses Z11.8
  myocardial infarction (acute) Z13.6
  neoplasm (malignant) (of) Z12.9
    bladder Z12.6
    blood Z12.89
    breast Z12.39
      routine mammogram Z12.31
    cervix Z12.4
    colon Z12.11
    genitourinary organs NEC Z12.79
      bladder Z12.6
      cervix Z12.4
      ovary Z12.73
      prostate Z12.5
      testis Z12.71
      vagina Z12.72
    hematopoietic system Z12.89
    intestinal tract Z12.10
      colon Z12.11
      rectum Z12.12
      small intestine Z12.13
    lung Z12.2
    lymph (glands) Z12.89
    nervous system Z12.82
    oral cavity Z12.81
    prostate Z12.5
    rectum Z12.12
    respiratory organs Z12.2
    skin Z12.83
    small intestine Z12.13
    specified site NEC Z12.89
    stomach Z12.0
  nephropathy Z13.89
  nervous system disorders NEC Z13.858
  neurological condition Z13.89
  osteoporosis Z13.820
  parasitic infestation Z11.9
    specified NEC Z11.8
  phenylketonuria Z13.228
  plague Z11.2
  poisoning (chemical) (heavy metal) Z13.88
  poliomyelitis Z11.59
  postnatal, chromosomal abnormalities Z13.89
  prenatal, of mother — *see also* Encounter, antenatal screening Z36.9
  protozoal disease Z11.6
    intestinal Z11.0
  pulmonary tuberculosis Z11.1
  radiation exposure Z13.88

☑ **Additional Character Required** — **Refer to the Tabular List for Character Selection**

Screening — *continued*
  respiratory condition Z13.83
  respiratory tuberculosis Z11.1
  rheumatoid arthritis Z13.828
  rubella Z11.59
  SARS-CoV-2 Z11.52
  schistosomiasis Z11.6
  sexually-transmitted disease NEC Z11.3
    human immunodeficiency virus (HIV) Z11.4
  sickle-cell disease or trait Z13.0
  skin condition Z13.89
  sleeping sickness Z11.6
  special Z13.9
    specified NEC Z13.89
  syphilis Z11.3
  tetanus Z11.2
  trachoma Z11.8
  traumatic brain injury Z13.850
  trypanosomiasis Z11.6
  tuberculosis, respiratory Z11.1
    active Z11.1
    latent Z11.7
  venereal disease Z11.3
  viral encephalitis (mosquito- or tick-borne) Z11.59
  whooping cough Z11.2
  worms, intestinal Z11.6
  yaws Z11.8
  yellow fever Z11.59
Scrofula, scrofulosis (tuberculosis of cervical lymph glands) A18.2
Scrofulide (primary) (tuberculous) A18.4
Scrofuloderma, scrofulodermia (any site) (primary) A18.4
Scrofulosus lichen (primary) (tuberculous) A18.4
Scrofulous — *see* condition
Scrotal tongue K14.5
Scrotum — *see* condition
Scurvy, scorbutic E54
  anemia D53.2
  gum E54
  infantile E54
  rickets E55.0 *[M90.80]*
Sealpox B08.62
Seasickness T75.3 ☑
Sebaceous — *see also* condition
  cyst — *see* Cyst, sebaceous
Seborrhea, seborrheic L21.9
  capillitii R23.8
  capitis L21.0
  dermatitis L21.9
    infantile L21.1
  eczema L21.9
    infantile L21.1
  sicca L21.0
Seckel's syndrome Q87.19
Seclusion, pupil — *see* Membrane, pupillary
Second hand tobacco smoke exposure (acute) (chronic) Z77.22
  in the perinatal period P96.81
Secondary
  dentin (in pulp) K04.3
  neoplasm, secondaries — *see* Table of Neoplasms, secondary
Secretion
  antidiuretic hormone, inappropriate E22.2
  catecholamine, by pheochromocytoma E27.5
  hormone
    antidiuretic, inappropriate (syndrome) E22.2
    by
      carcinoid tumor E34.0
      pheochromocytoma E27.5
    ectopic NEC E34.2
  urinary
    excessive R35.89
    suppression R34
Section
  nerve, traumatic — *see* Injury, nerve
Sedative, hypnotic, or anxiolytic-induced
  anxiety disorder F13.980
  bipolar and related disorder F13.94
  delirium F13.921
  depressive disorder F13.94
  major neurocognitive disorder F13.97
  mild neurocognitive disorder F13.988
  psychotic disorder F13.959
  sexual dysfunction F13.981
  sleep disorder F13.982

Segmentation, incomplete (congenital) — *see also* Fusion
  bone NEC Q78.8
  lumbosacral (joint) (vertebra) Q76.49
SEID (systemic exertion intolerance disease) G93.32
Seitelberger's syndrome (infantile neuraxonal dystrophy) G31.89
Seizure(s) — *see also* Convulsions R56.9
  absence G40.A- ☑ (*following* G40.3)
  akinetic — *see* Epilepsy, generalized, specified NEC
  atonic — *see* Epilepsy, generalized, specified NEC
  autonomic (hysterical) F44.5
  convulsive — *see* Convulsions
  cortical (focal) (motor) — *see* Epilepsy, localization-related, symptomatic, with simple partial seizures
  disorder — *see also* Epilepsy G40.909
  due to stroke — *see* Sequelae (of), disease, cerebrovascular, by type, specified NEC
  epileptic — *see* Epilepsy
  febrile (simple) R56.00
    with status epilepticus G40.901
    complex (atypical) (complicated) R56.01
      with status epilepticus G40.901
  grand mal G40.409
    intractable G40.419
      with status epilepticus G40.411
      without status epilepticus G40.419
    not intractable G40.409
      with status epilepticus G40.401
      without status epilepticus G40.409
  heart — *see* Disease, heart
  hysterical F44.5
  intractable G40.919
    with status epilepticus G40.911
  Jacksonian (focal) (motor type) (sensory type) — *see* Epilepsy, localization-related, symptomatic, with simple partial seizures
  newborn P90
  nonspecific epileptic
    atonic — *see* Epilepsy, generalized, specified NEC
    clonic — *see* Epilepsy, generalized, specified NEC
    myoclonic — *see* Epilepsy, generalized, specified NEC
    tonic — *see* Epilepsy, generalized, specified NEC
    tonic-clonic — *see* Epilepsy, generalized, specified NEC
  partial, developing into secondarily generalized seizures
    complex — *see* Epilepsy, localization-related, symptomatic, with complex partial seizures
    simple — *see* Epilepsy, localization-related, symptomatic, with simple partial seizures
  petit mal G40.A- ☑ (*following* G40.3)
    intractable G40.A1- ☑ (*following* G40.3)
      with status epilepticus G40.A11 (*following* G40.3)
      without status epilepticus G40.A19 (*following* G40.3)
    not intractable G40.A0- ☑ (*following* G40.3)
      with status epilepticus G40.A01 (*following* G40.3)
      without status epilepticus G40.A09 (*following* G40.3)
  post traumatic R56.1
  recurrent G40.909
  specified NEC G40.89
  uncinate — *see* Epilepsy, localization-related, symptomatic, with complex partial seizures
Selenium deficiency, dietary E59
Self-damaging behavior (life-style) Z72.89
Self-harm (attempted)
  history (personal)
    in family Z81.8
    nonsuicidal Z91.52
    suicidal Z91.51
  nonsuicidal R45.88
Self-injury, nonsuicidal R45.88
  personal history Z91.52
Self-mutilation (attempted)
  history (personal)
    in family Z81.8
    nonsuicidal Z91.52
    suicidal Z91.51
  nonsuicidal R45.88
Self-poisoning
  history (personal) Z91.51
    in family Z81.8
  observation following (alleged) attempt Z03.6
Semicoma R40.1
Seminal vesiculitis N49.0

Seminoma C62.9- ☑
  specified site — *see* Neoplasm, malignant, by site
Senear-Usher disease or syndrome L10.4
Senectus R54
Senescence (without mention of psychosis) R54
Senile, senility — *see also* condition R41.81
  with
    acute confusional state F05
    mental changes NOS F03 ☑
    psychosis NEC — *see* Psychosis, senile
  asthenia R54
  cervix (atrophic) N88.8
  debility R54
  endometrium (atrophic) N85.8
  fallopian tube (atrophic) — *see* Atrophy, fallopian tube
  heart (failure) R54
  ovary (atrophic) — *see* Atrophy, ovary
  premature E34.8
  vagina, vaginitis (atrophic) N95.2
  wart L82.1
Sensation
  burning (skin) R20.8
    tongue K14.6
  loss of R20.8
  prickling (skin) R20.2
  tingling (skin) R20.2
Sense loss
  smell — *see* Disturbance, sensation, smell
  taste — *see* Disturbance, sensation, taste
  touch R20.8
Sensibility disturbance (cortical) (deep) (vibratory) R20.9
Sensitive, sensitivity — *see also* Allergy
  carotid sinus G90.01
  child (excessive) F93.8
  cold, autoimmune D59.12
  dentin K03.89
  gluten (non-celiac) K90.41
  latex Z91.040
  methemoglobin D74.8
  tuberculin, without clinical or radiological symptoms R76.11
  visual
    glare H53.71
    impaired contrast H53.72
Sensitiver Beziehungswahn F22
Sensitization, auto-erythrocytic D69.2
Separation
  anxiety, abnormal (of childhood) F93.0
  apophysis, traumatic — *code as* Fracture, by site
  choroid — *see* Detachment, choroid
  epiphysis, epiphyseal
    nontraumatic — *see also* Osteochondropathy, specified type NEC
      upper femoral — *see* Slipped, epiphysis, upper femoral
    traumatic — *code as* Fracture, by site
  fracture — *see* Fracture
  infundibulum cardiac from right ventricle by a partition Q24.3
  joint (traumatic) (current) — *code by* site under Dislocation
  muscle (nontraumatic) — *see* Diastasis, muscle
  pubic bone, obstetrical trauma O71.6
  retina, retinal — *see* Detachment, retina
  symphysis pubis, obstetrical trauma O71.6
  tracheal ring, incomplete, congenital Q32.1
Sepsis (generalized) (unspecified organism) A41.9
  with
    organ dysfunction (acute) (multiple) R65.20
      with septic shock R65.21
  actinomycotic A42.7
  adrenal hemorrhage syndrome (meningococcal) A39.1
  anaerobic A41.4
  Bacillus anthracis A22.7
  Brucella — *see also* Brucellosis A23.9
  candidal B37.7
  cryptogenic A41.9
  due to device, implant or graft T85.79 ☑
    arterial graft NEC T82.7 ☑
    breast (implant) T85.79 ☑
    catheter NEC T85.79 ☑
      dialysis (renal) T82.7 ☑
        intraperitoneal T85.71 ☑
      infusion NEC T82.7 ☑
        spinal (cranial) (epidural) (intrathecal) (spinal) (subarachnoid) (subdural) T85.735 ☑
      urethral indwelling T83.511 ☑

☑ **Additional Character Required** — Refer to the Tabular List for Character Selection

Sepsis — *continued*
  due to device, implant or graft — *continued*
    catheter — *continued*
      urinary T83.518 ☑
    ectopic or molar pregnancy O08.82
    electronic (electrode) (pulse generator) (stimulator)
      bone T84.7 ☑
      cardiac T82.7 ☑
      nervous system T85.738 ☑
        brain T85.731 ☑
        neurostimulator generator T85.734 ☑
        peripheral nerve T85.732 ☑
        spinal cord T85.733 ☑
      urinary T83.590 ☑
    fixation, internal (orthopedic) — *see* Complication, fixation device, infection
    gastrointestinal (bile duct) (esophagus) T85.79 ☑
      neurostimulator electrode (lead) T85.732 ☑
    genital T83.69 ☑
    heart NEC T82.7 ☑
      valve (prosthesis) T82.6 ☑
      graft T82.7 ☑
    joint prosthesis — *see* Complication, joint prosthesis, infection
    ocular (corneal graft) (orbital implant) T85.79 ☑
    orthopedic NEC T84.7 ☑
      fixation device, internal — *see* Complication, fixation device, infection
    specified NEC T85.79 ☑
    vascular T82.7 ☑
    ventricular intracranial (communicating) shunt T85.730 ☑
  during labor O75.3
  Enterococcus A41.81
  Erysipelothrix (rhusiopathiae) (erysipeloid) A26.7
  Escherichia coli (E. coli) A41.5 ☑
  extraintestinal yersiniosis A28.2
  following
    abortion (subsequent episode) O08.0
      current episode — *see* Abortion
    ectopic or molar pregnancy O08.82
    immunization T88.0 ☑
    infusion, therapeutic injection or transfusion NEC T80.29 ☑
    obstetrical procedure O86.04
  gangrenous A41.9
  gonococcal A54.86
  Gram-negative (organism) A41.5 ☑
    anaerobic A41.4
  Haemophilus influenzae A41.3
  herpesviral B00.7
  intra-abdominal K65.1
  intraocular — *see* Endophthalmitis, purulent
  Listeria monocytogenes A32.7
  localized — *code to* specific localized infection
    in operation wound T81.49 ☑
    skin — *see* Abscess
  malleus A24.0
  melioidosis A24.1
  meningeal — *see* Meningitis
  meningococcal A39.4
    acute A39.2
    chronic A39.3
  MSSA (Methicillin susceptible Staphylococcus aureus) A41.01
  newborn P36.9
    due to
      anaerobes NEC P36.5
      Escherichia coli P36.4
      Staphylococcus P36.30
        aureus P36.2
        specified NEC P36.39
      Streptococcus P36.10
        group B P36.0
        specified NEC P36.19
      specified NEC P36.8
  Pasteurella multocida A28.0
  pelvic, puerperal, postpartum, childbirth O85
  pneumococcal A40.3
  postprocedural T81.44 ☑
  puerperal, postpartum, childbirth (pelvic) O85
  Salmonella (arizonae) (cholerae-suis) (enteritidis) (typhimurium) A02.1
  severe R65.20
    with septic shock R65.21
  Shigella — *see also* Dysentery, bacillary A03.9
  skin, localized — *see* Abscess

Sepsis — *continued*
  specified organism NEC A41.89
  Staphylococcus, staphylococcal A41.2
    aureus (methicillin susceptible) (MSSA) A41.01
      methicillin resistant (MRSA) A41.02
    coagulase-negative A41.1
    specified NEC A41.1
  Streptococcus, streptococcal A40.9
    agalactiae A40.1
    group
      A A40.0
      B A40.1
      D A41.81
    neonatal P36.10
      group B P36.0
      specified NEC P36.19
    pneumoniae A40.3
    pyogenes A40.0
    specified NEC A40.8
  tracheostomy stoma J95.02
  tularemic A21.7
  umbilical, umbilical cord (newborn) — *see* Sepsis, newborn
  Yersinia pestis A20.7
Septate — *see* Septum
Septic — *see* condition
  arm — *see* Cellulitis, upper limb
    with lymphangitis — *see* Lymphangitis, acute, upper limb
  embolus — *see* Embolism
  finger — *see* Cellulitis, digit
    with lymphangitis — *see* Lymphangitis, acute, digit
  foot — *see* Cellulitis, lower limb
    with lymphangitis — *see* Lymphangitis, acute, lower limb
  gallbladder (acute) K81.0
  hand — *see* Cellulitis, upper limb
    with lymphangitis — *see* Lymphangitis, acute, upper limb
  joint — *see* Arthritis, pyogenic or pyemic
  leg — *see* Cellulitis, lower limb
    with lymphangitis — *see* Lymphangitis, acute, lower limb
  nail — *see also* Cellulitis, digit
    with lymphangitis — *see* Lymphangitis, acute, digit
  sore — *see also* Abscess
    throat J02.0
      streptococcal J02.0
  spleen (acute) D73.89
  teeth, tooth (pulpal origin) K04.4
  throat — *see* Pharyngitis
  thrombus — *see* Thrombosis
  toe — *see* Cellulitis, digit
    with lymphangitis — *see* Lymphangitis, acute, digit
  tonsils, chronic J35.01
    with adenoiditis J35.03
  uterus — *see* Endometritis
Septicemia A41.9
  meaning sepsis — *see* Sepsis
Septum, septate (congenital) — *see also* Anomaly, by site
  anal Q42.3
    with fistula Q42.2
  aqueduct of Sylvius Q03.0
    with spina bifida — *see* Spina bifida, by site, with hydrocephalus
  uterus Q51.28
    complete Q51.21
    partial Q51.22
    specified NEC Q51.28
  vagina Q52.10
    in pregnancy — *see* Pregnancy, complicated by, abnormal vagina
      causing obstructed labor O65.5
    longitudinal Q52.129
      microperforate
        left side Q52.124
        right side Q52.123
      nonobstruction Q52.120
      obstructing Q52.129
        left side Q52.122
        right side Q52.121
    transverse Q52.11
Sequelae (of) — *see also* condition
  abscess, intracranial or intraspinal (conditions in G06) G09

Sequelae — *continued*
  amputation — *code to* injury with seventh character S
  burn and corrosion — *code to* injury with seventh character S
  calcium deficiency E64.8
  cerebrovascular disease — *see* Sequelae, disease, cerebrovascular
  childbirth O94
  contusion — *code to* injury with seventh character S
  corrosion — *see* Sequelae, burn and corrosion
  COVID-19 (post acute) U09.9
  crushing injury — *code to* injury with seventh character S
  disease
    cerebrovascular I69.90
      alteration of sensation I69.998
      aphasia I69.920
      apraxia I69.990
      ataxia I69.993
      cognitive deficits I69.91 ☑
      disturbance of vision I69.998
      dysarthria I69.922
      dysphagia I69.991
      dysphasia I69.921
      facial droop I69.992
      facial weakness I69.992
      fluency disorder I69.923
      hemiplegia I69.95- ☑
      hemorrhage
        intracerebral — *see* Sequelae, hemorrhage, intracerebral
        intracranial, nontraumatic NEC — *see* Sequelae, hemorrhage, intracranial, nontraumatic
        subarachnoid — *see* Sequelae, hemorrhage, subarachnoid
      language deficit I69.928
      monoplegia
        lower limb I69.94- ☑
        upper limb I69.93- ☑
      paralytic syndrome I69.96- ☑
      specified effect NEC I69.998
      specified type NEC I69.80
        alteration of sensation I69.898
        aphasia I69.820
        apraxia I69.890
        ataxia I69.893
        cognitive deficits I69.81 ☑
        disturbance of vision I69.898
        dysarthria I69.822
        dysphagia I69.891
        dysphasia I69.821
        facial droop I69.892
        facial weakness I69.892
        fluency disorder I69.823
        hemiplegia I69.85- ☑
        language deficit I69.828
        monoplegia
          lower limb I69.84- ☑
          upper limb I69.83- ☑
        paralytic syndrome I69.86- ☑
        specified effect NEC I69.898
      speech deficit I69.928
      speech deficit I69.828
      stroke NOS — *see* Sequelae, stroke NOS
  dislocation — *code to* injury with seventh character S
  encephalitis or encephalomyelitis (conditions in G04) G09
    in infectious disease NEC B94.8
    viral B94.1
  external cause — *code to* injury with seventh character S
  foreign body entering natural orifice — *code to* injury with seventh character S
  fracture — *code to* injury with seventh character S
  frostbite — *code to* injury with seventh character S
  Hansen's disease B92
  hemorrhage
    intracerebral I69.10
      alteration of sensation I69.198
      aphasia I69.120
      apraxia I69.190
      ataxia I69.193
      cognitive deficits I69.11 ☑
      disturbance of vision I69.198
      dysarthria I69.122
      dysphagia I69.191

Sequelae — *continued*
 hemorrhage — *continued*
  intracerebral — *continued*
   dysphasia I69.121
   facial droop I69.192
   facial weakness I69.192
   fluency disorder I69.123
   hemiplegia I69.15- ☑
   language deficit NEC I69.128
   monoplegia
    lower limb I69.14- ☑
    upper limb I69.13- ☑
   paralytic syndrome I69.16- ☑
   specified effect NEC I69.198
   speech deficit NEC I69.128
  intracranial, nontraumatic NEC I69.20
   alteration of sensation I69.298
   aphasia I69.220
   apraxia I69.290
   ataxia I69.293
   cognitive deficits I69.21 ☑
   disturbance of vision I69.298
   dysarthria I69.222
   dysphagia I69.291
   dysphasia I69.221
   facial droop I69.292
   facial weakness I69.292
   fluency disorder I69.223
   hemiplegia I69.25- ☑
   language deficit NEC I69.228
   monoplegia
    lower limb I69.24- ☑
    upper limb I69.23- ☑
   paralytic syndrome I69.26- ☑
   specified effect NEC I69.298
   speech deficit NEC I69.228
  subarachnoid I69.00
   alteration of sensation I69.098
   aphasia I69.020
   apraxia I69.090
   ataxia I69.093
   cognitive deficits — *see subcategory* I69.01- ☑
   disturbance of vision I69.098
   dysarthria I69.022
   dysphagia I69.091
   dysphasia I69.021
   facial droop I69.092
   facial weakness I69.092
   fluency disorder I69.023
   hemiplegia I69.05- ☑
   language deficit NEC I69.028
   monoplegia
    lower limb I69.04- ☑
    upper limb I69.03- ☑
   paralytic syndrome I69.06- ☑
   specified effect NEC I69.098
   speech deficit NEC I69.028
 infection, pyogenic, intracranial or intraspinal G09
 infectious disease B94.9
  specified NEC B94.8
 injury — *code to* injury with seventh character S
 leprosy B92
 meningitis
  bacterial (conditions in G00) G09

Sequelae — *continued*
 meningitis — *continued*
  other or unspecified cause (conditions in G03) G09
 muscle (and tendon) injury — *code to* injury with seventh character S
 myelitis — *see* Sequelae, encephalitis
 niacin deficiency E64.8
 nutritional deficiency E64.9
  specified NEC E64.8
 obstetrical condition O94
 parasitic disease B94.9
 phlebitis or thrombophlebitis of intracranial or intraspinal venous sinuses and veins (conditions in G08) G09
 poisoning — *code to* poisoning with seventh character S
  nonmedicinal substance — *see* Sequelae, toxic effect, nonmedicinal substance
 poliomyelitis (acute) B91
 pregnancy O94
 protein-energy malnutrition E64.0
 puerperium O94
 rickets E64.3
 SARS-CoV-2 (post acute) U09.9
 selenium deficiency E64.8
 sprain and strain — *code to* injury with seventh character S
 stroke NOS I69.30
  alteration in sensation I69.398
  aphasia I69.320
  apraxia I69.390
  ataxia I69.393
  cognitive deficits I69.31 ☑
  disturbance of vision I69.398
  dysarthria I69.322
  dysphagia I69.391
  dysphasia I69.321
  facial droop I69.392
  facial weakness I69.392
  hemiplegia I69.35- ☑
  language deficit NEC I69.328
  monoplegia
   lower limb I69.34- ☑
   upper limb I69.33- ☑
  paralytic syndrome I69.36- ☑
  specified effect NEC I69.398
  speech deficit NEC I69.328
 tendon and muscle injury — *code to* injury with seventh character S
 thiamine deficiency E64.8
 trachoma B94.0
 tuberculosis B90.9
  bones and joints B90.2
  central nervous system B90.0
  genitourinary B90.1
  pulmonary (respiratory) B90.9
  specified organs NEC B90.8
 viral
  encephalitis B94.1
  hepatitis B94.2
 vitamin deficiency NEC E64.8
  A E64.1
  B E64.8
  C E64.2
 wound, open — *code to* injury with seventh character S
Sequestration — *see also* Sequestrum
 disc — *see* Displacement, intervertebral disc
 lung, congenital Q33.2
Sequestrum
 bone — *see* Osteomyelitis, chronic
 dental M27.2
 jaw bone M27.2
 orbit — *see* Osteomyelitis, orbit
 sinus (accessory) (nasal) — *see* Sinusitis
Sequoiosis lung or pneumonitis J67.8
Serology for syphilis
 doubtful
  with signs or symptoms — *code by* site and stage under Syphilis
  follow-up of latent syphilis — *see* Syphilis, latent
 negative, with signs or symptoms — *code by* site and stage under Syphilis
 positive A53.0
  with signs or symptoms — *code by* site and stage under Syphilis
 reactivated A53.0
Seroma — *see also* Hematoma

Seroma — *continued*
 postprocedural — *see* Complication, postprocedural, seroma
 traumatic, secondary and recurrent T79.2 ☑
Seropurulent — *see* condition
Serositis, multiple K65.8
 pericardial I31.1
 peritoneal K65.8
Serous — *see* condition
Sertoli cell
 adenoma
  specified site — *see* Neoplasm, benign, by site
  unspecified site
   female D27.9
   male D29.20
 carcinoma
  specified site — *see* Neoplasm, malignant, by site
  unspecified site (male) C62.9- ☑
   female C56.9
 tumor
  with lipid storage
   specified site — *see* Neoplasm, benign, by site
   unspecified site
    female D27.9
    male D29.20
  specified site — *see* Neoplasm, benign, by site
  unspecified site
   female D27.9
   male D29.20
Sertoli-Leydig cell tumor — *see* Neoplasm, benign, by site
 specified site — *see* Neoplasm, benign, by site
 unspecified site
  female D27.9
  male D29.20
Serum
 allergy, allergic reaction — *see also* Reaction, serum T80.69 ☑
  shock — *see also* Shock, anaphylactic T80.59 ☑
 arthritis — *see also* Reaction, serum T80.69 ☑
 complication or reaction NEC — *see also* Reaction, serum T80.69 ☑
 disease NEC — *see also* Reaction, serum T80.69 ☑
 hepatitis — *see also* Hepatitis, viral, type B
  carrier (suspected) of B18.1
 intoxication — *see also* Reaction, serum T80.69 ☑
 neuritis — *see also* Reaction, serum T80.69 ☑
 neuropathy G61.1
 poisoning NEC — *see also* Reaction, serum T80.69 ☑
 rash NEC — *see also* Reaction, serum T80.69 ☑
 reaction NEC — *see also* Reaction, serum T80.69 ☑
 sickness NEC — *see also* Reaction, serum T80.69 ☑
 urticaria — *see also* Reaction, serum T80.69 ☑
Sesamoiditis M25.8- ☑
Severe sepsis R65.20
 with septic shock R65.21
Sever's disease or osteochondrosis — *see* Osteochondrosis, juvenile, tarsus
Sex
 chromosome mosaics Q97.8
  lines with various numbers of X chromosomes Q97.2
 education Z70.8
 reassignment surgery status Z87.890
Sextuplet pregnancy — *see* Pregnancy, sextuplet
Sexual
 function, disorder of (psychogenic) F52.9
 immaturity (female) E30.0
 impotence (psychogenic) organic origin NEC — *see* Dysfunction, sexual, male
 precocity (constitutional) (cryptogenic) (female) (idiopathic) (male) E30.1
Sexuality, pathologic — *see* Deviation, sexual
Sézary disease C84.1- ☑
Shadow, lung R91.8
Shaking palsy or paralysis — *see* Parkinsonism
Shallowness, acetabulum — *see* Derangement, joint, specified type NEC, hip
Shaver's disease J63.1
Sheath (tendon) — *see* condition
Sheathing, retinal vessels H35.01- ☑
Shedding
 nail L60.8
 premature, primary (deciduous) teeth K00.6
Sheehan's disease or syndrome E23.0
Shelf, rectal K62.89
Shell teeth K00.5
Shellshock (current) F43.0

Shellshock — *continued*
  lasting state — *see* Disorder, post-traumatic stress
Shield kidney Q63.1
Shift
  auditory threshold (temporary) H93.24- ☑
  mediastinal R93.89
Shifting sleep-work schedule (affecting sleep) G47.26
Shiga (-Kruse) **dysentery** A03.0
Shiga's bacillus A03.0
Shigella (dysentery) — *see* Dysentery, bacillary
Shigellosis A03.9
  Group A A03.0
  Group B A03.1
  Group C A03.2
  Group D A03.3
Shin splints S86.89- ☑
Shingles — *see* Herpes, zoster
Shipyard disease or eye B30.0
Shirodkar suture, in pregnancy — *see* Pregnancy, complicated by, incompetent cervix
Shock R57.9
  with ectopic or molar pregnancy O08.3
  adrenal (cortical) (Addisonian) E27.2
  adverse food reaction (anaphylactic) — *see* Shock, anaphylactic, due to food
  allergic — *see* Shock, anaphylactic
  anaphylactic T78.2 ☑
    chemical — *see* Table of Drugs and Chemicals
    due to drug or medicinal substance
      correct substance properly administered T88.6 ☑
      overdose or wrong substance given or taken (by accident) — *see* Table of Drugs and Chemicals, by drug, poisoning
    due to food (nonpoisonous) T78.00 ☑
      additives T78.06 ☑
      dairy products T78.07 ☑
      eggs T78.08 ☑
      fish T78.03 ☑
        shellfish T78.02 ☑
      fruit T78.04 ☑
      milk T78.07 ☑
      nuts T78.05 ☑
        multiple types T78.05 ☑
        peanuts T78.01 ☑
      peanuts T78.01 ☑
      seeds T78.05 ☑
      specified type NEC T78.09 ☑
      vegetable T78.04 ☑
    following sting(s) — *see* Venom
    immunization T80.52 ☑
    serum T80.59 ☑
      blood and blood products T80.51 ☑
      immunization T80.52 ☑
      specified NEC T80.59 ☑
      vaccination T80.52 ☑
  anaphylactoid — *see* Shock, anaphylactic
  anesthetic
    correct substance properly administered T88.2 ☑
    overdose or wrong substance given or taken — *see* Table of Drugs and Chemicals, by drug, poisoning
      specified anesthetic — *see* Table of Drugs and Chemicals, by drug, poisoning
  cardiogenic R57.0
  chemical substance — *see* Table of Drugs and Chemicals
  complicating ectopic or molar pregnancy O08.3
  culture — *see* Disorder, adjustment
  drug
    due to correct substance properly administered T88.6 ☑
    overdose or wrong substance given or taken (by accident) — *see* Table of Drugs and Chemicals, by drug, poisoning
  during or after labor and delivery O75.1
  electric T75.4 ☑
    (taser) T75.4 ☑
  endotoxic R65.21
    postprocedural (resulting from a procedure, not elsewhere classified) T81.12 ☑
  following
    ectopic or molar pregnancy O08.3
    injury (immediate) (delayed) T79.4 ☑
    labor and delivery O75.1
  food (anaphylactic) — *see* Shock, anaphylactic, due to food
  from electroshock gun (taser) T75.4 ☑

Shock — *continued*
  gram-negative R65.21
    postprocedural (resulting from a procedure, not elsewhere classified) T81.12 ☑
  hematologic R57.8
  hemorrhagic R57.8
    surgery (intraoperative) (postoperative) T81.19 ☑
    trauma T79.4 ☑
  hypovolemic R57.1
    surgical T81.19 ☑
    traumatic T79.4 ☑
  insulin E15
    therapeutic misadventure — *see* subcategory T38.3 ☑
  kidney N17.0
    traumatic (following crushing) T79.5 ☑
  lightning T75.01 ☑
  liver K72.00
  lung J80
  obstetric O75.1
    with ectopic or molar pregnancy O08.3
    following ectopic or molar pregnancy O08.3
  pleural (surgical) T81.19 ☑
    due to trauma T79.4 ☑
  postprocedural (postoperative) T81.10 ☑
    with ectopic or molar pregnancy O08.3
    cardiogenic T81.11 ☑
    endotoxic T81.12 ☑
    following ectopic or molar pregnancy O08.3
    gram-negative T81.12 ☑
    hypovolemic T81.19 ☑
    septic T81.12 ☑
    specified type NEC T81.19 ☑
  psychic F43.0
  septic (due to severe sepsis) R65.21
  specified NEC R57.8
  surgical T81.10 ☑
  taser gun (taser) T75.4 ☑
  therapeutic misadventure NEC T81.10 ☑
  thyroxin
    overdose or wrong substance given or taken — *see* Table of Drugs and Chemicals, by drug, poisoning
  toxic, syndrome A48.3
  transfusion — *see* Complications, transfusion
  traumatic (immediate) (delayed) T79.4 ☑
Shoemaker's chest M95.4
Short, shortening, shortness
  arm (acquired) — *see also* Deformity, limb, unequal length
    congenital Q71.81- ☑
    forearm — *see* Deformity, limb, unequal length
  bowel syndrome K91.2
  breath R06.02
  cervical (complicating pregnancy) O26.87- ☑
    non-gravid uterus N88.3
  common bile duct, congenital Q44.5
  cord (umbilical), complicating delivery O69.3 ☑
  cystic duct, congenital Q44.5
  esophagus (congenital) Q39.8
  femur (acquired) — *see* Deformity, limb, unequal length, femur
    congenital — *see* Defect, reduction, lower limb, longitudinal, femur
  frenum, frenulum, linguae (congenital) Q38.1
  hip (acquired) — *see also* Deformity, limb, unequal length
    congenital Q65.89
  leg (acquired) — *see also* Deformity, limb, unequal length
    congenital Q72.81- ☑
    lower leg — *see also* Deformity, limb, unequal length
  limbed stature, with immunodeficiency D82.2
  lower limb (acquired) — *see also* Deformity, limb, unequal length
    congenital Q72.81- ☑
  organ or site, congenital NEC — *see* Distortion
  palate, congenital Q38.5
  radius (acquired) — *see also* Deformity, limb, unequal length
    congenital — *see* Defect, reduction, upper limb, longitudinal, radius
  rib syndrome Q77.2
  stature (child) (hereditary) (idiopathic) NEC R62.52
    constitutional E34.31

Short, shortening, shortness — *continued*
  stature — *continued*
    due to
      endocrine disorder E34.30
        specified type NEC, due to endocrine dosorder E34.39
      genetic causes E34.329
        ACAN gene variant E34.328
        acid-labile subunit gene (IGFALS) defect E34.321
        aggrecan deficiency E34.328
        genetic syndrome with resistance to insulin-like growth factor-1 E34.322
        growth hormone gene 1 (GH1) defect with growth hormone neutralizing antibod-ies E34.321
        growth hormone insensitivity syndrome (GHIS) E34.321
        insulin-like growth factor 1 gene (IGF1) defect E34.321
        insulin-like growth factor-1 receptor (IGF-1R) defect E34.322
        insulin-like growth factor-1 (IGF-1) resistance E34.322
        NPR-2 gene variant E34.328
        post-insulin-like growth factor-1 receptor signaling defect E34.322
        primary insulin-like growth factor-1 (IGF-1) deficiency E34.321
        severe primary insulin-like growth factor-1 deficiency (SPIGFD) E34.321
        signal transducer and activator of transcrip-tion 5B gene (STAT5b) defect E34.321
        specified genetic cause NEC E34.328
    Laron-type E34.321
  tendon — *see also* Contraction, tendon
    with contracture of joint — *see* Contraction, joint
    Achilles (acquired) M67.0- ☑
      congenital Q66.89
    congenital Q79.8
  thigh (acquired) — *see also* Deformity, limb, unequal length, femur
    congenital — *see* Defect, reduction, lower limb, longitudinal, femur
  tibialis anterior (tendon) — *see* Contraction, tendon
  umbilical cord
    complicating delivery O69.3 ☑
  upper limb, congenital — *see* Defect, reduction, upper limb, specified type NEC
  urethra N36.8
  uvula, congenital Q38.5
  vagina (congenital) Q52.4
Shortsightedness — *see* Myopia
Shoshin (acute fulminating beriberi) E51.11
Shoulder — *see* condition
Shovel-shaped incisors K00.2
Shower, thromboembolic — *see* Embolism
Shunt
  arterial-venous (dialysis) Z99.2
  arteriovenous, pulmonary (acquired) I28.0
    congenital Q25.72
  cerebral ventricle (communicating) in situ Z98.2
  surgical, prosthetic, with complications — *see* Complications, cardiovascular, device or implant
Shutdown, renal N28.9
Shy-Drager syndrome G90.3
Sialadenitis, sialadenosis (any gland) (chronic) (period-ic) (suppurative) — *see* Sialoadenitis
Sialectasia K11.8
Sialidosis E77.1
Sialitis, silitis (any gland) (chronic) (suppurative) — *see* Sialoadenitis
Sialoadenitis (any gland) (periodic) (suppurative) K11.20
  acute K11.21
    recurrent K11.22
  chronic K11.23
Sialoadenopathy K11.9
Sialoangitis — *see* Sialoadenitis
Sialodochitis (fibrinosa) — *see* Sialoadenitis
Sialodocholithiasis K11.5
Sialolithiasis K11.5
Sialometaplasia, necrotizing K11.8
Sialorrhea — *see also* Ptyalism
  periodic — *see* Sialoadenitis
Sialosis K11.7
Siamese twin Q89.4
Sibling rivalry Z62.891
Sicard's syndrome G52.7

Sicca syndrome — *see* Syndrome, Sjögren
Sick R69
  or handicapped person in family Z63.79
    needing care at home Z63.6
  sinus (syndrome) I49.5
Sick-euthyroid syndrome E07.81
Sickle-cell
  anemia — *see* Disease, sickle-cell
  beta plus — *see* Disease, sickle-cell, thalassemia, beta
    plus
  beta zero — *see* Disease, sickle-cell, thalassemia, beta
    zero
  trait D57.3
Sicklemia — *see also* Disease, sickle-cell
  trait D57.3
Sickness
  air (travel) T75.3 ☑
  airplane T75.3 ☑
  alpine T70.29 ☑
  altitude T70.20 ☑
  Andes T70.29 ☑
  aviator's T70.29 ☑
  balloon T70.29 ☑
  car T75.3 ☑
  compressed air T70.3 ☑
  decompression T70.3 ☑
  green D50.8
  milk — *see* Poisoning, food, noxious
  motion T75.3 ☑
  mountain T70.29 ☑
    acute D75.1
  protein — *see also* Reaction, serum T80.69 ☑
  radiation T66 ☑
  roundabout (motion) T75.3 ☑
  sea T75.3 ☑
  serum NEC — *see also* Reaction, serum T80.69 ☑
  sleeping (African) B56.9
    by Trypanosoma B56.9
      brucei
        gambiense B56.0
        rhodesiense B56.1
      East African B56.1
      Gambian B56.0
      Rhodesian B56.1
      West African B56.0
  swing (motion) T75.3 ☑
  train (railway) (travel) T75.3 ☑
  travel (any vehicle) T75.3 ☑
Sideropenia — *see* Anemia, iron deficiency
Siderosilicosis J62.8
Siderosis (lung) J63.4
  brain G93.89
  eye (globe) — *see* Disorder, globe, degenerative,
    siderosis
Siemens' syndrome (ectodermal dysplasia) Q82.8
Sighing R06.89
  psychogenic F45.8
Sigmoid — *see also* condition
  flexure — *see* condition
  kidney Q63.1
Sigmoiditis — *see also* Enteritis K52.9
  infectious A09
  noninfectious K52.9
Silfversköld's syndrome Q78.9
Silicosiderosis J62.8
Silicosis, silicotic (simple) (complicated) J62.8
  with tuberculosis J65
Silicotuberculosis J65
Silo-fillers' disease J68.8
  bronchitis J68.0
  pneumonitis J68.0
  pulmonary edema J68.1
Silver's syndrome Q87.19
Simian malaria B53.1
Simmonds' cachexia or disease E23.0
Simons' disease or syndrome (progressive lipodystrophy) E88.1
Simple, simplex — *see* condition
Simulation, conscious (of illness) Z76.5
Simultanagnosia (asimultagnosia) R48.3
Sin Nombre virus disease (Hantavirus) (cardio)-pulmonary syndrome) B33.4
Sinding-Larsen disease or osteochondrosis — *see* Osteochondrosis, juvenile, patella
Singapore hemorrhagic fever A91
Singer's node or nodule J38.2

Single
  atrium Q21.20
  coronary artery Q24.5
  umbilical artery Q27.0
  ventricle Q20.4
Singultus R06.6
  epidemicus B33.0
Sinus — *see also* Fistula
  abdominal K63.89
  arrest I45.5
  arrhythmia I49.8
  bradycardia R00.1
  branchial cleft (internal) (external) Q18.0
  coccygeal — *see* Sinus, pilonidal
  dental K04.6
  dermal (congenital) Q06.8
    with abscess Q06.8
      coccygeal, pilonidal — *see* Sinus, coccygeal
  infected, skin NEC L08.89
  marginal, ruptured or bleeding — *see* Hemorrhage,
    antepartum, specified cause NEC
  medial, face and neck Q18.8
  pause I45.5
  pericranii Q01.9
  pilonidal (infected) (rectum) L05.92
    with abscess L05.02
  preauricular Q18.1
  rectovaginal N82.3
  Rokitansky-Aschoff (gallbladder) K82.8
  sacrococcygeal (dermoid) (infected) — *see* Sinus, pilonidal
  tachycardia R00.0
    paroxysmal I47.1
  tarsi syndrome M25.57- ☑
  testis N50.89
  tract (postinfective) — *see* Fistula
  urachus Q64.4
Sinusitis (accessory) (chronic) (hyperplastic) (nasal)
    (nonpurulent) (purulent) J32.9
  acute J01.90
    ethmoidal J01.20
      recurrent J01.21
    frontal J01.10
      recurrent J01.11
    involving more than one sinus, other than pansinusitis J01.80
      recurrent J01.81
    maxillary J01.00
      recurrent J01.01
    pansinusitis J01.40
      recurrent J01.41
    recurrent J01.91
    specified NEC J01.80
      recurrent J01.81
    sphenoidal J01.30
      recurrent J01.31
  allergic — *see* Rhinitis, allergic
  due to high altitude T70.1 ☑
  ethmoidal J32.2
    acute J01.20
      recurrent J01.21
  frontal J32.1
    acute J01.10
      recurrent J01.11
  influenzal — *see* Influenza, with, respiratory manifestations NEC
  involving more than one sinus but not pansinusitis J32.8
    acute J01.80
      recurrent J01.81
  maxillary J32.0
    acute J01.00
      recurrent J01.01
  sphenoidal J32.3
    acute J01.30
      recurrent J01.31
  tuberculous, any sinus A15.8
Sinusitis-bronchiectasis-situs inversus (syndrome)
    (triad) Q89.3
Sipple's syndrome E31.22
Sirenomelia (syndrome) Q87.2
Siriasis T67.01 ☑
Sirkari's disease B55.0
Siti A65
Situation, psychiatric F99
Situational
  disturbance (transient) — *see* Disorder, adjustment
    acute F43.0

Situational — *continued*
  maladjustment — *see* Disorder, adjustment
  reaction — *see* Disorder, adjustment
    acute F43.0
Situs inversus or transversus (abdominalis) (thoracis)
    Q89.3
Sixth disease B08.20
  due to human herpesvirus 6 B08.21
  due to human herpesvirus 7 B08.22
Sjögren-Larsson syndrome Q87.19
Sjögren's syndrome or disease — *see* Syndrome, Sjögren
Skeletal — *see* condition
Skene's gland — *see* condition
Skenitis — *see* Urethritis
Skerljevo A65
Skevas-Zerfus disease — *see* Toxicity, venom, marine
    animal, sea anemone
Skin — *see also* condition
  clammy R23.1
  donor — *see* Donor, skin
  dry L85.3
  hidebound M35.9
Slate-dressers' or slate-miners' lung J62.8
Sleep
  apnea — *see* Apnea, sleep
  deprivation Z72.820
  disorder or disturbance G47.9
    child F51.9
    nonorganic origin F51.9
    specified NEC G47.8
  disturbance G47.9
    nonorganic origin F51.9
  drunkenness F51.9
  rhythm inversion G47.2- ☑
  terrors F51.4
  walking F51.3
    hysterical F44.89
Sleep hygiene
  abuse Z72.821
  inadequate Z72.821
  poor Z72.821
Sleeping sickness — *see* Sickness, sleeping
Sleeplessness — *see* Insomnia
  menopausal N95.1
Sleep-wake schedule disorder G47.20
Slim disease (in HIV infection) B20
Slipped, slipping
  epiphysis (traumatic) — *see also* Osteochondropathy,
    specified type NEC
    capital femoral (traumatic) [SCFE]
      acute (on chronic) S79.01- ☑
      nontraumatic M93.00- ☑
    current traumatic — *code as* Fracture, by site
    upper femoral (nontraumatic) [SUFE] M93.00- ☑
      acute M93.01- ☑
        on chronic M93.03- ☑
      chronic M93.02- ☑
  intervertebral disc — *see* Displacement, intervertebral
    disc
  ligature, umbilical P51.8
  patella — *see* Disorder, patella, derangement NEC
  rib M89.8X8
  sacroiliac joint — *see* subcategory M53.2 ☑
  tendon — *see* Disorder, tendon
  ulnar nerve, nontraumatic — *see* Lesion, nerve, ulnar
  vertebra NEC — *see* Spondylolisthesis
Slocumb's syndrome E27.0
Sloughing (multiple) (phagedena) (skin) — *see also*
    Gangrene
  abscess — *see* Abscess
  appendix K38.8
  fascia — *see* Disorder, soft tissue, specified type NEC
  scrotum N50.89
  tendon — *see* Disorder, tendon
  transplanted organ — *see* Rejection, transplant
  ulcer — *see* Ulcer, skin
Slow
  feeding, newborn P92.2
  flow syndrome, coronary I20.8
  heart (beat) R00.1
Slowing, urinary stream R39.198
Sluder's neuralgia (syndrome) G44.89
Slurred, slurring speech R47.81
Small (ness)
  for gestational age — *see* Small for dates
  introitus, vagina N89.6

Small — *continued*
  kidney (unknown cause) N27.9
    bilateral N27.1
    unilateral N27.0
  ovary (congenital) Q50.39
  pelvis
    with disproportion (fetopelvic) O33.1
      causing obstructed labor O65.1
  uterus N85.8
  white kidney N03.9
Small-and-light-for-dates — *see* Small for dates
Small-for-dates (infant) P05.10
  with weight of
    499 grams or less P05.11
    500-749 grams P05.12
    750-999 grams P05.13
    1000-1249 grams P05.14
    1250-1499 grams P05.15
    1500-1749 grams P05.16
    1750-1999 grams P05.17
    2000-2499 grams P05.18
    2500 grams and over P05.19
  specified NEC P05.19
Smallpox B03
Smearing, fecal R15.1
SMEI (severe myoclonic epilepsy in infancy) G40.83- ☑
Smith-Lemli-Opitz syndrome E78.72
Smith's fracture S52.54- ☑
Smoker — *see* Dependence, drug, nicotine
Smoker's
  bronchitis J41.0
  cough J41.0
  palate K13.24
  throat J31.2
  tongue K13.24
Smoking
  passive Z77.22
Smothering spells R06.81
Snaggle teeth, tooth M26.39
Snapping
  finger — *see* Trigger finger
  hip — *see* Derangement, joint, specified type NEC, hip
    involving the iliotiblial band M76.3- ☑
  knee — *see* Derangement, knee
    involving the iliotiblial band M76.3- ☑
Sneddon-Wilkinson disease or syndrome (sub-corneal
    pustular dermatosis) L13.1
Sneezing (intractable) R06.7
Sniffing
  cocaine
    abuse — *see* Abuse, drug, cocaine
    dependence — *see* Dependence, drug, cocaine
  gasoline
    abuse — *see* Abuse, drug, inhalant
    dependence — *see* Dependence, drug, inhalant
  glue (airplane)
    abuse — *see* Abuse, drug, inhalant
    drug dependence — *see* Dependence, drug, in-
      halant
Sniffles
  newborn P28.89
Snoring R06.83
Snow blindness — *see* Photokeratitis
Snuffles (non-syphilitic) R06.5
  newborn P28.89
  syphilitic (infant) A50.05 *[J99]*
Social
  exclusion Z60.4
    due to discrimination or persecution (perceived)
      Z60.5
  migrant Z59.00
    acculturation difficulty Z60.3
  rejection Z60.4
    due to discrimination or persecution Z60.5
  role conflict NEC Z73.5
  skills inadequacy NEC Z73.4
  transplantation Z60.3
Sodoku A25.0
Soemmerring's ring — *see* Cataract, secondary
Soft — *see also* condition
  nails L60.3
Softening
  bone — *see* Osteomalacia
  brain (necrotic) (progressive) G93.89
    congenital Q04.8
    embolic I63.4- ☑

Softening — *continued*
  brain — *continued*
    hemorrhagic — *see* Hemorrhage, intracranial, intrac-
      erebral
      occlusive I63.5- ☑
      thrombotic I63.3- ☑
    cartilage M94.2- ☑
      patella M22.4- ☑
    cerebellar — *see* Softening, brain
    cerebral — *see* Softening, brain
    cerebrospinal — *see* Softening, brain
    myocardial, heart — *see* Degeneration, myocardial
    spinal cord G95.89
    stomach K31.89
Soldier's
  heart F45.8
  patches I31.0
Solitary
  cyst, kidney N28.1
  kidney, congenital Q60.0
Solvent abuse — *see* Abuse, drug, inhalant
  dependence — *see* Dependence, drug, inhalant
Somatization reaction, somatic reaction — *see* Disor-
    der, somatoform
Somnambulism F51.3
  hysterical F44.89
Somnolence R40.0
  nonorganic origin F51.11
Sonne dysentery A03.3
Soor B37.0
Sore
  bed — *see* Ulcer, pressure, by site
  chiclero B55.1
  Delhi B55.1
  desert — *see* Ulcer, skin
  eye H57.1- ☑
  Lahore B55.1
  mouth K13.79
    canker K12.0
  muscle M79.10
  Naga — *see* Ulcer, skin
  of skin — *see* Ulcer, skin
  oriental B55.1
  pressure — *see* Ulcer, pressure, by site
  skin L98.9
  soft A57
  throat (acute) — *see also* Pharyngitis
    with influenza, flu, or grippe — *see* Influenza, with,
      respiratory manifestations NEC
    chronic J31.2
    coxsackie (virus) B08.5
    diphtheritic A36.0
    herpesviral B00.2
    influenzal — *see* Influenza, with, respiratory mani-
      festations NEC
    septic J02.0
    streptococcal (ulcerative) J02.0
    viral NEC J02.8
      coxsackie B08.5
  tropical — *see* Ulcer, skin
  veldt — *see* Ulcer, skin
Soto's syndrome (cerebral gigantism) Q87.3
South African cardiomyopathy syndrome I42.8
Southeast Asian hemorrhagic fever A91
Spacing
  abnormal, tooth, teeth, fully erupted M26.30
  excessive, tooth, fully erupted M26.32
Spade-like hand (congenital) Q68.1
Spading nail L60.8
  congenital Q84.6
Spanish collar N47.1
Sparganosis B70.1
Spasm(s), **spastic, spasticity** — *see also* condition R25.2
  accommodation — *see* Spasm, of accommodation
  ampulla of Vater K83.4
  anus, ani (sphincter) (reflex) K59.4
    psychogenic F45.8
  artery I73.9
    cerebral G45.9
  Bell's G51.3- ☑
  bladder (sphincter, external or internal) N32.89
    psychogenic F45.8
  bronchus, bronchiole J98.01
  cardia K22.0
  cardiac I20.1
  carpopedal — *see* Tetany
  cerebral (arteries) (vascular) G45.9

Spasm(s), **spastic, spasticity** — *continued*
  cervix, complicating delivery O62.4
  ciliary body (of accommodation) — *see* Spasm, of ac-
    commodation
  colon — *see also* Irritable, bowel K58.9
    with diarrhea K58.0
    psychogenic F45.8
  common duct K83.8
  compulsive — *see* Tic
  conjugate H51.8
  coronary (artery) I20.1
  diaphragm (reflex) R06.6
    epidemic B33.0
    psychogenic F45.8
  duodenum K59.89
  epidemic diaphragmatic (transient) B33.0
  esophagus (diffuse) K22.4
    psychogenic F45.8
  facial G51.3- ☑
  fallopian tube N83.8
  gastrointestinal (tract) K31.89
    psychogenic F45.8
  glottis J38.5
    hysterical F44.4
    psychogenic F45.8
      conversion reaction F44.4
    reflex through recurrent laryngeal nerve J38.5
  habit — *see* Tic
  heart I20.1
  hemifacial (clonic) G51.3- ☑
  hourglass — *see* Contraction, hourglass
  hysterical F44.4
  infantile — *see* Epilepsy, spasms
  inferior oblique, eye H51.8
  intestinal — *see also* Syndrome, irritable bowel K58.9
    psychogenic F45.8
  larynx, laryngeal J38.5
    hysterical F44.4
    psychogenic F45.8
      conversion reaction F44.4
  levator palpebrae superioris — *see* Disorder, eyelid
    function
  muscle NEC M62.838
    back M62.830
  nerve, trigeminal G51.0
  nervous F45.8
  nodding F98.4
  occupational F48.8
  oculogyric H51.8
    psychogenic F45.8
  of accommodation H52.53- ☑
  ophthalmic artery — *see* Occlusion, artery, retina
  perineal, female N94.89
  peroneo-extensor — *see also* Deformity, limb, flat foot
  pharynx (reflex) J39.2
    hysterical F45.8
    psychogenic F45.8
  psychogenic F45.8
  pylorus NEC K31.3
    adult hypertrophic K31.89
    congenital or infantile Q40.0
    psychogenic F45.8
  rectum (sphincter) K59.4
    psychogenic F45.8
  retinal (artery) — *see* Occlusion, artery, retina
  sigmoid — *see also* Syndrome, irritable bowel K58.9
    psychogenic F45.8
  sphincter of Oddi K83.4
  stomach K31.89
    neurotic F45.8
  throat J39.2
    hysterical F45.8
    psychogenic F45.8
  tic F95.9
    chronic F95.1
    transient of childhood F95.0
  tongue K14.8
  torsion (progressive) G24.1
  trigeminal nerve — *see* Neuralgia, trigeminal
  ureter N13.5
  urethra (sphincter) N35.919
  uterus N85.8
    complicating labor O62.4
  vagina N94.2
    psychogenic F52.5
  vascular I73.9
  vasomotor I73.9
  vein NEC I87.8

☑ Additional Character Required — Refer to the Tabular List for Character Selection

Spasm(s), spastic, spasticity — *continued*
  viscera — *see* Pain, abdominal
Spasmodic — *see* condition
Spasmophilia — *see* Tetany
Spasmus nutans F98.4
Spastic, spasticity — *see also* Spasm
  child (cerebral) (congenital) (paralysis) G80.1
Speaker's throat R49.8
Specific, specified — *see* condition
Speech
  defect, disorder, disturbance, impediment — *see* Disorder, speech R47.9
    psychogenic, in childhood and adolescence F98.8
  slurring R47.81
  specified NEC R47.89
Spells, transient oxygen desaturation of newborn — *see also* Apnea, newborn P28.40
  during sleep — *see also* Apnea, newborn, sleep, primary P28.30
Spencer's disease A08.19
Spens' syndrome (syncope with heart block) I45.9
Sperm counts (fertility testing) Z31.41
  postvasectomy Z30.8
    reversal Z31.42
Spermatic cord — *see* condition
Spermatocele N43.40
  congenital Q55.4
  multiple N43.42
  single N43.41
Spermatocystitis N49.0
Spermatocytoma C62.9- ☑
  specified site — *see* Neoplasm, malignant, by site
Spermatorrhea N50.89
Sphacelus — *see* Gangrene
Sphenoidal — *see* condition
Sphenoiditis (chronic) — *see* Sinusitis, sphenoidal
Sphenopalatine ganglion neuralgia G90.09
Sphericity, increased, lens (congenital) Q12.4
Spherocytosis (congenital) (familial) (hereditary) D58.0
  hemoglobin disease D58.0
  sickle-cell (disease) D57.8- ☑
Spherophakia Q12.4
Sphincter — *see* condition
Sphincteritis, sphincter of Oddi — *see* Cholangitis
Sphingolipidosis E75.3
  specified NEC E75.29
Sphingomyelinosis E75.3
Spicule tooth K00.2
Spider
  bite — *see* Toxicity, venom, spider
    nonvenomous — *see* Bite, by site, superficial, insect
  fingers — *see* Syndrome, Marfan's
  nevus I78.1 *spider vein*
  toes — *see* Syndrome, Marfan's
  vascular I78.1
Spiegler-Fendt
  benign lymphocytoma L98.8
  sarcoid L08.89
Spielmeyer-Vogt disease E75.4
Spina bifida (aperta) Q05.9
  with hydrocephalus NEC Q05.4
  cervical Q05.5
    with hydrocephalus Q05.0
  dorsal Q05.6
    with hydrocephalus Q05.1
  lumbar Q05.7
    with hydrocephalus Q05.2
  lumbosacral Q05.7
    with hydrocephalus Q05.2
  occulta Q76.0
  sacral Q05.8
    with hydrocephalus Q05.3
  thoracic Q05.6
    with hydrocephalus Q05.1
  thoracolumbar Q05.6
    with hydrocephalus Q05.1
Spindle, Krukenberg's — *see* Pigmentation, cornea, posterior
Spine, spinal — *see* condition
Spiradenoma (eccrine) — *see* Neoplasm, skin, benign
Spirillosis A25.0
Spirillum
  minus A25.0
  obermeieri infection A68.0
Spirochetal — *see* condition
Spirochetosis A69.9
  arthritic, arthritica A69.9

Spirochetosis — *continued*
  bronchopulmonary A69.8
  icterohemorrhagic A27.0
  lung A69.8
Spirometrosis B70.1
Spitting blood — *see* Hemoptysis
Splanchnoptosis K63.4
Spleen, splenic — *see* condition
Splenectasis — *see* Splenomegaly
Splenitis (interstitial) (malignant) (nonspecific) D73.89
  malarial — *see also* Malaria B54 [D77]
  tuberculous A18.85
Splenocele D73.89
Splenomegaly, splenomegalia (Bengal) (cryptogenic) (idiopathic) (tropical) R16.1
  with hepatomegaly R16.2
  cirrhotic D73.2
  congenital Q89.09
  congestive, chronic D73.2
  Egyptian B65.1
  Gaucher's E75.22
  malarial — *see also* Malaria B54 [D77]
  neutropenic D73.81
  Niemann-Pick — *see* Niemann-Pick disease or syndrome
  sideritic D73.2
  syphilitic A52.79
    congenital (early) A50.08 [D77]
Splenopathy D73.9
Splenoptosis D73.89
Splenosis D73.89
Splinter — *see* Foreign body, superficial, by site
Split, splitting
  foot Q72.7- ☑
  hand Q71.6 ☑
  heart sounds R01.2
  lip, congenital — *see* Cleft, lip
  nails L60.3
  urinary stream R39.13
Spondylarthrosis — *see* Spondylosis
Spondylitis (chronic) — *see also* Spondylopathy, inflammatory
  ankylopoietica — *see* Spondylitis, ankylosing
  ankylosing (chronic) M45.9
    with lung involvement M45.9 [J99]
    cervical region M45.2
    cervicothoracic region M45.3
    juvenile M08.1
    lumbar region M45.6
    lumbosacral region M45.7
    multiple sites M45.0
    occipito-atlanto-axial region M45.1
    sacrococcygeal region M45.8
    thoracic region M45.4
    thoracolumbar region M45.5
  atrophic (ligamentous) — *see* Spondylitis, ankylosing
  deformans (chronic) — *see* Spondylosis
  gonococcal A54.41
  gouty — *see also* Gout, by type, vertebrae M10.08
  in (due to)
    brucellosis A23.9 [M49.80]
      cervical region A23.9 [M49.82]
      cervicothoracic region A23.9 [M49.83]
      lumbar region A23.9 [M49.86]
      lumbosacral region A23.9 [M49.87]
      multiple sites A23.9 [M49.89]
      occipito-atlanto-axial region A23.9 [M49.81]
      sacrococcygeal region A23.9 [M49.88]
      thoracic region A23.9 [M49.84]
      thoracolumbar region A23.9 [M49.85]
    enterobacteria — *see also* subcategory M49.8 A04.9
    tuberculosis A18.01
  infectious NEC — *see* Spondylopathy, infective
  juvenile ankylosing (chronic) M08.1
  Kümmell's — *see* Spondylopathy, traumatic
  Marie-Strümpell — *see* Spondylitis, ankylosing
  muscularis — *see* Spondylopathy, specified NEC
  psoriatic L40.53
  rheumatoid — *see* Spondylitis, ankylosing
  rhizomelica — *see* Spondylitis, ankylosing
  sacroiliac NEC M46.1
  senescent, senile — *see* Spondylosis
  traumatic (chronic) or post-traumatic — *see* Spondylopathy, traumatic
  tuberculous A18.01
  typhosa A01.05

Spondyloarthritis
  axial — *see also* Spondlyitis, ankylosing
    non-radiographic M45.A0
      cervical M45.A2
      cervicothoracic M45.A3
      lumbar M45.A6
      lumbosacral M45.A7
      multiple sites M45.AB
      occipito-atlanto-axial region M45.A1
      sacral and sacrococcygeal M45.A8
      thoracic M45.A4
      thoracolumbar M45.A5
Spondylolisthesis (acquired) (degenerative) M43.10
  with disproportion (fetopelvic) O33.0
    causing obstructed labor O65.0
  cervical region M43.12
  cervicothoracic region M43.13
  congenital Q76.2
  lumbar region M43.16
  lumbosacral region M43.17
  multiple sites M43.19
  occipito-atlanto-axial region M43.11
  sacrococcygeal region M43.18
  thoracic region M43.14
  thoracolumbar region M43.15
  traumatic (old) M43.10
    acute
      fifth cervical (displaced) S12.430 ☑
        nondisplaced S12.431 ☑
        specified type NEC (displaced) S12.450 ☑
          nondisplaced S12.451 ☑
        type III S12.44 ☑
      fourth cervical (displaced) S12.330 ☑
        nondisplaced S12.331 ☑
        specified type NEC (displaced) S12.350 ☑
          nondisplaced S12.351 ☑
        type III S12.34 ☑
      second cervical (displaced) S12.130 ☑
        nondisplaced S12.131 ☑
        specified type NEC (displaced) S12.150 ☑
          nondisplaced S12.151 ☑
        type III S12.14 ☑
      seventh cervical (displaced) S12.630 ☑
        nondisplaced S12.631 ☑
        specified type NEC (displaced) S12.650 ☑
          nondisplaced S12.651 ☑
        type III S12.64 ☑
      sixth cervical (displaced) S12.530 ☑
        nondisplaced S12.531 ☑
        specified type NEC (displaced) S12.550 ☑
          nondisplaced S12.551 ☑
        type III S12.54 ☑
      third cervical (displaced) S12.230 ☑
        nondisplaced S12.231 ☑
        specified type NEC (displaced) S12.250 ☑
          nondisplaced S12.251 ☑
        type III S12.24 ☑
Spondylolysis (acquired) M43.00
  cervical region M43.02
  cervicothoracic region M43.03
  congenital Q76.2
  lumbar region M43.06
  lumbosacral region M43.07
    with disproportion (fetopelvic) O33.0
    causing obstructed labor O65.8
  multiple sites M43.09
  occipito-atlanto-axial region M43.01
  sacrococcygeal region M43.08
  thoracic region M43.04
  thoracolumbar region M43.05
Spondylopathy M48.9
  infective NEC M46.50
    cervical region M46.52
    cervicothoracic region M46.53
    lumbar region M46.56
    lumbosacral region M46.57
    multiple sites M46.59
    occipito-atlanto-axial region M46.51
    sacrococcygeal region M46.58
    thoracic region M46.54
    thoracolumbar region M46.55
  inflammatory M46.90
    cervical region M46.92
    cervicothoracic region M46.93
    lumbar region M46.96
    lumbosacral region M46.97
    multiple sites M46.99

Spondylopathy — *continued*
  inflammatory — *continued*
    occipito-atlanto-axial region M46.91
    sacrococcygeal region M46.98
    specified type NEC M46.80
      cervical region M46.82
      cervicothoracic region M46.83
      lumbar region M46.86
      lumbosacral region M46.87
      multiple sites M46.89
      occipito-atlanto-axial region M46.81
      sacrococcygeal region M46.88
      thoracic region M46.84
      thoracolumbar region M46.85
    thoracic region M46.94
    thoracolumbar region M46.95
  neuropathic, in
    syringomyelia and syringobulbia G95.0
    tabes dorsalis A52.11
  specified NEC — *see subcategory* M48.8 ☑
  traumatic M48.30
    cervical region M48.32
    cervicothoracic region M48.33
    lumbar region M48.36
    lumbosacral region M48.37
    occipito-atlanto-axial region M48.31
    sacrococcygeal region M48.38
    thoracic region M48.34
    thoracolumbar region M48.35
Spondylosis M47.9
  with
    disproportion (fetopelvic) O33.0
      causing obstructed labor O65.0
    myelopathy NEC M47.10
      cervical region M47.12
      cervicothoracic region M47.13
      lumbar region M47.16
      occipito-atlanto-axial region M47.11
      thoracic region M47.14
      thoracolumbar region M47.15
    radiculopathy M47.20
      cervical region M47.22
      cervicothoracic region M47.23
      lumbar region M47.26
      lumbosacral region M47.27
      occipito-atlanto-axial region M47.21
      sacrococcygeal region M47.28
      thoracic region M47.24
      thoracolumbar region M47.25
  specified NEC M47.899
    cervical region M47.892
    cervicothoracic region M47.893
    facet joint — *see also* Spondylosis M47.819
    lumbar region M47.896
    lumbosacral region M47.897
    occipito-atlanto-axial region M47.891
    sacrococcygeal region M47.898
    thoracic region M47.894
    thoracolumbar region M47.895
  traumatic — *see* Spondylopathy, traumatic
  without myelopathy or radiculopathy M47.819
    cervical region M47.812
    cervicothoracic region M47.813
    lumbar region M47.816
    lumbosacral region M47.817
    occipito-atlanto-axial region M47.811
    sacrococcygeal region M47.818
    thoracic region M47.814
    thoracolumbar region M47.815
Sponge
  inadvertently left in operation wound — *see* Foreign body, accidentally left during a procedure
  kidney (medullary) Q61.5
Sponge-diver's disease — *see* Toxicity, venom, marine animal, sea anemone
Spongioblastoma (any type) — *see* Neoplasm, malignant, by site
  specified site — *see* Neoplasm, malignant, by site
  unspecified site C71.9
Spongioneuroblastoma — *see* Neoplasm, malignant, by site
Spontaneous — *see also* condition
  fracture (cause unknown) — *see* Fracture, pathological
Spoon nail L60.3
  congenital Q84.6
Sporadic — *see* condition
Sporothrix schenckii infection — *see* Sporotrichosis
Sporotrichosis B42.9

Sporotrichosis — *continued*
  arthritis B42.82
  disseminated B42.7
  generalized B42.7
  lymphocutaneous (fixed) (progressive) B42.1
  pulmonary B42.0
  specified NEC B42.89
Spots, spotting (in) (of)
  Bitot's — *see also* Pigmentation, conjunctiva
    in the young child E50.1
    vitamin A deficiency E50.1
  café, au lait L81.3
  Cayenne pepper I78.1
  cotton wool, retina — *see* Occlusion, artery, retina
  de Morgan's (senile angiomas) I78.1
  Fuchs' black (myopic) — *see also* Myopia, degenerative H44.2-
  intermenstrual (regular) N92.0
    irregular N92.1
  Koplik's B05.9
  liver L81.4
  pregnancy O26.85- ☑
  purpuric R23.3
  ruby I78.1
Spotted fever — *see* Fever, spotted A77.9
Sprain (joint) (ligament)
  acromioclavicular joint or ligament S43.5- ☑
  ankle S93.40- ☑
    calcaneofibular ligament S93.41- ☑
    deltoid ligament S93.42- ☑
    internal collateral ligament — *see* Sprain, ankle, specified ligament NEC
    specified ligament NEC S93.49- ☑
    talofibular ligament — *see* Sprain, ankle, specified ligament NEC
    tibiofibular ligament S93.43- ☑
  anterior longitudinal, cervical S13.4 ☑
  atlas, atlanto-axial, atlanto-occipital S13.4 ☑
  breast bone — *see* Sprain, sternum
  calcaneofibular — *see* Sprain, ankle
  carpal — *see* Sprain, wrist
  carpometacarpal — *see* Sprain, hand, specified site NEC
  cartilage
    costal S23.41 ☑
    semilunar (knee) — *see* Sprain, knee, specified site NEC
      with current tear — *see* Tear, meniscus
    thyroid region S13.5 ☑
    xiphoid — *see* Sprain, sternum
  cervical, cervicodorsal, cervicothoracic S13.4 ☑
  chondrosternal S23.421 ☑
  coracoclavicular S43.8- ☑
  coracohumeral S43.41- ☑
  coronary, knee — *see* Sprain, knee, specified site NEC
  costal cartilage S23.41 ☑
  cricoarytenoid articulation or ligament S13.5 ☑
  cricothyroid articulation S13.5 ☑
  cruciate, knee — *see* Sprain, knee, cruciate
  deltoid, ankle — *see* Sprain, ankle
  dorsal (spine) S23.3 ☑
  elbow S53.40- ☑
    radial collateral ligament S53.43- ☑
    radiohumeral S53.41- ☑
    rupture
      radial collateral ligament — *see* Rupture, traumatic, ligament, radial collateral
      ulnar collateral ligament — *see* Rupture, traumatic, ligament, ulnar collateral
    specified type NEC S53.49- ☑
    ulnar collateral ligament S53.44- ☑
    ulnohumeral S53.42- ☑
  femur, head — *see* Sprain, hip
  fibular collateral, knee — *see* Sprain, knee, collateral
  fibulocalcaneal — *see* Sprain, ankle
  finger(s) S63.61- ☑
    index S63.61- ☑
    interphalangeal (joint) S63.63- ☑
      index S63.63- ☑
      little S63.63- ☑
      middle S63.63- ☑
      ring S63.63- ☑
    little S63.61- ☑
    metacarpophalangeal (joint) S63.65- ☑
    middle S63.61- ☑
    ring S63.61- ☑

Sprain — *continued*
  finger(s) — *continued*
    specified site NEC S63.69- ☑
      index S63.69- ☑
      little S63.69- ☑
      middle S63.69- ☑
      ring S63.69- ☑
  foot S93.60- ☑
    specified ligament NEC S93.69- ☑
    tarsal ligament S93.61- ☑
    tarsometatarsal ligament S93.62- ☑
    toe — *see* Sprain, toe
  hand S63.9- ☑
    finger — *see* Sprain, finger
    specified site NEC — *see* subcategory S63.8 ☑
    thumb — *see* Sprain, thumb
  head S03.9 ☑
  hip S73.10- ☑
    iliofemoral ligament S73.11- ☑
    ischiocapsular (ligament) S73.12- ☑
    specified NEC S73.19- ☑
  iliofemoral — *see* Sprain, hip
  innominate
    acetabulum — *see* Sprain, hip
    sacral junction S33.6 ☑
  internal
    collateral, ankle — *see* Sprain, ankle
    semilunar cartilage — *see* Sprain, knee, specified site NEC
  interphalangeal
    finger — *see* Sprain, finger, interphalangeal (joint)
    toe — *see* Sprain, toe, interphalangeal joint
  ischiocapsular — *see* Sprain, hip
  ischiofemoral — *see* Sprain, hip
  jaw (articular disc) (cartilage) (meniscus) S03.4- ☑
    old M26.69
  knee S83.9- ☑
    collateral ligament S83.40- ☑
      lateral (fibular) S83.42- ☑
      medial (tibial) S83.41- ☑
    cruciate ligament S83.50- ☑
      anterior S83.51- ☑
      posterior S83.52- ☑
    lateral (fibular) collateral ligament S83.42- ☑
    medial (tibial) collateral ligament S83.41- ☑
    patellar ligament S76.11- ☑
    specified site NEC S83.8X- ☑
    superior tibiofibular joint (ligament) S83.6- ☑
  lateral collateral, knee — *see* Sprain, knee, collateral
  lumbar (spine) S33.5 ☑
  lumbosacral S33.9 ☑
  mandible (articular disc) S03.4- ☑
    old M26.69
  medial collateral, knee — *see* Sprain, knee, collateral
  meniscus
    jaw S03.4- ☑
      old M26.69
    knee — *see* Sprain, knee, specified site NEC
      with current tear — *see* Tear, meniscus
        old — *see* Derangement, knee, meniscus, due to old tear
    mandible S03.4- ☑
      old M26.69
  metacarpal (distal) (proximal) — *see* Sprain, hand, specified site NEC
  metacarpophalangeal — *see* Sprain, finger, metacarpophalangeal (joint)
  metatarsophalangeal — *see* Sprain, toe, metatarsophalangeal joint
  midcarpal — *see* Sprain, hand, specified site NEC
  midtarsal — *see* Sprain, foot, specified site NEC
  neck S13.9 ☑
    anterior longitudinal cervical ligament S13.4 ☑
    atlanto-axial joint S13.4 ☑
    atlanto-occipital joint S13.4 ☑
    cervical spine S13.4 ☑
    cricoarytenoid ligament S13.5 ☑
    cricothyroid ligament S13.5 ☑
    specified site NEC S13.8 ☑
    thyroid region (cartilage) S13.5 ☑
  nose S03.8 ☑
  orbicular, hip — *see* Sprain, hip
  patella — *see* Sprain, knee, specified site NEC
  patellar ligament S76.11- ☑
  pelvis NEC S33.8 ☑

Sprain — continued
- phalanx
  - finger — see Sprain, finger
  - toe — see Sprain, toe
- pubofemoral — see Sprain, hip
- radiocarpal — see Sprain, wrist
- radiohumeral — see Sprain, elbow
- radius, collateral — see Rupture, traumatic, ligament, radial collateral
- rib (cage) S23.41 ☑
- rotator cuff (capsule) S43.42- ☑
- sacroiliac (region)
  - chronic or old — see subcategory M53.2 ☑
  - joint S33.6 ☑
- scaphoid (hand) — see Sprain, hand, specified site NEC
- scapula (r) — see Sprain, shoulder girdle, specified site NEC
- semilunar cartilage (knee) — see Sprain, knee, specified site NEC
  - with current tear — see Tear, meniscus
    - old — see Derangement, knee, meniscus, due to old tear
- shoulder joint S43.40- ☑
  - acromioclavicular joint (ligament) — see Sprain, acromioclavicular joint
  - blade — see Sprain, shoulder, girdle, specified site NEC
  - coracoclavicular joint (ligament) — see Sprain, coracoclavicular joint
  - coracohumeral ligament — see Sprain, coracohumeral joint
  - girdle S43.9- ☑
    - specified site NEC S43.8- ☑
  - rotator cuff — see Sprain, rotator cuff
  - specified site NEC S43.49- ☑
  - sternoclavicular joint (ligament) — see Sprain, sternoclavicular joint
- spine
  - cervical S13.4 ☑
  - lumbar S33.5 ☑
  - thoracic S23.3 ☑
- sternoclavicular joint S43.6- ☑
- sternum S23.429 ☑
  - chondrosternal joint S23.421 ☑
  - specified site NEC S23.428 ☑
  - sternoclavicular (joint) (ligament) S23.420 ☑
- symphysis
  - jaw S03.4- ☑
    - old M26.69
  - mandibular S03.4- ☑
    - old M26.69
- talofibular — see Sprain, ankle
- tarsal — see Sprain, foot, specified site NEC
- tarsometatarsal — see Sprain, foot, specified site NEC
- temporomandibular S03.4- ☑
  - old M26.69
- thorax S23.9 ☑
  - ribs S23.41 ☑
  - specified site NEC S23.8 ☑
  - spine S23.3 ☑
  - sternum — see Sprain, sternum
- thumb S63.60- ☑
  - interphalangeal (joint) S63.62- ☑
  - metacarpophalangeal (joint) S63.64- ☑
  - specified site NEC S63.68- ☑
- thyroid cartilage or region S13.5 ☑
- tibia (proximal end) — see Sprain, knee, specified site NEC
- tibial collateral, knee — see Sprain, knee, collateral
- tibiofibular
  - distal — see Sprain, ankle
  - superior — see Sprain, knee, specified site NEC
- toe(s) S93.50- ☑
  - great S93.50- ☑
  - interphalangeal joint S93.51- ☑
    - great S93.51- ☑
    - lesser S93.51- ☑
  - lesser S93.50- ☑
  - metatarsophalangeal joint S93.52- ☑
    - great S93.52- ☑
    - lesser S93.52- ☑
- ulna, collateral — see Rupture, traumatic, ligament, ulnar collateral
- ulnohumeral — see Sprain, elbow
- wrist S63.50- ☑
  - carpal S63.51- ☑

Sprain — continued
- wrist — continued
  - radiocarpal S63.52- ☑
  - specified site NEC S63.59- ☑
- xiphoid cartilage — see Sprain, sternum

Sprengel's deformity (congenital) Q74.0
Sprue (tropical) K90.1
- celiac K90.0
- idiopathic K90.49
- meaning thrush B37.0
- nontropical K90.0
Spur, bone — see also Enthesopathy
- calcaneal M77.3- ☑
- iliac crest M76.2- ☑
- nose (septum) J34.89
Spurway's syndrome Q78.0
Sputum
- abnormal (amount) (color) (odor) (purulent) R09.3
- blood-stained R04.2
- excessive (cause unknown) R09.3
Squamous — see also condition
- epithelium in
  - cervical canal (congenital) Q51.828
  - uterine mucosa (congenital) Q51.818
Squashed nose M95.0
- congenital Q67.4
Squeeze, diver's T70.3 ☑
Squint — see also Strabismus
- accommodative — see Strabismus, convergent concomitant
SSADHD (succinic semialdehyde dehydrogenase deficiency) E72.81
St. Hubert's disease A82.9
Stab — see also Laceration
- internal organs — see Injury, by site
Stafne's cyst or cavity M27.0
Staggering gait R26.0
- hysterical F44.4
Staghorn calculus — see Calculus, kidney
Stähli's line (cornea) (pigment) — see Pigmentation, cornea, anterior
Stain, staining
- meconium (newborn) P96.83
- port wine Q82.5
- tooth, teeth (hard tissues) (extrinsic) K03.6
  - due to
    - accretions K03.6
    - deposits (betel) (black) (green) (materia alba) (orange) (soft) (tobacco) K03.6
    - metals (copper) (silver) K03.7
    - nicotine K03.6
    - pulpal bleeding K03.7
    - tobacco K03.6
  - intrinsic K00.8
Stammering — see also Disorder, fluency F80.81
Standstill
- auricular I45.5
- cardiac — see Arrest, cardiac
- sinoatrial I45.5
- ventricular — see Arrest, cardiac
Stannosis J63.5
Stanton's disease — see Melioidosis
Staphylitis (acute) (catarrhal) (chronic) (gangrenous) (membranous) (suppurative) (ulcerative) K12.2
Staphylococcal scalded skin syndrome L00
Staphylococcemia A41.2
Staphylococcus, staphylococcal — see also condition
- as cause of disease classified elsewhere B95.8
  - aureus (methicillin susceptible) (MSSA) B95.61
    - methicillin resistant (MRSA) B95.62
  - specified NEC, as cause of disease classified elsewhere B95.7
Staphyloma (sclera)
- cornea H18.72- ☑
- equatorial H15.81- ☑
- localized (anterior) H15.82- ☑
- posticum H15.83- ☑
- ring H15.85- ☑
Stargardt's disease — see Dystrophy, retina
Starvation (inanition) (due to lack of food) T73.0 ☑
- edema — see Malnutrition, severe
Stasis
- bile (noncalculous) K83.1
- bronchus J98.09
  - with infection — see Bronchitis
- cardiac — see Failure, heart, congestive
- cecum K59.89

Stasis — continued
- colon K59.89
- dermatitis I87.2
  - with
    - varicose ulcer — see Varix, leg, with ulcer, with inflammation
    - varicose veins — see Varix, leg, with, inflammation
  - due to postthrombotic syndrome — see Syndrome, postthrombotic
- duodenal K31.5
- eczema — see Varix, leg, with, inflammation
- edema — see Hypertension, venous (chronic), idiopathic
- foot T69.0- ☑
- ileocecal coil K59.89
- ileum K59.89
- intestinal K59.89
- jejunum K59.89
- kidney N19
- liver (cirrhotic) K76.1
- lymphatic I89.8
- pneumonia J18.2
- pulmonary — see Edema, lung
- rectal K59.89
- renal N19
  - tubular N17.0
- ulcer — see Varix, leg, with, ulcer
  - without varicose veins I87.2
- urine — see Retention, urine
- venous I87.8
State (of)
- affective and paranoid, mixed, organic psychotic F06.8
- agitated R45.1
  - acute reaction to stress F43.0
- anxiety (neurotic) F41.1
- apprehension F41.1
- burn-out Z73.0
- climacteric, female Z78.0
  - symptomatic N95.1
- compulsive F42.8
  - mixed with obsessional thoughts F42.2
- confusional (psychogenic) F44.89
  - acute — see also Delirium
    - with
      - arteriosclerotic dementia — see also Dementia, vascular F01.50
        - with behavioral disturbance — see Dementia, vascular
      - senility or dementia F05
    - alcoholic F10.231
  - epileptic F05
  - reactive (from emotional stress, psychological trauma) F44.89
  - subacute — see Delirium
- convulsive — see Convulsions
- crisis F43.0
- depressive F32.A
  - neurotic F34.1
- dissociative F44.9
- emotional shock (stress) R45.7
- hypercoagulation — see Hypercoagulable
- locked-in G83.5
- menopausal Z78.0
  - symptomatic N95.1
- neurotic F48.9
  - with depersonalization F48.1
- obsessional F42.8
- oneiroid (schizophrenia-like) F23
- organic
  - hallucinatory (nonalcoholic) F06.0
  - paranoid (-hallucinatory) F06.2
- panic F41.0
- paranoid F22
  - climacteric F22
  - involutional F22
  - menopausal F22
  - organic F06.2
  - senile F03 ☑
  - simple F22
- persistent vegetative R40.3
- phobic F40.9
- postleukotomy F07.0
- pregnant
  - gestational carrier Z33.3
  - incidental Z33.1
- psychogenic, twilight F44.89
- psychopathic (constitutional) F60.2

State — *continued*
- psychotic, organic — *see also* Psychosis, organic
  - mixed paranoid and affective F06.8
  - senile or presenile F03 ☑
  - transient NEC F06.8
    - with
      - depression F06.31
      - hallucinations F06.0
- residual schizophrenic F20.5
- restlessness R45.1
- stress (emotional) R45.7
- tension (mental) F48.9
  - specified NEC F48.8
- transient organic psychotic NEC F06.8
  - depressive type F06.31
  - hallucinatory type F06.0
- twilight
  - epileptic F05
  - psychogenic F44.89
- vegetative, persistent R40.3
- vital exhaustion Z73.0
- withdrawal, — *see* Withdrawal, state

Status (post) — *see also* Presence (of)
- absence, epileptic — *see* Epilepsy, by type, with status epilepticus
- administration of tPA (rtPA) in a different facility within the last 24 hours prior to admission to current facility Z92.82
- adrenalectomy (unilateral) (bilateral) E89.6
- anastomosis Z98.0
- anginosus I20.9
- angioplasty (peripheral) Z98.62
  - with implant Z95.820
  - coronary artery Z98.61
    - with implant Z95.5
- aortocoronary bypass Z95.1
- arthrodesis Z98.1
- artificial opening (of) Z93.9
  - gastrointestinal tract Z93.4
  - specified NEC Z93.8
  - urinary tract Z93.6
  - vagina Z93.8
- asthmaticus — *see* Asthma, by type, with status asthmaticus
- awaiting organ transplant Z76.82
- bariatric surgery Z98.84
- bed confinement Z74.01
- bleb, filtering (vitreous), after glaucoma surgery Z98.83
- breast implant Z98.82
  - removal Z98.86
- cataract extraction Z98.4- ☑
- cholecystectomy Z90.49
- clitorectomy N90.811
  - with excision of labia minora N90.812
- colectomy (complete) (partial) Z90.49
- colonization — *see* Carrier (suspected) of
- colostomy Z93.3
- convulsivus idiopathicus — *see* Epilepsy, by type, with status epilepticus
- coronary artery angioplasty — *see* Status, angioplasty, coronary artery
- coronary artery bypass graft Z95.1
- cystectomy (urinary bladder) Z90.6
- cystostomy Z93.50
  - appendico-vesicostomy Z93.52
  - cutaneous Z93.51
  - specified NEC Z93.59
- delinquent immunization Z28.39
  - COVID-19 Z28.31- ☑
- dental Z98.818
  - crown Z98.811
  - fillings Z98.811
  - restoration Z98.811
  - sealant Z98.810
  - specified NEC Z98.818
- deployment (current) (military) Z56.82
- dialysis (hemodialysis) (peritoneal) Z99.2
- do not resuscitate (DNR) Z66
- donor — *see* Donor
- embedded fragments — *see* Retained, foreign body fragments (type of)
- embedded splinter — *see* Retained, foreign body fragments (type of)
- enterostomy Z93.4
- epileptic, epilepticus — *see also* Epilepsy, by type, with status epilepticus G40.901
- estrogen receptor
  - negative Z17.1

Status — *continued*
- estrogen receptor — *continued*
  - positive Z17.0
- female genital cutting — *see* Female genital mutilation status
- female genital mutilation — *see* Female genital mutilation status
- filtering (vitreous) bleb after glaucoma surgery Z98.83
- gastrectomy (complete) (partial) Z90.3
- gastric banding Z98.84
- gastric bypass for obesity Z98.84
- gastrostomy Z93.1
- human immunodeficiency virus (HIV) infection, asymptomatic Z21
- hysterectomy (complete) (total) Z90.710
  - partial (with remaining cervial stump) Z90.711
- ileostomy Z93.2
- implant
  - breast Z98.82
- infibulation N90.813
- intestinal bypass Z98.0
- jejunostomy Z93.4
- lapsed immunization schedule Z28.39
- laryngectomy Z90.02
- lymphaticus E32.8
- malignancy
  - castrate resistant prostate Z19.2
  - hormone resistant Z19.2
  - hormone sensitive Z19.1
- marmoratus G80.3
- mastectomy (unilateral) (bilateral) Z90.1- ☑
- military deployment status (current) Z56.82
  - in theater or in support of military war, peacekeeping and humanitarian operations Z56.82
- nephrectomy (unilateral) (bilateral) Z90.5
- nephrostomy Z93.6
- obesity surgery Z98.84
- oophorectomy
  - bilateral Z90.722
  - unilateral Z90.721
- organ replacement
  - by artificial or mechanical device or prosthesis of
    - artery Z95.828
    - bladder Z96.0
    - blood vessel Z95.828
    - breast Z97.8
    - eye globe Z97.0
    - heart Z95.812
      - valve Z95.2
    - intestine Z97.8
    - joint Z96.60
      - hip — *see* Presence, hip joint implant
      - knee — *see* Presence, knee joint implant
      - specified site NEC Z96.698
    - kidney Z97.8
    - larynx Z96.3
    - lens Z96.1
    - limbs — *see* Presence, artificial, limb
    - liver Z97.8
    - lung Z97.8
    - pancreas Z97.8
  - by organ transplant (heterologous) (homologous) — *see* Transplant
- pacemaker
  - brain Z96.89
  - cardiac Z95.0
  - specified NEC Z96.89
- pancreatectomy Z90.410
  - complete Z90.410
  - partial Z90.411
  - total Z90.410
- physical restraint Z78.1
- pneumonectomy (complete) (partial) Z90.2
- pneumothorax, therapeutic Z98.3
- postcommotio cerebri F07.81
- postoperative (postprocedural) NEC Z98.890
  - breast implant Z98.82
  - dental Z98.818
    - crown Z98.811
    - fillings Z98.811
    - restoration Z98.811
    - sealant Z98.810
    - specified NEC Z98.818
  - pneumothorax, therapeutic Z98.3
  - uterine scar Z98.891
- postpartum (routine follow-up) Z39.2
  - care immediately after delivery Z39.0
- postsurgical (postprocedural) NEC Z98.890
  - pneumothorax, therapeutic Z98.3

Status — *continued*
- pregnancy, incidental Z33.1
- prosthesis coronary angioplasty Z95.5
- pseudophakia Z96.1
- renal dialysis (hemodialysis) (peritoneal) Z99.2
- retained foreign body — *see* Retained, foreign body fragments (type of)
- reversed jejunal transposition (for bypass) Z98.0
- salpingo-oophorectomy
  - bilateral Z90.722
  - unilateral Z90.721
- sex reassignment surgery status Z87.890
- shunt
  - arteriovenous (for dialysis) Z99.2
  - cerebrospinal fluid Z98.2
  - ventricular (communicating) (for drainage) Z98.2
- splenectomy Z90.81
- thymicolymphaticus E32.8
- thymicus E32.8
- thymolymphaticus E32.8
- thyroidectomy (hypothyroidism) E89.0
- tooth (teeth) extraction — *see also* Absence, teeth, acquired K08.409
- tPA (rtPA) administration in a different facility within the last 24 hours prior to admission to current facility Z92.82
- tracheostomy Z93.0
- transplant — *see* Transplant
  - organ removed Z98.85
- tubal ligation Z98.51
- underimmunization Z28.39
  - COVID-19 Z28.31- ☑
    - partially vaccinated (for) Z28.311
    - unvaccinated (for) Z28.310
- ureterostomy Z93.6
- urethrostomy Z93.6
- vagina, artificial Z93.8
- vasectomy Z98.52
- wheelchair confinement Z99.3

Stealing
- child problem F91.8
  - in company with others Z72.810
- pathological (compulsive) F63.2

Steam burn — *see* Burn

Steatocystoma multiplex L72.2

Steatohepatitis (nonalcoholic) (NASH) K75.81

Steatoma L72.3
- eyelid (cystic) — *see* Dermatosis, eyelid
  - infected — *see* Hordeolum

Steatorrhea (chronic) K90.9
- with lacteal obstruction K90.2
- idiopathic (adult) (infantile) K90.9
- pancreatic K90.3
- primary K90.0
- tropical K90.1

Steatosis E88.89
- heart — *see* Degeneration, myocardial
- kidney N28.89
- liver NEC K76.0

Steele-Richardson-Olszewski disease or syndrome G23.1

Steinbrocker's syndrome G90.8

Steinert's disease G71.11

Stein-Leventhal syndrome E28.2

Stein's syndrome E28.2

STEMI — *see also* Infarct, myocardium, ST elevation I21.3

Stenocardia I20.8

Stenocephaly Q75.8

Stenosis, stenotic (cicatricial) — *see also* Stricture
- ampulla of Vater K83.1
- anus, anal (canal) (sphincter) K62.4
  - and rectum K62.4
  - congenital Q42.3
    - with fistula Q42.2
- aorta (ascending) (supraventricular) (congenital) Q25.1
  - arteriosclerotic I70.0
  - calcified I70.0
  - supravalvular Q25.3
- aortic (valve) I35.0
  - with insufficiency I35.2
  - congenital Q23.0
  - rheumatic I06.0
    - with
      - incompetency, insufficiency or regurgitation I06.2
        - with mitral (valve) disease I08.0
          - with tricuspid (valve) disease I08.3
      - mitral (valve) disease I08.0

Stenosis, stenotic — *continued*
  aortic — *continued*
    rheumatic — *continued*
      with — *continued*
        mitral disease — *continued*
          with tricuspid (valve) disease I08.3
        tricuspid (valve) disease I08.2
          with mitral (valve) disease I08.3
    specified cause NEC I35.0
    syphilitic A52.03
  aqueduct of Sylvius (congenital) Q03.0
    with spina bifida — *see* Spina bifida, by site, with
      hydrocephalus
    acquired G91.1
  artery NEC — *see also* Arteriosclerosis I77.1
    celiac I77.4
    cerebral — *see* Occlusion, artery, cerebral
    extremities — *see* Arteriosclerosis, extremities
    precerebral — *see* Occlusion, artery, precerebral
    pulmonary (congenital) Q25.6
      acquired I28.8
    renal I70.1
    stent
      coronary T82.855 ☑
      peripheral T82.856 ☑
  bile duct (common) (hepatic) K83.1
    congenital Q44.3
  bladder-neck (acquired) N32.0
    congenital Q64.31
  brain G93.89
  bronchus J98.09
    congenital Q32.3
    syphilitic A52.72
  cardia (stomach) K22.2
    congenital Q39.3
  cardiovascular — *see* Disease, cardiovascular
  caudal M48.08
  cervix, cervical (canal) N88.2
    congenital Q51.828
    in pregnancy or childbirth — *see* Pregnancy, com-
      plicated by, abnormal cervix
  colon — *see also* Obstruction, intestine
    congenital Q42.9
      specified NEC Q42.8
  colostomy K94.03
  common (bile) duct K83.1
    congenital Q44.3
  coronary (artery) — *see* Disease, heart, ischemic,
    atherosclerotic
  cystic duct — *see* Obstruction, gallbladder
  due to presence of device, implant or graft — *see also*
    Complications, by site and type, specified NEC
    T85.858 ☑
    arterial graft NEC T82.858 ☑
    breast (implant) T85.858 ☑
    catheter T85.858 ☑
      dialysis (renal) T82.858 ☑
        intraperitoneal T85.858 ☑
      infusion NEC T82.858 ☑
        spinal (epidural) (subdural) T85.850 ☑
      urinary (indwelling) T83.85 ☑
    fixation, internal (orthopedic) NEC T84.85 ☑
    gastrointestinal (bile duct) (esophagus) T85.858 ☑
    genital NEC T83.85 ☑
    heart NEC T82.857 ☑
    joint prosthesis T84.85 ☑
    ocular (corneal graft) (orbital implant) NEC
      T85.858 ☑
    orthopedic NEC T84.85 ☑
    specified NEC T85.858 ☑
    urinary NEC T83.85 ☑
    vascular NEC T82.858 ☑
    ventricular intracranial shunt T85.850 ☑
  duodenum K31.5
    congenital Q41.0
  ejaculatory duct NEC N50.89
    stent
      vascular
        end stent
          adjacent to stent — *see* Arteriosclerosis
          within the stent
            coronary T82.855 ☑
            peripheral T82.856 ☑
        in stent
          coronary vessel T82.855 ☑
          peripheral vessel T82.856 ☑
  endocervical os — *see* Stenosis, cervix

Stenosis, stenotic — *continued*
  enterostomy K94.13
  esophagus K22.2
    congenital Q39.3
    syphilitic A52.79
      congenital A50.59 *[K23]*
  eustachian tube — *see* Obstruction, eustachian tube
  external ear canal (acquired) H61.30- ☑
    congenital Q16.1
    due to
      inflammation H61.32- ☑
      trauma H61.31- ☑
    postprocedural H95.81- ☑
    specified cause NEC H61.39- ☑
  gallbladder — *see* Obstruction, gallbladder
  glottis J38.6
  heart valve — *see also* Endocarditis I38
    aortic — *see* Stenosis, aortic
    congenital Q24.8
    mitral — *see* Stenosis, mitral
    pulmonary — *see* Stenosis, pulmonary valve
    tricuspid — *see* Stenosis, tricuspid
  hepatic duct K83.1
  hymen N89.6
  hypertrophic subaortic (idiopathic) I42.1
  ileum — *see also* Obstruction, intestine, specified NEC
    K56.699
    congenital Q41.2
  infundibulum cardia Q24.3
  intervertebral foramina — *see also* Lesion, biomechan-
    ical, specified NEC
    connective tissue M99.79
      abdomen M99.79
      cervical region M99.71
      cervicothoracic M99.71
      head region M99.70
      lumbar region M99.73
      lumbosacral M99.73
      occipitocervical M99.70
      sacral region M99.74
      sacrococcygeal M99.74
      sacroiliac M99.74
      specified NEC M99.79
      thoracic region M99.72
      thoracolumbar M99.72
    disc M99.79
      abdomen M99.79
      cervical region M99.71
      cervicothoracic M99.71
      head region M99.70
      lower extremity M99.76
      lumbar region M99.73
      lumbosacral M99.73
      occipitocervical M99.70
      pelvic M99.75
      rib cage M99.78
      sacral region M99.74
      sacrococcygeal M99.74
      sacroiliac M99.74
      specified NEC M99.79
      thoracic region M99.72
      thoracolumbar M99.72
      upper extremity M99.77
    osseous M99.69
      abdomen M99.69
      cervical region M99.61
      cervicothoracic M99.61
      head region M99.60
      lower extremity M99.66
      lumbar region M99.63
      lumbosacral M99.63
      occipitocervical M99.60
      pelvic M99.65
      rib cage M99.68
      sacral region M99.64
      sacrococcygeal M99.64
      sacroiliac M99.64
      specified NEC M99.69
      thoracic region M99.62
      thoracolumbar M99.62
      upper extremity M99.67
    subluxation — *see* Stenosis, intervertebral foramina,
      osseous
  intestine — *see also* Obstruction, intestine
    congenital (small) Q41.9
      large Q42.9
        specified NEC Q42.8
      specified NEC Q41.8

Stenosis, stenotic — *continued*
  jejunum — *see also* Obstruction, intestine, specified
    NEC K56.699
    congenital Q41.1
  lacrimal (passage)
    canaliculi H04.54- ☑
    congenital Q10.5
    duct H04.55- ☑
    punctum H04.56- ☑
    sac H04.57- ☑
  lacrimonasal duct — *see* Stenosis, lacrimal, duct
    congenital Q10.5
  larynx J38.6
    congenital NEC Q31.8
      subglottic Q31.1
    syphilitic A52.73
      congenital A50.59 *[J99]*
  mitral (chronic) (inactive) (valve) I05.0
    with
      aortic valve disease I08.0
      incompetency, insufficiency or regurgitation
        I05.2
    active or acute I01.1
      with rheumatic or Sydenham's chorea I02.0
    congenital Q23.2
    specified cause, except rheumatic I34.2
    syphilitic A52.03
  myocardium, myocardial — *see also* Degeneration,
    myocardial
    hypertrophic subaortic (idiopathic) I42.1
  nares (anterior) (posterior) J34.89
    congenital Q30.0
  nasal duct — *see also* Stenosis, lacrimal, duct
    congenital Q10.5
  nasolacrimal duct — *see also* Stenosis, lacrimal, duct
    congenital Q10.5
  neural canal — *see also* Lesion, biomechanical, speci-
    fied NEC
    connective tissue M99.49
      abdomen M99.49
      cervical region M99.41
      cervicothoracic M99.41
      head region M99.40
      lower extremity M99.46
      lumbar region M99.43
      lumbosacral M99.43
      occipitocervical M99.40
      pelvic M99.45
      rib cage M99.48
      sacral region M99.44
      sacrococcygeal M99.44
      sacroiliac M99.44
      specified NEC M99.49
      thoracic region M99.42
      thoracolumbar M99.42
      upper extremity M99.47
    intervertebral disc M99.59
      abdomen M99.59
      cervical region M99.51
      cervicothoracic M99.51
      head region M99.50
      lower extremity M99.56
      lumbar region M99.53
      lumbosacral M99.53
      occipitocervical M99.50
      pelvic M99.55
      rib cage M99.58
      sacral region M99.54
      sacrococcygeal M99.54
      sacroiliac M99.54
      specified NEC M99.59
      thoracic region M99.52
      thoracolumbar M99.52
      upper extremity M99.57
    osseous M99.39
      abdomen M99.39
      cervical region M99.31
      cervicothoracic M99.31
      head region M99.30
      lower extremity M99.36
      lumbar region M99.33
      lumbosacral M99.33
      occipitocervical M99.30
      pelvic M99.35
      rib cage M99.38
      sacral region M99.34
      sacrococcygeal M99.34
      sacroiliac M99.34

Stenosis, stenotic — *continued*
  neural canal — *see also* Lesion, biomechanical, specified — *continued*
    osseous — *continued*
      specified NEC M99.39
      thoracic region M99.32
      thoracolumbar M99.32
      upper extremity M99.37
    subluxation M99.29
      cervical region M99.21
      cervicothoracic M99.21
      head region M99.20
      lower extremity M99.26
      lumbar region M99.23
      lumbosacral M99.23
      occipitocervical M99.20
      pelvic M99.25
      rib cage M99.28
      sacral region M99.24
      sacrococcygeal M99.24
      sacroiliac M99.24
      specified NEC M99.29
      thoracic region M99.22
      thoracolumbar M99.22
      upper extremity M99.27
  organ or site, congenital NEC — *see* Atresia, by site
  papilla of Vater K83.1
  pulmonary (artery) (congenital) Q25.6
    with ventricular septal defect, transposition of aorta, and hypertrophy of right ventricle Q21.3
    acquired I28.8
    in tetralogy of Fallot Q21.3
    infundibular Q24.3
    subvalvular Q24.3
    supravalvular Q25.6
    valve I37.0
      with insufficiency I37.2
      congenital Q22.1
      rheumatic I09.89
        with aortic, mitral or tricuspid (valve) disease I08.8
    vein, acquired I28.8
    vessel NEC I28.8
  pulmonic (congenital) Q22.1
    infundibular Q24.3
    subvalvular Q24.3
  pylorus (hypertrophic) (acquired) K31.1
    adult K31.1
    congenital Q40.0
    infantile Q40.0
  rectum (sphincter) — *see* Stricture, rectum
  renal artery I70.1
    congenital Q27.1
  salivary duct (any) K11.8
  sphincter of Oddi K83.1
  spinal M48.00
    cervical region M48.02
    cervicothoracic region M48.03
    lumbar region (NOS) (without neurogenic claudication) M48.061
      with neurogenic claudication M48.062
    lumbosacral region M48.07
    occipito-atlanto-axial region M48.01
    sacrococcygeal region M48.08
    thoracic region M48.04
    thoracolumbar region M48.05
  stomach, hourglass K31.2
  subaortic (congenital) Q24.4
    hypertrophic (idiopathic) I42.1
  subglottic J38.6
    congenital Q31.1
    postprocedural J95.5
  trachea J39.8
    congenital Q32.1
    syphilitic A52.73
    tuberculous NEC A15.5
  tracheostomy J95.03
  tricuspid (valve) I07.0
    with
      aortic (valve) disease I08.2
      incompetency, insufficiency or regurgitation I07.2
        with aortic (valve) disease I08.2
          with mitral (valve) disease I08.3
      mitral (valve) disease I08.1
        with aortic (valve) disease I08.3
    congenital Q22.4
    nonrheumatic I36.0
      with insufficiency I36.2

Stenosis, stenotic — *continued*
  tubal N97.1
  ureter — *see* Atresia, ureter
  ureteropelvic junction, congenital Q62.11
  ureterovesical orifice, congenital Q62.12
  urethra (valve) *see also* Stricture, urethra
    congenital Q64.32
  urinary meatus, congenital Q64.33
  vagina N89.5
    congenital Q52.4
    in pregnancy — *see* Pregnancy, complicated by, abnormal vagina
      causing obstructed labor O65.5
  valve (cardiac) (heart) — *see also* Endocarditis I38
    congenital Q24.8
      aortic Q23.0
      mitral Q23.2
      pulmonary Q22.1
      tricuspid Q22.4
  vena cava (inferior) (superior) I87.1
    congenital Q26.0
  vesicourethral orifice Q64.31
  vulva N90.5
Stent jail T82.897 ☑
Stercolith (impaction) K56.41
  appendix K38.1
Stercoraceous, stercoral ulcer K63.3
  anus or rectum K62.6
Stereotypies NEC F98.4
Sterility — *see* Infertility
Sterilization — *see* Encounter (for), sterilization
Sternalgia — *see* Angina
Sternopagus Q89.4
Sternum bifidum Q76.7
Steroid
  effects (adverse) (adrenocortical) (iatrogenic)
    cushingoid E24.2
      correct substance properly administered — *see* Table of Drugs and Chemicals, by drug, adverse effect
      overdose or wrong substance given or taken — *see* Table of Drugs and Chemicals, by drug, poisoning
    diabetes — *see* subcategory E09 ☑
      correct substance properly administered — *see* Table of Drugs and Chemicals, by drug, adverse effect
      overdose or wrong substance given or taken — *see* Table of Drugs and Chemicals, by drug, poisoning
    fever R50.2
    insufficiency E27.3
      correct substance properly administered — *see* Table of Drugs and Chemicals, by drug, adverse effect
      overdose or wrong substance given or taken — *see* Table of Drugs and Chemicals, by drug, poisoning
  responder H40.04- ☑
Stevens-Johnson disease or syndrome L51.1
  toxic epidermal necrolysis overlap L51.3
Stewart-Morel syndrome M85.2
Sticker's disease B08.3
Sticky eye — *see* Conjunctivitis, acute, mucopurulent
Stieda's disease — *see* Bursitis, tibial collateral
Stiff neck — *see* Torticollis
Stiff-man syndrome G25.82
Stiffness, joint NEC M25.60
  ankle M25.67- ☑
  ankylosis — *see* Ankylosis, joint
  contracture — *see* Contraction, joint
  elbow M25.62- ☑
  foot M25.67- ☑
  hand M25.64- ☑
  hip M25.65- ☑
  knee M25.66- ☑
  shoulder M25.61- ☑
  specified site NEC M25.69
  wrist M25.63- ☑
Stigmata congenital syphilis A50.59
Stillbirth P95
Still-Felty syndrome — *see* Felty's syndrome
Still's disease or syndrome (juvenile) M08.20
  adult-onset M06.1
  ankle M08.27- ☑
  elbow M08.22- ☑
  foot joint M08.27- ☑

Still's disease or syndrome — *continued*
  hand joint M08.24- ☑
  hip M08.25- ☑
  knee M08.26- ☑
  multiple site M08.29
  shoulder M08.21- ☑
  specified site NEC M08.2A
  vertebra M08.28
  wrist M08.23- ☑
Stimulation, ovary E28.1
Sting (venomous) (with allergic or anaphylactic shock) — *see* Table of Drugs and Chemicals, by animal or substance, poisoning
Stippled epiphyses Q78.8
Stitch
  abscess T81.41 ☑
  burst (in operation wound) — *see* Disruption, wound, operation
Stokes' disease E05.00
  with thyroid storm E05.01
Stokes-Adams disease or syndrome I45.9
Stokvis (-Talma) **disease** D74.8
Stoma malfunction
  colostomy K94.03
  enterostomy K94.13
  gastrostomy K94.23
  ileostomy K94.13
  tracheostomy J95.03
Stomach — *see* condition
Stomatitis (denture) (ulcerative) K12.1
  angular K13.0
    due to dietary or vitamin deficiency E53.0
  aphthous K12.0
  bovine B08.61
  candidal B37.0
  catarrhal K12.1
  diphtheritic A36.89
  due to
    dietary deficiency E53.0
    thrush B37.0
    vitamin deficiency
      B group NEC E53.9
      B2 (riboflavin) E53.0
  epidemic B08.8
  epizootic B08.8
  follicular K12.1
  gangrenous A69.0
  Geotrichum B48.3
  herpesviral, herpetic B00.2
  herpetiformis K12.0
  malignant K12.1
  membranous acute K12.1
  monilial B37.0
  mycotic B37.0
  necrotizing ulcerative A69.0
  parasitic B37.0
  septic K12.1
  spirochetal A69.1
  suppurative (acute) K12.2
  ulceromembranous A69.1
  vesicular K12.1
    with exanthem (enteroviral) B08.4
    virus disease A93.8
  Vincent's A69.1
Stomatocytosis D58.8
Stomatomycosis B37.0
Stomatorrhagia K13.79
Stone(s) — *see also* Calculus
  bladder (diverticulum) N21.0
  cystine E72.09
  heart syndrome I50.1
  kidney N20.0
  prostate N42.0
  pulpal (dental) K04.2
  renal N20.0
  salivary gland or duct (any) K11.5
  urethra (impacted) N21.1
  urinary (duct) (impacted) (passage) N20.9
    bladder (diverticulum) N21.0
    lower tract N21.9
    specified NEC N21.8
  xanthine E79.8 *[N22]*
Stonecutter's lung J62.8
Stonemason's asthma, disease, lung or pneumoconiosis J62.8
Stoppage
  heart — *see* Arrest, cardiac
  urine — *see* Retention, urine

Storm, thyroid — see Thyrotoxicosis
Strabismus (congenital) (nonparalytic) H50.9
  concomitant H50.40
    convergent — see Strabismus, convergent concomitant
    divergent — see Strabismus, divergent concomitant
  convergent concomitant H50.00
    accommodative component H50.43
    alternating H50.05
      with
        A pattern H50.06
        specified nonconcomitances NEC H50.08
        V pattern H50.07
    monocular H50.01- ☑
      with
        A pattern H50.02- ☑
        specified nonconcomitances NEC H50.04- ☑
        V pattern H50.03- ☑
      intermittent H50.31- ☑
        alternating H50.32
  cyclotropia H50.41 ☑
  divergent concomitant H50.10
    alternating H50.15
      with
        A pattern H50.16
        specified noncomitances NEC H50.18
        V pattern H50.17
    monocular H50.11- ☑
      with
        A pattern H50.12- ☑
        specified noncomitances NEC H50.14- ☑
        V pattern H50.13- ☑
      intermittent H50.33 ☑
        alternating H50.34
  Duane's syndrome H50.81- ☑
  due to adhesions, scars H50.69
  heterophoria H50.50
    alternating H50.55
    cyclophoria H50.54
    esophoria H50.51
    exophoria H50.52
    vertical H50.53
  heterotropia H50.40
    intermittent H50.30
  hypertropia H50.2- ☑
  hypotropia — see Hypertropia
  latent H50.50
  mechanical H50.60
    Brown's sheath syndrome H50.61- ☑
    specified type NEC H50.69
  monofixation syndrome H50.42
  paralytic H49.9
    abducens nerve H49.2- ☑
    fourth nerve H49.1- ☑
    Kearns-Sayre syndrome H49.81- ☑
    ophthalmoplegia (external)
      progressive H49.4- ☑
        with pigmentary retinopathy H49.81- ☑
      total H49.3- ☑
    sixth nerve H49.2- ☑
    specified type NEC H49.88- ☑
    third nerve H49.0- ☑
    trochlear nerve H49.1- ☑
  specified type NEC H50.89
  vertical H50.2- ☑
Strain
  back S39.012 ☑
  cervical S16.1 ☑
  eye NEC — see Disturbance, vision, subjective
  heart — see Disease, heart
  low back S39.012 ☑
  mental NOS Z73.3
    work-related Z56.6
  muscle (tendon) — see Injury, muscle, by site, strain
  neck S16.1 ☑
  physical NOS Z73.3
    work-related Z56.6
  postural — see also Disorder, soft tissue, due to use
  psychological NEC Z73.3
  tendon — see Injury, muscle, by site, strain
Straining, on urination R39.16
Strand, vitreous — see Opacity, vitreous, membranes and strands
Strangulation, strangulated — see also Asphyxia, traumatic
  appendix K38.8
  bladder-neck N32.0

Strangulation, strangulated — continued
  bowel or colon K56.2
  food or foreign body — see Foreign body, by site
  hemorrhoids — see Hemorrhoids, with complication
  hernia — see also Hernia, by site, with obstruction
    with gangrene — see Hernia, by site, with gangrene
  intestine (large) (small) K56.2
    with hernia — see also Hernia, by site, with obstruction
      with gangrene — see Hernia, by site, with gangrene
  mesentery K56.2
  mucus — see Asphyxia, mucus
  omentum K56.2
  organ or site, congenital NEC — see Atresia, by site
  ovary — see Torsion, ovary
  penis N48.89
    foreign body T19.4 ☑
  rupture — see Hernia, by site, with obstruction
  stomach due to hernia — see also Hernia, by site, with obstruction
    with gangrene — see Hernia, by site, with gangrene
  vesicourethral orifice N32.0
Strangury R30.0
Straw itch B88.0
Strawberry
  gallbladder K82.4
  mark Q82.5
  tongue (red) (white) K14.3
Streak(s)
  macula, angioid H35.33
  ovarian Q50.32
Strephosymbolia F81.0
  secondary to organic lesion R48.8
Streptobacillary fever A25.1
Streptobacillosis A25.1
Streptobacillus moniliformis A25.1
Streptococcus, streptococcal — see also condition
  as cause of disease classified elsewhere B95.5
  group
    A, as cause of disease classified elsewhere B95.0
    B, as cause of disease classified elsewhere B95.1
    D, as cause of disease classified elsewhere B95.2
  pneumoniae, as cause of disease classified elsewhere B95.3
  specified NEC, as cause of disease classified elsewhere B95.4
Streptomycosis B47.1
Streptotrichosis A48.8
Stress F43.9
  family — see Disruption, family
  fetal P84
    complicating pregnancy O77.9
      due to drug administration O77.1
  mental NEC Z73.3
    work-related Z56.6
  physical NEC Z73.3
    work-related Z56.6
  polycythemia D75.1
  reaction — see also Reaction, stress F43.9
  work schedule Z56.3
Stretching, nerve — see Injury, nerve
Striae albicantes, atrophicae or distensae (cutis) L90.6
Stricture — see also Stenosis
  ampulla of Vater K83.1
  anus (sphincter) K62.4
    congenital Q42.3
      with fistula Q42.2
    infantile Q42.3
      with fistula Q42.2
  aorta (ascending) (congenital) Q25.1
    arteriosclerotic I70.0
    calcified I70.0
    supravalvular, congenital Q25.3
  aortic (valve) — see Stenosis, aortic
  aqueduct of Sylvius (congenital) Q03.0
    with spina bifida — see Spina bifida, by site, with hydrocephalus
    acquired G91.1
  artery I77.1
    basilar — see Occlusion, artery, basilar
    carotid — see Occlusion, artery, carotid
    celiac I77.4
    congenital (peripheral) Q27.8
      cerebral Q28.3
      coronary Q24.5
      digestive system Q27.8
      lower limb Q27.8

Stricture — continued
  artery — continued
    congenital — continued
      retinal Q14.1
      specified site NEC Q27.8
      umbilical Q27.0
      upper limb Q27.8
    coronary — see Disease, heart, ischemic, atherosclerotic
      congenital Q24.5
    precerebral — see Occlusion, artery, precerebral
    pulmonary (congenital) Q25.6
      acquired I28.8
    renal I70.1
    vertebral — see Occlusion, artery, vertebral
  auditory canal (external) (congenital)
    acquired — see Stenosis, external ear canal
  bile duct (common) (hepatic) K83.1
    congenital Q44.3
    postoperative K91.89
  bladder N32.89
    neck N32.0
  bowel — see Obstruction, intestine
  brain G93.89
  bronchus J98.09
    congenital Q32.3
    syphilitic A52.72
  cardia (stomach) K22.2
    congenital Q39.3
  cardiac — see also Disease, heart
    orifice (stomach) K22.2
  cecum — see Obstruction, intestine
  cervix, cervical (canal) N88.2
    congenital Q51.828
    in pregnancy — see Pregnancy, complicated by, abnormal cervix
      causing obstructed labor O65.5
  colon — see also Obstruction, intestine
    congenital Q42.9
      specified NEC Q42.8
  colostomy K94.03
  common (bile) duct K83.1
  coronary (artery) — see Disease, heart, ischemic, atherosclerotic
  cystic duct — see Obstruction, gallbladder
  digestive organs NEC, congenital Q45.8
  duodenum K31.5
    congenital Q41.0
  ear canal (external) (congenital) Q16.1
    acquired — see Stricture, auditory canal, acquired
  ejaculatory duct N50.89
  enterostomy K94.13
  esophagus K22.2
    congenital Q39.3
    syphilitic A52.79
      congenital A50.59 [K23]
  eustachian tube — see also Obstruction, eustachian tube
    congenital Q17.8
  fallopian tube N97.1
    gonococcal A54.24
    tuberculous A18.17
  gallbladder — see Obstruction, gallbladder
  glottis J38.6
  heart — see also Disease, heart
    valve — see also Endocarditis I38
      aortic Q23.0
      mitral Q23.2
      pulmonary Q22.1
      tricuspid Q22.4
  hepatic duct K83.1
  hourglass, of stomach K31.2
  hymen N89.6
  hypopharynx J39.2
  ileum — see also Obstruction, intestine, specified NEC K56.699
    congenital Q41.2
  intestine — see also Obstruction, intestine
    congenital (small) Q41.9
      large Q42.9
        specified NEC Q42.8
      specified NEC Q41.8
    ischemic K55.1
  jejunum — see also Obstruction, intestine, specified NEC K56.699
    congenital Q41.1
  lacrimal passages — see also Stenosis, lacrimal
    congenital Q10.5

Stricture — continued
  larynx J38.6
    congenital NEC Q31.8
      subglottic Q31.1
    syphilitic A52.73
      congenital A50.59 [J99]
  meatus
    ear (congenital) Q16.1
      acquired — see Stricture, auditory canal, acquired
    osseous (ear) (congenital) Q16.1
      acquired — see Stricture, auditory canal, acquired
    urinarius — see also Stricture, urethra
      congenital Q64.33
  mitral (valve) — see Stenosis, mitral
  myocardium, myocardial I51.5
    hypertrophic subaortic (idiopathic) I42.1
  nares (anterior) (posterior) J34.89
    congenital Q30.0
  nasal duct — see also Stenosis, lacrimal, duct
    congenital Q10.5
  nasolacrimal duct — see also Stenosis, lacrimal, duct
    congenital Q10.5
  nasopharynx J39.2
    syphilitic A52.73
  nose J34.89
    congenital Q30.0
  nostril (anterior) (posterior) J34.89
    congenital Q30.0
    syphilitic A52.73
      congenital A50.59 [J99]
  organ or site, congenital NEC — see Atresia, by site
  os uteri — see Stricture, cervix
  osseous meatus (ear) (congenital) Q16.1
    acquired — see Stricture, auditory canal, acquired
  oviduct — see Stricture, fallopian tube
  pelviureteric junction (congenital) Q62.11
    acquired, with hydronephrosis N13.0
  penis, by foreign body T19.4 ☑
  pharynx J39.2
  prostate N42.89
  pulmonary, pulmonic
    artery (congenital) Q25.6
      acquired I28.8
      noncongenital I28.8
    infundibulum (congenital) Q24.3
    valve I37.0
      congenital Q22.1
    vein, acquired I28.8
    vessel NEC I28.8
  punctum lacrimale — see also Stenosis, lacrimal, punctum
    congenital Q10.5
  pylorus (hypertrophic) K31.1
    adult K31.1
    congenital Q40.0
    infantile Q40.0
  rectosigmoid — see also Obstruction, intestine, specified NEC K56.699
  rectum (sphincter) K62.4
    congenital Q42.1
      with fistula Q42.0
    due to
      chlamydial lymphogranuloma A55
      irradiation K91.89
      lymphogranuloma venereum A55
    gonococcal A54.6
    inflammatory (chlamydial) A55
    syphilitic A52.74
    tuberculous A18.32
  renal artery I70.1
    congenital Q27.1
  salivary duct or gland (any) K11.8
  sigmoid (flexure) — see Obstruction, intestine
  spermatic cord N50.89
  stoma (following) (of)
    colostomy K94.03
    enterostomy K94.13
    gastrostomy K94.23
    ileostomy K94.13
    tracheostomy J95.03
  stomach K31.89
    congenital Q40.2
    hourglass K31.2
  subaortic Q24.4
    hypertrophic (acquired) (idiopathic) I42.1
  subglottic J38.6

Stricture — continued
  syphilitic NEC A52.79
  trachea J39.8
    congenital Q32.1
    syphilitic A52.73
    tuberculous NEC A15.5
  tracheostomy J95.03
  tricuspid (valve) — see Stenosis, tricuspid
  tunica vaginalis N50.89
  ureter (postoperative) N13.5
    with
      hydronephrosis N13.1
        with infection N13.6
      pyelonephritis (chronic) N11.1
    congenital — see Atresia, ureter
    tuberculous A18.11
  ureteropelvic junction (congenital) Q62.11
    acquired, with hydronephrosis N13.0
  ureterovesical orifice N13.5
    with infection N13.6
  urethra (organic) (spasmodic) — see also Stricture, urethra, male N35.919
    associated with schistosomiasis B65.0 [N37]
    congenital Q64.39
      valvular (posterior) Q64.2
    due to
      infection — see Stricture, urethra, postinfective
      trauma — see Stricture, urethra, post-traumatic
    female N35.92
    gonococcal, gonorrheal A54.01
    infective NEC — see Stricture, urethra, postinfective
    late effect (sequelae) of injury — see Stricture, urethra, post-traumatic
    male N35.919
      anterior urethra N35.914
      bulbous urethra N35.912
      meatal N35.911
      membranous urethra N35.913
      overlapping sites N35.916
    postcatheterization — see Stricture, urethra, postprocedural
    postinfective NEC
      female N35.12
      male N35.119
        anterior urethra N35.114
        bulbous urethra N35.112
        meatal N35.111
        membranous urethra N35.113
        overlapping sites N35.116
    postobstetric N35.021
    postoperative — see Stricture, urethra, postprocedural
    postprocedural
      female N99.12
      male N99.114
        anterior bulbous urethra N99.113
        bulbous urethra N99.111
        fossa navicularis N99.115
        meatal N99.110
        membranous urethra N99.112
        overlapping sites N99.116
    post-traumatic
      female N35.028
        due to childbirth N35.021
      male N35.014
        anterior urethra N35.013
        bulbous urethra N35.011
        meatal N35.010
        membranous urethra N35.012
        overlapping sites N35.016
    sequela (late effect) of
      childbirth N35.021
      injury — see Stricture, urethra, post-traumatic
    specified cause NEC
      female N35.82
      male N35.819
        anterior urethra N35.814
        bulbous urethra N35.812
        meatal N35.811
        membranous urethra N35.813
        overlapping sites N35.816
    syphilitic A52.76
    traumatic — see Stricture, urethra, post-traumatic
    valvular (posterior), congenital Q64.2
  urinary meatus — see Stricture, urethra
  uterus, uterine (synechiae) N85.6
    os (external) (internal) — see Stricture, cervix
  vagina (outlet) — see Stenosis, vagina

Stricture — continued
  valve (cardiac) (heart) — see also Endocarditis
    congenital
      aortic Q23.0
      mitral Q23.2
      pulmonary Q22.1
      tricuspid Q22.4
  vas deferens N50.89
    congenital Q55.4
  vein I87.1
  vena cava (inferior) (superior) NEC I87.1
    congenital Q26.0
  vesicourethral orifice N32.0
    congenital Q64.31
  vulva (acquired) N90.5
Stridor R06.1
  congenital (larynx) P28.89
Stridulous — see condition
Stroke (apoplectic) (brain) (embolic) (ischemic) (paralytic) (thrombotic) I63.9
  cerebral, perinatal P91.82- ☑
  cryptogenic — see also infarction, cerebral I63.9
  epileptic — see Epilepsy
  heat T67.01 ☑
    exertional T67.02 ☑
    specified NEC T67.09 ☑
  in evolution I63.9
  intraoperative
    during cardiac surgery I97.810
    during other surgery I97.811
  ischemic, perinatal arterial P91.82- ☑
  lightning — see Lightning
  meaning
    cerebral hemorrhage — code to Hemorrhage, intracranial
    cerebral infarction — code to Infarction, cerebral
  neonatal P91.82- ☑
  postprocedural
    following cardiac surgery I97.820
    following other surgery I97.821
  sun T67.01 ☑
    specified NEC T67.09 ☑
  unspecified (NOS) I63.9
Stromatosis, endometrial D39.0
Strongyloidiasis, strongyloidosis B78.9
  cutaneous B78.1
  disseminated B78.7
  intestinal B78.0
Strophulus pruriginosus L28.2
Struck by lightning — see Lightning
Struma — see also Goiter
  Hashimoto E06.3
  lymphomatosa E06.3
  nodosa (simplex) E04.9
    endemic E01.2
      multinodular E01.1
    multinodular E04.2
      iodine-deficiency related E01.1
    toxic or with hyperthyroidism E05.20
      with thyroid storm E05.21
      multinodular E05.20
        with thyroid storm E05.21
      uninodular E05.10
        with thyroid storm E05.11
    toxicosa E05.20
      with thyroid storm E05.21
      multinodular E05.20
        with thyroid storm E05.21
      uninodular E05.10
        with thyroid storm E05.11
    uninodular E04.1
  ovarii D27.- ☑
  Riedel's E06.5
Strumipriva cachexia E03.4
Strümpell-Marie spine — see Spondylitis, ankylosing
Strümpell-Westphal pseudosclerosis E83.01
Stuart deficiency disease (factor X) D68.2
Stuart-Prower factor deficiency (factor X) D68.2
Student's elbow — see Bursitis, elbow, olecranon
Stump — see Amputation
Stunting, nutritional E45
Stupor (catatonic) R40.1
  depressive (single episode) F32.89
    recurrent episode F33.8
  dissociative F44.2
  manic F30.2
  manic-depressive F31.89
  psychogenic (anergic) F44.2

☑ Additional Character Required — Refer to the Tabular List for Character Selection

Stupor — *continued*
   reaction to exceptional stress (transient) F43.0
Sturge (-Weber) (-Dimitri) (-Kalischer) **disease or syndrome** Q85.89
Stuttering F80.81
   adult onset F98.5
   childhood onset F80.81
   following cerebrovascular disease — *see* Disorder, fluency. following cerebrovascular disease
   in conditions classified elsewhere R47.82
Sty, stye (external) (internal) (meibomian) (zeisian) —
   see Hordeolum
Subacidity, gastric K31.89
   psychogenic F45.8
Subacute — *see* condition
Subarachnoid — *see* condition
Subcortical — *see* condition
Subcostal syndrome, nerve compression — *see*
   Mononeuropathy, upper limb, specified site NEC
Subcutaneous, subcuticular — *see* condition
Subdural — *see* condition
Subendocardium — *see* condition
Subependymoma
   specified site — *see* Neoplasm, uncertain behavior, by
      site
   unspecified site D43.2
Suberosis J67.3
Subglossitis — *see* Glossitis
Subhemophilia D66
Subinvolution
   breast (postlactational) (postpuerperal) N64.89
   puerperal O90.89
   uterus (chronic) (nonpuerperal) N85.3
      puerperal O90.89
Sublingual — *see* condition
Sublinguitis — *see* Sialoadenitis
Subluxatable hip Q65.6
Subluxation — *see also* Dislocation
   acromioclavicular S43.11- ☑
   ankle S93.0- ☑
   atlantoaxial, recurrent M43.4
      with myelopathy M43.3
   carpometacarpal (joint) NEC S63.05- ☑
      thumb S63.04- ☑
   complex, vertebral — *see* Complex, subluxation
   congenital — *see also* Malposition, congenital
      hip — *see* Dislocation, hip, congenital, partial
      joint (excluding hip)
         lower limb Q68.8
         shoulder Q68.8
         upper limb Q68.8
   elbow (traumatic) S53.10- ☑
      anterior S53.11- ☑
      lateral S53.14- ☑
      medial S53.13- ☑
      posterior S53.12- ☑
      specified type NEC S53.19- ☑
   finger S63.20- ☑
      index S63.20- ☑
      interphalangeal S63.22- ☑
         distal S63.24- ☑
            index S63.24- ☑
            little S63.24- ☑
            middle S63.24- ☑
            ring S63.24- ☑
         index S63.22- ☑
         little S63.22- ☑
         middle S63.22- ☑
         proximal S63.23- ☑
            index S63.23- ☑
            little S63.23- ☑
            middle S63.23- ☑
            ring S63.23- ☑
         ring S63.22- ☑
      little S63.20- ☑
      metacarpophalangeal S63.21- ☑
         index S63.21- ☑
         little S63.21- ☑
         middle S63.21- ☑
         ring S63.21- ☑
      middle S63.20- ☑
      ring S63.20- ☑
   foot S93.30- ☑
      specified site NEC S93.33- ☑
      tarsal joint S93.31- ☑
      tarsometatarsal joint S93.32- ☑

Subluxation — *continued*
   foot — *continued*
      toe — *see* Subluxation, toe
   hip S73.00- ☑
      anterior S73.03- ☑
         obturator S73.02- ☑
      central S73.04- ☑
      posterior S73.01- ☑
   interphalangeal (joint)
      finger S63.22- ☑
         distal joint S63.24- ☑
            index S63.24- ☑
            little S63.24- ☑
            middle S63.24- ☑
            ring S63.24- ☑
         index S63.22- ☑
         little S63.22- ☑
         middle S63.22- ☑
         proximal joint S63.23- ☑
            index S63.23- ☑
            little S63.23- ☑
            middle S63.23- ☑
            ring S63.23- ☑
         ring S63.22- ☑
      thumb S63.12- ☑
      toe S93.13- ☑
         great S93.13- ☑
         lesser S93.13- ☑
   joint prosthesis — *see* Complications, joint prosthesis,
      mechanical, displacement, by site
   knee S83.10- ☑
      cap — *see* Subluxation, patella
      patella — *see* Subluxation, patella
      proximal tibia
         anteriorly S83.11- ☑
         laterally S83.14- ☑
         medially S83.13- ☑
         posteriorly S83.12- ☑
      specified type NEC S83.19- ☑
   lens — *see* Dislocation, lens, partial
   ligament, traumatic — *see* Sprain, by site
   metacarpal (bone)
      proximal end S63.06- ☑
   metacarpophalangeal (joint)
      finger S63.21- ☑
         index S63.21- ☑
         little S63.21- ☑
         middle S63.21- ☑
         ring S63.21- ☑
      thumb S63.11- ☑
   metatarsophalangeal joint S93.14- ☑
      great toe S93.14- ☑
      lesser toe S93.14- ☑
   midcarpal (joint) S63.03- ☑
   patella S83.00- ☑
      lateral S83.01- ☑
      recurrent (nontraumatic) — *see* Dislocation, patella,
         recurrent, incomplete
      specified type NEC S83.09- ☑
   pathological — *see* Dislocation, pathological
   radial head S53.00- ☑
      anterior S53.01- ☑
      nursemaid's elbow S53.03- ☑
      posterior S53.02- ☑
      specified type NEC S53.09- ☑
   radiocarpal (joint) S63.02- ☑
   radioulnar (joint)
      distal S63.01- ☑
      proximal — *see* Subluxation, elbow
   shoulder
      congenital Q68.8
      girdle S43.30- ☑
         scapula S43.31- ☑
         specified site NEC S43.39- ☑
      traumatic S43.00- ☑
         anterior S43.01- ☑
         inferior S43.03- ☑
         posterior S43.02- ☑
         specified type NEC S43.08- ☑
   sternoclavicular (joint) S43.20- ☑
      anterior S43.21- ☑
      posterior S43.22- ☑
   symphysis (pubis) — *see also* Dislocation, symphysis
      pubis
   thumb S63.103 ☑

Subluxation — *continued*
   thumb — *continued*
      interphalangeal joint — *see* Subluxation, interphalangeal (joint), thumb
      metacarpophalangeal joint — *see* Subluxation,
         metacarpophalangeal (joint), thumb
   toe(s) S93.10- ☑
      great S93.10- ☑
         interphalangeal joint S93.13- ☑
         metatarsophalangeal joint S93.14- ☑
      interphalangeal joint S93.13- ☑
      lesser S93.10- ☑
         interphalangeal joint S93.13- ☑
         metatarsophalangeal joint S93.14- ☑
      metatarsophalangeal joint S93.149 ☑
   ulna
      distal end S63.07- ☑
      proximal end — *see* Subluxation, elbow
   ulnohumeral joint — *see* Subluxation, elbow
   vertebral
      recurrent NEC — *see* subcategory M43.5 ☑
      traumatic
         cervical S13.100 ☑
            atlantoaxial joint S13.120 ☑
            atlantooccipital joint S13.110 ☑
            atloidooccipital joint S13.110 ☑
            joint between
               C0 and C1 S13.110 ☑
               C1 and C2 S13.120 ☑
               C2 and C3 S13.130 ☑
               C3 and C4 S13.140 ☑
               C4 and C5 S13.150 ☑
               C5 and C6 S13.160 ☑
               C6 and C7 S13.170 ☑
               C7 and T1 S13.180 ☑
            occipitoatloid joint S13.110 ☑
         lumbar S33.100 ☑
            joint between
               L1 and L2 S33.110 ☑
               L2 and L3 S33.120 ☑
               L3 and L4 S33.130 ☑
               L4 and L5 S33.140 ☑
         thoracic S23.100 ☑
            joint between
               T1 and T2 S23.110 ☑
               T2 and T3 S23.120 ☑
               T3 and T4 S23.122 ☑
               T4 and T5 S23.130 ☑
               T5 and T6 S23.132 ☑
               T6 and T7 S23.140 ☑
               T7 and T8 S23.142 ☑
               T8 and T9 S23.150 ☑
               T9 and T10 S23.152 ☑
               T10 and T11 S23.160 ☑
               T11 and T12 S23.162 ☑
               T12 and L1 S23.170 ☑
   wrist (carpal bone) S63.00- ☑
      carpometacarpal joint — *see* Subluxation, carpometacarpal (joint)
      distal radioulnar joint — *see* Subluxation, radioulnar
         (joint), distal
      metacarpal bone, proximal — *see* Subluxation,
         metacarpal (bone), proximal end
      midcarpal — *see* Subluxation, midcarpal (joint)
      radiocarpal joint — *see* Subluxation, radiocarpal
         (joint)
      recurrent — *see* Dislocation, recurrent, wrist
      specified site NEC S63.09- ☑
      ulna — *see* Subluxation, ulna, distal end
Submaxillary — *see* condition
Submersion (fatal) (nonfatal) T75.1 ☑
Submucous — *see* condition
Subnormal, subnormality
   accommodation (old age) H52.4
   mental — *see* Disability, intellectual
   temperature (accidental) T68 ☑
Subphrenic — *see* condition
Subscapular nerve — *see* condition
Subseptus uterus Q51.28
Subsiding appendicitis K36
Substance (other psychoactive) **-induced**
   anxiety disorder F19.980
   bipolar and related disorder F19.94
   delirium F19.921
   depressive disorder F19.94
   major neurocognitive disorder F19.97

Substance (other psychoactive) **-induced** — *continued*
   mild neurocognitive disorder F19.988
   obsessive-compulsive and related disorder F19.988
   psychotic disorder F19.959
   sexual dysfunction F19.981
   sleep disorder F19.982
Substernal thyroid E04.9
   congenital Q89.2
Substitution disorder F44.9
Subtentorial — *see* condition
Subthyroidism (acquired) — *see also* Hypothyroidism
   congenital E03.1
Succenturiate placenta O43.19- ☑
Sucking thumb, child (excessive) F98.8
Sudamen, sudamina L74.1
Sudanese kala-azar B55.0
Sudden
   hearing loss — *see* Deafness, sudden
   heart failure — *see* Failure, heart
Sudeck's atrophy, disease, or syndrome — *see* Algoneurodystrophy
Suffocation — *see* Asphyxia, traumatic
Sugar
   blood
      high (transient) R73.9
      low (transient) E16.2
   in urine R81
Suicide, suicidal (attempted) T14.91 ☑
   by poisoning — *see* Table of Drugs and Chemicals
   history of (personal) Z91.51
      in family Z81.8
   ideation — *see* Ideation, suicidal
   risk
      meaning personal history of attempted suicide Z91.51
      meaning suicidal ideation — *see* Ideation, suicidal
   tendencies
      meaning personal history of attempted suicide Z91.51
      meaning suicidal ideation — *see* Ideation, suicidal
   trauma — *see* nature of injury by site
Suipestifer infection — *see* Infection, salmonella
Sulfhemoglobinemia, sulphemoglobinemia (acquired) (with methemoglobinemia) D74.8
Sumatran mite fever A75.3
Summer — *see* condition
Sunburn L55.9
   due to
      tanning bed (acute) L56.8
         chronic L57.8
      ultraviolet radiation (acute) L56.8
         chronic L57.8
   first degree L55.0
   second degree L55.1
   third degree L55.2
SUNCT (short lasting unilateral neuralgiform headache with conjunctival injection and tearing) G44.059
   intractable G44.051
   not intractable G44.059
Sundowning F05
Sunken acetabulum — *see* Derangement, joint, specified type NEC, hip
Sunstroke T67.01 ☑
   specified NEC T67.09 ☑
Superfecundation — *see* Pregnancy, multiple
Superfetation — *see* Pregnancy, multiple
Superinvolution (uterus) N85.8
Supernumerary (congenital)
   aortic cusps Q23.8
   auditory ossicles Q16.3
   bone Q79.8
   breast Q83.1
   carpal bones Q74.0
   cusps, heart valve NEC Q24.8
      aortic Q23.8
      mitral Q23.2
      pulmonary Q22.3
   digit(s) Q69.9
   ear (lobule) Q17.0
   fallopian tube Q50.6
   finger Q69.0
   hymen Q52.4
   kidney Q63.0
   lacrimonasal duct Q10.6
   lobule (ear) Q17.0
   mitral cusps Q23.2
   muscle Q79.8

Supernumerary — *continued*
   nipple(s) Q83.3
   organ or site not listed — *see* Accessory
   ossicles, auditory Q16.3
   ovary Q50.31
   oviduct Q50.6
   pulmonary, pulmonic cusps Q22.3
   rib Q76.6
      cervical or first (syndrome) Q76.5
   roots (of teeth) K00.2
   spleen Q89.09
   tarsal bones Q74.2
   teeth K00.1
   testis Q55.29
   thumb Q69.1
   toe Q69.2
   uterus Q51.28
   vagina Q52.1 ☑
   vertebra Q76.49
Supervision (of)
   contraceptive — *see* Prescription, contraceptives
   dietary (for) Z71.3
      allergy (food) Z71.3
      colitis Z71.3
      diabetes mellitus Z71.3
      food allergy or intolerance Z71.3
      gastritis Z71.3
      hypercholesterolemia Z71.3
      hypoglycemia Z71.3
      intolerance (food) Z71.3
      obesity Z71.3
      specified NEC Z71.3
   healthy infant or child Z76.2
      foundling Z76.1
   high-risk pregnancy — *see* Pregnancy, supervision of, high-risk
   lactation Z39.1
   pregnancy — *see* Pregnancy, supervision of
Supplemental teeth K00.1
Suppression
   binocular vision H53.34
   lactation O92.5
   menstruation N94.89
   ovarian secretion E28.39
   renal N28.9
   urine, urinary secretion R34
Suppuration, suppurative — *see also* condition
   accessory sinus (chronic) — *see* Sinusitis
   adrenal gland
   antrum (chronic) — *see* Sinusitis, maxillary
   bladder — *see* Cystitis
   brain G06.0
      sequelae G09
   breast N61.1
      puerperal, postpartum or gestational — *see* Mastitis, obstetric, purulent
   dental periosteum M27.3
   ear (middle) — *see also* Otitis, media
      external NEC — *see* Otitis, externa, infective
      internal — *see* subcategory H83.0 ☑
   ethmoidal (chronic) (sinus) — *see* Sinusitis, ethmoidal
   fallopian tube — *see* Salpingo-oophoritis
   frontal (chronic) (sinus) — *see* Sinusitis, frontal
   gallbladder (acute) K81.0
   gum K05.20
      generalized — *see* Periodontitis, aggressive, generalized
      localized — *see* Periodontitis, aggressive, localized
   intracranial G06.0
   joint — *see* Arthritis, pyogenic or pyemic
   labyrinthine — *see* subcategory H83.0 ☑
   lung — *see* Abscess, lung
   mammary gland N61.1
      puerperal, postpartum O91.12
         associated with lactation O91.13
   maxilla, maxillary M27.2
      sinus (chronic) — *see* Sinusitis, maxillary
   muscle — *see* Myositis, infective
   nasal sinus (chronic) — *see* Sinusitis
   pancreas, acute — *see also* Pancreatitis, acute K85.80
   parotid gland — *see* Sialoadenitis
   pelvis, pelvic
      female — *see* Disease, pelvis, inflammatory
      male K65.0
   pericranial — *see* Osteomyelitis
   salivary duct or gland (any) — *see* Sialoadenitis
   sinus (accessory) (chronic) (nasal) — *see* Sinusitis
   sphenoidal sinus (chronic) — *see* Sinusitis, sphenoidal

Suppuration, suppurative — *continued*
   thymus (gland) E32.1
   thyroid (gland) E06.0
   tonsil — *see* Tonsillitis
   uterus — *see* Endometritis
Supraeruption of tooth (teeth) M26.34
Supraglottitis J04.30
   with obstruction J04.31
Suprarenal (gland) — *see* condition
Suprascapular nerve — *see* condition
Suprasellar — *see* condition
Surfer's knots or nodules S89.8- ☑
Surgical
   emphysema T81.82 ☑
   procedures, complication or misadventure — *see* Complications, surgical procedures
   shock T81.10 ☑
Surveillance (of) (for) — *see also* Observation
   alcohol abuse Z71.41
   contraceptive — *see* Prescription, contraceptives
   dietary Z71.3
   drug abuse Z71.51
Susceptibility to disease, genetic Z15.89
   malignant neoplasm Z15.09
      breast Z15.01
      endometrium Z15.04
      ovary Z15.02
      prostate Z15.03
      specified NEC Z15.09
   multiple endocrine neoplasia Z15.81
Suspected condition, ruled out — *see also* Observation, suspected
   amniotic cavity and membrane Z03.71
   cervical shortening Z03.75
   fetal anomaly Z03.73
   fetal growth Z03.74
   maternal and fetal conditions NEC Z03.79
   newborn — *see also* Observation, newborn, suspected condition ruled out Z05.9
   oligohydramnios Z03.71
   placental problem Z03.72
   polyhydramnios Z03.71
Suspended uterus
   in pregnancy or childbirth — *see* Pregnancy, complicated by, abnormal uterus
Sutton's nevus D22.9
Suture
   burst (in operation wound) T81.31 ☑
      external operation wound T81.31 ☑
      internal operation wound T81.32 ☑
   inadvertently left in operation wound — *see* Foreign body, accidentally left during a procedure
   removal Z48.02
Swab inadvertently left in operation wound — *see* Foreign body, accidentally left during a procedure
Swallowed, swallowing
   difficulty — *see* Dysphagia
   foreign body — *see* Foreign body, alimentary tract
Swan-neck deformity (finger) — *see* Deformity, finger, swan-neck
Swearing, compulsive F42.8
   in Gilles de la Tourette's syndrome F95.2
Sweat, sweats
   fetid L75.0
   night R61
Sweating, excessive R61
Sweeley-Klionsky disease E75.21
Sweet's disease or dermatosis L98.2
Swelling (of) R60.9
   abdomen, abdominal (not referable to any particular organ) — *see* Mass, abdominal
   ankle — *see* Effusion, joint, ankle
   arm M79.89
      forearm M79.89
   breast — *see also* Lump, breast N63.0
   Calabar B74.3
   cervical gland R59.0
   chest, localized R22.2
   ear H93.8- ☑
   extremity (lower) (upper) — *see* Disorder, soft tissue, specified type NEC
   finger M79.89
   foot M79.89
   glands R59.9
      generalized R59.1
      localized R59.0
   hand M79.89

Swelling — *continued*
head (localized) R22.0
inflammatory — *see* Inflammation
intra-abdominal — *see* Mass, abdominal
joint — *see* Effusion, joint
leg M79.89
lower M79.89
limb — *see* Disorder, soft tissue, specified type NEC
localized (skin) R22.9
chest R22.2
head R22.0
limb
lower — *see* Mass, localized, limb, lower
upper — *see* Mass, localized, limb, upper
neck R22.1
trunk R22.2
neck (localized) R22.1
pelvic — *see* Mass, abdominal
scrotum N50.89
splenic — *see* Splenomegaly
testis N50.89
toe M79.89
umbilical R19.09
wandering, due to Gnathostoma (spinigerum) B83.1
white — *see* Tuberculosis, arthritis
Swift (-Feer) **disease**
overdose or wrong substance given or taken — *see* Table of Drugs and Chemicals, by drug, poisoning
Swimmer's
cramp T75.1 ☑
ear H60.33- ☑
itch B65.3
Swimming in the head R42
Swollen — *see* Swelling
Swyer syndrome Q99.1
Sycosis L73.8
barbae (not parasitic) L73.8
contagiosa (mycotic) B35.0
lupoides L73.8
mycotic B35.0
parasitic B35.0
vulgaris L73.8
Sydenham's chorea — *see* Chorea, Sydenham's
Sylvatic yellow fever A95.0
Sylvest's disease B33.0
Symblepharon H11.23- ☑
congenital Q10.3
Symond's syndrome G93.2
Sympathetic — *see* condition
Sympatheticotonia G90.8
Sympathicoblastoma
specified site — *see* Neoplasm, malignant, by site
unspecified site C74.90
Sympathogonioma — *see* Sympathicoblastoma
Symphalangy (fingers) (toes) Q70.9
Symptoms NEC R68.89
breast NEC N64.59
cold J00
development NEC R63.8
factitious, self-induced — *see* Disorder, factitious
genital organs, female R10.2
involving
abdomen NEC R19.8
appearance NEC R46.89
awareness R41.9
altered mental status R41.82
amnesia — *see* Amnesia
borderline intellectual functioning R41.83
coma — *see* Coma
disorientation R41.0
neurologic neglect syndrome R41.4
senile cognitive decline R41.81
specified symptom NEC R41.89
behavior NEC R46.89
cardiovascular system NEC R09.89
chest NEC R09.89
circulatory system NEC R09.89
cognitive functions R41.9
altered mental status R41.82
amnesia — *see* Amnesia
borderline intellectual functioning R41.83
coma — *see* Coma
disorientation R41.0
neurologic neglect syndrome R41.4
senile cognitive decline R41.81
specified symptom NEC R41.89
development NEC R62.50
digestive system NEC R19.8

Symptoms — *continued*
involving — *continued*
emotional state NEC R45.89
emotional lability R45.86
food and fluid intake R63.8
general perceptions and sensations R44.9
specified NEC R44.8
musculoskeletal system R29.91
specified NEC R29.898
nervous system R29.90
specified NEC R29.818
pelvis NEC R19.8
respiratory system NEC R09.89
skin and integument R23.9
urinary system R39.9
menopausal N95.1
metabolism NEC R63.8
neurotic F48.8
of infancy R68.19
pelvis NEC, female R10.2
skin and integument NEC R23.9
subcutaneous tissue NEC R23.9
viral cold J00
Sympus Q74.2
Syncephalus Q89.4
Synchondrosis
abnormal (congenital) Q78.8
ischiopubic M91.0
Synchysis (scintillans) (senile) (vitreous body) H43.89
Syncope (near) (pre-) R55
anginosa I20.8
bradycardia R00.1
cardiac R55
carotid sinus G90.01
due to spinal (lumbar) puncture G97.1
heart R55
heat T67.1 ☑
laryngeal R05.4
psychogenic F48.8
tussive R05.8
vasoconstriction R55
vasodepressor R55
vasomotor R55
vasovagal R55
Syndactylism, syndactyly Q70.9
complex (with synostosis)
fingers Q70.0- ☑
toes Q70.2- ☑
simple (without synostosis)
fingers Q70.1- ☑
toes Q70.3- ☑
Syndrome — *see also* Disease
5q minus NOS D46.C (*following* D46.2)
48,XXXX Q97.1
49,XXXXX Q97.1
abdominal
acute R10.0
muscle deficiency Q79.4
abnormal innervation H02.519
left H02.516
lower H02.515
upper H02.514
right H02.513
lower H02.512
upper H02.511
abstinence, neonatal P96.1
acid pulmonary aspiration, obstetric O74.0
acquired immunodeficiency — *see* Human, immunodeficiency virus (HIV) disease
activated phosphoinositide 3-kinase delta syndrome [APDS] D81.82
acute abdominal R10.0
acute respiratory distress (adult) (child) J80
idiopathic J84.114
Adair-Dighton Q78.0
Adams-Stokes (-Morgagni) I45.9
adiposogenital E23.6
adrenal
hemorrhage (meningococcal) A39.1
meningococcic A39.1
adrenocortical — *see* Cushing's, syndrome
adrenogenital E25.9
congenital, associated with enzyme deficiency E25.0
afferent loop NEC K91.89
Alagille's Q44.7
alcohol withdrawal (without convulsions) — *see* Dependence, alcohol, with, withdrawal
Alder's D72.0

Syndrome — *continued*
Aldrich (-Wiskott) D82.0
alien hand R41.4
Alport Q87.81
alveolar hypoventilation E66.2
alveolocapillary block J84.10
amnesic, amnestic (confabulatory) (due to) — *see* Disorder, amnesic
amyostatic (Wilson's disease) E83.01
androgen insensitivity E34.50
complete E34.51
partial E34.52
androgen resistance — *see also* Syndrome, androgen insensitivity E34.50
Angelman Q93.51
anginal — *see* Angina
ankyloglossia superior Q38.1
anterior
chest wall R07.89
cord G83.82
spinal artery G95.19
compression M47.019
cervical region M47.012
cervicothoracic region M47.013
lumbar region M47.016
occipito-atlanto-axial region M47.011
thoracic region M47.014
thoracolumbar region M47.015
tibial M76.81- ☑
antibody deficiency D80.9
agammaglobulinemic D80.1
hereditary D80.0
congenital D80.0
hypogammaglobulinemic D80.1
hereditary D80.0
anticardiolipin (-antibody) D68.61
antidepressant discontinuation T43.205 ☑
antiphospholipid (-antibody) D68.61
aortic
arch M31.4
bifurcation I74.09
aortomesenteric duodenum occlusion K31.5
apical ballooning (transient left ventricular) I51.81
arcuate ligament I77.4
argentaffin, argintaffinoma E34.0
Arnold-Chiari — *see* Arnold-Chiari disease
Arrillaga-Ayerza I27.0
arterial tortuosity Q87.82
arteriovenous steal T82.898- ☑
Asherman's N85.6
aspiration, of newborn — *see* Aspiration, by substance, with pneumonia
meconium P24.01
ataxia-telangiectasia G11.3
auriculotemporal G50.8
autoerythrocyte sensitization (Gardner-Diamond) D69.2
autoimmune lymphoproliferative [ALPS] D89.82
autoimmune polyglandular E31.0
autoinflammatory M04.9
specified type NEC M04.8
autosomal — *see* Abnormal, autosomes
Avellis' G46.8
Ayerza (-Arrillaga) I27.0
Babinski-Nageotte G83.89
Bakwin-Krida Q78.5
bare lymphocyte D81.6
Barré-Guillain G61.0
Barré-Liéou M53.0
Barrett's — *see* Barrett's, esophagus
Barsony-Polgar K22.4
Bársony-Teschendorf K22.4
Barth E78.71
Bartter's E26.81
basal cell nevus Q87.89
Basedow's E05.00
with thyroid storm E05.01
basilar artery G45.0
Batten-Steinert G71.11
battered
baby or child — *see* Maltreatment, child, physical abuse
spouse — *see* Maltreatment, adult, physical abuse
Beals Q87.40
Beau's I51.5
Beck's I65.8
Benedikt's G46.3
Béquez César (-Steinbrinck-Chédiak-Higashi) E70.330
Bernhardt-Roth — *see* Meralgia paresthetica

Syndrome — continued

Bernheim's — see Failure, heart, right
big spleen D73.1
bilateral polycystic ovarian E28.2
Bing-Horton's — see Horton's headache
Birt-Hogg-Dube syndrome Q87.89
Björck (-Thorsen) E34.0
black
  lung J60
  widow spider bite — see Toxicity, venom, spider, black widow
Blackfan-Diamond D61.01
Blau M04.8
blind loop K90.2
  congenital Q43.8
  postsurgical K91.2
blue sclera Q78.0
blue toe I75.02- ☑
Boder-Sedgewick G11.3
Boerhaave's K22.3
Borjeson Forssman Lehmann Q89.8
Bouillaud's I01.9
Bourneville (-Pringle) Q85.1
Bouveret (-Hoffman) I47.9
brachial plexus G54.0
bradycardia-tachycardia I49.5
brain (nonpsychotic) F09
  with psychosis, psychotic reaction F09
  acute or subacute — see Delirium
  congenital — see Disability, intellectual
  organic F09
    post-traumatic (nonpsychotic) F07.81
      psychotic F09
  personality change F07.0
  postcontusional F07.81
  post-traumatic, nonpsychotic F07.81
  psycho-organic F09
  psychotic F06.8
brain stem stroke G46.3
Brandt's (acrodermatitis enteropathica) E83.2
broad ligament laceration N83.8
Brock's J98.11
bronze baby P83.88
Brown-Sequard G83.81
Brugada I49.8
bubbly lung P27.0
Buchem's M85.2
Budd-Chiari I82.0
bulbar (progressive) G12.22
Bürger-Grütz E78.3
Burke's K86.89
Burnett's (milk-alkali) E83.52
burning feet E53.9
Bywaters' T79.5 ☑
Call-Fleming I67.841
carbohydrate-deficient glycoprotein (CDGS) E77.8
carcinogenic thrombophlebitis I82.1
carcinoid E34.0
cardiac asthma I50.1
cardiacos negros I27.0
cardiofaciocutaneous Q87.89
cardiopulmonary-obesity E66.2
cardiorenal — see Hypertension, cardiorenal
cardiorespiratory distress (idiopathic), newborn P22.0
cardiovascular renal — see Hypertension, cardiorenal
carotid
  artery (hemispheric) (internal) G45.1
  body G90.01
  sinus G90.01
carpal tunnel G56.0- ☑
Cassidy (-Scholte) E34.0
cat cry Q93.4
cat eye Q92.8
cauda equina G83.4
causalgia — see Causalgia
celiac K90.0
  artery compression I77.4
  axis I77.4
central pain G89.0
cerebellar
  hereditary G11.9
  stroke G46.4
cerebellomedullary malformation — see Spina bifida
cerebral
  artery
    anterior G46.1
    middle G46.0
    posterior G46.2

Syndrome — continued

cerebral — continued
  gigantism E22.0
cervical (root) M53.1
  disc — see Disorder, disc, cervical, with neuritis
  fusion Q76.1
  posterior, sympathicus M53.0
  rib Q76.5
  sympathetic paralysis G90.2
cervicobrachial (diffuse) M53.1
cervicocranial M53.0
cervicodorsal outlet G54.2
cervicothoracic outlet G54.0
Céstan (-Raymond) I65.8
Charcot's (angina cruris) (intermittent claudication) I73.9
Charcot-Weiss-Baker G90.09
CHARGE Q89.8
Chédiak-Higashi (-Steinbrinck) E70.330
chest wall R07.1
Chiari's (hepatic vein thrombosis) I82.0
Chilaiditi's Q43.3
child maltreatment — see Maltreatment, child
chondrocostal junction M94.0
chondroectodermal dysplasia Q77.6
chromosome 4 short arm deletion Q93.3
chromosome 5 short arm deletion Q93.4
chronic
  infantile neurological, cutaneous and articular (CINCA) M04.2
  pain G89.4
    personality F68.8
Churg-Strauss M30.1
Clarke-Hadfield K86.89
Clerambault's automatism G93.89
Clouston's (hidrotic ectodermal dysplasia) Q82.4
clumsiness, clumsy child F82
cluster headache G44.009
  intractable G44.001
  not intractable G44.009
Coffin-Lowry Q89.8
cold injury (newborn) P80.0
combined immunity deficiency D81.9
compartment (deep) (posterior) (traumatic) T79.A0 ☑ (following T79.7)
  abdomen T79.A3 ☑ (following T79.7)
  lower extremity (hip, buttock, thigh, leg, foot, toes) T79.A2 ☑ (following T79.7)
  nontraumatic
    abdomen M79.A3 (following M79.7)
    lower extremity (hip, buttock, thigh, leg, foot, toes) M79.A2- ☑ (following M79.7)
    specified site NEC M79.A9 (following M79.7)
    upper extremity (shoulder, arm, forearm, wrist, hand, fingers) M79.A1- ☑ (following M79.7)
  postprocedural — see Syndrome, compartment, nontraumatic
  specified site NEC T79.A9 ☑ (following T79.7)
  upper extremity (shoulder, arm, forearm, wrist, hand, fingers) T79.A1 ☑ (following T79.7)
complex regional pain — see Syndrome, pain, complex regional
compression T79.5 ☑
  anterior spinal — see Syndrome, anterior, spinal artery, compression
  cauda equina G83.4
  celiac artery I77.4
  vertebral artery M47.029
    cervical region M47.022
    occipito-atlanto-axial region M47.021
concussion F07.81
congenital
  affecting multiple systems NEC Q87.89
  central alveolar hypoventilation G47.35
  facial diplegia Q87.0
  muscular hypertrophy-cerebral Q87.89
  oculo-auriculovertebral Q87.0
  oculofacial diplegia (Moebius) Q87.0
  rubella (manifest) P35.0
congestion-fibrosis (pelvic), female N94.89
congestive dysmenorrhea N94.6
connective tissue M35.9
  overlap NEC M35.1
Conn's E26.01
conus medullaris G95.81
cord
  anterior G83.82

Syndrome — continued

cord — continued
  posterior G83.83
coronary
  acute NEC I24.9
  insufficiency or intermediate I20.0
  slow flow I20.8
Costen's (complex) M26.69
costochondral junction M94.0
costoclavicular G54.0
costovertebral E22.0
Cowden
  PTEN related Q85.81
  specified NEC Q85.82
craniovertebral M53.0
Creutzfeldt-Jakob — see Creutzfeldt-Jakob disease or syndrome
crib death R99
cricopharyngeal — see Dysphagia
cri-du-chat Q93.4
croup J05.0
CRPS I — see Syndrome, pain, complex regional I
crush T79.5 ☑
cryopyrin-associated perodic M04.2
cryptophthalmos Q87.0
cubital tunnel — see Lesion, nerve, ulnar
Curschmann (-Batten) (-Steinert) G71.11
Cushing's E24.9
  alcohol-induced E24.4
  due to
    alcohol
    drugs E24.2
    ectopic ACTH E24.3
    overproduction of pituitary ACTH E24.0
  drug-induced E24.2
  overdose or wrong substance given or taken — see Table of Drugs and Chemicals, by drug, poisoning
  pituitary-dependent E24.0
  specified type NEC E24.8
cystic duct stump K91.5
cytokine release D89.839
  grade 1 D89.831
  grade 2 D89.832
  grade 3 D89.833
  grade 4 D89.834
  grade 5 D89.835
Dana-Putnam D51.0
Danbolt (-Cross) (acrodermatitis enteropathica) E83.2
Dandy-Walker Q03.1
  with spina bifida Q07.01
Danlos' — see also Syndrome, Ehlers-Danlos Q79.60
De Quervain E34.51
de Toni-Fanconi (-Debré) E72.09
  with cystinosis E72.04
de Vivo syndrome E74.810
defibrination — see also Fibrinolysis
  with
    antepartum hemorrhage — see Hemorrhage, antepartum, with coagulation defect
    intrapartum hemorrhage — see Hemorrhage, complicating, delivery
  newborn P60
  postpartum O72.3
Degos' I77.89
Déjérine-Roussy G89.0
delayed sleep phase G47.21
demyelinating G37.9
dependence — see F10-F19 with fourth character .2
depersonalization (-derealization) F48.1
di George's D82.1
diabetes mellitus in newborn infant P70.2
diabetes mellitus-hypertension-nephrosis — see Diabetes, nephrosis
diabetes-nephrosis — see Diabetes, nephrosis
diabetic amyotrophy — see Diabetes, amyotrophy
dialysis associated steal T82.898- ☑
Diamond-Blackfan D61.01
Diamond-Gardener D69.2
DIC (diffuse or disseminated intravascular coagulopathy) D65
Dighton's Q78.0
disequilibrium E87.8
Döhle body-panmyelopathic D72.0
dorsolateral medullary G46.4
double athetosis G80.3
Down — see also Down syndrome Q90.9
Dravet (intractable) G40.834

Syndrome — *continued*
  Dravet — *continued*
    with status epilepticus G40.833
    without status epilepticus G40.834
  Dresbach's (elliptocytosis) D58.1
  DRESS (drug rash with eosinophilia and systemic symptoms) D72.12
  Dressler's (postmyocardial infarction) I24.1
    postcardiotomy I97.0
  drug rash with eosinophilia and systemic symptoms (DRESS) D72.12
  drug withdrawal, infant of dependent mother P96.1
  dry eye H04.12- ☑
  due to abnormality
    chromosomal Q99.9
      sex
        female phenotype Q97.9
        male phenotype Q98.9
      specified NEC Q99.8
  dumping (postgastrectomy) K91.1
    nonsurgical K31.89
  Dupré's (meningism) R29.1
  dysmetabolic X E88.81
  dyspraxia, developmental F82
  Eagle-Barrett Q79.4
  Eaton-Lambert — *see* Syndrome, Lambert-Eaton
  Ebstein's Q22.5
  ectopic ACTH E24.3
  eczema-thrombocytopenia D82.0
  Eddowes' Q78.0
  effort (psychogenic) F45.8
  Ehlers-Danlos Q79.60
    classical (cEDS) (classical EDS) Q79.61
    hypermobile (hEDS) (hypermobile EDS) Q79.62
    specified NEC Q79.69
    vascular (vascular EDS) (vEDS) Q79.63
  Eisenmenger's I27.83
  Ekman's Q78.0
  electric feet E53.8
  Ellis-van Creveld Q77.6
  empty nest Z60.0
  endocrine-hypertensive E27.0
  entrapment — *see* Neuropathy, entrapment
  eosinophilia-myalgia M35.89
  epileptic — *see also* Epilepsy, by type
    absence G40.A09 (*following* G40.3)
      intractable G40.A19 (*following* G40.3)
        with status epilepticus G40.A11 (*following* G40.3)
        without status epilepticus G40.A19 (*following* G40.3)
      not intractable G40.A09 (*following* G40.3)
        with status epilepticus G40.A01 (*following* G40.3)
        without status epilepticus G40.A09 (*following* G40.3)
  Erdheim-Chester (ECD) E88.89
  Erdheim's E22.0
  erythrocyte fragmentation D59.4
  Evans D69.41
  exhaustion F48.8
  extrapyramidal G25.9
    specified NEC G25.89
  eye retraction — *see* Strabismus
  eyelid-malar-mandible Q87.0
  Faber's D50.9
  facet M47.89- ☑
  facet joint — *see also* Spondylosis M47.819
  facial pain, paroxysmal G50.0
  Fallot's Q21.3
  familial cold autoinflammatory M04.2
  familial eczema-thrombocytopenia (Wiskott-Aldrich) D82.0
  Fanconi (-de Toni) (-Debré) E72.09
    with cystinosis E72.04
  Fanconi's (anemia) (congenital pancytopenia) D61.09
  fatigue
    chronic G93.32
    postviral G93.31
    psychogenic F48.8
  faulty bowel habit K59.39
  Feil-Klippel (brevicollis) Q76.1
  Felty's — *see* Felty's syndrome
  fertile eunuch E23.0
  fetal
    alcohol (dysmorphic) Q86.0
    hydantoin Q86.1
  Fiedler's I40.1

Syndrome — *continued*
  first arch Q87.0
  fish odor E72.89
  Fisher's G61.0
  Fitzhugh-Curtis
    due to
      Chlamydia trachomatis A74.81
      Neisseria gonorrhorea (gonococcal peritonitis) A54.85
  Fitz's — *see also* Pancreatitis, acute K85.80
  Flajani (-Basedow) E05.00
    with thyroid storm E05.01
  flatback — *see* Flatback syndrome
  floppy
    baby P94.2
    iris (intraoeprative) (IFIS) H21.81
    mitral valve I34.1
  flush E34.0
  Foix-Alajouanine G95.19
  Fong's Q87.2
  food protein-induced enterocolitis (FPIES) K52.21
  foramen magnum G93.5
  Foster-Kennedy H47.14- ☑
  Foville's (peduncular) G46.3
  fragile X Q99.2
  Franceschetti Q75.4
  Frey's
    auriculotemporal G50.8
    hyperhidrosis L74.52
  Friderichsen-Waterhouse A39.1
  Froin's G95.89
  frontal lobe F07.0
  Fukuhara E88.49
  functional
    bowel K59.9
    prepubertal castrate E29.1
  Gaisböck's D75.1
  ganglion (basal ganglia brain) G25.9
    geniculi G51.1
  Gardner-Diamond D69.2
  gastroesophageal
    junction K22.0
    laceration-hemorrhage K22.6
  gastrojejunal loop obstruction K91.89
  Gee-Herter-Heubner K90.0
  Gelineau's G47.419
    with cataplexy G47.411
  genito-anorectal A55
  Gerstmann-Sträussler-Scheinker (GSS) A81.82
  Gianotti-Crosti L44.4
  giant platelet (Bernard-Soulier) D69.1
  Gilles de la Tourette's F95.2
  Glass Q87.89
  Gleich's D72.118
  goiter-deafness E07.1
  Goldberg Q89.8
  Goldberg-Maxwell E34.51
  Good's D83.8
  Gopalan' (burning feet) E53.8
  Gorlin's Q87.89
  Gougerot-Blum L81.7
  Gouley's I31.1
  Gower's R55
  gray or grey (newborn) P93.0
    platelet D69.1
  Gubler-Millard G46.3
  Guillain-Barré (-Strohl) G61.0
  gustatory sweating G50.8
  Hadfield-Clarke K86.89
  hair tourniquet — *see* Constriction, external, by site
  Hamman's J98.19
  hand-foot L27.1
  hand-shoulder G90.8
  hantavirus (cardio)-pulmonary (HPS) (HCPS) B33.4
  happy puppet Q93.51
  Harada's H30.81- ☑
  Hayem-Faber D50.9
  headache NEC G44.89
    complicated NEC G44.59
  Heberden's I20.8
  Hedinger's E34.0
  Hegglin's D72.0
  HELLP (hemolysis, elevated liver enzymes and low platelet count) O14.2- ☑
    complicating
      childbirth O14.24
      puerperium O14.25
  hemolytic-uremic D59.30
    atypical D59.39

Syndrome — *continued*
  hemolytic-uremic — *continued*
    atypical — *continued*
      genetic D59.32
      hereditary D59.32
      infection-associated D59.31
      secondary D59.39
      specified NEC D59.39
    due to genetic disorder D59.32
    familial D59.32
    hereditary D59.32
    infection-associated D59.31
    secondary D59.39
    Shiga toxin-producing E. coli [STEC] related D59.31
    specified NEC D59.39
    typical D59.31
  hemophagocytic, infection-associated D76.2
  Henoch-Schönlein D69.0
  hepatic flexure K59.89
  hepatopulmonary K76.81
  hepatorenal K76.7
    following delivery O90.4
    postoperative or postprocedural K91.83
    postpartum, puerperal O90.4
  hepatourologic K76.7
  hereditary alpha tryptasemia D89.44
  Herter (-Gee) (nontropical sprue) K90.0
  Heubner-Herter K90.0
  Heyd's K76.7
  Hilger's G90.09
  histamine-like (fish poisoning) — *see* Poisoning, fish
  histiocytic D76.3
  histiocytosis NEC D76.3
  HIV infection, acute B20
  Hoffmann-Werdnig G12.0
  Hollander-Simons E88.1
  Hoppe-Goldflam G70.00
    with exacerbation (acute) G70.01
    in crisis G70.01
  Horner's G90.2
  hungry bone E83.81
  hunterian glossitis D51.0
  Hutchinson's triad A50.53
  hyperabduction G54.0
  hyperammonemia-hyperornithinemia-homocitrulline-mia E72.4
  hypereosinophilic (HES) D72.119
    idiopathic (IHES) D72.110
    lymphocytic variant (LHES) D72.111
    myeloid D72.118
    specified NEC D72.118
  hyperimmunoglobulin D M04.1
  hyperimmunoglobulin E (IgE) D82.4
  hyperkalemic E87.5
  hyperkinetic — *see* Hyperkinesia
  hypermobility M35.7
  hypernatremia E87.0
  hyperosmolarity E87.0
  hyperperfusion G97.82
  hypersplenic D73.1
  hypertransfusion, newborn P61.1
  hyperventilation F45.8
  hyperviscosity (of serum)
    polycythemic D75.1
    sclerothymic D58.8
  hypoglycemic (familial) (neonatal) E16.2
  hypokalemic E87.6
  hyponatremic E87.1
  hypopituitarism E23.0
  hypoplastic left-heart Q23.4
  hypopotassemia E87.6
  hyposmolality E87.1
  hypotension, maternal O26.5- ☑
  hypothenar hammer I73.89
  hypoventilation, obesity (OHS) E66.2
  ICF (intravascular coagulation-fibrinolysis) D65
  idiopathic
    cardiorespiratory distress, newborn P22.0
    nephrotic (infantile) N04.9
  iliotibial band M76.3- ☑
  immobility, immobilization (paraplegic) M62.3
  immune effector cell-associated neurotoxicity (ICANS) G92.00
    grade
      1 G92.01
      2 G92.02
      3 G92.03
      4 G92.04
      5 G92.05

Syndrome — *continued*
immune effector cell-associated neurotoxicity — *continued*
grade — *continued*
unspecified G92.00
immune reconstitution D89.3
immune reconstitution inflammatory [IRIS] D89.3
immunity deficiency, combined D81.9
immunodeficiency
acquired — *see* Human, immunodeficiency virus (HIV) disease
combined D81.9
impending coronary I20.0
impingement, shoulder M75.4- ☑
inappropriate secretion of antidiuretic hormone E22.2
infant
gestational diabetes P70.0
of diabetic mother P70.1
infantilism (pituitary) E23.0
inferior vena cava I87.1
inspissated bile (newborn) P59.1
institutional (childhood) F94.2
insufficient sleep F51.12
intermediate coronary (artery) I20.0
interspinous ligament — *see* Spondylopathy, specified NEC
intestinal
carcinoid E34.0
knot K56.2
intravascular coagulation-fibrinolysis (ICF) D65
iodine-deficiency, congenital E00.9
type
mixed E00.2
myxedematous E00.1
neurological E00.0
IRDS (idiopathic respiratory distress, newborn) P22.0
irritable
bowel K58.9
with
constipation K58.1
diarrhea K58.0
mixed K58.2
psychogenic F45.8
specified NEC K58.8
heart (psychogenic) F45.8
weakness F48.8
ischemic
bowel (transient) K55.9
chronic K55.1
due to mesenteric artery insufficiency K55.1
steal T82.898 ☑
IVC (intravascular coagulopathy) D65
Ivemark's Q89.01
Jaccoud's — *see* Arthropathy, postrheumatic, chronic
Jackson's G83.89
Jakob-Creutzfeldt — *see* Creutzfeldt-Jakob disease or syndrome
jaw-winking Q07.8
Jervell-Lange-Nielsen I45.81
jet lag G47.25
Job's D71
Joseph-Diamond-Blackfan D61.01
jugular foramen G52.7
Kabuki Q89.8
Kanner's (autism) F84.0
Kartagener's Q89.3
Kelly's D50.1
Kimmelsteil-Wilson — *see* Diabetes, specified type, with Kimmelstiel-Wilson disease
Klein (e)-Levine G47.13
Klippel-Feil (brevicollis) Q76.1
Köhler-Pellegrini-Steida — *see* Bursitis, tibial collateral
König's K59.89
Korsakoff (-Wernicke) (nonalcoholic) F04
alcoholic F10.26
Kostmann's D70.0
Krabbe's congenital muscle hypoplasia Q79.8
labyrinthine — *see* subcategory H83.2 ☑
lacunar NEC G46.7
Lambert-Eaton G70.80
in
neoplastic disease G73.1
specified disease NEC G70.81
Landau-Kleffner — *see* Epilepsy, specified NEC
Larsen's Q74.8
lateral
cutaneous nerve of thigh G57.1- ☑
medullary G46.4

Syndrome — *continued*
Launois' E22.0
lazy
leukocyte D70.8
posture M62.3
Lemiere I80.8
Lennox-Gastaut G40.812
intractable G40.814
with status epilepticus G40.813
without status epilepticus G40.814
not intractable G40.812
with status epilepticus G40.811
without status epilepticus G40.812
lenticular, progressive E83.01
Leopold-Levi's E05.90
Lev's I44.2
Lichtheim's D51.0
Li-Fraumeni Z15.01
Lightwood's N25.89
Lignac (de Toni) (-Fanconi) (-Debré) E72.09
with cystinosis E72.04
Likoff's I20.8
limbic epilepsy personality F07.0
liver-kidney K76.7
lobotomy F07.0
Löffler's J82.89
long arm 18 or 21 deletion Q93.89
long QT I45.81
Louis-Barré G11.3
low
atmospheric pressure T70.29 ☑
back M54.50
output (cardiac) I50.9
lower radicular, newborn (birth injury) P14.8
Luetscher's (dehydration) E86.0
Lupus anticoagulant D68.62
Lutembacher's Q21.19
macrophage activation D76.1
due to infection D76.2
magnesium-deficiency R29.0
Majeed M04.8
Mal de Debarquement R42
malabsorption K90.9
postsurgical K91.2
malformation, congenital, due to
alcohol Q86.0
exogenous cause NEC Q86.8
hydantoin Q86.1
warfarin Q86.2
malignant
carcinoid E34.0
neuroleptic G21.0
Mallory-Weiss K22.6
mandibulofacial dysostosis Q75.4
manic-depressive — *see* Disorder, bipolar
maple-syrup-urine E71.0
Marable's I77.4
Marfan's Q87.40
with
cardiovascular manifestations Q87.418
aortic dilation Q87.410
ocular manifestations Q87.42
skeletal manifestations Q87.43
Marie's (acromegaly) E22.0
mast cell activation — *see* Activation, mast cell
maternal hypotension — *see* Syndrome, hypotension, maternal
May (-Hegglin) D72.0
McArdle (-Schmidt) (-Pearson) E74.04
McQuarrie's E16.2
meconium plug (newborn) P76.0
median arcuate ligament I77.4
Meekeren-Ehlers-Danlos Q79.6 ☑
megavitamin-B6 E67.2
Meige G24.4
MELAS E88.41
Mendelson's O74.0
MERRF (myoclonic epilepsy associated with ragged-red fibers) E88.42
mesenteric
artery (superior) K55.1
vascular insufficiency K55.1
metabolic E88.81
metastatic carcinoid E34.0
micrognathia-glossoptosis Q87.0
midbrain NEC G93.89
middle lobe (lung) J98.19
middle radicular G54.0
migraine — *see also* Migraine G43.909

Syndrome — *continued*
Mikulicz' K11.8
milk-alkali E83.52
Millard-Gubler G46.3
Miller-Dieker Q93.88
Miller-Fisher G61.0
Minkowski-Chauffard D58.0
Mirizzi's K83.1
MNGIE (Mitochondrial Neurogastrointestinal Encephalopathy) E88.49
Möbius, ophthalmoplegic migraine — *see* Migraine, ophthalmoplegic
monofixation H50.42
Morel-Moore M85.2
Morel-Morgagni M85.2
Morgagni (-Morel) (-Stewart) M85.2
Morgagni-Adams-Stokes I45.9
Mounier-Kuhn Q32.4
with bronchiectasis J47.9
with
exacerbation (acute) J47.1
lower respiratory infection J47.0
acquired J98.09
with bronchiectasis J47.9
with
exacerbation (acute) J47.1
lower respiratory infection J47.0
Muckle-Wells M04.2
mucocutaneous lymph node (acute febrile) (MCLS) M30.3
multiple endocrine neoplasia (MEN) — *see* Neoplasia, endocrine, multiple (MEN)
multiple operations — *see* Disorder, factitious
multisystem inflammatory (in adults) (in children) M35.81
myasthenic G70.9
in
diabetes mellitus — *see* Diabetes, amyotrophy
endocrine disease NEC E34.9 *[G73.3]*
neoplastic disease — *see also* Neoplasm D49.9 *[G73.3]*
thyrotoxicosis (hyperthyroidism) E05.90 *[G73.3]*
with thyroid storm E05.91 *[G73.3]*
myelodysplastic D46.9
with
5q deletion D46.C (*following* D46.2)
isolated del (5q) chromosomal abnormality D46.C (*following* D46.2)
multilineage dysplasia D46.A (*following* D46.2)
with ringed sideroblasts D46.B (*following* D46.2)
lesions, low grade D46.20
specified NEC D46.Z (*following* D46.4)
myeloid hypereosinophilic D72.118
myelopathic pain G89.0
myeloproliferative (chronic) D47.1
myofascial pain M79.18
Naffziger's G54.0
nail patella Q87.2
NARP (Neuropathy, Ataxia and Retinitis pigmentosa) E88.49
neonatal abstinence P96.1
nephritic — *see also* Nephritis
with edema — *see* Nephrosis
acute N00.9
chronic N03.9
rapidly progressive N01.9
nephrotic (congenital) — *see also* Nephrosis N04.9
with
C3
glomerulonephritis N04.A
glomerulopathy N04.A
with dense deposit disease N04.6
dense deposit disease N04.6
diffuse
crescentic glomerulonephritis N04.7
endocapillary proliferative glomerulonephritis N04.4
membranous glomerulonephritis N04.2
mesangial proliferative glomerulonephritis N04.3
mesangiocapillary glomerulonephritis N04.5
focal and segmental glomerular lesions N04.1
minor glomerular abnormality N04.0
specified morphological changes NEC N04.8
diabetic — *see* Diabetes, nephrosis
neurologic neglect R41.4
Nezelof's D81.4

Syndrome — *continued*
- Nonne-Milroy-Meige Q82.0
- Nothnagel's vasomotor acroparesthesia I73.89
- obesity hypoventilation (OHS) E66.2
- oculomotor H51.9
- Ogilvie K59.81
- ophthalmoplegia-cerebellar ataxia — *see* Strabismus, paralytic, third nerve
- oral allergy T78.1 ☑
- oral-facial-digital Q87.0
- organic
  - affective F06.30
  - amnesic (not alcohol- or drug-induced) F04
  - brain F09
  - depressive F06.31
  - hallucinosis F06.0
  - personality F07.0
- Ormond's N13.5
- oro-facial-digital Q87.0
- os trigonum Q68.8
- Osler-Weber-Rendu I78.0
- osteoporosis-osteomalacia M83.8
- Osterreicher-Turner Q87.2
- otolith — *see* subcategory H81.8 ☑
- oto-palatal-digital Q87.0
- outlet (thoracic) G54.0
- ovary
  - polycystic E28.2
  - resistant E28.39
  - sclerocystic E28.2
- Owren's D68.2
- Paget-Schroetter I82.890
- pain — *see also* Pain
  - complex regional I G90.50
    - lower limb G90.52- ☑
    - specified site NEC G90.59
    - upper limb G90.51- ☑
  - complex regional II — *see* Causalgia
- painful
  - bruising D69.2
  - feet E53.8
  - prostate N42.81
- paralysis agitans — *see* Parkinsonism
- paralytic G83.9
  - specified NEC G83.89
- Parinaud's H51.0
- parkinsonian — *see* Parkinsonism
- Parkinson's — *see* Parkinsonism
- paroxysmal facial pain G50.0
- Parry's E05.00
  - with thyroid storm E05.01
- Parsonage (-Aldren)-Turner G54.5
- patella clunk M25.86- ☑
- Paterson (-Brown) (-Kelly) D50.1
- pectoral girdle I77.89
- pectoralis minor I77.89
- pediatric autoimmune neuropsychiatric disorders associated with streptococcal infections (PANDAS) D89.89
- pediatric inflammatory multisystem M35.81
- Pelger-Huet D72.0
- pellagra-cerebellar ataxia-renal aminoaciduria E72.02
- pellagroid E52
- Pellegrini-Stieda — *see* Bursitis, tibial collateral
- pelvic congestion-fibrosis, female N94.89
- penta X Q97.1
- peptic ulcer — *see* Ulcer, peptic
- perabduction I77.89
- periodic fever M04.1
- periodic fever, aphthous stomatitis, pharyngitis, and adenopathy [PFAPA] M04.8
- periodic headache, in adults and children — *see* Headache, periodic syndromes in adults and children
- periurethral fibrosis N13.5
- Peutz-Jeghers Q85.89
- phantom limb (without pain) G54.7
  - with pain G54.6
- pharyngeal pouch D82.1
- Pick's — *see* Disease, Pick's
- Pickwickian E66.2
- PIE (pulmonary infiltration with eosinophilia) — *see also* Eosinophilia, pulmonary J82.89
- pigmentary pallidal degeneration (progressive) G23.0
- pineal E34.8
- pituitary E22.0
- placental transfusion — *see* Pregnancy, complicated by, placental transfusion syndromes

Syndrome — *continued*
- plantar fascia M72.2
- plateau iris (post-iridectomy) (postprocedural) H21.82
- Plummer-Vinson D50.1
- pluricarential of infancy E40
- plurideficiency E40
- pluriglandular (compensatory) E31.8
  - autoimmune E31.0
- pneumatic hammer T75.21 ☑
- polyangiitis overlap M30.8
- polycarential of infancy E40
- polyglandular E31.8
  - autoimmune E31.0
- polysplenia Q89.09
- pontine NEC G93.89
- popliteal
  - artery entrapment I77.89
  - web Q87.89
- post chemoembolization — *code to* associated conditions
- post endometrial ablation N99.85
- postbacterial fatigue G93.39
- postcardiac injury
  - postcardiotomy I97.0
  - postmyocardial infarction I24.1
- postcardiotomy I97.0
- postcholecystectomy K91.5
- postcommissurotomy I97.0
- postconcussional F07.81
- postcontusional F07.81
- post-COVID (-19) U09.9
- postencephalitic F07.89
- posterior
  - cervical sympathetic M53.0
  - cord G83.83
  - fossa compression G93.5
  - reversible encephalopathy (PRES) I67.83
- postgastrectomy (dumping) K91.1
- postgastric surgery K91.1
- postinfarction I24.1
- postinfectious fatigue G93.39
- postlaminectomy NEC M96.1
- postleukotomy F07.0
- postmastectomy lymphedema I97.2
- postmyocardial infarction I24.1
- postoperative NEC T81.9 ☑
  - blind loop K90.2
- postpartum panhypopituitary (Sheehan) E23.0
- postpolio (myelitic) G14
- postthrombotic I87.009
  - with
    - inflammation I87.02- ☑
      - with ulcer I87.03- ☑
    - specified complication NEC I87.09- ☑
    - ulcer I87.01- ☑
      - with inflammation I87.03- ☑
  - asymptomatic I87.00- ☑
- postural
  - orthostatic tachycardia [POTS] G90.A
  - tachycardia G90.A
- postvagotomy K91.1
- postvalvulotomy I97.0
- postviral NEC G93.31
  - fatigue G93.31
- Potain's K31.0
- potassium intoxication E87.5
- Prader-Willi Q87.11
- Prader-Willi-like Q87.19
- precerebral artery (multiple) (bilateral) G45.2
- preinfarction I20.0
- preleukemic D46.9
- premature senility E34.8
- premenstrual dysphoric F32.81
- premenstrual tension N94.3
- Prinzmetal-Massumi R07.1
- prune belly Q79.4
- pseudo -Turner's Q87.19
- pseudocarpal tunnel (sublimis) — *see* Syndrome, carpal tunnel
- pseudoparalytica G70.00
  - with exacerbation (acute) G70.01
  - in crisis G70.01
- psycho-organic (nonpsychotic severity) F07.9
  - acute or subacute F05
  - depressive type F06.31
  - hallucinatory type F06.0
  - nonpsychotic severity F07.0
  - specified NEC F07.89

Syndrome — *continued*
- PTEN (hamartoma) tumor Q85.81
- pulmonary
  - arteriosclerosis I27.0
  - dysmaturity (Wilson-Mikity) P27.0
  - hypoperfusion (idiopathic) P22.0
  - renal (hemorrhagic) (Goodpasture's) M31.0
- pure
  - motor lacunar G46.5
  - sensory lacunar G46.6
- Putnam-Dana D51.0
- pyogenic arthritis, pyoderma gangrenosum, and acne [PAPA] M04.8
- pyramidopallidonigral G20
- pyriformis — *see* Lesion, nerve, sciatic
- QT interval prolongation I45.81
- radicular NEC — *see* Radiculopathy
  - upper limbs, newborn (birth injury) P14.3
- rapid time-zone change G47.25
- Rasmussen G04.81
- Raymond (-Céstan) I65.8
- Raynaud's I73.00
  - with gangrene I73.01
- RDS (respiratory distress syndrome, newborn) P22.0
- reactive airways dysfunction J68.3
- Refsum's G60.1
- Reifenstein E34.52
- renal glomerulohyalinosis-diabetic — *see* Diabetes, nephrosis
- Rendu-Osler-Weber I78.0
- residual ovary N99.83
- resistant ovary E28.39
- respiratory
  - distress
    - acute J80
      - adult J80
      - child J80
      - idiopathic J84.114
    - newborn (idiopathic) (type I) P22.0
    - type II P22.1
- restless legs G25.81
- retinoblastoma (familial) C69.2 ☑
- retroperitoneal fibrosis N13.5
- retroviral seroconversion (acute) Z21
- Reye's G93.7
- Richter — *see* Leukemia, chronic lymphocytic, B-cell type
- Ridley's I50.1
- right
  - heart, hypoplastic Q22.6
  - ventricular obstruction — *see* Failure, heart, right
- Romano-Ward (prolonged QT interval) I45.81
- rotator cuff, shoulder — *see also* Tear, rotator cuff M75.10- ☑
- Rotes Quérol — *see* Hyperostosis, ankylosing
- Roth — *see* Meralgia paresthetica
- rubella (congenital) P35.0
- Ruvalcaba-Myhre-Smith E71.440
- Rytand-Lipsitch I44.2
- salt
  - depletion E87.1
    - due to heat NEC T67.8 ☑
      - causing heat exhaustion or prostration T67.4 ☑
  - low E87.1
- salt-losing N28.89
- SATB2-associated Q87.89
- Scaglietti-Dagnini E22.0
- scalenus anticus (anterior) G54.0
- scapulocostal — *see* Mononeuropathy, upper limb, specified site NEC
- scapuloperoneal G71.09
- schizophrenic, of childhood NEC F84.5
- Schnitzler D47.2
- Scholte's E34.0
- Schroeder's E27.0
- Schüller-Christian C96.5
- Schwachman's — *see* Syndrome, Shwachman's
- Schwartz (-Jampel) G71.13
- Schwartz-Bartter E22.2
- scimitar Q26.8
- sclerocystic ovary E28.2
- Seitelberger's G31.89
- septicemic adrenal hemorrhage A39.1
- seroconversion, retroviral (acute) Z21
- serous meningitis G93.2
- severe acute respiratory (SARS) J12.81
  - coronavirus 2 (*see also* COVID-19) U07.1

Synostosis — *continued*
　radioulnar Q74.0
Synovial sarcoma — *see* Neoplasm, connective tissue, malignant
Synovioma (malignant) — *see also* Neoplasm, connective tissue, malignant
　benign — *see* Neoplasm, connective tissue, benign
Synoviosarcoma — *see* Neoplasm, connective tissue, malignant
Synovitis — *see also* Tenosynovitis M65.9
　crepitant
　　hand M70.0- ☑
　　wrist M70.03- ☑
　gonococcal A54.49
　gouty — *see* Gout
　in (due to)
　　crystals M65.8- ☑
　　gonorrhea A54.49
　　syphilis (late) A52.78
　　use, overuse, pressure — *see* Disorder, soft tissue, due to use
　infective NEC — *see* Tenosynovitis, infective NEC
　specified NEC — *see* Tenosynovitis, specified type NEC
　syphilitic A52.78
　　congenital (early) A50.02
　toxic — *see* Synovitis, transient
　transient M67.3- ☑
　　ankle M67.37- ☑
　　elbow M67.32- ☑
　　foot joint M67.37- ☑
　　hand joint M67.34- ☑
　　hip M67.35- ☑
　　knee M67.36- ☑
　　multiple site M67.39
　　pelvic region M67.35- ☑
　　shoulder M67.31- ☑
　　specified joint NEC M67.38
　　wrist M67.33- ☑
　traumatic, current — *see* Sprain
　tuberculous — *see* Tuberculosis, synovitis
　villonodular (pigmented) M12.2- ☑
　　ankle M12.27- ☑
　　elbow M12.22- ☑
　　foot joint M12.27- ☑
　　hand joint M12.24- ☑
　　hip M12.25- ☑
　　knee M12.26- ☑
　　multiple site M12.29
　　pelvic region M12.25- ☑
　　shoulder M12.21- ☑
　　specified joint NEC M12.28
　　vertebrae M12.28
　　wrist M12.23- ☑
Syphilid A51.39
　congenital A50.06
　newborn A50.06
　tubercular (late) A52.79
Syphilis, syphilitic (acquired) A53.9
　abdomen (late) A52.79
　acoustic nerve A52.15
　adenopathy (secondary) A51.49
　adrenal (gland) (with cortical hypofunction) A52.79
　age under 2 years NOS — *see also* Syphilis, congenital, early
　　acquired A51.9
　alopecia (secondary) A51.32
　anemia (late) A52.79 [D63.8]
　aneurysm (aorta) (ruptured) A52.01
　　central nervous system A52.05
　　congenital A50.54 [I79.0]
　anus (late) A52.74
　　primary A51.1
　　secondary A51.39
　aorta (arch) (abdominal) (thoracic) A52.02
　　aneurysm A52.01
　aortic (insufficiency) (regurgitation) (stenosis) A52.03
　　aneurysm A52.01
　arachnoid (adhesive) (cerebral) (spinal) A52.13
　asymptomatic — *see* Syphilis, latent
　ataxia (locomotor) A52.11
　atrophoderma maculatum A51.39
　auricular fibrillation A52.06
　bladder (late) A52.76
　bone A52.77
　　secondary A51.46
　brain A52.17
　breast (late) A52.79

Syphilis, syphilitic — *continued*
　bronchus (late) A52.72
　bubo (primary) A51.0
　bulbar palsy A52.19
　bursa (late) A52.78
　cardiac decompensation A52.06
　cardiovascular A52.00
　central nervous system (late) (recurrent) (relapse) (tertiary) A52.3
　　with
　　　ataxia A52.11
　　　general paralysis A52.17
　　　　juvenile A50.45
　　　paresis (general) A52.17
　　　　juvenile A50.45
　　　tabes (dorsalis) A52.11
　　　　juvenile A50.45
　　　taboparesis A52.17
　　　　juvenile A50.45
　　aneurysm A52.05
　　congenital A50.40
　　juvenile A50.40
　　remission in (sustained) A52.3
　　serology doubtful, negative, or positive A52.3
　　specified nature or site NEC A52.19
　　vascular A52.05
　cerebral A52.17
　　meningovascular A52.13
　　nerves (multiple palsies) A52.15
　　sclerosis A52.17
　　thrombosis A52.05
　cerebrospinal (tabetic type) A52.12
　cerebrovascular A52.05
　cervix (late) A52.76
　chancre (multiple) A51.0
　　extragenital A51.2
　　Rollet's A51.0
　Charcot's joint A52.16
　chorioretinitis A51.43
　　congenital A50.01
　　late A52.71
　　prenatal A50.01
　choroiditis — *see* Syphilitic chorioretinitis
　choroidoretinitis — *see* Syphilitic chorioretinitis
　ciliary body (secondary) A51.43
　　late A52.71
　colon (late) A52.74
　combined spinal sclerosis A52.11
　condyloma (latum) A51.31
　congenital A50.9
　　with
　　　paresis (general) A50.45
　　　tabes (dorsalis) A50.45
　　　taboparesis A50.45
　　chorioretinitis, choroiditis A50.01 [H32]
　　early, or less than 2 years after birth NEC A50.2
　　　with manifestations — *see* Syphilis, congenital, early, symptomatic
　　　latent (without manifestations) A50.1
　　　　negative spinal fluid test A50.1
　　　　serology positive A50.1
　　　symptomatic A50.09
　　　　cutaneous A50.06
　　　　mucocutaneous A50.07
　　　　oculopathy A50.01
　　　　osteochondropathy A50.02
　　　　pharyngitis A50.03
　　　　pneumonia A50.04
　　　　rhinitis A50.05
　　　　visceral A50.08
　　　interstitial keratitis A50.31
　　juvenile neurosyphilis A50.45
　　late, or 2 years or more after birth NEC A50.7
　　　chorioretinitis, choroiditis A50.32
　　　interstitial keratitis A50.31
　　　juvenile neurosyphilis A50.45
　　　latent (without manifestations) A50.6
　　　　negative spinal fluid test A50.6
　　　　serology positive A50.6
　　　symptomatic or with manifestations NEC A50.59
　　　　arthropathy A50.55
　　　　cardiovascular A50.54
　　　　Clutton's joints A50.51
　　　　Hutchinson's teeth A50.52
　　　　Hutchinson's triad A50.53
　　　　osteochondropathy A50.56
　　　　saddle nose A50.57
　conjugal A53.9
　　tabes A52.11

Syphilis, syphilitic — *continued*
　conjunctiva (late) A52.71
　contact Z20.2
　cord bladder A52.19
　cornea, late A52.71
　coronary (artery) (sclerosis) A52.06
　coryza, congenital A50.05
　cranial nerve A52.15
　　multiple palsies A52.15
　cutaneous — *see* Syphilis, skin
　dacryocystitis (late) A52.71
　degeneration, spinal cord A52.12
　dementia paralytica A52.17
　　juvenilis A50.45
　destruction of bone A52.77
　dilatation, aorta A52.01
　due to blood transfusion A53.9
　dura mater A52.13
　ear A52.79
　　inner A52.79
　　　nerve (eighth) A52.15
　　　neurorecurrence A52.15
　early A51.9
　　cardiovascular A52.00
　　central nervous system A52.3
　　latent (without manifestations) (less than 2 years after infection) A51.5
　　　negative spinal fluid test A51.5
　　　serological relapse after treatment A51.5
　　　serology positive A51.5
　　relapse (treated, untreated) A51.9
　　skin A51.39
　　symptomatic A51.9
　　　extragenital chancre A51.2
　　　primary, except extragenital chancre A51.0
　　　secondary — *see also* Syphilis, secondary A51.39
　　　　relapse (treated, untreated) A51.49
　　　ulcer A51.39
　eighth nerve (neuritis) A52.15
　endemic A65
　endocarditis A52.03
　　aortic A52.03
　　pulmonary A52.03
　epididymis (late) A52.76
　epiglottis (late) A52.73
　epiphysitis (congenital) (early) A50.02
　episcleritis (late) A52.71
　esophagus A52.79
　eustachian tube A52.73
　exposure to Z20.2
　eye A52.71
　eyelid (late) (with gumma) A52.71
　fallopian tube (late) A52.76
　fracture A52.77
　gallbladder (late) A52.74
　gastric (polyposis) (late) A52.74
　general A53.9
　　paralysis A52.17
　　　juvenile A50.45
　genital (primary) A51.0
　glaucoma A52.71
　gumma NEC A52.79
　　cardiovascular system A52.00
　　central nervous system A52.3
　　congenital A50.59
　heart (block) (decompensation) (disease) (failure) A52.06 [I52]
　　valve NEC A52.03
　hemianesthesia A52.19
　hemianopsia A52.71
　hemiparesis A52.17
　hemiplegia A52.17
　hepatic artery A52.09
　hepatis A52.74
　hepatomegaly, congenital A50.08
　hereditaria tarda — *see* Syphilis, congenital, late
　hereditary — *see* Syphilis, congenital
　Hutchinson's teeth A50.52
　hyalitis A52.71
　inactive — *see* Syphilis, latent
　infantum — *see* Syphilis, congenital
　inherited — *see* Syphilis, congenital
　internal ear A52.79
　intestine (late) A52.74
　iris, iritis (secondary) A51.43
　　late A52.71
　joint (late) A52.77
　keratitis (congenital) (interstitial) (late) A50.31

Syphilis, syphilitic — *continued*
kidney (late) A52.75
lacrimal passages (late) A52.71
larynx (late) A52.73
late A52.9
　cardiovascular A52.00
　central nervous system A52.3
　kidney A52.75
　latent or 2 years or more after infection (without manifestations) A52.8
　　negative spinal fluid test A52.8
　　serology positive A52.8
　paresis A52.17
　specified site NEC A52.79
　symptomatic or with manifestations A52.79
　tabes A52.11
latent A53.0
　with signs or symptoms — *code by* site and stage under Syphilis
　central nervous system A52.2
　date of infection unspecified A53.0
　early, or less than 2 years after infection A51.5
　follow-up of latent syphilis A53.0
　　date of infection unspecified A53.0
　　late, or 2 years or more after infection A52.8
　late, or 2 years or more after infection A52.8
　positive serology (only finding) A53.0
　　date of infection unspecified A53.0
　　early, or less than 2 years after infection A51.5
　　late, or 2 years or more after infection A52.8
lens (late) A52.71
leukoderma A51.39
　late A52.79
lienitis A52.79
lip A51.39
　chancre (primary) A51.2
　late A52.79
Lissauer's paralysis A52.17
liver A52.74
locomotor ataxia A52.11
lung A52.72
lymph gland (early) (secondary) A51.49
　late A52.79
lymphadenitis (secondary) A51.49
macular atrophy of skin A51.39
　striated A52.79
mediastinum (late) A52.73
meninges (adhesive) (brain) (spinal cord) A52.13
meningitis A52.13
　acute (secondary) A51.41
　congenital A50.41
meningoencephalitis A52.14
meningovascular A52.13
　congenital A50.41
mesarteritis A52.09
　brain A52.04
middle ear A52.77
mitral stenosis A52.03
monoplegia A52.17
mouth (secondary) A51.39
　late A52.79
mucocutaneous (secondary) A51.39
　late A52.79
mucous
　membrane (secondary) A51.39
　　late A52.79
　patches A51.39
　　congenital A50.07
mulberry molars A50.52
muscle A52.78
myocardium A52.06
nasal sinus (late) A52.73
neonatorum — *see* Syphilis, congenital
nephrotic syndrome (secondary) A51.44
nerve palsy (any cranial nerve) A52.15
　multiple A52.15
nervous system, central A52.3
neuritis A52.15
　acoustic A52.15
neurorecidive of retina A52.19
neuroretinitis A52.19
newborn — *see* Syphilis, congenital
nodular superficial (late) A52.79
nonvenereal A65
nose (late) A52.73
　saddle back deformity A50.57
occlusive arterial disease A52.09
oculopathy A52.71
ophthalmic (late) A52.71

Syphilis, syphilitic — *continued*
optic nerve (atrophy) (neuritis) (papilla) A52.15
orbit (late) A52.71
organic A53.9
osseous (late) A52.77
osteochondritis (congenital) (early) A50.02 [M90.80]
osteoporosis A52.77
ovary (late) A52.76
oviduct (late) A52.76
palate (late) A52.79
pancreas (late) A52.74
paralysis A52.17
　general A52.17
　　juvenile A50.45
paresis (general) A52.17
　juvenile A50.45
paresthesia A52.19
Parkinson's disease or syndrome A52.19
paroxysmal tachycardia A52.06
pemphigus (congenital) A50.06
penis (chancre) A51.0
　late A52.76
pericardium A52.06
perichondritis, larynx (late) A52.73
periosteum (late) A52.77
　congenital (early) A50.02 [M90.80]
　early (secondary) A51.46
peripheral nerve A52.79
petrous bone (late) A52.77
pharynx (late) A52.73
　secondary A51.39
pituitary (gland) A52.79
pleura (late) A52.73
pneumonia, white A50.04
pontine lesion A52.17
portal vein A52.09
primary A51.0
　anal A51.1
　and secondary — *see* Syphilis, secondary
　central nervous system A52.3
　extragenital chancre NEC A51.2
　fingers A51.2
　genital A51.0
　lip A51.2
　specified site NEC A51.2
　tonsils A51.2
prostate (late) A52.76
ptosis (eyelid) A52.71
pulmonary (late) A52.72
　artery A52.09
pyelonephritis (late) A52.75
recently acquired, symptomatic A51.9
rectum (late) A52.74
respiratory tract (late) A52.73
retina, late A52.71
retrobulbar neuritis A52.15
salpingitis A52.76
sclera (late) A52.71
sclerosis
　cerebral A52.17
　coronary A52.06
　multiple A52.11
scotoma (central) A52.71
scrotum (late) A52.76
secondary (and primary) A51.49
　adenopathy A51.49
　anus A51.39
　bone A51.46
　chorioretinitis, choroiditis A51.43
　hepatitis A51.45
　liver A51.45
　lymphadenitis A51.49
　meningitis (acute) A51.41
　mouth A51.39
　mucous membranes A51.39
　periosteum, periostitis A51.46
　pharynx A51.39
　relapse (treated, untreated) A51.49
　skin A51.39
　specified form NEC A51.49
　tonsil A51.39
　ulcer A51.39
　viscera NEC A51.49
　vulva A51.39
seminal vesicle (late) A52.76

Syphilis, syphilitic — *continued*
seronegative with signs or symptoms — *code by* site and stage under Syphilis
seropositive
　with signs or symptoms — *code by* site and stage under Syphilis
　follow-up of latent syphilis — *see* Syphilis, latent
　only finding — *see* Syphilis, latent
seventh nerve (paralysis) A52.15
sinus, sinusitis (late) A52.73
skeletal system A52.77
skin (with ulceration) (early) (secondary) A51.39
　late or tertiary A52.79
small intestine A52.74
spastic spinal paralysis A52.17
spermatic cord (late) A52.76
spinal (cord) A52.12
spleen A52.79
splenomegaly A52.79
spondylitis A52.77
staphyloma A52.71
stigmata (congenital) A50.59
stomach A52.74
synovium A52.78
tabes dorsalis (late) A52.11
　juvenile A50.45
tabetic type A52.11
　juvenile A50.45
taboparesis A52.17
　juvenile A50.45
tachycardia A52.06
tendon (late) A52.78
tertiary A52.9
　with symptoms NEC A52.79
　cardiovascular A52.00
　central nervous system A52.3
　multiple NEC A52.79
　specified site NEC A52.79
testis A52.76
thorax A52.73
throat A52.73
thymus (gland) (late) A52.79
thyroid (late) A52.79
tongue (late) A52.79
tonsil (lingual) (late) A52.73
　primary A51.2
　secondary A51.39
trachea (late) A52.73
tunica vaginalis (late) A52.76
ulcer (any site) (early) (secondary) A51.39
　late A52.79
　perforating A52.79
　　foot A52.11
urethra (late) A52.76
urogenital (late) A52.76
uterus (late) A52.76
uveal tract (secondary) A51.43
　late A52.71
uveitis (secondary) A51.43
　late A52.71
uvula (late) (perforated) A52.79
vagina A51.0
　late A52.76
valvulitis NEC A52.03
vascular A52.00
　brain (cerebral) A52.05
ventriculi A52.74
vesicae urinariae (late) A52.76
viscera (abdominal) (late) A52.74
　secondary A51.49
vitreous (opacities) (late) A52.71
　hemorrhage A52.71
vulva A51.0
　late A52.76
　secondary A51.39
Syphiloma A52.79
cardiovascular system A52.00
central nervous system A52.3
circulatory system A52.00
congenital A50.59
Syphilophobia F45.29
Syringadenoma — *see also* Neoplasm, skin, benign
papillary — *see* Neoplasm, skin, benign
Syringobulbia G95.0
Syringocystadenoma — *see* Neoplasm, skin, benign
papillary — *see* Neoplasm, skin, benign
Syringoma — *see also* Neoplasm, skin, benign
chondroid — *see* Neoplasm, skin, benign

Syringomyelia G95.0
Syringomyelitis — *see* Encephalitis
Syringomyelocele — *see* Spina bifida
Syringopontia G95.0

System, systemic — *see also* condition
  disease, combined — *see* Degeneration, combined
  inflammatory response syndrome (SIRS) of non-infectious origin (without organ dysfunction) R65.10
    with acute organ dysfunction R65.11

System, systemic — *continued*
  lupus erythematosus M32.9
    inhibitor present D68.62
Systemic exertion intolerance disease [SEID] G93.32

T

Tabacism, tabacosis, tabagism — *see also* Poisoning, tobacco
  meaning dependence (without remission) F17.200
    with
      disorder F17.299
        in remission F17.211
        specified disorder NEC F17.298
        withdrawal F17.203
Tabardillo A75.9
  flea-borne A75.2
  louse-borne A75.0
Tabes, tabetic A52.10
  with
    central nervous system syphilis A52.10
    Charcot's joint A52.16
    cord bladder A52.19
    crisis, viscera (any) A52.19
    paralysis, general A52.17
    paresis (general) A52.17
    perforating ulcer (foot) A52.19
  arthropathy (Charcot) A52.16
  bladder A52.19
  bone A52.11
  cerebrospinal A52.12
  congenital A50.45
  conjugal A52.10
  dorsalis A52.11
    juvenile A50.49
  juvenile A50.49
  latent A52.19
  mesenterica A18.39
  paralysis, insane, general A52.17
  spasmodic A52.17
  syphilis (cerebrospinal) A52.12
Taboparalysis A52.17
Taboparesis (remission) A52.17
  juvenile A50.45
TAC (trigeminal autonomic cephalgia) **NEC** G44.099
  intractable G44.091
  not intractable G44.099
Tache noir S60.22-✓
Tachyalimentation K91.2
Tachyarrhythmia, tachyrhythmia — *see* Tachycardia
Tachycardia R00.0
  atrial (paroxysmal) I47.1
  auricular I47.1
  AV nodal re-entry (re-entrant) I47.1
  junctional (paroxysmal) I47.1
  newborn P29.11
  nodal (paroxysmal) I47.1
  non-paroxysmal AV nodal I45.89
  paroxysmal (sustained) (nonsustained) I47.9
    with sinus bradycardia I49.5
    atrial (PAT) I47.1
    atrioventricular (AV) (re-entrant) I47.1
      psychogenic F54
    junctional I47.1
      ectopic I47.1
    nodal I47.1
    psychogenic (atrial) (supraventricular) (ventricular) F54
    supraventricular (sustained) I47.1
      psychogenic F54
    ventricular I47.20
      psychogenic F54
      specified type NEC I47.29
  psychogenic F45.8
  sick sinus I49.5
  sinoauricular NOS R00.0
    paroxysmal I47.1
  sinus [sinusal] NOS R00.0
    paroxysmal I47.1
  supraventricular I47.1
  ventricular (paroxysmal) (sustained) I47.20
    psychogenic F54
    specified NEC I47.29
Tachygastria K31.89
Tachypnea R06.82
  hysterical F45.8
  newborn (idiopathic) (transitory) P22.1
  psychogenic F45.8
  transitory, of newborn P22.1
TACO (transfusion associated circulatory overload) E87.71
TAD (transfusion-associated dyspnea) J95.87
Taenia (infection) (infestation) B68.9

Taenia — *continued*
  diminuta B71.0
  echinococcal infestation B67.90
  mediocanellata B68.1
  nana B71.0
  saginata B68.1
  solium (intestinal form) B68.0
    larval form — *see* Cysticercosis
Taeniasis (intestine) — *see* Taenia
Tag (hypertrophied skin) (infected) L91.8
  adenoid J35.8
  anus K64.4
  hemorrhoidal K64.4
  hymen N89.8
  perineal N90.89
  preauricular Q17.0
  sentinel K64.4
  skin L91.8
    accessory (congenital) Q82.8
    anus K64.4
    congenital Q82.8
    preauricular Q17.0
  tonsil J35.8
  urethra, urethral N36.8
  vulva N90.89
Tahyna fever B33.8
Takahara's disease E80.3
Takayasu's disease or syndrome M31.4
Talaromycosis B48.4
Talcosis (pulmonary) J62.0
Talipes (congenital) Q66.89
  acquired, planus — *see* Deformity, limb, flat foot
  asymmetric Q66.89
  calcaneovalgus Q66.4-✓
  calcaneovarus Q66.1-✓
  calcaneus Q66.89
  cavus Q66.7-✓
  equinovalgus Q66.6
  equinovarus Q66.0-✓
  equinus Q66.89
  percavus Q66.7-✓
  planovalgus Q66.6
  planus (acquired) (any degree) — *see also* Deformity, limb, flat foot
    congenital Q66.5-✓
    due to rickets (sequelae) E64.3
  valgus Q66.6
  varus Q66.3-✓
Tall stature, constitutional E34.4
Talma's disease M62.89
Talon noir S90.3-✓
  hand S60.22-✓
  heel S90.3-✓
  toe S90.1-✓
Tamponade, heart I31.4
Tanapox (virus disease) B08.71
Tangier disease E78.6
Tantrum, child problem F91.8
Tapeworm (infection) (infestation) — *see* Infestation, tapeworm
Tapia's syndrome G52.7
TAR (thrombocytopenia with absent radius) **syndrome** Q87.2
Tarral-Besnier disease L44.0
Tarsal tunnel syndrome — *see* Syndrome, tarsal tunnel
Tarsalgia — *see* Pain, limb, lower
Tarsitis (eyelid) H01.8
  syphilitic A52.71
  tuberculous A18.4
Tartar (teeth) (dental calculus) K03.6
Tattoo (mark) L81.8
Tauri's disease E74.09
Taurodontism K00.2
Taussig-Bing syndrome Q20.1
Taybi's syndrome Q87.2
Tay-Sachs amaurotic familial idiocy or disease E75.02
TBI (traumatic brain injury) S06.9✓
Teacher's node or nodule J38.2
Tear, torn (traumatic) — *see also* Laceration
  with abortion — *see* Abortion
  annular fibrosis M51.35
  anus, anal (sphincter) S31.831✓
    complicating delivery
      with third degree perineal laceration — *see also* Delivery, complicated, by, laceration, perineum, third degree O70.20
        with mucosa O70.3

Tear, torn — *continued*
  anus, anal — *continued*
    complicating delivery — *continued*
      without third degree perineal laceration O70.4
    nontraumatic (healed) (old) K62.81
  articular cartilage, old — *see* Derangement, joint, articular cartilage, by site
  bladder
    with ectopic or molar pregnancy O08.6
    following ectopic or molar pregnancy O08.6
    obstetrical O71.5
    traumatic — *see* Injury, bladder
  bowel
    with ectopic or molar pregnancy O08.6
    following ectopic or molar pregnancy O08.6
    obstetrical trauma O71.5
  broad ligament
    with ectopic or molar pregnancy O08.6
    following ectopic or molar pregnancy O08.6
    obstetrical trauma O71.6
  bucket handle (knee) (meniscus) — *see* Tear, meniscus
  capsule, joint — *see* Sprain
  cartilage — *see also* Sprain
    articular, old — *see* Derangement, joint, articular cartilage, by site
  cervix
    with ectopic or molar pregnancy O08.6
    following ectopic or molar pregnancy O08.6
    obstetrical trauma (current) O71.3
    old N88.1
    traumatic — *see* Injury, uterus
  dural G97.41
    nontraumatic G96.11
  internal organ — *see* Injury, by site
  knee cartilage
    articular (current) S83.3-✓
    old — *see* Derangement, knee, meniscus, due to old tear
  ligament — *see* Sprain
  meniscus (knee) (current injury) S83.209✓
    bucket-handle S83.20-✓
    lateral
      bucket-handle S83.25-✓
      complex S83.27-✓
      peripheral S83.26-✓
      specified type NEC S83.28-✓
    medial
      bucket-handle S83.21-✓
      complex S83.23-✓
      peripheral S83.22-✓
      specified type NEC S83.24-✓
    old — *see* Derangement, knee, meniscus, due to old tear
    site other than knee — *code as* Sprain
    specified type NEC S83.20-✓
  muscle — *see* Strain
  pelvic
    floor, complicating delivery O70.1
    organ NEC, obstetrical trauma O71.5
      with ectopic or molar pregnancy O08.6
      following ectopic or molar pregnancy O08.6
  perineal, secondary O90.1
  periurethral tissue, obstetrical trauma O71.82
    with ectopic or molar pregnancy O08.6
    following ectopic or molar pregnancy O08.6
  rectovaginal septum — *see* Laceration, vagina
  retina, retinal (without detachment) (horseshoe) — *see also* Break, retina, horseshoe
    with detachment — *see* Detachment, retina, with retinal, break
  rotator cuff (nontraumatic) M75.10-✓
    complete M75.12-✓
    incomplete M75.11-✓
    traumatic S46.01-✓
      capsule S43.42-✓
  semilunar cartilage, knee — *see* Tear, meniscus
  supraspinatus (complete) (incomplete) (nontraumatic) — *see also* Tear, rotator cuff M75.10-✓
  tendon — *see* Strain
  tentorial, at birth P10.4
  umbilical cord
    complicating delivery O69.89✓
  urethra
    with ectopic or molar pregnancy O08.6
    following ectopic or molar pregnancy O08.6
    obstetrical trauma O71.5
  uterus — *see* Injury, uterus

Tear, torn — *continued*
- vagina — *see* Laceration, vagina
- vessel, from catheter — *see* Puncture, accidental complicating surgery
- vulva, complicating delivery O70.0

Tear-stone — *see* Dacryolith

Teeth — *see also* condition
- grinding
  - psychogenic F45.8
  - sleep related G47.63

Teething (syndrome) K00.7

Telangiectasia, telangiectasis (verrucous) I78.1
- ataxic (cerebellar) (Louis-Bar) G11.3
- familial I78.0
- hemorrhagic, hereditary (congenital) (senile) I78.0
- hereditary, hemorrhagic (congenital) (senile) I78.0
- juxtafoveal H35.07- ☑
- macular H35.07- ☑
- macularis eruptiva perstans D47.01
- parafoveal H35.07- ☑
- retinal (idiopathic) (juxtafoveal) (macular) (parafoveal) H35.07- ☑
- spider I78.1

Telephone scatologia F65.89

Telescoped bowel or intestine K56.1
- congenital Q43.8

Temperature
- body, high (of unknown origin) R50.9
- cold, trauma from T69.9 ☑
  - newborn P80.0
  - specified effect NEC T69.8 ☑

Temple — *see* condition

Temporal — *see* condition

Temporomandibular joint pain-dysfunction syndrome M26.62- ☑

Temporosphenoidal — *see* condition

Tendency
- bleeding — *see* Defect, coagulation
- suicide
  - meaning personal history of attempted suicide Z91.51
  - meaning suicidal ideation — *see* Ideation, suicidal
- to fall R29.6

Tenderness, abdominal R10.819
- epigastric R10.816
- generalized R10.817
- left lower quadrant R10.814
- left upper quadrant R10.812
- periumbilic R10.815
- rebound R10.829
  - epigastric R10.826
  - generalized R10.827
  - left lower quadrant R10.824
  - left upper quadrant R10.822
  - periumbilic R10.825
  - right lower quadrant R10.823
  - right upper quadrant R10.821
- right lower quadrant R10.813
- right upper quadrant R10.811

Tendinitis, tendonitis — *see also* Enthesopathy
- Achilles M76.6- ☑
- adhesive — *see* Tenosynovitis, specified type NEC
  - shoulder — *see* Capsulitis, adhesive
- bicipital M75.2- ☑
- calcific M65.2- ☑
  - ankle M65.27- ☑
  - foot M65.27- ☑
  - forearm M65.23- ☑
  - hand M65.24- ☑
  - lower leg M65.26- ☑
  - multiple sites M65.29
  - pelvic region M65.25- ☑
  - shoulder M75.3- ☑
  - specified site NEC M65.28
  - thigh M65.25- ☑
  - upper arm M65.22- ☑
- due to use, overuse, pressure — *see also* Disorder, soft tissue, due to use
  - specified NEC — *see* Disorder, soft tissue, due to use, specified NEC
- gluteal M76.0- ☑
- patellar M76.5- ☑
- peroneal M76.7- ☑
- psoas M76.1- ☑
- tibial (posterior) M76.82- ☑
  - anterior M76.81- ☑
- trochanteric — *see* Bursitis, hip, trochanteric

Tendon — *see* condition

Tendosynovitis — *see* Tenosynovitis

Tenesmus (rectal) R19.8
- vesical R30.1

Tennis elbow — *see* Epicondylitis, lateral

Tenonitis — *see also* Tenosynovitis
- eye (capsule) H05.04- ☑

Tenontosynovitis — *see* Tenosynovitis

Tenontothecitis — *see* Tenosynovitis

Tenophyte — *see* Disorder, synovium, specified type NEC

Tenosynovitis — *see also* Synovitis M65.9
- adhesive — *see* Tenosynovitis, specified type NEC
  - shoulder — *see* Capsulitis, adhesive
- bicipital (calcifying) — *see* Tendinitis, bicipital
- gonococcal A54.49
- in (due to)
  - crystals M65.8- ☑
  - gonorrhea A54.49
  - syphilis (late) A52.78
  - use, overuse, pressure — *see also* Disorder, soft tissue, due to use
    - specified NEC — *see* Disorder, soft tissue, due to use, specified NEC
- infective NEC M65.1- ☑
  - ankle M65.17- ☑
  - foot M65.17- ☑
  - forearm M65.13- ☑
  - hand M65.14- ☑
  - lower leg M65.16- ☑
  - multiple sites M65.19
  - pelvic region M65.15- ☑
  - shoulder region M65.11- ☑
  - specified site NEC M65.18
  - thigh M65.15- ☑
  - upper arm M65.12- ☑
- radial styloid M65.4
- shoulder region M65.81- ☑
  - adhesive — *see* Capsulitis, adhesive
- specified type NEC M65.88
  - ankle M65.87- ☑
  - foot M65.87- ☑
  - forearm M65.83- ☑
  - hand M65.84- ☑
  - lower leg M65.86- ☑
  - multiple sites M65.89
  - pelvic region M65.85- ☑
  - shoulder region M65.81- ☑
  - specified site NEC M65.88
  - thigh M65.85- ☑
  - upper arm M65.82- ☑
- tuberculous — *see* Tuberculosis, tenosynovitis

Tenovaginitis — *see* Tenosynovitis

Tension
- arterial, high — *see also* Hypertension
  - without diagnosis of hypertension R03.0
- headache G44.209
  - intractable G44.201
  - not intractable G44.209
- nervous R45.0
- pneumothorax J93.0
- premenstrual N94.3
- state (mental) F48.9

Tentorium — *see* condition

Teratencephalus Q89.8

Teratism Q89.7

Teratoblastoma (malignant) — *see* Neoplasm, malignant, by site

Teratocarcinoma — *see also* Neoplasm, malignant, by site
- liver C22.7

Teratoma (solid) — *see also* Neoplasm, uncertain behavior, by site
- with embryonal carcinoma, mixed — *see* Neoplasm, malignant, by site
- with malignant transformation — *see* Neoplasm, malignant, by site
- adult (cystic) — *see* Neoplasm, benign, by site
- benign — *see* Neoplasm, benign, by site
- combined with choriocarcinoma — *see* Neoplasm, malignant, by site
- cystic (adult) — *see* Neoplasm, benign, by site
- differentiated — *see* Neoplasm, benign, by site
- embryonal — *see also* Neoplasm, malignant, by site
  - liver C22.7
- immature — *see* Neoplasm, malignant, by site
  - liver C22.7

Teratoma — *continued*
- liver — *continued*
  - adult, benign, cystic, differentiated type or mature D13.4
  - malignant — *see also* Neoplasm, malignant, by site
    - anaplastic — *see* Neoplasm, malignant, by site
    - intermediate — *see* Neoplasm, malignant, by site
    - specified site — *see* Neoplasm, malignant, by site
    - unspecified site C62.90
    - undifferentiated — *see* Neoplasm, malignant, by site
  - mature — *see* Neoplasm, uncertain behavior, by site
    - malignant — *see* Neoplasm, by site, malignant, by site
- ovary D27.- ☑
  - embryonal, immature or malignant C56- ☑
- solid — *see* Neoplasm, uncertain behavior, by site
- testis C62.9- ☑
  - adult, benign, cystic, differentiated type or mature D29.2- ☑
  - scrotal C62.1- ☑
  - undescended C62.0- ☑

Termination
- anomalous — *see also* Malposition, congenital
  - right pulmonary vein Q26.3
- pregnancy, elective Z33.2

Ternidens diminutus infestation B81.8

Ternidensiasis B81.8

Terror(s) night (child) F51.4

Terrorism, victim of Z65.4

Terry's syndrome — *see also* Myopia, degenerative H44.2- ☑

Tertiary — *see* condition

Test, tests, testing (for)
- adequacy (for dialysis)
  - hemodialysis Z49.31
  - peritoneal Z49.32
- blood pressure Z01.30
  - abnormal reading — *see* Blood, pressure
- blood typing Z01.83
  - Rh typing Z01.83
- blood-alcohol Z02.83
  - positive — *see* Findings, abnormal, in blood
- blood-drug Z02.83
  - positive — *see* Findings, abnormal, in blood
- cardiac pulse generator (battery) Z45.010
- fertility Z31.41
- genetic
  - disease carrier status for procreative management
    - female Z31.430
    - male Z31.440
  - male partner of patient with recurrent pregnancy loss Z31.441
  - procreative management NEC
    - female Z31.438
    - male Z31.448
- hearing Z01.10
  - with abnormal findings NEC Z01.118
  - infant or child (over 28 days old) Z00.129
    - with abnormal findings Z00.121
- HIV (human immunodeficiency virus)
  - nonconclusive (in infants) R75
  - positive Z21
  - seropositive Z21
- immunity status Z01.84
- intelligence NEC Z01.89
- laboratory (as part of a general medical examination) Z00.00
  - with abnormal finding Z00.01
  - for medicolegal reason NEC Z04.89
- male partner of patient with recurrent pregnancy loss Z31.441
- Mantoux (for tuberculosis) Z11.1
  - abnormal result R76.11
- pregnancy, positive first pregnancy — *see* Pregnancy, normal, first
- procreative Z31.49
  - fertility Z31.41
- skin, diagnostic
  - allergy Z01.82
    - special screening examination — *see* Screening, by name of disease
  - Mantoux Z11.1
  - tuberculin Z11.1
  - specified NEC Z01.89
- tuberculin Z11.1
  - abnormal result R76.11

Test, tests, testing — *continued*
  vision Z01.00
    with abnormal findings Z01.01
    following failed vision screening Z01.020
      with abnormal findings Z01.021
    infant or child (over 28 days old) Z00.129
      with abnormal findings Z00.121
  Wassermann Z11.3
    positive — *see* Serology for syphilis, positive
Testicle, testicular, testis — *see also* condition
  feminization syndrome — *see also* Syndrome, androgen insensitivity E34.51
  migrans Q55.29
Tetanus, tetanic (cephalic) (convulsions) A35
  with
    abortion A34
    ectopic or molar pregnancy O08.0
  following ectopic or molar pregnancy O08.0
  inoculation reaction (due to serum) — *see* Complications, vaccination
  neonatorum A33
  obstetrical A34
  puerperal, postpartum, childbirth A34
Tetany (due to) R29.0
  alkalosis E87.3
  associated with rickets E55.0
  convulsions R29.0
    hysterical F44.5
  functional (hysterical) F44.5
  hyperkinetic R29.0
    hysterical F44.5
  hyperpnea R06.4
    hysterical F44.5
    psychogenic F45.8
  hyperventilation — *see also* Hyperventilation R06.4
    hysterical F44.5
  neonatal (without calcium or magnesium deficiency) P71.3
  parathyroid (gland) E20.9
  parathyroprival E89.2
  post- (para)thyroidectomy E89.2
  postoperative E89.2
  pseudotetany R29.0
  psychogenic (conversion reaction) F44.5
Tetralogy of Fallot Q21.3
Tetraplegia (chronic) — *see also* Quadriplegia G82.50
Thailand hemorrhagic fever A91
Thalassanemia — *see* Thalassemia
Thalassemia (anemia) (disease) D56.9
  with other hemoglobinopathy D56.8
  alpha (major) (severe) (triple gene defect) D56.0
    minor D56.3
    silent carrier D56.3
    trait D56.3
  beta (severe) D56.1
    homozygous D56.1
    major D56.1
    minor D56.3
    trait D56.3
  delta-beta (homozygous) D56.2
    minor D56.3
    trait D56.3
  dominant D56.8
  hemoglobin
    C D56.8
    E-beta D56.5
  intermedia D56.1
  major D56.1
  minor D56.3
  mixed D56.8
  sickle-cell — *see* Disease, sickle-cell, thalassemia
  specified type NEC D56.8
  trait D56.3
  variants D56.8
Thanatophoric dwarfism or short stature Q77.1
Thaysen-Gee disease (nontropical sprue) K90.0
Thaysen's disease K90.0
Thecoma D27- ☑
  luteinized D27- ☑
  malignant C56- ☑
Thelarche, premature E30.8
Thelaziasis B83.8
Thelitis N61.0
  puerperal, postpartum or gestational — *see* Infection, nipple
Therapeutic — *see* condition

Therapy
  drug, long-term (current) (prophylactic)
    agents affecting estrogen receptors and estrogen levels NEC Z79.818
    anastrozole (Arimidex) Z79.811
    antibiotics Z79.2
      short-term use — *omit code*
    anticoagulants Z79.01
    anti-inflammatory Z79.1
    antiplatelet Z79.02
    antithrombotics Z79.02
    aromatase inhibitors Z79.811
    aspirin Z79.82
    birth control pill or patch Z79.3
    bisphosphonates Z79.83
    contraceptive, oral Z79.3
    drug, specified NEC Z79.899
    estrogen receptor downregulators Z79.818
    Evista Z79.810
    exemestane (Aromasin) Z79.811
    Fareston Z79.810
    fulvestrant (Faslodex) Z79.818
    gonadotropin-releasing hormone (GnRH) agonist Z79.818
    goserelin acetate (Zoladex) Z79.818
    hormone replacement Z79.890
    insulin Z79.4
    letrozole (Femara) Z79.811
    leuprolide acetate (leuprorelin) (Lupron) Z79.818
    megestrol acetate (Megace) Z79.818
    methadone
      for pain management Z79.891
      maintenance therapy F11.20
    Nolvadex Z79.810
    opiate analgesic Z79.891
    oral contraceptive Z79.3
    raloxifene (Evista) Z79.810
    selective estrogen receptor modulators (SERMs) Z79.810
    short term — *omit code*
    steroids
      inhaled Z79.51
      systemic Z79.52
    tamoxifen (Nolvadex) Z79.810
    toremifene (Fareston) Z79.810
Thermic — *see* condition
Thermography (abnormal) — *see also* Abnormal, diagnostic imaging R93.89
  breast R92.8
Thermoplegia T67.01 ☑
Thesaurismosis, glycogen — *see* Disease, glycogen storage
Thiamin deficiency E51.9
  specified NEC E51.8
Thiaminic deficiency with beriberi E51.11
Thibierge-Weissenbach syndrome — *see* Sclerosis, systemic
Thickening
  bone — *see* Hypertrophy, bone
  breast N64.59
  endometrium R93.89
  epidermal L85.9
    specified NEC L85.8
  hymen N89.6
  larynx J38.7
  nail L60.2
    congenital Q84.5
  periosteal — *see* Hypertrophy, bone
  pleura J92.9
    with asbestos J92.0
  skin R23.4
  subepiglottic J38.7
  tongue K14.8
  valve, heart — *see* Endocarditis
Thigh — *see* condition
Thinning vertebra — *see* Spondylopathy, specified NEC
Thirst, excessive R63.1
  due to deprivation of water T73.1 ☑
Thomsen disease G71.12
Thoracic — *see also* condition
  kidney Q63.2
  outlet syndrome G54.0
Thoracogastroschisis (congenital) Q79.8
Thoracopagus Q89.4
Thorax — *see* condition
Thorn's syndrome N28.89
Thorson-Björck syndrome E34.0
Threadworm (infection) (infestation) B80

Threatened
  abortion O20.0
    with subsequent abortion O03.9
  job loss, anxiety concerning Z56.2
  labor (without delivery) O47.9
    at or after 37 completed weeks of gestation O47.1
    before 37 completed weeks of gestation O47.0- ☑
  loss of job, anxiety concerning Z56.2
  miscarriage O20.0
  unemployment, anxiety concerning Z56.2
Three-day fever A93.1
Threshers' lung J67.0
Thrix annulata (congenital) Q84.1
Throat — *see* condition
Thrombasthenia (Glanzmann) (hemorrhagic) (hereditary) D69.1
Thromboangiitis I73.1
  obliterans (general) I73.1
    cerebral I67.89
    vessels
      brain I67.89
      spinal cord I67.89
Thromboarteritis — *see* Arteritis
Thromboasthenia (Glanzmann) (hemorrhagic) (hereditary) D69.1
Thrombocytasthenia (Glanzmann) D69.1
Thrombocythemia (hemorrhagic) *see also* Thrombocytosis D75.839
  essential D47.3
  idiopathic D47.3
  primary D47.3
Thrombocytopathy (dystrophic) (granulopenic) D69.1
Thrombocytopenia, thrombocytopenic D69.6
  with absent radius (TAR) Q87.2
  congenital D69.42
  dilutional D69.59
  due to
    (massive) blood transfusion D69.59
    drugs D69.59
    extracorporeal circulation of blood D69.59
    platelet alloimmunization D69.59
  essential D69.3
  heparin induced (HIT) D75.829
    delayed-onset D75.828
    immune-mediated D75.822
    non-immune D75.821
    persisting D75.828
    syndrome
      autoimmune D75.828
      specified NEC D75.828
      spontaneous (without heparin exposure) D75.84
    type 1 D75.821
    type 2 D75.822
  heparin-associated D75.821
  hereditary D69.42
  idiopathic D69.3
  neonatal, transitory P61.0
    due to
      exchange transfusion P61.0
      idiopathic maternal thrombocytopenia P61.0
      isoimmunization P61.0
  primary NEC D69.49
    idiopathic D69.3
  puerperal, postpartum O72.3
  secondary D69.59
  transient neonatal P61.0
  vaccine-induced thrombotic D75.84
Thrombocytosis D75.839
  essential D47.3
  idiopathic D47.3
  primary D47.3
  reactive D75.838
  secondary D75.838
  specified NEC D75.838
Thromboembolism — *see* Embolism
Thrombopathy (Bernard-Soulier) D69.1
  constitutional — *see* Disease, von Willebrand
  Willebrand-Jurgens — *see* Disease, von Willebrand
Thrombopenia — *see* Thrombocytopenia
Thrombophilia D68.59
  primary NEC D68.59
  secondary NEC D68.69
  specified NEC D68.69
Thrombophlebitis I80.9
  antepartum O22.2- ☑
    deep O22.3- ☑
    superficial O22.2- ☑
  calf muscular vein (NOS) I80.25- ☑

☑ **Additional Character Required — Refer to the Tabular List for Character Selection**

Thrombophlebitis — *continued*
cavernous (venous) sinus G08
  complicating pregnancy O22.5- ☑
  nonpyogenic I67.6
cerebral (sinus) (vein) G08
  nonpyogenic I67.6
  sequelae G09
due to implanted device — *see* Complications, by site and type, specified NEC
during or resulting from a procedure NEC T81.72 ☑
femoral vein (superficial) I80.1- ☑
femoropopliteal vein I80.0- ☑
gastrocnemial vein I80.25- ☑
hepatic (vein) I80.8
idiopathic, recurrent I82.1
iliac vein (common) (external) (internal) I80.21- ☑
iliofemoral I80.1- ☑
intracranial venous sinus (any) G08
  nonpyogenic I67.6
  sequelae G09
intraspinal venous sinuses and veins G08
  nonpyogenic G95.19
lateral (venous) sinus G08
  nonpyogenic I67.6
leg I80.3
  superficial I80.0- ☑
longitudinal (venous) sinus G08
  nonpyogenic I67.6
lower extremity I80.299
migrans, migrating I82.1
pelvic
  with ectopic or molar pregnancy O08.0
  following ectopic or molar pregnancy O08.0
  puerperal O87.1
peroneal vein I80.24- ☑
popliteal vein — *see* Phlebitis, leg, deep, popliteal
portal (vein) K75.1
postoperative T81.72 ☑
pregnancy — *see* Thrombophlebitis, antepartum
puerperal, postpartum, childbirth O87.0
  deep O87.1
  pelvic O87.1
  septic O86.81
  superficial O87.0
saphenous (greater) (lesser) I80.0- ☑
sinus (intracranial) G08
  nonpyogenic I67.6
soleal vein I80.25- ☑
specified site NEC I80.8
tibial vein (anterior) (posterior) I80.23- ☑

Thrombosis, thrombotic (bland) (multiple) (progressive) (silent) (vessel) I82.90
anal K64.5
antepartum — *see* Thrombophlebitis, antepartum
aorta, aortic I74.10
  abdominal I74.09
    saddle I74.01
  bifurcation I74.09
  saddle I74.01
  specified site NEC I74.19
  terminal I74.09
  thoracic I74.11
  valve — *see* Endocarditis, aortic
apoplexy I63.3- ☑
artery, arteries (postinfectional) I74.9
  auditory, internal — *see* Occlusion, artery, precerebral, specified NEC
  basilar — *see* Occlusion, artery, basilar
  carotid (common) (internal) — *see* Occlusion, artery, carotid
  cerebellar (anterior inferior) (posterior inferior) (superior) — *see* Occlusion, artery, cerebellar
  cerebral — *see* Occlusion, artery, cerebral
  choroidal (anterior) — *see* Occlusion, artery, precerebral, specified NEC
  communicating, posterior — *see* Occlusion, artery, precerebral, specified NEC
  coronary — *see also* Infarct, myocardium
    not resulting in infarction I24.0
  hepatic I74.8
  hypophyseal — *see* Occlusion, artery, precerebral, specified NEC
  iliac I74.5
  limb I74.4
    lower I74.3
    upper I74.2
  meningeal, anterior or posterior — *see* Occlusion, artery, cerebral, specified NEC

Thrombosis, thrombotic — *continued*
artery, arteries — *continued*
  mesenteric (with gangrene) — *see also* Infarct, intestine K55.069
  ophthalmic — *see* Occlusion, artery, retina
  pontine — *see* Occlusion, artery, precerebral, specified NEC
  precerebral — *see* Occlusion, artery, precerebral
  pulmonary (iatrogenic) — *see* Embolism, pulmonary
  renal N28.0
  retinal — *see* Occlusion, artery, retina
  spinal, anterior or posterior G95.11
  traumatic NEC T14.8 ☑
  vertebral — *see* Occlusion, artery, vertebral
atrium, auricular — *see also* Infarct, myocardium
  following acute myocardial infarction (current complication) I23.6
  not resulting in infarction I51.3
  old I51.3
basilar (artery) — *see* Occlusion, artery, basilar
brain (artery) (stem) — *see also* Occlusion, artery, cerebral
  due to syphilis A52.05
  puerperal O99.43
  sinus — *see* Thrombosis, intracranial venous sinus
capillary I78.8
cardiac — *see also* Infarct, myocardium
  not resulting in infarction I51.3
  old I51.3
  valve — *see* Endocarditis
carotid (artery) (common) (internal) — *see* Occlusion, artery, carotid
cavernous (venous) sinus — *see* Thrombosis, intracranial venous sinus
cerebellar artery (anterior inferior) (posterior inferior) (superior) I66.3
cerebral (artery) — *see* Occlusion, artery, cerebral
cerebrovenous sinus — *see also* Thrombosis, intracranial venous sinus
  puerperium O87.3
chronic I82.91
coronary (artery) (vein) — *see also* Infarct, myocardium
  not resulting in infarction I24.0
corpus cavernosum N48.89
cortical I66.9
deep — *see* Embolism, vein, lower extremity
due to device, implant or graft — *see also* Complications, by site and type, specified NEC T85.868 ☑
  arterial graft NEC T82.868 ☑
  breast (implant) T85.868 ☑
  catheter NEC T85.868 ☑
    dialysis (renal) T82.868 ☑
      intraperitoneal T85.868 ☑
    infusion NEC T82.868 ☑
      spinal (epidural) (subdural) T85.860 ☑
    urinary (indwelling) T83.86 ☑
  electronic (electrode) (pulse generator) (stimulator)
    bone T84.86 ☑
    cardiac T82.867 ☑
    nervous system (brain) (peripheral nerve) (spinal) T85.860 ☑
    urinary T83.86 ☑
  fixation, internal (orthopedic) NEC T84.86 ☑
  gastrointestinal (bile duct) (esophagus) T85.868 ☑
  genital NEC T83.86 ☑
  heart T82.867 ☑
  joint prosthesis T84.86 ☑
  ocular (corneal graft) (orbital implant) NEC T85.868 ☑
  orthopedic NEC T84.86 ☑
  specified NEC T85.868 ☑
  urinary NEC T83.86 ☑
  vascular NEC T82.868 ☑
  ventricular intracranial shunt T85.860 ☑
during the puerperium — *see* Thrombosis, puerperal
endocardial — *see also* Infarct, myocardium
  not resulting in infarction I51.3
eye — *see* Occlusion, retina
genital organ
  female NEC N94.89
    pregnancy — *see* Thrombophlebitis, antepartum
  male N50.1
gestational — *see* Phlebopathy, gestational
heart (chamber) — *see also* Infarct, myocardium
  not resulting in infarction I51.3
  old I51.3
hepatic (vein) I82.0

Thrombosis, thrombotic — *continued*
hepatic — *continued*
  artery I74.8
  history (of) Z86.718
  intestine (with gangrene) — *see also* Infarct, intestine K55.069
intracardiac NEC (apical) (atrial) (auricular) (ventricular) (old) I51.3
intracranial (arterial) I66.9
  venous sinus (any) G08
    nonpyogenic origin I67.6
    puerperium O87.3
intramural — *see also* Infarct, myocardium
  not resulting in infarction I51.3
  old I51.3
intraspinal venous sinuses and veins G08
  nonpyogenic G95.19
kidney (artery) N28.0
lateral (venous) sinus — *see* Thrombosis, intracranial venous sinus
leg — *see* Thrombosis, vein, lower extremity
  arterial I74.3
liver (venous) I82.0
  artery I74.8
  portal vein I81
longitudinal (venous) sinus — *see* Thrombosis, intracranial venous sinus
lower limb — *see* Thrombosis, vein, lower extremity
lung (iatrogenic) (postoperative) — *see* Embolism, pulmonary
meninges (brain) (arterial) I66.8
mesenteric (artery) (with gangrene) — *see also* Infarct, intestine K55.069
  vein (inferior) (superior) K55.0- ☑
mitral I34.89
mural — *see also* Infarct, myocardium
  due to syphilis A52.06
  not resulting in infarction I51.3
  old I51.3
omentum (with gangrene) — *see also* Infarct, intestine K55.069
ophthalmic — *see* Occlusion, retina
pampiniform plexus (male) N50.1
parietal — *see also* Infarct, myocardium
  not resulting in infarction I24.0
penis, superficial vein N48.81
perianal venous K64.5
peripheral arteries I74.4
  upper I74.2
personal history (of) Z86.718
portal I81
  due to syphilis A52.09
precerebral artery — *see* Occlusion, artery, precerebral
puerperal, postpartum O87.0
  brain (artery) O99.43
    venous (sinus) O87.3
  cardiac O99.43
  cerebral (artery) O99.43
    venous (sinus) O87.3
  superficial O87.0
pulmonary (artery) (iatrogenic) (postoperative) (vein) — *see* Embolism, pulmonary
renal (artery) N28.0
  vein I82.3
resulting from presence of device, implant or graft — *see* Complications, by site and type, specified NEC
retina, retinal — *see* Occlusion, retina
scrotum N50.1
seminal vesicle N50.1
sigmoid (venous) sinus — *see* Thrombosis, intracranial venous sinus
sinus, intracranial (any) — *see* Thrombosis, intracranial venous sinus
specified site NEC I82.890
  chronic I82.891
spermatic cord N50.1
spinal cord (arterial) G95.11
  due to syphilis A52.09
  pyogenic origin G06.1
spleen, splenic D73.5
  artery I74.8
testis N50.1
traumatic NEC T14.8 ☑
tricuspid I07.8
tumor — *see* Neoplasm, unspecified behavior, by site
tunica vaginalis N50.1
umbilical cord (vessels), complicating delivery O69.5 ☑

Thrombosis, thrombotic — continued
- vas deferens N50.1
- vein (acute) I82.90
  - antecubital I82.61- ☑
    - chronic I82.71- ☑
  - axillary I82.A1- ☑ (following I82.7)
    - chronic I82.A2- ☑ (following I82.7)
  - basilic I82.61- ☑
    - chronic I82.71- ☑
  - brachial I82.62- ☑
    - chronic I82.72- ☑
  - brachiocephalic (innominate) I82.290
    - chronic I82.291
  - cephalic I82.61- ☑
    - chronic I82.71- ☑
  - cerebral, nonpyogenic I67.6
  - chronic I82.91
  - deep (DVT) I82.40- ☑
    - calf I82.4Z- ☑
      - chronic I82.5Z- ☑
    - lower leg I82.4Z- ☑
      - chronic I82.5Z- ☑
    - thigh I82.4Y- ☑
      - chronic I82.5Y- ☑
    - upper leg I82.4Y- ☑
      - chronic I82.5Y- ☑
  - femoral I82.41- ☑
    - chronic I82.51- ☑
  - iliac (iliofemoral) I82.42- ☑
    - chronic I82.52- ☑
  - innominate I82.290
    - chronic I82.291
  - internal jugular I82.C1- ☑ (following I82.7)
    - chronic I82.C2- ☑ (following I82.7)
  - lower extremity
    - deep I82.40- ☑
      - chronic I82.50- ☑
      - specified NEC I82.49- ☑
        - chronic NEC I82.59- ☑
    - distal
      - deep I82.4Z- ☑
    - proximal
      - deep I82.4Y- ☑
        - chronic I82.5Y- ☑
    - superficial I82.81- ☑
  - perianal K64.5
  - popliteal I82.43- ☑
    - chronic I82.53- ☑
  - radial I82.62- ☑
    - chronic I82.72- ☑
  - renal I82.3
  - saphenous (greater) (lesser) I82.81- ☑
  - specified NEC I82.890
    - chronic NEC I82.891
  - subclavian I82.B1- ☑ (following I82.7)
    - chronic I82.B2- ☑ (following I82.7)
  - thoracic NEC I82.290
    - chronic I82.291
  - tibial I82.44- ☑
    - chronic I82.54- ☑
  - ulnar I82.62- ☑
    - chronic I82.72- ☑
  - upper extremity I82.60- ☑
    - chronic I82.70- ☑
    - deep I82.62- ☑
      - chronic I82.72- ☑
    - superficial I82.61- ☑
      - chronic I82.71- ☑
- vena cava
  - inferior I82.220
    - chronic I82.221
  - superior I82.210
    - chronic I82.211
- venous, perianal K64.5
- ventricle — see also Infarct, myocardium
  - following acute myocardial infarction (current complication) I23.6
  - not resulting in infarction I24.0
  - old I51.3

Thrombus — see Thrombosis
Thrush — see also Candidiasis
- newborn P37.5
- oral B37.0
- vaginal (acute) B37.31
  - chronic (recurrent) B37.32
Thumb — see also condition
- sucking (child problem) F98.8

Thymitis E32.8
Thymoma — see also Neoplasm, thymus, by type
- malignant C37
- metaplastic C37
- microscopic D15.0
- sclerosing C37
- type A C37
- type AB C37
- type B1 C37
- type B2 C37
- type B3 C37
Thymus, thymic (gland) — see condition
Thyrocele — see Goiter
Thyroglossal — see also condition
- cyst Q89.2
- duct, persistent Q89.2
Thyroid (gland) (body) — see also condition
- hormone resistance E07.89
- lingual Q89.2
- nodule (cystic) (nontoxic) (single) E04.1
Thyroiditis E06.9
- acute (nonsuppurative) (pyogenic) (suppurative) E06.0
- autoimmune E06.3
- chronic (nonspecific) (sclerosing) E06.5
  - with thyrotoxicosis, transient E06.2
  - fibrous E06.5
  - lymphadenoid E06.3
  - lymphocytic E06.3
  - lymphoid E06.3
- de Quervain's E06.1
- drug-induced E06.4
- fibrous (chronic) E06.5
- giant-cell (follicular) E06.1
- granulomatous (de Quervain) (subacute) E06.1
- Hashimoto's (struma lymphomatosa) E06.3
- iatrogenic E06.4
- ligneous E06.5
- lymphocytic (chronic) E06.3
- lymphoid E06.3
- lymphomatous E06.3
- nonsuppurative E06.1
- postpartum, puerperal O90.5
- pseudotuberculous E06.1
- pyogenic E06.0
- radiation E06.4
- Riedel's E06.5
- subacute (granulomatous) E06.1
- suppurative E06.0
- tuberculous A18.81
- viral E06.1
- woody E06.5
Thyrolingual duct, persistent Q89.2
Thyromegaly E01.0
Thyrotoxic
- crisis — see Thyrotoxicosis
- heart disease or failure — see also Thyrotoxicosis E05.90 [143]
  - with thyroid storm E05.91 [143]
- storm — see Thyrotoxicosis
Thyrotoxicosis (recurrent) E05.90
- with
  - goiter (diffuse) E05.00
    - with thyroid storm E05.01
    - adenomatous uninodular E05.10
      - with thyroid storm E05.11
    - multinodular E05.20
      - with thyroid storm E05.21
    - nodular E05.20
      - with thyroid storm E05.21
    - uninodular E05.10
      - with thyroid storm E05.11
  - infiltrative
    - dermopathy E05.00
      - with thyroid storm E05.01
    - ophthalmopathy E05.00
      - with thyroid storm E05.01
  - single thyroid nodule E05.10
    - with thyroid storm E05.11
  - thyroid storm E05.91
- due to
  - ectopic thyroid nodule or tissue E05.30
    - with thyroid storm E05.31
  - ingestion of (excessive) thyroid material E05.40
    - with thyroid storm E05.41
  - overproduction of thyroid-stimulating hormone E05.80
    - with thyroid storm E05.81
  - specified cause NEC E05.80

Thyrotoxicosis — continued
- due to — continued
  - specified cause — continued
    - with thyroid storm E05.81
  - factitia E05.40
    - with thyroid storm E05.41
  - heart — see also Failure, heart, high-output E05.90 [143]
    - with thyroid storm — see also Failure, heart, high-output E05.91 [143]
    - failure — see also Failure, heart, high-output E05.90 [143]
  - neonatal (transient) P72.1
  - transient with chronic thyroiditis E06.2
Tibia vara M92.51- ☑
Tic (disorder) F95.9
- breathing F95.8
- child problem F95.0
- compulsive F95.1
- de la Tourette F95.2
- degenerative (generalized) (localized) G25.69
  - facial G25.69
- disorder
  - chronic
    - motor F95.1
    - vocal F95.1
  - combined vocal and multiple motor F95.2
  - transient F95.0
- douloureux G50.0
  - atypical G50.1
  - postherpetic, postzoster B02.22
- drug-induced G25.61
- eyelid F95.8
- habit F95.9
  - chronic F95.1
  - transient of childhood F95.0
- lid, transient of childhood F95.0
- motor-verbal F95.2
- occupational F48.8
- orbicularis F95.8
  - transient of childhood F95.0
- organic origin G25.69
- postchoreic G25.69
- provisional F95.0
- psychogenic, compulsive F95.1
- salaam R25.8
- spasm (motor or vocal) F95.9
  - chronic F95.1
  - transient of childhood F95.0
- specified NEC F95.8
Tick-borne — see condition
Tietze's disease or syndrome M94.0
Tight, tightness
- anus K62.89
- chest R07.89
- fascia (lata) M62.89
- foreskin (congenital) N47.1
- hymen, hymenal ring N89.6
- introitus (acquired) (congenital) N89.6
- rectal sphincter K62.89
- tendon — see Short, tendon
- urethral sphincter N35.919
Tilting vertebra — see Dorsopathy, deforming, specified NEC
Timidity, child F93.8
Tinea (intersecta) (tarsi) B35.9
- amiantacea L44.8
- asbestina B35.0
- barbae B35.0
- beard B35.0
- black dot B35.0
- blanca B36.2
- capitis B35.0
- corporis B35.4
- cruris B35.6
- flava B36.0
- foot B35.3
- furfuracea B36.0
- imbricata (Tokelau) B35.5
- kerion B35.0
- manuum B35.2
- microsporic — see Dermatophytosis
- nigra B36.1
- nodosa — see Piedra
- pedis B35.3
- scalp B35.0
- specified NEC B35.8
- sycosis B35.0
- tonsurans B35.0

Tinea — *continued*
  trichophytic — *see* Dermatophytosis
  unguium B35.1
  versicolor B36.0
Tingling sensation (skin) R20.2
Tin-miner's lung J63.5
Tinnitus NOS H93.1- ☑
  audible H93.1- ☑
  aurium H93.1- ☑
  pulsatile H93.A- ☑
  subjective H93.1- ☑
Tipped tooth (teeth) M26.33
Tipping
  pelvis M95.5
    with disproportion (fetopelvic) O33.0
      causing obstructed labor O65.0
  tooth (teeth), fully erupted M26.33
Tiredness R53.83
Tissue — *see* condition
Tobacco (nicotine)
  abuse — *see* Tobacco, use
  dependence — *see* Dependence, drug, nicotine
  harmful use Z72.0
  heart — *see* Tobacco, toxic effect
  maternal use, affecting newborn P04.2
  toxic effect — *see* Table of Drugs and Chemicals, by
    substance, poisoning
    chewing tobacco — *see* Table of Drugs and Chemi-
      cals, by substance, poisoning
    cigarettes — *see* Table of Drugs and Chemicals, by
      substance, poisoning
  use Z72.0
    complicating
      childbirth O99.334
      pregnancy O99.33- ☑
      puerperium O99.335
    counseling and surveillance Z71.6
    history Z87.891
  withdrawal state — *see also* Dependence, drug, nico-
    tine F17.203
Tocopherol deficiency E56.0
Todd's
  cirrhosis K74.3
  paralysis (postepileptic) (transitory) G83.84
Toe — *see* condition
Toilet, artificial opening — *see* Attention to, artificial,
  opening
Tokelau (ringworm) B35.5
Tollwut — *see* Rabies
Tommaselli's disease R31.9
  correct substance properly administered — *see* Table
    of Drugs and Chemicals, by drug, adverse effect
  overdose or wrong substance given or taken — *see*
    Table of Drugs and Chemicals, by drug, poisoning
Tongue — *see also* condition
  tie Q38.1
Tonic pupil — *see* Anomaly, pupil, function, tonic pupil
Toni-Fanconi syndrome (cystinosis) E72.09
  with cystinosis E72.04
Tonsil — *see* condition
Tonsillitis (acute) (catarrhal) (croupous) (follicular) (gangrenous) (infective) (lacunar) (lingual) (malignant)
  (membranous) (parenchymatous) (phlegmonous)
  (pseudomembranous) (purulent) (septic) (subacute)
  (suppurative) (toxic) (ulcerative) (vesicular) (viral)
  J03.90
  chronic J35.01
    with adenoiditis J35.03
  diphtheritic A36.0
  hypertrophic J35.01
    with adenoiditis J35.03
  recurrent J03.91
  specified organism NEC J03.80
    recurrent J03.81
  staphylococcal J03.80
    recurrent J03.81
  streptococcal J03.00
    recurrent J03.01
  tuberculous A15.8
  Vincent's A69.1
Tooth, teeth — *see* condition
Toothache K08.89
Topagnosis R20.8
Tophi — *see* Gout, chronic
TORCH infection — *see* Infection, congenital
  without active infection P00.2
Torn — *see* Tear

Tornwaldt's cyst or disease J39.2
Torsades de pointes I47.21
Torsion
  accessory tube — *see* Torsion, fallopian tube
  adnexa (female) — *see* Torsion, fallopian tube
  aorta, acquired I77.1
  appendix epididymis N44.04
  appendix testis N44.03
  bile duct (common) (hepatic) K83.8
    congenital Q44.5
  bowel, colon or intestine K56.2
  cervix — *see* Malposition, uterus
  cystic duct K82.8
  dystonia — *see* Dystonia, torsion
  epididymis (appendix) N44.04
  fallopian tube N83.52- ☑
    with ovary N83.53
  gallbladder K82.8
    congenital Q44.1
  hydatid of Morgagni
    female N83.52- ☑
    male N44.03
  kidney (pedicle) (leading to infarction) N28.0
  Meckel's diverticulum (congenital) Q43.0
    malignant — *see* Table of Neoplasms, small intes-
      tine, malignant
  mesentery K56.2
  omentum K56.2
  organ or site, congenital NEC — *see* Anomaly, by site
  ovary (pedicle) N83.51- ☑
    with fallopian tube N83.53
    congenital Q50.2
  oviduct — *see* Torsion, fallopian tube
  penis (acquired) N48.82
    congenital Q55.63
  spasm — *see* Dystonia, torsion
  spermatic cord N44.02
    extravaginal N44.01
    intravaginal N44.02
  spleen D73.5
  testis, testicle N44.00
    appendix N44.03
  tibia — *see* Deformity, limb, specified type NEC, lower
    leg
  uterus — *see* Malposition, uterus
Torticollis (intermittent) (spastic) M43.6
  congenital (sternomastoid) Q68.0
  due to birth injury P15.8
  hysterical F44.4
  ocular R29.891
  psychogenic F45.8
    conversion reaction F44.4
  rheumatic M43.6
  rheumatoid M06.88
  spasmodic G24.3
  traumatic, current S13.4 ☑
Tortipelvis G24.1
Tortuous
  aortic arch Q25.46
  artery I77.1
  organ or site, congenital NEC — *see* Distortion
  retinal vessel, congenital Q14.1
  ureter N13.8
  urethra N36.8
  vein — *see* Varix
Torture, victim of Z65.4
Torula, torular (histolytica) (infection) — *see* Cryptococcosis
Torulosis — *see* Cryptococcosis
Torus (mandibularis) (palatinus) M27.0
  fracture — *see* Fracture, by site, torus
Touraine's syndrome Q79.8
Tourette's syndrome F95.2
Tourniquet syndrome — *see* Constriction, external, by
  site
Tower skull Q75.0
  with exophthalmos Q87.0
Toxemia R68.89
  bacterial — *see* Sepsis
  burn — *see* Burn
  eclamptic (with pre-existing hypertension) — *see*
    Eclampsia
  erysipelatous — *see* Erysipelas
  fatigue R68.89
  food — *see* Poisoning, food
  gastrointestinal K52.1
  intestinal K52.1
  kidney — *see* Uremia

Toxemia — *continued*
  malarial — *see* Malaria
  myocardial — *see* Myocarditis, toxic
  of pregnancy — *see* Pre-eclampsia
  pre-eclamptic — *see* Pre-eclampsia
  small intestine K52.1
  staphylococcal, due to food A05.0
  stasis R68.89
  uremic — *see* Uremia
  urinary — *see* Uremia
Toxemica cerebropathia psychica (nonalcoholic) F04
  alcoholic — *see* Alcohol, amnestic disorder
Toxic (poisoning) — *see also* condition T65.91 ☑
  effect — *see* Table of Drugs and Chemicals, by sub-
    stance, poisoning
  shock syndrome A48.3
  thyroid (gland) — *see* Thyrotoxicosis
Toxicemia — *see* Toxemia
Toxicity — *see* Table of Drugs and Chemicals, by sub-
    stance, poisoning
  fava bean D55.0
  food, noxious — *see* Poisoning, food
  from drug or nonmedicinal substance — *see* Table of
    Drugs and Chemicals, by drug
Toxicosis — *see also* Toxemia
  capillary, hemorrhagic D69.0
Toxinfection, gastrointestinal K52.1
Toxocariasis B83.0
Toxoplasma, toxoplasmosis (acquired) B58.9
  with
    hepatitis B58.1
    meningoencephalitis B58.2
    ocular involvement B58.00
    other organ involvement B58.89
    pneumonia, pneumonitis B58.3
  congenital (acute) (subacute) (chronic) P37.1
  maternal, manifest toxoplasmosis in infant (acute)
    (subacute) (chronic) P37.1
tPA (rtPA) **administration in a different facility within
  the last 24 hours prior to admission to current
  facility** Z92.82
Trabeculation, bladder N32.89
Trachea — *see* condition
Tracheitis (catarrhal) (infantile) (membranous) (plastic)
  (septal) (suppurative) (viral) J04.10
  with
    bronchitis (15 years of age and above) J40
      acute or subacute — *see* Bronchitis, acute
      chronic J42
      tuberculous NEC A15.5
      under 15 years of age J20.9
    laryngitis (acute) J04.2
      chronic J37.1
      tuberculous NEC A15.5
  acute J04.10
    with obstruction J04.11
  chronic J42
    with
      bronchitis (chronic) J42
      laryngitis (chronic) J37.1
  diphtheritic (membranous) A36.89
  due to external agent — *see* Inflammation, respiratory,
    upper, due to
  syphilitic A52.73
  tuberculous A15.5
Trachelitis (nonvenereal) — *see* Cervicitis
Tracheobronchial — *see* condition
Tracheobronchitis (15 years of age and above) — *see
  also* Bronchitis
  due to
    Bordetella bronchiseptica A37.80
      with pneumonia A37.81
    Francisella tularensis A21.8
Tracheobronchomegaly Q32.4
  with bronchiectasis J47.9
    with
      exacerbation (acute) J47.1
      lower respiratory infection J47.0
  acquired J98.09
    with bronchiectasis J47.9
      with
        exacerbation (acute) J47.1
        lower respiratory infection J47.0
Tracheobronchopneumonitis — *see* Pneumonia,
  broncho-
Tracheocele (external) (internal) J39.8
  congenital Q32.1
Tracheomalacia J39.8

Tracheomalacia — *continued*
congenital Q32.0
Tracheopharyngitis (acute) J06.9
chronic J42
due to external agent — *see* Inflammation, respiratory, upper, due to
Tracheostenosis J39.8
Tracheostomy
complication — *see* Complication, tracheostomy
status Z93.0
attention to Z43.0
malfunctioning J95.03
Trachoma, trachomatous A71.9
active (stage) A71.1
contraction of conjunctiva A71.1
dubium A71.0
healed or sequelae B94.0
initial (stage) A71.0
pannus A71.1
Türck's J37.0
Traction, vitreomacular H43.82- ☑
Train sickness T75.3 ☑
Trait(s)
Hb-S D57.3
hemoglobin
abnormal NEC D58.2
with thalassemia D56.3
C — *see* Disease, hemoglobin C
S (Hb-S) D57.3
Lepore D56.3
personality, accentuated Z73.1
sickle-cell D57.3
with elliptocytosis or spherocytosis D57.3
type A personality Z73.1
Tramp Z59.00
Trance R41.89
hysterical F44.89
Transaminasemia R74.01
Transection
abdomen (partial) S38.3 ☑
aorta (incomplete) — *see also* Injury, aorta
complete — *see* Injury, aorta, laceration, major
carotid artery (incomplete) — *see also* Injury, blood vessel, carotid, laceration
complete — *see* Injury, blood vessel, carotid, laceration, major
celiac artery (incomplete) S35.211 ☑
branch (incomplete) S35.291 ☑
complete S35.292 ☑
complete S35.212 ☑
innominate
artery (incomplete) — *see also* Injury, blood vessel, thoracic, innominate, artery, laceration
complete — *see* Injury, blood vessel, thoracic, innominate, artery, laceration, major
vein (incomplete) — *see also* Injury, blood vessel, thoracic, innominate, vein, laceration
complete — *see* Injury, blood vessel, thoracic, innominate, vein, laceration, major
jugular vein (external) (incomplete) — *see also* Injury, blood vessel, jugular vein, laceration
complete — *see* Injury, blood vessel, jugular vein, laceration, major
internal (incomplete) — *see also* Injury, blood vessel, jugular vein, internal, laceration
complete — *see* Injury, blood vessel, jugular vein, internal, laceration, major
mesenteric artery (incomplete) — *see also* Injury, mesenteric, artery, laceration
complete — *see* Injury, mesenteric artery, laceration, major
pulmonary vessel (incomplete) — *see also* Injury, blood vessel, thoracic, pulmonary, laceration
complete — *see* Injury, blood vessel, thoracic, pulmonary, laceration, major
subclavian — *see* Transection, innominate
vena cava (incomplete) — *see also* Injury, vena cava
complete — *see* Injury, vena cava, laceration, major
vertebral artery (incomplete) — *see also* Injury, blood vessel, vertebral, laceration
complete — *see* Injury, blood vessel, vertebral, laceration, major
Transfusion
associated (red blood cell) hemochromatosis E83.111
blood
ABO incompatible — *see* Complication(s), transfusion, incompatibility reaction, ABO

Transfusion — *continued*
blood — *continued*
minor blood group (Duffy) (E) (K) (Kell) (Kidd) (Lewis) (M) (N) (P) (S) T80.89 ☑
reaction or complication — *see* Complications, transfusion
fetomaternal (mother) — *see* Pregnancy, complicated by, placenta, transfusion syndrome
maternofetal (mother) — *see* Pregnancy, complicated by, placenta, transfusion syndrome
placental (syndrome) (mother) — *see* Pregnancy, complicated by, placenta, transfusion syndrome
reaction (adverse) — *see* Complications, transfusion
related acute lung injury (TRALI) J95.84
twin-to-twin — *see* Pregnancy, complicated by, placenta, transfusion syndrome, fetus to fetus
Transient (meaning homeless) — *see also* condition
Z59.00
Translocation
balanced autosomal Q95.9
in normal individual Q95.0
chromosomes NEC Q99.8
balanced and insertion in normal individual Q95.0
Down syndrome Q90.2
trisomy
13 Q91.6
18 Q91.2
21 Q90.2
Translucency, iris — *see* Degeneration, iris
Transmission of chemical substances through the placenta — *see* Absorption, chemical, through placenta
Transparency, lung, unilateral J43.0
Transplant (ed) (status) Z94.9
awaiting organ Z76.82
bone Z94.6
marrow Z94.81
candidate Z76.82
complication — *see* Complication, transplant
cornea Z94.7
heart Z94.1
and lung(s) Z94.3
valve Z95.2
prosthetic Z95.2
specified NEC Z95.4
xenogenic Z95.3
intestine Z94.82
kidney Z94.0
liver Z94.4
lung(s) Z94.2
and heart Z94.3
organ (failure) (infection) (rejection) Z94.9
removal status Z98.85
pancreas Z94.83
skin Z94.5
social Z60.3
specified organ or tissue NEC Z94.89
stem cells Z94.84
tissue Z94.9
Transplants, ovarian, endometrial N80.10- ☑
Transposed — *see* Transposition
Transposition (congenital) — *see also* Malposition, congenital
abdominal viscera Q89.3
aorta (dextra) Q20.3
appendix Q43.8
colon Q43.8
corrected Q20.5
great vessels (complete) (partial) Q20.3
heart Q24.0
with complete transposition of viscera Q89.3
intestine (large) (small) Q43.8
reversed jejunal (for bypass) (status) Z98.0
scrotum Q55.23
stomach Q40.2
with general transposition of viscera Q89.3
tooth, teeth, fully erupted M26.30
vessels, great (complete) (partial) Q20.3
viscera (abdominal) (thoracic) Q89.3
Transsexualism F64.0
Transverse — *see also* condition
arrest (deep), in labor O64.0 ☑
lie (mother) O32.2 ☑
causing obstructed labor O64.8 ☑
Transvestism, transvestitism (dual-role) F64.1
fetishistic F65.1
Trapped placenta (with hemorrhage) O72.0
without hemorrhage O73.0

TRAPS (tumor necrosis factor receptor associated periodic syndrome) M04.1
Trauma, traumatism — *see also* Injury
acoustic — *see* subcategory H83.3 ☑
birth — *see* Birth, injury
complicating ectopic or molar pregnancy O08.6
during delivery O71.9
following ectopic or molar pregnancy O08.6
obstetric O71.9
specified NEC O71.89
occusal
primary K08.81
secondary K08.82
Traumatic — *see also* condition
brain injury S06.9 ☑
Treacher Collins syndrome Q75.4
Treitz's hernia — *see* Hernia, abdomen, specified site NEC
Trematode infestation — *see* Infestation, fluke
Trematodiasis — *see* Infestation, fluke
Trembling paralysis — *see* Parkinsonism
Tremor(s) R25.1
drug induced G25.1
essential (benign) G25.0
familial G25.0
hereditary G25.0
hysterical F44.4
intention G25.2
medication induced postural G25.1
mercurial — *see* subcategory T56.1 ☑
Parkinson's — *see* Parkinsonism
psychogenic (conversion reaction) F44.4
senilis R54
specified type NEC G25.2
Trench
fever A79.0
foot — *see* Immersion, foot
mouth A69.1
Treponema pallidum infection — *see* Syphilis
Treponematosis
due to
T. pallidum — *see* Syphilis
T. pertenue — *see* Yaws
Triad
Hutchinson's (congenital syphilis) A50.53
Kartagener's Q89.3
Saint's — *see* Hernia, diaphragm
Trichiasis (eyelid) H02.059
with entropion — *see* Entropion
left H02.056
lower H02.055
upper H02.054
right H02.053
lower H02.052
upper H02.051
Trichinella spiralis (infection) (infestation) B75
Trichinellosis, trichiniasis, trichinelliasis, trichinosis B75
with muscle disorder B75 *[M63.80]*
ankle B75 *[M63.87-]* ☑
foot B75 *[M63.87-]* ☑
forearm B75 *[M63.83-]* ☑
hand B75 *[M63.84-]* ☑
lower leg B75 *[M63.86-]* ☑
multiple sites B75 *[M63.89]*
pelvic region B75 *[M63.85-]* ☑
shoulder region B75 *[M63.81-]* ☑
specified site NEC B75 *[M63.88]*
thigh B75 *[M63.85-]* ☑
upper arm B75 *[M63.82-]* ☑
Trichobezoar T18.9 ☑
intestine T18.3 ☑
stomach T18.2 ☑
Trichocephaliasis, trichocephalosis B79
Trichocephalus infestation B79
Trichoclasis L67.8
Trichoepithelioma — *see also* Neoplasm, skin, benign
malignant — *see* Neoplasm, skin, malignant
Trichofolliculoma — *see* Neoplasm, skin, benign
Tricholemmoma — *see* Neoplasm, skin, benign
Trichomoniasis A59.9
bladder A59.03
cervix A59.09
intestinal A07.8
prostate A59.02
seminal vesicles A59.09
specified site NEC A59.8

☑ **Additional Character Required — Refer to the Tabular List for Character Selection**

Trichomoniasis — *continued*
  urethra A59.03
  urogenitalis A59.00
  vagina A59.01
  vulva A59.01
Trichomycosis
  axillaris A48.8
  nodosa, nodularis B36.8
Trichonodosis L67.8
Trichophytid, trichophyton infection — *see* Dermatophytosis
Trichophytobezoar T18.9 ☑
  intestine T18.3 ☑
  stomach T18.2 ☑
Trichophytosis — *see* Dermatophytosis
Trichoptilosis L67.8
Trichorrhexis (nodosa) (invaginata) L67.0
Trichosis axillaris A48.8
Trichosporosis nodosa B36.2
Trichostasis spinulosa (congenital) Q84.1
Trichostrongyliasis, trichostrongylosis (small intestine) B81.2
Trichostrongylus infection B81.2
Trichotillomania F63.3
Trichromat, trichromatopsia, anomalous (congenital) H53.55
Trichuriasis B79
Trichuris trichiura (infection) (infestation) (any site) B79
Tricuspid (valve) — *see* condition
Trifid — *see also* Accessory
  kidney (pelvis) Q63.8
  tongue Q38.3
Trigeminal neuralgia — *see* Neuralgia, trigeminal
Trigeminy R00.8
Trigger finger (acquired) M65.30
  congenital Q74.0
  index finger M65.32- ☑
  little finger M65.35- ☑
  middle finger M65.33- ☑
  ring finger M65.34- ☑
  thumb M65.31- ☑
Trigonitis (bladder) (chronic) (pseudomembranous) N30.30
  with hematuria N30.31
Trigonocephaly Q75.0
Trilocular heart — *see* Cor triloculare
Trimethylaminuria E72.52
Tripartite placenta O43.19- ☑
Triphalangeal thumb Q74.0
Triple — *see also* Accessory
  kidneys Q63.0
  uteri Q51.818
  X, female Q97.0
Triple I O41.12- ☑
Triplegia G83.89
  congenital G80.8
Triplet (newborn) — *see also* Newborn, triplet
  complicating pregnancy — *see* Pregnancy, triplet
Triplication — *see* Accessory
Triploidy Q92.7
Trismus R25.2
  neonatorum A33
  newborn A33
Trisomy (syndrome) Q92.9
  13 (partial) Q91.7
    meiotic nondisjunction Q91.4
    mitotic nondisjunction Q91.5
    mosaicism Q91.5
    translocation Q91.6
  18 (partial) Q91.3
    meiotic nondisjunction Q91.0
    mitotic nondisjunction Q91.1
    mosaicism Q91.1
    translocation Q91.2
  20 Q92.8
  21 (partial) Q90.9
    meiotic nondisjunction Q90.0
    mitotic nondisjunction Q90.1
    mosaicism Q90.1
    translocation Q90.2
  22 Q92.8
  autosomes Q92.9
  chromosome specified NEC Q92.8
    partial Q92.2
      due to unbalanced translocation Q92.5
    specified NEC Q92.8

Trisomy — *continued*
  chromosome specified — *continued*
    whole (nonsex chromosome)
      meiotic nondisjunction Q92.0
      mitotic nondisjunction Q92.1
      mosaicism Q92.1
  due to
    dicentrics — *see* Extra, marker chromosomes
    extra rings — *see* Extra, marker chromosomes
    isochromosomes — *see* Extra, marker chromosomes
  specified NEC Q92.8
  whole chromosome Q92.9
    meiotic nondisjunction Q92.0
    mitotic nondisjunction Q92.1
    mosaicism Q92.1
    partial Q92.9
    specified NEC Q92.8
Tritanomaly, tritanopia H53.55
Trombiculosis, trombiculiasis, trombidiosis B88.0
Trophedema (congenital) (hereditary) Q82.0
Trophoblastic disease — *see also* Mole, hydatidiform O01.9
Tropholymphedema Q82.0
Trophoneurosis NEC G96.89
  disseminated M34.9
Tropical — *see* condition
Trouble — *see also* Disease
  heart — *see* Disease, heart
  kidney — *see* Disease, renal
  nervous R45.0
  sinus — *see* Sinusitis
Trousseau's syndrome (thrombophlebitis migrans) I82.1
Truancy, childhood
  from school Z72.810
Truncus
  arteriosus (persistent) Q20.0
  communis Q20.0
Trunk — *see* condition
Trypanosomiasis
  African B56.9
    by Trypanosoma brucei
      gambiense B56.0
      rhodesiense B56.1
  American — *see* Chagas' disease
  Brazilian — *see* Chagas' disease
  by Trypanosoma
    brucei gambiense B56.0
    brucei rhodesiense B56.1
    cruzi — *see* Chagas' disease
  gambiensis, Gambian B56.0
  rhodesiensis, Rhodesian B56.1
  South American — *see* Chagas' disease
  where
    African trypanosomiasis is prevalent B56.9
    Chagas' disease is prevalent B57.2
Tryptasemia, hereditary alpha D89.44
T-shaped incisors K00.2
Tsutsugamushi (disease) (fever) A75.3
Tube, tubal, tubular — *see* condition
Tubercle — *see also* Tuberculosis
  brain, solitary A17.81
  Darwin's Q17.8
  Ghon, primary infection A15.7
Tuberculid, tuberculide (indurating, subcutaneous) (lichenoid) (miliary) (papulonecrotic) (primary) (skin) A18.4
Tuberculoma — *see also* Tuberculosis
  brain A17.81
  meninges (cerebral) (spinal) A17.1
  spinal cord A17.81
Tuberculosis, tubercular, tuberculous (calcification) (calcified) (caseous) (chromogenic acid-fast bacilli) (degeneration) (fibrocaseous) (fistula) (interstitial) (isolated circumscribed lesions) (necrosis) (parenchymatous) (ulcerative) A15.9
  with pneumoconiosis (any condition in J60-J64) J65
  abdomen (lymph gland) A18.39
  abscess (respiratory) A15.9
    bone A18.03
      hip A18.02
      knee A18.02
      sacrum A18.01
      specified site NEC A18.03
      spinal A18.01
      vertebra A18.01
    brain A17.81
    breast A18.89
    Cowper's gland A18.15

Tuberculosis, tubercular, tuberculous — *continued*
  abscess — *continued*
    dura (mater) (cerebral) (spinal) A17.81
    epidural (cerebral) (spinal) A17.81
    female pelvis A18.17
    frontal sinus A15.8
    genital organs NEC A18.10
    genitourinary A18.10
    gland (lymphatic) — *see* Tuberculosis, lymph gland
    hip A18.02
    intestine A18.32
    ischiorectal A18.32
    joint NEC A18.02
      hip A18.02
      knee A18.02
      specified NEC A18.02
      vertebral A18.01
    kidney A18.11
    knee A18.02
    latent Z22.7
    lumbar (spine) A18.01
    lung — *see* Tuberculosis, pulmonary
    meninges (cerebral) (spinal) A17.0
    muscle A18.09
    perianal (fistula) A18.32
    perinephritic A18.11
    perirectal A18.32
    rectum A18.32
    retropharyngeal A15.8
    sacrum A18.01
    scrofulous A18.2
    scrotum A18.15
    skin (primary) A18.4
    spinal cord A17.81
    spine or vertebra (column) A18.01
    subdiaphragmatic A18.31
    testis A18.15
    urinary A18.13
    uterus A18.17
  accessory sinus — *see* Tuberculosis, sinus
  Addison's disease A18.7
  adenitis — *see* Tuberculosis, lymph gland
  adenoids A15.8
  adenopathy — *see* Tuberculosis, lymph gland
  adherent pericardium A18.84
  adnexa (uteri) A18.17
  adrenal (capsule) (gland) A18.7
  alimentary canal A18.32
  anemia A18.89
  ankle (joint) (bone) A18.02
  anus A18.32
  apex, apical — *see* Tuberculosis, pulmonary
  appendicitis, appendix A18.32
  arachnoid A17.0
  artery, arteritis A18.89
    cerebral A18.89
  arthritis (chronic) (synovial) A18.02
    spine or vertebra (column) A18.01
  articular — *see* Tuberculosis, joint
  ascites A18.31
  asthma — *see* Tuberculosis, pulmonary
  axilla, axillary (gland) A18.2
  bladder A18.12
  bone A18.03
    hip A18.02
    knee A18.02
    limb NEC A18.03
    sacrum A18.01
    spine or vertebral column A18.01
  bowel (miliary) A18.32
  brain A17.81
  breast A18.89
  broad ligament A18.17
  bronchi, bronchial, bronchus A15.5
    ectasia, ectasis (bronchiectasis) — *see* Tuberculosis, pulmonary
    fistula A15.5
      primary (progressive) A15.7
    gland or node A15.4
      primary (progressive) A15.7
    lymph gland or node A15.4
      primary (progressive) A15.7
  bronchiectasis — *see* Tuberculosis, pulmonary
  bronchitis A15.5
  bronchopleural A15.6
  bronchopneumonia, bronchopneumonic — *see* Tuberculosis, pulmonary
  bronchorrhagia A15.5

Tuberculosis, tubercular, tuberculous — *continued*
- bronchotracheal A15.5
- bronze disease A18.7
- buccal cavity A18.83
- bulbourethral gland A18.15
- bursa A18.09
- cachexia A15.9
- cardiomyopathy A18.84
- caries — *see* Tuberculosis, bone
- cartilage A18.02
  - intervertebral A18.01
- catarrhal — *see* Tuberculosis, respiratory
- cecum A18.32
- cellulitis (primary) A18.4
- cerebellum A17.81
- cerebral, cerebrum A17.81
- cerebrospinal A17.81
  - meninges A17.0
- cervical (lymph gland or node) A18.2
- cervicitis, cervix (uteri) A18.16
- chest — *see* Tuberculosis, respiratory
- chorioretinitis A18.53
- choroid, choroiditis A18.53
- ciliary body A18.54
- colitis A18.32
- collier's J65
- colliquativa (primary) A18.4
- colon A18.32
- complex, primary A15.7
- congenital P37.0
- conjunctiva A18.59
- connective tissue (systemic) A18.89
- contact Z20.1
- cornea (ulcer) A18.52
- Cowper's gland A18.15
- coxae A18.02
- coxalgia A18.02
- cul-de-sac of Douglas A18.17
- curvature, spine A18.01
- cutis (colliquativa) (primary) A18.4
- cyst, ovary A18.18
- cystitis A18.12
- dactylitis A18.03
- diarrhea A18.32
- diffuse — *see* Tuberculosis, miliary
- digestive tract A18.32
- disseminated — *see* Tuberculosis, miliary
- duodenum A18.32
- dura (mater) (cerebral) (spinal) A17.0
  - abscess (cerebral) (spinal) A17.81
- dysentery A18.32
- ear (inner) (middle) A18.6
  - bone A18.03
  - external (primary) A18.4
  - skin (primary) A18.4
- elbow A18.02
- emphysema — *see* Tuberculosis, pulmonary
- empyema A15.6
- encephalitis A17.82
- endarteritis A18.89
- endocarditis A18.84
  - aortic A18.84
  - mitral A18.84
  - pulmonary A18.84
  - tricuspid A18.84
- endocrine glands NEC A18.82
- endometrium A18.17
- enteric, enterica, enteritis A18.32
- enterocolitis A18.32
- epididymis, epididymitis A18.15
- epidural abscess (cerebral) (spinal) A17.81
- epiglottis A15.5
- episcleritis A18.51
- erythema (induratum) (nodosum) (primary) A18.4
- esophagus A18.83
- eustachian tube A18.6
- exposure (to) Z20.1
- exudative — *see* Tuberculosis, pulmonary
- eye A18.50
- eyelid (primary) (lupus) A18.4
- fallopian tube (acute) (chronic) A18.17
- fascia A18.09
- fauces A15.8
- female pelvic inflammatory disease A18.17
- finger A18.03
- first infection A15.7
- gallbladder A18.83
- ganglion A18.09

Tuberculosis, tubercular, tuberculous — *continued*
- gastritis A18.83
- gastrocolic fistula A18.32
- gastroenteritis A18.32
- gastrointestinal tract A18.32
- general, generalized — *see* Tuberculosis, miliary
- genital organs A18.10
- genitourinary A18.10
- genu A18.02
- glandula suprarenalis A18.7
- glandular, general A18.2
- glottis A15.5
- grinder's J65
- gum A18.83
- hand A18.03
- heart A18.84
- hematogenous — *see* Tuberculosis, miliary
- hemoptysis — *see* Tuberculosis, pulmonary
- hemorrhage NEC — *see* Tuberculosis, pulmonary
- hemothorax A15.6
- hepatitis A18.83
- hilar lymph nodes A15.4
  - primary (progressive) A15.7
- hip (joint) (disease) (bone) A18.02
- hydropneumothorax A15.6
- hydrothorax A15.6
- hypoadrenalism A18.7
- hypopharynx A15.8
- ileocecal (hyperplastic) A18.32
- ileocolitis A18.32
- ileum A18.32
- iliac spine (superior) A18.03
- immunological findings only A15.7
- indurativa (primary) A18.4
- infantile A15.7
- infection A15.9
  - without clinical manifestations A15.7
- infraclavicular gland A18.2
- inguinal gland A18.2
- inguinalis A18.2
- intestine (any part) A18.32
- iridocyclitis A18.54
- iris, iritis A18.54
- ischiorectal A18.32
- jaw A18.03
- jejunum A18.32
- joint A18.02
  - vertebral A18.01
- keratitis (interstitial) A18.52
- keratoconjunctivitis A18.52
- kidney A18.11
- knee (joint) A18.02
- kyphosis, kyphoscoliosis A18.01
- laryngitis A15.5
- larynx A15.5
- latent Z22.7
- leptomeninges, leptomeningitis (cerebral) (spinal) A17.0
- lichenoides (primary) A18.4
- linguae A18.83
- lip A18.83
- liver A18.83
- lordosis A18.01
- lung — *see* Tuberculosis, pulmonary
- lupus vulgaris A18.4
- lymph gland or node (peripheral) A18.2
  - abdomen A18.39
  - bronchial A15.4
    - primary (progressive) A15.7
  - cervical A18.2
  - hilar A15.4
    - primary (progressive) A15.7
  - intrathoracic A15.4
    - primary (progressive) A15.7
  - mediastinal A15.4
    - primary (progressive) A15.7
  - mesenteric A18.39
  - retroperitoneal A18.39
  - tracheobronchial A15.4
    - primary (progressive) A15.7
- lymphadenitis — *see* Tuberculosis, lymph gland
- lymphangitis — *see* Tuberculosis, lymph gland
- lymphatic (gland) (vessel) — *see* Tuberculosis, lymph gland
- mammary gland A18.89
- marasmus A15.9
- mastoiditis A18.03
- mediastinal lymph gland or node A15.4

Tuberculosis, tubercular, tuberculous — *continued*
- mediastinal lymph gland or node — *continued*
  - primary (progressive) A15.7
- mediastinitis A18.8
  - primary (progressive) A15.7
- mediastinum A18.8
  - primary (progressive) A15.7
- medulla A17.81
- melanosis, Addisonian A18.7
- meninges, meningitis (basilar) (cerebral) (cerebrospinal) (spinal) A17.0
- meningoencephalitis A17.82
- mesentery, mesenteric (gland or node) A18.39
- miliary A19.9
  - acute A19.2
    - multiple sites A19.1
    - single specified site A19.0
  - chronic A19.8
  - specified NEC A19.8
- millstone makers' J65
- miner's J65
- molder's J65
- mouth A18.83
- multiple A19.9
  - acute A19.1
  - chronic A19.8
- muscle A18.09
- myelitis A17.82
- myocardium, myocarditis A18.84
- nasal (passage) (sinus) A15.8
- nasopharynx A15.8
- neck gland A18.2
- nephritis A18.11
- nerve (mononeuropathy) A17.83
- nervous system A17.9
- nose (septum) A15.8
- ocular A18.50
- omentum A18.31
- oophoritis (acute) (chronic) A18.17
- optic (nerve trunk) (papilla) A18.59
- orbit A18.59
- orchitis A18.15
- organ, specified NEC A18.89
- osseous — *see* Tuberculosis, bone
- osteitis — *see* Tuberculosis, bone
- osteomyelitis — *see* Tuberculosis, bone
- otitis media A18.6
- ovary, ovaritis (acute) (chronic) A18.17
- oviduct (acute) (chronic) A18.17
- pachymeningitis A17.0
- palate (soft) A18.83
- pancreas A18.83
- papulonecrotic (a) (primary) A18.4
- parathyroid glands A18.82
- paronychia (primary) A18.4
- parotid gland or region A18.83
- pelvis (bony) A18.03
- penis A18.15
- peribronchitis A15.5
- pericardium, pericarditis A18.84
- perichondritis, larynx A15.5
- periostitis — *see* Tuberculosis, bone
- perirectal fistula A18.32
- peritoneum NEC A18.31
- peritonitis A18.31
- pharynx, pharyngitis A15.8
- phlyctenulosis (keratoconjunctivitis) A18.52
- phthisis NEC — *see* Tuberculosis, pulmonary
- pituitary gland A18.82
- pleura, pleural, pleurisy, pleuritis (fibrinous) (obliterative) (purulent) (simple plastic) (with effusion) A15.6
  - primary (progressive) A15.7
- pneumonia, pneumonic — *see* Tuberculosis, pulmonary
- pneumothorax (spontaneous) (tense valvular) — *see* Tuberculosis, pulmonary
- polyneuropathy A17.89
- polyserositis A19.9
  - acute A19.1
  - chronic A19.8
- potter's J65
- prepuce A18.15
- primary (complex) A15.7
- proctitis A18.32
- prostate, prostatitis A18.14
- pulmonalis — *see* Tuberculosis, pulmonary

☑ **Additional Character Required** — **Refer to the Tabular List for Character Selection**

Tuberculosis, tubercular, tuberculous — *continued*
pulmonary (cavitated) (fibrotic) (infiltrative) (nodular) A15.0
childhood type or first infection A15.7
primary (complex) A15.7
pyelitis A18.11
pyelonephritis A18.11
pyemia — *see* Tuberculosis, miliary
pyonephrosis A18.11
pyopneumothorax A15.6
pyothorax A15.6
rectum (fistula) (with abscess) A18.32
reinfection stage — *see* Tuberculosis, pulmonary
renal A18.11
renis A18.11
respiratory A15.9
primary A15.7
specified site NEC A15.8
retina, retinitis A18.53
retroperitoneal (lymph gland or node) A18.39
rheumatism NEC A18.09
rhinitis A15.8
sacroiliac (joint) A18.01
sacrum A18.01
salivary gland A18.83
salpingitis (acute) (chronic) A18.17
sandblaster's J65
sclera A18.51
scoliosis A18.01
scrofulous A18.2
scrotum A18.15
seminal tract or vesicle A18.15
senile A15.9
septic — *see* Tuberculosis, miliary
shoulder (joint) A18.02
blade A18.03
sigmoid A18.32
sinus (any nasal) A15.8
bone A18.03
epididymis A18.15
skeletal NEC A18.03
skin (any site) (primary) A18.4
small intestine A18.32
soft palate A18.83
spermatic cord A18.15
spine, spinal (column) A18.01
cord A17.81
medulla A17.81
membrane A17.0
meninges A17.0
spleen, splenitis A18.85
spondylitis A18.01
sternoclavicular joint A18.02
stomach A18.83
stonemason's J65
subcutaneous tissue (cellular) (primary) A18.4
subcutis (primary) A18.4
subdeltoid bursa A18.83
submaxillary (region) A18.83
supraclavicular gland A18.2
suprarenal (capsule) (gland) A18.7
swelling, joint (*see also* category M01) — *see also* Tuberculosis, joint A18.02
symphysis pubis A18.02
synovitis A18.09
articular A18.02
spine or vertebra A18.01
systemic — *see* Tuberculosis, miliary
tarsitis A18.4
tendon (sheath) — *see* Tuberculosis, tenosynovitis
tenosynovitis A18.09
spine or vertebra A18.01
testis A18.15
throat A15.8
thymus gland A18.82
thyroid gland A18.81
tongue A18.83
tonsil, tonsillitis A15.8
trachea, tracheal A15.5
lymph gland or node A15.4
primary (progressive) A15.7
tracheobronchial A15.5
lymph gland or node A15.4
primary (progressive) A15.7
tubal (acute) (chronic) A18.17
tunica vaginalis A18.15
ulcer (skin) (primary) A18.4
bowel or intestine A18.32

Tuberculosis, tubercular, tuberculous — *continued*
ulcer — *continued*
specified NEC — *see* Tuberculosis, by site
unspecified site A15.9
ureter A18.11
urethra, urethral (gland) A18.13
urinary organ or tract A18.13
uterus A18.17
uveal tract A18.54
uvula A18.83
vagina A18.18
vas deferens A18.15
verruca, verrucosa (cutis) (primary) A18.4
vertebra (column) A18.01
vesiculitis A18.15
vulva A18.18
wrist (joint) A18.02
Tuberculum
Carabelli — *see* Excludes Note at K00.2
occlusal — *see* Excludes Note at K00.2
paramolare K00.2
Tuberosity, enitre maxillary M26.07
Tuberous sclerosis (brain) Q85.1
Tubo-ovarian — *see* condition
Tuboplasty, after previous sterilization Z31.0
aftercare Z31.42
Tubotympanitis, catarrhal (chronic) — *see* Otitis, media, nonsuppurative, chronic, serous
Tularemia A21.9
with
conjunctivitis A21.1
pneumonia A21.2
abdominal A21.3
bronchopneumonic A21.2
conjunctivitis A21.1
cryptogenic A21.3
enteric A21.3
gastrointestinal A21.3
generalized A21.7
ingestion A21.3
intestinal A21.3
oculoglandular A21.1
ophthalmic A21.1
pneumonia (any), pneumonic A21.2
pulmonary A21.2
sepsis A21.7
specified NEC A21.8
typhoidal A21.7
ulceroglandular A21.0
Tularensis conjunctivitis A21.1
Tumefaction — *see also* Swelling
liver — *see* Hypertrophy, liver
Tumor — *see also* Neoplasm, unspecified behavior, by site
acinar cell — *see* Neoplasm, uncertain behavior, by site
acinic cell — *see* Neoplasm, uncertain behavior, by site
adenocarcinoid — *see* Neoplasm, malignant, by site
adenomatoid — *see also* Neoplasm, benign, by site
odontogenic — *see* Cyst, calcifying odontogenic
adnexal (skin) — *see* Neoplasm, skin, benign, by site
adrenal
cortical (benign) D35.0- ☑
malignant C74.0- ☑
rest — *see* Neoplasm, benign, by site
alpha-cell
malignant
pancreas C25.4
specified site NEC — *see* Neoplasm, malignant, by site
unspecified site C25.4
pancreas D13.7
specified site NEC — *see* Neoplasm, benign, by site
unspecified site D13.7
aneurysmal — *see* Aneurysm
aortic body D44.7
malignant C75.5
Askin's — *see* Neoplasm, connective tissue, malignant
basal cell — *see also* Neoplasm, skin, uncertain behavior D48.5
Bednar — *see* Neoplasm, skin, malignant
benign (unclassified) — *see* Neoplasm, benign, by site
beta-cell
malignant
pancreas C25.4
specified site NEC — *see* Neoplasm, malignant, by site
unspecified site C25.4
pancreas D13.7

Tumor — *continued*
beta-cell — *continued*
specified site NEC — *see* Neoplasm, benign, by site
unspecified site D13.7
Brenner D27.9
borderline malignancy D39.1- ☑
malignant C56- ☑
proliferating D39.1- ☑
bronchial alveolar, intravascular D38.1
Brooke's — *see* Neoplasm, skin, benign
brown fat — *see* Lipoma
Burkitt — *see* Lymphoma, Burkitt
calcifying epithelial odontogenic — *see* Cyst, calcifying odontogenic
carcinoid D3A.00 (*following* D36)
benign D3A.00 (*following* D36)
appendix D3A.020 (*following* D36)
ascending colon D3A.022 (*following* D36)
bronchus (lung) D3A.090 (*following* D36)
cecum D3A.021 (*following* D36)
colon D3A.029 (*following* D36)
descending colon D3A.024 (*following* D36)
duodenum D3A.010 (*following* D36)
foregut NOS D3A.094 (*following* D36)
hindgut NOS D3A.096 (*following* D36)
ileum D3A.012 (*following* D36)
jejunum D3A.011 (*following* D36)
kidney D3A.093 (*following* D36)
large intestine D3A.029 (*following* D36)
lung (bronchus) D3A.090 (*following* D36)
midgut NOS D3A.095 (*following* D36)
rectum D3A.026 (*following* D36)
sigmoid colon D3A.025 (*following* D36)
small intestine D3A.019 (*following* D36)
specified NEC D3A.098 (*following* D36)
stomach D3A.092 (*following* D36)
thymus D3A.091 (*following* D36)
transverse colon D3A.023 (*following* D36)
malignant C7A.00 (*following* C75)
appendix C7A.020 (*following* C75)
ascending colon C7A.022 (*following* C75)
bronchus (lung) C7A.090 (*following* C75)
cecum C7A.021 (*following* C75)
colon C7A.029 (*following* C75)
descending colon C7A.024 (*following* C75)
duodenum C7A.010 (*following* C75)
foregut NOS C7A.094 (*following* C75)
hindgut NOS C7A.096 (*following* C75)
ileum C7A.012 (*following* C75)
jejunum C7A.011 (*following* C75)
kidney C7A.093 (*following* C75)
large intestine C7A.029 (*following* C75)
lung (bronchus) C7A.090 (*following* C75)
midgut NOS C7A.095 (*following* C75)
rectum C7A.026 (*following* C75)
sigmoid colon C7A.025 (*following* C75)
small intestine C7A.019 (*following* C75)
specified NEC C7A.098 (*following* C75)
stomach C7A.092 (*following* C75)
thymus C7A.091 (*following* C75)
transverse colon C7A.023 (*following* C75)
mesentary metastasis C7B.04 (*following* C75)
secondary C7B.00 (*following* C75)
bone C7B.03 (*following* C75)
distant lymph nodes C7B.01 (*following* C75)
liver C7B.02 (*following* C75)
peritoneum C7B.04 (*following* C75)
specified NEC C7B.09 (*following* C75)
carotid body D44.6
malignant C75.4
cells — *see also* Neoplasm, unspecified behavior, by site
benign — *see* Neoplasm, benign, by site
malignant — *see* Neoplasm, malignant, by site
uncertain whether benign or malignant — *see* Neoplasm, uncertain behavior, by site
cervix, in pregnancy or childbirth — *see* Pregnancy, complicated by, tumor, cervix
chondromatous giant cell — *see* Neoplasm, bone, benign
chromaffin — *see also* Neoplasm, benign, by site
malignant — *see* Neoplasm, malignant, by site
Cock's peculiar L72.3
Codman's — *see* Neoplasm, bone, benign
dentigerous, mixed — *see* Cyst, calcifying odontogenic
dermoid — *see* Neoplasm, benign, by site
with malignant transformation C56- ☑

Tumor — continued

desmoid (extra-abdominal) — see also Neoplasm, connective tissue, uncertain behavior
  abdominal — see Neoplasm, connective tissue, uncertain behavior
embolus — see Neoplasm, secondary, by site
embryonal (mixed) — see also Neoplasm, uncertain behavior, by site
  liver C22.7
endodermal sinus
  specified site — see Neoplasm, malignant, by site
  unspecified site
    female C56.- ☑
    male C62.90
epithelial
  benign — see Neoplasm, benign, by site
  malignant — see Neoplasm, malignant, by site
Ewing's — see Neoplasm, bone, malignant, by site
fatty — see Lipoma
fibroid — see Leiomyoma
G cell
  malignant
    pancreas C25.4
    specified site NEC — see Neoplasm, malignant, by site
    unspecified site C25.4
  specified site — see Neoplasm, uncertain behavior, by site
  unspecified site D37.8
germ cell — see also Neoplasm, malignant, by site
  mixed — see Neoplasm, malignant, by site
ghost cell, odontogenic — see Cyst, calcifying odontogenic
giant cell — see also Neoplasm, uncertain behavior, by site
  bone D48.0
    malignant — see Neoplasm, bone, malignant
  chondromatous — see Neoplasm, bone, benign
  malignant — see Neoplasm, malignant, by site
  soft parts — see Neoplasm, connective tissue, uncertain behavior
    malignant — see Neoplasm, connective tissue, malignant
glomus D18.00
  intra-abdominal D18.03
  intracranial D18.02
  jugulare D44.7
    malignant C75.5
  skin D18.01
  specified site NEC D18.09
gonadal stromal — see Neoplasm, uncertain behavior, by site
granular cell — see also Neoplasm, connective tissue, benign
  malignant — see Neoplasm, connective tissue, malignant
granulosa cell D39.1- ☑
  juvenile D39.1- ☑
  malignant C56- ☑
granulosa cell-theca cell D39.1- ☑
  malignant C56- ☑
Grawitz's C64- ☑
hemorrhoidal — see Hemorrhoids
hilar cell D27- ☑
hilus cell D27- ☑
Hurthle cell (benign) D34
  malignant C73
hydatid — see Echinococcus
hypernephroid — see also Neoplasm, uncertain behavior, by site
interstitial cell — see also Neoplasm, uncertain behavior, by site
  benign — see Neoplasm, benign, by site
  malignant — see Neoplasm, malignant, by site
intravascular bronchial alveolar D38.1
islet cell — see Neoplasm, benign, by site
  malignant — see Neoplasm, malignant, by site
    pancreas C25.4
    specified site NEC — see Neoplasm, malignant, by site
    unspecified site C25.4
  pancreas D13.7
  specified site NEC — see Neoplasm, benign, by site
  unspecified site D13.7
juxtaglomerular D41.0- ☑
Klatskin's C22.1
Krukenberg's C79.6- ☑

Tumor — continued

Leydig cell — see Neoplasm, uncertain behavior, by site
  benign — see Neoplasm, benign, by site
    specified site — see Neoplasm, benign, by site
    unspecified site
      female D27.9
      male D29.20
  malignant — see Neoplasm, malignant, by site
    specified site — see Neoplasm, malignant, by site
    unspecified site
      female C56.9
      male C62.90
  specified site — see Neoplasm, uncertain behavior, by site
  unspecified site
    female D39.10
    male D40.10
lipid cell, ovary D27- ☑
lipoid cell, ovary D27- ☑
malignant — see also Neoplasm, malignant, by site C80.1
  fusiform cell (type) C80.1
  giant cell (type) C80.1
  localized, plasma cell — see Plasmacytoma, solitary
  mixed NEC C80.1
  small cell (type) C80.1
  spindle cell (type) C80.1
  unclassified C80.1
mast cell D47.09
melanotic, neuroectodermal — see Neoplasm, benign, by site
Merkel cell — see Carcinoma, Merkel cell
mesenchymal
  malignant — see Neoplasm, connective tissue, malignant
  mixed — see Neoplasm, connective tissue, uncertain behavior
mesodermal, mixed — see also Neoplasm, malignant, by site
  liver C22.4
mesonephric — see also Neoplasm, uncertain behavior, by site
  malignant — see Neoplasm, malignant, by site
metastatic
  from specified site — see Neoplasm, malignant, by site
  of specified site — see Neoplasm, malignant, by site
  to specified site — see Neoplasm, secondary, by site
mixed NEC — see also Neoplasm, benign, by site
  malignant — see Neoplasm, malignant, by site
mucinous of low malignant potential
  specified site — see Neoplasm, malignant, by site
  unspecified site C56.9
mucocarcinoid
  specified site — see Neoplasm, malignant, by site
  unspecified site C18.1
mucoepidermoid — see Neoplasm, uncertain behavior, by site
Müllerian, mixed
  specified site — see Neoplasm, malignant, by site
  unspecified site C54.9
myoepithelial — see Neoplasm, benign, by site
neuroectodermal (peripheral) — see Neoplasm, malignant, by site
  primitive
    specified site — see Neoplasm, malignant, by site
    unspecified site C71.9
neuroendocrine D3A.8 (following D36)
  malignant poorly differentiated C7A.1 (following C75)
  secondary NEC C7B.8 (following C75)
  specified NEC C7A.8 (following C75)
neurogenic olfactory C30.0
nonencapsulated sclerosing C73
odontogenic (adenomatoid) (benign) (calcifying epithelial) (keratocystic) (squamous) — see Cyst, calcifying odontogenic
  malignant C41.1
    upper jaw (bone) C41.0
ovarian stromal D39.1- ☑
ovary, in pregnancy — see Pregnancy, complicated by
pacinian — see Neoplasm, skin, benign
Pancoast's — see Pancoast's syndrome
papillary — see also Papilloma
  cystic D37.9

Tumor — continued

papillary — see also Papilloma — continued
  mucinous of low malignant potential C56- ☑
    specified site — see Neoplasm, malignant, by site
    unspecified site C56.9
  serous of low malignant potential
    specified site — see Neoplasm, malignant, by site
    unspecified site C56.9
pelvic, in pregnancy or childbirth — see Pregnancy, complicated by
phantom F45.8
phyllodes D48.6- ☑
  benign D24- ☑
  malignant — see Neoplasm, breast, malignant
Pindborg — see Cyst, calcifying odontogenic
placental site trophoblastic D39.2
plasma cell (malignant) (localized) — see Plasmacytoma, solitary
polyvesicular vitelline
  specified site — see Neoplasm, malignant, by site
  unspecified site
    female C56.9
    male C62.90
Pott's puffy — see Osteomyelitis, specified NEC
Rathke's pouch D44.3
retinal anlage — see Neoplasm, benign, by site
salivary gland type, mixed — see Neoplasm, salivary gland, benign
  malignant — see Neoplasm, salivary gland, malignant
Sampson's N80.10- ☑
Schmincke's — see Neoplasm, nasopharynx, malignant
sclerosing stromal D27- ☑
sebaceous — see Cyst, sebaceous
secondary — see Neoplasm, secondary, by site
  carcinoid C7B.00 (following C75)
    bone C7B.03 (following C75)
    distant lymph nodes C7B.01 (following C75)
    liver C7B.02 (following C75)
    peritoneum C7B.04 (following C75)
    specified NEC C7B.09 (following C75)
  neuroendocrine NEC C7B.8 (following C75)
serous of low malignant potential
  specified site — see Neoplasm, malignant, by site
  unspecified site C56.9
Sertoli cell — see Neoplasm, benign, by site
  with lipid storage
    specified site — see Neoplasm, benign, by site
    unspecified site
      female D27.9
      male D29.20
  specified site — see Neoplasm, benign, by site
  unspecified site
    female D27.9
    male D29.20
Sertoli-Leydig cell — see Neoplasm, benign, by site
  specified site — see Neoplasm, benign, by site
  unspecified site
    female D27.9
    male D29.20
sex cord (-stromal) — see Neoplasm, uncertain behavior, by site
  with annular tubules D39.1- ☑
skin appendage — see Neoplasm, skin, benign
smooth muscle — see Neoplasm, connective tissue, uncertain behavior
soft tissue
  benign — see Neoplasm, connective tissue, benign
  malignant — see Neoplasm, connective tissue, malignant
sternomastoid (congenital) Q68.0
stromal
  endometrial D39.0
  gastric D48.1
    benign D21.4
    malignant C16.9
    uncertain behavior D48.1
  gastrointestinal C49.A- ☑
    benign D21.4
    esophagus C49.A1
    malignant C49.A0
      colon C49.A4
      duodenum C49.A3
      esophagus C49.A1
      ileum C49.A3
      jejunum C49.A3

Tumor — *continued*
  stromal — *continued*
    gastrointestinal — *continued*
      malignant — *continued*
        large intestine C49.A4
        Meckel diverticulum C49.A3
        omentum C49.A9
        peritoneum C49.A9
        rectum C49.A5
        small intestine C49.A3
        specified site NEC C49.A9
        stomach C49.A2
      rectum C49.A5
      small intestine C49.A3
      specified site NEC C49.A9
      stomach C49.A2
      uncertain behavior D48.1
    intestine
      benign D21.4
      malignant
        large C49.A4
        small C49.A3
      uncertain behavior D48.1
    ovarian D39.1- ☑
    stomach C49.A2
      benign D21.4
      malignant C49.A2
      uncertain behavior D48.1
  sweat gland — *see also* Neoplasm, skin, uncertain behavior
    benign — *see* Neoplasm, skin, benign
    malignant — *see* Neoplasm, skin, malignant
  syphilitic, brain A52.17
  testicular D40.10
  testicular stromal D40.1- ☑
  theca cell D27.- ☑
  theca cell-granulosa cell D39.1- ☑
  Triton, malignant — *see* Neoplasm, nerve, malignant
  trophoblastic, placental site D39.2
  turban D23.4
  uterus (body), in pregnancy or childbirth — *see* Pregnancy, complicated by, tumor, uterus
  vagina, in pregnancy or childbirth — *see* Pregnancy, complicated by
  varicose — *see* Varix
  von Recklinghausen's — *see* Neurofibromatosis
  vulva or perineum, in pregnancy or childbirth — *see* Pregnancy, complicated by
    causing obstructed labor O65.5
  Warthin's — *see* Neoplasm, salivary gland, benign
  Wilms' C64- ☑
  yolk sac — *see* Neoplasm, malignant, by site
    specified site — *see* Neoplasm, malignant, by site
    unspecified site
      female C56.9
      male C62.90
Tumor lysis syndrome (following antineoplastic chemotherapy) (spontaneous) NEC E88.3
Tumorlet — *see* Neoplasm, uncertain behavior, by site
Tungiasis B88.1
Tunica vasculosa lentis Q12.2
Turban tumor D23.4
Türck's trachoma J37.0
Turner-Kieser syndrome Q87.2
Turner-like syndrome Q87.19
Turner's
  hypoplasia (tooth) K00.4
  syndrome Q96.9
    specified NEC Q96.8
  tooth K00.4
Turner-Ullrich syndrome Q96.9
Tussis convulsiva — *see* Whooping cough
Twiddler's syndrome (due to)
  automatic implantable defibrillator T82.198
  cardiac pacemaker T82.198 ☑
Twilight state
  epileptic F05
  psychogenic F44.89
Twin (newborn) — *see also* Newborn, twin
  conjoined Q89.4
  pregnancy — *see* Pregnancy, twin
Twinning, teeth K00.2
Twist, twisted
  bowel, colon or intestine K56.2
  hair (congenital) Q84.1
  mesentery K56.2
  omentum K56.2
  organ or site, congenital NEC — *see* Anomaly, by site

Twist, twisted — *continued*
  ovarian pedicle — *see* Torsion, ovary
Twitching R25.3
Tylosis (acquired) L84
  buccalis K13.29
  linguae K13.29
  palmaris et plantaris (congenital) (inherited) Q82.8
    acquired L85.1
Tympanism R14.0
Tympanites (abdominal) (intestinal) R14.0
Tympanitis — *see* Myringitis
Tympanosclerosis H74.0 ☑
Tympanum — *see* condition
Tympany
  abdomen R14.0
  chest R09.89
Type A behavior pattern Z73.1
Typhlitis — *see* Cecitis
Typhoenteritis — *see* Typhoid
Typhoid (abortive) (ambulant) (any site) (clinical) (fever) (hemorrhagic) (infection) (intermittent) (malignant) (rheumatic) (Widal negative) A01.00
  with pneumonia A01.03
  abdominal A01.09
  arthritis A01.04
  carrier (suspected) of Z22.0
  cholecystitis (current) A01.09
  endocarditis A01.02
  heart involvement A01.02
  inoculation reaction — *see* Complications, vaccination
  meningitis A01.01
  mesenteric lymph nodes A01.09
  myocarditis A01.02
  osteomyelitis A01.05
  perichondritis, larynx A01.09
  pneumonia A01.03
  specified NEC A01.09
  spine A01.05
  ulcer (perforating) A01.09
Typhomalaria (fever) — *see* Malaria
Typhomania A01.00
Typhoperitonitis A01.09
Typhus (fever) A75.9
  abdominal, abdominalis — *see* Typhoid
  African tick A77.1
  amarillic A95.9
  brain A75.9 *[G94]*
  cerebral A75.9 *[G94]*
  classical A75.0
  due to Rickettsia
    prowazekii A75.0
      recrudescent A75.1
    tsutsugamushi A75.3
    typhi A75.2
  endemic (flea-borne) A75.2
  epidemic (louse-borne) A75.0
  exanthematicus SAI A75.0
    brillii SAI A75.1
    mexicanus SAI A75.2
    typhus murinus A75.2
  exanthematic NEC A75.0
  flea-borne A75.2
  India tick A77.1
  Kenya (tick) A77.1
  louse-borne A75.0
  Mexican A75.2
  mite-borne A75.3
  murine A75.2
  North Asian tick-borne A77.2
  Orientia Tsutsugamushi (scrub typhus) A75.3
  petechial A75.9
  Queensland tick A77.3
  rat A75.2
  recrudescent A75.1
  recurrens — *see* Fever, relapsing
  Sao Paulo A77.0
  scrub (China) (India) (Malaysia) (New Guinea) A75.3
  shop (of Malaysia) A75.2
  Siberian tick A77.2
  tick-borne A77.9
  tropical (mite-borne) A75.3
Tyrosinemia E70.21
  newborn, transitory P74.5
Tyrosinosis E70.21
Tyrosinuria E70.29

U

Uhl's anomaly or disease Q24.8
Ulcer, ulcerated, ulcerating, ulceration, ulcerative
  alveolar process M27.3
  amebic (intestine) A06.1
    skin A06.7
  anastomotic — *see* Ulcer, gastrojejunal
  anorectal K62.6
  antral — *see* Ulcer, stomach
  anus (sphincter) (solitary) K62.6
  aorta — *see* Aneurysm
  aphthous (oral) (recurrent) K12.0
    genital organ(s)
      female N76.6
      male N50.89
  artery I77.2
  atrophic — *see* Ulcer, skin
    decubitus — *see* Ulcer, pressure, by site
  back L98.429
    with
      bone involvement without evidence of necrosis L98.426
      bone necrosis L98.424
      exposed fat layer L98.422
      muscle involvement without evidence of necrosis L98.425
      muscle necrosis L98.423
      skin breakdown only L98.421
      specified severity NEC L98.428
  Barrett's (esophagus) K22.10
    with bleeding K22.11
  bile duct (common) (hepatic) K83.8
  bladder (solitary) (sphincter) NEC N32.89
    bilharzial B65.9 *[N33]*
    in schistosomiasis (bilharzial) B65.9 *[N33]*
    submucosal — *see* Cystitis, interstitial
    tuberculous A18.12
  bleeding K27.4
  bone — *see* Osteomyelitis, specified type NEC
  bowel — *see* Ulcer, intestine
  breast N61.1
  bronchus J98.09
  buccal (cavity) (traumatic) K12.1
  Buruli A31.1
  buttock L98.419
    with
      bone involvement without evidence of necrosis L98.416
      bone necrosis L98.414
      exposed fat layer L98.412
      muscle involvement without evidence of necrosis L98.415
      muscle necrosis L98.413
      skin breakdown only L98.411
      specified severity NEC L98.418
  cancerous — *see* Neoplasm, malignant, by site
  cardia K22.10
    with bleeding K22.11
  cardioesophageal (peptic) K22.10
    with bleeding K22.11
  cecum — *see* Ulcer, intestine
  cervix (uteri) (decubitus) (trophic) N86
    with cervicitis N72
  chancroidal A57
  chiclero B55.1
  chronic (cause unknown) — *see* Ulcer, skin
  Cochin-China B55.1
  colon — *see* Ulcer, intestine
  conjunctiva H10.89
  cornea H16.00- ☑
    with hypopyon H16.03- ☑
    central H16.01- ☑
    dendritic (herpes simplex) B00.52
    marginal H16.04- ☑
    Mooren's H16.05- ☑
    mycotic H16.06- ☑
    perforated H16.07- ☑
    ring H16.02- ☑
    tuberculous (phlyctenular) A18.52
  corpus cavernosum (chronic) N48.5
  crural — *see* Ulcer, lower limb
  Curling's — *see* Ulcer, peptic, acute
  Cushing's — *see* Ulcer, peptic, acute
  cystic duct K82.8
  cystitis (interstitial) — *see* Cystitis, interstitial
  decubitus — *see* Ulcer, pressure, by site

Ulcer, ulcerated, ulcerating, ulceration, ulcerative
— *continued*
  dendritic, cornea (herpes simplex) B00.52
  diabetes, diabetic — *see* Diabetes, ulcer
  Dieulafoy's K25.0
  due to
    infection NEC — *see* Ulcer, skin
    radiation NEC L59.8
    trophic disturbance (any region) — *see* Ulcer, skin
    X-ray L58.1
  duodenum, duodenal (eroded) (peptic) K26.9
    with
      hemorrhage K26.4
        and perforation K26.6
      perforation K26.5
    acute K26.3
      with
        hemorrhage K26.0
          and perforation K26.2
        perforation K26.1
    chronic K26.7
      with
        hemorrhage K26.4
          and perforation K26.6
        perforation K26.5
  dysenteric A09
  elusive — *see* Cystitis, interstitial
  endocarditis (acute) (chronic) (subacute) I28.8
  epiglottis J38.7
  esophagus (peptic) K22.10
    with bleeding K22.11
    due to
      aspirin K22.10
        with bleeding K22.11
      gastrointestinal reflux disease (without bleeding) K21.00
        with bleeding K21.01
      ingestion of chemical or medicament K22.10
        with bleeding K22.11
      fungal K22.10
        with bleeding K22.11
      infective K22.10
        with bleeding K22.11
    varicose — *see* Varix, esophagus
  eyelid (region) H01.8
  fauces J39.2
  Fenwick (-Hunner) (solitary) — *see* Cystitis, interstitial
  fistulous — *see* Ulcer, skin
  foot (indolent) (trophic) — *see* Ulcer, lower limb
  frambesial, initial A66.0
  frenum (tongue) K14.0
  gallbladder or duct K82.8
  gangrenous — *see* Gangrene
  gastric — *see* Ulcer, stomach
  gastrocolic — *see* Ulcer, gastrojejunal
  gastroduodenal — *see* Ulcer, peptic
  gastroesophageal — *see* Ulcer, stomach
  gastrointestinal — *see* Ulcer, gastrojejunal
  gastrojejunal (peptic) K28.9
    with
      hemorrhage K28.4
        and perforation K28.6
      perforation K28.5
    acute K28.3
      with
        hemorrhage K28.0
          and perforation K28.2
        perforation K28.1
    chronic K28.7
      with
        hemorrhage K28.4
          and perforation K28.6
        perforation K28.5
  gastrojejunocolic — *see* Ulcer, gastrojejunal
  gingiva K06.8
  gingivitis K05.10
    nonplaque induced K05.11
    plaque induced K05.10
  glottis J38.7
  granuloma of pudenda A58
  gum K06.8
  gumma, due to yaws A66.4
  heel — *see* Ulcer, lower limb
  hemorrhoid — *see also* Hemorrhoids, by degree K64.8
  Hunner's — *see* Cystitis, interstitial
  hypopharynx J39.2
  hypopyon (chronic) (subacute) — *see* Ulcer, cornea, with hypopyon

Ulcer, ulcerated, ulcerating, ulceration, ulcerative
— *continued*
  hypostaticum — *see* Ulcer, varicose
  ileum — *see* Ulcer, intestine
  intestine, intestinal K63.3
    with perforation K63.1
    amebic A06.1
    duodenal — *see* Ulcer, duodenum
    granulocytopenic (with hemorrhage) — *see* Neutropenia
    marginal — *see* Ulcer, gastrojejunal
    perforating K63.1
      newborn P78.0
    primary, small intestine K63.3
    rectum K62.6
    stercoraceous, stercoral K63.3
    tuberculous A18.32
    typhoid (fever) — *see* Typhoid
    varicose I86.8
  jejunum, jejunal — *see* Ulcer, gastrojejunal
  keratitis — *see* Ulcer, cornea
  knee — *see* Ulcer, lower limb
  labium (majus) (minus) N76.6
  laryngitis — *see* Laryngitis
  larynx (aphthous) (contact) J38.7
    diphtheritic A36.2
  leg — *see* Ulcer, lower limb
  lip K13.0
  Lipschütz's N76.6
  lower limb (atrophic) (chronic) (neurogenic) (perforating) (pyogenic) (trophic) (tropical) L97.909
    with
      bone involvement without evidence of necrosis L97.906
      bone necrosis L97.904
      exposed fat layer L97.902
      muscle involvement without evidence of necrosis L97.905
      muscle necrosis L97.903
      skin breakdown only L97.901
      specified severity NEC L97.908
    ankle L97.309
      with
        bone involvement without evidence of necrosis L97.306
        bone necrosis L97.304
        exposed fat layer L97.302
        muscle involvement without evidence of necrosis L97.305
        muscle necrosis L97.303
        skin breakdown only L97.301
        specified severity NEC L97.308
      left L97.329
        with
          bone involvement without evidence of necrosis L97.326
          bone necrosis L97.324
          exposed fat layer L97.322
          muscle involvement without evidence of necrosis L97.325
          muscle necrosis L97.323
          skin breakdown only L97.321
          specified severity NEC L97.328
      right L97.319
        with
          bone involvement without evidence of necrosis L97.316
          bone necrosis L97.314
          exposed fat layer L97.312
          muscle involvement without evidence of necrosis L97.315
          muscle necrosis L97.313
          skin breakdown only L97.311
          specified severity NEC L97.318
    calf L97.209
      with
        bone involvement without evidence of necrosis L97.206
        bone necrosis L97.204
        exposed fat layer L97.202
        muscle involvement without evidence of necrosis L97.205
        muscle necrosis L97.203
        skin breakdown only L97.201
        specified severity NEC L97.208
      left L97.229

Ulcer, ulcerated, ulcerating, ulceration, ulcerative
— *continued*
  lower limb — *continued*
    calf — *continued*
      left — *continued*
        with
          bone involvement without evidence of necrosis L97.226
          bone necrosis L97.224
          exposed fat layer L97.222
          muscle involvement without evidence of necrosis L97.225
          muscle necrosis L97.223
          skin breakdown only L97.221
          specified severity NEC L97.228
      right L97.219
        with
          bone involvement without evidence of necrosis L97.216
          bone necrosis L97.214
          exposed fat layer L97.212
          muscle involvement without evidence of necrosis L97.215
          muscle necrosis L97.213
          skin breakdown only L97.211
          specified severity NEC L97.218
    decubitus — *see* Ulcer, pressure, by site
    foot specified NEC L97.509
      with
        bone involvement without evidence of necrosis L97.506
        bone necrosis L97.504
        exposed fat layer L97.502
        muscle involvement without evidence of necrosis L97.505
        muscle necrosis L97.503
        skin breakdown only L97.501
        specified severity NEC L97.508
      left L97.529
        with
          bone involvement without evidence of necrosis L97.526
          bone necrosis L97.524
          exposed fat layer L97.522
          muscle involvement without evidence of necrosis L97.525
          muscle necrosis L97.523
          skin breakdown only L97.521
          specified severity NEC L97.528
      right L97.519
        with
          bone involvement without evidence of necrosis L97.516
          bone necrosis L97.514
          exposed fat layer L97.512
          muscle involvement without evidence of necrosis L97.515
          muscle necrosis L97.513
          skin breakdown only L97.511
          specified severity NEC L97.518
    heel L97.409
      with
        bone involvement without evidence of necrosis L97.406
        bone necrosis L97.404
        exposed fat layer L97.402
        muscle involvement without evidence of necrosis L97.405
        muscle necrosis L97.403
        skin breakdown only L97.401
        specified severity NEC L97.408
      left L97.429
        with
          bone involvement without evidence of necrosis L97.426
          bone necrosis L97.424
          exposed fat layer L97.422
          muscle involvement without evidence of necrosis L97.425
          muscle necrosis L97.423
          skin breakdown only L97.421
          specified severity NEC L97.428
      right L97.419
        with
          bone involvement without evidence of necrosis L97.416
          bone necrosis L97.414
          exposed fat layer L97.412

Ulcer, ulcerated, ulcerating, ulceration, ulcerative
— *continued*
  lower limb — *continued*
    heel — *continued*
      right — *continued*
        with — *continued*
          muscle involvement without evidence of
            necrosis L97.415
          muscle necrosis L97.413
          skin breakdown only L97.411
          specified severity NEC L97.418
      left L97.929
        with
          bone involvement without evidence of
            necrosis L97.926
          bone necrosis L97.924
          exposed fat layer L97.922
          muscle involvement without evidence of
            necrosis L97.925
          muscle necrosis L97.923
          skin breakdown only L97.921
          specified severity NEC L97.928
      leprous A30.1
      lower leg NOS L97.909
        with
          bone involvement without evidence of
            necrosis L97.906
          bone necrosis L97.904
          exposed fat layer L97.902
          muscle involvement without evidence of
            necrosis L97.905
          muscle necrosis L97.903
          skin breakdown only L97.901
          specified severity NEC L97.908
      left L97.929
        with
          bone involvement without evidence of
            necrosis L97.926
          bone necrosis L97.924
          exposed fat layer L97.922
          muscle involvement without evidence of
            necrosis L97.925
          muscle necrosis L97.923
          skin breakdown only L97.921
          specified severity NEC L97.928
      right L97.919
        with
          bone involvement without evidence of
            necrosis L97.916
          bone necrosis L97.914
          exposed fat layer L97.912
          muscle involvement without evidence of
            necrosis L97.915
          muscle necrosis L97.913
          skin breakdown only L97.911
          specified severity NEC L97.918
      specified site NEC L97.809
        with
          bone involvement without evidence of
            necrosis L97.806
          bone necrosis L97.804
          exposed fat layer L97.802
          muscle involvement without evidence of
            necrosis L97.805
          muscle necrosis L97.803
          skin breakdown only L97.801
          specified severity NEC L97.808
      left L97.829
        with
          bone involvement without evidence
            of necrosis L97.826
          bone necrosis L97.824
          exposed fat layer L97.822
          muscle involvement without evidence
            of necrosis L97.825
          muscle necrosis L97.823
          skin breakdown only L97.821
          specified severity NEC L97.828
      right L97.819
        with
          bone involvement without evidence
            of necrosis L97.816
          bone necrosis L97.814
          exposed fat layer L97.812
          muscle involvement without evidence
            of necrosis L97.815
          muscle necrosis L97.813
          skin breakdown only L97.811
          specified severity NEC L97.818

Ulcer, ulcerated, ulcerating, ulceration, ulcerative
— *continued*
  lower limb — *continued*
    midfoot L97.409
      with
        bone involvement without evidence of
          necrosis L97.406
        bone necrosis L97.404
        exposed fat layer L97.402
        muscle involvement without evidence of
          necrosis L97.405
        muscle necrosis L97.403
        skin breakdown only L97.401
        specified severity NEC L97.408
    left L97.429
      with
        bone involvement without evidence of
          necrosis L97.426
        bone necrosis L97.424
        exposed fat layer L97.422
        muscle involvement without evidence of
          necrosis L97.425
        muscle necrosis L97.423
        skin breakdown only L97.421
        specified severity NEC L97.428
    right L97.419
      with
        bone involvement without evidence of
          necrosis L97.416
        bone necrosis L97.414
        exposed fat layer L97.412
        muscle involvement without evidence of
          necrosis L97.415
        muscle necrosis L97.413
        skin breakdown only L97.411
        specified severity NEC L97.418
    right L97.919
      with
        bone involvement without evidence of
          necrosis L97.916
        bone necrosis L97.914
        exposed fat layer L97.912
        muscle involvement without evidence of
          necrosis L97.915
        muscle necrosis L97.913
        skin breakdown only L97.911
        specified severity NEC L97.918
    syphilitic A52.19
    thigh L97.109
      with
        bone involvement without evidence of
          necrosis L97.106
        bone necrosis L97.104
        exposed fat layer L97.102
        muscle involvement without evidence of
          necrosis L97.105
        muscle necrosis L97.103
        skin breakdown only L97.101
        specified severity NEC L97.108
    left L97.129
      with
        bone involvement without evidence of
          necrosis L97.126
        bone necrosis L97.124
        exposed fat layer L97.122
        muscle involvement without evidence of
          necrosis L97.125
        muscle necrosis L97.123
        skin breakdown only L97.121
        specified severity NEC L97.128
    right L97.119
      with
        bone involvement without evidence of
          necrosis L97.116
        bone necrosis L97.114
        exposed fat layer L97.112
        muscle involvement without evidence of
          necrosis L97.115
        muscle necrosis L97.113
        skin breakdown only L97.111
        specified severity NEC L97.118
    toe L97.509
      with
        bone involvement without evidence of
          necrosis L97.506
        bone necrosis L97.504
        exposed fat layer L97.502
        muscle involvement without evidence of
          necrosis L97.505

Ulcer, ulcerated, ulcerating, ulceration, ulcerative
— *continued*
  lower limb — *continued*
    toe — *continued*
      with — *continued*
        muscle necrosis L97.503
        skin breakdown only L97.501
        specified severity NEC L97.508
      left L97.529
        with
          bone involvement without evidence of
            necrosis L97.526
          bone necrosis L97.524
          exposed fat layer L97.522
          muscle involvement without evidence of
            necrosis L97.525
          muscle necrosis L97.523
          skin breakdown only L97.521
          specified severity NEC L97.528
      right L97.519
        with
          bone involvement without evidence of
            necrosis L97.516
          bone necrosis L97.514
          exposed fat layer L97.512
          muscle involvement without evidence of
            necrosis L97.515
          muscle necrosis L97.513
          skin breakdown only L97.511
          specified severity NEC L97.518
    varicose — *see* Varix, leg, with, ulcer
  luetic — *see* Ulcer, syphilitic
  lung J98.4
    tuberculous — *see* Tuberculosis, pulmonary
  malignant — *see* Neoplasm, malignant, by site
  marginal NEC — *see* Ulcer, gastrojejunal
  meatus (urinarius) N34.2
  Meckel's diverticulum Q43.0
    malignant — *see* Table of Neoplasms, small intes-
      tine, malignant
  Meleney's (chronic undermining) — *see* Ulcer, skin
  Mooren's (cornea) — *see* Ulcer, cornea, Mooren's
  mycobacterial (skin) A31.1
  nasopharynx J39.2
  neck, uterus N86
  neurogenic NEC — *see* Ulcer, skin
  nose, nasal (passage) (infective) (septum) J34.0
    skin — *see* Ulcer, skin
    spirochetal A69.8
    varicose (bleeding) I86.8
  oral mucosa (traumatic) K12.1
  palate (soft) K12.1
  penis (chronic) N48.5
  peptic (site unspecified) K27.9
    with
      hemorrhage K27.4
        and perforation K27.6
      perforation K27.5
    acute K27.3
      with
        hemorrhage K27.0
          and perforation K27.2
        perforation K27.1
    chronic K27.7
      with
        hemorrhage K27.4
          and perforation K27.6
        perforation K27.5
    esophagus K22.10
      with bleeding K22.11
    newborn P78.82
  perforating K27.5
    skin — *see* Ulcer, skin
  peritonsillar J35.8
  phagedenic (tropical) — *see* Ulcer, skin
  pharynx J39.2
  phlebitis — *see* Phlebitis
  plaster — *see* Ulcer, pressure, by site
  popliteal space — *see* Ulcer, lower limb
  postpyloric — *see* Ulcer, duodenum
  prepuce N47.7
  prepyloric — *see* Ulcer, stomach
  pressure (pressure area) L89.9- ☑
    ankle L89.5- ☑
    back L89.1- ☑
    buttock L89.3- ☑
    coccyx L89.15- ☑
    contiguous site of back, buttock, hip L89.4- ☑

Ulcer, ulcerated, ulcerating, ulceration, ulcerative
— *continued*
pressure — *continued*
  elbow L89.0- ✓
  face L89.81- ✓
  head L89.81- ✓
  heel L89.6- ✓
  hip L89.2- ✓
  sacral region (tailbone) L89.15- ✓
  specified site NEC L89.89- ✓
  stage 1 (healing) (pre-ulcer skin changes limited to
      persistent focal edema)
    ankle L89.5- ✓
    back L89.1- ✓
    buttock L89.3- ✓
    coccyx L89.15- ✓
    contiguous site of back, buttock, hip L89.4- ✓
    elbow L89.0- ✓
    face L89.81- ✓
    head L89.81- ✓
    heel L89.6- ✓
    hip L89.2- ✓
    sacral region (tailbone) L89.15- ✓
    specified site NEC L89.89- ✓
  stage 2 (healing) (abrasion, blister, partial thickness
      skin loss involving epidermis and/or dermis)
    ankle L89.5- ✓
    back L89.1- ✓
    buttock L89.3- ✓
    coccyx L89.15- ✓
    contiguous site of back, buttock, hip L89.4- ✓
    elbow L89.0- ✓
    face L89.81- ✓
    head L89.81- ✓
    heel L89.6- ✓
    hip L89.2- ✓
    sacral region (tailbone) L89.15- ✓
    specified site NEC L89.89- ✓
  stage 3 (healing) (full thickness skin loss involving
      damage or necrosis of subcutaneous tissue)
    ankle L89.5- ✓
    back L89.1- ✓
    buttock L89.3- ✓
    coccyx L89.15- ✓
    contiguous site of back, buttock, hip L89.4- ✓
    elbow L89.0- ✓
    face L89.81- ✓
    head L89.81- ✓
    heel L89.6- ✓
    hip L89.2- ✓
    sacral region (tailbone) L89.15- ✓
    specified site NEC L89.89- ✓
  stage 4 (healing) (necrosis of soft tissues through
      to underlying muscle, tendon, or bone)
    ankle L89.5- ✓
    back L89.1- ✓
    buttock L89.3- ✓
    coccyx L89.15- ✓
    contiguous site of back, buttock, hip L89.4- ✓
    elbow L89.0- ✓
    face L89.81- ✓
    head L89.81- ✓
    heel L89.6- ✓
    hip L89.2- ✓
    sacral region (tailbone) L89.15- ✓
    specified site NEC L89.89- ✓
  unspecified stage
    ankle L89.5- ✓
    back L89.1- ✓
    buttock L89.3- ✓
    coccyx L89.15- ✓
    contiguous site of back, buttock, hip L89.4- ✓
    elbow L89.0- ✓
    face L89.81- ✓
    head L89.81- ✓
    heel L89.6- ✓
    hip L89.2- ✓
    sacral region (tailbone) L89.15- ✓
    specified site NEC L89.89- ✓
  unstageable
    ankle L89.5- ✓
    back L89.1- ✓
    buttock L89.3- ✓
    coccyx L89.15- ✓
    contiguous site of back, buttock, hip L89.4- ✓
    elbow L89.0- ✓

Ulcer, ulcerated, ulcerating, ulceration, ulcerative
— *continued*
pressure — *continued*
  unstageable — *continued*
    face L89.81- ✓
    head L89.81- ✓
    heel L89.6- ✓
    hip L89.2- ✓
    sacral region (tailbone) L89.15- ✓
    specified site NEC L89.89- ✓
  primary of intestine K63.3
    with perforation K63.1
  prostate N41.9
  pyloric — *see* Ulcer, stomach
  rectosigmoid K63.3
    with perforation K63.1
  rectum (sphincter) (solitary) K62.6
    stercoraceous, stercoral K62.6
  retina — *see* Inflammation, chorioretinal
  rodent — *see also* Neoplasm, skin, malignant
  sclera — *see* Scleritis
  scrofulous (tuberculous) A18.2
  scrotum N50.89
    tuberculous A18.15
    varicose I86.1
  seminal vesicle N50.89
  sigmoid — *see* Ulcer, intestine
  skin (atrophic) (chronic) (neurogenic) (non-healing)
      (perforating) (pyogenic) (trophic) (tropical)
      L98.499
    with gangrene — *see* Gangrene
    amebic A06.7
    back — *see* Ulcer, back
    buttock — *see* Ulcer, buttock
    decubitus — *see* Ulcer, pressure
    lower limb — *see* Ulcer, lower limb
    mycobacterial A31.1
    specified site NEC L98.499
      with
        bone involvement without evidence of
            necrosis L98.496
        bone necrosis L98.494
        exposed fat layer L98.492
        muscle involvement without evidence of
            necrosis L98.495
        muscle necrosis L98.493
        skin breakdown only L98.491
        specified severity NEC L98.498
    tuberculous (primary) A18.4
    varicose — *see* Ulcer, varicose
  sloughing — *see* Ulcer, skin
  solitary, anus or rectum (sphincter) K62.6
  sore throat J02.9
    streptococcal J02.0
  spermatic cord N50.89
  spine (tuberculous) A18.01
  stasis (venous) — *see* Varix, leg, with, ulcer
    without varicose veins I87.2
  stercoraceous, stercoral K63.3
    with perforation K63.1
    anus or rectum K62.6
  stoma, stomal — *see* Ulcer, gastrojejunal
  stomach (eroded) (peptic) (round) K25.9
    with
      hemorrhage K25.4
        and perforation K25.6
      perforation K25.5
    acute K25.3
      with
        hemorrhage K25.0
          and perforation K25.2
        perforation K25.1
    chronic K25.7
      with
        hemorrhage K25.4
          and perforation K25.6
        perforation K25.5
  stomal — *see* Ulcer, gastrojejunal
  stomatitis K12.1
  stress — *see* Ulcer, peptic
  strumous (tuberculous) A18.2
  submucosal, bladder — *see* Cystitis, interstitial
  syphilitic (any site) (early) (secondary) A51.39
    late A52.79
      perforating A52.79
        foot A52.11
  testis N50.89
  thigh — *see* Ulcer, lower limb

Ulcer, ulcerated, ulcerating, ulceration, ulcerative
— *continued*
  throat J39.2
    diphtheritic A36.0
  toe — *see* Ulcer, lower limb
  tongue (traumatic) K14.0
  tonsil J35.8
    diphtheritic A36.0
  trachea J39.8
  trophic — *see* Ulcer, skin
  tropical — *see* Ulcer, skin
  tuberculous — *see* Tuberculosis, ulcer
  tunica vaginalis N50.89
  turbinate J34.89
  typhoid (perforating) — *see* Typhoid
  unspecified site — *see* Ulcer, skin
  urethra (meatus) — *see* Urethritis
  uterus N85.8
    cervix N86
      with cervicitis N72
    neck N86
      with cervicitis N72
  vagina N76.5
    in Behçet's disease M35.2 *[N77.0]*
    pessary N89.8
  valve, heart I33.0
  varicose (lower limb, any part) — *see also* Varix, leg,
      with, ulcer
    broad ligament I86.2
    esophagus — *see* Varix, esophagus
    inflamed or infected — *see* Varix, leg, with ulcer,
        with inflammation
    nasal septum I86.8
    perineum I86.3
    scrotum I86.1
    specified site NEC I86.8
    sublingual I86.0
    vulva I86.3
  vas deferens N50.89
  vulva (acute) (infectional) N76.6
    in (due to)
      Behçet's disease M35.2 *[N77.0]*
      herpesviral (herpes simplex) infection A60.04
      tuberculosis A18.18
  vulvobuccal, recurring N76.6
  X-ray L58.1
  yaws A66.4
Ulcerosa scarlatina A38.8
Ulcus — *see also* Ulcer
  cutis tuberculosum A18.4
  duodeni — *see* Ulcer, duodenum
  durum (syphilitic) A51.0
    extragenital A51.2
  gastrojejunale — *see* Ulcer, gastrojejunal
  hypostaticum — *see* Ulcer, varicose
  molle (cutis) (skin) A57
  serpens corneae — *see* Ulcer, cornea, central
  ventriculi — *see* Ulcer, stomach
Ulegyria Q04.8
Ulerythema
  ophryogenes, congenital Q84.2
  sycosiforme L73.8
Ullrich (-Bonnevie) (-Turner) **syndrome** — *see also*
    Turner's syndrome Q87.19
Ullrich-Feichtiger syndrome Q87.0
Ulnar — *see* condition
Ulorrhagia, ulorrhea K06.8
Umbilicus, umbilical — *see* condition
Unable to
  make ends meet Z59.86
  obtain
    adequate
      childcare Z59.87
      clothing Z59.87
      utilities Z59.87
    basic needs Z59.87
Unacceptable
  contours of tooth K08.54
  morphology of tooth K08.54
Unaffordable transportation Z59.82
Unavailability (of)
  bed at medical facility Z75.1
  health service-related agencies Z75.4
  medical facilities (at) Z75.3
    due to
      investigation by social service agency Z75.2
      lack of services at home Z75.0
      remoteness from facility Z75.3

✓ **Additional Character Required** — **Refer to the Tabular List for Character Selection**

Unavailability — *continued*
  medical facilities — *continued*
    due to — *continued*
      waiting list Z75.1
    home Z75.0
    outpatient clinic Z75.3
  schooling Z55.1
  social service agencies Z75.4
Uncinaria americana infestation B76.1
Uncinariasis B76.9
Uncongenial work Z56.5
Unconscious (ness) — *see* Coma
Under observation — *see* Observation
Underachievement in school Z55.3
Underdevelopment — *see also* Undeveloped
  nose Q30.1
  sexual E30.0
Underdosing — *see also* Table of Drugs and Chemicals,
    categories T36-T50, with final character 6 Z91.14
  intentional NEC Z91.128
    due to financial hardship of patient Z91.120
  unintentional NEC Z91.138
    due to patient's age related debility Z91.130
Underfeeding, newborn P92.3
Underfill, endodontic M27.53
Underimmunization status Z28.39
  COVID-19 Z28.31- ☑
    partially vaccinated (for) Z28.311
    unvaccinated (for) Z28.310
Undernourishment — *see* Malnutrition
Undernutrition — *see* Malnutrition
Underweight R63.6
  for gestational age — *see* Light for dates
Underwood's disease P83.0
Undescended — *see also* Malposition, congenital
  cecum Q43.3
  colon Q43.3
  testicle — *see* Cryptorchid
Undeveloped, undevelopment — *see also* Hypoplasia
  brain (congenital) Q02
  cerebral (congenital) Q02
  heart Q24.8
  lung Q33.6
  testis E29.1
  uterus E30.0
Undiagnosed (disease) R69
Undulant fever — *see* Brucellosis
Unemployment, anxiety concerning Z56.0
  threatened Z56.2
Unequal length (acquired) (limb) — *see also* Deformity,
    limb, unequal length
  leg — *see also* Deformity, limb, unequal length
    congenital Q72.9- ☑
Unextracted dental root K08.3
Unguis incarnatus L60.0
Unhappiness R45.2
Unicornate uterus Q51.4
  in pregnancy or childbirth O34.00
Unilateral — *see also* condition
  development, breast N64.89
  organ or site, congenital NEC — *see* Agenesis, by site
Unilocular heart Q20.8
Unimmunized — *see also* Underimmunization status
  for COVID-19 Z28.310
Union, abnormal — *see also* Fusion
  larynx and trachea Q34.8
Universal mesentery Q43.3
Unreliable transportation Z59.82
Unrepairable overhanging of dental restorative
  materials K08.52
Unroofed coronary sinus Q21.13
Unsafe transportation Z59.82
Unsatisfactory
  restoration of tooth K08.50
    specified NEC K08.59
  sample of cytologic smear
    anus R85.615
    cervix R87.615
    vagina R87.625
  surroundings Z59.1
  work Z56.5
Unsoundness of mind — *see* Psychosis
Unstable
  back NEC — *see* Instability, joint, spine
  hip (congenital) Q65.6
    acquired — *see* Derangement, joint, specified type
      NEC, hip

Unstable — *continued*
  joint — *see* Instability, joint
    secondary to removal of joint prosthesis M96.89
  lie (mother) O32.0 ☑
  lumbosacral joint (congenital) — *see* subcategory
    M53.2
  sacroiliac — *see* subcategory M53.2 ☑
  spine NEC — *see* Instability, joint, spine
Unsteadiness on feet R26.81
Untruthfulness, child problem F91.8
Unvaccinated — *see also* Underimmunization status
  for COVID-19 Z28.310
Unverricht (-Lundborg) **disease or epilepsy** — *see*
  Epilepsy, generalized, idiopathic
Unwanted
  multiple moves in the last 12 months Z59.81- ☑
  pregnancy Z64.0
Upbringing, institutional Z62.22
  away from parents NEC Z62.29
  in care of non-parental family member Z62.21
  in foster care Z62.21
  in orphanage or group home Z62.22
  in welfare custody Z62.21
Upper respiratory — *see* condition
Upset
  gastric K30
  gastrointestinal K30
    psychogenic F45.8
  intestinal (large) (small) K59.9
    psychogenic F45.8
  menstruation N93.9
  mental F48.9
  stomach K30
    psychogenic F45.8
Urachus — *see also* condition
  patent or persistent Q64.4
Urbach-Oppenheim disease (necrobiosis lipoidica diabeticorum) — *see* E08-E13 with .620
Urbach's lipoid proteinosis E78.89
Urbach-Wiethe disease E78.89
Urban yellow fever A95.1
Urea
  blood, high — *see* Uremia
  cycle metabolism disorder — *see* Disorder, urea cycle
    metabolism
Uremia, uremic N19
  with
    ectopic or molar pregnancy O08.4
    polyneuropathy N18.9 *[G63]*
  chronic NOS — *see also* Disease, kidney, chronic N18.9
    due to hypertension — *see* Hypertensive, kidney
  complicating
    ectopic or molar pregnancy O08.4
  congenital P96.0
  extrarenal R39.2
  following ectopic or molar pregnancy O08.4
  newborn P96.0
  prerenal R39.2
Ureter, ureteral — *see* condition
Ureteralgia N23
Ureterectasis — *see* Hydroureter
Ureteritis N28.89
  cystica N28.86
  due to calculus N20.1
    with calculus, kidney N20.2
      with hydronephrosis N13.2
  gonococcal (acute) (chronic) A54.21
  nonspecific N28.89
Ureterocele N28.89
  congenital (orthotopic) Q62.31
    ectopic Q62.32
Ureterolith, ureterolithiasis — *see* Calculus, ureter
Ureterostomy
  attention to Z43.6
  status Z93.6
Urethra, urethral — *see* condition
Urethralgia R39.89
Urethritis (anterior) (posterior) N34.2
  calculous N21.1
  candidal B37.41
  chlamydial A56.01
  diplococcal (gonococcal) A54.01
    with abscess (accessory gland) (periurethral) A54.1
  gonococcal A54.01
    with abscess (accessory gland) (periurethral) A54.1
  nongonococcal N34.1
    Reiter's — *see* Reiter's disease

Urethritis — *continued*
  nonspecific N34.1
  nonvenereal N34.1
  postmenopausal N34.2
  puerperal O86.22
  Reiter's — *see* Reiter's disease
  specified NEC N34.2
  trichomonal or due to Trichomonas (vaginalis) A59.03
Urethrocele N81.0
  with
    cystocele — *see* Cystocele
    prolapse of uterus — *see* Prolapse, uterus
Urethrolithiasis (with colic or infection) N21.1
Urethrorectal — *see* condition
Urethrorrhagia N36.8
Urethrorrhea R36.9
Urethrostomy
  attention to Z43.6
  status Z93.6
Urethrotrigonitis — *see* Trigonitis
Urethrovaginal — *see* condition
Urgency
  fecal R15.2
  hypertensive — *see* Hypertension
  urinary R39.15
Urhidrosis, uridrosis L74.8
Uric acid in blood (increased) E79.0
Uricacidemia (asymptomatic) E79.0
Uricemia (asymptomatic) E79.0
Uricosuria R82.998
Urinary — *see* condition
Urination
  frequent R35.0
  painful R30.9
Urine
  blood in — *see* Hematuria
  discharge, excessive R35.89
  enuresis, nonorganic origin F98.0
  extravasation R39.0
  frequency R35.0
  incontinence R32
    nonorganic origin F98.0
  intermittent stream R39.198
  pus in N39.0
  retention or stasis R33.9
    organic R33.8
      drug-induced R33.0
    psychogenic F45.8
  secretion
    deficient R34
    excessive R35.89
    frequency R35.0
  stream
    intermittent R39.198
    slowing R39.198
    splitting R39.13
    weak R39.12
Urinemia — *see* Uremia
Urinoma, urethra N36.8
Uroarthritis, infectious (Reiter's) — *see* Reiter's disease
Urodialysis R34
Urolithiasis — *see* Calculus, urinary
Uronephrosis — *see* Hydronephrosis
Uropathy N39.9
  obstructive N13.9
    specified NEC N13.8
  reflux N13.9
    specified NEC N13.8
  vesicoureteral reflux-associated — *see* Reflux, vesi-
    coureteral
Urosepsis — *code to* condition
Urticaria L50.9
  with angioneurotic edema T78.3 ☑
    hereditary D84.1
  allergic L50.0
  cholinergic L50.5
  chronic L50.8
  cold, familial L50.2
  contact L50.6
  dermatographic L50.3
  due to
    cold or heat L50.2
    drugs L50.0
    food L50.0
    inhalants L50.0
    plants L50.6
    serum — *see also* Reaction, serum T80.69 ☑
  factitial L50.3

Urticaria — continued
familial cold M04.2
giant T78.3 ✓
  hereditary D84.1
gigantea T78.3 ✓
idiopathic L50.1
larynx T78.3 ✓
  hereditary D84.1
neonatorum P83.88
nonallergic L50.1
papulosa (Hebra) L28.2
pigmentosa D47.01
  congenital Q82.2
  of neonatal onset Q82.2
  of newborn onset Q82.2
recurrent periodic L50.8
serum — see also Reaction, serum T80.69 ✓
solar L56.3
specified type NEC L50.8
thermal (cold) (heat) L50.2
vibratory L50.4
xanthelasmoidea — see Urticaria pigmentosa

Use (of)
alcohol F10.90
  with
    intoxication F10.929
    sleep disorder F10.982
    withdrawal F10.939
      with
        perceptual disturbance F10.932
      delirium F10.931
      uncomplicated F10.930
  harmful — see Abuse, alcohol
  in remission F10.91
amphetamines — see Use, stimulant NEC
caffeine — see Use, stimulant NEC
cannabis F12.90
  with
    anxiety disorder F12.980
    intoxication F12.929
      with
        delirium F12.921
        perceptual disturbance F12.922
      uncomplicated F12.920
    other specified disorder F12.988
    psychosis F12.959
      delusions F12.950
      hallucinations F12.951
    unspecified disorder F12.99
    withdrawal F12.93
  in remission F12.91
cocaine F14.90
  with
    anxiety disorder F14.980
    intoxication F14.929
      with
        delirium F14.921
        perceptual disturbance F14.922
      uncomplicated F14.920
    other specified disorder F14.988
    psychosis F14.959
      delusions F14.950
      hallucinations F14.951
    sexual dysfunction F14.981
    sleep disorder F14.982
    unspecified disorder F14.99
    withdrawal F14.93
  harmful — see Abuse, drug, cocaine
  in remission F14.91
drug(s) NEC F19.90
  with sleep disorder F19.982
  harmful — see Abuse, drug, by type
hallucinogen NEC F16.90
  with
    anxiety disorder F16.980
    intoxication F16.929
      with
        delirium F16.921
      uncomplicated F16.920
    mood disorder F16.94
    other specified disorder F16.988
    perception disorder (flashbacks) F16.983
    psychosis F16.959
      delusions F16.950
      hallucinations F16.951
    unspecified disorder F16.99
  harmful — see Abuse, drug, hallucinogen NEC
  in remission F16.91

Use — continued
inhalants F18.90
  with
    anxiety disorder F18.980
    intoxication F18.929
      with delirium F18.921
      uncomplicated F18.920
    mood disorder F18.94
    other specified disorder F18.988
    persisting dementia F18.97
    psychosis F18.959
      delusions F18.950
      hallucinations F18.951
    unspecified disorder F18.99
  harmful — see Abuse, drug, inhalant
  in remission F18.91
methadone — see Use, opioid
nonprescribed drugs F19.90
  harmful — see Abuse, non-psychoactive substance
opioid F11.90
  with
    disorder F11.99
      mood F11.94
      sleep F11.982
      specified type NEC F11.988
    intoxication F11.929
      with
        delirium F11.921
        perceptual disturbance F11.922
      uncomplicated F11.920
    withdrawal F11.93
  harmful — see Abuse, drug, opioid
  in remission F11.91
patent medicines F19.90
  harmful — see Abuse, non-psychoactive substance
psychoactive drug NEC F19.90
  with
    anxiety disorder F19.980
    intoxication F19.929
      with
        delirium F19.921
        perceptual disturbance F19.922
      uncomplicated F19.920
    mood disorder F19.94
    other specified disorder F19.988
    persisting
      amnestic disorder F19.96
      dementia F19.97
    psychosis F19.959
      delusions F19.950
      hallucinations F19.951
    sexual dysfunction F19.981
    sleep disorder F19.982
    unspecified disorder F19.99
    withdrawal F19.939
      with
        delirium F19.931
        perceptual disturbance F19.932
      uncomplicated F19.930
  harmful — see Abuse, drug NEC, psychoactive NEC
  in remission F19.91
sedative, hypnotic, or anxiolytic F13.90
  with
    anxiety disorder F13.980
    intoxication F13.929
      with
        delirium F13.921
      uncomplicated F13.920
    other specified disorder F13.988
    persisting
      amnestic disorder F13.96
      dementia F13.97
    psychosis F13.959
      delusions F13.950
      hallucinations F13.951
    sexual dysfunction F13.981
    sleep disorder F13.982
    unspecified disorder F13.99
  harmful — see Abuse, drug, sedative, hypnotic, or anxiolytic
  in remission F13.91
stimulant NEC F15.90
  with
    anxiety disorder F15.980
    intoxication F15.929
      with
        delirium F15.921
        perceptual disturbance F15.922

Use — continued
stimulant — continued
  with — continued
    intoxication — continued
      uncomplicated F15.920
    mood disorder F15.94
    other specified disorder F15.988
    psychosis F15.959
      delusions F15.950
      hallucinations F15.951
    sexual dysfunction F15.981
    sleep disorder F15.982
    unspecified disorder F15.99
    withdrawal F15.93
  harmful — see Abuse, drug, stimulant NEC
  in remission F15.91
tobacco Z72.0
  with dependence — see Dependence, drug, nicotine
volatile solvents — see also Use, inhalant F18.90
  harmful — see Abuse, drug, inhalant

Usher-Senear disease or syndrome L10.4
Uta B55.1
Uteromegaly N85.2
Uterovaginal — see condition
Uterovesical — see condition
Uveal — see condition
Uveitis (anterior) — see also Iridocyclitis
  acute — see Iridocyclitis, acute
  chronic — see Iridocyclitis, chronic
  due to toxoplasmosis (acquired) B58.09
    congenital P37.1
  granulomatous — see Iridocyclitis, chronic
  heterochromic — see Cyclitis, Fuchs' heterochromic
  lens-induced — see Iridocyclitis, lens-induced
  posterior — see Chorioretinitis
  sympathetic H44.13- ✓
  syphilitic (secondary) A51.43
    congenital (early) A50.01
    late A52.71
  tuberculous A18.54
Uveoencephalitis — see Inflammation, chorioretinal
Uveokeratitis — see Iridocyclitis
Uveoparotitis D86.89
Uvula — see condition
Uvulitis (acute) (catarrhal) (chronic) (membranous) (suppurative) (ulcerative) K12.2

V

Vaccination (prophylactic)
  complication or reaction — see Complications, vaccination
  delayed Z28.9
  encounter for Z23
  not done — see Immunization, not done
  partial — see also Underimmunization status
    for COVID-19 Z28.311
Vaccinia (generalized) (localized) T88.1 ✓
  congenital P35.8
  without vaccination B08.011
Vacuum, in sinus (accessory) (nasal) J34.89
Vagabond, vagabondage Z59.00
Vagabond's disease B85.1
Vagina, vaginal — see condition
Vaginalitis (tunica) (testis) N49.1
Vaginismus (reflex) N94.2
  functional F52.5
  nonorganic F52.5
  psychogenic F52.5
  secondary N94.2
Vaginitis (acute) (circumscribed) (diffuse) (emphysematous) (nonvenereal) (ulcerative) N76.0
  with ectopic or molar pregnancy O08.0
  amebic A06.82
  atrophic, postmenopausal N95.2
  bacterial N76.0
  blennorrhagic (gonococcal) A54.02
  candidal (acute) B37.31
    chronic (recurrent) B37.32
  chlamydial A56.02
  chronic N76.1
  due to Trichomonas (vaginalis) A59.01
  following ectopic or molar pregnancy O08.0
  gonococcal A54.02
    with abscess (accessory gland) (periurethral) A54.1
  granuloma A58

Vaginitis — *continued*
- in (due to)
  - candidiasis (acute) B37.31
    - chronic (recurrent) B37.32
  - herpesviral (herpes simplex) infection A60.04
  - pinworm infection B80 *[N77.1]*
  - monilial (acute) B37.31
    - chronic (recurrent) B37.32
  - mycotic (candidal) (acute) B37.31
    - chronic (recurrent) B37.32
  - postmenopausal atrophic N95.2
  - puerperal (postpartum) O86.13
  - senile (atrophic) N95.2
  - subacute or chronic N76.1
  - syphilitic (early) A51.0
    - late A52.76
  - trichomonal A59.01
  - tuberculous A18.18

Vaginosis — *see* Vaginitis
Vagotonia G52.2
Vagrancy Z59.00
VAIN — *see* Neoplasia, intraepithelial, vagina
Vallecula — *see* condition
Valley fever B38.0
Valsuani's disease — *see* Anemia, obstetric
Valve, valvular (formation) — *see also* condition
- cerebral ventricle (communicating) in situ Z98.2
- cervix, internal os Q51.828
- congenital NEC — *see* Atresia, by site
- ureter (pelvic junction) (vesical orifice) Q62.39
- urethra (congenital) (posterior) Q64.2

Valvulitis (chronic) — *see* Endocarditis
Valvulopathy — *see* Endocarditis
Van Bogaert's leukoencephalopathy (sclerosing) (subacute) A81.1
Van Bogaert-Scherer-Epstein disease or syndrome E75.5
Van Buchem's syndrome M85.2
Van Creveld-von Gierke disease E74.01
Van der Hoeve (-de Kleyn) **syndrome** Q78.0
Van der Woude's syndrome Q38.0
Van Neck's disease or osteochondrosis M91.0
Vanishing lung J44.9
Vapor asphyxia or suffocation T59.9 ☑
- specified agent — *see* Table of Drugs and Chemicals

Variance, lethal ball, prosthetic heart valve T82.09 ☑
Variants, thalassemic D56.8
Variations in hair color L67.1
Varicella B01.9
- with
  - complications NEC B01.89
  - encephalitis B01.11
  - encephalomyelitis B01.11
  - meningitis B01.0
  - myelitis B01.12
  - pneumonia B01.2
- congenital P35.8

Varices — *see* Varix
Varicocele (scrotum) (thrombosed) I86.1
- ovary I86.2
- perineum I86.3
- spermatic cord (ulcerated) I86.1

Varicose
- aneurysm (ruptured) I77.0
- dermatitis — *see* Varix, leg, with, inflammation
- eczema — *see* Varix, leg, with, inflammation
- phlebitis — *see* Varix, with, inflammation
- tumor — *see* Varix
- ulcer (lower limb, any part) — *see also* Varix, leg, with, ulcer
  - anus — *see also* Hemorrhoids K64.8
  - esophagus — *see* Varix, esophagus
  - inflamed or infected — *see* Varix, leg, with ulcer, with inflammation
  - nasal septum I86.8
  - perineum I86.3
  - scrotum I86.1
  - specified site NEC I86.8
- vein — *see* Varix
- vessel — *see* Varix, leg

Varicosis, varicosities, varicosity — *see* Varix
Variola (major) (minor) B03
Varioloid B03
Varix (lower limb) I83.90
- with
  - bleeding I83.899
  - edema I83.899

Varix — *continued*
- with — *continued*
  - inflammation I83.10
    - with ulcer (venous) I83.209
  - pain I83.819
  - rupture I83.899
  - specified complication NEC I83.899
  - stasis dermatitis I83.10
    - with ulcer (venous) I83.209
  - swelling I83.899
  - ulcer I83.009
    - with inflammation I83.209
- aneurysmal I77.0
- asymptomatic I83.9- ☑
- bladder I86.2
- broad ligament I86.2
- complicating
  - childbirth (lower extremity) O87.4
    - anus or rectum O87.2
    - genital (vagina, vulva or perineum) O87.8
  - pregnancy (lower extremity) O22.0- ☑
    - anus or rectum O22.4- ☑
    - genital (vagina, vulva or perineum) O22.1- ☑
  - puerperium (lower extremity) O87.4
    - anus or rectum O87.2
    - genital (vagina, vulva, perineum) O87.8
- congenital (any site) Q27.8
- esophagus (idiopathic) (primary) (ulcerated) I85.00
  - bleeding I85.01
  - congenital Q27.8
  - in (due to)
    - alcoholic liver disease I85.10
      - bleeding I85.11
    - cirrhosis of liver I85.10
      - bleeding I85.11
    - portal hypertension I85.10
      - bleeding I85.11
    - schistosomiasis I85.10
      - bleeding I85.11
    - toxic liver disease I85.10
      - bleeding I85.11
  - secondary I85.10
    - bleeding I85.11
- gastric I86.4
- inflamed or infected I83.10
  - ulcerated I83.209
- labia (majora) I86.3
- leg (asymptomatic) I83.9- ☑
  - with
    - edema I83.899
    - inflammation I83.10
      - with ulcer — *see* Varix, leg, with, ulcer, with inflammation by site
    - pain I83.819
    - specified complication NEC I83.899
    - swelling I83.899
    - ulcer I83.0- ☑
      - with inflammation I83.2- ☑
      - ankle I83.003
        - with inflammation I83.203
      - calf I83.002
        - with inflammation I83.202
      - foot NEC I83.005
        - with inflammation I83.205
      - heel I83.004
        - with inflammation I83.204
      - lower leg NEC I83.008
        - with inflammation I83.208
      - midfoot I83.004
        - with inflammation I83.204
      - thigh I83.001
        - with inflammation I83.201
  - bilateral (asymptomatic) I83.93
    - with
      - edema I83.893
      - pain I83.813
      - specified complication NEC I83.893
      - swelling I83.893
      - ulcer I83.0- ☑
        - with inflammation I83.209
  - left (asymptomatic) I83.92
    - with
      - edema I83.892
      - inflammation I83.12
        - with ulcer — *see* Varix, leg, with, ulcer, with inflammation by site
      - pain I83.812
      - specified complication NEC I83.892

Varix — *continued*
- leg — *continued*
  - left — *continued*
    - with — *continued*
      - swelling I83.892
      - ulcer I83.029
        - with inflammation I83.229
        - ankle I83.023
          - with inflammation I83.223
        - calf I83.022
          - with inflammation I83.222
        - foot NEC I83.025
          - with inflammation I83.225
        - heel I83.024
          - with inflammation I83.224
        - lower leg NEC I83.028
          - with inflammation I83.228
        - midfoot I83.024
          - with inflammation I83.224
        - thigh I83.021
          - with inflammation I83.221
  - right (asymptomatic) I83.91
    - with
      - edema I83.891
      - inflammation I83.11
        - with ulcer — *see* Varix, leg, with, ulcer, with inflammation by site
      - pain I83.811
      - specified complication NEC I83.891
      - swelling I83.891
      - ulcer I83.019
        - with inflammation I83.219
        - ankle I83.013
          - with inflammation I83.213
        - calf I83.012
          - with inflammation I83.212
        - foot NEC I83.015
          - with inflammation I83.215
        - heel I83.014
          - with inflammation I83.214
        - lower leg NEC I83.018
          - with inflammation I83.218
        - midfoot I83.014
          - with inflammation I83.214
        - thigh I83.011
          - with inflammation I83.211
- nasal septum I86.8
- orbit I86.8
  - congenital Q27.8
- ovary I86.2
- papillary I78.1
- pelvis I86.2
- perineum I86.3
- pharynx I86.8
- placenta O43.89- ☑
- renal papilla I86.8
- retina H35.09
- scrotum (ulcerated) I86.1
- sigmoid colon I86.8
- specified site NEC I86.8
- spinal (cord) (vessels) I86.8
- spleen, splenic (vein) (with phlebolith) I86.8
- stomach I86.4
- sublingual I86.0
- ulcerated I83.009
  - inflamed or infected I83.209
- uterine ligament I86.2
- vagina I86.8
- vocal cord I86.8
- vulva I86.3

Vas deferens — *see* condition
Vas deferentitis N49.1
Vasa previa O69.4 ☑
- hemorrhage from, affecting newborn P50.0

Vascular — *see also* condition
- loop on optic papilla Q14.2
- spasm I73.9
- spider I78.1

Vascularization, cornea — *see* Neovascularization, cornea
Vasculitis I77.6
- allergic D69.0
- ANCA (antineutrophilic cytoplasmic antibody) associated I77.82
- ANCA (antineutrophilic cytoplasmic antibody) positive I77.82
- antineutrophilic cytoplasmic antibody [ANCA] I77.82
- cryoglobulinemic D89.1

Vasculitis — *continued*
  disseminated I77.6
  hypocomplementemic M31.8
  kidney I77.89
  leukocytoclastic M31.0
  livedoid L95.0
  nodular L95.8
  retina H35.06- ☑
  rheumatic — *see* Fever, rheumatic
  rheumatoid — *see* Rheumatoid, vasculitis
  skin (limited to) L95.9
    specified NEC L95.8
  systemic M31.8
Vasculopathy, necrotizing M31.9
  cardiac allograft T86.290
  specified NEC M31.8
Vasitis (nodosa) N49.1
  tuberculous A18.15
Vasodilation I73.9
Vasomotor — *see* condition
Vasoplasty, after previous sterilization Z31.0
  aftercare Z31.42
Vasospasm (vasoconstriction) I73.9
  cerebral (cerebrovascular) (artery) I67.848
    reversible I67.841
  coronary I20.1
  nerve
    arm — *see* Mononeuropathy, upper limb
    brachial plexus G54.0
    cervical plexus G54.2
    leg — *see* Mononeuropathy, lower limb
  peripheral NOS I73.9
  retina (artery) — *see* Occlusion, artery, retina
Vasospastic — *see* condition
Vasovagal attack (paroxysmal) R55
  psychogenic F45.8
VATER syndrome Q87.2
Vater's ampulla — *see* condition
Vegetation, vegetative
  adenoid (nasal fossa) J35.8
  endocarditis (acute) (any valve) (subacute) I33.0
  heart (mycotic) (valve) I33.0
Veil
  Jackson's Q43.3
Vein, venous — *see* condition
Veldt sore — *see* Ulcer, skin
Velpeau's hernia — *see* Hernia, femoral
Venereal
  bubo A55
  disease A64
  granuloma inguinale A58
  lymphogranuloma (Durand-Nicolas-Favre) A55
Venofibrosis I87.8
Venom, venomous — *see* Table of Drugs and Chemicals, by animal or substance, poisoning
Venous — *see* condition
Ventilator lung, newborn P27.8
Ventral — *see* condition
Ventricle, ventricular — *see also* condition
  escape I49.3
  inversion Q20.5
Ventriculitis (cerebral) — *see also* Encephalitis G04.90
Ventriculostomy status Z98.2
Vernet's syndrome G52.7
Verneuil's disease (syphilitic bursitis) A52.78
Verruca (due to HPV) (filiformis) (simplex) (viral) (vulgaris) B07.9
  acuminata A63.0
  necrogenica (primary) (tuberculosa) A18.4
  plana B07.8
  plantaris B07.0
  seborrheica L82.1
    inflamed L82.0
  senile (seborrheic) L82.1
    inflamed L82.0
  tuberculosa (primary) A18.4
  venereal A63.0
Verrucosities — *see* Verruca
Verruga peruana, peruviana A44.1
Version
  cervix — *see* Malposition, uterus
  uterus (postinfectional) (postpartal, old) — *see* Malposition, uterus
Vertebra, vertebral — *see* condition
Vertical talus (congenital) Q66.80
  left foot Q66.82
  right foot Q66.81

Vertigo R42
  auditory — *see* Vertigo, aural
  aural H81.31- ☑
  benign paroxysmal (positional) H81.1- ☑
  central (origin) H81.4
  cerebral H81.4
  Dix and Hallpike (epidemic) — *see* Neuronitis, vestibular
  due to infrasound T75.23 ☑
  epidemic A88.1
    Dix and Hallpike — *see* Neuronitis, vestibular
    Pedersen's — *see* Neuronitis, vestibular
    vestibular neuronitis — *see* Neuronitis, vestibular
  hysterical F44.89
  infrasound T75.23 ☑
  labyrinthine — *see* subcategory H81.0 ☑
  laryngeal R05.4
  malignant positional H81.4
  Ménière's — *see* subcategory H81.0 ☑
  menopausal N95.1
  otogenic — *see* Vertigo, aural
  paroxysmal positional, benign — *see* Vertigo, benign paroxysmal
  Pedersen's (epidemic) — *see* Neuronitis, vestibular
  peripheral NEC H81.39- ☑
  positional
    benign paroxysmal — *see* Vertigo, benign paroxysmal
    malignant H81.4
Very-low-density-lipoprotein-type (VLDL) **hyperlipoproteinemia** E78.1
Vesania — *see* Psychosis
Vesical — *see* condition
Vesicle
  cutaneous R23.8
  seminal — *see* condition
  skin R23.8
Vesicocolic — *see* condition
Vesicoperineal — *see* condition
Vesicorectal — *see* condition
Vesicourethrorectal — *see* condition
Vesicovaginal — *see* condition
Vesicular — *see* condition
Vesiculitis (seminal) N49.0
  amebic A06.82
  gonorrheal (acute) (chronic) A54.23
  trichomonal A59.09
  tuberculous A18.15
Vestibulitis (ear) — *see also* subcategory H83.0 ☑
  nose (external) J34.89
  vulvar N94.810
Vestibulopathy , acute peripheral (recurrent) — *see* Neuronitis, vestibular
Vestige, vestigial — *see also* Persistence
  branchial Q18.0
  structures in vitreous Q14.0
Vibration
  adverse effects T75.20 ☑
    pneumatic hammer syndrome T75.21 ☑
    specified effect NEC T75.29 ☑
    vasospastic syndrome T75.22 ☑
    vertigo from infrasound T75.23 ☑
  exposure (occupational) Z57.7
  vertigo T75.23 ☑
Vibriosis A28.9
Victim (of)
  crime Z65.4
  disaster Z65.5
  terrorism Z65.4
  torture Z65.4
  war Z65.5
Vidal's disease L28.0
Villaret's syndrome G52.7
Villous — *see* condition
VIN — *see* Neoplasia, intraepithelial, vulva
Vincent's infection (angina) (gingivitis) A69.1
  stomatitis NEC A69.1
Vinson-Plummer syndrome D50.1
Violence, physical R45.6
Viosterol deficiency — *see* Deficiency, calciferol
Vipoma — *see* Neoplasm, malignant, by site
Viremia B34.9
Virilism (adrenal) E25.9
  congenital E25.0
Virilization (female) (suprarenal) E25.9
  congenital E25.0
  isosexual E28.2

Virulent bubo A57
Virus, viral — *see also* condition
  as cause of disease classified elsewhere B97.89
    respiratory syncytial virus (RSV) — *see* Virus, respiratory syncytial (RSV)
  cytomegalovirus B25.9
  human immunodeficiency (HIV) — *see* Human, immunodeficiency virus (HIV) disease
  infection — *see* Infection, virus
  respiratory syncytial (RSV)
    as cause of disease classified elsewhere B97.4
    bronchiolitis J21.0
    bronchitis J20.5
    bronchopneumonia J12.1
    otitis media H65.- ☑ *[B97.4]*
    pneumonia J12.1
    upper respiratory infection J06.9 *[B97.4]*
  specified NEC B34.8
  swine influenza (viruses that normally cause infections in pigs) — *see also* Influenza, due to, identified novel influenza A virus J09.X2
  West Nile (fever) A92.30
    with
      complications NEC A92.39
      cranial nerve disorders A92.32
      encephalitis A92.31
      encephalomyelitis A92.31
      neurologic manifestation NEC A92.32
      optic neuritis A92.32
      polyradiculitis A92.32
Viscera, visceral — *see* condition
Visceroptosis K63.4
Visible peristalsis R19.2
Vision, visual
  binocular, suppression H53.34
  blurred, blurring H53.8
    hysterical F44.6
  defect, defective NEC H54.7
  disorientation (syndrome) H53.8
  disturbance H53.9
    hysterical F44.6
  double H53.2
  examination Z01.00
    with abnormal findings Z01.01
    following failed vision screening Z01.020
      with abnormal findings Z01.021
  field, limitation (defect) — *see* Defect, visual field
  hallucinations R44.1
  halos H53.19
  loss — *see* Loss, vision
    sudden — *see* Disturbance, vision, subjective, loss, sudden
  low (both eyes) — *see* Low, vision
  perception, simultaneous without fusion H53.33
Vitality, lack or want of R53.83
  newborn P96.89
Vitamin deficiency — *see* Deficiency, vitamin
Vitelline duct, persistent Q43.0
Vitiligo L80
  eyelid H02.739
    left H02.736
      lower H02.735
      upper H02.734
    right H02.733
      lower H02.732
      upper H02.731
  pinta A67.2
  vulva N90.89
Vitreal corneal syndrome H59.01- ☑
Vitreoretinopathy, proliferative — *see also* Retinopathy, proliferative
  with retinal detachment — *see* Detachment, retina, traction
Vitreous — *see also* condition
  touch syndrome — *see* Complication, postprocedural, following cataract surgery
Vocal cord — *see* condition
Vogt-Koyanagi syndrome H20.82- ☑
Vogt's disease or syndrome G80.3
Vogt-Spielmeyer amaurotic idiocy or disease E75.4
Voice
  change R49.9
    specified NEC R49.8
  loss — *see* Aphonia
Volhynian fever A79.0
Volkmann's ischemic contracture or paralysis (complicating trauma) T79.6 ☑
Volvulus (bowel) (colon) (intestine) K56.2

☑ Additional Character Required — Refer to the Tabular List for Character Selection

Volvulus — *continued*
  with perforation K56.2
  congenital Q43.8
  duodenum K31.5
  fallopian tube — *see* Torsion, fallopian tube
  oviduct — *see* Torsion, fallopian tube
  stomach (due to absence of gastrocolic ligament)
      K31.89
Vomiting R11.10
  with nausea R11.2
  asphyxia — *see* Foreign body, by site, causing asphyxia,
      gastric contents
  bilious (cause unknown) R11.14
      following gastro-intestinal surgery K91.0
      in newborn P92.01
  blood — *see* Hematemesis
  causing asphyxia, choking, or suffocation — *see* For-
      eign body, by site
  cyclical, in migraine G43.A0 (*following* G43.7)
      with refractory migraine G43.A1 (*following* G43.7)
      intractable G43.A1 (*following* G43.7)
      not intractable G43.A0 (*following* G43.7)
          psychogenic F50.89
          without refractory migraine G43.A0 (*following* G43.7)
  cyclical syndrome NOS (unrelated to migraine) R11.15
  fecal mater R11.13
  following gastrointestinal surgery K91.0
      psychogenic F50.89
  functional K31.89
  hysterical F50.89
  nervous F50.89
  neurotic F50.89
  newborn NEC P92.09
      bilious P92.01
  periodic R11.10
      psychogenic F50.89
  persistent R11.15
  projectile R11.12
  psychogenic F50.89
  uremic — *see* Uremia
  without nausea R11.11
Vomito negro — *see* Fever, yellow
Von Bezold's abscess — *see* Mastoiditis, acute
Von Economo-Cruchet disease A85.8
Von Eulenburg's disease G71.19
Von Gierke's disease E74.01
Von Hippel (-Lindau) **disease or syndrome** Q85.83
Von Jaksch's anemia or disease D64.89
Von Recklinghausen
  disease (neurofibromatosis) Q85.01
      bones E21.0
Von Schroetter's syndrome I82.890
Von Willebrand (-Jurgens) (-Minot) **disease or syn-
  drome** — *see* Disease, von Willebrand
Von Zumbusch's disease L40.1
Voyeurism F65.3
Vrolik's disease Q78.0
Vulva — *see* condition
Vulvismus N94.2
Vulvitis (acute) (allergic) (atrophic) (hypertrophic) (inter-
    triginous) (senile) N76.2
  with ectopic or molar pregnancy O08.0
  adhesive, congenital Q52.79
  blennorrhagic (gonococcal) A54.02
  candidal (acute) B37.31
      chronic (recurrent) B37.32
  chlamydial A56.02
  due to Haemophilus ducreyi A57
  following ectopic or molar pregnancy O08.0
  gonococcal A54.02
      with abscess (accessory gland) (periurethral) A54.1
  herpesviral A60.04
  leukoplakic N90.4
  monilial (acute) B37.31
      chronic (recurrent) B37.32
  puerperal (postpartum) O86.19
  subacute or chronic N76.3
  syphilitic (early) A51.0
      late A52.76
  trichomonal A59.01
  tuberculous A18.18
Vulvodynia N94.819
  specified NEC N94.818
Vulvorectal — *see* condition
Vulvovaginitis (acute) — *see* Vaginitis

W

Waiting list, person on Z75.1
  for organ transplant Z76.82
  undergoing social agency investigation Z75.2
Waldenström
  hypergammaglobulinemia D89.0
  syndrome or macroglobulinemia C88.0
Waldenström-Kjellberg syndrome D50.1
Walking
  difficulty R26.2
      psychogenic F44.4
  sleep F51.3
      hysterical F44.89
Wall, abdominal — *see* condition
Wallenberg's disease or syndrome G46.3
Wallgren's disease I87.8
Wandering
  gallbladder, congenital Q44.1
  in diseases classified elsewhere Z91.83
  kidney, congenital Q63.8
  organ or site, congenital NEC — *see* Malposition, con-
      genital, by site
  pacemaker (heart) I49.8
  spleen D73.89
War neurosis F48.8
Wart (due to HPV) (filiform) (infectious) (viral) B07.9
  anogenital region (venereal) A63.0
  common B07.8
  external genital organs (venereal) A63.0
  flat B07.8
  Hassal-Henle's (of cornea) H18.49
  Peruvian A44.1
  plantar B07.0
  prosector (tuberculous) A18.4
  seborrheic L82.1
      inflamed L82.0
  senile (seborrheic) L82.1
      inflamed L82.0
  tuberculous A18.4
  venereal A63.0
Warthin's tumor — *see* Neoplasm, salivary gland, benign
Wassilieff's disease A27.0
Wasting
  disease R64
      due to malnutrition E43
          with marasmus E41
  extreme (due to malnutrition) E43
      with marasmus E41
  muscle NEC — *see* Atrophy, muscle
Water
  clefts (senile cataract) — *see* Cataract, senile, incipient
  deprivation of T73.1 ☑
  intoxication E87.79
  itch B76.9
  lack of T73.1 ☑
      safe drinking Z58.6
  loading E87.70
  on
      brain — *see* Hydrocephalus
      chest J94.8
  poisoning E87.79
Waterbrash R12
Waterhouse (-Friderichsen) **syndrome or disease**
    (meningococcal) A39.1
Water-losing nephritis N25.89
Watermelon stomach K31.819
  with hemorrhage K31.811
  without hemorrhage K31.819
Watsoniasis B66.8
Wax in ear — *see* Impaction, cerumen
Weak, weakening, weakness (generalized) R53.1
  arches (acquired) — *see also* Deformity, limb, flat foot
  bladder (sphincter) R32
  facial R29.810
      following
          cerebrovascular disease I69.992
              cerebral infarction I69.392
              intracerebral hemorrhage I69.192
              nontraumatic intracranial hemorrhage NEC
                  I69.292
              specified disease NEC I69.892
              stroke I69.392
              subarachnoid hemorrhage I69.092
  foot (double) — *see also* Weak, arches
  heart, cardiac — *see* Failure, heart
  mind F70

Weak, weakening, weakness — *continued*
  muscle M62.81
  myocardium — *see* Failure, heart
  newborn P96.89
  pelvic fundus N81.89
  pubocervical tissue N81.82
  rectovaginal tissue N81.83
  senile R54
  urinary stream R39.12
  valvular — *see* Endocarditis
Wear, worn (with normal or routine use)
  articular bearing surface of internal joint prosthesis —
      see Complications, joint prosthesis, mechanical,
      wear of articular bearing surfaces, by site
  device, implant or graft — *see* Complications, by site,
      mechanical complication
  tooth, teeth (approximal) (hard tissues) (interproximal)
      (occlusal) K03.0
Weather, weathered
  effects of
      cold T69.9 ☑
          specified effect NEC T69.8 ☑
      hot — *see* Heat
  skin L57.8
Weaver's syndrome Q87.3
Web, webbed (congenital)
  duodenal Q43.8
  esophagus Q39.4
  fingers Q70.1- ☑
  larynx (glottic) (subglottic) Q31.0
  neck (pterygium colli) Q18.3
  Paterson-Kelly D50.1
  popliteal syndrome Q87.89
  toes Q70.3- ☑
Weber-Christian disease M35.6
Weber-Cockayne syndrome (epidermolysis bullosa)
    Q81.8
Weber-Gubler syndrome G46.3
Weber-Leyden syndrome G46.3
Weber-Osler syndrome I78.0
Weber's paralysis or syndrome G46.3
Wedge-shaped or wedging vertebra — *see* Collapse,
    vertebra NEC
Wegener's granulomatosis or syndrome M31.30
  with
      kidney involvement M31.31
      lung involvement M31.30
          with kidney involvement M31.31
Wegner's disease A50.02
Weight
  1000-2499 grams at birth (low) — *see* Low, birthweight
  999 grams or less at birth (extremely low) — *see* Low,
      birthweight, extreme
  and length below 10th percentile for gestational age
      P05.1- ☑
  below but length above 10th percentile for gestational
      age P05.0- ☑
  gain (abnormal) (excessive) R63.5
      in pregnancy — *see* Pregnancy, complicated by,
          excessive weight gain
      low — *see* Pregnancy, complicated by, insuffi-
          cient, weight gain
  loss (abnormal) (cause unknown) R63.4
Weightlessness (effect of) T75.82 ☑
Weil (I)-**Marchesani syndrome** Q87.19
Weil's disease A27.0
Weingarten's syndrome J82.89
Weir Mitchell's disease I73.81
Weiss-Baker syndrome G90.09
Wells' disease L98.3
Wen — *see* Cyst, sebaceous
Wenckebach's block or phenomenon I44.1
Werdnig-Hoffmann syndrome (muscular atrophy)
    G12.0
Werlhof's disease D69.3
Wermer's disease or syndrome E31.21
Werner-His disease A79.0
Werner's disease or syndrome E34.8
Wernicke-Korsakoff's syndrome or psychosis (alco-
    holic) F10.96
  with dependence F10.26
  drug-induced
      due to drug abuse — *see* Abuse, drug, by type, with
          amnestic disorder
      due to drug dependence — *see* Dependence, drug,
          by type, with amnestic disorder
  nonalcoholic F04

Wernicke-Posadas disease B38.9
Wernicke's
  developmental aphasia F80.2
  disease or syndrome E51.2
  encephalopathy E51.2
  polioencephalitis, superior E51.2
West African fever B50.8
Westphal-Strümpell syndrome E83.01
West's syndrome — *see* Epilepsy, spasms
Wet
  feet, tropical (maceration) (syndrome) — *see* Immersion, foot
  lung (syndrome), newborn P22.1
Wharton's duct — *see* condition
Wheal — *see* Urticaria
Wheezing R06.2
Whiplash injury S13.4 ☑
Whipple's disease — *see also* subcategory M14.8- K90.81
Whipworm (disease) (infection) (infestation) B79
Whistling face Q87.0
White — *see also* condition
  kidney, small N03.9
  leg, puerperal, postpartum, childbirth O87.1
  mouth B37.0
  patches of mouth K13.29
  spot lesions, teeth
    chewing surface K02.51
    pit and fissure surface K02.51
    smooth surface K02.61
Whitehead L70.0
Whitlow — *see also* Cellulitis, digit
  with lymphangitis — *see* Lymphangitis, acute, digit
  herpesviral B00.89
Whitmore's disease or fever — *see* Melioidosis
Whooping cough A37.90
  with pneumonia A37.91
    due to Bordetella
      bronchiseptica A37.81
      parapertussis A37.11
      pertussis A37.01
      specified organism NEC A37.81
  due to
    Bordetella
      bronchiseptica A37.80
        with pneumonia A37.81
      parapertussis A37.10
        with pneumonia A37.11
      pertussis A37.00
        with pneumonia A37.01
      specified NEC A37.80
        with pneumonia A37.81
Wichman's asthma J38.5
Wide cranial sutures, newborn P96.3
Widening aorta — *see* Ectasia, aorta
  with aneurysm — *see* Aneurysm, aorta
Wilkie's disease or syndrome K55.1
Wilkinson-Sneddon disease or syndrome L13.1
Willebrand (-Jürgens) **thrombopathy** — *see* Disease, von Willebrand
Williams syndrome Q93.82
Willige-Hunt disease or syndrome G23.1
Wilms' tumor C64- ☑
Wilson-Mikity syndrome P27.0
Wilson's
  disease or syndrome E83.01
  hepatolenticular degeneration E83.01
  lichen ruber L43.9
Window — *see also* Imperfect, closure
  aorticopulmonary Q21.4
Winter — *see* condition
Wiskott-Aldrich syndrome D82.0
Withdrawal state — *see also* Dependence, drug by type, with withdrawal
  alcohol
    with perceptual disturbances F10.232
      due to alcohol abuse F10.132
      due to alcohol use F10.932
    abuse — *see* Abuse, alcohol, with, withdrawal
    dependence — *see* Dependence, alcohol, with, withdrawal
    use — *see* Use, alcohol, with, withdrawal
    without perceptual disturbances F10.239
      due to alcohol abuse F10.139
      due to alcohol use F10.939
  caffeine F15.93
  cannabis F12.23

Withdrawal state — *continued*
  newborn
    correct therapeutic substance properly administered P96.2
    infant of dependent mother P96.1
  therapeutic substance, neonatal P96.2
Witts' anemia D50.8
Witzelsucht F07.0
Woakes' ethmoiditis or syndrome J33.1
Wolff-Hirschorn syndrome Q93.3
Wolff-Parkinson-White syndrome I45.6
Wolhynian fever A79.0
Wolman's disease E75.5
Wood lung or pneumonitis J67.8
Woolly, wooly hair (congenital) (nevus) Q84.1
Woolsorter's disease A22.1
Word
  blindness (congenital) (developmental) F81.0
  deafness (congenital) (developmental) H93.25
Worm(s) (infection) (infestation) — *see also* Infestation, helminth
  guinea B72
  in intestine NEC B82.0
Worm-eaten soles A66.3
Worn out — *see* Exhaustion
  cardiac
    defibrillator (with synchronous cardiac pacemaker) Z45.02
    pacemaker
      battery Z45.010
      lead Z45.018
  device, implant or graft — *see* Complications, by site, mechanical
Worried well Z71.1
Worries R45.82
Wound check Z48.0- ☑
  due to injury — *code to* Injury, by site, using appropriate seventh character for subsequent encounter
Wound, open T14.8- ☑
  abdomen, abdominal
    wall S31.109 ☑
      with penetration into peritoneal cavity S31.609 ☑
      bite — *see* Bite, abdomen, wall
      epigastric region S31.102 ☑
        with penetration into peritoneal cavity S31.602 ☑
        bite — *see* Bite, abdomen, wall, epigastric region
        laceration — *see* Laceration, abdomen, wall, epigastric region
        puncture — *see* Puncture, abdomen, wall, epigastric region
      laceration — *see* Laceration, abdomen, wall
      left
        lower quadrant S31.104 ☑
          with penetration into peritoneal cavity S31.604 ☑
          bite — *see* Bite, abdomen, wall, left, lower quadrant
          laceration — *see* Laceration, abdomen, wall, left, lower quadrant
          puncture — *see* Puncture, abdomen, wall, left, lower quadrant
        upper quadrant S31.101 ☑
          with penetration into peritoneal cavity S31.601 ☑
          bite — *see* Bite, abdomen, wall, left, upper quadrant
          laceration — *see* Laceration, abdomen, wall, left, upper quadrant
          puncture — *see* Puncture, abdomen, wall, left, upper quadrant
      periumbilic region S31.105 ☑
        with penetration into peritoneal cavity S31.605 ☑
        bite — *see* Bite, abdomen, wall, periumbilic region
        laceration — *see* Laceration, abdomen, wall, periumbilic region
        puncture — *see* Puncture, abdomen, wall, periumbilic region
      puncture — *see* Puncture, abdomen, wall
      right
        lower quadrant S31.103 ☑
          with penetration into peritoneal cavity S31.603 ☑

Wound, open — *continued*
  abdomen, abdominal — *continued*
    wall — *continued*
      right — *continued*
        lower quadrant — *continued*
          bite — *see* Bite, abdomen, wall, right, lower quadrant
          laceration — *see* Laceration, abdomen, wall, right, lower quadrant
          puncture — *see* Puncture, abdomen, wall, right, lower quadrant
        upper quadrant S31.100 ☑
          with penetration into peritoneal cavity S31.600 ☑
          bite — *see* Bite, abdomen, wall, right, upper quadrant
          laceration — *see* Laceration, abdomen, wall, right, upper quadrant
          puncture — *see* Puncture, abdomen, wall, right, upper quadrant
  alveolar (process) — *see* Wound, open, oral cavity
  ankle S91.00- ☑
    bite — *see* Bite, ankle
    laceration — *see* Laceration, ankle
    puncture — *see* Puncture, ankle
  antecubital space — *see* Wound, open, elbow
  anterior chamber, eye — *see* Wound, open, ocular
  anus S31.839 ☑
    bite S31.835 ☑
    laceration — *see* Laceration, anus
    puncture — *see* Puncture, anus
  arm (upper) S41.10- ☑
    with amputation — *see* Amputation, traumatic, arm
    bite — *see* Bite, arm
    forearm — *see* Wound, open, forearm
    laceration — *see* Laceration, arm
    puncture — *see* Puncture, arm
  auditory canal (external) (meatus) — *see* Wound, open, ear
  auricle, ear — *see* Wound, open, ear
  axilla — *see* Wound, open, arm
  back — *see also* Wound, open, thorax, back
    lower S31.000 ☑
      with penetration into retroperitoneal space S31.001 ☑
      bite — *see* Bite, back, lower
      laceration — *see* Laceration, back, lower
      puncture — *see* Puncture, back, lower
  bite — *see* Bite
  blood vessel — *see* Injury, blood vessel
  breast S21.00- ☑
    with amputation — *see* Amputation, traumatic, breast
    bite — *see* Bite, breast
    laceration — *see* Laceration, breast
    puncture — *see* Puncture, breast
  buttock S31.809 ☑
    bite — *see* Bite, buttock
    laceration — *see* Laceration, buttock
    left S31.829 ☑
    puncture — *see* Puncture, buttock
    right S31.819 ☑
  calf — *see* Wound, open, leg
  canaliculus lacrimalis — *see* Wound, open, eyelid
  canthus, eye — *see* Wound, open, eyelid
  cervical esophagus S11.20 ☑
    bite S11.25 ☑
    laceration — *see* Laceration, esophagus, traumatic, cervical
    puncture — *see* Puncture, cervical esophagus
  cheek (external) S01.40- ☑
    bite — *see* Bite, cheek
    internal — *see* Wound, open, oral cavity
    laceration — *see* Laceration, cheek
    puncture — *see* Puncture, cheek
  chest wall — *see* Wound, open, thorax
  chin — *see* Wound, open, head, specified site NEC
  choroid — *see* Wound, open, ocular
  ciliary body (eye) — *see* Wound, open, ocular
  clitoris S31.40 ☑
    with amputation — *see* Amputation, traumatic, clitoris
    bite S31.45 ☑
    laceration — *see* Laceration, vulva
    puncture — *see* Puncture, vulva
  conjunctiva — *see* Wound, open, ocular

Wound, open — *continued*
    cornea — *see* Wound, open, ocular
    costal region — *see* Wound, open, thorax
    Descemet's membrane — *see* Wound, open, ocular
    digit(s)
        foot — *see* Wound, open, toe
        hand — *see* Wound, open, finger
    ear (canal) (external) S01.30- ☑
        with amputation — *see* Amputation, traumatic, ear
        bite — *see* Bite, ear
        drum S09.2- ☑
        laceration — *see* Laceration, ear
        puncture — *see* Puncture, ear
    elbow S51.00- ☑
        bite — *see* Bite, elbow
        laceration — *see* Laceration, elbow
        puncture — *see* Puncture, elbow
    epididymis — *see* Wound, open, testis
    epigastric region S31.102 ☑
        with penetration into peritoneal cavity S31.602 ☑
        bite — *see* Bite, abdomen, wall, epigastric region
        laceration — *see* Laceration, abdomen, wall, epigastric region
        puncture — *see* Puncture, abdomen, wall, epigastric region
    epiglottis — *see* Wound, open, neck, specified site NEC
    esophagus (thoracic) S27.819 ☑
        cervical — *see* Wound, open, cervical esophagus
        laceration S27.813 ☑
        specified type NEC S27.818 ☑
    eye — *see* Wound, open, ocular
    eyeball — *see* Wound, open, ocular
    eyebrow — *see* Wound, open, eyelid
    eyelid S01.10- ☑
        bite — *see* Bite, eyelid
        laceration — *see* Laceration, eyelid
        puncture — *see* Puncture, eyelid
    face NEC — *see* Wound, open, head, specified site NEC
    finger(s) S61.209 ☑
        with
            amputation — *see* Amputation, traumatic, finger
            damage to nail S61.309 ☑
        bite — *see* Bite, finger
        index S61.208 ☑
            with
                damage to nail S61.308 ☑
            left S61.201 ☑
                with
                    damage to nail S61.301 ☑
            right S61.200 ☑
                with
                    damage to nail S61.300 ☑
        laceration — *see* Laceration, finger
        little S61.208 ☑
            with
                damage to nail S61.308 ☑
            left S61.207 ☑
                with damage to nail S61.307 ☑
            right S61.206 ☑
                with damage to nail S61.306 ☑
        middle S61.208 ☑
            with
                damage to nail S61.308 ☑
            left S61.203 ☑
                with damage to nail S61.303 ☑
            right S61.202 ☑
                with damage to nail S61.302 ☑
        puncture — *see* Puncture, finger
        ring S61.208 ☑
            with
                damage to nail S61.308 ☑
            left S61.205 ☑
                with damage to nail S61.305 ☑
            right S61.204 ☑
                with damage to nail S61.304 ☑
    flank — *see* Wound, open, abdomen, wall
    foot (except toe(s) alone) S91.30- ☑
        with amputation — *see* Amputation, traumatic, foot
        bite — *see* Bite, foot
        laceration — *see* Laceration, foot
        puncture — *see* Puncture, foot
        toe — *see* Wound, open, toe
    forearm S51.80- ☑
        with
            amputation — *see* Amputation, traumatic, forearm

Wound, open — *continued*
    forearm — *continued*
        bite — *see* Bite, forearm
        elbow only — *see* Wound, open, elbow
        laceration — *see* Laceration, forearm
        puncture — *see* Puncture, forearm
    forehead — *see* Wound, open, head, specified site NEC
    genital organs, external
        with amputation — *see* Amputation, traumatic, genital organs
        bite — *see* Bite, genital organ
        female S31.502 ☑
            vagina S31.40 ☑
            vulva S31.40 ☑
        laceration — *see* Laceration, genital organ
        male S31.501 ☑
            penis S31.20 ☑
            scrotum S31.30 ☑
            testes S31.30 ☑
        puncture — *see* Puncture, genital organ
    globe (eye) — *see* Wound, open, ocular
    groin — *see* Wound, open, abdomen, wall
    gum — *see* Wound, open, oral cavity
    hand S61.40- ☑
        with
            amputation — *see* Amputation, traumatic, hand
        bite — *see* Bite, hand
        finger(s) — *see* Wound, open, finger
        laceration — *see* Laceration, hand
        puncture — *see* Puncture, hand
        thumb — *see* Wound, open, thumb
    head S01.90 ☑
        bite — *see* Bite, head
        cheek — *see* Wound, open, cheek
        ear — *see* Wound, open, ear
        eyelid — *see* Wound, open, eyelid
        laceration — *see* Laceration, head
        lip — *see* Wound, open, lip
        nose S01.20 ☑
        oral cavity — *see* Wound, open, oral cavity
        puncture — *see* Puncture, head
        scalp — *see* Wound, open, scalp
        specified site NEC S01.80 ☑
        temporomandibular area — *see* Wound, open, cheek
    heel — *see* Wound, open, foot
    hip S71.00- ☑
        with amputation — *see* Amputation, traumatic, hip
        bite — *see* Bite, hip
        laceration — *see* Laceration, hip
        puncture — *see* Puncture, hip
    hymen S31.40 ☑
        bite — *see* Bite, vulva
        laceration — *see* Laceration, vagina
        puncture — *see* Puncture, vagina
    hypochondrium S31.109 ☑
        bite — *see* Bite, hypochondrium
        laceration — *see* Laceration, hypochondrium
        puncture — *see* Puncture, hypochondrium
    hypogastric region S31.109 ☑
        bite — *see* Bite, hypogastric region
        laceration — *see* Laceration, hypogastric region
        puncture — *see* Puncture, hypogastric region
    iliac (region) — *see* Wound, open, inguinal region
    inguinal region S31.109 ☑
        bite — *see* Bite, abdomen, wall, lower quadrant
        laceration — *see* Laceration, inguinal region
        puncture — *see* Puncture, inguinal region
    instep — *see* Wound, open, foot
    interscapular region — *see* Wound, open, thorax, back
    intraocular — *see* Wound, open, ocular
    iris — *see* Wound, open, ocular
    jaw — *see* Wound, open, head, specified site NEC
    knee S81.00- ☑
        bite — *see* Bite, knee
        laceration — *see* Laceration, knee
        puncture — *see* Puncture, knee
    labium (majus) (minus) — *see* Wound, open, vulva
    laceration — *see* Laceration, by site
    lacrimal duct — *see* Wound, open, eyelid
    larynx S11.019 ☑
        bite — *see* Bite, larynx
        laceration — *see* Laceration, larynx
        puncture — *see* Puncture, larynx
    left
        lower quadrant S31.104 ☑

Wound, open — *continued*
    left — *continued*
        lower quadrant — *continued*
            with penetration into peritoneal cavity S31.604 ☑
            bite — *see* Bite, abdomen, wall, left, lower quadrant
            laceration — *see* Laceration, abdomen, wall, left, lower quadrant
            puncture — *see* Puncture, abdomen, wall, left, lower quadrant
        upper quadrant S31.101 ☑
            with penetration into peritoneal cavity S31.601 ☑
            bite — *see* Bite, abdomen, wall, left, upper quadrant
            laceration — *see* Laceration, abdomen, wall, left, upper quadrant
            puncture — *see* Puncture, abdomen, wall, left, upper quadrant
    leg (lower) S81.80- ☑
        with amputation — *see* Amputation, traumatic, leg
        ankle — *see* Wound, open, ankle
        bite — *see* Bite, leg
        foot — *see* Wound, open, foot
        knee — *see* Wound, open, knee
        laceration — *see* Laceration, leg
        puncture — *see* Puncture, leg
        toe — *see* Wound, open, toe
        upper — *see* Wound, open, thigh
    lip S01.501 ☑
        bite — *see* Bite, lip
        laceration — *see* Laceration, lip
        puncture — *see* Puncture, lip
    loin S31.109 ☑
        bite — *see* Bite, abdomen, wall
        laceration — *see* Laceration, loin
        puncture — *see* Puncture, loin
    lower back — *see* Wound, open, back, lower
    lumbar region — *see* Wound, open, back, lower
    malar region — *see* Wound, open, head, specified site NEC
    mammary — *see* Wound, open, breast
    mastoid region — *see* Wound, open, head, specified site NEC
    mouth — *see* Wound, open, oral cavity
    nail
        finger — *see* Wound, open, finger, with damage to nail
        toe — *see* Wound, open, toe, with damage to nail
    nape (neck) — *see* Wound, open, neck
    nasal (septum) (sinus) — *see* Wound, open, nose
    nasopharynx — *see* Wound, open, head, specified site NEC
    neck S11.90 ☑
        bite — *see* Bite, neck
        involving
            cervical esophagus S11.20 ☑
            larynx — *see* Wound, open, larynx
            pharynx S11.20 ☑
            thyroid S11.10 ☑
            trachea (cervical) S11.029 ☑
                bite — *see* Bite, trachea
                laceration S11.021 ☑
                    with foreign body S11.022 ☑
                puncture S11.023 ☑
                    with foreign body S11.024 ☑
        laceration — *see* Laceration, neck
        puncture — *see* Puncture, neck
        specified site NEC S11.80 ☑
            specified type NEC S11.89 ☑
    nose (septum) (sinus) S01.20 ☑
        with amputation — *see* Amputation, traumatic, nose
        bite — *see* Bite, nose
        laceration — *see* Laceration, nose
        puncture — *see* Puncture, nose
    ocular S05.90 ☑
        avulsion (traumatic enucleation) S05.7- ☑
        eyeball S05.6- ☑
            with foreign body S05.5- ☑
        eyelid — *see* Wound, open, eyelid
        laceration and rupture S05.3- ☑
            with prolapse or loss of intraocular tissue S05.2- ☑

Wound, open — *continued*
  ocular — *continued*
    orbit (penetrating) (with or without foreign body) S05.4- ☑
    periocular area — *see* Wound, open, eyelid
    specified NEC S05.8X- ☑
  oral cavity S01.502 ☑
    bite S01.552 ☑
    laceration — *see* Laceration, oral cavity
    puncture — *see* Puncture, oral cavity
  orbit — *see* Wound, open, ocular, orbit
  palate — *see* Wound, open, oral cavity
  palm — *see* Wound, open, hand
  pelvis, pelvic — *see also* Wound, open, back, lower
    girdle — *see* Wound, open, hip
  penetrating — *see* Puncture, by site
  penis S31.20 ☑
    with amputation — *see* Amputation, traumatic, penis
    bite S31.25 ☑
    laceration — *see* Laceration, penis
    puncture — *see* Puncture, penis
  perineum
    bite — *see* Bite, perineum
    female S31.502 ☑
    laceration — *see* Laceration, perineum
    male S31.501 ☑
    puncture — *see* Puncture, perineum
  periocular area (with or without lacrimal passages) — *see* Wound, open, eyelid
  periumbilic region S31.105 ☑
    with penetration into peritoneal cavity S31.605 ☑
    bite — *see* Bite, abdomen, wall, periumbilic region
    laceration — *see* Laceration, abdomen, wall, periumbilic region
    puncture — *see* Puncture, abdomen, wall, periumbilic region
  phalanges
    finger — *see* Wound, open, finger
    toe — *see* Wound, open, toe
  pharynx S11.20 ☑
  pinna — *see* Wound, open, ear
  popliteal space — *see* Wound, open, knee
  prepuce — *see* Wound, open, penis
  pubic region — *see* Wound, open, back, lower
  pudendum — *see* Wound, open, genital organs, external
  puncture wound — *see* Puncture
  rectovaginal septum — *see* Wound, open, vagina
  right
    lower quadrant S31.103 ☑
      with penetration into peritoneal cavity S31.603 ☑
      bite — *see* Bite, abdomen, wall, right, lower quadrant
      laceration — *see* Laceration, abdomen, wall, right, lower quadrant
      puncture — *see* Puncture, abdomen, wall, right, lower quadrant
    upper quadrant S31.100 ☑
      with penetration into peritoneal cavity S31.600 ☑
      bite — *see* Bite, abdomen, wall, right, upper quadrant
      laceration — *see* Laceration, abdomen, wall, right, upper quadrant
      puncture — *see* Puncture, abdomen, wall, right, upper quadrant
  sacral region — *see* Wound, open, back, lower
  sacroiliac region — *see* Wound, open, back, lower
  salivary gland — *see* Wound, open, oral cavity
  scalp S01.00 ☑
    bite S01.05 ☑
    laceration — *see* Laceration, scalp
    puncture — *see* Puncture, scalp
  scalpel, newborn (birth injury) P15.8
  scapular region — *see* Wound, open, shoulder
  sclera — *see* Wound, open, ocular
  scrotum S31.30 ☑
    with amputation — *see* Amputation, traumatic, scrotum
    bite S31.35 ☑
    laceration — *see* Laceration, scrotum
    puncture — *see* Puncture, scrotum
  shin — *see* Wound, open, leg
  shoulder S41.00- ☑

Wound, open — *continued*
  shoulder — *continued*
    with amputation — *see* Amputation, traumatic, arm
    bite — *see* Bite, shoulder
    laceration — *see* Laceration, shoulder
    puncture — *see* Puncture, shoulder
  skin NOS T14.8 ☑
  spermatic cord — *see* Wound, open, testis
  sternal region — *see* Wound, open, thorax, front wall
  submaxillary region — *see* Wound, open, head, specified site NEC
  submental region — *see* Wound, open, head, specified site NEC
  subungual
    finger(s) — *see* Wound, open, finger
    toe(s) — *see* Wound, open, toe
  supraclavicular region — *see* Wound, open, neck, specified site NEC
  temple, temporal region — *see* Wound, open, head, specified site NEC
  temporomandibular area — *see* Wound, open, cheek
  testis S31.30 ☑
    with amputation — *see* Amputation, traumatic, testes
    bite S31.35 ☑
    laceration — *see* Laceration, testis
    puncture — *see* Puncture, testis
  thigh S71.10- ☑
    with amputation — *see* Amputation, traumatic, hip
    bite — *see* Bite, thigh
    laceration — *see* Laceration, thigh
    puncture — *see* Puncture, thigh
  thorax, thoracic (wall) S21.90 ☑
    back S21.20- ☑
      with penetration S21.40 ☑
    bite — *see* Bite, thorax
    breast — *see* Wound, open, breast
    front S21.10- ☑
      with penetration S21.30 ☑
    laceration — *see* Laceration, thorax
    puncture — *see* Puncture, thorax
  throat — *see* Wound, open, neck
  thumb S61.009 ☑
    with
      amputation — *see* Amputation, traumatic, thumb
      damage to nail S61.109 ☑
    bite — *see* Bite, thumb
    laceration — *see* Laceration, thumb
    left S61.002 ☑
      with
        damage to nail S61.102 ☑
    puncture — *see* Puncture, thumb
    right S61.001 ☑
      with
        damage to nail S61.101 ☑
  thyroid (gland) — *see* Wound, open, neck, thyroid
  toe(s) S91.109 ☑
    with
      amputation — *see* Amputation, traumatic, toe
      damage to nail S91.209 ☑
    bite — *see* Bite, toe
    great S91.103 ☑
      with
        damage to nail S91.203 ☑
      left S91.102 ☑
        with
          damage to nail S91.202 ☑
      right S91.101 ☑
        with
          damage to nail S91.201 ☑
    laceration — *see* Laceration, toe
    lesser S91.106 ☑
      with
        damage to nail S91.206 ☑
      left S91.105 ☑
        with
          damage to nail S91.205 ☑
      right S91.104 ☑
        with
          damage to nail S91.204 ☑
    puncture — *see* Puncture, toe
  tongue — *see* Wound, open, oral cavity
  trachea (cervical region) — *see* Wound, open, neck, trachea
  tunica vaginalis — *see* Wound, open, testis

Wound, open — *continued*
  tympanum, tympanic membrane S09.2- ☑
    laceration — *see* Laceration, ear, drum
    puncture — *see* Puncture, tympanum
  umbilical region — *see* Wound, open, abdomen, wall, periumbilic region
  uvula — *see* Wound, open, oral cavity
  vagina S31.40 ☑
    bite S31.45 ☑
    laceration — *see* Laceration, vagina
    puncture — *see* Puncture, vagina
  vitreous (humor) — *see* Wound, open, ocular
  vocal cord S11.039 ☑
    bite — *see* Bite, vocal cord
    laceration S11.031 ☑
      with foreign body S11.032 ☑
    puncture S11.033 ☑
      with foreign body S11.034 ☑
  vulva S31.40 ☑
    with amputation — *see* Amputation, traumatic, vulva
    bite S31.45 ☑
    laceration — *see* Laceration, vulva
    puncture — *see* Puncture, vulva
  wrist S61.50- ☑
    bite — *see* Bite, wrist
    laceration — *see* Laceration, wrist
    puncture — *see* Puncture, wrist
Wound, superficial — *see* Injury — *see also* specified injury type
Wright's syndrome G54.0
Wrist — *see* condition
Wrong drug (by accident) (given in error) — *see* Table of Drugs and Chemicals, by drug, poisoning
Wry neck — *see* Torticollis
Wuchereria (bancrofti) **infestation** B74.0
Wuchereriasis B74.0
Wuchernde Struma Langhans C73

X

Xanthelasma (eyelid) (palpebrarum) H02.60
  left H02.66
    lower H02.65
    upper H02.64
  right H02.63
    lower H02.62
    upper H02.61
Xanthelasmatosis (essential) E78.2
Xanthinuria, hereditary E79.8
Xanthoastrocytoma
  specified site — *see* Neoplasm, malignant, by site
  unspecified site C71.9
Xanthofibroma — *see* Neoplasm, connective tissue, benign
Xanthogranuloma D76.3
Xanthoma(s), xanthomatosis (primary) (familial) (hereditary) E75.5
  with
    hyperlipoproteinemia
      Type I E78.3
      Type III E78.2
      Type IV E78.1
      Type V E78.3
  bone (generalisata) C96.5
  cerebrotendinous E75.5
  cutaneotendinous E75.5
  disseminatum (skin) E78.2
  eruptive E78.2
  hypercholesterinemic E78.00
  hypercholesterolemic E78.00
  hyperlipidemic E78.5
  joint E75.5
  multiple (skin) E78.2
  tendon (sheath) E75.5
  tuberosum E78.2
  tuberous E78.2
  tubo-eruptive E78.2
  verrucous, oral mucosa K13.4
Xanthosis R23.8
Xenophobia F40.10
Xeroderma — *see also* Ichthyosis
  acquired L85.0
    eyelid H01.149
      left H01.146
        lower H01.145
        upper H01.144

☑ Additional Character Required — Refer to the Tabular List for Character Selection

Xeroderma — *continued*
  acquired — *continued*
    eyelid — *continued*
      right H01.143
        lower H01.142
        upper H01.141
  pigmentosum Q82.1
  vitamin A deficiency E50.8
Xerophthalmia (vitamin A deficiency) E50.7
  unrelated to vitamin A deficiency — *see* Keratoconjunctivitis
Xerosis
  conjunctiva H11.14- ☑
    with Bitot's spots — *see also* Pigmentation, conjunctiva
    vitamin A deficiency E50.1
    vitamin A deficiency E50.0
  cornea H18.89- ☑
    with ulceration — *see* Ulcer, cornea
    vitamin A deficiency E50.3
    vitamin A deficiency E50.2
  cutis (dry skin) L85.3
  skin L85.3
Xerostomia K11.7
Xiphopagus Q89.4
XO syndrome Q96.9
X-ray (of)
  abnormal findings — *see* Abnormal, diagnostic imaging
  breast (mammogram) (routine) Z12.31
  chest
    routine (as part of a general medical examination) Z00.00
      with abnormal findings Z00.01
    routine (as part of a general medical examination) Z00.00
      with abnormal findings Z00.01
XXXXY syndrome Q98.1
XXY syndrome Q98.0

Y

Yaba pox (virus disease) B08.72
Yatapoxvirus B08.70
  specified NEC B08.79
Yawning R06.89
  psychogenic F45.8
Yaws A66.9
  bone lesions A66.6
  butter A66.1
  chancre A66.0
  cutaneous, less than five years after infection A66.2
  early (cutaneous) (macular) (maculopapular) (micropapular) (papular) A66.2
    frambeside A66.2
    skin lesions NEC A66.2
  eyelid A66.2
  ganglion A66.6
  gangosis, gangosa A66.5
  gumma, gummata A66.4
    bone A66.6
  gummatous
    frambeside A66.4
    osteitis A66.6
    periostitis A66.6
  hydrarthrosis — *see also* subcategory M14.8- A66.6
  hyperkeratosis (early) (late) A66.3
  initial lesions A66.0
  joint lesions — *see also* subcategory M14.8- A66.6
  juxta-articular nodules A66.7
  late nodular (ulcerated) A66.4
  latent (without clinical manifestations) (with positive serology) A66.8
  mother A66.0
  mucosal A66.7
  multiple papillomata A66.1
  nodular, late (ulcerated) A66.4

Yaws — *continued*
  osteitis A66.6
  papilloma, plantar or palmar A66.1
  periostitis (hypertrophic) A66.6
  specified NEC A66.7
  ulcers A66.4
  wet crab A66.1
Yeast infection — *see also* Candidiasis B37.9
Yellow
  atrophy (liver) — *see* Failure, hepatic
  fever — *see* Fever, yellow
  jack — *see* Fever, yellow
  jaundice — *see* Jaundice
  nail syndrome L60.5
Yersiniosis — *see also* Infection, Yersinia
  extraintestinal A28.2
  intestinal A04.6

Z

Zahorsky's syndrome (herpangina) B08.5
Zellweger's syndrome E71.510
Zenker's diverticulum (esophagus) K22.5
Ziehen-Oppenheim disease G24.1
Zieve's syndrome K70.0
Zika NOS A92.5
  congenital P35.4
Zinc
  deficiency, dietary E60
  metabolism disorder E83.2
Zollinger-Ellison syndrome E16.4
Zona — *see* Herpes, zoster
Zoophobia F40.218
Zoster (herpes) — *see* Herpes, zoster
Zygomycosis B46.9
  specified NEC B46.8
Zymotic — *see* condition

Neoplasm Table

Neoplasm, abdomen, abdominal — Neoplasm, bile or biliary

Note: The list below gives the code number for neoplasms by anatomical site. For each site there are six possible code numbers according to whether the neoplasm in question is malignant, benign, in situ, of uncertain behavior, or of unspecified nature. The description of the neoplasm will often indicate which of the six columns is appropriate; e.g., malignant melanoma of skin, benign fibroadenoma of breast, carcinoma in situ of cervix uteri. Where such descriptors are not present, the remainder of the Index should be consulted where guidance is given to the appropriate column for each morphological (histological) variety listed; e.g., Mesonephroma – see Neoplasm, malignant; Embryoma — see also Neoplasm, uncertain behavior; Disease, Bowen's – see Neoplasm, skin, in situ. However, the guidance in the Index can be overridden if one of the descriptors mentioned above is present; e.g., malignant adenoma of colon is coded to C18.9 and not to D12.6 as the adjective "malignant" overrides the Index entry "Adenoma — see also Neoplasm, benign, by site." Codes listed with a dash -, following the code have a required additional character for laterality. The tabular list must be reviewed for the complete code.

	Malignant Primary	Malignant Secondary	Ca in situ	Benign	Uncertain Behavior	Unspecified Behavior
Neoplasm, neoplastic	C80.1	C79.9	D09.9	D36.9	D48.9	D49.9
abdomen, abdominal	C76.2	C79.8-☑	D09.8	D36.7	D48.7	D49.89
cavity	C76.2	C79.8-☑	D09.8	D36.7	D48.7	D49.89
organ	C76.2	C79.8-☑	D09.8	D36.7	D48.7	D49.89
viscera	C76.2	C79.8-☑	D09.8	D36.7	D48.7	D49.89
wall — *see also* Neoplasm, abdomen, wall, skin						
connective tissue	C49.4	C79.8-☑	—	D21.4	D48.1	D49.2
skin	C44.509	—	—	—	—	—
basal cell carcinoma	C44.519					
specified type NEC	C44.599					
squamous cell carcinoma	C44.529					
abdominopelvic	C76.8	C79.8-☑	—	D36.7	D48.7	D49.89
accessory sinus — *see* Neoplasm, sinus						
acoustic nerve	C72.4-☑	C79.49	—	D33.3	D43.3	D49.7
adenoid (pharynx) (tissue)	C11.1	C79.89	D00.08	D10.6	D37.05	D49.0
adipose tissue — *see also* Neoplasm, connective tissue	C49.4	C79.89	—	D21.9	D48.1	D49.2
adnexa (uterine)	C57.4	C79.89	D07.39	D28.7	D39.8	D49.59
adrenal	C74.9-☑	C79.7-☑	D09.3	D35.0-☑	D44.1-☑	D49.7
capsule	C74.9-☑	C79.7-☑	D09.3	D35.0-☑	D44.1-☑	D49.7
cortex	C74.0-☑	C79.7-☑	D09.3	D35.0-☑	D44.1-☑	D49.7
gland	C74.9-☑	C79.7-☑	D09.3	D35.0-☑	D44.1-☑	D49.7
medulla	C74.1-☑	C79.7-☑	D09.3	D35.0-☑	D44.1-☑	D49.7
ala nasi (external) — *see also* Neoplasm, skin, nose	C44.301	C79.2	D04.39	D23.39	D48.5	D49.2
alimentary canal or tract NEC	C26.9	C78.80	D01.9	D13.9	D37.9	D49.0
alveolar	C03.9	C79.89	D00.03	D10.39	D37.09	D49.0
mucosa	C03.9	C79.89	D00.03	D10.39	D37.09	D49.0
lower	C03.1	C79.89	D00.03	D10.39	D37.09	D49.0
upper	C03.0	C79.89	D00.03	D10.39	D37.09	D49.0
ridge or process	C41.1	C79.51	—	D16.5	D48.0	D49.2
carcinoma	C03.9	C79.8-☑	—	—	—	—
lower	C03.1	C79.8-☑	—	—	—	—
upper	C03.0	C79.8-☑	—	—	—	—
lower	C41.1	C79.51	—	D16.5	D48.0	D49.2
mucosa	C03.9	C79.89	D00.03	D10.39	D37.09	D49.0
lower	C03.1	C79.89	D00.03	D10.39	D37.09	D49.0
upper	C03.0	C79.89	D00.03	D10.39	D37.09	D49.0
upper	C41.0	C79.51	—	D16.4	D48.0	D49.2
sulcus	C06.1	C79.89	D00.02	D10.39	D37.09	D49.0
alveolus	C03.9	C79.89	D00.03	D10.39	D37.09	D49.0
lower	C03.1	C79.89	D00.03	D10.39	D37.09	D49.0
upper	C03.0	C79.89	D00.03	D10.39	D37.09	D49.0
ampulla of Vater	C24.1	C78.89	D01.5	D13.5	D37.6	D49.0
ankle NEC	C76.5-☑	C79.89	D04.7-☑	D36.7	D48.7	D49.89
anorectum, anorectal (junction)	C21.8	C78.5	D01.3	D12.9	D37.8	D49.0
antecubital fossa or space	C76.4-☑	C79.89	D04.6-☑	D36.7	D48.7	D49.89

	Malignant Primary	Malignant Secondary	Ca in situ	Benign	Uncertain Behavior	Unspecified Behavior
Neoplasm, neoplastic *— continued*						
antrum (Highmore) (maxillary)	C31.0	C78.39	D02.3	D14.0	D38.5	D49.1
pyloric	C16.3	C78.89	D00.2	D13.1	D37.1	D49.0
tympanicum	C30.1	C78.39	D02.3	D14.0	D38.5	D49.1
anus, anal	C21.0	C78.5	D01.3	D12.9	D37.8	D49.0
canal	C21.1	C78.5	D01.3	D12.9	D37.8	D49.0
cloacogenic zone	C21.2	C78.5	D01.3	D12.9	D37.8	D49.0
margin — *see also* Neoplasm, anus, skin	C44.500	C79.2	D04.5	D23.5	D48.5	D49.2
overlapping lesion with rectosigmoid junction or rectum	C21.8	—	—	—	—	—
skin	C44.500	C79.2	D04.5	D23.5	D48.5	D49.2
basal cell carcinoma	C44.510					
specified type NEC	C44.590					
squamous cell carcinoma	C44.520	—	—	—	—	—
sphincter	C21.1	C78.5	D01.3	D12.9	D37.8	D49.0
aorta (thoracic)	C49.3	C79.89	—	D21.3	D48.1	D49.2
abdominal	C49.4	C79.89	—	D21.4	D48.1	D49.2
aortic body	C75.5	C79.89	—	D35.6	D44.7	D49.7
aponeurosis	C49.9	C79.89	—	D21.9	D48.1	D49.2
palmar	C49.1-☑	C79.89	—	D21.1-☑	D48.1	D49.2
plantar	C49.2-☑	C79.89	—	D21.2-☑	D48.1	D49.2
appendix	C18.1	C78.5	D01.0	D12.1	D37.3	D49.0
arachnoid	C70.9	C79.49	—	D32.9	D42.9	D49.7
cerebral	C70.0	C79.32	—	D32.0	D42.0	D49.7
spinal	C70.1	C79.49	—	D32.1	D42.1	D49.7
areola	C50.0-☑	C79.81	D05-☑	D24-☑	D48.6-☑	D49.3
arm NEC	C76.4-☑	C79.89	D04.6-☑	D36.7	D48.7	D49.89
artery — *see* Neoplasm, connective tissue						
aryepiglottic fold	C13.1	C79.89	D00.08	D10.7	D37.05	D49.0
hypopharyngeal aspect	C13.1	C79.89	D00.08	D10.7	D37.05	D49.0
laryngeal aspect	C32.1	C78.39	D02.0	D14.1	D38.0	D49.1
marginal zone	C13.1	C79.89	D00.08	D10.7	D37.05	D49.0
arytenoid (cartilage)	C32.3	C78.39	D02.0	D14.1	D38.0	D49.1
fold — *see* Neoplasm, aryepiglottic						
associated with transplanted organ	C80.2	—	—	—	—	—
atlas	C41.2	C79.51	—	D16.6	D48.0	D49.2
atrium, cardiac	C38.0	C79.89	—	D15.1	D48.7	D49.89
auditory						
canal (external) (skin)	C44.20-☑	C79.2	D04.2-☑	D23.2-☑	D48.5	D49.2
internal	C30.1	C78.39	D02.3	D14.0	D38.5	D49.1
nerve	C72.4-☑	C79.49	—	D33.3	D43.3	D49.7
tube	C30.1	C78.39	D02.3	D14.0	D38.5	D49.1
opening	C11.2	C79.89	D00.08	D10.6	D37.05	D49.0
auricle, ear — *see also* Neoplasm, skin, ear	C44.20-☑	C79.2	D04.2-☑	D23.2-☑	D48.5	D49.2
auricular canal (external) — *see also* Neoplasm, skin, ear	C44.20-☑	C79.2	D04.2-☑	D23.2-☑	D48.5	D49.2
internal	C30.1	C78.39	D02.3	D14.0	D38.5	D49.2
autonomic nerve or nervous system NEC (see Neoplasm, nerve, peripheral)						
axilla, axillary	C76.1	C79.89	D09.8	D36.7	D48.7	D49.89
fold — *see also* Neoplasm, skin, trunk	C44.509	C79.2	D04.5	D23.5	D48.5	D49.2
back NEC	C76.8	C79.89	D04.5	D36.7	D48.7	D49.89
Bartholin's gland	C51.0	C79.82	D07.1	D28.0	D39.8	D49.59
basal ganglia	C71.0	C79.31	—	D33.0	D43.0	D49.6
basis pedunculi	C71.7	C79.31	—	D33.1	D43.1	D49.6
bile or biliary (tract)	C24.9	C78.89	D01.5	D13.5	D37.6	D49.0

☑ **Additional Character Required — Refer to the Tabular List for Character Selection**

Neoplasm, neoplastic	Malignant Primary	Malignant Secondary	Ca in situ	Benign	Uncertain Behavior	Unspecified Behavior
— continued						
bile or biliary — continued						
canaliculi (biliferi) (intrahepatic)	C22.1	C78.7	D01.5	D13.4	D37.6	D49.0
canals, interlobular	C22.1	C78.89	D01.5	D13.4	D37.6	D49.0
duct or passage (common) (cystic) (extrahepatic)	C24.0	C78.89	D01.5	D13.5	D37.6	D49.0
interlobular	C22.1	C78.89	D01.5	D13.4	D37.6	D49.0
intrahepatic	C22.1	C78.7	D01.5	D13.4	D37.6	D49.0
and extrahepatic	C24.8	C78.89	D01.5	D13.5	D37.6	D49.0
bladder (urinary)	C67.9	C79.11	D09.0	D30.3	D41.4	D49.4
dome	C67.1	C79.11	D09.0	D30.3	D41.4	D49.4
neck	C67.5	C79.11	D09.0	D30.3	D41.4	D49.4
orifice	C67.9	C79.11	D09.0	D30.3	D41.4	D49.4
ureteric	C67.6	C79.11	D09.0	D30.3	D41.4	D49.4
urethral	C67.5	C79.11	D09.0	D30.3	D41.4	D49.4
overlapping lesion	C67.8	—	—	—	—	—
sphincter	C67.8	C79.11	D09.0	D30.3	D41.4	D49.4
trigone	C67.0	C79.11	D09.0	D30.3	D41.4	D49.4
urachus	C67.7	C79.11	D09.0	D30.3	D41.4	D49.4
wall	C67.9	C79.11	D09.0	D30.3	D41.4	D49.4
anterior	C67.3	C79.11	D09.0	D30.3	D41.4	D49.4
lateral	C67.2	C79.11	D09.0	D30.3	D41.4	D49.4
posterior	C67.4	C79.11	D09.0	D30.3	D41.4	D49.4
blood vessel — see Neoplasm, connective tissue						
bone (periosteum)	C41.9	C79.51	—	D16.9-	D48.0	D49.2
acetabulum						
ankle	C40.3-☑	C79.51	—	D16.3-☑	—	—
arm NEC	C40.0-☑	C79.51	—	D16.0-☑	—	—
astragalus	C40.3-☑	C79.51	—	D16.3-☑	—	—
atlas	C41.2	C79.51	—	D16.6	D48.0	D49.2
axis	C41.2	C79.51	—	D16.6	D48.0	D49.2
back NEC	C41.2	C79.51	—	D16.6	D48.0	D49.2
calcaneus	C40.3-☑	C79.51	—	D16.3-☑	—	—
calvarium	C41.0	C79.51	—	D16.4	D48.0	D49.2
carpus (any)	C40.1-☑	C79.51	—	D16.1-☑	—	—
cartilage NEC	C41.9	C79.51	—	D16.9	D48.0	D49.2
clavicle	C41.3	C79.51	—	D16.7	D48.0	D49.2
clivus	C41.0	C79.51	—	D16.4	D48.0	D49.2
coccygeal vertebra	C41.4	C79.51	—	D16.8	D48.0	D49.2
coccyx	C41.4	C79.51	—	D16.8	D48.0	D49.2
costal cartilage	C41.3	C79.51	—	D16.7	D48.0	D49.2
costovertebral joint	C41.3	C79.51	—	D16.7	D48.0	D49.2
cranial	C41.0	C79.51	—	D16.4	D48.0	D49.2
cuboid	C40.3-☑	C79.51	—	D16.3-☑	—	—
cuneiform	C41.9	C79.51	—	D16.9	D48.0	D49.2
elbow	C40.0-☑	C79.51	—	D16.0-☑	—	—
ethmoid (labyrinth)	C41.0	C79.51	—	D16.4	D48.0	D49.2
face	C41.0	C79.51	—	D16.4	D48.0	D49.2
femur (any part)	C40.2-☑	C79.51	—	D16.2-☑	—	—
fibula (any part)	C40.2-☑	C79.51	—	D16.2-☑	—	—
finger (any)	C40.1-☑	C79.51	—	D16.1-☑	—	—
foot	C40.3-☑	C79.51	—	D16.3-☑	—	—
forearm	C40.0-☑	C79.51	—	D16.0-☑	—	—
frontal	C41.0	C79.51	—	D16.4	D48.0	D49.2
hand	C40.1-☑	C79.51	—	D16.1-☑	—	—
heel	C40.3-☑	C79.51	—	D16.3-☑	—	—
hip	C41.4	C79.51	—	D16.8	D48.0	D49.2
humerus (any part)	C40.0-☑	C79.51	—	D16.0-☑	—	—
hyoid	C41.0	C79.51	—	D16.4	D48.0	D49.2
ilium	C41.4	C79.51	—	D16.8	D48.0	D49.2
innominate	C41.4	C79.51	—	D16.8	D48.0	D49.2
intervertebral cartilage or disc	C41.2	C79.51	—	D16.6	D48.0	D49.2
ischium	C41.4	C79.51	—	D16.8	D48.0	D49.2
jaw (lower)	C41.1	C79.51	—	D16.5	D48.0	D49.2
knee	C40.2-☑	C79.51	—	D16.2-☑	—	—
leg NEC	C40.2-☑	C79.51	—	D16.2-☑	—	—
limb NEC	C40.9-☑	C79.51	—	D16.9	—	—

Neoplasm, neoplastic	Malignant Primary	Malignant Secondary	Ca in situ	Benign	Uncertain Behavior	Unspecified Behavior
— continued						
bone — continued						
limb — continued						
lower (long bones)	C40.2-☑	C79.51	—	D16.2-☑	—	—
short bones	C40.3-☑	C79.51	—	D16.3-☑	—	—
upper (long bones)	C40.0-☑	C79.51	—	D16.0-☑	—	—
short bones	C40.1-☑	C79.51	—	D16.1-☑	—	—
malar	C41.0	C79.51	—	D16.4	D48.0	D49.2
mandible	C41.1	C79.51	—	D16.5	D48.0	D49.2
marrow NEC (any bone)	C96.9	C79.52	—	—	D47.9	D49.89
mastoid	C41.0	C79.51	—	D16.4	D48.0	D49.2
maxilla, maxillary (superior)	C41.0	C79.51	—	D16.4	D48.0	D49.2
inferior	C41.1	C79.51	—	D16.5	D48.0	D49.2
metacarpus (any)	C40.1-☑	C79.51	—	D16.1-☑	—	—
metatarsus (any)	C40.3-☑	C79.51	—	D16.3-☑	—	—
navicular						
ankle	C40.3-☑	C79.51	—	—	—	—
hand	C40.1-☑	C79.51	—	—	—	—
nose, nasal	C41.0	C79.51	—	D16.4	D48.0	D49.2
occipital	C41.0	C79.51	—	D16.4	D48.0	D49.2
orbit	C41.0	C79.51	—	D16.4	D48.0	D49.2
overlapping sites	C40.8-☑	—	—	—	—	—
parietal	C41.0	C79.51	—	D16.4	D48.0	D49.2
patella	C40.2-☑	C79.51	—	—	—	D49.2
pelvic	C41.4	C79.51	—	D16.8	D48.0	D49.2
phalanges						
foot	C40.3-☑	C79.51	—	—	—	—
hand	C40.1-☑	C79.51	—	—	—	—
pubic	C41.4	C79.51	—	D16.8	D48.0	D49.2
radius (any part)	C40.0-☑	C79.51	—	D16.0-☑	—	—
rib	C41.3	C79.51	—	D16.7	D48.0	D49.2
sacral vertebra	C41.4	C79.51	—	D16.8	D48.0	D49.2
sacrum	C41.4	C79.51	—	D16.8	D48.0	D49.2
scaphoid						
of ankle	C40.3-☑	C79.51	—	—	—	—
of hand	C40.1-☑	C79.51	—	—	—	—
scapula (any part)	C40.0-☑	C79.51	—	D16.0-☑	—	—
sella turcica	C41.0	C79.51	—	D16.4	D48.0	D49.2
shoulder	C40.0-☑	C79.51	—	D16.0-☑	—	—
skull	C41.0	C79.51	—	D16.4	D48.0	D49.2
sphenoid	C41.0	C79.51	—	D16.4	D48.0	D49.2
spine, spinal (column)	C41.2	C79.51	—	D16.6	D48.0	D49.2
coccyx	C41.4	C79.51	—	D16.8	D48.0	D49.2
sacrum	C41.4	C79.51	—	D16.8	D48.0	D49.2
sternum	C41.3	C79.51	—	D16.7	D48.0	D49.2
tarsus (any)	C40.3-☑	C79.51	—	—	—	—
temporal	C41.0	C79.51	—	D16.4	D48.0	D49.2
thumb	C40.1-☑	C79.51	—	—	—	—
tibia (any part)	C40.2-☑	C79.51	—	—	—	—
toe (any)	C40.3-☑	C79.51	—	—	—	—
trapezium	C40.1-☑	C79.51	—	—	—	—
trapezoid	C40.1-☑	C79.51	—	—	—	—
turbinate	C41.0	C79.51	—	D16.4	D48.0	D49.2
ulna (any part)	C40.0-☑	C79.51	—	D16.0-☑	—	—
unciform	C40.1-☑	C79.51	—	—	—	—
vertebra (column)	C41.2	C79.51	—	D16.6	D48.0	D49.2
coccyx	C41.4	C79.51	—	D16.8	D48.0	D49.2
sacrum	C41.4	C79.51	—	D16.8	D48.0	D49.2
vomer	C41.0	C79.51	—	D16.4	D48.0	D49.2
wrist	C40.1-☑	C79.51	—	—	—	—
xiphoid process	C41.3	C79.51	—	D16.7	D48.0	D49.2
zygomatic	C41.0	C79.51	—	D16.4	D48.0	D49.2
book-leaf (mouth) — ventral surface of tongue and floor of mouth	C06.89	C79.89	D00.00	D10.39	D37.09	D49.0
bowel — see Neoplasm, intestine						
brachial plexus	C47.1-☑	C79.89	—	D36.12	D48.2	D49.2
brain NEC	C71.9	C79.31	—	D33.2	D43.2	D49.6

☑ Additional Character Required — Refer to the Tabular List for Character Selection

Neoplasm, neoplastic — continued	Malignant Primary	Malignant Secondary	Ca in situ	Benign	Uncertain Behavior	Unspecified Behavior
brain — continued						
basal ganglia	C71.0	C79.31	—	D33.0	D43.0	D49.6
cerebellopontine angle	C71.6	C79.31	—	D33.1	D43.1	D49.6
cerebellum NOS	C71.6	C79.31	—	D33.1	D43.1	D49.6
cerebrum	C71.0	C79.31	—	D33.0	D43.0	D49.6
choroid plexus	C71.7	C79.31	—	D33.1	D43.1	D49.6
corpus callosum	C71.8	C79.31	—	D33.2	D43.2	D49.6
corpus striatum	C71.0	C79.31	—	D33.0	D43.0	D49.6
cortex (cerebral)	C71.0	C79.31	—	D33.0	D43.0	D49.6
frontal lobe	C71.1	C79.31	—	D33.0	D43.0	D49.6
globus pallidus	C71.0	C79.31	—	D33.0	D43.0	D49.6
hippocampus	C71.2	C79.31	—	D33.0	D43.0	D49.6
hypothalamus	C71.0	C79.31	—	D33.0	D43.0	D49.6
internal capsule	C71.0	C79.31	—	D33.0	D43.0	D49.6
medulla oblongata	C71.7	C79.31	—	D33.1	D43.1	D49.6
meninges	C70.0	C79.32	—	D32.0	D42.0	D49.7
midbrain	C71.7	C79.31	—	D33.1	D43.1	D49.6
occipital lobe	C71.4	C79.31	—	D33.0	D43.0	D49.6
overlapping lesion	C71.8	C79.31	—	—	—	—
parietal lobe	C71.3	C79.31	—	D33.0	D43.0	D49.6
peduncle	C71.7	C79.31	—	D33.1	D43.1	D49.6
pons	C71.7	C79.31	—	D33.1	D43.1	D49.6
stem	C71.7	C79.31	—	D33.1	D43.1	D49.6
tapetum	C71.8	C79.31	—	D33.2	D43.2	D49.6
temporal lobe	C71.2	C79.31	—	D33.0	D43.0	D49.6
thalamus	C71.0	C79.31	—	D33.0	D43.0	D49.6
uncus	C71.2	C79.31	—	D33.0	D43.0	D49.6
ventricle (floor)	C71.5	C79.31	—	D33.0	D43.0	D49.6
fourth	C71.7	C79.31	—	D33.1	D43.1	D49.6
branchial (cleft) (cyst) (vestiges)	C10.4	C79.89	D00.08	D10.5	D37.05	D49.0
breast (connective tissue) (glandular tissue) (soft parts)	C50.9-☑	C79.81	D05.-☑	D24.-☑	D48.6-☑	D49.3
areola	C50.0-☑	C79.81	D05.-☑	D24.-☑	D48.6-☑	D49.3
axillary tail	C50.6-☑	C79.81	D05.-☑	D24.-☑	D48.6-☑	D49.3
central portion	C50.1-☑	C79.81	D05.-☑	D24.-☑	D48.6-☑	D49.3
inner	C50.8-☑	C79.81	D05.-☑	D24.-☑	D48.6-☑	D49.3
lower	C50.8-☑	C79.81	D05.-☑	D24.-☑	D48.6-☑	D49.3
lower-inner quadrant	C50.3-☑	C79.81	D05.-☑	D24.-☑	D48.6-☑	D49.3
lower-outer quadrant	C50.5-☑	C79.81	D05.-☑	D24.-☑	D48.6-☑	D49.3
mastectomy site (skin) — see also Neoplasm, breast, skin	C44.501	C79.2	—	—	—	—
specified as breast tissue	C50.8-☑	C79.81	—	—	—	—
midline	C50.8-☑	C79.81	D05.-☑	D24.-☑	D48.6-☑	D49.3
nipple	C50.0-☑	C79.81	D05.-☑	D24.-☑	D48.6-☑	D49.3
outer	C50.8-☑	C79.81	D05.-☑	D24.-☑	D48.6-☑	D49.3
overlapping lesion	C50.8-☑	—	—	—	—	—
skin	C44.501	C79.2	D04.5	D23.5	D48.5	D49.2
basal cell carcinoma	C44.511	—	—	—	—	—
specified type NEC	C44.591	—	—	—	—	—
squamous cell carcinoma	C44.521	—	—	—	—	—
tail (axillary)	C50.6-☑	C79.81	D05.-☑	D24.-☑	D48.6-☑	D49.3
upper	C50.8-☑	C79.81	D05.-☑	D24.-☑	D48.6-☑	D49.3
upper-inner quadrant	C50.2-☑	C79.81	D05.-☑	D24.-☑	D48.6-☑	D49.3
upper-outer quadrant	C50.4-☑	C79.81	D05.-☑	D24.-☑	D48.6-☑	D49.3
broad ligament	C57.1-☑	C79.82	D07.39	D28.2	D39.8	D49.59
bronchiogenic, bronchogenic (lung)	C34.9-☑	C78.0-☑	D02.2-☑	D14.3-☑	D38.1	D49.1
bronchiole	C34.9-☑	C78.0-☑	D02.2-☑	D14.3-☑	D38.1	D49.1
bronchus	C34.9-☑	C78.0-☑	D02.2-☑	D14.3-☑	D38.1	D49.1
carina	C34.0-☑	C78.0-☑	D02.2-☑	D14.3-☑	D38.1	D49.1
lower lobe of lung	C34.3-☑	C78.0-☑	D02.2-☑	D14.3-☑	D38.1	D49.1

Right table

Neoplasm, neoplastic — continued	Malignant Primary	Malignant Secondary	Ca in situ	Benign	Uncertain Behavior	Unspecified Behavior
bronchus — continued						
main	C34.0-☑	C78.0-☑	D02.2-☑	D14.3-☑	D38.1	D49.1
middle lobe of lung	C34.2	C78.0-☑	D02.21	D14.31	D38.1	D49.1
overlapping lesion	C34.8-☑	—	—	—	—	—
upper lobe of lung	C34.1-☑	C78.0-☑	D02.2-☑	D14.3-☑	D38.1	D49.1
brow	C44.309	C79.2	D04.39	D23.39	D48.5	D49.2
basal cell carcinoma	C44.319	—	—	—	—	—
specified type NEC	C44.399	—	—	—	—	—
squamous cell carcinoma	C44.329	—	—	—	—	—
buccal (cavity)	C06.9	C79.89	D00.00	D10.39	D37.09	D49.0
commissure	C06.0	C79.89	D00.02	D10.39	D37.09	D49.0
groove (lower) (upper)	C06.1	C79.89	D00.02	D10.39	D37.09	D49.0
mucosa	C06.0	C79.89	D00.02	D10.39	D37.09	D49.0
sulcus (lower) (upper)	C06.1	C79.89	D00.02	D10.39	D37.09	D49.0
bulbourethral gland	C68.0	C79.19	D09.19	D30.4	D41.3	D49.59
bursa — see Neoplasm, connective tissue						
buttock NEC	C76.3	C79.89	D04.5	D36.7	D48.7	D49.89
calf	C76.5-☑	C79.89	D04.7-☑	D36.7	D48.7	D49.89
calvarium	C41.0	C79.51	—	D16.4	D48.0	D49.2
calyx, renal	C65.-☑	C79.0-☑	D09.19	D30.1-☑	D41.1-☑	D49.51-☑
canal						
anal	C21.1	C78.5	D01.3	D12.9	D37.8	D49.0
auditory (external) — see also Neoplasm, skin, ear	C44.20-☑	C79.2	D04.2-☑	D23.2-☑	D48.5	D49.2
auricular (external) — see also Neoplasm, skin, ear	C44.20-☑	C79.2	D04.2-☑	D23.2-☑	D48.5	D49.2
canaliculi, biliary (biliferi) (intrahepatic)	C22.1	C78.7	D01.5	D13.4	D37.6	D49.0
canthus (eye) (inner) (outer)	C44.10-☑	C79.2	D04.1-☑	D23.1-☑	D48.5	D49.2
basal cell carcinoma	C44.11-☑	—	—	—	—	—
sebaceous cell	C44.13-☑	—	—	—	—	—
specified type NEC	C44.19-☑	—	—	—	—	—
squamous cell carcinoma	C44.12-☑	—	—	—	—	—
capillary — see Neoplasm, connective tissue						
caput coli	C18.0	C78.5	D01.0	D12.0	D37.4	D49.0
carcinoid — see Tumor, carcinoid						
cardia (gastric)	C16.0	C78.89	D00.2	D13.1	D37.1	D49.0
cardiac orifice (stomach)	C16.0	C78.89	D00.2	D13.1	D37.1	D49.0
cardio-esophageal junction	C16.0	C78.89	D00.2	D13.1	D37.1	D49.0
cardio-esophagus	C16.0	C78.89	D00.2	D13.1	D37.1	D49.0
carina (bronchus)	C34.0-☑	C78.0-☑	D02.2-☑	D14.3-☑	D38.1	D49.1
carotid (artery)	C49.0	C79.89	—	D21.0	D48.1	D49.2
body	C75.4	C79.89	—	D35.5	D44.6	D49.7
carpus (any bone)	C40.1-☑	C79.51	—	D16.1-☑	—	—
cartilage (articular) (joint) NEC — see also Neoplasm, bone	C41.9	C79.51	—	D16.9	D48.0	D49.2
arytenoid	C32.3	C78.39	D02.0	D14.1	D38.0	D49.1
auricular	C49.0	C79.89	—	D21.0	D48.1	D49.2
bronchi	C34.0-☑	C78.39	—	D14.3-☑	D38.1	D49.1
costal	C41.3	C79.51	—	D16.7	D48.0	D49.2
cricoid	C32.3	C78.39	D02.0	D14.1	D38.0	D49.1
cuneiform	C32.3	C78.39	D02.0	D14.1	D38.0	D49.1
ear (external)	C49.0	C79.89	—	D21.0	D48.1	D49.2
ensiform	C41.3	C79.51	—	D16.7	D48.0	D49.2
epiglottis	C32.1	C78.39	D02.0	D14.1	D38.0	D49.1

Neoplasm, neoplastic — continued	Malignant Primary	Malignant Secondary	Ca in situ	Benign	Uncertain Behavior	Unspecified Behavior
cartilage — see also Neoplasm, bone — continued						
epiglottis — continued						
anterior surface	C10.1	C79.89	D00.08	D10.5	D37.05	D49.0
eyelid	C49.0	C79.89	—	D21.0	D48.1	D49.2
intervertebral	C41.2	C79.51	—	D16.6	D48.0	D49.2
larynx, laryngeal	C32.3	C78.39	D02.0	D14.1	D38.0	D49.1
nose, nasal	C30.0	C78.39	D02.3	D14.0	D38.5	D49.1
pinna	C49.0	C79.89	—	D21.0	D48.1	D49.2
rib	C41.3	C79.51	—	D16.7	D48.0	D49.2
semilunar (knee)	C40.2-☑	C79.51	—	D16.2-☑	D48.0	D49.2
thyroid	C32.3	C78.39	D02.0	D14.1	D38.0	D49.1
trachea	C33	C78.39	D02.1	D14.2	D38.1	D49.1
cauda equina	C72.1	C79.49	—	D33.4	D43.4	D49.7
cavity						
buccal	C06.9	C79.89	D00.00	D10.30	D37.09	D49.0
nasal	C30.0	C78.39	D02.3	D14.0	D38.5	D49.1
oral	C06.9	C79.89	D00.00	D10.30	D37.09	D49.0
peritoneal	C48.2	C78.6	—	D20.0	D48.4	D49.0
tympanic	C30.1	C78.39	D02.3	D14.0	D38.5	D49.1
cecum	C18.0	C78.5	D01.0	D12.0	D37.4	D49.0
central nervous system	C72.9	C79.40	—	—	—	—
cerebellopontine (angle)	C71.6	C79.31	—	D33.1	D43.1	D49.6
cerebellum, cerebellar	C71.6	C79.31	—	D33.1	D43.1	D49.6
cerebrum, cerebra (cortex) (hemisphere) (white matter)	C71.0	C79.31	—	D33.0	D43.0	D49.6
meninges	C70.0	C79.32	—	D32.0	D42.0	D49.7
peduncle	C71.7	C79.31	—	D33.1	D43.1	D49.6
ventricle	C71.5	C79.31	—	D33.0	D43.0	D49.6
fourth	C71.7	C79.31	—	D33.1	D43.1	D49.6
cervical region	C76.0	C79.89	D09.8	D36.7	D48.7	D49.89
cervix (cervical) (uteri) (uterus)	C53.9	C79.82	D06.9	D26.0	D39.0	D49.59
canal	C53.0	C79.82	D06.0	D26.0	D39.0	D49.59
endocervix (canal) (gland)	C53.0	C79.82	D06.0	D26.0	D39.0	D49.59
exocervix	C53.1	C79.82	D06.1	D26.0	D39.0	D49.59
external os	C53.1	C79.82	D06.1	D26.0	D39.0	D49.59
internal os	C53.0	C79.82	D06.0	D26.0	D39.0	D49.59
nabothian gland	C53.0	C79.82	D06.0	D26.0	D39.0	D49.59
overlapping lesion	C53.8	—	—	—	—	—
squamocolumnar junction	C53.8	C79.82	D06.7	D26.0	D39.0	D49.59
stump	C53.8	C79.82	D06.7	D26.0	D39.0	D49.59
cheek	C76.0	C79.89	D09.8	D36.7	D48.7	D49.89
external	C44.309	C79.2	D04.39	D23.39	D48.5	D49.2
basal cell carcinoma	C44.319	—	—	—	—	—
specified type NEC	C44.399	—	—	—	—	—
squamous cell carcinoma	C44.329	—	—	—	—	—
inner aspect	C06.0	C79.89	D00.02	D10.39	D37.09	D49.0
internal	C06.0	C79.89	D00.02	D10.39	D37.09	D49.0
mucosa	C06.0	C79.89	D00.02	D10.39	D37.09	D49.0
chest (wall) NEC	C76.1	C79.89	D09.8	D36.7	D48.7	D49.89
chiasma opticum	C72.3-☑	C79.49	—	D33.3	D43.3	D49.7
chin	C44.309	C79.2	D04.39	D23.39	D48.5	D49.2
basal cell carcinoma	C44.319	—	—	—	—	—
specified type NEC	C44.399	—	—	—	—	—
squamous cell carcinoma	C44.329	—	—	—	—	—
choana	C11.3	C79.89	D00.08	D10.6	D37.05	D49.0
cholangiole	C22.1	C78.89	D01.5	D13.4	D37.6	D49.0
choledochal duct	C24.0	C78.89	D01.5	D13.5	D37.6	D49.0
choroid	C69.3-☑	C79.49	D09.2-☑	D31.3-☑	D48.7	D49.81
plexus	C71.5	C79.31	—	D33.0	D43.0	D49.6
ciliary body	C69.4-☑	C79.49	D09.2-☑	D31.4-☑	D48.7	D49.89
clavicle	C41.3	C79.51	—	D16.7	D48.0	D49.2

Neoplasm, neoplastic — continued	Malignant Primary	Malignant Secondary	Ca in situ	Benign	Uncertain Behavior	Unspecified Behavior
clitoris	C51.2	C79.82	D07.1	D28.0	D39.8	D49.59
clivus	C41.0	C79.51	—	D16.4	D48.0	D49.2
cloacogenic zone	C21.2	C78.5	D01.3	D12.9	D37.8	D49.0
coccygeal						
body or glomus	C49.5	C79.89	—	D21.5	D48.1	D49.2
vertebra	C41.4	C79.51	—	D16.8	D48.0	D49.2
coccyx	C41.4	C79.51	—	D16.8	D48.0	D49.2
colon — see also Neoplasm, intestine, large	C18.9	C78.5	—	—	—	—
with rectum	C19	C78.5	D01.1	D12.7	D37.5	D49.0
columnella — see also Neoplasm, skin, face	C44.390	C79.2	D04.39	D23.39	D48.5	D49.2
column, spinal — see Neoplasm, spine						
commissure						
labial, lip	C00.6	C79.89	D00.01	D10.39	D37.01	D49.0
laryngeal	C32.0	C78.39	D02.0	D14.1	D38.0	D49.1
common (bile) duct	C24.0	C78.89	D01.5	D13.5	D37.6	D49.0
concha — see also Neoplasm, skin, ear	C44.20-☑	C79.2	D04.2-☑	D23.2-☑	D48.5	D49.2
nose	C30.0	C78.39	D02.3	D14.0	D38.5	D49.1
conjunctiva	C69.0-☑	C79.49	D09.2-☑	D31.0-☑	D48.7	D49.89
connective tissue NEC	C49.9	C79.89	—	D21.9	D48.1	D49.2

Note: For neoplasms of connective tissue (blood vessel, bursa, fascia, ligament, muscle, peripheral nerves, sympathetic and parasympathetic nerves and ganglia, synovia, tendon, etc.) or of morphological types that indicate connective tissue, code according to the list under "Neoplasm, connective tissue". For sites that do not appear in this list, code to neoplasm of that site; e.g., fibrosarcoma, pancreas (C25.9)

Note: Morphological types that indicate connective tissue appear in their proper place in the alphabetic index with the instruction "see Neoplasm, connective tissue ...."

	Malignant Primary	Malignant Secondary	Ca in situ	Benign	Uncertain Behavior	Unspecified Behavior
abdomen	C49.4	C79.89	—	D21.4	D48.1	D49.2
abdominal wall	C49.4	C79.89	—	D21.4	D48.1	D49.2
ankle	C49.2-☑	C79.89	—	D21.2-☑	D48.1	D49.2
antecubital fossa or space	C49.1-☑	C79.89	—	D21.1-☑	D48.1	D49.2
arm	C49.1-☑	C79.89	—	D21.1-☑	D48.1	D49.2
auricle (ear)	C49.0	C79.89	—	D21.0	D48.1	D49.2
axilla	C49.3	C79.89	—	D21.3	D48.1	D49.2
back	C49.6	C79.89	—	D21.6	D48.1	D49.2
breast — see Neoplasm, breast						
buttock	C49.5	C79.89	—	D21.5	D48.1	D49.2
calf	C49.2-☑	C79.89	—	D21.2-☑	D48.1	D49.2
cervical region	C49.0	C79.89	—	D21.0	D48.1	D49.2
cheek	C49.0	C79.89	—	D21.0	D48.1	D49.2
chest (wall)	C49.3	C79.89	—	D21.3	D48.1	D49.2
chin	C49.0	C79.89	—	D21.0	D48.1	D49.2
diaphragm	C49.3	C79.89	—	D21.3	D48.1	D49.2
ear (external)	C49.0	C79.89	—	D21.0	D48.1	D49.2
elbow	C49.1-☑	C79.89	—	D21.1-☑	D48.1	D49.2
extrarectal	C49.5	C79.89	—	D21.5	D48.1	D49.2
extremity	C49.9	C79.89	—	D21.9	D48.1	D49.2
lower	C49.2-☑	C79.89	—	D21.2-☑	D48.1	D49.2
upper	C49.1-☑	C79.89	—	D21.1-☑	D48.1	D49.2
eyelid	C49.0	C79.89	—	D21.0	D48.1	D49.2
face	C49.0	C79.89	—	D21.0	D48.1	D49.2
finger	C49.1-☑	C79.89	—	D21.1-☑	D48.1	D49.2
flank	C49.6	C79.89	—	D21.6	D48.1	D49.2
foot	C49.2-☑	C79.89	—	D21.2-☑	D48.1	D49.2
forearm	C49.1-☑	C79.89	—	D21.1-☑	D48.1	D49.2
forehead	C49.0	C79.89	—	D21.0	D48.1	D49.2
gastric	C49.4	C79.89	—	D21.4	D48.1	D49.2
gastrointestinal	C49.4	C79.89	—	D21.4	D48.1	D49.2
gluteal region	C49.5	C79.89	—	D21.5	D48.1	D49.2
great vessels NEC	C49.3	C79.89	—	D21.3	D48.1	D49.2
groin	C49.5	C79.89	—	D21.5	D48.1	D49.2
hand	C49.1-☑	C79.89	—	D21.1-☑	D48.1	D49.2
head	C49.0	C79.89	—	D21.0	D48.1	D49.2

☑ Additional Character Required — Refer to the Tabular List for Character Selection

	Malignant Primary	Malignant Secondary	Ca in situ	Benign	Uncertain Behavior	Unspecified Behavior
Neoplasm, neoplastic						
— *continued*						
connective tissue —						
continued						
heel	C49.2-☑	C79.89	—	D21.2-☑	D48.1	D49.2
hip	C49.2-☑	C79.89	—	D21.2-☑	D48.1	D49.2
hypochondrium	C49.4	C79.89	—	D21.4	D48.1	D49.2
iliopsoas muscle	C49.5	C79.89	—	D21.5	D48.1	D49.2
infraclavicular						
region	C49.3	C79.89	—	D21.3	D48.1	D49.2
inguinal (canal)						
(region)	C49.5	C79.89	—	D21.5	D48.1	D49.2
intestinal	C49.4	C79.89	—	D21.4	D48.1	D49.2
intrathoracic	C49.3	C79.89	—	D21.3	D48.1	D49.2
ischiorectal						
fossa	C49.5	C79.89	—	D21.5	D48.1	D49.2
jaw	C03.9	C79.89	D00.03	D10.39	D48.1	D49.0
knee	C49.2-☑	C79.89	—	D21.2-☑	D48.1	D49.2
leg	C49.2-☑	C79.89	—	D21.2-☑	D48.1	D49.2
limb NEC	C49.9	C79.89	—	D21.9	D48.1	D49.2
lower	C49.2-☑	C79.89	—	D21.2-☑	D48.1	D49.2
upper	C49.1-☑	C79.89	—	D21.1-☑	D48.1	D49.2
nates	C49.5	C79.89	—	D21.5	D48.1	D49.2
neck	C49.0	C79.89	—	D21.0	D48.1	D49.2
orbit	C69.6-☑	C79.49	D09.2-☑	D31.6-☑	D48.1	D49.89
overlapping						
lesion	C49.8	—	—	—	—	—
pararectal	C49.5	C79.89	—	D21.5	D48.1	D49.2
para-urethral	C49.5	C79.89	—	D21.5	D48.1	D49.2
paravaginal	C49.5	C79.89	—	D21.5	D48.1	D49.2
pelvis (floor)	C49.5	C79.89	—	D21.5	D48.1	D49.2
pelvo-abdominal	C49.8	C79.89	—	D21.6	D48.1	D49.2
perineum	C49.5	C79.89	—	D21.5	D48.1	D49.2
perirectal						
(tissue)	C49.5	C79.89	—	D21.5	D48.1	D49.2
periurethral						
(tissue)	C49.5	C79.89	—	D21.5	D48.1	D49.2
popliteal fossa or						
space	C49.2-☑	C79.89	—	D21.2-☑	D48.1	D49.2
presacral	C49.5	C79.89	—	D21.5	D48.1	D49.2
psoas muscle	C49.4	C79.89	—	D21.4	D48.1	D49.2
pterygoid fossa	C49.0	C79.89	—	D21.0	D48.1	D49.2
rectovaginal septum						
or wall	C49.5	C79.89	—	D21.5	D48.1	D49.2
rectovesical	C49.5	C79.89	—	D21.5	D48.1	D49.2
retroperitoneum	C48.0	C78.6	—	D20.0	D48.3	D49.0
sacrococcygeal						
region	C49.5	C79.89	—	D21.5	D48.1	D49.2
scalp	C49.0	C79.89	—	D21.0	D48.1	D49.2
scapular region	C49.3	C79.89	—	D21.3	D48.1	D49.2
shoulder	C49.1-☑	C79.89	—	D21.1-☑	D48.1	D49.2
skin (dermis) NEC —						
see also						
Neoplasm, skin,						
by site	C44.90	C79.2	D04.9	D23.9	D48.5	D49.2
stomach	C49.4	C79.89	—	D21.4	D48.1	D49.2
submental	C49.0	C79.89	—	D21.0	D48.1	D49.2
supraclavicular						
region	C49.0	C79.89	—	D21.0	D48.1	D49.2
temple	C49.0	C79.89	—	D21.0	D48.1	D49.2
temporal region	C49.0	C79.89	—	D21.0	D48.1	D49.2
thigh	C49.2-☑	C79.89	—	D21.2-☑	D48.1	D49.2
thoracic (duct)						
(wall)	C49.3	C79.89	—	D21.3	D48.1	D49.2
thorax	C49.3	C79.89	—	D21.3	D48.1	D49.2
thumb	C49.1-☑	C79.89	—	D21.1-☑	D48.1	D49.2
toe	C49.2-☑	C79.89	—	D21.2-☑	D48.1	D49.2
trunk	C49.6	C79.89	—	D21.6	D48.1	D49.2
umbilicus	C49.4	C79.89	—	D21.4	D48.1	D49.2
vesicorectal	C49.5	C79.89	—	D21.5	D48.1	D49.2
wrist	C49.1-☑	C79.89	—	D21.1-☑	D48.1	D49.2
conus medullaris	C72.0	C79.49	—	D33.4	D43.4	D49.7
cord (true) (vocal)	C32.0	C78.39	D02.0	D14.1	D38.0	D49.1
false	C32.1	C78.39	D02.0	D14.1	D38.0	D49.1
spermatic	C63.1-☑	C79.82	D07.69	D29.8	D40.8	D49.59
spinal (cervical)						
(lumbar)						
(thoracic)	C72.0	C79.49	—	D33.4	D43.4	D49.7
cornea (limbus)	C69.1-☑	C79.49	D09.2-☑	D31.1-☑	D48.7	D49.89
corpus						
albicans	C56.-☑	C79.6-☑	D07.39	D27.-☑	D39.1-☑	D49.59
callosum, brain	C71.0	C79.31	—	D33.2	D43.2	D49.6

	Malignant Primary	Malignant Secondary	Ca in situ	Benign	Uncertain Behavior	Unspecified Behavior
Neoplasm, neoplastic						
— *continued*						
corpus — *continued*						
cavernosum	C60.2	C79.82	D07.4	D29.0	D40.8	D49.59
gastric	C16.2	C78.89	D00.2	D13.1	D37.1	D49.0
overlapping						
sites	C54.8	—	—	—	—	—
penis	C60.2	C79.82	D07.4	D29.0	D40.8	D49.59
striatum,						
cerebrum	C71.0	C79.31	—	D33.0	D43.0	D49.6
uteri	C54.9	C79.82	D07.0	D26.1	D39.0	D49.59
isthmus	C54.0	C79.82	D07.0	D26.1	D39.0	D49.59
cortex						
adrenal	C74.0-☑	C79.7-☑	D09.3	D35.0-☑	D44.1-☑	D49.7
cerebral	C71.0	C79.31	—	D33.0	D43.0	D49.6
costal cartilage	C41.3	C79.51	—	D16.7	D48.0	D49.2
costovertebral						
joint	C41.3	C79.51	—	D16.7	D48.0	D49.2
Cowper's gland	C68.0	C79.19	D09.19	D30.4	D41.3	D49.59
cranial (fossa, any)	C71.9	C79.31	—	D33.2	D43.2	D49.6
meninges	C70.0	C79.32	—	D32.0	D42.0	D49.7
nerve	C72.50	C79.49	—	D33.3	D43.3	D49.7
specified NEC	C72.59	C79.49	—	D33.3	D43.3	D49.7
craniobuccal						
pouch	C75.2	C79.89	D09.3	D35.2	D44.3	D49.7
craniopharyngeal (duct)						
(pouch)	C75.2	C79.89	D09.3	D35.3	D44.4	D49.7
cricoid	C13.0	C79.89	D00.08	D10.7	D37.05	D49.0
cartilage	C32.3	C78.39	D02.0	D14.1	D38.0	D49.1
cricopharynx	C13.0	C79.89	D00.08	D10.7	D37.05	D49.0
crypt of Morgagni	C21.8	C78.5	D01.3	D12.9	D37.8	D49.0
crystalline lens	C69.4-☑	C79.49	D09.2-☑	D31.4-☑	D48.7	D49.89
cul-de-sac						
(Douglas')	C48.1	C78.6	—	D20.1	D48.4	D49.0
cuneiform						
cartilage	C32.3	C78.39	D02.0	D14.1	D38.0	D49.1
cutaneous — *see*						
Neoplasm, skin						
cutis — *see* Neoplasm,						
skin						
cystic (bile) duct						
(common)	C24.0	C78.89	D01.5	D13.5	D37.6	D49.0
dermis — *see*						
Neoplasm, skin						
diaphragm	C49.3	C79.89	—	D21.3	D48.1	D49.2
digestive organs,						
system, tube, or						
tract NEC	C26.9	C78.89	D01.9	D13.9	D37.9	D49.0
disc,						
intervertebral	C41.2	C79.51	—	D16.6	D48.0	D49.2
disease,						
generalized	C80.0	—	—	—	—	—
disseminated	C80.0	—	—	—	—	—
Douglas' cul-de-sac or						
pouch	C48.1	C78.6	—	D20.1	D48.4	D49.0
duodenojejunal						
junction	C17.8	C78.4	D01.49	D13.39	D37.2	D49.0
duodenum	C17.0	C78.4	D01.49	D13.2	D37.2	D49.0
dura (cranial)						
(mater)	C70.9	C79.49	—	D32.9	D42.9	D49.7
cerebral	C70.0	C79.32	—	D32.0	D42.0	D49.7
spinal	C70.1	C79.49	—	D32.1	D42.1	D49.7
ear (external) — *see*						
also Neoplasm, skin,						
ear	C44.20-☑	C79.2	D04.2-☑	D23.2-☑	D48.5	D49.2
auricle or auris — *see*						
also Neoplasm,						
skin, ear	C44.20-☑	C79.2	D04.2-☑	D23.2-☑	D48.5	D49.2
canal, external — *see*						
also Neoplasm,						
skin, ear	C44.20-☑	C79.2	D04.2-☑	D23.2-☑	D48.5	D49.2
cartilage	C49.0	C79.89	—	D21.0	D48.1	D49.2
external meatus —						
see also						
Neoplasm, skin,						
ear	C44.20-☑	C79.2	D04.2-☑	D23.2-☑	D48.5	D49.2
inner	C30.1	C78.39	D02.3	D14.0	D38.5	D49.1
lobule — *see also*						
Neoplasm, skin,						
ear	C44.20-☑	C79.2	D04.2-☑	D23.2-☑	D48.5	D49.2
middle	C30.1	C78.39	D02.3	D14.0	D38.5	D49.1
overlapping lesion						
with accessory						
sinuses	C31.8	—	—	—	—	—

☑ **Additional Character Required — Refer to the Tabular List for Character Selection**

Neoplasm, neoplastic — continued	Malignant Primary	Malignant Secondary	Ca in situ	Benign	Uncertain Behavior	Unspecified Behavior
ear — see also Neoplasm, skin, ear — continued						
skin	C44.20-☑	C79.2	D04.2-☑	D23.2-☑	D48.5	D49.2
basal cell carcinoma	C44.21-☑	—	—	—	—	—
specified type NEC	C44.29-☑	—	—	—	—	—
squamous cell carcinoma	C44.22-☑	—	—	—	—	—
earlobe	C44.20-☑	C79.2	D04.2-☑	D23.2-☑	D48.5	D49.2
basal cell carcinoma	C44.21-☑	—	—	—	—	—
specified type NEC	C44.29-☑	—	—	—	—	—
squamous cell carcinoma	C44.22-☑	—	—	—	—	—
ejaculatory duct	C63.7	C79.82	D07.69	D29.8	D40.8	D49.59
elbow NEC	C76.4-☑	C79.89	D04.6-☑	D36.7	D48.7	D49.89
endocardium	C38.0	C79.89	—	D15.1	D48.7	D49.89
endocervix (canal) (gland)	C53.0	C79.82	D06.0	D26.0	D39.0	D49.59
endocrine gland NEC	C75.9	C79.89	D09.3	D35.9	D44.9	D49.7
pluriglandular	C75.8	C79.89	D09.3	D35.7	D44.9	D49.7
endometrium (gland) (stroma)	C54.1	C79.82	D07.0	D26.1	D39.0	D49.59
ensiform cartilage	C41.3	C79.51	—	D16.7	D48.0	D49.2
enteric — see Neoplasm, intestine						
ependyma (brain)	C71.5	C79.31	—	D33.0	D43.0	D49.6
fourth ventricle	C71.7	C79.31	—	D33.1	D43.1	D49.6
epicardium	C38.0	C79.89	—	D15.1	D48.7	D49.89
epididymis	C63.0-☑	C79.82	D07.69	D29.3-☑	D40.8	D49.59
epidural	C72.9	C79.49	—	D33.9	D43.9	D49.7
epiglottis	C32.1	C78.39	D02.0	D14.1	D38.0	D49.1
anterior aspect or surface	C10.1	C79.89	D00.08	D10.5	D37.05	D49.0
cartilage	C32.3	C78.39	D02.0	D14.1	D38.0	D49.1
free border (margin)	C10.1	C79.89	D00.08	D10.5	D37.05	D49.0
junctional region	C10.8	C79.89	D00.08	D10.5	D37.05	D49.0
posterior (laryngeal) surface	C32.1	C78.39	D02.0	D14.1	D38.0	D49.1
suprahyoid portion	C32.1	C78.39	D02.0	D14.1	D38.0	D49.1
esophagogastric junction	C16.0	C78.89	D00.2	D13.1	D37.1	D49.0
esophagus	C15.9	C78.89	D00.1	D13.0	D37.8	D49.0
abdominal	C15.5	C78.89	D00.1	D13.0	D37.8	D49.0
cervical	C15.3	C78.89	D00.1	D13.0	D37.8	D49.0
distal (third)	C15.5	C78.89	D00.1	D13.0	D37.8	D49.0
lower (third)	C15.5	C78.89	D00.1	D13.0	D37.8	D49.0
middle (third)	C15.4	C78.89	D00.1	D13.0	D37.8	D49.0
overlapping lesion	C15.8	—	—	—	—	—
proximal (third)	C15.3	C78.89	D00.1	D13.0	D37.8	D49.0
thoracic	C15.4	C78.89	D00.1	D13.0	D37.8	D49.0
upper (third)	C15.3	C78.89	D00.1	D13.0	D37.8	D49.0
ethmoid (sinus)	C31.1	C78.39	D02.3	D14.0	D38.5	D49.1
bone or labyrinth	C41.0	C79.51	—	D16.4	D48.0	D49.2
eustachian tube	C30.1	C78.39	D02.3	D14.0	D38.5	D49.1
exocervix	C53.1	C79.82	D06.1	D26.0	D39.0	D49.59
external						
meatus (ear) — see also Neoplasm, skin, ear	C44.20-☑	C79.2	D04.2-☑	D23.2-☑	D48.5	D49.2
os, cervix uteri	C53.1	C79.82	D06.1	D26.0	D39.0	D49.59
extradural	C72.9	C79.49	—	D33.9	D43.9	D49.7
extrahepatic (bile) duct	C24.0	C78.89	D01.5	D13.5	D37.6	D49.0
overlapping lesion with gallbladder	C24.8	—	—			
extraocular muscle	C69.6-☑	C79.49	D09.2-☑	D31.6-☑	D48.7	D49.89
extrarectal	C76.3	C79.89	D09.8	D36.7	D48.7	D49.89
extremity	C76.8	C79.89	D04.8	D36.7	D48.7	D49.89

Neoplasm, neoplastic — continued	Malignant Primary	Malignant Secondary	Ca in situ	Benign	Uncertain Behavior	Unspecified Behavior
extremity — continued						
lower	C76.5-☑	C79.89	D04.7-☑	D36.7	D48.7	D49.89
upper	C76.4-☑	C79.89	D04.6-☑	D36.7	D48.7	D49.89
eyeball	C69.9-☑	C79.49	D09.2-☑	D31.9-☑	D48.7	D49.89
eyebrow	C44.309	C79.2	D04.39	D23.39	D48.5	D49.2
basal cell carcinoma	C44.319	—	—	—	—	—
specified type NEC	C44.399	—	—	—	—	—
squamous cell carcinoma	C44.329	—	—	—	—	—
eyelid (lower) (skin) (upper)	C44.10-☑	—	—	—	—	—
basal cell carcinoma	C44.11-☑	—	—	—	—	—
cartilage	C49.0	C79.89	—	D21.0	D48.1	D49.2
sebaceous cell	C44.13-☑	—	—	—	—	—
specified type NEC	C44.19-☑	—	—	—	—	—
squamous cell carcinoma	C44.12-☑	—	—	—	—	—
eye NEC	C69.9-☑	C79.49	D09.2-☑	D31.9-☑	D48.7	D49.89
overlapping sites	C69.8-☑					
face NEC	C76.0	C79.89	D04.39	D36.7	D48.7	D49.89
fallopian tube (accessory)	C57.0-☑	C79.82	D07.39	D28.2	D39.8	D49.59
falx (cerebella) (cerebri)	C70.0	C79.32	—	D32.0	D42.0	D49.7
fascia — see also Neoplasm, connective tissue						
palmar	C49.1-☑	C79.89	—	D21.1-☑	D48.1	D49.2
plantar	C49.2-☑	C79.89	—	D21.2-☑	D48.1	D49.2
fatty tissue — see Neoplasm, connective tissue						
fauces, faucial NEC	C10.9	C79.89	D00.08	D10.5	D37.05	D49.0
pillars	C09.1	C79.89	D00.08	D10.5	D37.05	D49.0
tonsil	C09.9	C79.89	D00.08	D10.4	D37.05	D49.0
femur (any part)	C40.2-☑	—	—	D16.2-☑	—	—
fetal membrane	C58	C79.82	D07.0	D26.7	D39.2	D49.59
fibrous tissue — see Neoplasm, connective tissue						
fibula (any part)	C40.2-☑	C79.51	—	D16.2-☑	—	—
filum terminale	C72.0	C79.49	—	D33.4	D43.4	D49.7
finger NEC	C76.4-☑	C79.89	D04.6-☑	D36.7	D48.7	D49.89
flank NEC	C76.8	C79.89	D04.5	D36.7	D48.7	D49.89
follicle, nabothian	C53.0	C79.82	D06.0	D26.0	D39.0	D49.59
foot NEC	C76.5-☑	C79.89	D04.7-☑	D36.7	D48.7	D49.89
forearm NEC	C76.4-☑	C79.89	D04.6-☑	D36.7	D48.7	D49.89
forehead (skin)	C44.309	C79.2	D04.39	D23.39	D48.5	D49.2
basal cell carcinoma	C44.319	—	—	—	—	—
specified type NEC	C44.399	—	—	—	—	—
squamous cell carcinoma	C44.329	—	—	—	—	—
foreskin	C60.0	C79.82	D07.4	D29.0	D40.8	D49.59
fornix						
pharyngeal	C11.3	C79.89	D00.08	D10.6	D37.05	D49.0
vagina	C52	C79.82	D07.2	D28.1	D39.8	D49.59
fossa (of)						
anterior (cranial)	C71.9	C79.31	—	D33.2	D43.2	D49.6
cranial	C71.9	C79.31	—	D33.2	D43.2	D49.6
ischiorectal	C76.3	C79.89	D09.8	D36.7	D48.7	D49.89
middle (cranial)	C71.9	C79.31	—	D33.2	D43.2	D49.6
piriform	C12	C79.89	D00.08	D10.7	D37.05	D49.0
pituitary	C75.1	C79.89	D09.3	D35.2	D44.3	D49.7
posterior (cranial)	C71.9	C79.31	—	D33.2	D43.2	D49.6
pterygoid	C49.0	C79.89	—	D21.0	D48.1	D49.2
pyriform	C12	C79.89	D00.08	D10.7	D37.05	D49.0
Rosenmuller	C11.2	C79.89	D00.08	D10.6	D37.05	D49.0
tonsillar	C09.0	C79.89	D00.08	D10.5	D37.05	D49.0
fourchette	C51.9	C79.82	D07.1	D28.0	D39.8	D49.59
frenulum						
labii — see Neoplasm, lip, internal						

Neoplasm, frenulum — Neoplasm, intestine, intestinal

Neoplasm, neoplastic	Malignant Primary	Malignant Secondary	Ca in situ	Benign	Uncertain Behavior	Unspecified Behavior
— continued						
frenulum — continued						
linguae	C02.2	C79.89	D00.07	D10.1	D37.02	D49.0
frontal						
bone	C41.0	C79.51	—	D16.4	D48.0	D49.2
lobe, brain	C71.1	C79.31	—	D33.0	D43.0	D49.6
pole	C71.1	C79.31	—	D33.0	D43.0	D49.6
sinus	C31.2	C78.39	D02.3	D14.0	D38.5	D49.1
fundus						
stomach	C16.1	C78.89	D00.2	D13.1	D37.1	D49.0
uterus	C54.3	C79.82	D07.0	D26.1	D39.0	D49.59
gallbladder	C23	C78.89	D01.5	D13.5	D37.6	D49.0
overlapping lesion with extrahepatic bile ducts	C24.8	—	—	—	—	—
gall duct						
(extrahepatic)	C24.0	C78.89	D01.5	D13.5	D37.6	D49.0
intrahepatic	C22.1	C78.7	D01.5	D13.4	D37.6	D49.0
ganglia — see also						
Neoplasm, nerve, peripheral	C47.9	C79.89	—	D36.10	D48.2	D49.2
basal	C71.0	C79.31	—	D33.0	D43.0	D49.6
cranial nerve	C72.50	C79.49	—	D33.3	D43.3	D49.7
Gartner's duct	C52	C79.82	D07.2	D28.1	D39.8	D49.59
gastric — see Neoplasm, stomach						
gastrocolic	C26.9	C78.89	D01.9	D13.9	D37.9	D49.0
gastroesophageal junction	C16.0	C78.89	D00.2	D13.1	D37.1	D49.0
gastrointestinal (tract) NEC	C26.9	C78.89	D01.9	D13.9	D37.9	D49.0
generalized	C80.0	—	—	—	—	—
genital organ or tract						
female NEC	C57.9	C79.82	D07.30	D28.9	D39.9	D49.59
overlapping lesion	C57.8	—	—	—	—	—
specified site NEC	C57.7	C79.82	D07.39	D28.7	D39.8	D49.59
male NEC	C63.9	C79.82	D07.60	D29.9	D40.9	D49.59
overlapping lesion	C63.8	—	—	—	—	—
specified site NEC	C63.7	C79.82	D07.69	D29.8	D40.8	D49.59
genitourinary tract female	C57.9	C79.82	D07.30	D28.9	D39.9	D49.59
male	C63.9	C79.82	D07.60	D29.9	D40.9	D49.59
gingiva (alveolar) (marginal)	C03.9	C79.89	D00.03	D10.39	D37.09	D49.0
lower	C03.1	C79.89	D00.03	D10.39	D37.09	D49.0
mandibular	C03.1	C79.89	D00.03	D10.39	D37.09	D49.0
maxillary	C03.0	C79.89	D00.03	D10.39	D37.09	D49.0
upper	C03.0	C79.89	D00.03	D10.39	D37.09	D49.0
gland, glandular (lymphatic) (system) — see also Neoplasm, lymph gland						
endocrine NEC	C75.9	C79.89	D09.3	D35.9	D44.9	D49.7
salivary — see Neoplasm, salivary gland						
glans penis	C60.1	C79.82	D07.4	D29.0	D40.8	D49.59
globus pallidus	C71.0	C79.31	—	D33.0	D43.0	D49.6
glomus						
coccygeal	C49.5	C79.89	—	D21.5	D48.1	D49.2
jugularis	C75.5	C79.89	—	D35.6	D44.7	D49.7
glosso-epiglottic fold(s)	C10.1	C79.89	D00.08	D10.5	D37.05	D49.0
glossopalatine fold	C09.1	C79.89	D00.08	D10.5	D37.05	D49.0
glossopharyngeal sulcus	C09.0	C79.89	D00.08	D10.5	D37.05	D49.0
glottis	C32.0	C78.39	D02.0	D14.1	D38.0	D49.1
gluteal region	C76.3	C79.89	D04.5	D36.7	D48.7	D49.89
great vessels NEC	C49.3	C79.89	—	D21.3	D48.1	D49.2
groin NEC	C76.3	C79.89	D04.5	D36.7	D48.7	D49.89
gum	C03.9	C79.89	D00.03	D10.39	D37.09	D49.0
lower	C03.1	C79.89	D00.03	D10.39	D37.09	D49.0
upper	C03.0	C79.89	D00.03	D10.39	D37.09	D49.0
hand NEC	C76.4-☑	C79.89	D04.6-☑	D36.7	D48.7	D49.89
head NEC	C76.0	C79.89	D04.4	D36.7	D48.7	D49.89
heart	C38.0	C79.89	—	D15.1	D48.7	D49.89

Neoplasm, neoplastic	Malignant Primary	Malignant Secondary	Ca in situ	Benign	Uncertain Behavior	Unspecified Behavior
— continued						
heel NEC	C76.5-☑	C79.89	D04.7-☑	D36.7	D48.7	D49.89
helix — see also Neoplasm, skin, ear	C44.20-☑	C79.2	D04.2-☑	D23.2-☑	D48.5	D49.2
hematopoietic, hemopoietic tissue NEC	C96.9	—	—	—	—	—
specified NEC	C96.Z	—	—	—	—	—
hemisphere, cerebral	C71.0	C79.31	—	D33.0	D43.0	D49.6
hemorrhoidal zone	C21.1	C78.5	D01.3	D12.9	D37.8	D49.0
hepatic — see also Index to disease, by histology	C22.9	C78.7	D01.5	D13.4	D37.6	D49.0
duct (bile)	C24.0	C78.89	D01.5	D13.5	D37.6	D49.0
flexure (colon)	C18.3	C78.5	D01.0	D12.3	D37.4	D49.0
primary	C22.8	C78.7	D01.5	D13.4	D37.6	D49.0
hepatobiliary	C24.9	C78.89	D01.5	D13.5	D37.6	D49.0
hepatoblastoma	C22.2	C78.7	D01.5	D13.4	D37.6	D49.0
hepatoma	C22.0	C78.7	D01.5	D13.4	D37.6	D49.0
hilus of lung	C34.0-☑	C78.0-☑	D02.2-☑	D14.3-☑	D38.1	D49.1
hippocampus, brain	C71.2	C79.31	—	D33.0	D43.0	D49.6
hip NEC	C76.5-☑	C79.89	D04.7-☑	D36.7	D48.7	D49.89
humerus (any part)	C40.0-☑	C79.51	—	D16.0-☑	—	—
hymen	C52	C79.82	D07.2	D28.1	D39.8	D49.59
hypopharynx, hypopharyngeal NEC	C13.9	C79.89	D00.08	D10.7	D37.05	D49.0
overlapping lesion	C13.8	—	—	—	—	—
postcricoid region	C13.0	C79.89	D00.08	D10.7	D37.05	D49.0
posterior wall	C13.2	C79.89	D00.08	D10.7	D37.05	D49.0
pyriform fossa (sinus)	C12	C79.89	D00.08	D10.7	D37.05	D49.0
hypophysis	C75.1	C79.89	D09.3	D35.2	D44.3	D49.7
hypothalamus	C71.0	C79.31	—	D33.0	D43.0	D49.6
ileocecum, ileocecal (coil) (junction) (valve)	C18.0	C78.5	D01.0	D12.0	D37.4	D49.0
ileum	C17.2	C78.4	D01.49	D13.39	D37.2	D49.0
ilium	C41.4	C79.51	—	D16.8	D48.0	D49.2
immunoproliferative NEC	C88.9	—	—	—	—	—
infraclavicular (region)	C76.1	C79.89	D04.5	D36.7	D48.7	D49.89
inguinal (region)	C76.3	C79.89	D04.5	D36.7	D48.7	D49.89
insula	C71.0	C79.31	—	D33.0	D43.0	D49.6
insular tissue (pancreas)	C25.4	C78.89	D01.7	D13.7	D37.8	D49.0
brain	C71.0	C79.31	—	D33.0	D43.0	D49.6
interarytenoid fold	C13.1	C78.39	D00.08	D10.7	D37.05	D49.0
hypopharyngeal aspect	C13.1	C79.89	D00.08	D10.7	D37.05	D49.0
laryngeal aspect	C32.1	C78.39	D02.0	D14.1	D38.0	D49.1
marginal zone	C13.1	C79.89	D00.08	D10.7	D37.05	D49.0
interdental papillae	C03.9	C79.89	D00.03	D10.39	D37.09	D49.0
lower	C03.1	C79.89	D00.03	D10.39	D37.09	D49.0
upper	C03.0	C79.89	D00.03	D10.39	D37.09	D49.0
internal						
capsule	C71.0	C79.31	—	D33.0	D43.0	D49.6
os (cervix)	C53.0	C79.82	D06.0	D26.0	D39.0	D49.59
intervertebral cartilage or disc	C41.2	C79.51	—	D16.6	D48.0	D49.2
intestine, intestinal	C26.0	C78.80	D01.40	D13.9	D37.8	D49.0
large	C18.9	C78.5	D01.0	D12.6	D37.4	D49.0
appendix	C18.1	C78.5	D01.0	D12.1	D37.3	D49.0
caput coli	C18.0	C78.5	D01.0	D12.0	D37.4	D49.0
cecum	C18.0	C78.5	D01.0	D12.0	D37.4	D49.0
colon	C18.9	C78.5	D01.0	D12.6	D37.4	D49.0
and rectum	C19	C78.5	D01.1	D12.7	D37.5	D49.0
ascending	C18.2	C78.5	D01.0	D12.2	D37.4	D49.0
caput	C18.0	C78.5	D01.0	D12.0	D37.4	D49.0
descending	C18.6	C78.5	D01.0	D12.4	D37.4	D49.0
distal	C18.6	C78.5	D01.0	D12.4	D37.4	D49.0

☑ Additional Character Required — Refer to the Tabular List for Character Selection

	Malignant Primary	Malignant Secondary	Ca in situ	Benign	Uncertain Behavior	Unspecified Behavior
Neoplasm, neoplastic						
— *continued*						
intestine, intestinal — *continued*						
large — *continued*						
colon — *continued*						
left	C18.6	C78.5	D01.0	D12.4	D37.4	D49.0
overlapping lesion	C18.8	—	—	—	—	—
pelvic	C18.7	C78.5	D01.0	D12.5	D37.4	D49.0
right	C18.2	C78.5	D01.0	D12.2	D37.4	D49.0
sigmoid (flexure)	C18.7	C78.5	D01.0	D12.5	D37.4	D49.0
transverse	C18.4	C78.5	D01.0	D12.3	D37.4	D49.0
hepatic flexure	C18.3	C78.5	D01.0	D12.3	D37.4	D49.0
ileocecum, ileocecal (coil)						
(valve)	C18.0	C78.5	D01.0	D12.0	D37.4	D49.0
overlapping lesion	C18.8	—	—	—	—	—
sigmoid flexure (lower)						
(upper)	C18.7	C78.5	D01.0	D12.5	D37.4	D49.0
splenic flexure	C18.5	C78.5	D01.0	D12.3	D37.4	D49.0
small	C17.9	C78.4	D01.40	D13.30	D37.2	D49.0
duodenum	C17.0	C78.4	D01.49	D13.2	D37.2	D49.0
ileum	C17.2	C78.4	D01.49	D13.39	D37.2	D49.0
jejunum	C17.1	C78.4	D01.49	D13.39	D37.2	D49.0
overlapping lesion	C17.8	—	—	—	—	—
tract NEC	C26.0	C78.89	D01.40	D13.9	D37.8	D49.0
intra-abdominal	C76.2	C79.89	D09.8	D36.7	D48.7	D49.89
intracranial NEC	C71.9	C79.31	—	D33.2	D43.2	D49.6
intrahepatic (bile) duct	C22.1	C78.7	D01.5	D13.4	D37.6	D49.0
intraocular	C69.9-☑	C79.49	D09.2-☑	D31.9-☑	D48.7	D49.89
intraorbital	C69.6-☑	C79.49	D09.2-☑	D31.6-☑	D48.7	D49.89
intrasellar	C75.1	C79.89	D09.3	D35.2	D44.3	D49.7
intrathoracic (cavity) (organs)	C76.1	C79.89	D09.8	D15.9	D48.7	D49.89
specified NEC	C76.1	C79.89	D09.8	D15.7	—	—
iris	C69.4-☑	C79.49	D09.2-☑	D31.4-☑	D48.7	D49.89
ischiorectal (fossa)	C76.3	C79.89	D09.8	D36.7	D48.7	D49.89
ischium	C41.4	C79.51	—	D16.8	D48.0	D49.2
island of Reil	C71.0	C79.31	—	D33.0	D43.0	D49.6
islands or islets of Langerhans	C25.4	C78.89	D01.7	D13.7	D37.8	D49.0
isthmus uteri	C54.0	C79.82	D07.0	D26.1	D39.0	D49.59
jaw	C76.0	C79.89	D09.8	D36.7	D48.7	D49.89
bone	C41.1	C79.51	—	D16.5	D48.0	D49.2
lower	C41.1	C79.51	—	D16.5	—	—
upper	C41.0	C79.51	—	D16.4	—	—
carcinoma (any type) (lower)						
(upper)	C76.0	C79.89	—	—	—	—
skin — *see also* Neoplasm, skin, face	C44.309	C79.2	D04.39	D23.39	D48.5	D49.2
soft tissues	C03.9	C79.89	D00.03	D10.39	D37.09	D49.0
lower	C03.1	C79.89	D00.03	D10.39	D37.09	D49.0
upper	C03.0	C79.89	D00.03	D10.39	D37.09	D49.0
jejunum	C17.1	C78.4	D01.49	D13.39	D37.2	D49.0
joint NEC — *see also* Neoplasm, bone	C41.9	C79.51	—	D16.9	D48.0	D49.2
acromioclavicular	C40.0-☑	C79.51	—	D16.0-☑	—	—
bursa or synovial membrane — *see* Neoplasm, connective tissue						
costovertebral	C41.3	C79.51	—	D16.7	D48.0	D49.2
sternocostal	C41.3	C79.51	—	D16.7	D48.0	D49.2
temporomandibular	C41.1	C79.51	—	D16.5	D48.0	D49.2
junction						
anorectal	C21.8	C78.5	D01.3	D12.9	D37.8	D49.0
cardioesophageal	C16.0	C78.89	D00.2	D13.1	D37.1	D49.0
esophagogastric	C16.0	C78.89	D00.2	D13.1	D37.1	D49.0
gastroesophageal	C16.0	C78.89	D00.2	D13.1	D37.1	D49.0
hard and soft palate	C05.9	C79.89	D00.00	D10.39	D37.09	D49.0
ileocecal	C18.0	C78.5	D01.0	D12.0	D37.4	D49.0

	Malignant Primary	Malignant Secondary	Ca in situ	Benign	Uncertain Behavior	Unspecified Behavior
Neoplasm, neoplastic						
— *continued*						
junction — *continued*						
pelvirectal	C19	C78.5	D01.1	D12.7	D37.5	D49.0
pelviureteric	C65.-☑	C79.0-☑	D09.19	D30.1-☑	D41.1-☑	D49.59
rectosigmoid	C19	C78.5	D01.1	D12.7	D37.5	D49.0
squamocolumnar, of cervix	C53.8	C79.82	D06.7	D26.0	D39.0	D49.59
Kaposi's sarcoma — *see* Kaposi's, sarcoma						
kidney (parenchymal)	C64.-☑	C79.0-☑	D09.19	D30.0-☑	D41.0-☑	D49.51 ☑
calyx	C65.-☑	C79.0-☑	D09.19	D30.1-☑	D41.1-☑	D49.51 ☑
hilus	C65.-☑	C79.0-☑	D09.19	D30.1-☑	D41.1-☑	D49.51 ☑
pelvis	C65.-☑	C79.0-☑	D09.19	D30.1-☑	D41.1-☑	D49.51 ☑
knee NEC	C76.5-☑	C79.89	D04.7-☑	D36.7	D48.7	D49.89
labia (skin)	C51.9	C79.82	D07.1	D28.0	D39.8	D49.59
majora	C51.0	C79.82	D07.1	D28.0	D39.8	D49.59
minora	C51.1	C79.82	D07.1	D28.0	D39.8	D49.59
labial — *see also* Neoplasm, lip	C00.9	C79.89	D00.01	D10.0	D37.01	D49.0
sulcus (lower) (upper)	C06.1	C79.89	D00.02	D10.39	D37.09	D49.0
labium (skin)	C51.9	C79.82	D07.1	D28.0	D39.8	D49.59
majus	C51.0	C79.82	D07.1	D28.0	D39.8	D49.59
minus	C51.1	C79.82	D07.1	D28.0	D39.8	D49.59
lacrimal						
canaliculi	C69.5-☑	C79.49	D09.2-☑	D31.5-☑	D48.7	D49.89
duct (nasal)	C69.5-☑	C79.49	D09.2-☑	D31.5-☑	D48.7	D49.89
gland	C69.5-☑	C79.49	D09.2-☑	D31.5-☑	D48.7	D49.89
punctum	C69.5-☑	C79.49	D09.2-☑	D31.5-☑	D48.7	D49.89
sac	C69.5-☑	C79.49	D09.2-☑	D31.5-☑	D48.7	D49.89
Langerhans, islands or islets	C25.4	C78.89	D01.7	D13.7	D37.8	D49.0
laryngopharynx	C13.9	C79.89	D00.08	D10.7	D37.05	D49.0
larynx, laryngeal NEC	C32.9	C78.39	D02.0	D14.1	D38.0	D49.1
aryepiglottic fold	C32.1	C78.39	D02.0	D14.1	D38.0	D49.1
cartilage (arytenoid) (cricoid) (cuneiform) (thyroid)	C32.3	C78.39	D02.0	D14.1	D38.0	D49.1
commissure (anterior) (posterior)	C32.0	C78.39	D02.0	D14.1	D38.0	D49.1
extrinsic NEC	C32.1	C78.39	D02.0	D14.1	D38.0	D49.1
meaning hypopharynx	C13.9	C79.89	D00.08	D10.7	D37.05	D49.0
interarytenoid fold	C32.1	C78.39	D02.0	D14.1	D38.0	D49.1
intrinsic	C32.0	C78.39	D02.0	D14.1	D38.0	D49.1
overlapping lesion	C32.8	—	—	—	—	—
ventricular band	C32.1	C78.39	D02.0	D14.1	D38.0	D49.1
leg NEC	C76.5-☑	C79.89	D04.7-☑	D36.7	D48.7	D49.89
lens, crystalline	C69.4-☑	C79.49	D09.2-☑	D31.4-☑	D48.7	D49.89
lid (lower) (upper)	C44.10-☑	C79.2	D04.1-☑	D23.1-☑	D48.5	D49.2
basal cell carcinoma	C44.11-☑	—	—	—	—	—
sebaceous cell	C44.13-☑	—	—	—	—	—
specified type NEC	C44.19-☑	—	—	—	—	—
squamous cell carcinoma	C44.12-☑	—	—	—	—	—
ligament — *see also* Neoplasm, connective tissue						
broad	C57.1-☑	C79.82	D07.39	D28.2	D39.8	D49.59
Mackenrodt's	C57.7	C79.82	D07.39	D28.7	D39.8	D49.59
non-uterine — *see* Neoplasm, connective tissue						
round	C57.2-☑	C79.82	—	D28.2	D39.8	D49.59
sacro-uterine	C57.3	C79.82	—	D28.2	D39.8	D49.59
uterine	C57.3	C79.82	—	D28.2	D39.8	D49.59
utero-ovarian	C57.7	C79.82	D07.39	D28.2	D39.8	D49.59
uterosacral	C57.3	C79.82	—	D28.2	D39.8	D49.59
limb	C76.8	C79.89	D04.8		D48.7	D49.89
lower	C76.5-☑	C79.89	D04.7-☑	D36.7	D48.7	D49.89
upper	C76.4-☑	C79.89	D04.6-☑	D36.7	D48.7	D49.89
limbus of cornea	C69.1-☑	C79.49	D09.2-☑	D31.1-☑	D48.7	D49.89

Neoplasm Table

Neoplasm, neoplastic — continued	Malignant Primary	Malignant Secondary	Ca in situ	Benign	Uncertain Behavior	Unspecified Behavior
lingual NEC — see also Neoplasm, tongue	C02.9	C79.89	D00.07	D10.1	D37.02	D49.0
lingula, lung	C34.1-☑	C78.0-☑	D02.2-☑	D14.3-☑	D38.1	D49.1
lip	C00.9	C79.89	D00.01	D10.0	D37.01	D49.0
buccal aspect — see Neoplasm, lip, internal						
commissure	C00.6	C79.89	D00.01	D10.0	D37.01	D49.0
external	C00.2	C79.89	D00.01	D10.0	D37.01	D49.0
lower	C00.1	C79.89	D00.01	D10.0	D37.01	D49.0
upper	C00.0	C79.89	D00.01	D10.0	D37.01	D49.0
frenulum — see Neoplasm, lip, internal						
inner aspect — see Neoplasm, lip, internal						
internal	C00.5	C79.89	D00.01	D10.0	D37.01	D49.0
lower	C00.4	C79.89	D00.01	D10.0	D37.01	D49.0
upper	C00.3	C79.89	D00.01	D10.0	D37.01	D49.0
lipstick area	C00.2	C79.89	D00.01	D10.0	D37.01	D49.0
lower	C00.1	C79.89	D00.01	D10.0	D37.01	D49.0
upper	C00.0	C79.89	D00.01	D10.0	D37.01	D49.0
lower	C00.1	C79.89	D00.01	D10.0	D37.01	D49.0
internal	C00.4	C79.89	D00.01	D10.0	D37.01	D49.0
mucosa — see Neoplasm, lip, internal						
oral aspect — see Neoplasm, lip, internal						
overlapping lesion	C00.8	—	—	—	—	—
with oral cavity or pharynx	C14.8	—	—	—	—	—
skin (commissure) (lower) (upper)	C44.00	C79.2	D04.0	D23.0	D48.5	D49.2
basal cell carcinoma	C44.01	—	—	—	—	—
specified type NEC	C44.09	—	—	—	—	—
squamous cell carcinoma	C44.02	—	—	—	—	—
upper	C00.0	C79.89	D00.01	D10.0	D37.01	D49.0
internal	C00.3	C79.89	D00.01	D10.0	D37.01	D49.0
vermilion border	C00.2	C79.89	D00.01	D10.0	D37.01	D49.0
lower	C00.1	C79.89	D00.01	D10.0	D37.01	D49.0
upper	C00.0	C79.89	D00.01	D10.0	D37.01	D49.0
lipomatous — see Lipoma, by site						
liver — see also Index to disease, by histology	C22.9	C78.7	D01.5	D13.4	D37.6	D49.0
primary	C22.8	C78.7	D01.5	D13.4	D37.6	D49.0
lumbosacral plexus	C47.5	C79.89	—	D36.16	D48.2	D49.2
lung	C34.9-☑	C78.0-☑	D02.2-☑	D14.3-☑	D38.1	D49.1
azygos lobe	C34.1-☑	C78.0-☑	D02.2-☑	D14.3-☑	D38.1	D49.1
carina	C34.0-☑	C78.0-☑	D02.2-☑	D14.3-☑	D38.1	D49.1
hilus	C34.0-☑	C78.0-☑	D02.2-☑	D14.3-☑	D38.1	D49.1
linqula	C34.1-☑	C78.0-☑	D02.2-☑	D14.3-☑	D38.1	D49.1
lobe NEC	C34.9-☑	C78.0-☑	D02.2-☑	D14.3-☑	D38.1	D49.1
lower lobe	C34.3-☑	C78.0-☑	D02.2-☑	D14.3-☑	D38.1	D49.1
main bronchus	C34.0-☑	C78.0-☑	D02.2-☑	D14.3-☑	D38.1	D49.1
mesothelioma — see Mesothelioma						
middle lobe	C34.2	C78.0-☑	D02.21	D14.31	D38.1	D49.1
overlapping lesion	C34.8-☑	—	—	—	—	—
upper lobe	C34.1-☑	C78.0-☑	D02.2-☑	D14.3-☑	D38.1	D49.1
lymph, lymphatic channel NEC	C49.9	C79.89	—	D21.9	D48.1	D49.2
gland						
(secondary)	—	C77.9	—	D36.0	D48.7	D49.89
abdominal	—	C77.2	—	D36.0	D48.7	D49.89
aortic	—	C77.2	—	D36.0	D48.7	D49.89
arm	—	C77.3	—	D36.0	D48.7	D49.89

Neoplasm, neoplastic — continued lymph, lymphatic channel — continued gland — continued	Malignant Primary	Malignant Secondary	Ca in situ	Benign	Uncertain Behavior	Unspecified Behavior
auricular (anterior) (posterior)	—	C77.0	—	D36.0	D48.7	D49.89
axilla, axillary	—	C77.3	—	D36.0	D48.7	D49.89
brachial	—	C77.3	—	D36.0	D48.7	D49.89
bronchial	—	C77.1	—	D36.0	D48.7	D49.89
bronchopulmonary	—	C77.1	—	D36.0	D48.7	D49.89
celiac	—	C77.2	—	D36.0	D48.7	D49.89
cervical	—	C77.0	—	D36.0	D48.7	D49.89
cervicofacial	—	C77.0	—	D36.0	D48.7	D49.89
Cloquet	—	C77.4	—	D36.0	D48.7	D49.89
colic	—	C77.2	—	D36.0	D48.7	D49.89
common duct	—	C77.2	—	D36.0	D48.7	D49.89
cubital	—	C77.3	—	D36.0	D48.7	D49.89
diaphragmatic	—	C77.1	—	D36.0	D48.7	D49.89
epigastric, inferior	—	C77.1	—	D36.0	D48.7	D49.89
epitrochlear	—	C77.3	—	D36.0	D48.7	D49.89
esophageal	—	C77.1	—	D36.0	D48.7	D49.89
face	—	C77.0	—	D36.0	D48.7	D49.89
femoral	—	C77.4	—	D36.0	D48.7	D49.89
gastric	—	C77.2	—	D36.0	D48.7	D49.89
groin	—	C77.4	—	D36.0	D48.7	D49.89
head	—	C77.0	—	D36.0	D48.7	D49.89
hepatic	—	C77.2	—	D36.0	D48.7	D49.89
hilar (pulmonary)	—	C77.1	—	D36.0	D48.7	D49.89
splenic	—	C77.2	—	D36.0	D48.7	D49.89
hypogastric	—	C77.5	—	D36.0	D48.7	D49.89
ileocolic	—	C77.2	—	D36.0	D48.7	D49.89
iliac	—	C77.5	—	D36.0	D48.7	D49.89
infraclavicular	—	C77.3	—	D36.0	D48.7	D49.89
inguina, inguinal	—	C77.4	—	D36.0	D48.7	D49.89
innominate	—	C77.1	—	D36.0	D48.7	D49.89
intercostal	—	C77.1	—	D36.0	D48.7	D49.89
intestinal	—	C77.2	—	D36.0	D48.7	D49.89
intrabdominal	—	C77.2	—	D36.0	D48.7	D49.89
intrapelvic	—	C77.5	—	D36.0	D48.7	D49.89
intrathoracic	—	C77.1	—	D36.0	D48.7	D49.89
jugular	—	C77.0	—	D36.0	D48.7	D49.89
leg	—	C77.4	—	D36.0	D48.7	D49.89
limb						
lower	—	C77.4	—	D36.0	D48.7	D49.89
upper	—	C77.3	—	D36.0	D48.7	D49.89
lower limb	—	C77.4	—	D36.0	D48.7	D49.89
lumbar	—	C77.2	—	D36.0	D48.7	D49.89
mandibular	—	C77.0	—	D36.0	D48.7	D49.89
mediastinal	—	C77.1	—	D36.0	D48.7	
mesenteric (inferior) (superior)	—	C77.2	—	D36.0	D48.7	D49.89
midcolic	—	C77.2	—	D36.0	D48.7	D49.89
multiple sites in categories C77.0 - C77.5	—	C77.8	—	D36.0	D48.7	D49.89
neck	—	C77.0	—	D36.0	D48.7	D49.89
obturator	—	C77.5	—	D36.0	D48.7	D49.89
occipital	—	C77.0	—	D36.0	D48.7	D49.89
pancreatic	—	C77.2	—	D36.0	D48.7	D49.89
para-aortic	—	C77.2	—	D36.0	D48.7	D49.89
paracervical	—	C77.5	—	D36.0	D48.7	D49.89
parametrial	—	C77.5	—	D36.0	D48.7	D49.89
parasternal	—	C77.1	—	D36.0	D48.7	D49.89
parotid	—	C77.0	—	D36.0	D48.7	D49.89
pectoral	—	C77.3	—	D36.0	D48.7	D49.89
pelvic	—	C77.5	—	D36.0	D48.7	D49.89
peri-aortic	—	C77.2	—	D36.0	D48.7	D49.89
peripancreatic	—	C77.2	—	D36.0	D48.7	D49.89
popliteal	—	C77.4	—	D36.0	D48.7	D49.89
porta hepatis	—	C77.2	—	D36.0	D48.7	D49.89
portal	—	C77.2	—	D36.0	D48.7	D49.89
preauricular	—	C77.0	—	D36.0	D48.7	D49.89
prelaryngeal	—	C77.0	—	D36.0	D48.7	D49.89
presymphysial	—	C77.5	—	D36.0	D48.7	D49.89
pretracheal	—	C77.0	—	D36.0	D48.7	D49.89
primary (any site) NEC	C96.9	—	—	—	—	—

☑ Additional Character Required — Refer to the Tabular List for Character Selection

	Malignant Primary	Malignant Secondary	Ca in situ	Benign	Uncertain Behavior	Unspecified Behavior
Neoplasm, neoplastic						
— *continued*						
lymph, lymphatic						
channel —						
continued						
gland — *continued*						
pulmonary						
(hiler)	—	C77.1	—	D36.0	D48.7	D49.89
pyloric	—	C77.2	—	D36.0	D48.7	D49.89
retroperitoneal	—	C77.2	—	D36.0	D48.7	D49.89
retropharyngeal	—	C77.0	—	D36.0	D48.7	D49.89
Rosenmuller's	—	C77.4	—	D36.0	D48.7	D49.89
sacral	—	C77.5	—	D36.0	D48.7	D49.89
scalene	—	C77.0	—	D36.0	D48.7	D49.89
site NEC	—	C77.9	—	D36.0	D48.7	D49.89
splenic (hilar)	—	C77.2	—	D36.0	D48.7	D49.89
subclavicular	—	C77.3	—	D36.0	D48.7	D49.89
subinguinal	—	C77.4	—	D36.0	D48.7	D49.89
sublingual	—	C77.0	—	D36.0	D48.7	D49.89
submandibular	—	C77.0	—	D36.0	D48.7	D49.89
submaxillary	—	C77.0	—	D36.0	D48.7	D49.89
submental	—	C77.0	—	D36.0	D48.7	D49.89
subscapular	—	C77.3	—	D36.0	D48.7	D49.89
supraclavicular	—	C77.0	—	D36.0	D48.7	D49.89
thoracic	—	C77.1	—	D36.0	D48.7	D49.89
tibial	—	C77.4	—	D36.0	D48.7	D49.89
tracheal	—	C77.1	—	D36.0	D48.7	D49.89
tracheobronchial	—	C77.1	—	D36.0	D48.7	D49.89
upper limb	—	C77.3	—	D36.0	D48.7	D49.89
Virchow's	—	C77.0	—	D36.0	D48.7	D49.89
node — *see also*						
Neoplasm, lymph						
gland						
primary NEC	C96.9	—	—	—	—	—
vessel — *see also*						
Neoplasm,						
connective						
tissue	C49.9	C79.89	—	D21.9	D48.1	D49.2
Mackenrodt's						
ligament	C57.7	C79.82	D07.39	D28.7	D39.8	D49.59
malar	C41.0	C79.51		D16.4	D48.0	D49.2
region — *see*						
Neoplasm, cheek						
mammary gland — *see*						
Neoplasm, breast						
mandible	C41.1	C79.51	—	D16.5	D48.0	D49.2
alveolar						
mucosa						
(carcinoma)	C03.1	C79.89	D00.03	D10.39	D37.09	D49.0
ridge or						
process	C41.1	C79.51	—	D16.5	D48.0	D49.2
marrow (bone)						
NEC	C96.9	C79.52	—	—	D47.9	D49.89
mastectomy site (skin)						
— *see also*						
Neoplasm, breast,						
skin	C44.501	C79.2	—	—	—	—
specified as breast						
tissue	C50.8-☑	C79.81	—	—	—	—
mastoid (air cells)						
(antrum)						
(cavity)	C30.1	C78.39	D02.3	D14.0	D38.5	D49.1
bone or process	C41.0	C79.51	—	D16.4	D48.0	D49.2
maxilla, maxillary						
(superior)	C41.0	C79.51	—	D16.4	D48.0	D49.2
alveolar						
mucosa	C03.0	C79.89	D00.03	D10.39	D37.09	D49.0
ridge or process						
(carcinoma)	C41.0	C79.51	—	D16.4	D48.0	D49.2
antrum	C31.0	C78.39	D02.3	D14.0	D38.5	D49.1
carcinoma	C03.0	C79.51	—	—	—	—
inferior — *see*						
Neoplasm,						
mandible						
sinus	C31.0	C78.39	D02.3	D14.0	D38.5	D49.1
meatus external (ear)						
— *see also*						
Neoplasm, skin,						
ear	C44.20-☑	C79.2	D04.2-☑	D23.2-☑	D48.5	D49.2
Meckel diverticulum,						
malignant	C17.3	C78.4	D01.49	D13.39	D37.2	D49.0
mediastinum,						
mediastinal	C38.3	C78.1	—	D15.2	D38.3	D49.89
anterior	C38.1	C78.1	—	D15.2	D38.3	D49.89

	Malignant Primary	Malignant Secondary	Ca in situ	Benign	Uncertain Behavior	Unspecified Behavior
Neoplasm, neoplastic						
— *continued*						
mediastinum,						
mediastinal —						
continued						
posterior	C38.2	C78.1	—	D15.2	D38.3	D49.89
medulla						
adrenal	C74.1-☑	C79.7-☑	D09.3	D35.0-☑	D44.1-☑	D49.7
oblongata	C71.7	C79.31	—	D33.1	D43.1	D49.6
meibomian gland	C44.10-☑	C79.2	D04.1-☑	D23.1-☑	D48.5	D49.2
basal cell						
carcinoma	C44.11-☑	—	—	—	—	—
sebaceous cell	C44.13-☑	—	—	—	—	—
specified type						
NEC	C44.19-☑	—	—	—	—	—
squamous cell						
carcinoma	C44.12-☑	—	—	—	—	—
melanoma — *see*						
Melanoma						
meninges	C70.9	C79.49	—	D32.9	D42.9	D49.7
brain	C70.0	C79.32	—	D32.0	D42.0	D49.7
cerebral	C70.0	C79.32	—	D32.0	D42.0	D49.7
crainial	C70.0	C79.32	—	D32.0	D42.0	D49.7
intracranial	C70.0	C79.32	—	D32.0	D42.0	D49.7
spinal (cord)	C70.1	C79.49	—	D32.1	D42.1	D49.7
meniscus, knee joint						
(lateral)						
(medial)	C40.2-☑	C79.51	—	D16.2-☑	D48.0	D49.2
Merkel cell — *see*						
Carcinoma, Merkel						
cell						
mesentery,						
mesenteric	C48.1	C78.6	—	D20.1	D48.4	D49.0
mesoappendix	C48.1	C78.6	—	D20.1	D48.4	D49.0
mesocolon	C48.1	C78.6	—	D20.1	D48.4	D49.0
mesopharynx — *see*						
Neoplasm,						
oropharynx						
mesosalpinx	C57.1-☑	C79.82	D07.39	D28.2	D39.8	D49.59
mesothelial tissue —						
see Mesothelioma						
mesothelioma — *see*						
Mesothelioma						
mesovarium	C57.1-☑	C79.82	D07.39	D28.2	D39.8	D49.59
metacarpus (any						
bone)	C40.1-☑	C79.51	—	D16.1-☑	—	—
metastatic NEC — *see*						
also Neoplasm, by						
site,						
secondary	—	C79.9	—	—	—	—
metatarsus (any						
bone)	C40.3-☑	C79.51	—	D16.3-☑	—	—
midbrain	C71.7	C79.31	—	D33.1	D43.1	D49.6
milk duct — *see*						
Neoplasm, breast						
mons						
pubis	C51.9	C79.82	D07.1	D28.0	D39.8	D49.59
veneris	C51.9	C79.82	D07.1	D28.0	D39.8	D49.59
motor tract	C72.9	C79.49	—	D33.9	D43.9	D49.7
brain	C71.9	C79.31	—	D33.2	D43.2	D49.6
cauda equina	C72.1	C79.49	—	D33.4	D43.4	D49.7
spinal	C72.0	C79.49	—	D33.4	D43.4	D49.7
mouth	C06.9	C79.89	D00.00	D10.30	D37.09	D49.0
book-leaf	C06.89	C79.89	—	—	—	—
floor	C04.9	C79.89	D00.06	D10.2	D37.09	D49.0
anterior						
portion	C04.0	C79.89	D00.06	D10.2	D37.09	D49.0
lateral portion	C04.1	C79.89	D00.06	D10.2	D37.09	D49.0
overlapping						
lesion	C04.8	—	—	—	—	—
overlapping						
NEC	C06.80	—	—	—	—	—
roof	C05.9	C79.89	D00.00	D10.39	D37.09	D49.0
specified part						
NEC	C06.89	C79.89	D00.00	D10.39	D37.09	D49.0
vestibule	C06.1	C79.89	D00.00	D10.39	D37.09	D49.0
mucosa						
alveolar (ridge or						
process)	C03.9	C79.89	D00.03	D10.39	D37.09	D49.0
lower	C03.1	C79.89	D00.03	D10.39	D37.09	D49.0
upper	C03.0	C79.89	D00.03	D10.39	D37.09	D49.0
buccal	C06.0	C79.89	D00.02	D10.39	D37.09	D49.0
cheek	C06.0	C79.89	D00.02	D10.39	D37.09	D49.0

☑ **Additional Character Required — Refer to the Tabular List for Character Selection**

Neoplasm, neoplastic	Malignant Primary	Malignant Secondary	Ca in situ	Benign	Uncertain Behavior	Unspecified Behavior
— continued						
mucosa — continued						
lip — see Neoplasm, lip, internal						
nasal	C30.0	C78.39	D02.3	D14.0	D38.5	D49.1
oral	C06.0	C79.89	D00.02	D10.39	D37.09	D49.0
Mullerian duct						
female	C57.7	C79.82	D07.39	D28.7	D39.8	D49.59
male	C63.7	C79.82	D07.69	D29.8	D40.8	D49.59
muscle — see also Neoplasm, connective tissue						
extraocular	C69.6-☑	C79.49	D09.2-☑	D31.6-☑	D48.7	D49.89
myocardium	C38.0	C79.89	—	D15.1	D48.7	D49.89
myometrium	C54.2	C79.82	D07.0	D26.1	D39.0	D49.59
myopericardium	C38.0	C79.89	—	D15.1	D48.7	D49.89
nabothian gland (follicle)	C53.0	C79.82	D06.0	D26.0	D39.0	D49.59
nail — see also Neoplasm, skin, limb	C44.90	C79.2	D04.9	D23.9	D48.5	D49.2
finger — see also Neoplasm, skin, limb, upper	C44.60-☑	C79.2	D04.6-☑	D23.6-☑	D48.5	D49.2
toe — see also Neoplasm, skin, limb, lower	C44.70-☑	C79.2	D04.7-☑	D23.7-☑	D48.5	D49.2
nares, naris (anterior) (posterior)	C30.0	C78.39	D02.3	D14.0	D38.5	D49.1
nasal — see Neoplasm, nose						
nasolabial groove — see also Neoplasm, skin, face	C44.309	C79.2	D04.39	D23.39	D48.5	D49.2
nasolacrimal duct	C69.5-☑	C79.49	D09.2-☑	D31.5-☑	D48.7	D49.89
nasopharynx, nasopharyngeal	C11.9	C79.89	D00.08	D10.6	D37.05	D49.0
floor	C11.3	C79.89	D00.08	D10.6	D37.05	D49.0
overlapping lesion	C11.8	—	—	—	—	—
roof	C11.0	C79.89	D00.08	D10.6	D37.05	D49.0
wall	C11.9	C79.89	D00.08	D10.6	D37.05	D49.0
anterior	C11.3	C79.89	D00.08	D10.6	D37.05	D49.0
lateral	C11.2	C79.89	D00.08	D10.6	D37.05	D49.0
posterior	C11.1	C79.89	D00.08	D10.6	D37.05	D49.0
superior	C11.0	C79.89	D00.08	D10.6	D37.05	D49.0
nates — see also Neoplasm, skin, trunk	C44.509	C79.2	D04.5	D23.5	D48.5	D49.2
neck NEC	C76.0	C79.89	D09.8	D36.7	D48.7	D49.89
skin	C44.40	—	—	—	—	—
basal cell carcinoma	C44.41	—	—	—	—	—
specified type NEC	C44.49	—	—	—	—	—
squamous cell carcinoma	C44.42	—	—	—	—	—
nerve (ganglion)	C47.9	C79.89	—	D36.10	D48.2	D49.2
abducens	C72.59	C79.49	—	D33.3	D43.3	D49.7
accessory (spinal)	C72.59	C79.49	—	D33.3	D43.3	D49.7
acoustic	C72.4-☑	C79.49	—	D33.3	D43.3	D49.7
auditory	C72.4-☑	C79.49	—	D33.3	D43.3	D49.7
autonomic NEC — see also Neoplasm, nerve, peripheral	C47.9	C79.89	—	D36.10	D48.2	D49.2
brachial	C47.1-☑	C79.89	—	D36.12	D48.2	D49.2
cranial	C72.50	C79.49	—	D33.3	D43.3	D49.7
specified NEC	C72.59	C79.49	—	D33.3	D43.3	D49.7
facial	C72.59	C79.49	—	D33.3	D43.3	D49.7
femoral	C47.2-☑	C79.89	—	D36.13	D48.2	D49.2
ganglion NEC — see also Neoplasm, nerve, peripheral	C47.9	C79.89	—	D36.10	D48.2	D49.2
glossopharyngeal	C72.59	C79.49	—	D33.3	D43.3	D49.7
hypoglossal	C72.59	C79.49	—	D33.3	D43.3	D49.7
intercostal	C47.3	C79.89	—	D36.14	D48.2	D49.2
lumbar	C47.6	C79.89	—	D36.17	D48.2	D49.2
median	C47.1-☑	C79.89	—	D36.12	D48.2	D49.2
obturator	C47.2-☑	C79.89	—	D36.13	D48.2	D49.2
Neoplasm, neoplastic						
— continued						
nerve — continued						
oculomotor	C72.59	C79.49	—	D33.3	D43.3	D49.7
olfactory	C47.2-☑	C79.49	—	D33.3	D43.3	D49.7
optic	C72.3-☑	C79.49	—	D33.3	D43.3	D49.7
parasympathetic NEC	C47.9	C79.89	—	D36.10	D48.2	D49.2
peripheral NEC	C47.9	C79.89	—	D36.10	D48.2	D49.2
abdomen	C47.4	C79.89	—	D36.15	D48.2	D49.2
abdominal wall	C47.4	C79.89	—	D36.15	D48.2	D49.2
ankle	C47.2-☑	C79.89	—	D36.13	D48.2	D49.2
antecubital fossa or space	C47.1-☑	C79.89	—	D36.12	D48.2	D49.2
arm	C47.1-☑	C79.89	—	D36.12	D48.2	D49.2
auricle (ear)	C47.0	C79.89	—	D36.11	D48.2	D49.2
axilla	C47.3	C79.89	—	D36.12	D48.2	D49.2
back	C47.6	C79.89	—	D36.17	D48.2	D49.2
buttock	C47.5	C79.89	—	D36.16	D48.2	D49.2
calf	C47.2-☑	C79.89	—	D36.13	D48.2	D49.2
cervical region	C47.0	C79.89	—	D36.11	D48.2	D49.2
cheek	C47.0	C79.89	—	D36.11	D48.2	D49.2
chest (wall)	C47.3	C79.89	—	D36.14	D48.2	D49.2
chin	C47.0	C79.89	—	D36.11	D48.2	D49.2
ear (external)	C47.0	C79.89	—	D36.11	D48.2	D49.2
elbow	C47.1-☑	C79.89	—	D36.12	D48.2	D49.2
extrarectal	C47.5	C79.89	—	D36.16	D48.2	D49.2
extremity	C47.9	C79.89	—	D36.10	D48.2	D49.2
lower	C47.2-☑	C79.89	—	D36.13	D48.2	D49.2
upper	C47.1-☑	C79.89	—	D36.12	D48.2	D49.2
eyelid	C47.0	C79.89	—	D36.11	D48.2	D49.2
face	C47.0	C79.89	—	D36.11	D48.2	D49.2
finger	C47.1-☑	C79.89	—	D36.12	D48.2	D49.2
flank	C47.6	C79.89	—	D36.17	D48.2	D49.2
foot	C47.2-☑	C79.89	—	D36.13	D48.2	D49.2
forearm	C47.1-☑	C79.89	—	D36.12	D48.2	D49.2
forehead	C47.0	C79.89	—	D36.11	D48.2	D49.2
gluteal region	C47.5	C79.89	—	D36.16	D48.2	D49.2
groin	C47.5	C79.89	—	D36.16	D48.2	D49.2
hand	C47.1-☑	C79.89	—	D36.12	D48.2	D49.2
head	C47.0	C79.89	—	D36.11	D48.2	D49.2
heel	C47.2-☑	C79.89	—	D36.13	D48.2	D49.2
hip	C47.2-☑	C79.89	—	D36.13	D48.2	D49.2
infraclavicular region	C47.3	C79.89	—	D36.14	D48.2	D49.2
inguinal (canal) (region)	C47.5	C79.89	—	D36.16	D48.2	D49.2
intrathoracic	C47.3	C79.89	—	D36.14	D48.2	D49.2
ischiorectal fossa	C47.5	C79.89	—	D36.16	D48.2	D49.2
knee	C47.2-☑	C79.89	—	D36.13	D48.2	D49.2
leg	C47.2-☑	C79.89	—	D36.13	D48.2	D49.2
limb NEC	C47.9	C79.89	—	D36.10	D48.2	D49.2
lower	C47.2-☑	C79.89	—	D36.13	D48.2	D49.2
upper	C47.1-☑	C79.89	—	D36.12	D48.2	D49.2
nates	C47.5	C79.89	—	D36.16	D48.2	D49.2
neck	C47.0	C79.89	—	D36.11	D48.2	D49.2
orbit	C69.6-☑	C79.49	—	D31.6-☑	D48.7	D49.2
pararectal	C47.5	C79.89	—	D36.16	D48.2	D49.2
paraurethral	C47.5	C79.89	—	D36.16	D48.2	D49.2
paravaginal	C47.5	C79.89	—	D36.16	D48.2	D49.2
pelvis (floor)	C47.5	C79.89	—	D36.16	D48.2	D49.2
pelvoabdominal	C47.8	C79.89	—	D36.17	D48.2	D49.2
perineum	C47.5	C79.89	—	D36.16	D48.2	D49.2
perirectal (tissue)	C47.5	C79.89	—	D36.16	D48.2	D49.2
periurethral (tissue)	C47.5	C79.89	—	D36.16	D48.2	D49.2
popliteal fossa or space	C47.2-☑	C79.89	—	D36.13	D48.2	D49.2
presacral	C47.5	C79.89	—	D36.16	D48.2	D49.2
pterygoid fossa	C47.0	C79.89	—	D36.11	D48.2	D49.2
rectovaginal septum or wall	C47.5	C79.89	—	D36.16	D48.2	D49.2
rectovesical	C47.5	C79.89	—	D36.16	D48.2	D49.2
sacrococcygeal region	C47.5	C79.89	—	D36.16	D48.2	D49.2
scalp	C47.0	C79.89	—	D36.11	D48.2	D49.2

☑ Additional Character Required — Refer to the Tabular List for Character Selection

Neoplasm, neoplastic — continued	Malignant Primary	Malignant Secondary	Ca in situ	Benign	Uncertain Behavior	Unspecified Behavior
nerve — continued						
peripheral — continued						
scapular region	C47.3	C79.89	—	D36.14	D48.2	D49.2
shoulder	C47.1-☑	C79.89	—	D36.12	D48.2	D49.2
submental	C47.0	C79.89	—	D36.11	D48.2	D49.2
supraclavicular region	C47.0	C79.89	—	D36.11	D48.2	D49.2
temple	C47.0	C79.89	—	D36.11	D48.2	D49.2
temporal region	C47.0	C79.89	—	D36.11	D48.2	D49.2
thigh	C47.2-☑	C79.89	—	D36.13	D48.2	D49.2
thoracic (duct) (wall)	C47.3	C79.89	—	D36.14	D48.2	D49.2
thorax	C47.3	C79.89	—	D36.14	D48.2	D49.2
thumb	C47.1-☑	C79.89	—	D36.12	D48.2	D49.2
toe	C47.2-☑	C79.89	—	D36.13	D48.2	D49.2
trunk	C47.6	C79.89	—	D36.17	D48.2	D49.2
umbilicus	C47.4	C79.89	—	D36.15	D48.2	D49.2
vesicorectal	C47.5	C79.89	—	D36.16	D48.2	D49.2
wrist	C47.1-☑	C79.89	—	D36.12	D48.2	D49.2
radial	C47.1-☑	C79.89	—	D36.12	D48.2	D49.2
sacral	C47.5	C79.89	—	D36.16	D48.2	D49.2
sciatic	C47.2-☑	C79.89	—	D36.13	D48.2	D49.2
spinal NEC	C47.9	C79.89	—	D36.10	D48.2	D49.2
accessory	C72.59	C79.49	—	D33.3	D43.3	D49.7
sympathetic NEC — see also Neoplasm, nerve, peripheral	C47.9	C79.89	—	D36.10	D48.2	D49.2
trigeminal	C72.59	C79.49	—	D33.3	D43.3	D49.7
trochlear	C72.59	C79.49	—	D33.3	D43.3	D49.7
ulnar	C47.1-☑	C79.89	—	D36.12	D48.2	D49.2
vagus	C72.59	C79.49	—	D33.3	D43.3	D49.7
nervous system (central)	C72.9	C79.40	—	D33.9	D43.9	D49.7
autonomic — see Neoplasm, nerve, peripheral						
parasympathetic — see Neoplasm, nerve, peripheral						
specified site NEC	—	C79.49	—	D33.7	D43.8	—
sympathetic — see Neoplasm, nerve, peripheral						
nevus — see Nevus						
nipple	C50.0-☑	C79.81	D05.-☑	D24.-☑	—	—
nose, nasal	C76.0	C79.89	D09.8	D36.7	D48.7	D49.89
ala (external) (nasi) — see also Neoplasm, nose, skin	C44.301	C79.2	D04.39	D23.39	D48.5	D49.2
bone	C41.0	C79.51	—	D16.4	D48.0	D49.2
cartilage	C30.0	C78.39	D02.3	D14.0	D38.5	D49.1
cavity	C30.0	C78.39	D02.3	D14.0	D38.5	D49.1
choana	C11.3	C79.89	D00.08	D10.6	D37.05	D49.0
external (skin) — see also Neoplasm, nose, skin	C44.301	C79.2	D04.39	D23.39	D48.5	D49.2
fossa	C30.0	C78.39	D02.3	D14.0	D38.5	D49.1
internal	C30.0	C78.39	D02.3	D14.0	D38.5	D49.1
mucosa	C30.0	C78.39	D02.3	D14.0	D38.5	D49.1
septum	C30.0	C78.39	D02.3	D14.0	D38.5	D49.1
posterior margin	C11.3	C79.89	D00.08	D10.6	D37.05	D49.0
sinus — see Neoplasm, sinus						
skin	C44.301	C79.2	D04.39	D23.39	D48.5	D49.2
basal cell carcinoma	C44.311	—	—	—	—	—
specified type NEC	C44.391	—	—	—	—	—
squamous cell carcinoma	C44.321	—	—	—	—	—
turbinate (mucosa)	C30.0	C78.39	D02.3	D14.0	D38.5	D49.1
bone	C41.0	C79.51	—	D16.4	D48.0	D49.2
vestibule	C30.0	C78.39	D02.3	D14.0	D38.5	D49.1

Neoplasm, neoplastic — continued	Malignant Primary	Malignant Secondary	Ca in situ	Benign	Uncertain Behavior	Unspecified Behavior
nostril	C30.0	C78.39	D02.3	D14.0	D38.5	D49.1
nucleus pulposus	C41.2	C79.51	—	D16.6	D48.0	D49.2
occipital						
bone	C41.0	C79.51	—	D16.4	D48.0	D49.2
lobe or pole, brain	C71.4	C79.31	—	D33.0	D43.0	D49.6
odontogenic — see Neoplasm, jaw bone						
olfactory nerve or bulb	C72.2-☑	C79.49	—	D33.3	D43.3	D49.7
olive (brain)	C71.7	C79.31	—	D33.1	D43.1	D49.6
omentum	C48.1	C78.6	—	D20.1	D48.4	D49.0
operculum (brain)	C71.0	C79.31	—	D33.0	D43.0	D49.6
optic nerve, chiasm, or tract	C72.3-☑	C79.49	—	D33.3	D43.3	D49.7
oral (cavity)	C06.9	C79.89	D00.00	D10.30	D37.09	D49.0
ill-defined	C14.8	C79.89	D00.00	D10.30	D37.09	D49.0
mucosa	C06.0	C79.89	D00.02	D10.39	D37.09	D49.0
orbit	C69.6-☑	C79.49	D09.2-☑	D31.6-☑	D48.7	D49.89
autonomic nerve	C69.6-☑	C79.49	—	D31.6-☑	D48.7	D49.2
bone	C41.0	C79.51	—	D16.4	D48.0	D49.2
eye	C69.6-☑	C79.49	D09.2-☑	D31.6-☑	D48.7	D49.89
peripheral nerves	C69.6-☑	C79.49	—	D31.6-☑	D48.7	D49.2
soft parts	C69.6-☑	C79.49	D09.2-☑	D31.6-☑	D48.7	D49.89
organ of Zuckerkandl	C75.5	C79.89	—	D35.6	D44.7	D49.7
oropharynx	C10.9	C79.89	D00.08	D10.5	D37.05	D49.0
branchial cleft (vestige)	C10.4	C79.89	D00.08	D10.5	D37.05	D49.0
junctional region	C10.8	C79.89	D00.08	D10.5	D37.05	D49.0
lateral wall	C10.2	C79.89	D00.08	D10.5	D37.05	D49.0
overlapping lesion	C10.8	—	—	—	—	—
pillars or fauces	C09.1	C79.89	D00.08	D10.5	D37.05	D49.0
posterior wall	C10.3	C79.89	D00.08	D10.5	D37.05	D49.0
vallecula	C10.0	C79.89	D00.08	D10.5	D37.05	D49.0
os						
external	C53.1	C79.82	D06.1	D26.0	D39.0	D49.59
internal	C53.0	C79.82	D06.0	D26.0	D39.0	D49.59
ovary	C56.-☑	C79.6-☑	D07.39	D27.-☑	D39.1-☑	D49.59
oviduct	C57.0-☑	C79.82	D07.39	D28.2	D39.8	D49.59
palate	C05.9	C79.89	D00.00	D10.39	D37.09	D49.0
hard	C05.0	C79.89	D00.05	D10.39	D37.09	D49.0
junction of hard and soft palate	C05.9	C79.89	D00.00	D10.39	D37.09	D49.0
overlapping lesions	C05.8	—	—	—	—	—
soft	C05.1	C79.89	D00.04	D10.39	D37.09	D49.0
nasopharyngeal surface	C11.3	C79.89	D00.08	D10.6	D37.05	D49.0
posterior surface	C11.3	C79.89	D00.08	D10.6	D37.05	D49.0
superior surface	C11.3	C79.89	D00.08	D10.6	D37.05	D49.0
palatoglossal arch	C09.1	C79.89	D00.00	D10.5	D37.09	D49.0
palatopharyngeal arch	C09.1	C79.89	D00.00	D10.5	D37.09	D49.0
pallium	C71.0	C79.31	—	D33.0	D43.0	D49.6
palpebra	C44.10-☑	C79.2	D04.1-☑	D23.1-☑	D48.5	D49.2
basal cell carcinoma	C44.11-☑	—	—	—	—	—
sebaceous cell	C44.13-☑	—	—	—	—	—
specified type NEC	C44.19-☑	—	—	—	—	—
squamous cell carcinoma	C44.12-☑	—	—	—	—	—
pancreas	C25.9	C78.89	D01.7	D13.6	D37.8	D49.0
body	C25.1	C78.89	D01.7	D13.6	D37.8	D49.0
duct (of Santorini) (of Wirsung)	C25.3	C78.89	D01.7	D13.6	D37.8	D49.0
ectopic tissue	C25.7	C78.89	—	D13.6	D37.8	D49.0
head	C25.0	C78.89	D01.7	D13.6	D37.8	D49.0
islet cells	C25.4	C78.89	D01.7	D13.7	D37.8	D49.0
neck	C25.7	C78.89	D01.7	D13.6	D37.8	D49.0
overlapping lesion	C25.8	—	—	—	—	—
tail	C25.2	C78.89	D01.7	D13.6	D37.8	D49.0

☑ Additional Character Required — Refer to the Tabular List for Character Selection

Neoplasm Table

Neoplasm, para-aortic body — Neoplasm, rectum

Neoplasm, neoplastic	Malignant Primary	Malignant Secondary	Ca in situ	Benign	Uncertain Behavior	Unspecified Behavior
— continued						
para-aortic body	C75.5	C79.89	—	D35.6	D44.7	D49.7
paraganglion NEC	C75.5	C79.89	—	D35.6	D44.7	D49.7
parametrium	C57.3	C79.82	—	D28.2	D39.8	D49.59
paranephric	C48.0	C78.6	—	D20.0	D48.3	D49.0
pararectal	C76.3	C79.89	—	D36.7	D48.7	D49.89
parasagittal						
(region)	C76.0	C79.89	D09.8	D36.7	D48.7	D49.89
parasellar	C72.9	C79.49	—	D33.9	D43.8	D49.7
parathyroid						
(gland)	C75.0	C79.89	D09.3	D35.1	D44.2	D49.7
paraurethral	C76.3	C79.89	—	D36.7	D48.7	D49.89
gland	C68.1	C79.19	D09.19	D30.8	D41.8	D49.59
paravaginal	C76.3	C79.89	—	D36.7	D48.7	D49.89
parenchyma,						
kidney	C64.-☑	C79.0-☑	D09.19	D30.0-☑	D41.0-☑	D49.51-☑
parietal						
bone	C41.0	C79.51	—	D16.4	D48.0	D49.2
lobe, brain	C71.3	C79.31	—	D33.0	D43.0	D49.6
paroophoron	C57.1-☑	C79.82	D07.39	D28.2	D39.8	D49.59
parotid (duct)						
(gland)	C07	C79.89	D00.00	D11.0	D37.030	D49.0
parovarium	C57.1-☑	C79.82	D07.39	D28.2	D39.8	D49.59
patella	C40.20	C79.51	—	—	—	—
peduncle, cerebral	C71.7	C79.31	—	D33.1	D43.1	D49.6
pelvirectal						
junction	C19	C78.5	D01.1	D12.7	D37.5	D49.0
pelvis, pelvic	C76.3	C79.89	D09.8	D36.7	D48.7	D49.89
bone	C41.4	C79.51	—	D16.8	D48.0	D49.2
floor	C76.3	C79.89	D09.8	D36.7	D48.7	D49.89
renal	C65.-☑	C79.0-☑	D09.19	D30.1-☑	D41.1-☑	D49.51-☑
viscera	C76.3	C79.89	D09.8	D36.7	D48.7	D49.89
wall	C76.3	C79.89	D09.8	D36.7	D48.7	D49.89
pelvo-abdominal	C76.8	C79.89	D09.8	D36.7	D48.7	D49.89
penis	C60.9	C79.82	D07.4	D29.0	D40.8	D49.59
body	C60.2	C79.82	D07.4	D29.0	D40.8	D49.59
corpus						
(cavernosum)	C60.2	C79.82	D07.4	D29.0	D40.8	D49.59
glans	C60.1	C79.82	D07.4	D29.0	D40.8	D49.59
overlapping						
sites	C60.8	—	—	—	—	—
skin NEC	C60.9	C79.82	D07.4	D29.0	D40.8	D49.59
periadrenal						
(tissue)	C48.0	C78.6	—	D20.0	D48.3	D49.0
perianal (skin) — see						
also Neoplasm,						
anus, skin	C44.500	C79.2	D04.5	D23.5	D48.5	D49.2
pericardium	C38.0	C79.89	—	D15.1	D48.7	D49.89
perinephric	C48.0	C78.6	—	D20.0	D48.3	D49.0
perineum	C76.3	C79.89	D09.8	D36.7	D48.7	D49.89
periodontal tissue						
NEC	C03.9	C79.89	D00.03	D10.39	D37.09	D49.0
periosteum — see						
Neoplasm, bone						
peripancreatic	C48.0	C78.6	—	D20.0	D48.3	D49.0
peripheral nerve						
NEC	C47.9	C79.89	—	D36.10	D48.2	D49.2
perirectal (tissue)	C76.3	C79.89	—	D36.7	D48.7	D49.89
perirenal (tissue)	C48.0	C78.6	—	D20.0	D48.3	D49.0
peritoneum, peritoneal						
(cavity)	C48.2	C78.6	—	D20.1	D48.4	D49.0
benign mesothelial						
tissue — see						
Mesothelioma,						
benign						
overlapping						
lesion	C48.8	—	—	—	—	—
with digestive						
organs	C26.9	—	—	—	—	—
parietal	C48.1	C78.6	—	D20.1	D48.4	D49.0
pelvic	C48.1	C78.6	—	D20.1	D48.4	D49.0
specified part						
NEC	C48.1	C78.6	—	D20.1	D48.4	D49.0
peritonsillar						
(tissue)	C76.0	C79.89	D09.8	D36.7	D48.7	D49.89
periurethral tissue	C76.3	C79.89	—	D36.7	D48.7	D49.89
phalanges						
foot	C40.3-☑	C79.51	—	D16.3-☑	—	—
hand	C40.1-☑	C79.51	—	D16.1-☑	—	—
pharynx,						
pharyngeal	C14.0	C79.89	D00.08	D10.9	D37.05	D49.0
bursa	C11.1	C79.89	D00.08	D10.6	D37.05	D49.0

Neoplasm, neoplastic	Malignant Primary	Malignant Secondary	Ca in situ	Benign	Uncertain Behavior	Unspecified Behavior
— continued						
pharynx, pharyngeal						
— continued						
fornix	C11.3	C79.89	D00.08	D10.6	D37.05	D49.0
recess	C11.2	C79.89	D00.08	D10.6	D37.05	D49.0
region	C14.0	C79.89	D00.08	D10.9	D37.05	D49.0
tonsil	C11.1	C79.89	D00.08	D10.6	D37.05	D49.0
wall (lateral)						
(posterior)	C14.0	C79.89	D00.08	D10.9	D37.05	D49.0
pia mater	C70.9	C79.40	—	D32.9	D42.9	D49.7
cerebral	C70.0	C79.32	—	D32.0	D42.0	D49.7
cranial	C70.0	C79.32	—	D32.0	D42.0	D49.7
spinal	C70.1	C79.49	—	D32.1	D42.1	D49.7
pillars of fauces	C09.1	C79.89	D00.08	D10.5	D37.05	D49.0
pineal (body)						
(gland)	C75.3	C79.89	D09.3	D35.4	D44.5	D49.7
pinna (ear) NEC — see						
also Neoplasm, skin,						
ear	C44.20-☑	C79.2	D04.2-☑	D23.2-☑	D48.5	D49.2
piriform fossa or						
sinus	C12	C79.89	D00.08	D10.7	D37.05	D49.0
pituitary (body) (fossa)						
(gland) (lobe)	C75.1	C79.89	D09.3	D35.2	D44.3	D49.7
placenta	C58	C79.82	D07.0	D26.7	D39.2	D49.59
pleura, pleural						
(cavity)	C38.4	C78.2	—	D19.0	D38.2	D49.1
overlapping lesion						
with heart or						
mediastinum	C38.8	—	—	—	—	—
parietal	C38.4	C78.2	—	D19.0	D38.2	D49.1
visceral	C38.4	C78.2	—	D19.0	D38.2	D49.1
plexus						
brachial	C47.1-☑	C79.89	—	D36.12	D48.2	D49.2
cervical	C47.0	C79.89	—	D36.11	D48.2	D49.2
choroid	C71.5	C79.31	—	D33.0	D43.0	D49.6
lumbosacral	C47.5	C79.89	—	D36.16	D48.2	D49.2
sacral	C47.5	C79.89	—	D36.16	D48.2	D49.2
pluriendocrine	C75.8	C79.89	D09.3	D35.7	D44.9	D49.7
pole						
frontal	C71.1	C79.31	—	D33.0	D43.0	D49.6
occipital	C71.4	C79.31	—	D33.0	D43.0	D49.6
pons (varolii)	C71.7	C79.31	—	D33.1	D43.1	D49.6
popliteal fossa or						
space	C76.5-☑	C79.89	D04.7-☑	D36.7	D48.7	D49.89
postcricoid						
(region)	C13.0	C79.89	D00.08	D10.7	D37.05	D49.0
posterior fossa						
(cranial)	C71.9	C79.31	—	D33.2	D43.2	D49.6
postnasal space	C11.9	C79.89	D00.08	D10.6	D37.05	D49.0
prepuce	C60.0	C79.82	D07.4	D29.0	D40.8	D49.59
prepylorus	C16.4	C78.89	D00.2	D13.1	D37.1	D49.0
presacral (region)	C76.3	C79.89	—	D36.7	D48.7	D49.89
prostate (gland)	C61	C79.82	D07.5	D29.1	D40.0	D49.59
utricle	C68.0	C79.19	D09.19	D30.4	D41.3	D49.59
pterygoid fossa	C49.0	C79.89	—	D21.0	D48.1	D49.2
pubic bone	C41.4	C79.51	—	D16.8	D48.0	D49.2
pudenda, pudendum						
(female)	C51.9	C79.82	D07.1	D28.0	D39.8	D49.59
pulmonary — see also						
Neoplasm,						
lung	C34.9-☑	C78.0-☑	D02.2-☑	D14.3-☑	D38.1	D49.1
putamen	C71.0	C79.31	—	D33.0	D43.0	D49.6
pyloric						
antrum	C16.3	C78.89	D00.2	D13.1	D37.1	D49.0
canal	C16.4	C78.89	D00.2	D13.1	D37.1	D49.0
pylorus	C16.4	C78.89	D00.2	D13.1	D37.1	D49.0
pyramid (brain)	C71.7	C79.31	—	D33.1	D43.1	D49.6
pyriform fossa or						
sinus	C12	C79.89	D00.08	D10.7	D37.05	D49.0
radius (any part)	C40.0-☑	C79.51	—	D16.0-☑	—	—
Rathke's pouch	C75.1	C79.89	D09.3	D35.2	D44.3	D49.7
rectosigmoid						
(junction)	C19	C78.5	D01.1	D12.7	D37.5	D49.0
overlapping lesion						
with anus or						
rectum	C21.8	—	—	—	—	—
rectouterine						
pouch	C48.1	C78.6	—	D20.1	D48.4	D49.0
rectovaginal septum or						
wall	C76.3	C79.89	D09.8	D36.7	D48.7	D49.89
rectovesical						
septum	C76.3	C79.89	D09.8	D36.7	D48.7	D49.89
rectum (ampulla)	C20	C78.5	D01.2	D12.8	D37.5	D49.0

☑ **Additional Character Required — Refer to the Tabular List for Character Selection**

Neoplasm, neoplastic	Malignant Primary	Malignant Secondary	Ca in situ	Benign	Uncertain Behavior	Unspecified Behavior
— *continued*						
rectum — *continued*						
and colon	C19	C78.5	D01.1	D12.7	D37.5	D49.0
overlapping lesion with anus or rectosigmoid junction	C21.8	—	—	—	—	—
renal	C64.-☑	C79.0-☑	D09.19	D30.0-☑	D41.0-☑	D49.51-☑
calyx	C65.-☑	C79.0-☑	D09.19	D30.1-☑	D41.1-☑	D49.51-☑
hilus	C65.-☑	C79.0-☑	D09.19	D30.1-☑	D41.1-☑	D49.51-☑
parenchyma	C64.-☑	C79.0-☑	D09.19	D30.0-☑	D41.0-☑	D49.51-☑
pelvis	C65.-☑	C79.0-☑	D09.19	D30.1-☑	D41.1-☑	D49.51-☑
respiratory						
organs or system NEC	C39.9	C78.30	D02.4	D14.4	D38.6	D49.1
tract NEC	C39.9	C78.30	D02.4	D14.4	D38.5	D49.1
upper	C39.0	C78.30	D02.4	D14.4	D38.5	D49.1
retina	C69.2-☑	C79.49	D09.2-☑	D31.2-☑	D48.7	D49.81
retrobulbar	C69.6-☑	C79.49	—	D31.6-☑	D48.7	D49.89
retrocecal	C48.0	C78.6	—	D20.0	D48.3	D49.0
retromolar (area) (triangle) (trigone)	C06.2	C79.89	D00.00	D10.39	D37.09	D49.0
retro-orbital	C76.0	C79.89	D09.8	D36.7	D48.7	D49.89
retroperitoneal (space) (tissue)	C48.0	C78.6	—	D20.0	D48.3	D49.0
retroperitoneum	C48.0	C78.6	—	D20.0	D48.3	D49.0
retropharyngeal	C14.0	C79.89	D00.08	D10.9	D37.05	D49.0
retrovesical (septum)	C76.3	C79.89	D09.8	D36.7	D48.7	D49.89
rhinencephalon	C71.0	C79.31	—	D33.0	D43.0	D49.6
rib	C41.3	C79.51	—	D16.7	D48.0	D49.2
Rosenmuller's fossa	C11.2	C79.89	D00.08	D10.6	D37.05	D49.0
round ligament	C57.2-☑	C79.82	—	D28.2	D39.8	D49.59
sacrococcyx, sacrococcygeal	C41.4	C79.51	—	D16.8	D48.0	D49.2
region	C76.3	C79.89	D09.8	D36.7	D48.7	D49.89
sacrouterine ligament	C57.3	C79.82	—	D28.2	D39.8	D49.59
sacrum, sacral (vertebra)	C41.4	C79.51	—	D16.8	D48.0	D49.2
salivary gland or duct (major)	C08.9	C79.89	D00.00	D11.9	D37.039	D49.0
minor NEC	C06.9	C79.89	D00.00	D10.39	D37.04	D49.0
overlapping lesion	C08.9	—	—	—	—	—
parotid	C07	C79.89	D00.00	D11.0	D37.030	D49.0
pluriglandular	C08.9	C79.89	D00.00	D11.9	D37.039	D49.0
sublingual	C08.1	C79.89	D00.00	D11.7	D37.031	D49.0
submandibular	C08.0	C79.89	D00.00	D11.7	D37.032	D49.0
submaxillary	C08.0	C79.89	D00.00	D11.7	D37.032	D49.0
salpinx (uterine)	C57.0-☑	C79.82	D07.39	D28.2	D39.8	D49.59
Santorini's duct	C25.3	C78.89	D01.7	D13.6	D37.8	D49.0
scalp	C44.40	C79.2	D04.4	D23.4	D48.5	D49.2
basal cell carcinoma	C44.41	—	—	—	—	—
specified type NEC	C44.49	—	—	—	—	—
squamous cell carcinoma	C44.42	—	—	—	—	—
scapula (any part)	C40.0-☑	C79.51	—	D16.0-☑	—	—
scapular region	C76.1	C79.89	D09.8	D36.7	D48.7	D49.89
scar NEC — *see also* Neoplasm, skin, by site	C44.90	C79.2	D04.9	D23.9	D48.5	D49.2
sciatic nerve	C47.2-☑	C79.89	—	D36.13	D48.2	D49.2
sclera	C69.4-☑	C79.49	D09.2-☑	D31.4-☑	D48.7	D49.89
scrotum (skin)	C63.2	C79.82	D07.61	D29.4	D40.8	D49.59
sebaceous gland — *see* Neoplasm, skin						
sella turcica	C75.1	C79.89	D09.3	D35.2	D44.3	D49.7
bone	C41.0	C79.51	—	D16.4	D48.0	D49.2
semilunar cartilage (knee)	C40.2-☑	C79.51	—	D16.2-☑	D48.0	D49.2
seminal vesicle	C63.7	C79.82	D07.69	D29.8	D40.8	D49.59
septum						
nasal	C30.0	C78.39	D02.3	D14.0	D38.5	D49.1
posterior margin	C11.3	C79.89	D00.08	D10.6	D37.05	D49.0
rectovaginal	C76.3	C79.89	D09.8	D36.7	D48.7	D49.89
rectovesical	C76.3	C79.89	D09.8	D36.7	D48.7	D49.89

Neoplasm, neoplastic	Malignant Primary	Malignant Secondary	Ca in situ	Benign	Uncertain Behavior	Unspecified Behavior
— *continued*						
septum — *continued*						
urethrovaginal	C57.9	C79.82	D07.30	D28.9	D39.9	D49.59
vesicovaginal	C57.9	C79.82	D07.30	D28.9	D39.9	D49.59
shoulder NEC	C76.4-☑	C79.89	D04.6-☑	D36.7	D48.7	D49.89
sigmoid flexure (lower) (upper)	C18.7	C78.5	D01.0	D12.5	D37.4	D49.0
sinus (accessory)	C31.9	C78.39	D02.3	D14.0	D38.5	D49.1
bone (any)	C41.0	C79.51	—	D16.4	D48.0	D49.2
ethmoidal	C31.1	C78.39	D02.3	D14.0	D38.5	D49.1
frontal	C31.2	C78.39	D02.3	D14.0	D38.5	D49.1
maxillary	C31.0	C78.39	D02.3	D14.0	D38.5	D49.1
nasal, paranasal NEC	C31.9	C78.39	D02.3	D14.0	D38.5	D49.1
overlapping lesion	C31.8	—	—	—	—	—
pyriform	C12	C79.89	D00.08	D10.7	D37.05	D49.0
sphenoid	C31.3	C78.39	D02.3	D14.0	D38.5	D49.1
skeleton, skeletal NEC	C41.9	C79.51	—	D16.9	D48.0	D49.2
Skene's gland	C68.1	C79.19	D09.19	D30.8	D41.8	D49.59
skin NOS	C44.90	C79.2	D04.9	D23.9	D48.5	D49.2
abdominal wall	C44.509	C79.2	D04.5	D23.5	D48.5	D49.2
basal cell carcinoma	C44.519	—	—	—	—	—
specified type NEC	C44.599	—	—	—	—	—
squamous cell carcinoma	C44.529	—	—	—	—	—
ala nasi — *see also* Neoplasm, nose, skin	C44.301	C79.2	D04.39	D23.39	D48.5	D49.2
ankle — *see also* Neoplasm, skin, limb, lower	C44.70-☑	C79.2	D04.7-☑	D23.7-☑	D48.5	D49.2
antecubital space — *see also* Neoplasm, skin, limb, upper	C44.60-☑	C79.2	D04.6-☑	D23.6-☑	D48.5	D49.2
anus	C44.500	C79.2	D04.5	D23.5	D48.5	D49.2
basal cell carcinoma	C44.510	—	—	—	—	—
specified type NEC	C44.590	—	—	—	—	—
squamous cell carcinoma	C44.520	—	—	—	—	—
arm — *see also* Neoplasm, skin, limb, upper	C44.60-☑	C79.2	D04.6-☑	D23.6-☑	D48.5	D49.2
auditory canal (external) — *see also* Neoplasm, skin, ear	C44.20-☑	C79.2	D04.2-☑	D23.2-☑	D48.5	D49.2
auricle (ear) — *see also* Neoplasm, skin, ear	C44.20-☑	C79.2	D04.2-☑	D23.2-☑	D48.5	D49.2
auricular canal (external) — *see also* Neoplasm, skin, ear	C44.20-☑	C79.2	D04.2-☑	D23.2-☑	D48.5	D49.2
axilla, axillary fold — *see also* Neoplasm, skin, trunk	C44.509	C79.2	D04.5	D23.5	D48.5	D49.2
back — *see also* Neoplasm, skin, trunk	C44.509	C79.2	D04.5	D23.5	D48.5	D49.2
basal cell carcinoma	C44.91	—	—	—	—	—
breast	C44.501	C79.2	D04.5	D23.5	D48.5	D49.2
basal cell carcinoma	C44.511	—	—	—	—	—
specified type NEC	C44.591	—	—	—	—	—
squamous cell carcinoma	C44.521	—	—	—	—	—
brow — *see also* Neoplasm, skin, face	C44.309	C79.2	D04.39	D23.39	D48.5	D49.2
buttock — *see also* Neoplasm, skin, trunk	C44.509	C79.2	D04.5	D23.5	D48.5	D49.2

☑ **Additional Character Required** — **Refer to the Tabular List for Character Selection**

	Malignant Primary	Malignant Secondary	Ca in situ	Benign	Uncertain Behavior	Unspecified Behavior
Neoplasm, neoplastic						
— *continued*						
skin — *continued*						
calf — *see also*						
Neoplasm, skin,						
limb, lower	C44.70-☑	C79.2	D04.7-☑	D23.7-☑	D48.5	D49.2
canthus (eye) (inner)						
(outer)	C44.10-☑	C79.2	D04.1-☑	D23.1-☑	D48.5	D49.2
basal cell						
carcinoma	C44.11-☑	—	—	—	—	—
sebaceous cell	C44.13-☑	—	—	—	—	—
specified type						
NEC	C44.19-☑	—	—	—	—	—
squamous cell						
carcinoma	C44.12-☑	—	—	—	—	—
cervical region — *see*						
also Neoplasm,						
skin, neck	C44.40	C79.2	D04.4	D23.4	D48.5	D49.2
cheek (external) —						
see also						
Neoplasm, skin,						
face	C44.309	C79.2	D04.39	D23.39	D48.5	D49.2
chest (wall) — *see*						
also Neoplasm,						
skin, trunk	C44.509	C79.2	D04.5	D23.5	D48.5	D49.2
chin — *see also*						
Neoplasm, skin,						
face	C44.309	C79.2	D04.39	D23.39	D48.5	D49.2
clavicular area — *see*						
also Neoplasm,						
skin, trunk	C44.509	C79.2	D04.5	D23.5	D48.5	D49.2
clitoris	C51.2	C79.82	D07.1	D28.0	D39.8	D49.59
columnella — *see*						
also Neoplasm,						
skin, face	C44.309	C79.2	D04.39	D23.39	D48.5	D49.2
concha — *see also*						
Neoplasm, skin,						
ear	C44.20-☑	C79.2	D04.2-☑	D23.2-☑	D48.5	D49.2
ear (external)	C44.20-☑	C79.2	D04.2-☑	D23.2-☑	D48.5	D49.2
basal cell						
carcinoma	C44.21-☑	—	—	—	—	—
specified type						
NEC	C44.29-☑	—	—	—	—	—
squamous cell						
carcinoma	C44.22-☑	—	—	—	—	—
elbow — *see also*						
Neoplasm, skin,						
limb, upper	C44.60-☑	C79.2	D04.6-☑	D23.6-☑	D48.5	D49.2
eyebrow — *see also*						
Neoplasm, skin,						
face	C44.309	C79.2	D04.39	D23.39	D48.5	D49.2
eyelid	C44.10-☑	C79.2	D04.1-☑	D23.1-☑	D48.5	D49.2
basal cell						
carcinoma	C44.11-☑	—	—	—	—	—
sebaceous cell	C44.13-☑	—	—	—	—	—
specified type						
NEC	C44.19-☑	—	—	—	—	—
squamous cell						
carcinoma	C44.12-☑	—	—	—	—	—
face NOS	C44.300	C79.2	D04.30	D23.30	D48.5	D49.2
basal cell						
carcinoma	C44.310	—	—	—	—	—
specified type						
NEC	C44.390	—	—	—	—	—
squamous cell						
carcinoma	C44.320	—	—	—	—	—
female genital organs						
(external)	C51.9	C79.82	D07.1	D28.0	D39.8	D49.59
clitoris	C51.2	C79.82	D07.1	D28.0	D39.8	D49.59
labium NEC	C51.9	C79.82	D07.1	D28.0	D39.8	D49.59
majus	C51.0	C79.82	D07.1	D28.0	D39.8	D49.59
minus	C51.1	C79.82	D07.1	D28.0	D39.8	D49.59
pudendum	C51.9	C79.82	D07.1	D28.0	D39.8	D49.59
vulva	C51.9	C79.82	D07.1	D28.0	D39.8	D49.59
finger — *see also*						
Neoplasm, skin,						
limb, upper	C44.60-☑	C79.2	D04.6-☑	D23.6-☑	D48.5	D49.2
flank — *see also*						
Neoplasm, skin,						
trunk	C44.509	C79.2	D04.5	D23.5	D48.5	D49.2
foot — *see also*						
Neoplasm, skin,						
limb, lower	C44.70-☑	C79.2	D04.7-☑	D23.7-☑	D48.5	D49.2

	Malignant Primary	Malignant Secondary	Ca in situ	Benign	Uncertain Behavior	Unspecified Behavior
Neoplasm, neoplastic						
— *continued*						
skin — *continued*						
forearm — *see also*						
Neoplasm, skin,						
limb, upper	C44.60-☑	C79.2	D04.6-☑	D23.6-☑	D48.5	D49.2
forehead — *see also*						
Neoplasm, skin,						
face	C44.309	C79.2	D04.39	D23.39	D48.5	D49.2
glabella — *see also*						
Neoplasm, skin,						
face	C44.309	C79.2	D04.39	D23.39	D48.5	D49.2
gluteal region — *see*						
also Neoplasm,						
skin, trunk	C44.509	C79.2	D04.5	D23.5	D48.5	D49.2
groin — *see also*						
Neoplasm, skin,						
trunk	C44.509	C79.2	D04.5	D23.5	D48.5	D49.2
hand — *see also*						
Neoplasm, skin,						
limb, upper	C44.60-☑	C79.2	D04.6-☑	D23.6-☑	D48.5	D49.2
head NEC — *see also*						
Neoplasm, skin,						
scalp	C44.40	C79.2	D04.4	D23.4	D48.5	D49.2
heel — *see also*						
Neoplasm, skin,						
limb, lower	C44.70-☑	C79.2	D04.7-☑	D23.7-☑	D48.5	D49.2
helix — *see also*						
Neoplasm, skin,						
ear	C44.20-☑	C79.2	D04.2-☑	D23.2-☑	D48.5	D49.2
hip — *see also*						
Neoplasm, skin,						
limb, lower	C44.70-☑	C79.2	D04.7-☑	D23.7-☑	D48.5	D49.2
infraclavicular region						
— *see also*						
Neoplasm, skin,						
trunk	C44.509	C79.2	D04.5	D23.5	D48.5	D49.2
inguinal region — *see*						
also Neoplasm,						
skin, trunk	C44.509	C79.2	D04.5	D23.5	D48.5	D49.2
jaw — *see also*						
Neoplasm, skin,						
face	C44.309	C79.2	D04.39	D23.39	D48.5	D49.2
Kaposi's sarcoma —						
see Kaposi's,						
sarcoma, skin						
knee — *see also*						
Neoplasm, skin,						
limb, lower	C44.70-☑	C79.2	D04.7-☑	D23.7-☑	D48.5	D49.2
labia						
majora	C51.0	C79.82	D07.1	D28.0	D39.8	D49.59
minora	C51.1	C79.82	D07.1	D28.0	D39.8	D49.59
leg — *see also*						
Neoplasm, skin,						
limb, lower	C44.70-☑	C79.2	D04.7-☑	D23.7-☑	D48.5	D49.2
lid (lower)						
(upper)	C44.10-☑	C79.2	D04.1-☑	D23.1-☑	D48.5	D49.2
basal cell						
carcinoma	C44.11-☑	—	—	—	—	—
sebaceous cell	C44.13-☑	—	—	—	—	—
specified type						
NEC	C44.19-☑	—	—	—	—	—
squamous cell						
carcinoma	C44.12-☑	—	—	—	—	—
limb NEC	C44.90	C79.2	D04.9	D23.9	D48.5	D49.2
basal cell						
carcinoma	C44.91	—	—	—	—	—
lower	C44.70-☑	C79.2	D04.7-☑	D23.7-☑	D48.5	D49.2
basal cell						
carcinoma	C44.71-☑	—	—	—	—	—
specified type						
NEC	C44.79-☑	—	—	—	—	—
squamous cell						
carcinoma	C44.72-☑	—	—	—	—	—
upper	C44.60-☑	C79.2	D04.6-☑	D23.6-☑	D48.5	D49.2
basal cell						
carcinoma	C44.61-☑	—	—	—	—	—
specified type						
NEC	C44.69-☑	—	—	—	—	—
squamous cell						
carcinoma	C44.62-☑	—	—	—	—	—
lip (lower)						
(upper)	C44.00	C79.2	D04.0	D23.0	D48.5	D49.2

☑ **Additional Character Required — Refer to the Tabular List for Character Selection**

Neoplasm, neoplastic	Malignant Primary	Malignant Secondary	Ca in situ	Benign	Uncertain Behavior	Unspecified Behavior
— *continued*						
skin — *continued*						
lip — *continued*						
basal cell carcinoma	C44.01	—	—	—	—	—
specified type NEC	C44.09	—	—	—	—	—
squamous cell carcinoma	C44.02	—	—	—	—	—
male genital organs	C63.9	C79.82	D07.60	D29.9	D40.8	D49.59
penis	C60.9	C79.82	D07.4	D29.0	D40.8	D49.59
prepuce	C60.0	C79.82	D07.4	D29.0	D40.8	D49.59
scrotum	C63.2	C79.82	D07.61	D29.4	D40.8	D49.59
mastectomy site (skin) — *see also* Neoplasm, skin, breast	C44.501	C79.2		—		
specified as breast tissue	C50.8-☑	C79.81		—		
meatus, acoustic (external) — *see also* Neoplasm, skin, ear	C44.20-☑	C79.2	D04.2-☑	D23.2-☑	D48.5	D49.2
melanotic — *see* Melanoma						
Merkel cell — *see* Carcinoma, Merkel cell						
nates — *see also* Neoplasm, skin, trunk	C44.509	C79.2	D04.5	D23.5	D48.5	D49.2
neck	C44.40	C79.2	D04.4	D23.4	D48.5	D49.2
basal cell carcinoma	C44.41	—	—	—	—	—
specified type NEC	C44.49	—	—	—	—	—
squamous cell carcinoma	C44.42	—	—	—	—	—
nevus — *see* Nevus, skin						
nose (external) — *see also* Neoplasm, nose, skin	C44.301	C79.2	D04.39	D23.39	D48.5	D49.2
overlapping lesion	C44.80	—	—	—	—	—
basal cell carcinoma	C44.81	—	—	—	—	—
specified type NEC	C44.89	—	—	—	—	—
squamous cell carcinoma	C44.82	—	—	—	—	—
palm — *see also* Neoplasm, skin, limb, upper	C44.60-☑	C79.2	D04.6-☑	D23.6-☑	D48.5	D49.2
palpebra	C44.10-☑	C79.2	D04.1-☑	D23.1-☑	D48.5	D49.2
basal cell carcinoma	C44.11-☑	—	—	—	—	—
sebaceous cell	C44.13-☑	—	—	—	—	—
specified type NEC	C44.19-☑	—	—	—	—	—
squamous cell carcinoma	C44.12-☑	—	—	—	—	—
penis NEC	C60.9	C79.82	D07.4	D29.0	D40.8	D49.59
perianal — *see also* Neoplasm, skin, anus	C44.500	C79.2	D04.5	D23.5	D48.5	D49.2
perineum — *see also* Neoplasm, skin, anus	C44.500	C79.2	D04.5	D23.5	D48.5	D49.2
pinna — *see also* Neoplasm, skin, ear	C44.20-☑	C79.2	D04.2-☑	D23.2-☑	D48.5	D49.2
plantar — *see also* Neoplasm, skin, limb, lower	C44.70-☑	C79.2	D04.7-☑	D23.7-☑	D48.5	D49.2
popliteal fossa or space — *see also* Neoplasm, skin, limb, lower	C44.70-☑	C79.2	D04.7-☑	D23.7-☑	D48.5	D49.2
prepuce	C60.0	C79.82	D07.4	D29.0	D40.8	D49.59

Neoplasm, neoplastic	Malignant Primary	Malignant Secondary	Ca in situ	Benign	Uncertain Behavior	Unspecified Behavior
— *continued*						
skin — *continued*						
pubes — *see also* Neoplasm, skin, trunk	C44.509	C79.2	D04.5	D23.5	D48.5	D49.2
sacrococcygeal region — *see also* Neoplasm, skin, trunk	C44.509	C79.2	D04.5	D23.5	D48.5	D49.2
scalp	C44.40	C79.2	D04.4	D23.4	D48.5	D49.2
basal cell carcinoma	C44.41	—	—	—	—	—
specified type NEC	C44.49	—	—	—	—	—
squamous cell carcinoma	C44.42	—	—	—	—	—
scapular region — *see also* Neoplasm, skin, trunk	C44.509	C79.2	D04.5	D23.5	D48.5	D49.2
scrotum	C63.2	C79.82	D07.61	D29.4	D40.8	D49.59
shoulder — *see also* Neoplasm, skin, limb, upper	C44.60-☑	C79.2	D04.6-☑	D23.6-☑	D48.5	D49.2
sole (foot) — *see also* Neoplasm, skin, limb, lower	C44.70-☑	C79.2	D04.7-☑	D23.7-☑	D48.5	D49.2
specified sites NEC	C44.80	C79.2	D04.8	D23.9	D48.5	D49.2
basal cell carcinoma	C44.81	—	—	—	—	—
specified type NEC	C44.89	—	—	—	—	—
squamous cell carcinoma	C44.82	—	—	—	—	—
specified type NEC	C44.99	—	—	—	—	—
squamous cell carcinoma	C44.92	—	—	—	—	—
submammary fold — *see also* Neoplasm, skin, trunk	C44.509	C79.2	D04.5	D23.5	D48.5	D49.2
supraclavicular region — *see also* Neoplasm, skin, neck	C44.40	C79.2	D04.4	D23.4	D48.5	D49.2
temple — *see also* Neoplasm, skin, face	C44.309	C79.2	D04.39	D23.39	D48.5	D49.2
thigh — *see also* Neoplasm, skin, limb, lower	C44.70-☑	C79.2	D04.7-☑	D23.7-☑	D48.5	D49.2
thoracic wall — *see also* Neoplasm, skin, trunk	C44.509	C79.2	D04.5	D23.5	D48.5	D49.2
thumb — *see also* Neoplasm, skin, limb, upper	C44.60-☑	C79.2	D04.6-☑	D23.6-☑	D48.5	D49.2
toe — *see also* Neoplasm, skin, limb, lower	C44.70-☑	C79.2	D04.7-☑	D23.7-☑	D48.5	D49.2
tragus — *see also* Neoplasm, skin, ear	C44.20-☑	C79.2	D04.2-☑	D23.2-☑	D48.5	D49.2
trunk	C44.509	C79.2	D04.5	D23.5	D48.5	D49.2
basal cell carcinoma	C44.519	—	—	—	—	—
specified type NEC	C44.599	—	—	—	—	—
squamous cell carcinoma	C44.529	—	—	—	—	—
umbilicus — *see also* Neoplasm, skin, trunk	C44.509	C79.2	D04.5	D23.5	D48.5	D49.2
vulva	C51.9	C79.82	D07.1	D28.0	D39.8	D49.59
overlapping lesion	C51.8	—	—	—	—	—
wrist — *see also* Neoplasm, skin, limb, upper	C44.60-☑	C79.2	D04.6-☑	D23.6-☑	D48.5	D49.2
skull	C41.0	C79.51	—	D16.4	D48.0	D49.2

☑ **Additional Character Required** — Refer to the Tabular List for Character Selection

Neoplasm, neoplastic	Malignant Primary	Malignant Secondary	Ca in situ	Benign	Uncertain Behavior	Unspecified Behavior
— continued						
soft parts or tissues — see Neoplasm, connective tissue						
specified site NEC	C76.8	C79.89	D09.8	D36.7	D48.7	D49.89
spermatic cord	C63.1-☑	C79.82	D07.69	D29.8	D40.8	D49.59
sphenoid	C31.3	C78.39	D02.3	D14.0	D38.5	D49.1
bone	C41.0	C79.51	—	D16.4	D48.0	D49.2
sinus	C31.3	C78.39	D02.3	D14.0	D38.5	D49.1
sphincter						
anal	C21.1	C78.5	D01.3	D12.9	D37.8	D49.0
of Oddi	C24.0	C78.89	D01.5	D13.5	D37.6	D49.0
spine, spinal						
(column)	C41.2	C79.51	—	D16.6	D48.0	D49.2
bulb	C71.7	C79.31	—	D33.1	D43.1	D49.6
coccyx	C41.4	C79.51	—	D16.8	D48.0	D49.2
cord (cervical) (lumbar) (sacral) (thoracic)	C72.0	C79.49	—	D33.4	D43.4	D49.7
dura mater	C70.1	C79.49	—	D32.1	D42.1	D49.7
lumbosacral	C41.2	C79.51	—	D16.6	D48.0	D49.2
marrow NEC	C96.9	C79.52	—	—	D47.9	D49.89
membrane	C70.1	C79.49	—	D32.1	D42.1	D49.7
meninges	C70.1	C79.49	—	D32.1	D42.1	D49.7
nerve (root)	C47.9	C79.89	—	D36.10	D48.2	D49.2
pia mater	C70.1	C79.49	—	D32.1	D42.1	D49.7
root	C47.9	C79.89	—	D36.10	D48.2	D49.2
sacrum	C41.4	C79.51	—	D16.8	D48.0	D49.2
spleen, splenic						
NEC	C26.1	C78.89	D01.7	D13.9	D37.8	D49.0
flexure (colon)	C18.5	C78.5	D01.0	D12.3	D37.4	D49.0
stem, brain	C71.7	C79.31	—	D33.1	D43.1	D49.6
Stensen's duct	C07	C79.89	D00.00	D11.0	D37.030	D49.0
sternum	C41.3	C79.51	—	D16.7	D48.0	D49.2
stomach	C16.9	C78.89	D00.2	D13.1	D37.1	D49.0
antrum (pyloric)	C16.3	C78.89	D00.2	D13.1	D37.1	D49.0
body	C16.2	C78.89	D00.2	D13.1	D37.1	D49.0
cardia	C16.0	C78.89	D00.2	D13.1	D37.1	D49.0
cardiac orifice	C16.0	C78.89	D00.2	D13.1	D37.1	D49.0
corpus	C16.2	C78.89	D00.2	D13.1	D37.1	D49.0
fundus	C16.1	C78.89	D00.2	D13.1	D37.1	D49.0
greater curvature NEC	C16.6	C78.89	D00.2	D13.1	D37.1	D49.0
lesser curvature NEC	C16.5	C78.89	D00.2	D13.1	D37.1	D49.0
overlapping lesion	C16.8	—	—	—	—	—
prepylorus	C16.4	C78.89	D00.2	D13.1	D37.1	D49.0
pylorus	C16.4	C78.89	D00.2	D13.1	D37.1	D49.0
wall NEC	C16.9	C78.89	D00.2	D13.1	D37.1	D49.0
anterior NEC	C16.8	C78.89	D00.2	D13.1	D37.1	D49.0
posterior NEC	C16.8	C78.89	D00.2	D13.1	D37.1	D49.0
stroma, endometrial	C54.1	C79.82	D07.0	D26.1	D39.0	D49.59
stump, cervical	C53.8	C79.82	D06.7	D26.0	D39.0	D49.59
subcutaneous (nodule) (tissue) NEC — see Neoplasm, connective tissue						
subdural	C70.9	C79.32	—	D32.9	D42.9	D49.7
subglottis, subglottic	C32.2	C78.39	D02.0	D14.1	D38.0	D49.1
sublingual	C04.9	C79.89	D00.06	D10.2	D37.09	D49.0
gland or duct	C08.1	C79.89	D00.00	D11.7	D37.031	D49.0
submandibular gland	C08.0	C79.89	D00.00	D11.7	D37.032	D49.0
submaxillary gland or duct	C08.0	C79.89	D00.00	D11.7	D37.032	D49.0
submental	C76.0	C79.89	—	D36.7	D48.7	D49.89
subpleural	C34.9-☑	C78.0-☑	D02.2-☑	D14.3-☑	D38.1	D49.1
substernal	C38.1	C78.1	—	D15.2	D38.3	D49.89
sudoriferous, sudoriparous gland, site						
unspecified	C44.90	C79.2	D04.9	D23.9	D48.5	D49.2
specified site — see Neoplasm, skin						
supraclavicular region	C76.0	C79.89	D09.8	D36.7	D48.7	D49.89
supraglottis	C32.1	C78.39	D02.0	D14.1	D38.0	D49.1
suprarenal	C74.9-☑	C79.7-☑	D09.3	D35.0-☑	D44.1-☑	D49.7
capsule	C74.9-☑	C79.7-☑	D09.3	D35.0-☑	D44.1-☑	D49.7

Neoplasm, neoplastic	Malignant Primary	Malignant Secondary	Ca in situ	Benign	Uncertain Behavior	Unspecified Behavior
— continued						
suprarenal — continued						
cortex	C74.0-☑	C79.7-☑	D09.3	D35.0-☑	D44.1-☑	D49.7
gland	C74.9-☑	C79.7-☑	D09.3	D35.0-☑	D44.1-☑	D49.7
medulla	C74.1-☑	C79.7-☑	D09.3	D35.0-☑	D44.1-☑	D49.7
suprasellar (region)	C71.9	C79.31	—	D33.2	D43.2	D49.6
supratentorial (brain) NEC	C71.0	C79.31	—	D33.0	D43.0	D49.6
sweat gland (apocrine) (eccrine), site unspecified	C44.90	C79.2	D04.9	D23.9	D48.5	D49.2
specified site — see Neoplasm, skin						
sympathetic nerve or nervous system NEC	C47.9	C79.89	—	D36.10	D48.2	D49.2
symphysis pubis	C41.4	C79.51	—	D16.8	D48.0	D49.2
synovial membrane — see Neoplasm, connective tissue						
tapetum, brain	C71.8	C79.31	—	D33.2	D43.2	D49.6
tarsus (any bone)	C40.3-☑	C79.51	—	D16.3-☑	—	—
temple (skin) — see also Neoplasm, skin, face	C44.309	C79.2	D04.39	D23.39	D48.5	D49.2
temporal						
bone	C41.0	C79.51	—	D16.4	D48.0	D49.2
lobe or pole	C71.2	C79.31	—	D33.0	D43.0	D49.6
region	C76.0	C79.89	D09.8	D36.7	D48.7	D49.89
skin — see also Neoplasm, skin, face	C44.309	C79.2	D04.39	D23.39	D48.5	D49.2
tendon (sheath) — see Neoplasm, connective tissue						
tentorium (cerebelli)	C70.0	C79.32	—	D32.0	D42.0	D49.7
testis, testes	C62.9-☑	C79.82	D07.69	D29.2-☑	D40.1-☑	D49.59
descended	C62.1-☑	C79.82	D07.69	D29.2-☑	D40.1-☑	D49.59
ectopic	C62.0-☑	C79.82	D07.69	D29.2-☑	D40.1-☑	D49.59
retained	C62.0-☑	C79.82	D07.69	D29.2-☑	D40.1-☑	D49.59
scrotal	C62.1-☑	C79.82	D07.69	D29.2-☑	D40.1-☑	D49.59
undescended	C62.0-☑	C79.82	D07.69	D29.2-☑	D40.1-☑	D49.59
unspecified whether descended or undescended	C62.9-☑	C79.82	D07.69	D29.2-☑	D40.1-☑	D49.59
thalamus	C71.0	C79.31	—	D33.0	D43.0	D49.6
thigh NEC	C76.5-☑	C79.89	D04.7-☑	D36.7	D48.7	D49.89
thorax, thoracic (cavity) (organs NEC)	C76.1	C79.89	D09.8	D36.7	D48.7	D49.89
duct	C49.3	C79.89	—	D21.3	D48.1	D49.2
wall NEC	C76.1	C79.89	D09.8	D36.7	D48.7	D49.89
throat	C14.0	C79.89	D00.08	D10.9	D37.05	D49.0
thumb NEC	C76.4-☑	C79.89	D04.6-☑	D36.7	D48.7	D49.89
thymus (gland)	C37	C79.89	D09.3	D15.0	D38.4	D49.89
thyroglossal duct	C73	C79.89	D09.3	D34	D44.0	D49.7
thyroid (gland)	C73	C79.89	D09.3	D34	D44.0	D49.7
cartilage	C32.3	C78.39	D02.0	D14.1	D38.0	D49.1
tibia (any part)	C40.2-☑	C79.51	—	D16.2-☑	—	—
toe NEC	C76.5-☑	C79.89	D04.7-☑	D36.7	D48.7	D49.89
tongue	C02.9	C79.89	D00.07	D10.1	D37.02	D49.0
anterior (two-thirds) NEC	C02.3	C79.89	D00.07	D10.1	D37.02	D49.0
dorsal surface	C02.0	C79.89	D00.07	D10.1	D37.02	D49.0
ventral surface	C02.2	C79.89	D00.07	D10.1	D37.02	D49.0
base (dorsal surface)	C01	C79.89	D00.07	D10.1	D37.02	D49.0
border (lateral)	C02.1	C79.89	D00.07	D10.1	D37.02	D49.0
dorsal surface NEC	C02.0	C79.89	D00.07	D10.1	D37.02	D49.0
fixed part NEC	C01	C79.89	D00.07	D10.1	D37.02	D49.0
foreamen cecum	C02.0	C79.89	D00.07	D10.1	D37.02	D49.0
frenulum linguae	C02.2	C79.89	D00.07	D10.1	D37.02	D49.0
junctional zone	C02.8	C79.89	D00.07	D10.1	D37.02	D49.0
margin (lateral)	C02.1	C79.89	D00.07	D10.1	D37.02	D49.0
midline NEC	C02.0	C79.89	D00.07	D10.1	D37.02	D49.0
mobile part NEC	C02.3	C79.89	D00.07	D10.1	D37.02	D49.0

☑ Additional Character Required — Refer to the Tabular List for Character Selection

Neoplasm Table

Neoplasm, soft parts or tissues — Neoplasm, tongue

Neoplasm, neoplastic — continued

	Malignant Primary	Malignant Secondary	Ca in situ	Benign	Uncertain Behavior	Unspecified Behavior
tongue — continued						
overlapping lesion	C02.8	—	—	—	—	—
posterior (third)	C01	C79.89	D00.07	D10.1	D37.02	D49.0
root	C01	C79.89	D00.07	D10.1	D37.02	D49.0
surface (dorsal)	C02.0	C79.89	D00.07	D10.1	D37.02	D49.0
base	C01	C79.89	D00.07	D10.1	D37.02	D49.0
ventral	C02.2	C79.89	D00.07	D10.1	D37.02	D49.0
tip	C02.1	C79.89	D00.07	D10.1	D37.02	D49.0
tonsil	C02.4	C79.89	D00.07	D10.1	D37.02	D49.0
tonsil	C09.9	C79.89	D00.08	D10.4	D37.05	D49.0
fauces, faucial	C09.9	C79.89	D00.08	D10.4	D37.05	D49.0
lingual	C02.4	C79.89	D00.07	D10.1	D37.02	D49.0
overlapping sites	C09.8	—	—	—	—	—
palatine	C09.9	C79.89	D00.08	D10.4	D37.05	D49.0
pharyngeal	C11.1	C79.89	D00.08	D10.6	D37.05	D49.0
pillar (anterior) (posterior)	C09.1	C79.89	D00.08	D10.5	D37.05	D49.0
tonsillar fossa	C09.0	C79.89	D00.08	D10.5	D37.05	D49.0
tooth socket NEC	C03.9	C79.89	D00.03	D10.39	D37.09	D49.0
trachea (cartilage) (mucosa)	C33	C78.39	D02.1	D14.2	D38.1	D49.1
overlapping lesion with bronchus or lung	C34.8-☑	—	—	—	—	—
tracheobronchial	C34.8-☑	C78.39	D02.1	D14.2	D38.1	D49.1
overlapping lesion with lung	C34.8-☑	—	—	—	—	—
tragus — see also Neoplasm, skin, ear	C44.20-☑	C79.2	D04.2-☑	D23.2-☑	D48.5	D49.2
trunk NEC	C76.8	C79.89	D04.5	D36.7	D48.7	D49.89
tubo-ovarian	C57.8	C79.82	D07.39	D28.7	D39.8	D49.59
tunica vaginalis	C63.7	C79.82	D07.69	D29.8	D40.8	D49.59
turbinate (bone)	C41.0	C79.51	—	D16.4	D48.0	D49.2
nasal	C30.0	C78.39	D02.3	D14.0	D38.5	D49.1
tympanic cavity	C30.1	C78.39	D02.3	D14.0	D38.5	D49.1
ulna (any part)	C40.0-☑	C79.51	—	D16.0-☑	—	—
umbilicus, umbilical — see also Neoplasm, skin, trunk	C44.509	C79.2	D04.5	D23.5	D48.5	D49.2
uncus, brain	C71.2	C79.31	—	D33.0	D43.0	D49.6
unknown site or unspecified	C80.1	C79.9	D09.9	D36.9	D48.9	D49.9
urachus	C67.7	C79.11	D09.0	D30.3	D41.4	D49.4
ureter-bladder (junction)	C67.6	C79.11	D09.0	D30.3	D41.4	D49.4
ureter, ureteral	C66.-☑	C79.19	D09.19	D30.2-☑	D41.2-☑	D49.59
orifice (bladder)	C67.6	C79.11	D09.0	D30.3	D41.4	D49.4
urethra, urethral (gland)	C68.0	C79.19	D09.19	D30.4	D41.3	D49.59
orifice, internal	C67.5	C79.11	D09.0	D30.3	D41.4	D49.4
urethrovaginal (septum)	C57.9	C79.82	D07.30	D28.9	D39.8	D49.59
urinary organ or system	C68.9	C79.10	D09.10	D30.9	D41.9	D49.59
bladder — see Neoplasm, bladder						
overlapping lesion	C68.8	—	—	—	—	—
specified sites NEC	C68.8	C79.19	D09.19	D30.8	D41.8	D49.59
utero-ovarian	C57.8	C79.82	D07.39	D28.7	D39.8	D49.59
ligament	C57.1-☑	C79.82	D07.39	D28.2	D39.8	D49.59
uterosacral ligament	C57.3	C79.82	—	D28.2	D39.8	D49.59
uterus, uteri, uterine	C55	C79.82	D07.0	D26.9	D39.0	D49.59
adnexa NEC	C57.4	C79.82	D07.39	D28.7	D39.8	D49.59
body	C54.9	C79.82	D07.0	D26.1	D39.0	D49.59
cervix	C53.9	C79.82	D06.9	D26.0	D39.0	D49.59
cornu	C54.9	C79.82	D07.0	D26.1	D39.0	D49.59
corpus	C54.9	C79.82	D07.0	D26.1	D39.0	D49.59
endocervix (canal) (gland)	C53.0	C79.82	D06.0	D26.0	D39.0	D49.59
endometrium	C54.1	C79.82	D07.0	D26.1	D39.0	D49.59
exocervix	C53.1	C79.82	D06.1	D26.0	D39.0	D49.59
external os	C53.1	C79.82	D06.1	D26.0	D39.0	D49.59
fundus	C54.3	C79.82	D07.0	D26.1	D39.0	D49.59

Neoplasm, neoplastic — continued

	Malignant Primary	Malignant Secondary	Ca in situ	Benign	Uncertain Behavior	Unspecified Behavior
uterus, uteri, uterine — continued						
internal os	C53.0	C79.82	D06.0	D26.0	D39.0	D49.59
isthmus	C54.0	C79.82	D07.0	D26.1	D39.0	D49.59
ligament	C57.3	C79.82	—	D28.2	D39.8	D49.59
broad	C57.1-☑	C79.82	D07.39	D28.2	D39.8	D49.59
round	C57.2-☑	C79.82	—	D28.2	D39.8	D49.59
lower segment	C54.0	C79.82	D07.0	D26.1	D39.0	D49.59
myometrium	C54.2	C79.82	D07.0	D26.1	D39.0	D49.59
overlapping sites	C54.8	—	—	—	—	—
squamocolumnar junction	C53.8	C79.82	D06.7	D26.0	D39.0	D49.59
tube	C57.0-☑	C79.82	D07.39	D28.2	D39.8	D49.59
utricle, prostatic	C68.0	C79.19	D09.19	D30.4	D41.3	D49.59
uveal tract	C69.4-☑	C79.49	D09.2-☑	D31.4-☑	D48.7	D49.89
uvula	C05.2	C79.89	D00.04	D10.39	D37.09	D49.0
vagina, vaginal (fornix) (vault) (wall)	C52	C79.82	D07.2	D28.1	D39.8	D49.59
vaginovesical	C57.9	C79.82	D07.30	D28.9	D39.9	D49.59
septum	C57.9	C79.82	D07.30	D28.9	D39.9	D49.59
vallecula (epiglottis)	C10.0	C79.89	D00.08	D10.5	D37.05	D49.0
vascular — see Neoplasm, connective tissue						
vas deferens	C63.1-☑	C79.82	D07.69	D29.8	D40.8	D49.59
Vater's ampulla	C24.1	C78.89	D01.5	D13.5	D37.6	D49.0
vein, venous — see Neoplasm, connective tissue						
vena cava (abdominal) (inferior)	C49.4	C79.89	—	D21.4	D48.1	D49.2
superior	C49.3	C79.89	—	D21.3	D48.1	D49.2
ventricle (cerebral) (floor) (lateral) (third)	C71.5	C79.31	—	D33.0	D43.0	D49.6
cardiac (left) (right)	C38.0	C79.89	—	D15.1	D48.7	D49.89
fourth	C71.7	C79.31	—	D33.1	D43.1	D49.6
ventricular band of larynx	C32.1	C78.39	D02.0	D14.1	D38.0	D49.1
ventriculus — see Neoplasm, stomach						
vermillion border — see Neoplasm, lip						
vermis, cerebellum	C71.6	C79.31	—	D33.1	D43.1	D49.6
vertebra (column)	C41.2	C79.51	—	D16.6	D48.0	D49.2
coccyx	C41.4	C79.51	—	D16.8	D48.0	D49.2
marrow NEC	C96.9	C79.52	—	—	D47.9	D49.89
sacrum	C41.4	C79.51	—	D16.8	D48.0	D49.2
vesical — see Neoplasm, bladder						
vesicle, seminal	C63.7	C79.82	D07.69	D29.8	D40.8	D49.59
vesicocervical tissue	C57.9	C79.82	D07.30	D28.9	D39.9	D49.59
vesicorectal	C76.3	C79.82	D09.8	D36.7	D48.7	D49.89
vesicovaginal	C57.9	C79.82	D07.30	D28.9	D39.9	D49.59
septum	C57.9	C79.82	D07.30	D28.9	D39.8	D49.59
vessel (blood) — see Neoplasm, connective tissue						
vestibular gland, greater	C51.0	C79.82	D07.1	D28.0	D39.8	D49.59
vestibule mouth	C06.1	C79.89	D00.00	D10.39	D37.09	D49.0
nose	C30.0	C78.39	D02.3	D14.0	D38.5	D49.1
Virchow's gland	C77.0	C77.0	—	D36.0	D48.7	D49.89
viscera NEC	C76.8	C79.89	D09.8	D36.7	D48.7	D49.89
vocal cords (true)	C32.0	C78.39	D02.0	D14.1	D38.0	D49.1
false	C32.1	C78.39	D02.0	D14.1	D38.0	D49.1
vomer	C41.0	C79.51	—	D16.4	D48.0	D49.2
vulva	C51.9	C79.82	D07.1	D28.0	D39.8	D49.59
vulvovaginal gland	C51.0	C79.82	D07.1	D28.0	D39.8	D49.59
Waldeyer's ring	C14.2	C79.89	D00.08	D10.9	D37.05	D49.0
Wharton's duct	C08.0	C79.89	D00.00	D11.7	D37.032	D49.0
white matter (central) (cerebral)	C71.0	C79.31	—	D33.0	D43.0	D49.6

	Malignant Primary	Malignant Secondary	Ca in situ	Benign	Uncertain Behavior	Unspecified Behavior
Neoplasm, neoplastic						
— *continued*						
windpipe	C33	C78.39	D02.1	D14.2	D38.1	D49.1
Wirsung's duct	C25.3	C78.89	D01.7	D13.6	D37.8	D49.0
wolffian (body) (duct)						
female	C57.7	C79.82	D07.39	D28.7	D39.8	D49.59
male	C63.7	C79.82	D07.69	D29.8	D40.8	D49.59
womb — *see* Neoplasm, uterus						
wrist NEC	C76.4-☑	C79.89	D04.6-☑	D36.7	D48.7	D49.89
xiphoid process	C41.3	C79.51	—	D16.7	D48.0	D49.2
Zuckerkandl organ	C75.5	C79.89	—	D35.6	D44.7	D49.7

Substance	Poisoning, Accidental (unintentional)	Poisoning, Intentional Self-harm	Poisoning, Assault	Poisoning, Undetermined	Adverse Effect	Under-dosing
14-hydroxydihydro-morphinone	T40.2X1	T40.2X2	T40.2X3	T40.2X4	T40.2X5	T40.2X6
1-Propanol	T51.3X1	T51.3X2	T51.3X3	T51.3X4	—	—
2,3,7,8-Tetrachlorodibenzo-p-dioxin	T53.7X1	T53.7X2	T53.7X3	T53.7X4	—	—
2,4,5-T (trichloro-phenoxyacetic acid)	T60.1X1	T60.1X2	T60.1X3	T60.1X4	—	—
2,4,5-Trichlorophen-oxyacetic acid	T60.3X1	T60.3X2	T60.3X3	T60.3X4	—	—
2,4-D (dichlorophen-oxyacetic acid)	T60.3X1	T60.3X2	T60.3X3	T60.3X4	—	—
2,4-Toluene diisocyanate	T65.0X1	T65.0X2	T65.0X3	T65.0X4	—	—
2-Deoxy-5-fluorouridine	T45.1X1	T45.1X2	T45.1X3	T45.1X4	T45.1X5	T45.1X6
2-Ethoxyethanol	T52.3X1	T52.3X2	T52.3X3	T52.3X4	—	—
2-Methoxyethanol	T52.3X1	T52.3X2	T52.3X3	T52.3X4	—	—
2-Propanol	T51.2X1	T51.2X2	T51.2X3	T51.2X4	—	—
3,4-methylenedioxymeth-amphetamine	T43.641	T43.642	T43.643	T43.644	—	—
4-Aminobutyric acid	T43.8X1	T43.8X2	T43.8X3	T43.8X4	T43.8X5	T43.8X6
4-Aminophenol derivatives	T39.1X1	T39.1X2	T39.1X3	T39.1X4	T39.1X5	T39.1X6
5-Deoxy-5-fluorouridine	T45.1X1	T45.1X2	T45.1X3	T45.1X4	T45.1X5	T45.1X6
5-Methoxypsoralen (5-MOP)	T50.991	T50.992	T50.993	T50.994	T50.995	T50.996
8-Aminoquinoline drugs	T37.2X1	T37.2X2	T37.2X3	T37.2X4	T37.2X5	T37.2X6
8-Methoxypsoralen (8-MOP)	T50.991	T50.992	T50.993	T50.994	T50.995	T50.996
9-hydroxyrisperidone*	T43.591	T43.592	T43.593	T43.594	T43.595	T43.596
ABOB	T37.5X1	T37.5X2	T37.5X3	T37.5X4	T37.5X5	T37.5X6
Abrine	T62.2X1	T62.2X2	T62.2X3	T62.2X4	—	—
Abrus (seed)	T62.2X1	T62.2X2	T62.2X3	T62.2X4	—	—
Absinthe	T51.0X1	T51.0X2	T51.0X3	T51.0X4	—	—
beverage	T51.0X1	T51.0X2	T51.0X3	T51.0X4	—	—
Acaricide	T60.8X1	T60.8X2	T60.8X3	T60.8X4	—	—
Acebutolol	T44.7X1	T44.7X2	T44.7X3	T44.7X4	T44.7X5	T44.7X6
Acecarbromal	T42.6X1	T42.6X2	T42.6X3	T42.6X4	T42.6X5	T42.6X6
Aceclidine	T44.1X1	T44.1X2	T44.1X3	T44.1X4	T44.1X5	T44.1X6
Acedapsone	T37.0X1	T37.0X2	T37.0X3	T37.0X4	T37.0X5	T37.0X6
Acefylline piperazine	T48.6X1	T48.6X2	T48.6X3	T48.6X4	T48.6X5	T48.6X6
Acemorphan	T40.2X1	T40.2X2	T40.2X3	T40.2X4	—	—
Acenocoumarin	T45.511	T45.512	T45.513	T45.514	T45.515	T45.516
Acenocoumarol	T45.511	T45.512	T45.513	T45.514	T45.515	T45.516
Aceon*	T46.4X1	T46.4X2	T46.4X3	T46.4X4	T46.4X5	T46.4X6
Acepifylline	T48.6X1	T48.6X2	T48.6X3	T48.6X4	T48.6X5	T48.6X6
Acepromazine	T43.3X1	T43.3X2	T43.3X3	T43.3X4	T43.3X5	T43.3X6
Acesulfamethoxypyridazine	T37.0X1	T37.0X2	T37.0X3	T37.0X4	T37.0X5	T37.0X6
Acetal	T52.8X1	T52.8X2	T52.8X3	T52.8X4	—	—
Acetaldehyde (vapor)	T52.8X1	T52.8X2	T52.8X3	T52.8X4	—	—
liquid	T65.891	T65.892	T65.893	T65.894	—	—
Acetaminophen	T39.1X1	T39.1X2	T39.1X3	T39.1X4	T39.1X5	T39.1X6
Acetaminosalol	T39.1X1	T39.1X2	T39.1X3	T39.1X4	T39.1X5	T39.1X6
Acetanilide	T39.1X1	T39.1X2	T39.1X3	T39.1X4	T39.1X5	T39.1X6
Acetarsol	T37.3X1	T37.3X2	T37.3X3	T37.3X4	T37.3X5	T37.3X6
Acetazolamide	T50.2X1	T50.2X2	T50.2X3	T50.2X4	T50.2X5	T50.2X6
Acetiamine	T45.2X1	T45.2X2	T45.2X3	T45.2X4	T45.2X5	T45.2X6
Acetic						
acid	T54.2X1	T54.2X2	T54.2X3	T54.2X4	—	—
with sodium acetate (ointment)	T49.3X1	T49.3X2	T49.3X3	T49.3X4	T49.3X5	T49.3X6
ester (solvent)(vapor)	T52.8X1	T52.8X2	T52.8X3	T52.8X4	—	—
irrigating solution	T50.3X1	T50.3X2	T50.3X3	T50.3X4	T50.3X5	T50.3X6
medicinal (lotion)	T49.2X1	T49.2X2	T49.2X3	T49.2X4	T49.2X5	T49.2X6
anhydride	T65.891	T65.892	T65.893	T65.894	—	—
ether (vapor)	T52.8X1	T52.8X2	T52.8X3	T52.8X4	—	—
Acetohexamide	T38.3X1	T38.3X2	T38.3X3	T38.3X4	T38.3X5	T38.3X6
Acetohydroxamic acid	T50.991	T50.992	T50.993	T50.994	T50.995	T50.996
Acetomenaphthone	T45.7X1	T45.7X2	T45.7X3	T45.7X4	T45.7X5	T45.7X6
Acetomorphine	T40.1X1	T40.1X2	T40.1X3	T40.1X4	—	—
Acetone (oils)	T52.4X1	T52.4X2	T52.4X3	T52.4X4	—	—
chlorinated	T52.4X1	T52.4X2	T52.4X3	T52.4X4	—	—
vapor	T52.4X1	T52.4X2	T52.4X3	T52.4X4	—	—
Acetonitrile	T52.8X1	T52.8X2	T52.8X3	T52.8X4	—	—
Acetophenazine	T43.3X1	T43.3X2	T43.3X3	T43.3X4	T43.3X5	T43.3X6
Acetophenetedin	T39.1X1	T39.1X2	T39.1X3	T39.1X4	T39.1X5	T39.1X6
Acetophenone	T52.4X1	T52.4X2	T52.4X3	T52.4X4	—	—
Acetorphine	T40.2X1	T40.2X2	T40.2X3	T40.2X4	—	—
Acetosulfone (sodium)	T37.1X1	T37.1X2	T37.1X3	T37.1X4	T37.1X5	T37.1X6
Acetrizoate (sodium)	T50.8X1	T50.8X2	T50.8X3	T50.8X4	T50.8X5	T50.8X6
Acetrizoic acid	T50.8X1	T50.8X2	T50.8X3	T50.8X4	T50.8X5	T50.8X6
Acetyl						
bromide	T53.6X1	T53.6X2	T53.6X3	T53.6X4	—	—
chloride	T53.6X1	T53.6X2	T53.6X3	T53.6X4	—	—
Acetylcarbromal	T42.6X1	T42.6X2	T42.6X3	T42.6X4	T42.6X5	T42.6X6
Acetylcholine						
Acetylcholine — continued						
chloride	T44.1X1	T44.1X2	T44.1X3	T44.1X4	T44.1X5	T44.1X6
derivative	T44.1X1	T44.1X2	T44.1X3	T44.1X4	T44.1X5	T44.1X6
Acetylcysteine	T48.4X1	T48.4X2	T48.4X3	T48.4X4	T48.4X5	T48.4X6
Acetyldigitoxin	T46.0X1	T46.0X2	T46.0X3	T46.0X4	T46.0X5	T46.0X6
Acetyldigoxin	T46.0X1	T46.0X2	T46.0X3	T46.0X4	T46.0X5	T46.0X6
Acetyldihydrocodeine	T40.2X1	T40.2X2	T40.2X3	T40.2X4	—	—
Acetyldihydrocodeinone	T40.2X1	T40.2X2	T40.2X3	T40.2X4	—	—
Acetylene (gas)	T59.891	T59.892	T59.893	T59.894	—	—
dichloride	T53.6X1	T53.6X2	T53.6X3	T53.6X4	—	—
incomplete combustion of	T58.11	T58.12	T58.13	T58.14	—	—
industrial	T59.891	T59.892	T59.893	T59.894	—	—
tetrachloride	T53.6X1	T53.6X2	T53.6X3	T53.6X4	—	—
vapor	T53.6X1	T53.6X2	T53.6X3	T53.6X4	—	—
Acetylpheneturide	T42.6X1	T42.6X2	T42.6X3	T42.6X4	T42.6X5	T42.6X6
Acetylphenylhydrazine	T39.8X1	T39.8X2	T39.8X3	T39.8X4	T39.8X5	T39.8X6
Acetylsalicylic acid (salts)	T39.011	T39.012	T39.013	T39.014	T39.015	T39.016
enteric coated	T39.011	T39.012	T39.013	T39.014	T39.015	T39.016
Acetylsulfamethoxypyridazine	T37.0X1	T37.0X2	T37.0X3	T37.0X4	T37.0X5	T37.0X6
Achromycin	T36.4X1	T36.4X2	T36.4X3	T36.4X4	T36.4X5	T36.4X6
ophthalmic preparation	T49.5X1	T49.5X2	T49.5X3	T49.5X4	T49.5X5	T49.5X6
topical NEC	T49.0X1	T49.0X2	T49.0X3	T49.0X4	T49.0X5	T49.0X6
Aciclovir	T37.5X1	T37.5X2	T37.5X3	T37.5X4	T37.5X5	T37.5X6
Acidifying agent NEC	T50.901	T50.902	T50.903	T50.904	T50.905	T50.906
Acid (corrosive) NEC	T54.2X1	T54.2X2	T54.2X3	T54.2X4	—	—
AcipHex*	T47.1X1	T47.1X2	T47.1X3	T47.1X4	T47.1X5	T47.1X6
Acipimox	T46.6X1	T46.6X2	T46.6X3	T46.6X4	T46.6X5	T46.6X6
Acitretin	T50.991	T50.992	T50.993	T50.994	T50.995	T50.996
Aclarubicin	T45.1X1	T45.1X2	T45.1X3	T45.1X4	T45.1X5	T45.1X6
Aclatonium napadisilate	T48.1X1	T48.1X2	T48.1X3	T48.1X4	T48.1X5	T48.1X6
Aconite (wild)	T46.991	T46.992	T46.993	T46.994	T46.995	T46.996
Aconitine	T46.991	T46.992	T46.993	T46.994	T46.995	T46.996
Aconitum ferox	T46.991	T46.992	T46.993	T46.994	T46.995	T46.996
Acridine	T65.6X1	T65.6X2	T65.6X3	T65.6X4	—	—
vapor	T59.891	T59.892	T59.893	T59.894	—	—
Acriflavine	T37.91	T37.92	T37.93	T37.94	T37.95	T37.96
Acriflavinium chloride	T49.0X1	T49.0X2	T49.0X3	T49.0X4	T49.0X5	T49.0X6
Acrinol	T49.0X1	T49.0X2	T49.0X3	T49.0X4	T49.0X5	T49.0X6
Acrisorcin	T49.0X1	T49.0X2	T49.0X3	T49.0X4	T49.0X5	T49.0X6
Acrivastine	T45.0X1	T45.0X2	T45.0X3	T45.0X4	T45.0X5	T45.0X6
Acrolein (gas)	T59.891	T59.892	T59.893	T59.894	—	—
liquid	T54.1X1	T54.1X2	T54.1X3	T54.1X4	—	—
Acrylamide	T65.891	T65.892	T65.893	T65.894	—	—
Acrylic resin	T49.3X1	T49.3X2	T49.3X3	T49.3X4	T49.3X5	T49.3X6
Acrylonitrile	T65.891	T65.892	T65.893	T65.894	—	—
Actaea spicata	T62.2X1	T62.2X2	T62.2X3	T62.2X4	—	—
berry	T62.1X1	T62.1X2	T62.1X3	T62.1X4	—	—
Acterol	T37.3X1	T37.3X2	T37.3X3	T37.3X4	T37.3X5	T37.3X6
ACTH	T38.811	T38.812	T38.813	T38.814	T38.815	T38.816
Actinomycin C	T45.1X1	T45.1X2	T45.1X3	T45.1X4	T45.1X5	T45.1X6
Actinomycin D	T45.1X1	T45.1X2	T45.1X3	T45.1X4	T45.1X5	T45.1X6
Activated charcoal — see also Charcoal, medicinal	T47.6X1	T47.6X2	T47.6X3	T47.6X4	T47.6X5	T47.6X6
Activella*	T38.5X1	T38.5X2	T38.5X3	T38.5X4	T38.5X5	T38.5X6
Acyclovir	T37.5X1	T37.5X2	T37.5X3	T37.5X4	T37.5X5	T37.5X6
Adenine	T45.2X1	T45.2X2	T45.2X3	T45.2X4	T45.2X5	T45.2X6
arabinoside	T37.5X1	T37.5X2	T37.5X3	T37.5X4	T37.5X5	T37.5X6
Adenosine (phosphate)	T46.2X1	T46.2X2	T46.2X3	T46.2X4	T46.2X5	T46.2X6
ADH	T38.891	T38.892	T38.893	T38.894	T38.895	T38.896
Adhesive NEC	T65.891	T65.892	T65.893	T65.894	—	—
Adicillin	T36.0X1	T36.0X2	T36.0X3	T36.0X4	T36.0X5	T36.0X6
Adiphenine	T44.3X1	T44.3X2	T44.3X3	T44.3X4	T44.3X5	T44.3X6
Adipiodone	T50.8X1	T50.8X2	T50.8X3	T50.8X4	T50.8X5	T50.8X6
Adjunct, pharmaceutical	T50.901	T50.902	T50.903	T50.904	T50.905	T50.906
Adrenal (extract, cortex or medulla) (glucocorticoids) (hormones) (mineralocorticoids)	T38.0X1	T38.0X2	T38.0X3	T38.0X4	T38.0X5	T38.0X6
ENT agent	T49.6X1	T49.6X2	T49.6X3	T49.6X4	T49.6X5	T49.6X6
ophthalmic preparation	T49.5X1	T49.5X2	T49.5X3	T49.5X4	T49.5X5	T49.5X6
topical NEC	T49.0X1	T49.0X2	T49.0X3	T49.0X4	T49.0X5	T49.0X6
Adrenalin — see Adrenaline						
Adrenaline	T44.5X1	T44.5X2	T44.5X3	T44.5X4	T44.5X5	T44.5X6
Adrenergic NEC	T44.901	T44.902	T44.903	T44.904	T44.905	T44.906
blocking agent NEC	T44.8X1	T44.8X2	T44.8X3	T44.8X4	T44.8X5	T44.8X6
beta, heart	T44.7X1	T44.7X2	T44.7X3	T44.7X4	T44.7X5	T44.7X6
specified NEC	T44.991	T44.992	T44.993	T44.994	T44.995	T44.996
Adrenochrome						
derivative	T46.991	T46.992	T46.993	T46.994	T46.995	T46.996
(mono) semicarbazone	T46.991	T46.992	T46.993	T46.994	T46.995	T46.996
Adrenocorticotrophic hormone	T38.811	T38.812	T38.813	T38.814	T38.815	T38.816
Adrenocorticotrophin	T38.811	T38.812	T38.813	T38.814	T38.815	T38.816

Substance	Poisoning, Accidental (unintentional)	Poisoning, Intentional Self-harm	Poisoning, Assault	Poisoning, Undetermined	Adverse Effect	Under-dosing
Adriamycin	T45.1X1	T45.1X2	T45.1X3	T45.1X4	T45.1X5	T45.1X6
Adrucil*	T45.1X1	T45.1X2	T45.1X3	T45.1X4	T45.1X5	T45.1X6
Aerosol spray NEC	T65.91	T65.92	T65.93	T65.94	—	—
Aerosporin	T36.8X1	T36.8X2	T36.8X3	T36.8X4	T36.8X5	T36.8X6
ENT agent	T49.6X1	T49.6X2	T49.6X3	T49.6X4	T49.6X5	T49.6X6
ophthalmic preparation	T49.5X1	T49.5X2	T49.5X3	T49.5X4	T49.5X5	T49.5X6
topical NEC	T49.0X1	T49.0X2	T49.0X3	T49.0X4	T49.0X5	T49.0X6
Aethusa cynapium	T62.2X1	T62.2X2	T62.2X3	T62.2X4	—	—
Afghanistan black	T40.711	T40.712	T40.713	T40.714	T40.715	T40.716
Aflatoxin	T64.01	T64.02	T64.03	T64.04	—	—
Afloqualone	T42.8X1	T42.8X2	T42.8X3	T42.8X4	T42.8X5	T42.8X6
African boxwood	T62.2X1	T62.2X2	T62.2X3	T62.2X4	—	—
Agar	T47.4X1	T47.4X2	T47.4X3	T47.4X4	T47.4X5	T47.4X6
Agonist						
predominantly						
alpha-adrenoreceptor	T44.4X1	T44.4X2	T44.4X3	T44.4X4	T44.4X5	T44.4X6
beta-adrenoreceptor	T44.5X1	T44.5X2	T44.5X3	T44.5X4	T44.5X5	T44.5X6
Agricultural agent NEC	T65.91	T65.92	T65.93	T65.94	—	—
Agrypnal	T42.3X1	T42.3X2	T42.3X3	T42.3X4	T42.3X5	T42.3X6
AHLG	T50.Z11	T50.Z12	T50.Z13	T50.Z14	T50.Z15	T50.Z16
Air contaminant(s), source/type NOS	T65.91	T65.92	T65.93	T65.94	—	—
Ajmaline	T46.2X1	T46.2X2	T46.2X3	T46.2X4	T46.2X5	T46.2X6
Akee	T62.1X1	T62.1X2	T62.1X3	T62.1X4	—	—
Akne-Mycin*	T49.0X1	T49.0X2	T49.0X3	T49.0X4	T49.0X5	T49.0X6
Akrinol	T49.0X1	T49.0X2	T49.0X3	T49.0X4	T49.0X5	T49.0X6
Akritoin	T37.8X1	T37.8X2	T37.8X3	T37.8X4	T37.8X5	T37.8X6
Alacepril	T46.4X1	T46.4X2	T46.4X3	T46.4X4	T46.4X5	T46.4X6
Alantolactone	T37.4X1	T37.4X2	T37.4X3	T37.4X4	T37.4X5	T37.4X6
Albamycin	T36.8X1	T36.8X2	T36.8X3	T36.8X4	T36.8X5	T36.8X6
Albendazole	T37.4X1	T37.4X2	T37.4X3	T37.4X4	T37.4X5	T37.4X6
Albiglutide*	T38.3X1	T38.3X2	T38.3X3	T38.3X4	T38.3X5	T38.3X6
Albumin						
bovine	T45.8X1	T45.8X2	T45.8X3	T45.8X4	T45.8X5	T45.8X6
human serum	T45.8X1	T45.8X2	T45.8X3	T45.8X4	T45.8X5	T45.8X6
salt-poor	T45.8X1	T45.8X2	T45.8X3	T45.8X4	T45.8X5	T45.8X6
normal human serum	T45.8X1	T45.8X2	T45.8X3	T45.8X4	T45.8X5	T45.8X6
Albuterol	T48.6X1	T48.6X2	T48.6X3	T48.6X4	T48.6X5	T48.6X6
Albutoin	T42.0X1	T42.0X2	T42.0X3	T42.0X4	T42.0X5	T42.0X6
Alclometasone	T49.0X1	T49.0X2	T49.0X3	T49.0X4	T49.0X5	T49.0X6
Alcohol	T51.91	T51.92	T51.93	T51.94	—	—
absolute	T51.0X1	T51.0X2	T51.0X3	T51.0X4	—	—
beverage	T51.0X1	T51.0X2	T51.0X3	T51.0X4	—	—
allyl	T51.8X1	T51.8X2	T51.8X3	T51.8X4	—	—
amyl	T51.3X1	T51.3X2	T51.3X3	T51.3X4	—	—
antifreeze	T51.1X1	T51.1X2	T51.1X3	T51.1X4	—	—
beverage	T51.0X1	T51.0X2	T51.0X3	T51.0X4	—	—
butyl	T51.3X1	T51.3X2	T51.3X3	T51.3X4	—	—
dehydrated	T51.0X1	T51.0X2	T51.0X3	T51.0X4	—	—
beverage	T51.0X1	T51.0X2	T51.0X3	T51.0X4	—	—
denatured	T51.0X1	T51.0X2	T51.0X3	T51.0X4	—	—
deterrent NEC	T50.6X1	T50.6X2	T50.6X3	T50.6X4	T50.6X5	T50.6X6
diagnostic (gastric function)	T50.8X1	T50.8X2	T50.8X3	T50.8X4	T50.8X5	T50.8X6
ethyl	T51.0X1	T51.0X2	T51.0X3	T51.0X4	—	—
beverage	T51.0X1	T51.0X2	T51.0X3	T51.0X4	—	—
grain	T51.0X1	T51.0X2	T51.0X3	T51.0X4	—	—
beverage	T51.0X1	T51.0X2	T51.0X3	T51.0X4	—	—
industrial	T51.0X1	T51.0X2	T51.0X3	T51.0X4	—	—
isopropyl	T51.2X1	T51.2X2	T51.2X3	T51.2X4	—	—
methyl	T51.1X1	T51.1X2	T51.1X3	T51.1X4	—	—
preparation for consumption	T51.0X1	T51.0X2	T51.0X3	T51.0X4	—	—
propyl	T51.3X1	T51.3X2	T51.3X3	T51.3X4	—	—
secondary	T51.2X1	T51.2X2	T51.2X3	T51.2X4	—	—
radiator	T51.1X1	T51.1X2	T51.1X3	T51.1X4	—	—
rubbing	T51.2X1	T51.2X2	T51.2X3	T51.2X4	—	—
specified type NEC	T51.8X1	T51.8X2	T51.8X3	T51.8X4	—	—
surgical	T51.0X1	T51.0X2	T51.0X3	T51.0X4	—	—
vapor (from any type of Alcohol)	T59.891	T59.892	T59.893	T59.894	—	—
wood	T51.1X1	T51.1X2	T51.1X3	T51.1X4	—	—
Alcuronium (chloride)	T48.1X1	T48.1X2	T48.1X3	T48.1X4	T48.1X5	T48.1X6
Aldactone	T50.0X1	T50.0X2	T50.0X3	T50.0X4	T50.0X5	T50.0X6
Aldesulfone sodium	T37.1X1	T37.1X2	T37.1X3	T37.1X4	T37.1X5	T37.1X6
Aldicarb	T60.0X1	T60.0X2	T60.0X3	T60.0X4	—	—
Aldomet	T46.5X1	T46.5X2	T46.5X3	T46.5X4	T46.5X5	T46.5X6
Aldosterone	T50.0X1	T50.0X2	T50.0X3	T50.0X4	T50.0X5	T50.0X6
Aldrin (dust)	T60.1X1	T60.1X2	T60.1X3	T60.1X4	—	—
Aleve — see Naproxen						
Alexitol sodium	T47.1X1	T47.1X2	T47.1X3	T47.1X4	T47.1X5	T47.1X6
Alfacalcidol	T45.2X1	T45.2X2	T45.2X3	T45.2X4	T45.2X5	T45.2X6
Alfadolone	T41.1X1	T41.1X2	T41.1X3	T41.1X4	T41.1X5	T41.1X6

Substance	Poisoning, Accidental (unintentional)	Poisoning, Intentional Self-harm	Poisoning, Assault	Poisoning, Undetermined	Adverse Effect	Under-dosing
Alfaxalone	T41.1X1	T41.1X2	T41.1X3	T41.1X4	T41.1X5	T41.1X6
Alfentanil	T40.411	T40.412	T40.413	T40.414	T40.415	T40.416
Alfuzosin (hydrochloride)	T44.8X1	T44.8X2	T44.8X3	T44.8X4	T44.8X5	T44.8X6
Algae (harmful) (toxin)	T65.821	T65.822	T65.823	T65.824	—	—
Algeldrate	T47.1X1	T47.1X2	T47.1X3	T47.1X4	T47.1X5	T47.1X6
Algin	T47.8X1	T47.8X2	T47.8X3	T47.8X4	T47.8X5	T47.8X6
Alglucerase	T45.3X1	T45.3X2	T45.3X3	T45.3X4	T45.3X5	T45.3X6
Alidase	T45.3X1	T45.3X2	T45.3X3	T45.3X4	T45.3X5	T45.3X6
Alimemazine	T43.3X1	T43.3X2	T43.3X3	T43.3X4	T43.3X5	T43.3X6
Aliphatic thiocyanates	T65.0X1	T65.0X2	T65.0X3	T65.0X4	—	—
Alitretinoin*	T49.0X1	T49.0X2	T49.0X3	T49.0X4	T49.0X5	T49.0X6
Alizapride	T45.0X1	T45.0X2	T45.0X3	T45.0X4	T45.0X5	T45.0X6
Alkali (caustic)	T54.3X1	T54.3X2	T54.3X3	T54.3X4	—	—
Alkaline antiseptic solution (aromatic)	T49.6X1	T49.6X2	T49.6X3	T49.6X4	T49.6X5	T49.6X6
Alkalinizing agents (medicinal)	T50.901	T50.902	T50.903	T50.904	T50.905	T50.906
Alkalizing agent NEC	T50.901	T50.902	T50.903	T50.904	T50.905	T50.906
Alka-seltzer	T39.011	T39.012	T39.013	T39.014	T39.015	T39.016
Alkavervir	T46.5X1	T46.5X2	T46.5X3	T46.5X4	T46.5X5	T46.5X6
Alkeran*	T45.1X1	T45.1X2	T45.1X3	T45.1X4	T45.1X5	T45.1X6
Alkonium (bromide)	T49.0X1	T49.0X2	T49.0X3	T49.0X4	T49.0X5	T49.0X6
Alkylating drug NEC	T45.1X1	T45.1X2	T45.1X3	T45.1X4	T45.1X5	T45.1X6
antimyeloproliferative	T45.1X1	T45.1X2	T45.1X3	T45.1X4	T45.1X5	T45.1X6
lymphatic	T45.1X1	T45.1X2	T45.1X3	T45.1X4	T45.1X5	T45.1X6
Alkylisocyanate	T65.0X1	T65.0X2	T65.0X3	T65.0X4	—	—
Allantoin	T49.4X1	T49.4X2	T49.4X3	T49.4X4	T49.4X5	T49.4X6
Allegron	T43.011	T43.012	T43.013	T43.014	T43.015	T43.016
Allethrin	T49.0X1	T49.0X2	T49.0X3	T49.0X4	T49.0X5	T49.0X6
Allobarbital	T42.3X1	T42.3X2	T42.3X3	T42.3X4	T42.3X5	T42.3X6
Allopurinol	T50.4X1	T50.4X2	T50.4X3	T50.4X4	T50.4X5	T50.4X6
Allyl						
alcohol	T51.8X1	T51.8X2	T51.8X3	T51.8X4	—	—
disulfide	T46.6X1	T46.6X2	T46.6X3	T46.6X4	T46.6X5	T46.6X6
Allylestrenol	T38.5X1	T38.5X2	T38.5X3	T38.5X4	T38.5X5	T38.5X6
Allylisopropylacetylurea	T42.6X1	T42.6X2	T42.6X3	T42.6X4	T42.6X5	T42.6X6
Allylisopropylmalonylurea	T42.3X1	T42.3X2	T42.3X3	T42.3X4	T42.3X5	T42.3X6
Allylthiourea	T49.3X1	T49.3X2	T49.3X3	T49.3X4	T49.3X5	T49.3X6
Allyltribromide	T42.6X1	T42.6X2	T42.6X3	T42.6X4	T42.6X5	T42.6X6
Allypropymal	T42.3X1	T42.3X2	T42.3X3	T42.3X4	T42.3X5	T42.3X6
Almagate	T47.1X1	T47.1X2	T47.1X3	T47.1X4	T47.1X5	T47.1X6
Almasilate	T47.1X1	T47.1X2	T47.1X3	T47.1X4	T47.1X5	T47.1X6
Almitrine	T50.7X1	T50.7X2	T50.7X3	T50.7X4	T50.7X5	T50.7X6
Aloes	T47.2X1	T47.2X2	T47.2X3	T47.2X4	T47.2X5	T47.2X6
Aloglutamol	T47.1X1	T47.1X2	T47.1X3	T47.1X4	T47.1X5	T47.1X6
Aloin	T47.2X1	T47.2X2	T47.2X3	T47.2X4	T47.2X5	T47.2X6
Aloxidone	T42.2X1	T42.2X2	T42.2X3	T42.2X4	T42.2X5	T42.2X6
Alpha						
acetyldigoxin	T46.0X1	T46.0X2	T46.0X3	T46.0X4	T46.0X5	T46.0X6
adrenergic blocking drug	T44.6X1	T44.6X2	T44.6X3	T44.6X4	T44.6X5	T44.6X6
amylase	T45.3X1	T45.3X2	T45.3X3	T45.3X4	T45.3X5	T45.3X6
tocoferol (acetate)	T45.2X1	T45.2X2	T45.2X3	T45.2X4	T45.2X5	T45.2X6
tocopherol	T45.2X1	T45.2X2	T45.2X3	T45.2X4	T45.2X5	T45.2X6
Alphadolone	T41.1X1	T41.1X2	T41.1X3	T41.1X4	T41.1X5	T41.1X6
Alphaprodine	T40.491	T40.492	T40.493	T40.494	T40.495	T40.496
Alphaxalone	T41.1X1	T41.1X2	T41.1X3	T41.1X4	T41.1X5	T41.1X6
Alprazolam	T42.4X1	T42.4X2	T42.4X3	T42.4X4	T42.4X5	T42.4X6
Alprenolol	T44.7X1	T44.7X2	T44.7X3	T44.7X4	T44.7X5	T44.7X6
Alprostadil	T46.7X1	T46.7X2	T46.7X3	T46.7X4	T46.7X5	T46.7X6
Alsactide	T38.811	T38.812	T38.813	T38.814	T38.815	T38.816
Alseroxylon	T46.5X1	T46.5X2	T46.5X3	T46.5X4	T46.5X5	T46.5X6
Alteplase	T45.611	T45.612	T45.613	T45.614	T45.615	T45.616
Altizide	T50.2X1	T50.2X2	T50.2X3	T50.2X4	T50.2X5	T50.2X6
Altoprev*	T46.6X1	T46.6X2	T46.6X3	T46.6X4	T46.6X5	T46.6X6
Altretamine	T45.1X1	T45.1X2	T45.1X3	T45.1X4	T45.1X5	T45.1X6
Alum (medicinal)	T49.4X1	T49.4X2	T49.4X3	T49.4X4	T49.4X5	T49.4X6
nonmedicinal (ammonium) (potassium)	T56.891	T56.892	T56.893	T56.894	—	—
Aluminium, aluminum						
acetate	T49.2X1	T49.2X2	T49.2X3	T49.2X4	T49.2X5	T49.2X6
solution	T49.0X1	T49.0X2	T49.0X3	T49.0X4	T49.0X5	T49.0X6
aspirin	T39.011	T39.012	T39.013	T39.014	T39.015	T39.016
bis (acetylsalicylate)	T39.011	T39.012	T39.013	T39.014	T39.015	T39.016
carbonate (gel, basic)	T47.1X1	T47.1X2	T47.1X3	T47.1X4	T47.1X5	T47.1X6
chlorhydroxide-complex	T47.1X1	T47.1X2	T47.1X3	T47.1X4	T47.1X5	T47.1X6
chloride	T49.2X1	T49.2X2	T49.2X3	T49.2X4	T49.2X5	T49.2X6
clofibrate	T46.6X1	T46.6X2	T46.6X3	T46.6X4	T46.6X5	T46.6X6
diacetate	T49.2X1	T49.2X2	T49.2X3	T49.2X4	T49.2X5	T49.2X6
glycinate	T47.1X1	T47.1X2	T47.1X3	T47.1X4	T47.1X5	T47.1X6
hydroxide (gel)	T47.1X1	T47.1X2	T47.1X3	T47.1X4	T47.1X5	T47.1X6
hydroxide-magnesium carb. gel	T47.1X1	T47.1X2	T47.1X3	T47.1X4	T47.1X5	T47.1X6
magnesium silicate	T47.1X1	T47.1X2	T47.1X3	T47.1X4	T47.1X5	T47.1X6

☑ Additional Character May Be Required — Refer to the Tabular List for Character Selection

*Optum Value-Add

Substance	Poisoning, Accidental (unintentional)	Poisoning, Intentional Self-harm	Poisoning, Assault	Poisoning, Undetermined	Adverse Effect	Under-dosing
Aluminium, aluminum — continued						
nicotinate	T46.7X1	T46.7X2	T46.7X3	T46.7X4	T46.7X5	T46.7X6
ointment (surgical) (topical)	T49.3X1	T49.3X2	T49.3X3	T49.3X4	T49.3X5	T49.3X6
phosphate	T47.1X1	T47.1X2	T47.1X3	T47.1X4	T47.1X5	T47.1X6
salicylate	T39.091	T39.092	T39.093	T39.094	T39.095	T39.096
silicate	T47.1X1	T47.1X2	T47.1X3	T47.1X4	T47.1X5	T47.1X6
sodium silicate	T47.1X1	T47.1X2	T47.1X3	T47.1X4	T47.1X5	T47.1X6
subacetate	T49.2X1	T49.2X2	T49.2X3	T49.2X4	T49.2X5	T49.2X6
sulfate	T49.0X1	T49.0X2	T49.0X3	T49.0X4	T49.0X5	T49.0X6
tannate	T47.6X1	T47.6X2	T47.6X3	T47.6X4	T47.6X5	T47.6X6
topical NEC	T49.3X1	T49.3X2	T49.3X3	T49.3X4	T49.3X5	T49.3X6
Alurate	T42.3X1	T42.3X2	T42.3X3	T42.3X4	T42.3X5	T42.3X6
Alverine	T44.3X1	T44.3X2	T44.3X3	T44.3X4	T44.3X5	T44.3X6
Alvodine	T40.2X1	T40.2X2	T40.2X3	T40.2X4	T40.2X5	T40.2X6
Amanita phalloides	T62.0X1	T62.0X2	T62.0X3	T62.0X4	—	—
Amanitine	T62.0X1	T62.0X2	T62.0X3	T62.0X4	—	—
Amantadine	T42.8X1	T42.8X2	T42.8X3	T42.8X4	T42.8X5	T42.8X6
Ambazone	T49.6X1	T49.6X2	T49.6X3	T49.6X4	T49.6X5	T49.6X6
Ambenonium (chloride)	T44.0X1	T44.0X2	T44.0X3	T44.0X4	T44.0X5	T44.0X6
Ambroxol	T48.4X1	T48.4X2	T48.4X3	T48.4X4	T48.4X5	T48.4X6
Ambuphylline	T48.6X1	T48.6X2	T48.6X3	T48.6X4	T48.6X5	T48.6X6
Ambutonium bromide	T44.3X1	T44.3X2	T44.3X3	T44.3X4	T44.3X5	T44.3X6
Amcinonide	T49.0X1	T49.0X2	T49.0X3	T49.0X4	T49.0X5	T49.0X6
Amdinocilline	T36.0X1	T36.0X2	T36.0X3	T36.0X4	T36.0X5	T36.0X6
Americaine*	T41.3X1	T41.3X2	T41.3X3	T41.3X4	T41.3X5	T41.3X6
Ametazole	T50.8X1	T50.8X2	T50.8X3	T50.8X4	T50.8X5	T50.8X6
Amethocaine	T41.3X1	T41.3X2	T41.3X3	T41.3X4	T41.3X5	T41.3X6
regional	T41.3X1	T41.3X2	T41.3X3	T41.3X4	T41.3X5	T41.3X6
spinal	T41.3X1	T41.3X2	T41.3X3	T41.3X4	T41.3X5	T41.3X6
Amethopterin	T45.1X1	T45.1X2	T45.1X3	T45.1X4	T45.1X5	T45.1X6
Amezinium metilsulfate	T44.991	T44.992	T44.993	T44.994	T44.995	T44.996
Amfebutamone	T43.291	T43.292	T43.293	T43.294	T43.295	T43.296
Amfepramone	T50.5X1	T50.5X2	T50.5X3	T50.5X4	T50.5X5	T50.5X6
Amfetamine	T43.621	T43.622	T43.623	T43.624	T43.625	T43.626
Amfetaminil	T43.621	T43.622	T43.623	T43.624	T43.625	T43.626
Amfomycin	T36.8X1	T36.8X2	T36.8X3	T36.8X4	T36.8X5	T36.8X6
Amidefrine mesilate	T48.5X1	T48.5X2	T48.5X3	T48.5X4	T48.5X5	T48.5X6
Amidone	T40.3X1	T40.3X2	T40.3X3	T40.3X4	T40.3X5	T40.3X6
Amidopyrine	T39.2X1	T39.2X2	T39.2X3	T39.2X4	T39.2X5	T39.2X6
Amidotrizoate	T50.8X1	T50.8X2	T50.8X3	T50.8X4	T50.8X5	T50.8X6
Amiflamine	T43.1X1	T43.1X2	T43.1X3	T43.1X4	T43.1X5	T43.1X6
Amikacin	T36.5X1	T36.5X2	T36.5X3	T36.5X4	T36.5X5	T36.5X6
Amikhelline	T46.3X1	T46.3X2	T46.3X3	T46.3X4	T46.3X5	T46.3X6
Amiloride	T50.2X1	T50.2X2	T50.2X3	T50.2X4	T50.2X5	T50.2X6
Aminacrine	T49.0X1	T49.0X2	T49.0X3	T49.0X4	T49.0X5	T49.0X6
Amineptine	T43.011	T43.012	T43.013	T43.014	T43.015	T43.016
Aminitrozole	T37.3X1	T37.3X2	T37.3X3	T37.3X4	T37.3X5	T37.3X6
Aminoacetic acid (derivatives)	T50.3X1	T50.3X2	T50.3X3	T50.3X4	T50.3X5	T50.3X6
Amino acids	T50.3X1	T50.3X2	T50.3X3	T50.3X4	T50.3X5	T50.3X6
Aminoacridine	T49.0X1	T49.0X2	T49.0X3	T49.0X4	T49.0X5	T49.0X6
Aminobenzoic acid (-p)	T49.3X1	T49.3X2	T49.3X3	T49.3X4	T49.3X5	T49.3X6
Aminocaproic acid	T45.621	T45.622	T45.623	T45.624	T45.625	T45.626
Aminoethylisothiourium	T45.8X1	T45.8X2	T45.8X3	T45.8X4	T45.8X5	T45.8X6
Aminofenazone	T39.2X1	T39.2X2	T39.2X3	T39.2X4	T39.2X5	T39.2X6
Aminoglutethimide	T45.1X1	T45.1X2	T45.1X3	T45.1X4	T45.1X5	T45.1X6
Aminoglycosides*	T36.5X1	T36.5X2	T36.5X3	T36.5X4	T36.5X5	T36.5X6
Aminohippuric acid	T50.8X1	T50.8X2	T50.8X3	T50.8X4	T50.8X5	T50.8X6
Aminomethylbenzoic acid	T45.691	T45.692	T45.693	T45.694	T45.695	T45.696
Aminometradine	T50.2X1	T50.2X2	T50.2X3	T50.2X4	T50.2X5	T50.2X6
Aminopentamide	T44.3X1	T44.3X2	T44.3X3	T44.3X4	T44.3X5	T44.3X6
Aminophenazone	T39.2X1	T39.2X2	T39.2X3	T39.2X4	T39.2X5	T39.2X6
Aminophenol	T54.0X1	T54.0X2	T54.0X3	T54.0X4	—	—
Aminophenylpyridone	T43.591	T43.592	T43.593	T43.594	T43.595	T43.596
Aminophylline	T48.6X1	T48.6X2	T48.6X3	T48.6X4	T48.6X5	T48.6X6
Aminopterin sodium	T45.1X1	T45.1X2	T45.1X3	T45.1X4	T45.1X5	T45.1X6
Aminopyrine	T39.2X1	T39.2X2	T39.2X3	T39.2X4	T39.2X5	T39.2X6
Aminorex	T50.5X1	T50.5X2	T50.5X3	T50.5X4	T50.5X5	T50.5X6
Aminosalicylic acid	T37.1X1	T37.1X2	T37.1X3	T37.1X4	T37.1X5	T37.1X6
Aminosalylum	T37.1X1	T37.1X2	T37.1X3	T37.1X4	T37.1X5	T37.1X6
Amiodarone	T46.2X1	T46.2X2	T46.2X3	T46.2X4	T46.2X5	T46.2X6
Amiphenazole	T50.7X1	T50.7X2	T50.7X3	T50.7X4	T50.7X5	T50.7X6
Amiquinsin	T46.5X1	T46.5X2	T46.5X3	T46.5X4	T46.5X5	T46.5X6
Amisometradine	T50.2X1	T50.2X2	T50.2X3	T50.2X4	T50.2X5	T50.2X6
Amisulpride	T43.591	T43.592	T43.593	T43.594	T43.595	T43.596
Amitriptyline	T43.011	T43.012	T43.013	T43.014	T43.015	T43.016
Amitriptylinoxide	T43.011	T43.012	T43.013	T43.014	T43.015	T43.016
Amlexanox	T48.6X1	T48.6X2	T48.6X3	T48.6X4	T48.6X5	T48.6X6
Ammonia (fumes) (gas) (vapor)	T59.891	T59.892	T59.893	T59.894	—	—
aromatic spirit	T48.991	T48.992	T48.993	T48.994	T48.995	T48.996

Substance	Poisoning, Accidental (unintentional)	Poisoning, Intentional Self-harm	Poisoning, Assault	Poisoning, Undetermined	Adverse Effect	Under-dosing
Ammonia — continued						
liquid (household)	T54.3X1	T54.3X2	T54.3X3	T54.3X4	—	—
Ammoniated mercury	T49.0X1	T49.0X2	T49.0X3	T49.0X4	T49.0X5	T49.0X6
Ammonium						
acid tartrate	T49.5X1	T49.5X2	T49.5X3	T49.5X4	T49.5X5	T49.5X6
bromide	T42.6X1	T42.6X2	T42.6X3	T42.6X4	T42.6X5	T42.6X6
carbonate	T54.3X1	T54.3X2	T54.3X3	T54.3X4	—	—
chloride	T50.991	T50.992	T50.993	T50.994	T50.995	T50.996
expectorant	T48.4X1	T48.4X2	T48.4X3	T48.4X4	T48.4X5	T48.4X6
compounds (household) NEC	T54.3X1	T54.3X2	T54.3X3	T54.3X4	—	—
fumes (any usage)	T59.891	T59.892	T59.893	T59.894	—	—
industrial	T54.3X1	T54.3X2	T54.3X3	T54.3X4	—	—
ichthyosulronate	T49.4X1	T49.4X2	T49.4X3	T49.4X4	T49.4X5	T49.4X6
mandelate	T37.91	T37.92	T37.93	T37.94	T37.95	T37.96
sulfamate	T60.3X1	T60.3X2	T60.3X3	T60.3X4	—	—
sulfonate resin	T47.8X1	T47.8X2	T47.8X3	T47.8X4	T47.8X5	T47.8X6
Amobarbital (sodium)	T42.3X1	T42.3X2	T42.3X3	T42.3X4	T42.3X5	T42.3X6
Amodiaquine	T37.2X1	T37.2X2	T37.2X3	T37.2X4	T37.2X5	T37.2X6
Amopyroquin (e)	T37.2X1	T37.2X2	T37.2X3	T37.2X4	T37.2X5	T37.2X6
Amoxapine	T43.011	T43.012	T43.013	T43.014	T43.015	T43.016
Amoxicillin	T36.0X1	T36.0X2	T36.0X3	T36.0X4	T36.0X5	T36.0X6
Amperozide	T43.591	T43.592	T43.593	T43.594	T43.595	T43.596
Amphenidone	T43.591	T43.592	T43.593	T43.594	T43.595	T43.596
Amphetamine NEC	T43.621	T43.622	T43.623	T43.624	T43.625	T43.626
Amphogel*	T47.1X1	T47.1X2	T47.1X3	T47.1X4	T47.1X5	T47.1X6
Amphomycin	T36.8X1	T36.8X2	T36.8X3	T36.8X4	T36.8X5	T36.8X6
Amphotalide	T37.4X1	T37.4X2	T37.4X3	T37.4X4	T37.4X5	T37.4X6
Amphotericin B	T36.7X1	T36.7X2	T36.7X3	T36.7X4	T36.7X5	T36.7X6
topical	T49.0X1	T49.0X2	T49.0X3	T49.0X4	T49.0X5	T49.0X6
Ampicillin	T36.0X1	T36.0X2	T36.0X3	T36.0X4	T36.0X5	T36.0X6
Amprotropine	T44.3X1	T44.3X2	T44.3X3	T44.3X4	T44.3X5	T44.3X6
Amsacrine	T45.1X1	T45.1X2	T45.1X3	T45.1X4	T45.1X5	T45.1X6
Amygdaline	T62.2X1	T62.2X2	T62.2X3	T62.2X4	—	—
Amyl						
acetate	T52.8X1	T52.8X2	T52.8X3	T52.8X4	—	—
vapor	T59.891	T59.892	T59.893	T59.894	—	—
alcohol	T51.3X1	T51.3X2	T51.3X3	T51.3X4	—	—
chloride	T53.6X1	T53.6X2	T53.6X3	T53.6X4	—	—
formate	T52.8X1	T52.8X2	T52.8X3	T52.8X4	—	—
nitrite	T46.3X1	T46.3X2	T46.3X3	T46.3X4	T46.3X5	T46.3X6
propionate	T65.891	T65.892	T65.893	T65.894	—	—
Amylase	T47.5X1	T47.5X2	T47.5X3	T47.5X4	T47.5X5	T47.5X6
Amyleine, regional	T41.3X1	T41.3X2	T41.3X3	T41.3X4	T41.3X5	T41.3X6
Amylene						
dichloride	T53.6X1	T53.6X2	T53.6X3	T53.6X4	—	—
hydrate	T51.3X1	T51.3X2	T51.3X3	T51.3X4	—	—
Amylmetacresol	T49.6X1	T49.6X2	T49.6X3	T49.6X4	T49.6X5	T49.6X6
Amylobarbitone	T42.3X1	T42.3X2	T42.3X3	T42.3X4	T42.3X5	T42.3X6
Amylocaine, regional	T41.3X1	T41.3X2	T41.3X3	T41.3X4	T41.3X5	T41.3X6
infiltration (subcutaneous)	T41.3X1	T41.3X2	T41.3X3	T41.3X4	T41.3X5	T41.3X6
nerve block (peripheral) (plexus)	T41.3X1	T41.3X2	T41.3X3	T41.3X4	T41.3X5	T41.3X6
spinal	T41.3X1	T41.3X2	T41.3X3	T41.3X4	T41.3X5	T41.3X6
topical (surface)	T41.3X1	T41.3X2	T41.3X3	T41.3X4	T41.3X5	T41.3X6
Amylopectin	T47.6X1	T47.6X2	T47.6X3	T47.6X4	T47.6X5	T47.6X6
Amytal (sodium)	T42.3X1	T42.3X2	T42.3X3	T42.3X4	T42.3X5	T42.3X6
Anabolic steroid	T38.7X1	T38.7X2	T38.7X3	T38.7X4	T38.7X5	T38.7X6
Anacaine*	T41.3X1	T41.3X2	T41.3X3	T41.3X4	T41.3X5	T41.3X6
Analeptic NEC	T50.7X1	T50.7X2	T50.7X3	T50.7X4	T50.7X5	T50.7X6
Analgesic	T39.91	T39.92	T39.93	T39.94	T39.95	T39.96
anti-inflammatory NEC	T39.91	T39.92	T39.93	T39.94	T39.95	T39.96
propionic acid derivative	T39.311	T39.312	T39.313	T39.314	T39.315	T39.316
antirheumatic NEC	T39.4X1	T39.4X2	T39.4X3	T39.4X4	T39.4X5	T39.4X6
aromatic NEC	T39.1X1	T39.1X2	T39.1X3	T39.1X4	T39.1X5	T39.1X6
narcotic NEC	T40.601	T40.602	T40.603	T40.604	T40.605	T40.606
combination	T40.601	T40.602	T40.603	T40.604	T40.605	T40.606
obstetric	T40.601	T40.602	T40.603	T40.604	T40.605	T40.606
non-narcotic NEC	T39.91	T39.92	T39.93	T39.94	T39.95	T39.96
combination	T39.91	T39.92	T39.93	T39.94	T39.95	T39.96
pyrazole	T39.2X1	T39.2X2	T39.2X3	T39.2X4	T39.2X5	T39.2X6
specified NEC	T39.8X1	T39.8X2	T39.8X3	T39.8X4	T39.8X5	T39.8X6
Analgin	T39.2X1	T39.2X2	T39.2X3	T39.2X4	T39.2X5	T39.2X6
Anamirta cocculus	T62.1X1	T62.1X2	T62.1X3	T62.1X4	—	—
Ancillin	T36.0X1	T36.0X2	T36.0X3	T36.0X4	T36.0X5	T36.0X6
Ancrod	T45.691	T45.692	T45.693	T45.694	T45.695	T45.696
Androgen	T38.7X1	T38.7X2	T38.7X3	T38.7X4	T38.7X5	T38.7X6
Androgen-estrogen mixture	T38.7X1	T38.7X2	T38.7X3	T38.7X4	T38.7X5	T38.7X6
Androstalone	T38.7X1	T38.7X2	T38.7X3	T38.7X4	T38.7X5	T38.7X6
Androstanolone	T38.7X1	T38.7X2	T38.7X3	T38.7X4	T38.7X5	T38.7X6
Androsterone	T38.7X1	T38.7X2	T38.7X3	T38.7X4	T38.7X5	T38.7X6
Anemone pulsatilla	T62.2X1	T62.2X2	T62.2X3	T62.2X4	—	—

Substance	Poisoning, Accidental (unintentional)	Poisoning, Intentional Self-harm	Poisoning, Assault	Poisoning, Undetermined	Adverse Effect	Under-dosing
Anesthesia						
caudal	T41.3X1	T41.3X2	T41.3X3	T41.3X4	T41.3X5	T41.3X6
endotracheal	T41.0X1	T41.0X2	T41.0X3	T41.0X4	T41.0X5	T41.0X6
epidural	T41.3X1	T41.3X2	T41.3X3	T41.3X4	T41.3X5	T41.3X6
inhalation	T41.0X1	T41.0X2	T41.0X3	T41.0X4	T41.0X5	T41.0X6
local	T41.3X1	T41.3X2	T41.3X3	T41.3X4	T41.3X5	T41.3X6
mucosal	T41.3X1	T41.3X2	T41.3X3	T41.3X4	T41.3X5	T41.3X6
muscle relaxation	T48.1X1	T48.1X2	T48.1X3	T48.1X4	T48.1X5	T48.1X6
nerve blocking	T41.3X1	T41.3X2	T41.3X3	T41.3X4	T41.3X5	T41.3X6
plexus blocking	T41.3X1	T41.3X2	T41.3X3	T41.3X4	T41.3X5	T41.3X6
potentiated	T41.201	T41.202	T41.203	T41.204	T41.205	T41.206
rectal	T41.201	T41.202	T41.203	T41.204	T41.205	T41.206
general	T41.201	T41.202	T41.203	T41.204	T41.205	T41.206
local	T41.3X1	T41.3X2	T41.3X3	T41.3X4	T41.3X5	T41.3X6
regional	T41.3X1	T41.3X2	T41.3X3	T41.3X4	T41.3X5	T41.3X6
surface	T41.3X1	T41.3X2	T41.3X3	T41.3X4	T41.3X5	T41.3X6
Anesthetic NEC — *see also*	T41.41	T41.42	T41.43	T41.44	T41.45	T41.46
Anesthesia						
with muscle relaxant	T41.201	T41.202	T41.203	T41.204	T41.205	T41.206
general	T41.201	T41.202	T41.203	T41.204	T41.205	T41.206
local	T41.3X1	T41.3X2	T41.3X3	T41.3X4	T41.3X5	T41.3X6
gaseous NEC	T41.0X1	T41.0X2	T41.0X3	T41.0X4	T41.0X5	T41.0X6
general NEC	T41.201	T41.202	T41.203	T41.204	T41.205	T41.206
halogenated hydrocarbon derivatives NEC	T41.0X1	T41.0X2	T41.0X3	T41.0X4	T41.0X5	T41.0X6
infiltration NEC	T41.3X1	T41.3X2	T41.3X3	T41.3X4	T41.3X5	T41.3X6
intravenous NEC	T41.1X1	T41.1X2	T41.1X3	T41.1X4	T41.1X5	T41.1X6
local NEC	T41.3X1	T41.3X2	T41.3X3	T41.3X4	T41.3X5	T41.3X6
rectal	T41.201	T41.202	T41.203	T41.204	T41.205	T41.206
general	T41.201	T41.202	T41.203	T41.204	T41.205	T41.206
local	T41.3X1	T41.3X2	T41.3X3	T41.3X4	T41.3X5	T41.3X6
regional NEC	T41.3X1	T41.3X2	T41.3X3	T41.3X4	T41.3X5	T41.3X6
spinal NEC	T41.3X1	T41.3X2	T41.3X3	T41.3X4	T41.3X5	T41.3X6
thiobarbiturate	T41.1X1	T41.1X2	T41.1X3	T41.1X4	T41.1X5	T41.1X6
topical	T41.3X1	T41.3X2	T41.3X3	T41.3X4	T41.3X5	T41.3X6
Aneurine	T45.2X1	T45.2X2	T45.2X3	T45.2X4	T45.2X5	T45.2X6
Angelia*	T38.5X1	T38.5X2	T38.5X3	T38.5X4	T38.5X5	T38.5X6
Angio-Conray	T50.8X1	T50.8X2	T50.8X3	T50.8X4	T50.8X5	T50.8X6
Angiotensin	T44.5X1	T44.5X2	T44.5X3	T44.5X4	T44.5X5	T44.5X6
Angiotensinamide	T44.991	T44.992	T44.993	T44.994	T44.995	T44.996
Anhydrohydroxy-progesterone	T38.5X1	T38.5X2	T38.5X3	T38.5X4	T38.5X5	T38.5X6
Anhydron	T50.2X1	T50.2X2	T50.2X3	T50.2X4	T50.2X5	T50.2X6
Anileridine	T40.491	T40.492	T40.493	T40.494	T40.495	T40.496
Aniline (dye) (liquid)	T65.3X1	T65.3X2	T65.3X3	T65.3X4		
analgesic	T39.1X1	T39.1X2	T39.1X3	T39.1X4	T39.1X5	T39.1X6
derivatives, therapeutic NEC	T39.1X1	T39.1X2	T39.1X3	T39.1X4	T39.1X5	T39.1X6
vapor	T65.3X1	T65.3X2	T65.3X3	T65.3X4	—	—
Aniscoropine	T44.3X1	T44.3X2	T44.3X3	T44.3X4	T44.3X5	T44.3X6
Anise oil	T47.5X1	T47.5X2	T47.5X3	T47.5X4	T47.5X5	T47.5X6
Anisidine	T65.3X1	T65.3X2	T65.3X3	T65.3X4	—	—
Anisindione	T45.511	T45.512	T45.513	T45.514	T45.515	T45.516
Anisotropine methyl-bromide	T44.3X1	T44.3X2	T44.3X3	T44.3X4	T44.3X5	T44.3X6
Anistreplase	T45.611	T45.612	T45.613	T45.614	T45.615	T45.616
Anorexiant (central)	T50.5X1	T50.5X2	T50.5X3	T50.5X4	T50.5X5	T50.5X6
Anorexic agents	T50.5X1	T50.5X2	T50.5X3	T50.5X4	T50.5X5	T50.5X6
Ansaid*	T39.311	T39.312	T39.313	T39.314	T39.315	T39.316
Ansamycin	T36.6X1	T36.6X2	T36.6X3	T36.6X4	T36.6X5	T36.6X6
Ant (bite) (sting)	T63.421	T63.422	T63.423	T63.424	—	—
Antabuse	T50.6X1	T50.6X2	T50.6X3	T50.6X4	T50.6X5	T50.6X6
Antacid NEC	T47.1X1	T47.1X2	T47.1X3	T47.1X4	T47.1X5	T47.1X6
Antagonist						
Aldosterone	T50.0X1	T50.0X2	T50.0X3	T50.0X4	T50.0X5	T50.0X6
alpha-adrenoreceptor	T44.6X1	T44.6X2	T44.6X3	T44.6X4	T44.6X5	T44.6X6
anticoagulant	T45.7X1	T45.7X2	T45.7X3	T45.7X4	T45.7X5	T45.7X6
beta-adrenoreceptor	T44.7X1	T44.7X2	T44.7X3	T44.7X4	T44.7X5	T44.7X6
extrapyramidal NEC	T44.3X1	T44.3X2	T44.3X3	T44.3X4	T44.3X5	T44.3X6
folic acid	T45.1X1	T45.1X2	T45.1X3	T45.1X4	T45.1X5	T45.1X6
H2 receptor	T47.0X1	T47.0X2	T47.0X3	T47.0X4	T47.0X5	T47.0X6
heavy metal	T45.8X1	T45.8X2	T45.8X3	T45.8X4	T45.8X5	T45.8X6
narcotic analgesic	T50.7X1	T50.7X2	T50.7X3	T50.7X4	T50.7X5	T50.7X6
opiate	T50.7X1	T50.7X2	T50.7X3	T50.7X4	T50.7X5	T50.7X6
pyrimidine	T45.1X1	T45.1X2	T45.1X3	T45.1X4	T45.1X5	T45.1X6
serotonin	T46.5X1	T46.5X2	T46.5X3	T46.5X4	T46.5X5	T46.5X6
Antazolin (e)	T45.0X1	T45.0X2	T45.0X3	T45.0X4	T45.0X5	T45.0X6
Anterior pituitary hormone NEC	T38.811	T38.812	T38.813	T38.814	T38.815	T38.816
Anthelmintic NEC	T37.4X1	T37.4X2	T37.4X3	T37.4X4	T37.4X5	T37.4X6
Anthiolimine	T37.4X1	T37.4X2	T37.4X3	T37.4X4	T37.4X5	T37.4X6
Anthralin	T49.4X1	T49.4X2	T49.4X3	T49.4X4	T49.4X5	T49.4X6
Anthramycin	T45.1X1	T45.1X2	T45.1X3	T45.1X4	T45.1X5	T45.1X6
Antiadrenergic NEC	T44.8X1	T44.8X2	T44.8X3	T44.8X4	T44.8X5	T44.8X6

Substance	Poisoning, Accidental (unintentional)	Poisoning, Intentional Self-harm	Poisoning, Assault	Poisoning, Undetermined	Adverse Effect	Under-dosing
Antiallergic NEC	T45.0X1	T45.0X2	T45.0X3	T45.0X4	T45.0X5	T45.0X6
Antiandrogen NEC	T38.6X1	T38.6X2	T38.6X3	T38.6X4	T38.6X5	T38.6X6
Anti-anemic (drug)	T45.8X1	T45.8X2	T45.8X3	T45.8X4	T45.8X5	T45.8X6
(preparation)						
Antianxiety drug NEC	T43.501	T43.502	T43.503	T43.504	T43.505	T43.506
Antiaris toxicaria	T65.891	T65.892	T65.893	T65.894	—	—
Antiarteriosclerotic drug	T46.6X1	T46.6X2	T46.6X3	T46.6X4	T46.6X5	T46.6X6
Antiasthmatic drug NEC	T48.6X1	T48.6X2	T48.6X3	T48.6X4	T48.6X5	T48.6X6
Antibiotic Otic Suspension (Solution)*	T49.6X1	T49.6X2	T49.6X3	T49.6X4	T49.6X5	T49.6X6
Antibiotic NEC	T36.91	T36.92	T36.93	T36.94	T36.95	T36.96
aminoglycoside	T36.5X1	T36.5X2	T36.5X3	T36.5X4	T36.5X5	T36.5X6
anticancer	T45.1X1	T45.1X2	T45.1X3	T45.1X4	T45.1X5	T45.1X6
antifungal	T36.7X1	T36.7X2	T36.7X3	T36.7X4	T36.7X5	T36.7X6
antimycobacterial	T36.5X1	T36.5X2	T36.5X3	T36.5X4	T36.5X5	T36.5X6
antineoplastic	T45.1X1	T45.1X2	T45.1X3	T45.1X4	T45.1X5	T45.1X6
b-lactam NEC	T36.1X1	T36.1X2	T36.1X3	T36.1X4	T36.1X5	T36.1X6
cephalosporin (group)	T36.1X1	T36.1X2	T36.1X3	T36.1X4	T36.1X5	T36.1X6
chloramphenicol (group)	T36.2X1	T36.2X2	T36.2X3	T36.2X4	T36.2X5	T36.2X6
ENT	T49.6X1	T49.6X2	T49.6X3	T49.6X4	T49.6X5	T49.6X6
eye	T49.5X1	T49.5X2	T49.5X3	T49.5X4	T49.5X5	T49.5X6
fungicidal (local)	T49.0X1	T49.0X2	T49.0X3	T49.0X4	T49.0X5	T49.0X6
intestinal	T36.8X1	T36.8X2	T36.8X3	T36.8X4	T36.8X5	T36.8X6
local	T49.0X1	T49.0X2	T49.0X3	T49.0X4	T49.0X5	T49.0X6
macrolides	T36.3X1	T36.3X2	T36.3X3	T36.3X4	T36.3X5	T36.3X6
polypeptide	T36.8X1	T36.8X2	T36.8X3	T36.8X4	T36.8X5	T36.8X6
specified NEC	T36.8X1	T36.8X2	T36.8X3	T36.8X4	T36.8X5	T36.8X6
tetracycline (group)	T36.4X1	T36.4X2	T36.4X3	T36.4X4	T36.4X5	T36.4X6
throat	T49.6X1	T49.6X2	T49.6X3	T49.6X4	T49.6X5	T49.6X6
Anticancer agents NEC	T45.1X1	T45.1X2	T45.1X3	T45.1X4	T45.1X5	T45.1X6
Anticholesterolemic drug NEC	T46.6X1	T46.6X2	T46.6X3	T46.6X4	T46.6X5	T46.6X6
Anticholinergic NEC	T44.3X1	T44.3X2	T44.3X3	T44.3X4	T44.3X5	T44.3X6
Anticholinesterase	T44.0X1	T44.0X2	T44.0X3	T44.0X4	T44.0X5	T44.0X6
organophosphorus	T44.0X1	T44.0X2	T44.0X3	T44.0X4	T44.0X5	T44.0X6
insecticide	T60.0X1	T60.0X2	T60.0X3	T60.0X4		
nerve gas	T59.891	T59.892	T59.893	T59.894	—	—
reversible	T44.0X1	T44.0X2	T44.0X3	T44.0X4	T44.0X5	T44.0X6
ophthalmological	T49.5X1	T49.5X2	T49.5X3	T49.5X4	T49.5X5	T49.5X6
Anticoagulant NEC	T45.511	T45.512	T45.513	T45.514	T45.515	T45.516
Antagonist	T45.7X1	T45.7X2	T45.7X3	T45.7X4	T45.7X5	T45.7X6
Anti-common-cold drug NEC	T48.5X1	T48.5X2	T48.5X3	T48.5X4	T48.5X5	T48.5X6
Anticonvulsant	T42.71	T42.72	T42.73	T42.74	T42.75	T42.76
barbiturate	T42.3X1	T42.3X2	T42.3X3	T42.3X4	T42.3X5	T42.3X6
combination (with barbiturate)	T42.3X1	T42.3X2	T42.3X3	T42.3X4	T42.3X5	T42.3X6
hydantoin	T42.0X1	T42.0X2	T42.0X3	T42.0X4	T42.0X5	T42.0X6
hypnotic NEC	T42.6X1	T42.6X2	T42.6X3	T42.6X4	T42.6X5	T42.6X6
oxazolidinedione	T42.2X1	T42.2X2	T42.2X3	T42.2X4	T42.2X5	T42.2X6
pyrimidinedione	T42.6X1	T42.6X2	T42.6X3	T42.6X4	T42.6X5	T42.6X6
specified NEC	T42.6X1	T42.6X2	T42.6X3	T42.6X4	T42.6X5	T42.6X6
succinimide	T42.2X1	T42.2X2	T42.2X3	T42.2X4	T42.2X5	T42.2X6
Antidepressant	T43.201	T43.202	T43.203	T43.204	T43.205	T43.206
monoamine oxidase inhibitor	T43.1X1	T43.1X2	T43.1X3	T43.1X4	T43.1X5	T43.1X6
selective serotonin norepinephrine reuptake inhibitor	T43.211	T43.212	T43.213	T43.214	T43.215	T43.216
selective serotonin reuptake inhibitor	T43.221	T43.222	T43.223	T43.224	T43.225	T43.226
specified NEC	T43.291	T43.292	T43.293	T43.294	T43.295	T43.296
tetracyclic	T43.021	T43.022	T43.023	T43.024	T43.025	T43.026
triazolopyridine	T43.211	T43.212	T43.213	T43.214	T43.215	T43.216
tricyclic	T43.011	T43.012	T43.013	T43.014	T43.015	T43.016
Antidiabetic NEC	T38.3X1	T38.3X2	T38.3X3	T38.3X4	T38.3X5	T38.3X6
biguanide	T38.3X1	T38.3X2	T38.3X3	T38.3X4	T38.3X5	T38.3X6
and sulfonyl combined	T38.3X1	T38.3X2	T38.3X3	T38.3X4	T38.3X5	T38.3X6
combined	T38.3X1	T38.3X2	T38.3X3	T38.3X4	T38.3X5	T38.3X6
sulfonylurea	T38.3X1	T38.3X2	T38.3X3	T38.3X4	T38.3X5	T38.3X6
Antidiarrheal drug NEC	T47.6X1	T47.6X2	T47.6X3	T47.6X4	T47.6X5	T47.6X6
absorbent	T47.6X1	T47.6X2	T47.6X3	T47.6X4	T47.6X5	T47.6X6
Anti-D immunoglobulin (human)	T50.Z11	T50.Z12	T50.Z13	T50.Z14	T50.Z15	T50.Z16
Antidiphtheria serum	T50.Z11	T50.Z12	T50.Z13	T50.Z14	T50.Z15	T50.Z16
Antidiuretic hormone	T38.891	T38.892	T38.893	T38.894	T38.895	T38.896
Antidote NEC	T50.6X1	T50.6X2	T50.6X3	T50.6X4	T50.6X5	T50.6X6
heavy metal	T45.8X1	T45.8X2	T45.8X3	T45.8X4	T45.8X5	T45.8X6
Antidysrhythmic NEC	T46.2X1	T46.2X2	T46.2X3	T46.2X4	T46.2X5	T46.2X6
Antiemetic drug	T45.0X1	T45.0X2	T45.0X3	T45.0X4	T45.0X5	T45.0X6
Antiepilepsy agent	T42.71	T42.72	T42.73	T42.74	T42.75	T42.76
combination	T42.5X1	T42.5X2	T42.5X3	T42.5X4	T42.5X5	T42.5X6
mixed	T42.5X1	T42.5X2	T42.5X3	T42.5X4	T42.5X5	T42.5X6

☑ Additional Character May Be Required — Refer to the Tabular List for Character Selection

*Optum Value-Add

Substance	Poisoning, Accidental (unintentional)	Poisoning, Intentional Self-harm	Poisoning, Assault	Poisoning, Undetermined	Adverse Effect	Under-dosing
Antiepilepsy agent — *continued*						
specified, NEC	T42.6X1	T42.6X2	T42.6X3	T42.6X4	T42.6X5	T42.6X6
Antiestrogen NEC	T38.6X1	T38.6X2	T38.6X3	T38.6X4	T38.6X5	T38.6X6
Antifertility pill	T38.4X1	T38.4X2	T38.4X3	T38.4X4	T38.4X5	T38.4X6
Antifibrinolytic drug	T45.621	T45.622	T45.623	T45.624	T45.625	T45.626
Antifilarial drug	T37.4X1	T37.4X2	T37.4X3	T37.4X4	T37.4X5	T37.4X6
Antiflatulent	T47.5X1	T47.5X2	T47.5X3	T47.5X4	T47.5X5	T47.5X6
Antifreeze	T65.91	T65.92	T65.93	T65.94	—	—
alcohol	T51.1X1	T51.1X2	T51.1X3	T51.1X4	—	—
ethylene glycol	T51.8X1	T51.8X2	T51.8X3	T51.8X4	—	—
Antifungal						
antibiotic (systemic)	T36.7X1	T36.7X2	T36.7X3	T36.7X4	T36.7X5	T36.7X6
anti-infective NEC	T37.91	T37.92	T37.93	T37.94	T37.95	T37.96
disinfectant, local	T49.0X1	T49.0X2	T49.0X3	T49.0X4	T49.0X5	T49.0X6
nonmedicinal (spray)	T60.3X1	T60.3X2	T60.3X3	T60.3X4	—	—
topical	T49.0X1	T49.0X2	T49.0X3	T49.0X4	T49.0X5	T49.0X6
Anti-gastric-secretion drug NEC	T47.1X1	T47.1X2	T47.1X3	T47.1X4	T47.1X5	T47.1X6
Antigonadotrophin NEC	T38.6X1	T38.6X2	T38.6X3	T38.6X4	T38.6X5	T38.6X6
Antihallucinogen	T43.501	T43.502	T43.503	T43.504	T43.505	T43.506
Antihelmintics	T37.4X1	T37.4X2	T37.4X3	T37.4X4	T37.4X5	T37.4X6
Antihemophilic						
factor	T45.8X1	T45.8X2	T45.8X3	T45.8X4	T45.8X5	T45.8X6
fraction	T45.8X1	T45.8X2	T45.8X3	T45.8X4	T45.8X5	T45.8X6
globulin concentrate	T45.7X1	T45.7X2	T45.7X3	T45.7X4	T45.7X5	T45.7X6
human plasma	T45.8X1	T45.8X2	T45.8X3	T45.8X4	T45.8X5	T45.8X6
plasma, dried	T45.7X1	T45.7X2	T45.7X3	T45.7X4	T45.7X5	T45.7X6
Antihemorrhoidal preparation	T49.2X1	T49.2X2	T49.2X3	T49.2X4	T49.2X5	T49.2X6
Antiheparin drug	T45.7X1	T45.7X2	T45.7X3	T45.7X4	T45.7X5	T45.7X6
Antihistamine	T45.0X1	T45.0X2	T45.0X3	T45.0X4	T45.0X5	T45.0X6
Antihookworm drug	T37.4X1	T37.4X2	T37.4X3	T37.4X4	T37.4X5	T37.4X6
Anti-human lymphocytic globulin	T50.Z11	T50.Z12	T50.Z13	T50.Z14	T50.Z15	T50.Z16
Antihyperlipidemic drug	T46.6X1	T46.6X2	T46.6X3	T46.6X4	T46.6X5	T46.6X6
Antihypertensive drug NEC	T46.5X1	T46.5X2	T46.5X3	T46.5X4	T46.5X5	T46.5X6
Anti-infective NEC	T37.91	T37.92	T37.93	T37.94	T37.95	T37.96
anthelmintic	T37.4X1	T37.4X2	T37.4X3	T37.4X4	T37.4X5	T37.4X6
antibiotics	T36.91	T36.92	T36.93	T36.94	T36.95	T36.96
specified NEC	T36.8X1	T36.8X2	T36.8X3	T36.8X4	T36.8X5	T36.8X6
antimalarial	T37.2X1	T37.2X2	T37.2X3	T37.2X4	T37.2X5	T37.2X6
antimycobacterial NEC	T37.1X1	T37.1X2	T37.1X3	T37.1X4	T37.1X5	T37.1X6
antibiotics	T36.5X1	T36.5X2	T36.5X3	T36.5X4	T36.5X5	T36.5X6
antiprotozoal NEC	T37.3X1	T37.3X2	T37.3X3	T37.3X4	T37.3X5	T37.3X6
blood	T37.2X1	T37.2X2	T37.2X3	T37.2X4	T37.2X5	T37.2X6
antiviral	T37.5X1	T37.5X2	T37.5X3	T37.5X4	T37.5X5	T37.5X6
arsenical	T37.8X1	T37.8X2	T37.8X3	T37.8X4	T37.8X5	T37.8X6
bismuth, local	T49.0X1	T49.0X2	T49.0X3	T49.0X4	T49.0X5	T49.0X6
ENT	T49.6X1	T49.6X2	T49.6X3	T49.6X4	T49.6X5	T49.6X6
eye NEC	T49.5X1	T49.5X2	T49.5X3	T49.5X4	T49.5X5	T49.5X6
heavy metals NEC	T37.8X1	T37.8X2	T37.8X3	T37.8X4	T37.8X5	T37.8X6
local NEC	T49.0X1	T49.0X2	T49.0X3	T49.0X4	T49.0X5	T49.0X6
specified NEC	T49.0X1	T49.0X2	T49.0X3	T49.0X4	T49.0X5	T49.0X6
mixed	T37.91	T37.92	T37.93	T37.94	T37.95	T37.96
ophthalmic preparation	T49.5X1	T49.5X2	T49.5X3	T49.5X4	T49.5X5	T49.5X6
topical NEC	T49.0X1	T49.0X2	T49.0X3	T49.0X4	T49.0X5	T49.0X6
Anti-inflammatory drug NEC	T39.391	T39.392	T39.393	T39.394	T39.395	T39.396
local	T49.0X1	T49.0X2	T49.0X3	T49.0X4	T49.0X5	T49.0X6
nonsteroidal NEC	T39.391	T39.392	T39.393	T39.394	T39.395	T39.396
propionic acid derivative	T39.311	T39.312	T39.313	T39.314	T39.315	T39.316
specified NEC	T39.391	T39.392	T39.393	T39.394	T39.395	T39.396
Antikaluretic	T50.3X1	T50.3X2	T50.3X3	T50.3X4	T50.3X5	T50.3X6
Antiknock (tetraethyl lead)	T56.0X1	T56.0X2	T56.0X3	T56.0X4	—	—
Antilipemic drug NEC	T46.6X1	T46.6X2	T46.6X3	T46.6X4	T46.6X5	T46.6X6
Antilysin*	T45.621	T45.622	T45.623	T45.624	T45.625	T45.626
Antimalarial	T37.2X1	T37.2X2	T37.2X3	T37.2X4	T37.2X5	T37.2X6
prophylactic NEC	T37.2X1	T37.2X2	T37.2X3	T37.2X4	T37.2X5	T37.2X6
pyrimidine derivative	T37.2X1	T37.2X2	T37.2X3	T37.2X4	T37.2X5	T37.2X6
Antimetabolite	T45.1X1	T45.1X2	T45.1X3	T45.1X4	T45.1X5	T45.1X6
Antimitotic agent	T45.1X1	T45.1X2	T45.1X3	T45.1X4	T45.1X5	T45.1X6
Antimony (compounds) (vapor) NEC	T56.891	T56.892	T56.893	T56.894	—	—
anti-infectives	T37.8X1	T37.8X2	T37.8X3	T37.8X4	T37.8X5	T37.8X6
dimercaptosuccinate	T37.3X1	T37.3X2	T37.3X3	T37.3X4	T37.3X5	T37.3X6
hydride	T56.891	T56.892	T56.893	T56.894	—	—
pesticide (vapor)	T60.8X1	T60.8X2	T60.8X3	T60.8X4	—	—
potassium (sodium) tartrate	T37.8X1	T37.8X2	T37.8X3	T37.8X4	T37.8X5	T37.8X6
sodium dimercaptosuccinate	T37.3X1	T37.3X2	T37.3X3	T37.3X4	T37.3X5	T37.3X6
tartrated	T37.8X1	T37.8X2	T37.8X3	T37.8X4	T37.8X5	T37.8X6

Substance	Poisoning, Accidental (unintentional)	Poisoning, Intentional Self-harm	Poisoning, Assault	Poisoning, Undetermined	Adverse Effect	Under-dosing
Antimuscarinic NEC	T44.3X1	T44.3X2	T44.3X3	T44.3X4	T44.3X5	T44.3X6
Antimycobacterial drug NEC	T37.1X1	T37.1X2	T37.1X3	T37.1X4	T37.1X5	T37.1X6
antibiotics	T36.5X1	T36.5X2	T36.5X3	T36.5X4	T36.5X5	T36.5X6
combination	T37.1X1	T37.1X2	T37.1X3	T37.1X4	T37.1X5	T37.1X6
Antinausea drug	T45.0X1	T45.0X2	T45.0X3	T45.0X4	T45.0X5	T45.0X6
Antinematode drug	T37.4X1	T37.4X2	T37.4X3	T37.4X4	T37.4X5	T37.4X6
Antineoplastic NEC	T45.1X1	T45.1X2	T45.1X3	T45.1X4	T45.1X5	T45.1X6
alkaloidal	T45.1X1	T45.1X2	T45.1X3	T45.1X4	T45.1X5	T45.1X6
antibiotics	T45.1X1	T45.1X2	T45.1X3	T45.1X4	T45.1X5	T45.1X6
combination	T45.1X1	T45.1X2	T45.1X3	T45.1X4	T45.1X5	T45.1X6
estrogen	T38.5X1	T38.5X2	T38.5X3	T38.5X4	T38.5X5	T38.5X6
steroid	T38.7X1	T38.7X2	T38.7X3	T38.7X4	T38.7X5	T38.7X6
Antiparasitic drug (systemic)	T37.91	T37.92	T37.93	T37.94	T37.95	T37.96
local	T49.0X1	T49.0X2	T49.0X3	T49.0X4	T49.0X5	T49.0X6
specified NEC	T37.8X1	T37.8X2	T37.8X3	T37.8X4	T37.8X5	T37.8X6
Antiparkinsonism drug NEC	T42.8X1	T42.8X2	T42.8X3	T42.8X4	T42.8X5	T42.8X6
Antiperspirant NEC	T49.2X1	T49.2X2	T49.2X3	T49.2X4	T49.2X5	T49.2X6
Antiphlogistic NEC	T39.4X1	T39.4X2	T39.4X3	T39.4X4	T39.4X5	T39.4X6
Antiplatyhelmintic drug	T37.4X1	T37.4X2	T37.4X3	T37.4X4	T37.4X5	T37.4X6
Antiprotozoal drug NEC	T37.3X1	T37.3X2	T37.3X3	T37.3X4	T37.3X5	T37.3X6
blood	T37.2X1	T37.2X2	T37.2X3	T37.2X4	T37.2X5	T37.2X6
local	T49.0X1	T49.0X2	T49.0X3	T49.0X4	T49.0X5	T49.0X6
Antipruritic drug NEC	T49.1X1	T49.1X2	T49.1X3	T49.1X4	T49.1X5	T49.1X6
Antipsychotic drug	T43.501	T43.502	T43.503	T43.504	T43.505	T43.506
specified NEC	T43.591	T43.592	T43.593	T43.594	T43.595	T43.596
Antipyretic	T39.91	T39.92	T39.93	T39.94	T39.95	T39.96
specified NEC	T39.8X1	T39.8X2	T39.8X3	T39.8X4	T39.8X5	T39.8X6
Antipyrine	T39.2X1	T39.2X2	T39.2X3	T39.2X4	T39.2X5	T39.2X6
Antirabies hyperimmune serum	T50.Z11	T50.Z12	T50.Z13	T50.Z14	T50.Z15	T50.Z16
Antirheumatic NEC	T39.4X1	T39.4X2	T39.4X3	T39.4X4	T39.4X5	T39.4X6
Antirigidity drug NEC	T42.8X1	T42.8X2	T42.8X3	T42.8X4	T42.8X5	T42.8X6
Antischistosomal drug	T37.4X1	T37.4X2	T37.4X3	T37.4X4	T37.4X5	T37.4X6
Antiscorpion sera	T50.Z11	T50.Z12	T50.Z13	T50.Z14	T50.Z15	T50.Z16
Antiseborrheics	T49.4X1	T49.4X2	T49.4X3	T49.4X4	T49.4X5	T49.4X6
Antiseptics (external) (medicinal)	T49.0X1	T49.0X2	T49.0X3	T49.0X4	T49.0X5	T49.0X6
Antistine	T45.0X1	T45.0X2	T45.0X3	T45.0X4	T45.0X5	T45.0X6
Antitapeworm drug	T37.4X1	T37.4X2	T37.4X3	T37.4X4	T37.4X5	T37.4X6
Antitetanus immunoglobulin	T50.Z11	T50.Z12	T50.Z13	T50.Z14	T50.Z15	T50.Z16
Antithrombin III*	T45.511	T45.512	T45.513	T45.514	T45.515	T45.516
Antithrombotic	T45.521	T45.522	T45.523	T45.524	T45.525	T45.526
Antithyroid drug NEC	T38.2X1	T38.2X2	T38.2X3	T38.2X4	T38.2X5	T38.2X6
Antitoxin	T50.Z11	T50.Z12	T50.Z13	T50.Z14	T50.Z15	T50.Z16
diphtheria	T50.Z11	T50.Z12	T50.Z13	T50.Z14	T50.Z15	T50.Z16
gas gangrene	T50.Z11	T50.Z12	T50.Z13	T50.Z14	T50.Z15	T50.Z16
tetanus	T50.Z11	T50.Z12	T50.Z13	T50.Z14	T50.Z15	T50.Z16
Antitrichomonal drug	T37.3X1	T37.3X2	T37.3X3	T37.3X4	T37.3X5	T37.3X6
Antituberculars	T37.1X1	T37.1X2	T37.1X3	T37.1X4	T37.1X5	T37.1X6
antibiotics	T36.5X1	T36.5X2	T36.5X3	T36.5X4	T36.5X5	T36.5X6
Antitussive NEC	T48.3X1	T48.3X2	T48.3X3	T48.3X4	T48.3X5	T48.3X6
codeine mixture	T40.2X1	T40.2X2	T40.2X3	T40.2X4	T40.2X5	T40.2X6
opiate	T40.2X1	T40.2X2	T40.2X3	T40.2X4	T40.2X5	T40.2X6
Antivaricose drug	T46.8X1	T46.8X2	T46.8X3	T46.8X4	T46.8X5	T46.8X6
Antivenin, antivenom (sera)	T50.Z11	T50.Z12	T50.Z13	T50.Z14	T50.Z15	T50.Z16
crotaline	T50.Z11	T50.Z12	T50.Z13	T50.Z14	T50.Z15	T50.Z16
spider bite	T50.Z11	T50.Z12	T50.Z13	T50.Z14	T50.Z15	T50.Z16
Antivert*	T45.0X1	T45.0X2	T45.0X3	T45.0X4	T45.0X5	T45.0X6
Antivertigo drug	T45.0X1	T45.0X2	T45.0X3	T45.0X4	T45.0X5	T45.0X6
Antiviral drug NEC	T37.5X1	T37.5X2	T37.5X3	T37.5X4	T37.5X5	T37.5X6
eye	T49.5X1	T49.5X2	T49.5X3	T49.5X4	T49.5X5	T49.5X6
Antiwhipworm drug	T37.4X1	T37.4X2	T37.4X3	T37.4X4	T37.4X5	T37.4X6
Ant poison — *see* Insecticide						
Antrol — *see also* by specific chemical substance	T60.91	T60.92	T60.93	T60.94	—	—
fungicide	T60.91	T60.92	T60.93	T60.94	—	—
ANTU (alpha naphthylthiourea)	T60.4X1	T60.4X2	T60.4X3	T60.4X4	—	—
Apalcillin	T36.0X1	T36.0X2	T36.0X3	T36.0X4	T36.0X5	T36.0X6
APC	T48.5X1	T48.5X2	T48.5X3	T48.5X4	T48.5X5	T48.5X6
Aplonidine	T44.4X1	T44.4X2	T44.4X3	T44.4X4	T44.4X5	T44.4X6
Apomorphine	T47.7X1	T47.7X2	T47.7X3	T47.7X4	T47.7X5	T47.7X6
Appetite depressants, central	T50.5X1	T50.5X2	T50.5X3	T50.5X4	T50.5X5	T50.5X6
Apraclonidine (hydrochloride)	T44.4X1	T44.4X2	T44.4X3	T44.4X4	T44.4X5	T44.4X6
Apresoline	T46.5X1	T46.5X2	T46.5X3	T46.5X4	T46.5X5	T46.5X6
Apri*	T38.4X1	T38.4X2	T38.4X3	T38.4X4	T38.4X5	T38.4X6

Substance	Poisoning, Accidental (unintentional)	Poisoning, Intentional Self-harm	Poisoning, Assault	Poisoning, Undetermined	Adverse Effect	Under-dosing
Aprindine	T46.2X1	T46.2X2	T46.2X3	T46.2X4	T46.2X5	T46.2X6
Aprobarbital	T42.3X1	T42.3X2	T42.3X3	T42.3X4	T42.3X5	T42.3X6
Apronalide	T42.6X1	T42.6X2	T42.6X3	T42.6X4	T42.6X5	T42.6X6
Aprotinin	T45.621	T45.622	T45.623	T45.624	T45.625	T45.626
Aptocaine	T41.3X1	T41.3X2	T41.3X3	T41.3X4	T41.3X5	T41.3X6
Aqua fortis	T54.2X1	T54.2X2	T54.2X3	T54.2X4	—	—
Ara-A	T37.5X1	T37.5X2	T37.5X3	T37.5X4	T37.5X5	T37.5X6
Ara-C	T45.1X1	T45.1X2	T45.1X3	T45.1X4	T45.1X5	T45.1X6
Arachis oil	T49.3X1	T49.3X2	T49.3X3	T49.3X4	T49.3X5	T49.3X6
cathartic	T47.4X1	T47.4X2	T47.4X3	T47.4X4	T47.4X5	T47.4X6
Aralen	T37.2X1	T37.2X2	T37.2X3	T37.2X4	T37.2X5	T37.2X6
Arecoline	T44.1X1	T44.1X2	T44.1X3	T44.1X4	T44.1X5	T44.1X6
Arginine	T50.991	T50.992	T50.993	T50.994	T50.995	T50.996
glutamate	T50.991	T50.992	T50.993	T50.994	T50.995	T50.996
Argyrol	T49.0X1	T49.0X2	T49.0X3	T49.0X4	T49.0X5	T49.0X6
ENT agent	T49.6X1	T49.6X2	T49.6X3	T49.6X4	T49.6X5	T49.6X6
ophthalmic preparation	T49.5X1	T49.5X2	T49.5X3	T49.5X4	T49.5X5	T49.5X6
Aristocort	T38.0X1	T38.0X2	T38.0X3	T38.0X4	T38.0X5	T38.0X6
ENT agent	T49.6X1	T49.6X2	T49.6X3	T49.6X4	T49.6X5	T49.6X6
ophthalmic preparation	T49.5X1	T49.5X2	T49.5X3	T49.5X4	T49.5X5	T49.5X6
topical NEC	T49.0X1	T49.0X2	T49.0X3	T49.0X4	T49.0X5	T49.0X6
Aromatics, corrosive	T54.1X1	T54.1X2	T54.1X3	T54.1X4	—	—
disinfectants	T54.1X1	T54.1X2	T54.1X3	T54.1X4	—	—
Arsenate of lead	T57.0X1	T57.0X2	T57.0X3	T57.0X4	—	—
herbicide	T57.0X1	T57.0X2	T57.0X3	T57.0X4	—	—
Arsenic, arsenicals (compounds) (dust) (vapor) NEC	T57.0X1	T57.0X2	T57.0X3	T57.0X4	—	—
anti-infectives	T37.8X1	T37.8X2	T37.8X3	T37.8X4	T37.8X5	T37.8X6
pesticide (dust) (fumes)	T57.0X1	T57.0X2	T57.0X3	T57.0X4	—	—
Arsine (gas)	T57.0X1	T57.0X2	T57.0X3	T57.0X4	—	—
Arsobal*	T37.3X1	T37.3X2	T37.3X3	T37.3X4	T37.3X5	T37.3X6
Arsphenamine (silver)	T37.8X1	T37.8X2	T37.8X3	T37.8X4	T37.8X5	T37.8X6
Arsthinol	T37.3X1	T37.3X2	T37.3X3	T37.3X4	T37.3X5	T37.3X6
Artane	T44.3X1	T44.3X2	T44.3X3	T44.3X4	T44.3X5	T44.3X6
Arthropod (venomous) NEC	T63.481	T63.482	T63.483	T63.484	—	—
Articaine	T41.3X1	T41.3X2	T41.3X3	T41.3X4	T41.3X5	T41.3X6
Asbestos	T57.8X1	T57.8X2	T57.8X3	T57.8X4	—	—
Ascaridole	T37.4X1	T37.4X2	T37.4X3	T37.4X4	T37.4X5	T37.4X6
Ascorbic acid	T45.2X1	T45.2X2	T45.2X3	T45.2X4	T45.2X5	T45.2X6
Asiaticoside	T49.0X1	T49.0X2	T49.0X3	T49.0X4	T49.0X5	T49.0X6
Asparaginase	T45.1X1	T45.1X2	T45.1X3	T45.1X4	T45.1X5	T45.1X6
Aspidium (oleoresin)	T37.4X1	T37.4X2	T37.4X3	T37.4X4	T37.4X5	T37.4X6
Aspirin (aluminum) (soluble)	T39.011	T39.012	T39.013	T39.014	T39.015	T39.016
Aspoxicillin	T36.0X1	T36.0X2	T36.0X3	T36.0X4	T36.0X5	T36.0X6
Astemizole	T45.0X1	T45.0X2	T45.0X3	T45.0X4	T45.0X5	T45.0X6
Astringent (local)	T49.2X1	T49.2X2	T49.2X3	T49.2X4	T49.2X5	T49.2X6
specified NEC	T49.2X1	T49.2X2	T49.2X3	T49.2X4	T49.2X5	T49.2X6
Astromicin	T36.5X1	T36.5X2	T36.5X3	T36.5X4	T36.5X5	T36.5X6
Ataractic drug NEC	T43.501	T43.502	T43.503	T43.504	T43.505	T43.506
Atenolol	T44.7X1	T44.7X2	T44.7X3	T44.7X4	T44.7X5	T44.7X6
Atonia drug, intestinal	T47.4X1	T47.4X2	T47.4X3	T47.4X4	T47.4X5	T47.4X6
Atophan	T50.4X1	T50.4X2	T50.4X3	T50.4X4	T50.4X5	T50.4X6
Atracurium besilate	T48.1X1	T48.1X2	T48.1X3	T48.1X4	T48.1X5	T48.1X6
Atropine	T44.3X1	T44.3X2	T44.3X3	T44.3X4	T44.3X5	T44.3X6
derivative	T44.3X1	T44.3X2	T44.3X3	T44.3X4	T44.3X5	T44.3X6
methonitrate	T44.3X1	T44.3X2	T44.3X3	T44.3X4	T44.3X5	T44.3X6
Atrovent*	T48.6X1	T48.6X2	T48.6X3	T48.6X4	T48.6X5	T48.6X6
Attapulgite	T47.6X1	T47.6X2	T47.6X3	T47.6X4	T47.6X5	T47.6X6
Auramine	T65.891	T65.892	T65.893	T65.894	—	—
dye	T65.6X1	T65.6X2	T65.6X3	T65.6X4	—	—
fungicide	T60.3X1	T60.3X2	T60.3X3	T60.3X4	—	—
Auranofin	T39.4X1	T39.4X2	T39.4X3	T39.4X4	T39.4X5	T39.4X6
Aurantiin	T46.991	T46.992	T46.993	T46.994	T46.995	T46.996
Aureomycin	T36.4X1	T36.4X2	T36.4X3	T36.4X4	T36.4X5	T36.4X6
ophthalmic preparation	T49.5X1	T49.5X2	T49.5X3	T49.5X4	T49.5X5	T49.5X6
topical NEC	T49.0X1	T49.0X2	T49.0X3	T49.0X4	T49.0X5	T49.0X6
Aurothioglucose	T39.4X1	T39.4X2	T39.4X3	T39.4X4	T39.4X5	T39.4X6
Aurothioglycanide	T39.4X1	T39.4X2	T39.4X3	T39.4X4	T39.4X5	T39.4X6
Aurothiomalate sodium	T39.4X1	T39.4X2	T39.4X3	T39.4X4	T39.4X5	T39.4X6
Aurotioprol	T39.4X1	T39.4X2	T39.4X3	T39.4X4	T39.4X5	T39.4X6
Automobile fuel	T52.0X1	T52.0X2	T52.0X3	T52.0X4	—	—
Autonomic nervous system agent NEC	T44.901	T44.902	T44.903	T44.904	T44.905	T44.906
Avelox*	T36.8X1	T36.8X2	T36.8X3	T36.8X4	T36.8X5	T36.8X6
Avlosulfon	T37.1X1	T37.1X2	T37.1X3	T37.1X4	T37.1X5	T37.1X6
Avomine	T42.6X1	T42.6X2	T42.6X3	T42.6X4	T42.6X5	T42.6X6
Axerophthol	T45.2X1	T45.2X2	T45.2X3	T45.2X4	T45.2X5	T45.2X6
Azacitidine	T45.1X1	T45.1X2	T45.1X3	T45.1X4	T45.1X5	T45.1X6
Azacyclonol	T43.591	T43.592	T43.593	T43.594	T43.595	T43.596
Azadirachta	T60.2X1	T60.2X2	T60.2X3	T60.2X4	—	—
Azanidazole	T37.3X1	T37.3X2	T37.3X3	T37.3X4	T37.3X5	T37.3X6
Azapetine	T46.7X1	T46.7X2	T46.7X3	T46.7X4	T46.7X5	T46.7X6
Azapropazone	T39.2X1	T39.2X2	T39.2X3	T39.2X4	T39.2X5	T39.2X6
Azaribine	T45.1X1	T45.1X2	T45.1X3	T45.1X4	T45.1X5	T45.1X6
Azaserine	T45.1X1	T45.1X2	T45.1X3	T45.1X4	T45.1X5	T45.1X6
Azatadine	T45.0X1	T45.0X2	T45.0X3	T45.0X4	T45.0X5	T45.0X6
Azatepa	T45.1X1	T45.1X2	T45.1X3	T45.1X4	T45.1X5	T45.1X6
Azathioprine	T45.1X1	T45.1X2	T45.1X3	T45.1X4	T45.1X5	T45.1X6
Azelaic acid	T49.0X1	T49.0X2	T49.0X3	T49.0X4	T49.0X5	T49.0X6
Azelastine	T45.0X1	T45.0X2	T45.0X3	T45.0X4	T45.0X5	T45.0X6
Azidocillin	T36.0X1	T36.0X2	T36.0X3	T36.0X4	T36.0X5	T36.0X6
Azidothymidine	T37.5X1	T37.5X2	T37.5X3	T37.5X4	T37.5X5	T37.5X6
Azinphos (ethyl) (methyl)	T60.0X1	T60.0X2	T60.0X3	T60.0X4	—	—
Aziridine (chelating)	T54.1X1	T54.1X2	T54.1X3	T54.1X4	—	—
Azithromycin	T36.3X1	T36.3X2	T36.3X3	T36.3X4	T36.3X5	T36.3X6
Azlocillin	T36.0X1	T36.0X2	T36.0X3	T36.0X4	T36.0X5	T36.0X6
Azobenzene smoke	T65.3X1	T65.3X2	T65.3X3	T65.3X4	—	—
acaricide	T60.8X1	T60.8X2	T60.8X3	T60.8X4	—	—
Azo-Standard*	T49.0X1	T49.0X2	T49.0X3	T49.0X4	T49.0X5	T49.0X6
Azosulfamide	T37.0X1	T37.0X2	T37.0X3	T37.0X4	T37.0X5	T37.0X6
AZT	T37.5X1	T37.5X2	T37.5X3	T37.5X4	T37.5X5	T37.5X6
Aztreonam	T36.1X1	T36.1X2	T36.1X3	T36.1X4	T36.1X5	T36.1X6
Azulfidine	T37.0X1	T37.0X2	T37.0X3	T37.0X4	T37.0X5	T37.0X6
Azuresin	T50.8X1	T50.8X2	T50.8X3	T50.8X4	T50.8X5	T50.8X6
b-acetyldigoxin	T46.0X1	T46.0X2	T46.0X3	T46.0X4	T46.0X5	T46.0X6
P-Acetamidophenol	T39.1X1	T39.1X2	T39.1X3	T39.1X4	T39.1X5	T39.1X6
Bacampicillin	T36.0X1	T36.0X2	T36.0X3	T36.0X4	T36.0X5	T36.0X6
Bacillus						
lactobacillus	T47.8X1	T47.8X2	T47.8X3	T47.8X4	T47.8X5	T47.8X6
subtilis	T47.6X1	T47.6X2	T47.6X3	T47.6X4	T47.6X5	T47.6X6
Bacimycin	T49.0X1	T49.0X2	T49.0X3	T49.0X4	T49.0X5	T49.0X6
ophthalmic preparation	T49.5X1	T49.5X2	T49.5X3	T49.5X4	T49.5X5	T49.5X6
Bacitracin zinc	T49.0X1	T49.0X2	T49.0X3	T49.0X4	T49.0X5	T49.0X6
with neomycin	T49.0X1	T49.0X2	T49.0X3	T49.0X4	T49.0X5	T49.0X6
ENT agent	T49.6X1	T49.6X2	T49.6X3	T49.6X4	T49.6X5	T49.6X6
ophthalmic preparation	T49.5X1	T49.5X2	T49.5X3	T49.5X4	T49.5X5	T49.5X6
topical NEC	T49.0X1	T49.0X2	T49.0X3	T49.0X4	T49.0X5	T49.0X6
Baclofen	T42.8X1	T42.8X2	T42.8X3	T42.8X4	T42.8X5	T42.8X6
Baking soda	T50.991	T50.992	T50.993	T50.994	T50.995	T50.996
BAL	T45.8X1	T45.8X2	T45.8X3	T45.8X4	T45.8X5	T45.8X6
Bambuterol	T48.6X1	T48.6X2	T48.6X3	T48.6X4	T48.6X5	T48.6X6
Bamethan (sulfate)	T46.7X1	T46.7X2	T46.7X3	T46.7X4	T46.7X5	T46.7X6
Bamifylline	T48.6X1	T48.6X2	T48.6X3	T48.6X4	T48.6X5	T48.6X6
Bamipine	T45.0X1	T45.0X2	T45.0X3	T45.0X4	T45.0X5	T45.0X6
Baneberry — see Actaea spicata						
Banewort — see Belladonna						
Barbenyl	T42.3X1	T42.3X2	T42.3X3	T42.3X4	T42.3X5	T42.3X6
Barbexaclone	T42.6X1	T42.6X2	T42.6X3	T42.6X4	T42.6X5	T42.6X6
Barbital	T42.3X1	T42.3X2	T42.3X3	T42.3X4	T42.3X5	T42.3X6
sodium	T42.3X1	T42.3X2	T42.3X3	T42.3X4	T42.3X5	T42.3X6
Barbitone	T42.3X1	T42.3X2	T42.3X3	T42.3X4	T42.3X5	T42.3X6
Barbiturate NEC	T42.3X1	T42.3X2	T42.3X3	T42.3X4	T42.3X5	T42.3X6
with tranquilizer	T42.3X1	T42.3X2	T42.3X3	T42.3X4	T42.3X5	T42.3X6
anesthetic (intravenous)	T41.1X1	T41.1X2	T41.1X3	T41.1X4	T41.1X5	T41.1X6
Barium (carbonate) (chloride) (sulfite)	T57.8X1	T57.8X2	T57.8X3	T57.8X4	—	—
diagnostic agent	T50.8X1	T50.8X2	T50.8X3	T50.8X4	T50.8X5	T50.8X6
pesticide	T60.4X1	T60.4X2	T60.4X3	T60.4X4	—	—
rodenticide	T60.4X1	T60.4X2	T60.4X3	T60.4X4	—	—
sulfate (medicinal)	T50.8X1	T50.8X2	T50.8X3	T50.8X4	T50.8X5	T50.8X6
Barrier cream	T49.3X1	T49.3X2	T49.3X3	T49.3X4	T49.3X5	T49.3X6
Basic fuchsin	T49.0X1	T49.0X2	T49.0X3	T49.0X4	T49.0X5	T49.0X6
Basiliximab*	T45.1X1	T45.1X2	T45.1X3	T45.1X4	T45.1X5	T45.1X6
Battery acid or fluid	T54.2X1	T54.2X2	T54.2X3	T54.2X4	—	—
Bay rum	T51.8X1	T51.8X2	T51.8X3	T51.8X4	—	—
b-benzalbutyramide	T46.6X1	T46.6X2	T46.6X3	T46.6X4	T46.6X5	T46.6X6
BCG (vaccine)	T50.A91	T50.A92	T50.A93	T50.A94	T50.A95	T50.A96
BCNU	T45.1X1	T45.1X2	T45.1X3	T45.1X4	T45.1X5	T45.1X6
Bearsfoot	T62.2X1	T62.2X2	T62.2X3	T62.2X4	—	—
Beclamide	T42.6X1	T42.6X2	T42.6X3	T42.6X4	T42.6X5	T42.6X6
Beclomethasone	T44.5X1	T44.5X2	T44.5X3	T44.5X4	T44.5X5	T44.5X6
Bee (sting) (venom)	T63.441	T63.442	T63.443	T63.444	—	—
Befunolol	T49.5X1	T49.5X2	T49.5X3	T49.5X4	T49.5X5	T49.5X6
Bekanamycin	T36.5X1	T36.5X2	T36.5X3	T36.5X4	T36.5X5	T36.5X6
Belladonna — see also Nightshade						
alkaloids	T44.3X1	T44.3X2	T44.3X3	T44.3X4	T44.3X5	T44.3X6
extract	T44.3X1	T44.3X2	T44.3X3	T44.3X4	T44.3X5	T44.3X6
herb	T44.3X1	T44.3X2	T44.3X3	T44.3X4	T44.3X5	T44.3X6
Belviq*	T50.5X1	T50.5X2	T50.5X3	T50.5X4	T50.5X5	T50.5X6
Bemegride	T50.7X1	T50.7X2	T50.7X3	T50.7X4	T50.7X5	T50.7X6
Benactyzine	T44.3X1	T44.3X2	T44.3X3	T44.3X4	T44.3X5	T44.3X6
Benadryl	T45.0X1	T45.0X2	T45.0X3	T45.0X4	T45.0X5	T45.0X6
Benaprizine	T44.3X1	T44.3X2	T44.3X3	T44.3X4	T44.3X5	T44.3X6
Benazepril	T46.4X1	T46.4X2	T46.4X3	T46.4X4	T46.4X5	T46.4X6

☑ Additional Character May Be Required — Refer to the Tabular List for Character Selection *Optum Value-Add

Substance	Poisoning, Accidental (unintentional)	Poisoning, Intentional Self-harm	Poisoning, Assault	Poisoning, Undetermined	Adverse Effect	Under-dosing
Bencyclane	T46.7X1	T46.7X2	T46.7X3	T46.7X4	T46.7X5	T46.7X6
Bendazol	T46.3X1	T46.3X2	T46.3X3	T46.3X4	T46.3X5	T46.3X6
Bendrofluazide	T50.2X1	T50.2X2	T50.2X3	T50.2X4	T50.2X5	T50.2X6
Bendroflumethiazide	T50.2X1	T50.2X2	T50.2X3	T50.2X4	T50.2X5	T50.2X6
Benemid	T50.4X1	T50.4X2	T50.4X3	T50.4X4	T50.4X5	T50.4X6
Benethamine penicillin	T36.0X1	T36.0X2	T36.0X3	T36.0X4	T36.0X5	T36.0X6
Benexate	T47.1X1	T47.1X2	T47.1X3	T47.1X4	T47.1X5	T47.1X6
Benfluorex	T46.6X1	T46.6X2	T46.6X3	T46.6X4	T46.6X5	T46.6X6
Benfotiamine	T45.2X1	T45.2X2	T45.2X3	T45.2X4	T45.2X5	T45.2X6
Benisone	T49.0X1	T49.0X2	T49.0X3	T49.0X4	T49.0X5	T49.0X6
Benomyl	T60.0X1	T60.0X2	T60.0X3	T60.0X4	—	—
Benoquin	T49.8X1	T49.8X2	T49.8X3	T49.8X4	T49.8X5	T49.8X6
Benoxinate	T41.3X1	T41.3X2	T41.3X3	T41.3X4	T41.3X5	T41.3X6
Benperidol	T43.4X1	T43.4X2	T43.4X3	T43.4X4	T43.4X5	T43.4X6
Benproperine	T48.3X1	T48.3X2	T48.3X3	T48.3X4	T48.3X5	T48.3X6
Benserazide	T42.8X1	T42.8X2	T42.8X3	T42.8X4	T42.8X5	T42.8X6
Bentazepam	T42.4X1	T42.4X2	T42.4X3	T42.4X4	T42.4X5	T42.4X6
Bentiromide	T50.8X1	T50.8X2	T50.8X3	T50.8X4	T50.8X5	T50.8X6
Bentonite	T49.3X1	T49.3X2	T49.3X3	T49.3X4	T49.3X5	T49.3X6
Benzalbutyramide	T46.6X1	T46.6X2	T46.6X3	T46.6X4	T46.6X5	T46.6X6
Benzalkonium (chloride)	T49.0X1	T49.0X2	T49.0X3	T49.0X4	T49.0X5	T49.0X6
ophthalmic preparation	T49.5X1	T49.5X2	T49.5X3	T49.5X4	T49.5X5	T49.5X6
Benzamidosalicylate (calcium)	T37.1X1	T37.1X2	T37.1X3	T37.1X4	T37.1X5	T37.1X6
Benzamine	T41.3X1	T41.3X2	T41.3X3	T41.3X4	T41.3X5	T41.3X6
lactate	T49.1X1	T49.1X2	T49.1X3	T49.1X4	T49.1X5	T49.1X6
Benzamphetamine	T50.5X1	T50.5X2	T50.5X3	T50.5X4	T50.5X5	T50.5X6
Benzapril hydrochloride	T46.5X1	T46.5X2	T46.5X3	T46.5X4	T46.5X5	T46.5X6
Benzathine benzylpenicillin	T36.0X1	T36.0X2	T36.0X3	T36.0X4	T36.0X5	T36.0X6
Benzathine penicillin	T36.0X1	T36.0X2	T36.0X3	T36.0X4	T36.0X5	T36.0X6
Benzatropine	T42.8X1	T42.8X2	T42.8X3	T42.8X4	T42.8X5	T42.8X6
Benzbromarone	T50.4X1	T50.4X2	T50.4X3	T50.4X4	T50.4X5	T50.4X6
Benzcarbimine	T45.1X1	T45.1X2	T45.1X3	T45.1X4	T45.1X5	T45.1X6
Benzedrex	T44.991	T44.992	T44.993	T44.994	T44.995	T44.996
Benzedrine (amphetamine)	T43.621	T43.622	T43.623	T43.624	T43.625	T43.626
Benzenamine	T65.3X1	T65.3X2	T65.3X3	T65.3X4	—	—
Benzene	T52.1X1	T52.1X2	T52.1X3	T52.1X4	—	—
homologues (acetyl) (dimethyl) (methyl) (solvent)	T52.2X1	T52.2X2	T52.2X3	T52.2X4	—	—
Benzethonium (chloride)	T49.0X1	T49.0X2	T49.0X3	T49.0X4	T49.0X5	T49.0X6
Benzfetamine	T50.5X1	T50.5X2	T50.5X3	T50.5X4	T50.5X5	T50.5X6
Benzhexol	T44.3X1	T44.3X2	T44.3X3	T44.3X4	T44.3X5	T44.3X6
Benzhydramine (chloride)	T45.0X1	T45.0X2	T45.0X3	T45.0X4	T45.0X5	T45.0X6
Benzidine	T65.891	T65.892	T65.893	T65.894	—	—
Benzilonium bromide	T44.3X1	T44.3X2	T44.3X3	T44.3X4	T44.3X5	T44.3X6
Benzimidazole	T60.3X1	T60.3X2	T60.3X3	T60.3X4	—	—
Benzin (e) — see Ligroin						
Benziodarone	T46.3X1	T46.3X2	T46.3X3	T46.3X4	T46.3X5	T46.3X6
Benznidazole	T37.3X1	T37.3X2	T37.3X3	T37.3X4	T37.3X5	T37.3X6
Benzocaine	T41.3X1	T41.3X2	T41.3X3	T41.3X4	T41.3X5	T41.3X6
Benzocol*	T41.3X1	T41.3X2	T41.3X3	T41.3X4	T41.3X5	T41.3X6
Benzodiapin	T42.4X1	T42.4X2	T42.4X3	T42.4X4	T42.4X5	T42.4X6
Benzodiazepine NEC	T42.4X1	T42.4X2	T42.4X3	T42.4X4	T42.4X5	T42.4X6
Benzoic acid	T49.0X1	T49.0X2	T49.0X3	T49.0X4	T49.0X5	T49.0X6
with salicylic acid	T49.0X1	T49.0X2	T49.0X3	T49.0X4	T49.0X5	T49.0X6
Benzoin (tincture)	T48.5X1	T48.5X2	T48.5X3	T48.5X4	T48.5X5	T48.5X6
Benzol (benzene)	T52.1X1	T52.1X2	T52.1X3	T52.1X4	—	—
vapor	T52.0X1	T52.0X2	T52.0X3	T52.0X4	—	—
Benzomorphan	T40.2X1	T40.2X2	T40.2X3	T40.2X4	T40.2X5	T40.2X6
Benzonatate	T48.3X1	T48.3X2	T48.3X3	T48.3X4	T48.3X5	T48.3X6
Benzophenones	T49.3X1	T49.3X2	T49.3X3	T49.3X4	T49.3X5	T49.3X6
Benzopyrone	T46.991	T46.992	T46.993	T46.994	T46.995	T46.996
Benzothiadiazides	T50.2X1	T50.2X2	T50.2X3	T50.2X4	T50.2X5	T50.2X6
Benzoxonium chloride	T49.0X1	T49.0X2	T49.0X3	T49.0X4	T49.0X5	T49.0X6
Benzoylpas calcium	T37.1X1	T37.1X2	T37.1X3	T37.1X4	T37.1X5	T37.1X6
Benzoyl peroxide	T49.0X1	T49.0X2	T49.0X3	T49.0X4	T49.0X5	T49.0X6
Benzperidin	T43.591	T43.592	T43.593	T43.594	T43.595	T43.596
Benzperidol	T43.591	T43.592	T43.593	T43.594	T43.595	T43.596
Benzphetamine	T50.5X1	T50.5X2	T50.5X3	T50.5X4	T50.5X5	T50.5X6
Benzpyrinium bromide	T44.1X1	T44.1X2	T44.1X3	T44.1X4	T44.1X5	T44.1X6
Benzquinamide	T45.0X1	T45.0X2	T45.0X3	T45.0X4	T45.0X5	T45.0X6
Benzthiazide	T50.2X1	T50.2X2	T50.2X3	T50.2X4	T50.2X5	T50.2X6
Benztropine						
anticholinergic	T44.3X1	T44.3X2	T44.3X3	T44.3X4	T44.3X5	T44.3X6
antiparkinson	T42.8X1	T42.8X2	T42.8X3	T42.8X4	T42.8X5	T42.8X6
Benzydamine	T49.0X1	T49.0X2	T49.0X3	T49.0X4	T49.0X5	T49.0X6
Benzyl						
acetate	T52.8X1	T52.8X2	T52.8X3	T52.8X4	—	—
alcohol	T49.0X1	T49.0X2	T49.0X3	T49.0X4	T49.0X5	T49.0X6
benzoate	T49.0X1	T49.0X2	T49.0X3	T49.0X4	T49.0X5	T49.0X6
Benzoic acid	T49.0X1	T49.0X2	T49.0X3	T49.0X4	T49.0X5	T49.0X6
hydroquinone*	T49.4X1	T49.4X2	T49.4X3	T49.4X4	T49.4X5	T49.4X6
Benzyl — continued						
morphine	T40.2X1	T40.2X2	T40.2X3	T40.2X4	—	—
nicotinate	T46.6X1	T46.6X2	T46.6X3	T46.6X4	T46.6X5	T46.6X6
penicillin	T36.0X1	T36.0X2	T36.0X3	T36.0X4	T36.0X5	T36.0X6
Benzylhydrochlorthiazide	T50.2X1	T50.2X2	T50.2X3	T50.2X4	T50.2X5	T50.2X6
Benzylpenicillin	T36.0X1	T36.0X2	T36.0X3	T36.0X4	T36.0X5	T36.0X6
Benzylthiouracil	T38.2X1	T38.2X2	T38.2X3	T38.2X4	T38.2X5	T38.2X6
Bephenium hydroxynaphthoate	T37.4X1	T37.4X2	T37.4X3	T37.4X4	T37.4X5	T37.4X6
Bepridil	T46.1X1	T46.1X2	T46.1X3	T46.1X4	T46.1X5	T46.1X6
Bergamot oil	T65.891	T65.892	T65.893	T65.894	—	—
Bergapten	T50.991	T50.992	T50.993	T50.994	T50.995	T50.996
Berries, poisonous	T62.1X1	T62.1X2	T62.1X3	T62.1X4	—	—
Beryllium (compounds)	T56.7X1	T56.7X2	T56.7X3	T56.7X4	—	—
beta adrenergic blocking agent, heart	T44.7X1	T44.7X2	T44.7X3	T44.7X4	T44.7X5	T44.7X6
Betacarotene	T45.2X1	T45.2X2	T45.2X3	T45.2X4	T45.2X5	T45.2X6
Beta-Chlor	T42.6X1	T42.6X2	T42.6X3	T42.6X4	T42.6X5	T42.6X6
Betahistine	T46.7X1	T46.7X2	T46.7X3	T46.7X4	T46.7X5	T46.7X6
Betaine	T47.5X1	T47.5X2	T47.5X3	T47.5X4	T47.5X5	T47.5X6
Betamethasone	T49.0X1	T49.0X2	T49.0X3	T49.0X4	T49.0X5	T49.0X6
topical	T49.0X1	T49.0X2	T49.0X3	T49.0X4	T49.0X5	T49.0X6
Betamicin	T36.8X1	T36.8X2	T36.8X3	T36.8X4	T36.8X5	T36.8X6
Betanidine	T46.5X1	T46.5X2	T46.5X3	T46.5X4	T46.5X5	T46.5X6
Betaxolol	T44.7X1	T44.7X2	T44.7X3	T44.7X4	T44.7X5	T44.7X6
Betazole	T50.8X1	T50.8X2	T50.8X3	T50.8X4	T50.8X5	T50.8X6
Bethanechol	T44.1X1	T44.1X2	T44.1X3	T44.1X4	T44.1X5	T44.1X6
chloride	T44.1X1	T44.1X2	T44.1X3	T44.1X4	T44.1X5	T44.1X6
Bethanidine	T46.5X1	T46.5X2	T46.5X3	T46.5X4	T46.5X5	T46.5X6
Betoxycaine	T41.3X1	T41.3X2	T41.3X3	T41.3X4	T41.3X5	T41.3X6
Betula oil	T49.3X1	T49.3X2	T49.3X3	T49.3X4	T49.3X5	T49.3X6
Bevantolol	T44.7X1	T44.7X2	T44.7X3	T44.7X4	T44.7X5	T44.7X6
Bevonium metilsulfate	T44.3X1	T44.3X2	T44.3X3	T44.3X4	T44.3X5	T44.3X6
Bezafibrate	T46.6X1	T46.6X2	T46.6X3	T46.6X4	T46.6X5	T46.6X6
Bezitramide	T40.491	T40.492	T40.493	T40.494	T40.495	T40.496
BHA	T50.991	T50.992	T50.993	T50.994	T50.995	T50.996
Bhang	T40.711	T40.712	T40.713	T40.714	T40.715	T40.716
BHC (medicinal)	T49.0X1	T49.0X2	T49.0X3	T49.0X4	T49.0X5	T49.0X6
nonmedicinal (vapor)	T53.6X1	T53.6X2	T53.6X3	T53.6X4	—	—
Bialamicol	T37.3X1	T37.3X2	T37.3X3	T37.3X4	T37.3X5	T37.3X6
Bibenzonium bromide	T48.3X1	T48.3X2	T48.3X3	T48.3X4	T48.3X5	T48.3X6
Bibrocathol	T49.5X1	T49.5X2	T49.5X3	T49.5X4	T49.5X5	T49.5X6
Bichloride of mercury — see Mercury, chloride						
Bichromates (calcium) (potassium)(sodium) (crystals)	T57.8X1	T57.8X2	T57.8X3	T57.8X4		
fumes	T56.2X1	T56.2X2	T56.2X3	T56.2X4	—	—
Biclotymol	T49.6X1	T49.6X2	T49.6X3	T49.6X4	T49.6X5	T49.6X6
BiCNU*	T45.1X1	T45.1X2	T45.1X3	T45.1X4	T45.1X5	T45.1X6
Bicucculine	T50.7X1	T50.7X2	T50.7X3	T50.7X4	T50.7X5	T50.7X6
Bifemelane	T43.291	T43.292	T43.293	T43.294	T43.295	T43.296
Biguanide derivatives, oral	T38.3X1	T38.3X2	T38.3X3	T38.3X4	T38.3X5	T38.3X6
Bile salts	T47.5X1	T47.5X2	T47.5X3	T47.5X4	T47.5X5	T47.5X6
Biligrafin	T50.8X1	T50.8X2	T50.8X3	T50.8X4	T50.8X5	T50.8X6
Bilopaque	T50.8X1	T50.8X2	T50.8X3	T50.8X4	T50.8X5	T50.8X6
Binifibrate	T46.6X1	T46.6X2	T46.6X3	T46.6X4	T46.6X5	T46.6X6
Binitrobenzol	T65.3X1	T65.3X2	T65.3X3	T65.3X4	—	—
Bioflavonoid(s)	T46.991	T46.992	T46.993	T46.994	T46.995	T46.996
Biological substance NEC	T50.901	T50.902	T50.903	T50.904	T50.905	T50.906
Biotin	T45.2X1	T45.2X2	T45.2X3	T45.2X4	T45.2X5	T45.2X6
Biperiden	T44.3X1	T44.3X2	T44.3X3	T44.3X4	T44.3X5	T44.3X6
Bisacodyl	T47.2X1	T47.2X2	T47.2X3	T47.2X4	T47.2X5	T47.2X6
Bisbentiamine	T45.2X1	T45.2X2	T45.2X3	T45.2X4	T45.2X5	T45.2X6
Bisbutiamine	T45.2X1	T45.2X2	T45.2X3	T45.2X4	T45.2X5	T45.2X6
Bisdequalinium (salts) (diacetate)	T49.6X1	T49.6X2	T49.6X3	T49.6X4	T49.6X5	T49.6X6
Bishydroxycoumarin	T45.511	T45.512	T45.513	T45.514	T45.515	T45.516
Bismarsen	T37.8X1	T37.8X2	T37.8X3	T37.8X4	T37.8X5	T37.8X6
Bismuth salts	T47.6X1	T47.6X2	T47.6X3	T47.6X4	T47.6X5	T47.6X6
aluminate	T47.1X1	T47.1X2	T47.1X3	T47.1X4	T47.1X5	T47.1X6
anti-infectives	T37.8X1	T37.8X2	T37.8X3	T37.8X4	T37.8X5	T37.8X6
formic iodide	T49.0X1	T49.0X2	T49.0X3	T49.0X4	T49.0X5	T49.0X6
glycolylarsenate	T49.0X1	T49.0X2	T49.0X3	T49.0X4	T49.0X5	T49.0X6
nonmedicinal (compounds) NEC	T65.91	T65.92	T65.93	T65.94	—	—
subcarbonate	T47.6X1	T47.6X2	T47.6X3	T47.6X4	T47.6X5	T47.6X6
subsalicylate	T37.8X1	T37.8X2	T37.8X3	T37.8X4	T37.8X5	T37.8X6
sulfarsphenamine	T37.8X1	T37.8X2	T37.8X3	T37.8X4	T37.8X5	T37.8X6
Bisoprolol	T44.7X1	T44.7X2	T44.7X3	T44.7X4	T44.7X5	T44.7X6
Bisoxatin	T47.2X1	T47.2X2	T47.2X3	T47.2X4	T47.2X5	T47.2X6
Bisulepin (hydrochloride)	T45.0X1	T45.0X2	T45.0X3	T45.0X4	T45.0X5	T45.0X6

Table of Drugs and Chemicals

Bithionol — Butanol

Substance	Poisoning, Accidental (unintentional)	Poisoning, Intentional Self-harm	Poisoning, Assault	Poisoning, Undetermined	Adverse Effect	Under-dosing
Bithionol	T37.8X1	T37.8X2	T37.8X3	T37.8X4	T37.8X5	T37.8X6
anthelminthic	T37.4X1	T37.4X2	T37.4X3	T37.4X4	T37.4X5	T37.4X6
Bitolterol	T48.6X1	T48.6X2	T48.6X3	T48.6X4	T48.6X5	T48.6X6
Bitoscanate	T37.4X1	T37.4X2	T37.4X3	T37.4X4	T37.4X5	T37.4X6
Bitter almond oil	T62.8X1	T62.8X2	T62.8X3	T62.8X4	—	—
Bittersweet	T62.2X1	T62.2X2	T62.2X3	T62.2X4	—	—
Bivalirudin*	T45.511	T45.512	T45.513	T45.514	T45.515	T45.516
Black						
flag	T60.91	T60.92	T60.93	T60.94	—	—
henbane	T62.2X1	T62.2X2	T62.2X3	T62.2X4	—	—
leaf (40)	T60.91	T60.92	T60.93	T60.94	—	—
widow spider (bite)	T63.311	T63.312	T63.313	T63.314	—	—
antivenin	T50.Z11	T50.Z12	T50.Z13	T50.Z14	T50.Z15	T50.Z16
Blast furnace gas (carbon monoxide from)	T58.8X1	T58.8X2	T58.8X3	T58.8X4	—	—
Bleach	T54.91	T54.92	T54.93	T54.94	—	—
Bleaching agent (medicinal)	T49.4X1	T49.4X2	T49.4X3	T49.4X4	T49.4X5	T49.4X6
Bleomycin	T45.1X1	T45.1X2	T45.1X3	T45.1X4	T45.1X5	T45.1X6
Blockain	T41.3X1	T41.3X2	T41.3X3	T41.3X4	T41.3X5	T41.3X6
infiltration (subcutaneous)	T41.3X1	T41.3X2	T41.3X3	T41.3X4	T41.3X5	T41.3X6
nerve block (peripheral) (plexus)	T41.3X1	T41.3X2	T41.3X3	T41.3X4	T41.3X5	T41.3X6
topical (surface)	T41.3X1	T41.3X2	T41.3X3	T41.3X4	T41.3X5	T41.3X6
Blockers, calcium channel	T46.1X1	T46.1X2	T46.1X3	T46.1X4	T46.1X5	T46.1X6
Blood (derivatives) (natural) (plasma) (whole)	T45.8X1	T45.8X2	T45.8X3	T45.8X4	T45.8X5	T45.8X6
dried	T45.8X1	T45.8X2	T45.8X3	T45.8X4	T45.8X5	T45.8X6
drug affecting NEC	T45.91	T45.92	T45.93	T45.94	T45.95	T45.96
expander NEC	T45.8X1	T45.8X2	T45.8X3	T45.8X4	T45.8X5	T45.8X6
fraction NEC	T45.8X1	T45.8X2	T45.8X3	T45.8X4	T45.8X5	T45.8X6
substitute (macromolecular)	T45.8X1	T45.8X2	T45.8X3	T45.8X4	T45.8X5	T45.8X6
Blue velvet	T40.2X1	T40.2X2	T40.2X3	T40.2X4	—	—
Bone meal	T62.8X1	T62.8X2	T62.8X3	T62.8X4	—	—
Bonine	T45.0X1	T45.0X2	T45.0X3	T45.0X4	T45.0X5	T45.0X6
Bontril*	T50.5X1	T50.5X2	T50.5X3	T50.5X4	T50.5X5	T50.5X6
Bopindolol	T44.7X1	T44.7X2	T44.7X3	T44.7X4	T44.7X5	T44.7X6
Boracic acid	T49.0X1	T49.0X2	T49.0X3	T49.0X4	T49.0X5	T49.0X6
ENT agent	T49.6X1	T49.6X2	T49.6X3	T49.6X4	T49.6X5	T49.6X6
ophthalmic preparation	T49.5X1	T49.5X2	T49.5X3	T49.5X4	T49.5X5	T49.5X6
Borane complex	T57.8X1	T57.8X2	T57.8X3	T57.8X4	—	—
Borate(s)	T57.8X1	T57.8X2	T57.8X3	T57.8X4	—	—
buffer	T50.991	T50.992	T50.993	T50.994	T50.995	T50.996
cleanser	T54.91	T54.92	T54.93	T54.94	—	—
sodium	T57.8X1	T57.8X2	T57.8X3	T57.8X4	—	—
Borax (cleanser)	T54.91	T54.92	T54.93	T54.94	—	—
Bordeaux mixture	T60.3X1	T60.3X2	T60.3X3	T60.3X4	—	—
Boric acid	T49.0X1	T49.0X2	T49.0X3	T49.0X4	T49.0X5	T49.0X6
ENT agent	T49.6X1	T49.6X2	T49.6X3	T49.6X4	T49.6X5	T49.6X6
ophthalmic preparation	T49.5X1	T49.5X2	T49.5X3	T49.5X4	T49.5X5	T49.5X6
Bornaprine	T44.3X1	T44.3X2	T44.3X3	T44.3X4	T44.3X5	T44.3X6
Boron	T57.8X1	T57.8X2	T57.8X3	T57.8X4	—	—
hydride NEC	T57.8X1	T57.8X2	T57.8X3	T57.8X4	—	—
fumes or gas	T57.8X1	T57.8X2	T57.8X3	T57.8X4	—	—
trifluoride	T59.891	T59.892	T59.893	T59.894	—	—
Botox	T48.291	T48.292	T48.293	T48.294	T48.295	T48.296
Botulinus anti-toxin (type A, B)	T50.Z11	T50.Z12	T50.Z13	T50.Z14	T50.Z15	T50.Z16
Brake fluid vapor	T59.891	T59.892	T59.893	T59.894	—	—
Brallobarbital	T42.3X1	T42.3X2	T42.3X3	T42.3X4	T42.3X5	T42.3X6
Bran (wheat)	T47.4X1	T47.4X2	T47.4X3	T47.4X4	T47.4X5	T47.4X6
Brass (fumes)	T56.891	T56.892	T56.893	T56.894	—	—
Brasso	T52.0X1	T52.0X2	T52.0X3	T52.0X4	—	—
Bretylium tosilate	T46.2X1	T46.2X2	T46.2X3	T46.2X4	T46.2X5	T46.2X6
Brevital (sodium)	T41.1X1	T41.1X2	T41.1X3	T41.1X4	T41.1X5	T41.1X6
Brinase	T45.3X1	T45.3X2	T45.3X3	T45.3X4	T45.3X5	T45.3X6
British antilewisite	T45.8X1	T45.8X2	T45.8X3	T45.8X4	T45.8X5	T45.8X6
Brodalumab*	T50.991	T50.992	T50.993	T50.994	T50.995	T50.996
Brodifacoum	T60.4X1	T60.4X2	T60.4X3	T60.4X4	—	—
Bromal (hydrate)	T42.6X1	T42.6X2	T42.6X3	T42.6X4	T42.6X5	T42.6X6
Bromazepam	T42.4X1	T42.4X2	T42.4X3	T42.4X4	T42.4X5	T42.4X6
Bromazine	T45.0X1	T45.0X2	T45.0X3	T45.0X4	T45.0X5	T45.0X6
Brombenzylcyanide	T59.3X1	T59.3X2	T59.3X3	T59.3X4	—	—
Bromelains	T45.3X1	T45.3X2	T45.3X3	T45.3X4	T45.3X5	T45.3X6
Bromethalin	T60.4X1	T60.4X2	T60.4X3	T60.4X4	—	—
Bromhexine	T48.4X1	T48.4X2	T48.4X3	T48.4X4	T48.4X5	T48.4X6
Bromide salts	T42.6X1	T42.6X2	T42.6X3	T42.6X4	T42.6X5	T42.6X6
Bromindione	T45.511	T45.512	T45.513	T45.514	T45.515	T45.516
Bromine						
compounds (medicinal)	T42.6X1	T42.6X2	T42.6X3	T42.6X4	T42.6X5	T42.6X6
sedative	T42.6X1	T42.6X2	T42.6X3	T42.6X4	T42.6X5	T42.6X6
vapor	T59.891	T59.892	T59.893	T59.894	—	—
Bromisoval	T42.6X1	T42.6X2	T42.6X3	T42.6X4	T42.6X5	T42.6X6
Bromisovalum	T42.6X1	T42.6X2	T42.6X3	T42.6X4	T42.6X5	T42.6X6
Bromobenzylcyanide	T59.3X1	T59.3X2	T59.3X3	T59.3X4	—	—
Bromochlorosalicylani-lide	T49.0X1	T49.0X2	T49.0X3	T49.0X4	T49.0X5	T49.0X6
Bromocriptine	T42.8X1	T42.8X2	T42.8X3	T42.8X4	T42.8X5	T42.8X6
Bromodiphenhydramine	T45.0X1	T45.0X2	T45.0X3	T45.0X4	T45.0X5	T45.0X6
Bromoform	T42.6X1	T42.6X2	T42.6X3	T42.6X4	T42.6X5	T42.6X6
Bromophenol blue reagent	T50.991	T50.992	T50.993	T50.994	T50.995	T50.996
Bromopride	T47.8X1	T47.8X2	T47.8X3	T47.8X4	T47.8X5	T47.8X6
Bromosalicylchloranitide	T49.0X1	T49.0X2	T49.0X3	T49.0X4	T49.0X5	T49.0X6
Bromosalicylhydroxamic acid	T37.1X1	T37.1X2	T37.1X3	T37.1X4	T37.1X5	T37.1X6
Bromo-seltzer	T39.1X1	T39.1X2	T39.1X3	T39.1X4	T39.1X5	T39.1X6
Bromoxynil	T60.3X1	T60.3X2	T60.3X3	T60.3X4	—	—
Bromperidol	T43.4X1	T43.4X2	T43.4X3	T43.4X4	T43.4X5	T43.4X6
Brompheniramine	T45.0X1	T45.0X2	T45.0X3	T45.0X4	T45.0X5	T45.0X6
Bromsulfophthalein	T50.8X1	T50.8X2	T50.8X3	T50.8X4	T50.8X5	T50.8X6
Bromural	T42.6X1	T42.6X2	T42.6X3	T42.6X4	T42.6X5	T42.6X6
Bromvaletone	T42.6X1	T42.6X2	T42.6X3	T42.6X4	T42.6X5	T42.6X6
Bronchodilator NEC	T48.6X1	T48.6X2	T48.6X3	T48.6X4	T48.6X5	T48.6X6
Brotizolam	T42.4X1	T42.4X2	T42.4X3	T42.4X4	T42.4X5	T42.4X6
Brovincamine	T46.7X1	T46.7X2	T46.7X3	T46.7X4	T46.7X5	T46.7X6
Brown recluse spider (bite) (venom)	T63.331	T63.332	T63.333	T63.334	—	—
Brown spider (bite) (venom)	T63.391	T63.392	T63.393	T63.394	—	—
Broxaterol	T48.6X1	T48.6X2	T48.6X3	T48.6X4	T48.6X5	T48.6X6
Broxuridine	T45.1X1	T45.1X2	T45.1X3	T45.1X4	T45.1X5	T45.1X6
Broxyquinoline	T37.8X1	T37.8X2	T37.8X3	T37.8X4	T37.8X5	T37.8X6
Bruceine	T48.291	T48.292	T48.293	T48.294	T48.295	T48.296
Brucia	T62.2X1	T62.2X2	T62.2X3	T62.2X4	—	—
Brucine	T65.1X1	T65.1X2	T65.1X3	T65.1X4	—	—
Brunswick green — see Copper						
Bruten — see Ibuprofen						
Bryonia	T47.2X1	T47.2X2	T47.2X3	T47.2X4	T47.2X5	T47.2X6
Buclizine	T45.0X1	T45.0X2	T45.0X3	T45.0X4	T45.0X5	T45.0X6
Buclosamide	T49.0X1	T49.0X2	T49.0X3	T49.0X4	T49.0X5	T49.0X6
Budesonide	T44.5X1	T44.5X2	T44.5X3	T44.5X4	T44.5X5	T44.5X6
Budralazine	T46.5X1	T46.5X2	T46.5X3	T46.5X4	T46.5X5	T46.5X6
Bufferin	T39.011	T39.012	T39.013	T39.014	T39.015	T39.016
Buflomedil	T46.7X1	T46.7X2	T46.7X3	T46.7X4	T46.7X5	T46.7X6
Buformin	T38.3X1	T38.3X2	T38.3X3	T38.3X4	T38.3X5	T38.3X6
Bufotenine	T40.991	T40.992	T40.993	T40.994	—	—
Bufrolin	T48.6X1	T48.6X2	T48.6X3	T48.6X4	T48.6X5	T48.6X6
Bufylline	T48.6X1	T48.6X2	T48.6X3	T48.6X4	T48.6X5	T48.6X6
Bulgaricum IB*	T47.6X1	T47.6X2	T47.6X3	T47.6X4	T47.6X5	T47.6X6
Bulk filler	T50.5X1	T50.5X2	T50.5X3	T50.5X4	T50.5X5	T50.5X6
cathartic	T47.4X1	T47.4X2	T47.4X3	T47.4X4	T47.4X5	T47.4X6
Bumetanide	T50.1X1	T50.1X2	T50.1X3	T50.1X4	T50.1X5	T50.1X6
Bunaftine	T46.2X1	T46.2X2	T46.2X3	T46.2X4	T46.2X5	T46.2X6
Bunamiodyl	T50.8X1	T50.8X2	T50.8X3	T50.8X4	T50.8X5	T50.8X6
Bunazosin	T44.6X1	T44.6X2	T44.6X3	T44.6X4	T44.6X5	T44.6X6
Bunitrolol	T44.7X1	T44.7X2	T44.7X3	T44.7X4	T44.7X5	T44.7X6
Buphenine	T46.7X1	T46.7X2	T46.7X3	T46.7X4	T46.7X5	T46.7X6
Bupivacaine	T41.3X1	T41.3X2	T41.3X3	T41.3X4	T41.3X5	T41.3X6
infiltration (subcutaneous)	T41.3X1	T41.3X2	T41.3X3	T41.3X4	T41.3X5	T41.3X6
nerve block (peripheral) (plexus)	T41.3X1	T41.3X2	T41.3X3	T41.3X4	T41.3X5	T41.3X6
spinal	T41.3X1	T41.3X2	T41.3X3	T41.3X4	T41.3X5	T41.3X6
Bupranolol	T44.7X1	T44.7X2	T44.7X3	T44.7X4	T44.7X5	T44.7X6
Buprenorphine	T40.491	T40.492	T40.493	T40.494	T40.495	T40.496
Bupropion	T43.291	T43.292	T43.293	T43.294	T43.295	T43.296
Burimamide	T47.1X1	T47.1X2	T47.1X3	T47.1X4	T47.1X5	T47.1X6
Buserelin	T38.891	T38.892	T38.893	T38.894	T38.895	T38.896
Buspirone	T43.591	T43.592	T43.593	T43.594	T43.595	T43.596
Busulfan, busulphan	T45.1X1	T45.1X2	T45.1X3	T45.1X4	T45.1X5	T45.1X6
Busulfex*	T45.1X1	T45.1X2	T45.1X3	T45.1X4	T45.1X5	T45.1X6
Butabarbital (sodium)	T42.3X1	T42.3X2	T42.3X3	T42.3X4	T42.3X5	T42.3X6
Butabarbitone	T42.3X1	T42.3X2	T42.3X3	T42.3X4	T42.3X5	T42.3X6
Butabarpal	T42.3X1	T42.3X2	T42.3X3	T42.3X4	T42.3X5	T42.3X6
Butacaine	T41.3X1	T41.3X2	T41.3X3	T41.3X4	T41.3X5	T41.3X6
Butalamine	T46.7X1	T46.7X2	T46.7X3	T46.7X4	T46.7X5	T46.7X6
Butalbital	T42.3X1	T42.3X2	T42.3X3	T42.3X4	T42.3X5	T42.3X6
Butallylonal	T42.3X1	T42.3X2	T42.3X3	T42.3X4	T42.3X5	T42.3X6
Butamben	T41.3X1	T41.3X2	T41.3X3	T41.3X4	T41.3X5	T41.3X6
Butamirate	T48.3X1	T48.3X2	T48.3X3	T48.3X4	T48.3X5	T48.3X6
Butane (distributed in mobile container)	T59.891	T59.892	T59.893	T59.894	—	—
distributed through pipes	T59.891	T59.892	T59.893	T59.894	—	—
incomplete combustion	T58.11	T58.12	T58.13	T58.14	—	—
Butanilicaine	T41.3X1	T41.3X2	T41.3X3	T41.3X4	T41.3X5	T41.3X6
Butanol	T51.3X1	T51.3X2	T51.3X3	T51.3X4	—	—

☑ **Additional Character May Be Required — Refer to the Tabular List for Character Selection**
*Optum Value-Add

Substance	Poisoning, Accidental (unintentional)	Poisoning, Intentional Self-harm	Poisoning, Assault	Poisoning, Undetermined	Adverse Effect	Under-dosing
Butanone, 2-butanone	T52.4X1	T52.4X2	T52.4X3	T52.4X4	—	—
Butantrone	T49.4X1	T49.4X2	T49.4X3	T49.4X4	T49.4X5	T49.4X6
Butaperazine	T43.3X1	T43.3X2	T43.3X3	T43.3X4	T43.3X5	T43.3X6
Butazolidin	T39.2X1	T39.2X2	T39.2X3	T39.2X4	T39.2X5	T39.2X6
Butetamate	T48.6X1	T48.6X2	T48.6X3	T48.6X4	T48.6X5	T48.6X6
Butethal	T42.3X1	T42.3X2	T42.3X3	T42.3X4	T42.3X5	T42.3X6
Butethamate	T44.3X1	T44.3X2	T44.3X3	T44.3X4	T44.3X5	T44.3X6
Buthalitone (sodium)	T41.1X1	T41.1X2	T41.1X3	T41.1X4	T41.1X5	T41.1X6
Butisol (sodium)	T42.3X1	T42.3X2	T42.3X3	T42.3X4	T42.3X5	T42.3X6
Butizide	T50.2X1	T50.2X2	T50.2X3	T50.2X4	T50.2X5	T50.2X6
Butobarbital	T42.3X1	T42.3X2	T42.3X3	T42.3X4	T42.3X5	T42.3X6
sodium	T42.3X1	T42.3X2	T42.3X3	T42.3X4	T42.3X5	T42.3X6
Butobarbitone	T42.3X1	T42.3X2	T42.3X3	T42.3X4	T42.3X5	T42.3X6
Butoconazole (nitrate)	T49.0X1	T49.0X2	T49.0X3	T49.0X4	T49.0X5	T49.0X6
Butorphanol	T40.491	T40.492	T40.493	T40.494	T40.495	T40.496
Butriptyline	T43.011	T43.012	T43.013	T43.014	T43.015	T43.016
Butropium bromide	T44.3X1	T44.3X2	T44.3X3	T44.3X4	T44.3X5	T44.3X6
Buttercups	T62.2X1	T62.2X2	T62.2X3	T62.2X4	—	—
Butter of antimony — *see*						
Antimony						
Butyl						
acetate (secondary)	T52.8X1	T52.8X2	T52.8X3	T52.8X4	—	—
alcohol	T51.3X1	T51.3X2	T51.3X3	T51.3X4	—	—
aminobenzoate	T41.3X1	T41.3X2	T41.3X3	T41.3X4	T41.3X5	T41.3X6
butyrate	T52.8X1	T52.8X2	T52.8X3	T52.8X4	—	—
carbinol	T51.3X1	T51.3X2	T51.3X3	T51.3X4	—	—
carbitol	T52.3X1	T52.3X2	T52.3X3	T52.3X4	—	—
cellosolve	T52.3X1	T52.3X2	T52.3X3	T52.3X4	—	—
chloral (hydrate)	T42.6X1	T42.6X2	T42.6X3	T42.6X4	T42.6X5	T42.6X6
formate	T52.8X1	T52.8X2	T52.8X3	T52.8X4	—	—
lactate	T52.8X1	T52.8X2	T52.8X3	T52.8X4	—	—
propionate	T52.8X1	T52.8X2	T52.8X3	T52.8X4	—	—
scopolamine bromide	T44.3X1	T44.3X2	T44.3X3	T44.3X4	T44.3X5	T44.3X6
thiobarbital sodium	T41.1X1	T41.1X2	T41.1X3	T41.1X4	T41.1X5	T41.1X6
Butylated hydroxyanisole	T50.991	T50.992	T50.993	T50.994	T50.995	T50.996
Butylchloral hydrate	T42.6X1	T42.6X2	T42.6X3	T42.6X4	T42.6X5	T42.6X6
Butyltoluene	T52.2X1	T52.2X2	T52.2X3	T52.2X4	—	—
Butyn	T41.3X1	T41.3X2	T41.3X3	T41.3X4	T41.3X5	T41.3X6
Butyrophenone (-based tranquilizers)	T43.4X1	T43.4X2	T43.4X3	T43.4X4	T43.4X5	T43.4X6
Cabazitaxel*	T45.1X1	T45.1X2	T45.1X3	T45.1X4	T45.1X5	T45.1X6
Cabergoline	T42.8X1	T42.8X2	T42.8X3	T42.8X4	T42.8X5	T42.8X6
Cacodyl, cacodylic acid	T57.0X1	T57.0X2	T57.0X3	T57.0X4	—	—
Cactinomycin	T45.1X1	T45.1X2	T45.1X3	T45.1X4	T45.1X5	T45.1X6
Cade oil	T49.4X1	T49.4X2	T49.4X3	T49.4X4	T49.4X5	T49.4X6
Cadexomer iodine	T49.0X1	T49.0X2	T49.0X3	T49.0X4	T49.0X5	T49.0X6
Cadmium (chloride) (fumes) (oxide)	T56.3X1	T56.3X2	T56.3X3	T56.3X4	—	—
sulfide (medicinal) NEC	T49.4X1	T49.4X2	T49.4X3	T49.4X4	T49.4X5	T49.4X6
Cadralazine	T46.5X1	T46.5X2	T46.5X3	T46.5X4	T46.5X5	T46.5X6
Caffeine	T43.611	T43.612	T43.613	T43.614	T43.615	T43.616
Calabar bean	T62.2X1	T62.2X2	T62.2X3	T62.2X4	—	—
Caladium seguinum	T62.2X1	T62.2X2	T62.2X3	T62.2X4	—	—
Calamine (lotion)	T49.3X1	T49.3X2	T49.3X3	T49.3X4	T49.3X5	T49.3X6
Calcifediol	T45.2X1	T45.2X2	T45.2X3	T45.2X4	T45.2X5	T45.2X6
Calciferol	T45.2X1	T45.2X2	T45.2X3	T45.2X4	T45.2X5	T45.2X6
Calcijex*	T45.2X1	T45.2X2	T45.2X3	T45.2X4	T45.2X5	T45.2X6
Calcitonin	T50.991	T50.992	T50.993	T50.994	T50.995	T50.996
Calcitriol	T45.2X1	T45.2X2	T45.2X3	T45.2X4	T45.2X5	T45.2X6
Calcium	T50.3X1	T50.3X2	T50.3X3	T50.3X4	T50.3X5	T50.3X6
actylsalicylate	T39.011	T39.012	T39.013	T39.014	T39.015	T39.016
benzamidosalicylate	T37.1X1	T37.1X2	T37.1X3	T37.1X4	T37.1X5	T37.1X6
bromide	T42.6X1	T42.6X2	T42.6X3	T42.6X4	T42.6X5	T42.6X6
bromolactobionate	T42.6X1	T42.6X2	T42.6X3	T42.6X4	T42.6X5	T42.6X6
carbaspirin	T39.011	T39.012	T39.013	T39.014	T39.015	T39.016
carbimide	T50.6X1	T50.6X2	T50.6X3	T50.6X4	T50.6X5	T50.6X6
carbonate	T47.1X1	T47.1X2	T47.1X3	T47.1X4	T47.1X5	T47.1X6
chloride	T50.991	T50.992	T50.993	T50.994	T50.995	T50.996
anhydrous	T50.991	T50.992	T50.993	T50.994	T50.995	T50.996
cyanide	T57.8X1	T57.8X2	T57.8X3	T57.8X4	—	—
dioctyl sulfosuccinate	T47.4X1	T47.4X2	T47.4X3	T47.4X4	T47.4X5	T47.4X6
disodium edathamil	T45.8X1	T45.8X2	T45.8X3	T45.8X4	T45.8X5	T45.8X6
disodium edetate	T45.8X1	T45.8X2	T45.8X3	T45.8X4	T45.8X5	T45.8X6
dobesilate	T46.991	T46.992	T46.993	T46.994	T46.995	T46.996
EDTA	T45.8X1	T45.8X2	T45.8X3	T45.8X4	T45.8X5	T45.8X6
ferrous citrate	T45.4X1	T45.4X2	T45.4X3	T45.4X4	T45.4X5	T45.4X6
folinate	T45.8X1	T45.8X2	T45.8X3	T45.8X4	T45.8X5	T45.8X6
glubionate	T50.3X1	T50.3X2	T50.3X3	T50.3X4	T50.3X5	T50.3X6
gluconate	T50.3X1	T50.3X2	T50.3X3	T50.3X4	T50.3X5	T50.3X6
gluconogalactogluconate	T50.3X1	T50.3X2	T50.3X3	T50.3X4	T50.3X5	T50.3X6
hydrate, hydroxide	T54.3X1	T54.3X2	T54.3X3	T54.3X4	—	—
hypochlorite	T54.3X1	T54.3X2	T54.3X3	T54.3X4	—	—
iodide	T48.4X1	T48.4X2	T48.4X3	T48.4X4	T48.4X5	T48.4X6

Substance	Poisoning, Accidental (unintentional)	Poisoning, Intentional Self-harm	Poisoning, Assault	Poisoning, Undetermined	Adverse Effect	Under-dosing
Calcium — *continued*						
ipodate	T50.8X1	T50.8X2	T50.8X3	T50.8X4	T50.8X5	T50.8X6
lactate	T50.3X1	T50.3X2	T50.3X3	T50.3X4	T50.3X5	T50.3X6
leucovorin	T45.8X1	T45.8X2	T45.8X3	T45.8X4	T45.8X5	T45.8X6
mandelate	T37.91	T37.92	T37.93	T37.94	T37.95	T37.96
oxide	T54.3X1	T54.3X2	T54.3X3	T54.3X4	—	—
pantothenate	T45.2X1	T45.2X2	T45.2X3	T45.2X4	T45.2X5	T45.2X6
phosphate	T50.3X1	T50.3X2	T50.3X3	T50.3X4	T50.3X5	T50.3X6
salicylate	T39.091	T39.092	T39.093	T39.094	T39.095	T39.096
salts	T50.3X1	T50.3X2	T50.3X3	T50.3X4	T50.3X5	T50.3X6
Calculus-dissolving drug	T50.991	T50.992	T50.993	T50.994	T50.995	T50.996
Calomel	T49.0X1	T49.0X2	T49.0X3	T49.0X4	T49.0X5	T49.0X6
Caloric agent	T50.3X1	T50.3X2	T50.3X3	T50.3X4	T50.3X5	T50.3X6
Calusterone	T38.7X1	T38.7X2	T38.7X3	T38.7X4	T38.7X5	T38.7X6
Camazepam	T42.4X1	T42.4X2	T42.4X3	T42.4X4	T42.4X5	T42.4X6
Camomile	T49.0X1	T49.0X2	T49.0X3	T49.0X4	T49.0X5	T49.0X6
Camoquin	T37.2X1	T37.2X2	T37.2X3	T37.2X4	T37.2X5	T37.2X6
Camphor						
insecticide	T60.2X1	T60.2X2	T60.2X3	T60.2X4	—	—
medicinal	T49.8X1	T49.8X2	T49.8X3	T49.8X4	T49.8X5	T49.8X6
Camylofin	T44.3X1	T44.3X2	T44.3X3	T44.3X4	T44.3X5	T44.3X6
Cancer chemotherapy drug regimen	T45.1X1	T45.1X2	T45.1X3	T45.1X4	T45.1X5	T45.1X6
Candeptin	T49.0X1	T49.0X2	T49.0X3	T49.0X4	T49.0X5	T49.0X6
Candicidin	T49.0X1	T49.0X2	T49.0X3	T49.0X4	T49.0X5	T49.0X6
Cankaid*	T49.6X1	T49.6X2	T49.6X3	T49.6X4	T49.6X5	T49.6X6
Cannabinoids, synthetic	T40.721	T40.722	T40.723	T40.724	T40.725	T40.726
Cannabinol	T40.711	T40.712	T40.713	T40.714	T40.715	T40.716
Cannabis (derivatives)	T40.711	T40.712	T40.713	T40.714	T40.715	T40.716
Canned heat	T51.1X1	T51.1X2	T51.1X3	T51.1X4	—	—
Canrenoic acid	T50.0X1	T50.0X2	T50.0X3	T50.0X4	T50.0X5	T50.0X6
Canrenone	T50.0X1	T50.0X2	T50.0X3	T50.0X4	T50.0X5	T50.0X6
Cantharides, cantharidin, cantharis	T49.8X1	T49.8X2	T49.8X3	T49.8X4	T49.8X5	T49.8X6
Canthaxanthin	T50.991	T50.992	T50.993	T50.994	T50.995	T50.996
Capillary-active drug NEC	T46.901	T46.902	T46.903	T46.904	T46.905	T46.906
Capreomycin	T36.8X1	T36.8X2	T36.8X3	T36.8X4	T36.8X5	T36.8X6
Capresla*	T45.1X1	T45.1X2	T45.1X3	T45.1X4	T45.1X5	T45.1X6
Capsicum	T49.4X1	T49.4X2	T49.4X3	T49.4X4	T49.4X5	T49.4X6
Captafol	T60.3X1	T60.3X2	T60.3X3	T60.3X4	—	—
Captan	T60.3X1	T60.3X2	T60.3X3	T60.3X4	—	—
Captodiame, captodiamine	T43.591	T43.592	T43.593	T43.594	T43.595	T43.596
Captopril	T46.4X1	T46.4X2	T46.4X3	T46.4X4	T46.4X5	T46.4X6
Caramiphen	T44.3X1	T44.3X2	T44.3X3	T44.3X4	T44.3X5	T44.3X6
Carazolol	T44.7X1	T44.7X2	T44.7X3	T44.7X4	T44.7X5	T44.7X6
Carbachol	T44.1X1	T44.1X2	T44.1X3	T44.1X4	T44.1X5	T44.1X6
Carbacrylamine (resin)	T50.3X1	T50.3X2	T50.3X3	T50.3X4	T50.3X5	T50.3X6
Carbamate (insecticide)	T60.0X1	T60.0X2	T60.0X3	T60.0X4	—	—
Carbamate (sedative)	T42.6X1	T42.6X2	T42.6X3	T42.6X4	T42.6X5	T42.6X6
herbicide	T60.0X1	T60.0X2	T60.0X3	T60.0X4	—	—
insecticide	T60.0X1	T60.0X2	T60.0X3	T60.0X4	—	—
Carbamazepine	T42.1X1	T42.1X2	T42.1X3	T42.1X4	T42.1X5	T42.1X6
Carbamide	T47.3X1	T47.3X2	T47.3X3	T47.3X4	T47.3X5	T47.3X6
peroxide	T49.0X1	T49.0X2	T49.0X3	T49.0X4	T49.0X5	T49.0X6
topical	T49.8X1	T49.8X2	T49.8X3	T49.8X4	T49.8X5	T49.8X6
Carbamylcholine chloride	T44.1X1	T44.1X2	T44.1X3	T44.1X4	T44.1X5	T44.1X6
Carbaril	T60.0X1	T60.0X2	T60.0X3	T60.0X4	—	—
Carbarsone	T37.3X1	T37.3X2	T37.3X3	T37.3X4	T37.3X5	T37.3X6
Carbaryl	T60.0X1	T60.0X2	T60.0X3	T60.0X4	—	—
Carbaspirin	T39.011	T39.012	T39.013	T39.014	T39.015	T39.016
Carbastat*	T49.5X1	T49.5X2	T49.5X3	T49.5X4	T49.5X5	T49.5X6
Carbazochrome (salicylate) (sodium sulfonate)	T49.4X1	T49.4X2	T49.4X3	T49.4X4	T49.4X5	T49.4X6
Carbenicillin	T36.0X1	T36.0X2	T36.0X3	T36.0X4	T36.0X5	T36.0X6
Carbenoxolone	T47.1X1	T47.1X2	T47.1X3	T47.1X4	T47.1X5	T47.1X6
Carbetapentane	T48.3X1	T48.3X2	T48.3X3	T48.3X4	T48.3X5	T48.3X6
Carbethyl salicylate	T39.091	T39.092	T39.093	T39.094	T39.095	T39.096
Carbidopa (with levodopa)	T42.8X1	T42.8X2	T42.8X3	T42.8X4	T42.8X5	T42.8X6
Carbimazole	T38.2X1	T38.2X2	T38.2X3	T38.2X4	T38.2X5	T38.2X6
Carbinol	T51.1X1	T51.1X2	T51.1X3	T51.1X4	—	—
Carbinoxamine	T45.0X1	T45.0X2	T45.0X3	T45.0X4	T45.0X5	T45.0X6
Carbiphene	T39.8X1	T39.8X2	T39.8X3	T39.8X4	T39.8X5	T39.8X6
Carbitol	T52.3X1	T52.3X2	T52.3X3	T52.3X4	—	—
Carbocaine	T41.3X1	T41.3X2	T41.3X3	T41.3X4	T41.3X5	T41.3X6
infiltration (subcutaneous)	T41.3X1	T41.3X2	T41.3X3	T41.3X4	T41.3X5	T41.3X6
nerve block (peripheral) (plexus)	T41.3X1	T41.3X2	T41.3X3	T41.3X4	T41.3X5	T41.3X6
topical (surface)	T41.3X1	T41.3X2	T41.3X3	T41.3X4	T41.3X5	T41.3X6
Carbocisteine	T48.4X1	T48.4X2	T48.4X3	T48.4X4	T48.4X5	T48.4X6
Carbocromen	T46.3X1	T46.3X2	T46.3X3	T46.3X4	T46.3X5	T46.3X6
Carbol fuchsin	T49.0X1	T49.0X2	T49.0X3	T49.0X4	T49.0X5	T49.0X6

Substance	Poisoning, Accidental (unintentional)	Poisoning, Intentional Self-harm	Poisoning, Assault	Poisoning, Undetermined	Adverse Effect	Under-dosing
Carbolic acid — see also Phenol	T54.0X1	T54.0X2	T54.0X3	T54.0X4	—	—
Carbolonium (bromide)	T48.1X1	T48.1X2	T48.1X3	T48.1X4	T48.1X5	T48.1X6
Carbo medicinalis	T47.6X1	T47.6X2	T47.6X3	T47.6X4	T47.6X5	T47.6X6
Carbomycin	T36.8X1	T36.8X2	T36.8X3	T36.8X4	T36.8X5	T36.8X6
Carbon						
bisulfide (liquid)	T65.4X1	T65.4X2	T65.4X3	T65.4X4	—	—
vapor	T65.4X1	T65.4X2	T65.4X3	T65.4X4	—	—
dioxide (gas)	T59.7X1	T59.7X2	T59.7X3	T59.7X4	—	—
medicinal	T41.5X1	T41.5X2	T41.5X3	T41.5X4	T41.5X5	T41.5X6
nonmedicinal	T59.7X1	T59.7X2	T59.7X3	T59.7X4	—	—
snow	T49.4X1	T49.4X2	T49.4X3	T49.4X4	T49.4X5	T49.4X6
disulfide (liquid)	T65.4X1	T65.4X2	T65.4X3	T65.4X4	—	—
vapor	T65.4X1	T65.4X2	T65.4X3	T65.4X4	—	—
monoxide (from incomplete combustion)	T58.91	T58.92	T58.93	T58.94	—	—
blast furnace gas	T58.8X1	T58.8X2	T58.8X3	T58.8X4	—	—
butane (distributed in mobile container)	T58.11	T58.12	T58.13	T58.14	—	—
distributed through pipes	T58.11	T58.12	T58.13	T58.14	—	—
charcoal fumes	T58.2X1	T58.2X2	T58.2X3	T58.2X4	—	—
coal	T58.2X1	T58.2X2	T58.2X3	T58.2X4	—	—
coke (in domestic stoves, fireplaces)	T58.2X1	T58.2X2	T58.2X3	T58.2X4	—	—
exhaust gas (motor) not in transit	T58.01	T58.02	T58.03	T58.04	—	—
combustion engine, any not in watercraft	T58.01	T58.02	T58.03	T58.04	—	—
farm tractor, not in transit	T58.01	T58.02	T58.03	T58.04	—	—
gas engine	T58.01	T58.02	T58.03	T58.04	—	—
motor pump	T58.01	T58.02	T58.03	T58.04	—	—
motor vehicle, not in transit	T58.01	T58.02	T58.03	T58.04	—	—
fuel (in domestic use)	T58.2X1	T58.2X2	T58.2X3	T58.2X4	—	—
gas (piped)	T58.11	T58.12	T58.13	T58.14	—	—
in mobile container	T58.11	T58.12	T58.13	T58.14	—	—
piped (natural)	T58.11	T58.12	T58.13	T58.14	—	—
utility	T58.11	T58.12	T58.13	T58.14	—	—
in mobile container	T58.11	T58.12	T58.13	T58.14	—	—
gas (piped)	T58.11	T58.12	T58.13	T58.14	—	—
illuminating gas	T58.11	T58.12	T58.13	T58.14	—	—
industrial fuels or gases, any	T58.8X1	T58.8X2	T58.8X3	T58.8X4	—	—
kerosene (in domestic stoves, fireplaces)	T58.2X1	T58.2X2	T58.2X3	T58.2X4	—	—
kiln gas or vapor	T58.8X1	T58.8X2	T58.8X3	T58.8X4	—	—
motor exhaust gas, not in transit	T58.01	T58.02	T58.03	T58.04	—	—
piped gas (manufactured) (natural)	T58.11	T58.12	T58.13	T58.14	—	—
producer gas	T58.8X1	T58.8X2	T58.8X3	T58.8X4	—	—
propane (distributed in mobile container)	T58.11	T58.12	T58.13	T58.14	—	—
distributed through pipes	T58.11	T58.12	T58.13	T58.14	—	—
solid (in domestic stoves, fireplaces)	T58.2X1	T58.2X2	T58.2X3	T58.2X4	—	—
specified source NEC	T58.8X1	T58.8X2	T58.8X3	T58.8X4	—	—
stove gas	T58.11	T58.12	T58.13	T58.14	—	—
piped	T58.11	T58.12	T58.13	T58.14	—	—
utility gas	T58.11	T58.12	T58.13	T58.14	—	—
piped	T58.11	T58.12	T58.13	T58.14	—	—
water gas	T58.11	T58.12	T58.13	T58.14	—	—
wood (in domestic stoves, fireplaces)	T58.2X1	T58.2X2	T58.2X3	T58.2X4	—	—
tetrachloride (vapor) NEC	T53.0X1	T53.0X2	T53.0X3	T53.0X4	—	—
liquid (cleansing agent) NEC	T53.0X1	T53.0X2	T53.0X3	T53.0X4	—	—
solvent	T53.0X1	T53.0X2	T53.0X3	T53.0X4	—	—
Carbonic acid gas	T59.7X1	T59.7X2	T59.7X3	T59.7X4	—	—
anhydrase inhibitor NEC	T50.2X1	T50.2X2	T50.2X3	T50.2X4	T50.2X5	T50.2X6
Carbophenothion	T60.0X1	T60.0X2	T60.0X3	T60.0X4	—	—
Carboplatin	T45.1X1	T45.1X2	T45.1X3	T45.1X4	T45.1X5	T45.1X6
Carboprost	T48.0X1	T48.0X2	T48.0X3	T48.0X4	T48.0X5	T48.0X6
Carboquone	T45.1X1	T45.1X2	T45.1X3	T45.1X4	T45.1X5	T45.1X6
Carbowax	T49.3X1	T49.3X2	T49.3X3	T49.3X4	T49.3X5	T49.3X6
Carboxymethylcellulose	T47.4X1	T47.4X2	T47.4X3	T47.4X4	T47.4X5	T47.4X6
Carbrital	T42.3X1	T42.3X2	T42.3X3	T42.3X4	T42.3X5	T42.3X6
Carbromal	T42.6X1	T42.6X2	T42.6X3	T42.6X4	T42.6X5	T42.6X6
Carbutamide	T38.3X1	T38.3X2	T38.3X3	T38.3X4	T38.3X5	T38.3X6
Carbuterol	T48.6X1	T48.6X2	T48.6X3	T48.6X4	T48.6X5	T48.6X6

Substance	Poisoning, Accidental (unintentional)	Poisoning, Intentional Self-harm	Poisoning, Assault	Poisoning, Undetermined	Adverse Effect	Under-dosing
Cardiac						
depressants	T46.2X1	T46.2X2	T46.2X3	T46.2X4	T46.2X5	T46.2X6
rhythm regulator	T46.2X1	T46.2X2	T46.2X3	T46.2X4	T46.2X5	T46.2X6
specified NEC	T46.2X1	T46.2X2	T46.2X3	T46.2X4	T46.2X5	T46.2X6
Cardiografin	T50.8X1	T50.8X2	T50.8X3	T50.8X4	T50.8X5	T50.8X6
Cardiogreen	T50.8X1	T50.8X2	T50.8X3	T50.8X4	T50.8X5	T50.8X6
Cardiotonic (glycoside) NEC	T46.0X1	T46.0X2	T46.0X3	T46.0X4	T46.0X5	T46.0X6
Cardiovascular drug NEC	T46.901	T46.902	T46.903	T46.904	T46.905	T46.906
Cardizem*	T46.1X1	T46.1X2	T46.1X3	T46.1X4	T46.1X5	T46.1X6
Cardrase	T50.2X1	T50.2X2	T50.2X3	T50.2X4	T50.2X5	T50.2X6
Carfecillin	T36.0X1	T36.0X2	T36.0X3	T36.0X4	T36.0X5	T36.0X6
Carfenazine	T43.3X1	T43.3X2	T43.3X3	T43.3X4	T43.3X5	T43.3X6
Carfusin	T49.0X1	T49.0X2	T49.0X3	T49.0X4	T49.0X5	T49.0X6
Carindacillin	T36.0X1	T36.0X2	T36.0X3	T36.0X4	T36.0X5	T36.0X6
Carisoprodol	T42.8X1	T42.8X2	T42.8X3	T42.8X4	T42.8X5	T42.8X6
Carmellose	T47.4X1	T47.4X2	T47.4X3	T47.4X4	T47.4X5	T47.4X6
Carminative	T47.5X1	T47.5X2	T47.5X3	T47.5X4	T47.5X5	T47.5X6
Carmofur	T45.1X1	T45.1X2	T45.1X3	T45.1X4	T45.1X5	T45.1X6
Carmustine	T45.1X1	T45.1X2	T45.1X3	T45.1X4	T45.1X5	T45.1X6
Carotene	T45.2X1	T45.2X2	T45.2X3	T45.2X4	T45.2X5	T45.2X6
Carphenazine	T43.3X1	T43.3X2	T43.3X3	T43.3X4	T43.3X5	T43.3X6
Carpipramine	T42.4X1	T42.4X2	T42.4X3	T42.4X4	T42.4X5	T42.4X6
Carprofen	T39.311	T39.312	T39.313	T39.314	T39.315	T39.316
Carpronium chloride	T44.3X1	T44.3X2	T44.3X3	T44.3X4	T44.3X5	T44.3X6
Carrageenan	T47.8X1	T47.8X2	T47.8X3	T47.8X4	T47.8X5	T47.8X6
Carteolol	T44.7X1	T44.7X2	T44.7X3	T44.7X4	T44.7X5	T44.7X6
Carter's Little Pills	T47.2X1	T47.2X2	T47.2X3	T47.2X4	T47.2X5	T47.2X6
Cartia*	T46.1X1	T46.1X2	T46.1X3	T46.1X4	T46.1X5	T46.1X6
Cascara (sagrada)	T47.2X1	T47.2X2	T47.2X3	T47.2X4	T47.2X5	T47.2X6
Cassava	T62.2X1	T62.2X2	T62.2X3	T62.2X4	—	—
Castellani's paint	T49.0X1	T49.0X2	T49.0X3	T49.0X4	T49.0X5	T49.0X6
Castor						
bean	T62.2X1	T62.2X2	T62.2X3	T62.2X4	—	—
oil	T47.2X1	T47.2X2	T47.2X3	T47.2X4	T47.2X5	T47.2X6
Catalase	T45.3X1	T45.3X2	T45.3X3	T45.3X4	T45.3X5	T45.3X6
Caterpillar (sting)	T63.431	T63.432	T63.433	T63.434	—	—
Catha (edulis) (tea)	T43.691	T43.692	T43.693	T43.694	—	—
Cathartic NEC	T47.4X1	T47.4X2	T47.4X3	T47.4X4	T47.4X5	T47.4X6
anthacene derivative	T47.2X1	T47.2X2	T47.2X3	T47.2X4	T47.2X5	T47.2X6
bulk	T47.4X1	T47.4X2	T47.4X3	T47.4X4	T47.4X5	T47.4X6
contact	T47.2X1	T47.2X2	T47.2X3	T47.2X4	T47.2X5	T47.2X6
emollient NEC	T47.4X1	T47.4X2	T47.4X3	T47.4X4	T47.4X5	T47.4X6
irritant NEC	T47.2X1	T47.2X2	T47.2X3	T47.2X4	T47.2X5	T47.2X6
mucilage	T47.4X1	T47.4X2	T47.4X3	T47.4X4	T47.4X5	T47.4X6
saline	T47.3X1	T47.3X2	T47.3X3	T47.3X4	T47.3X5	T47.3X6
vegetable	T47.2X1	T47.2X2	T47.2X3	T47.2X4	T47.2X5	T47.2X6
Cathine	T50.5X1	T50.5X2	T50.5X3	T50.5X4	T50.5X5	T50.5X6
Cathomycin	T36.8X1	T36.8X2	T36.8X3	T36.8X4	T36.8X5	T36.8X6
Cation exchange resin	T50.3X1	T50.3X2	T50.3X3	T50.3X4	T50.3X5	T50.3X6
Caustic(s) NEC	T54.91	T54.92	T54.93	T54.94	—	—
alkali	T54.3X1	T54.3X2	T54.3X3	T54.3X4	—	—
hydroxide	T54.3X1	T54.3X2	T54.3X3	T54.3X4	—	—
potash	T54.3X1	T54.3X2	T54.3X3	T54.3X4	—	—
soda	T54.3X1	T54.3X2	T54.3X3	T54.3X4	—	—
specified NEC	T54.91	T54.92	T54.93	T54.94	—	—
Ceepryn	T49.0X1	T49.0X2	T49.0X3	T49.0X4	T49.0X5	T49.0X6
ENT agent	T49.6X1	T49.6X2	T49.6X3	T49.6X4	T49.6X5	T49.6X6
lozenges	T49.6X1	T49.6X2	T49.6X3	T49.6X4	T49.6X5	T49.6X6
Cefacetrile	T36.1X1	T36.1X2	T36.1X3	T36.1X4	T36.1X5	T36.1X6
Cefaclor	T36.1X1	T36.1X2	T36.1X3	T36.1X4	T36.1X5	T36.1X6
Cefadroxil	T36.1X1	T36.1X2	T36.1X3	T36.1X4	T36.1X5	T36.1X6
Cefalexin	T36.1X1	T36.1X2	T36.1X3	T36.1X4	T36.1X5	T36.1X6
Cefaloglycin	T36.1X1	T36.1X2	T36.1X3	T36.1X4	T36.1X5	T36.1X6
Cefaloridine	T36.1X1	T36.1X2	T36.1X3	T36.1X4	T36.1X5	T36.1X6
Cefalosporins	T36.1X1	T36.1X2	T36.1X3	T36.1X4	T36.1X5	T36.1X6
Cefalotin	T36.1X1	T36.1X2	T36.1X3	T36.1X4	T36.1X5	T36.1X6
Cefamandole	T36.1X1	T36.1X2	T36.1X3	T36.1X4	T36.1X5	T36.1X6
Cefamycin antibiotic	T36.1X1	T36.1X2	T36.1X3	T36.1X4	T36.1X5	T36.1X6
Cefapirin	T36.1X1	T36.1X2	T36.1X3	T36.1X4	T36.1X5	T36.1X6
Cefatrizine	T36.1X1	T36.1X2	T36.1X3	T36.1X4	T36.1X5	T36.1X6
Cefazedone	T36.1X1	T36.1X2	T36.1X3	T36.1X4	T36.1X5	T36.1X6
Cefazolin	T36.1X1	T36.1X2	T36.1X3	T36.1X4	T36.1X5	T36.1X6
Cefbuperazone	T36.1X1	T36.1X2	T36.1X3	T36.1X4	T36.1X5	T36.1X6
Cefetamet	T36.1X1	T36.1X2	T36.1X3	T36.1X4	T36.1X5	T36.1X6
Cefixime	T36.1X1	T36.1X2	T36.1X3	T36.1X4	T36.1X5	T36.1X6
Cefmenoxime	T36.1X1	T36.1X2	T36.1X3	T36.1X4	T36.1X5	T36.1X6
Cefmetazole	T36.1X1	T36.1X2	T36.1X3	T36.1X4	T36.1X5	T36.1X6
Cefminox	T36.1X1	T36.1X2	T36.1X3	T36.1X4	T36.1X5	T36.1X6
Cefonicid	T36.1X1	T36.1X2	T36.1X3	T36.1X4	T36.1X5	T36.1X6
Cefoperazone	T36.1X1	T36.1X2	T36.1X3	T36.1X4	T36.1X5	T36.1X6
Ceforanide	T36.1X1	T36.1X2	T36.1X3	T36.1X4	T36.1X5	T36.1X6
Cefotaxime	T36.1X1	T36.1X2	T36.1X3	T36.1X4	T36.1X5	T36.1X6
Cefotetan	T36.1X1	T36.1X2	T36.1X3	T36.1X4	T36.1X5	T36.1X6

Substance	Poisoning, Accidental (unintentional)	Poisoning, Intentional Self-harm	Poisoning, Assault	Poisoning, Undetermined	Adverse Effect	Under-dosing
Cefotiam	T36.1X1	T36.1X2	T36.1X3	T36.1X4	T36.1X5	T36.1X6
Cefoxitin	T36.1X1	T36.1X2	T36.1X3	T36.1X4	T36.1X5	T36.1X6
Cefpimizole	T36.1X1	T36.1X2	T36.1X3	T36.1X4	T36.1X5	T36.1X6
Cefpiramide	T36.1X1	T36.1X2	T36.1X3	T36.1X4	T36.1X5	T36.1X6
Cefradine	T36.1X1	T36.1X2	T36.1X3	T36.1X4	T36.1X5	T36.1X6
Cefroxadine	T36.1X1	T36.1X2	T36.1X3	T36.1X4	T36.1X5	T36.1X6
Cefsulodin	T36.1X1	T36.1X2	T36.1X3	T36.1X4	T36.1X5	T36.1X6
Ceftazidime	T36.1X1	T36.1X2	T36.1X3	T36.1X4	T36.1X5	T36.1X6
Cefteram	T36.1X1	T36.1X2	T36.1X3	T36.1X4	T36.1X5	T36.1X6
Ceftezole	T36.1X1	T36.1X2	T36.1X3	T36.1X4	T36.1X5	T36.1X6
Ceftin*	T36.1X1	T36.1X2	T36.1X3	T36.1X4	T36.1X5	T36.1X6
Ceftizoxime	T36.1X1	T36.1X2	T36.1X3	T36.1X4	T36.1X5	T36.1X6
Ceftriaxone	T36.1X1	T36.1X2	T36.1X3	T36.1X4	T36.1X5	T36.1X6
Cefuroxime	T36.1X1	T36.1X2	T36.1X3	T36.1X4	T36.1X5	T36.1X6
Cefuzonam	T36.1X1	T36.1X2	T36.1X3	T36.1X4	T36.1X5	T36.1X6
Celestone	T38.0X1	T38.0X2	T38.0X3	T38.0X4	T38.0X5	T38.0X6
topical	T49.0X1	T49.0X2	T49.0X3	T49.0X4	T49.0X5	T49.0X6
Celiprolol	T44.7X1	T44.7X2	T44.7X3	T44.7X4	T44.7X5	T44.7X6
Cellosolve	T52.91	T52.92	T52.93	T52.94	—	—
Cell stimulants and proliferants	T49.8X1	T49.8X2	T49.8X3	T49.8X4	T49.8X5	T49.8X6
Cellulose						
cathartic	T47.4X1	T47.4X2	T47.4X3	T47.4X4	T47.4X5	T47.4X6
hydroxyethyl	T47.4X1	T47.4X2	T47.4X3	T47.4X4	T47.4X5	T47.4X6
nitrates (topical)	T49.3X1	T49.3X2	T49.3X3	T49.3X4	T49.3X5	T49.3X6
oxidized	T49.4X1	T49.4X2	T49.4X3	T49.4X4	T49.4X5	T49.4X6
Centipede (bite)	T63.411	T63.412	T63.413	T63.414	—	—
Central nervous system						
depressants	T42.71	T42.72	T42.73	T42.74	T42.75	T42.76
anesthetic (general) NEC	T41.201	T41.202	T41.203	T41.204	T41.205	T41.206
gases NEC	T41.0X1	T41.0X2	T41.0X3	T41.0X4	T41.0X5	T41.0X6
intravenous	T41.1X1	T41.1X2	T41.1X3	T41.1X4	T41.1X5	T41.1X6
barbiturates	T42.3X1	T42.3X2	T42.3X3	T42.3X4	T42.3X5	T42.3X6
benzodiazepines	T42.4X1	T42.4X2	T42.4X3	T42.4X4	T42.4X5	T42.4X6
bromides	T42.6X1	T42.6X2	T42.6X3	T42.6X4	T42.6X5	T42.6X6
cannabis sativa	T40.711	T40.712	T40.713	T40.714	T40.715	T40.716
chloral hydrate	T42.6X1	T42.6X2	T42.6X3	T42.6X4	T42.6X5	T42.6X6
ethanol	T51.0X1	T51.0X2	T51.0X3	T51.0X4	—	—
hallucinogenics	T40.901	T40.902	T40.903	T40.904	T40.905	T40.906
hypnotics	T42.71	T42.72	T42.73	T42.74	T42.75	T42.76
specified NEC	T42.6X1	T42.6X2	T42.6X3	T42.6X4	T42.6X5	T42.6X6
muscle relaxants	T42.8X1	T42.8X2	T42.8X3	T42.8X4	T42.8X5	T42.8X6
paraldehyde	T42.6X1	T42.6X2	T42.6X3	T42.6X4	T42.6X5	T42.6X6
sedatives; sedative-hypnotics	T42.71	T42.72	T42.73	T42.74	T42.75	T42.76
mixed NEC	T42.6X1	T42.6X2	T42.6X3	T42.6X4	T42.6X5	T42.6X6
specified NEC	T42.6X1	T42.6X2	T42.6X3	T42.6X4	T42.6X5	T42.6X6
muscle-tone depressants	T42.8X1	T42.8X2	T42.8X3	T42.8X4	T42.8X5	T42.8X6
stimulants	T43.601	T43.602	T43.603	T43.604	T43.605	T43.606
amphetamines	T43.621	T43.622	T43.623	T43.624	T43.625	T43.626
analeptics	T50.7X1	T50.7X2	T50.7X3	T50.7X4	T50.7X5	T50.7X6
antidepressants	T43.201	T43.202	T43.203	T43.204	T43.205	T43.206
opiate antagonists	T50.7X1	T50.7X2	T50.7X3	T50.7X4	T50.7X5	T50.7X6
specified NEC	T43.691	T43.692	T43.693	T43.694	T43.695	T43.696
Cepacol*	T41.3X1	T41.3X2	T41.3X3	T41.3X4	T41.3X5	T41.3X6
Cephalexin	T36.1X1	T36.1X2	T36.1X3	T36.1X4	T36.1X5	T36.1X6
Cephaloglycin	T36.1X1	T36.1X2	T36.1X3	T36.1X4	T36.1X5	T36.1X6
Cephaloridine	T36.1X1	T36.1X2	T36.1X3	T36.1X4	T36.1X5	T36.1X6
Cephalosporins	T36.1X1	T36.1X2	T36.1X3	T36.1X4	T36.1X5	T36.1X6
N (adicillin)	T36.0X1	T36.0X2	T36.0X3	T36.0X4	T36.0X5	T36.0X6
Cephalothin	T36.1X1	T36.1X2	T36.1X3	T36.1X4	T36.1X5	T36.1X6
Cephalotin	T36.1X1	T36.1X2	T36.1X3	T36.1X4	T36.1X5	T36.1X6
Cephradine	T36.1X1	T36.1X2	T36.1X3	T36.1X4	T36.1X5	T36.1X6
Cerbera (odollam)	T62.2X1	T62.2X2	T62.2X3	T62.2X4	—	—
Cerberin	T46.0X1	T46.0X2	T46.0X3	T46.0X4	T46.0X5	T46.0X6
Cerebral stimulants	T43.601	T43.602	T43.603	T43.604	T43.605	T43.606
psychotherapeutic	T43.601	T43.602	T43.603	T43.604	T43.605	T43.606
specified NEC	T43.691	T43.692	T43.693	T43.694	T43.695	T43.696
Cerium oxalate	T45.0X1	T45.0X2	T45.0X3	T45.0X4	T45.0X5	T45.0X6
Cerous oxalate	T45.0X1	T45.0X2	T45.0X3	T45.0X4	T45.0X5	T45.0X6
Ceruletide	T50.8X1	T50.8X2	T50.8X3	T50.8X4	T50.8X5	T50.8X6
Cetacort*	T49.0X1	T49.0X2	T49.0X3	T49.0X4	T49.0X5	T49.0X6
Cetalkonium (chloride)	T49.0X1	T49.0X2	T49.0X3	T49.0X4	T49.0X5	T49.0X6
Cethexonium chloride	T49.0X1	T49.0X2	T49.0X3	T49.0X4	T49.0X5	T49.0X6
Cetiedil	T46.7X1	T46.7X2	T46.7X3	T46.7X4	T46.7X5	T46.7X6
Cetirizine	T45.0X1	T45.0X2	T45.0X3	T45.0X4	T45.0X5	T45.0X6
Cetomacrogol	T50.991	T50.992	T50.993	T50.994	T50.995	T50.996
Cetotiamine	T45.2X1	T45.2X2	T45.2X3	T45.2X4	T45.2X5	T45.2X6
Cetoxime	T45.0X1	T45.0X2	T45.0X3	T45.0X4	T45.0X5	T45.0X6
Cetraxate	T47.1X1	T47.1X2	T47.1X3	T47.1X4	T47.1X5	T47.1X6
Cetrimide	T49.0X1	T49.0X2	T49.0X3	T49.0X4	T49.0X5	T49.0X6
Cetrimonium (bromide)	T49.0X1	T49.0X2	T49.0X3	T49.0X4	T49.0X5	T49.0X6
Cetylpyridinium chloride	T49.0X1	T49.0X2	T49.0X3	T49.0X4	T49.0X5	T49.0X6

Substance	Poisoning, Accidental (unintentional)	Poisoning, Intentional Self-harm	Poisoning, Assault	Poisoning, Undetermined	Adverse Effect	Under-dosing
Cetylpyridinium chloride — continued						
ENT agent	T49.6X1	T49.6X2	T49.6X3	T49.6X4	T49.6X5	T49.6X6
lozenges	T49.6X1	T49.6X2	T49.6X3	T49.6X4	T49.6X5	T49.6X6
Cevadilla — see Sabadilla						
Cevitamic acid	T45.2X1	T45.2X2	T45.2X3	T45.2X4	T45.2X5	T45.2X6
Chalk, precipitated	T47.1X1	T47.1X2	T47.1X3	T47.1X4	T47.1X5	T47.1X6
Chamomile	T49.0X1	T49.0X2	T49.0X3	T49.0X4	T49.0X5	T49.0X6
Ch'an su	T46.0X1	T46.0X2	T46.0X3	T46.0X4	T46.0X5	T46.0X6
Charcoal	T47.6X1	T47.6X2	T47.6X3	T47.6X4	T47.6X5	T47.6X6
activated — see also Charcoal, medicinal	T47.6X1	T47.6X2	T47.6X3	T47.6X4	T47.6X5	T47.6X6
fumes (Carbon monoxide)	T58.2X1	T58.2X2	T58.2X3	T58.2X4	—	—
industrial	T58.8X1	T58.8X2	T58.8X3	T58.8X4	—	—
medicinal (activated)	T47.6X1	T47.6X2	T47.6X3	T47.6X4	T47.6X5	T47.6X6
antidiarrheal	T47.6X1	T47.6X2	T47.6X3	T47.6X4	T47.6X5	T47.6X6
poison control	T47.8X1	T47.8X2	T47.8X3	T47.8X4	T47.8X5	T47.8X6
specified use other than for diarrhea	T47.8X1	T47.8X2	T47.8X3	T47.8X4	T47.8X5	T47.8X6
topical	T49.8X1	T49.8X2	T49.8X3	T49.8X4	T49.8X5	T49.8X6
Chaulmosulfone	T37.1X1	T37.1X2	T37.1X3	T37.1X4	T37.1X5	T37.1X6
Chelating agent NEC	T50.6X1	T50.6X2	T50.6X3	T50.6X4	T50.6X5	T50.6X6
Chelidonium majus	T62.2X1	T62.2X2	T62.2X3	T62.2X4	—	—
Chemical substance NEC	T65.91	T65.92	T65.93	T65.94	—	—
Chenodeoxycholic acid	T45.5X1	T45.5X2	T45.5X3	T45.5X4	T45.5X5	T45.5X6
Chenodiol	T45.5X1	T45.5X2	T45.5X3	T45.5X4	T45.5X5	T45.5X6
Chenopodium	T37.4X1	T37.4X2	T37.4X3	T37.4X4	T37.4X5	T37.4X6
Cherry laurel	T62.2X1	T62.2X2	T62.2X3	T62.2X4	—	—
Chiggertox*	T41.3X1	T41.3X2	T41.3X3	T41.3X4	T41.3X5	T41.3X6
Chinidin (e)	T46.2X1	T46.2X2	T46.2X3	T46.2X4	T46.2X5	T46.2X6
Chiniofon	T37.8X1	T37.8X2	T37.8X3	T37.8X4	T37.8X5	T37.8X6
Chlophedianol	T48.3X1	T48.3X2	T48.3X3	T48.3X4	T48.3X5	T48.3X6
Chloral	T42.6X1	T42.6X2	T42.6X3	T42.6X4	T42.6X5	T42.6X6
derivative	T42.6X1	T42.6X2	T42.6X3	T42.6X4	T42.6X5	T42.6X6
hydrate	T42.6X1	T42.6X2	T42.6X3	T42.6X4	T42.6X5	T42.6X6
Chloralamide	T42.6X1	T42.6X2	T42.6X3	T42.6X4	T42.6X5	T42.6X6
Chloralodol	T42.6X1	T42.6X2	T42.6X3	T42.6X4	T42.6X5	T42.6X6
Chloralose	T60.4X1	T60.4X2	T60.4X3	T60.4X4	—	—
Chlorambucil	T45.1X1	T45.1X2	T45.1X3	T45.1X4	T45.1X5	T45.1X6
Chloramine	T57.8X1	T57.8X2	T57.8X3	T57.8X4	—	—
T	T49.0X1	T49.0X2	T49.0X3	T49.0X4	T49.0X5	T49.0X6
topical	T49.0X1	T49.0X2	T49.0X3	T49.0X4	T49.0X5	T49.0X6
Chloramphenicol	T36.2X1	T36.2X2	T36.2X3	T36.2X4	T36.2X5	T36.2X6
ENT agent	T49.6X1	T49.6X2	T49.6X3	T49.6X4	T49.6X5	T49.6X6
ophthalmic preparation	T49.5X1	T49.5X2	T49.5X3	T49.5X4	T49.5X5	T49.5X6
topical NEC	T49.0X1	T49.0X2	T49.0X3	T49.0X4	T49.0X5	T49.0X6
Chlorate (potassium) (sodium) NEC	T60.3X1	T60.3X2	T60.3X3	T60.3X4		
herbicide	T60.3X1	T60.3X2	T60.3X3	T60.3X4	—	—
Chlorazanil	T50.2X1	T50.2X2	T50.2X3	T50.2X4	T50.2X5	T50.2X6
Chlorbenzene, chlorbenzol	T53.7X1	T53.7X2	T53.7X3	T53.7X4		
Chlorbenzoxamine	T44.3X1	T44.3X2	T44.3X3	T44.3X4	T44.3X5	T44.3X6
Chlorbutol	T42.6X1	T42.6X2	T42.6X3	T42.6X4	T42.6X5	T42.6X6
Chlorcyclizine	T45.0X1	T45.0X2	T45.0X3	T45.0X4	T45.0X5	T45.0X6
Chlordan (e) (dust)	T60.1X1	T60.1X2	T60.1X3	T60.1X4	—	—
Chlordantoin	T49.0X1	T49.0X2	T49.0X3	T49.0X4	T49.0X5	T49.0X6
Chlordiazepoxide	T42.4X1	T42.4X2	T42.4X3	T42.4X4	T42.4X5	T42.4X6
Chlordiethyl benzamide	T49.3X1	T49.3X2	T49.3X3	T49.3X4	T49.3X5	T49.3X6
Chloresium	T49.8X1	T49.8X2	T49.8X3	T49.8X4	T49.8X5	T49.8X6
Chlorethiazol	T42.6X1	T42.6X2	T42.6X3	T42.6X4	T42.6X5	T42.6X6
Chlorethyl — see Ethyl, chloride						
Chloretone	T42.6X1	T42.6X2	T42.6X3	T42.6X4	T42.6X5	T42.6X6
Chlorex	T53.6X1	T53.6X2	T53.6X3	T53.6X4	—	—
insecticide	T60.1X1	T60.1X2	T60.1X3	T60.1X4	—	—
Chlorfenvinphos	T60.0X1	T60.0X2	T60.0X3	T60.0X4	—	—
Chlorhexadol	T42.6X1	T42.6X2	T42.6X3	T42.6X4	T42.6X5	T42.6X6
Chlorhexamide	T45.1X1	T45.1X2	T45.1X3	T45.1X4	T45.1X5	T45.1X6
Chlorhexidine	T49.0X1	T49.0X2	T49.0X3	T49.0X4	T49.0X5	T49.0X6
Chlorhexidine Gluconate Oral Rinse*	T49.6X1	T49.6X2	T49.6X3	T49.6X4	T49.6X5	T49.6X6
Chlorhydroxyquinolin	T49.0X1	T49.0X2	T49.0X3	T49.0X4	T49.0X5	T49.0X6
Chloride of lime (bleach)	T54.3X1	T54.3X2	T54.3X3	T54.3X4	—	—
Chlorimipramine	T43.011	T43.012	T43.013	T43.014	T43.015	T43.016
Chlorinated						
camphene	T53.6X1	T53.6X2	T53.6X3	T53.6X4	—	—
diphenyl	T53.7X1	T53.7X2	T53.7X3	T53.7X4	—	—
hydrocarbons NEC	T53.91	T53.92	T53.93	T53.94	—	—
solvents	T53.91	T53.92	T53.93	T53.94	—	—
lime (bleach)	T54.3X1	T54.3X2	T54.3X3	T54.3X4	—	—
and boric acid solution	T49.0X1	T49.0X2	T49.0X3	T49.0X4	T49.0X5	T49.0X6
naphthalene (insecticide)	T60.1X1	T60.1X2	T60.1X3	T60.1X4	—	—

Substance	Poisoning, Accidental (unintentional)	Poisoning, Intentional Self-harm	Poisoning, Assault	Poisoning, Undetermined	Adverse Effect	Under-dosing
Chlorinated — continued						
naphthalene — continued						
industrial (non-pesticide)	T53.7X1	T53.7X2	T53.7X3	T53.7X4	—	—
pesticide NEC	T60.8X1	T60.8X2	T60.8X3	T60.8X4	—	—
soda — see also sodium hypochlorite						
solution	T49.0X1	T49.0X2	T49.0X3	T49.0X4	T49.0X5	T49.0X6
Chlorine (fumes) (gas)	T59.4X1	T59.4X2	T59.4X3	T59.4X4	—	—
bleach	T54.3X1	T54.3X2	T54.3X3	T54.3X4	—	—
compound gas NEC	T59.4X1	T59.4X2	T59.4X3	T59.4X4	—	—
disinfectant	T59.4X1	T59.4X2	T59.4X3	T59.4X4	—	—
releasing agents NEC	T59.4X1	T59.4X2	T59.4X3	T59.4X4	—	—
Chlorisondamine chloride	T46.991	T46.992	T46.993	T46.994	T46.995	T46.996
Chlormadinone	T38.5X1	T38.5X2	T38.5X3	T38.5X4	T38.5X5	T38.5X6
Chlormephos	T60.0X1	T60.0X2	T60.0X3	T60.0X4	—	—
Chlormerodrin	T50.2X1	T50.2X2	T50.2X3	T50.2X4	T50.2X5	T50.2X6
Chlormethiazole	T42.6X1	T42.6X2	T42.6X3	T42.6X4	T42.6X5	T42.6X6
Chlormethine	T45.1X1	T45.1X2	T45.1X3	T45.1X4	T45.1X5	T45.1X6
Chlormethylenecycline	T36.4X1	T36.4X2	T36.4X3	T36.4X4	T36.4X5	T36.4X6
Chlormezanone	T42.6X1	T42.6X2	T42.6X3	T42.6X4	T42.6X5	T42.6X6
Chloroacetic acid	T60.3X1	T60.3X2	T60.3X3	T60.3X4	—	—
Chloroacetone	T59.3X1	T59.3X2	T59.3X3	T59.3X4	—	—
Chloroacetophenone	T59.3X1	T59.3X2	T59.3X3	T59.3X4	—	—
Chloroaniline	T53.7X1	T53.7X2	T53.7X3	T53.7X4	—	—
Chlorobenzene, chlorobenzol	T53.7X1	T53.7X2	T53.7X3	T53.7X4	—	—
Chlorobromomethane (fire extinguisher)	T53.6X1	T53.6X2	T53.6X3	T53.6X4	—	—
Chlorobutanol	T49.0X1	T49.0X2	T49.0X3	T49.0X4	T49.0X5	T49.0X6
Chlorocresol	T49.0X1	T49.0X2	T49.0X3	T49.0X4	T49.0X5	T49.0X6
Chlorodehydromethyltestosterone	T38.7X1	T38.7X2	T38.7X3	T38.7X4	T38.7X5	T38.7X6
Chlorodeoxyadenosine*	T45.1X1	T45.1X2	T45.1X3	T45.1X4	T45.1X5	T45.1X6
Chlorodinitrobenzene	T53.7X1	T53.7X2	T53.7X3	T53.7X4	—	—
dust or vapor	T53.7X1	T53.7X2	T53.7X3	T53.7X4	—	—
Chlorodiphenyl	T53.7X1	T53.7X2	T53.7X3	T53.7X4	—	—
Chloroethane — see Ethyl, chloride						
Chloroethylene	T53.6X1	T53.6X2	T53.6X3	T53.6X4	—	—
Chlorofluorocarbons	T53.5X1	T53.5X2	T53.5X3	T53.5X4	—	—
Chloroform (fumes) (vapor)	T53.1X1	T53.1X2	T53.1X3	T53.1X4	—	—
anesthetic	T41.0X1	T41.0X2	T41.0X3	T41.0X4	T41.0X5	T41.0X6
solvent	T53.1X1	T53.1X2	T53.1X3	T53.1X4	—	—
water, concentrated	T41.0X1	T41.0X2	T41.0X3	T41.0X4	T41.0X5	T41.0X6
Chloroguanide	T37.2X1	T37.2X2	T37.2X3	T37.2X4	T37.2X5	T37.2X6
Chloromycetin	T36.2X1	T36.2X2	T36.2X3	T36.2X4	T36.2X5	T36.2X6
ENT agent	T49.6X1	T49.6X2	T49.6X3	T49.6X4	T49.6X5	T49.6X6
ophthalmic preparation	T49.5X1	T49.5X2	T49.5X3	T49.5X4	T49.5X5	T49.5X6
otic solution	T49.6X1	T49.6X2	T49.6X3	T49.6X4	T49.6X5	T49.6X6
topical NEC	T49.0X1	T49.0X2	T49.0X3	T49.0X4	T49.0X5	T49.0X6
Chloronitrobenzene	T53.7X1	T53.7X2	T53.7X3	T53.7X4	—	—
dust or vapor	T53.7X1	T53.7X2	T53.7X3	T53.7X4	—	—
Chlorophacinone	T60.4X1	T60.4X2	T60.4X3	T60.4X4	—	—
Chlorophenol	T53.7X1	T53.7X2	T53.7X3	T53.7X4	—	—
Chlorophenothane	T60.1X1	T60.1X2	T60.1X3	T60.1X4	—	—
Chlorophyll	T50.991	T50.992	T50.993	T50.994	T50.995	T50.996
Chloropicrin (fumes)	T53.6X1	T53.6X2	T53.6X3	T53.6X4	—	—
fumigant	T60.8X1	T60.8X2	T60.8X3	T60.8X4	—	—
fungicide	T60.3X1	T60.3X2	T60.3X3	T60.3X4	—	—
pesticide	T60.8X1	T60.8X2	T60.8X3	T60.8X4	—	—
Chloroprocaine	T41.3X1	T41.3X2	T41.3X3	T41.3X4	T41.3X5	T41.3X6
infiltration (subcutaneous)	T41.3X1	T41.3X2	T41.3X3	T41.3X4	T41.3X5	T41.3X6
nerve block (peripheral) (plexus)	T41.3X1	T41.3X2	T41.3X3	T41.3X4	T41.3X5	T41.3X6
spinal	T41.3X1	T41.3X2	T41.3X3	T41.3X4	T41.3X5	T41.3X6
Chloroptic	T49.5X1	T49.5X2	T49.5X3	T49.5X4	T49.5X5	T49.5X6
Chloropurine	T45.1X1	T45.1X2	T45.1X3	T45.1X4	T45.1X5	T45.1X6
Chloropyramine	T45.0X1	T45.0X2	T45.0X3	T45.0X4	T45.0X5	T45.0X6
Chloropyrifos	T60.0X1	T60.0X2	T60.0X3	T60.0X4	—	—
Chloropyrilene	T45.0X1	T45.0X2	T45.0X3	T45.0X4	T45.0X5	T45.0X6
Chloroquine	T37.2X1	T37.2X2	T37.2X3	T37.2X4	T37.2X5	T37.2X6
Chlorostat*	T49.0X1	T49.0X2	T49.0X3	T49.0X4	T49.0X5	T49.0X6
Chlorothalonil	T60.3X1	T60.3X2	T60.3X3	T60.3X4	—	—
Chlorothen	T45.0X1	T45.0X2	T45.0X3	T45.0X4	T45.0X5	T45.0X6
Chlorothiazide	T50.2X1	T50.2X2	T50.2X3	T50.2X4	T50.2X5	T50.2X6
Chlorothymol	T49.4X1	T49.4X2	T49.4X3	T49.4X4	T49.4X5	T49.4X6
Chlorotrianisene	T38.5X1	T38.5X2	T38.5X3	T38.5X4	T38.5X5	T38.5X6
Chlorovinyldichloroarsine, not in war	T57.0X1	T57.0X2	T57.0X3	T57.0X4	—	—
Chloroxine	T49.4X1	T49.4X2	T49.4X3	T49.4X4	T49.4X5	T49.4X6
Chloroxylenol	T49.0X1	T49.0X2	T49.0X3	T49.0X4	T49.0X5	T49.0X6
Chlorphenamine	T45.0X1	T45.0X2	T45.0X3	T45.0X4	T45.0X5	T45.0X6

Substance	Poisoning, Accidental (unintentional)	Poisoning, Intentional Self-harm	Poisoning, Assault	Poisoning, Undetermined	Adverse Effect	Under-dosing
Chlorphenesin	T42.8X1	T42.8X2	T42.8X3	T42.8X4	T42.8X5	T42.8X6
topical (antifungal)	T49.0X1	T49.0X2	T49.0X3	T49.0X4	T49.0X5	T49.0X6
Chlorpheniramine	T45.0X1	T45.0X2	T45.0X3	T45.0X4	T45.0X5	T45.0X6
Chlorphenoxamine	T45.0X1	T45.0X2	T45.0X3	T45.0X4	T45.0X5	T45.0X6
Chlorphentermine	T50.5X1	T50.5X2	T50.5X3	T50.5X4	T50.5X5	T50.5X6
Chlorprocaine — see Chloroprocaine						
Chlorproguanil	T37.2X1	T37.2X2	T37.2X3	T37.2X4	T37.2X5	T37.2X6
Chlorpromazine	T43.3X1	T43.3X2	T43.3X3	T43.3X4	T43.3X5	T43.3X6
Chlorpropamide	T38.3X1	T38.3X2	T38.3X3	T38.3X4	T38.3X5	T38.3X6
Chlorprothixene	T43.4X1	T43.4X2	T43.4X3	T43.4X4	T43.4X5	T43.4X6
Chlorquinaldol	T49.0X1	T49.0X2	T49.0X3	T49.0X4	T49.0X5	T49.0X6
Chlorquinol	T49.0X1	T49.0X2	T49.0X3	T49.0X4	T49.0X5	T49.0X6
Chlortalidone	T50.2X1	T50.2X2	T50.2X3	T50.2X4	T50.2X5	T50.2X6
Chlortetracycline	T36.4X1	T36.4X2	T36.4X3	T36.4X4	T36.4X5	T36.4X6
Chlorthalidone	T50.2X1	T50.2X2	T50.2X3	T50.2X4	T50.2X5	T50.2X6
Chlorthion	T60.0X1	T60.0X2	T60.0X3	T60.0X4	—	—
Chlorthiophos	T60.0X1	T60.0X2	T60.0X3	T60.0X4	—	—
Chlortrianisene	T38.5X1	T38.5X2	T38.5X3	T38.5X4	T38.5X5	T38.5X6
Chlor-Trimeton	T45.0X1	T45.0X2	T45.0X3	T45.0X4	T45.0X5	T45.0X6
Chlorzoxazone	T42.8X1	T42.8X2	T42.8X3	T42.8X4	T42.8X5	T42.8X6
Choke damp	T59.7X1	T59.7X2	T59.7X3	T59.7X4	—	—
Cholagogues	T47.5X1	T47.5X2	T47.5X3	T47.5X4	T47.5X5	T47.5X6
Cholebrine	T50.8X1	T50.8X2	T50.8X3	T50.8X4	T50.8X5	T50.8X6
Cholecalciferol	T45.2X1	T45.2X2	T45.2X3	T45.2X4	T45.2X5	T45.2X6
Cholecystokinin	T50.8X1	T50.8X2	T50.8X3	T50.8X4	T50.8X5	T50.8X6
Cholera vaccine	T50.A91	T50.A92	T50.A93	T50.A94	T50.A95	T50.A96
Choleretic	T47.5X1	T47.5X2	T47.5X3	T47.5X4	T47.5X5	T47.5X6
Cholesterol-lowering agents	T46.6X1	T46.6X2	T46.6X3	T46.6X4	T46.6X5	T46.6X6
Cholestyramine (resin)	T46.6X1	T46.6X2	T46.6X3	T46.6X4	T46.6X5	T46.6X6
Cholic acid	T47.5X1	T47.5X2	T47.5X3	T47.5X4	T47.5X5	T47.5X6
Choline	T48.6X1	T48.6X2	T48.6X3	T48.6X4	T48.6X5	T48.6X6
chloride	T50.991	T50.992	T50.993	T50.994	T50.995	T50.996
dihydrogen citrate	T50.991	T50.992	T50.993	T50.994	T50.995	T50.996
salicylate	T39.091	T39.092	T39.093	T39.094	T39.095	T39.096
theophyllinate	T48.6X1	T48.6X2	T48.6X3	T48.6X4	T48.6X5	T48.6X6
Cholinergic (drug) NEC	T44.1X1	T44.1X2	T44.1X3	T44.1X4	T44.1X5	T44.1X6
muscle tone enhancer	T44.1X1	T44.1X2	T44.1X3	T44.1X4	T44.1X5	T44.1X6
organophosphorus						
insecticide	T60.0X1	T60.0X2	T60.0X3	T60.0X4	—	—
nerve gas	T59.891	T59.892	T59.893	T59.894	—	—
trimethyl ammonium propanediol	T44.1X1	T44.1X2	T44.1X3	T44.1X4	T44.1X5	T44.1X6
Cholinesterase reactivator	T50.6X1	T50.6X2	T50.6X3	T50.6X4	T50.6X5	T50.6X6
Cholografin	T50.8X1	T50.8X2	T50.8X3	T50.8X4	T50.8X5	T50.8X6
Chorionic gonadotropin	T38.891	T38.892	T38.893	T38.894	T38.895	T38.896
Chromate	T56.2X1	T56.2X2	T56.2X3	T56.2X4	—	—
dust or mist	T56.2X1	T56.2X2	T56.2X3	T56.2X4	—	—
lead — see also lead	T56.0X1	T56.0X2	T56.0X3	T56.0X4	—	—
paint	T56.0X1	T56.0X2	T56.0X3	T56.0X4	—	—
Chromelin*	T49.3X1	T49.3X2	T49.3X3	T49.3X4	T49.3X5	T49.3X6
Chromic						
acid	T56.2X1	T56.2X2	T56.2X3	T56.2X4	—	—
dust or mist	T56.2X1	T56.2X2	T56.2X3	T56.2X4	—	—
phosphate 32P	T45.1X1	T45.1X2	T45.1X3	T45.1X4	T45.1X5	T45.1X6
Chromium	T56.2X1	T56.2X2	T56.2X3	T56.2X4	—	—
compounds — see Chromate						
sesquioxide	T50.8X1	T50.8X2	T50.8X3	T50.8X4	T50.8X5	T50.8X6
Chromomycin A3	T45.1X1	T45.1X2	T45.1X3	T45.1X4	T45.1X5	T45.1X6
Chromonar	T46.3X1	T46.3X2	T46.3X3	T46.3X4	T46.3X5	T46.3X6
Chromyl chloride	T56.2X1	T56.2X2	T56.2X3	T56.2X4	—	—
Chrysarobin	T49.4X1	T49.4X2	T49.4X3	T49.4X4	T49.4X5	T49.4X6
Chrysazin	T47.2X1	T47.2X2	T47.2X3	T47.2X4	T47.2X5	T47.2X6
Chymar	T45.3X1	T45.3X2	T45.3X3	T45.3X4	T45.3X5	T45.3X6
ophthalmic preparation	T49.5X1	T49.5X2	T49.5X3	T49.5X4	T49.5X5	T49.5X6
Chymopapain	T45.3X1	T45.3X2	T45.3X3	T45.3X4	T45.3X5	T45.3X6
Chymotrypsin	T45.3X1	T45.3X2	T45.3X3	T45.3X4	T45.3X5	T45.3X6
ophthalmic preparation	T49.5X1	T49.5X2	T49.5X3	T49.5X4	T49.5X5	T49.5X6
Cianidanol	T50.991	T50.992	T50.993	T50.994	T50.995	T50.996
Cianopramine	T43.011	T43.012	T43.013	T43.014	T43.015	T43.016
Cibenzoline	T46.2X1	T46.2X2	T46.2X3	T46.2X4	T46.2X5	T46.2X6
Ciclacillin	T36.0X1	T36.0X2	T36.0X3	T36.0X4	T36.0X5	T36.0X6
Ciclobarbital — see Hexobarbital						
Ciclonicate	T46.7X1	T46.7X2	T46.7X3	T46.7X4	T46.7X5	T46.7X6
Ciclopirox (olamine)	T49.0X1	T49.0X2	T49.0X3	T49.0X4	T49.0X5	T49.0X6
Ciclosporin	T45.1X1	T45.1X2	T45.1X3	T45.1X4	T45.1X5	T45.1X6
Cicuta maculata or virosa	T62.2X1	T62.2X2	T62.2X3	T62.2X4	—	—
Cicutoxin	T62.2X1	T62.2X2	T62.2X3	T62.2X4	—	—
Cigarette lighter fluid	T52.0X1	T52.0X2	T52.0X3	T52.0X4	—	—
Cigarettes (tobacco)	T65.221	T65.222	T65.223	T65.224	—	—
Ciguatoxin	T61.01	T61.02	T61.03	T61.04	—	—

☑ Additional Character May Be Required — Refer to the Tabular List for Character Selection

*Optum Value-Add

Substance	Poisoning, Accidental (unintentional)	Poisoning, Intentional Self-harm	Poisoning, Assault	Poisoning, Undetermined	Adverse Effect	Under-dosing
Cilazapril	T46.4X1	T46.4X2	T46.4X3	T46.4X4	T46.4X5	T46.4X6
Cimetidine	T47.0X1	T47.0X2	T47.0X3	T47.0X4	T47.0X5	T47.0X6
Cimetropium bromide	T44.3X1	T44.3X2	T44.3X3	T44.3X4	T44.3X5	T44.3X6
Cinchocaine	T41.3X1	T41.3X2	T41.3X3	T41.3X4	T41.3X5	T41.3X6
topical (surface)	T41.3X1	T41.3X2	T41.3X3	T41.3X4	T41.3X5	T41.3X6
Cinchona	T37.2X1	T37.2X2	T37.2X3	T37.2X4	T37.2X5	T37.2X6
Cinchonine alkaloids	T37.2X1	T37.2X2	T37.2X3	T37.2X4	T37.2X5	T37.2X6
Cinchophen	T50.4X1	T50.4X2	T50.4X3	T50.4X4	T50.4X5	T50.4X6
Cinepazide	T46.7X1	T46.7X2	T46.7X3	T46.7X4	T46.7X5	T46.7X6
Cinnamedrine	T48.5X1	T48.5X2	T48.5X3	T48.5X4	T48.5X5	T48.5X6
Cinnarizine	T45.0X1	T45.0X2	T45.0X3	T45.0X4	T45.0X5	T45.0X6
Cinoxacin	T37.8X1	T37.8X2	T37.8X3	T37.8X4	T37.8X5	T37.8X6
Ciprofibrate	T46.6X1	T46.6X2	T46.6X3	T46.6X4	T46.6X5	T46.6X6
Ciprofloxacin	T36.8X1	T36.8X2	T36.8X3	T36.8X4	T36.8X5	T36.8X6
Cisapride	T47.8X1	T47.8X2	T47.8X3	T47.8X4	T47.8X5	T47.8X6
Cisplatin	T45.1X1	T45.1X2	T45.1X3	T45.1X4	T45.1X5	T45.1X6
Citalopram	T43.221	T43.222	T43.223	T43.224	T43.225	T43.226
Citanest	T41.3X1	T41.3X2	T41.3X3	T41.3X4	T41.3X5	T41.3X6
infiltration (subcutaneous)	T41.3X1	T41.3X2	T41.3X3	T41.3X4	T41.3X5	T41.3X6
nerve block (peripheral) (plexus)	T41.3X1	T41.3X2	T41.3X3	T41.3X4	T41.3X5	T41.3X6
Citracel*	T50.3X1	T50.3X2	T50.3X3	T50.3X4	T50.3X5	T50.3X6
Citric acid	T47.5X1	T47.5X2	T47.5X3	T47.5X4	T47.5X5	T47.5X6
Citrovorum (factor)	T45.8X1	T45.8X2	T45.8X3	T45.8X4	T45.8X5	T45.8X6
Claviceps purpurea	T62.2X1	T62.2X2	T62.2X3	T62.2X4	—	—
Clavulanic acid	T36.1X1	T36.1X2	T36.1X3	T36.1X4	T36.1X5	T36.1X6
Cleaner, cleansing agent, type not specified	T65.891	T65.892	T65.893	T65.894	—	—
of paint or varnish	T52.91	T52.92	T52.93	T52.94	—	—
specified type NEC	T65.891	T65.892	T65.893	T65.894	—	—
Clebopride	T47.8X1	T47.8X2	T47.8X3	T47.8X4	T47.8X5	T47.8X6
Clefamide	T37.3X1	T37.3X2	T37.3X3	T37.3X4	T37.3X5	T37.3X6
Clemastine	T45.0X1	T45.0X2	T45.0X3	T45.0X4	T45.0X5	T45.0X6
Clematis vitalba	T62.2X1	T62.2X2	T62.2X3	T62.2X4	—	—
Clemizole	T45.0X1	T45.0X2	T45.0X3	T45.0X4	T45.0X5	T45.0X6
penicillin	T36.0X1	T36.0X2	T36.0X3	T36.0X4	T36.0X5	T36.0X6
Clenbuterol	T48.6X1	T48.6X2	T48.6X3	T48.6X4	T48.6X5	T48.6X6
Clidinium bromide	T44.3X1	T44.3X2	T44.3X3	T44.3X4	T44.3X5	T44.3X6
Clinda-Derm*	T49.0X1	T49.0X2	T49.0X3	T49.0X4	T49.0X5	T49.0X6
Clindamycin	T36.8X1	T36.8X2	T36.8X3	T36.8X4	T36.8X5	T36.8X6
Clinofibrate	T46.6X1	T46.6X2	T46.6X3	T46.6X4	T46.6X5	T46.6X6
Clioquinol	T37.8X1	T37.8X2	T37.8X3	T37.8X4	T37.8X5	T37.8X6
Cliradon	T40.2X1	T40.2X2	T40.2X3	T40.2X4	—	—
Clobazam	T42.4X1	T42.4X2	T42.4X3	T42.4X4	T42.4X5	T42.4X6
Clobenzorex	T50.5X1	T50.5X2	T50.5X3	T50.5X4	T50.5X5	T50.5X6
Clobetasol	T49.0X1	T49.0X2	T49.0X3	T49.0X4	T49.0X5	T49.0X6
Clobetasone	T49.0X1	T49.0X2	T49.0X3	T49.0X4	T49.0X5	T49.0X6
Clobutinol	T48.3X1	T48.3X2	T48.3X3	T48.3X4	T48.3X5	T48.3X6
Clocortolone	T38.0X1	T38.0X2	T38.0X3	T38.0X4	T38.0X5	T38.0X6
Clodantoin	T49.0X1	T49.0X2	T49.0X3	T49.0X4	T49.0X5	T49.0X6
Clodronic acid	T50.991	T50.992	T50.993	T50.994	T50.995	T50.996
Clofazimine	T37.1X1	T37.1X2	T37.1X3	T37.1X4	T37.1X5	T37.1X6
Clofedanol	T48.3X1	T48.3X2	T48.3X3	T48.3X4	T48.3X5	T48.3X6
Clofenamide	T50.2X1	T50.2X2	T50.2X3	T50.2X4	T50.2X5	T50.2X6
Clofenotane	T49.0X1	T49.0X2	T49.0X3	T49.0X4	T49.0X5	T49.0X6
Clofezone	T39.2X1	T39.2X2	T39.2X3	T39.2X4	T39.2X5	T39.2X6
Clofibrate	T46.6X1	T46.6X2	T46.6X3	T46.6X4	T46.6X5	T46.6X6
Clofibride	T46.6X1	T46.6X2	T46.6X3	T46.6X4	T46.6X5	T46.6X6
Cloforex	T50.5X1	T50.5X2	T50.5X3	T50.5X4	T50.5X5	T50.5X6
Clomethiazole	T42.6X1	T42.6X2	T42.6X3	T42.6X4	T42.6X5	T42.6X6
Clometocillin	T36.0X1	T36.0X2	T36.0X3	T36.0X4	T36.0X5	T36.0X6
Clomifene	T38.5X1	T38.5X2	T38.5X3	T38.5X4	T38.5X5	T38.5X6
Clomiphene	T38.5X1	T38.5X2	T38.5X3	T38.5X4	T38.5X5	T38.5X6
Clomipramine	T43.011	T43.012	T43.013	T43.014	T43.015	T43.016
Clomocycline	T36.4X1	T36.4X2	T36.4X3	T36.4X4	T36.4X5	T36.4X6
Clonazepam	T42.4X1	T42.4X2	T42.4X3	T42.4X4	T42.4X5	T42.4X6
Clonidine	T46.5X1	T46.5X2	T46.5X3	T46.5X4	T46.5X5	T46.5X6
Clonixin	T39.8X1	T39.8X2	T39.8X3	T39.8X4	T39.8X5	T39.8X6
Clopamide	T50.2X1	T50.2X2	T50.2X3	T50.2X4	T50.2X5	T50.2X6
Clopenthixol	T43.4X1	T43.4X2	T43.4X3	T43.4X4	T43.4X5	T43.4X6
Cloperastine	T48.3X1	T48.3X2	T48.3X3	T48.3X4	T48.3X5	T48.3X6
Clophedianol	T48.3X1	T48.3X2	T48.3X3	T48.3X4	T48.3X5	T48.3X6
Cloponone	T36.2X1	T36.2X2	T36.2X3	T36.2X4	T36.2X5	T36.2X6
Cloprednol	T38.0X1	T38.0X2	T38.0X3	T38.0X4	T38.0X5	T38.0X6
Cloral betaine	T42.6X1	T42.6X2	T42.6X3	T42.6X4	T42.6X5	T42.6X6
Cloramfenicol	T36.2X1	T36.2X2	T36.2X3	T36.2X4	T36.2X5	T36.2X6
Clorazepate (dipotassium)	T42.4X1	T42.4X2	T42.4X3	T42.4X4	T42.4X5	T42.4X6
Clorexolone	T50.2X1	T50.2X2	T50.2X3	T50.2X4	T50.2X5	T50.2X6
Clorfenamine	T45.0X1	T45.0X2	T45.0X3	T45.0X4	T45.0X5	T45.0X6
Clorgiline	T43.1X1	T43.1X2	T43.1X3	T43.1X4	T43.1X5	T43.1X6
Clorotepine	T44.3X1	T44.3X2	T44.3X3	T44.3X4	T44.3X5	T44.3X6
Clorox (bleach)	T54.91	T54.92	T54.93	T54.94	—	—
Clorprenaline	T48.6X1	T48.6X2	T48.6X3	T48.6X4	T48.6X5	T48.6X6

Substance	Poisoning, Accidental (unintentional)	Poisoning, Intentional Self-harm	Poisoning, Assault	Poisoning, Undetermined	Adverse Effect	Under-dosing
Clortermine	T50.5X1	T50.5X2	T50.5X3	T50.5X4	T50.5X5	T50.5X6
Clotiapine	T43.591	T43.592	T43.593	T43.594	T43.595	T43.596
Clotiazepam	T42.4X1	T42.4X2	T42.4X3	T42.4X4	T42.4X5	T42.4X6
Clotibric acid	T46.6X1	T46.6X2	T46.6X3	T46.6X4	T46.6X5	T46.6X6
Clotrimazole	T49.0X1	T49.0X2	T49.0X3	T49.0X4	T49.0X5	T49.0X6
Cloxacillin	T36.0X1	T36.0X2	T36.0X3	T36.0X4	T36.0X5	T36.0X6
Cloxazolam	T42.4X1	T42.4X2	T42.4X3	T42.4X4	T42.4X5	T42.4X6
Cloxiquine	T49.0X1	T49.0X2	T49.0X3	T49.0X4	T49.0X5	T49.0X6
Clozapine	T42.4X1	T42.4X2	T42.4X3	T42.4X4	T42.4X5	T42.4X6
Coagulant NEC	T45.7X1	T45.7X2	T45.7X3	T45.7X4	T45.7X5	T45.7X6
Coal (carbon monoxide from) — see also Carbon, monoxide, coal	T58.2X1	T58.2X2	T58.2X3	T58.2X4		
oil — see Kerosene						
tar	T49.1X1	T49.1X2	T49.1X3	T49.1X4	T49.1X5	T49.1X6
fumes	T59.891	T59.892	T59.893	T59.894		
medicinal (ointment)	T49.4X1	T49.4X2	T49.4X3	T49.4X4	T49.4X5	T49.4X6
analgesics NEC	T39.2X1	T39.2X2	T39.2X3	T39.2X4	T39.2X5	T39.2X6
naphtha (solvent)	T52.0X1	T52.0X2	T52.0X3	T52.0X4		
Coartem*	T37.2X1	T37.2X2	T37.2X3	T37.2X4	T37.2X5	T37.2X6
Cobalamine	T45.2X1	T45.2X2	T45.2X3	T45.2X4	T45.2X5	T45.2X6
Cobalt (nonmedicinal) (fumes) (industrial)	T56.891	T56.892	T56.893	T56.894		
medicinal (trace) (chloride)	T45.8X1	T45.8X2	T45.8X3	T45.8X4	T45.8X5	T45.8X6
Cobra (venom)	T63.041	T63.042	T63.043	T63.044		
Coca (leaf)	T40.5X1	T40.5X2	T40.5X3	T40.5X4	T40.5X5	T40.5X6
Cocaine	T40.5X1	T40.5X2	T40.5X3	T40.5X4	T40.5X5	T40.5X6
topical anesthetic	T41.3X1	T41.3X2	T41.3X3	T41.3X4	T41.3X5	T41.3X6
Cocarboxylase	T45.3X1	T45.3X2	T45.3X3	T45.3X4	T45.3X5	T45.3X6
Coccidioidin	T50.8X1	T50.8X2	T50.8X3	T50.8X4	T50.8X5	T50.8X6
Cocculus indicus	T62.1X1	T62.1X2	T62.1X3	T62.1X4		
Cochineal	T65.6X1	T65.6X2	T65.6X3	T65.6X4		
medicinal products	T50.991	T50.992	T50.993	T50.994	T50.995	T50.996
Codeine	T40.2X1	T40.2X2	T40.2X3	T40.2X4	T40.2X5	T40.2X6
Cod-liver oil	T45.2X1	T45.2X2	T45.2X3	T45.2X4	T45.2X5	T45.2X6
Coenzyme A	T50.991	T50.992	T50.993	T50.994	T50.995	T50.996
Coffee	T62.8X1	T62.8X2	T62.8X3	T62.8X4		
Cogalactoisomerase	T50.991	T50.992	T50.993	T50.994	T50.995	T50.996
Cogentin	T44.3X1	T44.3X2	T44.3X3	T44.3X4	T44.3X5	T44.3X6
Coke fumes or gas (carbon monoxide)	T58.2X1	T58.2X2	T58.2X3	T58.2X4		
industrial use	T58.8X1	T58.8X2	T58.8X3	T58.8X4		
Colace	T47.4X1	T47.4X2	T47.4X3	T47.4X4	T47.4X5	T47.4X6
Colaspase	T45.1X1	T45.1X2	T45.1X3	T45.1X4	T45.1X5	T45.1X6
Colazal*	T47.8X1	T47.8X2	T47.8X3	T47.8X4	T47.8X5	T47.8X6
Colchicine	T50.4X1	T50.4X2	T50.4X3	T50.4X4	T50.4X5	T50.4X6
Colchicum	T62.2X1	T62.2X2	T62.2X3	T62.2X4		
Cold cream	T49.3X1	T49.3X2	T49.3X3	T49.3X4	T49.3X5	T49.3X6
Colecalciferol	T45.2X1	T45.2X2	T45.2X3	T45.2X4		T45.2X6
Colestipol	T46.6X1	T46.6X2	T46.6X3	T46.6X4	T46.6X5	T46.6X6
Colestyramine	T46.6X1	T46.6X2	T46.6X3	T46.6X4	T46.6X5	T46.6X6
Colimycin	T36.8X1	T36.8X2	T36.8X3	T36.8X4	T36.8X5	T36.8X6
Colistimethate	T36.8X1	T36.8X2	T36.8X3	T36.8X4	T36.8X5	T36.8X6
Colistin	T36.8X1	T36.8X2	T36.8X3	T36.8X4	T36.8X5	T36.8X6
sulfate (eye preparation)	T49.5X1	T49.5X2	T49.5X3	T49.5X4	T49.5X5	T49.5X6
Collagen	T50.991	T50.992	T50.993	T50.994	T50.995	T50.996
Collagenase	T49.4X1	T49.4X2	T49.4X3	T49.4X4	T49.4X5	T49.4X6
Collodion	T49.3X1	T49.3X2	T49.3X3	T49.3X4	T49.3X5	T49.3X6
Colocynth	T47.2X1	T47.2X2	T47.2X3	T47.2X4	T47.2X5	T47.2X6
Colophony adhesive	T49.3X1	T49.3X2	T49.3X3	T49.3X4	T49.3X5	T49.3X6
Colorant — see also Dye	T50.991	T50.992		T50.993	T50.995	T50.996
Coloring matter — see Dye(s)						
Combustion gas (after combustion) — see Carbon, monoxide						
prior to combustion	T59.891	T59.892	T59.893	T59.894		
Cometriq*	T45.1X1	T45.1X2	T45.1X3	T45.1X4	T45.1X5	T45.1X6
Compazine	T43.3X1	T43.3X2	T43.3X3	T43.3X4	T43.3X5	T43.3X6
Compound						
1080 (sodium fluoroacetate)	T60.4X1	T60.4X2	T60.4X3	T60.4X4	—	—
269 (endrin)	T60.1X1	T60.1X2	T60.1X3	T60.1X4	—	—
3422 (parathion)	T60.0X1	T60.0X2	T60.0X3	T60.0X4	—	—
3911 (phorate)	T60.0X1	T60.0X2	T60.0X3	T60.0X4	—	—
3956 (toxaphene)	T60.1X1	T60.1X2	T60.1X3	T60.1X4	—	—
4049 (malathion)	T60.0X1	T60.0X2	T60.0X3	T60.0X4	—	—
4069 (malathion)	T60.0X1	T60.0X2	T60.0X3	T60.0X4	—	—
4124 (dicapthon)	T60.0X1	T60.0X2	T60.0X3	T60.0X4	—	—
42 (warfarin)	T60.4X1	T60.4X2	T60.4X3	T60.4X4	—	—
497 (dieldrin)	T60.1X1	T60.1X2	T60.1X3	T60.1X4	—	—
E (cortisone)	T38.0X1	T38.0X2	T38.0X3	T38.0X4	T38.0X5	T38.0X6
F (hydrocortisone)	T38.0X1	T38.0X2	T38.0X3	T38.0X4	T38.0X5	T38.0X6
Comvax*	T50.A21	T50.A22	T50.A23	T50.A24	T50.A25	T50.A26

Substance	Poisoning, Accidental (unintentional)	Poisoning, Intentional Self-harm	Poisoning, Assault	Poisoning, Undetermined	Adverse Effect	Under-dosing
Congener, anabolic	T38.7X1	T38.7X2	T38.7X3	T38.7X4	T38.7X5	T38.7X6
Congo red	T50.8X1	T50.8X2	T50.8X3	T50.8X4	T50.8X5	T50.8X6
Coniine, conine	T62.2X1	T62.2X2	T62.2X3	T62.2X4	—	—
Conium (maculatum)	T62.2X1	T62.2X2	T62.2X3	T62.2X4	—	—
Conjugated estrogenic substances	T38.5X1	T38.5X2	T38.5X3	T38.5X4	T38.5X5	T38.5X6
Contac	T48.5X1	T48.5X2	T48.5X3	T48.5X4	T48.5X5	T48.5X6
Contact lens solution	T49.5X1	T49.5X2	T49.5X3	T49.5X4	T49.5X5	T49.5X6
Contraceptive (oral)	T38.4X1	T38.4X2	T38.4X3	T38.4X4	T38.4X5	T38.4X6
vaginal	T49.8X1	T49.8X2	T49.8X3	T49.8X4	T49.8X5	T49.8X6
Contrast medium, radiography	T50.8X1	T50.8X2	T50.8X3	T50.8X4	T50.8X5	T50.8X6
Convallaria glycosides	T46.0X1	T46.0X2	T46.0X3	T46.0X4	T46.0X5	T46.0X6
Convallaria majalis	T62.2X1	T62.2X2	T62.2X3	T62.2X4	—	—
berry	T62.1X1	T62.1X2	T62.1X3	T62.1X4	—	—
Copperhead snake (bite) (venom)	T63.061	T63.062	T63.063	T63.064	—	—
Copper (dust) (fumes) (nonmedicinal) NEC	T56.4X1	T56.4X2	T56.4X3	T56.4X4	—	—
arsenate, arsenite	T57.0X1	T57.0X2	T57.0X3	T57.0X4	—	—
insecticide	T60.2X1	T60.2X2	T60.2X3	T60.2X4	—	—
emetic	T47.7X1	T47.7X2	T47.7X3	T47.7X4	T47.7X5	T47.7X6
fungicide	T60.3X1	T60.3X2	T60.3X3	T60.3X4	—	—
gluconate	T49.0X1	T49.0X2	T49.0X3	T49.0X4	T49.0X5	T49.0X6
insecticide	T60.2X1	T60.2X2	T60.2X3	T60.2X4	—	—
medicinal (trace)	T45.8X1	T45.8X2	T45.8X3	T45.8X4	T45.8X5	T45.8X6
oleate	T49.0X1	T49.0X2	T49.0X3	T49.0X4	T49.0X5	T49.0X6
sulfate	T56.4X1	T56.4X2	T56.4X3	T56.4X4	—	—
cupric	T56.4X1	T56.4X2	T56.4X3	T56.4X4	—	—
fungicide	T60.3X1	T60.3X2	T60.3X3	T60.3X4	—	—
medicinal						
ear	T49.6X1	T49.6X2	T49.6X3	T49.6X4	T49.6X5	T49.6X6
emetic	T47.7X1	T47.7X2	T47.7X3	T47.7X4	T47.7X5	T47.7X6
eye	T49.5X1	T49.5X2	T49.5X3	T49.5X4	T49.5X5	T49.5X6
cuprous	T56.4X1	T56.4X2	T56.4X3	T56.4X4	—	—
fungicide	T60.3X1	T60.3X2	T60.3X3	T60.3X4	—	—
medicinal						
ear	T49.6X1	T49.6X2	T49.6X3	T49.6X4	T49.6X5	T49.6X6
emetic	T47.7X1	T47.7X2	T47.7X3	T47.7X4	T47.7X5	T47.7X6
eye	T49.5X1	T49.5X2	T49.5X3	T49.5X4	T49.5X5	T49.5X6
Coral (sting)	T63.691	T63.692	T63.693	T63.694	—	—
snake (bite) (venom)	T63.021	T63.022	T63.023	T63.024	—	—
Corbadrine	T49.6X1	T49.6X2	T49.6X3	T49.6X4	T49.6X5	T49.6X6
Cordite	T65.891	T65.892	T65.893	T65.894	—	—
vapor	T59.891	T59.892	T59.893	T59.894	—	—
Cordran	T49.0X1	T49.0X2	T49.0X3	T49.0X4	T49.0X5	T49.0X6
Cormax*	T49.0X1	T49.0X2	T49.0X3	T49.0X4	T49.0X5	T49.0X6
Corn cures	T49.4X1	T49.4X2	T49.4X3	T49.4X4	T49.4X5	T49.4X6
Cornhusker's lotion	T49.3X1	T49.3X2	T49.3X3	T49.3X4	T49.3X5	T49.3X6
Corn starch	T49.3X1	T49.3X2	T49.3X3	T49.3X4	T49.3X5	T49.3X6
Coronary vasodilator NEC	T46.3X1	T46.3X2	T46.3X3	T46.3X4	T46.3X5	T46.3X6
Corrosive NEC	T54.91	T54.92	T54.93	T54.94	—	—
acid NEC	T54.2X1	T54.2X2	T54.2X3	T54.2X4	—	—
aromatics	T54.1X1	T54.1X2	T54.1X3	T54.1X4	—	—
disinfectant	T54.1X1	T54.1X2	T54.1X3	T54.1X4	—	—
fumes NEC	T54.91	T54.92	T54.93	T54.94	—	—
specified NEC	T54.91	T54.92	T54.93	T54.94	—	—
sublimate	T56.1X1	T56.1X2	T56.1X3	T56.1X4	—	—
Cortate	T38.0X1	T38.0X2	T38.0X3	T38.0X4	T38.0X5	T38.0X6
Cort-Dome	T38.0X1	T38.0X2	T38.0X3	T38.0X4	T38.0X5	T38.0X6
ENT agent	T49.6X1	T49.6X2	T49.6X3	T49.6X4	T49.6X5	T49.6X6
ophthalmic preparation	T49.5X1	T49.5X2	T49.5X3	T49.5X4	T49.5X5	T49.5X6
topical NEC	T49.0X1	T49.0X2	T49.0X3	T49.0X4	T49.0X5	T49.0X6
Cortef	T38.0X1	T38.0X2	T38.0X3	T38.0X4	T38.0X5	T38.0X6
ENT agent	T49.6X1	T49.6X2	T49.6X3	T49.6X4	T49.6X5	T49.6X6
ophthalmic preparation	T49.5X1	T49.5X2	T49.5X3	T49.5X4	T49.5X5	T49.5X6
topical NEC	T49.0X1	T49.0X2	T49.0X3	T49.0X4	T49.0X5	T49.0X6
Corticosteroid	T38.0X1	T38.0X2	T38.0X3	T38.0X4	T38.0X5	T38.0X6
ENT agent	T49.6X1	T49.6X2	T49.6X3	T49.6X4	T49.6X5	T49.6X6
mineral	T50.0X1	T50.0X2	T50.0X3	T50.0X4	T50.0X5	T50.0X6
ophthalmic	T49.5X1	T49.5X2	T49.5X3	T49.5X4	T49.5X5	T49.5X6
topical NEC	T49.0X1	T49.0X2	T49.0X3	T49.0X4	T49.0X5	T49.0X6
Corticotropin	T38.811	T38.812	T38.813	T38.814	T38.815	T38.816
Cortisol	T49.0X1	T49.0X2	T49.0X3	T49.0X4	T49.0X5	T49.0X6
ENT agent	T49.6X1	T49.6X2	T49.6X3	T49.6X4	T49.6X5	T49.6X6
ophthalmic preparation	T49.5X1	T49.5X2	T49.5X3	T49.5X4	T49.5X5	T49.5X6
topical NEC	T49.0X1	T49.0X2	T49.0X3	T49.0X4	T49.0X5	T49.0X6
Cortisone (acetate)	T38.0X1	T38.0X2	T38.0X3	T38.0X4	T38.0X5	T38.0X6
ENT agent	T49.6X1	T49.6X2	T49.6X3	T49.6X4	T49.6X5	T49.6X6
ophthalmic preparation	T49.5X1	T49.5X2	T49.5X3	T49.5X4	T49.5X5	T49.5X6
topical NEC	T49.0X1	T49.0X2	T49.0X3	T49.0X4	T49.0X5	T49.0X6
Cortisporin*	T49.0X1	T49.0X2	T49.0X3	T49.0X4	T49.0X5	T49.0X6
Cortivazol	T38.0X1	T38.0X2	T38.0X3	T38.0X4	T38.0X5	T38.0X6
Cortogen	T38.0X1	T38.0X2	T38.0X3	T38.0X4	T38.0X5	T38.0X6
ENT agent	T49.6X1	T49.6X2	T49.6X3	T49.6X4	T49.6X5	T49.6X6
ophthalmic preparation	T49.5X1	T49.5X2	T49.5X3	T49.5X4	T49.5X5	T49.5X6
Cortone	T38.0X1	T38.0X2	T38.0X3	T38.0X4	T38.0X5	T38.0X6
ENT agent	T49.6X1	T49.6X2	T49.6X3	T49.6X4	T49.6X5	T49.6X6
ophthalmic preparation	T49.5X1	T49.5X2	T49.5X3	T49.5X4	T49.5X5	T49.5X6
Cortril	T38.0X1	T38.0X2	T38.0X3	T38.0X4	T38.0X5	T38.0X6
ENT agent	T49.6X1	T49.6X2	T49.6X3	T49.6X4	T49.6X5	T49.6X6
ophthalmic preparation	T49.5X1	T49.5X2	T49.5X3	T49.5X4	T49.5X5	T49.5X6
topical NEC	T49.0X1	T49.0X2	T49.0X3	T49.0X4	T49.0X5	T49.0X6
Corynebacterium parvum	T45.1X1	T45.1X2	T45.1X3	T45.1X4	T45.1X5	T45.1X6
Cosmetic preparation	T49.8X1	T49.8X2	T49.8X3	T49.8X4	T49.8X5	T49.8X6
Cosmetics	T49.8X1	T49.8X2	T49.8X3	T49.8X4	T49.8X5	T49.8X6
Cosyntropin	T38.811	T38.812	T38.813	T38.814	T38.815	T38.816
Cotarnine	T45.7X1	T45.7X2	T45.7X3	T45.7X4	T45.7X5	T45.7X6
Co-trimoxazole	T36.8X1	T36.8X2	T36.8X3	T36.8X4	T36.8X5	T36.8X6
Cottonseed oil	T49.3X1	T49.3X2	T49.3X3	T49.3X4	T49.3X5	T49.3X6
Cough mixture (syrup)	T48.4X1	T48.4X2	T48.4X3	T48.4X4	T48.4X5	T48.4X6
containing opiates	T40.2X1	T40.2X2	T40.2X3	T40.2X4	T40.2X5	T40.2X6
expectorants	T48.4X1	T48.4X2	T48.4X3	T48.4X4	T48.4X5	T48.4X6
Coumadin	T45.511	T45.512	T45.513	T45.514	T45.515	T45.516
rodenticide	T60.4X1	T60.4X2	T60.4X3	T60.4X4	—	—
Coumaphos	T60.0X1	T60.0X2	T60.0X3	T60.0X4	—	—
Coumarin	T45.511	T45.512	T45.513	T45.514	T45.515	T45.516
Coumetarol	T45.511	T45.512	T45.513	T45.514	T45.515	T45.516
Cowbane	T62.2X1	T62.2X2	T62.2X3	T62.2X4	—	—
Cozyme	T45.2X1	T45.2X2	T45.2X3	T45.2X4	T45.2X5	T45.2X6
Crack	T40.5X1	T40.5X2	T40.5X3	T40.5X4	—	—
Crataegus extract	T46.0X1	T46.0X2	T46.0X3	T46.0X4	T46.0X5	T46.0X6
Creolin	T54.1X1	T54.1X2	T54.1X3	T54.1X4	—	—
disinfectant	T54.1X1	T54.1X2	T54.1X3	T54.1X4	—	—
Creosol (compound)	T49.0X1	T49.0X2	T49.0X3	T49.0X4	T49.0X5	T49.0X6
Creosote (coal tar) (beechwood)	T49.0X1	T49.0X2	T49.0X3	T49.0X4	T49.0X5	T49.0X6
medicinal (expectorant)	T48.4X1	T48.4X2	T48.4X3	T48.4X4	T48.4X5	T48.4X6
syrup	T48.4X1	T48.4X2	T48.4X3	T48.4X4	T48.4X5	T48.4X6
Cresol(s)	T49.0X1	T49.0X2	T49.0X3	T49.0X4	T49.0X5	T49.0X6
and soap solution	T49.0X1	T49.0X2	T49.0X3	T49.0X4	T49.0X5	T49.0X6
Crestor*	T46.6X1	T46.6X2	T46.6X3	T46.6X4	T46.6X5	T46.6X6
Cresyl acetate	T49.0X1	T49.0X2	T49.0X3	T49.0X4	T49.0X5	T49.0X6
Cresylic acid	T49.0X1	T49.0X2	T49.0X3	T49.0X4	T49.0X5	T49.0X6
Crimidine	T60.4X1	T60.4X2	T60.4X3	T60.4X4	—	—
Croconazole	T37.8X1	T37.8X2	T37.8X3	T37.8X4	T37.8X5	T37.8X6
Cromoglicic acid	T48.6X1	T48.6X2	T48.6X3	T48.6X4	T48.6X5	T48.6X6
Cromolyn	T48.6X1	T48.6X2	T48.6X3	T48.6X4	T48.6X5	T48.6X6
Cromonar	T46.3X1	T46.3X2	T46.3X3	T46.3X4	T46.3X5	T46.3X6
Cropropamide	T39.8X1	T39.8X2	T39.8X3	T39.8X4	T39.8X5	T39.8X6
with crotethamide	T50.7X1	T50.7X2	T50.7X3	T50.7X4	T50.7X5	T50.7X6
Crotamiton	T49.0X1	T49.0X2	T49.0X3	T49.0X4	T49.0X5	T49.0X6
Crotethamide	T39.8X1	T39.8X2	T39.8X3	T39.8X4	T39.8X5	T39.8X6
with cropropamide	T50.7X1	T50.7X2	T50.7X3	T50.7X4	T50.7X5	T50.7X6
Croton (oil)	T47.2X1	T47.2X2	T47.2X3	T47.2X4	T47.2X5	T47.2X6
chloral	T42.6X1	T42.6X2	T42.6X3	T42.6X4	T42.6X5	T42.6X6
Crude oil	T52.0X1	T52.0X2	T52.0X3	T52.0X4	—	—
Cryogenine	T39.8X1	T39.8X2	T39.8X3	T39.8X4	T39.8X5	T39.8X6
Cryolite (vapor)	T60.1X1	T60.1X2	T60.1X3	T60.1X4	—	—
insecticide	T60.1X1	T60.1X2	T60.1X3	T60.1X4	—	—
Cryptenamine (tannates)	T46.5X1	T46.5X2	T46.5X3	T46.5X4	T46.5X5	T46.5X6
Crystal violet	T49.0X1	T49.0X2	T49.0X3	T49.0X4	T49.0X5	T49.0X6
Cuckoopint	T62.2X1	T62.2X2	T62.2X3	T62.2X4	—	—
Cumetharol	T45.511	T45.512	T45.513	T45.514	T45.515	T45.516
Cupric						
acetate	T60.3X1	T60.3X2	T60.3X3	T60.3X4	—	—
acetoarsenite	T57.0X1	T57.0X2	T57.0X3	T57.0X4	—	—
arsenate	T57.0X1	T57.0X2	T57.0X3	T57.0X4	—	—
gluconate	T49.0X1	T49.0X2	T49.0X3	T49.0X4	T49.0X5	T49.0X6
oleate	T49.0X1	T49.0X2	T49.0X3	T49.0X4	T49.0X5	T49.0X6
sulfate	T56.4X1	T56.4X2	T56.4X3	T56.4X4	—	—
Cuprimine*	T50.6X1	T50.6X2	T50.6X3	T50.6X4	T50.6X5	T50.6X6
Cuprous sulfate — see also Copper, sulfate	T56.4X1	T56.4X2	T56.4X3	T56.4X4	—	—
Curare, curarine	T48.1X1	T48.1X2	T48.1X3	T48.1X4	T48.1X5	T48.1X6
Cyamemazine	T43.3X1	T43.3X2	T43.3X3	T43.3X4	T43.3X5	T43.3X6
Cyamopsis tetragonoloba	T46.6X1	T46.6X2	T46.6X3	T46.6X4	T46.6X5	T46.6X6
Cyanacetic hydrazide	T37.1X1	T37.1X2	T37.1X3	T37.1X4	T37.1X5	T37.1X6
Cyanic acid (gas)	T59.891	T59.892	T59.893	T59.894	—	—
Cyanide(s) (compounds) (potassium) (sodium) NEC	T65.0X1	T65.0X2	T65.0X3	T65.0X4	—	—
dust or gas (inhalation) NEC	T57.3X1	T57.3X2	T57.3X3	T57.3X4	—	—
fumigant	T65.0X1	T65.0X2	T65.0X3	T65.0X4	—	—
hydrogen	T57.3X1	T57.3X2	T57.3X3	T57.3X4	—	—

☑ Additional Character May Be Required — Refer to the Tabular List for Character Selection   *Optum Value-Add

Substance	Poisoning, Accidental (unintentional)	Poisoning, Intentional Self-harm	Poisoning, Assault	Poisoning, Undetermined	Adverse Effect	Under-dosing
Cyanide(s) (compounds) (potassium) (sodium) NEC — continued						
mercuric — see Mercury						
pesticide (dust) (fumes)	T65.0X1	T65.0X2	T65.0X3	T65.0X4	—	—
Cyanoacrylate adhesive	T49.3X1	T49.3X2	T49.3X3	T49.3X4	T49.3X5	T49.3X6
Cyanocobalamin	T45.8X1	T45.8X2	T45.8X3	T45.8X4	T45.8X5	T45.8X6
Cyanogen (chloride) (gas) NEC	T59.891	T59.892	T59.893	T59.894		
Cyclacillin	T36.0X1	T36.0X2	T36.0X3	T36.0X4	T36.0X5	T36.0X6
Cyclaine	T41.3X1	T41.3X2	T41.3X3	T41.3X4	T41.3X5	T41.3X6
Cyclamate	T50.991	T50.992	T50.993	T50.994	T50.995	T50.996
Cyclamen europaeum	T62.2X1	T62.2X2	T62.2X3	T62.2X4	—	—
Cyclandelate	T46.7X1	T46.7X2	T46.7X3	T46.7X4	T46.7X5	T46.7X6
Cyclazocine	T50.7X1	T50.7X2	T50.7X3	T50.7X4	T50.7X5	T50.7X6
Cyclizine	T45.0X1	T45.0X2	T45.0X3	T45.0X4	T45.0X5	T45.0X6
Cyclobarbital	T42.3X1	T42.3X2	T42.3X3	T42.3X4	T42.3X5	T42.3X6
Cyclobarbitone	T42.3X1	T42.3X2	T42.3X3	T42.3X4	T42.3X5	T42.3X6
Cyclobenzaprine	T48.1X1	T48.1X2	T48.1X3	T48.1X4	T48.1X5	T48.1X6
Cyclodrine	T44.3X1	T44.3X2	T44.3X3	T44.3X4	T44.3X5	T44.3X6
Cycloguanil embonate	T37.2X1	T37.2X2	T37.2X3	T37.2X4	T37.2X5	T37.2X6
Cyclohexane	T52.8X1	T52.8X2	T52.8X3	T52.8X4	—	—
Cyclohexanol	T51.8X1	T51.8X2	T51.8X3	T51.8X4	—	—
Cyclohexanone	T52.4X1	T52.4X2	T52.4X3	T52.4X4	—	—
Cycloheximide	T60.3X1	T60.3X2	T60.3X3	T60.3X4	—	—
Cyclohexyl acetate	T52.8X1	T52.8X2	T52.8X3	T52.8X4	—	—
Cycloleucin	T45.1X1	T45.1X2	T45.1X3	T45.1X4	T45.1X5	T45.1X6
Cyclomethycaine	T41.3X1	T41.3X2	T41.3X3	T41.3X4	T41.3X5	T41.3X6
Cyclopentamine	T44.4X1	T44.4X2	T44.4X3	T44.4X4	T44.4X5	T44.4X6
Cyclopenthiazide	T50.2X1	T50.2X2	T50.2X3	T50.2X4	T50.2X5	T50.2X6
Cyclopentolate	T44.3X1	T44.3X2	T44.3X3	T44.3X4	T44.3X5	T44.3X6
Cyclophosphamide	T45.1X1	T45.1X2	T45.1X3	T45.1X4	T45.1X5	T45.1X6
Cycloplegic drug	T49.5X1	T49.5X2	T49.5X3	T49.5X4	T49.5X5	T49.5X6
Cyclopropane	T41.291	T41.292	T41.293	T41.294	T41.295	T41.296
Cyclopyrabital	T39.8X1	T39.8X2	T39.8X3	T39.8X4	T39.8X5	T39.8X6
Cycloserine	T37.1X1	T37.1X2	T37.1X3	T37.1X4	T37.1X5	T37.1X6
Cyclosporin	T45.1X1	T45.1X2	T45.1X3	T45.1X4	T45.1X5	T45.1X6
Cyclothiazide	T50.2X1	T50.2X2	T50.2X3	T50.2X4	T50.2X5	T50.2X6
Cycrimine	T44.3X1	T44.3X2	T44.3X3	T44.3X4	T44.3X5	T44.3X6
Cyhalothrin	T60.1X1	T60.1X2	T60.1X3	T60.1X4	—	—
Cymarin	T46.0X1	T46.0X2	T46.0X3	T46.0X4	T46.0X5	T46.0X6
Cypermethrin	T60.1X1	T60.1X2	T60.1X3	T60.1X4	—	—
Cyphenothrin	T60.2X1	T60.2X2	T60.2X3	T60.2X4	—	—
Cyproheptadine	T45.0X1	T45.0X2	T45.0X3	T45.0X4	T45.0X5	T45.0X6
Cyproterone	T38.6X1	T38.6X2	T38.6X3	T38.6X4	T38.6X5	T38.6X6
Cystaran*	T49.5X1	T49.5X2	T49.5X3	T49.5X4	T49.5X5	T49.5X6
Cysteamine	T50.6X1	T50.6X2	T50.6X3	T50.6X4	T50.6X5	T50.6X6
Cytarabine	T45.1X1	T45.1X2	T45.1X3	T45.1X4	T45.1X5	T45.1X6
Cytisus						
laburnum	T62.2X1	T62.2X2	T62.2X3	T62.2X4	—	—
scoparius	T62.2X1	T62.2X2	T62.2X3	T62.2X4	—	—
Cytochrome C	T47.5X1	T47.5X2	T47.5X3	T47.5X4	T47.5X5	T47.5X6
Cytomel	T38.1X1	T38.1X2	T38.1X3	T38.1X4	T38.1X5	T38.1X6
Cytosine arabinoside	T45.1X1	T45.1X2	T45.1X3	T45.1X4	T45.1X5	T45.1X6
Cytoxan	T45.1X1	T45.1X2	T45.1X3	T45.1X4	T45.1X5	T45.1X6
Cytozyme	T45.7X1	T45.7X2	T45.7X3	T45.7X4	T45.7X5	T45.7X6
S-Carboxymethylcysteine	T48.4X1	T48.4X2	T48.4X3	T48.4X4	T48.4X5	T48.4X6
Dabigatran*	T45.511	T45.512	T45.513	T45.514	T45.515	T45.516
Dacarbazine	T45.1X1	T45.1X2	T45.1X3	T45.1X4	T45.1X5	T45.1X6
Dactinomycin	T45.1X1	T45.1X2	T45.1X3	T45.1X4	T45.1X5	T45.1X6
DADPS	T37.1X1	T37.1X2	T37.1X3	T37.1X4	T37.1X5	T37.1X6
Dakin's solution	T49.0X1	T49.0X2	T49.0X3	T49.0X4	T49.0X5	T49.0X6
Dalapon (sodium)	T60.3X1	T60.3X2	T60.3X3	T60.3X4	—	—
Dalmane	T42.4X1	T42.4X2	T42.4X3	T42.4X4	T42.4X5	T42.4X6
Danazol	T38.6X1	T38.6X2	T38.6X3	T38.6X4	T38.6X5	T38.6X6
Danilone	T45.511	T45.512	T45.513	T45.514	T45.515	T45.516
Danthron	T47.2X1	T47.2X2	T47.2X3	T47.2X4	T47.2X5	T47.2X6
Dantrolene	T42.8X1	T42.8X2	T42.8X3	T42.8X4	T42.8X5	T42.8X6
Dantron	T47.2X1	T47.2X2	T47.2X3	T47.2X4	T47.2X5	T47.2X6
Daphne (gnidium) (mezereum)	T62.2X1	T62.2X2	T62.2X3	T62.2X4	—	—
berry	T37.1X1	T62.1X2	T62.1X3	T62.1X4	—	—
Dapsone	T37.1X1	T37.1X2	T37.1X3	T37.1X4	T37.1X5	T37.1X6
Daraprim	T37.2X1	T37.2X2	T37.2X3	T37.2X4	T37.2X5	T37.2X6
Darnel	T62.2X1	T62.2X2	T62.2X3	T62.2X4	—	—
Darvon	T39.8X1	T39.8X2	T39.8X3	T39.8X4	T39.8X5	T39.8X6
Daunomycin	T45.1X1	T45.1X2	T45.1X3	T45.1X4	T45.1X5	T45.1X6
Daunorubicin	T45.1X1	T45.1X2	T45.1X3	T45.1X4	T45.1X5	T45.1X6
DBI	T38.3X1	T38.3X2	T38.3X3	T38.3X4	T38.3X5	T38.3X6
D-Con	T60.91	T60.92	T60.93	T60.94	—	—
insecticide	T60.2X1	T60.2X2	T60.2X3	T60.2X4	—	—
rodenticide	T60.4X1	T60.4X2	T60.4X3	T60.4X4	—	—
DDAVP	T38.891	T38.892	T38.893	T38.894	T38.895	T38.896

Substance	Poisoning, Accidental (unintentional)	Poisoning, Intentional Self-harm	Poisoning, Assault	Poisoning, Undetermined	Adverse Effect	Under-dosing
DDE (bis(chlorophenyl)-dichloroethylene)	T60.2X1	T60.2X2	T60.2X3	T60.2X4	—	—
DDS	T37.1X1	T37.1X2	T37.1X3	T37.1X4	T37.1X5	T37.1X6
DDT (dust)	T60.1X1	T60.1X2	T60.1X3	T60.1X4	—	—
Deadly nightshade — see also Belladonna	T62.2X1	T62.2X2	T62.2X3	T62.2X4	—	—
berry	T62.1X1	T62.1X2	T62.1X3	T62.1X4	—	—
Deamino-D-arginine vasopressin	T38.891	T38.892	T38.893	T38.894	T38.895	T38.896
Deanol (aceglumate)	T50.991	T50.992	T50.993	T50.994	T50.995	T50.996
Debrisoquine	T46.5X1	T46.5X2	T46.5X3	T46.5X4	T46.5X5	T46.5X6
Decaborane	T57.8X1	T57.8X2	T57.8X3	T57.8X4	—	—
fumes	T59.891	T59.892	T59.893	T59.894		
Decadron	T38.0X1	T38.0X2	T38.0X3	T38.0X4	T38.0X5	T38.0X6
ENT agent	T49.6X1	T49.6X2	T49.6X3	T49.6X4	T49.6X5	T49.6X6
ophthalmic preparation	T49.5X1	T49.5X2	T49.5X3	T49.5X4	T49.5X5	T49.5X6
topical NEC	T49.0X1	T49.0X2	T49.0X3	T49.0X4	T49.0X5	T49.0X6
Decahydronaphthalene	T52.8X1	T52.8X2	T52.8X3	T52.8X4	—	—
Decalin	T52.8X1	T52.8X2	T52.8X3	T52.8X4	—	—
Decamethonium (bromide)	T48.1X1	T48.1X2	T48.1X3	T48.1X4	T48.1X5	T48.1X6
Decholin	T47.5X1	T47.5X2	T47.5X3	T47.5X4	T47.5X5	T47.5X6
Declomycin	T36.4X1	T36.4X2	T36.4X3	T36.4X4	T36.4X5	T36.4X6
Decongestant, nasal (mucosa)	T48.5X1	T48.5X2	T48.5X3	T48.5X4	T48.5X5	T48.5X6
combination	T48.5X1	T48.5X2	T48.5X3	T48.5X4	T48.5X5	T48.5X6
Deet	T60.8X1	T60.8X2	T60.8X3	T60.8X4	—	—
Deferoxamine	T45.8X1	T45.8X2	T45.8X3	T45.8X4	T45.8X5	T45.8X6
Deflazacort	T38.0X1	T38.0X2	T38.0X3	T38.0X4	T38.0X5	T38.0X6
Deglycyrrhizinized extract of licorice	T48.4X1	T48.4X2	T48.4X3	T48.4X4	T48.4X5	T48.4X6
Dehydrocholic acid	T47.5X1	T47.5X2	T47.5X3	T47.5X4	T47.5X5	T47.5X6
Dehydroemetine	T37.3X1	T37.3X2	T37.3X3	T37.3X4	T37.3X5	T37.3X6
Dekalin	T52.8X1	T52.8X2	T52.8X3	T52.8X4	—	—
Delafloxacin*	T36.8X1	T36.8X2	T36.8X3	T36.8X4	T36.8X5	T36.8X6
Delalutin	T38.5X1	T38.5X2	T38.5X3	T38.5X4	T38.5X5	T38.5X6
Delorazepam	T42.4X1	T42.4X2	T42.4X3	T42.4X4	T42.4X5	T42.4X6
Delphinium	T62.2X1	T62.2X2	T62.2X3	T62.2X4	—	—
Deltacortisone*	T38.0X1	T38.0X2	T38.0X3	T38.0X4	T38.0X5	T38.0X6
Deltamethrin	T60.1X1	T60.1X2	T60.1X3	T60.1X4	—	—
Deltasone	T38.0X1	T38.0X2	T38.0X3	T38.0X4	T38.0X5	T38.0X6
Deltra	T38.0X1	T38.0X2	T38.0X3	T38.0X4	T38.0X5	T38.0X6
Delvinal	T42.3X1	T42.3X2	T42.3X3	T42.3X4	T42.3X5	T42.3X6
Demecarium (bromide)	T49.5X1	T49.5X2	T49.5X3	T49.5X4	T49.5X5	T49.5X6
Demeclocycline	T36.4X1	T36.4X2	T36.4X3	T36.4X4	T36.4X5	T36.4X6
Demecolcine	T45.1X1	T45.1X2	T45.1X3	T45.1X4	T45.1X5	T45.1X6
Demecolcine	T45.1X1	T45.1X2	T45.1X3	T45.1X4	T45.1X5	T45.1X6
Demegestone	T38.5X1	T38.5X2	T38.5X3	T38.5X4	T38.5X5	T38.5X6
Demelanizing agents	T49.8X1	T49.8X2	T49.8X3	T49.8X4	T49.8X5	T49.8X6
Demephion -O and -S	T60.0X1	T60.0X2	T60.0X3	T60.0X4	—	—
Demerol	T40.2X1	T40.2X2	T40.2X3	T40.2X4	T40.2X5	T40.2X6
Demethylchlortetracycline	T36.4X1	T36.4X2	T36.4X3	T36.4X4	T36.4X5	T36.4X6
Demethyltetracycline	T36.4X1	T36.4X2	T36.4X3	T36.4X4	T36.4X5	T36.4X6
Demeton -O and -S	T60.0X1	T60.0X2	T60.0X3	T60.0X4	—	—
Demulcent (external)	T49.3X1	T49.3X2	T49.3X3	T49.3X4	T49.3X5	T49.3X6
specified NEC	T49.3X1	T49.3X2	T49.3X3	T49.3X4	T49.3X5	T49.3X6
Demulen	T38.4X1	T38.4X2	T38.4X3	T38.4X4	T38.4X5	T38.4X6
Denatured alcohol	T51.0X1	T51.0X2	T51.0X3	T51.0X4	—	—
Dendrid	T49.5X1	T49.5X2	T49.5X3	T49.5X4	T49.5X5	T49.5X6
Dental drug, topical application NEC	T49.7X1	T49.7X2	T49.7X3	T49.7X4	T49.7X5	T49.7X6
Dentifrice	T49.7X1	T49.7X2	T49.7X3	T49.7X4	T49.7X5	T49.7X6
Deodorant spray (feminine hygiene)	T49.8X1	T49.8X2	T49.8X3	T49.8X4	T49.8X5	T49.8X6
Deoxycortone	T50.0X1	T50.0X2	T50.0X3	T50.0X4	T50.0X5	T50.0X6
Deoxyribonuclease (pancreatic)	T45.3X1	T45.3X2	T45.3X3	T45.3X4	T45.3X5	T45.3X6
Depilatory	T49.4X1	T49.4X2	T49.4X3	T49.4X4	T49.4X5	T49.4X6
Deprenalin	T42.8X1	T42.8X2	T42.8X3	T42.8X4	T42.8X5	T42.8X6
Deprenyl	T42.8X1	T42.8X2	T42.8X3	T42.8X4	T42.8X5	T42.8X6
Depressant						
appetite (central)	T50.5X1	T50.5X2	T50.5X3	T50.5X4	T50.5X5	T50.5X6
cardiac	T46.2X1	T46.2X2	T46.2X3	T46.2X4	T46.2X5	T46.2X6
central nervous system (anesthetic) — see also Central nervous system, depressants	T42.71	T42.72	T42.73	T42.74	T42.75	T42.76
general anesthetic	T41.201	T41.202	T41.203	T41.204	T41.205	T41.206
muscle tone	T42.8X1	T42.8X2	T42.8X3	T42.8X4	T42.8X5	T42.8X6
muscle tone, central	T42.8X1	T42.8X2	T42.8X3	T42.8X4	T42.8X5	T42.8X6
psychotherapeutic	T43.501	T43.502	T43.503	T43.504	T43.505	T43.506
Depressant, appetite	T50.5X1	T50.5X2	T50.5X3	T50.5X4	T50.5X5	T50.5X6
Deptropine	T45.0X1	T45.0X2	T45.0X3	T45.0X4	T45.0X5	T45.0X6
Dequalinium (chloride)	T49.0X1	T49.0X2	T49.0X3	T49.0X4	T49.0X5	T49.0X6
Derris root	T60.2X1	T60.2X2	T60.2X3	T60.2X4	—	—

Substance	Poisoning, Accidental (unintentional)	Poisoning, Intentional Self-harm	Poisoning, Assault	Poisoning, Undetermined	Adverse Effect	Under-dosing
Deserpidine	T46.5X1	T46.5X2	T46.5X3	T46.5X4	T46.5X5	T46.5X6
Desferrioxamine	T45.8X1	T45.8X2	T45.8X3	T45.8X4	T45.8X5	T45.8X6
Desipramine	T43.011	T43.012	T43.013	T43.014	T43.015	T43.016
Deslanoside	T46.0X1	T46.0X2	T46.0X3	T46.0X4	T46.0X5	T46.0X6
Desloughing agent	T49.4X1	T49.4X2	T49.4X3	T49.4X4	T49.4X5	T49.4X6
Desmethylimipramine	T43.011	T43.012	T43.013	T43.014	T43.015	T43.016
Desmopressin	T38.891	T38.892	T38.893	T38.894	T38.895	T38.896
Desocodeine	T40.2X1	T40.2X2	T40.2X3	T40.2X4	T40.2X5	T40.2X6
Desogestrel	T38.5X1	T38.5X2	T38.5X3	T38.5X4	T38.5X5	T38.5X6
Desomorphine	T40.2X1	T40.2X2	T40.2X3	T40.2X4	—	—
Desonide	T49.0X1	T49.0X2	T49.0X3	T49.0X4	T49.0X5	T49.0X6
Desoximetasone	T49.0X1	T49.0X2	T49.0X3	T49.0X4	T49.0X5	T49.0X6
Desoxycorticosteroid	T50.0X1	T50.0X2	T50.0X3	T50.0X4	T50.0X5	T50.0X6
Desoxycortone	T50.0X1	T50.0X2	T50.0X3	T50.0X4	T50.0X5	T50.0X6
Desoxyephedrine	T43.651	T43.652	T43.652	T43.654	T43.655	T43.656
Detaxtran	T46.6X1	T46.6X2	T46.6X3	T46.6X4	T46.6X5	T46.6X6
Detergent	T49.2X1	T49.2X2	T49.2X3	T49.2X4	T49.2X5	T49.2X6
external medication	T49.2X1	T49.2X2	T49.2X3	T49.2X4	T49.2X5	T49.2X6
local	T49.2X1	T49.2X2	T49.2X3	T49.2X4	T49.2X5	T49.2X6
medicinal	T49.2X1	T49.2X2	T49.2X3	T49.2X4	T49.2X5	T49.2X6
nonmedicinal	T55.1X1	T55.1X2	T55.1X3	T55.1X4	—	—
specified NEC	T55.1X1	T55.1X2	T55.1X3	T55.1X4	—	—
Deterrent, alcohol	T50.6X1	T50.6X2	T50.6X3	T50.6X4	T50.6X5	T50.6X6
Detoxifying agent	T50.6X1	T50.6X2	T50.6X3	T50.6X4	T50.6X5	T50.6X6
Detrothyronine	T38.1X1	T38.1X2	T38.1X3	T38.1X4	T38.1X5	T38.1X6
Dettol (external medication)	T49.0X1	T49.0X2	T49.0X3	T49.0X4	T49.0X5	T49.0X6
Dexamethasone	T38.0X1	T38.0X2	T38.0X3	T38.0X4	T38.0X5	T38.0X6
ENT agent	T49.6X1	T49.6X2	T49.6X3	T49.6X4	T49.6X5	T49.6X6
ophthalmic preparation	T49.5X1	T49.5X2	T49.5X3	T49.5X4	T49.5X5	T49.5X6
topical NEC	T49.0X1	T49.0X2	T49.0X3	T49.0X4	T49.0X5	T49.0X6
Dexamfetamine	T43.621	T43.622	T43.623	T43.624	T43.625	T43.626
Dexamphetamine	T43.621	T43.622	T43.623	T43.624	T43.625	T43.626
Dexbrompheniramine	T45.0X1	T45.0X2	T45.0X3	T45.0X4	T45.0X5	T45.0X6
Dexchlorpheniramine	T45.0X1	T45.0X2	T45.0X3	T45.0X4	T45.0X5	T45.0X6
Dexedrine	T43.621	T43.622	T43.623	T43.624	T43.625	T43.626
Dexetimide	T44.3X1	T44.3X2	T44.3X3	T44.3X4	T44.3X5	T44.3X6
Dexfenfluramine	T50.5X1	T50.5X2	T50.5X3	T50.5X4	T50.5X5	T50.5X6
Dexpanthenol	T45.2X1	T45.2X2	T45.2X3	T45.2X4	T45.2X5	T45.2X6
Dextran (40) (70) (150)	T45.8X1	T45.8X2	T45.8X3	T45.8X4	T45.8X5	T45.8X6
Dextriferron	T45.4X1	T45.4X2	T45.4X3	T45.4X4	T45.4X5	T45.4X6
Dextroamphetamine	T43.621	T43.622	T43.623	T43.624	T43.625	T43.626
Dextro calcium pantothenate	T45.2X1	T45.2X2	T45.2X3	T45.2X4	T45.2X5	T45.2X6
Dextromethorphan	T48.3X1	T48.3X2	T48.3X3	T48.3X4	T48.3X5	T48.3X6
Dextromoramide	T40.491	T40.492	T40.493	T40.494	—	—
topical	T49.8X1	T49.8X2	T49.8X3	T49.8X4	T49.8X5	T49.8X6
Dextro pantothenyl alcohol	T45.2X1	T45.2X2	T45.2X3	T45.2X4	T45.2X5	T45.2X6
Dextropropoxyphene	T40.491	T40.492	T40.493	T40.494	T40.495	T40.496
Dextrorphan	T40.2X1	T40.2X2	T40.2X3	T40.2X4	T40.2X5	T40.2X6
Dextrose	T50.3X1	T50.3X2	T50.3X3	T50.3X4	T50.3X5	T50.3X6
concentrated solution, intravenous	T46.8X1	T46.8X2	T46.8X3	T46.8X4	T46.8X5	T46.8X6
Dextrothyroxin	T38.1X1	T38.1X2	T38.1X3	T38.1X4	T38.1X5	T38.1X6
Dextrothyroxine sodium	T38.1X1	T38.1X2	T38.1X3	T38.1X4	T38.1X5	T38.1X6
DFP	T44.0X1	T44.0X2	T44.0X3	T44.0X4	T44.0X5	T44.0X6
DHE	T37.3X1	T37.3X2	T37.3X3	T37.3X4	T37.3X5	T37.3X6
45	T46.5X1	T46.5X2	T46.5X3	T46.5X4	T46.5X5	I46.5X6
DiaBeta*	T38.3X1	T38.3X2	T38.3X3	T38.3X4	T38.3X5	T38.3X6
Diabinese	T38.3X1	T38.3X2	T38.3X3	T38.3X4	T38.3X5	T38.3X6
Diacetone alcohol	T52.4X1	T52.4X2	T52.4X3	T52.4X4	—	—
Diacetyl monoxime	T50.991	T50.992	T50.993	T50.994	—	—
Diacetylmorphine	T40.1X1	T40.1X2	T40.1X3	T40.1X4	—	—
Diachylon plaster	T49.4X1	T49.4X2	T49.4X3	T49.4X4	T49.4X5	T49.4X6
Diaethylstilboestrolum	T38.5X1	T38.5X2	T38.5X3	T38.5X4	T38.5X5	T38.5X6
Diagnostic agent NEC	T50.8X1	T50.8X2	T50.8X3	T50.8X4	T50.8X5	T50.8X6
Dial (soap)	T49.2X1	T49.2X2	T49.2X3	T49.2X4	T49.2X5	T49.2X6
sedative	T42.3X1	T42.3X2	T42.3X3	T42.3X4	T42.3X5	T42.3X6
Dialkyl carbonate	T52.91	T52.92	T52.93	T52.94	—	—
Diallylbarbituric acid	T42.3X1	T42.3X2	T42.3X3	T42.3X4	T42.3X5	T42.3X6
Diallymal	T42.3X1	T42.3X2	T42.3X3	T42.3X4	T42.3X5	T42.3X6
Dialysis solution (intraperitoneal)	T50.3X1	T50.3X2	T50.3X3	T50.3X4	T50.3X5	T50.3X6
Diaminodiphenylsulfone	T37.1X1	T37.1X2	T37.1X3	T37.1X4	T37.1X5	T37.1X6
Diamorphine	T40.1X1	T40.1X2	T40.1X3	T40.1X4	—	—
Diamox	T50.2X1	T50.2X2	T50.2X3	T50.2X4	T50.2X5	T50.2X6
Diamthazole	T49.0X1	T49.0X2	T49.0X3	T49.0X4	T49.0X5	T49.0X6
Dianthone	T47.2X1	T47.2X2	T47.2X3	T47.2X4	T47.2X5	T47.2X6
Diaphenylsulfone	T37.0X1	T37.0X2	T37.0X3	T37.0X4	T37.0X5	T37.0X6
Diasone (sodium)	T37.1X1	T37.1X2	T37.1X3	T37.1X4	T37.1X5	T37.1X6
Diastase	T47.5X1	T47.5X2	T47.5X3	T47.5X4	T47.5X5	T47.5X6
Diastat*	T42.4X1	T42.4X2	T42.4X3	T42.4X4	T42.4X5	T42.4X6
Diatrizoate	T50.8X1	T50.8X2	T50.8X3	T50.8X4	T50.8X5	T50.8X6

Substance	Poisoning, Accidental (unintentional)	Poisoning, Intentional Self-harm	Poisoning, Assault	Poisoning, Undetermined	Adverse Effect	Under-dosing
Diazepam	T42.4X1	T42.4X2	T42.4X3	T42.4X4	T42.4X5	T42.4X6
Diazinon	T60.0X1	T60.0X2	T60.0X3	T60.0X4	—	—
Diazomethane (gas)	T59.891	T59.892	T59.893	T59.894	—	—
Diazoxide	T46.5X1	T46.5X2	T46.5X3	T46.5X4	T46.5X5	T46.5X6
Dibekacin	T36.5X1	T36.5X2	T36.5X3	T36.5X4	T36.5X5	T36.5X6
Dibenamine	T44.6X1	T44.6X2	T44.6X3	T44.6X4	T44.6X5	T44.6X6
Dibenzepin	T43.011	T43.012	T43.013	T43.014	T43.015	T43.016
Dibenzheptropine	T45.0X1	T45.0X2	T45.0X3	T45.0X4	T45.0X5	T45.0X6
Dibenzyline	T44.6X1	T44.6X2	T44.6X3	T44.6X4	T44.6X5	T44.6X6
Diborane (gas)	T59.891	T59.892	T59.893	T59.894	—	—
Dibromochloropropane	T60.8X1	T60.8X2	T60.8X3	T60.8X4	—	—
Dibromodulcitol	T45.1X1	T45.1X2	T45.1X3	T45.1X4	T45.1X5	T45.1X6
Dibromoethane	T53.6X1	T53.6X2	T53.6X3	T53.6X4	—	—
Dibromomannitol	T45.1X1	T45.1X2	T45.1X3	T45.1X4	T45.1X5	T45.1X6
Dibromopropamidine isethionate	T49.0X1	T49.0X2	T49.0X3	T49.0X4	T49.0X5	T49.0X6
Dibropropamidine	T49.0X1	T49.0X2	T49.0X3	T49.0X4	T49.0X5	T49.0X6
Dibucaine	T41.3X1	T41.3X2	T41.3X3	T41.3X4	T41.3X5	T41.3X6
topical (surface)	T41.3X1	T41.3X2	T41.3X3	T41.3X4	T41.3X5	T41.3X6
Dibunate sodium	T48.3X1	T48.3X2	T48.3X3	T48.3X4	T48.3X5	T48.3X6
Dibutoline sulfate	T44.3X1	T44.3X2	T44.3X3	T44.3X4	T44.3X5	T44.3X6
Dicamba	T60.3X1	T60.3X2	T60.3X3	T60.3X4	—	—
Dicapthon	T60.0X1	T60.0X2	T60.0X3	T60.0X4	—	—
Dichlobenil	T60.3X1	T60.3X2	T60.3X3	T60.3X4	—	—
Dichlone	T60.3X1	T60.3X2	T60.3X3	T60.3X4	—	—
Dichloralphenozone	T42.6X1	T42.6X2	T42.6X3	T42.6X4	T42.6X5	T42.6X6
Dichlorbenzidine	T65.3X1	T65.3X2	T65.3X3	T65.3X4	—	—
Dichlorhydrin	T52.8X1	T52.8X2	T52.8X3	T52.8X4	—	—
Dichlorhydroxyquinoline	T37.8X1	T37.8X2	T37.8X3	T37.8X4	T37.8X5	T37.8X6
Dichlorobenzene	T53.7X1	T53.7X2	T53.7X3	T53.7X4	—	—
Dichlorobenzyl alcohol	T49.6X1	T49.6X2	T49.6X3	T49.6X4	T49.6X5	T49.6X6
Dichlorodifluoromethane	T53.5X1	T53.5X2	T53.5X3	T53.5X4	—	—
Dichloroethane	T52.8X1	T52.8X2	T52.8X3	T52.8X4	—	—
Dichloroethylene	T53.6X1	T53.6X2	T53.6X3	T53.6X4	—	—
Dichloroethyl sulfide, not in war	T59.891	T59.892	T59.893	T59.894	—	—
Dichloroformoxine, not in war	T59.891	T59.892	T59.893	T59.894	—	—
Dichlorohydrin, alpha-dichlorohydrin	T52.8X1	T52.8X2	T52.8X3	T52.8X4	—	—
Dichloromethane (solvent)	T53.4X1	T53.4X2	T53.4X3	T53.4X4	—	—
vapor	T53.4X1	T53.4X2	T53.4X3	T53.4X4	—	—
Dichloronaphthoquinone	T60.3X1	T60.3X2	T60.3X3	T60.3X4	—	—
Dichlorophen	T37.4X1	T37.4X2	T37.4X3	T37.4X4	T37.4X5	T37.4X6
Dichloropropene	T60.3X1	T60.3X2	T60.3X3	T60.3X4	—	—
Dichloropropionic acid	T60.3X1	T60.3X2	T60.3X3	T60.3X4	—	—
Dichlorphenamide	T50.2X1	T50.2X2	T50.2X3	T50.2X4	T50.2X5	T50.2X6
Dichlorvos	T60.0X1	T60.0X2	T60.0X3	T60.0X4	—	—
Dichysterol*	T45.2X1	T45.2X2	T45.2X3	T45.2X4	T45.2X5	T45.2X6
Diclofenac	T39.391	T39.392	T39.393	T39.394	T39.395	T39.396
Diclofenamide	T50.2X1	T50.2X2	T50.2X3	T50.2X4	T50.2X5	T50.2X6
Diclofensine	T43.291	T43.292	T43.293	T43.294	T43.295	T43.296
Diclonixine	T39.8X1	T39.8X2	T39.8X3	T39.8X4	T39.8X5	T39.8X6
Dicloxacillin	T36.0X1	T36.0X2	T36.0X3	T36.0X4	T36.0X5	T36.0X6
Dicophane	T49.0X1	T49.0X2	T49.0X3	T49.0X4	T49.0X5	T49.0X6
Dicoumarol, dicoumarin, dicumarol	T45.511	T45.512	T45.513	T45.514	T45.515	T45.516
Dicrotophos	T60.0X1	T60.0X2	T60.0X3	T60.0X4	—	—
Dicyanogen (gas)	T65.0X1	T65.0X2	T65.0X3	T65.0X4	—	—
Dicyclomine	T44.3X1	T44.3X2	T44.3X3	T44.3X4	T44.3X5	T44.3X6
Dicycloverine	T44.3X1	T44.3X2	T44.3X3	T44.3X4	T44.3X5	T44.3X6
Didanosine*	T37.5X1	T37.5X2	T37.5X3	T37.5X4	T37.5X5	T37.5X6
Dideoxycytidine	T37.5X1	T37.5X2	T37.5X3	T37.5X4	T37.5X5	T37.5X6
Dideoxyinosine	T37.5X1	T37.5X2	T37.5X3	T37.5X4	T37.5X5	T37.5X6
Dieldrin (vapor)	T60.1X1	T60.1X2	T60.1X3	T60.1X4	—	—
Diemal	T42.3X1	T42.3X2	T42.3X3	T42.3X4	T42.3X5	T42.3X6
Dienestrol	T38.5X1	T38.5X2	T38.5X3	T38.5X4	T38.5X5	T38.5X6
Dienoestrol	T38.5X1	T38.5X2	T38.5X3	T38.5X4	T38.5X5	T38.5X6
Dietetic drug NEC	T50.901	T50.902	T50.903	T50.904	T50.905	T50.906
Diethazine	T42.8X1	T42.8X2	T42.8X3	T42.8X4	T42.8X5	T42.8X6
Diethyl						
barbituric acid	T42.3X1	T42.3X2	T42.3X3	T42.3X4	T42.3X5	T42.3X6
carbamazine	T37.4X1	T37.4X2	T37.4X3	T37.4X4	T37.4X5	T37.4X6
carbinol	T51.3X1	T51.3X2	T51.3X3	T51.3X4	—	—
carbonate	T52.8X1	T52.8X2	T52.8X3	T52.8X4	—	—
ether (vapor) — see also ether	T41.0X1	T41.0X2	T41.0X3	T41.0X4	T41.0X5	T41.0X6
oxide	T52.8X1	T52.8X2	T52.8X3	T52.8X4	—	—
propion	T50.5X1	T50.5X2	T50.5X3	T50.5X4	T50.5X5	T50.5X6
stilbestrol	T38.5X1	T38.5X2	T38.5X3	T38.5X4	I38.5X5	T38.5X6
toluamide (nonmedicinal)	T60.8X1	T60.8X2	T60.8X3	T60.8X4	—	—
medicinal	T49.3X1	T49.3X2	T49.3X3	T49.3X4	T49.3X5	T49.3X6
Diethylcarbamazine	T37.4X1	T37.4X2	T37.4X3	T37.4X4	T37.4X5	T37.4X6

Substance	Poisoning, Accidental (unintentional)	Poisoning, Intentional Self-harm	Poisoning, Assault	Poisoning, Undetermined	Adverse Effect	Underdosing
Diethylene						
dioxide	T52.8X1	T52.8X2	T52.8X3	T52.8X4	—	—
glycol (monoacetate) (monobutyl ether) (monoethyl ether)	T52.3X1	T52.3X2	T52.3X3	T52.3X4	—	—
Diethylhexylphthalate	T65.891	T65.892	T65.893	T65.894	—	—
Diethylpropion	T50.5X1	T50.5X2	T50.5X3	T50.5X4	T50.5X5	T50.5X6
Diethylstilbestrol	T38.5X1	T38.5X2	T38.5X3	T38.5X4	T38.5X5	T38.5X6
Diethylstilboestrol	T38.5X1	T38.5X2	T38.5X3	T38.5X4	T38.5X5	T38.5X6
Diethylsulfone-diethyl-methane	T42.6X1	T42.6X2	T42.6X3	T42.6X4	T42.6X5	T42.6X6
Diethyltoluamide	T49.0X1	T49.0X2	T49.0X3	T49.0X4	T49.0X5	T49.0X6
Diethyltryptamine (DET)	T40.991	T40.992	T40.993	T40.994	—	—
Difebarbamate	T42.3X1	T42.3X2	T42.3X3	T42.3X4	T42.3X5	T42.3X6
Difencloxazine	T40.2X1	T40.2X2	T40.2X3	T40.2X4	T40.2X5	T40.2X6
Difenidol	T45.0X1	T45.0X2	T45.0X3	T45.0X4	T45.0X5	T45.0X6
Difenoxin	T47.6X1	T47.6X2	T47.6X3	T47.6X4	T47.6X5	T47.6X6
Difetarsone	T37.3X1	T37.3X2	T37.3X3	T37.3X4	T37.3X5	T37.3X6
Diffusin	T45.3X1	T45.3X2	T45.3X3	T45.3X4	T45.3X5	T45.3X6
Diflorasone	T49.0X1	T49.0X2	T49.0X3	T49.0X4	T49.0X5	T49.0X6
Diflos	T44.0X1	T44.0X2	T44.0X3	T44.0X4	T44.0X5	T44.0X6
Diflubenzuron	T60.1X1	T60.1X2	T60.1X3	T60.1X4	—	—
Diflucortolone	T49.0X1	T49.0X2	T49.0X3	T49.0X4	T49.0X5	T49.0X6
Diflunisal	T39.091	T39.092	T39.093	T39.094	T39.095	T39.096
Difluoromethyldopa	T42.8X1	T42.8X2	T42.8X3	T42.8X4	T42.8X5	T42.8X6
Difluorophate	T44.0X1	T44.0X2	T44.0X3	T44.0X4	T44.0X5	T44.0X6
Digestant NEC	T47.5X1	T47.5X2	T47.5X3	T47.5X4	T47.5X5	T47.5X6
Digitalin (e)	T46.0X1	T46.0X2	T46.0X3	T46.0X4	T46.0X5	T46.0X6
Digitalis (leaf)(glycoside)	T46.0X1	T46.0X2	T46.0X3	T46.0X4	T46.0X5	T46.0X6
lanata	T46.0X1	T46.0X2	T46.0X3	T46.0X4	T46.0X5	T46.0X6
purpurea	T46.0X1	T46.0X2	T46.0X3	T46.0X4	T46.0X5	T46.0X6
Digitoxin	T46.0X1	T46.0X2	T46.0X3	T46.0X4	T46.0X5	T46.0X6
Digitoxose	T46.0X1	T46.0X2	T46.0X3	T46.0X4	T46.0X5	T46.0X6
Digoxin	T46.0X1	T46.0X2	T46.0X3	T46.0X4	T46.0X5	T46.0X6
Digoxine	T46.0X1	T46.0X2	T46.0X3	T46.0X4	T46.0X5	T46.0X6
Dihydralazine	T46.5X1	T46.5X2	T46.5X3	T46.5X4	T46.5X5	T46.5X6
Dihydrazine	T46.5X1	T46.5X2	T46.5X3	T46.5X4	T46.5X5	T46.5X6
Dihydrocodeine	T40.2X1	T40.2X2	T40.2X3	T40.2X4	T40.2X5	T40.2X6
Dihydrocodeinone	T40.2X1	T40.2X2	T40.2X3	T40.2X4	T40.2X5	T40.2X6
Dihydroergocornine	T46.7X1	T46.7X2	T46.7X3	T46.7X4	T46.7X5	T46.7X6
Dihydroergocristine (mesilate)	T46.7X1	T46.7X2	T46.7X3	T46.7X4	T46.7X5	T46.7X6
Dihydroergokryptine	T46.7X1	T46.7X2	T46.7X3	T46.7X4	T46.7X5	T46.7X6
Dihydroergotamine	T46.5X1	T46.5X2	T46.5X3	T46.5X4	T46.5X5	T46.5X6
Dihydroergotoxine	T46.7X1	T46.7X2	T46.7X3	T46.7X4	T46.7X5	T46.7X6
mesilate	T46.7X1	T46.7X2	T46.7X3	T46.7X4	T46.7X5	T46.7X6
Dihydrohydroxycodeinone	T40.2X1	T40.2X2	T40.2X3	T40.2X4	T40.2X5	T40.2X6
Dihydrohydroxymorphinone	T40.2X1	T40.2X2	T40.2X3	T40.2X4	T40.2X5	T40.2X6
Dihydroisocodeine	T40.2X1	T40.2X2	T40.2X3	T40.2X4	T40.2X5	T40.2X6
Dihydromorphine	T40.2X1	T40.2X2	T40.2X3	T40.2X4	—	—
Dihydromorphinone	T40.2X1	T40.2X2	T40.2X3	T40.2X4	T40.2X5	T40.2X6
Dihydrostreptomycin	T36.5X1	T36.5X2	T36.5X3	T36.5X4	T36.5X5	T36.5X6
Dihydrotachysterol	T45.2X1	T45.2X2	T45.2X3	T45.2X4	T45.2X5	T45.2X6
Dihydroxyacetone*	T49.3X1	T49.3X2	T49.3X3	T49.3X4	T49.3X5	T49.3X6
Dihydroxyaluminum aminoacetate	T47.1X1	T47.1X2	T47.1X3	T47.1X4	T47.1X5	T47.1X6
Dihydroxyaluminum sodium carbonate	T47.1X1	T47.1X2	T47.1X3	T47.1X4	T47.1X5	T47.1X6
Dihydroxyanthraquinone	T47.2X1	T47.2X2	T47.2X3	T47.2X4	T47.2X5	T47.2X6
Dihydroxycodeinone	T40.2X1	T40.2X2	T40.2X3	T40.2X4	T40.2X5	T40.2X6
Dihydroxypropyl theophylline	T50.2X1	T50.2X2	T50.2X3	T50.2X4	T50.2X5	T50.2X6
Diiodohydroxyquin	T37.8X1	T37.8X2	T37.8X3	T37.8X4	T37.8X5	T37.8X6
topical	T49.0X1	T49.0X2	T49.0X3	T49.0X4	T49.0X5	T49.0X6
Diiodohydroxyquinoline	T37.8X1	T37.8X2	T37.8X3	T37.8X4	T37.8X5	T37.8X6
Diiodotyrosine	T38.2X1	T38.2X2	T38.2X3	T38.2X4	T38.2X5	T38.2X6
Diisopromine	T44.3X1	T44.3X2	T44.3X3	T44.3X4	T44.3X5	T44.3X6
Diisopropylamine	T46.3X1	T46.3X2	T46.3X3	T46.3X4	T46.3X5	T46.3X6
Diisopropylfluorophosphonate	T44.0X1	T44.0X2	T44.0X3	T44.0X4	T44.0X5	T44.0X6
Dilantin	T42.0X1	T42.0X2	T42.0X3	T42.0X4	T42.0X5	T42.0X6
Dilatrate*	T46.3X1	T46.3X2	T46.3X3	T46.3X4	T46.3X5	T46.3X6
Dilaudid	T40.2X1	T40.2X2	T40.2X3	T40.2X4	T40.2X5	T40.2X6
Dilazep	T46.3X1	T46.3X2	T46.3X3	T46.3X4	T46.3X5	T46.3X6
Dill	T47.5X1	T47.5X2	T47.5X3	T47.5X4	T47.5X5	T47.5X6
Diloxanide	T37.3X1	T37.3X2	T37.3X3	T37.3X4	T37.3X5	T37.3X6
Diltiazem	T46.1X1	T46.1X2	T46.1X3	T46.1X4	T46.1X5	T46.1X6
Dimazole	T49.0X1	T49.0X2	T49.0X3	T49.0X4	T49.0X5	T49.0X6
Dimefline	T50.7X1	T50.7X2	T50.7X3	T50.7X4	T50.7X5	T50.7X6
Dimefox	T60.0X1	T60.0X2	T60.0X3	T60.0X4	—	—
Dimemorfan	T48.3X1	T48.3X2	T48.3X3	T48.3X4	T48.3X5	T48.3X6
Dimenhydrinate	T45.0X1	T45.0X2	T45.0X3	T45.0X4	T45.0X5	T45.0X6
Dimercaprol (British anti-lewisite)	T45.8X1	T45.8X2	T45.8X3	T45.8X4	T45.8X5	T45.8X6
Dimercaptopropanol	T45.8X1	T45.8X2	T45.8X3	T45.8X4	T45.8X5	T45.8X6
Dimestrol	T38.5X1	T38.5X2	T38.5X3	T38.5X4	T38.5X5	T38.5X6
Dimetane	T45.0X1	T45.0X2	T45.0X3	T45.0X4	T45.0X5	T45.0X6
Dimethicone	T47.1X1	T47.1X2	T47.1X3	T47.1X4	T47.1X5	T47.1X6
Dimethindene	T45.0X1	T45.0X2	T45.0X3	T45.0X4	T45.0X5	T45.0X6
Dimethisoquin	T49.1X1	T49.1X2	T49.1X3	T49.1X4	T49.1X5	T49.1X6
Dimethisterone	T38.5X1	T38.5X2	T38.5X3	T38.5X4	T38.5X5	T38.5X6
Dimethoate	T60.0X1	T60.0X2	T60.0X3	T60.0X4	—	—
Dimethocaine	T41.3X1	T41.3X2	T41.3X3	T41.3X4	T41.3X5	T41.3X6
Dimethoxanate	T48.3X1	T48.3X2	T48.3X3	T48.3X4	T48.3X5	T48.3X6
Dimethyl						
arsine, arsinic acid	T57.0X1	T57.0X2	T57.0X3	T57.0X4	—	—
carbinol	T51.2X1	T51.2X2	T51.2X3	T51.2X4	—	—
carbonate	T52.8X1	T52.8X2	T52.8X3	T52.8X4	—	—
diguanide	T38.3X1	T38.3X2	T38.3X3	T38.3X4	T38.3X5	T38.3X6
ketone	T52.4X1	T52.4X2	T52.4X3	T52.4X4	—	—
vapor	T52.4X1	T52.4X2	T52.4X3	T52.4X4	—	—
meperidine	T40.2X1	T40.2X2	T40.2X3	T40.2X4	T40.2X5	T40.2X6
parathion	T60.0X1	T60.0X2	T60.0X3	T60.0X4	—	—
phthlate	T49.3X1	T49.3X2	T49.3X3	T49.3X4	T49.3X5	T49.3X6
polysiloxane	T47.8X1	T47.8X2	T47.8X3	T47.8X4	T47.8X5	T47.8X6
sulfate (fumes)	T59.891	T59.892	T59.893	T59.894		
liquid	T65.891	T65.892	T65.893	T65.894	—	—
sulfoxide (nonmedicinal)	T52.8X1	T52.8X2	T52.8X3	T52.8X4	—	—
medicinal	T49.4X1	T49.4X2	T49.4X3	T49.4X4	T49.4X5	T49.4X6
tryptamine	T40.991	T40.992	T40.993	T40.994	—	—
tubocurarine	T48.1X1	T48.1X2	T48.1X3	T48.1X4	T48.1X5	T48.1X6
Dimethylamine sulfate	T49.4X1	T49.4X2	T49.4X3	T49.4X4	T49.4X5	T49.4X6
Dimethylcysteine*	T50.6X1	T50.6X2	T50.6X3	T50.6X4	T50.6X5	T50.6X6
Dimethylformamide	T52.8X1	T52.8X2	T52.8X3	T52.8X4	—	—
Dimethyltubocurarinium chloride	T48.1X1	T48.1X2	T48.1X3	T48.1X4	T48.1X5	T48.1X6
Dimeticone	T47.1X1	T47.1X2	T47.1X3	T47.1X4	T47.1X5	T47.1X6
Dimetilan	T60.0X1	T60.0X2	T60.0X3	T60.0X4	—	—
Dimetindene	T45.0X1	T45.0X2	T45.0X3	T45.0X4	T45.0X5	T45.0X6
Dimetotiazine	T43.3X1	T43.3X2	T43.3X3	T43.3X4	T43.3X5	T43.3X6
Dimorpholamine	T50.7X1	T50.7X2	T50.7X3	T50.7X4	T50.7X5	T50.7X6
Dimoxyline	T46.3X1	T46.3X2	T46.3X3	T46.3X4	T46.3X5	T46.3X6
Dinitrobenzene	T65.3X1	T65.3X2	T65.3X3	T65.3X4	—	—
vapor	T59.891	T59.892	T59.893	T59.894		
Dinitrobenzol	T65.3X1	T65.3X2	T65.3X3	T65.3X4	—	—
vapor	T59.891	T59.892	T59.893	T59.894		
Dinitrobutylphenol	T65.3X1	T65.3X2	T65.3X3	T65.3X4	—	—
Dinitro (-ortho-)cresol (pesticide) (spray)	T65.3X1	T65.3X2	T65.3X3	T65.3X4	—	—
Dinitrocyclohexylphenol	T65.3X1	T65.3X2	T65.3X3	T65.3X4	—	—
Dinitrophenol	T65.3X1	T65.3X2	T65.3X3	T65.3X4	—	—
Dinoprost	T48.0X1	T48.0X2	T48.0X3	T48.0X4	T48.0X5	T48.0X6
Dinoprostone	T48.0X1	T48.0X2	T48.0X3	T48.0X4	T48.0X5	T48.0X6
Dinoseb	T60.3X1	T60.3X2	T60.3X3	T60.3X4	—	—
Dioctyl sulfosuccinate (calcium) (sodium)	T47.4X1	T47.4X2	T47.4X3	T47.4X4	T47.4X5	T47.4X6
Diodone	T50.8X1	T50.8X2	T50.8X3	T50.8X4	T50.8X5	T50.8X6
Diodoquin	T37.8X1	T37.8X2	T37.8X3	T37.8X4	T37.8X5	T37.8X6
Dionin	T40.2X1	T40.2X2	T40.2X3	T40.2X4	T40.2X5	T40.2X6
Diosmin	T46.991	T46.992	T46.993	T46.994	T46.995	T46.996
Diovan*	T46.5X1	T46.5X2	T46.5X3	T46.5X4	T46.5X5	T46.5X6
Dioxane	T52.8X1	T52.8X2	T52.8X3	T52.8X4	—	—
Dioxathion	T60.0X1	T60.0X2	T60.0X3	T60.0X4	—	—
Dioxin	T53.7X1	T53.7X2	T53.7X3	T53.7X4	—	—
Dioxopromethazine	T43.3X1	T43.3X2	T43.3X3	T43.3X4	T43.3X5	T43.3X6
Dioxyline	T46.3X1	T46.3X2	T46.3X3	T46.3X4	T46.3X5	T46.3X6
Dipentene	T52.8X1	T52.8X2	T52.8X3	T52.8X4	—	—
Diperodon	T41.3X1	T41.3X2	T41.3X3	T41.3X4	T41.3X5	T41.3X6
Diphacinone	T60.4X1	T60.4X2	T60.4X3	T60.4X4	—	—
Diphemanil	T44.3X1	T44.3X2	T44.3X3	T44.3X4	T44.3X5	T44.3X6
metilsulfate	T44.3X1	T44.3X2	T44.3X3	T44.3X4	T44.3X5	T44.3X6
Diphenadione	T45.511	T45.512	T45.513	T45.514	T45.515	T45.516
rodenticide	T60.4X1	T60.4X2	T60.4X3	T60.4X4	—	—
Diphenhydramine	T45.0X1	T45.0X2	T45.0X3	T45.0X4	T45.0X5	T45.0X6
Diphenidol	T45.0X1	T45.0X2	T45.0X3	T45.0X4	T45.0X5	T45.0X6
Diphenoxylate	T47.6X1	T47.6X2	T47.6X3	T47.6X4	T47.6X5	T47.6X6
Diphenylamine	T65.3X1	T65.3X2	T65.3X3	T65.3X4	—	—
Diphenylbutazone	T39.2X1	T39.2X2	T39.2X3	T39.2X4	T39.2X5	T39.2X6
Diphenylchloroarsine, not in war	T57.0X1	T57.0X2	T57.0X3	T57.0X4	—	—
Diphenylhydantoin	T42.0X1	T42.0X2	T42.0X3	T42.0X4	T42.0X5	T42.0X6
Diphenylmethane dye	T52.1X1	T52.1X2	T52.1X3	T52.1X4	—	—
Diphenylpyraline	T45.0X1	T45.0X2	T45.0X3	T45.0X4	T45.0X5	T45.0X6
Diphtheria						
antitoxin	T50.Z11	T50.Z12	T50.Z13	T50.Z14	T50.Z15	T50.Z16

Table of Drugs and Chemicals

Diphtheria — Enalapril

Substance	Poisoning, Accidental (unintentional)	Poisoning, Intentional Self-harm	Poisoning, Assault	Poisoning, Undetermined	Adverse Effect	Under-dosing
Diphtheria — continued						
toxoid	T50.A91	T50.A92	T50.A93	T50.A94	T50.A95	T50.A96
with tetanus toxoid	T50.A21	T50.A22	T50.A23	T50.A24	T50.A25	T50.A26
with pertussis component	T50.A11	T50.A12	T50.A13	T50.A14	T50.A15	T50.A16
vaccine	T50.A91	T50.A92	T50.A93	T50.A94	T50.A95	T50.A96
combination						
without pertussis	T50.A21	T50.A22	T50.A23	T50.A24	T50.A25	T50.A26
including pertussis	T50.A11	T50.A12	T50.A13	T50.A14	T50.A15	T50.A16
Diphylline	T50.2X1	T50.2X2	T50.2X3	T50.2X4	T50.2X5	T50.2X6
Dipipanone	T40.491	T40.492	T40.493	T40.494	—	—
Dipivefrine	T49.5X1	T49.5X2	T49.5X3	T49.5X4	T49.5X5	T49.5X6
Diplovax	T50.B91	T50.B92	T50.B93	T50.B94	T50.B95	T50.B96
Diprophylline	T50.2X1	T50.2X2	T50.2X3	T50.2X4	T50.2X5	T50.2X6
Dipropyline	T48.291	T48.292	T48.293	T48.294	T48.295	T48.296
Dipyridamole	T46.3X1	T46.3X2	T46.3X3	T46.3X4	T46.3X5	T46.3X6
Dipyrone	T39.2X1	T39.2X2	T39.2X3	T39.2X4	T39.2X5	T39.2X6
Diquat (dibromide)	T60.3X1	T60.3X2	T60.3X3	T60.3X4	—	—
Disinfectant	T65.891	T65.892	T65.893	T65.894	—	—
alkaline	T54.3X1	T54.3X2	T54.3X3	T54.3X4	—	—
aromatic	T54.1X1	T54.1X2	T54.1X3	T54.1X4	—	—
intestinal	T37.8X1	T37.8X2	T37.8X3	T37.8X4	T37.8X5	T37.8X6
Disipal	T42.8X1	T42.8X2	T42.8X3	T42.8X4	T42.8X5	T42.8X6
Disodium edetate	T50.6X1	T50.6X2	T50.6X3	T50.6X4	T50.6X5	T50.6X6
Disoprofol	T41.291	T41.292	T41.293	T41.294	T41.295	T41.296
Disopyramide*	T46.2X1	T46.2X2	T46.2X3	T46.2X4	T46.2X5	T46.2X6
Distigmine (bromide)	T44.0X1	T44.0X2	T44.0X3	T44.0X4	T44.0X5	T44.0X6
Disulfamide	T50.2X1	T50.2X2	T50.2X3	T50.2X4	T50.2X5	T50.2X6
Disulfanilamide	T37.0X1	T37.0X2	T37.0X3	T37.0X4	T37.0X5	T37.0X6
Disulfiram	T50.6X1	T50.6X2	T50.6X3	T50.6X4	T50.6X5	T50.6X6
Disulfoton	T60.0X1	T60.0X2	T60.0X3	T60.0X4	—	—
Dithiazanine iodide	T37.4X1	T37.4X2	T37.4X3	T37.4X4	T37.4X5	T37.4X6
Dithiocarbamate	T60.0X1	T60.0X2	T60.0X3	T60.0X4	—	—
Dithranol	T49.4X1	T49.4X2	T49.4X3	T49.4X4	T49.4X5	T49.4X6
Diucardin	T50.2X1	T50.2X2	T50.2X3	T50.2X4	T50.2X5	T50.2X6
Diupres	T50.2X1	T50.2X2	T50.2X3	T50.2X4	T50.2X5	T50.2X6
Diuretic NEC	T50.2X1	T50.2X2	T50.2X3	T50.2X4	T50.2X5	T50.2X6
benzothiadiazine	T50.2X1	T50.2X2	T50.2X3	T50.2X4	T50.2X5	T50.2X6
carbonic acid anhydrase inhibitors	T50.2X1	T50.2X2	T50.2X3	T50.2X4	T50.2X5	T50.2X6
furfuryl NEC	T50.2X1	T50.2X2	T50.2X3	T50.2X4	T50.2X5	T50.2X6
loop (high-ceiling)	T50.1X1	T50.1X2	T50.1X3	T50.1X4	T50.1X5	T50.1X6
mercurial NEC	T50.2X1	T50.2X2	T50.2X3	T50.2X4	T50.2X5	T50.2X6
osmotic	T50.2X1	T50.2X2	T50.2X3	T50.2X4	T50.2X5	T50.2X6
purine NEC	T50.2X1	T50.2X2	T50.2X3	T50.2X4	T50.2X5	T50.2X6
saluretic NEC	T50.2X1	T50.2X2	T50.2X3	T50.2X4	T50.2X5	T50.2X6
sulfonamide	T50.2X1	T50.2X2	T50.2X3	T50.2X4	T50.2X5	T50.2X6
thiazide NEC	T50.2X1	T50.2X2	T50.2X3	T50.2X4	T50.2X5	T50.2X6
xanthine	T50.2X1	T50.2X2	T50.2X3	T50.2X4	T50.2X5	T50.2X6
Diurgin	T50.2X1	T50.2X2	T50.2X3	T50.2X4	T50.2X5	T50.2X6
Diuril	T50.2X1	T50.2X2	T50.2X3	T50.2X4	T50.2X5	T50.2X6
Diuron	T60.3X1	T60.3X2	T60.3X3	T60.3X4	—	—
Divalproex	T42.6X1	T42.6X2	T42.6X3	T42.6X4	T42.6X5	T42.6X6
Divinyl ether	T41.0X1	T41.0X2	T41.0X3	T41.0X4	T41.0X5	T41.0X6
Dixanthogen	T49.0X1	T49.0X2	T49.0X3	T49.0X4	T49.0X5	T49.0X6
Dixyrazine	T43.3X1	T43.3X2	T43.3X3	T43.3X4	T43.3X5	T43.3X6
D-lysergic acid diethylamide	T40.8X1	T40.8X2	T40.8X3	T40.8X4	—	—
DMCT	T36.4X1	T36.4X2	T36.4X3	T36.4X4	T36.4X5	T36.4X6
DMSO — see Dimethyl, sulfoxide						
DNBP	T60.3X1	T60.3X2	T60.3X3	T60.3X4	—	—
DNOC	T65.3X1	T65.3X2	T65.3X3	T65.3X4	—	—
Dobutamine	T44.5X1	T44.5X2	T44.5X3	T44.5X4	T44.5X5	T44.5X6
DOCA	T38.0X1	T38.0X2	T38.0X3	T38.0X4	T38.0X5	T38.0X6
Docusate sodium	T47.4X1	T47.4X2	T47.4X3	T47.4X4	T47.4X5	T47.4X6
Dodicin	T49.0X1	T49.0X2	T49.0X3	T49.0X4	T49.0X5	T49.0X6
Dofamium chloride	T49.0X1	T49.0X2	T49.0X3	T49.0X4	T49.0X5	T49.0X6
Dolophine	T40.3X1	T40.3X2	T40.3X3	T40.3X4	T40.3X5	T40.3X6
Doloxene	T39.8X1	T39.8X2	T39.8X3	T39.8X4	T39.8X5	T39.8X6
Domestic gas (after combustion) — see Gas, utility						
prior to combustion	T59.891	T59.892	T59.893	T59.894	—	—
Domiodol	T48.4X1	T48.4X2	T48.4X3	T48.4X4	T48.4X5	T48.4X6
Domiphen (bromide)	T49.0X1	T49.0X2	T49.0X3	T49.0X4	T49.0X5	T49.0X6
Domperidone	T45.0X1	T45.0X2	T45.0X3	T45.0X4	T45.0X5	T45.0X6
Donepezil*	T44.0X1	T44.0X2	T44.0X3	T44.0X4	T44.0X5	T44.0X6
Dopa	T42.8X1	T42.8X2	T42.8X3	T42.8X4	T42.8X5	T42.8X6
Dopamine	T44.991	T44.992	T44.993	T44.994	T44.995	T44.996
Doriden	T42.6X1	T42.6X2	T42.6X3	T42.6X4	T42.6X5	T42.6X6
Dormiral	T42.3X1	T42.3X2	T42.3X3	T42.3X4	T42.3X5	T42.3X6
Dormison	T42.6X1	T42.6X2	T42.6X3	T42.6X4	T42.6X5	T42.6X6
Dornase	T48.4X1	T48.4X2	T48.4X3	T48.4X4	T48.4X5	T48.4X6
Dorsacaine	T41.3X1	T41.3X2	T41.3X3	T41.3X4	T41.3X5	T41.3X6
Dosulepin	T43.011	T43.012	T43.013	T43.014	T43.015	T43.016
Dothiepin	T43.011	T43.012	T43.013	T43.014	T43.015	T43.016
Doxantrazole	T48.6X1	T48.6X2	T48.6X3	T48.6X4	T48.6X5	T48.6X6
Doxapram	T50.7X1	T50.7X2	T50.7X3	T50.7X4	T50.7X5	T50.7X6
Doxazosin	T44.6X1	T44.6X2	T44.6X3	T44.6X4	T44.6X5	T44.6X6
Doxepin	T43.011	T43.012	T43.013	T43.014	T43.015	T43.016
Doxifluridine	T45.1X1	T45.1X2	T45.1X3	T45.1X4	T45.1X5	T45.1X6
Doxil*	T45.1X1	T45.1X2	T45.1X3	T45.1X4	T45.1X5	T45.1X6
Doxorubicin	T45.1X1	T45.1X2	T45.1X3	T45.1X4	T45.1X5	T45.1X6
Doxycycline	T36.4X1	T36.4X2	T36.4X3	T36.4X4	T36.4X5	T36.4X6
Doxylamine	T45.0X1	T45.0X2	T45.0X3	T45.0X4	T45.0X5	T45.0X6
Dramamine	T45.0X1	T45.0X2	T45.0X3	T45.0X4	T45.0X5	T45.0X6
Drano (drain cleaner)	T54.3X1	T54.3X2	T54.3X3	T54.3X4	—	—
Dressing, live pulp	T49.7X1	T49.7X2	T49.7X3	T49.7X4	T49.7X5	T49.7X6
Drocode	T40.2X1	T40.2X2	T40.2X3	T40.2X4	T40.2X5	T40.2X6
Dromoran	T40.2X1	T40.2X2	T40.2X3	T40.2X4	T40.2X5	T40.2X6
Dromostanolone	T38.7X1	T38.7X2	T38.7X3	T38.7X4	T38.7X5	T38.7X6
Dronabinol	T40.711	T40.712	T40.713	T40.714	T40.715	T40.716
Droperidol	T43.591	T43.592	T43.593	T43.594	T43.595	T43.596
Dropropizine	T48.3X1	T48.3X2	T48.3X3	T48.3X4	T48.3X5	T48.3X6
Drostanolone	T38.7X1	T38.7X2	T38.7X3	T38.7X4	T38.7X5	T38.7X6
Drotaverine	T44.3X1	T44.3X2	T44.3X3	T44.3X4	T44.3X5	T44.3X6
Drotrecogin alfa	T45.511	T45.512	T45.513	T45.514	T45.515	T45.516
Drug NEC	T50.901	T50.902	T50.903	T50.904	T50.905	T50.906
specified NEC	T50.991	T50.992	T50.993	T50.994	T50.995	T50.996
DTIC	T45.1X1	T45.1X2	T45.1X3	T45.1X4	T45.1X5	T45.1X6
Duboisine	T44.3X1	T44.3X2	T44.3X3	T44.3X4	T44.3X5	T44.3X6
Dulcolax	T47.2X1	T47.2X2	T47.2X3	T47.2X4	T47.2X5	T47.2X6
Duponol (C) (EP)	T49.2X1	T49.2X2	T49.2X3	T49.2X4	T49.2X5	T49.2X6
Durabolin	T38.7X1	T38.7X2	T38.7X3	T38.7X4	T38.7X5	T38.7X6
Durezol*	T49.5X1	T49.5X2	T49.5X3	T49.5X4	T49.5X5	T49.5X6
Dyclone	T41.3X1	T41.3X2	T41.3X3	T41.3X4	T41.3X5	T41.3X6
Dyclonine	T41.3X1	T41.3X2	T41.3X3	T41.3X4	T41.3X5	T41.3X6
Dydrogesterone	T38.5X1	T38.5X2	T38.5X3	T38.5X4	T38.5X5	T38.5X6
Dye NEC	T65.6X1	T65.6X2	T65.6X3	T65.6X4	—	—
antiseptic	T49.0X1	T49.0X2	T49.0X3	T49.0X4	T49.0X5	T49.0X6
diagnostic agents	T50.8X1	T50.8X2	T50.8X3	T50.8X4	T50.8X5	T50.8X6
pharmaceutical NEC	T50.901	T50.902	T50.903	T50.904	T50.905	T50.906
Dyflos	T44.0X1	T44.0X2	T44.0X3	T44.0X4	T44.0X5	T44.0X6
Dymelor	T38.3X1	T38.3X2	T38.3X3	T38.3X4	T38.3X5	T38.3X6
Dynamite	T65.3X1	T65.3X2	T65.3X3	T65.3X4	—	—
fumes	T59.891	T59.892	T59.893	T59.894	—	—
Dyphylline	T44.3X1	T44.3X2	T44.3X3	T44.3X4	T44.3X5	T44.3X6
b-eucaine	T49.1X1	T49.1X2	T49.1X3	T49.1X4	T49.1X5	T49.1X6
Ear drug NEC	T49.6X1	T49.6X2	T49.6X3	T49.6X4	T49.6X5	T49.6X6
Ear preparations	T49.6X1	T49.6X2	T49.6X3	T49.6X4	T49.6X5	T49.6X6
Echothiophate, echothiopate, ecothiopate	T49.5X1	T49.5X2	T49.5X3	T49.5X4	T49.5X5	T49.5X6
Econazole	T49.0X1	T49.0X2	T49.0X3	T49.0X4	T49.0X5	T49.0X6
Ecothiopate iodide	T49.5X1	T49.5X2	T49.5X3	T49.5X4	T49.5X5	T49.5X6
Ecstasy	T43.641	T43.642	T43.643	T43.644	—	—
Ectylurea	T42.6X1	T42.6X2	T42.6X3	T42.6X4	T42.6X5	T42.6X6
Edathamil disodium	T45.8X1	T45.8X2	T45.8X3	T45.8X4	T45.8X5	T45.8X6
Edecrin	T50.1X1	T50.1X2	T50.1X3	T50.1X4	T50.1X5	T50.1X6
Edetate, disodium (calcium)	T45.8X1	T45.8X2	T45.8X3	T45.8X4	T45.8X5	T45.8X6
Edoxudine	T49.5X1	T49.5X2	T49.5X3	T49.5X4	T49.5X5	T49.5X6
Edrophonium	T44.0X1	T44.0X2	T44.0X3	T44.0X4	T44.0X5	T44.0X6
chloride	T44.0X1	T44.0X2	T44.0X3	T44.0X4	T44.0X5	T44.0X6
EDTA	T50.6X1	T50.6X2	T50.6X3	T50.6X4	T50.6X5	T50.6X6
Eflornithine	T37.2X1	T37.2X2	T37.2X3	T37.2X4	T37.2X5	T37.2X6
Efloxate	T46.3X1	T46.3X2	T46.3X3	T46.3X4	T46.3X5	T46.3X6
Elase	T49.8X1	T49.8X2	T49.8X3	T49.8X4	T49.8X5	T49.8X6
Elastase	T47.5X1	T47.5X2	T47.5X3	T47.5X4	T47.5X5	T47.5X6
Elaterium	T47.2X1	T47.2X2	T47.2X3	T47.2X4	T47.2X5	T47.2X6
Elcatonin	T50.991	T50.992	T50.993	T50.994	T50.995	T50.996
Elder	T62.2X1	T62.2X2	T62.2X3	T62.2X4	—	—
berry, (unripe)	T62.1X1	T62.1X2	T62.1X3	T62.1X4	—	—
Electrolyte balance drug	T50.3X1	T50.3X2	T50.3X3	T50.3X4	T50.3X5	T50.3X6
Electrolytes NEC	T50.3X1	T50.3X2	T50.3X3	T50.3X4	T50.3X5	T50.3X6
Electrolytic agent NEC	T50.3X1	T50.3X2	T50.3X3	T50.3X4	T50.3X5	T50.3X6
Elemental diet	T50.901	T50.902	T50.903	T50.904	T50.905	T50.906
Elliptinium acetate	T45.1X1	T45.1X2	T45.1X3	T45.1X4	T45.1X5	T45.1X6
Elocon*	T49.0X1	T49.0X2	T49.0X3	T49.0X4	T49.0X5	T49.0X6
Embramine	T45.0X1	T45.0X2	T45.0X3	T45.0X4	T45.0X5	T45.0X6
Emepronium (salts)	T44.3X1	T44.3X2	T44.3X3	T44.3X4	T44.3X5	T44.3X6
bromide	T44.3X1	T44.3X2	T44.3X3	T44.3X4	T44.3X5	T44.3X6
Emetic NEC	T47.7X1	T47.7X2	T47.7X3	T47.7X4	T47.7X5	T47.7X6
Emetine	T37.3X1	T37.3X2	T37.3X3	T37.3X4	T37.3X5	T37.3X6
Emollient NEC	T49.3X1	T49.3X2	T49.3X3	T49.3X4	T49.3X5	T49.3X6
Emorfazone	T39.8X1	T39.8X2	T39.8X3	T39.8X4	T39.8X5	T39.8X6
Emylcamate	T43.591	T43.592	T43.593	T43.594	T43.595	T43.596
Enalapril	T46.4X1	T46.4X2	T46.4X3	T46.4X4	T46.4X5	T46.4X6

Substance	Poisoning, Accidental (unintentional)	Poisoning, Intentional Self-harm	Poisoning, Assault	Poisoning, Undetermined	Adverse Effect	Under-dosing
Enalaprilat	T46.4X1	T46.4X2	T46.4X3	T46.4X4	T46.4X5	T46.4X6
Enbrel*	T39.4X1	T39.4X2	T39.4X3	T39.4X4	T39.4X5	T39.4X6
Encainide	T46.2X1	T46.2X2	T46.2X3	T46.2X4	T46.2X5	T46.2X6
Endocaine	T41.3X1	T41.3X2	T41.3X3	T41.3X4	T41.3X5	T41.3X6
Endosulfan	T60.2X1	T60.2X2	T60.2X3	T60.2X4	—	—
Endothall	T60.3X1	T60.3X2	T60.3X3	T60.3X4	—	—
Endralazine	T46.5X1	T46.5X2	T46.5X3	T46.5X4	T46.5X5	T46.5X6
Endrin	T60.1X1	T60.1X2	T60.1X3	T60.1X4	—	—
Enflurane	T41.0X1	T41.0X2	T41.0X3	T41.0X4	T41.0X5	T41.0X6
Enfuvirtide*	T37.5X1	T37.5X2	T37.5X3	T37.5X4	T37.5X5	T37.5X6
Enhexymal	T42.3X1	T42.3X2	T42.3X3	T42.3X4	T42.3X5	T42.3X6
Enocitabine	T45.1X1	T45.1X2	T45.1X3	T45.1X4	T45.1X5	T45.1X6
Enovid	T38.4X1	T38.4X2	T38.4X3	T38.4X4	T38.4X5	T38.4X6
Enoxacin	T36.8X1	T36.8X2	T36.8X3	T36.8X4	T36.8X5	T36.8X6
Enoxaparin (sodium)	T45.511	T45.512	T45.513	T45.514	T45.515	T45.516
Enpiprazole	T43.591	T43.592	T43.593	T43.594	T43.595	T43.596
Enprofylline	T48.6X1	T48.6X2	T48.6X3	T48.6X4	T48.6X5	T48.6X6
Enprostil	T47.1X1	T47.1X2	T47.1X3	T47.1X4	T47.1X5	T47.1X6
Enterogastrone	T38.891	T38.892	T38.893	T38.894	T38.895	T38.896
ENT preparations (anti-infectives)	T49.6X1	T49.6X2	T49.6X3	T49.6X4	T49.6X5	T49.6X6
Enviomycin	T36.8X1	T36.8X2	T36.8X3	T36.8X4	T36.8X5	T36.8X6
Enzodase	T45.3X1	T45.3X2	T45.3X3	T45.3X4	T45.3X5	T45.3X6
Enzyme NEC	T45.3X1	T45.3X2	T45.3X3	T45.3X4	T45.3X5	T45.3X6
depolymerizing	T49.8X1	T49.8X2	T49.8X3	T49.8X4	T49.8X5	T49.8X6
fibrolytic	T45.3X1	T45.3X2	T45.3X3	T45.3X4	T45.3X5	T45.3X6
gastric	T47.5X1	T47.5X2	T47.5X3	T47.5X4	T47.5X5	T47.5X6
intestinal	T47.5X1	T47.5X2	T47.5X3	T47.5X4	T47.5X5	T47.5X6
local action	T49.4X1	T49.4X2	T49.4X3	T49.4X4	T49.4X5	T49.4X6
proteolytic	T49.4X1	T49.4X2	T49.4X3	T49.4X4	T49.4X5	T49.4X6
thrombolytic	T45.3X1	T45.3X2	T45.3X3	T45.3X4	T45.3X5	T45.3X6
EPAB	T41.3X1	T41.3X2	T41.3X3	T41.3X4	T41.3X5	T41.3X6
Epanutin	T42.0X1	T42.0X2	T42.0X3	T42.0X4	T42.0X5	T42.0X6
Ephedra	T44.991	T44.992	T44.993	T44.994	T44.995	T44.996
Ephedrine	T44.991	T44.992	T44.993	T44.994	T44.995	T44.996
Epichlorhydrin, epichlorohydrin	T52.8X1	T52.8X2	T52.8X3	T52.8X4	—	—
Epicillin	T36.0X1	T36.0X2	T36.0X3	T36.0X4	T36.0X5	T36.0X6
Epiestriol	T38.5X1	T38.5X2	T38.5X3	T38.5X4	T38.5X5	T38.5X6
Epilim — see Sodium, valproate						
Epimestrol	T38.5X1	T38.5X2	T38.5X3	T38.5X4	T38.5X5	T38.5X6
Epinephrine	T44.5X1	T44.5X2	T44.5X3	T44.5X4	T44.5X5	T44.5X6
EpiPen*	T44.5X1	T44.5X2	T44.5X3	T44.5X4	T44.5X5	T44.5X6
Epirubicin	T45.1X1	T45.1X2	T45.1X3	T45.1X4	T45.1X5	T45.1X6
Epitiostanol	T38.7X1	T38.7X2	T38.7X3	T38.7X4	T38.7X5	T38.7X6
Epitizide	T50.2X1	T50.2X2	T50.2X3	T50.2X4	T50.2X5	T50.2X6
EPN	T60.0X1	T60.0X2	T60.0X3	T60.0X4	—	—
EPO	T45.8X1	T45.8X2	T45.8X3	T45.8X4	T45.8X5	T45.8X6
Epoetin alpha	T45.8X1	T45.8X2	T45.8X3	T45.8X4	T45.8X5	T45.8X6
Epomediol	T50.991	T50.992	T50.993	T50.994	T50.995	T50.996
Epoprostenol	T45.521	T45.522	T45.523	T45.524	T45.525	T45.526
Epoxy resin	T65.891	T65.892	T65.893	T65.894	—	—
Eprazinone	T48.4X1	T48.4X2	T48.4X3	T48.4X4	T48.4X5	T48.4X6
Epsilon aminocaproic acid	T45.621	T45.622	T45.623	T45.624	T45.625	T45.626
Epsom salt	T47.3X1	T47.3X2	T47.3X3	T47.3X4	T47.3X5	T47.3X6
Eptazocine	T40.491	T40.492	T40.493	T40.494	T40.495	T40.496
Equanil	T43.591	T43.592	T43.593	T43.594	T43.595	T43.596
Equisetum	T62.2X1	T62.2X2	T62.2X3	T62.2X4	—	—
diuretic	T50.2X1	T50.2X2	T50.2X3	T50.2X4	T50.2X5	T50.2X6
Ergobasine	T48.0X1	T48.0X2	T48.0X3	T48.0X4	T48.0X5	T48.0X6
Ergocalciferol	T45.2X1	T45.2X2	T45.2X3	T45.2X4	T45.2X5	T45.2X6
Ergoloid mesylates	T46.7X1	T46.7X2	T46.7X3	T46.7X4	T46.7X5	T46.7X6
Ergometrine	T48.0X1	T48.0X2	T48.0X3	T48.0X4	T48.0X5	T48.0X6
Ergonovine	T48.0X1	T48.0X2	T48.0X3	T48.0X4	T48.0X5	T48.0X6
Ergotamine	T46.5X1	T46.5X2	T46.5X3	T46.5X4	T46.5X5	T46.5X6
Ergotocine	T48.0X1	T48.0X2	T48.0X3	T48.0X4	T48.0X5	T48.0X6
Ergotrate	T48.0X1	T48.0X2	T48.0X3	T48.0X4	T48.0X5	T48.0X6
Ergot NEC	T64.81	T64.82	T64.83	T64.84	—	—
derivative	T48.0X1	T48.0X2	T48.0X3	T48.0X4	T48.0X5	T48.0X6
medicinal (alkaloids)	T48.0X1	T48.0X2	T48.0X3	T48.0X4	T48.0X5	T48.0X6
prepared	T48.0X1	T48.0X2	T48.0X3	T48.0X4	T48.0X5	T48.0X6
Eritrityl tetranitrate	T46.3X1	T46.3X2	T46.3X3	T46.3X4	T46.3X5	T46.3X6
Erytrityl tetranitrate	T46.3X1	T46.3X2	T46.3X3	T46.3X4	T46.3X5	T46.3X6
Erythrol tetranitrate	T46.3X1	T46.3X2	T46.3X3	T46.3X4	T46.3X5	T46.3X6
Erythromycin (salts)	T36.3X1	T36.3X2	T36.3X3	T36.3X4	T36.3X5	T36.3X6
ophthalmic preparation	T49.5X1	T49.5X2	T49.5X3	T49.5X4	T49.5X5	T49.5X6
topical NEC	T49.0X1	T49.0X2	T49.0X3	T49.0X4	T49.0X5	T49.0X6
Erythropoietin	T45.8X1	T45.8X2	T45.8X3	T45.8X4	T45.8X5	T45.8X6
human	T45.8X1	T45.8X2	T45.8X3	T45.8X4	T45.8X5	T45.8X6
Esbriet*	T48.991	T48.992	T48.993	T48.994	T48.995	T48.996
Escin	T46.991	T46.992	T46.993	T46.994	T46.995	T46.996
Esculin	T45.2X1	T45.2X2	T45.2X3	T45.2X4	T45.2X5	T45.2X6
Esculoside	T45.2X1	T45.2X2	T45.2X3	T45.2X4	T45.2X5	T45.2X6
ESDT (ether-soluble tar distillate)	T49.1X1	T49.1X2	T49.1X3	T49.1X4	T49.1X5	T49.1X6
Eserine	T49.5X1	T49.5X2	T49.5X3	T49.5X4	T49.5X5	T49.5X6
Esflurbiprofen	T39.311	T39.312	T39.313	T39.314	T39.315	T39.316
Eskabarb	T42.3X1	T42.3X2	T42.3X3	T42.3X4	T42.3X5	T42.3X6
Eskalith	T43.8X1	T43.8X2	T43.8X3	T43.8X4	T43.8X5	T43.8X6
Esmolol	T44.7X1	T44.7X2	T44.7X3	T44.7X4	T44.7X5	T44.7X6
Estanozolol	T38.7X1	T38.7X2	T38.7X3	T38.7X4	T38.7X5	T38.7X6
Estazolam	T42.4X1	T42.4X2	T42.4X3	T42.4X4	T42.4X5	T42.4X6
Estradiol	T38.5X1	T38.5X2	T38.5X3	T38.5X4	T38.5X5	T38.5X6
with testosterone	T38.7X1	T38.7X2	T38.7X3	T38.7X4	T38.7X5	T38.7X6
benzoate	T38.5X1	T38.5X2	T38.5X3	T38.5X4	T38.5X5	T38.5X6
Estramustine	T45.1X1	T45.1X2	T45.1X3	T45.1X4	T45.1X5	T45.1X6
Estriol	T38.5X1	T38.5X2	T38.5X3	T38.5X4	T38.5X5	T38.5X6
Estrogen	T38.5X1	T38.5X2	T38.5X3	T38.5X4	T38.5X5	T38.5X6
with progesterone	T38.5X1	T38.5X2	T38.5X3	T38.5X4	T38.5X5	T38.5X6
conjugated	T38.5X1	T38.5X2	T38.5X3	T38.5X4	T38.5X5	T38.5X6
Estrone	T38.5X1	T38.5X2	T38.5X3	T38.5X4	T38.5X5	T38.5X6
Estropipate	T38.5X1	T38.5X2	T38.5X3	T38.5X4	T38.5X5	T38.5X6
Etacrynate sodium	T50.1X1	T50.1X2	T50.1X3	T50.1X4	T50.1X5	T50.1X6
Etacrynic acid	T50.1X1	T50.1X2	T50.1X3	T50.1X4	T50.1X5	T50.1X6
Etafedrine	T48.6X1	T48.6X2	T48.6X3	T48.6X4	T48.6X5	T48.6X6
Etafenone	T46.3X1	T46.3X2	T46.3X3	T46.3X4	T46.3X5	T46.3X6
Etambutol	T37.1X1	T37.1X2	T37.1X3	T37.1X4	T37.1X5	T37.1X6
Etamiphyllin	T48.6X1	T48.6X2	T48.6X3	T48.6X4	T48.6X5	T48.6X6
Etamivan	T50.7X1	T50.7X2	T50.7X3	T50.7X4	T50.7X5	T50.7X6
Etamsylate	T45.7X1	T45.7X2	T45.7X3	T45.7X4	T45.7X5	T45.7X6
Etebenecid	T50.4X1	T50.4X2	T50.4X3	T50.4X4	T50.4X5	T50.4X6
Ethacridine	T49.0X1	T49.0X2	T49.0X3	T49.0X4	T49.0X5	T49.0X6
Ethacrynate*	T50.1X1	T50.1X2	T50.1X3	T50.1X4	T50.1X5	T50.1X6
Ethacrynic acid	T50.1X1	T50.1X2	T50.1X3	T50.1X4	T50.1X5	T50.1X6
Ethadione	T42.2X1	T42.2X2	T42.2X3	T42.2X4	T42.2X5	T42.2X6
Ethambutol	T37.1X1	T37.1X2	T37.1X3	T37.1X4	T37.1X5	T37.1X6
Ethamide	T50.2X1	T50.2X2	T50.2X3	T50.2X4	T50.2X5	T50.2X6
Ethamivan	T50.7X1	T50.7X2	T50.7X3	T50.7X4	T50.7X5	T50.7X6
Ethamsylate	T45.7X1	T45.7X2	T45.7X3	T45.7X4	T45.7X5	T45.7X6
Ethanol	T51.0X1	T51.0X2	T51.0X3	T51.0X4	—	—
beverage	T51.0X1	T51.0X2	T51.0X3	T51.0X4	—	—
Ethanolamine oleate	T46.8X1	T46.8X2	T46.8X3	T46.8X4	T46.8X5	T46.8X6
Ethaverine	T44.3X1	T44.3X2	T44.3X3	T44.3X4	T44.3X5	T44.3X6
Ethchlorvynol	T42.6X1	T42.6X2	T42.6X3	T42.6X4	T42.6X5	T42.6X6
Ethebenecid	T50.4X1	T50.4X2	T50.4X3	T50.4X4	T50.4X5	T50.4X6
Ether (vapor)	T41.0X1	T41.0X2	T41.0X3	T41.0X4	T41.0X5	T41.0X6
anesthetic	T41.0X1	T41.0X2	T41.0X3	T41.0X4	T41.0X5	T41.0X6
divinyl	T41.0X1	T41.0X2	T41.0X3	T41.0X4	T41.0X5	T41.0X6
ethyl (medicinal)	T41.0X1	T41.0X2	T41.0X3	T41.0X4	T41.0X5	T41.0X6
nonmedicinal	T52.8X1	T52.8X2	T52.8X3	T52.8X4		
petroleum — see Ligroin						
solvent	T52.8X1	T52.8X2	T52.8X3	T52.8X4	—	—
Ethiazide	T50.2X1	T50.2X2	T50.2X3	T50.2X4	T50.2X5	T50.2X6
Ethidium chloride (vapor)	T59.891	T59.892	T59.893	T59.894	—	—
Ethinamate	T42.6X1	T42.6X2	T42.6X3	T42.6X4	T42.6X5	T42.6X6
Ethinylestradiol, ethinyloestradiol	T38.5X1	T38.5X2	T38.5X3	T38.5X4	T38.5X5	T38.5X6
with levonorgestrel	T38.4X1	T38.4X2	T38.4X3	T38.4X4	T38.4X5	T38.4X6
norethisterone	T38.4X1	T38.4X2	T38.4X3	T38.4X4	T38.4X5	T38.4X6
Ethiodized oil (131 l)	T50.8X1	T50.8X2	T50.8X3	T50.8X4	T50.8X5	T50.8X6
Ethiofos*	T50.991	T50.992	T50.993	T50.994	T50.995	T50.996
Ethion	T60.0X1	T60.0X2	T60.0X3	T60.0X4	—	—
Ethionamide	T37.1X1	T37.1X2	T37.1X3	T37.1X4	T37.1X5	T37.1X6
Ethioniamide	T37.1X1	T37.1X2	T37.1X3	T37.1X4	T37.1X5	T37.1X6
Ethisterone	T38.5X1	T38.5X2	T38.5X3	T38.5X4	T38.5X5	T38.5X6
Ethobral	T42.3X1	T42.3X2	T42.3X3	T42.3X4	T42.3X5	T42.3X6
Ethocaine (infiltration) (topical)	T41.3X1	T41.3X2	T41.3X3	T41.3X4	T41.3X5	T41.3X6
nerve block (peripheral) (plexus)	T41.3X1	T41.3X2	T41.3X3	T41.3X4	T41.3X5	T41.3X6
spinal	T41.3X1	T41.3X2	T41.3X3	T41.3X4	T41.3X5	T41.3X6
Ethoheptazine	T40.491	T40.492	T40.493	T40.494	T40.495	T40.496
Ethopropazine	T44.3X1	T44.3X2	T44.3X3	T44.3X4	T44.3X5	T44.3X6
Ethosuximide	T42.2X1	T42.2X2	T42.2X3	T42.2X4	T42.2X5	T42.2X6
Ethotoin	T42.0X1	T42.0X2	T42.0X3	T42.0X4	T42.0X5	T42.0X6
Ethoxazene	T37.91	T37.92	T37.93	T37.94	T37.95	T37.96
Ethoxazorutoside	T46.991	T46.992	T46.993	T46.994	T46.995	T46.996
Ethoxzolamide	T50.2X1	T50.2X2	T50.2X3	T50.2X4	T50.2X5	T50.2X6
Ethyl						
acetate	T52.8X1	T52.8X2	T52.8X3	T52.8X4	—	—
alcohol	T51.0X1	T51.0X2	T51.0X3	T51.0X4	—	—
beverage	T51.0X1	T51.0X2	T51.0X3	T51.0X4	—	—
aldehyde (vapor)	T59.891	T59.892	T59.893	T59.894	—	—
liquid	T52.8X1	T52.8X2	T52.8X3	T52.8X4	—	—
aminobenzoate	T41.3X1	T41.3X2	T41.3X3	T41.3X4	T41.3X5	T41.3X6

Table of Drugs and Chemicals

Substance	Poisoning, Accidental (unintentional)	Poisoning, Intentional Self-harm	Poisoning, Assault	Poisoning, Undetermined	Adverse Effect	Under-dosing
Ethyl — *continued*						
aminophenothiazine	T43.3X1	T43.3X2	T43.3X3	T43.3X4	T43.3X5	T43.3X6
benzoate	T52.8X1	T52.8X2	T52.8X3	T52.8X4	—	—
biscoumacetate	T45.511	T45.512	T45.513	T45.514	T45.515	T45.516
bromide (anesthetic)	T41.0X1	T41.0X2	T41.0X3	T41.0X4	T41.0X5	T41.0X6
carbamate	T45.1X1	T45.1X2	T45.1X3	T45.1X4	T45.1X5	T45.1X6
carbinol	T51.3X1	T51.3X2	T51.3X3	T51.3X4	—	—
carbonate	T52.8X1	T52.8X2	T52.8X3	T52.8X4	—	—
chaulmoograte	T37.1X1	T37.1X2	T37.1X3	T37.1X4	T37.1X5	T37.1X6
chloride (anesthetic)	T41.0X1	T41.0X2	T41.0X3	T41.0X4	T41.0X5	T41.0X6
anesthetic (local)	T41.3X1	T41.3X2	T41.3X3	T41.3X4	T41.3X5	T41.3X6
inhaled	T41.0X1	T41.0X2	T41.0X3	T41.0X4	T41.0X5	T41.0X6
local	T49.4X1	T49.4X2	T49.4X3	T49.4X4	T49.4X5	T49.4X6
solvent	T53.6X1	T53.6X2	T53.6X3	T53.6X4	—	—
dibunate	T48.3X1	T48.3X2	T48.3X3	T48.3X4	T48.3X5	T48.3X6
dichloroarsine (vapor)	T57.0X1	T57.0X2	T57.0X3	T57.0X4	—	—
estranol	T38.7X1	T38.7X2	T38.7X3	T38.7X4	T38.7X5	T38.7X6
ether — *see also* ether	T52.8X1	T52.8X2	T52.8X3	T52.8X4	—	—
formate NEC (solvent)	T52.0X1	T52.0X2	T52.0X3	T52.0X4	—	—
fumarate	T49.4X1	T49.4X2	T49.4X3	T49.4X4	T49.4X5	T49.4X6
hydroxyisobutyrate NEC (solvent)	T52.8X1	T52.8X2	T52.8X3	T52.8X4	—	—
iodoacetate	T59.3X1	T59.3X2	T59.3X3	T59.3X4	—	—
lactate NEC (solvent)	T52.8X1	T52.8X2	T52.8X3	T52.8X4	—	—
loflazepate	T42.4X1	T42.4X2	T42.4X3	T42.4X4	T42.4X5	T42.4X6
mercuric chloride	T56.1X1	T56.1X2	T56.1X3	T56.1X4	—	—
methylcarbinol	T51.8X1	T51.8X2	T51.8X3	T51.8X4	—	—
morphine	T40.2X1	T40.2X2	T40.2X3	T40.2X4	T40.2X5	T40.2X6
noradrenaline	T48.6X1	T48.6X2	T48.6X3	T48.6X4	T48.6X5	T48.6X6
oxybutyrate NEC (solvent)	T52.8X1	T52.8X2	T52.8X3	T52.8X4	—	—
Ethylene (gas)	T59.891	T59.892	T59.893	T59.894	—	—
anesthetic (general)	T41.0X1	T41.0X2	T41.0X3	T41.0X4	T41.0X5	T41.0X6
chlorohydrin	T52.8X1	T52.8X2	T52.8X3	T52.8X4	—	—
vapor	T53.6X1	T53.6X2	T53.6X3	T53.6X4	—	—
dichloride	T52.8X1	T52.8X2	T52.8X3	T52.8X4	—	—
vapor	T53.6X1	T53.6X2	T53.6X3	T53.6X4	—	—
dinitrate	T52.3X1	T52.3X2	T52.3X3	T52.3X4	—	—
glycol(s)	T52.8X1	T52.8X2	T52.8X3	T52.8X4	—	—
dinitrate	T52.3X1	T52.3X2	T52.3X3	T52.3X4	—	—
monobutyl ether	T52.3X1	T52.3X2	T52.3X3	T52.3X4	—	—
imine	T54.1X1	T54.1X2	T54.1X3	T54.1X4	—	—
oxide (fumigant) (nonmedicinal)	T59.891	T59.892	T59.893	T59.894	—	—
medicinal	T49.0X1	T49.0X2	T49.0X3	T49.0X4	T49.0X5	T49.0X6
Ethylenediaminetetra-acetic acid	T50.6X1	T50.6X2	T50.6X3	T50.6X4	T50.6X5	T50.6X6
Ethylenediamine theophylline	T48.6X1	T48.6X2	T48.6X3	T48.6X4	T48.6X5	T48.6X6
Ethylenedinitrilotetra-acetate	T50.6X1	T50.6X2	T50.6X3	T50.6X4	T50.6X5	T50.6X6
Ethylestrenol	T38.7X1	T38.7X2	T38.7X3	T38.7X4	T38.7X5	T38.7X6
Ethylhydroxycellulose	T47.4X1	T47.4X2	T47.4X3	T47.4X4	T47.4X5	T47.4X6
Ethylidene						
chloride NEC	T53.6X1	T53.6X2	T53.6X3	T53.6X4	—	—
diacetate	T60.3X1	T60.3X2	T60.3X3	T60.3X4	—	—
dicoumarin	T45.511	T45.512	T45.513	T45.514	T45.515	T45.516
dicoumarol	T45.511	T45.512	T45.513	T45.514	T45.515	T45.516
diethyl ether	T52.0X1	T52.0X2	T52.0X3	T52.0X4	—	—
Ethylmorphine	T40.2X1	T40.2X2	T40.2X3	T40.2X4	I40.2X5	T40.2X6
Ethylnorepinephrine	T48.6X1	T48.6X2	T48.6X3	T48.6X4	T48.6X5	T48.6X6
Ethylparachlorophen-oxyisobutyrate	T46.6X1	T46.6X2	T46.6X3	T46.6X4	T46.6X5	T46.6X6
Ethynodiol	T38.4X1	T38.4X2	T38.4X3	T38.4X4	T38.4X5	T38.4X6
with mestranol diacetate	T38.4X1	T38.4X2	T38.4X3	T38.4X4	T38.4X5	T38.4X6
Ethyol*	T50.991	T50.992	T50.993	T50.994	T50.995	T50.996
Etidocaine	T41.3X1	T41.3X2	T41.3X3	T41.3X4	T41.3X5	T41.3X6
infiltration (subcutaneous)	T41.3X1	T41.3X2	T41.3X3	T41.3X4	T41.3X5	T41.3X6
nerve (peripheral) (plexus)	T41.3X1	T41.3X2	T41.3X3	T41.3X4	T41.3X5	T41.3X6
Etidronate	T50.991	T50.992	T50.993	T50.994	T50.995	T50.996
Etidronic acid (disodium salt)	T50.991	T50.992	T50.993	T50.994	T50.995	T50.996
Etifoxine	T42.6X1	T42.6X2	T42.6X3	T42.6X4	T42.6X5	T42.6X6
Etilefrine	T44.4X1	T44.4X2	T44.4X3	T44.4X4	T44.4X5	T44.4X6
Etilfen	T42.3X1	T42.3X2	T42.3X3	T42.3X4	T42.3X5	T42.3X6
Etinodiol	T38.4X1	T38.4X2	T38.4X3	T38.4X4	T38.4X5	T38.4X6
Etiroxate	T46.6X1	T46.6X2	T46.6X3	T46.6X4	T46.6X5	T46.6X6
Etizolam	T42.4X1	T42.4X2	T42.4X3	T42.4X4	T42.4X5	T42.4X6
Etodolac	T39.391	T39.392	T39.393	T39.394	T39.395	T39.396
Etofamide	T37.3X1	T37.3X2	T37.3X3	T37.3X4	T37.3X5	T37.3X6
Etofibrate	T46.6X1	T46.6X2	T46.6X3	T46.6X4	T46.6X5	T46.6X6
Etofylline	T46.7X1	T46.7X2	T46.7X3	T46.7X4	T46.7X5	T46.7X6
clofibrate	T46.6X1	T46.6X2	T46.6X3	T46.6X4	T46.6X5	T46.6X6
Etoglucid	T45.1X1	T45.1X2	T45.1X3	T45.1X4	T45.1X5	T45.1X6
Etomidate	T41.1X1	T41.1X2	T41.1X3	T41.1X4	T41.1X5	T41.1X6
Etomide	T39.8X1	T39.8X2	T39.8X3	T39.8X4	T39.8X5	T39.8X6
Etomidoline	T44.3X1	T44.3X2	T44.3X3	T44.3X4	T44.3X5	T44.3X6
Etoposide	T45.1X1	T45.1X2	T45.1X3	T45.1X4	T45.1X5	T45.1X6
Etorphine	T40.2X1	T40.2X2	T40.2X3	T40.2X4	T40.2X5	T40.2X6
Etoval	T42.3X1	T42.3X2	T42.3X3	T42.3X4	T42.3X5	T42.3X6
Etozolin	T50.1X1	T50.1X2	T50.1X3	T50.1X4	T50.1X5	T50.1X6
Etravirine*	T37.5X1	T37.5X2	T37.5X3	T37.5X4	T37.5X5	T37.5X6
Etretinate	T50.991	T50.992	T50.993	T50.994	T50.995	T50.996
Etryptamine	T43.691	T43.692	T43.693	T43.694	T43.695	T43.696
Etybenzatropine	T44.3X1	T44.3X2	T44.3X3	T44.3X4	T44.3X5	T44.3X6
Etynodiol	T38.4X1	T38.4X2	T38.4X3	T38.4X4	T38.4X5	T38.4X6
Eucaine	T41.3X1	T41.3X2	T41.3X3	T41.3X4	T41.3X5	T41.3X6
Eucalyptus oil	T49.7X1	T49.7X2	T49.7X3	T49.7X4	T49.7X5	T49.7X6
Eucatropine	T49.5X1	T49.5X2	T49.5X3	T49.5X4	T49.5X5	T49.5X6
Eucodal	T40.2X1	T40.2X2	T40.2X3	T40.2X4	T40.2X5	T40.2X6
Euneryl	T42.3X1	T42.3X2	T42.3X3	T42.3X4	T42.3X5	T42.3X6
Euphthalmine	T44.3X1	T44.3X2	T44.3X3	T44.3X4	T44.3X5	T44.3X6
Eurax	T49.0X1	T49.0X2	T49.0X3	T49.0X4	T49.0X5	T49.0X6
Euresol	T49.4X1	T49.4X2	T49.4X3	T49.4X4	T49.4X5	T49.4X6
Euthroid	T38.1X1	T38.1X2	T38.1X3	T38.1X4	T38.1X5	T38.1X6
Evans blue	T50.8X1	T50.8X2	T50.8X3	T50.8X4	T50.8X5	T50.8X6
Evipal	T42.3X1	T42.3X2	T42.3X3	T42.3X4	T42.3X5	T42.3X6
sodium	T41.1X1	T41.1X2	T41.1X3	T41.1X4	T41.1X5	T41.1X6
Evipan	T42.3X1	T42.3X2	T42.3X3	T42.3X4	T42.3X5	T42.3X6
sodium	T41.1X1	T41.1X2	T41.1X3	T41.1X4	T41.1X5	T41.1X6
Exalamide	T49.0X1	T49.0X2	T49.0X3	T49.0X4	T49.0X5	T49.0X6
Exalgin	T39.1X1	T39.1X2	T39.1X3	T39.1X4	T39.1X5	T39.1X6
Excipients, pharmaceutical	T50.901	T50.902	T50.903	T50.904	T50.905	T50.906
Exhaust gas (engine) (motor vehicle)	T58.01	T58.02	T58.03	T58.04	—	—
Ex-Lax (phenolphthalein)	T47.2X1	T47.2X2	T47.2X3	T47.2X4	T47.2X5	T47.2X6
Expectorant NEC	T48.4X1	T48.4X2	T48.4X3	T48.4X4	T48.4X5	T48.4X6
Extended insulin zinc suspension	T38.3X1	T38.3X2	T38.3X3	T38.3X4	T38.3X5	T38.3X6
External medications (skin) (mucous membrane)	T49.91	T49.92	T49.93	T49.94	T49.95	T49.96
dental agent	T49.7X1	T49.7X2	T49.7X3	T49.7X4	T49.7X5	T49.7X6
ENT agent	T49.6X1	T49.6X2	T49.6X3	T49.6X4	T49.6X5	T49.6X6
ophthalmic preparation	T49.5X1	T49.5X2	T49.5X3	T49.5X4	T49.5X5	T49.5X6
specified NEC	T49.8X1	T49.8X2	T49.8X3	T49.8X4	T49.8X5	T49.8X6
Extina*	T49.0X1	T49.0X2	T49.0X3	T49.0X4	T49.0X5	T49.0X6
Extrapyramidal antagonist NEC	T44.3X1	T44.3X2	T44.3X3	T44.3X4	T44.3X5	T44.3X6
Eye agents (anti-infective)	T49.5X1	T49.5X2	T49.5X3	T49.5X4	T49.5X5	T49.5X6
Eye drug NEC	T49.5X1	T49.5X2	T49.5X3	T49.5X4	T49.5X5	T49.5X6
FAC (fluorouracil + doxorubicin + cyclophosphamide)	T45.1X1	T45.1X2	T45.1X3	T45.1X4	T45.1X5	T45.1X6
Factor						
I (fibrinogen)	T45.8X1	T45.8X2	T45.8X3	T45.8X4	T45.8X5	T45.0X6
III (thromboplastin)	T45.8X1	T45.8X2	T45.8X3	T45.8X4	T45.8X5	T45.8X6
IX complex	T45.7X1	T45.7X2	T45.7X3	T45.7X4	T45.7X5	T45.7X6
human	T45.8X1	T45.8X2	T45.8X3	T45.8X4	T45.8X5	T45.8X6
VIII (antihemophilic Factor) (concentrate)	T45.8X1	T45.8X2	T45.8X3	T45.8X4	T45.8X5	T45.8X6
Famotidine	T47.0X1	T47.0X2	T47.0X3	T47.0X4	T47.0X5	T47.0X6
Fat suspension, intravenous	T50.991	T50.992	T50.993	T50.994	T50.995	T50.996
Fazadinium bromide	T48.1X1	T48.1X2	T48.1X3	T48.1X4	T48.1X5	T48.1X6
Febarbamate	T42.3X1	T42.3X2	T42.3X3	T42.3X4	T42.3X5	T42.3X6
Fecal softener	T47.4X1	T47.4X2	T47.4X3	T47.4X4	T47.4X5	T47.4X6
Fedrilate	T48.3X1	T48.3X2	T48.3X3	T48.3X4	T48.3X5	T48.3X6
Felodipine	T46.1X1	T46.1X2	T46.1X3	T46.1X4	T46.1X5	T46.1X6
Felypressin	T38.891	T38.892	T38.893	T38.894	T38.895	T38.896
Femizol*	T49.0X1	T49.0X2	T49.0X3	T49.0X4	T49.0X5	T49.0X6
Femoxetine	T43.221	T43.222	T43.223	T43.224	T43.225	T43.226
Fenalcomine	T46.3X1	T46.3X2	T46.3X3	T46.3X4	T46.3X5	T46.3X6
Fenamisal	T37.1X1	T37.1X2	T37.1X3	T37.1X4	T37.1X5	T37.1X6
Fenazone	T39.2X1	T39.2X2	T39.2X3	T39.2X4	T39.2X5	T39.2X6
Fenbendazole	T37.4X1	T37.4X2	T37.4X3	T37.4X4	T37.4X5	T37.4X6
Fenbutrazate	T50.5X1	T50.5X2	T50.5X3	T50.5X4	T50.5X5	T50.5X6
Fencamfamine	T43.691	T43.692	T43.693	T43.694	T43.695	T43.696
Fendiline	T46.1X1	T46.1X2	T46.1X3	T46.1X4	T46.1X5	T46.1X6
Fenetylline	T43.691	T43.692	T43.693	T43.694	T43.695	T43.696
Fenflumizole	T39.391	T39.392	T39.393	T39.394	T39.395	T39.396
Fenfluramine	T50.5X1	T50.5X2	T50.5X3	T50.5X4	T50.5X5	T50.5X6
Fenobarbital	T42.3X1	T42.3X2	T42.3X3	T42.3X4	T42.3X5	T42.3X6
Fenofibrate	T46.6X1	T46.6X2	T46.6X3	T46.6X4	T46.6X5	T46.6X6
Fenoprofen	T39.311	T39.312	T39.313	T39.314	T39.315	T39.316
Fenoterol	T48.6X1	T48.6X2	T48.6X3	T48.6X4	T48.6X5	T48.6X6
Fenoverine	T44.3X1	T44.3X2	T44.3X3	T44.3X4	T44.3X5	T44.3X6
Fenoxazoline	T48.5X1	T48.5X2	T48.5X3	T48.5X4	T48.5X5	T48.5X6
Fenproporex	T50.5X1	T50.5X2	T50.5X3	T50.5X4	T50.5X5	T50.5X6

Substance	Poisoning, Accidental (unintentional)	Poisoning, Intentional Self-harm	Poisoning, Assault	Poisoning, Undetermined	Adverse Effect	Under-dosing
Fenquizone	T50.2X1	T50.2X2	T50.2X3	T50.2X4	T50.2X5	T50.2X6
Fentanyl (analogs)	T40.411	T40.412	T40.413	T40.414	T40.415	T40.416
Fentazin	T43.3X1	T43.3X2	T43.3X3	T43.3X4	T43.3X5	T43.3X6
Fenthion	T60.0X1	T60.0X2	T60.0X3	T60.0X4	—	—
Fenticlor	T49.0X1	T49.0X2	T49.0X3	T49.0X4	T49.0X5	T49.0X6
Fenylbutazone	T39.2X1	T39.2X2	T39.2X3	T39.2X4	T39.2X5	T39.2X6
Feprazone	T39.2X1	T39.2X2	T39.2X3	T39.2X4	T39.2X5	T39.2X6
Fer de lance (bite) (venom)	T63.061	T63.062	T63.063	T63.064	—	—
Ferrex*	T45.4X1	T45.4X2	T45.4X3	T45.4X4	T45.4X5	T45.4X6
Ferric — see also Iron						
chloride	T45.4X1	T45.4X2	T45.4X3	T45.4X4	T45.4X5	T45.4X6
citrate	T45.4X1	T45.4X2	T45.4X3	T45.4X4	T45.4X5	T45.4X6
hydroxide						
colloidal	T45.4X1	T45.4X2	T45.4X3	T45.4X4	T45.4X5	T45.4X6
polymaltose	T45.4X1	T45.4X2	T45.4X3	T45.4X4	T45.4X5	T45.4X6
pyrophosphate	T45.4X1	T45.4X2	T45.4X3	T45.4X4	T45.4X5	T45.4X6
Ferritin	T45.4X1	T45.4X2	T45.4X3	T45.4X4	T45.4X5	T45.4X6
Ferrocholinate	T45.4X1	T45.4X2	T45.4X3	T45.4X4	T45.4X5	T45.4X6
Ferrodextrane	T45.4X1	T45.4X2	T45.4X3	T45.4X4	T45.4X5	T45.4X6
Ferropolimaler	T45.4X1	T45.4X2	T45.4X3	T45.4X4	T45.4X5	T45.4X6
Ferrous — see also Iron						
phosphate	T45.4X1	T45.4X2	T45.4X3	T45.4X4	T45.4X5	T45.4X6
salt	T45.4X1	T45.4X2	T45.4X3	T45.4X4	T45.4X5	T45.4X6
with folic acid	T45.4X1	T45.4X2	T45.4X3	T45.4X4	T45.4X5	T45.4X6
Ferrous fumarate, gluconate, lactate, salt NEC, sulfate (medicinal)	T45.4X1	T45.4X2	T45.4X3	T45.4X4	T45.4X5	T45.4X6
Ferrovanadium (fumes)	T59.891	T59.892	T59.893	T59.894	—	—
Ferrum — see Iron						
Fertilizers NEC	T65.891	T65.892	T65.893	T65.894	—	—
with herbicide mixture	T60.3X1	T60.3X2	T60.3X3	T60.3X4	—	—
Fetoxilate	T47.6X1	T47.6X2	T47.6X3	T47.6X4	T47.6X5	T47.6X6
Fiber, dietary	T47.4X1	T47.4X2	T47.4X3	T47.4X4	T47.4X5	T47.4X6
Fiberglass	T65.831	T65.832	T65.833	T65.834	—	—
Fibrinogen (human)	T45.8X1	T45.8X2	T45.8X3	T45.8X4	T45.8X5	T45.8X6
Fibrinolysin (human)	T45.691	T45.692	T45.693	T45.694	T45.695	T45.696
Fibrinolysis						
affecting drug	T45.601	T45.602	T45.603	T45.604	T45.605	T45.606
inhibitor NEC	T45.621	T45.622	T45.623	T45.624	T45.625	T45.626
Fibrinolytic drug	T45.611	T45.612	T45.613	T45.614	T45.615	T45.616
Filix mas	T37.4X1	T37.4X2	T37.4X3	T37.4X4	T37.4X5	T37.4X6
Filtering cream	T49.3X1	T49.3X2	T49.3X3	T49.3X4	T49.3X5	T49.3X6
Finacea*	T49.0X1	T49.0X2	T49.0X3	T49.0X4	T49.0X5	T49.0X6
Fiorinal	T39.011	T39.012	T39.013	T39.014	T39.015	T39.016
Firedamp	T59.891	T59.892	T59.893	T59.894	—	—
Fish, noxious, nonbacterial	T61.91	T61.92	T61.93	T61.94	—	—
ciguatera	T61.01	T61.02	T61.03	T61.04	—	—
scombroid	T61.11	T61.12	T61.13	T61.14	—	—
shell	T61.781	T61.782	T61.783	T61.784	—	—
specified NEC	T61.771	T61.772	T61.773	T61.774	—	—
Flagyl	T37.3X1	T37.3X2	T37.3X3	T37.3X4	T37.3X5	T37.3X6
Flavine adenine dinucleotide	T45.2X1	T45.2X2	T45.2X3	T45.2X4	T45.2X5	T45.2X6
Flavodic acid	T46.991	T46.992	T46.993	T46.994	T46.995	T46.996
Flavoxate	T44.3X1	T44.3X2	T44.3X3	T44.3X4	T44.3X5	T44.3X6
Flaxedil	T48.1X1	T48.1X2	T48.1X3	T48.1X4	T48.1X5	T48.1X6
Flaxseed (medicinal)	T49.3X1	T49.3X2	T49.3X3	T49.3X4	T49.3X5	T49.3X6
Flecainide	T46.2X1	T46.2X2	T46.2X3	T46.2X4	T46.2X5	T46.2X6
Fleroxacin	T36.8X1	T36.8X2	T36.8X3	T36.8X4	T36.8X5	T36.8X6
Floctafenine	T39.8X1	T39.8X2	T39.8X3	T39.8X4	T39.8X5	T39.8X6
Flomax	T44.6X1	T44.6X2	T44.6X3	T44.6X4	T44.6X5	T44.6X6
Flomoxef	T36.1X1	T36.1X2	T36.1X3	T36.1X4	T36.1X5	T36.1X6
Flopropione	T44.3X1	T44.3X2	T44.3X3	T44.3X4	T44.3X5	T44.3X6
FLORAjen*	T47.6X1	T47.6X2	T47.6X3	T47.6X4	T47.6X5	T47.6X6
Florantyrone	T47.5X1	T47.5X2	T47.5X3	T47.5X4	T47.5X5	T47.5X6
Floraquin	T37.8X1	T37.8X2	T37.8X3	T37.8X4	T37.8X5	T37.8X6
Florinef	T38.0X1	T38.0X2	T38.0X3	T38.0X4	T38.0X5	T38.0X6
ENT agent	T49.6X1	T49.6X2	T49.6X3	T49.6X4	T49.6X5	T49.6X6
ophthalmic preparation	T49.5X1	T49.5X2	T49.5X3	T49.5X4	T49.5X5	T49.5X6
topical NEC	T49.0X1	T49.0X2	T49.0X3	T49.0X4	T49.0X5	T49.0X6
Flowers of sulfur	T49.4X1	T49.4X2	T49.4X3	T49.4X4	T49.4X5	T49.4X6
Floxuridine	T45.1X1	T45.1X2	T45.1X3	T45.1X4	T45.1X5	T45.1X6
Fluanisone	T43.4X1	T43.4X2	T43.4X3	T43.4X4	T43.4X5	T43.4X6
Flubendazole	T37.4X1	T37.4X2	T37.4X3	T37.4X4	T37.4X5	T37.4X6
Fluclorolone acetonide	T49.0X1	T49.0X2	T49.0X3	T49.0X4	T49.0X5	T49.0X6
Flucloxacillin	T36.0X1	T36.0X2	T36.0X3	T36.0X4	T36.0X5	T36.0X6
Fluconazole	T37.8X1	T37.8X2	T37.8X3	T37.8X4	T37.8X5	T37.8X6
Flucytosine	T37.8X1	T37.8X2	T37.8X3	T37.8X4	T37.8X5	T37.8X6
Fludeoxyglucose (18F)	T50.8X1	T50.8X2	T50.8X3	T50.8X4	T50.8X5	T50.8X6
Fludiazepam	T42.4X1	T42.4X2	T42.4X3	T42.4X4	T42.4X5	T42.4X6
Fludrocortisone	T50.0X1	T50.0X2	T50.0X3	T50.0X4	T50.0X5	T50.0X6
ENT agent	T49.6X1	T49.6X2	T49.6X3	T49.6X4	T49.6X5	T49.6X6

Substance	Poisoning, Accidental (unintentional)	Poisoning, Intentional Self-harm	Poisoning, Assault	Poisoning, Undetermined	Adverse Effect	Under-dosing
Fludrocortisone — continued						
ophthalmic preparation	T49.5X1	T49.5X2	T49.5X3	T49.5X4	T49.5X5	T49.5X6
topical NEC	T49.0X1	T49.0X2	T49.0X3	T49.0X4	T49.0X5	T49.0X6
Fludroxycortide	T49.0X1	T49.0X2	T49.0X3	T49.0X4	T49.0X5	T49.0X6
Flufenamic acid	T39.391	T39.392	T39.393	T39.394	T39.395	T39.396
Fluindione	T45.511	T45.512	T45.513	T45.514	T45.515	T45.516
Flumequine	T37.8X1	T37.8X2	T37.8X3	T37.8X4	T37.8X5	T37.8X6
Flumethasone	T49.0X1	T49.0X2	T49.0X3	T49.0X4	T49.0X5	T49.0X6
Flumethiazide	T50.2X1	T50.2X2	T50.2X3	T50.2X4	T50.2X5	T50.2X6
Flumidin	T37.5X1	T37.5X2	T37.5X3	T37.5X4	T37.5X5	T37.5X6
Flunarizine	T46.7X1	T46.7X2	T46.7X3	T46.7X4	T46.7X5	T46.7X6
Flunidazole	T37.8X1	T37.8X2	T37.8X3	T37.8X4	T37.8X5	T37.8X6
Flunisolide	T48.6X1	T48.6X2	T48.6X3	T48.6X4	T48.6X5	T48.6X6
Flunitrazepam	T42.4X1	T42.4X2	T42.4X3	T42.4X4	T42.4X5	T42.4X6
Fluocinolone (acetonide)	T49.0X1	T49.0X2	T49.0X3	T49.0X4	T49.0X5	T49.0X6
Fluocinonide	T49.0X1	T49.0X2	T49.0X3	T49.0X4	T49.0X5	T49.0X6
Fluocortin (butyl)	T49.0X1	T49.0X2	T49.0X3	T49.0X4	T49.0X5	T49.0X6
Fluocortolone	T49.0X1	T49.0X2	T49.0X3	T49.0X4	T49.0X5	T49.0X6
Fluohydrocortisone	T38.0X1	T38.0X2	T38.0X3	T38.0X4	T38.0X5	T38.0X6
ENT agent	T49.6X1	T49.6X2	T49.6X3	T49.6X4	T49.6X5	T49.6X6
ophthalmic preparation	T49.5X1	T49.5X2	T49.5X3	T49.5X4	T49.5X5	T49.5X6
topical NEC	T49.0X1	T49.0X2	T49.0X3	T49.0X4	T49.0X5	T49.0X6
Fluonid	T49.0X1	T49.0X2	T49.0X3	T49.0X4	T49.0X5	T49.0X6
Fluopromazine	T43.3X1	T43.3X2	T43.3X3	T43.3X4	T43.3X5	T43.3X6
Fluoracetate	T60.8X1	T60.8X2	T60.8X3	T60.8X4	—	—
Fluorescein	T50.8X1	T50.8X2	T50.8X3	T50.8X4	T50.8X5	T50.8X6
Fluorhydrocortisone	T50.0X1	T50.0X2	T50.0X3	T50.0X4	T50.0X5	T50.0X6
Fluoride (nonmedicinal) (pesticide) (sodium) NEC	T60.8X1	T60.8X2	T60.8X3	T60.8X4	—	—
hydrogen — see Hydrofluoric acid						
medicinal NEC	T50.991	T50.992	T50.993	T50.994	T50.995	T50.996
dental use	T49.7X1	T49.7X2	T49.7X3	T49.7X4	T49.7X5	T49.7X6
not pesticide NEC	T54.91	T54.92	T54.93	T54.94	—	—
stannous	T49.7X1	T49.7X2	T49.7X3	T49.7X4	T49.7X5	T49.7X6
Fluorigard*	T47.7X1	T47.7X2	T47.7X3	T47.7X4	T47.7X5	T47.7X6
Fluorinated corticosteroids	T38.0X1	T38.0X2	T38.0X3	T38.0X4	T38.0X5	T38.0X6
Fluorine (gas)	T59.5X1	T59.5X2	T59.5X3	T59.5X4	—	—
salt — see Fluoride(s)						
Fluoristan	T49.7X1	T49.7X2	T49.7X3	T49.7X4	T49.7X5	T49.7X6
Fluormetholone	T49.0X1	T49.0X2	T49.0X3	T49.0X4	T49.0X5	T49.0X6
Fluoroacetate	T60.8X1	T60.8X2	T60.8X3	T60.8X4	—	—
Fluorocarbon monomer	T53.6X1	T53.6X2	T53.6X3	T53.6X4	—	—
Fluorocytosine	T37.8X1	T37.8X2	T37.8X3	T37.8X4	T37.8X5	T37.8X6
Fluorodeoxyuridine	T45.1X1	T45.1X2	T45.1X3	T45.1X4	T45.1X5	T45.1X6
Fluorometholone	T49.0X1	T49.0X2	T49.0X3	T49.0X4	T49.0X5	T49.0X6
ophthalmic preparation	T49.5X1	T49.5X2	T49.5X3	T49.5X4	T49.5X5	T49.5X6
Fluorophosphate insecticide	T60.0X1	T60.0X2	T60.0X3	T60.0X4	—	—
Fluorosol	T46.3X1	T46.3X2	T46.3X3	T46.3X4	T46.3X5	T46.3X6
Fluorouracil	T45.1X1	T45.1X2	T45.1X3	T45.1X4	T45.1X5	T45.1X6
Fluorphenylalanine	T49.5X1	T49.5X2	T49.5X3	T49.5X4	T49.5X5	T49.5X6
Fluothane	T41.0X1	T41.0X2	T41.0X3	T41.0X4	T41.0X5	T41.0X6
Fluoxetine	T43.221	T43.222	T43.223	T43.224	T43.225	T43.226
Fluoxymesterone	T38.7X1	T38.7X2	T38.7X3	T38.7X4	T38.7X5	T38.7X6
Flupenthixol	T43.4X1	T43.4X2	T43.4X3	T43.4X4	T43.4X5	T43.4X6
Flupentixol	T43.4X1	T43.4X2	T43.4X3	T43.4X4	T43.4X5	T43.4X6
Fluphenazine	T43.3X1	T43.3X2	T43.3X3	T43.3X4	T43.3X5	T43.3X6
Fluprednidene	T49.0X1	T49.0X2	T49.0X3	T49.0X4	T49.0X5	T49.0X6
Fluprednisolone	T38.0X1	T38.0X2	T38.0X3	T38.0X4	T38.0X5	T38.0X6
Fluradoline	T39.8X1	T39.8X2	T39.8X3	T39.8X4	T39.8X5	T39.8X6
Flurandrenolide	T49.0X1	T49.0X2	T49.0X3	T49.0X4	T49.0X5	T49.0X6
Flurandrenolone	T49.0X1	T49.0X2	T49.0X3	T49.0X4	T49.0X5	T49.0X6
Flurazepam	T42.4X1	T42.4X2	T42.4X3	T42.4X4	T42.4X5	T42.4X6
Flurbiprofen	T39.311	T39.312	T39.313	T39.314	T39.315	T39.316
Flurobate	T49.0X1	T49.0X2	T49.0X3	T49.0X4	T49.0X5	T49.0X6
Fluroxene	T41.0X1	T41.0X2	T41.0X3	T41.0X4	T41.0X5	T41.0X6
Fluspirilene	T43.591	T43.592	T43.593	T43.594	T43.595	T43.596
Flutamide	T38.6X1	T38.6X2	T38.6X3	T38.6X4	T38.6X5	T38.6X6
Flutazolam	T38.0X1	T38.0X2	T38.0X3	T38.0X4	T38.0X5	T38.0X6
Fluticasone propionate	T38.0X1	T38.0X2	T38.0X3	T38.0X4	T38.0X5	T38.0X6
Flutoprazepam	T42.4X1	T42.4X2	T42.4X3	T42.4X4	T42.4X5	T42.4X6
Flutropium bromide	T48.6X1	T48.6X2	T48.6X3	T48.6X4	T48.6X5	T48.6X6
Fluvoxamine	T43.221	T43.222	T43.223	T43.224	T43.225	T43.226
Folacin	T45.8X1	T45.8X2	T45.8X3	T45.8X4	T45.8X5	T45.8X6
Folic acid	T45.8X1	T45.8X2	T45.8X3	T45.8X4	T45.8X5	T45.8X6
with ferrous salt	T45.2X1	T45.2X2	T45.2X3	T45.2X4	T45.2X5	T45.2X6
antagonist	T45.1X1	T45.1X2	T45.1X3	T45.1X4	T45.1X5	T45.1X6
Folinic acid	T45.8X1	T45.8X2	T45.8X3	T45.8X4	T45.8X5	T45.8X6
Folium stramoniae	T48.6X1	T48.6X2	T48.6X3	T48.6X4	T48.6X5	T48.6X6
Follicle-stimulating hormone, human	T38.811	T38.812	T38.813	T38.814	T38.815	T38.816

Substance	Poisoning, Accidental (unintentional)	Poisoning, Intentional Self-harm	Poisoning, Assault	Poisoning, Undetermined	Adverse Effect	Under-dosing
Folpet	T60.3X1	T60.3X2	T60.3X3	T60.3X4	—	—
Fomepizole*	T50.6X1	T50.6X2	T50.6X3	T50.6X4	T50.6X5	T50.6X6
Fominoben	T48.3X1	T48.3X2	T48.3X3	T48.3X4	T48.3X5	T48.3X6
Food, foodstuffs, noxious, nonbacterial, NEC	T62.91	T62.92	T62.93	T62.94	—	—
berries	T62.1X1	T62.1X2	T62.1X3	T62.1X4	—	—
fish — see also Fish	T61.91	T61.92	T61.93	T61.94	—	—
mushrooms	T62.0X1	T62.0X2	T62.0X3	T62.0X4	—	—
plants	T62.2X1	T62.2X2	T62.2X3	T62.2X4	—	—
seafood	T61.91	T61.92	T61.93	T61.94	—	—
specified NEC	T61.8X1	T61.8X2	T61.8X3	T61.8X4	—	—
seeds	T62.2X1	T62.2X2	T62.2X3	T62.2X4	—	—
shellfish	T61.781	T61.782	T61.783	T61.784	—	—
specified NEC	T62.8X1	T62.8X2	T62.8X3	T62.8X4	—	—
Fool's parsley	T62.2X1	T62.2X2	T62.2X3	T62.2X4	—	—
Formaldehyde (solution), gas or vapor	T59.2X1	T59.2X2	T59.2X3	T59.2X4	—	—
fungicide	T60.3X1	T60.3X2	T60.3X3	T60.3X4	—	—
Formalin	T59.2X1	T59.2X2	T59.2X3	T59.2X4	—	—
fungicide	T60.3X1	T60.3X2	T60.3X3	T60.3X4	—	—
vapor	T59.2X1	T59.2X2	T59.2X3	T59.2X4	—	—
Formic acid	T54.2X1	T54.2X2	T54.2X3	T54.2X4	—	—
vapor	T59.891	T59.892	T59.893	T59.894	—	—
Formoterol*	T48.6X1	T48.6X2	T48.6X3	T48.6X4	T48.6X5	T48.6X6
Fortaz*	T36.1X1	T36.1X2	T36.1X3	T36.1X4	T36.1X5	T36.1X6
Foscarnet sodium	T37.5X1	T37.5X2	T37.5X3	T37.5X4	T37.5X5	T37.5X6
Fosfestrol	T38.5X1	T38.5X2	T38.5X3	T38.5X4	T38.5X5	T38.5X6
Fosfomycin	T36.8X1	T36.8X2	T36.8X3	T36.8X4	T36.8X5	T36.8X6
Fosfonet sodium	T37.5X1	T37.5X2	T37.5X3	T37.5X4	T37.5X5	T37.5X6
Fosinopril	T46.4X1	T46.4X2	T46.4X3	T46.4X4	T46.4X5	T46.4X6
sodium	T46.4X1	T46.4X2	T46.4X3	T46.4X4	T46.4X5	T46.4X6
Fowler's solution	T57.0X1	T57.0X2	T57.0X3	T57.0X4	—	—
Foxglove	T62.2X1	T62.2X2	T62.2X3	T62.2X4	—	—
Framycetin	T36.5X1	T36.5X2	T36.5X3	T36.5X4	T36.5X5	T36.5X6
Frangula	T47.2X1	T47.2X2	T47.2X3	T47.2X4	T47.2X5	T47.2X6
extract	T47.2X1	T47.2X2	T47.2X3	T47.2X4	T47.2X5	T47.2X6
Frei antigen	T50.8X1	T50.8X2	T50.8X3	T50.8X4	T50.8X5	T50.8X6
Freon	T53.5X1	T53.5X2	T53.5X3	T53.5X4	—	—
Fructose	T50.3X1	T50.3X2	T50.3X3	T50.3X4	T50.3X5	T50.3X6
Frusemide	T50.1X1	T50.1X2	T50.1X3	T50.1X4	T50.1X5	T50.1X6
FSH	T38.811	T38.812	T38.813	T38.814	T38.815	T38.816
Ftorafur	T45.1X1	T45.1X2	T45.1X3	T45.1X4	T45.1X5	T45.1X6
Fuel						
automobile	T52.0X1	T52.0X2	T52.0X3	T52.0X4	—	—
exhaust gas, not in transit	T58.01	T58.02	T58.03	T58.04	—	—
vapor NEC	T52.0X1	T52.0X2	T52.0X3	T52.0X4	—	—
gas (domestic use) — see also Carbon, monoxide, fuel, utility	T59.891	T59.892	T59.893	T59.894	—	—
utility	T59.891	T59.892	T59.893	T59.894	—	—
incomplete combustion of — see Carbon, monoxide, fuel, utility						
in mobile container	T59.891	T59.892	T59.893	T59.894	—	—
piped (natural)	T59.891	T59.892	T59.893	T59.894	—	—
industrial, incomplete combustion	T58.8X1	T58.8X2	T58.8X3	T58.8X4	—	—
Fugillin	T36.8X1	T36.8X2	T36.8X3	T36.8X4	T36.8X5	T36.8X6
Fulminate of mercury	T56.1X1	T56.1X2	T56.1X3	T56.1X4	—	—
Fulvicin	T36.7X1	T36.7X2	T36.7X3	T36.7X4	T36.7X5	T36.7X6
Fumadil	T36.8X1	T36.8X2	T36.8X3	T36.8X4	T36.8X5	T36.8X6
Fumagillin	T36.8X1	T36.8X2	T36.8X3	T36.8X4	T36.8X5	T36.8X6
Fumaric acid	T49.4X1	T49.4X2	T49.4X3	T49.4X4	T49.4X5	T49.4X6
Fumes (from)	T59.91	T59.92	T59.93	T59.94	—	—
carbon monoxide — see Carbon, monoxide						
charcoal (domestic use) — see Charcoal, fumes						
chloroform — see Chloroform						
coke (in domestic stoves, fireplaces) — see Coke fumes						
corrosive NEC	T54.91	T54.92	T54.93	T54.94	—	—
ether — see ether						
freons	T53.5X1	T53.5X2	T53.5X3	T53.5X4	—	—
hydrocarbons	T59.891	T59.892	T59.893	T59.894	—	—
petroleum (liquefied)	T59.891	T59.892	T59.893	T59.894	—	—
distributed through pipes (pure or mixed with air)	T59.891	T59.892	T59.893	T59.894	—	—
lead — see lead						

Substance	Poisoning, Accidental (unintentional)	Poisoning, Intentional Self-harm	Poisoning, Assault	Poisoning, Undetermined	Adverse Effect	Under-dosing
Fumes — continued						
metal — see Metals, or the specified metal						
nitrogen dioxide	T59.0X1	T59.0X2	T59.0X3	T59.0X4	—	—
pesticides — see Pesticide						
petroleum (liquefied)	T59.891	T59.892	T59.893	T59.894	—	—
distributed through pipes (pure or mixed with air)	T59.891	T59.892	T59.893	T59.894	—	—
polyester	T59.891	T59.892	T59.893	T59.894	—	—
specified source NEC — see also substance specified	T59.891	T59.892	T59.893	T59.894	—	—
sulfur dioxide	T59.1X1	T59.1X2	T59.1X3	T59.1X4	—	—
Fumigant NEC	T60.91	T60.92	T60.93	T60.94	—	—
Fungicide NEC (nonmedicinal)	T60.3X1	T60.3X2	T60.3X3	T60.3X4	—	—
Fungi, noxious, used as food	T62.0X1	T62.0X2	T62.0X3	T62.0X4	—	—
Fungizone	T36.7X1	T36.7X2	T36.7X3	T36.7X4	T36.7X5	T36.7X6
topical	T49.0X1	T49.0X2	T49.0X3	T49.0X4	T49.0X5	T49.0X6
Fungoid*	T49.0X1	T49.0X2	T49.0X3	T49.0X4	T49.0X5	T49.0X6
Furacin	T49.0X1	T49.0X2	T49.0X3	T49.0X4	T49.0X5	T49.0X6
Furadantin	T37.91	T37.92	T37.93	T37.94	T37.95	T37.96
Furazolidone	T37.8X1	T37.8X2	T37.8X3	T37.8X4	T37.8X5	T37.8X6
Furazolium chloride	T49.0X1	T49.0X2	T49.0X3	T49.0X4	T49.0X5	T49.0X6
Furfural	T52.8X1	T52.8X2	T52.8X3	T52.8X4	—	—
Furnace (coal burning) (domestic), gas from	T58.2X1	T58.2X2	T58.2X3	T58.2X4	—	—
industrial	T58.8X1	T58.8X2	T58.8X3	T58.8X4	—	—
Furniture polish	T65.891	T65.892	T65.893	T65.894	—	—
Furosemide	T50.1X1	T50.1X2	T50.1X3	T50.1X4	T50.1X5	T50.1X6
Furoxone	T37.91	T37.92	T37.93	T37.94	T37.95	T37.96
Fursultiamine	T45.2X1	T45.2X2	T45.2X3	T45.2X4	T45.2X5	T45.2X6
Fusafungine	T36.8X1	T36.8X2	T36.8X3	T36.8X4	T36.8X5	T36.8X6
Fusel oil (any) (amyl) (butyl) (propyl), vapor	T51.3X1	T51.3X2	T51.3X3	T51.3X4	—	—
Fusidate (ethanolamine) (sodium)	T36.8X1	T36.8X2	T36.8X3	T36.8X4	T36.8X5	T36.8X6
Fusidic acid	T36.8X1	T36.8X2	T36.8X3	T36.8X4	T36.8X5	T36.8X6
Fytic acid, nonasodium	T50.6X1	T50.6X2	T50.6X3	T50.6X4	T50.6X5	T50.6X6
b-Galactosidase	T47.5X1	T47.5X2	T47.5X3	T47.5X4	T47.5X5	T47.5X6
GABA	T43.8X1	T43.8X2	T43.8X3	T43.8X4	T43.8X5	T43.8X6
Gabitril*	T42.6X1	T42.6X2	T42.6X3	T42.6X4	T42.6X5	T42.6X6
Gadopentetic acid	T50.8X1	T50.8X2	T50.8X3	T50.8X4	T50.8X5	T50.8X6
Galactose	T50.3X1	T50.3X2	T50.3X3	T50.3X4	T50.3X5	T50.3X6
Galantamine	T44.0X1	T44.0X2	T44.0X3	T44.0X4	T44.0X5	T44.0X6
Gallamine (triethiodide)	T48.1X1	T48.1X2	T48.1X3	T48.1X4	T48.1X5	T48.1X6
Gallium citrate	T50.991	T50.992	T50.993	T50.994	T50.995	T50.996
Gallopamil	T46.1X1	T46.1X2	T46.1X3	T46.1X4	T46.1X5	T46.1X6
Gamboge	T47.2X1	T47.2X2	T47.2X3	T47.2X4	T47.2X5	T47.2X6
Gamimune	T50.Z11	T50.Z12	T50.Z13	T50.Z14	T50.Z15	T50.Z16
Gamma-aminobutyric acid	T43.8X1	T43.8X2	T43.8X3	T43.8X4	T43.8X5	T43.8X6
Gamma-benzene hexachloride (medicinal)	T49.0X1	T49.0X2	T49.0X3	T49.0X4	T49.0X5	T49.0X6
nonmedicinal, vapor	T53.6X1	T53.6X2	T53.6X3	T53.6X4	—	—
Gamma-BHC (medicinal) — see also Gamma-benzene hexachloride	T49.0X1	T49.0X2	T49.0X3	T49.0X4	T49.0X5	T49.0X6
Gamma globulin	T50.Z11	T50.Z12	T50.Z13	T50.Z14	T50.Z15	T50.Z16
Gamulin	T50.Z11	T50.Z12	T50.Z13	T50.Z14	T50.Z15	T50.Z16
Ganciclovir (sodium)	T37.5X1	T37.5X2	T37.5X3	T37.5X4	T37.5X5	T37.5X6
Ganglionic blocking drug NEC	T44.2X1	T44.2X2	T44.2X3	T44.2X4	T44.2X5	T44.2X6
specified NEC	T44.2X1	T44.2X2	T44.2X3	T44.2X4	T44.2X5	T44.2X6
Ganja	T40.711	T40.712	T40.713	T40.714	T40.715	T40.716
Garamycin	T36.5X1	T36.5X2	T36.5X3	T36.5X4	T36.5X5	T36.5X6
ophthalmic preparation	T49.5X1	T49.5X2	T49.5X3	T49.5X4	T49.5X5	T49.5X6
topical NEC	T49.0X1	T49.0X2	T49.0X3	T49.0X4	T49.0X5	T49.0X6
Gardenal	T42.3X1	T42.3X2	T42.3X3	T42.3X4	T42.3X5	T42.3X6
Gardepanyl	T42.3X1	T42.3X2	T42.3X3	T42.3X4	T42.3X5	T42.3X6
Gaseous substance — see Gas						
Gasoline	T52.0X1	T52.0X2	T52.0X3	T52.0X4	—	—
vapor	T52.0X1	T52.0X2	T52.0X3	T52.0X4	—	—
Gastric enzymes	T47.5X1	T47.5X2	T47.5X3	T47.5X4	T47.5X5	T47.5X6
Gastrografin	T50.8X1	T50.8X2	T50.8X3	T50.8X4	T50.8X5	T50.8X6
Gastrointestinal drug	T47.91	T47.92	T47.93	T47.94	T47.95	T47.96
biological	T47.8X1	T47.8X2	T47.8X3	T47.8X4	T47.8X5	T47.8X6
specified NEC	T47.8X1	T47.8X2	T47.8X3	T47.8X4	T47.8X5	T47.8X6
Gas NEC	T59.91	T59.92	T59.93	T59.94	—	—
acetylene	T59.891	T59.892	T59.893	T59.894	—	—
incomplete combustion of	T58.11	T58.12	T58.13	T58.14	—	—

☑ Additional Character May Be Required — Refer to the Tabular List for Character Selection

*Optum Value-Add

Substance	Poisoning, Accidental (unintentional)	Poisoning, Intentional Self-harm	Poisoning, Assault	Poisoning, Undetermined	Adverse Effect	Under-dosing
Gas — *continued*						
air contaminants, source or type not specified	T59.91	T59.92	T59.93	T59.94	—	—
anesthetic	T41.0X1	T41.0X2	T41.0X3	T41.0X4	T41.0X5	T41.0X6
blast furnace	T58.8X1	T58.8X2	T58.8X3	T58.8X4	—	—
butane — *see* butane						
carbon monoxide — *see* Carbon, monoxide						
chlorine	T59.4X1	T59.4X2	T59.4X3	T59.4X4	—	—
coal	T58.2X1	T58.2X2	T58.2X3	T58.2X4	—	—
cyanide	T57.3X1	T57.3X2	T57.3X3	T57.3X4	—	—
dicyanogen	T65.0X1	T65.0X2	T65.0X3	T65.0X4	—	—
domestic — *see* Domestic gas						
exhaust	T58.01	T58.02	T58.03	T58.04		
from utility (for cooking, heating, or lighting) (after combustion) — *see* Carbon, monoxide, fuel, utility						
prior to combustion	T59.891	T59.892	T59.893	T59.894	—	—
from wood- or coal-burning stove or fireplace	T58.2X1	T58.2X2	T58.2X3	T58.2X4	—	—
fuel (domestic use) (after combustion) — *see also* Carbon, monoxide, fuel						
industrial use	T58.8X1	T58.8X2	T58.8X3	T58.8X4	—	—
prior to combustion	T59.891	T59.892	T59.893	T59.894	—	—
utility	T59.891	T59.892	T59.893	T59.894	—	—
incomplete combustion of — *see* Carbon, monoxide, fuel, utility						
in mobile container	T59.891	T59.892	T59.893	T59.894	—	—
piped (natural)	T59.891	T59.892	T59.893	T59.894	—	—
garage	T58.01	T58.02	T58.03	T58.04		
hydrocarbon NEC	T59.891	T59.892	T59.893	T59.894		
incomplete combustion of — *see* Carbon, monoxide, fuel, utility						
liquefied — *see* butane						
piped	T59.891	T59.892	T59.893	T59.894	—	—
hydrocyanic acid	T65.0X1	T65.0X2	T65.0X3	T65.0X4	—	—
illuminating (after combustion)	T58.11	T58.12	T58.13	T58.14		
prior to combustion	T59.891	T59.892	T59.893	T59.894	—	—
incomplete combustion, any — *see* Carbon, monoxide						
kiln	T58.8X1	T58.8X2	T58.8X3	T58.8X4	—	—
lacrimogenic	T59.3X1	T59.3X2	T59.3X3	T59.3X4	—	—
liquefied petroleum — *see* butane						
marsh	T59.891	T59.892	T59.893	T59.894	—	—
motor exhaust, not in transit	T58.01	T58.02	T58.03	T58.04		
mustard, not in war	T59.891	T59.892	T59.893	T59.894	—	—
natural	T59.891	T59.892	T59.893	T59.894	—	—
nerve, not in war	T59.91	T59.92	T59.93	T59.94	—	—
oil	T52.0X1	T52.0X2	T52.0X3	T52.0X4	—	—
petroleum (liquefied) (distributed in mobile containers)	T59.891	T59.892	T59.893	T59.894	—	—
piped (pure or mixed with air)	T59.891	T59.892	T59.893	T59.894	—	—
piped (manufactured) (natural) NEC	T59.891	T59.892	T59.893	T59.894	—	—
producer	T58.8X1	T58.8X2	T58.8X3	T58.8X4	—	—
propane — *see* propane						
refrigerant (chlorofluoro-carbon)	T53.5X1	T53.5X2	T53.5X3	T53.5X4	—	—
not chlorofluoro-carbon	T59.891	T59.892	T59.893	T59.894	—	—
sewer	T59.91	T59.92	T59.93	T59.94	—	—
specified source NEC	T59.91	T59.92	T59.93	T59.94	—	—
stove (after combustion)	T58.11	T58.12	T58.13	T58.14		
prior to combustion	T59.891	T59.892	T59.893	T59.894	—	—
tear	T59.3X1	T59.3X2	T59.3X3	T59.3X4	—	—
therapeutic	T41.5X1	T41.5X2	T41.5X3	T41.5X4	T41.5X5	T41.5X6
utility (for cooking, heating, or lighting) (piped) NEC	T59.891	T59.892	T59.893	T59.894	—	—
incomplete combustion of — *see* Carbon, monoxide, fuel, utility						
in mobile container	T59.891	T59.892	T59.893	T59.894	—	—
piped (natural)	T59.891	T59.892	T59.893	T59.894	—	—
water	T58.11	T58.12	T58.13	T58.14		

Substance	Poisoning, Accidental (unintentional)	Poisoning, Intentional Self-harm	Poisoning, Assault	Poisoning, Undetermined	Adverse Effect	Under-dosing
Gas — *continued*						
water — *continued*						
incomplete combustion of — *see* Carbon, monoxide, fuel, utility						
Gaultheria procumbens	T62.2X1	T62.2X2	T62.2X3	T62.2X4	—	—
Gaviscon*	T47.1X1	T47.1X2	T47.1X3	T47.1X4	T47.1X5	T47.1X6
Gefarnate	T44.3X1	T44.3X2	T44.3X3	T44.3X4	T44.3X5	T44.3X6
Gelatin (intravenous)	T45.8X1	T45.8X2	T45.8X3	T45.8X4	T45.8X5	T45.8X6
absorbable (sponge)	T45.7X1	T45.7X2	T45.7X3	T45.7X4	T45.7X5	T45.7X6
Gelfilm	T49.8X1	T49.8X2	T49.8X3	T49.8X4	T49.8X5	T49.8X6
Gelfoam	T45.7X1	T45.7X2	T45.7X3	T45.7X4	T45.7X5	T45.7X6
Gelsemine	T50.991	T50.992	T50.993	T50.994	T50.995	T50.996
Gelsemium (sempervirens)	T62.2X1	T62.2X2	T62.2X3	T62.2X4		
Gemeprost	T48.0X1	T48.0X2	T48.0X3	T48.0X4	T48.0X5	T48.0X6
Gemfibrozil	T46.6X1	T46.6X2	T46.6X3	T46.6X4	T46.6X5	T46.6X6
Gemonil	T42.3X1	T42.3X2	T42.3X3	T42.3X4	T42.3X5	T42.3X6
Gentamicin	T36.5X1	T36.5X2	T36.5X3	T36.5X4	T36.5X5	T36.5X6
ophthalmic preparation	T49.5X1	T49.5X2	T49.5X3	T49.5X4	T49.5X5	T49.5X6
topical NEC	T49.0X1	T49.0X2	T49.0X3	T49.0X4	T49.0X5	T49.0X6
Gentasol*	T49.5X1	T49.5X2	T49.5X3	T49.5X4	T49.5X5	T49.5X6
Gentian	T47.5X1	T47.5X2	T47.5X3	T47.5X4	T47.5X5	T47.5X6
violet	T49.0X1	T49.0X2	T49.0X3	T49.0X4	T49.0X5	T49.0X6
Gepefrine	T44.4X1	T44.4X2	T44.4X3	T44.4X4	T44.4X5	T44.4X6
Gestonorone caproate	T38.5X1	T38.5X2	T38.5X3	T38.5X4	T38.5X5	T38.5X6
Gexane	T49.0X1	T49.0X2	T49.0X3	T49.0X4	—	T49.0X6
Gila monster (venom)	T63.111	T63.112	T63.113	T63.114	—	—
Ginger	T47.5X1	T47.5X2	T47.5X3	T47.5X4	T47.5X5	T47.5X6
Jamaica — *see* Jamaica, ginger						
Gitalin	T46.0X1	T46.0X2	T46.0X3	T46.0X4	T46.0X5	T46.0X6
amorphous	T46.0X1	T46.0X2	T46.0X3	T46.0X4	T46.0X5	T46.0X6
Gitaloxin	T46.0X1	T46.0X2	T46.0X3	T46.0X4	T46.0X5	T46.0X6
Gitoxin	T46.0X1	T46.0X2	T46.0X3	T46.0X4	T46.0X5	T46.0X6
Glafenine	T39.8X1	T39.8X2	T39.8X3	T39.8X4	T39.8X5	T39.8X6
Glandular extract (medicinal) NEC	T50.Z91	T50.Z92	T50.Z93	T50.Z94	T50.Z95	T50.Z96
Glaucarubin	T37.3X1	T37.3X2	T37.3X3	T37.3X4	T37.3X5	T37.3X6
Glibenclamide	T38.3X1	T38.3X2	T38.3X3	T38.3X4	T38.3X5	T38.3X6
Glibornuride	T38.3X1	T38.3X2	T38.3X3	T38.3X4	T38.3X5	T38.3X6
Gliclazide	T38.3X1	T38.3X2	T38.3X3	T38.3X4	T38.3X5	T38.3X6
Glimidine	T38.3X1	T38.3X2	T38.3X3	T38.3X4	T38.3X5	T38.3X6
Glipizide	T38.3X1	T38.3X2	T38.3X3	T38.3X4	T38.3X5	T38.3X6
Gliquidone	T38.3X1	T38.3X2	T38.3X3	T38.3X4	T38.3X5	T38.3X6
Glisolamide	T38.3X1	T38.3X2	T38.3X3	T38.3X4	T38.3X5	T38.3X6
Glisoxepide	T38.3X1	T38.3X2	T38.3X3	T38.3X4	T38.3X5	T38.3X6
Globin zinc insulin	T38.3X1	T38.3X2	T38.3X3	T38.3X4	T38.3X5	T38.3X6
Globulin						
antilymphocytic	T50.Z11	T50.Z12	T50.Z13	T50.Z14	T50.Z15	T50.Z16
antirhesus	T50.Z11	T50.Z12	T50.Z13	T50.Z14	T50.Z15	T50.Z16
antivenin	T50.Z11	T50.Z12	T50.Z13	T50.Z14	T50.Z15	T50.Z16
antiviral	T50.Z11	T50.Z12	T50.Z13	T50.Z14	T50.Z15	T50.Z16
Glucagon	T38.3X1	T38.3X2	T38.3X3	T38.3X4	T38.3X5	T38.3X6
Glucocorticoids	T38.0X1	T38.0X2	T38.0X3	T38.0X4	T38.0X5	T38.0X6
Glucocorticosteroid	T38.0X1	T38.0X2	T38.0X3	T38.0X4	T38.0X5	T38.0X6
Gluconic acid	T50.991	T50.992	T50.993	T50.994	T50.995	T50.996
Glucosamine sulfate	T39.4X1	T39.4X2	T39.4X3	T39.4X4	T39.4X5	T39.4X6
Glucose	T50.3X1	T50.3X2	T50.3X3	T50.3X4	T50.3X5	T50.3X6
with sodium chloride	T50.3X1	T50.3X2	T50.3X3	T50.3X4	T50.3X5	T50.3X6
Glucosulfone sodium	T37.1X1	T37.1X2	T37.1X3	T37.1X4	T37.1X5	T37.1X6
Glucotrol*	T38.3X1	T38.3X2	T38.3X3	T38.3X4	T38.3X5	T38.3X6
Glucurolactone	T47.8X1	T47.8X2	T47.8X3	T47.8X4	T47.8X5	T47.8X6
Glue NEC	T52.8X1	T52.8X2	T52.8X3	T52.8X4	—	—
Glutamic acid	T47.5X1	T47.5X2	T47.5X3	T47.5X4	T47.5X5	T47.5X6
Glutaral (medicinal)	T49.0X1	T49.0X2	T49.0X3	T49.0X4	T49.0X5	T49.0X6
nonmedicinal	T65.891	T65.892	T65.893	T65.894	—	—
Glutaraldehyde (nonmedicinal)	T65.891	T65.892	T65.893	T65.894	—	—
medicinal	T49.0X1	T49.0X2	T49.0X3	T49.0X4	T49.0X5	T49.0X6
Glutathione	T50.6X1	T50.6X2	T50.6X3	T50.6X4	T50.6X5	T50.6X6
Glutethimide	T42.6X1	T42.6X2	T42.6X3	T42.6X4	T42.6X5	T42.6X6
Glyburide	T38.3X1	T38.3X2	T38.3X3	T38.3X4	T38.3X5	T38.3X6
Glycerin	T47.4X1	T47.4X2	T47.4X3	T47.4X4	T47.4X5	T47.4X6
Glycerol	T47.4X1	T47.4X2	T47.4X3	T47.4X4	T47.4X5	T47.4X6
borax	T49.6X1	T49.6X2	T49.6X3	T49.6X4	T49.6X5	T49.6X6
intravenous	T50.3X1	T50.3X2	T50.3X3	T50.3X4	T50.3X5	T50.3X6
iodinated	T48.4X1	T48.4X2	T48.4X3	T48.4X4	T48.4X5	T48.4X6
Glycerophosphate	T50.991	T50.992	T50.993	T50.994	T50.995	T50.996
Glyceryl						
gualacolate	T48.4X1	T48.4X2	T48.4X3	T48.4X4	T48.4X5	T48.4X6
nitrate	T46.3X1	T46.3X2	T46.3X3	T46.3X4	T46.3X5	T46.3X6
triacetate (topical)	T49.0X1	T49.0X2	T49.0X3	T49.0X4	T49.0X5	T49.0X6
trinitrate	T46.3X1	T46.3X2	T46.3X3	T46.3X4	T46.3X5	T46.3X6
Glycine	T50.3X1	T50.3X2	T50.3X3	T50.3X4	T50.3X5	T50.3X6

Substance	Poisoning, Accidental (unintentional)	Poisoning, Intentional Self-harm	Poisoning, Assault	Poisoning, Undetermined	Adverse Effect	Under-dosing
Glyclopyramide	T38.3X1	T38.3X2	T38.3X3	T38.3X4	T38.3X5	T38.3X6
Glycobiarsol	T37.3X1	T37.3X2	T37.3X3	T37.3X4	T37.3X5	T37.3X6
Glycols (ether)	T52.3X1	T52.3X2	T52.3X3	T52.3X4	—	—
Glyconiazide	T37.1X1	T37.1X2	T37.1X3	T37.1X4	T37.1X5	T37.1X6
Glycopyrrolate	T44.3X1	T44.3X2	T44.3X3	T44.3X4	T44.3X5	T44.3X6
Glycopyrronium	T44.3X1	T44.3X2	T44.3X3	T44.3X4	T44.3X5	T44.3X6
bromide	T44.3X1	T44.3X2	T44.3X3	T44.3X4	T44.3X5	T44.3X6
Glycoside, cardiac	T46.0X1	T46.0X2	T46.0X3	T46.0X4	T46.0X5	T46.0X6
(stimulant)						
Glycyclamide	T38.3X1	T38.3X2	T38.3X3	T38.3X4	T38.3X5	T38.3X6
Glycyrrhiza extract	T48.4X1	T48.4X2	T48.4X3	T48.4X4	T48.4X5	T48.4X6
Glycyrrhizic acid	T48.4X1	T48.4X2	T48.4X3	T48.4X4	T48.4X5	T48.4X6
Glycyrrhizinate potassium	T48.4X1	T48.4X2	T48.4X3	T48.4X4	T48.4X5	T48.4X6
Glymidine sodium	T38.3X1	T38.3X2	T38.3X3	T38.3X4	T38.3X5	T38.3X6
Glyphosate	T60.3X1	T60.3X2	T60.3X3	T60.3X4	—	—
Glyphylline	T48.6X1	T48.6X2	T48.6X3	T48.6X4	T48.6X5	T48.6X6
Gold						
colloidal (I98Au)	T45.1X1	T45.1X2	T45.1X3	T45.1X4	T45.1X5	T45.1X6
salts	T39.4X1	T39.4X2	T39.4X3	T39.4X4	T39.4X5	T39.4X6
Golden sulfide of antimony	T56.891	T56.892	T56.893	T56.894		
Goldylocks	T62.2X1	T62.2X2	T62.2X3	T62.2X4	—	—
Gonadal tissue extract	T38.901	T38.902	T38.903	T38.904	T38.905	T38.906
female	T38.5X1	T38.5X2	T38.5X3	T38.5X4	T38.5X5	T38.5X6
male	T38.7X1	T38.7X2	T38.7X3	T38.7X4	T38.7X5	T38.7X6
Gonadorelin	T38.891	T38.892	T38.893	T38.894	T38.895	T38.896
Gonadotropin	T38.891	T38.892	T38.893	T38.894	T38.895	T38.896
chorionic	T38.891	T38.892	T38.893	T38.894	T38.895	T38.896
pituitary	T38.811	T38.812	T38.813	T38.814	T38.815	T38.816
Goserelin	T45.1X1	T45.1X2	T45.1X3	T45.1X4	T45.1X5	T45.1X6
Grain alcohol	T51.0X1	T51.0X2	T51.0X3	T51.0X4		
Gralise*	T42.6X1	T42.6X2	T42.6X3	T42.6X4	T42.6X5	T42.6X6
Gramicidin	T49.0X1	T49.0X2	T49.0X3	T49.0X4	T49.0X5	T49.0X6
Granisetron	T45.0X1	T45.0X2	T45.0X3	T45.0X4	T45.0X5	T45.0X6
Gratiola officinalis	T62.2X1	T62.2X2	T62.2X3	T62.2X4	—	—
Grease	T65.891	T65.892	T65.893	T65.894	—	—
Green hellebore	T62.2X1	T62.2X2	T62.2X3	T62.2X4	—	—
Green soap	T49.2X1	T49.2X2	T49.2X3	T49.2X4	T49.2X5	T49.2X6
Grifulvin	T36.7X1	T36.7X2	T36.7X3	T36.7X4	T36.7X5	T36.7X6
Griseofulvin	T36.7X1	T36.7X2	T36.7X3	T36.7X4	T36.7X5	T36.7X6
Growth hormone	T38.811	T38.812	T38.813	T38.814	T38.815	T38.816
Guaiacol derivatives	T48.4X1	T48.4X2	T48.4X3	T48.4X4	T48.4X5	T48.4X6
Guaiac reagent	T50.991	T50.992	T50.993	T50.994	T50.995	T50.996
Guaifenesin	T48.4X1	T48.4X2	T48.4X3	T48.4X4	T48.4X5	T48.4X6
Guaimesal	T48.4X1	T48.4X2	T48.4X3	T48.4X4	T48.4X5	T48.4X6
Guaiphenesin	T48.4X1	T48.4X2	T48.4X3	T48.4X4	T48.4X5	T48.4X6
Guaituss*	T48.4X1	T48.4X2	T48.4X3	T48.4X4	T48.4X5	T48.4X6
Guamecycline	T36.4X1	T36.4X2	T36.4X3	T36.4X4	T36.4X5	T36.4X6
Guanabenz	T46.5X1	T46.5X2	T46.5X3	T46.5X4	T46.5X5	T46.5X6
Guanacline	T46.5X1	T46.5X2	T46.5X3	T46.5X4	T46.5X5	T46.5X6
Guanadrel	T46.5X1	T46.5X2	T46.5X3	T46.5X4	T46.5X5	T46.5X6
Guanatol	T37.2X1	T37.2X2	T37.2X3	T37.2X4	T37.2X5	T37.2X6
Guanethidine	T46.5X1	T46.5X2	T46.5X3	T46.5X4	T46.5X5	T46.5X6
Guanfacine	T46.5X1	T46.5X2	T46.5X3	T46.5X4	T46.5X5	T46.5X6
Guano	T65.891	T65.892	T65.893	T65.894	—	—
Guanochlor	T46.5X1	T46.5X2	T46.5X3	T46.5X4	T46.5X5	T46.5X6
Guanoclor	T46.5X1	T46.5X2	T46.5X3	T46.5X4	T46.5X5	T46.5X6
Guanoctine	T46.5X1	T46.5X2	T46.5X3	T46.5X4	T46.5X5	T46.5X6
Guanoxabenz	T46.5X1	T46.5X2	T46.5X3	T46.5X4	T46.5X5	T46.5X6
Guanoxan	T46.5X1	T46.5X2	T46.5X3	T46.5X4	T46.5X5	T46.5X6
Guar gum (medicinal)	T46.6X1	T46.6X2	T46.6X3	T46.6X4	T46.6X5	T46.6X6
Hachimycin	T36.7X1	T36.7X2	T36.7X3	T36.7X4	T36.7X5	T36.7X6
Hair						
dye	T49.4X1	T49.4X2	T49.4X3	T49.4X4	T49.4X5	T49.4X6
preparation NEC	T49.4X1	T49.4X2	T49.4X3	T49.4X4	T49.4X5	T49.4X6
Halazepam	T42.4X1	T42.4X2	T42.4X3	T42.4X4	T42.4X5	T42.4X6
Halcinolone	T49.0X1	T49.0X2	T49.0X3	T49.0X4	T49.0X5	T49.0X6
Halcinonide	T49.0X1	T49.0X2	T49.0X3	T49.0X4	T49.0X5	T49.0X6
Halethazole	T49.0X1	T49.0X2	T49.0X3	T49.0X4	T49.0X5	T49.0X6
Hallucinogen NOS	T40.901	T40.902	T40.903	T40.904	T40.905	T40.906
specified NEC	T40.991	T40.992	T40.993	T40.994	T40.995	T40.996
Halofantrine	T37.2X1	T37.2X2	T37.2X3	T37.2X4	T37.2X5	T37.2X6
Halofenate	T46.6X1	T46.6X2	T46.6X3	T46.6X4	T46.6X5	T46.6X6
Halometasone	T49.0X1	T49.0X2	T49.0X3	T49.0X4	T49.0X5	T49.0X6
Haloperidol	T43.4X1	T43.4X2	T43.4X3	T43.4X4	T43.4X5	T43.4X6
Haloprogin	T49.0X1	T49.0X2	T49.0X3	T49.0X4	T49.0X5	T49.0X6
Halotex	T49.0X1	T49.0X2	T49.0X3	T49.0X4	T49.0X5	T49.0X6
Halothane	T41.0X1	T41.0X2	T41.0X3	T41.0X4	T41.0X5	T41.0X6
Haloxazolam	T42.4X1	T42.4X2	T42.4X3	T42.4X4	T42.4X5	T42.4X6
Halquinols	T49.0X1	T49.0X2	T49.0X3	T49.0X4	T49.0X5	T49.0X6
Hamamelis	T49.2X1	T49.2X2	T49.2X3	T49.2X4	T49.2X5	T49.2X6
Haptendextran	T45.8X1	T45.8X2	T45.8X3	T45.8X4	T45.8X5	T45.8X6
Harmonyl	T46.5X1	T46.5X2	T46.5X3	T46.5X4	T46.5X5	T46.5X6

Substance	Poisoning, Accidental (unintentional)	Poisoning, Intentional Self-harm	Poisoning, Assault	Poisoning, Undetermined	Adverse Effect	Under-dosing
Hartmann's solution	T50.3X1	T50.3X2	T50.3X3	T50.3X4	T50.3X5	T50.3X6
Hashish	T40.711	T40.712	T40.713	T40.714	T40.715	T40.716
Havrix*	T50.B91	T50.B92	T50.B93	T50.B94	T50.B95	T50.B96
Hawaiian Woodrose seeds	T40.991	T40.992	T40.993	T40.994		
HCB	T60.3X1	T60.3X2	T60.3X3	T60.3X4		
HCH	T53.6X1	T53.6X2	T53.6X3	T53.6X4		
medicinal	T49.0X1	T49.0X2	T49.0X3	T49.0X4	T49.0X5	T49.0X6
HCN	T57.3X1	T57.3X2	T57.3X3	T57.3X4		
Headache cures, drugs, powders NEC	T50.901	T50.902	T50.903	T50.904	T50.905	T50.906
Heavenly Blue (morning glory)	T40.991	T40.992	T40.993	T40.994		
Heavy metal antidote	T45.8X1	T45.8X2	T45.8X3	T45.8X4	T45.8X5	T45.8X6
Hedaquinium	T49.0X1	T49.0X2	T49.0X3	T49.0X4	T49.0X5	T49.0X6
Hedge hyssop	T62.2X1	T62.2X2	T62.2X3	T62.2X4	—	—
Heet	T49.8X1	T49.8X2	T49.8X3	T49.8X4	T49.8X5	T49.8X6
Helenin	T37.4X1	T37.4X2	T37.4X3	T37.4X4	T37.4X5	T37.4X6
Helium (nonmedicinal) NEC	T59.891	T59.892	T59.893	T59.894		
medicinal	T48.991	T48.992	T48.993	T48.994	T48.995	T48.996
Helleborne (black) (green) (white)	T62.2X1	T62.2X2	T62.2X3	T62.2X4		
Hematin	T45.8X1	T45.8X2	T45.8X3	T45.8X4	T45.8X5	T45.8X6
Hematinic preparation	T45.8X1	T45.8X2	T45.8X3	T45.8X4	T45.8X5	T45.8X6
Hematological agent	T45.91	T45.92	T45.93	T45.94	T45.95	T45.96
specified NEC	T45.8X1	T45.8X2	T45.8X3	T45.8X4	T45.8X5	T45.8X6
Hemlock	T62.2X1	T62.2X2	T62.2X3	T62.2X4	—	—
Hemostatic	T45.621	T45.622	T45.623	T45.624	T45.625	T45.626
drug, systemic	T45.621	T45.622	T45.623	T45.624	T45.625	T45.626
Hemostyptic	T49.4X1	T49.4X2	T49.4X3	T49.4X4	T49.4X5	T49.4X6
Henbane	T62.2X1	T62.2X2	T62.2X3	T62.2X4	—	—
Heparin (sodium)	T45.511	T45.512	T45.513	T45.514	T45.515	T45.516
action reverser	T45.7X1	T45.7X2	T45.7X3	T45.7X4	T45.7X5	T45.7X6
Heparin-fraction	T45.511	T45.512	T45.513	T45.514	T45.515	T45.516
Heparinoid (systemic)	T45.511	T45.512	T45.513	T45.514	T45.515	T45.516
Hepatic secretion stimulant	T47.8X1	T47.8X2	T47.8X3	T47.8X4	T47.8X5	T47.8X6
Hepatitis A vaccine*	T50.B91	T50.B92	T50.B93	T50.B94	T50.B95	T50.B96
Hepatitis B						
immune globulin	T50.Z11	T50.Z12	T50.Z13	T50.Z14	T50.Z15	T50.Z16
vaccine	T50.B91	T50.B92	T50.B93	T50.B94	T50.B95	T50.B96
Hepronicate	T46.7X1	T46.7X2	T46.7X3	T46.7X4	T46.7X5	T46.7X6
Heptabarb	T42.3X1	T42.3X2	T42.3X3	T42.3X4	T42.3X5	T42.3X6
Heptabarbital	T42.3X1	T42.3X2	T42.3X3	T42.3X4	T42.3X5	T42.3X6
Heptabarbitone	T42.3X1	T42.3X2	T42.3X3	T42.3X4	T42.3X5	T42.3X6
Heptachlor	T60.1X1	T60.1X2	T60.1X3	T60.1X4	—	—
Heptalgin	T40.2X1	T40.2X2	T40.2X3	T40.2X4	T40.2X5	T40.2X6
Heptaminol	T46.3X1	T46.3X2	T46.3X3	T46.3X4	T46.3X5	T46.3X6
Herbicide NEC	T60.3X1	T60.3X2	T60.3X3	T60.3X4	—	—
Heroin	T40.1X1	T40.1X2	T40.1X3	T40.1X4	—	—
Herplex	T49.5X1	T49.5X2	T49.5X3	T49.5X4	T49.5X5	T49.5X6
HES	T45.8X1	T45.8X2	T45.8X3	T45.8X4	T45.8X5	T45.8X6
Hesperidin	T46.991	T46.992	T46.993	T46.994	T46.995	T46.996
Hetacillin	T36.0X1	T36.0X2	T36.0X3	T36.0X4	T36.0X5	T36.0X6
Hetastarch	T45.8X1	T45.8X2	T45.8X3	T45.8X4	T45.8X5	T45.8X6
HETP	T60.0X1	T60.0X2	T60.0X3	T60.0X4	—	—
Hexachlorobenzene (vapor)	T60.3X1	T60.3X2	T60.3X3	T60.3X4	—	—
Hexachlorocyclohexane	T53.6X1	T53.6X2	T53.6X3	T53.6X4	—	—
Hexachlorophene	T49.0X1	T49.0X2	T49.0X3	T49.0X4	T49.0X5	T49.0X6
Hexadiline	T46.3X1	T46.3X2	T46.3X3	T46.3X4	T46.3X5	T46.3X6
Hexadimethrine (bromide)	T45.7X1	T45.7X2	T45.7X3	T45.7X4	T45.7X5	T45.7X6
Hexadylamine	T46.3X1	T46.3X2	T46.3X3	T46.3X4	T46.3X5	T46.3X6
Hexaethyl tetraphosphate	T60.0X1	T60.0X2	T60.0X3	T60.0X4	—	—
Hexafluorenium bromide	T48.1X1	T48.1X2	T48.1X3	T48.1X4	T48.1X5	T48.1X6
Hexafluronium (bromide)	T48.1X1	T48.1X2	T48.1X3	T48.1X4	T48.1X5	T48.1X6
Hexa-germ	T49.2X1	T49.2X2	T49.2X3	T49.2X4	T49.2X5	T49.2X6
Hexahydrobenzol	T52.8X1	T52.8X2	T52.8X3	T52.8X4	—	—
Hexahydrocresol(s)	T51.8X1	T51.8X2	T51.8X3	T51.8X4		
arsenide	T57.0X1	T57.0X2	T57.0X3	T57.0X4		
arseniurated	T57.0X1	T57.0X2	T57.0X3	T57.0X4		
cyanide	T57.3X1	T57.3X2	T57.3X3	T57.3X4		
gas	T59.891	T59.892	T59.893	T59.894		
Fluoride (liquid)	T57.8X1	T57.8X2	T57.8X3	T57.8X4		
vapor	T59.891	T59.892	T59.893	T59.894		
phophorated	T60.0X1	T60.0X2	T60.0X3	T60.0X4	—	—
sulfate	T57.8X1	T57.8X2	T57.8X3	T57.8X4		
sulfide (gas)	T59.6X1	T59.6X2	T59.6X3	T59.6X4		
arseniurated	T57.0X1	T57.0X2	T57.0X3	T57.0X4		
sulfurated	T57.8X1	T57.8X2	T57.8X3	T57.8X4		
Hexahydrophenol	T51.8X1	T51.8X2	T51.8X3	T51.8X4		
Hexalen	T51.8X1	T51.8X2	T51.8X3	T51.8X4		
Hexamethonium bromide	T44.2X1	T44.2X2	T44.2X3	T44.2X4	T44.2X5	T44.2X6
Hexamethylene	T52.8X1	T52.8X2	T52.8X3	T52.8X4		

☑ Additional Character May Be Required — Refer to the Tabular List for Character Selection

*Optum Value-Add

Substance	Poisoning, Accidental (unintentional)	Poisoning, Intentional Self-harm	Poisoning, Assault	Poisoning, Undetermined	Adverse Effect	Under-dosing
Hexamethylmelamine	T45.1X1	T45.1X2	T45.1X3	T45.1X4	T45.1X5	T45.1X6
Hexamidine	T49.0X1	T49.0X2	T49.0X3	T49.0X4	T49.0X5	T49.0X6
Hexamine (mandelate)	T37.8X1	T37.8X2	T37.8X3	T37.8X4	T37.8X5	T37.8X6
Hexanone, 2-hexanone	T52.4X1	T52.4X2	T52.4X3	T52.4X4	—	—
Hexanuorenium	T48.1X1	T48.1X2	T48.1X3	T48.1X4	T48.1X5	T48.1X6
Hexapropymate	T42.6X1	T42.6X2	T42.6X3	T42.6X4	T42.6X5	T42.6X6
Hexasonium iodide	T44.3X1	T44.3X2	T44.3X3	T44.3X4	T44.3X5	T44.3X6
Hexcarbacholine bromide	T48.1X1	T48.1X2	T48.1X3	T48.1X4	T48.1X5	T48.1X6
Hexemal	T42.3X1	T42.3X2	T42.3X3	T42.3X4	T42.3X5	T42.3X6
Hexestrol	T38.5X1	T38.5X2	T38.5X3	T38.5X4	T38.5X5	T38.5X6
Hexethal (sodium)	T42.3X1	T42.3X2	T42.3X3	T42.3X4	T42.3X5	T42.3X6
Hexetidine	T37.8X1	T37.8X2	T37.8X3	T37.8X4	T37.8X5	T37.8X6
Hexobarbital	T42.3X1	T42.3X2	T42.3X3	T42.3X4	T42.3X5	T42.3X6
rectal	T41.291	T41.292	T41.293	T41.294	T41.295	T41.296
sodium	T41.1X1	T41.1X2	T41.1X3	T41.1X4	T41.1X5	T41.1X6
Hexobendine	T46.3X1	T46.3X2	T46.3X3	T46.3X4	T46.3X5	T46.3X6
Hexocyclium	T44.3X1	T44.3X2	T44.3X3	T44.3X4	T44.3X5	T44.3X6
metilsulfate	T44.3X1	T44.3X2	T44.3X3	T44.3X4	T44.3X5	T44.3X6
Hexoestrol	T38.5X1	T38.5X2	T38.5X3	T38.5X4	T38.5X5	T38.5X6
Hexone	T52.4X1	T52.4X2	T52.4X3	T52.4X4	—	—
Hexoprenaline	T48.6X1	T48.6X2	T48.6X3	T48.6X4	T48.6X5	T48.6X6
Hexylcaine	T41.3X1	T41.3X2	T41.3X3	T41.3X4	T41.3X5	T41.3X6
Hexylresorcinol	T52.2X1	T52.2X2	T52.2X3	T52.2X4	—	—
HGH (human growth hormone)	T38.811	T38.812	T38.813	T38.814	T38.815	T38.816
Hibistat*	T49.0X1	T49.0X2	T49.0X3	T49.0X4	T49.0X5	T49.0X6
Hinkle's pills	T47.2X1	T47.2X2	T47.2X3	T47.2X4	T47.2X5	T47.2X6
Histalog	T50.8X1	T50.8X2	T50.8X3	T50.8X4	T50.8X5	T50.8X6
Histamine (phosphate)	T50.8X1	T50.8X2	T50.8X3	T50.8X4	T50.8X5	T50.8X6
Histolyn*	T50.8X1	T50.8X2	T50.8X3	T50.8X4	T50.8X5	T50.8X6
Histoplasmin	T50.8X1	T50.8X2	T50.8X3	T50.8X4	T50.8X5	T50.8X6
Holly berries	T62.2X1	T62.2X2	T62.2X3	T62.2X4	—	—
Homatropine	T44.3X1	T44.3X2	T44.3X3	T44.3X4	T44.3X5	T44.3X6
methylbromide	T44.3X1	T44.3X2	T44.3X3	T44.3X4	T44.3X5	T44.3X6
Homochlorcyclizine	T45.0X1	T45.0X2	T45.0X3	T45.0X4	T45.0X5	T45.0X6
Homosalate	T49.3X1	T49.3X2	T49.3X3	T49.3X4	T49.3X5	T49.3X6
Homo-tet	T50.Z11	T50.Z12	T50.Z13	T50.Z14	T50.Z15	T50.Z16
Hormone	T38.801	T38.802	T38.803	T38.804	T38.805	T38.806
adrenal cortical steroids	T38.0X1	T38.0X2	T38.0X3	T38.0X4	T38.0X5	T38.0X6
androgenic	T38.7X1	T38.7X2	T38.7X3	T38.7X4	T38.7X5	T38.7X6
anterior pituitary NEC	T38.811	T38.812	T38.813	T38.814	T38.815	T38.816
antidiabetic agents	T38.3X1	T38.3X2	T38.3X3	T38.3X4	T38.3X5	T38.3X6
antidiuretic	T38.891	T38.892	T38.893	T38.894	T38.895	T38.896
cancer therapy	T45.1X1	T45.1X2	T45.1X3	T45.1X4	T45.1X5	T45.1X6
follicle stimulating	T38.811	T38.812	T38.813	T38.814	T38.815	T38.816
gonadotropic	T38.891	T38.892	T38.893	T38.894	T38.895	T38.896
pituitary	T38.811	T38.812	T38.813	T38.814	T38.815	T38.816
growth	T38.811	T38.812	T38.813	T38.814	T38.815	T38.816
luteinizing	T38.811	T38.812	T38.813	T38.814	T38.815	T38.816
ovarian	T38.5X1	T38.5X2	T38.5X3	T38.5X4	T38.5X5	T38.5X6
oxytocic	T48.0X1	T48.0X2	T48.0X3	T48.0X4	T48.0X5	T48.0X6
parathyroid (derivatives)	T50.991	T50.992	T50.993	T50.994	T50.995	T50.996
pituitary (posterior) NEC	T38.891	T38.892	T38.893	T38.894	T38.895	T38.896
anterior	T38.811	T38.812	T38.813	T38.814	T38.815	T38.816
specified, NEC	T38.891	T38.892	T38.893	T38.894	T38.895	T38.896
thyroid	T38.1X1	T38.1X2	T38.1X3	T38.1X4	T38.1X5	T38.1X6
Hornet (sting)	T63.451	T63.452	T63.453	T63.454	—	—
Horse anti-human lymphocytic serum	T50.Z11	T50.Z12	T50.Z13	T50.Z14	T50.Z15	T50.Z16
Horticulture agent NEC	T65.91	T65.92	T65.93	T65.94	—	—
with pesticide	T60.91	T60.92	T60.93	T60.94	—	—
Human						
albumin	T45.8X1	T45.8X2	T45.8X3	T45.8X4	T45.8X5	T45.8X6
growth hormone (HGH)	T38.811	T38.812	T38.813	T38.814	T38.815	T38.816
immune serum	T50.Z11	T50.Z12	T50.Z13	T50.Z14	T50.Z15	T50.Z16
Hyaluronidase	T45.3X1	T45.3X2	T45.3X3	T45.3X4	T45.3X5	T45.3X6
Hyazyme	T45.3X1	T45.3X2	T45.3X3	T45.3X4	T45.3X5	T45.3X6
Hycodan	T40.2X1	T40.2X2	T40.2X3	T40.2X4	T40.2X5	T40.2X6
Hydantoin derivative NEC	T42.0X1	T42.0X2	T42.0X3	T42.0X4	T42.0X5	T42.0X6
Hydeltra	T38.0X1	T38.0X2	T38.0X3	T38.0X4	T38.0X5	T38.0X6
Hydergine	T44.6X1	T44.6X2	T44.6X3	T44.6X4	T44.6X5	T44.6X6
Hydrabamine penicillin	T36.0X1	T36.0X2	T36.0X3	T36.0X4	T36.0X5	T36.0X6
Hydralazine	T46.5X1	T46.5X2	T46.5X3	T46.5X4	T46.5X5	T46.5X6
Hydrargaphen	T49.0X1	T49.0X2	T49.0X3	T49.0X4	T49.0X5	T49.0X6
Hydrargyri aminochloridum	T49.0X1	T49.0X2	T49.0X3	T49.0X4	T49.0X5	T49.0X6
Hydrastine	T48.291	T48.292	T48.293	T48.294	T48.295	T48.296
Hydrazine	T54.1X1	T54.1X2	T54.1X3	T54.1X4	—	—
monoamine oxidase inhibitors	T43.1X1	T43.1X2	T43.1X3	T43.1X4	T43.1X5	T43.1X6
Hydrazoic acid, azides	T54.2X1	T54.2X2	T54.2X3	T54.2X4	—	—
Hydriodic acid	T48.4X1	T48.4X2	T48.4X3	T48.4X4	T48.4X5	T48.4X6
Hydrisalic*	T49.4X1	T49.4X2	T49.4X3	T49.4X4	T49.4X5	T49.4X6
Hydrocarbon gas	T59.891	T59.892	T59.893	T59.894	—	—
incomplete combustion of — see Carbon, monoxide, fuel, utility						
liquefied (mobile container)	T59.891	T59.892	T59.893	T59.894	—	—
piped (natural)	T59.891	T59.892	T59.893	T59.894	—	—
Hydrochloric acid (liquid)	T54.2X1	T54.2X2	T54.2X3	T54.2X4	—	—
medicinal (digestant)	T47.5X1	T47.5X2	T47.5X3	T47.5X4	T47.5X5	T47.5X6
vapor	T59.891	T59.892	T59.893	T59.894	—	—
Hydrochlorothiazide	T50.2X1	T50.2X2	T50.2X3	T50.2X4	T50.2X5	T50.2X6
Hydrocodone	T40.2X1	T40.2X2	T40.2X3	T40.2X4	T40.2X5	T40.2X6
Hydrocortisone (derivatives)	T38.0X1	T38.0X2	T38.0X3	T38.0X4	T38.0X5	T38.0X6
aceponate	T49.0X1	T49.0X2	T49.0X3	T49.0X4	T49.0X5	T49.0X6
ENT agent	T49.6X1	T49.6X2	T49.6X3	T49.6X4	T49.6X5	T49.6X6
ophthalmic preparation	T49.5X1	T49.5X2	T49.5X3	T49.5X4	T49.5X5	T49.5X6
topical NEC	T49.0X1	T49.0X2	T49.0X3	T49.0X4	T49.0X5	T49.0X6
Hydrocortone	T38.0X1	T38.0X2	T38.0X3	T38.0X4	T38.0X5	T38.0X6
ENT agent	T49.6X1	T49.6X2	T49.6X3	T49.6X4	T49.6X5	T49.6X6
ophthalmic preparation	T49.5X1	T49.5X2	T49.5X3	T49.5X4	T49.5X5	T49.5X6
topical NEC	T49.0X1	T49.0X2	T49.0X3	T49.0X4	T49.0X5	T49.0X6
Hydrocyanic acid (liquid)	T57.3X1	T57.3X2	T57.3X3	T57.3X4	—	—
gas	T65.0X1	T65.0X2	T65.0X3	T65.0X4	—	—
Hydroflumethiazide	T50.2X1	T50.2X2	T50.2X3	T50.2X4	T50.2X5	T50.2X6
Hydrofluoric acid (liquid)	T54.2X1	T54.2X2	T54.2X3	T54.2X4	—	—
vapor	T59.891	T59.892	T59.893	T59.894	—	—
Hydrogen	T59.891	T59.892	T59.893	T59.894	—	—
arsenide	T57.0X1	T57.0X2	T57.0X3	T57.0X4	—	—
arseniureted	T57.0X1	T57.0X2	T57.0X3	T57.0X4	—	—
chloride	T57.8X1	T57.8X2	T57.8X3	T57.8X4	—	—
cyanide (salts)	T57.3X1	T57.3X2	T57.3X3	T57.3X4	—	—
gas	T57.3X1	T57.3X2	T57.3X3	T57.3X4	—	—
Fluoride	T59.5X1	T59.5X2	T59.5X3	T59.5X4	—	—
vapor	T59.5X1	T59.5X2	T59.5X3	T59.5X4	—	—
peroxide	T49.0X1	T49.0X2	T49.0X3	T49.0X4	T49.0X5	T49.0X6
phosphureted	T57.1X1	T57.1X2	T57.1X3	T57.1X4	—	—
sulfide	T59.6X1	T59.6X2	T59.6X3	T59.6X4	—	—
arseniureted	T57.0X1	T57.0X2	T57.0X3	T57.0X4	—	—
sulfureted	T59.6X1	T59.6X2	T59.6X3	T59.6X4	—	—
Hydromethylpyridine	T46.7X1	T46.7X2	T46.7X3	T46.7X4	T46.7X5	T46.7X6
Hydromorphinol	T40.2X1	T40.2X2	T40.2X3	T40.2X4	—	—
Hydromorphinone	T40.2X1	T40.2X2	T40.2X3	T40.2X4	T40.2X5	T40.2X6
Hydromorphone	T40.2X1	T40.2X2	T40.2X3	T40.2X4	T40.2X5	T40.2X6
Hydromox	T50.2X1	T50.2X2	T50.2X3	T50.2X4	T50.2X5	T50.2X6
Hydrophilic lotion	T49.3X1	T49.3X2	T49.3X3	T49.3X4	T49.3X5	T49.3X6
Hydroquinidine	T46.2X1	T46.2X2	T46.2X3	T46.2X4	T46.2X5	T46.2X6
Hydroquinone	T52.2X1	T52.2X2	T52.2X3	T52.2X4	—	—
vapor	T59.891	T59.892	T59.893	T59.894	—	—
Hydro-ride*	T50.2X1	T50.2X2	T50.2X3	T50.2X4	T50.2X5	T50.2X6
Hydrosulfuric acid (gas)	T59.6X1	T59.6X2	T59.6X3	T59.6X4	—	—
Hydrotalcite	T47.1X1	T47.1X2	T47.1X3	T47.1X4	T47.1X5	T47.1X6
Hydrous wool fat	T49.3X1	T49.3X2	T49.3X3	T49.3X4	T49.3X5	T49.3X6
Hydroxide, caustic	T54.3X1	T54.3X2	T54.3X3	T54.3X4	—	—
Hydroxocobalamin	T45.8X1	T45.8X2	T45.8X3	T45.8X4	T45.8X5	T45.8X6
Hydroxyamphetamine	T49.5X1	T49.5X2	T49.5X3	T49.5X4	T49.5X5	T49.5X6
Hydroxycarbamide	T45.1X1	T45.1X2	T45.1X3	T45.1X4	T45.1X5	T45.1X6
Hydroxychloroquine	T37.8X1	T37.8X2	T37.8X3	T37.8X4	T37.8X5	T37.8X6
Hydroxydaunorubicin*	T45.1X1	T45.1X2	T45.1X3	T45.1X4	T45.1X5	T45.1X6
Hydroxydihydrocodeinone	T40.2X1	T40.2X2	T40.2X3	T40.2X4	T40.2X5	T40.2X6
Hydroxyestrone	T38.5X1	T38.5X2	T38.5X3	T38.5X4	T38.5X5	T38.5X6
Hydroxyethyl starch	T45.8X1	T45.8X2	T45.8X3	T45.8X4	T45.8X5	T45.8X6
Hydroxymethylpentanone	T52.4X1	T52.4X2	T52.4X3	T52.4X4	—	—
Hydroxyphenamate	T43.591	T43.592	T43.593	T43.594	T43.595	T43.596
Hydroxyphenylbutazone	T39.2X1	T39.2X2	T39.2X3	T39.2X4	T39.2X5	T39.2X6
Hydroxyprogesterone	T38.5X1	T38.5X2	T38.5X3	T38.5X4	T38.5X5	T38.5X6
caproate	T38.5X1	T38.5X2	T38.5X3	T38.5X4	T38.5X5	T38.5X6
Hydroxyquinoline (derivatives) NEC	T37.8X1	T37.8X2	T37.8X3	T37.8X4	T37.8X5	T37.8X6
Hydroxystilbamidine	T37.3X1	T37.3X2	T37.3X3	T37.3X4	T37.3X5	T37.3X6
Hydroxytoluene (nonmedicinal)	T54.0X1	T54.0X2	T54.0X3	T54.0X4	—	—
medicinal	T49.0X1	T49.0X2	T49.0X3	T49.0X4	T49.0X5	T49.0X6
Hydroxyurea	T45.1X1	T45.1X2	T45.1X3	T45.1X4	T45.1X5	T45.1X6
Hydroxyzine	T43.591	T43.592	T43.593	T43.594	T43.595	T43.596
Hyoscine	T44.3X1	T44.3X2	T44.3X3	T44.3X4	T44.3X5	T44.3X6
Hyoscyamine	T44.3X1	T44.3X2	T44.3X3	T44.3X4	T44.3X5	T44.3X6
Hyoscyamus	T44.3X1	T44.3X2	T44.3X3	T44.3X4	T44.3X5	T44.3X6
dry extract	T44.3X1	T44.3X2	T44.3X3	T44.3X4	T44.3X5	T44.3X6
Hypaque	T50.8X1	T50.8X2	T50.8X3	T50.8X4	T50.8X5	T50.8X6
HyperRAB*	T50.Z11	T50.Z12	T50.Z13	T50.Z14	T50.Z15	T50.Z16
Hypertussis	T50.Z11	T50.Z12	T50.Z13	T50.Z14	T50.Z15	T50.Z16
Hypnotic	T42.71	T42.72	T42.73	T42.74	T42.75	T42.76

Substance	Poisoning, Accidental (unintentional)	Poisoning, Intentional Self-harm	Poisoning, Assault	Poisoning, Undetermined	Adverse Effect	Under-dosing
Hypnotic — continued						
anticonvulsant	T42.71	T42.72	T42.73	T42.74	T42.75	T42.76
specified NEC	T42.6X1	T42.6X2	T42.6X3	T42.6X4	T42.6X5	T42.6X6
Hypochlorite	T49.0X1	T49.0X2	T49.0X3	T49.0X4	T49.0X5	T49.0X6
Hypophysis, posterior	T38.891	T38.892	T38.893	T38.894	T38.895	T38.896
Hypotensive NEC	T46.5X1	T46.5X2	T46.5X3	T46.5X4	T46.5X5	T46.5X6
Hypromellose	T49.5X1	T49.5X2	T49.5X3	T49.5X4	T49.5X5	T49.5X6
Ibacitabine	T37.5X1	T37.5X2	T37.5X3	T37.5X4	T37.5X5	T37.5X6
Ibopamine	T44.991	T44.992	T44.993	T44.994	T44.995	T44.996
Ibufenac	T39.311	T39.312	T39.313	T39.314	T39.315	T39.316
Ibuprofen	T39.311	T39.312	T39.313	T39.314	T39.315	T39.316
Ibuproxam	T39.311	T39.312	T39.313	T39.314	T39.315	T39.316
Ibuterol	T48.6X1	T48.6X2	T48.6X3	T48.6X4	T48.6X5	T48.6X6
Ichthammol	T49.0X1	T49.0X2	T49.0X3	T49.0X4	T49.0X5	T49.0X6
Ichthyol	T49.4X1	T49.4X2	T49.4X3	T49.4X4	T49.4X5	T49.4X6
Idarubicin	T45.1X1	T45.1X2	T45.1X3	T45.1X4	T45.1X5	T45.1X6
Idrocilamide	T42.8X1	T42.8X2	T42.8X3	T42.8X4	T42.8X5	T42.8X6
Ifenprodil	T46.7X1	T46.7X2	T46.7X3	T46.7X4	T46.7X5	T46.7X6
Ifosfamide	T45.1X1	T45.1X2	T45.1X3	T45.1X4	T45.1X5	T45.1X6
Iletin	T38.3X1	T38.3X2	T38.3X3	T38.3X4	T38.3X5	T38.3X6
Ilex	T62.2X1	T62.2X2	T62.2X3	T62.2X4	—	—
Illuminating gas (after combustion)	T58.11	T58.12	T58.13	T58.14	—	—
prior to combustion	T59.891	T59.892	T59.893	T59.894	—	—
Ilopan	T45.2X1	T45.2X2	T45.2X3	T45.2X4	T45.2X5	T45.2X6
Iloprost	T46.7X1	T46.7X2	T46.7X3	T46.7X4	T46.7X5	T46.7X6
Ilotycin	T36.3X1	T36.3X2	T36.3X3	T36.3X4	T36.3X5	T36.3X6
ophthalmic preparation	T49.5X1	T49.5X2	T49.5X3	T49.5X4	T49.5X5	T49.5X6
topical NEC	T49.0X1	T49.0X2	T49.0X3	T49.0X4	T49.0X5	T49.0X6
Imdur*	T46.3X1	T46.3X2	T46.3X3	T46.3X4	T46.3X5	T46.3X6
Imidazole-4-carboxamide	T45.1X1	T45.1X2	T45.1X3	T45.1X4	T45.1X5	T45.1X6
Iminostilbene	T42.1X1	T42.1X2	T42.1X3	T42.1X4	T42.1X5	T42.1X6
Imipenem	T36.0X1	T36.0X2	T36.0X3	T36.0X4	T36.0X5	T36.0X6
Imipramine	T43.011	T43.012	T43.013	T43.014	T43.015	T43.016
Immu-G	T50.Z11	T50.Z12	T50.Z13	T50.Z14	T50.Z15	T50.Z16
Immuglobin	T50.Z11	T50.Z12	T50.Z13	T50.Z14	T50.Z15	T50.Z16
Immune						
globulin	T50.Z11	T50.Z12	T50.Z13	T50.Z14	T50.Z15	T50.Z16
serum globulin	T50.Z11	T50.Z12	T50.Z13	T50.Z14	T50.Z15	T50.Z16
Immunoglobin human (intravenous) (normal)	T50.Z11	T50.Z12	T50.Z13	T50.Z14	T50.Z15	T50.Z16
unmodified	T50.Z11	T50.Z12	T50.Z13	T50.Z14	T50.Z15	T50.Z16
Immunosuppressive drug	T45.1X1	T45.1X2	T45.1X3	T45.1X4	T45.1X5	T45.1X6
Immu-tetanus	T50.Z11	T50.Z12	T50.Z13	T50.Z14	T50.Z15	T50.Z16
Indalpine	T43.221	T43.222	T43.223	T43.224	T43.225	T43.226
Indanazoline	T48.5X1	T48.5X2	T48.5X3	T48.5X4	T48.5X5	T48.5X6
Indandione (derivatives)	T45.511	T45.512	T45.513	T45.514	T45.515	T45.516
Indapamide	T46.5X1	T46.5X2	T46.5X3	T46.5X4	T46.5X5	T46.5X6
Indendione (derivatives)	T45.511	T45.512	T45.513	T45.514	T45.515	T45.516
Indenolol	T44.7X1	T44.7X2	T44.7X3	T44.7X4	T44.7X5	T44.7X6
Inderal	T44.7X1	T44.7X2	T44.7X3	T44.7X4	T44.7X5	T44.7X6
Indian						
hemp	T40.711	T40.712	T40.713	T40.714	T40.715	T40.716
tobacco	T62.2X1	T62.2X2	T62.2X3	T62.2X4	—	—
Indigo carmine	T50.8X1	T50.8X2	T50.8X3	T50.8X4	T50.8X5	T50.8X6
Indobufen	T45.521	T45.522	T45.523	T45.524	T45.525	T45.526
Indocin	T39.2X1	T39.2X2	T39.2X3	T39.2X4	T39.2X5	T39.2X6
Indocyanine green	T50.8X1	T50.8X2	T50.8X3	T50.8X4	T50.8X5	T50.8X6
Indometacin	T39.391	T39.392	T39.393	T39.394	T39.395	T39.396
Indomethacin	T39.391	T39.392	T39.393	T39.394	T39.395	T39.396
farnesil	T39.4X1	T39.4X2	T39.4X3	T39.4X4	T39.4X5	T39.4X6
Indoramin	T44.6X1	T44.6X2	T44.6X3	T44.6X4	T44.6X5	T44.6X6
Industrial						
alcohol	T51.0X1	T51.0X2	T51.0X3	T51.0X4	—	—
fumes	T59.891	T59.892	T59.893	T59.894	—	—
solvents (fumes) (vapors)	T52.91	T52.92	T52.93	T52.94	—	—
Inflectra*	T39.4X1	T39.4X2	T39.4X3	T39.4X4	T39.4X5	T39.4X6
Influenza vaccine	T50.B91	T50.B92	T50.B93	T50.B94	T50.B95	T50.B96
Ingested substance NEC	T65.91	T65.92	T65.93	T65.94	—	—
INH	T37.1X1	T37.1X2	T37.1X3	T37.1X4	T37.1X5	T37.1X6
Inhalation, gas (noxious) — see Gas						
Inhibitor						
angiotensin-converting enzyme	T46.4X1	T46.4X2	T46.4X3	T46.4X4	T46.4X5	T46.4X6
carbonic anhydrase	T50.2X1	T50.2X2	T50.2X3	T50.2X4	T50.2X5	T50.2X6
fibrinolysis	T45.621	T45.622	T45.623	T45.624	T45.625	T45.626
monoamine oxidase NEC	T43.1X1	T43.1X2	T43.1X3	T43.1X4	T43.1X5	T43.1X6
hydrazine	T43.1X1	T43.1X2	T43.1X3	T43.1X4	T43.1X5	T43.1X6
postsynaptic	T43.8X1	T43.8X2	T43.8X3	T43.8X4	T43.8X5	T43.8X6
prothrombin synthesis	T45.511	T45.512	T45.513	T45.514	T45.515	T45.516
Ink	T65.891	T65.892	T65.893	T65.894	—	—
Innopran*	T44.7X1	T44.7X2	T44.7X3	T44.7X4	T44.7X5	T44.7X6

Substance	Poisoning, Accidental (unintentional)	Poisoning, Intentional Self-harm	Poisoning, Assault	Poisoning, Undetermined	Adverse Effect	Under-dosing
Inorganic substance NEC	T57.91	T57.92	T57.93	T57.94	—	—
Inosine pranobex	T37.5X1	T37.5X2	T37.5X3	T37.5X4	T37.5X5	T37.5X6
Inositol	T50.991	T50.992	T50.993	T50.994	T50.995	T50.996
nicotinate	T46.7X1	T46.7X2	T46.7X3	T46.7X4	T46.7X5	T46.7X6
Inproquone	T45.1X1	T45.1X2	T45.1X3	T45.1X4	T45.1X5	T45.1X6
Insecticide NEC	T60.91	T60.92	T60.93	T60.94	—	—
carbamate	T60.0X1	T60.0X2	T60.0X3	T60.0X4	—	—
chlorinated	T60.1X1	T60.1X2	T60.1X3	T60.1X4	—	—
mixed	T60.91	T60.92	T60.93	T60.94	—	—
organochlorine	T60.1X1	T60.1X2	T60.1X3	T60.1X4	—	—
organophosphorus	T60.0X1	T60.0X2	T60.0X3	T60.0X4	—	—
Insect (sting), venomous	T63.481	T63.482	T63.483	T63.484	—	—
ant	T63.421	T63.422	T63.423	T63.424	—	—
bee	T63.441	T63.442	T63.443	T63.444	—	—
caterpillar	T63.431	T63.432	T63.433	T63.434	—	—
hornet	T63.451	T63.452	T63.453	T63.454	—	—
wasp	T63.461	T63.462	T63.463	T63.464	—	—
Insular tissue extract	T38.3X1	T38.3X2	T38.3X3	T38.3X4	T38.3X5	T38.3X6
Insulin (amorphous) (globin) (isophane) (Lente) (NPH) (Semilente) (Ultralente)	T38.3X1	T38.3X2	T38.3X3	T38.3X4	T38.3X5	T38.3X6
defalan	T38.3X1	T38.3X2	T38.3X3	T38.3X4	T38.3X5	T38.3X6
human	T38.3X1	T38.3X2	T38.3X3	T38.3X4	T38.3X5	T38.3X6
injection, soluble	T38.3X1	T38.3X2	T38.3X3	T38.3X4	T38.3X5	T38.3X6
biphasic	T38.3X1	T38.3X2	T38.3X3	T38.3X4	T38.3X5	T38.3X6
intermediate acting	T38.3X1	T38.3X2	T38.3X3	T38.3X4	T38.3X5	T38.3X6
protamine zinc	T38.3X1	T38.3X2	T38.3X3	T38.3X4	T38.3X5	T38.3X6
slow acting	T38.3X1	T38.3X2	T38.3X3	T38.3X4	T38.3X5	T38.3X6
zinc						
protamine injection	T38.3X1	T38.3X2	T38.3X3	T38.3X4	T38.3X5	T38.3X6
suspension (amorphous) (crystalline)	T38.3X1	T38.3X2	T38.3X3	T38.3X4	T38.3X5	T38.3X6
Interferon (alpha) (beta) (gamma)	T37.5X1	T37.5X2	T37.5X3	T37.5X4	T37.5X5	T37.5X6
Intestinal motility control drug	T47.6X1	T47.6X2	T47.6X3	T47.6X4	T47.6X5	T47.6X6
biological	T47.8X1	T47.8X2	T47.8X3	T47.8X4	T47.8X5	T47.8X6
Intranarcon	T41.1X1	T41.1X2	T41.1X3	T41.1X4	T41.1X5	T41.1X6
Intravenous						
amino acids	T50.991	T50.992	T50.993	T50.994	T50.995	T50.996
fat suspension	T50.991	T50.992	T50.993	T50.994	T50.995	T50.996
Inulin	T50.8X1	T50.8X2	T50.8X3	T50.8X4	T50.8X5	T50.8X6
Invanz*	T36.1X1	T36.1X2	T36.1X3	T36.1X4	T36.1X5	T36.1X6
Invert sugar	T50.3X1	T50.3X2	T50.3X3	T50.3X4	T50.3X5	T50.3X6
Inza — see Naproxen						
Iobenzamic acid	T50.8X1	T50.8X2	T50.8X3	T50.8X4	T50.8X5	T50.8X6
Iocarmic acid	T50.8X1	T50.8X2	T50.8X3	T50.8X4	T50.8X5	T50.8X6
Iocetamic acid	T50.8X1	T50.8X2	T50.8X3	T50.8X4	T50.8X5	T50.8X6
Iodamide	T50.8X1	T50.8X2	T50.8X3	T50.8X4	T50.8X5	T50.8X6
Iodide NEC — see also Iodine	T49.0X1	T49.0X2	T49.0X3	T49.0X4	I49.0X5	I49.0X6
mercury (ointment)	T49.0X1	T49.0X2	T49.0X3	T49.0X4	T49.0X5	T49.0X6
methylate	T49.0X1	T49.0X2	T49.0X3	T49.0X4	T49.0X5	T49.0X6
potassium (expectorant) NEC	T48.4X1	T48.4X2	T48.4X3	T48.4X4	T48.4X5	T48.4X6
Iodinated						
contrast medium	T50.8X1	T50.8X2	T50.8X3	T50.8X4	T50.8X5	T50.8X6
glycerol	I48.4X1	I48.4X2	T48.4X3	T48.4X4	T48.4X5	T48.4X6
human serum albumin (131I)	T50.8X1	T50.8X2	T50.8X3	T50.8X4	T50.8X5	T50.8X6
Iodine (antiseptic, external) (tincture) **NEC**	T49.0X1	T49.0X2	T49.0X3	T49.0X4	T49.0X5	T49.0X6
125 — see also Radiation sickness, and Exposure to radioactive isotopes	T50.8X1	T50.8X2	T50.8X3	T50.8X4	T50.8X5	T50.8X6
therapeutic	T50.991	T50.992	T50.993	T50.994	T50.995	T50.996
131 — see also Radiation sickness, and Exposure to radioactive isotopes	T50.8X1	T50.8X2	T50.8X3	T50.8X4	T50.8X5	T50.8X6
therapeutic	T38.2X1	T38.2X2	T38.2X3	T38.2X4	T38.2X5	T38.2X6
diagnostic	T50.8X1	T50.8X2	T50.8X3	T50.8X4	T50.8X5	T50.8X6
for thyroid conditions (antithyroid)	T38.2X1	T38.2X2	T38.2X3	T38.2X4	T38.2X5	T38.2X6
solution	T49.0X1	T49.0X2	T49.0X3	T49.0X4	T49.0X5	T49.0X6
vapor	T59.891	T59.892	T59.893	T59.894	—	—
Iodipamide	T50.8X1	T50.8X2	T50.8X3	T50.8X4	T50.8X5	T50.8X6
Iodized (poppy seed) oil	T50.8X1	T50.8X2	T50.8X3	T50.8X4	T50.8X5	T50.8X6
Iodobismitol	T37.8X1	T37.8X2	T37.8X3	T37.8X4	T37.8X5	T37.8X6
Iodochlorhydroxyquin	T37.8X1	T37.8X2	T37.8X3	T37.8X4	T37.8X5	T37.8X6
topical	T49.0X1	T49.0X2	T49.0X3	T49.0X4	T49.0X5	T49.0X6
Iodochlorhydroxyquinoline	T37.8X1	T37.8X2	T37.8X3	T37.8X4	T37.8X5	T37.8X6
Iodocholesterol (131I)	T50.8X1	T50.8X2	T50.8X3	T50.8X4	T50.8X5	T50.8X6
Iodoform	T49.0X1	T49.0X2	T49.0X3	T49.0X4	T49.0X5	T49.0X6

☑ **Additional Character May Be Required — Refer to the Tabular List for Character Selection**

*Optum Value-Add

Substance	Poisoning, Accidental (unintentional)	Poisoning, Intentional Self-harm	Poisoning, Assault	Poisoning, Undetermined	Adverse Effect	Under-dosing
Iodohippuric acid	T50.8X1	T50.8X2	T50.8X3	T50.8X4	T50.8X5	T50.8X6
Iodopanoic acid	T50.8X1	T50.8X2	T50.8X3	T50.8X4	T50.8X5	T50.8X6
Iodophthalein (sodium)	T50.8X1	T50.8X2	T50.8X3	T50.8X4	T50.8X5	T50.8X6
Iodopyracet	T50.8X1	T50.8X2	T50.8X3	T50.8X4	T50.8X5	T50.8X6
Iodoquinol	T37.8X1	T37.8X2	T37.8X3	T37.8X4	T37.8X5	T37.8X6
Iodoxamic acid	T50.8X1	T50.8X2	T50.8X3	T50.8X4	T50.8X5	T50.8X6
Iofendylate	T50.8X1	T50.8X2	T50.8X3	T50.8X4	T50.8X5	T50.8X6
Ioglycamic acid	T50.8X1	T50.8X2	T50.8X3	T50.8X4	T50.8X5	T50.8X6
Iohexol	T50.8X1	T50.8X2	T50.8X3	T50.8X4	T50.8X5	T50.8X6
Ion exchange resin						
anion	T47.8X1	T47.8X2	T47.8X3	T47.8X4	T47.8X5	T47.8X6
cation	T50.3X1	T50.3X2	T50.3X3	T50.3X4	T50.3X5	T50.3X6
cholestyramine	T46.6X1	T46.6X2	T46.6X3	T46.6X4	T46.6X5	T46.6X6
intestinal	T47.8X1	T47.8X2	T47.8X3	T47.8X4	T47.8X5	T47.8X6
Iopamidol	T50.8X1	T50.8X2	T50.8X3	T50.8X4	T50.8X5	T50.8X6
Iopanoic acid	T50.8X1	T50.8X2	T50.8X3	T50.8X4	T50.8X5	T50.8X6
Iophenoic acid	T50.8X1	T50.8X2	T50.8X3	T50.8X4	T50.8X5	T50.8X6
Iopodate, sodium	T50.8X1	T50.8X2	T50.8X3	T50.8X4	T50.8X5	T50.8X6
Iopodic acid	T50.8X1	T50.8X2	T50.8X3	T50.8X4	T50.8X5	T50.8X6
Iopromide	T50.8X1	T50.8X2	T50.8X3	T50.8X4	T50.8X5	T50.8X6
Iopydol	T50.8X1	T50.8X2	T50.8X3	T50.8X4	T50.8X5	T50.8X6
Iotalamic acid	T50.8X1	T50.8X2	T50.8X3	T50.8X4	T50.8X5	T50.8X6
Iothalamate	T50.8X1	T50.8X2	T50.8X3	T50.8X4	T50.8X5	T50.8X6
Iothiouracil	T38.2X1	T38.2X2	T38.2X3	T38.2X4	T38.2X5	T38.2X6
Iotrol	T50.8X1	T50.8X2	T50.8X3	T50.8X4	T50.8X5	T50.8X6
Iotrolan	T50.8X1	T50.8X2	T50.8X3	T50.8X4	T50.8X5	T50.8X6
Iotroxate	T50.8X1	T50.8X2	T50.8X3	T50.8X4	T50.8X5	T50.8X6
Iotroxic acid	T50.8X1	T50.8X2	T50.8X3	T50.8X4	T50.8X5	T50.8X6
Ioversol	T50.8X1	T50.8X2	T50.8X3	T50.8X4	T50.8X5	T50.8X6
Ioxaglate	T50.8X1	T50.8X2	T50.8X3	T50.8X4	T50.8X5	T50.8X6
Ioxaglic acid	T50.8X1	T50.8X2	T50.8X3	T50.8X4	T50.8X5	T50.8X6
Ioxitalamic acid	T50.8X1	T50.8X2	T50.8X3	T50.8X4	T50.8X5	T50.8X6
Ipecac	T47.7X1	T47.7X2	T47.7X3	T47.7X4	T47.7X5	T47.7X6
Ipecacuanha	T48.4X1	T48.4X2	T48.4X3	T48.4X4	T48.4X5	T48.4X6
Ipodate, calcium	T50.8X1	T50.8X2	T50.8X3	T50.8X4	T50.8X5	T50.8X6
IPOL*	T50.B91	T50.B92	T50.B93	T50.B94	T50.B95	T50.B96
Ipral	T42.3X1	T42.3X2	T42.3X3	T42.3X4	T42.3X5	T42.3X6
Ipratropium (bromide)	T48.6X1	T48.6X2	T48.6X3	T48.6X4	T48.6X5	T48.6X6
Ipriflavone	T46.3X1	T46.3X2	T46.3X3	T46.3X4	T46.3X5	T46.3X6
Iprindole	T43.011	T43.012	T43.013	T43.014	T43.015	T43.016
Iproclozide	T43.1X1	T43.1X2	T43.1X3	T43.1X4	T43.1X5	T43.1X6
Iprofenin	T50.8X1	T50.8X2	T50.8X3	T50.8X4	T50.8X5	T50.8X6
Iproheptine	T49.2X1	T49.2X2	T49.2X3	T49.2X4	T49.2X5	T49.2X6
Iproniazid	T43.1X1	T43.1X2	T43.1X3	T43.1X4	T43.1X5	T43.1X6
Iproplatin	T45.1X1	T45.1X2	T45.1X3	T45.1X4	T45.1X5	T45.1X6
Iproveratril	T46.1X1	T46.1X2	T46.1X3	T46.1X4	T46.1X5	T46.1X6
Irinotecan*	T45.1X1	T45.1X2	T45.1X3	T45.1X4	T45.1X5	T45.1X6
Iron (compounds) (medicinal) NEC	T45.4X1	T45.4X2	T45.4X3	T45.4X4	T45.4X5	T45.4X6
ammonium	T45.4X1	T45.4X2	T45.4X3	T45.4X4	T45.4X5	T45.4X6
dextran injection	T45.4X1	T45.4X2	T45.4X3	T45.4X4	T45.4X5	T45.4X6
nonmedicinal	T56.891	T56.892	T56.893	T56.894	—	—
salts	T45.4X1	T45.4X2	T45.4X3	T45.4X4	T45.4X5	T45.4X6
sorbitex	T45.4X1	T45.4X2	T45.4X3	T45.4X4	T45.4X5	T45.4X6
sorbitol citric acid complex	T45.4X1	T45.4X2	T45.4X3	T45.4X4	T45.4X5	T45.4X6
Irrigating fluid (vaginal)	T49.8X1	T49.8X2	T49.8X3	T49.8X4	T49.8X5	T49.8X6
eye	T49.5X1	T49.5X2	T49.5X3	T49.5X4	T49.5X5	T49.5X6
Isepamicin	T36.5X1	T36.5X2	T36.5X3	T36.5X4	T36.5X5	T36.5X6
Isoaminile (citrate)	T48.3X1	T48.3X2	T48.3X3	T48.3X4	T48.3X5	T48.3X6
Isoamyl nitrite	T46.3X1	T46.3X2	T46.3X3	T46.3X4	T46.3X5	T46.3X6
Isobenzan	T60.1X1	T60.1X2	T60.1X3	T60.1X4	—	—
Isobutyl acetate	T52.8X1	T52.8X2	T52.8X3	T52.8X4	—	—
Isocarboxazid	T43.1X1	T43.1X2	T43.1X3	T43.1X4	T43.1X5	T43.1X6
Isoconazole	T49.0X1	T49.0X2	T49.0X3	T49.0X4	T49.0X5	T49.0X6
Isocyanate	T65.0X1	T65.0X2	T65.0X3	T65.0X4	—	—
Isoephedrine	T44.991	T44.992	T44.993	T44.994	T44.995	T44.996
Isoetarine	T48.6X1	T48.6X2	T48.6X3	T48.6X4	T48.6X5	T48.6X6
Isoethadione	T42.2X1	T42.2X2	T42.2X3	T42.2X4	T42.2X5	T42.2X6
Isoetharine	T44.5X1	T44.5X2	T44.5X3	T44.5X4	T44.5X5	T44.5X6
Isoflurane	T41.0X1	T41.0X2	T41.0X3	T41.0X4	T41.0X5	T41.0X6
Isoflurophate	T44.0X1	T44.0X2	T44.0X3	T44.0X4	T44.0X5	T44.0X6
Isomaltose, ferric complex	T45.4X1	T45.4X2	T45.4X3	T45.4X4	T45.4X5	T45.4X6
Isometheptene	T44.3X1	T44.3X2	T44.3X3	T44.3X4	T44.3X5	T44.3X6
Isoniazid	T37.1X1	T37.1X2	T37.1X3	T37.1X4	T37.1X5	T37.1X6
with						
rifampicin	T36.6X1	T36.6X2	T36.6X3	T36.6X4	T36.6X5	T36.6X6
thioacetazone	T37.1X1	T37.1X2	T37.1X3	T37.1X4	T37.1X5	T37.1X6
Isonicotinic acid hydrazide	T37.1X1	T37.1X2	T37.1X3	T37.1X4	T37.1X5	T37.1X6
Isonipecaine	T40.491	T40.492	T40.493	T40.494	T40.495	T40.496
Isopentaquine	T37.2X1	T37.2X2	T37.2X3	T37.2X4	T37.2X5	T37.2X6
Isophane insulin	T38.3X1	T38.3X2	T38.3X3	T38.3X4	T38.3X5	T38.3X6
Isophorone	T65.891	T65.892	T65.893	T65.894	—	—
Isophosphamide	T45.1X1	T45.1X2	T45.1X3	T45.1X4	T45.1X5	T45.1X6
Isopregnenone	T38.5X1	T38.5X2	T38.5X3	T38.5X4	T38.5X5	T38.5X6
Isoprenaline	T48.6X1	T48.6X2	T48.6X3	T48.6X4	T48.6X5	T48.6X6
Isopromethazine	T43.3X1	T43.3X2	T43.3X3	T43.3X4	T43.3X5	T43.3X6
Isopropamide	T44.3X1	T44.3X2	T44.3X3	T44.3X4	T44.3X5	T44.3X6
iodide	T44.3X1	T44.3X2	T44.3X3	T44.3X4	T44.3X5	T44.3X6
Isopropanol	T51.2X1	T51.2X2	T51.2X3	T51.2X4	—	—
Isopropyl						
acetate	T52.8X1	T52.8X2	T52.8X3	T52.8X4	—	—
alcohol	T51.2X1	T51.2X2	T51.2X3	T51.2X4	—	—
medicinal	T49.4X1	T49.4X2	T49.4X3	T49.4X4	T49.4X5	T49.4X6
ether	T52.8X1	T52.8X2	T52.8X3	T52.8X4	—	—
Isopropylaminophenazone	T39.2X1	T39.2X2	T39.2X3	T39.2X4	T39.2X5	T39.2X6
Isoproterenol	T48.6X1	T48.6X2	T48.6X3	T48.6X4	T48.6X5	T48.6X6
Isosorbide dinitrate	T46.3X1	T46.3X2	T46.3X3	T46.3X4	T46.3X5	T46.3X6
Isothipendyl	T45.0X1	T45.0X2	T45.0X3	T45.0X4	T45.0X5	T45.0X6
Isotretinoin	T50.991	T50.992	T50.993	T50.994	T50.995	T50.996
Isoxazolyl penicillin	T36.0X1	T36.0X2	T36.0X3	T36.0X4	T36.0X5	T36.0X6
Isoxicam	T39.391	T39.392	T39.393	T39.394	T39.395	T39.396
Isoxsuprine	T46.7X1	T46.7X2	T46.7X3	T46.7X4	T46.7X5	T46.7X6
Ispagula	T47.4X1	T47.4X2	T47.4X3	T47.4X4	T47.4X5	T47.4X6
husk	T47.4X1	T47.4X2	T47.4X3	T47.4X4	T47.4X5	T47.4X6
Isradipine	T46.1X1	T46.1X2	T46.1X3	T46.1X4	T46.1X5	T46.1X6
l-thyroxine sodium	T38.1X1	T38.1X2	T38.1X3	T38.1X4	T38.1X5	T38.1X6
Itraconazole	T37.8X1	T37.8X2	T37.8X3	T37.8X4	T37.8X5	T37.8X6
Itramin tosilate	T46.3X1	T46.3X2	T46.3X3	T46.3X4	T46.3X5	T46.3X6
Ivarest*	T41.3X1	T41.3X2	T41.3X3	T41.3X4	T41.3X5	T41.3X6
Ivermectin	T37.4X1	T37.4X2	T37.4X3	T37.4X4	T37.4X5	T37.4X6
Izoniazid	T37.1X1	T37.1X2	T37.1X3	T37.1X4	T37.1X5	T37.1X6
with thioacetazone	T37.1X1	T37.1X2	T37.1X3	T37.1X4	T37.1X5	T37.1X6
Jalap	T47.2X1	T47.2X2	T47.2X3	T47.2X4	T47.2X5	T47.2X6
Jamaica						
dogwood (bark)	T39.8X1	T39.8X2	T39.8X3	T39.8X4	T39.8X5	T39.8X6
ginger	T65.891	T65.892	T65.893	T65.894	—	—
root	T62.2X1	T62.2X2	T62.2X3	T62.2X4	—	—
Jantoven*	T45.511	T45.512	T45.513	T45.514	T45.515	T45.516
Jatropha	T62.2X1	T62.2X2	T62.2X3	T62.2X4	—	—
curcas	T62.2X1	T62.2X2	T62.2X3	T62.2X4	—	—
Jectofer	T45.4X1	T45.4X2	T45.4X3	T45.4X4	T45.4X5	T45.4X6
Jellyfish (sting)	T63.621	T63.622	T63.623	T63.624	—	—
Jequirity (bean)	T62.2X1	T62.2X2	T62.2X3	T62.2X4	—	—
Jimson weed (stramonium)	T62.2X1	T62.2X2	T62.2X3	T62.2X4	—	—
seeds	T62.2X1	T62.2X2	T62.2X3	T62.2X4	—	—
Josamycin	T36.3X1	T36.3X2	T36.3X3	T36.3X4	T36.3X5	T36.3X6
Juniper tar	T49.1X1	T49.1X2	T49.1X3	T49.1X4	T49.1X5	T49.1X6
Kaletra*	T37.5X1	T37.5X2	T37.5X3	T37.5X4	T37.5X5	T37.5X6
Kallidinogenase	T46.7X1	T46.7X2	T46.7X3	T46.7X4	T46.7X5	T46.7X6
Kallikrein	T46.7X1	T46.7X2	T46.7X3	T46.7X4	T46.7X5	T46.7X6
Kanamycin	T36.5X1	T36.5X2	T36.5X3	T36.5X4	T36.5X5	T36.5X6
Kantrex	T36.5X1	T36.5X2	T36.5X3	T36.5X4	T36.5X5	T36.5X6
Kaolin	T47.6X1	T47.6X2	T47.6X3	T47.6X4	T47.6X5	T47.6X6
light	T47.6X1	T47.6X2	T47.6X3	T47.6X4	T47.6X5	T47.6X6
Karaya (gum)	T47.4X1	T47.4X2	T47.4X3	T47.4X4	T47.4X5	T47.4X6
Kebuzone	T39.2X1	T39.2X2	T39.2X3	T39.2X4	T39.2X5	T39.2X6
Kelevan	T60.1X1	T60.1X2	T60.1X3	T60.1X4	—	—
Kemithal	T41.1X1	T41.1X2	T41.1X3	T41.1X4	T41.1X5	T41.1X6
Kenacort	T38.0X1	T38.0X2	T38.0X3	T38.0X4	T38.0X5	T38.0X6
Keratolytic drug NEC	T49.4X1	T49.4X2	T49.4X3	T49.4X4	T49.4X5	T49.4X6
anthracene	T49.4X1	T49.4X2	T49.4X3	T49.4X4	T49.4X5	T49.4X6
Keratoplastic NEC	T49.4X1	T49.4X2	T49.4X3	T49.4X4	T49.4X5	T49.4X6
Kerosene, kerosine (fuel) (solvent) NEC	T52.0X1	T52.0X2	T52.0X3	T52.0X4	—	—
insecticide	T52.0X1	T52.0X2	T52.0X3	T52.0X4	—	—
vapor	T52.0X1	T52.0X2	T52.0X3	T52.0X4	—	—
Ketamine	T41.291	T41.292	T41.293	T41.294	T41.295	T41.296
Ketazolam	T42.4X1	T42.4X2	T42.4X3	T42.4X4	T42.4X5	T42.4X6
Ketazon	T39.2X1	T39.2X2	T39.2X3	T39.2X4	T39.2X5	T39.2X6
Ketobemidone	T40.491	T40.492	T40.493	T40.494	—	—
Ketoconazole	T49.0X1	T49.0X2	T49.0X3	T49.0X4	T49.0X5	T49.0X6
Ketols	T52.4X1	T52.4X2	T52.4X3	T52.4X4	—	—
Ketone oils	T52.4X1	T52.4X2	T52.4X3	T52.4X4	—	—
Ketoprofen	T39.311	T39.312	T39.313	T39.314	T39.315	T39.316
Ketorolac	T39.8X1	T39.8X2	T39.8X3	T39.8X4	T39.8X5	T39.8X6
Ketotifen	T45.0X1	T45.0X2	T45.0X3	T45.0X4	T45.0X5	T45.0X6
Keytruda*	T45.1X1	T45.1X2	T45.1X3	T45.1X4	T45.1X5	T45.1X6
Khat	T43.691	T43.692	T43.693	T43.694	—	—
Khellin	T46.3X1	T46.3X2	T46.3X3	T46.3X4	T46.3X5	T46.3X6
Khelloside	T46.3X1	T46.3X2	T46.3X3	T46.3X4	T46.3X5	T46.3X6
Kiln gas or vapor (carbon monoxide)	T58.8X1	T58.8X2	T58.8X3	T58.8X4	—	—
Kineret*	T39.4X1	T39.4X2	T39.4X3	T39.4X4	T39.4X5	T39.4X6
Kitasamycin	T36.3X1	T36.3X2	T36.3X3	T36.3X4	T36.3X5	T36.3X6
Komgiblyze*	T38.3X1	T38.3X2	T38.3X3	T38.3X4	T38.3X5	T38.3X6
Konsyl	T47.4X1	T47.4X2	T47.4X3	T47.4X4	T47.4X5	T47.4X6

Table of Drugs and Chemicals

Substance	Poisoning, Accidental (unintentional)	Poisoning, Intentional Self-harm	Poisoning, Assault	Poisoning, Undetermined	Adverse Effect	Under-dosing
Kosam seed	T62.2X1	T62.2X2	T62.2X3	T62.2X4	—	—
Krait (venom)	T63.091	T63.092	T63.093	T63.094	—	—
Kwell (insecticide)	T60.1X1	T60.1X2	T60.1X3	T60.1X4	—	—
anti-infective (topical)	T49.0X1	T49.0X2	T49.0X3	T49.0X4	T49.0X5	T49.0X6
Labetalol	T44.8X1	T44.8X2	T44.8X3	T44.8X4	T44.8X5	T44.8X6
Laburnum (seeds)	T62.2X1	T62.2X2	T62.2X3	T62.2X4	—	—
leaves	T62.2X1	T62.2X2	T62.2X3	T62.2X4	—	—
Lachesine	T49.5X1	T49.5X2	T49.5X3	T49.5X4	T49.5X5	T49.5X6
Lacidipine	T46.5X1	T46.5X2	T46.5X3	T46.5X4	T46.5X5	T46.5X6
Lacquer	T65.6X1	T65.6X2	T65.6X3	T65.6X4	—	—
Lacrimogenic gas	T59.3X1	T59.3X2	T59.3X3	T59.3X4	—	—
Lactated potassic saline	T50.3X1	T50.3X2	T50.3X3	T50.3X4	T50.3X5	T50.3X6
Lactic acid	T49.8X1	T49.8X2	T49.8X3	T49.8X4	T49.8X5	T49.8X6
Lactobacillus						
acidophilus	T47.6X1	T47.6X2	T47.6X3	T47.6X4	T47.6X5	T47.6X6
compound	T47.6X1	T47.6X2	T47.6X3	T47.6X4	T47.6X5	T47.6X6
bifidus, lyophilized	T47.6X1	T47.6X2	T47.6X3	T47.6X4	T47.6X5	T47.6X6
bulgaricus	T47.6X1	T47.6X2	T47.6X3	T47.6X4	T47.6X5	T47.6X6
sporogenes	T47.6X1	T47.6X2	T47.6X3	T47.6X4	T47.6X5	T47.6X6
Lactoflavin	T45.2X1	T45.2X2	T45.2X3	T45.2X4	T45.2X5	T45.2X6
Lactose (as excipient)	T50.901	T50.902	T50.903	T50.904	T50.905	T50.906
Lactuca (virosa) (extract)	T42.6X1	T42.6X2	T42.6X3	T42.6X4	T42.6X5	T42.6X6
Lactucarium	T42.6X1	T42.6X2	T42.6X3	T42.6X4	T42.6X5	T42.6X6
Lactulose	T47.3X1	T47.3X2	T47.3X3	T47.3X4	T47.3X5	T47.3X6
Laevo — see Levo-						
Lanatosides	T46.0X1	T46.0X2	T46.0X3	T46.0X4	T46.0X5	T46.0X6
Lanolin	T49.3X1	T49.3X2	T49.3X3	T49.3X4	T49.3X5	T49.3X6
Lanoxin*	T46.0X1	T46.0X2	T46.0X3	T46.0X4	T46.0X5	T46.0X6
Largactil	T43.3X1	T43.3X2	T43.3X3	T43.3X4	T43.3X5	T43.3X6
Larkspur	T62.2X1	T62.2X2	T62.2X3	T62.2X4	—	—
Laroxyl	T43.011	T43.012	T43.013	T43.014	T43.015	T43.016
Lasix	T50.1X1	T50.1X2	T50.1X3	T50.1X4	T50.1X5	T50.1X6
Lassar's paste	T49.4X1	T49.4X2	T49.4X3	T49.4X4	T49.4X5	T49.4X6
Latamoxef	T36.1X1	T36.1X2	T36.1X3	T36.1X4	T36.1X5	T36.1X6
Latex	T65.811	T65.812	T65.813	T65.814	—	—
Lathyrus (seed)	T62.2X1	T62.2X2	T62.2X3	T62.2X4	—	—
Laudanum	T40.0X1	T40.0X2	T40.0X3	T40.0X4	T40.0X5	T40.0X6
Laudexium	T48.1X1	T48.1X2	T48.1X3	T48.1X4	T48.1X5	T48.1X6
Laughing gas	T41.0X1	T41.0X2	T41.0X3	T41.0X4	T41.0X5	T41.0X6
Laurel, black or cherry	T62.2X1	T62.2X2	T62.2X3	T62.2X4	—	—
Laurolinium	T49.0X1	T49.0X2	T49.0X3	T49.0X4	T49.0X5	T49.0X6
Lauryl sulfoacetate	T49.2X1	T49.2X2	T49.2X3	T49.2X4	T49.2X5	T49.2X6
Laxative NEC	T47.4X1	T47.4X2	T47.4X3	T47.4X4	T47.4X5	T47.4X6
osmotic	T47.3X1	T47.3X2	T47.3X3	T47.3X4	T47.3X5	T47.3X6
saline	T47.3X1	T47.3X2	T47.3X3	T47.3X4	T47.3X5	T47.3X6
stimulant	T47.2X1	T47.2X2	T47.2X3	T47.2X4	T47.2X5	T47.2X6
L-dopa	T42.8X1	T42.8X2	T42.8X3	T42.8X4	T42.8X5	T42.8X6
Lead (dust) (fumes) (vapor)	T56.0X1	T56.0X2	T56.0X3	T56.0X4	—	—
NFC						
acetate	T49.2X1	T49.2X2	T49.2X3	T49.2X4	T49.2X5	T49.2X6
alkyl (fuel additive)	T56.0X1	T56.0X2	T56.0X3	T56.0X4	—	—
anti-infectives	T37.8X1	T37.8X2	T37.8X3	T37.8X4	T37.8X5	T37.8X6
antiknock compound (tetraethyl)	T56.0X1	T56.0X2	T56.0X3	T56.0X4	—	—
arsenate, arsenite (dust)(herbicide) (insecticide) (vapor)	T57.0X1	T57.0X2	T57.0X3	T57.0X4	—	—
carbonate	T56.0X1	T56.0X2	T56.0X3	T56.0X4	—	—
paint	T56.0X1	T56.0X2	T56.0X3	T56.0X4	—	—
chromate	T56.0X1	T56.0X2	T56.0X3	T56.0X4	—	—
paint	T56.0X1	T56.0X2	T56.0X3	T56.0X4	—	—
dioxide	T56.0X1	T56.0X2	T56.0X3	T56.0X4	—	—
inorganic	T56.0X1	T56.0X2	T56.0X3	T56.0X4	—	—
iodide	T56.0X1	T56.0X2	T56.0X3	T56.0X4	—	—
pigment (paint)	T56.0X1	T56.0X2	T56.0X3	T56.0X4	—	—
monoxide (dust)	T56.0X1	T56.0X2	T56.0X3	T56.0X4	—	—
paint	T56.0X1	T56.0X2	T56.0X3	T56.0X4	—	—
organic	T56.0X1	T56.0X2	T56.0X3	T56.0X4	—	—
oxide	T56.0X1	T56.0X2	T56.0X3	T56.0X4	—	—
paint	T56.0X1	T56.0X2	T56.0X3	T56.0X4	—	—
paint	T56.0X1	T56.0X2	T56.0X3	T56.0X4	—	—
salts	T56.0X1	T56.0X2	T56.0X3	T56.0X4	—	—
specified compound NEC	T56.0X1	T56.0X2	T56.0X3	T56.0X4	—	—
tetra-ethyl	T56.0X1	T56.0X2	T56.0X3	T56.0X4	—	—
Lebanese red	T40.711	T40.712	T40.713	T40.714	T40.715	T40.716
Lefetamine	T39.8X1	T39.8X2	T39.8X3	T39.8X4	T39.8X5	T39.8X6
Lenperone	T43.4X1	T43.4X2	T43.4X3	T43.4X4	T43.4X5	T43.4X6
Lente lietin (insulin)	T38.3X1	T38.3X2	T38.3X3	T38.3X4	T38.3X5	T38.3X6
Leptazol	T50.7X1	T50.7X2	T50.7X3	T50.7X4	T50.7X5	T50.7X6
Leptophos	T60.0X1	T60.0X2	T60.0X3	T60.0X4	—	—
Leritine	T40.2X1	T40.2X2	T40.2X3	T40.2X4	T40.2X5	T40.2X6
Lescol*	T46.6X1	T46.6X2	T46.6X3	T46.6X4	T46.6X5	T46.6X6
Letosteine	T48.4X1	T48.4X2	T48.4X3	T48.4X4	T48.4X5	T48.4X6

Substance	Poisoning, Accidental (unintentional)	Poisoning, Intentional Self-harm	Poisoning, Assault	Poisoning, Undetermined	Adverse Effect	Under-dosing
Letter	T38.1X1	T38.1X2	T38.1X3	T38.1X4	T38.1X5	T38.1X6
Lettuce opium	T42.6X1	T42.6X2	T42.6X3	T42.6X4	T42.6X5	T42.6X6
Leucinocaine	T41.3X1	T41.3X2	T41.3X3	T41.3X4	T41.3X5	T41.3X6
Leucocianidol	T46.991	T46.992	T46.993	T46.994	T46.995	T46.996
Leucovorin (factor)	T45.8X1	T45.8X2	T45.8X3	T45.8X4	T45.8X5	T45.8X6
Leukeran	T45.1X1	T45.1X2	T45.1X3	T45.1X4	T45.1X5	T45.1X6
Leuprolide	T38.891	T38.892	T38.893	T38.894	T38.895	T38.896
Levalbuterol	T48.6X1	T48.6X2	T48.6X3	T48.6X4	T48.6X5	T48.6X6
Levallorphan	T50.7X1	T50.7X2	T50.7X3	T50.7X4	T50.7X5	T50.7X6
Levamisole	T37.4X1	T37.4X2	T37.4X3	T37.4X4	T37.4X5	T37.4X6
Levanil	T42.6X1	T42.6X2	T42.6X3	T42.6X4	T42.6X5	T42.6X6
Levarterenol	T44.4X1	T44.4X2	T44.4X3	T44.4X4	T44.4X5	T44.4X6
Levdropropizine	T48.3X1	T48.3X2	T48.3X3	T48.3X4	T48.3X5	T48.3X6
Levobunolol	T49.5X1	T49.5X2	T49.5X3	T49.5X4	T49.5X5	T49.5X6
Levocabastine (hydrochloride)	T45.0X1	T45.0X2	T45.0X3	T45.0X4	T45.0X5	T45.0X6
Levocarnitine	T50.991	T50.992	T50.993	T50.994	T50.995	T50.996
Levodopa	T42.8X1	T42.8X2	T42.8X3	T42.8X4	T42.8X5	T42.8X6
with carbidopa	T42.8X1	T42.8X2	T42.8X3	T42.8X4	T42.8X5	T42.8X6
Levo-dromoran	T40.2X1	T40.2X2	T40.2X3	T40.2X4	T40.2X5	T40.2X6
Levoglutamide	T50.991	T50.992	T50.993	T50.994	T50.995	T50.996
Levoid	T38.1X1	T38.1X2	T38.1X3	T38.1X4	T38.1X5	T38.1X6
Levo-isomethadone	T40.3X1	T40.3X2	T40.3X3	T40.3X4	T40.3X5	T40.3X6
Levomepromazine	T43.3X1	T43.3X2	T43.3X3	T43.3X4	T43.3X5	T43.3X6
Levonordefrin	T49.6X1	T49.6X2	T49.6X3	T49.6X4	T49.6X5	T49.6X6
Levonorgestrel	T38.4X1	T38.4X2	T38.4X3	T38.4X4	T38.4X5	T38.4X6
with ethinylestradiol	T38.5X1	T38.5X2	T38.5X3	T38.5X4	T38.5X5	T38.5X6
Levopromazine	T43.3X1	T43.3X2	T43.3X3	T43.3X4	T43.3X5	T43.3X6
Levoprome	T42.6X1	T42.6X2	T42.6X3	T42.6X4	T42.6X5	T42.6X6
Levopropoxyphene	T40.491	T40.492	T40.493	T40.494	T40.495	T40.496
Levopropylhexedrine	T50.5X1	T50.5X2	T50.5X3	T50.5X4	T50.5X5	T50.5X6
Levoproxyphylline	T48.6X1	T48.6X2	T48.6X3	T48.6X4	T48.6X5	T48.6X6
Levorphanol	T40.491	T40.492	T40.493	T40.494	T40.495	T40.496
Levothroid*	T38.1X1	T38.1X2	T38.1X3	T38.1X4	T38.1X5	T38.1X6
Levothyroxine	T38.1X1	T38.1X2	T38.1X3	T38.1X4	T38.1X5	T38.1X6
sodium	T38.1X1	T38.1X2	T38.1X3	T38.1X4	T38.1X5	T38.1X6
Levsin	T44.3X1	T44.3X2	T44.3X3	T44.3X4	T44.3X5	T44.3X6
Levulose	T50.3X1	T50.3X2	T50.3X3	T50.3X4	T50.3X5	T50.3X6
Lewisite (gas), not in war	T57.0X1	T57.0X2	T57.0X3	T57.0X4	—	—
Librium	T42.4X1	T42.4X2	T42.4X3	T42.4X4	T42.4X5	T42.4X6
Lidex	T49.0X1	T49.0X2	T49.0X3	T49.0X4	T49.0X5	T49.0X6
Lidocaine	T41.3X1	T41.3X2	T41.3X3	T41.3X4	T41.3X5	T41.3X6
regional	T41.3X1	T41.3X2	T41.3X3	T41.3X4	T41.3X5	T41.3X6
spinal	T41.3X1	T41.3X2	T41.3X3	T41.3X4	T41.3X5	T41.3X6
Lidofenin	T50.8X1	T50.8X2	T50.8X3	T50.8X4	T50.8X5	T50.8X6
Lidoflazine	T46.1X1	T46.1X2	T46.1X3	T46.1X4	T46.1X5	T46.1X6
Lighter fluid	T52.0X1	T52.0X2	T52.0X3	T52.0X4	—	—
Lignin hemicellulose	T47.6X1	T47.6X2	T47.6X3	T47.6X4	T47.6X5	T47.6X6
Lignocaine	T41.3X1	T41.3X2	T41.3X3	T41.3X4	T41.3X5	T41.3X6
regional	T41.3X1	T41.3X2	T41.3X3	T41.3X4	T41.3X5	T41.3X6
spinal	T41.3X1	T41.3X2	T41.3X3	T41.3X4	T41.3X5	T41.3X6
Ligroin(e) (solvent)	T52.0X1	T52.0X2	T52.0X3	T52.0X4	—	—
vapor	T59.891	T59.892	T59.893	T59.894	—	—
Ligustrum vulgare	T62.2X1	T62.2X2	T62.2X3	T62.2X4	—	—
Lily of the valley	T62.2X1	T62.2X2	T62.2X3	T62.2X4	—	—
Lime (chloride)	T54.3X1	T54.3X2	T54.3X3	T54.3X4	—	—
Limonene	T52.8X1	T52.8X2	T52.8X3	T52.8X4	—	—
Lincomycin	T36.8X1	T36.8X2	T36.8X3	T36.8X4	T36.8X5	T36.8X6
Lindane (insecticide) (nonmedicinal) (vapor)	T53.6X1	T53.6X2	T53.6X3	T53.6X4	—	—
medicinal	T49.0X1	T49.0X2	T49.0X3	T49.0X4	T49.0X5	T49.0X6
Liniments NEC	T49.91	T49.92	T49.93	T49.94	T49.95	T49.96
Linoleic acid	T46.6X1	T46.6X2	T46.6X3	T46.6X4	T46.6X5	T46.6X6
Linolenic acid	T46.6X1	T46.6X2	T46.6X3	T46.6X4	T46.6X5	T46.6X6
Linseed	T47.4X1	T47.4X2	T47.4X3	T47.4X4	T47.4X5	T47.4X6
Liothyronine	T38.1X1	T38.1X2	T38.1X3	T38.1X4	T38.1X5	T38.1X6
Liotrix	T38.1X1	T38.1X2	T38.1X3	T38.1X4	T38.1X5	T38.1X6
Lipancreatin	T47.5X1	T47.5X2	T47.5X3	T47.5X4	T47.5X5	T47.5X6
Lipo-alprostadil	T46.7X1	T46.7X2	T46.7X3	T46.7X4	T46.7X5	T46.7X6
Lipo-Lutin	T38.5X1	T38.5X2	T38.5X3	T38.5X4	T38.5X5	T38.5X6
Lipotropic drug NEC	T50.901	T50.902	T50.903	T50.904	T50.905	T50.906
Liquefied petroleum gases	T59.891	T59.892	T59.893	T59.894	—	—
piped (pure or mixed with air)	T59.891	T59.892	T59.893	T59.894	—	—
Liquid						
paraffin	T47.4X1	T47.4X2	T47.4X3	T47.4X4	T47.4X5	T47.4X6
petrolatum	T47.4X1	T47.4X2	T47.4X3	T47.4X4	T47.4X5	T47.4X6
topical	T49.3X1	T49.3X2	T49.3X3	T49.3X4	T49.3X5	T49.3X6
specified NEC	T65.891	T65.892	T65.893	T65.894	—	—
substance	T65.91	T65.92	T65.93	T65.94	—	—
Liquor creosolis compositus	T65.891	T65.892	T65.893	T65.894	—	—
Liquorice	T48.4X1	T48.4X2	T48.4X3	T48.4X4	T48.4X5	T48.4X6

☑ Additional Character May Be Required — Refer to the Tabular List for Character Selection

*Optum Value-Add

Kosam seed — Liquorice

Substance	Poisoning, Accidental (unintentional)	Poisoning, Intentional Self-harm	Poisoning, Assault	Poisoning, Undetermined	Adverse Effect	Under-dosing
Liquorice — *continued*						
extract	T47.8X1	T47.8X2	T47.8X3	T47.8X4	T47.8X5	T47.8X6
Liraglutide*	T38.3X1	T38.3X2	T38.3X3	T38.3X4	T38.3X5	T38.3X6
Lisinopril	T46.4X1	T46.4X2	T46.4X3	T46.4X4	T46.4X5	T46.4X6
Lisuride	T42.8X1	T42.8X2	T42.8X3	T42.8X4	T42.8X5	T42.8X6
Lithane	T43.8X1	T43.8X2	T43.8X3	T43.8X4	T43.8X5	T43.8X6
Lithium	T56.891	T56.892	T56.893	T56.894	—	—
gluconate	T43.591	T43.592	T43.593	T43.594	T43.595	T43.596
salts (carbonate)	T43.591	T43.592	T43.593	T43.594	T43.595	T43.596
Lithonate	T43.8X1	T43.8X2	T43.8X3	T43.8X4	T43.8X5	T43.8X6
Liver						
extract	T45.8X1	T45.8X2	T45.8X3	T45.8X4	T45.8X5	T45.8X6
for parenteral use	T45.8X1	T45.8X2	T45.8X3	T45.8X4	T45.8X5	T45.8X6
fraction 1	T45.8X1	T45.8X2	T45.8X3	T45.8X4	T45.8X5	T45.8X6
hydrolysate	T45.8X1	T45.8X2	T45.8X3	T45.8X4	T45.8X5	T45.8X6
Lizard (bite) (venom)	T63.121	T63.122	T63.123	T63.124	—	—
LMD	T45.8X1	T45.8X2	T45.8X3	T45.8X4	T45.8X5	T45.8X6
Lobelia	T62.2X1	T62.2X2	T62.2X3	T62.2X4	—	—
Lobeline	T50.7X1	T50.7X2	T50.7X3	T50.7X4	T50.7X5	T50.7X6
Local action drug NEC	T49.8X1	T49.8X2	T49.8X3	T49.8X4	T49.8X5	T49.8X6
Locorten	T49.0X1	T49.0X2	T49.0X3	T49.0X4	T49.0X5	T49.0X6
Lofepramine	T43.011	T43.012	T43.013	T43.014	T43.015	T43.016
Lolium temulentum	T62.2X1	T62.2X2	T62.2X3	T62.2X4	—	—
Lomotil	T47.6X1	T47.6X2	T47.6X3	T47.6X4	T47.6X5	T47.6X6
Lomustine	T45.1X1	T45.1X2	T45.1X3	T45.1X4	T45.1X5	T45.1X6
Lonidamine	T45.1X1	T45.1X2	T45.1X3	T45.1X4	T45.1X5	T45.1X6
LoOvral*	T38.4X1	T38.4X2	T38.4X3	T38.4X4	T38.4X5	T38.4X6
Loperamide	T47.6X1	T47.6X2	T47.6X3	T47.6X4	T47.6X5	T47.6X6
Loprazolam	T42.4X1	T42.4X2	T42.4X3	T42.4X4	T42.4X5	T42.4X6
Lorajmine	T46.2X1	T46.2X2	T46.2X3	T46.2X4	T46.2X5	T46.2X6
Loratidine	T45.0X1	T45.0X2	T45.0X3	T45.0X4	T45.0X5	T45.0X6
Lorazepam	T42.4X1	T42.4X2	T42.4X3	T42.4X4	T42.4X5	T42.4X6
Lorcainide	T46.2X1	T46.2X2	T46.2X3	T46.2X4	T46.2X5	T46.2X6
Lormetazepam	T42.4X1	T42.4X2	T42.4X3	T42.4X4	T42.4X5	T42.4X6
Lotions NEC	T49.91	T49.92	T49.93	T49.94	T49.95	T49.96
Lotrimin*	T49.0X1	T49.0X2	T49.0X3	T49.0X4	T49.0X5	T49.0X6
Lotusate	T42.3X1	T42.3X2	T42.3X3	T42.3X4	T42.3X5	T42.3X6
Lovastatin	T46.6X1	T46.6X2	T46.6X3	T46.6X4	T46.6X5	T46.6X6
Lowila	T49.2X1	T49.2X2	T49.2X3	T49.2X4	T49.2X5	T49.2X6
Loxapine	T43.591	T43.592	T43.593	T43.594	T43.595	T43.596
Lozenges (throat)	T49.6X1	T49.6X2	T49.6X3	T49.6X4	T49.6X5	T49.6X6
LSD	T40.8X1	T40.8X2	T40.8X3	T40.8X4	—	—
L-Tryptophan — *see* amino acid						
Lubricant, eye	T49.5X1	T49.5X2	T49.5X3	T49.5X4	T49.5X5	T49.5X6
Lubricating oil NEC	T52.0X1	T52.0X2	T52.0X3	T52.0X4	—	—
Lucanthone	T37.4X1	T37.4X2	T37.4X3	T37.4X4	T37.4X5	T37.4X6
Luminal	T42.3X1	T42.3X2	T42.3X3	T42.3X4	T42.3X5	T42.3X6
Lung irritant (gas) NEC	T59.91	T59.92	T59.93	T59.94		
Luteinizing hormone	T38.811	T38.812	T38.813	T38.814	T38.815	T38.816
Lutocylol	T38.5X1	T38.5X2	T38.5X3	T38.5X4	T38.5X5	T38.5X6
Lutromone	T38.5X1	T38.5X2	T38.5X3	T38.5X4	T38.5X5	T38.5X6
Lututrin	T48.291	T48.292	T48.293	T48.294	T48.295	T48.296
Luveris*	T38.891	T38.892	T38.893	T38.894	T38.895	T38.896
Lye (concentrated)	T54.3X1	T54.3X2	T54.3X3	T54.3X4	—	—
Lygranum (skin test)	T50.8X1	T50.8X2	T50.8X3	T50.8X4	T50.8X5	T50.8X6
Lymecycline	T36.4X1	T36.4X2	T36.4X3	T36.4X4	T36.4X5	T36.4X6
Lymphogranuloma venereum antigen	T50.8X1	T50.8X2	T50.8X3	T50.8X4	T50.8X5	T50.8X6
Lynestrenol	T38.4X1	T38.4X2	T38.4X3	T38.4X4	T38.4X5	T38.4X6
Lyovac Sodium Edecrin	T50.1X1	T50.1X2	T50.1X3	T50.1X4	T50.1X5	T50.1X6
Lypressin	T38.891	T38.892	T38.893	T38.894	T38.895	T38.896
Lysergic acid diethylamide	T40.8X1	T40.8X2	T40.8X3	T40.8X4	—	—
Lysergide	T40.8X1	T40.8X2	T40.8X3	T40.8X4	—	—
Lysine vasopressin	T38.891	T38.892	T38.893	T38.894	T38.895	T38.896
Lysol	T54.1X1	T54.1X2	T54.1X3	T54.1X4	—	—
Lysozyme	T49.0X1	T49.0X2	T49.0X3	T49.0X4	T49.0X5	T49.0X6
Lytta (vitatta)	T49.8X1	T49.8X2	T49.8X3	T49.8X4	T49.8X5	T49.8X6
Mace	T59.3X1	T59.3X2	T59.3X3	T59.3X4	—	—
Macrogol	T50.991	T50.992	T50.993	T50.994	T50.995	T50.996
Macrolide						
anabolic drug	T38.7X1	T38.7X2	T38.7X3	T38.7X4	T38.7X5	T38.7X6
antibiotic	T36.3X1	T36.3X2	T36.3X3	T36.3X4	T36.3X5	T36.3X6
Mafenide	T49.0X1	T49.0X2	T49.0X3	T49.0X4	T49.0X5	T49.0X6
Magaldrate	T47.1X1	T47.1X2	T47.1X3	T47.1X4	T47.1X5	T47.1X6
Magic mushroom	T40.991	T40.992	T40.993	T40.994	—	—
Magnamycin	T36.8X1	T36.8X2	T36.8X3	T36.8X4	T36.8X5	T36.8X6
Magnesia magma	T47.1X1	T47.1X2	T47.1X3	T47.1X4	T47.1X5	T47.1X6
Magnesium NEC	T56.891	T56.892	T56.893	T56.894	—	—
carbonate	T47.1X1	T47.1X2	T47.1X3	T47.1X4	T47.1X5	T47.1X6
citrate	T47.4X1	T47.4X2	T47.4X3	T47.4X4	T47.4X5	T47.4X6
hydroxide	T47.1X1	T47.1X2	T47.1X3	T47.1X4	T47.1X5	T47.1X6
oxide	T47.1X1	T47.1X2	T47.1X3	T47.1X4	T47.1X5	T47.1X6
peroxide	T49.0X1	T49.0X2	T49.0X3	T49.0X4	T49.0X5	T49.0X6

Substance	Poisoning, Accidental (unintentional)	Poisoning, Intentional Self-harm	Poisoning, Assault	Poisoning, Undetermined	Adverse Effect	Under-dosing
Magnesium — *continued*						
salicylate	T39.091	T39.092	T39.093	T39.094	T39.095	T39.096
silicofluoride	T50.3X1	T50.3X2	T50.3X3	T50.3X4	T50.3X5	T50.3X6
sulfate	T47.4X1	T47.4X2	T47.4X3	T47.4X4	T47.4X5	T47.4X6
thiosulfate	T45.0X1	T45.0X2	T45.0X3	T45.0X4	T45.0X5	T45.0X6
trisilicate	T47.1X1	T47.1X2	T47.1X3	T47.1X4	T47.1X5	T47.1X6
Malathion (medicinal)	T49.0X1	T49.0X2	T49.0X3	T49.0X4	T49.0X5	T49.0X6
insecticide	T60.0X1	T60.0X2	T60.0X3	T60.0X4	—	—
Male fern extract	T37.4X1	T37.4X2	T37.4X3	T37.4X4	T37.4X5	T37.4X6
M-AMSA	T45.1X1	T45.1X2	T45.1X3	T45.1X4	T45.1X5	T45.1X6
Mandelic acid	T37.8X1	T37.8X2	T37.8X3	T37.8X4	T37.8X5	T37.8X6
Manganese (dioxide) (salts)	T57.2X1	T57.2X2	T57.2X3	T57.2X4	—	—
medicinal	T50.991	T50.992	T50.993	T50.994	T50.995	T50.996
Mannitol	T47.3X1	T47.3X2	T47.3X3	T47.3X4	T47.3X5	T47.3X6
hexanitrate	T46.3X1	T46.3X2	T46.3X3	T46.3X4	T46.3X5	T46.3X6
Mannomustine	T45.1X1	T45.1X2	T45.1X3	T45.1X4	T45.1X5	T45.1X6
MAO inhibitors	T43.1X1	T43.1X2	T43.1X3	T43.1X4	T43.1X5	T43.1X6
Mapharsen	T37.8X1	T37.8X2	T37.8X3	T37.8X4	T37.8X5	T37.8X6
Maphenide	T49.0X1	T49.0X2	T49.0X3	T49.0X4	T49.0X5	T49.0X6
Maprotiline	T43.021	T43.022	T43.023	T43.024	T43.025	T43.026
Marcaine	T41.3X1	T41.3X2	T41.3X3	T41.3X4	T41.3X5	T41.3X6
infiltration (subcutaneous)	T41.3X1	T41.3X2	T41.3X3	T41.3X4	T41.3X5	T41.3X6
nerve block (peripheral) (plexus)	T41.3X1	T41.3X2	T41.3X3	T41.3X4	T41.3X5	T41.3X6
Marezine	T45.0X1	T45.0X2	T45.0X3	T45.0X4	T45.0X5	T45.0X6
Marihuana	T40.711	T40.712	T40.713	T40.714	T40.715	T40.716
Marijuana	T40.711	T40.712	T40.713	T40.714	T40.715	T40.716
Marine (sting)	T63.691	T63.692	T63.693	T63.694	—	—
animals (sting)	T63.691	T63.692	T63.693	T63.694	—	—
plants (sting)	T63.711	T63.712	T63.713	T63.714	—	—
Marplan	T43.1X1	T43.1X2	T43.1X3	T43.1X4	T43.1X5	T43.1X6
Marsh gas	T59.891	T59.892	T59.893	T59.894	—	—
Marsilid	T43.1X1	T43.1X2	T43.1X3	T43.1X4	T43.1X5	T43.1X6
Massengill*	T49.0X1	T49.0X2	T49.0X3	T49.0X4	T49.0X5	T49.0X6
Matulane	T45.1X1	T45.1X2	T45.1X3	T45.1X4	T45.1X5	T45.1X6
Mazindol	T50.5X1	T50.5X2	T50.5X3	T50.5X4	T50.5X5	T50.5X6
MCPA	T60.3X1	T60.3X2	T60.3X3	T60.3X4	—	—
MDMA	T43.641	T43.642	T43.643	T43.644	—	—
Meadow saffron	T62.2X1	T62.2X2	T62.2X3	T62.2X4	—	—
Measles virus vaccine (attenuated)	T50.B91	T50.B92	T50.B93	T50.B94	T50.B95	T50.B96
Meat, noxious	T62.8X1	T62.8X2	T62.8X3	T62.8X4	—	—
Meballymal	T42.3X1	T42.3X2	T42.3X3	T42.3X4	T42.3X5	T42.3X6
Mebanazine	T43.1X1	T43.1X2	T43.1X3	T43.1X4	T43.1X5	T43.1X6
Mebaral	T42.3X1	T42.3X2	T42.3X3	T42.3X4	T42.3X5	T42.3X6
Mebendazole	T37.4X1	T37.4X2	T37.4X3	T37.4X4	T37.4X5	T37.4X6
Mebeverine	T44.3X1	T44.3X2	T44.3X3	T44.3X4	T44.3X5	T44.3X6
Mebhydrolin	T45.0X1	T45.0X2	T45.0X3	T45.0X4	T45.0X5	T45.0X6
Mebumal	T42.3X1	T42.3X2	T42.3X3	T42.3X4	T42.3X5	T42.3X6
Mebutamate	T43.591	T43.592	T43.593	T43.594	T43.595	T43.596
Mecamylamine	T44.2X1	T44.2X2	T44.2X3	T44.2X4	T44.2X5	T44.2X6
Mechlorethamine	T45.1X1	T45.1X2	T45.1X3	T45.1X4	T45.1X5	T45.1X6
Mecillinam	T36.0X1	T36.0X2	T36.0X3	T36.0X4	T36.0X5	T36.0X6
Meclizine (hydrochloride)	T45.0X1	T45.0X2	T45.0X3	T45.0X4	T45.0X5	T45.0X6
Meclocycline	T36.4X1	T36.4X2	T36.4X3	T36.4X4	T36.4X5	T36.4X6
Meclofenamate	T39.391	T39.392	T39.393	T39.394	T39.395	T39.396
Meclofenamic acid	T39.391	T39.392	T39.393	T39.394	T39.395	T39.396
Meclofenoxate	T43.691	T43.692	T43.693	T43.694	T43.695	T43.696
Meclozine	T45.0X1	T45.0X2	T45.0X3	T45.0X4	T45.0X5	T45.0X6
Mecobalamin	T45.8X1	T45.8X2	T45.8X3	T45.8X4	T45.8X5	T45.8X6
Mecoprop	T60.3X1	T60.3X2	T60.3X3	T60.3X4	—	—
Mecrilate	T49.3X1	T49.3X2	T49.3X3	T49.3X4	T49.3X5	T49.3X6
Mecysteine	T48.4X1	T48.4X2	T48.4X3	T48.4X4	T48.4X5	T48.4X6
Medazepam	T42.4X1	T42.4X2	T42.4X3	T42.4X4	T42.4X5	T42.4X6
Medicament NEC	T50.901	T50.902	T50.903	T50.904	T50.905	T50.906
Medinal	T42.3X1	T42.3X2	T42.3X3	T42.3X4	T42.3X5	T42.3X6
Medomin	T42.3X1	T42.3X2	T42.3X3	T42.3X4	T42.3X5	T42.3X6
Medrogestone	T38.5X1	T38.5X2	T38.5X3	T38.5X4	T38.5X5	T38.5X6
Medroxalol	T44.8X1	T44.8X2	T44.8X3	T44.8X4	T44.8X5	T44.8X6
Medroxyprogesterone acetate (depot)	T38.5X1	T38.5X2	T38.5X3	T38.5X4	T38.5X5	T38.5X6
Medrysone	T49.0X1	T49.0X2	T49.0X3	T49.0X4	T49.0X5	T49.0X6
Mefenamic acid	T39.391	T39.392	T39.393	T39.394	T39.395	T39.396
Mefenorex	T50.5X1	T50.5X2	T50.5X3	T50.5X4	T50.5X5	T50.5X6
Mefloquine	T37.2X1	T37.2X2	T37.2X3	T37.2X4	T37.2X5	T37.2X6
Mefoxin*	T36.1X1	T36.1X2	T36.1X3	T36.1X4	T36.1X5	T36.1X6
Mefruside	T50.2X1	T50.2X2	T50.2X3	T50.2X4	T50.2X5	T50.2X6
Megahallucinogen	T40.901	T40.902	T40.903	T40.904	T40.905	T40.906
Megestrol	T38.5X1	T38.5X2	T38.5X3	T38.5X4	T38.5X5	T38.5X6
Meglumine						
antimoniate	T37.8X1	T37.8X2	T37.8X3	T37.8X4	T37.8X5	T37.8X6
diatrizoate	T50.8X1	T50.8X2	T50.8X3	T50.8X4	T50.8X5	T50.8X6
iodipamide	T50.8X1	T50.8X2	T50.8X3	T50.8X4	T50.8X5	T50.8X6

Table of Drugs and Chemicals

Substance	Poisoning, Accidental (unintentional)	Poisoning, Intentional Self-harm	Poisoning, Assault	Poisoning, Undetermined	Adverse Effect	Underdosing
Meglumine — continued						
iotroxate	T50.8X1	T50.8X2	T50.8X3	T50.8X4	T50.8X5	T50.8X6
MEK (methyl ethyl ketone)	T52.4X1	T52.4X2	T52.4X3	T52.4X4	—	—
Meladinin	T49.3X1	T49.3X2	T49.3X3	T49.3X4	T49.3X5	T49.3X6
Meladrazine	T44.3X1	T44.3X2	T44.3X3	T44.3X4	T44.3X5	T44.3X6
Melaleuca alternifolia oil	T49.0X1	T49.0X2	T49.0X3	T49.0X4	T49.0X5	T49.0X6
Melanizing agents	T49.3X1	T49.3X2	T49.3X3	T49.3X4	T49.3X5	T49.3X6
Melanocyte-stimulating hormone	T38.891	T38.892	T38.893	T38.894	T38.895	T38.896
Melarsonyl potassium	T37.3X1	T37.3X2	T37.3X3	T37.3X4	T37.3X5	T37.3X6
Melarsoprol	T37.3X1	T37.3X2	T37.3X3	T37.3X4	T37.3X5	T37.3X6
Melia azedarach	T62.2X1	T62.2X2	T62.2X3	T62.2X4	—	—
Melitracen	T43.011	T43.012	T43.013	T43.014	T43.015	T43.016
Mellaril	T43.3X1	T43.3X2	T43.3X3	T43.3X4	T43.3X5	T43.3X6
Meloxicam*	T39.391	T39.392	T39.393	T39.394	T39.395	T39.396
Meloxine	T49.3X1	T49.3X2	T49.3X3	T49.3X4	T49.3X5	T49.3X6
Melperone	T43.4X1	T43.4X2	T43.4X3	T43.4X4	T43.4X5	T43.4X6
Melphalan	T45.1X1	T45.1X2	T45.1X3	T45.1X4	T45.1X5	T45.1X6
Memantine	T43.8X1	T43.8X2	T43.8X3	T43.8X4	T43.8X5	T43.8X6
Menadiol	T45.7X1	T45.7X2	T45.7X3	T45.7X4	T45.7X5	T45.7X6
sodium sulfate	T45.7X1	T45.7X2	T45.7X3	T45.7X4	T45.7X5	T45.7X6
Menadione	T45.7X1	T45.7X2	T45.7X3	T45.7X4	T45.7X5	T45.7X6
sodium bisulfite	T45.7X1	T45.7X2	T45.7X3	T45.7X4	T45.7X5	T45.7X6
Menaphthone	T45.7X1	T45.7X2	T45.7X3	T45.7X4	T45.7X5	T45.7X6
Menaquinone	T45.7X1	T45.7X2	T45.7X3	T45.7X4	T45.7X5	T45.7X6
Menatetrenone	T45.7X1	T45.7X2	T45.7X3	T45.7X4	T45.7X5	T45.7X6
Meningococcal vaccine	T50.A91	T50.A92	T50.A93	T50.A94	T50.A95	T50.A96
Menningovax (-AC) (-C)	T50.A91	T50.A92	T50.A93	T50.A94	T50.A95	T50.A96
Menotropins	T38.811	T38.812	T38.813	T38.814	T38.815	T38.816
Menthol	T48.5X1	T48.5X2	T48.5X3	T48.5X4	T48.5X5	T48.5X6
Mepacrine	T37.2X1	T37.2X2	T37.2X3	T37.2X4	T37.2X5	T37.2X6
Meparfynol	T42.6X1	T42.6X2	T42.6X3	T42.6X4	T42.6X5	T42.6X6
Mepartricin	T36.7X1	T36.7X2	T36.7X3	T36.7X4	T36.7X5	T36.7X6
Mepazine	T43.3X1	T43.3X2	T43.3X3	T43.3X4	T43.3X5	T43.3X6
Mepenzolate	T44.3X1	T44.3X2	T44.3X3	T44.3X4	T44.3X5	T44.3X6
bromide	T44.3X1	T44.3X2	T44.3X3	T44.3X4	T44.3X5	T44.3X6
Meperidine	T40.491	T40.492	T40.493	T40.494	T40.495	T40.496
Mephebarbital	T42.3X1	T42.3X2	T42.3X3	T42.3X4	T42.3X5	T42.3X6
Mephenamin (e)	T42.8X1	T42.8X2	T42.8X3	T42.8X4	T42.8X5	T42.8X6
Mephenesin	T42.8X1	T42.8X2	T42.8X3	T42.8X4	T42.8X5	T42.8X6
Mephenhydramine	T45.0X1	T45.0X2	T45.0X3	T45.0X4	T45.0X5	T45.0X6
Mephenoxalone	T42.8X1	T42.8X2	T42.8X3	T42.8X4	T42.8X5	T42.8X6
Mephentermine	T44.991	T44.992	T44.993	T44.994	T44.995	T44.996
Mephenytoin	T42.0X1	T42.0X2	T42.0X3	T42.0X4	T42.0X5	T42.0X6
with phenobarbital	T42.3X1	T42.3X2	T42.3X3	T42.3X4	T42.3X5	T42.3X6
Mephobarbital	T42.3X1	T42.3X2	T42.3X3	T42.3X4	T42.3X5	T42.3X6
Mephosfolan	T60.0X1	T60.0X2	T60.0X3	T60.0X4	—	—
Mepindolol	T44.7X1	T44.7X2	T44.7X3	T44.7X4	T44.7X5	T44.7X6
Mepiperphenidol	T44.3X1	T44.3X2	T44.3X3	T44.3X4	T44.3X5	T44.3X6
Mepitiostane	T38.7X1	T38.7X2	T38.7X3	T38.7X4	T38.7X5	T38.7X6
Mepivacaine	T41.3X1	T41.3X2	T41.3X3	T41.3X4	T41.3X5	T41.3X6
epidural	T41.3X1	T41.3X2	T41.3X3	T41.3X4	T41.3X5	T41.3X6
Meprednisone	T38.0X1	T38.0X2	T38.0X3	T38.0X4	T38.0X5	T38.0X6
Meprobam	T43.591	T43.592	T43.593	T43.594	T43.595	T43.596
Meprobamate	T43.591	T43.592	T43.593	T43.594	T43.595	T43.596
Meproscillarin	T46.0X1	T46.0X2	T46.0X3	T46.0X4	T46.0X5	T46.0X6
Meprylcaine	T41.3X1	T41.3X2	T41.3X3	T41.3X4	T41.3X5	T41.3X6
Meptazinol	T39.8X1	T39.8X2	T39.8X3	T39.8X4	T39.8X5	T39.8X6
Mepyramine	T45.0X1	T45.0X2	T45.0X3	T45.0X4	T45.0X5	T45.0X6
Mequinol*	T49.8X1	T49.8X2	T49.8X3	T49.8X4	T49.8X5	T49.8X6
Mequitazine	T43.3X1	T43.3X2	T43.3X3	T43.3X4	T43.3X5	T43.3X6
Meralluride	T50.2X1	T50.2X2	T50.2X3	T50.2X4	T50.2X5	T50.2X6
Merbaphen	T50.2X1	T50.2X2	T50.2X3	T50.2X4	T50.2X5	T50.2X6
Merbromin	T49.0X1	T49.0X2	T49.0X3	T49.0X4	T49.0X5	T49.0X6
Mercaptobenzothiazole salts	T49.0X1	T49.0X2	T49.0X3	T49.0X4	T49.0X5	T49.0X6
Mercaptomerin	T50.2X1	T50.2X2	T50.2X3	T50.2X4	T50.2X5	T50.2X6
Mercaptopurine	T45.1X1	T45.1X2	T45.1X3	T45.1X4	T45.1X5	T45.1X6
Mercumatilin	T50.2X1	T50.2X2	T50.2X3	T50.2X4	T50.2X5	T50.2X6
Mercuramide	T50.2X1	T50.2X2	T50.2X3	T50.2X4	T50.2X5	T50.2X6
Mercurochrome	T49.0X1	T49.0X2	T49.0X3	T49.0X4	T49.0X5	T49.0X6
Mercurophylline	T50.2X1	T50.2X2	T50.2X3	T50.2X4	T50.2X5	T50.2X6
Mercury, mercurial, mercuric, mercurous (compounds) (cyanide) (fumes) (nonmedicinal) (vapor) **NEC**	T56.1X1	T56.1X2	T56.1X3	T56.1X4	—	—
ammoniated	T49.0X1	T49.0X2	T49.0X3	T49.0X4	T49.0X5	T49.0X6
anti-infective						
local	T49.0X1	T49.0X2	T49.0X3	T49.0X4	T49.0X5	T49.0X6
systemic	T37.8X1	T37.8X2	T37.8X3	T37.8X4	T37.8X5	T37.8X6
topical	T49.0X1	T49.0X2	T49.0X3	T49.0X4	T49.0X5	T49.0X6
chloride (ammoniated)	T49.0X1	T49.0X2	T49.0X3	T49.0X4	T49.0X5	T49.0X6
Mercury, mercurial, mercuric, mercurous (compounds) (cyanide) (fumes) (nonmedicinal) (vapor) **NEC** — continued						
chloride — continued						
fungicide	T56.1X1	T56.1X2	T56.1X3	T56.1X4	—	—
diuretic NEC	T50.2X1	T50.2X2	T50.2X3	T50.2X4	T50.2X5	T50.2X6
fungicide	T56.1X1	T56.1X2	T56.1X3	T56.1X4	—	—
organic (fungicide)	T56.1X1	T56.1X2	T56.1X3	T56.1X4	—	—
oxide, yellow	T49.0X1	T49.0X2	T49.0X3	T49.0X4	T49.0X5	T49.0X6
Mersalyl	T50.2X1	T50.2X2	T50.2X3	T50.2X4	T50.2X5	T50.2X6
Merthiolate	T49.0X1	T49.0X2	T49.0X3	T49.0X4	T49.0X5	T49.0X6
ophthalmic preparation	T49.5X1	T49.5X2	T49.5X3	T49.5X4	T49.5X5	T49.5X6
Meruvax	T50.B91	T50.B92	T50.B93	T50.B94	T50.B95	T50.B96
Mesalazine	T47.8X1	T47.8X2	T47.8X3	T47.8X4	T47.8X5	T47.8X6
Mescal buttons	T40.991	T40.992	T40.993	T40.994		
Mescaline	T40.991	T40.992	T40.993	T40.994		
Mesna	T48.4X1	T48.4X2	T48.4X3	T48.4X4	T48.4X5	T48.4X6
Mesoglycan	T46.6X1	T46.6X2	T46.6X3	T46.6X4	T46.6X5	T46.6X6
Mesoridazine	T43.3X1	T43.3X2	T43.3X3	T43.3X4	T43.3X5	T43.3X6
Mestanolone	T38.7X1	T38.7X2	T38.7X3	T38.7X4	T38.7X5	T38.7X6
Mesterolone	T38.7X1	T38.7X2	T38.7X3	T38.7X4	T38.7X5	T38.7X6
Mestranol	T38.5X1	T38.5X2	T38.5X3	T38.5X4	T38.5X5	T38.5X6
Mesulergine	T42.8X1	T42.8X2	T42.8X3	T42.8X4	T42.8X5	T42.8X6
Mesulfen	T49.0X1	T49.0X2	T49.0X3	T49.0X4	T49.0X5	T49.0X6
Mesuximide	T42.2X1	T42.2X2	T42.2X3	T42.2X4	T42.2X5	T42.2X6
Metabutethamine	T41.3X1	T41.3X2	T41.3X3	T41.3X4	T41.3X5	T41.3X6
Metactesylacetate	T49.0X1	T49.0X2	T49.0X3	T49.0X4	T49.0X5	T49.0X6
Metacycline	T36.4X1	T36.4X2	T36.4X3	T36.4X4	T36.4X5	T36.4X6
Metaldehyde (snail killer) **NEC**	T60.8X1	T60.8X2	T60.8X3	T60.8X4	—	—
Metals (heavy) (nonmedicinal)	T56.91	T56.92	T56.93	T56.94	—	—
dust, fumes, or vapor NEC	T56.91	T56.92	T56.93	T56.94		
light NEC	T56.91	T56.92	T56.93	T56.94		
dust, fumes, or vapor NEC	T56.91	T56.92	T56.93	T56.94		
specified NEC	T56.891	T56.892	T56.893	T56.894	—	—
thallium	T56.811	T56.812	T56.813	T56.814		
Metamfetamine	T43.651	T43.652	T43.653	T43.654	T43.655	T43.656
Metamizole sodium	T39.2X1	T39.2X2	T39.2X3	T39.2X4	T39.2X5	T39.2X6
Metampicillin	T36.0X1	T36.0X2	T36.0X3	T36.0X4	T36.0X5	T36.0X6
Metamucil	T47.4X1	T47.4X2	T47.4X3	T47.4X4	T47.4X5	T47.4X6
Metandienone	T38.7X1	T38.7X2	T38.7X3	T38.7X4	T38.7X5	T38.7X6
Metandrostenolone	T38.7X1	T38.7X2	T38.7X3	T38.7X4	T38.7X5	T38.7X6
Metaphen	T49.0X1	T49.0X2	T49.0X3	T49.0X4	T49.0X5	T49.0X6
Metaphos	T60.0X1	T60.0X2	T60.0X3	T60.0X4	—	—
Metapramine	T43.011	T43.012	T43.013	T43.014	T43.015	T43.016
Metaproterenol	T48.291	T48.292	T48.293	T48.294	T48.295	T48.296
Metaraminol	T44.4X1	T44.4X2	T44.4X3	T44.4X4	T44.4X5	T44.4X6
Metaxalone	T42.8X1	T42.8X2	T42.8X3	T42.8X4	T42.8X5	T42.8X6
Meted*	T49.4X1	T49.4X2	T49.4X3	T49.4X4	T49.4X5	T49.4X6
Metenolone	T38.7X1	T38.7X2	T38.7X3	T38.7X4	T38.7X5	T38.7X6
Metergoline	T42.8X1	T42.8X2	T42.8X3	T42.8X4	T42.8X5	T42.8X6
Metescufylline	T46.991	T46.992	T46.993	T46.994	T46.995	T46.996
Metetoin	T42.0X1	T42.0X2	T42.0X3	T42.0X4	T42.0X5	T42.0X6
Metformin	T38.3X1	T38.3X2	T38.3X3	T38.3X4	T38.3X5	T38.3X6
Methacholine	T44.1X1	T44.1X2	T44.1X3	T44.1X4	T44.1X5	T44.1X6
Methacycline	T36.4X1	T36.4X2	T36.4X3	T36.4X4	T36.4X5	T36.4X6
Methadone	T40.3X1	T40.3X2	T40.3X3	T40.3X4	T40.3X5	T40.3X6
Methadose*	T40.3X1	T40.3X2	T40.3X3	T40.3X4	T40.3X5	T40.3X6
Methallenestril	T38.5X1	T38.5X2	T38.5X3	T38.5X4	T38.5X5	T38.5X6
Methallenoestril	T38.5X1	T38.5X2	T38.5X3	T38.5X4	T38.5X5	T38.5X6
Methamphetamine	T43.651	T43.652	T43.653	T43.654	T43.655	T43.656
Methampyrone	T39.2X1	T39.2X2	T39.2X3	T39.2X4	T39.2X5	T39.2X6
Methandienone	T38.7X1	T38.7X2	T38.7X3	T38.7X4	T38.7X5	T38.7X6
Methandriol	T38.7X1	T38.7X2	T38.7X3	T38.7X4	T38.7X5	T38.7X6
Methandrostenolone	T38.7X1	T38.7X2	T38.7X3	T38.7X4	T38.7X5	T38.7X6
Methane	T59.891	T59.892	T59.893	T59.894	—	—
Methanethiol	T59.891	T59.892	T59.893	T59.894	—	—
Methaniazide	T37.1X1	T37.1X2	T37.1X3	T37.1X4	T37.1X5	T37.1X6
Methanol (vapor)	T51.1X1	T51.1X2	T51.1X3	T51.1X4	—	—
Methantheline	T44.3X1	T44.3X2	T44.3X3	T44.3X4	T44.3X5	T44.3X6
Methanthelinium bromide	T44.3X1	T44.3X2	T44.3X3	T44.3X4	T44.3X5	T44.3X6
Methaphenilene	T45.0X1	T45.0X2	T45.0X3	T45.0X4	T45.0X5	T45.0X6
Methapyrilene	T45.0X1	T45.0X2	T45.0X3	T45.0X4	T45.0X5	T45.0X6
Methaqualone (compound)	T42.6X1	T42.6X2	T42.6X3	T42.6X4	T42.6X5	T42.6X6
Metharbital	T42.3X1	T42.3X2	T42.3X3	T42.3X4	T42.3X5	T42.3X6
Methazolamide	T50.2X1	T50.2X2	T50.2X3	T50.2X4	T50.2X5	T50.2X6
Methdilazine	T43.3X1	T43.3X2	T43.3X3	T43.3X4	T43.3X5	T43.3X6
Methedrine	T43.651	T43.652	T43.653	T43.654	T43.655	T43.656
Methenamine (mandelate)	T37.8X1	T37.8X2	T37.8X3	T37.8X4	T37.8X5	T37.8X6
Methenolone	T38.7X1	T38.7X2	T38.7X3	T38.7X4	T38.7X5	T38.7X6

Substance	Poisoning, Accidental (unintentional)	Poisoning, Intentional Self-harm	Poisoning, Assault	Poisoning, Undetermined	Adverse Effect	Under-dosing
Methergine	T48.0X1	T48.0X2	T48.0X3	T48.0X4	T48.0X5	T48.0X6
Methetoin	T42.0X1	T42.0X2	T42.0X3	T42.0X4	T42.0X5	T42.0X6
Methiacil	T38.2X1	T38.2X2	T38.2X3	T38.2X4	T38.2X5	T38.2X6
Methicillin	T36.0X1	T36.0X2	T36.0X3	T36.0X4	T36.0X5	T36.0X6
Methimazole	T38.2X1	T38.2X2	T38.2X3	T38.2X4	T38.2X5	T38.2X6
Methiodal sodium	T50.8X1	T50.8X2	T50.8X3	T50.8X4	T50.8X5	T50.8X6
Methionine	T50.991	T50.992	T50.993	T50.994	T50.995	T50.996
Methisazone	T37.5X1	T37.5X2	T37.5X3	T37.5X4	T37.5X5	T37.5X6
Methisoprinol	T37.5X1	T37.5X2	T37.5X3	T37.5X4	T37.5X5	T37.5X6
Methitural	T42.3X1	T42.3X2	T42.3X3	T42.3X4	T42.3X5	T42.3X6
Methixene	T44.3X1	T44.3X2	T44.3X3	T44.3X4	T44.3X5	T44.3X6
Methobarbital, methobarbitone	T42.3X1	T42.3X2	T42.3X3	T42.3X4	T42.3X5	T42.3X6
Methocarbamol	T42.8X1	T42.8X2	T42.8X3	T42.8X4	T42.8X5	T42.8X6
skeletal muscle relaxant	T48.1X1	T48.1X2	T48.1X3	T48.1X4	T48.1X5	T48.1X6
Methohexital	T41.1X1	T41.1X2	T41.1X3	T41.1X4	T41.1X5	T41.1X6
Methohexitone	T41.1X1	T41.1X2	T41.1X3	T41.1X4	T41.1X5	T41.1X6
Methoin	T42.0X1	T42.0X2	T42.0X3	T42.0X4	T42.0X5	T42.0X6
Methopholine	T39.8X1	T39.8X2	T39.8X3	T39.8X4	T39.8X5	T39.8X6
Methopromazine	T43.3X1	T43.3X2	T43.3X3	T43.3X4	T43.3X5	T43.3X6
Methorate	T48.3X1	T48.3X2	T48.3X3	T48.3X4	T48.3X5	T48.3X6
Methoserpidine	T46.5X1	T46.5X2	T46.5X3	T46.5X4	T46.5X5	T46.5X6
Methotrexate	T45.1X1	T45.1X2	T45.1X3	T45.1X4	T45.1X5	T45.1X6
Methotrimeprazine	T43.3X1	T43.3X2	T43.3X3	T43.3X4	T43.3X5	T43.3X6
Methoxa-Dome	T49.3X1	T49.3X2	T49.3X3	T49.3X4	T49.3X5	T49.3X6
Methoxamine	T44.4X1	T44.4X2	T44.4X3	T44.4X4	T44.4X5	T44.4X6
Methoxsalen	T50.991	T50.992	T50.993	T50.994	T50.995	T50.996
Methoxyaniline	T65.3X1	T65.3X2	T65.3X3	T65.3X4	—	—
Methoxybenzyl penicillin	T36.0X1	T36.0X2	T36.0X3	T36.0X4	T36.0X5	T36.0X6
Methoxychlor	T53.7X1	T53.7X2	T53.7X3	T53.7X4	—	—
Methoxy-DDT	T53.7X1	T53.7X2	T53.7X3	T53.7X4	—	—
Methoxyflurane	T41.0X1	T41.0X2	T41.0X3	T41.0X4	T41.0X5	T41.0X6
Methoxyphenamine	T48.6X1	T48.6X2	T48.6X3	T48.6X4	T48.6X5	T48.6X6
Methoxypromazine	T43.3X1	T43.3X2	T43.3X3	T43.3X4	T43.3X5	T43.3X6
Methscopolamine bromide	T44.3X1	T44.3X2	T44.3X3	T44.3X4	T44.3X5	T44.3X6
Methsuximide	T42.2X1	T42.2X2	T42.2X3	T42.2X4	T42.2X5	T42.2X6
Methyclothiazide	T50.2X1	T50.2X2	T50.2X3	T50.2X4	T50.2X5	T50.2X6
Methyl						
acetate	T52.4X1	T52.4X2	T52.4X3	T52.4X4	—	—
acetone	T52.4X1	T52.4X2	T52.4X3	T52.4X4	—	—
acrylate	T65.891	T65.892	T65.893	T65.894	—	—
alcohol	T51.1X1	T51.1X2	T51.1X3	T51.1X4	—	—
aminophenol	T65.3X1	T65.3X2	T65.3X3	T65.3X4	—	—
amphetamine	T43.651	T43.652	T43.652	T43.654	T43.655	T43.656
androstanolone	T38.7X1	T38.7X2	T38.7X3	T38.7X4	T38.7X5	T38.7X6
atropine	T44.3X1	T44.3X2	T44.3X3	T44.3X4	T44.3X5	T44.3X6
benzene	T52.2X1	T52.2X2	T52.2X3	T52.2X4	—	—
benzoate	T52.8X1	T52.8X2	T52.8X3	T52.8X4	—	—
benzol	T52.2X1	T52.2X2	T52.2X3	T52.2X4	—	—
bromide (gas)	T59.891	T59.892	T59.893	T59.894	—	—
fumigant	T60.8X1	T60.8X2	T60.8X3	T60.8X4	—	—
butanol	T51.3X1	T51.3X2	T51.3X3	T51.3X4	—	—
carbinol	T51.1X1	T51.1X2	T51.1X3	T51.1X4	—	—
carbonate	T52.8X1	T52.8X2	T52.8X3	T52.8X4	—	—
CCNU	T45.1X1	T45.1X2	T45.1X3	T45.1X4	T45.1X5	T45.1X6
cellosolve	T52.91	T52.92	T52.93	T52.94	—	—
cellulose	T47.4X1	T47.4X2	T47.4X3	T47.4X4	T47.4X5	T47.4X6
chloride (gas)	T59.891	T59.892	T59.893	T59.894	—	—
chloroformate	T59.3X1	T59.3X2	T59.3X3	T59.3X4	—	—
cyclohexane	T52.8X1	T52.8X2	T52.8X3	T52.8X4	—	—
cyclohexanol	T51.8X1	T51.8X2	T51.8X3	T51.8X4	—	—
cyclohexanone	T52.8X1	T52.8X2	T52.8X3	T52.8X4	—	—
cyclohexyl acetate	T52.8X1	T52.8X2	T52.8X3	T52.8X4	—	—
demeton	T60.0X1	T60.0X2	T60.0X3	T60.0X4	—	—
dihydromorphinone	T40.2X1	T40.2X2	T40.2X3	T40.2X4	T40.2X5	T40.2X6
ergometrine	T48.0X1	T48.0X2	T48.0X3	T48.0X4	T48.0X5	T48.0X6
ergonovine	T48.0X1	T48.0X2	T48.0X3	T48.0X4	T48.0X5	T48.0X6
ethyl ketone	T52.4X1	T52.4X2	T52.4X3	T52.4X4	—	—
glucamine antimonate	T37.8X1	T37.8X2	T37.8X3	T37.8X4	T37.8X5	T37.8X6
hydrazine	T65.891	T65.892	T65.893	T65.894	—	—
iodide	T65.891	T65.892	T65.893	T65.894	—	—
isobutyl ketone	T52.4X1	T52.4X2	T52.4X3	T52.4X4	—	—
isothiocyanate	T60.3X1	T60.3X2	T60.3X3	T60.3X4	—	—
mercaptan	T59.891	T59.892	T59.893	T59.894	—	—
morphine NEC	T40.2X1	T40.2X2	T40.2X3	T40.2X4	T40.2X5	T40.2X6
nicotinate	T49.4X1	T49.4X2	T49.4X3	T49.4X4	T49.4X5	T49.4X6
paraben	T49.0X1	T49.0X2	T49.0X3	T49.0X4	T49.0X5	T49.0X6
parafynol	T42.6X1	T42.6X2	T42.6X3	T42.6X4	T42.6X5	T42.6X6
parathion	T60.0X1	T60.0X2	T60.0X3	T60.0X4	—	—
peridol	T43.4X1	T43.4X2	T43.4X3	T43.4X4	T43.4X5	T43.4X6
phenidate	T43.631	T43.632	T43.633	T43.634	T43.635	T43.636
prednisolone	T38.0X1	T38.0X2	T38.0X3	T38.0X4	T38.0X5	T38.0X6

Substance	Poisoning, Accidental (unintentional)	Poisoning, Intentional Self-harm	Poisoning, Assault	Poisoning, Undetermined	Adverse Effect	Under-dosing
Methyl — continued						
prednisolone — continued						
ENT agent	T49.6X1	T49.6X2	T49.6X3	T49.6X4	T49.6X5	T49.6X6
ophthalmic preparation	T49.5X1	T49.5X2	T49.5X3	T49.5X4	T49.5X5	T49.5X6
topical NEC	T49.0X1	T49.0X2	T49.0X3	T49.0X4	T49.0X5	T49.0X6
propylcarbinol	T51.3X1	T51.3X2	T51.3X3	T51.3X4		
rosaniline NEC	T49.0X1	T49.0X2	T49.0X3	T49.0X4	T49.0X5	T49.0X6
salicylate	T49.2X1	T49.2X2	T49.2X3	T49.2X4	T49.2X5	T49.2X6
sulfate (fumes)	T59.891	T59.892	T59.893	T59.894	—	—
liquid	T52.8X1	T52.8X2	T52.8X3	T52.8X4	—	—
sulfonal	T42.6X1	T42.6X2	T42.6X3	T42.6X4	T42.6X5	T42.6X6
testosterone	T38.7X1	T38.7X2	T38.7X3	T38.7X4	T38.7X5	T38.7X6
thiouracil	T38.2X1	T38.2X2	T38.2X3	T38.2X4	T38.2X5	T38.2X6
Methylacetoxyprogesterone*	T38.5X1	T38.5X2	T38.5X3	T38.5X4	T38.5X5	T38.5X6
Methylamphetamine	T43.651	T43.652	T43.652	T43.654	T43.655	T43.656
Methylated spirit	T51.1X1	T51.1X2	T51.1X3	T51.1X4	—	—
Methylatropine nitrate	T44.3X1	T44.3X2	T44.3X3	T44.3X4	T44.3X5	T44.3X6
Methylbenactyzium bromide	T44.3X1	T44.3X2	T44.3X3	T44.3X4	T44.3X5	T44.3X6
Methylbenzethonium chloride	T49.0X1	T49.0X2	T49.0X3	T49.0X4	T49.0X5	T49.0X6
Methylcellulose	T47.4X1	T47.4X2	T47.4X3	T47.4X4	T47.4X5	T47.4X6
laxative	T47.4X1	T47.4X2	T47.4X3	T47.4X4	T47.4X5	T47.4X6
Methylchlorophenoxyacetic acid	T60.3X1	T60.3X2	T60.3X3	T60.3X4	—	—
Methyldopa	T46.5X1	T46.5X2	T46.5X3	T46.5X4	T46.5X5	T46.5X6
Methyldopate	T46.5X1	T46.5X2	T46.5X3	T46.5X4	T46.5X5	T46.5X6
Methylene						
blue	T50.6X1	T50.6X2	T50.6X3	T50.6X4	T50.6X5	T50.6X6
chloride or dichloride (solvent)	T53.4X1	T53.4X2	T53.4X3	T53.4X4	—	—
NEC						
Methylenedioxyamphetamine	T43.621	T43.622	T43.623	T43.624	T43.625	T43.626
Methylenedioxymeth-amphetamine	T43.641	T43.642	T43.643	T43.644	—	—
Methylergometrine	T48.0X1	T48.0X2	T48.0X3	T48.0X4	T48.0X5	T48.0X6
Methylergonovine	T48.0X1	T48.0X2	T48.0X3	T48.0X4	T48.0X5	T48.0X6
Methylestrenolone	T38.5X1	T38.5X2	T38.5X3	T38.5X4	T38.5X5	T38.5X6
Methylethyl cellulose	T50.991	T50.992	T50.993	T50.994	T50.995	T50.996
Methylhexabital	T42.3X1	T42.3X2	T42.3X3	T42.3X4	T42.3X5	T42.3X6
Methylmorphine	T40.2X1	T40.2X2	T40.2X3	T40.2X4	T40.2X5	T40.2X6
Methylparaben (ophthalmic)	T49.5X1	T49.5X2	T49.5X3	T49.5X4	T49.5X5	T49.5X6
Methylparafynol	T42.6X1	T42.6X2	T42.6X3	T42.6X4	T42.6X5	T42.6X6
Methylpentynol, methylpenthynol	T42.6X1	T42.6X2	T42.6X3	T42.6X4	T42.6X5	T42.6X6
Methylphenidate	T43.631	T43.632	T43.633	T43.634	T43.635	T43.636
Methylphenobarbital	T42.3X1	T42.3X2	T42.3X3	T42.3X4	T42.3X5	T42.3X6
Methylpolysiloxane	T47.1X1	T47.1X2	T47.1X3	T47.1X4	T47.1X5	T47.1X6
Methylprednisolone — see Methyl, prednisolone						
Methylrosaniline	T49.0X1	T49.0X2	T49.0X3	T49.0X4	T49.0X5	T49.0X6
Methylrosanilinium chloride	T49.0X1	T49.0X2	T49.0X3	T49.0X4	T49.0X5	T49.0X6
Methyltestosterone	T38.7X1	T38.7X2	T38.7X3	T38.7X4	T38.7X5	T38.7X6
Methylthionine chloride	T50.6X1	T50.6X2	T50.6X3	T50.6X4	T50.6X5	T50.6X6
Methylthioninium chloride	T50.6X1	T50.6X2	T50.6X3	T50.6X4	T50.6X5	T50.6X6
Methylthiouracil	T38.2X1	T38.2X2	T38.2X3	T38.2X4	T38.2X5	T38.2X6
Methyprylon	T42.6X1	T42.6X2	T42.6X3	T42.6X4	T42.6X5	T42.6X6
Methysergide	T46.5X1	T46.5X2	T46.5X3	T46.5X4	T46.5X5	T46.5X6
Metiamide	T47.1X1	T47.1X2	T47.1X3	T47.1X4	T47.1X5	T47.1X6
Meticillin	T36.0X1	T36.0X2	T36.0X3	T36.0X4	T36.0X5	T36.0X6
Meticrane	T50.2X1	T50.2X2	T50.2X3	T50.2X4	T50.2X5	T50.2X6
Metildigoxin	T46.0X1	T46.0X2	T46.0X3	T46.0X4	T46.0X5	T46.0X6
Metipranolol	T49.5X1	T49.5X2	T49.5X3	T49.5X4	T49.5X5	T49.5X6
Metirosine	T46.5X1	T46.5X2	T46.5X3	T46.5X4	T46.5X5	T46.5X6
Metisazone	T37.5X1	T37.5X2	T37.5X3	T37.5X4	T37.5X5	T37.5X6
Metixene	T44.3X1	T44.3X2	T44.3X3	T44.3X4	T44.3X5	T44.3X6
Metizoline	T48.5X1	T48.5X2	T48.5X3	T48.5X4	T48.5X5	T48.5X6
Metoclopramide	T45.0X1	T45.0X2	T45.0X3	T45.0X4	T45.0X5	T45.0X6
Metofenazate	T43.3X1	T43.3X2	T43.3X3	T43.3X4	T43.3X5	T43.3X6
Metofoline	T39.8X1	T39.8X2	T39.8X3	T39.8X4	T39.8X5	T39.8X6
Metolazone	T50.2X1	T50.2X2	T50.2X3	T50.2X4	T50.2X5	T50.2X6
Metopon	T40.2X1	T40.2X2	T40.2X3	T40.2X4	T40.2X5	T40.2X6
Metoprine	T45.1X1	T45.1X2	T45.1X3	T45.1X4	T45.1X5	T45.1X6
Metoprolol	T44.7X1	T44.7X2	T44.7X3	T44.7X4	T44.7X5	T44.7X6
Metrifonate	T60.0X1	T60.0X2	T60.0X3	T60.0X4		
Metrizamide	T50.8X1	T50.8X2	T50.8X3	T50.8X4	T50.8X5	T50.8X6
Metrizoic acid	T50.8X1	T50.8X2	T50.8X3	T50.8X4	T50.8X5	T50.8X6
Metronidazole	T37.8X1	T37.8X2	T37.8X3	T37.8X4	T37.8X5	T37.8X6
Metycaine	T41.3X1	T41.3X2	T41.3X3	T41.3X4	T41.3X5	T41.3X6
infiltration (subcutaneous)	T41.3X1	T41.3X2	T41.3X3	T41.3X4	T41.3X5	T41.3X6

Table of Drugs and Chemicals

Substance	Poisoning, Accidental (unintentional)	Poisoning, Intentional Self-harm	Poisoning, Assault	Poisoning, Undetermined	Adverse Effect	Under-dosing
Metycaine — *continued*						
nerve block (peripheral) (plexus)	T41.3X1	T41.3X2	T41.3X3	T41.3X4	T41.3X5	T41.3X6
topical (surface)	T41.3X1	T41.3X2	T41.3X3	T41.3X4	T41.3X5	T41.3X6
Metyrapone	T50.8X1	T50.8X2	T50.8X3	T50.8X4	T50.8X5	T50.8X6
Mevacor*	T46.6X1	T46.6X2	T46.6X3	T46.6X4	T46.6X5	T46.6X6
Mevinphos	T60.0X1	T60.0X2	T60.0X3	T60.0X4	—	—
Mexazolam	T42.4X1	T42.4X2	T42.4X3	T42.4X4	T42.4X5	T42.4X6
Mexenone	T49.3X1	T49.3X2	T49.3X3	T49.3X4	T49.3X5	T49.3X6
Mexiletine	T46.2X1	T46.2X2	T46.2X3	T46.2X4	T46.2X5	T46.2X6
Mezereon	T62.2X1	T62.2X2	T62.2X3	T62.2X4	—	—
berries	T62.1X1	T62.1X2	T62.1X3	T62.1X4	—	—
Mezlocillin	T36.0X1	T36.0X2	T36.0X3	T36.0X4	T36.0X5	T36.0X6
Mianserin	T43.021	T43.022	T43.023	T43.024	T43.025	T43.026
Micatin	T49.0X1	T49.0X2	T49.0X3	T49.0X4	T49.0X5	T49.0X6
Miconazole	T49.0X1	T49.0X2	T49.0X3	T49.0X4	T49.0X5	T49.0X6
Micronomicin	T36.5X1	T36.5X2	T36.5X3	T36.5X4	T36.5X5	T36.5X6
Microzide*	T50.2X1	T50.2X2	T50.2X3	T50.2X4	T50.2X5	T50.2X6
Midazolam	T42.4X1	T42.4X2	T42.4X3	T42.4X4	T42.4X5	T42.4X6
Midecamycin	T36.3X1	T36.3X2	T36.3X3	T36.3X4	T36.3X5	T36.3X6
Mifepristone	T38.6X1	T38.6X2	T38.6X3	T38.6X4	T38.6X5	T38.6X6
Milk of magnesia	T47.1X1	T47.1X2	T47.1X3	T47.1X4	T47.1X5	T47.1X6
Millipede (tropical) (venomous)	T63.411	T63.412	T63.413	T63.414	—	—
Miltown	T43.591	T43.592	T43.593	T43.594	T43.595	T43.596
Milverine	T44.3X1	T44.3X2	T44.3X3	T44.3X4	T44.3X5	T44.3X6
Minaprine	T43.291	T43.292	T43.293	T43.294	T43.295	T43.296
Minaxolone	T41.291	T41.292	T41.293	T41.294	T41.295	T41.296
Mineral						
acids	T54.2X1	T54.2X2	T54.2X3	T54.2X4	—	—
oil (laxative)(medicinal)	T47.4X1	T47.4X2	T47.4X3	T47.4X4	T47.4X5	T47.4X6
emulsion	T47.2X1	T47.2X2	T47.2X3	T47.2X4	T47.2X5	T47.2X6
nonmedicinal	T52.0X1	T52.0X2	T52.0X3	T52.0X4	—	—
topical	T49.3X1	T49.3X2	T49.3X3	T49.3X4	T49.3X5	T49.3X6
salt NEC	T50.3X1	T50.3X2	T50.3X3	T50.3X4	T50.3X5	T50.3X6
spirits	T52.0X1	T52.0X2	T52.0X3	T52.0X4	—	—
Mineralocorticosteroid	T50.0X1	T50.0X2	T50.0X3	T50.0X4	T50.0X5	T50.0X6
Minocycline	T36.4X1	T36.4X2	T36.4X3	T36.4X4	T36.4X5	T36.4X6
Minoxidil	T46.7X1	T46.7X2	T46.7X3	T46.7X4	T46.7X5	T46.7X6
Miokamycin	T36.3X1	T36.3X2	T36.3X3	T36.3X4	T36.3X5	T36.3X6
Miotic drug	T49.5X1	T49.5X2	T49.5X3	T49.5X4	T49.5X5	T49.5X6
Mipafox	T60.0X1	T60.0X2	T60.0X3	T60.0X4	—	—
Mipomersen*	T46.6X1	T46.6X2	T46.6X3	T46.6X4	T46.6X5	T46.6X6
Mirex	T60.1X1	T60.1X2	T60.1X3	T60.1X4	—	—
Mirtazapine	T43.021	T43.022	T43.023	T43.024	T43.025	T43.026
Misonidazole	T37.3X1	T37.3X2	T37.3X3	T37.3X4	T37.3X5	T37.3X6
Misoprostol	T47.1X1	T47.1X2	T47.1X3	T47.1X4	T47.1X5	T47.1X6
Mithramycin	T45.1X1	T45.1X2	T45.1X3	T45.1X4	T45.1X5	T45.1X6
Mitobronitol	T45.1X1	T45.1X2	T45.1X3	T45.1X4	T45.1X5	T45.1X6
Mitoguazone	T45.1X1	T45.1X2	T45.1X3	T45.1X4	T45.1X5	T45.1X6
Mitolactol	T45.1X1	T45.1X2	T45.1X3	T45.1X4	T45.1X5	T45.1X6
Mitomycin	T45.1X1	T45.1X2	T45.1X3	T45.1X4	T45.1X5	T45.1X6
Mitopodozide	T45.1X1	T45.1X2	T45.1X3	T45.1X4	T45.1X5	T45.1X6
Mitotane	T45.1X1	T45.1X2	T45.1X3	T45.1X4	T45.1X5	T45.1X6
Mitoxantrone	T45.1X1	T45.1X2	T45.1X3	T45.1X4	T45.1X5	T45.1X6
Mivacurium chloride	T48.1X1	T48.1X2	T48.1X3	T48.1X4	T48.1X5	T48.1X6
Miyari bacteria	T47.6X1	T47.6X2	T47.6X3	T47.6X4	T47.6X5	T47.6X6
Moclobemide	T43.1X1	T43.1X2	T43.1X3	T43.1X4	T43.1X5	T43.1X6
Moderil	T46.5X1	T46.5X2	T46.5X3	T46.5X4	T46.5X5	T46.5X6
Mofebutazone	T39.2X1	T39.2X2	T39.2X3	T39.2X4	T39.2X5	T39.2X6
Mogadon — *see* Nitrazepam						
Molindone	T43.591	T43.592	T43.593	T43.594	T43.595	T43.596
Molsidomine	T46.3X1	T46.3X2	T46.3X3	T46.3X4	T46.3X5	T46.3X6
Mometasone	T49.0X1	T49.0X2	T49.0X3	T49.0X4	T49.0X5	T49.0X6
Monistat	T49.0X1	T49.0X2	T49.0X3	T49.0X4	T49.0X5	T49.0X6
Monkshood	T62.2X1	T62.2X2	T62.2X3	T62.2X4	—	—
Monoamine oxidase inhibitor NEC	T43.1X1	T43.1X2	T43.1X3	T43.1X4	T43.1X5	T43.1X6
hydrazine	T43.1X1	T43.1X2	T43.1X3	T43.1X4	T43.1X5	T43.1X6
Monobenzone	T49.4X1	T49.4X2	T49.4X3	T49.4X4	T49.4X5	T49.4X6
Monochloroacetic acid	T60.3X1	T60.3X2	T60.3X3	T60.3X4	—	—
Monochlorobenzene	T53.7X1	T53.7X2	T53.7X3	T53.7X4	—	—
Monoethanolamine	T46.8X1	T46.8X2	T46.8X3	T46.8X4	T46.8X5	T46.8X6
oleate	T46.8X1	T46.8X2	T46.8X3	T46.8X4	T46.8X5	T46.8X6
Monooctanoin	T50.991	T50.992	T50.993	T50.994	T50.995	T50.996
Monophenylbutazone	T39.2X1	T39.2X2	T39.2X3	T39.2X4	T39.2X5	T39.2X6
Monopril*	T46.4X1	T46.4X2	T46.4X3	T46.4X4	T46.4X5	T46.4X6
Monosodium glutamate	T65.891	T65.892	T65.893	T65.894	—	—
Monosulfiram	T49.0X1	T49.0X2	T49.0X3	T49.0X4	T49.0X5	T49.0X6
Monoxide, carbon — *see* Carbon, monoxide						
Monoxidine hydrochloride	T46.1X1	T46.1X2	T46.1X3	T46.1X4	T46.1X5	T46.1X6
Monuron	T60.3X1	T60.3X2	T60.3X3	T60.3X4	—	—

Substance	Poisoning, Accidental (unintentional)	Poisoning, Intentional Self-harm	Poisoning, Assault	Poisoning, Undetermined	Adverse Effect	Under-dosing
Moperone	T43.4X1	T43.4X2	T43.4X3	T43.4X4	T43.4X5	T43.4X6
Mopidamol	T45.1X1	T45.1X2	T45.1X3	T45.1X4	T45.1X5	T45.1X6
MOPP (mechloreth-amine + vincristine + prednisone + procarba-zine)	T45.1X1	T45.1X2	T45.1X3	T45.1X4	T45.1X5	T45.1X6
Morfin	T40.2X1	T40.2X2	T40.2X3	T40.2X4	T40.2X5	T40.2X6
Morinamide	T37.1X1	T37.1X2	T37.1X3	T37.1X4	T37.1X5	T37.1X6
Morning glory seeds	T40.991	T40.992	T40.993	T40.994	—	—
Moroxydine	T37.5X1	T37.5X2	T37.5X3	T37.5X4	T37.5X5	T37.5X6
Morphazinamide	T37.1X1	T37.1X2	T37.1X3	T37.1X4	T37.1X5	T37.1X6
Morphine	T40.2X1	T40.2X2	T40.2X3	T40.2X4	T40.2X5	T40.2X6
antagonist	T50.7X1	T50.7X2	T50.7X3	T50.7X4	T50.7X5	T50.7X6
Morpholinylethylmorphine	T40.2X1	T40.2X2	T40.2X3	T40.2X4		
Morsuximide	T42.2X1	T42.2X2	T42.2X3	T42.2X4	T42.2X5	T42.2X6
Mosapramine	T43.591	T43.592	T43.593	T43.594	T43.595	T43.596
Moth balls — *see also* Pesticide	T60.2X1	T60.2X2	T60.2X3	T60.2X4	—	—
naphthalene	T60.2X1	T60.2X2	T60.2X3	T60.2X4	—	—
paradichlorobenzene	T60.1X1	T60.1X2	T60.1X3	T60.1X4	—	—
Motor exhaust gas	T58.01	T58.02	T58.03	T58.04		
Motrin*	T39.311	T39.312	T39.313	T39.314	T39.315	T39.316
Mouthwash (antiseptic) (zinc chloride)	T49.6X1	T49.6X2	T49.6X3	T49.6X4	T49.6X5	T49.6X6
Moxastine	T45.0X1	T45.0X2	T45.0X3	T45.0X4	T45.0X5	T45.0X6
Moxaverine	T44.3X1	T44.3X2	T44.3X3	T44.3X4	T44.3X5	T44.3X6
Moxisylyte	T46.7X1	T46.7X2	T46.7X3	T46.7X4	T46.7X5	T46.7X6
Mucilage, plant	T47.4X1	T47.4X2	T47.4X3	T47.4X4	T47.4X5	T47.4X6
Mucolytic drug	T48.4X1	T48.4X2	T48.4X3	T48.4X4	T48.4X5	T48.4X6
Mucomyst	T48.4X1	T48.4X2	T48.4X3	T48.4X4	T48.4X5	T48.4X6
Mucous membrane agents (external)	T49.91	T49.92	T49.93	T49.94	T49.95	T49.96
specified NEC	T49.8X1	T49.8X2	T49.8X3	T49.8X4	T49.8X5	T49.8X6
Multaq*	T46.2X1	T46.2X2	T46.2X3	T46.2X4	T46.2X5	T46.2X6
Multiple unspecified drugs, medicaments and biological substances	T50.911	T50.912	T50.913	T50.914	T50.915	T50.916
Mumps						
immune globulin (human)	T50.Z11	T50.Z12	T50.Z13	T50.Z14	T50.Z15	T50.Z16
skin test antigen	T50.8X1	T50.8X2	T50.8X3	T50.8X4	T50.8X5	T50.8X6
vaccine	T50.B91	T50.B92	T50.B93	T50.B94	T50.B95	T50.B96
Mumpsvax	T50.B91	T50.B92	T50.B93	T50.B94	T50.B95	T50.B96
Mupirocin	T49.0X1	T49.0X2	T49.0X3	T49.0X4	T49.0X5	T49.0X6
Muriatic acid — *see* Hydrochloric acid						
Muromonab-CD3	T45.1X1	T45.1X2	T45.1X3	T45.1X4	T45.1X5	T45.1X6
Muscle-action drug NEC	T48.201	T48.202	T48.203	T48.204	T48.205	T48.206
Muscle affecting agents NEC	T48.201	T48.202	T48.203	T48.204	T48.205	T48.206
oxytocic	T48.0X1	T48.0X2	T48.0X3	T48.0X4	T48.0X5	T48.0X6
relaxants	T48.201	T48.202	T48.203	T48.204	T48.205	T48.206
central nervous system	T42.8X1	T42.8X2	T42.8X3	T42.8X4	T42.8X5	T42.8X6
skeletal	T48.1X1	T48.1X2	T48.1X3	T48.1X4	T48.1X5	T48.1X6
smooth	T44.3X1	T44.3X2	T44.3X3	T44.3X4	T44.3X5	T44.3X6
Muscle relaxant — *see* Relaxant, muscle						
Muscle-tone depressant, central NEC	T42.8X1	T42.8X2	T42.8X3	T42.8X4	T42.8X5	T42.8X6
specified NEC	T42.8X1	T42.8X2	T42.8X3	T42.8X4	T42.8X5	T42.8X6
Mushroom, noxious	T62.0X1	T62.0X2	T62.0X3	T62.0X4	—	—
Mussel, noxious	T61.781	T61.782	T61.783	T61.784	—	—
Mustard (emetic)	T47.7X1	T47.7X2	T47.7X3	T47.7X4	T47.7X5	T47.7X6
black	T47.7X1	T47.7X2	T47.7X3	T47.7X4	T47.7X5	T47.7X6
gas, not in war	T59.91	T59.92	T59.93	T59.94	—	—
nitrogen	T45.1X1	T45.1X2	T45.1X3	T45.1X4	T45.1X5	T45.1X6
Mustine	T45.1X1	T45.1X2	T45.1X3	T45.1X4	T45.1X5	T45.1X6
M-vac	T45.1X1	T45.1X2	T45.1X3	T45.1X4	T45.1X5	T45.1X6
Mycifradin	T36.5X1	T36.5X2	T36.5X3	T36.5X4	T36.5X5	T36.5X6
topical	T49.0X1	T49.0X2	T49.0X3	T49.0X4	T49.0X5	T49.0X6
Mycitracin	T36.8X1	T36.8X2	T36.8X3	T36.8X4	T36.8X5	T36.8X6
ophthalmic preparation	T49.5X1	T49.5X2	T49.5X3	T49.5X4	T49.5X5	T49.5X6
Mycostatin	T36.7X1	T36.7X2	T36.7X3	T36.7X4	T36.7X5	T36.7X6
topical	T49.0X1	T49.0X2	T49.0X3	T49.0X4	T49.0X5	T49.0X6
Mycotoxins	T64.81	T64.82	T64.83	T64.84	—	—
aflatoxin	T64.01	T64.02	T64.03	T64.04	—	—
specified NEC	T64.81	T64.82	T64.83	T64.84	—	—
Mydriacyl	T44.3X1	T44.3X2	T44.3X3	T44.3X4	T44.3X5	T44.3X6
Mydriatic drug	T49.5X1	T49.5X2	T49.5X3	T49.5X4	T49.5X5	T49.5X6
Myelobromal	T45.1X1	T45.1X2	T45.1X3	T45.1X4	T45.1X5	T45.1X6
Myleran	T45.1X1	T45.1X2	T45.1X3	T45.1X4	T45.1X5	T45.1X6
Myochrysin (e)	T39.2X1	T39.2X2	T39.2X3	T39.2X4	T39.2X5	T39.2X6
Myoneural blocking agents	T48.1X1	T48.1X2	T48.1X3	T48.1X4	T48.1X5	T48.1X6
Myrac*	T36.4X1	T36.4X2	T36.4X3	T36.4X4	T36.4X5	T36.4X6

☑ Additional Character May Be Required — Refer to the Tabular List for Character Selection   *Optum Value-Add

Substance	Poisoning, Accidental (unintentional)	Poisoning, Intentional Self-harm	Poisoning, Assault	Poisoning, Undetermined	Adverse Effect	Under-dosing
Myralact	T49.0X1	T49.0X2	T49.0X3	T49.0X4	T49.0X5	T49.0X6
Myristica fragrans	T62.2X1	T62.2X2	T62.2X3	T62.2X4	—	—
Myristicin	T65.891	T65.892	T65.893	T65.894	—	—
Mysoline	T42.3X1	T42.3X2	T42.3X3	T42.3X4	T42.3X5	T42.3X6
Nabilone	T40.711	T40.712	T40.713	T40.714	T40.715	T40.716
Nabumetone	T39.391	T39.392	T39.393	T39.394	T39.395	T39.396
Nadolol	T44.7X1	T44.7X2	T44.7X3	T44.7X4	T44.7X5	T44.7X6
Nafcillin	T36.0X1	T36.0X2	T36.0X3	T36.0X4	T36.0X5	T36.0X6
Nafoxidine	T38.6X1	T38.6X2	T38.6X3	T38.6X4	T38.6X5	T38.6X6
Naftazone	T46.991	T46.992	T46.993	T46.994	T46.995	T46.996
Naftidrofuryl (oxalate)	T46.7X1	T46.7X2	T46.7X3	T46.7X4	T46.7X5	T46.7X6
Naftifine	T49.0X1	T49.0X2	T49.0X3	T49.0X4	T49.0X5	T49.0X6
Nail polish remover	T52.91	T52.92	T52.93	T52.94	—	—
Nalbuphine	T40.491	T40.492	T40.493	T40.494	T40.495	T40.496
Naled	T60.0X1	T60.0X2	T60.0X3	T60.0X4	—	—
Nalidixic acid	T37.8X1	T37.8X2	T37.8X3	T37.8X4	T37.8X5	T37.8X6
Nalorphine	T50.7X1	T50.7X2	T50.7X3	T50.7X4	T50.7X5	T50.7X6
Naloxone	T50.7X1	T50.7X2	T50.7X3	T50.7X4	T50.7X5	T50.7X6
Naltrexone	T50.7X1	T50.7X2	T50.7X3	T50.7X4	T50.7X5	T50.7X6
Namenda	T43.8X1	T43.8X2	T43.8X3	T43.8X4	T43.8X5	T43.8X6
Nandrolone	T38.7X1	T38.7X2	T38.7X3	T38.7X4	T38.7X5	T38.7X6
Naphazoline	T48.5X1	T48.5X2	T48.5X3	T48.5X4	T48.5X5	T48.5X6
Naphtha (painters') (petroleum)	T52.0X1	T52.0X2	T52.0X3	T52.0X4	—	—
solvent	T52.0X1	T52.0X2	T52.0X3	T52.0X4	—	—
vapor	T52.0X1	T52.0X2	T52.0X3	T52.0X4	—	—
Naphthalene (non-chlorinated)	T60.2X1	T60.2X2	T60.2X3	T60.2X4	—	—
chlorinated	T60.1X1	T60.1X2	T60.1X3	T60.1X4	—	—
vapor	T60.1X1	T60.1X2	T60.1X3	T60.1X4	—	—
insecticide or moth repellent	T60.2X1	T60.2X2	T60.2X3	T60.2X4	—	—
chlorinated	T60.1X1	T60.1X2	T60.1X3	T60.1X4	—	—
vapor	T60.2X1	T60.2X2	T60.2X3	T60.2X4	—	—
chlorinated	T60.1X1	T60.1X2	T60.1X3	T60.1X4	—	—
Naphthol	T65.891	T65.892	T65.893	T65.894	—	—
Naphthylamine	T65.891	T65.892	T65.893	T65.894	—	—
Naphthylthiourea (ANTU)	T60.4X1	T60.4X2	T60.4X3	T60.4X4	—	—
Naprosyn — see Naproxen						
Naproxen	T39.311	T39.312	T39.313	T39.314	T39.315	T39.316
Narcotic (drug)	T40.601	T40.602	T40.603	T40.604	T40.605	T40.606
analgesic NEC	T40.601	T40.602	T40.603	T40.604	T40.605	T40.606
antagonist	T50.7X1	T50.7X2	T50.7X3	T50.7X4	T50.7X5	T50.7X6
specified NEC	T40.691	T40.692	T40.693	T40.694	T40.695	T40.696
synthetic	T40.491	T40.492	T40.493	T40.494	T40.495	T40.496
Narcotine	T48.3X1	T48.3X2	T48.3X3	T48.3X4	T48.3X5	T48.3X6
Nardil	T43.1X1	T43.1X2	T43.1X3	T43.1X4	T43.1X5	T43.1X6
Nasacort*	T49.5X1	T49.5X2	T49.5X3	T49.5X4	T49.5X5	T49.5X6
Nasal drug NEC	T49.6X1	T49.6X2	T49.6X3	T49.6X4	T49.6X5	T49.6X6
Natamycin	T49.0X1	T49.0X2	T49.0X3	T49.0X4	T49.0X5	T49.0X6
Natrium cyanide — see Cyanide(s)						
Natural						
blood (product)	T45.8X1	T45.8X2	T45.8X3	T45.8X4	T45.8X5	T45.8X6
gas (piped)	T59.891	T59.892	T59.893	T59.894	—	—
incomplete combustion	T58.11	T58.12	T58.13	T58.14	—	—
Nealbarbital	T42.3X1	T42.3X2	T42.3X3	T42.3X4	T42.3X5	T42.3X6
Nectadon	T48.3X1	T48.3X2	T48.3X3	T48.3X4	T48.3X5	T48.3X6
Nedocromil	T48.6X1	T48.6X2	T48.6X3	T48.6X4	T48.6X5	T48.6X6
Nefopam	T39.8X1	T39.8X2	T39.8X3	T39.8X4	T39.8X5	T39.8X6
Nematocyst (sting)	T63.691	T63.692	T63.693	T63.694	—	—
Nembutal	T42.3X1	T42.3X2	T42.3X3	T42.3X4	T42.3X5	T42.3X6
Nemonapride	T43.591	T43.592	T43.593	T43.594	T43.595	T43.596
Neoarsphenamine	T37.8X1	T37.8X2	T37.8X3	T37.8X4	T37.8X5	T37.8X6
Neocinchophen	T50.4X1	T50.4X2	T50.4X3	T50.4X4	T50.4X5	T50.4X6
Neomycin (derivatives)	T36.5X1	T36.5X2	T36.5X3	T36.5X4	T36.5X5	T36.5X6
with						
bacitracin	T49.0X1	T49.0X2	T49.0X3	T49.0X4	T49.0X5	T49.0X6
neostigmine	T44.0X1	T44.0X2	T44.0X3	T44.0X4	T44.0X5	T44.0X6
ENT agent	T49.6X1	T49.6X2	T49.6X3	T49.6X4	T49.6X5	T49.6X6
ophthalmic preparation	T49.5X1	T49.5X2	T49.5X3	T49.5X4	T49.5X5	T49.5X6
topical NEC	T49.0X1	T49.0X2	T49.0X3	T49.0X4	T49.0X5	T49.0X6
Neonal	T42.3X1	T42.3X2	T42.3X3	T42.3X4	T42.3X5	T42.3X6
Neopham*	T50.3X1	T50.3X2	T50.3X3	T50.3X4	T50.3X5	T50.3X6
Neoprontosil	T37.0X1	T37.0X2	T37.0X3	T37.0X4	T37.0X5	T37.0X6
Neosalvarsan	T37.8X1	T37.8X2	T37.8X3	T37.8X4	T37.8X5	T37.8X6
Neosilversalvarsan	T37.8X1	T37.8X2	T37.8X3	T37.8X4	T37.8X5	T37.8X6
Neosporin	T36.8X1	T36.8X2	T36.8X3	T36.8X4	T36.8X5	T36.8X6
ENT agent	T49.6X1	T49.6X2	T49.6X3	T49.6X4	T49.6X5	T49.6X6
opthalmic preparation	T49.5X1	T49.5X2	T49.5X3	T49.5X4	T49.5X5	T49.5X6
topical NEC	T49.0X1	T49.0X2	T49.0X3	T49.0X4	T49.0X5	T49.0X6
Neostigmine bromide	T44.0X1	T44.0X2	T44.0X3	T44.0X4	T44.0X5	T44.0X6
Neraval	T42.3X1	T42.3X2	T42.3X3	T42.3X4	T42.3X5	T42.3X6
Neravan	T42.3X1	T42.3X2	T42.3X3	T42.3X4	T42.3X5	T42.3X6
Nerium oleander	T62.2X1	T62.2X2	T62.2X3	T62.2X4	—	—
Nerlynx*	T45.1X1	T45.1X2	T45.1X3	T45.1X4	T45.1X5	T45.1X6
Nerve gas, not in war	T59.91	T59.92	T59.93	T59.94	—	—
Nesacaine	T41.3X1	T41.3X2	T41.3X3	T41.3X4	T41.3X5	T41.3X6
infiltration (subcutaneous)	T41.3X1	T41.3X2	T41.3X3	T41.3X4	T41.3X5	T41.3X6
nerve block (peripheral) (plexus)	T41.3X1	T41.3X2	T41.3X3	T41.3X4	T41.3X5	T41.3X6
Netilmicin	T36.5X1	T36.5X2	T36.5X3	T36.5X4	T36.5X5	T36.5X6
Neurobarb	T42.3X1	T42.3X2	T42.3X3	T42.3X4	T42.3X5	T42.3X6
Neuroleptic drug NEC	T43.501	T43.502	T43.503	T43.504	T43.505	T43.506
Neuromuscular blocking drug	T48.1X1	T48.1X2	T48.1X3	T48.1X4	T48.1X5	T48.1X6
Neutral insulin injection	T38.3X1	T38.3X2	T38.3X3	T38.3X4	T38.3X5	T38.3X6
Neutral spirits	T51.0X1	T51.0X2	T51.0X3	T51.0X4	—	—
beverage	T51.0X1	T51.0X2	T51.0X3	T51.0X4	—	—
Niacin	T46.7X1	T46.7X2	T46.7X3	T46.7X4	T46.7X5	T46.7X6
Niacinamide	T45.2X1	T45.2X2	T45.2X3	T45.2X4	T45.2X5	T45.2X6
Nialamide	T43.1X1	T43.1X2	T43.1X3	T43.1X4	T43.1X5	T43.1X6
Niaprazine	T42.6X1	T42.6X2	T42.6X3	T42.6X4	T42.6X5	T42.6X6
Nicametate	T46.7X1	T46.7X2	T46.7X3	T46.7X4	T46.7X5	T46.7X6
Nicardipine	T46.1X1	T46.1X2	T46.1X3	T46.1X4	T46.1X5	T46.1X6
Nicergoline	T46.7X1	T46.7X2	T46.7X3	T46.7X4	T46.7X5	T46.7X6
Nickel (carbonyl) (tetra-carbonyl) (fumes) (vapor)	T56.891	T56.892	T56.893	T56.894	—	—
Nickelocene	T56.891	T56.892	T56.893	T56.894	—	—
Niclosamide	T37.4X1	T37.4X2	T37.4X3	T37.4X4	T37.4X5	T37.4X6
Nicofuranose	T46.7X1	T46.7X2	T46.7X3	T46.7X4	T46.7X5	T46.7X6
Nicomorphine	T40.2X1	T40.2X2	T40.2X3	T40.2X4	—	—
Nicorandil	T46.3X1	T46.3X2	T46.3X3	T46.3X4	T46.3X5	T46.3X6
Nicotiana (plant)	T62.2X1	T62.2X2	T62.2X3	T62.2X4	—	—
Nicotinamide	T45.2X1	T45.2X2	T45.2X3	T45.2X4	T45.2X5	T45.2X6
Nicotine (insecticide) (spray) (sulfate) NEC	T60.2X1	T60.2X2	T60.2X3	T60.2X4	—	—
from tobacco	T65.291	T65.292	T65.293	T65.294	—	—
cigarettes	T65.221	T65.222	T65.223	T65.224	—	—
not insecticide	T65.291	T65.292	T65.293	T65.294	—	—
Nicotinic acid	T46.7X1	T46.7X2	T46.7X3	T46.7X4	T46.7X5	T46.7X6
Nicotinyl alcohol	T46.7X1	T46.7X2	T46.7X3	T46.7X4	T46.7X5	T46.7X6
Nicoumalone	T45.511	T45.512	T45.513	T45.514	T45.515	T45.516
Nifedipine	T46.1X1	T46.1X2	T46.1X3	T46.1X4	T46.1X5	T46.1X6
Nifenazone	T39.2X1	T39.2X2	T39.2X3	T39.2X4	T39.2X5	T39.2X6
Nifuraldezone	T37.91	T37.92	T37.93	T37.94	T37.95	T37.96
Nifuratel	T37.8X1	T37.8X2	T37.8X3	T37.8X4	T37.8X5	T37.8X6
Nifurtimox	T37.3X1	T37.3X2	T37.3X3	T37.3X4	T37.3X5	T37.3X6
Nifurtoinol	T37.8X1	T37.8X2	T37.8X3	T37.8X4	T37.8X5	T37.8X6
Nightshade, deadly (solanum) — see also Belladonna	T62.2X1	T62.2X2	T62.2X3	T62.2X4	—	—
berry	T62.1X1	T62.1X2	T62.1X3	T62.1X4	—	—
Nikethamide	T50.7X1	T50.7X2	T50.7X3	T50.7X4	T50.7X5	T50.7X6
Nilstat	T36.7X1	T36.7X2	T36.7X3	T36.7X4	T36.7X5	T36.7X6
topical	T49.0X1	T49.0X2	T49.0X3	T49.0X4	T49.0X5	T49.0X6
Nilutamide	T38.6X1	T38.6X2	T38.6X3	T38.6X4	T38.6X5	T38.6X6
Nimesulide	T39.391	T39.392	T39.393	T39.394	T39.395	T39.396
Nimetazepam	T42.4X1	T42.4X2	T42.4X3	T42.4X4	T42.4X5	T42.4X6
Nimodipine	T46.1X1	T46.1X2	T46.1X3	T46.1X4	T46.1X5	T46.1X6
Nimorazole	T37.3X1	T37.3X2	T37.3X3	T37.3X4	T37.3X5	T37.3X6
Nimustine	T45.1X1	T45.1X2	T45.1X3	T45.1X4	T45.1X5	T45.1X6
Nipent*	T45.1X1	T45.1X2	T45.1X3	T45.1X4	T45.1X5	T45.1X6
Niridazole	T37.4X1	T37.4X2	T37.4X3	T37.4X4	T37.4X5	T37.4X6
Nisentil	T40.2X1	T40.2X2	T40.2X3	T40.2X4	T40.2X5	T40.2X6
Nisoldipine	T46.1X1	T46.1X2	T46.1X3	T46.1X4	T46.1X5	T46.1X6
Nitramine	T65.3X1	T65.3X2	T65.3X3	T65.3X4	—	—
Nitrate, organic	T46.3X1	T46.3X2	T46.3X3	T46.3X4	T46.3X5	T46.3X6
Nitrazepam	T42.4X1	T42.4X2	T42.4X3	T42.4X4	T42.4X5	T42.4X6
Nitrefazole	T50.6X1	T50.6X2	T50.6X3	T50.6X4	T50.6X5	T50.6X6
Nitrendipine	T46.1X1	T46.1X2	T46.1X3	T46.1X4	T46.1X5	T46.1X6
Nitric						
acid (liquid)	T54.2X1	T54.2X2	T54.2X3	T54.2X4	—	—
vapor	T59.891	T59.892	T59.893	T59.894	—	—
oxide (gas)	T59.0X1	T59.0X2	T59.0X3	T59.0X4	—	—
Nitrimidazine	T37.3X1	T37.3X2	T37.3X3	T37.3X4	T37.3X5	T37.3X6
Nitrite, amyl (medicinal) (vapor)	T46.3X1	T46.3X2	T46.3X3	T46.3X4	T46.3X5	T46.3X6
Nitroaniline	T65.3X1	T65.3X2	T65.3X3	T65.3X4	—	—
vapor	T59.891	T59.892	T59.893	T59.894	—	—
Nitrobenzene, nitrobenzol	T65.3X1	T65.3X2	T65.3X3	T65.3X4	—	—
vapor	T65.3X1	T65.3X2	T65.3X3	T65.3X4	—	—
Nitrocellulose	T65.891	T65.892	T65.893	T65.894	—	—
lacquer	T65.891	T65.892	T65.893	T65.894	—	—
Nitrodiphenyl	T65.3X1	T65.3X2	T65.3X3	T65.3X4	—	—
Nitrofural	T49.0X1	T49.0X2	T49.0X3	T49.0X4	T49.0X5	T49.0X6
Nitrofurantoin	T37.8X1	T37.8X2	T37.8X3	T37.8X4	T37.8X5	T37.8X6

Table of Drugs and Chemicals

Substance	Poisoning, Accidental (unintentional)	Poisoning, Intentional Self-harm	Poisoning, Assault	Poisoning, Undetermined	Adverse Effect	Under-dosing
Nitrofurazone	T49.0X1	T49.0X2	T49.0X3	T49.0X4	T49.0X5	T49.0X6
Nitrogen	T59.0X1	T59.0X2	T59.0X3	T59.0X4	—	—
mustard	T45.1X1	T45.1X2	T45.1X3	T45.1X4	T45.1X5	T45.1X6
Nitroglycerin, nitroglycerol (medicinal)	T46.3X1	T46.3X2	T46.3X3	T46.3X4	T46.3X5	T46.3X6
nonmedicinal	T65.5X1	T65.5X2	T65.5X3	T65.5X4	—	—
fumes	T65.5X1	T65.5X2	T65.5X3	T65.5X4	—	—
Nitroglycol	T52.3X1	T52.3X2	T52.3X3	T52.3X4	—	—
Nitrohydrochloric acid	T54.2X1	T54.2X2	T54.2X3	T54.2X4	—	—
Nitromersol	T49.0X1	T49.0X2	T49.0X3	T49.0X4	T49.0X5	T49.0X6
Nitronaphthalene	T65.891	T65.892	T65.893	T65.894	—	—
Nitrophenol	T54.0X1	T54.0X2	T54.0X3	T54.0X4	—	—
Nitropropane	T52.8X1	T52.8X2	T52.8X3	T52.8X4	—	—
Nitroprusside	T46.5X1	T46.5X2	T46.5X3	T46.5X4	T46.5X5	T46.5X6
Nitrosodimethylamine	T65.3X1	T65.3X2	T65.3X3	T65.3X4	—	—
Nitrothiazol	T37.4X1	T37.4X2	T37.4X3	T37.4X4	T37.4X5	T37.4X6
Nitrotoluene, nitrotoluol	T65.3X1	T65.3X2	T65.3X3	T65.3X4	—	—
vapor	T65.3X1	T65.3X2	T65.3X3	T65.3X4	—	—
Nitrous						
acid (liquid)	T54.2X1	T54.2X2	T54.2X3	T54.2X4	—	—
fumes	T59.891	T59.892	T59.893	T59.894	—	—
ether spirit	T46.3X1	T46.3X2	T46.3X3	T46.3X4	T46.3X5	T46.3X6
oxide	T41.0X1	T41.0X2	T41.0X3	T41.0X4	T41.0X5	T41.0X6
Nitroxoline	T37.8X1	T37.8X2	T37.8X3	T37.8X4	T37.8X5	T37.8X6
Nitrozone	T49.0X1	T49.0X2	T49.0X3	T49.0X4	T49.0X5	T49.0X6
Nizatidine	T47.0X1	T47.0X2	T47.0X3	T47.0X4	T47.0X5	T47.0X6
Nizofenone	T43.8X1	T43.8X2	T43.8X3	T43.8X4	T43.8X5	T43.8X6
Noctec	T42.6X1	T42.6X2	T42.6X3	T42.6X4	T42.6X5	T42.6X6
No Doz*	T43.611	T43.612	T43.613	T43.614	T43.615	T43.616
Noludar	T42.6X1	T42.6X2	T42.6X3	T42.6X4	T42.6X5	T42.6X6
Nomegestrol	T38.5X1	T38.5X2	T38.5X3	T38.5X4	T38.5X5	T38.5X6
Nomifensine	T43.291	T43.292	T43.293	T43.294	T43.295	T43.296
Nonoxinol	T49.8X1	T49.8X2	T49.8X3	T49.8X4	T49.8X5	T49.8X6
Nonylphenoxy (polyethoxyethanol)	T49.8X1	T49.8X2	T49.8X3	T49.8X4	T49.8X5	T49.8X6
Noptil	T42.3X1	T42.3X2	T42.3X3	T42.3X4	T42.3X5	T42.3X6
Noradrenaline	T44.4X1	T44.4X2	T44.4X3	T44.4X4	T44.4X5	T44.4X6
Noramidopyrine	T39.2X1	T39.2X2	T39.2X3	T39.2X4	T39.2X5	T39.2X6
methanesulfonate sodium	T39.2X1	T39.2X2	T39.2X3	T39.2X4	T39.2X5	T39.2X6
Norbormide	T60.4X1	T60.4X2	T60.4X3	T60.4X4	—	—
Nordazepam	T42.4X1	T42.4X2	T42.4X3	T42.4X4	T42.4X5	T42.4X6
Norepinephrine	T44.4X1	T44.4X2	T44.4X3	T44.4X4	T44.4X5	T44.4X6
Norethandrolone	T38.7X1	T38.7X2	T38.7X3	T38.7X4	T38.7X5	T38.7X6
Norethindrone	T38.4X1	T38.4X2	T38.4X3	T38.4X4	T38.4X5	T38.4X6
Norethisterone (acetate) (enantate)	T38.4X1	T38.4X2	T38.4X3	T38.4X4	T38.4X5	T38.4X6
with ethinylestradiol	T38.5X1	T38.5X2	T38.5X3	T38.5X4	T38.5X5	T38.5X6
Noretynodrel	T38.5X1	T38.5X2	T38.5X3	T38.5X4	T38.5X5	T38.5X6
Norfenefrine	T44.4X1	T44.4X2	T44.4X3	T44.4X4	T44.4X5	T44.4X6
Norfloxacin	T36.8X1	T36.8X2	T36.8X3	T36.8X4	T36.8X5	T36.8X6
Norgestrel	T38.4X1	T38.4X2	T38.4X3	T38.4X4	T38.4X5	T38.4X6
Norgestrienone	T38.4X1	T38.4X2	T38.4X3	T38.4X4	T38.4X5	T38.4X6
Norlestrin	T38.4X1	T38.4X2	T38.4X3	T38.4X4	T38.4X5	T38.4X6
Norlutin	T38.4X1	T38.4X2	T38.4X3	T38.4X4	T38.4X5	T38.4X6
Normal serum albumin (human), salt-poor	T45.8X1	T45.8X2	T45.8X3	T45.8X4	T45.8X5	T45.8X6
Normethandrone	T38.5X1	T38.5X2	T38.5X3	T38.5X4	T38.5X5	T38.5X6
Normison — *see* Benzodiazepines						
Normorphine	T40.2X1	T40.2X2	T40.2X3	T40.2X4	—	—
Norpseudoephedrine	T50.5X1	T50.5X2	T50.5X3	T50.5X4	T50.5X5	T50.5X6
Nortestosterone (furanpropionate)	T38.7X1	T38.7X2	T38.7X3	T38.7X4	T38.7X5	T38.7X6
Nortriptyline	T43.011	T43.012	T43.013	T43.014	T43.015	T43.016
Norvasc*	T46.1X1	T46.1X2	T46.1X3	T46.1X4	T46.1X5	T46.1X6
Noscapine	T48.3X1	T48.3X2	T48.3X3	T48.3X4	T48.3X5	T48.3X6
Nose preparations	T49.6X1	T49.6X2	T49.6X3	T49.6X4	T49.6X5	T49.6X6
Novobiocin	T36.5X1	T36.5X2	T36.5X3	T36.5X4	T36.5X5	T36.5X6
Novocain (infiltration) (topical)	T41.3X1	T41.3X2	T41.3X3	T41.3X4	T41.3X5	T41.3X6
nerve block (peripheral) (plexus)	T41.3X1	T41.3X2	T41.3X3	T41.3X4	T41.3X5	T41.3X6
spinal	T41.3X1	T41.3X2	T41.3X3	T41.3X4	T41.3X5	T41.3X6
Noxious foodstuff	T62.91	T62.92	T62.93	T62.94	—	—
specified NEC	T62.8X1	T62.8X2	T62.8X3	T62.8X4	—	—
Noxiptiline	T43.011	T43.012	T43.013	T43.014	T43.015	T43.016
Noxytiolin	T49.0X1	T49.0X2	T49.0X3	T49.0X4	T49.0X5	T49.0X6
NPH Iletin (insulin)	T38.3X1	T38.3X2	T38.3X3	T38.3X4	T38.3X5	T38.3X6
Numorphan	T40.2X1	T40.2X2	T40.2X3	T40.2X4	T40.2X5	T40.2X6
Nunol	T42.3X1	T42.3X2	T42.3X3	T42.3X4	T42.3X5	T42.3X6
Nupercaine (spinal anesthetic)	T41.3X1	T41.3X2	T41.3X3	T41.3X4	T41.3X5	T41.3X6
topical (surface)	T41.3X1	T41.3X2	T41.3X3	T41.3X4	T41.3X5	T41.3X6
Nutmeg oil (liniment)	T49.3X1	T49.3X2	T49.3X3	T49.3X4	T49.3X5	T49.3X6
Nutrilipid*	T50.991	T50.992	T50.993	T50.994	T50.995	T50.996
Nutritional supplement	T50.901	T50.902	T50.903	T50.904	T50.905	T50.906
Nux vomica	T65.1X1	T65.1X2	T65.1X3	T65.1X4	—	—
Nydrazid	T37.1X1	T37.1X2	T37.1X3	T37.1X4	T37.1X5	T37.1X6
Nylidrin	T46.7X1	T46.7X2	T46.7X3	T46.7X4	T46.7X5	T46.7X6
Nystatin	T36.7X1	T36.7X2	T36.7X3	T36.7X4	T36.7X5	T36.7X6
topical	T49.0X1	T49.0X2	T49.0X3	T49.0X4	T49.0X5	T49.0X6
Nytol	T45.0X1	T45.0X2	T45.0X3	T45.0X4	T45.0X5	T45.0X6
Obidoxime chloride	T50.6X1	T50.6X2	T50.6X3	T50.6X4	T50.6X5	T50.6X6
Octafonium (chloride)	T49.3X1	T49.3X2	T49.3X3	T49.3X4	T49.3X5	T49.3X6
Octamethyl pyrophosphoramide	T60.0X1	T60.0X2	T60.0X3	T60.0X4	—	—
Octanoin	T50.991	T50.992	T50.993	T50.994	T50.995	T50.996
Octatropine methylbromide	T44.3X1	T44.3X2	T44.3X3	T44.3X4	T44.3X5	T44.3X6
Octotiamine	T45.2X1	T45.2X2	T45.2X3	T45.2X4	T45.2X5	T45.2X6
Octoxinol (9)	T49.8X1	T49.8X2	T49.8X3	T49.8X4	T49.8X5	T49.8X6
Octreotide	T38.991	T38.992	T38.993	T38.994	T38.995	T38.996
Octyl nitrite	T46.3X1	T46.3X2	T46.3X3	T46.3X4	T46.3X5	T46.3X6
Oestradiol	T38.5X1	T38.5X2	T38.5X3	T38.5X4	T38.5X5	T38.5X6
Oestriol	T38.5X1	T38.5X2	T38.5X3	T38.5X4	T38.5X5	T38.5X6
Oestrogen	T38.5X1	T38.5X2	T38.5X3	T38.5X4	T38.5X5	T38.5X6
Oestrone	T38.5X1	T38.5X2	T38.5X3	T38.5X4	T38.5X5	T38.5X6
Ofloxacin	T36.8X1	T36.8X2	T36.8X3	T36.8X4	T36.8X5	T36.8X6
Oil (of)	T65.891	T65.892	T65.893	T65.894	—	—
bitter almond	T62.8X1	T62.8X2	T62.8X3	T62.8X4	—	—
cloves	T49.7X1	T49.7X2	T49.7X3	T49.7X4	T49.7X5	T49.7X6
colors	T65.6X1	T65.6X2	T65.6X3	T65.6X4	—	—
fumes	T59.891	T59.892	T59.893	T59.894	—	—
lubricating	T52.0X1	T52.0X2	T52.0X3	T52.0X4	—	—
Niobe	T52.8X1	T52.8X2	T52.8X3	T52.8X4	—	—
vitriol (liquid)	T54.2X1	T54.2X2	T54.2X3	T54.2X4	—	—
fumes	T54.2X1	T54.2X2	T54.2X3	T54.2X4	—	—
wintergreen (bitter) NEC	T49.3X1	T49.3X2	T49.3X3	T49.3X4	T49.3X5	T49.3X6
Oily preparation (for skin)	T49.3X1	T49.3X2	T49.3X3	T49.3X4	T49.3X5	T49.3X6
Ointment NEC	T49.3X1	T49.3X2	T49.3X3	T49.3X4	T49.3X5	T49.3X6
Olanzapine	T43.591	T43.592	T43.593	T43.594	T43.595	T43.596
Oleander	T62.2X1	T62.2X2	T62.2X3	T62.2X4	—	—
Oleandomycin	T36.3X1	T36.3X2	T36.3X3	T36.3X4	T36.3X5	T36.3X6
Oleandrin	T46.0X1	T46.0X2	T46.0X3	T46.0X4	T46.0X5	T46.0X6
Oleic acid	T46.6X1	T46.6X2	T46.6X3	T46.6X4	T46.6X5	T46.6X6
Oleovitamin A	T45.2X1	T45.2X2	T45.2X3	T45.2X4	T45.2X5	T45.2X6
Oleum ricini	T47.2X1	T47.2X2	T47.2X3	T47.2X4	T47.2X5	T47.2X6
Olive oil (medicinal) NEC	T47.4X1	T47.4X2	T47.4X3	T47.4X4	T47.4X5	T47.4X6
Olivomycin	T45.1X1	T45.1X2	T45.1X3	T45.1X4	T45.1X5	T45.1X6
Olodaterol*	T48.6X1	T48.6X2	T48.6X3	T48.6X4	T48.6X5	T48.6X6
Olsalazine	T47.8X1	T47.8X2	T47.8X3	T47.8X4	T47.8X5	T47.8X6
Omeprazole	T47.1X1	T47.1X2	T47.1X3	T47.1X4	T47.1X5	T47.1X6
OMPA	T60.0X1	T60.0X2	T60.0X3	T60.0X4	—	—
Oncovin	T45.1X1	T45.1X2	T45.1X3	T45.1X4	T45.1X5	T45.1X6
Ondansetron	T45.0X1	T45.0X2	T45.0X3	T45.0X4	T45.0X5	T45.0X6
Ophthaine	T41.3X1	T41.3X2	T41.3X3	T41.3X4	T41.3X5	T41.3X6
Ophthetic	T41.3X1	T41.3X2	T41.3X3	T41.3X4	T41.3X5	T41.3X6
Opiate NEC	T40.601	T40.602	T40.603	T40.604	T40.605	T40.606
antagonists	T50.7X1	T50.7X2	T50.7X3	T50.7X4	T50.7X5	T50.7X6
Opioid NEC	T40.2X1	T40.2X2	T40.2X3	T40.2X4	T40.2X5	T40.2X6
Opipramol	T43.011	T43.012	T43.013	T43.014	T43.015	T43.016
Opium alkaloids (total)	T40.0X1	T40.0X2	T40.0X3	T40.0X4	T40.0X5	T40.0X6
standardized powdered	T40.0X1	T40.0X2	T40.0X3	T40.0X4	T40.0X5	T40.0X6
tincture (camphorated)	T40.0X1	T40.0X2	T40.0X3	T40.0X4	T40.0X5	T40.0X6
Optivar*	T49.5X1	T49.5X2	T49.5X3	T49.5X4	T49.5X5	T49.5X6
Oracon	T38.4X1	T38.4X2	T38.4X3	T38.4X4	T38.4X5	T38.4X6
Oragrafin	T50.8X1	T50.8X2	T50.8X3	T50.8X4	T50.8X5	T50.8X6
Oral contraceptives	T38.4X1	T38.4X2	T38.4X3	T38.4X4	T38.4X5	T38.4X6
Oral rehydration salts	T50.3X1	T50.3X2	T50.3X3	T50.3X4	T50.3X5	T50.3X6
Orazamide	T50.991	T50.992	T50.993	T50.994	T50.995	T50.996
Orciprenaline	T48.291	T48.292	T48.293	T48.294	T48.295	T48.296
Organidin	T48.4X1	T48.4X2	T48.4X3	T48.4X4	T48.4X5	T48.4X6
Organonitrate NEC	T46.3X1	T46.3X2	T46.3X3	T46.3X4	T46.3X5	T46.3X6
Organophosphates	T60.0X1	T60.0X2	T60.0X3	T60.0X4	—	—
Orimune	T50.B91	T50.B92	T50.B93	T50.B94	T50.B95	T50.B96
Orinase	T38.3X1	T38.3X2	T38.3X3	T38.3X4	T38.3X5	T38.3X6
Ormeloxifene	T38.6X1	T38.6X2	T38.6X3	T38.6X4	T38.6X5	T38.6X6
Ornidazole	T37.3X1	T37.3X2	T37.3X3	T37.3X4	T37.3X5	T37.3X6
Ornithine aspartate	T50.991	T50.992	T50.993	T50.994	T50.995	T50.996
Ornoprostil	T47.1X1	T47.1X2	T47.1X3	T47.1X4	T47.1X5	T47.1X6
Orphenadrine (hydrochloride)	T42.8X1	T42.8X2	T42.8X3	T42.8X4	T42.8X5	T42.8X6
Ortal (sodium)	T42.3X1	T42.3X2	T42.3X3	T42.3X4	T42.3X5	T42.3X6
Orthoboric acid	T49.0X1	T49.0X2	T49.0X3	T49.0X4	T49.0X5	T49.0X6
ENT agent	T49.6X1	T49.6X2	T49.6X3	T49.6X4	T49.6X5	T49.6X6
ophthalmic preparation	T49.5X1	T49.5X2	T49.5X3	T49.5X4	T49.5X5	T49.5X6

☑ **Additional Character May Be Required — Refer to the Tabular List for Character Selection**

*Optum Value-Add

Nitrofurazone — Orthoboric acid

Substance	Poisoning, Accidental (unintentional)	Poisoning, Intentional Self-harm	Poisoning, Assault	Poisoning, Undetermined	Adverse Effect	Under-dosing
Orthocaine	T41.3X1	T41.3X2	T41.3X3	T41.3X4	T41.3X5	T41.3X6
Orthodichlorobenzene	T53.7X1	T53.7X2	T53.7X3	T53.7X4	—	—
Ortho-Novum	T38.4X1	T38.4X2	T38.4X3	T38.4X4	T38.4X5	T38.4X6
Orthotolidine (reagent)	T54.2X1	T54.2X2	T54.2X3	T54.2X4	—	—
Osmic acid (liquid)	T54.2X1	T54.2X2	T54.2X3	T54.2X4	—	—
fumes	T54.2X1	T54.2X2	T54.2X3	T54.2X4	—	—
Osmotic diuretics	T50.2X1	T50.2X2	T50.2X3	T50.2X4	T50.2X5	T50.2X6
Otilonium bromide	T44.3X1	T44.3X2	T44.3X3	T44.3X4	T44.3X5	T44.3X6
Otorhinolaryngological drug NEC	T49.6X1	T49.6X2	T49.6X3	T49.6X4	T49.6X5	T49.6X6
Ouabain (e)	T46.0X1	T46.0X2	T46.0X3	T46.0X4	T46.0X5	T46.0X6
Ovarian						
hormone	T38.5X1	T38.5X2	T38.5X3	T38.5X4	T38.5X5	T38.5X6
stimulant	T38.5X1	T38.5X2	T38.5X3	T38.5X4	T38.5X5	T38.5X6
Ovide*	T49.0X1	T49.0X2	T49.0X3	T49.0X4	T49.0X5	T49.0X6
Ovral	T38.4X1	T38.4X2	T38.4X3	T38.4X4	T38.4X5	T38.4X6
Ovulen	T38.4X1	T38.4X2	T38.4X3	T38.4X4	T38.4X5	T38.4X6
Oxacillin	T36.0X1	T36.0X2	T36.0X3	T36.0X4	T36.0X5	T36.0X6
Oxalic acid	T54.2X1	T54.2X2	T54.2X3	T54.2X4	—	—
ammonium salt	T50.991	T50.992	T50.993	T50.994	T50.995	T50.996
Oxamniquine	T37.4X1	T37.4X2	T37.4X3	T37.4X4	T37.4X5	T37.4X6
Oxanamide	T43.591	T43.592	T43.593	T43.595	T43.595	T43.596
Oxandrolone	T38.7X1	T38.7X2	T38.7X3	T38.7X4	T38.7X5	T38.7X6
Oxantel	T37.4X1	T37.4X2	T37.4X3	T37.4X4	T37.4X5	T37.4X6
Oxapium iodide	T44.3X1	T44.3X2	T44.3X3	T44.3X4	T44.3X5	T44.3X6
Oxaprotiline	T43.021	T43.022	T43.023	T43.024	T43.025	T43.026
Oxaprozin	T39.311	T39.312	T39.313	T39.314	T39.315	T39.316
Oxatomide	T45.0X1	T45.0X2	T45.0X3	T45.0X4	T45.0X5	T45.0X6
Oxazepam	T42.4X1	T42.4X2	T42.4X3	T42.4X4	T42.4X5	T42.4X6
Oxazimedrine	T50.5X1	T50.5X2	T50.5X3	T50.5X4	T50.5X5	T50.5X6
Oxazolam	T42.4X1	T42.4X2	T42.4X3	T42.4X4	T42.4X5	T42.4X6
Oxazolidine derivatives	T42.2X1	T42.2X2	T42.2X3	T42.2X4	T42.2X5	T42.2X6
Oxazolidinedione (derivative)	T42.2X1	T42.2X2	T42.2X3	T42.2X4	T42.2X5	T42.2X6
Ox bile extract	T47.5X1	T47.5X2	T47.5X3	T47.5X4	T47.5X5	T47.5X6
Oxcarbazepine	T42.1X1	T42.1X2	T42.1X3	T42.1X4	T42.1X5	T42.1X6
Oxedrine	T44.4X1	T44.4X2	T44.4X3	T44.4X4	T44.4X5	T44.4X6
Oxeladin (citrate)	T48.3X1	T48.3X2	T48.3X3	T48.3X4	T48.3X5	T48.3X6
Oxendolone	T38.5X1	T38.5X2	T38.5X3	T38.5X4	T38.5X5	T38.5X6
Oxetacaine	T41.3X1	T41.3X2	T41.3X3	T41.3X4	T41.3X5	T41.3X6
Oxethazine	T41.3X1	T41.3X2	T41.3X3	T41.3X4	T41.3X5	T41.3X6
Oxetorone	T39.8X1	T39.8X2	T39.8X3	T39.8X4	T39.8X5	T39.8X6
Oxiconazole	T49.0X1	T49.0X2	T49.0X3	T49.0X4	T49.0X5	T49.0X6
Oxidizing agent NEC	T54.91	T54.92	T54.93	T54.94	—	—
Oxipurinol	T50.4X1	T50.4X2	T50.4X3	T50.4X4	T50.4X5	T50.4X6
Oxitriptan	T43.291	T43.292	T43.293	T43.294	T43.295	T43.296
Oxitropium bromide	T48.6X1	T48.6X2	T48.6X3	T48.6X4	T48.6X5	T48.6X6
Oxodipine	T46.1X1	T46.1X2	T46.1X3	T46.1X4	T46.1X5	T46.1X6
Oxolamine	T48.3X1	T48.3X2	T48.3X3	T48.3X4	T48.3X5	T48.3X6
Oxolinic acid	T37.8X1	T37.8X2	T37.8X3	T37.8X4	T37.8X5	T37.8X6
Oxomemazine	T43.3X1	T43.3X2	T43.3X3	T43.3X4	T43.3X5	T43.3X6
Oxophenarsine	T37.3X1	T37.3X2	T37.3X3	T37.3X4	T37.3X5	T37.3X6
Oxprenolol	T44.7X1	T44.7X2	T44.7X3	T44.7X4	T44.7X5	T44.7X6
Oxsoralen	T49.3X1	T49.3X2	T49.3X3	T49.3X4	T49.3X5	T49.3X6
Oxtriphylline	T48.6X1	T48.6X2	T48.6X3	T48.6X4	T48.6X5	T48.6X6
Oxybate sodium	T41.291	T41.292	T41.293	T41.294	T41.295	T41.296
Oxybuprocaine	T41.3X1	T41.3X2	T41.3X3	T41.3X4	T41.3X5	T41.3X6
Oxybutynin	T44.3X1	T44.3X2	T44.3X3	T44.3X4	T44.3X5	T44.3X6
Oxychlorosene	T49.0X1	T49.0X2	T49.0X3	T49.0X4	T49.0X5	T49.0X6
Oxycodone	T40.2X1	T40.2X2	T40.2X3	T40.2X4	T40.2X5	T40.2X6
OxyContin*	T40.2X1	T40.2X2	T40.2X3	T40.2X4	T40.2X5	T40.2X6
Oxyfedrine	T46.3X1	T46.3X2	T46.3X3	T46.3X4	T46.3X5	T46.3X6
Oxygen	T41.5X1	T41.5X2	T41.5X3	T41.5X4	T41.5X5	T41.5X6
Oxylone	T49.0X1	T49.0X2	T49.0X3	T49.0X4	T49.0X5	T49.0X6
ophthalmic preparation	T49.5X1	T49.5X2	T49.5X3	T49.5X4	T49.5X5	T49.5X6
Oxymesterone	T38.7X1	T38.7X2	T38.7X3	T38.7X4	T38.7X5	T38.7X6
Oxymetazoline	T48.5X1	T48.5X2	T48.5X3	T48.5X4	T48.5X5	T48.5X6
Oxymetholone	T38.7X1	T38.7X2	T38.7X3	T38.7X4	T38.7X5	T38.7X6
Oxymorphone	T40.2X1	T40.2X2	T40.2X3	T40.2X4	T40.2X5	T40.2X6
Oxypertine	T43.591	T43.592	T43.593	T43.594	T43.595	T43.596
Oxyphenbutazone	T39.2X1	T39.2X2	T39.2X3	T39.2X4	T39.2X5	T39.2X6
Oxyphencyclimine	T44.3X1	T44.3X2	T44.3X3	T44.3X4	T44.3X5	T44.3X6
Oxyphenisatine	T47.2X1	T47.2X2	T47.2X3	T47.2X4	T47.2X5	T47.2X6
Oxyphenonium bromide	T44.3X1	T44.3X2	T44.3X3	T44.3X4	T44.3X5	T44.3X6
Oxypolygelatin	T45.8X1	T45.8X2	T45.8X3	T45.8X4	T45.8X5	T45.8X6
Oxyquinoline (derivatives)	T37.8X1	T37.8X2	T37.8X3	T37.8X4	T37.8X5	T37.8X6
Oxytetracycline	T36.4X1	T36.4X2	T36.4X3	T36.4X4	T36.4X5	T36.4X6
Oxytocic drug NEC	T48.0X1	T48.0X2	T48.0X3	T48.0X4	T48.0X5	T48.0X6
Oxytocin (synthetic)	T48.0X1	T48.0X2	T48.0X3	T48.0X4	T48.0X5	T48.0X6
Oxytrol*	T44.3X1	T44.3X2	T44.3X3	T44.3X4	T44.3X5	T44.3X6
Ozone	T59.891	T59.892	T59.893	T59.894	—	—
PABA	T49.3X1	T49.3X2	T49.3X3	T49.3X4	T49.3X5	T49.3X6
Packed red cells	T45.8X1	T45.8X2	T45.8X3	T45.8X4	T45.8X5	T45.8X6

Substance	Poisoning, Accidental (unintentional)	Poisoning, Intentional Self-harm	Poisoning, Assault	Poisoning, Undetermined	Adverse Effect	Under-dosing
Padimate	T49.3X1	T49.3X2	T49.3X3	T49.3X4	T49.3X5	T49.3X6
Paint NEC	T65.6X1	T65.6X2	T65.6X3	T65.6X4	—	—
cleaner	T52.91	T52.92	T52.93	T52.94	—	—
fumes NEC	T59.891	T59.892	T59.893	T59.894	—	—
lead (fumes)	T56.0X1	T56.0X2	T56.0X3	T56.0X4	—	—
solvent NEC	T52.8X1	T52.8X2	T52.8X3	T52.8X4	—	—
stripper	T52.8X1	T52.8X2	T52.8X3	T52.8X4	—	—
Palfium	T40.2X1	T40.2X2	T40.2X3	T40.2X4	—	—
Palm kernel oil	T50.991	T50.992	T50.993	T50.994	T50.995	T50.996
Paludrine	T37.2X1	T37.2X2	T37.2X3	T37.2X4	T37.2X5	T37.2X6
PAM (pralidoxime)	T50.6X1	T50.6X2	T50.6X3	T50.6X4	T50.6X5	T50.6X6
Pamaquine (naphthoute)	T37.2X1	T37.2X2	T37.2X3	T37.2X4	T37.2X5	T37.2X6
Panadol	T39.1X1	T39.1X2	T39.1X3	T39.1X4	T39.1X5	T39.1X6
Pancreatic						
digestive secretion stimulant	T47.8X1	T47.8X2	T47.8X3	T47.8X4	T47.8X5	T47.8X6
dornase	T45.3X1	T45.3X2	T45.3X3	T45.3X4	T45.3X5	T45.3X6
Pancreatin	T47.5X1	T47.5X2	T47.5X3	T47.5X4	T47.5X5	T47.5X6
Pancrelipase	T47.5X1	T47.5X2	T47.5X3	T47.5X4	T47.5X5	T47.5X6
Pancuronium (bromide)	T48.1X1	T48.1X2	T48.1X3	T48.1X4	T48.1X5	T48.1X6
Pangamic acid	T45.2X1	T45.2X2	T45.2X3	T45.2X4	T45.2X5	T45.2X6
Panthenol	T45.2X1	T45.2X2	T45.2X3	T45.2X4	T45.2X5	T45.2X6
topical	T49.8X1	T49.8X2	T49.8X3	T49.8X4	T49.8X5	T49.8X6
Pantopon	T40.0X1	T40.0X2	T40.0X3	T40.0X4	T40.0X5	T40.0X6
Pantoprazole*	T47.1X1	T47.1X2	T47.1X3	T47.1X4	T47.1X5	T47.1X6
Pantothenic acid	T45.2X1	T45.2X2	T45.2X3	T45.2X4	T45.2X5	T45.2X6
Panwarfin	T45.511	T45.512	T45.513	T45.514	T45.515	T45.516
Papain	T47.5X1	T47.5X2	T47.5X3	T47.5X4	T47.5X5	T47.5X6
digestant	T47.5X1	T47.5X2	T47.5X3	T47.5X4	T47.5X5	T47.5X6
Papaveretum	T40.0X1	T40.0X2	T40.0X3	T40.0X4	T40.0X5	T40.0X6
Papaverine	T44.3X1	T44.3X2	T44.3X3	T44.3X4	T44.3X5	T44.3X6
Para-acetamidophenol	T39.1X1	T39.1X2	T39.1X3	T39.1X4	T39.1X5	T39.1X6
Para-aminobenzoic acid	T49.3X1	T49.3X2	T49.3X3	T49.3X4	T49.3X5	T49.3X6
Para-aminophenol derivatives	T39.1X1	T39.1X2	T39.1X3	T39.1X4	T39.1X5	T39.1X6
Para-aminosalicylic acid	T37.1X1	T37.1X2	T37.1X3	T37.1X4	T37.1X5	T37.1X6
Paracetaldehyde	T42.6X1	T42.6X2	T42.6X3	T42.6X4	T42.6X5	T42.6X6
Paracetamol	T39.1X1	T39.1X2	T39.1X3	T39.1X4	T39.1X5	T39.1X6
Parachlorophenol (camphorated)	T49.0X1	T49.0X2	T49.0X3	T49.0X4	T49.0X5	T49.0X6
Paracodin	T40.2X1	T40.2X2	T40.2X3	T40.2X4	T40.2X5	T40.2X6
Paradione	T42.2X1	T42.2X2	T42.2X3	T42.2X4	T42.2X5	T42.2X6
Paraffin(s) (wax)	T52.0X1	T52.0X2	T52.0X3	T52.0X4	—	—
liquid (medicinal)	T47.4X1	T47.4X2	T47.4X3	T47.4X4	T47.4X5	T47.4X6
nonmedicinal	T52.0X1	T52.0X2	T52.0X3	T52.0X4	—	—
Paraformaldehyde	T60.3X1	T60.3X2	T60.3X3	T60.3X4	—	—
Paraldehyde	T42.6X1	T42.6X2	T42.6X3	T42.6X4	T42.6X5	T42.6X6
Paramethadione	T42.2X1	T42.2X2	T42.2X3	T42.2X4	T42.2X5	T42.2X6
Paramethasone	T38.0X1	T38.0X2	T38.0X3	T38.0X4	T38.0X5	T38.0X6
acetate	T49.0X1	T49.0X2	T49.0X3	T49.0X4	T49.0X5	T49.0X6
Paraoxon	T60.0X1	T60.0X2	T60.0X3	T60.0X4	—	—
Paraquat	T60.3X1	T60.3X2	T60.3X3	T60.3X4	—	—
Parasympatholytic NEC	T44.3X1	T44.3X2	T44.3X3	T44.3X4	T44.3X5	T44.3X6
Parasympathomimetic drug NEC	T44.1X1	T44.1X2	T44.1X3	T44.1X4	T44.1X5	T44.1X6
Parathion	T60.0X1	T60.0X2	T60.0X3	T60.0X4	—	—
Parathormone	T50.991	T50.992	T50.993	T50.994	T50.995	T50.996
Parathyroid extract	T50.991	T50.992	T50.993	T50.994	T50.995	T50.996
Paratyphoid vaccine	T50.A91	T50.A92	T50.A93	T50.A94	T50.A95	T50.A96
Paredrine	T44.4X1	T44.4X2	T44.4X3	T44.4X4	T44.4X5	T44.4X6
Paregoric	T40.0X1	T40.0X2	T40.0X3	T40.0X4	T40.0X5	T40.0X6
Pargyline	T46.5X1	T46.5X2	T46.5X3	T46.5X4	T46.5X5	T46.5X6
Paris green	T57.0X1	T57.0X2	T57.0X3	T57.0X4	—	—
insecticide	T57.0X1	T57.0X2	T57.0X3	T57.0X4	—	—
Parnate	T43.1X1	T43.1X2	T43.1X3	T43.1X4	T43.1X5	T43.1X6
Paromomycin	T36.5X1	T36.5X2	T36.5X3	T36.5X4	T36.5X5	T36.5X6
Paroxypropione	T45.1X1	T45.1X2	T45.1X3	T45.1X4	T45.1X5	T45.1X6
Parsabiv*	T50.991	T50.992	T50.993	T50.994	T50.995	T50.996
Parzone	T40.2X1	T40.2X2	T40.2X3	T40.2X4	T40.2X5	T40.2X6
PAS	T37.1X1	T37.1X2	T37.1X3	T37.1X4	T37.1X5	T37.1X6
Pasiniazid	T37.1X1	T37.1X2	T37.1X3	T37.1X4	T37.1X5	T37.1X6
PBB (polybrominated biphenyls)	T65.891	T65.892	T65.893	T65.894	—	—
PCB	T65.891	T65.892	T65.893	T65.894	—	—
PCP						
meaning pentachlorophenol	T60.1X1	T60.1X2	T60.1X3	T60.1X4	—	—
fungicide	T60.3X1	T60.3X2	T60.3X3	T60.3X4	—	—
herbicide	T60.3X1	T60.3X2	T60.3X3	T60.3X4	—	—
insecticide	T60.1X1	T60.1X2	T60.1X3	T60.1X4	—	—
meaning phencyclidine	T40.991	T40.992	T40.993	T40.994	—	—
Peach kernel oil (emulsion)	T47.4X1	T47.4X2	T47.4X3	T47.4X4	T47.4X5	T47.4X6
Peanut oil (emulsion) NEC	T47.4X1	T47.4X2	T47.4X3	T47.4X4	T47.4X5	T47.4X6

*Optum Value-Add   ☑ Additional Character May Be Required — Refer to the Tabular List for Character Selection

Table of Drugs and Chemicals

Substance	Poisoning, Accidental (unintentional)	Poisoning, Intentional Self-harm	Poisoning, Assault	Poisoning, Undetermined	Adverse Effect	Under-dosing
Peanut oil (emulsion) **NEC** — continued						
topical	T49.3X1	T49.3X2	T49.3X3	T49.3X4	T49.3X5	T49.3X6
Pearly Gates (morning glory seeds)	T40.991	T40.992	T40.993	T40.994	—	—
Pecazine	T43.3X1	T43.3X2	T43.3X3	T43.3X4	T43.3X5	T43.3X6
Pectin	T47.6X1	T47.6X2	T47.6X3	T47.6X4	T47.6X5	T47.6X6
Pediaflor*	T49.7X1	T49.7X2	T49.7X3	T49.7X4	T49.7X5	T49.7X6
Pefloxacin	T37.8X1	T37.8X2	T37.8X3	T37.8X4	T37.8X5	T37.8X6
Pegademase, bovine	T50.Z91	T50.Z92	T50.Z93	T50.Z94	T50.Z95	T50.Z96
Pelletierine tannate	T37.4X1	T37.4X2	T37.4X3	T37.4X4	T37.4X5	T37.4X6
Pemirolast (potassium)	T48.6X1	T48.6X2	T48.6X3	T48.6X4	T48.6X5	T48.6X6
Pemoline	T50.7X1	T50.7X2	T50.7X3	T50.7X4	T50.7X5	T50.7X6
Pempidine	T44.2X1	T44.2X2	T44.2X3	T44.2X4	T44.2X5	T44.2X6
Penamecillin	T36.0X1	T36.0X2	T36.0X3	T36.0X4	T36.0X5	T36.0X6
Penbutolol	T44.7X1	T44.7X2	T44.7X3	T44.7X4	T44.7X5	T44.7X6
Penethamate	T36.0X1	T36.0X2	T36.0X3	T36.0X4	T36.0X5	T36.0X6
Penfluridol	T43.591	T43.592	T43.593	T43.594	T43.595	T43.596
Penflutizide	T50.2X1	T50.2X2	T50.2X3	T50.2X4	T50.2X5	T50.2X6
Pengitoxin	T46.0X1	T46.0X2	T46.0X3	T46.0X4	T46.0X5	T46.0X6
Penicillamine	T50.6X1	T50.6X2	T50.6X3	T50.6X4	T50.6X5	T50.6X6
Penicillin (any)	T36.0X1	T36.0X2	T36.0X3	T36.0X4	T36.0X5	T36.0X6
Penicillinase	T45.3X1	T45.3X2	T45.3X3	T45.3X4	T45.3X5	T45.3X6
Penicilloyl polylysine	T50.8X1	T50.8X2	T50.8X3	T50.8X4	T50.8X5	T50.8X6
Penimepicycline	T36.4X1	T36.4X2	T36.4X3	T36.4X4	T36.4X5	T36.4X6
Pentacel*	T50.A11	T50.A12	T50.A13	T50.A14	T50.A15	T50.A16
Pentachloroethane	T53.6X1	T53.6X2	T53.6X3	T53.6X4	—	—
Pentachloronaphthalene	T53.7X1	T53.7X2	T53.7X3	T53.7X4	—	—
Pentachlorophenol (pesticide)	T60.1X1	T60.1X2	T60.1X3	T60.1X4	—	—
fungicide	T60.3X1	T60.3X2	T60.3X3	T60.3X4	—	—
herbicide	T60.3X1	T60.3X2	T60.3X3	T60.3X4	—	—
insecticide	T60.1X1	T60.1X2	T60.1X3	T60.1X4	—	—
Pentaerythritol	T46.3X1	T46.3X2	T46.3X3	T46.3X4	T46.3X5	T46.3X6
chloral	T42.6X1	T42.6X2	T42.6X3	T42.6X4	T42.6X5	T42.6X6
tetranitrate NEC	T46.3X1	T46.3X2	T46.3X3	T46.3X4	T46.3X5	T46.3X6
Pentaerythrityl tetranitrate	T46.3X1	T46.3X2	T46.3X3	T46.3X4	T46.3X5	T46.3X6
Pentagastrin	T50.8X1	T50.8X2	T50.8X3	T50.8X4	T50.8X5	T50.8X6
Pentalin	T53.6X1	T53.6X2	T53.6X3	T53.6X4	—	—
Pentamethonium bromide	T44.2X1	T44.2X2	T44.2X3	T44.2X4	T44.2X5	T44.2X6
Pentamidine	T37.3X1	T37.3X2	T37.3X3	T37.3X4	T37.3X5	T37.3X6
Pentanol	T51.3X1	T51.3X2	T51.3X3	T51.3X4	—	—
Pentapyrrolinium (bitartrate)	T44.2X1	T44.2X2	T44.2X3	T44.2X4	T44.2X5	T44.2X6
Pentaquine	T37.2X1	T37.2X2	T37.2X3	T37.2X4	T37.2X5	T37.2X6
Pentazocine	T40.491	T40.492	T40.493	T40.494	T40.495	T40.496
Pentetrazole	T50.7X1	T50.7X2	T50.7X3	T50.7X4	T50.7X5	T50.7X6
Penthienate bromide	T44.3X1	T44.3X2	T44.3X3	T44.3X4	T44.3X5	T44.3X6
Pentifylline	T46.7X1	T46.7X2	T46.7X3	T46.7X4	T46.7X5	T46.7X6
Pentobarbital	T42.3X1	T42.3X2	T42.3X3	T42.3X4	T42.3X5	T42.3X6
sodium	T42.3X1	T42.3X2	T42.3X3	T42.3X4	T42.3X5	T42.3X6
Pentobarbitone	T42.3X1	T42.3X2	T42.3X3	T42.3X4	T42.3X5	T42.3X6
Pentolonium tartrate	T44.2X1	T44.2X2	T44.2X3	T44.2X4	T44.2X5	T44.2X6
Pentosan polysulfate (sodium)	T39.8X1	T39.8X2	T39.8X3	T39.8X4	T39.8X5	T39.8X6
Pentostatin	T45.1X1	T45.1X2	T45.1X3	T45.1X4	T45.1X5	T45.1X6
Pentothal	T41.1X1	T41.1X2	T41.1X3	T41.1X4	T41.1X5	T41.1X6
Pentoxifylline	T46.7X1	T46.7X2	T46.7X3	T46.7X4	T46.7X5	T46.7X6
Pentoxyverine	T48.3X1	T48.3X2	T48.3X3	T48.3X4	T48.3X5	T48.3X6
Pentrinat	T46.3X1	T46.3X2	T46.3X3	T46.3X4	T46.3X5	T46.3X6
Pentylenetetrazole	T50.7X1	T50.7X2	T50.7X3	T50.7X4	T50.7X5	T50.7X6
Pentylsalicylamide	T37.1X1	T37.1X2	T37.1X3	T37.1X4	T37.1X5	T37.1X6
Pentymal	T42.3X1	T42.3X2	T42.3X3	T42.3X4	T42.3X5	T42.3X6
Pepcid*	T47.0X1	T47.0X2	T47.0X3	T47.0X4	T47.0X5	T47.0X6
Peplomycin	T45.1X1	T45.1X2	T45.1X3	T45.1X4	T45.1X5	T45.1X6
Peppermint (oil)	T47.5X1	T47.5X2	T47.5X3	T47.5X4	T47.5X5	T47.5X6
Pepsin	T47.5X1	T47.5X2	T47.5X3	T47.5X4	T47.5X5	T47.5X6
digestant	T47.5X1	T47.5X2	T47.5X3	T47.5X4	T47.5X5	T47.5X6
Pepstatin	T47.1X1	T47.1X2	T47.1X3	T47.1X4	T47.1X5	T47.1X6
Peptavlon	T50.8X1	T50.8X2	T50.8X3	T50.8X4	T50.8X5	T50.8X6
Perazine	T43.3X1	T43.3X2	T43.3X3	T43.3X4	T43.3X5	T43.3X6
Percaine (spinal)	T41.3X1	T41.3X2	T41.3X3	T41.3X4	T41.3X5	T41.3X6
topical (surface)	T41.3X1	T41.3X2	T41.3X3	T41.3X4	T41.3X5	T41.3X6
Perchloroethylene	T53.3X1	T53.3X2	T53.3X3	T53.3X4	—	—
medicinal	T37.4X1	T37.4X2	T37.4X3	T37.4X4	T37.4X5	T37.4X6
vapor	T53.3X1	T53.3X2	T53.3X3	T53.3X4	—	—
Percodan	T40.2X1	T40.2X2	T40.2X3	T40.2X4	T40.2X5	T40.2X6
Percogesic — see also acetaminophen	T45.0X1	T45.0X2	T45.0X3	T45.0X4	T45.0X5	T45.0X6
Percorten	T38.0X1	T38.0X2	T38.0X3	T38.0X4	T38.0X5	T38.0X6
Pergolide	T42.8X1	T42.8X2	T42.8X3	T42.8X4	T42.8X5	T42.8X6
Pergonal	T38.811	T38.812	T38.813	T38.814	T38.815	T38.816

Substance	Poisoning, Accidental (unintentional)	Poisoning, Intentional Self-harm	Poisoning, Assault	Poisoning, Undetermined	Adverse Effect	Under-dosing
Perhexilene	T46.3X1	T46.3X2	T46.3X3	T46.3X4	T46.3X5	T46.3X6
Perhexiline (maleate)	T46.3X1	T46.3X2	T46.3X3	T46.3X4	T46.3X5	T46.3X6
Periactin	T45.0X1	T45.0X2	T45.0X3	T45.0X4	T45.0X5	T45.0X6
Periciazine	T43.3X1	T43.3X2	T43.3X3	T43.3X4	T43.3X5	T43.3X6
Periclor	T42.6X1	T42.6X2	T42.6X3	T42.6X4	T42.6X5	T42.6X6
Perindopril	T46.4X1	T46.4X2	T46.4X3	T46.4X4	T46.4X5	T46.4X6
Perisoxal	T39.8X1	T39.8X2	T39.8X3	T39.8X4	T39.8X5	T39.8X6
Peritoneal dialysis solution	T50.3X1	T50.3X2	T50.3X3	T50.3X4	T50.3X5	T50.3X6
Peritrate	T46.3X1	T46.3X2	T46.3X3	T46.3X4	T46.3X5	T46.3X6
Perlapine	T42.4X1	T42.4X2	T42.4X3	T42.4X4	T42.4X5	T42.4X6
Permanganate	T65.891	T65.892	T65.893	T65.894	—	—
Permapen*	T36.0X1	T36.0X2	T36.0X3	T36.0X4	T36.0X5	T36.0X6
Permethrin	T60.1X1	T60.1X2	T60.1X3	T60.1X4	—	—
Pernocton	T42.3X1	T42.3X2	T42.3X3	T42.3X4	T42.3X5	T42.3X6
Pernoston	T42.3X1	T42.3X2	T42.3X3	T42.3X4	T42.3X5	T42.3X6
Peronine	T40.2X1	T40.2X2	T40.2X3	T40.2X4	—	—
Perphenazine	T43.3X1	T43.3X2	T43.3X3	T43.3X4	T43.3X5	T43.3X6
Pertofrane	T43.011	T43.012	T43.013	T43.014	T43.015	T43.016
Pertussis						
immune serum (human)	T50.Z11	T50.Z12	T50.Z13	T50.Z14	T50.Z15	T50.Z16
vaccine (with diphtheria toxoid) (with tetanus toxoid)	T50.A11	T50.A12	T50.A13	T50.A14	T50.A15	T50.A16
Peruvian balsam	T49.0X1	T49.0X2	T49.0X3	T49.0X4	T49.0X5	T49.0X6
Peruvoside	T46.0X1	T46.0X2	T46.0X3	T46.0X4	T46.0X5	T46.0X6
Pesticide (dust) (fumes) (vapor) **NEC**	T60.91	T60.92	T60.93	T60.94		
arsenic	T57.0X1	T57.0X2	T57.0X3	T57.0X4	—	—
chlorinated	T60.1X1	T60.1X2	T60.1X3	T60.1X4	—	—
cyanide	T65.0X1	T65.0X2	T65.0X3	T65.0X4	—	—
kerosene	T52.0X1	T52.0X2	T52.0X3	T52.0X4	—	—
mixture (of compounds)	T60.91	T60.92	T60.93	T60.94	—	—
naphthalene	T60.2X1	T60.2X2	T60.2X3	T60.2X4	—	—
organochlorine (compounds)	T60.1X1	T60.1X2	T60.1X3	T60.1X4	—	—
petroleum (distillate) (products) NEC	T60.8X1	T60.8X2	T60.8X3	T60.8X4	—	—
specified ingredient NEC	T60.8X1	T60.8X2	T60.8X3	T60.8X4	—	—
strychnine	T65.1X1	T65.1X2	T65.1X3	T65.1X4	—	—
thallium	T60.4X1	T60.4X2	T60.4X3	T60.4X4	—	—
Pethidine	T40.491	T40.492	T40.493	T40.494	T40.495	T40.496
Petrichloral	T42.6X1	T42.6X2	T42.6X3	T42.6X4	T42.6X5	T42.6X6
Petrol	T52.0X1	T52.0X2	T52.0X3	T52.0X4	—	—
vapor	T52.0X1	T52.0X2	T52.0X3	T52.0X4	—	—
Petrolatum	T49.3X1	T49.3X2	T49.3X3	T49.3X4	T49.3X5	T49.3X6
hydrophilic	T49.3X1	T49.3X2	T49.3X3	T49.3X4	T49.3X5	T49.3X6
liquid	T47.4X1	T47.4X2	T47.4X3	T47.4X4	T47.4X5	T47.4X6
topical	T49.3X1	T49.3X2	T49.3X3	T49.3X4	T49.3X5	T49.3X6
nonmedicinal	T52.0X1	T52.0X2	T52.0X3	T52.0X4	—	—
red veterinary	T49.3X1	T49.3X2	T49.3X3	T49.3X4	T49.3X5	T49.3X6
white	T49.3X1	T49.3X2	T49.3X3	T49.3X4	T49.3X5	T49.3X6
Petroleum (products) **NEC**	T52.0X1	T52.0X2	T52.0X3	T52.0X4	—	—
benzine(s) — see Ligroin						
ether — see Ligroin						
jelly — see Petrolatum						
naphtha — see Ligroin						
pesticide	T60.8X1	T60.8X2	T60.8X3	T60.8X4	—	—
solids	T52.0X1	T52.0X2	T52.0X3	T52.0X4	—	—
solvents	T52.0X1	T52.0X2	T52.0X3	T52.0X4	—	—
vapor	T52.0X1	T52.0X2	T52.0X3	T52.0X4	—	—
Peyote	T40.991	T40.992	T40.993	T40.994	—	—
Phanodorm, phanodorn	T42.3X1	T42.3X2	T42.3X3	T42.3X4	T42.3X5	T42.3X6
Phanquinone	T37.3X1	T37.3X2	T37.3X3	T37.3X4	T37.3X5	T37.3X6
Phanquone	T37.3X1	T37.3X2	T37.3X3	T37.3X4	T37.3X5	T37.3X6
Pharmaceutical						
adjunct NEC	T50.901	T50.902	T50.903	T50.904	T50.905	T50.906
excipient NEC	T50.901	T50.902	T50.903	T50.904	T50.905	T50.906
sweetener	T50.901	T50.902	T50.903	T50.904	T50.905	T50.906
viscous agent	T50.901	T50.902	T50.903	T50.904	T50.905	T50.906
Phazyme*	T47.1X1	T47.1X2	T47.1X3	T47.1X4	T47.1X5	T47.1X6
Phemitone	T42.3X1	T42.3X2	T42.3X3	T42.3X4	T42.3X5	T42.3X6
Phenacaine	T41.3X1	T41.3X2	T41.3X3	T41.3X4	T41.3X5	T41.3X6
Phenacemide	T42.6X1	T42.6X2	T42.6X3	T42.6X4	T42.6X5	T42.6X6
Phenacetin	T39.1X1	T39.1X2	T39.1X3	T39.1X4	T39.1X5	T39.1X6
Phenadoxone	T40.2X1	T40.2X2	T40.2X3	T40.2X4	—	—
Phenaglycodol	T43.591	T43.592	T43.593	T43.594	T43.595	T43.596
Phenantoin	T42.0X1	T42.0X2	T42.0X3	T42.0X4	T42.0X5	T42.0X6
Phenaphthazine reagent	T50.991	T50.992	T50.993	T50.994	T50.995	T50.996
Phenazocine	T40.491	T40.492	T40.493	T40.494	T40.495	T40.496
Phenazone	T39.2X1	T39.2X2	T39.2X3	T39.2X4	T39.2X5	T39.2X6
Phenazopyridine	T39.8X1	T39.8X2	T39.8X3	T39.8X4	T39.8X5	T39.8X6
Phenbenicillin	T36.0X1	T36.0X2	T36.0X3	T36.0X4	T36.0X5	T36.0X6
Phenbutrazate	T50.5X1	T50.5X2	T50.5X3	T50.5X4	T50.5X5	T50.5X6

Substance	Poisoning, Accidental (unintentional)	Poisoning, Intentional Self-harm	Poisoning, Assault	Poisoning, Undetermined	Adverse Effect	Under-dosing
Phencyclidine	T40.991	T40.992	T40.993	T40.994	T40.995	T40.996
Phendimetrazine	T50.5X1	T50.5X2	T50.5X3	T50.5X4	T50.5X5	T50.5X6
Phenelzine	T43.1X1	T43.1X2	T43.1X3	T43.1X4	T43.1X5	T43.1X6
Phenemal	T42.3X1	T42.3X2	T42.3X3	T42.3X4	T42.3X5	T42.3X6
Phenergan	T42.6X1	T42.6X2	T42.6X3	T42.6X4	T42.6X5	T42.6X6
Pheneticillin	T36.0X1	T36.0X2	T36.0X3	T36.0X4	T36.0X5	T36.0X6
Pheneturide	T42.6X1	T42.6X2	T42.6X3	T42.6X4	T42.6X5	T42.6X6
Phenformin	T38.3X1	T38.3X2	T38.3X3	T38.3X4	T38.3X5	T38.3X6
Phenglutarimide	T44.3X1	T44.3X2	T44.3X3	T44.3X4	T44.3X5	T44.3X6
Phenicarbazide	T39.8X1	T39.8X2	T39.8X3	T39.8X4	T39.8X5	T39.8X6
Phenindamine	T45.0X1	T45.0X2	T45.0X3	T45.0X4	T45.0X5	T45.0X6
Phenindione	T45.511	T45.512	T45.513	T45.514	T45.515	T45.516
Pheniprazine	T43.1X1	T43.1X2	T43.1X3	T43.1X4	T43.1X5	T43.1X6
Pheniramine	T45.0X1	T45.0X2	T45.0X3	T45.0X4	T45.0X5	T45.0X6
Phenisatin	T47.2X1	T47.2X2	T47.2X3	T47.2X4	T47.2X5	T47.2X6
Phenmetrazine	T50.5X1	T50.5X2	T50.5X3	T50.5X4	T50.5X5	T50.5X6
Phenobal	T42.3X1	T42.3X2	T42.3X3	T42.3X4	T42.3X5	T42.3X6
Phenobarbital	T42.3X1	T42.3X2	T42.3X3	T42.3X4	T42.3X5	T42.3X6
with						
mephenytoin	T42.3X1	T42.3X2	T42.3X3	T42.3X4	T42.3X5	T42.3X6
phenytoin	T42.3X1	T42.3X2	T42.3X3	T42.3X4	T42.3X5	T42.3X6
sodium	T42.3X1	T42.3X2	T42.3X3	T42.3X4	T42.3X5	T42.3X6
Phenobarbitone	T42.3X1	T42.3X2	T42.3X3	T42.3X4	T42.3X5	T42.3X6
Phenobutiodil	T50.8X1	T50.8X2	T50.8X3	T50.8X4	T50.8X5	T50.8X6
Phenoctide	T49.0X1	T49.0X2	T49.0X3	T49.0X4	T49.0X5	T49.0X6
Phenol	T49.0X1	T49.0X2	T49.0X3	T49.0X4	T49.0X5	T49.0X6
disinfectant	T54.0X1	T54.0X2	T54.0X3	T54.0X4	—	—
in oil injection	T46.8X1	T46.8X2	T46.8X3	T46.8X4	T46.8X5	T46.8X6
medicinal	T49.1X1	T49.1X2	T49.1X3	T49.1X4	T49.1X5	T49.1X6
nonmedicinal NEC	T54.0X1	T54.0X2	T54.0X3	T54.0X4	—	—
pesticide	T60.8X1	T60.8X2	T60.8X3	T60.8X4	—	—
red	T50.8X1	T50.8X2	T50.8X3	T50.8X4	T50.8X5	T50.8X6
Phenolic preparation	T49.1X1	T49.1X2	T49.1X3	T49.1X4	T49.1X5	T49.1X6
Phenolphthalein	T47.2X1	T47.2X2	T47.2X3	T47.2X4	T47.2X5	T47.2X6
Phenolsulfonphthalein	T50.8X1	T50.8X2	T50.8X3	T50.8X4	T50.8X5	T50.8X6
Phenomorphan	T40.2X1	T40.2X2	T40.2X3	T40.2X4		
Phenonyl	T42.3X1	T42.3X2	T42.3X3	T42.3X4	T42.3X5	T42.3X6
Phenoperidine	T40.491	T40.492	T40.493	T40.494		
Phenopyrazone	T46.991	T46.992	T46.993	T46.994	T46.995	T46.996
Phenoquin	T50.4X1	T50.4X2	T50.4X3	T50.4X4	T50.4X5	T50.4X6
Phenothiazine (psychotropic)	T43.3X1	T43.3X2	T43.3X3	T43.3X4	T43.3X5	T43.3X6
NEC						
insecticide	T60.2X1	T60.2X2	T60.2X3	T60.2X4	—	—
Phenothrin	T49.0X1	T49.0X2	T49.0X3	T49.0X4	T49.0X5	T49.0X6
Phenoxybenzamine	T46.7X1	T46.7X2	T46.7X3	T46.7X4	T46.7X5	T46.7X6
Phenoxyethanol	T49.0X1	T49.0X2	T49.0X3	T49.0X4	T49.0X5	T49.0X6
Phenoxymethyl penicillin	T36.0X1	T36.0X2	T36.0X3	T36.0X4	T36.0X5	T36.0X6
Phenprobamate	T42.8X1	T42.8X2	T42.8X3	T42.8X4	T42.8X5	T42.8X6
Phenprocoumon	T45.511	T45.512	T45.513	T45.514	T45.515	T45.516
Phensuximide	T42.2X1	T42.2X2	T42.2X3	T42.2X4	T42.2X5	T42.2X6
Phentermine	T50.5X1	T50.5X2	T50.5X3	T50.5X4	T50.5X5	T50.5X6
Phenthicillin	T36.0X1	T36.0X2	T36.0X3	T36.0X4	T36.0X5	T36.0X6
Phentolamine	T46.7X1	T46.7X2	T46.7X3	T46.7X4	T46.7X5	T46.7X6
Phenyl						
butazone	T39.2X1	T39.2X2	T39.2X3	T39.2X4	T39.2X5	T39.2X6
enediamine	T65.3X1	T65.3X2	T65.3X3	T65.3X4	—	—
hydrazine	T65.3X1	T65.3X2	T65.3X3	T65.3X4	—	—
antineoplastic	T45.1X1	T45.1X2	T45.1X3	T45.1X4	T45.1X5	T45.1X6
mercuric compounds — see						
Mercury						
salicylate	T49.3X1	T49.3X2	T49.3X3	T49.3X4	T49.3X5	T49.3X6
Phenylalanine mustard	T45.1X1	T45.1X2	T45.1X3	T45.1X4	T45.1X5	T45.1X6
Phenylbutazone	T39.2X1	T39.2X2	T39.2X3	T39.2X4	T39.2X5	T39.2X6
Phenylenediamine	T65.3X1	T65.3X2	T65.3X3	T65.3X4	—	—
Phenylephrine	T44.4X1	T44.4X2	T44.4X3	T44.4X4	T44.4X5	T44.4X6
Phenylethylbiguanide	T38.3X1	T38.3X2	T38.3X3	T38.3X4	T38.3X5	T38.3X6
Phenylmercuric						
acetate	T49.0X1	T49.0X2	T49.0X3	T49.0X4	T49.0X5	T49.0X6
borate	T49.0X1	T49.0X2	T49.0X3	T49.0X4	T49.0X5	T49.0X6
nitrate	T49.0X1	T49.0X2	T49.0X3	T49.0X4	T49.0X5	T49.0X6
Phenylmethylbarbitone	T42.3X1	T42.3X2	T42.3X3	T42.3X4	T42.3X5	T42.3X6
Phenylpropanol	T47.5X1	T47.5X2	T47.5X3	T47.5X4	T47.5X5	T47.5X6
Phenylpropanolamine	T44.991	T44.992	T44.993	T44.994	T44.995	T44.996
Phenylsulfthion	T60.0X1	T60.0X2	T60.0X3	T60.0X4	—	—
Phenyltoloxamine	T45.0X1	T45.0X2	T45.0X3	T45.0X4	T45.0X5	T45.0X6
Phenyramidol, phenyramidon	T39.8X1	T39.8X2	T39.8X3	T39.8X4	T39.8X5	T39.8X6
Phenytek*	T42.0X1	T42.0X2	T42.0X3	T42.0X4	T42.0X5	T42.0X6
Phenytoin	T42.0X1	T42.0X2	T42.0X3	T42.0X4	T42.0X5	T42.0X6
with Phenobarbital	T42.3X1	T42.3X2	T42.3X3	T42.3X4	T42.3X5	T42.3X6
pHisoHex	T49.2X1	T49.2X2	T49.2X3	T49.2X4	T49.2X5	T49.2X6
Pholcodine	T48.3X1	T48.3X2	T48.3X3	T48.3X4	T48.3X5	T48.3X6
Pholedrine	T46.991	T46.992	T46.993	T46.994	T46.995	T46.996

Substance	Poisoning, Accidental (unintentional)	Poisoning, Intentional Self-harm	Poisoning, Assault	Poisoning, Undetermined	Adverse Effect	Under-dosing
Phorate	T60.0X1	T60.0X2	T60.0X3	T60.0X4	—	—
Phosdrin	T60.0X1	T60.0X2	T60.0X3	T60.0X4	—	—
Phosfolan	T60.0X1	T60.0X2	T60.0X3	T60.0X4	—	—
Phosgene (gas)	T59.891	T59.892	T59.893	T59.894		
Phosphamidon	T60.0X1	T60.0X2	T60.0X3	T60.0X4		
Phosphate	T65.891	T65.892	T65.893	T65.894	—	—
laxative	T47.4X1	T47.4X2	T47.4X3	T47.4X4	T47.4X5	T47.4X6
organic	T60.0X1	T60.0X2	T60.0X3	T60.0X4	—	—
solvent	T52.91	T52.92	T52.93	T52.94		
tricresyl	T65.891	T65.892	T65.893	T65.894		
Phosphine	T57.1X1	T57.1X2	T57.1X3	T57.1X4		
fumigant	T57.1X1	T57.1X2	T57.1X3	T57.1X4		
Phospholine	T49.5X1	T49.5X2	T49.5X3	T49.5X4	T49.5X5	T49.5X6
Phosphoric acid	T54.2X1	T54.2X2	T54.2X3	T54.2X4		
Phosphorus (compound) NEC	T57.1X1	T57.1X2	T57.1X3	T57.1X4		
pesticide	T60.0X1	T60.0X2	T60.0X3	T60.0X4		
Photrexa*	T49.5X1	T49.5X2	T49.5X3	T49.5X4	T49.5X5	T49.5X6
Phthalates	T65.891	T65.892	T65.893	T65.894		
Phthalic anhydride	T65.891	T65.892	T65.893	T65.894		
Phthalimidoglutarimide	T42.6X1	T42.6X2	T42.6X3	T42.6X4	T42.6X5	T42.6X6
Phthalylsulfathiazole	T37.0X1	T37.0X2	T37.0X3	T37.0X4	T37.0X5	T37.0X6
Phylloquinone	T45.7X1	T45.7X2	T45.7X3	T45.7X4	T45.7X5	T45.7X6
Physeptone	T40.3X1	T40.3X2	T40.3X3	T40.3X4	T40.3X5	T40.3X6
Physostigma venenosum	T62.2X1	T62.2X2	T62.2X3	T62.2X4		
Physostigmine	T49.5X1	T49.5X2	T49.5X3	T49.5X4	T49.5X5	T49.5X6
Phytolacca decandra	T62.2X1	T62.2X2	T62.2X3	T62.2X4		
berries	T62.1X1	T62.1X2	T62.1X3	T62.1X4		
Phytomenadione	T45.7X1	T45.7X2	T45.7X3	T45.7X4	T45.7X5	T45.7X6
Phytonadione	T45.7X1	T45.7X2	T45.7X3	T45.7X4	T45.7X5	T45.7X6
Picoperine	T48.3X1	T48.3X2	T48.3X3	T48.3X4	T48.3X5	T48.3X6
Picosulfate (sodium)	T47.2X1	T47.2X2	T47.2X3	T47.2X4	T47.2X5	T47.2X6
Picric (acid)	T54.2X1	T54.2X2	T54.2X3	T54.2X4		
Picrotoxin	T50.7X1	T50.7X2	T50.7X3	T50.7X4	T50.7X5	T50.7X6
Piketoprofen	T49.0X1	T49.0X2	T49.0X3	T49.0X4	T49.0X5	T49.0X6
Pilocarpine	T44.1X1	T44.1X2	T44.1X3	T44.1X4	T44.1X5	T44.1X6
Pilocarpus (jaborandi) extract	T44.1X1	T44.1X2	T44.1X3	T44.1X4	T44.1X5	T44.1X6
Pilsicainide (hydrochloride)	T46.2X1	T46.2X2	T46.2X3	T46.2X4	T46.2X5	T46.2X6
Pimaricin	T36.7X1	T36.7X2	T36.7X3	T36.7X4	T36.7X5	T36.7X6
Pimeclone	T50.7X1	T50.7X2	T50.7X3	T50.7X4	T50.7X5	T50.7X6
Pimelic ketone	T52.8X1	T52.8X2	T52.8X3	T52.8X4		
Pimethixene	T45.0X1	T45.0X2	T45.0X3	T45.0X4	T45.0X5	T45.0X6
Piminodine	T40.2X1	T40.2X2	T40.2X3	T40.2X4	T40.2X5	T40.2X6
Pimozide	T43.591	T43.592	T43.593	T43.594	T43.595	T43.596
Pinacidil	T46.5X1	T46.5X2	T46.5X3	T46.5X4	T46.5X5	T46.5X6
Pinaverium bromide	T44.3X1	T44.3X2	T44.3X3	T44.3X4	T44.3X5	T44.3X6
Pinazepam	T42.4X1	T42.4X2	T42.4X3	T42.4X4	T42.4X5	T42.4X6
Pindolol	T44.7X1	T44.7X2	T44.7X3	T44.7X4	T44.7X5	T44.7X6
Pindone	T60.4X1	T60.4X2	T60.4X3	T60.4X4	—	—
Pine oil (disinfectant)	T65.891	T65.892	T65.893	T65.894		
Pinkroot	T37.4X1	T37.4X2	T37.4X3	T37.4X4	T37.4X5	T37.4X6
Pipadone	T40.2X1	T40.2X2	T40.2X3	T40.2X4		
Pipamazine	T45.0X1	T45.0X2	T45.0X3	T45.0X4	T45.0X5	T45.0X6
Pipamperone	T43.4X1	T43.4X2	T43.4X3	T43.4X4	T43.4X5	T43.4X6
Pipazetate	T48.3X1	T48.3X2	T48.3X3	T48.3X4	T48.3X5	T48.3X6
Pipemidic acid	T37.8X1	T37.8X2	T37.8X3	T37.8X4	T37.8X5	T37.8X6
Pipenzolate bromide	T44.3X1	T44.3X2	T44.3X3	T44.3X4	T44.3X5	T44.3X6
Piperacetazine	T43.3X1	T43.3X2	T43.3X3	T43.3X4	T43.3X5	T43.3X6
Piperacillin	T36.0X1	T36.0X2	T36.0X3	T36.0X4	T36.0X5	T36.0X6
Piperazine	T37.4X1	T37.4X2	T37.4X3	T37.4X4	T37.4X5	T37.4X6
estrone sulfate	T38.5X1	T38.5X2	T38.5X3	T38.5X4	T38.5X5	T38.5X6
Piper cubeba	T62.2X1	T62.2X2	T62.2X3	T62.2X4		
Piperidione	T48.3X1	T48.3X2	T48.3X3	T48.3X4	T48.3X5	T48.3X6
Piperidolate	T44.3X1	T44.3X2	T44.3X3	T44.3X4	T44.3X5	T44.3X6
Piperocaine	T41.3X1	T41.3X2	T41.3X3	T41.3X4	T41.3X5	T41.3X6
infiltration (subcutaneous)	T41.3X1	T41.3X2	T41.3X3	T41.3X4	T41.3X5	T41.3X6
nerve block (peripheral) (plexus)	T41.3X1	T41.3X2	T41.3X3	T41.3X4	T41.3X5	T41.3X6
topical (surface)	T41.3X1	T41.3X2	T41.3X3	T41.3X4	T41.3X5	T41.3X6
Piperonyl butoxide	T60.8X1	T60.8X2	T60.8X3	T60.8X4		
Pipethanate	T44.3X1	T44.3X2	T44.3X3	T44.3X4	T44.3X5	T44.3X6
Pipobroman	T45.1X1	T45.1X2	T45.1X3	T45.1X4	T45.1X5	T45.1X6
Pipotiazine	T43.3X1	T43.3X2	T43.3X3	T43.3X4	T43.3X5	T43.3X6
Pipoxizine	T45.0X1	T45.0X2	T45.0X3	T45.0X4	T45.0X5	T45.0X6
Pipradrol	T43.691	T43.692	T43.693	T43.694	T43.695	T43.696
Piprinhydrinate	T45.0X1	T45.0X2	T45.0X3	T45.0X4	T45.0X5	T45.0X6
Pirarubicin	T45.1X1	T45.1X2	T45.1X3	T45.1X4	T45.1X5	T45.1X6
Pirazinamide	T37.1X1	T37.1X2	T37.1X3	T37.1X4	T37.1X5	T37.1X6
Pirbuterol	T48.6X1	T48.6X2	T48.6X3	T48.6X4	T48.6X5	T48.6X6
Pirenzepine	T47.1X1	T47.1X2	T47.1X3	T47.1X4	T47.1X5	T47.1X6
Piretanide	T50.1X1	T50.1X2	T50.1X3	T50.1X4	T50.1X5	T50.1X6
Pirfenidone*	T48.991	T48.992	T48.993	T48.994	T48.995	T48.996

Table of Drugs and Chemicals

Piribedil — Preparation, local

Substance	Poisoning, Accidental (unintentional)	Poisoning, Intentional Self-harm	Poisoning, Assault	Poisoning, Undetermined	Adverse Effect	Under-dosing
Piribedil	T42.8X1	T42.8X2	T42.8X3	T42.8X4	T42.8X5	T42.8X6
Piridoxilate	T46.3X1	T46.3X2	T46.3X3	T46.3X4	T46.3X5	T46.3X6
Piritramide	T40.491	T40.492	T40.493	T40.494	—	—
Piromidic acid	T37.8X1	T37.8X2	T37.8X3	T37.8X4	T37.8X5	T37.8X6
Piroxicam	T39.391	T39.392	T39.393	T39.394	T39.395	T39.396
beta-cyclodextrin complex	T39.8X1	T39.8X2	T39.8X3	T39.8X4	T39.8X5	T39.8X6
Pirozadil	T46.6X1	T46.6X2	T46.6X3	T46.6X4	T46.6X5	T46.6X6
Piscidia (bark) (erythrina)	T39.8X1	T39.8X2	T39.8X3	T39.8X4	T39.8X5	T39.8X6
Pitch	T65.891	T65.892	T65.893	T65.894	—	—
Pitkin's solution	T41.3X1	T41.3X2	T41.3X3	T41.3X4	T41.3X5	T41.3X6
Pitocin	T48.0X1	T48.0X2	T48.0X3	T48.0X4	T48.0X5	T48.0X6
Pitressin (tannate)	T38.891	T38.892	T38.893	T38.894	T38.895	T38.896
Pituitary extracts (posterior)	T38.891	T38.892	T38.893	T38.894	T38.895	T38.896
anterior	T38.811	T38.812	T38.813	T38.814	T38.815	T38.816
Pituitrin	T38.891	T38.892	T38.893	T38.894	T38.895	T38.896
Pivampicillin	T36.0X1	T36.0X2	T36.0X3	T36.0X4	T36.0X5	T36.0X6
Pivmecillinam	T36.0X1	T36.0X2	T36.0X3	T36.0X4	T36.0X5	T36.0X6
Placental hormone	T38.891	T38.892	T38.893	T38.894	T38.895	T38.896
Placidyl	T42.6X1	T42.6X2	T42.6X3	T42.6X4	T42.6X5	T42.6X6
Plague vaccine	T50.A91	T50.A92	T50.A93	T50.A94	T50.A95	T50.A96
Plant						
food or fertilizer NEC	T65.891	T65.892	T65.893	T65.894	—	—
containing herbicide	T60.3X1	T60.3X2	T60.3X3	T60.3X4	—	—
noxious, used as food	T62.2X1	T62.2X2	T62.2X3	T62.2X4	—	—
berries	T62.1X1	T62.1X2	T62.1X3	T62.1X4	—	—
seeds	T62.2X1	T62.2X2	T62.2X3	T62.2X4	—	—
specified type NEC	T62.2X1	T62.2X2	T62.2X3	T62.2X4	—	—
Plasma	T45.8X1	T45.8X2	T45.8X3	T45.8X4	T45.8X5	T45.8X6
expander NEC	T45.8X1	T45.8X2	T45.8X3	T45.8X4	T45.8X5	T45.8X6
protein fraction (human)	T45.8X1	T45.8X2	T45.8X3	T45.8X4	T45.8X5	T45.8X6
Plasmanate	T45.8X1	T45.8X2	T45.8X3	T45.8X4	T45.8X5	T45.8X6
Plasminogen (tissue)	T45.611	T45.612	T45.613	T45.614	T45.615	T45.616
activator	T45.611	T45.612	T45.613	T45.614	T45.615	T45.616
Plaster dressing	T49.3X1	T49.3X2	T49.3X3	T49.3X4	T49.3X5	T49.3X6
Plastic dressing	T49.3X1	T49.3X2	T49.3X3	T49.3X4	T49.3X5	T49.3X6
Plavix*	T45.521	T45.522	T45.523	T45.524	T45.525	T45.526
Plegicil	T43.3X1	T43.3X2	T43.3X3	T43.3X4	T43.3X5	T43.3X6
Plicamycin	T45.1X1	T45.1X2	T45.1X3	T45.1X4	T45.1X5	T45.1X6
Podophyllotoxin	T49.8X1	T49.8X2	T49.8X3	T49.8X4	T49.8X5	T49.8X6
Podophyllum (resin)	T49.4X1	T49.4X2	T49.4X3	T49.4X4	T49.4X5	T49.4X6
Poisonous berries	T62.1X1	T62.1X2	T62.1X3	T62.1X4	—	—
Poison NEC	T65.91	T65.92	T65.93	T65.94	—	—
Pokeweed (any part)	T62.2X1	T62.2X2	T62.2X3	T62.2X4	—	—
Poldine metilsulfate	T44.3X1	T44.3X2	T44.3X3	T44.3X4	T44.3X5	T44.3X6
Polidexide (sulfate)	T46.6X1	T46.6X2	T46.6X3	T46.6X4	T46.6X5	T46.6X6
Polidocanol	T46.8X1	T46.8X2	T46.8X3	T46.8X4	T46.8X5	T46.8X6
Poliomyelitis vaccine	T50.B91	T50.B92	T50.B93	T50.B94	T50.B95	T50.B96
Polish (car) (floor) (furniture) (metal) (porcelain) (silver)	T65.891	T65.892	T65.893	T65.894	—	—
abrasive	T65.891	T65.892	T65.893	T65.894	—	—
porcelain	T65.891	T65.892	T65.893	T65.894	—	—
Poloxalkol	T47.4X1	T47.4X2	T47.4X3	T47.4X4	T47.4X5	T47.4X6
Poloxamer	T47.4X1	T47.4X2	T47.4X3	T47.4X4	T47.4X5	T47.4X6
Polyaminostyrene resins	T50.3X1	T50.3X2	T50.3X3	T50.3X4	T50.3X5	T50.3X6
Polycarbophil	T47.4X1	T47.4X2	T47.4X3	T47.4X4	T47.4X5	T47.4X6
Polychlorinated biphenyl	T65.891	T65.892	T65.893	T65.894	—	—
Polycycline	T36.4X1	T36.4X2	T36.4X3	T36.4X4	T36.4X5	T36.4X6
Polyester fumes	T59.891	T59.892	T59.893	T59.894	—	—
Polyester resin hardener	T52.91	T52.92	T52.93	T52.94	—	—
fumes	T59.891	T59.892	T59.893	T59.894	—	—
Polyestradiol phosphate	T38.5X1	T38.5X2	T38.5X3	T38.5X4	T38.5X5	T38.5X6
Polyethanolamine alkyl sulfate	T49.2X1	T49.2X2	T49.2X3	T49.2X4	T49.2X5	T49.2X6
Polyethylene adhesive	T49.3X1	T49.3X2	T49.3X3	T49.3X4	T49.3X5	T49.3X6
Polyferose	T45.4X1	T45.4X2	T45.4X3	T45.4X4	T45.4X5	T45.4X6
Polygeline	T45.8X1	T45.8X2	T45.8X3	T45.8X4	T45.8X5	T45.8X6
Polymyxin	T36.8X1	T36.8X2	T36.8X3	T36.8X4	T36.8X5	T36.8X6
B	T36.8X1	T36.8X2	T36.8X3	T36.8X4	T36.8X5	T36.8X6
ENT agent	T49.6X1	T49.6X2	T49.6X3	T49.6X4	T49.6X5	T49.6X6
ophthalmic preparation	T49.5X1	T49.5X2	T49.5X3	T49.5X4	T49.5X5	T49.5X6
topical NEC	T49.0X1	T49.0X2	T49.0X3	T49.0X4	T49.0X5	T49.0X6
E sulfate (eye preparation)	T49.5X1	T49.5X2	T49.5X3	T49.5X4	T49.5X5	T49.5X6
Polynoxylin	T49.0X1	T49.0X2	T49.0X3	T49.0X4	T49.0X5	T49.0X6
Polyoestradiol phosphate	T38.5X1	T38.5X2	T38.5X3	T38.5X4	T38.5X5	T38.5X6
Polyoxymethyleneurea	T49.0X1	T49.0X2	T49.0X3	T49.0X4	T49.0X5	T49.0X6
Poly-Pred*	T49.5X1	T49.5X2	T49.5X3	T49.5X4	T49.5X5	T49.5X6
Polysilane	T47.8X1	T47.8X2	T47.8X3	T47.8X4	T47.8X5	T47.8X6
Polytetrafluoroethylene (inhaled)	T59.891	T59.892	T59.893	T59.894	—	—
Polythiazide	T50.2X1	T50.2X2	T50.2X3	T50.2X4	T50.2X5	T50.2X6
Polyvidone	T45.8X1	T45.8X2	T45.8X3	T45.8X4	T45.8X5	T45.8X6
Polyvinylpyrrolidone	T45.8X1	T45.8X2	T45.8X3	T45.8X4	T45.8X5	T45.8X6
Pontocaine (hydrochloride) (infiltration) (topical)	T41.3X1	T41.3X2	T41.3X3	T41.3X4	T41.3X5	T41.3X6
nerve block (peripheral) (plexus)	T41.3X1	T41.3X2	T41.3X3	T41.3X4	T41.3X5	T41.3X6
spinal	T41.3X1	T41.3X2	T41.3X3	T41.3X4	T41.3X5	T41.3X6
Porfiromycin	T45.1X1	T45.1X2	T45.1X3	T45.1X4	T45.1X5	T45.1X6
Portactant alfa*	T48.991	T48.992	T48.993	T48.994	T48.995	T48.996
Posterior pituitary hormone NEC	T38.891	T38.892	T38.893	T38.894	T38.895	T38.896
Pot	T40.711	T40.712	T40.713	T40.714	T40.715	T40.716
Potash (caustic)	T54.3X1	T54.3X2	T54.3X3	T54.3X4	—	—
Potassic saline injection (lactated)	T50.3X1	T50.3X2	T50.3X3	T50.3X4	T50.3X5	T50.3X6
Potassium (salts) NEC	T50.3X1	T50.3X2	T50.3X3	T50.3X4	T50.3X5	T50.3X6
aminobenzoate	T45.8X1	T45.8X2	T45.8X3	T45.8X4	T45.8X5	T45.8X6
aminosalicylate	T37.1X1	T37.1X2	T37.1X3	T37.1X4	T37.1X5	T37.1X6
antimony ' tartrate'	T37.8X1	T37.8X2	T37.8X3	T37.8X4	T37.8X5	T37.8X6
arsenite (solution)	T57.0X1	T57.0X2	T57.0X3	T57.0X4	—	—
bichromate	T56.2X1	T56.2X2	T56.2X3	T56.2X4	—	—
bisulfate	T47.3X1	T47.3X2	T47.3X3	T47.3X4	T47.3X5	T47.3X6
bromide	T42.6X1	T42.6X2	T42.6X3	T42.6X4	T42.6X5	T42.6X6
canrenoate	T50.0X1	T50.0X2	T50.0X3	T50.0X4	T50.0X5	T50.0X6
carbonate	T54.3X1	T54.3X2	T54.3X3	T54.3X4	—	—
chlorate NEC	T65.891	T65.892	T65.893	T65.894	—	—
chloride	T50.3X1	T50.3X2	T50.3X3	T50.3X4	T50.3X5	T50.3X6
citrate	T50.991	T50.992	T50.993	T50.994	T50.995	T50.996
cyanide	T65.0X1	T65.0X2	T65.0X3	T65.0X4	—	—
ferric hexacyanoferrate (medicinal)	T50.6X1	T50.6X2	T50.6X3	T50.6X4	T50.6X5	T50.6X6
nonmedicinal	T65.891	T65.892	T65.893	T65.894	—	—
Fluoride	T57.8X1	T57.8X2	T57.8X3	T57.8X4	—	—
glucaldrate	T47.1X1	T47.1X2	T47.1X3	T47.1X4	T47.1X5	T47.1X6
hydroxide	T54.3X1	T54.3X2	T54.3X3	T54.3X4	—	—
iodate	T49.0X1	T49.0X2	T49.0X3	T49.0X4	T49.0X5	T49.0X6
iodide	T48.4X1	T48.4X2	T48.4X3	T48.4X4	T48.4X5	T48.4X6
nitrate	T57.8X1	T57.8X2	T57.8X3	T57.8X4	—	—
oxalate	T65.891	T65.892	T65.893	T65.894	—	—
perchlorate (nonmedicinal) NEC	T65.891	T65.892	T65.893	T65.894	—	—
antithyroid	T38.2X1	T38.2X2	T38.2X3	T38.2X4	T38.2X5	T38.2X6
medicinal	T38.2X1	T38.2X2	T38.2X3	T38.2X4	T38.2X5	T38.2X6
Permanganate (nonmedicinal)	T65.891	T65.892	T65.893	T65.894	—	—
medicinal	T49.0X1	T49.0X2	T49.0X3	T49.0X4	T49.0X5	T49.0X6
sulfate	T47.2X1	T47.2X2	T47.2X3	T47.2X4	T47.2X5	T47.2X6
Potassium-removing resin	T50.3X1	T50.3X2	T50.3X3	T50.3X4	T50.3X5	T50.3X6
Potassium-retaining drug	T50.3X1	T50.3X2	T50.3X3	T50.3X4	T50.3X5	T50.3X6
Povidone	T45.8X1	T45.8X2	T45.8X3	T45.8X4	T45.8X5	T45.8X6
iodine	T49.0X1	T49.0X2	T49.0X3	T49.0X4	T49.0X5	T49.0X6
Practolol	T44.7X1	T44.7X2	T44.7X3	T44.7X4	T44.7X5	T44.7X6
Prajmalium bitartrate	T46.2X1	T46.2X2	T46.2X3	T46.2X4	T46.2X5	T46.2X6
Pralidoxime (iodide)	T50.6X1	T50.6X2	T50.6X3	T50.6X4	T50.6X5	T50.6X6
chloride	T50.6X1	T50.6X2	T50.6X3	T50.6X4	T50.6X5	T50.6X6
Pramiverine	T44.3X1	T44.3X2	T44.3X3	T44.3X4	T44.3X5	T44.3X6
Pramlintide*	T38.3X1	T38.3X2	T38.3X3	T38.3X4	T38.3X5	T38.3X6
Pramocaine	T49.1X1	T49.1X2	T49.1X3	T49.1X4	T49.1X5	T49.1X6
Pramoxine	T49.1X1	T49.1X2	T49.1X3	T49.1X4	T49.1X5	T49.1X6
Prasterone	T38.7X1	T38.7X2	T38.7X3	T38.7X4	T38.7X5	T38.7X6
Pravastatin	T46.6X1	T46.6X2	T46.6X3	T46.6X4	T46.6X5	T46.6X6
Prazepam	T42.4X1	T42.4X2	T42.4X3	T42.4X4	T42.4X5	T42.4X6
Praziquantel	T37.4X1	T37.4X2	T37.4X3	T37.4X4	T37.4X5	T37.4X6
Prazitone	T43.291	T43.292	T43.293	T43.294	T43.295	T43.296
Prazosin	T44.6X1	T44.6X2	T44.6X3	T44.6X4	T44.6X5	T44.6X6
Prednicarbate	T49.0X1	T49.0X2	T49.0X3	T49.0X4	T49.0X5	T49.0X6
Prednimustine	T45.1X1	T45.1X2	T45.1X3	T45.1X4	T45.1X5	T45.1X6
Prednisolone	T38.0X1	T38.0X2	T38.0X3	T38.0X4	T38.0X5	T38.0X6
ENT agent	T49.6X1	T49.6X2	T49.6X3	T49.6X4	T49.6X5	T49.6X6
ophthalmic preparation	T49.5X1	T49.5X2	T49.5X3	T49.5X4	T49.5X5	T49.5X6
steaglate	T49.0X1	T49.0X2	T49.0X3	T49.0X4	T49.0X5	T49.0X6
topical NEC	T49.0X1	T49.0X2	T49.0X3	T49.0X4	T49.0X5	T49.0X6
Prednisone	T38.0X1	T38.0X2	T38.0X3	T38.0X4	T38.0X5	T38.0X6
Prednylidene	T38.0X1	T38.0X2	T38.0X3	T38.0X4	T38.0X5	T38.0X6
Pregnandiol	T38.5X1	T38.5X2	T38.5X3	T38.5X4	T38.5X5	T38.5X6
Pregneninolone	T38.5X1	T38.5X2	T38.5X3	T38.5X4	T38.5X5	T38.5X6
Preludin	T43.691	T43.692	T43.693	T43.694	T43.695	T43.696
Premarin	T38.5X1	T38.5X2	T38.5X3	T38.5X4	T38.5X5	T38.5X6
Premedication anesthetic	T41.201	T41.202	T41.203	T41.204	T41.205	T41.206
Prenalterol	T44.5X1	T44.5X2	T44.5X3	T44.5X4	T44.5X5	T44.5X6
Prenoxdiazine	T48.3X1	T48.3X2	T48.3X3	T48.3X4	T48.3X5	T48.3X6
Prenylamine	T46.3X1	T46.3X2	T46.3X3	T46.3X4	T46.3X5	T46.3X6
Preparation H	T49.8X1	T49.8X2	T49.8X3	T49.8X4	T49.8X5	T49.8X6
Preparation, local	T49.4X1	T49.4X2	T49.4X3	T49.4X4	T49.4X5	T49.4X6

Substance	Poisoning, Accidental (unintentional)	Poisoning, Intentional Self-harm	Poisoning, Assault	Poisoning, Undetermined	Adverse Effect	Under-dosing
Preservative	T65.891	T65.892	T65.893	T65.894	—	—
(nonmedicinal)						
medicinal	T50.901	T50.902	T50.903	T50.904	T50.905	T50.906
wood	T60.91	T60.92	T60.93	T60.94		
Prethcamide	T50.7X1	T50.7X2	T50.7X3	T50.7X4	T50.7X5	T50.7X6
Prevacid*	T47.1X1	T47.1X2	T47.1X3	T47.1X4	T47.1X5	T47.1X6
Pride of China	T62.2X1	T62.2X2	T62.2X3	T62.2X4		
Pridinol	T44.3X1	T44.3X2	T44.3X3	T44.3X4	T44.3X5	T44.3X6
Prifinium bromide	T44.3X1	T44.3X2	T44.3X3	T44.3X4	T44.3X5	T44.3X6
Prilocaine	T41.3X1	T41.3X2	T41.3X3	T41.3X4	T41.3X5	T41.3X6
infiltration (subcutaneous)	T41.3X1	T41.3X2	T41.3X3	T41.3X4	T41.3X5	T41.3X6
nerve block (peripheral) (plexus)	T41.3X1	T41.3X2	T41.3X3	T41.3X4	T41.3X5	T41.3X6
regional	T41.3X1	T41.3X2	T41.3X3	T41.3X4	T41.3X5	T41.3X6
Primaquine	T37.2X1	T37.2X2	T37.2X3	T37.2X4	T37.2X5	T37.2X6
Primidone	T42.6X1	T42.6X2	T42.6X3	T42.6X4	T42.6X5	T42.6X6
Primula (veris)	T62.2X1	T62.2X2	T62.2X3	T62.2X4		
Prinadol	T40.2X1	T40.2X2	T40.2X3	T40.2X4	T40.2X5	T40.2X6
Priscol, Priscoline	T44.6X1	T44.6X2	T44.6X3	T44.6X4	T44.6X5	T44.6X6
Pristinamycin	T36.3X1	T36.3X2	T36.3X3	T36.3X4	T36.3X5	T36.3X6
Pristiq*	T43.211	T43.212	T43.213	T43.214	T43.215	T43.216
Privet	T62.2X1	T62.2X2	T62.2X3	T62.2X4		
berries	T62.1X1	T62.1X2	T62.1X3	T62.1X4		
Privine	T44.4X1	T44.4X2	T44.4X3	T44.4X4	T44.4X5	T44.4X6
Pro-Banthine	T44.3X1	T44.3X2	T44.3X3	T44.3X4	T44.3X5	T44.3X6
Probarbital	T42.3X1	T42.3X2	T42.3X3	T42.3X4	T42.3X5	T42.3X6
Probenecid	T50.4X1	T50.4X2	T50.4X3	T50.4X4	T50.4X5	T50.4X6
Probucol	T46.6X1	T46.6X2	T46.6X3	T46.6X4	T46.6X5	T46.6X6
Procainamide	T46.2X1	T46.2X2	T46.2X3	T46.2X4	T46.2X5	T46.2X6
Procaine	T41.3X1	T41.3X2	T41.3X3	T41.3X4	T41.3X5	T41.3X6
benzylpenicillin	T36.0X1	T36.0X2	T36.0X3	T36.0X4	T36.0X5	T36.0X6
nerve block (periphreal) (plexus)	T41.3X1	T41.3X2	T41.3X3	T41.3X4	T41.3X5	T41.3X6
penicillin G	T36.0X1	T36.0X2	T36.0X3	T36.0X4	T36.0X5	T36.0X6
regional	T41.3X1	T41.3X2	T41.3X3	T41.3X4	T41.3X5	T41.3X6
spinal	T41.3X1	T41.3X2	T41.3X3	T41.3X4	T41.3X5	T41.3X6
Procalmidol	T43.591	T43.592	T43.593	T43.594	T43.595	T43.596
Procarbazine	T45.1X1	T45.1X2	T45.1X3	T45.1X4	T45.1X5	T45.1X6
Procaterol	T44.5X1	T44.5X2	T44.5X3	T44.5X4	T44.5X5	T44.5X6
Prochlorperazine	T43.3X1	T43.3X2	T43.3X3	T43.3X4	T43.3X5	T43.3X6
Procyclidine	T44.3X1	T44.3X2	T44.3X3	T44.3X4	T44.3X5	T44.3X6
Producer gas	T58.8X1	T58.8X2	T58.8X3	T58.8X4	—	—
Profadol	T40.491	T40.492	T40.493	T40.494	T40.495	T40.496
Profenamine	T44.3X1	T44.3X2	T44.3X3	T44.3X4	T44.3X5	T44.3X6
Profenil	T44.3X1	T44.3X2	T44.3X3	T44.3X4	T44.3X5	T44.3X6
Proflavine	T49.0X1	T49.0X2	T49.0X3	T49.0X4	T49.0X5	T49.0X6
Progabide	T42.6X1	T42.6X2	T42.6X3	T42.6X4	T42.6X5	T42.6X6
Progesterone	T38.5X1	T38.5X2	T38.5X3	T38.5X4	T38.5X5	T38.5X6
Progestin	T38.5X1	T38.5X2	T38.5X3	T38.5X4	T38.5X5	T38.5X6
oral contraceptive	T38.4X1	T38.4X2	T38.4X3	T38.4X4	T38.4X5	T38.4X6
Progestogen NEC	T38.5X1	T38.5X2	T38.5X3	T38.5X4	T38.5X5	T38.5X6
Progestone	T38.5X1	T38.5X2	T38.5X3	T38.5X4	T38.5X5	T38.5X6
Proglumide	T47.1X1	T47.1X2	T47.1X3	T47.1X4	T47.1X5	T47.1X6
Prograf*	T45.1X1	T45.1X2	T45.1X3	T45.1X4	T45.1X5	T45.1X6
Proguanil	T37.2X1	T37.2X2	T37.2X3	T37.2X4	T37.2X5	T37.2X6
Prolactin	T38.811	T38.812	T38.813	T38.814	T38.815	T38.816
Prolintane	T43.691	T43.692	T43.693	T43.694	T43.695	T43.696
Proloid	T38.1X1	T38.1X2	T38.1X3	T38.1X4	T38.1X5	T38.1X6
Proluton	T38.5X1	T38.5X2	T38.5X3	T38.5X4	T38.5X5	T38.5X6
Promacetin	T37.1X1	T37.1X2	T37.1X3	T37.1X4	T37.1X5	T37.1X6
Promazine	T43.3X1	T43.3X2	T43.3X3	T43.3X4	T43.3X5	T43.3X6
Promedol	T40.2X1	T40.2X2	T40.2X3	T40.2X4	—	—
Promegestone	T38.5X1	T38.5X2	T38.5X3	T38.5X4	T38.5X5	T38.5X6
Promethazine (teoclate)	T43.3X1	T43.3X2	T43.3X3	T43.3X4	T43.3X5	T43.3X6
Promin	T37.1X1	T37.1X2	T37.1X3	T37.1X4	T37.1X5	T37.1X6
Pronase	T45.3X1	T45.3X2	T45.3X3	T45.3X4	T45.3X5	T45.3X6
Pronestyl (hydrochloride)	T46.2X1	T46.2X2	T46.2X3	T46.2X4	T46.2X5	T46.2X6
Pronetalol	T44.7X1	T44.7X2	T44.7X3	T44.7X4	T44.7X5	T44.7X6
Prontosil	T37.0X1	T37.0X2	T37.0X3	T37.0X4	T37.0X5	T37.0X6
Propachlor	T60.3X1	T60.3X2	T60.3X3	T60.3X4	—	—
Propafenone	T46.2X1	T46.2X2	T46.2X3	T46.2X4	T46.2X5	T46.2X6
Propallylonal	T42.3X1	T42.3X2	T42.3X3	T42.3X4	T42.3X5	T42.3X6
Propamidine	T49.0X1	T49.0X2	T49.0X3	T49.0X4	T49.0X5	T49.0X6
Propane (distributed in mobile container)	T59.891	T59.892	T59.893	T59.894	—	—
distributed through pipes	T59.891	T59.892	T59.893	T59.894	—	—
incomplete combustion	T58.11	T58.12	T58.13	T58.14	—	—
Propanidid	T41.291	T41.292	T41.293	T41.294	T41.295	T41.296
Propanil	T60.3X1	T60.3X2	T60.3X3	T60.3X4	—	—
Propantheline	T44.3X1	T44.3X2	T44.3X3	T44.3X4	T44.3X5	T44.3X6
bromide	T44.3X1	T44.3X2	T44.3X3	T44.3X4	T44.3X5	T44.3X6
Proparacaine	T41.3X1	T41.3X2	T41.3X3	T41.3X4	T41.3X5	T41.3X6
Propatylnitrate	T46.3X1	T46.3X2	T46.3X3	T46.3X4	T46.3X5	T46.3X6

Substance	Poisoning, Accidental (unintentional)	Poisoning, Intentional Self-harm	Poisoning, Assault	Poisoning, Undetermined	Adverse Effect	Under-dosing
Propicillin	T36.0X1	T36.0X2	T36.0X3	T36.0X4	T36.0X5	T36.0X6
Propine*	T49.5X1	T49.5X2	T49.5X3	T49.5X4	T49.5X5	T49.5X6
Propiolactone	T49.0X1	T49.0X2	T49.0X3	T49.0X4	T49.0X5	T49.0X6
Propiomazine	T45.0X1	T45.0X2	T45.0X3	T45.0X4	T45.0X5	T45.0X6
Propionaldehyde (medicinal)	T42.6X1	T42.6X2	T42.6X3	T42.6X4	T42.6X5	T42.6X6
Propionate (calcium) (sodium)	T49.0X1	T49.0X2	T49.0X3	T49.0X4	T49.0X5	T49.0X6
Propion gel	T49.0X1	T49.0X2	T49.0X3	T49.0X4	T49.0X5	T49.0X6
Propitocaine	T41.3X1	T41.3X2	T41.3X3	T41.3X4	T41.3X5	T41.3X6
infiltration (subcutaneous)	T41.3X1	T41.3X2	T41.3X3	T41.3X4	T41.3X5	T41.3X6
nerve block (peripheral) (plexus)	T41.3X1	T41.3X2	T41.3X3	T41.3X4	T41.3X5	T41.3X6
Propofol	T41.291	T41.292	T41.293	T41.294	T41.295	T41.296
Propoxur	T60.0X1	T60.0X2	T60.0X3	T60.0X4	—	—
Propoxycaine	T41.3X1	T41.3X2	T41.3X3	T41.3X4	T41.3X5	T41.3X6
infiltration (subcutaneous)	T41.3X1	T41.3X2	T41.3X3	T41.3X4	T41.3X5	T41.3X6
nerve block (peripheral) (plexus)	T41.3X1	T41.3X2	T41.3X3	T41.3X4	T41.3X5	T41.3X6
topical (surface)	T41.3X1	T41.3X2	T41.3X3	T41.3X4	T41.3X5	T41.3X6
Propoxyphene	T40.491	T40.492	T40.493	T40.494	T40.495	T40.496
Propranolol	T44.7X1	T44.7X2	T44.7X3	T44.7X4	T44.7X5	T44.7X6
Propyl						
alcohol	T51.3X1	T51.3X2	T51.3X3	T51.3X4	—	—
carbinol	T51.3X1	T51.3X2	T51.3X3	T51.3X4	—	—
hexadrine	T44.4X1	T44.4X2	T44.4X3	T44.4X4	T44.4X5	T44.4X6
iodone	T50.8X1	T50.8X2	T50.8X3	T50.8X4	T50.8X5	T50.8X6
thiouracil	T38.2X1	T38.2X2	T38.2X3	T38.2X4	T38.2X5	T38.2X6
Propylaminophenothiazine	T43.3X1	T43.3X2	T43.3X3	T43.3X4	T43.3X5	T43.3X6
Propylene	T59.891	T59.892	T59.893	T59.894	—	—
Propylhexedrine	T48.5X1	T48.5X2	T48.5X3	T48.5X4	T48.5X5	T48.5X6
Propyliodone	T50.8X1	T50.8X2	T50.8X3	T50.8X4	T50.8X5	T50.8X6
Propylparaben (ophthalmic)	T49.5X1	T49.5X2	T49.5X3	T49.5X4	T49.5X5	T49.5X6
Propylthiouracil	T38.2X1	T38.2X2	T38.2X3	T38.2X4	T38.2X5	T38.2X6
Propyphenazone	T39.2X1	T39.2X2	T39.2X3	T39.2X4	T39.2X5	T39.2X6
Proquazone	T39.391	T39.392	T39.393	T39.394	T39.395	T39.396
Proscar*	T38.6X1	T38.6X2	T38.6X3	T38.6X4	T38.6X5	T38.6X6
Proscillaridin	T46.0X1	T46.0X2	T46.0X3	T46.0X4	T46.0X5	T46.0X6
Prostacyclin	T45.521	T45.522	T45.523	T45.524	T45.525	T45.526
Prostaglandin (I2)	T45.521	T45.522	T45.523	T45.524	T45.525	T45.526
E1	T46.7X1	T46.7X2	T46.7X3	T46.7X4	T46.7X5	T46.7X6
E2	T48.0X1	T48.0X2	T48.0X3	T48.0X4	T48.0X5	T48.0X6
F2 alpha	T48.0X1	T48.0X2	T48.0X3	T48.0X4	T48.0X5	T48.0X6
Prostigmin	T44.0X1	T44.0X2	T44.0X3	T44.0X4	T44.0X5	T44.0X6
Prosultiamine	T45.2X1	T45.2X2	T45.2X3	T45.2X4	T45.2X5	T45.2X6
Protamine sulfate	T45.7X1	T45.7X2	T45.7X3	T45.7X4	T45.7X5	T45.7X6
zinc insulin	T38.3X1	T38.3X2	T38.3X3	T38.3X4	T38.3X5	T38.3X6
Protease	T47.5X1	T47.5X2	T47.5X3	T47.5X4	T47.5X5	T47.5X6
Protectant, skin NEC	T49.3X1	T49.3X2	T49.3X3	T49.3X4	T49.3X5	T49.3X6
Protein hydrolysate	T50.991	T50.992	T50.993	T50.994	T50.995	T50.996
Prothiaden — see Dothiepin hydrochloride						
Prothionamide	T37.1X1	T37.1X2	T37.1X3	T37.1X4	T37.1X5	T37.1X6
Prothipendyl	T43.591	T43.592	T43.593	T43.594	T43.595	T43.596
Prothoate	T60.0X1	T60.0X2	T60.0X3	T60.0X4		
Prothrombin						
activator	T45.7X1	T45.7X2	T45.7X3	T45.7X4	T45.7X5	T45.7X6
synthesis inhibitor	T45.511	T45.512	T45.513	T45.514	T45.515	T45.516
Protionamide	T37.1X1	T37.1X2	T37.1X3	T37.1X4	T37.1X5	T37.1X6
Protirelin	T38.891	T38.892	T38.893	T38.894	T38.895	T38.896
Protokylol	T48.6X1	T48.6X2	T48.6X3	T48.6X4	T48.6X5	T48.6X6
Protopam	T50.6X1	T50.6X2	T50.6X3	T50.6X4	T50.6X5	T50.6X6
Protoveratrine(s) (A) (B)	T46.5X1	T46.5X2	T46.5X3	T46.5X4	T46.5X5	T46.5X6
Protriptyline	T43.011	T43.012	T43.013	T43.014	T43.015	T43.016
Proventil*	T48.6X1	T48.6X2	T48.6X3	T48.6X4	T48.6X5	T48.6X6
Provera	T38.5X1	T38.5X2	T38.5X3	T38.5X4	T38.5X5	T38.5X6
Provitamin A	T45.2X1	T45.2X2	T45.2X3	T45.2X4	T45.2X5	T45.2X6
Proxibarbal	T42.3X1	T42.3X2	T42.3X3	T42.3X4	T42.3X5	T42.3X6
Proxymetacaine	T41.3X1	T41.3X2	T41.3X3	T41.3X4	T41.3X5	T41.3X6
Proxyphylline	T48.6X1	T48.6X2	T48.6X3	T48.6X4	T48.6X5	T48.6X6
Prozac — see Fluoxetine hydrochloride						
Prunus						
laurocerasus	T62.2X1	T62.2X2	T62.2X3	T62.2X4		
virginiana	T62.2X1	T62.2X2	T62.2X3	T62.2X4		
Prussian blue						
commercial	T65.891	T65.892	T65.893	T65.894		
therapeutic	T50.6X1	T50.6X2	T50.6X3	T50.6X4	T50.6X5	T50.6X6
Prussic acid	T65.0X1	T65.0X2	T65.0X3	T65.0X4		
vapor	T57.3X1	T57.3X2	T57.3X3	T57.3X4		
Pseudoephedrine	T44.991	T44.992	T44.993	T44.994	T44.995	T44.996
Psilocin	T40.991	T40.992	T40.993	T40.994	—	—

Table of Drugs and Chemicals

Psilocybin — Respiratory drug NEC

Substance	Poisoning, Accidental (unintentional)	Poisoning, Intentional Self-harm	Poisoning, Assault	Poisoning, Undetermined	Adverse Effect	Under-dosing
Psilocybin	T40.991	T40.992	T40.993	T40.994	—	—
Psilocybine	T40.991	T40.992	T40.993	T40.994	—	—
Psoralene (nonmedicinal)	T65.891	T65.892	T65.893	T65.894	—	—
Psoralens (medicinal)	T50.991	T50.992	T50.993	T50.994	T50.995	T50.996
PSP	T50.8X1	T50.8X2	T50.8X3	T50.8X4	T50.8X5	T50.8X6
(phenolsulfonphthalein)						
Psychodysleptic drug NOS	T40.901	T40.902	T40.903	T40.904	T40.905	T40.906
specified NEC	T40.991	T40.992	T40.993	T40.994	T40.995	T40.996
Psychostimulant	T43.601	T43.602	T43.603	T43.604	T43.605	T43.606
amphetamine	T43.621	T43.622	T43.623	T43.624	T43.625	T43.626
caffeine	T43.611	T43.612	T43.613	T43.614	T43.615	T43.616
methylphenidate	T43.631	T43.632	T43.633	T43.634	T43.635	T43.636
specified NEC	T43.691	T43.692	T43.693	T43.694	T43.695	T43.696
Psychotherapeutic drug NEC	T43.91	T43.92	T43.93	T43.94	T43.95	T43.96
antidepressants — see also Antidepressant	T43.201	T43.202	T43.203	T43.204	T43.205	T43.206
specified NEC	T43.8X1	T43.8X2	T43.8X3	T43.8X4	T43.8X5	T43.8X6
tranquilizers NEC	T43.501	T43.502	T43.503	T43.504	T43.505	T43.506
Psychotomimetic agents	T40.901	T40.902	T40.903	T40.904	T40.905	T40.906
Psychotropic drug NEC	T43.91	T43.92	T43.93	T43.94	T43.95	T43.96
specified NEC	T43.8X1	T43.8X2	T43.8X3	T43.8X4	T43.8X5	T43.8X6
Psyllium hydrophilic mucilloid	T47.4X1	T47.4X2	T47.4X3	T47.4X4	T47.4X5	T47.4X6
Pteroylglutamic acid	T45.8X1	T45.8X2	T45.8X3	T45.8X4	T45.8X5	T45.8X6
Pteroyltriglutamate	T45.1X1	T45.1X2	T45.1X3	T45.1X4	T45.1X5	T45.1X6
PTFE — see Polytetrafluoroethylene						
Pulmicort*	T44.5X1	T44.5X2	T44.5X3	T44.5X4	T44.5X5	T44.5X6
Pulp						
devitalizing paste	T49.7X1	T49.7X2	T49.7X3	T49.7X4	T49.7X5	T49.7X6
dressing	T49.7X1	T49.7X2	T49.7X3	T49.7X4	T49.7X5	T49.7X6
Pulsatilla	T62.2X1	T62.2X2	T62.2X3	T62.2X4	—	—
Pumpkin seed extract	T37.4X1	T37.4X2	T37.4X3	T37.4X4	T37.4X5	T37.4X6
Purex (bleach)	T54.91	T54.92	T54.93	T54.94	—	—
Purgative NEC — see also Cathartic	T47.4X1	T47.4X2	T47.4X3	T47.4X4	T47.4X5	T47.4X6
Purine analogue (antineoplastic)	T45.1X1	T45.1X2	T45.1X3	T45.1X4	T45.1X5	T45.1X6
Purine diuretics	T50.2X1	T50.2X2	T50.2X3	T50.2X4	T50.2X5	T50.2X6
Purinethol	T45.1X1	T45.1X2	T45.1X3	T45.1X4	T45.1X5	T45.1X6
PVP	T45.8X1	T45.8X2	T45.8X3	T45.8X4	T45.8X5	T45.8X6
Pyrabital	T39.8X1	T39.8X2	T39.8X3	T39.8X4	T39.8X5	T39.8X6
Pyramidon	T39.2X1	T39.2X2	T39.2X3	T39.2X4	T39.2X5	T39.2X6
Pyrantel	T37.4X1	T37.4X2	T37.4X3	T37.4X4	T37.4X5	T37.4X6
Pyrathiazine	T45.0X1	T45.0X2	T45.0X3	T45.0X4	T45.0X5	T45.0X6
Pyrazinamide	T37.1X1	T37.1X2	T37.1X3	T37.1X4	T37.1X5	T37.1X6
Pyrazinoic acid (amide)	T37.1X1	T37.1X2	T37.1X3	T37.1X4	T37.1X5	T37.1X6
Pyrazole (derivatives)	T39.2X1	T39.2X2	T39.2X3	T39.2X4	T39.2X5	T39.2X6
Pyrazolone analgesic NEC	T39.2X1	T39.2X2	T39.2X3	T39.2X4	T39.2X5	T39.2X6
Pyrethrin, pyrethrum (nonmedicinal)	T60.2X1	T60.2X2	T60.2X3	T60.2X4	—	—
Pyrethrum extract	T49.0X1	T49.0X2	T49.0X3	T49.0X4	T49.0X5	T49.0X6
Pyribenzamine	T45.0X1	T45.0X2	T45.0X3	T45.0X4	T45.0X5	T45.0X6
Pyridine	T52.8X1	T52.8X2	T52.8X3	T52.8X4	—	—
aldoxime methiodide	T50.6X1	T50.6X2	T50.6X3	T50.6X4	T50.6X5	T50.6X6
aldoxime methyl chloride	T50.6X1	T50.6X2	T50.6X3	T50.6X4	T50.6X5	T50.6X6
vapor	T59.891	T59.892	T59.893	T59.894	—	—
Pyridium	T39.8X1	T39.8X2	T39.8X3	T39.8X4	T39.8X5	T39.8X6
Pyridostigmine bromide	T44.0X1	T44.0X2	T44.0X3	T44.0X4	T44.0X5	T44.0X6
Pyridoxal phosphate	T45.2X1	T45.2X2	T45.2X3	T45.2X4	T45.2X5	T45.2X6
Pyridoxine	T45.2X1	T45.2X2	T45.2X3	T45.2X4	T45.2X5	T45.2X6
Pyrilamine	T45.0X1	T45.0X2	T45.0X3	T45.0X4	T45.0X5	T45.0X6
Pyrimethamine	T37.2X1	T37.2X2	T37.2X3	T37.2X4	T37.2X5	T37.2X6
with sulfadoxine	T37.2X1	T37.2X2	T37.2X3	T37.2X4	T37.2X5	T37.2X6
Pyrimidine antagonist	T45.1X1	T45.1X2	T45.1X3	T45.1X4	T45.1X5	T45.1X6
Pyriminil	T60.4X1	T60.4X2	T60.4X3	T60.4X4	—	—
Pyrithione zinc	T49.4X1	T49.4X2	T49.4X3	T49.4X4	T49.4X5	T49.4X6
Pyrithyldione	T42.6X1	T42.6X2	T42.6X3	T42.6X4	T42.6X5	T42.6X6
Pyrogallic acid	T49.0X1	T49.0X2	T49.0X3	T49.0X4	T49.0X5	T49.0X6
Pyrogallol	T49.0X1	T49.0X2	T49.0X3	T49.0X4	T49.0X5	T49.0X6
Pyroxylin	T49.3X1	T49.3X2	T49.3X3	T49.3X4	T49.3X5	T49.3X6
Pyrrobutamine	T45.0X1	T45.0X2	T45.0X3	T45.0X4	T45.0X5	T45.0X6
Pyrrolizidine alkaloids	T62.8X1	T62.8X2	T62.8X3	T62.8X4	—	—
Pyrvinium chloride	T37.4X1	T37.4X2	T37.4X3	T37.4X4	T37.4X5	T37.4X6
PZI	T38.3X1	T38.3X2	T38.3X3	T38.3X4	T38.3X5	T38.3X6
Qbrelis*	T46.4X1	T46.4X2	T46.4X3	T46.4X4	T46.4X5	T46.4X6
Quaalude	T42.6X1	T42.6X2	T42.6X3	T42.6X4	T42.6X5	T42.6X6
Quarternary ammonium						
anti-infective	T49.0X1	T49.0X2	T49.0X3	T49.0X4	T49.0X5	T49.0X6
ganglion blocking	T44.2X1	T44.2X2	T44.2X3	T44.2X4	T44.2X5	T44.2X6
parasympatholytic	T44.3X1	T44.3X2	T44.3X3	T44.3X4	T44.3X5	T44.3X6
Quazepam	T42.4X1	T42.4X2	T42.4X3	T42.4X4	T42.4X5	T42.4X6
Quicklime	T54.3X1	T54.3X2	T54.3X3	T54.3X4	—	—
Quilbron-T*	T48.6X1	T48.6X2	T48.6X3	T48.6X4	T48.6X5	T48.6X6
Quillaja extract	T48.4X1	T48.4X2	T48.4X3	T48.4X4	T48.4X5	T48.4X6
Quinacrine	T37.2X1	T37.2X2	T37.2X3	T37.2X4	T37.2X5	T37.2X6
Quinaglute	T46.2X1	T46.2X2	T46.2X3	T46.2X4	T46.2X5	T46.2X6
Quinalbarbital	T42.3X1	T42.3X2	T42.3X3	T42.3X4	T42.3X5	T42.3X6
Quinalbarbitone sodium	T42.3X1	T42.3X2	T42.3X3	T42.3X4	T42.3X5	T42.3X6
Quinalphos	T60.0X1	T60.0X2	T60.0X3	T60.0X4	—	—
Quinapril	T46.4X1	T46.4X2	T46.4X3	T46.4X4	T46.4X5	T46.4X6
Quinestradiol	T38.5X1	T38.5X2	T38.5X3	T38.5X4	T38.5X5	T38.5X6
Quinestradol	T38.5X1	T38.5X2	T38.5X3	T38.5X4	T38.5X5	T38.5X6
Quinestrol	T38.5X1	T38.5X2	T38.5X3	T38.5X4	T38.5X5	T38.5X6
Quinethazone	T50.2X1	T50.2X2	T50.2X3	T50.2X4	T50.2X5	T50.2X6
Quingestanol	T38.4X1	T38.4X2	T38.4X3	T38.4X4	T38.4X5	T38.4X6
Quinidine	T46.2X1	T46.2X2	T46.2X3	T46.2X4	T46.2X5	T46.2X6
Quinine	T37.2X1	T37.2X2	T37.2X3	T37.2X4	T37.2X5	T37.2X6
Quiniobine	T37.8X1	T37.8X2	T37.8X3	T37.8X4	T37.8X5	T37.8X6
Quinisocaine	T49.1X1	T49.1X2	T49.1X3	T49.1X4	T49.1X5	T49.1X6
Quinocide	T37.2X1	T37.2X2	T37.2X3	T37.2X4	T37.2X5	T37.2X6
Quinoline (derivatives) **NEC**	T37.8X1	T37.8X2	T37.8X3	T37.8X4	T37.8X5	T37.8X6
Quinupramine	T43.011	T43.012	T43.013	T43.014	T43.015	T43.016
Quixin*	T49.5X1	T49.5X2	T49.5X3	T49.5X4	T49.5X5	T49.5X6
Quotane	T41.3X1	T41.3X2	T41.3X3	T41.3X4	T41.3X5	T41.3X6
Rabies						
immune globulin (human)	T50.Z11	T50.Z12	T50.Z13	T50.Z14	T50.Z15	T50.Z16
vaccine	T50.B91	T50.B92	T50.B93	T50.B94	T50.B95	T50.B96
Racemoramide	T40.2X1	T40.2X2	T40.2X3	T40.2X4	—	—
Racemorphan	T40.2X1	T40.2X2	T40.2X3	T40.2X4	T40.2X5	T40.2X6
Racepinefrin	T44.5X1	T44.5X2	T44.5X3	T44.5X4	T44.5X5	T44.5X6
Raclopride	T43.591	T43.592	T43.593	T43.594	T43.595	T43.596
Radiator alcohol	T51.1X1	T51.1X2	T51.1X3	T51.1X4	—	—
Radioactive drug NEC	T50.8X1	T50.8X2	T50.8X3	T50.8X4	T50.8X5	T50.8X6
Radio-opaque (drugs) (materials)	T50.8X1	T50.8X2	T50.8X3	T50.8X4	T50.8X5	T50.8X6
Ramifenazone	T39.2X1	T39.2X2	T39.2X3	T39.2X4	T39.2X5	T39.2X6
Ramipril	T46.4X1	T46.4X2	T46.4X3	T46.4X4	T46.4X5	T46.4X6
Ranitidine	T47.0X1	T47.0X2	T47.0X3	T47.0X4	T47.0X5	T47.0X6
Ranunculus	T62.2X1	T62.2X2	T62.2X3	T62.2X4	—	—
Rat poison NEC	T60.4X1	T60.4X2	T60.4X3	T60.4X4	—	—
Rattlesnake (venom)	T63.011	T63.012	T63.013	T63.014	—	—
Raubasine	T46.7X1	T46.7X2	T46.7X3	T46.7X4	T46.7X5	T46.7X6
Raudixin	T46.5X1	T46.5X2	T46.5X3	T46.5X4	T46.5X5	T46.5X6
Rautensin	T46.5X1	T46.5X2	T46.5X3	T46.5X4	T46.5X5	T46.5X6
Rautina	T46.5X1	T46.5X2	T46.5X3	T46.5X4	T46.5X5	T46.5X6
Rautotal	T46.5X1	T46.5X2	T46.5X3	T46.5X4	T46.5X5	T46.5X6
Rauwiloid	T46.5X1	T46.5X2	T46.5X3	T46.5X4	T46.5X5	T46.5X6
Rauwoldin	T46.5X1	T46.5X2	T46.5X3	T46.5X4	T46.5X5	T46.5X6
Rauwolfia (alkaloids)	T46.5X1	T46.5X2	T46.5X3	T46.5X4	T46.5X5	T46.5X6
Razadyne*	T44.0X1	T44.0X2	T44.0X3	T44.0X4	T44.0X5	T44.0X6
Razoxane	T45.1X1	T45.1X2	T45.1X3	T45.1X4	T45.1X5	T45.1X6
Realgar	T57.0X1	T57.0X2	T57.0X3	T57.0X4	—	—
Recombinant (R) — see specific protein						
Red blood cells, packed	T45.8X1	T45.8X2	T45.8X3	T45.8X4	T45.8X5	T45.8X6
Red squill (scilliroside)	T60.4X1	T60.4X2	T60.4X3	T60.4X4	—	—
Reducing agent, industrial NEC	T65.891	T65.892	T65.893	T65.894	—	—
Refrigerant gas (chlorofluorocarbon)	T53.5X1	T53.5X2	T53.5X3	T53.5X4	—	—
not chlorofluorocarbon	T59.891	T59.892	T59.893	T59.894	—	—
Regroton	T50.2X1	T50.2X2	T50.2X3	T50.2X4	T50.2X5	T50.2X6
Rehydration salts (oral)	T50.3X1	T50.3X2	T50.3X3	T50.3X4	T50.3X5	T50.3X6
Rela	T42.8X1	T42.8X2	T42.8X3	T42.8X4	T42.8X5	T42.8X6
Relaxant, muscle						
anesthetic	T48.1X1	T48.1X2	T48.1X3	T48.1X4	T48.1X5	T48.1X6
central nervous system	T42.8X1	T42.8X2	T42.8X3	T42.8X4	T42.8X5	T42.8X6
skeletal NEC	T48.1X1	T48.1X2	T48.1X3	T48.1X4	T48.1X5	T48.1X6
smooth NEC	T44.3X1	T44.3X2	T44.3X3	T44.3X4	T44.3X5	T44.3X6
Remoxipride	T43.591	T43.592	T43.593	T43.594	T43.595	T43.596
Renese	T50.2X1	T50.2X2	T50.2X3	T50.2X4	T50.2X5	T50.2X6
Renografin	T50.8X1	T50.8X2	T50.8X3	T50.8X4	T50.8X5	T50.8X6
Replacement solution	T50.3X1	T50.3X2	T50.3X3	T50.3X4	T50.3X5	T50.3X6
Reproterol	T48.6X1	T48.6X2	T48.6X3	T48.6X4	T48.6X5	T48.6X6
Rescinnamine	T46.5X1	T46.5X2	T46.5X3	T46.5X4	T46.5X5	T46.5X6
Reserpin (e)	T46.5X1	T46.5X2	T46.5X3	T46.5X4	T46.5X5	T46.5X6
Resorcin, resorcinol (nonmedicinal)	T65.891	T65.892	T65.893	T65.894	—	—
medicinal	T49.4X1	T49.4X2	T49.4X3	T49.4X4	T49.4X5	T49.4X6
Respaire	T48.4X1	T48.4X2	T48.4X3	T48.4X4	T48.4X5	T48.4X6
Respiratory drug NEC	T48.901	T48.902	T48.903	T48.904	T48.905	T48.906
antiasthmatic NEC	T48.6X1	T48.6X2	T48.6X3	T48.6X4	T48.6X5	T48.6X6
anti-common-cold NEC	T48.5X1	T48.5X2	T48.5X3	T48.5X4	T48.5X5	T48.5X6
expectorant NEC	T48.4X1	T48.4X2	T48.4X3	T48.4X4	T48.4X5	T48.4X6

☑ Additional Character May Be Required — Refer to the Tabular List for Character Selection

*Optum Value-Add

Substance	Poisoning, Accidental (unintentional)	Poisoning, Intentional Self-harm	Poisoning, Assault	Poisoning, Undetermined	Adverse Effect	Under-dosing
Respiratory drug — *continued*						
stimulant	T48.901	T48.902	T48.903	T48.904	T48.905	T48.906
Restoril*	T42.4X1	T42.4X2	T42.4X3	T42.4X4	T42.4X5	T42.4X6
Retinoic acid	T49.0X1	T49.0X2	T49.0X3	T49.0X4	T49.0X5	T49.0X6
Retinol	T45.2X1	T45.2X2	T45.2X3	T45.2X4	T45.2X5	T45.2X6
Rh (D) immune globulin	T50.Z11	T50.Z12	T50.Z13	T50.Z14	T50.Z15	T50.Z16
(human)						
Rhodine	T39.011	T39.012	T39.013	T39.014	T39.015	T39.016
RhoGAM	T50.Z11	T50.Z12	T50.Z13	T50.Z14	T50.Z15	T50.Z16
Rhubarb						
dry extract	T47.2X1	T47.2X2	T47.2X3	T47.2X4	T47.2X5	T47.2X6
tincture, compound	T47.2X1	T47.2X2	T47.2X3	T47.2X4	T47.2X5	T47.2X6
Ribavirin	T37.5X1	T37.5X2	T37.5X3	T37.5X4	T37.5X5	T37.5X6
Riboflavin	T45.2X1	T45.2X2	T45.2X3	T45.2X4	T45.2X5	T45.2X6
Ribostamycin	T36.5X1	T36.5X2	T36.5X3	T36.5X4	T36.5X5	T36.5X6
Ricin	T62.2X1	T62.2X2	T62.2X3	T62.2X4	—	—
Ricinus communis	T62.2X1	T62.2X2	T62.2X3	T62.2X4	—	—
Rickettsial vaccine NEC	T50.A91	T50.A92	T50.A93	T50.A94	T50.A95	T50.A96
Rifabutin	T36.6X1	T36.6X2	T36.6X3	T36.6X4	T36.6X5	T36.6X6
Rifamide	T36.6X1	T36.6X2	T36.6X3	T36.6X4	T36.6X5	T36.6X6
Rifampicin	T36.6X1	T36.6X2	T36.6X3	T36.6X4	T36.6X5	T36.6X6
with isoniazid	T37.1X1	T37.1X2	T37.1X3	T37.1X4	T37.1X5	T37.1X6
Rifampin	T36.6X1	T36.6X2	T36.6X3	T36.6X4	T36.6X5	T36.6X6
Rifamycin	T36.6X1	T36.6X2	T36.6X3	T36.6X4	T36.6X5	T36.6X6
Rifaximin	T36.6X1	T36.6X2	T36.6X3	T36.6X4	T36.6X5	T36.6X6
Rimantadine	T37.5X1	T37.5X2	T37.5X3	T37.5X4	T37.5X5	T37.5X6
Rimazolium metilsulfate	T39.8X1	T39.8X2	T39.8X3	T39.8X4	T39.8X5	T39.8X6
Rimifon	T37.1X1	T37.1X2	T37.1X3	T37.1X4	T37.1X5	T37.1X6
Rimiterol	T48.6X1	T48.6X2	T48.6X3	T48.6X4	T48.6X5	T48.6X6
Ringer (lactate) **solution**	T50.3X1	T50.3X2	T50.3X3	T50.3X4	T50.3X5	T50.3X6
Risperdal*	T43.591	T43.592	T43.593	T43.594	T43.595	T43.596
Ristocetin	T36.8X1	T36.8X2	T36.8X3	T36.8X4	T36.8X5	T36.8X6
Ritalin	T43.631	T43.632	T43.633	T43.634	T43.635	T43.636
Ritodrine	T44.5X1	T44.5X2	T44.5X3	T44.5X4	T44.5X5	T44.5X6
Roach killer — *see* Insecticide						
Robitussin*	T48.3X1	T48.3X2	T48.3X3	T48.3X4	T48.3X5	T48.3X6
Rociverine	T44.3X1	T44.3X2	T44.3X3	T44.3X4	T44.3X5	T44.3X6
Rocky Mountain spotted fever vaccine	T50.A91	T50.A92	T50.A93	T50.A94	T50.A95	T50.A96
Rodenticide NEC	T60.4X1	T60.4X2	T60.4X3	T60.4X4	—	—
Rohypnol	T42.4X1	T42.4X2	T42.4X3	T42.4X4	T42.4X5	T42.4X6
Rokitamycin	T36.3X1	T36.3X2	T36.3X3	T36.3X4	T36.3X5	T36.3X6
Rolaids	T47.1X1	T47.1X2	T47.1X3	T47.1X4	T47.1X5	T47.1X6
Rolitetracycline	T36.4X1	T36.4X2	T36.4X3	T36.4X4	T36.4X5	T36.4X6
Romilar	T48.3X1	T48.3X2	T48.3X3	T48.3X4	T48.3X5	T48.3X6
Ronifibrate	T46.6X1	T46.6X2	T46.6X3	T46.6X4	T46.6X5	T46.6X6
Rosaprostol	T47.1X1	T47.1X2	T47.1X3	T47.1X4	T47.1X5	T47.1X6
Rose bengal sodium (131I)	T50.8X1	T50.8X2	T50.8X3	T50.8X4	T50.8X5	T50.8X6
Rose water ointment	T49.3X1	T49.3X2	T49.3X3	T49.3X4	T49.3X5	T49.3X6
Rosoxacin	T37.8X1	T37.8X2	T37.8X3	T37.8X4	T37.8X5	T37.8X6
Rotenone	T60.2X1	T60.2X2	T60.2X3	T60.2X4	—	—
Rotoxamine	T45.0X1	T45.0X2	T45.0X3	T45.0X4	T45.0X5	T45.0X6
Rough-on-rats	T60.4X1	T60.4X2	T60.4X3	T60.4X4	—	—
Roxatidine	T47.0X1	T47.0X2	T47.0X3	T47.0X4	T47.0X5	T47.0X6
Roxithromycin	T36.3X1	T36.3X2	T36.3X3	T36.3X4	T36.3X5	T36.3X6
Rt-PA	T45.611	T45.612	T45.613	T45.614	T45.615	T45.616
Rubbing alcohol	T51.2X1	T51.2X2	T51.2X3	T51.2X4	—	—
Rubefacient	T49.4X1	T49.4X2	T49.4X3	T49.4X4	T49.4X5	T49.4X6
Rubella vaccine	T50.B91	T50.B92	T50.B93	T50.B94	T50.B95	T50.B96
Rubeola vaccine	T50.B91	T50.B92	T50.B93	T50.B94	T50.B95	T50.B96
Rubidium chloride Rb82	T50.8X1	T50.8X2	T50.8X3	T50.8X4	T50.8X5	T50.8X6
Rubidomycin	T45.1X1	T45.1X2	T45.1X3	T45.1X4	T45.1X5	T45.1X6
Rue	T62.2X1	T62.2X2	T62.2X3	T62.2X4	—	—
Rufocromomycin	T45.1X1	T45.1X2	T45.1X3	T45.1X4	T45.1X5	T45.1X6
Russel's viper venin	T45.7X1	T45.7X2	T45.7X3	T45.7X4	T45.7X5	T45.7X6
Ruta (graveolens)	T62.2X1	T62.2X2	T62.2X3	T62.2X4	—	—
Rutinum	T46.991	T46.992	T46.993	T46.994	T46.995	T46.996
Rutoside	T46.991	T46.992	T46.993	T46.994	T46.995	T46.996
b-sitosterol(s)	T46.6X1	T46.6X2	T46.6X3	T46.6X4	T46.6X5	T46.6X6
Sabadilla (plant)	T62.2X1	T62.2X2	T62.2X3	T62.2X4	—	—
pesticide	T60.2X1	T60.2X2	T60.2X3	T60.2X4	—	—
Sabril*	T42.6X1	T42.6X2	T42.6X3	T42.6X4	T42.6X5	T42.6X6
Saccharated iron oxide	T45.8X1	T45.8X2	T45.8X3	T45.8X4	T45.8X5	T45.8X6
Saccharin	T50.901	T50.902	T50.903	T50.904	T50.905	T50.906
Saccharomyces boulardii	T47.6X1	T47.6X2	T47.6X3	T47.6X4	T47.6X5	T47.6X6
Safflower oil	T46.6X1	T46.6X2	T46.6X3	T46.6X4	T46.6X5	T46.6X6
Safrazine	T43.1X1	T43.1X2	T43.1X3	T43.1X4	T43.1X5	T43.1X6
Salazosulfapyridine	T37.0X1	T37.0X2	T37.0X3	T37.0X4	T37.0X5	T37.0X6
Salbutamol	T48.6X1	T48.6X2	T48.6X3	T48.6X4	T48.6X5	T48.6X6
Salicylamide	T39.091	T39.092	T39.093	T39.094	T39.095	T39.096
Salicylate NEC	T39.091	T39.092	T39.093	T39.094	T39.095	T39.096
methyl	T49.3X1	T49.3X2	T49.3X3	T49.3X4	T49.3X5	T49.3X6
theobromine calcium	T50.2X1	T50.2X2	T50.2X3	T50.2X4	T50.2X5	T50.2X6

Substance	Poisoning, Accidental (unintentional)	Poisoning, Intentional Self-harm	Poisoning, Assault	Poisoning, Undetermined	Adverse Effect	Under-dosing
Salicylazosulfapyridine	T37.0X1	T37.0X2	T37.0X3	T37.0X4	T37.0X5	T37.0X6
Salicylhydroxamic acid	T49.0X1	T49.0X2	T49.0X3	T49.0X4	T49.0X5	T49.0X6
Salicylic acid	T49.4X1	T49.4X2	T49.4X3	T49.4X4	T49.4X5	T49.4X6
with benzoic acid	T49.4X1	T49.4X2	T49.4X3	T49.4X4	T49.4X5	T49.4X6
congeners	T39.091	T39.092	T39.093	T39.094	T39.095	T39.096
derivative	T39.091	T39.092	T39.093	T39.094	T39.095	T39.096
salts	T39.091	T39.092	T39.093	T39.094	T39.095	T39.096
Salinazid	T37.1X1	T37.1X2	T37.1X3	T37.1X4	T37.1X5	T37.1X6
Salmeterol	T48.6X1	T48.6X2	T48.6X3	T48.6X4	T48.6X5	T48.6X6
Salol	T49.3X1	T49.3X2	T49.3X3	T49.3X4	T49.3X5	T49.3X6
Salsalate	T39.091	T39.092	T39.093	T39.094	T39.095	T39.096
Salt-replacing drug	T50.901	T50.902	T50.903	T50.904	T50.905	T50.906
Salt-retaining mineralocorticoid	T50.0X1	T50.0X2	T50.0X3	T50.0X4	T50.0X5	T50.0X6
Salt substitute	T50.901	T50.902	T50.903	T50.904	T50.905	T50.906
Saluretic NEC	T50.2X1	T50.2X2	T50.2X3	T50.2X4	T50.2X5	T50.2X6
Saluron	T50.2X1	T50.2X2	T50.2X3	T50.2X4	T50.2X5	T50.2X6
Salvarsan 606 (neosilver) (silver)	T37.8X1	T37.8X2	T37.8X3	T37.8X4	T37.8X5	T37.8X6
Sambucus canadensis	T62.2X1	T62.2X2	T62.2X3	T62.2X4	—	—
berry	T62.1X1	T62.1X2	T62.1X3	T62.1X4	—	—
Sandril	T46.5X1	T46.5X2	T46.5X3	T46.5X4	T46.5X5	T46.5X6
Sanguinaria canadensis	T62.2X1	T62.2X2	T62.2X3	T62.2X4	—	—
Saniflush (cleaner)	T54.2X1	T54.2X2	T54.2X3	T54.2X4	—	—
Santonin	T37.4X1	T37.4X2	T37.4X3	T37.4X4	T37.4X5	T37.4X6
Santyl	T49.8X1	T49.8X2	T49.8X3	T49.8X4	T49.8X5	T49.8X6
Saralasin	T46.5X1	T46.5X2	T46.5X3	T46.5X4	T46.5X5	T46.5X6
Sarcolysin	T45.1X1	T45.1X2	T45.1X3	T45.1X4	T45.1X5	T45.1X6
Sarilumab*	T39.4X1	T39.4X2	T39.4X3	T39.4X4	T39.4X5	T39.4X6
Sarkomycin	T45.1X1	T45.1X2	T45.1X3	T45.1X4	T45.1X5	T45.1X6
Saroten	T43.011	T43.012	T43.013	T43.014	T43.015	T43.016
Saturnine — *see* Lead						
Savin (oil)	T49.4X1	T49.4X2	T49.4X3	T49.4X4	T49.4X5	T49.4X6
Scammony	T47.2X1	T47.2X2	T47.2X3	T47.2X4	T47.2X5	T47.2X6
Scarlet red	T49.8X1	T49.8X2	T49.8X3	T49.8X4	T49.8X5	T49.8X6
Scheele's green	T57.0X1	T57.0X2	T57.0X3	T57.0X4	—	—
insecticide	T57.0X1	T57.0X2	T57.0X3	T57.0X4	—	—
Schizontozide (blood) (tissue)	T37.2X1	T37.2X2	T37.2X3	T37.2X4	T37.2X5	T37.2X6
Schradan	T60.0X1	T60.0X2	T60.0X3	T60.0X4	—	—
Schweinfurth green	T57.0X1	T57.0X2	T57.0X3	T57.0X4	—	—
insecticide	T57.0X1	T57.0X2	T57.0X3	T57.0X4	—	—
Scilla, rat poison	T60.4X1	T60.4X2	T60.4X3	T60.4X4	—	—
Scillaren	T60.4X1	T60.4X2	T60.4X3	T60.4X4	—	—
Sclerosing agent	T46.8X1	T46.8X2	T46.8X3	T46.8X4	T46.8X5	T46.8X6
Scombrotoxin	T61.11	T61.12	T61.13	T61.14	—	—
Scopolamine	T44.3X1	T44.3X2	T44.3X3	T44.3X4	T44.3X5	T44.3X6
Scopolia extract	T44.3X1	T44.3X2	T44.3X3	T44.3X4	T44.3X5	T44.3X6
Scouring powder	T65.891	T65.892	T65.893	T65.894	—	—
Sea						
anemone (sting)	T63.631	T63.632	T63.633	T63.634	—	—
cucumber (sting)	T63.691	T63.692	T63.693	T63.694	—	—
snake (bite) (venom)	T63.091	T63.092	T63.093	T63.094	—	—
urchin spine (puncture)	T63.691	T63.692	T63.693	T63.694	—	—
Seafood	T61.91	T61.92	T61.93	T61.94	—	—
specified NEC	T61.8X1	T61.8X2	T61.8X3	T61.8X4	—	—
Secbutabarbital	T42.3X1	T42.3X2	T42.3X3	T42.3X4	T42.3X5	T42.3X6
Secbutabarbitone	T42.3X1	T42.3X2	T42.3X3	T42.3X4	T42.3X5	T42.3X6
Secnidazole	T37.3X1	T37.3X2	T37.3X3	T37.3X4	T37.3X5	T37.3X6
Secobarbital	T42.3X1	T42.3X2	T42.3X3	T42.3X4	T42.3X5	T42.3X6
Seconal	T42.3X1	T42.3X2	T42.3X3	T42.3X4	T42.3X5	T42.3X6
Secretin	T50.8X1	T50.8X2	T50.8X3	T50.8X4	T50.8X5	T50.8X6
Sectral*	T44.7X1	T44.7X2	T44.7X3	T44.7X4	T44.7X5	T44.7X6
Sedative NEC	T42.71	T42.72	T42.73	T42.74	T42.75	T42.76
mixed NEC	T42.6X1	T42.6X2	T42.6X3	T42.6X4	T42.6X5	T42.6X6
Sedormid	T42.6X1	T42.6X2	T42.6X3	T42.6X4	T42.6X5	T42.6X6
Seed disinfectant or dressing	T60.8X1	T60.8X2	T60.8X3	T60.8X4	—	—
Seeds (poisonous)	T62.2X1	T62.2X2	T62.2X3	T62.2X4	—	—
Selegiline	T42.8X1	T42.8X2	T42.8X3	T42.8X4	T42.8X5	T42.8X6
Selenium NEC	T56.891	T56.892	T56.893	T56.894	—	—
disulfide or sulfide	T49.4X1	T49.4X2	T49.4X3	T49.4X4	T49.4X5	T49.4X6
fumes	T59.891	T59.892	T59.893	T59.894	—	—
sulfide	T49.4X1	T49.4X2	T49.4X3	T49.4X4	T49.4X5	T49.4X6
Selenomethionine (75Se)	T50.8X1	T50.8X2	T50.8X3	T50.8X4	T50.8X5	T50.8X6
Selsun	T49.4X1	T49.4X2	T49.4X3	T49.4X4	T49.4X5	T49.4X6
Semustine	T45.1X1	T45.1X2	T45.1X3	T45.1X4	T45.1X5	T45.1X6
Senega syrup	T48.4X1	T48.4X2	T48.4X3	T48.4X4	T48.4X5	T48.4X6
Senna	T47.2X1	T47.2X2	T47.2X3	T47.2X4	T47.2X5	T47.2X6
Sennoside A+B	T47.2X1	T47.2X2	T47.2X3	T47.2X4	T47.2X5	T47.2X6
Septisol	T49.2X1	T49.2X2	T49.2X3	T49.2X4	T49.2X5	T49.2X6
Seractide	T38.811	T38.812	T38.813	T38.814	T38.815	T38.816
Serax	T42.4X1	T42.4X2	T42.4X3	T42.4X4	T42.4X5	T42.4X6

Table of Drugs and Chemicals

Respiratory drug NEC — Serax

Substance	Poisoning, Accidental (unintentional)	Poisoning, Intentional Self-harm	Poisoning, Assault	Poisoning, Undetermined	Adverse Effect	Under-dosing
Serenesil	T42.6X1	T42.6X2	T42.6X3	T42.6X4	T42.6X5	T42.6X6
Serenium (hydrochloride)	T37.91	T37.92	T37.93	T37.94	T37.95	T37.96
Serepax — see Oxazepam						
Serevent*	T48.6X1	T48.6X2	T48.6X3	T48.6X4	T48.6X5	T48.6X6
Sermorelin	T38.891	T38.892	T38.893	T38.894	T38.895	T38.896
Sernyl	T41.1X1	T41.1X2	T41.1X3	T41.1X4	T41.1X5	T41.1X6
Serotonin	T50.991	T50.992	T50.993	T50.994	T50.995	T50.996
Serpasil	T46.5X1	T46.5X2	T46.5X3	T46.5X4	T46.5X5	T46.5X6
Serrapeptase	T45.3X1	T45.3X2	T45.3X3	T45.3X4	T45.3X5	T45.3X6
Serum						
antibotulinus	T50.Z11	T50.Z12	T50.Z13	T50.Z14	T50.Z15	T50.Z16
anticytotoxic	T50.Z11	T50.Z12	T50.Z13	T50.Z14	T50.Z15	T50.Z16
antidiphtheria	T50.Z11	T50.Z12	T50.Z13	T50.Z14	T50.Z15	T50.Z16
antimeningococcus	T50.Z11	T50.Z12	T50.Z13	T50.Z14	T50.Z15	T50.Z16
anti-Rh	T50.Z11	T50.Z12	T50.Z13	T50.Z14	T50.Z15	T50.Z16
anti-snake-bite	T50.Z11	T50.Z12	T50.Z13	T50.Z14	T50.Z15	T50.Z16
antitetanic	T50.Z11	T50.Z12	T50.Z13	T50.Z14	T50.Z15	T50.Z16
antitoxic	T50.Z11	T50.Z12	T50.Z13	T50.Z14	T50.Z15	T50.Z16
complement (inhibitor)	T45.8X1	T45.8X2	T45.8X3	T45.8X4	T45.8X5	T45.8X6
convalescent	T50.Z11	T50.Z12	T50.Z13	T50.Z14	T50.Z15	T50.Z16
hemolytic complement	T45.8X1	T45.8X2	T45.8X3	T45.8X4	T45.8X5	T45.8X6
immune (human)	T50.Z11	T50.Z12	T50.Z13	T50.Z14	T50.Z15	T50.Z16
protective NEC	T50.Z11	T50.Z12	T50.Z13	T50.Z14	T50.Z15	T50.Z16
Setastine	T45.0X1	T45.0X2	T45.0X3	T45.0X4	T45.0X5	T45.0X6
Setoperone	T43.591	T43.592	T43.593	T43.594	T43.595	T43.596
Sewer gas	T59.91	T59.92	T59.93	T59.94	—	—
Shampoo	T55.0X1	T55.0X2	T55.0X3	T55.0X4	—	—
Shellfish, noxious, nonbacterial	T61.781	T61.782	T61.783	T61.784	—	—
Sildenafil	T46.7X1	T46.7X2	T46.7X3	T46.7X4	T46.7X5	T46.7X6
Silibinin	T50.991	T50.992	T50.993	T50.994	T50.995	T50.996
Silicone NEC	T65.891	T65.892	T65.893	T65.894	—	—
medicinal	T49.3X1	T49.3X2	T49.3X3	T49.3X4	T49.3X5	T49.3X6
Silvadene	T49.0X1	T49.0X2	T49.0X3	T49.0X4	T49.0X5	T49.0X6
Silver	T49.0X1	T49.0X2	T49.0X3	T49.0X4	T49.0X5	T49.0X6
anti-infectives	T49.0X1	T49.0X2	T49.0X3	T49.0X4	T49.0X5	T49.0X6
arsphenamine	T37.8X1	T37.8X2	T37.8X3	T37.8X4	T37.8X5	T37.8X6
colloidal	T49.0X1	T49.0X2	T49.0X3	T49.0X4	T49.0X5	T49.0X6
nitrate	T49.0X1	T49.0X2	T49.0X3	T49.0X4	T49.0X5	T49.0X6
ophthalmic preparation	T49.5X1	T49.5X2	T49.5X3	T49.5X4	T49.5X5	T49.5X6
toughened (keratolytic)	T49.4X1	T49.4X2	T49.4X3	T49.4X4	T49.4X5	T49.4X6
nonmedicinal (dust)	T56.891	T56.892	T56.893	T56.894	—	—
protein	T49.5X1	T49.5X2	T49.5X3	T49.5X4	T49.5X5	T49.5X6
salvarsan	T37.8X1	T37.8X2	T37.8X3	T37.8X4	T37.8X5	T37.8X6
sulfadiazine	T49.4X1	T49.4X2	T49.4X3	T49.4X4	T49.4X5	T49.4X6
Silymarin	T50.991	T50.992	T50.993	T50.994	T50.995	T50.996
Simaldrate	T47.1X1	T47.1X2	T47.1X3	T47.1X4	T47.1X5	T47.1X6
Simazine	T60.3X1	T60.3X2	T60.3X3	T60.3X4	—	—
Simethicone	T47.1X1	T47.1X2	T47.1X3	T47.1X4	T47.1X5	T47.1X6
Simfibrate	T46.6X1	T46.6X2	T46.6X3	T46.6X4	T46.6X5	T46.6X6
Simvastatin	T46.6X1	T46.6X2	T46.6X3	T46.6X4	T46.6X5	T46.6X6
Sincalide	T50.8X1	T50.8X2	T50.8X3	T50.8X4	T50.8X5	T50.8X6
Sinequan	T43.011	T43.012	T43.013	T43.014	T43.015	T43.016
Singoserp	T46.5X1	T46.5X2	T46.5X3	T46.5X4	T46.5X5	T46.5X6
Singulair*	T48.6X1	T48.6X2	T48.6X3	T48.6X4	T48.6X5	T48.6X6
Sintrom	T45.511	T45.512	T45.513	T45.514	T45.515	T45.516
Sisomicin	T36.5X1	T36.5X2	T36.5X3	T36.5X4	T36.5X5	T36.5X6
Sitosterols	T46.6X1	T46.6X2	T46.6X3	T46.6X4	T46.6X5	T46.6X6
Skeletal muscle relaxants	T48.1X1	T48.1X2	T48.1X3	T48.1X4	T48.1X5	T48.1X6
Skin						
agents (external)	T49.91	T49.92	T49.93	T49.94	T49.95	T49.96
specified NEC	T49.8X1	T49.8X2	T49.8X3	T49.8X4	T49.8X5	T49.8X6
test antigen	T50.8X1	T50.8X2	T50.8X3	T50.8X4	T50.8X5	T50.8X6
Sleep-eze	T45.0X1	T45.0X2	T45.0X3	T45.0X4	T45.0X5	T45.0X6
Sleeping draught, pill	T42.71	T42.72	T42.73	T42.74	T42.75	T42.76
Smallpox vaccine	T50.B11	T50.B12	T50.B13	T50.B14	T50.B15	T50.B16
Smelter fumes NEC	T56.91	T56.92	T56.93	T56.94	—	—
Smog	T59.1X1	T59.1X2	T59.1X3	T59.1X4	—	—
Smoke NEC	T59.811	T59.812	T59.813	T59.814	—	—
Smooth muscle relaxant	T44.3X1	T44.3X2	T44.3X3	T44.3X4	T44.3X5	T44.3X6
Snail killer NEC	T60.8X1	T60.8X2	T60.8X3	T60.8X4	—	—
Snake venom or bite	T63.001	T63.002	T63.003	T63.004	—	—
hemocoagulase	T45.7X1	T45.7X2	T45.7X3	T45.7X4	T45.7X5	T45.7X6
Snuff	T65.211	T65.212	T65.213	T65.214	—	—
Soap (powder) (product)	T55.0X1	T55.0X2	T55.0X3	T55.0X4	—	—
enema	T47.4X1	T47.4X2	T47.4X3	T47.4X4	T47.4X5	T47.4X6
medicinal, soft	T49.2X1	T49.2X2	T49.2X3	T49.2X4	T49.2X5	T49.2X6
superfatted	T49.2X1	T49.2X2	T49.2X3	T49.2X4	T49.2X5	T49.2X6
Sobrerol	T48.4X1	T48.4X2	T48.4X3	T48.4X4	T48.4X5	T48.4X6
Soda (caustic)	T54.3X1	T54.3X2	T54.3X3	T54.3X4	—	—
bicarb	T47.1X1	T47.1X2	T47.1X3	T47.1X4	T47.1X5	T47.1X6
chlorinated — see Sodium, hypochlorite						

Substance	Poisoning, Accidental (unintentional)	Poisoning, Intentional Self-harm	Poisoning, Assault	Poisoning, Undetermined	Adverse Effect	Under-dosing
Sodium						
acetosulfone	T37.1X1	T37.1X2	T37.1X3	T37.1X4	T37.1X5	T37.1X6
acetrizoate	T50.8X1	T50.8X2	T50.8X3	T50.8X4	T50.8X5	T50.8X6
acid phosphate	T50.3X1	T50.3X2	T50.3X3	T50.3X4	T50.3X5	T50.3X6
alginate	T47.8X1	T47.8X2	T47.8X3	T47.8X4	T47.8X5	T47.8X6
amidotrizoate	T50.8X1	T50.8X2	T50.8X3	T50.8X4	T50.8X5	T50.8X6
aminohippurate*	T50.8X1	T50.8X2	T50.8X3	T50.8X4	T50.8X5	T50.8X6
aminopterin	T45.1X1	T45.1X2	T45.1X3	T45.1X4	T45.1X5	T45.1X6
amylosulfate	T47.8X1	T47.8X2	T47.8X3	T47.8X4	T47.8X5	T47.8X6
amytal	T42.3X1	T42.3X2	T42.3X3	T42.3X4	T42.3X5	T42.3X6
antimony gluconate	T37.3X1	T37.3X2	T37.3X3	T37.3X4	T37.3X5	T37.3X6
arsenate	T57.0X1	T57.0X2	T57.0X3	T57.0X4	—	—
aurothiomalate	T39.4X1	T39.4X2	T39.4X3	T39.4X4	T39.4X5	T39.4X6
aurothiosulfate	T39.4X1	T39.4X2	T39.4X3	T39.4X4	T39.4X5	T39.4X6
barbiturate	T42.3X1	T42.3X2	T42.3X3	T42.3X4	T42.3X5	T42.3X6
basic phosphate	T47.4X1	T47.4X2	T47.4X3	T47.4X4	T47.4X5	T47.4X6
bicarbonate	T47.1X1	T47.1X2	T47.1X3	T47.1X4	T47.1X5	T47.1X6
bichromate	T57.8X1	T57.8X2	T57.8X3	T57.8X4	—	—
biphosphate	T50.3X1	T50.3X2	T50.3X3	T50.3X4	T50.3X5	T50.3X6
bisulfate	T65.891	T65.892	T65.893	T65.894	—	—
borate						
cleanser	T57.8X1	T57.8X2	T57.8X3	T57.8X4	—	—
eye	T49.5X1	T49.5X2	T49.5X3	T49.5X4	T49.5X5	T49.5X6
therapeutic	T49.8X1	T49.8X2	T49.8X3	T49.8X4	T49.8X5	T49.8X6
bromide	T42.6X1	T42.6X2	T42.6X3	T42.6X4	T42.6X5	T42.6X6
cacodylate (nonmedicinal) NEC	T50.8X1	T50.8X2	T50.8X3	T50.8X4	T50.8X5	T50.8X6
anti-infective	T37.8X1	T37.8X2	T37.8X3	T37.8X4	T37.8X5	T37.8X6
herbicide	T60.3X1	T60.3X2	T60.3X3	T60.3X4	—	—
calcium edetate	T45.8X1	T45.8X2	T45.8X3	T45.8X4	T45.8X5	T45.8X6
carbonate NEC	T54.3X1	T54.3X2	T54.3X3	T54.3X4	—	—
chlorate NEC	T65.891	T65.892	T65.893	T65.894	—	—
herbicide	T54.91	T54.92	T54.93	T54.94	—	—
chloride	T50.3X1	T50.3X2	T50.3X3	T50.3X4	T50.3X5	T50.3X6
with glucose	T50.3X1	T50.3X2	T50.3X3	T50.3X4	T50.3X5	T50.3X6
chromate	T65.891	T65.892	T65.893	T65.894	—	—
citrate	T50.991	T50.992	T50.993	T50.994	T50.995	T50.996
cromoglicate	T48.6X1	T48.6X2	T48.6X3	T48.6X4	T48.6X5	T48.6X6
cyanide	T65.0X1	T65.0X2	T65.0X3	T65.0X4	—	—
cyclamate	T50.3X1	T50.3X2	T50.3X3	T50.3X4	T50.3X5	T50.3X6
dehydrocholate	T45.8X1	T45.8X2	T45.8X3	T45.8X4	T45.8X5	T45.8X6
diatrizoate	T50.8X1	T50.8X2	T50.8X3	T50.8X4	T50.8X5	T50.8X6
dibunate	T48.4X1	T48.4X2	T48.4X3	T48.4X4	T48.4X5	T48.4X6
dioctyl sulfosuccinate	T47.4X1	T47.4X2	T47.4X3	T47.4X4	T47.4X5	T47.4X6
dipantoyl ferrate	T45.8X1	T45.8X2	T45.8X3	T45.8X4	T45.8X5	T45.8X6
edetate	T45.8X1	T45.8X2	T45.8X3	T45.8X4	T45.8X5	T45.8X6
ethacrynate	T50.1X1	T50.1X2	T50.1X3	T50.1X4	T50.1X5	T50.1X6
etidronate*	T50.991	T50.992	T50.993	T50.994	T50.995	T50.996
feredetate	T45.8X1	T45.8X2	T45.8X3	T45.8X4	T45.8X5	T45.8X6
Fluoride — see Fluoride						
fluoroacetate (dust) (pesticide)	T60.4X1	T60.4X2	T60.4X3	T60.4X4	—	—
free salt	T50.3X1	T50.3X2	T50.3X3	T50.3X4	T50.3X5	T50.3X6
fusidate	T36.8X1	T36.8X2	T36.8X3	T36.8X4	T36.8X5	T36.8X6
glucaldrate	T47.1X1	T47.1X2	T47.1X3	T47.1X4	T47.1X5	T47.1X6
glucosulfone	T37.1X1	T37.1X2	T37.1X3	T37.1X4	T37.1X5	T37.1X6
glutamate	T45.8X1	T45.8X2	T45.8X3	T45.8X4	T45.8X5	T45.8X6
hydrogen carbonate	T50.3X1	T50.3X2	T50.3X3	T50.3X4	T50.3X5	T50.3X6
hydroxide	T54.3X1	T54.3X2	T54.3X3	T54.3X4	—	—
hypochlorite (bleach) NEC	T54.3X1	T54.3X2	T54.3X3	T54.3X4	—	—
disinfectant	T54.3X1	T54.3X2	T54.3X3	T54.3X4	—	—
medicinal (anti-infective) (external)	T49.0X1	T49.0X2	T49.0X3	T49.0X4	T49.0X5	T49.0X6
vapor	T54.3X1	T54.3X2	T54.3X3	T54.3X4	—	—
hyposulfite	T49.0X1	T49.0X2	T49.0X3	T49.0X4	T49.0X5	T49.0X6
indigotin disulfonate	T50.8X1	T50.8X2	T50.8X3	T50.8X4	T50.8X5	T50.8X6
iodide	T50.991	T50.992	T50.993	T50.994	T50.995	T50.996
I-131	T50.8X1	T50.8X2	T50.8X3	T50.8X4	T50.8X5	T50.8X6
therapeutic	T38.2X1	T38.2X2	T38.2X3	T38.2X4	T38.2X5	T38.2X6
iodohippurate (131I)	T50.8X1	T50.8X2	T50.8X3	T50.8X4	T50.8X5	T50.8X6
iopodate	T50.8X1	T50.8X2	T50.8X3	T50.8X4	T50.8X5	T50.8X6
iothalamate	T50.8X1	T50.8X2	T50.8X3	T50.8X4	T50.8X5	T50.8X6
iron edetate	T45.4X1	T45.4X2	T45.4X3	T45.4X4	T45.4X5	T45.4X6
lactate (compound solution)	T45.8X1	T45.8X2	T45.8X3	T45.8X4	T45.8X5	T45.8X6
lauryl (sulfate)	T49.2X1	T49.2X2	T49.2X3	T49.2X4	T49.2X5	T49.2X6
L-triiodothyronine	T38.1X1	T38.1X2	T38.1X3	T38.1X4	T38.1X5	T38.1X6
magnesium citrate	T50.991	T50.992	T50.993	T50.994	T50.995	T50.996
mersalate	T50.2X1	T50.2X2	T50.2X3	T50.2X4	T50.2X5	T50.2X6
metasilicate	T65.891	T65.892	T65.893	T65.894	—	—
metrizoate	T50.8X1	T50.8X2	T50.8X3	T50.8X4	T50.8X5	T50.8X6
monofluoroacetate (pesticide)	T60.1X1	T60.1X2	T60.1X3	T60.1X4	—	—

Substance	Poisoning, Accidental (unintentional)	Poisoning, Intentional Self-harm	Poisoning, Assault	Poisoning, Undetermined	Adverse Effect	Under-dosing
Sodium — *continued*						
morrhuate	T46.8X1	T46.8X2	T46.8X3	T46.8X4	T46.8X5	T46.8X6
nafcillin	T36.0X1	T36.0X2	T36.0X3	T36.0X4	T36.0X5	T36.0X6
nitrate (oxidizing agent)	T65.891	T65.892	T65.893	T65.894	—	—
nitrite	T50.6X1	T50.6X2	T50.6X3	T50.6X4	T50.6X5	T50.6X6
nitroferricyanide	T46.5X1	T46.5X2	T46.5X3	T46.5X4	T46.5X5	T46.5X6
nitroprusside	T46.5X1	T46.5X2	T46.5X3	T46.5X4	T46.5X5	T46.5X6
oxalate	T65.891	T65.892	T65.893	T65.894	—	—
oxide/peroxide	T65.891	T65.892	T65.893	T65.894	—	—
oxybate	T41.291	T41.292	T41.293	T41.294	T41.295	T41.296
para-aminohippurate	T50.8X1	T50.8X2	T50.8X3	T50.8X4	T50.8X5	T50.8X6
perborate (nonmedicinal) NEC	T65.891	T65.892	T65.893	T65.894	—	—
medicinal	T49.0X1	T49.0X2	T49.0X3	T49.0X4	T49.0X5	T49.0X6
soap	T55.0X1	T55.0X2	T55.0X3	T55.0X4	—	—
percarbonate — *see* Sodium, perborate						
pertechnetate Tc99m	T50.8X1	T50.8X2	T50.8X3	T50.8X4	T50.8X5	T50.8X6
phosphate						
cellulose	T45.8X1	T45.8X2	T45.8X3	T45.8X4	T45.8X5	T45.8X6
dibasic	T47.2X1	T47.2X2	T47.2X3	T47.2X4	T47.2X5	T47.2X6
monobasic	T47.2X1	T47.2X2	T47.2X3	T47.2X4	T47.2X5	T47.2X6
phytate	T50.6X1	T50.6X2	T50.6X3	T50.6X4	T50.6X5	T50.6X6
picosulfate	T47.2X1	T47.2X2	T47.2X3	T47.2X4	T47.2X5	T47.2X6
polyhydroxyaluminium monocarbonate	T47.1X1	T47.1X2	T47.1X3	T47.1X4	T47.1X5	T47.1X6
polystyrene sulfonate	T50.3X1	T50.3X2	T50.3X3	T50.3X4	T50.3X5	T50.3X6
propionate	T49.0X1	T49.0X2	T49.0X3	T49.0X4	T49.0X5	T49.0X6
propyl hydroxybenzoate	T50.991	T50.992	T50.993	T50.994	T50.995	T50.996
psylliate	T46.8X1	T46.8X2	T46.8X3	T46.8X4	T46.8X5	T46.8X6
removing resins	T50.3X1	T50.3X2	T50.3X3	T50.3X4	T50.3X5	T50.3X6
salicylate	T39.091	T39.092	T39.093	T39.094	T39.095	T39.096
salt NEC	T50.3X1	T50.3X2	T50.3X3	T50.3X4	T50.3X5	T50.3X6
selenate	T60.2X1	T60.2X2	T60.2X3	T60.2X4	—	—
stibogluconate	T37.3X1	T37.3X2	T37.3X3	T37.3X4	T37.3X5	T37.3X6
sulfate	T47.4X1	T47.4X2	T47.4X3	T47.4X4	T47.4X5	T47.4X6
sulfoxone	T37.1X1	T37.1X2	T37.1X3	T37.1X4	T37.1X5	T37.1X6
tetradecyl sulfate	T46.8X1	T46.8X2	T46.8X3	T46.8X4	T46.8X5	T46.8X6
thiopental	T41.1X1	T41.1X2	T41.1X3	T41.1X4	T41.1X5	T41.1X6
thiosalicylate	T39.091	T39.092	T39.093	T39.094	T39.095	T39.096
thiosulfate	T50.6X1	T50.6X2	T50.6X3	T50.6X4	T50.6X5	T50.6X6
tolbutamide	T38.3X1	T38.3X2	T38.3X3	T38.3X4	T38.3X5	T38.3X6
(L)-triiodothyronine	T38.1X1	T38.1X2	T38.1X3	T38.1X4	T38.1X5	T38.1X6
tyropanoate	T50.8X1	T50.8X2	T50.8X3	T50.8X4	T50.8X5	T50.8X6
valproate	T42.6X1	T42.6X2	T42.6X3	T42.6X4	T42.6X5	T42.6X6
versenate	T50.6X1	T50.6X2	T50.6X3	T50.6X4	T50.6X5	T50.6X6
Sodium-free salt	T50.901	T50.902	T50.903	T50.904	T50.905	T50.906
Sodium-removing resin	T50.3X1	T50.3X2	T50.3X3	T50.3X4	T50.3X5	T50.3X6
Soft soap	T55.0X1	T55.0X2	T55.0X3	T55.0X4	—	—
Solanine	T62.2X1	T62.2X2	T62.2X3	T62.2X4	—	—
berries	T62.1X1	T62.1X2	T62.1X3	T62.1X4	—	—
Solanum dulcamara	T62.2X1	T62.2X2	T62.2X3	T62.2X4	—	—
berries	T62.1X1	T62.1X2	T62.1X3	T62.1X4	—	—
Solapsone	T37.1X1	T37.1X2	T37.1X3	T37.1X4	T37.1X5	T37.1X6
Solaquin*	T49.8X1	T49.8X2	T49.8X3	T49.8X4	T49.8X5	T49.8X6
Solar lotion	T49.3X1	T49.3X2	T49.3X3	T49.3X4	T49.3X5	T49.3X6
Solasulfone	T37.1X1	T37.1X2	T37.1X3	T37.1X4	T37.1X5	T37.1X6
Soldering fluid	T65.891	T65.892	T65.893	T65.894	—	—
Solid substance	T65.91	T65.92	T65.93	T65.94	—	—
specified NEC	T65.891	T65.892	T65.893	T65.894	—	—
Solvent, industrial NEC	T52.91	T52.92	T52.93	T52.94	—	—
naphtha	T52.0X1	T52.0X2	T52.0X3	T52.0X4	—	—
petroleum	T52.0X1	T52.0X2	T52.0X3	T52.0X4	—	—
specified NEC	T52.8X1	T52.8X2	T52.8X3	T52.8X4	—	—
Soma	T42.8X1	T42.8X2	T42.8X3	T42.8X4	T42.8X5	T42.8X6
Somatorelin	T38.891	T38.892	T38.893	T38.894	T38.895	T38.896
Somatostatin	T38.991	T38.992	T38.993	T38.994	T38.995	T38.996
Somatotropin	T38.811	T38.812	T38.813	T38.814	T38.815	T38.816
Somatrem	T38.811	T38.812	T38.813	T38.814	T38.815	T38.816
Somatropin	T38.811	T38.812	T38.813	T38.814	T38.815	T38.816
Sominex	T45.0X1	T45.0X2	T45.0X3	T45.0X4	T45.0X5	T45.0X6
Somnos	T42.6X1	T42.6X2	T42.6X3	T42.6X4	T42.6X5	T42.6X6
Somonal	T42.3X1	T42.3X2	T42.3X3	T42.3X4	T42.3X5	T42.3X6
Soneryl	T42.3X1	T42.3X2	T42.3X3	T42.3X4	T42.3X5	T42.3X6
Soothing syrup	T50.901	T50.902	T50.903	T50.904	T50.905	T50.906
Sopor	T42.6X1	T42.6X2	T42.6X3	T42.6X4	T42.6X5	T42.6X6
Soporific	T42.71	T42.72	T42.73	T42.74	T42.75	T42.76
Soporific drug	T42.71	T42.72	T42.73	T42.74	T42.75	T42.76
specified type NEC	T42.6X1	T42.6X2	T42.6X3	T42.6X4	T42.6X5	T42.6X6
Sorbide nitrate	T46.3X1	T46.3X2	T46.3X3	T46.3X4	T46.3X5	T46.3X6
Sorbitol	T47.4X1	T47.4X2	T47.4X3	T47.4X4	T47.4X5	T47.4X6
Sotalol	T44.7X1	T44.7X2	T44.7X3	T44.7X4	T44.7X5	T44.7X6
Sotradecol	T46.8X1	T46.8X2	T46.8X3	T46.8X4	T46.8X5	T46.8X6
Soysterol	T46.6X1	T46.6X2	T46.6X3	T46.6X4	T46.6X5	T46.6X6
Spacoline	T44.3X1	T44.3X2	T44.3X3	T44.3X4	T44.3X5	T44.3X6
Spanish fly	T49.8X1	T49.8X2	T49.8X3	T49.8X4	T49.8X5	T49.8X6
Sparine	T43.3X1	T43.3X2	T43.3X3	T43.3X4	T43.3X5	T43.3X6
Sparteine	T48.0X1	T48.0X2	T48.0X3	T48.0X4	T48.0X5	T48.0X6
Spasmolytic						
anticholinergics	T44.3X1	T44.3X2	T44.3X3	T44.3X4	T44.3X5	T44.3X6
autonomic	T44.3X1	T44.3X2	T44.3X3	T44.3X4	T44.3X5	T44.3X6
bronchial NEC	T48.6X1	T48.6X2	T48.6X3	T48.6X4	T48.6X5	T48.6X6
quaternary ammonium	T44.3X1	T44.3X2	T44.3X3	T44.3X4	T44.3X5	T44.3X6
skeletal muscle NEC	T48.1X1	T48.1X2	T48.1X3	T48.1X4	T48.1X5	T48.1X6
Spectinomycin	T36.5X1	T36.5X2	T36.5X3	T36.5X4	T36.5X5	T36.5X6
Spectracef*	T36.1X1	T36.1X2	T36.1X3	T36.1X4	T36.1X5	T36.1X6
Speed	T43.651	T43.652	T43.652	T43.654	T43.655	T43.656
Spermicide	T49.8X1	T49.8X2	T49.8X3	T49.8X4	T49.8X5	T49.8X6
Spider (bite) (venom)	T63.391	T63.392	T63.393	T63.394	—	—
antivenin	T50.Z11	T50.Z12	T50.Z13	T50.Z14	T50.Z15	T50.Z16
Spigelia (root)	T37.4X1	T37.4X2	T37.4X3	T37.4X4	T37.4X5	T37.4X6
Spindle inactivator	T50.4X1	T50.4X2	T50.4X3	T50.4X4	T50.4X5	T50.4X6
Spiperone	T43.4X1	T43.4X2	T43.4X3	T43.4X4	T43.4X5	T43.4X6
Spiramycin	T36.3X1	T36.3X2	T36.3X3	T36.3X4	T36.3X5	T36.3X6
Spirapril	T46.4X1	T46.4X2	T46.4X3	T46.4X4	T46.4X5	T46.4X6
Spirilene	T43.591	T43.592	T43.593	T43.594	T43.595	T43.596
Spirit(s) (neutral) **NEC**	T51.0X1	T51.0X2	T51.0X3	T51.0X4	—	—
beverage	T51.0X1	T51.0X2	T51.0X3	T51.0X4	—	—
industrial	T51.0X1	T51.0X2	T51.0X3	T51.0X4	—	—
mineral	T52.0X1	T52.0X2	T52.0X3	T52.0X4	—	—
of salt — *see* Hydrochloric acid						
surgical	T51.0X1	T51.0X2	T51.0X3	T51.0X4	—	—
Spiriva*	T44.3X1	T44.3X2	T44.3X3	T44.3X4	T44.3X5	T44.3X6
Spironolactone	T50.0X1	T50.0X2	T50.0X3	T50.0X4	T50.0X5	T50.0X6
Spiroperidol	T43.4X1	T43.4X2	T43.4X3	T43.4X4	T43.4X5	T43.4X6
Sponge, absorbable (gelatin)	T45.7X1	T45.7X2	T45.7X3	T45.7X4	T45.7X5	T45.7X6
Sporostacin	T49.0X1	T49.0X2	T49.0X3	T49.0X4	T49.0X5	T49.0X6
Spray (aerosol)	T65.91	T65.92	T65.93	T65.94	—	—
cosmetic	T65.891	T65.892	T65.893	T65.894	—	—
medicinal NEC	T50.901	T50.902	T50.903	T50.904	T50.905	T50.906
pesticides — *see* Pesticide						
specified content — *see* specific substance						
Spurge flax	T62.2X1	T62.2X2	T62.2X3	T62.2X4	—	—
Spurges	T62.2X1	T62.2X2	T62.2X3	T62.2X4	—	—
Sputum viscosity-lowering drug	T48.4X1	T48.4X2	T48.4X3	T48.4X4	T48.4X5	T48.4X6
Squill	T46.0X1	T46.0X2	T46.0X3	T46.0X4	T46.0X5	T46.0X6
rat poison	T60.4X1	T60.4X2	T60.4X3	T60.4X4	—	—
Squirting cucumber (cathartic)	T47.2X1	T47.2X2	T47.2X3	T47.2X4	T47.2X5	T47.2X6
Stains	T65.6X1	T65.6X2	T65.6X3	T65.6X4	—	—
Stannous fluoride	T49.7X1	T49.7X2	T49.7X3	T49.7X4	T49.7X5	T49.7X6
Stanolone	T38.7X1	T38.7X2	T38.7X3	T38.7X4	T38.7X5	T38.7X6
Stanozolol	T38.7X1	T38.7X2	T38.7X3	T38.7X4	T38.7X5	T38.7X6
Staphisagria or stavesacre (pediculicide)	T49.0X1	T49.0X2	T49.0X3	T49.0X4	T49.0X5	T49.0X6
Starch	T50.901	T50.902	T50.903	T50.904	T50.905	T50.906
Stavzor*	T42.6X1	T42.6X2	T42.6X3	T42.6X4	T42.6X5	T42.6X6
Stelazine	T43.3X1	T43.3X2	T43.3X3	T43.3X4	T43.3X5	T43.3X6
Stemetil	T43.3X1	T43.3X2	T43.3X3	T43.3X4	T43.3X5	T43.3X6
Stepronin	T48.4X1	T48.4X2	T48.4X3	T48.4X4	T48.4X5	T48.4X6
Sterculia	T47.4X1	T47.4X2	T47.4X3	T47.4X4	T47.4X5	T47.4X6
Sternutator gas	T59.891	T59.892	T59.893	T59.894	—	—
Steroid	T38.0X1	T38.0X2	T38.0X3	T38.0X4	T38.0X5	T38.0X6
anabolic	T38.7X1	T38.7X2	T38.7X3	T38.7X4	T38.7X5	T38.7X6
androgenic	T38.7X1	T38.7X2	T38.7X3	T38.7X4	T38.7X5	T38.7X6
antineoplastic, hormone	T38.7X1	T38.7X2	T38.7X3	T38.7X4	T38.7X5	T38.7X6
estrogen	T38.5X1	T38.5X2	T38.5X3	T38.5X4	T38.5X5	T38.5X6
ENT agent	T49.6X1	T49.6X2	T49.6X3	T49.6X4	T49.6X5	T49.6X6
ophthalmic preparation	T49.5X1	T49.5X2	T49.5X3	T49.5X4	T49.5X5	T49.5X6
topical NEC	T49.0X1	T49.0X2	T49.0X3	T49.0X4	T49.0X5	T49.0X6
Stibine	T56.891	T56.892	T56.893	T56.894	—	—
Stibogluconate	T37.3X1	T37.3X2	T37.3X3	T37.3X4	T37.3X5	T37.3X6
Stibophen	T37.4X1	T37.4X2	T37.4X3	T37.4X4	T37.4X5	T37.4X6
Stilbamidine (isetionate)	T37.3X1	T37.3X2	T37.3X3	T37.3X4	T37.3X5	T37.3X6
Stilbestrol	T38.5X1	T38.5X2	T38.5X3	T38.5X4	T38.5X5	T38.5X6
Stilboestrol	T38.5X1	T38.5X2	T38.5X3	T38.5X4	T38.5X5	T38.5X6
Stimulant						
central nervous system — *see also* Psychostimulant	T43.601	T43.602	T43.603	T43.604	T43.605	T43.606
analeptics	T50.7X1	T50.7X2	T50.7X3	T50.7X4	T50.7X5	T50.7X6
opiate antagonist	T50.7X1	T50.7X2	T50.7X3	T50.7X4	T50.7X5	T50.7X6

Table of Drugs and Chemicals

Stimulant — Sulprostone

Substance	Poisoning, Accidental (unintentional)	Poisoning, Intentional Self-harm	Poisoning, Assault	Poisoning, Undetermined	Adverse Effect	Under-dosing
Stimulant — continued						
central nervous system — see also Psychostimulant — continued						
psychotherapeutic NEC — see also Psychotherapeutic drug	T43.601	T43.602	T43.603	T43.604	T43.605	T43.606
specified NEC	T43.691	T43.692	T43.693	T43.694	T43.695	T43.696
respiratory	T48.901	T48.902	T48.903	T48.904	T48.905	T48.906
Stone-dissolving drug	T50.901	T50.902	T50.903	T50.904	T50.905	T50.906
Storage battery (cells) (acid)	T54.2X1	T54.2X2	T54.2X3	T54.2X4	—	—
Stovaine	T41.3X1	T41.3X2	T41.3X3	T41.3X4	T41.3X5	T41.3X6
infiltration (subcutaneous)	T41.3X1	T41.3X2	T41.3X3	T41.3X4	T41.3X5	T41.3X6
nerve block (peripheral) (plexus)	T41.3X1	T41.3X2	T41.3X3	T41.3X4	T41.3X5	T41.3X6
spinal	T41.3X1	T41.3X2	T41.3X3	T41.3X4	T41.3X5	T41.3X6
topical (surface)	T41.3X1	T41.3X2	T41.3X3	T41.3X4	T41.3X5	T41.3X6
Stovarsal	T37.8X1	T37.8X2	T37.8X3	T37.8X4	T37.8X5	T37.8X6
Stove gas — see Gas, stove						
Stoxil	T49.5X1	T49.5X2	T49.5X3	T49.5X4	T49.5X5	T49.5X6
Stramonium	T48.6X1	T48.6X2	T48.6X3	T48.6X4	T48.6X5	T48.6X6
natural state	T62.2X1	T62.2X2	T62.2X3	T62.2X4	—	—
Streptodornase	T45.3X1	T45.3X2	T45.3X3	T45.3X4	T45.3X5	T45.3X6
Streptoduocin	T36.5X1	T36.5X2	T36.5X3	T36.5X4	T36.5X5	T36.5X6
Streptokinase	T45.611	T45.612	T45.613	T45.614	T45.615	T45.616
Streptomycin (derivative)	T36.5X1	T36.5X2	T36.5X3	T36.5X4	T36.5X5	T36.5X6
Streptonivicin	T36.5X1	T36.5X2	T36.5X3	T36.5X4	T36.5X5	T36.5X6
Streptovarycin	T36.5X1	T36.5X2	T36.5X3	T36.5X4	T36.5X5	T36.5X6
Streptozocin	T45.1X1	T45.1X2	T45.1X3	T45.1X4	T45.1X5	T45.1X6
Streptozotocin	T45.1X1	T45.1X2	T45.1X3	T45.1X4	T45.1X5	T45.1X6
Stripper (paint) (solvent)	T52.8X1	T52.8X2	T52.8X3	T52.8X4	—	—
Strobane	T60.1X1	T60.1X2	T60.1X3	T60.1X4	—	—
Strofantina	T46.0X1	T46.0X2	T46.0X3	T46.0X4	T46.0X5	T46.0X6
Stromectol*	T37.4X1	T37.4X2	T37.4X3	T37.4X4	T37.4X5	T37.4X6
Strophanthin (g) (k)	T46.0X1	T46.0X2	T46.0X3	T46.0X4	T46.0X5	T46.0X6
Strophanthus	T46.0X1	T46.0X2	T46.0X3	T46.0X4	T46.0X5	T46.0X6
Strophantin	T46.0X1	T46.0X2	T46.0X3	T46.0X4	T46.0X5	T46.0X6
Strophantin-g	T46.0X1	T46.0X2	T46.0X3	T46.0X4	T46.0X5	T46.0X6
Strychnine (nonmedicinal) (pesticide) (salts)	T65.1X1	T65.1X2	T65.1X3	T65.1X4	—	—
medicinal	T48.291	T48.292	T48.293	T48.294	T48.295	T48.296
Strychnos (ignatii) — see Strychnine						
Styramate	T42.8X1	T42.8X2	T42.8X3	T42.8X4	T42.8X5	T42.8X6
Styrene	T65.891	T65.892	T65.893	T65.894	—	—
Succinimide, antiepileptic or anticonvulsant	T42.2X1	T42.2X2	T42.2X3	T42.2X4	T42.2X5	T42.2X6
mercuric — see Mercury						
Succinylcholine	T48.1X1	T48.1X2	T48.1X3	T48.1X4	T48.1X5	T48.1X6
Succinylsulfathiazole	T37.0X1	T37.0X2	T37.0X3	T37.0X4	T37.0X5	T37.0X6
Sucralfate	T47.1X1	T47.1X2	T47.1X3	T47.1X4	T47.1X5	T47.1X6
Sucrose	T50.3X1	T50.3X2	T50.3X3	T50.3X4	T50.3X5	T50.3X6
Sufentanil	T40.411	T40.412	T40.413	T40.414	T40.415	T40.416
Sulbactam	T36.0X1	T36.0X2	T36.0X3	T36.0X4	T36.0X5	T36.0X6
Sulbenicillin	T36.0X1	T36.0X2	T36.0X3	T36.0X4	T36.0X5	T36.0X6
Sulbentine	T49.0X1	T49.0X2	T49.0X3	T49.0X4	T49.0X5	T49.0X6
Sulconazole*	T49.0X1	T49.0X2	T49.0X3	T49.0X4	T49.0X5	T49.0X6
Sulfacetamide	T49.0X1	T49.0X2	T49.0X3	T49.0X4	T49.0X5	T49.0X6
ophthalmic preparation	T49.5X1	T49.5X2	T49.5X3	T49.5X4	T49.5X5	T49.5X6
Sulfachlorpyridazine	T37.0X1	T37.0X2	T37.0X3	T37.0X4	T37.0X5	T37.0X6
Sulfacitine	T37.0X1	T37.0X2	T37.0X3	T37.0X4	T37.0X5	T37.0X6
Sulfadiasulfone sodium	T37.0X1	T37.0X2	T37.0X3	T37.0X4	T37.0X5	T37.0X6
Sulfadiazine	T37.0X1	T37.0X2	T37.0X3	T37.0X4	T37.0X5	T37.0X6
silver (topical)	T49.0X1	T49.0X2	T49.0X3	T49.0X4	T49.0X5	T49.0X6
Sulfadimethoxine	T37.0X1	T37.0X2	T37.0X3	T37.0X4	T37.0X5	T37.0X6
Sulfadimidine	T37.0X1	T37.0X2	T37.0X3	T37.0X4	T37.0X5	T37.0X6
Sulfadoxine	T37.0X1	T37.0X2	T37.0X3	T37.0X4	T37.0X5	T37.0X6
with pyrimethamine	T37.2X1	T37.2X2	T37.2X3	T37.2X4	T37.2X5	T37.2X6
Sulfaethidole	T37.0X1	T37.0X2	T37.0X3	T37.0X4	T37.0X5	T37.0X6
Sulfafurazole	T37.0X1	T37.0X2	T37.0X3	T37.0X4	T37.0X5	T37.0X6
Sulfaguanidine	T37.0X1	T37.0X2	T37.0X3	T37.0X4	T37.0X5	T37.0X6
Sulfalene	T37.0X1	T37.0X2	T37.0X3	T37.0X4	T37.0X5	T37.0X6
Sulfaloxate	T37.0X1	T37.0X2	T37.0X3	T37.0X4	T37.0X5	T37.0X6
Sulfaloxic acid	T37.0X1	T37.0X2	T37.0X3	T37.0X4	T37.0X5	T37.0X6
Sulfamazone	T39.2X1	T39.2X2	T39.2X3	T39.2X4	T39.2X5	T39.2X6
Sulfamerazine	T37.0X1	T37.0X2	T37.0X3	T37.0X4	T37.0X5	T37.0X6
Sulfameter	T37.0X1	T37.0X2	T37.0X3	T37.0X4	T37.0X5	T37.0X6
Sulfamethazine	T37.0X1	T37.0X2	T37.0X3	T37.0X4	T37.0X5	T37.0X6
Sulfamethizole	T37.0X1	T37.0X2	T37.0X3	T37.0X4	T37.0X5	T37.0X6
Sulfamethoxazole	T37.0X1	T37.0X2	T37.0X3	T37.0X4	T37.0X5	T37.0X6
with trimethoprim	T36.8X1	T36.8X2	T36.8X3	T36.8X4	T36.8X5	T36.8X6
Sulfamethoxydiazine	T37.0X1	T37.0X2	T37.0X3	T37.0X4	T37.0X5	T37.0X6
Sulfamethoxypyridazine	T37.0X1	T37.0X2	T37.0X3	T37.0X4	T37.0X5	T37.0X6
Sulfamethylthiazole	T37.0X1	T37.0X2	T37.0X3	T37.0X4	T37.0X5	T37.0X6
Sulfametoxydiazine	T37.0X1	T37.0X2	T37.0X3	T37.0X4	T37.0X5	T37.0X6
Sulfamidopyrine	T39.2X1	T39.2X2	T39.2X3	T39.2X4	T39.2X5	T39.2X6
Sulfamonomethoxine	T37.0X1	T37.0X2	T37.0X3	T37.0X4	T37.0X5	T37.0X6
Sulfamoxole	T37.0X1	T37.0X2	T37.0X3	T37.0X4	T37.0X5	T37.0X6
Sulfamylon	T49.0X1	T49.0X2	T49.0X3	T49.0X4	T49.0X5	T49.0X6
Sulfan blue (diagnostic dye)	T50.8X1	T50.8X2	T50.8X3	T50.8X4	T50.8X5	T50.8X6
Sulfanilamide	T37.0X1	T37.0X2	T37.0X3	T37.0X4	T37.0X5	T37.0X6
Sulfanilylguanidine	T37.0X1	T37.0X2	T37.0X3	T37.0X4	T37.0X5	T37.0X6
Sulfaperin	T37.0X1	T37.0X2	T37.0X3	T37.0X4	T37.0X5	T37.0X6
Sulfaphenazole	T37.0X1	T37.0X2	T37.0X3	T37.0X4	T37.0X5	T37.0X6
Sulfaphenylthiazole	T37.0X1	T37.0X2	T37.0X3	T37.0X4	T37.0X5	T37.0X6
Sulfaproxyline	T37.0X1	T37.0X2	T37.0X3	T37.0X4	T37.0X5	T37.0X6
Sulfapyridine	T37.0X1	T37.0X2	T37.0X3	T37.0X4	T37.0X5	T37.0X6
Sulfapyrimidine	T37.0X1	T37.0X2	T37.0X3	T37.0X4	T37.0X5	T37.0X6
Sulfarsphenamine	T37.8X1	T37.8X2	T37.8X3	T37.8X4	T37.8X5	T37.8X6
Sulfasalazine	T37.0X1	T37.0X2	T37.0X3	T37.0X4	T37.0X5	T37.0X6
Sulfasuxidine	T37.0X1	T37.0X2	T37.0X3	T37.0X4	T37.0X5	T37.0X6
Sulfasymazine	T37.0X1	T37.0X2	T37.0X3	T37.0X4	T37.0X5	T37.0X6
Sulfated amylopectin	T47.8X1	T47.8X2	T47.8X3	T47.8X4	T47.8X5	T47.8X6
Sulfathiazole	T37.0X1	T37.0X2	T37.0X3	T37.0X4	T37.0X5	T37.0X6
Sulfatostearate	T49.2X1	T49.2X2	T49.2X3	T49.2X4	T49.2X5	T49.2X6
Sulfatrim*	T36.8X1	T36.8X2	T36.8X3	T36.8X4	T36.8X5	T36.8X6
Sulfinpyrazone	T50.4X1	T50.4X2	T50.4X3	T50.4X4	T50.4X5	T50.4X6
Sulfiram	T49.0X1	T49.0X2	T49.0X3	T49.0X4	T49.0X5	T49.0X6
Sulfisomidine	T37.0X1	T37.0X2	T37.0X3	T37.0X4	T37.0X5	T37.0X6
Sulfisoxazole	T37.0X1	T37.0X2	T37.0X3	T37.0X4	T37.0X5	T37.0X6
ophthalmic preparation	T49.5X1	T49.5X2	T49.5X3	T49.5X4	T49.5X5	T49.5X6
Sulfobromophthalein (sodium)	T50.8X1	T50.8X2	T50.8X3	T50.8X4	T50.8X5	T50.8X6
Sulfobromphthalein	T50.8X1	T50.8X2	T50.8X3	T50.8X4	T50.8X5	T50.8X6
Sulfogaiacol	T48.4X1	T48.4X2	T48.4X3	T48.4X4	T48.4X5	T48.4X6
Sulfomyxin	T36.8X1	T36.8X2	T36.8X3	T36.8X4	T36.8X5	T36.8X6
Sulfonal	T42.6X1	T42.6X2	T42.6X3	T42.6X4	T42.6X5	T42.6X6
Sulfonamide NEC	T37.0X1	T37.0X2	T37.0X3	T37.0X4	T37.0X5	T37.0X6
eye	T49.5X1	T49.5X2	T49.5X3	T49.5X4	T49.5X5	T49.5X6
Sulfonazide	T37.1X1	T37.1X2	T37.1X3	T37.1X4	T37.1X5	T37.1X6
Sulfones	T37.1X1	T37.1X2	T37.1X3	T37.1X4	T37.1X5	T37.1X6
Sulfonethylmethane	T42.6X1	T42.6X2	T42.6X3	T42.6X4	T42.6X5	T42.6X6
Sulfonmethane	T42.6X1	T42.6X2	T42.6X3	T42.6X4	T42.6X5	T42.6X6
Sulfonphthal, sulfonphthol	T50.8X1	T50.8X2	T50.8X3	T50.8X4	T50.8X5	T50.8X6
Sulfonylurea derivatives, oral	T38.3X1	T38.3X2	T38.3X3	T38.3X4	T38.3X5	T38.3X6
Sulforidazine	T43.3X1	T43.3X2	T43.3X3	T43.3X4	T43.3X5	T43.3X6
Sulfoxone	T37.1X1	T37.1X2	T37.1X3	T37.1X4	T37.1X5	T37.1X6
Sulfuric acid	T54.2X1	T54.2X2	T54.2X3	T54.2X4	—	—
Sulfur, sulfurated, sulfuric, sulfurous, sulfuryl (compounds NEC) (medicinal)	T49.4X1	T49.4X2	T49.4X3	T49.4X4	T49.4X5	T49.4X6
acid	T54.2X1	T54.2X2	T54.2X3	T54.2X4	—	—
dioxide (gas)	T59.1X1	T59.1X2	T59.1X3	T59.1X4	—	—
ether — see Ether(s)						
hydrogen	T59.6X1	T59.6X2	T59.6X3	T59.6X4	—	—
medicinal (keratolytic) (ointment) NEC	T49.4X1	T49.4X2	T49.4X3	T49.4X4	T49.4X5	T49.4X6
ointment	T49.0X1	T49.0X2	T49.0X3	T49.0X4	T49.0X5	T49.0X6
pesticide (vapor)	T60.91	T60.92	T60.93	T60.94	—	—
vapor NEC	T59.891	T59.892	T59.893	T59.894	—	—
Sulglicotide	T47.1X1	T47.1X2	T47.1X3	T47.1X4	T47.1X5	T47.1X6
Sulindac	T39.391	T39.392	T39.393	T39.394	T39.395	T39.396
Sulisatin	T47.2X1	T47.2X2	T47.2X3	T47.2X4	T47.2X5	T47.2X6
Sulisobenzone	T49.3X1	T49.3X2	T49.3X3	T49.3X4	T49.3X5	T49.3X6
Sulkowitch's reagent	T50.8X1	T50.8X2	T50.8X3	T50.8X4	T50.8X5	T50.8X6
Sulmetozine	T44.3X1	T44.3X2	T44.3X3	T44.3X4	T44.3X5	T44.3X6
Suloctidil	T46.7X1	T46.7X2	T46.7X3	T46.7X4	T46.7X5	T46.7X6
Sulph- — see also Sulf-						
Sulphadiazine	T37.0X1	T37.0X2	T37.0X3	T37.0X4	T37.0X5	T37.0X6
Sulphadimethoxine	T37.0X1	T37.0X2	T37.0X3	T37.0X4	T37.0X5	T37.0X6
Sulphadimidine	T37.0X1	T37.0X2	T37.0X3	T37.0X4	T37.0X5	T37.0X6
Sulphadione	T37.1X1	T37.1X2	T37.1X3	T37.1X4	T37.1X5	T37.1X6
Sulphafurazole	T37.0X1	T37.0X2	T37.0X3	T37.0X4	T37.0X5	T37.0X6
Sulphamethizole	T37.0X1	T37.0X2	T37.0X3	T37.0X4	T37.0X5	T37.0X6
Sulphamethoxazole	T37.0X1	T37.0X2	T37.0X3	T37.0X4	T37.0X5	T37.0X6
Sulphan blue	T50.8X1	T50.8X2	T50.8X3	T50.8X4	T50.8X5	T50.8X6
Sulphaphenazole	T37.0X1	T37.0X2	T37.0X3	T37.0X4	T37.0X5	T37.0X6
Sulphapyridine	T37.0X1	T37.0X2	T37.0X3	T37.0X4	T37.0X5	T37.0X6
Sulphasalazine	T37.0X1	T37.0X2	T37.0X3	T37.0X4	T37.0X5	T37.0X6
Sulphinpyrazone	T50.4X1	T50.4X2	T50.4X3	T50.4X4	T50.4X5	T50.4X6
Sulpiride	T43.591	T43.592	T43.593	T43.594	T43.595	T43.596
Sulprostone	T48.0X1	T48.0X2	T48.0X3	T48.0X4	T48.0X5	T48.0X6

☑ Additional Character May Be Required — Refer to the Tabular List for Character Selection

*Optum Value-Add

Substance	Poisoning, Accidental (unintentional)	Poisoning, Intentional Self-harm	Poisoning, Assault	Poisoning, Undetermined	Adverse Effect	Under-dosing
Sulpyrine	T39.2X1	T39.2X2	T39.2X3	T39.2X4	T39.2X5	T39.2X6
Sultamicillin	T36.0X1	T36.0X2	T36.0X3	T36.0X4	T36.0X5	T36.0X6
Sulthiame	T42.6X1	T42.6X2	T42.6X3	T42.6X4	T42.6X5	T42.6X6
Sultiame	T42.6X1	T42.6X2	T42.6X3	T42.6X4	T42.6X5	T42.6X6
Sultopride	T43.591	T43.592	T43.593	T43.594	T43.595	T43.596
Sumatriptan	T39.8X1	T39.8X2	T39.8X3	T39.8X4	T39.8X5	T39.8X6
Sumavel*	T39.8X1	T39.8X2	T39.8X3	T39.8X4	T39.8X5	T39.8X6
Sunflower seed oil	T46.6X1	T46.6X2	T46.6X3	T46.6X4	T46.6X5	T46.6X6
Superinone	T48.4X1	T48.4X2	T48.4X3	T48.4X4	T48.4X5	T48.4X6
Suprofen	T39.311	T39.312	T39.313	T39.314	T39.315	T39.316
Suramin (sodium)	T37.4X1	T37.4X2	T37.4X3	T37.4X4	T37.4X5	T37.4X6
Surfacaine	T41.3X1	T41.3X2	T41.3X3	T41.3X4	T41.3X5	T41.3X6
Surital	T41.1X1	T41.1X2	T41.1X3	T41.1X4	T41.1X5	T41.1X6
Sutilains	T45.3X1	T45.3X2	T45.3X3	T45.3X4	T45.3X5	T45.3X6
Suxamethonium (chloride)	T48.1X1	T48.1X2	T48.1X3	T48.1X4	T48.1X5	T48.1X6
Suxethonium (chloride)	T48.1X1	T48.1X2	T48.1X3	T48.1X4	T48.1X5	T48.1X6
Suxibuzone	T39.2X1	T39.2X2	T39.2X3	T39.2X4	T39.2X5	T39.2X6
Sweetener	T50.901	T50.902	T50.903	T50.904	T50.905	T50.906
Sweet niter spirit	T46.3X1	T46.3X2	T46.3X3	T46.3X4	T46.3X5	T46.3X6
Sweet oil (birch)	T49.3X1	T49.3X2	T49.3X3	T49.3X4	T49.3X5	T49.3X6
Sylvant*	T45.1X1	T45.1X2	T45.1X3	T45.1X4	T45.1X5	T45.1X6
Sym-dichloroethyl ether	T53.6X1	T53.6X2	T53.6X3	T53.6X4	—	—
Sympatholytic NEC	T44.8X1	T44.8X2	T44.8X3	T44.8X4	T44.8X5	T44.8X6
haloalkylamine	T44.8X1	T44.8X2	T44.8X3	T44.8X4	T44.8X5	T44.8X6
Sympathomimetic NEC	T44.901	T44.902	T44.903	T44.904	T44.905	T44.906
anti-common-cold	T48.5X1	T48.5X2	T48.5X3	T48.5X4	T48.5X5	T48.5X6
bronchodilator	T48.6X1	T48.6X2	T48.6X3	T48.6X4	T48.6X5	T48.6X6
specified NEC	T44.991	T44.992	T44.993	T44.994	T44.995	T44.996
Synagis	T50.B91	T50.B92	T50.B93	T50.B94	T50.B95	T50.B96
Synalar	T49.0X1	T49.0X2	T49.0X3	T49.0X4	T49.0X5	T49.0X6
Synthetic cannabinoids	T40.721	T40.722	T40.723	T40.724	T40.725	T40.726
Synthroid	T38.1X1	T38.1X2	T38.1X3	T38.1X4	T38.1X5	T38.1X6
Syntocinon	T48.0X1	T48.0X2	T48.0X3	T48.0X4	T48.0X5	T48.0X6
Syrosingopine	T46.5X1	T46.5X2	T46.5X3	T46.5X4	T46.5X5	T46.5X6
Systemic drug	T45.91	T45.92	T45.93	T45.94	T45.95	T45.96
specified NEC	T45.8X1	T45.8X2	T45.8X3	T45.8X4	T45.8X5	T45.8X6
Tablets — see also specified substance	T50.901	T50.902	T50.903	T50.904	T50.905	T50.906
Tace	T38.5X1	T38.5X2	T38.5X3	T38.5X4	T38.5X5	T38.5X6
Tacrine	T44.0X1	T44.0X2	T44.0X3	T44.0X4	T44.0X5	T44.0X6
Tadalafil	T46.7X1	T46.7X2	T46.7X3	T46.7X4	T46.7X5	T46.7X6
Talampicillin	T36.0X1	T36.0X2	T36.0X3	T36.0X4	T36.0X5	T36.0X6
Talbutal	T42.3X1	T42.3X2	T42.3X3	T42.3X4	T42.3X5	T42.3X6
Talc powder	T49.3X1	T49.3X2	T49.3X3	T49.3X4	T49.3X5	T49.3X6
Talcum	T49.3X1	T49.3X2	T49.3X3	T49.3X4	T49.3X5	T49.3X6
Taleranol	T38.6X1	T38.6X2	T38.6X3	T38.6X4	T38.6X5	T38.6X6
Taltz*	T39.391	T39.392	T39.393	T39.394	T39.395	T39.396
Tamoxifen	T38.6X1	T38.6X2	T38.6X3	T38.6X4	T38.6X5	T38.6X6
Tamsulosin	T44.6X1	T44.6X2	T44.6X3	T44.6X4	T44.6X5	T44.6X6
Tandearil, tanderil	T39.2X1	T39.2X2	T39.2X3	T39.2X4	T39.2X5	T39.2X6
Tannic acid	T49.2X1	T49.2X2	T49.2X3	T49.2X4	T49.2X5	T49.2X6
medicinal (astringent)	T49.2X1	T49.2X2	T49.2X3	T49.2X4	T49.2X5	T49.2X6
Tannin — see Tannic acid						
Tansy	T62.2X1	T62.2X2	T62.2X3	T62.2X4	—	—
TAO	T36.3X1	T36.3X2	T36.3X3	T36.3X4	T36.3X5	T36.3X6
Tapazole	T38.2X1	T38.2X2	T38.2X3	T38.2X4	T38.2X5	T38.2X6
Taractan	T43.591	T43.592	T43.593	T43.594	T43.595	T43.596
Tarantula (venomous)	T63.321	T63.322	T63.323	T63.324	—	—
Tartar emetic	T37.8X1	T37.8X2	T37.8X3	T37.8X4	T37.8X5	T37.8X6
Tartaric acid	T65.891	T65.892	T65.893	T65.894	—	—
Tartrated antimony (anti-infective)	T37.8X1	T37.8X2	T37.8X3	T37.8X4	T37.8X5	T37.8X6
Tartrate, laxative	T47.4X1	T47.4X2	T47.4X3	T47.4X4	T47.4X5	T47.4X6
Tar NEC	T52.0X1	T52.0X2	T52.0X3	T52.0X4	—	—
camphor	T60.1X1	T60.1X2	T60.1X3	T60.1X4	—	—
distillate	T49.1X1	T49.1X2	T49.1X3	T49.1X4	T49.1X5	T49.1X6
fumes	T59.891	T59.892	T59.893	T59.894	—	—
medicinal	T49.1X1	T49.1X2	T49.1X3	T49.1X4	T49.1X5	T49.1X6
ointment	T49.1X1	T49.1X2	T49.1X3	T49.1X4	T49.1X5	T49.1X6
Tauromustine	T45.1X1	T45.1X2	T45.1X3	T45.1X4	T45.1X5	T45.1X6
TCA — see Trichloroacetic acid						
TCDD	T53.7X1	T53.7X2	T53.7X3	T53.7X4	—	—
TDI (vapor)	T65.0X1	T65.0X2	T65.0X3	T65.0X4	—	—
Tear						
gas	T59.3X1	T59.3X2	T59.3X3	T59.3X4	—	—
solution	T49.5X1	T49.5X2	T49.5X3	T49.5X4	T49.5X5	T49.5X6
Tecentriq*	T45.1X1	T45.1X2	T45.1X3	T45.1X4	T45.1X5	T45.1X6
Teclothiazide	T50.2X1	T50.2X2	T50.2X3	T50.2X4	T50.2X5	T50.2X6
Teclozan	T37.3X1	T37.3X2	T37.3X3	T37.3X4	T37.3X5	T37.3X6
Tegafur	T45.1X1	T45.1X2	T45.1X3	T45.1X4	T45.1X5	T45.1X6
Tegretol	T42.1X1	T42.1X2	T42.1X3	T42.1X4	T42.1X5	T42.1X6
Teicoplanin	T36.8X1	T36.8X2	T36.8X3	T36.8X4	T36.8X5	T36.8X6
Telepaque	T50.8X1	T50.8X2	T50.8X3	T50.8X4	T50.8X5	T50.8X6
Tellurium	T56.891	T56.892	T56.893	T56.894	—	—
fumes	T56.891	T56.892	T56.893	T56.894	—	—
TEM	T45.1X1	T45.1X2	T45.1X3	T45.1X4	T45.1X5	T45.1X6
Temazepam	T42.4X1	T42.4X2	T42.4X3	T42.4X4	T42.4X5	T42.4X6
Temocillin	T36.0X1	T36.0X2	T36.0X3	T36.0X4	T36.0X5	T36.0X6
Tenamfetamine	T43.621	T43.622	T43.623	T43.624	T43.625	T43.626
Tenecteplase*	T45.611	T45.612	T45.613	T45.614	T45.615	T45.616
Teniposide	T45.1X1	T45.1X2	T45.1X3	T45.1X4	T45.1X5	T45.1X6
Tenitramine	T46.3X1	T46.3X2	T46.3X3	T46.3X4	T46.3X5	T46.3X6
Tenoglicin	T48.4X1	T48.4X2	T48.4X3	T48.4X4	T48.4X5	T48.4X6
Tenonitrozole	T37.3X1	T37.3X2	T37.3X3	T37.3X4	T37.3X5	T37.3X6
Tenoxicam	T39.391	T39.392	T39.393	T39.394	T39.395	T39.396
TEPA	T45.1X1	T45.1X2	T45.1X3	T45.1X4	T45.1X5	T45.1X6
TEPP	T60.0X1	T60.0X2	T60.0X3	T60.0X4	—	—
Teprotide	T46.5X1	T46.5X2	T46.5X3	T46.5X4	T46.5X5	T46.5X6
Terazosin	T44.6X1	T44.6X2	T44.6X3	T44.6X4	T44.6X5	T44.6X6
Terbufos	T60.0X1	T60.0X2	T60.0X3	T60.0X4	—	—
Terbutaline	T48.6X1	T48.6X2	T48.6X3	T48.6X4	T48.6X5	T48.6X6
Terconazole	T49.0X1	T49.0X2	T49.0X3	T49.0X4	T49.0X5	T49.0X6
Terfenadine	T45.0X1	T45.0X2	T45.0X3	T45.0X4	T45.0X5	T45.0X6
Teriparatide (acetate)	T50.991	T50.992	T50.993	T50.994	T50.995	T50.996
Terizidone	T37.1X1	T37.1X2	T37.1X3	T37.1X4	T37.1X5	T37.1X6
Terlipressin	T38.891	T38.892	T38.893	T38.894	T38.895	T38.896
Terodiline	T46.3X1	T46.3X2	T46.3X3	T46.3X4	T46.3X5	T46.3X6
Teroxalene	T37.4X1	T37.4X2	T37.4X3	T37.4X4	T37.4X5	T37.4X6
Terpin (cis) hydrate	T48.4X1	T48.4X2	T48.4X3	T48.4X4	T48.4X5	T48.4X6
Terramycin	T36.4X1	T36.4X2	T36.4X3	T36.4X4	T36.4X5	T36.4X6
Tertatolol	T44.7X1	T44.7X2	T44.7X3	T44.7X4	T44.7X5	T44.7X6
Tessalon	T48.3X1	T48.3X2	T48.3X3	T48.3X4	T48.3X5	T48.3X6
Testolactone	T38.7X1	T38.7X2	T38.7X3	T38.7X4	T38.7X5	T38.7X6
Testosterone	T38.7X1	T38.7X2	T38.7X3	T38.7X4	T38.7X5	T38.7X6
Tetanus toxoid or vaccine	T50.A91	T50.A92	T50.A93	T50.A94	T50.A95	T50.A96
antitoxin	T50.Z11	T50.Z12	T50.Z13	T50.Z14	T50.Z15	T50.Z16
immune globulin (human)	T50.Z11	T50.Z12	T50.Z13	T50.Z14	T50.Z15	T50.Z16
toxoid	T50.A91	T50.A92	T50.A93	T50.A94	T50.A95	T50.A96
with diphtheria toxoid	T50.A21	T50.A22	T50.A23	T50.A24	T50.A25	T50.A26
with pertussis	T50.A11	T50.A12	T50.A13	T50.A14	T50.A15	T50.A16
Tetrabenazine	T43.591	T43.592	T43.593	T43.594	T43.595	T43.596
Tetracaine	T41.3X1	T41.3X2	T41.3X3	T41.3X4	T41.3X5	T41.3X6
nerve block (peripheral) (plexus)	T41.3X1	T41.3X2	T41.3X3	T41.3X4	T41.3X5	T41.3X6
regional	T41.3X1	T41.3X2	T41.3X3	T41.3X4	T41.3X5	T41.3X6
spinal	T41.3X1	T41.3X2	T41.3X3	T41.3X4	T41.3X5	T41.3X6
Tetrachlorethylene — see Tetrachloroethylene						
Tetrachlormethiazide	T50.2X1	T50.2X2	T50.2X3	T50.2X4	T50.2X5	T50.2X6
Tetrachloroethane	T53.6X1	T53.6X2	T53.6X3	T53.6X4	—	—
vapor	T53.6X1	T53.6X2	T53.6X3	T53.6X4	—	—
paint or varnish	T53.6X1	T53.6X2	T53.6X3	T53.6X4	—	—
Tetrachloroethylene (liquid)	T53.3X1	T53.3X2	T53.3X3	T53.3X4	—	—
medicinal	T37.4X1	T37.4X2	T37.4X3	T37.4X4	T37.4X5	T37.4X6
vapor	T53.3X1	T53.3X2	T53.3X3	T53.3X4	—	—
Tetrachloromethane — see Carbon tetrachloride						
Tetracosactide	T38.811	T38.812	T38.813	T38.814	T38.815	T38.816
Tetracosactrin	T38.811	T38.812	T38.813	T38.814	T38.815	T38.816
Tetracycline	T36.4X1	T36.4X2	T36.4X3	T36.4X4	T36.4X5	T36.4X6
ophthalmic preparation	T49.5X1	T49.5X2	T49.5X3	T49.5X4	T49.5X5	T49.5X6
topical NEC	T49.0X1	T49.0X2	T49.0X3	T49.0X4	T49.0X5	T49.0X6
Tetradifon	T60.8X1	T60.8X2	T60.8X3	T60.8X4	—	—
Tetradotoxin	T61.771	T61.772	T61.773	T61.774	—	—
Tetraethyl						
lead	T56.0X1	T56.0X2	T56.0X3	T56.0X4	—	—
pyrophosphate	T60.0X1	T60.0X2	T60.0X3	T60.0X4	—	—
Tetraethylammonium chloride	T44.2X1	T44.2X2	T44.2X3	T44.2X4	T44.2X5	T44.2X6
Tetraethylthiuram disulfide	T50.6X1	T50.6X2	T50.6X3	T50.6X4	T50.6X5	T50.6X6
Tetrahydroaminoacridine	T44.0X1	T44.0X2	T44.0X3	T44.0X4	T44.0X5	T44.0X6
Tetrahydrocannabinol	T40.711	T40.712	T40.713	T40.714	T40.715	T40.716
Tetrahydrofuran	T52.8X1	T52.8X2	T52.8X3	T52.8X4	—	—
Tetrahydrolipstatin*	T47.8X1	T47.8X2	T47.8X3	T47.8X4	T47.8X5	T47.8X6
Tetrahydronaphthalene	T52.8X1	T52.8X2	T52.8X3	T52.8X4	—	—
Tetrahydrozoline	T49.5X1	T49.5X2	T49.5X3	T49.5X4	T49.5X5	T49.5X6
Tetralin	T52.8X1	T52.8X2	T52.8X3	T52.8X4	—	—
Tetramethrin	T60.2X1	T60.2X2	T60.2X3	T60.2X4	—	—
Tetramethylthiuram (disulfide) NEC	T60.3X1	T60.3X2	T60.3X3	T60.3X4	—	—
medicinal	T49.0X1	T49.0X2	T49.0X3	T49.0X4	T49.0X5	T49.0X6
Tetramisole	T37.4X1	T37.4X2	T37.4X3	T37.4X4	T37.4X5	T37.4X6
Tetranicotinoyl fructose	T46.7X1	T46.7X2	T46.7X3	T46.7X4	T46.7X5	T46.7X6
Tetrazepam	T42.4X1	T42.4X2	T42.4X3	T42.4X4	T42.4X5	T42.4X6

Table of Drugs and Chemicals

Tetronal — Tofisopam

Substance	Poisoning, Accidental (unintentional)	Poisoning, Intentional Self-harm	Poisoning, Assault	Poisoning, Undetermined	Adverse Effect	Under-dosing
Tetronal	T42.6X1	T42.6X2	T42.6X3	T42.6X4	T42.6X5	T42.6X6
Tetryl	T65.3X1	T65.3X2	T65.3X3	T65.3X4	—	—
Tetrylammonium chloride	T44.2X1	T44.2X2	T44.2X3	T44.2X4	T44.2X5	T44.2X6
Tetryzoline	T49.5X1	T49.5X2	T49.5X3	T49.5X4	T49.5X5	T49.5X6
Thalidomide	T45.1X1	T45.1X2	T45.1X3	T45.1X4	T45.1X5	T45.1X6
Thallium (compounds) (dust) NEC	T56.811	T56.812	T56.813	T56.814	—	—
pesticide	T60.4X1	T60.4X2	T60.4X3	T60.4X4	—	—
THC	T40.711	T40.712	T40.713	T40.714	T40.715	T40.716
Thebacon	T48.3X1	T48.3X2	T48.3X3	T48.3X4	T48.3X5	T48.3X6
Thebaine	T40.2X1	T40.2X2	T40.2X3	T40.2X4	T40.2X5	T40.2X6
Thenoic acid	T49.6X1	T49.6X2	T49.6X3	T49.6X4	T49.6X5	T49.6X6
Thenyldiamine	T45.0X1	T45.0X2	T45.0X3	T45.0X4	T45.0X5	T45.0X6
Theobromine (calcium salicylate)	T48.6X1	T48.6X2	T48.6X3	T48.6X4	T48.6X5	T48.6X6
sodium salicylate	T48.6X1	T48.6X2	T48.6X3	T48.6X4	T48.6X5	T48.6X6
Theolair*	T48.6X1	T48.6X2	T48.6X3	T48.6X4	T48.6X5	T48.6X6
Theophyllamine	T48.6X1	T48.6X2	T48.6X3	T48.6X4	T48.6X5	T48.6X6
Theophylline	T48.6X1	T48.6X2	T48.6X3	T48.6X4	T48.6X5	T48.6X6
aminobenzoic acid	T48.6X1	T48.6X2	T48.6X3	T48.6X4	T48.6X5	T48.6X6
ethylenediamine	T48.6X1	T48.6X2	T48.6X3	T48.6X4	T48.6X5	T48.6X6
piperazine	T48.6X1	T48.6X2	T48.6X3	T48.6X4	T48.6X5	T48.6X6
p-amino-benzoate						
Therevac*	T47.4X1	T47.4X2	T47.4X3	T47.4X4	T47.4X5	T47.4X6
Thiabendazole	T37.4X1	T37.4X2	T37.4X3	T37.4X4	T37.4X5	T37.4X6
Thialbarbital	T41.1X1	T41.1X2	T41.1X3	T41.1X4	T41.1X5	T41.1X6
Thiamazole	T38.2X1	T38.2X2	T38.2X3	T38.2X4	T38.2X5	T38.2X6
Thiambutosine	T37.1X1	T37.1X2	T37.1X3	T37.1X4	T37.1X5	T37.1X6
Thiamine	T45.2X1	T45.2X2	T45.2X3	T45.2X4	T45.2X5	T45.2X6
Thiamphenicol	T36.2X1	T36.2X2	T36.2X3	T36.2X4	T36.2X5	T36.2X6
Thiamylal	T41.1X1	T41.1X2	T41.1X3	T41.1X4	T41.1X5	T41.1X6
sodium	T41.1X1	T41.1X2	T41.1X3	T41.1X4	T41.1X5	T41.1X6
Thiazesim	T43.291	T43.292	T43.293	T43.294	T43.295	T43.296
Thiazides (diuretics)	T50.2X1	T50.2X2	T50.2X3	T50.2X4	T50.2X5	T50.2X6
Thiazinamium metilsulfate	T43.3X1	T43.3X2	T43.3X3	T43.3X4	T43.3X5	T43.3X6
Thiethylperazine	T43.3X1	T43.3X2	T43.3X3	T43.3X4	T43.3X5	T43.3X6
Thimerosal	T49.0X1	T49.0X2	T49.0X3	T49.0X4	T49.0X5	T49.0X6
ophthalmic preparation	T49.5X1	T49.5X2	T49.5X3	T49.5X4	T49.5X5	T49.5X6
Thioacetazone	T37.1X1	T37.1X2	T37.1X3	T37.1X4	T37.1X5	T37.1X6
with isoniazid	T37.1X1	T37.1X2	T37.1X3	T37.1X4	T37.1X5	T37.1X6
Thiobarbital sodium	T41.1X1	T41.1X2	T41.1X3	T41.1X4	T41.1X5	T41.1X6
Thiobarbiturate anesthetic	T41.1X1	T41.1X2	T41.1X3	T41.1X4	T41.1X5	T41.1X6
Thiobismol	T37.8X1	T37.8X2	T37.8X3	T37.8X4	T37.8X5	T37.8X6
Thiobutabarbital sodium	T41.1X1	T41.1X2	T41.1X3	T41.1X4	T41.1X5	T41.1X6
Thiocarbamate (insecticide)	T60.0X1	T60.0X2	T60.0X3	T60.0X4	—	—
Thiocarbamide	T38.2X1	T38.2X2	T38.2X3	T38.2X4	T38.2X5	T38.2X6
Thiocarbarsone	T37.8X1	T37.8X2	T37.8X3	T37.8X4	T37.8X5	T37.8X6
Thiocarlide	T37.1X1	T37.1X2	T37.1X3	T37.1X4	T37.1X5	T37.1X6
Thioctamide	T50.991	T50.992	T50.993	T50.994	T50.995	T50.996
Thioctic acid	T50.991	T50.992	T50.993	T50.994	T50.995	T50.996
Thiofos	T60.0X1	T60.0X2	T60.0X3	T60.0X4	—	—
Thioglycolate	T49.4X1	T49.4X2	T49.4X3	T49.4X4	T49.4X5	T49.4X6
Thioglycolic acid	T65.891	T65.892	T65.893	T65.894	—	—
Thioguanine	T45.1X1	T45.1X2	T45.1X3	T45.1X4	T45.1X5	T45.1X6
Thiomercaptomerin	T50.2X1	T50.2X2	T50.2X3	T50.2X4	T50.2X5	T50.2X6
Thiomerin	T50.2X1	T50.2X2	T50.2X3	T50.2X4	T50.2X5	T50.2X6
Thiomersal	T49.0X1	T49.0X2	T49.0X3	T49.0X4	T49.0X5	T49.0X6
Thionazin	T60.0X1	T60.0X2	T60.0X3	T60.0X4	—	—
Thiopental (sodium)	T41.1X1	T41.1X2	T41.1X3	T41.1X4	T41.1X5	T41.1X6
Thiopentone (sodium)	T41.1X1	T41.1X2	T41.1X3	T41.1X4	T41.1X5	T41.1X6
Thiopropazate	T43.3X1	T43.3X2	T43.3X3	T43.3X4	T43.3X5	T43.3X6
Thioproperazine	T43.3X1	T43.3X2	T43.3X3	T43.3X4	T43.3X5	T43.3X6
Thioridazine	T43.3X1	T43.3X2	T43.3X3	T43.3X4	T43.3X5	T43.3X6
Thiosinamine	T49.3X1	T49.3X2	T49.3X3	T49.3X4	T49.3X5	T49.3X6
Thiotepa	T45.1X1	T45.1X2	T45.1X3	T45.1X4	T45.1X5	T45.1X6
Thiothixene	T43.4X1	T43.4X2	T43.4X3	T43.4X4	T43.4X5	T43.4X6
Thiouracil (benzyl) (methyl) (propyl)	T38.2X1	T38.2X2	T38.2X3	T38.2X4	T38.2X5	T38.2X6
Thiourea	T38.2X1	T38.2X2	T38.2X3	T38.2X4	T38.2X5	T38.2X6
Thiphenamil	T44.3X1	T44.3X2	T44.3X3	T44.3X4	T44.3X5	T44.3X6
Thiram	T60.3X1	T60.3X2	T60.3X3	T60.3X4	—	—
medicinal	T49.2X1	T49.2X2	T49.2X3	T49.2X4	T49.2X5	T49.2X6
Thonzylamine (systemic)	T45.0X1	T45.0X2	T45.0X3	T45.0X4	T45.0X5	T45.0X6
mucosal decongestant	T48.5X1	T48.5X2	T48.5X3	T48.5X4	T48.5X5	T48.5X6
Thorazine	T43.3X1	T43.3X2	T43.3X3	T43.3X4	T43.3X5	T43.3X6
Thorium dioxide suspension	T50.8X1	T50.8X2	T50.8X3	T50.8X4	T50.8X5	T50.8X6
Thornapple	T62.2X1	T62.2X2	T62.2X3	T62.2X4	—	—
Throat drug NEC	T49.6X1	T49.6X2	T49.6X3	T49.6X4	T49.6X5	T49.6X6
Thrombate 111*	T45.511	T45.512	T45.513	T45.514	T45.515	T45.516

Substance	Poisoning, Accidental (unintentional)	Poisoning, Intentional Self-harm	Poisoning, Assault	Poisoning, Undetermined	Adverse Effect	Under-dosing
Thrombin	T45.7X1	T45.7X2	T45.7X3	T45.7X4	T45.7X5	T45.7X6
Thrombolysin	T45.611	T45.612	T45.613	T45.614	T45.615	T45.616
Thromboplastin	T45.7X1	T45.7X2	T45.7X3	T45.7X4	T45.7X5	T45.7X6
Thurfyl nicotinate	T46.7X1	T46.7X2	T46.7X3	T46.7X4	T46.7X5	T46.7X6
Thymol	T49.0X1	T49.0X2	T49.0X3	T49.0X4	T49.0X5	T49.0X6
Thymopentin	T37.5X1	T37.5X2	T37.5X3	T37.5X4	T37.5X5	T37.5X6
Thymoxamine	T46.7X1	T46.7X2	T46.7X3	T46.7X4	T46.7X5	T46.7X6
Thymus extract	T38.891	T38.892	T38.893	T38.894	T38.895	T38.896
Thyreotrophic hormone	T38.811	T38.812	T38.813	T38.814	T38.815	T38.816
Thyroglobulin	T38.1X1	T38.1X2	T38.1X3	T38.1X4	T38.1X5	T38.1X6
Thyroid (hormone)	T38.1X1	T38.1X2	T38.1X3	T38.1X4	T38.1X5	T38.1X6
Thyrolar	T38.1X1	T38.1X2	T38.1X3	T38.1X4	T38.1X5	T38.1X6
Thyrotrophin	T38.811	T38.812	T38.813	T38.814	T38.815	T38.816
Thyrotropic hormone	T38.811	T38.812	T38.813	T38.814	T38.815	T38.816
Thyroxine	T38.1X1	T38.1X2	T38.1X3	T38.1X4	T38.1X5	T38.1X6
Tiabendazole	T37.4X1	T37.4X2	T37.4X3	T37.4X4	T37.4X5	T37.4X6
Tiamizide	T50.2X1	T50.2X2	T50.2X3	T50.2X4	T50.2X5	T50.2X6
Tianeptine	T43.291	T43.292	T43.293	T43.294	T43.295	T43.296
Tiapamil	T46.1X1	T46.1X2	T46.1X3	T46.1X4	T46.1X5	T46.1X6
Tiapride	T43.591	T43.592	T43.593	T43.594	T43.595	T43.596
Tiaprofenic acid	T39.311	T39.312	T39.313	T39.314	T39.315	T39.316
Tiaramide	T39.8X1	T39.8X2	T39.8X3	T39.8X4	T39.8X5	T39.8X6
Ticagrelor*	T45.521	T45.522	T45.523	T45.524	T45.525	T45.526
Ticarcillin	T36.0X1	T36.0X2	T36.0X3	T36.0X4	T36.0X5	T36.0X6
Ticlatone	T49.0X1	T49.0X2	T49.0X3	T49.0X4	T49.0X5	T49.0X6
Ticlopidine	T45.521	T45.522	T45.523	T45.524	T45.525	T45.526
Ticrynafen	T50.1X1	T50.1X2	T50.1X3	T50.1X4	T50.1X5	T50.1X6
Tidiacic	T50.991	T50.992	T50.993	T50.994	T50.995	T50.996
Tiemonium	T44.3X1	T44.3X2	T44.3X3	T44.3X4	T44.3X5	T44.3X6
iodide	T44.3X1	T44.3X2	T44.3X3	T44.3X4	T44.3X5	T44.3X6
Tienilic acid	T50.1X1	T50.1X2	T50.1X3	T50.1X4	T50.1X5	T50.1X6
Tifenamil	T44.3X1	T44.3X2	T44.3X3	T44.3X4	T44.3X5	T44.3X6
Tigan	T45.0X1	T45.0X2	T45.0X3	T45.0X4	T45.0X5	T45.0X6
Tigloidine	T44.3X1	T44.3X2	T44.3X3	T44.3X4	T44.3X5	T44.3X6
Tilactase	T47.5X1	T47.5X2	T47.5X3	T47.5X4	T47.5X5	T47.5X6
Tiletamine	T41.291	T41.292	T41.293	T41.294	T41.295	T41.296
Tilidine	T40.491	T40.492	T40.493	T40.494	—	—
Timepidium bromide	T44.3X1	T44.3X2	T44.3X3	T44.3X4	T44.3X5	T44.3X6
Timiperone	T43.4X1	T43.4X2	T43.4X3	T43.4X4	T43.4X5	T43.4X6
Timolol	T44.7X1	T44.7X2	T44.7X3	T44.7X4	T44.7X5	T44.7X6
Tincture, iodine — see Iodine						
Tindal	T43.3X1	T43.3X2	T43.3X3	T43.3X4	T43.3X5	T43.3X6
Tinidazole	T37.3X1	T37.3X2	T37.3X3	T37.3X4	T37.3X5	T37.3X6
Tin (chloride) (dust) (oxide) NEC	T56.6X1	T56.6X2	T56.6X3	T56.6X4	—	—
anti-infectives	T37.8X1	T37.8X2	T37.8X3	T37.8X4	T37.8X5	T37.8X6
Tinoridine	T39.8X1	T39.8X2	T39.8X3	T39.8X4	T39.8X5	T39.8X6
Tiocarlide	T37.1X1	T37.1X2	T37.1X3	T37.1X4	T37.1X5	T37.1X6
Tioclomarol	T45.511	T45.512	T45.513	T45.514	T45.515	T45.516
Tioconazole	T49.0X1	T49.0X2	T49.0X3	T49.0X4	T49.0X5	T49.0X6
Tioguanine	T45.1X1	T45.1X2	T45.1X3	T45.1X4	T45.1X5	T45.1X6
Tiopronin	T50.991	T50.992	T50.993	T50.994	T50.995	T50.996
Tiotixene	T43.4X1	T43.4X2	T43.4X3	T43.4X4	T43.4X5	T43.4X6
Tioxolone	T49.4X1	T49.4X2	T49.4X3	T49.4X4	T49.4X5	T49.4X6
Tipepidine	T48.3X1	T48.3X2	T48.3X3	T48.3X4	T48.3X5	T48.3X6
Tiquizium bromide	T44.3X1	T44.3X2	T44.3X3	T44.3X4	T44.3X5	T44.3X6
Tiratricol	T38.1X1	T38.1X2	T38.1X3	T38.1X4	T38.1X5	T38.1X6
Tisopurine	T50.4X1	T50.4X2	T50.4X3	T50.4X4	T50.4X5	T50.4X6
Titanium (compounds) (vapor)	T56.891	T56.892	T56.893	T56.894	—	—
dioxide	T49.3X1	T49.3X2	T49.3X3	T49.3X4	T49.3X5	T49.3X6
ointment	T49.3X1	T49.3X2	T49.3X3	T49.3X4	T49.3X5	T49.3X6
oxide	T49.3X1	T49.3X2	T49.3X3	T49.3X4	T49.3X5	T49.3X6
tetrachloride	T56.891	T56.892	T56.893	T56.894	—	—
Titanocene	T56.891	T56.892	T56.893	T56.894	—	—
Titroid	T38.1X1	T38.1X2	T38.1X3	T38.1X4	T38.1X5	T38.1X6
Tizanidine	T42.8X1	T42.8X2	T42.8X3	T42.8X4	T42.8X5	T42.8X6
TMTD	T60.3X1	T60.3X2	T60.3X3	T60.3X4	—	—
TNT (fumes)	T65.3X1	T65.3X2	T65.3X3	T65.3X4	—	—
Toadstool	T62.0X1	T62.0X2	T62.0X3	T62.0X4	—	—
Tobacco NEC	T65.291	T65.292	T65.293	T65.294	—	—
cigarettes	T65.221	T65.222	T65.223	T65.224	—	—
Indian	T62.2X1	T62.2X2	T62.2X3	T62.2X4	—	—
smoke, second-hand	T65.221	T65.222	T65.223	T65.224	—	—
Tobraflex*	T49.5X1	T49.5X2	T49.5X3	T49.5X4	T49.5X5	T49.5X6
Tobramycin	T36.5X1	T36.5X2	T36.5X3	T36.5X4	T36.5X5	T36.5X6
Tocainide	T46.2X1	T46.2X2	T46.2X3	T46.2X4	T46.2X5	T46.2X6
Tocoferol	T45.2X1	T45.2X2	T45.2X3	T45.2X4	T45.2X5	T45.2X6
Tocopherol	T45.2X1	T45.2X2	T45.2X3	T45.2X4	T45.2X5	T45.2X6
acetate	T45.2X1	T45.2X2	T45.2X3	T45.2X4	T45.2X5	T45.2X6
Tocosamine	T48.0X1	T48.0X2	T48.0X3	T48.0X4	T48.0X5	T48.0X6
Todralazine	T46.5X1	T46.5X2	T46.5X3	T46.5X4	T46.5X5	T46.5X6
Tofisopam	T42.4X1	T42.4X2	T42.4X3	T42.4X4	T42.4X5	T42.4X6

☑ Additional Character May Be Required — Refer to the Tabular List for Character Selection

*Optum Value-Add

Substance	Poisoning, Accidental (unintentional)	Poisoning, Intentional Self-harm	Poisoning, Assault	Poisoning, Undetermined	Adverse Effect	Under-dosing
Tofranil	T43.011	T43.012	T43.013	T43.014	T43.015	T43.016
Toilet deodorizer	T65.891	T65.892	T65.893	T65.894	—	—
Tolamolol	T44.7X1	T44.7X2	T44.7X3	T44.7X4	T44.7X5	T44.7X6
Tolazamide	T38.3X1	T38.3X2	T38.3X3	T38.3X4	T38.3X5	T38.3X6
Tolazoline	T46.7X1	T46.7X2	T46.7X3	T46.7X4	T46.7X5	T46.7X6
Tolbutamide (sodium)	T38.3X1	T38.3X2	T38.3X3	T38.3X4	T38.3X5	T38.3X6
Tolciclate	T49.0X1	T49.0X2	T49.0X3	T49.0X4	T49.0X5	T49.0X6
Tolmetin	T39.391	T39.392	T39.393	T39.394	T39.395	T39.396
Tolnaftate	T49.0X1	T49.0X2	T49.0X3	T49.0X4	T49.0X5	T49.0X6
Tolonidine	T46.5X1	T46.5X2	T46.5X3	T46.5X4	T46.5X5	T46.5X6
Toloxatone	T42.6X1	T42.6X2	T42.6X3	T42.6X4	T42.6X5	T42.6X6
Tolperisone	T44.3X1	T44.3X2	T44.3X3	T44.3X4	T44.3X5	T44.3X6
Tolserol	T42.8X1	T42.8X2	T42.8X3	T42.8X4	T42.8X5	T42.8X6
Toluene (liquid)	T52.2X1	T52.2X2	T52.2X3	T52.2X4	—	—
diisocyanate	T65.0X1	T65.0X2	T65.0X3	T65.0X4	—	—
Toluidine	T65.891	T65.892	T65.893	T65.894	—	—
vapor	T59.891	T59.892	T59.893	T59.894	—	—
Toluol (liquid)	T52.2X1	T52.2X2	T52.2X3	T52.2X4	—	—
vapor	T52.2X1	T52.2X2	T52.2X3	T52.2X4	—	—
Toluylenediamine	T65.3X1	T65.3X2	T65.3X3	T65.3X4	—	—
Tolylene-2,4-diisocyanate	T65.0X1	T65.0X2	T65.0X3	T65.0X4	—	—
Tonic NEC	T50.901	T50.902	T50.903	T50.904	T50.905	T50.906
Topical action drug NEC	T49.91	T49.92	T49.93	T49.94	T49.95	T49.96
ear, nose or throat	T49.6X1	T49.6X2	T49.6X3	T49.6X4	T49.6X5	T49.6X6
eye	T49.5X1	T49.5X2	T49.5X3	T49.5X4	T49.5X5	T49.5X6
skin	T49.91	T49.92	T49.93	T49.94	T49.95	T49.96
specified NEC	T49.8X1	T49.8X2	T49.8X3	T49.8X4	T49.8X5	T49.8X6
Toprol*	T44.7X1	T44.7X2	T44.7X3	T44.7X4	T44.7X5	T44.7X6
Toquizine	T44.3X1	T44.3X2	T44.3X3	T44.3X4	T44.3X5	T44.3X6
Toremifene	T38.6X1	T38.6X2	T38.6X3	T38.6X4	T38.6X5	T38.6X6
Tosylchloramide sodium	T49.8X1	T49.8X2	T49.8X3	T49.8X4	T49.8X5	T49.8X6
Toxaphene (dust) (spray)	T60.1X1	T60.1X2	T60.1X3	T60.1X4	—	—
Toxin, diphtheria (Schick Test)	T50.8X1	T50.8X2	T50.8X3	T50.8X4	T50.8X5	T50.8X6
Toxoid						
combined	T50.A21	T50.A22	T50.A23	T50.A24	T50.A25	T50.A26
diphtheria	T50.A91	T50.A92	T50.A93	T50.A94	T50.A95	T50.A96
tetanus	T50.A91	T50.A92	T50.A93	T50.A94	T50.A95	T50.A96
Trace element NEC	T45.8X1	T45.8X2	T45.8X3	T45.8X4	T45.8X5	T45.8X6
Tractor fuel NEC	T52.0X1	T52.0X2	T52.0X3	T52.0X4	—	—
Tragacanth	T50.991	T50.992	T50.993	T50.994	T50.995	T50.996
Tramadol	T40.421	T40.422	T40.423	T40.424	T40.425	T40.426
Tramazoline	T48.5X1	T48.5X2	T48.5X3	T48.5X4	T48.5X5	T48.5X6
Tranexamic acid	T45.621	T45.622	T45.623	T45.624	T45.625	T45.626
Tranilast	T45.0X1	T45.0X2	T45.0X3	T45.0X4	T45.0X5	T45.0X6
Tranquilizer NEC	T43.501	T43.502	T43.503	T43.504	T43.505	T43.506
with hypnotic or sedative	T42.6X1	T42.6X2	T42.6X3	T42.6X4	T42.6X5	T42.6X6
benzodiazepine NEC	T42.4X1	T42.4X2	T42.4X3	T42.4X4	T42.4X5	T42.4X6
butyrophenone NEC	T43.4X1	T43.4X2	T43.4X3	T43.4X4	T43.4X5	T43.4X6
carbamate	T43.591	T43.592	T43.593	T43.594	T43.595	T43.596
dimethylamine	T43.3X1	T43.3X2	T43.3X3	T43.3X4	T43.3X5	T43.3X6
ethylamine	T43.3X1	T43.3X2	T43.3X3	T43.3X4	T43.3X5	T43.3X6
hydroxyzine	T43.591	T43.592	T43.593	T43.594	T43.595	T43.596
major NEC	T43.501	T43.502	T43.503	T43.504	T43.505	T43.506
penothiazine NEC	T43.3X1	T43.3X2	T43.3X3	T43.3X4	T43.3X5	T43.3X6
phenothiazine-based	T43.3X1	T43.3X2	T43.3X3	T43.3X4	T43.3X5	T43.3X6
piperazine NEC	T43.3X1	T43.3X2	T43.3X3	T43.3X4	T43.3X5	T43.3X6
piperidine	T43.3X1	T43.3X2	T43.3X3	T43.3X4	T43.3X5	T43.3X6
propylamine	T43.3X1	T43.3X2	T43.3X3	T43.3X4	T43.3X5	T43.3X6
specified NEC	T43.591	T43.592	T43.593	T43.594	T43.595	T43.596
thioxanthene NEC	T43.591	T43.592	T43.593	T43.594	T43.595	T43.596
Tranxene	T42.4X1	T42.4X2	T42.4X3	T42.4X4	T42.4X5	T42.4X6
Tranylcypromine	T43.1X1	T43.1X2	T43.1X3	T43.1X4	T43.1X5	T43.1X6
Trapidil	T46.3X1	T46.3X2	T46.3X3	T46.3X4	T46.3X5	T46.3X6
Trasentine	T44.3X1	T44.3X2	T44.3X3	T44.3X4	T44.3X5	T44.3X6
Travert	T50.3X1	T50.3X2	T50.3X3	T50.3X4	T50.3X5	T50.3X6
Trazodone	T43.211	T43.212	T43.213	T43.214	T43.215	T43.216
Treanda*	T45.1X1	T45.1X2	T45.1X3	T45.1X4	T45.1X5	T45.1X6
Trecator	T37.1X1	T37.1X2	T37.1X3	T37.1X4	T37.1X5	T37.1X6
Treosulfan	T45.1X1	T45.1X2	T45.1X3	T45.1X4	T45.1X5	T45.1X6
Tretamine	T45.1X1	T45.1X2	T45.1X3	T45.1X4	T45.1X5	T45.1X6
Tretinoin	T49.0X1	T49.0X2	T49.0X3	T49.0X4	T49.0X5	T49.0X6
Tretoquinol	T48.6X1	T48.6X2	T48.6X3	T48.6X4	T48.6X5	T48.6X6
Triacetin	T49.0X1	T49.0X2	T49.0X3	T49.0X4	T49.0X5	T49.0X6
Triacetoxyanthracene	T49.4X1	T49.4X2	T49.4X3	T49.4X4	T49.4X5	T49.4X6
Triacetyloleandomycin	T36.3X1	T36.3X2	T36.3X3	T36.3X4	T36.3X5	T36.3X6
Triamcinolone	T38.0X1	T38.0X2	T38.0X3	T38.0X4	T38.0X5	T38.0X6
ENT agent	T49.6X1	T49.6X2	T49.6X3	T49.6X4	T49.6X5	T49.6X6
hexacetonide	T49.0X1	T49.0X2	T49.0X3	T49.0X4	T49.0X5	T49.0X6
ophthalmic preparation	T49.5X1	T49.5X2	T49.5X3	T49.5X4	T49.5X5	T49.5X6
topical NEC	T49.0X1	T49.0X2	T49.0X3	T49.0X4	T49.0X5	T49.0X6
Triampyzine	T44.3X1	T44.3X2	T44.3X3	T44.3X4	T44.3X5	T44.3X6
Triamterene	T50.2X1	T50.2X2	T50.2X3	T50.2X4	T50.2X5	T50.2X6

Substance	Poisoning, Accidental (unintentional)	Poisoning, Intentional Self-harm	Poisoning, Assault	Poisoning, Undetermined	Adverse Effect	Under-dosing
Triazine (herbicide)	T60.3X1	T60.3X2	T60.3X3	T60.3X4	—	—
Triaziquone	T45.1X1	T45.1X2	T45.1X3	T45.1X4	T45.1X5	T45.1X6
Triazolam	T42.4X1	T42.4X2	T42.4X3	T42.4X4	T42.4X5	T42.4X6
Triazole (herbicide)	T60.3X1	T60.3X2	T60.3X3	T60.3X4	—	—
Tribavirin*	T37.5X1	T37.5X2	T37.5X3	T37.5X4	T37.5X5	T37.5X6
Tribenoside	T46.991	T46.992	T46.993	T46.994	T46.995	T46.996
Tribromacetaldehyde	T42.6X1	T42.6X2	T42.6X3	T42.6X4	T42.6X5	T42.6X6
Tribromoethanol, rectal	T41.291	T41.292	T41.293	T41.294	T41.295	T41.296
Tribromomethane	T42.6X1	T42.6X2	T42.6X3	T42.6X4	T42.6X5	T42.6X6
Trichlorethane	T53.2X1	T53.2X2	T53.2X3	T53.2X4	—	—
Trichlorethylene	T53.2X1	T53.2X2	T53.2X3	T53.2X4	—	—
Trichlorfon	T60.0X1	T60.0X2	T60.0X3	T60.0X4	—	—
Trichlormethiazide	T50.2X1	T50.2X2	T50.2X3	T50.2X4	T50.2X5	T50.2X6
Trichlormethine	T45.1X1	T45.1X2	T45.1X3	T45.1X4	T45.1X5	T45.1X6
Trichloroacetic acid, Trichloracetic acid	T54.2X1	T54.2X2	T54.2X3	T54.2X4	—	—
medicinal	T49.4X1	T49.4X2	T49.4X3	T49.4X4	T49.4X5	T49.4X6
Trichloroethane	T53.2X1	T53.2X2	T53.2X3	T53.2X4	—	—
Trichloroethanol	T42.6X1	T42.6X2	T42.6X3	T42.6X4	T42.6X5	T42.6X6
Trichloroethylene (liquid) (vapor)	T53.2X1	T53.2X2	T53.2X3	T53.2X4	—	—
anesthetic (gas)	T41.0X1	T41.0X2	T41.0X3	T41.0X4	T41.0X5	T41.0X6
vapor NEC	T53.2X1	T53.2X2	T53.2X3	T53.2X4	—	—
Trichloroethyl phosphate	T42.6X1	T42.6X2	T42.6X3	T42.6X4	T42.6X5	T42.6X6
Trichlorofluoromethane NEC	T53.5X1	T53.5X2	T53.5X3	T53.5X4	—	—
Trichloronate	T60.0X1	T60.0X2	T60.0X3	T60.0X4	—	—
Trichloropropane	T53.6X1	T53.6X2	T53.6X3	T53.6X4	—	—
Trichlorotriethylamine	T45.1X1	T45.1X2	T45.1X3	T45.1X4	T45.1X5	T45.1X6
Trichomonacides NEC	T37.3X1	T37.3X2	T37.3X3	T37.3X4	T37.3X5	T37.3X6
Trichomycin	T36.7X1	T36.7X2	T36.7X3	T36.7X4	T36.7X5	T36.7X6
Triclobisonium chloride	T49.0X1	T49.0X2	T49.0X3	T49.0X4	T49.0X5	T49.0X6
Triclocarban	T49.0X1	T49.0X2	T49.0X3	T49.0X4	T49.0X5	T49.0X6
Triclofos	T42.6X1	T42.6X2	T42.6X3	T42.6X4	T42.6X5	T42.6X6
Triclosan	T49.0X1	T49.0X2	T49.0X3	T49.0X4	T49.0X5	T49.0X6
Tricosal*	T39.091	T39.092	T39.093	T39.094	T39.095	T39.096
Tricresyl phosphate	T65.891	T65.892	T65.893	T65.894	—	—
solvent	T52.91	T52.92	T52.93	T52.94	—	—
Tricyclamol chloride	T44.3X1	T44.3X2	T44.3X3	T44.3X4	T44.3X5	T44.3X6
Tridesilon	T49.0X1	T49.0X2	T49.0X3	T49.0X4	T49.0X5	T49.0X6
Tridihexethyl iodide	T44.3X1	T44.3X2	T44.3X3	T44.3X4	T44.3X5	T44.3X6
Tridione	T42.2X1	T42.2X2	T42.2X3	T42.2X4	T42.2X5	T42.2X6
Trientine	T45.8X1	T45.8X2	T45.8X3	T45.8X4	T45.8X5	T45.8X6
Triethanolamine NEC	T54.3X1	T54.3X2	T54.3X3	T54.3X4	—	—
detergent	T54.3X1	T54.3X2	T54.3X3	T54.3X4	—	—
trinitrate (biphosphate)	T46.3X1	T46.3X2	T46.3X3	T46.3X4	T46.3X5	T46.3X6
Triethanomelamine	T45.1X1	T45.1X2	T45.1X3	T45.1X4	T45.1X5	T45.1X6
Triethylenemelamine	T45.1X1	T45.1X2	T45.1X3	T45.1X4	T45.1X5	T45.1X6
Triethylenephosphoramide	T45.1X1	T45.1X2	T45.1X3	T45.1X4	T45.1X5	T45.1X6
Triethylenethiophosphora-mide	T45.1X1	T45.1X2	T45.1X3	T45.1X4	T45.1X5	T45.1X6
Trifluoperazine	T43.3X1	T43.3X2	T43.3X3	T43.3X4	T43.3X5	T43.3X6
Trifluoroethyl vinyl ether	T41.0X1	T41.0X2	T41.0X3	T41.0X4	T41.0X5	T41.0X6
Trifluperidol	T43.4X1	T43.4X2	T43.4X3	T43.4X4	T43.4X5	T43.4X6
Triflupromazine	T43.3X1	T43.3X2	T43.3X3	T43.3X4	T43.3X5	T43.3X6
Trifluridine	T37.5X1	T37.5X2	T37.5X3	T37.5X4	T37.5X5	T37.5X6
Triflusal	T45.521	T45.522	T45.523	T45.524	T45.525	T45.526
Trihexyphenidyl	T44.3X1	T44.3X2	T44.3X3	T44.3X4	T44.3X5	T44.3X6
Triiodothyronine	T38.1X1	T38.1X2	T38.1X3	T38.1X4	T38.1X5	T38.1X6
Trilene	T41.0X1	T41.0X2	T41.0X3	T41.0X4	T41.0X5	T41.0X6
Trilostane	T38.991	T38.992	T38.993	T38.994	T38.995	T38.996
Trimebutine	T44.3X1	T44.3X2	T44.3X3	T44.3X4	T44.3X5	T44.3X6
Trimecaine	T41.3X1	T41.3X2	T41.3X3	T41.3X4	T41.3X5	T41.3X6
Trimeprazine (tartrate)	T44.3X1	T44.3X2	T44.3X3	T44.3X4	T44.3X5	T44.3X6
Trimetaphan camsilate	T44.2X1	T44.2X2	T44.2X3	T44.2X4	T44.2X5	T44.2X6
Trimetazidine	T46.7X1	T46.7X2	T46.7X3	T46.7X4	T46.7X5	T46.7X6
Trimethadione	T42.2X1	T42.2X2	T42.2X3	T42.2X4	T42.2X5	T42.2X6
Trimethaphan	T44.2X1	T44.2X2	T44.2X3	T44.2X4	T44.2X5	T44.2X6
Trimethidinium	T44.2X1	T44.2X2	T44.2X3	T44.2X4	T44.2X5	T44.2X6
Trimethobenzamide	T45.0X1	T45.0X2	T45.0X3	T45.0X4	T45.0X5	T45.0X6
Trimethoprim	T37.8X1	T37.8X2	T37.8X3	T37.8X4	T37.8X5	T37.8X6
with sulfamethoxazole	T36.8X1	T36.8X2	T36.8X3	T36.8X4	T36.8X5	T36.8X6
Trimethylcarbinol	T51.3X1	T51.3X2	T51.3X3	T51.3X4	—	—
Trimethylpsoralen	T49.3X1	T49.3X2	T49.3X3	T49.3X4	T49.3X5	T49.3X6
Trimeton	T45.0X1	T45.0X2	T45.0X3	T45.0X4	T45.0X5	T45.0X6
Trimetrexate	T45.1X1	T45.1X2	T45.1X3	T45.1X4	T45.1X5	T45.1X6
Trimipramine	T43.011	T43.012	T43.013	T43.014	T43.015	T43.016
Trimox*	T36.0X1	T36.0X2	T36.0X3	T36.0X4	T36.0X5	T36.0X6
Trimustine	T45.1X1	T45.1X2	T45.1X3	T45.1X4	T45.1X5	T45.1X6
Trinitrine	T46.3X1	T46.3X2	T46.3X3	T46.3X4	T46.3X5	T46.3X6
Trinitrobenzol	T65.3X1	T65.3X2	T65.3X3	T65.3X4	—	—
Trinitrophenol	T65.3X1	T65.3X2	T65.3X3	T65.3X4	—	—
Trinitrotoluene (fumes)	T65.3X1	T65.3X2	T65.3X3	T65.3X4	—	—

Substance	Poisoning, Accidental (unintentional)	Poisoning, Intentional Self-harm	Poisoning, Assault	Poisoning, Undetermined	Adverse Effect	Under-dosing
Trional	T42.6X1	T42.6X2	T42.6X3	T42.6X4	T42.6X5	T42.6X6
Triorthocresyl phosphate	T65.891	T65.892	T65.893	T65.894	—	—
Trioxide of arsenic	T57.0X1	T57.0X2	T57.0X3	T57.0X4	—	—
Trioxysalen	T49.4X1	T49.4X2	T49.4X3	T49.4X4	T49.4X5	T49.4X6
Tripamide	T50.2X1	T50.2X2	T50.2X3	T50.2X4	T50.2X5	T50.2X6
Triparanol	T46.6X1	T46.6X2	T46.6X3	T46.6X4	T46.6X5	T46.6X6
Tripelennamine	T45.0X1	T45.0X2	T45.0X3	T45.0X4	T45.0X5	T45.0X6
Triperiden	T44.3X1	T44.3X2	T44.3X3	T44.3X4	T44.3X5	T44.3X6
Triperidol	T43.4X1	T43.4X2	T43.4X3	T43.4X4	T43.4X5	T43.4X6
Triphenylphosphate	T65.891	T65.892	T65.893	T65.894	—	—
Triple						
bromides	T42.6X1	T42.6X2	T42.6X3	T42.6X4	T42.6X5	T42.6X6
carbonate	T47.1X1	T47.1X2	T47.1X3	T47.1X4	T47.1X5	T47.1X6
vaccine						
DPT	T50.A11	T50.A12	T50.A13	T50.A14	T50.A15	T50.A16
including pertussis	T50.A11	T50.A12	T50.A13	T50.A14	T50.A15	T50.A16
MMR	T50.B91	T50.B92	T50.B93	T50.B94	T50.B95	T50.B96
Triprolidine	T45.0X1	T45.0X2	T45.0X3	T45.0X4	T45.0X5	T45.0X6
Trisodium hydrogen edetate	T50.6X1	T50.6X2	T50.6X3	T50.6X4	T50.6X5	T50.6X6
Trisoralen	T49.3X1	T49.3X2	T49.3X3	T49.3X4	T49.3X5	T49.3X6
Trisulfapyrimidines	T37.0X1	T37.0X2	T37.0X3	T37.0X4	T37.0X5	T37.0X6
Trithiozine	T44.3X1	T44.3X2	T44.3X3	T44.3X4	T44.3X5	T44.3X6
Tritiozine	T44.3X1	T44.3X2	T44.3X3	T44.3X4	T44.3X5	T44.3X6
Tritoqualine	T45.0X1	T45.0X2	T45.0X3	T45.0X4	T45.0X5	T45.0X6
Trizivir*	T37.5X1	T37.5X2	T37.5X3	T37.5X4	T37.5X5	T37.5X6
Trofosfamide	T45.1X1	T45.1X2	T45.1X3	T45.1X4	T45.1X5	T45.1X6
Troleandomycin	T36.3X1	T36.3X2	T36.3X3	T36.3X4	T36.3X5	T36.3X6
Trolnitrate (phosphate)	T46.3X1	T46.3X2	T46.3X3	T46.3X4	T46.3X5	T46.3X6
Tromantadine	T37.5X1	T37.5X2	T37.5X3	T37.5X4	T37.5X5	T37.5X6
Trometamol	T50.2X1	T50.2X2	T50.2X3	T50.2X4	T50.2X5	T50.2X6
Tromethamine	T50.2X1	T50.2X2	T50.2X3	T50.2X4	T50.2X5	T50.2X6
Tronothane	T41.3X1	T41.3X2	T41.3X3	T41.3X4	T41.3X5	T41.3X6
Tropacine	T44.3X1	T44.3X2	T44.3X3	T44.3X4	T44.3X5	T44.3X6
Tropatepine	T44.3X1	T44.3X2	T44.3X3	T44.3X4	T44.3X5	T44.3X6
Tropicamide	T44.3X1	T44.3X2	T44.3X3	T44.3X4	T44.3X5	T44.3X6
Trospium chloride	T44.3X1	T44.3X2	T44.3X3	T44.3X4	T44.3X5	T44.3X6
Troxerutin	T46.991	T46.992	T46.993	T46.994	T46.995	T46.996
Troxidone	T42.2X1	T42.2X2	T42.2X3	T42.2X4	T42.2X5	T42.2X6
Tryparsamide	T37.3X1	T37.3X2	T37.3X3	T37.3X4	T37.3X5	T37.3X6
Trypsin	T45.3X1	T45.3X2	T45.3X3	T45.3X4	T45.3X5	T45.3X6
Tryptizol	T43.011	T43.012	T43.013	T43.014	T43.015	T43.016
TSH	T38.811	T38.812	T38.813	T38.814	T38.815	T38.816
Tuaminoheptane	T48.5X1	T48.5X2	T48.5X3	T48.5X4	T48.5X5	T48.5X6
Tuberculin, purified protein derivative (PPD)	T50.8X1	T50.8X2	T50.8X3	T50.8X4	T50.8X5	T50.8X6
Tubocurare	T48.1X1	T48.1X2	T48.1X3	T48.1X4	T48.1X5	T48.1X6
Tubocurarine (chloride)	T48.1X1	T48.1X2	T48.1X3	T48.1X4	T48.1X5	T48.1X6
Tulobuterol	T48.6X1	T48.6X2	T48.6X3	T48.6X4	T48.6X5	T48.6X6
Turpentine (spirits of)	T52.8X1	T52.8X2	T52.8X3	T52.8X4	—	—
vapor	T52.8X1	T52.8X2	T52.8X3	T52.8X4	—	—
Twinrix*	T50.B91	T50.B92	T50.B93	T50.B94	T50.B95	T50.B96
Tybamate	T43.591	T43.592	T43.593	T43.594	T43.595	T43.596
Tygacil*	T36.4X1	T36.4X2	T36.4X3	T36.4X4	T36.4X5	T36.4X6
Tyloxapol	T48.4X1	T48.4X2	T48.4X3	T48.4X4	T48.4X5	T48.4X6
Tymazoline	T48.5X1	T48.5X2	T48.5X3	T48.5X4	T48.5X5	T48.5X6
Tymlos*	T50.991	T50.992	T50.993	T50.994	T50.995	T50.996
Typhoid-paratyphoid vaccine	T50.A91	T50.A92	T50.A93	T50.A94	T50.A95	T50.A96
Typhus vaccine	T50.A91	T50.A92	T50.A93	T50.A94	T50.A95	T50.A96
Tyropanoate	T50.8X1	T50.8X2	T50.8X3	T50.8X4	T50.8X5	T50.8X6
Tyrothricin	T49.6X1	T49.6X2	T49.6X3	T49.6X4	T49.6X5	T49.6X6
ENT agent	T49.6X1	T49.6X2	T49.6X3	T49.6X4	T49.6X5	T49.6X6
ophthalmic preparation	T49.5X1	T49.5X2	T49.5X3	T49.5X4	T49.5X5	T49.5X6
Ufenamate	T39.391	T39.392	T39.393	T39.394	T39.395	T39.396
Ultraviolet light protectant	T49.3X1	T49.3X2	T49.3X3	T49.3X4	T49.3X5	T49.3X6
Unasyn*	T36.0X1	T36.0X2	T36.0X3	T36.0X4	T36.0X5	T36.0X6
Undecenoic acid	T49.0X1	T49.0X2	T49.0X3	T49.0X4	T49.0X5	T49.0X6
Undecoylium	T49.0X1	T49.0X2	T49.0X3	T49.0X4	T49.0X5	T49.0X6
Undecylenic acid (derivatives)	T49.0X1	T49.0X2	T49.0X3	T49.0X4	T49.0X5	T49.0X6
Unna's boot	T49.3X1	T49.3X2	T49.3X3	T49.3X4	T49.3X5	T49.3X6
Unsaturated fatty acid	T46.6X1	T46.6X2	T46.6X3	T46.6X4	T46.6X5	T46.6X6
Uracil mustard	T45.1X1	T45.1X2	T45.1X3	T45.1X4	T45.1X5	T45.1X6
Uramustine	T45.1X1	T45.1X2	T45.1X3	T45.1X4	T45.1X5	T45.1X6
Urapidil	T46.5X1	T46.5X2	T46.5X3	T46.5X4	T46.5X5	T46.5X6
Urari	T48.1X1	T48.1X2	T48.1X3	T48.1X4	T48.1X5	T48.1X6
Urate oxidase	T50.4X1	T50.4X2	T50.4X3	T50.4X4	T50.4X5	T50.4X6
Urea	T47.3X1	T47.3X2	T47.3X3	T47.3X4	T47.3X5	T47.3X6
peroxide	T49.0X1	T49.0X2	T49.0X3	T49.0X4	T49.0X5	T49.0X6
stibamine	T37.4X1	T37.4X2	T37.4X3	T37.4X4	T37.4X5	T37.4X6
topical	T49.8X1	T49.8X2	T49.8X3	T49.8X4	T49.8X5	T49.8X6

Substance	Poisoning, Accidental (unintentional)	Poisoning, Intentional Self-harm	Poisoning, Assault	Poisoning, Undetermined	Adverse Effect	Under-dosing
Ureaphil*	T48.0X1	T48.0X2	T48.0X3	T48.0X4	T48.0X5	T48.0X6
Urethane	T45.1X1	T45.1X2	T45.1X3	T45.1X4	T45.1X5	T45.1X6
Urginea (maritima) (scilla) — see Squill						
Uric acid metabolism drug NEC	T50.4X1	T50.4X2	T50.4X3	T50.4X4	T50.4X5	T50.4X6
Uricosuric agent	T50.4X1	T50.4X2	T50.4X3	T50.4X4	T50.4X5	T50.4X6
Urinary anti-infective	T37.8X1	T37.8X2	T37.8X3	T37.8X4	T37.8X5	T37.8X6
Urofollitropin	T38.811	T38.812	T38.813	T38.814	T38.815	T38.816
Urokinase	T45.611	T45.612	T45.613	T45.614	T45.615	T45.616
Urokon	T50.8X1	T50.8X2	T50.8X3	T50.8X4	T50.8X5	T50.8X6
Ursodeoxycholic acid	T50.991	T50.992	T50.993	T50.994	T50.995	T50.996
Ursodiol	T50.991	T50.992	T50.993	T50.994	T50.995	T50.996
Urtica	T62.2X1	T62.2X2	T62.2X3	T62.2X4	—	—
Utility gas — see Gas, utility						
Vaccine NEC	T50.Z91	T50.Z92	T50.Z93	T50.Z94	T50.Z95	T50.Z96
antineoplastic	T50.Z91	T50.Z92	T50.Z93	T50.Z94	T50.Z95	T50.Z96
bacterial NEC	T50.A91	T50.A92	T50.A93	T50.A94	T50.A95	T50.A96
with						
other bacterial component	T50.A21	T50.A22	T50.A23	T50.A24	T50.A25	T50.A26
pertussis component	T50.A11	T50.A12	T50.A13	T50.A14	T50.A15	T50.A16
viral-rickettsial component	T50.A21	T50.A22	T50.A23	T50.A24	T50.A25	T50.A26
mixed NEC	T50.A21	T50.A22	T50.A23	T50.A24	T50.A25	T50.A26
BCG	T50.A91	T50.A92	T50.A93	T50.A94	T50.A95	T50.A96
cholera	T50.A91	T50.A92	T50.A93	T50.A94	T50.A95	T50.A96
diphtheria	T50.A91	T50.A92	T50.A93	T50.A94	T50.A95	T50.A96
with tetanus	T50.A21	T50.A22	T50.A23	T50.A24	T50.A25	T50.A26
and pertussis	T50.A11	T50.A12	T50.A13	T50.A14	T50.A15	T50.A16
influenza	T50.B91	T50.B92	T50.B93	T50.B94	T50.B95	T50.B96
measles	T50.B91	T50.B92	T50.B93	T50.B94	T50.B95	T50.B96
with mumps and rubella	T50.B91	T50.B92	T50.B93	T50.B94	T50.B95	T50.B96
meningococcal	T50.A91	T50.A92	T50.A93	T50.A94	T50.A95	T50.A96
mumps	T50.B91	T50.B92	T50.B93	T50.B94	T50.B95	T50.B96
paratyphoid	T50.A91	T50.A92	T50.A93	T50.A94	T50.A95	T50.A96
pertussis	T50.A11	T50.A12	T50.A13	T50.A14	T50.A15	T50.A16
with diphtheria	T50.A11	T50.A12	T50.A13	T50.A14	T50.A15	T50.A16
and tetanus	T50.A11	T50.A12	T50.A13	T50.A14	T50.A15	T50.A16
with other component	T50.A11	T50.A12	T50.A13	T50.A14	T50.A15	T50.A16
plague	T50.A91	T50.A92	T50.A93	T50.A94	T50.A95	T50.A96
poliomyelitis	T50.B91	T50.B92	T50.B93	T50.B94	T50.B95	T50.B96
poliovirus	T50.B91	T50.B92	T50.B93	T50.B94	T50.B95	T50.B96
rabies	T50.B91	T50.B92	T50.B93	T50.B94	T50.B95	T50.B96
respiratory syncytial virus	T50.B91	T50.B92	T50.B93	T50.B94	T50.B95	T50.B96
rickettsial NEC	T50.A91	T50.A92	T50.A93	T50.A94	T50.A95	T50.A96
with						
bacterial component	T50.A21	T50.A22	T50.A23	T50.A24	T50.A25	T50.A26
Rocky Mountain spotted fever	T50.A91	T50.A92	T50.A93	T50.A94	T50.A95	T50.A96
rubella	T50.B91	T50.B92	T50.B93	T50.B94	T50.B95	T50.B96
sabin oral	T50.B91	T50.B92	T50.B93	T50.B94	T50.B95	T50.B96
smallpox	T50.B11	T50.B12	T50.B13	T50.B14	T50.B15	T50.B16
TAB	T50.A91	T50.A92	T50.A93	T50.A94	T50.A95	T50.A96
tetanus	T50.A91	T50.A92	T50.A93	T50.A94	T50.A95	T50.A96
typhoid	T50.A91	T50.A92	T50.A93	T50.A94	T50.A95	T50.A96
typhus	T50.A91	T50.A92	T50.A93	T50.A94	T50.A95	T50.A96
viral NEC	T50.B91	T50.B92	T50.B93	T50.B94	T50.B95	T50.B96
yellow fever	T50.B91	T50.B92	T50.B93	T50.B94	T50.B95	T50.B96
Vaccinia immune globulin	T50.Z11	T50.Z12	T50.Z13	T50.Z14	T50.Z15	T50.Z16
Vaginal contraceptives	T49.8X1	T49.8X2	T49.8X3	T49.8X4	T49.8X5	T49.8X6
Valacyclovir*	T37.5X1	T37.5X2	T37.5X3	T37.5X4	T37.5X5	T37.5X6
Valerian						
root	T42.6X1	T42.6X2	T42.6X3	T42.6X4	T42.6X5	T42.6X6
tincture	T42.6X1	T42.6X2	T42.6X3	T42.6X4	T42.6X5	T42.6X6
Valethamate bromide	T44.3X1	T44.3X2	T44.3X3	T44.3X4	T44.3X5	T44.3X6
Valisone	T49.0X1	T49.0X2	T49.0X3	T49.0X4	T49.0X5	T49.0X6
Valium	T42.4X1	T42.4X2	T42.4X3	T42.4X4	T42.4X5	T42.4X6
Valmid	T42.6X1	T42.6X2	T42.6X3	T42.6X4	T42.6X5	T42.6X6
Valnoctamide	T42.6X1	T42.6X2	T42.6X3	T42.6X4	T42.6X5	T42.6X6
Valproate (sodium)	T42.6X1	T42.6X2	T42.6X3	T42.6X4	T42.6X5	T42.6X6
Valproic acid	T42.6X1	T42.6X2	T42.6X3	T42.6X4	T42.6X5	T42.6X6
Valpromide	T42.6X1	T42.6X2	T42.6X3	T42.6X4	T42.6X5	T42.6X6
Vanadium	T56.891	T56.892	T56.893	T56.894	—	—
Vancomycin	T36.8X1	T36.8X2	T36.8X3	T36.8X4	T36.8X5	T36.8X6
Vandazole*	T49.0X1	T49.0X2	T49.0X3	T49.0X4	T49.0X5	T49.0X6
Vapor — see also Gas	T59.91	T59.92	T59.93	T59.94	—	—
kiln (carbon monoxide)	T58.8X1	T58.8X2	T58.8X3	T58.8X4	—	—
lead — see lead						
specified source NEC	T59.891	T59.892	T59.893	T59.894	—	—
Vardenafil	T46.7X1	T46.7X2	T46.7X3	T46.7X4	T46.7X5	T46.7X6
Varicose reduction drug	T46.8X1	T46.8X2	T46.8X3	T46.8X4	T46.8X5	T46.8X6
Varnish	T65.4X1	T65.4X2	T65.4X3	T65.4X4	—	—

☑ Additional Character May Be Required — Refer to the Tabular List for Character Selection

*Optum Value-Add

Substance	Poisoning, Accidental (unintentional)	Poisoning, Intentional Self-harm	Poisoning, Assault	Poisoning, Undetermined	Adverse Effect	Under-dosing
Varnish — *continued*						
cleaner	T52.91	T52.92	T52.93	T52.94	—	—
Vaseline	T49.3X1	T49.3X2	T49.3X3	T49.3X4	T49.3X5	T49.3X6
Vasodilan	T46.7X1	T46.7X2	T46.7X3	T46.7X4	T46.7X5	T46.7X6
Vasodilator						
coronary NEC	T46.3X1	T46.3X2	T46.3X3	T46.3X4	T46.3X5	T46.3X6
peripheral NEC	T46.7X1	T46.7X2	T46.7X3	T46.7X4	T46.7X5	T46.7X6
Vasopressin	T38.891	T38.892	T38.893	T38.894	T38.895	T38.896
Vasopressor drugs	T38.891	T38.892	T38.893	T38.894	T38.895	T38.896
Vecuronium bromide	T48.1X1	T48.1X2	T48.1X3	T48.1X4	T48.1X5	T48.1X6
Vegetable extract, astringent	T49.2X1	T49.2X2	T49.2X3	T49.2X4	T49.2X5	T49.2X6
Venlafaxine	T43.211	T43.212	T43.213	T43.214	T43.215	T43.216
Venom, venomous (bite) (sting)	T63.91	T63.92	T63.93	T63.94	—	—
amphibian NEC	T63.831	T63.832	T63.833	T63.834	—	—
animal NEC	T63.891	T63.892	T63.893	T63.894	—	—
ant	T63.421	T63.422	T63.423	T63.424	—	—
arthropod NEC	T63.481	T63.482	T63.483	T63.484	—	—
bee	T63.441	T63.442	T63.443	T63.444	—	—
centipede	T63.411	T63.412	T63.413	T63.414	—	—
fish	T63.591	T63.592	T63.593	T63.594	—	—
frog	T63.811	T63.812	T63.813	T63.814	—	—
hornet	T63.451	T63.452	T63.453	T63.454	—	—
insect NEC	T63.481	T63.482	T63.483	T63.484	—	—
lizard	T63.121	T63.122	T63.123	T63.124	—	—
marine						
animals	T63.691	T63.692	T63.693	T63.694	—	—
bluebottle	T63.611	T63.612	T63.613	T63.614	—	—
jellyfish NEC	T63.621	T63.622	T63.623	T63.624	—	—
Portuguese Man-o-war	T63.611	T63.612	T63.613	T63.614	—	—
sea anemone	T63.631	T63.632	T63.633	T63.634	—	—
specified NEC	T63.691	T63.692	T63.693	T63.694	—	—
fish	T63.591	T63.592	T63.593	T63.594	—	—
plants	T63.711	T63.712	T63.713	T63.714	—	—
sting ray	T63.511	T63.512	T63.513	T63.514	—	—
millipede (tropical)	T63.411	T63.412	T63.413	T63.414	—	—
plant NEC	T63.791	T63.792	T63.793	T63.794	—	—
marine	T63.711	T63.712	T63.713	T63.714	—	—
reptile	T63.191	T63.192	T63.193	T63.194	—	—
gila monster	T63.111	T63.112	T63.113	T63.114	—	—
lizard NEC	T63.121	T63.122	T63.123	T63.124	—	—
scorpion	T63.2X1	T63.2X2	T63.2X3	T63.2X4	—	—
snake	T63.001	T63.002	T63.003	T63.004	—	—
African NEC	T63.081	T63.082	T63.083	T63.084	—	—
American (North) (South) NEC	T63.061	T63.062	T63.063	T63.064	—	—
Asian	T63.081	T63.082	T63.083	T63.084	—	—
Australian	T63.071	T63.072	T63.073	T63.074	—	—
cobra	T63.041	T63.042	T63.043	T63.044	—	—
coral snake	T63.021	T63.022	T63.023	T63.024	—	—
rattlesnake	T63.011	T63.012	T63.013	T63.014	—	—
specified NEC	T63.091	T63.092	T63.093	T63.094	—	—
taipan	T63.031	T63.032	T63.033	T63.034	—	—
specified NEC	T63.891	T63.892	T63.893	T63.894	—	—
spider	T63.301	T63.302	T63.303	T63.304	—	—
black widow	T63.311	T63.312	T63.313	T63.314	—	—
brown recluse	T63.331	T63.332	T63.333	T63.334	—	—
specified NEC	T63.391	T63.392	T63.393	T63.394	—	—
tarantula	T63.321	T63.322	T63.323	T63.324	—	—
sting ray	T63.511	T63.512	T63.513	T63.514	—	—
toad	T63.821	T63.822	T63.823	T63.824	—	—
wasp	T63.461	T63.462	T63.463	T63.464	—	—
Venous sclerosing drug NEC	T46.8X1	T46.8X2	T46.8X3	T46.8X4	T46.8X5	T46.8X6
Ventavis*	T46.7X1	T46.7X2	T46.7X3	T46.7X4	T46.7X5	T46.7X6
Ventolin — *see* Albuterol						
Veramon	T42.3X1	T42.3X2	T42.3X3	T42.3X4	T42.3X5	T42.3X6
Verapamil	T46.1X1	T46.1X2	T46.1X3	T46.1X4	T46.1X5	T46.1X6
Veratrine	T46.5X1	T46.5X2	T46.5X3	T46.5X4	T46.5X5	T46.5X6
Veratrum						
album	T62.2X1	T62.2X2	T62.2X3	T62.2X4	—	—
alkaloids	T46.5X1	T46.5X2	T46.5X3	T46.5X4	T46.5X5	T46.5X6
viride	T62.2X1	T62.2X2	T62.2X3	T62.2X4	—	—
Verdigris	T60.3X1	T60.3X2	T60.3X3	T60.3X4	—	—
Veronal	T42.3X1	T42.3X2	T42.3X3	T42.3X4	T42.3X5	T42.3X6
Veroxil	T37.4X1	T37.4X2	T37.4X3	T37.4X4	T37.4X5	T37.4X6
Versenate	T50.6X1	T50.6X2	T50.6X3	T50.6X4	T50.6X5	T50.6X6
Versidyne	T39.8X1	T39.8X2	T39.8X3	T39.8X4	T39.8X5	T39.8X6
Vetrabutine	T48.0X1	T48.0X2	T48.0X3	T48.0X4	T48.0X5	T48.0X6
Vexol*	T49.5X1	T49.5X2	T49.5X3	T49.5X4	T49.5X5	T49.5X6
Victrelis*	T37.5X1	T37.5X2	T37.5X3	T37.5X4	T37.5X5	T37.5X6
Vidarabine	T37.5X1	T37.5X2	T37.5X3	T37.5X4	T37.5X5	T37.5X6
Vienna						
green	T57.0X1	T57.0X2	T57.0X3	T57.0X4	—	—
insecticide	T60.2X1	T60.2X2	T60.2X3	T60.2X4	—	—
red	T57.0X1	T57.0X2	T57.0X3	T57.0X4	—	—
pharmaceutical dye	T50.991	T50.992	T50.993	T50.994	T50.995	T50.996
Vigabatrin	T42.6X1	T42.6X2	T42.6X3	T42.6X4	T42.6X5	T42.6X6
Viloxazine	T43.291	T43.292	T43.293	T43.294	T43.295	T43.296
Viminol	T39.8X1	T39.8X2	T39.8X3	T39.8X4	T39.8X5	T39.8X6
Vinbarbital, vinbarbitone	T42.3X1	T42.3X2	T42.3X3	T42.3X4	T42.3X5	T42.3X6
Vinblastine	T45.1X1	T45.1X2	T45.1X3	T45.1X4	T45.1X5	T45.1X6
Vinburnine	T46.7X1	T46.7X2	T46.7X3	T46.7X4	T46.7X5	T46.7X6
Vincamine	T45.1X1	T45.1X2	T45.1X3	T45.1X4	T45.1X5	T45.1X6
Vincristine	T45.1X1	T45.1X2	T45.1X3	T45.1X4	T45.1X5	T45.1X6
Vindesine	T45.1X1	T45.1X2	T45.1X3	T45.1X4	T45.1X5	T45.1X6
Vinesthene, vinethene	T41.0X1	T41.0X2	T41.0X3	T41.0X4	T41.0X5	T41.0X6
Vinorelbine tartrate	T45.1X1	T45.1X2	T45.1X3	T45.1X4	T45.1X5	T45.1X6
Vinpocetine	T46.7X1	T46.7X2	T46.7X3	T46.7X4	T46.7X5	T46.7X6
Vinyl						
acetate	T65.891	T65.892	T65.893	T65.894	—	—
bital	T42.3X1	T42.3X2	T42.3X3	T42.3X4	T42.3X5	T42.3X6
bromide	T65.891	T65.892	T65.893	T65.894	—	—
chloride	T59.891	T59.892	T59.893	T59.894	—	—
ether	T41.0X1	T41.0X2	T41.0X3	T41.0X4	T41.0X5	T41.0X6
Vinylbital	T42.3X1	T42.3X2	T42.3X3	T42.3X4	T42.3X5	T42.3X6
Vinylidene chloride	T65.891	T65.892	T65.893	T65.894	—	—
Vioform	T37.8X1	T37.8X2	T37.8X3	T37.8X4	T37.8X5	T37.8X6
topical	T49.0X1	T49.0X2	T49.0X3	T49.0X4	T49.0X5	T49.0X6
Viokase*	T47.5X1	T47.5X2	T47.5X3	T47.5X4	T47.5X5	T47.5X6
Viomycin	T36.8X1	T36.8X2	T36.8X3	T36.8X4	T36.8X5	T36.8X6
Viosterol	T45.2X1	T45.2X2	T45.2X3	T45.2X4	T45.2X5	T45.2X6
Viper (venom)	T63.091	T63.092	T63.093	T63.094	—	—
Viprynium	T37.4X1	T37.4X2	T37.4X3	T37.4X4	T37.4X5	T37.4X6
Viquidil	T46.7X1	T46.7X2	T46.7X3	T46.7X4	T46.7X5	T46.7X6
Viral vaccine NEC	T50.B91	T50.B92	T50.B93	T50.B94	T50.B95	T50.B96
Virginiamycin	T36.8X1	T36.8X2	T36.8X3	T36.8X4	T36.8X5	T36.8X6
Virugon	T37.5X1	T37.5X2	T37.5X3	T37.5X4	T37.5X5	T37.5X6
Viscous agent	T50.901	T50.902	T50.903	T50.904	T50.905	T50.906
Visine	T49.5X1	T49.5X2	T49.5X3	T49.5X4	T49.5X5	T49.5X6
Visnadine	T46.3X1	T46.3X2	T46.3X3	T46.3X4	T46.3X5	T46.3X6
Vitamin NEC	T45.2X1	T45.2X2	T45.2X3	T45.2X4	T45.2X5	T45.2X6
A	T45.2X1	T45.2X2	T45.2X3	T45.2X4	T45.2X5	T45.2X6
B1	T45.2X1	T45.2X2	T45.2X3	T45.2X4	T45.2X5	T45.2X6
B2	T45.2X1	T45.2X2	T45.2X3	T45.2X4	T45.2X5	T45.2X6
B6	T45.2X1	T45.2X2	T45.2X3	T45.2X4	T45.2X5	T45.2X6
B12	T45.2X1	T45.2X2	T45.2X3	T45.2X4	T45.2X5	T45.2X6
B15	T45.2X1	T45.2X2	T45.2X3	T45.2X4	T45.2X5	T45.2X6
B NEC	T45.2X1	T45.2X2	T45.2X3	T45.2X4	T45.2X5	T45.2X6
nicotinic acid	T46.7X1	T46.7X2	T46.7X3	T46.7X4	T46.7X5	T46.7X6
C	T45.2X1	T45.2X2	T45.2X3	T45.2X4	T45.2X5	T45.2X6
D	T45.2X1	T45.2X2	T45.2X3	T45.2X4	T45.2X5	T45.2X6
D2	T45.2X1	T45.2X2	T45.2X3	T45.2X4	T45.2X5	T45.2X6
D3	T45.2X1	T45.2X2	T45.2X3	T45.2X4	T45.2X5	T45.2X6
E	T45.2X1	T45.2X2	T45.2X3	T45.2X4	T45.2X5	T45.2X6
E acetate	T45.2X1	T45.2X2	T45.2X3	T45.2X4	T45.2X5	T45.2X6
hematopoietic	T45.8X1	T45.8X2	T45.8X3	T45.8X4	T45.8X5	T45.8X6
K1	T45.7X1	T45.7X2	T45.7X3	T45.7X4	T45.7X5	T45.7X6
K2	T45.7X1	T45.7X2	T45.7X3	T45.7X4	T45.7X5	T45.7X6
K NEC	T45.7X1	T45.7X2	T45.7X3	T45.7X4	T45.7X5	T45.7X6
PP	T45.2X1	T45.2X2	T45.2X3	T45.2X4	T45.2X5	T45.2X6
ulceroprotectant	T47.1X1	T47.1X2	T47.1X3	T47.1X4	T47.1X5	T47.1X6
Vleminckx's solution	T49.4X1	T49.4X2	T49.4X3	T49.4X4	T49.4X5	T49.4X6
Voltaren — *see* Diclofenac sodium						
Voraxaze*	T50.6X1	T50.6X2	T50.6X3	T50.6X4	T50.6X5	T50.6X6
Warfarin	T45.511	T45.512	T45.513	T45.514	T45.515	T45.516
rodenticide	T60.4X1-	T60.4X2-	T60.4X3-	T60.4X4-	—	—
sodium	T45.511	T45.512	T45.513	T45.514	T45.515	T45.516
Wasp (sting)	T63.461	T63.462	T63.463	T63.464	—	—
Water						
balance drug	T50.3X1	T50.3X2	T50.3X3	T50.3X4	T50.3X5	T50.3X6
distilled	T50.3X1	T50.3X2	T50.3X3	T50.3X4	T50.3X5	T50.3X6
gas — *see* Gas, water						
incomplete combustion of — *see* Carbon, monoxide, fuel, utility						
hemlock	T62.2X1	T62.2X2	T62.2X3	T62.2X4	—	—
moccasin (venom)	T63.061	T63.062	T63.063	T63.064	—	—
purified	T50.3X1	T50.3X2	T50.3X3	T50.3X4	T50.3X5	T50.3X6
Wax (paraffin) (petroleum)	T52.0X1	T52.0X2	T52.0X3	T52.0X4	—	—
automobile	T65.891	T65.892	T65.893	T65.894	—	—
floor	T52.0X1	T52.0X2	T52.0X3	T52.0X4	—	—
Weed killers NEC	T60.3X1	T60.3X2	T60.3X3	T60.3X4	—	—
Wellbutrin*	T43.291	T43.292	T43.293	T43.294	T43.295	T43.296

Table of Drugs and Chemicals

Varnish — Wellbutrin*

Table of Drugs and Chemicals

Welldorm — Zyzal*

Substance	Poisoning, Accidental (unintentional)	Poisoning, Intentional Self-harm	Poisoning, Assault	Poisoning, Undetermined	Adverse Effect	Under-dosing
Welldorm	T42.6X1	T42.6X2	T42.6X3	T42.6X4	T42.6X5	T42.6X6
Westcort*	T49.0X1	T49.0X2	T49.0X3	T49.0X4	T49.0X5	T49.0X6
White						
arsenic	T57.0X1	T57.0X2	T57.0X3	T57.0X4	—	—
hellebore	T62.2X1	T62.2X2	T62.2X3	T62.2X4	—	—
lotion (keratolytic)	T49.4X1	T49.4X2	T49.4X3	T49.4X4	T49.4X5	T49.4X6
spirit	T52.0X1	T52.0X2	T52.0X3	T52.0X4	—	—
Whitewash	T65.891	T65.892	T65.893	T65.894	—	—
Whole blood (human)	T45.8X1	T45.8X2	T45.8X3	T45.8X4	T45.8X5	T45.8X6
Wild						
black cherry	T62.2X1	T62.2X2	T62.2X3	T62.2X4	—	—
poisonous plants NEC	T62.2X1	T62.2X2	T62.2X3	T62.2X4	—	—
Window cleaning fluid	T65.891	T65.892	T65.893	T65.894	—	—
Wintergreen (oil)	T49.3X1	T49.3X2	T49.3X3	T49.3X4	T49.3X5	T49.3X6
Wisterine	T62.2X1	T62.2X2	T62.2X3	T62.2X4	—	—
Witch hazel	T49.2X1	T49.2X2	T49.2X3	T49.2X4	T49.2X5	T49.2X6
Wood alcohol or spirit	T51.1X1	T51.1X2	T51.1X3	T51.1X4	—	—
Wool fat (hydrous)	T49.3X1	T49.3X2	T49.3X3	T49.3X4	T49.3X5	T49.3X6
Woorali	T48.1X1	T48.1X2	T48.1X3	T48.1X4	T48.1X5	T48.1X6
Wormseed, American	T37.4X1	T37.4X2	T37.4X3	T37.4X4	T37.4X5	T37.4X6
Xamoterol	T44.5X1	T44.5X2	T44.5X3	T44.5X4	T44.5X5	T44.5X6
Xanax*	T42.4X1	T42.4X2	T42.4X3	T42.4X4	T42.4X5	T42.4X6
Xanthine diuretics	T50.2X1	T50.2X2	T50.2X3	T50.2X4	T50.2X5	T50.2X6
Xanthinol nicotinate	T46.7X1	T46.7X2	T46.7X3	T46.7X4	T46.7X5	T46.7X6
Xanthotoxin	T49.3X1	T49.3X2	T49.3X3	T49.3X4	T49.3X5	T49.3X6
Xantinol nicotinate	T46.7X1	T46.7X2	T46.7X3	T46.7X4	T46.7X5	T46.7X6
Xantocillin	T36.0X1	T36.0X2	T36.0X3	T36.0X4	T36.0X5	T36.0X6
Xenon (127Xe) (133Xe)	T50.8X1	T50.8X2	T50.8X3	T50.8X4	T50.8X5	T50.8X6
Xenysalate	T49.4X1	T49.4X2	T49.4X3	T49.4X4	T49.4X5	T49.4X6
Xibornol	T37.8X1	T37.8X2	T37.8X3	T37.8X4	T37.8X5	T37.8X6
Xigris	T45.511	T45.512	T45.513	T45.514	T45.515	T45.516
Xipamide	T50.2X1	T50.2X2	T50.2X3	T50.2X4	T50.2X5	T50.2X6
Xylene (vapor)	T52.2X1	T52.2X2	T52.2X3	T52.2X4	—	—
Xylocaine (infiltration) (topical)	T41.3X1	T41.3X2	T41.3X3	T41.3X4	T41.3X5	T41.3X6
nerve block (peripheral) (plexus)	T41.3X1	T41.3X2	T41.3X3	T41.3X4	T41.3X5	T41.3X6
spinal	T41.3X1	T41.3X2	T41.3X3	T41.3X4	T41.3X5	T41.3X6
Xylol (vapor)	T52.2X1	T52.2X2	T52.2X3	T52.2X4	—	—
Xylometazoline	T48.5X1	T48.5X2	T48.5X3	T48.5X4	T48.5X5	T48.5X6
Xylose*	T50.8X1	T50.8X2	T50.8X3	T50.8X4	T50.8X5	T50.8X6
Yaz*	T38.4X1	T38.4X2	T38.4X3	T38.4X4	T38.4X5	T38.4X6
Yeast	T45.2X1	T45.2X2	T45.2X3	T45.2X4	T45.2X5	T45.2X6
dried	T45.2X1	T45.2X2	T45.2X3	T45.2X4	T45.2X5	T45.2X6
Yellow						
fever vaccine	T50.B91	T50.B92	T50.B93	T50.B94	T50.B95	T50.B96
jasmine	T62.2X1	T62.2X2	T62.2X3	T62.2X4	—	—
phenolphthalein	T47.2X1	T47.2X2	T47.2X3	T47.2X4	T47.2X5	T47.2X6
Yervoy*	T45.1X1	T45.1X2	T45.1X3	T45.1X4	T45.1X5	T45.1X6
Yew	T62.2X1	T62.2X2	T62.2X3	T62.2X4	—	—
Yohimbic acid	T40.991	T40.992	T40.993	T40.994	T40.995	T40.996
Zactane	T39.8X1	T39.8X2	T39.8X3	T39.8X4	T39.8X5	T39.8X6
Zalcitabine	T37.5X1	T37.5X2	T37.5X3	T37.5X4	T37.5X5	T37.5X6
Zanaflex*	T48.1X1	T48.1X2	T48.1X3	T48.1X4	T48.1X5	T48.1X6
Zaroxolyn	T50.2X1	T50.2X2	T50.2X3	T50.2X4	T50.2X5	T50.2X6
Zephiran (topical)	T49.0X1	T49.0X2	T49.0X3	T49.0X4	T49.0X5	T49.0X6
ophthalmic preparation	T49.5X1	T49.5X2	T49.5X3	T49.5X4	T49.5X5	T49.5X6
Zeranol	T38.7X1	T38.7X2	T38.7X3	T38.7X4	T38.7X5	T38.7X6
Zerone	T51.1X1	T51.1X2	T51.1X3	T51.1X4	—	—
Zidovudine	T37.5X1	T37.5X2	T37.5X3	T37.5X4	T37.5X5	T37.5X6
Zilactin*	T41.3X1	T41.3X2	T41.3X3	T41.3X4	T41.3X5	T41.3X6
Zimeldine	T43.221	T43.222	T43.223	T43.224	T43.225	T43.226
Zinc (compounds) (fumes) (vapor)	T56.5X1	T56.5X2	T56.5X3	T56.5X4	—	—
NEC						
anti-infectives	T49.0X1	T49.0X2	T49.0X3	T49.0X4	T49.0X5	T49.0X6
antivaricose	T46.8X1	T46.8X2	T46.8X3	T46.8X4	T46.8X5	T46.8X6
bacitracin	T49.0X1	T49.0X2	T49.0X3	T49.0X4	T49.0X5	T49.0X6
chloride (mouthwash)	T49.6X1	T49.6X2	T49.6X3	T49.6X4	T49.6X5	T49.6X6
chromate	T56.5X1	T56.5X2	T56.5X3	T56.5X4	—	—
gelatin	T49.3X1	T49.3X2	T49.3X3	T49.3X4	T49.3X5	T49.3X6
oxide	T49.3X1	T49.3X2	T49.3X3	T49.3X4	T49.3X5	T49.3X6
plaster	T49.3X1	T49.3X2	T49.3X3	T49.3X4	T49.3X5	T49.3X6
peroxide	T49.0X1	T49.0X2	T49.0X3	T49.0X4	T49.0X5	T49.0X6
pesticides	T56.5X1	T56.5X2	T56.5X3	T56.5X4	—	—
phosphide	T60.4X1	T60.4X2	T60.4X3	T60.4X4	—	—
pyrithionate	T49.4X1	T49.4X2	T49.4X3	T49.4X4	T49.4X5	T49.4X6
stearate	T49.3X1	T49.3X2	T49.3X3	T49.3X4	T49.3X5	T49.3X6
sulfate	T49.5X1	T49.5X2	T49.5X3	T49.5X4	T49.5X5	T49.5X6
ENT agent	T49.6X1	T49.6X2	T49.6X3	T49.6X4	T49.6X5	T49.6X6
ophthalmic solution	T49.5X1	T49.5X2	T49.5X3	T49.5X4	T49.5X5	T49.5X6
topical NEC	T49.0X1	T49.0X2	T49.0X3	T49.0X4	T49.0X5	T49.0X6
undecylenate	T49.0X1	T49.0X2	T49.0X3	T49.0X4	T49.0X5	T49.0X6
Zineb	T60.0X1	T60.0X2	T60.0X3	T60.0X4	—	—

Substance	Poisoning, Accidental (unintentional)	Poisoning, Intentional Self-harm	Poisoning, Assault	Poisoning, Undetermined	Adverse Effect	Under-dosing
Zinostatin	T45.1X1	T45.1X2	T45.1X3	T45.1X4	T45.1X5	T45.1X6
Zipeprol	T48.3X1	T48.3X2	T48.3X3	T48.3X4	T48.3X5	T48.3X6
Zofenopril	T46.4X1	T46.4X2	T46.4X3	T46.4X4	T46.4X5	T46.4X6
Zolpidem	T42.6X1	T42.6X2	T42.6X3	T42.6X4	T42.6X5	T42.6X6
Zomepirac	T39.391	T39.392	T39.393	T39.394	T39.395	T39.396
Zopiclone	T42.6X1	T42.6X2	T42.6X3	T42.6X4	T42.6X5	T42.6X6
Zorubicin	T45.1X1	T45.1X2	T45.1X3	T45.1X4	T45.1X5	T45.1X6
Zotepine	T43.591	T43.592	T43.593	T43.594	T43.595	T43.596
Zovant	T45.511	T45.512	T45.513	T45.514	T45.515	T45.516
Zoxazolamine	T42.8X1	T42.8X2	T42.8X3	T42.8X4	T42.8X5	T42.8X6
Zuclopenthixol	T43.4X1	T43.4X2	T43.4X3	T43.4X4	T43.4X5	T43.4X6
Zyflo*	T48.6X1	T48.6X2	T48.6X3	T48.6X4	T48.6X5	T48.6X6
Zygadenus (venenosus)	T62.2X1	T62.2X2	T62.2X3	T62.2X4	—	—
Zyprexa	T43.591	T43.592	T43.593	T43.594	T43.595	T43.596
Zyzal*	T45.0X1	T45.0X2	T45.0X3	T45.0X4	T45.0X5	T45.0X6

☑ Additional Character May Be Required — Refer to the Tabular List for Character Selection

*Optum Value-Add

A

Abandonment (causing exposure to weather conditions) (with intent to injure or kill) NEC X58 ☑
Abuse (adult) (child) (mental) (physical) (sexual) X58 ☑
Accident (to) X58 ☑
  aircraft (in transit) (powered) — *see also* Accident, transport, aircraft
    due to, caused by cataclysm — *see* Forces of nature, by type
  animal-drawn vehicle — *see* Accident, transport, animal-drawn vehicle occupant
  animal-rider — *see* Accident, transport, animal-rider
  automobile — *see* Accident, transport, car occupant
  bare foot water skier V94.4 ☑
  boat, boating — *see also* Accident, watercraft
    striking swimmer
      powered V94.11 ☑
      unpowered V94.12 ☑
  bus — *see* Accident, transport, bus occupant
  cable car, not on rails V98.0 ☑
    on rails — *see* Accident, transport, streetcar occupant
  car — *see* Accident, transport, car occupant
  caused by, due to
    animal NEC W64 ☑
    chain hoist W24.0 ☑
    cold (excessive) — *see* Exposure, cold
    corrosive liquid, substance — *see* Table of Drugs and Chemicals
    cutting or piercing instrument — *see* Contact, with, by type of instrument
    drive belt W24.0 ☑
    electric
      current — *see* Exposure, electric current
      motor — *see also* Contact, with, by type of machine W31.3 ☑
      current (of) W86.8 ☑
    environmental factor NEC X58 ☑
    explosive material — *see* Explosion
    fire, flames — *see* Exposure, fire
    firearm missile — *see* Discharge, firearm by type
    heat (excessive) — *see* Heat
    hot — *see* Contact, with, hot
    ignition — *see* Ignition
    lifting device W24.0 ☑
    lightning — *see* subcategory T75.0 ☑
      causing fire — *see* Exposure, fire
    machine, machinery — *see* Contact, with, by type of machine
    natural factor NEC X58 ☑
    pulley (block) W24.0 ☑
    radiation — *see* Radiation
    steam X13.1 ☑
      inhalation X13.0 ☑
      pipe X16 ☑
    thunderbolt — *see* subcategory T75.0 ☑
      causing fire — *see* Exposure, fire
    transmission device W24.1 ☑
  coach — *see* Accident, transport, bus occupant
  coal car — *see* Accident, transport, industrial vehicle occupant
  diving — *see also* Fall, into, water
    with
      drowning or submersion — *see* Drowning
  forklift — *see* Accident, transport, industrial vehicle occupant
  heavy transport vehicle NOS — *see* Accident, transport, truck occupant
  ice yacht V98.2 ☑
  in
    medical, surgical procedure
      as, or due to misadventure — *see* Misadventure
      causing an abnormal reaction or later complication without mention of misadventure — *see also* Complication of or following, by type of procedure Y84.9
  land yacht V98.1 ☑
  late effect of — *see* W00-X58 with 7th character S
  logging car — *see* Accident, transport, industrial vehicle occupant
  machine, machinery — *see also* Contact, with, by type of machine
    on board watercraft V93.69 ☑
      explosion — *see* Explosion, in, watercraft

Accident — *continued*
  machine, machinery — *see also* Contact, with, by type of machine — *continued*
    on board watercraft — *continued*
      fire — *see* Burn, on board watercraft
      powered craft V93.63 ☑
        ferry boat V93.61 ☑
        fishing boat V93.62 ☑
        jetskis V93.63 ☑
        liner V93.61 ☑
        merchant ship V93.60 ☑
        passenger ship V93.61 ☑
        sailboat V93.64 ☑
  mine tram — *see* Accident, transport, industrial vehicle occupant
  mobility scooter (motorized) — *see* Accident, transport, pedestrian, conveyance, specified type NEC
  motor scooter — *see* Accident, transport, motorcyclist
  motor vehicle NOS (traffic) — *see also* Accident, transport V89.2 ☑
    nontraffic V89.0 ☑
    three-wheeled NOS — *see* Accident, transport, three-wheeled motor vehicle occupant
  motorcycle NOS — *see* Accident, transport, motorcyclist
  nonmotor vehicle NOS (nontraffic) — *see also* Accident, transport V89.1 ☑
    traffic NOS V89.3 ☑
  nontraffic (victim's mode of transport NOS) V88.9 ☑
    collision (between) V88.7 ☑
      bus and truck V88.5 ☑
      car and:
        bus V88.3 ☑
        pickup V88.2 ☑
        three-wheeled motor vehicle V88.0 ☑
        train V88.6 ☑
        truck V88.4 ☑
        two-wheeled motor vehicle V88.0 ☑
        van V88.2 ☑
      specified vehicle NEC and:
        three-wheeled motor vehicle V88.1 ☑
        two-wheeled motor vehicle V88.1 ☑
    known mode of transport — *see* Accident, transport, by type of vehicle
    noncollision V88.8 ☑
  on board watercraft V93.89 ☑
    powered craft V93.83 ☑
      ferry boat V93.81 ☑
      fishing boat V93.82 ☑
      jetskis V93.83 ☑
      liner V93.81 ☑
      merchant ship V93.80 ☑
      passenger ship V93.81 ☑
    unpowered craft V93.88 ☑
      canoe V93.85 ☑
      inflatable V93.86 ☑
        in tow
          recreational V94.31 ☑
          specified NEC V94.32 ☑
      kayak V93.85 ☑
      sailboat V93.84 ☑
      surf-board V93.88 ☑
      water skis V93.87 ☑
      windsurfer V93.88 ☑
  parachutist V97.29 ☑
    entangled in object V97.21 ☑
    injured on landing V97.22 ☑
  pedal cycle — *see* Accident, transport, pedal cyclist
  pedestrian (on foot)
    with
      another pedestrian W51 ☑
        on pedestrian conveyance NEC V00.09 ☑
      with fall W03 ☑
        due to ice or snow W00.0 ☑
      rider of
        hoverboard V00.038 ☑
        Segway V00.038 ☑
        standing
          electric scooter V00.031 ☑
          micro-mobility pedestrian conveyance NEC V00.038 ☑
      roller skater (in-line) V00.01 ☑
      skate boarder V00.02 ☑
    transport vehicle — *see* Accident, transport
    on pedestrian conveyance — *see* Accident, transport, pedestrian, conveyance

Accident — *continued*
  pick-up truck or van — *see* Accident, transport, pickup truck occupant
  quarry truck — *see* Accident, transport, industrial vehicle occupant
  railway vehicle (any) (in motion) — *see* Accident, transport, railway vehicle occupant
    due to cataclysm — *see* Forces of nature, by type
  scooter (non-motorized) — *see* Accident, transport, pedestrian, conveyance, scooter
  sequelae of — *see* categories W00-X58 with 7th character S
  skateboard — *see* Accident, transport, pedestrian, conveyance, skateboard
  ski(ing) — *see* Accident, transport, pedestrian, conveyance
    lift V98.3 ☑
  specified cause NEC X58 ☑
  streetcar — *see* Accident, transport, streetcar occupant
  traffic (victim's mode of transport NOS) V87.9 ☑
    collision (between) V87.7 ☑
      bus and truck V87.5 ☑
      car and:
        bus V87.3 ☑
        pickup V87.2 ☑
        three-wheeled motor vehicle V87.0 ☑
        train V87.1 ☑
        truck V87.4 ☑
        two-wheeled motor vehicle V87.0 ☑
        van V87.2 ☑
      specified vehicle NEC V86.39 ☑
      and
        three-wheeled motor vehicle V87.1 ☑
        two-wheeled motor vehicle V87.1 ☑
      driver V86.09 ☑
      passenger V86.19 ☑
      person on outside V86.29 ☑
      while boarding or alighting V86.49 ☑
    known mode of transport — *see* Accident, transport, by type of vehicle
    noncollision V87.8 ☑
  transport (involving injury to) V99 ☑
    18 wheeler — *see* Accident, transport, truck occupant
    agricultural vehicle occupant (nontraffic) V84.9 ☑
      driver V84.5 ☑
      hanger-on V84.7 ☑
      passenger V84.6 ☑
      traffic V84.3 ☑
        driver V84.0 ☑
        hanger-on V84.2 ☑
        passenger V84.1 ☑
      while boarding or alighting V84.4 ☑
    aircraft NEC V97.89 ☑
      military NEC V97.818 ☑
        civilian injured by V97.811 ☑
        with civilian aircraft V97.810 ☑
      occupant injured (in)
        nonpowered craft accident V96.9 ☑
          balloon V96.00 ☑
            collision V96.03 ☑
            crash V96.01 ☑
            explosion V96.05 ☑
            fire V96.04 ☑
            forced landing V96.02 ☑
            specified type NEC V96.09 ☑
          glider V96.20 ☑
            collision V96.23 ☑
            crash V96.21 ☑
            explosion V96.25 ☑
            fire V96.24 ☑
            forced landing V96.22 ☑
            specified type NEC V96.29 ☑
          hang glider V96.10 ☑
            collision V96.13 ☑
            crash V96.11 ☑
            explosion V96.15 ☑
            fire V96.14 ☑
            forced landing V96.12 ☑
            specified type NEC V96.19 ☑
          specified craft NEC V96.8 ☑
        powered craft accident V95.9 ☑
          fixed wing NEC
            commercial V95.30 ☑
              collision V95.33 ☑
              crash V95.31 ☑

Accident — *continued*
  transport — *continued*
    aircraft — *continued*
      occupant injured — *continued*
        powered craft accident — *continued*
          fixed wing — *continued*
            commercial — *continued*
              explosion V95.35 ☑
              fire V95.34 ☑
              forced landing V95.32 ☑
              specified type NEC V95.39 ☑
            private V95.20 ☑
              collision V95.23 ☑
              crash V95.21 ☑
              explosion V95.25 ☑
              fire V95.24 ☑
              forced landing V95.22 ☑
              specified type NEC V95.29 ☑
          glider V95.10 ☑
            collision V95.13 ☑
            crash V95.11 ☑
            explosion V95.15 ☑
            fire V95.14 ☑
            forced landing V95.12 ☑
            specified type NEC V95.19 ☑
          helicopter V95.00 ☑
            collision V95.03 ☑
            crash V95.01 ☑
            explosion V95.05 ☑
            fire V95.04 ☑
            forced landing V95.02 ☑
            specified type NEC V95.09 ☑
          spacecraft V95.40 ☑
            collision V95.43 ☑
            crash V95.41 ☑
            explosion V95.45 ☑
            fire V95.44 ☑
            forced landing V95.42 ☑
            specified type NEC V95.49 ☑
          specified craft NEC V95.8 ☑
          ultralight V95.10 ☑
            collision V95.13 ☑
            crash V95.11 ☑
            explosion V95.15 ☑
            fire V95.14 ☑
            forced landing V95.12 ☑
            specified type NEC V95.19 ☑
      specified accident NEC V97.0 ☑
      while boarding or alighting V97.1 ☑
     person (injured by)
      falling from, in or on aircraft V97.0 ☑
      machinery on aircraft V97.89 ☑
      on ground with aircraft involvement
        V97.39 ☑
      rotating propeller V97.32 ☑
      struck by object falling from aircraft V97.31 ☑
      sucked into aircraft jet V97.33 ☑
      while boarding or alighting aircraft V97.1 ☑
    airport (battery-powered) passenger vehicle — *see* Accident, transport, industrial vehicle occupant
    all-terrain vehicle occupant (nontraffic) V86.95 ☑
      driver V86.55 ☑
      dune buggy — *see* Accident, transport, dune buggy occupant
      hanger-on V86.75 ☑
      passenger V86.65 ☑
      snowmobile — *see* Accident, transport, snowmobile occupant
      specified type NEC V86.99 ☑
        driver V86.59 ☑
        passenger V86.69 ☑
        person on outside V86.79 ☑
      traffic V86.35 ☑
        driver V86.05 ☑
        hanger-on V86.25 ☑
        passenger V86.15 ☑
      while boarding or alighting V86.45 ☑
    ambulance occupant (traffic) V86.31 ☑
      driver V86.01 ☑
      hanger-on V86.21 ☑
      nontraffic V86.91 ☑
        driver V86.51 ☑
        hanger-on V86.71 ☑
        passenger V86.61 ☑
      passenger V86.11 ☑

Accident — *continued*
  transport — *continued*
    ambulance occupant — *continued*
      while boarding or alighting V86.41 ☑
    animal-drawn vehicle occupant (in) V80.929 ☑
      collision (with)
        animal V80.12 ☑
          being ridden V80.711 ☑
        animal-drawn vehicle V80.721 ☑
        bus V80.42 ☑
        car V80.42 ☑
        fixed or stationary object V80.82 ☑
        military vehicle V80.920 ☑
        nonmotor vehicle V80.791 ☑
        pedal cycle V80.22 ☑
        pedestrian V80.12 ☑
        pickup V80.42 ☑
        railway train or vehicle V80.62 ☑
        specified motor vehicle NEC V80.52 ☑
        streetcar V80.731 ☑
        truck V80.42 ☑
        two- or three-wheeled motor vehicle V80.32 ☑
        van V80.42 ☑
      noncollision V80.02 ☑
      specified circumstance NEC V80.928 ☑
    animal-rider V80.919 ☑
      collision (with)
        animal V80.11 ☑
          being ridden V80.710 ☑
        animal-drawn vehicle V80.720 ☑
        bus V80.41 ☑
        car V80.41 ☑
        fixed or stationary object V80.81 ☑
        military vehicle V80.910 ☑
        nonmotor vehicle V80.790 ☑
        pedal cycle V80.21 ☑
        pedestrian V80.11 ☑
        pickup V80.41 ☑
        railway train or vehicle V80.61 ☑
        specified motor vehicle NEC V80.51 ☑
        streetcar V80.730 ☑
        truck V80.41 ☑
        two- or three-wheeled motor vehicle V80.31 ☑
        van V80.41 ☑
      noncollision V80.018 ☑
        specified as horse rider V80.010 ☑
      specified circumstance NEC V80.918 ☑
    armored car — *see* Accident, transport, truck occupant
    battery-powered truck (baggage) (mail) — *see* Accident, transport, industrial vehicle occupant
    bus occupant V79.9 ☑
      collision (with)
        animal (traffic) V70.9 ☑
          being ridden (traffic) V76.9 ☑
            nontraffic V76.3 ☑
            while boarding or alighting V76.4 ☑
          nontraffic V70.3 ☑
          while boarding or alighting V70.4 ☑
        animal-drawn vehicle (traffic) V76.9 ☑
          nontraffic V76.3 ☑
          while boarding or alighting V76.4 ☑
        bus (traffic) V74.9 ☑
          nontraffic V74.3 ☑
          while boarding or alighting V74.4 ☑
        car (traffic) V73.9 ☑
          nontraffic V73.3 ☑
          while boarding or alighting V73.4 ☑
        motor vehicle NOS (traffic) V79.60 ☑
          nontraffic V79.20 ☑
          specified type NEC (traffic) V79.69 ☑
            nontraffic V79.29 ☑
        pedal cycle (traffic) V71.9 ☑
          nontraffic V71.3 ☑
          while boarding or alighting V71.4 ☑
        pickup truck (traffic) V73.9 ☑
          nontraffic V73.3 ☑
          while boarding or alighting V73.4 ☑
        railway vehicle (traffic) V75.9 ☑
          nontraffic V75.3 ☑
          while boarding or alighting V75.4 ☑
        specified vehicle NEC (traffic) V76.9 ☑
          nontraffic V76.3 ☑
          while boarding or alighting V76.4 ☑

Accident — *continued*
  transport — *continued*
    bus occupant — *continued*
      collision — *continued*
        stationary object (traffic) V77.9 ☑
          nontraffic V77.3 ☑
          while boarding or alighting V77.4 ☑
        streetcar (traffic) V76.9 ☑
          nontraffic V76.3 ☑
          while boarding or alighting V76.4 ☑
        three wheeled motor vehicle (traffic) V72.9 ☑
          nontraffic V72.3 ☑
          while boarding or alighting V72.4 ☑
        truck (traffic) V74.9 ☑
          nontraffic V74.3 ☑
          while boarding or alighting V74.4 ☑
        two wheeled motor vehicle (traffic) V72.9 ☑
          nontraffic V72.3 ☑
          while boarding or alighting V72.4 ☑
        van (traffic) V73.9 ☑
          nontraffic V73.3 ☑
          while boarding or alighting V73.4 ☑
      driver
        collision (with)
          animal (traffic) V70.5 ☑
            being ridden (traffic) V76.5 ☑
              nontraffic V76.0 ☑
            nontraffic V70.0 ☑
          animal-drawn vehicle (traffic) V76.5 ☑
            nontraffic V76.0 ☑
          bus (traffic) V74.5 ☑
            nontraffic V74.0 ☑
          car (traffic) V73.5 ☑
            nontraffic V73.0 ☑
          motor vehicle NOS (traffic) V79.40 ☑
            nontraffic V79.00 ☑
            specified type NEC (traffic) V79.49 ☑
              nontraffic V79.09 ☑
          pedal cycle (traffic) V71.5 ☑
            nontraffic V71.0 ☑
          pickup truck (traffic) V73.5 ☑
            nontraffic V73.0 ☑
          railway vehicle (traffic) V75.5 ☑
            nontraffic V75.0 ☑
          specified vehicle NEC (traffic) V76.5 ☑
            nontraffic V76.0 ☑
          stationary object (traffic) V77.5 ☑
            nontraffic V77.0 ☑
          streetcar (traffic) V76.5 ☑
            nontraffic V76.0 ☑
          three wheeled motor vehicle (traffic) V72.5 ☑
            nontraffic V72.0 ☑
          truck (traffic) V74.5 ☑
            nontraffic V74.0 ☑
          two wheeled motor vehicle (traffic) V72.5 ☑
            nontraffic V72.0 ☑
          van (traffic) V73.5 ☑
            nontraffic V73.0 ☑
        noncollision accident (traffic) V78.5 ☑
          nontraffic V78.0 ☑
      hanger-on
        collision (with)
          animal (traffic) V70.7 ☑
            being ridden (traffic) V76.7 ☑
              nontraffic V76.2 ☑
            nontraffic V70.2 ☑
          animal-drawn vehicle (traffic) V76.7 ☑
            nontraffic V76.2 ☑
          bus (traffic) V74.7 ☑
            nontraffic V74.2 ☑
          car (traffic) V73.7 ☑
            nontraffic V73.2 ☑
          pedal cycle (traffic) V71.7 ☑
            nontraffic V71.2 ☑
          pickup truck (traffic) V73.7 ☑
            nontraffic V73.2 ☑
          railway vehicle (traffic) V75.7 ☑
            nontraffic V75.2 ☑
          specified vehicle NEC (traffic) V76.7 ☑
            nontraffic V76.2 ☑
          stationary object (traffic) V77.7 ☑
            nontraffic V77.2 ☑
          streetcar (traffic) V76.7 ☑
            nontraffic V76.2 ☑

Accident — *continued*
  transport — *continued*
    bus occupant — *continued*
      hanger-on — *continued*
        collision — *continued*
          three wheeled motor vehicle (traffic)
            V72.7 ☑
            nontraffic V72.2 ☑
          truck (traffic) V74.7 ☑
            nontraffic V74.2 ☑
          two wheeled motor vehicle (traffic)
            V72.7 ☑
            nontraffic V72.2 ☑
          van (traffic) V73.7 ☑
            nontraffic V73.2 ☑
        noncollision accident (traffic) V78.7 ☑
          nontraffic V78.2 ☑
      noncollision accident (traffic) V78.9 ☑
        nontraffic V78.3 ☑
        while boarding or alighting V78.4 ☑
      nontraffic V79.3 ☑
      passenger
        collision (with)
          animal (traffic) V70.6 ☑
            being ridden (traffic) V76.6 ☑
              nontraffic V76.1 ☑
            nontraffic V70.1 ☑
            animal-drawn vehicle (traffic) V76.6 ☑
              nontraffic V76.1 ☑
            bus (traffic) V74.6 ☑
              nontraffic V74.1 ☑
            car (traffic) V73.6 ☑
              nontraffic V73.1 ☑
            motor vehicle NOS (traffic) V79.50 ☑
              nontraffic V79.10 ☑
              specified type NEC (traffic) V79.59 ☑
                nontraffic V79.19 ☑
            pedal cycle (traffic) V71.6 ☑
              nontraffic V71.1 ☑
            pickup truck (traffic) V73.6 ☑
              nontraffic V73.1 ☑
            railway vehicle (traffic) V75.6 ☑
              nontraffic V75.1 ☑
            specified vehicle NEC (traffic) V76.6 ☑
              nontraffic V76.1 ☑
            stationary object (traffic) V77.6 ☑
              nontraffic V77.1 ☑
            streetcar (traffic) V76.6 ☑
              nontraffic V76.1 ☑
            three wheeled motor vehicle (traffic)
              V72.6 ☑
              nontraffic V72.1 ☑
            truck (traffic) V74.6 ☑
              nontraffic V74.1 ☑
            two wheeled motor vehicle (traffic)
              V72.6 ☑
              nontraffic V72.1 ☑
            van (traffic) V73.6 ☑
              nontraffic V73.1 ☑
          noncollision accident (traffic) V78.6 ☑
            nontraffic V78.1 ☑
    specified type NEC V79.88 ☑
      military vehicle V79.81 ☑
  cable car, not on rails V98.0 ☑
    on rails — *see* Accident, transport, streetcar oc-
      cupant
  car occupant V49.9 ☑
    ambulance occupant — *see* Accident, transport,
      ambulance occupant
    collision (with)
      animal (traffic) V40.9 ☑
        being ridden (traffic) V46.9 ☑
          nontraffic V46.3 ☑
          while boarding or alighting V46.4 ☑
        nontraffic V40.3 ☑
        while boarding or alighting V40.4 ☑
      animal-drawn vehicle (traffic) V46.9 ☑
        nontraffic V46.3 ☑
        while boarding or alighting V46.4 ☑
      bus (traffic) V44.9 ☑
        nontraffic V44.3 ☑
        while boarding or alighting V44.4 ☑
      car (traffic) V43.92 ☑
        nontraffic V43.32 ☑
        while boarding or alighting V43.42 ☑
      motor vehicle NOS (traffic) V49.60 ☑

Accident — *continued*
  transport — *continued*
    car occupant — *continued*
      collision — *continued*
        motor vehicle — *continued*
          nontraffic V49.20 ☑
          specified type NEC (traffic) V49.69 ☑
            nontraffic V49.29 ☑
        pedal cycle (traffic) V41.9 ☑
          nontraffic V41.3 ☑
          while boarding or alighting V41.4 ☑
        pickup truck (traffic) V43.93 ☑
          nontraffic V43.33 ☑
          while boarding or alighting V43.43 ☑
        railway vehicle (traffic) V45.9 ☑
          nontraffic V45.3 ☑
          while boarding or alighting V45.4 ☑
        specified vehicle NEC (traffic) V46.9 ☑
          nontraffic V46.3 ☑
          while boarding or alighting V46.4 ☑
        sport utility vehicle (traffic) V43.91 ☑
          nontraffic V43.31 ☑
          while boarding or alighting V43.41 ☑
        stationary object (traffic) V47.9 ☑
          nontraffic V47.3 ☑
          while boarding or alighting V47.4 ☑
        streetcar (traffic) V46.9 ☑
          nontraffic V46.3 ☑
          while boarding or alighting V46.4 ☑
        three wheeled motor vehicle (traffic) V42.9 ☑
          nontraffic V42.3 ☑
          while boarding or alighting V42.4 ☑
        truck (traffic) V44.9 ☑
          nontraffic V44.3 ☑
          while boarding or alighting V44.4 ☑
        two wheeled motor vehicle (traffic) V42.9 ☑
          nontraffic V42.3 ☑
          while boarding or alighting V42.4 ☑
        van (traffic) V43.94 ☑
          nontraffic V43.34 ☑
          while boarding or alighting V43.44 ☑
      driver
        collision (with)
          animal (traffic) V40.5 ☑
            being ridden (traffic) V46.5 ☑
              nontraffic V46.0 ☑
            nontraffic V40.0 ☑
          animal-drawn vehicle (traffic) V46.5 ☑
            nontraffic V46.0 ☑
          bus (traffic) V44.5 ☑
            nontraffic V44.0 ☑
          car (traffic) V43.52 ☑
            nontraffic V43.02 ☑
          motor vehicle NOS (traffic) V49.40 ☑
            nontraffic V49.00 ☑
            specified type NEC (traffic) V49.49 ☑
              nontraffic V49.09 ☑
          pedal cycle (traffic) V41.5 ☑
            nontraffic V41.0 ☑
          pickup truck (traffic) V43.53 ☑
            nontraffic V43.03 ☑
          railway vehicle (traffic) V45.5 ☑
            nontraffic V45.0 ☑
          specified vehicle NEC (traffic) V46.5 ☑
            nontraffic V46.0 ☑
          sport utility vehicle (traffic) V43.51 ☑
            nontraffic V43.01 ☑
          stationary object (traffic) V47.5 ☑
            nontraffic V47.0 ☑
          streetcar (traffic) V46.5 ☑
            nontraffic V46.0 ☑
          three wheeled motor vehicle (traffic)
            V42.5 ☑
            nontraffic V42.0 ☑
          truck (traffic) V44.5 ☑
            nontraffic V44.0 ☑
          two wheeled motor vehicle (traffic)
            V42.5 ☑
            nontraffic V42.0 ☑
          van (traffic) V43.54 ☑
            nontraffic V43.04 ☑
        noncollision accident (traffic) V48.5 ☑
          nontraffic V48.0 ☑
      hanger-on
        collision (with)
          animal (traffic) V40.7 ☑

Accident — *continued*
  transport — *continued*
    car occupant — *continued*
      hanger-on — *continued*
        collision — *continued*
          animal — *continued*
            being ridden (traffic) V46.7 ☑
              nontraffic V46.2 ☑
            nontraffic V40.2 ☑
          animal-drawn vehicle (traffic) V46.7 ☑
            nontraffic V46.2 ☑
          bus (traffic) V44.7 ☑
            nontraffic V44.2 ☑
          car (traffic) V43.72 ☑
            nontraffic V43.22 ☑
          pedal cycle (traffic) V41.7 ☑
            nontraffic V41.2 ☑
          pickup truck (traffic) V43.73 ☑
            nontraffic V43.23 ☑
          railway vehicle (traffic) V45.7 ☑
            nontraffic V45.2 ☑
          specified vehicle NEC (traffic) V46.7 ☑
            nontraffic V46.2 ☑
          sport utility vehicle (traffic) V43.71 ☑
            nontraffic V43.21 ☑
          stationary object (traffic) V47.7 ☑
            nontraffic V47.2 ☑
          streetcar (traffic) V46.7 ☑
            nontraffic V46.2 ☑
          three wheeled motor vehicle (traffic)
            V42.7 ☑
            nontraffic V42.2 ☑
          truck (traffic) V44.7 ☑
            nontraffic V44.2 ☑
          two wheeled motor vehicle (traffic)
            V42.7 ☑
            nontraffic V42.2 ☑
          van (traffic) V43.74 ☑
            nontraffic V43.24 ☑
        noncollision accident (traffic) V48.7 ☑
          nontraffic V48.2 ☑
      noncollision accident (traffic) V48.9 ☑
        nontraffic V48.3 ☑
        while boarding or alighting V48.4 ☑
      nontraffic V49.3 ☑
      passenger
        collision (with)
          animal (traffic) V40.6 ☑
            being ridden (traffic) V46.6 ☑
              nontraffic V46.1 ☑
            nontraffic V40.1 ☑
          animal-drawn vehicle (traffic) V46.6 ☑
            nontraffic V46.1 ☑
          bus (traffic) V44.6 ☑
            nontraffic V44.1 ☑
          car (traffic) V43.62 ☑
            nontraffic V43.12 ☑
          motor vehicle NOS (traffic) V49.50 ☑
            nontraffic V49.10 ☑
            specified type NEC (traffic) V49.59 ☑
              nontraffic V49.19 ☑
          pedal cycle (traffic) V41.6 ☑
            nontraffic V41.1 ☑
          pickup truck (traffic) V43.63 ☑
            nontraffic V43.13 ☑
          railway vehicle (traffic) V45.6 ☑
            nontraffic V45.1 ☑
          specified vehicle NEC (traffic) V46.6 ☑
            nontraffic V46.1 ☑
          sport utility vehicle (traffic) V43.61 ☑
            nontraffic V43.11 ☑
          stationary object (traffic) V47.6 ☑
            nontraffic V47.1 ☑
          streetcar (traffic) V46.6 ☑
            nontraffic V46.1 ☑
          three wheeled motor vehicle (traffic)
            V42.6 ☑
            nontraffic V42.1 ☑
          truck (traffic) V44.6 ☑
            nontraffic V44.1 ☑
          two wheeled motor vehicle (traffic)
            V42.6 ☑
            nontraffic V42.1 ☑
          van (traffic) V43.64 ☑
            nontraffic V43.14 ☑
        noncollision accident (traffic) V48.6 ☑

Accident — *continued*
 transport — *continued*
  car occupant — *continued*
   passenger — *continued*
    noncollision accident — *continued*
     nontraffic V48.1 ☑
    specified type NEC V49.88 ☑
    military vehicle V49.81 ☑
   coal car — *see* Accident, transport, industrial vehicle occupant
   construction vehicle occupant (nontraffic) V85.9 ☑
    driver V85.5 ☑
    hanger-on V85.7 ☑
    passenger V85.6 ☑
    traffic V85.3 ☑
     driver V85.0 ☑
     hanger-on V85.2 ☑
     passenger V85.1 ☑
    while boarding or alighting V85.4 ☑
   dirt bike rider (nontraffic) V86.96 ☑
    driver V86.56 ☑
    hanger-on V86.76 ☑
    passenger V86.66 ☑
    traffic V86.36 ☑
     driver V86.06 ☑
     hanger-on V86.26 ☑
     passenger V86.16 ☑
    while boarding or alighting V86.46 ☑
   due to cataclysm — *see* Forces of nature, by type
   dune buggy occupant (nontraffic) V86.93 ☑
    driver V86.53 ☑
    hanger-on V86.73 ☑
    passenger V86.63 ☑
    traffic V86.33 ☑
     driver V86.03 ☑
     hanger-on V86.23 ☑
     passenger V86.13 ☑
    while boarding or alighting V86.43 ☑
   e-bicycle — *see* Accident, transport, electric (assisted) bicyclist
   e-bike — *see* Accident, transport, electric (assisted) bicyclist
   electric (assisted) bicyclist V29.91 ☑
    collision (with)
     animal (traffic) V20.91 ☑
      being ridden (traffic) V26.91 ☑
       nontraffic V26.21 ☑
        while boarding or alighting V26.31 ☑
      nontraffic V20.21 ☑
       while boarding or alighting V20.31 ☑
     animal-drawn vehicle (traffic) V26.91 ☑
      nontraffic V26.21 ☑
      while boarding or alighting V26.31 ☑
     bus (traffic) V24.91 ☑
      nontraffic V24.21 ☑
      while boarding or alighting V24.31 ☑
     car (traffic) V23.91 ☑
      nontraffic V23.21 ☑
      while boarding or alighting V23.31 ☑
     motor vehicle NOS (traffic) V29.601 ☑
      nontraffic V29.201 ☑
      specified type NEC (traffic) V29.691 ☑
       nontraffic V29.291 ☑
     pedal cycle (traffic) V21.91 ☑
      nontraffic V21.21 ☑
      while boarding or alighting V21.31 ☑
     pedestrian V20.91 ☑
      nontraffic V20.01 ☑
      while boarding or alighting V20.31 ☑
     pickup truck (traffic) V23.91 ☑
      nontraffic V23.21 ☑
      while boarding or alighting V23.31 ☑
     railway vehicle (traffic) V25.91 ☑
      nontraffic V25.21 ☑
      while boarding or alighting V25.31 ☑
     specified vehicle NEC (traffic) V26.91 ☑
      nontraffic V26.21 ☑
      while boarding or alighting V26.31 ☑
     stationary object (traffic) V27.91 ☑
      nontraffic V27.21 ☑
      while boarding or alighting V27.31 ☑
     streetcar (traffic) V26.91 ☑
      nontraffic V26.21 ☑
      while boarding or alighting V26.31 ☑
     three wheeled motor vehicle (traffic) V22.91 ☑

Accident — *continued*
 transport — *continued*
  electric bicyclist — *continued*
   collision — *continued*
    three wheeled motor vehicle — *continued*
     nontraffic V22.21 ☑
     while boarding or alighting V22.31 ☑
    truck (traffic) V24.91 ☑
     nontraffic V24.21 ☑
     while boarding or alighting V24.31 ☑
    two wheeled motor vehicle (traffic) V22.91 ☑
     nontraffic V22.21 ☑
     while boarding or alighting V22.31 ☑
    van (traffic) V23.91 ☑
     nontraffic V23.21 ☑
     while boarding or alighting V23.31 ☑
   driver
    collision (with)
     animal (traffic) V20.41 ☑
      being ridden (traffic) V26.41 ☑
       nontraffic V26.01 ☑
      nontraffic V20.01 ☑
     animal-drawn vehicle (traffic) V26.41 ☑
      nontraffic V26.01 ☑
     bus (traffic) V24.41 ☑
      nontraffic V24.01 ☑
     car (traffic) V23.41 ☑
      nontraffic V23.01 ☑
     motor vehicle NOS (traffic) V29.401 ☑
      nontraffic V29.001 ☑
      specified type NEC (traffic) V29.491 ☑
       nontraffic V29.091 ☑
     pedal cycle (traffic) V21.41 ☑
      nontraffic V21.01 ☑
     pedestrian
      nontraffic V20.01 ☑
      traffic V20.41 ☑
     pickup truck (traffic) V23.41 ☑
      nontraffic V23.01 ☑
     railway vehicle (traffic) V25.41 ☑
      nontraffic V25.01 ☑
     specified vehicle NEC (traffic) V26.41 ☑
      nontraffic V26.01 ☑
     stationary object (traffic) V27.41 ☑
      nontraffic V27.01 ☑
     streetcar (traffic) V26.41 ☑
      nontraffic V26.01 ☑
     three wheeled motor vehicle (traffic) V22.41 ☑
      nontraffic V22.01 ☑
     truck (traffic) V24.41 ☑
      nontraffic V24.01 ☑
     two wheeled motor vehicle (traffic) V22.41 ☑
      nontraffic V22.01 ☑
     van (traffic) V23.41 ☑
      nontraffic V23.01 ☑
    noncollision accident (traffic) V28.41 ☑
     nontraffic V28.01 ☑
   noncollision accident (traffic) V28.91 ☑
    nontraffic V28.21 ☑
    while boarding or alighting V28.31 ☑
   nontraffic V29.31 ☑
   passenger
    collision (with)
     animal (traffic) V20.51 ☑
      being ridden (traffic) V26.51 ☑
       nontraffic V26.11 ☑
      nontraffic V20.11 ☑
     animal-drawn vehicle (traffic) V26.51 ☑
      nontraffic V26.11 ☑
     bus (traffic) V24.51 ☑
      nontraffic V24.11 ☑
     car (traffic) V23.51 ☑
      nontraffic V23.11 ☑
     motor vehicle NOS (traffic) V29.501 ☑
      nontraffic V29.101 ☑
      specified type NEC (traffic) V29.591 ☑
       nontraffic V29.191 ☑
     pedal cycle (traffic) V21.51 ☑
      nontraffic V21.11 ☑
     pedestrian
      nontraffic V20.11 ☑
      traffic V20.51 ☑
     pickup truck (traffic) V23.51 ☑
      nontraffic V23.11 ☑

Accident — *continued*
 transport — *continued*
  electric bicyclist — *continued*
   passenger — *continued*
    collision — *continued*
     railway vehicle (traffic) V25.51 ☑
      nontraffic V25.11 ☑
     specified vehicle NEC (traffic) V26.51 ☑
      nontraffic V26.11 ☑
     stationary object (traffic) V27.51 ☑
      nontraffic V27.11 ☑
     streetcar (traffic) V26.51 ☑
      nontraffic V26.11 ☑
     three wheeled motor vehicle (traffic) V22.51 ☑
      nontraffic V22.11 ☑
     truck (traffic) V24.51 ☑
      nontraffic V24.11 ☑
     two wheeled motor vehicle (traffic) V22.51 ☑
      nontraffic V22.11 ☑
     van (traffic) V23.51 ☑
      nontraffic V23.11 ☑
    noncollision accident (traffic) V28.51 ☑
     nontraffic V28.11 ☑
    specified type NEC V29.881 ☑
    military vehicle V29.811 ☑
   forklift — *see* Accident, transport, industrial vehicle occupant
   go cart — *see* Accident, transport, all-terrain vehicle occupant
   golf cart — *see* Accident, transport, all-terrain vehicle occupant
   heavy transport vehicle occupant — *see* Accident, transport, truck occupant
   hoverboard V00.848 ☑
   ice yacht V98.2 ☑
   industrial vehicle occupant (nontraffic) V83.9 ☑
    driver V83.5 ☑
    hanger-on V83.7 ☑
    passenger V83.6 ☑
    traffic V83.3 ☑
     driver V83.0 ☑
     hanger-on V83.2 ☑
     passenger V83.1 ☑
    while boarding or alighting V83.4 ☑
   interurban electric car — *see* Accident, transport, streetcar
   land yacht V98.1 ☑
   logging car — *see* Accident, transport, industrial vehicle occupant
   military vehicle occupant (traffic) V86.34 ☑
    driver V86.04 ☑
    hanger-on V86.24 ☑
    nontraffic V86.94 ☑
     driver V86.54 ☑
     hanger-on V86.74 ☑
     passenger V86.64 ☑
    passenger V86.14 ☑
    while boarding or alighting V86.44 ☑
   mine tram — *see* Accident, transport, industrial vehicle occupant
   motor vehicle NEC occupant (traffic) V89.2 ☑
   motorcoach — *see* Accident, transport, bus occupant
   motor/cross bike rider — *see also* Accident, transport, dirt bike rider V86.96 ☑
   motorcyclist V29.99 ☑
    collision (with)
     animal (traffic) V20.99 ☑
      being ridden (traffic) V26.99 ☑
       nontraffic V26.29 ☑
        while boarding or alighting V26.39 ☑
      nontraffic V20.29 ☑
       while boarding or alighting V20.39 ☑
     animal-drawn vehicle (traffic) V26.99 ☑
      nontraffic V26.29 ☑
       while boarding or alighting V26.39 ☑
     bus (traffic) V24.99 ☑
      nontraffic V24.29 ☑
       while boarding or alighting V24.39 ☑
     car (traffic) V23.99 ☑
      nontraffic V23.29 ☑
       while boarding or alighting V23.39 ☑
     motor vehicle NOS (traffic) V29.608 ☑
      nontraffic V29.208 ☑

☑ Additional Character Required — Refer to the Tabular List for Character Selection

Accident — *continued*
  transport — *continued*
    motorcyclist — *continued*
      collision — *continued*
        motor vehicle — *continued*
          specified type NEC (traffic) V29.698 ☑
            nontraffic V29.298 ☑
          pedal cycle (traffic) V21.99 ☑
            nontraffic V21.29 ☑
            while boarding or alighting V21.39 ☑
          pickup truck (traffic) V23.99 ☑
            nontraffic V23.29 ☑
            while boarding or alighting V23.39 ☑
          railway vehicle (traffic) V25.99 ☑
            nontraffic V25.29 ☑
            while boarding or alighting V25.39 ☑
          specified vehicle NEC (traffic) V26.99 ☑
            nontraffic V26.29 ☑
            while boarding or alighting V26.39 ☑
          stationary object (traffic) V27.99 ☑
            nontraffic V27.29 ☑
            while boarding or alighting V27.39 ☑
          streetcar (traffic) V26.99 ☑
            nontraffic V26.29 ☑
            while boarding or alighting V26.39 ☑
          three wheeled motor vehicle (traffic)
              V22.99 ☑
            nontraffic V22.29 ☑
            while boarding or alighting V22.39 ☑
          truck (traffic) V24.99 ☑
            nontraffic V24.29 ☑
            while boarding or alighting V24.39 ☑
          two wheeled motor vehicle (traffic) V22.99 ☑
            nontraffic V22.29 ☑
            while boarding or alighting V22.39 ☑
          van (traffic) V23.99 ☑
            nontraffic V23.29 ☑
            while boarding or alighting V23.39 ☑
      driver
        collision (with)
          animal (traffic) V20.49 ☑
            being ridden (traffic) V26.49 ☑
              nontraffic V26.09 ☑
            nontraffic V20.09 ☑
          animal-drawn vehicle (traffic) V26.49 ☑
            nontraffic V26.09 ☑
          bus (traffic) V24.49 ☑
            nontraffic V24.09 ☑
          car (traffic) V23.49 ☑
            nontraffic V23.09 ☑
          motor vehicle NOS (traffic) V29.408 ☑
            nontraffic V29.008 ☑
            specified type NEC (traffic) V29.498 ☑
              nontraffic V29.098 ☑
          pedal cycle (traffic) V21.49 ☑
            nontraffic V21.09 ☑
          pedestrian
            nontraffic V20.09 ☑
            traffic V20.49 ☑
          pickup truck (traffic) V23.49 ☑
            nontraffic V23.09 ☑
          railway vehicle (traffic) V25.49 ☑
            nontraffic V25.09 ☑
          specified vehicle NEC (traffic) V26.49 ☑
            nontraffic V26.09 ☑
          stationary object (traffic) V27.49 ☑
            nontraffic V27.09 ☑
          streetcar (traffic) V26.49 ☑
            nontraffic V26.09 ☑
          three wheeled motor vehicle (traffic)
              V22.49 ☑
            nontraffic V22.09 ☑
          truck (traffic) V24.49 ☑
            nontraffic V24.09 ☑
          two wheeled motor vehicle (traffic)
              V22.49 ☑
            nontraffic V22.09 ☑
          van (traffic) V23.49 ☑
            nontraffic V23.09 ☑
        noncollision accident (traffic) V28.49 ☑
          nontraffic V28.09 ☑
      noncollision accident (traffic) V28.99 ☑
        nontraffic V28.29 ☑
        while boarding or alighting V28.39 ☑
      nontraffic V29.39 ☑

Accident — *continued*
  transport — *continued*
    motorcyclist — *continued*
      passenger
        collision (with)
          animal (traffic) V20.59 ☑
            being ridden (traffic) V26.59 ☑
              nontraffic V26.19 ☑
            nontraffic V20.19 ☑
          animal-drawn vehicle (traffic) V26.59 ☑
            nontraffic V26.19 ☑
          bus (traffic) V24.59 ☑
            nontraffic V24.19 ☑
          car (traffic) V23.59 ☑
            nontraffic V23.19 ☑
          motor vehicle NOS (traffic) V29.508 ☑
            nontraffic V29.108 ☑
            specified type NEC (traffic) V29.598 ☑
              nontraffic V29.198 ☑
          pedal cycle (traffic) V21.59 ☑
            nontraffic V21.19 ☑
          pedestrian
            nontraffic V20.19 ☑
            traffic V20.59 ☑
          pickup truck (traffic) V23.59 ☑
            nontraffic V23.19 ☑
          railway vehicle (traffic) V25.59 ☑
            nontraffic V25.19 ☑
          specified vehicle NEC (traffic) V26.59 ☑
            nontraffic V26.19 ☑
          stationary object (traffic) V27.59 ☑
            nontraffic V27.19 ☑
          streetcar (traffic) V26.59 ☑
            nontraffic V26.19 ☑
          three wheeled motor vehicle (traffic)
              V22.59 ☑
            nontraffic V22.19 ☑
          truck (traffic) V24.59 ☑
            nontraffic V24.19 ☑
          two wheeled motor vehicle (traffic)
              V22.59 ☑
            nontraffic V22.19 ☑
          van (traffic) V23.59 ☑
            nontraffic V23.19 ☑
        noncollision accident (traffic) V28.59 ☑
          nontraffic V28.19 ☑
      specified type NEC V29.888 ☑
      military vehicle V29.818 ☑
    occupant (of)
      aircraft (powered) V95.9 ☑
        fixed wing
          commercial — *see* Accident, transport,
              aircraft, occupant, powered, fixed
              wing, commercial
          private — *see* Accident, transport, air-
              craft, occupant, powered, fixed
              wing, private
        nonpowered V96.9 ☑
        specified NEC V95.8 ☑
      airport battery-powered vehicle — *see* Accident,
          transport, industrial vehicle occupant
      all-terrain vehicle (ATV) — *see* Accident, trans-
          port, all-terrain vehicle occupant
      animal-drawn vehicle — *see* Accident, transport,
          animal-drawn vehicle occupant
      automobile — *see* Accident, transport, car occu-
          pant
      balloon V96.00 ☑
      battery-powered vehicle — *see* Accident, trans-
          port, industrial vehicle occupant
      bicycle — *see* Accident, transport, pedal cyclist
        motorized — *see* Accident, transport, motor-
            cycle rider
      boat NEC — *see* Accident, watercraft
      bulldozer — *see* Accident, transport, construction
          vehicle occupant
      bus — *see* Accident, transport, bus occupant
      cable car (on rails) — *see also* Accident, transport,
          streetcar occupant
        not on rails V98.0 ☑
      car — *see also* Accident, transport, car occupant
        cable (on rails) — *see also* Accident, transport,
            streetcar occupant
        not on rails V98.0 ☑
      coach — *see* Accident, transport, bus occupant

Accident — *continued*
  transport — *continued*
    occupant — *continued*
      coal-car — *see* Accident, transport, industrial
          vehicle occupant
      digger — *see* Accident, transport, construction
          vehicle occupant
      dump truck — *see* Accident, transport, construc-
          tion vehicle occupant
      earth-leveler — *see* Accident, transport, construc-
          tion vehicle occupant
      farm machinery (self-propelled) — *see* Accident,
          transport, agricultural vehicle occupant
      forklift — *see* Accident, transport, industrial ve-
          hicle occupant
      glider (unpowered) V96.20 ☑
        hang V96.10 ☑
        powered (microlight) (ultralight) — *see* Acci-
            dent, transport, aircraft, occupant,
            powered, glider
      glider (unpowered) NEC V96.20 ☑
      hang-glider V96.10 ☑
      harvester — *see* Accident, transport, agricultural
          vehicle occupant
      heavy (transport) vehicle — *see* Accident, trans-
          port, truck occupant
      helicopter — *see* Accident, transport, aircraft,
          occupant, helicopter
      ice-yacht V98.2 ☑
      kite (carrying person) V96.8 ☑
      land-yacht V98.1 ☑
      logging car — *see* Accident, transport, industrial
          vehicle occupant
      mechanical shovel — *see* Accident, transport,
          construction vehicle occupant
      microlight — *see* Accident, transport, aircraft,
          occupant, powered, glider
      minibus — *see* Accident, transport, pickup truck
          occupant
      minivan — *see* Accident, transport, pickup truck
          occupant
      moped — *see* Accident, transport, motorcycle
      motor scooter — *see* Accident, transport, motor-
          cycle
      motorcycle (with sidecar) — *see* Accident,
          transport, motorcycle
      off-road motor-vehicle — *see also* Accident,
          transport, all-terrain vehicle occupant
          V86.99 ☑
      pedal cycle — *see also* Accident, transport, pedal
          cyclist
      pick-up (truck) — *see* Accident, transport, pickup
          truck occupant
      railway (train) (vehicle) (subterranean) (elevated)
          — *see* Accident, transport, railway vehicle
          occupant
      rickshaw — *see* Accident, transport, pedal cycle
        motorized — *see* Accident, transport, three-
            wheeled motor vehicle
        pedal driven — *see* Accident, transport, pedal
            cyclist
      road-roller — *see* Accident, transport, construc-
          tion vehicle occupant
      ship NOS V94.9 ☑
      ski-lift (chair) (gondola) V98.3 ☑
      snowmobile — *see* Accident, transport, snowmo-
          bile occupant
      spacecraft, spaceship — *see* Accident, transport,
          aircraft, occupant, spacecraft
      sport utility vehicle — *see* Accident, transport,
          pickup truck occupant
      streetcar (interurban) (operating on public street
          or highway) — *see* Accident, transport,
          streetcar occupant
      SUV — *see* Accident, transport, pickup truck oc-
          cupant
      téléférique V98.0 ☑
      three-wheeled vehicle (motorized) — *see also*
          Accident, transport, three-wheeled motor
          vehicle occupant
        nonmotorized — *see* Accident, transport,
            pedal cycle
      tractor (farm) (and trailer) — *see* Accident,
          transport, agricultural vehicle occupant
      train — *see* Accident, transport, railway vehicle
          occupant

Accident — *continued*
  transport — *continued*
    occupant — *continued*
      tram — *see* Accident, transport, streetcar occupant
        in mine or quarry — *see* Accident, transport, industrial vehicle occupant
      tricycle — *see* Accident, transport, pedal cycle
        motorized — *see* Accident, transport, three-wheeled motor vehicle
      trolley — *see* Accident, transport, streetcar occupant
        in mine or quarry — *see* Accident, transport, industrial vehicle occupant
      tub, in mine or quarry — *see* Accident, transport, industrial vehicle occupant
      ultralight — *see* Accident, transport, aircraft, occupant, powered, glider
      van — *see* Accident, transport, van occupant
      vehicle NEC V89.9 ☑
        heavy transport — *see* Accident, transport, truck occupant
        motor (traffic) NEC V89.2 ☑
          nontraffic NEC V89.0 ☑
      watercraft NOS V94.9 ☑
        causing drowning — *see* Drowning, resulting from accident to boat
      off-road motor-vehicle — *see also* Accident, transport, all-terrain vehicle occupant V86.99 ☑
    parachutist V97.29 ☑
      after accident to aircraft — *see* Accident, transport, aircraft
      entangled in object V97.21 ☑
      injured on landing V97.22 ☑
    pedal cyclist V19.9 ☑
      collision (with)
        animal (traffic) V10.9 ☑
          being ridden (traffic) V16.9 ☑
            nontraffic V16.2 ☑
              while boarding or alighting V16.3 ☑
          nontraffic V10.2 ☑
            while boarding or alighting V10.3 ☑
        animal-drawn vehicle (traffic) V16.9 ☑
          nontraffic V16.2 ☑
            while boarding or alighting V16.3 ☑
        bus (traffic) V14.9 ☑
          nontraffic V14.2 ☑
            while boarding or alighting V14.3 ☑
        car (traffic) V13.9 ☑
          nontraffic V13.2 ☑
            while boarding or alighting V13.3 ☑
        motor vehicle NOS (traffic) V19.60 ☑
          nontraffic V19.20 ☑
          specified type NEC (traffic) V19.69 ☑
            nontraffic V19.29 ☑
        pedal cycle (traffic) V11.9 ☑
          nontraffic V11.2 ☑
            while boarding or alighting V11.3 ☑
        pickup truck (traffic) V13.9 ☑
          nontraffic V13.2 ☑
            while boarding or alighting V13.3 ☑
        railway vehicle (traffic) V15.9 ☑
          nontraffic V15.2 ☑
            while boarding or alighting V15.3 ☑
        specified vehicle NEC (traffic) V16.9 ☑
          nontraffic V16.2 ☑
            while boarding or alighting V16.3 ☑
        stationary object (traffic) V17.9 ☑
          nontraffic V17.2 ☑
            while boarding or alighting V17.3 ☑
        streetcar (traffic) V16.9 ☑
          nontraffic V16.2 ☑
            while boarding or alighting V16.3 ☑
        three wheeled motor vehicle (traffic) V12.9 ☑
          nontraffic V12.2 ☑
            while boarding or alighting V12.3 ☑
        truck (traffic) V14.9 ☑
          nontraffic V14.2 ☑
            while boarding or alighting V14.3 ☑
        two wheeled motor vehicle (traffic) V12.9 ☑
          nontraffic V12.2 ☑
            while boarding or alighting V12.3 ☑
        van (traffic) V13.9 ☑
          nontraffic V13.2 ☑
            while boarding or alighting V13.3 ☑

Accident — *continued*
  transport — *continued*
    pedal cyclist — *continued*
      driver
        collision (with)
          animal (traffic) V10.4 ☑
            being ridden (traffic) V16.4 ☑
              nontraffic V16.0 ☑
            nontraffic V10.0 ☑
          animal-drawn vehicle (traffic) V16.4 ☑
            nontraffic V16.0 ☑
          bus (traffic) V14.4 ☑
            nontraffic V14.0 ☑
          car (traffic) V13.4 ☑
            nontraffic V13.0 ☑
          motor vehicle NOS (traffic) V19.40 ☑
            nontraffic V19.00 ☑
            specified type NEC (traffic) V19.49 ☑
              nontraffic V19.09 ☑
          pedal cycle (traffic) V11.4 ☑
            nontraffic V11.0 ☑
          pickup truck (traffic) V13.4 ☑
            nontraffic V13.0 ☑
          railway vehicle (traffic) V15.4 ☑
            nontraffic V15.0 ☑
          specified vehicle NEC (traffic) V16.4 ☑
            nontraffic V16.0 ☑
          stationary object (traffic) V17.4 ☑
            nontraffic V17.0 ☑
          streetcar (traffic) V16.4 ☑
            nontraffic V16.0 ☑
          three wheeled motor vehicle (traffic) V12.4 ☑
            nontraffic V12.0 ☑
          truck (traffic) V14.4 ☑
            nontraffic V14.0 ☑
          two wheeled motor vehicle (traffic) V12.4 ☑
            nontraffic V12.0 ☑
          van (traffic) V13.4 ☑
            nontraffic V13.0 ☑
        noncollision accident (traffic) V18.4 ☑
          nontraffic V18.0 ☑
      noncollision accident (traffic) V18.9 ☑
        nontraffic V18.2 ☑
          while boarding or alighting V18.3 ☑
      nontraffic V19.3 ☑
      passenger
        collision (with)
          animal (traffic) V10.5 ☑
            being ridden (traffic) V16.5 ☑
              nontraffic V16.1 ☑
            nontraffic V10.1 ☑
          animal-drawn vehicle (traffic) V16.5 ☑
            nontraffic V16.1 ☑
          bus (traffic) V14.5 ☑
            nontraffic V14.1 ☑
          car (traffic) V13.5 ☑
            nontraffic V13.1 ☑
          motor vehicle NOS (traffic) V19.50 ☑
            nontraffic V19.10 ☑
            specified type NEC (traffic) V19.59 ☑
              nontraffic V19.19 ☑
          pedal cycle (traffic) V11.5 ☑
            nontraffic V11.1 ☑
          pickup truck (traffic) V13.5 ☑
            nontraffic V13.1 ☑
          railway vehicle (traffic) V15.5 ☑
            nontraffic V15.1 ☑
          specified vehicle NEC (traffic) V16.5 ☑
            nontraffic V16.1 ☑
          stationary object (traffic) V17.5 ☑
            nontraffic V17.1 ☑
          streetcar (traffic) V16.5 ☑
            nontraffic V16.1 ☑
          three wheeled motor vehicle (traffic) V12.5 ☑
            nontraffic V12.1 ☑
          truck (traffic) V14.5 ☑
            nontraffic V14.1 ☑
          two wheeled motor vehicle (traffic) V12.5 ☑
            nontraffic V12.1 ☑
          van (traffic) V13.5 ☑
            nontraffic V13.1 ☑
        noncollision accident (traffic) V18.5 ☑

Accident — *continued*
  transport — *continued*
    pedal cyclist — *continued*
      passenger — *continued*
        noncollision accident — *continued*
          nontraffic V18.1 ☑
        specified type NEC V19.88 ☑
        military vehicle V19.81 ☑
    pedestrian
      conveyance (occupant) V09.9 ☑
        baby stroller V00.828 ☑
          collision (with) V09.9 ☑
            animal being ridden or animal drawn vehicle V06.99 ☑
              nontraffic V06.09 ☑
              traffic V06.19 ☑
            bus or heavy transport V04.99 ☑
              nontraffic V04.09 ☑
              traffic V04.19 ☑
            car V03.99 ☑
              nontraffic V03.09 ☑
              traffic V03.19 ☑
            pedal cycle V01.99 ☑
              nontraffic V01.09 ☑
              traffic V01.19 ☑
            pick-up truck or van V03.99 ☑
              nontraffic V03.09 ☑
              traffic V03.19 ☑
            railway (train) (vehicle) V05.99 ☑
              nontraffic V05.09 ☑
              traffic V05.19 ☑
            stationary object V00.822 ☑
            streetcar V06.99 ☑
              nontraffic V06.09 ☑
              traffic V06.19 ☑
            two- or three-wheeled motor vehicle V02.99 ☑
              nontraffic V02.09 ☑
              traffic V02.19 ☑
            vehicle V09.9 ☑
              animal-drawn V06.99 ☑
                nontraffic V06.09 ☑
                traffic V06.19 ☑
              motor
                nontraffic V09.00 ☑
                traffic V09.20 ☑
        fall V00.821 ☑
        nontraffic V09.1 ☑
          involving motor vehicle NEC V09.00 ☑
        traffic V09.3 ☑
          involving motor vehicle NEC V09.20 ☑
      flat-bottomed NEC V00.388 ☑
        collision (with) V09.9 ☑
          animal being ridden or animal drawn vehicle V06.99 ☑
            nontraffic V06.09 ☑
            traffic V06.19 ☑
          bus or heavy transport V04.99 ☑
            nontraffic V04.09 ☑
            traffic V04.19 ☑
          car V03.99 ☑
            nontraffic V03.09 ☑
            traffic V03.19 ☑
          pedal cycle V01.99 ☑
            nontraffic V01.09 ☑
            traffic V01.19 ☑
          pick-up truck or van V03.99 ☑
            nontraffic V03.09 ☑
            traffic V03.19 ☑
          railway (train) (vehicle) V05.99 ☑
            nontraffic V05.09 ☑
            traffic V05.19 ☑
          stationary object V00.382 ☑
          streetcar V06.99 ☑
            nontraffic V06.09 ☑
            traffic V06.19 ☑
          two- or three-wheeled motor vehicle V02.99 ☑
            nontraffic V02.09 ☑
            traffic V02.19 ☑
          vehicle V09.9 ☑
            animal-drawn V06.99 ☑
              nontraffic V06.09 ☑
              traffic V06.19 ☑
            motor
              nontraffic V09.00 ☑

☑ **Additional Character Required — Refer to the Tabular List for Character Selection**

Accident — *continued*
  transport — *continued*
    pedestrian — *continued*
      conveyance — *continued*
        flat-bottomed — *continued*
          collision — *continued*
            vehicle — *continued*
              motor — *continued*
                traffic V09.20 ☑
          fall V00.381 ☑
          nontraffic V09.1 ☑
            involving motor vehicle NEC V09.00 ☑
        snow
          board — *see* Accident, transport,
              pedestrian, conveyance, snow
              board
          ski — *see* Accident, transport, pedes-
              trian, conveyance, skis (snow)
          traffic V09.3 ☑
            involving motor vehicle NEC V09.20 ☑
        gliding type NEC V00.288 ☑
          collision (with) V09.9 ☑
            animal being ridden or animal drawn
                vehicle V06.99 ☑
              nontraffic V06.09 ☑
              traffic V06.19 ☑
            bus or heavy transport V04.99 ☑
              nontraffic V04.09 ☑
              traffic V04.19 ☑
            car V03.99 ☑
              nontraffic V03.09 ☑
              traffic V03.19 ☑
            pedal cycle V01.99 ☑
              nontraffic V01.09 ☑
              traffic V01.19 ☑
            pick-up truck or van V03.99 ☑
              nontraffic V03.09 ☑
              traffic V03.19 ☑
            railway (train) (vehicle) V05.99 ☑
              nontraffic V05.09 ☑
              traffic V05.19 ☑
            stationary object V00.282 ☑
            streetcar V06.99 ☑
              nontraffic V06.09 ☑
              traffic V02.19 ☑
            two- or three-wheeled motor vehicle
                V02.99 ☑
              nontraffic V02.09 ☑
              traffic V02.19 ☑
            vehicle V09.9 ☑
              animal-drawn V06.99 ☑
                nontraffic V06.09 ☑
                traffic V06.19 ☑
              motor
                nontraffic V09.00 ☑
                traffic V09.20 ☑
          fall V00.281 ☑
        heelies — *see* Accident, transport,
            pedestrian, conveyance, heelies
        ice skate — *see* Accident, transport,
            pedestrian, conveyance, ice skate
        nontraffic V09.1 ☑
          involving motor vehicle NEC V09.00 ☑
        sled — *see* Accident, transport, pedestri-
            an, conveyance, sled
        traffic V09.3 ☑
          involving motor vehicle NEC V09.20 ☑
          wheelies — *see* Accident, transport,
              pedestrian, conveyance, heelies
      heelies V00.158 ☑
        colliding with stationary object
            V00.152 ☑
        fall V00.151 ☑
      hoverboard
        collision with
          animal being ridden or animal drawn
              vehicle V06.938 ☑
            nontraffic V06.038 ☑
            traffic V06.138 ☑
          bus or heavy transport V04.938 ☑
            nontraffic V04.038 ☑
            traffic V04.138 ☑
          car V03.938 ☑
            nontraffic V03.038 ☑
            traffic V03.138 ☑
          pedal cycle V01.938 ☑

Accident — *continued*
  transport — *continued*
    pedestrian — *continued*
      conveyance — *continued*
        hoverboard — *continued*
          collision with — *continued*
            pedal cycle — *continued*
              nontraffic V01.038 ☑
              traffic V01.138 ☑
            pick-up or van V03.938 ☑
              nontraffic V03.038 ☑
              traffic V03.138 ☑
            railway (train) (vehicle) V05.938 ☑
              nontraffic V05.038 ☑
              traffic V05.138 ☑
            streetcar V06.938 ☑
              nontraffic V06.038 ☑
              traffic V06.138 ☑
            three-wheeled motor vehicle
                V02.938 ☑
              nontraffic V02.038 ☑
              traffic V02.138 ☑
            two-wheeled motor vehicle
                V02.938 ☑
              nontraffic V02.038 ☑
              traffic V02.138 ☑
            vehicle, nonmotor, specified NEC
                V06.938 ☑
              nontraffic V06.038 ☑
              traffic V06.138 ☑
          fall V00.848 ☑
        ice skates V00.218 ☑
          collision (with) V09.9 ☑
            animal being ridden or animal drawn
                vehicle V06.99 ☑
              nontraffic V06.09 ☑
              traffic V06.19 ☑
            bus or heavy transport V04.99 ☑
              nontraffic V04.09 ☑
              traffic V04.19 ☑
            car V03.99 ☑
              nontraffic V03.09 ☑
              traffic V03.19 ☑
            pedal cycle V01.99 ☑
              nontraffic V01.09 ☑
              traffic V01.19 ☑
            pick-up truck or van V03.99 ☑
              nontraffic V03.09 ☑
              traffic V03.19 ☑
            railway (train) (vehicle) V05.99 ☑
              nontraffic V05.09 ☑
              traffic V05.19 ☑
            stationary object V00.212 ☑
            streetcar V06.99 ☑
              nontraffic V06.09 ☑
              traffic V06.19 ☑
            two- or three-wheeled motor vehicle
                V02.99 ☑
              nontraffic V02.09 ☑
              traffic V02.19 ☑
            vehicle V09.9 ☑
              animal-drawn V06.99 ☑
                nontraffic V06.09 ☑
                traffic V06.19 ☑
              motor
                nontraffic V09.00 ☑
                traffic V09.20 ☑
          fall V00.211 ☑
          nontraffic V09.1 ☑
            involving motor vehicle NEC V09.00 ☑
          traffic V09.3 ☑
            involving motor vehicle NEC V09.20 ☑
        motorized mobility scooter V00.838 ☑
          collision with stationary object
              V00.832 ☑
          fall from V00.831 ☑
        nontraffic V09.1 ☑
          involving motor vehicle V09.00 ☑
            military V09.01 ☑
            specified type NEC V09.09 ☑
        roller skates (non in-line) V00.128 ☑
          collision (with) V09.9 ☑
            animal being ridden or animal drawn
                vehicle V06.91 ☑
              nontraffic V06.01 ☑
              traffic V06.11 ☑

Accident — *continued*
  transport — *continued*
    pedestrian — *continued*
      conveyance — *continued*
        roller skates — *continued*
          collision — *continued*
            bus or heavy transport V04.91 ☑
              nontraffic V04.01 ☑
              traffic V04.11 ☑
            car V03.91 ☑
              nontraffic V03.01 ☑
              traffic V03.11 ☑
            pedal cycle V01.91 ☑
              nontraffic V01.01 ☑
              traffic V01.11 ☑
            pick-up truck or van V03.91 ☑
              nontraffic V03.01 ☑
              traffic V03.11 ☑
            railway (train) (vehicle) V05.91 ☑
              nontraffic V05.01 ☑
              traffic V05.11 ☑
            stationary object V00.122 ☑
            streetcar V06.91 ☑
              nontraffic V06.01 ☑
              traffic V06.11 ☑
            two- or three-wheeled motor vehicle
                V02.91 ☑
              nontraffic V02.01 ☑
              traffic V02.11 ☑
            vehicle V09.9 ☑
              animal-drawn V06.91 ☑
                nontraffic V06.01 ☑
                traffic V06.11 ☑
              motor
                nontraffic V09.00 ☑
                traffic V09.20 ☑
          fall V00.121 ☑
          in-line V00.118 ☑
            collision — *see also* Accident, trans-
                port, pedestrian, conveyance
                occupant, roller skates, collision
                with stationary object V00.112 ☑
            fall V00.111 ☑
          nontraffic V09.1 ☑
            involving motor vehicle NEC V09.00 ☑
          traffic V09.3 ☑
            involving motor vehicle NEC V09.20 ☑
        rolling shoes V00.158 ☑
          colliding with stationary object
              V00.152 ☑
          fall V00.151 ☑
        rolling type NEC V00.188 ☑
          collision (with) V09.9 ☑
            animal being ridden or animal drawn
                vehicle V06.99 ☑
              nontraffic V06.09 ☑
              traffic V06.19 ☑
            bus or heavy transport V04.99 ☑
              nontraffic V04.09 ☑
              traffic V04.19 ☑
            car V03.99 ☑
              nontraffic V03.09 ☑
              traffic V03.19 ☑
            pedal cycle V01.99 ☑
              nontraffic V01.09 ☑
              traffic V01.19 ☑
            pick-up truck or van V03.99 ☑
              nontraffic V03.09 ☑
              traffic V03.19 ☑
            railway (train) (vehicle) V05.99 ☑
              nontraffic V05.09 ☑
              traffic V05.19 ☑
            stationary object V00.182 ☑
            streetcar V06.99 ☑
              nontraffic V06.09 ☑
              traffic V06.19 ☑
            two- or three-wheeled motor vehicle
                V02.99 ☑
              nontraffic V02.09 ☑
              traffic V02.19 ☑
            vehicle V09.9 ☑
              animal-drawn V06.99 ☑
                nontraffic V06.09 ☑
                traffic V06.19 ☑
              motor
                nontraffic V09.00 ☑

Accident — *continued*
 transport — *continued*
  pedestrian — *continued*
   conveyance — *continued*
    rolling type — *continued*
     collision — *continued*
      vehicle — *continued*
       motor — *continued*
        traffic V09.20 ☑
     fall V00.181 ☑
     in-line roller skate — *see* Accident, transport, pedestrian, conveyance, roller skate, in-line
     nontraffic V09.1 ☑
      involving motor vehicle NEC V09.00 ☑
     roller skate — *see* Accident, transport, pedestrian, conveyance, roller skate
     scooter (non-motorized) — *see* Accident, transport, pedestrian, conveyance, scooter
     skateboard — *see* Accident, transport, pedestrian, conveyance, skateboard
     traffic V09.3 ☑
      involving motor vehicle NEC V09.20 ☑
    scooter (non-motorized) V00.148 ☑
     collision (with) V09.9 ☑
      animal being ridden or animal drawn vehicle V06.99 ☑
       nontraffic V06.09 ☑
       traffic V06.19 ☑
      bus or heavy transport V04.99 ☑
       nontraffic V04.09 ☑
       traffic V04.19 ☑
      car V03.99 ☑
       nontraffic V03.09 ☑
       traffic V03.19 ☑
      pedal cycle V01.99 ☑
       nontraffic V01.09 ☑
       traffic V01.19 ☑
      pick-up truck or van V03.99 ☑
       nontraffic V03.09 ☑
       traffic V03.19 ☑
      railway (train) (vehicle) V05.99 ☑
       nontraffic V05.09 ☑
       traffic V05.19 ☑
      stationary object V00.142 ☑
      streetcar V06.99 ☑
       nontraffic V06.09 ☑
       traffic V06.19 ☑
      two- or three-wheeled motor vehicle V02.99 ☑
       nontraffic V02.09 ☑
       traffic V02.19 ☑
      vehicle V09.9 ☑
       animal-drawn V06.99 ☑
        nontraffic V06.09 ☑
        traffic V06.19 ☑
       motor
        nontraffic V09.00 ☑
        traffic V09.20 ☑
     fall V00.141 ☑
     nontraffic V09.1 ☑
      involving motor vehicle NEC V09.00 ☑
     traffic V09.3 ☑
      involving motor vehicle NEC V09.20 ☑
    Segway
     collision with
      animal being ridden or animal drawn vehicle V06.938 ☑
       nontraffic V06.038 ☑
       traffic V06.138 ☑
      bus or heavy transport V04.938 ☑
       nontraffic V04.038 ☑
       traffic V04.138 ☑
      car V03.938 ☑
       nontraffic V03.038 ☑
       traffic V03.138 ☑
      pedal cycle V01.938 ☑
       nontraffic V01.038 ☑
       traffic V01.138 ☑
      pick-up or van V03.938 ☑
       nontraffic V03.038 ☑
       traffic V03.138 ☑
      railway (train) (vehicle) V05.938

Accident — *continued*
 transport — *continued*
  pedestrian — *continued*
   conveyance — *continued*
    Segway — *continued*
     collision with — *continued*
      railway V05.938 ☑
       nontraffic V05.038 ☑
       traffic V05.138 ☑
      streetcar V06.938 ☑
       nontraffic V06.038 ☑
       traffic V06.138 ☑
      three-wheeled vehicle V02.938 ☑
       nontraffic V02.038 ☑
       traffic V02.138 ☑
      two-wheeled vehicle V02.938 ☑
       nontraffic V02.038 ☑
       traffic V02.138 ☑
      vehicle, nonmotor, specified NEC V06.938 ☑
       nontraffic V06.038 ☑
       traffic V06.138 ☑
     fall V00.848 ☑
    skateboard V00.138 ☑
     collision (with) V09.9 ☑
      animal being ridden or animal drawn vehicle V06.92 ☑
       nontraffic V06.02 ☑
       traffic V06.12 ☑
      bus or heavy transport V04.92 ☑
       nontraffic V04.02 ☑
       traffic V04.12 ☑
      car V03.92 ☑
       nontraffic V03.02 ☑
       traffic V03.12 ☑
      pedal cycle V01.92 ☑
       nontraffic V01.02 ☑
       traffic V01.12 ☑
      pick-up truck or van V03.92 ☑
       nontraffic V03.02 ☑
       traffic V03.12 ☑
      railway (train) (vehicle) V05.92 ☑
       nontraffic V05.02 ☑
       traffic V05.12 ☑
      stationary object V00.132 ☑
      streetcar V06.92 ☑
       nontraffic V06.02 ☑
       traffic V06.12 ☑
      two- or three-wheeled motor vehicle V02.92 ☑
       nontraffic V02.02 ☑
       traffic V02.12 ☑
      vehicle V09.9 ☑
       animal-drawn V06.92 ☑
        nontraffic V06.02 ☑
        traffic V06.12 ☑
       motor
        nontraffic V09.00 ☑
        traffic V09.20 ☑
     fall V00.131 ☑
     nontraffic V09.1 ☑
      involving motor vehicle NEC V09.00 ☑
     traffic V09.3 ☑
      involving motor vehicle NEC V09.20 ☑
    skis (snow) V00.328 ☑
     collision (with) V09.9 ☑
      animal being ridden or animal drawn vehicle V06.99 ☑
       nontraffic V06.09 ☑
       traffic V06.19 ☑
      bus or heavy transport V04.99 ☑
       nontraffic V04.09 ☑
       traffic V04.19 ☑
      car V03.99 ☑
       nontraffic V03.09 ☑
       traffic V03.19 ☑
      pedal cycle V01.99 ☑
       nontraffic V01.09 ☑
       traffic V01.19 ☑
      pick-up truck or van V03.99 ☑
       nontraffic V03.09 ☑
       traffic V03.19 ☑
      railway (train) (vehicle) V05.99 ☑
       nontraffic V05.09 ☑
       traffic V05.19 ☑
      stationary object V00.322 ☑

Accident — *continued*
 transport — *continued*
  pedestrian — *continued*
   conveyance — *continued*
    skis — *continued*
     collision — *continued*
      streetcar V06.99 ☑
       nontraffic V06.09 ☑
       traffic V06.19 ☑
      two- or three-wheeled motor vehicle V02.99 ☑
       nontraffic V02.09 ☑
       traffic V02.19 ☑
      vehicle V09.9 ☑
       animal-drawn V06.99 ☑
        nontraffic V06.09 ☑
        traffic V06.19 ☑
       motor
        nontraffic V09.00 ☑
        traffic V09.20 ☑
     fall V00.321 ☑
     nontraffic V09.1 ☑
      involving motor vehicle NEC V09.00 ☑
     traffic V09.3 ☑
      involving motor vehicle NEC V09.20 ☑
    sled V00.228 ☑
     collision (with) V09.9 ☑
      animal being ridden or animal drawn vehicle V06.99 ☑
       nontraffic V06.09 ☑
       traffic V06.19 ☑
      bus or heavy transport V04.99 ☑
       nontraffic V04.09 ☑
       traffic V04.19 ☑
      car V03.99 ☑
       nontraffic V03.09 ☑
       traffic V03.19 ☑
      pedal cycle V01.99 ☑
       nontraffic V01.09 ☑
       traffic V01.19 ☑
      pick-up truck or van V03.99 ☑
       nontraffic V03.09 ☑
       traffic V03.19 ☑
      railway (train) (vehicle) V05.99 ☑
       nontraffic V05.09 ☑
       traffic V05.19 ☑
      stationary object V00.222 ☑
      streetcar V06.99 ☑
       nontraffic V06.09 ☑
       traffic V06.19 ☑
      two- or three-wheeled motor vehicle V02.99 ☑
       nontraffic V02.09 ☑
       traffic V02.19 ☑
      vehicle V09.9 ☑
       animal-drawn V06.99 ☑
        nontraffic V06.09 ☑
        traffic V06.19 ☑
       motor
        nontraffic V09.00 ☑
        traffic V09.20 ☑
     fall V00.221 ☑
     nontraffic V09.1 ☑
      involving motor vehicle NEC V09.00 ☑
     traffic V09.3 ☑
      involving motor vehicle NEC V09.20 ☑
    snow board V00.318 ☑
     collision (with) V09.9 ☑
      animal being ridden or animal drawn vehicle V06.99 ☑
       nontraffic V06.09 ☑
       traffic V06.19 ☑
      bus or heavy transport V04.99 ☑
       nontraffic V04.09 ☑
       traffic V04.19 ☑
      car V03.99 ☑
       nontraffic V03.09 ☑
       traffic V03.19 ☑
      pedal cycle V01.99 ☑
       nontraffic V01.09 ☑
       traffic V01.19 ☑
      pick-up truck or van V03.99 ☑
       nontraffic V03.09 ☑
       traffic V03.19 ☑
      railway (train) (vehicle) V05.99 ☑
       nontraffic V05.09 ☑

☑ Additional Character Required — Refer to the Tabular List for Character Selection

Accident — *continued*
  transport — *continued*
    pedestrian — *continued*
      conveyance — *continued*
        snow board — *continued*
          collision — *continued*
            railway — *continued*
              traffic V05.19 ☑
            stationary object V00.312 ☑
            streetcar V06.99 ☑
              nontraffic V06.09 ☑
              traffic V06.19 ☑
            two- or three-wheeled motor vehicle V02.99 ☑
              nontraffic V02.09 ☑
              traffic V02.19 ☑
            vehicle V09.9 ☑
              animal-drawn V06.99 ☑
                nontraffic V06.09 ☑
                traffic V06.19 ☑
              motor
                nontraffic V09.00 ☑
                traffic V09.20 ☑
           fall V00.311 ☑
          nontraffic V09.1 ☑
            involving motor vehicle NEC V09.00 ☑
          traffic V09.3 ☑
            involving motor vehicle NEC V09.20 ☑
        specified type NEC V00.898 ☑
          collision (with) V09.9 ☑
            animal being ridden or animal drawn vehicle V06.99 ☑
              nontraffic V06.09 ☑
              traffic V06.19 ☑
            bus or heavy transport V04.99 ☑
              nontraffic V04.09 ☑
              traffic V04.19 ☑
            car V03.99 ☑
              nontraffic V03.09 ☑
              traffic V03.19 ☑
            pedal cycle V01.99 ☑
              nontraffic V01.09 ☑
              traffic V01.19 ☑
            pick-up truck or van V03.99 ☑
              nontraffic V03.09 ☑
              traffic V03.19 ☑
            railway (train) (vehicle) V05.99 ☑
              nontraffic V05.09 ☑
              traffic V05.19 ☑
            stationary object V00.892 ☑
            streetcar V06.99 ☑
              nontraffic V06.09 ☑
              traffic V06.19 ☑
            two- or three-wheeled motor vehicle V02.99 ☑
              nontraffic V02.09 ☑
              traffic V02.19 ☑
            vehicle V09.9 ☑
              animal-drawn V06.99 ☑
                nontraffic V06.09 ☑
                traffic V06.19 ☑
              motor
                nontraffic V09.00 ☑
                traffic V09.20 ☑
          fall V00.891 ☑
         nontraffic V09.1 ☑
           involving motor vehicle NEC V09.00 ☑
        traffic V09.3 ☑
           involving motor vehicle NEC V09.20 ☑
      standing
        electric scooter
          collision with
            animal being ridden or animal drawn vehicle V06.931 ☑
              nontraffic V06.031 ☑
              traffic V06.131 ☑
            bus or heavy transport V04.931 ☑
              nontraffic V04.031 ☑
              traffic V04.131 ☑
            car V03.931 ☑
              nontraffic V04.031 ☑
              traffic V04.131 ☑
            pedal cycle V01.931 ☑
              nontraffic V01.031 ☑
              traffic V01.131 ☑
            pick-up or van V03.931 ☑

Accident — *continued*
  transport — *continued*
    pedestrian — *continued*
      conveyance — *continued*
        standing — *continued*
          electric scooter — *continued*
            collision with — *continued*
              pick-up or van — *continued*
                nontraffic V03.031 ☑
                traffic V03.131 ☑
              railway (train) (vehicle) V05.931 ☑
                nontraffic V05.031 ☑
                traffic V05.131 ☑
              streetcar V06.931 ☑
                nontraffic V06.031 ☑
                traffic V06.131 ☑
              three-wheeled motor vehicle V02.931 ☑
                nontraffic V02.031 ☑
                traffic V02.131 ☑
              two-wheeled motor vehicle V02.931 ☑
                nontraffic V02.031 ☑
                traffic V02.131 ☑
              vehicle, nonmotor, specified NEC V06.931 ☑
                nontraffic V06.031 ☑
                traffic V06.131 ☑
           fall V00.841 ☑
        micro-mobility pedestrian conveyance
          collision with
            animal being ridden or animal drawn vehicle V06.938 ☑
              nontraffic V06.038 ☑
              traffic V06.138 ☑
            bus or heavy transport V04.938 ☑
              nontraffic V04.038 ☑
              traffic V04.138 ☑
            car V03.938 ☑
              nontraffic V03.038 ☑
              traffic V03.138 ☑
            pedal cycle V01.938 ☑
              nontraffic V01.038 ☑
              traffic V01.138 ☑
            pick-up or van V03.938 ☑
              nontraffic V03.038 ☑
              traffic V03.138 ☑
            railway (train) (vehicle) V05.938 ☑
              nontraffic V05.038 ☑
              traffic V05.138 ☑
            stationary object V00.842 ☑
            streetcar V06.938 ☑
              nontraffic V06.038 ☑
              traffic V06.138 ☑
            three-wheeled motor vehicle V02.938 ☑
              nontraffic V02.038 ☑
              traffic V02.138 ☑
            two-wheeled motor vehicle V02.938 ☑
              nontraffic V02.038 ☑
              traffic V02.138 ☑
            vehicle, nonmotor, specified NEC V06.938 ☑
              nontraffic V06.038 ☑
              traffic V06.138 ☑
          fall V00.848 ☑
      traffic V09.3 ☑
        involving motor vehicle V09.20 ☑
          military V09.21 ☑
          specified type NEC V09.29 ☑
      wheelchair (powered) V00.818 ☑
        collision (with) V09.9 ☑
          animal being ridden or animal drawn vehicle V06.99 ☑
            nontraffic V06.09 ☑
            traffic V06.19 ☑
          bus or heavy transport V04.99 ☑
            nontraffic V04.09 ☑
            traffic V04.19 ☑
          car V03.99 ☑
            nontraffic V03.09 ☑
            traffic V03.19 ☑
          pedal cycle V01.99 ☑
            nontraffic V01.09 ☑
            traffic V01.19 ☑

Accident — *continued*
  transport — *continued*
    pedestrian — *continued*
      conveyance — *continued*
        wheelchair — *continued*
          collision — *continued*
            pick-up truck or van V03.99 ☑
              nontraffic V03.09 ☑
              traffic V03.19 ☑
            railway (train) (vehicle) V05.99 ☑
              nontraffic V05.09 ☑
              traffic V05.19 ☑
            stationary object V00.812 ☑
            streetcar V06.99 ☑
              nontraffic V06.09 ☑
              traffic V06.19 ☑
            two- or three-wheeled motor vehicle V02.99 ☑
              nontraffic V02.09 ☑
              traffic V02.19 ☑
            vehicle V09.9 ☑
              animal-drawn V06.99 ☑
                nontraffic V06.09 ☑
                traffic V06.19 ☑
              motor
                nontraffic V09.00 ☑
                traffic V09.20 ☑
          fall V00.811 ☑
        nontraffic V09.1 ☑
          involving motor vehicle NEC V09.00 ☑
        traffic V09.3 ☑
          involving motor vehicle NEC V09.20 ☑
      wheeled shoe V00.158 ☑
        colliding with stationary object V00.152 ☑
        fall V00.151 ☑
    on foot — *see also* Accident, pedestrian
      collision (with)
        animal being ridden or animal drawn vehicle V06.90 ☑
          nontraffic V06.00 ☑
          traffic V06.10 ☑
        bus or heavy transport V04.90 ☑
          nontraffic V04.00 ☑
          traffic V04.10 ☑
        car V03.90 ☑
          nontraffic V03.00 ☑
          traffic V03.10 ☑
        pedal cycle V01.90 ☑
          nontraffic V01.00 ☑
          traffic V01.10 ☑
        pick-up truck or van V03.90 ☑
          nontraffic V03.00 ☑
          traffic V03.10 ☑
        railway (train) (vehicle) V05.90 ☑
          nontraffic V05.00 ☑
          traffic V05.10 ☑
        streetcar V06.90 ☑
          nontraffic V06.00 ☑
          traffic V06.10 ☑
        two- or three-wheeled motor vehicle V02.90 ☑
          nontraffic V02.00 ☑
          traffic V02.10 ☑
        vehicle V09.9 ☑
          animal-drawn V06.90 ☑
           nontraffic V06.00 ☑
           traffic V06.10 ☑
          motor
      nontraffic V09.1 ☑
        involving motor vehicle V09.00 ☑
          military V09.01 ☑
          specified type NEC V09.09 ☑
      traffic V09.3 ☑
        involving motor vehicle V09.20 ☑
          military V09.21 ☑
          specified type NEC V09.29 ☑
    person NEC (unknown way or transportation) V99 ☑
      collision (between)
        bus (with)
          heavy transport vehicle (traffic) V87.5 ☑
          nontraffic V88.5 ☑
        car (with)
          bus (traffic) V87.3 ☑
           nontraffic V88.3 ☑
          heavy transport vehicle (traffic) V87.4 ☑

Accident — *continued*
  transport — *continued*
    person — *continued*
      collision — *continued*
        car — *continued*
          heavy transport vehicle — *continued*
            nontraffic V88.4 ☑
            nontraffic V88.5 ☑
          pick-up truck or van (traffic) V87.2 ☑
            nontraffic V88.2 ☑
          train or railway vehicle (traffic) V87.6 ☑
            nontraffic V88.6 ☑
          two-or three-wheeled motor vehicle
            (traffic) V87.0 ☑
            nontraffic V88.0 ☑
        motor vehicle (traffic) NEC V87.7 ☑
          nontraffic V88.7 ☑
        two-or three-wheeled vehicle (with) (traffic)
          motor vehicle NEC V87.1 ☑
          nontraffic V88.1 ☑
        nonmotor vehicle (collision) (noncollision) (traffic) V87.9 ☑
          nontraffic V88.9 ☑
    pickup truck occupant V59.9 ☑
      collision (with)
        animal (traffic) V50.9 ☑
          being ridden (traffic) V56.9 ☑
            nontraffic V56.3 ☑
              while boarding or alighting V56.4 ☑
          nontraffic V50.3 ☑
          while boarding or alighting V50.4 ☑
        animal-drawn vehicle (traffic) V56.9 ☑
          nontraffic V56.3 ☑
          while boarding or alighting V56.4 ☑
        bus (traffic) V54.9 ☑
          nontraffic V54.3 ☑
          while boarding or alighting V54.4 ☑
        car (traffic) V53.9 ☑
          nontraffic V53.3 ☑
          while boarding or alighting V53.4 ☑
        motor vehicle NOS (traffic) V59.60 ☑
          nontraffic V59.20 ☑
          specified type NEC (traffic) V59.69 ☑
            nontraffic V59.29 ☑
        pedal cycle (traffic) V51.9 ☑
          nontraffic V51.3 ☑
          while boarding or alighting V51.4 ☑
        pickup truck (traffic) V53.9 ☑
          nontraffic V53.3 ☑
          while boarding or alighting V53.4 ☑
        railway vehicle (traffic) V55.9 ☑
          nontraffic V55.3 ☑
          while boarding or alighting V55.4 ☑
        specified vehicle NEC (traffic) V56.9 ☑
          nontraffic V56.3 ☑
          while boarding or alighting V56.4 ☑
        stationary object (traffic) V57.9 ☑
          nontraffic V57.3 ☑
          while boarding or alighting V57.4 ☑
        streetcar (traffic) V56.9 ☑
          nontraffic V56.3 ☑
          while boarding or alighting V56.4 ☑
        three wheeled motor vehicle (traffic) V52.9 ☑
          nontraffic V52.3 ☑
          while boarding or alighting V52.4 ☑
        truck (traffic) V54.9 ☑
          nontraffic V54.3 ☑
          while boarding or alighting V54.4 ☑
        two wheeled motor vehicle (traffic) V52.9 ☑
          nontraffic V52.3 ☑
          while boarding or alighting V52.4 ☑
        van (traffic) V53.9 ☑
          nontraffic V53.3 ☑
          while boarding or alighting V53.4 ☑
      driver
        collision (with)
          animal (traffic) V50.5 ☑
            being ridden (traffic) V56.5 ☑
              nontraffic V56.0 ☑
            nontraffic V50.0 ☑
          animal-drawn vehicle (traffic) V56.5 ☑
            nontraffic V56.0 ☑
          bus (traffic) V54.5 ☑
            nontraffic V54.0 ☑
          car (traffic) V53.5 ☑
            nontraffic V53.0 ☑

Accident — *continued*
  transport — *continued*
    pickup truck occupant — *continued*
      driver — *continued*
        collision — *continued*
          motor vehicle NOS (traffic) V59.40 ☑
            nontraffic V59.00 ☑
            specified type NEC (traffic) V59.49 ☑
              nontraffic V59.09 ☑
          pedal cycle (traffic) V51.5 ☑
            nontraffic V51.0 ☑
          pickup truck (traffic) V53.5 ☑
            nontraffic V53.0 ☑
          railway vehicle (traffic) V55.5 ☑
            nontraffic V55.0 ☑
          specified vehicle NEC (traffic) V56.5 ☑
            nontraffic V56.0 ☑
          stationary object (traffic) V57.5 ☑
            nontraffic V57.0 ☑
          streetcar (traffic) V56.5 ☑
            nontraffic V56.0 ☑
          three wheeled motor vehicle (traffic)
            V52.5 ☑
            nontraffic V52.0 ☑
          truck (traffic) V54.5 ☑
            nontraffic V54.0 ☑
          two wheeled motor vehicle (traffic)
            V52.5 ☑
            nontraffic V52.0 ☑
          van (traffic) V53.5 ☑
            nontraffic V53.0 ☑
        noncollision accident (traffic) V58.5 ☑
          nontraffic V58.0 ☑
      hanger-on
        collision (with)
          animal (traffic) V50.7 ☑
            being ridden (traffic) V56.7 ☑
              nontraffic V56.2 ☑
            nontraffic V50.2 ☑
          animal-drawn vehicle (traffic) V56.7 ☑
            nontraffic V56.2 ☑
          bus (traffic) V54.7 ☑
            nontraffic V54.2 ☑
          car (traffic) V53.7 ☑
            nontraffic V53.2 ☑
          pedal cycle (traffic) V51.7 ☑
            nontraffic V51.2 ☑
          pickup truck (traffic) V53.7 ☑
            nontraffic V53.2 ☑
          railway vehicle (traffic) V55.7 ☑
            nontraffic V55.2 ☑
          specified vehicle NEC (traffic) V56.7 ☑
            nontraffic V56.2 ☑
          stationary object (traffic) V57.7 ☑
            nontraffic V57.2 ☑
          streetcar (traffic) V56.7 ☑
            nontraffic V56.2 ☑
          three wheeled motor vehicle (traffic)
            V52.7 ☑
            nontraffic V52.2 ☑
          truck (traffic) V54.7 ☑
            nontraffic V54.2 ☑
          two wheeled motor vehicle (traffic)
            V52.7 ☑
            nontraffic V52.2 ☑
          van (traffic) V53.7 ☑
            nontraffic V53.2 ☑
        noncollision accident (traffic) V58.7 ☑
          nontraffic V58.2 ☑
      noncollision accident (traffic) V58.9 ☑
        nontraffic V58.3 ☑
        while boarding or alighting V58.4 ☑
      nontraffic V59.3 ☑
      passenger
        collision (with)
          animal (traffic) V50.6 ☑
            being ridden (traffic) V56.6 ☑
              nontraffic V56.1 ☑
            nontraffic V50.1 ☑
          animal-drawn vehicle (traffic) V56.6 ☑
            nontraffic V56.1 ☑
          bus (traffic) V54.6 ☑
            nontraffic V54.1 ☑
          car (traffic) V53.6 ☑
            nontraffic V53.1 ☑
          motor vehicle NOS (traffic) V59.50 ☑

Accident — *continued*
  transport — *continued*
    pickup truck occupant — *continued*
      passenger — *continued*
        collision — *continued*
          motor vehicle — *continued*
            nontraffic V59.10 ☑
            specified type NEC (traffic) V59.59 ☑
              nontraffic V59.19 ☑
          pedal cycle (traffic) V51.6 ☑
            nontraffic V51.1 ☑
          pickup truck (traffic) V53.6 ☑
            nontraffic V53.1 ☑
          railway vehicle (traffic) V55.6 ☑
            nontraffic V55.1 ☑
          specified vehicle NEC (traffic) V56.6 ☑
            nontraffic V56.1 ☑
          stationary object (traffic) V57.6 ☑
            nontraffic V57.1 ☑
          streetcar (traffic) V56.6 ☑
            nontraffic V56.1 ☑
          three wheeled motor vehicle (traffic)
            V52.6 ☑
            nontraffic V52.1 ☑
          truck (traffic) V54.6 ☑
            nontraffic V54.1 ☑
          two wheeled motor vehicle (traffic)
            V52.6 ☑
            nontraffic V52.1 ☑
          van (traffic) V53.6 ☑
            nontraffic V53.1 ☑
        noncollision accident (traffic) V58.6 ☑
          nontraffic V58.1 ☑
      specified type NEC V59.88 ☑
      military vehicle V59.81 ☑
    quarry truck — *see* Accident, transport, industrial
      vehicle occupant
    race car — *see* Accident, transport, motor vehicle
      NEC occupant
    railway vehicle occupant V81.9 ☑
      collision (with) V81.3 ☑
        motor vehicle (non-military) (traffic) V81.1 ☑
          military V81.83 ☑
          nontraffic V81.0 ☑
        rolling stock V81.2 ☑
        specified object NEC V81.3 ☑
      during derailment V81.7 ☑
        with antecedent collision — *see* Accident,
          transport, railway vehicle occupant,
          collision
      explosion V81.81 ☑
      fall (in railway vehicle) V81.5 ☑
        during derailment V81.7 ☑
          with antecedent collision — *see* Accident,
            transport, railway vehicle occupant,
            collision
        from railway vehicle V81.6 ☑
          during derailment V81.7 ☑
            with antecedent collision — *see* Accident, transport, railway vehicle
              occupant, collision
        while boarding or alighting V81.4 ☑
      fire V81.81 ☑
      object falling onto train V81.82 ☑
      specified type NEC V81.89 ☑
      while boarding or alighting V81.4 ☑
    Segway V00.848 ☑
    ski lift V98.3 ☑
    snowmobile occupant (nontraffic) V86.92 ☑
      driver V86.52 ☑
      hanger-on V86.72 ☑
      passenger V86.62 ☑
      traffic V86.32 ☑
        driver V86.02 ☑
        hanger-on V86.22 ☑
        passenger V86.12 ☑
      while boarding or alighting V86.42 ☑
    specified NEC V98.8 ☑
    sport utility vehicle occupant — *see also* Accident,
      transport, pickup truck occupant
    streetcar occupant V82.9 ☑
      collision (with) V82.3 ☑
        motor vehicle (traffic) V82.1 ☑
          nontraffic V82.0 ☑
        rolling stock V82.2 ☑
      during derailment V82.7 ☑

Accident — *continued*
  transport — *continued*
    streetcar occupant — *continued*
      during derailment — *continued*
        with antecedent collision — *see* Accident,
          transport, streetcar occupant, collision
      fall (in streetcar) V82.5 ☑
        during derailment V82.7 ☑
          with antecedent collision — *see* Accident,
            transport, streetcar occupant, colli-
            sion
        from streetcar V82.6 ☑
          during derailment V82.7 ☑
            with antecedent collision — *see* Acci-
              dent, transport, streetcar occu-
              pant, collision
        while boarding or alighting V82.4 ☑
      while boarding or alighting V82.4 ☑
      specified type NEC V82.8 ☑
      while boarding or alighting V82.4 ☑
    three-wheeled motor vehicle occupant V39.9 ☑
      collision (with)
        animal (traffic) V30.9 ☑
          being ridden (traffic) V36.9 ☑
            nontraffic V36.3 ☑
            while boarding or alighting V36.4 ☑
          nontraffic V30.3 ☑
          while boarding or alighting V30.4 ☑
        animal-drawn vehicle (traffic) V36.9 ☑
          nontraffic V36.3 ☑
          while boarding or alighting V36.4 ☑
        bus (traffic) V34.9 ☑
          nontraffic V34.3 ☑
          while boarding or alighting V34.4 ☑
        car (traffic) V33.9 ☑
          nontraffic V33.3 ☑
          while boarding or alighting V33.4 ☑
        motor vehicle NOS (traffic) V39.60 ☑
          nontraffic V39.20 ☑
          specified type NEC (traffic) V39.69 ☑
            nontraffic V39.29 ☑
        pedal cycle (traffic) V31.9 ☑
          nontraffic V31.3 ☑
          while boarding or alighting V31.4 ☑
        pickup truck (traffic) V33.9 ☑
          nontraffic V33.3 ☑
          while boarding or alighting V33.4 ☑
        railway vehicle (traffic) V35.9 ☑
          nontraffic V35.3 ☑
          while boarding or alighting V35.4 ☑
        specified vehicle NEC (traffic) V36.9 ☑
          nontraffic V36.3 ☑
          while boarding or alighting V36.4 ☑
        stationary object (traffic) V37.9 ☑
          nontraffic V37.3 ☑
          while boarding or alighting V37.4 ☑
        streetcar (traffic) V36.9 ☑
          nontraffic V36.3 ☑
          while boarding or alighting V36.4 ☑
        three wheeled motor vehicle (traffic) V32.9 ☑
          nontraffic V32.3 ☑
          while boarding or alighting V32.4 ☑
        truck (traffic) V34.9 ☑
          nontraffic V34.3 ☑
          while boarding or alighting V34.4 ☑
        two wheeled motor vehicle (traffic) V32.9 ☑
          nontraffic V32.3 ☑
          while boarding or alighting V32.4 ☑
        van (traffic) V33.9 ☑
          nontraffic V33.3 ☑
          while boarding or alighting V33.4 ☑
      driver
        collision (with)
          animal (traffic) V30.5 ☑
            being ridden (traffic) V36.5 ☑
              nontraffic V36.0 ☑
            nontraffic V30.0 ☑
          animal-drawn vehicle (traffic) V36.5 ☑
            nontraffic V36.0 ☑
          bus (traffic) V34.5 ☑
            nontraffic V34.0 ☑
          car (traffic) V33.5 ☑
            nontraffic V33.0 ☑
          motor vehicle NOS (traffic) V39.40 ☑
            nontraffic V39.00 ☑
            specified type NEC (traffic) V39.49 ☑

Accident — *continued*
  transport — *continued*
    three-wheeled motor vehicle occupant — *contin-
ued*
      driver — *continued*
        collision — *continued*
          motor vehicle — *continued*
            specified type — *continued*
              nontraffic V39.09 ☑
          pedal cycle (traffic) V31.5 ☑
            nontraffic V31.0 ☑
          pickup truck (traffic) V33.5 ☑
            nontraffic V33.0 ☑
          railway vehicle (traffic) V35.5 ☑
            nontraffic V35.0 ☑
          specified vehicle NEC (traffic) V36.5 ☑
            nontraffic V36.0 ☑
          stationary object (traffic) V37.5 ☑
            nontraffic V37.0 ☑
          streetcar (traffic) V36.5 ☑
            nontraffic V36.0 ☑
          three wheeled motor vehicle (traffic)
            V32.5 ☑
            nontraffic V32.0 ☑
          truck (traffic) V34.5 ☑
            nontraffic V34.0 ☑
          two wheeled motor vehicle (traffic)
            V32.5 ☑
            nontraffic V32.0 ☑
          van (traffic) V33.5 ☑
            nontraffic V33.0 ☑
        noncollision accident (traffic) V38.5 ☑
          nontraffic V38.0 ☑
      hanger-on
        collision (with)
          animal (traffic) V30.7 ☑
            being ridden (traffic) V36.7 ☑
              nontraffic V36.2 ☑
            nontraffic V30.2 ☑
          animal-drawn vehicle (traffic) V36.7 ☑
            nontraffic V36.2 ☑
          bus (traffic) V34.7 ☑
            nontraffic V34.2 ☑
          car (traffic) V33.7 ☑
            nontraffic V33.2 ☑
          pedal cycle (traffic) V31.7 ☑
            nontraffic V31.2 ☑
          pickup truck (traffic) V33.7 ☑
            nontraffic V33.2 ☑
          railway vehicle (traffic) V35.7 ☑
            nontraffic V35.2 ☑
          specified vehicle NEC (traffic) V36.7 ☑
            nontraffic V36.2 ☑
          stationary object (traffic) V37.7 ☑
            nontraffic V37.2 ☑
          streetcar (traffic) V36.7 ☑
            nontraffic V36.2 ☑
          three wheeled motor vehicle (traffic)
            V32.7 ☑
            nontraffic V32.2 ☑
          truck (traffic) V34.7 ☑
            nontraffic V34.2 ☑
          two wheeled motor vehicle (traffic)
            V32.7 ☑
            nontraffic V32.2 ☑
          van (traffic) V33.7 ☑
            nontraffic V33.2 ☑
        noncollision accident (traffic) V38.7 ☑
          nontraffic V38.2 ☑
      noncollision accident (traffic) V38.9 ☑
        nontraffic V38.3 ☑
        while boarding or alighting V38.4 ☑
      nontraffic V39.3 ☑
      passenger
        collision (with)
          animal (traffic) V30.6 ☑
            being ridden (traffic) V36.6 ☑
              nontraffic V36.1 ☑
            nontraffic V30.1 ☑
          animal-drawn vehicle (traffic) V36.6 ☑
            nontraffic V36.1 ☑
          bus (traffic) V34.6 ☑
            nontraffic V34.1 ☑
          car (traffic) V33.6 ☑
            nontraffic V33.1 ☑
          motor vehicle NOS (traffic) V39.50 ☑

Accident — *continued*
  transport — *continued*
    three-wheeled motor vehicle occupant — *contin-
ued*
      passenger — *continued*
        collision — *continued*
          motor vehicle — *continued*
            nontraffic V39.10 ☑
            specified type NEC (traffic) V39.59 ☑
              nontraffic V39.19 ☑
          pedal cycle (traffic) V31.6 ☑
            nontraffic V31.1 ☑
          pickup truck (traffic) V33.6 ☑
            nontraffic V33.1 ☑
          railway vehicle (traffic) V35.6 ☑
            nontraffic V35.1 ☑
          specified vehicle NEC (traffic) V36.6 ☑
            nontraffic V36.1 ☑
          stationary object (traffic) V37.6 ☑
            nontraffic V37.1 ☑
          streetcar (traffic) V36.6 ☑
            nontraffic V36.1 ☑
          three wheeled motor vehicle (traffic)
            V32.6 ☑
            nontraffic V32.1 ☑
          truck (traffic) V34.6 ☑
            nontraffic V34.1 ☑
          two wheeled motor vehicle (traffic)
            V32.6 ☑
            nontraffic V32.1 ☑
          van (traffic) V33.6 ☑
            nontraffic V33.1 ☑
        noncollision accident (traffic) V38.6 ☑
          nontraffic V38.1 ☑
      specified type NEC V39.89 ☑
      military vehicle V39.81 ☑
    tractor (farm) (and trailer) — *see* Accident, transport,
      agricultural vehicle occupant
    tram — *see* Accident, transport, streetcar
      in mine or quarry — *see* Accident, transport, in-
        dustrial vehicle occupant
    trolley — *see* Accident, transport, streetcar
      in mine or quarry — *see* Accident, transport, in-
        dustrial vehicle occupant
    truck (heavy) occupant V69.9 ☑
      collision (with)
        animal (traffic) V60.9 ☑
          being ridden (traffic) V66.9 ☑
            nontraffic V66.3 ☑
            while boarding or alighting V66.4 ☑
          nontraffic V60.3 ☑
          while boarding or alighting V60.4 ☑
        animal-drawn vehicle (traffic) V66.9 ☑
          nontraffic V66.3 ☑
          while boarding or alighting V66.4 ☑
        bus (traffic) V64.9 ☑
          nontraffic V64.3 ☑
          while boarding or alighting V64.4 ☑
        car (traffic) V63.9 ☑
          nontraffic V63.3 ☑
          while boarding or alighting V63.4 ☑
        motor vehicle NOS (traffic) V69.60 ☑
          nontraffic V69.20 ☑
          specified type NEC (traffic) V69.69 ☑
            nontraffic V69.29 ☑
        pedal cycle (traffic) V61.9 ☑
          nontraffic V61.3 ☑
          while boarding or alighting V61.4 ☑
        pickup truck (traffic) V63.9 ☑
          nontraffic V63.3 ☑
          while boarding or alighting V63.4 ☑
        railway vehicle (traffic) V65.9 ☑
          nontraffic V65.3 ☑
          while boarding or alighting V65.4 ☑
        specified vehicle NEC (traffic) V66.9 ☑
          nontraffic V66.3 ☑
          while boarding or alighting V66.4 ☑
        stationary object (traffic) V67.9 ☑
          nontraffic V67.3 ☑
          while boarding or alighting V67.4 ☑
        streetcar (traffic) V66.9 ☑
          nontraffic V66.3 ☑
          while boarding or alighting V66.4 ☑
        three wheeled motor vehicle (traffic) V62.9 ☑
          nontraffic V62.3 ☑
          while boarding or alighting V62.4 ☑

Accident — *continued*
  transport — *continued*
    truck occupant — *continued*
      collision — *continued*
        truck (traffic) V64.9 ✓
          nontraffic V64.3 ✓
          while boarding or alighting V64.4 ✓
        two wheeled motor vehicle (traffic) V62.9 ✓
          nontraffic V62.3 ✓
          while boarding or alighting V62.4 ✓
        van (traffic) V63.9 ✓
          nontraffic V63.3 ✓
          while boarding or alighting V63.4 ✓
      driver
        collision (with)
          animal (traffic) V60.5 ✓
            being ridden (traffic) V66.5 ✓
              nontraffic V66.0 ✓
            nontraffic V60.0 ✓
          animal-drawn vehicle (traffic) V66.5 ✓
            nontraffic V66.0 ✓
          bus (traffic) V64.5 ✓
            nontraffic V64.0 ✓
          car (traffic) V63.5 ✓
            nontraffic V63.0 ✓
          motor vehicle NOS (traffic) V69.40 ✓
            nontraffic V69.00 ✓
            specified type NEC (traffic) V69.49 ✓
              nontraffic V69.09 ✓
          pedal cycle (traffic) V61.5 ✓
            nontraffic V61.0 ✓
          pickup truck (traffic) V63.5 ✓
            nontraffic V63.0 ✓
          railway vehicle (traffic) V65.5 ✓
            nontraffic V65.0 ✓
          specified vehicle NEC (traffic) V66.5 ✓
            nontraffic V66.0 ✓
          stationary object (traffic) V67.5 ✓
            nontraffic V67.0 ✓
          streetcar (traffic) V66.5 ✓
            nontraffic V66.0 ✓
          three wheeled motor vehicle (traffic)
            V62.5 ✓
            nontraffic V62.0 ✓
          truck (traffic) V64.5 ✓
            nontraffic V64.0 ✓
          two wheeled motor vehicle (traffic)
            V62.5 ✓
            nontraffic V62.0 ✓
          van (traffic) V63.5 ✓
            nontraffic V63.0 ✓
        noncollision accident (traffic) V68.5 ✓
          nontraffic V68.0 ✓
      dump — *see* Accident, transport, construction
        vehicle occupant
      hanger-on
        collision (with)
          animal (traffic) V60.7 ✓
            being ridden (traffic) V66.7 ✓
              nontraffic V66.2 ✓
            nontraffic V60.2 ✓
          animal-drawn vehicle (traffic) V66.7 ✓
            nontraffic V66.2 ✓
          bus (traffic) V64.7 ✓
            nontraffic V64.2 ✓
          car (traffic) V63.7 ✓
            nontraffic V63.2 ✓
          pedal cycle (traffic) V61.7 ✓
            nontraffic V61.2 ✓
          pickup truck (traffic) V63.7 ✓
            nontraffic V63.2 ✓
          railway vehicle (traffic) V65.7 ✓
            nontraffic V65.2 ✓
          specified vehicle NEC (traffic) V66.7 ✓
            nontraffic V66.2 ✓
          stationary object (traffic) V67.7 ✓
            nontraffic V67.2 ✓
          streetcar (traffic) V66.7 ✓
            nontraffic V66.2 ✓
          three wheeled motor vehicle (traffic)
            V62.7 ✓
            nontraffic V62.2 ✓
          truck (traffic) V64.7 ✓
            nontraffic V64.2 ✓
          two wheeled motor vehicle (traffic)
            V62.7 ✓

Accident — *continued*
  transport — *continued*
    truck occupant — *continued*
      hanger-on — *continued*
        collision — *continued*
          two wheeled motor vehicle — *continued*
            nontraffic V62.2 ✓
          van (traffic) V63.7 ✓
            nontraffic V63.2 ✓
        noncollision accident (traffic) V68.7 ✓
          nontraffic V68.2 ✓
      noncollision accident (traffic) V68.9 ✓
        nontraffic V68.3 ✓
        while boarding or alighting V68.4 ✓
      nontraffic V69.3 ✓
      passenger
        collision (with)
          animal (traffic) V60.6 ✓
            being ridden (traffic) V66.6 ✓
              nontraffic V66.1- ✓
            nontraffic V60.1 ✓
          animal-drawn vehicle (traffic) V66.6 ✓
            nontraffic V66.1 ✓
          bus (traffic) V64.6 ✓
            nontraffic V64.1 ✓
          car (traffic) V63.6 ✓
            nontraffic V63.1 ✓
          motor vehicle NOS (traffic) V69.50 ✓
            nontraffic V69.10 ✓
            specified type NEC (traffic) V69.59 ✓
              nontraffic V69.19 ✓
          pedal cycle (traffic) V61.6 ✓
            nontraffic V61.1 ✓
          pickup truck (traffic) V63.6 ✓
            nontraffic V63.1 ✓
          railway vehicle (traffic) V65.6 ✓
            nontraffic V65.1 ✓
          specified vehicle NEC (traffic) V66.6 ✓
            nontraffic V66.1 ✓
          stationary object (traffic) V67.6 ✓
            nontraffic V67.1 ✓
          streetcar (traffic) V66.6 ✓
            nontraffic V66.1 ✓
          three wheeled motor vehicle (traffic)
            V62.6 ✓
            nontraffic V62.1 ✓
          truck (traffic) V64.6 ✓
            nontraffic V64.1 ✓
          two wheeled motor vehicle (traffic)
            V62.6 ✓
            nontraffic V62.1 ✓
          van (traffic) V63.6 ✓
            nontraffic V63.1 ✓
        noncollision accident (traffic) V68.6 ✓
          nontraffic V68.1 ✓
      pickup — *see* Accident, transport, pickup truck
        occupant
      specified type NEC V69.88 ✓
        military vehicle V69.81 ✓
    van occupant V59.9 ✓
      collision (with)
        animal (traffic) V50.9 ✓
          being ridden (traffic) V56.9 ✓
            nontraffic V56.3 ✓
            while boarding or alighting V56.4 ✓
          nontraffic V50.3 ✓
          while boarding or alighting V50.4 ✓
          animal-drawn vehicle (traffic) V56.9 ✓
            nontraffic V56.3 ✓
            while boarding or alighting V56.4 ✓
          bus (traffic) V54.9 ✓
            nontraffic V54.3 ✓
            while boarding or alighting V54.4 ✓
          car (traffic) V53.9 ✓
            nontraffic V53.3 ✓
            while boarding or alighting V53.4 ✓
          motor vehicle NOS (traffic) V59.60 ✓
            nontraffic V59.20 ✓
            specified type NEC (traffic) V59.69 ✓
              nontraffic V59.29 ✓
          pedal cycle (traffic) V51.9 ✓
            nontraffic V51.3 ✓
            while boarding or alighting V51.4 ✓
          pickup truck (traffic) V53.9 ✓
            nontraffic V53.3 ✓

Accident — *continued*
  transport — *continued*
    van occupant — *continued*
      collision — *continued*
        pickup truck — *continued*
          while boarding or alighting V53.4 ✓
        railway vehicle (traffic) V55.9 ✓
          nontraffic V55.3 ✓
          while boarding or alighting V55.4 ✓
        specified vehicle NEC (traffic) V56.9 ✓
          nontraffic V56.3 ✓
          while boarding or alighting V56.4 ✓
        stationary object (traffic) V57.9 ✓
          nontraffic V57.3 ✓
          while boarding or alighting V57.4 ✓
        streetcar (traffic) V56.9 ✓
          nontraffic V56.3 ✓
          while boarding or alighting V56.4 ✓
        three wheeled motor vehicle (traffic) V52.9 ✓
          nontraffic V52.3 ✓
          while boarding or alighting V52.4 ✓
        truck (traffic) V54.9 ✓
          nontraffic V54.3 ✓
          while boarding or alighting V54.4 ✓
        two wheeled motor vehicle (traffic) V52.9 ✓
          nontraffic V52.3 ✓
          while boarding or alighting V52.4 ✓
        van (traffic) V53.9 ✓
          nontraffic V53.3 ✓
          while boarding or alighting V53.4 ✓
      driver
        collision (with)
          animal (traffic) V50.5 ✓
            being ridden (traffic) V56.5 ✓
              nontraffic V56.0 ✓
            nontraffic V50.0 ✓
          animal-drawn vehicle (traffic) V56.5 ✓
            nontraffic V56.0 ✓
          bus (traffic) V54.5 ✓
            nontraffic V54.0 ✓
          car (traffic) V53.5 ✓
            nontraffic V53.0 ✓
          motor vehicle NOS (traffic) V59.40 ✓
            nontraffic V59.00 ✓
            specified type NEC (traffic) V59.49 ✓
              nontraffic V59.09 ✓
          pedal cycle (traffic) V51.5 ✓
            nontraffic V51.0 ✓
          pickup truck (traffic) V53.5 ✓
            nontraffic V53.0 ✓
          railway vehicle (traffic) V55.5 ✓
            nontraffic V55.0 ✓
          specified vehicle NEC (traffic) V56.5 ✓
            nontraffic V56.0 ✓
          stationary object (traffic) V57.5 ✓
            nontraffic V57.0 ✓
          streetcar (traffic) V56.5 ✓
            nontraffic V56.0 ✓
          three wheeled motor vehicle (traffic)
            V52.5 ✓
            nontraffic V52.0 ✓
          truck (traffic) V54.5 ✓
            nontraffic V54.0 ✓
          two wheeled motor vehicle (traffic)
            V52.5 ✓
            nontraffic V52.0 ✓
          van (traffic) V53.5 ✓
            nontraffic V53.0 ✓
        noncollision accident (traffic) V58.5 ✓
          nontraffic V58.0 ✓
      hanger-on
        collision (with)
          animal (traffic) V50.7 ✓
            being ridden (traffic) V56.7 ✓
              nontraffic V56.2 ✓
            nontraffic V50.2 ✓
          animal-drawn vehicle (traffic) V56.7 ✓
            nontraffic V56.2 ✓
          bus (traffic) V54.7 ✓
            nontraffic V54.2 ✓
          car (traffic) V53.7 ✓
            nontraffic V53.2 ✓
          pedal cycle (traffic) V51.7 ✓
            nontraffic V51.2 ✓
          pickup truck (traffic) V53.7 ✓
            nontraffic V53.2 ✓

✓ Additional Character Required — Refer to the Tabular List for Character Selection

Accident — continued
  transport — continued
    van occupant — continued
      hanger-on — continued
        collision — continued
          railway vehicle (traffic) V55.7 ☑
            nontraffic V55.2 ☑
          specified vehicle NEC (traffic) V56.7 ☑
            nontraffic V56.2 ☑
          stationary object (traffic) V57.7 ☑
            nontraffic V57.2 ☑
          streetcar (traffic) V56.7 ☑
            nontraffic V56.2 ☑
          three wheeled motor vehicle (traffic)
            V52.7 ☑
            nontraffic V52.2 ☑
          truck (traffic) V54.7 ☑
            nontraffic V54.2 ☑
          two wheeled motor vehicle (traffic)
            V52.7 ☑
            nontraffic V52.2 ☑
          van (traffic) V53.7 ☑
            nontraffic V53.2 ☑
        noncollision accident (traffic) V58.7 ☑
          nontraffic V58.2 ☑
      noncollision accident (traffic) V58.9 ☑
        nontraffic V58.3 ☑
      while boarding or alighting V58.4 ☑
    nontraffic V59.3 ☑
    passenger
      collision (with)
        animal (traffic) V50.6 ☑
          being ridden (traffic) V56.6 ☑
            nontraffic V56.1 ☑
          nontraffic V50.1 ☑
        animal-drawn vehicle (traffic) V56.6 ☑
          nontraffic V56.1 ☑
        bus (traffic) V54.6 ☑
          nontraffic V54.1 ☑
        car (traffic) V53.6 ☑
          nontraffic V53.1 ☑
        motor vehicle NOS (traffic) V59.50 ☑
          nontraffic V59.10 ☑
          specified type NEC (traffic) V59.59 ☑
            nontraffic V59.19 ☑
        pedal cycle (traffic) V51.6 ☑
          nontraffic V51.1 ☑
        pickup truck (traffic) V53.6 ☑
          nontraffic V53.1 ☑
        railway vehicle (traffic) V55.6 ☑
          nontraffic V55.1 ☑
        specified vehicle NEC (traffic) V56.6 ☑
          nontraffic V56.1 ☑
        stationary object (traffic) V57.6 ☑
          nontraffic V57.1 ☑
        streetcar (traffic) V56.6 ☑
          nontraffic V56.1 ☑
        three wheeled motor vehicle (traffic)
          V52.6 ☑
          nontraffic V52.1 ☑
        truck (traffic) V54.6 ☑
          nontraffic V54.1 ☑
        two wheeled motor vehicle (traffic)
          V52.6 ☑
          nontraffic V52.1 ☑
        van (traffic) V53.6 ☑
          nontraffic V53.1 ☑
      noncollision accident (traffic) V58.6 ☑
        nontraffic V58.1 ☑
  specified type NEC V59.88 ☑
    military vehicle V59.81 ☑
  watercraft occupant — see Accident, watercraft
vehicle NEC V89.9 ☑
  animal-drawn NEC — see Accident, transport, ani-
    mal-drawn vehicle occupant
  special
    agricultural — see Accident, transport, agricultur-
      al vehicle occupant
    construction — see Accident, transport, construc-
      tion vehicle occupant
    industrial — see Accident, transport, industrial
      vehicle occupant
    three-wheeled NEC (motorized) — see Accident,
      transport, three-wheeled motor vehicle occu-
      pant
  watercraft V94.9 ☑

Accident — continued
  watercraft — continued
    causing
      drowning — see Drowning, due to, accident to,
        watercraft
      injury NEC V91.89 ☑
        crushed between craft and object V91.19 ☑
          powered craft V91.13 ☑
            ferry boat V91.11 ☑
            fishing boat V91.12 ☑
            jetskis V91.13 ☑
            liner V91.11 ☑
            merchant ship V91.10 ☑
            passenger ship V91.11 ☑
          unpowered craft V91.18 ☑
            canoe V91.15 ☑
            inflatable V91.16 ☑
            kayak V91.15 ☑
            sailboat V91.14 ☑
            surf-board V91.18 ☑
            windsurfer V91.18 ☑
        fall on board V91.29 ☑
          powered craft V91.23 ☑
            ferry boat V91.21 ☑
            fishing boat V91.22 ☑
            jetskis V91.23 ☑
            liner V91.21 ☑
            merchant ship V91.20 ☑
            passenger ship V91.21 ☑
          unpowered craft
            canoe V91.25 ☑
            inflatable V91.26 ☑
            kayak V91.25 ☑
            sailboat V91.24 ☑
        fire on board causing burn V91.09 ☑
          powered craft V91.03 ☑
            ferry boat V91.01 ☑
            fishing boat V91.02 ☑
            jetskis V91.03 ☑
            liner V91.01 ☑
            merchant ship V91.00 ☑
            passenger ship V91.01 ☑
          unpowered craft V91.08 ☑
            canoe V91.05 ☑
            inflatable V91.06 ☑
            kayak V91.05 ☑
            sailboat V91.04 ☑
            surf-board V91.08 ☑
            water skis V91.07 ☑
            windsurfer V91.08 ☑
        hit by falling object V91.39 ☑
          powered craft V91.33 ☑
            ferry boat V91.31 ☑
            fishing boat V91.32 ☑
            jetskis V91.33 ☑
            liner V91.31 ☑
            merchant ship V91.30 ☑
            passenger ship V91.31 ☑
          unpowered craft V91.38 ☑
            canoe V91.35 ☑
            inflatable V91.36 ☑
            kayak V91.35 ☑
            sailboat V91.34 ☑
            surf-board V91.38 ☑
            water skis V91.37 ☑
            windsurfer V91.38 ☑
        specified type NEC V91.89 ☑
          powered craft V91.83 ☑
            ferry boat V91.81 ☑
            fishing boat V91.82 ☑
            jetskis V91.83 ☑
            liner V91.81 ☑
            merchant ship V91.80 ☑
            passenger ship V91.81 ☑
          unpowered craft V91.88 ☑
            canoe V91.85 ☑
            inflatable V91.86 ☑
            kayak V91.85 ☑
            sailboat V91.84 ☑
            surf-board V91.88 ☑
            water skis V91.87 ☑
            windsurfer V91.88 ☑
    due to, caused by cataclysm — see Forces of nature,
      by type
    military NEC V94.818 ☑
      civilian in water injured by V94.811 ☑

Accident — continued
  watercraft — continued
    military — continued
      with civilian watercraft V94.810 ☑
    nonpowered, struck by
      nonpowered vessel V94.22 ☑
      powered vessel V94.21 ☑
      specified type NEC V94.89 ☑
    striking swimmer
      powered V94.11 ☑
      unpowered V94.12 ☑
Acid throwing (assault) Y08.89 ☑
Activity (involving) (of victim at time of event) Y93.9
  aerobic and step exercise (class) Y93.A3 (following
    Y93.7)
  alpine skiing Y93.23
  animal care NEC Y93.K9 (following Y93.7)
  arts and handcrafts NEC Y93.D9 (following Y93.7)
  athletics played as a team or group NEC Y93.69
  athletics played individually NEC Y93.59
  athletics NEC Y93.79
  baking Y93.G3 (following Y93.7)
  ballet Y93.41
  barbells Y93.B3 (following Y93.7)
  BASE (Building, Antenna, Span, Earth) jumping Y93.33
  baseball Y93.64
  basketball Y93.67
  bathing (personal) Y93.E1 (following Y93.7)
  beach volleyball Y93.68
  bike riding Y93.55
  blackout game Y93.85
  boogie boarding Y93.18
  bowling Y93.54
  boxing Y93.71
  brass instrument playing Y93.J4 (following Y93.7)
  building construction Y93.H3 (following Y93.7)
  bungee jumping Y93.34
  calisthenics Y93.A2 (following Y93.7)
  canoeing (in calm and turbulent water) Y93.16
  capture the flag Y93.6A
  cardiorespiratory exercise NEC Y93.A9 (following Y93.7)
  caregiving (providing) NEC Y93.F9 (following Y93.7)
    bathing Y93.F1 (following Y93.7)
    lifting Y93.F2 (following Y93.7)
  cellular
    communication device Y93.C2 (following Y93.7)
    telephone Y93.C2 (following Y93.7)
  challenge course Y93.A5 (following Y93.7)
  cheerleading Y93.45
  choking game Y93.85
  circuit training Y93.A4 (following Y93.7)
  cleaning
    floor Y93.E5 (following Y93.7)
  climbing NEC Y93.39
    mountain Y93.31
    rock Y93.31
    wall Y93.31
  clothing care and maintenance NEC Y93.E9 (following
    Y93.7)
  combatives Y93.75
  computer
    keyboarding Y93.C1 (following Y93.7)
    technology NEC Y93.C9 (following Y93.7)
  confidence course Y93.A5 (following Y93.7)
  construction (building) Y93.H3 (following Y93.7)
  cooking and baking Y93.G3 (following Y93.7)
  cool down exercises Y93.A2 (following Y93.7)
  cricket Y93.69
  crocheting Y93.D1 (following Y93.7)
  cross country skiing Y93.24
  dancing (all types) Y93.41
  digging
    dirt Y93.H1 (following Y93.7)
  dirt digging Y93.H1 (following Y93.7)
  dishwashing Y93.G1 (following Y93.7)
  diving (platform) (springboard) Y93.12
    underwater Y93.15
  dodge ball Y93.6A
  downhill skiing Y93.23
  drum playing Y93.J2 (following Y93.7)
  dumbbells Y93.B3 (following Y93.7)
  electronic
    devices NEC Y93.C9 (following Y93.7)
      hand held interactive Y93.C2 (following Y93.7)
    game playing (using) (with)
      interactive device Y93.C2 (following Y93.7)
      keyboard or other stationary device Y93.C1 (fol-
        lowing Y93.7)

Activity — *continued*
elliptical machine Y93.A1 (*following* Y93.7)
exercise(s)
  machines ((primarily) for)
    cardiorespiratory conditioning Y93.A1 (*following* Y93.7)
    muscle strengthening Y93.B1 (*following* Y93.7)
    muscle strengthening (non-machine) NEC Y93.B9 (*following* Y93.7)
  external motion NEC Y93.I9 (*following* Y93.7)
  rollercoaster Y93.I1 (*following* Y93.7)
fainting game Y93.85
field hockey Y93.65
figure skating (pairs) (singles) Y93.21
flag football Y93.62
floor mopping and cleaning Y93.E5 (*following* Y93.7)
food preparation and clean up Y93.G1 (*following* Y93.7)
football (American) NOS Y93.61
  flag Y93.62
  tackle Y93.61
  touch Y93.62
four square Y93.6A
free weights Y93.B3 (*following* Y93.7)
frisbee (ultimate) Y93.74
furniture
  building Y93.D3 (*following* Y93.7)
  finishing Y93.D3 (*following* Y93.7)
  repair Y93.D3 (*following* Y93.7)
game playing (electronic)
  using interactive device Y93.C2 (*following* Y93.7)
  using keyboard or other stationary device Y93.C1 (*following* Y93.7)
gardening Y93.H2 (*following* Y93.7)
golf Y93.53
grass drills Y93.A6 (*following* Y93.7)
grilling and smoking food Y93.G2 (*following* Y93.7)
grooming and shearing an animal Y93.K3 (*following* Y93.7)
guerilla drills Y93.A6 (*following* Y93.7)
gymnastics (rhythmic) Y93.43
hand held interactive electronic device Y93.C2 (*following* Y93.7)
handball Y93.73
handcrafts NEC Y93.D9 (*following* Y93.7)
hang gliding Y93.35
hiking (on level or elevated terrain) Y93.01
hockey (ice) Y93.22
  field Y93.65
horseback riding Y93.52
household (interior) maintenance NEC Y93.E9 (*following* Y93.7)
ice NEC Y93.29
  dancing Y93.21
  hockey Y93.22
  skating Y93.21
inline roller skating Y93.51
ironing Y93.E4 (*following* Y93.7)
judo Y93.75
jumping jacks Y93.A2 (*following* Y93.7)
jumping rope Y93.56
jumping (off) NEC Y93.39
  BASE (Building, Antenna, Span, Earth) Y93.33
  bungee Y93.34
  jacks Y93.A2 (*following* Y93.7)
  rope Y93.56
karate Y93.75
kayaking (in calm and turbulent water) Y93.16
keyboarding (computer) Y93.C1 (*following* Y93.7)
kickball Y93.6A
knitting Y93.D1 (*following* Y93.7)
lacrosse Y93.65
land maintenance NEC Y93.H9 (*following* Y93.7)
landscaping Y93.H2 (*following* Y93.7)
laundry Y93.E2 (*following* Y93.7)
machines (exercise)
  primarily for cardiorespiratory conditioning Y93.A1 (*following* Y93.7)
  primarily for muscle strengthening Y93.B1 (*following* Y93.7)
maintenance
  exterior building NEC Y93.H9 (*following* Y93.7)
  household (interior) NEC Y93.E9 (*following* Y93.7)
  land Y93.H9 (*following* Y93.7)
  property Y93.H9 (*following* Y93.7)
marching (on level or elevated terrain) Y93.01
martial arts Y93.75
microwave oven Y93.G3 (*following* Y93.7)
milking an animal Y93.K2 (*following* Y93.7)
mopping (floor) Y93.E5 (*following* Y93.7)

Activity — *continued*
mountain climbing Y93.31
muscle strengthening
  exercises (non-machine) NEC Y93.B9 (*following* Y93.7)
  machines Y93.B1 (*following* Y93.7)
musical keyboard (electronic) playing Y93.J1 (*following* Y93.7)
nordic skiing Y93.24
obstacle course Y93.A5 (*following* Y93.7)
oven (microwave) Y93.G3 (*following* Y93.7)
packing up and unpacking in moving to a new residence Y93.E6 (*following* Y93.7)
parasailing Y93.19
pass out game Y93.85
percussion instrument playing NEC Y93.J2 (*following* Y93.7)
personal
  bathing and showering Y93.E1 (*following* Y93.7)
  hygiene NEC Y93.E8 (*following* Y93.7)
  showering Y93.E1 (*following* Y93.7)
physical games generally associated with school recess, summer camp and children Y93.6A
physical training NEC Y93.A9 (*following* Y93.7)
piano playing Y93.J1 (*following* Y93.7)
pilates Y93.B4 (*following* Y93.7)
platform diving Y93.12
playing musical instrument
  brass instrument Y93.J4 (*following* Y93.7)
  drum Y93.J2 (*following* Y93.7)
  musical keyboard (electronic) Y93.J1 (*following* Y93.7)
  percussion instrument NEC Y93.J2 (*following* Y93.7)
  piano Y93.J1 (*following* Y93.7)
  string instrument Y93.J3 (*following* Y93.7)
  winds instrument Y93.J4 (*following* Y93.7)
property maintenance
  exterior NEC Y93.H9 (*following* Y93.7)
  interior NEC Y93.E9 (*following* Y93.7)
pruning (garden and lawn) Y93.H2 (*following* Y93.7)
pull-ups Y93.B2 (*following* Y93.7)
push-ups Y93.B2 (*following* Y93.7)
racquetball Y93.73
rafting (in calm and turbulent water) Y93.16
raking (leaves) Y93.H1 (*following* Y93.7)
rappelling Y93.32
refereeing a sports activity Y93.81
residential relocation Y93.E6 (*following* Y93.7)
rhythmic gymnastics Y93.43
rhythmic movement NEC Y93.49
riding
  horseback Y93.52
  rollercoaster Y93.I1 (*following* Y93.7)
rock climbing Y93.31
roller skating (inline) Y93.51
rollercoaster riding Y93.I1 (*following* Y93.7)
rough housing and horseplay Y93.83
rowing (in calm and turbulent water) Y93.16
rugby Y93.63
running Y93.02
SCUBA diving Y93.15
sewing Y93.D2 (*following* Y93.7)
shoveling Y93.H1 (*following* Y93.7)
  dirt Y93.H1 (*following* Y93.7)
  snow Y93.H1 (*following* Y93.7)
showering (personal) Y93.E1 (*following* Y93.7)
sit-ups Y93.B2 (*following* Y93.7)
skateboarding Y93.51
skating (ice) Y93.21
  roller Y93.51
skiing (alpine) (downhill) Y93.23
  cross country Y93.24
  nordic Y93.24
  water Y93.17
sledding (snow) Y93.23
sleeping (sleep) Y93.84
smoking and grilling food Y93.G2 (*following* Y93.7)
snorkeling Y93.15
snow NEC Y93.29
  boarding Y93.23
  shoveling Y93.H1 (*following* Y93.7)
  sledding Y93.23
  tubing Y93.23
soccer Y93.66
softball Y93.64
specified NEC Y93.89
spectator at an event Y93.82
sports NEC Y93.79
  sports played as a team or group NEC Y93.69

Activity — *continued*
sports — *continued*
  sports played individually NEC Y93.59
springboard diving Y93.12
squash Y93.73
stationary bike Y93.A1 (*following* Y93.7)
step (stepping) exercise (class) Y93.A3 (*following* Y93.7)
stepper machine Y93.A1 (*following* Y93.7)
stove Y93.G3 (*following* Y93.7)
string instrument playing Y93.J3 (*following* Y93.7)
surfing Y93.18
  wind Y93.18
swimming Y93.11
tackle football Y93.61
tap dancing Y93.41
tennis Y93.73
tobogganing Y93.23
touch football Y93.62
track and field events (non-running) Y93.57
  running Y93.02
trampoline Y93.44
treadmill Y93.A1 (*following* Y93.7)
trimming shrubs Y93.H2 (*following* Y93.7)
tubing (in calm and turbulent water) Y93.16
  snow Y93.23
ultimate frisbee Y93.74
underwater diving Y93.15
unpacking in moving to a new residence Y93.E6 (*following* Y93.7)
use of stove, oven and microwave oven Y93.G3 (*following* Y93.7)
vacuuming Y93.E3 (*following* Y93.7)
volleyball (beach) (court) Y93.68
wake boarding Y93.17
walking (on level or elevated terrain) Y93.01
  an animal Y93.K1 (*following* Y93.7)
walking an animal Y93.K1 (*following* Y93.7)
wall climbing Y93.31
warm up and cool down exercises Y93.A2 (*following* Y93.7)
water NEC Y93.19
  aerobics Y93.14
  craft NEC Y93.19
  exercise Y93.14
  polo Y93.13
  skiing Y93.17
  sliding Y93.18
  survival training and testing Y93.19
weeding (garden and lawn) Y93.H2 (*following* Y93.7)
wind instrument playing Y93.J4 (*following* Y93.7)
windsurfing Y93.18
wrestling Y93.72
yoga Y93.42
Adverse effect of drugs — *see* Table of Drugs and Chemicals
Aerosinusitis — *see* Air, pressure
After-effect, late — *see* Sequelae
Air
  blast in war operations — *see* War operations, air blast
  pressure
    change, rapid
      during
        ascent W94.29 ☑
          while (in) (surfacing from)
            aircraft W94.23 ☑
            deep water diving W94.21 ☑
            underground W94.22 ☑
        descent W94.39 ☑
          in
            aircraft W94.31 ☑
            water W94.32 ☑
      high, prolonged W94.0 ☑
      low, prolonged W94.12 ☑
        due to residence or long visit at high altitude W94.11 ☑
Alpine sickness W94.11 ☑
Altitude sickness W94.11 ☑
Anaphylactic shock, anaphylaxis — *see* Table of Drugs and Chemicals
Andes disease W94.11 ☑
Arachnidism, arachnoidism X58 ☑
Arson (with intent to injure or kill) X97 ☑
Asphyxia, asphyxiation
  by
    food (bone) (seed) — *see* categories T17 and T18 ☑
    gas — *see also* Table of Drugs and Chemicals
      legal
        execution — *see* Legal, intervention, gas

☑ **Additional Character Required** — **Refer to the Tabular List for Character Selection**

Asphyxia, asphyxiation — *continued*
  by — *continued*
    gas — *see also* Table of Drugs and Chemicals —
        continued
      legal — *continued*
        intervention — *see* Legal, intervention, gas
    from
      fire — *see also* Exposure, fire
        in war operations — *see* War operations, fire
      ignition — *see* Ignition
      vomitus T17.81 ☑
    in war operations — *see* War operations, restriction of
      airway
Aspiration
  food (any type) (into respiratory tract) (with asphyxia,
      obstruction respiratory tract, suffocation) —
      see categories T17 and T18
  foreign body — *see* Foreign body, aspiration
  vomitus (with asphyxia, obstruction respiratory tract,
      suffocation) T17.81 ☑
Assassination (attempt) — *see* Assault
Assault (homicidal) (by) (in) Y09
  arson X97 ☑
  bite (of human being) Y04.1 ☑
  bodily force Y04.8 ☑
    bite Y04.1 ☑
    bumping into Y04.2 ☑
    sexual — *see* subcategories T74.0, T76.0 ☑
    unarmed fight Y04.0 ☑
  bomb X96.9 ☑
    antipersonnel X96.0 ☑
    fertilizer X96.3 ☑
    gasoline X96.1 ☑
    letter X96.2 ☑
    petrol X96.1 ☑
    pipe X96.3 ☑
    specified NEC X96.8 ☑
  brawl (hand) (fists) (foot) (unarmed) Y04.0 ☑
  burning, burns (by fire) NEC X97 ☑
    acid Y08.89 ☑
    caustic, corrosive substance Y08.89 ☑
    chemical from swallowing caustic, corrosive sub-
        stance — *see* Table of Drugs and Chemicals
    cigarette(s) X97 ☑
    hot object X98.9 ☑
      fluid NEC X98.2 ☑
      household appliance X98.3 ☑
      specified NEC X98.8 ☑
      steam X98.0 ☑
      tap water X98.1 ☑
      vapors X98.0 ☑
    scalding — *see* Assault, burning
    steam X98.0 ☑
    vitriol Y08.89 ☑
  caustic, corrosive substance (gas) Y08.89 ☑
  crashing of
    aircraft Y08.81 ☑
    motor vehicle Y03.8 ☑
      pushed in front of Y02.0 ☑
      run over Y03.0 ☑
      specified NEC Y03.8 ☑
  cutting or piercing instrument X99.9 ☑
    dagger X99.2 ☑
    glass X99.0 ☑
    knife X99.1 ☑
    specified NEC X99.8 ☑
    sword X99.2 ☑
  dagger X99.2 ☑
  drowning (in) X92.9 ☑
    bathtub X92.0 ☑
    natural water X92.3 ☑
    specified NEC X92.8 ☑
    swimming pool X92.1 ☑
      following fall X92.2 ☑
  dynamite X96.8 ☑
  explosive(s) (material) X96.9 ☑
  fight (hand) (fists) (foot) (unarmed) Y04.0 ☑
    with weapon — *see* Assault, by type of weapon
  fire X97 ☑
  firearm X95.9 ☑
    airgun X95.01 ☑
    handgun X93 ☑
    hunting rifle X94.1 ☑
    larger X94.9 ☑
      specified NEC X94.8 ☑
    machine gun X94.2 ☑

Assault — *continued*
  firearm — *continued*
    shotgun X94.0 ☑
    specified NEC X95.8 ☑
  from high place Y01 ☑
  gunshot (wound) NEC — *see* Assault, firearm, by type
  incendiary device X97 ☑
  injury Y09
    to child due to criminal abortion attempt NEC
        Y08.89 ☑
  knife X99.1 ☑
  late effect of — *see* categories X92-Y08 with 7th char-
      acter S
  placing before moving object NEC Y02.8 ☑
    motor vehicle Y02.0 ☑
  poisoning — *see* categories T36-T65 with 7th character
      S
  puncture, any part of body — *see* Assault, cutting or
      piercing instrument
  pushing
    before moving object NEC Y02.8 ☑
      motor vehicle Y02.0 ☑
      subway train Y02.1 ☑
      train Y02.1 ☑
    from high place Y01 ☑
  rape T74.2- ☑
  scalding — *see* Assault, burning
  sequelae of — *see* categories X92-Y08 with 7th charac-
      ter S
  sexual (by bodily force) T74.2- ☑
  shooting — *see* Assault, firearm
  specified means NEC Y08.89 ☑
  stab, any part of body — *see* Assault, cutting or piercing
      instrument
  steam X98.0 ☑
  striking against
    other person Y04.2 ☑
    sports equipment Y08.09 ☑
      baseball bat Y08.02 ☑
      hockey stick Y08.01 ☑
  struck by
    sports equipment Y08.09 ☑
      baseball bat Y08.02 ☑
      hockey stick Y08.01 ☑
  submersion — *see* Assault, drowning
  violence Y09
  weapon Y09
    blunt Y00 ☑
    cutting or piercing — *see* Assault, cutting or piercing
        instrument
    firearm — *see* Assault, firearm
  wound Y09
    cutting — *see* Assault, cutting or piercing instru-
        ment
    gunshot — *see* Assault, firearm
    knife X99.1 ☑
    piercing — *see* Assault, cutting or piercing instru-
        ment
    puncture — *see* Assault, cutting or piercing instru-
        ment
    stab — *see* Assault, cutting or piercing instrument
Attack by mammals NEC W55.89 ☑
Avalanche — *see* Landslide
Aviator's disease — *see* Air, pressure

B

Barotitis, barodontalgia, barosinusitis, barotrauma
    (otitic) (sinus) — *see* Air, pressure
Battered (baby) (child) (person) (syndrome) X58 ☑
Bayonet wound W26.1 ☑
  in
    legal intervention — *see* Legal, intervention, sharp
        object, bayonet
    war operations — *see* War operations, combat
  stated as undetermined whether accidental or inten-
      tional Y28.8 ☑
  suicide (attempt) X78.2 ☑
Bean in nose — *see* categories T17 and T18
Bed set on fire NEC — *see* Exposure, fire, uncontrolled,
    building, bed
Beheading (by guillotine)
  homicide X99.9 ☑
  legal execution — *see* Legal, intervention
Bending, injury in (prolonged) (static) X50.1 ☑
Bends — *see* Air, pressure, change

Bite, bitten by
  alligator W58.01 ☑
  arthropod (nonvenomous) NEC W57 ☑
  bull W55.21 ☑
  cat W55.01 ☑
  cow W55.21 ☑
  crocodile W58.11 ☑
  dog W54.0 ☑
  goat W55.31 ☑
  hoof stock NEC W55.31 ☑
  horse W55.11 ☑
  human being (accidentally) W50.3 ☑
    with intent to injure or kill Y04.1 ☑
    as, or caused by, a crowd or human stampede (with
        fall) W52 ☑
    assault Y04.1 ☑
    homicide (attempt) Y04.1 ☑
    in
      fight Y04.1 ☑
  insect (nonvenomous) W57 ☑
  lizard (nonvenomous) W59.01 ☑
  mammal NEC W55.81 ☑
    marine W56.31 ☑
  marine animal (nonvenomous) W56.81 ☑
  millipede W57 ☑
  moray eel W56.51 ☑
  mouse W53.01 ☑
  person(s) (accidentally) W50.3 ☑
    with intent to injure or kill Y04.1 ☑
    as, or caused by, a crowd or human stampede (with
        fall) W52 ☑
    assault Y04.1 ☑
    homicide (attempt) Y04.1 ☑
    in
      fight Y04.1 ☑
  pig W55.41 ☑
  raccoon W55.51 ☑
  rat W53.11 ☑
  reptile W59.81 ☑
    lizard W59.01 ☑
    snake W59.11 ☑
    turtle W59.21 ☑
      terrestrial W59.81 ☑
  rodent W53.81 ☑
    mouse W53.01 ☑
    rat W53.11 ☑
    specified NEC W53.81 ☑
    squirrel W53.21 ☑
  shark W56.41 ☑
  sheep W55.31 ☑
  snake (nonvenomous) W59.11 ☑
  spider (nonvenomous) W57 ☑
  squirrel W53.21 ☑
Blast (air) in war operations — *see* War operations, blast
Blizzard X37.2 ☑
Blood alcohol level Y90.9
  less than 20mg/100ml Y90.0
  presence in blood, level not specified Y90.9
  20-39mg/100ml Y90.1
  40-59mg/100ml Y90.2
  60-79mg/100ml Y90.3
  80-99mg/100ml Y90.4
  100-119mg/100ml Y90.5
  120-199mg/100ml Y90.6
  200-239mg/100ml Y90.7
Blow X58 ☑
  by law-enforcing agent, police (on duty) — *see* Legal,
      intervention, manhandling
    blunt object — *see* Legal, intervention, blunt object
Blowing up — *see* Explosion
Brawl (hand) (fists) (foot) Y04.0 ☑
Breakage (accidental) (part of)
  ladder (causing fall) W11 ☑
  scaffolding (causing fall) W12 ☑
Broken
  glass, contact with — *see* Contact, with, glass
  power line (causing electric shock) W85 ☑
Bumping against, into (accidentally)
  object NEC W22.8 ☑
    caused by crowd or human stampede (with fall)
        W52 ☑
    sports equipment W21.9 ☑
    with fall — *see* Fall, due to, bumping against, object
  person(s) W51 ☑
    with fall W03 ☑
      due to ice or snow W00.0 ☑

Bumping against, into — *continued*
  person(s) — *continued*
    assault Y04.2 ☑
    caused by, a crowd or human stampede (with fall)
      W52 ☑
    homicide (attempt) Y04.2 ☑
  sports equipment W21.9 ☑
Burn, burned, burning (accidental) (by) (from) (on)
  acid NEC — *see* Table of Drugs and Chemicals
  bed linen — *see* Exposure, fire, uncontrolled, in building, bed
  blowtorch X08.8 ☑
    with ignition of clothing NEC X06.2 ☑
      nightwear X05 ☑
  bonfire, campfire (controlled) — *see also* Exposure, fire, controlled, not in building)
    uncontrolled — *see* Exposure, fire, uncontrolled, not in building
  candle X08.8 ☑
    with ignition of clothing NEC X06.2 ☑
      nightwear X05 ☑
  caustic liquid, substance (external) (internal) NEC — *see* Table of Drugs and Chemicals
  chemical (external) (internal) — *see also* Table of Drugs and Chemicals
    in war operations — *see* War operations. fire
  cigar(s) or cigarette(s) X08.8 ☑
    with ignition of clothing NEC X06.2 ☑
      nightwear X05 ☑
  clothes, clothing NEC (from controlled fire) X06.2 ☑
    with conflagration — *see* Exposure, fire, uncontrolled, building
    not in building or structure — *see* Exposure, fire, uncontrolled, not in building
  cooker (hot) X15.8 ☑
    stated as undetermined whether accidental or intentional Y27.3 ☑
    suicide (attempt) X77.3 ☑
  electric blanket X16 ☑
  engine (hot) X17 ☑
  fire, flames — *see* Exposure, fire
  flare, Very pistol — *see* Discharge, firearm NEC
  heat
    from appliance (electrical) (household) X15.8 ☑
      cooker X15.8 ☑
      hotplate X15.2 ☑
      kettle X15.8 ☑
      light bulb X15.8 ☑
      saucepan X15.3 ☑
      skillet X15.3 ☑
      stated as undetermined whether accidental or intentional Y27.3 ☑
      stove X15.0 ☑
      suicide (attempt) X77.3 ☑
      toaster X15.1 ☑
    in local application or packing during medical or surgical procedure Y63.5
  heating
    appliance, radiator or pipe X16 ☑
  homicide (attempt) — *see* Assault, burning
  hot
    air X14.1 ☑
    cooker X15.8 ☑
    drink X10.0 ☑
    engine X17 ☑
    fat X10.2 ☑
    fluid NEC X12 ☑
    food X10.1 ☑
    gases X14.1 ☑
    heating appliance X16 ☑
    household appliance NEC X15.8 ☑
    kettle X15.8 ☑
    liquid NEC X12 ☑
    machinery X17 ☑
    metal (molten) (liquid) NEC X18 ☑
    object (not producing fire or flames) NEC X19 ☑
    oil (cooking) X10.2 ☑
    pipe(s) X16 ☑
    radiator X16 ☑
    saucepan (glass) (metal) X15.3 ☑
    stove (kitchen) X15.0 ☑
    substance NEC X19 ☑
      caustic or corrosive NEC — *see* Table of Drugs and Chemicals
    toaster X15.1 ☑
    tool X17 ☑

Burn, burned, burning — *continued*
  hot — *continued*
    vapor X13.1 ☑
    water (tap) — *see* Contact, with, hot, tap water
  hotplate X15.2 ☑
    suicide (attempt) X77.3 ☑
  ignition — *see* Ignition
  in war operations — *see* War operations, fire
  inflicted by other person X97 ☑
    by hot objects, hot vapor, and steam — *see* Assault, burning, hot object
  internal, from swallowed caustic, corrosive liquid, substance — *see* Table of Drugs and Chemicals
  iron (hot) X15.8 ☑
    stated as undetermined whether accidental or intentional Y27.3 ☑
    suicide (attempt) X77.3 ☑
  kettle (hot) X15.8 ☑
    stated as undetermined whether accidental or intentional Y27.3 ☑
    suicide (attempt) X77.3 ☑
  lamp (flame) X08.8 ☑
    with ignition of clothing NEC X06.2 ☑
      nightwear X05 ☑
  lighter (cigar) (cigarette) X08.8 ☑
    with ignition of clothing NEC X06.2 ☑
      nightwear X05 ☑
  lightning — *see* subcategory T75.0 ☑
    causing fire — *see* Exposure, fire
  liquid (boiling) (hot) NEC X12 ☑
    stated as undetermined whether accidental or intentional Y27.2 ☑
    suicide (attempt) X77.2 ☑
  local application of externally applied substance in medical or surgical care Y63.5
  machinery (hot) X17 ☑
  matches X08.8 ☑
    with ignition of clothing NEC X06.2 ☑
      nightwear X05 ☑
  mattress — *see* Exposure, fire, uncontrolled, building, bed
  medicament, externally applied Y63.5
  metal (hot) (liquid) (molten) NEC X18 ☑
  nightwear (nightclothes, nightdress, gown, pajamas, robe) X05 ☑
  object (hot) NEC X19 ☑
  on board watercraft
    due to
      accident to watercraft V91.09 ☑
        powered craft V91.03 ☑
          ferry boat V91.01 ☑
          fishing boat V91.02 ☑
          jetskis V91.03 ☑
          liner V91.01 ☑
          merchant ship V91.00 ☑
          passenger ship V91.01 ☑
        unpowered craft V91.08 ☑
          canoe V91.05 ☑
          inflatable V91.06 ☑
          kayak V91.05 ☑
          sailboat V91.04 ☑
          surf-board V91.08 ☑
          water skis V91.07 ☑
          windsurfer V91.08 ☑
      fire on board V93.09 ☑
        ferry boat V93.01 ☑
        fishing boat V93.02 ☑
        jetskis V93.03 ☑
        liner V93.01 ☑
        merchant ship V93.00 ☑
        passenger ship V93.01 ☑
        powered craft NEC V93.03 ☑
        sailboat V93.04 ☑
      specified heat source NEC on board V93.19 ☑
        ferry boat V93.11 ☑
        fishing boat V93.12 ☑
        jetskis V93.13 ☑
        liner V93.11 ☑
        merchant ship V93.10 ☑
        passenger ship V93.11 ☑
        powered craft NEC V93.13 ☑
        sailboat V93.14 ☑
  pipe (hot) X16 ☑
    smoking X08.8 ☑
      with ignition of clothing NEC X06.2 ☑
        nightwear X05 ☑

Burn, burned, burning — *continued*
  powder — *see* Powder burn
  radiator (hot) X16 ☑
  saucepan (hot) (glass) (metal) X15.3 ☑
    stated as undetermined whether accidental or intentional Y27.3 ☑
    suicide (attempt) X77.3 ☑
  self-inflicted X76 ☑
    stated as undetermined whether accidental or intentional Y26 ☑
  stated as undetermined whether accidental or intentional Y27.0 ☑
  steam X13.1 ☑
    pipe X16 ☑
      stated as undetermined whether accidental or intentional Y27.8 ☑
      stated as undetermined whether accidental or intentional Y27.0 ☑
    suicide (attempt) X77.0 ☑
  stove (hot) (kitchen) X15.0 ☑
    stated as undetermined whether accidental or intentional Y27.3 ☑
    suicide (attempt) X77.3 ☑
  substance (hot) NEC X19 ☑
    boiling X12 ☑
      stated as undetermined whether accidental or intentional Y27.2 ☑
      suicide (attempt) X77.2 ☑
    molten (metal) X18 ☑
  suicide (attempt) NEC X76 ☑
    hot
      household appliance X77.3 ☑
      object X77.9 ☑
  therapeutic misadventure
    heat in local application or packing during medical or surgical procedure Y63.5
    overdose of radiation Y63.2
  toaster (hot) X15.1 ☑
    stated as undetermined whether accidental or intentional Y27.3 ☑
    suicide (attempt) X77.3 ☑
  tool (hot) X17 ☑
  torch, welding X08.8 ☑
    with ignition of clothing NEC X06.2 ☑
      nightwear X05 ☑
  trash fire (controlled) — *see* Exposure, fire, controlled, not in building
    uncontrolled — *see* Exposure, fire, uncontrolled, not in building
  vapor (hot) X13.1 ☑
    stated as undetermined whether accidental or intentional Y27.0 ☑
    suicide (attempt) X77.0 ☑
  Very pistol — *see* Discharge, firearm NEC
Butted by animal W55.82 ☑
  bull W55.22 ☑
  cow W55.22 ☑
  goat W55.32 ☑
  horse W55.12 ☑
  pig W55.42 ☑
  sheep W55.32 ☑

C

Caisson disease — *see* Air, pressure, change
Campfire (exposure to) (controlled) — *see also* Exposure, fire, controlled, not in building
  uncontrolled — *see* Exposure, fire, uncontrolled, not in building
Capital punishment (any means) — *see* Legal, intervention
Car sickness T75.3 ☑
Casualty (not due to war) NEC X58 ☑
  war — *see* War operations
Cat
  bite W55.01 ☑
  scratch W55.03 ☑
Cataclysm, cataclysmic (any injury) NEC — *see* Forces of nature
Catching fire — *see* Exposure, fire
Caught
  between
    folding object W23.0 ☑
    objects (moving) W23.0 ☑

☑ Additional Character Required — Refer to the Tabular List for Character Selection

Caught — *continued*
between — *continued*
objects — *continued*
and
machinery — *see* Contact, with, by type of machine
stationary
stationary W23.1 ☑
and moving
sliding door and door frame W23.0 ☑
by, in
machinery (moving parts of) — *see* Contact, with, by type of machine
washing-machine wringer W23.0 ☑
under packing crate (due to losing grip) W23.1 ☑
Cave-in caused by cataclysmic earth surface movement or eruption — *see* Landslide
Change(s) in air pressure — *see* Air, pressure, change
Choked, choking (on) (any object except food or vomitus)
food (bone) (seed) — *see* categories T17 and T18 ☑
vomitus T17.81- ☑
Civil insurrection — *see* War operations
Cloudburst (any injury) X37.8 ☑
Cold, exposure to (accidental) (excessive) (extreme) (natural) (place) NEC — *see* Exposure, cold
Collapse
building W20.1 ☑
burning (uncontrolled fire) X00.2 ☑
dam or man-made structure (causing earth movement) X36.0 ☑
machinery — *see* Contact, with, by type of machine
structure W20.1 ☑
burning (uncontrolled fire) X00.2 ☑
Collision (accidental) NEC — *see also* Accident, transport V89.9 ☑
pedestrian W51 ☑
with fall W03 ☑
due to ice or snow W00.0 ☑
involving pedestrian conveyance — *see* Accident, transport, pedestrian, conveyance
and
crowd or human stampede (with fall) W52 ☑
object W22.8 ☑
with fall — *see* Fall, due to, bumping against, object
person(s) — *see* Collision, pedestrian
transport vehicle NEC V89.9 ☑
and
avalanche, fallen or not moving — *see* Accident, transport
falling or moving — *see* Landslide
landslide, fallen or not moving — *see* Accident, transport
falling or moving — *see* Landslide
due to cataclysm — *see* Forces of nature, by type
intentional, purposeful suicide (attempt) — *see* Suicide, collision
Combustion, spontaneous — *see* Ignition
Complication (delayed) **of or following** (medical or surgical procedure) Y84.9
with misadventure — *see* Misadventure
amputation of limb(s) Y83.5
anastomosis (arteriovenous) (blood vessel) (gastrojejunal) (tendon) (natural or artificial material) Y83.2
aspiration (of fluid) Y84.4
tissue Y84.8
biopsy Y84.8
blood
sampling Y84.7
transfusion
procedure Y84.8
bypass Y83.2
catheterization (urinary) Y84.6
cardiac Y84.0
colostomy Y83.3
cystostomy Y83.3
dialysis (kidney) Y84.1
drug — *see* Table of Drugs and Chemicals
due to misadventure — *see* Misadventure
duodenostomy Y83.3
electroshock therapy Y84.3
external stoma, creation of Y83.3
formation of external stoma Y83.3
graft Y83.2
hypothermia (medically-induced) Y84.8

Complication (delayed) **of or following** — *continued*
implant, implantation (of)
artificial
internal device (cardiac pacemaker) (electrodes in brain) (heart valve prosthesis) (orthopedic) Y83.1
material or tissue (for anastomosis or bypass) Y83.2
with creation of external stoma Y83.3
natural tissues (for anastomosis or bypass) Y83.2
with creation of external stoma Y83.3
infusion
procedure Y84.8
injection — *see* Table of Drugs and Chemicals
procedure Y84.8
insertion of gastric or duodenal sound Y84.5
insulin-shock therapy Y84.3
paracentesis (abdominal) (thoracic) (aspirative) Y84.4
procedures other than surgical operation — *see* Complication of or following, by type of procedure
radiological procedure or therapy Y84.2
removal of organ (partial) (total) NEC Y83.6
sampling
blood Y84.7
fluid NEC Y84.4
tissue Y84.8
shock therapy Y84.3
surgical operation NEC — *see also* Complication of or following, by type of operation Y83.9
reconstructive NEC Y83.4
with
anastomosis, bypass or graft Y83.2
formation of external stoma Y83.3
specified NEC Y83.8
transfusion — *see also* Table of Drugs and Chemicals
procedure Y84.8
transplant, transplantation (heart) (kidney) (liver) (whole organ, any) Y83.0
partial organ Y83.4
ureterostomy Y83.3
vaccination — *see also* Table of Drugs and Chemicals
procedure Y84.8
Compression
divers' squeeze — *see* Air, pressure, change
trachea by
food (lodged in esophagus) — *see* categories T17 and T18 ☑
vomitus (lodged in esophagus) T17.81- ☑
Conflagration — *see* Exposure, fire, uncontrolled
Constriction (external)
hair W49.01 ☑
jewelry W49.04 ☑
ring W49.04 ☑
rubber band W49.03 ☑
specified item NEC W49.09 ☑
string W49.02 ☑
thread W49.02 ☑
Contact (accidental)
with
abrasive wheel (metalworking) W31.1 ☑
alligator W58.09 ☑
bite W58.01 ☑
crushing W58.03 ☑
strike W58.02 ☑
amphibian W62.9 ☑
frog W62.0 ☑
toad W62.1 ☑
animal (nonvenomous) NEC W64 ☑
marine W56.89 ☑
bite W56.81 ☑
dolphin — *see* Contact, with, dolphin
fish NEC — *see* Contact, with, fish
mammal — *see* Contact, with, mammal, marine
orca — *see* Contact, with, orca
sea lion — *see* Contact, with, sea lion
shark — *see* Contact, with, shark
strike W56.82 ☑
animate mechanical force NEC W64 ☑
arrow W21.89 ☑
not thrown, projected or falling W45.8 ☑
arthropods (nonvenomous) W57 ☑
axe W27.0 ☑
band-saw (industrial) W31.2 ☑
bayonet — *see* Bayonet wound
bee(s) X58 ☑

Contact — *continued*
with — *continued*
bench-saw (industrial) W31.2 ☑
bird W61.99 ☑
bite W61.91 ☑
chicken — *see* Contact, with, chicken
duck — *see* Contact, with, duck
goose — *see* Contact, with, goose
macaw — *see* Contact, with, macaw
parrot — *see* Contact, with, parrot
psittacine — *see* Contact, with, psittacine
strike W61.92 ☑
turkey — *see* Contact, with, turkey
blender W29.0 ☑
boiling water X12 ☑
stated as undetermined whether accidental or intentional Y27.2 ☑
suicide (attempt) X77.2 ☑
bore, earth-drilling or mining (land) (seabed) W31.0 ☑
buffalo — *see* Contact, with, hoof stock NEC
bull W55.29 ☑
bite W55.21 ☑
gored W55.22 ☑
strike W55.22 ☑
bumper cars W31.81 ☑
camel — *see* Contact, with, hoof stock NEC
can
lid W26.8 ☑
opener W27.4 ☑
powered W29.0 ☑
cat W55.09 ☑
bite W55.01 ☑
scratch W55.03 ☑
caterpillar (venomous) X58 ☑
centipede (venomous) X58 ☑
chain
hoist W24.0 ☑
agricultural operations W30.89 ☑
saw W29.3 ☑
chicken W61.39 ☑
peck W61.33 ☑
strike W61.32 ☑
chisel W27.0 ☑
circular saw W31.2 ☑
cobra X58 ☑
combine (harvester) W30.0 ☑
conveyer belt W24.1 ☑
cooker (hot) X15.8 ☑
stated as undetermined whether accidental or intentional Y27.3 ☑
suicide (attempt) X77.3 ☑
coral X58 ☑
cotton gin W31.82 ☑
cow W55.29 ☑
bite W55.21 ☑
strike W55.22 ☑
crane W24.0 ☑
agricultural operations W30.89 ☑
crocodile W58.19 ☑
bite W58.11 ☑
crushing W58.13 ☑
strike W58.12 ☑
dagger W26.1 ☑
stated as undetermined whether accidental or intentional Y28.2 ☑
suicide (attempt) X78.2 ☑
dairy equipment W31.82 ☑
dart W21.89 ☑
not thrown, projected or falling W45.8 ☑
deer — *see* Contact, with, hoof stock NEC
derrick W24.0 ☑
agricultural operations W30.89 ☑
hay W30.2 ☑
dog W54.8 ☑
bite W54.0 ☑
strike W54.1 ☑
dolphin W56.09 ☑
bite W56.01 ☑
strike W56.02 ☑
donkey — *see* Contact, with, hoof stock NEC
drill (powered) W29.8 ☑
earth (land) (seabed) W31.0 ☑
nonpowered W27.8 ☑
drive belt W24.0 ☑
agricultural operations W30.89 ☑

Contact — *continued*
  with — *continued*
    dry ice — *see* Exposure, cold, man-made
    dryer (clothes) (powered) (spin) W29.2 ☑
    duck W61.69 ☑
      bite W61.61 ☑
      strike W61.62 ☑
    earth (-)
      drilling machine (industrial) W31.0 ☑
      scraping machine in stationary use W31.83 ☑
    edge of stiff paper W26.2 ☑
    electric
      beater W29.0 ☑
      blanket X16 ☑
      fan W29.2 ☑
        commercial W31.82 ☑
      knife W29.1 ☑
      mixer W29.0 ☑
    elevator (building) W24.0 ☑
      agricultural operations W30.89 ☑
        grain W30.3 ☑
    engine(s), hot NEC X17 ☑
    excavating machine W31.0 ☑
    farm machine W30.9 ☑
    feces — *see* Contact, with, by type of animal
    fer de lance X58 ☑
    fish W56.59 ☑
      bite W56.51 ☑
      shark — *see* Contact, with, shark
      strike W56.52 ☑
    flying horses W31.81 ☑
    forging (metalworking) machine W31.1 ☑
    fork W27.4 ☑
    forklift (truck) W24.0 ☑
      agricultural operations W30.89 ☑
    frog W62.0 ☑
    garden
      cultivator (powered) W29.3 ☑
        riding W30.89 ☑
      fork W27.1 ☑
    gas turbine W31.3 ☑
    Gila monster X58 ☑
    giraffe — *see* Contact, with, hoof stock NEC
    glass (sharp) (broken) W25 ☑
      assault X99.0 ☑
      due to fall — *see* Fall, by type
      stated as undetermined whether accidental or
        intentional Y28.0 ☑
      suicide (attempt) X78.0 ☑
      with subsequent fall W18.02 ☑
    goat W55.39 ☑
      bite W55.31 ☑
      strike W55.32 ☑
    goose W61.59 ☑
      bite W61.51 ☑
      strike W61.52 ☑
    hand
      saw W27.0 ☑
      tool (not powered) NEC W27.8 ☑
        powered W29.8 ☑
    harvester W30.0 ☑
    hay-derrick W30.2 ☑
    heating
      appliance (hot) X16 ☑
      pad (electric) X16 ☑
    heat NEC X19 ☑
      from appliance (electrical) (household) — *see*
        Contact, with, hot, household appliance
      heating appliance X16 ☑
    hedge-trimmer (powered) W29.3 ☑
    hoe W27.1 ☑
    hoist (chain) (shaft) NEC W24.0 ☑
      agricultural W30.89 ☑
    hoof stock NEC W55.39 ☑
      bite W55.31 ☑
      strike W55.32 ☑
    hornet(s) X58 ☑
    horse W55.19 ☑
      bite W55.11 ☑
      strike W55.12 ☑
    hot
      air X14.1 ☑
        inhalation X14.0 ☑
      cooker X15.8 ☑
      cooking
        pan X15.3 ☑

Contact — *continued*
  with — *continued*
    hot — *continued*
      cooking — *continued*
        pot X15.3 ☑
      drinks X10.0 ☑
      engine X17 ☑
      fats X10.2 ☑
      fluids NEC X12 ☑
        assault X98.2 ☑
        suicide (attempt) X77.2 ☑
        undetermined whether accidental or inten-
          tional Y27.2 ☑
      food X10.1 ☑
      gases X14.1 ☑
        inhalation X14.0 ☑
      heating appliance X16 ☑
      household appliance X15.8 ☑
        assault X98.3 ☑
        cooker X15.8 ☑
        hotplate X15.2 ☑
        kettle X15.8 ☑
        light bulb X15.8 ☑
        object NEC X19 ☑
          assault X98.8 ☑
          stated as undetermined whether acciden-
            tal or intentional Y27.9 ☑
          suicide (attempt) X77.8 ☑
        saucepan X15.3 ☑
        skillet X15.3 ☑
        stated as undetermined whether accidental
          or intentional Y27.3 ☑
        stove X15.0 ☑
        suicide (attempt) X77.3 ☑
        toaster X15.1 ☑
      kettle X15.8 ☑
      light bulb X15.8 ☑
      liquid NEC — *see also* Burn X12 ☑
        drinks X10.0 ☑
        stated as undetermined whether accidental
          or intentional Y27.2 ☑
        suicide (attempt) X77.2 ☑
        tap water X11.8 ☑
          stated as undetermined whether acciden-
            tal or intentional Y27.1 ☑
          suicide (attempt) X77.1 ☑
      machinery X17 ☑
      metal (molten) (liquid) NEC X18 ☑
      object (not producing fire or flames) NEC X19 ☑
      oil (cooking) X10.2 ☑
      pipe X16 ☑
      plate X15.2 ☑
      radiator X16 ☑
      saucepan (glass) (metal) X15.3 ☑
      skillet X15.3 ☑
      stove (kitchen) X15.0 ☑
      substance NEC X19 ☑
      tap-water X11.8 ☑
        assault X98.1 ☑
        heated on stove X12 ☑
          stated as undetermined whether acciden-
            tal or intentional Y27.2 ☑
          suicide (attempt) X77.2 ☑
        in bathtub X11.0 ☑
        running X11.1 ☑
        stated as undetermined whether accidental
          or intentional Y27.1 ☑
        suicide (attempt) X77.1 ☑
      toaster X15.1 ☑
      tool X17 ☑
      vapors X13.1 ☑
        inhalation X13.0 ☑
      water (tap) X11.8 ☑
        boiling X12 ☑
          stated as undetermined whether acciden-
            tal or intentional Y27.2 ☑
          suicide (attempt) X77.2 ☑
        heated on stove X12 ☑
          stated as undetermined whether acciden-
            tal or intentional Y27.2 ☑
          suicide (attempt) X77.2 ☑
        in bathtub X11.0 ☑
        running X11.1 ☑
        stated as undetermined whether accidental
          or intentional Y27.1 ☑
        suicide (attempt) X77.1 ☑

Contact — *continued*
  with — *continued*
    hotplate X15.2 ☑
    ice-pick W27.4 ☑
    insect (nonvenomous) NEC W57 ☑
    kettle (hot) X15.8 ☑
    knife W26.0 ☑
      assault X99.1 ☑
      electric W29.1 ☑
      stated as undetermined whether accidental or
        intentional Y28.1 ☑
      suicide (attempt) X78.1 ☑
    lathe (metalworking) W31.1 ☑
      turnings W45.8 ☑
      woodworking W31.2 ☑
    lawnmower (powered) (ridden) W28 ☑
      causing electrocution W86.8 ☑
        suicide (attempt) X83.1 ☑
      unpowered W27.1 ☑
    lift, lifting (devices) W24.0 ☑
      agricultural operations W30.89 ☑
      shaft W24.0 ☑
    liquefied gas — *see* Exposure, cold, man-made
    liquid air, hydrogen, nitrogen — *see* Exposure, cold,
      man-made
    lizard (nonvenomous) W59.09 ☑
      bite W59.01 ☑
      strike W59.02 ☑
    llama — *see* Contact, with, hoof stock NEC
    macaw W61.19 ☑
      bite W61.11 ☑
      strike W61.12 ☑
    machine, machinery W31.9 ☑
      abrasive wheel W31.1 ☑
      agricultural including animal-powered W30.9 ☑
        combine harvester W30.0 ☑
        grain storage elevator W30.3 ☑
        hay derrick W30.2 ☑
        power take-off device W30.1 ☑
        reaper W30.0 ☑
        specified NEC W30.89 ☑
        thresher W30.0 ☑
        transport vehicle, stationary W30.81 ☑
      band saw W31.2 ☑
      bench saw W31.2 ☑
      circular saw W31.2 ☑
      commercial NEC W31.82 ☑
      drilling, metal (industrial) W31.1 ☑
      earth-drilling W31.0 ☑
      earthmoving or scraping W31.89 ☑
      excavating W31.89 ☑
      forging machine W31.1 ☑
      gas turbine W31.3 ☑
      hot X17 ☑
      internal combustion engine W31.3 ☑
      land drill W31.0 ☑
      lathe W31.1 ☑
      lifting (devices) W24.0 ☑
      metal drill W31.1 ☑
      metalworking (industrial) W31.1 ☑
      milling, metal W31.1 ☑
      mining W31.0 ☑
      molding W31.2 ☑
      overhead plane W31.2 ☑
      power press, metal W31.1 ☑
      prime mover W31.3 ☑
      printing W31.89 ☑
      radial saw W31.2 ☑
      recreational W31.81 ☑
      roller-coaster W31.81 ☑
      rolling mill, metal W31.1 ☑
      sander W31.2 ☑
      seabed drill W31.0 ☑
      shaft
        hoist W31.0 ☑
        lift W31.0 ☑
      specified NEC W31.89 ☑
      spinning W31.89 ☑
      steam engine W31.3 ☑
      transmission W24.1 ☑
      undercutter W31.0 ☑
      water driven turbine W31.3 ☑
      weaving W31.89 ☑
      woodworking or forming (industrial) W31.2 ☑
    mammal (feces) (urine) W55.89 ☑
      bull — *see* Contact, with, bull

☑ **Additional Character Required** — **Refer to the Tabular List for Character Selection**

Contact — *continued*
  with — *continued*
    mammal — *continued*
      cat — *see* Contact, with, cat
      cow — *see* Contact, with, cow
      goat — *see* Contact, with, goat
      hoof stock — *see* Contact, with, hoof stock
      horse — *see* Contact, with, horse
      marine W56.39 ☑
        dolphin — *see* Contact, with, dolphin
        orca — *see* Contact, with, orca
        sea lion — *see* Contact, with, sea lion
        specified NEC W56.39 ☑
          bite W56.31 ☑
          strike W56.32 ☑
      pig — *see* Contact, with, pig
      raccoon — *see* Contact, with, raccoon
      rodent — *see* Contact, with, rodent
      sheep — *see* Contact, with, sheep
      specified NEC W55.89 ☑
        bite W55.81 ☑
        strike W55.82 ☑
    marine
      animal W56.89 ☑
        bite W56.81 ☑
        dolphin — *see* Contact, with, dolphin
        fish NEC — *see* Contact, with, fish
        mammal — *see* Contact, with, mammal, marine
        orca — *see* Contact, with, orca
        sea lion — *see* Contact, with, sea lion
        shark — *see* Contact, with, shark
        strike W56.82 ☑
    meat
      grinder (domestic) W29.0 ☑
        industrial W31.82 ☑
        nonpowered W27.4 ☑
      slicer (domestic) W29.0 ☑
        industrial W31.82 ☑
    merry go round W31.81 ☑
    metal, hot (liquid) (molten) NEC X18 ☑
    millipede W57 ☑
    nail W45.0 ☑
      gun W29.4 ☑
    needle (sewing) W27.3 ☑
      hypodermic W46.0 ☑
        contaminated W46.1 ☑
    object (blunt) NEC
      hot NEC X19 ☑
      legal intervention — *see* Legal, intervention, blunt object
      sharp NEC W45.8 ☑
        inflicted by other person NEC W45.8 ☑
          stated as
            intentional homicide (attempt) — *see* Assault, cutting or piercing instrument
        legal intervention — *see* Legal, intervention, sharp object
        self-inflicted X78.9 ☑
    orca W56.29 ☑
      bite W56.21 ☑
      strike W56.22 ☑
    overhead plane W31.2 ☑
    paper (as sharp object) W26.2 ☑
    paper-cutter W27.5 ☑
    parrot W61.09 ☑
      bite W61.01 ☑
      strike W61.02 ☑
    pig W55.49 ☑
      bite W55.41 ☑
      strike W55.42 ☑
    pipe, hot X16 ☑
    pitchfork W27.1 ☑
    plane (metal) (wood) W27.0 ☑
      overhead W31.2 ☑
    plant thorns, spines, sharp leaves or other mechanisms W60 ☑
    powered
      garden cultivator W29.3 ☑
      household appliance, implement, or machine W29.8 ☑
      saw (industrial) W31.2 ☑
        hand W29.8 ☑
    printing machine W31.89 ☑
    psittacine bird W61.29 ☑

Contact — *continued*
  with — *continued*
    psittacine bird — *continued*
      bite W61.21 ☑
      macaw — *see* Contact, with, macaw
      parrot — *see* Contact, with, parrot
      strike W61.22 ☑
    pulley (block) (transmission) W24.0 ☑
      agricultural operations W30.89 ☑
    raccoon W55.59 ☑
      bite W55.51 ☑
      strike W55.52 ☑
    radial-saw (industrial) W31.2 ☑
    radiator (hot) X16 ☑
    rake W27.1 ☑
    rattlesnake X58 ☑
    reaper W30.0 ☑
    reptile W59.89 ☑
      lizard — *see* Contact, with, lizard
      snake — *see* Contact, with, snake
      specified NEC W59.89 ☑
        bite W59.81 ☑
        crushing W59.83 ☑
        strike W59.82 ☑
      turtle — *see* Contact, with, turtle
    rivet gun (powered) W29.4 ☑
    road scraper — *see* Accident, transport, construction vehicle
    rodent (feces) (urine) W53.89 ☑
      bite W53.81 ☑
      mouse W53.09 ☑
        bite W53.01 ☑
      rat W53.19 ☑
        bite W53.11 ☑
      specified NEC W53.89 ☑
        bite W53.81 ☑
      squirrel W53.29 ☑
        bite W53.21 ☑
    roller coaster W31.81 ☑
    rope NEC W24.0 ☑
      agricultural operations W30.89 ☑
    saliva — *see* Contact, with, by type of animal
    sander W29.8 ☑
      industrial W31.2 ☑
    saucepan (hot) (glass) (metal) X15.3 ☑
    saw W27.0 ☑
      band (industrial) W31.2 ☑
      bench (industrial) W31.2 ☑
      chain W29.3 ☑
      hand W27.0 ☑
    sawing machine, metal W31.1 ☑
    scissors W27.2 ☑
    scorpion X58 ☑
    screwdriver W27.0 ☑
      powered W29.8 ☑
    sea
      anemone, cucumber or urchin (spine) X58 ☑
      lion W56.19 ☑
        bite W56.11 ☑
        strike W56.12 ☑
    serpent — *see* Contact, with, snake, by type
    sewing-machine (electric) (powered) W29.2 ☑
      not powered W27.8 ☑
    shaft (hoist) (lift) (transmission) NEC W24.0 ☑
      agricultural W30.89 ☑
    shark W56.49 ☑
      bite W56.41 ☑
      strike W56.42 ☑
    sharp object(s) W26.9 ☑
      specified NEC W26.8 ☑
    shears (hand) W27.2 ☑
      powered (industrial) W31.1 ☑
        domestic W29.2 ☑
    sheep W55.39 ☑
      bite W55.31 ☑
      strike W55.32 ☑
    shovel W27.8 ☑
      steam — *see* Accident, transport, construction vehicle
    snake (nonvenomous) W59.19 ☑
      bite W59.11 ☑
      crushing W59.13 ☑
      strike W59.12 ☑
    spade W27.1 ☑
    spider (venomous) X58 ☑
    spin-drier W29.2 ☑

Contact — *continued*
  with — *continued*
    spinning machine W31.89 ☑
    splinter W45.8 ☑
    sports equipment W21.9 ☑
    staple gun (powered) W29.8 ☑
    steam X13.1 ☑
      engine W31.3 ☑
      inhalation X13.0 ☑
      pipe X16 ☑
      shovel W31.89 ☑
    stove (hot) (kitchen) X15.0 ☑
    substance, hot NEC X19 ☑
      molten (metal) X18 ☑
    sword W26.1 ☑
      assault X99.2 ☑
      stated as undetermined whether accidental or intentional Y28.2 ☑
      suicide (attempt) X78.2 ☑
    tarantula X58 ☑
    thresher W30.0 ☑
    tin can lid W26.8 ☑
    toad W62.1 ☑
    toaster (hot) X15.1 ☑
    tool W27.8 ☑
      hand (not powered) W27.8 ☑
        auger W27.0 ☑
        axe W27.0 ☑
        can opener W27.4 ☑
        chisel W27.0 ☑
        fork W27.4 ☑
        garden W27.1 ☑
        handsaw W27.0 ☑
        hoe W27.1 ☑
        ice-pick W27.4 ☑
        kitchen utensil W27.4 ☑
        manual
          lawn mower W27.1 ☑
          sewing machine W27.8 ☑
        meat grinder W27.4 ☑
        needle (sewing) W27.3 ☑
          hypodermic W46.0 ☑
            contaminated W46.1 ☑
        paper cutter W27.5 ☑
        pitchfork W27.1 ☑
        rake W27.1 ☑
        scissors W27.2 ☑
        screwdriver W27.0 ☑
        specified NEC W27.8 ☑
        workbench W27.0 ☑
      hot X17 ☑
      powered W29.8 ☑
        blender W29.0 ☑
          commercial W31.82 ☑
        can opener W29.0 ☑
          commercial W31.82 ☑
        chainsaw W29.3 ☑
        clothes dryer W29.2 ☑
          commercial W31.82 ☑
        dishwasher W29.2 ☑
          commercial W31.82 ☑
        edger W29.3 ☑
        electric fan W29.2 ☑
          commercial W31.82 ☑
        electric knife W29.1 ☑
        food processor W29.0 ☑
          commercial W31.82 ☑
        garbage disposal W29.0 ☑
          commercial W31.82 ☑
        garden tool W29.3 ☑
        hedge trimmer W29.3 ☑
        ice maker W29.0 ☑
          commercial W31.82 ☑
        kitchen appliance W29.0 ☑
          commercial W31.82 ☑
        lawn mower W28
        meat grinder W29.0 ☑
          commercial W31.82 ☑
        mixer W29.0 ☑
          commercial W31.82 ☑
        rototiller W29.3 ☑
        sewing machine W29.2 ☑
          commercial W31.82 ☑
        washing machine W29.2 ☑
          commercial W31.82 ☑

Contact — *continued*
  with — *continued*
    transmission device (belt, cable, chain, gear, pinion, shaft) W24.1 ☑
      agricultural operations W30.89 ☑
    turbine (gas) (water-driven) W31.3 ☑
    turkey W61.49 ☑
      peck W61.43 ☑
      strike W61.42 ☑
    turtle (nonvenomous) W59.29 ☑
      bite W59.21 ☑
      strike W59.22 ☑
      terrestrial W59.89 ☑
        bite W59.81 ☑
        crushing W59.83 ☑
        strike W59.82 ☑
    under-cutter W31.0 ☑
    urine — *see* Contact, with, by type of animal
    vehicle
      agricultural use (transport) — *see* Accident, transport, agricultural vehicle
        not on public highway W30.81 ☑
      industrial use (transport) — *see* Accident, transport, industrial vehicle
        not on public highway W31.83 ☑
      off-road use (transport) — *see* Accident, transport, all-terrain or off-road vehicle
        not on public highway W31.83 ☑
      special construction use (transport) — *see* Accident, transport, construction vehicle
        not on public highway W31.83 ☑
    venomous
      animal X58 ☑
      arthropods X58 ☑
      lizard X58 ☑
      marine animal NEC X58 ☑
      marine plant NEC X58 ☑
      millipedes (tropical) X58 ☑
      plant(s) X58 ☑
      snake X58 ☑
      spider X58 ☑
      viper X58 ☑
    washing-machine (powered) W29.2 ☑
    wasp X58 ☑
    weaving-machine W31.89 ☑
    winch W24.0 ☑
      agricultural operations W30.89 ☑
    wire NEC W24.0 ☑
      agricultural operations W30.89 ☑
    wood slivers W45.8 ☑
    yellow jacket X58 ☑
    zebra — *see* Contact, with, hoof stock NEC
  pressure X50.9 ☑
  stress X50.9 ☑
Coup de soleil X32 ☑
Crash
  aircraft (in transit) (powered) V95.9 ☑
    balloon V96.01 ☑
    fixed wing NEC (private) V95.21 ☑
      commercial V95.31 ☑
    glider V96.21 ☑
      hang V96.11 ☑
      powered V95.11 ☑
    helicopter V95.01 ☑
    in war operations — *see* War operations, destruction of aircraft
    microlight V95.11 ☑
    nonpowered V96.9 ☑
      specified NEC V96.8 ☑
    powered NEC V95.8 ☑
    stated as
      homicide (attempt) Y08.81 ☑
      suicide (attempt) X83.0 ☑
    ultralight V95.11 ☑
  spacecraft V95.41 ☑
  transport vehicle NEC — *see also* Accident, transport V89.9 ☑
    homicide (attempt) Y03.8 ☑
    motor NEC (traffic) V89.2 ☑
      homicide (attempt) Y03.8 ☑
      suicide (attempt) — *see* Suicide, collision
Cruelty (mental) (physical) (sexual) X58 ☑
Crushed (accidentally) X58 ☑
  between objects (moving) (stationary and moving) W23.0 ☑
    stationary W23.1 ☑

Crushed — *continued*
  by
    alligator W58.03 ☑
    avalanche NEC — *see* Landslide
    cave-in W20.0 ☑
      caused by cataclysmic earth surface movement — *see* Landslide
    crocodile W58.13 ☑
    crowd or human stampede W52 ☑
    falling
      aircraft V97.39 ☑
        in war operations — *see* War operations, destruction of aircraft
      earth, material W20.0 ☑
        caused by cataclysmic earth surface movement — *see* Landslide
      object NEC W20.8 ☑
    landslide NEC — *see* Landslide
    lizard (nonvenomous) W59.09 ☑
    machinery — *see* Contact, with, by type of machine
    reptile NEC W59.89 ☑
    snake (nonvenomous) W59.13 ☑
  in
    machinery — *see* Contact, with, by type of machine
Cut, cutting (any part of body) (accidental) — *see also* Contact, with, by object or machine
  during medical or surgical treatment as misadventure — *see* Index to Diseases and Injuries, Complications
  homicide (attempt) — *see* Assault, cutting or piercing instrument
  inflicted by other person — *see* Assault, cutting or piercing instrument
  legal
    execution — *see* Legal, intervention
    intervention — *see* Legal, intervention, sharp object
  machine NEC — *see also* Contact, with, by type of machine W31.9 ☑
  self-inflicted — *see* Suicide, cutting or piercing instrument
  suicide (attempt) — *see* Suicide, cutting or piercing instrument
Cyclone (any injury) X37.1 ☑

D

Decapitation (accidental circumstances) NEC X58 ☑
  homicide X99.9 ☑
  legal execution — *see* Legal, intervention
Dehydration from lack of water X58 ☑
Deprivation X58 ☑
Derailment (accidental)
  railway (rolling stock) (train) (vehicle) (without antecedent collision) V81.7 ☑
    with antecedent collision — *see* Accident, transport, railway vehicle occupant
  streetcar (without antecedent collision) V82.7 ☑
    with antecedent collision — *see* Accident, transport, streetcar occupant
Descent
  parachute (voluntary) (without accident to aircraft) V97.29 ☑
    due to accident to aircraft — *see* Accident, transport, aircraft
Desertion X58 ☑
Destitution X58 ☑
Disability, late effect or sequela of injury — *see* Sequelae
Discharge (accidental)
  airgun W34.010 ☑
    assault X95.01 ☑
    homicide (attempt) X95.01 ☑
    stated as undetermined whether accidental or intentional Y24.0 ☑
    suicide (attempt) X74.01 ☑
  BB gun — *see* Discharge, airgun
  firearm (accidental) W34.00 ☑
    assault X95.9 ☑
    handgun (pistol) (revolver) W32.0 ☑
      assault X93 ☑
      homicide (attempt) X93 ☑
      legal intervention — *see* Legal, intervention, firearm, handgun
      stated as undetermined whether accidental or intentional Y22 ☑
      suicide (attempt) X72 ☑

Discharge — *continued*
  firearm — *continued*
    homicide (attempt) X95.9 ☑
    hunting rifle W33.02 ☑
      assault X94.1 ☑
      homicide (attempt) X94.1 ☑
      legal intervention
        injuring
          bystander Y35.032 ☑
          law enforcement personnel Y35.031 ☑
          suspect Y35.033 ☑
          unspecified person Y35.039 ☑
      stated as undetermined whether accidental or intentional Y23.1 ☑
      suicide (attempt) X73.1 ☑
    larger W33.00 ☑
      assault X94.9 ☑
      homicide (attempt) X94.9 ☑
      hunting rifle — *see* Discharge, firearm, hunting rifle
      legal intervention — *see* Legal, intervention, firearm by type of firearm
      machine gun — *see* Discharge, firearm, machine gun
      shotgun — *see* Discharge, firearm, shotgun
      specified NEC W33.09 ☑
        assault X94.8 ☑
        homicide (attempt) X94.8 ☑
        legal intervention
          injuring
            bystander Y35.092 ☑
            law enforcement personnel Y35.091 ☑
            suspect Y35.093 ☑
            unspecified person Y35.099 ☑
        stated as undetermined whether accidental or intentional Y23.8 ☑
        suicide (attempt) X73.8 ☑
      stated as undetermined whether accidental or intentional Y23.9 ☑
      suicide (attempt) X73.9 ☑
    legal intervention
      injuring
        bystander Y35.002 ☑
        law enforcement personnel Y35.001 ☑
        suspect Y35.03 ☑
        unspecified person Y35.009 ☑
      using rubber bullet
        injuring
          bystander Y35.042 ☑
          law enforcement personnel Y35.041 ☑
          suspect Y35.043 ☑
          unspecified person Y35.049 ☑
    machine gun W33.03 ☑
      assault X94.2 ☑
      homicide (attempt) X94.2 ☑
      legal intervention — *see* Legal, intervention, firearm, machine gun
      stated as undetermined whether accidental or intentional Y23.3 ☑
      suicide (attempt) X73.2 ☑
    pellet gun — *see* Discharge, airgun
    shotgun W33.01 ☑
      assault X94.0 ☑
      homicide (attempt) X94.0 ☑
      legal intervention — *see* Legal, intervention, firearm, specified NEC
      stated as undetermined whether accidental or intentional Y23.0 ☑
      suicide (attempt) X73.0 ☑
    specified NEC W34.09 ☑
      assault X95.8 ☑
      homicide (attempt) X95.8 ☑
      legal intervention — *see* Legal, intervention, firearm, specified NEC
      stated as undetermined whether accidental or intentional Y24.8 ☑
      suicide (attempt) X74.8 ☑
    stated as undetermined whether accidental or intentional Y24.9 ☑
    suicide (attempt) X74.9 ☑
    Very pistol W34.09 ☑
      assault X95.8 ☑
      homicide (attempt) X95.8 ☑
      stated as undetermined whether accidental or intentional Y24.8 ☑

☑ **Additional Character Required — Refer to the Tabular List for Character Selection**

Discharge — *continued*
  firearm — *continued*
    Very pistol — *continued*
      suicide (attempt) X74.8 ☑
  firework(s) W39 ☑
    stated as undetermined whether accidental or intentional Y25 ☑
  gas-operated gun NEC W34.018 ☑
    airgun — *see* Discharge, airgun
    assault X95.09 ☑
    homicide (attempt) X95.09 ☑
    paintball gun — *see* Discharge, paintball gun
    stated as undetermined whether accidental or intentional Y24.8 ☑
    suicide (attempt) X74.09 ☑
  gun NEC — *see also* Discharge, firearm NEC
    air — *see* Discharge, airgun
    BB — *see* Discharge, airgun
    for single hand use — *see* Discharge, firearm, handgun
    hand — *see* Discharge, firearm, handgun
    machine — *see* Discharge, firearm, machine gun
    other specified — *see* Discharge, firearm NEC
    paintball — *see* Discharge, paintball gun
    pellet — *see* Discharge, airgun
  handgun — *see* Discharge, firearm, handgun
  machine gun — *see* Discharge, firearm, machine gun
  paintball gun W34.011 ☑
    assault X95.02 ☑
    homicide (attempt) X95.02 ☑
    stated as undetermined whether accidental or intentional Y24.8 ☑
    suicide (attempt) X74.02 ☑
  pistol — *see* Discharge, firearm, handgun
    flare — *see* Discharge, firearm, Very pistol
    pellet — *see* Discharge, airgun
    Very — *see* Discharge, firearm, Very pistol
  revolver — *see* Discharge, firearm, handgun
  rifle (hunting) — *see* Discharge, firearm, hunting rifle
  shotgun — *see* Discharge, firearm, shotgun
  spring-operated gun NEC W34.018 ☑
    assault X95.09 ☑
    homicide (attempt) X95.09 ☑
    stated as undetermined whether accidental or intentional Y24.8 ☑
    suicide (attempt) X74.09 ☑

Disease
  Andes W94.11 ☑
  aviator's — *see* Air, pressure
  range W94.11 ☑

Diver's disease, palsy, paralysis, squeeze — *see* Air, pressure

Diving (into water) — *see* Accident, diving

Dog bite W54.0 ☑

Dragged by transport vehicle NEC — *see also* Accident, transport V09.9 ☑

Drinking poison (accidental) — *see* Table of Drugs and Chemicals

Dropped (accidentally) **while being carried or supported by other person** W04 ☑

Drowning (accidental) W74 ☑
  assault X92.9 ☑
  due to
    accident (to)
      machinery — *see* Contact, with, by type of machine
      watercraft V90.89 ☑
        burning V90.29 ☑
          powered V90.23 ☑
            fishing boat V90.22 ☑
            jetskis V90.23 ☑
            merchant ship V90.20 ☑
            passenger ship V90.21 ☑
          unpowered V90.28 ☑
            canoe V90.25 ☑
            inflatable V90.26 ☑
            kayak V90.25 ☑
            sailboat V90.24 ☑
            water skis V90.27 ☑
        crushed V90.39 ☑
          powered V90.33 ☑
            fishing boat V90.32 ☑
            jetskis V90.33 ☑
            merchant ship V90.30 ☑
            passenger ship V90.31 ☑
          unpowered V90.38 ☑

Drowning — *continued*
  due to — *continued*
    accident — *continued*
      watercraft — *continued*
        crushed — *continued*
          unpowered — *continued*
            canoe V90.35 ☑
            inflatable V90.36 ☑
            kayak V90.35 ☑
            sailboat V90.34 ☑
            water skis V90.37 ☑
        overturning V90.09 ☑
          powered V90.03 ☑
            fishing boat V90.02 ☑
            jetskis V90.03 ☑
            merchant ship V90.00 ☑
            passenger ship V90.01 ☑
          unpowered V90.08 ☑
            canoe V90.05 ☑
            inflatable V90.06 ☑
            kayak V90.05 ☑
            sailboat V90.04 ☑
        sinking V90.19 ☑
          powered V90.13 ☑
            fishing boat V90.12 ☑
            jetskis V90.13 ☑
            merchant ship V90.10 ☑
            passenger ship V90.11 ☑
          unpowered V90.18 ☑
            canoe V90.15 ☑
            inflatable V90.16 ☑
            kayak V90.15 ☑
            sailboat V90.14 ☑
        specified type NEC V90.89 ☑
          powered V90.83 ☑
            fishing boat V90.82 ☑
            jetskis V90.83 ☑
            merchant ship V90.80 ☑
            passenger ship V90.81 ☑
          unpowered V90.88 ☑
            canoe V90.85 ☑
            inflatable V90.86 ☑
            kayak V90.85 ☑
            sailboat V90.84 ☑
            water skis V90.87 ☑
    avalanche — *see* Landslide
    cataclysmic
      earth surface movement NEC — *see* Forces of nature, earth movement
      storm — *see* Forces of nature, cataclysmic storm
    cloudburst X37.8 ☑
    cyclone X37.1 ☑
    fall overboard (from) V92.09 ☑
      powered craft V92.03 ☑
        ferry boat V92.01 ☑
        fishing boat V92.02 ☑
        jetskis V92.03 ☑
        liner V92.01 ☑
        merchant ship V92.00 ☑
        passenger ship V92.01 ☑
      resulting from
        accident to watercraft — *see* Drowning, due to, accident to, watercraft
        being washed overboard (from) V92.29 ☑
          powered craft V92.23 ☑
            ferry boat V92.21 ☑
            fishing boat V92.22 ☑
            jetskis V92.23 ☑
            liner V92.21 ☑
            merchant ship V92.20 ☑
            passenger ship V92.21 ☑
          unpowered craft V92.28 ☑
            canoe V92.25 ☑
            inflatable V92.26 ☑
            kayak V92.25 ☑
            sailboat V92.24 ☑
            surf-board V92.28 ☑
            water skis V92.27 ☑
            windsurfer V92.28 ☑
        motion of watercraft V92.19 ☑
          powered craft V92.13 ☑
            ferry boat V92.11 ☑
            fishing boat V92.12 ☑
            jetskis V92.13 ☑
            liner V92.11 ☑
            merchant ship V92.10 ☑

Drowning — *continued*
  due to — *continued*
    fall overboard — *continued*
      resulting from — *continued*
        motion of watercraft — *continued*
          powered craft — *continued*
            passenger ship V92.11 ☑
          unpowered craft
            canoe V92.15 ☑
            inflatable V92.16 ☑
            kayak V92.15 ☑
            sailboat V92.14 ☑
        unpowered craft V92.08 ☑
          canoe V92.05 ☑
          inflatable V92.06 ☑
          kayak V92.05 ☑
          sailboat V92.04 ☑
          surf-board V92.08 ☑
          water skis V92.07 ☑
          windsurfer V92.08 ☑
    hurricane X37.0 ☑
    jumping into water from watercraft (involved in accident) — *see also* Drowning, due to, accident to, watercraft
      without accident to or on watercraft W16.711 ☑
    tidal wave NEC — *see* Forces of nature, tidal wave
    torrential rain X37.8 ☑
  following
    fall
      into
        bathtub W16.211 ☑
        bucket W16.221 ☑
        fountain — *see* Drowning, following, fall, into, water, specified NEC
        quarry — *see* Drowning, following, fall, into, water, specified NEC
        reservoir — *see* Drowning, following, fall, into, water, specified NEC
        swimming-pool W16.011 ☑
          stated as undetermined whether accidental or intentional Y21.3 ☑
          striking
            bottom W16.021 ☑
            wall W16.031 ☑
          suicide (attempt) X71.2 ☑
        water NOS W16.41 ☑
          natural (lake) (open sea) (river) (stream) (pond) W16.111 ☑
            striking
              bottom W16.121 ☑
              side W16.131 ☑
          specified NEC W16.311 ☑
            striking
              bottom W16.321 ☑
              wall W16.331 ☑
    overboard NEC — *see* Drowning, due to, fall overboard
    jump or dive
      from boat W16.711 ☑
        striking bottom W16.721 ☑
      into
        fountain — *see* Drowning, following, jump or dive, into, water, specified NEC
        quarry — *see* Drowning, following, jump or dive, into, water, specified NEC
        reservoir — *see* Drowning, following, jump or dive, into, water, specified NEC
        swimming-pool W16.511 ☑
          striking
            bottom W16.521 ☑
            wall W16.531 ☑
          suicide (attempt) X71.2 ☑
        water NOS W16.91 ☑
          natural (lake) (open sea) (river) (stream) (pond) W16.611 ☑
          specified NEC W16.811 ☑
            bottom W16.821 ☑
            striking
              bottom W16.821 ☑
              wall W16.831 ☑
          striking
            bottom W16.821 ☑
            wall W16.831 ☑
          striking bottom W16.621 ☑
  homicide (attempt) X92.9 ☑
  in
    bathtub (accidental) W65 ☑

Drowning — continued
in — continued
  bathtub — continued
    assault X92.0 ☑
    following fall W16.211 ☑
      stated as undetermined whether accidental
        or intentional Y21.1 ☑
      stated as undetermined whether accidental or
        intentional Y21.0 ☑
    suicide (attempt) X71.0 ☑
  lake — see Drowning, in, natural water
  natural water (lake) (open sea) (river) (stream)
    (pond) W69 ☑
    assault X92.3 ☑
    following
      dive or jump W16.611 ☑
        striking bottom W16.621 ☑
      fall W16.111 ☑
        striking
          bottom W16.121 ☑
          side W16.131 ☑
      stated as undetermined whether accidental or
        intentional Y21.4 ☑
    suicide (attempt) X71.3 ☑
  quarry — see Drowning, in, specified place NEC
  quenching tank — see Drowning, in, specified place
    NEC
  reservoir — see Drowning, in, specified place NEC
  river — see Drowning, in, natural water
  sea — see Drowning, in, natural water
  specified place NEC W73 ☑
    assault X92.8 ☑
    following
      dive or jump W16.811 ☑
        striking
          bottom W16.821 ☑
          wall W16.831 ☑
      fall W16.311 ☑
        striking
          bottom W16.321 ☑
          wall W16.331 ☑
      stated as undetermined whether accidental or
        intentional Y21.8 ☑
    suicide (attempt) X71.8 ☑
  stream — see Drowning, in, natural water
  swimming-pool W67 ☑
    assault X92.1 ☑
      following fall X92.2 ☑
    following
      dive or jump W16.511 ☑
        striking
          bottom W16.521 ☑
          wall W16.531 ☑
      fall W16.011 ☑
        striking
          bottom W16.021 ☑
          wall W16.031 ☑
      stated as undetermined whether accidental or
        intentional Y21.2 ☑
      following fall Y21.3 ☑
    suicide (attempt) X71.1 ☑
      following fall X71.2 ☑
  war operations — see War operations, restriction
    of airway
resulting from accident to watercraft — see Drowning,
  due to, accident, watercraft
self-inflicted X71.9 ☑
stated as undetermined whether accidental or intentional Y21.9 ☑
suicide (attempt) X71.9 ☑

E

Earth falling (on) W20.0 ☑
caused by cataclysmic earth surface movement or
  eruption — see Landslide
Earth (surface) **movement NEC** — see Forces of nature,
  earth movement
Earthquake (any injury) X34 ☑
Effect(s) (adverse) **of**
air pressure (any) — see Air, pressure
cold, excessive (exposure to) — see Exposure, cold
heat (excessive) — see Heat
hot place (weather) — see Heat
insolation X30 ☑
late — see Sequelae

Effect(s) (adverse) **of** — continued
motion — see Motion
nuclear explosion or weapon in war operations — see
  War operations, nuclear weapon
radiation — see Radiation
travel — see Travel
Electric shock (accidental) (by) (in) — see Exposure,
  electric current
Electrocution (accidental) — see Exposure, electric current
Endotracheal tube wrongly placed during anesthetic
  procedure
Entanglement
in
  bed linen, causing suffocation T71 ☑
  wheel of pedal cycle V19.88 ☑
Entry of foreign body or material — see Foreign body
Environmental pollution related condition — see
  category Z57 ☑
Execution, legal (any method) — see Legal, intervention
Exhaustion
cold — see Exposure, cold
due to excessive exertion — see also Overexertion
  X50.9 ☑
heat — see Heat
Explosion (accidental) (of) (with secondary fire) W40.9 ☑
acetylene W40.1 ☑
aerosol can W36.1 ☑
air tank (compressed) (in machinery) W36.2 ☑
aircraft (in transit) (powered) NEC V95.9 ☑
  balloon V96.05 ☑
  fixed wing NEC (private) V95.25 ☑
    commercial V95.35 ☑
  glider V96.25 ☑
    hang V96.15 ☑
    powered V95.15 ☑
  helicopter V95.05 ☑
  in war operations — see War operations, destruction
    of aircraft
  microlight V95.15 ☑
  nonpowered V96.9 ☑
    specified NEC V96.8 ☑
  powered NEC V95.8 ☑
  stated as
    homicide (attempt) Y03.8 ☑
    suicide (attempt) X83.0 ☑
  ultralight V95.15 ☑
anesthetic gas in operating room W40.1 ☑
antipersonnel bomb W40.8 ☑
  assault X96.0 ☑
  homicide (attempt) X96.0 ☑
  suicide (attempt) X75 ☑
assault X96.9 ☑
bicycle tire W37.0 ☑
blasting (cap) (materials) W40.0 ☑
boiler (machinery), not on transport vehicle W35 ☑
  on watercraft — see Explosion, in, watercraft
butane W40.1 ☑
caused by other person X96.9 ☑
coal gas W40.1 ☑
detonator W40.0 ☑
dump (munitions) W40.8 ☑
dynamite W40.0 ☑
  in
    assault X96.8 ☑
    homicide (attempt) X96.8 ☑
    legal intervention
      injuring
        bystander Y35.112 ☑
        law enforcement personnel Y35.111 ☑
        suspect Y35.113 ☑
        unspecified person Y35.119 ☑
    suicide (attempt) X75 ☑
explosive (material) W40.9 ☑
  gas W40.1 ☑
  in blasting operation W40.0 ☑
  specified NEC W40.8 ☑
    in
      assault X96.8 ☑
      homicide (attempt) X96.8 ☑
      legal intervention
        injuring
          bystander Y35.192 ☑
          law enforcement personnel
            Y35.191 ☑
          suspect Y35.193 ☑

Explosion — continued
explosive — continued
  specified — continued
    in — continued
      legal intervention — continued
        injuring — continued
          unspecified person Y35.199 ☑
        suicide (attempt) X75 ☑
factory (munitions) W40.8 ☑
fertilizer bomb W40.8 ☑
  assault X96.3 ☑
  homicide (attempt) X96.3 ☑
  suicide (attempt) X75 ☑
firearm (parts) NEC W34.19 ☑
  airgun W34.110 ☑
  BB gun W34.110 ☑
  gas, air or spring-operated gun NEC W34.118 ☑
  hangun W32.1 ☑
  hunting rifle W33.12 ☑
  larger firearm W33.10 ☑
    specified NEC W33.19 ☑
  machine gun W33.13 ☑
  paintball gun W34.111 ☑
  pellet gun W34.110 ☑
  shotgun W33.11 ☑
  Very pistol [flare] W34.19 ☑
fire-damp W40.1 ☑
fireworks W39 ☑
gas (coal) (explosive) W40.1 ☑
  cylinder W36.9 ☑
    aerosol can W36.1 ☑
    air tank W36.2 ☑
    pressurized W36.3 ☑
    specified NEC W36.8 ☑
gasoline (fumes) (tank) not in moving motor vehicle
  W40.1 ☑
  bomb W40.8 ☑
    assault X96.1 ☑
    homicide (attempt) X96.1 ☑
    suicide (attempt) X75 ☑
  in motor vehicle — see Accident, transport, by type
    of vehicle
grain store W40.8 ☑
grenade W40.8 ☑
  in
    assault X96.8 ☑
    homicide (attempt) X96.8 ☑
    legal intervention
      injuring
        bystander Y35.192 ☑
        law enforcement personnel Y35.191 ☑
        suspect Y35.193 ☑
        unspecified person Y35.199 ☑
    suicide (attempt) X75 ☑
handgun (parts) — see Explosion, firearm, hangun
  (parts)
homicide (attempt) X96.9 ☑
  antipersonnel bomb — see Explosion, antipersonnel
    bomb
  fertilizer bomb — see Explosion, fertilizer bomb
  gasoline bomb — see Explosion, gasoline bomb
  letter bomb — see Explosion, letter bomb
  pipe bomb — see Explosion, pipe bomb
  specified NEC X96.8 ☑
hose, pressurized W37.8 ☑
hot water heater, tank (in machinery) W35 ☑
  on watercraft — see Explosion, in, watercraft
in, on
  dump W40.8 ☑
  factory W40.8 ☑
  mine (of explosive gases) NEC W40.1 ☑
  watercraft V93.59 ☑
    powered craft V93.53 ☑
      ferry boat V93.51 ☑
      fishing boat V93.52 ☑
      jetskis V93.53 ☑
      liner V93.51 ☑
      merchant ship V93.50 ☑
      passenger ship V93.51 ☑
      sailboat V93.54 ☑
letter bomb W40.8 ☑
  assault X96.2 ☑
  homicide (attempt) X96.2 ☑
  suicide (attempt) X75 ☑
machinery — see also Contact, with, by type of machine

☑ Additional Character Required — Refer to the Tabular List for Character Selection

Explosion — *continued*
  machinery — *see also* Contact, with, by type of machine — *continued*
    on board watercraft — *see* Explosion, in, watercraft
    pressure vessel — *see* Explosion, by type of vessel
  methane W40.1 ☑
  mine W40.1 ☑
  missile NEC W40.8 ☑
  mortar bomb W40.8 ☑
    in
      assault X96.8 ☑
      homicide (attempt) X96.8 ☑
      legal intervention
        injuring
          bystander Y35.192 ☑
          law enforcement personnel Y35.191 ☑
          suspect Y35.193 ☑
          unspecified person Y35.199 ☑
      suicide (attempt) X75 ☑
  munitions (dump) (factory) W40.8 ☑
  pipe, pressurized W37.8 ☑
    bomb W40.8 ☑
      assault X96.4 ☑
      homicide (attempt) X96.4 ☑
      suicide (attempt) X75 ☑
  pressure, pressurized
    cooker W38 ☑
    gas tank (in machinery) W36.3 ☑
    hose W37.8 ☑
    pipe W37.8 ☑
    specified device NEC W38 ☑
    tire W37.8 ☑
      bicycle W37.0 ☑
    vessel (in machinery) W38 ☑
  propane W40.1 ☑
  self-inflicted X75 ☑
  shell (artillery) NEC W40.8 ☑
    during war operations — *see* War operations, explosion
    in
      legal intervention
        injuring
          bystander Y35.122 ☑
          law enforcement personnel Y35.121 ☑
          suspect Y35.123 ☑
          unspecified person Y35.129 ☑
    war — *see* War operations, explosion
  spacecraft V95.45 ☑
  stated as undetermined whether accidental or intentional Y25 ☑
  steam or water lines (in machinery) W37.8 ☑
  stove W40.9 ☑
  suicide (attempt) X75 ☑
  tire, pressurized W37.8 ☑
    bicycle W37.0 ☑
  undetermined whether accidental or intentional Y25 ☑
  vehicle tire NEC W37.8 ☑
    bicycle W37.0 ☑
  war operations — *see* War operations, explosion
Exposure (to) X58 ☑
  air pressure change — *see* Air, pressure
  cold (accidental) (excessive) (extreme) (natural) (place) X31 ☑
    assault Y08.89 ☑
    due to
      man-made conditions W93.8 ☑
        dry ice (contact) W93.01 ☑
          inhalation W93.02 ☑
        liquid air (contact) (hydrogen) (nitrogen) W93.11 ☑
          inhalation W93.12 ☑
        refrigeration unit (deep freeze) W93.2 ☑
        suicide (attempt) X83.2 ☑
      weather (conditions) X31 ☑
    homicide (attempt) Y08.89 ☑
    self-inflicted X83.2 ☑
  due to abandonment or neglect X58 ☑
  electric current W86.8 ☑
    appliance (faulty) W86.8 ☑
      domestic W86.0 ☑
    caused by other person Y08.89 ☑
    conductor (faulty) W86.1 ☑
    control apparatus (faulty) W86.1 ☑
    electric power generating plant, distribution station W86.1 ☑

Exposure — *continued*
  electric current — *continued*
    electroshock gun — *see* Exposure, electric current, taser
    high-voltage cable W85 ☑
    homicide (attempt) Y08.89 ☑
    legal execution — *see* Legal, intervention, specified means NEC
    lightning — *see* subcategory T75.0 ☑
    live rail W86.8 ☑
    misadventure in medical or surgical procedure in electroshock therapy Y63.4
    motor (electric) (faulty) W86.8 ☑
      domestic W86.0 ☑
    self-inflicted X83.1 ☑
    specified NEC W86.8 ☑
      domestic W86.0 ☑
    stun gun — *see* Exposure, electric current, taser
    suicide (attempt) X83.1 ☑
    taser W86.8 ☑
      assault Y08.89 ☑
      legal intervention — *see* category Y35
      self-harm (intentional) X83.8 ☑
      undetermined intent Y33 ☑
    third rail W86.8 ☑
    transformer (faulty) W86.1 ☑
    transmission lines W85 ☑
  environmental tobacco smoke X58 ☑
  excessive
    cold — *see* Exposure, cold
    heat (natural) NEC X30 ☑
      man-made W92 ☑
  factor(s) NOS X58 ☑
    environmental NEC X58 ☑
    man-made NEC W99 ☑
    natural NEC — *see* Forces of nature
    specified NEC X58 ☑
  fire, flames (accidental) X08.8 ☑
    assault X97 ☑
    campfire — *see* Exposure, fire, controlled, not in building
    controlled (in)
      with ignition (of) clothing — *see also* Ignition, clothes X06.2 ☑
        nightwear X05 ☑
      bonfire — *see* Exposure, fire, controlled, not in building
      brazier (in building or structure) — *see also* Exposure, fire, controlled, building
        not in building or structure — *see* Exposure, fire, controlled, not in building
      building or structure X02.0 ☑
        with
          fall from building X02.3 ☑
          from building X02.5 ☑
          injury due to building collapse X02.2 ☑
          smoke inhalation X02.1 ☑
        hit by object from building X02.4 ☑
        specified mode of injury NEC X02.8 ☑
      fireplace, furnace or stove — *see* Exposure, fire, controlled, building
      not in building or structure X03.0 ☑
        with
          fall X03.3 ☑
          smoke inhalation X03.1 ☑
        hit by object X03.4 ☑
        specified mode of injury NEC X03.8 ☑
      trash — *see* Exposure, fire, controlled, not in building
    fireplace — *see* Exposure, fire, controlled, building
    fittings or furniture (in building or structure) (uncontrolled) — *see* Exposure, fire, uncontrolled, building
    forest (uncontrolled) — *see* Exposure, fire, uncontrolled, not in building
    grass (uncontrolled) — *see* Exposure, fire, uncontrolled, not in building
    hay (uncontrolled) — *see* Exposure, fire, uncontrolled, not in building
    homicide (attempt) X97 ☑
    ignition of highly flammable material X04 ☑
    in, of, on, starting in
      machinery — *see* Contact, with, by type of machine

Exposure — *continued*
  fire, flames — *continued*
    in, of, on, starting in — *continued*
      motor vehicle (in motion) — *see also* Accident, transport, occupant by type of vehicle V87.8 ☑
        with collision — *see* Collision
      railway rolling stock, train, vehicle V81.81 ☑
        with collision — *see* Accident, transport, railway vehicle occupant
      street car (in motion) V82.8 ☑
        with collision — *see* Accident, transport, streetcar occupant
      transport vehicle NEC — *see also* Accident, transport
        with collision — *see* Collision
      war operations — *see also* War operations, fire
        from nuclear explosion — *see* War operations, nuclear weapons
      watercraft (in transit) (not in transit) V91.09 ☑
        localized — *see* Burn, on board watercraft, due to, fire on board
        powered craft V91.03 ☑
          ferry boat V91.01 ☑
          fishing boat V91.02 ☑
          jet skis V91.03 ☑
          liner V91.01 ☑
          merchant ship V91.00 ☑
          passenger ship V91.01 ☑
        unpowered craft V91.08 ☑
          canoe V91.05 ☑
          inflatable V91.06 ☑
          kayak V91.05 ☑
          sailboat V91.04 ☑
          surf-board V91.08 ☑
          waterskis V91.07 ☑
          windsurfer V91.08 ☑
    lumber (uncontrolled) — *see* Exposure, fire, uncontrolled, not in building
    mine (uncontrolled) — *see* Exposure, fire, uncontrolled, not in building
    prairie (uncontrolled) — *see* Exposure, fire, uncontrolled, not in building
    resulting from
      explosion — *see* Explosion
      lightning X08.8 ☑
    self-inflicted X76 ☑
    specified NEC X08.8 ☑
    started by other person X97 ☑
    stated as undetermined whether accidental or intentional Y26 ☑
    stove — *see* Exposure, fire, controlled, building
    suicide (attempt) X76 ☑
    tunnel (uncontrolled) — *see* Exposure, fire, uncontrolled, not in building
    uncontrolled
      in building or structure X00.0 ☑
        with
          fall from building X00.3 ☑
          injury due to building collapse X00.2 ☑
          jump from building X00.5 ☑
          smoke inhalation X00.1 ☑
        bed X08.00 ☑
          due to
            cigarette X08.01 ☑
            specified material NEC X08.09 ☑
        furniture NEC X08.20 ☑
          due to
            cigarette X08.21 ☑
            specified material NEC X08.29 ☑
        hit by object from building X00.4 ☑
        sofa X08.10 ☑
          due to
            cigarette X08.11 ☑
            specified material NEC X08.19 ☑
        specified mode of injury NEC X00.8 ☑
      not in building or structure (any) X01.0 ☑
        with
          fall X01.3 ☑
          smoke inhalation X01.1 ☑
        hit by object X01.4 ☑
        specified mode of injury NEC X01.8 ☑
    undetermined whether accidental or intentional Y26 ☑
  forces of nature NEC — *see* Forces of nature
  G-forces (abnormal) W49.9 ☑

External Causes Index

Exposure — Fall, falling

Exposure — *continued*
  gravitational forces (abnormal) W49.9 ☑
  heat (natural) NEC — *see* Heat
  high-pressure jet (hydraulic) (pneumatic) W49.9 ☑
  hydraulic jet W49.9 ☑
  inanimate mechanical force W49.9 ☑
  jet, high-pressure (hydraulic) (pneumatic) W49.9 ☑
  lightning — *see* subcategory T75.0 ☑
    causing fire — *see* Exposure, fire
  mechanical forces NEC W49.9 ☑
    animate NEC W64 ☑
    inanimate NEC W49.9 ☑
  noise W42.9 ☑
    supersonic W42.0 ☑
  noxious substance — *see* Table of Drugs and Chemicals
  pneumatic jet W49.9 ☑
  prolonged in deep-freeze unit or refrigerator W93.2 ☑
  radiation — *see* Radiation
  smoke — *see also* Exposure, fire
    tobacco, second hand Z77.22
  specified factors NEC X58 ☑
  sunlight X32 ☑
    man-made (sun lamp) W89.8 ☑
      tanning bed W89.1 ☑
  supersonic waves W42.0 ☑
  transmission line(s), electric W85 ☑
  vibration W49.9 ☑
  waves
    infrasound W49.9 ☑
    sound W42.9 ☑
    supersonic W42.0 ☑
  weather NEC — *see* Forces of nature
External cause status Y99.9
  child assisting in compensated work for family Y99.8
  civilian activity done for financial or other compensation Y99.0
  civilian activity done for income or pay Y99.0
  family member assisting in compensated work for other family member Y99.8
  hobby not done for income Y99.8
  leisure activity Y99.8
  military activity Y99.1
  off-duty activity of military personnel Y99.8
  recreation or sport not for income or while a student Y99.8
  specified NEC Y99.8
  student activity Y99.8
  volunteer activity Y99.2

F

Factors, supplemental
  alcohol
    blood level
      less than 20mg/100ml Y90.0
      presence in blood, level not specified Y90.9
      20-39mg/100ml Y90.1
      40-59mg/100ml Y90.2
      60-79mg/100ml Y90.3
      80-99mg/100ml Y90.4
      100-119mg/100ml Y90.5
      120-199mg/100ml Y90.6
      200-239mg/100ml Y90.7
      240mg/100ml or more Y90.8
    presence in blood, but level not specified Y90.9
  environmental-pollution-related condition- see Z57 ☑
  nosocomial condition Y95
  work-related condition Y99.0
Failure
  in suture or ligature during surgical procedure Y65.2
  mechanical, of instrument or apparatus (any) (during any medical or surgical procedure) Y65.8
  sterile precautions (during medical and surgical care) — *see* Misadventure, failure, sterile precautions, by type of procedure
  to
    introduce tube or instrument Y65.4
      endotracheal tube during anesthesia Y65.3
    make curve (transport vehicle) NEC — *see* Accident, transport
    remove tube or instrument Y65.4
Fall, falling (accidental) W19 ☑
  building W20.1 ☑
    burning (uncontrolled fire) X00.3 ☑
  down
    embankment W17.81 ☑
    escalator W10.0 ☑

Fall, falling — *continued*
  down — *continued*
    hill W17.81 ☑
    ladder W11 ☑
    ramp W10.2 ☑
    stairs, steps W10.9 ☑
  due to
    bumping against
      object W18.00 ☑
        sharp glass W18.02 ☑
        specified NEC W18.09 ☑
        sports equipment W18.01 ☑
      person W03 ☑
        due to ice or snow W00.0 ☑
        on pedestrian conveyance — *see* Accident, transport, pedestrian, conveyance
    collision with another person W03 ☑
      due to ice or snow W00.0 ☑
      involving pedestrian conveyance — *see* Accident, transport, pedestrian, conveyance
    grocery cart tipping over W17.82 ☑
    ice or snow W00.9 ☑
      from one level to another W00.2 ☑
      on stairs or steps W00.1 ☑
      involving pedestrian conveyance — *see* Accident, transport, pedestrian, conveyance
      on same level W00.0 ☑
    slipping (on moving sidewalk) W01.0 ☑
      with subsequent striking against object W01.10 ☑
        furniture W01.190 ☑
        sharp object W01.119 ☑
          glass W01.110 ☑
          power tool or machine W01.111 ☑
          specified NEC W01.118 ☑
        specified NEC W01.198 ☑
    striking against
      object W18.00 ☑
        sharp glass W18.02 ☑
        specified NEC W18.09 ☑
        sports equipment W18.01 ☑
      person W03 ☑
        due to ice or snow W00.0 ☑
        on pedestrian conveyance — *see* Accident, transport, pedestrian, conveyance
  earth (with asphyxia or suffocation (by pressure)) — *see* Earth, falling
  from, off, out of
    aircraft NEC (with accident to aircraft NEC) V97.0 ☑
      while boarding or alighting V97.1 ☑
    balcony W13.0 ☑
    bed W06 ☑
    boat, ship, watercraft NEC (with drowning or submersion) — *see* Drowning, due to, fall overboard
      with hitting bottom or object V94.0 ☑
    bridge W13.1 ☑
    building W13.9 ☑
      burning (uncontrolled fire) X00.3 ☑
    cavity W17.2 ☑
    chair W07 ☑
    cherry picker W17.89 ☑
    cliff W15 ☑
    dock W17.4 ☑
    embankment W17.81 ☑
    escalator W10.0 ☑
    flagpole W13.8 ☑
    furniture NEC W08 ☑
    grocery cart W17.82 ☑
    haystack W17.89 ☑
    high place NEC W17.89 ☑
      stated as undetermined whether accidental or intentional Y30 ☑
    hole W17.2 ☑
    incline W10.2 ☑
    ladder W11 ☑
    lifting device W17.89 ☑
    machine, machinery — *see also* Contact, with, by type of machine
      not in operation W17.89 ☑
    manhole W17.1 ☑
    mobile elevated work platform [MEWP] W17.89 ☑
    motorized mobility scooter W05.2 ☑
    one level to another NEC W17.89 ☑
      intentional, purposeful, suicide (attempt) X80 ☑

Fall, falling — *continued*
  from, off, out of — *continued*
    one level to another — *continued*
      stated as undetermined whether accidental or intentional Y30 ☑
    pit W17.2 ☑
    playground equipment W09.8 ☑
      jungle gym W09.2 ☑
      slide W09.0 ☑
      swing W09.1 ☑
    quarry W17.89 ☑
    railing W13.9 ☑
    ramp W10.2 ☑
    roof W13.2 ☑
    scaffolding W12 ☑
    scooter (nonmotorized) W05.1 ☑
      motorized mobility W05.2 ☑
    sky lift W17.89 ☑
    stairs, steps W10.9 ☑
      curb W10.1 ☑
      due to ice or snow W00.1 ☑
      escalator W10.0 ☑
      incline W10.2 ☑
      ramp W10.2 ☑
      sidewalk curb W10.1 ☑
      specified NEC W10.8 ☑
      standing
        electric scooter V00.841 ☑
        micro-mobility pedestrian conveyance V00.848 ☑
    stepladder W11 ☑
    stool W08 ☑
    storm drain W17.1 ☑
    streetcar NEC V82.6 ☑
      while boarding or alighting V82.4 ☑
      with antecedent collision — *see* Accident, transport, streetcar occupant
    structure NEC W13.8 ☑
      burning (uncontrolled fire) X00.3 ☑
    table W08 ☑
    toilet W18.11 ☑
      with subsequent striking against object W18.12 ☑
    train NEC V81.6 ☑
      during derailment (without antecedent collision) V81.7 ☑
      with antecedent collision — *see* Accident, transport, railway vehicle occupant
      while boarding or alighting V81.4 ☑
    transport vehicle after collision — *see* Accident, transport, by type of vehicle, collision
    tree W14 ☑
    vehicle (in motion) NEC — *see also* Accident, transport V89.9 ☑
      motor NEC — *see also* Accident, transport, occupant, by type of vehicle V87.8 ☑
      stationary W17.89 ☑
        while boarding or alighting — *see* Accident, transport, by type of vehicle, while boarding or alighting
    viaduct W13.8 ☑
    wall W13.8 ☑
    watercraft — *see also* Drowning, due to, fall overboard
      with hitting bottom or object V94.0 ☑
    well W17.0 ☑
    wheelchair, non-moving W05.0 ☑
      powered — *see* Accident, transport, pedestrian, conveyance occupant, specified type NEC
    window W13.4 ☑
  in, on
    aircraft NEC V97.0 ☑
      while boarding or alighting V97.1 ☑
      with accident to aircraft V97.0 ☑
    bathtub (empty) W18.2 ☑
      filled W16.212 ☑
        causing drowning W16.211 ☑
    escalator W10.0 ☑
    incline W10.2 ☑
    ladder W11 ☑
    machine, machinery — *see* Contact, with, by type of machine
    object, edged, pointed or sharp (with cut) — *see* Fall, by type
    playground equipment W09.8 ☑
      jungle gym W09.2 ☑

Fall, falling — *continued*
in, on — *continued*
  playground equipment — *continued*
    slide W09.0 ☑
    swing W09.1 ☑
  ramp W10.2 ☑
  scaffolding W12 ☑
  shower W18.2 ☑
    causing drowning W16.211 ☑
  staircase, stairs, steps W10.9 ☑
    curb W10.1 ☑
    due to ice or snow W00.1 ☑
    escalator W10.0 ☑
    incline W10.2 ☑
    specified NEC W10.8 ☑
  streetcar (without antecedent collision) V82.5 ☑
    with antecedent collision — *see* Accident, transport, streetcar occupant
    while boarding or alighting V82.4 ☑
  train (without antecedent collision) V81.5 ☑
    with antecedent collision — *see* Accident, transport, railway vehicle occupant
    during derailment (without antecedent collision) V81.7 ☑
      with antecedent collision — *see* Accident, transport, railway vehicle occupant
    while boarding or alighting V81.4 ☑
  transport vehicle after collision — *see* Accident, transport, by type of vehicle, collision
  watercraft V93.39 ☑
    due to
      accident to craft V91.29 ☑
        powered craft V91.23 ☑
          ferry boat V91.21 ☑
          fishing boat V91.22 ☑
          jetskis V91.23 ☑
          liner V91.21 ☑
          merchant ship V91.20 ☑
          passenger ship V91.21 ☑
        unpowered craft
          canoe V91.25 ☑
          inflatable V91.26 ☑
          kayak V91.25 ☑
          sailboat V91.24 ☑
      powered craft V93.33 ☑
        ferry boat V93.31 ☑
        fishing boat V93.32 ☑
        jetskis V93.33 ☑
        liner V93.31 ☑
        merchant ship V93.30 ☑
        passenger ship V93.31 ☑
      unpowered craft V93.38 ☑
        canoe V93.35 ☑
        inflatable V93.36 ☑
        kayak V93.35 ☑
        sailboat V93.34 ☑
        surf-board V93.38 ☑
        windsurfer V93.38 ☑
into
  cavity W17.2 ☑
  dock W17.4 ☑
  fire — *see* Exposure, fire, by type
  haystack W17.89 ☑
  hole W17.2 ☑
  lake — *see* Fall, into, water
  manhole W17.1 ☑
  moving part of machinery — *see* Contact, with, by type of machine
  ocean — *see* Fall, into, water
  opening in surface NEC W17.89 ☑
  pit W17.2 ☑
  pond — *see* Fall, into, water
  quarry W17.89 ☑
  river — *see* Fall, into, water
  shaft W17.89 ☑
  storm drain W17.1 ☑
  stream — *see* Fall, into, water
  swimming pool — *see also* Fall, into, water, in, swimming pool
    empty W17.3 ☑
  tank W17.89 ☑
  water W16.42 ☑
    causing drowning W16.41 ☑
    from watercraft — *see* Drowning, due to, fall overboard
    hitting diving board W21.4 ☑

Fall, falling — *continued*
into — *continued*
  water — *continued*
    in
      bathtub W16.212 ☑
        causing drowning W16.211 ☑
      bucket W16.222 ☑
        causing drowning W16.221 ☑
      natural body of water W16.112 ☑
        causing drowning W16.111 ☑
        striking
          bottom W16.122 ☑
            causing drowning W16.121 ☑
          side W16.132 ☑
            causing drowning W16.131 ☑
      specified water NEC W16.312 ☑
      causing drowning W16.311 ☑
        striking
          bottom W16.322 ☑
            causing drowning W16.321 ☑
          wall W16.332 ☑
            causing drowning W16.331 ☑
      swimming pool W16.012 ☑
        causing drowning W16.011 ☑
        striking
          bottom W16.022 ☑
            causing drowning W16.031 ☑
          wall W16.032 ☑
            causing drowning W16.021 ☑
      utility bucket W16.222 ☑
        causing drowning W16.221 ☑
    well W17.0 ☑
  involving
    bed W06 ☑
    chair W07 ☑
    furniture NEC W08 ☑
    glass — *see* Fall, by type
    playground equipment W09.8 ☑
      jungle gym W09.2 ☑
      slide W09.0 ☑
      swing W09.1 ☑
    roller blades — *see* Accident, transport, pedestrian, conveyance
    skateboard(s) — *see* Accident, transport, pedestrian, conveyance
    skates (ice) (in line) (roller) — *see* Accident, transport, pedestrian, conveyance
    skis — *see* Accident, transport, pedestrian, conveyance
    table W08 ☑
    wheelchair, non-moving W05.0 ☑
      powered — *see* Accident, transport, pedestrian, conveyance, specified type NEC
object — *see* Struck by, object, falling
off
  toilet W18.11 ☑
    with subsequent striking against object W18.12 ☑
on same level W18.30 ☑
  due to
    specified NEC W18.39 ☑
    stepping on an object W18.31 ☑
out of
  bed W06 ☑
  building NEC W13.8 ☑
  chair W07 ☑
  furniture NEC W08 ☑
  wheelchair, non-moving W05.0 ☑
    powered — *see* Accident, transport, pedestrian, conveyance, specified type NEC
  window W13.4 ☑
over
  animal W01.0 ☑
  cliff W15 ☑
  embankment W17.81 ☑
  small object W01.0 ☑
rock W20.8 ☑
same level W18.30 ☑
  from
    being crushed, pushed, or stepped on by a crowd or human stampede W52 ☑
    collision, pushing, shoving, by or with other person W03 ☑
    slipping, stumbling, tripping W01.0 ☑
  involving ice or snow W00.0 ☑

Fall, falling — *continued*
same level — *continued*
  involving ice or snow — *continued*
    involving skates (ice) (roller), skateboard, skis — *see* Accident, transport, pedestrian, conveyance
  snowslide (avalanche) — *see* Landslide
  stone W20.8 ☑
  structure W20.1 ☑
    burning (uncontrolled fire) X00.3 ☑
  through
    bridge W13.1 ☑
    floor W13.3 ☑
    roof W13.2 ☑
    wall W13.8 ☑
    window W13.4 ☑
  timber W20.8 ☑
  tree (caused by lightning) W20.8 ☑
  while being carried or supported by other person(s) W04 ☑
Fallen on by
  animal (not being ridden) NEC W55.89 ☑
Felo-de-se — *see* Suicide
Fight (hand) (fists) (foot) — *see* Assault, fight
Fire (accidental) — *see* Exposure, fire
Firearm discharge — *see* Discharge, firearm
Fireball effects from nuclear explosion in war operations — *see* War operations, nuclear weapons
Fireworks (explosion) W39
Flash burns from explosion — *see* Explosion
Flood (any injury) (caused by) X38 ☑
  collapse of man-made structure causing earth movement X36.0 ☑
  tidal wave — *see* Forces of nature, tidal wave
Food (any type) **in**
  air passages (with asphyxia, obstruction, or suffocation) — *see* categories T17 and T18 ☑
  alimentary tract causing asphyxia (due to compression of trachea) — *see* categories T17 and T18 ☑
Forces of nature X39.8 ☑
  avalanche X36.1 ☑
    causing transport accident — *see* Accident, transport, by type of vehicle
  blizzard X37.2 ☑
  cataclysmic storm X37.9 ☑
    with flood X38
    blizzard X37.2 ☑
    cloudburst X37.8 ☑
    cyclone X37.1 ☑
    dust storm X37.3 ☑
    hurricane X37.0 ☑
    specified storm NEC X37.8 ☑
    storm surge X37.0 ☑
    tornado X37.1 ☑
    twister X37.1 ☑
    typhoon X37.0 ☑
  cloudburst X37.8 ☑
  cold (natural) X31
  cyclone X37.1 ☑
  dam collapse causing earth movement X36.0 ☑
  dust storm X37.3 ☑
  earth movement X36.1 ☑
    caused by dam or structure collapse X36.0 ☑
    earthquake X34 ☑
  earthquake X34 ☑
  flood (caused by) X38 ☑
    dam collapse X36.0 ☑
    tidal wave — *see* Forces of nature, tidal wave
  heat (natural) X30 ☑
  hurricane X37.0 ☑
  landslide X36.1 ☑
    causing transport accident — *see* Accident, transport, by type of vehicle
  lightning — *see* subcategory T75.0 ☑
    causing fire — *see* Exposure, fire
  mudslide X36.1 ☑
    causing transport accident — *see* Accident, transport, by type of vehicle
  radiation (natural) X39.08 ☑
    radon X39.01 ☑
  radon X39.01 ☑
  specified force NEC X39.8 ☑
  storm surge X37.0 ☑
  structure collapse causing earth movement X36.0 ☑
  sunlight X32
  tidal wave X37.41 ☑

Forces of nature — *continued*
  tidal wave — *continued*
    due to
      earthquake X37.41 ☑
      landslide X37.43 ☑
      storm X37.42 ☑
      volcanic eruption X37.41 ☑
  tornado X37.1 ☑
  tsunami X37.41 ☑
  twister X37.1 ☑
  typhoon X37.0 ☑
  volcanic eruption X35 ☑
Foreign body
  aspiration — *see* Index to Diseases and Injuries, Foreign body, respiratory tract
  embedded in skin W45 ☑
  entering through skin W45.8 ☑
    can lid W26.8 ☑
    nail W45.0 ☑
    paper W26.2 ☑
    specified NEC W45.8 ☑
    splinter W45.8 ☑
Forest fire (exposure to) — *see* Exposure, fire, uncontrolled, not in building
Found injured X58 ☑
  from exposure (to) — *see* Exposure
  on
    highway, road(way), street V89.9 ☑
    railway right of way V81.9 ☑
Fracture (circumstances unknown or unspecified) X58 ☑
  due to specified cause NEC X58 ☑
Freezing — *see* Exposure, cold
Frostbite X31 ☑
  due to man-made conditions — *see* Exposure, cold, man-made
Frozen — *see* Exposure, cold

G

Gored by bull W55.22 ☑
Gunshot wound W34.00 ☑

H

Hailstones, injured by X39.8 ☑
Hanged herself or himself — *see* Hanging, self-inflicted
Hanging (accidental) — *see also* category T71 ☑
  legal execution — *see* Legal, intervention, specified means NEC
Heat (effects of) (excessive) X30 ☑
  due to
    man-made conditions W92 ☑
      on board watercraft V93.29 ☑
        fishing boat V93.22 ☑
        merchant ship V93.20 ☑
        passenger ship V93.21 ☑
        sailboat V93.24 ☑
        specified powered craft NEC V93.23 ☑
    weather (conditions) X30 ☑
  from
    electric heating apparatus causing burning X16 ☑
    nuclear explosion in war operations — *see* War operations, nuclear weapons
  inappropriate in local application or packing in medical or surgical procedure Y63.5
Hemorrhage
  delayed following medical or surgical treatment without mention of misadventure — *see* Index to Diseases and Injuries, Complication(s)
  during medical or surgical treatment as misadventure — *see* Index to Diseases and Injuries, Complication(s)
High
  altitude (effects) — *see* Air, pressure, low
  level of radioactivity, effects — *see* Radiation
  pressure (effects) — *see* Air, pressure, high
  temperature, effects — *see* Heat
Hit, hitting (accidental) by — *see* Struck by
Hitting against — *see* Striking against
Homicide (attempt) (justifiable) — *see* Assault
Hot
  place, effects — *see also* Heat
  weather, effects X30 ☑
House fire (uncontrolled) — *see* Exposure, fire, uncontrolled, building
Humidity, causing problem X39.8 ☑

Hunger X58 ☑
Hurricane (any injury) X37.0 ☑
Hypobarism, hypobaropathy — *see* Air, pressure, low

I

Ictus
  caloris — *see also* Heat
  solaris X30 ☑
Ignition (accidental) — *see also* Exposure, fire X08.8 ☑
  anesthetic gas in operating room W40.1 ☑
  apparel X06.2 ☑
    from highly flammable material X04 ☑
    nightwear X05 ☑
  bed linen (sheets) (spreads) (pillows) (mattress) — *see* Exposure, fire, uncontrolled, building, bed
  benzine X04 ☑
  clothes, clothing NEC (from controlled fire) X06.2 ☑
    from
      highly flammable material X04 ☑
  ether X04 ☑
    in operating room W40.1 ☑
  explosive material — *see* Explosion
  gasoline X04 ☑
  jewelry (plastic) (any) X06.0 ☑
  kerosene X04 ☑
  material
    explosive — *see* Explosion
    highly flammable with secondary explosion X04 ☑
  nightwear X05 ☑
  paraffin X04 ☑
  petrol X04 ☑
Immersion (accidental) — *see also* Drowning
  hand or foot due to cold (excessive) X31 ☑
Implantation of quills of porcupine W55.89 ☑
Inanition (from) (hunger) X58 ☑
  thirst X58 ☑
Inappropriate operation performed
  correct operation on wrong side or body part (wrong side) (wrong site) Y65.53
  operation intended for another patient done on wrong patient Y65.52
  wrong operation performed on correct patient Y65.51
Inattention after, at birth (homicidal intent) (infanticidal intent) X58 ☑
Incident, adverse
  device
    anesthesiology Y70.8
      accessory Y70.2
      diagnostic Y70.0
      miscellaneous Y70.8
      monitoring Y70.0
      prosthetic Y70.2
      rehabilitative Y70.1
      surgical Y70.3
      therapeutic Y70.1
    cardiovascular Y71.8
      accessory Y71.2
      diagnostic Y71.0
      miscellaneous Y71.8
      monitoring Y71.0
      prosthetic Y71.2
      rehabilitative Y71.1
      surgical Y71.3
      therapeutic Y71.1
    gastroenterology Y73.8
      accessory Y73.2
      diagnostic Y73.0
      miscellaneous Y73.8
      monitoring Y73.0
      prosthetic Y73.2
      rehabilitative Y73.1
      surgical Y73.3
      therapeutic Y73.1
    general
      hospital Y74.8
        accessory Y74.2
        diagnostic Y74.0
        miscellaneous Y74.8
        monitoring Y74.0
        prosthetic Y74.2
        rehabilitative Y74.1
        surgical Y74.3
        therapeutic Y74.1
      surgical Y81.8
        accessory Y81.2
        diagnostic Y81.0

Incident, adverse — *continued*
  device — *continued*
    general — *continued*
      surgical — *continued*
        miscellaneous Y81.8
        monitoring Y81.0
        prosthetic Y81.2
        rehabilitative Y81.1
        surgical Y81.3
        therapeutic Y81.1
    gynecological Y76.8
      accessory Y76.2
      diagnostic Y76.0
      miscellaneous Y76.8
      monitoring Y76.0
      prosthetic Y76.2
      rehabilitative Y76.1
      surgical Y76.3
      therapeutic Y76.1
    medical Y82.9
      specified type NEC Y82.8
    neurological Y75.8
      accessory Y75.2
      diagnostic Y75.0
      miscellaneous Y75.8
      monitoring Y75.0
      prosthetic Y75.2
      rehabilitative Y75.1
      surgical Y75.3
      therapeutic Y75.1
    obstetrical Y76.8
      accessory Y76.2
      diagnostic Y76.0
      miscellaneous Y76.8
      monitoring Y76.0
      prosthetic Y76.2
      rehabilitative Y76.1
      surgical Y76.3
      therapeutic Y76.1
    ophthalmic Y77.8
      accessory Y77.2
      contact lens (rigid gas permeable) (soft (hydrophilic)) Y77.11
      diagnostic Y77.0
      miscellaneous Y77.8
      monitoring Y77.0
      prosthetic Y77.2
      rehabilitative Y77.19
      surgical Y77.3
      therapeutic Y77.19
    orthopedic Y79.8
      accessory Y79.2
      diagnostic Y79.0
      miscellaneous Y79.8
      monitoring Y79.0
      prosthetic Y79.2
      rehabilitative Y79.1
      surgical Y79.3
      therapeutic Y79.1
    otorhinolaryngological Y72.8
      accessory Y72.2
      diagnostic Y72.0
      miscellaneous Y72.8
      monitoring Y72.0
      prosthetic Y72.2
      rehabilitative Y72.1
      surgical Y72.3
      therapeutic Y72.1
    personal use Y74.8
      accessory Y74.2
      diagnostic Y74.0
      miscellaneous Y74.8
      monitoring Y74.0
      prosthetic Y74.2
      rehabilitative Y74.1
      surgical Y74.3
      therapeutic Y74.1
    physical medicine Y80.8
      accessory Y80.2
      diagnostic Y80.0
      miscellaneous Y80.8
      monitoring Y80.0
      prosthetic Y80.2
      rehabilitative Y80.1
      surgical Y80.3
      therapeutic Y80.1
    plastic surgical Y81.8
      accessory Y81.2
      diagnostic Y81.0

Incident, adverse — *continued*
  device — *continued*
    plastic surgical — *continued*
      miscellaneous Y81.8
      monitoring Y81.0
      prosthetic Y81.2
      rehabilitative Y81.1
      surgical Y81.3
      therapeutic Y81.1
    radiological Y78.8
      accessory Y78.2
      diagnostic Y78.0
      miscellaneous Y78.8
      monitoring Y78.0
      prosthetic Y78.2
      rehabilitative Y78.1
      surgical Y78.3
      therapeutic Y78.1
    urology Y73.8
      accessory Y73.2
      diagnostic Y73.0
      miscellaneous Y73.8
      monitoring Y73.0
      prosthetic Y73.2
      rehabilitative Y73.1
      surgical Y73.3
      therapeutic Y73.1
Incineration (accidental) — *see* Exposure, fire
Infanticide — *see* Assault
Infrasound waves (causing injury) W49.9 ☑
Ingestion
  foreign body (causing injury) (with obstruction) — *see* Foreign body, alimentary canal
  poisonous
    plant(s) X58 ☑
    substance NEC — *see* Table of Drugs and Chemicals
Inhalation
  excessively cold substance, man-made — *see* Exposure, cold, man-made
  food (any type) (into respiratory tract) (with asphyxia, obstruction respiratory tract, suffocation) — *see* categories T17 and T18 ☑
  foreign body — *see* Foreign body, aspiration
  gastric contents (with asphyxia, obstruction respiratory passage, suffocation) T17.81- ☑
  hot air or gases X14.0 ☑
  liquid air, hydrogen, nitrogen W93.12 ☑
    suicide (attempt) X83.2 ☑
  steam X13.0 ☑
    assault X98.0 ☑
    stated as undetermined whether accidental or intentional Y27.0 ☑
    suicide (attempt) X77.0 ☑
  toxic gas — *see* Table of Drugs and Chemicals
  vomitus (with asphyxia, obstruction respiratory passage, suffocation) T17.81- ☑
Injury, injured (accidental(ly)) NOS X58 ☑
  by, caused by, from
    assault — *see* Assault
    law-enforcing agent, police, in course of legal intervention — *see* Legal intervention
    suicide (attempt) X83.8 ☑
  due to, in
    civil insurrection — *see* War operations
    fight — *see also* Assault, fight Y04.0 ☑
    war operations — *see* War operations
  homicide — *see also* Assault Y09
  inflicted (by)
    in course of arrest (attempted), suppression of disturbance, maintenance of order, by law-enforcing agents — *see* Legal intervention
    other person
      stated as
        accidental X58 ☑
        intentional, homicide (attempt) — *see* Assault
        undetermined whether accidental or intentional Y33 ☑
    purposely (inflicted) by other person(s) — *see* Assault
  self-inflicted X83.8 ☑
    stated as accidental X58 ☑
  specified cause NEC X58 ☑
  undetermined whether accidental or intentional Y33 ☑
Insolation, effects X30 ☑
Insufficient nourishment X58 ☑
Interruption of respiration (by)
  food (lodged in esophagus) — *see* categories T17 and T18 ☑

Interruption of respiration — *continued*
  vomitus (lodged in esophagus) T17.81- ☑
Intervention, legal — *see* Legal intervention
Intoxication
  drug — *see* Table of Drugs and Chemicals
  poison — *see* Table of Drugs and Chemicals

J

Jammed (accidentally)
  between objects (moving) (stationary and moving) W23.0 ☑
    stationary W23.1 ☑
Jumped, jumping
  before moving object NEC X81.8 ☑
    motor vehicle X81.0 ☑
    subway train X81.1 ☑
    train X81.1 ☑
    undetermined whether accidental or intentional Y31 ☑
  from
    boat (into water) voluntarily, without accident (to or on boat) W16.712 ☑
      striking bottom W16.722 ☑
        causing drowning W16.721 ☑
      with
        accident to or on boat — *see* Accident, watercraft
        drowning or submersion W16.711 ☑
          suicide (attempt) X71.3 ☑
    building — *see also* Jumped, from, high place W13.9 ☑
      burning (uncontrolled fire) X00.5 ☑
    high place NEC W17.89 ☑
      suicide (attempt) X80 ☑
      undetermined whether accidental or intentional Y30 ☑
    structure — *see also* Jumped, from, high place W13.9 ☑
      burning (uncontrolled fire) X00.5 ☑
  into water W16.92 ☑
    causing drowning W16.91 ☑
    from, off watercraft — *see* Jumped, from, boat
    in
      natural body W16.612 ☑
        causing drowning W16.611 ☑
        striking bottom W16.622 ☑
          causing drowning W16.621 ☑
      specified place NEC W16.812 ☑
        causing drowning W16.811 ☑
        striking
          bottom W16.822 ☑
            causing drowning W16.821 ☑
          wall W16.832 ☑
            causing drowning W16.831 ☑
      swimming pool W16.512 ☑
        causing drowning W16.511 ☑
        striking
          bottom W16.522 ☑
            causing drowning W16.521 ☑
          wall W16.532 ☑
            causing drowning W16.531 ☑
    suicide (attempt) X71.3 ☑

K

Kicked by
  animal NEC W55.82 ☑
  person(s) (accidentally) W50.1 ☑
    with intent to injure or kill Y04.0 ☑
    as, or caused by, a crowd or human stampede (with fall) W52 ☑
    assault Y04.0 ☑
    homicide (attempt) Y04.0 ☑
    in
      fight Y04.0 ☑
      legal intervention
        injuring
          bystander Y35.812 ☑
          law enforcement personnel Y35.811 ☑
          suspect Y35.813 ☑
          unspecified person Y35.819 ☑
Kicking
  against
    object W22.8 ☑
      sports equipment W21.9 ☑

Kicking — *continued*
  against — *continued*
    object — *continued*
      stationary W22.09 ☑
        sports equipment W21.89 ☑
      person — *see* Striking against, person
      sports equipment W21.9 ☑
  carpet stretcher with knee X50.3 ☑
Killed, killing (accidentally) NOS — *see also* Injury X58 ☑
  in
    action — *see* War operations
    brawl, fight (hand) (fists) (foot) Y04.0 ☑
      by weapon — *see also* Assault
        cutting, piercing — *see* Assault, cutting or piercing instrument
        firearm — *see* Discharge, firearm, by type, homicide
  self
    stated as
      accident NOS X58 ☑
      suicide — *see* Suicide
      undetermined whether accidental or intentional Y33 ☑
Kneeling (prolonged) (static) X50.1 ☑
Knocked down (accidentally) (by) NOS X58 ☑
  animal (not being ridden) NEC — *see also* Struck by, by type of animal
  crowd or human stampede W52 ☑
  person W51 ☑
    in brawl, fight Y04.0 ☑
  transport vehicle NEC — *see also* Accident, transport V09.9 ☑

L

Laceration NEC — *see* Injury
Lack of
  care (helpless person) (infant) (newborn) X58 ☑
  food except as result of abandonment or neglect X58 ☑
    due to abandonment or neglect X58 ☑
  water except as result of transport accident X58 ☑
    due to transport accident — *see* Accident, transport, by type
  helpless person, infant, newborn X58 ☑
Landslide (falling on transport vehicle) X36.1 ☑
  caused by collapse of man-made structure X36.0 ☑
Late effect — *see* Sequelae
Legal
  execution (any method) — *see* Legal, intervention
  intervention (by)
    baton — *see* Legal, intervention, blunt object, baton
    bayonet — *see* Legal, intervention, sharp object, bayonet
    blow — *see* Legal, intervention, manhandling
    blunt object
      baton
        injuring
          bystander Y35.312 ☑
          law enforcement personnel Y35.311 ☑
          suspect Y35.313 ☑
          unspecified person Y35.319 ☑
      injuring
        bystander Y35.302 ☑
        law enforcement personnel Y35.301 ☑
        suspect Y35.303 ☑
        unspecified person Y35.309 ☑
      specified NEC
        injuring
          bystander Y35.392 ☑
          law enforcement personnel Y35.391 ☑
          suspect Y35.393 ☑
          unspecified person Y35.399 ☑
      stave
        injuring
          bystander Y35.392 ☑
          law enforcement personnel Y35.391 ☑
          suspect Y35.393 ☑
          unspecified person Y35.399 ☑
    bomb — *see* Legal, intervention, explosive
    conducted energy device
      injuring
        bystander Y35.832 ☑
        law enforcement personnel Y35.831 ☑
        suspect Y35.833 ☑
        unspecified person Y35.839 ☑

Legal — *continued*
  intervention — *continued*
    cutting or piercing instrument — *see* Legal, intervention, sharp object
    dynamite — *see* Legal, intervention, explosive, dynamite
    electroshock device (taser)
      injuring
        bystander Y35.832 ☑
        law enforcement personnel Y35.831 ☑
        suspect Y35.833 ☑
        unspecified person Y35.839 ☑
    explosive(s)
      dynamite
        injuring
          bystander Y35.112 ☑
          law enforcement personnel Y35.111 ☑
          suspect Y35.113 ☑
          unspecified person Y35.119 ☑
      grenade
        injuring
          bystander Y35.192 ☑
          law enforcement personnel Y35.191 ☑
          suspect Y35.193 ☑
          unspecified person Y35.199 ☑
      injuring
        bystander Y35.102 ☑
        law enforcement personnel Y35.101 ☑
        suspect Y35.103 ☑
        unspecified person Y35.109 ☑
      mortar bomb
        injuring
          bystander Y35.192 ☑
          law enforcement personnel Y35.191 ☑
          suspect Y35.193 ☑
          unspecified person Y35.199 ☑
      shell
        injuring
          bystander Y35.122 ☑
          law enforcement personnel Y35.121 ☑
          suspect Y35.123 ☑
          unspecified person Y35.129 ☑
      specified NEC
        injuring
          bystander Y35.192 ☑
          law enforcement personnel Y35.191 ☑
          suspect Y35.193 ☑
          unspecified person Y35.199 ☑
    firearm(s) (discharge)
      handgun
        injuring
          bystander Y35.022 ☑
          law enforcement personnel Y35.021 ☑
          suspect Y35.023 ☑
          unspecified person Y35.029 ☑
      injuring
        bystander Y35.002 ☑
        law enforcement personnel Y35.001 ☑
        suspect Y35.003 ☑
        unspecified person Y35.009 ☑
      machine gun
        injuring
          bystander Y35.012 ☑
          law enforcement personnel Y35.011 ☑
          suspect Y35.013 ☑
          unspecified person Y35.019 ☑
      rifle pellet
        injuring
          bystander Y35.032 ☑
          law enforcement personnel Y35.031 ☑
          suspect Y35.033 ☑
          unspecified person Y35.039 ☑
      rubber bullet
        injuring
          bystander Y35.042 ☑
          law enforcement personnel Y35.041 ☑
          suspect Y35.043 ☑
          unspecified person Y35.049 ☑
      shotgun — *see* Legal, intervention, firearm, specified NEC
      specified NEC
        injuring
          bystander Y35.092 ☑
          law enforcement personnel Y35.091 ☑
          suspect Y35.093 ☑
          unspecified person Y35.099 ☑

Legal — *continued*
  intervention — *continued*
    gas (asphyxiation) (poisoning)
      injuring
        bystander Y35.202 ☑
        law enforcement personnel Y35.201 ☑
        suspect Y35.203 ☑
        unspecified person Y35.209 ☑
      specified NEC
        injuring
          bystander Y35.292 ☑
          law enforcement personnel Y35.291 ☑
          suspect Y35.293 ☑
          unspecified person Y35.299 ☑
      tear gas
        injuring
          bystander Y35.212 ☑
          law enforcement personnel Y35.211 ☑
          suspect Y35.213 ☑
          unspecified person Y35.219 ☑
    grenade — *see* Legal, intervention, explosive, grenade
    injuring
      bystander Y35.92 ☑
      law enforcement personnel Y35.91 ☑
      suspect Y35.93 ☑
      unspecified person Y35.99 ☑
    late effect (of) — *see* with 7th character S Y35 ☑
    manhandling
      injuring
        bystander Y35.812 ☑
        law enforcement personnel Y35.811 ☑
        suspect Y35.813 ☑
        unspecified person Y35.819 ☑
    sequelae (of) — *see* with 7th character S Y35 ☑
    sharp objects
      bayonet
        injuring
          bystander Y35.412 ☑
          law enforcement personnel Y35.411 ☑
          suspect Y35.413 ☑
          unspecified person Y35.419 ☑
      injuring
        bystander Y35.402 ☑
        law enforcement personnel Y35.401 ☑
        suspect Y35.403 ☑
        unspecified person Y35.409 ☑
      specified NEC
        injuring
          bystander Y35.492 ☑
          law enforcement personnel Y35.491 ☑
          suspect Y35.493 ☑
          unspecified person Y35.499 ☑
    specified means NEC
      injuring
        bystander Y35.892 ☑
        law enforcement personnel Y35.891 ☑
        suspect Y35.893 ☑
        unspecified person Y35.899 ☑
    stabbing — *see* Legal, intervention, sharp object
    stave — *see* Legal, intervention, blunt object, stave
    stun gun
      injuring
        bystander Y35.832 ☑
        law enforcement personnel Y35.831 ☑
        suspect Y35.833 ☑
        unspecified person Y35.839 ☑
    taser
      injuring
        bystander Y35.832 ☑
        law enforcement personnel Y35.831 ☑
        suspect Y35.833 ☑
        unspecified person Y35.839 ☑
    tear gas — *see* Legal, intervention, gas, tear gas
    truncheon — *see* Legal, intervention, blunt object, stave

Lifting — *see also* Overexertion
  heavy objects X50.0 ☑
  weights X50.0 ☑
Lightning (shock) (stroke) (struck by) — *see* subcategory T75.0 ☑
  causing fire — *see* Exposure, fire
Loss of control (transport vehicle) NEC — *see* Accident, transport
Lost at sea NOS — *see* Drowning, due to, fall overboard

Low
  pressure (effects) — *see* Air, pressure, low
  temperature (effects) — *see* Exposure, cold
Lying before train, vehicle or other moving object
  X81.8 ☑
  subway train X81.1 ☑
  train X81.1 ☑
  undetermined whether accidental or intentional Y31 ☑
Lynching — *see* Assault

M

Malfunction (mechanism or component) (of)
  firearm W34.10 ☑
    airgun W34.110 ☑
    BB gun W34.110 ☑
    gas, air or spring-operated gun NEC W34.118 ☑
    handgun W32.1 ☑
    hunting rifle W33.12 ☑
    larger firearm W33.10 ☑
      specified NEC W33.19 ☑
    machine gun W33.13 ☑
    paintball gun W34.111 ☑
    pellet gun W34.110 ☑
    shotgun W33.11 ☑
    specified NEC W34.19 ☑
    Very pistol [flare] W34.19 ☑
  handgun — *see* Malfunction, firearm, handgun
Maltreatment — *see* Perpetrator
Mangled (accidentally) NOS X58 ☑
Manhandling (in brawl, fight) Y04.0 ☑
  legal intervention — *see* Legal, intervention, manhandling
Manslaughter (nonaccidental) — *see* Assault
Mauled by animal NEC W55.89 ☑
Medical procedure, complication of (delayed or as an abnormal reaction without mention of misadventure) — *see* Complication of or following, by specified type of procedure
  due to or as a result of misadventure — *see* Misadventure
Melting (due to fire) — *see also* Exposure, fire
  apparel NEC X06.3 ☑
  clothes, clothing NEC X06.3 ☑
    nightwear X05 ☑
  fittings or furniture (burning building) (uncontrolled fire) X00.8 ☑
  nightwear X05 ☑
  plastic jewelry X06.1 ☑
Mental cruelty X58 ☑
Military operations (injuries to military and civilians occuring during peacetime on military property and during routine military exercises and operations) (by) (from) (involving) Y37.90- ☑
  air blast Y37.20- ☑
  aircraft
    destruction — *see* Military operations, destruction of aircraft
    airway restriction — *see* Military operations, restriction of airways
    asphyxiation — *see* Military operations, restriction of airways
  biological weapons Y37.6X- ☑
  blast Y37.20- ☑
  blast fragments Y37.20- ☑
  blast wave Y37.20- ☑
  blast wind Y37.20- ☑
  bomb Y37.20- ☑
    dirty Y37.50- ☑
    gasoline Y37.31- ☑
    incendiary Y37.31- ☑
    petrol Y37.31- ☑
  bullet Y37.43- ☑
    incendiary Y37.32- ☑
    rubber Y37.41- ☑
  chemical weapons Y37.7X- ☑
  combat
    hand to hand (unarmed) combat Y37.44- ☑
    using blunt or piercing object Y37.45- ☑
  conflagration — *see* Military operations, fire
  conventional warfare NEC Y37.49- ☑
  depth-charge Y37.01- ☑
  destruction of aircraft Y37.10- ☑
    due to
      air to air missile Y37.11- ☑
      collision with other aircraft Y37.12- ☑

Military operations — *continued*
  destruction of aircraft — *continued*
    due to — *continued*
      detonation (accidental) of onboard munitions
        and explosives Y37.14- ☑
      enemy fire or explosives Y37.11- ☑
      explosive placed on aircraft Y37.11- ☑
      onboard fire Y37.13- ☑
      rocket propelled grenade [RPG] Y37.11- ☑
      small arms fire Y37.11- ☑
      surface to air missile Y37.11- ☑
    specified NEC Y37.19- ☑
  detonation (accidental) of
    onboard marine weapons Y37.05- ☑
    own munitions or munitions launch device
      Y37.24- ☑
  dirty bomb Y37.50- ☑
  explosion (of) Y37.20- ☑
    aerial bomb Y37.21- ☑
    bomb NOS — *see also* Military operations, bomb(s)
      Y37.20- ☑
    fragments Y37.20- ☑
    grenade Y37.29- ☑
    guided missile Y37.22- ☑
    improvised explosive device [IED] (person-borne)
      (roadside) (vehicle-borne) Y37.23- ☑
    land mine Y37.29- ☑
    marine mine (at sea) (in harbor) Y37.02- ☑
    marine weapon Y37.00- ☑
      specified NEC Y37.09- ☑
    own munitions or munitions launch device (acciden-
      tal) Y37.24- ☑
    sea-based artillery shell Y37.03- ☑
    specified NEC Y37.29- ☑
    torpedo Y37.04- ☑
  fire Y37.30- ☑
    specified NEC Y37.39- ☑
  firearms
    discharge Y37.43- ☑
    pellets Y37.42- ☑
  flamethrower Y37.33- ☑
  fragments (from) (of)
    improvised explosive device [IED] (person-borne)
      (roadside) (vehicle-borne) Y37.26- ☑
    munitions Y37.25- ☑
    specified NEC Y37.29- ☑
    weapons Y37.27- ☑
  friendly fire Y37.92- ☑
  hand to hand (unarmed) combat Y37.44- ☑
  hot substances — *see* Military operations, fire
  incendiary bullet Y37.32- ☑
  nuclear weapon (effects of) Y37.50- ☑
    acute radiation exposure Y37.54- ☑
    blast pressure Y37.51- ☑
    direct blast Y37.51- ☑
    direct heat Y37.53- ☑
    fallout exposure Y37.54- ☑
    fireball Y37.53- ☑
    indirect blast (struck or crushed by blast debris)
      (being thrown by blast) Y37.52- ☑
    ionizing radiation (immediate exposure) Y37.54- ☑
    nuclear radiation Y37.54- ☑
    radiation
      ionizing (immediate exposure) Y37.54- ☑
      nuclear Y37.54- ☑
      thermal Y37.53- ☑
    secondary effects Y37.54- ☑
    specified NEC Y37.59- ☑
    thermal radiation Y37.53- ☑
  restriction of air (airway)
    intentional Y37.46- ☑
    unintentional Y37.47- ☑
  rubber bullets Y37.41- ☑
  shrapnel NOS Y37.29- ☑
  suffocation — *see* Military operations, restriction of
    airways
  unconventional warfare NEC Y37.7X- ☑
  underwater blast NOS Y37.00- ☑
  warfare
    conventional NEC Y37.49- ☑
    unconventional NEC Y37.7X- ☑
  weapon of mass destruction [WMD] Y37.91- ☑
  weapons
    biological weapons Y37.6X- ☑
    chemical Y37.7X- ☑
    nuclear (effects of) Y37.50- ☑

Military operations — *continued*
  weapons — *continued*
    nuclear — *continued*
      acute radiation exposure Y37.54- ☑
      blast pressure Y37.51- ☑
      direct blast Y37.51- ☑
      direct heat Y37.53- ☑
      fallout exposure Y37.54- ☑
      fireball Y37.53- ☑
      radiation
        ionizing (immediate exposure) Y37.54- ☑
        nuclear Y37.54- ☑
        thermal Y37.53- ☑
      secondary effects Y37.54- ☑
      specified NEC Y37.59- ☑
    of mass destruction [WMD] Y37.91- ☑
Misadventure(s) **to patient**(s) **during surgical or
medical care** Y69
  contaminated medical or biological substance (blood,
    drug, fluid) Y64.9
    administered (by) NEC Y64.9
      immunization Y64.1
      infusion Y64.0
      injection Y64.1
      specified means NEC Y64.8
      transfusion Y64.0
      vaccination Y64.1
  excessive amount of blood or other fluid during trans-
    fusion or infusion Y63.0
  failure
    in dosage Y63.9
      electroshock therapy Y63.4
      inappropriate temperature (too hot or too cold)
        in local application and packing Y63.5
      infusion
        excessive amount of fluid Y63.0
        incorrect dilution of fluid Y63.1
      insulin-shock therapy Y63.4
      nonadministration of necessary drug or biologi-
        cal substance Y63.6
      overdose — *see* Table of Drugs and Chemicals
        radiation, in therapy Y63.2
      radiation
        overdose Y63.2
      specified procedure NEC Y63.8
      transfusion
        excessive amount of blood Y63.0
    mechanical, of instrument or apparatus (any) (during
      any procedure) Y65.8
    sterile precautions (during procedure) Y62.9
      aspiration of fluid or tissue (by puncture or
        catheterization, except heart) Y62.6
      biopsy (except needle aspiration) Y62.8
        needle (aspirating) Y62.6
      blood sampling Y62.6
      catheterization Y62.6
        heart Y62.5
      dialysis (kidney) Y62.2
      endoscopic examination Y62.4
      enema Y62.8
      immunization Y62.3
      infusion Y62.1
      injection Y62.3
      needle biopsy Y62.6
      paracentesis (abdominal) (thoracic) Y62.6
      perfusion Y62.2
      puncture (lumbar) Y62.6
      removal of catheter or packing Y62.8
      specified procedure NEC Y62.8
      surgical operation Y62.0
      transfusion Y62.1
      vaccination Y62.3
    suture or ligature during surgical procedure Y65.2
    to introduce or to remove tube or instrument —
      see Failure, to
  hemorrhage — *see* Index to Diseases and Injuries,
    Complication(s)
  inadvertent exposure of patient to radiation Y63.3
  inappropriate
    operation performed — *see* Inappropriate operation
      performed
    temperature (too hot or too cold) in local application
      or packing Y63.5
  infusion — *see also* Misadventure, by type, infusion
    Y69
    excessive amount of fluid Y63.0
    incorrect dilution of fluid Y63.1
    wrong fluid Y65.1

Misadventure(s) **to patient**(s) **during surgical or
medical care** — *continued*
  mismatched blood in transfusion Y65.0
  nonadministration of necessary drug or biological
    substance Y63.6
  overdose — *see* Table of Drugs and Chemicals
    radiation (in therapy) Y63.2
  perforation — *see* Index to Diseases and Injuries,
    Complication(s)
  performance of inappropriate operation — *see* Inap-
    propriate operation performed
  puncture — *see* Index to Diseases and Injuries, Compli-
    cation(s)
  specified type NEC Y65.8
    failure
      suture or ligature during surgical operation Y65.2
      to introduce or to remove tube or instrument —
        see Failure, to
    infusion of wrong fluid Y65.1
    performance of inappropriate operation — *see* In-
      appropriate operation performed
    transfusion of mismatched blood Y65.0
    wrong
      fluid in infusion Y65.1
      placement of endotracheal tube during anesthet-
        ic procedure Y65.3
  transfusion — *see* Misadventure, by type, transfusion
    excessive amount of blood Y63.0
    mismatched blood Y65.0
  wrong
    drug given in error — *see* Table of Drugs and
      Chemicals
    fluid in infusion Y65.1
    placement of endotracheal tube during anesthetic
      procedure Y65.3
Mismatched blood in transfusion Y65.0
Motion sickness T75.3 ☑
Mountain sickness W94.11 ☑
Mudslide (of cataclysmic nature) — *see* Landslide
Murder (attempt) — *see* Assault

N

Nail
  contact with W45.0 ☑
    gun W29.4 ☑
  embedded in skin W45.0 ☑
Neglect (criminal) (homicidal intent) X58 ☑
Noise (causing injury) (pollution) W42.9 ☑
  supersonic W42.0 ☑
Nonadministration (of)
  drug or biological substance (necessary) Y63.6
  surgical and medical care Y66
Nosocomial condition Y95

O

Object
  falling
    from, in, on, hitting
      machinery — *see* Contact, with, by type of ma-
        chine
  set in motion by
    accidental explosion or rupture of pressure vessel
      W38 ☑
    firearm — *see* Discharge, firearm, by type
    machine(ry) — *see* Contact, with, by type of ma-
      chine
Overdose (drug) — *see* Table of Drugs and Chemicals
  radiation Y63.2
Overexertion X50.9 ☑
  from
    prolonged static or awkward postures X50.1 ☑
    repetitive movements X50.3 ☑
    specified strenuous movements or postures NEC
      X50.9 ☑
    strenuous movement or load X50.0 ☑
Overexposure (accidental) (to)
  cold — *see also* Exposure, cold X31 ☑
    due to man-made conditions — *see* Exposure, cold,
      man-made
  heat — *see also* Heat X30 ☑
  radiation — *see* Radiation
  radioactivity W88.0 ☑
  sun (sunburn) X32 ☑
  weather NEC — *see* Forces of nature
  wind NEC — *see* Forces of nature

☑ **Additional Character Required — Refer to the Tabular List for Character Selection**

Overheated — *see* Heat
Overturning (accidental)
machinery — *see* Contact, with, by type of machine
transport vehicle NEC — *see also* Accident, transport
V89.9 ☑
watercraft (causing drowning, submersion) — *see also*
Drowning, due to, accident to, watercraft, overturning
causing injury except drowning or submersion —
see Accident, watercraft, causing, injury NEC

P

Parachute descent (voluntary) (without accident to aircraft) V97.29 ☑
due to accident to aircraft — *see* Accident, transport, aircraft
Pecked by bird W61.99 ☑
Perforation during medical or surgical treatment as misadventure — *see* Index to Diseases and Injuries, Complication(s)
Perpetrator, perpetration, of assault, maltreatment and neglect (by) Y07.9
boyfriend Y07.03
brother Y07.410
stepbrother Y07.435
coach Y07.53
cousin
female Y07.491
male Y07.490
daycare provider Y07.519
at-home
adult care Y07.512
childcare Y07.510
care center
adult care Y07.513
childcare Y07.511
family member NEC Y07.499
father Y07.11
adoptive Y07.13
foster Y07.420
stepfather Y07.430
foster father Y07.420
foster mother Y07.421
girl friend Y07.04
healthcare provider Y07.529
mental health Y07.521
specified NEC Y07.528
husband Y07.01
instructor Y07.53
mother Y07.12
adoptive Y07.14
foster Y07.421
stepmother Y07.433
multiple perpetrators Y07.6
nonfamily member Y07.50
specified NEC Y07.59
nurse Y07.528
occupational therapist Y07.528
partner of parent
female Y07.434
male Y07.432
physical therapist Y07.528
sister Y07.411
speech therapist Y07.528
stepbrother Y07.435
stepfather Y07.430
stepmother Y07.433
stepsister Y07.436
teacher Y07.53
wife Y07.02
Piercing — *see* Contact, with, by type of object or machine
Pinched
between objects (moving) (stationary and moving)
W23.0 ☑
stationary W23.1 ☑
Pinned under machine(ry) — *see* Contact, with, by type of machine
Place of occurrence Y92.9
abandoned house Y92.89
airplane Y92.813
airport Y92.520
ambulatory health services establishment NEC Y92.538
ambulatory surgery center Y92.530
amusement park Y92.831
apartment (co-op) — *see* Place of occurrence, residence, apartment

Place of occurrence — *continued*
assembly hall Y92.29
bank Y92.510
barn Y92.71
baseball field Y92.320
basketball court Y92.310
beach Y92.832
boarding house — *see* Place of occurrence, residence, boarding house
boat Y92.814
bowling alley Y92.39
bridge Y92.89
building under construction Y92.61
bus Y92.811
station Y92.521
cafe Y92.511
campsite Y92.833
campus — *see* Place of occurrence, school
canal Y92.89
car Y92.810
casino Y92.59
children's home — *see* Place of occurrence, residence, institutional, orphanage
church Y92.22
cinema Y92.26
clubhouse Y92.29
coal pit Y92.64
college (community) Y92.214
condominium — *see* Place of occurrence, residence, apartment
construction area — *see* Place of occurrence, industrial and construction area
convalescent home — *see* Place of occurrence, residence, institutional, nursing home
court-house Y92.240
cricket ground Y92.328
cultural building Y92.258
art gallery Y92.250
museum Y92.251
music hall Y92.252
opera house Y92.253
specified NEC Y92.258
theater Y92.254
dancehall Y92.252
day nursery Y92.210
dentist office Y92.531
derelict house Y92.89
desert Y92.820
dockyard Y92.62
dock NOS Y92.89
doctor's office Y92.531
dormitory — *see* Place of occurrence, residence, institutional, school dormitory
dry dock Y92.62
factory (building) (premises) Y92.63
farm (land under cultivation) (outbuildings) Y92.79
barn Y92.71
chicken coop Y92.72
field Y92.73
hen house Y92.72
house — *see* Place of occurrence, residence, house
orchard Y92.74
specified NEC Y92.79
football field Y92.321
forest Y92.821
freeway Y92.411
gallery Y92.250
garage (commercial) Y92.59
boarding house Y92.044
military base Y92.135
mobile home Y92.025
nursing home Y92.124
orphanage Y92.114
private house Y92.015
reform school Y92.155
gas station Y92.524
gasworks Y92.69
golf course Y92.39
gravel pit Y92.64
grocery Y92.512
gymnasium Y92.39
handball court Y92.318
harbor Y92.89
harness racing course Y92.39
healthcare provider office Y92.531
highway Y92.410
interstate Y92.411
hill Y92.828

Place of occurrence — *continued*
hockey rink Y92.330
home — *see* Place of occurrence, residence
hospice — *see* Place of occurrence, residence, institutional, nursing home
hospital Y92.239
cafeteria Y92.233
corridor Y92.232
operating room Y92.234
patient
bathroom Y92.231
room Y92.230
specified NEC Y92.238
hotel Y92.59
house — *see also* Place of occurrence, residence
abandoned Y92.89
under construction Y92.61
industrial and construction area (yard) Y92.69
building under construction Y92.61
dock Y92.62
dry dock Y92.62
factory Y92.63
gasworks Y92.69
mine Y92.64
oil rig Y92.65
pit Y92.64
power station Y92.69
shipyard Y92.62
specified NEC Y92.69
tunnel under construction Y92.69
workshop Y92.69
interstate Y92.411
kindergarten Y92.211
lacrosse field Y92.328
lake Y92.838
wilderness Y92.828
library Y92.241
mall Y92.59
market Y92.512
marsh Y92.828
military
base — *see* Place of occurrence, residence, institutional, military base
training ground Y92.84
mine Y92.64
mosque Y92.22
motel Y92.59
motorway (interstate) Y92.411
mountain Y92.828
movie-house Y92.26
museum Y92.251
music-hall Y92.252
not applicable Y92.9
nuclear power station Y92.69
nursing home — *see* Place of occurrence, residence, institutional, nursing home
office building Y92.59
offshore installation Y92.65
oil rig Y92.65
old people's home — *see* Place of occurrence, residence, institutional, specified NEC
opera-house Y92.253
orphanage — *see* Place of occurrence, residence, institutional, orphanage
outpatient surgery center Y92.530
park (public) Y92.830
amusement Y92.831
parking garage Y92.89
lot Y92.481
pavement Y92.480
physician office Y92.531
polo field Y92.328
pond Y92.828
post office Y92.242
power station Y92.69
prairie Y92.828
prison — *see* Place of occurrence, residence, institutional, prison
public
administration building Y92.248
city hall Y92.243
courthouse Y92.240
library Y92.241
post office Y92.242
specified NEC Y92.248
building NEC Y92.29
hall Y92.29
place NOS Y92.89

Place of occurrence — *continued*
  race course Y92.39
  radio station Y92.59
  railway line (bridge) Y92.85
  ranch (outbuildings) — *see* Place of occurrence, farm
  recreation area Y92.838
    amusement park Y92.831
    beach Y92.832
    campsite Y92.833
    park (public) Y92.830
    seashore Y92.832
    specified NEC Y92.838
  reform school - — *see* Place of occurrence, residence, institutional, reform school
  religious institution Y92.22
  residence (non-institutional) (private) Y92.009
    apartment Y92.039
      bathroom Y92.031
      bedroom Y92.032
      kitchen Y92.030
      specified NEC Y92.038
    bathroom Y92.002
    bedroom Y92.003
    boarding house Y92.049
      bathroom Y92.041
      bedroom Y92.042
      driveway Y92.043
      garage Y92.044
      garden Y92.046
      kitchen Y92.040
      specified NEC Y92.048
      swimming pool Y92.045
      yard Y92.046
    dining room Y92.001
    garden Y92.007
    home Y92.009
    house, single family Y92.019
      bathroom Y92.012
      bedroom Y92.013
      dining room Y92.011
      driveway Y92.014
      garage Y92.015
      garden Y92.017
      kitchen Y92.010
      specified NEC Y92.018
      swimming pool Y92.016
      yard Y92.017
    institutional Y92.10
      children's home — *see* Place of occurrence, residence, institutional, orphanage
      hospice — *see* Place of occurrence, residence, institutional, nursing home
      military base Y92.139
        barracks Y92.133
        garage Y92.135
        garden Y92.137
        kitchen Y92.130
        mess hall Y92.131
        specified NEC Y92.138
        swimming pool Y92.136
        yard Y92.137
      nursing home Y92.129
        bathroom Y92.121
        bedroom Y92.122
        driveway Y92.123
        garage Y92.124
        garden Y92.126
        kitchen Y92.120
        specified NEC Y92.128
        swimming pool Y92.125
        yard Y92.126
      orphanage Y92.119
        bathroom Y92.111
        bedroom Y92.112
        driveway Y92.113
        garage Y92.114
        garden Y92.116
        kitchen Y92.110
        specified NEC Y92.118
        swimming pool Y92.115
        yard Y92.116
      prison Y92.149
        bathroom Y92.142
        cell Y92.143
        courtyard Y92.147
        dining room Y92.141
        kitchen Y92.140
        specified NEC Y92.148
        swimming pool Y92.146

Place of occurrence — *continued*
  residence — *continued*
    institutional — *continued*
      reform school Y92.159
        bathroom Y92.152
        bedroom Y92.153
        dining room Y92.151
        driveway Y92.154
        garage Y92.155
        garden Y92.157
        kitchen Y92.150
        specified NEC Y92.158
        swimming pool Y92.156
        yard Y92.157
      school dormitory Y92.169
        bathroom Y92.162
        bedroom Y92.163
        dining room Y92.161
        kitchen Y92.160
        specified NEC Y92.168
      specified NEC Y92.199
        bathroom Y92.192
        bedroom Y92.193
        dining room Y92.191
        driveway Y92.194
        garage Y92.195
        garden Y92.197
        kitchen Y92.190
        specified NEC Y92.198
        swimming pool Y92.196
        yard Y92.197
    kitchen Y92.000
    mobile home Y92.029
      bathroom Y92.022
      bedroom Y92.023
      dining room Y92.021
      driveway Y92.024
      garage Y92.025
      garden Y92.027
      kitchen Y92.020
      specified NEC Y92.028
      swimming pool Y92.026
      yard Y92.027
    specified place in residence NEC Y92.008
    specified residence type NEC Y92.099
      bathroom Y92.091
      bedroom Y92.092
      driveway Y92.093
      garage Y92.094
      garden Y92.096
      kitchen Y92.090
      specified NEC Y92.098
      swimming pool Y92.095
      yard Y92.096
  restaurant Y92.511
  riding school Y92.39
  river Y92.828
  road Y92.410
  rodeo ring Y92.39
  rugby field Y92.328
  same day surgery center Y92.530
  sand pit Y92.64
  school (private) (public) (state) Y92.219
    college Y92.214
    daycare center Y92.210
    elementary school Y92.211
    high school Y92.213
    kindergarten Y92.211
    middle school Y92.212
    specified NEC Y92.218
    trace school Y92.215
    university Y92.214
    vocational school Y92.215
  sea (shore) Y92.832
  senior citizen center Y92.29
  service area
    airport Y92.520
    bus station Y92.521
    gas station Y92.524
    highway rest stop Y92.523
    railway station Y92.522
  shipyard Y92.62
  shop (commercial) Y92.513
  sidewalk Y92.480
  silo Y92.79
  skating rink (roller) Y92.331
    ice Y92.330
  slaughter house Y92.86
  soccer field Y92.322

Place of occurrence — *continued*
  specified place NEC Y92.89
  sports area Y92.39
    athletic
      court Y92.318
        basketball Y92.310
        specified NEC Y92.318
        squash Y92.311
        tennis Y92.312
      field Y92.328
        baseball Y92.320
        cricket ground Y92.328
        football Y92.321
        hockey Y92.328
        soccer Y92.322
        specified NEC Y92.328
    golf course Y92.39
    gymnasium Y92.39
    riding school Y92.39
    skating rink (roller) Y92.331
      ice Y92.330
    stadium Y92.39
    swimming pool Y92.34
  squash court Y92.311
  stadium Y92.39
  steeplechasing course Y92.39
  store Y92.512
  stream Y92.828
  street and highway Y92.410
    bike path Y92.482
    freeway Y92.411
    highway ramp Y92.415
    interstate highway Y92.411
    local residential or business street Y92.414
    motorway Y92.411
    parking lot Y92.481
    parkway Y92.412
    sidewalk Y92.480
    specified NEC Y92.488
    state road Y92.413
  subway car Y92.816
  supermarket Y92.512
  swamp Y92.828
  swimming pool (public) Y92.34
    private (at) Y92.095
      boarding house Y92.045
      military base Y92.136
      mobile home Y92.026
      nursing home Y92.125
      orphanage Y92.115
      prison Y92.146
      reform school Y92.156
      single family residence Y92.016
  synagogue Y92.22
  television station Y92.59
  tennis court Y92.312
  theater Y92.254
  trade area Y92.59
    bank Y92.510
    cafe Y92.511
    casino Y92.59
    garage Y92.59
    hotel Y92.59
    market Y92.512
    office building Y92.59
    radio station Y92.59
    restaurant Y92.511
    shop Y92.513
    shopping mall Y92.59
    store Y92.512
    supermarket Y92.512
    television station Y92.59
    warehouse Y92.59
  trailer park, residential — *see* Place of occurrence, residence, mobile home
  trailer site NOS Y92.89
  train Y92.815
    station Y92.522
  truck Y92.812
  tunnel under construction Y92.69
  university Y92.214
  urgent (health) care center Y92.532
  vehicle (transport) Y92.818
    airplane Y92.813
    boat Y92.814
    bus Y92.811
    car Y92.810
    specified NEC Y92.818
    subway car Y92.816

☑ **Additional Character Required — Refer to the Tabular List for Character Selection**

External Causes Index

Place of occurrence — Scald, scalding

Place of occurrence — *continued*
  vehicle — *continued*
    train Y92.815
    truck Y92.812
  warehouse Y92.59
  water reservoir Y92.89
  wilderness area Y92.828
    desert Y92.820
    forest Y92.821
    marsh Y92.828
    mountain Y92.828
    prairie Y92.828
    specified NEC Y92.828
    swamp Y92.828
  workshop Y92.69
  yard, private Y92.096
    boarding house Y92.046
    mobile home Y92.027
    single family house Y92.017
  youth center Y92.29
  zoo (zoological garden) Y92.834
Plumbism — *see* Table of Drugs and Chemicals, lead
Poisoning (accidental) (by) — *see also* Table of Drugs
    and Chemicals
  by plant, thorns, spines, sharp leaves or other mecha-
    nisms NEC X58 ☑
  carbon monoxide
    generated by
      motor vehicle — *see* Accident, transport
      watercraft (in transit) (not in transit) V93.89 ☑
        ferry boat V93.81 ☑
        fishing boat V93.82 ☑
        jet skis V93.83 ☑
        liner V93.81 ☑
        merchant ship V93.80 ☑
        passenger ship V93.81 ☑
        powered craft NEC V93.83 ☑
  caused by injection of poisons into skin by plant thorns,
    spines, sharp leaves X58 ☑
    marine or sea plants (venomous) X58 ☑
  execution — *see* Legal, intervention, gas
  intervention
    by gas — *see* Legal, intervention, gas
    other specified means — *see* Legal, intervention,
      specified means NEC
  exhaust gas
    generated by
      motor vehicle — *see* Accident, transport
      watercraft (in transit) (not in transit) V93.89 ☑
        ferry boat V93.81 ☑
        fishing boat V93.82 ☑
        jet skis V93.83 ☑
        liner V93.81 ☑
        merchant ship V93.80 ☑
        passenger ship V93.81 ☑
        powered craft NEC V93.83 ☑
  fumes or smoke due to
    explosion — *see also* Explosion W40.9 ☑
    fire — *see* Exposure, fire
    ignition — *see* Ignition
  gas
    in legal intervention — *see* Legal, intervention, gas
    legal execution — *see* Legal, intervention, gas
  in war operations — *see* War operations
  legal
Powder burn (by) (from)
  airgun W34.110 ☑
  BB gun W34.110 ☑
  firearm NEC W34.19 ☑
  gas, air or spring-operated gun NEC W34.118 ☑
  handgun W32.1 ☑
  hunting rifle W33.12 ☑
  larger firearm W33.10 ☑
    specified NEC W33.19 ☑
  machine gun W33.13 ☑
  paintball gun W34.111 ☑
  pellet gun W34.110 ☑
  shotgun W33.11 ☑
  Very pistol [flare] W34.19 ☑
Premature cessation (of) **surgical and medical care**
  Y66
Privation (food) (water) X58 ☑
Procedure (operation)
  correct, on wrong side or body part (wrong side)
    (wrong site) Y65.53
  intended for another patient done on wrong patient
    Y65.52

Procedure — *continued*
  performed on patient not scheduled for surgery Y65.52
  performed on wrong patient Y65.52
  wrong, performed on correct patient Y65.51
Prolonged
  sitting in transport vehicle — *see* Travel, by type of
    vehicle
  stay in
    high altitude as cause of anoxia, barodontalgia,
      barotitis or hypoxia W94.11 ☑
    weightless environment X52 ☑
Pulling, excessive — *see also* Overexertion X50.9- ☑
Puncture, puncturing — *see also* Contact, with, by type
    of object or machine
  by
    plant thorns, spines, sharp leaves or other mecha-
      nisms NEC W60 ☑
  during medical or surgical treatment as misadventure
    — *see* Index to Diseases and Injuries, Complica-
    tion(s)
Pushed, pushing (accidental) (injury in)
  by other person(s) (accidental) W51 ☑
    as, or caused by, a crowd or human stampede (with
      fall) W52 ☑
    before moving object NEC Y02.8 ☑
      motor vehicle Y02.0 ☑
      subway train Y02.1 ☑
      train Y02.1 ☑
    from
      high place NEC
        in accidental circumstances W17.89 ☑
        stated as
          intentional, homicide (attempt) Y01 ☑
          undetermined whether accidental or in-
            tentional Y30 ☑
      transport vehicle NEC — *see also* Accident,
        transport V89.9 ☑
        stated as
          intentional, homicide (attempt) Y08.89 ☑
    with fall W03 ☑
      due to ice or snow W00.0 ☑
  overexertion X50.9 ☑

R

Radiation (exposure to)
  arc lamps W89.0 ☑
  atomic power plant (malfunction) NEC W88.1 ☑
  complication of or abnormal reaction to medical radio-
    therapy Y84.2
  electromagnetic, ionizing W88.0 ☑
  gamma rays W88.1 ☑
  in
    war operations (from or following nuclear explosion)
      — *see* War operations
  inadvertent exposure of patient (receiving test or
    therapy) Y63.3
  infrared (heaters and lamps) W90.1 ☑
    excessive heat from W92 ☑
  ionized, ionizing (particles, artificially accelerated)
    radioisotopes W88.1 ☑
    specified NEC W88.8 ☑
    x-rays W88.0 ☑
  isotopes, radioactive — *see* Radiation, radioactive iso-
    topes
  laser(s) W90.2 ☑
    in war operations — *see* War operations
    misadventure in medical care Y63.2
  light sources (man-made visible and ultraviolet)
    W89.9 ☑
    natural X32 ☑
    specified NEC W89.8 ☑
    tanning bed W89.1 ☑
    welding light W89.0 ☑
  man-made visible light W89.9 ☑
    specified NEC W89.8 ☑
    tanning bed W89.1 ☑
    welding light W89.0 ☑
  microwave W90.8 ☑
  misadventure in medical or surgical procedure Y63.2
  natural NEC X39.08 ☑
    radon X39.01 ☑
  overdose (in medical or surgical procedure) Y63.2
  radar W90.0 ☑
  radioactive isotopes (any) W88.1 ☑
    atomic power plant malfunction W88.1 ☑
    misadventure in medical or surgical treatment Y63.2

Radiation — *continued*
  radiofrequency W90.0 ☑
  radium NEC W88.1 ☑
  sun X32 ☑
  ultraviolet (light) (man-made) W89.9 ☑
    natural X32 ☑
    specified NEC W89.8 ☑
    tanning bed W89.1 ☑
    welding light W89.0 ☑
  welding arc, torch, or light W89.0 ☑
    excessive heat from W92 ☑
  x-rays (hard) (soft) W88.0 ☑
Range disease W94.11 ☑
Rape (attempted) T74.2- ☑
Rat bite W53.11 ☑
Reaching (prolonged) (static) X50.1 ☑
Reaction, abnormal to medical procedure — *see also*
    Complication of or following, by type of procedure
    Y84.9
  biologicals — *see* Table of Drugs and Chemicals
  drugs — *see* Table of Drugs and Chemicals
  vaccine — *see* Table of Drugs and Chemicals
  with misadventure — *see* Misadventure
Recoil
  airgun W34.110 ☑
  BB gun W34.110 ☑
  firearm NEC W34.19 ☑
  gas, air or spring-operated gun NEC W34.118 ☑
  handgun W32.1 ☑
  hunting rifle W33.12 ☑
  larger firearm W33.10 ☑
    specified NEC W33.19 ☑
  machine gun W33.13 ☑
  paintball gun W34.111 ☑
  pellet W34.110 ☑
  shotgun W33.11 ☑
  Very pistol [flare] W34.19 ☑
Reduction in
  atmospheric pressure — *see* Air, pressure, change
Rock falling on or hitting (accidentally) (person)
  W20.8 ☑
  in cave-in W20.0 ☑
Run over (accidentally) (by)
  animal (not being ridden) NEC W55.89 ☑
  machinery — *see* Contact, with, by specified type of
    machine
  transport vehicle NEC — *see also* Accident, transport
    V09.9 ☑
    intentional homicide (attempt) Y03.0 ☑
    motor NEC V09.20 ☑
      intentional homicide (attempt) Y03.0 ☑
Running
  before moving object X81.8 ☑
    motor vehicle X81.0 ☑
Running off, away
  animal (being ridden) — *see also* Accident, transport
    V80.918 ☑
    not being ridden W55.89 ☑
  animal-drawn vehicle NEC — *see also* Accident, trans-
    port V80.928 ☑
  highway, road(way), street
    transport vehicle NEC — *see also* Accident, transport
      V89.9 ☑
Rupture pressurized devices — *see* Explosion, by type
    of device

S

Saturnism — *see* Table of Drugs and Chemicals, lead
Scald, scalding (accidental) (by) (from) (in) X19 ☑
  air (hot) X14.1 ☑
  gases (hot) X14.1 ☑
  homicide (attempt) — *see* Assault, burning, hot object
  inflicted by other person
    stated as intentional, homicide (attempt) — *see*
      Assault, burning, hot object
  liquid (boiling) (hot) NEC X12 ☑
    stated as undetermined whether accidental or inten-
      tional Y27.2 ☑
    suicide (attempt) X77.2 ☑
  local application of externally applied substance in
    medical or surgical care Y63.5
  metal (molten) (liquid) (hot) NEC X18 ☑
  self-inflicted X77.9 ☑
  stated as undetermined whether accidental or inten-
    tional Y27.8 ☑

Scald, scalding — *continued*
  steam X13.1 ☑
    assault X98.0 ☑
    stated as undetermined whether accidental or inten-
      tional Y27.0 ☑
    suicide (attempt) X77.0 ☑
  suicide (attempt) X77.9 ☑
  vapor (hot) X13.1 ☑
    assault X98.0 ☑
    stated as undetermined whether accidental or inten-
      tional Y27.0 ☑
    suicide (attempt) X77.0 ☑
Scratched by
  cat W55.03 ☑
  person(s) (accidentally) W50.4 ☑
    with intent to injure or kill Y04.0 ☑
    as, or caused by, a crowd or human stampede (with
      fall) W52
    assault Y04.0 ☑
    homicide (attempt) Y04.0 ☑
    in
      fight Y04.0 ☑
      legal intervention
        injuring
          bystander Y35.892 ☑
          law enforcement personnel Y35.891 ☑
          suspect Y35.893 ☑
          unspecified person Y35.899 ☑
Seasickness T75.3 ☑
Self-harm NEC — *see also* External cause by type, undetermined whether accidental or intentional
  intentional — *see* Suicide
  poisoning NEC — *see* Table of Drugs and Chemicals,
    poisoning, accidental
Self-inflicted (injury) **NEC** — *see also* External cause by
  type, undetermined whether accidental or intentional
  intentional — *see* Suicide
  poisoning NEC — *see* Table of Drugs and Chemicals,
    poisoning, accidental
Sequelae (of)
  accident NEC — *see* W00-X58 with 7th character S
  assault (homicidal) (any means) — *see* X92-Y08 with
    7th character S
  homicide, attempt (any means) — *see* X92-Y08 with
    7th character S
  injury undetermined whether accidentally or purposely
    inflicted — *see* Y21-Y33 with 7th character S
  intentional self-harm (classifiable to X71-X83) — *see*
    X71-X83 with 7th character S
  legal intervention — *see* with 7th character S Y35 ☑
  motor vehicle accident — *see* V00-V99 with 7th char-
    acter S
  suicide, attempt (any means) — *see* X71-X83 with 7th
    character S
  transport accident — *see* V00-V99 with 7th character
    S
  war operations — *see* War operations
Shock
  electric — *see* Exposure, electric current
  from electric appliance (any) (faulty) W86.8 ☑
    domestic W86.0 ☑
    suicide (attempt) X83.1 ☑
Shooting, shot (accidental(ly)) — *see also* Discharge,
  firearm, by type
  herself or himself — *see* Discharge, firearm by type,
    self-inflicted
  homicide (attempt) — *see* Discharge, firearm by type,
    homicide
  in war operations — *see* War operations
  inflicted by other person — *see* Discharge, firearm by
    type, homicide
    accidental — *see* Discharge, firearm, by type of
      firearm
  legal
    execution — *see* Legal, intervention, firearm
    intervention — *see* Legal, intervention, firearm
  self-inflicted — *see* Discharge, firearm by type, suicide
    accidental — *see* Discharge, firearm, by type of
      firearm
  suicide (attempt) — *see* Discharge, firearm by type,
    suicide
Shoving (accidentally) **by other person** — *see* Pushed,
  by other person
Sickness
  alpine W94.11 ☑
  motion — *see* Motion

Sickness — *continued*
  mountain W94.11 ☑
Sinking (accidental)
  watercraft (causing drowning, submersion) — *see also*
    Drowning, due to, accident to, watercraft, sinking
    causing injury except drowning or submersion —
      see Accident, watercraft, causing, injury NEC
Siriasis X32
Sitting (prolonged) (static) X50.1 ☑
Slashed wrists — *see* Cut, self-inflicted
Slipping (accidental) (on same level) (with fall) W01.0 ☑
  on
    ice W00.0 ☑
      with skates — *see* Accident, transport, pedestri-
        an, conveyance
    mud W01.0 ☑
    oil W01.0 ☑
    snow W00.0 ☑
      with skis — *see* Accident, transport, pedestrian,
        conveyance
    surface (slippery) (wet) NEC W01.0 ☑
  without fall W18.40 ☑
    due to
      specified NEC W18.49 ☑
      stepping from one level to another W18.43 ☑
      stepping into hole or opening W18.42 ☑
      stepping on object W18.41 ☑
Sliver, wood, contact with W45.8 ☑
Smoldering (due to fire) — *see* Exposure, fire
Sodomy (attempted) **by force** T74.2 ☑
Sound waves (causing injury) W42.9 ☑
  supersonic W42.0 ☑
Splinter, contact with W45.8 ☑
Stab, stabbing — *see* Cut
Standing (prolonged) (static) X50.1 ☑
Starvation X58 ☑
Status of external cause Y99.9
  child assisting in compensated work for family Y99.8
  civilian activity done for financial or other compensa-
    tion Y99.0
  civilian activity done for income or pay Y99.0
  family member assisting in compensated work for
    other family member Y99.8
  hobby not done for income Y99.8
  leisure activity Y99.8
  military activity Y99.1
  off-duty activity of military personnel Y99.8
  recreation or sport not for income or while a student
    Y99.8
  specified NEC Y99.8
  student activity Y99.8
  volunteer activity Y99.2
Stepped on
  by
    animal (not being ridden) NEC W55.89 ☑
    crowd or human stampede W52 ☑
    person W50.0 ☑
Stepping on
  object W22.8 ☑
    sports equipment W21.9 ☑
    stationary W22.09 ☑
      sports equipment W21.89 ☑
    with fall W18.31 ☑
  person W51 ☑
    by crowd or human stampede W52 ☑
  sports equipment W21.9 ☑
Sting
  arthropod, nonvenomous W57 ☑
  insect, nonvenomous W57 ☑
Storm (cataclysmic) — *see* Forces of nature, cataclysmic
  storm
Straining, excessive — *see also* Overexertion X50.9 ☑
Strangling — *see* Strangulation
Strangulation (accidental) T71 ☑
Strenuous movements — *see also* Overexertion
  X50.9 ☑
Striking against
  airbag (automobile) W22.10 ☑
    driver side W22.11 ☑
    front passenger side W22.12 ☑
    specified NEC W22.19 ☑
  bottom when
    diving or jumping into water (in) W16.822 ☑
      causing drowning W16.821 ☑
      from boat W16.722 ☑
        causing drowning W16.721 ☑

Striking against — *continued*
  bottom when — *continued*
    diving or jumping into water — *continued*
      natural body W16.822 ☑
        causing drowning W16.821 ☑
      swimming pool W16.522 ☑
        causing drowning W16.521 ☑
    falling into water (in) W16.322 ☑
      causing drowning W16.321 ☑
      fountain — *see* Striking against, bottom when,
        falling into water, specified NEC
      natural body W16.122 ☑
        causing drowning W16.121 ☑
      reservoir — *see* Striking against, bottom when,
        falling into water, specified NEC
      specified NEC W16.322 ☑
        causing drowning W16.321 ☑
      swimming pool W16.022 ☑
        causing drowning W16.021 ☑
  diving board (swimming-pool) W21.4 ☑
  object W22.8 ☑
    caused by crowd or human stampede (with fall)
      W52
    furniture W22.03 ☑
    lamppost W22.02 ☑
    sports equipment W21.9 ☑
    stationary W22.09 ☑
      sports equipment W21.89 ☑
    wall W22.01 ☑
    with
      drowning or submersion — *see* Drowning
      fall — *see* Fall, due to, bumping against, object
  person(s) W51 ☑
    as, or caused by, a crowd or human stampede (with
      fall) W52 ☑
    assault Y04.2 ☑
    homicide (attempt) Y04.2 ☑
    with fall W03 ☑
      due to ice or snow W00.0 ☑
  sports equipment W21.9 ☑
  wall (when) W22.01 ☑
    diving or jumping into water (in) W16.832 ☑
      causing drowning W16.831 ☑
      swimming pool W16.532 ☑
        causing drowning W16.531 ☑
    falling into water (in) W16.332 ☑
      causing drowning W16.331 ☑
      fountain — *see* Striking against, wall when,
        falling into water, specified NEC
      natural body W16.132 ☑
        causing drowning W16.131 ☑
      reservoir — *see* Striking against, wall when,
        falling into water, specified NEC
      specified NEC W16.332 ☑
        causing drowning W16.331 ☑
      swimming pool W16.032 ☑
        causing drowning W16.031 ☑
    swimming pool (when) W22.042 ☑
      causing drowning W22.041 ☑
      diving or jumping into water W16.532 ☑
        causing drowning W16.531 ☑
      falling into water W16.032 ☑
        causing drowning W16.031 ☑
Struck (accidentally) **by**
  airbag (automobile) W22.10 ☑
    driver side W22.11 ☑
    front passenger side W22.12 ☑
    specified NEC W22.19 ☑
  alligator W58.02 ☑
  animal (not being ridden) NEC W55.89 ☑
  avalanche — *see* Landslide
  ball (hit) (thrown) W21.00 ☑
    assault Y08.09 ☑
    baseball W21.03 ☑
    basketball W21.05 ☑
    football W21.01 ☑
    golf ball W21.04 ☑
    soccer W21.02 ☑
    softball W21.07 ☑
    specified NEC W21.09 ☑
    volleyball W21.06 ☑
  bat or racquet
    baseball bat W21.11 ☑
      assault Y08.02 ☑
    golf club W21.13 ☑
      assault Y08.09 ☑

Struck (accidentally) **by** — *continued*
  bat or racquet — *continued*
    specified NEC W21.19 ☑
      assault Y08.09 ☑
    tennis racquet W21.12 ☑
      assault Y08.09 ☑
  bullet — *see also* Discharge, firearm by type
    in war operations — *see* War operations
  crocodile W58.12 ☑
  dog W54.1 ☑
  flare, Very pistol — *see* Discharge, firearm NEC
  hailstones X39.8 ☑
  hockey (ice)
    field
      puck W21.221 ☑
      stick W21.211 ☑
    puck W21.220 ☑
    stick W21.210 ☑
      assault Y08.01 ☑
  landslide — *see* Landslide
  law-enforcement agent (on duty) — *see* Legal, inter-
      vention, manhandling
    with blunt object — *see* Legal, intervention, blunt
        object
  lightning T75.0 ☑
    causing fire — *see* Exposure, fire
  machine — *see* Contact, with, by type of machine
  mammal NEC W55.89 ☑
    marine W56.32 ☑
  marine animal W56.82 ☑
  missile
    firearm — *see* Discharge, firearm by type
    in war operations — *see* War operations, missile
  object W22.8 ☑
    blunt W22.8 ☑
      assault Y00 ☑
      suicide (attempt) X79 ☑
      undetermined whether accidental or intentional
          Y29 ☑
    falling W20.8 ☑
      from, in, on
        building W20.1 ☑
          burning (uncontrolled fire) X00.4 ☑
        cataclysmic
          earth surface movement NEC — *see*
              Landslide
          storm — *see* Forces of nature, cataclysmic
              storm
        cave-in W20.0 ☑
        earthquake X34 ☑
        machine (in operation) — *see* Contact, with,
            by type of machine
        structure W20.1 ☑
          burning X00.4 ☑
        transport vehicle (in motion) — *see* Accident,
            transport, by type of vehicle
        watercraft V93.49 ☑
          due to
            accident to craft V91.39 ☑
              powered craft V91.33 ☑
                ferry boat V91.31 ☑
                fishing boat V91.32 ☑
                jetskis V91.33 ☑
                liner V91.31 ☑
                merchant ship V91.30 ☑
                passenger ship V91.31 ☑
              unpowered craft V91.38 ☑
                canoe V91.35 ☑
                inflatable V91.36 ☑
                kayak V91.35 ☑
                sailboat V91.34 ☑
                surf-board V91.38 ☑
                windsurfer V91.38 ☑
            powered craft V93.43 ☑
              ferry boat V93.41 ☑
              fishing boat V93.42 ☑
              jetskis V93.43 ☑
              liner V93.41 ☑
              merchant ship V93.40 ☑
              passenger ship V93.41 ☑
            unpowered craft V93.48 ☑
              sailboat V93.44 ☑
              surf-board V93.48 ☑
              windsurfer V93.48 ☑
      moving NEC W20.8 ☑
      projected W20.8 ☑

Struck (accidentally) **by** — *continued*
  object — *continued*
    projected — *continued*
      assault Y00 ☑
      in sports W21.9 ☑
        assault Y08.09 ☑
        ball W21.00 ☑
          baseball W21.03 ☑
          basketball W21.05 ☑
          football W21.01 ☑
          golf ball W21.04 ☑
          soccer W21.02 ☑
          softball W21.07 ☑
          specified NEC W21.09 ☑
          volleyball W21.06 ☑
        bat or racquet
          baseball bat W21.11 ☑
            assault Y08.02 ☑
          golf club W21.13 ☑
            assault Y08.09 ☑
          specified NEC W21.19 ☑
            assault Y08.09 ☑
          tennis racquet W21.12 ☑
            assault Y08.09 ☑
        hockey (ice)
          field
            puck W21.221 ☑
            stick W21.211 ☑
          puck W21.220 ☑
          stick W21.210 ☑
            assault Y08.01 ☑
        specified NEC W21.89 ☑
    set in motion by explosion — *see* Explosion
    thrown W20.8 ☑
      assault Y00 ☑
      in sports W21.9 ☑
        assault Y08.09 ☑
        ball W21.00 ☑
          baseball W21.03 ☑
          basketball W21.05 ☑
          football W21.01 ☑
          golf ball W21.04 ☑
          soccer W21.02 ☑
          soft ball W21.07 ☑
          specified NEC W21.09 ☑
          volleyball W21.06 ☑
        bat or racquet
          baseball bat W21.11 ☑
            assault Y08.02 ☑
          golf club W21.13 ☑
            assault Y08.09 ☑
          specified NEC W21.19 ☑
            assault Y08.09 ☑
          tennis racquet W21.12 ☑
            assault Y08.09 ☑
        hockey (ice)
          field
            puck W21.221 ☑
            stick W21.211 ☑
          puck W21.220 ☑
          stick W21.210 ☑
            assault Y08.01 ☑
        specified NEC W21.89 ☑
  other person(s) W50.0 ☑
    with
      blunt object W22.8 ☑
        intentional, homicide (attempt) Y00 ☑
        sports equipment W21.9 ☑
        undetermined whether accidental or inten-
            tional Y29 ☑
      fall W03 ☑
        due to ice or snow W00.0 ☑
    as, or caused by, a crowd or human stampede (with
        fall) W52 ☑
    assault Y04.2 ☑
    homicide (attempt) Y04.2 ☑
    in legal intervention
      injuring
        bystander Y35.812 ☑
        law enforcement personnel Y35.811 ☑
        suspect Y35.813 ☑
        unspecified person Y35.819 ☑
    sports equipment W21.9 ☑
  police (on duty) — *see* Legal, intervention, manhan-
      dling

Struck (accidentally) **by** — *continued*
  police — *see* Legal, intervention, manhandling —
      continued
    with blunt object — *see* Legal, intervention, blunt
        object
  sports equipment W21.9 ☑
    assault Y08.09 ☑
    ball W21.00 ☑
      baseball W21.03 ☑
      basketball W21.05 ☑
      football W21.01 ☑
      golf ball W21.04 ☑
      soccer W21.02 ☑
      soft ball W21.07 ☑
      specified NEC W21.09 ☑
      volleyball W21.06 ☑
    bat or racquet
      baseball bat W21.11 ☑
        assault Y08.02 ☑
      golf club W21.13 ☑
        assault Y08.09 ☑
      specified NEC W21.19 ☑
        assault Y08.09 ☑
      tennis racquet W21.12 ☑
        assault Y08.09 ☑
    cleats (shoe) W21.31 ☑
    foot wear NEC W21.39 ☑
    football helmet W21.81 ☑
    hockey (ice)
      field
        puck W21.221 ☑
        stick W21.211 ☑
      puck W21.220 ☑
      stick W21.210 ☑
        assault Y08.01 ☑
    skate blades W21.32 ☑
    specified NEC W21.89 ☑
      assault Y08.09 ☑
  thunderbolt — *see* subcategory T75.0 ☑
    causing fire — *see* Exposure, fire
  transport vehicle NEC — *see also* Accident, transport
      V09.9 ☑
    intentional, homicide (attempt) Y03.0 ☑
    motor NEC — *see also* Accident, transport V09.20 ☑
      homicide Y03.0 ☑
  vehicle (transport) NEC — *see* Accident, transport, by
      type of vehicle
    stationary (falling from jack, hydraulic lift, ramp)
        W20.8 ☑

Stumbling
  over
    animal NEC W01.0 ☑
      with fall W18.09 ☑
    carpet, rug or (small) object W22.8 ☑
      with fall W18.09 ☑
    person W51 ☑
      with fall W03 ☑
        due to ice or snow W00.0 ☑
  without fall W18.40 ☑
    due to
      specified NEC W18.49 ☑
      stepping from one level to another W18.43 ☑
      stepping into hole or opening W18.42 ☑
      stepping on object W18.41 ☑
Submersion (accidental) — *see* Drowning
Suffocation (accidental) (by external means) (by pressure)
    (mechanical) — *see also* category T71 ☑
  due to, by
    avalanche — *see* Landslide
    explosion — *see* Explosion
    fire — *see* Exposure, fire
    food, any type (aspiration) (ingestion) (inhalation)
        — *see* categories T17 and T18 ☑
    ignition — *see* Ignition
    landslide — *see* Landslide
    machine(ry) — *see* Contact, with, by type of ma-
        chine
    vomitus (aspiration) (inhalation) T17.81- ☑
  in
    burning building X00.8 ☑
Suicide, suicidal (attempted) (by) X83.8 ☑
  blunt object X79 ☑
  burning, burns X76 ☑
    hot object X77.9 ☑
      fluid NEC X77.2 ☑
      household appliance X77.3 ☑
      specified NEC X77.8 ☑

☑ **Additional Character Required — Refer to the Tabular List for Character Selection**

Suicide, suicidal — continued
burning, burns — continued
  hot object — continued
    steam X77.0
    tap water X77.1
    vapors X77.0
  caustic substance — see Table of Drugs and Chemicals
  cold, extreme X83.2
  collision of motor vehicle with
    motor vehicle X82.0
    specified NEC X82.8
    train X82.1
    tree X82.2
  crashing of aircraft X83.0
  cut (any part of body) X78.9
  cutting or piercing instrument X78.9
    dagger X78.2
    glass X78.0
    knife X78.1
    specified NEC X78.8
    sword X78.2
  drowning (in) X71.9
    bathtub X71.0
    natural water X71.3
    specified NEC X71.8
    swimming pool X71.1
      following fall X71.2
  electrocution X83.1
  explosive(s) (material) X75
  fire, flames X76
  firearm X74.9
    airgun X74.01
    handgun X72
    hunting rifle X73.1
    larger X73.9
      specified NEC X73.8
    machine gun X73.2
    shotgun X73.0
    specified NEC X74.8
  hanging X83.8
  hot object — see Suicide, burning, hot object
  jumping
    before moving object X81.8
      motor vehicle X81.0
      subway train X81.1
      train X81.1
    from high place X80
  late effect of attempt — see X71-X83 with 7th character S
  lying before moving object, train, vehicle X81.8
  poisoning — see Table of Drugs and Chemicals
  puncture (any part of body) — see Suicide, cutting or piercing instrument
  scald — see Suicide, burning, hot object
  sequelae of attempt — see X71-X83 with 7th character S
  sharp object (any) — see Suicide, cutting or piercing instrument
  shooting — see Suicide, firearm
  specified means NEC X83.8
  stab (any part of body) — see Suicide, cutting or piercing instrument
  steam, hot vapors X77.0
  strangulation X83.8
  submersion — see Suicide, drowning
  suffocation X83.8
  wound NEC X83.8
Sunstroke X32
Supersonic waves (causing injury) W42.0
Surgical procedure, complication of (delayed or as an abnormal reaction without mention of misadventure) — see also Complication of or following, by type of procedure
  due to or as a result of misadventure — see Misadventure
Swallowed, swallowing
  foreign body — see Foreign body, alimentary canal
  poison — see Table of Drugs and Chemicals
  substance
    caustic or corrosive — see Table of Drugs and Chemicals
    poisonous — see Table of Drugs and Chemicals

T

Tackle in sport W03

Terrorism (involving) Y38.80
  biological weapons Y38.6X-
  chemical weapons Y38.7X-
  conflagration Y38.3X-
  drowning and submersion Y38.89-
  explosion Y38.2X-
    destruction of aircraft Y38.1X-
    marine weapons Y38.0X-
  fire Y38.3X-
  firearms Y38.4X-
  hot substances Y38.3X-
  lasers Y38.89-
  nuclear weapons Y38.5X-
  piercing or stabbing instruments Y38.89-
  secondary effects Y38.9X-
  specified method NEC Y38.89-
  suicide bomber Y38.81-
Thirst X58
Threat to breathing
  aspiration — see Aspiration
  due to cave-in, falling earth or substance NEC T71
Thrown (accidentally)
  against part (any) of or object in transport vehicle (in motion) NEC — see also Accident, transport
  from
    high place, homicide (attempt) Y01
    machinery — see Contact, with, by type of machine
    transport vehicle NEC — see also Accident, transport V89.9
  off — see Thrown, from
Thunderbolt — see subcategory T75.0
  causing fire — see Exposure, fire
Tidal wave (any injury) NEC — see Forces of nature, tidal wave
Took
  overdose (drug) — see Table of Drugs and Chemicals
  poison — see Table of Drugs and Chemicals
Tornado (any injury) X37.1
Torrential rain (any injury) X37.8
Torture X58
Trampled by animal NEC W55.89
Trapped (accidentally)
  between objects (moving) (stationary and moving) — see Caught
  by part (any) of
    electric (assisted) bicycle V29.881
    motorcycle V29.888
    pedal cycle V19.88
    transport vehicle NEC — see also Accident, transport V89.9
Travel (effects) (sickness) T75.3
Tree falling on or hitting (accidentally) (person) W20.8
Tripping
  over
    animal W01.0
      with fall W01.0
    carpet, rug or (small) object W22.8
      with fall W18.09
    person W51
      with fall W03
        due to ice or snow W00.0
    without fall W18.40
      due to
        specified NEC W18.49
        stepping from one level to another W18.43
        stepping into hole or opening W18.42
        stepping on object W18.41
Twisted by person(s) (accidentally) W50.2
  with intent to injure or kill Y04.0
  as, or caused by, a crowd or human stampede (with fall) W52
  assault Y04.0
  homicide (attempt) Y04.0
  in
    fight Y04.0
    legal intervention — see Legal, intervention, manhandling
Twisting (prolonged) (static) X50.1-

U

Underdosing of necessary drugs, medicaments or biological substances Y63.6
Undetermined intent (contact) (exposure)
  automobile collision Y32

Undetermined intent — continued
  blunt object Y29
  drowning (submersion) (in) Y21.9
    bathtub Y21.0
      after fall Y21.1
    natural water (lake) (ocean) (pond) (river) (stream) Y21.4
    specified place NEC Y21.8
    swimming pool Y21.2
      after fall Y21.3
  explosive material Y25
  fall, jump or push from high place Y30
  falling, lying or running before moving object Y31
  fire Y26
  firearm discharge Y24.9
    airgun (BB) (pellet) Y24.0
    handgun (pistol) (revolver) Y22
    hunting rifle Y23.1
    larger Y23.9
      hunting rifle Y23.1
      machine gun Y23.3
      military Y23.2
      shotgun Y23.0
      specified type NEC Y23.8
    machine gun Y23.3
    military Y23.2
    shotgun Y23.0
    specified type NEC Y24.8
    Very pistol Y24.8
  hot object Y27.9
    fluid NEC Y27.2
    household appliance Y27.3
    specified object NEC Y27.8
    steam Y27.0
    tap water Y27.1
    vapor Y27.0
  jump, fall or push from high place Y30
  lying, falling or running before moving object Y31
  motor vehicle crash Y32
  push, fall or jump from high place Y30
  running, falling or lying before moving object Y31
  sharp object Y28.9
    dagger Y28.2
    glass Y28.0
    knife Y28.1
    specified object NEC Y28.8
    sword Y28.2
  smoke Y26
  specified event NEC Y33
Use of hand as hammer X50.3

V

Vibration (causing injury) W49.9
Victim (of)
  avalanche — see Landslide
  earth movements NEC — see Forces of nature, earth movement
  earthquake X34
  flood — see Flood
  landslide — see Landslide
  lightning — see subcategory T75.0
    causing fire — see Exposure, fire
  storm (cataclysmic) NEC — see Forces of nature, cataclysmic storm
  volcanic eruption X35
Volcanic eruption (any injury) X35
Vomitus, gastric contents in air passages (with asphyxia, obstruction or suffocation) T17.81-

W

Walked into stationary object (any) W22.09
  furniture W22.03
  lamppost W22.02
  wall W22.01
War operations (injuries to military personnel and civilians during war, civil insurrection and peacekeeping missions) (by) (from) (involving) Y36.90
  after cessation of hostilities Y36.89-
    explosion Y36.89-
      bomb placed during war operations Y36.82-
      mine placed during war operations Y36.81-
    specified NEC Y36.88-
  air blast Y36.20-

War operations — *continued*
  aircraft
    destruction — *see* War operations, destruction of aircraft
  airway restriction — *see* War operations, restriction of airways
  asphyxiation — *see* War operations, restriction of airways
  biological weapons Y36.6X- ☑
  blast Y36.20- ☑
  blast fragments Y36.20- ☑
  blast wave Y36.20- ☑
  blast wind Y36.20- ☑
  bomb Y36.20- ☑
    dirty Y36.50- ☑
    gasoline Y36.31- ☑
    incendiary Y36.31- ☑
    petrol Y36.31- ☑
  bullet Y36.43- ☑
    incendiary Y36.32- ☑
    rubber Y36.41- ☑
  chemical weapons Y36.7X- ☑
  combat
    hand to hand (unarmed) combat Y36.44- ☑
    using blunt or piercing object Y36.45- ☑
  conflagration — *see* War operations, fire
  conventional warfare NEC Y36.49- ☑
  depth-charge Y36.01- ☑
  destruction of aircraft Y36.10- ☑
    due to
      air to air missile Y36.11- ☑
      collision with other aircraft Y36.12- ☑
      detonation (accidental) of onboard munitions and explosives Y36.14- ☑
      enemy fire or explosives Y36.11- ☑
      explosive placed on aircraft Y36.11- ☑
      onboard fire Y36.13- ☑
      rocket propelled grenade [RPG] Y36.11- ☑
      small arms fire Y36.11- ☑
      surface to air missile Y36.11- ☑
    specified NEC Y36.19- ☑
  detonation (accidental) of
    onboard marine weapons Y36.05- ☑
    own munitions or munitions launch device Y36.24- ☑
  dirty bomb Y36.50- ☑
  explosion (of) Y36.20- ☑
    aerial bomb Y36.21- ☑
    after cessation of hostilities
      bomb placed during war operations Y36.82- ☑
      mine placed during war operations Y36.81- ☑

War operations — *continued*
  explosion — *continued*
    bomb NOS — *see also* War operations, bomb(s) Y36.20- ☑
    fragments Y36.20- ☑
    grenade Y36.29- ☑
    guided missile Y36.22- ☑
    improvised explosive device [IED] (person-borne) (roadside) (vehicle-borne) Y36.23- ☑
    land mine Y36.29- ☑
    marine mine (at sea) (in harbor) Y36.02- ☑
    marine weapon Y36.00- ☑
      specified NEC Y36.09- ☑
    own munitions or munitions launch device (accidental) Y36.24- ☑
    sea-based artillery shell Y36.03- ☑
    specified NEC Y36.29- ☑
    torpedo Y36.04- ☑
  fire Y36.30- ☑
    specified NEC Y36.39- ☑
  firearms
    discharge Y36.43- ☑
    pellets Y36.42- ☑
  flamethrower Y36.33- ☑
  fragments (from) (of)
    improvised explosive device [IED] (person-borne) (roadside) (vehicle-borne) Y36.26- ☑
    munitions Y36.25- ☑
    specified NEC Y36.29- ☑
    weapons Y36.27- ☑
  friendly fire Y36.92
  hand to hand (unarmed) combat Y36.44- ☑
  hot substances — *see* War operations, fire
  incendiary bullet Y36.32- ☑
  nuclear weapon (effects of) Y36.50- ☑
    acute radiation exposure Y36.54- ☑
    blast pressure Y36.51- ☑
    direct blast Y36.51- ☑
    direct heat Y36.53- ☑
    fallout exposure Y36.54- ☑
    fireball Y36.53- ☑
    indirect blast (struck or crushed by blast debris) (being thrown by blast) Y36.52- ☑
    ionizing radiation (immediate exposure) Y36.54- ☑
    nuclear radiation Y36.54- ☑
    radiation
      ionizing (immediate exposure) Y36.54- ☑
      nuclear Y36.54- ☑
      thermal Y36.53- ☑
    secondary effects Y36.54- ☑

War operations — *continued*
  nuclear weapon — *continued*
    specified NEC Y36.59- ☑
    thermal radiation Y36.53- ☑
  restriction of air (airway)
    intentional Y36.46- ☑
    unintentional Y36.47- ☑
  rubber bullets Y36.41- ☑
  shrapnel NOS Y36.29- ☑
  suffocation — *see* War operations, restriction of airways
  unconventional warfare NEC Y36.7X- ☑
  underwater blast NOS Y36.00- ☑
  warfare
    conventional NEC Y36.49- ☑
    unconventional NEC Y36.7X- ☑
  weapon of mass destruction [WMD] Y36.91 ☑
  weapons
    biological weapons Y36.6X- ☑
    chemical Y36.7X- ☑
    nuclear (effects of) Y36.50- ☑
      acute radiation exposure Y36.54- ☑
      blast pressure Y36.51- ☑
      direct blast Y36.51- ☑
      direct heat Y36.53- ☑
      fallout exposure Y36.54- ☑
      fireball Y36.53- ☑
      radiation
        ionizing (immediate exposure) Y36.54- ☑
        nuclear Y36.54- ☑
        thermal Y36.53- ☑
      secondary effects Y36.54- ☑
      specified NEC Y36.59- ☑
    of mass destruction [WMD] Y36.91 ☑
Washed
  away by flood — *see* Flood
  off road by storm (transport vehicle) — *see* Forces of nature, cataclysmic storm
Weather exposure NEC — *see* Forces of nature
Weightlessness (causing injury) (effects of) (in spacecraft, real or simulated) X52 ☑
Work related condition Y99.0
Wound (accidental) NEC — *see also* Injury X58 ☑
  battle — *see also* War operations Y36.90 ☑
  gunshot — *see* Discharge, firearm by type
Wreck transport vehicle NEC — *see also* Accident, transport V89.9 ☑
Wrong
  device implanted into correct surgical site Y65.51
  fluid in infusion Y65.1
  patient, procedure performed on Y65.52
  procedure (operation) on correct patient Y65.51

ICD-10-CM Tabular List of Diseases and Injuries

Chapter 1. Certain Infectious and Parasitic Diseases (A00–B99)

Chapter-specific Guidelines with Coding Examples

The chapter-specific guidelines from the ICD-10-CM Official Guidelines for Coding and Reporting have been provided below. Along with these guidelines are coding examples, contained in the shaded boxes, that have been developed to help illustrate the coding and/or sequencing guidance found in these guidelines.

a. Human immunodeficiency virus (HIV) infections

1) Code only confirmed cases

Code only confirmed cases of HIV infection/illness. This is an exception to the hospital inpatient guideline Section II, H.

In this context, "confirmation" does not require documentation of positive serology or culture for HIV; the provider's diagnostic statement that the patient is HIV positive or has an HIV-related illness is sufficient.

> Patient being seen for hypothyroidism with possible HIV infection
>
> **E03.9   Hypothyroidism, unspecified**
>
> *Explanation:* Only the hypothyroidism is coded in this scenario because it has not been confirmed that an HIV infection is present.

2) Selection and sequencing of HIV codes

(a) Patient admitted for HIV-related condition

If a patient is admitted for an HIV-related condition, the principal diagnosis should be B20, Human immunodeficiency virus [HIV] disease followed by additional diagnosis codes for all reported HIV-related conditions.

An exception to this guideline is if the reason for admission is hemolytic-uremic syndrome associated with HIV disease. Assign code D59.31, Infection-associated hemolytic-uremic syndrome, followed by code B20, Human immunodeficiency virus [HIV] disease.

> HIV with CMV
>
> **B20   Human immunodeficiency virus [HIV] disease**
>
> **B25.9   Cytomegaloviral disease, unspecified**
>
> *Explanation:* Cytomegaloviral infection is an HIV related condition, so the HIV diagnosis code is reported first, followed by the code for the CMV.

(b) Patient with HIV disease admitted for unrelated condition

If a patient with HIV disease is admitted for an unrelated condition (such as a traumatic injury), the code for the unrelated condition (e.g., the nature of injury code) should be the principal diagnosis. Other diagnoses would be B20 followed by additional diagnosis codes for all reported HIV-related conditions.

> Sprain of the internal collateral ligament, right ankle; HIV
>
> **S93.491A   Sprain of other ligament of right ankle, initial encounter**
>
> **B20   Human immunodeficiency virus [HIV] disease**
>
> *Explanation:* The ankle sprain is not related to HIV, so it is the first-listed diagnosis code, and HIV is reported secondarily.

(c) Whether the patient is newly diagnosed

Whether the patient is newly diagnosed or has had previous admissions/encounters for HIV conditions is irrelevant to the sequencing decision.

> Newly diagnosed multiple cutaneous Kaposi's sarcoma lesions in previously diagnosed HIV disease
>
> **B20   Human immunodeficiency virus [HIV] disease**
>
> **C46.0   Kaposi's sarcoma of skin**
>
> *Explanation:* Even though the HIV was diagnosed on a previous encounter, it is still sequenced first when coded with an HIV-related condition. Kaposi's sarcoma is an HIV-related condition.

(d) Asymptomatic human immunodeficiency virus

Z21, Asymptomatic human immunodeficiency virus [HIV] infection status, is to be applied when the patient without any documentation of symptoms is listed as being "HIV positive," "known HIV," "HIV test positive," or similar terminology. Do not use this code if the term "AIDS" or "HIV disease" is used or if the patient is treated for any HIV-related illness or is described as having any condition(s) resulting from his/her HIV positive status; use B20 in these cases.

(e) Patients with inconclusive HIV serology

Patients with inconclusive HIV serology, but no definitive diagnosis or manifestations of the illness, may be assigned code R75, Inconclusive laboratory evidence of human immunodeficiency virus [HIV].

(f) Previously diagnosed HIV-related illness

Patients with any known prior diagnosis of an HIV-related illness should be coded to B20. Once a patient has developed an HIV-related illness, the patient should always be assigned code B20 on every subsequent admission/encounter. Patients previously diagnosed with any HIV illness (B20) should never be assigned to R75 or Z21, Asymptomatic human immunodeficiency virus [HIV] infection status.

(g) HIV infection in pregnancy, childbirth and the puerperium

During pregnancy, childbirth or the puerperium, a patient admitted (or presenting for a health care encounter) because of an HIV-related illness should receive a principal diagnosis code of O98.7-, Human immunodeficiency [HIV] disease complicating pregnancy, childbirth and the puerperium, followed by B20 and the code(s) for the HIV-related illness(es). Codes from Chapter 15 always take sequencing priority.

Patients with asymptomatic HIV infection status admitted (or presenting for a health care encounter) during pregnancy, childbirth, or the puerperium should receive codes of O98.7- and Z21.

(h) Encounters for testing for HIV

If a patient is being seen to determine his/her HIV status, use code Z11.4, Encounter for screening for human immunodeficiency virus [HIV]. Use additional codes for any associated high-risk behavior, if applicable.

If a patient with signs or symptoms is being seen for HIV testing, code the signs and symptoms. An additional counseling code Z71.7, Human immunodeficiency virus [HIV] counseling, may be used if counseling is provided during the encounter for the test.

When a patient returns to be informed of his/her HIV test results and the test result is negative, use code Z71.7, Human immunodeficiency virus [HIV] counseling.

If the results are positive, see previous guidelines and assign codes as appropriate.

(i) HIV managed by antiretroviral medication

If a patient with documented HIV disease, **HIV-related illness or AIDS** is currently managed on antiretroviral medications, assign code B20, Human immunodeficiency virus [HIV] disease. Code Z79.899, Other long term (current) drug therapy, may be assigned as an additional code to identify the long-term (current) use of antiretroviral medications.

b. Infectious agents as the cause of diseases classified to other chapters

Certain infections are classified in chapters other than Chapter 1 and no organism is identified as part of the infection code. In these instances, it is necessary to use an additional code from Chapter 1 to identify the organism. A code from category B95, Streptococcus, Staphylococcus, and Enterococcus as the cause of diseases classified to other chapters, B96, Other bacterial agents as the cause of diseases classified to other chapters, or B97, Viral agents as the cause of diseases classified to other chapters, is to be used as an additional code to identify the organism. An instructional note will be found at the infection code advising that an additional organism code is required.

> Acute *E. coli* cystitis
>
> **N30.00   Acute cystitis without hematuria**
>
> **B96.20   Unspecified Escherichia coli [E.coli] as the cause of diseases classified elsewhere**
>
> *Explanation:* An instructional note under the category for the cystitis indicates to code also the specific organism.

c. Infections resistant to antibiotics

Many bacterial infections are resistant to current antibiotics. It is necessary to identify all infections documented as antibiotic resistant. Assign a code from category Z16, Resistance to antimicrobial drugs, following the infection code only if the infection code does not identify drug resistance.

Penicillin-resistant *Streptococcus pneumoniae* pneumonia

J13	Pneumonia due to Streptococcus pneumoniae
Z16.11	Resistance to penicillins

Explanation: Code Z16.11 is assigned as a secondary code to represent the penicillin resistance. This code includes resistance to amoxicillin and ampicillin.

d. Sepsis, severe sepsis, and septic shock

1) Coding of Sepsis and Severe Sepsis

(a) Sepsis

For a diagnosis of sepsis, assign the appropriate code for the underlying systemic infection. If the type of infection or causal organism is not further specified, assign code A41.9, Sepsis, unspecified organism.

A code from subcategory R65.2, Severe sepsis, should not be assigned unless severe sepsis or an associated acute organ dysfunction is documented.

Gram-negative sepsis

A41.50	Gram-negative sepsis, unspecified

Staphylococcal sepsis

A41.2	Sepsis due to unspecified staphylococcus

Explanation: In both examples above the organism causing the sepsis is identified, therefore A41.9 Sepsis, unspecified organism, would not be appropriate as this code would not capture the highest degree of specificity found in the documentation. Do not use an additional code for severe sepsis unless an acute organ dysfunction was also documented as "associated with" or "due to" the sepsis or the sepsis was documented as "severe."

(i) Negative or inconclusive blood cultures and sepsis

Negative or inconclusive blood cultures do not preclude a diagnosis of sepsis in patients with clinical evidence of the condition; however, the provider should be queried.

(ii) Urosepsis

The term urosepsis is a nonspecific term. It is not to be considered synonymous with sepsis. It has no default code in the Alphabetic Index. Should a provider use this term, he/she must be queried for clarification.

(iii) Sepsis with organ dysfunction

If a patient has sepsis and associated acute organ dysfunction or multiple organ dysfunction (MOD), follow the instructions for coding severe sepsis.

(iv) Acute organ dysfunction that is not clearly associated with the sepsis

If a patient has sepsis and an acute organ dysfunction, but the medical record documentation indicates that the acute organ dysfunction is related to a medical condition other than the sepsis, do not assign a code from subcategory R65.2, Severe sepsis. An acute organ dysfunction must be associated with the sepsis in order to assign the severe sepsis code. If the documentation is not clear as to whether an acute organ dysfunction is related to the sepsis or another medical condition, query the provider.

Sepsis and acute respiratory failure due to COPD exacerbation

A41.9	Sepsis, unspecified organism
J44.1	Chronic obstructive pulmonary disease with (acute) exacerbation
J96.00	Acute respiratory failure, unspecified whether with hypoxia or hypercapnia

Explanation: Although acute organ dysfunction is present in the form of acute respiratory failure, severe sepsis (R65.2) is not coded in this example, as the acute respiratory failure is attributed to the COPD exacerbation rather than the sepsis. Sequencing of these codes would be determined by the reason for the encounter.

(b) Severe sepsis

The coding of severe sepsis requires a minimum of 2 codes: first a code for the underlying systemic infection, followed by a code from subcategory R65.2, Severe sepsis. If the causal organism is not documented, assign code A41.9, Sepsis, unspecified organism, for the infection. Additional code(s) for the associated acute organ dysfunction are also required.

Due to the complex nature of severe sepsis, some cases may require querying the provider prior to assignment of the codes.

2) Septic shock

Septic shock generally refers to circulatory failure associated with severe sepsis, and therefore, it represents a type of acute organ dysfunction.

For cases of septic shock, the code for the systemic infection should be sequenced first, followed by code R65.21, Severe sepsis with septic shock or code T81.12, Postprocedural septic shock. Any additional codes for the other acute organ dysfunctions should also be assigned. As noted in the sequencing instructions in the Tabular List, the code for septic shock cannot be assigned as a principal diagnosis.

Sepsis with septic shock

A41.9	Sepsis, unspecified organism
R65.21	Severe sepsis with septic shock

Explanation: Documentation of septic shock automatically implies severe sepsis as it is a form of acute organ dysfunction. Septic shock is not coded as the first-listed diagnosis; it is always preceded by the code for the systemic infection.

3) Sequencing of severe sepsis

If severe sepsis is present on admission, and meets the definition of principal diagnosis, the underlying systemic infection should be assigned as principal diagnosis followed by the appropriate code from subcategory R65.2 as required by the sequencing rules in the Tabular List. A code from subcategory R65.2 can never be assigned as a principal diagnosis.

When severe sepsis develops during an encounter (it was not present on admission), the underlying systemic infection and the appropriate code from subcategory R65.2 should be assigned as secondary diagnoses.

Severe sepsis may be present on admission, but the diagnosis may not be confirmed until sometime after admission. If the documentation is not clear whether severe sepsis was present on admission, the provider should be queried.

For infection-associated hemolytic-uremic syndrome with severe sepsis, see guideline I.C.1.d.9.

4) Sepsis or severe sepsis with a localized infection

If the reason for admission is sepsis or severe sepsis and a localized infection, such as pneumonia or cellulitis, a code(s) for the underlying systemic infection should be assigned first and the code for the localized infection should be assigned as a secondary diagnosis. If the patient has severe sepsis, a code from subcategory R65.2 should also be assigned as a secondary diagnosis. If the patient is admitted with a localized infection, such as pneumonia, and sepsis/severe sepsis doesn't develop until after admission, the localized infection should be assigned first, followed by the appropriate sepsis/severe sepsis codes.

For hemolytic-uremic syndrome associated with sepsis, see guideline I.C.1.d.9.

Patient presents with acute renal failure due to severe sepsis from *Pseudomonas pneumonia*

A41.52	Sepsis due to Pseudomonas
J15.1	Pneumonia due to Pseudomonas
R65.20	Severe sepsis without septic shock
N17.9	Acute kidney failure, unspecified

Explanation: If all conditions are present, the systemic infection (sepsis) is sequenced first followed by the codes for the localized infection (pneumonia), severe sepsis and any organ dysfunction.

5) Sepsis due to a postprocedural infection

(a) Documentation of causal relationship

As with all postprocedural complications, code assignment is based on the provider's documentation of the relationship between the infection and the procedure.

(b) Sepsis due to a postprocedural infection

For infections following a procedure, a code from T81.40, to T81.43 Infection following a procedure, or a code from O86.00 to O86.03, Infection of obstetric surgical wound, that identifies the site of the infection should be coded first, if known. Assign an additional code for sepsis following a procedure (T81.44) or sepsis following an obstetrical procedure (O86.04). Use an additional code to identify the infectious agent. If the patient has severe sepsis, the appropriate code from subcategory R65.2 should also be assigned with the additional code(s) for any acute organ dysfunction.

For infections following infusion, transfusion, therapeutic injection, or immunization, a code from subcategory T80.2, Infections following infusion, transfusion, and therapeutic injection, or code T88.0-,

Infection following immunization, should be coded first, followed by the code for the specific infection. If the patient has severe sepsis, the appropriate code from subcategory R65.2 should also be assigned, with the additional codes(s) for any acute organ dysfunction.

(c) Postprocedural infection and postprocedural septic shock

If a postprocedural infection has resulted in postprocedural septic shock, assign the codes indicated above for sepsis due to a postprocedural infection, followed by code T81.12-, Postprocedural septic shock. Do not assign code R65.21, Severe sepsis with septic shock. Additional code(s) should be assigned for any acute organ dysfunction.

6) Sepsis and severe sepsis associated with a noninfectious process (condition)

In some cases, a noninfectious process (condition) such as trauma, may lead to an infection which can result in sepsis or severe sepsis. If sepsis or severe sepsis is documented as associated with a noninfectious condition, such as a burn or serious injury, and this condition meets the definition for principal diagnosis, the code for the noninfectious condition should be sequenced first, followed by the code for the resulting infection. If severe sepsis is present, a code from subcategory R65.2 should also be assigned with any associated organ dysfunction(s) codes. It is not necessary to assign a code from subcategory R65.1, Systemic inflammatory response syndrome (SIRS) of non-infectious origin, for these cases.

If the infection meets the definition of principal diagnosis, it should be sequenced before the non-infectious condition. When both the associated non-infectious condition and the infection meet the definition of principal diagnosis, either may be assigned as principal diagnosis.

Only one code from category R65, Symptoms and signs specifically associated with systemic inflammation and infection, should be assigned. Therefore, when a non-infectious condition leads to an infection resulting in severe sepsis, assign the appropriate code from subcategory R65.2, Severe sepsis. Do not additionally assign a code from subcategory R65.1, Systemic inflammatory response syndrome (SIRS) of non-infectious origin.

See Section I.C.18. SIRS due to non-infectious process

7) Sepsis and septic shock complicating abortion, pregnancy, childbirth, and the puerperium

See Section I.C.15. Sepsis and septic shock complicating abortion, pregnancy, childbirth and the puerperium

8) Newborn sepsis

See Section I.C.16. f. Bacterial sepsis of Newborn

9) Hemolytic-uremic syndrome associated with sepsis

If the reason for admission is hemolytic-uremic syndrome that is associated with sepsis, assign code D59.31, Infection-associated hemolytic-uremic syndrome, as the principal diagnosis. Codes for the underlying systemic infection and any other conditions (such as severe sepsis) should be assigned as secondary diagnoses.

e. Methicillin resistant Staphylococcus aureus (MRSA) conditions

1) Selection and sequencing of MRSA codes

(a) Combination codes for MRSA infection

When a patient is diagnosed with an infection that is due to methicillin resistant *Staphylococcus aureus* (MRSA), and that infection has a combination code that includes the causal organism (e.g., sepsis, pneumonia) assign the appropriate combination code for the condition (e.g., code A41.02, Sepsis due to Methicillin resistant Staphylococcus aureus or code J15.212, Pneumonia due to Methicillin resistant Staphylococcus aureus). Do not assign code B95.62, Methicillin resistant Staphylococcus aureus infection as the cause of diseases classified elsewhere, as an additional code, because the combination code includes the type of infection and the MRSA organism. Do not assign a code from subcategory Z16.11, Resistance to penicillins, as an additional diagnosis.

See Section C.1. for instructions on coding and sequencing of sepsis and severe sepsis.

(b) Other codes for MRSA infection

When there is documentation of a current infection (e.g., wound infection, stitch abscess, urinary tract infection) due to MRSA, and that infection does not have a combination code that includes the causal organism, assign the appropriate code to identify the condition along with code B95.62, Methicillin resistant Staphylococcus aureus infection as the cause of diseases classified elsewhere for the MRSA infection. Do not assign a code from subcategory Z16.11, Resistance to penicillins.

(c) Methicillin susceptible Staphylococcus aureus (MSSA) and MRSA colonization

The condition or state of being colonized or carrying MSSA or MRSA is called colonization or carriage, while an individual person is described as being colonized or being a carrier.

Colonization means that MSSA or MSRA is present on or in the body without necessarily causing illness. A positive MRSA colonization test might be documented by the provider as "MRSA screen positive" or "MRSA nasal swab positive".

Assign code Z22.322, Carrier or suspected carrier of Methicillin resistant Staphylococcus aureus, for patients documented as having MRSA colonization. Assign code Z22.321, Carrier or suspected carrier of Methicillin susceptible Staphylococcus aureus, for patient**s** documented as having MSSA colonization. Colonization is not necessarily indicative of a disease process or as the cause of a specific condition the patient may have unless documented as such by the provider.

(d) MRSA colonization and infection

If a patient is documented as having both MRSA colonization and infection during a hospital admission, code Z22.322, Carrier or suspected carrier of Methicillin resistant Staphylococcus aureus, and a code for the MRSA infection may both be assigned.

f. Zika virus infections

1) Code only confirmed cases

Code only a confirmed diagnosis of Zika virus (A92.5, Zika virus disease) as documented by the provider. This is an exception to the hospital inpatient guideline Section II, H. In this context, "confirmation" does not require documentation of the type of test performed; the provider's diagnostic statement that the condition is confirmed is sufficient. This code should be assigned regardless of the stated mode of transmission.

If the provider documents "suspected", "possible" or "probable" Zika, do not assign code A92.5. Assign a code(s) explaining the reason for encounter (such as fever, rash, or joint pain) or Z20.821, Contact with and (suspected) exposure to Zika virus.

g. Coronavirus infections

1) COVID-19 infection (infection due to SARS-CoV-2)

(a) Code only confirmed cases

Code only a confirmed diagnosis of the 2019 novel coronavirus disease (COVID-19) as documented by the provider, or documentation of a positive COVID-19 test result. For a confirmed diagnosis, assign code U07.1, COVID-19. This is an exception to the hospital inpatient guideline Section II, H. In this context, "confirmation" does not require documentation of a positive test result for COVID-19; the provider's documentation that the individual has COVID-19 is sufficient.

> Physician documentation states the patient has tested positive for the 2019 novel coronavirus disease.
>
> **U07.1   COVID-19**
>
> *Explanation*: The type of test is not required; physician documentation that states the patient has COVID-19 or a documented positive COVID-19 test result is sufficient.

If the provider documents "suspected," "possible," "probable," or "inconclusive" COVID-19, do not assign code U07.1. Instead, code the signs and symptoms reported. See guideline I.C.1.g.1.g**.**

> Patient presents with cough and a slight fever and fear they were exposed to the coronavirus. The provider documents cough, temperature of 99.4, lungs clear, rule out COVID-19.
>
> **R50.9   Fever, unspecified**
>
> **R05.9   Cough, unspecified**
>
> **Z20.822   Contact with and (suspected) exposure to COVID-19**
>
> *Explanation*: For patients who have been exposed or fear they have been exposed to coronavirus, report codes for signs and symptoms, followed by the Z code. Report U07.1 COVID-19, only when the diagnosis is confirmed through provider documentation or a documented positive test result.

(b) Sequencing of codes

When COVID-19 meets the definition of principal diagnosis, code U07.1, COVID-19, should be sequenced first, followed by the appropriate codes for associated manifestations, except when another guideline requires that certain codes be sequenced first, such as obstetrics, sepsis, or transplant complications.

For a COVID-19 infection that progresses to sepsis, see Section I.C.1.d. Sepsis, Severe Sepsis, and Septic Shock

See Section I.C.15.s. for COVID-19 infection in pregnancy, childbirth, and the puerperium

See Section I.C.16.h. for COVID-19 infection in newborn

For a COVID-19 infection in a lung transplant patient, see Section I.C.19.g.3.a. Transplant complications other than kidney.

(c) Acute respiratory manifestations of COVID-19

When the reason for the encounter/admission is a respiratory manifestation of COVID-19, assign code U07.1, COVID-19, as the principal/first-listed diagnosis and assign code(s) for the respiratory manifestation(s) as additional diagnoses.

The following conditions are examples of common respiratory manifestations of COVID-19.

(i) Pneumonia

For a patient with pneumonia confirmed as due to COVID-19, assign codes U07.1, COVID-19, and J12.82, Pneumonia due to coronavirus disease 2019.

(ii) Acute bronchitis

For a patient with acute bronchitis confirmed as due to COVID-19, assign codes U07.1, and J20.8, Acute bronchitis due to other specified organisms.

Bronchitis not otherwise specified (NOS) due to COVID-19 should be coded using code U07.1 and J40, Bronchitis, not specified as acute or chronic.

(iii) Lower respiratory infection

If the COVID-19 is documented as being associated with a lower respiratory infection, not otherwise specified (NOS), or an acute respiratory infection, NOS, codes U07.1 and J22, Unspecified acute lower respiratory infection, should be assigned.

If the COVID-19 is documented as being associated with a respiratory infection, NOS, codes U07.1 and J98.8, Other specified respiratory disorders, should be assigned.

(iv) Acute respiratory distress syndrome

For acute respiratory distress syndrome (ARDS) due to COVID-19, assign codes U07.1, and J80, Acute respiratory distress syndrome.

(v) Acute respiratory failure

For acute respiratory failure due to COVID-19, assign code U07.1, and code J96.0-, Acute respiratory failure.

(d) Non-respiratory manifestations of COVID-19

When the reason for the encounter/admission is a non-respiratory manifestation (e.g., viral enteritis) of COVID-19, assign code U07.1, COVID-19, as the principal/first-listed diagnosis and assign code(s) for the manifestation(s) as additional diagnoses.

(e) Exposure to COVID-19

For asymptomatic individuals with actual or suspected exposure to COVID-19, assign code Z20.822, Contact with and (suspected) exposure to COVID-19.

For symptomatic individuals with actual or suspected exposure to COVID-19 and the infection has been ruled out, or test results are inconclusive or unknown, assign code Z20.822, Contact with and (suspected) exposure to COVID-19. See guideline I.C.21.c.1, Contact/Exposure, for additional guidance regarding the use of category Z20 codes.

If COVID-19 is confirmed, see guideline I.C.1.g.1.a.

> Patient was exposed to COVID-19 by a family member. They are asymptomatic and their test result is negative.
>
> **Z20.822   Contact with and (suspected) exposure to COVID-19**
>
> *Explanation*: Report Z20.822 for patients who have a negative test result but have known exposure to someone who has tested positive for COVID-19.

(f) Screening for COVID-19

During the COVID-19 pandemic, a screening code is generally not appropriate. Do not assign code Z11.52, Encounter for screening for COVID-19. For encounters for COVID-19 testing, including preoperative testing, code as exposure to COVID-19 (guideline I.C.1.g.1.e).

Coding guidance will be updated as new information concerning changes in the pandemic status becomes available.

(g) Signs and symptoms without definitive diagnosis of COVID-19

For patients presenting with any signs/symptoms associated with COVID-19 (such as fever, etc.) but a definitive diagnosis has not been established, assign the appropriate code(s) for each of the presenting signs and symptoms such as:

- R05.1, Acute cough, or R05.9, Cough, unspecified
- R06.02 Shortness of breath
- R50.9 Fever, unspecified

If a patient with signs/symptoms associated with COVID-19 also has an actual or suspected contact with or exposure to COVID-19, assign Z20.822, Contact with and (suspected) exposure to COVID19, as an additional code.

(h) Asymptomatic individuals who test positive for COVID-19

For asymptomatic individuals who test positive for COVID-19, see guideline I.C.1.g.1.a. Although the individual is asymptomatic, the individual has tested positive and is considered to have the COVID-19 infection.

(i) Personal history of COVID-19

For patients with a history of COVID-19, assign code Z86.16, Personal history of COVID-19.

(j) Follow-up visits after COVID-19 infection has resolved

For individuals who previously had COVID-19, without residual symptom(s) or condition(s), and are being seen for follow-up evaluation, and COVID-19 test results are negative, assign codes Z09, Encounter for follow-up examination after completed treatment for conditions other than malignant neoplasm, and Z86.16, Personal history of COVID-19.

For follow-up visits for individuals with symptom(s) or condition(s) related to a previous COVID-19 infection, see guideline I.C.1.g.1.m.

See Section I.C.21.c.8, Factors influencing health states and contact with health services, Follow-up

(k) Encounter for antibody testing

For an encounter for antibody testing that is not being performed to confirm a current COVID-19 infection, nor is a follow-up test after resolution of COVID-19, assign Z01.84, Encounter for antibody response examination.

Follow the applicable guidelines above if the individual is being tested to confirm a current COVID-19 infection.

For follow-up testing after a COVID-19 infection, see guideline I.C.1.g.1.j.

(l) Multisystem inflammatory syndrome

For individuals with multisystem inflammatory syndrome (MIS) and COVID-19, assign code U07.1, COVID-19, as the principal/first-listed diagnosis and assign code M35.81, Multisystem inflammatory syndrome, as an additional diagnosis.

If an individual with a history of COVID-19 develops MIS, assign codes M35.81, Multisystem inflammatory syndrome, and U09.9, Post COVID-19 condition, unspecified.

If an individual with a known or suspected exposure to COVID-19, and no current COVID-19 infection or history of COVID-19, develops MIS, assign codes M35.81, Multisystem inflammatory syndrome, and Z20.822, Contact with and (suspected) exposure to COVID-19.

Additional codes should be assigned for any associated complications of MIS.

(m) Post COVID-19 condition

For sequela of COVID-19, or associated symptoms or conditions that develop following a previous COVID-19 infection, assign a code(s) for the specific symptom(s) or condition(s) related to the previous COVID-19 infection, if known, and code U09.9, Post COVID-19 condition, unspecified.

Code U09.9 should not be assigned for manifestations of an active (current) COVID-19 infection.

If a patient has a condition(s) associated with a previous COVID-19 infection and develops a new active (current) COVID-19 infection, code U09.9 may be assigned in conjunction with code U07.1, COVID-19, to identify that the patient also has a condition(s) associated with a previous COVID-19 infection. Code(s) for the specific condition(s) associated with the previous COVID-19 infection and code(s) for manifestation(s) of the new active (current) COVID-19 infection should also be assigned.

(n) Underimmunization for COVID-19 Status

Code Z28.310, Unvaccinated for COVID-19, may be assigned when the patient has not received a COVID-19 vaccine of any type. Code Z28.311, Partially vaccinated for COVID-19, may be assigned when the patient has been partially vaccinated for COVID-19 as per the recommendations of the Centers for Disease Control and Prevention (CDC) in place at the time of the encounter. For information, visit the CDC's website https://www.cdc.gov/coronavirus/2019-ncov/vaccines/.

See Section I.B.14. for underimmunization documentation by clinicians other than patient's provider.

Chapter 1. Certain Infectious and Parasitic Diseases (A00-B99)

INCLUDES diseases generally recognized as communicable or transmissible
Use additional code to identify resistance to antimicrobial drugs (Z16.-)
EXCLUDES 1 certain localized infections - see body system-related chapters
EXCLUDES 2 carrier or suspected carrier of infectious disease (Z22.-)
infectious and parasitic diseases complicating pregnancy, childbirth and the puerperium (O98.-)
infectious and parasitic diseases specific to the perinatal period (P35-P39)
influenza and other acute respiratory infections (J00-J22)

This chapter contains the following blocks:

A00-A09   Intestinal infectious diseases
A15-A19   Tuberculosis
A20-A28   Certain zoonotic bacterial diseases
A30-A49   Other bacterial diseases
A50-A64   Infections with a predominantly sexual mode of transmission
A65-A69   Other spirochetal diseases
A70-A74   Other diseases caused by chlamydiae
A75-A79   Rickettsioses
A80-A89   Viral and prion infections of the central nervous system
A90-A99   Arthropod-borne viral fevers and viral hemorrhagic fevers
B00-B09   Viral infections characterized by skin and mucous membrane lesions
B10   Other human herpesviruses
B15-B19   Viral hepatitis
B20   Human immunodeficiency virus [HIV] disease
B25-B34   Other viral diseases
B35-B49   Mycoses
B50-B64   Protozoal diseases
B65-B83   Helminthiases
B85-B89   Pediculosis, acariasis and other infestations
B90-B94   Sequelae of infectious and parasitic diseases
B95-B97   Bacterial and viral infectious agents
B99   Other infectious diseases

Intestinal infectious diseases (A00-A09)

✓4ᵗʰ A00 Cholera

DEF: Acute infection of the bowel due to *Vibrio cholerae* that presents with profuse diarrhea, cramps, and vomiting, resulting in severe dehydration, electrolyte imbalance, and death. It is spread through ingestion of food or water contaminated with feces of infected persons.

A00.0 Cholera due to Vibrio cholerae 01, biovar cholerae
Classical cholera

A00.1 Cholera due to Vibrio cholerae 01, biovar eltor
Cholera eltor

A00.9 Cholera, unspecified

✓4ᵗʰ A01 Typhoid and paratyphoid fevers

DEF: Typhoid fever: Acute generalized illness caused by *Salmonella typhi*. Clinical features include fever, headache, abdominal pain, cough, toxemia, leukopenia, abnormal pulse, rose spots on the skin, bacteremia, hyperplasia of intestinal lymph nodes, mesenteric lymphadenopathy, and Peyer's patches in the intestines.
DEF: Paratyphoid fever: Prolonged febrile illness, caused by *Salmonella* serotypes other than *S. typhi*, especially *S. enterica* serotypes paratyphi A, B, and C.

✓5ᵗʰ A01.0 Typhoid fever
Infection due to Salmonella typhi

A01.00 Typhoid fever, unspecified
A01.01 Typhoid meningitis COM
A01.02 Typhoid fever with heart involvement COM
Typhoid endocarditis
Typhoid myocarditis
A01.03 Typhoid pneumonia HCC ESR
A01.04 Typhoid arthritis HCC ESR COM
A01.05 Typhoid osteomyelitis HCC ESR COM
A01.09 Typhoid fever with other complications

A01.1 Paratyphoid fever A
A01.2 Paratyphoid fever B
A01.3 Paratyphoid fever C
A01.4 Paratyphoid fever, unspecified
Infection due to Salmonella paratyphi NOS

✓4ᵗʰ A02 Other salmonella infections

INCLUDES infection or foodborne intoxication due to any Salmonella species other than S. typhi and S. paratyphi

A02.0 Salmonella enteritis
Salmonellosis
TIP: Dehydration (E86.0) is a complication of salmonella enteritis and may be reported separately.

A02.1 Salmonella sepsis HCC ESR COM

✓5ᵗʰ A02.2 Localized salmonella infections

A02.20 Localized salmonella infection, unspecified
A02.21 Salmonella meningitis COM
A02.22 Salmonella pneumonia HCC ESR
A02.23 Salmonella arthritis HCC ESR COM
A02.24 Salmonella osteomyelitis HCC ESR COM
A02.25 Salmonella pyelonephritis
Salmonella tubulo-interstitial nephropathy
A02.29 Salmonella with other localized infection

A02.8 Other specified salmonella infections
A02.9 Salmonella infection, unspecified

✓4ᵗʰ A03 Shigellosis

DEF: Infection caused by the genus *Shigella*, of the family *Enterobacteriaceae* that is known to cause an acute dysenteric infection of the bowel with fever, drowsiness, anorexia, nausea, vomiting, bloody diarrhea, abdominal cramps, and distention.

A03.0 Shigellosis due to Shigella dysenteriae
Group A shigellosis [Shiga-Kruse dysentery]

A03.1 Shigellosis due to Shigella flexneri
Group B shigellosis

A03.2 Shigellosis due to Shigella boydii
Group C shigellosis

A03.3 Shigellosis due to Shigella sonnei
Group D shigellosis

A03.8 Other shigellosis
A03.9 Shigellosis, unspecified
Bacillary dysentery NOS

✓4ᵗʰ A04 Other bacterial intestinal infections

EXCLUDES 1 bacterial foodborne intoxications, NEC (A05.-)
tuberculous enteritis (A18.32)

DEF: *Escherichia coli*: Gram-negative, anaerobic bacteria of the family *Enterobacteriaceae* found in the large intestine of warm-blooded animals, generally as a nonpathologic entity aiding in digestion. They become pathogenic when an opportunity to grow somewhere outside this relationship presents itself, such as ingestion of fecal-contaminated food or water.

A04.0 Enteropathogenic Escherichia coli infection
A04.1 Enterotoxigenic Escherichia coli infection
A04.2 Enteroinvasive Escherichia coli infection
A04.3 Enterohemorrhagic Escherichia coli infection
DEF: *E. coli* infection penetrating the intestinal mucosa, producing microscopic ulceration and bleeding.
A04.4 Other intestinal Escherichia coli infections
Escherichia coli enteritis NOS
A04.5 Campylobacter enteritis
TIP: For Guillain-Barre syndrome occurring as a sequela of *Campylobacter enteritis*, assign code G61.0 as the first-listed diagnosis followed by B94.8 for the sequelae.
A04.6 Enteritis due to Yersinia enterocolitica
EXCLUDES 1 extraintestinal yersiniosis (A28.2)

✓5ᵗʰ A04.7 Enterocolitis due to Clostridium difficile
Foodborne intoxication by Clostridium difficile
Pseudomembraneous colitis
AHA: 2017,4Q,4
A04.71 Enterocolitis due to Clostridium difficile, recurrent
AHA: 2020,1Q,18
A04.72 Enterocolitis due to Clostridium difficile, not specified as recurrent

A04.8 Other specified bacterial intestinal infections
A04.9 Bacterial intestinal infection, unspecified
Bacterial enteritis NOS

| ☑ Additional Character Required | ✓x7ᵗʰ Placeholder Alert | Manifestation | Unspecified Dx | 🄠 QPP | UPD Unacceptable PDx |

ICD-10-CM 2023   451

✓4ᵗʰ **A05   Other bacterial foodborne intoxications, not elsewhere classified**

> **EXCLUDES 1**   Clostridium difficile foodborne intoxication and infection (A04.7-)
> Escherichia coli infection (A04.0-A04.4)
> listeriosis (A32.-)
> salmonella foodborne intoxication and infection (A02.-)
> toxic effect of noxious foodstuffs (T61-T62)

A05.0   Foodborne staphylococcal intoxication
> **TIP:** Assign code A04.8 to report a staphylococcal infection when it is caused by the ingestion of contaminated food but not caused by *S. aureus* toxins.

A05.1   Botulism food poisoning
> Botulism NOS
> Classical foodborne intoxication due to Clostridium botulinum
> **EXCLUDES 1**   infant botulism (A48.51)
> wound botulism (A48.52)
> **DEF:** Muscle-paralyzing neurotoxic disease caused by ingesting pre-formed toxin from the bacterium *Clostridium botulinum*. It causes vomiting and diarrhea, vision problems, slurred speech, difficulty swallowing, paralysis, and death.

A05.2   Foodborne Clostridium perfringens [Clostridium welchii] intoxication
> Enteritis necroticans
> Pig-bel

A05.3   Foodborne Vibrio parahaemolyticus intoxication

A05.4   Foodborne Bacillus cereus intoxication

A05.5   Foodborne Vibrio vulnificus intoxication

A05.8   Other specified bacterial foodborne intoxications

A05.9   Bacterial foodborne intoxication, unspecified

✓4ᵗʰ **A06   Amebiasis**

> **INCLUDES**   infection due to Entamoeba histolytica
> **EXCLUDES 1**   other protozoal intestinal diseases (A07.-)
> **EXCLUDES 2**   acanthamebiasis (B60.1-)
> Naegleriasis (B60.2)
> **DEF:** Infection with a single cell protozoan known as the amoeba. Transmission occurs through ingestion of feces, contaminated food or water, use of human feces as fertilizer, or person-to-person contact.

A06.0   Acute amebic dysentery
> Acute amebiasis
> Intestinal amebiasis NOS

A06.1   Chronic intestinal amebiasis

A06.2   Amebic nondysenteric colitis

A06.3   Ameboma of intestine
> Ameboma NOS

A06.4   Amebic liver abscess   COM
> Hepatic amebiasis

A06.5   Amebic lung abscess   HCC ESR COM
> Amebic abscess of lung (and liver)

A06.6   Amebic brain abscess   COM
> Amebic abscess of brain (and liver) (and lung)

A06.7   Cutaneous amebiasis

✓5ᵗʰ **A06.8   Amebic infection of other sites**

> **A06.81   Amebic cystitis**

> **A06.82   Other amebic genitourinary infections**
> Amebic balanitis
> Amebic vesiculitis
> Amebic vulvovaginitis

> **A06.89   Other amebic infections**
> Amebic appendicitis
> Amebic splenic abscess

A06.9   Amebiasis, unspecified

✓4ᵗʰ **A07   Other protozoal intestinal diseases**

> **DEF:** Protozoa: Group comprised of the simplest, single celled organisms, ranging in size from micro to macroscopic. They can live alone or in colonies, and do not show any differentiation in tissues. Most are motile and can live free in nature, but some are parasitic, causing disease in the variety of hosts they inhabit.

A07.0   Balantidiasis
> Balantidial dysentery

A07.1   Giardiasis [lambliasis]
> **DEF:** Infection caused by the flagellate protozoan *Giardia lamblia* causing gastrointestinal problems such as vomiting, chronic diarrhea, and weight loss. The most common parasite in the U.S., this is usually transmitted by ingesting contaminated water while in the cyst state, after which it latches onto the wall of the small intestine.

A07.2   Cryptosporidiosis   HCC Rx ESR COM
> **DEF:** Microscopic parasite found in water and one of the most common causes of waterborne gastrointestinal infectious disease in the United States. It is usually transmitted by ingesting contaminated drinking water or recreational water and causes profuse watery diarrhea, flatulence, abdominal pain, and cramping.

A07.3   Isosporiasis
> Infection due to Isospora belli and Isospora hominis
> Intestinal coccidiosis
> Isosporosis

A07.4   Cyclosporiasis

A07.8   Other specified protozoal intestinal diseases
> Intestinal microsporidiosis
> Intestinal trichomoniasis
> Sarcocystosis
> Sarcosporidiosis

A07.9   Protozoal intestinal disease, unspecified
> Flagellate diarrhea
> Protozoal colitis
> Protozoal diarrhea
> Protozoal dysentery

✓4ᵗʰ **A08   Viral and other specified intestinal infections**

> **EXCLUDES 1**   influenza with involvement of gastrointestinal tract (J09.X3, J10.2, J11.2)

A08.0   Rotaviral enteritis

✓5ᵗʰ **A08.1   Acute gastroenteropathy due to Norwalk agent and other small round viruses**

> **A08.11   Acute gastroenteropathy due to Norwalk agent**
> Acute gastroenteropathy due to Norovirus
> Acute gastroenteropathy due to Norwalk-like agent

> **A08.19   Acute gastroenteropathy due to other small round viruses**
> Acute gastroenteropathy due to small round virus [SRV] NOS

A08.2   Adenoviral enteritis

✓5ᵗʰ **A08.3   Other viral enteritis**

> **A08.31   Calicivirus enteritis**

> **A08.32   Astrovirus enteritis**

> **A08.39   Other viral enteritis**
> Coxsackie virus enteritis
> Echovirus enteritis
> Enterovirus enteritis NEC
> Torovirus enteritis

A08.4   Viral intestinal infection, unspecified
> Viral enteritis NOS
> Viral gastroenteritis NOS
> Viral gastroenteropathy NOS
> **AHA:** 2016,3Q,12

[handwritten: Stomach flu]

A08.8   Other specified intestinal infections

A09   Infectious gastroenteritis and colitis, unspecified
> Infectious colitis NOS
> Infectious enteritis NOS
> Infectious gastroenteritis NOS
> **EXCLUDES 1**   colitis NOS (K52.9)
> diarrhea NOS (R19.7)
> enteritis NOS (K52.9)
> gastroenteritis NOS (K52.9)
> noninfective gastroenteritis and colitis, unspecified (K52.9)
> **DEF:** Colitis: Inflammation of mucous membranes of the colon.
> **DEF:** Enteritis: Inflammation of mucous membranes of the small intestine.
> **DEF:** Gastroenteritis: Inflammation of mucous membranes of the stomach and intestines.

Tuberculosis (A15-A19)

INCLUDES   infections due to Mycobacterium tuberculosis and Mycobacterium bovis

EXCLUDES 1   *congenital tuberculosis (P37.0)*
nonspecific reaction to test for tuberculosis without active tuberculosis (R76.1-)
pneumoconiosis associated with tuberculosis, any type in A15 (J65)
positive PPD (R76.11)
positive tuberculin skin test without active tuberculosis (R76.11)
sequelae of tuberculosis (B90.-)
silicotuberculosis (J65)

DEF: Bacterial infection that typically spreads by inhalation of an airborne agent that usually attacks the lungs, but may also affect other organs.

☑4ᵗʰ **A15**   **Respiratory tuberculosis**

   A15.0   **Tuberculosis of lung**
      Tuberculous bronchiectasis
      Tuberculous fibrosis of lung
      Tuberculous pneumonia
      Tuberculous pneumothorax

Tuberculosis of Lung

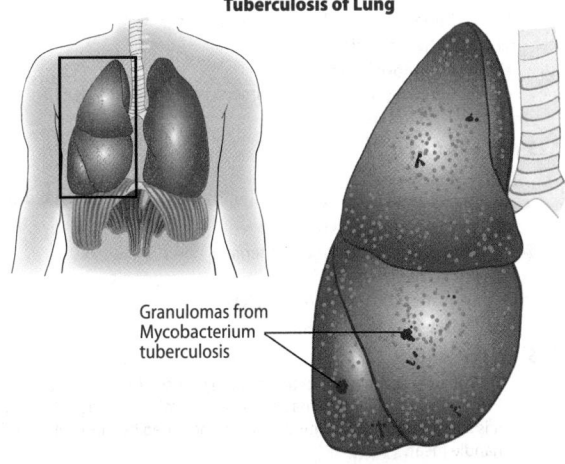

Granulomas from Mycobacterium tuberculosis

   A15.4   **Tuberculosis of intrathoracic lymph nodes**
      Tuberculosis of hilar lymph nodes
      Tuberculosis of mediastinal lymph nodes
      Tuberculosis of tracheobronchial lymph nodes
      EXCLUDES 1   *tuberculosis specified as primary (A15.7)*

   A15.5   **Tuberculosis of larynx, trachea and bronchus**
      Tuberculosis of bronchus
      Tuberculosis of glottis
      Tuberculosis of larynx
      Tuberculosis of trachea

   A15.6   **Tuberculous pleurisy**
      Tuberculosis of pleura Tuberculous empyema
      EXCLUDES 1   *primary respiratory tuberculosis (A15.7)*

   A15.7   **Primary respiratory tuberculosis**
   A15.8   **Other respiratory tuberculosis**
      Mediastinal tuberculosis
      Nasopharyngeal tuberculosis
      Tuberculosis of nose
      Tuberculosis of sinus [any nasal]
   A15.9   **Respiratory tuberculosis unspecified**

☑4ᵗʰ **A17**   **Tuberculosis of nervous system**

   A17.0   **Tuberculous meningitis**   COM
      Tuberculosis of meninges (cerebral)(spinal)
      Tuberculous leptomeningitis
      EXCLUDES 1   *tuberculous meningoencephalitis (A17.82)*

   A17.1   **Meningeal tuberculoma**   COM
      Tuberculoma of meninges (cerebral) (spinal)
      EXCLUDES 2   *tuberculoma of brain and spinal cord (A17.81)*

  ☑5ᵗʰ **A17.8**   **Other tuberculosis of nervous system**
      A17.81   **Tuberculoma of brain and spinal cord**   COM
         Tuberculous abscess of brain and spinal cord
      A17.82   **Tuberculous meningoencephalitis**   COM
         Tuberculous myelitis
      A17.83   **Tuberculous neuritis**   COM
         Tuberculous mononeuropathy

      A17.89   **Other tuberculosis of nervous system**   COM
         Tuberculous polyneuropathy
   A17.9   **Tuberculosis of nervous system, unspecified**   COM

☑4ᵗʰ **A18**   **Tuberculosis of other organs**

  ☑5ᵗʰ **A18.0**   **Tuberculosis of bones and joints**
      A18.01   **Tuberculosis of spine**
         Pott's disease or curvature of spine
         Tuberculous arthritis
         Tuberculous osteomyelitis of spine
         Tuberculous spondylitis
      A18.02   **Tuberculous arthritis of other joints**
         Tuberculosis of hip (joint)
         Tuberculosis of knee (joint)
      A18.03   **Tuberculosis of other bones**
         Tuberculous mastoiditis
         Tuberculous osteomyelitis
      A18.09   **Other musculoskeletal tuberculosis**
         Tuberculous myositis
         Tuberculous synovitis
         Tuberculous tenosynovitis

  ☑5ᵗʰ **A18.1**   **Tuberculosis of genitourinary system**
      A18.10   **Tuberculosis of genitourinary system, unspecified**
      A18.11   **Tuberculosis of kidney and ureter**
      A18.12   **Tuberculosis of bladder**
      A18.13   **Tuberculosis of other urinary organs**
         Tuberculous urethritis
      A18.14   **Tuberculosis of prostate**   A ♂
      A18.15   **Tuberculosis of other male genital organs**   ♂
      A18.16   **Tuberculosis of cervix**   ♀
      A18.17   **Tuberculous female pelvic inflammatory disease**   ♀
         Tuberculous endometritis
         Tuberculous oophoritis and salpingitis
      A18.18   **Tuberculosis of other female genital organs**   ♀
         Tuberculous ulceration of vulva

   A18.2   **Tuberculous peripheral lymphadenopathy**
      Tuberculous adenitis
      EXCLUDES 2   *tuberculosis of bronchial and mediastinal lymph nodes (A15.4)*
               tuberculosis of mesenteric and retroperitoneal lymph nodes (A18.39)
               tuberculous tracheobronchial adenopathy (A15.4)

  ☑5ᵗʰ **A18.3**   **Tuberculosis of intestines, peritoneum and mesenteric glands**
      A18.31   **Tuberculous peritonitis**
         Tuberculous ascites
         DEF: Tuberculous inflammation of the membrane lining the abdomen.
      A18.32   **Tuberculous enteritis**
         Tuberculosis of anus and rectum
         Tuberculosis of intestine (large) (small)
      A18.39   **Retroperitoneal tuberculosis**
         Tuberculosis of mesenteric glands
         Tuberculosis of retroperitoneal (lymph glands)

   A18.4   **Tuberculosis of skin and subcutaneous tissue**
      Erythema induratum, tuberculous
      Lupus excedens
      Lupus vulgaris NOS
      Lupus vulgaris of eyelid
      Scrofuloderma
      Tuberculosis of external ear
      EXCLUDES 2   *lupus erythematosus (L93.-)*
               systemic lupus erythematosus (M32.-)

  ☑5ᵗʰ **A18.5**   **Tuberculosis of eye**
      EXCLUDES 2   *lupus vulgaris of eyelid (A18.4)*
      A18.50   **Tuberculosis of eye, unspecified**
      A18.51   **Tuberculous episcleritis**
      A18.52   **Tuberculous keratitis**
         Tuberculous interstitial keratitis
         Tuberculous keratoconjunctivitis (interstitial) (phlyctenular)
      A18.53   **Tuberculous chorioretinitis**
      A18.54   **Tuberculous iridocyclitis**
      A18.59   **Other tuberculosis of eye**
         Tuberculous conjunctivitis

Chapter 1. Certain Infectious and Parasitic Diseases

A18.6   Tuberculosis of (inner) (middle) ear
Tuberculous otitis media
EXCLUDES 2   *tuberculosis of external ear (A18.4)*
tuberculous mastoiditis (A18.03)

A18.7   Tuberculosis of adrenal glands
Tuberculous Addison's disease

✓5ᵗʰ **A18.8   Tuberculosis of other specified organs**

A18.81   Tuberculosis of thyroid gland

A18.82   Tuberculosis of other endocrine glands
Tuberculosis of pituitary gland
Tuberculosis of thymus gland

A18.83   Tuberculosis of digestive tract organs, not elsewhere classified
EXCLUDES 1   *tuberculosis of intestine (A18.32)*

A18.84   Tuberculosis of heart
Tuberculous cardiomyopathy
Tuberculous endocarditis
Tuberculous myocarditis
Tuberculous pericarditis

A18.85   Tuberculosis of spleen

A18.89   Tuberculosis of other sites
Tuberculosis of muscle
Tuberculous cerebral arteritis

✓4ᵗʰ **A19   Miliary tuberculosis**
INCLUDES   disseminated tuberculosis
generalized tuberculosis
tuberculous polyserositis

A19.0   Acute miliary tuberculosis of a single specified site

A19.1   Acute miliary tuberculosis of multiple sites

A19.2   Acute miliary tuberculosis, unspecified

A19.8   Other miliary tuberculosis

A19.9   Miliary tuberculosis, unspecified

Certain zoonotic bacterial diseases (A20-A28)

✓4ᵗʰ **A20   Plague**
INCLUDES   infection due to Yersinia pestis

A20.0   Bubonic plague

A20.1   Cellulocutaneous plague

A20.2   Pneumonic plague   HCC ESR

A20.3   Plague meningitis   COM

A20.7   Septicemic plague   HCC ESR COM

A20.8   Other forms of plague
Abortive plague
Asymptomatic plague
Pestis minor

A20.9   Plague, unspecified

✓4ᵗʰ **A21   Tularemia**
INCLUDES   deer-fly fever
infection due to Francisella tularensis
rabbit fever
DEF: Febrile disease transmitted to humans by the bites of deer flies, fleas, and ticks, by inhaling aerosolized *F. tularensis*, or by ingesting contaminated food or water. Patients quickly develop fever, chills, weakness, headache, backache, and malaise.

A21.0   Ulceroglandular tularemia

A21.1   Oculoglandular tularemia
Ophthalmic tularemia

A21.2   Pulmonary tularemia   HCC ESR

A21.3   Gastrointestinal tularemia
Abdominal tularemia

A21.7   Generalized tularemia

A21.8   Other forms of tularemia

A21.9   Tularemia, unspecified

✓4ᵗʰ **A22   Anthrax**
INCLUDES   infection due to Bacillus anthracis

A22.0   Cutaneous anthrax
Malignant carbuncle
Malignant pustule

A22.1   Pulmonary anthrax   HCC ESR
Inhalation anthrax
Ragpicker's disease
Woolsorter's disease

A22.2   Gastrointestinal anthrax

A22.7   Anthrax sepsis   HCC ESR COM

A22.8   Other forms of anthrax
Anthrax meningitis

A22.9   Anthrax, unspecified

✓4ᵗʰ **A23   Brucellosis**
INCLUDES   Malta fever
Mediterranean fever
undulant fever

A23.0   Brucellosis due to Brucella melitensis

A23.1   Brucellosis due to Brucella abortus

A23.2   Brucellosis due to Brucella suis

A23.3   Brucellosis due to Brucella canis

A23.8   Other brucellosis

A23.9   Brucellosis, unspecified

✓4ᵗʰ **A24   Glanders and melioidosis**

A24.0   Glanders
Infection due to Pseudomonas mallei
Malleus

A24.1   Acute and fulminating melioidosis
Melioidosis pneumonia
Melioidosis sepsis

A24.2   Subacute and chronic melioidosis

A24.3   Other melioidosis

A24.9   Melioidosis, unspecified
Infection due to Pseudomonas pseudomallei NOS
Whitmore's disease

✓4ᵗʰ **A25   Rat-bite fevers**

A25.0   Spirillosis
Sodoku

A25.1   Streptobacillosis
Epidemic arthritic erythema
Haverhill fever
Streptobacillary rat-bite fever

A25.9   Rat-bite fever, unspecified

✓4ᵗʰ **A26   Erysipeloid**
DEF: Acute cutaneous infection typically caused by trauma to the skin. Presenting as cellulitis, it may become systemic, affecting other organs. It is a gram-positive bacillus and mainly acquired by those who routinely handle meat.

A26.0   Cutaneous erysipeloid
Erythema migrans

A26.7   Erysipelothrix sepsis   HCC ESR COM

A26.8   Other forms of erysipeloid

A26.9   Erysipeloid, unspecified

✓4ᵗʰ **A27   Leptospirosis**

A27.0   Leptospirosis icterohemorrhagica
Leptospiral or spirochetal jaundice (hemorrhagic)
Weil's disease

✓5ᵗʰ **A27.8   Other forms of leptospirosis**

A27.81   Aseptic meningitis in leptospirosis   COM

A27.89   Other forms of leptospirosis

A27.9   Leptospirosis, unspecified

✓4ᵗʰ **A28   Other zoonotic bacterial diseases, not elsewhere classified**

A28.0   Pasteurellosis

A28.1   Cat-scratch disease
Cat-scratch fever

A28.2   Extraintestinal yersiniosis
EXCLUDES 1   *enteritis due to Yersinia enterocolitica (A04.6)*
plague (A20.-)

A28.8   Other specified zoonotic bacterial diseases, not elsewhere classified

A28.9   Zoonotic bacterial disease, unspecified

Other bacterial diseases (A30-A49)

AHA: 2016,3Q,8-14

✓4ᵗʰ **A30   Leprosy [Hansen's disease]**
INCLUDES   infection due to Mycobacterium leprae
EXCLUDES 1   *sequelae of leprosy (B92)*

A30.0   Indeterminate leprosy
I leprosy

A30.1   Tuberculoid leprosy
TT leprosy

A30.2 Borderline tuberculoid **leprosy**
BT leprosy

A30.3 Borderline **leprosy**
BB leprosy

A30.4 Borderline lepromatous **leprosy**
BL leprosy

A30.5 Lepromatous **leprosy**
LL leprosy

A30.8 Other forms of leprosy

A30.9 Leprosy, unspecified

✓4ᵗʰ **A31 Infection due to other mycobacteria**

EXCLUDES 2   leprosy (A30.-)
tuberculosis (A15-A19)

A31.0 Pulmonary **mycobacterial infection**   HCC Rx ESR COM
Infection due to Mycobacterium avium
Infection due to Mycobacterium intracellulare [Battey bacillus]
Infection due to Mycobacterium kansasii

A31.1 Cutaneous **mycobacterial infection**
Buruli ulcer
Infection due to Mycobacterium marinum
Infection due to Mycobacterium ulcerans

A31.2 Disseminated mycobacterium avium-intracellulare complex **(DMAC)**   HCC Rx ESR COM
MAC sepsis

A31.8 Other mycobacterial infections

A31.9 Mycobacterial infection, unspecified
Atypical mycobacterial infection NOS
Mycobacteriosis NOS

✓4ᵗʰ **A32 Listeriosis**

INCLUDES   listerial foodborne infection
EXCLUDES 1   neonatal (disseminated) listeriosis (P37.2)

A32.0 Cutaneous **listeriosis**

✓5ᵗʰ **A32.1** Listerial **meningitis and meningoencephalitis**

A32.11 Listerial **meningitis**   COM

A32.12 Listerial **meningoencephalitis**   COM

A32.7 Listerial **sepsis**   HCC ESR COM

✓5ᵗʰ **A32.8** Other forms of listeriosis

A32.81 Oculoglandular **listeriosis**

A32.82 Listerial **endocarditis**   COM

A32.89 Other forms of listeriosis
Listerial cerebral arteritis

A32.9 Listeriosis, unspecified

A33 Tetanus neonatorum   N

A34 Obstetrical tetanus   COM M ♀

A35 Other tetanus   COM
Tetanus NOS
EXCLUDES 1   obstetrical tetanus (A34)
tetanus neonatorum (A33)

DEF: Tetanus: Acute, often fatal, infectious disease caused by the anaerobic, spore-forming bacillus *Clostridium tetani*. The bacillus enters the body through a contaminated wound, burns, surgical wounds, or cutaneous ulcers. Symptoms include lockjaw, spasms, seizures, and paralysis.

✓4ᵗʰ **A36 Diphtheria**

A36.0 Pharyngeal **diphtheria**
Diphtheritic membranous angina
Tonsillar diphtheria

A36.1 Nasopharyngeal **diphtheria**

A36.2 Laryngeal **diphtheria**
Diphtheritic laryngotracheitis

A36.3 Cutaneous **diphtheria**
EXCLUDES 2   erythrasma (L08.1)

✓5ᵗʰ **A36.8** Other diphtheria

A36.81 Diphtheritic **cardiomyopathy**   HCC Rx ESR COM
Diphtheritic myocarditis

A36.82 Diphtheritic **radiculomyelitis**

A36.83 Diphtheritic **polyneuritis**

A36.84 Diphtheritic **tubulo-interstitial nephropathy**

A36.85 Diphtheritic **cystitis**

A36.86 Diphtheritic **conjunctivitis**

A36.89 Other **diphtheritic complications**
Diphtheritic peritonitis

A36.9 Diphtheria, unspecified

✓4ᵗʰ **A37 Whooping cough**

DEF: Acute, highly contagious respiratory tract infection caused by *Bordetella pertussis* and *B. bronchiseptica*. Whooping cough is known by its characteristic paroxysmal cough.

✓5ᵗʰ **A37.0** Whooping cough due to Bordetella pertussis

A37.00 Whooping cough due to Bordetella pertussis **without pneumonia**
Paroxysmal cough due to Bordetella pertussis without pneumonia

A37.01 Whooping cough due to Bordetella pertussis **with pneumonia**
Paroxysmal cough due to Bordetella pertussis with pneumonia

✓5ᵗʰ **A37.1** Whooping cough due to Bordetella parapertussis

A37.10 Whooping cough due to Bordetella parapertussis **without pneumonia**

A37.11 Whooping cough due to Bordetella parapertussis **with pneumonia**

✓5ᵗʰ **A37.8** Whooping cough due to other Bordetella species

A37.80 Whooping cough due to other Bordetella species **without pneumonia**

A37.81 Whooping cough due to other Bordetella species **with pneumonia**

✓5ᵗʰ **A37.9** Whooping cough, unspecified species

A37.90 Whooping cough, unspecified species **without pneumonia**

A37.91 Whooping cough, unspecified species **with pneumonia**

✓4ᵗʰ **A38 Scarlet fever**

INCLUDES   scarlatina
EXCLUDES 2   streptococcal sore throat (J02.0)

DEF: Acute contagious disease caused by Group A bacteria, the same bacterium that causes strep throat. Individuals with strep throat can develop scarlet fever particularly if the infection is not treated with antibiotics. It is characterized by a red blush to the skin of the chest and abdomen and swelling of the nose, throat, and mouth.

A38.0 Scarlet fever with otitis media

A38.1 Scarlet fever with myocarditis   COM

A38.8 Scarlet fever with other complications

A38.9 Scarlet fever, uncomplicated
Scarlet fever, NOS

✓4ᵗʰ **A39 Meningococcal infection**

DEF: Condition caused by *Neisseria meningitidis*, a bacteria that may invade the spinal cord, brain, heart, joints, optic nerve, or bloodstream.

A39.0 Meningococcal **meningitis**   COM

A39.1 Waterhouse-Friderichsen **syndrome**   HCC Rx ESR COM
Meningococcal hemorrhagic adrenalitis
Meningococcic adrenal syndrome

A39.2 Acute **meningococcemia**   HCC ESR COM

A39.3 Chronic **meningococcemia**   HCC ESR COM

A39.4 Meningococcemia, unspecified   HCC ESR COM

✓5ᵗʰ **A39.5** Meningococcal **heart disease**

A39.50 Meningococcal carditis, unspecified   COM

A39.51 Meningococcal **endocarditis**   COM

A39.52 Meningococcal **myocarditis**   COM

A39.53 Meningococcal **pericarditis**   COM

✓5ᵗʰ **A39.8** Other meningococcal infections

A39.81 Meningococcal **encephalitis**   COM

A39.82 Meningococcal **retrobulbar neuritis**

A39.83 Meningococcal **arthritis**   HCC ESR COM

A39.84 Postmeningococcal **arthritis**   HCC ESR COM

A39.89 Other meningococcal infections
Meningococcal conjunctivitis

A39.9 Meningococcal infection, unspecified
Meningococcal disease NOS

(handwritten left margin: Chapter 1. Certain Infectious and Parasitic Diseases / A40–A48.51)

✓4th A40 Streptococcal sepsis

(handwritten: ∅ 085 ✗)

Code first:
  postprocedural streptococcal sepsis (T81.4-)
  streptococcal sepsis during labor (O75.3)
  streptococcal sepsis following abortion or ectopic or molar pregnancy (O03-O07, O08.0)
  streptococcal sepsis following immunization (T88.0)
  streptococcal sepsis following infusion, transfusion or therapeutic injection (T80.2-)

  EXCLUDES 1 neonatal (P36.0-P36.1)
  puerperal sepsis (O85)
  sepsis due to Streptococcus, group D (A41.81)

  AHA: 2020,2Q,8,28; 2019,4Q,65; 2018,4Q,89; 2018,1Q,16; 2016,1Q,32

A40.0 Sepsis due to streptococcus, group A HCC ESR COM

A40.1 Sepsis due to streptococcus, group B HCC ESR COM
  AHA: 2019,1Q,14

A40.3 Sepsis due to Streptococcus pneumoniae HCC ESR COM
  Pneumococcal sepsis

A40.8 Other streptococcal sepsis HCC ESR COM

A40.9 Streptococcal sepsis, unspecified HCC ESR COM

✓4th A41 Other sepsis

(handwritten: do not use if patient pregnant / ↑ sepsis use O85)

Code first:
  postprocedural sepsis (T81.4-)
  sepsis during labor (O75.3)
  sepsis following abortion, ectopic or molar pregnancy (O03-O07, O08.0)
  sepsis following immunization (T88.0)
  sepsis following infusion, transfusion or therapeutic injection (T80.2-)

(handwritten left margin: do not use for puerperal sepsis / ∅ O85 ✗)

  EXCLUDES 1 bacteremia NOS (R78.81)
  neonatal (P36.-)
  puerperal sepsis (O85)
  streptococcal sepsis (A40.-)

  EXCLUDES 2 sepsis (due to) (in) actinomycotic (A42.7)
  sepsis (due to) (in) anthrax (A22.7)
  sepsis (due to) (in) candidal (B37.7)
  sepsis (due to) (in) Erysipelothrix (A26.7)
  sepsis (due to) (in) extraintestinal yersiniosis (A28.2)
  sepsis (due to) (in) gonococcal (A54.86)
  sepsis (due to) (in) herpesviral (B00.7)
  sepsis (due to) (in) listerial (A32.7)
  sepsis (due to) (in) melioidosis (A24.1)
  sepsis (due to) (in) meningococcal (A39.2-A39.4)
  sepsis (due to) (in) plague (A20.7)
  sepsis (due to) (in) tularemia (A21.7)
  toxic shock syndrome (A48.3)

  AHA: 2020,2Q,8,28; 2019,4Q,65; 2019,3Q,17; 2018,4Q,18; 2018,1Q,16; 2016,1Q,32; 2014,2Q,13

✓5th A41.0 Sepsis due to Staphylococcus aureus

(handwritten: With sepsis shock add R65.21)

A41.01 Sepsis due to Methicillin susceptible Staphylococcus aureus HCC ESR COM
  MSSA sepsis
  Staphylococcus aureus sepsis NOS
  AHA: 2020,2Q,17

A41.02 Sepsis due to Methicillin resistant Staphylococcus aureus HCC ESR COM

A41.1 Sepsis due to other specified staphylococcus HCC ESR COM
  Coagulase negative staphylococcus sepsis

A41.2 Sepsis due to unspecified staphylococcus HCC ESR COM

A41.3 Sepsis due to Hemophilus influenzae HCC ESR COM

A41.4 Sepsis due to anaerobes HCC ESR COM
  EXCLUDES 1 gas gangrene (A48.0)

✓5th A41.5 Sepsis due to other Gram-negative organisms

(handwritten: organ disfunction / metabolic encephalopathy add R65.20 / G93.41)

A41.50 Gram-negative sepsis, unspecified HCC ESR COM
  Gram-negative sepsis NOS
  AHA: 2020,2Q,28

A41.51 Sepsis due to Escherichia coli [E. coli] HCC ESR COM
  AHA: 2020,2Q,17

A41.52 Sepsis due to Pseudomonas HCC ESR COM
  Pseudomonas aeroginosa

A41.53 Sepsis due to Serratia HCC ESR COM

A41.59 Other Gram-negative sepsis HCC ESR COM

(handwritten bottom: Septic shock due to Enterococcus infection follow appendectomy)

✓5th A41.8 Other specified sepsis

(handwritten: streptococcus group D)

A41.81 Sepsis due to Enterococcus HCC ESR COM
  TIP: E. faecium, is a species of Enterococcus that is highly resistant to multiple antibiotics. Assign a code from category Z16 when resistance to antimicrobial drugs is documented.

A41.89 Other specified sepsis HCC ESR COM

(handwritten: viral sepsis)
  AHA: 2020,2Q,8; 2017,1Q,51; 2016,3Q,8-14

A41.9 Sepsis, unspecified organism HCC ESR COM
  Septicemia NOS
  (handwritten: No organ failure)
  AHA: 2022,2Q,5; 2022,1Q,35; 2020,2Q,28

✓4th A42 Actinomycosis

  EXCLUDES 1 actinomycetoma (B47.1)

A42.0 Pulmonary actinomycosis HCC ESR

A42.1 Abdominal actinomycosis

A42.2 Cervicofacial actinomycosis

A42.7 Actinomycotic sepsis HCC ESR COM

✓5th A42.8 Other forms of actinomycosis

A42.81 Actinomycotic meningitis OOM

A42.82 Actinomycotic encephalitis COM

A42.89 Other forms of actinomycosis

A42.9 Actinomycosis, unspecified

✓4th A43 Nocardiosis

  DEF: Rare bacterial infection occurring most often in those with weakened immune systems. Can be acquired in soil, decaying plants, or standing water. It typically begins in the lungs and has a tendency to spread to other body systems.

A43.0 Pulmonary nocardiosis HCC ESR

A43.1 Cutaneous nocardiosis

A43.8 Other forms of nocardiosis

A43.9 Nocardiosis, unspecified

✓4th A44 Bartonellosis

A44.0 Systemic bartonellosis
  Oroya fever

A44.1 Cutaneous and mucocutaneous bartonellosis
  Verruga peruana

A44.8 Other forms of bartonellosis

A44.9 Bartonellosis, unspecified

A46 Erysipelas

  EXCLUDES 1 postpartum or puerperal erysipelas (O86.89)

  DEF: Skin infection affecting the upper dermis and superficial dermal lymphatics. Lesion edges are well-demarcated with distinct raised borders. It is often caused by group A Streptococci.

✓4th A48 Other bacterial diseases, not elsewhere classified

  EXCLUDES 1 actinomycetoma (B47.1)

A48.0 Gas gangrene HCC ESR COM
  Clostridial cellulitis
  Clostridial myonecrosis
  AHA: 2017,4Q,102

A48.1 Legionnaires' disease HCC ESR COM
  DEF: Severe and often fatal infection by Legionella pneumophila. Symptoms include high fever, gastrointestinal pain, headache, myalgia, dry cough, and pneumonia and it is usually transmitted through airborne water droplets via air conditioning systems or hot tubs.

A48.2 Nonpneumonic Legionnaires' disease [Pontiac fever]

A48.3 Toxic shock syndrome HCC ESR COM
  Use additional code to identify the organism (B95, B96)
  EXCLUDES 1 endotoxic shock NOS (R57.8)
    sepsis NOS (A41.9)
  AHA: 2022,1Q,35
  DEF: Bacteria producing an endotoxin, such as Staphylococci, flood the body with the toxins producing a high fever, vomiting and diarrhea, decreasing blood pressure, a skin rash, and shock. Synonym(s): TSS.

A48.4 Brazilian purpuric fever
  Systemic Hemophilus aegyptius infection

✓5th A48.5 Other specified botulism

  Non-foodborne intoxication due to toxins of Clostridium botulinum [C. botulinum]
  EXCLUDES 1 food poisoning due to toxins of Clostridium botulinum (A05.1)

A48.51 Infant botulism P

(handwritten bottom: T81.4XXA . A41.81 . R65.21)

A48.52 **Wound botulism**
Non-foodborne botulism NOS
Use additional code for associated wound

A48.8 **Other specified bacterial diseases**

✓4th A49 **Bacterial infection of unspecified site**

> EXCLUDES 1   *bacterial agents as the cause of diseases classified elsewhere (B95-B96)*
> *chlamydial infection NOS (A74.9)*
> *meningococcal infection NOS (A39.9)*
> *rickettsial infection NOS (A79.9)*
> *spirochetal infection NOS (A69.9)*

✓5th A49.0 **Staphylococcal infection, unspecified site**

A49.01 **Methicillin susceptible Staphylococcus aureus infection, unspecified site**
Methicillin susceptible Staphylococcus aureus (MSSA) infection
Staphylococcus aureus infection NOS

A49.02 **Methicillin resistant Staphylococcus aureus infection, unspecified site**
Methicillin resistant Staphylococcus aureus (MRSA) infection

A49.1 **Streptococcal infection, unspecified site**

A49.2 **Hemophilus influenzae infection, unspecified site**

A49.3 **Mycoplasma infection, unspecified site**

A49.8 **Other bacterial infections of unspecified site**

A49.9 **Bacterial infection, unspecified**
> EXCLUDES 1   *bacteremia NOS (R78.81)*

Infections with a predominantly sexual mode of transmission (A50-A64)

> EXCLUDES 1   *human immunodeficiency virus [HIV] disease (B20)*
> *nonspecific and nongonococcal urethritis (N34.1)*
> *Reiter's disease (M02.3-)*

AHA: 2021,2Q,6

✓4th A50 **Congenital syphilis**

✓5th A50.0 **Early congenital syphilis, symptomatic**
Any congenital syphilitic condition specified as early or manifest less than two years after birth.

A50.01 **Early congenital syphilitic oculopathy**

A50.02 **Early congenital syphilitic osteochondropathy**

A50.03 **Early congenital syphilitic pharyngitis**
Early congenital syphilitic laryngitis

A50.04 **Early congenital syphilitic pneumonia** COM

A50.05 **Early congenital syphilitic rhinitis**

A50.06 **Early cutaneous congenital syphilis**

A50.07 **Early mucocutaneous congenital syphilis**

A50.08 **Early visceral congenital syphilis**

A50.09 **Other early congenital syphilis, symptomatic**

A50.1 **Early congenital syphilis, latent**
Congenital syphilis without clinical manifestations, with positive serological reaction and negative spinal fluid test, less than two years after birth.

A50.2 **Early congenital syphilis, unspecified**
Congenital syphilis NOS less than two years after birth.

✓5th A50.3 **Late congenital syphilitic oculopathy**
> EXCLUDES 1   *Hutchinson's triad (A50.53)*

A50.30 **Late congenital syphilitic oculopathy, unspecified**

A50.31 **Late congenital syphilitic interstitial keratitis**

A50.32 **Late congenital syphilitic chorioretinitis**

A50.39 **Other late congenital syphilitic oculopathy**

✓5th A50.4 **Late congenital neurosyphilis [juvenile neurosyphilis]**
Use additional code to identify any associated mental disorder
> EXCLUDES 1   *Hutchinson's triad (A50.53)*

A50.40 **Late congenital neurosyphilis, unspecified** COM
Juvenile neurosyphilis NOS

A50.41 **Late congenital syphilitic meningitis** COM

A50.42 **Late congenital syphilitic encephalitis** COM

A50.43 **Late congenital syphilitic polyneuropathy** COM

A50.44 **Late congenital syphilitic optic nerve atrophy** COM

A50.45 **Juvenile general paresis** COM
Dementia paralytica juvenilis
Juvenile tabetoparetic neurosyphilis

A50.49 **Other late congenital neurosyphilis** COM
Juvenile tabes dorsalis

✓5th A50.5 **Other late congenital syphilis, symptomatic**
Any congenital syphilitic condition specified as late or manifest two years or more after birth.

A50.51 **Clutton's joints**

A50.52 **Hutchinson's teeth**

A50.53 **Hutchinson's triad**

A50.54 **Late congenital cardiovascular syphilis** COM

A50.55 **Late congenital syphilitic arthropathy** HCC ESR COM

A50.56 **Late congenital syphilitic osteochondropathy**

A50.57 **Syphilitic saddle nose**

A50.59 **Other late congenital syphilis, symptomatic**

A50.6 **Late congenital syphilis, latent**
Congenital syphilis without clinical manifestations, with positive serological reaction and negative spinal fluid test, two years or more after birth.

A50.7 **Late congenital syphilis, unspecified**
Congenital syphilis NOS two years or more after birth.

A50.9 **Congenital syphilis, unspecified**

✓4th A51 **Early syphilis**
DEF: Syphilis: Sexually transmitted disease caused by the *Treponema pallidum* spirochete. Syphilis usually exhibits cutaneous manifestations and may exist for years without symptoms.

A51.0 **Primary genital syphilis**
Syphilitic chancre NOS

syphilitic vulvitis A51.0

A51.1 **Primary anal syphilis**

A51.2 **Primary syphilis of other sites**

✓5th A51.3 **Secondary syphilis of skin and mucous membranes**
DEF: Transitory or chronic cutaneous eruptions that present within two to 10 weeks following an initial syphilis infection that may include nontender lymphadenopathy along with alopecia and condylomata lata.

A51.31 **Condyloma latum**

A51.32 **Syphilitic alopecia**

A51.39 **Other secondary syphilis of skin**
Syphilitic leukoderma
Syphilitic mucous patch
> EXCLUDES 1   *late syphilitic leukoderma (A52.79)*

✓5th A51.4 **Other secondary syphilis**

A51.41 **Secondary syphilitic meningitis** COM

A51.42 **Secondary syphilitic female pelvic disease** ♀

A51.43 **Secondary syphilitic oculopathy**
Secondary syphilitic chorioretinitis
Secondary syphilitic iridocyclitis, iritis
Secondary syphilitic uveitis

A51.44 **Secondary syphilitic nephritis**

A51.45 **Secondary syphilitic hepatitis**

A51.46 **Secondary syphilitic osteopathy**

A51.49 **Other secondary syphilitic conditions**
Secondary syphilitic lymphadenopathy
Secondary syphilitic myositis

A51.5 **Early syphilis, latent**
Syphilis (acquired) without clinical manifestations, with positive serological reaction and negative spinal fluid test, less than two years after infection.

A51.9 **Early syphilis, unspecified**

✓4th A52 **Late syphilis**

✓5th A52.0 **Cardiovascular and cerebrovascular syphilis**

A52.00 **Cardiovascular syphilis, unspecified** COM

A52.01 **Syphilitic aneurysm of aorta** COM

A52.02 **Syphilitic aortitis** COM

A52.03 **Syphilitic endocarditis** COM
Syphilitic aortic valve incompetence or stenosis
Syphilitic mitral valve stenosis
Syphilitic pulmonary valve regurgitation

A52.04 **Syphilitic cerebral arteritis**

A52.05 **Other cerebrovascular syphilis** COM
Syphilitic cerebral aneurysm (ruptured) (non-ruptured)
Syphilitic cerebral thrombosis

A52.06　Other syphilitic heart involvement `COM`
Syphilitic coronary artery disease
Syphilitic myocarditis
Syphilitic pericarditis

A52.09　Other cardiovascular syphilis `COM`

✓5ᵗʰ **A52.1　Symptomatic neurosyphilis**

A52.10　Symptomatic neurosyphilis, unspecified `COM`

A52.11　Tabes dorsalis `COM`
Locomotor ataxia (progressive)
Tabetic neurosyphilis

A52.12　Other cerebrospinal syphilis `COM`

A52.13　Late syphilitic meningitis `COM`

A52.14　Late syphilitic encephalitis `COM`

A52.15　Late syphilitic neuropathy `COM`
Late syphilitic acoustic neuritis
Late syphilitic optic (nerve) atrophy
Late syphilitic polyneuropathy
Late syphilitic retrobulbar neuritis

A52.16　Charcôt's arthropathy (tabetic) `COM`
DEF: Progressive neurologic arthropathy in which chronic degeneration of joints in the weight-bearing areas with peripheral hypertrophy occurs as a complication of a neuropathy disorder. Supporting structures relax from a loss of sensation resulting in chronic joint instability.

A52.17　General paresis `COM`
Dementia paralytica

A52.19　Other symptomatic neurosyphilis `COM`
Syphilitic parkinsonism

A52.2　Asymptomatic neurosyphilis `COM`

A52.3　Neurosyphilis, unspecified `COM`
Gumma (syphilitic)
Syphilis (late)
Syphiloma
AHA: 2021,2Q,6

✓5ᵗʰ **A52.7　Other symptomatic late syphilis**

A52.71　Late syphilitic oculopathy
Late syphilitic chorioretinitis
Late syphilitic episcleritis

A52.72　Syphilis of lung and bronchus

A52.73　Symptomatic late syphilis of other respiratory organs

A52.74　Syphilis of liver and other viscera
Late syphilitic peritonitis

A52.75　Syphilis of kidney and ureter
Syphilitic glomerular disease

A52.76　Other genitourinary symptomatic late syphilis
Late syphilitic female pelvic inflammatory disease

A52.77　Syphilis of bone and joint

A52.78　Syphilis of other musculoskeletal tissue
Late syphilitic bursitis
Syphilis [stage unspecified] of bursa
Syphilis [stage unspecified] of muscle
Syphilis [stage unspecified] of synovium
Syphilis [stage unspecified] of tendon

A52.79　Other symptomatic late syphilis
Late syphilitic leukoderma
Syphilis of adrenal gland
Syphilis of pituitary gland
Syphilis of thyroid gland
Syphilitic splenomegaly
EXCLUDES 1 *syphilitic leukoderma (secondary) (A51.39)*

A52.8　Late syphilis, latent
Syphilis (acquired) without clinical manifestations, with positive serological reaction and negative spinal fluid test, two years or more after infection

A52.9　Late syphilis, unspecified

✓4ᵗʰ **A53　Other and unspecified syphilis**

A53.0　Latent syphilis, unspecified as early or late
Latent syphilis NOS
Positive serological reaction for syphilis

A53.9　Syphilis, unspecified
Infection due to Treponema pallidum NOS
Syphilis (acquired) NOS
EXCLUDES 1 *syphilis NOS under two years of age (A50.2)*

✓4ᵗʰ **A54　Gonococcal infection**
DEF: Sexually transmitted bacterial infection caused by *Neisseria gonorrhoeae*. Women are often asymptomatic, while men tend to develop urinary symptoms quickly.

✓5ᵗʰ **A54.0　Gonococcal infection of lower genitourinary tract without periurethral or accessory gland abscess**
EXCLUDES 1 *gonococcal infection with genitourinary gland abscess (A54.1)*
gonococcal infection with periurethral abscess (A54.1)

A54.00　Gonococcal infection of lower genitourinary tract, unspecified

A54.01　Gonococcal cystitis and urethritis, unspecified

A54.02　Gonococcal vulvovaginitis, unspecified ♀

A54.03　Gonococcal cervicitis, unspecified ♀

A54.09　Other gonococcal infection of lower genitourinary tract

A54.1　Gonococcal infection of lower genitourinary tract with periurethral and accessory gland abscess
Gonococcal Bartholin's gland abscess

✓5ᵗʰ **A54.2　Gonococcal pelviperitonitis and other gonococcal genitourinary infection**

A54.21　Gonococcal infection of kidney and ureter

A54.22　Gonococcal prostatitis ♂

A54.23　Gonococcal infection of other male genital organs ♂
Gonococcal epididymitis
Gonococcal orchitis

A54.24　Gonococcal female pelvic inflammatory disease ♀
Gonococcal pelviperitonitis
EXCLUDES 1 *gonococcal peritonitis (A54.85)*

A54.29　Other gonococcal genitourinary infections

✓5ᵗʰ **A54.3　Gonococcal infection of eye**

A54.30　Gonococcal infection of eye, unspecified

A54.31　Gonococcal conjunctivitis
Ophthalmia neonatorum due to gonococcus

A54.32　Gonococcal iridocyclitis

A54.33　Gonococcal keratitis

A54.39　Other gonococcal eye infection
Gonococcal endophthalmia

✓5ᵗʰ **A54.4　Gonococcal infection of musculoskeletal system**

A54.40　Gonococcal infection of musculoskeletal system, unspecified `HCC` `ESR` `COM`

A54.41　Gonococcal spondylopathy `HCC` `ESR` `COM`

A54.42　Gonococcal arthritis `HCC` `ESR` `COM`
EXCLUDES 2 *gonococcal infection of spine (A54.41)*

A54.43　Gonococcal osteomyelitis `HCC` `ESR` `COM`
EXCLUDES 2 *gonococcal infection of spine (A54.41)*

A54.49　Gonococcal infection of other musculoskeletal tissue `HCC` `ESR` `COM`
Gonococcal bursitis
Gonococcal myositis
Gonococcal synovitis
Gonococcal tenosynovitis

A54.5　Gonococcal pharyngitis

A54.6　Gonococcal infection of anus and rectum

✓5ᵗʰ **A54.8　Other gonococcal infections**

A54.81　Gonococcal meningitis `COM`

A54.82　Gonococcal brain abscess `COM`

A54.83　Gonococcal heart infection `COM`
Gonococcal endocarditis
Gonococcal myocarditis
Gonococcal pericarditis

A54.84　Gonococcal pneumonia `HCC` `ESR`

A54.85　Gonococcal peritonitis `HCC` `ESR` `COM`
EXCLUDES 1 *gonococcal pelviperitonitis (A54.24)*

A54.86　Gonococcal sepsis `HCC` `ESR` `COM`

A54.89　Other gonococcal infections
Gonococcal keratoderma
Gonococcal lymphadenitis

A54.9　Gonococcal infection, unspecified

`HCC` CMS-HCC　　`Rx` Rx HCC　　`ESR` ESRD HCC　　`COM` Commercial HCC　　　`N` Newborn: 0　　`P` Pediatric: 0-17　　`M` Maternity: 9-64　　`A` Adult: 15-124

458　　　ICD-10-CM 2023

A55 Chlamydial lymphogranuloma (venereum)
Climatic or tropical bubo
Durand-Nicolas-Favre disease
Esthiomene
Lymphogranuloma inguinale

☑4ᵗʰ **A56 Other sexually transmitted chlamydial diseases**
INCLUDES   sexually transmitted diseases due to Chlamydia trachomatis
EXCLUDES 1   neonatal chlamydial conjunctivitis (P39.1)
neonatal chlamydial pneumonia (P23.1)
EXCLUDES 2   chlamydial lymphogranuloma (A55)
conditions classified to A74.-

DEF: *Chlamydia trachomatis*: Bacterium that causes a common venereal disease. Symptoms of chlamydia are usually mild or absent, however, serious complications may cause irreversible damage, including cystitis, pelvic inflammatory disease, and infertility in women and discharge from the penis, prostatitis, and infertility in men. Genital chlamydial infection can cause arthritis, skin lesions, and inflammation of the eye and urethra. *Synonym(s): Reiter's syndrome.*

☑5ᵗʰ **A56.0 Chlamydial infection of** lower genitourinary tract
    A56.00 Chlamydial infection of lower genitourinary tract, unspecified
    A56.01 Chlamydial cystitis and urethritis
    A56.02 Chlamydial vulvovaginitis   ♀
    A56.09 Other chlamydial infection of lower genitourinary tract
       Chlamydial cervicitis

☑5ᵗʰ **A56.1 Chlamydial infection of** pelviperitoneum **and other** genitourinary organs
    A56.11 Chlamydial female pelvic inflammatory disease   ♀
    A56.19 Other chlamydial genitourinary infection
       Chlamydial epididymitis
       Chlamydial orchitis

    A56.2 Chlamydial infection of genitourinary tract, unspecified
    A56.3 Chlamydial infection of anus and rectum
    A56.4 Chlamydial infection of pharynx
    A56.8 Sexually transmitted chlamydial infection of other sites

A57 Chancroid
Ulcus molle
DEF: Localized infection by *Haemophilus ducreyi,* causing genital ulcers and infecting the inguinal lymph nodes.

A58 Granuloma inguinale
Donovanosis

☑4ᵗʰ **A59 Trichomoniasis**
EXCLUDES 2   intestinal trichomoniasis (A07.8)
DEF: Infection with the parasitic, flagellated protozoa of the genus *Trichomonas.* This protozoon is found in the intestinal and genitourinary tracts of humans and in the mouth around tartar, cavities, and areas of periodontal disease.

☑5ᵗʰ **A59.0 Urogenital trichomoniasis**
    A59.00 Urogenital trichomoniasis, unspecified
       Fluor (vaginalis) due to Trichomonas
       Leukorrhea (vaginalis) due to Trichomonas
    A59.01 Trichomonal vulvovaginitis   *[handwritten: vaginitis]*   ♀
    A59.02 Trichomonal prostatitis   ♂
    A59.03 Trichomonal cystitis and urethritis
    A59.09 Other urogenital trichomoniasis
       Trichomonas cervicitis

    A59.8 Trichomoniasis of other sites
    A59.9 Trichomoniasis, unspecified

☑4ᵗʰ **A60 Anogenital herpesviral [herpes simplex] infections**
☑5ᵗʰ **A60.0 Herpesviral infection of** genitalia and urogenital tract
    A60.00 Herpesviral infection of urogenital system, unspecified
    A60.01 Herpesviral infection of penis   ♂
    A60.02 Herpesviral infection of other male genital organs   ♂
    A60.03 Herpesviral cervicitis   ♀
    A60.04 Herpesviral vulvovaginitis   ♀
       Herpesviral [herpes simplex] ulceration
       Herpesviral [herpes simplex] vaginitis
       Herpesviral [herpes simplex] vulvitis
    A60.09 Herpesviral infection of other urogenital tract
       AHA: 2020,1Q,20

    A60.1 Herpesviral infection of perianal skin and rectum

A60.9 Anogenital herpesviral infection, unspecified

☑4ᵗʰ **A63 Other predominantly sexually transmitted diseases, not elsewhere classified**
EXCLUDES 2   molluscum contagiosum (B08.1)
papilloma of cervix (D26.0)

[handwritten: Condylomata genital warts.]

A63.0 Anogenital (venereal) warts
[handwritten: vagina]
Anogenital warts due to (human) papillomavirus [HPV]
Condyloma acuminatum

A63.8 Other specified predominantly sexually transmitted diseases

A64 Unspecified sexually transmitted disease

Other spirochetal diseases (A65-A69)

EXCLUDES 2   leptospirosis (A27.-)
syphilis (A50-A53)

A65 Nonvenereal syphilis
Bejel
Endemic syphilis
Njovera

☑4ᵗʰ **A66 Yaws**
INCLUDES   bouba
frambesia (tropica)
pian

A66.0 Initial lesions of yaws
Chancre of yaws
Frambesia, initial or primary
Initial frambesial ulcer
Mother yaw

A66.1 Multiple papillomata and wet crab yaws
Frambesioma
Pianoma
Plantar or palmar papilloma of yaws

A66.2 Other early skin lesions of yaws
Cutaneous yaws, less than five years after infection
Early yaws (cutaneous) (macular) (maculopapular) (micropapular) (papular)
Frambeside of early yaws

A66.3 Hyperkeratosis of yaws
Ghoul hand
Hyperkeratosis, palmar or plantar (early) (late) due to yaws
Worm-eaten soles

A66.4 Gummata and ulcers of yaws
Gummatous frambeside
Nodular late yaws (ulcerated)

A66.5 Gangosa
Rhinopharyngitis mutilans

A66.6 Bone and joint lesions of yaws   HCC ESR COM
Yaws ganglion
Yaws goundou
Yaws gumma, bone
Yaws gummatous osteitis or periostitis
Yaws hydrarthrosis
Yaws osteitis
Yaws periostitis (hypertrophic)

A66.7 Other manifestations of yaws
Juxta-articular nodules of yaws
Mucosal yaws

A66.8 Latent yaws
Yaws without clinical manifestations, with positive serology

A66.9 Yaws, unspecified

☑4ᵗʰ **A67 Pinta [carate]**
A67.0 Primary lesions of pinta
Chancre (primary) of pinta
Papule (primary) of pinta

A67.1 Intermediate lesions of pinta
Erythematous plaques of pinta
Hyperchromic lesions of pinta
Hyperkeratosis of pinta
Pintids

A67.2 Late lesions of pinta
Achromic skin lesions of pinta
Cicatricial skin lesions of pinta
Dyschromic skin lesions of pinta

A67.3 Mixed lesions of pinta
Achromic with hyperchromic skin lesions of pinta [carate]

A67.9 Pinta, unspecified

A68 Relapsing fevers

> **INCLUDES** recurrent fever
> **EXCLUDES 2** Lyme disease (A69.2-)

A68.0 Louse-borne relapsing fever
Relapsing fever due to Borrelia recurrentis

A68.1 Tick-borne relapsing fever
Relapsing fever due to any Borrelia species other than Borrelia recurrentis

A68.9 Relapsing fever, unspecified

A69 Other spirochetal infections

A69.0 Necrotizing ulcerative stomatitis
Cancrum oris
Fusospirochetal gangrene
Noma
Stomatitis gangrenosa

A69.1 Other Vincent's infections
Fusospirochetal pharyngitis
Necrotizing ulcerative (acute) gingivitis
Necrotizing ulcerative (acute) gingivostomatitis
Spirochetal stomatitis
Trench mouth
Vincent's angina
Vincent's gingivitis

A69.2 Lyme disease
Erythema chronicum migrans due to Borrelia burgdorferi
DEF: Recurrent multisystem disorder through tick bites that begins with lesions of erythema chronicum migrans and is followed by arthritis of the large joints, myalgia, malaise, and neurological and cardiac manifestations.

A69.20 Lyme disease, unspecified
AHA: 2021,4Q,5

A69.21 Meningitis due to Lyme disease   COM

A69.22 Other neurologic disorders in Lyme disease
Cranial neuritis
Meningoencephalitis
Polyneuropathy

A69.23 Arthritis due to Lyme disease   HCC ESR COM

A69.29 Other conditions associated with Lyme disease
Myopericarditis due to Lyme disease
AHA: 2016,3Q,12

A69.8 Other specified spirochetal infections

A69.9 Spirochetal infection, unspecified

Other diseases caused by chlamydiae (A70-A74)

> **EXCLUDES 1** sexually transmitted chlamydial diseases (A55-A56)

A70 Chlamydia psittaci infections
Ornithosis
Parrot fever
Psittacosis

A71 Trachoma

> **EXCLUDES 1** sequelae of trachoma (B94.0)

A71.0 Initial stage of trachoma
Trachoma dubium

A71.1 Active stage of trachoma
Granular conjunctivitis (trachomatous)
Trachomatous follicular conjunctivitis
Trachomatous pannus

A71.9 Trachoma, unspecified

A74 Other diseases caused by chlamydiae

> **EXCLUDES 1** neonatal chlamydial conjunctivitis (P39.1)
> neonatal chlamydial pneumonia (P23.1)
> Reiter's disease (M02.3-)
> sexually transmitted chlamydial diseases (A55-A56)
> **EXCLUDES 2** chlamydial pneumonia (J16.0)

A74.0 Chlamydial conjunctivitis
Paratrachoma

A74.8 Other chlamydial diseases

A74.81 Chlamydial peritonitis
A74.89 Other chlamydial diseases

A74.9 Chlamydial infection, unspecified
Chlamydiosis NOS

Rickettsioses (A75-A79)

DEF: Rickettsia: Condition caused by bacteria that live in lice/ticks transmitted to humans through bites.

A75 Typhus fever

> **EXCLUDES 1** rickettsiosis due to Ehrlichia sennetsu (A79.81)

A75.0 Epidemic louse-borne typhus fever due to Rickettsia prowazekii
Classical typhus (fever)
Epidemic (louse-borne) typhus

A75.1 Recrudescent typhus [Brill's disease]
Brill-Zinsser disease

A75.2 Typhus fever due to Rickettsia typhi
Murine (flea-borne) typhus

A75.3 Typhus fever due to Rickettsia tsutsugamushi
Scrub (mite-borne) typhus
Tsutsugamushi fever
Typhus fever due to Orientia Tsutsugamushi (scrub typhus)

A75.9 Typhus fever, unspecified
Typhus (fever) NOS

A77 Spotted fever [tick-borne rickettsioses]

A77.0 Spotted fever due to Rickettsia rickettsii
Rocky Mountain spotted fever
Sao Paulo fever

A77.1 Spotted fever due to Rickettsia conorii
African tick typhus
Boutonneuse fever
India tick typhus
Kenya tick typhus
Marseilles fever
Mediterranean tick fever

A77.2 Spotted fever due to Rickettsia siberica
North Asian tick fever
Siberian tick typhus

A77.3 Spotted fever due to Rickettsia australis
Queensland tick typhus

A77.4 Ehrlichiosis

> **EXCLUDES 1** anaplasmosis [A. phagocytophilum] (A79.82)
> rickettsiosis due to Ehrlichia sennetsu (A79.81)

AHA: 2021,4Q,5

A77.40 Ehrlichiosis, unspecified
A77.41 Ehrlichiosis chafeensis [E. chafeensis]
A77.49 Other ehrlichiosis
Ehrlichiosis due to E. ewingii
Ehrlichiosis due to E. muris euclairensis

A77.8 Other spotted fevers
Rickettsia 364D/R. philipii (Pacific Coast tick fever)
Spotted fever due to Rickettsia africae (African tick bite fever)
Spotted fever due to Rickettsia parkeri

A77.9 Spotted fever, unspecified
Tick-borne typhus NOS

A78 Q fever
Infection due to Coxiella burnetii
Nine Mile fever
Quadrilateral fever

A79 Other rickettsioses

A79.0 Trench fever
Quintan fever
Wolhynian fever

A79.1 Rickettsialpox due to Rickettsia akari
Kew Garden fever
Vesicular rickettsiosis

A79.8 Other specified rickettsioses

A79.81 Rickettsiosis due to Ehrlichia sennetsu
Rickettsiosis due to Neorickettsia sennetsu

A79.82 Anaplasmosis [A. phagocytophilum]
Transfusion transmitted A. phagocytophilum
AHA: 2021,4Q,4-5

A79.89 Other specified rickettsioses

A79.9 Rickettsiosis, unspecified
Rickettsial infection NOS

Viral and prion infections of the central nervous system (A80-A89)

EXCLUDES 1   *postpolio syndrome (G14)*
sequelae of poliomyelitis (B91)
sequelae of viral encephalitis (B94.1)

✓4ᵗʰ **A80 Acute poliomyelitis**

EXCLUDES 1   *acute flaccid myelitis (G04.82)*

A80.0 Acute paralytic poliomyelitis, vaccine-associated   COM

A80.1 Acute paralytic poliomyelitis, wild virus, imported   COM

A80.2 Acute paralytic poliomyelitis, wild virus, indigenous   COM

✓5ᵗʰ **A80.3 Acute paralytic poliomyelitis, other and unspecified**

A80.30 Acute paralytic poliomyelitis, unspecified   COM

A80.39 Other acute paralytic poliomyelitis   COM

A80.4 Acute nonparalytic poliomyelitis   COM

A80.9 Acute poliomyelitis, unspecified   COM

✓4ᵗʰ **A81 Atypical virus infections of central nervous system**

INCLUDES   diseases of the central nervous system caused by prions

▶Use additional code, if applicable, to identify:◀

▶dementia with anxiety (F02.84, F02.A4, F02.B4, F02.C4)◀

dementia with behavioral disturbance ▶(F02.81-, F02.A1-, F02.B1-, F02.C1-)◀

▶dementia with mood disturbance (F02.83, F02.A3, F02.B3, F02.C3)◀

▶dementia with psychotic disturbance (F02.82, F02.A2, F02.B2, F02.C2)◀

dementia without behavioral disturbance ▶(F02.80, F02.A0, F02.B0, F02.C0)◀

▶mild neurocognitive disorder due to known physiological condition (F06.7-)◀

✓5ᵗʰ **A81.0 Creutzfeldt-Jakob disease**

DEF: Communicable, rare spongiform encephalopathy occurring later in life with progressive destruction of the pyramidal and extrapyramidal systems eventually leading to death. Progressive dementia, wasting of muscles, tremor, and other symptoms are present.

A81.00 Creutzfeldt-Jakob disease, unspecified   HCC Rx ESR
Jakob-Creutzfeldt disease, unspecified

A81.01 Variant Creutzfeldt-Jakob disease   HCC Rx ESR
vCJD

A81.09 Other Creutzfeldt-Jakob disease   HCC Rx ESR
CJD
Familial Creutzfeldt-Jakob disease
Iatrogenic Creutzfeldt-Jakob disease
Sporadic Creutzfeldt-Jakob disease
Subacute spongiform encephalopathy (with dementia)

A81.1 Subacute sclerosing panencephalitis   HCC Rx ESR
Dawson's inclusion body encephalitis
Van Bogaert's sclerosing leukoencephalopathy

A81.2 Progressive multifocal leukoencephalopathy   HCC Rx ESR
Multifocal leukoencephalopathy NOS

✓5ᵗʰ **A81.8 Other atypical virus infections of central nervous system**

A81.81 Kuru   HCC Rx ESR

A81.82 Gerstmann-Sträussler-Scheinker syndrome   HCC Rx ESR
GSS syndrome

A81.83 Fatal familial insomnia   HCC Rx ESR
FFI

A81.89 Other atypical virus infections of central nervous system   HCC Rx ESR

A81.9 Atypical virus infection of central nervous system, unspecified   HCC Rx ESR
Prion diseases of the central nervous system NOS

✓4ᵗʰ **A82 Rabies**

A82.0 Sylvatic rabies   COM

A82.1 Urban rabies   COM

A82.9 Rabies, unspecified   COM

✓4ᵗʰ **A83 Mosquito-borne viral encephalitis**

INCLUDES   mosquito-borne viral meningoencephalitis

EXCLUDES 2   *Venezuelan equine encephalitis (A92.2)*
West Nile fever (A92.3-)
West Nile virus (A92.3-)

A83.0 Japanese encephalitis   COM

A83.1 Western equine encephalitis   COM

A83.2 Eastern equine encephalitis   COM

A83.3 St Louis encephalitis   COM

A83.4 Australian encephalitis   COM
Kunjin virus disease

A83.5 California encephalitis   COM
California meningoencephalitis
La Crosse encephalitis

A83.6 Rocio virus disease   COM

A83.8 Other mosquito-borne viral encephalitis   COM

A83.9 Mosquito-borne viral encephalitis, unspecified   COM

✓4ᵗʰ **A84 Tick-borne viral encephalitis**

INCLUDES   tick-borne viral meningoencephalitis

A84.0 Far Eastern tick-borne encephalitis [Russian spring-summer encephalitis]   COM

A84.1 Central European tick-borne encephalitis   COM

✓5ᵗʰ **A84.8 Other tick-borne viral encephalitis**

AHA: 2020,4Q,4-5

A84.81 Powassan virus disease   COM

A84.89 Other tick-borne viral encephalitis   COM
Louping ill
Code first, if applicable, transfusion related infection (T80.22-)

A84.9 Tick-borne viral encephalitis, unspecified   COM

✓4ᵗʰ **A85 Other viral encephalitis, not elsewhere classified**

INCLUDES   specified viral encephalomyelitis NEC
specified viral meningoencephalitis NEC

EXCLUDES 1   *benign myalgic encephalomyelitis (G93.3)*
encephalitis due to cytomegalovirus (B25.8)
encephalitis due to herpesvirus NEC (B10.0-)
encephalitis due to herpesvirus [herpes simplex] (B00.4)
encephalitis due to measles virus (B05.0)
encephalitis due to mumps virus (B26.2)
encephalitis due to poliomyelitis virus (A80.-)
encephalitis due to zoster (B02.0)
lymphocytic choriomeningitis (A87.2)
▶*myalgic encephalomyelitis (G93.32)*◀

A85.0 Enteroviral encephalitis   COM
Enteroviral encephalomyelitis

A85.1 Adenoviral encephalitis   COM
Adenoviral meningoencephalitis

A85.2 Arthropod-borne viral encephalitis, unspecified   COM
EXCLUDES 1   *West nile virus with encephalitis (A92.31)*

A85.8 Other specified viral encephalitis   COM
Encephalitis lethargica
Von Economo-Cruchet disease

A86 Unspecified viral encephalitis   COM
Viral encephalomyelitis NOS
Viral meningoencephalitis NOS

✓4ᵗʰ **A87 Viral meningitis**

EXCLUDES 1   *meningitis due to herpesvirus [herpes simplex] (B00.3)*
meningitis due to measles virus (B05.1)
meningitis due to mumps virus (B26.1)
meningitis due to poliomyelitis virus (A80.-)
meningitis due to zoster (B02.1)

DEF: Meningitis: Inflammation of the meningeal layers of the brain and spine.

A87.0 Enteroviral meningitis   COM
Coxsackievirus meningitis
Echovirus meningitis

A87.1 Adenoviral meningitis   COM

A87.2 Lymphocytic choriomeningitis   COM
Lymphocytic meningoencephalitis

A87.8 Other viral meningitis   COM

A87.9 Viral meningitis, unspecified   COM

☑ Additional Character Required   ✓x7ᵗʰ Placeholder Alert   Manifestation   Unspecified Dx   Q QPP   UPD Unacceptable PDx

Chapter 1. Certain Infectious and Parasitic Diseases *(left margin, vertical)*

✓4ᵗʰ **A88 Other viral infections of central nervous system, not elsewhere classified**

　　EXCLUDES 1　*viral encephalitis NOS (A86)*
　　　　　　　　viral meningitis NOS (A87.9)

　　A88.0 Enteroviral exanthematous fever [Boston exanthem] **COM**
　　A88.1 Epidemic vertigo
　　A88.8 Other specified viral infections of central nervous system **COM**

A89 Unspecified viral infection of central nervous system **COM**

Arthropod-borne viral fevers and viral hemorrhagic fevers (A90-A99)

A90 Dengue fever [classical dengue]

　　EXCLUDES 1　*dengue hemorrhagic fever (A91)*
　　AHA: 2016,3Q,13

A91 Dengue hemorrhagic fever

✓4ᵗʰ **A92 Other mosquito-borne viral fevers**

　　EXCLUDES 1　*Ross River disease (B33.1)*

　　A92.0 Chikungunya virus disease
　　　　Chikungunya (hemorrhagic) fever
　　A92.1 O'nyong-nyong fever
　　A92.2 Venezuelan equine fever **COM**
　　　　Venezuelan equine encephalitis
　　　　Venezuelan equine encephalomyelitis virus disease

✓5ᵗʰ **A92.3 West Nile virus infection**
　　　　West Nile fever
　　　　AHA: 2016,3Q,12

　　　　A92.30 West Nile virus infection, unspecified **COM**
　　　　　　West Nile fever NOS
　　　　　　West Nile fever without complications
　　　　　　West Nile virus NOS
　　　　A92.31 West Nile virus infection with encephalitis **COM**
　　　　　　West Nile encephalitis
　　　　　　West Nile encephalomyelitis
　　　　A92.32 West Nile virus infection with other neurologic manifestation **COM**
　　　　　　Use additional code to specify the neurologic manifestation
　　　　A92.39 West Nile virus infection with other complications **COM**
　　　　　　Use additional code to specify the other conditions

　　A92.4 Rift Valley fever
　　A92.5 Zika virus disease
　　　　Zika virus fever
　　　　Zika virus infection
　　　　Zika NOS
　　　　EXCLUDES 1　*congenital Zika virus disease (P35.4)*
　　　　AHA: 2016,4Q,4-7
　　　　DEF: Virus transmitted via a bite from an infected Aedes species mosquito. Common symptoms of the virus include fever, rash, joint pain, and conjunctivitis; they are usually mild in nature and may last from several days to a week. Most people who have the Zika virus do not require medical attention; however, in pregnant women, the Zika virus can cause a serious birth defect called microcephaly, as well as other severe fetal brain defects.
　　　　TIP: Assign code Z71.1, when a patient requests testing for Zika virus but in the absence of symptoms or recent exposure to the virus.
　　　　TIP: Code only confirmed diagnoses of Zika virus; documentation by the physician that the disease is confirmed is sufficient.
　　A92.8 Other specified mosquito-borne viral fevers
　　A92.9 Mosquito-borne viral fever, unspecified

✓4ᵗʰ **A93 Other arthropod-borne viral fevers, not elsewhere classified**

　　A93.0 Oropouche virus disease
　　　　Oropouche fever
　　A93.1 Sandfly fever
　　　　Pappataci fever
　　　　Phlebotomus fever
　　A93.2 Colorado tick fever
　　A93.8 Other specified arthropod-borne viral fevers
　　　　Piry virus disease
　　　　Vesicular stomatitis virus disease [Indiana fever]

A94 Unspecified arthropod-borne viral fever
　　Arboviral fever NOS
　　Arbovirus infection NOS

✓4ᵗʰ **A95 Yellow fever**
　　A95.0 Sylvatic yellow fever
　　　　Jungle yellow fever
　　A95.1 Urban yellow fever
　　A95.9 Yellow fever, unspecified

✓4ᵗʰ **A96 Arenaviral hemorrhagic fever**
　　A96.0 Junin hemorrhagic fever
　　　　Argentinian hemorrhagic fever
　　A96.1 Machupo hemorrhagic fever
　　　　Bolivian hemorrhagic fever
　　A96.2 Lassa fever
　　A96.8 Other arenaviral hemorrhagic fevers
　　A96.9 Arenaviral hemorrhagic fever, unspecified

✓4ᵗʰ **A98 Other viral hemorrhagic fevers, not elsewhere classified**
　　EXCLUDES 1　*chikungunya hemorrhagic fever (A92.0)*
　　　　　　　　dengue hemorrhagic fever (A91)

　　A98.0 Crimean-Congo hemorrhagic fever
　　　　Central Asian hemorrhagic fever
　　A98.1 Omsk hemorrhagic fever
　　A98.2 Kyasanur Forest disease
　　A98.3 Marburg virus disease
　　A98.4 Ebola virus disease
　　A98.5 Hemorrhagic fever with renal syndrome
　　　　Epidemic hemorrhagic fever
　　　　Korean hemorrhagic fever
　　　　Russian hemorrhagic fever
　　　　Hantaan virus disease
　　　　Hantavirus disease with renal manifestations
　　　　Nephropathia epidemica
　　　　Songo fever
　　　　EXCLUDES 1　*hantavirus (cardio)-pulmonary syndrome (B33.4)*
　　A98.8 Other specified viral hemorrhagic fevers

A99 Unspecified viral hemorrhagic fever

Viral infections characterized by skin and mucous membrane lesions (B00-B09)

✓4ᵗʰ **B00 Herpesviral [herpes simplex] infections**
　　EXCLUDES 1　*congenital herpesviral infections (P35.2)*
　　EXCLUDES 2　*anogenital herpesviral infection (A60.-)*
　　　　　　　　gammaherpesviral mononucleosis (B27.0-)
　　　　　　　　herpangina (B08.5)

　　B00.0 Eczema herpeticum
　　　　Kaposi's varicelliform eruption
　　B00.1 Herpesviral vesicular dermatitis
　　　　Herpes simplex facialis
　　　　Herpes simplex labialis
　　　　Herpes simplex otitis externa
　　　　Vesicular dermatitis of ear
　　　　Vesicular dermatitis of lip
　　B00.2 Herpesviral gingivostomatitis and pharyngotonsillitis
　　　　Herpesviral pharyngitis
　　B00.3 Herpesviral meningitis **COM**
　　B00.4 Herpesviral encephalitis **COM**
　　　　Herpesviral meningoencephalitis
　　　　Simian B disease
　　　　EXCLUDES 1　*herpesviral encephalitis due to herpesvirus 6 and 7 (B10.01, B10.09)*
　　　　　　　　non-simplex herpesviral encephalitis (B10.0-)

✓5ᵗʰ **B00.5 Herpesviral ocular disease**
　　　　B00.50 Herpesviral ocular disease, unspecified
　　　　B00.51 Herpesviral iridocyclitis
　　　　　　Herpesviral iritis
　　　　　　Herpesviral uveitis, anterior
　　　　B00.52 Herpesviral keratitis
　　　　　　Herpesviral keratoconjunctivitis
　　　　B00.53 Herpesviral conjunctivitis
　　　　B00.59 Other herpesviral disease of eye
　　　　　　Herpesviral dermatitis of eyelid
　　B00.7 Disseminated herpesviral disease **HCC ESR COM**
　　　　Herpesviral sepsis

HCC CMS-HCC　　**Rx** Rx HCC　　**ESR** ESRD HCC　　**COM** Commercial HCC　　　**N** Newborn: 0　　**P** Pediatric: 0-17　　**M** Maternity: 9-64　　**A** Adult: 15-124

462　　　ICD-10-CM 2023

*(left margin, vertical)* A88–B00.7

☑5ᵗʰ B00.8 Other forms of herpesviral infections
- **B00.81 Herpesviral hepatitis**
- **B00.82 Herpes simplex myelitis** `HCC` `Rx` `ESR` `COM`
- **B00.89 Other herpesviral infection**
  - Herpesviral whitlow
- **B00.9 Herpesviral infection, unspecified**
  - Herpes simplex infection NOS

☑4ᵗʰ B01 Varicella [chickenpox]
- **B01.0 Varicella meningitis** `COM`
- **☑5ᵗʰ B01.1 Varicella encephalitis, myelitis and encephalomyelitis**
  - Postchickenpox encephalitis, myelitis and encephalomyelitis
  - **B01.11 Varicella encephalitis and encephalomyelitis** `COM`
    - Postchickenpox encephalitis and encephalomyelitis
  - **B01.12 Varicella myelitis** `HCC` `Rx` `ESR` `COM`
    - Postchickenpox myelitis
- **B01.2 Varicella pneumonia**
- **☑5ᵗʰ B01.8 Varicella with other complications**
  - **B01.81 Varicella keratitis**
  - **B01.89 Other varicella complications**
- **B01.9 Varicella without complication**
  - Varicella NOS

☑4ᵗʰ B02 Zoster [herpes zoster]
- `INCLUDES` shingles
  - zona
- **B02.0 Zoster encephalitis** `COM`
  - Zoster meningoencephalitis
- **B02.1 Zoster meningitis** `COM`
  - AHA: 2019,1Q,18
- **☑5ᵗʰ B02.2 Zoster with other nervous system involvement**
  - **B02.21 Postherpetic geniculate ganglionitis** `Rx`
  - **B02.22 Postherpetic trigeminal neuralgia** `Rx`
  - **B02.23 Postherpetic polyneuropathy** `Rx`
  - **B02.24 Postherpetic myelitis** `HCC` `Rx` `ESR` `COM`
    - Herpes zoster myelitis
  - **B02.29 Other postherpetic nervous system involvement** `Rx`
    - Postherpetic radiculopathy
- **☑5ᵗʰ B02.3 Zoster ocular disease**
  - **B02.30 Zoster ocular disease, unspecified**
  - **B02.31 Zoster conjunctivitis**
  - **B02.32 Zoster iridocyclitis**
  - **B02.33 Zoster keratitis**
    - Herpes zoster keratoconjunctivitis
  - **B02.34 Zoster scleritis**
  - **B02.39 Other herpes zoster eye disease**
    - Zoster blepharitis
- **B02.7 Disseminated zoster**
- **B02.8 Zoster with other complications**
  - Herpes zoster otitis externa
- **B02.9 Zoster without complications**
  - Zoster NOS

B03 Smallpox
- `NOTE` In 1980 the 33rd World Health Assembly declared that smallpox had been eradicated.
  - The classification is maintained for surveillance purposes.

B04 Monkeypox

☑4ᵗʰ B05 Measles
- `INCLUDES` morbilli
- `EXCLUDES 1` subacute sclerosing panencephalitis (A81.1)
- **B05.0 Measles complicated by encephalitis** `COM`
  - Postmeasles encephalitis
- **B05.1 Measles complicated by meningitis** `COM`
  - Postmeasles meningitis
- **B05.2 Measles complicated by pneumonia**
  - Postmeasles pneumonia
- **B05.3 Measles complicated by otitis media**
  - Postmeasles otitis media
- **B05.4 Measles with intestinal complications**
- **☑5ᵗʰ B05.8 Measles with other complications**
  - **B05.81 Measles keratitis and keratoconjunctivitis**
  - **B05.89 Other measles complications**

- **B05.9 Measles without complication**
  - Measles NOS

☑4ᵗʰ B06 Rubella [German measles]
- `EXCLUDES 1` congenital rubella (P35.0)
- **DEF:** Highly contagious virus in which the symptoms are mild and short-lived in most people. Rubella during pregnancy, however, can result in abortion, stillbirth, or congenital defects.
- **☑5ᵗʰ B06.0 Rubella with neurological complications**
  - **B06.00 Rubella with neurological complication, unspecified**
  - **B06.01 Rubella encephalitis** `COM`
    - Rubella meningoencephalitis
  - **B06.02 Rubella meningitis** `COM`
  - **B06.09 Other neurological complications of rubella**
- **☑5ᵗʰ B06.8 Rubella with other complications**
  - **B06.81 Rubella pneumonia**
  - **B06.82 Rubella arthritis** `HCC` `ESR` `COM`
  - **B06.89 Other rubella complications**
- **B06.9 Rubella without complication**
  - Rubella NOS

☑4ᵗʰ B07 Viral warts
- `INCLUDES` verruca simplex
  - verruca vulgaris
  - viral warts due to human papillomavirus
- `EXCLUDES 2` anogenital (venereal) warts (A63.0)
  - papilloma of bladder (D41.4)
  - papilloma of cervix (D26.0)
  - papilloma larynx (D14.1)
- **B07.0 Plantar wart**
  - Verruca plantaris
- **B07.8 Other viral warts**
  - Common wart
  - Flat wart
  - Verruca plana
- **B07.9 Viral wart, unspecified**

☑4ᵗʰ B08 Other viral infections characterized by skin and mucous membrane lesions, not elsewhere classified
- `EXCLUDES 1` vesicular stomatitis virus disease (A93.8)
- **☑5ᵗʰ B08.0 Other orthopoxvirus infections**
  - `EXCLUDES 2` monkeypox (B04)
  - **☑6ᵗʰ B08.01 Cowpox and vaccinia not from vaccine**
    - **B08.010 Cowpox**
      - **DEF:** Disease contracted by milking infected cows. The vesicles usually appear on the fingers, hands, and adjacent areas and usually disappear without scarring. Other symptoms include local edema, lymphangitis, and regional lymphadenitis with or without fever.
    - **B08.011 Vaccinia not from vaccine**
      - `EXCLUDES 1` vaccinia (from vaccination) (generalized) (T88.1)
  - **B08.02 Orf virus disease**
    - Contagious pustular dermatitis
    - Ecthyma contagiosum
  - **B08.03 Pseudocowpox [milker's node]**
  - **B08.04 Paravaccinia, unspecified**
  - **B08.09 Other orthopoxvirus infections**
    - Orthopoxvirus infection NOS
- **B08.1 Molluscum contagiosum**
  - **DEF:** Benign poxvirus infection causing small bumps on the skin or conjunctiva, transmitted by close contact.
- **☑5ᵗʰ B08.2 Exanthema subitum [sixth disease]**
  - Roseola infantum
  - **B08.20 Exanthema subitum [sixth disease], unspecified** `P`
    - Roseola infantum, unspecified
  - **B08.21 Exanthema subitum [sixth disease] due to human herpesvirus 6** `P`
    - Roseola infantum due to human herpesvirus 6
  - **B08.22 Exanthema subitum [sixth disease] due to human herpesvirus 7** `P`
    - Roseola infantum due to human herpesvirus 7

Chapter 1. Certain Infectious and Parasitic Diseases *(side tab)*

B08.3   Erythema infectiosum [fifth disease]
DEF: Infection with human parvovirus B19, mainly occurring in children. Symptoms include a low-grade fever, malaise, or a "cold" a few days before the appearance of a mild rash illness that presents as a "slapped-cheek" rash on the face and a lacy red rash on the trunk and limbs.

B08.4   Enteroviral vesicular stomatitis with exanthem
Hand, foot and mouth disease

B08.5   Enteroviral vesicular pharyngitis
Herpangina
DEF: Acute infectious Coxsackie virus infection causing throat lesions, fever, and vomiting that generally affects children in the summer.

✓5ᵗʰ **B08.6   Parapoxvirus infections**
B08.60   Parapoxvirus infection, unspecified
B08.61   Bovine stomatitis
B08.62   Sealpox
B08.69   Other parapoxvirus infections

✓5ᵗʰ **B08.7   Yatapoxvirus infections**
B08.70   Yatapoxvirus infection, unspecified
B08.71   Tanapox virus disease
B08.72   Yaba pox virus disease
Yaba monkey tumor disease
B08.79   Other yatapoxvirus infections

B08.8   Other specified viral infections characterized by skin and mucous membrane lesions
Enteroviral lymphonodular pharyngitis
Foot-and-mouth disease
Poxvirus NEC

B09   Unspecified viral infection characterized by skin and mucous membrane lesions
Viral enanthema NOS
Viral exanthema NOS

Other human herpesviruses (B10)

✓4ᵗʰ **B10   Other human herpesviruses**
EXCLUDES 2   cytomegalovirus (B25.9)
Epstein-Barr virus (B27.0-)
herpes NOS (B00.9)
herpes simplex (B00.-)
herpes zoster (B02.-)
human herpesvirus NOS (B00.-)
human herpesvirus 1 and 2 (B00.-)
human herpesvirus 3 (B01.-, B02.-)
human herpesvirus 4 (B27.0-)
human herpesvirus 5 (B25.-)
varicella (B01.-)
zoster (B02.-)

✓5ᵗʰ **B10.0   Other human herpesvirus encephalitis**
EXCLUDES 2   herpes encephalitis NOS (B00.4)
herpes simplex encephalitis (B00.4)
human herpesvirus encephalitis (B00.4)
simian B herpes virus encephalitis (B00.4)
B10.01   Human herpesvirus 6 encephalitis COM
B10.09   Other human herpesvirus encephalitis COM
Human herpesvirus 7 encephalitis

✓5ᵗʰ **B10.8   Other human herpesvirus infection**
B10.81   Human herpesvirus 6 infection
B10.82   Human herpesvirus 7 infection
B10.89   Other human herpesvirus infection
Human herpesvirus 8 infection
Kaposi's sarcoma-associated herpesvirus infection

Viral hepatitis (B15-B19)

EXCLUDES 1   sequelae of viral hepatitis (B94.2)
EXCLUDES 2   cytomegaloviral hepatitis (B25.1)
herpesviral [herpes simplex] hepatitis (B00.81)
DEF: Hepatitis A: HAV infection that is self-limiting with flulike symptoms. Transmission is fecal-oral.
DEF: Hepatitis B: HBV infection that can be chronic and systemic. Transmission is bodily fluids.
DEF: Hepatitis C: HCV infection that can be chronic and systemic. Transmission is blood transfusion and unidentified agents.
DEF: Hepatitis D (delta): HDV that occurs only in the presence of hepatitis B virus. Transmission is contaminated blood in contact with mucous membranes.
DEF: Hepatitis E: HEV is an epidemic form. Transmission is fecal-oral, most often from contaminated water.

✓4ᵗʰ **B15   Acute hepatitis A**
B15.0   Hepatitis A with hepatic coma COM
B15.9   Hepatitis A without hepatic coma
Hepatitis A (acute)(viral) NOS

✓4ᵗʰ **B16   Acute hepatitis B**
AHA: 2016,3Q,13
B16.0   Acute hepatitis B with delta-agent with hepatic coma COM
B16.1   Acute hepatitis B with delta-agent without hepatic coma
B16.2   Acute hepatitis B without delta-agent with hepatic coma COM
B16.9   Acute hepatitis B without delta-agent and without hepatic coma
Hepatitis B (acute) (viral) NOS

✓4ᵗʰ **B17   Other acute viral hepatitis**
B17.0   Acute delta-(super) infection of hepatitis B carrier
✓5ᵗʰ **B17.1   Acute hepatitis C**
B17.10   Acute hepatitis C without hepatic coma Rx
Acute hepatitis C NOS
B17.11   Acute hepatitis C with hepatic coma Rx COM
B17.2   Acute hepatitis E
B17.8   Other specified acute viral hepatitis
Hepatitis non-A non-B (acute) (viral) NEC
B17.9   Acute viral hepatitis, unspecified
Acute hepatitis NOS
Acute infectious hepatitis NOS

✓4ᵗʰ **B18   Chronic viral hepatitis**
INCLUDES   carrier of viral hepatitis
AHA: 2017,1Q,41
B18.0   Chronic viral hepatitis B with delta-agent HCC Rx ESR COM
B18.1   Chronic viral hepatitis B without delta-agent HCC Rx ESR COM
Carrier of viral hepatitis B
Chronic (viral) hepatitis B
B18.2   Chronic viral hepatitis C HCC Rx ESR COM
Carrier of viral hepatitis C
AHA: 2018,1Q,4
B18.8   Other chronic viral hepatitis HCC Rx ESR COM
Carrier of other viral hepatitis
B18.9   Chronic viral hepatitis, unspecified HCC ESR COM
Carrier of unspecified viral hepatitis

✓4ᵗʰ **B19   Unspecified viral hepatitis**
B19.0   Unspecified viral hepatitis with hepatic coma COM
✓5ᵗʰ **B19.1   Unspecified viral hepatitis B**
B19.10   Unspecified viral hepatitis B without hepatic coma
Unspecified viral hepatitis B NOS
B19.11   Unspecified viral hepatitis B with hepatic coma COM
✓5ᵗʰ **B19.2   Unspecified viral hepatitis C**
B19.20   Unspecified viral hepatitis C without hepatic coma Rx
Viral hepatitis C NOS
B19.21   Unspecified viral hepatitis C with hepatic coma Rx COM
B19.9   Unspecified viral hepatitis without hepatic coma
Viral hepatitis NOS

Human immunodeficiency virus [HIV] disease (B20)

B20 **Human immunodeficiency virus [HIV] disease** `HCC` `Rx` `ESR` `COM`

     `INCLUDES`   acquired immune deficiency syndrome [AIDS]
              AIDS-related complex [ARC]
              HIV infection, symptomatic

     Code first Human immunodeficiency virus [HIV] disease complicating pregnancy, childbirth and the puerperium, if applicable (O98.7-)

     Use additional code(s) to identify all manifestations of HIV infection

     `EXCLUDES 1`   *asymptomatic human immunodeficiency virus [HIV] infection status (Z21)*
              exposure to HIV virus (Z20.6)
              inconclusive serologic evidence of HIV (R75)

     AHA: 2022,1Q,36; 2021,2Q,6; 2021,1Q,52; 2020,4Q,97; 2020,2Q,12; 2019,1Q,8-11

Other viral diseases (B25-B34)

✓4ᵗʰ **B25** **Cytomegaloviral disease**

     `EXCLUDES 1`   *congenital cytomegalovirus infection (P35.1)*
              cytomegaloviral mononucleosis (B27.1-)

     B25.0 **Cytomegaloviral** pneumonitis   `HCC` `Rx` `ESR` `COM`

     B25.1 **Cytomegaloviral** hepatitis   `HCC` `Rx` `ESR` `COM`

     B25.2 **Cytomegaloviral** pancreatitis   `HCC` `Rx` `ESR` `COM`

     B25.8 **Other cytomegaloviral diseases**   `HCC` `Rx` `ESR` `COM`
              Cytomegaloviral encephalitis

     B25.9 **Cytomegaloviral disease, unspecified**   `HCC` `Rx` `ESR` `COM`

✓4ᵗʰ **B26** **Mumps**

     `INCLUDES`   epidemic parotitis
              infectious parotitis

     B26.0 **Mumps** orchitis   ♂

     B26.1 **Mumps** meningitis   `COM`

     B26.2 **Mumps** encephalitis   `COM`

     B26.3 **Mumps** pancreatitis   `COM`

✓5ᵗʰ   **B26.8** **Mumps with other complications**

         B26.81 **Mumps** hepatitis

         B26.82 **Mumps** myocarditis   `COM`

         B26.83 **Mumps** nephritis

         B26.84 **Mumps** polyneuropathy

         B26.85 **Mumps** arthritis   `HCC` `ESR` `COM`

         B26.89 **Other mumps complications**

     B26.9 **Mumps without complication**
              Mumps NOS
              Mumps parotitis NOS

✓4ᵗʰ **B27** **Infectious mononucleosis**

     `INCLUDES`   glandular fever
              monocytic angina
              Pfeiffer's disease

✓5ᵗʰ   **B27.0** **Gammaherpesviral mononucleosis**
              Mononucleosis due to Epstein-Barr virus

         B27.00 **Gammaherpesviral mononucleosis** without complication

         B27.01 **Gammaherpesviral mononucleosis** with polyneuropathy

         B27.02 **Gammaherpesviral mononucleosis** with meningitis   `COM`

         B27.09 **Gammaherpesviral mononucleosis with other complications**
              Hepatomegaly in gammaherpesviral mononucleosis

✓5ᵗʰ   **B27.1** **Cytomegaloviral mononucleosis**

         B27.10 **Cytomegaloviral mononucleosis** without complications

         B27.11 **Cytomegaloviral mononucleosis** with polyneuropathy

         B27.12 **Cytomegaloviral mononucleosis** with meningitis   `COM`

         B27.19 **Cytomegaloviral mononucleosis** with other complication
              Hepatomegaly in cytomegaloviral mononucleosis

✓5ᵗʰ   **B27.8** **Other infectious mononucleosis**

         B27.80 **Other infectious mononucleosis** without complication

         B27.81 **Other infectious mononucleosis** with polyneuropathy

         B27.82 **Other infectious mononucleosis** with meningitis   `COM`

         B27.89 **Other infectious mononucleosis with other complication**
              Hepatomegaly in other infectious mononucleosis

✓5ᵗʰ   **B27.9** **Infectious mononucleosis, unspecified**

         B27.90 **Infectious mononucleosis, unspecified** without complication

         B27.91 **Infectious mononucleosis, unspecified** with polyneuropathy

         B27.92 **Infectious mononucleosis, unspecified** with meningitis   `COM`

         B27.99 **Infectious mononucleosis, unspecified with other complication**
              Hepatomegaly in unspecified infectious mononucleosis

✓4ᵗʰ **B30** **Viral conjunctivitis**

     `EXCLUDES 1`   *herpesviral [herpes simplex] ocular disease (B00.5)*
              ocular zoster (B02.3)

Viral Conjunctivitis

Normal conjunctiva

Inflamed conjunctiva

     B30.0 **Keratoconjunctivitis** due to adenovirus
              Epidemic keratoconjunctivitis
              Shipyard eye

     B30.1 **Conjunctivitis** due to adenovirus
              Acute adenoviral follicular conjunctivitis
              Swimming-pool conjunctivitis

     B30.2 **Viral** pharyngoconjunctivitis

     B30.3 **Acute epidemic hemorrhagic conjunctivitis (enteroviral)**
              Conjunctivitis due to coxsackievirus 24
              Conjunctivitis due to enterovirus 70
              Hemorrhagic conjunctivitis (acute)(epidemic)

     B30.8 **Other viral conjunctivitis**
              Newcastle conjunctivitis

     B30.9 **Viral conjunctivitis, unspecified**

✓4ᵗʰ **B33** **Other viral diseases, not elsewhere classified**

     B33.0 **Epidemic myalgia**
              Bornholm disease

     B33.1 **Ross River disease**
              Epidemic polyarthritis and exanthema
              Ross River fever

✓5ᵗʰ   **B33.2** **Viral carditis**
              Coxsackie (virus) carditis

         B33.20 **Viral carditis, unspecified**   `COM`

         B33.21 **Viral endocarditis**   `COM`

         B33.22 **Viral myocarditis**   `COM`

         B33.23 **Viral pericarditis**   `COM`

         B33.24 **Viral cardiomyopathy**   `HCC` `Rx` `ESR` `COM`

     B33.3 **Retrovirus infections, not elsewhere classified**
              Retrovirus infection NOS

     B33.4 **Hantavirus (cardio)-pulmonary syndrome [HPS] [HCPS]**
              Hantavirus disease with pulmonary manifestations
              Sin nombre virus disease
              Use additional code to identify any associated acute kidney failure (N17.9)

         `EXCLUDES 1`   *hantavirus disease with renal manifestations (A98.5)*
                  hemorrhagic fever with renal manifestations (A98.5)

     B33.8 **Other specified viral diseases**

         `EXCLUDES 1`   *anogenital human papillomavirus infection (A63.0)*
                  viral warts due to human papillomavirus infection (B07)

✅ Additional Character Required   ✓x7ᵗʰ Placeholder Alert   Manifestation   Unspecified Dx   Ⓠ QPP   `UPD` Unacceptable PDx

Chapter 1. Certain Infectious and Parasitic Diseases

B34–B38.9

✓4ᵗʰ **B34 Viral infection of unspecified site**

    EXCLUDES 1   anogenital human papillomavirus infection (A63.0)
                 cytomegaloviral disease NOS (B25.9)
                 herpesvirus [herpes simplex] infection NOS (B00.9)
                 retrovirus infection NOS (B33.3)
                 viral agents as the cause of diseases classified elsewhere
                    (B97.-)
                 viral warts due to human papillomavirus infection (B07)

B34.0 Adenovirus infection, unspecified

B34.1 Enterovirus infection, unspecified
    Coxsackievirus infection NOS
    Echovirus infection NOS

B34.2 Coronavirus infection, unspecified
    EXCLUDES 1   COVID-19 (U07.1)
              pneumonia due to SARS-associated coronavirus
                (J12.81)
    AHA: 2020,1Q,34-36

B34.3 Parvovirus infection, unspecified

B34.4 Papovavirus infection, unspecified

B34.8 Other viral infections of unspecified site

B34.9 Viral infection, unspecified
    Viremia NOS
    AHA: 2016,3Q,10

Mycoses (B35-B49)

    EXCLUDES 2   hypersensitivity pneumonitis due to organic dust (J67.-)
              mycosis fungoides (C84.0-)

✓4ᵗʰ **B35 Dermatophytosis**

    INCLUDES   favus
              infections due to species of Epidermophyton, Micro-sporum
                 and Trichophyton
              tinea, any type except those in B36.-
    DEF: Contagious superficial fungal infection of the skin that invades and
    grows in dead keratin.

B35.0 Tinea barbae and tinea capitis
    Beard ringworm
    Kerion
    Scalp ringworm
    Sycosis, mycotic

B35.1 Tinea unguium
    Dermatophytic onychia
    Dermatophytosis of nail
    Onychomycosis
    Ringworm of nails

B35.2 Tinea manuum
    Dermatophytosis of hand
    Hand ringworm

B35.3 Tinea pedis
    Athlete's foot
    Dermatophytosis of foot
    Foot ringworm

B35.4 Tinea corporis
    Ringworm of the body

B35.5 Tinea imbricata
    Tokelau

B35.6 Tinea cruris
    Dhobi itch
    Groin ringworm
    Jock itch

B35.8 Other dermatophytoses
    Disseminated dermatophytosis
    Granulomatous dermatophytosis

B35.9 Dermatophytosis, unspecified
    Ringworm NOS

✓4ᵗʰ **B36 Other superficial mycoses**

B36.0 Pityriasis versicolor
    Tinea flava
    Tinea versicolor

B36.1 Tinea nigra
    Keratomycosis nigricans palmaris
    Microsporosis nigra
    Pityriasis nigra

B36.2 White piedra
    Tinea blanca

B36.3 Black piedra

B36.8 Other specified superficial mycoses

B36.9 Superficial mycosis, unspecified

✓4ᵗʰ **B37 Candidiasis**

    INCLUDES   candidosis
              moniliasis
    EXCLUDES 1   neonatal candidiasis (P37.5)
    DEF: Candida: Genus of yeast-like fungi that are commonly found in the
    mouth, skin, intestinal tract, and vagina. It may cause a white, cheesy
    discharge.

B37.0 Candidal stomatitis
    Oral thrush

B37.1 Pulmonary candidiasis   HCC Rx ESR COM
    Candidal bronchitis
    Candidal pneumonia

B37.2 Candidiasis of skin and nail
    Candidal onychia
    Candidal paronychia
    EXCLUDES 2   diaper dermatitis (L22)

▲ ✓5ᵗʰ **B37.3 Candidiasis of vulva and vagina** [vaginitis]
    Candidal vulvovaginitis
    Monilial vulvovaginitis
    Vaginal thrush

●   **B37.31 Acute candidiasis of vulva and vagina**
        Candidiasis of vulva and vagina NOS

● [monilia]   **B37.32 Chronic candidiasis of vulva and vagina**
        Recurrent candidiasis of vulva and vagina

✓5ᵗʰ **B37.4 Candidiasis of other urogenital sites**

    B37.41 Candidal cystitis and urethritis

    B37.42 Candidal balanitis   ♂

    B37.49 Other urogenital candidiasis
        Candidal pyelonephritis

B37.5 Candidal meningitis   COM

B37.6 Candidal endocarditis   COM

B37.7 Candidal sepsis   HCC Rx ESR COM
    Disseminated candidiasis
    Systemic candidiasis
    AHA: 2014,4Q,46
    TIP: This code is assigned when sepsis is documented as due to
    any Candida type. If the nonspecific term "non-Candida albicans"
    is documented, code B48.8 Other specified mycoses, is assigned.

✓5ᵗʰ **B37.8 Candidiasis of other sites**

    B37.81 Candidal esophagitis   HCC Rx ESR COM

    B37.82 Candidal enteritis
        Candidal proctitis

    B37.83 Candidal cheilitis

    B37.84 Candidal otitis externa

    B37.89 Other sites of candidiasis
        Candidal osteomyelitis

B37.9 Candidiasis, unspecified
    Thrush NOS

✓4ᵗʰ **B38 Coccidioidomycosis**

B38.0 Acute pulmonary coccidioidomycosis   HCC ESR COM

B38.1 Chronic pulmonary coccidioidomycosis   HCC ESR COM

B38.2 Pulmonary coccidioidomycosis, unspecified   HCC ESR COM

B38.3 Cutaneous coccidioidomycosis

B38.4 Coccidioidomycosis meningitis   COM
    DEF: Coccidioides immitis infection of the lining of the brain and/or
    spinal cord.

B38.7 Disseminated coccidioidomycosis
    Generalized coccidioidomycosis

✓5ᵗʰ **B38.8 Other forms of coccidioidomycosis**

    B38.81 Prostatic coccidioidomycosis   ♂

    B38.89 Other forms of coccidioidomycosis

B38.9 Coccidioidomycosis, unspecified

| HCC CMS-HCC | Rx Rx HCC | ESR ESRD HCC | COM Commercial HCC | N Newborn: 0 | P Pediatric: 0-17 | M Maternity: 9-64 | A Adult: 15-124 |

466   ICD-10-CM 2023

B39 Histoplasmosis ✓4ᵗʰ
Code first associated AIDS (B20)
Use additional code for any associated manifestations, such as:
  endocarditis (I39)
  meningitis (G02)
  pericarditis (I32)
  retinitis (H32)
DEF: Type of lung infection caused by breathing in fungal spores often found in the droppings of bats and birds or soil contaminated by their droppings.

Histoplasmosis

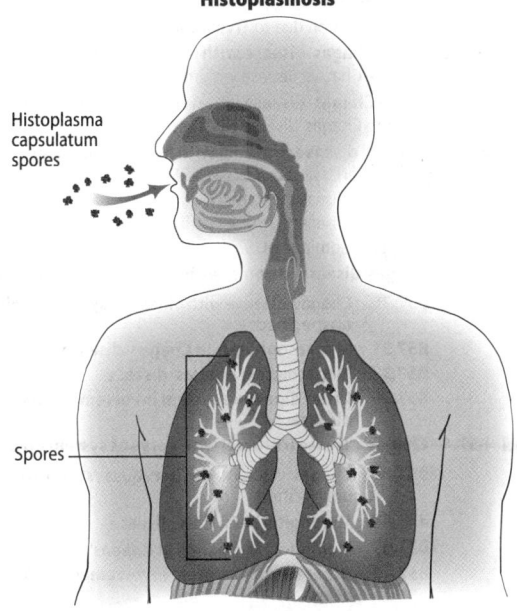

Histoplasma capsulatum spores

Spores

B39.0 Acute pulmonary histoplasmosis capsulati HCC ESR COM
B39.1 Chronic pulmonary histoplasmosis capsulati HCC ESR COM
B39.2 Pulmonary histoplasmosis capsulati, unspecified HCC ESR COM
B39.3 Disseminated histoplasmosis capsulati
  Generalized histoplasmosis capsulati
B39.4 Histoplasmosis capsulati, unspecified
  American histoplasmosis
B39.5 Histoplasmosis duboisii
  African histoplasmosis
B39.9 Histoplasmosis, unspecified

B40 Blastomycosis ✓4ᵗʰ
EXCLUDES 1   Brazilian blastomycosis (B41.-)
             keloidal blastomycosis (B48.0)
B40.0 Acute pulmonary blastomycosis HCC ESR COM
B40.1 Chronic pulmonary blastomycosis HCC ESR COM
B40.2 Pulmonary blastomycosis, unspecified HCC ESR COM
B40.3 Cutaneous blastomycosis
B40.7 Disseminated blastomycosis
  Generalized blastomycosis
B40.8 Other forms of blastomycosis ✓5ᵗʰ
  B40.81 Blastomycotic meningoencephalitis COM
    Meningomyelitis due to blastomycosis
  B40.89 Other forms of blastomycosis
B40.9 Blastomycosis, unspecified

B41 Paracoccidioidomycosis ✓4ᵗʰ
INCLUDES   Brazilian blastomycosis
           Lutz' disease
B41.0 Pulmonary paracoccidioidomycosis HCC ESR COM
B41.7 Disseminated paracoccidioidomycosis
  Generalized paracoccidioidomycosis
B41.8 Other forms of paracoccidioidomycosis
B41.9 Paracoccidioidomycosis, unspecified

B42 Sporotrichosis ✓4ᵗʰ
B42.0 Pulmonary sporotrichosis
B42.1 Lymphocutaneous sporotrichosis

B42.7 Disseminated sporotrichosis
  Generalized sporotrichosis
B42.8 Other forms of sporotrichosis ✓5ᵗʰ
  B42.81 Cerebral sporotrichosis COM
    Meningitis due to sporotrichosis
  B42.82 Sporotrichosis arthritis HCC ESR COM
  B42.89 Other forms of sporotrichosis
B42.9 Sporotrichosis, unspecified

B43 Chromomycosis and pheomycotic abscess ✓4ᵗʰ
B43.0 Cutaneous chromomycosis
  Dermatitis verrucosa
B43.1 Pheomycotic brain abscess COM
  Cerebral chromomycosis
B43.2 Subcutaneous pheomycotic abscess and cyst
B43.8 Other forms of chromomycosis
B43.9 Chromomycosis, unspecified

B44 Aspergillosis ✓4ᵗʰ
INCLUDES   aspergilloma
B44.0 Invasive pulmonary aspergillosis HCC Rx ESR COM
B44.1 Other pulmonary aspergillosis HCC Rx ESR COM
B44.2 Tonsillar aspergillosis HCC Rx ESR COM
B44.7 Disseminated aspergillosis HCC Rx ESR COM
  Generalized aspergillosis
B44.8 Other forms of aspergillosis ✓5ᵗʰ
  B44.81 Allergic bronchopulmonary aspergillosis HCC Rx ESR COM
  B44.89 Other forms of aspergillosis HCC Rx ESR COM
B44.9 Aspergillosis, unspecified HCC Rx ESR COM

B45 Cryptococcosis ✓4ᵗʰ
B45.0 Pulmonary cryptococcosis HCC Rx COM
B45.1 Cerebral cryptococcosis HCC Rx ESR COM
  Cryptococcal meningitis
  Cryptococcosis meningocerebralis
B45.2 Cutaneous cryptococcosis HCC Rx ESR COM
B45.3 Osseous cryptococcosis HCC Rx ESR COM
B45.7 Disseminated cryptococcosis HCC Rx ESR COM
  Generalized cryptococcosis
B45.8 Other forms of cryptococcosis HCC Rx ESR COM
B45.9 Cryptococcosis, unspecified HCC Rx ESR COM

B46 Zygomycosis ✓4ᵗʰ
B46.0 Pulmonary mucormycosis HCC Rx ESR COM
B46.1 Rhinocerebral mucormycosis HCC Rx ESR COM
B46.2 Gastrointestinal mucormycosis HCC Rx ESR COM
B46.3 Cutaneous mucormycosis
  Subcutaneous mucormycosis
B46.4 Disseminated mucormycosis HCC Rx ESR COM
  Generalized mucormycosis
B46.5 Mucormycosis, unspecified HCC Rx ESR COM
B46.8 Other zygomycoses HCC Rx ESR COM
  Entomophthoromycosis
B46.9 Zygomycosis, unspecified HCC Rx ESR COM
  Phycomycosis NOS

B47 Mycetoma ✓4ᵗʰ
B47.0 Eumycetoma
  Madura foot, mycotic
  Maduromycosis
B47.1 Actinomycetoma
B47.9 Mycetoma, unspecified
  Madura foot NOS

B48 Other mycoses, not elsewhere classified ✓4ᵗʰ
B48.0 Lobomycosis
  Keloidal blastomycosis
  Lobo's disease
B48.1 Rhinosporidiosis
B48.2 Allescheriasis
  Infection due to Pseudallescheria boydii
  EXCLUDES 1   eumycetoma (B47.0)
B48.3 Geotrichosis
  Geotrichum stomatitis

Chapter 1. Certain Infectious and Parasitic Diseases

B48.4 **Penicillosis** `HCC` `Rx` `ESR` `COM`
　　Talaromycosis

B48.8 **Other specified mycoses** `HCC` `Rx` `ESR` `COM`
　　Adiaspiromycosis
　　Infection of tissue and organs by Alternaria
　　Infection of tissue and organs by Drechslera
　　Infection of tissue and organs by Fusarium
　　Infection of tissue and organs by saprophytic fungi NEC
　　AHA: 2014,4Q,46; 2014,2Q,13
　　TIP: This code is assigned when the nonspecific term
　　"non-*Candida albicans*" sepsis is documented. If sepsis is
　　documented as due to any *Candida* type, code B37.7 Candidal
　　sepsis, is assigned.

B49 **Unspecified mycosis**
　　Fungemia NOS

Protozoal diseases (B5Ø-B64)

EXCLUDES 1　amebiasis (AØ6.-)
　　　　　　　other protozoal intestinal diseases (AØ7.-)

✓4ᵗʰ **B5Ø** **Plasmodium falciparum malaria**
　　INCLUDES　mixed infections of Plasmodium falciparum with any other
　　　　　　　Plasmodium species

B5Ø.Ø **Plasmodium falciparum malaria with cerebral complications**
　　Cerebral malaria NOS

B5Ø.8 **Other severe and complicated Plasmodium falciparum malaria**
　　Severe or complicated Plasmodium falciparum malaria NOS

B5Ø.9 **Plasmodium falciparum malaria, unspecified**

✓4ᵗʰ **B51** **Plasmodium vivax malaria**
　　INCLUDES　mixed infections of Plasmodium vivax with other
　　　　　　　Plasmodium species, except Plasmodium falciparum
　　EXCLUDES 1　*Plasmodium vivax with Plasmodium falciparum (B5Ø.-)*

B51.Ø **Plasmodium vivax malaria with rupture of spleen**

B51.8 **Plasmodium vivax malaria with other complications**

B51.9 **Plasmodium vivax malaria without complication**
　　Plasmodium vivax malaria NOS

✓4ᵗʰ **B52** **Plasmodium malariae malaria**
　　INCLUDES　mixed infections of Plasmodium malariae with other
　　　　　　　Plasmodium species, except Plasmodium falciparum
　　　　　　　and Plasmodium vivax
　　EXCLUDES 1　*Plasmodium falciparum (B5Ø.-)*
　　　　　　　Plasmodium vivax (B51.-)

B52.Ø **Plasmodium malariae malaria with nephropathy**

B52.8 **Plasmodium malariae malaria with other complications**

B52.9 **Plasmodium malariae malaria without complication**
　　Plasmodium malariae malaria NOS

✓4ᵗʰ **B53** **Other specified malaria**

B53.Ø **Plasmodium ovale malaria**
　　EXCLUDES 1　*Plasmodium ovale with Plasmodium falciparum (B5Ø.-)*
　　　　　　　Plasmodium ovale with Plasmodium malariae (B52.-)
　　　　　　　Plasmodium ovale with Plasmodium vivax (B51.-)

B53.1 **Malaria due to simian plasmodia**
　　EXCLUDES 1　*malaria due to simian plasmodia with Plasmodium falciparum (B5Ø.-)*
　　　　　　　malaria due to simian plasmodia with Plasmodium malariae (B52.-)
　　　　　　　malaria due to simian plasmodia with Plasmodium ovale (B53.Ø)
　　　　　　　malaria due to simian plasmodia with Plasmodium vivax (B51.-)

B53.8 **Other malaria, not elsewhere classified**

B54 **Unspecified malaria**

✓4ᵗʰ **B55** **Leishmaniasis**

B55.Ø **Visceral leishmaniasis**
　　Kala-azar
　　Post-kala-azar dermal leishmaniasis

B55.1 **Cutaneous leishmaniasis**

B55.2 **Mucocutaneous leishmaniasis**

B55.9 **Leishmaniasis, unspecified**

✓4ᵗʰ **B56** **African trypanosomiasis**

B56.Ø **Gambiense trypanosomiasis**
　　Infection due to Trypanosoma brucei gambiense
　　West African sleeping sickness

B56.1 **Rhodesiense trypanosomiasis**
　　East African sleeping sickness
　　Infection due to Trypanosoma brucei rhodesiense

B56.9 **African trypanosomiasis, unspecified**
　　Sleeping sickness NOS

✓4ᵗʰ **B57** **Chagas' disease**
　　INCLUDES　American trypanosomiasis
　　　　　　　infection due to Trypanosoma cruzi

B57.Ø **Acute Chagas' disease with heart involvement**
　　Acute Chagas' disease with myocarditis

B57.1 **Acute Chagas' disease without heart involvement**
　　Acute Chagas' disease NOS

B57.2 **Chagas' disease (chronic) with heart involvement**
　　American trypanosomiasis NOS
　　Chagas' disease (chronic) NOS
　　Chagas' disease (chronic) with myocarditis
　　Trypanosomiasis NOS

✓5ᵗʰ **B57.3** **Chagas' disease (chronic) with digestive system involvement**

B57.3Ø **Chagas' disease with digestive system involvement, unspecified**

B57.31 **Megaesophagus in Chagas' disease**

B57.32 **Megacolon in Chagas' disease**

B57.39 **Other digestive system involvement in Chagas' disease**

✓5ᵗʰ **B57.4** **Chagas' disease (chronic) with nervous system involvement**

B57.4Ø **Chagas' disease with nervous system involvement, unspecified**

B57.41 **Meningitis in Chagas' disease** `COM`

B57.42 **Meningoencephalitis in Chagas' disease** `COM`

B57.49 **Other nervous system involvement in Chagas' disease**

B57.5 **Chagas' disease (chronic) with other organ involvement**

✓4ᵗʰ **B58** **Toxoplasmosis**
　　INCLUDES　infection due to Toxoplasma gondii
　　EXCLUDES 1　*congenital toxoplasmosis (P37.1)*

✓5ᵗʰ **B58.Ø** **Toxoplasma oculopathy**

B58.ØØ **Toxoplasma oculopathy, unspecified**

B58.Ø1 **Toxoplasma chorioretinitis**

B58.Ø9 **Other toxoplasma oculopathy**
　　Toxoplasma uveitis

B58.1 **Toxoplasma hepatitis**

B58.2 **Toxoplasma meningoencephalitis** `HCC` `Rx` `ESR` `COM`

B58.3 **Pulmonary toxoplasmosis** `HCC` `Rx` `ESR` `COM`

✓5ᵗʰ **B58.8** **Toxoplasmosis with other organ involvement**

B58.81 **Toxoplasma myocarditis** `COM`

B58.82 **Toxoplasma myositis**

B58.83 **Toxoplasma tubulo-interstitial nephropathy**
　　Toxoplasma pyelonephritis

B58.89 **Toxoplasmosis with other organ involvement**

B58.9 **Toxoplasmosis, unspecified**

B59 **Pneumocystosis** `HCC` `Rx` `ESR` `COM`
　　Pneumonia due to Pneumocystis carinii
　　Pneumonia due to Pneumocystis jiroveci

✓4ᵗʰ **B6Ø** **Other protozoal diseases, not elsewhere classified**
　　EXCLUDES 1　*cryptosporidiosis (AØ7.2)*
　　　　　　　intestinal microsporidiosis (AØ7.8)
　　　　　　　isosporiasis (AØ7.3)

✓5ᵗʰ **B6Ø.Ø** **Babesiosis**
　　AHA: 2020,4Q,5-6

B6Ø.ØØ **Babesiosis, unspecified**
　　Babesiosis due to unspecified Babesia species
　　Piroplasmosis, unspecified

B6Ø.Ø1 **Babesiosis due to Babesia microti**
　　Infection due to B. microti

B6Ø.Ø2 **Babesiosis due to Babesia duncani**
　　Infection due to B. duncani and B. duncani-type species

| `HCC` CMS-HCC | `Rx` Rx HCC | `ESR` ESRD HCC | `COM` Commercial HCC | `N` Newborn: 0 | `P` Pediatric: 0-17 | `M` Maternity: 9-64 | `A` Adult: 15-124 |

B60.03 Babesiosis due to Babesia divergens
Babesiosis due to Babesia MO-1
Infection due to B. divergens and B. divergens-like strains

B60.09 Other babesiosis
Babesiosis due to Babesia KO-1
Babesiosis due to Babesia venatorum
Infection due to other Babesia species
Infection due to other protozoa of the order Piroplasmida
Other piroplasmosis

✓5ᵗʰ **B60.1 Acanthamebiasis**

B60.10 Acanthamebiasis, unspecified

B60.11 Meningoencephalitis due to Acanthamoeba (culbertsoni) `COM`

B60.12 Conjunctivitis due to Acanthamoeba

B60.13 Keratoconjunctivitis due to Acanthamoeba

B60.19 Other acanthamebic disease

B60.2 Naegleriasis
Primary amebic meningoencephalitis

B60.8 Other specified protozoal diseases
Microsporidiosis

B64 Unspecified protozoal disease

Helminthiases (B65-B83)

✓4ᵗʰ **B65 Schistosomiasis [bilharziasis]**

`INCLUDES` snail fever

B65.0 Schistosomiasis due to Schistosoma haematobium [urinary schistosomiasis]

B65.1 Schistosomiasis due to Schistosoma mansoni [intestinal schistosomiasis]

B65.2 Schistosomiasis due to Schistosoma japonicum
Asiatic schistosomiasis

B65.3 Cercarial dermatitis
Swimmer's itch

B65.8 Other schistosomiasis
Infection due to Schistosoma intercalatum
Infection due to Schistosoma mattheei
Infection due to Schistosoma mekongi

B65.9 Schistosomiasis, unspecified

✓4ᵗʰ **B66 Other fluke infections**

B66.0 Opisthorchiasis
Infection due to cat liver fluke
Infection due to Opisthorchis (felineus)(viverrini)

B66.1 Clonorchiasis
Chinese liver fluke disease
Infection due to Clonorchis sinensis
Oriental liver fluke disease

B66.2 Dicroceliasis
Infection due to Dicrocoelium dendriticum
Lancet fluke infection

B66.3 Fascioliasis
Infection due to Fasciola gigantica
Infection due to Fasciola hepatica
Infection due to Fasciola indica
Sheep liver fluke disease

B66.4 Paragonimiasis `HCC` `ESR` `COM`
Infection due to Paragonimus species
Lung fluke disease
Pulmonary distomiasis

B66.5 Fasciolopsiasis
Infection due to Fasciolopsis buski
Intestinal distomiasis

B66.8 Other specified fluke infections
Echinostomiasis
Heterophyiasis
Metagonimiasis
Nanophyetiasis
Watsoniasis

B66.9 Fluke infection, unspecified

✓4ᵗʰ **B67 Echinococcosis**

`INCLUDES` hydatidosis

B67.0 Echinococcus granulosus infection of liver

B67.1 Echinococcus granulosus infection of lung `HCC` `ESR` `COM`

B67.2 Echinococcus granulosus infection of bone

✓5ᵗʰ **B67.3 Echinococcus granulosus infection, other and multiple sites**

B67.31 Echinococcus granulosus infection, thyroid gland

B67.32 Echinococcus granulosus infection, multiple sites

B67.39 Echinococcus granulosus infection, other sites

B67.4 Echinococcus granulosus infection, unspecified
Dog tapeworm (infection)

B67.5 Echinococcus multilocularis infection of liver

✓5ᵗʰ **B67.6 Echinococcus multilocularis infection, other and multiple sites**

B67.61 Echinococcus multilocularis infection, multiple sites

B67.69 Echinococcus multilocularis infection, other sites

B67.7 Echinococcus multilocularis infection, unspecified

B67.8 Echinococcosis, unspecified, of liver

✓5ᵗʰ **B67.9 Echinococcosis, other and unspecified**

B67.90 Echinococcosis, unspecified
Echinococcosis NOS

B67.99 Other echinococcosis

✓4ᵗʰ **B68 Taeniasis**

`EXCLUDES 1` cysticercosis (B69.-)

B68.0 Taenia solium taeniasis
Pork tapeworm (infection)

B68.1 Taenia saginata taeniasis
Beef tapeworm (infection)
Infection due to adult tapeworm Taenia saginata

B68.9 Taeniasis, unspecified

✓4ᵗʰ **B69 Cysticercosis**

`INCLUDES` cysticerciasis infection due to larval form of Taenia solium

DEF: Condition that is developed when larvae or eggs of the tapeworm *Taenia solium* are ingested, most commonly in fecally contaminated water or undercooked pork.

B69.0 Cysticercosis of central nervous system

B69.1 Cysticercosis of eye

✓5ᵗʰ **B69.8 Cysticercosis of other sites**

B69.81 Myositis in cysticercosis

B69.89 Cysticercosis of other sites

B69.9 Cysticercosis, unspecified

✓4ᵗʰ **B70 Diphyllobothriasis and sparganosis**

B70.0 Diphyllobothriasis
Diphyllobothrium (adult) (latum) (pacificum) infection
Fish tapeworm (infection)
`EXCLUDES 2` larval diphyllobothriasis (B70.1)

B70.1 Sparganosis
Infection due to Sparganum (mansoni) (proliferum)
Infection due to Spirometra larva
Larval diphyllobothriasis
Spirometrosis

✓4ᵗʰ **B71 Other cestode infections**

B71.0 Hymenolepiasis
Dwarf tapeworm infection
Rat tapeworm (infection)

B71.1 Dipylidiasis

B71.8 Other specified cestode infections
Coenurosis

B71.9 Cestode infection, unspecified
Tapeworm (infection) NOS

B72 Dracunculiasis

`INCLUDES` guinea worm infection
infection due to Dracunculus medinensis

✓4ᵗʰ **B73 Onchocerciasis**

`INCLUDES` onchocerca volvulus infection
onchocercosis
river blindness

✓5ᵗʰ **B73.0 Onchocerciasis with eye disease**

B73.00 Onchocerciasis with eye involvement, unspecified

B73.01 Onchocerciasis with endophthalmitis

B73.02 Onchocerciasis with glaucoma

B73.09 Onchocerciasis with other eye involvement
Infestation of eyelid due to onchocerciasis

B73.1 Onchocerciasis without eye disease

✓4ᵗʰ B74 Filariasis

EXCLUDES 2   onchocerciasis (B73)
            tropical (pulmonary) eosinophilia NOS (J82.89)

B74.0 Filariasis due to Wuchereria bancrofti
Bancroftian elephantiasis
Bancroftian filariasis

B74.1 Filariasis due to Brugia malayi

B74.2 Filariasis due to Brugia timori

B74.3 Loiasis
Calabar swelling
Eyeworm disease of Africa
Loa loa infection

B74.4 Mansonelliasis
Infection due to Mansonella ozzardi
Infection due to Mansonella perstans
Infection due to Mansonella streptocerca

B74.8 Other filariases
Dirofilariasis

B74.9 Filariasis, unspecified

B75 Trichinellosis

INCLUDES   infection due to Trichinella species
           trichiniasis

DEF: Infection by *Trichinella spiralis,* the smallest of the parasitic nematodes, that is transmitted by eating undercooked pork or bear meat. ***Synonym(s):*** *Trichinosis.*

✓4ᵗʰ B76 Hookworm diseases

INCLUDES   uncinariasis

B76.0 Ancylostomiasis
Infection due to Ancylostoma species

B76.1 Necatoriasis
Infection due to Necator americanus

B76.8 Other hookworm diseases

B76.9 Hookworm disease, unspecified
Cutaneous larva migrans NOS

✓4ᵗʰ B77 Ascariasis

INCLUDES   ascaridiasis
           roundworm infection

B77.0 Ascariasis with intestinal complications

✓5ᵗʰ B77.8 Ascariasis with other complications

B77.81 Ascariasis pneumonia

B77.89 Ascariasis with other complications

B77.9 Ascariasis, unspecified

✓4ᵗʰ B78 Strongyloidiasis

EXCLUDES 1   trichostrongyliasis (B81.2)

B78.0 Intestinal strongyloidiasis

B78.1 Cutaneous strongyloidiasis

B78.7 Disseminated strongyloidiasis

B78.9 Strongyloidiasis, unspecified

B79 Trichuriasis

INCLUDES   trichocephaliasis
           whipworm (disease)(infection)

B80 Enterobiasis

INCLUDES   oxyuriasis
           pinworm infection
           threadworm infection

✓4ᵗʰ B81 Other intestinal helminthiases, not elsewhere classified

EXCLUDES 1   angiostrongyliasis due to:
            angiostrongylus cantonensis (B83.2)
            parastrongylus cantonensis (B83.2)

B81.0 Anisakiasis
Infection due to Anisakis larva

B81.1 Intestinal capillariasis
Capillariasis NOS
Infection due to Capillaria philippinensis
EXCLUDES 2   hepatic capillariasis (B83.8)

B81.2 Trichostrongyliasis

B81.3 Intestinal angiostrongyliasis
Angiostrongyliasis due to:
Angiostrongylus costaricensis
Parastrongylus costaricensis

B81.4 Mixed intestinal helminthiases
Infection due to intestinal helminths classified to more than one of the categories B65.0-B81.3 and B81.8
Mixed helminthiasis NOS

B81.8 Other specified intestinal helminthiases
Infection due to Oesophagostomum species [esophagostomiasis]
Infection due to Ternidens diminutus [ternidensiasis]

✓4ᵗʰ B82 Unspecified intestinal parasitism

B82.0 Intestinal helminthiasis, unspecified

B82.9 Intestinal parasitism, unspecified

✓4ᵗʰ B83 Other helminthiases

EXCLUDES 1   capillariasis NOS (B81.1)
EXCLUDES 2   intestinal capillariasis (B81.1)

B83.0 Visceral larva migrans
Toxocariasis

B83.1 Gnathostomiasis
Wandering swelling

B83.2 Angiostrongyliasis due to Parastrongylus cantonensis
Eosinophilic meningoencephalitis due to Parastrongylus cantonensis
EXCLUDES 2   intestinal angiostrongyliasis (B81.3)

B83.3 Syngamiasis
Syngamosis

B83.4 Internal hirudiniasis
EXCLUDES 2   external hirudiniasis (B88.3)

B83.8 Other specified helminthiases
Acanthocephaliasis
Gongylonemiasis
Hepatic capillariasis
Metastrongyliasis
Thelaziasis

B83.9 Helminthiasis, unspecified
Worms NOS
EXCLUDES 1   intestinal helminthiasis NOS (B82.0)

Pediculosis, acariasis and other infestations (B85-B89)

✓4ᵗʰ B85 Pediculosis and phthiriasis

B85.0 Pediculosis due to Pediculus humanus capitis
Head-louse infestation

B85.1 Pediculosis due to Pediculus humanus corporis
Body-louse infestation

B85.2 Pediculosis, unspecified

B85.3 Phthiriasis   *crabs*
Infestation by crab-louse
Infestation by Phthirus pubis

pediculosis pubic

B85.4 Mixed pediculosis and phthiriasis
Infestation classifiable to more than one of the categories B85.0-B85.3

B86 Scabies   *bugs*
Sarcoptic itch
DEF: Mite infestation that is caused by *Sarcoptes scabiei.* Scabies causes intense itching and sometimes secondary infection.

✓4ᵗʰ B87 Myiasis

INCLUDES   infestation by larva of flies

B87.0 Cutaneous myiasis
Creeping myiasis

B87.1 Wound myiasis
Traumatic myiasis

B87.2 Ocular myiasis

B87.3 Nasopharyngeal myiasis
Laryngeal myiasis

B87.4 Aural myiasis

✓5ᵗʰ B87.8 Myiasis of other sites

B87.81 Genitourinary myiasis

B87.82 Intestinal myiasis

B87.89 Myiasis of other sites

B87.9 Myiasis, unspecified

✓4ᵗʰ **B88** **Other infestations**

   B88.0 **Other acariasis**
       Acarine dermatitis
       Dermatitis due to Demodex species
       Dermatitis due to Dermanyssus gallinae
       Dermatitis due to Liponyssoides sanguineus
       Trombiculosis
       EXCLUDES 2   *scabies (B86)*

   B88.1 **Tungiasis [sandflea infestation]**

   B88.2 **Other arthropod infestations**
       Scarabiasis

   B88.3 **External hirudiniasis**
       Leech infestation NOS
       EXCLUDES 2   *internal hirudiniasis (B83.4)*

   B88.8 **Other specified infestations**
       Ichthyoparasitism due to Vandellia cirrhosa
       Linguatulosis
       Porocephaliasis

   B88.9 **Infestation, unspecified**
       Infestation (skin) NOS
       Infestation by mites NOS
       Skin parasites NOS

B89 **Unspecified parasitic disease**

Sequelae of infectious and parasitic diseases (B90-B94)

NOTE   Categories B90-B94 are to be used to indicate conditions in categories A00-B89 as the cause of sequelae, which are themselves classified elsewhere. The "sequelae" include conditions specified as such; they also include residuals of diseases classifiable to the above categories if there is evidence that the disease itself is no longer present. Codes from these categories are not to be used for chronic infections. Code chronic current infections to active infectious disease as appropriate.

Code first condition resulting from (sequela) the infectious or parasitic disease

✓4ᵗʰ **B90** **Sequelae of tuberculosis**

   B90.0 **Sequelae of central nervous system tuberculosis**

   B90.1 **Sequelae of genitourinary tuberculosis** kidney.

   B90.2 **Sequelae of tuberculosis of bones and joints**

   B90.8 **Sequelae of tuberculosis of other organs**
       EXCLUDES 2   *sequelae of respiratory tuberculosis (B90.9)*

   B90.9 **Sequelae of respiratory and unspecified tuberculosis**
       Sequelae of tuberculosis NOS

B91 **Sequelae of poliomyelitis**
       EXCLUDES 1   *postpolio syndrome (G14)*

B92 **Sequelae of leprosy**

✓4ᵗʰ **B94** **Sequelae of other and unspecified infectious and parasitic diseases**

   B94.0 **Sequelae of trachoma**

   B94.1 **Sequelae of viral encephalitis**

   B94.2 **Sequelae of viral hepatitis**

   B94.8 **Sequelae of other specified infectious and parasitic diseases**
       AHA: 2021,1Q,25-30,31-49; 2020,3Q,10-14; 2017,4Q,109

   B94.9 **Sequelae of unspecified infectious and parasitic disease**
       EXCLUDES 2   *post COVID-19 condition (U09.9)*

Bacterial and viral infectious agents (B95-B97)

NOTE   These categories are provided for use as supplementary or additional codes to identify the infectious agent(s) in diseases classified elsewhere.

AHA: 2020,2Q,18; 2018,4Q,34; 2018,1Q,16

✓4ᵗʰ **B95** **Streptococcus, Staphylococcus, and Enterococcus as the cause of diseases classified elsewhere**

   B95.0 **Streptococcus, group A, as the cause of diseases classified elsewhere** UPD

   B95.1 **Streptococcus, group B, as the cause of diseases classified elsewhere** UPD
       AHA: 2020,1Q,10; 2019,2Q,8-10

   B95.2 **Enterococcus as the cause of diseases classified elsewhere** UPD

   B95.3 **Streptococcus pneumoniae as the cause of diseases classified elsewhere** UPD

   B95.4 **Other streptococcus as the cause of diseases classified elsewhere** UPD

   B95.5 **Unspecified streptococcus as the cause of diseases classified elsewhere** UPD

✓5ᵗʰ **B95.6** **Staphylococcus aureus as the cause of diseases classified elsewhere**

     B95.61 **Methicillin susceptible Staphylococcus aureus infection as the cause of diseases classified elsewhere** UPD
         Methicillin susceptible Staphylococcus aureus (MSSA) infection as the cause of diseases classified elsewhere
         Staphylococcus aureus infection NOS as the cause of diseases classified elsewhere

MSSA

     B95.62 **Methicillin resistant Staphylococcus aureus infection as the cause of diseases classified elsewhere** UPD
         Methicillin resistant staphylococcus aureus (MRSA) infection as the cause of diseases classified elsewhere

     AHA: 2016,1Q,12

   B95.7 **Other staphylococcus as the cause of diseases classified elsewhere** UPD

   B95.8 **Unspecified staphylococcus as the cause of diseases classified elsewhere** UPD

✓4ᵗʰ **B96** **Other bacterial agents as the cause of diseases classified elsewhere**

   B96.0 **Mycoplasma pneumoniae [M. pneumoniae] as the cause of diseases classified elsewhere** UPD
       Pleuro-pneumonia-like-organism [PPLO]

   B96.1 **Klebsiella pneumoniae [K. pneumoniae] as the cause of diseases classified elsewhere** UPD

✓5ᵗʰ **B96.2** **Escherichia coli [E. coli] as the cause of diseases classified elsewhere**
       AHA: 2022,1Q,31

     B96.20 **Unspecified Escherichia coli [E. coli] as the cause of diseases classified elsewhere** UPD
         Escherichia coli [E. coli] NOS

     B96.21 **Shiga toxin-producing Escherichia coli [E. coli] [STEC] O157 as the cause of diseases classified elsewhere** UPD
         E. coli O157:H- (nonmotile) with confirmation of Shiga toxin
         E. coli O157 with confirmation of Shiga toxin when H antigen is unknown, or is not H7
         O157:H7 Escherichia coli [E.coli] with or without confirmation of Shiga toxin-production
         Shiga toxin-producing Escherichia coli [E.coli] O157:H7 with or without confirmation of Shiga toxin-production
         STEC O157:H7 with or without confirmation of Shiga toxin-production

     B96.22 **Other specified Shiga toxin-producing Escherichia coli [E. coli] [STEC] as the cause of diseases classified elsewhere** UPD
         Non-O157 Shiga toxin-producing Escherichia coli [E.coli]
         Non-O157 Shiga toxin-producing Escherichia coli [E.coli] with known O group

     B96.23 **Unspecified Shiga toxin-producing Escherichia coli [E. coli] [STEC] as the cause of diseases classified elsewhere** UPD
         Shiga toxin-producing Escherichia coli [E. coli] with unspecified O group
         STEC NOS

     B96.29 **Other Escherichia coli [E. coli] as the cause of diseases classified elsewhere** UPD
         Non-Shiga toxin-producing E. coli

   B96.3 **Hemophilus influenzae [H. influenzae] as the cause of diseases classified elsewhere** UPD

   B96.4 **Proteus (mirabilis) (morganii) as the cause of diseases classified elsewhere** UPD

   B96.5 **Pseudomonas (aeruginosa) (mallei) (pseudomallei) as the cause of diseases classified elsewhere** UPD
       AHA: 2015,1Q,18

   B96.6 **Bacteroides fragilis [B. fragilis] as the cause of diseases classified elsewhere** UPD

   B96.7 **Clostridium perfringens [C. perfringens] as the cause of diseases classified elsewhere** UPD

✓6ᵗʰ **B96.8** **Other specified bacterial agents as the cause of diseases classified elsewhere**

     B96.81 **Helicobacter pylori [H. pylori] as the cause of diseases classified elsewhere** UPD

B96.82　Vibrio vulnificus as the cause of diseases classified elsewhere **UPD**

B96.89　Other specified bacterial agents as the cause of diseases classified elsewhere **UPD**

✓4ᵗʰ **B97　Viral agents as the cause of diseases classified elsewhere**
AHA: 2016,3Q,8-10,14

B97.0　**Adenovirus** as the cause of diseases classified elsewhere **UPD**

✓5ᵗʰ B97.1　**Enterovirus** as the cause of diseases classified elsewhere

B97.10　Unspecified enterovirus as the cause of diseases classified elsewhere **UPD**

B97.11　**Coxsackievirus** as the cause of diseases classified elsewhere **UPD**

B97.12　**Echovirus** as the cause of diseases classified elsewhere **UPD**

B97.19　Other enterovirus as the cause of diseases classified elsewhere **UPD**

✓5ᵗʰ B97.2　**Coronavirus** as the cause of diseases classified elsewhere
TIP: Do not report a code from this subcategory for COVID-19; refer to U07.1.

B97.21　**SARS-associated** coronavirus as the cause of diseases classified elsewhere **UPD**
　　EXCLUDES 1　pneumonia due to SARS-associated coronavirus (J12.81)

B97.29　Other coronavirus as the cause of diseases classified elsewhere **UPD**
AHA: 2020,2Q,5; 2020,1Q,34-36

✓5ᵗʰ B97.3　**Retrovirus** as the cause of diseases classified elsewhere
EXCLUDES 1　human immunodeficiency virus [HIV] disease (B20)

B97.30　Unspecified retrovirus as the cause of diseases classified elsewhere **UPD**

B97.31　**Lentivirus** as the cause of diseases classified elsewhere **UPD**

B97.32　**Oncovirus** as the cause of diseases classified elsewhere **UPD**

B97.33　**Human T-cell lymphotrophic virus, type I [HTLV-I]** as the cause of diseases classified elsewhere **UPD**

B97.34　**Human T-cell lymphotrophic virus, type II [HTLV-II]** as the cause of diseases classified elsewhere **UPD**

B97.35　**Human immunodeficiency virus, type 2 [HIV 2]** as the cause of diseases classified elsewhere **HCC** **Rx** **ESR** **COM** **UPD**

B97.39　Other retrovirus as the cause of diseases classified elsewhere **UPD**

B97.4　**Respiratory syncytial** virus as the cause of diseases classified elsewhere **UPD**
RSV as the cause of diseases classified elsewhere
Code first related disorders, such as:
　otitis media (H65.-)
　upper respiratory infection (J06.9)
　EXCLUDES 1　acute bronchiolitis due to respiratory syncytial virus (RSV) (J21.0)
　　　acute bronchitis due to respiratory syncytial virus (RSV) (J20.5)
　　　respiratory syncytial virus (RSV) pneumonia (J12.1)

B97.5　**Reovirus** as the cause of diseases classified elsewhere **UPD**

B97.6　**Parvovirus** as the cause of diseases classified elsewhere **UPD**

HPV B97.7　**Papillomavirus** as the cause of diseases classified elsewhere **UPD**

✓5ᵗʰ B97.8　**Other viral agents** as the cause of diseases classified elsewhere

B97.81　**Human metapneumovirus** as the cause of diseases classified elsewhere **UPD**

B97.89　Other viral agents as the cause of diseases classified elsewhere **UPD**

Other infectious diseases (B99)

✓4ᵗʰ **B99　Other and unspecified infectious diseases**

B99.8　Other infectious disease

B99.9　Unspecified infectious disease

Chapter 2. Neoplasms (C00–D49)

Chapter-specific Guidelines with Coding Examples

The chapter-specific guidelines from the ICD-10-CM Official Guidelines for Coding and Reporting have been provided below. Along with these guidelines are coding examples, contained in the shaded boxes, that have been developed to help illustrate the coding and/or sequencing guidance found in these guidelines.

General guidelines

Chapter 2 of the ICD-10-CM contains the codes for most benign and all malignant neoplasms. Certain benign neoplasms, such as prostatic adenomas, may be found in the specific body system chapters. To properly code a neoplasm, it is necessary to determine from the record if the neoplasm is benign, in-situ, malignant, or of uncertain histologic behavior. If malignant, any secondary (metastatic) sites should also be determined.

Primary malignant neoplasms overlapping site boundaries

A primary malignant neoplasm that overlaps two or more contiguous (next to each other) sites should be classified to the subcategory/code .8 ('overlapping lesion'), unless the combination is specifically indexed elsewhere. For multiple neoplasms of the same site that are not contiguous such as tumors in different quadrants of the same breast, codes for each site should be assigned.

> A 62-year-old female with a malignant lesion of the upper lip that extends from the lipstick area to the labial frenulum
>
> **C00.8**   **Malignant neoplasm of overlapping sites of lip**
>
> *Explanation*: Because this is a single lesion that overlaps two contiguous sites, a single code for overlapping sites is assigned.

> A 74-year-old male is treated for two distinct malignant lesions, one in the mucosa of the upper lip and a second in the mucosa of the lower lip.
>
> **C00.3**   **Malignant neoplasm of upper lip, inner aspect**
>
> **C00.4**   **Malignant neoplasm of lower lip, inner aspect**
>
> *Explanation*: This patient has two distinct malignant lesions of the upper and lower lips. Because the lesions are not contiguous, two codes are reported.

Malignant neoplasm of ectopic tissue

Malignant neoplasms of ectopic tissue are to be coded to the site of origin mentioned, e.g., ectopic pancreatic malignant neoplasms involving the stomach are coded to malignant neoplasm of pancreas, unspecified (C25.9).

The neoplasm table in the Alphabetic Index should be referenced first. However, if the histological term is documented, that term should be referenced first, rather than going immediately to the Neoplasm Table, in order to determine which column in the Neoplasm Table is appropriate. For example, if the documentation indicates "adenoma," refer to the term in the Alphabetic Index to review the entries under this term and the instructional note to "see also neoplasm, by site, benign." The table provides the proper code based on the type of neoplasm and the site. It is important to select the proper column in the table that corresponds to the type of neoplasm. The Tabular List should then be referenced to verify that the correct code has been selected from the table and that a more specific site code does not exist.

See Section I.C.21. Factors influencing health status and contact with health services, Status, for information regarding Z15.0, codes for genetic susceptibility to cancer.

a. *Admission/Encounter for treatment of primary site*

If the malignancy **is chiefly responsible for occasioning the patient admission/encounter and treatment is directed at the primary site**, designate the **primary** malignancy as the principal/**first-listed** diagnosis.

The only exception to this guideline is if the administration of chemotherapy, immunotherapy or external beam radiation therapy **is chiefly responsible for occasioning the admission/encounter.** In that case, assign the appropriate Z51.-- code as the first-listed or principal diagnosis, and the **underlying** diagnosis or problem for which the service is being performed as a secondary diagnosis.

b. *Admission/Encounter for treatment of secondary site*

When a patient is admitted because of a primary neoplasm with metastasis and treatment is directed toward the secondary site only, the secondary

neoplasm is designated as the principal diagnosis even though the primary malignancy is still present.

> Patient with primary prostate cancer with metastasis to lungs presents for wedge resection of mass in right lung
>
> **C78.01**   **Secondary malignant neoplasm of right lung**
>
> **C61**   **Malignant neoplasm of prostate**
>
> *Explanation*: Since the encounter is for treatment of the lung metastasis, the secondary lung metastasis is sequenced before the primary prostate cancer.

c. Coding and sequencing of complications

Coding and sequencing of complications associated with the malignancies or with the therapy thereof are subject to the following guidelines:

1) Anemia associated with malignancy

When admission/encounter is for management of an anemia associated with the malignancy, and the treatment is only for anemia, the appropriate code for the malignancy is sequenced as the principal or first-listed diagnosis followed by the appropriate code for the anemia (such as code D63.0, Anemia in neoplastic disease).

> Patient is seen for treatment of anemia in advanced primary liver cancer
>
> **C22.8**   **Malignant neoplasm of liver, primary, unspecified as to type**
>
> **D63.0**   **Anemia in neoplastic disease**
>
> *Explanation*: Even though the admission was solely to treat the anemia, this guideline indicates that the code for the malignancy is sequenced first.

2) Anemia associated with chemotherapy, immunotherapy and radiation therapy

When the admission/encounter is for management of an anemia associated with an adverse effect of the administration of chemotherapy or immunotherapy and the only treatment is for the anemia, the anemia code is sequenced first followed by the appropriate codes for the neoplasm and the adverse effect (T45.1X5, Adverse effect of antineoplastic and immunosuppressive drugs).

When the admission/encounter is for management of an anemia associated with an adverse effect of radiotherapy, the anemia code should be sequenced first, followed by the appropriate neoplasm code and code Y84.2, Radiological procedure and radiotherapy as the cause of abnormal reaction of the patient, or of later complication, without mention of misadventure at the time of the procedure.

> A 55-year-old male with a large malignant rectal tumor has been receiving external radiation therapy to shrink the tumor prior to planned surgery. He is referred today for a blood transfusion to treat anemia related to radiation therapy.
>
> **D64.89**   **Other specified anemias**
>
> **C20**   **Malignant neoplasm of rectum**
>
> **Y84.2**   **Radiological procedure and radiotherapy as the cause of abnormal reaction of the patient, or of later complication, without mention of misadventure at the time of the procedure**
>
> *Explanation*: The code for the anemia is sequenced first, followed by the code for the malignancy, and lastly the code for the abnormal reaction due to radiotherapy.

3) Management of dehydration due to the malignancy

When the admission/encounter is for management of dehydration due to the malignancy and only the dehydration is being treated (intravenous rehydration), the dehydration is sequenced first, followed by the code(s) for the malignancy.

4) Treatment of a complication resulting from a surgical procedure

When the admission/encounter is for treatment of a complication resulting from a surgical procedure, designate the complication as the principal or first-listed diagnosis if treatment is directed at resolving the complication.

Chapter 2. Neoplasms

d. Primary malignancy previously excised

When a primary malignancy has been previously excised or eradicated from its site and there is no further treatment directed to that site and there is no evidence of any existing primary malignancy at that site, a code from category Z85, Personal history of malignant neoplasm, should be used to indicate the former site of the malignancy. Any mention of extension, invasion, or metastasis to another site is coded as a secondary malignant neoplasm to that site. The secondary site may be the principal or first-listed diagnosis with the Z85 code used as a secondary code.

See section I.C.2.t. Secondary malignant neoplasm of lymphoid tissue.

History of lung cancer, left upper lobectomy 18 months ago with no current treatment; MRI of the brain shows metastatic disease in the brain

C79.31	Secondary malignant neoplasm of brain
Z85.118	Personal history of other malignant neoplasm of bronchus and lung

Explanation: The patient has undergone a diagnostic procedure that revealed metastatic lung cancer in the brain. The code for the secondary (metastatic) site is sequenced first, followed by a personal history code to identify the former site of the primary malignancy.

e. Admissions/encounters involving chemotherapy, immunotherapy and radiation therapy

1) Episode of care involves surgical removal of neoplasm

When an episode of care involves the surgical removal of a neoplasm, primary or secondary site, followed by adjunct chemotherapy or radiation treatment during the same episode of care, the code for the neoplasm should be assigned as principal or first-listed diagnosis.

2) Patient admission/encounter solely for administration of chemotherapy, immunotherapy and radiation therapy

If a patient admission/encounter is solely for the administration of chemotherapy, immunotherapy or external beam radiation therapy assign code Z51.0, Encounter for antineoplastic radiation therapy, or Z51.11, Encounter for antineoplastic chemotherapy, or Z51.12, Encounter for antineoplastic immunotherapy as the first-listed or principal diagnosis. If a patient receives more than one of these therapies during the same admission more than one of these codes may be assigned, in any sequence.

The malignancy for which the therapy is being administered should be assigned as a secondary diagnosis.

If a patient admission/encounter is for the insertion or implantation of radioactive elements (e.g., brachytherapy) the appropriate code for the malignancy is sequenced as the principal or first-listed diagnosis. Code Z51.0 should not be assigned.

Patient presents for second round of rituximab and fludarabine for his chronic B cell lymphocytic leukemia

Z51.11	Encounter for antineoplastic chemotherapy
Z51.12	Encounter for antineoplastic immunotherapy
C91.10	Chronic lymphocytic leukemia of B-cell type not having achieved remission

Explanation: Rituximab is an antineoplastic immunotherapy while fludarabine is an antineoplastic chemotherapy. The two treatments are often used together. The encounter was solely for the purpose of administering this treatment and either can be sequenced first, before the neoplastic condition.

3) Patient admitted for radiation therapy, chemotherapy or immunotherapy and develops complications

When a patient is admitted for the purpose of external beam radiotherapy, immunotherapy or chemotherapy and develops complications such as uncontrolled nausea and vomiting or dehydration, the principal or first-listed diagnosis is Z51.0, Encounter for antineoplastic radiation therapy, or Z51.11, Encounter for antineoplastic chemotherapy, or Z51.12, Encounter for antineoplastic immunotherapy followed by any codes for the complications.

When a patient is admitted for the purpose of insertion or implantation of radioactive elements (e.g., brachytherapy) and develops complications such as uncontrolled nausea and vomiting or dehydration, the principal or first-listed diagnosis is the appropriate code for the malignancy followed by any codes for the complications.

f. Admission/encounter to determine extent of malignancy

When the reason for admission/encounter is to determine the extent of the malignancy, or for a procedure such as paracentesis or thoracentesis, the primary malignancy or appropriate metastatic site is designated as the principal or first-listed diagnosis, even though chemotherapy or radiotherapy is administered.

Patient with left lung cancer with malignant pleural effusion being seen for paracentesis and initiation/administration of chemotherapy

C34.92	Malignant neoplasm of unspecified part of left bronchus or lung
J91.0	Malignant pleural effusion
Z51.11	Encounter for antineoplastic chemotherapy

Explanation: The lung cancer is sequenced before the chemotherapy in this instance because the paracentesis for the malignant effusion is also being performed. An instructional note under the malignant effusion instructs that the lung cancer be sequenced first.

g. Symptoms, signs, and abnormal findings listed in Chapter 18 associated with neoplasms

Symptoms, signs, and ill-defined conditions listed in Chapter 18 characteristic of, or associated with, an existing primary or secondary site malignancy cannot be used to replace the malignancy as principal or first-listed diagnosis, regardless of the number of admissions or encounters for treatment and care of the neoplasm.

See Section I.C.21. Factors influencing health status and contact with health services, Encounter for prophylactic organ removal.

h. Admission/encounter for pain control/management

See Section I.C.6. for information on coding admission/encounter for pain control/management.

i. Malignancy in two or more noncontiguous sites

A patient may have more than one malignant tumor in the same organ. These tumors may represent different primaries or metastatic disease, depending on the site. Should the documentation be unclear, the provider should be queried as to the status of each tumor so that the correct codes can be assigned.

j. Disseminated malignant neoplasm, unspecified

Code C80.0, Disseminated malignant neoplasm, unspecified, is for use only in those cases where the patient has advanced metastatic disease and no known primary or secondary sites are specified. It should not be used in place of assigning codes for the primary site and all known secondary sites.

k. Malignant neoplasm without specification of site

Code C80.1, Malignant (primary) neoplasm, unspecified, equates to Cancer, unspecified. This code should only be used when no determination can be made as to the primary site of a malignancy. This code should rarely be used in the inpatient setting.

Evaluation of painful hip leads to diagnosis of a metastatic bone lesion from an unknown primary neoplasm source

C79.51	Secondary malignant neoplasm of bone
C80.1	Malignant (primary) neoplasm, unspecified

Explanation: If only the secondary site is known, use code C80.1 for the unknown primary site.

l. Sequencing of neoplasm codes

1) Encounter for treatment of primary malignancy

If the reason for the encounter is for treatment of a primary malignancy, assign the malignancy as the principal/first-listed diagnosis. The primary site is to be sequenced first, followed by any metastatic sites.

2) Encounter for treatment of secondary malignancy

When an encounter is for a primary malignancy with metastasis and treatment is directed toward the metastatic (secondary) site(s) only, the metastatic site(s) is designated as the principal/first-listed diagnosis. The primary malignancy is coded as an additional code.

> Patient has primary colon cancer with metastasis to rib and is evaluated for possible excision of portion of rib bone
>
> | C79.51 | Secondary malignant neoplasm of bone |
> |---|---|
> | C18.9 | Malignant neoplasm of colon, unspecified |
>
> *Explanation*: The treatment for this encounter is focused on the metastasis to the rib bone rather than the primary colon cancer, thus indicating that the bone metastasis is sequenced as the first-listed code.

3) Malignant neoplasm in a pregnant patient

When a pregnant patient has a malignant neoplasm, a code from subcategory O9A.1-, Malignant neoplasm complicating pregnancy, childbirth, and the puerperium, should be sequenced first, followed by the appropriate code from Chapter 2 to indicate the type of neoplasm.

> A 30-year-old pregnant female in first trimester evaluated for pituitary gland malignancy
>
> | O9A.111 | Malignant neoplasm complicating pregnancy, first trimester |
> |---|---|
> | C75.1 | Malignant neoplasm of pituitary gland |
>
> *Explanation*: Codes from chapter 15 describing complications of pregnancy are sequenced as first-listed codes, further specified by codes from other chapters such as neoplastic, unless the pregnancy is documented as incidental to the condition. See also guideline 1.C.15.a.1.

4) Encounter for complication associated with a neoplasm

When an encounter is for management of a complication associated with a neoplasm, such as dehydration, and the treatment is only for the complication, the complication is coded first, followed by the appropriate code(s) for the neoplasm.

The exception to this guideline is anemia. When the admission/encounter is for management of an anemia associated with the malignancy, and the treatment is only for anemia, the appropriate code for the malignancy is sequenced as the principal or first-listed diagnosis followed by code D63.0, Anemia in neoplastic disease.

> Patient with pancreatic cancer is seen for initiation of TPN for cancer-related moderate protein-calorie malnutrition
>
> | E44.0 | Moderate protein-calorie malnutrition |
> |---|---|
> | C25.9 | Malignant neoplasm of pancreas, unspecified |
>
> *Explanation*: The encounter is to initiate treatment for malnutrition, a common complication of many types of neoplasms, and is sequenced first.

5) Complication from surgical procedure for treatment of a neoplasm

When an encounter is for treatment of a complication resulting from a surgical procedure performed for the treatment of the neoplasm, designate the complication as the principal/first-listed diagnosis. See the guideline regarding the coding of a current malignancy versus personal history to determine if the code for the neoplasm should also be assigned.

6) Pathologic fracture due to a neoplasm

When an encounter is for a pathological fracture due to a neoplasm, and the focus of treatment is the fracture, a code from subcategory M84.5, Pathological fracture in neoplastic disease, should be sequenced first, followed by the code for the neoplasm.

If the focus of treatment is the neoplasm with an associated pathological fracture, the neoplasm code should be sequenced first, followed by a code from M84.5 for the pathological fracture.

m. Current malignancy versus personal history of malignancy

When a primary malignancy has been excised but further treatment, such as an additional surgery for the malignancy, radiation therapy or chemotherapy is directed to that site, the primary malignancy code should be used until treatment is completed.

> Female patient with ongoing chemotherapy after right mastectomy for breast cancer
>
> | C50.911 | Malignant neoplasm of unspecified site of right female breast |
> |---|---|
> | Z90.11 | Acquired absence of right breast and nipple |
>
> *Explanation*: Even though the breast has been removed, the breast cancer is still being treated with chemotherapy and therefore is still coded as a current condition rather than personal history.

When a primary malignancy has been previously excised or eradicated from its site, there is no further treatment (of the malignancy) directed to that site, and there is no evidence of any existing primary malignancy at that site, a code from category Z85, Personal history of malignant neoplasm, should be used to indicate the former site of the malignancy.

Codes from subcategories Z85.0 – Z85.85 should only be assigned for the former site of a primary malignancy, not the site of a secondary malignancy. Code Z85.89 may be assigned for the former site(s) of either a primary or secondary malignancy.

See Section I.C.21. Factors influencing health status and contact with health services, History (of)

n. Leukemia, multiple myeloma, and malignant plasma cell neoplasms in remission versus personal history

The categories for leukemia, and category C90, Multiple myeloma and malignant plasma cell neoplasms, have codes indicating whether or not the leukemia has achieved remission. There are also codes Z85.6, Personal history of leukemia, and Z85.79, Personal history of other malignant neoplasms of lymphoid, hematopoietic and related tissues. If the documentation is unclear as to whether the leukemia has achieved remission, the provider should be queried.

See Section I.C.21. Factors influencing health status and contact with health services, History (of)

o. Aftercare following surgery for neoplasm

See Section I.C.21. Factors influencing health status and contact with health services, Aftercare

p. Follow-up care for completed treatment of a malignancy

See Section I.C.21. Factors influencing health status and contact with health services, Follow-up

q. Prophylactic organ removal for prevention of malignancy

See Section I.C. 21, Factors influencing health status and contact with health services, Prophylactic organ removal

r. Malignant neoplasm associated with transplanted organ

A malignant neoplasm of a transplanted organ should be coded as a transplant complication. Assign first the appropriate code from category T86.-, Complications of transplanted organs and tissue, followed by code C80.2, Malignant neoplasm associated with transplanted organ. Use an additional code for the specific malignancy.

s. Breast implant associated anaplastic large cell lymphoma

Breast implant associated anaplastic large cell lymphoma (BIA-ALCL) is a type of lymphoma that can develop around breast implants. Assign code C84.7A, Anaplastic large cell lymphoma, ALK-negative, breast, for BIA-ALCL. Do not assign a complication code from chapter 19.

t. Secondary malignant neoplasm of lymphoid tissue

When a malignant neoplasm of lymphoid tissue metastasizes beyond the lymph nodes, a code from categories C81-C85 with a final character "9" should be assigned identifying "extranodal and solid organ sites" rather than a code for the secondary neoplasm of the affected solid organ. For example, for metastasis of B-cell lymphoma to the lung, brain and left adrenal gland, assign code C83.39, Diffuse large B-cell lymphoma, extranodal and solid organ sites.

Chapter 2. Neoplasms

Chapter 2. Neoplasms (C00-D49)

NOTE

Functional activity

All neoplasms are classified in this chapter, whether they are functionally active or not. An additional code from Chapter 4 may be used, to identify functional activity associated with any neoplasm.

Morphology [Histology]

Chapter 2 classifies neoplasms primarily by site (topography), with broad groupings for behavior, malignant, in situ, benign, etc. The Table of Neoplasms should be used to identify the correct topography code. In a few cases, such as for malignant melanoma and certain neuroendocrine tumors, the morphology (histologic type) is included in the category and codes.

Primary malignant neoplasms overlapping site boundaries

A primary malignant neoplasm that overlaps two or more contiguous (next to each other) sites should be classified to the subcategory/code .8 ("overlapping lesion"), unless the combination is specifically indexed elsewhere. For multiple neoplasms of the same site that are not contiguous, such as tumors in different quadrants of the same breast, codes for each site should be assigned.

Malignant neoplasm of ectopic tissue

Malignant neoplasms of ectopic tissue are to be coded to the site mentioned, e.g., ectopic pancreatic malignant neoplasms are coded to pancreas, unspecified (C25.9).

AHA: 2017,4Q,103; 2017,1Q,4,5-6,8

This chapter contains the following blocks:

C00-C14	Malignant neoplasms of lip, oral cavity and pharynx
C15-C26	Malignant neoplasms of digestive organs
C30-C39	Malignant neoplasms of respiratory and intrathoracic organs
C40-C41	Malignant neoplasms of bone and articular cartilage
C43-C44	Melanoma and other malignant neoplasms of skin
C45-C49	Malignant neoplasms of mesothelial and soft tissue
C50	Malignant neoplasms of breast
C51-C58	Malignant neoplasms of female genital organs
C60-C63	Malignant neoplasms of male genital organs
C64-C68	Malignant neoplasms of urinary tract
C69-C72	Malignant neoplasms of eye, brain and other parts of central nervous system
C73-C75	Malignant neoplasms of thyroid and other endocrine glands
C7A	Malignant neuroendocrine tumors
C7B	Secondary neuroendocrine tumors
C76-C80	Malignant neoplasms of ill-defined, other secondary and unspecified sites
C81-C96	Malignant neoplasms of lymphoid, hematopoietic and related tissue
D00-D09	In situ neoplasms
D10-D36	Benign neoplasms, except benign neuroendocrine tumors
D3A	Benign neuroendocrine tumors
D37-D48	Neoplasms of uncertain behavior, polycythemia vera and myelodysplastic syndromes
D49	Neoplasms of unspecified behavior

MALIGNANT NEOPLASMS (C00-C96)

Malignant neoplasms, stated or presumed to be primary (of specified sites), and certain specified histologies, except neuroendocrine, and of lymphoid, hematopoietic and related tissue (C00-C75)

AHA: 2022,1Q,16

TIP: Codes from this code block can be assigned for outpatient encounters based on the diagnosis listed in a pathology or cytology report when authenticated by a pathologist and available at the time of code assignment.

Malignant neoplasms of lip, oral cavity and pharynx (C00-C14)

✓4ᵗʰ **C00 Malignant neoplasm of lip**

Use additional code to identify:
    alcohol abuse and dependence (F10.-)
    history of tobacco dependence (Z87.891)
    tobacco dependence (F17.-)
    tobacco use (Z72.0)

    EXCLUDES 1   malignant melanoma of lip (C43.0)
                 Merkel cell carcinoma of lip (C4A.0)
                 other and unspecified malignant neoplasm of skin of lip (C44.0-)

    C00.0 Malignant neoplasm of external upper lip
         Malignant neoplasm of lipstick area of upper lip
         Malignant neoplasm of upper lip NOS
         Malignant neoplasm of vermilion border of upper lip

    C00.1 Malignant neoplasm of external lower lip
         Malignant neoplasm of lower lip NOS
         Malignant neoplasm of lipstick area of lower lip
         Malignant neoplasm of vermilion border of lower lip

    C00.2 Malignant neoplasm of external lip, unspecified
         Malignant neoplasm of vermilion border of lip NOS

    C00.3 Malignant neoplasm of upper lip, inner aspect
         Malignant neoplasm of buccal aspect of upper lip
         Malignant neoplasm of frenulum of upper lip
         Malignant neoplasm of mucosa of upper lip
         Malignant neoplasm of oral aspect of upper lip

    C00.4 Malignant neoplasm of lower lip, inner aspect
         Malignant neoplasm of buccal aspect of lower lip
         Malignant neoplasm of frenulum of lower lip
         Malignant neoplasm of mucosa of lower lip
         Malignant neoplasm of oral aspect of lower lip

    C00.5 Malignant neoplasm of lip, unspecified, inner aspect
         Malignant neoplasm of buccal aspect of lip, unspecified
         Malignant neoplasm of frenulum of lip, unspecified
         Malignant neoplasm of mucosa of lip, unspecified
         Malignant neoplasm of oral aspect of lip, unspecified

    C00.6 Malignant neoplasm of commissure of lip, unspecified

    C00.8 Malignant neoplasm of overlapping sites of lip

    C00.9 Malignant neoplasm of lip, unspecified

C01 Malignant neoplasm of base of tongue   HCC Rx ESR COM

     Malignant neoplasm of dorsal surface of base of tongue
     Malignant neoplasm of fixed part of tongue NOS
     Malignant neoplasm of posterior third of tongue
     Use additional code to identify:
         alcohol abuse and dependence (F10.-)
         history of tobacco dependence (Z87.891)
         tobacco dependence (F17.-)
         tobacco use (Z72.0)

Malignant Neoplasm of Tongue

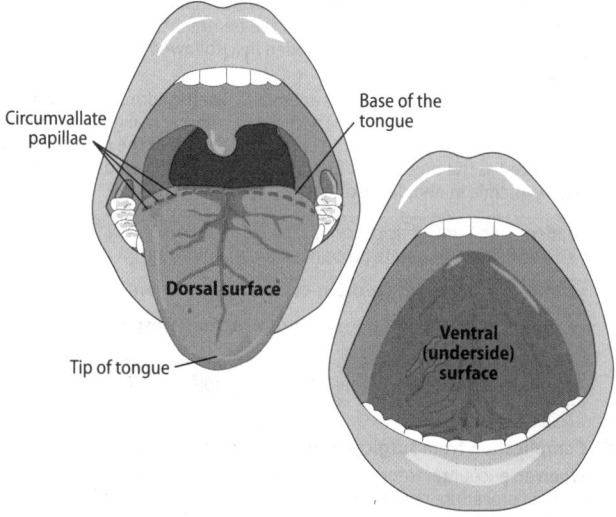

Circumvallate papillae   Base of the tongue   Dorsal surface   Tip of tongue   Ventral (underside) surface

✓4ᵗʰ **C02 Malignant neoplasm of other and unspecified parts of tongue**

     Use additional code to identify:
         alcohol abuse and dependence (F10.-)
         history of tobacco dependence (Z87.891)
         tobacco dependence (F17.-)
         tobacco use (Z72.0)

    C02.0 Malignant neoplasm of dorsal surface of tongue   HCC Rx ESR COM
         Malignant neoplasm of anterior two-thirds of tongue, dorsal surface
         EXCLUDES 2   malignant neoplasm of dorsal surface of base of tongue (C01)

    C02.1 Malignant neoplasm of border of tongue   HCC Rx ESR COM
         Malignant neoplasm of tip of tongue

    C02.2 Malignant neoplasm of ventral surface of tongue   HCC Rx ESR COM
         Malignant neoplasm of anterior two-thirds of tongue, ventral surface
         Malignant neoplasm of frenulum linguae

    C02.3 Malignant neoplasm of anterior two-thirds of tongue, part unspecified   HCC Rx ESR COM
         Malignant neoplasm of middle third of tongue NOS
         Malignant neoplasm of mobile part of tongue NOS

C02.4 **Malignant neoplasm of** lingual tonsil `HCC` `Rx` `ESR` `COM`
    EXCLUDES 2 *malignant neoplasm of tonsil NOS (C09.9)*

C02.8 **Malignant neoplasm of** overlapping sites **of** tongue `HCC` `Rx` `ESR` `COM`
    Malignant neoplasm of two or more contiguous sites of tongue

C02.9 **Malignant neoplasm of** tongue, unspecified `HCC` `Rx` `ESR` `COM`

✓4ᵗʰ **C03** **Malignant neoplasm of** gum
    `INCLUDES` malignant neoplasm of alveolar (ridge) mucosa
               malignant neoplasm of gingiva
    Use additional code to identify:
      alcohol abuse and dependence (F10.-)
      history of tobacco dependence (Z87.891)
      tobacco dependence (F17.-)
      tobacco use (Z72.0)
    EXCLUDES 2 *malignant odontogenic neoplasms (C41.0-C41.1)*

C03.0 **Malignant neoplasm of** upper gum `HCC` `Rx` `ESR` `COM`

C03.1 **Malignant neoplasm of** lower gum `HCC` `Rx` `ESR` `COM`

C03.9 **Malignant neoplasm of** gum, unspecified `HCC` `Rx` `ESR` `COM`

✓4ᵗʰ **C04** **Malignant neoplasm of** floor of mouth
    Use additional code to identify:
      alcohol abuse and dependence (F10.-)
      history of tobacco dependence (Z87.891)
      tobacco dependence (F17.-)
      tobacco use (Z72.0)

C04.0 **Malignant neoplasm of** anterior **floor of mouth** `HCC` `Rx` `ESR` `COM`
    Malignant neoplasm of anterior to the premolar-canine junction

C04.1 **Malignant neoplasm of** lateral **floor of mouth** `HCC` `Rx` `ESR` `COM`

C04.8 **Malignant neoplasm of** overlapping sites **of floor of mouth** `HCC` `Rx` `ESR` `COM`

C04.9 **Malignant neoplasm of** floor of mouth, unspecified `HCC` `Rx` `ESR` `COM`

✓4ᵗʰ **C05** **Malignant neoplasm of** palate
    Use additional code to identify:
      alcohol abuse and dependence (F10.-)
      history of tobacco dependence (Z87.891)
      tobacco dependence (F17.-)
      tobacco use (Z72.0)
    EXCLUDES 1 *Kaposi's sarcoma of palate (C46.2)*

C05.0 **Malignant neoplasm of** hard palate `HCC` `Rx` `ESR` `COM`

C05.1 **Malignant neoplasm of** soft palate `HCC` `Rx` `ESR` `COM`
    EXCLUDES 2 *malignant neoplasm of nasopharyngeal surface of soft palate (C11.3)*

C05.2 **Malignant neoplasm of** uvula `HCC` `Rx` `ESR` `COM`

C05.8 **Malignant neoplasm of** overlapping sites **of** palate `HCC` `Rx` `ESR` `COM`

C05.9 **Malignant neoplasm of** palate, unspecified `HCC` `Rx` `ESR` `COM`
    Malignant neoplasm of roof of mouth

✓4ᵗʰ **C06** **Malignant neoplasm of** other and unspecified parts of mouth
    Use additional code to identify:
      alcohol abuse and dependence (F10.-)
      history of tobacco dependence (Z87.891)
      tobacco dependence (F17.-)
      tobacco use (Z72.0)

C06.0 **Malignant neoplasm of** cheek mucosa `HCC` `Rx` `ESR` `COM`
    Malignant neoplasm of buccal mucosa NOS
    Malignant neoplasm of internal cheek

C06.1 **Malignant neoplasm of** vestibule **of mouth** `HCC` `Rx` `ESR` `COM`
    Malignant neoplasm of buccal sulcus (upper) (lower)
    Malignant neoplasm of labial sulcus (upper) (lower)

C06.2 **Malignant neoplasm of** retromolar area `HCC` `Rx` `ESR` `COM`

✓5ᵗʰ **C06.8** **Malignant neoplasm of** overlapping sites **of other and unspecified parts of mouth**

    C06.80 **Malignant neoplasm of overlapping sites of unspecified parts of mouth** `HCC` `Rx` `ESR` `COM`

    C06.89 **Malignant neoplasm of overlapping sites of other parts of mouth** `HCC` `Rx` `ESR` `COM`
        "book leaf" neoplasm [ventral surface of tongue and floor of mouth]

C06.9 **Malignant neoplasm of** mouth, unspecified `HCC` `Rx` `ESR` `COM`
    Malignant neoplasm of minor salivary gland, unspecified site
    Malignant neoplasm of oral cavity NOS

C07 **Malignant neoplasm of** parotid gland `HCC` `Rx` `ESR` `COM`
    Use additional code to identify:
      alcohol abuse and dependence (F10.-)
      exposure to environmental tobacco smoke (Z77.22)
      exposure to tobacco smoke in the perinatal period (P96.81)
      history of tobacco dependence (Z87.891)
      occupational exposure to environmental tobacco smoke (Z57.31)
      tobacco dependence (F17.-)
      tobacco use (Z72.0)

✓4ᵗʰ **C08** **Malignant neoplasm of** other and unspecified major salivary glands
    `INCLUDES` malignant neoplasm of salivary ducts
    Use additional code to identify:
      alcohol abuse and dependence (F10.-)
      exposure to environmental tobacco smoke (Z77.22)
      exposure to tobacco smoke in the perinatal period (P96.81)
      history of tobacco dependence (Z87.891)
      occupational exposure to environmental tobacco smoke (Z57.31)
      tobacco dependence (F17.-)
      tobacco use (Z72.0)
    EXCLUDES 1 *malignant neoplasms of specified minor salivary glands which are classified according to their anatomical location*
    EXCLUDES 2 *malignant neoplasms of minor salivary glands NOS (C06.9)*
               malignant neoplasm of parotid gland (C07)

C08.0 **Malignant neoplasm of** submandibular gland `HCC` `Rx` `ESR` `COM`
    Malignant neoplasm of submaxillary gland

C08.1 **Malignant neoplasm of** sublingual gland `HCC` `Rx` `ESR` `COM`

C08.9 **Malignant neoplasm of** major salivary gland, unspecified `HCC` `Rx` `ESR` `COM`
    Malignant neoplasm of salivary gland (major) NOS

✓4ᵗʰ **C09** **Malignant neoplasm of** tonsil
    Use additional code to identify:
      alcohol abuse and dependence (F10.-)
      exposure to environmental tobacco smoke (Z77.22)
      exposure to tobacco smoke in the perinatal period (P96.81)
      history of tobacco dependence (Z87.891)
      occupational exposure to environmental tobacco smoke (Z57.31)
      tobacco dependence (F17.-)
      tobacco use (Z72.0)
    EXCLUDES 2 *malignant neoplasm of lingual tonsil (C02.4)*
               malignant neoplasm of pharyngeal tonsil (C11.1)

C09.0 **Malignant neoplasm of** tonsillar fossa `HCC` `ESR` `COM`

C09.1 **Malignant neoplasm of** tonsillar pillar (anterior) (posterior) `HCC` `ESR` `COM`

C09.8 **Malignant neoplasm of** overlapping sites **of** tonsil `HCC` `ESR` `COM`

C09.9 **Malignant neoplasm of** tonsil, unspecified `HCC` `ESR` `COM`
    Malignant neoplasm of tonsil NOS
    Malignant neoplasm of faucial tonsils
    Malignant neoplasm of palatine tonsils

✓4ᵗʰ **C10** **Malignant neoplasm of** oropharynx
    Use additional code to identify:
      alcohol abuse and dependence (F10.-)
      exposure to environmental tobacco smoke (Z77.22)
      exposure to tobacco smoke in the perinatal period (P96.81)
      history of tobacco dependence (Z87.891)
      occupational exposure to environmental tobacco smoke (Z57.31)
      tobacco dependence (F17.-)
      tobacco use (Z72.0)
    EXCLUDES 2 *malignant neoplasm of tonsil (C09.-)*
    DEF: Oropharynx: Middle portion of pharynx (throat); communicates with the oral cavity, nasopharynx and laryngopharynx.

C10.0 **Malignant neoplasm of** vallecula `HCC` `ESR` `COM`

C10.1 **Malignant neoplasm of** anterior surface of epiglottis `HCC` `ESR` `COM`
    Malignant neoplasm of epiglottis, free border [margin]
    Malignant neoplasm of glossoepiglottic fold(s)
    EXCLUDES 2 *malignant neoplasm of epiglottis (suprahyoid portion) NOS (C32.1)*

C10.2 **Malignant neoplasm of** lateral wall **of** oropharynx `HCC` `ESR` `COM`

C10.3 **Malignant neoplasm of** posterior wall **of** oropharynx `HCC` `ESR` `COM`

☑ Additional Character Required   ✓x7ᵗʰ Placeholder Alert   Manifestation   Unspecified Dx   Q QPP   UPD Unacceptable PDx

Chapter 2. Neoplasms

C02.4–C10.3

C10.4 Malignant neoplasm of branchial cleft   HCC ESR COM
Malignant neoplasm of branchial cyst [site of neoplasm]

C10.8 Malignant neoplasm of overlapping sites of oropharynx   HCC ESR COM
Malignant neoplasm of junctional region of oropharynx

C10.9 Malignant neoplasm of oropharynx, unspecified   HCC ESR COM

✓4ᵗʰ **C11 Malignant neoplasm of** nasopharynx
Use additional code to identify:
  exposure to environmental tobacco smoke (Z77.22)
  exposure to tobacco smoke in the perinatal period (P96.81)
  history of tobacco dependence (Z87.891)
  occupational exposure to environmental tobacco smoke (Z57.31)
  tobacco dependence (F17.-)
  tobacco use (Z72.0)
DEF: Nasopharynx: Upper portion of pharynx (throat); communicates with the nasal cavities, oropharynx and tympanic cavities.

C11.0 Malignant neoplasm of superior wall of nasopharynx   HCC ESR COM
Malignant neoplasm of roof of nasopharynx

C11.1 Malignant neoplasm of posterior wall of nasopharynx   HCC ESR COM
Malignant neoplasm of adenoid
Malignant neoplasm of pharyngeal tonsil

C11.2 Malignant neoplasm of lateral wall of nasopharynx   HCC ESR COM
Malignant neoplasm of fossa of Rosenmüller
Malignant neoplasm of opening of auditory tube
Malignant neoplasm of pharyngeal recess

C11.3 Malignant neoplasm of anterior wall of nasopharynx   HCC ESR COM
Malignant neoplasm of floor of nasopharynx
Malignant neoplasm of nasopharyngeal (anterior) (posterior) surface of soft palate
Malignant neoplasm of posterior margin of nasal choana
Malignant neoplasm of posterior margin of nasal septum

C11.8 Malignant neoplasm of overlapping sites of nasopharynx   HCC ESR COM

C11.9 Malignant neoplasm of nasopharynx, unspecified   HCC ESR COM
Malignant neoplasm of nasopharyngeal wall NOS

C12 Malignant neoplasm of pyriform sinus   HCC ESR COM
Malignant neoplasm of pyriform fossa
Use additional code to identify:
  exposure to environmental tobacco smoke (Z77.22)
  exposure to tobacco smoke in the perinatal period (P96.81)
  history of tobacco dependence (Z87.891)
  occupational exposure to environmental tobacco smoke (Z57.31)
  tobacco dependence (F17.-)
  tobacco use (Z72.0)

✓4ᵗʰ **C13 Malignant neoplasm of** hypopharynx
Use additional code to identify:
  exposure to environmental tobacco smoke (Z77.22)
  exposure to tobacco smoke in the perinatal period (P96.81)
  history of tobacco dependence (Z87.891)
  occupational exposure to environmental tobacco smoke (Z57.31)
  tobacco dependence (F17.-)
  tobacco use (Z72.0)
EXCLUDES 2   malignant neoplasm of pyriform sinus (C12)
DEF: Hypopharynx: Lower portion of pharynx (throat); communicates with the oropharynx and the esophagus. **Synonym(s):** laryngopharynx.

C13.0 Malignant neoplasm of postcricoid region   HCC ESR COM

C13.1 Malignant neoplasm of aryepiglottic fold, hypopharyngeal aspect   HCC ESR COM
Malignant neoplasm of aryepiglottic fold, marginal zone
Malignant neoplasm of aryepiglottic fold NOS
Malignant neoplasm of interarytenoid fold, marginal zone
Malignant neoplasm of interarytenoid fold NOS
EXCLUDES 2   malignant neoplasm of aryepiglottic fold or interarytenoid fold, laryngeal aspect (C32.1)

C13.2 Malignant neoplasm of posterior wall of hypopharynx   HCC ESR COM

C13.8 Malignant neoplasm of overlapping sites of hypopharynx   HCC ESR COM

C13.9 Malignant neoplasm of hypopharynx, unspecified   HCC ESR COM
Malignant neoplasm of hypopharyngeal wall NOS

✓4ᵗʰ **C14 Malignant neoplasm of** other and ill-defined sites in the lip, oral cavity and pharynx
Use additional code to identify:
  alcohol abuse and dependence (F10.-)
  exposure to environmental tobacco smoke (Z77.22)
  exposure to tobacco smoke in the perinatal period (P96.81)
  history of tobacco dependence (Z87.891)
  occupational exposure to environmental tobacco smoke (Z57.31)
  tobacco dependence (F17.-)
  tobacco use (Z72.0)
EXCLUDES 1   malignant neoplasm of oral cavity NOS (C06.9)

C14.0 Malignant neoplasm of pharynx, unspecified   HCC ESR COM

C14.2 Malignant neoplasm of Waldeyer's ring   HCC ESR COM
DEF: Waldeyer's ring: Ring of lymphoid tissue that is made up of the two palatine tonsils, the pharyngeal tonsil (adenoid), and the lingual tonsil. It functions as the defense against infection and assists with the development of the immune system.

C14.8 Malignant neoplasm of overlapping sites of lip, oral cavity and pharynx   HCC ESR COM
Primary malignant neoplasm of two or more contiguous sites of lip, oral cavity and pharynx
EXCLUDES 1   "book leaf" neoplasm [ventral surface of tongue and floor of mouth] (C06.89)

Malignant neoplasms of digestive organs (C15-C26)

EXCLUDES 1   Kaposi's sarcoma of gastrointestinal sites (C46.4)
EXCLUDES 2   gastrointestinal stromal tumors (C49.A-)

✓4ᵗʰ **C15 Malignant neoplasm of** esophagus
Use additional code to identify:
  alcohol abuse and dependence (F10.-)

proximal

C15.3 Malignant neoplasm of ~~upper third~~ of esophagus   HCC ESR COM

C15.4 Malignant neoplasm of middle third of esophagus   HCC ESR COM

C15.5 Malignant neoplasm of lower third of esophagus   HCC ESR COM
EXCLUDES 1   malignant neoplasm of cardio-esophageal junction (C16.0)

C15.8 Malignant neoplasm of overlapping sites of esophagus   HCC ESR COM

C15.9 Malignant neoplasm of esophagus, unspecified   HCC ESR COM

✓4ᵗʰ **C16 Malignant neoplasm of** stomach
Use additional code to identify:
  alcohol abuse and dependence (F10.-)
EXCLUDES 2   malignant carcinoid tumor of the stomach (C7A.092)

C16.0 Malignant neoplasm of cardia   HCC Rx ESR COM
Malignant neoplasm of cardiac orifice
Malignant neoplasm of cardio-esophageal junction
Malignant neoplasm of esophagus and stomach
Malignant neoplasm of gastro-esophageal junction

C16.1 Malignant neoplasm of fundus of stomach   HCC Rx ESR COM

C16.2 Malignant neoplasm of body of stomach   HCC Rx ESR COM

C16.3 Malignant neoplasm of pyloric antrum   HCC Rx ESR COM
Malignant neoplasm of gastric antrum

C16.4 Malignant neoplasm of pylorus   HCC Rx ESR COM
Malignant neoplasm of prepylorus
Malignant neoplasm of pyloric canal

C16.5 Malignant neoplasm of lesser curvature of stomach, unspecified   HCC Rx ESR COM
Malignant neoplasm of lesser curvature of stomach, not classifiable to C16.1-C16.4

C16.6 Malignant neoplasm of greater curvature of stomach, unspecified   HCC Rx ESR COM
Malignant neoplasm of greater curvature of stomach, not classifiable to C16.0-C16.4

C16.8 Malignant neoplasm of overlapping sites of stomach   HCC Rx ESR COM

C16.9 Malignant neoplasm of stomach, unspecified   HCC Rx ESR COM
Gastric cancer NOS

✓4ᵗʰ C17   Malignant neoplasm of small intestine
    EXCLUDES 1   malignant carcinoid tumors of the small intestine (C7A.Ø1)
    AHA: 2016,1Q,19

   C17.Ø   Malignant neoplasm of duodenum   `HCC` `Rx` `ESR` `COM`
   C17.1   Malignant neoplasm of jejunum   `HCC` `Rx` `ESR` `COM`
   C17.2   Malignant neoplasm of ileum   `HCC` `Rx` `ESR` `COM`
      EXCLUDES 1   malignant neoplasm of ileocecal valve (C18.Ø)
   C17.3   Meckel's diverticulum, malignant   `HCC` `Rx` `ESR` `COM`
      EXCLUDES 1   Meckel's diverticulum, congenital (Q43.Ø)
      DEF: Congenital, abnormal remnant of embryonic digestive system development that leaves a sacculation or outpouching from the wall of the small intestine near the terminal part of the ileum made of acid-secreting tissue as in the stomach.
   C17.8   Malignant neoplasm of overlapping sites of small intestine   `HCC` `Rx` `ESR` `COM`
   C17.9   Malignant neoplasm of small intestine, unspecified   `HCC` `Rx` `ESR` `COM`

✓4ᵗʰ C18   Malignant neoplasm of colon
    EXCLUDES 1   malignant carcinoid tumors of the colon (C7A.Ø2-)

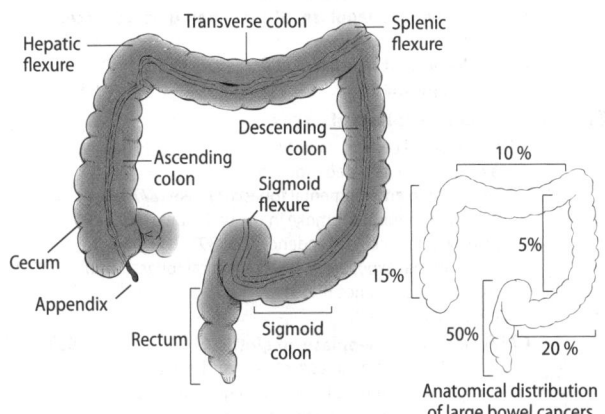

Colon

Anatomical distribution of large bowel cancers

   C18.Ø   Malignant neoplasm of cecum   `HCC` `ESR` `COM`
      Malignant neoplasm of ileocecal valve
   C18.1   Malignant neoplasm of appendix   `HCC` `ESR` `COM`
   C18.2   Malignant neoplasm of ascending colon   `HCC` `ESR` `COM`
   C18.3   Malignant neoplasm of hepatic flexure   `HCC` `ESR` `COM`
   C18.4   Malignant neoplasm of transverse colon   `HCC` `ESR` `COM`
   C18.5   Malignant neoplasm of splenic flexure   `HCC` `ESR` `COM`
   C18.6   Malignant neoplasm of descending colon   `HCC` `ESR` `COM`
   C18.7   Malignant neoplasm of sigmoid colon   `HCC` `ESR` `COM`
      Malignant neoplasm of sigmoid (flexure)
      EXCLUDES 1   malignant neoplasm of rectosigmoid junction (C19)
   C18.8   Malignant neoplasm of overlapping sites of colon   `HCC` `ESR` `COM`
   C18.9   Malignant neoplasm of colon, unspecified   `HCC` `ESR` `COM`
      Malignant neoplasm of large intestine NOS

C19   Malignant neoplasm of rectosigmoid junction   `HCC` `ESR` `COM`
    Malignant neoplasm of colon with rectum
    Malignant neoplasm of rectosigmoid (colon)
    EXCLUDES 1   malignant carcinoid tumors of the colon (C7A.Ø2-)

C2Ø   Malignant neoplasm of rectum   `HCC` `ESR` `COM`
    Malignant neoplasm of rectal ampulla
    EXCLUDES 1   malignant carcinoid tumor of the rectum (C7A.Ø26)

✓4ᵗʰ C21   Malignant neoplasm of anus and anal canal
    EXCLUDES 2   malignant carcinoid tumors of the colon (C7A.Ø2-)
              malignant melanoma of anal margin (C43.51)
              malignant melanoma of anal skin (C43.51)
              malignant melanoma of perianal skin (C43.51)
              other and unspecified malignant neoplasm of anal margin (C44.5ØØ, C44.51Ø, C44.52Ø, C44.59Ø)
              other and unspecified malignant neoplasm of anal skin (C44.5ØØ, C44.51Ø, C44.52Ø, C44.59Ø)
              other and unspecified malignant neoplasm of perianal skin (C44.5ØØ, C44.51Ø, C44.52Ø, C44.59Ø)

   C21.Ø   Malignant neoplasm of anus, unspecified   `HCC` `ESR` `COM`

   C21.1   Malignant neoplasm of anal canal   `HCC` `ESR` `COM`
      Malignant neoplasm of anal sphincter
   C21.2   Malignant neoplasm of cloacogenic zone   `HCC` `ESR` `COM`
   C21.8   Malignant neoplasm of overlapping sites of rectum, anus and anal canal   `HCC` `ESR` `COM`
      Malignant neoplasm of anorectal junction
      Malignant neoplasm of anorectum
      Primary malignant neoplasm of two or more contiguous sites of rectum, anus and anal canal

✓4ᵗʰ C22   Malignant neoplasm of liver and intrahepatic bile ducts
    EXCLUDES 1   malignant neoplasm of biliary tract NOS (C24.9)
              secondary malignant neoplasm of liver and intrahepatic bile duct (C78.7)
    Use additional code to identify:
     alcohol abuse and dependence (F1Ø.-)
     hepatitis B (B16.-, B18.Ø-B18.1)
     hepatitis C (B17.1-, B18.2)

   C22.Ø   Liver cell carcinoma   `HCC` `Rx` `ESR` `COM`
      Hepatocellular carcinoma
      Hepatoma
      AHA: 2016,1Q,18
   C22.1   Intrahepatic bile duct carcinoma   `HCC` `Rx` `ESR` `COM`
      Cholangiocarcinoma
      EXCLUDES 1   malignant neoplasm of hepatic duct (C24.Ø)
   C22.2   Hepatoblastoma   `HCC` `Rx` `ESR` `COM`
   C22.3   Angiosarcoma of liver   `HCC` `Rx` `ESR` `COM`
      Kupffer cell sarcoma
   C22.4   Other sarcomas of liver   `HCC` `Rx` `ESR` `COM`
   C22.7   Other specified carcinomas of liver   `HCC` `Rx` `ESR` `COM`
   C22.8   Malignant neoplasm of liver, primary, unspecified as to type   `HCC` `Rx` `ESR` `COM`
   C22.9   Malignant neoplasm of liver, not specified as primary or secondary   `HCC` `Rx` `ESR` `COM`

C23   Malignant neoplasm of gallbladder   `HCC` `Rx` `ESR` `COM`

✓4ᵗʰ C24   Malignant neoplasm of other and unspecified parts of biliary tract
    EXCLUDES 1   malignant neoplasm of intrahepatic bile duct (C22.1)

   C24.Ø   Malignant neoplasm of extrahepatic bile duct   `HCC` `Rx` `ESR` `COM`
      Malignant neoplasm of biliary duct or passage NOS
      Malignant neoplasm of common bile duct
      Malignant neoplasm of cystic duct
      Malignant neoplasm of hepatic duct
   C24.1   Malignant neoplasm of ampulla of Vater   `HCC` `Rx` `ESR` `COM`
      DEF: Malignant neoplasm in the area of dilation at the juncture of the common bile and pancreatic ducts near the opening into the lumen of the duodenum.
   C24.8   Malignant neoplasm of overlapping sites of biliary tract   `HCC` `Rx` `ESR` `COM`
      Malignant neoplasm involving both intrahepatic and extrahepatic bile ducts
      Primary malignant neoplasm of two or more contiguous sites of biliary tract
   C24.9   Malignant neoplasm of biliary tract, unspecified   `HCC` `Rx` `ESR` `COM`

✓4ᵗʰ C25 Malignant neoplasm of pancreas

Code also if applicable exocrine pancreatic insufficiency (K86.81)
Use additional code to identify:
    alcohol abuse and dependence (F1Ø.-)

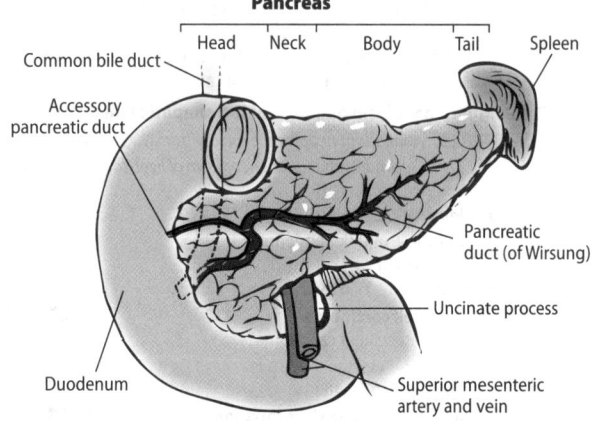

Pancreas

- **C25.Ø** Malignant neoplasm of head of pancreas `HCC` `Rx` `ESR` `COM`
- **C25.1** Malignant neoplasm of body of pancreas `HCC` `Rx` `ESR` `COM`
- **C25.2** Malignant neoplasm of tail of pancreas `HCC` `Rx` `ESR` `COM`
- **C25.3** Malignant neoplasm of pancreatic duct `HCC` `Rx` `ESR` `COM`
- **C25.4** Malignant neoplasm of endocrine pancreas `HCC` `Rx` `ESR` `COM`
  Malignant neoplasm of islets of Langerhans
  Use additional code to identify any functional activity
- **C25.7** Malignant neoplasm of other parts of pancreas `HCC` `Rx` `ESR` `COM`
  Malignant neoplasm of neck of pancreas
- **C25.8** Malignant neoplasm of overlapping sites of pancreas `HCC` `Rx` `ESR` `COM`
- **C25.9** Malignant neoplasm of pancreas, unspecified `HCC` `Rx` `ESR` `COM`

✓4ᵗʰ C26 Malignant neoplasm of other and ill-defined digestive organs

EXCLUDES 1   malignant neoplasm of peritoneum and retroperitoneum (C48.-)

- **C26.Ø** Malignant neoplasm of intestinal tract, part unspecified `HCC` `ESR` `COM`
  Malignant neoplasm of intestine NOS
- **C26.1** Malignant neoplasm of spleen `HCC` `ESR` `COM`
  EXCLUDES 1   Hodgkin lymphoma (C81.-)
             non-Hodgkin lymphoma (C82-C85)
- **C26.9** Malignant neoplasm of ill-defined sites within the digestive system `HCC` `ESR` `COM`
  Malignant neoplasm of alimentary canal or tract NOS
  Malignant neoplasm of gastrointestinal tract NOS
  EXCLUDES 1   malignant neoplasm of abdominal NOS (C76.2)
             malignant neoplasm of intra-abdominal NOS (C76.2)

Malignant neoplasms of respiratory and intrathoracic organs (C3Ø-C39)

INCLUDES   malignant neoplasm of middle ear
EXCLUDES 1   mesothelioma (C45.-)

✓4ᵗʰ C3Ø Malignant neoplasm of nasal cavity and middle ear

- **C3Ø.Ø** Malignant neoplasm of nasal cavity `HCC` `Rx` `ESR` `COM`
  Malignant neoplasm of cartilage of nose
  Malignant neoplasm of nasal concha
  Malignant neoplasm of internal nose
  Malignant neoplasm of septum of nose
  Malignant neoplasm of vestibule of nose
  EXCLUDES 1   malignant neoplasm of nasal bone (C41.Ø)
          malignant neoplasm of nose NOS (C76.Ø)
          malignant neoplasm of olfactory bulb (C72.2-)
          malignant neoplasm of posterior margin of nasal septum and choana (C11.3)
          malignant melanoma of skin of nose (C43.31)
          malignant neoplasm of turbinates (C41.Ø)
          other and unspecified malignant neoplasm of skin of nose (C44.3Ø1, C44.311, C44.321, C44.391)

- **C3Ø.1** Malignant neoplasm of middle ear `HCC` `Rx` `ESR` `COM`
  Malignant neoplasm of antrum tympanicum
  Malignant neoplasm of auditory tube
  Malignant neoplasm of eustachian tube
  Malignant neoplasm of inner ear
  Malignant neoplasm of mastoid air cells
  Malignant neoplasm of tympanic cavity
  EXCLUDES 1   malignant neoplasm of auricular canal (external) (C43.2-,C44.2-)
          malignant neoplasm of bone of ear (meatus) (C41.Ø)
          malignant neoplasm of cartilage of ear (C49.Ø)
          malignant melanoma of skin of (external) ear (C43.2-)
          other and unspecified malignant neoplasm of skin of (external) ear (C44.2-)

✓4ᵗʰ C31 Malignant neoplasm of accessory sinuses

- **C31.Ø** Malignant neoplasm of maxillary sinus `HCC` `Rx` `ESR` `COM`
  Malignant neoplasm of antrum (Highmore) (maxillary)
- **C31.1** Malignant neoplasm of ethmoidal sinus `HCC` `Rx` `ESR` `COM`
- **C31.2** Malignant neoplasm of frontal sinus `HCC` `Rx` `ESR` `COM`
- **C31.3** Malignant neoplasm of sphenoid sinus `HCC` `Rx` `ESR` `COM`
- **C31.8** Malignant neoplasm of overlapping sites of accessory sinuses `HCC` `Rx` `ESR` `COM`
- **C31.9** Malignant neoplasm of accessory sinus, unspecified `HCC` `Rx` `ESR` `COM`

✓4ᵗʰ C32 Malignant neoplasm of larynx

Use additional code to identify:
alcohol abuse and dependence (F1Ø.-)
exposure to environmental tobacco smoke (Z77.22)
exposure to tobacco smoke in the perinatal period (P96.81)
history of tobacco dependence (Z87.891)
occupational exposure to environmental tobacco smoke (Z57.31)
tobacco dependence (F17.-)
tobacco use (Z72.Ø)

- **C32.Ø** Malignant neoplasm of glottis `HCC` `ESR` `COM`
  Malignant neoplasm of intrinsic larynx
  Malignant neoplasm of laryngeal commissure (anterior)(posterior)
  Malignant neoplasm of vocal cord (true) NOS
- **C32.1** Malignant neoplasm of supraglottis `HCC` `ESR` `COM`
  Malignant neoplasm of aryepiglottic fold or interarytenoid fold, laryngeal aspect
  Malignant neoplasm of epiglottis (suprahyoid portion) NOS
  Malignant neoplasm of extrinsic larynx
  Malignant neoplasm of false vocal cord
  Malignant neoplasm of posterior (laryngeal) surface of epiglottis
  Malignant neoplasm of ventricular bands
  EXCLUDES 2   malignant neoplasm of anterior surface of epiglottis (C1Ø.1)
          malignant neoplasm of aryepiglottic fold or interarytenoid fold, hypopharyngeal aspect (C13.1)
          malignant neoplasm of aryepiglottic fold or interarytenoid fold, marginal zone (C13.1)
          malignant neoplasm of aryepiglottic fold or interarytenoid fold NOS (C13.1)
- **C32.2** Malignant neoplasm of subglottis `HCC` `ESR` `COM`
- **C32.3** Malignant neoplasm of laryngeal cartilage `HCC` `ESR` `COM`
- **C32.8** Malignant neoplasm of overlapping sites of larynx `HCC` `ESR` `COM`
- **C32.9** Malignant neoplasm of larynx, unspecified `HCC` `ESR` `COM`

C33 Malignant neoplasm of trachea `HCC` `Rx` `ESR` `COM`

Use additional code to identify:
exposure to environmental tobacco smoke (Z77.22)
exposure to tobacco smoke in the perinatal period (P96.81)
history of tobacco dependence (Z87.891)
occupational exposure to environmental tobacco smoke (Z57.31)
tobacco dependence (F17.-)
tobacco use (Z72.Ø)

☑4ᵗʰ **C34 Malignant neoplasm of** bronchus and lung

Use additional code to identify:
    exposure to environmental tobacco smoke (Z77.22)
    exposure to tobacco smoke in the perinatal period (P96.81)
    history of tobacco dependence (Z87.891)
    occupational exposure to environmental tobacco smoke (Z57.31)
    tobacco dependence (F17.-)
    tobacco use (Z72.0)

EXCLUDES 1   Kaposi's sarcoma of lung (C46.5-)
       malignant carcinoid tumor of the bronchus and lung
        (C7A.090)

AHA: 2019,1Q,16

TIP: When documented, assign code I31.3 for associated malignant pericardial effusion. If the sole reason for admission is to treat the effusion with no treatment of the lung malignancy rendered, code I31.3 may be sequenced first.

☑5ᵗʰ **C34.0 Malignant neoplasm of** main bronchus

    Malignant neoplasm of carina
    Malignant neoplasm of hilus (of lung)

    C34.00 Malignant neoplasm of unspecified main bronchus HCC Rx ESR COM Q

    C34.01 Malignant neoplasm of right **main bronchus** HCC Rx ESR COM Q

    C34.02 Malignant neoplasm of left **main bronchus** HCC Rx ESR COM Q

☑5ᵗʰ **C34.1 Malignant neoplasm of** upper lobe, **bronchus or lung**

    C34.10 Malignant neoplasm of upper lobe, unspecified bronchus or lung HCC Rx ESR COM Q

    C34.11 Malignant neoplasm of upper lobe, right **bronchus or lung** HCC Rx ESR COM Q

    C34.12 Malignant neoplasm of upper lobe, left **bronchus or lung** HCC Rx ESR COM Q

C34.2 Malignant neoplasm of middle lobe, **bronchus or lung** HCC Rx ESR COM Q

☑5ᵗʰ **C34.3 Malignant neoplasm of** lower lobe, **bronchus or lung**

    C34.30 Malignant neoplasm of lower lobe, unspecified bronchus or lung HCC Rx ESR COM Q

    C34.31 Malignant neoplasm of lower lobe, right **bronchus or lung** HCC Rx ESR COM Q

    C34.32 Malignant neoplasm of lower lobe, left **bronchus or lung** HCC Rx ESR COM Q

☑5ᵗʰ **C34.8 Malignant neoplasm of** overlapping sites **of bronchus and lung**

    C34.80 Malignant neoplasm of overlapping sites of unspecified bronchus and lung HCC Rx ESR COM Q

    C34.81 Malignant neoplasm of overlapping sites of right **bronchus and lung** HCC Rx ESR COM Q

    C34.82 Malignant neoplasm of overlapping sites of left **bronchus and lung** HCC Rx ESR COM Q

☑5ᵗʰ **C34.9 Malignant neoplasm of unspecified part of bronchus or lung**

    C34.90 Malignant neoplasm of unspecified part of unspecified bronchus or lung HCC Rx ESR COM Q
       Lung cancer NOS

    C34.91 Malignant neoplasm of unspecified part of right **bronchus or lung** HCC Rx ESR COM Q

    C34.92 Malignant neoplasm of unspecified part of left **bronchus or lung** HCC Rx ESR COM Q

C37 Malignant neoplasm of thymus   HCC Rx ESR COM

    EXCLUDES 1   malignant carcinoid tumor of the thymus (C7A.091)

☑4ᵗʰ **C38 Malignant neoplasm of** heart, mediastinum and pleura

    EXCLUDES 1   mesothelioma (C45.-)

C38.0 Malignant neoplasm of heart   HCC Rx ESR COM
    Malignant neoplasm of pericardium
    EXCLUDES 1   malignant neoplasm of great vessels (C49.3)

C38.1 Malignant neoplasm of anterior mediastinum   HCC Rx ESR COM

C38.2 Malignant neoplasm of posterior mediastinum   HCC Rx ESR COM

C38.3 Malignant neoplasm of mediastinum, **part unspecified**   HCC Rx ESR COM

C38.4 Malignant neoplasm of pleura   HCC Rx ESR COM

C38.8 Malignant neoplasm of overlapping sites **of heart, mediastinum and pleura**   HCC Rx ESR COM

☑4ᵗʰ **C39 Malignant neoplasm of other and ill-defined sites in the** respiratory system and intrathoracic organs

Use additional code to identify:
    exposure to environmental tobacco smoke (Z77.22)
    exposure to tobacco smoke in the perinatal period (P96.81)
    history of tobacco dependence (Z87.891)
    occupational exposure to environmental tobacco smoke (Z57.31)
    tobacco dependence (F17.-)
    tobacco use (Z72.0)

EXCLUDES 1   intrathoracic malignant neoplasm NOS (C76.1)
       thoracic malignant neoplasm NOS (C76.1)

C39.0 Malignant neoplasm of upper **respiratory tract, part unspecified**   HCC Rx ESR COM

C39.9 Malignant neoplasm of lower **respiratory tract, part unspecified**   HCC Rx ESR COM
    Malignant neoplasm of respiratory tract NOS

Malignant neoplasms of bone and articular cartilage (C40-C41)

INCLUDES   malignant neoplasm of cartilage (articular) (joint)
       malignant neoplasm of periosteum
EXCLUDES 1   malignant neoplasm of bone marrow NOS (C96.9)
       malignant neoplasm of synovia (C49.-)

☑4ᵗʰ **C40 Malignant neoplasm of** bone and articular cartilage of limbs

Use additional code to identify major osseous defect, if applicable (M89.7-)

☑5ᵗʰ **C40.0 Malignant neoplasm of** scapula and long bones of upper limb

    C40.00 Malignant neoplasm of scapula and long bones of unspecified upper limb HCC Rx ESR COM

    C40.01 Malignant neoplasm of scapula and long bones of right **upper limb** HCC Rx ESR COM

    C40.02 Malignant neoplasm of scapula and long bones of left **upper limb** HCC Rx ESR COM

☑5ᵗʰ **C40.1 Malignant neoplasm of** short bones of upper limb

    C40.10 Malignant neoplasm of short bones of unspecified upper limb HCC Rx ESR COM

    C40.11 Malignant neoplasm of short bones of right **upper limb** HCC Rx ESR COM

    C40.12 Malignant neoplasm of short bones of left **upper limb** HCC Rx ESR COM

☑5ᵗʰ **C40.2 Malignant neoplasm of** long bones of lower limb

    C40.20 Malignant neoplasm of long bones of unspecified lower limb HCC Rx ESR COM

    C40.21 Malignant neoplasm of long bones of right **lower limb** HCC Rx ESR COM

    C40.22 Malignant neoplasm of long bones of left **lower limb** HCC Rx ESR COM

☑5ᵗʰ **C40.3 Malignant neoplasm of** short bones of lower limb

    C40.30 Malignant neoplasm of short bones of unspecified lower limb HCC Rx ESR COM

    C40.31 Malignant neoplasm of short bones of right **lower limb** HCC Rx ESR COM

    C40.32 Malignant neoplasm of short bones of left **lower limb** HCC Rx ESR COM

☑5ᵗʰ **C40.8 Malignant neoplasm of** overlapping sites **of bone and articular cartilage of limb**

    C40.80 Malignant neoplasm of overlapping sites of bone and articular cartilage of unspecified limb HCC Rx ESR COM

    C40.81 Malignant neoplasm of overlapping sites of bone and articular cartilage of right **limb** HCC Rx ESR COM

    C40.82 Malignant neoplasm of overlapping sites of bone and articular cartilage of left **limb** HCC Rx ESR COM

☑5ᵗʰ **C40.9 Malignant neoplasm of unspecified bones and articular cartilage of limb**

    C40.90 Malignant neoplasm of unspecified bones and articular cartilage of unspecified limb HCC Rx ESR COM

    C40.91 Malignant neoplasm of unspecified bones and articular cartilage of right **limb** HCC Rx ESR COM

    C40.92 Malignant neoplasm of unspecified bones and articular cartilage of left **limb** HCC Rx ESR COM

(handwritten note: longbones = tibia)

☑ Additional Character Required   ✓x7ᵗʰ Placeholder Alert   Manifestation   Unspecified Dx   Q QPP   UPD Unacceptable PDx

√4ᵗʰ **C41 Malignant neoplasm of bone and articular cartilage of other and unspecified sites**

     EXCLUDES 1   malignant neoplasm of bones of limbs (C40.-)
                malignant neoplasm of cartilage of ear (C49.0)
                malignant neoplasm of cartilage of eyelid (C49.0)
                malignant neoplasm of cartilage of larynx (C32.3)
                malignant neoplasm of cartilage of limbs (C40.-)
                malignant neoplasm of cartilage of nose (C30.0)

C41.0 Malignant neoplasm of bones of skull and face HCC Rx ESR COM
     Malignant neoplasm of maxilla (superior)
     Malignant neoplasm of orbital bone
     EXCLUDES 2   carcinoma, any type except intraosseous or odontogenic of:
                maxillary sinus (C31.0)
                upper jaw (C03.0)
                malignant neoplasm of jaw bone (lower) (C41.1)

C41.1 Malignant neoplasm of mandible HCC Rx ESR COM
     Malignant neoplasm of inferior maxilla
     Malignant neoplasm of lower jaw bone
     EXCLUDES 2   carcinoma, any type except intraosseous or odontogenic of:
                jaw NOS (C03.9)
                lower (C03.1)
                malignant neoplasm of upper jaw bone (C41.0)

C41.2 Malignant neoplasm of vertebral column HCC Rx ESR COM
     EXCLUDES 1   malignant neoplasm of sacrum and coccyx (C41.4)

C41.3 Malignant neoplasm of ribs, sternum and clavicle HCC Rx ESR COM

C41.4 Malignant neoplasm of pelvic bones, sacrum and coccyx HCC Rx ESR COM

C41.9 Malignant neoplasm of bone and articular cartilage, unspecified HCC Rx ESR COM

Melanoma and other malignant neoplasms of skin (C43-C44)

√4ᵗʰ **C43 Malignant melanoma of skin**

     EXCLUDES 1   melanoma in situ (D03.-)
     EXCLUDES 2   malignant melanoma of skin of genital organs (C51-C52, C60.-, C63.-)
                Merkel cell carcinoma (C4A.-)
                sites other than skin - code to malignant neoplasm of the site

C43.0 Malignant melanoma of lip HCC Rx ESR COM Q
     EXCLUDES 1   malignant neoplasm of vermilion border of lip (C00.0-C00.2)

√5ᵗʰ **C43.1 Malignant melanoma of eyelid, including canthus**
     AHA: 2018,4Q,4

     C43.10 Malignant melanoma of unspecified eyelid, including canthus HCC Rx ESR COM

     √6ᵗʰ **C43.11 Malignant melanoma of right eyelid, including canthus**
         C43.111 Malignant melanoma of right upper eyelid, including canthus HCC Rx ESR COM
         C43.112 Malignant melanoma of right lower eyelid, including canthus HCC Rx ESR COM

     √6ᵗʰ **C43.12 Malignant melanoma of left eyelid, including canthus**
         C43.121 Malignant melanoma of left upper eyelid, including canthus HCC Rx ESR COM
         C43.122 Malignant melanoma of left lower eyelid, including canthus HCC Rx ESR COM

√5ᵗʰ **C43.2 Malignant melanoma of ear and external auricular canal**

     C43.20 Malignant melanoma of unspecified ear and external auricular canal HCC Rx ESR COM Q
     C43.21 Malignant melanoma of right ear and external auricular canal HCC Rx ESR COM Q
     C43.22 Malignant melanoma of left ear and external auricular canal HCC Rx ESR COM Q

√5ᵗʰ **C43.3 Malignant melanoma of other and unspecified parts of face**

     C43.30 Malignant melanoma of unspecified part of face HCC Rx ESR COM Q
     C43.31 Malignant melanoma of nose HCC Rx ESR COM Q
     C43.39 Malignant melanoma of other parts of face HCC Rx ESR COM Q

C43.4 Malignant melanoma of scalp and neck HCC Rx ESR COM Q

√5ᵗʰ **C43.5 Malignant melanoma of trunk**
     EXCLUDES 2   malignant neoplasm of anus NOS (C21.0)
                malignant neoplasm of scrotum (C63.2)

     C43.51 Malignant melanoma of anal skin HCC Rx ESR COM Q
         Malignant melanoma of anal margin
         Malignant melanoma of perianal skin
     C43.52 Malignant melanoma of skin of breast HCC Rx ESR COM Q
     C43.59 Malignant melanoma of other part of trunk HCC Rx ESR COM Q

√5ᵗʰ **C43.6 Malignant melanoma of upper limb, including shoulder**

     C43.60 Malignant melanoma of unspecified upper limb, including shoulder HCC Rx ESR COM Q
     C43.61 Malignant melanoma of right upper limb, including shoulder HCC Rx ESR COM Q
     C43.62 Malignant melanoma of left upper limb, including shoulder HCC Rx ESR COM Q

√5ᵗʰ **C43.7 Malignant melanoma of lower limb, including hip**

     C43.70 Malignant melanoma of unspecified lower limb, including hip HCC Rx ESR COM Q
     C43.71 Malignant melanoma of right lower limb, including hip HCC Rx ESR COM Q
     C43.72 Malignant melanoma of left lower limb, including hip HCC Rx ESR COM Q

C43.8 Malignant melanoma of overlapping sites of skin HCC Rx ESR COM Q

C43.9 Malignant melanoma of skin, unspecified HCC Rx ESR COM Q
     Malignant melanoma of unspecified site of skin
     Melanoma (malignant) NOS

√4ᵗʰ **C4A Merkel cell carcinoma**

     DEF: Malignant cutaneous cancer predominantly found in elderly patients with sun exposure that usually presents as a flesh-colored or bluish-red lump typically seen on the neck, head, and face.

C4A.0 Merkel cell carcinoma of lip HCC Rx ESR COM
     EXCLUDES 1   malignant neoplasm of vermilion border of lip (C00.0-C00.2)

√5ᵗʰ **C4A.1 Merkel cell carcinoma of eyelid, including canthus**
     AHA: 2018,4Q,4

     C4A.10 Merkel cell carcinoma of unspecified eyelid, including canthus HCC Rx ESR COM

     √6ᵗʰ **C4A.11 Merkel cell carcinoma of right eyelid, including canthus**
         C4A.111 Merkel cell carcinoma of right upper eyelid, including canthus HCC Rx ESR COM
         C4A.112 Merkel cell carcinoma of right lower eyelid, including canthus HCC Rx ESR COM

     √6ᵗʰ **C4A.12 Merkel cell carcinoma of left eyelid, including canthus**
         C4A.121 Merkel cell carcinoma of left upper eyelid, including canthus HCC Rx ESR COM
         C4A.122 Merkel cell carcinoma of left lower eyelid, including canthus HCC Rx ESR COM

√5ᵗʰ **C4A.2 Merkel cell carcinoma of ear and external auricular canal**

     C4A.20 Merkel cell carcinoma of unspecified ear and external auricular canal HCC Rx ESR COM
     C4A.21 Merkel cell carcinoma of right ear and external auricular canal HCC Rx ESR COM
     C4A.22 Merkel cell carcinoma of left ear and external auricular canal HCC Rx ESR COM

√5ᵗʰ **C4A.3 Merkel cell carcinoma of other and unspecified parts of face**

     C4A.30 Merkel cell carcinoma of unspecified part of face HCC Rx ESR COM
     C4A.31 Merkel cell carcinoma of nose HCC Rx ESR COM
     C4A.39 Merkel cell carcinoma of other parts of face HCC Rx ESR COM

C4A.4 Merkel cell carcinoma of scalp and neck HCC Rx ESR COM

✓5ᵗʰ **C4A.5** **Merkel cell carcinoma of** trunk

    EXCLUDES 2   malignant neoplasm of anus NOS (C21.0)

                 malignant neoplasm of scrotum (C63.2)

    C4A.51   **Merkel cell carcinoma of** anal skin   HCC Rx ESR COM

           Merkel cell carcinoma of anal margin

           Merkel cell carcinoma of perianal skin

    C4A.52   **Merkel cell carcinoma of** skin of breast   HCC Rx ESR COM

    C4A.59   **Merkel cell carcinoma of other part of trunk**   HCC Rx ESR COM

✓5ᵗʰ **C4A.6** **Merkel cell carcinoma of** upper limb, including shoulder

    C4A.60   **Merkel cell carcinoma of unspecified upper limb, including shoulder**   HCC Rx ESR COM

    C4A.61   **Merkel cell carcinoma of** right **upper limb, including shoulder**   HCC Rx ESR COM

    C4A.62   **Merkel cell carcinoma of** left **upper limb, including shoulder**   HCC Rx ESR COM

✓5ᵗʰ **C4A.7** **Merkel cell carcinoma of** lower limb, including hip

    C4A.70   **Merkel cell carcinoma of unspecified lower limb, including hip**   HCC Rx ESR COM

    C4A.71   **Merkel cell carcinoma of** right **lower limb, including hip**   HCC Rx ESR COM

    C4A.72   **Merkel cell carcinoma of** left **lower limb, including hip**   HCC Rx ESR COM

  C4A.8   **Merkel cell carcinoma of** overlapping sites   HCC Rx ESR COM

  C4A.9   **Merkel cell carcinoma, unspecified**   HCC Rx ESR COM

          Merkel cell carcinoma of unspecified site

          Merkel cell carcinoma NOS

✓4ᵗʰ **C44** **Other and unspecified malignant neoplasm of skin**

    INCLUDES   malignant neoplasm of sebaceous glands

              malignant neoplasm of sweat glands

    EXCLUDES 1   Kaposi's sarcoma of skin (C46.0)

              malignant melanoma of skin (C43.-)

              malignant neoplasm of skin of genital organs (C51-C52, C60.-, C63.2)

              Merkel cell carcinoma (C4A.-)

    DEF: Basal cell carcinoma: Abnormal growth of skin cells that arises from the deepest layer of the epidermis and may present as an open sore, red patches, pink growth, or scar. Typically caused by sun exposure, it is one of the most common forms of skin cancer.

    DEF: Squamous cell carcinoma: Uncontrolled growth of abnormal skin cells that arises from the outer layers of the skin (epidermis) and may present as an open sore. It is characterized by a firm, red nodule, elevated growth with a central depression, or a flat sore with a scaly crust.

✓5ᵗʰ **C44.0** **Other and unspecified malignant neoplasm of skin of** lip

    EXCLUDES 1   malignant neoplasm of lip (C00.-)

    C44.00   **Unspecified malignant neoplasm of skin of lip**

    C44.01   **Basal cell carcinoma of skin of lip**

    C44.02   **Squamous cell carcinoma of skin of lip**

    C44.09   **Other specified malignant neoplasm of skin of lip**

✓5ᵗʰ **C44.1** **Other and unspecified malignant neoplasm of skin of** eyelid, including canthus

    EXCLUDES 1   connective tissue of eyelid (C49.0)

    AHA: 2018,4Q,4

  ✓6ᵗʰ **C44.10**   **Unspecified malignant neoplasm of skin of eyelid, including canthus**

      C44.101   **Unspecified malignant neoplasm of skin of unspecified eyelid, including canthus**

     ✓7ᵗʰ **C44.102**   **Unspecified malignant neoplasm of skin of right eyelid, including canthus**

          C44.1021   **Unspecified malignant neoplasm of skin of right upper eyelid, including canthus**

          C44.1022   **Unspecified malignant neoplasm of skin of right lower eyelid, including canthus**

     ✓7ᵗʰ **C44.109**   **Unspecified malignant neoplasm of skin of left eyelid, including canthus**

          C44.1091   **Unspecified malignant neoplasm of skin of left upper eyelid, including canthus**

          C44.1092   **Unspecified malignant neoplasm of skin of left lower eyelid, including canthus**

  ✓6ᵗʰ **C44.11**   **Basal cell carcinoma of skin of eyelid, including canthus**

      C44.111   **Basal cell carcinoma of skin of unspecified eyelid, including canthus**

     ✓7ᵗʰ **C44.112**   **Basal cell carcinoma of skin of** right **eyelid, including canthus**

          C44.1121   **Basal cell carcinoma of skin of right upper eyelid, including canthus**

          C44.1122   **Basal cell carcinoma of skin of right lower eyelid, including canthus**

     ✓7ᵗʰ **C44.119**   **Basal cell carcinoma of skin of** left **eyelid, including canthus**

          C44.1191   **Basal cell carcinoma of skin of left upper eyelid, including canthus**

          C44.1192   **Basal cell carcinoma of skin of left lower eyelid, including canthus**

  ✓6ᵗʰ **C44.12**   Squamous cell carcinoma **of skin of eyelid, including canthus**

      C44.121   **Squamous cell carcinoma of skin of unspecified eyelid, including canthus**

     ✓7ᵗʰ **C44.122**   **Squamous cell carcinoma of skin of** right **eyelid, including canthus**

          C44.1221   **Squamous cell carcinoma of skin of right upper eyelid, including canthus**

          C44.1222   **Squamous cell carcinoma of skin of right lower eyelid, including canthus**

     ✓7ᵗʰ **C44.129**   **Squamous cell carcinoma of skin of** left **eyelid, including canthus**

          C44.1291   **Squamous cell carcinoma of skin of left upper eyelid, including canthus**

          C44.1292   **Squamous cell carcinoma of skin of left lower eyelid, including canthus**

  ✓6ᵗʰ **C44.13**   Sebaceous cell carcinoma **of skin of eyelid, including canthus**

      C44.131   **Sebaceous cell carcinoma of skin of unspecified eyelid, including canthus**

     ✓7ᵗʰ **C44.132**   **Sebaceous cell carcinoma of skin of** right **eyelid, including canthus**

          C44.1321   **Sebaceous cell carcinoma of skin of right upper eyelid, including canthus**

          C44.1322   **Sebaceous cell carcinoma of skin of right lower eyelid, including canthus**

     ✓7ᵗʰ **C44.139**   **Sebaceous cell carcinoma of skin of** left **eyelid, including canthus**

          C44.1391   **Sebaceous cell carcinoma of skin of left upper eyelid, including canthus**

          C44.1392   **Sebaceous cell carcinoma of skin of left lower eyelid, including canthus**

  ✓6ᵗʰ **C44.19**   **Other specified malignant neoplasm of skin of eyelid, including canthus**

      C44.191   **Other specified malignant neoplasm of skin of unspecified eyelid, including canthus**

     ✓7ᵗʰ **C44.192**   **Other specified malignant neoplasm of skin of** right **eyelid, including canthus**

          C44.1921   **Other specified malignant neoplasm of skin of right upper eyelid, including canthus**

          C44.1922   **Other specified malignant neoplasm of skin of right lower eyelid, including canthus**

     ✓7ᵗʰ **C44.199**   **Other specified malignant neoplasm of skin of** left **eyelid, including canthus**

          C44.1991   **Other specified malignant neoplasm of skin of left upper eyelid, including canthus**

          C44.1992   **Other specified malignant neoplasm of skin of left lower eyelid, including canthus**

Chapter 2. Neoplasms

C44.2–C44.699

✓5ᵗʰ **C44.2** Other and unspecified malignant neoplasm of skin of ear and external auricular canal
> EXCLUDES 1   connective tissue of ear (C49.0)

   ✓6ᵗʰ **C44.20** Unspecified malignant neoplasm of skin of ear and external auricular canal
     C44.201 Unspecified malignant neoplasm of skin of unspecified ear and external auricular canal
     C44.202 Unspecified malignant neoplasm of skin of right ear and external auricular canal
     C44.209 Unspecified malignant neoplasm of skin of left ear and external auricular canal

   ✓6ᵗʰ **C44.21** Basal cell carcinoma of skin of ear and external auricular canal
     C44.211 Basal cell carcinoma of skin of unspecified ear and external auricular canal
     C44.212 Basal cell carcinoma of skin of right ear and external auricular canal
     C44.219 Basal cell carcinoma of skin of left ear and external auricular canal

   ✓6ᵗʰ **C44.22** Squamous cell carcinoma of skin of ear and external auricular canal

SCC ↙ (handwritten annotation)

     C44.221 Squamous cell carcinoma of skin of unspecified ear and external auricular canal
     C44.222 Squamous cell carcinoma of skin of right ear and external auricular canal
     C44.229 Squamous cell carcinoma of skin of left ear and external auricular canal

   ✓6ᵗʰ **C44.29** Other specified malignant neoplasm of skin of ear and external auricular canal
     C44.291 Other specified malignant neoplasm of skin of unspecified ear and external auricular canal
     C44.292 Other specified malignant neoplasm of skin of right ear and external auricular canal
     C44.299 Other specified malignant neoplasm of skin of left ear and external auricular canal

✓5ᵗʰ **C44.3** Other and unspecified malignant neoplasm of skin of other and unspecified parts of face

   ✓6ᵗʰ **C44.30** Unspecified malignant neoplasm of skin of other and unspecified parts of face
     C44.300 Unspecified malignant neoplasm of skin of unspecified part of face
     C44.301 Unspecified malignant neoplasm of skin of nose
     C44.309 Unspecified malignant neoplasm of skin of other parts of face

   ✓6ᵗʰ **C44.31** Basal cell carcinoma of skin of other and unspecified parts of face
     C44.310 Basal cell carcinoma of skin of unspecified parts of face
     C44.311 Basal cell carcinoma of skin of nose
     C44.319 Basal cell carcinoma of skin of other parts of face

   ✓6ᵗʰ **C44.32** Squamous cell carcinoma of skin of other and unspecified parts of face
     C44.320 Squamous cell carcinoma of skin of unspecified parts of face
     C44.321 Squamous cell carcinoma of skin of nose
     C44.329 Squamous cell carcinoma of skin of other parts of face

   ✓6ᵗʰ **C44.39** Other specified malignant neoplasm of skin of other and unspecified parts of face
     C44.390 Other specified malignant neoplasm of skin of unspecified parts of face
     C44.391 Other specified malignant neoplasm of skin of nose
     C44.399 Other specified malignant neoplasm of skin of other parts of face

✓5ᵗʰ **C44.4** Other and unspecified malignant neoplasm of skin of scalp and neck
   C44.40 Unspecified malignant neoplasm of skin of scalp and neck
   C44.41 Basal cell carcinoma of skin of scalp and neck
   C44.42 Squamous cell carcinoma of skin of scalp and neck
   C44.49 Other specified malignant neoplasm of skin of scalp and neck

✓5ᵗʰ **C44.5** Other and unspecified malignant neoplasm of skin of trunk
> EXCLUDES 1   anus NOS (C21.0)
> scrotum (C63.2)

   ✓6ᵗʰ **C44.50** Unspecified malignant neoplasm of skin of trunk
     C44.500 Unspecified malignant neoplasm of anal skin
       Unspecified malignant neoplasm of anal margin
       Unspecified malignant neoplasm of perianal skin
     C44.501 Unspecified malignant neoplasm of skin of breast
     C44.509 Unspecified malignant neoplasm of skin of other part of trunk

   ✓6ᵗʰ **C44.51** Basal cell carcinoma of skin of trunk
     C44.510 Basal cell carcinoma of anal skin
       Basal cell carcinoma of anal margin
       Basal cell carcinoma of perianal skin
     C44.511 Basal cell carcinoma of skin of breast
     C44.519 Basal cell carcinoma of skin of other part of trunk

   ✓6ᵗʰ **C44.52** Squamous cell carcinoma of skin of trunk
     C44.520 Squamous cell carcinoma of anal skin
       Squamous cell carcinoma of anal margin
       Squamous cell carcinoma of perianal skin
     C44.521 Squamous cell carcinoma of skin of breast
     C44.529 Squamous cell carcinoma of skin of other part of trunk

   ✓6ᵗʰ **C44.59** Other specified malignant neoplasm of skin of trunk
     C44.590 Other specified malignant neoplasm of anal skin
       Other specified malignant neoplasm of anal margin
       Other specified malignant neoplasm of perianal skin
     C44.591 Other specified malignant neoplasm of skin of breast
     C44.599 Other specified malignant neoplasm of skin of other part of trunk

✓5ᵗʰ **C44.6** Other and unspecified malignant neoplasm of skin of upper limb, including shoulder

   ✓6ᵗʰ **C44.60** Unspecified malignant neoplasm of skin of upper limb, including shoulder
     C44.601 Unspecified malignant neoplasm of skin of unspecified upper limb, including shoulder
     C44.602 Unspecified malignant neoplasm of skin of right upper limb, including shoulder
     C44.609 Unspecified malignant neoplasm of skin of left upper limb, including shoulder

   ✓6ᵗʰ **C44.61** Basal cell carcinoma of skin of upper limb, including shoulder
     C44.611 Basal cell carcinoma of skin of unspecified upper limb, including shoulder
     C44.612 Basal cell carcinoma of skin of right upper limb, including shoulder
     C44.619 Basal cell carcinoma of skin of left upper limb, including shoulder

   ✓6ᵗʰ **C44.62** Squamous cell carcinoma of skin of upper limb, including shoulder
     C44.621 Squamous cell carcinoma of skin of unspecified upper limb, including shoulder
     C44.622 Squamous cell carcinoma of skin of right upper limb, including shoulder
     C44.629 Squamous cell carcinoma of skin of left upper limb, including shoulder

   ✓6ᵗʰ **C44.69** Other specified malignant neoplasm of skin of upper limb, including shoulder
     C44.691 Other specified malignant neoplasm of skin of unspecified upper limb, including shoulder
     C44.692 Other specified malignant neoplasm of skin of right upper limb, including shoulder
     C44.699 Other specified malignant neoplasm of skin of left upper limb, including shoulder

☑5ᵗʰ **C44.7** **Other and unspecified malignant neoplasm of skin of** lower limb, including hip

   ☑6ᵗʰ **C44.70** **Unspecified malignant neoplasm of skin of lower limb, including hip**

       C44.701 **Unspecified malignant neoplasm of skin of unspecified lower limb, including hip**

       C44.702 **Unspecified malignant neoplasm of skin of** right **lower limb, including hip**

       C44.709 **Unspecified malignant neoplasm of skin of** left **lower limb, including hip**

   ☑6ᵗʰ **C44.71** Basal cell carcinoma **of skin of lower limb, including hip**

       C44.711 **Basal cell carcinoma of skin of unspecified lower limb, including hip**

       C44.712 **Basal cell carcinoma of skin of** right **lower limb, including hip**

       C44.719 **Basal cell carcinoma of skin of** left **lower limb, including hip**

   ☑6ᵗʰ **C44.72** Squamous cell carcinoma **of skin of lower limb, including hip**

       C44.721 **Squamous cell carcinoma of skin of unspecified lower limb, including hip**

       C44.722 **Squamous cell carcinoma of skin of** right **lower limb, including hip**

       C44.729 **Squamous cell carcinoma of skin of** left **lower limb, including hip**

   ☑6ᵗʰ **C44.79** **Other specified malignant neoplasm of skin of lower limb, including hip**

       C44.791 **Other specified malignant neoplasm of skin of unspecified lower limb, including hip**

       C44.792 **Other specified malignant neoplasm of skin of** right **lower limb, including hip**

       C44.799 **Other specified malignant neoplasm of skin of** left **lower limb, including hip**

☑5ᵗʰ **C44.8** **Other and unspecified malignant neoplasm of** overlapping sites of skin

    C44.80 **Unspecified malignant neoplasm of overlapping sites of skin**

    C44.81 Basal cell carcinoma **of overlapping sites of skin**

    C44.82 Squamous cell carcinoma **of overlapping sites of skin**

    C44.89 **Other specified malignant neoplasm of overlapping sites of skin**

☑5ᵗʰ **C44.9** **Other and unspecified malignant neoplasm of skin, unspecified**

    C44.90 **Unspecified malignant neoplasm of skin, unspecified**

      Malignant neoplasm of unspecified site of skin

    C44.91 Basal cell carcinoma **of skin, unspecified**

    C44.92 Squamous cell carcinoma **of skin, unspecified**

    C44.99 **Other specified malignant neoplasm of skin, unspecified**

Malignant neoplasms of mesothelial and soft tissue (C45-C49)

☑4ᵗʰ **C45** **Mesothelioma**

    DEF: Rare type of cancer that forms in the thin layer of protective tissue that covers the majority of internal organs (mesothelium).

    C45.0 **Mesothelioma of** pleura   HCC Rx ESR COM

      EXCLUDES 1   *other malignant neoplasm of pleura (C38.4)*

      AHA: 2017,2Q,11

      TIP: For pleural mesothelioma that has metastasized to the chest wall, assign this code for the primary site along with C79.89 for metastatic cancer in the chest wall.

    C45.1 **Mesothelioma of** peritoneum   HCC Rx ESR COM

      Mesothelioma of cul-de-sac

      Mesothelioma of mesentery

      Mesothelioma of mesocolon

      Mesothelioma of omentum

      Mesothelioma of peritoneum (parietal) (pelvic)

      EXCLUDES 1   *other malignant neoplasm of soft tissue of peritoneum (C48.-)*

    C45.2 **Mesothelioma of** pericardium   HCC Rx ESR COM

      EXCLUDES 1   *other malignant neoplasm of pericardium (C38.0)*

    C45.7 **Mesothelioma of other sites**   HCC Rx ESR COM

    C45.9 **Mesothelioma, unspecified**   HCC Rx ESR COM

☑4ᵗʰ **C46** **Kaposi's sarcoma**

    Code first any human immunodeficiency virus [HIV] disease (B20)

    DEF: Malignant neoplasm that causes patches of abnormal tissue to grow under the skin, in the lining of the mouth, nose, and throat, in lymph nodes, or in other visceral organs. Kaposi's sarcoma is caused by human herpesvirus8 (HHV8).

    C46.0 **Kaposi's sarcoma of** skin   HCC Rx ESR COM

    C46.1 **Kaposi's sarcoma of** soft tissue   HCC Rx ESR COM

      Kaposi's sarcoma of blood vessel

      Kaposi's sarcoma of connective tissue

      Kaposi's sarcoma of fascia

      Kaposi's sarcoma of ligament

      Kaposi's sarcoma of lymphatic(s) NEC

      Kaposi's sarcoma of muscle

      EXCLUDES 2   *Kaposi's sarcoma of lymph glands and nodes (C46.3)*

    C46.2 **Kaposi's sarcoma of** palate   HCC Rx ESR COM

    C46.3 **Kaposi's sarcoma of** lymph nodes   HCC Rx ESR COM

    C46.4 **Kaposi's sarcoma of** gastrointestinal sites   HCC Rx ESR COM

   ☑5ᵗʰ **C46.5** **Kaposi's sarcoma of** lung

      AHA: 2019,1Q,16

      TIP: When associated malignant pericardial effusion is documented, assign code I31.3. If the sole reason for admission is to treat the effusion with no treatment of the lung malignancy rendered, code I31.3 may be sequenced first.

      C46.50 **Kaposi's sarcoma of unspecified lung**   HCC Rx ESR COM

      C46.51 **Kaposi's sarcoma of** right **lung**   HCC Rx ESR COM

      C46.52 **Kaposi's sarcoma of** left **lung**   HCC Rx ESR COM

    C46.7 **Kaposi's sarcoma of other sites**   HCC Rx ESR COM

    C46.9 **Kaposi's sarcoma, unspecified**   HCC Rx ESR COM

      Kaposi's sarcoma of unspecified site

☑4ᵗʰ **C47** **Malignant neoplasm of peripheral nerves and autonomic nervous system**

    INCLUDES   malignant neoplasm of sympathetic and parasympathetic nerves and ganglia

    EXCLUDES 1   *Kaposi's sarcoma of soft tissue (C46.1)*

    C47.0 **Malignant neoplasm of peripheral nerves of** head, face and neck   HCC Rx ESR COM

      EXCLUDES 1   *malignant neoplasm of peripheral nerves of orbit (C69.6-)*

   ☑5ᵗʰ **C47.1** **Malignant neoplasm of peripheral nerves of** upper limb, including shoulder

      C47.10 **Malignant neoplasm of peripheral nerves of unspecified upper limb, including shoulder**   HCC Rx ESR COM

      C47.11 **Malignant neoplasm of peripheral nerves of** right **upper limb, including shoulder**   HCC Rx ESR COM

      C47.12 **Malignant neoplasm of peripheral nerves of** left **upper limb, including shoulder**   HCC Rx ESR COM

   ☑5ᵗʰ **C47.2** **Malignant neoplasm of peripheral nerves of** lower limb, including hip

      C47.20 **Malignant neoplasm of peripheral nerves of unspecified lower limb, including hip**   HCC Rx ESR COM

      C47.21 **Malignant neoplasm of peripheral nerves of** right **lower limb, including hip**   HCC Rx ESR COM

      C47.22 **Malignant neoplasm of peripheral nerves of** left **lower limb, including hip**   HCC Rx ESR COM

    C47.3 **Malignant neoplasm of peripheral nerves of** thorax   HCC Rx ESR COM

    C47.4 **Malignant neoplasm of peripheral nerves of** abdomen   HCC Rx ESR COM

    C47.5 **Malignant neoplasm of peripheral nerves of** pelvis   HCC Rx ESR COM

    C47.6 **Malignant neoplasm of peripheral nerves of** trunk, unspecified   HCC Rx ESR COM

      Malignant neoplasm of peripheral nerves of unspecified part of trunk

    C47.8 **Malignant neoplasm of** overlapping sites **of peripheral nerves and autonomic nervous system**   HCC Rx ESR COM

    C47.9 **Malignant neoplasm of peripheral nerves and autonomic nervous system, unspecified**   HCC Rx ESR COM

      Malignant neoplasm of unspecified site of peripheral nerves and autonomic nervous system

✓4ᵗʰ **C48** **Malignant neoplasm of** retroperitoneum and peritoneum

> EXCLUDES 1   Kaposi's sarcoma of connective tissue (C46.1)
> mesothelioma (C45.-)

C48.0 **Malignant neoplasm of** retroperitoneum   HCC Rx ESR COM

C48.1 **Malignant neoplasm of** specified parts of peritoneum   HCC Rx ESR COM

> Malignant neoplasm of cul-de-sac
> Malignant neoplasm of mesentery
> Malignant neoplasm of mesocolon
> Malignant neoplasm of omentum
> Malignant neoplasm of parietal peritoneum
> Malignant neoplasm of pelvic peritoneum

[handwritten: uterus liomosarcoma]

C48.2 **Malignant neoplasm of** peritoneum, unspecified   HCC Rx ESR COM

C48.8 **Malignant neoplasm of** overlapping sites of retroperitoneum and peritoneum   HCC Rx ESR COM

✓4ᵗʰ **C49** **Malignant neoplasm of** other connective and soft tissue

> INCLUDES   malignant neoplasm of blood vessel
> malignant neoplasm of bursa
> malignant neoplasm of cartilage
> malignant neoplasm of fascia
> malignant neoplasm of fat
> malignant neoplasm of ligament, except uterine
> malignant neoplasm of lymphatic vessel
> malignant neoplasm of muscle
> malignant neoplasm of synovia
> malignant neoplasm of tendon (sheath)

> EXCLUDES 1   malignant neoplasm of cartilage (of):
>   articular (C40-C41)
>   larynx (C32.3)
>   nose (C30.0)
> malignant neoplasm of connective tissue of breast (C50.-)

> EXCLUDES 2   Kaposi's sarcoma of soft tissue (C46.1)
> malignant neoplasm of heart (C38.0)
> malignant neoplasm of peripheral nerves and autonomic nervous system (C47.-)
> malignant neoplasm of peritoneum (C48.2)
> malignant neoplasm of retroperitoneum (C48.0)
> malignant neoplasm of uterine ligament (C57.3)
> mesothelioma (C45.-)

C49.0 **Malignant neoplasm of connective and soft tissue of** head, face and neck   HCC Rx ESR COM

> Malignant neoplasm of connective tissue of ear
> Malignant neoplasm of connective tissue of eyelid
> > EXCLUDES 1   connective tissue of orbit (C69.6-)

✓5ᵗʰ **C49.1** **Malignant neoplasm of connective and soft tissue of** upper limb, including shoulder

> **C49.10** **Malignant neoplasm of connective and soft tissue of unspecified upper limb, including shoulder**   HCC Rx ESR COM
>
> **C49.11** **Malignant neoplasm of connective and soft tissue of** right **upper limb, including shoulder**   HCC Rx ESR COM
>
> **C49.12** **Malignant neoplasm of connective and soft tissue of** left **upper limb, including shoulder**   HCC Rx ESR COM

✓5ᵗʰ **C49.2** **Malignant neoplasm of connective and soft tissue of** lower limb, including hip

> **C49.20** **Malignant neoplasm of connective and soft tissue of unspecified lower limb, including hip**   HCC Rx ESR COM
>
> **C49.21** **Malignant neoplasm of connective and soft tissue of** right **lower limb, including hip**   HCC Rx ESR COM
>
> **C49.22** **Malignant neoplasm of connective and soft tissue of** left **lower limb, including hip**   HCC Rx ESR COM

C49.3 **Malignant neoplasm of connective and soft tissue of** thorax   HCC Rx ESR COM

> Malignant neoplasm of axilla
> Malignant neoplasm of diaphragm
> Malignant neoplasm of great vessels
> > EXCLUDES 1   malignant neoplasm of breast (C50.-)
> > malignant neoplasm of heart (C38.0)
> > malignant neoplasm of mediastinum (C38.1-C38.3)
> > malignant neoplasm of thymus (C37)

> **AHA:** 2015,3Q,19

C49.4 **Malignant neoplasm of connective and soft tissue of** abdomen   HCC Rx ESR COM

> Malignant neoplasm of abdominal wall
> Malignant neoplasm of hypochondrium

C49.5 **Malignant neoplasm of connective and soft tissue of** pelvis   HCC Rx ESR COM

> Malignant neoplasm of buttock
> Malignant neoplasm of groin
> Malignant neoplasm of perineum

C49.6 **Malignant neoplasm of connective and soft tissue of** trunk, **unspecified**   HCC Rx ESR COM

> Malignant neoplasm of back NOS

C49.8 **Malignant neoplasm of** overlapping sites **of connective and soft tissue**   HCC Rx ESR COM

> Primary malignant neoplasm of two or more contiguous sites of connective and soft tissue

C49.9 **Malignant neoplasm of connective and soft tissue, unspecified**   HCC Rx ESR COM

✓5ᵗʰ **C49.A** **Gastrointestinal stromal tumor**

> **AHA:** 2016,4Q,8
> **DEF:** Uncommon malignant tumor found in the GI tract that originates from interstitial cells of the autonomic nervous system. Most occur in the stomach or small intestine but can originate anywhere in the GI tract.

> **C49.A0** **Gastrointestinal stromal tumor, unspecified site**   HCC Rx ESR COM
>
> **C49.A1** **Gastrointestinal stromal tumor of** esophagus   HCC Rx ESR COM
>
> **C49.A2** **Gastrointestinal stromal tumor of** stomach   HCC Rx ESR COM
>
> **C49.A3** **Gastrointestinal stromal tumor of** small intestine   HCC Rx ESR COM
>
> **C49.A4** **Gastrointestinal stromal tumor of** large intestine   HCC Rx ESR COM
>
> **C49.A5** **Gastrointestinal stromal tumor of** rectum   HCC Rx ESR COM
>
> **C49.A9** **Gastrointestinal stromal tumor of other** sites   HCC Rx ESR COM

Malignant neoplasms of breast (C50)

✓4ᵗʰ **C50** **Malignant neoplasm of** breast

> INCLUDES   connective tissue of breast
> Paget's disease of breast
> Paget's disease of nipple
> Use additional code to identify estrogen receptor status (Z17.0, Z17.1)
> EXCLUDES 1   skin of breast (C44.501, C44.511, C44.521, C44.591)
> **AHA:** 2017,4Q,19

Female Breast

Upper outer quadrant · Upper inner quadrant · Midline · Areola · Nipple · Axillary tail · Mammary gland · Lower outer quadrant · Lower inner quadrant · Right Breast

✓5ᵗʰ **C50.0** **Malignant neoplasm of** nipple and areola

> ✓6ᵗʰ **C50.01** **Malignant neoplasm of nipple and areola,** female
>
> > **C50.011** **Malignant neoplasm of nipple and areola,** right **female breast**   HCC Rx ESR COM ♀
> >
> > **C50.012** **Malignant neoplasm of nipple and areola,** left **female breast**   HCC Rx ESR COM ♀

C50.019 Malignant neoplasm of nipple and areola, unspecified female breast HCC Rx ESR COM ♀

✓6th **C50.02** Malignant neoplasm of nipple and areola, male

     C50.021 Malignant neoplasm of nipple and areola, right male breast HCC Rx ESR COM ♂

     C50.022 Malignant neoplasm of nipple and areola, left male breast HCC Rx ESR COM ♂

     C50.029 Malignant neoplasm of nipple and areola, unspecified male breast HCC Rx ESR COM ♂

✓5th **C50.1** Malignant neoplasm of central portion of breast

   ✓6th **C50.11** Malignant neoplasm of central portion of breast, female

     C50.111 Malignant neoplasm of central portion of right female breast HCC Rx ESR COM ♀

     C50.112 Malignant neoplasm of central portion of left female breast HCC Rx ESR COM ♀

     C50.119 Malignant neoplasm of central portion of unspecified female breast HCC Rx ESR COM ♀

   ✓6th **C50.12** Malignant neoplasm of central portion of breast, male

     C50.121 Malignant neoplasm of central portion of right male breast HCC Rx ESR COM ♂

     C50.122 Malignant neoplasm of central portion of left male breast HCC Rx ESR COM ♂

     C50.129 Malignant neoplasm of central portion of unspecified male breast HCC Rx ESR COM ♂

✓5th **C50.2** Malignant neoplasm of upper-inner quadrant of breast

   ✓6th **C50.21** Malignant neoplasm of upper-inner quadrant of breast, female

     C50.211 Malignant neoplasm of upper-inner quadrant of right female breast HCC Rx ESR COM ♀

     C50.212 Malignant neoplasm of upper-inner quadrant of left female breast HCC Rx ESR COM ♀

     C50.219 Malignant neoplasm of upper-inner quadrant of unspecified female breast HCC Rx ESR COM ♀

   ✓6th **C50.22** Malignant neoplasm of upper-inner quadrant of breast, male

     C50.221 Malignant neoplasm of upper-inner quadrant of right male breast HCC Rx ESR COM ♂

     C50.222 Malignant neoplasm of upper-inner quadrant of left male breast HCC Rx ESR COM ♂

     C50.229 Malignant neoplasm of upper-inner quadrant of unspecified male breast HCC Rx ESR COM ♂

✓5th **C50.3** Malignant neoplasm of lower-inner quadrant of breast

   ✓6th **C50.31** Malignant neoplasm of lower-inner quadrant of breast, female

     C50.311 Malignant neoplasm of lower-inner quadrant of right female breast HCC Rx ESR COM ♀

     C50.312 Malignant neoplasm of lower-inner quadrant of left female breast HCC Rx ESR COM ♀

     C50.319 Malignant neoplasm of lower-inner quadrant of unspecified female breast HCC Rx ESR COM ♀

   ✓6th **C50.32** Malignant neoplasm of lower-inner quadrant of breast, male

     C50.321 Malignant neoplasm of lower-inner quadrant of right male breast HCC Rx ESR COM ♂

     C50.322 Malignant neoplasm of lower-inner quadrant of left male breast HCC Rx ESR COM ♂

     C50.329 Malignant neoplasm of lower-inner quadrant of unspecified male breast HCC Rx ESR COM ♂

✓5th **C50.4** Malignant neoplasm of upper-outer quadrant of breast

   ✓6th **C50.41** Malignant neoplasm of upper-outer quadrant of breast, female

     C50.411 Malignant neoplasm of upper-outer quadrant of right female breast HCC Rx ESR COM ♀

     C50.412 Malignant neoplasm of upper-outer quadrant of left female breast HCC Rx ESR COM ♀

     C50.419 Malignant neoplasm of upper-outer quadrant of unspecified female breast HCC Rx ESR COM ♀

   ✓6th **C50.42** Malignant neoplasm of upper-outer quadrant of breast, male

     C50.421 Malignant neoplasm of upper-outer quadrant of right male breast HCC Rx ESR COM ♂

     C50.422 Malignant neoplasm of upper-outer quadrant of left male breast HCC Rx ESR COM ♂

     C50.429 Malignant neoplasm of upper-outer quadrant of unspecified male breast HCC Rx ESR COM ♂

✓5th **C50.5** Malignant neoplasm of lower-outer quadrant of breast

   ✓6th **C50.51** Malignant neoplasm of lower-outer quadrant of breast, female

     C50.511 Malignant neoplasm of lower-outer quadrant of right female breast HCC Rx ESR COM ♀

     C50.512 Malignant neoplasm of lower-outer quadrant of left female breast HCC Rx ESR COM ♀

     C50.519 Malignant neoplasm of lower-outer quadrant of unspecified female breast HCC Rx ESR COM ♀

   ✓6th **C50.52** Malignant neoplasm of lower-outer quadrant of breast, male

     C50.521 Malignant neoplasm of lower-outer quadrant of right male breast HCC Rx ESR COM ♂

     C50.522 Malignant neoplasm of lower-outer quadrant of left male breast HCC Rx ESR COM ♂

     C50.529 Malignant neoplasm of lower-outer quadrant of unspecified male breast HCC Rx ESR COM ♂

✓5th **C50.6** Malignant neoplasm of axillary tail of breast

   ✓6th **C50.61** Malignant neoplasm of axillary tail of breast, female

     C50.611 Malignant neoplasm of axillary tail of right female breast HCC Rx ESR COM ♀

     C50.612 Malignant neoplasm of axillary tail of left female breast HCC Rx ESR COM ♀

     C50.619 Malignant neoplasm of axillary tail of unspecified female breast HCC Rx ESR COM ♀

   ✓6th **C50.62** Malignant neoplasm of axillary tail of breast, male

     C50.621 Malignant neoplasm of axillary tail of right male breast HCC Rx ESR COM ♂

     C50.622 Malignant neoplasm of axillary tail of left male breast HCC Rx ESR COM ♂

     C50.629 Malignant neoplasm of axillary tail of unspecified male breast HCC Rx ESR COM ♂

✓5th **C50.8** Malignant neoplasm of overlapping sites of breast

   ✓6th **C50.81** Malignant neoplasm of overlapping sites of breast, female

     C50.811 Malignant neoplasm of overlapping sites of right female breast HCC Rx ESR COM ♀

     C50.812 Malignant neoplasm of overlapping sites of left female breast HCC Rx ESR COM ♀

     C50.819 Malignant neoplasm of overlapping sites of unspecified female breast HCC Rx ESR COM ♀

   ✓6th **C50.82** Malignant neoplasm of overlapping sites of breast, male

     C50.821 Malignant neoplasm of overlapping sites of right male breast HCC Rx ESR COM ♂

     C50.822 Malignant neoplasm of overlapping sites of left male breast HCC Rx ESR COM ♂

✔ Additional Character Required   ✓x7th Placeholder Alert   Manifestation   Unspecified Dx   Q QPP   UPD Unacceptable PDx

Chapter 2. Neoplasms

√5ᵗʰ **C50.829** Malignant neoplasm of overlapping sites of unspecified male breast HCC Rx ESR COM ♂

√5ᵗʰ **C50.9** Malignant neoplasm of breast of unspecified site

√6ᵗʰ **C50.91** Malignant neoplasm of breast of unspecified site, female

C50.911 Malignant neoplasm of unspecified site of right female breast HCC Rx ESR COM ♀

C50.912 Malignant neoplasm of unspecified site of left female breast HCC Rx ESR COM ♀

C50.919 Malignant neoplasm of unspecified site of unspecified female breast HCC Rx ESR COM ♀

√6ᵗʰ **C50.92** Malignant neoplasm of breast of unspecified site, male

C50.921 Malignant neoplasm of unspecified site of right male breast HCC Rx ESR COM ♂

C50.922 Malignant neoplasm of unspecified site of left male breast HCC Rx ESR COM ♂

C50.929 Malignant neoplasm of unspecified site of unspecified male breast HCC Rx ESR COM ♂

Malignant neoplasms of female genital organs (C51-C58)

INCLUDES malignant neoplasm of skin of female genital organs

√4ᵗʰ **C51** Malignant neoplasm of vulva

EXCLUDES 1 carcinoma in situ of vulva (D07.1)

C51.0 Malignant neoplasm of labium majus HCC ESR COM ♀
Malignant neoplasm of Bartholin's [greater vestibular] gland

C51.1 Malignant neoplasm of labium minus HCC ESR COM ♀

C51.2 Malignant neoplasm of clitoris HCC ESR COM ♀

C51.8 Malignant neoplasm of overlapping sites of vulva HCC ESR COM ♀

C51.9 Malignant neoplasm of vulva, unspecified HCC ESR COM ♀
Paget's disease Malignant neoplasm of external female genitalia NOS
Malignant neoplasm of pudendum

√4ᵗʰ **C52** Malignant neoplasm of vagina HCC ESR COM ♀
Vagina EXCLUDES 1 carcinoma in situ of vagina (D07.2)

√4ᵗʰ **C53** Malignant neoplasm of cervix uteri
EXCLUDES 1 carcinoma in situ of cervix uteri (D06.-)
AHA: 2017,4Q,103

C53.0 Malignant neoplasm of endocervix HCC ESR COM ♀

C53.1 Malignant neoplasm of exocervix HCC ESR COM ♀

C53.8 Malignant neoplasm of overlapping sites of cervix uteri HCC ESR COM ♀

C53.9 Malignant neoplasm of cervix uteri, unspecified HCC ESR COM ♀

√4ᵗʰ **C54** Malignant neoplasm of corpus uteri

C54.0 Malignant neoplasm of isthmus uteri HCC ESR COM ♀
Malignant neoplasm of lower uterine segment

C54.1 Malignant neoplasm of endometrium HCC ESR COM ♀

C54.2 Malignant neoplasm of myometrium HCC ESR COM ♀

C54.3 Malignant neoplasm of fundus uteri HCC ESR COM ♀

C54.8 Malignant neoplasm of overlapping sites of corpus uteri HCC ESR COM ♀

C54.9 Malignant neoplasm of corpus uteri, unspecified HCC ESR COM ♀

C55 Malignant neoplasm of uterus, part unspecified HCC ESR COM ♀

√4ᵗʰ **C56** Malignant neoplasm of ovary
Use additional code to identify any functional activity
malignant ovary

C56.1 Malignant neoplasm of right ovary HCC Rx ESR COM ♀

C56.2 Malignant neoplasm of left ovary HCC Rx ESR COM ♀

C56.3 Malignant neoplasm of bilateral ovaries HCC Rx ESR COM ♀

C56.9 Malignant neoplasm of unspecified ovary HCC Rx ESR COM ♀

√4ᵗʰ **C57** Malignant neoplasm of other and unspecified female genital organs

√5ᵗʰ **C57.0** Malignant neoplasm of fallopian tube
Malignant neoplasm of oviduct
Malignant neoplasm of uterine tube

C57.00 Malignant neoplasm of unspecified fallopian tube HCC Rx ESR COM ♀

C57.01 Malignant neoplasm of right fallopian tube HCC Rx ESR COM ♀

C57.02 Malignant neoplasm of left fallopian tube HCC Rx ESR COM ♀

√5ᵗʰ **C57.1** Malignant neoplasm of broad ligament

C57.10 Malignant neoplasm of unspecified broad ligament HCC Rx ESR COM ♀

C57.11 Malignant neoplasm of right broad ligament HCC Rx ESR COM ♀

C57.12 Malignant neoplasm of left broad ligament HCC Rx ESR COM ♀

√5ᵗʰ **C57.2** Malignant neoplasm of round ligament

C57.20 Malignant neoplasm of unspecified round ligament HCC Rx ESR COM ♀

C57.21 Malignant neoplasm of right round ligament HCC Rx ESR COM ♀

C57.22 Malignant neoplasm of left round ligament HCC Rx ESR COM ♀

C57.3 Malignant neoplasm of parametrium HCC Rx ESR COM ♀
Malignant neoplasm of uterine ligament NOS

C57.4 Malignant neoplasm of uterine adnexa, unspecified HCC Rx ESR COM ♀

C57.7 Malignant neoplasm of other specified female genital organs HCC ESR COM ♀
Malignant neoplasm of wolffian body or duct

C57.8 Malignant neoplasm of overlapping sites of female genital organs HCC ESR COM ♀
Primary malignant neoplasm of two or more contiguous sites of the female genital organs whose point of origin cannot be determined
Primary tubo-ovarian malignant neoplasm whose point of origin cannot be determined
Primary utero-ovarian malignant neoplasm whose point of origin cannot be determined

C57.9 Malignant neoplasm of female genital organ, unspecified HCC ESR COM ♀
Malignant neoplasm of female genitourinary tract NOS

C58 Malignant neoplasm of placenta HCC Rx ESR COM M ♀
INCLUDES choriocarcinoma NOS
chorionepithelioma NOS
EXCLUDES 1 chorioadenoma (destruens) (D39.2)
hydatidiform mole NOS (O01.9)
invasive hydatidiform mole (D39.2)
male choriocarcinoma NOS (C62.9-)
malignant hydatidiform mole (D39.2)

Malignant neoplasms of male genital organs (C60-C63)

INCLUDES malignant neoplasm of skin of male genital organs

√4ᵗʰ **C60** Malignant neoplasm of penis

C60.0 Malignant neoplasm of prepuce HCC Rx ESR COM ♂
Malignant neoplasm of foreskin

C60.1 Malignant neoplasm of glans penis HCC Rx ESR COM ♂

C60.2 Malignant neoplasm of body of penis HCC Rx ESR COM ♂
Malignant neoplasm of corpus cavernosum

C60.8 Malignant neoplasm of overlapping sites of penis HCC Rx ESR COM ♂

C60.9 Malignant neoplasm of penis, unspecified HCC Rx ESR COM ♂
Malignant neoplasm of skin of penis NOS

C61 Malignant neoplasm of prostate HCC Rx ESR COM Q ♂
►Use additional code, if applicable, to identify:◄
hormone sensitivity status (Z19.1-Z19.2)
rising PSA following treatment for malignant neoplasm of prostate (R97.21)
EXCLUDES 1 malignant neoplasm of seminal vesicle (C63.7)
AHA: 2017,1Q,17

√4ᵗʰ **C62** Malignant neoplasm of testis
Use additional code to identify any functional activity

√5ᵗʰ **C62.0** Malignant neoplasm of undescended testis
Malignant neoplasm of ectopic testis
Malignant neoplasm of retained testis

C62.00 Malignant neoplasm of unspecified undescended testis HCC Rx ESR COM ♂

C62.01 Malignant neoplasm of undescended right testis HCC Rx ESR COM ♂

C62.02 Malignant neoplasm of undescended left testis `HCC` `Rx` `ESR` `COM` ♂

✓5ᵗʰ **C62.1** Malignant neoplasm of descended testis
Malignant neoplasm of scrotal testis

  C62.10 Malignant neoplasm of unspecified descended testis `HCC` `Rx` `ESR` `COM` ♂

  C62.11 Malignant neoplasm of descended right testis `HCC` `Rx` `ESR` `COM` ♂

  C62.12 Malignant neoplasm of descended left testis `HCC` `Rx` `ESR` `COM` ♂

✓5ᵗʰ **C62.9** Malignant neoplasm of testis, unspecified whether descended or undescended

  C62.90 Malignant neoplasm of unspecified testis, unspecified whether descended or undescended `HCC` `Rx` `ESR` `COM` ♂
Malignant neoplasm of testis NOS

  C62.91 Malignant neoplasm of right testis, unspecified whether descended or undescended `HCC` `Rx` `ESR` `COM` ♂

  C62.92 Malignant neoplasm of left testis, unspecified whether descended or undescended `HCC` `Rx` `ESR` `COM` ♂

✓4ᵗʰ **C63** Malignant neoplasm of other and unspecified male genital organs

✓5ᵗʰ **C63.0** Malignant neoplasm of epididymis

  C63.00 Malignant neoplasm of unspecified epididymis `HCC` `Rx` `ESR` `COM` ♂

  C63.01 Malignant neoplasm of right epididymis `HCC` `Rx` `ESR` `COM` ♂

  C63.02 Malignant neoplasm of left epididymis `HCC` `Rx` `ESR` `COM` ♂

✓5ᵗʰ **C63.1** Malignant neoplasm of spermatic cord

  C63.10 Malignant neoplasm of unspecified spermatic cord `HCC` `Rx` `ESR` `COM` ♂

  C63.11 Malignant neoplasm of right spermatic cord `HCC` `Rx` `ESR` `COM` ♂

  C63.12 Malignant neoplasm of left spermatic cord `HCC` `Rx` `ESR` `COM` ♂

C63.2 Malignant neoplasm of scrotum `HCC` `Rx` `ESR` `COM` ♂
Malignant neoplasm of skin of scrotum

C63.7 Malignant neoplasm of other specified male genital organs `HCC` `Rx` `ESR` `COM` ♂
Malignant neoplasm of seminal vesicle
Malignant neoplasm of tunica vaginalis

C63.8 Malignant neoplasm of overlapping sites of male genital organs `HCC` `Rx` `ESR` `COM` ♂
Primary malignant neoplasm of two or more contiguous sites of male genital organs whose point of origin cannot be determined

C63.9 Malignant neoplasm of male genital organ, unspecified `HCC` `Rx` `ESR` `COM` ♂
Malignant neoplasm of male genitourinary tract NOS

Malignant neoplasms of urinary tract (C64-C68)

✓4ᵗʰ **C64** Malignant neoplasm of kidney, except renal pelvis
  EXCLUDES 1   malignant carcinoid tumor of the kidney (C7A.093)
    malignant neoplasm of renal calyces (C65.-)
    malignant neoplasm of renal pelvis (C65.-)

C64.1 Malignant neoplasm of right kidney, except renal pelvis `HCC` `Rx` `ESR` `COM`

C64.2 Malignant neoplasm of left kidney, except renal pelvis `HCC` `Rx` `ESR` `COM`

C64.9 Malignant neoplasm of unspecified kidney, except renal pelvis `HCC` `Rx` `ESR` `COM`

✓4ᵗʰ **C65** Malignant neoplasm of renal pelvis
  INCLUDES   malignant neoplasm of pelviureteric junction
    malignant neoplasm of renal calyces

C65.1 Malignant neoplasm of right renal pelvis `HCC` `Rx` `ESR` `COM`

C65.2 Malignant neoplasm of left renal pelvis `HCC` `Rx` `ESR` `COM`

C65.9 Malignant neoplasm of unspecified renal pelvis `HCC` `Rx` `ESR` `COM`

✓4ᵗʰ **C66** Malignant neoplasm of ureter
  EXCLUDES 1   malignant neoplasm of ureteric orifice of bladder (C67.6)

C66.1 Malignant neoplasm of right ureter `HCC` `Rx` `ESR` `COM`

C66.2 Malignant neoplasm of left ureter `HCC` `Rx` `ESR` `COM`

C66.9 Malignant neoplasm of unspecified ureter `HCC` `Rx` `ESR` `COM`

✓4ᵗʰ **C67** Malignant neoplasm of bladder

C67.0 Malignant neoplasm of trigone of bladder `HCC` `Rx` `ESR` `COM`

C67.1 Malignant neoplasm of dome of bladder `HCC` `Rx` `ESR` `COM`

C67.2 Malignant neoplasm of lateral wall of bladder `HCC` `Rx` `ESR` `COM`

C67.3 Malignant neoplasm of anterior wall of bladder `HCC` `Rx` `ESR` `COM`

C67.4 Malignant neoplasm of posterior wall of bladder `HCC` `Rx` `ESR` `COM`

C67.5 Malignant neoplasm of bladder neck `HCC` `Rx` `ESR` `COM`
Malignant neoplasm of internal urethral orifice

C67.6 Malignant neoplasm of ureteric orifice `HCC` `Rx` `ESR` `COM`

C67.7 Malignant neoplasm of urachus `HCC` `Rx` `ESR` `COM`

C67.8 Malignant neoplasm of overlapping sites of bladder `HCC` `Rx` `ESR` `COM`

C67.9 Malignant neoplasm of bladder, unspecified `HCC` `Rx` `ESR` `COM`
AHA: 2016,1Q,19

✓4ᵗʰ **C68** Malignant neoplasm of other and unspecified urinary organs
  EXCLUDES 1   malignant neoplasm of female genitourinary tract NOS (C57.9)
    malignant neoplasm of male genitourinary tract NOS (C63.9)

C68.0 Malignant neoplasm of urethra `HCC` `Rx` `ESR` `COM`
  EXCLUDES 1   malignant neoplasm of urethral orifice of bladder (C67.5)

C68.1 Malignant neoplasm of paraurethral glands `HCC` `Rx` `ESR` `COM`

C68.8 Malignant neoplasm of overlapping sites of urinary organs `HCC` `Rx` `ESR` `COM`
Primary malignant neoplasm of two or more contiguous sites of urinary organs whose point of origin cannot be determined

C68.9 Malignant neoplasm of urinary organ, unspecified `HCC` `Rx` `ESR` `COM`
Malignant neoplasm of urinary system NOS

Malignant neoplasms of eye, brain and other parts of central nervous system (C69-C72)

✓4ᵗʰ **C69** Malignant neoplasm of eye and adnexa
  EXCLUDES 1   malignant neoplasm of connective tissue of eyelid (C49.0)
    malignant neoplasm of eyelid (skin) (C43.1-, C44.1-)
    malignant neoplasm of optic nerve (C72.3-)

✓5ᵗʰ **C69.0** Malignant neoplasm of conjunctiva

  C69.00 Malignant neoplasm of unspecified conjunctiva `HCC` `Rx` `ESR` `COM`

  C69.01 Malignant neoplasm of right conjunctiva `HCC` `Rx` `ESR` `COM`

  C69.02 Malignant neoplasm of left conjunctiva `HCC` `Rx` `ESR` `COM`

✓5ᵗʰ **C69.1** Malignant neoplasm of cornea

  C69.10 Malignant neoplasm of unspecified cornea `HCC` `Rx` `ESR` `COM`

  C69.11 Malignant neoplasm of right cornea `HCC` `Rx` `ESR` `COM`

  C69.12 Malignant neoplasm of left cornea `HCC` `Rx` `ESR` `COM`

✓5ᵗʰ **C69.2** Malignant neoplasm of retina
  EXCLUDES 1   dark area on retina (D49.81)
    neoplasm of unspecified behavior of retina and choroid (D49.81)
    retinal freckle (D49.81)

  C69.20 Malignant neoplasm of unspecified retina `HCC` `Rx` `ESR` `COM`

  C69.21 Malignant neoplasm of right retina `HCC` `Rx` `ESR` `COM`

  C69.22 Malignant neoplasm of left retina `HCC` `Rx` `ESR` `COM`

✓5ᵗʰ **C69.3** Malignant neoplasm of choroid

  C69.30 Malignant neoplasm of unspecified choroid `HCC` `Rx` `ESR` `COM`

  C69.31 Malignant neoplasm of right choroid `HCC` `Rx` `ESR` `COM`

  C69.32 Malignant neoplasm of left choroid `HCC` `Rx` `ESR` `COM`

√5ᵗʰ **C69.4 Malignant neoplasm of** ciliary body

　C69.40 Malignant neoplasm of unspecified ciliary body `HCC` `Rx` `ESR` `COM`

　C69.41 Malignant neoplasm of right **ciliary body** `HCC` `Rx` `ESR` `COM`

　C69.42 Malignant neoplasm of left **ciliary body** `HCC` `Rx` `ESR` `COM`

√5ᵗʰ **C69.5 Malignant neoplasm of** lacrimal gland and duct

　Malignant neoplasm of lacrimal sac
　Malignant neoplasm of nasolacrimal duct

　C69.50 Malignant neoplasm of unspecified lacrimal gland and duct `HCC` `Rx` `ESR` `COM`

　C69.51 Malignant neoplasm of right **lacrimal gland and duct** `HCC` `Rx` `ESR` `COM`

　C69.52 Malignant neoplasm of left **lacrimal gland and duct** `HCC` `Rx` `ESR` `COM`

√5ᵗʰ **C69.6 Malignant neoplasm of** orbit

　Malignant neoplasm of connective tissue of orbit
　Malignant neoplasm of extraocular muscle
　Malignant neoplasm of peripheral nerves of orbit
　Malignant neoplasm of retrobulbar tissue
　Malignant neoplasm of retro-ocular tissue

　　EXCLUDES 1　malignant neoplasm of orbital bone (C41.0)

　C69.60 Malignant neoplasm of unspecified orbit `HCC` `Rx` `ESR` `COM`

　C69.61 Malignant neoplasm of right **orbit** `HCC` `Rx` `ESR` `COM`

　C69.62 Malignant neoplasm of left **orbit** `HCC` `Rx` `ESR` `COM`

√5ᵗʰ **C69.8 Malignant neoplasm of** overlapping sites **of eye and adnexa**

　C69.80 Malignant neoplasm of overlapping sites of unspecified eye and adnexa `HCC` `Rx` `ESR` `COM`

　C69.81 Malignant neoplasm of overlapping sites of right **eye and adnexa** `HCC` `Rx` `ESR` `COM`

　C69.82 Malignant neoplasm of overlapping sites of left **eye and adnexa** `HCC` `Rx` `ESR` `COM`

√5ᵗʰ **C69.9 Malignant neoplasm of unspecified site of eye**

　Malignant neoplasm of eyeball

　C69.90 Malignant neoplasm of unspecified site of unspecified eye `HCC` `Rx` `ESR` `COM`

　C69.91 Malignant neoplasm of unspecified site of right **eye** `HCC` `Rx` `ESR` `COM`

　C69.92 Malignant neoplasm of unspecified site of left **eye** `HCC` `Rx` `ESR` `COM`

√4ᵗʰ **C70 Malignant neoplasm of** meninges

　C70.0 Malignant neoplasm of cerebral **meninges** `HCC` `Rx` `ESR` `COM`

　C70.1 Malignant neoplasm of spinal **meninges** `HCC` `Rx` `ESR` `COM`

　C70.9 Malignant neoplasm of meninges, unspecified `HCC` `Rx` `ESR` `COM`

√4ᵗʰ **C71 Malignant neoplasm of** brain

　　EXCLUDES 1　*malignant neoplasm of cranial nerves (C72.2-C72.5)*
　　　　　　　retrobulbar malignant neoplasm (C69.6-)

Lobes of the Brain

C71.0 **Malignant neoplasm of** cerebrum, except lobes and ventricles `HCC` `Rx` `ESR` `COM`
　Malignant neoplasm of supratentorial NOS

C71.1 **Malignant neoplasm of** frontal **lobe** `HCC` `Rx` `ESR` `COM`

C71.2 **Malignant neoplasm of** temporal **lobe** `HCC` `Rx` `ESR` `COM`

C71.3 **Malignant neoplasm of** parietal **lobe** `HCC` `Rx` `ESR` `COM`

C71.4 **Malignant neoplasm of** occipital **lobe** `HCC` `Rx` `ESR` `COM`

C71.5 **Malignant neoplasm of** cerebral **ventricle** `HCC` `Rx` `ESR` `COM`
　　EXCLUDES 1　*malignant neoplasm of fourth cerebral ventricle (C71.7)*

C71.6 **Malignant neoplasm of** cerebellum `HCC` `Rx` `ESR` `COM`

C71.7 **Malignant neoplasm of** brain stem `HCC` `Rx` `ESR` `COM`
　Malignant neoplasm of fourth cerebral ventricle
　Infratentorial malignant neoplasm NOS

C71.8 **Malignant neoplasm of** overlapping sites **of brain** `HCC` `Rx` `ESR` `COM`

C71.9 **Malignant neoplasm of brain, unspecified** `HCC` `Rx` `ESR` `COM`
　AHA: 2014,3Q,3

√4ᵗʰ **C72 Malignant neoplasm of** spinal cord, cranial nerves **and other parts of** central nervous system

　　EXCLUDES 1　*malignant neoplasm of meninges (C70.-)*
　　　　　　　malignant neoplasm of peripheral nerves and autonomic nervous system (C47.-)

C72.0 **Malignant neoplasm of** spinal cord `HCC` `Rx` `ESR` `COM`

C72.1 **Malignant neoplasm of** cauda equina `HCC` `Rx` `ESR` `COM`

√5ᵗʰ C72.2 **Malignant neoplasm of** olfactory nerve
　Malignant neoplasm of olfactory bulb

　C72.20 Malignant neoplasm of unspecified olfactory nerve `HCC` `Rx` `ESR` `COM`

　C72.21 Malignant neoplasm of right **olfactory nerve** `HCC` `Rx` `ESR` `COM`

　C72.22 Malignant neoplasm of left **olfactory nerve** `HCC` `Rx` `ESR` `COM`

√5ᵗʰ C72.3 **Malignant neoplasm of** optic nerve

　C72.30 Malignant neoplasm of unspecified optic nerve `HCC` `Rx` `ESR` `COM`

　C72.31 Malignant neoplasm of right **optic nerve** `HCC` `Rx` `ESR` `COM`

　C72.32 Malignant neoplasm of left **optic nerve** `HCC` `Rx` `ESR` `COM`

√5ᵗʰ C72.4 **Malignant neoplasm of** acoustic nerve

　C72.40 Malignant neoplasm of unspecified acoustic nerve `HCC` `Rx` `ESR` `COM`

　C72.41 Malignant neoplasm of right **acoustic nerve** `HCC` `Rx` `ESR` `COM`

　C72.42 Malignant neoplasm of left **acoustic nerve** `HCC` `Rx` `ESR` `COM`

√5ᵗʰ **C72.5** Malignant neoplasm of other and unspecified cranial nerves

    C72.50 Malignant neoplasm of unspecified cranial nerve   HCC Rx ESR COM

         Malignant neoplasm of cranial nerve NOS

    C72.59 Malignant neoplasm of other cranial nerves   HCC Rx ESR COM

C72.9 Malignant neoplasm of central nervous system, unspecified

     Malignant neoplasm of unspecified site of central nervous system

     Malignant neoplasm of nervous system NOS

Malignant neoplasms of thyroid and other endocrine glands (C73-C75)

C73 Malignant neoplasm of thyroid gland   HCC Rx ESR COM

     Use additional code to identify any functional activity

√4ᵗʰ **C74** Malignant neoplasm of adrenal gland

     TIP: If an adrenal gland tumor is described as functioning (producing too much of a hormone), additional codes should be assigned to report the functional activity.

√5ᵗʰ **C74.0** Malignant neoplasm of cortex of adrenal gland

    C74.00 Malignant neoplasm of cortex of unspecified adrenal gland   HCC Rx ESR COM

    C74.01 Malignant neoplasm of cortex of right adrenal gland   HCC Rx ESR COM

    C74.02 Malignant neoplasm of cortex of left adrenal gland   HCC Rx ESR COM

√5ᵗʰ **C74.1** Malignant neoplasm of medulla of adrenal gland

    C74.10 Malignant neoplasm of medulla of unspecified adrenal gland   HCC Rx ESR COM

    C74.11 Malignant neoplasm of medulla of right adrenal gland   HCC Rx ESR COM

    C74.12 Malignant neoplasm of medulla of left adrenal gland   HCC Rx ESR COM

√5ᵗʰ **C74.9** Malignant neoplasm of unspecified part of adrenal gland

    C74.90 Malignant neoplasm of unspecified part of unspecified adrenal gland   HCC Rx ESR COM

    C74.91 Malignant neoplasm of unspecified part of right adrenal gland   HCC Rx ESR COM

    C74.92 Malignant neoplasm of unspecified part of left adrenal gland   HCC Rx ESR COM

√4ᵗʰ **C75** Malignant neoplasm of other endocrine glands and related structures

     EXCLUDES 1   malignant carcinoid tumors (C7A.0-)

         malignant neoplasm of adrenal gland (C74.-)

         malignant neoplasm of endocrine pancreas (C25.4)

         malignant neoplasm of islets of Langerhans (C25.4)

         malignant neoplasm of ovary (C56.-)

         malignant neoplasm of testis (C62.-)

         malignant neoplasm of thymus (C37)

         malignant neoplasm of thyroid gland (C73)

         malignant neuroendocrine tumors (C7A.-)

C75.0 Malignant neoplasm of parathyroid gland   HCC Rx ESR COM

C75.1 Malignant neoplasm of pituitary gland   HCC Rx ESR COM

C75.2 Malignant neoplasm of craniopharyngeal duct   HCC Rx ESR COM

C75.3 Malignant neoplasm of pineal gland   HCC Rx ESR COM

C75.4 Malignant neoplasm of carotid body   HCC Rx ESR COM

C75.5 Malignant neoplasm of aortic body and other paraganglia   HCC Rx ESR COM

C75.8 Malignant neoplasm with pluriglandular involvement, unspecified

C75.9 Malignant neoplasm of endocrine gland, unspecified   HCC Rx ESR COM

Malignant neuroendocrine tumors (C7A)

√4ᵗʰ **C7A** Malignant neuroendocrine tumors

     Code also any associated multiple endocrine neoplasia [MEN] syndromes (E31.2-)

     Use additional code to identify any associated endocrine syndrome, such as:

     carcinoid syndrome (E34.0)

     EXCLUDES 2   malignant pancreatic islet cell tumors (C25.4)

         Merkel cell carcinoma (C4A.-)

     AHA: 2019,3Q,7

     DEF: Tumors comprised of cells that are capable of producing hormonal syndromes in which the normal hormonal balance required to support body system function is adversely affected.

√5ᵗʰ **C7A.0** Malignant carcinoid tumors

     AHA: 2019,3Q,7

     DEF: Specific type of slow-growing neuroendocrine tumors. Carcinoid tumors occur most commonly in the hormone producing cells of the gastrointestinal tracts and can also occur in the pancreas, testes, ovaries, or lungs.

    C7A.00 Malignant carcinoid tumor of unspecified site   HCC Rx ESR COM

√6ᵗʰ **C7A.01** Malignant carcinoid tumors of the small intestine

    C7A.010 Malignant carcinoid tumor of the duodenum   HCC Rx ESR COM

    C7A.011 Malignant carcinoid tumor of the jejunum   HCC Rx ESR COM

    C7A.012 Malignant carcinoid tumor of the ileum   HCC Rx ESR COM

    C7A.019 Malignant carcinoid tumor of the small intestine, unspecified portion   HCC Rx ESR COM

√6ᵗʰ **C7A.02** Malignant carcinoid tumors of the appendix, large intestine, and rectum

    C7A.020 Malignant carcinoid tumor of the appendix   HCC Rx ESR COM

    C7A.021 Malignant carcinoid tumor of the cecum   HCC Rx ESR COM

    C7A.022 Malignant carcinoid tumor of the ascending colon   HCC Rx ESR COM

    C7A.023 Malignant carcinoid tumor of the transverse colon   HCC Rx ESR COM

    C7A.024 Malignant carcinoid tumor of the descending colon   HCC Rx ESR COM

    C7A.025 Malignant carcinoid tumor of the sigmoid colon   HCC Rx ESR COM

    C7A.026 Malignant carcinoid tumor of the rectum   HCC Rx ESR COM

    C7A.029 Malignant carcinoid tumor of the large intestine, unspecified portion   HCC Rx ESR COM

         Malignant carcinoid tumor of the colon NOS

√6ᵗʰ **C7A.09** Malignant carcinoid tumors of other sites

    C7A.090 Malignant carcinoid tumor of the bronchus and lung   HCC Rx ESR COM

         AHA: 2019,1Q,16

         TIP: When associated malignant pericardial effusion is documented, assign code I31.3. If the sole reason for admission is to treat the effusion with no treatment of the lung malignancy rendered, code I31.3 may be sequenced first.

    C7A.091 Malignant carcinoid tumor of the thymus   HCC Rx ESR COM

    C7A.092 Malignant carcinoid tumor of the stomach   HCC Rx ESR COM

    C7A.093 Malignant carcinoid tumor of the kidney   HCC Rx ESR COM

    C7A.094 Malignant carcinoid tumor of the foregut, unspecified   HCC Rx ESR COM

    C7A.095 Malignant carcinoid tumor of the midgut, unspecified   HCC Rx ESR COM

    C7A.096 Malignant carcinoid tumor of the hindgut, unspecified   HCC Rx ESR COM

    C7A.098 Malignant carcinoid tumors of other sites   HCC Rx ESR COM

C7A.1   **Malignant poorly differentiated neuroendocrine tumors** `HCC` `Rx` `ESR` `COM`
    Malignant poorly differentiated neuroendocrine tumor NOS
    Malignant poorly differentiated neuroendocrine carcinoma, any site
    High grade neuroendocrine carcinoma, any site

C7A.8   **Other malignant neuroendocrine tumors** `HCC` `Rx` `ESR` `COM`
    AHA: 2019,3Q,7

Secondary neuroendocrine tumors (C7B)

✓4th **C7B**   **Secondary neuroendocrine tumors**
    Use additional code to identify any functional activity

✓5th **C7B.Ø**   **Secondary carcinoid tumors**
    AHA: 2019,3Q,7
    DEF: Specific type of slow-growing neuroendocrine tumors. Carcinoid tumors occur most commonly in the hormone producing cells of the gastrointestinal tracts and can also occur in the pancreas, testes, ovaries, or lungs.

    C7B.ØØ   **Secondary carcinoid tumors, unspecified site** `HCC` `Rx` `ESR` `COM`

    C7B.Ø1   **Secondary carcinoid tumors of distant lymph nodes** `HCC` `Rx` `ESR` `COM`

    C7B.Ø2   **Secondary carcinoid tumors of liver** `HCC` `Rx` `ESR` `COM`

    C7B.Ø3   **Secondary carcinoid tumors of bone** `HCC` `Rx` `ESR` `COM`

    C7B.Ø4   **Secondary carcinoid tumors of peritoneum** `HCC` `Rx` `ESR` `COM`
       Mesentary metastasis of carcinoid tumor

    C7B.Ø9   **Secondary carcinoid tumors of other sites** `HCC` `Rx` `ESR` `COM`

C7B.1   **Secondary Merkel cell carcinoma** `HCC` `Rx` `ESR` `COM`
    Merkel cell carcinoma nodal presentation
    Merkel cell carcinoma visceral metastatic presentation

C7B.8   **Other secondary neuroendocrine tumors** `HCC` `Rx` `ESR` `COM`
    AHA: 2019,3Q,7

Malignant neoplasms of ill-defined, other secondary and unspecified sites (C76-C8Ø)

✓4th **C76**   **Malignant neoplasm of other and ill-defined sites**
    EXCLUDES 1   _malignant neoplasm of female genitourinary tract NOS (C57.9)_
          malignant neoplasm of male genitourinary tract NOS (C63.9)
          malignant neoplasm of lymphoid, hematopoietic and related tissue (C81-C96)
          malignant neoplasm of skin (C44.-)
          malignant neoplasm of unspecified site NOS (C8Ø.1)

C76.Ø   **Malignant neoplasm of head, face and neck** `HCC` `Rx` `ESR` `COM`
    Malignant neoplasm of cheek NOS
    Malignant neoplasm of nose NOS

C76.1   **Malignant neoplasm of thorax** `HCC` `Rx` `ESR` `COM`
    Intrathoracic malignant neoplasm NOS
    Malignant neoplasm of axilla NOS
    Thoracic malignant neoplasm NOS

C76.2   **Malignant neoplasm of abdomen** `HCC` `Rx` `ESR` `COM`

C76.3   **Malignant neoplasm of pelvis** `HCC` `Rx` `ESR` `COM`
    Malignant neoplasm of groin NOS
    Malignant neoplasm of sites overlapping systems within the pelvis
    Rectovaginal (septum) malignant neoplasm
    Rectovesical (septum) malignant neoplasm

✓5th **C76.4**   **Malignant neoplasm of upper limb**

    C76.4Ø   **Malignant neoplasm of unspecified upper limb** `HCC` `Rx` `ESR` `COM`

    C76.41   **Malignant neoplasm of right upper limb** `HCC` `Rx` `ESR` `COM`

    C76.42   **Malignant neoplasm of left upper limb** `HCC` `Rx` `ESR` `COM`

✓5th **C76.5**   **Malignant neoplasm of lower limb**

    C76.5Ø   **Malignant neoplasm of unspecified lower limb** `HCC` `Rx` `ESR` `COM`

    C76.51   **Malignant neoplasm of right lower limb** `HCC` `Rx` `ESR` `COM`

    C76.52   **Malignant neoplasm of left lower limb** `HCC` `Rx` `ESR` `COM`

C76.8   **Malignant neoplasm of other specified ill-defined sites** `HCC` `Rx` `ESR` `COM`
    Malignant neoplasm of overlapping ill-defined sites

✓4th **C77**   **Secondary and unspecified malignant neoplasm of lymph nodes**
    EXCLUDES 1   _malignant neoplasm of lymph nodes, specified as primary (C81-C86, C88, C96.-)_
          mesentary metastasis of carcinoid tumor (C7B.Ø4)
          secondary carcinoid tumors of distant lymph nodes (C7B.Ø1)

C77.Ø   **Secondary and unspecified malignant neoplasm of lymph nodes of head, face and neck** `HCC` `Rx` `ESR` `COM`
    Secondary and unspecified malignant neoplasm of supraclavicular lymph nodes

C77.1   **Secondary and unspecified malignant neoplasm of intrathoracic lymph nodes** `HCC` `Rx` `ESR` `COM`

C77.2   **Secondary and unspecified malignant neoplasm of intra-abdominal lymph nodes** `HCC` `Rx` `ESR` `COM`

C77.3   **Secondary and unspecified malignant neoplasm of axilla and upper limb lymph nodes** `HCC` `Rx` `ESR` `COM`
    Secondary and unspecified malignant neoplasm of pectoral lymph nodes

C77.4   **Secondary and unspecified malignant neoplasm of inguinal and lower limb lymph nodes** `HCC` `Rx` `ESR` `COM`

C77.5   **Secondary and unspecified malignant neoplasm of intrapelvic lymph nodes** `HCC` `Rx` `ESR` `COM`

C77.8   **Secondary and unspecified malignant neoplasm of lymph nodes of multiple regions** `HCC` `Rx` `ESR` `COM`

C77.9   **Secondary and unspecified malignant neoplasm of lymph node, unspecified** `HCC` `Rx` `ESR` `COM`

✓4th **C78**   **Secondary malignant neoplasm of respiratory and digestive organs**
    EXCLUDES 1   _secondary carcinoid tumors of liver (C7B.Ø2)_
          secondary carcinoid tumors of peritoneum (C7B.Ø4)
    EXCLUDES 2   _lymph node metastases (C77.Ø)_

✓5th **C78.Ø**   **Secondary malignant neoplasm of lung**
    AHA: 2019,1Q,16

    C78.ØØ   **Secondary malignant neoplasm of unspecified lung** `HCC` `Rx` `ESR` `COM`

    C78.Ø1   **Secondary malignant neoplasm of right lung** `HCC` `Rx` `ESR` `COM`

    C78.Ø2   **Secondary malignant neoplasm of left lung** `HCC` `Rx` `ESR` `COM`

C78.1   **Secondary malignant neoplasm of mediastinum** `HCC` `Rx` `ESR` `COM`

C78.2   **Secondary malignant neoplasm of pleura** `HCC` `Rx` `ESR` `COM`

✓5th **C78.3**   **Secondary malignant neoplasm of other and unspecified respiratory organs**

    C78.3Ø   **Secondary malignant neoplasm of unspecified respiratory organ** `HCC` `Rx` `ESR` `COM`

    C78.39   **Secondary malignant neoplasm of other respiratory organs** `HCC` `Rx` `ESR` `COM`

C78.4   **Secondary malignant neoplasm of small intestine** `HCC` `Rx` `ESR` `COM`

C78.5   **Secondary malignant neoplasm of large intestine and rectum** `HCC` `Rx` `ESR` `COM`

C78.6   **Secondary malignant neoplasm of retroperitoneum and peritoneum** `HCC` `Rx` `ESR` `COM`
    AHA: 2017,2Q,12

C78.7   **Secondary malignant neoplasm of liver and intrahepatic bile duct** `HCC` `Rx` `ESR` `COM`

✓5th **C78.8**   **Secondary malignant neoplasm of other and unspecified digestive organs**

    C78.8Ø   **Secondary malignant neoplasm of unspecified digestive organ** `HCC` `Rx` `ESR` `COM`

    C78.89   **Secondary malignant neoplasm of other digestive organs** `HCC` `Rx` `ESR` `COM`
       Code also exocrine pancreatic insufficiency (K86.81)

✓4th **C79**   **Secondary malignant neoplasm of other and unspecified sites**
    EXCLUDES 1   _secondary carcinoid tumors (C7B.-)_
          secondary neuroendocrine tumors (C7B.-)

✓5th **C79.Ø**   **Secondary malignant neoplasm of kidney and renal pelvis**

    C79.ØØ   **Secondary malignant neoplasm of unspecified kidney and renal pelvis** `HCC` `Rx` `ESR` `COM`

    C79.Ø1   **Secondary malignant neoplasm of right kidney and renal pelvis** `HCC` `Rx` `ESR` `COM`

    C79.Ø2   **Secondary malignant neoplasm of left kidney and renal pelvis** `HCC` `Rx` `ESR` `COM`

`HCC` CMS-HCC   `Rx` Rx HCC   `ESR` ESRD HCC   `COM` Commercial HCC   `N` Newborn: 0   `P` Pediatric: 0-17   `M` Maternity: 9-64   `A` Adult: 15-124

492   ICD-10-CM 2023

√6ᵗʰ **C79.1** **Secondary malignant neoplasm of** bladder **and other and unspecified** urinary organs

     C79.10 **Secondary malignant neoplasm of unspecified urinary organs** `HCC` `Rx` `ESR` `COM`

     C79.11 **Secondary malignant neoplasm of** bladder `HCC` `Rx` `ESR` `COM`

         EXCLUDES 2   lymph node metastases (C77.0)

     C79.19 **Secondary malignant neoplasm of other urinary organs** `HCC` `Rx` `ESR` `COM`

C79.2 **Secondary malignant neoplasm of** skin `HCC` `Rx` `ESR` `COM`

     EXCLUDES 1   secondary Merkel cell carcinoma (C7B.1)

√5ᵗʰ **C79.3** **Secondary malignant neoplasm of** brain and cerebral meninges

     C79.31 **Secondary malignant neoplasm of** brain `HCC` `Rx` `ESR` `COM`

     C79.32 **Secondary malignant neoplasm of** cerebral meninges `HCC` `Rx` `ESR` `COM`

         AHA: 2020,1Q,13

√5ᵗʰ **C79.4** **Secondary malignant neoplasm of other and unspecified** parts of nervous system

     C79.40 **Secondary malignant neoplasm of unspecified part of nervous system** `HCC` `Rx` `ESR` `COM`

     C79.49 **Secondary malignant neoplasm of other parts of nervous system** `HCC` `Rx` `ESR` `COM`

√5ᵗʰ **C79.5** **Secondary malignant neoplasm of** bone and bone marrow

     EXCLUDES 1   secondary carcinoid tumors of bone (C7B.03)

     C79.51 **Secondary malignant neoplasm of** bone `HCC` `Rx` `ESR` `COM`

         TIP: Do not assign in addition to a code from subcategory C90.0 when multiple myeloma is described as metastatic to the bone; bone involvement is integral to multiple myeloma.

     C79.52 **Secondary malignant neoplasm of** bone marrow `HCC` `Rx` `ESR` `COM`

√5ᵗʰ **C79.6** **Secondary malignant neoplasm of** ovary

     C79.60 **Secondary malignant neoplasm of unspecified** ovary `HCC` `Rx` `ESR` `COM` ♀

     C79.61 **Secondary malignant neoplasm of** right ovary `HCC` `Rx` `ESR` `COM` ♀

     C79.62 **Secondary malignant neoplasm of** left ovary `HCC` `Rx` `ESR` `COM` ♀

     C79.63 **Secondary malignant neoplasm of** bilateral ovaries `HCC` `Rx` `ESR` `COM` ♀

√5ᵗʰ **C79.7** **Secondary malignant neoplasm of** adrenal gland

     C79.70 **Secondary malignant neoplasm of unspecified adrenal gland** `HCC` `Rx` `ESR` `COM`

     C79.71 **Secondary malignant neoplasm of** right **adrenal gland** `HCC` `Rx` `ESR` `COM`

     C79.72 **Secondary malignant neoplasm of** left **adrenal gland** `HCC` `Rx` `ESR` `COM`

√5ᵗʰ **C79.8** **Secondary malignant neoplasm of other specified sites**

     C79.81 **Secondary malignant neoplasm of** breast `HCC` `Rx` `ESR` `COM`

     C79.82 **Secondary malignant neoplasm of** genital organs `HCC` `Rx` `ESR` `COM`

     C79.89 **Secondary malignant neoplasm of other specified sites** `HCC` `Rx` `ESR` `COM`

         AHA: 2017,2Q,11

C79.9 **Secondary malignant neoplasm of unspecified site** `HCC` `Rx` `ESR` `COM`

     Metastatic cancer NOS

     Metastatic disease NOS

     EXCLUDES 1   carcinomatosis NOS (C80.0)

         generalized cancer NOS (C80.0)

         malignant (primary) neoplasm of unspecified site (C80.1)

√4ᵗʰ **C80** **Malignant neoplasm** without specification of site

     EXCLUDES 1   malignant carcinoid tumor of unspecified site (C7A.00)

         malignant neoplasm of specified multiple sites - code to each site

     C80.0 **Disseminated malignant neoplasm,** *[handwritten: secondary site]* **unspecified** *[handwritten: no known primary]* `HCC` `Rx` `ESR` `COM`

     Carcinomatosis NOS

     Generalized cancer, unspecified site (primary) (secondary)

     Generalized malignancy, unspecified site (primary) (secondary)

C80.1 **Malignant** (primary) **neoplasm, unspecified** `HCC` `ESR` `COM`

     Cancer NOS

     Cancer unspecified site (primary)

     Carcinoma unspecified site (primary)

     Malignancy unspecified site (primary)

     EXCLUDES 1   secondary malignant neoplasm of unspecified site (C79.9)

C80.2 **Malignant neoplasm associated with** transplanted organ `HCC` `Rx` `ESR` `COM` `UPD`

     Code first complication of transplanted organ (T86.-)

     Use additional code to identify the specific malignancy

Malignant neoplasms of lymphoid, hematopoietic and related tissue (C81-C96)

     EXCLUDES 2   Kaposi's sarcoma of lymph nodes (C46.3)

         secondary and unspecified neoplasm of lymph nodes (C77.-)

         secondary neoplasm of bone marrow (C79.52)

         secondary neoplasm of spleen (C78.89)

√4ᵗʰ **C81** **Hodgkin lymphoma**

     EXCLUDES 1   personal history of Hodgkin lymphoma (Z85.71)

     DEF: Malignant disorder of lymphoid cells characterized by the presence of progressively swollen lymph nodes and spleen that may also involve the liver. A diagnosis of Hodgkin's lymphoma can be confirmed by the presence of Reed-Sternberg cells. *Synonym(s): Hodgkin disease.*

√5ᵗʰ **C81.0** **Nodular lymphocyte predominant Hodgkin lymphoma**

     C81.00 **Nodular lymphocyte predominant Hodgkin lymphoma, unspecified site** `HCC` `Rx` `ESR` `COM`

     C81.01 **Nodular lymphocyte predominant Hodgkin lymphoma, lymph nodes of** head, face, and neck `HCC` `Rx` `ESR` `COM`

     C81.02 **Nodular lymphocyte predominant Hodgkin lymphoma,** intrathoracic **lymph nodes** `HCC` `Rx` `ESR` `COM`

     C81.03 **Nodular lymphocyte predominant Hodgkin lymphoma,** intra-abdominal **lymph nodes** `HCC` `Rx` `ESR` `COM`

     C81.04 **Nodular lymphocyte predominant Hodgkin lymphoma, lymph nodes of** axilla and upper limb `HCC` `Rx` `ESR` `COM`

     C81.05 **Nodular lymphocyte predominant Hodgkin lymphoma, lymph nodes of** inguinal region and lower limb `HCC` `Rx` `ESR` `COM`

     C81.06 **Nodular lymphocyte predominant Hodgkin lymphoma,** intrapelvic **lymph nodes** `HCC` `Rx` `ESR` `COM`

     C81.07 **Nodular lymphocyte predominant Hodgkin lymphoma,** spleen `HCC` `Rx` `ESR` `COM`

     C81.08 **Nodular lymphocyte predominant Hodgkin lymphoma, lymph nodes of** multiple sites `HCC` `Rx` `ESR` `COM`

     C81.09 **Nodular lymphocyte predominant Hodgkin lymphoma,** extranodal and solid organ sites `HCC` `Rx` `ESR` `COM`

√5ᵗʰ **C81.1** **Nodular sclerosis Hodgkin lymphoma**

     Nodular sclerosis classical Hodgkin lymphoma

     C81.10 **Nodular sclerosis Hodgkin lymphoma, unspecified site** `HCC` `Rx` `ESR` `COM`

     C81.11 **Nodular sclerosis Hodgkin lymphoma, lymph nodes of** head, face, and neck `HCC` `Rx` `ESR` `COM`

     C81.12 **Nodular sclerosis Hodgkin lymphoma,** intrathoracic **lymph nodes** `HCC` `Rx` `ESR` `COM`

     C81.13 **Nodular sclerosis Hodgkin lymphoma,** intra-abdominal **lymph nodes** `HCC` `Rx` `ESR` `COM`

     C81.14 **Nodular sclerosis Hodgkin lymphoma, lymph nodes of** axilla and upper limb `HCC` `Rx` `ESR` `COM`

     C81.15 **Nodular sclerosis Hodgkin lymphoma, lymph nodes of** inguinal region and lower limb `HCC` `Rx` `ESR` `COM`

     C81.16 **Nodular sclerosis Hodgkin lymphoma,** intrapelvic **lymph nodes** `HCC` `Rx` `ESR` `COM`

     C81.17 **Nodular sclerosis Hodgkin lymphoma,** spleen `HCC` `Rx` `ESR` `COM`

     C81.18 **Nodular sclerosis Hodgkin lymphoma, lymph nodes of** multiple sites `HCC` `Rx` `ESR` `COM`

     C81.19 **Nodular sclerosis Hodgkin lymphoma,** extranodal and solid organ sites `HCC` `Rx` `ESR` `COM`

√5ᵗʰ **C81.2** **Mixed cellularity Hodgkin lymphoma**

     Mixed cellularity classical Hodgkin lymphoma

     C81.20 **Mixed cellularity Hodgkin lymphoma, unspecified site** `HCC` `Rx` `ESR` `COM`

Chapter 2. Neoplasms

C81.21 Mixed cellularity Hodgkin lymphoma, lymph nodes of head, face, and neck `HCC` `Rx` `ESR` `COM`

C81.22 Mixed cellularity Hodgkin lymphoma, intrathoracic lymph nodes `HCC` `Rx` `ESR` `COM`

C81.23 Mixed cellularity Hodgkin lymphoma, intra-abdominal lymph nodes `HCC` `Rx` `ESR` `COM`

C81.24 Mixed cellularity Hodgkin lymphoma, lymph nodes of axilla and upper limb `HCC` `Rx` `ESR` `COM`

C81.25 Mixed cellularity Hodgkin lymphoma, lymph nodes of inguinal region and lower limb `HCC` `Rx` `ESR` `COM`

C81.26 Mixed cellularity Hodgkin lymphoma, intrapelvic lymph nodes `HCC` `Rx` `ESR` `COM`

C81.27 Mixed cellularity Hodgkin lymphoma, spleen `HCC` `Rx` `ESR` `COM`

C81.28 Mixed cellularity Hodgkin lymphoma, lymph nodes of multiple sites `HCC` `Rx` `ESR` `COM`

C81.29 Mixed cellularity Hodgkin lymphoma, extranodal and solid organ sites `HCC` `Rx` `ESR` `COM`

✓5ᵗʰ **C81.3** Lymphocyte depleted Hodgkin lymphoma

Lymphocyte depleted classical Hodgkin lymphoma

C81.30 Lymphocyte depleted Hodgkin lymphoma, unspecified site `HCC` `Rx` `ESR` `COM`

C81.31 Lymphocyte depleted Hodgkin lymphoma, lymph nodes of head, face, and neck `HCC` `Rx` `ESR` `COM`

C81.32 Lymphocyte depleted Hodgkin lymphoma, intrathoracic lymph nodes `HCC` `Rx` `ESR` `COM`

C81.33 Lymphocyte depleted Hodgkin lymphoma, intra-abdominal lymph nodes `HCC` `Rx` `ESR` `COM`

C81.34 Lymphocyte depleted Hodgkin lymphoma, lymph nodes of axilla and upper limb `HCC` `Rx` `ESR` `COM`

C81.35 Lymphocyte depleted Hodgkin lymphoma, lymph nodes of inguinal region and lower limb `HCC` `Rx` `ESR` `COM`

C81.36 Lymphocyte depleted Hodgkin lymphoma, intrapelvic lymph nodes `HCC` `Rx` `ESR` `COM`

C81.37 Lymphocyte depleted Hodgkin lymphoma, spleen `HCC` `Rx` `ESR` `COM`

C81.38 Lymphocyte depleted Hodgkin lymphoma, lymph nodes of multiple sites `HCC` `Rx` `ESR` `COM`

C81.39 Lymphocyte depleted Hodgkin lymphoma, extranodal and solid organ sites `HCC` `Rx` `ESR` `COM`

✓5ᵗʰ **C81.4** Lymphocyte-rich Hodgkin lymphoma

Lymphocyte-rich classical Hodgkin lymphoma

EXCLUDES 1 nodular lymphocyte predominant Hodgkin lymphoma (C81.0-)

C81.40 Lymphocyte-rich Hodgkin lymphoma, unspecified site `HCC` `Rx` `ESR` `COM`

C81.41 Lymphocyte-rich Hodgkin lymphoma, lymph nodes of head, face, and neck `HCC` `Rx` `ESR` `COM`

C81.42 Lymphocyte-rich Hodgkin lymphoma, intrathoracic lymph nodes `HCC` `Rx` `ESR` `COM`

C81.43 Lymphocyte-rich Hodgkin lymphoma, intra-abdominal lymph nodes `HCC` `Rx` `ESR` `COM`

C81.44 Lymphocyte-rich Hodgkin lymphoma, lymph nodes of axilla and upper limb `HCC` `Rx` `ESR` `COM`

C81.45 Lymphocyte-rich Hodgkin lymphoma, lymph nodes of inguinal region and lower limb `HCC` `Rx` `ESR` `COM`

C81.46 Lymphocyte-rich Hodgkin lymphoma, intrapelvic lymph nodes `HCC` `Rx` `ESR` `COM`

C81.47 Lymphocyte-rich Hodgkin lymphoma, spleen `HCC` `Rx` `ESR` `COM`

C81.48 Lymphocyte-rich Hodgkin lymphoma, lymph nodes of multiple sites `HCC` `Rx` `ESR` `COM`

C81.49 Lymphocyte-rich Hodgkin lymphoma, extranodal and solid organ sites `HCC` `Rx` `ESR` `COM`

✓5ᵗʰ **C81.7** Other Hodgkin lymphoma

Classical Hodgkin lymphoma NOS
Other classical Hodgkin lymphoma

C81.70 Other Hodgkin lymphoma, unspecified site `HCC` `Rx` `ESR` `COM`

C81.71 Other Hodgkin lymphoma, lymph nodes of head, face, and neck `HCC` `Rx` `ESR` `COM`

C81.72 Other Hodgkin lymphoma, intrathoracic lymph nodes `HCC` `Rx` `ESR` `COM`

C81.73 Other Hodgkin lymphoma, intra-abdominal lymph nodes `HCC` `Rx` `ESR` `COM`

C81.74 Other Hodgkin lymphoma, lymph nodes of axilla and upper limb `HCC` `Rx` `ESR` `COM`

C81.75 Other Hodgkin lymphoma, lymph nodes of inguinal region and lower limb `HCC` `Rx` `ESR` `COM`

C81.76 Other Hodgkin lymphoma, intrapelvic lymph nodes `HCC` `Rx` `ESR` `COM`

C81.77 Other Hodgkin lymphoma, spleen `HCC` `Rx` `ESR` `COM`

C81.78 Other Hodgkin lymphoma, lymph nodes of multiple sites `HCC` `Rx` `ESR` `COM`

C81.79 Other Hodgkin lymphoma, extranodal and solid organ sites `HCC` `Rx` `ESR` `COM`

✓5ᵗʰ **C81.9** Hodgkin lymphoma, unspecified

C81.90 Hodgkin lymphoma, unspecified, unspecified site `HCC` `Rx` `ESR` `COM`

C81.91 Hodgkin lymphoma, unspecified, lymph nodes of head, face, and neck `HCC` `Rx` `ESR` `COM`

C81.92 Hodgkin lymphoma, unspecified, intrathoracic lymph nodes `HCC` `Rx` `ESR` `COM`

C81.93 Hodgkin lymphoma, unspecified, intra-abdominal lymph nodes `HCC` `Rx` `ESR` `COM`

C81.94 Hodgkin lymphoma, unspecified, lymph nodes of axilla and upper limb `HCC` `Rx` `ESR` `COM`

C81.95 Hodgkin lymphoma, unspecified, lymph nodes of inguinal region and lower limb `HCC` `Rx` `ESR` `COM`

C81.96 Hodgkin lymphoma, unspecified, intrapelvic lymph nodes `HCC` `Rx` `ESR` `COM`

C81.97 Hodgkin lymphoma, unspecified, spleen `HCC` `Rx` `ESR` `COM`

C81.98 Hodgkin lymphoma, unspecified, lymph nodes of multiple sites `HCC` `Rx` `ESR` `COM`

C81.99 Hodgkin lymphoma, unspecified, extranodal and solid organ sites `HCC` `Rx` `ESR` `COM`

✓4ᵗʰ **C82** Follicular lymphoma

INCLUDES follicular lymphoma with or without diffuse areas
EXCLUDES 1 mature T/NK-cell lymphomas (C84.-)
personal history of non-Hodgkin lymphoma (Z85.72)

DEF: Most common subgroup of non-Hodgkin lymphomas (NHL), accounting for 20 to 30 percent of all NHLs. NHL is a B-cell lymphoma that is slow growing and characterized by the circular pattern of malignant cell growth with the cells clustered into identifiable nodules or follicles.

✓5ᵗʰ **C82.0** Follicular lymphoma grade I

C82.00 Follicular lymphoma grade I, unspecified site `HCC` `Rx` `ESR` `COM`

C82.01 Follicular lymphoma grade I, lymph nodes of head, face, and neck `HCC` `Rx` `ESR` `COM`

C82.02 Follicular lymphoma grade I, intrathoracic lymph nodes `HCC` `Rx` `ESR` `COM`

C82.03 Follicular lymphoma grade I, intra-abdominal lymph nodes `HCC` `Rx` `ESR` `COM`

C82.04 Follicular lymphoma grade I, lymph nodes of axilla and upper limb `HCC` `Rx` `ESR` `COM`

C82.05 Follicular lymphoma grade I, lymph nodes of inguinal region and lower limb `HCC` `Rx` `ESR` `COM`

C82.06 Follicular lymphoma grade I, intrapelvic lymph nodes `HCC` `Rx` `ESR` `COM`

C82.07 Follicular lymphoma grade I, spleen `HCC` `Rx` `ESR` `COM`

C82.08 Follicular lymphoma grade I, lymph nodes of multiple sites `HCC` `Rx` `ESR` `COM`

C82.09 Follicular lymphoma grade I, extranodal and solid organ sites `HCC` `Rx` `ESR` `COM`

✓5ᵗʰ **C82.1** Follicular lymphoma grade II

C82.10 Follicular lymphoma grade II, unspecified site `HCC` `Rx` `ESR` `COM`

C82.11 Follicular lymphoma grade II, lymph nodes of head, face, and neck `HCC` `Rx` `ESR` `COM`

C82.12 Follicular lymphoma grade II, intrathoracic lymph nodes `HCC` `Rx` `ESR` `COM`

C82.13 Follicular lymphoma grade II, intra-abdominal lymph nodes `HCC` `Rx` `ESR` `COM`

C82.14 Follicular lymphoma grade II, lymph nodes of axilla and upper limb `HCC` `Rx` `ESR` `COM`

C82.15 Follicular lymphoma grade II, lymph nodes of inguinal region and lower limb `HCC` `Rx` `ESR` `COM`

C82.16 Follicular lymphoma grade II, intrapelvic lymph nodes `HCC` `Rx` `ESR` `COM`

C82.17 Follicular lymphoma grade II, spleen `HCC` `Rx` `ESR` `COM`

`HCC` CMS-HCC　　`Rx` Rx HCC　　`ESR` ESRD HCC　　`COM` Commercial HCC　　　N Newborn: 0　　P Pediatric: 0-17　　M Maternity: 9-64　　A Adult: 15-124

494　　　　　ICD-10-CM 2023

C82.18   Follicular lymphoma grade II, lymph nodes of multiple sites `HCC` `Rx` `ESR` `COM`

C82.19   Follicular lymphoma grade II, extranodal and solid organ sites `HCC` `Rx` `ESR` `COM`

✓5th **C82.2**   Follicular lymphoma grade III, unspecified

C82.20   Follicular lymphoma grade III, unspecified, unspecified site `HCC` `Rx` `ESR` `COM`

C82.21   Follicular lymphoma grade III, unspecified, lymph nodes of head, face, and neck `HCC` `Rx` `ESR` `COM`

C82.22   Follicular lymphoma grade III, unspecified, intrathoracic lymph nodes `HCC` `Rx` `ESR` `COM`

C82.23   Follicular lymphoma grade III, unspecified, intra-abdominal lymph nodes `HCC` `Rx` `ESR` `COM`

C82.24   Follicular lymphoma grade III, unspecified, lymph nodes of axilla and upper limb `HCC` `Rx` `ESR` `COM`

C82.25   Follicular lymphoma grade III, unspecified, lymph nodes of inguinal region and lower limb `HCC` `Rx` `ESR` `COM`

C82.26   Follicular lymphoma grade III, unspecified, intrapelvic lymph nodes `HCC` `Rx` `ESR` `COM`

C82.27   Follicular lymphoma grade III, unspecified, spleen `HCC` `Rx` `ESR` `COM`

C82.28   Follicular lymphoma grade III, unspecified, lymph nodes of multiple sites `HCC` `Rx` `ESR` `COM`

C82.29   Follicular lymphoma grade III, unspecified, extranodal and solid organ sites `HCC` `Rx` `ESR` `COM`

✓5th **C82.3**   Follicular lymphoma grade IIIa

C82.30   Follicular lymphoma grade IIIa, unspecified site `HCC` `Rx` `ESR` `COM`

C82.31   Follicular lymphoma grade IIIa, lymph nodes of head, face, and neck

C82.32   Follicular lymphoma grade IIIa, intrathoracic lymph nodes `HCC` `Rx` `ESR` `COM`

C82.33   Follicular lymphoma grade IIIa, intra-abdominal lymph nodes `HCC` `Rx` `ESR` `COM`

C82.34   Follicular lymphoma grade IIIa, lymph nodes of axilla and upper limb `HCC` `Rx` `ESR` `COM`

C82.35   Follicular lymphoma grade IIIa, lymph nodes of inguinal region and lower limb `HCC` `Rx` `ESR` `COM`

C82.36   Follicular lymphoma grade IIIa, intrapelvic lymph nodes `HCC` `Rx` `ESR` `COM`

C82.37   Follicular lymphoma grade IIIa, spleen `HCC` `Rx` `ESR` `COM`

C82.38   Follicular lymphoma grade IIIa, lymph nodes of multiple sites `HCC` `Rx` `ESR` `COM`

C82.39   Follicular lymphoma grade IIIa, extranodal and solid organ sites `HCC` `Rx` `ESR` `COM`

✓5th **C82.4**   Follicular lymphoma grade IIIb

C82.40   Follicular lymphoma grade IIIb, unspecified site `HCC` `Rx` `ESR` `COM`

C82.41   Follicular lymphoma grade IIIb, lymph nodes of head, face, and neck `HCC` `Rx` `ESR` `COM`

C82.42   Follicular lymphoma grade IIIb, intrathoracic lymph nodes `HCC` `Rx` `ESR` `COM`

C82.43   Follicular lymphoma grade IIIb, intra-abdominal lymph nodes `HCC` `Rx` `ESR` `COM`

C82.44   Follicular lymphoma grade IIIb, lymph nodes of axilla and upper limb `HCC` `Rx` `ESR` `COM`

C82.45   Follicular lymphoma grade IIIb, lymph nodes of inguinal region and lower limb `HCC` `Rx` `ESR` `COM`

C82.46   Follicular lymphoma grade IIIb, intrapelvic lymph nodes `HCC` `Rx` `ESR` `COM`

C82.47   Follicular lymphoma grade IIIb, spleen `HCC` `Rx` `ESR` `COM`

C82.48   Follicular lymphoma grade IIIb, lymph nodes of multiple sites `HCC` `Rx` `ESR` `COM`

C82.49   Follicular lymphoma grade IIIb, extranodal and solid organ sites `HCC` `Rx` `ESR` `COM`

✓5th **C82.5**   Diffuse follicle center lymphoma

C82.50   Diffuse follicle center lymphoma, unspecified site `HCC` `Rx` `ESR` `COM`

C82.51   Diffuse follicle center lymphoma, lymph nodes of head, face, and neck `HCC` `Rx` `ESR` `COM`

C82.52   Diffuse follicle center lymphoma, intrathoracic lymph nodes `HCC` `Rx` `ESR` `COM`

C82.53   Diffuse follicle center lymphoma, intra-abdominal lymph nodes `HCC` `Rx` `ESR` `COM`

C82.54   Diffuse follicle center lymphoma, lymph nodes of axilla and upper limb `HCC` `Rx` `ESR` `COM`

C82.55   Diffuse follicle center lymphoma, lymph nodes of inguinal region and lower limb `HCC` `Rx` `ESR` `COM`

C82.56   Diffuse follicle center lymphoma, intrapelvic lymph nodes `HCC` `Rx` `ESR` `COM`

C82.57   Diffuse follicle center lymphoma, spleen `HCC` `Rx` `ESR` `COM`

C82.58   Diffuse follicle center lymphoma, lymph nodes of multiple sites `HCC` `Rx` `ESR` `COM`

C82.59   Diffuse follicle center lymphoma, extranodal and solid organ sites `HCC` `Rx` `ESR` `COM`

✓5th **C82.6**   Cutaneous follicle center lymphoma

C82.60   Cutaneous follicle center lymphoma, unspecified site `HCC` `Rx` `ESR` `COM`

C82.61   Cutaneous follicle center lymphoma, lymph nodes of head, face, and neck

C82.62   Cutaneous follicle center lymphoma, intrathoracic lymph nodes

C82.63   Cutaneous follicle center lymphoma, intra-abdominal lymph nodes `HCC` `Rx` `ESR` `COM`

C82.64   Cutaneous follicle center lymphoma, lymph nodes of axilla and upper limb

C82.65   Cutaneous follicle center lymphoma, lymph nodes of inguinal region and lower limb `HCC` `Rx` `ESR` `COM`

C82.66   Cutaneous follicle center lymphoma, intrapelvic lymph nodes

C82.67   Cutaneous follicle center lymphoma, spleen

C82.68   Cutaneous follicle center lymphoma, lymph nodes of multiple sites `HCC` `Rx` `ESR` `COM`

C82.69   Cutaneous follicle center lymphoma, extranodal and solid organ sites `HCC` `Rx` `ESR` `COM`

✓5th **C82.8**   Other types of follicular lymphoma

C82.80   Other types of follicular lymphoma, unspecified site `HCC` `Rx` `ESR` `COM`

C82.81   Other types of follicular lymphoma, lymph nodes of head, face, and neck `HCC` `Rx` `ESR` `COM`

C82.82   Other types of follicular lymphoma, intrathoracic lymph nodes

C82.83   Other types of follicular lymphoma, intra-abdominal lymph nodes `HCC` `Rx` `ESR` `COM`

C82.84   Other types of follicular lymphoma, lymph nodes of axilla and upper limb `HCC` `Rx` `ESR` `COM`

C82.85   Other types of follicular lymphoma, lymph nodes of inguinal region and lower limb `HCC` `Rx` `ESR` `COM`

C82.86   Other types of follicular lymphoma, intrapelvic lymph nodes `HCC` `Rx` `ESR` `COM`

C82.87   Other types of follicular lymphoma, spleen `HCC` `Rx` `ESR` `COM`

C82.88   Other types of follicular lymphoma, lymph nodes of multiple sites `HCC` `Rx` `ESR` `COM`

C82.89   Other types of follicular lymphoma, extranodal and solid organ sites `HCC` `Rx` `ESR` `COM`

✓5th **C82.9**   Follicular lymphoma, unspecified

C82.90   Follicular lymphoma, unspecified, unspecified site `HCC` `Rx` `ESR` `COM`

C82.91   Follicular lymphoma, unspecified, lymph nodes of head, face, and neck `HCC` `Rx` `ESR` `COM`

C82.92   Follicular lymphoma, unspecified, intrathoracic lymph nodes `HCC` `Rx` `ESR` `COM`

C82.93   Follicular lymphoma, unspecified, intra-abdominal lymph nodes `HCC` `Rx` `ESR` `COM`

C82.94   Follicular lymphoma, unspecified, lymph nodes of axilla and upper limb `HCC` `Rx` `ESR` `COM`

C82.95   Follicular lymphoma, unspecified, lymph nodes of inguinal region and lower limb `HCC` `Rx` `ESR` `COM`

C82.96   Follicular lymphoma, unspecified, intrapelvic lymph nodes `HCC` `Rx` `ESR` `COM`

C82.97   Follicular lymphoma, unspecified, spleen `HCC` `Rx` `ESR` `COM`

C82.98   Follicular lymphoma, unspecified, lymph nodes of multiple sites `HCC` `Rx` `ESR` `COM`

C82.99   Follicular lymphoma, unspecified, extranodal and solid organ sites `HCC` `Rx` `ESR` `COM`

✅ Additional Character Required   ✓x7th Placeholder Alert   Manifestation   Unspecified Dx   🄠 QPP   UPD Unacceptable PDx

✓4ᵗʰ **C83** Non-follicular **lymphoma**

　　　EXCLUDES 1　　*personal history of non-Hodgkin lymphoma (Z85.72)*

✓5ᵗʰ **C83.Ø** Small cell B-cell **lymphoma**

　　Lymphoplasmacytic lymphoma
　　Nodal marginal zone lymphoma
　　Non-leukemic variant of B-CLL
　　Splenic marginal zone lymphoma
　　　EXCLUDES 1　　*chronic lymphocytic leukemia (C91.1)*
　　　　　　　　mature T/NK-cell lymphomas (C84.-)
　　　　　　　　Waldenström macroglobulinemia (C88.Ø)
　　DEF: Nonfollicular lymphoma that is rare, slow growing, and
　　usually found in the older population.

　　C83.ØØ **Small cell B-cell lymphoma, unspecified
　　　　site** HCC Rx ESR COM

　　C83.Ø1 Small cell B-cell **lymphoma, lymph nodes of** head,
　　　　face, and neck HCC Rx ESR COM

　　C83.Ø2 Small cell B-cell **lymphoma,** intrathoracic **lymph
　　　　nodes** HCC Rx ESR COM

　　C83.Ø3 Small cell B-cell **lymphoma,** intra-abdominal **lymph
　　　　nodes** HCC Rx ESR COM

　　C83.Ø4 Small cell B-cell **lymphoma, lymph nodes of** axilla
　　　　and upper limb HCC Rx ESR COM

　　C83.Ø5 Small cell B-cell **lymphoma, lymph nodes of** inguinal
　　　　region and lower limb HCC Rx ESR COM

　　C83.Ø6 Small cell B-cell **lymphoma,** intrapelvic **lymph
　　　　nodes** HCC Rx ESR COM

　　C83.Ø7 Small cell B-cell **lymphoma,**
　　　　spleen HCC Rx ESR COM

　　C83.Ø8 Small cell B-cell **lymphoma, lymph nodes of**
　　　　multiple sites HCC Rx ESR COM

　　C83.Ø9 Small cell B-cell **lymphoma,** extranodal and solid
　　　　organ sites HCC Rx ESR COM

✓5ᵗʰ **C83.1** Mantle cell **lymphoma**

　　Centrocytic lymphoma
　　Malignant lymphomatous polyposis
　　DEF: Rare form of B-cell non-Hodgkin lymphoma named for the
　　location of the tumor cell production, the mantle zone of the
　　lymph nodes.

　　C83.1Ø **Mantle cell lymphoma, unspecified
　　　　site** HCC Rx ESR COM

　　C83.11 Mantle cell **lymphoma, lymph nodes of** head, face,
　　　　and neck HCC Rx ESR COM

　　C83.12 Mantle cell **lymphoma,** intrathoracic **lymph
　　　　nodes** HCC Rx ESR COM

　　C83.13 Mantle cell **lymphoma,** intra-abdominal **lymph
　　　　nodes** HCC Rx ESR COM

　　C83.14 Mantle cell **lymphoma, lymph nodes of** axilla and
　　　　upper limb HCC Rx ESR COM

　　C83.15 Mantle cell **lymphoma, lymph nodes of** inguinal
　　　　region and lower limb HCC Rx ESR COM

　　C83.16 Mantle cell **lymphoma,** intrapelvic **lymph
　　　　nodes** HCC Rx ESR COM

　　C83.17 Mantle cell **lymphoma,** spleen HCC Rx ESR COM

　　C83.18 Mantle cell **lymphoma, lymph nodes of** multiple
　　　　sites HCC Rx ESR COM

　　C83.19 Mantle cell **lymphoma,** extranodal and solid organ
　　　　sites HCC Rx ESR COM

✓5ᵗʰ **C83.3** Diffuse large B-cell **lymphoma**

　　Anaplastic diffuse large B-cell lymphoma
　　CD3Ø-positive diffuse large B-cell lymphoma
　　Centroblastic diffuse large B-cell lymphoma
　　Diffuse large B-cell lymphoma, subtype not specified
　　Immunoblastic diffuse large B-cell lymphoma
　　Plasmablastic diffuse large B-cell lymphoma
　　T-cell rich diffuse large B-cell lymphoma
　　　EXCLUDES 1　　*mediastinal (thymic) large B-cell lymphoma (C85.2-)*
　　　　　　　　mature T/NK-cell lymphomas (C84.-)
　　DEF: Nonfollicular lymphoma that is one of the more common
　　types of lymphoma. This cancer is fast growing and affects any
　　age and is found mostly in the older population.

　　C83.3Ø **Diffuse large B-cell lymphoma, unspecified
　　　　site** HCC Rx ESR COM

　　C83.31 Diffuse large B-cell **lymphoma, lymph nodes of**
　　　　head, face, and neck HCC Rx ESR COM

　　C83.32 Diffuse large B-cell **lymphoma,** intrathoracic **lymph
　　　　nodes** HCC Rx ESR COM

　　C83.33 Diffuse large B-cell **lymphoma,** intra-abdominal
　　　　lymph nodes HCC Rx ESR COM

C83.34 Diffuse large B-cell **lymphoma, lymph nodes of**
　　axilla and upper limb HCC Rx ESR COM

C83.35 Diffuse large B-cell **lymphoma, lymph nodes of**
　　inguinal region and lower limb HCC Rx ESR COM

C83.36 Diffuse large B-cell **lymphoma,** intrapelvic **lymph
　　nodes** HCC Rx ESR COM

C83.37 Diffuse large B-cell **lymphoma,**
　　spleen HCC Rx ESR COM

C83.38 Diffuse large B-cell **lymphoma, lymph nodes of**
　　multiple sites HCC Rx ESR COM

C83.39 Diffuse large B-cell **lymphoma,** extranodal and solid
　　organ sites HCC Rx ESR COM

✓5ᵗʰ **C83.5** Lymphoblastic (diffuse) **lymphoma**

　　B-precursor lymphoma
　　Lymphoblastic B-cell lymphoma
　　Lymphoblastic lymphoma NOS
　　Lymphoblastic T-cell lymphoma
　　T-precursor lymphoma
　　DEF: Type of non-Hodgkin lymphoma considered lymphoma or
　　leukemia—the determination is made based on the amount of
　　bone marrow involvement. The cells are small to medium
　　immature T-cells that often originate in the thymus where many
　　of the T-cells are made.

　　C83.5Ø **Lymphoblastic (diffuse) lymphoma, unspecified
　　　　site** HCC Rx ESR COM

　　C83.51 Lymphoblastic (diffuse) **lymphoma, lymph nodes
　　　　of** head, face, and neck HCC Rx ESR COM

　　C83.52 Lymphoblastic (diffuse) **lymphoma,** intrathoracic
　　　　lymph nodes HCC Rx ESR COM

　　C83.53 Lymphoblastic (diffuse) **lymphoma,**
　　　　intra-abdominal **lymph nodes** HCC Rx ESR COM

　　C83.54 Lymphoblastic (diffuse) **lymphoma, lymph nodes
　　　　of** axilla and upper limb HCC Rx ESR COM

　　C83.55 Lymphoblastic (diffuse) **lymphoma, lymph nodes
　　　　of** inguinal region and lower limb HCC Rx ESR COM

　　C83.56 Lymphoblastic (diffuse) **lymphoma,** intrapelvic
　　　　lymph nodes HCC Rx ESR COM

　　C83.57 Lymphoblastic (diffuse) **lymphoma,**
　　　　spleen HCC Rx ESR COM

　　C83.58 Lymphoblastic (diffuse) **lymphoma, lymph nodes
　　　　of** multiple sites HCC Rx ESR COM

　　C83.59 Lymphoblastic (diffuse) **lymphoma,** extranodal and
　　　　solid organ sites HCC Rx ESR COM

✓5ᵗʰ **C83.7** Burkitt **lymphoma**

　　Atypical Burkitt lymphoma
　　Burkitt-like lymphoma
　　　EXCLUDES 1　　*mature B-cell leukemia Burkitt type (C91.A-)*
　　DEF: Malignancy of the lymphatic system, most often seen as a
　　large bone-deteriorating lesion within the jaw or as an abdominal
　　mass. It is a form of non-Hodgkin's lymphoma and is recognized
　　as the fastest growing human tumor.

　　C83.7Ø **Burkitt lymphoma, unspecified
　　　　site** HCC Rx ESR COM

　　C83.71 Burkitt **lymphoma, lymph nodes of** head, face, and
　　　　neck HCC Rx ESR COM

　　C83.72 Burkitt **lymphoma,** intrathoracic **lymph
　　　　nodes** HCC Rx ESR COM

　　C83.73 Burkitt **lymphoma,** intra-abdominal **lymph
　　　　nodes** HCC Rx ESR COM

　　C83.74 Burkitt **lymphoma, lymph nodes of** axilla and upper
　　　　limb HCC Rx ESR COM

　　C83.75 Burkitt **lymphoma, lymph nodes of** inguinal region
　　　　and lower limb HCC Rx ESR COM

　　C83.76 Burkitt **lymphoma,** intrapelvic **lymph
　　　　nodes** HCC Rx ESR COM

　　C83.77 Burkitt **lymphoma,** spleen HCC Rx ESR COM

　　C83.78 Burkitt **lymphoma, lymph nodes of** multiple
　　　　sites HCC Rx ESR COM

　　C83.79 Burkitt **lymphoma,** extranodal and solid organ
　　　　sites HCC Rx ESR COM

✓5ᵗʰ **C83.8** Other non-follicular **lymphoma**

　　Intravascular large B-cell lymphoma
　　Lymphoid granulomatosis
　　Primary effusion B-cell lymphoma
　　　EXCLUDES 1　　*mediastinal (thymic) large B-cell lymphoma (C85.2-)*
　　　　　　　　T-cell rich B-cell lymphoma (C83.3-)

　　C83.8Ø **Other non-follicular lymphoma, unspecified
　　　　site** HCC Rx ESR COM

C83.81   Other non-follicular lymphoma, lymph nodes of head, face, and neck   `HCC` `Rx` `ESR` `COM`

C83.82   Other non-follicular lymphoma, intrathoracic lymph nodes   `HCC` `Rx` `ESR` `COM`

C83.83   Other non-follicular lymphoma, intra-abdominal lymph nodes   `HCC` `Rx` `ESR` `COM`

C83.84   Other non-follicular lymphoma, lymph nodes of axilla and upper limb   `HCC` `Rx` `ESR` `COM`

C83.85   Other non-follicular lymphoma, lymph nodes of inguinal region and lower limb   `HCC` `Rx` `ESR` `COM`

C83.86   Other non-follicular lymphoma, intrapelvic lymph nodes   `HCC` `Rx` `ESR` `COM`

C83.87   Other non-follicular lymphoma, spleen   `HCC` `Rx` `ESR` `COM`

C83.88   Other non-follicular lymphoma, lymph nodes of multiple sites   `HCC` `Rx` `ESR` `COM`

C83.89   Other non-follicular lymphoma, extranodal and solid organ sites   `HCC` `Rx` `ESR` `COM`

√5ᵗʰ **C83.9**   Non-follicular (diffuse) lymphoma, unspecified

C83.90   Non-follicular (diffuse) lymphoma, unspecified, unspecified site   `HCC` `Rx` `ESR` `COM`

C83.91   Non-follicular (diffuse) lymphoma, unspecified, lymph nodes of head, face, and neck   `HCC` `Rx` `ESR` `COM`

C83.92   Non-follicular (diffuse) lymphoma, unspecified, intrathoracic lymph nodes   `HCC` `Rx` `ESR` `COM`

C83.93   Non-follicular (diffuse) lymphoma, unspecified, intra-abdominal lymph nodes   `HCC` `Rx` `ESR` `COM`

C83.94   Non-follicular (diffuse) lymphoma, unspecified, lymph nodes of axilla and upper limb   `HCC` `Rx` `ESR` `COM`

C83.95   Non-follicular (diffuse) lymphoma, unspecified, lymph nodes of inguinal region and lower limb   `HCC` `Rx` `ESR` `COM`

C83.96   Non-follicular (diffuse) lymphoma, unspecified, intrapelvic lymph nodes   `HCC` `Rx` `ESR` `COM`

C83.97   Non-follicular (diffuse) lymphoma, unspecified, spleen   `HCC` `Rx` `ESR` `COM`

C83.98   Non-follicular (diffuse) lymphoma, unspecified, lymph nodes of multiple sites   `HCC` `Rx` `ESR` `COM`

C83.99   Non-follicular (diffuse) lymphoma, unspecified, extranodal and solid organ sites   `HCC` `Rx` `ESR` `COM`

√4ᵗʰ **C84**   **Mature T/NK-cell lymphomas**

> `EXCLUDES 1`   personal history of non-Hodgkin lymphoma (Z85.72)

√5ᵗʰ **C84.0**   Mycosis fungoides

> `EXCLUDES 1`   ►peripheral T-cell lymphoma, not elsewhere classified◄ (C84.4-)
>
> **DEF:** Most common form of cutaneous T-cell lymphoma. A type of non-Hodgkin lymphoma in which white blood cells become cancerous and affect the skin and sometimes internal organs.
> ***Synonym(s):*** *Alibert-Bazin syndrome.*

C84.00   Mycosis fungoides, unspecified site   `HCC` `Rx` `ESR` `COM`

C84.01   Mycosis fungoides, lymph nodes of head, face, and neck   `HCC` `Rx` `ESR` `COM`

C84.02   Mycosis fungoides, intrathoracic lymph nodes   `HCC` `Rx` `ESR` `COM`

C84.03   Mycosis fungoides, intra-abdominal lymph nodes   `HCC` `Rx` `ESR` `COM`

C84.04   Mycosis fungoides, lymph nodes of axilla and upper limb   `HCC` `Rx` `ESR` `COM`

C84.05   Mycosis fungoides, lymph nodes of inguinal region and lower limb   `HCC` `Rx` `ESR` `COM`

C84.06   Mycosis fungoides, intrapelvic lymph nodes   `HCC` `Rx` `ESR` `COM`

C84.07   Mycosis fungoides, spleen   `HCC` `Rx` `ESR` `COM`

C84.08   Mycosis fungoides, lymph nodes of multiple sites   `HCC` `Rx` `ESR` `COM`

C84.09   Mycosis fungoides, extranodal and solid organ sites   `HCC` `Rx` `ESR` `COM`

√5ᵗʰ **C84.1**   Sézary disease

> **DEF:** Extension of mycosis fungoides that affects the blood and all of the skin, appearing as sunburn, rather than patches. It spreads to the lymph nodes and is often linked to a weakened immune system.

C84.10   Sézary disease, unspecified site   `HCC` `Rx` `ESR` `COM`

C84.11   Sézary disease, lymph nodes of head, face, and neck   `HCC` `Rx` `ESR` `COM`

C84.12   Sézary disease, intrathoracic lymph nodes   `HCC` `Rx` `ESR` `COM`

C84.13   Sézary disease, intra-abdominal lymph nodes   `HCC` `Rx` `ESR` `COM`

C84.14   Sézary disease, lymph nodes of axilla and upper limb   `HCC` `Rx` `ESR` `COM`

C84.15   Sézary disease, lymph nodes of inguinal region and lower limb   `HCC` `Rx` `ESR` `COM`

C84.16   Sézary disease, intrapelvic lymph nodes   `HCC` `Rx` `ESR` `COM`

C84.17   Sézary disease, spleen   `HCC` `Rx` `ESR` `COM`

C84.18   Sézary disease, lymph nodes of multiple sites   `HCC` `Rx` `ESR` `COM`

C84.19   Sézary disease, extranodal and solid organ sites   `HCC` `Rx` `ESR` `COM`

▲ √5ᵗʰ **C84.4**   Peripheral T-cell lymphoma, not elsewhere classified

> Lennert's lymphoma
> Lymphoepithelioid lymphoma
> Mature T-cell lymphoma, not elsewhere classified

▲ **C84.40**   Peripheral T-cell lymphoma, not elsewhere classified, unspecified site   `HCC` `Rx` `ESR` `COM`

▲ **C84.41**   Peripheral T-cell lymphoma, not elsewhere classified, lymph nodes of head, face, and neck   `HCC` `Rx` `ESR` `COM`

▲ **C84.42**   Peripheral T-cell lymphoma, not elsewhere classified, intrathoracic lymph nodes   `HCC` `Rx` `ESR` `COM`

▲ **C84.43**   Peripheral T-cell lymphoma, not elsewhere classified, intra-abdominal lymph nodes   `HCC` `Rx` `ESR` `COM`

▲ **C84.44**   Peripheral T-cell lymphoma, not elsewhere classified, lymph nodes of axilla and upper limb   `HCC` `Rx` `ESR` `COM`

▲ **C84.45**   Peripheral T-cell lymphoma, not elsewhere classified, lymph nodes of inguinal region and lower limb   `HCC` `Rx` `ESR` `COM`

▲ **C84.46**   Peripheral T-cell lymphoma, not elsewhere classified, intrapelvic lymph nodes   `HCC` `Rx` `ESR` `COM`

▲ **C84.47**   Peripheral T-cell lymphoma, not elsewhere classified, spleen   `HCC` `Rx` `ESR` `COM`

▲ **C84.48**   Peripheral T-cell lymphoma, not elsewhere classified, lymph nodes of multiple sites   `HCC` `Rx` `ESR` `COM`

▲ **C84.49**   Peripheral T-cell lymphoma, not elsewhere classified, extranodal and solid organ sites   `HCC` `Rx` `ESR` `COM`

√5ᵗʰ **C84.6**   Anaplastic large cell lymphoma, ALK-positive

> Anaplastic large cell lymphoma, CD30-positive

C84.60   Anaplastic large cell lymphoma, ALK-positive, unspecified site   `HCC` `Rx` `ESR` `COM`

C84.61   Anaplastic large cell lymphoma, ALK-positive, lymph nodes of head, face, and neck   `HCC` `Rx` `ESR` `COM`

C84.62   Anaplastic large cell lymphoma, ALK-positive, intrathoracic lymph nodes   `HCC` `Rx` `ESR` `COM`

C84.63   Anaplastic large cell lymphoma, ALK-positive, intra-abdominal lymph nodes   `HCC` `Rx` `ESR` `COM`

C84.64   Anaplastic large cell lymphoma, ALK-positive, lymph nodes of axilla and upper limb   `HCC` `Rx` `ESR` `COM`

C84.65   Anaplastic large cell lymphoma, ALK-positive, lymph nodes of inguinal region and lower limb   `HCC` `Rx` `ESR` `COM`

C84.66   Anaplastic large cell lymphoma, ALK-positive, intrapelvic lymph nodes   `HCC` `Rx` `ESR` `COM`

C84.67   Anaplastic large cell lymphoma, ALK-positive, spleen   `HCC` `Rx` `ESR` `COM`

C84.68   Anaplastic large cell lymphoma, ALK-positive, lymph nodes of multiple sites   `HCC` `Rx` `ESR` `COM`

C84.69   Anaplastic large cell lymphoma, ALK-positive, extranodal and solid organ sites   `HCC` `Rx` `ESR` `COM`

√5ᵗʰ **C84.7**   Anaplastic large cell lymphoma, ALK-negative

> `EXCLUDES 1`   primary cutaneous CD30-positive T-cell proliferations (C86.6-)

C84.70   Anaplastic large cell lymphoma, ALK-negative, unspecified site   `HCC` `Rx` `ESR` `COM`

C84.71 Anaplastic large cell lymphoma, ALK-negative, lymph nodes of head, face, and neck `HCC` `Rx` `ESR` `COM`

C84.72 Anaplastic large cell lymphoma, ALK-negative, intrathoracic lymph nodes `HCC` `Rx` `ESR` `COM`

C84.73 Anaplastic large cell lymphoma, ALK-negative, intra-abdominal lymph nodes `HCC` `Rx` `ESR` `COM`

C84.74 Anaplastic large cell lymphoma, ALK-negative, lymph nodes of axilla and upper limb `HCC` `Rx` `ESR` `COM`

C84.75 Anaplastic large cell lymphoma, ALK-negative, lymph nodes of inguinal region and lower limb `HCC` `Rx` `ESR` `COM`

C84.76 Anaplastic large cell lymphoma, ALK-negative, intrapelvic lymph nodes `HCC` `Rx` `ESR` `COM`

C84.77 Anaplastic large cell lymphoma, ALK-negative, spleen `HCC` `Rx` `ESR` `COM`

C84.78 Anaplastic large cell lymphoma, ALK-negative, lymph nodes of multiple sites `HCC` `Rx` `ESR` `COM`

C84.79 Anaplastic large cell lymphoma, ALK-negative, extranodal and solid organ sites `HCC` `Rx` `ESR` `COM`

C84.7A Anaplastic large cell lymphoma, ALK-negative, breast `HCC` `Rx` `ESR` `COM`
Breast implant associated anaplastic large cell lymphoma (BIA-ALCL)
Use additional code to identify:
  breast implant status (Z98.82)
  personal history of breast implant removal (Z98.86)
AHA: 2021,4Q,6

√5ᵗʰ **C84.A** Cutaneous T-cell lymphoma, unspecified
AHA: 2021,2Q,6

C84.A0 Cutaneous T-cell lymphoma, unspecified, unspecified site `HCC` `Rx` `ESR` `COM`

C84.A1 Cutaneous T-cell lymphoma, unspecified lymph nodes of head, face, and neck `HCC` `Rx` `ESR` `COM`

C84.A2 Cutaneous T-cell lymphoma, unspecified, intrathoracic lymph nodes `HCC` `Rx` `ESR` `COM`

C84.A3 Cutaneous T-cell lymphoma, unspecified, intra-abdominal lymph nodes `HCC` `Rx` `ESR` `COM`

C84.A4 Cutaneous T-cell lymphoma, unspecified, lymph nodes of axilla and upper limb `HCC` `Rx` `ESR` `COM`

C84.A5 Cutaneous T-cell lymphoma, unspecified, lymph nodes of inguinal region and lower limb `HCC` `Rx` `ESR` `COM`

C84.A6 Cutaneous T-cell lymphoma, unspecified, intrapelvic lymph nodes `HCC` `Rx` `ESR` `COM`

C84.A7 Cutaneous T-cell lymphoma, unspecified, spleen `HCC` `Rx` `ESR` `COM`

C84.A8 Cutaneous T-cell lymphoma, unspecified, lymph nodes of multiple sites `HCC` `Rx` `ESR` `COM`

C84.A9 Cutaneous T-cell lymphoma, unspecified, extranodal and solid organ sites `HCC` `Rx` `ESR` `COM`

√5ᵗʰ **C84.Z** Other mature T/NK-cell lymphomas

NOTE If T-cell lineage or involvement is mentioned in conjunction with a specific lymphoma, code to the more specific description.

EXCLUDES 1 angioimmunoblastic T-cell lymphoma (C86.5)
blastic NK-cell lymphoma (C86.4)
enteropathy-type T-cell lymphoma (C86.2)
extranodal NK-cell lymphoma, nasal type (C86.0)
hepatosplenic T-cell lymphoma (C86.1)
primary cutaneous CD30-positive T-cell proliferations (C86.6)
subcutaneous panniculitis-like T-cell lymphoma (C86.3)
T-cell leukemia (C91.1-)

C84.Z0 Other mature T/NK-cell lymphomas, unspecified site `HCC` `Rx` `ESR` `COM`

C84.Z1 Other mature T/NK-cell lymphomas, lymph nodes of head, face, and neck `HCC` `Rx` `ESR` `COM`

C84.Z2 Other mature T/NK-cell lymphomas, intrathoracic lymph nodes `HCC` `Rx` `ESR` `COM`

C84.Z3 Other mature T/NK-cell lymphomas, intra-abdominal lymph nodes `HCC` `Rx` `ESR` `COM`

C84.Z4 Other mature T/NK-cell lymphomas, lymph nodes of axilla and upper limb `HCC` `Rx` `ESR` `COM`

C84.Z5 Other mature T/NK-cell lymphomas, lymph nodes of inguinal region and lower limb `HCC` `Rx` `ESR` `COM`

C84.Z6 Other mature T/NK-cell lymphomas, intrapelvic lymph nodes `HCC` `Rx` `ESR` `COM`

C84.Z7 Other mature T/NK-cell lymphomas, spleen `HCC` `Rx` `ESR` `COM`

C84.Z8 Other mature T/NK-cell lymphomas, lymph nodes of multiple sites `HCC` `Rx` `ESR` `COM`

C84.Z9 Other mature T/NK-cell lymphomas, extranodal and solid organ sites `HCC` `Rx` `ESR` `COM`

√5ᵗʰ **C84.9** Mature T/NK-cell lymphomas, unspecified
NK/T cell lymphoma NOS
EXCLUDES 1 mature T-cell lymphoma, not elsewhere classified (C84.4-)

C84.90 Mature T/NK-cell lymphomas, unspecified, unspecified site `HCC` `Rx` `ESR` `COM`

C84.91 Mature T/NK-cell lymphomas, unspecified, lymph nodes of head, face, and neck `HCC` `Rx` `ESR` `COM`

C84.92 Mature T/NK-cell lymphomas, unspecified, intrathoracic lymph nodes `HCC` `Rx` `ESR` `COM`

C84.93 Mature T/NK-cell lymphomas, unspecified, intra-abdominal lymph nodes `HCC` `Rx` `ESR` `COM`

C84.94 Mature T/NK-cell lymphomas, unspecified, lymph nodes of axilla and upper limb `HCC` `Rx` `ESR` `COM`

C84.95 Mature T/NK-cell lymphomas, unspecified, lymph nodes of inguinal region and lower limb `HCC` `Rx` `ESR` `COM`

C84.96 Mature T/NK-cell lymphomas, unspecified, intrapelvic lymph nodes `HCC` `Rx` `ESR` `COM`

C84.97 Mature T/NK-cell lymphomas, unspecified, spleen `HCC` `Rx` `ESR` `COM`

C84.98 Mature T/NK-cell lymphomas, unspecified, lymph nodes of multiple sites `HCC` `Rx` `ESR` `COM`

C84.99 Mature T/NK-cell lymphomas, unspecified, extranodal and solid organ sites `HCC` `Rx` `ESR` `COM`

√4ᵗʰ **C85** Other specified and unspecified types of non-Hodgkin lymphoma
EXCLUDES 1 other specified types of T/NK-cell lymphoma (C86.-)
personal history of non-Hodgkin lymphoma (Z85.72)

√5ᵗʰ **C85.1** Unspecified B-cell lymphoma

NOTE If B-cell lineage or involvement is mentioned in conjunction with a specific lymphoma, code to the more specific description.

C85.10 Unspecified B-cell lymphoma, unspecified site `HCC` `Rx` `ESR` `COM`

C85.11 Unspecified B-cell lymphoma, lymph nodes of head, face, and neck `HCC` `Rx` `ESR` `COM`

C85.12 Unspecified B-cell lymphoma, intrathoracic lymph nodes `HCC` `Rx` `ESR` `COM`

C85.13 Unspecified B-cell lymphoma, intra-abdominal lymph nodes `HCC` `Rx` `ESR` `COM`

C85.14 Unspecified B-cell lymphoma, lymph nodes of axilla and upper limb `HCC` `Rx` `ESR` `COM`

C85.15 Unspecified B-cell lymphoma, lymph nodes of inguinal region and lower limb `HCC` `Rx` `ESR` `COM`

C85.16 Unspecified B-cell lymphoma, intrapelvic lymph nodes `HCC` `Rx` `ESR` `COM`

C85.17 Unspecified B-cell lymphoma, spleen `HCC` `Rx` `ESR` `COM`

C85.18 Unspecified B-cell lymphoma, lymph nodes of multiple sites `HCC` `Rx` `ESR` `COM`

C85.19 Unspecified B-cell lymphoma, extranodal and solid organ sites `HCC` `Rx` `ESR` `COM`

√5ᵗʰ **C85.2** Mediastinal (thymic) large B-cell lymphoma

C85.20 Mediastinal (thymic) large B-cell lymphoma, unspecified site `HCC` `Rx` `ESR` `COM`

C85.21 Mediastinal (thymic) large B-cell lymphoma, lymph nodes of head, face, and neck `HCC` `Rx` `ESR` `COM`

C85.22 Mediastinal (thymic) large B-cell lymphoma, intrathoracic lymph nodes `HCC` `Rx` `ESR` `COM`

C85.23 Mediastinal (thymic) large B-cell lymphoma, intra-abdominal lymph nodes `HCC` `Rx` `ESR` `COM`

C85.24 Mediastinal (thymic) large B-cell lymphoma, lymph nodes of axilla and upper limb `HCC` `Rx` `ESR` `COM`

C85.25 Mediastinal (thymic) large B-cell lymphoma, lymph nodes of inguinal region and lower limb `HCC` `Rx` `ESR` `COM`

C85.26 Mediastinal (thymic) large B-cell lymphoma, intrapelvic lymph nodes `HCC` `Rx` `ESR` `COM`

C85.27   **Mediastinal (thymic) large B-cell lymphoma, spleen**   `HCC` `Rx` `ESR` `COM`

C85.28   **Mediastinal (thymic) large B-cell lymphoma, lymph nodes of** multiple sites   `HCC` `Rx` `ESR` `COM`

C85.29   **Mediastinal (thymic) large B-cell lymphoma, extranodal and solid organ sites**   `HCC` `Rx` `ESR` `COM`

✓5ᵗʰ **C85.8**   **Other specified types of non-Hodgkin lymphoma**

    C85.80   **Other specified types of non-Hodgkin lymphoma, unspecified site**   `HCC` `Rx` `ESR` `COM`

    C85.81   **Other specified types of non-Hodgkin lymphoma, lymph nodes of** head, face, and neck   `HCC` `Rx` `ESR` `COM`

    C85.82   **Other specified types of non-Hodgkin lymphoma,** intrathoracic **lymph nodes**   `HCC` `Rx` `ESR` `COM`

    C85.83   **Other specified types of non-Hodgkin lymphoma,** intra-abdominal **lymph nodes**   `HCC` `Rx` `ESR` `COM`

    C85.84   **Other specified types of non-Hodgkin lymphoma, lymph nodes of** axilla and upper limb   `HCC` `Rx` `ESR` `COM`

    C85.85   **Other specified types of non-Hodgkin lymphoma, lymph nodes of** inguinal region and lower limb   `HCC` `Rx` `ESR` `COM`

    C85.86   **Other specified types of non-Hodgkin lymphoma,** intrapelvic **lymph nodes**   `HCC` `Rx` `ESR` `COM`

    C85.87   **Other specified types of non-Hodgkin lymphoma, spleen**   `HCC` `Rx` `ESR` `COM`

    C85.88   **Other specified types of non-Hodgkin lymphoma, lymph nodes of** multiple sites   `HCC` `Rx` `ESR` `COM`

    C85.89   **Other specified types of non-Hodgkin lymphoma, extranodal and solid organ sites**   `HCC` `Rx` `ESR` `COM`

✓5ᵗʰ **C85.9**   **Non-Hodgkin lymphoma, unspecified**

Lymphoma NOS
Malignant lymphoma NOS
Non-Hodgkin lymphoma NOS

    C85.90   **Non-Hodgkin lymphoma, unspecified, unspecified site**   `HCC` `Rx` `ESR` `COM`

    C85.91   **Non-Hodgkin lymphoma, unspecified, lymph nodes of** head, face, and neck   `HCC` `Rx` `ESR` `COM`

    C85.92   **Non-Hodgkin lymphoma, unspecified,** intrathoracic **lymph nodes**   `HCC` `Rx` `ESR` `COM`

    C85.93   **Non-Hodgkin lymphoma, unspecified,** intra-abdominal **lymph nodes**   `HCC` `Rx` `ESR` `COM`

    C85.94   **Non-Hodgkin lymphoma, unspecified, lymph nodes of** axilla and upper limb   `HCC` `Rx` `ESR` `COM`

    C85.95   **Non-Hodgkin lymphoma, unspecified, lymph nodes of** inguinal region and lower limb   `HCC` `Rx` `ESR` `COM`

    C85.96   **Non-Hodgkin lymphoma, unspecified,** intrapelvic **lymph nodes**   `HCC` `Rx` `ESR` `COM`

    C85.97   **Non-Hodgkin lymphoma, unspecified, spleen**   `HCC` `Rx` `ESR` `COM`

    C85.98   **Non-Hodgkin lymphoma, unspecified, lymph nodes of** multiple sites   `HCC` `Rx` `ESR` `COM`

    C85.99   **Non-Hodgkin lymphoma, unspecified,** extranodal and solid organ sites   `HCC` `Rx` `ESR` `COM`

✓4ᵗʰ **C86**   **Other specified types of T/NK-cell lymphoma**

    EXCLUDES 1   *anaplastic large cell lymphoma, ALK negative (C84.7-)*
                anaplastic large cell lymphoma, ALK positive (C84.6-)
                mature T/NK-cell lymphomas (C84.-)
                other specified types of non-Hodgkin lymphoma (C85.8-)

C86.0   **Extranodal NK/T-cell lymphoma, nasal type**   `HCC` `Rx` `ESR` `COM`

C86.1   **Hepatosplenic T-cell lymphoma**   `HCC` `Rx` `ESR` `COM`

Alpha-beta and gamma delta types

C86.2   **Enteropathy-type (intestinal) T-cell lymphoma**   `HCC` `Rx` `ESR` `COM`

Enteropathy associated T-cell lymphoma

C86.3   **Subcutaneous panniculitis-like T-cell lymphoma**   `HCC` `Rx` `ESR` `COM`

C86.4   **Blastic NK-cell lymphoma**   `HCC` `Rx` `ESR` `COM`

Blastic plasmacytoid dendritic cell neoplasm (BPDCN)

C86.5   **Angioimmunoblastic T-cell lymphoma**   `HCC` `Rx` `ESR` `COM`

Angioimmunoblastic lymphadenopathy with dysproteinemia (AILD)

C86.6   **Primary cutaneous CD30-positive T-cell proliferations**   `HCC` `Rx` `ESR` `COM`

Lymphomatoid papulosis
Primary cutaneous anaplastic large cell lymphoma
Primary cutaneous CD30-positive large T-cell lymphoma

✓4ᵗʰ **C88**   **Malignant immunoproliferative diseases and certain other B-cell lymphomas**

    EXCLUDES 1   *B-cell lymphoma, unspecified (C85.1-)*
                personal history of other malignant neoplasms of lymphoid, hematopoietic and related tissues (Z85.79)

C88.0   **Waldenström macroglobulinemia**   `HCC` `Rx` `ESR` `COM`

Lymphoplasmacytic lymphoma with IgM-production
Macroglobulinemia (idiopathic) (primary)
    EXCLUDES 1   *small cell B-cell lymphoma (C83.0)*

C88.2   **Heavy chain disease**   `HCC` `Rx` `ESR` `COM`

Franklin disease
Gamma heavy chain disease
Mu heavy chain disease

C88.3   **Immunoproliferative small intestinal disease**   `HCC` `Rx` `ESR` `COM`

Alpha heavy chain disease
Mediterranean lymphoma

C88.4   **Extranodal marginal zone B-cell lymphoma of mucosa-associated lymphoid tissue [MALT-lymphoma]**   `HCC` `Rx` `ESR` `COM`

Lymphoma of skin-associated lymphoid tissue [SALT-lymphoma]
Lymphoma of bronchial-associated lymphoid tissue [BALT-lymphoma]
    EXCLUDES 1   *high malignant (diffuse large B-cell) lymphoma (C83.3-)*

C88.8   **Other malignant immunoproliferative diseases**   `HCC` `Rx` `ESR` `COM`

C88.9   **Malignant immunoproliferative disease, unspecified**   `HCC` `Rx` `ESR` `COM`

Immunoproliferative disease NOS

✓4ᵗʰ **C90**   **Multiple myeloma and malignant plasma cell neoplasms**

    EXCLUDES 1   *personal history of other malignant neoplasms of lymphoid, hematopoietic and related tissues (Z85.79)*

AHA: 2019,2Q,30

✓5ᵗʰ **C90.0**   **Multiple myeloma**

Kahler's disease
Medullary plasmacytoma
Myelomatosis
Plasma cell myeloma
    EXCLUDES 1   *solitary myeloma (C90.3-)*
                solitary plasmactyoma (C90.3-)

AHA: 2021,3Q,5

TIP: Smoldering multiple myeloma (SMM) is a plasma cell disorder that has not yet progressed to active multiple myeloma. Code D47.2 should be used when only SMM is documented.

TIP: Do not assign an additional code for bone metastasis (C79.51) when multiple myeloma is described as metastatic to the bone; bone involvement is integral to this disease process.

    C90.00   **Multiple myeloma** not having achieved remission   `HCC` `Rx` `ESR` `COM`

Multiple myeloma with failed remission
Multiple myeloma NOS

    C90.01   **Multiple myeloma** in remission   `HCC` `Rx` `ESR` `COM`

    C90.02   **Multiple myeloma** in relapse   `HCC` `Rx` `ESR` `COM`

✓5ᵗʰ **C90.1**   **Plasma cell leukemia**

Plasmacytic leukemia
AHA: 2019,2Q,30

    C90.10   **Plasma cell leukemia** not having achieved remission   `HCC` `Rx` `ESR` `COM`

Plasma cell leukemia with failed remission
Plasma cell leukemia NOS

    C90.11   **Plasma cell leukemia** in remission   `HCC` `Rx` `ESR` `COM`

    C90.12   **Plasma cell leukemia** in relapse   `HCC` `Rx` `ESR` `COM`

✓5ᵗʰ **C90.2**   **Extramedullary plasmacytoma**

    C90.20   **Extramedullary plasmacytoma** not having achieved remission   `HCC` `Rx` `ESR` `COM`

Extramedullary plasmacytoma with failed remission
Extramedullary plasmacytoma NOS

    C90.21   **Extramedullary plasmacytoma** in remission   `HCC` `Rx` `ESR` `COM`

☑ Additional Character Required   ✓x7ᵗʰ Placeholder Alert   Manifestation   Unspecified Dx   Q QPP   UPD Unacceptable PDx

Chapter 2. Neoplasms

C90.22   **Extramedullary plasmacytoma** in relapse   HCC Rx ESR COM

✓5ᵗʰ **C90.3**   **Solitary plasmacytoma**

     Localized malignant plasma cell tumor NOS
     Plasmacytoma NOS
     Solitary myeloma

     C90.30   **Solitary plasmacytoma** not having achieved remission   HCC Rx ESR COM
         Solitary plasmacytoma with failed remission
         Solitary plasmacytoma NOS

     C90.31   **Solitary plasmacytoma** in remission   HCC Rx ESR COM

     C90.32   **Solitary plasmacytoma** in relapse   HCC Rx ESR COM

✓4ᵗʰ **C91**   **Lymphoid leukemia**

     EXCLUDES 1   personal history of leukemia (Z85.6)

     AHA: 2020,1Q,13
     DEF: Malignant proliferation of immature lymphocytes (white blood cells that make up lymphoid tissue), called lymphoblasts, that originate in the bone marrow. Can be acute (ALL) or chronic (CLL).

✓5ᵗʰ **C91.0**   **Acute lymphoblastic** leukemia [ALL]

     NOTE   Codes in subcategory C91.0- should only be used for T-cell and B-cell precursor leukemia

     C91.00   **Acute lymphoblastic leukemia** not having achieved remission   HCC Rx ESR COM
         Acute lymphoblastic leukemia with failed remission
         Acute lymphoblastic leukemia NOS

     C91.01   **Acute lymphoblastic leukemia,** in remission   HCC Rx ESR COM

     C91.02   **Acute lymphoblastic leukemia,** in relapse   HCC Rx ESR COM

✓5ᵗʰ **C91.1**   **Chronic lymphocytic** leukemia of B-cell type

     Lymphoplasmacytic leukemia
     Richter syndrome
     EXCLUDES 1   lymphoplasmacytic lymphoma (C83.0-)

     C91.10   **Chronic lymphocytic leukemia of B-cell type** not having achieved remission   HCC Rx ESR COM
         Chronic lymphocytic leukemia of B-cell type with failed remission
         Chronic lymphocytic leukemia of B-cell type NOS

     C91.11   **Chronic lymphocytic leukemia of B-cell type** in remission   HCC Rx ESR COM

     C91.12   **Chronic lymphocytic leukemia of B-cell type** in relapse   HCC Rx ESR COM

✓5ᵗʰ **C91.3**   **Prolymphocytic** leukemia of B-cell type

     C91.30   **Prolymphocytic leukemia of B-cell type** not having achieved remission   HCC Rx ESR COM
         Prolymphocytic leukemia of B-cell type with failed remission
         Prolymphocytic leukemia of B-cell type NOS

     C91.31   **Prolymphocytic leukemia of B-cell type,** in remission   HCC Rx ESR COM

     C91.32   **Prolymphocytic leukemia of B-cell type,** in relapse   HCC Rx ESR COM

✓5ᵗʰ **C91.4**   **Hairy cell** leukemia

     Leukemic reticuloendotheliosis
     DEF: Rare type of leukemia that is slow growing and often also considered a type of lymphoma. The small B-cell lymphocytes appear with "hairy" projections under a microscope and are found mostly in the bone marrow, spleen, and blood.

     C91.40   **Hairy cell leukemia** not having achieved remission   HCC Rx ESR COM
         Hairy cell leukemia with failed remission
         Hairy cell leukemia NOS

     C91.41   **Hairy cell leukemia,** in remission   HCC Rx ESR COM

     C91.42   **Hairy cell leukemia,** in relapse   HCC Rx ESR COM

✓5ᵗʰ **C91.5**   **Adult T-cell** lymphoma/leukemia (HTLV-1-associated)

     Acute variant of adult T-cell lymphoma/leukemia (HTLV-1-associated)
     Chronic variant of adult T-cell lymphoma/leukemia (HTLV-1-associated)
     Lymphomatoid variant of adult T-cell lymphoma/leukemia (HTLV-1-associated)
     Smouldering variant of adult T-cell lymphoma/leukemia (HTLV-1-associated)

     C91.50   **Adult T-cell lymphoma/leukemia (HTLV-1-associated)** not having achieved remission   HCC Rx ESR COM A
         Adult T-cell lymphoma/leukemia (HTLV-1-associated) with failed remission
         Adult T-cell lymphoma/leukemia (HTLV-1-associated) NOS

     C91.51   **Adult T-cell lymphoma/leukemia (HTLV-1-associated),** in remission   HCC Rx ESR COM A

     C91.52   **Adult T-cell lymphoma/leukemia (HTLV-1-associated),** in relapse   HCC Rx ESR COM A

✓5ᵗʰ **C91.6**   **Prolymphocytic** leukemia of T-cell type

     C91.60   **Prolymphocytic leukemia of T-cell type** not having achieved remission   HCC Rx ESR COM
         Prolymphocytic leukemia of T-cell type with failed remission
         Prolymphocytic leukemia of T-cell type NOS

     C91.61   **Prolymphocytic leukemia of T-cell type,** in remission   HCC Rx ESR COM

     C91.62   **Prolymphocytic leukemia of T-cell type,** in relapse   HCC Rx ESR COM

✓5ᵗʰ **C91.A**   **Mature B-cell** leukemia Burkitt-type

     EXCLUDES 1   Burkitt lymphoma (C83.7-)

     C91.A0   **Mature B-cell leukemia Burkitt-type** not having achieved remission   HCC Rx ESR COM
         Mature B-cell leukemia Burkitt-type with failed remission
         Mature B-cell leukemia Burkitt-type NOS

     C91.A1   **Mature B-cell leukemia Burkitt-type,** in remission   HCC Rx ESR COM

     C91.A2   **Mature B-cell leukemia Burkitt-type,** in relapse   HCC Rx ESR COM

✓5ᵗʰ **C91.Z**   **Other lymphoid leukemia**

     T-cell large granular lymphocytic leukemia (associated with rheumatoid arthritis)

     C91.Z0   **Other lymphoid leukemia** not having achieved remission   HCC Rx ESR COM
         Other lymphoid leukemia with failed remission
         Other lymphoid leukemia NOS

     C91.Z1   **Other lymphoid leukemia,** in remission   HCC Rx ESR COM

     C91.Z2   **Other lymphoid leukemia,** in relapse   HCC Rx ESR COM

✓5ᵗʰ **C91.9**   **Lymphoid leukemia, unspecified**

     C91.90   **Lymphoid leukemia, unspecified** not having achieved remission   HCC Rx ESR COM
         Lymphoid leukemia with failed remission
         Lymphoid leukemia NOS

     C91.91   **Lymphoid leukemia, unspecified,** in remission   HCC Rx ESR COM

     C91.92   **Lymphoid leukemia, unspecified,** in relapse   HCC Rx ESR COM

✓4ᵗʰ C92 Myeloid leukemia

    INCLUDES   granulocytic leukemia
               myelogenous leukemia
    EXCLUDES 1 *personal history of leukemia (Z85.6)*

    AHA: 2020,1Q,13; 2019,1Q,16
    DEF: Cancer that develops in immature myelocytes called myeloblasts. These are the cells that become white blood cells (except lymphocytes), red blood cells, or platelet-making cells. Can be acute (AML) or chronic (CML).
    TIP: Pancytopenia, although common in some types of myeloid leukemias, is not always inherent. When it is documented, code D61.818 can be assigned in addition to a code from this category.

  ✓5ᵗʰ C92.0 Acute myeloblastic leukemia

    Acute myeloblastic leukemia, minimal differentiation
    Acute myeloblastic leukemia (with maturation)
    Acute myeloblastic leukemia 1/ETO
    Acute myeloblastic leukemia M0
    Acute myeloblastic leukemia M1
    Acute myeloblastic leukemia M2
    Acute myeloblastic leukemia with t(8;21)
    Acute myeloblastic leukemia (without a FAB classification) NOS
    Refractory anemia with excess blasts in transformation [RAEBT]
      EXCLUDES 1 *acute exacerbation of chronic myeloid leukemia (C92.10)*
                  refractory anemia with excess of blasts not in transformation (D46.2-)

      AHA: 2018,4Q,87

    C92.00 Acute myeloblastic leukemia, not having achieved remission HCC Rx ESR COM
          Acute myeloblastic leukemia with failed remission
          Acute myeloblastic leukemia NOS
    C92.01 Acute myeloblastic leukemia, in remission HCC Rx ESR COM
          AHA: 2021,3Q,4
    C92.02 Acute myeloblastic leukemia, in relapse HCC Rx ESR COM

  ✓5ᵗʰ C92.1 Chronic myeloid leukemia, BCR/ABL-positive

    Chronic myelogenous leukemia, Philadelphia chromosome (Ph1) positive
    Chronic myelogenous leukemia, t(9;22) (q34;q11)
    Chronic myelogenous leukemia with crisis of blast cells
      EXCLUDES 1 *atypical chronic myeloid leukemia BCR/ABL-negative (C92.2-)*
                  chronic myelomonocytic leukemia (C93.1-)
                  chronic myeloproliferative disease (D47.1)

    C92.10 Chronic myeloid leukemia, BCR/ABL-positive, not having achieved remission HCC Rx ESR COM
          Chronic myeloid leukemia, BCR/ABL-positive with failed remission
          Chronic myeloid leukemia, BCR/ABL-positive NOS
    C92.11 Chronic myeloid leukemia, BCR/ABL-positive, in remission HCC Rx ESR COM
    C92.12 Chronic myeloid leukemia, BCR/ABL-positive, in relapse HCC Rx ESR COM

  ✓5ᵗʰ C92.2 Atypical chronic myeloid leukemia, BCR/ABL-negative

    C92.20 Atypical chronic myeloid leukemia, BCR/ABL-negative, not having achieved remission HCC Rx ESR COM
          Atypical chronic myeloid leukemia, BCR/ABL-negative with failed remission
          Atypical chronic myeloid leukemia, BCR/ABL-negative NOS
    C92.21 Atypical chronic myeloid leukemia, BCR/ABL-negative, in remission HCC Rx ESR COM
    C92.22 Atypical chronic myeloid leukemia, BCR/ABL-negative, in relapse HCC Rx ESR COM

  ✓5ᵗʰ C92.3 Myeloid sarcoma

    A malignant tumor of immature myeloid cells
    Chloroma
    Granulocytic sarcoma
    C92.30 Myeloid sarcoma, not having achieved remission HCC Rx ESR COM
          Myeloid sarcoma with failed remission
          Myeloid sarcoma NOS
    C92.31 Myeloid sarcoma, in remission HCC Rx ESR COM
    C92.32 Myeloid sarcoma, in relapse HCC Rx ESR COM

  ✓5ᵗʰ C92.4 Acute promyelocytic leukemia

    AML M3
    AML Me with t(15;17) and variants
    C92.40 Acute promyelocytic leukemia, not having achieved remission HCC Rx ESR COM
          Acute promyelocytic leukemia with failed remission
          Acute promyelocytic leukemia NOS
    C92.41 Acute promyelocytic leukemia, in remission HCC Rx ESR COM
    C92.42 Acute promyelocytic leukemia, in relapse HCC Rx ESR COM

  ✓5ᵗʰ C92.5 Acute myelomonocytic leukemia

    AML M4
    AML M4 Eo with inv(16) or t(16;16)
    C92.50 Acute myelomonocytic leukemia, not having achieved remission HCC Rx ESR COM
          Acute myelomonocytic leukemia with failed remission
          Acute myelomonocytic leukemia NOS
    C92.51 Acute myelomonocytic leukemia, in remission HCC Rx ESR COM
    C92.52 Acute myelomonocytic leukemia, in relapse HCC Rx ESR COM

  ✓5ᵗʰ C92.6 Acute myeloid leukemia with 11q23-abnormality

    Acute myeloid leukemia with variation of MLL-gene
    C92.60 Acute myeloid leukemia with 11q23-abnormality not having achieved remission HCC Rx ESR COM
          Acute myeloid leukemia with 11q23-abnormality with failed remission
          Acute myeloid leukemia with 11q23-abnormality NOS
    C92.61 Acute myeloid leukemia with 11q23-abnormality in remission HCC Rx ESR COM
    C92.62 Acute myeloid leukemia with 11q23-abnormality in relapse HCC Rx ESR COM

  ✓5ᵗʰ C92.A Acute myeloid leukemia with multilineage dysplasia

    Acute myeloid leukemia with dysplasia of remaining hematopoesis and/or myelodysplastic disease in its history
    C92.A0 Acute myeloid leukemia with multilineage dysplasia, not having achieved remission HCC Rx ESR COM
          Acute myeloid leukemia with multilineage dysplasia with failed remission
          Acute myeloid leukemia with multilineage dysplasia NOS
    C92.A1 Acute myeloid leukemia with multilineage dysplasia, in remission HCC Rx ESR COM
    C92.A2 Acute myeloid leukemia with multilineage dysplasia, in relapse HCC Rx ESR COM

  ✓5ᵗʰ C92.Z Other myeloid leukemia

    C92.Z0 Other myeloid leukemia not having achieved remission HCC Rx ESR COM
          Myeloid leukemia NEC with failed remission
          Myeloid leukemia NEC
    C92.Z1 Other myeloid leukemia, in remission HCC Rx ESR COM
    C92.Z2 Other myeloid leukemia, in relapse HCC Rx ESR COM

  ✓5ᵗʰ C92.9 Myeloid leukemia, unspecified

    C92.90 Myeloid leukemia, unspecified, not having achieved remission HCC Rx ESR COM
          Myeloid leukemia, unspecified with failed remission
          Myeloid leukemia, unspecified NOS
    C92.91 Myeloid leukemia, unspecified in remission HCC Rx ESR COM
    C92.92 Myeloid leukemia, unspecified in relapse HCC Rx ESR COM

✔ Additional Character Required   ✓x7ᵗʰ Placeholder Alert   Manifestation   Unspecified Dx   Q QPP   UPD Unacceptable PDx

Chapter 2. Neoplasms *(side tab)*

✓4ᵗʰ **C93 Monocytic leukemia**

INCLUDES monocytoid leukemia

EXCLUDES 1 *personal history of leukemia (Z85.6)*

AHA: 2020,1Q,13

✓5ᵗʰ **C93.0 Acute monoblastic/monocytic leukemia**

AML M5
AML M5a
AML M5b

C93.00 Acute monoblastic/monocytic leukemia, not having achieved remission HCC Rx ESR COM

Acute monoblastic/monocytic leukemia with failed remission
Acute monoblastic/monocytic leukemia NOS

C93.01 Acute monoblastic/monocytic leukemia, in remission HCC Rx ESR COM

C93.02 Acute monoblastic/monocytic leukemia, in relapse HCC Rx ESR COM

✓5ᵗʰ **C93.1 Chronic myelomonocytic leukemia**

Chronic monocytic leukemia
CMML-1
CMML-2
CMML with eosinophilia
Code also, if applicable, eosinophilia (D72.18)

C93.10 Chronic myelomonocytic leukemia not having achieved remission HCC Rx ESR COM

Chronic myelomonocytic leukemia with failed remission
Chronic myelomonocytic leukemia NOS

C93.11 Chronic myelomonocytic leukemia, in remission HCC Rx ESR COM

C93.12 Chronic myelomonocytic leukemia, in relapse HCC Rx ESR COM

✓5ᵗʰ **C93.3 Juvenile myelomonocytic leukemia**

C93.30 Juvenile myelomonocytic leukemia, not having achieved remission HCC Rx ESR COM P

Juvenile myelomonocytic leukemia with failed remission
Juvenile myelomonocytic leukemia NOS

C93.31 Juvenile myelomonocytic leukemia, in remission HCC Rx ESR COM P

C93.32 Juvenile myelomonocytic leukemia, in relapse HCC Rx ESR COM P

✓5ᵗʰ **C93.Z Other monocytic leukemia**

C93.Z0 Other monocytic leukemia, not having achieved remission HCC Rx ESR COM

Other monocytic leukemia NOS

C93.Z1 Other monocytic leukemia, in remission HCC Rx ESR COM

C93.Z2 Other monocytic leukemia, in relapse HCC Rx ESR COM

✓5ᵗʰ **C93.9 Monocytic leukemia, unspecified**

C93.90 Monocytic leukemia, unspecified, not having achieved remission HCC Rx ESR COM

Monocytic leukemia, unspecified with failed remission
Monocytic leukemia, unspecified NOS

C93.91 Monocytic leukemia, unspecified in remission HCC Rx ESR COM

C93.92 Monocytic leukemia, unspecified in relapse HCC Rx ESR COM

✓4ᵗʰ **C94 Other leukemias of specified cell type**

EXCLUDES 1 *leukemic reticuloendotheliosis (C91.4-)*
myelodysplastic syndromes (D46.-)
personal history of leukemia (Z85.6)
plasma cell leukemia (C90.1-)

AHA: 2020,1Q,13

✓5ᵗʰ **C94.0 Acute erythroid leukemia**

Acute myeloid leukemia M6(a)(b)
Erythroleukemia
DEF: Erythroleukemia: Malignant blood dyscrasia (a myeloproliferative disorder).

C94.00 Acute erythroid leukemia, not having achieved remission HCC Rx ESR COM

Acute erythroid leukemia with failed remission
Acute erythroid leukemia NOS

C94.01 Acute erythroid leukemia, in remission HCC Rx ESR COM

C94.02 Acute erythroid leukemia, in relapse HCC Rx ESR COM

✓5ᵗʰ **C94.2 Acute megakaryoblastic leukemia**

Acute myeloid leukemia M7
Acute megakaryocytic leukemia

C94.20 Acute megakaryoblastic leukemia not having achieved remission HCC Rx ESR COM

Acute megakaryoblastic leukemia with failed remission
Acute megakaryoblastic leukemia NOS

C94.21 Acute megakaryoblastic leukemia, in remission HCC Rx ESR COM

C94.22 Acute megakaryoblastic leukemia, in relapse HCC Rx ESR COM

✓5ᵗʰ **C94.3 Mast cell leukemia**

AHA: 2017,4Q,5

C94.30 Mast cell leukemia not having achieved remission HCC Rx ESR COM

Mast cell leukemia with failed remission
Mast cell leukemia NOS

C94.31 Mast cell leukemia, in remission HCC Rx ESR COM

C94.32 Mast cell leukemia, in relapse HCC Rx ESR COM

✓5ᵗʰ **C94.4 Acute panmyelosis with myelofibrosis**

Acute myelofibrosis
EXCLUDES 1 *myelofibrosis NOS (D75.81)*
secondary myelofibrosis NOS (D75.81)

C94.40 Acute panmyelosis with myelofibrosis not having achieved remission HCC Rx ESR COM

Acute myelofibrosis NOS
Acute panmyelosis with myelofibrosis with failed remission
Acute panmyelosis NOS

C94.41 Acute panmyelosis with myelofibrosis, in remission HCC Rx ESR COM

C94.42 Acute panmyelosis with myelofibrosis, in relapse HCC Rx ESR COM

▲ **C94.6 Myelodysplastic disease, not elsewhere classified** HCC Rx ESR COM

▶Myelodysplastic/myeloproliferative neoplasm, unclassifiable◀
▶Myeloproliferative disease, not elsewhere classified◀

✓5ᵗʰ **C94.8 Other specified leukemias**

Aggressive NK-cell leukemia
Acute basophilic leukemia

C94.80 Other specified leukemias not having achieved remission HCC Rx ESR COM

Other specified leukemia with failed remission
Other specified leukemias NOS

C94.81 Other specified leukemias, in remission HCC Rx ESR COM

C94.82 Other specified leukemias, in relapse HCC Rx ESR COM

✓4ᵗʰ **C95 Leukemia of unspecified cell type**

EXCLUDES 1 *personal history of leukemia (Z85.6)*

AHA: 2020,1Q,13

✓5ᵗʰ **C95.0 Acute leukemia of unspecified cell type**

Acute bilineal leukemia
Acute mixed lineage leukemia
Biphenotypic acute leukemia
Stem cell leukemia of unclear lineage
EXCLUDES 1 *acute exacerbation of unspecified chronic leukemia (C95.10)*

C95.00 Acute leukemia of unspecified cell type not having achieved remission HCC Rx ESR COM

Acute leukemia of unspecified cell type with failed remission
Acute leukemia NOS

C95.01 Acute leukemia of unspecified cell type, in remission HCC Rx ESR COM

C95.02 Acute leukemia of unspecified cell type, in relapse HCC Rx ESR COM

(side tab) C93–C95.02

☑5ᵗʰ **C95.1** Chronic **leukemia of unspecified cell type**

    C95.10 **Chronic leukemia of unspecified cell type** not having achieved remission   `HCC` `Rx` `ESR` `COM`
        Chronic leukemia of unspecified cell type with failed remission
        Chronic leukemia NOS

    C95.11 **Chronic leukemia of unspecified cell type, in remission**   `HCC` `Rx` `ESR` `COM`

    C95.12 **Chronic leukemia of unspecified cell type, in relapse**   `HCC` `Rx` `ESR` `COM`

☑5ᵗʰ **C95.9** **Leukemia, unspecified**

    C95.90 **Leukemia, unspecified** not having achieved remission   `HCC` `Rx` `ESR` `COM`
        Leukemia, unspecified with failed remission
        Leukemia NOS

    C95.91 **Leukemia, unspecified, in remission**   `HCC` `Rx` `ESR` `COM`

    C95.92 **Leukemia, unspecified, in relapse**   `HCC` `Rx` `ESR` `COM`

☑4ᵗʰ **C96** **Other and unspecified malignant neoplasms of lymphoid, hematopoietic and related tissue**

    EXCLUDES 1   personal history of other malignant neoplasms of lymphoid, hematopoietic and related tissues (Z85.79)

    C96.0 **Multifocal and multisystemic (disseminated) Langerhans-cell histiocytosis**   `HCC` `Rx` `ESR` `COM`
        Histiocytosis X, multisystemic
        Letterer-Siwe disease
        EXCLUDES 1   adult pulmonary Langerhans cell histiocytosis (J84.82)
                 multifocal and unisystemic Langerhans-cell histiocytosis (C96.5)
                 unifocal Langerhans-cell histiocytosis (C96.6)

    ☑5ᵗʰ **C96.2** **Malignant mast cell neoplasm**
        EXCLUDES 1   indolent mastocytosis (D47.02)
                 mast cell leukemia (C94.30)
                 mastocytosis (congenital) (cutaneous) (Q82.2)

        AHA: 2017,4Q,5
        DEF: Mast cell: Type of white blood cell found in the loose connective tissue of blood vessels and bronchioles responsible for acute hypersensitivity reactions, including anaphylactic shock. The IgE receptors on these cells bind with allergens causing cell degranulation and diffuse, widespread histamine release that results in airway constriction and vasodilation with decreased systemic blood pressure.

        C96.20 **Malignant mast cell neoplasm, unspecified**   `HCC` `Rx` `ESR` `COM`
        C96.21 **Aggressive systemic mastocytosis**   `HCC` `Rx` `ESR` `COM`
        C96.22 **Mast cell sarcoma**   `HCC` `Rx` `ESR` `COM`
        C96.29 **Other malignant mast cell neoplasm**   `HCC` `Rx` `ESR` `COM`

    C96.4 **Sarcoma of dendritic cells (accessory cells)**   `HCC` `Rx` `ESR` `COM`
        Follicular dendritic cell sarcoma
        Interdigitating dendritic cell sarcoma
        Langerhans cell sarcoma

    C96.5 **Multifocal and unisystemic Langerhans-cell histiocytosis**   `HCC` `Rx` `ESR` `COM`
        Hand-Schüller-Christian disease
        Histiocytosis X, multifocal
        EXCLUDES 1   multifocal and multisystemic (disseminated) Langerhans-cell histiocytosis (C96.0)
                 unifocal Langerhans-cell histiocytosis (C96.6)

    C96.6 **Unifocal Langerhans-cell histiocytosis**   `HCC` `Rx` `ESR` `COM`
        Eosinophilic granuloma
        Histiocytosis X, unifocal
        Histiocytosis X NOS
        Langerhans-cell histiocytosis NOS
        EXCLUDES 1   multifocal and multisysemic (disseminated) Langerhans-cell histiocytosis (C96.0)
                 multifocal and unisystemic Langerhans-cell histiocytosis (C96.5)

    C96.A **Histicytic sarcoma**   `HCC` `Rx` `ESR` `COM`
        Malignant histiocytosis

    C96.Z **Other specified malignant neoplasms of lymphoid, hematopoietic and related tissue**   `HCC` `Rx` `ESR` `COM`

    C96.9 **Malignant neoplasm of lymphoid, hematopoietic and related tissue, unspecified**   `HCC` `Rx` `ESR` `COM`

In situ neoplasms (D00-D09)

`INCLUDES`   Bowen's disease
               erythroplasia
               grade III intraepithelial neoplasia
               Queyrat's erythroplasia

☑4ᵗʰ **D00** **Carcinoma in situ of** oral cavity, esophagus and stomach
    EXCLUDES 1   melanoma in situ (D03.-)

    ☑5ᵗʰ **D00.0** **Carcinoma in situ of** lip, oral cavity and pharynx
        Use additional code to identify:
           exposure to environmental tobacco smoke (Z77.22)
           exposure to tobacco smoke in the perinatal period (P96.81)
           history of tobacco dependence (Z87.891)
           occupational exposure to environmental tobacco smoke (Z57.31)
           tobacco dependence (F17.-)
           tobacco use (Z72.0)
        EXCLUDES 1   carcinoma in situ of aryepiglottic fold or interarytenoid fold, laryngeal aspect (D02.0)
                 carcinoma in situ of epiglottis NOS (D02.0)
                 carcinoma in situ of epiglottis suprahyoid portion (D02.0)
                 carcinoma in situ of skin of lip (D03.0, D04.0)

        D00.00 **Carcinoma in situ of oral cavity, unspecified site**
        D00.01 **Carcinoma in situ of** labial mucosa and vermilion border
        D00.02 **Carcinoma in situ of** buccal mucosa
        D00.03 **Carcinoma in situ of** gingiva and edentulous alveolar ridge
        D00.04 **Carcinoma in situ of** soft palate
        D00.05 **Carcinoma in situ of** hard palate
        D00.06 **Carcinoma in situ of** floor of mouth
        D00.07 **Carcinoma in situ of** tongue
        D00.08 **Carcinoma in situ of** pharynx
           Carcinoma in situ of aryepiglottic fold NOS
           Carcinoma in situ of hypopharyngeal aspect of aryepiglottic fold
           Carcinoma in situ of marginal zone of aryepiglottic fold

    D00.1 **Carcinoma in situ of** esophagus
    D00.2 **Carcinoma in situ of** stomach

☑4ᵗʰ **D01** **Carcinoma in situ of other and unspecified** digestive organs
    EXCLUDES 1   melanoma in situ (D03.-)

    D01.0 **Carcinoma in situ of** colon
        EXCLUDES 1   carcinoma in situ of rectosigmoid junction (D01.1)

    D01.1 **Carcinoma in situ of** rectosigmoid junction
    D01.2 **Carcinoma in situ of** rectum
    D01.3 **Carcinoma in situ of** anus and anal canal
        Anal intraepithelial neoplasia III [AIN III]
        Severe dysplasia of anus
        EXCLUDES 1   anal intraepithelial neoplasia I and II [AIN I and AIN II] (K62.82)
                 carcinoma in situ of anal margin (D04.5)
                 carcinoma in situ of anal skin (D04.5)
                 carcinoma in situ of perianal skin (D04.5)

    ☑5ᵗʰ **D01.4** **Carcinoma in situ of other and unspecified parts of** intestine
        EXCLUDES 1   carcinoma in situ of ampulla of Vater (D01.5)
        D01.40 **Carcinoma in situ of unspecified part of intestine**
        D01.49 **Carcinoma in situ of other parts of intestine**

    D01.5 **Carcinoma in situ of** liver, gallbladder and bile ducts
        Carcinoma in situ of ampulla of Vater

    D01.7 **Carcinoma in situ of other specified digestive organs**
        Carcinoma in situ of pancreas

    D01.9 **Carcinoma in situ of digestive organ, unspecified**

☑4ᵗʰ D02 Carcinoma in situ of middle ear and respiratory system
  Use additional code to identify:
    exposure to environmental tobacco smoke (Z77.22)
    exposure to tobacco smoke in the perinatal period (P96.81)
    history of tobacco dependence (Z87.891)
    occupational exposure to environmental tobacco smoke (Z57.31)
    tobacco dependence (F17.-)
    tobacco use (Z72.0)
    EXCLUDES 1   melanoma in situ (D03.-)

  D02.0 Carcinoma in situ of larynx
    Carcinoma in situ of aryepiglottic fold or interarytenoid fold, laryngeal aspect
    Carcinoma in situ of epiglottis (suprahyoid portion)
      EXCLUDES 1   carcinoma in situ of aryepiglottic fold or interarytenoid fold NOS (D00.08)
              carcinoma in situ of hypopharyngeal aspect (D00.08)
              carcinoma in situ of marginal zone (D00.08)

  D02.1 Carcinoma in situ of trachea
  ☑5ᵗʰ D02.2 Carcinoma in situ of bronchus and lung
    D02.20 Carcinoma in situ of unspecified bronchus and lung
    D02.21 Carcinoma in situ of right bronchus and lung
    D02.22 Carcinoma in situ of left bronchus and lung
  D02.3 Carcinoma in situ of other parts of respiratory system
    Carcinoma in situ of accessory sinuses
    Carcinoma in situ of middle ear
    Carcinoma in situ of nasal cavities
      EXCLUDES 1   carcinoma in situ of ear (external) (skin) (D04.2-)
              carcinoma in situ of nose NOS (D09.8)
              carcinoma in situ of skin of nose (D04.3)

  D02.4 Carcinoma in situ of respiratory system, unspecified

☑4ᵗʰ D03 Melanoma in situ

  D03.0 Melanoma in situ of lip   HCC Rx ESR COM
  ☑5ᵗʰ D03.1 Melanoma in situ of eyelid, including canthus
    AHA: 2018,4Q,4
    D03.10 Melanoma in situ of unspecified eyelid, including canthus   HCC Rx ESR COM
    ☑6ᵗʰ D03.11 Melanoma in situ of right eyelid, including canthus
      D03.111 Melanoma in situ of right upper eyelid, including canthus   HCC Rx ESR COM
      D03.112 Melanoma in situ of right lower eyelid, including canthus   HCC Rx ESR COM
    ☑6ᵗʰ D03.12 Melanoma in situ of left eyelid, including canthus
      D03.121 Melanoma in situ of left upper eyelid, including canthus   HCC Rx ESR COM
      D03.122 Melanoma in situ of left lower eyelid, including canthus   HCC Rx ESR COM
  ☑5ᵗʰ D03.2 Melanoma in situ of ear and external auricular canal
    D03.20 Melanoma in situ of unspecified ear and external auricular canal   HCC Rx ESR COM
    D03.21 Melanoma in situ of right ear and external auricular canal   HCC Rx ESR COM
    D03.22 Melanoma in situ of left ear and external auricular canal   HCC Rx ESR COM
  ☑5ᵗʰ D03.3 Melanoma in situ of other and unspecified parts of face
    D03.30 Melanoma in situ of unspecified part of face   HCC Rx ESR COM
    D03.39 Melanoma in situ of other parts of face   HCC Rx ESR COM
  D03.4 Melanoma in situ of scalp and neck   HCC Rx ESR COM
  ☑5ᵗʰ D03.5 Melanoma in situ of trunk
    D03.51 Melanoma in situ of anal skin   HCC Rx ESR COM
      Melanoma in situ of anal margin
      Melanoma in situ of perianal skin
    D03.52 Melanoma in situ of breast (skin) (soft tissue)   HCC Rx ESR COM
    D03.59 Melanoma in situ of other part of trunk   HCC Rx ESR COM
  ☑5ᵗʰ D03.6 Melanoma in situ of upper limb, including shoulder
    D03.60 Melanoma in situ of unspecified upper limb, including shoulder   HCC Rx ESR COM
    D03.61 Melanoma in situ of right upper limb, including shoulder   HCC Rx ESR COM
    D03.62 Melanoma in situ of left upper limb, including shoulder   HCC Rx ESR COM

  ☑5ᵗʰ D03.7 Melanoma in situ of lower limb, including hip
    D03.70 Melanoma in situ of unspecified lower limb, including hip   HCC Rx ESR COM
    D03.71 Melanoma in situ of right lower limb, including hip   HCC Rx ESR COM
    D03.72 Melanoma in situ of left lower limb, including hip   HCC Rx ESR COM
  D03.8 Melanoma in situ of other sites   HCC Rx ESR COM
    Melanoma in situ of scrotum
      EXCLUDES 1   carcinoma in situ of scrotum (D07.61)
  D03.9 Melanoma in situ, unspecified   HCC Rx COM

☑4ᵗʰ D04 Carcinoma in situ of skin
    EXCLUDES 1   erythroplasia of Queyrat (penis) NOS (D07.4)
            melanoma in situ (D03.-)

  D04.0 Carcinoma in situ of skin of lip
    EXCLUDES 2   carcinoma in situ of vermilion border of lip (D00.01)
  ☑5ᵗʰ D04.1 Carcinoma in situ of skin of eyelid, including canthus
    AHA: 2018,4Q,4
    D04.10 Carcinoma in situ of skin of unspecified eyelid, including canthus
    ☑6ᵗʰ D04.11 Carcinoma in situ of skin of right eyelid, including canthus
      D04.111 Carcinoma in situ of skin of right upper eyelid, including canthus
      D04.112 Carcinoma in situ of skin of right lower eyelid, including canthus
    ☑6ᵗʰ D04.12 Carcinoma in situ of skin of left eyelid, including canthus
      D04.121 Carcinoma in situ of skin of left upper eyelid, including canthus
      D04.122 Carcinoma in situ of skin of left lower eyelid, including canthus
  ☑5ᵗʰ D04.2 Carcinoma in situ of skin of ear and external auricular canal
    D04.20 Carcinoma in situ of skin of unspecified ear and external auricular canal
    D04.21 Carcinoma in situ of skin of right ear and external auricular canal
    D04.22 Carcinoma in situ of skin of left ear and external auricular canal
  ☑5ᵗʰ D04.3 Carcinoma in situ of skin of other and unspecified parts of face
    D04.30 Carcinoma in situ of skin of unspecified part of face
    D04.39 Carcinoma in situ of skin of other parts of face
  D04.4 Carcinoma in situ of skin of scalp and neck
  D04.5 Carcinoma in situ of skin of trunk
    Carcinoma in situ of anal margin
    Carcinoma in situ of anal skin
    Carcinoma in situ of perianal skin
    Carcinoma in situ of skin of breast
      EXCLUDES 1   carcinoma in situ of anus NOS (D01.3)
              carcinoma in situ of scrotum (D07.61)
              carcinoma in situ of skin of genital organs (D07.-)
  ☑5ᵗʰ D04.6 Carcinoma in situ of skin of upper limb, including shoulder
    D04.60 Carcinoma in situ of skin of unspecified upper limb, including shoulder
    D04.61 Carcinoma in situ of skin of right upper limb, including shoulder
    D04.62 Carcinoma in situ of skin of left upper limb, including shoulder
  ☑5ᵗʰ D04.7 Carcinoma in situ of skin of lower limb, including hip
    D04.70 Carcinoma in situ of skin of unspecified lower limb, including hip
    D04.71 Carcinoma in situ of skin of right lower limb, including hip
    D04.72 Carcinoma in situ of skin of left lower limb, including hip
  D04.8 Carcinoma in situ of skin of other sites
  D04.9 Carcinoma in situ of skin, unspecified

☑4ᵗʰ D05 Carcinoma in situ of breast
    EXCLUDES 1   carcinoma in situ of skin of breast (D04.5)
            melanoma in situ of breast (skin) (D03.5)
            Paget's disease of breast or nipple (C50.-)

  ☑5ᵗʰ D05.0 Lobular carcinoma in situ of breast
    D05.00 Lobular carcinoma in situ of unspecified breast
    D05.01 Lobular carcinoma in situ of right breast
    D05.02 Lobular carcinoma in situ of left breast

✓5ᵗʰ **D05.1** Intraductal carcinoma in situ of breast

    D05.10 Intraductal carcinoma in situ of unspecified breast

    D05.11 Intraductal carcinoma in situ of right breast

    D05.12 Intraductal carcinoma in situ of left breast

✓5ᵗʰ **D05.8** Other specified type of carcinoma in situ of breast

    D05.80 Other specified type of carcinoma in situ of unspecified breast

    D05.81 Other specified type of carcinoma in situ of right breast

    D05.82 Other specified type of carcinoma in situ of left breast

✓5ᵗʰ **D05.9** Unspecified type of carcinoma in situ of breast

    D05.90 Unspecified type of carcinoma in situ of unspecified breast

    D05.91 Unspecified type of carcinoma in situ of right breast

    D05.92 Unspecified type of carcinoma in situ of left breast

✓4ᵗʰ **D06** Carcinoma in situ of cervix uteri

    INCLUDES   cervical adenocarcinoma in situ

                 cervical intraepithelial glandular neoplasia

                 cervical intraepithelial neoplasia III [CIN III]

                 severe dysplasia of cervix uteri

    EXCLUDES 1   *cervical intraepithelial neoplasia II [CIN II] (N87.1)*

                 cytologic evidence of malignancy of cervix without histologic confirmation (R87.614)

                 high grade squamous intraepithelial lesion (HGSIL) of cervix (R87.613)

                 melanoma in situ of cervix (D03.5)

                 moderate cervical dysplasia (N87.1)

    D06.0 Carcinoma in situ of endocervix ♀

    D06.1 Carcinoma in situ of exocervix ♀

    D06.7 Carcinoma in situ of other parts of cervix ♀

    D06.9 Carcinoma in situ of cervix, unspecified ♀

✓4ᵗʰ **D07** Carcinoma in situ of other and unspecified genital organs

    EXCLUDES 1   *melanoma in situ of trunk (D03.5)*

    D07.0 Carcinoma in situ of endometrium ♀

    D07.1 Carcinoma in situ of vulva ♀

        Severe dysplasia of vulva

        Vulvar intraepithelial neoplasia III [VIN III]

        EXCLUDES 1   *moderate dysplasia of vulva (N90.1)*

                 vulvar intraepithelial neoplasia II [VIN II] (N90.1)

    D07.2 Carcinoma in situ of vagina ♀

        Severe dysplasia of vagina

        Vaginal intraepithelial neoplasia III [VAIN III]

        EXCLUDES 1   *moderate dysplasia of vagina (N89.1)*

                 vaginal intraepithelial neoplasia II [VIN II] (N89.1)

✓5ᵗʰ **D07.3** Carcinoma in situ of other and unspecified female genital organs

    D07.30 Carcinoma in situ of unspecified female genital organs ♀

    D07.39 Carcinoma in situ of other female genital organs ♀

    D07.4 Carcinoma in situ of penis ♂

        Erythroplasia of Queyrat NOS

    D07.5 Carcinoma in situ of prostate ♂

        Prostatic intraepithelial neoplasia III (PIN III)

        Severe dysplasia of prostate

        EXCLUDES 1   *dysplasia (mild) (moderate) of prostate (N42.3-)*

                 prostatic intraepithelial neoplasia II [PIN II] (N42.3-)

✓5ᵗʰ **D07.6** Carcinoma in situ of other and unspecified male genital organs

    D07.60 Carcinoma in situ of unspecified male genital organs ♂

    D07.61 Carcinoma in situ of scrotum ♂

    D07.69 Carcinoma in situ of other male genital organs ♂

✓4ᵗʰ **D09** Carcinoma in situ of other and unspecified sites

    EXCLUDES 1   *melanoma in situ (D03.-)*

    D09.0 Carcinoma in situ of bladder

✓5ᵗʰ **D09.1** Carcinoma in situ of other and unspecified urinary organs

    D09.10 Carcinoma in situ of unspecified urinary organ

    D09.19 Carcinoma in situ of other urinary organs

✓5ᵗʰ **D09.2** Carcinoma in situ of eye

    EXCLUDES 1   *carcinoma in situ of skin of eyelid (D04.1-)*

    D09.20 Carcinoma in situ of unspecified eye

    D09.21 Carcinoma in situ of right eye

    D09.22 Carcinoma in situ of left eye

    D09.3 Carcinoma in situ of thyroid and other endocrine glands

        EXCLUDES 1   *carcinoma in situ of endocrine pancreas (D01.7)*

                 carcinoma in situ of ovary (D07.39)

                 carcinoma in situ of testis (D07.69)

    D09.8 Carcinoma in situ of other specified sites

    D09.9 Carcinoma in situ, unspecified

Benign neoplasms, except benign neuroendocrine tumors (D10-D36)

✓4ᵗʰ **D10** Benign neoplasm of mouth and pharynx

    D10.0 Benign neoplasm of lip

        Benign neoplasm of lip (frenulum) (inner aspect) (mucosa) (vermilion border)

        EXCLUDES 1   *benign neoplasm of skin of lip (D22.0, D23.0)*

    D10.1 Benign neoplasm of tongue

        Benign neoplasm of lingual tonsil

    D10.2 Benign neoplasm of floor of mouth

✓5ᵗʰ **D10.3** Benign neoplasm of other and unspecified parts of mouth

    D10.30 Benign neoplasm of unspecified part of mouth

    D10.39 Benign neoplasm of other parts of mouth

        Benign neoplasm of minor salivary gland NOS

        EXCLUDES 1   *benign odontogenic neoplasms (D16.4-D16.5)*

                 benign neoplasm of mucosa of lip (D10.0)

                 benign neoplasm of nasopharyngeal surface of soft palate (D10.6)

    D10.4 Benign neoplasm of tonsil

        Benign neoplasm of tonsil (faucial) (palatine)

        EXCLUDES 1   *benign neoplasm of lingual tonsil (D10.1)*

                 benign neoplasm of pharyngeal tonsil (D10.6)

                 benign neoplasm of tonsillar fossa (D10.5)

                 benign neoplasm of tonsillar pillars (D10.5)

    D10.5 Benign neoplasm of other parts of oropharynx

        Benign neoplasm of epiglottis, anterior aspect

        Benign neoplasm of tonsillar fossa

        Benign neoplasm of tonsillar pillars

        Benign neoplasm of vallecula

        EXCLUDES 1   *benign neoplasm of epiglottis NOS (D14.1)*

                 benign neoplasm of epiglottis, suprahyoid portion (D14.1)

        DEF: Oropharynx: Middle portion of pharynx (throat); communicates with the oral cavity, nasopharynx and laryngopharynx.

    D10.6 Benign neoplasm of nasopharynx

        Benign neoplasm of pharyngeal tonsil

        Benign neoplasm of posterior margin of septum and choanae

        DEF: Nasopharynx: Upper portion of pharynx (throat); communicates with the nasal cavities, oropharynx and tympanic cavities.

    D10.7 Benign neoplasm of hypopharynx

        DEF: Hypopharynx: Lower portion of pharynx (throat); communicates with the oropharynx and the esophagus.

        Synonym(s): laryngopharynx.

    D10.9 Benign neoplasm of pharynx, unspecified

✓4ᵗʰ **D11** Benign neoplasm of major salivary glands

    EXCLUDES 1   *benign neoplasms of specified minor salivary glands which are classified according to their anatomical location*

                 benign neoplasms of minor salivary glands NOS (D10.39)

    D11.0 Benign neoplasm of parotid gland

    D11.7 Benign neoplasm of other major salivary glands

        Benign neoplasm of sublingual salivary gland

        Benign neoplasm of submandibular salivary gland

    D11.9 Benign neoplasm of major salivary gland, unspecified

✓4ᵗʰ **D12** Benign neoplasm of colon, rectum, anus and anal canal

    EXCLUDES 1   *benign carcinoid tumors of the large intestine, and rectum (D3A.02-)*

                 polyp of colon NOS (K63.5)

    AHA: 2018,2Q,14; 2017,1Q,15; 2015,2Q,14

    TIP: Code K63.5 Polyp of colon, is assigned when documentation states hyperplastic colon polyps, regardless of the site in the colon. Slow-growing, hyperplastic polyps are not precancerous and are classified differently from benign or adenomatous polyps.

    D12.0 Benign neoplasm of cecum

        Benign neoplasm of ileocecal valve

D12.1   **Benign neoplasm of** appendix
    EXCLUDES 1   *benign carcinoid tumor of the appendix (D3A.Ø2Ø)*

D12.2   **Benign neoplasm of** ascending colon

D12.3   **Benign neoplasm of** transverse colon
    Benign neoplasm of hepatic flexure
    Benign neoplasm of splenic flexure
    AHA: 2017,1Q,16

D12.4   **Benign neoplasm of** descending colon

D12.5   **Benign neoplasm of** sigmoid colon

D12.6   **Benign neoplasm of colon, unspecified**
    Adenomatosis of colon
    Benign neoplasm of large intestine NOS
    Polyposis (hereditary) of colon
    EXCLUDES 1   *inflammatory polyp of colon (K51.4-)*

D12.7   **Benign neoplasm of** rectosigmoid junction

D12.8   **Benign neoplasm of** rectum   *hyperplastic*
    EXCLUDES 1   *benign carcinoid tumor of the rectum (D3A.Ø26)*
    AHA: 2018,1Q,6

D12.9   **Benign neoplasm of** anus and anal canal
    Benign neoplasm of anus NOS
    EXCLUDES 1   *benign neoplasm of anal margin (D22.5, D23.5)*
             benign neoplasm of anal skin (D22.5, D23.5)
             benign neoplasm of perianal skin (D22.5, D23.5)

✓4ᵗʰ **D13**   **Benign neoplasm of other and ill-defined parts of** digestive system
    EXCLUDES 1   *benign stromal tumors of digestive system (D21.4)*

D13.Ø   **Benign neoplasm of** esophagus

D13.1   **Benign neoplasm of** stomach
    EXCLUDES 1   *benign carcinoid tumor of the stomach (D3A.Ø92)*

D13.2   **Benign neoplasm of** duodenum
    EXCLUDES 1   *benign carcinoid tumor of the duodenum (D3A.Ø1Ø)*

✓5ᵗʰ **D13.3**   **Benign neoplasm of other and unspecified parts of** small intestine
    EXCLUDES 1   *benign carcinoid tumors of the small intestine (D3A.Ø1-)*
             benign neoplasm of ileocecal valve (D12.Ø)

    D13.3Ø   **Benign neoplasm of unspecified part of small intestine**

    D13.39   **Benign neoplasm of other parts of small intestine**

D13.4   **Benign neoplasm of** liver
    Benign neoplasm of intrahepatic bile ducts

D13.5   **Benign neoplasm of** extrahepatic bile ducts

D13.6   **Benign neoplasm of** pancreas
    EXCLUDES 1   *benign neoplasm of endocrine pancreas (D13.7)*

D13.7   **Benign neoplasm of** endocrine pancreas
    Benign neoplasm of islets of Langerhans
    Islet cell tumor
    Use additional code to identify any functional activity

D13.9   **Benign neoplasm of** ill-defined sites **within the digestive system**
    Benign neoplasm of digestive system NOS
    Benign neoplasm of intestine NOS
    Benign neoplasm of spleen

✓4ᵗʰ **D14**   **Benign neoplasm of** middle ear and respiratory system

D14.Ø   **Benign neoplasm of** middle ear, nasal cavity and accessory sinuses
    Benign neoplasm of cartilage of nose
    EXCLUDES 1   *benign neoplasm of auricular canal (external) (D22.2-, D23.2-)*
             benign neoplasm of bone of ear (D16.4)
             benign neoplasm of bone of nose (D16.4)
             benign neoplasm of cartilage of ear (D21.Ø)
             benign neoplasm of ear (external)(skin) (D22.2-, D23.2-)
             benign neoplasm of nose NOS (D36.7)
             benign neoplasm of skin of nose (D22.39, D23.39)
             benign neoplasm of olfactory bulb (D33.3)
             benign neoplasm of posterior margin of septum and choanae (D1Ø.6)
             polyp of accessory sinus (J33.8)
             polyp of ear (middle) (H74.4)
             polyp of nasal (cavity) (J33.-)

D14.1   **Benign neoplasm of** larynx
    Adenomatous polyp of larynx
    Benign neoplasm of epiglottis (suprahyoid portion)
    EXCLUDES 1   *benign neoplasm of epiglottis, anterior aspect (D1Ø.5)*
             polyp (nonadenomatous) of vocal cord or larynx (J38.1)

D14.2   **Benign neoplasm of** trachea

✓5ᵗʰ **D14.3**   **Benign neoplasm of** bronchus and lung
    EXCLUDES 1   *benign carcinoid tumor of the bronchus and lung (D3A.Ø9Ø)*

    D14.3Ø   **Benign neoplasm of unspecified bronchus and lung**

    D14.31   **Benign neoplasm of** right **bronchus and lung**

    D14.32   **Benign neoplasm of** left **bronchus and lung**

D14.4   **Benign neoplasm of respiratory system, unspecified**

✓4ᵗʰ **D15**   **Benign neoplasm of other and unspecified** intrathoracic organs
    EXCLUDES 1   *benign neoplasm of mesothelial tissue (D19.-)*

D15.Ø   **Benign neoplasm of** thymus
    EXCLUDES 1   *benign carcinoid tumor of the thymus (D3A.Ø91)*

D15.1   **Benign neoplasm of** heart   COM
    EXCLUDES 1   *benign neoplasm of great vessels (D21.3)*

D15.2   **Benign neoplasm of** mediastinum

D15.7   **Benign neoplasm of other specified intrathoracic organs**

D15.9   **Benign neoplasm of intrathoracic organ, unspecified**

✓4ᵗʰ **D16**   **Benign neoplasm of** bone and articular cartilage
    EXCLUDES 1   *benign neoplasm of connective tissue of ear (D21.Ø)*
             benign neoplasm of connective tissue of eyelid (D21.Ø)
             benign neoplasm of connective tissue of larynx (D14.1)
             benign neoplasm of connective tissue of nose (D14.Ø)
             benign neoplasm of synovia (D21.-)

✓5ᵗʰ **D16.Ø**   **Benign neoplasm of** scapula and long bones of upper limb

    D16.ØØ   **Benign neoplasm of scapula and long bones of unspecified upper limb**

    D16.Ø1   **Benign neoplasm of scapula and long bones of** right **upper limb**

    D16.Ø2   **Benign neoplasm of scapula and long bones of** left **upper limb**

✓5ᵗʰ **D16.1**   **Benign neoplasm of** short bones of upper limb

    D16.1Ø   **Benign neoplasm of short bones of unspecified upper limb**

    D16.11   **Benign neoplasm of short bones of** right **upper limb**

    D16.12   **Benign neoplasm of short bones of** left **upper limb**

✓5ᵗʰ **D16.2**   **Benign neoplasm of** long bones of lower limb

    D16.2Ø   **Benign neoplasm of long bones of unspecified lower limb**

    D16.21   **Benign neoplasm of long bones of** right **lower limb**

    D16.22   **Benign neoplasm of long bones of** left **lower limb**

✓5ᵗʰ **D16.3**   **Benign neoplasm of** short bones of lower limb

    D16.3Ø   **Benign neoplasm of short bones of unspecified lower limb**

    D16.31   **Benign neoplasm of short bones of** right **lower limb**

    D16.32   **Benign neoplasm of short bones of** left **lower limb**

D16.4   **Benign neoplasm of bones of** skull and face
    Benign neoplasm of maxilla (superior)
    Benign neoplasm of orbital bone
    Keratocyst of maxilla
    Keratocystic odontogenic tumor of maxilla
    EXCLUDES 2   *benign neoplasm of lower jaw bone (D16.5)*

D16.5   **Benign neoplasm of** lower jaw bone
    Keratocyst of mandible
    Keratocystic odontogenic tumor of mandible

D16.6   **Benign neoplasm of** vertebral column
    EXCLUDES 1   *benign neoplasm of sacrum and coccyx (D16.8)*

D16.7   **Benign neoplasm of** ribs, sternum and clavicle

D16.8   **Benign neoplasm of** pelvic bones, sacrum and coccyx

D16.9   **Benign neoplasm of bone and articular cartilage, unspecified**

✓4ᵗʰ **D17**   **Benign** lipomatous **neoplasm**

D17.Ø   **Benign lipomatous neoplasm of** skin and subcutaneous tissue of head, face and neck

D17.1   **Benign lipomatous neoplasm of** skin and subcutaneous tissue of trunk   *Flank*

✓5ᵗʰ **D17.2**   **Benign lipomatous neoplasm of** skin and subcutaneous tissue of limb

    D17.2Ø   **Benign lipomatous neoplasm of skin and subcutaneous tissue of unspecified limb**

D17.21 Benign lipomatous neoplasm of skin and subcutaneous tissue of right arm

D17.22 Benign lipomatous neoplasm of skin and subcutaneous tissue of left arm

D17.23 Benign lipomatous neoplasm of skin and subcutaneous tissue of right leg

D17.24 Benign lipomatous neoplasm of skin and subcutaneous tissue of left leg

√5ᵗʰ **D17.3** Benign lipomatous neoplasm of skin and subcutaneous tissue of other and unspecified sites

    D17.30 Benign lipomatous neoplasm of skin and subcutaneous tissue of unspecified sites

    D17.39 Benign lipomatous neoplasm of skin and subcutaneous tissue of other sites

D17.4 Benign lipomatous neoplasm of intrathoracic organs

D17.5 Benign lipomatous neoplasm of intra-abdominal organs

    EXCLUDES 1   *benign lipomatous neoplasm of peritoneum and retroperitoneum (D17.79)*

D17.6 Benign lipomatous neoplasm of spermatic cord   ♂

√5ᵗʰ **D17.7** Benign lipomatous neoplasm of other sites

    D17.71 Benign lipomatous neoplasm of kidney

    D17.72 Benign lipomatous neoplasm of other genitourinary organ

    D17.79 Benign lipomatous neoplasm of other sites
         Benign lipomatous neoplasm of peritoneum
         Benign lipomatous neoplasm of retroperitoneum

D17.9 Benign lipomatous neoplasm, unspecified
     Lipoma NOS

√4ᵗʰ **D18** Hemangioma and lymphangioma, any site

    EXCLUDES 1   *benign neoplasm of glomus jugulare (D35.6)*
           blue or pigmented nevus (D22.-)
           nevus NOS (D22.-)
           vascular nevus (Q82.5)

√5ᵗʰ **D18.0** Hemangioma
     Angioma NOS
     Cavernous nevus
     DEF: Common benign tumor usually occurring in infancy that is composed of newly formed blood vessels due to malformation of the angioblastic tissue.

    D18.00 Hemangioma unspecified site

    D18.01 Hemangioma of skin and subcutaneous tissue

    D18.02 Hemangioma of intracranial structures   HCC Rx ESR COM

    D18.03 Hemangioma of intra-abdominal structures

    D18.09 Hemangioma of other sites

D18.1 Lymphangioma, any site *Vulva.*
     AHA: 2018,3Q,31; 2018,2Q,13

√4ᵗʰ **D19** Benign neoplasm of mesothelial tissue

D19.0 Benign neoplasm of mesothelial tissue of pleura

D19.1 Benign neoplasm of mesothelial tissue of peritoneum

D19.7 Benign neoplasm of mesothelial tissue of other sites

D19.9 Benign neoplasm of mesothelial tissue, unspecified
     Benign mesothelioma NOS

√4ᵗʰ **D20** Benign neoplasm of soft tissue of retroperitoneum and peritoneum

    EXCLUDES 1   *benign lipomatous neoplasm of peritoneum and retroperitoneum (D17.79)*
           benign neoplasm of mesothelial tissue (D19.-)

D20.0 Benign neoplasm of soft tissue of retroperitoneum

D20.1 Benign neoplasm of soft tissue of peritoneum

√4ᵗʰ **D21** Other benign neoplasms of connective and other soft tissue

    INCLUDES   benign neoplasm of blood vessel
           benign neoplasm of bursa
           benign neoplasm of cartilage
           benign neoplasm of fascia
           benign neoplasm of fat
           benign neoplasm of ligament, except uterine
           benign neoplasm of lymphatic channel
           benign neoplasm of muscle
           benign neoplasm of synovia
           benign neoplasm of tendon (sheath)
           benign stromal tumors

    EXCLUDES 1   *benign neoplasm of articular cartilage (D16.-)*
           benign neoplasm of cartilage of larynx (D14.1)
           benign neoplasm of cartilage of nose (D14.0)
           benign neoplasm of connective tissue of breast (D24.-)
           benign neoplasm of peripheral nerves and autonomic nervous system (D36.1-)
           benign neoplasm of peritoneum (D20.1)
           benign neoplasm of retroperitoneum (D20.0)
           benign neoplasm of uterine ligament, any (D28.2)
           benign neoplasm of vascular tissue (D18.-)
           hemangioma (D18.0-)
           lipomatous neoplasm (D17.-)
           lymphangioma (D18.1)
           uterine leiomyoma (D25.-)

D21.0 Benign neoplasm of connective and other soft tissue of head, face and neck
     Benign neoplasm of connective tissue of ear
     Benign neoplasm of connective tissue of eyelid
    EXCLUDES 1   *benign neoplasm of connective tissue of orbit (D31.6-)*

√5ᵗʰ **D21.1** Benign neoplasm of connective and other soft tissue of upper limb, including shoulder

    D21.10 Benign neoplasm of connective and other soft tissue of unspecified upper limb, including shoulder

    D21.11 Benign neoplasm of connective and other soft tissue of right upper limb, including shoulder

    D21.12 Benign neoplasm of connective and other soft tissue of left upper limb, including shoulder

√5ᵗʰ **D21.2** Benign neoplasm of connective and other soft tissue of lower limb, including hip

    D21.20 Benign neoplasm of connective and other soft tissue of unspecified lower limb, including hip

    D21.21 Benign neoplasm of connective and other soft tissue of right lower limb, including hip

    D21.22 Benign neoplasm of connective and other soft tissue of left lower limb, including hip

D21.3 Benign neoplasm of connective and other soft tissue of thorax
     Benign neoplasm of axilla
     Benign neoplasm of diaphragm
     Benign neoplasm of great vessels
    EXCLUDES 1   *benign neoplasm of heart (D15.1)*
           benign neoplasm of mediastinum (D15.2)
           benign neoplasm of thymus (D15.0)

D21.4 Benign neoplasm of connective and other soft tissue of abdomen
     Benign stromal tumors of abdomen

D21.5 Benign neoplasm of connective and other soft tissue of pelvis
    EXCLUDES 1   *benign neoplasm of any uterine ligament (D28.2)*
           uterine leiomyoma (D25.-)

D21.6 Benign neoplasm of connective and other soft tissue of trunk, unspecified
     Benign neoplasm of connective and other soft tissue of back NOS

D21.9 Benign neoplasm of connective and other soft tissue, unspecified

√4ᵗʰ **D22** Melanocytic nevi

    INCLUDES   atypical nevus
           blue hairy pigmented nevus
           nevus NOS

D22.0 Melanocytic nevi of lip

√5ᵗʰ **D22.1** Melanocytic nevi of eyelid, including canthus
     AHA: 2018,4Q,4

    D22.10 Melanocytic nevi of unspecified eyelid, including canthus

✓6ᵗʰ **D22.11** Melanocytic nevi of right eyelid, including canthus

     D22.111 Melanocytic nevi of right upper eyelid, including canthus

     D22.112 Melanocytic nevi of right lower eyelid, including canthus

✓6ᵗʰ **D22.12** Melanocytic nevi of left eyelid, including canthus

     D22.121 Melanocytic nevi of left upper eyelid, including canthus

     D22.122 Melanocytic nevi of left lower eyelid, including canthus

✓5ᵗʰ **D22.2** Melanocytic nevi of ear and external auricular canal

     D22.20 Melanocytic nevi of unspecified ear and external auricular canal

     D22.21 Melanocytic nevi of right ear and external auricular canal

     D22.22 Melanocytic nevi of left ear and external auricular canal

✓5ᵗʰ **D22.3** Melanocytic nevi of other and unspecified parts of face

[handwritten: nevus]

     D22.30 Melanocytic nevi of unspecified part of face

     D22.39 Melanocytic nevi of other parts of face

D22.4 Melanocytic nevi of scalp and neck

D22.5 Melanocytic nevi of trunk

     Melanocytic nevi of anal margin

     Melanocytic nevi of anal skin

     Melanocytic nevi of perianal skin

     Melanocytic nevi of skin of breast

✓5ᵗʰ **D22.6** Melanocytic nevi of upper limb, including shoulder

     D22.60 Melanocytic nevi of unspecified upper limb, including shoulder

     D22.61 Melanocytic nevi of right upper limb, including shoulder

     D22.62 Melanocytic nevi of left upper limb, including shoulder

✓5ᵗʰ **D22.7** Melanocytic nevi of lower limb, including hip

     D22.70 Melanocytic nevi of unspecified lower limb, including hip

     D22.71 Melanocytic nevi of right lower limb, including hip

     D22.72 Melanocytic nevi of left lower limb, including hip

     D22.9 Melanocytic nevi, unspecified

✓4ᵗʰ **D23** Other benign neoplasms of skin

     INCLUDES   benign neoplasm of hair follicles

               benign neoplasm of sebaceous glands

               benign neoplasm of sweat glands

     EXCLUDES 1   benign lipomatous neoplasms of skin (D17.0-D17.3)

     EXCLUDES 2   melanocytic nevi (D22.-)

D23.0 Other benign neoplasm of skin of lip

     EXCLUDES 1   benign neoplasm of vermilion border of lip (D10.0)

✓5ᵗʰ **D23.1** Other benign neoplasm of skin of eyelid, including canthus

     AHA: 2018,4Q,4

     D23.10 Other benign neoplasm of skin of unspecified eyelid, including canthus

     ✓6ᵗʰ **D23.11** Other benign neoplasm of skin of right eyelid, including canthus

         D23.111 Other benign neoplasm of skin of right upper eyelid, including canthus

         D23.112 Other benign neoplasm of skin of right lower eyelid, including canthus

     ✓6ᵗʰ **D23.12** Other benign neoplasm of skin of left eyelid, including canthus

         D23.121 Other benign neoplasm of skin of left upper eyelid, including canthus

         D23.122 Other benign neoplasm of skin of left lower eyelid, including canthus

✓5ᵗʰ **D23.2** Other benign neoplasm of skin of ear and external auricular canal

     D23.20 Other benign neoplasm of skin of unspecified ear and external auricular canal

     D23.21 Other benign neoplasm of skin of right ear and external auricular canal

     D23.22 Other benign neoplasm of skin of left ear and external auricular canal

✓5ᵗʰ **D23.3** Other benign neoplasm of skin of other and unspecified parts of face

     D23.30 Other benign neoplasm of skin of unspecified part of face

     D23.39 Other benign neoplasm of skin of other parts of face

D23.4 Other benign neoplasm of skin of scalp and neck

D23.5 Other benign neoplasm of skin of trunk

     Other benign neoplasm of anal margin

     Other benign neoplasm of anal skin

     Other benign neoplasm of perianal skin

     Other benign neoplasm of skin of breast

     EXCLUDES 1   benign neoplasm of anus NOS (D12.9)

✓5ᵗʰ **D23.6** Other benign neoplasm of skin of upper limb, including shoulder

     D23.60 Other benign neoplasm of skin of unspecified upper limb, including shoulder

     D23.61 Other benign neoplasm of skin of right upper limb, including shoulder

     D23.62 Other benign neoplasm of skin of left upper limb, including shoulder

✓5ᵗʰ **D23.7** Other benign neoplasm of skin of lower limb, including hip

     D23.70 Other benign neoplasm of skin of unspecified lower limb, including hip

     D23.71 Other benign neoplasm of skin of right lower limb, including hip

     D23.72 Other benign neoplasm of skin of left lower limb, including hip

     D23.9 Other benign neoplasm of skin, unspecified

✓4ᵗʰ **D24** Benign neoplasm of breast

     INCLUDES   benign neoplasm of connective tissue of breast

               benign neoplasm of soft parts of breast

               fibroadenoma of breast

     EXCLUDES 2   adenofibrosis of breast (N60.2)

               benign cyst of breast (N60.-)

               benign mammary dysplasia (N60.-)

               benign neoplasm of skin of breast (D22.5, D23.5)

               fibrocystic disease of breast (N60.-)

[handwritten: Papilloma] **D24.1** Benign neoplasm of right breast

D24.2 Benign neoplasm of left breast

D24.9 Benign neoplasm of unspecified breast

✓4ᵗʰ **D25** Leiomyoma of uterus

     INCLUDES   uterine fibroid

               uterine fibromyoma

               uterine myoma

Uterine Leiomyomas (Fibroids)

Cornual — Pedunculated

Uterine cavity — Intramural

Subserosal — Submucosal

Cervical

D25.0 Submucous leiomyoma of uterus ♀

D25.1 Intramural leiomyoma of uterus ♀ *[handwritten: hysteroscope]*

     Interstitial leiomyoma of uterus

D25.2 Subserosal leiomyoma of uterus ♀

     Subperitoneal leiomyoma of uterus

D25.9 Leiomyoma of uterus, unspecified ♀

✓4ᵗʰ **D26** Other benign neoplasms of uterus

D26.0 Other benign neoplasm of cervix uteri ♀

D26.1 Other benign neoplasm of corpus uteri ♀

D26.7 Other benign neoplasm of other parts of uterus ♀

D26.9 Other benign neoplasm of uterus, unspecified ♀

[handwritten: D25.9 leiomyoma, unspecified]

✓4ᵗʰ **D27**   **Benign neoplasm of** ovary
> Use additional code to identify any functional activity
> EXCLUDES 2   *corpus albicans cyst (N83.2-)*
>   *corpus luteum cyst (N83.1-)*
>   *endometrial cyst ▶(N80.1-)◀*
>   *follicular (atretic) cyst (N83.0-)*
>   *graafian follicle cyst (N83.0-)*
>   *ovarian cyst NEC (N83.2-)*
>   *ovarian retention cyst (N83.2-)*

   D27.0   **Benign neoplasm of** right **ovary**   ♀
   D27.1   **Benign neoplasm of** left **ovary**   ♀
   D27.9   **Benign neoplasm of unspecified ovary**   ♀

✓4ᵗʰ **D28**   **Benign neoplasm of other and unspecified** female genital organs
> INCLUDES   adenomatous polyp
>   benign neoplasm of skin of female genital organs
>   benign teratoma
> EXCLUDES 1   *epoophoron cyst (Q50.5)*
>   *fimbrial cyst (Q50.4)*
>   *Gartner's duct cyst (Q52.4)*
>   *parovarian cyst (Q50.5)*

   D28.0   **Benign neoplasm of** vulva   ♀
   D28.1   **Benign neoplasm of** vagina   ♀
   D28.2   **Benign neoplasm of** uterine tubes and ligaments   ♀
>   Benign neoplasm of fallopian tube
>   Benign neoplasm of uterine ligament (broad) (round)

   D28.7   **Benign neoplasm of other specified female genital organs**   ♀
   D28.9   **Benign neoplasm of female genital organ, unspecified**   ♀

✓4ᵗʰ **D29**   **Benign neoplasm of** male genital organs
> INCLUDES   benign neoplasm of skin of male genital organs

   D29.0   **Benign neoplasm of** penis   ♂
   D29.1   **Benign neoplasm of** prostate   ♂
> EXCLUDES 1   *enlarged prostate (N40.-)*

✓5ᵗʰ   **D29.2**   **Benign neoplasm of** testis
> Use additional code to identify any functional activity

     D29.20   **Benign neoplasm of unspecified testis**   ♂
     D29.21   **Benign neoplasm of** right **testis**   ♂
     D29.22   **Benign neoplasm of** left **testis**   ♂

✓5ᵗʰ   **D29.3**   **Benign neoplasm of** epididymis

     D29.30   **Benign neoplasm of unspecified epididymis**   ♂
     D29.31   **Benign neoplasm of** right **epididymis**   ♂
     D29.32   **Benign neoplasm of** left **epididymis**   ♂

   D29.4   **Benign neoplasm of** scrotum   ♂
>   Benign neoplasm of skin of scrotum

   D29.8   **Benign neoplasm of other specified male genital organs**   ♂
>   Benign neoplasm of seminal vesicle
>   Benign neoplasm of spermatic cord
>   Benign neoplasm of tunica vaginalis

   D29.9   **Benign neoplasm of male genital organ, unspecified**   ♂

✓4ᵗʰ **D30**   **Benign neoplasm of** urinary organs

✓5ᵗʰ   **D30.0**   **Benign neoplasm of** kidney
> EXCLUDES 1   *benign carcinoid tumor of the kidney (D3A.093)*
>   *benign neoplasm of renal calyces (D30.1-)*
>   *benign neoplasm of renal pelvis (D30.1-)*

     D30.00   **Benign neoplasm of unspecified kidney**
     D30.01   **Benign neoplasm of** right **kidney**
     D30.02   **Benign neoplasm of** left **kidney**

✓5ᵗʰ   **D30.1**   **Benign neoplasm of** renal pelvis

     D30.10   **Benign neoplasm of unspecified renal pelvis**
     D30.11   **Benign neoplasm of** right **renal pelvis**
     D30.12   **Benign neoplasm of** left **renal pelvis**

✓5ᵗʰ   **D30.2**   **Benign neoplasm of** ureter
> EXCLUDES 1   *benign neoplasm of ureteric orifice of bladder (D30.3)*

     D30.20   **Benign neoplasm of unspecified ureter**
     D30.21   **Benign neoplasm of** right **ureter**
     D30.22   **Benign neoplasm of** left **ureter**

   D30.3   **Benign neoplasm of** bladder
>   Benign neoplasm of ureteric orifice of bladder
>   Benign neoplasm of urethral orifice of bladder

   D30.4   **Benign neoplasm of** urethra
> EXCLUDES 1   *benign neoplasm of urethral orifice of bladder (D30.3)*

   D30.8   **Benign neoplasm of other specified urinary organs**
>   Benign neoplasm of paraurethral glands

   D30.9   **Benign neoplasm of urinary organ, unspecified**
>   Benign neoplasm of urinary system NOS

✓4ᵗʰ **D31**   **Benign neoplasm of** eye and adnexa
> EXCLUDES 1   *benign neoplasm of connective tissue of eyelid (D21.0)*
>   *benign neoplasm of optic nerve (D33.3)*
>   *benign neoplasm of skin of eyelid (D22.1-, D23.1-)*

✓5ᵗʰ   **D31.0**   **Benign neoplasm of** conjunctiva

     D31.00   **Benign neoplasm of unspecified conjunctiva**
     D31.01   **Benign neoplasm of** right **conjunctiva**
     D31.02   **Benign neoplasm of** left **conjunctiva**

✓5ᵗʰ   **D31.1**   **Benign neoplasm of** cornea

     D31.10   **Benign neoplasm of unspecified cornea**
     D31.11   **Benign neoplasm of** right **cornea**
     D31.12   **Benign neoplasm of** left **cornea**

✓5ᵗʰ   **D31.2**   **Benign neoplasm of** retina
> EXCLUDES 1   *dark area on retina (D49.81)*
>   *hemangioma of retina (D49.81)*
>   *neoplasm of unspecified behavior of retina and*
>   *choroid (D49.81)*
>   *retinal freckle (D49.81)*

     D31.20   **Benign neoplasm of unspecified retina**
     D31.21   **Benign neoplasm of** right **retina**
     D31.22   **Benign neoplasm of** left **retina**

✓5ᵗʰ   **D31.3**   **Benign neoplasm of** choroid

     D31.30   **Benign neoplasm of unspecified choroid**
     D31.31   **Benign neoplasm of** right **choroid**
     D31.32   **Benign neoplasm of** left **choroid**

✓5ᵗʰ   **D31.4**   **Benign neoplasm of** ciliary body

     D31.40   **Benign neoplasm of unspecified ciliary body**
     D31.41   **Benign neoplasm of** right **ciliary body**
     D31.42   **Benign neoplasm of** left **ciliary body**

✓5ᵗʰ   **D31.5**   **Benign neoplasm of** lacrimal gland and duct
>   Benign neoplasm of lacrimal sac
>   Benign neoplasm of nasolacrimal duct

     D31.50   **Benign neoplasm of unspecified lacrimal gland and duct**
     D31.51   **Benign neoplasm of** right **lacrimal gland and duct**
     D31.52   **Benign neoplasm of** left **lacrimal gland and duct**

✓5ᵗʰ   **D31.6**   **Benign neoplasm of unspecified site of** orbit
>   Benign neoplasm of connective tissue of orbit
>   Benign neoplasm of extraocular muscle
>   Benign neoplasm of peripheral nerves of orbit
>   Benign neoplasm of retrobulbar tissue
>   Benign neoplasm of retro-ocular tissue
> EXCLUDES 1   *benign neoplasm of orbital bone (D16.4)*

     D31.60   **Benign neoplasm of unspecified site of unspecified orbit**
     D31.61   **Benign neoplasm of unspecified site of** right **orbit**
     D31.62   **Benign neoplasm of unspecified site of** left **orbit**

✓5ᵗʰ   **D31.9**   **Benign neoplasm of unspecified** part of eye
>   Benign neoplasm of eyeball

     D31.90   **Benign neoplasm of unspecified part of unspecified eye**
     D31.91   **Benign neoplasm of unspecified part of right eye**
     D31.92   **Benign neoplasm of unspecified part of left eye**

✓4ᵗʰ **D32**   **Benign neoplasm of** meninges

   D32.0   **Benign neoplasm of** cerebral **meninges**   HCC Rx ESR COM
   D32.1   **Benign neoplasm of** spinal **meninges**   HCC Rx ESR COM
   D32.9   **Benign neoplasm of meninges, unspecified**   HCC Rx ESR COM
>   Meningioma NOS

✓4ᵗʰ **D33 Benign neoplasm of brain and other parts of central nervous system**
> EXCLUDES 1   angioma (D18.0-)
> benign neoplasm of meninges (D32.-)
> benign neoplasm of peripheral nerves and autonomic nervous system (D36.1-)
> hemangioma (D18.0-)
> neurofibromatosis (Q85.0-)
> retro-ocular benign neoplasm (D31.6-)

D33.0 Benign neoplasm of brain, supratentorial HCC Rx ESR COM
> Benign neoplasm of cerebral ventricle
> Benign neoplasm of cerebrum
> Benign neoplasm of frontal lobe
> Benign neoplasm of occipital lobe
> Benign neoplasm of parietal lobe
> Benign neoplasm of temporal lobe
> EXCLUDES 1   benign neoplasm of fourth ventricle (D33.1)

D33.1 Benign neoplasm of brain, infratentorial HCC Rx ESR COM
> Benign neoplasm of brain stem
> Benign neoplasm of cerebellum
> Benign neoplasm of fourth ventricle

D33.2 Benign neoplasm of brain, unspecified HCC Rx ESR COM

D33.3 Benign neoplasm of cranial nerves HCC Rx ESR COM
> Benign neoplasm of olfactory bulb

D33.4 Benign neoplasm of spinal cord HCC Rx ESR COM

D33.7 Benign neoplasm of other specified parts of central nervous system HCC Rx ESR COM

D33.9 Benign neoplasm of central nervous system, unspecified HCC Rx ESR COM
> Benign neoplasm of nervous system (central) NOS

D34 Benign neoplasm of thyroid gland
> Use additional code to identify any functional activity

✓4ᵗʰ **D35 Benign neoplasm of other and unspecified endocrine glands**
> Use additional code to identify any functional activity
> EXCLUDES 1   benign neoplasm of endocrine pancreas (D13.7)
> benign neoplasm of ovary (D27.-)
> benign neoplasm of testis (D29.2.-)
> benign neoplasm of thymus (D15.0)

✓5ᵗʰ **D35.0 Benign neoplasm of adrenal gland**
> **D35.00 Benign neoplasm of unspecified adrenal gland**
> **D35.01 Benign neoplasm of right adrenal gland**
> **D35.02 Benign neoplasm of left adrenal gland**

D35.1 Benign neoplasm of parathyroid gland

D35.2 Benign neoplasm of pituitary gland HCC Rx ESR COM
> AHA: 2014,3Q,22

D35.3 Benign neoplasm of craniopharyngeal duct HCC Rx ESR COM

D35.4 Benign neoplasm of pineal gland HCC Rx ESR COM

D35.5 Benign neoplasm of carotid body

D35.6 Benign neoplasm of aortic body and other paraganglia
> Benign tumor of glomus jugulare

D35.7 Benign neoplasm of other specified endocrine glands

D35.9 Benign neoplasm of endocrine gland, unspecified
> Benign neoplasm of unspecified endocrine gland

✓4ᵗʰ **D36 Benign neoplasm of other and unspecified sites**

D36.0 Benign neoplasm of lymph nodes
> EXCLUDES 1   lymphangioma (D18.1)

✓5ᵗʰ **D36.1 Benign neoplasm of peripheral nerves and autonomic nervous system**
> EXCLUDES 1   benign neoplasm of peripheral nerves of orbit (D31.6-)
> neurofibromatosis (Q85.0-)

> **D36.10 Benign neoplasm of peripheral nerves and autonomic nervous system, unspecified**
> **D36.11 Benign neoplasm of peripheral nerves and autonomic nervous system of face, head, and neck**
> **D36.12 Benign neoplasm of peripheral nerves and autonomic nervous system, upper limb, including shoulder**
> **D36.13 Benign neoplasm of peripheral nerves and autonomic nervous system of lower limb, including hip**
> **D36.14 Benign neoplasm of peripheral nerves and autonomic nervous system of thorax**
> **D36.15 Benign neoplasm of peripheral nerves and autonomic nervous system of abdomen**

> **D36.16 Benign neoplasm of peripheral nerves and autonomic nervous system of pelvis**
> **D36.17 Benign neoplasm of peripheral nerves and autonomic nervous system of trunk, unspecified**

D36.7 Benign neoplasm of other specified sites
> Benign neoplasm of back NOS
> Benign neoplasm of nose NOS

D36.9 Benign neoplasm, unspecified site

Benign neuroendocrine tumors (D3A)

✓4ᵗʰ **D3A Benign neuroendocrine tumors**
> Code also any associated multiple endocrine neoplasia [MEN] syndromes (E31.2-)
> Use additional code to identify any associated endocrine syndrome, such as:
> carcinoid syndrome (E34.0)
> EXCLUDES 2   benign pancreatic islet cell tumors (D13.7)

✓5ᵗʰ **D3A.0 Benign carcinoid tumors**
> **DEF:** Specific type of slow-growing neuroendocrine tumors. Carcinoid tumors occur most commonly in the hormone producing cells of the gastrointestinal tracts and can also occur in the pancreas, testes, ovaries, or lungs.

> **D3A.00 Benign carcinoid tumor of unspecified site** Rx
> Carcinoid tumor NOS

✓6ᵗʰ **D3A.01 Benign carcinoid tumors of the small intestine**
> **D3A.010 Benign carcinoid tumor of the duodenum** Rx
> **D3A.011 Benign carcinoid tumor of the jejunum** Rx
> **D3A.012 Benign carcinoid tumor of the ileum** Rx
> **D3A.019 Benign carcinoid tumor of the small intestine, unspecified portion** Rx

✓6ᵗʰ **D3A.02 Benign carcinoid tumors of the appendix, large intestine, and rectum**
> **D3A.020 Benign carcinoid tumor of the appendix** Rx
> **D3A.021 Benign carcinoid tumor of the cecum** Rx
> **D3A.022 Benign carcinoid tumor of the ascending colon** Rx
> **D3A.023 Benign carcinoid tumor of the transverse colon** Rx
> **D3A.024 Benign carcinoid tumor of the descending colon** Rx
> **D3A.025 Benign carcinoid tumor of the sigmoid colon** Rx
> **D3A.026 Benign carcinoid tumor of the rectum** Rx
> **D3A.029 Benign carcinoid tumor of the large intestine, unspecified portion** Rx
> Benign carcinoid tumor of the colon NOS

✓6ᵗʰ **D3A.09 Benign carcinoid tumors of other sites**
> **D3A.090 Benign carcinoid tumor of the bronchus and lung** Rx
> **D3A.091 Benign carcinoid tumor of the thymus** Rx
> **D3A.092 Benign carcinoid tumor of the stomach** Rx
> **D3A.093 Benign carcinoid tumor of the kidney** Rx
> **D3A.094 Benign carcinoid tumor of the foregut, unspecified** Rx
> **D3A.095 Benign carcinoid tumor of the midgut, unspecified** Rx
> **D3A.096 Benign carcinoid tumor of the hindgut, unspecified** Rx
> **D3A.098 Benign carcinoid tumors of other sites** Rx

D3A.8 Other benign neuroendocrine tumors Rx
> Neuroendocrine tumor NOS

Neoplasms of uncertain behavior, polycythemia vera and myelodysplastic syndromes (D37-D48)

NOTE   Categories D37-D44, and D48 classify by site neoplasms of uncertain behavior, i.e., histologic confirmation whether the neoplasm is malignant or benign cannot be made.

EXCLUDES 1   *neoplasms of unspecified behavior (D49.-)*

☑4ᵗʰ D37 Neoplasm of uncertain behavior of oral cavity and digestive organs

     EXCLUDES 1   *stromal tumors of uncertain behavior of digestive system (D48.1)*

   ☑5ᵗʰ D37.0 Neoplasm of uncertain behavior of lip, oral cavity and pharynx

     EXCLUDES 1   *neoplasm of uncertain behavior of aryepiglottic fold or interarytenoid fold, laryngeal aspect (D38.0)*
        neoplasm of uncertain behavior of epiglottis NOS (D38.0)
        neoplasm of uncertain behavior of skin of lip (D48.5)
        neoplasm of uncertain behavior of suprahyoid portion of epiglottis (D38.0)

     D37.01 Neoplasm of uncertain behavior of lip
        Neoplasm of uncertain behavior of vermilion border of lip

     D37.02 Neoplasm of uncertain behavior of tongue

     ☑6ᵗʰ D37.03 Neoplasm of uncertain behavior of the major salivary glands

        D37.030 Neoplasm of uncertain behavior of the parotid salivary glands

        D37.031 Neoplasm of uncertain behavior of the sublingual salivary glands

        D37.032 Neoplasm of uncertain behavior of the submandibular salivary glands

        D37.039 Neoplasm of uncertain behavior of the major salivary glands, unspecified

     D37.04 Neoplasm of uncertain behavior of the minor salivary glands
        Neoplasm of uncertain behavior of submucosal salivary glands of lip
        Neoplasm of uncertain behavior of submucosal salivary glands of cheek
        Neoplasm of uncertain behavior of submucosal salivary glands of hard palate
        Neoplasm of uncertain behavior of submucosal salivary glands of soft palate

     D37.05 Neoplasm of uncertain behavior of pharynx
        Neoplasm of uncertain behavior of aryepiglottic fold of pharynx NOS
        Neoplasm of uncertain behavior of hypopharyngeal aspect of aryepiglottic fold of pharynx
        Neoplasm of uncertain behavior of marginal zone of aryepiglottic fold of pharynx

     D37.09 Neoplasm of uncertain behavior of other specified sites of the oral cavity

   D37.1 Neoplasm of uncertain behavior of stomach

   D37.2 Neoplasm of uncertain behavior of small intestine

   D37.3 Neoplasm of uncertain behavior of appendix

   D37.4 Neoplasm of uncertain behavior of colon

   D37.5 Neoplasm of uncertain behavior of rectum
     Neoplasm of uncertain behavior of rectosigmoid junction

   D37.6 Neoplasm of uncertain behavior of liver, gallbladder and bile ducts
     Neoplasm of uncertain behavior of ampulla of Vater

   D37.8 Neoplasm of uncertain behavior of other specified digestive organs
     Neoplasm of uncertain behavior of anal canal
     Neoplasm of uncertain behavior of anal sphincter
     Neoplasm of uncertain behavior of anus NOS
     Neoplasm of uncertain behavior of esophagus
     Neoplasm of uncertain behavior of intestine NOS
     Neoplasm of uncertain behavior of pancreas
     EXCLUDES 1   *neoplasm of uncertain behavior of anal margin (D48.5)*
        neoplasm of uncertain behavior of anal skin (D48.5)
        neoplasm of uncertain behavior of perianal skin (D48.5)

   D37.9 Neoplasm of uncertain behavior of digestive organ, unspecified

☑4ᵗʰ D38 Neoplasm of uncertain behavior of middle ear and respiratory and intrathoracic organs

     EXCLUDES 1   *neoplasm of uncertain behavior of heart (D48.7)*

   D38.0 Neoplasm of uncertain behavior of larynx
     Neoplasm of uncertain behavior of aryepiglottic fold or interarytenoid fold, laryngeal aspect
     Neoplasm of uncertain behavior of epiglottis (suprahyoid portion)
     EXCLUDES 1   *neoplasm of uncertain behavior of aryepiglottic fold or interarytenoid fold NOS (D37.05)*
        neoplasm of uncertain behavior of hypopharyngeal aspect of aryepiglottic fold (D37.05)
        neoplasm of uncertain behavior of marginal zone of aryepiglottic fold (D37.05)

   D38.1 Neoplasm of uncertain behavior of trachea, bronchus and lung

   D38.2 Neoplasm of uncertain behavior of pleura

   D38.3 Neoplasm of uncertain behavior of mediastinum

   D38.4 Neoplasm of uncertain behavior of thymus

   D38.5 Neoplasm of uncertain behavior of other respiratory organs
     Neoplasm of uncertain behavior of accessory sinuses
     Neoplasm of uncertain behavior of cartilage of nose
     Neoplasm of uncertain behavior of middle ear
     Neoplasm of uncertain behavior of nasal cavities
     EXCLUDES 1   *neoplasm of uncertain behavior of ear (external) (skin) (D48.5)*
        neoplasm of uncertain behavior of nose NOS (D48.7)
        neoplasm of uncertain behavior of skin of nose (D48.5)

   D38.6 Neoplasm of uncertain behavior of respiratory organ, unspecified

☑4ᵗʰ D39 Neoplasm of uncertain behavior of female genital organs

   D39.0 Neoplasm of uncertain behavior of uterus   ♀

   ☑5ᵗʰ D39.1 Neoplasm of uncertain behavior of ovary
     Use additional code to identify any functional activity

     D39.10 Neoplasm of uncertain behavior of unspecified ovary   ♀

     D39.11 Neoplasm of uncertain behavior of right ovary   ♀

     D39.12 Neoplasm of uncertain behavior of left ovary   ♀

   D39.2 Neoplasm of uncertain behavior of placenta   M ♀
     Chorioadenoma destruens
     Invasive hydatidiform mole
     Malignant hydatidiform mole
     EXCLUDES 1   *hydatidiform mole NOS (O01.9)*

   D39.8 Neoplasm of uncertain behavior of other specified female genital organs   ♀
     Neoplasm of uncertain behavior of skin of female genital organs

   D39.9 Neoplasm of uncertain behavior of female genital organ, unspecified   ♀

☑4ᵗʰ D40 Neoplasm of uncertain behavior of male genital organs

   D40.0 Neoplasm of uncertain behavior of prostate   ♂

   ☑5ᵗʰ D40.1 Neoplasm of uncertain behavior of testis

     D40.10 Neoplasm of uncertain behavior of unspecified testis   ♂

     D40.11 Neoplasm of uncertain behavior of right testis   ♂

     D40.12 Neoplasm of uncertain behavior of left testis   ♂

   D40.8 Neoplasm of uncertain behavior of other specified male genital organs   ♂
     Neoplasm of uncertain behavior of skin of male genital organs

   D40.9 Neoplasm of uncertain behavior of male genital organ, unspecified   ♂

☑4ᵗʰ D41 Neoplasm of uncertain behavior of urinary organs

   ☑5ᵗʰ D41.0 Neoplasm of uncertain behavior of kidney

     EXCLUDES 1   *neoplasm of uncertain behavior of renal pelvis (D41.1-)*

     D41.00 Neoplasm of uncertain behavior of unspecified kidney

     D41.01 Neoplasm of uncertain behavior of right kidney

     D41.02 Neoplasm of uncertain behavior of left kidney

   ☑5ᵗʰ D41.1 Neoplasm of uncertain behavior of renal pelvis

     D41.10 Neoplasm of uncertain behavior of unspecified renal pelvis

     D41.11 Neoplasm of uncertain behavior of right renal pelvis

     D41.12 Neoplasm of uncertain behavior of left renal pelvis

Chapter 2. Neoplasms

✓5ᵗʰ **D41.2 Neoplasm of uncertain behavior of** ureter

     D41.20 Neoplasm of uncertain behavior of unspecified ureter

     D41.21 Neoplasm of uncertain behavior of right **ureter**

     D41.22 Neoplasm of uncertain behavior of left **ureter**

D41.3 Neoplasm of uncertain behavior of urethra

D41.4 Neoplasm of uncertain behavior of bladder

D41.8 Neoplasm of uncertain behavior of other specified urinary organs

D41.9 Neoplasm of uncertain behavior of unspecified urinary organ

✓4ᵗʰ **D42 Neoplasm of uncertain behavior of** meninges

   D42.0 Neoplasm of uncertain behavior of cerebral meninges HCC Rx ESR COM

   D42.1 Neoplasm of uncertain behavior of spinal meninges HCC Rx ESR COM

   D42.9 Neoplasm of uncertain behavior of meninges, unspecified HCC Rx ESR COM

✓4ᵗʰ **D43 Neoplasm of uncertain behavior of** brain and central nervous system

    EXCLUDES 1   *neoplasm of uncertain behavior of peripheral nerves and autonomic nervous system (D48.2)*

   D43.0 Neoplasm of uncertain behavior of brain, supratentorial HCC Rx ESR COM

      Neoplasm of uncertain behavior of cerebral ventricle

      Neoplasm of uncertain behavior of cerebrum

      Neoplasm of uncertain behavior of frontal lobe

      Neoplasm of uncertain behavior of occipital lobe

      Neoplasm of uncertain behavior of parietal lobe

      Neoplasm of uncertain behavior of temporal lobe

      EXCLUDES 1   *neoplasm of uncertain behavior of fourth ventricle (D43.1)*

   D43.1 Neoplasm of uncertain behavior of brain, infratentorial HCC Rx ESR COM

      Neoplasm of uncertain behavior of brain stem

      Neoplasm of uncertain behavior of cerebellum

      Neoplasm of uncertain behavior of fourth ventricle

   D43.2 Neoplasm of uncertain behavior of brain, unspecified HCC Rx ESR COM

   D43.3 Neoplasm of uncertain behavior of cranial nerves HCC Rx ESR COM

   D43.4 Neoplasm of uncertain behavior of spinal cord HCC Rx ESR COM

   D43.8 Neoplasm of uncertain behavior of other specified parts of central nervous system HCC Rx ESR COM

   D43.9 Neoplasm of uncertain behavior of central nervous system, unspecified HCC Rx ESR COM

      Neoplasm of uncertain behavior of nervous system (central) NOS

✓4ᵗʰ **D44 Neoplasm of uncertain behavior of** endocrine glands

    EXCLUDES 1   *multiple endocrine adenomatosis (E31.2-)*

        multiple endocrine neoplasia (E31.2-)

        neoplasm of uncertain behavior of endocrine pancreas (D37.8)

        neoplasm of uncertain behavior of ovary (D39.1-)

        neoplasm of uncertain behavior of testis (D40.1-)

        neoplasm of uncertain behavior of thymus (D38.4)

   D44.0 Neoplasm of uncertain behavior of thyroid gland

✓5ᵗʰ **D44.1 Neoplasm of uncertain behavior of** adrenal gland

      Use additional code to identify any functional activity

     D44.10 Neoplasm of uncertain behavior of unspecified adrenal gland

     D44.11 Neoplasm of uncertain behavior of right **adrenal gland**

     D44.12 Neoplasm of uncertain behavior of left **adrenal gland**

   D44.2 Neoplasm of uncertain behavior of parathyroid gland

   D44.3 Neoplasm of uncertain behavior of pituitary gland HCC Rx ESR COM

      Use additional code to identify any functional activity

   D44.4 Neoplasm of uncertain behavior of craniopharyngeal duct HCC Rx ESR COM

   D44.5 Neoplasm of uncertain behavior of pineal gland HCC Rx ESR COM

   D44.6 Neoplasm of uncertain behavior of carotid body HCC Rx ESR COM

   D44.7 Neoplasm of uncertain behavior of aortic body and other paraganglia HCC Rx ESR COM

      AHA: 2021,2Q,7; 2016,4Q,26

   D44.9 Neoplasm of uncertain behavior of unspecified endocrine gland

D45 Polycythemia vera HCC Rx ESR COM

    EXCLUDES 1   *familial polycythemia (D75.0)*

        secondary polycythemia (D75.1)

   DEF: Abnormal proliferation of all bone marrow elements, increased red cell mass, and total blood volume. The etiology is unknown, but it is frequently associated with splenomegaly, leukocytosis, and thrombocythemia.

✓4ᵗʰ **D46 Myelodysplastic syndromes**

      Use additional code for adverse effect, if applicable, to identify drug (T36-T50 with fifth or sixth character 5)

    EXCLUDES 2   *drug-induced aplastic anemia (D61.1)*

   D46.0 Refractory anemia without ring sideroblasts, **so stated** HCC Rx ESR COM

      Refractory anemia without sideroblasts, without excess of blasts

   D46.1 Refractory anemia with ring sideroblasts HCC Rx ESR COM

      RARS

✓5ᵗʰ **D46.2 Refractory anemia** with excess of blasts [RAEB]

     D46.20 Refractory anemia with excess of blasts, unspecified HCC Rx ESR COM

       RAEB NOS

     D46.21 Refractory anemia with excess of blasts 1 HCC Rx ESR COM

       RAEB 1

     D46.22 Refractory anemia with excess of blasts 2 HCC Rx ESR COM

       RAEB 2

   D46.A Refractory cytopenia with multilineage dysplasia HCC Rx ESR COM

   D46.B Refractory cytopenia with multilineage dysplasia and ring sideroblasts HCC Rx ESR COM

      RCMD RS

   D46.C Myelodysplastic syndrome with isolated del(5q) chromosomal abnormality HCC Rx ESR COM

      Myelodysplastic syndrome with 5q deletion

      5q minus syndrome NOS

   D46.4 Refractory anemia, unspecified HCC Rx ESR COM

   D46.Z Other myelodysplastic syndromes HCC Rx ESR COM

    EXCLUDES 1   *chronic myelomonocytic leukemia (C93.1-)*

   D46.9 Myelodysplastic syndrome, unspecified HCC Rx ESR COM

      Myelodysplasia NOS

✓4ᵗʰ **D47 Other neoplasms of uncertain behavior of** lymphoid, hematopoietic and related tissue

✓5ᵗʰ **D47.0 Mast cell neoplasms of uncertain behavior**

    EXCLUDES 1   *congenital cutaneous mastocytosis (Q82.2)*

        histiocytic neoplasms of uncertain behavior (D47.Z9)

        malignant mast cell neoplasm (C96.2-)

      AHA: 2017,4Q,5

     D47.01 Cutaneous mastocytosis Rx

       Diffuse cutaneous mastocytosis

       Maculopapular cutaneous mastocytosis

       Solitary mastocytoma

       Telangiectasia macularis eruptiva perstans

       Urticaria pigmentosa

       EXCLUDES 1   *congenital (diffuse) (maculopapular) cutaneous mastocytosis (Q82.2)*

          congenital urticaria pigmentosa (Q82.2)

          extracutaneous mastocytoma (D47.09)

D47.02 Systemic **mastocytosis** `Rx`
  Indolent systemic mastocytosis
  Isolated bone marrow mastocytosis
  Smoldering systemic mastocytosis
  Systemic mastocytosis, with an associated
    hematological non-mast cell lineage disease
    (SM-AHNMD)
  Code also, if applicable, any associated hematological
    non-mast cell lineage disease, such as:
    acute myeloid leukemia (C92.6-, C92.A-)
    chronic myelomonocytic leukemia (C93.1-)
    essential thrombocytosis (D47.3)
    hypereosinophilic syndrome (D72.1)
    myelodysplastic syndrome (D46.9)
    myeloproliferative syndrome (D47.1)
    non-Hodgkin lymphoma (C82-C85)
    plasma cell myeloma (C90.0-)
    polycythemia vera (D45)
    EXCLUDES 1   aggressive systemic mastocytosis (C96.21)
           mast cell leukemia (C94.3-)

D47.09 Other mast cell neoplasms of uncertain
  behavior `Rx`
  Extracutaneous mastocytoma
  Mast cell tumor NOS
  Mastocytoma NOS
  Mastocytosis NOS

D47.1 **Chronic myeloproliferative disease** `HCC` `Rx` `ESR` `COM`
  Chronic neutrophilic leukemia
  Myeloproliferative disease, unspecified
  EXCLUDES 1   atypical chronic myeloid leukemia BCR/ABL-negative
    (C92.2-)
         chronic myeloid leukemia BCR/ABL-positive (C92.1-)
         myelofibrosis NOS (D75.81)
         myelophthisic anemia (D61.82)
         myelophthisis (D61.82)
         secondary myelofibrosis NOS (D75.81)

D47.2 **Monoclonal gammopathy**
  Monoclonal gammopathy of undetermined significance [MGUS]
  AHA: 2021,3Q,5
  TIP: Smoldering multiple myeloma (SMM) is coded here.

D47.3 **Essential (hemorrhagic) thrombocythemia** `HCC` `Rx` `ESR` `COM`
  Essential thrombocytosis
  Idiopathic hemorrhagic thrombocythemia
  Primary thrombocytosis
  EXCLUDES 2   reactive thrombocytosis (D75.838)
         secondary thrombocytosis (D75.838)
         thrombocythemia NOS (D75.839)
         thrombocytosis NOS (D75.839)
  DEF: Chronic myeloproliferative neoplasm involving production
  of excess blood platelets that may result in abnormal clotting or
  hemorrhaging.

D47.4 **Osteomyelofibrosis** `HCC` `Rx` `ESR` `COM`
  Chronic idiopathic myelofibrosis
  Myelofibrosis (idiopathic) (with myeloid metaplasia)
  Myelosclerosis (megakaryocytic) with myeloid metaplasia
  Secondary myelofibrosis in myeloproliferative disease
  EXCLUDES 1   acute myelofibrosis (C94.4-)

✓5ᵗʰ **D47.Z** **Other specified neoplasms of uncertain behavior of
  lymphoid, hematopoietic and related tissue**
  AHA: 2016,4Q,8

  D47.Z1 **Post-transplant lymphoproliferative disorder
    (PTLD)** `HCC` `ESR` `COM` `UPD`
    Code first complications of transplanted organs and
      tissue (T86.-)
    DEF: Excessive proliferation of B-cell lymphocytes
    following Epstein-Barr virus infection in organ
    transplant patients. It may progress to non-Hodgkin
    lymphoma.

  D47.Z2 **Castleman disease** `HCC` `Rx` `ESR` `COM`
    Code also, if applicable, human herpesvirus 8 infection
      (B10.89)
    EXCLUDES 2   Kaposi's sarcoma (C46.-)
    DEF: Rare disease of the lymph nodes and lymphoid
    tissues that closely mimics lymphoma.

  D47.Z9 **Other specified neoplasms of uncertain behavior
    of lymphoid, hematopoietic and related
    tissue** `HCC` `Rx` `ESR` `COM`
    Histiocytic tumors of uncertain behavior

D47.9 **Neoplasm of uncertain behavior of lymphoid, hematopoietic
  and related tissue, unspecified** `HCC` `Rx` `ESR` `COM`
  Lymphoproliferative disease NOS

✓4ᵗʰ **D48** **Neoplasm of uncertain behavior of other and unspecified sites**
  EXCLUDES 1   neurofibromatosis (nonmalignant) (Q85.0-)

D48.0 **Neoplasm of uncertain behavior of** bone and articular
  cartilage
  EXCLUDES 1   neoplasm of uncertain behavior of cartilage of ear
    (D48.1)
         neoplasm of uncertain behavior of cartilage of larynx
    (D38.0)
         neoplasm of uncertain behavior of cartilage of nose
    (D38.5)
         neoplasm of uncertain behavior of connective tissue
    of eyelid (D48.1)
         neoplasm of uncertain behavior of synovia (D48.1)

D48.1 **Neoplasm of uncertain behavior of** connective and other
  soft tissue
  Neoplasm of uncertain behavior of connective tissue of ear
  Neoplasm of uncertain behavior of connective tissue of eyelid
  Stromal tumors of uncertain behavior of digestive system
  EXCLUDES 1   neoplasm of uncertain behavior of articular cartilage
    (D48.0)
         neoplasm of uncertain behavior of cartilage of larynx
    (D38.0)
         neoplasm of uncertain behavior of cartilage of nose
    (D38.5)
         neoplasm of uncertain behavior of connective tissue
    of breast (D48.6-)

D48.2 **Neoplasm of uncertain behavior of** peripheral nerves and
  autonomic nervous system
  EXCLUDES 1   neoplasm of uncertain behavior of peripheral nerves
    of orbit (D48.7)

D48.3 **Neoplasm of uncertain behavior of** retroperitoneum

D48.4 **Neoplasm of uncertain behavior of** peritoneum

D48.5 **Neoplasm of uncertain behavior of** skin
  Neoplasm of uncertain behavior of anal margin
  Neoplasm of uncertain behavior of anal skin
  Neoplasm of uncertain behavior of perianal skin
  Neoplasm of uncertain behavior of skin of breast
  EXCLUDES 1   neoplasm of uncertain behavior of anus NOS (D37.8)
         neoplasm of uncertain behavior of skin of genital
    organs (D39.8, D40.8)
         neoplasm of uncertain behavior of vermilion border
    of lip (D37.0)

✓5ᵗʰ **D48.6** **Neoplasm of uncertain behavior of** breast
  Neoplasm of uncertain behavior of connective tissue of breast
  Cystosarcoma phyllodes
  EXCLUDES 1   neoplasm of uncertain behavior of skin of breast
    (D48.5)

  D48.60 **Neoplasm of uncertain behavior of unspecified
    breast**

  D48.61 **Neoplasm of uncertain behavior of** right **breast**

  D48.62 **Neoplasm of uncertain behavior of** left **breast**

D48.7 **Neoplasm of uncertain behavior of other specified sites**
  Neoplasm of uncertain behavior of eye
  Neoplasm of uncertain behavior of heart
  Neoplasm of uncertain behavior of peripheral nerves of orbit
  EXCLUDES 1   neoplasm of uncertain behavior of connective tissue
    (D48.1)
         neoplasm of uncertain behavior of skin of eyelid
    (D48.5)

D48.9 **Neoplasm of uncertain behavior, unspecified**

Chapter 2. Neoplasms

Neoplasms of unspecified behavior (D49)

☑4ᵗʰ D49 Neoplasms of unspecified behavior

> **NOTE**   Category D49 classifies by site neoplasms of unspecified morphology and behavior. The term "mass", unless otherwise stated, is not to be regarded as a neoplastic growth.
>
> **INCLUDES**   "growth" NOS
> neoplasm NOS
> new growth NOS
> tumor NOS
>
> **EXCLUDES 1**   neoplasms of uncertain behavior (D37-D44, D48)

D49.0 Neoplasm of unspecified behavior of digestive system

> **EXCLUDES 1**   neoplasm of unspecified behavior of margin of anus (D49.2)
> neoplasm of unspecified behavior of perianal skin (D49.2)
> neoplasm of unspecified behavior of skin of anus (D49.2)

D49.1 Neoplasm of unspecified behavior of respiratory system

D49.2 Neoplasm of unspecified behavior of bone, soft tissue, and skin

> **EXCLUDES 1**   neoplasm of unspecified behavior of anal canal (D49.0)
> neoplasm of unspecified behavior of anus NOS (D49.0)
> neoplasm of unspecified behavior of bone marrow (D49.89)
> neoplasm of unspecified behavior of cartilage of larynx (D49.1)
> neoplasm of unspecified behavior of cartilage of nose (D49.1)
> neoplasm of unspecified behavior of connective tissue of breast (D49.3)
> neoplasm of unspecified behavior of skin of genital organs (D49.59)
> neoplasm of unspecified behavior of vermilion border of lip (D49.0)

D49.3 Neoplasm of unspecified behavior of breast

> **EXCLUDES 1**   neoplasm of unspecified behavior of skin of breast (D49.2)

D49.4 Neoplasm of unspecified behavior of bladder

☑5ᵗʰ D49.5 Neoplasm of unspecified behavior of other genitourinary organs

> AHA: 2016,4Q,9

> **☑6ᵗʰ D49.51 Neoplasm of unspecified behavior of kidney**
>
> > **D49.511 Neoplasm of unspecified behavior of right kidney**
> > **D49.512 Neoplasm of unspecified behavior of left kidney**
> > **D49.519 Neoplasm of unspecified behavior of unspecified kidney**
>
> **D49.59 Neoplasm of unspecified behavior of other genitourinary organ**

D49.6 Neoplasm of unspecified behavior of brain HCC Rx ESR COM

> **EXCLUDES 1**   neoplasm of unspecified behavior of cerebral meninges (D49.7)
> neoplasm of unspecified behavior of cranial nerves (D49.7)

D49.7 Neoplasm of unspecified behavior of endocrine glands and other parts of nervous system

> **EXCLUDES 1**   neoplasm of unspecified behavior of peripheral, sympathetic, and parasympathetic nerves and ganglia (D49.2)

☑5ᵗʰ D49.8 Neoplasm of unspecified behavior of other specified sites

> **EXCLUDES 1**   neoplasm of unspecified behavior of eyelid (skin) (D49.2)
> neoplasm of unspecified behavior of eyelid cartilage (D49.2)
> neoplasm of unspecified behavior of great vessels (D49.2)
> neoplasm of unspecified behavior of optic nerve (D49.7)

> **D49.81 Neoplasm of unspecified behavior of retina and choroid**
>
> > Dark area on retina
> > Retinal freckle
>
> **D49.89 Neoplasm of unspecified behavior of other specified sites**

D49.9 Neoplasm of unspecified behavior of unspecified site

Chapter 3. Disease of the Blood and Blood-Forming Organs and Certain Disorders Involving the Immune Mechanism (D50–D89)

Chapter-specific Guidelines with Coding Examples
Reserved for future guideline expansion.

Chapter 3. Diseases of the Blood and Blood-forming Organs and Certain Disorders Involving the Immune Mechanism (D50-D89)

EXCLUDES 2   *autoimmune disease (systemic) NOS (M35.9)*
certain conditions originating in the perinatal period (P00-P96)
complications of pregnancy, childbirth and the puerperium (O00-O9A)
congenital malformations, deformations and chromosomal abnormalities (Q00-Q99)
endocrine, nutritional and metabolic diseases (E00-E88)
human immunodeficiency virus [HIV] disease (B20)
injury, poisoning and certain other consequences of external causes (S00-T88)
neoplasms (C00-D49)
symptoms, signs and abnormal clinical and laboratory findings, not elsewhere classified (R00-R94)

This chapter contains the following blocks:

D50-D53   Nutritional anemias
D55-D59   Hemolytic anemias
D60-D64   Aplastic and other anemias and other bone marrow failure syndromes
D65-D69   Coagulation defects, purpura and other hemorrhagic conditions
D70-D77   Other disorders of blood and blood-forming organs
D78   Intraoperative and postprocedural complications of the spleen
D80-D89   Certain disorders involving the immune mechanism

Nutritional anemias (D50-D53)

DEF: Nutritional anemia: The result of inadequate intake or absorption of a vitamin or mineral that impacts the production of red blood cells or causes them to develop abnormally affecting the size and shape.
TIP: Documentation must identify a link between anemia and the nutritional deficiency; low levels of a particular nutrient may occur concurrently with anemia but not cause the anemia.

✓4ᵗʰ **D50**   Iron **deficiency anemia**
    INCLUDES   asiderotic anemia
              hypochromic anemia

    D50.0   **Iron deficiency anemia** secondary to blood loss (chronic)
         Posthemorrhagic anemia (chronic)
         EXCLUDES 1   *acute posthemorrhagic anemia (D62)*
                     congenital anemia from fetal blood loss (P61.3)
         AHA: 2019,3Q,17

[handwritten margin note: regular bleeding]

    D50.1   Sideropenic dysphagia
         Kelly-Paterson syndrome
         Plummer-Vinson syndrome

    D50.8   **Other iron deficiency anemias**
         Iron deficiency anemia due to inadequate dietary iron intake

    D50.9   **Iron deficiency anemia, unspecified**

✓4ᵗʰ **D51**   Vitamin B12 **deficiency anemia**
         EXCLUDES 1   *vitamin B12 deficiency (E53.8)*

    D51.0   **Vitamin B12 deficiency anemia due to** intrinsic factor deficiency
         Addison anemia
         Biermer anemia
         Pernicious (congenital) anemia
         Congenital intrinsic factor deficiency
         DEF: Chronic progressive anemia due to vitamin B12 malabsorption, caused by lack of secretion of intrinsic factor, which is produced by the gastric mucosa of the stomach.

    D51.1   **Vitamin B12 deficiency anemia due to** selective vitamin B12 malabsorption with proteinuria
         Imerslund (Gräsbeck) syndrome
         Megaloblastic hereditary anemia

    D51.2   Transcobalamin II **deficiency**

    D51.3   **Other dietary vitamin B12 deficiency anemia**
         Vegan anemia

    D51.8   **Other vitamin B12 deficiency anemias**

    D51.9   **Vitamin B12 deficiency anemia, unspecified**

✓4ᵗʰ **D52**   Folate **deficiency anemia**
         EXCLUDES 1   *folate deficiency without anemia (E53.8)*
         DEF: Deficiency in a B complex vitamin needed for the production of healthy red blood cells. Lack of folate, or folic acid, and other absorption conditions can cause anemia resulting in large, misshapen red blood cells called megaloblasts.

    D52.0   Dietary **folate deficiency anemia**
         Nutritional megaloblastic anemia
         DEF: Result of a poor diet with inadequate intake of folate, which is needed to produce healthy red blood cells.

    D52.1   **Drug-induced** folate deficiency anemia
         Use additional code for adverse effect, if applicable, to identify drug (T36-T50 with fifth or sixth character 5)

    D52.8   **Other folate deficiency anemias**

    D52.9   **Folate deficiency anemia, unspecified**
         Folic acid deficiency anemia NOS

✓4ᵗʰ **D53**   Other nutritional anemias
         INCLUDES   megaloblastic anemia unresponsive to vitamin B12 or folate therapy

    D53.0   Protein **deficiency anemia**
         Amino-acid deficiency anemia
         Orotaciduric anemia
         EXCLUDES 1   *Lesch-Nyhan syndrome (E79.1)*

    D53.1   **Other** megaloblastic **anemias, not elsewhere classified**
         Megaloblastic anemia NOS
         EXCLUDES 1   *Di Guglielmo's disease (C94.0)*

    D53.2   Scorbutic **anemia**
         EXCLUDES 1   *scurvy (E54)*

    D53.8   **Other specified nutritional anemias**
         Anemia associated with deficiency of copper
         Anemia associated with deficiency of molybdenum
         Anemia associated with deficiency of zinc
         EXCLUDES 1   *nutritional deficiencies without anemia, such as:*
                   copper deficiency NOS (E61.0)
                   molybdenum deficiency NOS (E61.5)
                   zinc deficiency NOS (E60)

    D53.9   **Nutritional anemia, unspecified**
         Simple chronic anemia
         EXCLUDES 1   *anemia NOS (D64.9)*
         AHA: 2018,4Q,88

Hemolytic anemias (D55-D59)

✓4ᵗʰ **D55**   Anemia due to enzyme disorders
         EXCLUDES 1   *drug-induced enzyme deficiency anemia (D59.2)*

    D55.0   **Anemia due to** glucose-6-phosphate dehydrogenase [G6PD] deficiency   HCC ESR
         Favism
         G6PD deficiency anemia
         EXCLUDES 1   *glucose-6-phosphate dehydrogenase (G6PD) deficiency without anemia (D75.A)*

    D55.1   **Anemia due to other disorders of** glutathione metabolism   HCC ESR
         Anemia (due to) enzyme deficiencies, except G6PD, related to the hexose monophosphate [HMP] shunt pathway
         Anemia (due to) hemolytic nonspherocytic (hereditary), type I

✓5ᵗʰ **D55.2**   **Anemia due to disorders of** glycolytic enzymes
         EXCLUDES 1   *disorders of glycolysis not associated with anemia (E74.81-)*
         AHA: 2021,4Q,6-7

         D55.21   **Anemia due to** pyruvate kinase deficiency   HCC ESR
                 PK deficiency anemia
                 Pyruvate kinase deficiency anemia

         D55.29   **Anemia due to other disorders of glycolytic enzymes**   HCC ESR
                 Hexokinase deficiency anemia
                 Triose-phosphate isomerase deficiency anemia

    D55.3   **Anemia due to disorders of** nucleotide metabolism   HCC ESR

    D55.8   **Other anemias due to enzyme disorders**   HCC ESR

    D55.9   **Anemia due to enzyme disorder, unspecified**   HCC ESR

✓4th D56 Thalassemia

> **EXCLUDES 1**   *sickle-cell thalassemia (D57.4-)*

DEF: Group of inherited disorders of hemoglobin metabolism causing mild to severe anemia. It is usually found in people of Mediterranean, African, Chinese, or Asian descent.

Thalassemia

Misshapen RBC

Misshapen RBC   Healthy RBC

D56.0   Alpha thalassemia   `HCC` `ESR`

Alpha thalassemia major
Hemoglobin H Constant Spring
Hemoglobin H disease
Hydrops fetalis due to alpha thalassemia
Severe alpha thalassemia
Triple gene defect alpha thalassemia
Use additional code, if applicable, for hydrops fetalis due to alpha thalassemia (P56.99)

> **EXCLUDES 1**   *alpha thalassemia trait or minor (D56.3)*
> *asymptomatic alpha thalassemia (D56.3)*
> *hydrops fetalis due to isoimmunization (P56.0)*
> *hydrops fetalis not due to immune hemolysis (P83.2)*

DEF: HBA1 and HBA2 genetic variant of chromosome 16 prevalent among those of African and Southeast Asian descent. Alpha thalassemia is associated with a wide spectrum of anemic presentation and includes hemoglobin H disease subtypes.

D56.1   Beta thalassemia   `HCC` `ESR` `COM`

Beta thalassemia major
Cooley's anemia
Homozygous beta thalassemia
Severe beta thalassemia
Thalassemia intermedia
Thalassemia major

> **EXCLUDES 1**   *beta thalassemia minor (D56.3)*
> *beta thalassemia trait (D56.3)*
> *delta-beta thalassemia (D56.2)*
> *hemoglobin E-beta thalassemia (D56.5)*
> *sickle-cell beta thalassemia (D57.4-)*

D56.2   Delta-beta thalassemia   `HCC` `ESR` `COM`

Homozygous delta-beta thalassemia

> **EXCLUDES 1**   *delta-beta thalassemia minor (D56.3)*
> *delta-beta thalassemia trait (D56.3)*

D56.3   Thalassemia minor

Alpha thalassemia minor
Alpha thalassemia silent carrier
Alpha thalassemia trait
Beta thalassemia minor
Beta thalassemia trait
Delta-beta thalassemia minor
Delta-beta thalassemia trait
Thalassemia trait NOS

> **EXCLUDES 1**   *alpha thalassemia (D56.0)*
> *beta thalassemia (D56.1)*
> *delta-beta thalassemia (D56.2)*
> *hemoglobin E-beta thalassemia (D56.5)*
> *sickle-cell trait (D57.3)*

DEF: Solitary abnormal gene that identifies a carrier of the disease, yet with an absence of symptoms or a clinically mild anemic presentation.

D56.4   Hereditary persistence of fetal hemoglobin [HPFH]   `HCC` `ESR`

D56.5   Hemoglobin E-beta thalassemia   `HCC` `ESR` `COM`

> **EXCLUDES 1**   *beta thalassemia (D56.1)*
> *beta thalassemia minor (D56.3)*
> *beta thalassemia trait (D56.3)*
> *delta-beta thalassemia (D56.2)*
> *delta-beta thalassemia trait (D56.3)*
> *hemoglobin E disease (D58.2)*
> *other hemoglobinopathies (D58.2)*
> *sickle-cell beta thalassemia (D57.4-)*

D56.8   Other thalassemias   `HCC` `ESR`

Dominant thalassemia
Hemoglobin C thalassemia
Mixed thalassemia
Thalassemia with other hemoglobinopathy

> **EXCLUDES 1**   *hemoglobin C disease (D58.2)*
> *hemoglobin E disease (D58.2)*
> *other hemoglobinopathies (D58.2)*
> *sickle-cell anemia (D57.-)*
> *sickle-cell thalassemia (D57.4)*

D56.9   Thalassemia, unspecified

Mediterranean anemia (with other hemoglobinopathy)

✓4th D57 Sickle-cell disorders

Use additional code for any associated fever (R50.81)

> **EXCLUDES 1**   *other hemoglobinopathies (D58.-)*

AHA: 2022,2Q,28

DEF: Severe, chronic inherited diseases caused by a genetic variation in hemoglobin protein of the red blood cell. The gene mutation causes the red blood cell to become hard, sticky, and crescent or sickle shaped, making it harder for red blood cells to travel through the bloodstream, disrupting blood flow and decreasing oxygen transport to tissues.

Sickle cell

Sickle cells

Normal RBCs

✓5th D57.0   Hb-SS disease with crisis

Sickle-cell disease with crisis
Hb-SS disease with vasoocclusive pain
AHA: 2020,4Q,6-7

D57.00   Hb-SS disease with crisis, unspecified   `HCC` `Rx` `ESR` `COM`

Hb-SS disease with (painful) crisis NOS
Hb-SS disease with vasoocclusive pain NOS

D57.01   Hb-SS disease with acute chest syndrome   `HCC` `Rx` `ESR` `COM`

D57.02   Hb-SS disease with splenic sequestration   `HCC` `Rx` `ESR` `COM`

D57.03   Hb-SS disease with cerebral vascular involvement   `HCC` `Rx` `ESR` `COM`

Code also, if applicable, cerebral infarction (I63.-)

D57.09   Hb-SS disease with crisis with other specified complication   `HCC` `Rx` `ESR` `COM`

Use additional code to identify complications, such as:
cholelithiasis (K80.-)
priapism (N48.32)

D57.1   Sickle-cell disease without crisis   `HCC` `Rx` `ESR` `COM`

Hb-SS disease without crisis
Sickle-cell anemia NOS
Sickle-cell disease NOS
Sickle-cell disorder NOS

✓5th D57.2   Sickle-cell/Hb-C disease

Hb-SC disease
Hb-S/Hb-C disease
AHA: 2020,4Q,6-7

D57.20   Sickle-cell/Hb-C disease without crisis   `HCC` `ESR`

Chapter 3. Diseases of the Blood and Blood-forming Organs

D57.21–D57.459

✓6ᵗʰ **D57.21** **Sickle-cell/Hb-C disease** with crisis

D57.211 **Sickle-cell/Hb-C disease** with acute chest syndrome `HCC` `ESR`

D57.212 **Sickle-cell/Hb-C disease** with splenic sequestration `HCC` `ESR`

D57.213 **Sickle-cell/Hb-C disease** with cerebral vascular involvement `HCC` `ESR`
　Code also, if applicable, cerebral infarction (I63.-)

D57.218 **Sickle-cell/Hb-C disease with crisis with other specified complication** `HCC` `ESR`
　Use additional code to identify complications, such as:
　　cholelithiasis (K80.-)
　　priapism (N48.32)

D57.219 **Sickle-cell/Hb-C disease with crisis, unspecified** `HCC` `ESR`
　Sickle-cell/Hb-C disease with crisis NOS
　Sickle-cell/Hb-C disease with vasoocclusive pain NOS

D57.3 **Sickle-cell** trait `HCC` `ESR`
Hb-S trait
Heterozygous hemoglobin S
DEF: Heterozygous genetic makeup characterized by one gene for normal hemoglobin and one for sickle-cell hemoglobin. The clinical disease is rarely present.

✓6ᵗʰ **D57.4** **Sickle-cell** thalassemia
Sickle-cell beta thalassemia
Thalassemia Hb-S disease
AHA: 2020,4Q,6-7

D57.40 **Sickle-cell thalassemia** without crisis `HCC` `ESR`
　Microdrepanocytosis
　Sickle-cell thalassemia NOS

✓6ᵗʰ **D57.41** **Sickle-cell thalassemia, unspecified, with crisis**
　Sickle-cell thalassemia with (painful) crisis NOS
　Sickle-cell thalassemia with vasoocclusive pain NOS

D57.411 **Sickle-cell thalassemia, unspecified,** with acute chest syndrome `HCC` `ESR`

D57.412 **Sickle-cell thalassemia, unspecified,** with splenic sequestration `HCC` `ESR`

D57.413 **Sickle-cell thalassemia, unspecified,** with cerebral vascular involvement `HCC` `ESR`
　Code also, if applicable cerebral infarction (I63.-)

D57.418 **Sickle-cell thalassemia, unspecified, with crisis with other specified complication** `HCC` `ESR`
　Use additional code to identify complications, such as:
　　cholelithiasis (K80.-)
　　priapism (N48.32)

D57.419 **Sickle-cell thalassemia, unspecified, with crisis** `HCC` `ESR`
　Sickle-cell thalassemia with (painful) crisis NOS
　Sickle-cell thalassemia with vasoocclusive pain NOS

D57.42 **Sickle-cell thalassemia** beta zero without crisis `HCC` `Rx` `ESR` `COM`
　HbS-beta zero without crisis
　Sickle-cell beta zero without crisis

✓6ᵗʰ **D57.43** **Sickle-cell thalassemia** beta zero with crisis
　HbS-beta zero with crisis
　Sickle-cell beta zero with crisis

D57.431 **Sickle-cell thalassemia beta zero** with acute chest syndrome `HCC` `Rx` `ESR` `COM`
　HbS-beta zero with acute chest syndrome
　Sickle-cell beta zero with acute chest syndrome

D57.432 **Sickle-cell thalassemia beta zero** with splenic sequestration `HCC` `Rx` `ESR` `COM`
　HbS-beta zero with splenic sequestration
　Sickle-cell beta zero with splenic sequestration

D57.433 **Sickle-cell thalassemia beta zero** with cerebral vascular involvement `HCC` `Rx` `ESR` `COM`
　HbS-beta zero with cerebral vascular involvement
　Sickle-cell beta zero with cerebral vascular involvement
　Code also, if applicable cerebral infarction (I63.-)

D57.438 **Sickle-cell thalassemia beta zero with crisis with other specified complication** `HCC` `Rx` `ESR` `COM`
　HbS-beta zero with other specified complication
　Sickle-cell beta zero with other specified complication
　Use additional code to identify complications, such as:
　　cholelithiasis (K80.-)
　　priapism (N48.32)

D57.439 **Sickle-cell thalassemia beta zero with crisis, unspecified** `HCC` `Rx` `ESR` `COM`
　HbS-beta zero with other specified complication
　Sickle-cell beta zero with crisis unspecified
　Sickle-cell thalassemia beta zero with (painful) crisis NOS
　Sickle-cell thalassemia beta zero with vasoocclusive pain NOS

D57.44 **Sickle-cell thalassemia** beta plus without crisis `HCC` `ESR`
　HbS-beta plus without crisis
　Sickle-cell beta plus without crisis

✓6ᵗʰ **D57.45** **Sickle-cell thalassemia** beta plus with crisis
　HbS-beta plus with crisis
　Sickle-cell beta plus with crisis

D57.451 **Sickle-cell thalassemia beta plus** with acute chest syndrome `HCC` `ESR`
　HbS-beta plus with acute chest syndrome
　Sickle-cell beta plus with acute chest syndrome

D57.452 **Sickle-cell thalassemia beta plus** with splenic sequestration `HCC` `ESR`
　HbS-beta plus with splenic sequestration
　Sickle-cell beta plus with splenic sequestration

D57.453 **Sickle-cell thalassemia beta plus** with cerebral vascular involvement `HCC` `ESR`
　HbS-beta plus with cerebral vascular involvement
　Sickle-cell beta plus with cerebral vascular involvement
　Code also, if applicable cerebral infarction (I63.-)

D57.458 **Sickle-cell thalassemia beta plus with crisis with other specified complication** `HCC` `ESR`
　HbS-beta plus with crisis with other specified complication
　Sickle-cell beta plus with crisis with other specified complication
　Use additional code to identify complications, such as:
　　cholelithiasis (K80.-)
　　priapism (N48.32)

D57.459 **Sickle-cell thalassemia beta plus with crisis, unspecified** `HCC` `ESR`
　HbS-beta plus with crisis with unspecified complication
　Sickle-cell beta plus with crisis with unspecified complication
　Sickle-cell thalassemia beta plus with (painful) crisis NOS
　Sickle-cell thalassemia beta plus with vasoocclusive pain NOS

`HCC` CMS-HCC　　`Rx` Rx HCC　　`ESR` ESRD HCC　　`COM` Commercial HCC　　`N` Newborn: 0　　`P` Pediatric: 0-17　　`M` Maternity: 9-64　　`A` Adult: 15-124

518
ICD-10-CM 2023

✓5th **D57.8 Other sickle-cell disorders**
- Hb-SD disease
- Hb-SE disease
- **AHA:** 2020,4Q,6-7

     D57.80 Other sickle-cell disorders without crisis `HCC` `ESR`

✓6th   **D57.81 Other sickle-cell disorders** with crisis

       D57.811 Other sickle-cell disorders with acute chest syndrome `HCC` `ESR`

       D57.812 Other sickle-cell disorders with splenic sequestration `HCC` `ESR`

       D57.813 Other sickle-cell disorders with cerebral vascular involvement `HCC` `ESR`
- Code also, if applicable: cerebral infarction (I63.-)

       D57.818 Other sickle-cell disorders with crisis with other specified complication `HCC` `ESR`
- Use additional code to identify complications, such as:
  - cholelithiasis (K80.-)
  - priapism (N48.32)

       D57.819 Other sickle-cell disorders with crisis, unspecified `HCC` `ESR`
- Other sickle-cell disorders with crisis NOS
- Other sickle-cell disorders with vasooclusive pain NOS

✓4th **D58 Other** hereditary **hemolytic anemias**

     EXCLUDES 1   hemolytic anemia of the newborn (P55.-)

     D58.0 Hereditary spherocytosis `HCC` `ESR`
- Acholuric (familial) jaundice
- Congenital (spherocytic) hemolytic icterus
- Minkowski-Chauffard syndrome
- **DEF:** Inherited condition caused by mutations to genes responsible for the production of proteins that form the membranes of red blood cells. The shape and flexibility of the red blood cell membrane is altered, diminishing the cell's ability to traverse the spleen, therefore becoming trapped and destroyed before the red blood cell has reached maturity.

     D58.1 Hereditary elliptocytosis `HCC` `ESR`
- Elliptocytosis (congenital)
- Ovalocytosis (congenital) (hereditary)

     D58.2 Other hemoglobinopathies `HCC` `ESR`
- Abnormal hemoglobin NOS
- Congenital Heinz body anemia
- Hb-C disease
- Hb-D disease
- Hb-E disease
- Hemoglobinopathy NOS
- Unstable hemoglobin hemolytic disease
- EXCLUDES 1   familial polycythemia (D75.0)
  - Hb-M disease (D74.0)
  - hemoglobin E-beta thalassemia (D56.5)
  - hereditary persistence of fetal hemoglobin [HPFH] (D56.4)
  - high-altitude polycythemia (D75.1)
  - methemoglobinemia (D74.-)
  - other hemoglobinopathies with thalassemia (D56.8)

     D58.8 Other specified hereditary hemolytic anemias `HCC` `ESR`
- Stomatocytosis

     D58.9 Hereditary hemolytic anemia, unspecified `HCC` `ESR`

✓4th **D59 Acquired** hemolytic anemia
- **DEF:** Non-hereditary anemia characterized by premature destruction of red blood cells caused by infectious organisms, poisons, and physical agents.

     D59.0 Drug-induced autoimmune hemolytic **anemia** `HCC` `Rx` `ESR` `COM`
- Use additional code for adverse effect, if applicable, to identify drug (T36-T50 with fifth or sixth character 5)

✓5th   **D59.1 Other** autoimmune **hemolytic anemias**
- EXCLUDES 2   Evans syndrome (D69.41)
  - hemolytic disease of newborn (P55.-)
  - paroxysmal cold hemoglobinuria (D59.6)
- **AHA:** 2020,4Q,7-8

       D59.10 Autoimmune hemolytic anemia, unspecified `HCC` `Rx` `ESR` `COM`

       D59.11 Warm autoimmune hemolytic anemia `HCC` `Rx` `ESR` `COM`
- Warm type (primary) (secondary) (symptomatic) autoimmune hemolytic anemia
- Warm type autoimmune hemolytic disease

       D59.12 Cold autoimmune hemolytic anemia `HCC` `Rx` `ESR` `COM`
- Chronic cold hemagglutinin disease
- Cold agglutinin disease
- Cold agglutinin hemoglobinuria
- Cold type (primary) (secondary) (symptomatic) autoimmune hemolytic anemia
- Cold type autoimmune hemolytic disease

       D59.13 Mixed type autoimmune hemolytic anemia `HCC` `Rx` `ESR` `COM`
- Mixed type autoimmune hemolytic disease
- Mixed type, cold and warm, (primary) (secondary) (symptomatic) autoimmune hemolytic anemia

       D59.19 Other autoimmune hemolytic anemia `HCC` `Rx` `ESR` `COM`

     D59.2 Drug-induced nonautoimmune hemolytic **anemia** `HCC` `Rx` `ESR` `COM`
- Drug-induced enzyme deficiency anemia
- Use additional code for adverse effect, if applicable, to identify drug (T36-T50 with fifth or sixth character 5)

▲ ✓5th **D59.3 Hemolytic-uremic syndrome**
- ~~Use additional code to identify associated:~~
  - ~~E. coli infection (B96.2-)~~
  - ~~Pneumococcal pneumonia (J13)~~
  - ~~Shigella dysenteriae (A03.9)~~
- ►Code also, if applicable, any associated:◄
  - ►acute kidney failure (N17.-)◄
  - ►chronic kidney disease (N18.-)◄
- **DEF:** Condition typically precipitated by infection causing low platelets and destruction of red blood cells resulting in hemolytic anemia. This cell damage and blockage of renal capillaries lead to kidney failure. Mainly affects children.

       ● **D59.30 Hemolytic-uremic syndrome, unspecified**
- Hemolytic-uremic syndrome NOS

       ● **D59.31 Infection-associated hemolytic-uremic syndrome**
- Shiga toxin-producing E. coli [STEC] related hemolytic uremic syndrome
- Typical hemolytic uremic syndrome
- Use additional code to identify associated infection, such as:
  - E. coli infection (B96.2-)
  - human immunodeficiency virus [HIV] disease (B20)
  - pneumococcal meningitis (G00.1)
  - pneumococcal pneumonia (J13)
  - sepsis due to Streptococcus pneumoniae (A40.3)
  - Shigella dysenteriae (A03.9)
  - streptococcus pneumoniae as the cause of diseases classified elsewhere (B95.3)

       ● **D59.32 Hereditary hemolytic-uremic syndrome**
- Atypical hemolytic uremic syndrome with an identified genetic cause
- Code also, if applicable:
  - defects in the complement system (D84.1)
  - methylmalonic acidemia (E71.120)

       ● **D59.39 Other hemolytic-uremic syndrome**
- Atypical (nongenetic) hemolytic uremic syndrome
- Secondary hemolytic-uremic syndrome
- Code first, if applicable, any associated:
  - COVID-19 (U07.1)
  - complications of kidney transplant (T86.1-)
  - complications of heart transplant (T86.2-)
  - complications of liver transplant (T86.4-)
- Code also, if applicable, any associated condition, such as:
  - hypertensive emergency (I16.1)
  - malignant neoplasm (C00-C96)
  - systemic lupus erythematosus (M32.-)
- Use additional code, if applicable, for adverse effect to identify drug (T36-T50 with fifth or sixth character 5)

Chapter 3. Diseases of the Blood and Blood-forming Organs

D59.4 Other nonautoimmune hemolytic anemias `HCC` `Rx` `ESR` `COM`
     Mechanical hemolytic anemia
     Microangiopathic hemolytic anemia
     Toxic hemolytic anemia

D59.5 Paroxysmal nocturnal hemoglobinuria [Marchiafava-Micheli] `HCC` `Rx` `ESR` `COM`
     EXCLUDES 1   *hemoglobinuria NOS (R82.3)*

D59.6 Hemoglobinuria due to hemolysis from other external causes `HCC` `Rx` `ESR` `COM`
     Hemoglobinuria from exertion
     March hemoglobinuria
     Paroxysmal cold hemoglobinuria
     Use additional code (Chapter 20) to identify external cause
     EXCLUDES 1   *hemoglobinuria NOS (R82.3)*

D59.8 Other acquired hemolytic anemias `HCC` `Rx` `ESR` `COM`

D59.9 Acquired hemolytic anemia, unspecified `HCC` `Rx` `ESR` `COM`
     Idiopathic hemolytic anemia, chronic

Aplastic and other anemias and other bone marrow failure syndromes (D60-D64)

✓4ᵗʰ D60 Acquired pure red cell aplasia [erythroblastopenia]
     INCLUDES   red cell aplasia (acquired) (adult) (with thymoma)
     EXCLUDES 1   *congenital red cell aplasia (D61.01)*
     DEF: Bone marrow failure characterized by underproduction of red blood cells while white blood cell and platelet production remains normal.

D60.0 Chronic acquired pure red cell aplasia `HCC` `Rx` `ESR` `COM`

D60.1 Transient acquired pure red cell aplasia `HCC` `Rx` `ESR` `COM`

D60.8 Other acquired pure red cell aplasias `HCC` `Rx` `ESR` `COM`

D60.9 Acquired pure red cell aplasia, unspecified `HCC` `Rx` `ESR` `COM`

✓4ᵗʰ D61 Other aplastic anemias and other bone marrow failure syndromes
     EXCLUDES 2   *neutropenia (D70.-)*
     AHA: 2020,3Q,22; 2014,4Q,22
     DEF: Aplastic anemia: Bone marrow failure characterized by underproduction of red bloods cells, white blood cells and platelets.

✓5ᵗʰ D61.0 Constitutional aplastic anemia

     D61.01 Constitutional (pure) red blood cell aplasia `HCC` `Rx` `ESR` `COM`
         Blackfan-Diamond syndrome
         Congenital (pure) red cell aplasia
         Familial hypoplastic anemia
         Primary (pure) red cell aplasia
         Red cell (pure) aplasia of infants
         EXCLUDES 1   *acquired red cell aplasia (D60.9)*

     D61.09 Other constitutional aplastic anemia `HCC` `Rx` `ESR` `COM`
         Fanconi's anemia *[handwritten: Congenital]*
         Pancytopenia with malformations

D61.1 Drug-induced aplastic anemia `HCC` `Rx` `ESR` `COM`
     Use additional code for adverse effect, if applicable, to identify drug (T36-T50 with fifth or sixth character 5)

D61.2 Aplastic anemia due to other external agents `HCC` `Rx` `ESR` `COM`
     Code first, if applicable, toxic effects of substances chiefly nonmedicinal as to source (T51-T65)

D61.3 Idiopathic aplastic anemia `HCC` `Rx` `ESR` `COM`

[handwritten: not for acute exacerbation of a chronic condition]

✓5ᵗʰ D61.8 Other specified aplastic anemias and other bone marrow failure syndromes

     ✓6ᵗʰ D61.81 Pancytopenia
         EXCLUDES 1   *pancytopenia (due to) (with) aplastic anemia (D61.9)*
                 pancytopenia (due to) (with) bone marrow infiltration (D61.82)
                 pancytopenia (due to) (with) congenital (pure) red cell aplasia (D61.01)
                 pancytopenia (due to) (with) hairy cell leukemia (C91.4-)
                 pancytopenia (due to) (with) human immunodeficiency virus disease (B20)
                 pancytopenia (due to) (with) leukoerythroblastic anemia (D61.82)
                 pancytopenia (due to) (with) myeloproliferative disease (D47.1)
         EXCLUDES 2   *pancytopenia (due to) (with) myelodysplastic syndromes (D46.-)*
         DEF: Shortage of all three blood cells: white, red, and platelets.

     D61.810 Antineoplastic chemotherapy induced pancytopenia `HCC` `ESR`
         EXCLUDES 2   *aplastic anemia due to antineoplastic chemotherapy (D61.1)*
         AHA: 2020,3Q,22

     D61.811 Other drug-induced pancytopenia `HCC` `ESR`
         EXCLUDES 2   *aplastic anemia due to drugs (D61.1)*

     D61.818 Other pancytopenia `HCC` `ESR`
         AHA: 2020,3Q,24; 2019,1Q,16
         TIP: Assign this code in addition to myeloid leukemia codes (C92.-) when pancytopenia is documented. Although common in some types of myeloid leukemia, pancytopenia is not always inherent.

     D61.82 Myelophthisis `HCC` `Rx` `ESR` `COM`
         Leukoerythroblastic anemia
         Myelophthisic anemia
         Panmyelophthisis
         Code also the underlying disorder, such as:
            malignant neoplasm of breast (C50.-)
            tuberculosis (A15.-)
         EXCLUDES 1   *idiopathic myelofibrosis (D47.1)*
                 myelofibrosis NOS (D75.81)
                 myelofibrosis with myeloid metaplasia (D47.4)
                 primary myelofibrosis (D47.1)
                 secondary myelofibrosis (D75.81)
         DEF: Condition that occurs when normal hematopoietic tissue in the bone marrow is replaced with abnormal tissue, such as fibrous tissue or tumors. Most commonly seen during the advanced stages of cancer.

     D61.89 Other specified aplastic anemias and other bone marrow failure syndromes `HCC` `Rx` `ESR` `COM`

D61.9 Aplastic anemia, unspecified `HCC` `Rx` `ESR` `COM`
     Hypoplastic anemia NOS
     Medullary hypoplasia

D62 Acute posthemorrhagic anemia
     EXCLUDES 1   *anemia due to chronic blood loss (D50.0)*
               blood loss anemia NOS (D50.0)
               congenital anemia from fetal blood loss (P61.3)
     AHA: 2019,3Q,11,17

[handwritten: GSW surgical hemorr]

✓4ᵗʰ D63 Anemia in chronic diseases classified elsewhere

D63.0 Anemia in neoplastic disease
     Code first neoplasm (C00-D49)
     EXCLUDES 1   *aplastic anemia due to antineoplastic chemotherapy (D61.1)*
     EXCLUDES 2   *anemia due to antineoplastic chemotherapy (D64.81)*

[handwritten: ① malignancy ② anemia]

D63.1 Anemia in chronic kidney disease
     Erythropoietin resistant anemia (EPO resistant anemia)
     Code first underlying chronic kidney disease (CKD) (N18.-)

`HCC` CMS-HCC   `Rx` Rx HCC   `ESR` ESRD HCC   `COM` Commercial HCC   N Newborn: 0   P Pediatric: 0-17   M Maternity: 9-64   A Adult: 15-124

520   ICD-10-CM 2023

D63.8 **Anemia in other** *chronic diseases classified elsewhere*

Code first underlying disease, such as:
- diphyllobothriasis (B70.0)
- hookworm disease (B76.0-B76.9)
- hypothyroidism (E00.0-E03.9)
- malaria (B50.0-B54)
- symptomatic late syphilis (A52.79)
- tuberculosis (A18.89)

✔4ᵗʰ **D64 Other anemias**

EXCLUDES 1   refractory anemia (D46.-)
refractory anemia with excess blasts in transformation [RAEB T] (C92.0-)

DEF: Sideroblastic anemia: Hereditary or secondary disorder in which the red blood cells cannot effectively use iron, a nutrient needed to make hemoglobin. Although the iron can enter the red blood cell it is not assimilated into the hemoglobin molecule and builds up ringed sideroblasts around the cell nucleus.

D64.0 Hereditary sideroblastic anemia   HCC Rx ESR COM
Sex-linked hypochromic sideroblastic anemia

D64.1 **Secondary sideroblastic** *anemia due to disease*   HCC Rx ESR COM
Code first underlying disease

D64.2 Secondary sideroblastic anemia due to drugs and toxins   HCC Rx ESR COM
Code first poisoning due to drug or toxin, if applicable (T36-T65 with fifth or sixth character 1-4 or 6)
Use additional code for adverse effect, if applicable, to identify drug (T36-T50 with fifth or sixth character 5)

D64.3 Other sideroblastic anemias   HCC Rx ESR COM
Sideroblastic anemia NOS
Pyridoxine-responsive sideroblastic anemia NEC

D64.4 Congenital dyserythropoietic anemia
Dyshematopoietic anemia (congenital)
EXCLUDES 1   Blackfan-Diamond syndrome (D61.01)
Di Guglielmo's disease (C94.0)

✔5ᵗʰ **D64.8 Other specified anemias**

D64.81 Anemia due to antineoplastic chemotherapy
Antineoplastic chemotherapy induced anemia
EXCLUDES 2   anemia in neoplastic disease (D63.0)
aplastic anemia due to antineoplastic chemotherapy (D61.1)
AHA: 2021,3Q,4; 2014,4Q,22

D64.89 Other specified anemias
Infantile pseudoleukemia

D64.9 Anemia, unspecified
AHA: 2020,3Q,24; 2018,4Q,88; 2017,1Q,7

Coagulation defects, purpura and other hemorrhagic conditions (D65-D69)

D65 Disseminated intravascular coagulation [defibrination syndrome]   HCC ESR COM
Afibrinogenemia, acquired
Consumption coagulopathy
Diffuse or disseminated intravascular coagulation [DIC]
Fibrinolytic hemorrhage, acquired
Fibrinolytic purpura
Purpura fulminans
EXCLUDES 1   disseminated intravascular coagulation (complicating):
abortion or ectopic or molar pregnancy (O00-O07, O08.1)
in newborn (P60)
pregnancy, childbirth and the puerperium (O45.0, O46.0, O67.0, O72.3)
AHA: 2021,1Q,39

Coagulation

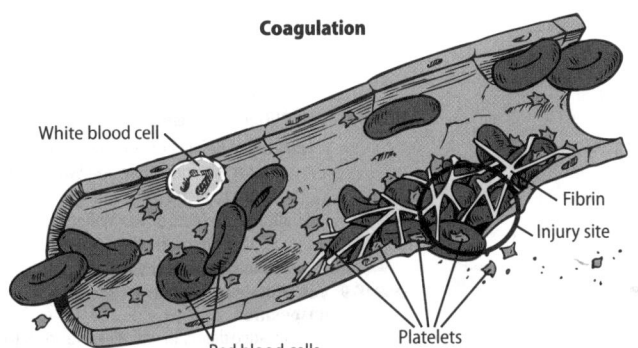

White blood cell
Fibrin
Injury site
Red blood cells
Platelets

D66 Hereditary factor VIII deficiency   HCC ESR COM
Classical hemophilia
Deficiency factor VIII (with functional defect)
Hemophilia NOS
Hemophilia A
EXCLUDES 1   factor VIII deficiency with vascular defect ▶(D68.0-)◀
DEF: Hereditary, sex-linked lack of antihemophilic globulin (AHG) (factor VIII) that causes abnormal coagulation characterized by increased bleeding; large bruises of skin; bleeding in the mouth, nose, and gastrointestinal tract; and hemorrhages into joints, resulting in swelling and impaired function.

D67 Hereditary factor IX deficiency   HCC ESR COM
Christmas disease
Factor IX deficiency (with functional defect)
Hemophilia B
Plasma thromboplastin component [PTC] deficiency

✔4ᵗʰ **D68 Other coagulation defects**
EXCLUDES 1   ▶abnormal coagulation profile NOS◀ (R79.1)
~~coagulation defects complicating abortion or ectopic or molar pregnancy (O00-O07, O08.1)~~
~~coagulation defects complicating pregnancy, childbirth and the puerperium (O45.0, O46.0, O67.0, O72.3)~~
EXCLUDES 2   ▶coagulation defects complicating abortion or ectopic or molar pregnancy (O00-O07, O08.1)◀
▶coagulation defects complicating pregnancy, childbirth and the puerperium (O45.0, O46.0, O67.0, O72.3)◀
AHA: 2016,1Q,14

▲ ✔5ᵗʰ **D68.0 Von Willebrand disease**
~~Angiohemophilia~~
~~Factor VIII deficiency with vascular defect~~
~~Vascular hemophilia~~
EXCLUDES 1   capillary fragility (hereditary) (D69.8)
factor VIII deficiency NOS (D66)
factor VIII deficiency with functional defect (D66)
DEF: Congenital, abnormal blood coagulation caused by deficient blood factor VII. Symptoms include excess or prolonged bleeding.

● **D68.00 Von Willebrand disease, unspecified**

● **D68.01 Von Willebrand disease, type 1**
Partial quantitative deficiency of von Willebrand factor
Type 1C von Willebrand disease

● ✓6ᵗʰ **D68.02** **Von Willebrand disease, type 2**
Qualitative defects of von Willebrand factor

● **D68.020** **Von Willebrand disease, type 2A**
Qualitative defects of von Willebrand factor with decreased platelet adhesion and selective deficiency of high-molecular-weight multimers

● **D68.021** **Von Willebrand disease, type 2B**
Qualitative defects of von Willebrand factor with high-molecular-weight von Willebrand factor loss
Qualitative defects of von Willebrand factor with hyper-adhesive forms
Qualitative defects of von Willebrand factor with increased affinity for platelet glycoprotein lb

● **D68.022** **Von Willebrand disease, type 2M**
Qualitative defects of von Willebrand factor with defective platelet adhesion with a normal size distribution of von Willebrand factor multimers

● **D68.023** **Von Willebrand disease, type 2N**
Qualitative defects of von Willebrand factor with defective von Willebrand factor to factor VIII binding
Qualitative defects of von Willebrand factor with markedly decreased affinity for factor VIII

● **D68.029** **Von Willebrand disease, type 2, unspecified**
Qualitative defect in von Willebrand factor function, with no further subtyping

● **D68.03** **Von Willebrand disease, type 3**
(Near) complete absence of von Willebrand factor
Total quantitative deficiency of von Willebrand factor

● **D68.04** **Acquired von Willebrand disease**
Acquired von Willebrand syndrome

● **D68.09** **Other von Willebrand disease**
Platelet-type von Willebrand disease
Pseudo-von Willebrand disease
Code also, if applicable, qualitative platelet defects (D69.1)

D68.1 **Hereditary factor XI deficiency** `HCC` `ESR` `COM`
Hemophilia C
Plasma thromboplastin antecedent [PTA] deficiency
Rosenthal's disease

D68.2 **Hereditary deficiency of other clotting factors** `HCC` `ESR` `COM`
AC globulin deficiency
Congenital afibrinogenemia
Deficiency of factor I [fibrinogen]
Deficiency of factor II [prothrombin]
Deficiency of factor V [labile]
Deficiency of factor VII [stable]
Deficiency of factor X [Stuart-Prower]
Deficiency of factor XII [Hageman]
Deficiency of factor XIII [fibrin stabilizing]
Dysfibrinogenemia (congenital)
Hypoproconvertinemia
Owren's disease
Proaccelerin deficiency

✓5ᵗʰ **D68.3** **Hemorrhagic disorder due to circulating anticoagulants**

✓6ᵗʰ **D68.31** **Hemorrhagic disorder due to intrinsic circulating anticoagulants, antibodies, or inhibitors**

D68.311 **Acquired hemophilia** `HCC` `ESR` `COM`
Autoimmune hemophilia
Autoimmune inhibitors to clotting factors
Secondary hemophilia

D68.312 **Antiphospholipid antibody with hemorrhagic disorder** `HCC` `ESR` `COM`
Lupus anticoagulant (LAC) with hemorrhagic disorder
Systemic lupus erythematosus [SLE] inhibitor with hemorrhagic disorder
EXCLUDES 1   *antiphospholipid antibody, finding without diagnosis (R76.0)*
antiphospholipid antibody syndrome (D68.61)
antiphospholipid antibody with hypercoagulable state (D68.61)
lupus anticoagulant (LAC) finding without diagnosis (R76.0)
lupus anticoagulant (LAC) with hypercoagulable state (D68.62)
systemic lupus erythematosus [SLE] inhibitor finding without diagnosis (R76.0)
systemic lupus erythematosus [SLE] inhibitor with hypercoagulable state (D68.62)

D68.318 **Other hemorrhagic disorder due to intrinsic circulating anticoagulants, antibodies, or inhibitors** `HCC` `ESR` `COM`
Antithromboplastinemia
Antithromboplastinogenemia
Hemorrhagic disorder due to intrinsic increase in antithrombin
Hemorrhagic disorder due to intrinsic increase in anti-VIIIa
Hemorrhagic disorder due to intrinsic increase in anti-IXa
Hemorrhagic disorder due to intrinsic increase in anti-XIa

D68.32 **Hemorrhagic disorder due to extrinsic circulating anticoagulants** `HCC` `ESR` `COM`
Drug-induced hemorrhagic disorder
Hemorrhagic disorder due to increase in anti-IIa
Hemorrhagic disorder due to increase in anti-Xa
Hyperheparinemia
Use additional code for adverse effect, if applicable, to identify drug (T45.515, T45.525)
AHA: 2021,1Q,4; 2016,1Q,14-15
TIP: Do not assign to identify routine therapeutic anticoagulation effects; assign only for documented adverse effects.

D68.4 **Acquired coagulation factor deficiency** `HCC` `ESR` `COM`
Deficiency of coagulation factor due to liver disease
Deficiency of coagulation factor due to vitamin K deficiency
EXCLUDES 1   *vitamin K deficiency of newborn (P53)*

✓5ᵗʰ **D68.5** **Primary thrombophilia**
Primary hypercoagulable states
EXCLUDES 1   *antiphospholipid syndrome (D68.61)*
lupus anticoagulant (D68.62)
secondary activated protein C resistance (D68.69)
secondary antiphospholipid antibody syndrome (D68.69)
secondary lupus anticoagulant with hypercoagulable state (D68.69)
secondary systemic lupus erythematosus [SLE] inhibitor with hypercoagulable state (D68.69)
systemic lupus erythematosus [SLE] inhibitor finding without diagnosis (R76.0)
systemic lupus erythematosus [SLE] inhibitor with hemorrhagic disorder (D68.312)
thrombotic thrombocytopenic purpura (M31.19)
DEF: Thrombophilia: Increased tendency of the blood to clot, which can lead to thrombus or embolus formation.

D68.51 **Activated protein C resistance** `HCC` `ESR` `COM`
Factor V Leiden mutation

D68.52 **Prothrombin gene mutation** `HCC` `ESR` `COM`

D68.59   **Other primary thrombophilia** `HCC` `ESR` `COM`
Antithrombin III deficiency
Hypercoagulable state NOS
Primary hypercoagulable state NEC
Primary thrombophilia NEC
Protein C deficiency
Protein S deficiency
Thrombophilia NOS
AHA: 2021,2Q,8

☑5ᵗʰ **D68.6**   **Other thrombophilia**
Other hypercoagulable states
> *EXCLUDES 1*   diffuse or disseminated intravascular coagulation [DIC] (D65)
> heparin induced thrombocytopenia (HIT) ►(D75.82-)◄
> hyperhomocysteinemia (E72.11)

D68.61   **Antiphospholipid syndrome** `HCC` `ESR` `COM`
Anticardiolipin syndrome
Antiphospholipid antibody syndrome
> *EXCLUDES 1*   anti-phospholipid antibody, finding without diagnosis (R76.0)
> anti-phospholipid antibody with hemorrhagic disorder (D68.312)
> lupus anticoagulant syndrome (D68.62)

D68.62   **Lupus anticoagulant syndrome** `HCC` `ESR` `COM`
Lupus anticoagulant
Presence of systemic lupus erythematosus [SLE] inhibitor
> *EXCLUDES 1*   anticardiolipin syndrome (D68.61)
> antiphospholipid syndrome (D68.61)
> lupus anticoagulant (LAC) finding without diagnosis (R76.0)
> lupus anticoagulant (LAC) with hemorrhagic disorder (D68.312)

D68.69   **Other thrombophilia** `HCC` `ESR` `COM`
Hypercoagulable states NEC
Secondary hypercoagulable state NOS
AHA: 2021,2Q,8

D68.8   **Other specified coagulation defects** `HCC` `ESR` `COM`
> *EXCLUDES 1*   hemorrhagic disease of newborn (P53)

AHA: 2021,1Q,39

D68.9   **Coagulation defect, unspecified** `HCC` `ESR` `COM`

☑4ᵗʰ **D69**   **Purpura and other hemorrhagic conditions**
> *EXCLUDES 1*   benign hypergammaglobulinemic purpura (D89.0)
> cryoglobulinemic purpura (D89.1)
> essential (hemorrhagic) thrombocythemia (D47.3)
> hemorrhagic thrombocythemia (D47.3)
> purpura fulminans (D65)
> thrombotic thrombocytopenic purpura (M31.19)
> Waldenström hypergammaglobulinemic purpura (D89.0)

D69.0   **Allergic purpura** `HCC` `ESR`
Allergic vasculitis
Nonthrombocytopenic hemorrhagic purpura
Nonthrombocytopenic idiopathic purpura
Purpura anaphylactoid
Purpura Henoch(-Schönlein)
Purpura rheumatica
Vascular purpura
> *EXCLUDES 1*   thrombocytopenic hemorrhagic purpura (D69.3)

AHA: 2020,3Q,26
DEF: Any hemorrhagic condition, thrombocytic or nonthrombocytopenic in origin, caused by a presumed allergic reaction.

D69.1   **Qualitative platelet defects** `HCC` `ESR` `COM`
Bernard-Soulier [giant platelet] syndrome
Glanzmann's disease
Grey platelet syndrome
Thromboasthenia (hemorrhagic) (hereditary)
Thrombocytopathy
> *EXCLUDES 1*   ►hemolytic-uremic syndrome (D59.3-)◄
> von Willebrand's disease (D68.0)
> *EXCLUDES 2*   ►von Willebrand disease (D68.0-)◄

D69.2   **Other nonthrombocytopenic purpura** `HCC` `ESR`
Purpura NOS
Purpura simplex
Senile purpura

D69.3   **Immune thrombocytopenic purpura** `HCC` `Rx` `ESR` `COM`
Hemorrhagic (thrombocytopenic) purpura
Idiopathic thrombocytopenic purpura
Tidal platelet dysgenesis
DEF: Tidal platelet dysgenesis: Fluctuation of platelet counts from normal to very low within periods of 20 to 40 days and may involve autoimmune platelet destruction.

☑5ᵗʰ **D69.4**   **Other primary thrombocytopenia**
> *EXCLUDES 1*   transient neonatal thrombocytopenia (P61.0)
> Wiskott-Aldrich syndrome (D82.0)

D69.41   **Evans syndrome** `HCC` `ESR` `COM`

D69.42   **Congenital and hereditary thrombocytopenia purpura** `HCC` `ESR` `COM`
Congenital thrombocytopenia
Hereditary thrombocytopenia
Code first congenital or hereditary disorder, such as:
   thrombocytopenia with absent radius (TAR syndrome) (Q87.2)

D69.49   **Other primary thrombocytopenia** `HCC` `ESR` `COM`
Megakaryocytic hypoplasia
Primary thrombocytopenia NOS

☑5ᵗʰ **D69.5**   **Secondary thrombocytopenia**
> *EXCLUDES 1*   heparin induced thrombocytopenia (HIT) ►(D75.82-)◄
> transient thrombocytopenia of newborn (P61.0)

D69.51   **Posttransfusion purpura**
Posttransfusion purpura from whole blood (fresh) or blood products
PTP

D69.59   **Other secondary thrombocytopenia**
AHA: 2014,4Q,22

D69.6   **Thrombocytopenia, unspecified** `HCC` `ESR`
AHA: 2020,3Q,24

D69.8   **Other specified hemorrhagic conditions** `HCC` `ESR`
Capillary fragility (hereditary)
Vascular pseudohemophilia

D69.9   **Hemorrhagic condition, unspecified** `HCC` `ESR`

Other disorders of blood and blood-forming organs (D70-D77)

☑4ᵗʰ **D70**   **Neutropenia**
> *INCLUDES*   agranulocytosis
> decreased absolute neurophile count (ANC)

Use additional code for any associated:
   fever (R50.81)
   mucositis (J34.81, K12.3-, K92.81, N76.81)
> *EXCLUDES 1*   neutropenic splenomegaly (D73.81)
> transient neonatal neutropenia (P61.5)

DEF: Abnormally low number of neutrophils. Neutrophils are phagocytic, meaning they surround and consume harmful pathogens, primarily bacteria. When neutrophil counts decrease the risk of infection increases.

D70.0   **Congenital agranulocytosis** `HCC` `ESR` `COM`
Congenital neutropenia
Infantile genetic agranulocytosis
Kostmann's disease

D70.1   **Agranulocytosis secondary to cancer chemotherapy** `HCC` `ESR`
Code also underlying neoplasm
Use additional code for adverse effect, if applicable, to identify drug (T45.1X5)
AHA: 2020,3Q,22; 2014,4Q,22

D70.2   **Other drug-induced agranulocytosis** `HCC` `ESR`
Use additional code for adverse effect, if applicable, to identify drug (T36-T50 with fifth or sixth character 5)

D70.3   **Neutropenia due to infection** `HCC` `ESR`

D70.4   **Cyclic neutropenia** `HCC` `ESR` `COM`
Cyclic hematopoiesis
Periodic neutropenia

D70.8   **Other neutropenia** `HCC` `ESR`

D70.9   **Neutropenia, unspecified** `HCC` `ESR`
AHA: 2020,3Q,24

Chapter 3. Diseases of the Blood and Blood-forming Organs

D71   Functional disorders of polymorphonuclear neutrophils   HCC ESR COM
 Cell membrane receptor complex [CR3] defect
 Chronic (childhood) granulomatous disease
 Congenital dysphagocytosis
 Progressive septic granulomatosis

✓4ᵗʰ **D72   Other disorders of white blood cells**
 EXCLUDES 1   basophilia (D72.824)
         immunity disorders (D80-D89)
         neutropenia (D70)
         preleukemia (syndrome) (D46.9)

D72.0   Genetic anomalies of leukocytes   HCC ESR COM
 Alder (granulation) (granulocyte) anomaly
 Alder syndrome
 Hereditary leukocytic hypersegmentation
 Hereditary leukocytic hyposegmentation
 Hereditary leukomelanopathy
 May-Hegglin (granulation) (granulocyte) anomaly
 May-Hegglin syndrome
 Pelger-Huët (granulation) (granulocyte) anomaly
 Pelger-Huët syndrome
 EXCLUDES 1   Chédiak (-Steinbrinck)-Higashi syndrome (E70.330)

✓5ᵗʰ **D72.1   Eosinophilia**
 EXCLUDES 2   Löffler's syndrome (J82.89)
         pulmonary eosinophilia (J82.-)
 AHA: 2020,4Q,8-10
 DEF: Abnormally large accumulation or formation of eosinophils (nucleated, granular leukocytes) in the blood, characteristic of allergic states and infection.
 D72.10   Eosinophilia, unspecified
✓6ᵗʰ **D72.11   Hypereosinophilic syndrome [HES]**
  D72.110   Idiopathic hypereosinophilic syndrome [IHES]
  D72.111   Lymphocytic Variant Hypereosinophilic Syndrome [LHES]
   Lymphocyte variant hypereosinophilia
   Code also, if applicable, any associated lymphocytic neoplastic disorder
  D72.118   Other hypereosinophilic syndrome
   Episodic angioedema with eosinophilia
   Gleich's syndrome
  D72.119   Hypereosinophilic syndrome [HES], unspecified
 D72.12   Drug rash with eosinophilia and systemic symptoms syndrome
  DRESS syndrome
  Use additional code for adverse effect, if applicable, to identify drug (T36-T50 with fifth or sixth character 5)
 D72.18   Eosinophilia in diseases classified elsewhere
  Code first underlying disease, such as:
   chronic myelomonocytic leukemia (C93.1-)
 D72.19   Other eosinophilia
  Familial eosinophilia
  Hereditary eosinophilia
✓5ᵗʰ **D72.8   Other specified disorders of white blood cells**
 EXCLUDES 1   leukemia (C91-C95)
 ✓6ᵗʰ **D72.81   Decreased white blood cell count**
  EXCLUDES 1   neutropenia (D70.-)
  D72.810   Lymphocytopenia
   Decreased lymphocytes
  D72.818   Other decreased white blood cell count
   Basophilic leukopenia
   Eosinophilic leukopenia
   Monocytopenia
   Other decreased leukocytes
   Plasmacytopenia
  D72.819   Decreased white blood cell count, unspecified
   Decreased leukocytes, unspecified
   Leukocytopenia, unspecified
   Leukopenia
   EXCLUDES 1   malignant leukopenia (D70.9)

✓6ᵗʰ **D72.82   Elevated white blood cell count**
 EXCLUDES 1   eosinophilia (D72.1)
 D72.820   Lymphocytosis (symptomatic)
  Elevated lymphocytes
 D72.821   Monocytosis (symptomatic)
  EXCLUDES 1   infectious mononucleosis (B27.-)
 D72.822   Plasmacytosis
 D72.823   Leukemoid reaction
  Basophilic leukemoid reaction
  Leukemoid reaction NOS
  Lymphocytic leukemoid reaction
  Monocytic leukemoid reaction
  Myelocytic leukemoid reaction
  Neutrophilic leukemoid reaction
 D72.824   Basophilia
  DEF: Increase in the basophils of the blood, a type of white blood cell, often seen in conjunction with neoplastic disorders.
 D72.825   Bandemia
  Bandemia without diagnosis of specific infection
  EXCLUDES 1   confirmed infection - code to infection
         leukemia (C91.-, C92.-, C93.-, C94.-, C95.-)
  DEF: Increase in early neutrophil cells, called band cells, that may indicate infection.
 D72.828   Other elevated white blood cell count
 D72.829   Elevated white blood cell count, unspecified
  Elevated leukocytes, unspecified
  Leukocytosis, unspecified
 D72.89   Other specified disorders of white blood cells
  Abnormality of white blood cells NEC
D72.9   Disorder of white blood cells, unspecified
 Abnormal leukocyte differential NOS

✓4ᵗʰ **D73   Diseases of spleen**
 D73.0   Hyposplenism
  Atrophy of spleen
  EXCLUDES 1   asplenia (congenital) (Q89.01)
         postsurgical absence of spleen (Z90.81)
 D73.1   Hypersplenism
  EXCLUDES 1   neutropenic splenomegaly (D73.81)
         primary splenic neutropenia (D73.81)
         splenitis, splenomegaly in late syphilis (A52.79)
         splenitis, splenomegaly in tuberculosis (A18.85)
         splenomegaly NOS (R16.1)
         splenomegaly congenital (Q89.0)
 D73.2   Chronic congestive splenomegaly
 D73.3   Abscess of spleen
 D73.4   Cyst of spleen
 D73.5   Infarction of spleen
  Splenic rupture, nontraumatic
  Torsion of spleen
  EXCLUDES 1   rupture of spleen due to Plasmodium vivax malaria (B51.0)
         traumatic rupture of spleen (S36.03-)
✓5ᵗʰ **D73.8   Other diseases of spleen**
 D73.81   Neutropenic splenomegaly
  Werner-Schultz disease
 D73.89   Other diseases of spleen
  Fibrosis of spleen NOS
  Perisplenitis
  Splenitis NOS
D73.9   Disease of spleen, unspecified

✓4ᵗʰ **D74   Methemoglobinemia**
 D74.0   Congenital methemoglobinemia
  Congenital NADH-methemoglobin reductase deficiency
  Hemoglobin-M [Hb-M] disease
  Methemoglobinemia, hereditary
 D74.8   Other methemoglobinemias
  Acquired methemoglobinemia (with sulfhemoglobinemia)
  Toxic methemoglobinemia
D74.9   Methemoglobinemia, unspecified

☑4ᵗʰ **D75 Other and unspecified diseases of blood and blood-forming organs**

     EXCLUDES 2   *acute lymphadenitis (L04.-)*
            chronic lymphadenitis (I88.1)
            enlarged lymph nodes (R59.-)
            hypergammaglobulinemia NOS (D89.2)
            lymphadenitis NOS (I88.9)
            mesenteric lymphadenitis (acute) (chronic) (I88.0)

    D75.0 Familial erythrocytosis
        Benign polycythemia
        Familial polycythemia
        EXCLUDES 1   *hereditary ovalocytosis (D58.1)*

    D75.1 Secondary polycythemia
        Acquired polycythemia
        Emotional polycythemia
        Erythrocytosis NOS
        Hypoxemic polycythemia
        Nephrogenous polycythemia
        Polycythemia due to erythropoietin
        Polycythemia due to fall in plasma volume
        Polycythemia due to high altitude
        Polycythemia due to stress
        Polycythemia NOS
        Relative polycythemia
        EXCLUDES 1   *polycythemia neonatorum (P61.1)*
                   polycythemia vera (D45)
        DEF: Elevated number of red blood cells in circulating blood as a result of reduced oxygen supply to the tissues.

☑5ᵗʰ **D75.8 Other specified diseases of blood and blood-forming organs**

    D75.81 Myelofibrosis   HCC Rx ESR COM
        Myelofibrosis NOS
        Secondary myelofibrosis NOS
        Code first the underlying disorder, such as:
           malignant neoplasm of breast (C50.-)
        Use additional code, if applicable, for associated therapy-related myelodysplastic syndrome (D46.-)
        Use additional code for adverse effect, if applicable, to identify drug (T45.1X5)
        EXCLUDES 1   *acute myelofibrosis (C94.4-)*
                   idiopathic myelofibrosis (D47.1)
                   leukoerythroblastic anemia (D61.82)
                   myelofibrosis with myeloid metaplasia (D47.4)
                   myelophthisic anemia (D61.82)
                   myelophthisis (D61.82)
                   primary myelofibrosis (D47.1)

▲   ☑6ᵗʰ **D75.82 Heparin induced thrombocytopenia (HIT)**
        ▶Use additional code, if applicable, for adverse effect of heparin (T45.515-)◀
        DEF: Immune-mediated reaction to heparin therapy causing an abrupt fall in platelet count and serious complications such as pulmonary embolism, stroke, AMI, or DVT.

●   **D75.821 Non-immune heparin-induced thrombocytopenia**
           Non-immune HIT
           Type 1 heparin-induced thrombocytopenia

●   **D75.822 Immune-mediated heparin-induced thrombocytopenia**
           Immune-mediated HIT
           Type 2 heparin-induced thrombocytopenia

●   **D75.828 Other heparin-induced thrombocytopenia syndrome**
           Autoimmune heparin-induced thrombocytopenia syndrome
           Delayed-onset heparin-induced thrombocytopenia
           Persisting heparin-induced thrombocytopenia

●   **D75.829 Heparin-induced thrombocytopenia, unspecified**

√6ᵗʰ **D75.83 Thrombocytosis**
        EXCLUDES 2   *essential thrombocythemia (D47.3)*
        AHA: 2021,4Q,7-8

    D75.838 Other thrombocytosis
           Reactive thrombocytosis
           Secondary thrombocytosis
           Code also underlying condition, if known and applicable

    D75.839 Thrombocytosis, unspecified
           Thrombocythemia NOS
           Thrombocytosis NOS

●   **D75.84 Other platelet-activating anti-PF4 disorders**
        Spontaneous heparin-induced thrombocytopenia syndrome (without heparin exposure)
        Thrombosis with thrombocytopenia syndrome
        Vaccine-induced thrombotic thrombocytopenia
        Use additional code, if applicable, for adverse effect of other viral vaccine (T50.B95-)

    D75.89 Other specified diseases of blood and blood-forming organs

D75.9 Disease of blood and blood-forming organs, unspecified

D75.A Glucose-6-phosphate dehydrogenase (G6PD) deficiency without anemia
        EXCLUDES 1   *glucose-6-phosphate dehydrogenase (G6PD) deficiency with anemia (D55.0)*
        AHA: 2019,4Q,4-5

☑4ᵗʰ **D76 Other specified diseases with participation of lymphoreticular and reticulohistiocytic tissue**
        EXCLUDES 1   *(Abt-) Letterer-Siwe disease (C96.0)*
                   eosinophilic granuloma (C96.6)
                   Hand-Schüller-Christian disease (C96.5)
                   histiocytic medullary reticulosis (C96.9)
                   histiocytic sarcoma (C96.A)
                   histiocytosis X, multifocal (C96.5)
                   histiocytosis X, unifocal (C96.6)
                   Langerhans-cell histiocytosis, multifocal (C96.5)
                   Langerhans-cell histiocytosis NOS (C96.6)
                   Langerhans-cell histiocytosis, unifocal (C96.6)
                   leukemic reticuloendotheliosis (C91.4-)
                   lipomelanotic reticulosis (I89.8)
                   malignant histiocytosis (C96.A)
                   malignant reticulosis (C86.0)
                   nonlipid reticuloendotheliosis (C96.0)

    D76.1 Hemophagocytic lymphohistiocytosis   HCC ESR COM
        Familial hemophagocytic reticulosis
        Histiocytoses of mononuclear phagocytes

    D76.2 Hemophagocytic syndrome, infection-associated   HCC ESR COM
        Use additional code to identify infectious agent or disease

    D76.3 Other histiocytosis syndromes   HCC ESR COM
        Reticulohistiocytoma (giant-cell)
        Sinus histiocytosis with massive lymphadenopathy
        Xanthogranuloma

D77 Other disorders of blood and blood-forming organs in diseases classified elsewhere
        Code first underlying disease, such as:
        amyloidosis (E85.-)
        congenital early syphilis (A50.0)
        echinococcosis (B67.0-B67.9)
        malaria (B50.0-B54)
        schistosomiasis [bilharziasis] (B65.0-B65.9)
        vitamin C deficiency (E54)
        EXCLUDES 1   *rupture of spleen due to Plasmodium vivax malaria (B51.0)*
                   splenitis, splenomegaly in late syphilis (A52.79)
                   splenitis, splenomegaly in tuberculosis (A18.85)

Intraoperative and postprocedural complications of the spleen (D78)

✓4ᵗʰ D78 Intraoperative and postprocedural complications of the spleen
> AHA: 2016,4Q,9-10

✓5ᵗʰ D78.0 Intraoperative hemorrhage and hematoma of the spleen complicating a procedure
> EXCLUDES 1   intraoperative hemorrhage and hematoma of the spleen due to accidental puncture or laceration during a procedure (D78.1-)

    D78.01 Intraoperative hemorrhage and hematoma of the spleen complicating a procedure on the spleen

    D78.02 Intraoperative hemorrhage and hematoma of the spleen complicating other procedure

✓5ᵗʰ D78.1 Accidental puncture and laceration of the spleen during a procedure

    D78.11 Accidental puncture and laceration of the spleen during a procedure on the spleen

    D78.12 Accidental puncture and laceration of the spleen during other procedure
>   AHA: 2022,1Q,22

✓5ᵗʰ D78.2 Postprocedural hemorrhage of the spleen following a procedure

    D78.21 Postprocedural hemorrhage of the spleen following a procedure on the spleen

    D78.22 Postprocedural hemorrhage of the spleen following other procedure

✓5ᵗʰ D78.3 Postprocedural hematoma and seroma of the spleen following a procedure

    D78.31 Postprocedural hematoma of the spleen following a procedure on the spleen

    D78.32 Postprocedural hematoma of the spleen following other procedure

    D78.33 Postprocedural seroma of the spleen following a procedure on the spleen

    D78.34 Postprocedural seroma of the spleen following other procedure

✓5ᵗʰ D78.8 Other intraoperative and postprocedural complications of the spleen
> Use additional code, if applicable, to further specify disorder

    D78.81 Other intraoperative complications of the spleen

    D78.89 Other postprocedural complications of the spleen

Certain disorders involving the immune mechanism (D80-D89)

> **INCLUDES**   defects in the complement system
> immunodeficiency disorders, except human immunodeficiency virus [HIV] disease
> sarcoidosis
> **EXCLUDES 1**   autoimmune disease (systemic) NOS (M35.9)
> functional disorders of polymorphonuclear neutrophils (D71)
> human immunodeficiency virus [HIV] disease (B20)

✓4ᵗʰ D80 Immunodeficiency with predominantly antibody defects

D80.0 Hereditary hypogammaglobulinemia   HCC Rx ESR COM
> Autosomal recessive agammaglobulinemia (Swiss type)
> X-linked agammaglobulinemia [Bruton] (with growth hormone deficiency)

D80.1 Nonfamilial hypogammaglobulinemia   HCC Rx ESR COM
> Agammaglobulinemia with immunoglobulin-bearing B-lymphocytes
> Common variable agammaglobulinemia [CVAgamma]
> Hypogammaglobulinemia NOS

D80.2 Selective deficiency of immunoglobulin A [IgA]   HCC Rx ESR COM

D80.3 Selective deficiency of immunoglobulin G [IgG] subclasses   HCC Rx ESR COM

D80.4 Selective deficiency of immunoglobulin M [IgM]   HCC Rx ESR COM

D80.5 Immunodeficiency with increased immunoglobulin M [IgM]   HCC Rx ESR COM

D80.6 Antibody deficiency with near-normal immunoglobulins or with hyperimmunoglobulinemia   HCC Rx ESR COM

D80.7 Transient hypogammaglobulinemia of infancy   HCC Rx ESR COM

D80.8 Other immunodeficiencies with predominantly antibody defects   HCC Rx ESR COM
> Kappa light chain deficiency

D80.9 Immunodeficiency with predominantly antibody defects, unspecified   HCC Rx ESR COM

✓4ᵗʰ D81 Combined immunodeficiencies
> **EXCLUDES 1**   autosomal recessive agammaglobulinemia (Swiss type) (D80.0)

D81.0 Severe combined immunodeficiency [SCID] with reticular dysgenesis   HCC Rx ESR COM

D81.1 Severe combined immunodeficiency [SCID] with low T- and B-cell numbers   HCC Rx ESR COM

D81.2 Severe combined immunodeficiency [SCID] with low or normal B-cell numbers   HCC Rx ESR COM

✓5ᵗʰ D81.3 Adenosine deaminase [ADA] deficiency
> AHA: 2019,4Q,5-6

    D81.30 Adenosine deaminase deficiency, unspecified   HCC Rx ESR COM
> ADA deficiency NOS

    D81.31 Severe combined immunodeficiency due to adenosine deaminase deficiency   HCC Rx ESR COM
> ADA deficiency with SCID
> Adenosine deaminase [ADA] deficiency with severe combined immunodeficiency

    D81.32 Adenosine deaminase 2 deficiency   HCC Rx ESR COM
> ADA2 deficiency
> Adenosine deaminase deficiency type 2
> Code also, if applicable, any associated manifestations, such as:
>   polyarteritis nodosa (M30.0)
>   stroke (I63.-)

    D81.39 Other adenosine deaminase deficiency   HCC Rx ESR COM
> Adenosine deaminase [ADA] deficiency type 1, NOS
> Adenosine deaminase [ADA] deficiency type 1, without SCID
> Adenosine deaminase [ADA] deficiency type 1, without severe combined immunodeficiency
> Partial ADA deficiency (type 1)
> Partial adenosine deaminase deficiency (type 1)

D81.4 Nezelof's syndrome   HCC Rx ESR COM

D81.5 Purine nucleoside phosphorylase [PNP] deficiency   HCC Rx ESR COM

D81.6 Major histocompatibility complex class I deficiency   HCC Rx ESR COM
> Bare lymphocyte syndrome

D81.7 Major histocompatibility complex class II deficiency   HCC Rx ESR COM

✓5ᵗʰ D81.8 Other combined immunodeficiencies

    ✓6ᵗʰ D81.81 Biotin-dependent carboxylase deficiency
> Multiple carboxylase deficiency
> **EXCLUDES 1**   biotin-dependent carboxylase deficiency due to dietary deficiency of biotin (E53.8)

        D81.810 Biotinidase deficiency

        D81.818 Other biotin-dependent carboxylase deficiency
> Holocarboxylase synthetase deficiency
> Other multiple carboxylase deficiency

        D81.819 Biotin-dependent carboxylase deficiency, unspecified
> Multiple carboxylase deficiency, unspecified

    D81.82 Activated Phosphoinositide 3-kinase Delta Syndrome [APDS]
> p110d-activating mutation causing senescent T cells, lymphadenopathy, and immunodeficiency [PASLI] disease
> Code also, if applicable, any associated manifestations, such as:
>   bronchiectasis (J47.-)
>   herpes virus infections (B00.-)
>   other acute respiratory tract infections (J00-J06; J20-J22)
>   other infections (A00-B99)
>   pneumonia (J12-J18)

    D81.89 Other combined immunodeficiencies   HCC Rx ESR COM

D81.9 Combined immunodeficiency, unspecified   HCC Rx ESR COM
> Severe combined immunodeficiency disorder [SCID] NOS

☑4ᵗʰ **D82 Immunodeficiency associated with other major defects**
    EXCLUDES 1   ataxia telangiectasia [Louis-Bar] (G11.3)

D82.0 Wiscott-Aldrich syndrome   HCC Rx ESR COM
    Immunodeficiency with thrombocytopenia and eczema

D82.1 Di George's syndrome   HCC Rx ESR COM
    Pharyngeal pouch syndrome
    Thymic alymphoplasia
    Thymic aplasia or hypoplasia with immunodeficiency
    AHA: 2019,3Q,14

D82.2 Immunodeficiency with short-limbed stature   HCC Rx ESR COM

D82.3 Immunodeficiency following hereditary defective response to Epstein-Barr virus   HCC Rx ESR COM
    X-linked lymphoproliferative disease

D82.4 Hyperimmunoglobulin E [IgE] syndrome   HCC Rx ESR COM

D82.8 Immunodeficiency associated with other specified major defects   HCC Rx ESR COM

D82.9 Immunodeficiency associated with major defect, unspecified   HCC Rx ESR COM

☑4ᵗʰ **D83 Common variable immunodeficiency**

D83.0 Common variable immunodeficiency with predominant abnormalities of B-cell numbers and function   HCC Rx ESR COM

D83.1 Common variable immunodeficiency with predominant immunoregulatory T-cell disorders   HCC Rx ESR COM

D83.2 Common variable immunodeficiency with autoantibodies to B- or T-cells   HCC Rx ESR COM

D83.8 Other common variable immunodeficiencies   HCC Rx ESR COM

D83.9 Common variable immunodeficiency, unspecified   HCC Rx ESR COM

☑4ᵗʰ **D84 Other immunodeficiencies**

D84.0 Lymphocyte function antigen-1 [LFA-1] defect   HCC Rx ESR COM

D84.1 Defects in the complement system   HCC Rx ESR COM
    C1 esterase inhibitor [C1-INH] deficiency

☑5ᵗʰ **D84.8 Other specified immunodeficiencies**
    AHA: 2020,4Q,10-12

  D84.81 *Immunodeficiency due to conditions classified elsewhere*   HCC Rx ESR COM
    Code first underlying condition, such as:
      chromosomal abnormalities (Q90-Q99)
      diabetes mellitus (E08-E13)
      malignant neoplasms (C00-C96)
      EXCLUDES 1   certain disorders involving the immune mechanism (D80-D83, D84.0, D84.1, D84.9)
            human immunodeficiency virus [HIV] disease (B20)
    AHA: 2021,1Q,52

☑6ᵗʰ **D84.82 Immunodeficiency due to drugs and external causes**

  D84.821 Immunodeficiency due to drugs   HCC Rx ESR COM
    Immunodeficiency due to (current or past) medication
    Use additional code for adverse effect if applicable, to identify adverse effect of drug (T36-T50 with fifth or six character 5)
    Use additional code, if applicable, for associated long term (current) drug therapy drug or medication such as:
      long term (current) drug therapy systemic steroids (Z79.52)
      other long term (current) drug therapy (Z79.899)

  D84.822 Immunodeficiency due to external causes   HCC Rx ESR COM
    Code also, if applicable, radiological procedure and radiotherapy (Y84.2)
    Use additional code for external cause such as:
      exposure to ionizing radiation (W88)

  D84.89 Other immunodeficiencies   HCC Rx ESR COM

D84.9 Immunodeficiency, unspecified   HCC Rx ESR COM
    Immunocompromised NOS
    Immunodeficient NOS
    Immunosuppressed NOS
    AHA: 2020,4Q,10

☑4ᵗʰ **D86 Sarcoidosis**
    DEF: Clustering of immune cells resulting in granuloma formation. Often affects the lungs and lymphatic system but can occur in other body sites.

D86.0 Sarcoidosis of lung   HCC Rx ESR COM

D86.1 Sarcoidosis of lymph nodes

D86.2 Sarcoidosis of lung with sarcoidosis of lymph nodes   HCC Rx ESR COM

D86.3 Sarcoidosis of skin

☑5ᵗʰ **D86.8 Sarcoidosis of other sites**

  D86.81 Sarcoid meningitis   COM

  D86.82 Multiple cranial nerve palsies in sarcoidosis   HCC Rx ESR COM

  D86.83 Sarcoid iridocyclitis

  D86.84 Sarcoid pyelonephritis
    Tubulo-interstitial nephropathy in sarcoidosis

  D86.85 Sarcoid myocarditis   COM

  D86.86 Sarcoid arthropathy
    Polyarthritis in sarcoidosis

  D86.87 Sarcoid myositis

  D86.89 Sarcoidosis of other sites
    Hepatic granuloma
    Uveoparotid fever [Heerfordt]

D86.9 Sarcoidosis, unspecified

☑4ᵗʰ **D89 Other disorders involving the immune mechanism, not elsewhere classified**
    EXCLUDES 1   hyperglobulinemia NOS (R77.1)
                monoclonal gammopathy (of undetermined significance) (D47.2)
    EXCLUDES 2   transplant failure and rejection (T86.-)

D89.0 Polyclonal hypergammaglobulinemia   Rx
    Benign hypergammaglobulinemic purpura
    Polyclonal gammopathy NOS

D89.1 Cryoglobulinemia   HCC Rx ESR
    Cryoglobulinemic purpura
    Cryoglobulinemic vasculitis
    Essential cryoglobulinemia
    Idiopathic cryoglobulinemia
    Mixed cryoglobulinemia
    Primary cryoglobulinemia
    Secondary cryoglobulinemia

D89.2 Hypergammaglobulinemia, unspecified

D89.3 Immune reconstitution syndrome   HCC Rx ESR COM
    Immune reconstitution inflammatory syndrome [IRIS]
    Use additional code for adverse effect, if applicable, to identify drug (T36-T50 with fifth or sixth character 5)

☑5ᵗʰ **D89.4 Mast cell activation syndrome and related disorders**
    EXCLUDES 1   aggressive systemic mastocytosis (C96.21)
                congenital cutaneous mastocytosis (Q82.2)
                (non-congenital) cutaneous mastocytosis (D47.01)
                (indolent) systemic mastocytosis (D47.02)
                malignant mast cell neoplasm (C96.2-)
                malignant mastocytoma (C96.29)
                mast cell leukemia (C94.3-)
                mast cell sarcoma (C96.22)
                mastocytoma NOS (D47.09)
                other mast cell neoplasms of uncertain behavior (D47.09)
                systemic mastocytosis associated with a clonal hematologic non-mast cell lineage disease (SM-AHNMD) (D47.02)
    AHA: 2016,4Q,11

D89.40 Mast cell activation, unspecified   HCC Rx ESR COM
    Mast cell activation disorder, unspecified
    Mast cell activation syndrome, NOS

D89.41 Monoclonal mast cell activation syndrome   HCC Rx ESR COM

D89.42 Idiopathic mast cell activation syndrome   HCC Rx ESR COM

☑ Additional Character Required   ✓x7ᵗʰ Placeholder Alert   Manifestation   Unspecified Dx   Q QPP   UPD Unacceptable PDx

Chapter 3. Diseases of the Blood and Blood-forming Organs

D89.43   Secondary **mast cell activation** `HCC` `Rx` `ESR` `COM`
  Secondary mast cell activation syndrome
  Code also underlying etiology, if known

D89.44   Hereditary alpha tryptasemia `HCC` `Rx` `ESR` `COM`
  Use additional code, if applicable, for:
    allergy status, other than to drugs and biological substances (Z91.0-)
    personal history of anaphylaxis (Z87.892)
  AHA: 2021,4Q,8

D89.49   **Other mast cell activation disorder** `HCC` `Rx` `ESR` `COM`
  Other mast cell activation syndrome

✓5th **D89.8**   **Other specified disorders involving the immune mechanism, not elsewhere classified**

  ✓6th **D89.81**   **Graft-versus-host disease**
    Code first underlying cause, such as:
      complications of transplanted organs and tissue (T86.-)
      complications of blood transfusion (T80.89)
    Use additional code to identify associated manifestations, such as:
      desquamative dermatitis (L30.8)
      diarrhea (R19.7)
      elevated bilirubin (R17)
      hair loss (L65.9)

    D89.810   Acute **graft-versus-host disease** `HCC` `Rx` `ESR` `COM` `UPD`
    D89.811   Chronic **graft-versus-host disease** `HCC` `Rx` `ESR` `COM` `UPD`
    D89.812   Acute on chronic **graft-versus-host disease** `HCC` `Rx` `ESR` `COM` `UPD`
    D89.813   **Graft-versus-host disease, unspecified** `HCC` `Rx` `ESR` `COM` `UPD`

  D89.82   **Autoimmune lymphoproliferative syndrome [ALPS]** `HCC` `ESR` `COM`
    DEF: Rare genetic alteration of the Fas protein that impairs normal cellular apoptosis (normal cell death), causing abnormal accumulation of lymphocytes in the lymph glands, liver, and spleen. Symptoms include neutropenia, anemia, and thrombocytopenia.

  ✓6th **D89.83**   **Cytokine release syndrome**
    Code first underlying cause, such as:
      complications following infusion, transfusion and therapeutic injection (T80.89-)
      complications of transplanted organs and tissue (T86.-)
    Use additional code to identify associated manifestations
    AHA: 2020,4Q,12-15
    DEF: Form of systemic inflammatory response syndrome (SIRS) in which immune substances (cytokines) are released rapidly and in large amounts from the affected immune cells into the blood. The severity of associated symptoms or manifestations varies based on the underlying cause. This syndrome occurs as a complication of a disease, infection, or drug (often an adverse effect of immunotherapy in the form of treatment receiving monoclonal antibodies or Chimeric Antigen Receptor T [CAR-T] cells).

    D89.831   Cytokine release syndrome, grade 1 `UPD`
    D89.832   Cytokine release syndrome, grade 2 `UPD`
    D89.833   Cytokine release syndrome, grade 3 `UPD`
    D89.834   Cytokine release syndrome, grade 4 `UPD`
    D89.835   Cytokine release syndrome, grade 5 `UPD`
    D89.839   Cytokine release syndrome, grade unspecified `UPD`

  D89.89   **Other specified disorders involving the immune mechanism, not elsewhere classified** `HCC` `Rx` `ESR` `COM`
    `EXCLUDES 1`   human immunodeficiency virus disease (B20)
    AHA: 2017,4Q,109

D89.9   **Disorder involving the immune mechanism, unspecified** `HCC` `Rx` `ESR` `COM`
  Immune disease NOS
  AHA: 2015,3Q,22

`HCC` CMS-HCC   `Rx` Rx HCC   `ESR` ESRD HCC   `COM` Commercial HCC   `N` Newborn: 0   `P` Pediatric: 0-17   `M` Maternity: 9-64   `A` Adult: 15-124

528   ICD-10-CM 2023

Chapter 4. Endocrine, Nutritional, and Metabolic Diseases (E00–E89)

Chapter-specific Guidelines with Coding Examples

The chapter-specific guidelines from the ICD-10-CM Official Guidelines for Coding and Reporting have been provided below. Along with these guidelines are coding examples, contained in the shaded boxes, that have been developed to help illustrate the coding and/or sequencing guidance found in these guidelines.

a. Diabetes mellitus

The diabetes mellitus codes are combination codes that include the type of diabetes mellitus, the body system affected, and the complications affecting that body system. As many codes within a particular category as are necessary to describe all of the complications of the disease may be used. They should be sequenced based on the reason for a particular encounter. Assign as many codes from categories E08–E13 as needed to identify all of the associated conditions that the patient has.

> Patient is seen for uncontrolled diabetes, type 2, with hyperglycemia diabetic nephropathy, and diabetic gastroparesis
>
> **E11.65**   **Type 2 diabetes mellitus with hyperglycemia**
>
> **E11.21**   **Type 2 diabetes mellitus with diabetic nephropathy**
>
> **E11.43**   **Type 2 diabetes mellitus with diabetic autonomic (poly)neuropathy**
>
> **K31.84**   **Gastroparesis**
>
> *Explanation*: Use as many codes to describe the diabetic complications as needed. Many are combination codes that describe more than one condition. Code first the reason for the encounter. The term "uncontrolled" can refer to either hyperglycemia or hypoglycemia. In this case, "uncontrolled" is described as "with hyperglycemia."

1) Type of diabetes

The age of a patient is not the sole determining factor, though most type 1 diabetics develop the condition before reaching puberty. For this reason, type 1 diabetes mellitus is also referred to as juvenile diabetes.

> A 45-year-old patient is diagnosed with type 1 diabetes
>
> **E10.9**   **Type 1 diabetes mellitus without complications**
>
> *Explanation*: Although most type 1 diabetics are diagnosed in childhood or adolescence, it can also begin in adults.

2) Type of diabetes mellitus not documented

If the type of diabetes mellitus is not documented in the medical record the default is E11.-, Type 2 diabetes mellitus.

> Office visit lists diabetic retinopathy with macular edema and hypertension on patient problem list
>
> **E11.311**   **Type 2 diabetes mellitus with unspecified diabetic retinopathy with macular edema**
>
> **I10**   **Essential (primary) hypertension**
>
> *Explanation*: Since the type of diabetes was not documented, default to category E11.

3) Diabetes mellitus and the use of insulin, oral hypoglycemics, and injectable non-insulin drugs

If the documentation in a medical record does not indicate the type of diabetes but does indicate that the patient uses insulin, code E11-, Type 2 diabetes mellitus, should be assigned. Additional code(s) should be assigned from category Z79 to identify the long-term (current) use of insulin, oral hypoglycemic drugs, or injectable non-insulin antidiabetic, as follows:

If the patient is treated with both oral **hypoglycemic drugs** and insulin, both code Z79.4, Long term (current) use of insulin, and code Z79.84, Long term (current) use of oral hypoglycemic drugs, should be assigned.

If the patient is treated with both insulin and an injectable non-insulin antidiabetic drug, assign codes Z79.4, Long term (current) use of insulin, and **Z79.85, Long-term (current) use of injectable non-insulin antidiabetic drugs.**

If the patient is treated with both oral hypoglycemic drugs and an injectable non-insulin antidiabetic drug, assign codes Z79.84, Long term (current) use of oral hypoglycemic drugs, and **Z79.85, Long-term (current) use of injectable non-insulin antidiabetic drugs.**

Code Z79.4 should not be assigned if insulin is given temporarily to bring a type 2 patient's blood sugar under control during an encounter.

> Office visit lists chronic diabetes with daily insulin use on patient problem list
>
> **E11.9**   **Type 2 diabetes mellitus without complications**
>
> **Z79.4**   **Long term (current) use of insulin**
>
> *Explanation*: Do not assume that a patient on insulin must have type 1 diabetes. The default for diabetes without further specification defaults to type 2. Add the code for long term use of insulin.

4) Diabetes mellitus in pregnancy and gestational diabetes

See Section I.C.15. Diabetes mellitus in pregnancy.

See Section I.C.15. Gestational (pregnancy induced) diabetes

5) Complications due to insulin pump malfunction

(a) Underdose of insulin due to insulin pump failure

An underdose of insulin due to an insulin pump failure should be assigned to a code from subcategory T85.6, Mechanical complication of other specified internal and external prosthetic devices, implants and grafts, that specifies the type of pump malfunction, as the principal or first-listed code, followed by code T38.3X6-, Underdosing of insulin and oral hypoglycemic [antidiabetic] drugs. Additional codes for the type of diabetes mellitus and any associated complications due to the underdosing should also be assigned.

> A 24-year-old type 1 diabetic male treated in for hyperglycemia; insulin pump found to be malfunctioning and underdosing
>
> **T85.614A**   **Breakdown (mechanical) of insulin pump, initial encounter**
>
> **T38.3X6A**   **Underdosing of insulin and oral hypoglycemic [antidiabetic] drugs, initial encounter**
>
> **E10.65**   **Type 1 diabetes mellitus with hyperglycemia**
>
> *Explanation*: The complication code for the mechanical breakdown of the pump is sequenced first, followed by the underdosing code and type of diabetes with complication. Code all other diabetic complication codes necessary to describe the patient's condition.

(b) Overdose of insulin due to insulin pump failure

The principal or first-listed code for an encounter due to an insulin pump malfunction resulting in an overdose of insulin, should also be T85.6-, Mechanical complication of other specified internal and external prosthetic devices, implants and grafts, followed by code T38.3X1-, Poisoning by insulin and oral hypoglycemic [antidiabetic] drugs, accidental (unintentional).

> A 24-year-old type 1 diabetic male found down with diabetic coma, brought into ED and treated for hypoglycemia; insulin pump found to be malfunctioning and overdosing
>
> **T85.614A**   **Breakdown (mechanical) of insulin pump, initial encounter**
>
> **T38.3X1A**   **Poisoning by insulin and oral hypoglycemic [antidiabetic] drugs, accidental (unintentional), initial encounter**
>
> **E10.641**   **Type 1 diabetes mellitus with hypoglycemia with coma**
>
> *Explanation*: The complication code for the mechanical breakdown of the pump is sequenced first, followed by the poisoning code and type of diabetes with complication. All the characters in the combination code must be used to form a valid code and to fully describe the type of diabetes, the hypoglycemia, and the coma.

6) Secondary diabetes mellitus

Codes under categories E08, Diabetes mellitus due to underlying condition, E09, Drug or chemical induced diabetes mellitus, and E13, Other specified diabetes mellitus, identify complications/manifestations associated with secondary diabetes mellitus. Secondary diabetes is always caused by another condition or event (e.g., cystic fibrosis,

Chapter 4. Endocrine, Nutritional, and Metabolic Diseases

malignant neoplasm of pancreas, pancreatectomy, adverse effect of drug, or poisoning).

(a) Secondary diabetes mellitus and the use of insulin or oral hypoglycemic drugs

For patients with secondary diabetes mellitus who routinely use insulin, oral hypoglycemic drugs, or injectable non-insulin drugs, additional code(s) from category Z79 should be assigned to identify the long-term (current) use of insulin, oral hypoglycemic drugs, or non-injectable non-insulin drugs as follows:

If the patient is treated with both oral **hypoglycemic drugs** and insulin, both code Z79.4, Long term (current) use of insulin, and code Z79.84, Long term (current) use of oral hypoglycemic drugs, should be assigned.

If the patient is treated with both insulin and an injectable non-insulin antidiabetic drug, assign codes Z79.4, Long-term (current) use of insulin, and **Z79.85, Long-term (current) use of injectable non-insulin antidiabetic drugs**.

If the patient is treated with both oral hypoglycemic drugs and an injectable non-insulin antidiabetic drug, assign codes Z79.84, Long-term (current) use of oral hypoglycemic drugs, and **Z79.85, Long-term (current) use of injectable non-insulin antidiabetic drugs.**

Code Z79.4 should not be assigned if insulin is given temporarily to bring a secondary diabetic patient's blood sugar under control during an encounter.

Type 2 diabetic with no complications, normally only on oral metformin, is given insulin for three days to maintain glucose control while in the hospital recovering from surgery

E11.9	Type 2 diabetes mellitus without complications
Z79.84	Long term (current) use of oral hypoglycemic drugs

Explanation: Although the patient was given insulin for a short time during his hospital stay, the intent was only to maintain the patient's glucose levels while off his regular oral hypoglycemic medication, not for long term use. No code is needed for long term use of insulin, but a Z code for long term use of an oral hypoglycemic should be added to identify the chronic use of this drug.

Type 2 diabetic with diabetic polyneuropathy on insulin

E11.42	Type 2 diabetes mellitus with diabetic polyneuropathy
Z79.4	Long term (current) use of insulin

Explanation: Add a Z code for the long term use of insulin and the long term use of metformin because both are taken chronically.

(b) Assigning and sequencing secondary diabetes codes and its causes

The sequencing of the secondary diabetes codes in relationship to codes for the cause of the diabetes is based on the Tabular List instructions for categories E08, E09 and E13.

(i) Secondary diabetes mellitus due to pancreatectomy

For postpancreatectomy diabetes mellitus (lack of insulin due to the surgical removal of all or part of the pancreas), assign code E89.1, Postprocedural hypoinsulinemia. Assign a code from category E13 and a code from subcategory Z90.41-, Acquired absence of pancreas, as additional codes.

Patient with newly diagnosed diabetes after surgical removal of part of pancreas

E89.1	Postprocedural hypoinsulinemia
E13.9	Other specified diabetes mellitus without complications
Z90.411	Acquired partial absence of pancreas

Explanation: Sequence the postprocedural complication of the hypoinsulinemia due to the partial removal of the pancreas as the first-listed code, followed by codes for other specified diabetes (NEC) without complications and partial acquired absence of the pancreas.

(ii) Secondary diabetes due to drugs

Secondary diabetes may be caused by an adverse effect of correctly administered medications, poisoning or sequela of poisoning.

See section I.C.19.e. for coding of adverse effects and poisoning, and section I.C.20 for external cause code reporting.

Initial encounter for corticosteroid-induced diabetes mellitus

E09.9	Drug or chemical induced diabetes mellitus without complications
T38.0X5A	Adverse effect of glucocorticoids and synthetic analogues, initial encounter

Explanation: If the diabetes is caused by an adverse effect of a drug, the diabetic condition is coded first. If it occurs from a poisoning or overdose, the poisoning code causing the diabetes is sequenced first.

Chapter 4. Endocrine, Nutritional and Metabolic Diseases (E00-E89) *E00-E07 thyroid*

NOTE All neoplasms, whether functionally active or not, are classified in Chapter 2. Appropriate codes in this chapter (i.e. E05.8, E07.0, E16-E31, E34.-) may be used as additional codes to indicate either functional activity by neoplasms and ectopic endocrine tissue or hyperfunction and hypofunction of endocrine glands associated with neoplasms and other conditions classified elsewhere.

EXCLUDES 1   transitory endocrine and metabolic disorders specific to newborn (P70-P74)

AHA: 2018,2Q,6

This chapter contains the following blocks:

E00-E07   Disorders of thyroid gland
E08-E13   Diabetes mellitus
E15-E16   Other disorders of glucose regulation and pancreatic internal secretion
E20-E35   Disorders of other endocrine glands
E36   Intraoperative complications of endocrine system
E40-E46   Malnutrition
E50-E64   Other nutritional deficiencies
E65-E68   Overweight, obesity and other hyperalimentation
E70-E88   Metabolic disorders
E89   Postprocedural endocrine and metabolic complications and disorders, not elsewhere classified

Disorders of thyroid gland (E00-E07)

✓4ᵗʰ E00 Congenital iodine-deficiency syndrome

Use additional code (F70-F79) to identify associated intellectual disabilities

EXCLUDES 1   subclinical iodine-deficiency hypothyroidism (E02)

E00.0 Congenital iodine-deficiency syndrome, neurological type   Rx
Endemic cretinism, neurological type

E00.1 Congenital iodine-deficiency syndrome, myxedematous type   Rx
Endemic hypothyroid cretinism
Endemic cretinism, myxedematous type

E00.2 Congenital iodine-deficiency syndrome, mixed type   Rx
Endemic cretinism, mixed type

E00.9 Congenital iodine-deficiency syndrome, unspecified   Rx
Congenital iodine-deficiency hypothyroidism NOS
Endemic cretinism NOS

✓4ᵗʰ E01 Iodine-deficiency related thyroid disorders and allied conditions

EXCLUDES 1   congenital iodine-deficiency syndrome (E00.-)
subclinical iodine-deficiency hypothyroidism (E02)

E01.0 Iodine-deficiency related diffuse (endemic) goiter   Rx

E01.1 Iodine-deficiency related multinodular (endemic) goiter   Rx
Iodine-deficiency related nodular goiter

E01.2 Iodine-deficiency related (endemic) goiter, unspecified   Rx
Endemic goiter NOS

E01.8 Other iodine-deficiency related thyroid disorders and allied conditions   Rx
Acquired iodine-deficiency hypothyroidism NOS

E02 Subclinical iodine-deficiency hypothyroidism
AHA: 2021,1Q,8   *borderline*

✓4ᵗʰ E03 Other hypothyroidism

EXCLUDES 1   iodine-deficiency related hypothyroidism (E00-E02)
postprocedural hypothyroidism (E89.0)

DEF: Hypothyroidism: Underproduction of thyroid hormone.

E03.0 Congenital hypothyroidism with diffuse goiter   Rx
Congenital parenchymatous goiter (nontoxic)
Congenital goiter (nontoxic) NOS
EXCLUDES 1   transitory congenital goiter with normal function (P72.0)

E03.1 Congenital hypothyroidism without goiter   Rx
Aplasia of thyroid (with myxedema)
Congenital atrophy of thyroid
Congenital hypothyroidism NOS

E03.2 Hypothyroidism due to medicaments and other exogenous substances   Rx
Code first poisoning due to drug or toxin, if applicable (T36-T65 with fifth or sixth character 1-4 or 6)
Use additional code for adverse effect, if applicable, to identify drug (T36-T50 with fifth or sixth character 5)

E03.3 Postinfectious hypothyroidism   Rx

E03.4 Atrophy of thyroid (acquired)   Rx
EXCLUDES 1   congenital atrophy of thyroid (E03.1)

E03.5 Myxedema coma   HCC Rx ESR COM

E03.8 Other specified hypothyroidism   Rx
AHA: 2021,1Q,8

E03.9 Hypothyroidism, unspecified   Rx
Myxedema NOS

✓4ᵗʰ E04 Other nontoxic goiter

EXCLUDES 1   congenital goiter (NOS) (diffuse) (parenchymatous) (E03.0)
iodine-deficiency related goiter (E00-E02)

E04.0 Nontoxic diffuse goiter   Rx
Diffuse (colloid) nontoxic goiter
Simple nontoxic goiter

E04.1 Nontoxic single thyroid nodule   Rx
Colloid nodule (cystic) (thyroid)
Nontoxic uninodular goiter
Thyroid (cystic) nodule NOS
DEF: Enlarged thyroid, commonly due to decreased thyroid production, with a single nodule. No clinical hypothyroidism.

E04.2 Nontoxic multinodular goiter   Rx
Cystic goiter NOS
Multinodular (cystic) goiter NOS
DEF: Enlarged thyroid, commonly due to decreased thyroid production with multiple nodules. No clinical hypothyroidism.

E04.8 Other specified nontoxic goiter   Rx

E04.9 Nontoxic goiter, unspecified   Rx
Goiter NOS
Nodular goiter (nontoxic) NOS

✓4ᵗʰ E05 Thyrotoxicosis [hyperthyroidism]

EXCLUDES 1   chronic thyroiditis with transient thyrotoxicosis (E06.2)
neonatal thyrotoxicosis (P72.1)

DEF: Excessive quantities of hormones from the thyroid gland caused by overproduction or loss of storage ability.

✓5ᵗʰ E05.0 Thyrotoxicosis with diffuse goiter
Exophthalmic or toxic goiter NOS
Graves' disease
Toxic diffuse goiter
DEF: Diffuse thyroid enlargement accompanied by hyperthyroidism, bulging eyes, and dermopathy.

E05.00 Thyrotoxicosis with diffuse goiter without thyrotoxic crisis or storm   Rx

E05.01 Thyrotoxicosis with diffuse goiter with thyrotoxic crisis or storm   Rx

Goiter

Pyramidal lobe
Thyroid cartilage
Healthy thyroid
Goiter (hyperfunctioning thyroid)

✓5ᵗʰ E05.1 Thyrotoxicosis with toxic single thyroid nodule
Thyrotoxicosis with toxic uninodular goiter
DEF: Symptomatic hyperthyroidism with a single nodule on the enlarged thyroid gland. Onset of symptoms can be abrupt and include extreme nervousness, insomnia, weight loss, tremors, and psychosis or coma.

E05.10 Thyrotoxicosis with toxic single thyroid nodule without thyrotoxic crisis or storm   Rx

E05.11 Thyrotoxicosis with toxic single thyroid nodule with thyrotoxic crisis or storm   Rx

✓5ᵗʰ E05.2 Thyrotoxicosis with toxic multinodular goiter
Toxic nodular goiter NOS

E05.20 Thyrotoxicosis with toxic multinodular goiter without thyrotoxic crisis or storm   Rx

E05.21 Thyrotoxicosis with toxic multinodular goiter with thyrotoxic crisis or storm   Rx

√5ᵗʰ **E05.3** Thyrotoxicosis from ectopic thyroid tissue

  E05.30 **Thyrotoxicosis from ectopic thyroid tissue** without thyrotoxic crisis or storm ▪Rx

  E05.31 **Thyrotoxicosis from ectopic thyroid tissue** with thyrotoxic crisis or storm ▪Rx

√5ᵗʰ **E05.4** Thyrotoxicosis factitia

  E05.40 **Thyrotoxicosis factitia** without thyrotoxic crisis or storm ▪Rx

  E05.41 **Thyrotoxicosis factitia** with thyrotoxic crisis or storm ▪Rx

√5ᵗʰ **E05.8** **Other thyrotoxicosis**

  Overproduction of thyroid-stimulating hormone

  E05.80 **Other thyrotoxicosis** without thyrotoxic crisis or storm ▪Rx

  E05.81 **Other thyrotoxicosis** with thyrotoxic crisis or storm ▪Rx

√5ᵗʰ **E05.9** **Thyrotoxicosis, unspecified**

  Hyperthyroidism NOS

  E05.90 **Thyrotoxicosis, unspecified** without thyrotoxic crisis or storm ▪Rx

  E05.91 **Thyrotoxicosis, unspecified** with thyrotoxic crisis or storm ▪Rx

√4ᵗʰ **E06** **Thyroiditis**

  EXCLUDES 1   postpartum thyroiditis (O90.5)

  DEF: Inflammation of the thyroid gland.

  E06.0 **Acute thyroiditis** ▪Rx

    Abscess of thyroid
    Pyogenic thyroiditis
    Suppurative thyroiditis
    Use additional code (B95-B97) to identify infectious agent

  E06.1 **Subacute thyroiditis** ▪Rx

    de Quervain thyroiditis
    Giant-cell thyroiditis
    Granulomatous thyroiditis
    Nonsuppurative thyroiditis
    Viral thyroiditis
    EXCLUDES 1   autoimmune thyroiditis (E06.3)

  E06.2 **Chronic thyroiditis with transient thyrotoxicosis** ▪Rx
    EXCLUDES 1   autoimmune thyroiditis (E06.3)

  E06.3 **Autoimmune thyroiditis** ▪Rx
    Hashimoto's thyroiditis
    Hashitoxicosis (transient)
    Lymphadenoid goiter
    Lymphocytic thyroiditis
    Struma lymphomatosa

  E06.4 **Drug-induced thyroiditis** ▪Rx
    Use additional code for adverse effect, if applicable, to identify drug (T36-T50 with fifth or sixth character 5)

  E06.5 **Other chronic thyroiditis** ▪Rx
    Chronic fibrous thyroiditis
    Chronic thyroiditis NOS
    Ligneous thyroiditis
    Riedel thyroiditis

  E06.9 **Thyroiditis, unspecified** ▪Rx

√4ᵗʰ **E07** **Other disorders of thyroid**

  E07.0 **Hypersecretion of calcitonin** ▪Rx
    C-cell hyperplasia of thyroid
    Hypersecretion of thyrocalcitonin

  E07.1 **Dyshormogenetic goiter** ▪Rx
    Familial dyshormogenetic goiter
    Pendred's syndrome
    EXCLUDES 1   transitory congenital goiter with normal function (P72.0)

√5ᵗʰ **E07.8** **Other specified disorders of thyroid**

  E07.81 **Sick-euthyroid syndrome**
    Euthyroid sick-syndrome
    DEF: Thyroid dysfunction caused by abnormal levels of thyroid hormones T3 and/or T4. This syndrome is often associated with starvation or critical illness.

  E07.89 **Other specified disorders of thyroid** ▪Rx
    Abnormality of thyroid-binding globulin
    Hemorrhage of thyroid
    Infarction of thyroid

  E07.9 **Disorder of thyroid, unspecified** ▪Rx

Diabetes mellitus (E08-E13)

AHA: 2020,1Q,12; 2018,2Q,6; 2017,4Q,100-101; 2016,2Q,36; 2016,1Q,11-13; 2013,4Q,114; 2013,3Q,20

TIP: There is no default code for diabetes mellitus documented only as uncontrolled. The provider must indicate whether the diabetic patient is hypoglycemic or hyperglycemic to determine the appropriate code.

√4ᵗʰ **E08** **Diabetes mellitus** due to underlying condition

  Code first the underlying condition, such as:
    congenital rubella (P35.0)
    Cushing's syndrome (E24.-)
    cystic fibrosis (E84.-)
    malignant neoplasm (C00-C96)
    malnutrition (E40-E46)
    pancreatitis and other diseases of the pancreas (K85-K86.-)
  Use additional code to identify control using:
    insulin (Z79.4)
    oral antidiabetic drugs (Z79.84)
    oral hypoglycemic drugs (Z79.84)
    EXCLUDES 1   drug or chemical induced diabetes mellitus (E09.-)
              gestational diabetes (O24.4-)
              neonatal diabetes mellitus (P70.2)
              postpancreatectomy diabetes mellitus (E13.-)
              postprocedural diabetes mellitus (E13.-)
              secondary diabetes mellitus NEC (E13.-)
              type 1 diabetes mellitus (E10.-)
              type 2 diabetes mellitus (E11.-)

[handwritten: ✗ Secondary DM]

√5ᵗʰ **E08.0** **Diabetes mellitus due to underlying condition with hyperosmolarity**
    DEF: Diabetic hyperosmolarity: Extremely high levels of glucose in the blood without ketones.

  E08.00 ***Diabetes mellitus due to underlying condition with hyperosmolarity without nonketotic hyperglycemic-hyperosmolar coma (NKHHC)*** HCC Rx ESR COM

  E08.01 ***Diabetes mellitus due to underlying condition with hyperosmolarity with coma*** HCC Rx ESR COM

√5ᵗʰ **E08.1** **Diabetes mellitus due to underlying condition with ketoacidosis**
    DEF: Diabetic ketoacidosis: Potentially life-threatening complication due to a shortage of insulin in which the body switches to burning fatty acids and producing acidic ketone bodies.

  E08.10 ***Diabetes mellitus due to underlying condition with ketoacidosis without coma*** HCC Rx ESR COM

  E08.11 ***Diabetes mellitus due to underlying condition with ketoacidosis with coma*** HCC Rx ESR COM

√5ᵗʰ **E08.2** **Diabetes mellitus due to underlying condition with kidney complications**
    AHA: 2019,3Q,3; 2018,4Q,88

  E08.21 ***Diabetes mellitus due to underlying condition with diabetic nephropathy*** HCC Rx ESR COM
    Diabetes mellitus due to underlying condition with intercapillary glomerulosclerosis
    Diabetes mellitus due to underlying condition with intracapillary glomerulonephrosis
    Diabetes mellitus due to underlying condition with Kimmelstiel-Wilson disease

  E08.22 ***Diabetes mellitus due to underlying condition with diabetic chronic kidney disease*** HCC Rx ESR COM
    Use additional code to identify stage of chronic kidney disease (N18.1-N18.6)

  E08.29 ***Diabetes mellitus due to underlying condition with other diabetic kidney complication*** HCC Rx ESR COM
    Renal tubular degeneration in diabetes mellitus due to underlying condition

✓5ʰ **E08.3 Diabetes mellitus due to underlying condition with ophthalmic complications**
AHA: 2016,4Q,11-13

One of the following 7th characters is to be assigned to codes in subcategories E08.32, E08.33, E08.34, E08.35, and E08.37 to designate laterality of the disease:
1   right eye
2   left eye
3   bilateral
9   unspecified eye

✓6ʰ **E08.31 Diabetes mellitus due to underlying condition with unspecified diabetic retinopathy**
DEF: Diabetic retinopathy: Diabetic complication from damage to the retinal vessels resulting in vision problems that can progress to blindness.

E08.311 Diabetes mellitus due to underlying condition with unspecified diabetic retinopathy with macular edema HCC Rx ESR COM

E08.319 Diabetes mellitus due to underlying condition with unspecified diabetic retinopathy without macular edema HCC Rx ESR COM

✓6ʰ **E08.32 Diabetes mellitus due to underlying condition with mild nonproliferative diabetic retinopathy**
Diabetes mellitus due to underlying condition with nonproliferative diabetic retinopathy NOS

✓7ʰ *E08.321 Diabetes mellitus due to underlying condition with mild nonproliferative diabetic retinopathy with macular edema* HCC Rx ESR COM

✓7ʰ *E08.329 Diabetes mellitus due to underlying condition with mild nonproliferative diabetic retinopathy without macular edema* HCC Rx ESR COM

✓6ʰ **E08.33 Diabetes mellitus due to underlying condition with moderate nonproliferative diabetic retinopathy**

✓7ʰ *E08.331 Diabetes mellitus due to underlying condition with moderate nonproliferative diabetic retinopathy with macular edema* HCC Rx ESR COM

✓7ʰ *E08.339 Diabetes mellitus due to underlying condition with moderate nonproliferative diabetic retinopathy without macular edema* HCC Rx ESR COM

✓6ʰ **E08.34 Diabetes mellitus due to underlying condition with severe nonproliferative diabetic retinopathy**

✓7ʰ *E08.341 Diabetes mellitus due to underlying condition with severe nonproliferative diabetic retinopathy with macular edema* HCC Rx ESR COM

✓7ʰ *E08.349 Diabetes mellitus due to underlying condition with severe nonproliferative diabetic retinopathy without macular edema* HCC Rx ESR COM

✓6ʰ **E08.35 Diabetes mellitus due to underlying condition with proliferative diabetic retinopathy**

✓7ʰ *E08.351 Diabetes mellitus due to underlying condition with proliferative diabetic retinopathy with macular edema* HCC Rx ESR COM

✓7ʰ *E08.352 Diabetes mellitus due to underlying condition with proliferative diabetic retinopathy with traction retinal detachment involving the macula* HCC Rx ESR COM

✓7ʰ *E08.353 Diabetes mellitus due to underlying condition with proliferative diabetic retinopathy with traction retinal detachment not involving the macula* HCC Rx ESR COM

✓7ʰ *E08.354 Diabetes mellitus due to underlying condition with proliferative diabetic retinopathy with combined traction retinal detachment and rhegmatogenous retinal detachment* HCC Rx ESR COM

✓7ʰ *E08.355 Diabetes mellitus due to underlying condition with stable proliferative diabetic retinopathy* HCC Rx ESR COM

✓7ʰ *E08.359 Diabetes mellitus due to underlying condition with proliferative diabetic retinopathy without macular edema* HCC Rx ESR COM

E08.36 Diabetes mellitus due to underlying condition with diabetic cataract HCC Rx ESR COM
AHA: 2019,2Q,30-31; 2016,4Q,142

✓x7ʰ **E08.37 Diabetes mellitus due to underlying condition with diabetic macular edema, resolved following treatment** HCC Rx ESR COM

E08.39 Diabetes mellitus due to underlying condition with other diabetic ophthalmic complication HCC Rx ESR COM
Use additional code to identify manifestation, such as:
diabetic glaucoma (H40-H42)

✓5ʰ **E08.4 Diabetes mellitus due to underlying condition with neurological complications**

E08.40 Diabetes mellitus due to underlying condition with diabetic neuropathy, unspecified HCC Rx ESR COM

E08.41 Diabetes mellitus due to underlying condition with diabetic mononeuropathy HCC Rx ESR COM

E08.42 Diabetes mellitus due to underlying condition with diabetic polyneuropathy HCC Rx ESR COM
Diabetes mellitus due to underlying condition with diabetic neuralgia

E08.43 Diabetes mellitus due to underlying condition with diabetic autonomic (poly)neuropathy HCC Rx ESR COM
Diabetes mellitus due to underlying condition with diabetic gastroparesis
AHA: 2013,4Q,114

E08.44 Diabetes mellitus due to underlying condition with diabetic amyotrophy HCC Rx ESR COM

E08.49 Diabetes mellitus due to underlying condition with other diabetic neurological complication HCC Rx ESR COM

✓5ʰ **E08.5 Diabetes mellitus due to underlying condition with circulatory complications**

E08.51 Diabetes mellitus due to underlying condition with diabetic peripheral angiopathy without gangrene HCC Rx ESR COM
AHA: 2018,3Q,3-4; 2018,2Q,7

E08.52 Diabetes mellitus due to underlying condition with diabetic peripheral angiopathy with gangrene
Diabetes mellitus due to underlying condition with diabetic gangrene
AHA: 2020,2Q,18; 2018,3Q,3; 2018,2Q,7; 2017,4Q,102

E08.59 Diabetes mellitus due to underlying condition with other circulatory complications HCC Rx ESR COM

✓5ʰ **E08.6 Diabetes mellitus due to underlying condition with other specified complications**

✓6ʰ **E08.61 Diabetes mellitus due to underlying condition with diabetic arthropathy**

E08.610 Diabetes mellitus due to underlying condition with diabetic neuropathic arthropathy HCC Rx ESR COM
Diabetes mellitus due to underlying condition with Charcôt's joints
DEF: Charcot's joint: Progressive neurologic arthropathy in which chronic degeneration of joints in the weight-bearing areas with peripheral hypertrophy occurs as a complication of a neuropathy disorder. Supporting structures relax from a loss of sensation resulting in chronic joint instability.

E08.618 Diabetes mellitus due to underlying condition with other diabetic arthropathy HCC Rx ESR COM
AHA: 2018,2Q,6

✓6ʰ **E08.62 Diabetes mellitus due to underlying condition with skin complications**

E08.620 Diabetes mellitus due to underlying condition with diabetic dermatitis HCC Rx ESR COM
Diabetes mellitus due to underlying condition with diabetic necrobiosis lipoidica

E08.621 *Diabetes mellitus due to underlying condition with foot ulcer* `HCC` `Rx` `ESR` `COM`
Use additional code to identify site of ulcer (L97.4-, L97.5-)
AHA: 2020,2Q,19
TIP: Do not assign a code for diabetic ulcer when the ulcer is closed/resolved or to report history of diabetic ulcers; Z86.31 Personal history of diabetic foot ulcer, may be assigned.

E08.622 *Diabetes mellitus due to underlying condition with other skin ulcer* `HCC` `Rx` `ESR` `COM`
Use additional code to identify site of ulcer (L97.1-L97.9, L98.41-L98.49)
AHA: 2021,1Q,7; 2017,4Q,17

E08.628 *Diabetes mellitus due to underlying condition with other skin complications* `HCC` `Rx` `ESR` `COM`

✓6ᵗʰ **E08.63** **Diabetes mellitus due to underlying condition with oral complications**

E08.630 *Diabetes mellitus due to underlying condition with periodontal disease* `HCC` `Rx` `ESR` `COM`

E08.638 *Diabetes mellitus due to underlying condition with other oral complications* `HCC` `Rx` `ESR` `COM`

✓6ᵗʰ **E08.64** **Diabetes mellitus due to underlying condition with hypoglycemia**
AHA: 2017,1Q,42

E08.641 *Diabetes mellitus due to underlying condition with hypoglycemia with coma* `HCC` `Rx` `ESR` `COM`

E08.649 *Diabetes mellitus due to underlying condition with hypoglycemia without coma* `HCC` `Rx` `ESR` `COM`
AHA: 2016,3Q,42; 2015,3Q,21

E08.65 *Diabetes mellitus due to underlying condition with hyperglycemia* `HCC` `Rx` `ESR` `COM`
AHA: 2017,1Q,42; 2013,3Q,20

E08.69 *Diabetes mellitus due to underlying condition with other specified complication* `HCC` `Rx` `ESR` `COM`
Use additional code to identify complication
AHA: 2016,4Q,141; 2016,1Q,13

E08.8 *Diabetes mellitus due to underlying condition with unspecified complications* `HCC` `Rx` `ESR` `COM`

E08.9 *Diabetes mellitus due to underlying condition without complications* `HCC` `Rx` `ESR` `COM`
AHA: 2020,2Q,18

✓4ᵗʰ **E09** **Drug or chemical induced diabetes mellitus**

[handwritten: Secondary DM]

Code first poisoning due to drug or toxin, if applicable (T36-T65 with fifth or sixth character 1-4 or 6)
Use additional code for adverse effect, if applicable, to identify drug (T36-T50 with fifth or sixth character 5)
Use additional code to identify control using:
insulin (Z79.4)
oral antidiabetic drugs (Z79.84)
oral hypoglycemic drugs (Z79.84)
`EXCLUDES 1` diabetes mellitus due to underlying condition (E08.-)
gestational diabetes (O24.4-)
neonatal diabetes mellitus (P70.2)
postpancreatectomy diabetes mellitus (E13.-)
postprocedural diabetes mellitus (E13.-)
secondary diabetes mellitus NEC (E13.-)
type 1 diabetes mellitus (E10.-)
type 2 diabetes mellitus (E11.-)

✓5ᵗʰ **E09.0** **Drug or chemical induced diabetes mellitus with hyperosmolarity**
DEF: Diabetic hyperosmolarity: Extremely high levels of glucose in the blood without ketones.

E09.00 **Drug or chemical induced diabetes mellitus with hyperosmolarity without nonketotic hyperglycemic-hyperosmolar coma (NKHHC)** `HCC` `Rx` `ESR` `COM`

E09.01 **Drug or chemical induced diabetes mellitus with hyperosmolarity with coma** `HCC` `Rx` `ESR` `COM`

✓5ᵗʰ **E09.1** **Drug or chemical induced diabetes mellitus with ketoacidosis**
DEF: Diabetic ketoacidosis: Potentially life-threatening complication due to a shortage of insulin in which the body switches to burning fatty acids and producing acidic ketone bodies.

E09.10 **Drug or chemical induced diabetes mellitus with ketoacidosis without coma** `HCC` `Rx` `ESR` `COM`

E09.11 **Drug or chemical induced diabetes mellitus with ketoacidosis with coma** `HCC` `Rx` `ESR` `COM`

✓5ᵗʰ **E09.2** **Drug or chemical induced diabetes mellitus with kidney complications**
AHA: 2019,3Q,3; 2018,4Q,88

E09.21 **Drug or chemical induced diabetes mellitus with diabetic nephropathy** `HCC` `Rx` `ESR` `COM`
Drug or chemical induced diabetes mellitus with intercapillary glomerulosclerosis
Drug or chemical induced diabetes mellitus with intracapillary glomerulonephrosis
Drug or chemical induced diabetes mellitus with Kimmelstiel-Wilson disease

E09.22 **Drug or chemical induced diabetes mellitus with diabetic chronic kidney disease** `HCC` `Rx` `ESR` `COM`
Use additional code to identify stage of chronic kidney disease (N18.1-N18.6)

E09.29 **Drug or chemical induced diabetes mellitus with other diabetic kidney complication** `HCC` `Rx` `ESR` `COM`
Drug or chemical induced diabetes mellitus with renal tubular degeneration

✓5ᵗʰ **E09.3** **Drug or chemical induced diabetes mellitus with ophthalmic complications**
AHA: 2016,4Q,11-13

[handwritten: adverse effect code second]

> One of the following 7th characters is to be assigned to codes in subcategories E09.32, E09.33, E09.34, E09.35, and E09.37 to designate laterality of the disease:
> 1　right eye
> 2　left eye
> 3　bilateral
> 9　unspecified eye

✓6ᵗʰ **E09.31** **Drug or chemical induced diabetes mellitus with unspecified diabetic retinopathy**
DEF: Diabetic retinopathy: Diabetic complication from damage to the retinal vessels resulting in vision problems that can progress to blindness.

E09.311 **Drug or chemical induced diabetes mellitus with unspecified diabetic retinopathy with macular edema** `HCC` `Rx` `ESR` `COM`

E09.319 **Drug or chemical induced diabetes mellitus with unspecified diabetic retinopathy without macular edema** `HCC` `Rx` `ESR` `COM`

✓6ᵗʰ **E09.32** **Drug or chemical induced diabetes mellitus with mild nonproliferative diabetic retinopathy**
Drug or chemical induced diabetes mellitus with nonproliferative diabetic retinopathy NOS

✓7ᵗʰ **E09.321** **Drug or chemical induced diabetes mellitus with mild nonproliferative diabetic retinopathy with macular edema** `HCC` `Rx` `ESR` `COM`

✓7ᵗʰ **E09.329** **Drug or chemical induced diabetes mellitus with mild nonproliferative diabetic retinopathy without macular edema** `HCC` `Rx` `ESR` `COM`

✓6ᵗʰ **E09.33** **Drug or chemical induced diabetes mellitus with moderate nonproliferative diabetic retinopathy**

✓7ᵗʰ **E09.331** **Drug or chemical induced diabetes mellitus with moderate nonproliferative diabetic retinopathy with macular edema** `HCC` `Rx` `ESR` `COM`

✓7ᵗʰ **E09.339** **Drug or chemical induced diabetes mellitus with moderate nonproliferative diabetic retinopathy without macular edema** `HCC` `Rx` `ESR` `COM`

✓6ᵗʰ **E09.34** **Drug or chemical induced diabetes mellitus with severe nonproliferative diabetic retinopathy**

✓7ᵗʰ **E09.341** **Drug or chemical induced diabetes mellitus with severe nonproliferative diabetic retinopathy with macular edema** `HCC` `Rx` `ESR` `COM`

√7ᵗʰ **E09.349** Drug or chemical induced diabetes mellitus with severe nonproliferative diabetic retinopathy without macular edema   `HCC` `Rx` `ESR` `COM`

√6ᵗʰ **E09.35** Drug or chemical induced diabetes mellitus with proliferative diabetic retinopathy

  √7ᵗʰ **E09.351** Drug or chemical induced diabetes mellitus with proliferative diabetic retinopathy with macular edema   `HCC` `Rx` `ESR` `COM`

  √7ᵗʰ **E09.352** Drug or chemical induced diabetes mellitus with proliferative diabetic retinopathy with traction retinal detachment involving the macula   `HCC` `Rx` `ESR` `COM`

  √7ᵗʰ **E09.353** Drug or chemical induced diabetes mellitus with proliferative diabetic retinopathy with traction retinal detachment not involving the macula   `HCC` `Rx` `ESR` `COM`

  √7ᵗʰ **E09.354** Drug or chemical induced diabetes mellitus with proliferative diabetic retinopathy with combined traction retinal detachment and rhegmatogenous retinal detachment   `HCC` `Rx` `ESR` `COM`

  √7ᵗʰ **E09.355** Drug or chemical induced diabetes mellitus with stable proliferative diabetic retinopathy   `HCC` `Rx` `ESR` `COM`

  √7ᵗʰ **E09.359** Drug or chemical induced diabetes mellitus with proliferative diabetic retinopathy without macular edema   `HCC` `Rx` `ESR` `COM`

E09.36 Drug or chemical induced diabetes mellitus with diabetic cataract   `HCC` `Rx` `ESR` `COM`
    AHA: 2019,2Q,30-31; 2016,4Q,142

√x7ᵗʰ **E09.37** Drug or chemical induced diabetes mellitus with diabetic macular edema, resolved following treatment   `HCC` `Rx` `ESR` `COM`

E09.39 Drug or chemical induced diabetes mellitus with other diabetic ophthalmic complication   `HCC` `Rx` `ESR` `COM`
    Use additional code to identify manifestation, such as:
      diabetic glaucoma (H40-H42)

√5ᵗʰ **E09.4** Drug or chemical induced diabetes mellitus with neurological complications

E09.40 Drug or chemical induced diabetes mellitus with neurological complications with diabetic neuropathy, unspecified   `HCC` `Rx` `ESR` `COM`

E09.41 Drug or chemical induced diabetes mellitus with neurological complications with diabetic mononeuropathy   `HCC` `Rx` `ESR` `COM`

E09.42 Drug or chemical induced diabetes mellitus with neurological complications with diabetic polyneuropathy   `HCC` `Rx` `ESR` `COM`
    Drug or chemical induced diabetes mellitus with diabetic neuralgia

E09.43 Drug or chemical induced diabetes mellitus with neurological complications with diabetic autonomic (poly)neuropathy   `HCC` `Rx` `ESR` `COM`
    Drug or chemical induced diabetes mellitus with diabetic gastroparesis
    AHA: 2013,4Q,114

E09.44 Drug or chemical induced diabetes mellitus with neurological complications with diabetic amyotrophy   `HCC` `Rx` `ESR` `COM`

E09.49 Drug or chemical induced diabetes mellitus with neurological complications with other diabetic neurological complication   `HCC` `Rx` `ESR` `COM`

√5ᵗʰ **E09.5** Drug or chemical induced diabetes mellitus with circulatory complications

E09.51 Drug or chemical induced diabetes mellitus with diabetic peripheral angiopathy without gangrene   `HCC` `Rx` `ESR` `COM`
    AHA: 2018,3Q,3-4; 2018,2Q,7

E09.52 Drug or chemical induced diabetes mellitus with diabetic peripheral angiopathy with gangrene   `HCC` `Rx` `ESR` `COM`
    Drug or chemical induced diabetes mellitus with diabetic gangrene
    AHA: 2020,2Q,18; 2018,3Q,3; 2018,2Q,7; 2017,4Q,102

E09.59 Drug or chemical induced diabetes mellitus with other circulatory complications   `HCC` `Rx` `ESR` `COM`

√5ᵗʰ **E09.6** Drug or chemical induced diabetes mellitus with other specified complications

√6ᵗʰ **E09.61** Drug or chemical induced diabetes mellitus with diabetic arthropathy

E09.610 Drug or chemical induced diabetes mellitus with diabetic neuropathic arthropathy   `HCC` `Rx` `ESR` `COM`
    Drug or chemical induced diabetes mellitus with Charcôt's joints
    DEF: Charcot's joint: Progressive neurologic arthropathy in which chronic degeneration of joints in the weight-bearing areas with peripheral hypertrophy occurs as a complication of a neuropathy disorder. Supporting structures relax from a loss of sensation resulting in chronic joint instability.

E09.618 Drug or chemical induced diabetes mellitus with other diabetic arthropathy   `HCC` `Rx` `ESR` `COM`
    AHA: 2018,2Q,6

√6ᵗʰ **E09.62** Drug or chemical induced diabetes mellitus with skin complications

E09.620 Drug or chemical induced diabetes mellitus with diabetic dermatitis   `HCC` `Rx` `ESR` `COM`
    Drug or chemical induced diabetes mellitus with diabetic necrobiosis lipoidica

E09.621 Drug or chemical induced diabetes mellitus with foot ulcer   `HCC` `Rx` `ESR` `COM`
    Use additional code to identify site of ulcer (L97.4-, L97.5-)
    AHA: 2020,2Q,19
    TIP: Do not assign a code for diabetic ulcer when the ulcer is closed/resolved or to report history of diabetic ulcers; Z86.31 Personal history of diabetic foot ulcer, may be assigned.

E09.622 Drug or chemical induced diabetes mellitus with other skin ulcer   `HCC` `Rx` `ESR` `COM`
    Use additional code to identify site of ulcer (L97.1-L97.9, L98.41-L98.49)
    AHA: 2021,1Q,7; 2017,4Q,17

E09.628 Drug or chemical induced diabetes mellitus with other skin complications   `HCC` `Rx` `ESR` `COM`

√6ᵗʰ **E09.63** Drug or chemical induced diabetes mellitus with oral complications

E09.630 Drug or chemical induced diabetes mellitus with periodontal disease   `HCC` `Rx` `ESR` `COM`

E09.638 Drug or chemical induced diabetes mellitus with other oral complications   `HCC` `Rx` `ESR` `COM`

√6ᵗʰ **E09.64** Drug or chemical induced diabetes mellitus with hypoglycemia
    AHA: 2017,1Q,42

E09.641 Drug or chemical induced diabetes mellitus with hypoglycemia with coma   `HCC` `Rx` `ESR` `COM`

E09.649 Drug or chemical induced diabetes mellitus with hypoglycemia without coma   `HCC` `Rx` `ESR` `COM`
    AHA: 2016,3Q,42; 2015,3Q,21

E09.65 Drug or chemical induced diabetes mellitus with hyperglycemia   `HCC` `Rx` `ESR` `COM`
    AHA: 2017,1Q,42; 2013,3Q,20

E09.69 Drug or chemical induced diabetes mellitus with other specified complication   `HCC` `Rx` `ESR` `COM`
    Use additional code to identify complication
    AHA: 2016,4Q,141; 2016,1Q,13

E09.8 Drug or chemical induced diabetes mellitus with unspecified complications   `HCC` `Rx` `ESR` `COM`

E09.9 Drug or chemical induced diabetes mellitus without complications   `HCC` `Rx` `ESR` `COM`
    AHA: 2020,2Q,18

☑ Additional Character Required   √x7ᵗʰ Placeholder Alert   Manifestation   Unspecified Dx   Ⓠ QPP   UPD Unacceptable PDx

☑4ᵗʰ **E10 Type 1 diabetes mellitus**

INCLUDES brittle diabetes (mellitus)
diabetes (mellitus) due to autoimmune process
diabetes (mellitus) due to immune mediated pancreatic islet beta-cell destruction
idiopathic diabetes (mellitus)
juvenile onset diabetes (mellitus)
ketosis-prone diabetes (mellitus)

EXCLUDES 1 *diabetes mellitus due to underlying condition (E08.-)*
drug or chemical induced diabetes mellitus (E09.-)
gestational diabetes (O24.4-)
hyperglycemia NOS (R73.9)
neonatal diabetes mellitus (P70.2)
postpancreatectomy diabetes mellitus (E13.-)
postprocedural diabetes mellitus (E13.-)
secondary diabetes mellitus NEC (E13.-)
type 2 diabetes mellitus (E11.-)

AHA: 2020,3Q,30

☑5ᵗʰ **E10.1 Type 1 diabetes mellitus with ketoacidosis**
AHA: 2013,3Q,20
DEF: Diabetic ketoacidosis: Potentially life-threatening complication due to a shortage of insulin in which the body switches to burning fatty acids and producing acidic ketone bodies.
E10.10 Type 1 diabetes mellitus with ketoacidosis without coma HCC Rx ESR COM Q
E10.11 Type 1 diabetes mellitus with ketoacidosis with coma HCC Rx ESR COM Q

☑5ᵗʰ **E10.2 Type 1 diabetes mellitus with kidney complications**
AHA: 2019,3Q,3; 2018,4Q,88
E10.21 Type 1 diabetes mellitus with diabetic nephropathy HCC Rx ESR COM Q
Type 1 diabetes mellitus with intercapillary glomerulosclerosis
Type 1 diabetes mellitus with intracapillary glomerulonephrosis
Type 1 diabetes mellitus with Kimmelstiel-Wilson disease
E10.22 Type 1 diabetes mellitus with diabetic chronic kidney disease HCC Rx ESR COM Q
Use additional code to identify stage of chronic kidney disease (N18.1-N18.6)
E10.29 Type 1 diabetes mellitus with other diabetic kidney complication HCC Rx ESR COM Q
Type 1 diabetes mellitus with renal tubular degeneration
AHA: 2016,1Q,13

☑5ᵗʰ **E10.3 Type 1 diabetes mellitus with ophthalmic complications**
AHA: 2016,4Q,11-13
One of the following 7th characters is to be assigned to codes in subcategories E10.32, E10.33, E10.34, E10.35, and E10.37 to designate laterality of the disease:
1 right eye
2 left eye
3 bilateral
9 unspecified eye

☑6ᵗʰ E10.31 Type 1 diabetes mellitus with unspecified diabetic retinopathy
DEF: Diabetic retinopathy: Diabetic complication from damage to the retinal vessels resulting in vision problems that can progress to blindness.
E10.311 Type 1 diabetes mellitus with unspecified diabetic retinopathy with macular edema HCC Rx ESR COM Q
E10.319 Type 1 diabetes mellitus with unspecified diabetic retinopathy without macular edema HCC Rx ESR COM Q
☑6ᵗʰ E10.32 Type 1 diabetes mellitus with mild nonproliferative diabetic retinopathy
Type 1 diabetes mellitus with nonproliferative diabetic retinopathy NOS
E10.321 Type 1 diabetes mellitus with mild nonproliferative diabetic retinopathy with macular edema HCC Rx ESR COM Q
E10.329 Type 1 diabetes mellitus with mild nonproliferative diabetic retinopathy without macular edema HCC Rx ESR COM Q

☑6ᵗʰ E10.33 Type 1 diabetes mellitus with moderate nonproliferative diabetic retinopathy
E10.331 Type 1 diabetes mellitus with moderate nonproliferative diabetic retinopathy with macular edema HCC Rx ESR COM Q
E10.339 Type 1 diabetes mellitus with moderate nonproliferative diabetic retinopathy without macular edema HCC Rx ESR COM Q
☑6ᵗʰ E10.34 Type 1 diabetes mellitus with severe nonproliferative diabetic retinopathy
E10.341 Type 1 diabetes mellitus with severe nonproliferative diabetic retinopathy with macular edema HCC Rx ESR COM Q
E10.349 Type 1 diabetes mellitus with severe nonproliferative diabetic retinopathy without macular edema HCC Rx ESR COM Q
☑6ᵗʰ E10.35 Type 1 diabetes mellitus with proliferative diabetic retinopathy
E10.351 Type 1 diabetes mellitus with proliferative diabetic retinopathy with macular edema HCC Rx ESR COM Q
E10.352 Type 1 diabetes mellitus with proliferative diabetic retinopathy with traction retinal detachment involving the macula HCC Rx ESR COM Q
E10.353 Type 1 diabetes mellitus with proliferative diabetic retinopathy with traction retinal detachment not involving the macula HCC Rx ESR COM Q
E10.354 Type 1 diabetes mellitus with proliferative diabetic retinopathy with combined traction retinal detachment and rhegmatogenous retinal detachment HCC Rx ESR COM Q
E10.355 Type 1 diabetes mellitus with stable proliferative diabetic retinopathy HCC Rx ESR COM Q
E10.359 Type 1 diabetes mellitus with proliferative diabetic retinopathy without macular edema HCC Rx ESR COM Q
E10.36 Type 1 diabetes mellitus with diabetic cataract HCC Rx ESR COM Q
AHA: 2019,2Q,30-31; 2016,4Q,142
☑x7ᵗʰ E10.37 Type 1 diabetes mellitus with diabetic macular edema, resolved following treatment HCC Rx ESR COM Q
E10.39 Type 1 diabetes mellitus with other diabetic ophthalmic complication HCC Rx ESR COM Q
Use additional code to identify manifestation, such as:
diabetic glaucoma (H40-H42)
☑5ᵗʰ **E10.4 Type 1 diabetes mellitus with neurological complications**
E10.40 Type 1 diabetes mellitus with diabetic neuropathy, unspecified HCC Rx ESR COM Q
E10.41 Type 1 diabetes mellitus with diabetic mononeuropathy HCC Rx ESR COM Q
E10.42 Type 1 diabetes mellitus with diabetic polyneuropathy HCC Rx ESR COM Q
Type 1 diabetes mellitus with diabetic neuralgia
E10.43 Type 1 diabetes mellitus with diabetic autonomic (poly)neuropathy HCC Rx ESR COM Q
Type 1 diabetes mellitus with diabetic gastroparesis
AHA: 2013,4Q,114
E10.44 Type 1 diabetes mellitus with diabetic amyotrophy HCC Rx ESR COM Q
E10.49 Type 1 diabetes mellitus with other diabetic neurological complication HCC Rx ESR COM Q
☑5ᵗʰ **E10.5 Type 1 diabetes mellitus with circulatory complications**
E10.51 Type 1 diabetes mellitus with diabetic peripheral angiopathy without gangrene HCC Rx ESR COM Q
AHA: 2018,3Q,3-4; 2018,2Q,7
E10.52 Type 1 diabetes mellitus with diabetic peripheral angiopathy with gangrene HCC Rx ESR COM Q
Type 1 diabetes mellitus with diabetic gangrene
AHA: 2020,2Q,18; 2018,3Q,3; 2018,2Q,7; 2017,4Q,102
E10.59 Type 1 diabetes mellitus with other circulatory complications HCC Rx ESR COM Q

✓5ᵗʰ **E10.6**   **Type 1 diabetes mellitus with other specified complications**

✓6ᵗʰ   **E10.61**   **Type 1 diabetes mellitus with diabetic arthropathy**

E10.610   **Type 1 diabetes mellitus with diabetic neuropathic arthropathy**   HCC Rx ESR COM Q

Type 1 diabetes mellitus with Charcôt's joints

DEF: Charcot's joint: Progressive neurologic arthropathy in which chronic degeneration of joints in the weight-bearing areas with peripheral hypertrophy occurs as a complication of a neuropathy disorder. Supporting structures relax from a loss of sensation resulting in chronic joint instability.

E10.618   **Type 1 diabetes mellitus with other diabetic arthropathy**   HCC Rx ESR COM Q

AHA: 2018,2Q,6

✓6ᵗʰ   **E10.62**   **Type 1 diabetes mellitus with skin complications**

E10.620   **Type 1 diabetes mellitus with diabetic dermatitis**   HCC Rx ESR COM Q

Type 1 diabetes mellitus with diabetic necrobiosis lipoidica

E10.621   **Type 1 diabetes mellitus with foot ulcer**   HCC Rx ESR COM Q

Use additional code to identify site of ulcer (L97.4-, L97.5-)

AHA: 2020,2Q,19

TIP: Do not assign a code for diabetic ulcer when the ulcer is closed/resolved or to report history of diabetic ulcers; Z86.31 Personal history of diabetic foot ulcer, may be assigned.

E10.622   **Type 1 diabetes mellitus with other skin ulcer**   HCC Rx ESR COM Q

Use additional code to identify site of ulcer (L97.1-L97.9, L98.41-L98.49)

AHA: 2021,1Q,7; 2017,4Q,17

E10.628   **Type 1 diabetes mellitus with other skin complications**   HCC Rx ESR COM Q

✓6ᵗʰ   **E10.63**   **Type 1 diabetes mellitus with oral complications**

E10.630   **Type 1 diabetes mellitus with periodontal disease**   HCC Rx ESR COM Q

E10.638   **Type 1 diabetes mellitus with other oral complications**   HCC Rx ESR COM Q

✓6ᵗʰ   **E10.64**   **Type 1 diabetes mellitus with hypoglycemia**

AHA: 2017,1Q,42

E10.641   **Type 1 diabetes mellitus with hypoglycemia with coma**   HCC Rx ESR COM Q

E10.649   **Type 1 diabetes mellitus with hypoglycemia without coma**   HCC Rx ESR COM Q

AHA: 2016,3Q,42; 2016,1Q,13; 2015,3Q,21

E10.65   **Type 1 diabetes mellitus with hyperglycemia**   HCC Rx ESR COM Q

AHA: 2022,1Q,28; 2017,1Q,42; 2013,3Q,20

E10.69   **Type 1 diabetes mellitus with other specified complication**   HCC Rx ESR COM Q

Use additional code to identify complication

AHA: 2022,1Q,28; 2016,4Q,141; 2016,1Q,13

[handwritten margin note: adhesive Capsulitis]

E10.8   **Type 1 diabetes mellitus with unspecified complications**   HCC Rx ESR COM Q

E10.9   **Type 1 diabetes mellitus without complications**   HCC Rx ESR COM Q

AHA: 2020,2Q,18

✓4ᵗʰ **E11**   **Type 2 diabetes mellitus**   *[handwritten: unspecified]*

INCLUDES   diabetes (mellitus) due to insulin secretory defect
diabetes NOS
insulin resistant diabetes (mellitus)

Use additional code to identify control using:
insulin (Z79.4)
oral antidiabetic drugs (Z79.84)
oral hypoglycemic drugs (Z79.84)

EXCLUDES 1   *diabetes mellitus due to underlying condition (E08.-)*
drug or chemical induced diabetes mellitus (E09.-)
gestational diabetes (O24.4-)
neonatal diabetes mellitus (P70.2)
postpancreatectomy diabetes mellitus (E13.-)
postprocedural diabetes mellitus (E13.-)
secondary diabetes mellitus NEC (E13.-)
type 1 diabetes mellitus (E10.-)

AHA: 2020,3Q,30; 2020,1Q,12; 2016,2Q,10; 2013,1Q,26

✓5ᵗʰ **E11.0**   **Type 2 diabetes mellitus with hyperosmolarity**

DEF: Diabetic hyperosmolarity: Extremely high levels of glucose in the blood without ketones.

E11.00   **Type 2 diabetes mellitus with hyperosmolarity without nonketotic hyperglycemic-hyperosmolar coma (NKHHC)**   HCC Rx ESR COM Q

AHA: 2022,1Q,28

E11.01   **Type 2 diabetes mellitus with hyperosmolarity with coma**   HCC Rx ESR COM Q

✓5ᵗʰ **E11.1**   **Type 2 diabetes mellitus with ketoacidosis**

AHA: 2017,4Q,6

DEF: Diabetic ketoacidosis: Potentially life-threatening complication due to a shortage of insulin in which the body switches to burning fatty acids and producing acidic ketone bodies.

E11.10   **Type 2 diabetes mellitus with ketoacidosis without coma**   HCC Rx ESR COM

E11.11   **Type 2 diabetes mellitus with ketoacidosis with coma**   HCC Rx ESR COM

✓5ᵗʰ **E11.2**   **Type 2 diabetes mellitus with kidney complications**

AHA: 2019,3Q,3; 2018,4Q,88

E11.21   **Type 2 diabetes mellitus with diabetic nephropathy**   HCC Rx ESR COM Q

Type 2 diabetes mellitus with intercapillary glomerulosclerosis

Type 2 diabetes mellitus with intracapillary glomerulonephrosis

Type 2 diabetes mellitus with Kimmelstiel-Wilson disease

E11.22   **Type 2 diabetes mellitus with diabetic chronic kidney disease**   HCC Rx ESR COM Q

Use additional code to identify stage of chronic kidney disease (N18.1-N18.6)

E11.29   **Type 2 diabetes mellitus with other diabetic kidney complication**   HCC Rx ESR COM Q

Type 2 diabetes mellitus with renal tubular degeneration

✓5ᵗʰ **E11.3**   **Type 2 diabetes mellitus with ophthalmic complications**

AHA: 2016,4Q,11-13

One of the following 7th characters is to be assigned to codes in subcategories E11.32, E11.33, E11.34, E11.35, and E11.37 to designate laterality of the disease:

1   right eye
2   left eye
3   bilateral
9   unspecified eye

✓6ᵗʰ   **E11.31**   **Type 2 diabetes mellitus with unspecified diabetic retinopathy**

DEF: Diabetic retinopathy: Diabetic complication from damage to the retinal vessels resulting in vision problems that can progress to blindness.

E11.311   **Type 2 diabetes mellitus with unspecified diabetic retinopathy with macular edema**   HCC Rx ESR COM Q

E11.319   **Type 2 diabetes mellitus with unspecified diabetic retinopathy without macular edema**   HCC Rx ESR COM Q

Chapter 4. Endocrine, Nutritional and Metabolic Diseases

E11.32–E11.9

✓6ᵗʰ **E11.32 Type 2 diabetes mellitus with** mild nonproliferative **diabetic** retinopathy
Type 2 diabetes mellitus with nonproliferative diabetic retinopathy NOS

✓7ᵗʰ **E11.321 Type 2 diabetes mellitus with mild nonproliferative diabetic retinopathy** with macular edema HCC Rx ESR COM Q

✓7ᵗʰ **E11.329 Type 2 diabetes mellitus with mild nonproliferative diabetic retinopathy** without macular edema HCC Rx ESR COM Q

✓6ᵗʰ **E11.33 Type 2 diabetes mellitus with** moderate nonproliferative **diabetic** retinopathy

✓7ᵗʰ **E11.331 Type 2 diabetes mellitus with moderate nonproliferative diabetic retinopathy** with macular edema HCC Rx ESR COM Q

✓7ᵗʰ **E11.339 Type 2 diabetes mellitus with moderate nonproliferative diabetic retinopathy** without macular edema HCC Rx ESR COM Q

✓6ᵗʰ **E11.34 Type 2 diabetes mellitus with** severe nonproliferative **diabetic** retinopathy

✓7ᵗʰ **E11.341 Type 2 diabetes mellitus with severe nonproliferative diabetic retinopathy** with macular edema HCC Rx ESR COM Q

✓7ᵗʰ **E11.349 Type 2 diabetes mellitus with severe nonproliferative diabetic retinopathy** without macular edema HCC Rx ESR COM Q

✓6ᵗʰ **E11.35 Type 2 diabetes mellitus with** proliferative **diabetic** retinopathy

✓7ᵗʰ **E11.351 Type 2 diabetes mellitus with proliferative diabetic retinopathy** with macular edema HCC Rx ESR COM Q

✓7ᵗʰ **E11.352 Type 2 diabetes mellitus with proliferative diabetic retinopathy** with traction retinal detachment involving the macula HCC Rx ESR COM Q

✓7ᵗʰ **E11.353 Type 2 diabetes mellitus with proliferative diabetic retinopathy** with traction retinal detachment not involving the macula HCC Rx ESR COM Q

✓7ᵗʰ **E11.354 Type 2 diabetes mellitus with proliferative diabetic retinopathy** with combined traction retinal detachment and rhegmatogenous retinal detachment HCC Rx ESR COM Q

✓7ᵗʰ **E11.355 Type 2 diabetes mellitus** with stable proliferative diabetic retinopathy HCC Rx ESR COM Q

✓7ᵗʰ **E11.359 Type 2 diabetes mellitus with proliferative diabetic retinopathy** without macular edema HCC Rx ESR COM Q

E11.36 Type 2 diabetes mellitus with diabetic cataract HCC Rx ESR COM Q
AHA: 2019,2Q,30-31; 2016,4Q,142

✓x7ᵗʰ **E11.37 Type 2 diabetes mellitus with diabetic** macular edema, resolved following treatment HCC Rx ESR COM Q

E11.39 Type 2 diabetes mellitus with other diabetic ophthalmic complication HCC Rx ESR COM Q
Use additional code to identify manifestation, such as:
diabetic glaucoma (H40-H42)

✓5ᵗʰ **E11.4 Type 2 diabetes mellitus with** neurological complications

E11.40 Type 2 diabetes mellitus with diabetic neuropathy, unspecified HCC Rx ESR COM Q
AHA: 2013,4Q,129

E11.41 Type 2 diabetes mellitus with diabetic mononeuropathy HCC Rx ESR COM Q

E11.42 Type 2 diabetes mellitus with diabetic polyneuropathy HCC Rx ESR COM Q
Type 2 diabetes mellitus with diabetic neuralgia
AHA: 2020,1Q,12

E11.43 Type 2 diabetes mellitus with diabetic autonomic (poly)neuropathy HCC Rx ESR COM Q
Type 2 diabetes mellitus with diabetic gastroparesis
AHA: 2013,4Q,114

E11.44 Type 2 diabetes mellitus with diabetic amyotrophy HCC Rx ESR COM Q

E11.49 Type 2 diabetes mellitus with other diabetic neurological complication HCC Rx ESR COM Q

✓5ᵗʰ **E11.5 Type 2 diabetes mellitus with** circulatory complications

E11.51 Type 2 diabetes mellitus with diabetic peripheral angiopathy without gangrene HCC Rx ESR COM Q
AHA: 2018,3Q,3-4; 2018,2Q,7

E11.52 Type 2 diabetes mellitus with diabetic peripheral angiopathy with gangrene HCC Rx ESR COM Q
Type 2 diabetes mellitus with diabetic gangrene
AHA: 2020,2Q,18; 2018,3Q,3; 2018,2Q,7; 2017,4Q,102

E11.59 Type 2 diabetes mellitus with other circulatory complications HCC Rx ESR COM Q

✓5ᵗʰ **E11.6 Type 2 diabetes mellitus with other specified complications**

✓6ᵗʰ **E11.61 Type 2 diabetes mellitus with diabetic** arthropathy

E11.610 Type 2 diabetes mellitus with diabetic neuropathic arthropathy HCC Rx ESR COM Q
Type 2 diabetes mellitus with Charcôt's joints
DEF: Charcot's joint: Progressive neurologic arthropathy in which chronic degeneration of joints in the weight-bearing areas with peripheral hypertrophy occurs as a complication of a neuropathy disorder. Supporting structures relax from a loss of sensation resulting in chronic joint instability.

E11.618 Type 2 diabetes mellitus with other diabetic arthropathy HCC Rx ESR COM Q
AHA: 2018,2Q,6

✓6ᵗʰ **E11.62 Type 2 diabetes mellitus with** skin complications

E11.620 Type 2 diabetes mellitus with diabetic dermatitis HCC Rx ESR COM Q
Type 2 diabetes mellitus with diabetic necrobiosis lipoidica

E11.621 Type 2 diabetes mellitus with foot ulcer HCC Rx ESR COM Q
Use additional code to identify site of ulcer (L97.4-, L97.5-)
AHA: 2020,2Q,19; 2020,1Q,12
TIP: Do not assign a code for diabetic ulcer when the ulcer is closed/resolved or to report history of diabetic ulcers; Z86.31 Personal history of diabetic foot ulcer, may be assigned.

E11.622 Type 2 diabetes mellitus with other skin ulcer HCC Rx ESR COM Q
Use additional code to identify site of ulcer (L97.1-L97.9, L98.41-L98.49)
AHA: 2021,1Q,7; 2017,4Q,17

E11.628 Type 2 diabetes mellitus with other skin complications HCC Rx ESR COM Q

✓6ᵗʰ **E11.63 Type 2 diabetes mellitus with** oral complications

E11.630 Type 2 diabetes mellitus with periodontal disease HCC Rx ESR COM Q

E11.638 Type 2 diabetes mellitus with other oral complications HCC Rx ESR COM Q

✓6ᵗʰ **E11.64 Type 2 diabetes mellitus with** hypoglycemia
AHA: 2017,1Q,42

E11.641 Type 2 diabetes mellitus with hypoglycemia with coma HCC Rx ESR COM Q

E11.649 Type 2 diabetes mellitus with hypoglycemia without coma HCC Rx ESR COM Q
AHA: 2016,3Q,42; 2015,3Q,21

E11.65 Type 2 diabetes mellitus with hyperglycemia HCC Rx ESR COM Q
AHA: 2022,1Q,28; 2017,1Q,42; 2013,3Q,20

E11.69 Type 2 diabetes mellitus with other specified complication HCC Rx ESR COM Q
Use additional code to identify complication
AHA: 2020,1Q,12; 2016,4Q,141; 2016,1Q,13

E11.8 Type 2 diabetes mellitus with unspecified complications HCC Rx ESR COM Q

E11.9 Type 2 diabetes mellitus without complications HCC Rx ESR COM Q
AHA: 2020,2Q,18

[handwritten: Foot Ulcer]

✓4th **E13** **Other specified diabetes mellitus**

Secondary DM

   [INCLUDES] diabetes mellitus due to genetic defects of beta-cell function
   diabetes mellitus due to genetic defects in insulin action
   postpancreatectomy diabetes mellitus
   postprocedural diabetes mellitus
   secondary diabetes mellitus NEC

Use additional code to identify control using:
   insulin (Z79.4)
   oral antidiabetic drugs (Z79.84)
   oral hypoglycemic drugs (Z79.84)

[EXCLUDES 1] diabetes (mellitus) due to autoimmune process (E10.-)
   diabetes (mellitus) due to immune mediated pancreatic islet beta-cell destruction (E10.-)
   diabetes mellitus due to underlying condition (E08.-)
   drug or chemical induced diabetes mellitus (E09.-)
   gestational diabetes (O24.4-)
   neonatal diabetes mellitus (P70.2)
   type 1 diabetes mellitus (E10.-)

AHA: 2018,3Q,4; 2016,1Q,11-13

TIP: Use this category when the diabetes is documented as diabetes type 1.5. Synonymous terms used in the documentation may also include combined diabetes type 1 and type 2, latent autoimmune diabetes of adults (LADA), slow-progressing type 1 diabetes, or double diabetes.

TIP: When postprocedural or postpancreatectomy hypoinsulinemia (E89.1) is documented with postprocedural or postpancreatectomy diabetes mellitus (E13.-), code E89.1 should be sequenced first.

✓5th **E13.0** **Other specified diabetes mellitus with** hyperosmolarity
   DEF: Diabetic hyperosmolarity: Extremely high levels of glucose in the blood without ketones.

   E13.00 **Other specified diabetes mellitus with hyperosmolarity** without nonketotic hyperglycemic-hyperosmolar coma (NKHHC) HCC Rx ESR COM Q
      [EXCLUDES 2] type 2 diabetes mellitus (E11.-)

   E13.01 **Other specified diabetes mellitus with hyperosmolarity** with coma HCC Rx ESR COM Q

✓5th **E13.1** **Other specified diabetes mellitus with** ketoacidosis
   AHA: 2016,2Q,10; 2013,1Q,26
   DEF: Diabetic ketoacidosis: Potentially life-threatening complication due to a shortage of insulin in which the body switches to burning fatty acids and producing acidic ketone bodies.

   E13.10 **Other specified diabetes mellitus with ketoacidosis** without coma HCC Rx ESR COM Q

   E13.11 **Other specified diabetes mellitus with ketoacidosis** with coma HCC Rx ESR COM Q

✓5th **E13.2** **Other specified diabetes mellitus with** kidney complications
   AHA: 2019,3Q,3; 2018,4Q,88

   E13.21 **Other specified diabetes mellitus with diabetic nephropathy** HCC Rx ESR COM Q
      Other specified diabetes mellitus with intercapillary glomerulosclerosis
      Other specified diabetes mellitus with intracapillary glomerulonephrosis
      Other specified diabetes mellitus with Kimmelstiel-Wilson disease

   E13.22 **Other specified diabetes mellitus with diabetic chronic kidney disease** HCC Rx ESR COM Q
      Use additional code to identify stage of chronic kidney disease (N18.1-N18.6)

   E13.29 **Other specified diabetes mellitus with other diabetic kidney complication** HCC Rx ESR COM Q
      Other specified diabetes mellitus with renal tubular degeneration

✓5th **E13.3** **Other specified diabetes mellitus with** ophthalmic complications
   AHA: 2016,4Q,11-13

   One of the following 7th characters is to be assigned to codes in subcategories E13.32, E13.33, E13.34, E13.35, and E13.37 to designate laterality of the disease:
   1 right eye
   2 left eye
   3 bilateral
   9 unspecified eye

✓6th **E13.31** **Other specified diabetes mellitus with unspecified diabetic** retinopathy
   DEF: Diabetic retinopathy: Diabetic complication from damage to the retinal vessels resulting in vision problems that can progress to blindness.

   E13.311 **Other specified diabetes mellitus with unspecified diabetic retinopathy** with macular edema HCC Rx ESR COM Q

   E13.319 **Other specified diabetes mellitus with unspecified diabetic retinopathy** without macular edema HCC Rx ESR COM Q

✓6th **E13.32** **Other specified diabetes mellitus with** mild nonproliferative **diabetic** retinopathy
   Other specified diabetes mellitus with nonproliferative diabetic retinopathy NOS

   ✓7th **E13.321** **Other specified diabetes mellitus with mild nonproliferative diabetic retinopathy** with macular edema HCC Rx ESR COM Q

   ✓7th **E13.329** **Other specified diabetes mellitus with mild nonproliferative diabetic retinopathy** without macular edema HCC Rx ESR COM Q

✓6th **E13.33** **Other specified diabetes mellitus with** moderate nonproliferative **diabetic** retinopathy

   ✓7th **E13.331** **Other specified diabetes mellitus with moderate nonproliferative diabetic retinopathy** with macular edema HCC Rx ESR COM Q

   ✓7th **E13.339** **Other specified diabetes mellitus with moderate nonproliferative diabetic retinopathy** without macular edema HCC Rx ESR COM Q

✓6th **E13.34** **Other specified diabetes mellitus with** severe nonproliferative **diabetic** retinopathy

   ✓7th **E13.341** **Other specified diabetes mellitus with severe nonproliferative diabetic retinopathy** with macular edema HCC Rx ESR COM Q

   ✓7th **E13.349** **Other specified diabetes mellitus with severe nonproliferative diabetic retinopathy** without macular edema HCC Rx ESR COM Q

✓6th **E13.35** **Other specified diabetes mellitus with** proliferative **diabetic** retinopathy

   ✓7th **E13.351** **Other specified diabetes mellitus with proliferative diabetic retinopathy** with macular edema HCC Rx ESR COM Q

   ✓7th **E13.352** **Other specified diabetes mellitus with proliferative diabetic retinopathy** with traction retinal detachment involving the macula HCC Rx ESR COM Q

   ✓7th **E13.353** **Other specified diabetes mellitus with proliferative diabetic retinopathy** with traction retinal detachment not involving the macula HCC Rx ESR COM Q

   ✓7th **E13.354** **Other specified diabetes mellitus with proliferative diabetic retinopathy** with combined traction retinal detachment and rhegmatogenous retinal detachment HCC Rx ESR COM Q

   ✓7th **E13.355** **Other specified diabetes mellitus with** stable **proliferative diabetic retinopathy** HCC Rx ESR COM Q

   ✓7th **E13.359** **Other specified diabetes mellitus with proliferative diabetic retinopathy** without macular edema HCC Rx ESR COM Q

   E13.36 **Other specified diabetes mellitus with diabetic cataract** HCC Rx ESR COM Q
      AHA: 2019,2Q,30-31; 2016,4Q,142

☑ Additional Character Required   ✓x7th Placeholder Alert   Manifestation   Unspecified Dx   Q QPP   UPD Unacceptable PDx

Chapter 4. Endocrine, Nutritional and Metabolic Diseases   E13.37–E16.4

✓x 7th   **E13.37**   **Other specified diabetes mellitus with diabetic macular edema, resolved following treatment**   HCC Rx ESR COM Q

E13.39   **Other specified diabetes mellitus with other diabetic ophthalmic complication**   HCC Rx ESR COM Q
- Use additional code to identify manifestation, such as:
  - diabetic glaucoma (H40-H42)

✓5th   **E13.4**   **Other specified diabetes mellitus with neurological complications**

   E13.40   **Other specified diabetes mellitus with diabetic neuropathy, unspecified**   HCC Rx ESR COM Q

   E13.41   **Other specified diabetes mellitus with diabetic mononeuropathy**   HCC Rx ESR COM Q

   E13.42   **Other specified diabetes mellitus with diabetic polyneuropathy**   HCC Rx ESR COM Q
- Other specified diabetes mellitus with diabetic neuralgia

   E13.43   **Other specified diabetes mellitus with diabetic autonomic (poly)neuropathy**   HCC Rx ESR COM Q
- Other specified diabetes mellitus with diabetic gastroparesis
- **AHA:** 2013,4Q,114

   E13.44   **Other specified diabetes mellitus with diabetic amyotrophy**   HCC Rx ESR COM Q

   E13.49   **Other specified diabetes mellitus with other diabetic neurological complication**   HCC Rx ESR COM Q

✓5th   **E13.5**   **Other specified diabetes mellitus with circulatory complications**

   E13.51   **Other specified diabetes mellitus with diabetic peripheral angiopathy without gangrene**   HCC Rx ESR COM Q
- **AHA:** 2018,3Q,3-4; 2018,2Q,7

   E13.52   **Other specified diabetes mellitus with diabetic peripheral angiopathy with gangrene**   HCC Rx ESR COM Q
- Other specified diabetes mellitus with diabetic gangrene
- **AHA:** 2020,2Q,18; 2018,3Q,3; 2018,2Q,7; 2017,4Q,102

   E13.59   **Other specified diabetes mellitus with other circulatory complications**   HCC Rx ESR COM Q

✓5th   **E13.6**   **Other specified diabetes mellitus with other specified complications**

✓6th   **E13.61**   **Other specified diabetes mellitus with diabetic arthropathy**

     E13.610   **Other specified diabetes mellitus with diabetic neuropathic arthropathy**   HCC Rx ESR COM Q
- Other specified diabetes mellitus with Charcôt's joints
- **DEF:** Charcôt's joint: Progressive neurologic arthropathy in which chronic degeneration of joints in the weight-bearing areas with peripheral hypertrophy occurs as a complication of a neuropathy disorder. Supporting structures relax from a loss of sensation resulting in chronic joint instability.

     E13.618   **Other specified diabetes mellitus with other diabetic arthropathy**   HCC Rx ESR COM Q
- **AHA:** 2018,2Q,6

✓6th   **E13.62**   **Other specified diabetes mellitus with skin complications**

     E13.620   **Other specified diabetes mellitus with diabetic dermatitis**   HCC Rx ESR COM Q
- Other specified diabetes mellitus with diabetic necrobiosis lipoidica

     E13.621   **Other specified diabetes mellitus with foot ulcer**   HCC Rx ESR COM Q
- Use additional code to identify site of ulcer (L97.4-, L97.5-)
- **AHA:** 2020,2Q,19
- **TIP:** Do not assign a code for diabetic ulcer when the ulcer is closed/resolved or to report history of diabetic ulcers; Z86.31 Personal history of diabetic foot ulcer, may be assigned.

     E13.622   **Other specified diabetes mellitus with other skin ulcer**   HCC Rx ESR COM Q
- Use additional code to identify site of ulcer (L97.1-L97.9, L98.41-L98.49)
- **AHA:** 2021,1Q,7; 2017,4Q,17

     E13.628   **Other specified diabetes mellitus with other skin complications**   HCC Rx ESR COM Q

✓6th   **E13.63**   **Other specified diabetes mellitus with oral complications**

     E13.630   **Other specified diabetes mellitus with periodontal disease**   HCC Rx ESR COM Q

     E13.638   **Other specified diabetes mellitus with other oral complications**   HCC Rx ESR COM Q

✓6th   **E13.64**   **Other specified diabetes mellitus with hypoglycemia**
- **AHA:** 2017,1Q,42

     E13.641   **Other specified diabetes mellitus with hypoglycemia with coma**   HCC Rx ESR COM Q

     E13.649   **Other specified diabetes mellitus with hypoglycemia without coma**   HCC Rx ESR COM Q
- **AHA:** 2016,3Q,42; 2015,3Q,21

   E13.65   **Other specified diabetes mellitus with hyperglycemia**   HCC Rx ESR COM Q
- **AHA:** 2017,1Q,42; 2013,3Q,20

   E13.69   **Other specified diabetes mellitus with other specified complication**   HCC Rx ESR COM Q
- Use additional code to identify complication
- **AHA:** 2016,4Q,141; 2016,1Q,13

E13.8   **Other specified diabetes mellitus with unspecified complications**   HCC Rx ESR COM Q

E13.9   **Other specified diabetes mellitus without complications**   HCC Rx ESR COM Q
- **AHA:** 2020,2Q,18

Other disorders of glucose regulation and pancreatic internal secretion (E15-E16)

E15   **Nondiabetic hypoglycemic coma**   HCC ESR COM
- INCLUDES   drug-induced insulin coma in nondiabetic
  - hyperinsulinism with hypoglycemic coma
  - hypoglycemic coma NOS

✓4th   **E16**   **Other disorders of pancreatic internal secretion**

   E16.0   **Drug-induced hypoglycemia without coma**
- EXCLUDES 1   diabetes with hypoglycemia without coma (E09.649)
- Use additional code for adverse effect, if applicable, to identify drug (T36-T50 with fifth or sixth character 5)

   E16.1   **Other hypoglycemia**
- Functional hyperinsulinism
- Functional nonhyperinsulinemic hypoglycemia
- Hyperinsulinism NOS
- Hyperplasia of pancreatic islet beta cells NOS
- EXCLUDES 1   diabetes with hypoglycemia (E08.649, E10.649, E11.649, E13.649)
  - hypoglycemia in infant of diabetic mother (P70.1)
  - neonatal hypoglycemia (P70.4)

   E16.2   **Hypoglycemia, unspecified**
- EXCLUDES 1   diabetes with hypoglycemia (E08.649, E10.649, E11.649, E13.649)
- **AHA:** 2016,3Q,42
- **TIP:** Assign for nondiabetic hypoglycemic encephalopathy not further clarified in the documentation.

   E16.3   **Increased secretion of glucagon**   Rx
- Hyperplasia of pancreatic endocrine cells with glucagon excess

   E16.4   **Increased secretion of gastrin**   Rx
- Hypergastrinemia
- Hyperplasia of pancreatic endocrine cells with gastrin excess
- Zollinger-Ellison syndrome

E16.8 Other specified disorders of pancreatic internal secretion `Rx`
  Increased secretion from endocrine pancreas of growth hormone-releasing hormone
  Increased secretion from endocrine pancreas of pancreatic polypeptide
  Increased secretion from endocrine pancreas of somatostatin
  Increased secretion from endocrine pancreas of vasoactive-intestinal polypeptide

E16.9 Disorder of pancreatic internal secretion, unspecified `Rx`
  Islet-cell hyperplasia NOS
  Pancreatic endocrine cell hyperplasia NOS

Disorders of other endocrine glands (E20-E35)

  EXCLUDES 1   galactorrhea (N64.3)
                gynecomastia (N62)

✓4ᵗʰ **E20 Hypoparathyroidism**
  EXCLUDES 1   Di George's syndrome (D82.1)
                postprocedural hypoparathyroidism (E89.2)
                tetany NOS (R29.0)
                transitory neonatal hypoparathyroidism (P71.4)

E20.0 Idiopathic hypoparathyroidism `HCC` `Rx` `ESR` `COM`
  DEF: Abnormally low secretion of parathyroid hormones, with unknown cause, which triggers decreased calcium and increased phosphorus in the blood that can result in cataracts, muscle cramps, tetany, tingling, or burning in the lips, fingers, and toes.

E20.1 Pseudohypoparathyroidism
E20.8 Other hypoparathyroidism `HCC` `Rx` `ESR` `COM`
E20.9 Hypoparathyroidism, unspecified `HCC` `Rx` `ESR` `COM`
  Parathyroid tetany

✓4ᵗʰ **E21 Hyperparathyroidism and other disorders of parathyroid gland**
  EXCLUDES 1   adult osteomalacia (M83.-)
                ectopic hyperparathyroidism (E34.2)
                hungry bone syndrome (E83.81)
                infantile and juvenile osteomalacia (E55.0)
  EXCLUDES 2   familial hypocalciuric hypercalcemia (E83.52)

E21.0 Primary hyperparathyroidism `HCC` `Rx` `ESR` `COM`
  Hyperplasia of parathyroid
  Osteitis fibrosa cystica generalisata [von Recklinghausen's disease of bone]
  DEF: Parathyroid dysfunction commonly caused by hyperplasia of two or more glands. Symptoms include hypercalcemia and increased parathyroid hormone levels.

E21.1 Secondary hyperparathyroidism, not elsewhere classified `HCC` `Rx` `ESR` `COM`
  EXCLUDES 1   secondary hyperparathyroidism of renal origin (N25.81)

E21.2 Other hyperparathyroidism `HCC` `Rx` `ESR` `COM`
  Tertiary hyperparathyroidism
  EXCLUDES 1   familial hypocalciuric hypercalcemia (E83.52)

E21.3 Hyperparathyroidism, unspecified `HCC` `Rx` `ESR` `COM`
E21.4 Other specified disorders of parathyroid gland `HCC` `Rx` `ESR` `COM`
E21.5 Disorder of parathyroid gland, unspecified `HCC` `Rx` `ESR` `COM`

✓4ᵗʰ **E22 Hyperfunction of pituitary gland**
  EXCLUDES 1   Cushing's syndrome (E24.-)
                Nelson's syndrome (E24.1)
                overproduction of ACTH not associated with Cushing's disease (E27.0)
                overproduction of pituitary ACTH (E24.0)
                overproduction of thyroid-stimulating hormone (E05.8-)

E22.0 Acromegaly and pituitary gigantism `HCC` `Rx` `ESR` `COM`
  Overproduction of growth hormone
  EXCLUDES 1   constitutional gigantism (E34.4)
                constitutional tall stature (E34.4)
                increased secretion from endocrine pancreas of growth hormone-releasing hormone (E16.8)
  DEF: Acromegaly: Chronic condition caused by overproduction of the pituitary growth hormone resulting in enlarged skeletal parts and facial features.

E22.1 Hyperprolactinemia `HCC` `Rx` `ESR` `COM`
  Use additional code for adverse effect, if applicable, to identify drug (T36-T50 with fifth or sixth character 5)

E22.2 Syndrome of inappropriate secretion of antidiuretic hormone `HCC` `Rx` `ESR` `COM`

E22.8 Other hyperfunction of pituitary gland `HCC` `Rx` `ESR` `COM`
  Central precocious puberty

E22.9 Hyperfunction of pituitary gland, unspecified `HCC` `Rx` `ESR` `COM`

✓4ᵗʰ **E23 Hypofunction and other disorders of the pituitary gland**
  INCLUDES   the listed conditions whether the disorder is in the pituitary or the hypothalamus
  EXCLUDES 1   postprocedural hypopituitarism (E89.3)
              ▶short stature due to endocrine disorder (E34.3-)◀

E23.0 Hypopituitarism `HCC` `Rx` `ESR` `COM`
  Fertile eunuch syndrome
  Hypogonadotropic hypogonadism
  Idiopathic growth hormone deficiency
  Isolated deficiency of gonadotropin
  Isolated deficiency of growth hormone
  Isolated deficiency of pituitary hormone
  Kallmann's syndrome
  Lorain-Levi short stature
  Necrosis of pituitary gland (postpartum)
  Panhypopituitarism
  Pituitary cachexia
  Pituitary insufficiency NOS
  Pituitary short stature
  Sheehan's syndrome
  Simmonds' disease

E23.1 Drug-induced hypopituitarism `HCC` `Rx` `ESR` `COM`
  Use additional code for adverse effect, if applicable, to identify drug (T36-T50 with fifth or sixth character 5)

E23.2 Diabetes insipidus `HCC` `Rx` `ESR` `COM`
  EXCLUDES 1   nephrogenic diabetes insipidus (N25.1)

E23.3 Hypothalamic dysfunction, not elsewhere classified `HCC` `Rx` `ESR` `COM`
  EXCLUDES 1   Prader-Willi syndrome (Q87.11)
                Russell-Silver syndrome (Q87.19)

E23.6 Other disorders of pituitary gland `HCC` `Rx` `ESR` `COM`
  Abscess of pituitary
  Adiposogenital dystrophy

E23.7 Disorder of pituitary gland, unspecified `HCC` `Rx` `ESR` `COM`

✓4ᵗʰ **E24 Cushing's syndrome**
  EXCLUDES 1   congenital adrenal hyperplasia (E25.0)
  DEF: Abdominal striae, acne, hypertension, decreased carbohydrate tolerance, moon face, obesity, protein catabolism, and psychiatric disturbances resulting from increased adrenocortical secretion of cortisol caused by ACTH-dependent adrenocortical hyperplasia or tumor, or by steroid effects.

E24.0 Pituitary-dependent Cushing's disease `HCC` `Rx` `ESR` `COM`
  Overproduction of pituitary ACTH
  Pituitary-dependent hypercorticalism

E24.1 Nelson's syndrome `HCC` `Rx` `ESR` `COM`
E24.2 Drug-induced Cushing's syndrome `HCC` `Rx` `ESR` `COM`
  Use additional code for adverse effect, if applicable, to identify drug (T36-T50 with fifth or sixth character 5)

E24.3 Ectopic ACTH syndrome `HCC` `Rx` `ESR` `COM`
E24.4 Alcohol-induced pseudo-Cushing's syndrome `HCC` `Rx` `ESR` `COM`
E24.8 Other Cushing's syndrome `HCC` `Rx` `ESR` `COM`
E24.9 Cushing's syndrome, unspecified `HCC` `Rx` `ESR` `COM`

✓4ᵗʰ E25 Adrenogenital disorders

INCLUDES   adrenogenital syndromes, virilizing or feminizing, whether acquired or due to adrenal hyperplasia
consequent on inborn enzyme defects in hormone synthesis
female adrenal pseudohermaphroditism
female heterosexual precocious pseudopuberty
male isosexual precocious pseudopuberty
male macrogenitosomia praecox
male sexual precocity with adrenal hyperplasia
male virilization (female)

EXCLUDES 1   *indeterminate sex and pseudohermaphroditism (Q56)*
chromosomal abnormalities (Q90-Q99)

E25.0 Congenital adrenogenital disorders associated with enzyme deficiency   HCC Rx ESR COM
Congenital adrenal hyperplasia
21-Hydroxylase deficiency
Salt-losing congenital adrenal hyperplasia

E25.8 Other adrenogenital disorders   HCC Rx ESR COM
Idiopathic adrenogenital disorder
Use additional code for adverse effect, if applicable, to identify drug (T36-T50 with fifth or sixth character 5)

E25.9 Adrenogenital disorder, unspecified   HCC Rx ESR COM
Adrenogenital syndrome NOS

✓4ᵗʰ E26 Hyperaldosteronism

✓5ᵗʰ E26.0 Primary hyperaldosteronism

E26.01 Conn's syndrome   HCC Rx ESR COM
Code also adrenal adenoma (D35.0-)

E26.02 Glucocorticoid-remediable aldosteronism   HCC Rx ESR COM
Familial aldosteronism type I
DEF: Rare autosomal dominant familial form of primary aldosteronism in which the secretion of aldosterone is under the influence of adrenocorticotrophic hormone (ACTH) rather than the renin-angiotensin mechanism. Moderate hypersecretion of aldosterone and suppressed plasma renin activity that are rapidly reversed by administration of glucosteroids. Symptoms include hypertension and mild hypokalemia.

E26.09 Other primary hyperaldosteronism   HCC Rx ESR COM
Primary aldosteronism due to adrenal hyperplasia (bilateral)

E26.1 Secondary hyperaldosteronism   HCC Rx ESR COM

✓5ᵗʰ E26.8 Other hyperaldosteronism

E26.81 Bartter's syndrome   HCC Rx ESR COM
E26.89 Other hyperaldosteronism   HCC Rx ESR COM

E26.9 Hyperaldosteronism, unspecified   HCC Rx ESR COM
Aldosteronism NOS
Hyperaldosteronism NOS

✓4ᵗʰ E27 Other disorders of adrenal gland

E27.0 Other adrenocortical overactivity   HCC Rx ESR COM
Overproduction of ACTH, not associated with Cushing's disease
Premature adrenarche
EXCLUDES 1   *Cushing's syndrome (E24.-)*

E27.1 Primary adrenocortical insufficiency   HCC Rx ESR COM
Addison's disease
Autoimmune adrenalitis
EXCLUDES 1   *Addison only phenotype adrenoleukodystrophy (E71.528)*
amyloidosis (E85.-)
tuberculous Addison's disease (A18.7)
Waterhouse-Friderichsen syndrome (A39.1)

E27.2 Addisonian crisis   HCC Rx ESR COM
Adrenal crisis
Adrenocortical crisis
DEF: Life-threatening condition that occurs when there is not enough cortisol excreted from the adrenal glands. This condition may be due to injury to the adrenal glands or to the pituitary gland, which controls adrenal hormone secretion, or when a patient stops hydrocortisone treatment too quickly or too early.

E27.3 Drug-induced adrenocortical insufficiency   HCC Rx ESR COM
Use additional code for adverse effect, if applicable, to identify drug (T36-T50 with fifth or sixth character 5)

✓5ᵗʰ E27.4 Other and unspecified adrenocortical insufficiency
EXCLUDES 1   *adrenoleukodystrophy [Addison-Schilder] (E71.528)*
Waterhouse-Friderichsen syndrome (A39.1)

E27.40 Unspecified adrenocortical insufficiency   HCC Rx ESR COM
Adrenocortical insufficiency NOS
Hypoaldosteronism

E27.49 Other adrenocortical insufficiency   HCC Rx ESR COM
Adrenal hemorrhage
Adrenal infarction

E27.5 Adrenomedullary hyperfunction   HCC Rx ESR COM
Adrenomedullary hyperplasia
Catecholamine hypersecretion

E27.8 Other specified disorders of adrenal gland   HCC Rx ESR COM
Abnormality of cortisol-binding globulin

E27.9 Disorder of adrenal gland, unspecified   HCC Rx ESR COM

✓4ᵗʰ E28 Ovarian dysfunction
EXCLUDES 1   *isolated gonadotropin deficiency (E23.0)*
postprocedural ovarian failure (E89.4-)

E28.0 Estrogen excess   ♀
Use additional code for adverse effect, if applicable, to identify drug (T36-T50 with fifth or sixth character 5)

E28.1 Androgen excess   ♀
Hypersecretion of ovarian androgens
Use additional code for adverse effect, if applicable, to identify drug (T36-T50 with fifth or sixth character 5)

E28.2 Polycystic ovarian syndrome   ♀
Sclerocystic ovary syndrome
Stein-Leventhal syndrome
AHA: 2022,2Q,16
DEF: Common hormonal disorder among women of reproductive age that involves enlarged ovaries with numerous small cysts located along the outer ovarian edge.

✓5ᵗʰ E28.3 Primary ovarian failure
EXCLUDES 1   *pure gonadal dysgenesis (Q99.1)*
Turner's syndrome (Q96.-)

✓6ᵗʰ E28.31 Premature menopause

E28.310 Symptomatic premature menopause   A ♀
Symptoms such as flushing, sleeplessness, headache, lack of concentration, associated with premature menopause

E28.319 Asymptomatic premature menopause   A ♀
Premature menopause NOS

E28.39 Other primary ovarian failure   ♀
Decreased estrogen
Resistant ovary syndrome

E28.8 Other ovarian dysfunction   ♀
Ovarian hyperfunction NOS
EXCLUDES 1   *postprocedural ovarian failure (E89.4-)*

E28.9 Ovarian dysfunction, unspecified   ♀

✓4ᵗʰ E29 Testicular dysfunction
EXCLUDES 1   *androgen insensitivity syndrome (E34.5-)*
azoospermia or oligospermia NOS (N46.0-N46.1)
isolated gonadotropin deficiency (E23.0)
Klinefelter's syndrome (Q98.0-Q98.1, Q98.4)

E29.0 Testicular hyperfunction   ♂
Hypersecretion of testicular hormones

E29.1 Testicular hypofunction   ♂
Defective biosynthesis of testicular androgen NOS
5-delta-Reductase deficiency (with male pseudohermaphroditism)
Testicular hypogonadism NOS
Use additional code for adverse effect, if applicable, to identify drug (T36-T50 with fifth or sixth character 5)
EXCLUDES 1   *postprocedural testicular hypofunction (E89.5)*

E29.8 Other testicular dysfunction   ♂

E29.9 Testicular dysfunction, unspecified   ♂

✓4ᵗʰ E30 Disorders of puberty, not elsewhere classified

E30.0 Delayed puberty
Constitutional delay of puberty
Delayed sexual development

E30.1 Precocious puberty   P
Precocious menstruation
EXCLUDES 1   Albright (-McCune) (-Sternberg) syndrome (Q78.1)
central precocious puberty (E22.8)
congenital adrenal hyperplasia (E25.0)
female heterosexual precocious pseudopuberty (E25.-)
male isosexual precocious pseudopuberty (E25.-)

E30.8 Other disorders of puberty   P
Premature thelarche

E30.9 Disorder of puberty, unspecified

✓4ᵗʰ E31 Polyglandular dysfunction
EXCLUDES 1   ataxia telangiectasia [Louis-Bar] (G11.3)
dystrophia myotonica [Steinert] (G71.11)
pseudohypoparathyroidism (E20.1)

E31.0 Autoimmune polyglandular failure   HCC Rx ESR COM
Schmidt's syndrome

E31.1 Polyglandular hyperfunction   HCC Rx ESR COM
EXCLUDES 1   multiple endocrine adenomatosis (E31.2-)
multiple endocrine neoplasia (E31.2-)

✓5ᵗʰ E31.2 Multiple endocrine neoplasia [MEN] syndromes
Multiple endocrine adenomatosis
Code also any associated malignancies and other conditions associated with the syndromes
DEF: Group of conditions in which several endocrine glands grow excessively (such as in adenomatous hyperplasia) and/or develop benign or malignant tumors. Tumors and hyperplasia associated with MEN often produce excess hormones, which impede normal physiology. There is no comprehensive cure known for MEN syndrome. Treatment is directed at the hyperplasia or tumors in each individual gland. Tumors are usually surgically removed and oral medications or hormonal injections are used to correct hormone imbalances.

E31.20 Multiple endocrine neoplasia [MEN] syndrome, unspecified   HCC Rx ESR COM
Multiple endocrine adenomatosis NOS
Multiple endocrine neoplasia [MEN] syndrome NOS

E31.21 Multiple endocrine neoplasia [MEN] type I   HCC Rx ESR COM
Wermer's syndrome

E31.22 Multiple endocrine neoplasia [MEN] type IIA   HCC Rx ESR COM
Sipple's syndrome

E31.23 Multiple endocrine neoplasia [MEN] type IIB   HCC Rx ESR COM

E31.8 Other polyglandular dysfunction   HCC Rx ESR COM

E31.9 Polyglandular dysfunction, unspecified   HCC Rx ESR COM

✓4ᵗʰ E32 Diseases of thymus
EXCLUDES 1   aplasia or hypoplasia of thymus with immunodeficiency (D82.1)
myasthenia gravis (G70.0)

E32.0 Persistent hyperplasia of thymus   HCC Rx ESR COM
Hypertrophy of thymus

E32.1 Abscess of thymus   HCC Rx ESR COM

E32.8 Other diseases of thymus   HCC Rx ESR COM
EXCLUDES 1   aplasia or hypoplasia with immunodeficiency (D82.1)
thymoma (D15.0)

E32.9 Disease of thymus, unspecified   HCC Rx ESR COM

✓4ᵗʰ E34 Other endocrine disorders
EXCLUDES 1   pseudohypoparathyroidism (E20.1)

E34.0 Carcinoid syndrome   HCC Rx ESR COM
NOTE   May be used as an additional code to identify functional activity associated with a carcinoid tumor.

E34.1 Other hypersecretion of intestinal hormones

E34.2 Ectopic hormone secretion, not elsewhere classified
EXCLUDES 1   ectopic ACTH syndrome (E24.3)

▲ **✓5ᵗʰ E34.3 Short stature due to** endocrine disorder
~~Constitutional short stature~~
~~Laron-type short stature~~
EXCLUDES 1   achondroplastic short stature (Q77.4)
hypochondroplastic short stature (Q77.4)
nutritional short stature (E45)
pituitary short stature (E23.0)
progeria (E34.8)
renal short stature (N25.0)
Russell-Silver syndrome (Q87.19)
short-limbed stature with immunodeficiency (D82.2)
►short stature (child) (R62.52)◄
short stature in specific dysmorphic syndromes - code to syndrome - see Alphabetical Index
short stature NOS (R62.52)

E34.30 Short stature due to endocrine disorder, unspecified

E34.31 Constitutional short stature
Constitutional delay of growth, puberty, or maturation

✓6ᵗʰ E34.32 Genetic causes of short stature

E34.321 Primary insulin-like growth factor-1 (IGF-1) deficiency
Acid-labile subunit gene (IGFALS) defect
Growth hormone gene 1 (GH1) defect with growth hormone neutralizing antibodies
Growth hormone insensitivity syndrome (GHIS)
Insulin-like growth factor 1 gene (IGF1) defect
Laron type short stature
Severe primary insulin-like growth factor-1 deficiency (SPIGFD)
Signal transducer and activator of transcription 5B gene (STAT5b) defect

E34.322 Insulin-like growth factor-1 (IGF-1) resistance
Genetic syndrome with resistance to insulin-like growth factor-1
Insulin-like growth factor-1 receptor (IGF-1R) defect
Post-insulin-like growth factor-1 receptor signaling defect

E34.328 Other genetic causes of short stature
Short stature due to ACAN gene variant
Short stature due to aggrecan deficiency
Short stature due to NPR-2 gene variant

E34.329 Unspecified genetic causes of short stature

E34.39 Other short stature due to endocrine disorder

E34.4 Constitutional tall stature   HCC Rx ESR COM
Constitutional gigantism

✓5ᵗʰ E34.5 Androgen insensitivity syndrome
DEF: X-linked recessive condition in which individuals that are chromosomally male fail to develop normal male external genitalia due to an abnormality on the X chromosome that prohibits the body, completely or in part, from recognizing the androgens produced. **Synonym(s):** AIS

E34.50 Androgen insensitivity syndrome, unspecified
Androgen insensitivity NOS

E34.51 Complete androgen insensitivity syndrome
Complete androgen insensitivity
de Quervain syndrome
Goldberg-Maxwell syndrome

E34.52 Partial androgen insensitivity syndrome
Partial androgen insensitivity
Reifenstein syndrome

E34.8 Other specified endocrine disorders
Pineal gland dysfunction
Progeria
EXCLUDES 2   pseudohypoparathyroidism (E20.1)

E34.9 Endocrine disorder, unspecified
Endocrine disturbance NOS
Hormone disturbance NOS

☑ Additional Character Required   ✓x7ᵗʰ Placeholder Alert   Manifestation   Unspecified Dx   Q QPP   UPD Unacceptable PDx

Chapter 4. Endocrine, Nutritional and Metabolic Diseases

E35–E53.9

E35 Disorders of endocrine glands in diseases classified elsewhere

Code first underlying disease, such as:
late congenital syphilis of thymus gland [Dubois disease] (A50.5)
Use additional code, if applicable, to identify:
sequelae of tuberculosis of other organs (B90.8)

EXCLUDES 1   *Echinococcus granulosus infection of thyroid gland (B67.3)*
meningococcal hemorrhagic adrenalitis (A39.1)
syphilis of endocrine gland (A52.79)
tuberculosis of adrenal gland, except calcification (A18.7)
tuberculosis of endocrine gland NEC (A18.82)
tuberculosis of thyroid gland (A18.81)
Waterhouse-Friderichsen syndrome (A39.1)

Intraoperative complications of endocrine system (E36)

✓4ᵗʰ E36 Intraoperative complications of endocrine system

EXCLUDES 2   *postprocedural endocrine and metabolic complications and disorders, not elsewhere classified (E89.-)*

✓5ᵗʰ E36.0 Intraoperative hemorrhage and hematoma of an endocrine system organ or structure complicating a procedure

EXCLUDES 1   *intraoperative hemorrhage and hematoma of an endocrine system organ or structure due to accidental puncture or laceration during a procedure (E36.1-)*

E36.01 Intraoperative hemorrhage and hematoma of an endocrine system organ or structure complicating an endocrine system procedure
AHA: 2020,1Q,19

E36.02 Intraoperative hemorrhage and hematoma of an endocrine system organ or structure complicating other procedure

✓5ᵗʰ E36.1 Accidental puncture and laceration of an endocrine system organ or structure during a procedure

E36.11 Accidental puncture and laceration of an endocrine system organ or structure during an endocrine system procedure

E36.12 Accidental puncture and laceration of an endocrine system organ or structure during other procedure

E36.8 Other intraoperative complications of endocrine system
Use additional code, if applicable, to further specify disorder

Malnutrition (E40-E46)

EXCLUDES 1   *intestinal malabsorption (K90.-)*
sequelae of protein-calorie malnutrition (E64.0)
EXCLUDES 2   *nutritional anemias (D50-D53)*
starvation (T73.0)
AHA: 2020,1Q,4-7; 2017,4Q,108; 2017,3Q,25
TIP: Assign additional code for BMI from category Z68, when documented. BMI can be based on documentation from clinicians who are not the patient's provider.
TIP: Malnutrition is not considered integral to cancer; assign the appropriate code in addition to the code for the specific type of cancer.

E40 Kwashiorkor   HCC ESR COM
Severe malnutrition with nutritional edema with dyspigmentation of skin and hair
EXCLUDES 1   *marasmic kwashiorkor (E42)*

E41 Nutritional marasmus   HCC ESR COM
Severe malnutrition with marasmus
EXCLUDES 1   *marasmic kwashiorkor (E42)*
AHA: 2017,3Q,24
DEF: Protein-calorie malabsorption or malnutrition in children characterized by tissue wasting, dehydration, and subcutaneous fat depletion. It may occur with infectious disease.

E42 Marasmic kwashiorkor   HCC ESR COM
Intermediate form severe protein-calorie malnutrition
Severe protein-calorie malnutrition with signs of both kwashiorkor and marasmus

E43 Unspecified severe protein-calorie malnutrition   HCC ESR COM
Starvation edema
AHA: 2022,1Q,13; 2020,1Q,5,6; 2017,4Q,108
TIP: Assign code R64 when emaciation is documented without documentation of malnutrition.

✓4ᵗʰ E44 Protein-calorie malnutrition of moderate and mild degree
AHA: 2020,1Q,5

E44.0 Moderate protein-calorie malnutrition   HCC ESR COM

E44.1 Mild protein-calorie malnutrition   HCC ESR COM

E45 Retarded development following protein-calorie malnutrition   HCC ESR COM
Nutritional short stature
Nutritional stunting
Physical retardation due to malnutrition

E46 Unspecified protein-calorie malnutrition   HCC ESR COM
Malnutrition NOS
Protein-calorie imbalance NOS
EXCLUDES 1   *nutritional deficiency NOS (E63.9)*
AHA: 2018,4Q,82

Other nutritional deficiencies (E50-E64)

EXCLUDES 2   *nutritional anemias (D50-D53)*

✓4ᵗʰ E50 Vitamin A deficiency
EXCLUDES 1   *sequelae of vitamin A deficiency (E64.1)*

E50.0 Vitamin A deficiency with conjunctival xerosis

E50.1 Vitamin A deficiency with Bitot's spot and conjunctival xerosis
Bitot's spot in the young child
DEF: Vitamin A deficiency with conjunctival dryness and superficial spots of keratinized epithelium.

E50.2 Vitamin A deficiency with corneal xerosis

E50.3 Vitamin A deficiency with corneal ulceration and xerosis

E50.4 Vitamin A deficiency with keratomalacia
DEF: Vitamin A deficiency creating corneal dryness that progresses to corneal insensitivity, softness, and necrosis. It is usually bilateral.

E50.5 Vitamin A deficiency with night blindness

E50.6 Vitamin A deficiency with xerophthalmic scars of cornea

E50.7 Other ocular manifestations of vitamin A deficiency
Xerophthalmia NOS

E50.8 Other manifestations of vitamin A deficiency
Follicular keratosis
Xeroderma

E50.9 Vitamin A deficiency, unspecified
Hypovitaminosis A NOS

✓4ᵗʰ E51 Thiamine deficiency
EXCLUDES 1   *sequelae of thiamine deficiency (E64.8)*

✓5ᵗʰ E51.1 Beriberi

E51.11 Dry beriberi
Beriberi NOS
Beriberi with polyneuropathy

E51.12 Wet beriberi
Beriberi with cardiovascular manifestations
Cardiovascular beriberi
Shoshin disease

E51.2 Wernicke's encephalopathy
DEF: Deficiency of vitamin B1 resulting in a triad of acute mental confusion, ataxia, and ophthalmoplegia. The vast majority of affected patients are alcoholics.

E51.8 Other manifestations of thiamine deficiency

E51.9 Thiamine deficiency, unspecified

E52 Niacin deficiency [pellagra]
Niacin (-tryptophan) deficiency
Nicotinamide deficiency
Pellagra (alcoholic)
EXCLUDES 1   *sequelae of niacin deficiency (E64.8)*

✓4ᵗʰ E53 Deficiency of other B group vitamins
EXCLUDES 1   *sequelae of vitamin B deficiency (E64.8)*

E53.0 Riboflavin deficiency
Ariboflavinosis
Vitamin B2 deficiency

E53.1 Pyridoxine deficiency
Vitamin B6 deficiency
EXCLUDES 1   *pyridoxine-responsive sideroblastic anemia (D64.3)*

E53.8 Deficiency of other specified B group vitamins
Biotin deficiency
Cyanocobalamin deficiency
Folate deficiency
Folic acid deficiency
Pantothenic acid deficiency
Vitamin B12 deficiency
EXCLUDES 1   *folate deficiency anemia (D52.-)*
vitamin B12 deficiency anemia (D51.-)

E53.9 Vitamin B deficiency, unspecified

E54 Ascorbic acid deficiency
Deficiency of vitamin C
Scurvy
EXCLUDES 1   *scorbutic anemia (D53.2)*
       sequelae of vitamin C deficiency (E64.2)
DEF: Vitamin C deficiency causing swollen gums, myalgia, weight loss, and weakness.

✓4ᵗʰ **E55 Vitamin D deficiency**
EXCLUDES 1   *adult osteomalacia (M83.-)*
       osteoporosis (M80.-)
       sequelae of rickets (E64.3)

    E55.0 Rickets, active   Rx
       Infantile osteomalacia
       Juvenile osteomalacia
       EXCLUDES 1   *celiac rickets (K90.0)*
          Crohn's rickets (K50.-)
          hereditary vitamin D-dependent rickets (E83.32)
          inactive rickets (E64.3)
          renal rickets (N25.0)
          sequelae of rickets (E64.3)
          vitamin D-resistant rickets (E83.31)
       DEF: Rickets: Softening or weakening of the bones due to a lack of vitamin D, calcium, and phosphate.
    E55.9 Vitamin D deficiency, unspecified
       Avitaminosis D

✓4ᵗʰ **E56 Other vitamin deficiencies**
EXCLUDES 1   *sequelae of other vitamin deficiencies (E64.8)*

    E56.0 Deficiency of vitamin E
    E56.1 Deficiency of vitamin K
       EXCLUDES 1   *deficiency of coagulation factor due to vitamin K deficiency (D68.4)*
          vitamin K deficiency of newborn (P53)
    E56.8 Deficiency of other vitamins
    E56.9 Vitamin deficiency, unspecified

E58 Dietary calcium deficiency
EXCLUDES 1   *disorders of calcium metabolism (E83.5-)*
       sequelae of calcium deficiency (E64.8)

E59 Dietary selenium deficiency
Keshan disease
EXCLUDES 1   *sequelae of selenium deficiency (E64.8)*

E60 Dietary zinc deficiency

✓4ᵗʰ **E61 Deficiency of other nutrient elements**
Use additional code for adverse effect, if applicable, to identify drug (T36-T50 with fifth or sixth character 5)
EXCLUDES 1   *disorders of mineral metabolism (E83.-)*
       iodine deficiency related thyroid disorders (E00-E02)
       sequelae of malnutrition and other nutritional deficiencies (E64.-)

    E61.0 Copper deficiency
    E61.1 Iron deficiency
       EXCLUDES 1   *iron deficiency anemia (D50.-)*
    E61.2 Magnesium deficiency
    E61.3 Manganese deficiency
    E61.4 Chromium deficiency
    E61.5 Molybdenum deficiency
    E61.6 Vanadium deficiency
    E61.7 Deficiency of multiple nutrient elements
    E61.8 Deficiency of other specified nutrient elements
    E61.9 Deficiency of nutrient element, unspecified

✓4ᵗʰ **E63 Other nutritional deficiencies**
EXCLUDES 2   *dehydration (E86.0)*
       failure to thrive, adult (R62.7)
       failure to thrive, child (R62.51)
       feeding problems in newborn (P92.-)
       sequelae of malnutrition and other nutritional deficiencies (E64.-)

    E63.0 Essential fatty acid [EFA] deficiency
    E63.1 Imbalance of constituents of food intake
    E63.8 Other specified nutritional deficiencies
    E63.9 Nutritional deficiency, unspecified

✓4ᵗʰ **E64 Sequelae of malnutrition and other nutritional deficiencies**
    NOTE   This category is to be used to indicate conditions in categories E43, E44, E46, E50-E63 as the cause of sequelae, which are themselves classified elsewhere. The 'sequelae' include conditions specified as such; they also include the late effects of diseases classifiable to the above categories if the disease itself is no longer present
    Code first condition resulting from (sequela) of malnutrition and other nutritional deficiencies

    E64.0 Sequelae of protein-calorie malnutrition   HCC ESR
       EXCLUDES 2   *retarded development following protein-calorie malnutrition (E45)*
    E64.1 Sequelae of vitamin A deficiency
    E64.2 Sequelae of vitamin C deficiency
    E64.3 Sequelae of rickets
    E64.8 Sequelae of other nutritional deficiencies
    E64.9 Sequelae of unspecified nutritional deficiency

Overweight, obesity and other hyperalimentation (E65-E68)

E65 Localized adiposity
Fat pad

✓4ᵗʰ **E66 Overweight and obesity**
Code first obesity complicating pregnancy, childbirth and the puerperium, if applicable (O99.21-)
Use additional code to identify body mass index (BMI), if known (Z68.-)
EXCLUDES 1   *adiposogenital dystrophy (E23.6)*
       lipomatosis NOS (E88.2)
       lipomatosis dolorosa [Dercum] (E88.2)
       Prader-Willi syndrome (Q87.11)
AHA: 2018,4Q,77,79-80
TIP: Do not assign a BMI code (Z68.-) when a pregnant patient is documented as being overweight or obese. Only a code from subcategory O99.21- and a code from this category should be assigned.

✓5ᵗʰ   **E66.0 Obesity due to excess calories**
       E66.01 Morbid (severe) obesity due to excess calories   HCC ESR
          EXCLUDES 1   *morbid (severe) obesity with alveolar hypoventilation (E66.2)*
          AHA: 2022,2Q,9
       E66.09 Other obesity due to excess calories
    E66.1 Drug-induced obesity
       Use additional code for adverse effect, if applicable, to identify drug (T36-T50 with fifth or sixth character 5)
    E66.2 Morbid (severe) obesity with alveolar hypoventilation   HCC ESR
       Obesity hypoventilation syndrome (OHS)
       Pickwickian syndrome
    E66.3 Overweight
       AHA: 2018,4Q,78
    E66.8 Other obesity
    E66.9 Obesity, unspecified
       Obesity NOS
       AHA: 2021,2Q,10

✓4ᵗʰ **E67 Other hyperalimentation**
EXCLUDES 1   *hyperalimentation NOS (R63.2)*
       sequelae of hyperalimentation (E68)

    E67.0 Hypervitaminosis A
    E67.1 Hypercarotenemia
       DEF: Elevated blood carotene level as a result of excessive carotenoid ingestion or an inability to convert carotenoids to vitamin A. Characteristics often include yellow discoloration of the skin, which may follow overeating of carotenoid-rich foods such as carrots, sweet potatoes, or squash.
    E67.2 Megavitamin-B6 syndrome
    E67.3 Hypervitaminosis D
    E67.8 Other specified hyperalimentation

E68 Sequelae of hyperalimentation
Code first condition resulting from (sequela) of hyperalimentation

Metabolic disorders (E70-E88)

EXCLUDES 1   androgen insensitivity syndrome (E34.5-)
congenital adrenal hyperplasia (E25.0)
hemolytic anemias attributable to enzyme disorders (D55.-)
Marfan's syndrome (Q87.4)
5-alpha-reductase deficiency (E29.1)
EXCLUDES 2   Ehlers-Danlos syndromes (Q79.6-)
AHA: 2018,2Q,6

✓4ᵗʰ E70 Disorders of aromatic amino-acid metabolism

E70.0 Classical phenylketonuria   HCC Rx ESR COM

E70.1 Other hyperphenylalaninemias   HCC Rx ESR COM

✓5ᵗʰ E70.2 Disorders of tyrosine metabolism

EXCLUDES 1   transitory tyrosinemia of newborn (P74.5)

E70.20 Disorder of tyrosine metabolism, unspecified   HCC Rx ESR COM

E70.21 Tyrosinemia   HCC Rx ESR COM
Hypertyrosinemia

E70.29 Other disorders of tyrosine metabolism   HCC Rx ESR COM
Alkaptonuria
Ochronosis

✓5ᵗʰ E70.3 Albinism

DEF: Absence of pigment in skin, hair, and eyes. This genetic condition is often accompanied by astigmatism, photophobia, and nystagmus.

E70.30 Albinism, unspecified   HCC Rx ESR COM

✓6ᵗʰ E70.31 Ocular albinism

E70.310 X-linked ocular albinism   HCC Rx ESR COM

E70.311 Autosomal recessive ocular albinism   HCC Rx ESR COM

E70.318 Other ocular albinism   HCC Rx ESR COM

E70.319 Ocular albinism, unspecified   HCC Rx ESR COM

✓6ᵗʰ E70.32 Oculocutaneous albinism

EXCLUDES 1   Chediak-Higashi syndrome (E70.330)
Hermansky-Pudlak syndrome (E70.331)

E70.320 Tyrosinase negative oculocutaneous albinism   HCC Rx ESR COM
Albinism I
Oculocutaneous albinism ty-neg

E70.321 Tyrosinase positive oculocutaneous albinism   HCC Rx ESR COM
Albinism II
Oculocutaneous albinism ty-pos

E70.328 Other oculocutaneous albinism   HCC Rx ESR COM
Cross syndrome

E70.329 Oculocutaneous albinism, unspecified   HCC Rx ESR COM

✓6ᵗʰ E70.33 Albinism with hematologic abnormality

E70.330 Chediak-Higashi syndrome   HCC Rx ESR COM

E70.331 Hermansky-Pudlak syndrome   HCC Rx ESR COM

E70.338 Other albinism with hematologic abnormality   HCC Rx ESR COM

E70.339 Albinism with hematologic abnormality, unspecified   HCC Rx ESR COM

E70.39 Other specified albinism   HCC Rx ESR COM
Piebaldism

✓5ᵗʰ E70.4 Disorders of histidine metabolism

E70.40 Disorders of histidine metabolism, unspecified   HCC Rx ESR COM

E70.41 Histidinemia   HCC Rx ESR COM

E70.49 Other disorders of histidine metabolism   HCC Rx ESR COM

E70.5 Disorders of tryptophan metabolism   HCC Rx ESR COM

✓5ᵗʰ E70.8 Other disorders of aromatic amino-acid metabolism

AHA: 2020,4Q,15-16

E70.81 Aromatic L-amino acid decarboxylase deficiency   HCC Rx ESR COM
AADC deficiency

E70.89 Other disorders of aromatic amino-acid metabolism   HCC Rx ESR COM

E70.9 Disorder of aromatic amino-acid metabolism, unspecified   HCC Rx ESR COM

✓4ᵗʰ E71 Disorders of branched-chain amino-acid metabolism and fatty-acid metabolism

E71.0 Maple-syrup-urine disease   HCC Rx ESR COM

✓5ᵗʰ E71.1 Other disorders of branched-chain amino-acid metabolism

✓6ᵗʰ E71.11 Branched-chain organic acidurias

E71.110 Isovaleric acidemia   HCC Rx ESR COM

E71.111 3-methylglutaconic aciduria   HCC Rx ESR COM

E71.118 Other branched-chain organic acidurias   HCC Rx ESR COM

✓6ᵗʰ E71.12 Disorders of propionate metabolism

E71.120 Methylmalonic acidemia   HCC Rx ESR COM

E71.121 Propionic acidemia   HCC Rx ESR COM

E71.128 Other disorders of propionate metabolism   HCC Rx ESR COM

E71.19 Other disorders of branched-chain amino-acid metabolism   HCC Rx ESR COM
Hyperleucine-isoleucinemia
Hypervalinemia

E71.2 Disorder of branched-chain amino-acid metabolism, unspecified   HCC Rx ESR COM

✓5ᵗʰ E71.3 Disorders of fatty-acid metabolism

EXCLUDES 1   peroxisomal disorders (E71.5)
Refsum's disease (G60.1)
Schilder's disease (G37.0)
EXCLUDES 2   carnitine deficiency due to inborn error of metabolism (E71.42)

E71.30 Disorder of fatty-acid metabolism, unspecified   Rx COM

✓6ᵗʰ E71.31 Disorders of fatty-acid oxidation

E71.310 Long chain/very long chain acyl CoA dehydrogenase deficiency   HCC Rx ESR COM
LCAD
VLCAD

E71.311 Medium chain acyl CoA dehydrogenase deficiency   HCC Rx ESR COM
MCAD

E71.312 Short chain acyl CoA dehydrogenase deficiency   HCC Rx ESR COM
SCAD

E71.313 Glutaric aciduria type II   HCC Rx ESR COM
Glutaric aciduria type II A
Glutaric aciduria type II B
Glutaric aciduria type II C
EXCLUDES 1   glutaric aciduria (type 1) NOS (E72.3)

E71.314 Muscle carnitine palmitoyltransferase deficiency   HCC Rx ESR COM

E71.318 Other disorders of fatty-acid oxidation   HCC Rx ESR COM

E71.32 Disorders of ketone metabolism   HCC Rx ESR COM

E71.39 Other disorders of fatty-acid metabolism   HCC Rx ESR COM

✓5ᵗʰ E71.4 Disorders of carnitine metabolism

EXCLUDES 1   muscle carnitine palmitoyltransferase deficiency (E71.314)

E71.40 Disorder of carnitine metabolism, unspecified   HCC Rx ESR COM

E71.41 Primary carnitine deficiency   HCC Rx ESR COM

E71.42 Carnitine deficiency due to inborn errors of metabolism   HCC Rx ESR COM
Code also associated inborn error or metabolism

E71.43 Iatrogenic carnitine deficiency   HCC Rx ESR COM
Carnitine deficiency due to hemodialysis
Carnitine deficiency due to Valproic acid therapy

✓6ᵗʰ E71.44 Other secondary carnitine deficiency

E71.440 Ruvalcaba-Myhre-Smith syndrome   HCC Rx ESR COM

E71.448 Other secondary carnitine deficiency   HCC Rx ESR COM

HCC CMS-HCC   Rx Rx HCC   ESR ESRD HCC   COM Commercial HCC   N Newborn: 0   P Pediatric: 0-17   M Maternity: 9-64   A Adult: 15-124

√5ᵗʰ **E71.5** **Peroxisomal** disorders
> *EXCLUDES 1*   Schilder's disease (G37.0)

    E71.50 **Peroxisomal disorder, unspecified** `HCC` `Rx` `ESR` `COM`

√6ᵗʰ **E71.51** **Disorders of peroxisome** biogenesis
> Group 1 peroxisomal disorders
> *EXCLUDES 1*   Refsum's disease (G60.1)

    E71.510 **Zellweger syndrome** `HCC` `Rx` `ESR` `COM`
    E71.511 **Neonatal adrenoleukodystrophy** `HCC` `Rx` `ESR` `COM`
> *EXCLUDES 1*   X-linked adrenoleukodystrophy (E71.42-)

    E71.518 **Other disorders of peroxisome biogenesis** `HCC` `Rx` `ESR` `COM`

√6ᵗʰ **E71.52** **X-linked adrenoleukodystrophy**

    E71.520 **Childhood cerebral X-linked adrenoleukodystrophy** `HCC` `Rx` `ESR` `COM`
    E71.521 **Adolescent X-linked adrenoleukodystrophy** `HCC` `Rx` `ESR` `COM`
    E71.522 **Adrenomyeloneuropathy** `HCC` `Rx` `ESR` `COM`
    E71.528 **Other X-linked adrenoleukodystrophy**
> Addison only phenotype adrenoleukodystrophy
> Addison-Schilder adrenoleukodystrophy

    E71.529 **X-linked adrenoleukodystrophy, unspecified type** `HCC` `Rx` `ESR` `COM`

    E71.53 **Other** group 2 peroxisomal disorders `HCC` `Rx` `ESR` `COM`

√6ᵗʰ **E71.54** **Other peroxisomal disorders**

    E71.540 **Rhizomelic chondrodysplasia punctata** `HCC` `Rx` `ESR` `COM`
> *EXCLUDES 1*   chondrodysplasia punctata NOS (Q77.3)

    E71.541 **Zellweger-like syndrome** `HCC` `Rx` `ESR` `COM`
    E71.542 **Other group 3 peroxisomal disorders** `HCC` `Rx` `ESR` `COM`
    E71.548 **Other peroxisomal disorders** `HCC` `Rx` `ESR` `COM`

√4ᵗʰ **E72** **Other disorders of amino-acid metabolism**
> *EXCLUDES 1*   disorders of:
> aromatic amino-acid metabolism (E70.-)
> branched-chain amino-acid metabolism (E71.0-E71.2)
> fatty-acid metabolism (E71.3)
> purine and pyrimidine metabolism (E79.-)
> gout (M1A.-, M10.-)

√5ᵗʰ **E72.0** **Disorders of amino-acid** transport
> *EXCLUDES 1*   disorders of tryptophan metabolism (E70.5)

    E72.00 **Disorders of amino-acid transport, unspecified** `HCC` `Rx` `ESR` `COM`
    E72.01 **Cystinuria** `HCC` `Rx` `ESR` `COM`
    E72.02 **Hartnup's disease** `HCC` `Rx` `ESR` `COM`
    E72.03 **Lowe's syndrome** `HCC` `Rx` `ESR` `COM`
> Use additional code for associated glaucoma (H42)

    E72.04 **Cystinosis** `HCC` `Rx` `ESR` `COM`
> Fanconi (-de Toni) (-Debré) syndrome with cystinosis
> *EXCLUDES 1*   Fanconi (-de Toni) (-Debré) syndrome without cystinosis (E72.09)

    E72.09 **Other disorders of amino-acid transport** `HCC` `Rx` `ESR` `COM`
> Fanconi (-de Toni) (-Debré) syndrome, unspecified

√5ᵗʰ **E72.1** **Disorders of** sulfur-bearing **amino-acid metabolism**
> *EXCLUDES 1*   cystinosis (E72.04)
> cystinuria (E72.01)
> transcobalamin II deficiency (D51.2)

    E72.10 **Disorders of sulfur-bearing amino-acid metabolism, unspecified** `HCC` `Rx` `ESR` `COM`
    E72.11 **Homocystinuria** `HCC` `Rx` `ESR` `COM`
> Cystathionine synthase deficiency
> **AHA:** 2021,4Q,28

    E72.12 **Methylenetetrahydrofolate reductase deficiency** `HCC` `Rx` `ESR` `COM`

    E72.19 **Other disorders of sulfur-bearing amino-acid metabolism** `HCC` `Rx` `ESR` `COM`
> Cystathioninuria
> Methioninemia
> Sulfite oxidase deficiency

√5ᵗʰ **E72.2** **Disorders of** urea cycle **metabolism**
> *EXCLUDES 1*   disorders of ornithine metabolism (E72.4)

    E72.20 **Disorder of urea cycle metabolism, unspecified** `HCC` `Rx` `ESR` `COM`
> Hyperammonemia
> *EXCLUDES 1*   hyperammonemia- hyperornithinemia-homocitrullinemia syndrome E72.4
> transient hyperammonemia of newborn (P74.6)

    E72.21 **Argininemia** `HCC` `Rx` `ESR` `COM`
    E72.22 **Arginosuccinic aciduria** `HCC` `Rx` `ESR` `COM`
    E72.23 **Citrullinemia** `HCC` `Rx` `ESR` `COM`
    E72.29 **Other disorders of urea cycle metabolism** `HCC` `Rx` `ESR` `COM`

E72.3 **Disorders of** lysine and hydroxylysine metabolism `HCC` `Rx` `ESR` `COM`
> Glutaric aciduria NOS
> Glutaric aciduria (type I)
> Hydroxylysinemia
> Hyperlysinemia
> *EXCLUDES 1*   glutaric aciduria type II (E71.313)
> Refsum's disease (G60.1)
> Zellweger syndrome (E71.510)

E72.4 **Disorders of** ornithine metabolism `HCC` `Rx` `ESR` `COM`
> Hyperammonemia-Hyperornithinemia-Homocitrullinemia syndrome
> Ornithinemia (types I, II)
> Ornithine transcarbamylase deficiency
> *EXCLUDES 1*   hereditary choroidal dystrophy (H31.2-)

√5ᵗʰ **E72.5** **Disorders of** glycine metabolism

    E72.50 **Disorder of glycine metabolism, unspecified** `HCC` `Rx` `ESR` `COM`
    E72.51 **Non-ketotic hyperglycinemia** `HCC` `Rx` `ESR` `COM`
    E72.52 **Trimethylaminuria** `HCC` `Rx` `ESR` `COM`
    E72.53 **Primary hyperoxaluria** `HCC` `Rx` `ESR` `COM`
> Oxalosis
> Oxaluria
> **AHA:** 2018,4Q,29

    E72.59 **Other disorders of glycine metabolism** `HCC` `Rx` `ESR` `COM`
> D-glycericacidemia
> Hyperhydroxyprolinemia
> Hyperprolinemia (types I, II)
> Sarcosinemia

√5ᵗʰ **E72.8** **Other specified disorders of amino-acid metabolism**
> **AHA:** 2018,4Q,5

    E72.81 **Disorders of** gamma aminobutyric **acid metabolism** `HCC` `Rx` `ESR` `COM`
> 4-hydroxybutyric aciduria
> Disorders of GABA metabolism
> GABA metabolic defect
> GABA transaminase deficiency
> GABA-T deficiency
> Gamma-hydroxybutyric aciduria
> SSADHD
> Succinic semialdehyde dehydrogenase deficiency

    E72.89 **Other specified disorders of amino-acid metabolism** `HCC` `Rx` `ESR` `COM`
> Disorders of beta-amino-acid metabolism
> Disorders of gamma-glutamyl cycle

E72.9 **Disorder of amino-acid metabolism, unspecified** `HCC` `Rx` `ESR` `COM`

√4ᵗʰ **E73** **Lactose intolerance**
> **DEF:** Inability to break down sugar in dairy products due to a deficiency in the enzyme lactase.

    E73.0 **Congenital** lactase deficiency
    E73.1 **Secondary** lactase deficiency
    E73.8 **Other lactose intolerance**
    E73.9 **Lactose intolerance, unspecified**

✓4ᵗʰ **E74 Other disorders of carbohydrate metabolism**

EXCLUDES 1   *diabetes mellitus (E08-E13)*
    hypoglycemia NOS (E16.2)
    increased secretion of glucagon (E16.3)
    mucopolysaccharidosis (E76.0-E76.3)

✓5ᵗʰ **E74.0 Glycogen storage disease**

  E74.00 Glycogen storage disease, unspecified `HCC` `Rx` `ESR` `COM`

  E74.01 von Gierke disease `HCC` `Rx` `ESR` `COM`
    Type I glycogen storage disease

  E74.02 Pompe disease `HCC` `Rx` `ESR` `COM`
    Cardiac glycogenosis
    Type II glycogen storage disease

  E74.03 Cori disease `HCC` `Rx` `ESR` `COM`
    Forbes disease
    Type III glycogen storage disease

  E74.04 McArdle disease `HCC` `Rx` `ESR` `COM`
    Type V glycogen storage disease

  E74.09 Other glycogen storage disease `HCC` `Rx` `ESR` `COM`
    Andersen disease
    Hers disease
    Tauri disease
    Glycogen storage disease, types Ø, IV, VI-XI
    Liver phosphorylase deficiency
    Muscle phosphofructokinase deficiency

✓5ᵗʰ **E74.1 Disorders of fructose metabolism**

EXCLUDES 1   *muscle phosphofructokinase deficiency (E74.09)*

  E74.10 Disorder of fructose metabolism, unspecified

  E74.11 Essential fructosuria
    Fructokinase deficiency

  E74.12 Hereditary fructose intolerance
    Fructosemia

  E74.19 Other disorders of fructose metabolism
    Fructose-1, 6-diphosphatase deficiency

✓5ᵗʰ **E74.2 Disorders of galactose metabolism**

  E74.20 Disorders of galactose metabolism, unspecified `HCC` `Rx` `ESR` `COM`

  E74.21 Galactosemia `HCC` `Rx` `ESR` `COM`
    DEF: Any of three genetic disorders caused by a defective galactose metabolism. Symptoms include failure to thrive in infancy, jaundice, liver and spleen damage, cataracts, and mental retardation.

  E74.29 Other disorders of galactose metabolism `HCC` `Rx` `ESR` `COM`
    Galactokinase deficiency

✓5ᵗʰ **E74.3 Other disorders of intestinal carbohydrate absorption**

EXCLUDES 2   *lactose intolerance (E73.-)*

  E74.31 Sucrase-isomaltase deficiency `Rx`

  E74.39 Other disorders of intestinal carbohydrate absorption
    Disorder of intestinal carbohydrate absorption NOS
    Glucose-galactose malabsorption
    Sucrase deficiency

E74.4 Disorders of pyruvate metabolism and gluconeogenesis `HCC` `Rx` `ESR` `COM`
  Deficiency of phosphoenolpyruvate carboxykinase
  Deficiency of pyruvate carboxylase
  Deficiency of pyruvate dehydrogenase

EXCLUDES 1   *disorders of pyruvate metabolism and gluconeogenesis with anemia (D55.-)*
    Leigh's syndrome (G31.82)

✓5ᵗʰ **E74.8 Other specified disorders of carbohydrate metabolism**

AHA: 2020,4Q,16

✓6ᵗʰ **E74.81 Disorders of glucose transport, not elsewhere classified**

  E74.810 Glucose transporter protein type 1 deficiency `HCC` `Rx` `ESR` `COM`
    De Vivo syndrome
    Glucose transport defect, blood-brain barrier
    Glut1 deficiency
    GLUT1 deficiency syndrome 1, infantile onset
    GLUT1 deficiency syndrome 2, childhood onset

  E74.818 Other disorders of glucose transport `HCC` `Rx` `ESR` `COM`
    (Familial) renal glycosuria

  E74.819 Disorders of glucose transport, unspecified `HCC` `Rx` `ESR` `COM`

  E74.89 Other specified disorders of carbohydrate metabolism `HCC` `Rx` `ESR` `COM`
    Essential pentosuria

  E74.9 Disorder of carbohydrate metabolism, unspecified `HCC` `Rx` `ESR` `COM`

✓4ᵗʰ **E75 Disorders of sphingolipid metabolism and other lipid storage disorders**

EXCLUDES 1   *mucolipidosis, types I-III (E77.0-E77.1)*
    Refsum's disease (G60.1)

✓5ᵗʰ **E75.0 GM2 gangliosidosis**

  E75.00 GM2 gangliosidosis, unspecified `HCC` `Rx` `ESR` `COM`

  E75.01 Sandhoff disease `HCC` `Rx` `ESR` `COM`

  E75.02 Tay-Sachs disease
    DEF: Genetic mutation of the HEXA gene that inhibits the breakdown of a toxic substance called ganglioside. The accumulation of ganglioside results in destruction of the neurons in the brain and spinal cord.

Tay-Sachs Disease

  E75.09 Other GM2 gangliosidosis `HCC` `Rx` `ESR` `COM`
    Adult GM2 gangliosidosis
    Juvenile GM2 gangliosidosis

✓5ᵗʰ **E75.1 Other and unspecified gangliosidosis**

  E75.10 Unspecified gangliosidosis `HCC` `Rx` `ESR` `COM`
    Gangliosidosis NOS

  E75.11 Mucolipidosis IV `HCC` `Rx` `ESR` `COM`

  E75.19 Other gangliosidosis `HCC` `Rx` `ESR` `COM`
    GM1 gangliosidosis
    GM3 gangliosidosis

✓5ᵗʰ **E75.2 Other sphingolipidosis**

EXCLUDES 1   *adrenoleukodystrophy [Addison-Schilder] (E71.528)*

  E75.21 Fabry (-Anderson) disease `HCC` `Rx` `ESR` `COM`

  E75.22 Gaucher disease `HCC` `Rx` `ESR` `COM`

  E75.23 Krabbe disease `HCC` `Rx` `ESR` `COM`

✓6ᵗʰ **E75.24 Niemann-Pick disease**
    Acid sphingomyelinase deficiency (ASMD)

  E75.240 Niemann-Pick disease type A `HCC` `Rx` `ESR` `COM`
    Acid sphingomyelinase deficiency type A (ASMD type A)
    Infantile neurovisceral acid sphingomyelinase deficiency

  E75.241 Niemann-Pick disease type B `HCC` `Rx` `ESR` `COM`
    Acid sphingomyelinase deficiency type B (ASMD type B)
    Chronic visceral acid sphingomyelinase deficiency

`HCC` CMS-HCC   `Rx` Rx HCC   `ESR` ESRD HCC   `COM` Commercial HCC   🆖 Newborn: 0   🅿 Pediatric: 0-17   🅼 Maternity: 9-64   🅰 Adult: 15-124

548

ICD-10-CM 2023

E75.242 **Niemann-Pick disease** type C `HCC` `Rx` `ESR` `COM`

E75.243 **Niemann-Pick disease** type D `HCC` `Rx` `ESR` `COM`

E75.244 **Niemann-Pick disease** type A/B `HCC` `Rx` `ESR` `COM`
> Acid sphingomyelinase deficiency type A/B (ASMD type A/B)
> Chronic neurovisceral acid sphingomyelinase deficiency
> **AHA:** 2021,4Q,8-9

E75.248 **Other Niemann-Pick disease** `HCC` `Rx` `ESR` `COM`

E75.249 **Niemann-Pick disease, unspecified** `HCC` `Rx` `ESR` `COM`
> Acid sphingomyelinase deficiency (ASMD) NOS

E75.25 **Metachromatic leukodystrophy** `HCC` `Rx` `ESR` `COM`

E75.26 **Sulfatase deficiency** `HCC` `Rx` `ESR` `COM`
> Multiple sulfatase deficiency (MSD)
> **AHA:** 2018,4Q,5-6

E75.29 **Other sphingolipidosis** `HCC` `Rx` `ESR` `COM`
> Farber's syndrome
> Sulfatide lipidosis

E75.3 **Sphingolipidosis, unspecified** `HCC` `Rx` `ESR` `COM`

E75.4 **Neuronal ceroid lipofuscinosis** `HCC` `Rx` `ESR` `COM`
> Batten disease
> Bielschowsky-Jansky disease
> Kufs disease
> Spielmeyer-Vogt disease

E75.5 **Other lipid storage disorders** `Rx`
> Cerebrotendinous cholesterosis [van Bogaert-Scherer-Epstein]
> Wolman's disease

E75.6 **Lipid storage disorder, unspecified** `Rx`

✓4ᵗʰ **E76 Disorders of glycosaminoglycan metabolism**

  ✓5ᵗʰ **E76.0 Mucopolysaccharidosis, type I**

    E76.01 **Hurler's syndrome** `HCC` `Rx` `ESR` `COM`

    E76.02 **Hurler-Scheie syndrome** `HCC` `Rx` `ESR` `COM`

    E76.03 **Scheie's syndrome** `HCC` `Rx` `ESR` `COM`

  E76.1 **Mucopolysaccharidosis, type II**
> Hunter's syndrome

  ✓5ᵗʰ **E76.2 Other mucopolysaccharidoses**

    ✓6ᵗʰ **E76.21 Morquio mucopolysaccharidoses**

      E76.210 **Morquio A mucopolysaccharidoses** `HCC` `Rx` `ESR` `COM`
> Classic Morquio syndrome
> Morquio syndrome A
> Mucopolysaccharidosis, type IVA

      E76.211 **Morquio B mucopolysaccharidoses** `HCC` `Rx` `ESR` `COM`
> Morquio-like mucopolysaccharidoses
> Morquio-like syndrome
> Morquio syndrome B
> Mucopolysaccharidosis, type IVB

      E76.219 **Morquio mucopolysaccharidoses, unspecified** `HCC` `Rx` `ESR` `COM`
> Morquio syndrome
> Mucopolysaccharidosis, type IV

    E76.22 **Sanfilippo mucopolysaccharidoses** `HCC` `Rx` `ESR` `COM`
> Mucopolysaccharidosis, type III (A) (B) (C) (D)
> Sanfilippo A syndrome
> Sanfilippo B syndrome
> Sanfilippo C syndrome
> Sanfilippo D syndrome

    E76.29 **Other mucopolysaccharidoses** `HCC` `Rx` `ESR` `COM`
> beta-Glucuronidase deficiency
> Maroteaux-Lamy (mild) (severe) syndrome
> Mucopolysaccharidosis, types VI, VII

  E76.3 **Mucopolysaccharidosis, unspecified** `HCC` `Rx` `ESR` `COM`

  E76.8 **Other disorders of glucosaminoglycan metabolism** `HCC` `Rx` `ESR` `COM`

  E76.9 **Glucosaminoglycan metabolism disorder, unspecified** `HCC` `Rx` `ESR` `COM`

✓4ᵗʰ **E77 Disorders of glycoprotein metabolism**

  E77.0 **Defects in post-translational modification of lysosomal enzymes** `HCC` `Rx` `ESR` `COM`
> Mucolipidosis II [I-cell disease]
> Mucolipidosis III [pseudo-Hurler polydystrophy]

  E77.1 **Defects in glycoprotein degradation** `HCC` `Rx` `ESR` `COM`
> Aspartylglucosaminuria
> Fucosidosis
> Mannosidosis
> Sialidosis [mucolipidosis I]

  E77.8 **Other disorders of glycoprotein metabolism** `HCC` `Rx` `ESR` `COM`

  E77.9 **Disorder of glycoprotein metabolism, unspecified** `HCC` `Rx` `ESR` `COM`

✓4ᵗʰ **E78 Disorders of lipoprotein metabolism and other lipidemias**
> **EXCLUDES 1**   *sphingolipidosis (E75.0-E75.3)*

  ✓5ᵗʰ **E78.0 Pure hypercholesterolemia**
> **AHA:** 2016,4Q,13-14

    E78.00 **Pure hypercholesterolemia, unspecified** `Rx`
> Fredrickson's hyperlipoproteinemia, type IIa
> Hyperbetalipoproteinemia
> Low-density-lipoprotein-type [LDL] hyperlipoproteinemia
> (Pure) hypercholesterolemia NOS
> **AHA:** 2022,2Q,5-6

    E78.01 **Familial hypercholesterolemia** `Rx`

  E78.1 **Pure hyperglyceridemia** `Rx`
> Elevated fasting triglycerides
> Endogenous hyperglyceridemia
> Fredrickson's hyperlipoproteinemia, type IV
> Hyperlipidemia, group B
> Hyperprebetalipoproteinemia
> Very-low-density-lipoprotein-type [VLDL] hyperlipoproteinemia

  E78.2 **Mixed hyperlipidemia** `Rx`
> Broad- or floating-betalipoproteinemia
> Combined hyperlipidemia NOS
> Elevated cholesterol with elevated triglycerides NEC
> Fredrickson's hyperlipoproteinemia, type IIb or III
> Hyperbetalipoproteinemia with prebetalipoproteinemia
> Hypercholesteremia with endogenous hyperglyceridemia
> Hyperlipidemia, group C
> Tubo-eruptive xanthoma
> Xanthoma tuberosum
>
> **EXCLUDES 1**   *cerebrotendinous cholesterosis [van Bogaert-Scherer-Epstein] (E75.5)*
>   *familial combined hyperlipidemia (E78.49)*
>
> **AHA:** 2022,2Q,6

  E78.3 **Hyperchylomicronemia** `Rx`
> Chylomicron retention disease
> Fredrickson's hyperlipoproteinemia, type I or V
> Hyperlipidemia, group D
> Mixed hyperglyceridemia

  ✓5ᵗʰ **E78.4 Other hyperlipidemia**
> **AHA:** 2018,4Q,6

    E78.41 **Elevated Lipoprotein(a)** `Rx`
> Elevated Lp(a)

    E78.49 **Other hyperlipidemia** `Rx`
> Familial combined hyperlipidemia

  E78.5 **Hyperlipidemia, unspecified** `Rx`
> **AHA:** 2022,2Q,5

  E78.6 **Lipoprotein deficiency** `Rx`
> Abetalipoproteinemia
> Depressed HDL cholesterol
> High-density lipoprotein deficiency
> Hypoalphalipoproteinemia
> Hypobetalipoproteinemia (familial)
> Lecithin cholesterol acyltransferase deficiency
> Tangier disease

  ✓5ᵗʰ **E78.7 Disorders of bile acid and cholesterol metabolism**
> **EXCLUDES 1**   *Niemann-Pick disease type C (E75.242)*

    E78.70 **Disorder of bile acid and cholesterol metabolism, unspecified** `Rx`

    E78.71 **Barth syndrome** `COM`

    E78.72 **Smith-Lemli-Opitz syndrome** `COM`

E78.79   **Other disorders of bile acid and cholesterol metabolism**   `Rx`

√5th   E78.8   **Other disorders of lipoprotein metabolism**

    E78.81   **Lipoid dermatoarthritis**   `Rx`

    E78.89   **Other lipoprotein metabolism disorders**   `Rx`

   E78.9   **Disorder of lipoprotein metabolism, unspecified**   `Rx`

√4th   **E79   Disorders of purine and pyrimidine metabolism**

    `EXCLUDES 1`   Ataxia-telangiectasia (Q87.19)

          Bloom's syndrome (Q82.8)

          Cockayne's syndrome (Q87.19)

          calculus of kidney (N20.0)

          combined immunodeficiency disorders (D81.-)

          Fanconi's anemia (D61.09)

          gout (M1A.-, M10.-)

          orotaciduric anemia (D53.0)

          progeria (E34.8)

          Werner's syndrome (E34.8)

          xeroderma pigmentosum (Q82.1)

   E79.0   **Hyperuricemia without signs of inflammatory arthritis and tophaceous disease**

       Asymptomatic hyperuricemia

   E79.1   **Lesch-Nyhan syndrome**   `HCC` `Rx` `ESR` `COM`

       HGPRT deficiency

   E79.2   **Myoadenylate deaminase deficiency**   `HCC` `Rx` `ESR` `COM`

   E79.8   **Other disorders of purine and pyrimidine metabolism**   `HCC` `Rx` `ESR` `COM`

       Hereditary xanthinuria

   E79.9   **Disorder of purine and pyrimidine metabolism, unspecified**   `HCC` `Rx` `ESR` `COM`

√4th   **E80   Disorders of porphyrin and bilirubin metabolism**

    `INCLUDES`   defects of catalase and peroxidase

   E80.0   **Hereditary erythropoietic porphyria**   `HCC` `Rx` `ESR` `COM`

       Congenital erythropoietic porphyria

       Erythropoietic protoporphyria

   E80.1   **Porphyria cutanea tarda**   `HCC` `Rx` `ESR` `COM`

√5th   E80.2   **Other and unspecified porphyria**

    E80.20   **Unspecified porphyria**   `HCC` `Rx` `ESR` `COM`

       Porphyria NOS

    E80.21   **Acute intermittent (hepatic) porphyria**   `HCC` `Rx` `ESR` `COM`

    E80.29   **Other porphyria**   `HCC` `Rx` `ESR` `COM`

       Hereditary coproporphyria

   E80.3   **Defects of catalase and peroxidase**   `HCC` `Rx` `ESR` `COM`

       Acatalasia [Takahara]

   E80.4   **Gilbert syndrome**

   E80.5   **Crigler-Najjar syndrome**

   E80.6   **Other disorders of bilirubin metabolism**

       Dubin-Johnson syndrome

       Rotor's syndrome

   E80.7   **Disorder of bilirubin metabolism, unspecified**

√4th   **E83   Disorders of mineral metabolism**

    `EXCLUDES 1`   dietary mineral deficiency (E58-E61)

          parathyroid disorders (E20-E21)

          vitamin D deficiency (E55.-)

√5th   E83.0   **Disorders of copper metabolism**

    E83.00   **Disorder of copper metabolism, unspecified**   `Rx` `COM`

    E83.01   **Wilson's disease**   `Rx` `COM`

       Code also associated Kayser Fleischer ring (H18.04-)

    E83.09   **Other disorders of copper metabolism**   `Rx` `COM`

       Menkes' (kinky hair) (steely hair) disease

√5th   E83.1   **Disorders of iron metabolism**

    `EXCLUDES 1`   iron deficiency anemia (D50.-)

          sideroblastic anemia (D64.0-D64.3)

    E83.10   **Disorder of iron metabolism, unspecified**   `Rx`

√6th   E83.11   **Hemochromatosis**

      `EXCLUDES 1`   GALD (P78.84)

            gestational alloimmune liver disease (P78.84)

            neonatal hemochromatosis (P78.84)

     E83.110   **Hereditary hemochromatosis**   `HCC` `Rx` `ESR`

       Bronzed diabetes

       Pigmentary cirrhosis (of liver)

       Primary (hereditary) hemochromatosis

     E83.111   **Hemochromatosis due to repeated red blood cell transfusions**

       Iron overload due to repeated red blood cell transfusions

       Transfusion (red blood cell) associated hemochromatosis

     E83.118   **Other hemochromatosis**   `Rx`

     E83.119   **Hemochromatosis, unspecified**   `Rx`

    E83.19   **Other disorders of iron metabolism**   `Rx`

       Use additional code, if applicable, for idiopathic pulmonary hemosiderosis (J84.03)

   E83.2   **Disorders of zinc metabolism**

       Acrodermatitis enteropathica

√5th   E83.3   **Disorders of phosphorus metabolism and phosphatases**

    `EXCLUDES 1`   adult osteomalacia (M83.-)

          osteoporosis (M80.-)

    E83.30   **Disorder of phosphorus metabolism, unspecified**   `Rx`

    E83.31   **Familial hypophosphatemia**   `Rx`

       Vitamin D-resistant osteomalacia

       Vitamin D-resistant rickets

      `EXCLUDES 1`   vitamin D-deficiency rickets (E55.0)

    E83.32   **Hereditary vitamin D-dependent rickets (type 1) (type 2)**   `Rx`

       25-hydroxyvitamin D 1-alpha-hydroxylase deficiency

       Pseudovitamin D deficiency

       Vitamin D receptor defect

    E83.39   **Other disorders of phosphorus metabolism**   `Rx`

       Acid phosphatase deficiency

       Hypophosphatasia

√5th   E83.4   **Disorders of magnesium metabolism**

    E83.40   **Disorders of magnesium metabolism, unspecified**

    E83.41   **Hypermagnesemia**

       AHA: 2016,4Q,54

    E83.42   **Hypomagnesemia**

    E83.49   **Other disorders of magnesium metabolism**

√5th   E83.5   **Disorders of calcium metabolism**

    `EXCLUDES 1`   chondrocalcinosis (M11.1-M11.2)

          hungry bone syndrome (E83.81)

          hyperparathyroidism (E21.0-E21.3)

    E83.50   **Unspecified disorder of calcium metabolism**

    E83.51   **Hypocalcemia**

    E83.52   **Hypercalcemia**

       Familial hypocalciuric hypercalcemia

    E83.59   **Other disorders of calcium metabolism**

√5th   E83.8   **Other disorders of mineral metabolism**

    E83.81   **Hungry bone syndrome**

    E83.89   **Other disorders of mineral metabolism**

   E83.9   **Disorder of mineral metabolism, unspecified**

√4th   **E84   Cystic fibrosis**

    `INCLUDES`   mucoviscidosis

    Code also exocrine pancreatic insufficiency (K86.81)

    DEF: Genetic disorder affecting the respiratory, digestive, and reproductive systems in infants to young adults by disturbing exocrine gland function and causing chronic pulmonary disease with excess mucus production and pancreatic deficiency.

   E84.0   **Cystic fibrosis with pulmonary manifestations**   `HCC` `Rx` `ESR` `COM`

       Use additional code to identify any infectious organism present, such as:

       Pseudomonas (B96.5)

       AHA: 2021,1Q,23

`HCC` CMS-HCC   `Rx` Rx HCC   `ESR` ESRD HCC   `COM` Commercial HCC   `N` Newborn: 0   `P` Pediatric: 0-17   `M` Maternity: 9-64   `A` Adult: 15-124

550   ICD-10-CM 2023

✓5ᵗʰ **E84.1** **Cystic fibrosis with** intestinal manifestations

    E84.11 **Meconium ileus in cystic fibrosis** `HCC` `Rx` `ESR` `COM` `N`

        EXCLUDES 1   *meconium ileus not due to cystic fibrosis (P76.0)*

    E84.19 **Cystic fibrosis with other intestinal manifestations** `HCC` `Rx` `ESR` `COM`

        Distal intestinal obstruction syndrome

E84.8 **Cystic fibrosis with other manifestations** `HCC` `Rx` `ESR` `COM`

E84.9 **Cystic fibrosis, unspecified** `HCC` `Rx` `ESR` `COM`

✓4ᵗʰ **E85** **Amyloidosis**

    EXCLUDES 2   *Alzheimer's disease (G30.0-)*

    DEF: Conditions of diverse etiologies characterized by the accumulation of insoluble fibrillar proteins (amyloid) in various organs and tissues of the body, compromising vital functions.

    E85.0 **Non-neuropathic heredofamilial amyloidosis** `HCC` `ESR` `COM`

        Hereditary amyloid nephropathy

        Code also associated disorders, such as:

          autoinflammatory syndromes (M04.-)

        EXCLUDES 2   *transthyretin-related (ATTR) familial amyloid cardiomyopathy (E85.4)*

    E85.1 **Neuropathic heredofamilial amyloidosis** `HCC` `ESR` `COM`

        Amyloid polyneuropathy (Portuguese)

        Transthyretin-related (ATTR) familial amyloid polyneuropathy

        AHA: 2012,4Q,99

    E85.2 **Heredofamilial amyloidosis, unspecified** `HCC` `ESR` `COM`

    E85.3 **Secondary systemic amyloidosis** `HCC` `ESR` `COM`

        Hemodialysis-associated amyloidosis

    E85.4 **Organ-limited amyloidosis** `HCC` `ESR` `COM`

        Localized amyloidosis

        Transthyretin-related (ATTR) familial amyloid cardiomyopathy

    ✓5ᵗʰ **E85.8** **Other amyloidosis**

        AHA: 2017,4Q,7

        E85.81 **Light chain (AL) amyloidosis** `HCC` `ESR` `COM`

        E85.82 **Wild-type transthyretin-related (ATTR) amyloidosis** `HCC` `ESR` `COM`

          Senile systemic amyloidosis (SSA)

        E85.89 **Other amyloidosis** `HCC` `ESR` `COM`

    E85.9 **Amyloidosis, unspecified** `HCC` `ESR` `COM`

✓4ᵗʰ **E86** **Volume depletion**

    Use additional code(s) for any associated disorders of electrolyte and acid-base balance (E87.-)

    EXCLUDES 1   *dehydration of newborn (P74.1)*

               postprocedural hypovolemic shock (T81.19)

               traumatic hypovolemic shock (T79.4)

    EXCLUDES 2   *hypovolemic shock NOS (R57.1)*

    AHA: 2019,2Q,7; 2018,2Q,6

    E86.0 **Dehydration**

        AHA: 2019,2Q,7; 2019,1Q,12; 2014,1Q,7

        TIP: Can be assigned in addition to hypernatremia (E87.0) or hyponatremia (E87.1), when documented.

    E86.1 **Hypovolemia**

        Depletion of volume of plasma

    E86.9 **Volume depletion, unspecified**

        DEF: Depletion of total body water (dehydration) and/or contraction of total intravascular plasma (hypovolemia).

✓4ᵗʰ **E87** **Other disorders of fluid, electrolyte and acid-base balance**

    EXCLUDES 1   *diabetes insipidus (E23.2)*

               electrolyte imbalance associated with hyperemesis gravidarum (O21.1)

               electrolyte imbalance following ectopic or molar pregnancy (O08.5)

               familial periodic paralysis (G72.3)

    AHA: 2018,2Q,6

    E87.0 **Hyperosmolality and hypernatremia**

        Sodium [Na] excess

        Sodium [Na] overload

        AHA: 2022,1Q,28; 2014,1Q,7

        TIP: Assign an additional code for dehydration (E86.0), when documented.

E87.1 **Hypo-osmolality and hyponatremia**

    Sodium [Na] deficiency

    EXCLUDES 1   *syndrome of inappropriate secretion of antidiuretic hormone (E22.2)*

    AHA: 2014,1Q,7

    TIP: Assign an additional code for dehydration (E86.0), when documented.

▲ ✓5ᵗʰ **E87.2** **Acidosis**

    ~~Acidosis NOS~~

    ~~Lactic acidosis~~

    ~~Metabolic acidosis~~

    ~~Respiratory acidosis~~

    EXCLUDES 1   *diabetic acidosis - see categories E08-E10, E11, E13 with ketoacidosis*

    AHA: 2020,3Q,30

    DEF: Reduction of alkaline in the blood and tissues caused by an increase in acid and decrease in bicarbonate.

    ● **E87.20** **Acidosis, unspecified**

        Lactic acidosis NOS

        Metabolic acidosis NOS

        Code also, if applicable, respiratory failure with hypercapnia (J96. with 5th character 2)

    ● **E87.21** **Acute metabolic acidosis**

        Acute lactic acidosis

    ● **E87.22** **Chronic metabolic acidosis**

        Chronic lactic acidosis

        Code first underlying etiology, if applicable

    ● **E87.29** **Other acidosis**

        Respiratory acidosis NOS

        EXCLUDES 2   *acute respiratory acidosis (J96.02)*

                           chronic respiratory acidosis (J96.12)

E87.3 **Alkalosis**

    Alkalosis NOS

    Metabolic alkalosis

    Respiratory alkalosis

E87.4 **Mixed disorder of acid-base balance**

E87.5 **Hyperkalemia**

    Potassium [K] excess

    Potassium [K] overload

E87.6 **Hypokalemia**

    Potassium [K] deficiency

✓5ᵗʰ **E87.7** **Fluid overload**

    EXCLUDES 1   *edema NOS (R60.9)*

               fluid retention (R60.9)

    E87.70 **Fluid overload, unspecified**

    E87.71 **Transfusion associated circulatory overload**

        Fluid overload due to transfusion (blood) (blood components)

        TACO

    E87.79 **Other fluid overload**

E87.8 **Other disorders of electrolyte and fluid balance, not elsewhere classified**

    Electrolyte imbalance NOS

    Hyperchloremia

    Hypochloremia

✓4ᵗʰ **E88** **Other and unspecified metabolic disorders**

    Use additional codes for associated conditions

    EXCLUDES 1   *histiocytosis X (chronic) (C96.6)*

✓5ᵗʰ **E88.0** **Disorders of plasma-protein metabolism, not elsewhere classified**

    EXCLUDES 1   *monoclonal gammopathy (of undetermined significance) (D47.2)*

               polyclonal hypergammaglobulinemia (D89.0)

               Waldenström macroglobulinemia (C88.0)

    EXCLUDES 2   *disorder of lipoprotein metabolism (E78.-)*

    E88.01 **Alpha-1-antitrypsin deficiency** `HCC` `Rx` `ESR` `COM`

        AAT deficiency

☑ Additional Character Required   ✓x7ᵗʰ Placeholder Alert   Manifestation   Unspecified Dx   ◻ QPP   UPD Unacceptable PDx

Chapter 4. Endocrine, Nutritional and Metabolic Diseases

E88.02–E89.89

E88.02 Plasminogen deficiency
Dysplasminogenemia
Hypoplasminogenemia
Type 1 plasminogen deficiency
Type 2 plasminogen deficiency
Code also, if applicable, ligneous conjunctivitis
(H10.51)
Use additional code for associated findings, such as:
hydrocephalus (G91.4)
otitis media (H67.-)
respiratory disorder related to plasminogen
deficiency (J99)
AHA: 2018,4Q,6-7

E88.09 Other disorders of plasma-protein metabolism, not elsewhere classified
Bisalbuminemia

E88.1 Lipodystrophy, not elsewhere classified
Lipodystrophy NOS
EXCLUDES 1   Whipple's disease (K90.81)

E88.2 Lipomatosis, not elsewhere classified   Rx
Lipomatosis NOS
Lipomatosis (Check) dolorosa [Dercum]

E88.3 Tumor lysis syndrome   COM
Tumor lysis syndrome (spontaneous)
Tumor lysis syndrome following antineoplastic drug
chemotherapy
Use additional code for adverse effect, if applicable, to identify
drug (T45.1X5)
AHA: 2020,1Q,37; 2019,2Q,24
DEF: Potentially fatal metabolic complication of tumor necrosis
caused by spontaneous or treatment-related accumulation of
byproducts from dying cancer cells. Symptoms include
hyperkalemia, hyperphosphatemia, hypocalcemia, hyperuricemia,
and hyperuricosuria.

✓5ᵗʰ E88.4 Mitochondrial metabolism disorders
EXCLUDES 1   disorders of pyruvate metabolism (E74.4)
Kearns-Sayre syndrome (H49.81)
Leber's disease (H47.22)
Leigh's encephalopathy (G31.82)
mitochondrial myopathy, NEC (G71.3)
Reye's syndrome (G93.7)

E88.40 Mitochondrial metabolism disorder, unspecified   HCC Rx ESR COM

E88.41 MELAS syndrome   HCC Rx ESR COM
Mitochondrial myopathy, encephalopathy, lactic
acidosis and stroke-like episodes

E88.42 MERRF syndrome   HCC Rx ESR COM
Myoclonic epilepsy associated with ragged-red fibers
Code also progressive myoclonic epilepsy (G40.3-)

E88.49 Other mitochondrial metabolism disorders   HCC Rx ESR COM

✓5ᵗʰ E88.8 Other specified metabolic disorders

E88.81 Metabolic syndrome
Dysmetabolic syndrome X
Use additional codes for associated manifestations,
such as:
obesity (E66.-)
DEF: Group of health risks that increase the likelihood
of developing heart disease, stroke, and diabetes. These
risks include certain parameters for blood pressure,
cholesterol, and glucose levels.

E88.89 Other specified metabolic disorders   HCC Rx ESR COM
Launois-Bensaude adenolipomatosis
EXCLUDES 1   adult pulmonary Langerhans cell
histiocytosis (J84.82)

E88.9 Metabolic disorder, unspecified

Postprocedural endocrine and metabolic complications and disorders, not elsewhere classified (E89)

✓4ᵗʰ E89 Postprocedural endocrine and metabolic complications and disorders, not elsewhere classified
EXCLUDES 2   intraoperative complications of endocrine system organ or
structure (E36.0-, E36.1-, E36.8)

E89.0 Postprocedural hypothyroidism   Rx
Postirradiation hypothyroidism
Postsurgical hypothyroidism

E89.1 Postprocedural hypoinsulinemia
Postpancreatectomy hyperglycemia
Postsurgical hypoinsulinemia
Use additional code, if applicable, to identify:
acquired absence of pancreas (Z90.41-)
diabetes mellitus (postpancreatectomy) (postprocedural)
(E13.-)
insulin use (Z79.4)
EXCLUDES 1   transient postprocedural hyperglycemia (R73.9)
transient postprocedural hypoglycemia (E16.2)

[handwritten annotations: ① ② E13.— ③ Z90.41— post pancreatectomy]

E89.2 Postprocedural hypoparathyroidism   HCC Rx ESR COM
Parathyroprival tetany

E89.3 Postprocedural hypopituitarism   HCC Rx ESR COM
Postirradiation hypopituitarism

✓5ᵗʰ E89.4 Postprocedural ovarian failure

E89.40 Asymptomatic postprocedural ovarian failure   ♀
Postprocedural ovarian failure NOS

E89.41 Symptomatic postprocedural ovarian failure   ♀
Symptoms such as flushing, sleeplessness, headache,
lack of concentration, associated with
postprocedural menopause

E89.5 Postprocedural testicular hypofunction   ♂

E89.6 Postprocedural adrenocortical (-medullary) hypofunction   HCC Rx ESR COM

✓5ᵗʰ E89.8 Other postprocedural endocrine and metabolic complications and disorders
AHA: 2016,4Q,9-10

✓6ᵗʰ E89.81 Postprocedural hemorrhage of an endocrine system organ or structure following a procedure

E89.810 Postprocedural hemorrhage of an endocrine system organ or structure following an endocrine system procedure

E89.811 Postprocedural hemorrhage of an endocrine system organ or structure following other procedure

✓6ᵗʰ E89.82 Postprocedural hematoma and seroma of an endocrine system organ or structure

E89.820 Postprocedural hematoma of an endocrine system organ or structure following an endocrine system procedure

E89.821 Postprocedural hematoma of an endocrine system organ or structure following other procedure

E89.822 Postprocedural seroma of an endocrine system organ or structure following an endocrine system procedure

E89.823 Postprocedural seroma of an endocrine system organ or structure following other procedure

E89.89 Other postprocedural endocrine and metabolic complications and disorders
Use additional code, if applicable, to further specify
disorder

Chapter 5. Mental, Behavioral and Neurodevelopmental Disorders (F01–F99)

Chapter-specific Guidelines with Coding Examples

The chapter-specific guidelines from the ICD-10-CM Official Guidelines for Coding and Reporting have been provided below. Along with these guidelines are coding examples, contained in the shaded boxes, that have been developed to help illustrate the coding and/or sequencing guidance found in these guidelines.

a. Pain disorders related to psychological factors

Assign code F45.41, for pain that is exclusively related to psychological disorders. As indicated by the Excludes 1 note under category G89, a code from category G89 should not be assigned with code F45.41.

> Chest pain determined to be persistent somatoform pain disorder
>
> **F45.41   Pain disorder exclusively related to psychological factors**
>
> *Explanation*: This pain was diagnosed as being exclusively psychological; therefore, no code from category G89 is added.

Code F45.42, Pain disorders with related psychological factors, should be used with a code from category G89, Pain, not elsewhere classified, if there is documentation of a psychological component for a patient with acute or chronic pain.

See Section I.C.6. Pain

b. Mental and behavioral disorders due to psychoactive substance use

1) In remission

Selection of codes **describing** "in remission" for categories F10-F19, Mental and behavioral disorders due to psychoactive substance use (categories F10-F19 with -.11, -.21, **-.91**) requires the provider's clinical judgment **and** are assigned only on the basis of provider documentation (as defined in the Official Guidelines for Coding and Reporting), unless otherwise instructed by the classification.

Mild substance use disorders in early or sustained remission are classified to the appropriate codes for substance abuse in remission, and moderate or severe substance use disorders in early or sustained remission are classified to the appropriate codes for substance dependence in remission.

> Physician documentation indicates the patient is seen to monitor progress on quitting cigarette smoking. The problem list indicates mild tobacco use disorder that is currently in remission.
>
> **F17.211   Nicotine dependence, cigarettes, in remission**
>
> *Explanation*: According to the index, Disorder, tobacco use, cigarettes (mild) (moderate) (severe), in remission (early) (sustained) is categorized to dependence (F17.211). Since the physician clearly documents mild cigarette use "disorder" and that the disorder is in remission, a code for nicotine dependence "in remission" is appropriate.

2) Psychoactive substance use, abuse and dependence

When the provider documentation refers to use, abuse and dependence of the same substance (e.g. alcohol, opioid, cannabis, etc.), only one code should be assigned to identify the pattern of use based on the following hierarchy:

- If both use and abuse are documented, assign only the code for abuse
- If both abuse and dependence are documented, assign only the code for dependence
- If use, abuse and dependence are all documented, assign only the code for dependence
- If both use and dependence are documented, assign only the code for dependence.

> History and physical notes cannabis dependence and ongoing cannabis abuse
>
> **F12.20   Cannabis dependence, uncomplicated**
>
> *Explanation*: In the hierarchy, the dependence code is used if both abuse and dependence are documented.

> Current problem list indicates daily opioid use with opioid abuse.
>
> **F11.10   Opioid abuse, uncomplicated**
>
> *Explanation*: In the hierarchy, the abuse code is used if both abuse and use are documented.

3) Psychoactive substance use, unspecified

As with all other unspecified diagnoses, the codes for unspecified psychoactive substance use (F10.9-, F11.9-, F12.9-, F13.9-, F14.9-, F15.9-, F16.9-, F18.9-, F19.9-) should only be assigned based on provider documentation and when they meet the definition of a reportable diagnosis (see Section III, Reporting Additional Diagnoses). These codes are to be used only when the psychoactive substance use is associated with a substance related disorder (chapter 5 disorders such as sexual dysfunction, sleep disorder, or a mental or behavioral disorder) or medical condition, and such a relationship is documented by the provider.

4) Medical conditions due to psychoactive substance use, abuse and dependence

Medical conditions due to substance use, abuse, and dependence are not classified as substance-induced disorders. Assign the diagnosis code for the medical condition as directed by the Alphabetical Index along with the appropriate psychoactive substance use, abuse or dependence code. For example, for alcoholic pancreatitis due to alcohol dependence, assign the appropriate code from subcategory K85.2, Alcohol induced acute pancreatitis, and the appropriate code from subcategory F10.2, such as code F10.20, Alcohol dependence, uncomplicated. It would not be appropriate to assign code F10.288, Alcohol dependence with other alcohol-induced disorder.

5) Blood alcohol level

A code from category Y90, Evidence of alcohol involvement determined by blood alcohol level, may be assigned when this information is documented and the patient's provider has documented a condition classifiable to category F10, Alcohol related disorders. The blood alcohol level does not need to be documented by the patient's provider in order for it to be coded.

See Section I.B.14. for blood alcohol level documentation by clinicians other than patient's provider.

c. Factitious disorder

Factitious disorder imposed on self or Munchausen's syndrome is a disorder in which a person falsely reports or causes his or her own physical or psychological signs or symptoms. For patients with documented factitious disorder on self or Munchausen's syndrome, assign the appropriate code from subcategory F68.1-, Factitious disorder imposed on self.

Munchausen's syndrome by proxy (MSBP) is a disorder in which a caregiver (perpetrator) falsely reports or causes an illness or injury in another person (victim) under his or her care, such as a child, an elderly adult, or a person who has a disability. The condition is also referred to as "factitious disorder imposed on another" or "factitious disorder by proxy." The perpetrator, not the victim, receives this diagnosis. Assign code F68.A, Factitious disorder imposed on another, to the perpetrator's record. For the victim of a patient suffering from MSBP, assign the appropriate code from categories T74, Adult and child abuse, neglect and other maltreatment, confirmed, or T76, Adult and child abuse, neglect and other maltreatment, suspected.

See Section I.C.19.f. Adult and child abuse, neglect and other maltreatment

d. Dementia

The ICD-10-CM classifies dementia (categories F01, F02, and F03) on the basis of the etiology and severity (unspecified, mild, moderate or severe). Selection of the appropriate severity level requires the provider's clinical judgment and codes should be assigned only on the basis of provider documentation (as defined in the *Official Guidelines for Coding and Reporting*), unless otherwise instructed by the classification. If the documentation does not provide information about the severity of the dementia, assign the appropriate code for unspecified severity.

If a patient is admitted to an inpatient acute care hospital or other inpatient facility setting with dementia at one severity level and it progresses to a higher severity level, assign one code for the highest severity level reported during the stay.

Chapter 5. Mental, Behavioral and Neurodevelopmental Disorders

Chapter 5. Mental, Behavioral and Neurodevelopmental Disorders (F01-F99)

> **INCLUDES**   disorders of psychological development
>
> **EXCLUDES 2**   symptoms, signs and abnormal clinical laboratory findings, not elsewhere classified (R00-R99)

This chapter contains the following blocks:

F01-F09	Mental disorders due to known physiological conditions
F10-F19	Mental and behavioral disorders due to psychoactive substance use
F20-F29	Schizophrenia, schizotypal, delusional, and other non-mood psychotic disorders
F30-F39	Mood [affective] disorders
F40-F48	Anxiety, dissociative, stress-related, somatoform and other nonpsychotic mental disorders
F50-F59	Behavioral syndromes associated with physiological disturbances and physical factors
F60-F69	Disorders of adult personality and behavior
F70-F79	Intellectual disabilities
F80-F89	Pervasive and specific developmental disorders
F90-F98	Behavioral and emotional disorders with onset usually occurring in childhood and adolescence
F99	Unspecified mental disorder

Mental disorders due to known physiological conditions (F01-F09)

> **NOTE**   This block comprises a range of mental disorders grouped together on the basis of their having in common a demonstrable etiology in cerebral disease, brain injury, or other insult leading to cerebral dysfunction. The dysfunction may be primary, as in diseases, injuries, and insults that affect the brain directly and selectively; or secondary, as in systemic diseases and disorders that attack the brain only as one of the multiple organs or systems of the body that are involved.

✓4ᵗʰ **F01   Vascular dementia**

Vascular dementia as a result of infarction of the brain due to vascular disease, including hypertensive cerebrovascular disease.

> **INCLUDES**   arteriosclerotic dementia
> ▶major neurocognitive disorder due to vascular disease◄
> ▶multi-infarct dementia◄

Code first the underlying physiological condition or sequelae of cerebrovascular disease.

▲   ✓5ᵗʰ **F01.5   Vascular dementia, unspecified severity**

▲   **F01.50   Vascular dementia, unspecified severity, without behavioral disturbance, psychotic disturbance, mood disturbance, and anxiety**   HCC Rx ESR A
▶Major neurocognitive disorder due to vascular disease NOS◄
▶Vascular dementia NOS◄
AHA: 2021,2Q,4

▲   ✓6ᵗʰ **F01.51   Vascular dementia, unspecified severity, with behavioral disturbance**
~~Major neurocognitive disorder due to vascular disease, with behavioral disturbance~~
~~Major neurocognitive disorder with aggressive behavior~~
~~Major neurocognitive disorder with combative behavior~~
~~Major neurocognitive disorder with violent behavior~~
~~Vascular dementia with aggressive behavior~~
~~Vascular dementia with combative behavior~~
~~Vascular dementia with violent behavior~~
~~Use additional code, if applicable, to identify wandering in vascular dementia (Z91.83)~~

●   **F01.511   Vascular dementia, unspecified severity, with agitation**
Major neurocognitive disorder due to vascular disease, unspecified severity, with aberrant motor behavior such as restlessness, rocking, pacing, or exit-seeking
Major neurocognitive disorder due to vascular disease, unspecified severity, with verbal or physical behaviors such as profanity, shouting, threatening, anger, aggression, combativeness, or violence
Vascular dementia, unspecified severity, with aberrant motor behavior such as restlessness, rocking, pacing, or exit-seeking
Vascular dementia, unspecified severity, with verbal or physical behaviors such as profanity, shouting, threatening, anger, aggression, combativeness, or violence

●   **F01.518   Vascular dementia, unspecified severity, with other behavioral disturbance**
Major neurocognitive disorder due to vascular disease, unspecified severity, with behavioral disturbances such as sleep disturbance, social disinhibition, or sexual disinhibition
Vascular dementia, unspecified severity, with behavioral disturbances such as sleep disturbance, social disinhibition, or sexual disinhibition
Use additional code, if applicable, to identify wandering in vascular dementia (Z91.83)

●   **F01.52   Vascular dementia, unspecified severity, with psychotic disturbance**
Major neurocognitive disorder due to vascular disease, unspecified severity, with psychotic disturbance such as hallucinations, paranoia, suspiciousness, or delusional state
Vascular dementia, unspecified severity, with psychotic disturbance such as hallucinations, paranoia, suspiciousness, or delusional state

●   **F01.53   Vascular dementia, unspecified severity, with mood disturbance**
Major neurocognitive disorder due to vascular disease, unspecified severity, with mood disturbance such as depression, apathy, or anhedonia
Vascular dementia, unspecified severity, with mood disturbance such as depression, apathy, or anhedonia

●   **F01.54   Vascular dementia, unspecified severity, with anxiety**
Major neurocognitive disorder due to vascular disease, unspecified severity, with anxiety

- ☑5ᵗʰ **F01.A Vascular dementia, mild**

  > **EXCLUDES 1** *mild neurocognitive disorder due to known physiological condition with or without behavioral disturbance (F06.7-)*

  - **F01.A0 Vascular dementia, mild, without behavioral disturbance, psychotic disturbance, mood disturbance, and anxiety**
    Major neurocognitive disorder due to vascular disease, mild, NOS
    Vascular dementia, mild, NOS

  - ☑6ᵗʰ **F01.A1 Vascular dementia, mild, with behavioral disturbance**
    - **F01.A11 Vascular dementia, mild, with agitation**
      Major neurocognitive disorder due to vascular disease, mild, with aberrant motor behavior such as restlessness, rocking, pacing, or exit-seeking
      Major neurocognitive disorder due to vascular disease, mild, with verbal or physical behaviors such as profanity, shouting, threatening, anger, aggression, combativeness, or violence
      Vascular dementia, mild, with aberrant motor behavior such as restlessness, rocking, pacing, or exit-seeking
      Vascular dementia, mild, with verbal or physical behaviors such as profanity, shouting, threatening, anger, aggression, combativeness, or violence

    - **F01.A18 Vascular dementia, mild, with other behavioral disturbance**
      Major neurocognitive disorder due to vascular disease, mild, with behavioral disturbances such as sleep disturbance, social disinhibition, or sexual disinhibition
      Vascular dementia, mild, with behavioral disturbances such as sleep disturbance, social disinhibition, or sexual disinhibition
      Use additional code, if applicable, to identify wandering in vascular dementia (Z91.83)

  - **F01.A2 Vascular dementia, mild, with psychotic disturbance**
    Major neurocognitive disorder due to vascular disease, mild, with psychotic disturbance such as hallucinations, paranoia, suspiciousness, or delusional state
    Vascular dementia, mild, with psychotic disturbance such as hallucinations, paranoia, suspiciousness, or delusional state

  - **F01.A3 Vascular dementia, mild, with mood disturbance**
    Major neurocognitive disorder due to vascular disease, mild, with mood disturbance such as depression, apathy, or anhedonia
    Vascular dementia, mild, with mood disturbance such as depression, apathy, or anhedonia

  - **F01.A4 Vascular dementia, mild, with anxiety**
    Major neurocognitive disorder due to vascular disease, mild, with anxiety

- ☑5ᵗʰ **F01.B Vascular dementia, moderate**

  - **F01.B0 Vascular dementia, moderate, without behavioral disturbance, psychotic disturbance, mood disturbance, and anxiety**
    Major neurocognitive disorder due to vascular disease, moderate, NOS
    Vascular dementia, moderate, NOS

  - ☑6ᵗʰ **F01.B1 Vascular dementia, moderate, with behavioral disturbance**
    - **F01.B11 Vascular dementia, moderate, with agitation**
      Major neurocognitive disorder due to vascular disease, moderate, with aberrant motor behavior such as restlessness, rocking, pacing, or exit-seeking
      Major neurocognitive disorder due to vascular disease, moderate, with verbal or physical behaviors such as profanity, shouting, threatening, anger, aggression, combativeness, or violence
      Vascular dementia, moderate, with aberrant motor behavior such as restlessness, rocking, pacing, or exit-seeking
      Vascular dementia, moderate, with verbal or physical behaviors such as profanity, shouting, threatening, anger, aggression, combativeness, or violence

    - **F01.B18 Vascular dementia, moderate, with other behavioral disturbance**
      Major neurocognitive disorder due to vascular disease, moderate, with behavioral disturbances such as sleep disturbance, social disinhibition, or sexual disinhibition
      Vascular dementia, moderate, with behavioral disturbances such as sleep disturbance, social disinhibition, or sexual disinhibition
      Use additional code, if applicable, to identify wandering in vascular dementia (Z91.83)

  - **F01.B2 Vascular dementia, moderate, with psychotic disturbance**
    Major neurocognitive disorder due to vascular disease, moderate, with psychotic disturbance such as hallucinations, paranoia, suspiciousness, or delusional state
    Vascular dementia, moderate, with psychotic disturbance such as hallucinations, paranoia, suspiciousness, or delusional state

  - **F01.B3 Vascular dementia, moderate, with mood disturbance**
    Major neurocognitive disorder due to vascular disease, moderate, with mood disturbance such as depression, apathy, or anhedonia
    Vascular dementia, moderate, with mood disturbance such as depression, apathy, or anhedonia

  - **F01.B4 Vascular dementia, moderate, with anxiety**
    Major neurocognitive disorder due to vascular disease, moderate, with anxiety

- ☑5ᵗʰ **F01.C Vascular dementia, severe**

  - **F01.C0 Vascular dementia, severe, without behavioral disturbance, psychotic disturbance, mood disturbance, and anxiety**
    Major neurocognitive disorder due to vascular disease, severe, NOS
    Vascular dementia, severe, NOS

Chapter 5. Mental, Behavioral and Neurodevelopmental Disorders

√6ᵗʰ **F01.C1 Vascular dementia, severe, with behavioral disturbance**

    F01.C11 Vascular dementia, severe, with agitation

         Major neurocognitive disorder due to vascular disease, severe, with aberrant motor behavior such as restlessness, rocking, pacing, or exit-seeking

         Major neurocognitive disorder due to vascular disease, severe, with verbal or physical behaviors such as profanity, shouting, threatening, anger, aggression, combativeness, or violence

         Vascular dementia, severe, with aberrant motor behavior such as restlessness, rocking, pacing, or exit-seeking

         Vascular dementia, severe, with verbal or physical behaviors such as profanity, shouting, threatening, anger, aggression, combativeness, or violence

    F01.C18 Vascular dementia, severe, with other behavioral disturbance

         Major neurocognitive disorder due to vascular disease, severe, with behavioral disturbances such as sleep disturbance, social disinhibition, or sexual disinhibition

         Vascular dementia, severe, with behavioral disturbances such as sleep disturbance, social disinhibition, or sexual disinhibition

         Use additional code, if applicable, to identify wandering in vascular dementia (Z91.83)

F01.C2 Vascular dementia, severe, with psychotic disturbance

     Major neurocognitive disorder due to vascular disease, severe, with psychotic disturbance such as hallucinations, paranoia, suspiciousness, or delusional state

     Vascular dementia, severe, with psychotic disturbance such as hallucinations, paranoia, suspiciousness, or delusional state

F01.C3 Vascular dementia, severe, with mood disturbance

     Major neurocognitive disorder due to vascular disease, severe, with mood disturbance such as depression, apathy, or anhedonia

     Vascular dementia, severe, with mood disturbance such as depression, apathy, or anhedonia

F01.C4 Vascular dementia, severe, with anxiety

     Major neurocognitive disorder due to vascular disease, severe, with anxiety

√4ᵗʰ **F02 Dementia in other diseases classified elsewhere**

    INCLUDES major neurocognitive disorder in other diseases classified elsewhere

     Code first the underlying physiological condition, such as:
       Alzheimer's (G30.-)
       cerebral lipidosis (E75.4)
       Creutzfeldt-Jakob disease (A81.0-)
       dementia with Lewy bodies (G31.83)
       dementia with Parkinsonism (G31.83)
       epilepsy and recurrent seizures (G40.-)
       frontotemporal dementia (G31.09)
       hepatolenticular degeneration (E83.0)
       human immunodeficiency virus [HIV] disease (B20)
       Huntington's disease (G10)
       hypercalcemia (E83.52)
       hypothyroidism, acquired (E00-E03.-)
       intoxications (T36-T65)
       Jakob-Creutzfeldt disease (A81.0-)
       multiple sclerosis (G35)
       neurosyphilis (A52.17)
       niacin deficiency [pellagra] (E52)
       Parkinson's disease (G20)
       Pick's disease (G31.01)
       polyarteritis nodosa (M30.0)
       prion disease (A81.9)
       systemic lupus erythematosus (M32.-)
       traumatic brain injury (S06.-)
       trypanosomiasis (B56.-, B57.-)
       vitamin B deficiency (E53.8)

    EXCLUDES 1 ▶mild neurocognitive disorder due to known physiological condition with or without behavioral disturbance (F06.7-)◀

    EXCLUDES 2 dementia in alcohol and psychoactive substance disorders (F10-F19, with .17, .27, .97)

         vascular dementia ▶(F01.5-, F01.A-, F01.B-, F01.C-)◀

▲ √5ᵗʰ **F02.8 Dementia in other diseases classified elsewhere, unspecified severity**

    AHA: 2022,1Q,25; 2017,2Q,7; 2016,4Q,141; 2016,2Q,6

    TIP: A code from this subcategory should always be assigned with a code from category G30 when Alzheimer's disease is documented, even in the absence of documented dementia.

▲   *F02.80 Dementia in other diseases classified elsewhere, unspecified severity, without behavioral disturbance, psychotic disturbance, mood disturbance, and anxiety*   HCC Rx ESR

         Dementia in other diseases classified elsewhere NOS

         ▶Major neurocognitive disorder in other diseases classified elsewhere NOS◀

▲   ✓6ᵗʰ   **F02.81   Dementia in other diseases classified elsewhere, unspecified severity, with behavioral disturbance**
~~Dementia in other diseases classified elsewhere with aggressive behavior~~
~~Dementia in other diseases classified elsewhere with combative behavior~~
~~Dementia in other diseases classified elsewhere with violent behavior~~
~~Major neurocognitive disorder in other diseases classified elsewhere with aggressive behavior~~
~~Major neurocognitive disorder in other diseases classified elsewhere with combative behavior~~
~~Major neurocognitive disorder in other diseases classified elsewhere with violent behavior~~
~~Use additional code, if applicable, to identify wandering in dementia in conditions classified elsewhere (Z91.83)~~

● **F02.811   Dementia in other diseases classified elsewhere, unspecified severity, with agitation**
Dementia in other diseases classified elsewhere, unspecified severity, with aberrant motor behavior such as restlessness, rocking, pacing, or exit-seeking
Dementia in other diseases classified elsewhere, unspecified severity, with verbal or physical behaviors such as profanity, shouting, threatening, anger, aggression, combativeness, or violence
Major neurocognitive disorder in other diseases classified elsewhere, unspecified severity, with aberrant motor behavior such as restlessness, rocking, pacing, or exit-seeking
Major neurocognitive disorder in other diseases classified elsewhere, unspecified severity, with verbal or physical behaviors such as profanity, shouting, threatening, anger, aggression, combativeness, or violence

● **F02.818   Dementia in other diseases classified elsewhere, unspecified severity, with other behavioral disturbance**
Dementia in other diseases classified elsewhere with sleep disturbance, social disinhibition, or sexual disinhibition
Major neurocognitive disorder in other diseases classified elsewhere with sleep disturbance, social disinhibition, or sexual disinhibition
Use additional code, if applicable, to identify wandering in dementia in conditions classified elsewhere (Z91.83)

● **F02.82   Dementia in other diseases classified elsewhere, unspecified severity, with psychotic disturbance**
Dementia in other diseases classified elsewhere, unspecified severity, with psychotic disturbance such as hallucinations, paranoia, suspiciousness, or delusional state
Major neurocognitive disorder in other diseases classified elsewhere, unspecified, with psychotic disturbance such as hallucinations, paranoia, suspiciousness, or delusional state

● **F02.83   Dementia in other diseases classified elsewhere, unspecified severity, with mood disturbance**
Dementia in other diseases classified elsewhere, unspecified severity, with mood disturbance such as depression, apathy, or anhedonia
Major neurocognitive disorder in other diseases classified elsewhere unspecified severity, with mood disturbance such as with depression, apathy, or anhedonia

● **F02.84   Dementia in other diseases classified elsewhere, unspecified severity, with anxiety**
Major neurocognitive disorder in other diseases classified elsewhere unspecified severity, with anxiety

● ✓5ᵗʰ **F02.A   Dementia in other diseases classified elsewhere, mild**
EXCLUDES 1   *mild neurocognitive disorder due to known physiological condition with or without behavioral disturbance (F06.7-)*

● **F02.A0   Dementia in other diseases classified elsewhere, mild, without behavioral disturbance, psychotic disturbance, mood disturbance, and anxiety**
Dementia in other diseases classified elsewhere, mild, NOS
Major neurocognitive disorder in other diseases classified elsewhere, mild, NOS

● ✓6ᵗʰ **F02.A1   Dementia in other diseases classified elsewhere, mild, with behavioral disturbance**
F02.A11   Dementia in other diseases classified elsewhere, mild, with agitation
Dementia in other diseases classified elsewhere, mild, with aberrant motor behavior such as restlessness, rocking, pacing, or exit-seeking
Dementia in other diseases classified elsewhere, mild, with verbal or physical behaviors such as profanity, shouting, threatening, anger, aggression, combativeness, or violence
Major neurocognitive disorder in other diseases classified elsewhere, mild, with aberrant motor behavior such as restlessness, rocking, pacing, or exit-seeking
Major neurocognitive disorder in other diseases classified elsewhere, mild, with verbal or physical behaviors such as profanity, shouting, threatening, anger, aggression, combativeness, or violence

● **F02.A18   Dementia in other diseases classified elsewhere, mild, with other behavioral disturbance**
Dementia in other diseases classified elsewhere, mild, with behavioral disturbances such as sleep disturbance, social disinhibition, or sexual disinhibition
Major neurocognitive disorder in other diseases classified elsewhere, mild, with behavioral disturbances such as sleep disturbance, social disinhibition, or sexual disinhibition
Use additional code, if applicable, to identify wandering in dementia in conditions classified elsewhere (Z91.83)

● **F02.A2   Dementia in other diseases classified elsewhere, mild, with psychotic disturbance**
Dementia in other diseases classified elsewhere, mild, with psychotic disturbance such as hallucinations, paranoia, suspiciousness, or delusional state
Major neurocognitive disorder in other diseases classified elsewhere, mild, with psychotic disturbance such as hallucinations, paranoia, suspiciousness, or delusional state

● **F02.A3   Dementia in other diseases classified elsewhere, mild, with mood disturbance**
Dementia in other diseases classified elsewhere, mild, with mood disturbance such as depression, apathy, or anhedonia
Major neurocognitive disorder in other diseases classified elsewhere, mild, with mood disturbance such as depression, apathy, or anhedonia

● **F02.A4** **Dementia in other diseases classified elsewhere, mild, with anxiety**
Major neurocognitive disorder in other diseases classified elsewhere, mild, with anxiety

● ✓5ᵗʰ **F02.B** **Dementia in other diseases classified elsewhere, moderate**

● **F02.B0** **Dementia in other diseases classified elsewhere, moderate, without behavioral disturbance, psychotic disturbance, mood disturbance, and anxiety**
Dementia in other diseases classified elsewhere, moderate, NOS
Major neurocognitive disorder in other diseases classified elsewhere, moderate, NOS

● ✓6ᵗʰ **F02.B1** **Dementia in other diseases classified elsewhere, moderate, with behavioral disturbance**

● **F02.B11** **Dementia in other diseases classified elsewhere, moderate, with agitation**
Dementia in other diseases classified elsewhere, moderate, with aberrant motor behavior such as restlessness, rocking, pacing, or exit-seeking
Dementia in other diseases classified elsewhere, moderate, with verbal or physical behaviors such as profanity, shouting, threatening, anger, aggression, combativeness, or violence
Major neurocognitive disorder in other diseases classified elsewhere, moderate, with aberrant motor behavior such as restlessness, rocking, pacing, or exit-seeking
Major neurocognitive disorder in other diseases classified elsewhere, moderate, with verbal or physical behaviors such as profanity, shouting, threatening, anger, aggression, combativeness, or violence

● **F02.B18** **Dementia in other diseases classified elsewhere, moderate, with other behavioral disturbance**
Dementia in other diseases classified elsewhere, moderate, with behavioral disturbances such as sleep disturbance, social disinhibition, or sexual disinhibition
Major neurocognitive disorder in other diseases classified elsewhere, moderate, with behavioral disturbance such as sleep disturbance, social disinhibition, or sexual disinhibition
Use additional code, if applicable, to identify wandering in dementia in conditions classified elsewhere (Z91.83)

● **F02.B2** **Dementia in other diseases classified elsewhere, moderate, with psychotic disturbance**
Dementia in other diseases classified elsewhere, moderate, with psychotic disturbance such as hallucinations, paranoia, suspiciousness, or delusional state
Major neurocognitive disorder in other diseases classified elsewhere, moderate, with psychotic disturbance such as hallucinations, paranoia, suspiciousness, or delusional state

● **F02.B3** **Dementia in other diseases classified elsewhere, moderate, with mood disturbance**
Dementia in other diseases classified elsewhere, moderate, with mood disturbance such as depression, apathy, or anhedonia
Major neurocognitive disorder in other diseases classified elsewhere, moderate, with mood disturbance such as depression, apathy, or anhedonia

● **F02.B4** **Dementia in other diseases classified elsewhere, moderate, with anxiety**
Major neurocognitive disorder in other diseases classified elsewhere, moderate, with anxiety

● ✓5ᵗʰ **F02.C** **Dementia in other diseases classified elsewhere, severe**

● **F02.C0** **Dementia in other diseases classified elsewhere, severe, without behavioral disturbance, psychotic disturbance, mood disturbance, and anxiety**
Dementia in other diseases classified elsewhere, severe, NOS
Major neurocognitive disorder in other diseases classified elsewhere, severe, NOS

● ✓6ᵗʰ **F02.C1** **Dementia in other diseases classified elsewhere, severe, with behavioral disturbance**

● **F02.C11** **Dementia in other diseases classified elsewhere, severe, with agitation**
Dementia in other diseases classified elsewhere, severe, with aberrant motor behavior such as restlessness, rocking, pacing, or exit-seeking
Dementia in other diseases classified elsewhere, severe, with verbal or physical behaviors such as profanity, shouting, threatening, anger, aggression, combativeness, or violence
Major neurocognitive disorder in other diseases classified elsewhere, severe, with aberrant motor behavior such as restlessness, rocking, pacing, or exit-seeking
Major neurocognitive disorder in other diseases classified elsewhere, severe, with verbal or physical behaviors such as profanity, shouting, threatening, anger, aggression, combativeness, or violence

● **F02.C18** **Dementia in other diseases classified elsewhere, severe, with other behavioral disturbance**
Dementia in other diseases classified elsewhere, severe, with behavioral disturbances such as sleep disturbance, social disinhibition, or sexual disinhibition
Major neurocognitive disorder in other diseases classified elsewhere, severe, with behavioral disturbances such as sleep disturbance, social disinhibition, or sexual disinhibition
Use additional code, if applicable, to identify wandering in dementia in conditions classified elsewhere (Z91.83)

● **F02.C2** **Dementia in other diseases classified elsewhere, severe, with psychotic disturbance**
Dementia in other diseases classified elsewhere, severe, with psychotic disturbance such as hallucinations, paranoia, suspiciousness, or delusional state
Major neurocognitive disorder in other diseases classified elsewhere, severe, with psychotic disturbance such as hallucinations, paranoia, suspiciousness, or delusional state

● **F02.C3** **Dementia in other diseases classified elsewhere, severe, with mood disturbance**
Dementia in other diseases classified elsewhere, severe, with mood disturbance such as depression, apathy, or anhedonia
Major neurocognitive disorder in other diseases classified elsewhere, severe, with mood disturbance such as depression, apathy, or anhedonia

● **F02.C4** **Dementia in other diseases classified elsewhere, severe, with anxiety**
Major neurocognitive disorder in other diseases classified elsewhere, severe, with anxiety

✓4ᵗʰ **F03** Unspecified dementia
  ▶Major neurocognitive disorder NOS◀
  Presenile dementia NOS
  Presenile psychosis NOS
  Primary degenerative dementia NOS
  Senile dementia NOS
  Senile dementia depressed or paranoid type
  Senile psychosis NOS
  EXCLUDES 1   senility NOS (R41.81)
  EXCLUDES 2   mild memory disturbance due to known physiological
         condition (F06.8)
         senile dementia with delirium or acute confusional state (F05)

▲   ✓5ᵗʰ   **F03.9**   **Unspecified dementia, unspecified severity**

▲   **F03.90**   **Unspecified dementia, unspecified severity,** without
        behavioral disturbance, psychotic disturbance,
        mood disturbance, and anxiety   HCC Rx ESR A
        Dementia NOS
        AHA: 2021,2Q,4; 2012,4Q,92

▲   ✓6ᵗʰ   **F03.91**   **Unspecified dementia, unspecified severity, with**
        behavioral disturbance
        ~~Unspecified dementia with aggressive behavior~~
        ~~Unspecified dementia with combative behavior~~
        ~~Unspecified dementia with violent behavior~~
        ~~Use additional code, if applicable, to identify~~
        ~~wandering in unspecified dementia (Z91.83)~~

  ●   **F03.911**   **Unspecified dementia, unspecified**
          severity, with agitation
          Unspecified dementia, unspecified
           severity, with aberrant motor
           behavior such as restlessness, rocking,
           pacing, or exit-seeking
          Unspecified dementia, unspecified
           severity, with verbal or physical
           behaviors such as profanity, shouting,
           threatening, anger, aggression,
           combativeness, or violence

  ●   **F03.918**   **Unspecified dementia, unspecified**
          severity, with other behavioral
          disturbance
          Unspecified dementia, unspecified
           severity, with behavioral disturbances
           such as sleep disturbance, social
           disinhibition, or sexual disinhibition
          Use additional code, if applicable, to
           identify wandering in unspecified
           dementia (Z91.83)

  ●   **F03.92**   **Unspecified dementia, unspecified severity,** with
        psychotic disturbance
        Unspecified dementia, unspecified severity, with
         psychotic disturbance such as hallucinations,
         paranoia, suspiciousness, or delusional state

  ●   **F03.93**   **Unspecified dementia, unspecified severity,** with
        mood disturbance
        Unspecified dementia, unspecified severity, with
         mood disturbance such as depression, apathy,
         or anhedonia

  ●   **F03.94**   **Unspecified dementia, unspecified severity,** with
        anxiety

  ●   ✓5ᵗʰ   **F03.A**   **Unspecified dementia,** mild
        EXCLUDES 1   mild neurocognitive disorder due to known
            physiological condition with or without
            behavioral disturbance (F06.7-)

  ●   **F03.A0**   **Unspecified dementia, mild,** without behavioral
        disturbance, psychotic disturbance, mood
        disturbance, and anxiety
        Dementia, mild, NOS

  ●   ✓6ᵗʰ   **F03.A1**   **Unspecified dementia, mild, with behavioral**
        disturbance

  ●   **F03.A11**   **Unspecified dementia, mild,** with
          agitation
          Unspecified dementia, mild, with aberrant
           motor behavior such as restlessness,
           rocking, pacing, or exit-seeking
          Unspecified dementia, mild, with verbal
           or physical behaviors such as
           profanity, shouting, threatening,
           anger, aggression, combativeness, or
           violence

  ●   **F03.A18**   **Unspecified dementia, mild, with other**
          behavioral disturbance
          Unspecified dementia, mild, with
           behavioral disturbances such as sleep
           disturbance, social disinhibition, or
           sexual disinhibition
          Use additional code, if applicable, to
           identify wandering in unspecified
           dementia (Z91.83)

  ●   **F03.A2**   **Unspecified dementia, mild,** with psychotic
        disturbance
        Unspecified dementia, mild, with psychotic
         disturbance such as hallucinations, paranoia,
         suspiciousness, or delusional state

  ●   **F03.A3**   **Unspecified dementia, mild,** with mood disturbance
        Unspecified dementia, mild, with mood disturbance
         such as depression, apathy, or anhedonia

  ●   **F03.A4**   **Unspecified dementia, mild,** with anxiety

  ●   ✓5ᵗʰ   **F03.B**   **Unspecified dementia,** moderate

  ●   **F03.B0**   **Unspecified dementia, moderate,** without
        behavioral disturbance, psychotic disturbance,
        mood disturbance, and anxiety
        Dementia, moderate, NOS

     ✓6ᵗʰ   **F03.B1**   **Unspecified dementia, moderate, with behavioral**
        disturbance

         F03.B11   **Unspecified dementia, moderate,** with
          agitation
          Unspecified dementia, moderate, with
           aberrant motor behavior such as
           restlessness, rocking, pacing, or
           exit-seeking
          Unspecified dementia, moderate, with
           verbal or physical behaviors such as
           profanity, shouting, threatening,
           anger, aggression, combativeness, or
           violence

         F03.B18   **Unspecified dementia, moderate, with**
          other behavioral disturbance
          Unspecified dementia, moderate, with
           behavioral disturbances such as sleep
           disturbance, social disinhibition, or
           sexual disinhibition
          Use additional code, if applicable, to
           identify wandering in unspecified
           dementia (Z91.83)

  ●   **F03.B2**   **Unspecified dementia, moderate,** with psychotic
        disturbance
        Unspecified dementia, moderate, with psychotic
         disturbance such as hallucinations, paranoia,
         suspiciousness, or delusional state

  ●   **F03.B3**   **Unspecified dementia, moderate,** with mood
        disturbance
        Unspecified dementia, moderate, with mood
         disturbance such as depression, apathy, or
         anhedonia

  ●   **F03.B4**   **Unspecified dementia, moderate,** with anxiety

  ●   ✓5ᵗʰ   **F03.C**   **Unspecified dementia,** severe

  ●   **F03.C0**   **Unspecified dementia, severe,** without behavioral
        disturbance, psychotic disturbance, mood
        disturbance, and anxiety
        Dementia, severe, NOS

  ●   ✓6ᵗʰ   **F03.C1**   **Unspecified dementia, severe, with behavioral**
        disturbance

  ●   **F03.C11**   **Unspecified dementia, severe,** with
          agitation
          Unspecified dementia, severe, with
           aberrant motor behavior such as
           restlessness, rocking, pacing, or
           exit-seeking
          Unspecified dementia, severe, with verbal
           or physical behaviors such as
           profanity, shouting, threatening,
           anger, aggression, combativeness, or
           violence

● **F03.C18** **Unspecified dementia, severe, with other behavioral disturbance**
  Unspecified dementia, severe, with behavioral disturbances such as sleep disturbance, social disinhibition, or sexual disinhibition
  Use additional code, if applicable, to identify wandering in unspecified dementia (Z91.83)

● **F03.C2** **Unspecified dementia, severe, with psychotic disturbance**
  Unspecified dementia, severe, with psychotic disturbance such as hallucinations, paranoia, suspiciousness, or delusional state

● **F03.C3** **Unspecified dementia, severe, with mood disturbance**
  Unspecified dementia, severe, with mood disturbance such as depression, apathy, or anhedonia

● **F03.C4** **Unspecified dementia, severe, with anxiety**

F04 **Amnestic disorder due to known physiological condition**   `HCC` `Rx` `ESR`
  Korsakov's psychosis or syndrome, nonalcoholic
  Code first the underlying physiological condition
  EXCLUDES 1   amnesia NOS (R41.3)
  anterograde amnesia (R41.1)
  dissociative amnesia (F44.0)
  retrograde amnesia (R41.2)
  EXCLUDES 2   alcohol-induced or unspecified Korsakov's syndrome (F10.26, F10.96)
  Korsakov's syndrome induced by other psychoactive substances (F13.26, F13.96, F19.16, F19.26, F19.96)

F05 **Delirium due to known physiological condition**
  Acute or subacute brain syndrome
  Acute or subacute confusional state (nonalcoholic)
  Acute or subacute infective psychosis
  Acute or subacute organic reaction
  Acute or subacute psycho-organic syndrome
  Delirium of mixed etiology
  Delirium superimposed on dementia
  Sundowning
  Code first the underlying physiological condition
  EXCLUDES 1   delirium NOS (R41.0)
  EXCLUDES 2   delirium tremens alcohol-induced or unspecified (F10.231, F10.921)
  AHA: 2019,2Q,34

☑4ᵗʰ **F06** **Other mental disorders due to known physiological condition**
  `INCLUDES`   mental disorders due to endocrine disorder
  mental disorders due to exogenous hormone
  mental disorders due to exogenous toxic substance
  mental disorders due to primary cerebral disease
  mental disorders due to somatic illness
  mental disorders due to systemic disease affecting the brain
  Code first the underlying physiological condition
  EXCLUDES 1   unspecified dementia (F03)
  EXCLUDES 2   delirium due to known physiological condition (F05)
  dementia as classified in F01-F02
  other mental disorders associated with alcohol and other psychoactive substances (F10-F19)

F06.0 **Psychotic disorder with hallucinations due to known physiological condition**
  Organic hallucinatory state (nonalcoholic)
  EXCLUDES 2   hallucinations and perceptual disturbance induced by alcohol and other psychoactive substances (F10-F19 with .151, .251, .951)
  schizophrenia (F20.-)

F06.1 **Catatonic disorder due to known physiological condition**
  Catatonia associated with another mental disorder
  Catatonia NOS
  EXCLUDES 1   catatonic stupor (R40.1)
  stupor NOS (R40.1)
  EXCLUDES 2   catatonic schizophrenia (F20.2)
  dissociative stupor (F44.2)
  DEF: Catatonic: Abnormal neuropsychiatric state characterized by stupor, immobility or purposeless movements, or unresponsiveness in a person who otherwise appears awake.

F06.2 **Psychotic disorder with delusions due to known physiological condition**
  Paranoid and paranoid-hallucinatory organic states
  Schizophrenia-like psychosis in epilepsy
  EXCLUDES 2   alcohol and drug-induced psychotic disorder (F10-F19 with .150, .250, .950)
  brief psychotic disorder (F23)
  delusional disorder (F22)
  schizophrenia (F20.-)

☑5ᵗʰ **F06.3** **Mood disorder due to known physiological condition**
  EXCLUDES 2   mood disorders due to alcohol and other psychoactive substances (F10-F19 with .14, .24, .94)
  mood disorders, not due to known physiological condition or unspecified (F30-F39)

F06.30 **Mood disorder due to known physiological condition, unspecified**

F06.31 **Mood disorder due to known physiological condition with depressive features**
  Depressive disorder due to known physiological condition, with depressive features

F06.32 **Mood disorder due to known physiological condition with major depressive-like episode**
  Depressive disorder due to known physiological condition, with major depressive-like episode

F06.33 **Mood disorder due to known physiological condition with manic features**
  Bipolar and related disorder due to a known physiological condition, with manic features
  Bipolar and related disorder due to known physiological condition, with manic- or hypomanic-like episodes

F06.34 **Mood disorder due to known physiological condition with mixed features**
  Bipolar and related disorder due to known physiological condition, with mixed features
  Depressive disorder due to known physiological condition, with mixed features

F06.4 **Anxiety disorder due to known physiological condition**
  EXCLUDES 2   anxiety disorders due to alcohol and other psychoactive substances (F10-F19 with .180, .280, .980)
  anxiety disorders, not due to known physiological condition or unspecified (F40.-, F41.-)

● ☑5ᵗʰ **F06.7** **Mild neurocognitive disorder due to known physiological condition**
  Mild neurocognitive impairment due to a known physiological condition
  Code first the underlying physiological condition, such as:
  Alzheimer's disease (G30.-)
  frontotemporal neurocognitive disorder (G31.09)
  human immunodeficiency virus [HIV] disease (B20)
  Huntington's disease (G10)
  neurocognitive disorder with Lewy bodies (G31.83)
  Parkinson's disease (G20)
  systemic lupus erythematosus (M32.-)
  traumatic brain injury (S06.-)
  vitamin B deficiency (E53-)
  EXCLUDES 1   age related cognitive decline (R41.81)
  altered mental status (R41.82)
  cerebral degeneration (G31.9)
  change in mental status (R41.82)
  cognitive deficits following (sequelae of) cerebral hemorrhage or infarction (I69.01-I69.11-, I69.21-I69.31-, I69.81- I69.91-)
  dementia (F01.-, F02.-, F03)
  mild cognitive impairment due to unknown or unspecified etiology (G31.84)
  neurologic neglect syndrome (R41.4)
  personality change, nonpsychotic (F68.8)

● **F06.70** **Mild neurocognitive disorder due to known physiological condition without behavioral disturbance**
  Mild neurocognitive disorder due to known physiological condition, NOS

● **F06.71** **Mild neurocognitive disorder due to known physiological condition with behavioral disturbance**

`HCC` CMS-HCC   `Rx` Rx HCC   `ESR` ESRD HCC   `COM` Commercial HCC   `N` Newborn: 0   `P` Pediatric: 0-17   `M` Maternity: 9-64   `A` Adult: 15-124

560

ICD-10-CM 2023

F06.8   **Other specified mental disorders due to known physiological condition**
Epileptic psychosis NOS
Obsessive-compulsive and related disorder due to a known physiological condition
Organic dissociative disorder
Organic emotionally labile [asthenic] disorder

✓4ᵗʰ **F07**   **Personality and behavioral disorders due to known physiological condition**
Code first the underlying physiological condition

     F07.0   **Personality change due to known physiological condition**
Frontal lobe syndrome
Limbic epilepsy personality syndrome
Lobotomy syndrome
Organic personality disorder
Organic pseudopsychopathic personality
Organic pseudoretarded personality
Postleucotomy syndrome
~~Code first underlying physiological condition~~
     EXCLUDES 1   mild cognitive impairment (G31.84)
                 postconcussional syndrome (F07.81)
                 postencephalitic syndrome (F07.89)
                 signs and symptoms involving emotional state (R45.-)
     EXCLUDES 2   specific personality disorder (F60.-)

✓5ᵗʰ **F07.8**   **Other personality and behavioral disorders due to known physiological condition**
     F07.81   **Postconcussional syndrome**
Postcontusional syndrome (encephalopathy)
Post-traumatic brain syndrome, nonpsychotic
Use additional code to identify associated post-traumatic headache, if applicable (G44.3-)
     EXCLUDES 1   current concussion (brain) (S06.0-)
                 postencephalitic syndrome (F07.89)
DEF: Concussion symptoms that persist for weeks or months after a head injury. These symptoms may include headache, giddiness, fatigue, insomnia, mood fluctuation, and a subjective feeling of impaired intellectual function with extreme reaction to normal stressors.
     F07.89   **Other personality and behavioral disorders due to known physiological condition**
Postencephalitic syndrome
Right hemispheric organic affective disorder

     F07.9   **Unspecified personality and behavioral disorder due to known physiological condition**
Organic psychosyndrome

F09   **Unspecified mental disorder due to known physiological condition**
Mental disorder NOS due to known physiological condition
Organic brain syndrome NOS
Organic mental disorder NOS
Organic psychosis NOS
Symptomatic psychosis NOS
Code first the underlying physiological condition
     EXCLUDES 1   ▶mild neurocognitive disorder due to known physiological condition (F06.7-)◀
                 psychosis NOS (F29)

Mental and behavioral disorders due to psychoactive substance use (F10–F19)

AHA: 2022,1Q,34; 2020,1Q,9; 2018,4Q,69-70; 2017,4Q,8; 2017,2Q,27
TIP: Psychoactive substance withdrawal can occur in individuals who do not have a diagnosis of dependence but who use the substance regularly (i.e., use or abuse) and then reduce or cease the use.

✓4ᵗʰ **F10**   **Alcohol related disorders**
Use additional code for blood alcohol level, if applicable (Y90.-)
AHA: 2019,3Q,8

✓5ᵗʰ **F10.1**   **Alcohol abuse**
     EXCLUDES 1   alcohol dependence (F10.2-)
                 alcohol use, unspecified (F10.9-)
     AHA: 2018,1Q,16; 2015,2Q,15
     F10.10   **Alcohol abuse, uncomplicated**
Alcohol use disorder, mild
     F10.11   **Alcohol abuse, in remission**
Alcohol use disorder, mild, in early remission
Alcohol use disorder, mild, in sustained remission
         AHA: 2022,1Q,25

✓6ᵗʰ **F10.12**   **Alcohol abuse with intoxication**
     F10.120   **Alcohol abuse with intoxication, uncomplicated**   HCC ESR
     F10.121   **Alcohol abuse with intoxication delirium**   HCC ESR
     F10.129   **Alcohol abuse with intoxication, unspecified**   HCC ESR

✓6ᵗʰ **F10.13**   **Alcohol abuse, with withdrawal**
     AHA: 2020,4Q,16-17
     F10.130   **Alcohol abuse with withdrawal, uncomplicated**   HCC ESR COM
     F10.131   **Alcohol abuse with withdrawal delirium**   HCC ESR COM
     F10.132   **Alcohol abuse with withdrawal with perceptual disturbance**   HCC ESR COM
     F10.139   **Alcohol abuse with withdrawal, unspecified**   HCC ESR COM
     F10.14   **Alcohol abuse with alcohol-induced mood disorder**   HCC ESR COM
Alcohol use disorder, mild, with alcohol-induced bipolar or related disorder
Alcohol use disorder, mild, with alcohol-induced depressive disorder

✓6ᵗʰ **F10.15**   **Alcohol abuse with alcohol-induced psychotic disorder**
     F10.150   **Alcohol abuse with alcohol-induced psychotic disorder with delusions**   HCC ESR COM
     F10.151   **Alcohol abuse with alcohol-induced psychotic disorder with hallucinations**   HCC ESR COM
         DEF: Psychosis lasting less than six months with slight or no clouding of consciousness in which auditory hallucinations predominate.
     F10.159   **Alcohol abuse with alcohol-induced psychotic disorder, unspecified**   HCC ESR COM

✓6ᵗʰ **F10.18**   **Alcohol abuse with other alcohol-induced disorders**
     AHA: 2022,1Q,33
     F10.180   **Alcohol abuse with alcohol-induced anxiety disorder**   HCC ESR COM
         AHA: 2022,1Q,25,33
     F10.181   **Alcohol abuse with alcohol-induced sexual dysfunction**   HCC ESR COM
     F10.182   **Alcohol abuse with alcohol-induced sleep disorder**   HCC ESR COM
     F10.188   **Alcohol abuse with other alcohol-induced disorder**   HCC ESR COM
         AHA: 2022,1Q,25

     F10.19   **Alcohol abuse with unspecified alcohol-induced disorder**   HCC ESR

✓5ᵗʰ **F10.2**   **Alcohol dependence**
     EXCLUDES 1   alcohol abuse (F10.1-)
                 alcohol use, unspecified (F10.9-)
     EXCLUDES 2   toxic effect of alcohol (T51.0-)
     F10.20   **Alcohol dependence, uncomplicated**   HCC ESR COM
Alcohol use disorder, moderate
Alcohol use disorder, severe
         AHA: 2020,1Q,9
     F10.21   **Alcohol dependence, in remission**   HCC ESR COM
Alcohol use disorder, moderate, in early remission
Alcohol use disorder, moderate, in sustained remission
Alcohol use disorder, severe, in early remission
Alcohol use disorder, severe, in sustained remission

✓6ᵗʰ **F10.22**   **Alcohol dependence with intoxication**
Acute drunkenness (in alcoholism)
     EXCLUDES 2   alcohol dependence with withdrawal (F10.23-)
     F10.220   **Alcohol dependence with intoxication, uncomplicated**   HCC ESR COM
     F10.221   **Alcohol dependence with intoxication delirium**   HCC ESR COM
     F10.229   **Alcohol dependence with intoxication, unspecified**   HCC ESR COM

√6ᵗʰ **F10.23 Alcohol dependence with** withdrawal

> EXCLUDES 2   *alcohol dependence with intoxication (F10.22-)*

> **AHA:** 2018,1Q,16; 2015,2Q,15

F10.230 Alcohol dependence with withdrawal, uncomplicated HCC ESR COM

F10.231 Alcohol dependence with withdrawal delirium HCC ESR COM

F10.232 Alcohol dependence with withdrawal with perceptual disturbance HCC ESR COM

F10.239 Alcohol dependence with withdrawal, unspecified

F10.24 Alcohol dependence with alcohol-induced mood disorder HCC ESR COM

> Alcohol use disorder, moderate, with alcohol-induced bipolar or related disorder
> Alcohol use disorder, moderate, with alcohol-induced depressive disorder
> Alcohol use disorder, severe, with alcohol-induced bipolar or related disorder
> Alcohol use disorder, severe, with alcohol-induced depressive disorder

√6ᵗʰ **F10.25 Alcohol dependence with alcohol-induced** psychotic disorder

F10.250 Alcohol dependence with alcohol-induced psychotic disorder with delusions HCC ESR COM

F10.251 Alcohol dependence with alcohol-induced psychotic disorder with hallucinations HCC ESR COM

F10.259 Alcohol dependence with alcohol-induced psychotic disorder, unspecified HCC ESR COM

F10.26 Alcohol dependence with alcohol-induced persisting amnestic disorder HCC ESR COM

> Alcohol use disorder, moderate, with alcohol-induced major neurocognitive disorder, amnestic-confabulatory type
> Alcohol use disorder, severe, with alcohol-induced major neurocognitive disorder, amnestic-confabulatory type

> **DEF:** Prominent and lasting reduced memory span and disordered time appreciation and confabulation that occurs in alcoholics as sequel to acute alcoholic psychosis.

F10.27 Alcohol dependence with alcohol-induced persisting dementia HCC ESR COM

> Alcohol use disorder, moderate, with alcohol-induced major neurocognitive disorder, nonamnestic-confabulatory type
> Alcohol use disorder, severe, with alcohol-induced major neurocognitive disorder, nonamnestic-confabulatory type

√6ᵗʰ **F10.28 Alcohol dependence with other alcohol-induced disorders**

F10.280 Alcohol dependence with alcohol-induced anxiety disorder HCC ESR COM

F10.281 Alcohol dependence with alcohol-induced sexual dysfunction HCC ESR COM

F10.282 Alcohol dependence with alcohol-induced sleep disorder HCC ESR COM

F10.288 Alcohol dependence with other alcohol-induced disorder HCC ESR COM

> Alcohol use disorder, moderate, with alcohol-induced mild neurocognitive disorder
> Alcohol use disorder, severe, with alcohol-induced mild neurocognitive disorder

> **AHA:** 2020,1Q,9

F10.29 Alcohol dependence with unspecified alcohol-induced disorder HCC ESR COM

√5ᵗʰ **F10.9 Alcohol** use, **unspecified**

> EXCLUDES 1   *alcohol abuse (F10.1-)*
> *alcohol dependence (F10.2-)*

> **AHA:** 2018,2Q,10-11

> **TIP:** Assign a substance use code only when the provider documents a relationship between the use and an associated physical, mental, or behavioral disorder. As with all diagnoses, substance use codes must meet the definition of a reportable diagnosis.

● **F10.90 Alcohol use, unspecified, uncomplicated**

● **F10.91 Alcohol use, unspecified,** in remission

√6ᵗʰ **F10.92 Alcohol use, unspecified with** intoxication

F10.920 Alcohol use, unspecified with intoxication, uncomplicated HCC ESR

> **AHA:** 2018,2Q,10-11

F10.921 Alcohol use, unspecified with intoxication delirium HCC ESR

F10.929 Alcohol use, unspecified with intoxication, unspecified HCC ESR

√6ᵗʰ **F10.93 Alcohol use, unspecified with** withdrawal

> **AHA:** 2020,4Q,16-17

F10.930 Alcohol use, unspecified with withdrawal, uncomplicated HCC ESR COM

F10.931 Alcohol use, unspecified with withdrawal delirium HCC ESR COM

F10.932 Alcohol use, unspecified with withdrawal with perceptual disturbance HCC ESR COM

F10.939 Alcohol use, unspecified with withdrawal, unspecified HCC ESR COM

F10.94 Alcohol use, unspecified with alcohol-induced mood disorder HCC ESR COM

> Alcohol induced bipolar or related disorder, without use disorder
> Alcohol induced depressive disorder, without use disorder

√6ᵗʰ **F10.95 Alcohol use, unspecified with alcohol-induced** psychotic disorder

F10.950 Alcohol use, unspecified with alcohol-induced psychotic disorder with delusions HCC ESR COM

F10.951 Alcohol use, unspecified with alcohol-induced psychotic disorder with hallucinations HCC ESR COM

F10.959 Alcohol use, unspecified with alcohol-induced psychotic disorder, unspecified HCC ESR COM

> Alcohol-induced psychotic disorder without use disorder

F10.96 Alcohol use, unspecified with alcohol-induced persisting amnestic disorder HCC ESR COM

> Alcohol-induced major neurocognitive disorder, amnestic-confabulatory type, without use disorder

F10.97 Alcohol use, unspecified with alcohol-induced persisting dementia HCC ESR COM

> Alcohol-induced major neurocognitive disorder, nonamnestic-confabulatory type, without use disorder

√6ᵗʰ **F10.98 Alcohol use, unspecified with other alcohol-induced disorders**

F10.980 Alcohol use, unspecified with alcohol-induced anxiety disorder HCC ESR COM

> Alcohol induced anxiety disorder, without use disorder

F10.981 Alcohol use, unspecified with alcohol-induced sexual dysfunction HCC ESR COM

> Alcohol induced sexual dysfunction, without use disorder

F10.982 Alcohol use, unspecified with alcohol-induced sleep disorder HCC ESR COM

> Alcohol induced sleep disorder, without use disorder

F10.988   Alcohol use, unspecified with other alcohol-induced disorder   `HCC` `ESR` `COM`
> Alcohol induced mild neurocognitive disorder, without use disorder

F10.99   Alcohol use, unspecified with unspecified alcohol-induced disorder   `HCC` `ESR`

√4ᵗʰ **F11**   Opioid related disorders

√5ᵗʰ **F11.1**   Opioid abuse
> *EXCLUDES 1*   opioid dependence (F11.2-)
> opioid use, unspecified (F11.9-)

F11.10   Opioid abuse, uncomplicated   `HCC` `ESR`
> Opioid use disorder, mild

F11.11   Opioid abuse, in remission   `HCC` `ESR`
> Opioid use disorder, mild, in early remission
> Opioid use disorder, mild, in sustained remission

√6ᵗʰ **F11.12**   Opioid abuse with intoxication

     F11.120   Opioid abuse with intoxication, uncomplicated   `HCC` `ESR` `COM`

     F11.121   Opioid abuse with intoxication delirium   `HCC` `ESR` `COM`

     F11.122   Opioid abuse with intoxication with perceptual disturbance   `HCC` `ESR` `COM`

     F11.129   Opioid abuse with intoxication, unspecified   `HCC` `ESR` `COM`

F11.13   Opioid abuse with withdrawal   `HCC` `ESR` `COM`
> **AHA:** 2020,4Q,16-17

F11.14   Opioid abuse with opioid-induced mood disorder   `HCC` `ESR` `COM`
> Opioid use disorder, mild, with opioid-induced depressive disorder

√6ᵗʰ **F11.15**   Opioid abuse with opioid-induced psychotic disorder

     F11.150   Opioid abuse with opioid-induced psychotic disorder with delusions   `HCC` `ESR` `COM`

     F11.151   Opioid abuse with opioid-induced psychotic disorder with hallucinations   `HCC` `ESR` `COM`

     F11.159   Opioid abuse with opioid-induced psychotic disorder, unspecified   `HCC` `ESR` `COM`

√6ᵗʰ **F11.18**   Opioid abuse with other opioid-induced disorder

     F11.181   Opioid abuse with opioid-induced sexual dysfunction   `HCC` `ESR` `COM`

     F11.182   Opioid abuse with opioid-induced sleep disorder   `HCC` `ESR` `COM`

     F11.188   Opioid abuse with other opioid-induced disorder   `HCC` `ESR` `COM`

F11.19   Opioid abuse with unspecified opioid-induced disorder   `HCC` `ESR` `COM`

√5ᵗʰ **F11.2**   Opioid dependence
> *EXCLUDES 1*   opioid abuse (F11.1-)
> opioid use, unspecified (F11.9-)
> *EXCLUDES 2*   opioid poisoning (T40.0-T40.2-)

F11.20   Opioid dependence, uncomplicated   `HCC` `ESR` `COM`
> Opioid use disorder, moderate
> Opioid use disorder, severe

F11.21   Opioid dependence, in remission   `HCC` `ESR` `COM`
> Opioid use disorder, moderate, in early remission
> Opioid use disorder, moderate, in sustained remission
> Opioid use disorder, severe, in early remission
> Opioid use disorder, severe, in sustained remission

√6ᵗʰ **F11.22**   Opioid dependence with intoxication
> *EXCLUDES 1*   opioid dependence with withdrawal (F11.23)

     F11.220   Opioid dependence with intoxication, uncomplicated   `HCC` `ESR` `COM`

     F11.221   Opioid dependence with intoxication delirium   `HCC` `ESR` `COM`

     F11.222   Opioid dependence with intoxication with perceptual disturbance   `HCC` `ESR` `COM`

     F11.229   Opioid dependence with intoxication, unspecified   `HCC` `ESR` `COM`

F11.23   Opioid dependence with withdrawal   `HCC` `ESR` `COM`
> *EXCLUDES 1*   opioid dependence with intoxication (F11.22-)

F11.24   Opioid dependence with opioid-induced mood disorder   `HCC` `ESR` `COM`
> Opioid use disorder, moderate, with opioid induced depressive disorder

√6ᵗʰ **F11.25**   Opioid dependence with opioid-induced psychotic disorder

     F11.250   Opioid dependence with opioid-induced psychotic disorder with delusions   `HCC` `ESR` `COM`

     F11.251   Opioid dependence with opioid-induced psychotic disorder with hallucinations   `HCC` `ESR` `COM`

     F11.259   Opioid dependence with opioid-induced psychotic disorder, unspecified   `HCC` `ESR` `COM`

√6ᵗʰ **F11.28**   Opioid dependence with other opioid-induced disorder

     F11.281   Opioid dependence with opioid-induced sexual dysfunction   `HCC` `ESR` `COM`

     F11.282   Opioid dependence with opioid-induced sleep disorder   `HCC` `ESR` `COM`

     F11.288   Opioid dependence with other opioid-induced disorder   `HCC` `ESR` `COM`

F11.29   Opioid dependence with unspecified opioid-induced disorder   `HCC` `ESR` `COM`

√5ᵗʰ **F11.9**   Opioid use, unspecified
> *EXCLUDES 1*   opioid abuse (F11.1-)
> opioid dependence (F11.2-)

> **TIP:** Assign a substance use code only when the provider documents a relationship between the use and an associated physical, mental, or behavioral disorder. As with all diagnoses, substance use codes must meet the definition of a reportable diagnosis.

F11.90   Opioid use, unspecified, uncomplicated
> **AHA:** 2018,2Q,10-11

F11.91   Opioid use, unspecified, in remission

√6ᵗʰ **F11.92**   Opioid use, unspecified with intoxication
> *EXCLUDES 1*   opioid use, unspecified with withdrawal (F11.93)

     F11.920   Opioid use, unspecified with intoxication, uncomplicated   `HCC` `ESR` `COM`

     F11.921   Opioid use, unspecified with intoxication delirium   `HCC` `ESR` `COM`
> Opioid-induced delirium

     F11.922   Opioid use, unspecified with intoxication with perceptual disturbance   `HCC` `ESR` `COM`

     F11.929   Opioid use, unspecified with intoxication, unspecified   `HCC` `ESR` `COM`

F11.93   Opioid use, unspecified with withdrawal   `HCC` `ESR` `COM`
> *EXCLUDES 1*   opioid use, unspecified with intoxication (F11.92-)

F11.94   Opioid use, unspecified with opioid-induced mood disorder   `HCC` `ESR` `COM`
> Opioid induced depressive disorder, without use disorder

√6ᵗʰ **F11.95**   Opioid use, unspecified with opioid-induced psychotic disorder

     F11.950   Opioid use, unspecified with opioid-induced psychotic disorder with delusions   `HCC` `ESR` `COM`

     F11.951   Opioid use, unspecified with opioid-induced psychotic disorder with hallucinations   `HCC` `ESR` `COM`

     F11.959   Opioid use, unspecified with opioid-induced psychotic disorder, unspecified   `HCC` `ESR` `COM`

√6ᵗʰ **F11.98**   Opioid use, unspecified with other specified opioid-induced disorder

     F11.981   Opioid use, unspecified with opioid-induced sexual dysfunction   `HCC` `ESR` `COM`
> Opioid induced sexual dysfunction, without use disorder

F11.982 Opioid use, unspecified with opioid-induced sleep disorder `HCC` `ESR` `COM`
> Opioid induced sleep disorder, without use disorder

F11.988 Opioid use, unspecified with other opioid-induced disorder `HCC` `ESR` `COM`
> Opioid induced anxiety disorder, without use disorder

F11.99 Opioid use, unspecified with unspecified opioid-induced disorder `HCC` `ESR` `COM`

✓4th **F12** Cannabis related disorders
    `INCLUDES` marijuana
    AHA: 2020,1Q,8

✓5th **F12.1** Cannabis abuse
    `EXCLUDES 1` *cannabis dependence (F12.2-)*
         cannabis use, unspecified (F12.9-)

[handwritten: habitual abuse]

  F12.10 Cannabis abuse, uncomplicated
> Cannabis use disorder, mild

  F12.11 Cannabis abuse, in remission
> Cannabis use disorder, mild, in early remission
> Cannabis use disorder, mild, in sustained remission

✓6th   **F12.12** Cannabis abuse with intoxication
    F12.120 Cannabis abuse with intoxication, uncomplicated `HCC` `ESR` `COM`
    F12.121 Cannabis abuse with intoxication delirium `HCC` `ESR` `COM`
    F12.122 Cannabis abuse with intoxication with perceptual disturbance `HCC` `ESR` `COM`
    F12.129 Cannabis abuse with intoxication, unspecified `HCC` `ESR` `COM`

  F12.13 Cannabis abuse with withdrawal `HCC` `ESR` `COM`
    AHA: 2020,4Q,16-17

✓6th   **F12.15** Cannabis abuse with psychotic disorder
    F12.150 Cannabis abuse with psychotic disorder with delusions `HCC` `ESR` `COM`
    F12.151 Cannabis abuse with psychotic disorder with hallucinations `HCC` `ESR` `COM`
    F12.159 Cannabis abuse with psychotic disorder, unspecified `HCC` `ESR` `COM`

✓6th   **F12.18** Cannabis abuse with other cannabis-induced disorder
    F12.180 Cannabis abuse with cannabis-induced anxiety disorder `HCC` `ESR` `COM`
    F12.188 Cannabis abuse with other cannabis-induced disorder `HCC` `ESR` `COM`
> Cannabis use disorder, mild, with cannabis-induced sleep disorder

  F12.19 Cannabis abuse with unspecified cannabis-induced disorder `HCC` `ESR` `COM`

✓5th **F12.2** Cannabis dependence
    `EXCLUDES 1` *cannabis abuse (F12.1-)*
         cannabis use, unspecified (F12.9-)
    `EXCLUDES 2` *cannabis poisoning (T40.7-)*

  F12.20 Cannabis dependence, uncomplicated `HCC` `ESR` `COM`
> Cannabis use disorder, moderate
> Cannabis use disorder, severe

  F12.21 Cannabis dependence, in remission `HCC` `ESR` `COM`
> Cannabis use disorder, moderate, in early remission
> Cannabis use disorder, moderate, in sustained remission
> Cannabis use disorder, severe, in early remission
> Cannabis use disorder, severe, in sustained remission

✓6th   **F12.22** Cannabis dependence with intoxication
    F12.220 Cannabis dependence with intoxication, uncomplicated `HCC` `ESR` `COM`
    F12.221 Cannabis dependence with intoxication delirium `HCC` `ESR` `COM`
    F12.222 Cannabis dependence with intoxication with perceptual disturbance `HCC` `ESR` `COM`
    F12.229 Cannabis dependence with intoxication, unspecified `HCC` `ESR` `COM`

  F12.23 Cannabis dependence with withdrawal `HCC` `ESR` `COM`
    AHA: 2018,4Q,7

✓6th   **F12.25** Cannabis dependence with psychotic disorder
    F12.250 Cannabis dependence with psychotic disorder with delusions `HCC` `ESR` `COM`
    F12.251 Cannabis dependence with psychotic disorder with hallucinations `HCC` `ESR` `COM`
    F12.259 Cannabis dependence with psychotic disorder, unspecified `HCC` `ESR` `COM`

✓6th   **F12.28** Cannabis dependence with other cannabis-induced disorder
    F12.280 Cannabis dependence with cannabis-induced anxiety disorder `HCC` `ESR` `COM`
    F12.288 Cannabis dependence with other cannabis-induced disorder `HCC` `ESR` `COM`
> Cannabis use disorder, moderate, with cannabis-induced sleep disorder
> Cannabis use disorder, severe, with cannabis-induced sleep disorder

  F12.29 Cannabis dependence with unspecified cannabis-induced disorder `HCC` `ESR` `COM`

✓5th **F12.9** Cannabis use, unspecified
    `EXCLUDES 1` *cannabis abuse (F12.1-)*
         cannabis dependence (F12.2-)

    TIP: Assign a substance use code only when the provider documents a relationship between the use and an associated physical, mental, or behavioral disorder. As with all diagnoses, substance use codes must meet the definition of a reportable diagnosis.

  F12.90 Cannabis use, unspecified, uncomplicated
    AHA: 2018,2Q,10-11

  F12.91 Cannabis use, unspecified, in remission

✓6th   **F12.92** Cannabis use, unspecified with intoxication
    F12.920 Cannabis use, unspecified with intoxication, uncomplicated `HCC` `ESR` `COM`
    F12.921 Cannabis use, unspecified with intoxication delirium `HCC` `ESR` `COM`
    F12.922 Cannabis use, unspecified with intoxication with perceptual disturbance `HCC` `ESR` `COM`
    F12.929 Cannabis use, unspecified with intoxication, unspecified `HCC` `ESR` `COM`

  F12.93 Cannabis use, unspecified with withdrawal `HCC` `ESR` `COM`
    AHA: 2018,4Q,7

✓6th   **F12.95** Cannabis use, unspecified with psychotic disorder
    F12.950 Cannabis use, unspecified with psychotic disorder with delusions `HCC` `ESR` `COM`
    F12.951 Cannabis use, unspecified with psychotic disorder with hallucinations `HCC` `ESR` `COM`
    F12.959 Cannabis use, unspecified with psychotic disorder, unspecified `HCC` `ESR` `COM`
> Cannabis induced psychotic disorder, without use disorder

✓6th   **F12.98** Cannabis use, unspecified with other cannabis-induced disorder
    F12.980 Cannabis use, unspecified with anxiety disorder `HCC` `ESR` `COM`
> Cannabis induced anxiety disorder, without use disorder
    F12.988 Cannabis use, unspecified with other cannabis-induced disorder `HCC` `ESR` `COM`
> Cannabis induced sleep disorder, without use disorder

  F12.99 Cannabis use, unspecified with unspecified cannabis-induced disorder `HCC` `ESR` `COM`

`HCC` CMS-HCC   `Rx` Rx HCC   `ESR` ESRD HCC   `COM` Commercial HCC   `N` Newborn: 0   `P` Pediatric: 0-17   `M` Maternity: 9-64   `A` Adult: 15-124

564   ICD-10-CM 2023

☑4ᵗʰ **F13** Sedative, hypnotic, or anxiolytic related disorders

  ☑5ᵗʰ **F13.1** **Sedative, hypnotic or anxiolytic-related** abuse

    EXCLUDES 1   *sedative, hypnotic or anxiolytic-related dependence (F13.2-)*

                sedative, hypnotic, or anxiolytic use, unspecified (F13.9-)

    F13.10 **Sedative, hypnotic or anxiolytic abuse, uncomplicated** `HCC` `ESR`

         Sedative, hypnotic, or anxiolytic use disorder, mild

    F13.11 **Sedative, hypnotic or anxiolytic abuse, in remission** `HCC` `ESR`

         Sedative, hypnotic or anxiolytic use disorder, mild, in early remission

         Sedative, hypnotic or anxiolytic use disorder, mild, in sustained remission

  ☑6ᵗʰ **F13.12** **Sedative, hypnotic or anxiolytic abuse with intoxication**

    F13.120 **Sedative, hypnotic or anxiolytic abuse with intoxication, uncomplicated** `HCC` `ESR` `COM`

    F13.121 **Sedative, hypnotic or anxiolytic abuse with intoxication** delirium `HCC` `ESR` `COM`

    F13.129 **Sedative, hypnotic or anxiolytic abuse with intoxication, unspecified** `HCC` `ESR` `COM`

  ☑6ᵗʰ **F13.13** **Sedative, hypnotic or anxiolytic abuse with withdrawal**

         AHA: 2020,4Q,16-17

    F13.130 **Sedative, hypnotic or anxiolytic abuse with withdrawal, uncomplicated** `HCC` `ESR` `COM`

    F13.131 **Sedative, hypnotic or anxiolytic abuse with withdrawal** delirium `HCC` `ESR` `COM`

    F13.132 **Sedative, hypnotic or anxiolytic abuse with withdrawal with** perceptual disturbance `HCC` `ESR` `COM`

    F13.139 **Sedative, hypnotic or anxiolytic abuse with withdrawal, unspecified** `HCC` `ESR` `COM`

    F13.14 **Sedative, hypnotic or anxiolytic abuse with sedative, hypnotic or anxiolytic-induced** mood **disorder** `HCC` `ESR` `COM`

         Sedative, hypnotic, or anxiolytic use disorder, mild, with sedative, hypnotic, or anxiolytic-induced bipolar or related disorder

         Sedative, hypnotic, or anxiolytic use disorder, mild, with sedative, hypnotic, or anxiolytic-induced depressive disorder

  ☑6ᵗʰ **F13.15** **Sedative, hypnotic or anxiolytic abuse with sedative, hypnotic or anxiolytic-induced** psychotic **disorder**

    F13.150 **Sedative, hypnotic or anxiolytic abuse with sedative, hypnotic or anxiolytic-induced psychotic disorder with** delusions `HCC` `ESR` `COM`

    F13.151 **Sedative, hypnotic or anxiolytic abuse with sedative, hypnotic or anxiolytic-induced psychotic disorder with** hallucinations `HCC` `ESR` `COM`

    F13.159 **Sedative, hypnotic or anxiolytic abuse with sedative, hypnotic or anxiolytic-induced psychotic disorder, unspecified** `HCC` `ESR` `COM`

  ☑6ᵗʰ **F13.18** **Sedative, hypnotic or anxiolytic abuse with other sedative, hypnotic or anxiolytic-induced disorders**

    F13.180 **Sedative, hypnotic or anxiolytic abuse with sedative, hypnotic or anxiolytic-induced** anxiety **disorder** `HCC` `ESR` `COM`

    F13.181 **Sedative, hypnotic or anxiolytic abuse with sedative, hypnotic or anxiolytic-induced** sexual **dysfunction** `HCC` `ESR` `COM`

    F13.182 **Sedative, hypnotic or anxiolytic abuse with sedative, hypnotic or anxiolytic-induced** sleep **disorder** `HCC` `ESR` `COM`

    F13.188 **Sedative, hypnotic or anxiolytic abuse with other sedative, hypnotic or anxiolytic-induced disorder** `HCC` `ESR` `COM`

    F13.19 **Sedative, hypnotic or anxiolytic abuse with unspecified sedative, hypnotic or anxiolytic-induced disorder** `HCC` `ESR` `COM`

  ☑5ᵗʰ **F13.2** **Sedative, hypnotic or anxiolytic-related** dependence

    EXCLUDES 1   *sedative, hypnotic or anxiolytic-related abuse (F13.1-)*

                sedative, hypnotic, or anxiolytic use, unspecified (F13.9-)

    EXCLUDES 2   *sedative, hypnotic, or anxiolytic poisoning (T42.-)*

    F13.20 **Sedative, hypnotic or anxiolytic dependence, uncomplicated** `HCC` `ESR` `COM`

    F13.21 **Sedative, hypnotic or anxiolytic dependence, in remission** `HCC` `ESR` `COM`

         Sedative, hypnotic or anxiolytic use disorder, moderate, in early remission

         Sedative, hypnotic or anxiolytic use disorder, moderate, in sustained remission

         Sedative, hypnotic or anxiolytic use disorder, severe, in early remission

         Sedative, hypnotic or anxiolytic use disorder, severe, in sustained remission

  ☑6ᵗʰ **F13.22** **Sedative, hypnotic or anxiolytic dependence with intoxication**

    EXCLUDES 1   *sedative, hypnotic or anxiolytic dependence with withdrawal (F13.23-)*

    F13.220 **Sedative, hypnotic or anxiolytic dependence with intoxication, uncomplicated** `HCC` `ESR` `COM`

    F13.221 **Sedative, hypnotic or anxiolytic dependence with intoxication** delirium `HCC` `ESR` `COM`

    F13.229 **Sedative, hypnotic or anxiolytic dependence with intoxication, unspecified** `HCC` `ESR` `COM`

  ☑6ᵗʰ **F13.23** **Sedative, hypnotic or anxiolytic dependence with withdrawal**

         Sedative, hypnotic, or anxiolytic use disorder, moderate

         Sedative, hypnotic, or anxiolytic use disorder, severe

    EXCLUDES 1   *sedative, hypnotic or anxiolytic dependence with intoxication (F13.22-)*

    F13.230 **Sedative, hypnotic or anxiolytic dependence with withdrawal, uncomplicated** `HCC` `ESR` `COM`

    F13.231 **Sedative, hypnotic or anxiolytic dependence with withdrawal** delirium `HCC` `ESR` `COM`

    F13.232 **Sedative, hypnotic or anxiolytic dependence with withdrawal with** perceptual disturbance `HCC` `ESR` `COM`

         Sedative, hypnotic, or anxiolytic withdrawal with perceptual disturbances

    F13.239 **Sedative, hypnotic or anxiolytic dependence with withdrawal, unspecified** `HCC` `ESR` `COM`

         Sedative, hypnotic, or anxiolytic withdrawal without perceptual disturbances

    F13.24 **Sedative, hypnotic or anxiolytic dependence with sedative, hypnotic or anxiolytic-induced** mood **disorder** `HCC` `ESR` `COM`

         Sedative, hypnotic, or anxiolytic use disorder, moderate, with sedative, hypnotic, or anxiolytic-induced bipolar or related disorder

         Sedative, hypnotic, or anxiolytic use disorder, moderate, with sedative, hypnotic, or anxiolytic-induced depressive disorder

         Sedative, hypnotic, or anxiolytic use disorder, severe, with sedative, hypnotic, or anxiolytic-induced bipolar or related disorder

         Sedative, hypnotic, or anxiolytic use disorder, severe, with sedative, hypnotic, or anxiolytic-induced depressive disorder

Chapter 5. Mental, Behavioral and Neurodevelopmental Disorders

F13.25–F13.982

✓6ᵗʰ **F13.25** **Sedative, hypnotic or anxiolytic dependence with sedative, hypnotic or anxiolytic-induced** psychotic disorder

    F13.250 **Sedative, hypnotic or anxiolytic dependence with sedative, hypnotic or anxiolytic-induced psychotic disorder with** delusions   HCC ESR COM

    F13.251 **Sedative, hypnotic or anxiolytic dependence with sedative, hypnotic or anxiolytic-induced psychotic disorder with** hallucinations   HCC ESR COM

    F13.259 **Sedative, hypnotic or anxiolytic dependence with sedative, hypnotic or anxiolytic-induced psychotic disorder, unspecified**   HCC ESR COM

F13.26 **Sedative, hypnotic or anxiolytic dependence with sedative, hypnotic or anxiolytic-induced** persisting amnestic disorder   HCC ESR COM

F13.27 **Sedative, hypnotic or anxiolytic dependence with sedative, hypnotic or anxiolytic-induced** persisting dementia   HCC ESR COM

    Sedative, hypnotic, or anxiolytic use disorder, moderate, with sedative, hypnotic, or anxiolytic induced major neurocognitive disorder

    Sedative, hypnotic, or anxiolytic use disorder, severe, with sedative, hypnotic, or anxiolytic-induced major neurocognitive disorder

✓6ᵗʰ **F13.28** **Sedative, hypnotic or anxiolytic dependence with other sedative, hypnotic or anxiolytic-induced disorders**

    F13.280 **Sedative, hypnotic or anxiolytic dependence with sedative, hypnotic or anxiolytic-induced** anxiety disorder   HCC ESR COM

    F13.281 **Sedative, hypnotic or anxiolytic dependence with sedative, hypnotic or anxiolytic-induced** sexual dysfunction   HCC ESR COM

    F13.282 **Sedative, hypnotic or anxiolytic dependence with sedative, hypnotic or anxiolytic-induced** sleep disorder   HCC ESR COM

    F13.288 **Sedative, hypnotic or anxiolytic dependence with other sedative, hypnotic or anxiolytic-induced disorder**   HCC ESR COM

        Sedative, hypnotic, or anxiolytic use disorder, moderate, with sedative, hypnotic, or anxiolytic-induced mild neurocognitive disorder

        Sedative, hypnotic, or anxiolytic use disorder, severe, with sedative, hypnotic, or anxiolytic-induced mild neurocognitive disorder

F13.29 **Sedative, hypnotic or anxiolytic dependence with unspecified sedative, hypnotic or anxiolytic-induced disorder**   HCC ESR COM

✓5ᵗʰ **F13.9** **Sedative, hypnotic or anxiolytic-related use, unspecified**

    EXCLUDES 1   *sedative, hypnotic or anxiolytic-related abuse (F13.1-)*

                 sedative, hypnotic or anxiolytic-related dependence (F13.2-)

    TIP: Assign a substance use code only when the provider documents a relationship between the use and an associated physical, mental, or behavioral disorder. As with all diagnoses, substance use codes must meet the definition of a reportable diagnosis.

    F13.90 **Sedative, hypnotic, or anxiolytic use, unspecified, uncomplicated**

        AHA: 2018,2Q,10-11

    F13.91 **Sedative, hypnotic or anxiolytic use, unspecified, in remission**

✓6ᵗʰ **F13.92** **Sedative, hypnotic or anxiolytic use, unspecified with** intoxication

    EXCLUDES 1   *sedative, hypnotic or anxiolytic use, unspecified with withdrawal (F13.93-)*

    F13.920 **Sedative, hypnotic or anxiolytic use, unspecified with intoxication, uncomplicated**   HCC ESR COM

    F13.921 **Sedative, hypnotic or anxiolytic use, unspecified with intoxication** delirium   HCC ESR COM

        Sedative, hypnotic, or anxiolytic-induced delirium

    F13.929 **Sedative, hypnotic or anxiolytic use, unspecified with intoxication, unspecified**   HCC ESR COM

✓6ᵗʰ **F13.93** **Sedative, hypnotic or anxiolytic use, unspecified with** withdrawal

    EXCLUDES 1   *sedative, hypnotic or anxiolytic use, unspecified with intoxication (F13.92-)*

    F13.930 **Sedative, hypnotic or anxiolytic use, unspecified with withdrawal, uncomplicated**   HCC ESR COM

    F13.931 **Sedative, hypnotic or anxiolytic use, unspecified with withdrawal** delirium   HCC ESR COM

    F13.932 **Sedative, hypnotic or anxiolytic use, unspecified with withdrawal with** perceptual disturbances   HCC ESR COM

    F13.939 **Sedative, hypnotic or anxiolytic use, unspecified with withdrawal, unspecified**   HCC ESR COM

F13.94 **Sedative, hypnotic or anxiolytic use, unspecified with sedative, hypnotic or anxiolytic-induced** mood disorder   HCC ESR COM

    Sedative, hypnotic, or anxiolytic-induced bipolar or related disorder, without use disorder

    Sedative, hypnotic, or anxiolytic-induced depressive disorder, without use disorder

✓6ᵗʰ **F13.95** **Sedative, hypnotic or anxiolytic use, unspecified with sedative, hypnotic or anxiolytic-induced** psychotic disorder

    F13.950 **Sedative, hypnotic or anxiolytic use, unspecified with sedative, hypnotic or anxiolytic-induced psychotic disorder with** delusions   HCC ESR COM

    F13.951 **Sedative, hypnotic or anxiolytic use, unspecified with sedative, hypnotic or anxiolytic-induced psychotic disorder with** hallucinations   HCC ESR COM

    F13.959 **Sedative, hypnotic or anxiolytic use, unspecified with sedative, hypnotic or anxiolytic-induced psychotic disorder, unspecified**   HCC ESR COM

        Sedative, hypnotic, or anxiolytic-induced psychotic disorder, without use disorder

F13.96 **Sedative, hypnotic or anxiolytic use, unspecified with sedative, hypnotic or anxiolytic-induced** persisting amnestic disorder   HCC ESR COM

F13.97 **Sedative, hypnotic or anxiolytic use, unspecified with sedative, hypnotic or anxiolytic-induced** persisting dementia   HCC ESR COM

    Sedative, hypnotic, or anxiolytic-induced major neurocognitive disorder, without use disorder

✓6ᵗʰ **F13.98** **Sedative, hypnotic or anxiolytic use, unspecified with other sedative, hypnotic or anxiolytic-induced disorders**

    F13.980 **Sedative, hypnotic or anxiolytic use, unspecified with sedative, hypnotic or anxiolytic-induced** anxiety disorder   HCC ESR COM

        Sedative, hypnotic, or anxiolytic-induced anxiety disorder, without use disorder

    F13.981 **Sedative, hypnotic or anxiolytic use, unspecified with sedative, hypnotic or anxiolytic-induced** sexual dysfunction   HCC ESR COM

        Sedative, hypnotic, or anxiolytic-induced sexual dysfunction disorder, without use disorder

    F13.982 **Sedative, hypnotic or anxiolytic use, unspecified with sedative, hypnotic or anxiolytic-induced** sleep disorder   HCC ESR COM

        Sedative, hypnotic, or anxiolytic-induced sleep disorder, without use disorder

F13.988   Sedative, hypnotic or anxiolytic use, unspecified with other sedative, hypnotic or anxiolytic-induced disorder   HCC ESR COM
Sedative, hypnotic, or anxiolytic-induced mild neurocognitive disorder

F13.99   Sedative, hypnotic or anxiolytic use, unspecified with unspecified sedative, hypnotic or anxiolytic-induced disorder   HCC ESR COM

✓4th **F14**   Cocaine related disorders
    EXCLUDES 2   other stimulant-related disorders (F15.-)

✓5th **F14.1**   Cocaine abuse
    EXCLUDES 1   cocaine dependence (F14.2-)
            cocaine use, unspecified (F14.9-)

   F14.10   Cocaine abuse, uncomplicated   HCC ESR
Cocaine use disorder, mild

   F14.11   Cocaine abuse, in remission   HCC ESR
Cocaine use disorder, mild, in early remission
Cocaine use disorder, mild, in sustained remission

✓6th   **F14.12**   Cocaine abuse with intoxication

     F14.120   Cocaine abuse with intoxication, uncomplicated   HCC ESR COM

     F14.121   Cocaine abuse with intoxication with delirium   HCC ESR COM

     F14.122   Cocaine abuse with intoxication with perceptual disturbance   HCC ESR COM

     F14.129   Cocaine abuse with intoxication, unspecified   HCC ESR COM

   F14.13   Cocaine abuse, unspecified with withdrawal   HCC ESR COM
      AHA: 2020,4Q,16-17

   F14.14   Cocaine abuse with cocaine-induced mood disorder   HCC ESR COM
Cocaine use disorder, mild, with cocaine-induced bipolar or related disorder
Cocaine use disorder, mild, with cocaine-induced depressive disorder

✓6th   **F14.15**   Cocaine abuse with cocaine-induced psychotic disorder

     F14.150   Cocaine abuse with cocaine-induced psychotic disorder with delusions   HCC ESR COM

     F14.151   Cocaine abuse with cocaine-induced psychotic disorder with hallucinations   HCC ESR COM

     F14.159   Cocaine abuse with cocaine-induced psychotic disorder, unspecified   HCC ESR COM

✓6th   **F14.18**   Cocaine abuse with other cocaine-induced disorder

     F14.180   Cocaine abuse with cocaine-induced anxiety disorder   HCC ESR COM

     F14.181   Cocaine abuse with cocaine-induced sexual dysfunction   HCC ESR COM

     F14.182   Cocaine abuse with cocaine-induced sleep disorder   HCC ESR COM

     F14.188   Cocaine abuse with other cocaine-induced disorder   HCC ESR COM
Cocaine use disorder, mild, with cocaine-induced obsessive compulsive or related disorder

   F14.19   Cocaine abuse with unspecified cocaine-induced disorder   HCC ESR COM

✓5th **F14.2**   Cocaine dependence
    EXCLUDES 1   cocaine abuse (F14.1-)
            cocaine use, unspecified (F14.9-)
    EXCLUDES 2   cocaine poisoning (T40.5-)

   F14.20   Cocaine dependence, uncomplicated   HCC ESR COM
Cocaine use disorder, moderate
Cocaine use disorder, severe

   F14.21   Cocaine dependence, in remission   HCC ESR COM
Cocaine use disorder, moderate, in early remission
Cocaine use disorder, moderate, in sustained remission
Cocaine use disorder, severe, in early remission
Cocaine use disorder, severe, in sustained remission

✓6th   **F14.22**   Cocaine dependence with intoxication
     EXCLUDES 1   cocaine dependence with withdrawal (F14.23)

     F14.220   Cocaine dependence with intoxication, uncomplicated   HCC ESR COM

     F14.221   Cocaine dependence with intoxication delirium   HCC ESR COM

     F14.222   Cocaine dependence with intoxication with perceptual disturbance   HCC ESR COM

     F14.229   Cocaine dependence with intoxication, unspecified   HCC ESR COM

   F14.23   Cocaine dependence with withdrawal   HCC ESR COM
     EXCLUDES 1   cocaine dependence with intoxication (F14.22-)

   F14.24   Cocaine dependence with cocaine-induced mood disorder   HCC ESR COM
Cocaine use disorder, moderate, with cocaine-induced bipolar or related disorder
Cocaine use disorder, moderate, with cocaine-induced depressive disorder
Cocaine use disorder, severe, with cocaine-induced bipolar or related disorder
Cocaine use disorder, severe, with cocaine-induced depressive disorder

✓6th   **F14.25**   Cocaine dependence with cocaine-induced psychotic disorder

     F14.250   Cocaine dependence with cocaine-induced psychotic disorder with delusions   HCC ESR COM

     F14.251   Cocaine dependence with cocaine-induced psychotic disorder with hallucinations   HCC ESR COM

     F14.259   Cocaine dependence with cocaine-induced psychotic disorder, unspecified   HCC ESR COM

✓6th   **F14.28**   Cocaine dependence with other cocaine-induced disorder

     F14.280   Cocaine dependence with cocaine-induced anxiety disorder   HCC ESR COM

     F14.281   Cocaine dependence with cocaine-induced sexual dysfunction   HCC ESR COM

     F14.282   Cocaine dependence with cocaine-induced sleep disorder   HCC ESR COM

     F14.288   Cocaine dependence with other cocaine-induced disorder   HCC ESR COM
Cocaine use disorder, moderate, with cocaine-induced obsessive compulsive or related disorder
Cocaine use disorder, severe, with cocaine-induced obsessive compulsive or related disorder

   F14.29   Cocaine dependence with unspecified cocaine-induced disorder   HCC ESR COM

✓5th **F14.9**   Cocaine use, unspecified
    EXCLUDES 1   cocaine abuse (F14.1-)
            cocaine dependence (F14.2-)

    TIP: Assign a substance use code only when the provider documents a relationship between the use and an associated physical, mental, or behavioral disorder. As with all diagnoses, substance use codes must meet the definition of a reportable diagnosis.

   F14.90   Cocaine use, unspecified, uncomplicated
      AHA: 2018,2Q,10-11

   F14.91   Cocaine use, unspecified, in remission

✓6th   **F14.92**   Cocaine use, unspecified with intoxication

     F14.920   Cocaine use, unspecified with intoxication, uncomplicated   HCC ESR COM

     F14.921   Cocaine use, unspecified with intoxication delirium   HCC ESR COM

     F14.922   Cocaine use, unspecified with intoxication with perceptual disturbance   HCC ESR COM

     F14.929   Cocaine use, unspecified with intoxication, unspecified   HCC ESR COM

Chapter 5. Mental, Behavioral and Neurodevelopmental Disorders

F14.93 Cocaine use, unspecified with withdrawal   HCC ESR COM
   AHA: 2020,4Q,16-17

F14.94 Cocaine use, unspecified with cocaine-induced mood disorder   HCC ESR COM
   Cocaine induced bipolar or related disorder, without use disorder
   Cocaine induced depressive disorder, without use disorder

✓6th **F14.95** Cocaine use, unspecified with cocaine-induced psychotic disorder
   F14.950 Cocaine use, unspecified with cocaine-induced psychotic disorder with delusions   HCC ESR COM
   F14.951 Cocaine use, unspecified with cocaine-induced psychotic disorder with hallucinations   HCC ESR COM
   F14.959 Cocaine use, unspecified with cocaine-induced psychotic disorder, unspecified   HCC ESR COM
     Cocaine induced psychotic disorder, without use disorder

✓6th **F14.98** Cocaine use, unspecified with other specified cocaine-induced disorder
   F14.980 Cocaine use, unspecified with cocaine-induced anxiety disorder   HCC ESR COM
     Cocaine induced anxiety disorder, without use disorder
   F14.981 Cocaine use, unspecified with cocaine-induced sexual dysfunction   HCC ESR COM
     Cocaine induced sexual dysfunction, without use disorder
   F14.982 Cocaine use, unspecified with cocaine-induced sleep disorder   HCC ESR COM
     Cocaine induced sleep disorder, without use disorder
   F14.988 Cocaine use, unspecified with other cocaine-induced disorder   HCC ESR COM
     Cocaine induced obsessive compulsive or related disorder

F14.99 Cocaine use, unspecified with unspecified cocaine-induced disorder   HCC ESR COM

✓4th **F15** Other stimulant related disorders
   INCLUDES   amphetamine-related disorders
            caffeine
   EXCLUDES 2   cocaine-related disorders (F14.-)

✓5th **F15.1** Other stimulant abuse
   EXCLUDES 1   other stimulant dependence (F15.2-)
              other stimulant use, unspecified (F15.9-)
   F15.10 Other stimulant abuse, uncomplicated   HCC ESR
     Amphetamine type substance use disorder, mild
     Other or unspecified stimulant use disorder, mild
   F15.11 Other stimulant abuse, in remission   HCC ESR
     Amphetamine type substance use disorder, mild, in early remission
     Amphetamine type substance use disorder, mild, in sustained remission
     Other or unspecified stimulant use disorder, mild, in early remission
     Other or unspecified stimulant use disorder, mild, in sustained remission
     AHA: 2021,3Q,8

✓6th **F15.12** Other stimulant abuse with intoxication
   F15.120 Other stimulant abuse with intoxication, uncomplicated   HCC ESR COM
   F15.121 Other stimulant abuse with intoxication delirium   HCC ESR COM
   F15.122 Other stimulant abuse with intoxication with perceptual disturbance   HCC ESR COM
     Amphetamine or other stimulant use disorder, mild, with amphetamine or other stimulant intoxication, with perceptual disturbances

F15.129 Other stimulant abuse with intoxication, unspecified   HCC ESR COM
     Amphetamine or other stimulant use disorder, mild, with amphetamine or other stimulant intoxication, without perceptual disturbances

F15.13 Other stimulant abuse with withdrawal   HCC ESR COM
   AHA: 2020,4Q,16-17

F15.14 Other stimulant abuse with stimulant-induced mood disorder   HCC ESR COM
   Amphetamine or other stimulant use disorder, mild, with amphetamine or other stimulant induced bipolar or related disorder
   Amphetamine or other stimulant use disorder, mild, with amphetamine or other stimulant induced depressive disorder

✓6th **F15.15** Other stimulant abuse with stimulant-induced psychotic disorder
   F15.150 Other stimulant abuse with stimulant-induced psychotic disorder with delusions   HCC ESR COM
   F15.151 Other stimulant abuse with stimulant-induced psychotic disorder with hallucinations   HCC ESR COM
   F15.159 Other stimulant abuse with stimulant-induced psychotic disorder, unspecified   HCC ESR COM

✓6th **F15.18** Other stimulant abuse with other stimulant-induced disorder
   F15.180 Other stimulant abuse with stimulant-induced anxiety disorder   HCC ESR COM
   F15.181 Other stimulant abuse with stimulant-induced sexual dysfunction   HCC ESR COM
   F15.182 Other stimulant abuse with stimulant-induced sleep disorder   HCC ESR COM
   F15.188 Other stimulant abuse with other stimulant-induced disorder   HCC ESR COM
     Amphetamine or other stimulant use disorder, mild, with amphetamine or other stimulant induced obsessive-compulsive or related disorder

F15.19 Other stimulant abuse with unspecified stimulant-induced disorder   HCC ESR COM

✓5th **F15.2** Other stimulant dependence
   EXCLUDES 1   other stimulant abuse (F15.1-)
              other stimulant use, unspecified (F15.9-)
   F15.20 Other stimulant dependence, uncomplicated   HCC ESR COM
     Amphetamine type substance use disorder, moderate
     Amphetamine type substance use disorder, severe
     Other or unspecified stimulant use disorder, moderate
     Other or unspecified stimulant use disorder, severe
   F15.21 Other stimulant dependence, in remission   HCC ESR COM
     Amphetamine type substance use disorder, moderate, in early remission
     Amphetamine type substance use disorder, moderate, in sustained remission
     Amphetamine type substance use disorder, severe, in early remission
     Amphetamine type substance use disorder, severe, in sustained remission
     Other or unspecified stimulant use disorder, moderate, in early remission
     Other or unspecified stimulant use disorder, moderate, in sustained remission
     Other or unspecified stimulant use disorder, severe, in early remission
     Other or unspecified stimulant use disorder, severe, in sustained remission

√6ᵗʰ **F15.22 Other stimulant dependence with** intoxication

> EXCLUDES 1   *other stimulant dependence with withdrawal (F15.23)*

F15.220 Other stimulant dependence with intoxication, uncomplicated   HCC ESR COM

F15.221 Other stimulant dependence with intoxication delirium   HCC ESR COM

F15.222 Other stimulant dependence with intoxication with perceptual disturbance   HCC ESR COM

> Amphetamine or other stimulant use disorder, moderate, with amphetamine or other stimulant intoxication, with perceptual disturbances
>
> Amphetamine or other stimulant use disorder, severe, with amphetamine or other stimulant intoxication, with perceptual disturbances

F15.229 Other stimulant dependence with intoxication, unspecified   HCC ESR COM

> Amphetamine or other stimulant use disorder, moderate, with amphetamine or other stimulant intoxication, without perceptual disturbances
>
> Amphetamine or other stimulant use disorder, severe, with amphetamine or other stimulant intoxication, without perceptual disturbances

F15.23 Other stimulant dependence with withdrawal   HCC ESR COM

> Amphetamine or other stimulant withdrawal

> EXCLUDES 1   *other stimulant dependence with intoxication (F15.22-)*

F15.24 Other stimulant dependence with stimulant-induced mood disorder   HCC ESR COM

> Amphetamine or other stimulant use disorder, moderate, with amphetamine or other stimulant-induced bipolar or related disorder
>
> Amphetamine or other stimulant use disorder, moderate, with amphetamine or other stimulant induced depressive disorder
>
> Amphetamine or other stimulant use disorder, severe, with amphetamine or other stimulant-induced bipolar or related disorder
>
> Amphetamine or other stimulant use disorder, severe, with amphetamine or other stimulant-induced depressive disorder

√6ᵗʰ **F15.25 Other stimulant dependence with stimulant-induced** psychotic disorder

F15.250 Other stimulant dependence with stimulant-induced psychotic disorder with delusions   HCC ESR COM

F15.251 Other stimulant dependence with stimulant-induced psychotic disorder with hallucinations   HCC ESR COM

F15.259 Other stimulant dependence with stimulant-induced psychotic disorder, unspecified   HCC ESR COM

√6ᵗʰ **F15.28 Other stimulant dependence with other stimulant-induced disorder**

F15.280 Other stimulant dependence with stimulant-induced anxiety disorder   HCC ESR COM

F15.281 Other stimulant dependence with stimulant-induced sexual dysfunction   HCC ESR COM

F15.282 Other stimulant dependence with stimulant-induced sleep disorder   HCC ESR COM

F15.288 Other stimulant dependence with other stimulant-induced disorder   HCC ESR COM

> Amphetamine or other stimulant use disorder, moderate, with amphetamine or other stimulant induced obsessive compulsive or related disorder
>
> Amphetamine or other stimulant use disorder, severe, with amphetamine or other stimulant induced obsessive compulsive or related disorder

F15.29 Other stimulant dependence with unspecified stimulant-induced disorder   HCC ESR COM

√5ᵗʰ **F15.9 Other stimulant** use, unspecified

> EXCLUDES 1   *other stimulant abuse (F15.1-)*
>   *other stimulant dependence (F15.2-)*

TIP: Assign a substance use code only when the provider documents a relationship between the use and an associated physical, mental, or behavioral disorder. As with all diagnoses, substance use codes must meet the definition of a reportable diagnosis.

F15.90 Other stimulant use, unspecified, uncomplicated

> **AHA:** 2018,2Q,10-11

F15.91 Other stimulant use, unspecified, in remission

√6ᵗʰ **F15.92 Other stimulant use, unspecified with** intoxication

> EXCLUDES 1   *other stimulant use, unspecified with withdrawal (F15.93)*

F15.920 Other stimulant use, unspecified with intoxication, uncomplicated   HCC ESR COM

F15.921 Other stimulant use, unspecified with intoxication delirium   HCC ESR COM

> Amphetamine or other stimulant-induced delirium

F15.922 Other stimulant use, unspecified with intoxication with perceptual disturbance   HCC ESR COM

F15.929 Other stimulant use, unspecified with intoxication, unspecified   HCC ESR COM

> Caffeine intoxication

F15.93 Other stimulant use, unspecified with withdrawal   HCC ESR COM

> Caffeine withdrawal

> EXCLUDES 1   *other stimulant use, unspecified with intoxication (F15.92-)*

F15.94 Other stimulant use, unspecified with stimulant-induced mood disorder   HCC ESR COM

> Amphetamine or other stimulant-induced bipolar or related disorder, without use disorder
>
> Amphetamine or other stimulant-induced depressive disorder, without use disorder

√6ᵗʰ **F15.95 Other stimulant use, unspecified with stimulant-induced** psychotic disorder

F15.950 Other stimulant use, unspecified with stimulant-induced psychotic disorder with delusions   HCC ESR COM

F15.951 Other stimulant use, unspecified with stimulant-induced psychotic disorder with hallucinations   HCC ESR COM

F15.959 Other stimulant use, unspecified with stimulant-induced psychotic disorder, unspecified   HCC ESR COM

> Amphetamine or other stimulant-induced psychotic disorder, without use disorder

√6ᵗʰ **F15.98 Other stimulant use, unspecified with other stimulant-induced disorder**

F15.980 Other stimulant use, unspecified with stimulant-induced anxiety disorder   HCC ESR COM

> Amphetamine or other stimulant-induced anxiety disorder, without use disorder
>
> Caffeine induced anxiety disorder, without use disorder

F15.981 Other stimulant use, unspecified with stimulant-induced sexual dysfunction `HCC` `ESR` `COM`
  Amphetamine or other stimulant-induced sexual dysfunction, without use disorder

F15.982 Other stimulant use, unspecified with stimulant-induced sleep disorder `HCC` `ESR` `COM`
  Amphetamine or other stimulant-induced sleep disorder, without use disorder
  Caffeine induced sleep disorder, without use disorder

F15.988 Other stimulant use, unspecified with other stimulant-induced disorder `HCC` `ESR` `COM`
  Amphetamine or other stimulant-induced obsessive compulsive or related disorder, without use disorder

F15.99 Other stimulant use, unspecified with unspecified stimulant-induced disorder `HCC` `ESR` `COM`

✓4ᵗʰ **F16 Hallucinogen related disorders**
  INCLUDES   ecstasy
             PCP
             phencyclidine
  AHA: 2018,4Q,31

✓5ᵗʰ **F16.1 Hallucinogen abuse**
  EXCLUDES 1   *hallucinogen dependence (F16.2-)*
              hallucinogen use, unspecified (F16.9-)

  F16.10 Hallucinogen abuse, uncomplicated `HCC` `ESR`
    Other hallucinogen use disorder, mild
    Phencyclidine use disorder, mild

  F16.11 Hallucinogen abuse, in remission `HCC` `ESR`
    Other hallucinogen use disorder, mild, in early remission
    Other hallucinogen use disorder, mild, in sustained remission
    Phencyclidine use disorder, mild, in early remission
    Phencyclidine use disorder, mild, in sustained remission

  ✓6ᵗʰ **F16.12 Hallucinogen abuse with intoxication**
    F16.120 Hallucinogen abuse with intoxication, uncomplicated `HCC` `ESR` `COM`
    F16.121 Hallucinogen abuse with intoxication with delirium `HCC` `ESR` `COM`
    F16.122 Hallucinogen abuse with intoxication with perceptual disturbance `HCC` `ESR` `COM`
    F16.129 Hallucinogen abuse with intoxication, unspecified `HCC` `ESR` `COM`

  F16.14 Hallucinogen abuse with hallucinogen-induced mood disorder `HCC` `ESR` `COM`
    Other hallucinogen use disorder, mild, with other hallucinogen induced bipolar or related disorder
    Other hallucinogen use disorder, mild, with other hallucinogen induced depressive disorder
    Phencyclidine use disorder, mild, with phencyclidine induced bipolar or related disorder
    Phencyclidine use disorder, mild, with phencyclidine induced depressive disorder

  ✓6ᵗʰ **F16.15 Hallucinogen abuse with hallucinogen-induced psychotic disorder**
    F16.150 Hallucinogen abuse with hallucinogen-induced psychotic disorder with delusions `HCC` `ESR` `COM`
    F16.151 Hallucinogen abuse with hallucinogen-induced psychotic disorder with hallucinations `HCC` `ESR` `COM`
    F16.159 Hallucinogen abuse with hallucinogen-induced psychotic disorder, unspecified `HCC` `ESR` `COM`

  ✓6ᵗʰ **F16.18 Hallucinogen abuse with other hallucinogen-induced disorder**
    F16.180 Hallucinogen abuse with hallucinogen-induced anxiety disorder `HCC` `ESR` `COM`
    F16.183 Hallucinogen abuse with hallucinogen persisting perception disorder (flashbacks) `HCC` `ESR` `COM`

  F16.188 Hallucinogen abuse with other hallucinogen-induced disorder `HCC` `ESR` `COM`

  F16.19 Hallucinogen abuse with unspecified hallucinogen-induced disorder `HCC` `ESR` `COM`

✓5ᵗʰ **F16.2 Hallucinogen dependence**
  EXCLUDES 1   *hallucinogen abuse (F16.1-)*
              hallucinogen use, unspecified (F16.9-)

  F16.20 Hallucinogen dependence, uncomplicated `HCC` `ESR` `COM`
    Other hallucinogen use disorder, moderate
    Other hallucinogen use disorder, severe
    Phencyclidine use disorder, moderate
    Phencyclidine use disorder, severe

  F16.21 Hallucinogen dependence, in remission `HCC` `ESR` `COM`
    Other hallucinogen use disorder, moderate, in early remission
    Other hallucinogen use disorder, moderate, in sustained remission
    Other hallucinogen use disorder, severe, in early remission
    Other hallucinogen use disorder, severe, in sustained remission
    Phencyclidine use disorder, moderate, in early remission
    Phencyclidine use disorder, moderate, in sustained remission
    Phencyclidine use disorder, severe, in early remission
    Phencyclidine use disorder, severe, in sustained remission

  ✓6ᵗʰ **F16.22 Hallucinogen dependence with intoxication**
    F16.220 Hallucinogen dependence with intoxication, uncomplicated `HCC` `ESR` `COM`
    F16.221 Hallucinogen dependence with intoxication with delirium `HCC` `ESR` `COM`
    F16.229 Hallucinogen dependence with intoxication, unspecified `HCC` `ESR` `COM`

  F16.24 Hallucinogen dependence with hallucinogen-induced mood disorder `HCC` `ESR` `COM`
    Other hallucinogen use disorder, moderate, with other hallucinogen induced bipolar or related disorder
    Other hallucinogen use disorder, moderate, with other hallucinogen induced depressive disorder
    Other hallucinogen use disorder, severe, with other hallucinogen-induced bipolar or related disorder
    Other hallucinogen use disorder, severe, with other hallucinogen-induced depressive disorder
    Phencyclidine use disorder, moderate, with phencyclidine induced bipolar or related disorder
    Phencyclidine use disorder, moderate, with phencyclidine induced depressive disorder
    Phencyclidine use disorder, severe, with phencyclidine induced bipolar or related disorder
    Phencyclidine use disorder, severe, with phencyclidine-induced depressive disorder

  ✓6ᵗʰ **F16.25 Hallucinogen dependence with hallucinogen-induced psychotic disorder**
    F16.250 Hallucinogen dependence with hallucinogen-induced psychotic disorder with delusions `HCC` `ESR` `COM`
    F16.251 Hallucinogen dependence with hallucinogen-induced psychotic disorder with hallucinations `HCC` `ESR` `COM`
    F16.259 Hallucinogen dependence with hallucinogen-induced psychotic disorder, unspecified `HCC` `ESR` `COM`

  ✓6ᵗʰ **F16.28 Hallucinogen dependence with other hallucinogen-induced disorder**
    F16.280 Hallucinogen dependence with hallucinogen-induced anxiety disorder `HCC` `ESR` `COM`
    F16.283 Hallucinogen dependence with hallucinogen persisting perception disorder (flashbacks) `HCC` `ESR` `COM`

`HCC` CMS-HCC   `Rx` Rx HCC   `ESR` ESRD HCC   `COM` Commercial HCC   `N` Newborn: 0   `P` Pediatric: 0-17   `M` Maternity: 9-64   `A` Adult: 15-124

570
ICD-10-CM 2023

F16.288 Hallucinogen dependence with other hallucinogen-induced disorder `HCC` `ESR` `COM`

F16.29 Hallucinogen dependence with unspecified hallucinogen-induced disorder `HCC` `ESR` `COM`

√5th **F16.9 Hallucinogen use, unspecified**

     EXCLUDES 1   *hallucinogen abuse (F16.1-)*
                      hallucinogen dependence (F16.2-)

     TIP: Assign a substance use code only when the provider documents a relationship between the use and an associated physical, mental, or behavioral disorder. As with all diagnoses, substance use codes must meet the definition of a reportable diagnosis.

F16.90 Hallucinogen use, unspecified, uncomplicated
     AHA: 2018,2Q,10-11

F16.91 Hallucinogen use, unspecified, in remission

√6th **F16.92 Hallucinogen use, unspecified with intoxication**

F16.920 Hallucinogen use, unspecified with intoxication, uncomplicated `HCC` `ESR` `COM`

F16.921 Hallucinogen use, unspecified with intoxication with delirium `HCC` `ESR` `COM`
     Other hallucinogen intoxication delirium

F16.929 Hallucinogen use, unspecified with intoxication, unspecified `HCC` `ESR` `COM`

F16.94 Hallucinogen use, unspecified with hallucinogen-induced mood disorder `HCC` `ESR` `COM`
     Other hallucinogen induced bipolar or related disorder, without use disorder
     Other hallucinogen induced depressive disorder, without use disorder
     Phencyclidine induced bipolar or related disorder, without use disorder
     Phencyclidine induced depressive disorder, without use disorder

√6th **F16.95 Hallucinogen use, unspecified with hallucinogen-induced psychotic disorder**

F16.950 Hallucinogen use, unspecified with hallucinogen-induced psychotic disorder with delusions `HCC` `ESR` `COM`

F16.951 Hallucinogen use, unspecified with hallucinogen-induced psychotic disorder with hallucinations `HCC` `ESR` `COM`

F16.959 Hallucinogen use, unspecified with hallucinogen-induced psychotic disorder, unspecified `HCC` `ESR` `COM`
     Other hallucinogen induced psychotic disorder, without use disorder
     Phencyclidine induced psychotic disorder, without use disorder

√6th **F16.98 Hallucinogen use, unspecified with other specified hallucinogen-induced disorder**

F16.980 Hallucinogen use, unspecified with hallucinogen-induced anxiety disorder `HCC` `ESR` `COM`
     Other hallucinogen-induced anxiety disorder, without use disorder
     Phencyclidine induced anxiety disorder, without use disorder

F16.983 Hallucinogen use, unspecified with hallucinogen persisting perception disorder (flashbacks) `HCC` `ESR` `COM`

F16.988 Hallucinogen use, unspecified with other hallucinogen-induced disorder `HCC` `ESR` `COM`

F16.99 Hallucinogen use, unspecified with unspecified hallucinogen-induced disorder `HCC` `ESR` `COM`

√4th **F17 Nicotine dependence**

     EXCLUDES 1   *history of tobacco dependence (Z87.891)*
                     tobacco use NOS (Z72.0)
     EXCLUDES 2   *tobacco use (smoking) during pregnancy, childbirth and the puerperium (O99.33-)*
                     toxic effect of nicotine (T65.2-)

     AHA: 2013,4Q,108-109

√5th **F17.2 Nicotine dependence**

√6th **F17.20 Nicotine dependence, unspecified**

F17.200 Nicotine dependence, unspecified, uncomplicated
     Tobacco use disorder, mild
     Tobacco use disorder, moderate
     Tobacco use disorder, severe
     AHA: 2016,1Q,36
     TIP: Assign when provider documentation indicates "smoker" without further specification.

F17.201 Nicotine dependence, unspecified, in remission
     Tobacco use disorder, mild, in early remission
     Tobacco use disorder, mild, in sustained remission
     Tobacco use disorder, moderate, in early remission
     Tobacco use disorder, moderate, in sustained remission
     Tobacco use disorder, severe, in early remission
     Tobacco use disorder, severe, in sustained remission

F17.203 Nicotine dependence unspecified, with withdrawal
     Tobacco withdrawal

F17.208 Nicotine dependence, unspecified, with other nicotine-induced disorders

F17.209 Nicotine dependence, unspecified, with unspecified nicotine-induced disorders

√6th **F17.21 Nicotine dependence, cigarettes**

F17.210 Nicotine dependence, cigarettes, uncomplicated
     AHA: 2017,2Q,28-29

F17.211 Nicotine dependence, cigarettes, in remission
     Tobacco use disorder, cigarettes, mild, in early remission
     Tobacco use disorder, cigarettes, mild, in sustained remission
     Tobacco use disorder, cigarettes, moderate, in early remission
     Tobacco use disorder, cigarettes, moderate, in sustained remission
     Tobacco use disorder, cigarettes, severe, in early remission
     Tobacco use disorder, cigarettes, severe, in sustained remission

F17.213 Nicotine dependence, cigarettes, with withdrawal

F17.218 Nicotine dependence, cigarettes, with other nicotine-induced disorders

F17.219 Nicotine dependence, cigarettes, with unspecified nicotine-induced disorders

√6th **F17.22 Nicotine dependence, chewing tobacco**

F17.220 Nicotine dependence, chewing tobacco, uncomplicated

☑ Additional Character Required   √x7th Placeholder Alert   Manifestation   Unspecified Dx   Q QPP   UPD Unacceptable PDx

Chapter 5. Mental, Behavioral and Neurodevelopmental Disorders

F17.221   Nicotine dependence, chewing tobacco, in remission
> Tobacco use disorder, chewing tobacco, mild, in early remission
> Tobacco use disorder, chewing tobacco, mild, in sustained remission
> Tobacco use disorder, chewing tobacco, moderate, in early remission
> Tobacco use disorder, chewing tobacco, moderate, in sustained remission
> Tobacco use disorder, chewing tobacco, severe, in early remission
> Tobacco use disorder, chewing tobacco, severe, in sustained remission

F17.223   Nicotine dependence, chewing tobacco, with withdrawal

F17.228   Nicotine dependence, chewing tobacco, with other nicotine-induced disorders

F17.229   Nicotine dependence, chewing tobacco, with unspecified nicotine-induced disorders

✓6ᵗʰ **F17.29**   Nicotine dependence, other tobacco product

F17.290   Nicotine dependence, other tobacco product, uncomplicated
> **AHA:** 2017,2Q,28-29

F17.291   Nicotine dependence, other tobacco product, in remission
> Tobacco use disorder, other tobacco product, mild, in early remission
> Tobacco use disorder, other tobacco product, mild, in sustained remission
> Tobacco use disorder, other tobacco product, moderate, in early remission
> Tobacco use disorder, other tobacco product, moderate, in sustained remission
> Tobacco use disorder, other tobacco product, severe, in early remission
> Tobacco use disorder, other tobacco product, severe, in sustained remission

F17.293   Nicotine dependence, other tobacco product, with withdrawal

F17.298   Nicotine dependence, other tobacco product, with other nicotine-induced disorders

F17.299   Nicotine dependence, other tobacco product, with unspecified nicotine-induced disorders

✓4ᵗʰ **F18**   Inhalant related disorders
> **INCLUDES**   volatile solvents

✓5ᵗʰ **F18.1**   Inhalant abuse
> **EXCLUDES 1**   inhalant dependence (F18.2-)
> inhalant use, unspecified (F18.9-)

F18.10   Inhalant abuse, uncomplicated   `HCC` `ESR`
> Inhalant use disorder, mild

F18.11   Inhalant abuse, in remission   `HCC` `ESR`
> Inhalant use disorder, mild, in early remission
> Inhalant use disorder, mild, in sustained remission

✓6ᵗʰ **F18.12**   Inhalant abuse with intoxication

F18.120   Inhalant abuse with intoxication, uncomplicated   `HCC` `ESR` `COM`

F18.121   Inhalant abuse with intoxication delirium   `HCC` `ESR` `COM`

F18.129   Inhalant abuse with intoxication, unspecified   `HCC` `ESR` `COM`

F18.14   Inhalant abuse with inhalant-induced mood disorder   `HCC` `ESR` `COM`
> Inhalant use disorder, mild, with inhalant induced depressive disorder

✓6ᵗʰ **F18.15**   Inhalant abuse with inhalant-induced psychotic disorder

F18.150   Inhalant abuse with inhalant-induced psychotic disorder with delusions   `HCC` `ESR` `COM`

F18.151   Inhalant abuse with inhalant-induced psychotic disorder with hallucinations   `HCC` `ESR` `COM`

F18.159   Inhalant abuse with inhalant-induced psychotic disorder, unspecified   `HCC` `ESR` `COM`

F18.17   Inhalant abuse with inhalant-induced dementia   `HCC` `ESR` `COM`
> Inhalant use disorder, mild, with inhalant induced major neurocognitive disorder

✓6ᵗʰ **F18.18**   Inhalant abuse with other inhalant-induced disorders

F18.180   Inhalant abuse with inhalant-induced anxiety disorder   `HCC` `ESR` `COM`

F18.188   Inhalant abuse with other inhalant-induced disorder   `HCC` `ESR` `COM`
> Inhalant use disorder, mild, with inhalant induced mild neurocognitive disorder

F18.19   Inhalant abuse with unspecified inhalant-induced disorder   `HCC` `ESR` `COM`

✓5ᵗʰ **F18.2**   Inhalant dependence
> **EXCLUDES 1**   inhalant abuse (F18.1-)
> inhalant use, unspecified (F18.9-)

F18.20   Inhalant dependence, uncomplicated   `HCC` `ESR` `COM`
> Inhalant use disorder, moderate
> Inhalant use disorder, severe

F18.21   Inhalant dependence, in remission   `HCC` `ESR` `COM`
> Inhalant use disorder, moderate, in early remission
> Inhalant use disorder, moderate, in sustained remission
> Inhalant use disorder, severe, in early remission
> Inhalant use disorder, severe, in sustained remission

✓6ᵗʰ **F18.22**   Inhalant dependence with intoxication

F18.220   Inhalant dependence with intoxication, uncomplicated   `HCC` `ESR` `COM`

F18.221   Inhalant dependence with intoxication delirium   `HCC` `ESR` `COM`

F18.229   Inhalant dependence with intoxication, unspecified   `HCC` `ESR` `COM`

F18.24   Inhalant dependence with inhalant-induced mood disorder   `HCC` `ESR` `COM`
> Inhalant use disorder, moderate, with inhalant induced depressive disorder
> Inhalant use disorder, severe, with inhalant induced depressive disorder

✓6ᵗʰ **F18.25**   Inhalant dependence with inhalant-induced psychotic disorder

F18.250   Inhalant dependence with inhalant-induced psychotic disorder with delusions   `HCC` `ESR` `COM`

F18.251   Inhalant dependence with inhalant-induced psychotic disorder with hallucinations   `HCC` `ESR` `COM`

F18.259   Inhalant dependence with inhalant-induced psychotic disorder, unspecified   `HCC` `ESR` `COM`

F18.27   Inhalant dependence with inhalant-induced dementia   `HCC` `ESR` `COM`
> Inhalant use disorder, moderate, with inhalant induced major neurocognitive disorder
> Inhalant use disorder, severe, with inhalant induced major neurocognitive disorder

✓6ᵗʰ **F18.28**   Inhalant dependence with other inhalant-induced disorders

F18.280   Inhalant dependence with inhalant-induced anxiety disorder   `HCC` `ESR` `COM`

F18.288   Inhalant dependence with other inhalant-induced disorder   `HCC` `ESR` `COM`
> Inhalant use disorder, moderate, with inhalant-induced mild neurocognitive disorder
> Inhalant use disorder, severe, with inhalant-induced mild neurocognitive disorder

F18.29   Inhalant dependence with unspecified inhalant-induced disorder   `HCC` `ESR` `COM`

`HCC` CMS-HCC   `Rx` Rx HCC   `ESR` ESRD HCC   `COM` Commercial HCC   `N` Newborn: 0   `P` Pediatric: 0-17   `M` Maternity: 9-64   `A` Adult: 15-124

572

ICD-10-CM 2023

Chapter 5. Mental, Behavioral and Neurodevelopmental Disorders

✓5ᵗʰ F18.9 Inhalant use, unspecified

> EXCLUDES 1   *inhalant abuse (F18.1-)*
> *inhalant dependence (F18.2-)*

> **TIP:** Assign a substance use code only when the provider documents a relationship between the use and an associated physical, mental, or behavioral disorder. As with all diagnoses, substance use codes must meet the definition of a reportable diagnosis.

> **F18.90 Inhalant use, unspecified, uncomplicated**
> AHA: 2018,2Q,10-11

> **F18.91 Inhalant use, unspecified, in remission**

✓6ᵗʰ F18.92 Inhalant use, unspecified with intoxication

> **F18.920 Inhalant use, unspecified with intoxication, uncomplicated** HCC ESR COM

> **F18.921 Inhalant use, unspecified with intoxication with delirium** HCC ESR COM

> **F18.929 Inhalant use, unspecified with intoxication, unspecified** HCC ESR COM

F18.94 Inhalant use, unspecified with inhalant-induced mood disorder
> Inhalant induced depressive disorder

✓6ᵗʰ F18.95 Inhalant use, unspecified with inhalant-induced psychotic disorder

> **F18.950 Inhalant use, unspecified with inhalant-induced psychotic disorder with delusions** HCC ESR COM

> **F18.951 Inhalant use, unspecified with inhalant-induced psychotic disorder with hallucinations** HCC ESR COM

> **F18.959 Inhalant use, unspecified with inhalant-induced psychotic disorder, unspecified** HCC ESR COM

F18.97 Inhalant use, unspecified with inhalant-induced persisting dementia HCC ESR COM
> Inhalant-induced major neurocognitive disorder

✓6ᵗʰ F18.98 Inhalant use, unspecified with other inhalant-induced disorders

> **F18.980 Inhalant use, unspecified with inhalant-induced anxiety disorder** HCC ESR COM

> **F18.988 Inhalant use, unspecified with other inhalant-induced disorder** HCC ESR COM
> > Inhalant-induced mild neurocognitive disorder

> **F18.99 Inhalant use, unspecified with unspecified inhalant-induced disorder** HCC ESR COM

✓4ᵗʰ F19 Other psychoactive substance related disorders

> INCLUDES   polysubstance drug use (indiscriminate drug use)

✓5ᵗʰ F19.1 Other psychoactive substance abuse

> EXCLUDES 1   *other psychoactive substance dependence (F19.2-)*
> *other psychoactive substance use, unspecified (F19.9-)*

> **F19.10 Other psychoactive substance abuse, uncomplicated** HCC ESR
> > Other (or unknown) substance use disorder, mild

> **F19.11 Other psychoactive substance abuse, in remission** HCC ESR
> > Other (or unknown) substance use disorder, mild, in early remission
> > Other (or unknown) substance use disorder, mild, in sustained remission

✓6ᵗʰ F19.12 Other psychoactive substance abuse with intoxication

> **F19.120 Other psychoactive substance abuse with intoxication, uncomplicated** HCC ESR COM

> **F19.121 Other psychoactive substance abuse with intoxication delirium** HCC ESR COM

> **F19.122 Other psychoactive substance abuse with intoxication with perceptual disturbances** HCC ESR COM

> **F19.129 Other psychoactive substance abuse with intoxication, unspecified** HCC ESR COM

✓6ᵗʰ F19.13 Other psychoactive substance abuse with withdrawal
> AHA: 2020,4Q,16-17

> **F19.130 Other psychoactive substance abuse with withdrawal, uncomplicated** HCC ESR COM

> **F19.131 Other psychoactive substance abuse with withdrawal delirium** HCC ESR COM

> **F19.132 Other psychoactive substance abuse with withdrawal with perceptual disturbance** HCC ESR COM

> **F19.139 Other psychoactive substance abuse with withdrawal, unspecified** HCC ESR COM

F19.14 Other psychoactive substance abuse with psychoactive substance-induced mood disorder HCC ESR COM
> Other (or unknown) substance use disorder, mild, with other (or unknown) substance-induced bipolar or related disorder
> Other (or unknown) substance use disorder, mild, with other (or unknown) substance-induced depressive disorder

✓6ᵗʰ F19.15 Other psychoactive substance abuse with psychoactive substance-induced psychotic disorder

> **F19.150 Other psychoactive substance abuse with psychoactive substance-induced psychotic disorder with delusions** HCC ESR COM

> **F19.151 Other psychoactive substance abuse with psychoactive substance-induced psychotic disorder with hallucinations** HCC ESR COM

> **F19.159 Other psychoactive substance abuse with psychoactive substance-induced psychotic disorder, unspecified** HCC ESR COM

F19.16 Other psychoactive substance abuse with psychoactive substance-induced persisting amnestic disorder HCC ESR COM

F19.17 Other psychoactive substance abuse with psychoactive substance-induced persisting dementia HCC ESR COM
> Other (or unknown) substance use disorder, mild, with other (or unknown) substance-induced major neurocognitive disorder

✓6ᵗʰ F19.18 Other psychoactive substance abuse with other psychoactive substance-induced disorders

> **F19.180 Other psychoactive substance abuse with psychoactive substance-induced anxiety disorder** HCC ESR COM

> **F19.181 Other psychoactive substance abuse with psychoactive substance-induced sexual dysfunction** HCC ESR COM

> **F19.182 Other psychoactive substance abuse with psychoactive substance-induced sleep disorder** HCC ESR COM

> **F19.188 Other psychoactive substance abuse with other psychoactive substance-induced disorder** HCC ESR COM
> > Other (or unknown) substance use disorder, mild, with other (or unknown) substance induced mild neurocognitive disorder
> > Other (or unknown) substance use disorder, mild, with other (or unknown) substance induced obsessive-compulsive or related disorder

> **F19.19 Other psychoactive substance abuse with unspecified psychoactive substance-induced disorder** HCC ESR COM

✓5ᵗʰ F19.2 Other psychoactive substance dependence

> EXCLUDES 1   *other psychoactive substance abuse (F19.1-)*
> *other psychoactive substance use, unspecified (F19.9-)*

> **F19.20 Other psychoactive substance dependence, uncomplicated** HCC ESR COM
> > Other (or unknown) substance use disorder, moderate
> > Other (or unknown) substance use disorder, severe

✔ Additional Character Required   ✔x7ᵗʰ Placeholder Alert   Manifestation   Unspecified Dx   Q QPP   UPD Unacceptable PDx

Chapter 5. Mental, Behavioral and Neurodevelopmental Disorders

F19.21 Other psychoactive substance dependence, in remission `HCC` `ESR` `COM`
  Other (or unknown) substance use disorder, moderate, in early remission
  Other (or unknown) substance use disorder, moderate, in sustained remission
  Other (or unknown) substance use disorder, severe, in early remission
  Other (or unknown) substance use disorder, severe, in sustained remission

✓6ᵗʰ **F19.22** Other psychoactive substance dependence with intoxication
  `EXCLUDES 1` *other psychoactive substance dependence with withdrawal (F19.23-)*
  F19.220 Other psychoactive substance dependence with intoxication, uncomplicated `HCC` `ESR` `COM`
  F19.221 Other psychoactive substance dependence with intoxication delirium `HCC` `ESR` `COM`
  F19.222 Other psychoactive substance dependence with intoxication with perceptual disturbance `HCC` `ESR` `COM`
  F19.229 Other psychoactive substance dependence with intoxication, unspecified `HCC` `ESR` `COM`

✓6ᵗʰ **F19.23** Other psychoactive substance dependence with withdrawal
  `EXCLUDES 1` *other psychoactive substance dependence with intoxication (F19.22-)*
  F19.230 Other psychoactive substance dependence with withdrawal, uncomplicated `HCC` `ESR` `COM`
  F19.231 Other psychoactive substance dependence with withdrawal delirium `HCC` `ESR` `COM`
  F19.232 Other psychoactive substance dependence with withdrawal with perceptual disturbance `HCC` `ESR` `COM`
  F19.239 Other psychoactive substance dependence with withdrawal, unspecified `HCC` `ESR` `COM`

F19.24 Other psychoactive substance dependence with psychoactive substance-induced mood disorder `HCC` `ESR` `COM`
  Other (or unknown) substance use disorder, moderate, with other (or unknown) substance induced bipolar or related disorder
  Other (or unknown) substance use disorder, moderate, with other (or unknown) substance induced depressive disorder
  Other (or unknown) substance use disorder, severe, with other (or unknown) substance induced bipolar or related disorder
  Other (or unknown) substance use disorder, severe, with other (or unknown) substance induced depressive disorder

✓6ᵗʰ **F19.25** Other psychoactive substance dependence with psychoactive substance-induced psychotic disorder
  F19.250 Other psychoactive substance dependence with psychoactive substance-induced psychotic disorder with delusions `HCC` `ESR` `COM`
  F19.251 Other psychoactive substance dependence with psychoactive substance-induced psychotic disorder with hallucinations `HCC` `ESR` `COM`
  F19.259 Other psychoactive substance dependence with psychoactive substance-induced psychotic disorder, unspecified `HCC` `ESR` `COM`

F19.26 Other psychoactive substance dependence with psychoactive substance-induced persisting amnestic disorder `HCC` `ESR` `COM`

F19.27 Other psychoactive substance dependence with psychoactive substance-induced persisting dementia `HCC` `ESR` `COM`
  Other (or unknown) substance use disorder, moderate, with other (or unknown) substance induced major neurocognitive disorder
  Other (or unknown) substance use disorder, severe, with other (or unknown) substance induced major neurocognitive disorder

✓6ᵗʰ **F19.28** Other psychoactive substance dependence with other psychoactive substance-induced disorders
  F19.280 Other psychoactive substance dependence with psychoactive substance-induced anxiety disorder `HCC` `ESR` `COM`
  F19.281 Other psychoactive substance dependence with psychoactive substance-induced sexual dysfunction `HCC` `ESR` `COM`
  F19.282 Other psychoactive substance dependence with psychoactive substance-induced sleep disorder `HCC` `ESR` `COM`
  F19.288 Other psychoactive substance dependence with other psychoactive substance-induced disorder `HCC` `ESR` `COM`
    Other (or unknown) substance use disorder, moderate, with other (or unknown) substance induced mild neurocognitive disorder
    Other (or unknown) substance use disorder, severe, with other (or unknown) substance induced mild neurocognitive disorder
    Other (or unknown) substance use disorder, moderate, with other (or unknown) substance induced obsessive compulsive or related disorder
    Other (or unknown) substance use disorder, severe, with other (or unknown) substance induced obsessive-compulsive or related disorder

F19.29 Other psychoactive substance dependence with unspecified psychoactive substance-induced disorder `HCC` `ESR` `COM`

✓5ᵗʰ **F19.9** Other psychoactive substance use, unspecified
  `EXCLUDES 1` *other psychoactive substance abuse (F19.1-)*
    other psychoactive substance dependence (F19.2-)
  TIP: Assign a substance use code only when the provider documents a relationship between the use and an associated physical, mental, or behavioral disorder. As with all diagnoses, substance use codes must meet the definition of a reportable diagnosis.

F19.90 Other psychoactive substance use, unspecified, uncomplicated
  AHA: 2018,2Q,10-11

F19.91 Other psychoactive substance use, unspecified, in remission

✓6ᵗʰ **F19.92** Other psychoactive substance use, unspecified with intoxication
  `EXCLUDES 1` *other psychoactive substance use, unspecified with withdrawal (F19.93)*
  F19.920 Other psychoactive substance use, unspecified with intoxication, uncomplicated `HCC` `ESR` `COM`
  F19.921 Other psychoactive substance use, unspecified with intoxication with delirium `HCC` `ESR` `COM`
    Other (or unknown) substance-induced delirium
  F19.922 Other psychoactive substance use, unspecified with intoxication with perceptual disturbance `HCC` `ESR` `COM`
  F19.929 Other psychoactive substance use, unspecified with intoxication, unspecified `HCC` `ESR` `COM`

`HCC` CMS-HCC   `Rx` Rx HCC   `ESR` ESRD HCC   `COM` Commercial HCC   `N` Newborn: 0   `P` Pediatric: 0-17   `M` Maternity: 9-64   `A` Adult: 15-124

574   ICD-10-CM 2023

✓6ᵗʰ F19.93 Other psychoactive substance use, unspecified with withdrawal

     EXCLUDES 1   *other psychoactive substance use, unspecified with intoxication (F19.92-)*

     F19.930 **Other psychoactive substance use, unspecified with withdrawal, uncomplicated**   HCC ESR COM

     F19.931 **Other psychoactive substance use, unspecified with withdrawal delirium**   HCC ESR COM

     F19.932 **Other psychoactive substance use, unspecified with withdrawal with perceptual disturbance**   HCC ESR COM

     F19.939 **Other psychoactive substance use, unspecified with withdrawal, unspecified**   HCC ESR COM

F19.94 Other psychoactive substance use, unspecified with psychoactive substance-induced mood disorder   HCC ESR COM

     Other (or unknown) substance-induced bipolar or related disorder, without use disorder

     Other (or unknown) substance-induced depressive disorder, without use disorder

✓6ᵗʰ F19.95 Other psychoactive substance use, unspecified with psychoactive substance-induced psychotic disorder

     F19.950 **Other psychoactive substance use, unspecified with psychoactive substance-induced psychotic disorder with delusions**   HCC ESR COM

     F19.951 **Other psychoactive substance use, unspecified with psychoactive substance-induced psychotic disorder with hallucinations**   HCC ESR COM

     F19.959 **Other psychoactive substance use, unspecified with psychoactive substance-induced psychotic disorder, unspecified**   HCC ESR COM

        Other or unknown substance-induced psychotic disorder, without use disorder

F19.96 Other psychoactive substance use, unspecified with psychoactive substance-induced persisting amnestic disorder   HCC ESR COM

F19.97 Other psychoactive substance use, unspecified with psychoactive substance-induced persisting dementia   HCC ESR COM

     Other (or unknown) substance-induced major neurocognitive disorder, without use disorder

✓6ᵗʰ F19.98 Other psychoactive substance use, unspecified with other psychoactive substance-induced disorders

     F19.980 **Other psychoactive substance use, unspecified with psychoactive substance-induced anxiety disorder**   HCC ESR COM

        Other (or unknown) substance-induced anxiety disorder, without use disorder

     F19.981 **Other psychoactive substance use, unspecified with psychoactive substance-induced sexual dysfunction**   HCC ESR COM

        Other (or unknown) substance-induced sexual dysfunction, without use disorder

     F19.982 **Other psychoactive substance use, unspecified with psychoactive substance-induced sleep disorder**   HCC ESR COM

        Other (or unknown) substance-induced sleep disorder, without use disorder

     F19.988 **Other psychoactive substance use, unspecified with other psychoactive substance-induced disorder**   HCC ESR COM

        Other (or unknown) substance-induced mild neurocognitive disorder, without use disorder

        Other (or unknown) substance-induced obsessive-compulsive or related disorder, without use disorder

F19.99 Other psychoactive substance use, unspecified with unspecified psychoactive substance-induced disorder   HCC ESR COM

Schizophrenia, schizotypal, delusional, and other non-mood psychotic disorders (F20-F29)

✓4ᵗʰ F20 Schizophrenia

     EXCLUDES 1   *brief psychotic disorder (F23)*

        cyclic schizophrenia (F25.0)

        mood [affective] disorders with psychotic symptoms (F30.2, F31.2, F31.5, F31.64, F32.3, F33.3)

        schizoaffective disorder (F25.-)

        schizophrenic reaction NOS (F23)

     EXCLUDES 2   *schizophrenic reaction in:*

        alcoholism (F10.15-, F10.25-, F10.95-)

        brain disease (F06.2)

        epilepsy (F06.2)

        psychoactive drug use (F11-F19 with .15. .25, .95)

        schizotypal disorder (F21)

DEF: Group of disorders with disturbances in thought (delusions, hallucinations), mood (blunted, flattened, inappropriate affect), and sense of self. Schizophrenia also includes bizarre, purposeless behavior, repetitious activity, or inactivity.

F20.0 Paranoid schizophrenia   HCC Rx ESR COM

     Paraphrenic schizophrenia

     EXCLUDES 1   *involutional paranoid state (F22)*

        paranoia (F22)

     DEF: Preoccupied with delusional suspicions and auditory hallucinations related to a single theme. This type of schizophrenia is usually hostile, grandiose, threatening, persecutory, and occasionally hypochondriacal.

F20.1 Disorganized schizophrenia   HCC Rx ESR COM

     Hebephrenic schizophrenia

     Hebephrenia

F20.2 Catatonic schizophrenia   HCC Rx ESR COM

     Schizophrenic catalepsy

     Schizophrenic catatonia

     Schizophrenic flexibilitas cerea

     EXCLUDES 1   *catatonic stupor (R40.1)*

     DEF: Extreme changes in motor activity. One extreme is a decreased response or reaction to the environment and the other is spontaneous activity.

F20.3 Undifferentiated schizophrenia   HCC Rx ESR COM

     Atypical schizophrenia

     EXCLUDES 1   *acute schizophrenia-like psychotic disorder (F23)*

     EXCLUDES 2   *post-schizophrenic depression (F32.89)*

F20.5 Residual schizophrenia   HCC Rx ESR COM

     Restzustand (schizophrenic)

     Schizophrenic residual state

✓5ᵗʰ F20.8 Other schizophrenia

     F20.81 **Schizophreniform disorder**   HCC Rx ESR COM

        Schizophreniform psychosis NOS

     F20.89 **Other schizophrenia**   HCC Rx ESR COM

        Cenesthopathic schizophrenia

        Simple schizophrenia

F20.9 Schizophrenia, unspecified   HCC Rx ESR COM

     AHA: 2019,2Q,32   *a cute exacerbation*

F21 Schizotypal disorder   HCC Rx ESR COM

     Borderline schizophrenia

     Latent schizophrenia

     Latent schizophrenic reaction

     Prepsychotic schizophrenia

     Prodromal schizophrenia

     Pseudoneurotic schizophrenia

     Pseudopsychopathic schizophrenia

     Schizotypal personality disorder

     EXCLUDES 2   *Asperger's syndrome (F84.5)*

        schizoid personality disorder (F60.1)

     DEF: Disorder characterized by various oddities of thinking, perception, communication, and behavior that may be manifested as magical thinking, ideas of reference, paranoid ideation, recurrent illusions and derealization (depersonalization), or social isolation.

Chapter 5. Mental, Behavioral and Neurodevelopmental Disorders

F19.93–F21

Chapter 5. Mental, Behavioral and Neurodevelopmental Disorders *(side tab)*

F22 Delusional disorders `HCC` `Rx` `ESR` `COM`
Delusional dysmorphophobia
Involutional paranoid state
Paranoia
Paranoia querulans
Paranoid psychosis
Paranoid state
Paraphrenia (late)
Sensitiver Beziehungswahn
　EXCLUDES 1 mood [affective] disorders with psychotic symptoms (F30.2, F31.2, F31.5, F31.64, F32.3, F33.3)
　　　paranoid schizophrenia (F20.0)
　EXCLUDES 2 paranoid personality disorder (F60.0)
　　　paranoid psychosis, psychogenic (F23)
　　　paranoid reaction (F23)

F23 Brief psychotic disorder `HCC` `Rx` `ESR` `COM`
Paranoid reaction
Psychogenic paranoid psychosis
　EXCLUDES 2 mood [affective] disorders with psychotic symptoms (F30.2, F31.2, F31.5, F31.64, F32.3, F33.3)
AHA: 2019,2Q,32

F24 Shared psychotic disorder `HCC` `Rx` `ESR` `COM`
Folie à deux
Induced paranoid disorder
Induced psychotic disorder

√4ᵗʰ F25 Schizoaffective disorders
　EXCLUDES 1 mood [affective] disorders with psychotic symptoms (F30.2, F31.2, F31.5, F31.64, F32.3, F33.3)
　　　schizophrenia (F20.-)

F25.0 Schizoaffective disorder, bipolar type `HCC` `Rx` `ESR` `COM`
Cyclic schizophrenia
Schizoaffective disorder, manic type
Schizoaffective disorder, mixed type
Schizoaffective psychosis, bipolar type

F25.1 Schizoaffective disorder, depressive type `HCC` `Rx` `ESR` `COM`
Schizoaffective psychosis, depressive type

F25.8 Other schizoaffective disorders `HCC` `Rx` `ESR` `COM`

F25.9 Schizoaffective disorder, unspecified `HCC` `Rx` `ESR` `COM`
Schizoaffective psychosis NOS

F28 Other psychotic disorder not due to a substance or known physiological condition `HCC` `Rx` `ESR` `COM`
Chronic hallucinatory psychosis
Other specified schizophrenia spectrum and other psychotic disorder

F29 Unspecified psychosis not due to a substance or known physiological condition `HCC` `Rx` `ESR` `COM`
Psychosis NOS
Unspecified schizophrenia spectrum and other psychotic disorder
　EXCLUDES 1 mental disorder NOS (F99)
　　　unspecified mental disorder due to known physiological condition (F09)

Mood [affective] disorders (F30-F39)

√4ᵗʰ F30 Manic episode
　INCLUDES bipolar disorder, single manic episode
　　　mixed affective episode
　EXCLUDES 1 bipolar disorder (F31.-)
　　　major depressive disorder, recurrent (F33.-)
　　　major depressive disorder, single episode (F32.-)
DEF: Mania: Characterized by abnormal states of elation or excitement out of keeping with the individual's circumstances and varying from enhanced liveliness (hypomania) to violent, almost uncontrollable, excitement. Aggression and anger, flight of ideas, distractibility, impaired judgment, and grandiose ideas are common.

√5ᵗʰ F30.1 Manic episode without psychotic symptoms
F30.10 Manic episode without psychotic symptoms, unspecified `HCC` `Rx` `ESR` `COM`
F30.11 Manic episode without psychotic symptoms, mild `HCC` `Rx` `ESR` `COM`
F30.12 Manic episode without psychotic symptoms, moderate `HCC` `Rx` `ESR` `COM`
F30.13 Manic episode, severe, without psychotic symptoms `HCC` `Rx` `ESR` `COM`

F30.2 Manic episode, severe with psychotic symptoms `HCC` `Rx` `ESR` `COM`
Manic stupor
Mania with mood-congruent psychotic symptoms
Mania with mood-incongruent psychotic symptoms

F30.3 Manic episode in partial remission `HCC` `Rx` `ESR` `COM`
F30.4 Manic episode in full remission `HCC` `Rx` `ESR` `COM`
F30.8 Other manic episodes `HCC` `Rx` `ESR` `COM`
Hypomania
F30.9 Manic episode, unspecified `HCC` `Rx` `ESR` `COM`
Mania NOS

√4ᵗʰ F31 Bipolar disorder
　INCLUDES bipolar I disorder
　　　bipolar type I disorder
　　　manic-depressive illness
　　　manic-depressive psychosis
　　　manic-depressive reaction
　　　▶seasonal bipolar disorder◀
　EXCLUDES 1 bipolar disorder, single manic episode (F30.-)
　　　major depressive disorder, recurrent (F33.-)
　　　major depressive disorder, single episode (F32.-)
　EXCLUDES 2 cyclothymia (F34.0)
AHA: 2020,1Q,23

F31.0 Bipolar disorder, current episode hypomanic `HCC` `Rx` `ESR` `COM`

√5ᵗʰ F31.1 Bipolar disorder, current episode manic without psychotic features
F31.10 Bipolar disorder, current episode manic without psychotic features, unspecified `HCC` `Rx` `ESR` `COM` `Q`
F31.11 Bipolar disorder, current episode manic without psychotic features, mild `HCC` `Rx` `ESR` `COM` `Q`
F31.12 Bipolar disorder, current episode manic without psychotic features, moderate `HCC` `Rx` `ESR` `COM` `Q`
F31.13 Bipolar disorder, current episode manic without psychotic features, severe `HCC` `Rx` `ESR` `COM` `Q`

F31.2 Bipolar disorder, current episode manic severe with psychotic features `HCC` `Rx` `ESR` `COM` `Q`
Bipolar disorder, current episode manic with mood-congruent psychotic symptoms
Bipolar disorder, current episode manic with mood-incongruent psychotic symptoms
Bipolar I disorder, current or most recent episode manic with psychotic features

√5ᵗʰ F31.3 Bipolar disorder, current episode depressed, mild or moderate severity
F31.30 Bipolar disorder, current episode depressed, mild or moderate severity, unspecified `HCC` `Rx` `ESR` `COM` `Q`
F31.31 Bipolar disorder, current episode depressed, mild `HCC` `Rx` `ESR` `COM` `Q`
F31.32 Bipolar disorder, current episode depressed, moderate `HCC` `Rx` `ESR` `COM` `Q`

F31.4 Bipolar disorder, current episode depressed, severe, without psychotic features `HCC` `Rx` `ESR` `COM`
F31.5 Bipolar disorder, current episode depressed, severe, with psychotic features `HCC` `Rx` `ESR` `COM`
Bipolar disorder, current episode depressed with mood-congruent psychotic symptoms
Bipolar disorder, current episode depressed with mood-incongruent psychotic symptoms
Bipolar I disorder, current or most recent episode depressed, with psychotic features

√5ᵗʰ F31.6 Bipolar disorder, current episode mixed
F31.60 Bipolar disorder, current episode mixed, unspecified `HCC` `Rx` `ESR` `COM` `Q`
F31.61 Bipolar disorder, current episode mixed, mild `HCC` `Rx` `ESR` `COM` `Q`
F31.62 Bipolar disorder, current episode mixed, moderate `HCC` `Rx` `ESR` `COM` `Q`
F31.63 Bipolar disorder, current episode mixed, severe, without psychotic features `HCC` `Rx` `ESR` `COM` `Q`

F31.64 Bipolar disorder, current episode mixed, severe, with psychotic features `HCC` `Rx` `ESR` `COM` `Q`
Bipolar disorder, current episode mixed with mood-congruent psychotic symptoms
Bipolar disorder, current episode mixed with mood-incongruent psychotic symptoms

✓5ᵗʰ F31.7 Bipolar disorder, currently in remission

F31.70 Bipolar disorder, currently in remission, most recent episode unspecified `HCC` `Rx` `ESR` `COM` `Q`

F31.71 Bipolar disorder, in partial remission, most recent episode hypomanic `HCC` `Rx` `ESR` `COM` `Q`

F31.72 Bipolar disorder, in full remission, most recent episode hypomanic `HCC` `Rx` `ESR` `COM` `Q`

F31.73 Bipolar disorder, in partial remission, most recent episode manic `HCC` `Rx` `ESR` `COM` `Q`

F31.74 Bipolar disorder, in full remission, most recent episode manic `HCC` `Rx` `ESR` `COM` `Q`

F31.75 Bipolar disorder, in partial remission, most recent episode depressed `HCC` `Rx` `ESR` `COM` `Q`

F31.76 Bipolar disorder, in full remission, most recent episode depressed `HCC` `Rx` `ESR` `COM` `Q`

F31.77 Bipolar disorder, in partial remission, most recent episode mixed `HCC` `Rx` `ESR` `COM` `Q`

F31.78 Bipolar disorder, in full remission, most recent episode mixed `HCC` `Rx` `ESR` `COM` `Q`

✓5ᵗʰ F31.8 Other bipolar disorders

F31.81 Bipolar II disorder `HCC` `Rx` `ESR` `COM` `Q`
Bipolar disorder, type 2

F31.89 Other bipolar disorder `HCC` `Rx` `ESR` `COM` `Q`
Recurrent manic episodes NOS

F31.9 Bipolar disorder, unspecified `HCC` `Rx` `ESR` `COM` `Q`
Manic depression
AHA: 2020,1Q,23

✓4ᵗʰ F32 Depressive episode
`INCLUDES` single episode of agitated depression
single episode of depressive reaction
single episode of major depression
single episode of psychogenic depression
single episode of reactive depression
single episode of vital depression
`EXCLUDES 1` bipolar disorder (F31.-)
manic episode (F30.-)
recurrent depressive disorder (F33.-)
`EXCLUDES 2` adjustment disorder (F43.2)
AHA: 2020,1Q,23
DEF: Mood disorder that produces depression that may exhibit as sadness, low self-esteem, or guilt feelings. Other manifestations may be withdrawal from friends and family and interrupted sleep.

F32.0 Major depressive disorder, single episode, mild `HCC` `Rx` `ESR` `Q`

F32.1 Major depressive disorder, single episode, moderate `HCC` `Rx` `ESR` `Q`

F32.2 Major depressive disorder, single episode, severe without psychotic features `HCC` `Rx` `ESR` `COM` `Q`

F32.3 Major depressive disorder, single episode, severe with psychotic features `HCC` `Rx` `ESR` `COM` `Q`
Single episode of major depression with mood-congruent psychotic symptoms
Single episode of major depression with mood-incongruent psychotic symptoms
Single episode of major depression with psychotic symptoms
Single episode of psychogenic depressive psychosis
Single episode of psychotic depression
Single episode of reactive depressive psychosis

F32.4 Major depressive disorder, single episode, in partial remission `HCC` `Rx` `ESR` `Q`

F32.5 Major depressive disorder, single episode, in full remission `HCC` `Rx` `ESR` `Q`

✓5ᵗʰ F32.8 Other depressive episodes
AHA: 2016,4Q,14

F32.81 Premenstrual dysphoric disorder `Rx` ♀
`EXCLUDES 1` premenstrual tension syndrome (N94.3)
DEF: Severe manifestation of premenstrual syndrome (PMS) that can be disabling and destructive to day-to-day activities. It can exacerbate pre-existing emotional disorders, like depression and anxiety, and cause feelings of loss of control, fatigue, and irritability.

F32.89 Other specified depressive episodes `Rx` `Q`
Atypical depression
Post-schizophrenic depression
Single episode of 'masked' depression NOS

F32.9 Major depressive disorder, single episode, unspecified `Rx` `Q`
Major depression NOS
AHA: 2021,4Q,10; 2021,1Q,10; 2013,4Q,107

F32.A Depression, unspecified `Rx` `Q`
Depression NOS
Depressive disorder NOS
AHA: 2021,4Q,9-10

✓4ᵗʰ F33 Major depressive disorder, recurrent
`INCLUDES` recurrent episodes of depressive reaction
recurrent episodes of endogenous depression
recurrent episodes of major depression
recurrent episodes of psychogenic depression
recurrent episodes of reactive depression
▶recurrent episodes of seasonal affective disorder◀
recurrent episodes of seasonal depressive disorder
recurrent episodes of vital depression
`EXCLUDES 1` bipolar disorder (F31.-)
manic episode (F30.-)
AHA: 2020,1Q,23
DEF: Mood disorder that produces depression that may exhibit as sadness, low self-esteem, or guilt feelings. Other manifestations may be withdrawal from friends and family and interrupted sleep.

F33.0 Major depressive disorder, recurrent, mild `HCC` `Rx` `ESR` `Q`

F33.1 Major depressive disorder, recurrent, moderate `HCC` `Rx` `ESR` `Q`

F33.2 Major depressive disorder, recurrent, severe without psychotic features `HCC` `Rx` `ESR` `COM` `Q`

F33.3 Major depressive disorder, recurrent, severe with psychotic symptoms `HCC` `Rx` `ESR` `COM` `Q`
Endogenous depression with psychotic symptoms
Major depressive disorder, recurrent, with psychotic features
Recurrent severe episodes of major depression with mood-congruent psychotic symptoms
Recurrent severe episodes of major depression with mood-incongruent psychotic symptoms
Recurrent severe episodes of major depression with psychotic symptoms
Recurrent severe episodes of psychogenic depressive psychosis
Recurrent severe episodes of psychotic depression
Recurrent severe episodes of reactive depressive psychosis

✓5ᵗʰ F33.4 Major depressive disorder, recurrent, in remission

F33.40 Major depressive disorder, recurrent, in remission, unspecified `HCC` `Rx` `ESR` `Q`

F33.41 Major depressive disorder, recurrent, in partial remission `HCC` `Rx` `ESR` `Q`

F33.42 Major depressive disorder, recurrent, in full remission `HCC` `Rx` `ESR` `Q`

F33.8 Other recurrent depressive disorders `HCC` `Rx` `ESR` `Q`
Recurrent brief depressive episodes

F33.9 Major depressive disorder, recurrent, unspecified `HCC` `Rx` `ESR` `Q`
Monopolar depression NOS

✓4ᵗʰ F34 Persistent mood [affective] disorders

F34.0 Cyclothymic disorder `Rx`
Affective personality disorder
Cycloid personality
Cyclothymia
Cyclothymic personality
DEF: Mood disorder characterized by fast and repeated alterations between hypomanic and depressed moods.

F34.1 **Dysthymic disorder** `Rx` `0`
Depressive neurosis
Depressive personality disorder
Dysthymia
Neurotic depression
Persistent anxiety depression
Persistent depressive disorder
EXCLUDES 2 anxiety depression (mild or not persistent) (F41.8)
DEF: Depression without psychosis. It is a less severe but persistent depression and is considered a mild to moderate chronic form of depression.

✓5th **F34.8** **Other persistent mood [affective] disorders**
AHA: 2016,4Q,14

F34.81 **Disruptive mood dysregulation disorder** `HCC` `Rx` `ESR` `COM` `0`

F34.89 **Other specified persistent mood disorders** `HCC` `Rx` `ESR` `0`

F34.9 **Persistent mood [affective] disorder, unspecified** `HCC` `Rx` `ESR`

F39 **Unspecified mood [affective] disorder** `HCC` `Rx` `ESR`
Affective psychosis NOS

Anxiety, dissociative, stress-related, somatoform and other nonpsychotic mental disorders (F40-F48)

✓4th **F40** **Phobic anxiety disorders**
DEF: Phobia: Broad-range anxiety with abnormally intense dread of certain objects or specific situations that would not normally have that effect.

✓5th **F40.0** **Agoraphobia**
DEF: Profound anxiety or fear of leaving familiar settings like home, or being in unfamiliar locations or with strangers or crowds. Agoraphobia may or may not be preceded by recurrent panic attacks.

F40.00 **Agoraphobia, unspecified** `Rx`

F40.01 **Agoraphobia with panic disorder** `Rx`
Panic disorder with agoraphobia
EXCLUDES 1 panic disorder without agoraphobia (F41.0)

F40.02 **Agoraphobia without panic disorder** `Rx`

✓5th **F40.1** **Social phobias**
Anthropophobia
Social anxiety disorder
Social anxiety disorder of childhood
Social neurosis

F40.10 **Social phobia, unspecified** `Rx`

F40.11 **Social phobia, generalized** `Rx`

✓5th **F40.2** **Specific (isolated) phobias**
EXCLUDES 2 dysmorphophobia (nondelusional) (F45.22)
nosophobia (F45.22)

✓6th **F40.21** **Animal type phobia**

F40.210 **Arachnophobia** `Rx`
Fear of spiders

F40.218 **Other animal type phobia** `Rx`

✓6th **F40.22** **Natural environment type phobia**

F40.220 **Fear of thunderstorms** `Rx`

F40.228 **Other natural environment type phobia** `Rx`

✓6th **F40.23** **Blood, injection, injury type phobia**

F40.230 **Fear of blood** `Rx`

F40.231 **Fear of injections and transfusions** `Rx`

F40.232 **Fear of other medical care** `Rx`

F40.233 **Fear of injury** `Rx`

✓6th **F40.24** **Situational type phobia**

F40.240 **Claustrophobia** `Rx`

F40.241 **Acrophobia** `Rx`

F40.242 **Fear of bridges** `Rx`

F40.243 **Fear of flying** `Rx`

F40.248 **Other situational type phobia** `Rx`

✓6th **F40.29** **Other specified phobia**

F40.290 **Androphobia** `Rx`
Fear of men

F40.291 **Gynephobia** `Rx`
Fear of women

F40.298 **Other specified phobia** `Rx`

F40.8 **Other phobic anxiety disorders** `Rx`
Phobic anxiety disorder of childhood

F40.9 **Phobic anxiety disorder, unspecified** `Rx`
Phobia NOS
Phobic state NOS

✓4th **F41** **Other anxiety disorders**
EXCLUDES 2 anxiety in:
acute stress reaction (F43.0)
neurasthenia (F48.8)
psychophysiologic disorders (F45.-)
transient adjustment reaction (F43.2)
separation anxiety (F93.0)

F41.0 **Panic disorder [episodic paroxysmal anxiety]** `Rx`
Panic attack
Panic state
EXCLUDES 1 panic disorder with agoraphobia (F40.01)
DEF: Neurotic disorder characterized by recurrent panic or anxiety, apprehension, fear, or terror. Symptoms include shortness of breath, palpitations, dizziness, and shakiness; fear of dying may persist.

F41.1 **Generalized anxiety disorder** `Rx`
Anxiety neurosis
Anxiety reaction
Anxiety state
Overanxious disorder
EXCLUDES 2 neurasthenia (F48.8)

F41.3 **Other mixed anxiety disorders**

F41.8 **Other specified anxiety disorders**
Anxiety depression (mild or not persistent)
Anxiety hysteria
Mixed anxiety and depressive disorder
AHA: 2021,1Q,10

F41.9 **Anxiety disorder, unspecified**
Anxiety NOS
AHA: 2021,1Q,10

✓4th **F42** **Obsessive-compulsive disorder**
EXCLUDES 2 obsessive-compulsive personality (disorder) (F60.5)
obsessive-compulsive symptoms occurring in depression (F32-F33)
obsessive-compulsive symptoms occurring in schizophrenia (F20.-)
AHA: 2016,4Q,14-15

F42.2 **Mixed obsessional thoughts and acts** `Rx`

F42.3 **Hoarding disorder** `Rx`

F42.4 **Excoriation (skin-picking) disorder** `Rx`
EXCLUDES 1 factitial dermatitis (L98.1)
other specified behavioral and emotional disorders with onset usually occurring in early childhood and adolescence (F98.8)

F42.8 **Other obsessive-compulsive disorder** `Rx`
Anancastic neurosis
Obsessive-compulsive neurosis

F42.9 **Obsessive-compulsive disorder, unspecified** `Rx`

✓4th **F43** **Reaction to severe stress, and adjustment disorders**

F43.0 **Acute stress reaction**
Acute crisis reaction
Acute reaction to stress
Combat and operational stress reaction
Combat fatigue
Crisis state
Psychic shock

✓5th **F43.1** **Post-traumatic stress disorder (PTSD)**
Traumatic neurosis
DEF: Preoccupation with traumatic events beyond normal experience (i.e., rape, personal assault, etc.) that may also include recurring flashbacks of the trauma. Symptoms include difficulty remembering, sleeping, or concentrating, and guilt feelings for surviving.

F43.10 **Post-traumatic stress disorder, unspecified** `Rx`

F43.11 **Post-traumatic stress disorder, acute** `Rx`

F43.12 **Post-traumatic stress disorder, chronic** `Rx`

`HCC` CMS-HCC   `Rx` Rx HCC   `ESR` ESRD HCC   `COM` Commercial HCC   `N` Newborn: 0   `P` Pediatric: 0-17   `M` Maternity: 9-64   `A` Adult: 15-124

578

ICD-10-CM 2023

☑5ᵗʰ F43.2 Adjustment disorders
Culture shock
Grief reaction
Hospitalism in children
EXCLUDES 2   separation anxiety disorder of childhood (F93.0)

    F43.20 Adjustment disorder, unspecified   Rx

    F43.21 Adjustment disorder with depressed mood   Rx Q
       AHA: 2014,1Q,25

    F43.22 Adjustment disorder with anxiety   Rx

    F43.23 Adjustment disorder with mixed anxiety and depressed mood   Rx Q

    F43.24 Adjustment disorder with disturbance of conduct   Rx

    F43.25 Adjustment disorder with mixed disturbance of emotions and conduct   Rx

    F43.29 Adjustment disorder with other symptoms   Rx

▲ ☑5ᵗʰ **F43.8 Other reactions to severe stress**
Other specified trauma and stressor-related disorder

    ● **F43.81 Prolonged grief disorder**
       Complicated grief
       Complicated grief disorder
       Persistent complex bereavement disorder

    ● **F43.89 Other reactions to severe stress**

    F43.9 Reaction to severe stress, unspecified
Trauma and stressor-related disorder, NOS
►Unspecified trauma and stressor-related disorder◄

☑4ᵗʰ F44 Dissociative and conversion disorders
INCLUDES   conversion hysteria
          conversion reaction
          hysteria
          hysterical psychosis
EXCLUDES 2   malingering [conscious simulation] (Z76.5)

    F44.0 Dissociative amnesia   HCC Rx ESR COM
EXCLUDES 1   amnesia NOS (R41.3)
          anterograde amnesia (R41.1)
          dissociative amnesia with dissociative fugue (F44.1)
          retrograde amnesia (R41.2)
EXCLUDES 2   alcohol-or other psychoactive substance-induced amnestic disorder (F10, F13, F19 with .26, .96)
          amnestic disorder due to known physiological condition (F04)
          postictal amnesia in epilepsy (G40.-)

    F44.1 Dissociative fugue   HCC Rx ESR COM
Dissociative amnesia with dissociative fugue
EXCLUDES 1   postictal fugue in epilepsy (G40.-)
DEF: Dissociative hysteria identified by memory loss and flight from familiar surroundings to a completely separate environment. Episodes may last hours or days. Conscious activity is not associated with perception of surroundings and there is no later memory of the episode.

    F44.2 Dissociative stupor   Rx
EXCLUDES 1   catatonic stupor (R40.1)
          stupor NOS (R40.1)
EXCLUDES 2   catatonic disorder due to known physiological condition (F06.1)
          depressive stupor (F32, F33)
          manic stupor (F30, F31)

    F44.4 Conversion disorder with motor symptom or deficit   Rx
Conversion disorder with abnormal movement
Conversion disorder with speech symptoms
Conversion disorder with swallowing symptoms
Conversion disorder with weakness/paralysis
Dissociative motor disorders
Psychogenic aphonia
Psychogenic dysphonia

    F44.5 Conversion disorder with seizures or convulsions   Rx
Conversion disorder with attacks or seizures
Dissociative convulsions
AHA: 2021,1Q,3; 2019,1Q,19

    F44.6 Conversion disorder with sensory symptom or deficit   Rx
Conversion disorder with anesthesia or sensory loss
Conversion disorder with special sensory symptoms
Dissociative anesthesia and sensory loss
Psychogenic deafness

    F44.7 Conversion disorder with mixed symptom presentation   Rx

☑5ᵗʰ F44.8 Other dissociative and conversion disorders

    F44.81 Dissociative identity disorder   HCC Rx ESR COM
       Multiple personality disorder

    F44.89 Other dissociative and conversion disorders   Rx
       Ganser's syndrome
       Psychogenic confusion
       Psychogenic twilight state
       Trance and possession disorders

    F44.9 Dissociative and conversion disorder, unspecified   Rx
Dissociative disorder NOS

☑4ᵗʰ F45 Somatoform disorders
EXCLUDES 2   dissociative and conversion disorders (F44.-)
          factitious disorders (F68.1-, F68.A)
          hair-plucking (F63.3)
          lalling (F80.0)
          lisping (F80.0)
          malingering [conscious simulation] (Z76.5)
          nail-biting (F98.8)
          psychological or behavioral factors associated with disorders or diseases classified elsewhere (F54)
          sexual dysfunction, not due to a substance or known physiological condition (F52.-)
          thumb-sucking (F98.8)
          tic disorders (in childhood and adolescence) (F95.-)
          Tourette's syndrome (F95.2)
          trichotillomania (F63.3)
DEF: Types of disorders causing inconsistent physical symptoms that cannot be explained.

    F45.0 Somatization disorder   Rx
Briquet's disorder
Multiple psychosomatic disorder

    F45.1 Undifferentiated somatoform disorder   Rx
Somatic symptom disorder
Undifferentiated psychosomatic disorder

☑5ᵗʰ F45.2 Hypochondriacal disorders
EXCLUDES 2   delusional dysmorphophobia (F22)
          fixed delusions about bodily functions or shape (F22)

    F45.20 Hypochondriacal disorder, unspecified   Rx

    F45.21 Hypochondriasis   Rx
       Hypochondriacal neurosis
       Illness anxiety disorder

    F45.22 Body dysmorphic disorder   Rx
       Dysmorphophobia (nondelusional)
       Nosophobia

    F45.29 Other hypochondriacal disorders   Rx

☑5ᵗʰ F45.4 Pain disorders related to psychological factors
EXCLUDES 1   pain NOS (R52)

    F45.41 Pain disorder exclusively related to psychological factors
Somatoform pain disorder (persistent)

    F45.42 Pain disorder with related psychological factors
Code also associated acute or chronic pain (G89.-)

    F45.8 Other somatoform disorders   Rx
Psychogenic dysmenorrhea
Psychogenic dysphagia, including 'globus hystericus'
Psychogenic pruritus
Psychogenic torticollis
Somatoform autonomic dysfunction
Teeth grinding
EXCLUDES 1   sleep related teeth grinding (G47.63)

    F45.9 Somatoform disorder, unspecified   Rx
Psychosomatic disorder NOS

☑4ᵗʰ F48 Other nonpsychotic mental disorders

    F48.1 Depersonalization-derealization syndrome   HCC Rx ESR COM

    F48.2 Pseudobulbar affect
Involuntary emotional expression disorder
Code first underlying cause, if known, such as:
    amyotrophic lateral sclerosis (G12.21)
    multiple sclerosis (G35)
    sequelae of cerebrovascular disease (I69.-)
    sequelae of traumatic intracranial injury (S06.-)

Chapter 5. Mental, Behavioral and Neurodevelopmental Disorders

F48.8–F52.5

F48.8   Other specified nonpsychotic mental disorders
Dhat syndrome
Neurasthenia
Occupational neurosis, including writer's cramp
Psychasthenia
Psychasthenic neurosis
Psychogenic syncope

F48.9   Nonpsychotic mental disorder, unspecified
Neurosis NOS

Behavioral syndromes associated with physiological disturbances and physical factors (F50-F59)

✓4ᵗʰ **F50   Eating disorders**
> *EXCLUDES 1*   *anorexia NOS (R63.0)*
> *feeding problems of newborn (P92.-)*
> *polyphagia (R63.2)*
> *EXCLUDES 2*   *feeding difficulties (R63.3)*
> *feeding disorder in infancy or childhood (F98.2-)*
> **AHA:** 2022,1Q,13; 2018,4Q,82
> **TIP:** Assign additional code for BMI from category Z68, when documented. BMI can be based on documentation from clinicians who are not the patient's provider.

✓5ᵗʰ **F50.0   Anorexia nervosa**
> *EXCLUDES 1*   *loss of appetite (R63.0)*
> *psychogenic loss of appetite (F50.89)*
> **DEF:** Psychological eating disorder characterized by an intense fear of gaining weight and an unrealistic perception of body image that perpetuates the feeling of being fat or having too much fat. Avoidance of food and restrictive or unhealthy eating are common.

    F50.00   Anorexia nervosa, unspecified   `Rx` `COM`
    F50.01   Anorexia nervosa, restricting type   `Rx` `COM`
    F50.02   Anorexia nervosa, binge eating/purging type   `Rx` `COM`
> *EXCLUDES 1*   *bulimia nervosa (F50.2)*

F50.2   Bulimia nervosa   `Rx` `COM`
Bulimia NOS
Hyperorexia nervosa
> *EXCLUDES 1*   *anorexia nervosa, binge eating/purging type (F50.02)*
> **DEF:** Episodic pattern of overeating (binge eating) followed by purging or extreme exercise accompanied by an awareness of the abnormal eating pattern with a fear of not being able to stop eating.

✓5ᵗʰ **F50.8   Other eating disorders**
> *EXCLUDES 2*   *pica of infancy and childhood (F98.3)*
> **AHA:** 2017,4Q,9; 2016,4Q,15-16

    F50.81   Binge eating disorder   `Rx`
    F50.82   Avoidant/restrictive food intake disorder   `Rx`
    F50.89   Other specified eating disorder   `Rx`
       Pica in adults
       Psychogenic loss of appetite

F50.9   Eating disorder, unspecified   `Rx`
Atypical anorexia nervosa
Atypical bulimia nervosa
Feeding or eating disorder, unspecified
Other specified feeding disorder

✓4ᵗʰ **F51   Sleep disorders not due to a substance or known physiological condition**
> *EXCLUDES 2*   *organic sleep disorders (G47.-)*

✓5ᵗʰ **F51.0   Insomnia not due to a substance or known physiological condition**
> *EXCLUDES 2*   *alcohol related insomnia (F10.182, F10.282, F10.982)*
> *drug-related insomnia (F11.182, F11.282, F11.982, F13.182, F13.282, F13.982, F14.182, F14.282, F14.982, F15.182, F15.282, F15.982, F19.182, F19.282, F19.982)*
> *insomnia NOS (G47.0-)*
> *insomnia due to known physiological condition (G47.0-)*
> *organic insomnia (G47.0-)*
> *sleep deprivation (Z72.820)*

    F51.01   Primary insomnia
       Idiopathic insomnia
    F51.02   Adjustment insomnia
    F51.03   Paradoxical insomnia
    F51.04   Psychophysiologic insomnia

    F51.05   Insomnia due to other mental disorder
       Code also associated mental disorder
    F51.09   Other insomnia not due to a substance or known physiological condition

✓5ᵗʰ **F51.1   Hypersomnia not due to a substance or known physiological condition**
> *EXCLUDES 2*   *alcohol related hypersomnia (F10.182, F10.282, F10.982)*
> *drug-related hypersomnia (F11.182, F11.282, F11.982, F13.182, F13.282, F13.982, F14.182, F14.282, F14.982, F15.182, F15.282, F15.982, F19.182, F19.282, F19.982)*
> *hypersomnia NOS (G47.10)*
> *hypersomnia due to known physiological condition (G47.10)*
> *idiopathic hypersomnia (G47.11, G47.12)*
> *narcolepsy (G47.4-)*

    F51.11   Primary hypersomnia
    F51.12   Insufficient sleep syndrome
> *EXCLUDES 1*   *sleep deprivation (Z72.820)*

    F51.13   Hypersomnia due to other mental disorder
       Code also associated mental disorder
    F51.19   Other hypersomnia not due to a substance or known physiological condition

F51.3   Sleepwalking [somnambulism]
Non-rapid eye movement sleep arousal disorders, sleepwalking type

F51.4   Sleep terrors [night terrors]
Non-rapid eye movement sleep arousal disorders, sleep terror type

F51.5   Nightmare disorder
Dream anxiety disorder

F51.8   Other sleep disorders not due to a substance or known physiological condition

F51.9   Sleep disorder not due to a substance or known physiological condition, unspecified
Emotional sleep disorder NOS

✓4ᵗʰ **F52   Sexual dysfunction not due to a substance or known physiological condition**
> *EXCLUDES 2*   *Dhat syndrome (F48.8)*

F52.0   Hypoactive sexual desire disorder
Lack or loss of sexual desire
Male hypoactive sexual desire disorder
Sexual anhedonia
> *EXCLUDES 1*   *decreased libido (R68.82)*

F52.1   Sexual aversion disorder
Sexual aversion and lack of sexual enjoyment

✓5ᵗʰ **F52.2   Sexual arousal disorders**
Failure of genital response

    F52.21   Male erectile disorder   ♂
       Erectile disorder
       Psychogenic impotence
> *EXCLUDES 1*   *impotence of organic origin (N52.-)*
> *impotence NOS (N52.-)*

    F52.22   Female sexual arousal disorder   ♀
       Female sexual interest/arousal disorder

✓5ᵗʰ **F52.3   Orgasmic disorder**
Inhibited orgasm
Psychogenic anorgasmy

    F52.31   Female orgasmic disorder   ♀
    F52.32   Male orgasmic disorder   ♂
       Delayed ejaculation

F52.4   Premature ejaculation   ♂

F52.5   Vaginismus not due to a substance or known physiological condition   ♀
Psychogenic vaginismus
> *EXCLUDES 2*   *vaginismus (due to a known physiological condition) (N94.2)*
> **DEF:** Psychogenic response resulting in painful contractions of the vaginal canal muscles. This condition can be severe enough to prevent sexual intercourse.

`HCC` CMS-HCC   `Rx` Rx HCC   `ESR` ESRD HCC   `COM` Commercial HCC   `N` Newborn: 0   `P` Pediatric: 0-17   `M` Maternity: 9-64   `A` Adult: 15-124

580   ICD-10-CM 2023

F52.6 Dyspareunia not due to a substance or known physiological condition
Genito-pelvic pain penetration disorder
Psychogenic dyspareunia
EXCLUDES 2 dyspareunia (due to a known physiological condition) (N94.1-)

F52.8 Other sexual dysfunction not due to a substance or known physiological condition
Excessive sexual drive
Nymphomania
Satyriasis

F52.9 Unspecified sexual dysfunction not due to a substance or known physiological condition
Sexual dysfunction NOS

F53 Mental and behavioral disorders associated with the puerperium, not elsewhere classified
EXCLUDES 1 mood disorders with psychotic features (F30.2, F31.2, F31.5, F31.64, F32.3, F33.3)
postpartum dysphoria (O90.6)
psychosis in schizophrenia, schizotypal, delusional, and other psychotic disorders (F20-F29)
AHA: 2018,4Q,8

F53.0 Postpartum depression
Postnatal depression, NOS
Postpartum depression, NOS

F53.1 Puerperal psychosis
Postpartum psychosis
Puerperal psychosis, NOS

F54 Psychological and behavioral factors associated with disorders or diseases classified elsewhere
Psychological factors affecting physical conditions
Code first the associated physical disorder, such as:
asthma (J45.-)
dermatitis (L23-L25)
gastric ulcer (K25.-)
mucous colitis (K58.-)
ulcerative colitis (K51.-)
urticaria (L50.-)
EXCLUDES 2 tension-type headache (G44.2)

F55 Abuse of non-psychoactive substances
EXCLUDES 2 abuse of psychoactive substances (F10-F19)

F55.0 Abuse of antacids
F55.1 Abuse of herbal or folk remedies
F55.2 Abuse of laxatives
F55.3 Abuse of steroids or hormones
F55.4 Abuse of vitamins
F55.8 Abuse of other non-psychoactive substances

F59 Unspecified behavioral syndromes associated with physiological disturbances and physical factors
Psychogenic physiological dysfunction NOS

Disorders of adult personality and behavior (F60-F69)

F60 Specific personality disorders

F60.0 Paranoid personality disorder
Expansive paranoid personality (disorder)
Fanatic personality (disorder)
Paranoid personality (disorder)
Querulant personality (disorder)
Sensitive paranoid personality (disorder)
EXCLUDES 2 paranoia (F22)
paranoia querulans (F22)
paranoid psychosis (F22)
paranoid schizophrenia (F20.0)
paranoid state (F22)

F60.1 Schizoid personality disorder
EXCLUDES 2 Asperger's syndrome (F84.5)
delusional disorder (F22)
schizoid disorder of childhood (F84.5)
schizophrenia (F20.-)
schizotypal disorder (F21)

F60.2 Antisocial personality disorder
Amoral personality (disorder)
Asocial personality (disorder)
Dissocial personality disorder
Psychopathic personality (disorder)
Sociopathic personality (disorder)
EXCLUDES 1 conduct disorders (F91.-)
EXCLUDES 2 borderline personality disorder (F60.3)

F60.3 Borderline personality disorder
Aggressive personality (disorder)
Emotionally unstable personality disorder
Explosive personality (disorder)
EXCLUDES 2 antisocial personality disorder (F60.2)

F60.4 Histrionic personality disorder
Hysterical personality (disorder)
Psychoinfantile personality (disorder)

F60.5 Obsessive-compulsive personality disorder
Anankastic personality (disorder)
Compulsive personality (disorder)
Obsessional personality (disorder)
EXCLUDES 2 obsessive-compulsive disorder (F42.-)

F60.6 Avoidant personality disorder
Anxious personality disorder

F60.7 Dependent personality disorder
Asthenic personality (disorder)
Inadequate personality (disorder)
Passive personality (disorder)
DEF: Lack of self-confidence, fear of abandonment, and an obsessive need to be taken care of.

F60.8 Other specific personality disorders

F60.81 Narcissistic personality disorder

F60.89 Other specific personality disorders
Eccentric personality disorder
"Haltlose" type personality disorder
Immature personality disorder
Passive-aggressive personality disorder
Psychoneurotic personality disorder
Self-defeating personality disorder

F60.9 Personality disorder, unspecified
Character disorder NOS
Character neurosis NOS
Pathological personality NOS

F63 Impulse disorders
EXCLUDES 2 habitual excessive use of alcohol or psychoactive substances (F10-F19)
impulse disorders involving sexual behavior (F65.-)

F63.0 Pathological gambling
Compulsive gambling
Gambling disorder
EXCLUDES 1 gambling and betting NOS (Z72.6)
EXCLUDES 2 excessive gambling by manic patients (F30, F31)
gambling in antisocial personality disorder (F60.2)

F63.1 Pyromania
Pathological fire-setting
EXCLUDES 2 fire-setting (by) (in):
adult with antisocial personality disorder (F60.2)
alcohol or psychoactive substance intoxication (F10-F19)
conduct disorders (F91.-)
mental disorders due to known physiological condition (F01-F09)
schizophrenia (F20.-)

F63.2 Kleptomania
Pathological stealing
EXCLUDES 1 shoplifting as the reason for observation for suspected mental disorder (Z03.8)
EXCLUDES 2 depressive disorder with stealing (F31-F33)
stealing due to underlying mental condition - code to mental condition
stealing in mental disorders due to known physiological condition (F01-F09)

F63.3 Trichotillomania `Rx`
Hair plucking
EXCLUDES 2 other stereotyped movement disorder (F98.4)

✓5ᵗʰ **F63.8 Other impulse disorders**
F63.81 Intermittent explosive disorder `Rx`
F63.89 Other impulse disorders `Rx`
F63.9 Impulse disorder, unspecified `Rx`
Impulse control disorder NOS

✓4ᵗʰ **F64 Gender identity disorders**
AHA: 2016,4Q,16
F64.0 Transsexualism
Gender identity disorder in adolescence and adulthood
Gender dysphoria in adolescents and adults
F64.1 Dual role transvestism
Use additional code to identify sex reassignment status (Z87.890)
EXCLUDES 1 gender identity disorder in childhood (F64.2)
EXCLUDES 2 fetishistic transvestism (F65.1)
F64.2 Gender identity disorder of childhood `P`
Gender dysphoria in children
EXCLUDES 1 gender identity disorder in adolescence and adulthood (F64.0)
EXCLUDES 2 sexual maturation disorder (F66)
F64.8 Other gender identity disorders
Other specified gender dysphoria
F64.9 Gender identity disorder, unspecified
Gender dysphoria, unspecified
Gender-role disorder NOS

✓4ᵗʰ **F65 Paraphilias**
F65.0 Fetishism
Fetishistic disorder
F65.1 Transvestic fetishism
Fetishistic transvestism
Transvestic disorder
F65.2 Exhibitionism
Exhibitionistic disorder
F65.3 Voyeurism
Voyeuristic disorder
F65.4 Pedophilia
Pedophilic disorder
✓5ᵗʰ **F65.5 Sadomasochism**
F65.50 Sadomasochism, unspecified
F65.51 Sexual masochism
Sexual masochism disorder
F65.52 Sexual sadism
Sexual sadism disorder
✓5ᵗʰ **F65.8 Other paraphilias**
F65.81 Frotteurism
Frotteuristic disorder
F65.89 Other paraphilias
Necrophilia
Other specified paraphilic disorder
F65.9 Paraphilia, unspecified
Paraphilic disorder, unspecified
Sexual deviation NOS

F66 Other sexual disorders
Sexual maturation disorder
Sexual relationship disorder

✓4ᵗʰ **F68 Other disorders of adult personality and behavior**
AHA: 2018,4Q,9,65
✓5ᵗʰ **F68.1 Factitious disorder imposed on self**
Compensation neurosis
Elaboration of physical symptoms for psychological reasons
Hospital hopper syndrome
Münchausen's syndrome
Peregrinating patient
EXCLUDES 2 factitial dermatitis (L98.1)
person feigning illness (with obvious motivation) (Z76.5)
F68.10 Factitious disorder imposed on self, unspecified `Rx`
F68.11 Factitious disorder imposed on self, with predominantly psychological signs and symptoms `Rx`

F68.12 Factitious disorder imposed on self, with predominantly physical signs and symptoms `Rx`
F68.13 Factitious disorder imposed on self, with combined psychological and physical signs and symptoms `Rx`
F68.A Factitious disorder imposed on another `Rx`
Factitious disorder by proxy
Münchausen's by proxy
F68.8 Other specified disorders of adult personality and behavior
F69 Unspecified disorder of adult personality and behavior `A`

Intellectual disabilities (F70-F79)
Code first any associated physical or developmental disorders
EXCLUDES 1 borderline intellectual functioning, IQ above 70 to 84 (R41.83)

F70 Mild intellectual disabilities `Rx`
IQ level 50-55 to approximately 70
Mild mental subnormality
F71 Moderate intellectual disabilities `Rx`
IQ level 35-40 to 50-55
Moderate mental subnormality
F72 Severe intellectual disabilities `Rx`
IQ 20-25 to 35-40
Severe mental subnormality
F73 Profound intellectual disabilities `Rx`
IQ level below 20-25
Profound mental subnormality
✓4ᵗʰ **F78 Other intellectual disabilities** `Rx`
✓5ᵗʰ **F78.A Other genetic related intellectual disabilities**
AHA: 2021,4Q,10-11
F78.A1 SYNGAP1-related intellectual disability `Rx`
Code also, if applicable, any associated:
autism spectrum disorder (F84.0)
autistic disorder (F84.0)
encephalopathy (G93.4-)
epilepsy and recurrent seizures (G40.-)
other pervasive developmental disorders (F84.8)
pervasive developmental disorder, NOS (F84.9)
F78.A9 Other genetic related intellectual disability `Rx`
Code also, if applicable, any associated disorders
F79 Unspecified intellectual disabilities `Rx`
Mental deficiency NOS
Mental subnormality NOS

Pervasive and specific developmental disorders (F80-F89)
✓4ᵗʰ **F80 Specific developmental disorders of speech and language**
F80.0 Phonological disorder
Dyslalia
Functional speech articulation disorder
Lalling
Lisping
Phonological developmental disorder
Speech articulation developmental disorder
Speech-sound disorder
EXCLUDES 1 speech articulation impairment due to aphasia NOS (R47.01)
speech articulation impairment due to apraxia (R48.2)
EXCLUDES 2 speech articulation impairment due to hearing loss (F80.4)
speech articulation impairment due to intellectual disabilities (F70-F79)
speech articulation impairment with expressive language developmental disorder (F80.1)
speech articulation impairment with mixed receptive expressive language developmental disorder (F80.2)

F80.1 Expressive language disorder
Developmental dysphasia or aphasia, expressive type
> EXCLUDES 1   *mixed receptive-expressive language disorder (F80.2)*
> *dysphasia and aphasia NOS (R47.-)*
> EXCLUDES 2   *acquired aphasia with epilepsy [Landau-Kleffner]*
> *(G40.80-)*
> *selective mutism (F94.0)*
> *intellectual disabilities (F70-F79)*
> *pervasive developmental disorders (F84.-)*

F80.2 Mixed receptive-expressive language disorder
Developmental dysphasia or aphasia, receptive type
Developmental Wernicke's aphasia
> EXCLUDES 1   *central auditory processing disorder (H93.25)*
> *dysphasia or aphasia NOS (R47.-)*
> *expressive language disorder (F80.1)*
> *expressive type dysphasia or aphasia (F80.1)*
> *word deafness (H93.25)*
> EXCLUDES 2   *acquired aphasia with epilepsy [Landau-Kleffner]*
> *(G40.80-)*
> *pervasive developmental disorders (F84.-)*
> *selective mutism (F94.0)*
> *intellectual disabilities (F70-F79)*

F80.4 Speech and language development delay due to hearing loss
Code also type of hearing loss (H90.-, H91.-)

✓5ᵗʰ **F80.8** Other developmental disorders of speech and language
AHA: 2017,1Q,27

F80.81 Childhood onset fluency disorder
Cluttering NOS
Stuttering NOS
> EXCLUDES 1   *adult onset fluency disorder (F98.5)*
> *fluency disorder in conditions classified*
> *elsewhere (R47.82)*
> *fluency disorder (stuttering) following*
> *cerebrovascular disease (I69. with*
> *final characters -23)*

F80.82 Social pragmatic communication disorder
> EXCLUDES 1   *Asperger's syndrome (F84.5)*
> *autistic disorder (F84.0)*

AHA: 2016,4Q,16

F80.89 Other developmental disorders of speech and language

F80.9 Developmental disorder of speech and language, unspecified
Communication disorder NOS
Language disorder NOS

✓4ᵗʰ **F81** Specific developmental disorders of scholastic skills

F81.0 Specific reading disorder
"Backward reading"
Developmental dyslexia
Specific learning disorder, with impairment in reading
Specific reading retardation
> EXCLUDES 1   *alexia NOS (R48.0)*
> *dyslexia NOS (R48.0)*

DEF: Serious impairment of reading skills unexplained in relation to general intelligence and teaching processes.

F81.2 Mathematics disorder
Developmental acalculia
Developmental arithmetical disorder
Developmental Gerstmann's syndrome
Specific learning disorder, with impairment in mathematics
> EXCLUDES 1   *acalculia NOS (R48.8)*
> EXCLUDES 2   *arithmetical difficulties associated with a reading*
> *disorder (F81.0)*
> *arithmetical difficulties associated with a spelling*
> *disorder (F81.81)*
> *arithmetical difficulties due to inadequate teaching*
> *(Z55.8)*

✓5ᵗʰ **F81.8** Other developmental disorders of scholastic skills

F81.81 Disorder of written expression
Specific learning disorder, with impairment in written expression
Specific spelling disorder

F81.89 Other developmental disorders of scholastic skills

F81.9 Developmental disorder of scholastic skills, unspecified
Knowledge acquisition disability NOS
Learning disability NOS
Learning disorder NOS

F82 Specific developmental disorder of motor function
Clumsy child syndrome
Developmental coordination disorder
Developmental dyspraxia
> EXCLUDES 1   *abnormalities of gait and mobility (R26.-)*
> *lack of coordination (R27.-)*
> EXCLUDES 2   *lack of coordination secondary to intellectual disabilities*
> *(F70-F79)*

✓4ᵗʰ **F84** Pervasive developmental disorders
Code also any associated medical condition and intellectual disabilities

F84.0 Autistic disorder   Rx COM
Autism spectrum disorder
Infantile autism
Infantile psychosis
Kanner's syndrome
> EXCLUDES 1   *Asperger's syndrome (F84.5)*

AHA: 2017,1Q,27
TIP: When the encounter is focused on treatment of conditions related to autism spectrum disorder, first assign codes to identify the problem or manifestation receiving therapeutic services.

F84.2 Rett's syndrome   Rx COM
> EXCLUDES 1   *Asperger's syndrome (F84.5)*
> *autistic disorder (F84.0)*
> *other childhood disintegrative disorder (F84.3)*

F84.3 Other childhood disintegrative disorder   Rx COM P
Dementia infantilis
Disintegrative psychosis
Heller's syndrome
Symbiotic psychosis
Use additional code to identify any associated neurological condition
> EXCLUDES 1   *Asperger's syndrome (F84.5)*
> *autistic disorder (F84.0)*
> *Rett's syndrome (F84.2)*

F84.5 Asperger's syndrome   Rx COM
Asperger's disorder
Autistic psychopathy
Schizoid disorder of childhood
DEF: High-functioning form of autism. Children with this syndrome usually develop speech on schedule, are generally very intelligent, and communicate well, but have considerable social shortcomings. *Synonym(s):* AS.

F84.8 Other pervasive developmental disorders   Rx COM
Overactive disorder associated with intellectual disabilities and stereotyped movements

F84.9 Pervasive developmental disorder, unspecified   Rx COM
Atypical autism

F88 Other disorders of psychological development
Developmental agnosia
Global developmental delay
Other specified neurodevelopmental disorder

F89 Unspecified disorder of psychological development
Developmental disorder NOS
Neurodevelopmental disorder NOS

Chapter 5. Mental, Behavioral and Neurodevelopmental Disorders

F90–F98.3

Behavioral and emotional disorders with onset usually occurring in childhood and adolescence (F90-F98)

NOTE   Codes within categories F90-F98 may be used regardless of the age of a patient. These disorders generally have onset within the childhood or adolescent years, but may continue throughout life or not be diagnosed until adulthood

✓4ᵗʰ **F90 Attention-deficit hyperactivity disorders**
- INCLUDES   attention deficit disorder with hyperactivity
  - attention deficit syndrome with hyperactivity
- EXCLUDES 2   anxiety disorders (F40.-, F41.-)
  - mood [affective] disorders (F30-F39)
  - pervasive developmental disorders (F84.-)
  - schizophrenia (F20.-)

F90.0 Attention-deficit hyperactivity disorder, predominantly inattentive type Rx
- Attention-deficit/hyperactivity disorder, predominantly inattentive presentation

F90.1 Attention-deficit hyperactivity disorder, predominantly hyperactive type Rx
- Attention-deficit/hyperactivity disorder, predominantly hyperactive impulsive presentation

F90.2 Attention-deficit hyperactivity disorder, combined type Rx
- Attention-deficit/hyperactivity disorder, combined presentation

F90.8 Attention-deficit hyperactivity disorder, other type Rx

F90.9 Attention-deficit hyperactivity disorder, unspecified type Rx
- Attention-deficit hyperactivity disorder of childhood or adolescence NOS
- Attention-deficit hyperactivity disorder NOS

✓4ᵗʰ **F91 Conduct disorders**
- EXCLUDES 1   antisocial behavior (Z72.81-)
  - antisocial personality disorder (F60.2)
- EXCLUDES 2   conduct problems associated with attention-deficit hyperactivity disorder (F90.-)
  - mood [affective] disorders (F30-F39)
  - pervasive developmental disorders (F84.-)
  - schizophrenia (F20.-)

F91.0 Conduct disorder confined to family context Rx

F91.1 Conduct disorder, childhood-onset type Rx
- Unsocialized conduct disorder
- Conduct disorder, solitary aggressive type
- Unsocialized aggressive disorder

F91.2 Conduct disorder, adolescent-onset type Rx
- Socialized conduct disorder
- Conduct disorder, group type

F91.3 Oppositional defiant disorder Rx

F91.8 Other conduct disorders Rx
- Other specified conduct disorder
- Other specified disruptive disorder

F91.9 Conduct disorder, unspecified Rx
- Behavioral disorder NOS
- Conduct disorder NOS
- Disruptive behavior disorder NOS
- Disruptive disorder NOS

✓4ᵗʰ **F93 Emotional disorders with onset specific to childhood**

F93.0 Separation anxiety disorder of childhood Rx
- EXCLUDES 2   mood [affective] disorders (F30-F39)
  - nonpsychotic mental disorders (F40-F48)
  - phobic anxiety disorder of childhood (F40.8)
  - social phobia (F40.1)

F93.8 Other childhood emotional disorders
- Identity disorder
- EXCLUDES 2   gender identity disorder of childhood (F64.2)

F93.9 Childhood emotional disorder, unspecified

✓4ᵗʰ **F94 Disorders of social functioning with onset specific to childhood and adolescence**

F94.0 Selective mutism
- Elective mutism
- EXCLUDES 2   pervasive developmental disorders (F84.-)
  - schizophrenia (F20.-)
  - specific developmental disorders of speech and language (F80.-)
  - transient mutism as part of separation anxiety in young children (F93.0)

F94.1 Reactive attachment disorder of childhood
- Use additional code to identify any associated failure to thrive or growth retardation
- EXCLUDES 1   disinhibited attachment disorder of childhood (F94.2)
  - normal variation in pattern of selective attachment
- EXCLUDES 2   Asperger's syndrome (F84.5)
  - maltreatment syndromes (T74.-)
  - sexual or physical abuse in childhood, resulting in psychosocial problems (Z62.81-)

F94.2 Disinhibited attachment disorder of childhood
- Affectionless psychopathy
- Institutional syndrome
- EXCLUDES 1   reactive attachment disorder of childhood (F94.1)
- EXCLUDES 2   Asperger's syndrome (F84.5)
  - attention-deficit hyperactivity disorders (F90.-)
  - hospitalism in children (F43.2-)

F94.8 Other childhood disorders of social functioning

F94.9 Childhood disorder of social functioning, unspecified

✓4ᵗʰ **F95 Tic disorder**

F95.0 Transient tic disorder Rx
- Provisional tic disorder

F95.1 Chronic motor or vocal tic disorder Rx

F95.2 Tourette's disorder Rx
- Combined vocal and multiple motor tic disorder [de la Tourette]
- Tourette's syndrome

F95.8 Other tic disorders Rx

F95.9 Tic disorder, unspecified Rx
- Tic NOS

✓4ᵗʰ **F98 Other behavioral and emotional disorders with onset usually occurring in childhood and adolescence**
- EXCLUDES 2   breath-holding spells (R06.89)
  - gender identity disorder of childhood (F64.2)
  - Kleine-Levin syndrome (G47.13)
  - obsessive-compulsive disorder (F42.-)
  - sleep disorders not due to a substance or known physiological condition (F51.-)

F98.0 Enuresis not due to a substance or known physiological condition
- Enuresis (primary) (secondary) of nonorganic origin
- Functional enuresis
- Psychogenic enuresis
- Urinary incontinence of nonorganic origin
- EXCLUDES 1   enuresis NOS (R32)

F98.1 Encopresis not due to a substance or known physiological condition
- Functional encopresis
- Incontinence of feces of nonorganic origin
- Psychogenic encopresis
- Use additional code to identify the cause of any coexisting constipation
- EXCLUDES 1   encopresis NOS (R15.-)

✓5ᵗʰ **F98.2 Other feeding disorders of infancy and childhood**
- EXCLUDES 2   anorexia nervosa and other eating disorders (F50.-)
  - feeding difficulties (R63.3)
  - feeding problems of newborn (P92.-)
  - pica of infancy or childhood (F98.3)

F98.21 Rumination disorder of infancy Rx

F98.29 Other feeding disorders of infancy and early childhood Rx

F98.3 Pica of infancy and childhood Rx

F98.4   **Stereotyped movement disorders**   `Rx`

Stereotype/habit disorder

   EXCLUDES 1   abnormal involuntary movements (R25.-)

   EXCLUDES 2   compulsions in obsessive-compulsive disorder (F42.-)

          hair plucking (F63.3)

          movement disorders of organic origin (G20-G25)

          nail-biting (F98.8)

          nose-picking (F98.8)

          stereotypies that are part of a broader psychiatric condition (F01-F95)

          thumb-sucking (F98.8)

          tic disorders (F95.-)

          trichotillomania (F63.3)

F98.5   **Adult onset fluency disorder**

   EXCLUDES 1   childhood onset fluency disorder (F80.81)

          dysphasia (R47.02)

          fluency disorder in conditions classified elsewhere (R47.82)

          fluency disorder (stuttering) following cerebrovascular disease (I69. with final characters -23)

          tic disorders (F95.-)

F98.8   **Other specified behavioral and emotional disorders with onset usually occurring in childhood and adolescence**

Excessive masturbation

Nail-biting

Nose-picking

Thumb-sucking

F98.9   **Unspecified behavioral and emotional disorders with onset usually occurring in childhood and adolescence**

Unspecified mental disorder (F99)

F99   **Mental disorder, not otherwise specified**

Mental illness NOS

   EXCLUDES 1   unspecified mental disorder due to known physiological condition (F09)

Chapter 6. Diseases of the Nervous System (G00-G99)

Chapter-specific Guidelines with Coding Examples

The chapter-specific guidelines from the ICD-10-CM Official Guidelines for Coding and Reporting have been provided below. Along with these guidelines are coding examples, contained in the shaded boxes, that have been developed to help illustrate the coding and/or sequencing guidance found in these guidelines.

a. Dominant/nondominant side

Codes from category G81, Hemiplegia and hemiparesis, and subcategories G83.1, Monoplegia of lower limb, G83.2, Monoplegia of upper limb, and G83.3, Monoplegia, unspecified, identify whether the dominant or nondominant side is affected. Should the affected side be documented, but not specified as dominant or nondominant, and the classification system does not indicate a default, code selection is as follows:

- For ambidextrous patients, the default should be dominant.
- If the left side is affected, the default is non-dominant.
- If the right side is affected, the default is dominant.

Hemiplegia affecting left side of ambidextrous patient

G81.92   Hemiplegia, unspecified affecting left dominant side

Explanation: Documentation states that the left side is affected and dominant is used for ambidextrous persons.

Right spastic hemiplegia, unknown whether patient is right- or left-handed

G81.11   Spastic hemiplegia affecting right dominant side

Explanation: Since it is unknown whether the patient is right- or left-handed, if the right side is affected, the default is dominant.

---

b. Pain—Category G89

1) General coding information

Codes in category G89, Pain, not elsewhere classified, may be used in conjunction with codes from other categories and chapters to provide more detail about acute or chronic pain and neoplasm-related pain, unless otherwise indicated below.

If the pain is not specified as acute or chronic, post-thoracotomy, postprocedural, or neoplasm-related, do not assign codes from category G89.

A code from category G89 should not be assigned if the underlying (definitive) diagnosis is known, unless the reason for the encounter is pain control/ management and not management of the underlying condition.

When an admission or encounter is for a procedure aimed at treating the underlying condition (e.g., spinal fusion, kyphoplasty), a code for the underlying condition (e.g., vertebral fracture, spinal stenosis) should be assigned as the principal diagnosis. No code from category G89 should be assigned.

Elderly patient with back pain is admitted for outpatient kyphoplasty for age-related osteopathic compression fracture at vertebra T3

M80.08XA   Age-related osteoporosis with current pathological fracture, vertebra(e), initial encounter for fracture

Explanation: No code is assigned for the pain as it is inherent in the underlying condition being treated.

(a) Category G89 codes as principal or first-listed diagnosis

Category G89 codes are acceptable as principal diagnosis or the first-listed code:

- When pain control or pain management is the reason for the admission/encounter (e.g., a patient with displaced intervertebral disc, nerve impingement and severe back pain presents for injection of steroid into the spinal canal). The underlying cause of the pain should be reported as an additional diagnosis, if known.

Patient presents for steroid injection in the right elbow due to chronic pain associated with primary degenerative joint disease.

G89.29   Other chronic pain

M19.021   Primary osteoarthritis, right elbow

Explanation: Since the encounter is for control of pain, not treating the underlying condition, the pain code is sequenced first followed by the underlying condition. The M25 pain code is not necessary as the underlying condition code represents the specific site.

- When a patient is admitted for the insertion of a neurostimulator for pain control, assign the appropriate pain code as the principal or first-listed diagnosis. When an admission or encounter is for a procedure aimed at treating the underlying condition and a neurostimulator is inserted for pain control during the same admission/encounter, a code for the underlying condition should be assigned as the principal diagnosis and the appropriate pain code should be assigned as a secondary diagnosis.

(b) Use of category G89 codes in conjunction with site specific pain codes

(i) Assigning category G89 and site-specific pain codes

Codes from category G89 may be used in conjunction with codes that identify the site of pain (including codes from chapter 18) if the category G89 code provides additional information. For example, if the code describes the site of the pain, but does not fully describe whether the pain is acute or chronic, then both codes should be assigned.

Patient is seen to evaluate chronic right knee pain

M25.561   Pain in right knee

G89.29   Other chronic pain

Explanation: No underlying condition has been determined yet so the pain would be the reason for the visit. The M25 pain code in this instance does not fully describe the condition as it does not represent that the pain is chronic. The G89 chronic pain code is assigned to provide specificity.

(ii) Sequencing of category G89 codes with site-specific pain codes

The sequencing of category G89 codes with site-specific pain codes (including chapter 18 codes), is dependent on the circumstances of the encounter/admission as follows:

- If the encounter is for pain control or pain management, assign the code from category G89 followed by the code identifying the specific site of pain (e.g., encounter for pain management for acute neck pain from trauma is assigned code G89.11, Acute pain due to trauma, followed by code M54.2, Cervicalgia, to identify the site of pain).

Management of acute, traumatic left shoulder pain

G89.11   Acute pain due to trauma

M25.512   Pain in left shoulder

Explanation: The reason for the encounter is to manage or control the pain, not to treat or evaluate an underlying condition. The G89 pain code is assigned as the first-listed diagnosis but in this instance does not fully describe the condition as it does not include the site and laterality. The M25 pain code is added to provide this information.

- If the encounter is for any other reason except pain control or pain management, and a related definitive diagnosis has not been established (confirmed) by the provider, assign the code for the specific site of pain first, followed by the appropriate code from category G89.

Chapter 6. Diseases of the Nervous System

> Tests are performed to investigate the source of the patient's chronic epigastric abdominal pain
>
> **R10.13**   **Epigastric pain**
>
> **G89.29**   **Other chronic pain**
>
> *Explanation*: In this instance the patient's epigastric pain is not being treated; rather the source of the pain is being investigated. A code from chapter 18 for epigastric pain is sequenced before the additional specificity of the G89 code for the chronic pain.

2) **Pain due to devices, implants and grafts**

     See Section I.C.19. Pain due to medical devices

3) **Postoperative Pain**

     The provider's documentation should be used to guide the coding of postoperative pain, as well as *Section III. Reporting Additional Diagnoses* and *Section IV. Diagnostic Coding and Reporting in the Outpatient Setting*.

     The default for post-thoracotomy and other postoperative pain not specified as acute or chronic is the code for the acute form.

     Routine or expected postoperative pain immediately after surgery should not be coded.

> Pain pump dose is increased for the patient's unexpected, extreme pain post-thoracotomy
>
> **G89.12**   **Acute post-thoracotomy pain**
>
> *Explanation*: When acute or chronic is not documented, default to acute. The use of "unexpected, extreme" and the increase of medication dosage indicate that the pain was more than routine or expected.

     (a) **Postoperative pain not associated with specific postoperative complication**

         Postoperative pain not associated with a specific postoperative complication is assigned to the appropriate postoperative pain code in category G89.

     (b) **Postoperative pain associated with specific postoperative complication**

         Postoperative pain associated with a specific postoperative complication (such as painful wire sutures) is assigned to the appropriate code(s) found in Chapter 19, Injury, poisoning, and certain other consequences of external causes. If appropriate, use additional code(s) from category G89 to identify acute or chronic pain (G89.18 or G89.28).

4) **Chronic pain**

     Chronic pain is classified to subcategory G89.2. There is no time frame defining when pain becomes chronic pain. The provider's documentation should be used to guide use of these codes.

5) **Neoplasm related pain**

     Code G89.3 is assigned to pain documented as being related, associated or due to cancer, primary or secondary malignancy, or tumor. This code is assigned regardless of whether the pain is acute or chronic.

     This code may be assigned as the principal or first-listed code when the stated reason for the admission/encounter is documented as pain control/pain management. The underlying neoplasm should be reported as an additional diagnosis.

> Patient referred today for pain management due to acute pain related to malignancy of the right breast.
>
> **G89.3**   **Neoplasm related pain (acute)(chronic)**
>
> **C50.911**   **Malignant neoplasm of unspecified site of right female breast**
>
> *Explanation*: Since the encounter was for pain medication management, the pain, rather than the neoplasm, was the reason for the encounter and is sequenced first. This "neoplasm-related pain" code includes both acute and chronic pain.

     When the reason for the admission/encounter is management of the neoplasm and the pain associated with the neoplasm is also documented, code G89.3 may be assigned as an additional diagnosis. It is not necessary to assign an additional code for the site of the pain.

     See Section I.C.2. for instructions on the sequencing of neoplasms for all other stated reasons or the admission/encounter (except for pain control/pain management).

> Patient with lung cancer presents with acute hip pain and is evaluated and found to have iliac bone metastasis
>
> **C79.51**   **Secondary malignant neoplasm of bone**
>
> **C34.90**   **Malignant neoplasm of unspecified part of unspecified bronchus or lung**
>
> **G89.3**   **Neoplasm related pain (acute)(chronic)**
>
> *Explanation*: The reason for the encounter was the evaluation and diagnosis of the bone metastasis, whose code would be assigned as first-listed, followed by codes for the primary neoplasm and the pain due to the iliac bone metastasis.

6) **Chronic pain syndrome**

     Central pain syndrome (G89.0) and chronic pain syndrome (G89.4) are different than the term "chronic pain," and therefore codes should only be used when the provider has specifically documented this condition.

     See Section I.C.5. Pain disorders related to psychological factors

Chapter 6. Diseases of the Nervous System (G00-G99)

EXCLUDES 2   certain conditions originating in the perinatal period (P04-P96)
certain infectious and parasitic diseases (A00-B99)
complications of pregnancy, childbirth and the puerperium (O00-O9A)
congenital malformations, deformations, and chromosomal abnormalities (Q00-Q99)
endocrine, nutritional and metabolic diseases (E00-E88)
injury, poisoning and certain other consequences of external causes (S00-T88)
neoplasms (C00-D49)
symptoms, signs and abnormal clinical and laboratory findings, not elsewhere classified (R00-R94)

This chapter contains the following blocks:

G00-G09   Inflammatory diseases of the central nervous system
G10-G14   Systemic atrophies primarily affecting the central nervous system
G20-G26   Extrapyramidal and movement disorders
G30-G32   Other degenerative diseases of the nervous system
G35-G37   Demyelinating diseases of the central nervous system
G40-G47   Episodic and paroxysmal disorders
G50-G59   Nerve, nerve root and plexus disorders
G60-G65   Polyneuropathies and other disorders of the peripheral nervous system
G70-G73   Diseases of myoneural junction and muscle
G80-G83   Cerebral palsy and other paralytic syndromes
G89-G99   Other disorders of the nervous system

Inflammatory diseases of the central nervous system (G00-G09)

✓4ᵗʰ G00 Bacterial meningitis, not elsewhere classified

INCLUDES   bacterial arachnoiditis
bacterial leptomeningitis
bacterial meningitis
bacterial pachymeningitis

EXCLUDES 1   bacterial meningoencephalitis (G04.2)
bacterial meningomyelitis (G04.2)

DEF: Inflammation of meningeal layers of the brain and spinal cord due to a bacterial infection.

G00.0 Hemophilus meningitis   COM
Meningitis due to Hemophilus influenzae

G00.1 Pneumococcal meningitis   COM
Meningtitis due to Streptococcal pneumoniae

G00.2 Streptococcal meningitis   COM
Use additional code to further identify organism (B95.0-B95.5)

G00.3 Staphylococcal meningitis   COM
Use additional code to further identify organism (B95.61-B95.8)

G00.8 Other bacterial meningitis   COM
Meningitis due to Escherichia coli
Meningitis due to Friedländer's bacillus
Meningitis due to Klebsiella
Use additional code to further identify organism (B96.-)

G00.9 Bacterial meningitis, unspecified   COM
Meningitis due to gram-negative bacteria, unspecified
Purulent meningitis NOS
Pyogenic meningitis NOS
Suppurative meningitis NOS

G01 Meningitis in bacterial diseases classified elsewhere   COM
Code first underlying disease

EXCLUDES 1   meningitis (in):
gonococcal (A54.81)
leptospirosis (A27.81)
listeriosis (A32.11)
Lyme disease (A69.21)
meningococcal (A39.0)
neurosyphilis (A52.13)
tuberculosis (A17.0)
meningoencephalitis and meningomyelitis in bacterial diseases classified elsewhere (G05)

G02 Meningitis in other infectious and parasitic diseases classified elsewhere   COM
Code first underlying disease, such as:
African trypanosomiasis (B56.-)
poliovirus infection (A80.-)

EXCLUDES 1   candidal meningitis (B37.5)
coccidioidomycosis meningitis (B38.4)
cryptococcal meningitis (B45.1)
herpesviral [herpes simplex] meningitis (B00.3)
infectious mononucleosis complicated by meningitis (B27.- with fifth character 2)
measles complicated by meningitis (B05.1)
meningoencephalitis and meningomyelitis in other infectious and parasitic diseases classified elsewhere (G05)
mumps meningitis (B26.1)
rubella meningitis (B06.02)
varicella [chickenpox] meningitis (B01.0)
zoster meningitis (B02.1)

✓4ᵗʰ G03 Meningitis due to other and unspecified causes

INCLUDES   arachnoiditis NOS
leptomeningitis NOS
meningitis NOS
pachymeningitis NOS

EXCLUDES 1   meningoencephalitis (G04.-)
meningomyelitis (G04.-)

G03.0 Nonpyogenic meningitis   COM
Aseptic meningitis
Nonbacterial meningitis
DEF: Type of meningitis where no bacterial, viral, or other infectious source exists that explains the meningitis symptomology.

G03.1 Chronic meningitis   COM

G03.2 Benign recurrent meningitis [Mollaret]   COM
DEF: Aseptic or noninfectious inflammation of the meninges with the presence of Mollaret cells in the spinal fluid. The patient experiences recurrent bouts of inflammation, lasting anywhere from two to five days.

G03.8 Meningitis due to other specified causes   COM

G03.9 Meningitis, unspecified   COM
Arachnoiditis (spinal) NOS

✓4ᵗʰ G04 Encephalitis, myelitis and encephalomyelitis

INCLUDES   acute ascending myelitis
meningoencephalitis
meningomyelitis

EXCLUDES 1   encephalopathy NOS (G93.40)

EXCLUDES 2   acute transverse myelitis (G37.3-)
alcoholic encephalopathy (G31.2)
benign myalgic encephalomyelitis (G93.3)
multiple sclerosis (G35)
▶myalgic encephalomyelitis (G93.32)◀
subacute necrotizing myelitis (G37.4)
toxic encephalitis (G92.8)
toxic encephalopathy (G92.8)

DEF: Encephalitis: Inflammation of the brain, often caused by viral or bacterial infection.
DEF: Encephalomyelitis: Inflammatory disease, often viral in nature, that affects the brain and spinal cord.
DEF: Myelitis: Inflammation of the spinal cord.

✓5ᵗʰ G04.0 Acute disseminated encephalitis and encephalomyelitis (ADEM)

EXCLUDES 1   acute necrotizing hemorrhagic encephalopathy (G04.3-)
other noninfectious acute disseminated encephalomyelitis (noninfectious ADEM) (G04.81)

G04.00 Acute disseminated encephalitis and encephalomyelitis, unspecified   COM

G04.01 Postinfectious acute disseminated encephalitis and encephalomyelitis (postinfectious ADEM)   COM
EXCLUDES 1   post chickenpox encephalitis (B01.1)
post measles encephalitis (B05.0)
post measles myelitis (B05.1)

☑ Additional Character Required   ✓x7ᵗʰ Placeholder Alert   Manifestation   Unspecified Dx   Q QPP   UPD Unacceptable PDx

Chapter 6. Diseases of the Nervous System

G04.02   **Postimmunization** acute disseminated encephalitis, myelitis and encephalomyelitis   COM
     Encephalitis, post immunization
     Encephalomyelitis, post immunization
     Use additional code to identify the vaccine (T50.A-, T50.B-, T50.Z-)

G04.1   **Tropical spastic paraplegia**   HCC   Rx   ESR   COM

G04.2   **Bacterial meningoencephalitis and meningomyelitis, not elsewhere classified**   COM

✓5ᵗʰ   **G04.3**   **Acute necrotizing hemorrhagic encephalopathy**
     EXCLUDES 1   acute disseminated encephalitis and encephalomyelitis (G04.0-)

     G04.30   **Acute necrotizing hemorrhagic encephalopathy, unspecified**   COM

     G04.31   **Postinfectious** acute necrotizing hemorrhagic encephalopathy   COM

     G04.32   **Postimmunization** acute necrotizing hemorrhagic encephalopathy   COM
         Use additional code to identify the vaccine (T50.A-, T50.B-, T50.Z-)

     G04.39   **Other acute necrotizing hemorrhagic encephalopathy**   COM
         Code also underlying etiology, if applicable

✓5ᵗʰ   **G04.8**   **Other encephalitis, myelitis and encephalomyelitis**
     Code also any associated seizure (G40.-, R56.9)

     G04.81   **Other encephalitis and encephalomyelitis**   COM
         Noninfectious acute disseminated encephalomyelitis (noninfectious ADEM)

     G04.82   **Acute flaccid myelitis**   HCC   Rx   ESR   COM
         EXCLUDES 1   transverse myelitis (G37.3)
         AHA: 2021,4Q,11

     G04.89   **Other myelitis**   HCC   Rx   ESR   COM
         AHA: 2020,1Q,14

✓5ᵗʰ   **G04.9**   **Encephalitis, myelitis and encephalomyelitis, unspecified**

     G04.90   **Encephalitis and encephalomyelitis, unspecified**   COM
         Ventriculitis (cerebral) NOS

     G04.91   **Myelitis, unspecified**   HCC   Rx   ESR   COM

✓4ᵗʰ   **G05**   **Encephalitis, myelitis and encephalomyelitis in diseases classified elsewhere**
     Code first underlying disease, such as:
       congenital toxoplasmosis encephalitis, myelitis and encephalomyelitis (P37.1)
       cytomegaloviral encephalitis, myelitis and encephalomyelitis (B25.8)
       encephalitis, myelitis and encephalomyelitis (in) systemic lupus erythematosus (M32.19)
       eosinophilic meningoencephalitis (B83.2)
       human immunodeficiency virus [HIV] disease (B20)
       poliovirus (A80.-)
       suppurative otitis media (H66.01-H66.4)
       trichinellosis (B75)
     EXCLUDES 1   adenoviral encephalitis, myelitis and encephalomyelitis (A85.1)
         encephalitis, myelitis and encephalomyelitis (in) measles (B05.0)
         enteroviral encephalitis, myelitis and encephalomyelitis (A85.0)
         herpesviral [herpes simplex] encephalitis, myelitis and encephalomyelitis (B00.4)
         listerial encephalitis, myelitis and encephalomyelitis (A32.12)
         meningococcal encephalitis, myelitis and encephalomyelitis (A39.81)
         mumps encephalitis, myelitis and encephalomyelitis (B26.2)
         postchickenpox encephalitis, myelitis and encephalomyelitis (B01.1-)
         rubella encephalitis, myelitis and encephalomyelitis (B06.01)
         toxoplasmosis encephalitis, myelitis and encephalomyelitis (B58.2)
         zoster encephalitis, myelitis and encephalomyelitis (B02.0)

     G05.3   *Encephalitis and encephalomyelitis in diseases classified elsewhere*   COM
         Meningoencephalitis in diseases classified elsewhere

     G05.4   *Myelitis in diseases classified elsewhere*   HCC   Rx   ESR   COM
         Meningomyelitis in diseases classified elsewhere

✓4ᵗʰ   **G06**   **Intracranial and intraspinal abscess and granuloma**
     Use additional code (B95-B97) to identify infectious agent
     DEF: Abscess: Circumscribed collection of pus resulting from bacteria, frequently associated with swelling and other signs of inflammation.
     DEF: Granuloma: Abnormal, dense collections of cells forming a mass or nodule of chronically inflamed tissue with granulations that is usually associated with an infective process.

     G06.0   **Intracranial** abscess and granuloma   COM
         Brain [any part] abscess (embolic)
         Cerebellar abscess (embolic)
         Cerebral abscess (embolic)
         Intracranial epidural abscess or granuloma
         Intracranial extradural abscess or granuloma
         Intracranial subdural abscess or granuloma
         Otogenic abscess (embolic)
         EXCLUDES 1   tuberculous intracranial abscess and granuloma (A17.81)

     G06.1   **Intraspinal** abscess and granuloma   COM
         Abscess (embolic) of spinal cord [any part]
         Intraspinal epidural abscess or granuloma
         Intraspinal extradural abscess or granuloma
         Intraspinal subdural abscess or granuloma
         EXCLUDES 1   tuberculous intraspinal abscess and granuloma (A17.81)

     G06.2   **Extradural and subdural abscess, unspecified**   COM

G07   *Intracranial and intraspinal abscess and granuloma in diseases classified elsewhere*   COM
     Code first underlying disease, such as:
       schistosomiasis granuloma of brain (B65.-)
     EXCLUDES 1   abscess of brain:
           amebic (A06.6)
           chromomycotic (B43.1)
           gonococcal (A54.82)
           tuberculous (A17.81)
         tuberculoma of meninges (A17.1)

G08   **Intracranial and intraspinal phlebitis and thrombophlebitis**   COM
     Septic embolism of intracranial or intraspinal venous sinuses and veins
     Septic endophlebitis of intracranial or intraspinal venous sinuses and veins
     Septic phlebitis of intracranial or intraspinal venous sinuses and veins
     Septic thrombophlebitis of intracranial or intraspinal venous sinuses and veins
     Septic thrombosis of intracranial or intraspinal venous sinuses and veins
     EXCLUDES 1   intracranial phlebitis and thrombophlebitis complicating:
         abortion, ectopic or molar pregnancy (O00-O07, O08.7)
         pregnancy, childbirth and the puerperium (O22.5, O87.3)
         nonpyogenic intracranial phlebitis and thrombophlebitis (I67.6)
     EXCLUDES 2   intracranial phlebitis and thrombophlebitis complicating nonpyogenic intraspinal phlebitis and thrombophlebitis (G95.1)
     DEF: Inflammation and formation of a blood clot in a vein within the brain or spine, or their linings.

G09   **Sequelae of inflammatory diseases of central nervous system**
     NOTE   Category G09 is to be used to indicate conditions whose primary classification is to G00-G08 as the cause of sequelae, themselves classifiable elsewhere. The "sequelae" include conditions specified as residuals.
     Code first condition resulting from (sequela) of inflammatory diseases of central nervous system

old bacterial meningitis.

Systemic atrophies primarily affecting the central nervous system (G10-G14)

G10 Huntington's disease `HCC` `Rx` `ESR` `COM`
Huntington's chorea
Huntington's dementia
▶Use additional code, if applicable, to identify:◄
▶dementia with anxiety (F02.84, F02.A4, F02.B4, F02.C4)◄
▶dementia with behavioral disturbance (F02.81-, F02.A1-, F02.B1-, F02.C1-)◄
▶dementia with mood disturbance (F02.83, F02.A3, F02.B3, F02.C3)◄
▶dementia with psychotic disturbance (F02.82, F02.A2, F02.B2, F02.C2)◄
▶dementia without behavioral disturbance (F02.80, F02.A0, F02.B0, F02.C0)◄
▶mild neurocognitive disorder due to known physiological condition (F06.7-)◄
~~Code also dementia in other diseases classified elsewhere without behavioral disturbance (F02.80)~~
DEF: Genetic disease caused by degeneration of nerve cells in the brain, characterized by chronic progressive mental deterioration. Dementia and death occur within 15 to 20 years of onset.

✓4ᵗʰ **G11 Hereditary ataxia**
     EXCLUDES 2   *cerebral palsy (G80.-)*
                 hereditary and idiopathic neuropathy (G60.-)
                 metabolic disorders (E70-E88)
     DEF: Ataxia: Defect in muscular control or coordination due to a central nervous system disorder, particularly when voluntary muscular movements are attempted.
G11.0 Congenital nonprogressive ataxia `HCC` `ESR` `COM`
✓5ᵗʰ **G11.1 Early-onset cerebellar ataxia**
     AHA: 2020,4Q,17-18
     G11.10 Early-onset cerebellar ataxia, unspecified `HCC` `ESR` `COM`
     G11.11 Friedreich ataxia `HCC` `ESR` `COM`
         Autosomal recessive Friedreich ataxia
         Friedreich ataxia with retained reflexes
     G11.19 Other early-onset cerebellar ataxia `HCC` `ESR` `COM`
         Early-onset cerebellar ataxia with essential tremor
         Early-onset cerebellar ataxia with myoclonus [Hunt's ataxia]
         Early-onset cerebellar ataxia with retained tendon reflexes
         X-linked recessive spinocerebellar ataxia
G11.2 Late-onset cerebellar ataxia `HCC` `ESR` `COM` `A`
G11.3 Cerebellar ataxia with defective DNA repair `HCC` `ESR` `COM`
     Ataxia telangiectasia [Louis-Bar]
     EXCLUDES 2   *Cockayne's syndrome (Q87.19)*
                other disorders of purine and pyrimidine metabolism (E79.-)
                xeroderma pigmentosum (Q82.1)
G11.4 Hereditary spastic paraplegia `HCC` `ESR` `COM`
G11.8 Other hereditary ataxias `HCC` `ESR` `COM`
G11.9 Hereditary ataxia, unspecified `HCC` `ESR` `COM`
     Hereditary cerebellar ataxia NOS
     Hereditary cerebellar degeneration
     Hereditary cerebellar disease
     Hereditary cerebellar syndrome

✓4ᵗʰ **G12 Spinal muscular atrophy and related syndromes**
G12.0 Infantile spinal muscular atrophy, type I [Werdnig-Hoffman] `HCC` `Rx` `ESR` `COM`
G12.1 Other inherited spinal muscular atrophy `HCC` `Rx` `ESR` `COM`
     Adult form spinal muscular atrophy
     Childhood form, type II spinal muscular atrophy
     Distal spinal muscular atrophy
     Juvenile form, type III spinal muscular atrophy [Kugelberg-Welander]
     Progressive bulbar palsy of childhood [Fazio-Londe]
     Scapuloperoneal form spinal muscular atrophy
✓5ᵗʰ **G12.2 Motor neuron disease**
     AHA: 2017,4Q,9-10
     G12.20 Motor neuron disease, unspecified `HCC` `Rx` `ESR` `COM`
     G12.21 Amyotrophic lateral sclerosis `HCC` `Rx` `ESR` `COM` `A`
     G12.22 Progressive bulbar palsy `HCC` `Rx` `ESR` `COM`

G12.23 Primary lateral sclerosis `HCC` `Rx` `ESR` `COM`
G12.24 Familial motor neuron disease `HCC` `Rx` `ESR` `COM`
G12.25 Progressive spinal muscle atrophy `HCC` `Rx` `ESR` `COM`
G12.29 Other motor neuron disease `HCC` `Rx` `ESR` `COM`
G12.8 Other spinal muscular atrophies and related syndromes `HCC` `Rx` `ESR` `COM`
G12.9 Spinal muscular atrophy, unspecified `HCC` `Rx` `ESR` `COM`

✓4ᵗʰ **G13 Systemic atrophies primarily affecting central nervous system in diseases classified elsewhere**
G13.0 Paraneoplastic neuromyopathy and neuropathy `HCC` `Rx` `ESR` `COM`
     Carcinomatous neuromyopathy
     Sensorial paraneoplastic neuropathy [Denny Brown]
     Code first underlying neoplasm (C00-D49)
G13.1 Other systemic atrophy primarily affecting central nervous system in neoplastic disease `HCC` `Rx` `ESR` `COM`
     Paraneoplastic limbic encephalopathy
     Code first underlying neoplasm (C00-D49)
G13.2 Systemic atrophy primarily affecting the central nervous system in myxedema `HCC` `Rx` `ESR`
     Code first underlying disease, such as:
         hypothyroidism (E03.-)
         myxedematous congenital iodine deficiency (E00.1)
G13.8 Systemic atrophy primarily affecting central nervous system in other diseases classified elsewhere `HCC` `Rx` `ESR`
     Code first underlying disease

G14 Postpolio syndrome
     INCLUDES   postpolio myelitic syndrome
     EXCLUDES 1   *sequelae of poliomyelitis (B91)*

Extrapyramidal and movement disorders (G20-G26)

G20 Parkinson's disease `HCC` `Rx` `ESR` `COM`

[handwritten: G20 A. G20.B. G20.C unspecified]

     Hemiparkinsonism
     Idiopathic Parkinsonism or Parkinson's disease
     Paralysis agitans
     Parkinsonism or Parkinson's disease NOS
     Primary Parkinsonism or Parkinson's disease
▶Use additional code, if applicable, to identify:◄
▶dementia with anxiety (F02.84, F02.A4, F02.B4, F02.C4)◄
dementia with behavioral disturbance ▶(F02.81-, F02.A1-, F02.B1-, F02.C1-)◄
▶dementia with mood disturbance (F02.83, F02.A3, F02.B3, F02.C3)◄
▶dementia with psychotic disturbance (F02.82, F02.A2, F02.B2, F02.C2)◄
dementia without behavioral disturbance ▶(F02.80, F02.A0, F02.B0, F02.C0)◄
▶mild neurocognitive disorder due to known physiological condition (F06.7-)◄
     EXCLUDES 1   *dementia with Parkinsonism (G31.83)*
AHA: 2017,2Q,7; 2016,2Q,6
TIP: Repeated falls (R29.6) are not integral to Parkinson's disease and can be separately coded.

✓4ᵗʰ **G21 Secondary parkinsonism**
     EXCLUDES 1   *dementia with Parkinsonism (G31.83)*
               Huntington's disease (G10)
               Shy-Drager syndrome (G90.3)
               syphilitic Parkinsonism (A52.19)

G21.0 Malignant neuroleptic syndrome
     Use additional code for adverse effect, if applicable, to identify drug (T43.3X5, T43.4X5, T43.505, T43.595)
     EXCLUDES 1   *neuroleptic induced parkinsonism (G21.11)*
✓5ᵗʰ **G21.1 Other drug-induced secondary parkinsonism**
     G21.11 Neuroleptic induced parkinsonism `HCC` `Rx` `ESR` `COM`
         Use additional code for adverse effect, if applicable, to identify drug (T43.3X5, T43.4X5, T43.505, T43.595)
         EXCLUDES 1   *malignant neuroleptic syndrome (G21.0)*
     G21.19 Other drug induced secondary parkinsonism `HCC` `Rx` `ESR` `COM`
         Other medication-induced parkinsonism
         Use additional code for adverse effect, if applicable, to identify drug (T36-T50 with fifth or sixth character 5)

G21.2 **Secondary parkinsonism due to other external agents** `HCC` `Rx` `ESR` `COM`
> Code first (T51-T65) to identify external agent

G21.3 **Postencephalitic** parkinsonism `HCC` `Rx` `ESR` `COM`

G21.4 Vascular **parkinsonism** `HCC` `Rx` `ESR` `COM`

G21.8 **Other secondary parkinsonism** `HCC` `Rx` `ESR` `COM`

G21.9 Secondary parkinsonism, **unspecified** `HCC` `Rx` `ESR` `COM`

☑4ᵗʰ **G23** **Other degenerative diseases of basal ganglia**
> `EXCLUDES 2` *multi-system degeneration of the autonomic nervous system (G90.3)*

G23.0 **Hallervorden-Spatz disease** `HCC` `Rx` `ESR` `COM`
> Pigmentary pallidal degeneration

G23.1 **Progressive supranuclear ophthalmoplegia [Steele-Richardson-Olszewski]** `HCC` `Rx` `ESR` `COM`
> Progressive supranuclear palsy

G23.2 **Striatonigral degeneration** `HCC` `Rx` `ESR` `COM`

G23.8 **Other specified degenerative diseases of basal ganglia** `HCC` `Rx` `ESR` `COM`
> Calcification of basal ganglia

G23.9 **Degenerative disease of basal ganglia, unspecified** `HCC` `Rx` `ESR` `COM`

☑4ᵗʰ **G24** **Dystonia**
> `INCLUDES` dyskinesia
> `EXCLUDES 2` *athetoid cerebral palsy (G80.3)*
> **DEF:** Disorder of abnormal muscle tone, excessive or inadequate. Involuntary movements and prolonged muscle contractions result in tremors, abnormalities in posture, and twisting body motions that affect an isolated area or the whole body.

☑5ᵗʰ **G24.0** Drug induced **dystonia**
> Use additional code for adverse effect, if applicable, to identify drug (T36-T50 with fifth or sixth character 5)

G24.01 Drug induced subacute **dyskinesia**
> Drug induced blepharospasm
> Drug induced orofacial dyskinesia
> Neuroleptic induced tardive dyskinesia
> Tardive dyskinesia

G24.02 Drug induced acute **dystonia**
> Acute dystonic reaction to drugs
> Neuroleptic induced acute dystonia

G24.09 **Other drug induced dystonia**

G24.1 Genetic torsion **dystonia**
> Dystonia deformans progressiva
> Dystonia musculorum deformans
> Familial torsion dystonia
> Idiopathic familial dystonia
> Idiopathic (torsion) dystonia NOS
> (Schwalbe-) Ziehen-Oppenheim disease

G24.2 Idiopathic nonfamilial **dystonia**

G24.3 Spasmodic **torticollis**
> `EXCLUDES 1` *congenital torticollis (Q68.0)*
> *hysterical torticollis (F44.4)*
> *ocular torticollis (R29.891)*
> *psychogenic torticollis (F45.8)*
> *torticollis NOS (M43.6)*
> *traumatic recurrent torticollis (S13.4)*
> **DEF:** Twisted, unnatural position of the neck due to contracted cervical muscles that pull the head to one side or cause involuntary shaking of the head.

G24.4 Idiopathic orofacial **dystonia**
> Orofacial dyskinesia
> `EXCLUDES 1` *drug induced orofacial dyskinesia (G24.01)*

G24.5 Blepharospasm
> `EXCLUDES 1` *drug induced blepharospasm (G24.01)*
> **DEF:** Involuntary contraction of the orbicularis oculi muscle, resulting in the eyelids being completely closed.

G24.8 **Other dystonia**
> Acquired torsion dystonia NOS

G24.9 **Dystonia, unspecified**
> Dyskinesia NOS

☑4ᵗʰ **G25** **Other extrapyramidal and movement disorders**
> `EXCLUDES 2` *sleep related movement disorders (G47.6-)*

G25.0 Essential **tremor**
> Familial tremor
> `EXCLUDES 1` *tremor NOS (R25.1)*

G25.1 Drug-induced **tremor**
> Use additional code for adverse effect, if applicable, to identify drug (T36-T50 with fifth or sixth character 5)

G25.2 **Other specified forms of tremor**
> Intention tremor

G25.3 Myoclonus
> Drug-induced myoclonus
> Palatal myoclonus
> Use additional code for adverse effect, if applicable, to identify drug (T36-T50 with fifth or sixth character 5)
> `EXCLUDES 1` *facial myokymia (G51.4)*
> *myoclonic epilepsy (G40.-)*
> **DEF:** Spasmodic, brief, involuntary muscle contractions that can be due to an undetermined etiology, drug-induced, or caused by a disease process.

G25.4 Drug-induced **chorea**
> Use additional code for adverse effect, if applicable, to identify drug (T36-T50 with fifth or sixth character 5)

G25.5 **Other chorea**
> Chorea NOS
> `EXCLUDES 1` *chorea NOS with heart involvement (I02.0)*
> *Huntington's chorea (G10)*
> *rheumatic chorea (I02.-)*
> *Sydenham's chorea (I02.-)*

☑5ᵗʰ **G25.6** **Drug induced tics and other tics of organic origin**

G25.61 Drug induced **tics**
> Use additional code for adverse effect, if applicable, to identify drug (T36-T50 with fifth or sixth character 5)

G25.69 **Other tics of organic origin**
> `EXCLUDES 1` *habit spasm (F95.9)*
> *tic NOS (F95.9)*
> *Tourette's syndrome (F95.2)*

☑5ᵗʰ **G25.7** **Other and unspecified drug induced movement disorders**
> Use additional code for adverse effect, if applicable, to identify drug (T36-T50 with fifth or sixth character 5)

G25.70 **Drug induced movement disorder, unspecified**

G25.71 **Drug induced akathisia**
> Drug induced acathisia
> Neuroleptic induced acute akathisia
> Tardive akathisia

G25.79 **Other drug induced movement disorders**

☑5ᵗʰ **G25.8** **Other specified extrapyramidal and movement disorders**

G25.81 Restless legs syndrome
> **DEF:** Neurological disorder of unknown etiology creating an irresistible urge to move the legs, which may temporarily relieve the symptoms. This syndrome is accompanied by motor restlessness and sensations of pain, burning, prickling, or tingling.

G25.82 **Stiff-man syndrome**

G25.83 **Benign shuddering attacks**

G25.89 **Other specified extrapyramidal and movement disorders**

G25.9 Extrapyramidal and movement disorder, **unspecified**

G26 *Extrapyramidal and movement disorders in diseases classified elsewhere*
> Code first underlying disease

`HCC` CMS-HCC   `Rx` Rx HCC   `ESR` ESRD HCC   `COM` Commercial HCC   `N` Newborn: 0   `P` Pediatric: 0-17   `M` Maternity: 9-64   `A` Adult: 15-124

592   ICD-10-CM 2023

Other degenerative diseases of the nervous system (G30-G32)

☑️4ᵗʰ G30 Alzheimer's disease

INCLUDES Alzheimer's dementia senile and presenile forms

▶Use additional code, if applicable, to identify:◀

delirium, if applicable (F05)

▶dementia with anxiety (F02.84, F02.A4, F02.B4, F02.C4)◀

dementia with behavioral disturbance ▶(F02.81-, F02.A1-, F02.B1-, F02.C1-)◀

▶dementia with mood disturbance (F02.83, F02.A3, F02.B3, F02.C3)◀

▶dementia with psychotic disturbance (F02.82, F02.A2, F02.B2, F02.C2)◀

dementia without behavioral disturbance ▶(F02.80, F02.A0, F02.B0, F02.C0)◀

▶mild neurocognitive disorder due to known physiological condition (F06.7-)◀

EXCLUDES 1   senile degeneration of brain NEC (G31.1)

senile dementia NOS (F03)

senility NOS (R41.81)

AHA: 2017,1Q,43

TIP: A code from subcategory F02.8 should always be assigned with a code from this category, even in the absence of documented dementia.
TIP: Functional quadriplegia (R53.2) is not integral to Alzheimer's disease and can be coded in addition to codes from category G30.

G30.0   **Alzheimer's disease with** early onset   HCC Rx ESR

G30.1   **Alzheimer's disease with** late onset   HCC Rx ESR A

G30.8   **Other Alzheimer's disease**   HCC Rx ESR

G30.9   **Alzheimer's disease, unspecified**   HCC Rx ESR
     AHA: 2016,2Q,6; 2012,4Q,95

☑️4ᵗʰ G31 Other degenerative diseases of nervous system, not elsewhere classified

For codes G31.0 - G31.83, G31.85 - G31.9, use additional code, if applicable, to identify:

▶dementia with anxiety (F02.84, F02.A4, F02.B4, F02.C4)◀

dementia with behavioral disturbance ▶(F02.81-, F02.A1-, F02.B1-, F02.C1-)◀

▶dementia with mood disturbance (F02.83, F02.A3, F02.B3, F02.C3)◀

▶dementia with psychotic disturbance (F02.82, F02.A2, F02.B2, F02.C2)◀

dementia without behavioral disturbance ▶(F02.80, F02.A0, F02.B0, F02.C0)◀

▶mild neurocognitive disorder due to known physiological condition (F06.7-)◀

EXCLUDES 2   Reye's syndrome (G93.7)

☑️5ᵗʰ G31.0 Frontotemporal dementia

G31.01   **Pick's disease**   HCC Rx ESR

Primary progressive aphasia

Progressive isolated aphasia

DEF: Progressive frontotemporal dementia with asymmetrical atrophy of the frontal and temporal regions of the cerebral cortex and abnormal rounded brain cells called Pick cells with the presence of abnormal staining of protein (called tau). Symptoms include prominent apathy, behavioral changes such as disinhibition and restlessness, echolalia, impairment of language, memory, and intellect, increased carelessness, poor personal hygiene, and decreased attention span.

G31.09   **Other frontotemporal neurocognitive disorder**   HCC Rx ESR

Frontal dementia

▶Use additional code, if applicable, to identify mild neurocognitive disorders due to known physiological condition (F06.7-)◀

G31.1 Senile degeneration of brain, not elsewhere classified   HCC Rx ESR

EXCLUDES 1   Alzheimer's disease (G30.-)

senility NOS (R41.81)

G31.2 Degeneration of nervous system due to alcohol   HCC Rx ESR

Alcoholic cerebellar ataxia

Alcoholic cerebellar degeneration

Alcoholic cerebral degeneration

Alcoholic encephalopathy

Dysfunction of the autonomic nervous system due to alcohol

Code also associated alcoholism (F10.-)

☑️5ᵗʰ G31.8 Other specified degenerative diseases of nervous system

G31.81   **Alpers disease**   HCC Rx ESR COM

Grey-matter degeneration

G31.82   **Leigh's disease**   HCC Rx ESR COM

Subacute necrotizing encephalopathy

G31.83   **Neurocognitive disorder with Lewy bodies**   HCC Rx ESR

~~Dementia with Parkinsonism~~

Lewy body dementia

Lewy body disease

▶Use additional code, if applicable, to identify mild neurocognitive disorders due to known physiological condition (F06.7-)◀

AHA: 2017,2Q,7; 2016,4Q,141

DEF: Cerebral dementia with neurophysiologic changes, increased hippocampal volume, hypoperfusion in the occipital lobes, beta amyloid deposits with neurofibrillary tangles, and atrophy of the cortex and brainstem. Hallmark neuropsychological characteristics include fluctuating cognition with pronounced variation in attention and alertness, recurrent hallucinations, and Parkinsonism.

G31.84   **Mild cognitive impairment of uncertain or unknown etiology**

▶Mild cognitive disorder NOS◀

~~Mild neurocognitive disorder~~

▶Mild neurocognitive disorder of uncertain or unknown etiology◀

▶Use additional code to identify presence of:◀

▶alcohol abuse and dependence (F10.-)◀

▶exposure to environmental tobacco smoke (Z77.22)◀

▶history of tobacco dependence (Z87.891)◀

▶hypertension (I10-I16)◀

▶occupational exposure to environmental tobacco smoke (Z57.31)◀

▶tobacco dependence (F17.-)◀

▶tobacco use (Z72.0)◀

EXCLUDES 1   age related cognitive decline (R41.81)

altered mental status (R41.82)

cerebral degeneration (G31.9)

▶cerebrovascular diseases (I60-I69)◀

change in mental status (R41.82)

cognitive deficits following (sequelae of) cerebral hemorrhage or infarction (I69.01-, I69.11-, I69.21-, I69.31-, I69.81-, I69.91-)

cognitive impairment due to intracranial or head injury (S06.-)

dementia (F01.-, F02.-, F03)

~~mild memory disturbance (F06.8)~~

▶mild neurocognitive disorder due to a known physiological condition (F06.7-)◀

neurologic neglect syndrome (R41.4)

personality change, nonpsychotic (F68.8)

AHA: 2021,3Q,3

G31.85   **Corticobasal degeneration**   HCC Rx ESR

G31.89   **Other specified degenerative diseases of nervous system**   HCC Rx ESR

G31.9 Degenerative disease of nervous system, unspecified   HCC Rx ESR

AHA: 2021,3Q,3

☑️4ᵗʰ G32 Other degenerative disorders of nervous system in diseases classified elsewhere

G32.0 *Subacute combined degeneration of spinal cord in diseases classified elsewhere*   HCC Rx ESR COM

Dana-Putnam syndrome

Sclerosis of spinal cord (combined) (dorsolateral) (posterolateral)

Code first underlying disease, such as:

anemia (D51.9)

dietary (D51.3)

pernicious (D51.0)

vitamin B12 deficiency (E53.8)

EXCLUDES 1   syphilitic combined degeneration of spinal cord (A52.11)

✓5ᵗʰ **G32.8** **Other specified degenerative disorders of nervous system in diseases classified elsewhere**
Code first underlying disease, such as:
amyloidosis cerebral degeneration (E85.-)
cerebral degeneration (due to) hypothyroidism (E00.0-E03.9)
cerebral degeneration (due to) neoplasm (C00-D49)
cerebral degeneration (due to) vitamin B deficiency, except thiamine (E52-E53.-)
EXCLUDES 1   *superior hemorrhagic polioencephalitis [Wernicke's encephalopathy] (E51.2)*

G32.81 *Cerebellar ataxia in diseases classified elsewhere* HCC ESR COM
Code first underlying disease, such as:
celiac disease (with gluten ataxia) (K90.0)
cerebellar ataxia (in) neoplastic disease (paraneoplastic cerebellar degeneration) (C00-D49)
non-celiac gluten ataxia (M35.9)
EXCLUDES 1   *systemic atrophy primarily affecting the central nervous system in alcoholic cerebellar ataxia (G31.2)*
systemic atrophy primarily affecting the central nervous system in myxedema (G13.2)

G32.89 *Other specified degenerative disorders of nervous system in diseases classified elsewhere*
Degenerative encephalopathy in diseases classified elsewhere

Demyelinating diseases of the central nervous system (G35-G37)

G35 Multiple sclerosis HCC Rx ESR COM
Disseminated multiple sclerosis
Generalized multiple sclerosis
Multiple sclerosis NOS
Multiple sclerosis of brain stem
Multiple sclerosis of cord
AHA: 2021,1Q,7

✓4ᵗʰ **G36** **Other acute disseminated demyelination**
EXCLUDES 1   *postinfectious encephalitis and encephalomyelitis NOS (G04.01)*
DEF: Demyelination: Abnormal loss of myelin, the protective white matter that insulates nerve endings and facilitates neuroreception and neurotransmission. When this substance is damaged, the nerve is short-circuited, resulting in impaired or loss of function.

G36.0 **Neuromyelitis optica [Devic]** HCC Rx ESR COM
Demyelination in optic neuritis
EXCLUDES 1   *optic neuritis NOS (H46)*

G36.1 **Acute and subacute hemorrhagic leukoencephalitis [Hurst]** HCC ESR

G36.8 **Other specified acute disseminated demyelination** HCC ESR

G36.9 **Acute disseminated demyelination, unspecified** HCC ESR

✓4ᵗʰ **G37** **Other demyelinating diseases of central nervous system**

G37.0 **Diffuse sclerosis of central nervous system** HCC Rx ESR COM
Periaxial encephalitis
Schilder's disease
EXCLUDES 1   *X linked adrenoleukodystrophy (E71.52-)*

G37.1 **Central demyelination of corpus callosum** HCC ESR

G37.2 **Central pontine myelinolysis** HCC ESR
AHA: 2022,2Q,10

G37.3 **Acute transverse myelitis in demyelinating disease of central nervous system** HCC Rx ESR COM
Acute transverse myelitis NOS
Acute transverse myelopathy
EXCLUDES 1   *acute flaccid myelitis (G04.82)*
multiple sclerosis (G35)
neuromyelitis optica [Devic] (G36.0)

G37.4 **Subacute necrotizing myelitis of central nervous system** HCC Rx ESR COM

G37.5 **Concentric sclerosis [Balo] of central nervous system** HCC Rx ESR COM

G37.8 **Other specified demyelinating diseases of central nervous system** HCC ESR

G37.9 **Demyelinating disease of central nervous system, unspecified** HCC ESR

Episodic and paroxysmal disorders (G40-G47)

✓4ᵗʰ **G40** **Epilepsy and recurrent seizures**
NOTE   The following terms are to be considered equivalent to intractable: pharmacoresistant (pharmacologically resistant), treatment resistant, refractory (medically) and poorly controlled
EXCLUDES 1   *conversion disorder with seizures (F44.5)*
convulsions NOS (R56.9)
post traumatic seizures (R56.1)
seizure (convulsive) NOS (R56.9)
seizure of newborn (P90)
EXCLUDES 2   *hippocampal sclerosis (G93.81)*
mesial temporal sclerosis (G93.81)
temporal sclerosis (G93.81)
Todd's paralysis (G83.84)

✓5ᵗʰ **G40.0** **Localization-related (focal) (partial) idiopathic epilepsy and epileptic syndromes with** seizures of localized onset
Benign childhood epilepsy with centrotemporal EEG spikes
Childhood epilepsy with occipital EEG paroxysms
EXCLUDES 1   *adult onset localization-related epilepsy (G40.1-, G40.2-)*

✓6ᵗʰ **G40.00** **Localization-related (focal) (partial) idiopathic epilepsy and epileptic syndromes with seizures of localized onset,** not intractable
Localization-related (focal) (partial) idiopathic epilepsy and epileptic syndromes with seizures of localized onset without intractability

G40.001 **Localization-related (focal) (partial) idiopathic epilepsy and epileptic syndromes with seizures of localized onset, not intractable,** with status epilepticus HCC Rx ESR COM

G40.009 **Localization-related (focal) (partial) idiopathic epilepsy and epileptic syndromes with seizures of localized onset, not intractable,** without status epilepticus HCC Rx ESR COM
Localization-related (focal) (partial) idiopathic epilepsy and epileptic syndromes with seizures of localized onset NOS

✓6ᵗʰ **G40.01** **Localization-related (focal) (partial) idiopathic epilepsy and epileptic syndromes with seizures of localized onset,** intractable

G40.011 **Localization-related (focal) (partial) idiopathic epilepsy and epileptic syndromes with seizures of localized onset, intractable,** with status epilepticus HCC Rx ESR COM

G40.019 **Localization-related (focal) (partial) idiopathic epilepsy and epileptic syndromes with seizures of localized onset, intractable,** without status epilepticus HCC Rx ESR COM

✓5ᵗʰ **G40.1** **Localization-related (focal) (partial) symptomatic epilepsy and epileptic syndromes with** simple partial seizures
Attacks without alteration of consciousness
Epilepsia partialis continua [Kozhevnikof]
Simple partial seizures developing into secondarily generalized seizures

✓6ᵗʰ **G40.10** **Localization-related (focal) (partial) symptomatic epilepsy and epileptic syndromes with simple partial seizures,** not intractable
Localization-related (focal) (partial) symptomatic epilepsy and epileptic syndromes with simple partial seizures without intractability

G40.101 **Localization-related (focal) (partial) symptomatic epilepsy and epileptic syndromes with simple partial seizures, not intractable,** with status epilepticus HCC Rx ESR COM

G40.109   Localization-related (focal) (partial) symptomatic epilepsy and epileptic syndromes with simple partial seizures, not intractable, without status epilepticus   `HCC` `Rx` `ESR` `COM`

Localization-related (focal) (partial) symptomatic epilepsy and epileptic syndromes with simple partial seizures NOS

✓6th G40.11   Localization-related (focal) (partial) symptomatic epilepsy and epileptic syndromes with simple partial seizures, intractable

G40.111   Localization-related (focal) (partial) symptomatic epilepsy and epileptic syndromes with simple partial seizures, intractable, with status epilepticus   `HCC` `Rx` `ESR` `COM`

G40.119   Localization-related (focal) (partial) symptomatic epilepsy and epileptic syndromes with simple partial seizures, intractable, without status epilepticus   `HCC` `Rx` `ESR` `COM`

✓5th G40.2   Localization-related (focal) (partial) symptomatic epilepsy and epileptic syndromes with complex partial seizures

Attacks with alteration of consciousness, often with automatisms

Complex partial seizures developing into secondarily generalized seizures

✓6th G40.20   Localization-related (focal) (partial) symptomatic epilepsy and epileptic syndromes with complex partial seizures, not intractable

Localization-related (focal) (partial) symptomatic epilepsy and epileptic syndromes with complex partial seizures without intractability

G40.201   Localization-related (focal) (partial) symptomatic epilepsy and epileptic syndromes with complex partial seizures, not intractable, with status epilepticus   `HCC` `Rx` `ESR` `COM`

G40.209   Localization-related (focal) (partial) symptomatic epilepsy and epileptic syndromes with complex partial seizures, not intractable, without status epilepticus   `HCC` `Rx` `ESR` `COM`

Localization-related (focal) (partial) symptomatic epilepsy and epileptic syndromes with complex partial seizures NOS

✓6th G40.21   Localization-related (focal) (partial) symptomatic epilepsy and epileptic syndromes with complex partial seizures, intractable

G40.211   Localization-related (focal) (partial) symptomatic epilepsy and epileptic syndromes with complex partial seizures, intractable, with status epilepticus   `HCC` `Rx` `ESR` `COM`

G40.219   Localization-related (focal) (partial) symptomatic epilepsy and epileptic syndromes with complex partial seizures, intractable, without status epilepticus   `HCC` `Rx` `ESR` `COM`

✓5th G40.3   Generalized idiopathic epilepsy and epileptic syndromes

Code also MERRF syndrome, if applicable (E88.42)

✓6th G40.30   Generalized idiopathic epilepsy and epileptic syndromes, not intractable

Generalized idiopathic epilepsy and epileptic syndromes without intractability

G40.301   Generalized idiopathic epilepsy and epileptic syndromes, not intractable, with status epilepticus   `HCC` `Rx` `ESR` `COM`

G40.309   Generalized idiopathic epilepsy and epileptic syndromes, not intractable, without status epilepticus   `HCC` `Rx` `ESR` `COM`

Generalized idiopathic epilepsy and epileptic syndromes NOS

✓6th G40.31   Generalized idiopathic epilepsy and epileptic syndromes, intractable

G40.311   Generalized idiopathic epilepsy and epileptic syndromes, intractable, with status epilepticus   `HCC` `Rx` `ESR` `COM`

G40.319   Generalized idiopathic epilepsy and epileptic syndromes, intractable, without status epilepticus   `HCC` `Rx` `ESR` `COM`

✓5th G40.A   Absence epileptic syndrome

Childhood absence epilepsy [pyknolepsy]
Juvenile absence epilepsy
Absence epileptic syndrome, NOS

✓6th G40.A0   Absence epileptic syndrome, not intractable

G40.A01   Absence epileptic syndrome, not intractable, with status epilepticus   `HCC` `Rx` `ESR` `COM`

G40.A09   Absence epileptic syndrome, not intractable, without status epilepticus   `HCC` `Rx` `ESR` `COM`

✓6th G40.A1   Absence epileptic syndrome, intractable

G40.A11   Absence epileptic syndrome, intractable, with status epilepticus   `HCC` `Rx` `ESR` `COM`

G40.A19   Absence epileptic syndrome, intractable, without status epilepticus   `HCC` `Rx` `ESR` `COM`

✓5th G40.B   Juvenile myoclonic epilepsy [impulsive petit mal]

✓6th G40.B0   Juvenile myoclonic epilepsy, not intractable

G40.B01   Juvenile myoclonic epilepsy, not intractable, with status epilepticus   `HCC` `Rx` `ESR` `COM`

G40.B09   Juvenile myoclonic epilepsy, not intractable, without status epilepticus   `HCC` `Rx` `ESR` `COM`

✓6th G40.B1   Juvenile myoclonic epilepsy, intractable

G40.B11   Juvenile myoclonic epilepsy, intractable, with status epilepticus   `HCC` `Rx` `ESR` `COM`

G40.B19   Juvenile myoclonic epilepsy, intractable, without status epilepticus   `HCC` `Rx` `ESR` `COM`

✓5th G40.4   Other generalized epilepsy and epileptic syndromes

Epilepsy with grand mal seizures on awakening
Epilepsy with myoclonic absences
Epilepsy with myoclonic-astatic seizures
Grand mal seizure NOS
Nonspecific atonic epileptic seizures
Nonspecific clonic epileptic seizures
Nonspecific myoclonic epileptic seizures
Nonspecific tonic epileptic seizures
Nonspecific tonic-clonic epileptic seizures
Symptomatic early myoclonic encephalopathy

✓6th G40.40   Other generalized epilepsy and epileptic syndromes, not intractable

Other generalized epilepsy and epileptic syndromes without intractability

Other generalized epilepsy and epileptic syndromes NOS

G40.401   Other generalized epilepsy and epileptic syndromes, not intractable, with status epilepticus   `HCC` `Rx` `ESR` `COM`

G40.409   Other generalized epilepsy and epileptic syndromes, not intractable, without status epilepticus   `HCC` `Rx` `ESR` `COM`

✓6th G40.41   Other generalized epilepsy and epileptic syndromes, intractable

G40.411   Other generalized epilepsy and epileptic syndromes, intractable, with status epilepticus   `HCC` `Rx` `ESR` `COM`

G40.419   Other generalized epilepsy and epileptic syndromes, intractable, without status epilepticus   `HCC` `Rx` `ESR` `COM`

G40.42   Cyclin-Dependent Kinase-Like 5 Deficiency Disorder   `HCC` `Rx` `ESR` `COM`

CDKL5

Use additional code, if known, to identify associated manifestations, such as:
cortical blindness (H47.61-)
global development delay (F88)

AHA: 2020,4Q,18-19

✓5ᵗʰ G40.5 Epileptic seizures related to external causes

Epileptic seizures related to alcohol
Epileptic seizures related to drugs
Epileptic seizures related to hormonal changes
Epileptic seizures related to sleep deprivation
Epileptic seizures related to stress
Code also, if applicable, associated epilepsy and recurrent seizures (G40.-)
Use additional code for adverse effect, if applicable, to identify drug (T36-T50 with fifth or sixth character 5)

✓6ᵗʰ G40.50 Epileptic seizures related to external causes, not intractable

G40.501 Epileptic seizures related to external causes, not intractable, with status epilepticus HCC Rx ESR COM

G40.509 Epileptic seizures related to external causes, not intractable, without status epilepticus HCC Rx ESR COM
Epileptic seizures related to external causes, NOS

✓5ᵗʰ G40.8 Other epilepsy and recurrent seizures

Epilepsies and epileptic syndromes undetermined as to whether they are focal or generalized
Landau-Kleffner syndrome

✓6ᵗʰ G40.80 Other epilepsy

G40.801 Other epilepsy, not intractable, with status epilepticus HCC Rx ESR COM
Other epilepsy without intractability with status epilepticus

G40.802 Other epilepsy, not intractable, without status epilepticus HCC Rx ESR COM
Other epilepsy NOS
Other epilepsy without intractability without status epilepticus

G40.803 Other epilepsy, intractable, with status epilepticus HCC Rx ESR COM

G40.804 Other epilepsy, intractable, without status epilepticus HCC Rx ESR COM

✓6ᵗʰ G40.81 Lennox-Gastaut syndrome

DEF: Severe form of epilepsy with usual onset in early childhood. Seizures are frequent and difficult to treat, causing falls and intellectual impairment.

G40.811 Lennox-Gastaut syndrome, not intractable, with status epilepticus HCC Rx ESR COM

G40.812 Lennox-Gastaut syndrome, not intractable, without status epilepticus HCC Rx ESR COM

G40.813 Lennox-Gastaut syndrome, intractable, with status epilepticus HCC Rx ESR COM

G40.814 Lennox-Gastaut syndrome, intractable, without status epilepticus HCC Rx ESR COM

✓6ᵗʰ G40.82 Epileptic spasms

Infantile spasms
Salaam attacks
West's syndrome

G40.821 Epileptic spasms, not intractable, with status epilepticus HCC Rx ESR COM

G40.822 Epileptic spasms, not intractable, without status epilepticus HCC Rx ESR COM

G40.823 Epileptic spasms, intractable, with status epilepticus HCC Rx ESR COM

G40.824 Epileptic spasms, intractable, without status epilepticus HCC Rx ESR COM

✓6ᵗʰ G40.83 Dravet syndrome

Polymorphic epilepsy in infancy (PMEI)
Severe myoclonic epilepsy in infancy (SMEI)
AHA: 2020,4Q,19

G40.833 Dravet syndrome, intractable, with status epilepticus HCC Rx ESR COM

G40.834 Dravet syndrome, intractable, without status epilepticus HCC Rx ESR COM
Dravet syndrome NOS

G40.89 Other seizures HCC Rx ESR COM
EXCLUDES 1 post traumatic seizures (R56.1)
recurrent seizures NOS (G40.909)
seizure NOS (R56.9)

✓5ᵗʰ G40.9 Epilepsy, unspecified
AHA: 2019,1Q,19

✓6ᵗʰ G40.90 Epilepsy, unspecified, not intractable
Epilepsy, unspecified, without intractability

G40.901 Epilepsy, unspecified, not intractable, with status epilepticus HCC Rx ESR COM

G40.909 Epilepsy, unspecified, not intractable, without status epilepticus HCC Rx ESR COM
Epilepsy NOS
Epileptic convulsions NOS
Epileptic fits NOS
Epileptic seizures NOS
Recurrent seizures NOS
Seizure disorder NOS
AHA: 2021,2Q,3; 2021,1Q,3

✓6ᵗʰ G40.91 Epilepsy, unspecified, intractable
Intractable seizure disorder NOS

G40.911 Epilepsy, unspecified, intractable, with status epilepticus HCC Rx ESR COM

G40.919 Epilepsy, unspecified, intractable, without status epilepticus HCC Rx ESR COM

✓4ᵗʰ G43 Migraine

NOTE The following terms are to be considered equivalent to intractable: pharmacoresistant (pharmacologically resistant), treatment resistant, refractory (medically) and poorly controlled

Use additional code for adverse effect, if applicable, to identify drug (T36-T50 with fifth or sixth character 5)
EXCLUDES 1 headache NOS (R51.9)
lower half migraine (G44.00)
EXCLUDES 2 headache syndromes (G44.-)
DEF: Headaches that occur periodically on one or both sides of the head that may be associated with nausea and vomiting, sensitivity to light and sound, dizziness, distorted vision, and cognitive disturbances.

✓5ᵗʰ G43.0 Migraine without aura
Common migraine
EXCLUDES 1 chronic migraine without aura (G43.7-)

✓6ᵗʰ G43.00 Migraine without aura, not intractable
Migraine without aura without mention of refractory migraine

G43.001 Migraine without aura, not intractable, with status migrainosus Rx

G43.009 Migraine without aura, not intractable, without status migrainosus Rx
Migraine without aura NOS

✓6ᵗʰ G43.01 Migraine without aura, intractable
Migraine without aura with refractory migraine

G43.011 Migraine without aura, intractable, with status migrainosus Rx

G43.019 Migraine without aura, intractable, without status migrainosus Rx

✓5ᵗʰ G43.1 Migraine with aura
Basilar migraine
Classical migraine
Migraine equivalents
Migraine preceded or accompanied by transient focal neurological phenomena
Migraine triggered seizures
Migraine with acute-onset aura
Migraine with aura without headache (migraine equivalents)
Migraine with prolonged aura
Migraine with typical aura
Retinal migraine
Code also any associated seizure (G40.-, R56.9)
EXCLUDES 1 persistent migraine aura (G43.5-, G43.6-)

✓6ᵗʰ G43.10 Migraine with aura, not intractable
Migraine with aura without mention of refractory migraine

G43.101 Migraine with aura, not intractable, with status migrainosus Rx *classical migraine.* [handwritten]

G43.109   **Migraine with aura, not intractable, without status migrainosus**   Rx
     Migraine with aura NOS

√6ᵗʰ   **G43.11**   **Migraine with aura,** intractable
     Migraine with aura with refractory migraine

G43.111   **Migraine with aura, intractable,** with status migrainosus   Rx

G43.119   **Migraine with aura, intractable,** without status migrainosus   Rx

√5ᵗʰ   **G43.4**   **Hemiplegic migraine**
     Familial migraine
     Sporadic migraine

√6ᵗʰ   **G43.40**   **Hemiplegic migraine,** not intractable
     Hemiplegic migraine without refractory migraine

G43.401   **Hemiplegic migraine, not intractable, with status migrainosus**   Rx

G43.409   **Hemiplegic migraine, not intractable, without status migrainosus**   Rx
     Hemiplegic migraine NOS

√6ᵗʰ   **G43.41**   **Hemiplegic migraine,** intractable
     Hemiplegic migraine with refractory migraine

G43.411   **Hemiplegic migraine, intractable,** with status migrainosus   Rx

G43.419   **Hemiplegic migraine, intractable,** without status migrainosus   Rx

√5ᵗʰ   **G43.5**   **Persistent migraine aura without cerebral infarction**

√6ᵗʰ   **G43.50**   **Persistent migraine aura without cerebral infarction,** not intractable
     Persistent migraine aura without cerebral infarction, without refractory migraine

G43.501   **Persistent migraine aura without cerebral infarction, not intractable,** with status migrainosus   Rx

G43.509   **Persistent migraine aura without cerebral infarction, not intractable,** without status migrainosus   Rx
     Persistent migraine aura NOS

√6ᵗʰ   **G43.51**   **Persistent migraine aura without cerebral infarction,** intractable
     Persistent migraine aura without cerebral infarction, with refractory migraine

G43.511   **Persistent migraine aura without cerebral infarction, intractable,** with status migrainosus   Rx

G43.519   **Persistent migraine aura without cerebral infarction, intractable,** without status migrainosus   Rx

√5ᵗʰ   **G43.6**   **Persistent migraine aura with cerebral infarction**
     Code also the type of cerebral infarction (I63.-)

√6ᵗʰ   **G43.60**   **Persistent migraine aura with cerebral infarction, not intractable**
     Persistent migraine aura with cerebral infarction, without refractory migraine

G43.601   **Persistent migraine aura with cerebral infarction, not intractable,** with status migrainosus   Rx

G43.609   **Persistent migraine aura with cerebral infarction, not intractable,** without status migrainosus   Rx

√6ᵗʰ   **G43.61**   **Persistent migraine aura with cerebral infarction, intractable**
     Persistent migraine aura with cerebral infarction, with refractory migraine

G43.611   **Persistent migraine aura with cerebral infarction, intractable,** with status migrainosus   Rx

G43.619   **Persistent migraine aura with cerebral infarction, intractable,** without status migrainosus   Rx

√5ᵗʰ   **G43.7**   **Chronic migraine** without aura
     Transformed migraine
     EXCLUDES 1   *migraine without aura (G43.0-)*

√6ᵗʰ   **G43.70**   **Chronic migraine without aura,** not intractable
     Chronic migraine without aura, without refractory migraine

G43.701   **Chronic migraine without aura, not intractable,** with status migrainosus   Rx

G43.709   **Chronic migraine without aura, not intractable,** without status migrainosus   Rx
     Chronic migraine without aura NOS

√6ᵗʰ   **G43.71**   **Chronic migraine without aura,** intractable
     Chronic migraine without aura, with refractory migraine

G43.711   **Chronic migraine without aura, intractable,** with status migrainosus   Rx

G43.719   **Chronic migraine without aura, intractable,** without status migrainosus   Rx

√5ᵗʰ   **G43.A**   **Cyclical vomiting**
     EXCLUDES 1   *cyclical vomiting syndrome unrelated to migraine (R11.15)*
     AHA: 2019,4Q,15

G43.A0   **Cyclical vomiting, in migraine,** not intractable
     Cyclical vomiting, without refractory migraine

G43.A1   **Cyclical vomiting, in migraine,** intractable   Rx
     Cyclical vomiting, with refractory migraine

√5ᵗʰ   **G43.B**   **Ophthalmoplegic migraine**

G43.B0   **Ophthalmoplegic migraine,** not intractable   Rx
     Ophthalmoplegic migraine, without refractory migraine

G43.B1   **Ophthalmoplegic migraine,** intractable   Rx
     Ophthalmoplegic migraine, with refractory migraine

√5ᵗʰ   **G43.C**   **Periodic headache syndromes in child or adult**

G43.C0   **Periodic headache syndromes in child or adult,** not intractable   Rx
     Periodic headache syndromes in child or adult, without refractory migraine

G43.C1   **Periodic headache syndromes in child or adult,** intractable   Rx
     Periodic headache syndromes in child or adult, with refractory migraine

√5ᵗʰ   **G43.D**   **Abdominal migraine**

G43.D0   **Abdominal migraine,** not intractable   Rx
     Abdominal migraine, without refractory migraine

G43.D1   **Abdominal migraine,** intractable   Rx
     Abdominal migraine, with refractory migraine

√5ᵗʰ   **G43.8**   **Other migraine**

√6ᵗʰ   **G43.80**   **Other migraine,** not intractable
     Other migraine, without refractory migraine

G43.801   **Other migraine, not intractable,** with status migrainosus   Rx

G43.809   **Other migraine, not intractable,** without status migrainosus   Rx

√6ᵗʰ   **G43.81**   **Other migraine,** intractable
     Other migraine, with refractory migraine

G43.811   **Other migraine, intractable,** with status migrainosus   Rx

G43.819   **Other migraine, intractable,** without status migrainosus   Rx

√6ᵗʰ   **G43.82**   **Menstrual migraine,** not intractable
     Menstrual headache, not intractable
     Menstrual migraine, without refractory migraine
     Menstrually related migraine, not intractable
     Pre-menstrual headache, not intractable
     Pre-menstrual migraine, not intractable
     Pure menstrual migraine, not intractable
     Code also associated premenstrual tension syndrome (N94.3)

G43.821   **Menstrual migraine, not intractable,** with status migrainosus   Rx ♀

G43.829   **Menstrual migraine, not intractable,** without status migrainosus   Rx ♀
     Menstrual migraine NOS

✔ Additional Character Required   √x7ᵗʰ Placeholder Alert   Manifestation   Unspecified Dx   Q QPP   UPD Unacceptable PDx

Chapter 6. Diseases of the Nervous System

✓6ᵗʰ **G43.83** Menstrual migraine, intractable

Menstrual headache, intractable

Menstrual migraine, with refractory migraine

Menstrually related migraine, intractable

Pre-menstrual headache, intractable

Pre-menstrual migraine, intractable

Pure menstrual migraine, intractable

Code also associated premenstrual tension syndrome (N94.3)

G43.831 **Menstrual migraine, intractable, with status migrainosus** Rx ♀

G43.839 **Menstrual migraine, intractable, without status migrainosus** Rx ♀

✓5ᵗʰ **G43.9** Migraine, unspecified

✓6ᵗʰ **G43.90** Migraine, unspecified, not intractable

Migraine, unspecified, without refractory migraine

G43.901 **Migraine, unspecified, not intractable, with status migrainosus** Rx

Status migrainosus NOS

G43.909 **Migraine, unspecified, not intractable, without status migrainosus** Rx

Migraine NOS

✓6ᵗʰ **G43.91** Migraine, unspecified, intractable

Migraine, unspecified, with refractory migraine

G43.911 **Migraine, unspecified, intractable, with status migrainosus** Rx

G43.919 **Migraine, unspecified, intractable, without status migrainosus** Rx

✓4ᵗʰ **G44** **Other headache syndromes**

EXCLUDES 1 headache NOS (R51.9)

EXCLUDES 2 atypical facial pain (G50.1)

headache due to lumbar puncture (G97.1)

migraines (G43.-)

trigeminal neuralgia (G50.0)

✓5ᵗʰ **G44.0** **Cluster headaches and other trigeminal autonomic cephalgias (TAC)**

DEF: Cluster headache: Characteristic grouping or clustering of headaches that can last for a number of weeks or months and then completely disappear for months or years. They are typically not associated with gastrointestinal upset or light sensitivity as experienced in migraines.

✓6ᵗʰ **G44.00** Cluster headache syndrome, unspecified

Ciliary neuralgia

Cluster headache NOS

Histamine cephalgia

Lower half migraine

Migrainous neuralgia

G44.001 **Cluster headache syndrome, unspecified, intractable**

G44.009 **Cluster headache syndrome, unspecified, not intractable**

Cluster headache syndrome NOS

✓6ᵗʰ **G44.01** Episodic cluster headache

G44.011 **Episodic cluster headache, intractable**

G44.019 **Episodic cluster headache, not intractable**

Episodic cluster headache NOS

✓6ᵗʰ **G44.02** Chronic cluster headache

G44.021 **Chronic cluster headache, intractable**

G44.029 **Chronic cluster headache, not intractable**

Chronic cluster headache NOS

✓6ᵗʰ **G44.03** Episodic paroxysmal hemicrania

Paroxysmal hemicrania NOS

G44.031 **Episodic paroxysmal hemicrania, intractable**

G44.039 **Episodic paroxysmal hemicrania, not intractable**

Episodic paroxysmal hemicrania NOS

✓6ᵗʰ **G44.04** Chronic paroxysmal hemicrania

G44.041 **Chronic paroxysmal hemicrania, intractable**

G44.049 **Chronic paroxysmal hemicrania, not intractable**

Chronic paroxysmal hemicrania NOS

✓6ᵗʰ **G44.05** Short lasting unilateral neuralgiform headache with conjunctival injection and tearing (SUNCT)

G44.051 **Short lasting unilateral neuralgiform headache with conjunctival injection and tearing (SUNCT), intractable**

G44.059 **Short lasting unilateral neuralgiform headache with conjunctival injection and tearing (SUNCT), not intractable**

Short lasting unilateral neuralgiform headache with conjunctival injection and tearing (SUNCT) NOS

✓6ᵗʰ **G44.09** Other trigeminal autonomic cephalgias (TAC)

G44.091 **Other trigeminal autonomic cephalgias (TAC), intractable**

G44.099 **Other trigeminal autonomic cephalgias (TAC), not intractable**

G44.1 Vascular headache, not elsewhere classified

EXCLUDES 2 cluster headache (G44.0)

complicated headache syndromes (G44.5-)

drug-induced headache (G44.4-)

migraine (G43.-)

other specified headache syndromes (G44.8-)

post-traumatic headache (G44.3-)

tension-type headache (G44.2-)

✓5ᵗʰ **G44.2** Tension-type headache

✓6ᵗʰ **G44.20** Tension-type headache, unspecified

G44.201 **Tension-type headache, unspecified, intractable**

G44.209 **Tension-type headache, unspecified, not intractable**

Tension headache NOS

✓6ᵗʰ **G44.21** Episodic tension-type headache

G44.211 **Episodic tension-type headache, intractable**

G44.219 **Episodic tension-type headache, not intractable**

Episodic tension-type headache NOS

✓6ᵗʰ **G44.22** Chronic tension-type headache

G44.221 **Chronic tension-type headache, intractable**

G44.229 **Chronic tension-type headache, not intractable**

Chronic tension-type headache NOS

✓5ᵗʰ **G44.3** Post-traumatic headache

✓6ᵗʰ **G44.30** Post-traumatic headache, unspecified

G44.301 **Post-traumatic headache, unspecified, intractable**

G44.309 **Post-traumatic headache, unspecified, not intractable**

Post-traumatic headache NOS

✓6ᵗʰ **G44.31** Acute post-traumatic headache

G44.311 **Acute post-traumatic headache, intractable**

G44.319 **Acute post-traumatic headache, not intractable**

Acute post-traumatic headache NOS

✓6ᵗʰ **G44.32** Chronic post-traumatic headache

G44.321 **Chronic post-traumatic headache, intractable**

G44.329 **Chronic post-traumatic headache, not intractable**

Chronic post-traumatic headache NOS

✓5ᵗʰ **G44.4** Drug-induced headache, not elsewhere classified

Medication overuse headache

Use additional code for adverse effect, if applicable, to identify drug (T36-T50 with fifth or sixth character 5)

G44.40 **Drug-induced headache, not elsewhere classified, not intractable**

G44.41 **Drug-induced headache, not elsewhere classified, intractable**

✓5ᵗʰ **G44.5** Complicated headache syndromes

G44.51 Hemicrania continua

DEF: Persistent primary headache of unknown causation occurring on one side of the face and head. May last for more than three months, with daily and continuous pain of moderate intensity with severe exacerbations.

G44.52 New daily persistent headache (NDPH)

G44.53 Primary thunderclap **headache**

G44.59 Other complicated headache syndrome

✓5ᵗʰ **G44.8** Other specified headache syndromes

> EXCLUDES 2   headache with orthostatic or positional component, not elsewhere classifed (R51.0)

G44.81 Hypnic **headache**

G44.82 Headache associated with sexual activity
Orgasmic headache
Preorgasmic headache

G44.83 Primary cough **headache**

G44.84 Primary exertional **headache**

G44.85 Primary stabbing **headache**

G44.86 Cervicogenic **headache**
Code also associated cervical spinal condition, if known
AHA: 2021,4Q,11-12

G44.89 Other headache syndrome

✓4ᵗʰ **G45** Transient cerebral ischemic attacks and related syndromes

> EXCLUDES 1   neonatal cerebral ischemia (P91.0)
> transient retinal artery occlusion (H34.0-)

AHA: 2018,2Q,9
DEF: Transient cerebral ischemic attack: Intermittent or brief cerebral dysfunction from lack of oxygenation with no persistent neurological deficits associated with occlusive vascular disease. TIA may denote an impending cerebrovascular accident.

G45.0 Vertebro-basilar artery syndrome

G45.1 Carotid artery syndrome (hemispheric)

G45.2 Multiple and bilateral precerebral artery syndromes

G45.3 Amaurosis fugax

G45.4 Transient global amnesia
> EXCLUDES 1   amnesia NOS (R41.3)

G45.8 Other transient cerebral ischemic attacks and related syndromes

G45.9 Transient cerebral ischemic attack, unspecified
Spasm of cerebral artery
TIA
Transient cerebral ischemia NOS

✓4ᵗʰ **G46** Vascular syndromes of brain in cerebrovascular diseases
Code first underlying cerebrovascular disease (I60-I69)

G46.0 Middle **cerebral artery syndrome**

G46.1 Anterior **cerebral artery syndrome**

G46.2 Posterior **cerebral artery syndrome**

G46.3 Brain stem stroke **syndrome**
Benedikt syndrome
Claude syndrome
Foville syndrome
Millard-Gubler syndrome
Wallenberg syndrome
Weber syndrome

G46.4 Cerebellar stroke **syndrome**

G46.5 Pure motor lacunar **syndrome**

G46.6 Pure sensory lacunar **syndrome**

G46.7 Other lacunar **syndromes**

G46.8 Other vascular syndromes of brain in cerebrovascular diseases

✓4ᵗʰ **G47** Sleep disorders

> EXCLUDES 2   nightmares (F51.5)
> nonorganic sleep disorders (F51.-)
> sleep terrors (F51.4)
> sleepwalking (F51.3)

✓5ᵗʰ **G47.0** Insomnia

> EXCLUDES 2   alcohol related insomnia (F10.182, F10.282, F10.982)
> drug-related insomnia (F11.182, F11.282, F11.982, F13.182, F13.282, F13.982, F14.182, F14.282, F14.982, F15.182, F15.282, F15.982, F19.182, F19.282, F19.982)
> idiopathic insomnia (F51.01)
> insomnia due to a mental disorder (F51.05)
> insomnia not due to a substance or known physiological condition (F51.0-)
> nonorganic insomnia (F51.0-)
> primary insomnia (F51.01)
> sleep apnea (G47.3-)

G47.00 Insomnia, unspecified
Insomnia NOS

G47.01 Insomnia due to medical condition
Code also associated medical condition

G47.09 Other insomnia

✓5ᵗʰ **G47.1** Hypersomnia

> EXCLUDES 2   alcohol-related hypersomnia (F10.182, F10.282, F10.982)
> drug-related hypersomnia (F11.182, F11.282, F11.982, F13.182, F13.282, F13.982, F14.182, F14.282, F14.982, F15.182, F15.282, F15.982, F19.182, F19.282, F19.982)
> hypersomnia due to a mental disorder (F51.13)
> hypersomnia not due to a substance or known physiological condition (F51.1-)
> primary hypersomnia (F51.11)
> sleep apnea (G47.3-)

G47.10 Hypersomnia, unspecified
Hypersomnia NOS

G47.11 Idiopathic **hypersomnia** with long sleep time
Idiopathic hypersomnia NOS

G47.12 Idiopathic **hypersomnia** without long sleep time

G47.13 Recurrent **hypersomnia**
Kleine-Levin syndrome
Menstrual related hypersomnia

G47.14 Hypersomnia due to medical condition
Code also associated medical condition

G47.19 Other hypersomnia

✓5ᵗʰ **G47.2** Circadian rhythm sleep disorders
Disorders of the sleep wake schedule
Inversion of nyctohemeral rhythm
Inversion of sleep rhythm
DEF: Circadian rhythm: Daily cycle (24-hour period) of physical, mental, and behavioral changes. It is largely influenced by environmental cues, such as changes in light or temperature.
Synonym(s): sleep/wake cycle.

G47.20 Circadian rhythm sleep disorder, unspecified type
Sleep wake schedule disorder NOS

G47.21 Circadian rhythm sleep disorder, delayed sleep phase type
Delayed sleep phase syndrome

G47.22 Circadian rhythm sleep disorder, advanced sleep phase type

G47.23 Circadian rhythm sleep disorder, irregular sleep wake type
Irregular sleep-wake pattern

G47.24 Circadian rhythm sleep disorder, free running type
Circadian rhythm sleep disorder, non-24-hour sleep-wake type

G47.25 Circadian rhythm sleep disorder, jet lag type

G47.26 Circadian rhythm sleep disorder, shift work type

G47.27 Circadian rhythm sleep disorder in conditions classified elsewhere
Code first underlying condition

G47.29 Other circadian rhythm sleep disorder

☑ Additional Character Required   ✓x7ᵗʰ Placeholder Alert   Manifestation   Unspecified Dx   Q QPP   UPD Unacceptable PDx

Chapter 6. Diseases of the Nervous System

G47.3–G53

✓5ᵗʰ **G47.3　Sleep apnea**

Code also any associated underlying condition

EXCLUDES 1　*apnea NOS (R06.81)*

Cheyne-Stokes breathing (R06.3)

pickwickian syndrome (E66.2)

sleep apnea of newborn ▶(P28.3-)◀

G47.30　Sleep apnea, unspecified

Sleep apnea NOS

G47.31　Primary central sleep apnea

Idiopathic central sleep apnea

G47.32　High altitude periodic breathing

G47.33　Obstructive sleep apnea (adult) (pediatric)

Obstructive sleep apnea hypopnea

EXCLUDES 1　*obstructive sleep apnea of newborn*
　　　　　▶(P28.3-)◀

G47.34　Idiopathic sleep related nonobstructive alveolar hypoventilation

Sleep related hypoxia

G47.35　Congenital central alveolar hypoventilation syndrome

G47.36　Sleep related hypoventilation in conditions classified elsewhere

Sleep related hypoxemia in conditions classified elsewhere

Code first underlying condition

G47.37　Central sleep apnea in conditions classified elsewhere

Code first underlying condition

G47.39　Other sleep apnea

✓5ᵗʰ **G47.4　Narcolepsy and cataplexy**

✓6ᵗʰ **G47.41　Narcolepsy**

G47.411　Narcolepsy with cataplexy Rx COM

G47.419　Narcolepsy without cataplexy Rx COM

Narcolepsy NOS

✓6ᵗʰ **G47.42　Narcolepsy in conditions classified elsewhere**

Code first underlying condition

G47.421　Narcolepsy in conditions classified elsewhere with cataplexy Rx COM

G47.429　Narcolepsy in conditions classified elsewhere without cataplexy Rx COM

✓5ᵗʰ **G47.5　Parasomnia**

EXCLUDES 1　*alcohol induced parasomnia (F10.182, F10.282, F10.982)*

drug induced parasomnia (F11.182, F11.282, F11.982, F13.182, F13.282, F13.982, F14.182, F14.282, F14.982, F15.182, F15.282, F15.982, F19.182, F19.282, F19.982)

parasomnia not due to a substance or known physiological condition (F51.8)

G47.50　Parasomnia, unspecified

Parasomnia NOS

G47.51　Confusional arousals

G47.52　REM sleep behavior disorder

G47.53　Recurrent isolated sleep paralysis

G47.54　Parasomnia in conditions classified elsewhere

Code first underlying condition

G47.59　Other parasomnia

✓5ᵗʰ **G47.6　Sleep related movement disorders**

EXCLUDES 2　*restless legs syndrome (G25.81)*

G47.61　Periodic limb movement disorder

G47.62　Sleep related leg cramps

G47.63　Sleep related bruxism

EXCLUDES 1　*psychogenic bruxism (F45.8)*

G47.69　Other sleep related movement disorders

G47.8　Other sleep disorders

Other specified sleep-wake disorder

G47.9　Sleep disorder, unspecified

Sleep disorder NOS

Unspecified sleep-wake disorder

Nerve, nerve root and plexus disorders (G50-G59)

EXCLUDES 1　*current traumatic nerve, nerve root and plexus disorders - see Injury, nerve by body region*

neuralgia NOS (M79.2)

neuritis NOS (M79.2)

peripheral neuritis in pregnancy (O26.82-)

radiculitis NOS (M54.1-)

✓4ᵗʰ **G50　Disorders of trigeminal nerve**

INCLUDES　disorders of 5th cranial nerve

G50.0　Trigeminal neuralgia Rx

Syndrome of paroxysmal facial pain

Tic douloureux

G50.1　Atypical facial pain Rx

G50.8　Other disorders of trigeminal nerve Rx

G50.9　Disorder of trigeminal nerve, unspecified Rx

✓4ᵗʰ **G51　Facial nerve disorders**

INCLUDES　disorders of 7th cranial nerve

G51.0　Bell's palsy

Facial palsy

G51.1　Geniculate ganglionitis

EXCLUDES 1　*postherpetic geniculate ganglionitis (B02.21)*

G51.2　Melkersson's syndrome

Melkersson-Rosenthal syndrome

✓5ᵗʰ **G51.3　Clonic hemifacial spasm**

AHA: 2018,4Q,10

G51.31　Clonic hemifacial spasm, right

G51.32　Clonic hemifacial spasm, left

G51.33　Clonic hemifacial spasm, bilateral

G51.39　Clonic hemifacial spasm, unspecified

G51.4　Facial myokymia

G51.8　Other disorders of facial nerve

G51.9　Disorder of facial nerve, unspecified

✓4ᵗʰ **G52　Disorders of other cranial nerves**

EXCLUDES 2　*disorders of acoustic [8th] nerve (H93.3)*

disorders of optic [2nd] nerve (H46, H47.0)

paralytic strabismus due to nerve palsy (H49.0-H49.2)

G52.0　Disorders of olfactory nerve

Disorders of 1st cranial nerve

G52.1　Disorders of glossopharyngeal nerve

Disorder of 9th cranial nerve

Glossopharyngeal neuralgia

G52.2　Disorders of vagus nerve

Disorders of pneumogastric [10th] nerve

G52.3　Disorders of hypoglossal nerve

Disorders of 12th cranial nerve

G52.7　Disorders of multiple cranial nerves

Polyneuritis cranialis

G52.8　Disorders of other specified cranial nerves

G52.9　Cranial nerve disorder, unspecified

G53　Cranial nerve disorders in diseases classified elsewhere

Code first underlying disease, such as:

neoplasm (C00-D49)

EXCLUDES 1　*multiple cranial nerve palsy in sarcoidosis (D86.82)*

multiple cranial nerve palsy in syphilis (A52.15)

postherpetic geniculate ganglionitis (B02.21)

postherpetic trigeminal neuralgia (B02.22)

✓4ᵗʰ **G54 Nerve root and plexus disorders**

> EXCLUDES 1   current traumatic nerve root and plexus disorders - see nerve injury by body region
> intervertebral disc disorders (M50-M51)
> neuralgia or neuritis NOS (M79.2)
> neuritis or radiculitis brachial NOS (M54.13)
> neuritis or radiculitis lumbar NOS (M54.16)
> neuritis or radiculitis lumbosacral NOS (M54.17)
> neuritis or radiculitis thoracic NOS (M54.14)
> radiculitis NOS (M54.10)
> radiculopathy NOS (M54.10)
> spondylosis (M47.-)

G54.0 Brachial plexus disorders
Thoracic outlet syndrome
DEF: Acquired disorder affecting the spinal nerves that send signals to the shoulder, arm, and hand, causing corresponding motor and sensory dysfunction. This disorder is characterized by regional paresthesia, pain, muscle weakness, and in severe cases paralysis.

G54.1 Lumbosacral plexus disorders

G54.2 Cervical root disorders, not elsewhere classified

G54.3 Thoracic root disorders, not elsewhere classified

G54.4 Lumbosacral root disorders, not elsewhere classified

G54.5 Neuralgic amyotrophy
Parsonage-Aldren-Turner syndrome
Shoulder-girdle neuritis
> EXCLUDES 1   neuralgic amyotrophy in diabetes mellitus (E08-E13 with .44)

G54.6 Phantom limb syndrome with pain   HCC ESR COM

G54.7 Phantom limb syndrome without pain   HCC ESR COM
Phantom limb syndrome NOS

G54.8 Other nerve root and plexus disorders

G54.9 Nerve root and plexus disorder, unspecified

G55 Nerve root and plexus compressions in diseases classified elsewhere
Code first underlying disease, such as:
neoplasm (C00-D49)
> EXCLUDES 1   nerve root compression (due to) (in) ankylosing spondylitis (M45.-)
> nerve root compression (due to) (in) dorsopathies (M53.-, M54.-)
> nerve root compression (due to) (in) intervertebral disc disorders (M50.1.-, M51.1.-)
> nerve root compression (due to) (in) spondylopathies (M46.-, M48.-)
> nerve root compression (due to) (in) spondylosis (M47.0-, M47.2-)

✓4ᵗʰ **G56 Mononeuropathies of upper limb**
> EXCLUDES 1   current traumatic nerve disorder - see nerve injury by body region

AHA: 2016,4Q,17-18

✓5ᵗʰ **G56.0 Carpal tunnel syndrome**
DEF: Swelling and inflammation in the tendons or bursa surrounding the median nerve caused by repetitive activity. The resulting compression on the nerve causes pain, numbness, and tingling especially to the palm, index, middle finger, and thumb.
   G56.00 Carpal tunnel syndrome, unspecified upper limb
   G56.01 Carpal tunnel syndrome, right upper limb
   G56.02 Carpal tunnel syndrome, left upper limb
   G56.03 Carpal tunnel syndrome, bilateral upper limbs

✓6ᵗʰ **G56.1 Other lesions of median nerve**
   G56.10 Other lesions of median nerve, unspecified upper limb
   G56.11 Other lesions of median nerve, right upper limb
   G56.12 Other lesions of median nerve, left upper limb
   G56.13 Other lesions of median nerve, bilateral upper limbs

✓5ᵗʰ **G56.2 Lesion of ulnar nerve**
Tardy ulnar nerve palsy
   G56.20 Lesion of ulnar nerve, unspecified upper limb
   G56.21 Lesion of ulnar nerve, right upper limb
   G56.22 Lesion of ulnar nerve, left upper limb
   G56.23 Lesion of ulnar nerve, bilateral upper limbs

✓5ᵗʰ **G56.3 Lesion of radial nerve**
   G56.30 Lesion of radial nerve, unspecified upper limb
   G56.31 Lesion of radial nerve, right upper limb
   G56.32 Lesion of radial nerve, left upper limb
   G56.33 Lesion of radial nerve, bilateral upper limbs

[handwritten margin note: Cubital tunnel syndrome.]

✓5ᵗʰ **G56.4 Causalgia of upper limb**
Complex regional pain syndrome II of upper limb
> EXCLUDES 1   complex regional pain syndrome I of lower limb (G90.52-)
> complex regional pain syndrome I of upper limb (G90.51-)
> complex regional pain syndrome II of lower limb (G57.7-)
> reflex sympathetic dystrophy of lower limb (G90.52-)
> reflex sympathetic dystrophy of upper limb (G90.51-)
   G56.40 Causalgia of unspecified upper limb
   G56.41 Causalgia of right upper limb
   G56.42 Causalgia of left upper limb
   G56.43 Causalgia of bilateral upper limbs

✓5ᵗʰ **G56.8 Other specified mononeuropathies of upper limb**
Interdigital neuroma of upper limb
   G56.80 Other specified mononeuropathies of unspecified upper limb
   G56.81 Other specified mononeuropathies of right upper limb
   G56.82 Other specified mononeuropathies of left upper limb
   G56.83 Other specified mononeuropathies of bilateral upper limbs

✓5ᵗʰ **G56.9 Unspecified mononeuropathy of upper limb**
   G56.90 Unspecified mononeuropathy of unspecified upper limb
   G56.91 Unspecified mononeuropathy of right upper limb
   G56.92 Unspecified mononeuropathy of left upper limb
   G56.93 Unspecified mononeuropathy of bilateral upper limbs

✓4ᵗʰ **G57 Mononeuropathies of lower limb**
> EXCLUDES 1   current traumatic nerve disorder - see nerve injury by body region

AHA: 2016,4Q,17-18

✓5ᵗʰ **G57.0 Lesion of sciatic nerve**
> EXCLUDES 1   sciatica NOS (M54.3-)
> EXCLUDES 2   sciatica attributed to intervertebral disc disorder (M51.1.-)
   G57.00 Lesion of sciatic nerve, unspecified lower limb
   G57.01 Lesion of sciatic nerve, right lower limb
   G57.02 Lesion of sciatic nerve, left lower limb
   G57.03 Lesion of sciatic nerve, bilateral lower limbs

✓5ᵗʰ **G57.1 Meralgia paresthetica**
Lateral cutaneous nerve of thigh syndrome
   G57.10 Meralgia paresthetica, unspecified lower limb
   G57.11 Meralgia paresthetica, right lower limb
   G57.12 Meralgia paresthetica, left lower limb
   G57.13 Meralgia paresthetica, bilateral lower limbs

✓5ᵗʰ **G57.2 Lesion of femoral nerve**
   G57.20 Lesion of femoral nerve, unspecified lower limb
   G57.21 Lesion of femoral nerve, right lower limb
   G57.22 Lesion of femoral nerve, left lower limb
   G57.23 Lesion of femoral nerve, bilateral lower limbs

✓5ᵗʰ **G57.3 Lesion of lateral popliteal nerve**
Peroneal nerve palsy
AHA: 2020,3Q,12
   G57.30 Lesion of lateral popliteal nerve, unspecified lower limb
   G57.31 Lesion of lateral popliteal nerve, right lower limb
   G57.32 Lesion of lateral popliteal nerve, left lower limb
   G57.33 Lesion of lateral popliteal nerve, bilateral lower limbs

✓5ᵗʰ **G57.4 Lesion of medial popliteal nerve**
   G57.40 Lesion of medial popliteal nerve, unspecified lower limb
   G57.41 Lesion of medial popliteal nerve, right lower limb
   G57.42 Lesion of medial popliteal nerve, left lower limb
   G57.43 Lesion of medial popliteal nerve, bilateral lower limbs

✓5ᵗʰ **G57.5 Tarsal tunnel syndrome**
   G57.50 Tarsal tunnel syndrome, unspecified lower limb
   G57.51 Tarsal tunnel syndrome, right lower limb
   G57.52 Tarsal tunnel syndrome, left lower limb
   G57.53 Tarsal tunnel syndrome, bilateral lower limbs

Chapter 6. Diseases of the Nervous System

G57.6-G65.2

✓5ᵗʰ **G57.6** **Lesion of** plantar nerve
     Morton's metatarsalgia
     G57.60 **Lesion of plantar nerve, unspecified lower limb**
     G57.61 **Lesion of plantar nerve, right lower limb**
     G57.62 **Lesion of plantar nerve, left lower limb**
     G57.63 **Lesion of plantar nerve, bilateral lower limbs**

✓5ᵗʰ **G57.7** **Causalgia of** lower limb
     Complex regional pain syndrome II of lower limb
     EXCLUDES 1   *complex regional pain syndrome I of lower limb (G90.52-)*
              complex regional pain syndrome I of upper limb (G90.51-)
              complex regional pain syndrome II of upper limb (G56.4-)
              reflex sympathetic dystrophy of lower limb (G90.52-)
              reflex sympathetic dystrophy of upper limb (G90.51-)
     G57.70 **Causalgia of unspecified lower limb**
     G57.71 **Causalgia of right lower limb**
     G57.72 **Causalgia of left lower limb**
     G57.73 **Causalgia of bilateral lower limbs**

✓5ᵗʰ **G57.8** **Other specified mononeuropathies of lower limb**
     Interdigital neuroma of lower limb
     G57.80 **Other specified mononeuropathies of unspecified lower limb**
     G57.81 **Other specified mononeuropathies of right lower limb**
     G57.82 **Other specified mononeuropathies of left lower limb**
     G57.83 **Other specified mononeuropathies of bilateral lower limbs**

✓5ᵗʰ **G57.9** **Unspecified mononeuropathy of lower limb**
     G57.90 **Unspecified mononeuropathy of unspecified lower limb**
     G57.91 **Unspecified mononeuropathy of right lower limb**
     G57.92 **Unspecified mononeuropathy of left lower limb**
     G57.93 **Unspecified mononeuropathy of bilateral lower limbs**

✓4ᵗʰ **G58** **Other mononeuropathies**
     G58.0 **Intercostal neuropathy**
     G58.7 **Mononeuritis multiplex**
     G58.8 **Other specified mononeuropathies**
     G58.9 **Mononeuropathy, unspecified**

G59 *Mononeuropathy in diseases classified elsewhere*
     Code first underlying disease
     EXCLUDES 1   *diabetic mononeuropathy (E08-E13 with .41)*
              syphilitic nerve paralysis (A52.19)
              syphilitic neuritis (A52.15)
              tuberculous mononeuropathy (A17.83)

Polyneuropathies and other disorders of the peripheral nervous system (G60-G65)

     EXCLUDES 1   *neuralgia NOS (M79.2)*
              neuritis NOS (M79.2)
              peripheral neuritis in pregnancy (O26.82-)
              radiculitis NOS (M54.10)

✓4ᵗʰ **G60** **Hereditary and idiopathic** neuropathy
     G60.0 **Hereditary motor and sensory neuropathy**
     Charcôt-Marie-Tooth disease
     Déjérine-Sottas disease
     Hereditary motor and sensory neuropathy, types I-IV
     Hypertrophic neuropathy of infancy
     Peroneal muscular atrophy (axonal type) (hypertrophic type)
     Roussy-Levy syndrome
     G60.1 **Refsum's disease**
     Infantile Refsum disease
     DEF: Genetic disorder of the lipid metabolism characterized by retinitis pigmentosa, degenerative nerve disease, ataxia, and dry, rough, scaly skin.
     G60.2 **Neuropathy in association with hereditary ataxia**
     G60.3 **Idiopathic progressive neuropathy**
     G60.8 **Other hereditary and idiopathic neuropathies**
     Dominantly inherited sensory neuropathy
     Morvan's disease
     Nelaton's syndrome
     Recessively inherited sensory neuropathy
     G60.9 **Hereditary and idiopathic neuropathy, unspecified**

✓4ᵗʰ **G61** **Inflammatory** polyneuropathy
     G61.0 **Guillain-Barre syndrome**   HCC Rx ESR COM
     Acute (post-)infective polyneuritis
     Miller Fisher syndrome
     AHA: 2020,3Q,12; 2014,2Q,4
     DEF: Autoimmune disorder due to an immune response to foreign antigens with paraplegia of limbs, flaccid paralysis, ophthalmoplegia, ataxia, and areflexia. In most cases, this disorder is triggered by a mild viral infection, surgery, or following an immunization.
     TIP: Guillain-Barre syndrome can occur as a sequela of *Campylobacter* enteritis. Assign code B94.8 for the sequelae as an additional diagnosis.
     G61.1 **Serum neuropathy**   HCC Rx ESR COM
     Use additional code for adverse effect, if applicable, to identify serum (T50.-)

✓5ᵗʰ **G61.8** **Other inflammatory polyneuropathies**
     G61.81 **Chronic inflammatory demyelinating polyneuritis**   HCC Rx ESR COM
     G61.82 **Multifocal motor neuropathy**   HCC Rx ESR COM
     MMN
     AHA: 2016,4Q,18
     G61.89 **Other inflammatory polyneuropathies**   HCC Rx ESR COM
     G61.9 **Inflammatory polyneuropathy, unspecified**   HCC Rx ESR COM

✓4ᵗʰ **G62** **Other and unspecified polyneuropathies**
     G62.0 **Drug-induced polyneuropathy**   HCC Rx ESR COM
     Use additional code for adverse effect, if applicable, to identify drug (T36-T50 with fifth or sixth character 5)
     G62.1 **Alcoholic polyneuropathy**   HCC Rx ESR COM
     AHA: 2019,3Q,8
     G62.2 **Polyneuropathy due to other toxic agents**   HCC Rx ESR COM
     Code first (T51-T65) to identify toxic agent

✓5ᵗʰ **G62.8** **Other specified polyneuropathies**
     G62.81 **Critical illness polyneuropathy**   HCC Rx ESR COM
     Acute motor neuropathy
     G62.82 **Radiation-induced polyneuropathy**   HCC Rx ESR COM
     Use additional external cause code (W88-W90, X39.0-) to identify cause
     G62.89 **Other specified polyneuropathies**
     AHA: 2016,2Q,11
     G62.9 **Polyneuropathy, unspecified**
     Neuropathy NOS

G63 *Polyneuropathy in diseases classified elsewhere*   HCC Rx ESR COM
     Code first underlying disease, such as:
     amyloidosis (E85.-)
     endocrine disease, except diabetes (E00-E07, E15-E16, E20-E34)
     metabolic diseases (E70-E88)
     neoplasm (C00-D49)
     nutritional deficiency (E40-E64)
     EXCLUDES 1   *polyneuropathy (in):*
              diabetes mellitus (E08-E13 with .42)
              diphtheria (A36.83)
              infectious mononucleosis complicated by polyneuropathy (B27.0-B27.9 with fifth character 1)
              Lyme disease (A69.22)
              mumps (B26.84)
              postherpetic (B02.23)
              rheumatoid arthritis (M05.5-)
              scleroderma (M34.83)
              systemic lupus erythematosus (M32.19)
     AHA: 2021,1Q,7; 2012,4Q,99

G64 **Other disorders of peripheral nervous system**
     Disorder of peripheral nervous system NOS

✓4ᵗʰ **G65** **Sequelae of inflammatory and toxic polyneuropathies**
     Code first condition resulting from (sequela) of inflammatory and toxic polyneuropathies
     G65.0 **Sequelae of Guillain-Barré syndrome**   HCC Rx ESR COM
     G65.1 **Sequelae of other inflammatory polyneuropathy**   HCC Rx ESR COM
     G65.2 **Sequelae of toxic polyneuropathy**   HCC Rx ESR COM

Diseases of myoneural junction and muscle (G70-G73)

✓4ᵗʰ G70 Myasthenia gravis and other myoneural disorders

    EXCLUDES 1   botulism (A05.1, A48.51-A48.52)
               transient neonatal myasthenia gravis (P94.0)

  ✓5ᵗʰ G70.0 Myasthenia gravis

    DEF: Autoimmune neuromuscular disorder caused by antibodies to the acetylcholine receptors at the neuromuscular junction, interfering with proper binding of the neurotransmitter from the neuron to the target muscle, causing muscle weakness, fatigue, and exhaustion, without pain or atrophy.

    G70.00 Myasthenia gravis without (acute) exacerbation `HCC` `Rx` `ESR` `COM`
         Myasthenia gravis NOS

    G70.01 Myasthenia gravis with (acute) exacerbation `HCC` `Rx` `ESR` `COM`
         Myasthenia gravis in crisis

  G70.1 Toxic myoneural disorders `HCC` `Rx` `ESR` `COM`
     Code first (T51-T65) to identify toxic agent

  G70.2 Congenital and developmental myasthenia `HCC` `Rx` `ESR` `COM`

  ✓5ᵗʰ G70.8 Other specified myoneural disorders

    G70.80 Lambert-Eaton syndrome, unspecified `HCC` `Rx` `ESR` `COM`
         Lambert-Eaton syndrome NOS

    G70.81 *Lambert-Eaton syndrome in disease classified elsewhere* `HCC` `Rx` `ESR` `COM`
         Code first underlying disease
           EXCLUDES 1   Lambert-Eaton syndrome in neoplastic disease (G73.1)

    G70.89 Other specified myoneural disorders `HCC` `Rx` `ESR` `COM`

  G70.9 Myoneural disorder, unspecified `HCC` `Rx` `ESR` `COM`

✓4ᵗʰ G71 Primary disorders of muscles

    EXCLUDES 2   arthrogryposis multiplex congenita (Q74.3)
              metabolic disorders (E70-E88)
              myositis (M60.-)

  ✓5ᵗʰ G71.0 Muscular dystrophy

    AHA: 2018,4Q,11-12

    G71.00 Muscular dystrophy, unspecified `HCC` `ESR` `COM`

    G71.01 Duchenne or Becker muscular dystrophy `HCC` `ESR` `COM`
         Autosomal recessive, childhood type, muscular dystrophy resembling Duchenne or Becker muscular dystrophy
         Benign [Becker] muscular dystrophy
         Severe [Duchenne] muscular dystrophy

    G71.02 Facioscapulohumeral muscular dystrophy `HCC` `ESR` `COM`
         Scapulohumeral muscular dystrophy

    ✓6ᵗʰ G71.03 Limb girdle muscular dystrophies

      G71.031 Autosomal dominant limb girdle muscular dystrophy
           LGMD D4 calpain-3-related
           LGMD D5 collagen 6-related
           Limb girdle muscular dystrophy type 1

      G71.032 Autosomal recessive limb girdle muscular dystrophy due to calpain-3 dysfunction
           Limb girdle muscular dystrophy type 2A
           LGMD R1 calpain-3-related
           Primary calpainopathy

      G71.033 Limb girdle muscular dystrophy due to dysferlin dysfunction
           Dysferlinopathy
           LGMD R2 dysferlin-related
           Limb girdle muscular dystrophy type 2B
           Miyoshi Myopathy type 1

      ✓7ᵗʰ G71.034 Limb girdle muscular dystrophy due to sarcoglycan dysfunction

        G71.0340 Limb girdle muscular dystrophy due to sarcoglycan dysfunction, unspecified
             Sarcoglycanopathy, NOS

        G71.0341 Limb girdle muscular dystrophy due to alpha sarcoglycan dysfunction
             Alpha sarcoglycanopathy
             Limb-girdle muscular dystrophy due to alpha-sarcoglycan deficiency
             Limb girdle muscular dystrophy type 2D

        G71.0342 Limb girdle muscular dystrophy due to beta sarcoglycan dysfunction
             Beta sarcoglycanopathy
             Limb girdle muscular dystrophy due to beta-sarcoglycan deficiency
             Limb girdle muscular dystrophy type 2E

        G71.0349 Limb girdle muscular dystrophy due to other sarcoglycan dysfunction
             Delta sarcoglycanopathy
             Delta-sarcoglycan-related LGMD R6
             Gamma sarcoglycanopathy
             Gamma-sarcoglycan-related LGMD R5
             Limb girdle muscular dystrophy type 2C
             Limb girdle muscular dystrophy type 2F

      G71.035 Limb girdle muscular dystrophy due to anoctamin-5 dysfunction
           Anoctamin-5-related LGMD R12
           Anoctaminopathy
           Autosomal recessive limb girdle muscular dystrophy type 2L
           Miyoshi myopathy type 3

      G71.038 Other limb girdle muscular dystrophy
           LGMD R9 FKRP-related
           LGMD R22 collagen 6-related
           Limb girdle muscular dystrophy due to fukutin related protein dysfunction
           Limb girdle muscular dystrophy type 2I
           Other autosomal recessive limb girdle muscular dystrophy

      G71.039 Limb girdle muscular dystrophy, unspecified

    G71.09 Other specified muscular dystrophies `HCC` `ESR` `COM`
         Benign scapuloperoneal muscular dystrophy with early contractures [Emery-Dreifuss]
         Congenital muscular dystrophy NOS
         Congenital muscular dystrophy with specific morphological abnormalities of the muscle fiber
         Distal muscular dystrophy
         ~~Limb-girdle muscular dystrophy~~
         Ocular muscular dystrophy
         Oculopharyngeal muscular dystrophy
         Scapuloperoneal muscular dystrophy

  ✓5ᵗʰ G71.1 Myotonic disorders

    G71.11 Myotonic muscular dystrophy `HCC` `ESR` `COM`
         Dystrophia myotonica [Steinert]
         Myotonia atrophica
         Myotonic dystrophy
         Proximal myotonic myopathy (PROMM)
         Steinert disease

    G71.12 Myotonia congenita
         Acetazolamide responsive myotonia congenita
         Dominant myotonia congenita [Thomsen disease]
         Myotonia levior
         Recessive myotonia congenita [Becker disease]

    G71.13 Myotonic chondrodystrophy
         Chondrodystrophic myotonia
         Congenital myotonic chondrodystrophy
         Schwartz-Jampel disease

Chapter 6. Diseases of the Nervous System

G71.14   **Drug induced myotonia**
Use additional code for adverse effect, if applicable, to identify drug (T36-T50 with fifth or sixth character 5)

G71.19   **Other specified myotonic disorders**
Myotonia fluctuans
Myotonia permanens
Neuromyotonia [Isaacs]
Paramyotonia congenita (of von Eulenburg)
Pseudomyotonia
Symptomatic myotonia

✓5ᵗʰ **G71.2**   **Congenital myopathies**

EXCLUDES 2   arthrogryposis multiplex congenita (Q74.3)

AHA: 2020,4Q,19-21

G71.20   **Congenital myopathy, unspecified**   HCC ESR COM

G71.21   **Nemaline myopathy**   HCC ESR COM

✓6ᵗʰ G71.22   **Centronuclear myopathy**

G71.220   **X-linked myotubular myopathy**   HCC ESR COM
Myotubular (centronuclear) myopathy

G71.228   **Other centronuclear myopathy**   HCC ESR COM
Autosomal centronuclear myopathy
Autosomal dominant centronuclear myopathy
Autosomal recessive centronuclear myopathy
Centronuclear myopathy, NOS

G71.29   **Other congenital myopathy**   HCC ESR COM
Central core disease
Minicore disease
Multicore disease
Multiminicore disease

G71.3   **Mitochondrial myopathy, not elsewhere classified**

EXCLUDES 1   Kearns-Sayre syndrome (H49.81)
Leber's disease (H47.21)
Leigh's encephalopathy (G31.82)
mitochondrial metabolism disorders (E88.4.-)
Reye's syndrome (G93.7)

G71.8   **Other primary disorders of muscles**

G71.9   **Primary disorder of muscle, unspecified**
Hereditary myopathy NOS

✓4ᵗʰ **G72**   **Other and unspecified myopathies**

EXCLUDES 1   arthrogryposis multiplex congenita (Q74.3)
dermatopolymyositis (M33.-)
ischemic infarction of muscle (M62.2-)
myositis (M60.-)
polymyositis (M33.2.-)

G72.0   **Drug-induced myopathy**
Use additional code for adverse effect, if applicable, to identify drug (T36-T50 with fifth or sixth character 5)

G72.1   **Alcoholic myopathy**
Use additional code to identify alcoholism (F10.-)

G72.2   **Myopathy due to other toxic agents**
Code first (T51-T65) to identify toxic agent

G72.3   **Periodic paralysis**
Familial periodic paralysis
Hyperkalemic periodic paralysis (familial)
Hypokalemic periodic paralysis (familial)
Myotonic periodic paralysis (familial)
Normokalemic paralysis (familial)
Potassium sensitive periodic paralysis

EXCLUDES 1   paramyotonia congenita (of von Eulenburg) (G71.19)

✓5ᵗʰ **G72.4**   **Inflammatory and immune myopathies, not elsewhere classified**

G72.41   **Inclusion body myositis [IBM]**

G72.49   **Other inflammatory and immune myopathies, not elsewhere classified**
Inflammatory myopathy NOS

✓5ᵗʰ G72.8   **Other specified myopathies**

G72.81   **Critical illness myopathy**
Acute necrotizing myopathy
Acute quadriplegic myopathy
Intensive care (ICU) myopathy
Myopathy of critical illness
AHA: 2020,3Q,12

G72.89   **Other specified myopathies**

G72.9   **Myopathy, unspecified**

✓4ᵗʰ **G73**   **Disorders of myoneural junction and muscle in diseases classified elsewhere**

G73.1   *Lambert-Eaton syndrome in neoplastic disease*   HCC Rx ESR COM UPD
Code first underlying neoplasm (C00-D49)

EXCLUDES 1   Lambert-Eaton syndrome not associated with neoplasm (G70.80-G70.81)

G73.3   *Myasthenic syndromes in other diseases classified elsewhere*   HCC Rx ESR COM
Code first underlying disease, such as:
neoplasm (C00-D49)
thyrotoxicosis (E05.-)

G73.7   *Myopathy in diseases classified elsewhere*
Code first underlying disease, such as:
hyperparathyroidism (E21.0, E21.3)
hypoparathyroidism (E20.-)
glycogen storage disease (E74.0)
lipid storage disorders (E75.-)

EXCLUDES 1   myopathy in:
rheumatoid arthritis (M05.32)
sarcoidosis (D86.87)
scleroderma (M34.82)
Sjögren syndrome (M35.03)
systemic lupus erythematosus (M32.19)

Cerebral palsy and other paralytic syndromes (G80-G83)

✓4ᵗʰ **G80**   **Cerebral palsy**

EXCLUDES 1   hereditary spastic paraplegia (G11.4)

G80.0   **Spastic quadriplegic cerebral palsy**   HCC ESR COM
Congenital spastic paralysis (cerebral)

G80.1   **Spastic diplegic cerebral palsy**   HCC ESR COM
Spastic cerebral palsy NOS

G80.2   **Spastic hemiplegic cerebral palsy**   HCC ESR COM

G80.3   **Athetoid cerebral palsy**   HCC ESR COM
Double athetosis (syndrome)
Dyskinetic cerebral palsy
Dystonic cerebral palsy
Vogt disease

G80.4   **Ataxic cerebral palsy**   HCC ESR COM

G80.8   **Other cerebral palsy**   HCC ESR COM
Mixed cerebral palsy syndromes

G80.9   **Cerebral palsy, unspecified**   HCC ESR COM
Cerebral palsy NOS

✓4ᵗʰ **G81**   **Hemiplegia and hemiparesis**

NOTE   This category is to be used only when hemiplegia (complete)(incomplete) is reported without further specification, or is stated to be old or longstanding but of unspecified cause. The category is also for use in multiple coding to identify these types of hemiplegia resulting from any cause.

EXCLUDES 1   congenital cerebral palsy (G80.-)
hemiplegia and hemiparesis due to sequela of cerebrovascular disease (I69.05-, I69.15-, I69.25-, I69.35-, I69.85-, I69.95-)

AHA: 2015,1Q,25

TIP: If the documentation specifies the affected side but not whether it is the dominant or nondominant side, the default is as follows: for ambidextrous patients, the default is dominant; when the left side is affected, the default is nondominant; and when the right side is affected, the default is dominant.

✓5ᵗʰ **G81.0**   **Flaccid hemiplegia**

G81.00   **Flaccid hemiplegia affecting unspecified side**   HCC ESR COM

G81.01   **Flaccid hemiplegia affecting right dominant side**   HCC ESR COM

G81.02   **Flaccid hemiplegia affecting left dominant side**   HCC ESR COM

G81.Ø3   **Flaccid hemiplegia affecting** right nondominant **side** `HCC` `ESR` `COM`

G81.Ø4   **Flaccid hemiplegia affecting** left nondominant **side** `HCC` `ESR` `COM`

✓5ᵗʰ **G81.1**   Spastic **hemiplegia**

G81.1Ø   **Spastic hemiplegia affecting unspecified side** `HCC` `Rx` `ESR` `COM`

G81.11   **Spastic hemiplegia affecting** right dominant **side** `HCC` `Rx` `ESR` `COM`

G81.12   **Spastic hemiplegia affecting** left dominant **side** `HCC` `Rx` `ESR` `COM`

G81.13   **Spastic hemiplegia affecting** right nondominant **side** `HCC` `Rx` `ESR` `COM`

G81.14   **Spastic hemiplegia affecting** left nondominant **side** `HCC` `Rx` `ESR` `COM`

✓5ᵗʰ **G81.9**   Hemiplegia, unspecified

     AHA: 2014,1Q,23   *Hemiparesis.*

G81.9Ø   **Hemiplegia, unspecified affecting unspecified side** `HCC` `ESR` `COM`

G81.91   **Hemiplegia, unspecified affecting** right dominant **side** `HCC` `ESR` `COM`

G81.92   **Hemiplegia, unspecified affecting** left dominant **side** `HCC` `ESR` `COM`

G81.93   **Hemiplegia, unspecified affecting** right nondominant **side** `HCC` `ESR` `COM`

G81.94   **Hemiplegia, unspecified affecting** left nondominant **side** `HCC` `ESR` `COM`

✓4ᵗʰ **G82**   **Paraplegia (paraparesis) and quadriplegia (quadriparesis)**

> `NOTE`   This category is to be used only when the listed conditions are reported without further specification, or are stated to be old or longstanding but of unspecified cause. The category is also for use in multiple coding to identify these conditions resulting from any cause

> `EXCLUDES 1`   congenital cerebral palsy (G8Ø.-)
> functional quadriplegia (R53.2)
> hysterical paralysis (F44.4)

✓5ᵗʰ **G82.2**   Paraplegia

     Paralysis of both lower limbs NOS
     Paraparesis (lower) NOS
     Paraplegia (lower) NOS
     AHA: 2017,3Q,3

G82.2Ø   **Paraplegia, unspecified** `HCC` `ESR` `COM`

G82.21   **Paraplegia,** complete `HCC` `ESR` `COM`

G82.22   **Paraplegia,** incomplete `HCC` `ESR` `COM`

✓5ᵗʰ **G82.5**   Quadriplegia

G82.5Ø   **Quadriplegia, unspecified** `HCC` `ESR` `COM`

G82.51   **Quadriplegia,** C1-C4 complete `HCC` `ESR` `COM`

G82.52   **Quadriplegia,** C1-C4 incomplete `HCC` `ESR` `COM`

G82.53   **Quadriplegia,** C5-C7 complete `HCC` `ESR` `COM`

G82.54   **Quadriplegia,** C5-C7 incomplete `HCC` `ESR` `COM`

✓4ᵗʰ **G83**   **Other paralytic syndromes**

> `NOTE`   This category is to be used only when the listed conditions are reported without further specification, or are stated to be old or longstanding but of unspecified cause. The category is also for use in multiple coding to identify these conditions resulting from any cause.

> `INCLUDES`   paralysis (complete) (incomplete), except as in G8Ø-G82

G83.Ø   **Diplegia of upper limbs** `HCC` `ESR` `COM`
     Diplegia (upper)
     Paralysis of both upper limbs

✓5ᵗʰ **G83.1**   Monoplegia of lower limb

     Paralysis of lower limb
> `EXCLUDES 1`   monoplegia of lower limbs due to sequela of cerebrovascular disease (I69.Ø4-, I69.14-, I69.24-, I69.34-, I69.84-, I69.94-)

     TIP: If the documentation specifies the affected side but not whether it is the dominant or nondominant side, the default is as follows: for ambidextrous patients, the default is dominant; when the left side is affected, the default is nondominant; and when the right side is affected, the default is dominant.

G83.1Ø   **Monoplegia of lower limb affecting unspecified side** `HCC` `ESR` `COM`

G83.11   **Monoplegia of lower limb affecting** right dominant **side** `HCC` `ESR` `COM`

G83.12   **Monoplegia of lower limb affecting** left dominant **side** `HCC` `ESR` `COM`

G83.13   **Monoplegia of lower limb affecting** right nondominant **side** `HCC` `ESR` `COM`

G83.14   **Monoplegia of lower limb affecting** left nondominant **side** `HCC` `ESR` `COM`

✓5ᵗʰ **G83.2**   Monoplegia of upper limb

     Paralysis of upper limb
> `EXCLUDES 1`   monoplegia of upper limbs due to sequela of cerebrovascular disease (I69.Ø3-, I69.13-, I69.23-, I69.33-, I69.83-, I69.93-)

     TIP: If the documentation specifies the affected side but not whether it is the dominant or nondominant side, the default is as follows: for ambidextrous patients, the default is dominant; when the left side is affected, the default is nondominant; and when the right side is affected, the default is dominant.

G83.2Ø   **Monoplegia of upper limb affecting unspecified side** `HCC` `ESR` `COM`

G83.21   **Monoplegia of upper limb affecting** right dominant **side** `HCC` `ESR` `COM`

G83.22   **Monoplegia of upper limb affecting** left dominant **side** `HCC` `ESR` `COM`

G83.23   **Monoplegia of upper limb affecting** right nondominant **side** `HCC` `ESR` `COM`

G83.24   **Monoplegia of upper limb affecting** left nondominant **side** `HCC` `ESR` `COM`

✓5ᵗʰ **G83.3**   Monoplegia, unspecified

     TIP: If the documentation specifies the affected side but not whether it is the dominant or nondominant side, the default is as follows: for ambidextrous patients, the default is dominant; when the left side is affected, the default is nondominant; and when the right side is affected, the default is dominant.

G83.3Ø   **Monoplegia, unspecified affecting unspecified side** `HCC` `ESR` `COM`

G83.31   **Monoplegia, unspecified affecting** right dominant **side** `HCC` `ESR` `COM`

G83.32   **Monoplegia, unspecified affecting** left dominant **side** `HCC` `ESR` `COM`

G83.33   **Monoplegia, unspecified affecting** right nondominant **side** `HCC` `ESR` `COM`

G83.34   **Monoplegia, unspecified affecting** left nondominant **side** `HCC` `ESR` `COM`

G83.4   **Cauda equina syndrome** `HCC` `Rx` `ESR` `COM`
     Neurogenic bladder due to cauda equina syndrome
> `EXCLUDES 1`   cord bladder NOS (G95.89)
> neurogenic bladder NOS (N31.9)

     AHA: 2020,3Q,24
     DEF: Compression of the spinal nerve roots presenting with pain and tingling radiating down the buttocks, back of the thigh and calf, and into the foot in a sciatic manner with aching in the bladder, perineum, and sacrum. Loss of bowel and bladder control may also occur.

G83.5   **Locked-in state** `HCC` `ESR` `COM`
     AHA: 2022,2Q,10

✓5ᵗʰ **G83.8**   Other specified paralytic syndromes

> `EXCLUDES 1`   paralytic syndromes due to current spinal cord injury - code to spinal cord injury (S14, S24, S34)

G83.81   **Brown-Séquard syndrome** `HCC` `ESR` `COM`

G83.82   **Anterior cord syndrome** `HCC` `ESR` `COM`

G83.83   **Posterior cord syndrome** `HCC` `ESR` `COM`

G83.84   **Todd's paralysis (postepileptic)** `HCC` `ESR` `COM`

G83.89   **Other specified paralytic syndromes** `HCC` `ESR` `COM`

G83.9   **Paralytic syndrome, unspecified** `HCC` `ESR` `COM`

Other disorders of the nervous system (G89-G99)

✓4ᵗʰ G89 Pain, not elsewhere classified

Code also related psychological factors associated with pain (F45.42)

EXCLUDES 1 *generalized pain NOS (R52)*

pain disorders exclusively related to psychological factors (F45.41)

pain NOS (R52)

EXCLUDES 2 *atypical face pain (G50.1)*

headache syndromes (G44.-)

localized pain, unspecified type - code to pain by site, such as:

abdomen pain (R10.-)

back pain (M54.9)

breast pain (N64.4)

chest pain (R07.1-R07.9)

ear pain (H92.0-)

eye pain (H57.1)

headache (R51.9)

joint pain (M25.5-)

limb pain (M79.6-)

lumbar region pain (M54.5-)

painful urination (R30.9)

pelvic and perineal pain (R10.2)

renal colic (N23)

shoulder pain (M25.51-)

spine pain (M54.-)

throat pain (R07.0)

tongue pain (K14.6)

tooth pain (K08.8)

migraines (G43.-)

myalgia (M79.1-)

pain from prosthetic devices, implants, and grafts (T82.84, T83.84, T84.84, T85.84-)

phantom limb syndrome with pain (G54.6)

vulvar vestibulitis (N94.810)

vulvodynia (N94.81-)

G89.0 Central pain syndrome

Déjérine-Roussy syndrome

Myelopathic pain syndrome

Thalamic pain syndrome (hyperesthetic)

✓5ᵗʰ G89.1 Acute pain, not elsewhere classified

G89.11 Acute pain due to trauma

G89.12 Acute post-thoracotomy pain

Post-thoracotomy pain NOS

G89.18 Other acute postprocedural pain

Postoperative pain NOS

Postprocedural pain NOS

✓5ᵗʰ G89.2 Chronic pain, not elsewhere classified

EXCLUDES 1 *causalgia, lower limb (G57.7-)*

causalgia, upper limb (G56.4-)

central pain syndrome (G89.0)

chronic pain syndrome (G89.4)

complex regional pain syndrome II, lower limb (G57.7-)

complex regional pain syndrome II, upper limb (G56.4-)

neoplasm related chronic pain (G89.3)

reflex sympathetic dystrophy (G90.5-)

G89.21 Chronic pain due to trauma

G89.22 Chronic post-thoracotomy pain

G89.28 Other chronic postprocedural pain

Other chronic postoperative pain

G89.29 Other chronic pain

G89.3 Neoplasm related pain (acute) (chronic)

Cancer associated pain

Pain due to malignancy (primary) (secondary)

Tumor associated pain

G89.4 Chronic pain syndrome

Chronic pain associated with significant psychosocial dysfunction

✓4ᵗʰ G90 Disorders of autonomic nervous system

EXCLUDES 1 *dysfunction of the autonomic nervous system due to alcohol (G31.2)*

✓5ᵗʰ G90.0 Idiopathic peripheral autonomic neuropathy

G90.01 Carotid sinus syncope

Carotid sinus syndrome

DEF: Vagal activation caused by pressure on the carotid sinus baroreceptors. Sympathetic nerve impulses may cause sinus arrest or AV block.

G90.09 Other idiopathic peripheral autonomic neuropathy

Idiopathic peripheral autonomic neuropathy NOS

G90.1 Familial dysautonomia [Riley-Day]   HCC Rx ESR COM

G90.2 Horner's syndrome

Bernard(-Horner) syndrome

Cervical sympathetic dystrophy or paralysis

G90.3 Multi-system degeneration of the autonomic nervous system   HCC Rx ESR COM

Neurogenic orthostatic hypotension [Shy-Drager]

EXCLUDES 1 *orthostatic hypotension NOS (I95.1)*

G90.4 Autonomic dysreflexia

Use additional code to identify the cause, such as:

fecal impaction (K56.41)

pressure ulcer (pressure area) (L89.-)

urinary tract infection (N39.0)

✓5ᵗʰ G90.5 Complex regional pain syndrome I (CRPS I)

Reflex sympathetic dystrophy

EXCLUDES 1 *causalgia of lower limb (G57.7-)*

causalgia of upper limb (G56.4-)

complex regional pain syndrome II of lower limb (G57.7-)

complex regional pain syndrome II of upper limb (G56.4-)

G90.50 Complex regional pain syndrome I, unspecified

✓6ᵗʰ G90.51 Complex regional pain syndrome I of upper limb

G90.511 Complex regional pain syndrome I of right upper limb

G90.512 Complex regional pain syndrome I of left upper limb

G90.513 Complex regional pain syndrome I of upper limb, bilateral

G90.519 Complex regional pain syndrome I of unspecified upper limb

✓6ᵗʰ G90.52 Complex regional pain syndrome I of lower limb

G90.521 Complex regional pain syndrome I of right lower limb

G90.522 Complex regional pain syndrome I of left lower limb

G90.523 Complex regional pain syndrome I of lower limb, bilateral

G90.529 Complex regional pain syndrome I of unspecified lower limb

G90.59 Complex regional pain syndrome I of other specified site

G90.8 Other disorders of autonomic nervous system

G90.9 Disorder of the autonomic nervous system, unspecified

G90.A Postural orthostatic tachycardia syndrome [POTS]

Chronic orthostatic intolerance

Postural tachycardia syndrome

☑4ᵗʰ **G91 Hydrocephalus**

> INCLUDES acquired hydrocephalus
> EXCLUDES 1 *Arnold-Chiari syndrome with hydrocephalus (Q07.-)*
> *congenital hydrocephalus (Q03.-)*
> *spina bifida with hydrocephalus (Q05.-)*

DEF: Abnormal buildup of cerebrospinal fluid in the brain causing dilation of the ventricles.

Hydrocephalus (Acquired)

Normal ventricles   Hydrocephalic ventricles

G91.0 Communicating hydrocephalus   HCC ESR COM
Secondary normal pressure hydrocephalus

G91.1 Obstructive hydrocephalus   HCC ESR COM
DEF: Obstruction of the cerebrospinal fluid passage from the brain into the spinal canal characterized by headaches, drowsiness, poor coordination, urinary incontinence, nausea, vomiting, and papilledema.

G91.2 (Idiopathic) normal pressure hydrocephalus HCC ESR COM
Normal pressure hydrocephalus NOS

G91.3 Post-traumatic hydrocephalus, unspecified HCC ESR COM

G91.4 Hydrocephalus in diseases classified elsewhere HCC ESR COM
Code first underlying condition, such as:
congenital syphilis (A50.4-)
neoplasm (C00-D49)
plasminogen deficiency (E88.02)
> EXCLUDES 1 *hydrocephalus due to congenital toxoplasmosis (P37.1)*

AHA: 2014,3Q,3

G91.8 Other hydrocephalus   HCC ESR COM

G91.9 Hydrocephalus, unspecified   HCC ESR COM

☑4ᵗʰ **G92 Toxic encephalopathy**
AHA: 2022,1Q,52; 2021,4Q,12-14; 2021,1Q,13; 2017,1Q,39-40
DEF: Brain tissue degeneration due to a toxic substance.

☑5ᵗʰ **G92.0 Immune effector cell-associated neurotoxicity syndrome**

Code first underlying cause such as:
complications of immune effector cellular therapy (T80.82)
Code also associated signs and symptoms, such as seizures and cerebral edema
Code also, if applicable:
cerebral edema (G93.6)
unspecified convulsions (R56.9)

G92.00 Immune effector cell-associated neurotoxicity syndrome, grade unspecified UPD
ICANS, grade unspecified

G92.01 Immune effector cell-associated neurotoxicity syndrome, grade 1 UPD
ICANS, grade 1

G92.02 Immune effector cell-associated neurotoxicity syndrome, grade 2 UPD
ICANS, grade 2

G92.03 Immune effector cell-associated neurotoxicity syndrome, grade 3 UPD
ICANS, grade 3

G92.04 Immune effector cell-associated neurotoxicity syndrome, grade 4 UPD
ICANS, grade 4

G92.05 Immune effector cell-associated neurotoxicity syndrome, grade 5 UPD
ICANS, grade 5

G92.8 Other toxic encephalopathy
Toxic encephalitis
Toxic metabolic encephalopathy
Code first poisoning due to drug or toxin, if applicable, (T36-T65 with fifth or sixth character 1-4 or 6)
Use additional code for adverse effect, if applicable, to identify drug (T36-T50 with fifth or sixth character 5)
AHA: 2022,1Q,52

G92.9 Unspecified toxic encephalopathy
Code first poisoning due to drug or toxin, if applicable, (T36-T65 with fifth or sixth character 1-4 or 6)
Use additional code for adverse effect, if applicable, to identify drug (T36-T50 with fifth or sixth character 5)

☑4ᵗʰ **G93 Other disorders of brain**

G93.0 Cerebral cysts
Arachnoid cyst
Porencephalic cyst, acquired
> EXCLUDES 1 *acquired periventricular cysts of newborn (P91.1)*
> *congenital cerebral cysts (Q04.6)*

G93.1 Anoxic brain damage, not elsewhere classified HCC ESR COM
> EXCLUDES 1 *cerebral anoxia due to anesthesia during labor and delivery (O74.3)*
> *cerebral anoxia due to anesthesia during the puerperium (O89.2)*
> *neonatal anoxia (P84)*

DEF: Brain injury not resulting from birth trauma that is due to lack of oxygen. Brain cells, when deprived of oxygen, begin to expire after four minutes.

G93.2 Benign intracranial hypertension
Pseudotumor
> EXCLUDES 1 *hypertensive encephalopathy (I67.4)*
> *obstructive hydrocephalus (G91.1)*

▲ ☑5ᵗʰ **G93.3 Postviral and related fatigue syndromes**
~~Benign myalgic encephalomyelitis~~
▶Use additional code, if applicable, for post COVID-19 condition, unspecified (U09.9)◀
> EXCLUDES 1 *chronic fatigue syndrome NOS (R53.82)*
> ▶*neurasthenia (F48.8)*◀

● **G93.31 Postviral fatigue syndrome**

● **G93.32 Myalgic encephalomyelitis/chronic fatigue syndrome**
Chronic fatigue syndrome
ME/CFS
Myalgic encephalomyelitis

● **G93.39 Other post infection and related fatigue syndromes**

☑5ᵗʰ **G93.4 Other and unspecified encephalopathy**
> EXCLUDES 1 *alcoholic encephalopathy (G31.2)*
> *encephalopathy in diseases classified elsewhere (G94)*
> *hypertensive encephalopathy (I67.4)*
> EXCLUDES 2 *toxic (metabolic) encephalopathy (G92.8)*

G93.40 Encephalopathy, unspecified
AHA: 2017,2Q,8

G93.41 Metabolic encephalopathy
Septic encephalopathy
AHA: 2017,2Q,8; 2016,3Q,42; 2015,3Q,21
TIP: Assign separately when documented with diabetic hypoglycemia (E08.649, E09.649, E10.649, E11.649, E13.649).

G93.49 Other encephalopathy
Encephalopathy NEC
AHA: 2021,2Q,3; 2018,4Q,16; 2018,2Q,22,24; 2017,2Q,9

G93.5 Compression of brain   HCC ESR COM
Arnold-Chiari type 1 compression of brain
Compression of brain (stem)
Herniation of brain (stem)
> EXCLUDES 1 *traumatic compression of brain (S06.A-)*
AHA: 2020,2Q,31

G93.6 Cerebral edema   HCC ESR COM
> EXCLUDES 1 *cerebral edema due to birth injury (P11.0)*
> *traumatic cerebral edema (S06.1-)*

Chapter 6. Diseases of the Nervous System

G93.7 Reye's syndrome `HCC` `Rx` `ESR` `COM` `P`

Code first poisoning due to salicylates, if applicable (T39.0-, with sixth character 1-4)

Use additional code for adverse effect due to salicylates, if applicable (T39.0-, with sixth character 5)

DEF: Rare childhood illness often developed after a viral upper respiratory infection. Symptoms include vomiting, elevated serum transaminase, brain swelling, disturbances of consciousness, seizures, and changes in liver and other viscera; it can be fatal.

✓5ᵗʰ **G93.8 Other specified disorders of brain**

G93.81 Temporal sclerosis
Hippocampal sclerosis
Mesial temporal sclerosis

G93.82 Brain death

G93.89 Other specified disorders of brain
Postradiation encephalopathy
AHA: 2020,2Q,24; 2019,3Q,8

G93.9 Disorder of brain, unspecified

G94 *Other disorders of brain in diseases classified elsewhere*
Code first underlying disease
EXCLUDES 1   *encephalopathy in congenital syphilis (A50.49)*
encephalopathy in influenza (J09.X9, J10.81, J11.81)
encephalopathy in syphilis (A52.19)
hydrocephalus in diseases classified elsewhere (G91.4)
AHA: 2018,2Q,22; 2017,2Q,8-9

✓4ᵗʰ **G95 Other and unspecified diseases of spinal cord**
EXCLUDES 2   *myelitis (G04.-)*

G95.0 Syringomyelia and syringobulbia `HCC` `Rx` `ESR` `COM`

✓5ᵗʰ **G95.1 Vascular myelopathies**
EXCLUDES 2   *intraspinal phlebitis and thrombophlebitis, except non-pyogenic (G08)*

G95.11 Acute infarction of spinal cord (embolic) (nonembolic) `HCC` `Rx` `ESR` `COM`
Anoxia of spinal cord
Arterial thrombosis of spinal cord

G95.19 Other vascular myelopathies `HCC` `Rx` `ESR` `COM`
Edema of spinal cord
Hematomyelia
Nonpyogenic intraspinal phlebitis and thrombophlebitis
Subacute necrotic myelopathy

✓5ᵗʰ **G95.2 Other and unspecified cord compression**

G95.20 Unspecified cord compression `HCC` `Rx` `ESR` `COM`

G95.29 Other cord compression `HCC` `Rx` `ESR` `COM`

✓5ᵗʰ **G95.8 Other specified diseases of spinal cord**
EXCLUDES 1   *neurogenic bladder NOS (N31.9)*
neurogenic bladder due to cauda equina syndrome (G83.4)
neuromuscular dysfunction of bladder without spinal cord lesion (N31.-)

G95.81 Conus medullaris syndrome `HCC` `Rx` `ESR` `COM`

G95.89 Other specified diseases of spinal cord `HCC` `Rx` `ESR` `COM`
Cord bladder NOS
Drug-induced myelopathy
Radiation-induced myelopathy
EXCLUDES 1   *myelopathy NOS (G95.9)*

G95.9 Disease of spinal cord, unspecified `HCC` `Rx` `ESR` `COM`
Myelopathy NOS

✓4ᵗʰ **G96 Other disorders of central nervous system**

✓5ᵗʰ **G96.0 Cerebrospinal fluid leak**
Code also if applicable:
intracranial hypotension (G96.81-)
EXCLUDES 1   *cerebrospinal fluid leak from spinal puncture (G97.0)*
AHA: 2020,4Q,21-22; 2018,2Q,13

G96.00 Cerebrospinal fluid leak, unspecified
Code also if applicable:
head injury ▶(S00-S09)◀

G96.01 Cranial cerebrospinal fluid leak, spontaneous
Otorrhea due to spontaneous cerebrospinal fluid CSF leak
Rhinorrhea due to spontaneous cerebrospinal fluid CSF leak
Spontaneous cerebrospinal fluid leak from skull base

G96.02 Spinal cerebrospinal fluid leak, spontaneous
Spontaneous cerebrospinal fluid leak from spine

G96.08 Other cranial cerebrospinal fluid leak
Postoperative cranial cerebrospinal fluid leak
Traumatic cranial cerebrospinal fluid leak
Code also if applicable:
head injury (S00.- to S09.-)

G96.09 Other spinal cerebrospinal fluid leak
Other spinal CSF leak
Postoperative spinal cerebrospinal fluid leak
Traumatic spinal cerebrospinal fluid leak
Code also if applicable:
head injury (S00.- to S09.-)

✓5ᵗʰ **G96.1 Disorders of meninges, not elsewhere classified**

G96.11 Dural tear
Code also intracranial hypotension, if applicable (G96.81-)
EXCLUDES 1   *accidental puncture or laceration of dura during a procedure (G97.41)*
AHA: 2014,4Q,24

G96.12 Meningeal adhesions (cerebral) (spinal)

✓6ᵗʰ **G96.19 Other disorders of meninges, not elsewhere classified**
AHA: 2020,4Q,22

G96.191 Perineural cyst
Cervical nerve root cyst
Lumbar nerve root cyst
Sacral nerve root cyst
Tarlov cyst
Thoracic nerve root cyst

G96.198 Other disorders of meninges, not elsewhere classified

✓5ᵗʰ **G96.8 Other specified disorders of central nervous system**
AHA: 2020,4Q,21,23-24

✓6ᵗʰ **G96.81 Intracranial hypotension**
Code also any associated diagnoses, such as:
brachial amyotrophy (G54.5)
cerebrospinal fluid leak from spine (G96.02)
cranial nerve disorders in diseases classified elsewhere (G53)
nerve root and compressions in diseases classified elsewhere (G55)
nonpyogenic thrombosis of intracranial venous system (I67.6)
nontraumatic intracerebral hemorrhage (I61.-)
nontraumatic subdural hemorrhage (I62.0-)
other and unspecified cord compression (G95.2-)
other secondary parkinsonism (G21.8)
reversible cerebrovascular vasoconstriction syndrome (I67.841)
spinal cord herniation (G95.89)
stroke (I63.-)
syringomyelia (G95.0)
DEF: Central nervous system disorder resulting from a loss of cerebrospinal fluid (CSF) volume. More often associated with CSF leak at the level of the spine rather than the skull base, causes can be spontaneous, iatrogenic or traumatic spinal dura defects or holes, or overdrainage of CSF shunt devices. The most common symptom is headache.

G96.810 Intracranial hypotension, unspecified
G96.811 Intracranial hypotension, spontaneous
G96.819 Other intracranial hypotension

G96.89 Other specified disorders of central nervous system

G96.9 Disorder of central nervous system, unspecified

`HCC` CMS-HCC   `Rx` Rx HCC   `ESR` ESRD HCC   `COM` Commercial HCC   `N` Newborn: 0   `P` Pediatric: 0-17   `M` Maternity: 9-64   `A` Adult: 15-124

608   ICD-10-CM 2023

☑4ᵗʰ **G97** **Intraoperative and postprocedural complications and disorders of nervous system, not elsewhere classified**

     EXCLUDES 2   *intraoperative and postprocedural cerebrovascular infarction (I97.81-, I97.82-)*

   AHA: 2016,4Q,9-10

G97.0 **Cerebrospinal fluid leak from spinal puncture**
     Code also any associated diagnoses or complications, such as: intracranial hypotension following a procedure (G97.83-G97.84)

Spinal Puncture

Spinal cord
Epidural space
Subarachnoid space
Vertebra
Spinal needle

Lumbar area

G97.1 **Other reaction to spinal and lumbar puncture**
     Headache due to lumbar puncture
     Other reaction to spinal dural puncture
     Code also, if applicable, any associated headache with orthostatic component (R51.0)

G97.2 **Intracranial hypotension following ventricular shunting**
     Code also any associated diagnoses or complications

☑5ᵗʰ **G97.3** **Intraoperative hemorrhage and hematoma of a nervous system organ or structure complicating a procedure**
     EXCLUDES 1   *intraoperative hemorrhage and hematoma of a nervous system organ or structure due to accidental puncture and laceration during a procedure (G97.4-)*

   G97.31 **Intraoperative hemorrhage and hematoma of a nervous system organ or structure complicating a nervous system procedure**

   G97.32 **Intraoperative hemorrhage and hematoma of a nervous system organ or structure complicating other procedure**

☑5ᵗʰ **G97.4** **Accidental puncture and laceration of a nervous system organ or structure during a procedure**

   G97.41 **Accidental puncture or laceration of dura during a procedure**
       Incidental (inadvertent) durotomy
       Code also any associated diagnoses or complications
       AHA: 2014,4Q,24

   G97.48 **Accidental puncture and laceration of other nervous system organ or structure during a nervous system procedure**

   G97.49 **Accidental puncture and laceration of other nervous system organ or structure during other procedure**

☑5ᵗʰ **G97.5** **Postprocedural hemorrhage of a nervous system organ or structure following a procedure**

   G97.51 **Postprocedural hemorrhage of a nervous system organ or structure following a nervous system procedure**

   G97.52 **Postprocedural hemorrhage of a nervous system organ or structure following other procedure**

☑5ᵗʰ **G97.6** **Postprocedural hematoma and seroma of a nervous system organ or structure following a procedure**

   G97.61 **Postprocedural hematoma of a nervous system organ or structure following a nervous system procedure**
       AHA: 2020,3Q,24

   G97.62 **Postprocedural hematoma of a nervous system organ or structure following other procedure**

   G97.63 **Postprocedural seroma of a nervous system organ or structure following a nervous system procedure**

   G97.64 **Postprocedural seroma of a nervous system organ or structure following other procedure**

☑5ᵗʰ **G97.8** **Other intraoperative and postprocedural complications and disorders of nervous system**
     Use additional code to further specify disorder
     AHA: 2020,4Q,23

   G97.81 **Other intraoperative complications of nervous system**

   G97.82 **Other postprocedural complications and disorders of nervous system**
       AHA: 2022,1Q,34

   G97.83 **Intracranial hypotension following lumbar cerebrospinal fluid shunting**
       Code also any associated diagnoses or complications

   G97.84 **Intracranial hypotension following other procedure**
       Code also, if applicable:
         accidental puncture or laceration of dura during a procedure (G97.41)
         cerebrospinal fluid leak from spinal puncture (G97.0)

☑4ᵗʰ **G98** **Other disorders of nervous system not elsewhere classified**
     INCLUDES   nervous system disorder NOS

G98.0 **Neurogenic arthritis, not elsewhere classified**
     Nonsyphilitic neurogenic arthropathy NEC
     Nonsyphilitic neurogenic spondylopathy NEC
     EXCLUDES 1   *spondylopathy (in):*
         syringomyelia and syringobulbia (G95.0)
         tabes dorsalis (A52.11)

G98.8 **Other disorders of nervous system**
     Nervous system disorder NOS

☑4ᵗʰ **G99** **Other disorders of nervous system in diseases classified elsewhere**

G99.0 *Autonomic neuropathy in diseases classified elsewhere*
     Code first underlying disease, such as:
     amyloidosis (E85.-)
     gout (M1A.-, M10.-)
     hyperthyroidism (E05.-)
     EXCLUDES 1   *diabetic autonomic neuropathy (E08-E13 with .43)*

G99.2 *Myelopathy in diseases classified elsewhere*   HCC   Rx   ESR   COM
     Code first underlying disease, such as:
     neoplasm (C00-D49)
     EXCLUDES 1   *myelopathy in:*
         intervertebral disease (M50.0-, M51.0-)
         spondylosis (M47.0-, M47.1-)
     AHA: 2018,3Q,18-19
     TIP: Use this code in addition to a spondylolisthesis code (M43.1-) or a spinal stenosis code (M48.0-) when either of these disorders is documented as the cause of the myelopathy.

G99.8 *Other specified disorders of nervous system in diseases classified elsewhere*
     Code first underlying disorder, such as:
     amyloidosis (E85.-)
     avitaminosis (E56.9)
     EXCLUDES 1   *nervous system involvement in:*
         cysticercosis (B69.0)
         rubella (B06.0-)
         syphilis (A52.1-)

☑ Additional Character Required   ✔x7ᵗʰ Placeholder Alert   Manifestation   Unspecified Dx   Q QPP   UPD Unacceptable PDx

Chapter 7. Diseases of the Eye and Adnexa (HØØ–H59)

Chapter-specific Guidelines with Coding Examples

The chapter-specific guidelines from the ICD-10-CM Official Guidelines for Coding and Reporting have been provided below. Along with these guidelines are coding examples, contained in the shaded boxes, that have been developed to help illustrate the coding and/or sequencing guidance found in these guidelines.

a. Glaucoma

1) **Assigning glaucoma codes**

   Assign as many codes from category H4Ø, Glaucoma, as needed to identify the type of glaucoma, the affected eye, and the glaucoma stage.

2) **Bilateral glaucoma with same type and stage**

   When a patient has bilateral glaucoma and both eyes are documented as being the same type and stage, and there is a code for bilateral glaucoma, report only the code for the type of glaucoma, bilateral, with the seventh character for the stage.

   > Bilateral mild stage primary open-angle glaucoma
   >
   > **H4Ø.1131**   **Primary open-angle glaucoma, bilateral, mild stage**
   >
   > *Explanation*: In this scenario, the patient has the same type and stage of glaucoma in both eyes. As this type of glaucoma has a code for bilateral, assign only the code for the bilateral glaucoma with the seventh character for the stage.

   When a patient has bilateral glaucoma and both eyes are documented as being the same type and stage, and the classification does not provide a code for bilateral glaucoma (i.e. subcategories H4Ø.1Ø and H4Ø.2Ø) report only one code for the type of glaucoma with the appropriate seventh character for the stage.

   > Bilateral open-angle glaucoma, severe stage; not specified as to type
   >
   > **H4Ø.1ØX3**   **Unspecified open-angle glaucoma, severe stage**
   >
   > *Explanation*: In this scenario, the patient has glaucoma of the same type and stage of both eyes, but there is no code specifically for bilateral glaucoma. Only one code is assigned with the appropriate seventh character for the stage.

3) **Bilateral glaucoma stage with different types or stages**

   When a patient has bilateral glaucoma and each eye is documented as having a different type or stage, and the classification distinguishes laterality, assign the appropriate code for each eye rather than the code for bilateral glaucoma.

   > Bilateral chronic angle-closure glaucoma; right eye is documented as mild stage and left eye as moderate stage
   >
   > **H4Ø.2211**   **Chronic angle-closure glaucoma, right eye, mild stage**
   >
   > **H4Ø.2222**   **Chronic angle-closure glaucoma, left eye, moderate stage**
   >
   > *Explanation*: In this scenario the patient has the same type of glaucoma in both eyes, but each eye is at a different stage. Because the subcategory for this condition identifies laterality, one code is assigned for the right eye and one code is assigned for the left eye, each with the appropriate seventh character for the stage appended.

When a patient has bilateral glaucoma and each eye is documented as having a different type, and the classification does not distinguish laterality (i.e. subcategories H4Ø.1Ø and H4Ø.2Ø), assign one code for each type of glaucoma with the appropriate seventh character for the stage.

> Documentation relates mild, unspecified primary angle-closure glaucoma of the left eye with mild unspecified open-angle glaucoma of the right eye
>
> **H4Ø.2ØX1**   **Unspecified primary angle-closure glaucoma, mild stage**
>
> **H4Ø.1ØX1**   **Unspecified open-angle glaucoma, mild stage**
>
> *Explanation*: In this scenario the patient has a different type of glaucoma in each eye and the classification does not distinguish laterality. A code for each type of glaucoma is assigned, each with the appropriate seventh character for the stage.

When a patient has bilateral glaucoma and each eye is documented as having the same type, but different stage, and the classification does not distinguish laterality (i.e. subcategories H4Ø.1Ø and H4Ø.2Ø), assign a code for the type of glaucoma for each eye with the seventh character for the specific glaucoma stage documented for each eye.

> Bilateral open-angle glaucoma, not specified as to type; the right eye is documented to be in mild stage and the left eye as being in moderate stage
>
> **H4Ø.1ØX1**   **Unspecified open-angle glaucoma, mild stage**
>
> **H4Ø.1ØX2**   **Unspecified open-angle glaucoma, moderate stage**
>
> *Explanation*: In this scenario the patient has the same type of glaucoma in each eye but each eye is at a different stage, and the classification does not distinguish laterality at this subcategory level. Two codes are assigned; both codes represent the same type of glaucoma but each has a different seventh character identifying the appropriate stage for each eye.

4) **Patient admitted with glaucoma and stage evolves during the admission**

   If a patient is admitted with glaucoma and the stage progresses during the admission, assign the code for highest stage documented.

5) **Indeterminate stage glaucoma**

   Assignment of the seventh character "4" for "indeterminate stage" should be based on the clinical documentation. The seventh character "4" is used for glaucomas whose stage cannot be clinically determined. This seventh character should not be confused with the seventh character "Ø", unspecified, which should be assigned when there is no documentation regarding the stage of the glaucoma.

b. Blindness

If "blindness" or "low vision" of both eyes is documented but the visual impairment category is not documented, assign code H54.3, Unqualified visual loss, both eyes. If "blindness" or "low vision" in one eye is documented but the visual impairment category is not documented, assign a code from H54.6-, Unqualified visual loss, one eye. If "blindness" or "visual loss" is documented without any information about whether one or both eyes are affected, assign code H54.7, Unspecified visual loss.

> Patient assessment indicates moderately impaired/low vision in the left eye with no visual impairments in the right eye
>
> **H54.62**   **Unqualified visual loss, left eye, normal vision right eye**
>
> Report unqualified visual loss when the visual impairment category is not specified. In this case, only the left eye is impacted by visual loss with normal vision of the right eye documented.

Chapter 7. Diseases of the Eye and Adnexa (H00-H59)

NOTE Use an external cause code following the code for the eye condition, if applicable, to identify the cause of the eye condition

EXCLUDES 2   certain conditions originating in the perinatal period (P04-P96)
certain infectious and parasitic diseases (A00-B99)
complications of pregnancy, childbirth and the puerperium (O00-O9A)
congenital malformations, deformations, and chromosomal abnormalities (Q00-Q99)
diabetes mellitus related eye conditions (E09.3-, E10.3-, E11.3-, E13.3-)
endocrine, nutritional and metabolic diseases (E00-E88)
injury (trauma) of eye and orbit (S05.-)
injury, poisoning and certain other consequences of external causes (S00-T88)
neoplasms (C00-D49)
symptoms, signs and abnormal clinical and laboratory findings, not elsewhere classified (R00-R94)
syphilis related eye disorders (A50.01, A50.3-, A51.43, A52.71)

This chapter contains the following blocks:

H00-H05   Disorders of eyelid, lacrimal system and orbit
H10-H11   Disorders of conjunctiva
H15-H22   Disorders of sclera, cornea, iris and ciliary body
H25-H28   Disorders of lens
H30-H36   Disorders of choroid and retina
H40-H42   Glaucoma
H43-H44   Disorders of vitreous body and globe
H46-H47   Disorders of optic nerve and visual pathways
H49-H52   Disorders of ocular muscles, binocular movement, accommodation and refraction
H53-H54   Visual disturbances and blindness
H55-H57   Other disorders of eye and adnexa
H59   Intraoperative and postprocedural complications and disorders of eye and adnexa, not elsewhere classified

Disorders of eyelid, lacrimal system and orbit (H00-H05)

EXCLUDES 2   open wound of eyelid (S01.1-)
superficial injury of eyelid (S00.1-, S00.2-)

✓4ᵗʰ H00 Hordeolum and chalazion

✓5ᵗʰ H00.0 Hordeolum (externum) (internum) of eyelid

DEF: Acute localized infection of the gland of Zeis (external hordeolum) or Molt or of the meibomian glands (internal hordeolum) of the orbit.

✓6ᵗʰ H00.01 Hordeolum externum

Hordeolum NOS
Stye

H00.011   Hordeolum externum right upper eyelid
H00.012   Hordeolum externum right lower eyelid
H00.013   Hordeolum externum right eye, unspecified eyelid
H00.014   Hordeolum externum left upper eyelid
H00.015   Hordeolum externum left lower eyelid
H00.016   Hordeolum externum left eye, unspecified eyelid
H00.019   Hordeolum externum unspecified eye, unspecified eyelid

✓6ᵗʰ H00.02 Hordeolum internum

Infection of meibomian gland

H00.021   Hordeolum internum right upper eyelid
H00.022   Hordeolum internum right lower eyelid
H00.023   Hordeolum internum right eye, unspecified eyelid
H00.024   Hordeolum internum left upper eyelid
H00.025   Hordeolum internum left lower eyelid
H00.026   Hordeolum internum left eye, unspecified eyelid
H00.029   Hordeolum internum unspecified eye, unspecified eyelid

✓6ᵗʰ H00.03 Abscess of eyelid

Furuncle of eyelid

H00.031   Abscess of right upper eyelid
H00.032   Abscess of right lower eyelid
H00.033   Abscess of eyelid right eye, unspecified eyelid
H00.034   Abscess of left upper eyelid
H00.035   Abscess of left lower eyelid
H00.036   Abscess of eyelid left eye, unspecified eyelid
H00.039   Abscess of eyelid unspecified eye, unspecified eyelid

✓5ᵗʰ H00.1 Chalazion

Meibomian (gland) cyst

EXCLUDES 2   infected meibomian gland (H00.02-)

DEF: Noninfectious, obstructive mass in the oil gland of the eyelid that results in a small chronic lump or inflammation.

H00.11   Chalazion right upper eyelid
H00.12   Chalazion right lower eyelid
H00.13   Chalazion right eye, unspecified eyelid
H00.14   Chalazion left upper eyelid
H00.15   Chalazion left lower eyelid
H00.16   Chalazion left eye, unspecified eyelid
H00.19   Chalazion unspecified eye, unspecified eyelid

✓4ᵗʰ H01 Other inflammation of eyelid

✓5ᵗʰ H01.0 Blepharitis

EXCLUDES 1   blepharoconjunctivitis (H10.5-)

✓6ᵗʰ H01.00 Unspecified blepharitis

AHA: 2018,4Q,13

H01.001   Unspecified blepharitis right upper eyelid
H01.002   Unspecified blepharitis right lower eyelid
H01.003   Unspecified blepharitis right eye, unspecified eyelid
H01.004   Unspecified blepharitis left upper eyelid
H01.005   Unspecified blepharitis left lower eyelid
H01.006   Unspecified blepharitis left eye, unspecified eyelid
H01.009   Unspecified blepharitis unspecified eye, unspecified eyelid
H01.00A   Unspecified blepharitis right eye, upper and lower eyelids
H01.00B   Unspecified blepharitis left eye, upper and lower eyelids

✓6ᵗʰ H01.01 Ulcerative blepharitis

AHA: 2018,4Q,13

H01.011   Ulcerative blepharitis right upper eyelid
H01.012   Ulcerative blepharitis right lower eyelid
H01.013   Ulcerative blepharitis right eye, unspecified eyelid
H01.014   Ulcerative blepharitis left upper eyelid
H01.015   Ulcerative blepharitis left lower eyelid
H01.016   Ulcerative blepharitis left eye, unspecified eyelid
H01.019   Ulcerative blepharitis unspecified eye, unspecified eyelid
H01.01A   Ulcerative blepharitis right eye, upper and lower eyelids
H01.01B   Ulcerative blepharitis left eye, upper and lower eyelids

✓6ᵗʰ H01.02 Squamous blepharitis

AHA: 2018,4Q,13

H01.021   Squamous blepharitis right upper eyelid
H01.022   Squamous blepharitis right lower eyelid
H01.023   Squamous blepharitis right eye, unspecified eyelid
H01.024   Squamous blepharitis left upper eyelid
H01.025   Squamous blepharitis left lower eyelid
H01.026   Squamous blepharitis left eye, unspecified eyelid
H01.029   Squamous blepharitis unspecified eye, unspecified eyelid
H01.02A   Squamous blepharitis right eye, upper and lower eyelids
H01.02B   Squamous blepharitis left eye, upper and lower eyelids

✓5ᵗʰ H01.1 Noninfectious dermatoses of eyelid

✓6ᵗʰ H01.11 Allergic dermatitis of eyelid

Contact dermatitis of eyelid

H01.111   Allergic dermatitis of right upper eyelid
H01.112   Allergic dermatitis of right lower eyelid
H01.113   Allergic dermatitis of right eye, unspecified eyelid
H01.114   Allergic dermatitis of left upper eyelid
H01.115   Allergic dermatitis of left lower eyelid
H01.116   Allergic dermatitis of left eye, unspecified eyelid
H01.119   Allergic dermatitis of unspecified eye, unspecified eyelid

✓6ᵗʰ **H01.12** Discoid lupus erythematosus of eyelid

    H01.121 Discoid lupus erythematosus of right upper eyelid Rx

    H01.122 Discoid lupus erythematosus of right lower eyelid Rx

    H01.123 Discoid lupus erythematosus of right eye, unspecified eyelid

    H01.124 Discoid lupus erythematosus of left upper eyelid Rx

    H01.125 Discoid lupus erythematosus of left lower eyelid

    H01.126 Discoid lupus erythematosus of left eye, unspecified eyelid Rx

    H01.129 Discoid lupus erythematosus of unspecified eye, unspecified eyelid Rx

✓6ᵗʰ **H01.13** Eczematous dermatitis of eyelid

    H01.131 Eczematous dermatitis of right upper eyelid

    H01.132 Eczematous dermatitis of right lower eyelid

    H01.133 Eczematous dermatitis of right eye, unspecified eyelid

    H01.134 Eczematous dermatitis of left upper eyelid

    H01.135 Eczematous dermatitis of left lower eyelid

    H01.136 Eczematous dermatitis of left eye, unspecified eyelid

    H01.139 Eczematous dermatitis of unspecified eye, unspecified eyelid

✓6ᵗʰ **H01.14** Xeroderma of eyelid

    H01.141 Xeroderma of right upper eyelid

    H01.142 Xeroderma of right lower eyelid

    H01.143 Xeroderma of right eye, unspecified eyelid

    H01.144 Xeroderma of left upper eyelid

    H01.145 Xeroderma of left lower eyelid

    H01.146 Xeroderma of left eye, unspecified eyelid

    H01.149 Xeroderma of unspecified eye, unspecified eyelid

H01.8 Other specified inflammations of eyelid

H01.9 Unspecified inflammation of eyelid
    Inflammation of eyelid NOS

✓4ᵗʰ **H02** Other disorders of eyelid

    EXCLUDES 1 congenital malformations of eyelid (Q10.0-Q10.3)

Entropion and Ectropion

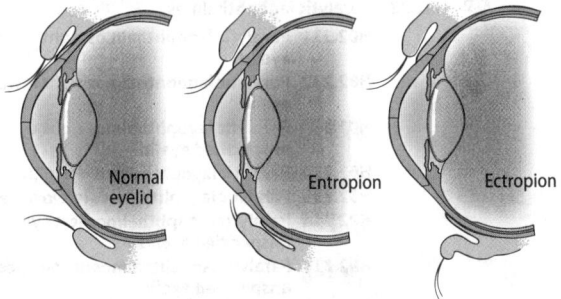

Normal eyelid   Entropion   Ectropion

✓5ᵗʰ **H02.0** Entropion and trichiasis of eyelid

    DEF: Entropion: Inversion of the eyelid, turning the edge in toward the eyeball and causing irritation from contact of the lashes with the surface of the eye.

    DEF: Trichiasis: Condition wherein the eyelid is in a normal position but lashes are ingrown or misdirected in their growth so that they irritate the tissues of the eye.

✓6ᵗʰ **H02.00** Unspecified entropion of eyelid

    H02.001 Unspecified entropion of right upper eyelid

    H02.002 Unspecified entropion of right lower eyelid

    H02.003 Unspecified entropion of right eye, unspecified eyelid

    H02.004 Unspecified entropion of left upper eyelid

    H02.005 Unspecified entropion of left lower eyelid

    H02.006 Unspecified entropion of left eye, unspecified eyelid

    H02.009 Unspecified entropion of unspecified eye, unspecified eyelid

✓6ᵗʰ **H02.01** Cicatricial entropion of eyelid

    H02.011 Cicatricial entropion of right upper eyelid

    H02.012 Cicatricial entropion of right lower eyelid

    H02.013 Cicatricial entropion of right eye, unspecified eyelid

    H02.014 Cicatricial entropion of left upper eyelid

    H02.015 Cicatricial entropion of left lower eyelid

    H02.016 Cicatricial entropion of left eye, unspecified eyelid

    H02.019 Cicatricial entropion of unspecified eye, unspecified eyelid

✓6ᵗʰ **H02.02** Mechanical entropion of eyelid

    H02.021 Mechanical entropion of right upper eyelid

    H02.022 Mechanical entropion of right lower eyelid

    H02.023 Mechanical entropion of right eye, unspecified eyelid

    H02.024 Mechanical entropion of left upper eyelid

    H02.025 Mechanical entropion of left lower eyelid

    H02.026 Mechanical entropion of left eye, unspecified eyelid

    H02.029 Mechanical entropion of unspecified eye, unspecified eyelid

✓6ᵗʰ **H02.03** Senile entropion of eyelid

    H02.031 Senile entropion of right upper eyelid A

    H02.032 Senile entropion of right lower eyelid A

    H02.033 Senile entropion of right eye, unspecified eyelid A

    H02.034 Senile entropion of left upper eyelid A

    H02.035 Senile entropion of left lower eyelid A

    H02.036 Senile entropion of left eye, unspecified eyelid A

    H02.039 Senile entropion of unspecified eye, unspecified eyelid A

✓6ᵗʰ **H02.04** Spastic entropion of eyelid

    H02.041 Spastic entropion of right upper eyelid

    H02.042 Spastic entropion of right lower eyelid

    H02.043 Spastic entropion of right eye, unspecified eyelid

    H02.044 Spastic entropion of left upper eyelid

    H02.045 Spastic entropion of left lower eyelid

    H02.046 Spastic entropion of left eye, unspecified eyelid

    H02.049 Spastic entropion of unspecified eye, unspecified eyelid

✓6ᵗʰ **H02.05** Trichiasis without entropion

    H02.051 Trichiasis without entropion right upper eyelid

    H02.052 Trichiasis without entropion right lower eyelid

    H02.053 Trichiasis without entropion right eye, unspecified eyelid

    H02.054 Trichiasis without entropion left upper eyelid

    H02.055 Trichiasis without entropion left lower eyelid

    H02.056 Trichiasis without entropion left eye, unspecified eyelid

    H02.059 Trichiasis without entropion unspecified eye, unspecified eyelid

✓5ᵗʰ **H02.1** Ectropion of eyelid

    DEF: Drooping of the lower eyelid away from the eye or outward turning or eversion of the edge of the eyelid, exposing the palpebral conjunctiva and causing irritation.

✓6ᵗʰ **H02.10** Unspecified ectropion of eyelid

    H02.101 Unspecified ectropion of right upper eyelid

    H02.102 Unspecified ectropion of right lower eyelid

    H02.103 Unspecified ectropion of right eye, unspecified eyelid

    H02.104 Unspecified ectropion of left upper eyelid

    H02.105 Unspecified ectropion of left lower eyelid

    H02.106 Unspecified ectropion of left eye, unspecified eyelid

H02.109 Unspecified ectropion of unspecified eye, unspecified eyelid

✓6th **H02.11** Cicatricial ectropion of eyelid

H02.111 Cicatricial ectropion of right upper eyelid

H02.112 Cicatricial ectropion of right lower eyelid

H02.113 Cicatricial ectropion of right eye, unspecified eyelid

H02.114 Cicatricial ectropion of left upper eyelid

H02.115 Cicatricial ectropion of left lower eyelid

H02.116 Cicatricial ectropion of left eye, unspecified eyelid

H02.119 Cicatricial ectropion of unspecified eye, unspecified eyelid

✓6th **H02.12** Mechanical ectropion of eyelid

H02.121 Mechanical ectropion of right upper eyelid

H02.122 Mechanical ectropion of right lower eyelid

H02.123 Mechanical ectropion of right eye, unspecified eyelid

H02.124 Mechanical ectropion of left upper eyelid

H02.125 Mechanical ectropion of left lower eyelid

H02.126 Mechanical ectropion of left eye, unspecified eyelid

H02.129 Mechanical ectropion of unspecified eye, unspecified eyelid

✓6th **H02.13** Senile ectropion of eyelid

H02.131 Senile ectropion of right upper eyelid   A

H02.132 Senile ectropion of right lower eyelid   A

H02.133 Senile ectropion of right eye, unspecified eyelid   A

H02.134 Senile ectropion of left upper eyelid   A

H02.135 Senile ectropion of left lower eyelid   A

H02.136 Senile ectropion of left eye, unspecified eyelid   A

H02.139 Senile ectropion of unspecified eye, unspecified eyelid   A

✓6th **H02.14** Spastic ectropion of eyelid

H02.141 Spastic ectropion of right upper eyelid

H02.142 Spastic ectropion of right lower eyelid

H02.143 Spastic ectropion of right eye, unspecified eyelid

H02.144 Spastic ectropion of left upper eyelid

H02.145 Spastic ectropion of left lower eyelid

H02.146 Spastic ectropion of left eye, unspecified eyelid

H02.149 Spastic ectropion of unspecified eye, unspecified eyelid

✓6th **H02.15** Paralytic ectropion of eyelid

AHA: 2018,4Q,13

H02.151 Paralytic ectropion of right upper eyelid

H02.152 Paralytic ectropion of right lower eyelid

H02.153 Paralytic ectropion of right eye, unspecified eyelid

H02.154 Paralytic ectropion of left upper eyelid

H02.155 Paralytic ectropion of left lower eyelid

H02.156 Paralytic ectropion of left eye, unspecified eyelid

H02.159 Paralytic ectropion of unspecified eye, unspecified eyelid

✓5th **H02.2** Lagophthalmos

AHA: 2018,4Q,14

DEF: Condition of the eye that prevents it from closing completely.

✓6th **H02.20** Unspecified lagophthalmos

H02.201 Unspecified lagophthalmos right upper eyelid

H02.202 Unspecified lagophthalmos right lower eyelid

H02.203 Unspecified lagophthalmos right eye, unspecified eyelid

H02.204 Unspecified lagophthalmos left upper eyelid

H02.205 Unspecified lagophthalmos left lower eyelid

H02.206 Unspecified lagophthalmos left eye, unspecified eyelid

H02.209 Unspecified lagophthalmos unspecified eye, unspecified eyelid

H02.20A Unspecified lagophthalmos right eye, upper and lower eyelids

H02.20B Unspecified lagophthalmos left eye, upper and lower eyelids

H02.20C Unspecified lagophthalmos, bilateral, upper and lower eyelids

✓6th **H02.21** Cicatricial lagophthalmos

H02.211 Cicatricial lagophthalmos right upper eyelid

H02.212 Cicatricial lagophthalmos right lower eyelid

H02.213 Cicatricial lagophthalmos right eye, unspecified eyelid

H02.214 Cicatricial lagophthalmos left upper eyelid

H02.215 Cicatricial lagophthalmos left lower eyelid

H02.216 Cicatricial lagophthalmos left eye, unspecified eyelid

H02.219 Cicatricial lagophthalmos unspecified eye, unspecified eyelid

H02.21A Cicatricial lagophthalmos right eye, upper and lower eyelids

H02.21B Cicatricial lagophthalmos left eye, upper and lower eyelids

H02.21C Cicatricial lagophthalmos, bilateral, upper and lower eyelids

✓6th **H02.22** Mechanical lagophthalmos

H02.221 Mechanical lagophthalmos right upper eyelid

H02.222 Mechanical lagophthalmos right lower eyelid

H02.223 Mechanical lagophthalmos right eye, unspecified eyelid

H02.224 Mechanical lagophthalmos left upper eyelid

H02.225 Mechanical lagophthalmos left lower eyelid

H02.226 Mechanical lagophthalmos left eye, unspecified eyelid

H02.229 Mechanical lagophthalmos unspecified eye, unspecified eyelid

H02.22A Mechanical lagophthalmos right eye, upper and lower eyelids

H02.22B Mechanical lagophthalmos left eye, upper and lower eyelids

H02.22C Mechanical lagophthalmos, bilateral, upper and lower eyelids

✓6th **H02.23** Paralytic lagophthalmos

H02.231 Paralytic lagophthalmos right upper eyelid

H02.232 Paralytic lagophthalmos right lower eyelid

H02.233 Paralytic lagophthalmos right eye, unspecified eyelid

H02.234 Paralytic lagophthalmos left upper eyelid

H02.235 Paralytic lagophthalmos left lower eyelid

H02.236 Paralytic lagophthalmos left eye, unspecified eyelid

H02.239 Paralytic lagophthalmos unspecified eye, unspecified eyelid

H02.23A Paralytic lagophthalmos right eye, upper and lower eyelids

H02.23B Paralytic lagophthalmos left eye, upper and lower eyelids

H02.23C Paralytic lagophthalmos, bilateral, upper and lower eyelids

✓5th **H02.3** Blepharochalasis

Pseudoptosis

DEF: Loss of elasticity and relaxation of skin of the eyelid, thickened or indurated skin on the eyelid associated with recurrent episodes of edema, and intracellular atrophy.

H02.30 Blepharochalasis unspecified eye, unspecified eyelid

H02.31 Blepharochalasis right upper eyelid

H02.32 Blepharochalasis right lower eyelid

H02.33 Blepharochalasis right eye, unspecified eyelid

H02.34 Blepharochalasis left upper eyelid

H02.35 Blepharochalasis left lower eyelid

H02.36 Blepharochalasis left eye, unspecified eyelid

✓5ᵗʰ **H02.4 Ptosis of eyelid**

  ✓6ᵗʰ **H02.40 Unspecified ptosis of eyelid**

    H02.401 Unspecified ptosis of right **eyelid**
    H02.402 Unspecified ptosis of left **eyelid**
    H02.403 Unspecified ptosis of bilateral **eyelids**
    H02.409 Unspecified ptosis of unspecified eyelid

  ✓6ᵗʰ **H02.41 Mechanical ptosis of eyelid**

    H02.411 Mechanical ptosis of right **eyelid**
    H02.412 Mechanical ptosis of left **eyelid**
    H02.413 Mechanical ptosis of bilateral **eyelids**
    H02.419 Mechanical ptosis of unspecified eyelid

  ✓6ᵗʰ **H02.42 Myogenic ptosis of eyelid**

    H02.421 Myogenic ptosis of right **eyelid**
    H02.422 Myogenic ptosis of left **eyelid**
    H02.423 Myogenic ptosis of bilateral **eyelids**
    H02.429 Myogenic ptosis of unspecified eyelid

  ✓6ᵗʰ **H02.43 Paralytic ptosis of eyelid**

    Neurogenic ptosis of eyelid
    H02.431 Paralytic ptosis of right **eyelid**
    H02.432 Paralytic ptosis of left **eyelid**
    H02.433 Paralytic ptosis of bilateral **eyelids**
    H02.439 Paralytic ptosis unspecified eyelid

✓5ᵗʰ **H02.5 Other disorders affecting eyelid function**

    EXCLUDES 2   *blepharospasm (G24.5)*
              organic tic (G25.69)
              psychogenic tic (F95.-)

  ✓6ᵗʰ **H02.51 Abnormal innervation syndrome**

    H02.511 Abnormal innervation syndrome right **upper eyelid**
    H02.512 Abnormal innervation syndrome right **lower eyelid**
    H02.513 Abnormal innervation syndrome right **eye, unspecified eyelid**
    H02.514 Abnormal innervation syndrome left **upper eyelid**
    H02.515 Abnormal innervation syndrome left **lower eyelid**
    H02.516 Abnormal innervation syndrome left eye, **unspecified eyelid**
    H02.519 Abnormal innervation syndrome unspecified eye, unspecified eyelid

  ✓6ᵗʰ **H02.52 Blepharophimosis**

    Ankyloblepharon
    H02.521 Blepharophimosis right upper **eyelid**
    H02.522 Blepharophimosis right lower **eyelid**
    H02.523 Blepharophimosis right eye, **unspecified eyelid**
    H02.524 Blepharophimosis left upper **eyelid**
    H02.525 Blepharophimosis left lower **eyelid**
    H02.526 Blepharophimosis left eye, **unspecified eyelid**
    H02.529 Blepharophimosis unspecified eye, unspecified lid

  ✓6ᵗʰ **H02.53 Eyelid retraction**

    Eyelid lag
    H02.531 Eyelid retraction right upper **eyelid**
    H02.532 Eyelid retraction right lower **eyelid**
    H02.533 Eyelid retraction right eye, **unspecified eyelid**
    H02.534 Eyelid retraction left upper **eyelid**
    H02.535 Eyelid retraction left lower **eyelid**
    H02.536 Eyelid retraction left eye, **unspecified eyelid**
    H02.539 Eyelid retraction unspecified eye, unspecified lid

  H02.59 Other disorders affecting eyelid function
    Deficient blink reflex
    Sensory disorders

✓5ᵗʰ **H02.6 Xanthelasma of eyelid**

    DEF: Condition in which there are small yellow tumors that occur on the eyelid, usually appearing near the nose.

    H02.60 Xanthelasma of unspecified eye, unspecified eyelid
    H02.61 Xanthelasma of right upper **eyelid**
    H02.62 Xanthelasma of right lower **eyelid**
    H02.63 Xanthelasma of right eye, **unspecified eyelid**
    H02.64 Xanthelasma of left upper **eyelid**
    H02.65 Xanthelasma of left lower **eyelid**
    H02.66 Xanthelasma of left eye, **unspecified eyelid**

✓5ᵗʰ **H02.7 Other and unspecified degenerative disorders of eyelid and periocular area**

    H02.70 Unspecified degenerative disorders of eyelid and periocular area

  ✓6ᵗʰ **H02.71 Chloasma of eyelid and periocular area**

    Dyspigmentation of eyelid
    Hyperpigmentation of eyelid
    H02.711 Chloasma of right upper **eyelid and periocular area**
    H02.712 Chloasma of right lower **eyelid and periocular area**
    H02.713 Chloasma of right eye, unspecified eyelid **and periocular area**
    H02.714 Chloasma of left upper **eyelid and periocular area**
    H02.715 Chloasma of left lower **eyelid and periocular area**
    H02.716 Chloasma of left eye, unspecified eyelid **and periocular area**
    H02.719 Chloasma of unspecified eye, unspecified eyelid and periocular area

  ✓6ᵗʰ **H02.72 Madarosis of eyelid and periocular area**

    Hypotrichosis of eyelid
    H02.721 Madarosis of right upper **eyelid and periocular area**
    H02.722 Madarosis of right lower **eyelid and periocular area**
    H02.723 Madarosis of right eye, unspecified eyelid **and periocular area**
    H02.724 Madarosis of left upper **eyelid and periocular area**
    H02.725 Madarosis of left lower **eyelid and periocular area**
    H02.726 Madarosis of left eye, unspecified eyelid **and periocular area**
    H02.729 Madarosis of unspecified eye, unspecified eyelid and periocular area

  ✓6ᵗʰ **H02.73 Vitiligo of eyelid and periocular area**

    Hypopigmentation of eyelid
    H02.731 Vitiligo of right upper **eyelid and periocular area**
    H02.732 Vitiligo of right lower **eyelid and periocular area**
    H02.733 Vitiligo of right eye, unspecified eyelid **and periocular area**
    H02.734 Vitiligo of left upper **eyelid and periocular area**
    H02.735 Vitiligo of left lower **eyelid and periocular area**
    H02.736 Vitiligo of left eye, unspecified eyelid **and periocular area**
    H02.739 Vitiligo of unspecified eye, unspecified eyelid and periocular area

  H02.79 Other degenerative disorders of eyelid and periocular area

✓5ᵗʰ **H02.8 Other specified disorders of eyelid**

  ✓6ᵗʰ **H02.81 Retained foreign body in eyelid**

    Use additional code to identify the type of retained foreign body (Z18.-)
    EXCLUDES 1   *laceration of eyelid with foreign body (S01.12-)*
              retained intraocular foreign body (H44.6-, H44.7-)
              superficial foreign body of eyelid and periocular area (S00.25-)
    H02.811 Retained foreign body in right upper **eyelid**
    H02.812 Retained foreign body in right lower **eyelid**
    H02.813 Retained foreign body in right eye, **unspecified eyelid**
    H02.814 Retained foreign body in left upper **eyelid**
    H02.815 Retained foreign body in left lower **eyelid**
    H02.816 Retained foreign body in left eye, **unspecified eyelid**
    H02.819 Retained foreign body in unspecified eye, unspecified eyelid

  ✓6ᵗʰ **H02.82 Cysts of eyelid**

    Sebaceous cyst of eyelid
    H02.821 Cysts of right upper **eyelid**
    H02.822 Cysts of right lower **eyelid**

Chapter 7. Diseases of the Eye and Adnexa

H02.823–H04.151

      H02.823 Cysts of right eye, unspecified eyelid
      H02.824 Cysts of left upper **eyelid**
      H02.825 Cysts of left lower **eyelid**
      H02.826 Cysts of left eye, unspecified eyelid
      H02.829 Cysts of unspecified eye, unspecified eyelid

✓6ᵗʰ **H02.83** Dermatochalasis **of eyelid**

    DEF: Acquired form of connective tissue disorder associated with decreased elastic tissue and abnormal elastin formation, resulting in loss of elasticity of the skin of the eyelid. It is generally associated with aging.

      H02.831 Dermatochalasis of right upper **eyelid**
      H02.832 Dermatochalasis of right lower **eyelid**
      H02.833 Dermatochalasis of right eye, unspecified eyelid
      H02.834 Dermatochalasis of left upper **eyelid**
      H02.835 Dermatochalasis of left lower **eyelid**
      H02.836 Dermatochalasis of left eye, unspecified eyelid
      H02.839 Dermatochalasis of unspecified eye, unspecified eyelid

✓6ᵗʰ **H02.84** Edema **of eyelid**

    Hyperemia of eyelid

      H02.841 Edema of right upper **eyelid**
      H02.842 Edema of right lower **eyelid**
      H02.843 Edema of right eye, unspecified eyelid
      H02.844 Edema of left upper **eyelid**
      H02.845 Edema of left lower **eyelid**
      H02.846 Edema of left eye, unspecified eyelid
      H02.849 Edema of unspecified eye, unspecified eyelid

✓6ᵗʰ **H02.85** Elephantiasis **of eyelid**

      H02.851 Elephantiasis of right upper **eyelid**
      H02.852 Elephantiasis of right lower **eyelid**
      H02.853 Elephantiasis of right eye, unspecified eyelid
      H02.854 Elephantiasis of left upper **eyelid**
      H02.855 Elephantiasis of left lower **eyelid**
      H02.856 Elephantiasis of left eye, unspecified eyelid
      H02.859 Elephantiasis of unspecified eye, unspecified eyelid

✓6ᵗʰ **H02.86** Hypertrichosis **of eyelid**

      H02.861 Hypertrichosis of right upper **eyelid**
      H02.862 Hypertrichosis of right lower **eyelid**
      H02.863 Hypertrichosis of right eye, unspecified eyelid
      H02.864 Hypertrichosis of left upper **eyelid**
      H02.865 Hypertrichosis of left lower **eyelid**
      H02.866 Hypertrichosis of left eye, unspecified eyelid
      H02.869 Hypertrichosis of unspecified eye, unspecified eyelid

✓6ᵗʰ **H02.87** Vascular anomalies **of eyelid**

      H02.871 Vascular anomalies of right upper **eyelid**
      H02.872 Vascular anomalies of right lower **eyelid**
      H02.873 Vascular anomalies of right eye, unspecified eyelid
      H02.874 Vascular anomalies of left upper **eyelid**
      H02.875 Vascular anomalies of left lower **eyelid**
      H02.876 Vascular anomalies of left eye, unspecified eyelid
      H02.879 Vascular anomalies of unspecified eye, unspecified eyelid

✓6ᵗʰ **H02.88** Meibomian gland dysfunction **of eyelid**

    AHA: 2018,4Q,14-15

      H02.881 Meibomian gland dysfunction right upper **eyelid**
      H02.882 Meibomian gland dysfunction right lower **eyelid**
      H02.883 Meibomian gland dysfunction of right eye, unspecified eyelid
      H02.884 Meibomian gland dysfunction left upper **eyelid**
      H02.885 Meibomian gland dysfunction left lower **eyelid**
      H02.886 Meibomian gland dysfunction of left eye, unspecified eyelid
      H02.889 Meibomian gland dysfunction of unspecified eye, unspecified eyelid

      H02.88A Meibomian gland dysfunction right eye, upper and lower **eyelids**
      H02.88B Meibomian gland dysfunction left eye, upper and lower **eyelids**
    H02.89 Other specified disorders of eyelid
      Hemorrhage of eyelid
  H02.9 Unspecified disorder of eyelid
    Disorder of eyelid NOS

✓4ᵗʰ **H04 Disorders of lacrimal system**

    EXCLUDES 1   congenital malformations of lacrimal system (Q10.4-Q10.6)

  ✓5ᵗʰ **H04.0 Dacryoadenitis**

    DEF: Inflammation of the lacrimal gland.

    ✓6ᵗʰ **H04.00 Unspecified dacryoadenitis**

      H04.001 Unspecified dacryoadenitis, right **lacrimal gland**
      H04.002 Unspecified dacryoadenitis, left **lacrimal gland**
      H04.003 Unspecified dacryoadenitis, bilateral **lacrimal glands**
      H04.009 Unspecified dacryoadenitis, unspecified **lacrimal gland**

    ✓6ᵗʰ **H04.01** Acute **dacryoadenitis**

      H04.011 Acute dacryoadenitis, right **lacrimal gland**
      H04.012 Acute dacryoadenitis, left **lacrimal gland**
      H04.013 Acute dacryoadenitis, bilateral **lacrimal glands**
      H04.019 Acute dacryoadenitis, unspecified **lacrimal gland**

    ✓6ᵗʰ **H04.02** Chronic **dacryoadenitis**

      H04.021 Chronic dacryoadenitis, right **lacrimal gland**
      H04.022 Chronic dacryoadenitis, left **lacrimal gland**
      H04.023 Chronic dacryoadenitis, bilateral **lacrimal gland**
      H04.029 Chronic dacryoadenitis, unspecified **lacrimal gland**

    ✓6ᵗʰ **H04.03 Chronic enlargement of lacrimal gland**

      H04.031 Chronic enlargement of right **lacrimal gland**
      H04.032 Chronic enlargement of left **lacrimal gland**
      H04.033 Chronic enlargement of bilateral **lacrimal glands**
      H04.039 Chronic enlargement of unspecified **lacrimal gland**

  ✓5ᵗʰ **H04.1 Other disorders of lacrimal gland**

    ✓6ᵗʰ **H04.11 Dacryops**

      H04.111 Dacryops of right **lacrimal gland**
      H04.112 Dacryops of left **lacrimal gland**
      H04.113 Dacryops of bilateral **lacrimal glands**
      H04.119 Dacryops of unspecified **lacrimal gland**

    ✓6ᵗʰ **H04.12 Dry eye syndrome**

    Tear film insufficiency, NOS

      H04.121 Dry eye syndrome of right **lacrimal gland**
      H04.122 Dry eye syndrome of left **lacrimal gland**
      H04.123 Dry eye syndrome of bilateral **lacrimal glands**
      H04.129 Dry eye syndrome of unspecified **lacrimal gland**

    ✓6ᵗʰ **H04.13 Lacrimal cyst**

    Lacrimal cystic degeneration

      H04.131 Lacrimal cyst, right **lacrimal gland**
      H04.132 Lacrimal cyst, left **lacrimal gland**
      H04.133 Lacrimal cyst, bilateral **lacrimal glands**
      H04.139 Lacrimal cyst, unspecified **lacrimal gland**

    ✓6ᵗʰ **H04.14** Primary **lacrimal gland atrophy**

      H04.141 Primary lacrimal gland atrophy, right **lacrimal gland**
      H04.142 Primary lacrimal gland atrophy, left **lacrimal gland**
      H04.143 Primary lacrimal gland atrophy, bilateral **lacrimal glands**
      H04.149 Primary lacrimal gland atrophy, unspecified **lacrimal gland**

    ✓6ᵗʰ **H04.15** Secondary **lacrimal gland atrophy**

      H04.151 Secondary lacrimal gland atrophy, right **lacrimal gland**

H04.152 Secondary lacrimal gland atrophy, left lacrimal gland
H04.153 Secondary lacrimal gland atrophy, bilateral lacrimal glands
H04.159 Secondary lacrimal gland atrophy, unspecified lacrimal gland

√6ᵗʰ **H04.16** Lacrimal gland dislocation
H04.161 Lacrimal gland dislocation, right lacrimal gland
H04.162 Lacrimal gland dislocation, left lacrimal gland
H04.163 Lacrimal gland dislocation, bilateral lacrimal glands
H04.169 Lacrimal gland dislocation, unspecified lacrimal gland
H04.19 Other specified disorders of lacrimal gland

√5ᵗʰ **H04.2** Epiphora
DEF: Excessive tearing or overflow of tears down the cheeks often due to a stricture in the lacrimal passages but can be caused by other conditions.

√6ᵗʰ **H04.20** Unspecified epiphora
H04.201 Unspecified epiphora, right side
H04.202 Unspecified epiphora, left side
H04.203 Unspecified epiphora, bilateral
H04.209 Unspecified epiphora, unspecified side

√6ᵗʰ **H04.21** Epiphora due to excess lacrimation
H04.211 Epiphora due to excess lacrimation, right lacrimal gland
H04.212 Epiphora due to excess lacrimation, left lacrimal gland
H04.213 Epiphora due to excess lacrimation, bilateral lacrimal glands
H04.219 Epiphora due to excess lacrimation, unspecified lacrimal gland

√6ᵗʰ **H04.22** Epiphora due to insufficient drainage
H04.221 Epiphora due to insufficient drainage, right side
H04.222 Epiphora due to insufficient drainage, left side
H04.223 Epiphora due to insufficient drainage, bilateral
H04.229 Epiphora due to insufficient drainage, unspecified side

√5ᵗʰ **H04.3** Acute and unspecified inflammation of lacrimal passages
EXCLUDES 1   neonatal dacryocystitis (P39.1)

√6ᵗʰ **H04.30** Unspecified dacryocystitis
H04.301 Unspecified dacryocystitis of right lacrimal passage
H04.302 Unspecified dacryocystitis of left lacrimal passage
H04.303 Unspecified dacryocystitis of bilateral lacrimal passages
H04.309 Unspecified dacryocystitis of unspecified lacrimal passage

√6ᵗʰ **H04.31** Phlegmonous dacryocystitis
H04.311 Phlegmonous dacryocystitis of right lacrimal passage
H04.312 Phlegmonous dacryocystitis of left lacrimal passage
H04.313 Phlegmonous dacryocystitis of bilateral lacrimal passages
H04.319 Phlegmonous dacryocystitis of unspecified lacrimal passage

√6ᵗʰ **H04.32** Acute dacryocystitis
Acute dacryopericystitis
H04.321 Acute dacryocystitis of right lacrimal passage
H04.322 Acute dacryocystitis of left lacrimal passage
H04.323 Acute dacryocystitis of bilateral lacrimal passages
H04.329 Acute dacryocystitis of unspecified lacrimal passage

√6ᵗʰ **H04.33** Acute lacrimal canaliculitis
H04.331 Acute lacrimal canaliculitis of right lacrimal passage
H04.332 Acute lacrimal canaliculitis of left lacrimal passage
H04.333 Acute lacrimal canaliculitis of bilateral lacrimal passages

H04.339 Acute lacrimal canaliculitis of unspecified lacrimal passage

√5ᵗʰ **H04.4** Chronic inflammation of lacrimal passages
√6ᵗʰ **H04.41** Chronic dacryocystitis
H04.411 Chronic dacryocystitis of right lacrimal passage
H04.412 Chronic dacryocystitis of left lacrimal passage
H04.413 Chronic dacryocystitis of bilateral lacrimal passages
H04.419 Chronic dacryocystitis of unspecified lacrimal passage

√6ᵗʰ **H04.42** Chronic lacrimal canaliculitis
H04.421 Chronic lacrimal canaliculitis of right lacrimal passage
H04.422 Chronic lacrimal canaliculitis of left lacrimal passage
H04.423 Chronic lacrimal canaliculitis of bilateral lacrimal passages
H04.429 Chronic lacrimal canaliculitis of unspecified lacrimal passage

√6ᵗʰ **H04.43** Chronic lacrimal mucocele
H04.431 Chronic lacrimal mucocele of right lacrimal passage
H04.432 Chronic lacrimal mucocele of left lacrimal passage
H04.433 Chronic lacrimal mucocele of bilateral lacrimal passages
H04.439 Chronic lacrimal mucocele of unspecified lacrimal passage

√5ᵗʰ **H04.5** Stenosis and insufficiency of lacrimal passages
√6ᵗʰ **H04.51** Dacryolith
H04.511 Dacryolith of right lacrimal passage
H04.512 Dacryolith of left lacrimal passage
H04.513 Dacryolith of bilateral lacrimal passages
H04.519 Dacryolith of unspecified lacrimal passage

√6ᵗʰ **H04.52** Eversion of lacrimal punctum
H04.521 Eversion of right lacrimal punctum
H04.522 Eversion of left lacrimal punctum
H04.523 Eversion of bilateral lacrimal punctum
H04.529 Eversion of unspecified lacrimal punctum

√6ᵗʰ **H04.53** Neonatal obstruction of nasolacrimal duct
EXCLUDES 1   congenital stenosis and stricture of lacrimal duct (Q10.5)
H04.531 Neonatal obstruction of right nasolacrimal duct N
H04.532 Neonatal obstruction of left nasolacrimal duct N
H04.533 Neonatal obstruction of bilateral nasolacrimal duct N
H04.539 Neonatal obstruction of unspecified nasolacrimal duct N

√6ᵗʰ **H04.54** Stenosis of lacrimal canaliculi
H04.541 Stenosis of right lacrimal canaliculi
H04.542 Stenosis of left lacrimal canaliculi
H04.543 Stenosis of bilateral lacrimal canaliculi
H04.549 Stenosis of unspecified lacrimal canaliculi

√6ᵗʰ **H04.55** Acquired stenosis of nasolacrimal duct
H04.551 Acquired stenosis of right nasolacrimal duct
H04.552 Acquired stenosis of left nasolacrimal duct
H04.553 Acquired stenosis of bilateral nasolacrimal duct
H04.559 Acquired stenosis of unspecified nasolacrimal duct

√6ᵗʰ **H04.56** Stenosis of lacrimal punctum
H04.561 Stenosis of right lacrimal punctum
H04.562 Stenosis of left lacrimal punctum
H04.563 Stenosis of bilateral lacrimal punctum
H04.569 Stenosis of unspecified lacrimal punctum

√6ᵗʰ **H04.57** Stenosis of lacrimal sac
H04.571 Stenosis of right lacrimal sac
H04.572 Stenosis of left lacrimal sac
H04.573 Stenosis of bilateral lacrimal sac
H04.579 Stenosis of unspecified lacrimal sac

✓5ᵗʰ **H04.6**   **Other changes of lacrimal passages**
    ✓6ᵗʰ **H04.61**   **Lacrimal** fistula
       H04.611   **Lacrimal fistula** right **lacrimal passage**
       H04.612   **Lacrimal fistula** left **lacrimal passage**
       H04.613   **Lacrimal fistula** bilateral **lacrimal passages**
       H04.619   **Lacrimal fistula unspecified lacrimal passage**
    H04.69   **Other changes of lacrimal passages**
✓5ᵗʰ **H04.8**   **Other disorders of lacrimal system**
    ✓6ᵗʰ **H04.81**   **Granuloma of lacrimal passages**
       H04.811   **Granuloma of** right **lacrimal passage**
       H04.812   **Granuloma of** left **lacrimal passage**
       H04.813   **Granuloma of** bilateral **lacrimal passages**
       H04.819   **Granuloma of unspecified lacrimal passage**
    H04.89   **Other disorders of lacrimal system**
H04.9   **Disorder of lacrimal system, unspecified**

✓4ᵗʰ **H05**   **Disorders of orbit**
    EXCLUDES 1   congenital malformation of orbit (Q10.7)
    ✓5ᵗʰ **H05.0**   **Acute inflammation** of orbit
       H05.00   **Unspecified acute inflammation of orbit**
      ✓6ᵗʰ **H05.01**   **Cellulitis** of orbit
        Abscess of orbit
       H05.011   **Cellulitis of** right **orbit**
       H05.012   **Cellulitis of** left **orbit**
       H05.013   **Cellulitis of** bilateral **orbits**
       H05.019   **Cellulitis of unspecified orbit**
      ✓6ᵗʰ **H05.02**   **Osteomyelitis** of orbit
       H05.021   **Osteomyelitis of** right **orbit**
       H05.022   **Osteomyelitis of** left **orbit**
       H05.023   **Osteomyelitis of** bilateral **orbits**
       H05.029   **Osteomyelitis of unspecified orbit**
      ✓6ᵗʰ **H05.03**   **Periostitis** of orbit
       H05.031   **Periostitis of** right **orbit**
       H05.032   **Periostitis of** left **orbit**
       H05.033   **Periostitis of** bilateral **orbits**
       H05.039   **Periostitis of unspecified orbit**
      ✓6ᵗʰ **H05.04**   **Tenonitis** of orbit
       H05.041   **Tenonitis of** right **orbit**
       H05.042   **Tenonitis of** left **orbit**
       H05.043   **Tenonitis of** bilateral **orbits**
       H05.049   **Tenonitis of unspecified orbit**
    ✓5ᵗʰ **H05.1**   **Chronic inflammatory disorders of orbit**
       H05.10   **Unspecified chronic inflammatory disorders of orbit**
      ✓6ᵗʰ **H05.11**   **Granuloma** of orbit
        Pseudotumor (inflammatory) of orbit
       H05.111   **Granuloma of** right **orbit**
       H05.112   **Granuloma of** left **orbit**
       H05.113   **Granuloma of** bilateral **orbits**
       H05.119   **Granuloma of unspecified orbit**
      ✓6ᵗʰ **H05.12**   **Orbital** myositis
       H05.121   **Orbital myositis,** right **orbit**
       H05.122   **Orbital myositis,** left **orbit**
       H05.123   **Orbital myositis,** bilateral
       H05.129   **Orbital myositis, unspecified orbit**
    ✓5ᵗʰ **H05.2**   **Exophthalmic conditions**
       H05.20   **Unspecified exophthalmos**
      ✓6ᵗʰ **H05.21**   **Displacement (lateral) of globe**
       H05.211   **Displacement (lateral) of globe,** right **eye**
       H05.212   **Displacement (lateral) of globe,** left **eye**
       H05.213   **Displacement (lateral) of globe,** bilateral
       H05.219   **Displacement (lateral) of globe, unspecified eye**
      ✓6ᵗʰ **H05.22**   **Edema of orbit**
        Orbital congestion
       H05.221   **Edema of** right **orbit**
       H05.222   **Edema of** left **orbit**
       H05.223   **Edema of** bilateral **orbit**
       H05.229   **Edema of unspecified orbit**
      ✓6ᵗʰ **H05.23**   **Hemorrhage of orbit**
       H05.231   **Hemorrhage of** right **orbit**
       H05.232   **Hemorrhage of** left **orbit**
       H05.233   **Hemorrhage of** bilateral **orbit**
       H05.239   **Hemorrhage of unspecified orbit**

      ✓6ᵗʰ **H05.24**   **Constant** exophthalmos
       H05.241   **Constant exophthalmos,** right **eye**
       H05.242   **Constant exophthalmos,** left **eye**
       H05.243   **Constant exophthalmos,** bilateral
       H05.249   **Constant exophthalmos, unspecified eye**
      ✓6ᵗʰ **H05.25**   **Intermittent** exophthalmos
       H05.251   **Intermittent exophthalmos,** right **eye**
       H05.252   **Intermittent exophthalmos,** left **eye**
       H05.253   **Intermittent exophthalmos,** bilateral
       H05.259   **Intermittent exophthalmos, unspecified eye**
      ✓6ᵗʰ **H05.26**   **Pulsating** exophthalmos
       H05.261   **Pulsating exophthalmos,** right **eye**
       H05.262   **Pulsating exophthalmos,** left **eye**
       H05.263   **Pulsating exophthalmos,** bilateral
       H05.269   **Pulsating exophthalmos, unspecified eye**
    ✓5ᵗʰ **H05.3**   **Deformity of orbit**
       EXCLUDES 1   congenital deformity of orbit (Q10.7)
                 hypertelorism (Q75.2)
       H05.30   **Unspecified deformity of orbit**
      ✓6ᵗʰ **H05.31**   **Atrophy** of orbit
       H05.311   **Atrophy of** right **orbit**
       H05.312   **Atrophy of** left **orbit**
       H05.313   **Atrophy of** bilateral **orbit**
       H05.319   **Atrophy of unspecified orbit**
      ✓6ᵗʰ **H05.32**   **Deformity of orbit** due to bone disease
        Code also associated bone disease
       H05.321   **Deformity of** right **orbit due to bone disease**
       H05.322   **Deformity of** left **orbit due to bone disease**
       H05.323   **Deformity of** bilateral **orbits due to bone disease**
       H05.329   **Deformity of unspecified orbit due to bone disease**
      ✓6ᵗʰ **H05.33**   **Deformity of orbit** due to trauma or surgery
       H05.331   **Deformity of** right **orbit due to trauma or surgery**
       H05.332   **Deformity of** left **orbit due to trauma or surgery**
       H05.333   **Deformity of** bilateral **orbits due to trauma or surgery**
       H05.339   **Deformity of unspecified orbit due to trauma or surgery**
      ✓6ᵗʰ **H05.34**   **Enlargement** of orbit
       H05.341   **Enlargement of** right **orbit**
       H05.342   **Enlargement of** left **orbit**
       H05.343   **Enlargement of** bilateral **orbits**
       H05.349   **Enlargement of unspecified orbit**
      ✓6ᵗʰ **H05.35**   **Exostosis** of orbit
       H05.351   **Exostosis of** right **orbit**
       H05.352   **Exostosis of** left **orbit**
       H05.353   **Exostosis of** bilateral **orbits**
       H05.359   **Exostosis of unspecified orbit**
    ✓5ᵗʰ **H05.4**   **Enophthalmos**
      ✓6ᵗʰ **H05.40**   **Unspecified enophthalmos**
       H05.401   **Unspecified enophthalmos,** right **eye**
       H05.402   **Unspecified enophthalmos,** left **eye**
       H05.403   **Unspecified enophthalmos,** bilateral
       H05.409   **Unspecified enophthalmos, unspecified eye**
      ✓6ᵗʰ **H05.41**   **Enophthalmos** due to atrophy of orbital tissue
       H05.411   **Enophthalmos due to atrophy of orbital tissue,** right **eye**
       H05.412   **Enophthalmos due to atrophy of orbital tissue,** left **eye**
       H05.413   **Enophthalmos due to atrophy of orbital tissue,** bilateral
       H05.419   **Enophthalmos due to atrophy of orbital tissue, unspecified eye**
      ✓6ᵗʰ **H05.42**   **Enophthalmos** due to trauma or surgery
       H05.421   **Enophthalmos due to trauma or surgery,** right **eye**
       H05.422   **Enophthalmos due to trauma or surgery,** left **eye**
       H05.423   **Enophthalmos due to trauma or surgery,** bilateral

H05.429 **Enophthalmos due to trauma or surgery, unspecified eye**

√5ᵗʰ H05.5 **Retained (old) foreign body following penetrating wound of orbit**
Retrobulbar foreign body
Use additional code to identify the type of retained foreign body (Z18.-)
EXCLUDES 1   current penetrating wound of orbit (S05.4-)
EXCLUDES 2   retained foreign body of eyelid (H02.81-)
           retained intraocular foreign body (H44.6-, H44.7-)

H05.50   **Retained (old) foreign body following penetrating wound of unspecified orbit**
H05.51   **Retained (old) foreign body following penetrating wound of right orbit**
H05.52   **Retained (old) foreign body following penetrating wound of left orbit**
H05.53   **Retained (old) foreign body following penetrating wound of bilateral orbits**

√5ᵗʰ H05.8 **Other disorders of orbit**

√6ᵗʰ H05.81   **Cyst of orbit**
Encephalocele of orbit
H05.811   **Cyst of right orbit**
H05.812   **Cyst of left orbit**
H05.813   **Cyst of bilateral orbits**
H05.819   **Cyst of unspecified orbit**

√6ᵗʰ H05.82   **Myopathy of extraocular muscles**
H05.821   **Myopathy of extraocular muscles, right orbit**
H05.822   **Myopathy of extraocular muscles, left orbit**
H05.823   **Myopathy of extraocular muscles, bilateral**
H05.829   **Myopathy of extraocular muscles, unspecified orbit**

H05.89   **Other disorders of orbit**
H05.9   **Unspecified disorder of orbit**

Disorders of conjunctiva (H10-H11)

√4ᵗʰ H10 **Conjunctivitis**
EXCLUDES 1   keratoconjunctivitis (H16.2-)

√5ᵗʰ H10.0 **Mucopurulent conjunctivitis**

√6ᵗʰ H10.01   **Acute follicular conjunctivitis**
H10.011   **Acute follicular conjunctivitis, right eye**
H10.012   **Acute follicular conjunctivitis, left eye**
H10.013   **Acute follicular conjunctivitis, bilateral**
H10.019   **Acute follicular conjunctivitis, unspecified eye**

√6ᵗʰ H10.02   **Other mucopurulent conjunctivitis**
H10.021   **Other mucopurulent conjunctivitis, right eye**
H10.022   **Other mucopurulent conjunctivitis, left eye**
H10.023   **Other mucopurulent conjunctivitis, bilateral**
H10.029   **Other mucopurulent conjunctivitis, unspecified eye**

√5ᵗʰ H10.1 **Acute atopic conjunctivitis**
Acute papillary conjunctivitis
H10.10   **Acute atopic conjunctivitis, unspecified eye**
H10.11   **Acute atopic conjunctivitis, right eye**
H10.12   **Acute atopic conjunctivitis, left eye**
H10.13   **Acute atopic conjunctivitis, bilateral**

√5ᵗʰ H10.2 **Other acute conjunctivitis**

√6ᵗʰ H10.21   **Acute toxic conjunctivitis**
Acute chemical conjunctivitis
Code first (T51-T65) to identify chemical and intent
EXCLUDES 1   burn and corrosion of eye and adnexa (T26.-)
H10.211   **Acute toxic conjunctivitis, right eye**
H10.212   **Acute toxic conjunctivitis, left eye**
H10.213   **Acute toxic conjunctivitis, bilateral**
H10.219   **Acute toxic conjunctivitis, unspecified eye**

√6ᵗʰ H10.22   **Pseudomembranous conjunctivitis**
H10.221   **Pseudomembranous conjunctivitis, right eye**

H10.222   **Pseudomembranous conjunctivitis, left eye**
H10.223   **Pseudomembranous conjunctivitis, bilateral**
H10.229   **Pseudomembranous conjunctivitis, unspecified eye**

√6ᵗʰ H10.23 **Serous conjunctivitis, except viral**
EXCLUDES 1   viral conjunctivitis (B30.-)
H10.231   **Serous conjunctivitis, except viral, right eye**
H10.232   **Serous conjunctivitis, except viral, left eye**
H10.233   **Serous conjunctivitis, except viral, bilateral**
H10.239   **Serous conjunctivitis, except viral, unspecified eye**

√5ᵗʰ H10.3 **Unspecified acute conjunctivitis**
EXCLUDES 1   ophthalmia neonatorum NOS (P39.1)
H10.30   **Unspecified acute conjunctivitis, unspecified eye**
H10.31   **Unspecified acute conjunctivitis, right eye**
H10.32   **Unspecified acute conjunctivitis, left eye**
H10.33   **Unspecified acute conjunctivitis, bilateral**

√5ᵗʰ H10.4 **Chronic conjunctivitis**

√6ᵗʰ H10.40   **Unspecified chronic conjunctivitis**
H10.401   **Unspecified chronic conjunctivitis, right eye**
H10.402   **Unspecified chronic conjunctivitis, left eye**
H10.403   **Unspecified chronic conjunctivitis, bilateral**
H10.409   **Unspecified chronic conjunctivitis, unspecified eye**

√6ᵗʰ H10.41   **Chronic giant papillary conjunctivitis**
H10.411   **Chronic giant papillary conjunctivitis, right eye**
H10.412   **Chronic giant papillary conjunctivitis, left eye**
H10.413   **Chronic giant papillary conjunctivitis, bilateral**
H10.419   **Chronic giant papillary conjunctivitis, unspecified eye**

√6ᵗʰ H10.42   **Simple chronic conjunctivitis**
H10.421   **Simple chronic conjunctivitis, right eye**
H10.422   **Simple chronic conjunctivitis, left eye**
H10.423   **Simple chronic conjunctivitis, bilateral**
H10.429   **Simple chronic conjunctivitis, unspecified eye**

√6ᵗʰ H10.43   **Chronic follicular conjunctivitis**
H10.431   **Chronic follicular conjunctivitis, right eye**
H10.432   **Chronic follicular conjunctivitis, left eye**
H10.433   **Chronic follicular conjunctivitis, bilateral**
H10.439   **Chronic follicular conjunctivitis, unspecified eye**

H10.44   **Vernal conjunctivitis**
EXCLUDES 1   vernal keratoconjunctivitis with limbar and corneal involvement (H16.26-)

H10.45   **Other chronic allergic conjunctivitis**

√5ᵗʰ H10.5 **Blepharoconjunctivitis**

√6ᵗʰ H10.50   **Unspecified blepharoconjunctivitis**
H10.501   **Unspecified blepharoconjunctivitis, right eye**
H10.502   **Unspecified blepharoconjunctivitis, left eye**
H10.503   **Unspecified blepharoconjunctivitis, bilateral**
H10.509   **Unspecified blepharoconjunctivitis, unspecified eye**

√6ᵗʰ H10.51   **Ligneous conjunctivitis**
Code also underlying condition if known, such as: plasminogen deficiency (E88.02)
H10.511   **Ligneous conjunctivitis, right eye**
H10.512   **Ligneous conjunctivitis, left eye**
H10.513   **Ligneous conjunctivitis, bilateral**
H10.519   **Ligneous conjunctivitis, unspecified eye**

√6ᵗʰ H10.52   **Angular blepharoconjunctivitis**
H10.521   **Angular blepharoconjunctivitis, right eye**
H10.522   **Angular blepharoconjunctivitis, left eye**
H10.523   **Angular blepharoconjunctivitis, bilateral**

H10.529   Angular blepharoconjunctivitis, unspecified eye

☑6ᵗʰ H10.53   Contact blepharoconjunctivitis

     H10.531   Contact blepharoconjunctivitis, right eye
     H10.532   Contact blepharoconjunctivitis, left eye
     H10.533   Contact blepharoconjunctivitis, bilateral
     H10.539   Contact blepharoconjunctivitis, unspecified eye

☑5ᵗʰ H10.8   Other conjunctivitis

☑6ᵗʰ H10.81   Pingueculitis

     EXCLUDES 1   *pinguecula (H11.15-)*

     H10.811   Pingueculitis, right eye
     H10.812   Pingueculitis, left eye
     H10.813   Pingueculitis, bilateral
     H10.819   Pingueculitis, unspecified eye

☑6ᵗʰ H10.82   Rosacea conjunctivitis

     Code first underlying rosacea dermatitis (L71.-)
     AHA: 2018,4Q,15

     H10.821   Rosacea conjunctivitis, right eye
     H10.822   Rosacea conjunctivitis, left eye
     H10.823   Rosacea conjunctivitis, bilateral
     H10.829   Rosacea conjunctivitis, unspecified eye

   H10.89   Other conjunctivitis

H10.9   Unspecified conjunctivitis

☑4ᵗʰ **H11   Other disorders of conjunctiva**

     EXCLUDES 1   *keratoconjunctivitis (H16.2-)*

☑5ᵗʰ H11.0   Pterygium of eye

     EXCLUDES 1   *pseudopterygium (H11.81-)*
     DEF: Benign, wedge-shaped, conjunctival thickening that advances from the inner corner of the eye toward the cornea.

Pterygium

Pterygium

☑6ᵗʰ H11.00   Unspecified pterygium of eye

     H11.001   Unspecified pterygium of right eye
     H11.002   Unspecified pterygium of left eye
     H11.003   Unspecified pterygium of eye, bilateral
     H11.009   Unspecified pterygium of unspecified eye

☑6ᵗʰ H11.01   Amyloid pterygium

     H11.011   Amyloid pterygium of right eye
     H11.012   Amyloid pterygium of left eye
     H11.013   Amyloid pterygium of eye, bilateral
     H11.019   Amyloid pterygium of unspecified eye

☑6ᵗʰ H11.02   Central pterygium of eye

     H11.021   Central pterygium of right eye
     H11.022   Central pterygium of left eye
     H11.023   Central pterygium of eye, bilateral
     H11.029   Central pterygium of unspecified eye

☑6ᵗʰ H11.03   Double pterygium of eye

     H11.031   Double pterygium of right eye
     H11.032   Double pterygium of left eye
     H11.033   Double pterygium of eye, bilateral
     H11.039   Double pterygium of unspecified eye

☑6ᵗʰ H11.04   Peripheral pterygium of eye, stationary

     H11.041   Peripheral pterygium, stationary, right eye
     H11.042   Peripheral pterygium, stationary, left eye
     H11.043   Peripheral pterygium, stationary, bilateral
     H11.049   Peripheral pterygium, stationary, unspecified eye

☑6ᵗʰ H11.05   Peripheral pterygium of eye, progressive

     H11.051   Peripheral pterygium, progressive, right eye

     H11.052   Peripheral pterygium, progressive, left eye
     H11.053   Peripheral pterygium, progressive, bilateral
     H11.059   Peripheral pterygium, progressive, unspecified eye

☑6ᵗʰ H11.06   Recurrent pterygium of eye

     H11.061   Recurrent pterygium of right eye
     H11.062   Recurrent pterygium of left eye
     H11.063   Recurrent pterygium of eye, bilateral
     H11.069   Recurrent pterygium of unspecified eye

☑5ᵗʰ H11.1   Conjunctival degenerations and deposits

     EXCLUDES 2   *pseudopterygium (H11.81)*

   H11.10   Unspecified conjunctival degenerations

☑6ᵗʰ H11.11   Conjunctival deposits

     H11.111   Conjunctival deposits, right eye
     H11.112   Conjunctival deposits, left eye
     H11.113   Conjunctival deposits, bilateral
     H11.119   Conjunctival deposits, unspecified eye

☑6ᵗʰ H11.12   Conjunctival concretions

     H11.121   Conjunctival concretions, right eye
     H11.122   Conjunctival concretions, left eye
     H11.123   Conjunctival concretions, bilateral
     H11.129   Conjunctival concretions, unspecified eye

☑6ᵗʰ H11.13   Conjunctival pigmentations

     Conjunctival argyrosis [argyria]

     H11.131   Conjunctival pigmentations, right eye
     H11.132   Conjunctival pigmentations, left eye
     H11.133   Conjunctival pigmentations, bilateral
     H11.139   Conjunctival pigmentations, unspecified eye

☑6ᵗʰ H11.14   Conjunctival xerosis, unspecified

     EXCLUDES 1   *xerosis of conjunctiva due to vitamin A deficiency (E50.0, E50.1)*
     DEF: Abnormal dryness of the conjunctiva due to lack of sufficient tears or conjunctival secretions.

     H11.141   Conjunctival xerosis, unspecified, right eye
     H11.142   Conjunctival xerosis, unspecified, left eye
     H11.143   Conjunctival xerosis, unspecified, bilateral
     H11.149   Conjunctival xerosis, unspecified, unspecified eye

☑6ᵗʰ H11.15   Pinguecula

     EXCLUDES 1   *pingueculitis (H10.81-)*
     DEF: Proliferation on the conjunctiva near the sclerocorneal junction, usually of the side of the nose and usually in older patients.

Pinguecula

Pinguecula

     H11.151   Pinguecula, right eye
     H11.152   Pinguecula, left eye
     H11.153   Pinguecula, bilateral
     H11.159   Pinguecula, unspecified eye

☑5ᵗʰ H11.2   Conjunctival scars

☑6ᵗʰ H11.21   Conjunctival adhesions and strands (localized)

     H11.211   Conjunctival adhesions and strands (localized), right eye
     H11.212   Conjunctival adhesions and strands (localized), left eye
     H11.213   Conjunctival adhesions and strands (localized), bilateral
     H11.219   Conjunctival adhesions and strands (localized), unspecified eye

☑6ᵗʰ H11.22   Conjunctival granuloma

     H11.221   Conjunctival granuloma, right eye
     H11.222   Conjunctival granuloma, left eye

          H11.223   Conjunctival granuloma, bilateral
          H11.229   Conjunctival granuloma, unspecified

✓6th   H11.23   **Symblepharon**
          H11.231   Symblepharon, right eye
          H11.232   Symblepharon, left eye
          H11.233   Symblepharon, bilateral
          H11.239   Symblepharon, unspecified eye

✓6th   H11.24   **Scarring of conjunctiva**
          H11.241   Scarring of conjunctiva, right eye
          H11.242   Scarring of conjunctiva, left eye
          H11.243   Scarring of conjunctiva, bilateral
          H11.249   Scarring of conjunctiva, unspecified eye

✓5th   **H11.3   Conjunctival hemorrhage**
      Subconjunctival hemorrhage
        H11.30   Conjunctival hemorrhage, unspecified eye
        H11.31   Conjunctival hemorrhage, right eye
        H11.32   Conjunctival hemorrhage, left eye
        H11.33   Conjunctival hemorrhage, bilateral

✓5th   **H11.4   Other conjunctival vascular disorders and cysts**

✓6th   H11.41   Vascular abnormalities of conjunctiva
          Conjunctival aneurysm
          H11.411   Vascular abnormalities of conjunctiva, right eye
          H11.412   Vascular abnormalities of conjunctiva, left eye
          H11.413   Vascular abnormalities of conjunctiva, bilateral
          H11.419   Vascular abnormalities of conjunctiva, unspecified eye

✓6th   H11.42   **Conjunctival** edema
          H11.421   Conjunctival edema, right eye
          H11.422   Conjunctival edema, left eye
          H11.423   Conjunctival edema, bilateral
          H11.429   Conjunctival edema, unspecified eye

✓6th   H11.43   **Conjunctival** hyperemia
          H11.431   Conjunctival hyperemia, right eye
          H11.432   Conjunctival hyperemia, left eye
          H11.433   Conjunctival hyperemia, bilateral
          H11.439   Conjunctival hyperemia, unspecified eye

✓6th   H11.44   **Conjunctival** cysts
          H11.441   Conjunctival cysts, right eye
          H11.442   Conjunctival cysts, left eye
          H11.443   Conjunctival cysts, bilateral
          H11.449   Conjunctival cysts, unspecified eye

✓5th   **H11.8   Other specified disorders of conjunctiva**

✓6th   H11.81   **Pseudopterygium of conjunctiva**
          H11.811   Pseudopterygium of conjunctiva, right eye
          H11.812   Pseudopterygium of conjunctiva, left eye
          H11.813   Pseudopterygium of conjunctiva, bilateral
          H11.819   Pseudopterygium of conjunctiva, unspecified eye

✓6th   H11.82   **Conjunctivochalasis**
          H11.821   Conjunctivochalasis, right eye
          H11.822   Conjunctivochalasis, left eye
          H11.823   Conjunctivochalasis, bilateral
          H11.829   Conjunctivochalasis, unspecified eye

        H11.89   Other specified disorders of conjunctiva

    H11.9   Unspecified disorder of conjunctiva

Disorders of sclera, cornea, iris and ciliary body (H15-H22)

✓4th   **H15   Disorders of sclera**

✓5th   **H15.0   Scleritis**

✓6th   H15.00   **Unspecified scleritis**
          H15.001   Unspecified scleritis, right eye
          H15.002   Unspecified scleritis, left eye
          H15.003   Unspecified scleritis, bilateral
          H15.009   Unspecified scleritis, unspecified eye

✓6th   H15.01   Anterior scleritis
          H15.011   Anterior scleritis, right eye
          H15.012   Anterior scleritis, left eye
          H15.013   Anterior scleritis, bilateral
          H15.019   Anterior scleritis, unspecified eye

✓6th   H15.02   Brawny scleritis
          H15.021   Brawny scleritis, right eye
          H15.022   Brawny scleritis, left eye
          H15.023   Brawny scleritis, bilateral
          H15.029   Brawny scleritis, unspecified eye

✓6th   H15.03   Posterior scleritis
      Sclerotenonitis
          H15.031   Posterior scleritis, right eye
          H15.032   Posterior scleritis, left eye
          H15.033   Posterior scleritis, bilateral
          H15.039   Posterior scleritis, unspecified eye

✓6th   H15.04   **Scleritis with** corneal involvement
          H15.041   Scleritis with corneal involvement, right eye
          H15.042   Scleritis with corneal involvement, left eye
          H15.043   Scleritis with corneal involvement, bilateral
          H15.049   Scleritis with corneal involvement, unspecified eye

✓6th   H15.05   Scleromalacia perforans
          H15.051   Scleromalacia perforans, right eye
          H15.052   Scleromalacia perforans, left eye
          H15.053   Scleromalacia perforans, bilateral
          H15.059   Scleromalacia perforans, unspecified eye

✓6th   H15.09   **Other scleritis**
      Scleral abscess
          H15.091   Other scleritis, right eye
          H15.092   Other scleritis, left eye
          H15.093   Other scleritis, bilateral
          H15.099   Other scleritis, unspecified eye

✓5th   **H15.1   Episcleritis**

✓6th   H15.10   **Unspecified episcleritis**
          H15.101   Unspecified episcleritis, right eye
          H15.102   Unspecified episcleritis, left eye
          H15.103   Unspecified episcleritis, bilateral
          H15.109   Unspecified episcleritis, unspecified eye

✓6th   H15.11   **Episcleritis** periodica fugax
          H15.111   Episcleritis periodica fugax, right eye
          H15.112   Episcleritis periodica fugax, left eye
          H15.113   Episcleritis periodica fugax, bilateral
          H15.119   Episcleritis periodica fugax, unspecified eye

✓6th   H15.12   Nodular episcleritis
          H15.121   Nodular episcleritis, right eye
          H15.122   Nodular episcleritis, left eye
          H15.123   Nodular episcleritis, bilateral
          H15.129   Nodular episcleritis, unspecified eye

✓5th   **H15.8   Other disorders of sclera**
       EXCLUDES 2   blue sclera (Q13.5)
                    degenerative myopia (H44.2-)

✓6th   H15.81   Equatorial staphyloma
          H15.811   Equatorial staphyloma, right eye
          H15.812   Equatorial staphyloma, left eye
          H15.813   Equatorial staphyloma, bilateral
          H15.819   Equatorial staphyloma, unspecified eye

✓6th   H15.82   Localized anterior staphyloma
          H15.821   Localized anterior staphyloma, right eye
          H15.822   Localized anterior staphyloma, left eye
          H15.823   Localized anterior staphyloma, bilateral
          H15.829   Localized anterior staphyloma, unspecified eye

✓6th   H15.83   **Staphyloma posticum**
          H15.831   Staphyloma posticum, right eye
          H15.832   Staphyloma posticum, left eye
          H15.833   Staphyloma posticum, bilateral
          H15.839   Staphyloma posticum, unspecified eye

✓6th   H15.84   Scleral ectasia
          H15.841   Scleral ectasia, right eye
          H15.842   Scleral ectasia, left eye
          H15.843   Scleral ectasia, bilateral
          H15.849   Scleral ectasia, unspecified eye

✓6th   H15.85   Ring staphyloma
          H15.851   Ring staphyloma, right eye
          H15.852   Ring staphyloma, left eye
          H15.853   Ring staphyloma, bilateral

H15.859   Ring staphyloma, unspecified eye
H15.89   Other disorders of sclera
H15.9   Unspecified disorder of sclera
✓4ᵗʰ H16   Keratitis
DEF: Condition in which the cornea becomes inflamed and irritated.
✓5ᵗʰ H16.0   Corneal ulcer
✓6ᵗʰ H16.00   Unspecified corneal ulcer
H16.001   Unspecified corneal ulcer, right eye
H16.002   Unspecified corneal ulcer, left eye
H16.003   Unspecified corneal ulcer, bilateral
H16.009   Unspecified corneal ulcer, unspecified eye
✓6ᵗʰ H16.01   Central corneal ulcer
H16.011   Central corneal ulcer, right eye
H16.012   Central corneal ulcer, left eye
H16.013   Central corneal ulcer, bilateral
H16.019   Central corneal ulcer, unspecified eye
✓6ᵗʰ H16.02   Ring corneal ulcer
H16.021   Ring corneal ulcer, right eye
H16.022   Ring corneal ulcer, left eye
H16.023   Ring corneal ulcer, bilateral
H16.029   Ring corneal ulcer, unspecified eye
✓6ᵗʰ H16.03   Corneal ulcer with hypopyon
H16.031   Corneal ulcer with hypopyon, right eye
H16.032   Corneal ulcer with hypopyon, left eye
H16.033   Corneal ulcer with hypopyon, bilateral
H16.039   Corneal ulcer with hypopyon, unspecified eye
✓6ᵗʰ H16.04   Marginal corneal ulcer
H16.041   Marginal corneal ulcer, right eye
H16.042   Marginal corneal ulcer, left eye
H16.043   Marginal corneal ulcer, bilateral
H16.049   Marginal corneal ulcer, unspecified eye
✓6ᵗʰ H16.05   Mooren's corneal ulcer
H16.051   Mooren's corneal ulcer, right eye
H16.052   Mooren's corneal ulcer, left eye
H16.053   Mooren's corneal ulcer, bilateral
H16.059   Mooren's corneal ulcer, unspecified eye
✓6ᵗʰ H16.06   Mycotic corneal ulcer
H16.061   Mycotic corneal ulcer, right eye
H16.062   Mycotic corneal ulcer, left eye
H16.063   Mycotic corneal ulcer, bilateral
H16.069   Mycotic corneal ulcer, unspecified eye
✓6ᵗʰ H16.07   Perforated corneal ulcer
H16.071   Perforated corneal ulcer, right eye
H16.072   Perforated corneal ulcer, left eye
H16.073   Perforated corneal ulcer, bilateral
H16.079   Perforated corneal ulcer, unspecified eye
✓5ᵗʰ H16.1   Other and unspecified superficial keratitis without conjunctivitis
✓6ᵗʰ H16.10   Unspecified superficial keratitis
H16.101   Unspecified superficial keratitis, right eye
H16.102   Unspecified superficial keratitis, left eye
H16.103   Unspecified superficial keratitis, bilateral
H16.109   Unspecified superficial keratitis, unspecified eye
✓6ᵗʰ H16.11   Macular keratitis
Areolar keratitis
Nummular keratitis
Stellate keratitis
Striate keratitis
H16.111   Macular keratitis, right eye
H16.112   Macular keratitis, left eye
H16.113   Macular keratitis, bilateral
H16.119   Macular keratitis, unspecified eye
✓6ᵗʰ H16.12   Filamentary keratitis
H16.121   Filamentary keratitis, right eye
H16.122   Filamentary keratitis, left eye
H16.123   Filamentary keratitis, bilateral
H16.129   Filamentary keratitis, unspecified eye
✓6ᵗʰ H16.13   Photokeratitis
Snow blindness
Welders keratitis
H16.131   Photokeratitis, right eye
H16.132   Photokeratitis, left eye
H16.133   Photokeratitis, bilateral

H16.139   Photokeratitis, unspecified eye
✓6ᵗʰ H16.14   Punctate keratitis
H16.141   Punctate keratitis, right eye
H16.142   Punctate keratitis, left eye
H16.143   Punctate keratitis, bilateral
H16.149   Punctate keratitis, unspecified eye
✓5ᵗʰ H16.2   Keratoconjunctivitis
✓6ᵗʰ H16.20   Unspecified keratoconjunctivitis
Superficial keratitis with conjunctivitis NOS
H16.201   Unspecified keratoconjunctivitis, right eye
H16.202   Unspecified keratoconjunctivitis, left eye
H16.203   Unspecified keratoconjunctivitis, bilateral
H16.209   Unspecified keratoconjunctivitis, unspecified eye
✓6ᵗʰ H16.21   Exposure keratoconjunctivitis
H16.211   Exposure keratoconjunctivitis, right eye
H16.212   Exposure keratoconjunctivitis, left eye
H16.213   Exposure keratoconjunctivitis, bilateral
H16.219   Exposure keratoconjunctivitis, unspecified eye
✓6ᵗʰ H16.22   Keratoconjunctivitis sicca, not specified as Sjögren's
EXCLUDES 1   Sjögren's syndrome (M35.01)
H16.221   Keratoconjunctivitis sicca, not specified as Sjögren's, right eye
H16.222   Keratoconjunctivitis sicca, not specified as Sjögren's, left eye
H16.223   Keratoconjunctivitis sicca, not specified as Sjögren's, bilateral
H16.229   Keratoconjunctivitis sicca, not specified as Sjögren's, unspecified eye
✓6ᵗʰ H16.23   Neurotrophic keratoconjunctivitis
H16.231   Neurotrophic keratoconjunctivitis, right eye
H16.232   Neurotrophic keratoconjunctivitis, left eye
H16.233   Neurotrophic keratoconjunctivitis, bilateral
H16.239   Neurotrophic keratoconjunctivitis, unspecified eye
✓6ᵗʰ H16.24   Ophthalmia nodosa
H16.241   Ophthalmia nodosa, right eye
H16.242   Ophthalmia nodosa, left eye
H16.243   Ophthalmia nodosa, bilateral
H16.249   Ophthalmia nodosa, unspecified eye
✓6ᵗʰ H16.25   Phlyctenular keratoconjunctivitis
H16.251   Phlyctenular keratoconjunctivitis, right eye
H16.252   Phlyctenular keratoconjunctivitis, left eye
H16.253   Phlyctenular keratoconjunctivitis, bilateral
H16.259   Phlyctenular keratoconjunctivitis, unspecified eye
✓6ᵗʰ H16.26   Vernal keratoconjunctivitis, with limbar and corneal involvement
EXCLUDES 1   vernal conjunctivitis without limbar and corneal involvement (H10.44)
H16.261   Vernal keratoconjunctivitis, with limbar and corneal involvement, right eye
H16.262   Vernal keratoconjunctivitis, with limbar and corneal involvement, left eye
H16.263   Vernal keratoconjunctivitis, with limbar and corneal involvement, bilateral
H16.269   Vernal keratoconjunctivitis, with limbar and corneal involvement, unspecified eye
✓6ᵗʰ H16.29   Other keratoconjunctivitis
H16.291   Other keratoconjunctivitis, right eye
H16.292   Other keratoconjunctivitis, left eye
H16.293   Other keratoconjunctivitis, bilateral
H16.299   Other keratoconjunctivitis, unspecified eye
✓5ᵗʰ H16.3   Interstitial and deep keratitis
✓6ᵗʰ H16.30   Unspecified interstitial keratitis
H16.301   Unspecified interstitial keratitis, right eye
H16.302   Unspecified interstitial keratitis, left eye
H16.303   Unspecified interstitial keratitis, bilateral

H16.309   Unspecified interstitial keratitis, unspecified eye

✓6th H16.31   Corneal abscess

H16.311   Corneal abscess, right eye
H16.312   Corneal abscess, left eye
H16.313   Corneal abscess, bilateral
H16.319   Corneal abscess, unspecified eye

✓6th H16.32   Diffuse interstitial keratitis

Cogan's syndrome

H16.321   Diffuse interstitial keratitis, right eye
H16.322   Diffuse interstitial keratitis, left eye
H16.323   Diffuse interstitial keratitis, bilateral
H16.329   Diffuse interstitial keratitis, unspecified eye

✓6th H16.33   Sclerosing keratitis

H16.331   Sclerosing keratitis, right eye
H16.332   Sclerosing keratitis, left eye
H16.333   Sclerosing keratitis, bilateral
H16.339   Sclerosing keratitis, unspecified eye

✓6th H16.39   Other interstitial and deep keratitis

H16.391   Other interstitial and deep keratitis, right eye
H16.392   Other interstitial and deep keratitis, left eye
H16.393   Other interstitial and deep keratitis, bilateral
H16.399   Other interstitial and deep keratitis, unspecified eye

✓5th H16.4   Corneal neovascularization

✓6th H16.40   Unspecified corneal neovascularization

H16.401   Unspecified corneal neovascularization, right eye
H16.402   Unspecified corneal neovascularization, left eye
H16.403   Unspecified corneal neovascularization, bilateral
H16.409   Unspecified corneal neovascularization, unspecified eye

✓6th H16.41   Ghost vessels (corneal)

H16.411   Ghost vessels (corneal), right eye
H16.412   Ghost vessels (corneal), left eye
H16.413   Ghost vessels (corneal), bilateral
H16.419   Ghost vessels (corneal), unspecified eye

✓6th H16.42   Pannus (corneal)

H16.421   Pannus (corneal), right eye
H16.422   Pannus (corneal), left eye
H16.423   Pannus (corneal), bilateral
H16.429   Pannus (corneal), unspecified eye

✓6th H16.43   Localized vascularization of cornea

H16.431   Localized vascularization of cornea, right eye
H16.432   Localized vascularization of cornea, left eye
H16.433   Localized vascularization of cornea, bilateral
H16.439   Localized vascularization of cornea, unspecified eye

✓6th H16.44   Deep vascularization of cornea

H16.441   Deep vascularization of cornea, right eye
H16.442   Deep vascularization of cornea, left eye
H16.443   Deep vascularization of cornea, bilateral
H16.449   Deep vascularization of cornea, unspecified eye

H16.8   Other keratitis
H16.9   Unspecified keratitis

✓4th H17   Corneal scars and opacities

✓5th H17.0   Adherent leukoma

H17.00   Adherent leukoma, unspecified eye
H17.01   Adherent leukoma, right eye
H17.02   Adherent leukoma, left eye
H17.03   Adherent leukoma, bilateral

✓5th H17.1   Central corneal opacity

H17.10   Central corneal opacity, unspecified eye
H17.11   Central corneal opacity, right eye
H17.12   Central corneal opacity, left eye
H17.13   Central corneal opacity, bilateral

✓5th H17.8   Other corneal scars and opacities

✓6th H17.81   Minor opacity of cornea

Corneal nebula

H17.811   Minor opacity of cornea, right eye
H17.812   Minor opacity of cornea, left eye
H17.813   Minor opacity of cornea, bilateral
H17.819   Minor opacity of cornea, unspecified eye

✓6th H17.82   Peripheral opacity of cornea

H17.821   Peripheral opacity of cornea, right eye
H17.822   Peripheral opacity of cornea, left eye
H17.823   Peripheral opacity of cornea, bilateral
H17.829   Peripheral opacity of cornea, unspecified eye

H17.89   Other corneal scars and opacities

H17.9   Unspecified corneal scar and opacity

✓4th H18   Other disorders of cornea

✓5th H18.0   Corneal pigmentations and deposits

✓6th H18.00   Unspecified corneal deposit

H18.001   Unspecified corneal deposit, right eye
H18.002   Unspecified corneal deposit, left eye
H18.003   Unspecified corneal deposit, bilateral
H18.009   Unspecified corneal deposit, unspecified eye

✓6th H18.01   Anterior corneal pigmentations

Staehli's line

H18.011   Anterior corneal pigmentations, right eye
H18.012   Anterior corneal pigmentations, left eye
H18.013   Anterior corneal pigmentations, bilateral
H18.019   Anterior corneal pigmentations, unspecified eye

✓6th H18.02   Argentous corneal deposits

H18.021   Argentous corneal deposits, right eye
H18.022   Argentous corneal deposits, left eye
H18.023   Argentous corneal deposits, bilateral
H18.029   Argentous corneal deposits, unspecified eye

✓6th H18.03   Corneal deposits in metabolic disorders

Code also associated metabolic disorder

H18.031   Corneal deposits in metabolic disorders, right eye
H18.032   Corneal deposits in metabolic disorders, left eye
H18.033   Corneal deposits in metabolic disorders, bilateral
H18.039   Corneal deposits in metabolic disorders, unspecified eye

✓6th H18.04   Kayser-Fleischer ring

Code also associated Wilson's disease (E83.01)

H18.041   Kayser-Fleischer ring, right eye
H18.042   Kayser-Fleischer ring, left eye
H18.043   Kayser-Fleischer ring, bilateral
H18.049   Kayser-Fleischer ring, unspecified eye

✓6th H18.05   Posterior corneal pigmentations

Krukenberg's spindle

H18.051   Posterior corneal pigmentations, right eye
H18.052   Posterior corneal pigmentations, left eye
H18.053   Posterior corneal pigmentations, bilateral
H18.059   Posterior corneal pigmentations, unspecified eye

✓6th H18.06   Stromal corneal pigmentations

Hematocornea

H18.061   Stromal corneal pigmentations, right eye
H18.062   Stromal corneal pigmentations, left eye
H18.063   Stromal corneal pigmentations, bilateral
H18.069   Stromal corneal pigmentations, unspecified eye

✓5th H18.1   Bullous keratopathy

DEF: Corneal swelling due to a damaged corneal endothelium. Bullous keratopathy is characterized by recurring, rupturing epithelial blisters causing glaucoma, iridocyclitis, and Fuchs' dystrophy.

H18.10   Bullous keratopathy, unspecified eye
H18.11   Bullous keratopathy, right eye
H18.12   Bullous keratopathy, left eye
H18.13   Bullous keratopathy, bilateral

Chapter 7. Diseases of the Eye and Adnexa

H18.2–H18.619

√5ᵗʰ **H18.2 Other and unspecified corneal edema**

  H18.20 Unspecified corneal edema

√6ᵗʰ **H18.21 Corneal edema** secondary to contact lens

    EXCLUDES 2   *other corneal disorders due to contact lens (H18.82-)*

    H18.211 Corneal edema secondary to contact lens, right eye

    H18.212 Corneal edema secondary to contact lens, left eye

    H18.213 Corneal edema secondary to contact lens, bilateral

    H18.219 Corneal edema secondary to contact lens, unspecified eye

√6ᵗʰ **H18.22 Idiopathic** corneal edema

    H18.221 Idiopathic corneal edema, right eye

    H18.222 Idiopathic corneal edema, left eye

    H18.223 Idiopathic corneal edema, bilateral

    H18.229 Idiopathic corneal edema, unspecified eye

√6ᵗʰ **H18.23 Secondary** corneal edema

    H18.231 Secondary corneal edema, right eye

    H18.232 Secondary corneal edema, left eye

    H18.233 Secondary corneal edema, bilateral

    H18.239 Secondary corneal edema, unspecified eye

√5ᵗʰ **H18.3 Changes of corneal membranes**

  H18.30 Unspecified corneal membrane change

√6ᵗʰ **H18.31 Folds and rupture in** Bowman's membrane

    H18.311 Folds and rupture in Bowman's membrane, right eye

    H18.312 Folds and rupture in Bowman's membrane, left eye

    H18.313 Folds and rupture in Bowman's membrane, bilateral

    H18.319 Folds and rupture in Bowman's membrane, unspecified eye

√6ᵗʰ **H18.32 Folds** in Descemet's membrane

    H18.321 Folds in Descemet's membrane, right eye

    H18.322 Folds in Descemet's membrane, left eye

    H18.323 Folds in Descemet's membrane, bilateral

    H18.329 Folds in Descemet's membrane, unspecified eye

√6ᵗʰ **H18.33 Rupture** in Descemet's membrane

    H18.331 Rupture in Descemet's membrane, right eye

    H18.332 Rupture in Descemet's membrane, left eye

    H18.333 Rupture in Descemet's membrane, bilateral

    H18.339 Rupture in Descemet's membrane, unspecified eye

√5ᵗʰ **H18.4 Corneal degeneration**

    EXCLUDES 1   *Mooren's ulcer (H16.0-)*

                 recurrent erosion of cornea (H18.83-)

  H18.40 Unspecified corneal degeneration

√6ᵗʰ **H18.41 Arcus senilis**

    Senile corneal changes

    H18.411 Arcus senilis, right eye

    H18.412 Arcus senilis, left eye

    H18.413 Arcus senilis, bilateral

    H18.419 Arcus senilis, unspecified eye

√6ᵗʰ **H18.42 Band keratopathy**

    H18.421 Band keratopathy, right eye

    H18.422 Band keratopathy, left eye

    H18.423 Band keratopathy, bilateral

    H18.429 Band keratopathy, unspecified eye

  H18.43 Other calcerous corneal degeneration

√6ᵗʰ **H18.44 Keratomalacia**

    EXCLUDES 1   *keratomalacia due to vitamin A deficiency (E50.4)*

    H18.441 Keratomalacia, right eye

    H18.442 Keratomalacia, left eye

    H18.443 Keratomalacia, bilateral

    H18.449 Keratomalacia, unspecified eye

√6ᵗʰ **H18.45 Nodular corneal degeneration**

    H18.451 Nodular corneal degeneration, right eye

    H18.452 Nodular corneal degeneration, left eye

    H18.453 Nodular corneal degeneration, bilateral

    H18.459 Nodular corneal degeneration, unspecified eye

√6ᵗʰ **H18.46 Peripheral corneal degeneration**

    H18.461 Peripheral corneal degeneration, right eye

    H18.462 Peripheral corneal degeneration, left eye

    H18.463 Peripheral corneal degeneration, bilateral

    H18.469 Peripheral corneal degeneration, unspecified eye

  H18.49 Other corneal degeneration

√5ᵗʰ **H18.5 Hereditary corneal dystrophies**

    AHA: 2020,4Q,24

√6ᵗʰ **H18.50 Unspecified hereditary corneal dystrophies**

    H18.501 Unspecified hereditary corneal dystrophies, right eye

    H18.502 Unspecified hereditary corneal dystrophies, left eye

    H18.503 Unspecified hereditary corneal dystrophies, bilateral

    H18.509 Unspecified hereditary corneal dystrophies, unspecified eye

√6ᵗʰ **H18.51 Endothelial corneal dystrophy**

    Fuchs' dystrophy

    H18.511 Endothelial corneal dystrophy, right eye

    H18.512 Endothelial corneal dystrophy, left eye

    H18.513 Endothelial corneal dystrophy, bilateral

    H18.519 Endothelial corneal dystrophy, unspecified eye

√6ᵗʰ **H18.52 Epithelial (juvenile) corneal dystrophy**

    H18.521 Epithelial (juvenile) corneal dystrophy, right eye

    H18.522 Epithelial (juvenile) corneal dystrophy, left eye

    H18.523 Epithelial (juvenile) corneal dystrophy, bilateral

    H18.529 Epithelial (juvenile) corneal dystrophy, unspecified eye

√6ᵗʰ **H18.53 Granular corneal dystrophy**

    H18.531 Granular corneal dystrophy, right eye

    H18.532 Granular corneal dystrophy, left eye

    H18.533 Granular corneal dystrophy, bilateral

    H18.539 Granular corneal dystrophy, unspecified eye

√6ᵗʰ **H18.54 Lattice corneal dystrophy**

    H18.541 Lattice corneal dystrophy, right eye

    H18.542 Lattice corneal dystrophy, left eye

    H18.543 Lattice corneal dystrophy, bilateral

    H18.549 Lattice corneal dystrophy, unspecified eye

√6ᵗʰ **H18.55 Macular corneal dystrophy**

    H18.551 Macular corneal dystrophy, right eye

    H18.552 Macular corneal dystrophy, left eye

    H18.553 Macular corneal dystrophy, bilateral

    H18.559 Macular corneal dystrophy, unspecified eye

√6ᵗʰ **H18.59 Other hereditary corneal dystrophies**

    H18.591 Other hereditary corneal dystrophies, right eye

    H18.592 Other hereditary corneal dystrophies, left eye

    H18.593 Other hereditary corneal dystrophies, bilateral

    H18.599 Other hereditary corneal dystrophies, unspecified eye

√5ᵗʰ **H18.6 Keratoconus**

√6ᵗʰ **H18.60 Keratoconus, unspecified**

    H18.601 Keratoconus, unspecified, right eye

    H18.602 Keratoconus, unspecified, left eye

    H18.603 Keratoconus, unspecified, bilateral

    H18.609 Keratoconus, unspecified, unspecified eye

√6ᵗʰ **H18.61 Keratoconus, stable**

    H18.611 Keratoconus, stable, right eye

    H18.612 Keratoconus, stable, left eye

    H18.613 Keratoconus, stable, bilateral

    H18.619 Keratoconus, stable, unspecified eye

✓6ᵗʰ **H18.62**   **Keratoconus,** unstable
Acute hydrops
H18.621   **Keratoconus, unstable, right eye**
H18.622   **Keratoconus, unstable, left eye**
H18.623   **Keratoconus, unstable, bilateral**
H18.629   **Keratoconus, unstable, unspecified eye**

✓5ᵗʰ **H18.7**   **Other and unspecified corneal deformities**
> EXCLUDES 1   congenital malformations of cornea (Q13.3-Q13.4)

H18.70   **Unspecified corneal deformity**

✓6ᵗʰ **H18.71**   **Corneal** ectasia
H18.711   **Corneal ectasia, right eye**
H18.712   **Corneal ectasia, left eye**
H18.713   **Corneal ectasia, bilateral**
H18.719   **Corneal ectasia, unspecified eye**

✓6ᵗʰ **H18.72**   **Corneal** staphyloma
H18.721   **Corneal staphyloma, right eye**
H18.722   **Corneal staphyloma, left eye**
H18.723   **Corneal staphyloma, bilateral**
H18.729   **Corneal staphyloma, unspecified eye**

✓6ᵗʰ **H18.73**   Descemetocele
H18.731   **Descemetocele, right eye**
H18.732   **Descemetocele, left eye**
H18.733   **Descemetocele, bilateral**
H18.739   **Descemetocele, unspecified eye**

✓6ᵗʰ **H18.79**   **Other corneal deformities**
H18.791   **Other corneal deformities, right eye**
H18.792   **Other corneal deformities, left eye**
H18.793   **Other corneal deformities, bilateral**
H18.799   **Other corneal deformities, unspecified eye**

✓5ᵗʰ **H18.8**   **Other specified disorders of cornea**

✓6ᵗʰ **H18.81**   **Anesthesia and hypoesthesia of cornea**
H18.811   **Anesthesia and hypoesthesia of cornea, right eye**
H18.812   **Anesthesia and hypoesthesia of cornea, left eye**
H18.813   **Anesthesia and hypoesthesia of cornea, bilateral**
H18.819   **Anesthesia and hypoesthesia of cornea, unspecified eye**

✓6ᵗʰ **H18.82**   **Corneal disorder due to contact lens**
> EXCLUDES 2   corneal edema due to contact lens (H18.21-)

H18.821   **Corneal disorder due to contact lens, right eye**
H18.822   **Corneal disorder due to contact lens, left eye**
H18.823   **Corneal disorder due to contact lens, bilateral**
H18.829   **Corneal disorder due to contact lens, unspecified eye**

✓6ᵗʰ **H18.83**   **Recurrent erosion of cornea**
H18.831   **Recurrent erosion of cornea, right eye**
H18.832   **Recurrent erosion of cornea, left eye**
H18.833   **Recurrent erosion of cornea, bilateral**
H18.839   **Recurrent erosion of cornea, unspecified eye**

✓6ᵗʰ **H18.89**   **Other specified disorders of cornea**
H18.891   **Other specified disorders of cornea, right eye**
H18.892   **Other specified disorders of cornea, left eye**
H18.893   **Other specified disorders of cornea, bilateral**
H18.899   **Other specified disorders of cornea, unspecified eye**

H18.9   **Unspecified disorder of cornea**

✓4ᵗʰ **H20**   **Iridocyclitis**

✓5ᵗʰ **H20.0**   **Acute and subacute iridocyclitis**
Acute anterior uveitis
Acute cyclitis
Acute iritis
Subacute anterior uveitis
Subacute cyclitis
Subacute iritis
> EXCLUDES 1   iridocyclitis, iritis, uveitis (due to) (in) diabetes mellitus (E08-E13 with .39)
> iridocyclitis, iritis, uveitis (due to) (in) diphtheria (A36.89)
> iridocyclitis, iritis, uveitis (due to) (in) gonococcal (A54.32)
> iridocyclitis, iritis, uveitis (due to) (in) herpes (simplex) (B00.51)
> iridocyclitis, iritis, uveitis (due to) (in) herpes zoster (B02.32)
> iridocyclitis, iritis, uveitis (due to) (in) late congenital syphilis (A50.39)
> iridocyclitis, iritis, uveitis (due to) (in) late syphilis (A52.71)
> iridocyclitis, iritis, uveitis (due to) (in) sarcoidosis (D86.83)
> iridocyclitis, iritis, uveitis (due to) (in) syphilis (A51.43)
> iridocyclitis, iritis, uveitis (due to) (in) toxoplasmosis (B58.09)
> iridocyclitis, iritis, uveitis (due to) (in) tuberculosis (A18.54)

H20.00   **Unspecified acute and subacute iridocyclitis**

✓6ᵗʰ **H20.01**   Primary **iridocyclitis**
H20.011   **Primary iridocyclitis, right eye**
H20.012   **Primary iridocyclitis, left eye**
H20.013   **Primary iridocyclitis, bilateral**
H20.019   **Primary iridocyclitis, unspecified eye**

✓6ᵗʰ **H20.02**   Recurrent acute **iridocyclitis**
H20.021   **Recurrent acute iridocyclitis, right eye**
H20.022   **Recurrent acute iridocyclitis, left eye**
H20.023   **Recurrent acute iridocyclitis, bilateral**
H20.029   **Recurrent acute iridocyclitis, unspecified eye**

✓6ᵗʰ **H20.03**   Secondary infectious **iridocyclitis**
H20.031   **Secondary infectious iridocyclitis, right eye**
H20.032   **Secondary infectious iridocyclitis, left eye**
H20.033   **Secondary infectious iridocyclitis, bilateral**
H20.039   **Secondary infectious iridocyclitis, unspecified eye**

✓6ᵗʰ **H20.04**   Secondary noninfectious **iridocyclitis**
H20.041   **Secondary noninfectious iridocyclitis, right eye**
H20.042   **Secondary noninfectious iridocyclitis, left eye**
H20.043   **Secondary noninfectious iridocyclitis, bilateral**
H20.049   **Secondary noninfectious iridocyclitis, unspecified eye**

✓6ᵗʰ **H20.05**   Hypopyon
H20.051   **Hypopyon, right eye**
H20.052   **Hypopyon, left eye**
H20.053   **Hypopyon, bilateral**
H20.059   **Hypopyon, unspecified eye**

✓5ᵗʰ **H20.1**   Chronic **iridocyclitis**
Use additional code for any associated cataract (H26.21-)
> EXCLUDES 2   posterior cyclitis (H30.2-)

H20.10   **Chronic iridocyclitis, unspecified eye**
H20.11   **Chronic iridocyclitis, right eye**
H20.12   **Chronic iridocyclitis, left eye**
H20.13   **Chronic iridocyclitis, bilateral**

✓6ᵗʰ **H20.2**   Lens-induced **iridocyclitis**
H20.20   **Lens-induced iridocyclitis, unspecified eye**
H20.21   **Lens-induced iridocyclitis, right eye**
H20.22   **Lens-induced iridocyclitis, left eye**
H20.23   **Lens-induced iridocyclitis, bilateral**

✓5ᵗʰ **H20.8 Other iridocyclitis**

     EXCLUDES 2   *glaucomatocyclitis crises (H40.4-)*
                       posterior cyclitis (H30.2-)
                       sympathetic uveitis (H44.13-)

   ✓6ᵗʰ **H20.81 Fuchs' heterochromic cyclitis**

       H20.811 Fuchs' heterochromic cyclitis, right eye
       H20.812 Fuchs' heterochromic cyclitis, left eye
       H20.813 Fuchs' heterochromic cyclitis, bilateral
       H20.819 Fuchs' heterochromic cyclitis, unspecified eye

   ✓6ᵗʰ **H20.82 Vogt-Koyanagi syndrome**

       H20.821 Vogt-Koyanagi syndrome, right eye
       H20.822 Vogt-Koyanagi syndrome, left eye
       H20.823 Vogt-Koyanagi syndrome, bilateral
       H20.829 Vogt-Koyanagi syndrome, unspecified eye

H20.9 Unspecified iridocyclitis
     Uveitis NOS

✓4ᵗʰ **H21 Other disorders of iris and ciliary body**

     EXCLUDES 2   *sympathetic uveitis (H44.1-)*

   ✓5ᵗʰ **H21.0 Hyphema**

     EXCLUDES 1   *traumatic hyphema (S05.1-)*

Hyphema

- Iris
- Cornea
- Hyphema

     H21.00 Hyphema, unspecified eye
     H21.01 Hyphema, right eye
     H21.02 Hyphema, left eye
     H21.03 Hyphema, bilateral

   ✓5ᵗʰ **H21.1 Other vascular disorders of iris and ciliary body**

     Neovascularization of iris or ciliary body
     Rubeosis iridis
     Rubeosis of iris

   ✓6ᵗʰ **H21.1X Other vascular disorders of iris and ciliary body**

       H21.1X1 Other vascular disorders of iris and ciliary body, right eye
       H21.1X2 Other vascular disorders of iris and ciliary body, left eye
       H21.1X3 Other vascular disorders of iris and ciliary body, bilateral
       H21.1X9 Other vascular disorders of iris and ciliary body, unspecified eye

   ✓5ᵗʰ **H21.2 Degeneration of iris and ciliary body**

   ✓6ᵗʰ **H21.21 Degeneration of chamber angle**

       H21.211 Degeneration of chamber angle, right eye
       H21.212 Degeneration of chamber angle, left eye
       H21.213 Degeneration of chamber angle, bilateral
       H21.219 Degeneration of chamber angle, unspecified eye

   ✓6ᵗʰ **H21.22 Degeneration of ciliary body**

       H21.221 Degeneration of ciliary body, right eye
       H21.222 Degeneration of ciliary body, left eye
       H21.223 Degeneration of ciliary body, bilateral
       H21.229 Degeneration of ciliary body, unspecified eye

   ✓6ᵗʰ **H21.23 Degeneration of iris (pigmentary)**
     Translucency of iris

       H21.231 Degeneration of iris (pigmentary), right eye
       H21.232 Degeneration of iris (pigmentary), left eye
       H21.233 Degeneration of iris (pigmentary), bilateral

       H21.239 Degeneration of iris (pigmentary), unspecified eye

   ✓6ᵗʰ **H21.24 Degeneration of pupillary margin**

       H21.241 Degeneration of pupillary margin, right eye
       H21.242 Degeneration of pupillary margin, left eye
       H21.243 Degeneration of pupillary margin, bilateral
       H21.249 Degeneration of pupillary margin, unspecified eye

   ✓6ᵗʰ **H21.25 Iridoschisis**

       H21.251 Iridoschisis, right eye
       H21.252 Iridoschisis, left eye
       H21.253 Iridoschisis, bilateral
       H21.259 Iridoschisis, unspecified eye

   ✓6ᵗʰ **H21.26 Iris atrophy (essential) (progressive)**

       H21.261 Iris atrophy (essential) (progressive), right eye
       H21.262 Iris atrophy (essential) (progressive), left eye
       H21.263 Iris atrophy (essential) (progressive), bilateral
       H21.269 Iris atrophy (essential) (progressive), unspecified eye

   ✓6ᵗʰ **H21.27 Miotic pupillary cyst**

       H21.271 Miotic pupillary cyst, right eye
       H21.272 Miotic pupillary cyst, left eye
       H21.273 Miotic pupillary cyst, bilateral
       H21.279 Miotic pupillary cyst, unspecified eye

     H21.29 Other iris atrophy

   ✓5ᵗʰ **H21.3 Cyst of iris, ciliary body and anterior chamber**

     EXCLUDES 2   *miotic pupillary cyst (H21.27-)*

   ✓6ᵗʰ **H21.30 Idiopathic cysts of iris, ciliary body or anterior chamber**
     Cyst of iris, ciliary body or anterior chamber NOS

       H21.301 Idiopathic cysts of iris, ciliary body or anterior chamber, right eye
       H21.302 Idiopathic cysts of iris, ciliary body or anterior chamber, left eye
       H21.303 Idiopathic cysts of iris, ciliary body or anterior chamber, bilateral
       H21.309 Idiopathic cysts of iris, ciliary body or anterior chamber, unspecified eye

   ✓6ᵗʰ **H21.31 Exudative cysts of iris or anterior chamber**

       H21.311 Exudative cysts of iris or anterior chamber, right eye
       H21.312 Exudative cysts of iris or anterior chamber, left eye
       H21.313 Exudative cysts of iris or anterior chamber, bilateral
       H21.319 Exudative cysts of iris or anterior chamber, unspecified eye

   ✓6ᵗʰ **H21.32 Implantation cysts of iris, ciliary body or anterior chamber**

       H21.321 Implantation cysts of iris, ciliary body or anterior chamber, right eye
       H21.322 Implantation cysts of iris, ciliary body or anterior chamber, left eye
       H21.323 Implantation cysts of iris, ciliary body or anterior chamber, bilateral
       H21.329 Implantation cysts of iris, ciliary body or anterior chamber, unspecified eye

   ✓6ᵗʰ **H21.33 Parasitic cyst of iris, ciliary body or anterior chamber**

       H21.331 Parasitic cyst of iris, ciliary body or anterior chamber, right eye
       H21.332 Parasitic cyst of iris, ciliary body or anterior chamber, left eye
       H21.333 Parasitic cyst of iris, ciliary body or anterior chamber, bilateral
       H21.339 Parasitic cyst of iris, ciliary body or anterior chamber, unspecified eye

   ✓6ᵗʰ **H21.34 Primary cyst of pars plana**

       H21.341 Primary cyst of pars plana, right eye
       H21.342 Primary cyst of pars plana, left eye
       H21.343 Primary cyst of pars plana, bilateral
       H21.349 Primary cyst of pars plana, unspecified eye

√6ᵗʰ H21.35 Exudative cyst of pars plana

DEF: Protein, fatty-filled bullous elevation of the nonpigmented outermost ciliary epithelium of pars plana, due to fluid leak from blood vessels.

- H21.351 Exudative cyst of pars plana, right eye
- H21.352 Exudative cyst of pars plana, left eye
- H21.353 Exudative cyst of pars plana, bilateral
- H21.359 Exudative cyst of pars plana, unspecified eye

√5ᵗʰ H21.4 Pupillary membranes

Iris bombé
Pupillary occlusion
Pupillary seclusion

EXCLUDES 1   congenital pupillary membranes (Q13.8)

- H21.40 Pupillary membranes, unspecified eye
- H21.41 Pupillary membranes, right eye
- H21.42 Pupillary membranes, left eye
- H21.43 Pupillary membranes, bilateral

√5ᵗʰ H21.5 Other and unspecified adhesions and disruptions of iris and ciliary body

EXCLUDES 1   corectopia (Q13.2)

√6ᵗʰ H21.50 Unspecified adhesions of iris

Synechia (iris) NOS

- H21.501 Unspecified adhesions of iris, right eye
- H21.502 Unspecified adhesions of iris, left eye
- H21.503 Unspecified adhesions of iris, bilateral
- H21.509 Unspecified adhesions of iris and ciliary body, unspecified eye

√6ᵗʰ H21.51 Anterior synechiae (iris)

- H21.511 Anterior synechiae (iris), right eye
- H21.512 Anterior synechiae (iris), left eye
- H21.513 Anterior synechiae (iris), bilateral
- H21.519 Anterior synechiae (iris), unspecified eye

√6ᵗʰ H21.52 Goniosynechiae

- H21.521 Goniosynechiae, right eye
- H21.522 Goniosynechiae, left eye
- H21.523 Goniosynechiae, bilateral
- H21.529 Goniosynechiae, unspecified eye

√6ᵗʰ H21.53 Iridodialysis

- H21.531 Iridodialysis, right eye
- H21.532 Iridodialysis, left eye
- H21.533 Iridodialysis, bilateral
- H21.539 Iridodialysis, unspecified eye

√6ᵗʰ H21.54 Posterior synechiae (iris)

- H21.541 Posterior synechiae (iris), right eye
- H21.542 Posterior synechiae (iris), left eye
- H21.543 Posterior synechiae (iris), bilateral
- H21.549 Posterior synechiae (iris), unspecified eye

√6ᵗʰ H21.55 Recession of chamber angle

- H21.551 Recession of chamber angle, right eye
- H21.552 Recession of chamber angle, left eye
- H21.553 Recession of chamber angle, bilateral
- H21.559 Recession of chamber angle, unspecified eye

√6ᵗʰ H21.56 Pupillary abnormalities

Deformed pupil
Ectopic pupil
Rupture of sphincter, pupil

EXCLUDES 1   congenital deformity of pupil (Q13.2-)

- H21.561 Pupillary abnormality, right eye
- H21.562 Pupillary abnormality, left eye
- H21.563 Pupillary abnormality, bilateral
- H21.569 Pupillary abnormality, unspecified eye

√5ᵗʰ H21.8 Other specified disorders of iris and ciliary body

H21.81 Floppy iris syndrome

Intraoperative floppy iris syndrome (IFIS)
Use additional code for adverse effect, if applicable, to identify drug (T36-T50 with fifth or sixth character 5)

H21.82 Plateau iris syndrome (post-iridectomy) (postprocedural)

H21.89 Other specified disorders of iris and ciliary body

H21.9 Unspecified disorder of iris and ciliary body

H22 Disorders of iris and ciliary body in diseases classified elsewhere

Code first underlying disease, such as:
gout (M1A.-, M10.-)
leprosy (A30.-)
parasitic disease (B89)

Disorders of lens (H25-H28)

√4ᵗʰ H25 Age-related cataract

Senile cataract

EXCLUDES 2   capsular glaucoma with pseudoexfoliation of lens (H40.1-)

Cataracts

Iris / Cornea / Pupil / Lens / Vitreous / Retina / Normal lens / Clouded lens / Lens affected by cataracts

√5ᵗʰ H25.0 Age-related incipient cataract

√6ᵗʰ H25.01 Cortical age-related cataract

- H25.011 Cortical age-related cataract, right eye [A]
- H25.012 Cortical age-related cataract, left eye [A]
- H25.013 Cortical age-related cataract, bilateral [A]
- H25.019 Cortical age-related cataract, unspecified eye [A]

√6ᵗʰ H25.03 Anterior subcapsular polar age-related cataract

- H25.031 Anterior subcapsular polar age-related cataract, right eye [A]
- H25.032 Anterior subcapsular polar age-related cataract, left eye [A]
- H25.033 Anterior subcapsular polar age-related cataract, bilateral [A]
- H25.039 Anterior subcapsular polar age-related cataract, unspecified eye [A]

√6ᵗʰ H25.04 Posterior subcapsular polar age-related cataract

- H25.041 Posterior subcapsular polar age-related cataract, right eye [A]
- H25.042 Posterior subcapsular polar age-related cataract, left eye [A]
- H25.043 Posterior subcapsular polar age-related cataract, bilateral [A]
- H25.049 Posterior subcapsular polar age-related cataract, unspecified eye [A]

√6ᵗʰ H25.09 Other age-related incipient cataract

Coronary age-related cataract
Punctate age-related cataract
Water clefts

- H25.091 Other age-related incipient cataract, right eye [A]
- H25.092 Other age-related incipient cataract, left eye [A]
- H25.093 Other age-related incipient cataract, bilateral [A]
- H25.099 Other age-related incipient cataract, unspecified eye [A]

√5ᵗʰ H25.1 Age-related nuclear cataract

Cataracta brunescens
Nuclear sclerosis cataract

AHA: 2019,2Q,31; 2016,1Q,32

- H25.10 Age-related nuclear cataract, unspecified eye [A]
- H25.11 Age-related nuclear cataract, right eye [A]
- H25.12 Age-related nuclear cataract, left eye [A]
- H25.13 Age-related nuclear cataract, bilateral [A]

√5ᵗʰ **H25.2 Age-related cataract,** morgagnian type
Age-related hypermature cataract
- H25.20 **Age-related cataract, morgagnian type, unspecified eye** Ⓐ
- H25.21 **Age-related cataract, morgagnian type,** right **eye** Ⓐ
- H25.22 **Age-related cataract, morgagnian type,** left **eye** Ⓐ
- H25.23 **Age-related cataract, morgagnian type,** bilateral Ⓐ

√5ᵗʰ **H25.8 Other age-related cataract**
√6ᵗʰ H25.81 **Combined forms** of age-related cataract
AHA: 2019,2Q,30
- H25.811 **Combined forms of age-related cataract,** right **eye** Ⓐ
- H25.812 **Combined forms of age-related cataract,** left **eye** Ⓐ
- H25.813 **Combined forms of age-related cataract,** bilateral Ⓐ
- H25.819 **Combined forms of age-related cataract, unspecified eye** Ⓐ
- H25.89 **Other age-related cataract** Ⓐ
H25.9 Unspecified age-related cataract Ⓐ

√4ᵗʰ **H26 Other cataract**
EXCLUDES 1   congenital cataract (Q12.0)

√5ᵗʰ **H26.0 Infantile and juvenile cataract**
√6ᵗʰ H26.00 **Unspecified infantile and juvenile cataract**
- H26.001 **Unspecified infantile and juvenile cataract,** right **eye** Ⓟ
- H26.002 **Unspecified infantile and juvenile cataract,** left **eye** Ⓟ
- H26.003 **Unspecified infantile and juvenile cataract,** bilateral Ⓟ
- H26.009 **Unspecified infantile and juvenile cataract, unspecified eye** Ⓟ
√6ᵗʰ H26.01 **Infantile and juvenile** cortical, lamellar, or zonular **cataract**
- H26.011 **Infantile and juvenile cortical, lamellar, or zonular cataract,** right **eye** Ⓟ
- H26.012 **Infantile and juvenile cortical, lamellar, or zonular cataract,** left **eye** Ⓟ
- H26.013 **Infantile and juvenile cortical, lamellar, or zonular cataract,** bilateral Ⓟ
- H26.019 **Infantile and juvenile cortical, lamellar, or zonular cataract, unspecified eye** Ⓟ
√6ᵗʰ H26.03 **Infantile and juvenile** nuclear **cataract**
- H26.031 **Infantile and juvenile nuclear cataract,** right **eye** Ⓟ
- H26.032 **Infantile and juvenile nuclear cataract,** left **eye** Ⓟ
- H26.033 **Infantile and juvenile nuclear cataract,** bilateral Ⓟ
- H26.039 **Infantile and juvenile nuclear cataract, unspecified eye** Ⓟ
√6ᵗʰ H26.04 **Anterior subcapsular polar** infantile and juvenile **cataract**
- H26.041 **Anterior subcapsular polar infantile and juvenile cataract,** right **eye** Ⓟ
- H26.042 **Anterior subcapsular polar infantile and juvenile cataract,** left **eye** Ⓟ
- H26.043 **Anterior subcapsular polar infantile and juvenile cataract,** bilateral Ⓟ
- H26.049 **Anterior subcapsular polar infantile and juvenile cataract, unspecified eye** Ⓟ
√6ᵗʰ H26.05 **Posterior subcapsular polar** infantile and juvenile **cataract**
- H26.051 **Posterior subcapsular polar infantile and juvenile cataract,** right **eye** Ⓟ
- H26.052 **Posterior subcapsular polar infantile and juvenile cataract,** left **eye** Ⓟ
- H26.053 **Posterior subcapsular polar infantile and juvenile cataract,** bilateral Ⓟ
- H26.059 **Posterior subcapsular polar infantile and juvenile cataract, unspecified eye** Ⓟ
√6ᵗʰ H26.06 **Combined forms** of infantile and juvenile cataract
- H26.061 **Combined forms of infantile and juvenile cataract,** right **eye** Ⓟ

- H26.062 **Combined forms of infantile and juvenile cataract,** left **eye** Ⓟ
- H26.063 **Combined forms of infantile and juvenile cataract,** bilateral Ⓟ
- H26.069 **Combined forms of infantile and juvenile cataract, unspecified eye** Ⓟ
- H26.09 **Other infantile and juvenile cataract** Ⓟ
√5ᵗʰ **H26.1 Traumatic cataract**
Use additional code (Chapter 20) to identify external cause
√6ᵗʰ H26.10 **Unspecified traumatic cataract**
- H26.101 **Unspecified traumatic cataract,** right **eye**
- H26.102 **Unspecified traumatic cataract,** left **eye**
- H26.103 **Unspecified traumatic cataract,** bilateral
- H26.109 **Unspecified traumatic cataract, unspecified eye**
√6ᵗʰ H26.11 **Localized** traumatic opacities
- H26.111 **Localized traumatic opacities,** right **eye**
- H26.112 **Localized traumatic opacities,** left **eye**
- H26.113 **Localized traumatic opacities,** bilateral
- H26.119 **Localized traumatic opacities, unspecified eye**
√6ᵗʰ H26.12 **Partially resolved** traumatic cataract
- H26.121 **Partially resolved traumatic cataract,** right **eye**
- H26.122 **Partially resolved traumatic cataract,** left **eye**
- H26.123 **Partially resolved traumatic cataract,** bilateral
- H26.129 **Partially resolved traumatic cataract, unspecified eye**
√6ᵗʰ H26.13 **Total** traumatic cataract
- H26.131 **Total traumatic cataract,** right **eye**
- H26.132 **Total traumatic cataract,** left **eye**
- H26.133 **Total traumatic cataract,** bilateral
- H26.139 **Total traumatic cataract, unspecified eye**
√5ᵗʰ **H26.2 Complicated cataract**
- H26.20 **Unspecified complicated cataract**
Cataracta complicata NOS
√6ᵗʰ H26.21 **Cataract** with neovascularization
Code also associated condition, such as: chronic iridocyclitis (H20.1-)
- H26.211 **Cataract with neovascularization,** right **eye**
- H26.212 **Cataract with neovascularization,** left **eye**
- H26.213 **Cataract with neovascularization,** bilateral
- H26.219 **Cataract with neovascularization, unspecified eye**
√6ᵗʰ H26.22 **Cataract** secondary to ocular disorders **(degenerative) (inflammatory)**
Code also associated ocular disorder
- H26.221 **Cataract secondary to ocular disorders (degenerative) (inflammatory),** right **eye**
- H26.222 **Cataract secondary to ocular disorders (degenerative) (inflammatory),** left **eye**
- H26.223 **Cataract secondary to ocular disorders (degenerative) (inflammatory),** bilateral
- H26.229 **Cataract secondary to ocular disorders (degenerative) (inflammatory), unspecified eye**
√6ᵗʰ H26.23 **Glaucomatous flecks (subcapsular)**
Code first underlying glaucoma (H40-H42)
- H26.231 **Glaucomatous flecks (subcapsular),** right **eye**
- H26.232 **Glaucomatous flecks (subcapsular),** left **eye**
- H26.233 **Glaucomatous flecks (subcapsular),** bilateral
- H26.239 **Glaucomatous flecks (subcapsular), unspecified eye**
√5ᵗʰ **H26.3 Drug-induced cataract**
Toxic cataract
Use additional code for adverse effect, if applicable, to identify drug (T36-T50 with fifth or sixth character 5)
- H26.30 **Drug-induced cataract, unspecified eye**
- H26.31 **Drug-induced cataract,** right **eye**
- H26.32 **Drug-induced cataract,** left **eye**
- H26.33 **Drug-induced cataract,** bilateral

✓5th **H26.4** Secondary **cataract**

     H26.40   **Unspecified secondary cataract**

     ✓6th **H26.41**   Soemmering's ring

         H26.411   **Soemmering's ring, right eye**

         H26.412   **Soemmering's ring, left eye**

         H26.413   **Soemmering's ring, bilateral**

         H26.419   **Soemmering's ring, unspecified eye**

     ✓6th **H26.49**   **Other secondary cataract**

         AHA: 2018,2Q,14

         H26.491   **Other secondary cataract, right eye**

         H26.492   **Other secondary cataract, left eye**

         H26.493   **Other secondary cataract, bilateral**

         H26.499   **Other secondary cataract, unspecified eye**

H26.8   **Other specified cataract**

H26.9   **Unspecified cataract**

✓4th **H27**   **Other disorders of lens**

     EXCLUDES 1   *congenital lens malformations (Q12.-)*

         mechanical complications of intraocular lens implant (T85.2)

         pseudophakia (Z96.1)

   ✓5th **H27.0**   **Aphakia**

     Acquired absence of lens

     Acquired aphakia

     Aphakia due to trauma

       EXCLUDES 1   *cataract extraction status (Z98.4-)*

           congenital absence of lens (Q12.3)

           congenital aphakia (Q12.3)

     H27.00   **Aphakia, unspecified eye**

     H27.01   **Aphakia, right eye**

     H27.02   **Aphakia, left eye**

     H27.03   **Aphakia, bilateral**

   ✓5th **H27.1**   **Dislocation of lens**

     H27.10   **Unspecified dislocation of lens**

     ✓6th **H27.11**   **Subluxation of lens**

         H27.111   **Subluxation of lens, right eye**

         H27.112   **Subluxation of lens, left eye**

         H27.113   **Subluxation of lens, bilateral**

         H27.119   **Subluxation of lens, unspecified eye**

     ✓6th **H27.12**   **Anterior dislocation of lens**

         H27.121   **Anterior dislocation of lens, right eye**

         H27.122   **Anterior dislocation of lens, left eye**

         H27.123   **Anterior dislocation of lens, bilateral**

         H27.129   **Anterior dislocation of lens, unspecified eye**

     ✓6th **H27.13**   **Posterior dislocation of lens**

         H27.131   **Posterior dislocation of lens, right eye**

         H27.132   **Posterior dislocation of lens, left eye**

         H27.133   **Posterior dislocation of lens, bilateral**

         H27.139   **Posterior dislocation of lens, unspecified eye**

   H27.8   **Other specified disorders of lens**

   H27.9   **Unspecified disorder of lens**

H28   *Cataract in diseases classified elsewhere*

     Code first underlying disease, such as:

       hypoparathyroidism (E20.-)

       myotonia (G71.1-)

       myxedema (E03.-)

       protein-calorie malnutrition (E40-E46)

       EXCLUDES 1   *cataract in diabetes mellitus (E08.36, E09.36, E10.36, E11.36, E13.36)*

Disorders of choroid and retina (H30-H36)

✓4th **H30**   **Chorioretinal inflammation**

   ✓5th **H30.0**   Focal **chorioretinal inflammation**

     Focal chorioretinitis

     Focal choroiditis

     Focal retinitis

     Focal retinochoroiditis

     ✓6th **H30.00**   **Unspecified focal chorioretinal inflammation**

       Focal chorioretinitis NOS

       Focal choroiditis NOS

       Focal retinitis NOS

       Focal retinochoroiditis NOS

       H30.001   **Unspecified focal chorioretinal inflammation, right eye**

       H30.002   **Unspecified focal chorioretinal inflammation, left eye**

       H30.003   **Unspecified focal chorioretinal inflammation, bilateral**

       H30.009   **Unspecified focal chorioretinal inflammation, unspecified eye**

     ✓6th **H30.01**   **Focal chorioretinal inflammation, juxtapapillary**

       H30.011   **Focal chorioretinal inflammation, juxtapapillary, right eye**

       H30.012   **Focal chorioretinal inflammation, juxtapapillary, left eye**

       H30.013   **Focal chorioretinal inflammation, juxtapapillary, bilateral**

       H30.019   **Focal chorioretinal inflammation, juxtapapillary, unspecified eye**

     ✓6th **H30.02**   **Focal chorioretinal inflammation of posterior pole**

       H30.021   **Focal chorioretinal inflammation of posterior pole, right eye**

       H30.022   **Focal chorioretinal inflammation of posterior pole, left eye**

       H30.023   **Focal chorioretinal inflammation of posterior pole, bilateral**

       H30.029   **Focal chorioretinal inflammation of posterior pole, unspecified eye**

     ✓6th **H30.03**   **Focal chorioretinal inflammation, peripheral**

       H30.031   **Focal chorioretinal inflammation, peripheral, right eye**

       H30.032   **Focal chorioretinal inflammation, peripheral, left eye**

       H30.033   **Focal chorioretinal inflammation, peripheral, bilateral**

       H30.039   **Focal chorioretinal inflammation, peripheral, unspecified eye**

     ✓6th **H30.04**   **Focal chorioretinal inflammation, macular or paramacular**

       H30.041   **Focal chorioretinal inflammation, macular or paramacular, right eye**

       H30.042   **Focal chorioretinal inflammation, macular or paramacular, left eye**

       H30.043   **Focal chorioretinal inflammation, macular or paramacular, bilateral**

       H30.049   **Focal chorioretinal inflammation, macular or paramacular, unspecified eye**

   ✓5th **H30.1**   Disseminated **chorioretinal inflammation**

     Disseminated chorioretinitis

     Disseminated choroiditis

     Disseminated retinitis

     Disseminated retinochoroiditis

       EXCLUDES 2   *exudative retinopathy (H35.02-)*

     ✓6th **H30.10**   **Unspecified disseminated chorioretinal inflammation**

       Disseminated chorioretinitis NOS

       Disseminated choroiditis NOS

       Disseminated retinitis NOS

       Disseminated retinochoroiditis NOS

       H30.101   **Unspecified disseminated chorioretinal inflammation, right eye**

       H30.102   **Unspecified disseminated chorioretinal inflammation, left eye**

       H30.103   **Unspecified disseminated chorioretinal inflammation, bilateral**

       H30.109   **Unspecified disseminated chorioretinal inflammation, unspecified eye**

     ✓6th **H30.11**   **Disseminated chorioretinal inflammation of posterior pole**

       H30.111   **Disseminated chorioretinal inflammation of posterior pole, right eye**

       H30.112   **Disseminated chorioretinal inflammation of posterior pole, left eye**

       H30.113   **Disseminated chorioretinal inflammation of posterior pole, bilateral**

       H30.119   **Disseminated chorioretinal inflammation of posterior pole, unspecified eye**

     ✓6th **H30.12**   **Disseminated chorioretinal inflammation, peripheral**

       H30.121   **Disseminated chorioretinal inflammation, peripheral right eye**

       H30.122   **Disseminated chorioretinal inflammation, peripheral, left eye**

       H30.123   **Disseminated chorioretinal inflammation, peripheral, bilateral**

Chapter 7. Diseases of the Eye and Adnexa

H30.129–H31.402

H30.129   Disseminated chorioretinal inflammation, peripheral, unspecified eye

✓6ᵗʰ H30.13   Disseminated chorioretinal inflammation, generalized

H30.131   Disseminated chorioretinal inflammation, generalized, right eye

H30.132   Disseminated chorioretinal inflammation, generalized, left eye

H30.133   Disseminated chorioretinal inflammation, generalized, bilateral

H30.139   Disseminated chorioretinal inflammation, generalized, unspecified eye

✓6ᵗʰ H30.14   Acute posterior multifocal placoid pigment epitheliopathy

H30.141   Acute posterior multifocal placoid pigment epitheliopathy, right eye

H30.142   Acute posterior multifocal placoid pigment epitheliopathy, left eye

H30.143   Acute posterior multifocal placoid pigment epitheliopathy, bilateral

H30.149   Acute posterior multifocal placoid pigment epitheliopathy, unspecified eye

✓5ᵗʰ H30.2   Posterior cyclitis

Pars planitis

H30.20   Posterior cyclitis, unspecified eye

H30.21   Posterior cyclitis, right eye

H30.22   Posterior cyclitis, left eye

H30.23   Posterior cyclitis, bilateral

✓5ᵗʰ H30.8   Other chorioretinal inflammations

✓6ᵗʰ H30.81   Harada's disease

H30.811   Harada's disease, right eye

H30.812   Harada's disease, left eye

H30.813   Harada's disease, bilateral

H30.819   Harada's disease, unspecified eye

✓6ᵗʰ H30.89   Other chorioretinal inflammations

H30.891   Other chorioretinal inflammations, right eye

H30.892   Other chorioretinal inflammations, left eye

H30.893   Other chorioretinal inflammations, bilateral

H30.899   Other chorioretinal inflammations, unspecified eye

✓5ᵗʰ H30.9   Unspecified chorioretinal inflammation

Chorioretinitis NOS
Choroiditis NOS
Neuroretinitis NOS
Retinitis NOS
Retinochoroiditis NOS

H30.90   Unspecified chorioretinal inflammation, unspecified eye

H30.91   Unspecified chorioretinal inflammation, right eye

H30.92   Unspecified chorioretinal inflammation, left eye

H30.93   Unspecified chorioretinal inflammation, bilateral

✓4ᵗʰ **H31**   **Other disorders of choroid**

✓5ᵗʰ H31.0   Chorioretinal scars

EXCLUDES 2   postsurgical chorioretinal scars (H59.81-)

✓6ᵗʰ H31.00   Unspecified chorioretinal scars

H31.001   Unspecified chorioretinal scars, right eye

H31.002   Unspecified chorioretinal scars, left eye

H31.003   Unspecified chorioretinal scars, bilateral

H31.009   Unspecified chorioretinal scars, unspecified eye

✓6ᵗʰ H31.01   Macula scars of posterior pole (postinflammatory) (post-traumatic)

EXCLUDES 1   postprocedural chorioretinal scar (H59.81-)

H31.011   Macula scars of posterior pole (postinflammatory) (post-traumatic), right eye

H31.012   Macula scars of posterior pole (postinflammatory) (post-traumatic), left eye

H31.013   Macula scars of posterior pole (postinflammatory) (post-traumatic), bilateral

H31.019   Macula scars of posterior pole (postinflammatory) (post-traumatic), unspecified eye

✓6ᵗʰ H31.02   Solar retinopathy

H31.021   Solar retinopathy, right eye

H31.022   Solar retinopathy, left eye

H31.023   Solar retinopathy, bilateral

H31.029   Solar retinopathy, unspecified eye

✓6ᵗʰ H31.09   Other chorioretinal scars

H31.091   Other chorioretinal scars, right eye

H31.092   Other chorioretinal scars, left eye

H31.093   Other chorioretinal scars, bilateral

H31.099   Other chorioretinal scars, unspecified eye

✓5ᵗʰ H31.1   Choroidal degeneration

EXCLUDES 2   angioid streaks of macula (H35.33)

✓6ᵗʰ H31.10   Unspecified choroidal degeneration

Choroidal sclerosis NOS

H31.101   Choroidal degeneration, unspecified, right eye

H31.102   Choroidal degeneration, unspecified, left eye

H31.103   Choroidal degeneration, unspecified, bilateral

H31.109   Choroidal degeneration, unspecified, unspecified eye

✓6ᵗʰ H31.11   Age-related choroidal atrophy

H31.111   Age-related choroidal atrophy, right eye   Ⓐ

H31.112   Age-related choroidal atrophy, left eye   Ⓐ

H31.113   Age-related choroidal atrophy, bilateral   Ⓐ

H31.119   Age-related choroidal atrophy, unspecified eye   Ⓐ

✓6ᵗʰ H31.12   Diffuse secondary atrophy of choroid

H31.121   Diffuse secondary atrophy of choroid, right eye

H31.122   Diffuse secondary atrophy of choroid, left eye

H31.123   Diffuse secondary atrophy of choroid, bilateral

H31.129   Diffuse secondary atrophy of choroid, unspecified eye

✓5ᵗʰ H31.2   Hereditary choroidal dystrophy

EXCLUDES 2   hyperornithinemia (E72.4)
ornithinemia (E72.4)

H31.20   Hereditary choroidal dystrophy, unspecified

H31.21   Choroideremia

H31.22   Choroidal dystrophy (central areolar) (generalized) (peripapillary)

H31.23   Gyrate atrophy, choroid

H31.29   Other hereditary choroidal dystrophy

✓5ᵗʰ H31.3   Choroidal hemorrhage and rupture

✓6ᵗʰ H31.30   Unspecified choroidal hemorrhage

H31.301   Unspecified choroidal hemorrhage, right eye

H31.302   Unspecified choroidal hemorrhage, left eye

H31.303   Unspecified choroidal hemorrhage, bilateral

H31.309   Unspecified choroidal hemorrhage, unspecified eye

✓6ᵗʰ H31.31   Expulsive choroidal hemorrhage

H31.311   Expulsive choroidal hemorrhage, right eye

H31.312   Expulsive choroidal hemorrhage, left eye

H31.313   Expulsive choroidal hemorrhage, bilateral

H31.319   Expulsive choroidal hemorrhage, unspecified eye

✓6ᵗʰ H31.32   Choroidal rupture

H31.321   Choroidal rupture, right eye

H31.322   Choroidal rupture, left eye

H31.323   Choroidal rupture, bilateral

H31.329   Choroidal rupture, unspecified eye

✓5ᵗʰ H31.4   Choroidal detachment

✓6ᵗʰ H31.40   Unspecified choroidal detachment

H31.401   Unspecified choroidal detachment, right eye

H31.402   Unspecified choroidal detachment, left eye

Chapter 7. Diseases of the Eye and Adnexa

H31.403 Unspecified choroidal detachment, bilateral

H31.409 Unspecified choroidal detachment, unspecified eye

√6ᵗʰ **H31.41** Hemorrhagic choroidal detachment

H31.411 Hemorrhagic choroidal detachment, right eye

H31.412 Hemorrhagic choroidal detachment, left eye

H31.413 Hemorrhagic choroidal detachment, bilateral

H31.419 Hemorrhagic choroidal detachment, unspecified eye

√6ᵗʰ **H31.42** Serous choroidal detachment

H31.421 Serous choroidal detachment, right eye

H31.422 Serous choroidal detachment, left eye

H31.423 Serous choroidal detachment, bilateral

H31.429 Serous choroidal detachment, unspecified eye

H31.8 Other specified disorders of choroid

H31.9 Unspecified disorder of choroid

H32 *Chorioretinal disorders in diseases classified elsewhere*

Code first underlying disease, such as:

congenital toxoplasmosis (P37.1)

histoplasmosis (B39.-)

leprosy (A30.-)

EXCLUDES 1 *chorioretinitis (in):*

toxoplasmosis (acquired) (B58.01)

tuberculosis (A18.53)

√4ᵗʰ H33 Retinal detachments and breaks

EXCLUDES 1 *detachment of retinal pigment epithelium (H35.72-, H35.73-)*

Retinal Detachment

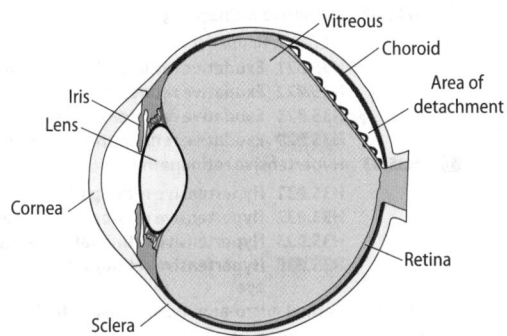

√5ᵗʰ **H33.0** Retinal detachment with retinal break

Rhegmatogenous retinal detachment

EXCLUDES 1 *serous retinal detachment (without retinal break) (H33.2-)*

√6ᵗʰ **H33.00** Unspecified retinal detachment with retinal break

H33.001 Unspecified retinal detachment with retinal break, right eye

H33.002 Unspecified retinal detachment with retinal break, left eye

H33.003 Unspecified retinal detachment with retinal break, bilateral

H33.009 Unspecified retinal detachment with retinal break, unspecified eye

√6ᵗʰ **H33.01** Retinal detachment with single break

H33.011 Retinal detachment with single break, right eye

H33.012 Retinal detachment with single break, left eye

H33.013 Retinal detachment with single break, bilateral

H33.019 Retinal detachment with single break, unspecified eye

√6ᵗʰ **H33.02** Retinal detachment with multiple breaks

H33.021 Retinal detachment with multiple breaks, right eye

H33.022 Retinal detachment with multiple breaks, left eye

H33.023 Retinal detachment with multiple breaks, bilateral

H33.029 Retinal detachment with multiple breaks, unspecified eye

√6ᵗʰ **H33.03** Retinal detachment with giant retinal tear

H33.031 Retinal detachment with giant retinal tear, right eye

H33.032 Retinal detachment with giant retinal tear, left eye

H33.033 Retinal detachment with giant retinal tear, bilateral

H33.039 Retinal detachment with giant retinal tear, unspecified eye

√6ᵗʰ **H33.04** Retinal detachment with retinal dialysis

H33.041 Retinal detachment with retinal dialysis, right eye

H33.042 Retinal detachment with retinal dialysis, left eye

H33.043 Retinal detachment with retinal dialysis, bilateral

H33.049 Retinal detachment with retinal dialysis, unspecified eye

√6ᵗʰ **H33.05** Total retinal detachment

H33.051 Total retinal detachment, right eye

H33.052 Total retinal detachment, left eye

H33.053 Total retinal detachment, bilateral

H33.059 Total retinal detachment, unspecified eye

√5ᵗʰ **H33.1** Retinoschisis and retinal cysts

EXCLUDES 1 *congenital retinoschisis (Q14.1)*

microcystoid degeneration of retina (H35.42-)

√6ᵗʰ **H33.10** Unspecified retinoschisis

H33.101 Unspecified retinoschisis, right eye

H33.102 Unspecified retinoschisis, left eye

H33.103 Unspecified retinoschisis, bilateral

H33.109 Unspecified retinoschisis, unspecified eye

√6ᵗʰ **H33.11** Cyst of ora serrata

H33.111 Cyst of ora serrata, right eye

H33.112 Cyst of ora serrata, left eye

H33.113 Cyst of ora serrata, bilateral

H33.119 Cyst of ora serrata, unspecified eye

√6ᵗʰ **H33.12** Parasitic cyst of retina

H33.121 Parasitic cyst of retina, right eye

H33.122 Parasitic cyst of retina, left eye

H33.123 Parasitic cyst of retina, bilateral

H33.129 Parasitic cyst of retina, unspecified eye

√6ᵗʰ **H33.19** Other retinoschisis and retinal cysts

Pseudocyst of retina

H33.191 Other retinoschisis and retinal cysts, right eye

H33.192 Other retinoschisis and retinal cysts, left eye

H33.193 Other retinoschisis and retinal cysts, bilateral

H33.199 Other retinoschisis and retinal cysts, unspecified eye

√5ᵗʰ **H33.2** Serous retinal detachment

Retinal detachment NOS

Retinal detachment without retinal break

EXCLUDES 1 *central serous chorioretinopathy (H35.71-)*

H33.20 Serous retinal detachment, unspecified eye

H33.21 Serous retinal detachment, right eye

H33.22 Serous retinal detachment, left eye

H33.23 Serous retinal detachment, bilateral

√5ᵗʰ **H33.3** Retinal breaks without detachment

EXCLUDES 1 *chorioretinal scars after surgery for detachment (H59.81-)*

peripheral retinal degeneration without break (H35.4-)

√6ᵗʰ **H33.30** Unspecified retinal break

H33.301 Unspecified retinal break, right eye

H33.302 Unspecified retinal break, left eye

H33.303 Unspecified retinal break, bilateral

H33.309 Unspecified retinal break, unspecified eye

√6ᵗʰ **H33.31** Horseshoe tear of retina without detachment

Operculum of retina without detachment

H33.311 Horseshoe tear of retina without detachment, right eye

H33.312 Horseshoe tear of retina without detachment, left eye

H31.403–H33.312

Chapter 7. Diseases of the Eye and Adnexa

        H33.313   **Horseshoe tear of retina without detachment,** bilateral

        H33.319   **Horseshoe tear of retina without detachment, unspecified eye**

   ✓6th   H33.32   Round hole **of retina without detachment**

        H33.321   **Round hole,** right eye

        H33.322   **Round hole,** left eye

        H33.323   **Round hole,** bilateral

        H33.329   **Round hole, unspecified eye**

   ✓6th   H33.33   Multiple defects **of retina without detachment**

        H33.331   **Multiple defects of retina without detachment,** right eye

        H33.332   **Multiple defects of retina without detachment,** left eye

        H33.333   **Multiple defects of retina without detachment,** bilateral

        H33.339   **Multiple defects of retina without detachment, unspecified eye**

  ✓5th   H33.4   Traction **detachment of retina**

      Proliferative vitreo-retinopathy with retinal detachment

      H33.40   **Traction detachment of retina, unspecified eye**

      H33.41   **Traction detachment of retina,** right eye

      H33.42   **Traction detachment of retina,** left eye

      H33.43   **Traction detachment of retina,** bilateral

     H33.8   **Other retinal detachments**

✓4th   **H34   Retinal vascular occlusions**

    EXCLUDES 1   *amaurosis fugax (G45.3)*

  ✓5th   H34.0   Transient **retinal artery occlusion**

      H34.00   **Transient retinal artery occlusion, unspecified eye**

      H34.01   **Transient retinal artery occlusion,** right eye

      H34.02   **Transient retinal artery occlusion,** left eye

      H34.03   **Transient retinal artery occlusion,** bilateral

  ✓5th   H34.1   Central **retinal artery occlusion**

      H34.10   **Central retinal artery occlusion, unspecified eye**

      H34.11   **Central retinal artery occlusion,** right eye

      H34.12   **Central retinal artery occlusion,** left eye

      H34.13   **Central retinal artery occlusion,** bilateral

  ✓5th   H34.2   **Other retinal artery occlusions**

   ✓6th   H34.21   Partial **retinal artery occlusion**

        Hollenhorst's plaque

        Retinal microembolism

        H34.211   **Partial retinal artery occlusion,** right eye

        H34.212   **Partial retinal artery occlusion,** left eye

        H34.213   **Partial retinal artery occlusion,** bilateral

        H34.219   **Partial retinal artery occlusion, unspecified eye**

   ✓6th   H34.23   **Retinal artery** branch occlusion

        H34.231   **Retinal artery branch occlusion,** right eye

        H34.232   **Retinal artery branch occlusion,** left eye

        H34.233   **Retinal artery branch occlusion,** bilateral

        H34.239   **Retinal artery branch occlusion, unspecified eye**

  ✓5th   H34.8   **Other retinal vascular occlusions**

      AHA: 2016,4Q,19

   ✓6th   H34.81   **Central retinal vein occlusion**

> One of the following 7th characters is to be assigned to codes in subcategory H34.81 to designate the severity of the occlusion:
> Ø   with macular edema
> 1   with retinal neovascularization
> 2   stable
>   old central retinal vein occlusion

        ✓7th   H34.811   **Central retinal vein occlusion,** right eye

        ✓7th   H34.812   **Central retinal vein occlusion,** left eye

        ✓7th   H34.813   **Central retinal vein occlusion,** bilateral

        ✓7th   H34.819   **Central retinal vein occlusion, unspecified eye**

   ✓6th   H34.82   **Venous engorgement**

        Incipient retinal vein occlusion

        Partial retinal vein occlusion

        H34.821   **Venous engorgement,** right eye

        H34.822   **Venous engorgement,** left eye

        H34.823   **Venous engorgement,** bilateral

        H34.829   **Venous engorgement, unspecified eye**

   ✓6th   H34.83   **Tributary (branch) retinal vein occlusion**

> One of the following 7th characters is to be assigned to codes in subcategory H34.83 to designate the severity of the occlusion:
> Ø   with macular edema
> 1   with retinal neovascularization
> 2   stable
>   old tributary (branch) retinal vein occlusion

        ✓7th   H34.831   **Tributary (branch) retinal vein occlusion,** right eye

        ✓7th   H34.832   **Tributary (branch) retinal vein occlusion,** left eye

        ✓7th   H34.833   **Tributary (branch) retinal vein occlusion,** bilateral

        ✓7th   H34.839   **Tributary (branch) retinal vein occlusion, unspecified eye**

     H34.9   **Unspecified retinal vascular occlusion**

✓4th   **H35   Other retinal disorders**

    EXCLUDES 2   *diabetic retinal disorders (E08.311-E08.359, E09.311-E09.359, E10.311-E10.359, E11.311-E11.359, E13.311-E13.359)*

  ✓5th   H35.0   **Background retinopathy and retinal vascular changes**

      Code also any associated hypertension (I10)

      H35.00   **Unspecified background retinopathy**

   ✓6th   H35.01   **Changes in retinal vascular appearance**

        Retinal vascular sheathing

        H35.011   **Changes in retinal vascular appearance,** right eye

        H35.012   **Changes in retinal vascular appearance,** left eye

        H35.013   **Changes in retinal vascular appearance,** bilateral

        H35.019   **Changes in retinal vascular appearance, unspecified eye**

   ✓6th   H35.02   Exudative **retinopathy**

        Coats retinopathy

        H35.021   **Exudative retinopathy,** right eye

        H35.022   **Exudative retinopathy,** left eye

        H35.023   **Exudative retinopathy,** bilateral

        H35.029   **Exudative retinopathy, unspecified eye**

   ✓6th   H35.03   Hypertensive **retinopathy**

        H35.031   **Hypertensive retinopathy,** right eye

        H35.032   **Hypertensive retinopathy,** left eye

        H35.033   **Hypertensive retinopathy,** bilateral

        H35.039   **Hypertensive retinopathy, unspecified eye**

   ✓6th   H35.04   **Retinal** micro-aneurysms, unspecified

        H35.041   **Retinal micro-aneurysms, unspecified,** right eye

        H35.042   **Retinal micro-aneurysms, unspecified,** left eye

        H35.043   **Retinal micro-aneurysms, unspecified,** bilateral

        H35.049   **Retinal micro-aneurysms, unspecified, unspecified eye**

   ✓6th   H35.05   **Retinal** neovascularization, unspecified

        H35.051   **Retinal neovascularization, unspecified,** right eye

        H35.052   **Retinal neovascularization, unspecified,** left eye

        H35.053   **Retinal neovascularization, unspecified,** bilateral

        H35.059   **Retinal neovascularization, unspecified, unspecified eye**

   ✓6th   H35.06   **Retinal** vasculitis

        Eales disease

        Retinal perivasculitis

        DEF: Sight-threatening intraocular inflammation of the retinal blood vessels that causes minimal, partial, or even complete blindness.

        H35.061   **Retinal vasculitis,** right eye

        H35.062   **Retinal vasculitis,** left eye

        H35.063   **Retinal vasculitis,** bilateral

        H35.069   **Retinal vasculitis, unspecified eye**

   ✓6th   H35.07   **Retinal** telangiectasis

        H35.071   **Retinal telangiectasis,** right eye

        H35.072   **Retinal telangiectasis,** left eye

        H35.073   **Retinal telangiectasis,** bilateral

        H35.079   **Retinal telangiectasis, unspecified eye**

H35.Ø9   **Other intraretinal microvascular abnormalities**
      Retinal varices

☑5ᵗʰ   **H35.1**   **Retinopathy of prematurity**

    ☑6ᵗʰ   **H35.1Ø**   **Retinopathy of prematurity, unspecified**
         Retinopathy of prematurity NOS

        H35.1Ø1   **Retinopathy of prematurity, unspecified, right eye**
        H35.1Ø2   **Retinopathy of prematurity, unspecified, left eye**
        H35.1Ø3   **Retinopathy of prematurity, unspecified, bilateral**
        H35.1Ø9   **Retinopathy of prematurity, unspecified, unspecified eye**

    ☑6ᵗʰ   **H35.11**   **Retinopathy of prematurity, stage Ø**

        H35.111   **Retinopathy of prematurity, stage Ø, right eye**
        H35.112   **Retinopathy of prematurity, stage Ø, left eye**
        H35.113   **Retinopathy of prematurity, stage Ø, bilateral**
        H35.119   **Retinopathy of prematurity, stage Ø, unspecified eye**

    ☑6ᵗʰ   **H35.12**   **Retinopathy of prematurity, stage 1**

        H35.121   **Retinopathy of prematurity, stage 1, right eye**
        H35.122   **Retinopathy of prematurity, stage 1, left eye**
        H35.123   **Retinopathy of prematurity, stage 1, bilateral**
        H35.129   **Retinopathy of prematurity, stage 1, unspecified eye**

    ☑6ᵗʰ   **H35.13**   **Retinopathy of prematurity, stage 2**

        H35.131   **Retinopathy of prematurity, stage 2, right eye**
        H35.132   **Retinopathy of prematurity, stage 2, left eye**
        H35.133   **Retinopathy of prematurity, stage 2, bilateral**
        H35.139   **Retinopathy of prematurity, stage 2, unspecified eye**

    ☑6ᵗʰ   **H35.14**   **Retinopathy of prematurity, stage 3**

        H35.141   **Retinopathy of prematurity, stage 3, right eye**
        H35.142   **Retinopathy of prematurity, stage 3, left eye**
        H35.143   **Retinopathy of prematurity, stage 3, bilateral**
        H35.149   **Retinopathy of prematurity, stage 3, unspecified eye**

    ☑6ᵗʰ   **H35.15**   **Retinopathy of prematurity, stage 4**

        H35.151   **Retinopathy of prematurity, stage 4, right eye**
        H35.152   **Retinopathy of prematurity, stage 4, left eye**
        H35.153   **Retinopathy of prematurity, stage 4, bilateral**
        H35.159   **Retinopathy of prematurity, stage 4, unspecified eye**

    ☑6ᵗʰ   **H35.16**   **Retinopathy of prematurity, stage 5**

        H35.161   **Retinopathy of prematurity, stage 5, right eye**
        H35.162   **Retinopathy of prematurity, stage 5, left eye**
        H35.163   **Retinopathy of prematurity, stage 5, bilateral**
        H35.169   **Retinopathy of prematurity, stage 5, unspecified eye**

    ☑6ᵗʰ   **H35.17**   **Retrolental fibroplasia**

        H35.171   **Retrolental fibroplasia, right eye**
        H35.172   **Retrolental fibroplasia, left eye**
        H35.173   **Retrolental fibroplasia, bilateral**
        H35.179   **Retrolental fibroplasia, unspecified eye**

☑5ᵗʰ   **H35.2**   **Other non-diabetic proliferative retinopathy**
      Proliferative vitreo-retinopathy
      EXCLUDES 1   *proliferative vitreo-retinopathy with retinal detachment (H33.4-)*

    H35.2Ø   **Other non-diabetic proliferative retinopathy, unspecified eye**
    H35.21   **Other non-diabetic proliferative retinopathy, right eye**

H35.22   **Other non-diabetic proliferative retinopathy, left eye**

H35.23   **Other non-diabetic proliferative retinopathy, bilateral**

☑5ᵗʰ   **H35.3**   **Degeneration of macula and posterior pole**

    H35.3Ø   **Unspecified macular degeneration**   Ⓐ
         Age-related macular degeneration

    ☑6ᵗʰ   **H35.31**   **Nonexudative age-related macular degeneration**
         Atrophic age-related macular degeneration
         Dry age-related macular degeneration
         AHA: 2016,4Q,20-21

> One of the following 7th characters is to be assigned to each code in subcategory H35.31 to designate the stage of the disease:
> Ø   stage unspecified
> 1   early dry stage
> 2   intermediate dry stage
> 3   advanced atrophic without subfoveal involvement
>   advanced dry stage
> 4   advanced atrophic with subfoveal involvement

      ☑7ᵗʰ   H35.311   **Nonexudative age-related macular degeneration, right eye**   Ⓐ
      ☑7ᵗʰ   H35.312   **Nonexudative age-related macular degeneration, left eye**   Ⓐ
      ☑7ᵗʰ   H35.313   **Nonexudative age-related macular degeneration, bilateral**   Ⓐ
      ☑7ᵗʰ   H35.319   **Nonexudative age-related macular degeneration, unspecified eye**   Ⓐ

    ☑6ᵗʰ   **H35.32**   **Exudative age-related macular degeneration**
         Wet age-related macular degeneration
         AHA: 2016,4Q,20-21

> One of the following 7th characters is to be assigned to each code in subcategory H35.32 to designate the stage of the disease:
> Ø   stage unspecified
> 1   with active choroidal neovascularization
> 2   with inactive choroidal neovascularization
>   with involuted or regressed neovascularization
> 3   with inactive scar

      ☑7ᵗʰ   H35.321   **Exudative age-related macular degeneration, right eye**   HCC ESR COM Ⓐ
      ☑7ᵗʰ   H35.322   **Exudative age-related macular degeneration, left eye**   HCC ESR COM Ⓐ
      ☑7ᵗʰ   H35.323   **Exudative age-related macular degeneration, bilateral**   HCC ESR COM Ⓐ
      ☑7ᵗʰ   H35.329   **Exudative age-related macular degeneration, unspecified eye**   HCC ESR COM Ⓐ

    H35.33   **Angioid streaks of macula**
         DEF: Degeneration of the choroid, characterized by broad, irregular, dark brown streaks radiating from the optic disc; occurs with pseudoxanthoma elasticum or Paget's disease.

    ☑6ᵗʰ   **H35.34**   **Macular cyst, hole, or pseudohole**

        H35.341   **Macular cyst, hole, or pseudohole, right eye**
        H35.342   **Macular cyst, hole, or pseudohole, left eye**
        H35.343   **Macular cyst, hole, or pseudohole, bilateral**
        H35.349   **Macular cyst, hole, or pseudohole, unspecified eye**

    ☑6ᵗʰ   **H35.35**   **Cystoid macular degeneration**
         EXCLUDES 1   *cystoid macular edema following cataract surgery (H59.Ø3-)*

        H35.351   **Cystoid macular degeneration, right eye**
        H35.352   **Cystoid macular degeneration, left eye**
        H35.353   **Cystoid macular degeneration, bilateral**
        H35.359   **Cystoid macular degeneration, unspecified eye**

    ☑6ᵗʰ   **H35.36**   **Drusen (degenerative) of macula**
         AHA: 2017,1Q,51; 2016,4Q,21

        H35.361   **Drusen (degenerative) of macula, right eye**
        H35.362   **Drusen (degenerative) of macula, left eye**
        H35.363   **Drusen (degenerative) of macula, bilateral**

Chapter 7. Diseases of the Eye and Adnexa

H35.369–H36

H35.369 Drusen (degenerative) of macula, unspecified eye

√6ᵗʰ **H35.37** Puckering of macula

H35.371 Puckering of macula, right eye

H35.372 Puckering of macula, left eye

H35.373 Puckering of macula, bilateral

H35.379 Puckering of macula, unspecified eye

√6ᵗʰ **H35.38** Toxic maculopathy

Code first poisoning due to drug or toxin, if applicable (T36-T65 with fifth or sixth character 1-4 or 6)

Use additional code for adverse effect, if applicable, to identify drug (T36-T50 with fifth or sixth character 5)

H35.381 Toxic maculopathy, right eye

H35.382 Toxic maculopathy, left eye

H35.383 Toxic maculopathy, bilateral

H35.389 Toxic maculopathy, unspecified eye

√5ᵗʰ **H35.4** Peripheral retinal degeneration

EXCLUDES 1   *hereditary retinal degeneration (dystrophy) (H35.5-)*

peripheral retinal degeneration with retinal break (H33.3-)

H35.40 Unspecified peripheral retinal degeneration

√6ᵗʰ **H35.41** Lattice degeneration of retina

Palisade degeneration of retina

DEF: Degeneration of the retina, often bilateral, that is usually benign. It is characterized by lines intersecting at irregular intervals in the peripheral retina. Retinal thinning and retinal holes may occur.

H35.411 Lattice degeneration of retina, right eye

H35.412 Lattice degeneration of retina, left eye

H35.413 Lattice degeneration of retina, bilateral

H35.419 Lattice degeneration of retina, unspecified eye

√6ᵗʰ **H35.42** Microcystoid degeneration of retina

H35.421 Microcystoid degeneration of retina, right eye

H35.422 Microcystoid degeneration of retina, left eye

H35.423 Microcystoid degeneration of retina, bilateral

H35.429 Microcystoid degeneration of retina, unspecified eye

√6ᵗʰ **H35.43** Paving stone degeneration of retina

H35.431 Paving stone degeneration of retina, right eye

H35.432 Paving stone degeneration of retina, left eye

H35.433 Paving stone degeneration of retina, bilateral

H35.439 Paving stone degeneration of retina, unspecified eye

√6ᵗʰ **H35.44** Age-related reticular degeneration of retina

H35.441 Age-related reticular degeneration of retina, right eye   Ⓐ

H35.442 Age-related reticular degeneration of retina, left eye   Ⓐ

H35.443 Age-related reticular degeneration of retina, bilateral   Ⓐ

H35.449 Age-related reticular degeneration of retina, unspecified eye   Ⓐ

√6ᵗʰ **H35.45** Secondary pigmentary degeneration

H35.451 Secondary pigmentary degeneration, right eye

H35.452 Secondary pigmentary degeneration, left eye

H35.453 Secondary pigmentary degeneration, bilateral

H35.459 Secondary pigmentary degeneration, unspecified eye

√6ᵗʰ **H35.46** Secondary vitreoretinal degeneration

H35.461 Secondary vitreoretinal degeneration, right eye

H35.462 Secondary vitreoretinal degeneration, left eye

H35.463 Secondary vitreoretinal degeneration, bilateral

H35.469 Secondary vitreoretinal degeneration, unspecified eye

√5ᵗʰ **H35.5** Hereditary retinal dystrophy

EXCLUDES 1   *dystrophies primarily involving Bruch's membrane (H31.1-)*

H35.50 Unspecified hereditary retinal dystrophy

H35.51 Vitreoretinal dystrophy

H35.52 Pigmentary retinal dystrophy

Albipunctate retinal dystrophy

Retinitis pigmentosa

Tapetoretinal dystrophy

H35.53 Other dystrophies primarily involving the sensory retina

Stargardt's disease

H35.54 Dystrophies primarily involving the retinal pigment epithelium

Vitelliform retinal dystrophy

√5ᵗʰ **H35.6** Retinal hemorrhage

H35.60 Retinal hemorrhage, unspecified eye

H35.61 Retinal hemorrhage, right eye

H35.62 Retinal hemorrhage, left eye

H35.63 Retinal hemorrhage, bilateral

√5ᵗʰ **H35.7** Separation of retinal layers

EXCLUDES 1   *retinal detachment (serous) (H33.2-)*

rhegmatogenous retinal detachment (H33.0-)

H35.70 Unspecified separation of retinal layers

√6ᵗʰ **H35.71** Central serous chorioretinopathy

H35.711 Central serous chorioretinopathy, right eye

H35.712 Central serous chorioretinopathy, left eye

H35.713 Central serous chorioretinopathy, bilateral

H35.719 Central serous chorioretinopathy, unspecified eye

√6ᵗʰ **H35.72** Serous detachment of retinal pigment epithelium

H35.721 Serous detachment of retinal pigment epithelium, right eye

H35.722 Serous detachment of retinal pigment epithelium, left eye

H35.723 Serous detachment of retinal pigment epithelium, bilateral

H35.729 Serous detachment of retinal pigment epithelium, unspecified eye

√6ᵗʰ **H35.73** Hemorrhagic detachment of retinal pigment epithelium

H35.731 Hemorrhagic detachment of retinal pigment epithelium, right eye

H35.732 Hemorrhagic detachment of retinal pigment epithelium, left eye

H35.733 Hemorrhagic detachment of retinal pigment epithelium, bilateral

H35.739 Hemorrhagic detachment of retinal pigment epithelium, unspecified eye

√5ᵗʰ **H35.8** Other specified retinal disorders

EXCLUDES 2   *retinal hemorrhage (H35.6-)*

H35.81 Retinal edema

Retinal cotton wool spots

H35.82 Retinal ischemia

H35.89 Other specified retinal disorders

H35.9 Unspecified retinal disorder

H36 *Retinal disorders in diseases classified elsewhere*

Code first underlying disease, such as:

lipid storage disorders (E75.-)

sickle-cell disorders (D57.-)

EXCLUDES 1   *arteriosclerotic retinopathy (H35.0-)*

diabetic retinopathy (E08.3-, E09.3-, E10.3-, E11.3-, E13.3-)

HCC CMS-HCC   **Rx** Rx HCC   **ESR** ESRD HCC   **COM** Commercial HCC   Ⓝ Newborn: 0   Ⓟ Pediatric: 0-17   Ⓜ Maternity: 9-64   Ⓐ Adult: 15-124

634   ICD-10-CM 2023

Glaucoma (H40-H42)

✓4ᵗʰ H40 Glaucoma

> **EXCLUDES 1**   absolute glaucoma (H44.51-)
> congenital glaucoma (Q15.0)
> traumatic glaucoma due to birth injury (P15.3)

Open Angle/Angle Closure Glaucoma

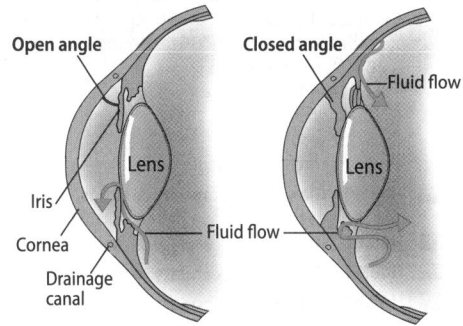

✓5ᵗʰ H40.0 Glaucoma suspect

✓6ᵗʰ H40.00 Preglaucoma, unspecified
- H40.001 Preglaucoma, unspecified, right eye
- H40.002 Preglaucoma, unspecified, left eye
- H40.003 Preglaucoma, unspecified, bilateral
- H40.009 Preglaucoma, unspecified, unspecified eye

✓6ᵗʰ H40.01 Open angle with borderline findings, low risk
Open angle, low risk
- H40.011 Open angle with borderline findings, low risk, right eye
- H40.012 Open angle with borderline findings, low risk, left eye
- H40.013 Open angle with borderline findings, low risk, bilateral
- H40.019 Open angle with borderline findings, low risk, unspecified eye

✓6ᵗʰ H40.02 Open angle with borderline findings, high risk
Open angle, high risk
- H40.021 Open angle with borderline findings, high risk, right eye
- H40.022 Open angle with borderline findings, high risk, left eye
- H40.023 Open angle with borderline findings, high risk, bilateral
- H40.029 Open angle with borderline findings, high risk, unspecified eye

✓6ᵗʰ H40.03 Anatomical narrow angle
Primary angle closure suspect
- H40.031 Anatomical narrow angle, right eye
- H40.032 Anatomical narrow angle, left eye
- H40.033 Anatomical narrow angle, bilateral
- H40.039 Anatomical narrow angle, unspecified eye

✓6ᵗʰ H40.04 Steroid responder
- H40.041 Steroid responder, right eye
- H40.042 Steroid responder, left eye
- H40.043 Steroid responder, bilateral
- H40.049 Steroid responder, unspecified eye

✓6ᵗʰ H40.05 Ocular hypertension
- H40.051 Ocular hypertension, right eye
- H40.052 Ocular hypertension, left eye
- H40.053 Ocular hypertension, bilateral
- H40.059 Ocular hypertension, unspecified eye

✓6ᵗʰ H40.06 Primary angle closure without glaucoma damage
- H40.061 Primary angle closure without glaucoma damage, right eye
- H40.062 Primary angle closure without glaucoma damage, left eye
- H40.063 Primary angle closure without glaucoma damage, bilateral
- H40.069 Primary angle closure without glaucoma damage, unspecified eye

✓5ᵗʰ H40.1 Open-angle glaucoma

> One of the following 7th characters is to be assigned to each code in subcategories H40.10, H40.11, H40.12, H40.13, and H40.14 to designate the stage of glaucoma.
> 0   stage unspecified
> 1   mild stage
> 2   moderate stage
> 3   severe stage
> 4   indeterminate stage

✓x7ᵗʰ H40.10 Unspecified open-angle glaucoma   Rx
> **TIP:** Only one code from this subcategory should be assigned when both left and right eyes are the same stage.

✓6ᵗʰ H40.11 Primary open-angle glaucoma
Chronic simple glaucoma
AHA: 2016,4Q,22
- ✓7ᵗʰ H40.111 Primary open-angle glaucoma, right eye   Rx Q
- ✓7ᵗʰ H40.112 Primary open-angle glaucoma, left eye   Rx Q
- ✓7ᵗʰ H40.113 Primary open-angle glaucoma, bilateral   Rx Q
- ✓7ᵗʰ H40.119 Primary open-angle glaucoma, unspecified eye   Rx

✓6ᵗʰ H40.12 Low-tension glaucoma
- ✓7ᵗʰ H40.121 Low-tension glaucoma, right eye   Rx Q
- ✓7ᵗʰ H40.122 Low-tension glaucoma, left eye   Rx Q
- ✓7ᵗʰ H40.123 Low-tension glaucoma, bilateral   Rx Q
- ✓7ᵗʰ H40.129 Low-tension glaucoma, unspecified eye   Rx

✓6ᵗʰ H40.13 Pigmentary glaucoma
- ✓7ᵗʰ H40.131 Pigmentary glaucoma, right eye   Rx
- ✓7ᵗʰ H40.132 Pigmentary glaucoma, left eye   Rx
- ✓7ᵗʰ H40.133 Pigmentary glaucoma, bilateral   Rx
- ✓7ᵗʰ H40.139 Pigmentary glaucoma, unspecified eye   Rx

✓6ᵗʰ H40.14 Capsular glaucoma with pseudoexfoliation of lens
- ✓7ᵗʰ H40.141 Capsular glaucoma with pseudoexfoliation of lens, right eye   Rx
- ✓7ᵗʰ H40.142 Capsular glaucoma with pseudoexfoliation of lens, left eye   Rx
- ✓7ᵗʰ H40.143 Capsular glaucoma with pseudoexfoliation of lens, bilateral   Rx
- ✓7ᵗʰ H40.149 Capsular glaucoma with pseudoexfoliation of lens, unspecified eye   Rx

✓6ᵗʰ H40.15 Residual stage of open-angle glaucoma
- H40.151 Residual stage of open-angle glaucoma, right eye   Rx Q
- H40.152 Residual stage of open-angle glaucoma, left eye   Rx Q
- H40.153 Residual stage of open-angle glaucoma, bilateral   Rx Q
- H40.159 Residual stage of open-angle glaucoma, unspecified eye   Rx

✓5ᵗʰ H40.2 Primary angle-closure glaucoma

> **EXCLUDES 1**   aqueous misdirection (H40.83-)
> malignant glaucoma (H40.83-)

> One of the following 7th characters is to be assigned to code H40.20 and H40.22 to designate the stage of glaucoma.
> 0   stage unspecified
> 1   mild stage
> 2   moderate stage
> 3   severe stage
> 4   indeterminate stage

✓x7ᵗʰ H40.20 Unspecified primary angle-closure glaucoma   Rx
> **TIP:** Only one code from this subcategory should be assigned when both left and right eyes are the same stage.

✓6ᵗʰ H40.21 Acute angle-closure glaucoma
Acute angle-closure glaucoma attack
Acute angle-closure glaucoma crisis
- H40.211 Acute angle-closure glaucoma, right eye
- H40.212 Acute angle-closure glaucoma, left eye

Chapter 7. Diseases of the Eye and Adnexa

H40.213–H43.12

H40.213   **Acute angle-closure glaucoma,** bilateral

H40.219   **Acute angle-closure glaucoma, unspecified eye**

✓6ᵗʰ **H40.22**   Chronic **angle-closure glaucoma**

Chronic primary angle closure glaucoma

✓7ᵗʰ H40.221   **Chronic angle-closure glaucoma,** right **eye**   Rx

✓7ᵗʰ H40.222   **Chronic angle-closure glaucoma,** left **eye**   Rx

✓7ᵗʰ H40.223   **Chronic angle-closure glaucoma,** bilateral   Rx

✓7ᵗʰ H40.229   **Chronic angle-closure glaucoma, unspecified eye**   Rx

✓6ᵗʰ **H40.23**   Intermittent **angle-closure glaucoma**

H40.231   **Intermittent angle-closure glaucoma,** right **eye**   Rx

H40.232   **Intermittent** angle-closure glaucoma, left **eye**   Rx

H40.233   **Intermittent angle-closure glaucoma,** bilateral   Rx

H40.239   **Intermittent angle-closure glaucoma, unspecified eye**   Rx

✓6ᵗʰ **H40.24**   Residual stage **of angle-closure glaucoma**

H40.241   **Residual stage of angle-closure glaucoma,** right **eye**   Rx

H40.242   **Residual stage of angle-closure glaucoma,** left **eye**   Rx

H40.243   **Residual stage of angle-closure glaucoma,** bilateral   Rx

H40.249   **Residual stage of angle-closure glaucoma, unspecified eye**   Rx

✓5ᵗʰ **H40.3**   **Glaucoma** secondary to eye trauma

Code also underlying condition

One of the following 7th characters is to be assigned to each code in subcategory H40.3 to designate the stage of glaucoma.
- Ø   stage unspecified
- 1   mild stage
- 2   moderate stage
- 3   severe stage
- 4   indeterminate stage

✓x7ᵗʰ **H40.30**   **Glaucoma secondary to eye trauma, unspecified eye**   Rx

✓x7ᵗʰ **H40.31**   **Glaucoma secondary to eye trauma,** right **eye**   Rx

✓x7ᵗʰ **H40.32**   **Glaucoma secondary to eye trauma,** left **eye**   Rx

✓x7ᵗʰ **H40.33**   **Glaucoma secondary to eye trauma,** bilateral   Rx

✓5ᵗʰ **H40.4**   **Glaucoma** secondary to eye inflammation

Code also underlying condition

One of the following 7th characters is to be assigned to each code in subcategory H40.4 to designate the stage of glaucoma.
- Ø   stage unspecified
- 1   mild stage
- 2   moderate stage
- 3   severe stage
- 4   indeterminate stage

✓x7ᵗʰ **H40.40**   **Glaucoma secondary to eye inflammation, unspecified eye**   Rx

✓x7ᵗʰ **H40.41**   **Glaucoma secondary to eye inflammation,** right **eye**   Rx

✓x7ᵗʰ **H40.42**   **Glaucoma secondary to eye inflammation,** left **eye**   Rx

✓x7ᵗʰ **H40.43**   **Glaucoma secondary to eye inflammation,** bilateral   Rx

✓5ᵗʰ **H40.5**   **Glaucoma** secondary to other eye disorders

Code also underlying eye disorder

One of the following 7th characters is to be assigned to each code in subcategory H40.5 to designate the stage of glaucoma.
- Ø   stage unspecified
- 1   mild stage
- 2   moderate stage
- 3   severe stage
- 4   indeterminate stage

✓x7ᵗʰ **H40.50**   **Glaucoma secondary to other eye disorders, unspecified eye**   Rx

✓x7ᵗʰ **H40.51**   **Glaucoma secondary to other eye disorders,** right **eye**   Rx

✓x7ᵗʰ **H40.52**   **Glaucoma secondary to other eye disorders,** left **eye**   Rx

✓x7ᵗʰ **H40.53**   **Glaucoma secondary to other eye disorders,** bilateral   Rx

✓5ᵗʰ **H40.6**   **Glaucoma** secondary to drugs

Use additional code for adverse effect, if applicable, to identify drug (T36-T50 with fifth or sixth character 5)

One of the following 7th characters is to be assigned to each code in subcategory H40.6 to designate the stage of glaucoma
- Ø   stage unspecified
- 1   mild stage
- 2   moderate stage
- 3   severe stage
- 4   indeterminate stage

✓x7ᵗʰ **H40.60**   **Glaucoma secondary to drugs, unspecified eye**   Rx

✓x7ᵗʰ **H40.61**   **Glaucoma secondary to drugs,** right **eye**   Rx

✓x7ᵗʰ **H40.62**   **Glaucoma secondary to drugs,** left **eye**   Rx

✓x7ᵗʰ **H40.63**   **Glaucoma secondary to drugs,** bilateral   Rx

✓5ᵗʰ **H40.8**   **Other glaucoma**

✓6ᵗʰ **H40.81**   **Glaucoma with** increased episcleral venous pressure

H40.811   **Glaucoma with increased episcleral venous pressure,** right **eye**   Rx

H40.812   **Glaucoma with increased episcleral venous pressure,** left **eye**   Rx

H40.813   **Glaucoma with increased episcleral venous pressure,** bilateral   Rx

H40.819   **Glaucoma with increased episcleral venous pressure, unspecified eye**   Rx

✓6ᵗʰ **H40.82**   Hypersecretion **glaucoma**

H40.821   **Hypersecretion glaucoma,** right **eye**   Rx

H40.822   **Hypersecretion glaucoma,** left **eye**   Rx

H40.823   **Hypersecretion glaucoma,** bilateral   Rx

H40.829   **Hypersecretion glaucoma, unspecified eye**   Rx

✓6ᵗʰ **H40.83**   Aqueous misdirection

Malignant glaucoma

H40.831   **Aqueous misdirection,** right **eye**   Rx

H40.832   **Aqueous misdirection,** left **eye**   Rx

H40.833   **Aqueous misdirection,** bilateral   Rx

H40.839   **Aqueous misdirection, unspecified eye**   Rx

H40.89   **Other specified glaucoma**   Rx

H40.9   **Unspecified glaucoma**   Rx

H42   ***Glaucoma in diseases classified elsewhere***   Rx

Code first underlying condition, such as:
- amyloidosis (E85.-)
- aniridia (Q13.1)
- glaucoma (in) diabetes mellitus (E08.39, E09.39, E10.39, E11.39, E13.39)
- Lowe's syndrome (E72.03)
- Reiger's anomaly (Q13.81)
- specified metabolic disorder (E70-E88)

EXCLUDES 1   *glaucoma (in) onchocerciasis (B73.02)*
         glaucoma (in) syphilis (A52.71)
         glaucoma (in) tuberculous (A18.59)

Disorders of vitreous body and globe (H43-H44)

✓4ᵗʰ **H43**   **Disorders of vitreous body**

✓5ᵗʰ **H43.0**   **Vitreous** prolapse

EXCLUDES 1   *traumatic vitreous prolapse (S05.2-)*
         vitreous syndrome following cataract surgery (H59.0-)

H43.00   **Vitreous prolapse, unspecified eye**

H43.01   **Vitreous prolapse,** right **eye**

H43.02   **Vitreous prolapse,** left **eye**

H43.03   **Vitreous prolapse,** bilateral

✓5ᵗʰ **H43.1**   **Vitreous** hemorrhage

H43.10   **Vitreous hemorrhage, unspecified eye**   HCC ESR

H43.11   **Vitreous hemorrhage,** right **eye**   HCC ESR

H43.12   **Vitreous hemorrhage,** left **eye**   HCC ESR

H43.13   **Vitreous hemorrhage,** bilateral   `HCC` `ESR`

√5ᵗʰ   **H43.2**   Crystalline deposits in vitreous body

    `H43.20`   **Crystalline deposits in vitreous body, unspecified eye**

    H43.21   **Crystalline deposits in vitreous body,** right **eye**

    H43.22   **Crystalline deposits in vitreous body,** left **eye**

    H43.23   **Crystalline deposits in vitreous body,** bilateral

√5ᵗʰ   **H43.3**   Other vitreous opacities

   √6ᵗʰ   **H43.31**   **Vitreous** membranes and strands

      H43.311   **Vitreous membranes and strands,** right **eye**

      H43.312   **Vitreous membranes and strands,** left **eye**

      H43.313   **Vitreous membranes and strands,** bilateral

      `H43.319`   **Vitreous membranes and strands, unspecified eye**

   √6ᵗʰ   **H43.39**   **Other vitreous opacities**

     Vitreous floaters

      H43.391   **Other vitreous opacities,** right **eye**

      H43.392   **Other vitreous opacities,** left **eye**

      H43.393   **Other vitreous opacities,** bilateral

      `H43.399`   **Other vitreous opacities, unspecified eye**

√5ᵗʰ   **H43.8**   Other disorders of vitreous body

    EXCLUDES 1   *proliferative vitreo-retinopathy with retinal detachment (H33.4-)*

    EXCLUDES 2   *vitreous abscess (H44.02-)*

   √6ᵗʰ   **H43.81**   **Vitreous** degeneration

     Vitreous detachment

      H43.811   **Vitreous degeneration,** right **eye**

      H43.812   **Vitreous degeneration,** left **eye**

      H43.813   **Vitreous degeneration,** bilateral

      `H43.819`   **Vitreous degeneration, unspecified eye**

   √6ᵗʰ   **H43.82**   **Vitreomacular** adhesion

     Vitreomacular traction

      H43.821   **Vitreomacular adhesion,** right **eye**   `A`

      H43.822   **Vitreomacular adhesion,** left **eye**   `A`

      H43.823   **Vitreomacular adhesion,** bilateral   `A`

      `H43.829`   **Vitreomacular adhesion, unspecified eye**   `A`

    H43.89   **Other disorders of vitreous body**

   `H43.9`   **Unspecified disorder of vitreous body**

√4ᵗʰ   **H44**   **Disorders of globe**

    `INCLUDES`   disorders affecting multiple structures of eye

  √5ᵗʰ   **H44.0**   Purulent endophthalmitis

    Use additional code to identify organism

    EXCLUDES 1   *bleb associated endophthalmitis (H59.4-)*

   √6ᵗʰ   **H44.00**   **Unspecified purulent endophthalmitis**

      `H44.001`   **Unspecified purulent endophthalmitis,** right **eye**

      `H44.002`   **Unspecified purulent endophthalmitis,** left **eye**

      `H44.003`   **Unspecified purulent endophthalmitis,** bilateral

      `H44.009`   **Unspecified purulent endophthalmitis, unspecified eye**

   √6ᵗʰ   **H44.01**   **Panophthalmitis (acute)**

      H44.011   **Panophthalmitis (acute),** right **eye**

      H44.012   **Panophthalmitis (acute),** left **eye**

      H44.013   **Panophthalmitis (acute),** bilateral

      `H44.019`   **Panophthalmitis (acute), unspecified eye**

   √6ᵗʰ   **H44.02**   **Vitreous abscess (chronic)**

      H44.021   **Vitreous abscess (chronic),** right **eye**

      H44.022   **Vitreous abscess (chronic),** left **eye**

      H44.023   **Vitreous abscess (chronic),** bilateral

      `H44.029`   **Vitreous abscess (chronic), unspecified eye**

  √5ᵗʰ   **H44.1**   Other endophthalmitis

    EXCLUDES 1   *bleb associated endophthalmitis (H59.4-)*

    EXCLUDES 2   *ophthalmia nodosa (H16.2-)*

   √6ᵗʰ   **H44.11**   **Panuveitis**

     DEF: Inflammation of all layers of the uvea of the eye, including the choroid, iris, and ciliary body. It also typically involves the lens, retina, optic nerve, and vitreous and causes reduced vision or blindness.

      H44.111   **Panuveitis,** right **eye**

      H44.112   **Panuveitis,** left **eye**

      H44.113   **Panuveitis,** bilateral

      `H44.119`   **Panuveitis, unspecified eye**

   √6ᵗʰ   **H44.12**   **Parasitic endophthalmitis, unspecified**

      `H44.121`   **Parasitic endophthalmitis, unspecified,** right **eye**

      `H44.122`   **Parasitic endophthalmitis, unspecified,** left **eye**

      `H44.123`   **Parasitic endophthalmitis, unspecified,** bilateral

      `H44.129`   **Parasitic endophthalmitis, unspecified, unspecified eye**

   √6ᵗʰ   **H44.13**   **Sympathetic uveitis**

      H44.131   **Sympathetic uveitis,** right **eye**

      H44.132   **Sympathetic uveitis,** left **eye**

      H44.133   **Sympathetic uveitis,** bilateral

      `H44.139`   **Sympathetic uveitis, unspecified eye**

    H44.19   **Other endophthalmitis**

  √5ᵗʰ   **H44.2**   Degenerative myopia

    Malignant myopia

    AHA: 2017,4Q,10-11

    `H44.20`   **Degenerative myopia, unspecified eye**

    H44.21   **Degenerative myopia,** right **eye**

    H44.22   **Degenerative myopia,** left **eye**

    H44.23   **Degenerative myopia,** bilateral

   √6ᵗʰ   **H44.2A**   **Degenerative myopia with** choroidal neovascularization

     Use additional code for any associated choroid disorders (H31.-)

      H44.2A1   **Degenerative myopia with choroidal neovascularization,** right **eye**

      H44.2A2   **Degenerative myopia with choroidal neovascularization,** left **eye**

      H44.2A3   **Degenerative myopia with choroidal neovascularization,** bilateral **eye**

      `H44.2A9`   **Degenerative myopia with choroidal neovascularization, unspecified eye**

   √6ᵗʰ   **H44.2B**   **Degenerative myopia** with macular hole

      H44.2B1   **Degenerative myopia with macular hole,** right **eye**

      H44.2B2   **Degenerative myopia with macular hole,** left **eye**

      H44.2B3   **Degenerative myopia with macular hole,** bilateral **eye**

      `H44.2B9`   **Degenerative myopia with macular hole, unspecified eye**

   √6ᵗʰ   **H44.2C**   **Degenerative myopia** with retinal detachment

     Use additional code to identify the retinal detachment (H33.-)

      H44.2C1   **Degenerative myopia with retinal detachment,** right **eye**

      H44.2C2   **Degenerative myopia with retinal detachment,** left **eye**

      H44.2C3   **Degenerative myopia with retinal detachment,** bilateral **eye**

      `H44.2C9`   **Degenerative myopia with retinal detachment, unspecified eye**

   √6ᵗʰ   **H44.2D**   **Degenerative myopia** with foveoschisis

      H44.2D1   **Degenerative myopia with foveoschisis,** right **eye**

      H44.2D2   **Degenerative myopia with foveoschisis,** left **eye**

      H44.2D3   **Degenerative myopia with foveoschisis,** bilateral **eye**

      `H44.2D9`   **Degenerative myopia with foveoschisis, unspecified eye**

   √6ᵗʰ   **H44.2E**   **Degenerative myopia with other maculopathy**

      H44.2E1   **Degenerative myopia with other maculopathy,** right **eye**

      H44.2E2   **Degenerative myopia with other maculopathy,** left **eye**

      H44.2E3   **Degenerative myopia with other maculopathy,** bilateral **eye**

      `H44.2E9`   **Degenerative myopia with other maculopathy, unspecified eye**

   √6ᵗʰ   **H44.3**   **Other and unspecified degenerative disorders of globe**

    `H44.30`   **Unspecified degenerative disorder of globe**

   √6ᵗʰ   **H44.31**   **Chalcosis**

      H44.311   **Chalcosis,** right **eye**

      H44.312   **Chalcosis,** left **eye**

☑ Additional Character Required   √x7ᵗʰ Placeholder Alert   Manifestation   Unspecified Dx   Q QPP   UPD Unacceptable PDx

H44.313 **Chalcosis,** bilateral
H44.319 **Chalcosis, unspecified eye**

✓6ᵗʰ **H44.32 Siderosis of eye**

DEF: Iron pigment deposits within tissue of the eyeball caused by high iron content of the blood. Symptoms include cataracts, rust-colored anterior subcapsular deposits, iris heterochromia, pupillary mydriasis, and depressed electroretinogram amplitudes.

H44.321 **Siderosis of eye,** right eye
H44.322 **Siderosis of eye,** left eye
H44.323 **Siderosis of eye,** bilateral
H44.329 **Siderosis of eye, unspecified eye**

✓6ᵗʰ **H44.39 Other degenerative disorders of globe**

H44.391 **Other degenerative disorders of globe,** right eye
H44.392 **Other degenerative disorders of globe,** left eye
H44.393 **Other degenerative disorders of globe,** bilateral
H44.399 **Other degenerative disorders of globe, unspecified eye**

✓5ᵗʰ **H44.4 Hypotony of eye**

H44.40 **Unspecified hypotony of eye**

✓6ᵗʰ **H44.41 Flat anterior chamber hypotony of eye**

H44.411 **Flat anterior chamber hypotony of** right eye
H44.412 **Flat anterior chamber hypotony of** left eye
H44.413 **Flat anterior chamber hypotony of eye,** bilateral
H44.419 **Flat anterior chamber hypotony of unspecified eye**

✓6ᵗʰ **H44.42 Hypotony of eye due to** ocular fistula

H44.421 **Hypotony of** right **eye due to ocular fistula**
H44.422 **Hypotony of** left **eye due to ocular fistula**
H44.423 **Hypotony of eye due to ocular fistula,** bilateral
H44.429 **Hypotony of unspecified eye due to ocular fistula**

✓6ᵗʰ **H44.43 Hypotony of eye due to other ocular disorders**

H44.431 **Hypotony of eye due to other ocular disorders,** right eye
H44.432 **Hypotony of eye due to other ocular disorders,** left eye
H44.433 **Hypotony of eye due to other ocular disorders,** bilateral
H44.439 **Hypotony of eye due to other ocular disorders, unspecified eye**

✓6ᵗʰ **H44.44 Primary hypotony of eye**

H44.441 **Primary hypotony of** right **eye**
H44.442 **Primary hypotony of** left **eye**
H44.443 **Primary hypotony of eye,** bilateral
H44.449 **Primary hypotony of unspecified eye**

✓5ᵗʰ **H44.5 Degenerated conditions of globe**

H44.50 **Unspecified degenerated conditions of globe**

✓6ᵗʰ **H44.51 Absolute glaucoma**

H44.511 **Absolute glaucoma,** right eye
H44.512 **Absolute glaucoma,** left eye
H44.513 **Absolute glaucoma,** bilateral
H44.519 **Absolute glaucoma, unspecified eye**

✓6ᵗʰ **H44.52 Atrophy of globe**

Phthisis bulbi
H44.521 **Atrophy of globe,** right eye
H44.522 **Atrophy of globe,** left eye
H44.523 **Atrophy of globe,** bilateral
H44.529 **Atrophy of globe, unspecified eye**

✓6ᵗʰ **H44.53 Leucocoria**

H44.531 **Leucocoria,** right eye
H44.532 **Leucocoria,** left eye
H44.533 **Leucocoria,** bilateral
H44.539 **Leucocoria, unspecified eye**

✓5ᵗʰ **H44.6 Retained (old) intraocular foreign body,** magnetic

Use additional code to identify magnetic foreign body (Z18.11)
EXCLUDES 1 *current intraocular foreign body (S05.-)*
EXCLUDES 2 *retained foreign body in eyelid (H02.81-)*
retained (old) foreign body following penetrating wound of orbit (H05.5-)
retained (old) intraocular foreign body, nonmagnetic (H44.7-)

✓6ᵗʰ **H44.60 Unspecified retained (old) intraocular foreign body, magnetic**

H44.601 **Unspecified retained (old) intraocular foreign body, magnetic,** right eye
H44.602 **Unspecified retained (old) intraocular foreign body, magnetic,** left eye
H44.603 **Unspecified retained (old) intraocular foreign body, magnetic,** bilateral
H44.609 **Unspecified retained (old) intraocular foreign body, magnetic, unspecified eye**

✓6ᵗʰ **H44.61 Retained (old) magnetic foreign body in** anterior chamber

H44.611 **Retained (old) magnetic foreign body in anterior chamber,** right eye
H44.612 **Retained (old) magnetic foreign body in anterior chamber,** left eye
H44.613 **Retained (old) magnetic foreign body in anterior chamber,** bilateral
H44.619 **Retained (old) magnetic foreign body in anterior chamber, unspecified eye**

✓6ᵗʰ **H44.62 Retained (old) magnetic foreign body in** iris or ciliary body

H44.621 **Retained (old) magnetic foreign body in iris or ciliary body,** right eye
H44.622 **Retained (old) magnetic foreign body in iris or ciliary body,** left eye
H44.623 **Retained (old) magnetic foreign body in iris or ciliary body,** bilateral
H44.629 **Retained (old) magnetic foreign body in iris or ciliary body, unspecified eye**

✓6ᵗʰ **H44.63 Retained (old) magnetic foreign body in** lens

H44.631 **Retained (old) magnetic foreign body in lens,** right eye
H44.632 **Retained (old) magnetic foreign body in lens,** left eye
H44.633 **Retained (old) magnetic foreign body in lens,** bilateral
H44.639 **Retained (old) magnetic foreign body in lens, unspecified eye**

✓6ᵗʰ **H44.64 Retained (old) magnetic foreign body in** posterior wall of globe

H44.641 **Retained (old) magnetic foreign body in posterior wall of globe,** right eye
H44.642 **Retained (old) magnetic foreign body in posterior wall of globe,** left eye
H44.643 **Retained (old) magnetic foreign body in posterior wall of globe,** bilateral
H44.649 **Retained (old) magnetic foreign body in posterior wall of globe, unspecified eye**

✓6ᵗʰ **H44.65 Retained (old) magnetic foreign body in** vitreous body

H44.651 **Retained (old) magnetic foreign body in vitreous body,** right eye
H44.652 **Retained (old) magnetic foreign body in vitreous body,** left eye
H44.653 **Retained (old) magnetic foreign body in vitreous body,** bilateral
H44.659 **Retained (old) magnetic foreign body in vitreous body, unspecified eye**

✓6ᵗʰ **H44.69 Retained (old) intraocular foreign body, magnetic, in other or multiple sites**

H44.691 **Retained (old) intraocular foreign body, magnetic, in other or multiple sites,** right eye
H44.692 **Retained (old) intraocular foreign body, magnetic, in other or multiple sites,** left eye
H44.693 **Retained (old) intraocular foreign body, magnetic, in other or multiple sites,** bilateral
H44.699 **Retained (old) intraocular foreign body, magnetic, in other or multiple sites, unspecified eye**

HCC CMS-HCC   **Rx** Rx HCC   **ESR** ESRD HCC   **COM** Commercial HCC   **N** Newborn: 0   **P** Pediatric: 0-17   **M** Maternity: 9-64   **A** Adult: 15-124

638
ICD-10-CM 2023

✓5ᵗʰ **H44.7 Retained (old) intraocular foreign body, nonmagnetic**

Use additional code to identify nonmagnetic foreign body (Z18.01-Z18.10, Z18.12, Z18.2-Z18.9)

EXCLUDES 1   current intraocular foreign body (S05.-)

EXCLUDES 2   retained foreign body in eyelid (H02.81-)

retained (old) foreign body following penetrating wound of orbit (H05.5-)

retained (old) intraocular foreign body, magnetic (H44.6-)

✓6ᵗʰ **H44.70 Unspecified retained (old) intraocular foreign body, nonmagnetic**

H44.701 Unspecified retained (old) intraocular foreign body, nonmagnetic, right eye

H44.702 Unspecified retained (old) intraocular foreign body, nonmagnetic, left eye

H44.703 Unspecified retained (old) intraocular foreign body, nonmagnetic, bilateral

H44.709 Unspecified retained (old) intraocular foreign body, nonmagnetic, unspecified eye

Retained (old) intraocular foreign body NOS

✓6ᵗʰ **H44.71 Retained (nonmagnetic) (old) foreign body in anterior chamber**

H44.711 Retained (nonmagnetic) (old) foreign body in anterior chamber, right eye

H44.712 Retained (nonmagnetic) (old) foreign body in anterior chamber, left eye

H44.713 Retained (nonmagnetic) (old) foreign body in anterior chamber, bilateral

H44.719 Retained (nonmagnetic) (old) foreign body in anterior chamber, unspecified eye

✓6ᵗʰ **H44.72 Retained (nonmagnetic) (old) foreign body in iris or ciliary body**

H44.721 Retained (nonmagnetic) (old) foreign body in iris or ciliary body, right eye

H44.722 Retained (nonmagnetic) (old) foreign body in iris or ciliary body, left eye

H44.723 Retained (nonmagnetic) (old) foreign body in iris or ciliary body, bilateral

H44.729 Retained (nonmagnetic) (old) foreign body in iris or ciliary body, unspecified eye

✓6ᵗʰ **H44.73 Retained (nonmagnetic) (old) foreign body in lens**

H44.731 Retained (nonmagnetic) (old) foreign body in lens, right eye

H44.732 Retained (nonmagnetic) (old) foreign body in lens, left eye

H44.733 Retained (nonmagnetic) (old) foreign body in lens, bilateral

H44.739 Retained (nonmagnetic) (old) foreign body in lens, unspecified eye

✓6ᵗʰ **H44.74 Retained (nonmagnetic) (old) foreign body in posterior wall of globe**

H44.741 Retained (nonmagnetic) (old) foreign body in posterior wall of globe, right eye

H44.742 Retained (nonmagnetic) (old) foreign body in posterior wall of globe, left eye

H44.743 Retained (nonmagnetic) (old) foreign body in posterior wall of globe, bilateral

H44.749 Retained (nonmagnetic) (old) foreign body in posterior wall of globe, unspecified eye

✓6ᵗʰ **H44.75 Retained (nonmagnetic) (old) foreign body in vitreous body**

H44.751 Retained (nonmagnetic) (old) foreign body in vitreous body, right eye

H44.752 Retained (nonmagnetic) (old) foreign body in vitreous body, left eye

H44.753 Retained (nonmagnetic) (old) foreign body in vitreous body, bilateral

H44.759 Retained (nonmagnetic) (old) foreign body in vitreous body, unspecified eye

✓6ᵗʰ **H44.79 Retained (old) intraocular foreign body, nonmagnetic, in other or multiple sites**

H44.791 Retained (old) intraocular foreign body, nonmagnetic, in other or multiple sites, right eye

H44.792 Retained (old) intraocular foreign body, nonmagnetic, in other or multiple sites, left eye

H44.793 Retained (old) intraocular foreign body, nonmagnetic, in other or multiple sites, bilateral

H44.799 Retained (old) intraocular foreign body, nonmagnetic, in other or multiple sites, unspecified eye

✓5ᵗʰ **H44.8 Other disorders of globe**

✓6ᵗʰ **H44.81 Hemophthalmos**

DEF: Pool of blood within the eyeball, not from a current injury.

H44.811 Hemophthalmos, right eye

H44.812 Hemophthalmos, left eye

H44.813 Hemophthalmos, bilateral

H44.819 Hemophthalmos, unspecified eye

✓6ᵗʰ **H44.82 Luxation of globe**

H44.821 Luxation of globe, right eye

H44.822 Luxation of globe, left eye

H44.823 Luxation of globe, bilateral

H44.829 Luxation of globe, unspecified eye

H44.89 Other disorders of globe

AHA: 2022,1Q,33

H44.9 Unspecified disorder of globe

Disorders of optic nerve and visual pathways (H46-H47)

✓4ᵗʰ **H46 Optic neuritis**

EXCLUDES 2   ischemic optic neuropathy (H47.01-)

neuromyelitis optica [Devic] (G36.0)

✓5ᵗʰ **H46.0 Optic papillitis**

H46.00 Optic papillitis, unspecified eye

H46.01 Optic papillitis, right eye

H46.02 Optic papillitis, left eye

H46.03 Optic papillitis, bilateral

✓5ᵗʰ **H46.1 Retrobulbar neuritis**

Retrobulbar neuritis NOS

EXCLUDES 1   syphilitic retrobulbar neuritis (A52.15)

H46.10 Retrobulbar neuritis, unspecified eye

H46.11 Retrobulbar neuritis, right eye

H46.12 Retrobulbar neuritis, left eye

H46.13 Retrobulbar neuritis, bilateral

H46.2 Nutritional optic neuropathy

H46.3 Toxic optic neuropathy

Code first (T51-T65) to identify cause

H46.8 Other optic neuritis

H46.9 Unspecified optic neuritis

✓4ᵗʰ **H47 Other disorders of optic [2nd] nerve and visual pathways**

✓5ᵗʰ **H47.0 Disorders of optic nerve, not elsewhere classified**

✓6ᵗʰ **H47.01 Ischemic optic neuropathy**

H47.011 Ischemic optic neuropathy, right eye

H47.012 Ischemic optic neuropathy, left eye

H47.013 Ischemic optic neuropathy, bilateral

H47.019 Ischemic optic neuropathy, unspecified eye

✓6ᵗʰ **H47.02 Hemorrhage in optic nerve sheath**

H47.021 Hemorrhage in optic nerve sheath, right eye

H47.022 Hemorrhage in optic nerve sheath, left eye

H47.023 Hemorrhage in optic nerve sheath, bilateral

H47.029 Hemorrhage in optic nerve sheath, unspecified eye

✓6ᵗʰ **H47.03 Optic nerve hypoplasia**

H47.031 Optic nerve hypoplasia, right eye

H47.032 Optic nerve hypoplasia, left eye

H47.033 Optic nerve hypoplasia, bilateral

H47.039 Optic nerve hypoplasia, unspecified eye

✓6ᵗʰ **H47.09 Other disorders of optic nerve, not elsewhere classified**

Compression of optic nerve

H47.091 Other disorders of optic nerve, not elsewhere classified, right eye

H47.092 Other disorders of optic nerve, not elsewhere classified, left eye

H47.093 Other disorders of optic nerve, not elsewhere classified, bilateral

---

☑ Additional Character Required   ✓x7ᵗʰ Placeholder Alert   Manifestation   Unspecified Dx   Q QPP   UPD Unacceptable PDx

H47.Ø99   **Other disorders of optic nerve, not elsewhere classified, unspecified eye**

☑5ᵗʰ **H47.1**   **Papilledema**

DEF: Swelling of the optic papilla, the raised area connected to the optic disk made up of nerves that enter the eyeball. It may be caused by increased intracranial pressure, decreased ocular pressure, or a retinal disorder.

H47.1Ø   **Unspecified papilledema**

H47.11   **Papilledema associated with** increased intracranial pressure

H47.12   **Papilledema associated with** decreased ocular pressure

H47.13   **Papilledema associated with** retinal disorder

☑6ᵗʰ **H47.14**   **Foster-Kennedy syndrome**

H47.141   **Foster-Kennedy syndrome,** right **eye**
H47.142   **Foster-Kennedy syndrome,** left **eye**
H47.143   **Foster-Kennedy syndrome,** bilateral
H47.149   **Foster-Kennedy syndrome, unspecified eye**

☑5ᵗʰ **H47.2**   **Optic atrophy**

H47.2Ø   **Unspecified optic atrophy**

☑6ᵗʰ **H47.21**   **Primary** optic atrophy

H47.211   **Primary optic atrophy,** right **eye**
H47.212   **Primary optic atrophy,** left **eye**
H47.213   **Primary optic atrophy,** bilateral
H47.219   **Primary optic atrophy, unspecified eye**

H47.22   **Hereditary** optic atrophy

Leber's optic atrophy

☑6ᵗʰ **H47.23**   **Glaucomatous** optic atrophy

H47.231   **Glaucomatous optic atrophy,** right **eye**
H47.232   **Glaucomatous optic atrophy,** left **eye**
H47.233   **Glaucomatous optic atrophy,** bilateral
H47.239   **Glaucomatous optic atrophy, unspecified eye**

☑6ᵗʰ **H47.29**   **Other optic atrophy**

Temporal pallor of optic disc

H47.291   **Other optic atrophy,** right **eye**
H47.292   **Other optic atrophy,** left **eye**
H47.293   **Other optic atrophy,** bilateral
H47.299   **Other optic atrophy, unspecified eye**

☑5ᵗʰ **H47.3**   **Other disorders of optic disc**

☑6ᵗʰ **H47.31**   **Coloboma** of optic disc

H47.311   **Coloboma of optic disc,** right **eye**
H47.312   **Coloboma of optic disc,** left **eye**
H47.313   **Coloboma of optic disc,** bilateral
H47.319   **Coloboma of optic disc, unspecified eye**

☑6ᵗʰ **H47.32**   **Drusen** of optic disc

H47.321   **Drusen of optic disc,** right **eye**
H47.322   **Drusen of optic disc,** left **eye**
H47.323   **Drusen of optic disc,** bilateral
H47.329   **Drusen of optic disc, unspecified eye**

☑6ᵗʰ **H47.33**   **Pseudopapilledema** of optic disc

H47.331   **Pseudopapilledema of optic disc,** right **eye**
H47.332   **Pseudopapilledema of optic disc,** left **eye**
H47.333   **Pseudopapilledema of optic disc,** bilateral
H47.339   **Pseudopapilledema of optic disc, unspecified eye**

☑6ᵗʰ **H47.39**   **Other disorders of optic disc**

H47.391   **Other disorders of optic disc,** right **eye**
H47.392   **Other disorders of optic disc,** left **eye**
H47.393   **Other disorders of optic disc,** bilateral
H47.399   **Other disorders of optic disc, unspecified eye**

☑5ᵗʰ **H47.4**   **Disorders of optic chiasm**

Code also underlying condition

H47.41   **Disorders of optic chiasm in (due to)** inflammatory disorders

H47.42   **Disorders of optic chiasm in (due to)** neoplasm

H47.43   **Disorders of optic chiasm in (due to)** vascular disorders

H47.49   **Disorders of optic chiasm in (due to) other disorders**

☑5ᵗʰ **H47.5**   **Disorders of other visual pathways**

Disorders of optic tracts, geniculate nuclei and optic radiations
Code also underlying condition

☑6ᵗʰ **H47.51**   **Disorders of visual pathways in (due to)** inflammatory disorders

H47.511   **Disorders of visual pathways in (due to) inflammatory disorders,** right **side**
H47.512   **Disorders of visual pathways in (due to) inflammatory disorders,** left **side**
H47.519   **Disorders of visual pathways in (due to) inflammatory disorders, unspecified side**

☑6ᵗʰ **H47.52**   **Disorders of visual pathways in (due to)** neoplasm

H47.521   **Disorders of visual pathways in (due to) neoplasm,** right **side**
H47.522   **Disorders of visual pathways in (due to) neoplasm,** left **side**
H47.529   **Disorders of visual pathways in (due to) neoplasm, unspecified side**

☑6ᵗʰ **H47.53**   **Disorders of visual pathways in (due to)** vascular disorders

H47.531   **Disorders of visual pathways in (due to) vascular disorders,** right **side**
H47.532   **Disorders of visual pathways in (due to) vascular disorders,** left **side**
H47.539   **Disorders of visual pathways in (due to) vascular disorders, unspecified side**

☑5ᵗʰ **H47.6**   **Disorders of visual cortex**

Code also underlying condition

EXCLUDES 1   injury to visual cortex SØ4.Ø4-

☑6ᵗʰ **H47.61**   **Cortical blindness**

H47.611   **Cortical blindness,** right **side of brain**
H47.612   **Cortical blindness,** left **side of brain**
H47.619   **Cortical blindness, unspecified side of brain**

☑6ᵗʰ **H47.62**   **Disorders of visual cortex in (due to)** inflammatory disorders

H47.621   **Disorders of visual cortex in (due to) inflammatory disorders,** right **side of brain**
H47.622   **Disorders of visual cortex in (due to) inflammatory disorders,** left **side of brain**
H47.629   **Disorders of visual cortex in (due to) inflammatory disorders, unspecified side of brain**

☑6ᵗʰ **H47.63**   **Disorders of visual cortex in (due to)** neoplasm

H47.631   **Disorders of visual cortex in (due to) neoplasm,** right **side of brain**
H47.632   **Disorders of visual cortex in (due to) neoplasm,** left **side of brain**
H47.639   **Disorders of visual cortex in (due to) neoplasm, unspecified side of brain**

☑6ᵗʰ **H47.64**   **Disorders of visual cortex in (due to)** vascular disorders

H47.641   **Disorders of visual cortex in (due to) vascular disorders,** right **side of brain**
H47.642   **Disorders of visual cortex in (due to) vascular disorders,** left **side of brain**
H47.649   **Disorders of visual cortex in (due to) vascular disorders, unspecified side of brain**

H47.9   **Unspecified disorder of visual pathways**

Disorders of ocular muscles, binocular movement, accommodation and refraction (H49-H52)

EXCLUDES 2   nystagmus and other irregular eye movements (H55)

☑4ᵗʰ **H49**   **Paralytic strabismus**

EXCLUDES 2   internal ophthalmoplegia (H52.51-)
internuclear ophthalmoplegia (H51.2-)
progressive supranuclear ophthalmoplegia (G23.1)

DEF: Strabismus: Misalignment of the eyes with the inability to move and focus in the same direction due to conditions affecting the muscles controlling them.

☑5ᵗʰ **H49.Ø**   **Third [oculomotor] nerve palsy**

H49.ØØ   **Third [oculomotor] nerve palsy, unspecified eye**
H49.Ø1   **Third [oculomotor] nerve palsy,** right **eye**
H49.Ø2   **Third [oculomotor] nerve palsy,** left **eye**
H49.Ø3   **Third [oculomotor] nerve palsy,** bilateral

☑5ᵗʰ **H49.1**   **Fourth [trochlear] nerve palsy**

H49.1Ø   **Fourth [trochlear] nerve palsy, unspecified eye**

HCC CMS-HCC   **Rx** Rx HCC   **ESR** ESRD HCC   **COM** Commercial HCC   **N** Newborn: 0   **P** Pediatric: 0-17   **M** Maternity: 9-64   **A** Adult: 15-124

640   ICD-10-CM 2023

        H49.11   Fourth [trochlear] nerve palsy, **right** eye
        H49.12   Fourth [trochlear] nerve palsy, **left** eye
        H49.13   Fourth [trochlear] nerve palsy, **bilateral**

✓5ᵗʰ **H49.2**   Sixth [abducent] nerve palsy
        H49.20   Sixth [abducent] nerve palsy, unspecified eye
        H49.21   Sixth [abducent] nerve palsy, **right** eye
        H49.22   Sixth [abducent] nerve palsy, **left** eye
        H49.23   Sixth [abducent] nerve palsy, **bilateral**

✓5ᵗʰ **H49.3**   Total (external) ophthalmoplegia
        H49.30   Total (external) ophthalmoplegia, unspecified eye
        H49.31   Total (external) ophthalmoplegia, **right** eye
        H49.32   Total (external) ophthalmoplegia, **left** eye
        H49.33   Total (external) ophthalmoplegia, **bilateral**

✓5ᵗʰ **H49.4**   Progressive external ophthalmoplegia
      EXCLUDES 1   *Kearns-Sayre syndrome (H49.81-)*
        H49.40   Progressive external ophthalmoplegia, unspecified eye
        H49.41   Progressive external ophthalmoplegia, **right** eye
        H49.42   Progressive external ophthalmoplegia, **left** eye
        H49.43   Progressive external ophthalmoplegia, **bilateral**

✓5ᵗʰ **H49.8**   Other paralytic strabismus
     ✓6ᵗʰ   **H49.81**   Kearns-Sayre syndrome
          Progressive external ophthalmoplegia with pigmentary retinopathy
          Use additional code for other manifestation, such as: heart block (I45.9)
          H49.811   Kearns-Sayre syndrome, **right** eye   HCC Rx ESR COM
          H49.812   Kearns-Sayre syndrome, **left** eye   HCC Rx ESR COM
          H49.813   Kearns-Sayre syndrome, **bilateral**   HCC Rx ESR COM
          H49.819   Kearns-Sayre syndrome, unspecified eye   HCC Rx ESR COM
     ✓6ᵗʰ   **H49.88**   Other paralytic strabismus
          External ophthalmoplegia NOS
          H49.881   Other paralytic strabismus, **right** eye
          H49.882   Other paralytic strabismus, **left** eye
          H49.883   Other paralytic strabismus, **bilateral**
          H49.889   Other paralytic strabismus, unspecified eye

     H49.9   Unspecified paralytic strabismus

✓4ᵗʰ **H50**   Other strabismus
     DEF: Strabismus: Misalignment of the eyes with the inability to move and focus in the same direction due to conditions affecting the muscles controlling them.

✓5ᵗʰ **H50.0**   Esotropia
     Convergent concomitant strabismus
      EXCLUDES 1   *intermittent esotropia (H50.31-, H50.32)*
        H50.00   Unspecified esotropia
     ✓6ᵗʰ   **H50.01**   Monocular esotropia
          H50.011   Monocular esotropia, **right** eye
          H50.012   Monocular esotropia, **left** eye
     ✓6ᵗʰ   **H50.02**   Monocular esotropia with **A pattern**
          H50.021   Monocular esotropia with A pattern, **right** eye
          H50.022   Monocular esotropia with A pattern, **left** eye
     ✓6ᵗʰ   **H50.03**   Monocular esotropia with **V pattern**
          H50.031   Monocular esotropia with V pattern, **right** eye
          H50.032   Monocular esotropia with V pattern, **left** eye
     ✓6ᵗʰ   **H50.04**   Monocular esotropia with **other noncomitancies**
          H50.041   Monocular esotropia with other noncomitancies, **right** eye
          H50.042   Monocular esotropia with other noncomitancies, **left** eye
        H50.05   Alternating esotropia
        H50.06   Alternating esotropia with **A pattern**
        H50.07   Alternating esotropia with **V pattern**

        H50.08   Alternating esotropia with other noncomitancies

Eye Muscle Diseases

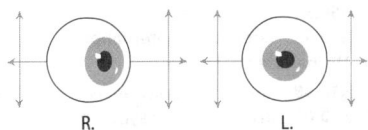

Monocular (one eye only) esotropia (inward)

Monocular exotropia (outward)

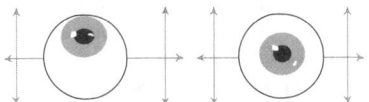

Monocular hypertropia (upward)

✓5ᵗʰ **H50.1**   Exotropia
     Divergent concomitant strabismus
      EXCLUDES 1   *intermittent exotropia (H50.33-, H50.34)*
        H50.10   Unspecified exotropia
     ✓6ᵗʰ   **H50.11**   Monocular exotropia
          H50.111   Monocular exotropia, **right** eye
          H50.112   Monocular exotropia, **left** eye
     ✓6ᵗʰ   **H50.12**   Monocular exotropia with **A pattern**
          H50.121   Monocular exotropia with A pattern, **right** eye
          H50.122   Monocular exotropia with A pattern, **left** eye
     ✓6ᵗʰ   **H50.13**   Monocular exotropia with **V pattern**
          H50.131   Monocular exotropia with V pattern, **right** eye
          H50.132   Monocular exotropia with V pattern, **left** eye
     ✓6ᵗʰ   **H50.14**   Monocular exotropia with **other noncomitancies**
          H50.141   Monocular exotropia with other noncomitancies, **right** eye
          H50.142   Monocular exotropia with other noncomitancies, **left** eye
        H50.15   Alternating exotropia
        H50.16   Alternating exotropia with **A pattern**
        H50.17   Alternating exotropia with **V pattern**
        H50.18   Alternating exotropia with other noncomitancies

✓5ᵗʰ **H50.2**   Vertical strabismus
     Hypertropia
        H50.21   Vertical strabismus, **right** eye
        H50.22   Vertical strabismus, **left** eye

✓5ᵗʰ **H50.3**   Intermittent heterotropia
        H50.30   Unspecified intermittent heterotropia
     ✓6ᵗʰ   **H50.31**   Intermittent monocular esotropia
          H50.311   Intermittent monocular esotropia, **right** eye
          H50.312   Intermittent monocular esotropia, **left** eye
        H50.32   Intermittent alternating esotropia
     ✓6ᵗʰ   **H50.33**   Intermittent monocular exotropia
          H50.331   Intermittent monocular exotropia, **right** eye
          H50.332   Intermittent monocular exotropia, **left** eye
        H50.34   Intermittent alternating exotropia

✓5ᵗʰ **H50.4**   Other and unspecified heterotropia
        H50.40   Unspecified heterotropia
     ✓6ᵗʰ   **H50.41**   Cyclotropia
          H50.411   Cyclotropia, **right** eye
          H50.412   Cyclotropia, **left** eye
        H50.42   Monofixation syndrome
        H50.43   Accommodative component in esotropia

✓5ᵗʰ **H50.5**   Heterophoria
        H50.50   Unspecified heterophoria

H50.51 **Esophoria**
H50.52 **Exophoria**
H50.53 **Vertical heterophoria**
H50.54 **Cyclophoria**
H50.55 **Alternating heterophoria**
√5ᵗʰ H50.6 **Mechanical strabismus**
H50.60 **Mechanical strabismus, unspecified**
√6ᵗʰ H50.61 **Brown's sheath syndrome**
H50.611 **Brown's sheath syndrome, right eye**
H50.612 **Brown's sheath syndrome, left eye**
H50.69 **Other mechanical strabismus**
Strabismus due to adhesions
Traumatic limitation of duction of eye muscle
√5ᵗʰ H50.8 **Other specified strabismus**
√6ᵗʰ H50.81 **Duane's syndrome**
H50.811 **Duane's syndrome, right eye**
H50.812 **Duane's syndrome, left eye**
H50.89 **Other specified strabismus**
H50.9 **Unspecified strabismus**
√4ᵗʰ H51 **Other disorders of binocular movement**
H51.0 **Palsy (spasm) of conjugate gaze**
√5ᵗʰ H51.1 **Convergence insufficiency and excess**
H51.11 **Convergence insufficiency**
H51.12 **Convergence excess**
√5ᵗʰ H51.2 **Internuclear ophthalmoplegia**
H51.20 **Internuclear ophthalmoplegia, unspecified eye**
H51.21 **Internuclear ophthalmoplegia, right eye**
H51.22 **Internuclear ophthalmoplegia, left eye**
H51.23 **Internuclear ophthalmoplegia, bilateral**
H51.8 **Other specified disorders of binocular movement**
H51.9 **Unspecified disorder of binocular movement**
√4ᵗʰ H52 **Disorders of refraction and accommodation**
√5ᵗʰ H52.0 **Hypermetropia**
H52.00 **Hypermetropia, unspecified eye**
H52.01 **Hypermetropia, right eye**
H52.02 **Hypermetropia, left eye**
H52.03 **Hypermetropia, bilateral**
√5ᵗʰ H52.1 **Myopia**
EXCLUDES 1 *degenerative myopia (H44.2-)*
H52.10 **Myopia, unspecified eye**
H52.11 **Myopia, right eye**
H52.12 **Myopia, left eye**
H52.13 **Myopia, bilateral**
√5ᵗʰ H52.2 **Astigmatism**
√6ᵗʰ H52.20 **Unspecified astigmatism**
H52.201 **Unspecified astigmatism, right eye**
H52.202 **Unspecified astigmatism, left eye**
H52.203 **Unspecified astigmatism, bilateral**
H52.209 **Unspecified astigmatism, unspecified eye**
√6ᵗʰ H52.21 **Irregular astigmatism**
H52.211 **Irregular astigmatism, right eye**
H52.212 **Irregular astigmatism, left eye**
H52.213 **Irregular astigmatism, bilateral**
H52.219 **Irregular astigmatism, unspecified eye**
√6ᵗʰ H52.22 **Regular astigmatism**
H52.221 **Regular astigmatism, right eye**
H52.222 **Regular astigmatism, left eye**
H52.223 **Regular astigmatism, bilateral**
H52.229 **Regular astigmatism, unspecified eye**
√5ᵗʰ H52.3 **Anisometropia and aniseikonia**
H52.31 **Anisometropia**
H52.32 **Aniseikonia**
H52.4 **Presbyopia**
√5ᵗʰ H52.5 **Disorders of accommodation**
√6ᵗʰ H52.51 **Internal ophthalmoplegia (complete) (total)**
H52.511 **Internal ophthalmoplegia (complete) (total), right eye**
H52.512 **Internal ophthalmoplegia (complete) (total), left eye**
H52.513 **Internal ophthalmoplegia (complete) (total), bilateral**
H52.519 **Internal ophthalmoplegia (complete) (total), unspecified eye**

√6ᵗʰ H52.52 **Paresis of accommodation**
H52.521 **Paresis of accommodation, right eye**
H52.522 **Paresis of accommodation, left eye**
H52.523 **Paresis of accommodation, bilateral**
H52.529 **Paresis of accommodation, unspecified eye**
√6ᵗʰ H52.53 **Spasm of accommodation**
H52.531 **Spasm of accommodation, right eye**
H52.532 **Spasm of accommodation, left eye**
H52.533 **Spasm of accommodation, bilateral**
H52.539 **Spasm of accommodation, unspecified eye**
H52.6 **Other disorders of refraction**
H52.7 **Unspecified disorder of refraction**

Visual disturbances and blindness (H53-H54)

√4ᵗʰ H53 **Visual disturbances**
√5ᵗʰ H53.0 **Amblyopia ex anopsia**
EXCLUDES 1 *amblyopia due to vitamin A deficiency (E50.5)*
√6ᵗʰ H53.00 **Unspecified amblyopia**
H53.001 **Unspecified amblyopia, right eye**
H53.002 **Unspecified amblyopia, left eye**
H53.003 **Unspecified amblyopia, bilateral**
H53.009 **Unspecified amblyopia, unspecified eye**
√6ᵗʰ H53.01 **Deprivation amblyopia**
H53.011 **Deprivation amblyopia, right eye**
H53.012 **Deprivation amblyopia, left eye**
H53.013 **Deprivation amblyopia, bilateral**
H53.019 **Deprivation amblyopia, unspecified eye**
√6ᵗʰ H53.02 **Refractive amblyopia**
H53.021 **Refractive amblyopia, right eye**
H53.022 **Refractive amblyopia, left eye**
H53.023 **Refractive amblyopia, bilateral**
H53.029 **Refractive amblyopia, unspecified eye**
√6ᵗʰ H53.03 **Strabismic amblyopia**
EXCLUDES 1 *strabismus (H50.-)*
H53.031 **Strabismic amblyopia, right eye**
H53.032 **Strabismic amblyopia, left eye**
H53.033 **Strabismic amblyopia, bilateral**
H53.039 **Strabismic amblyopia, unspecified eye**
√6ᵗʰ H53.04 **Amblyopia suspect**
AHA: 2016,4Q,22-23
H53.041 **Amblyopia suspect, right eye**
H53.042 **Amblyopia suspect, left eye**
H53.043 **Amblyopia suspect, bilateral**
H53.049 **Amblyopia suspect, unspecified eye**
√5ᵗʰ H53.1 **Subjective visual disturbances**
EXCLUDES 1 *subjective visual disturbances due to vitamin A deficiency (E50.5)*
visual hallucinations (R44.1)
H53.10 **Unspecified subjective visual disturbances**
H53.11 **Day blindness**
Hemeralopia
√6ᵗʰ H53.12 **Transient visual loss**
Scintillating scotoma
EXCLUDES 1 *amaurosis fugax (G45.3-)*
transient retinal artery occlusion (H34.0-)
AHA: 2022,1Q,30
H53.121 **Transient visual loss, right eye**
H53.122 **Transient visual loss, left eye**
H53.123 **Transient visual loss, bilateral**
H53.129 **Transient visual loss, unspecified eye**
√6ᵗʰ H53.13 **Sudden visual loss**
H53.131 **Sudden visual loss, right eye**
H53.132 **Sudden visual loss, left eye**
H53.133 **Sudden visual loss, bilateral**
H53.139 **Sudden visual loss, unspecified eye**
√6ᵗʰ H53.14 **Visual discomfort**
Asthenopia
Photophobia
H53.141 **Visual discomfort, right eye**
H53.142 **Visual discomfort, left eye**
H53.143 **Visual discomfort, bilateral**
H53.149 **Visual discomfort, unspecified**

H53.15 **Visual** distortions **of shape and size**
     Metamorphopsia

H53.16 **Psychophysical visual disturbances**

H53.19 **Other subjective visual disturbances**
     Visual halos
     AHA: 2022,1Q,30

H53.2 **Diplopia**
     Double vision

√6ᵗʰ H53.3 **Other and unspecified disorders of binocular vision**

   H53.30 **Unspecified disorder of binocular vision**

   H53.31 **Abnormal retinal correspondence**

   H53.32 **Fusion with defective stereopsis**

   H53.33 **Simultaneous visual perception without fusion**

   H53.34 **Suppression of binocular vision**

√5ᵗʰ H53.4 **Visual field defects**

   H53.40 **Unspecified visual field defects**

   √6ᵗʰ H53.41 **Scotoma involving** central area
       Central scotoma
       AHA: 2022,1Q,30

     H53.411 **Scotoma involving central area, right eye**

     H53.412 **Scotoma involving central area, left eye**

     H53.413 **Scotoma involving central area, bilateral**

     H53.419 **Scotoma involving central area, unspecified eye**

   √6ᵗʰ H53.42 **Scotoma of** blind spot **area**
       Enlarged blind spot

     H53.421 **Scotoma of blind spot area, right eye**

     H53.422 **Scotoma of blind spot area, left eye**

     H53.423 **Scotoma of blind spot area, bilateral**

     H53.429 **Scotoma of blind spot area, unspecified eye**

   √6ᵗʰ H53.43 **Sector or arcuate defects**
       Arcuate scotoma
       Bjerrum scotoma

     H53.431 **Sector or arcuate defects, right eye**

     H53.432 **Sector or arcuate defects, left eye**

     H53.433 **Sector or arcuate defects, bilateral**

     H53.439 **Sector or arcuate defects, unspecified eye**

   √6ᵗʰ H53.45 **Other localized visual field defect**
       Peripheral visual field defect
       Ring scotoma NOS
       Scotoma NOS

     H53.451 **Other localized visual field defect, right eye**

     H53.452 **Other localized visual field defect, left eye**

     H53.453 **Other localized visual field defect, bilateral**

     H53.459 **Other localized visual field defect, unspecified eye**

   √6ᵗʰ H53.46 **Homonymous bilateral field defects**
       Homonymous hemianopia
       Homonymous hemianopsia
       Quadrant anopia
       Quadrant anopsia

     H53.461 **Homonymous bilateral field defects, right side**

     H53.462 **Homonymous bilateral field defects, left side**

     H53.469 **Homonymous bilateral field defects, unspecified side**
       Homonymous bilateral field defects NOS

   H53.47 **Heteronymous bilateral field defects**
     Heteronymous hemianop(s)ia

   √6ᵗʰ H53.48 **Generalized contraction of visual field**

     H53.481 **Generalized contraction of visual field, right eye**

     H53.482 **Generalized contraction of visual field, left eye**

     H53.483 **Generalized contraction of visual field, bilateral**

     H53.489 **Generalized contraction of visual field, unspecified eye**

√5ᵗʰ H53.5 **Color vision deficiencies**
     Color blindness
     EXCLUDES 2   day blindness (H53.11)

   H53.50 **Unspecified color vision deficiencies**
     Color blindness NOS

   H53.51 **Achromatopsia**
     DEF: Nonprogressive genetic visual disorder characterized by complete color blindness, decreased vision, and light sensitivity.

   H53.52 **Acquired color vision deficiency**

   H53.53 **Deuteranomaly**
     Deuteranopia
     DEF: Male-only genetic disorder causing difficulty in distinguishing green and red; no shortened spectrum.

   H53.54 **Protanomaly**
     Protanopia

   H53.55 **Tritanomaly**
     Tritanopia

   H53.59 **Other color vision deficiencies**

√5ᵗʰ H53.6 **Night blindness**
     EXCLUDES 1   night blindness due to vitamin A deficiency (E50.5)

   H53.60 **Unspecified night blindness**

   H53.61 **Abnormal dark adaptation curve**

   H53.62 **Acquired night blindness**

   H53.63 **Congenital night blindness**

   H53.69 **Other night blindness**

√5ᵗʰ H53.7 **Vision** sensitivity **deficiencies**

   H53.71 **Glare sensitivity**

   H53.72 **Impaired contrast sensitivity**

H53.8 **Other visual disturbances**

H53.9 **Unspecified visual disturbance**

√4ᵗʰ H54 **Blindness and low vision**

   NOTE   For definition of visual impairment categories see table below

   Code first any associated underlying cause of the blindness
   EXCLUDES 1   amaurosis fugax (G45.3)
   AHA: 2017,4Q,11-12

√5ᵗʰ H54.0 **Blindness,** both eyes
     Visual impairment categories 3, 4, 5 in both eyes.

   √6ᵗʰ H54.0X **Blindness, both eyes, different category levels**

     √7ᵗʰ H54.0X3 **Blindness right eye, category 3**

       H54.0X33 **Blindness right eye category 3, blindness left eye category 3**

       H54.0X34 **Blindness right eye category 3, blindness left eye category 4**

       H54.0X35 **Blindness right eye category 3, blindness left eye category 5**

     √7ᵗʰ H54.0X4 **Blindness right eye, category 4**

       H54.0X43 **Blindness right eye category 4, blindness left eye category 3**

       H54.0X44 **Blindness right eye category 4, blindness left eye category 4**

       H54.0X45 **Blindness right eye category 4, blindness left eye category 5**

     √7ᵗʰ H54.0X5 **Blindness right eye, category 5**

       H54.0X53 **Blindness right eye category 5, blindness left eye category 3**

       H54.0X54 **Blindness right eye category 5, blindness left eye category 4**

       H54.0X55 **Blindness right eye category 5, blindness left eye category 5**

   √6ᵗʰ H54.1 **Blindness, one eye, low vision other eye**
     Visual impairment categories 3, 4, 5 in one eye, with categories 1 or 2 in the other eye.

   H54.10 **Blindness, one eye, low vision other eye, unspecified eyes**

   √6ᵗʰ H54.11 **Blindness, right eye, low vision left eye**

     √7ᵗʰ H54.113 **Blindness right eye category 3, low vision left eye**

       H54.1131 **Blindness right eye category 3, low vision left eye category 1**

       H54.1132 **Blindness right eye category 3, low vision left eye category 2**

     √7ᵗʰ H54.114 **Blindness right eye category 4, low vision left eye**

       H54.1141 **Blindness right eye category 4, low vision left eye category 1**

           H54.1142 Blindness right eye category 4, low vision left eye category 2
     ✓7ᵗʰ **H54.115** Blindness right eye category 5, low vision left eye
           H54.1151 Blindness right eye category 5, low vision left eye category 1
           H54.1152 Blindness right eye category 5, low vision left eye category 2

   ✓6ᵗʰ **H54.12** Blindness, left eye, low vision right eye
     ✓7ᵗʰ **H54.121** Low vision right eye category 1, blindness left eye
           H54.1213 Low vision right eye category 1, blindness left eye category 3
           H54.1214 Low vision right eye category 1, blindness left eye category 4
           H54.1215 Low vision right eye category 1, blindness left eye category 5
     ✓7ᵗʰ **H54.122** Low vision right eye category 2, blindness left eye
           H54.1223 Low vision right eye category 2, blindness left eye category 3
           H54.1224 Low vision right eye category 2, blindness left eye category 4
           H54.1225 Low vision right eye category 2, blindness left eye category 5

✓5ᵗʰ **H54.2** Low vision, both eyes
     Visual impairment categories 1 or 2 in both eyes.
   ✓6ᵗʰ **H54.2X** Low vision, both eyes, different category levels
     ✓7ᵗʰ **H54.2X1** Low vision, right eye, category 1
           H54.2X11 Low vision right eye category 1, low vision left eye category 1
           H54.2X12 Low vision right eye category 1, low vision left eye category 2
     ✓7ᵗʰ **H54.2X2** Low vision, right eye, category 2
           H54.2X21 Low vision right eye category 2, low vision left eye category 1
           H54.2X22 Low vision right eye category 2, low vision left eye category 2

H54.3 Unqualified visual loss, both eyes
     Visual impairment category 9 in both eyes.
     TIP: Assign only when both eyes are documented as affected by blindness or low vision but the visual impairment category is not documented.

✓5ᵗʰ **H54.4** Blindness, one eye
     Visual impairment categories 3, 4, 5 in one eye [normal vision in other eye]
   H54.40 Blindness, one eye, unspecified eye
   ✓6ᵗʰ **H54.41** Blindness, right eye, normal vision left eye
     ✓7ᵗʰ **H54.413** Blindness, right eye, category 3
           H54.413A Blindness right eye category 3, normal vision left eye
     ✓7ᵗʰ **H54.414** Blindness, right eye, category 4
           H54.414A Blindness right eye category 4, normal vision left eye
     ✓7ᵗʰ **H54.415** Blindness, right eye, category 5
           H54.415A Blindness right eye category 5, normal vision left eye
   ✓6ᵗʰ **H54.42** Blindness, left eye, normal vision right eye
     ✓7ᵗʰ **H54.42A** Blindness, left eye, category 3-5
           H54.42A3 Blindness left eye category 3, normal vision right eye
           H54.42A4 Blindness left eye category 4, normal vision right eye
           H54.42A5 Blindness left eye category 5, normal vision right eye

✓5ᵗʰ **H54.5** Low vision, one eye
     Visual impairment categories 1 or 2 in one eye [normal vision in other eye].
   H54.50 Low vision, one eye, unspecified eye

✓6ᵗʰ **H54.51** Low vision, right eye, normal vision left eye
     ✓7ᵗʰ **H54.511** Low vision, right eye, category 1-2
           H54.511A Low vision right eye category 1, normal vision left eye
           H54.512A Low vision right eye category 2, normal vision left eye
✓7ᵗʰ **H54.52** Low vision, left eye, normal vision right eye
     ✓7ᵗʰ **H54.52A** Low vision, left eye, category 1-2
           H54.52A1 Low vision left eye category 1, normal vision right eye
           H54.52A2 Low vision left eye category 2, normal vision right eye

✓5ᵗʰ **H54.6** Unqualified visual loss, one eye
     Visual impairment category 9 in one eye [normal vision in other eye].
     TIP: Assign a code from this category only when one eye is documented as affected by blindness or low vision but the visual impairment category is not documented.
   H54.60 Unqualified visual loss, one eye, unspecified
   H54.61 Unqualified visual loss, right eye, normal vision left eye
   H54.62 Unqualified visual loss, left eye, normal vision right eye

H54.7 Unspecified visual loss
     Visual impairment category 9 NOS
     TIP: Assign only when documentation specifies blindness, visual loss, or low vision but not whether one or both eyes are affected or the visual impairment category.

H54.8 Legal blindness, as defined in USA
     Blindness NOS according to USA definition
     EXCLUDES 1   legal blindness with specification of impairment level (H54.0-H54.7)

     NOTE   The table below gives a classification of severity of visual impairment recommended by a WHO Study Group on the Prevention of Blindness, Geneva, 6-10 November 1972.

     The term "low vision" in category H54 comprises categories 1 and 2 of the table, the term "blindness" categories 3, 4 and 5, and the term "unqualified visual loss" category 9.

     If the extent of the visual field is taken into account, patients with a field no greater than 10 but greater than 5 around central fixation should be placed in category 3 and patients with a field no greater than 5 around central fixation should be placed in category 4, even if the central acuity is not impaired.

[handwritten note: category 2 is low vision]

Category of visual impairment	Visual acuity with best possible correction	
	Maximum less than:	**Minimum equal to or better than:**
1	6/18 3/10 (0.3) 20/70	6/60 1/10 (0.1) 20/200
2	6/60 1/10 (0.1) 20/200	3/60 1/20 (0.05) 20/400
3	3/60 1/200 (0.05) 20/400	1/60 (finger counting at one meter) 1/50 (0.02) 5/300 (20/1200)
4	1/60 (finger counting at one meter) 1/50 (0.02) 5/300	Light perception
5	No light perception	
9	Undetermined or unspecified	

Other disorders of eye and adnexa (H55-H57)

✓4ᵗʰ H55 Nystagmus and other irregular eye movements

  ✓5ᵗʰ H55.0 Nystagmus

    DEF: Rapid, rhythmic, involuntary movements of the eyeball in vertical, horizontal, rotational, or mixed directions.

    H55.00 Unspecified nystagmus

    H55.01 **Congenital nystagmus**

    H55.02 **Latent nystagmus**

    H55.03 **Visual deprivation nystagmus**

    H55.04 **Dissociated nystagmus**

    H55.09 **Other forms of nystagmus**

  ✓5ᵗʰ H55.8 Other irregular eye movements

    AHA: 2020,4Q,25

    H55.81 **Deficient saccadic eye movements**

    H55.82 **Deficient smooth pursuit eye movements**

    H55.89 **Other irregular eye movements**

✓4ᵗʰ H57 Other disorders of eye and adnexa

  ✓5ᵗʰ H57.0 Anomalies of pupillary function

    H57.00 Unspecified anomaly of pupillary function

    H57.01 **Argyll Robertson pupil, atypical**

      EXCLUDES 1   *syphilitic Argyll Robertson pupil (A52.19)*

    H57.02 **Anisocoria**

    H57.03 **Miosis**

    H57.04 **Mydriasis**

    ✓6ᵗʰ H57.05 Tonic pupil

      H57.051 **Tonic pupil, right eye**

      H57.052 **Tonic pupil, left eye**

      H57.053 **Tonic pupil, bilateral**

      H57.059 Tonic pupil, unspecified eye

    H57.09 **Other anomalies of pupillary function**

  ✓5ᵗʰ H57.1 Ocular pain

    H57.10 Ocular pain, unspecified eye

    H57.11 **Ocular pain, right eye**

    H57.12 **Ocular pain, left eye**

    H57.13 **Ocular pain, bilateral**

  ✓6ᵗʰ H57.8 Other specified disorders of eye and adnexa

    AHA: 2018,4Q,15-16

    ✓6ᵗʰ H57.81 Brow ptosis

      H57.811 **Brow ptosis, right**

      H57.812 **Brow ptosis, left**

      H57.813 **Brow ptosis, bilateral**

      H57.819 Brow ptosis, unspecified

    H57.89 **Other specified disorders of eye and adnexa**

  H57.9 Unspecified disorder of eye and adnexa

Intraoperative and postprocedural complications and disorders of eye and adnexa, not elsewhere classified (H59)

✓4ᵗʰ H59 Intraoperative and postprocedural complications and disorders of eye and adnexa, not elsewhere classified

    EXCLUDES 1   *mechanical complication of intraocular lens (T85.2)*

        mechanical complication of other ocular prosthetic devices, implants and grafts (T85.3)

        pseudophakia (Z96.1)

        secondary cataracts (H26.4-)

  ✓5ᵗʰ H59.0 Disorders of the eye following cataract surgery

    ✓6ᵗʰ H59.01 Keratopathy (bullous aphakic) following cataract surgery

      Vitreal corneal syndrome

      Vitreous (touch) syndrome

      H59.011 **Keratopathy (bullous aphakic) following cataract surgery, right eye**

      H59.012 **Keratopathy (bullous aphakic) following cataract surgery, left eye**

      H59.013 **Keratopathy (bullous aphakic) following cataract surgery, bilateral**

      H59.019 Keratopathy (bullous aphakic) following cataract surgery, unspecified eye

    ✓6ᵗʰ H59.02 Cataract (lens) fragments in eye following cataract surgery

      H59.021 **Cataract (lens) fragments in eye following cataract surgery, right eye**

      H59.022 **Cataract (lens) fragments in eye following cataract surgery, left eye**

      H59.023 **Cataract (lens) fragments in eye following cataract surgery, bilateral**

      H59.029 Cataract (lens) fragments in eye following cataract surgery, unspecified eye

    ✓6ᵗʰ H59.03 Cystoid macular edema following cataract surgery

      H59.031 **Cystoid macular edema following cataract surgery, right eye**

      H59.032 **Cystoid macular edema following cataract surgery, left eye**

      H59.033 **Cystoid macular edema following cataract surgery, bilateral**

      H59.039 Cystoid macular edema following cataract surgery, unspecified eye

    ✓6ᵗʰ H59.09 Other disorders of the eye following cataract surgery

      H59.091 **Other disorders of the right eye following cataract surgery**

      H59.092 **Other disorders of the left eye following cataract surgery**

      H59.093 **Other disorders of the eye following cataract surgery, bilateral**

      H59.099 Other disorders of unspecified eye following cataract surgery

  ✓5ᵗʰ H59.1 Intraoperative hemorrhage and hematoma of eye and adnexa complicating a procedure

    EXCLUDES 1   *intraoperative hemorrhage and hematoma of eye and adnexa due to accidental puncture or laceration during a procedure (H59.2-)*

    ✓6ᵗʰ H59.11 Intraoperative hemorrhage and hematoma of eye and adnexa complicating an ophthalmic procedure

      H59.111 **Intraoperative hemorrhage and hematoma of right eye and adnexa complicating an ophthalmic procedure**

      H59.112 **Intraoperative hemorrhage and hematoma of left eye and adnexa complicating an ophthalmic procedure**

      H59.113 **Intraoperative hemorrhage and hematoma of eye and adnexa complicating an ophthalmic procedure, bilateral**

      H59.119 Intraoperative hemorrhage and hematoma of unspecified eye and adnexa complicating an ophthalmic procedure

    ✓6ᵗʰ H59.12 Intraoperative hemorrhage and hematoma of eye and adnexa complicating other procedure

      H59.121 **Intraoperative hemorrhage and hematoma of right eye and adnexa complicating other procedure**

      H59.122 **Intraoperative hemorrhage and hematoma of left eye and adnexa complicating other procedure**

      H59.123 **Intraoperative hemorrhage and hematoma of eye and adnexa complicating other procedure, bilateral**

      H59.129 Intraoperative hemorrhage and hematoma of unspecified eye and adnexa complicating other procedure

  ✓5ᵗʰ H59.2 Accidental puncture and laceration of eye and adnexa during a procedure

    ✓6ᵗʰ H59.21 Accidental puncture and laceration of eye and adnexa during an ophthalmic procedure

      H59.211 **Accidental puncture and laceration of right eye and adnexa during an ophthalmic procedure**

      H59.212 **Accidental puncture and laceration of left eye and adnexa during an ophthalmic procedure**

      H59.213 **Accidental puncture and laceration of eye and adnexa during an ophthalmic procedure, bilateral**

      H59.219 Accidental puncture and laceration of unspecified eye and adnexa during an ophthalmic procedure

    ✓6ᵗʰ H59.22 Accidental puncture and laceration of eye and adnexa during other procedure

      H59.221 **Accidental puncture and laceration of right eye and adnexa during other procedure**

      H59.222 **Accidental puncture and laceration of left eye and adnexa during other procedure**

      H59.223 **Accidental puncture and laceration of eye and adnexa during other procedure, bilateral**

Chapter 7. Diseases of the Eye and Adnexa

    H59.229   Accidental puncture and laceration of unspecified eye and adnexa during other procedure

✓5ᵗʰ **H59.3**   Postprocedural hemorrhage, hematoma, and seroma of eye and adnexa following a procedure
    AHA: 2016,4Q,9-10

  ✓6ᵗʰ **H59.31**   Postprocedural hemorrhage of eye and adnexa following an ophthalmic procedure
      H59.311   Postprocedural hemorrhage of right eye and adnexa following an ophthalmic procedure
      H59.312   Postprocedural hemorrhage of left eye and adnexa following an ophthalmic procedure
      H59.313   Postprocedural hemorrhage of eye and adnexa following an ophthalmic procedure, bilateral
      H59.319   Postprocedural hemorrhage of unspecified eye and adnexa following an ophthalmic procedure

  ✓6ᵗʰ **H59.32**   Postprocedural hemorrhage of eye and adnexa following other procedure
      H59.321   Postprocedural hemorrhage of right eye and adnexa following other procedure
      H59.322   Postprocedural hemorrhage of left eye and adnexa following other procedure
      H59.323   Postprocedural hemorrhage of eye and adnexa following other procedure, bilateral
      H59.329   Postprocedural hemorrhage of unspecified eye and adnexa following other procedure

  ✓6ᵗʰ **H59.33**   Postprocedural hematoma of eye and adnexa following an ophthalmic procedure
      H59.331   Postprocedural hematoma of right eye and adnexa following an ophthalmic procedure
      H59.332   Postprocedural hematoma of left eye and adnexa following an ophthalmic procedure
      H59.333   Postprocedural hematoma of eye and adnexa following an ophthalmic procedure, bilateral
      H59.339   Postprocedural hematoma of unspecified eye and adnexa following an ophthalmic procedure

  ✓6ᵗʰ **H59.34**   Postprocedural hematoma of eye and adnexa following other procedure
      H59.341   Postprocedural hematoma of right eye and adnexa following other procedure
      H59.342   Postprocedural hematoma of left eye and adnexa following other procedure
      H59.343   Postprocedural hematoma of eye and adnexa following other procedure, bilateral
      H59.349   Postprocedural hematoma of unspecified eye and adnexa following other procedure

  ✓6ᵗʰ **H59.35**   Postprocedural seroma of eye and adnexa following an ophthalmic procedure
      H59.351   Postprocedural seroma of right eye and adnexa following an ophthalmic procedure
      H59.352   Postprocedural seroma of left eye and adnexa following an ophthalmic procedure
      H59.353   Postprocedural seroma of eye and adnexa following an ophthalmic procedure, bilateral
      H59.359   Postprocedural seroma of unspecified eye and adnexa following an ophthalmic procedure

  ✓6ᵗʰ **H59.36**   Postprocedural seroma of eye and adnexa following other procedure
      H59.361   Postprocedural seroma of right eye and adnexa following other procedure
      H59.362   Postprocedural seroma of left eye and adnexa following other procedure
      H59.363   Postprocedural seroma of eye and adnexa following other procedure, bilateral
      H59.369   Postprocedural seroma of unspecified eye and adnexa following other procedure

✓5ᵗʰ **H59.4**   Inflammation (infection) of postprocedural bleb
    Postprocedural blebitis
    EXCLUDES 1   filtering (vitreous) bleb after glaucoma surgery status (Z98.83)

  H59.40   Inflammation (infection) of postprocedural bleb, unspecified
  H59.41   Inflammation (infection) of postprocedural bleb, stage 1
  H59.42   Inflammation (infection) of postprocedural bleb, stage 2
  H59.43   Inflammation (infection) of postprocedural bleb, stage 3
    Bleb endophthalmitis

✓5ᵗʰ **H59.8**   Other intraoperative and postprocedural complications and disorders of eye and adnexa, not elsewhere classified

  ✓6ᵗʰ **H59.81**   Chorioretinal scars after surgery for detachment
      H59.811   Chorioretinal scars after surgery for detachment, right eye
      H59.812   Chorioretinal scars after surgery for detachment, left eye
      H59.813   Chorioretinal scars after surgery for detachment, bilateral
      H59.819   Chorioretinal scars after surgery for detachment, unspecified eye

  H59.88   Other intraoperative complications of eye and adnexa, not elsewhere classified
  H59.89   Other postprocedural complications and disorders of eye and adnexa, not elsewhere classified
    AHA: 2020,3Q,29

Chapter 8. Diseases of the Ear and Mastoid Process (H60–H95)

Chapter-specific Guidelines with Coding Examples
Reserved for future guideline expansion.

Chapter 8. Diseases of the Ear and Mastoid Process (H60–H95)

> **NOTE**   Use an external cause code following the code for the ear condition, if applicable, to identify the cause of the ear condition
>
> **EXCLUDES 2**   *certain conditions originating in the perinatal period (P04-P96)*
> *certain infectious and parasitic diseases (A00-B99)*
> *complications of pregnancy, childbirth and the puerperium (O00-O9A)*
> *congenital malformations, deformations and chromosomal abnormalities (Q00-Q99)*
> *endocrine, nutritional and metabolic diseases (E00-E88)*
> *injury, poisoning and certain other consequences of external causes (S00-T88)*
> *neoplasms (C00-D49)*
> *symptoms, signs and abnormal clinical and laboratory findings, not elsewhere classified (R00-R94)*

This chapter contains the following blocks:

H60-H62   Diseases of external ear
H65-H75   Diseases of middle ear and mastoid
H80-H83   Diseases of inner ear
H90-H94   Other disorders of ear
H95   Intraoperative and postprocedural complications and disorders of ear and mastoid process, not elsewhere classified

Diseases of external ear (H60-H62)

✓4ᵗʰ H60 Otitis externa

> **TIP:** When the specific infectious agent is identified, a code from Chapter 1 is assigned instead of a code from this category.

✓5ᵗʰ H60.0 Abscess of external ear

> Boil of external ear
> Carbuncle of auricle or external auditory canal
> Furuncle of external ear

     H60.00   Abscess of external ear, unspecified ear
     H60.01   Abscess of right external ear
     H60.02   Abscess of left external ear
     H60.03   Abscess of external ear, bilateral

✓5ᵗʰ H60.1 Cellulitis of external ear

> Cellulitis of auricle
> Cellulitis of external auditory canal

     H60.10   Cellulitis of external ear, unspecified ear
     H60.11   Cellulitis of right external ear
     H60.12   Cellulitis of left external ear
     H60.13   Cellulitis of external ear, bilateral

✓5ᵗʰ H60.2 Malignant otitis externa

     H60.20   Malignant otitis externa, unspecified ear
     H60.21   Malignant otitis externa, right ear
     H60.22   Malignant otitis externa, left ear
     H60.23   Malignant otitis externa, bilateral

✓5ᵗʰ H60.3 Other infective otitis externa

✓6ᵗʰ H60.31 Diffuse otitis externa

     H60.311   Diffuse otitis externa, right ear
     H60.312   Diffuse otitis externa, left ear
     H60.313   Diffuse otitis externa, bilateral
     H60.319   Diffuse otitis externa, unspecified ear

✓6ᵗʰ H60.32 Hemorrhagic otitis externa

     H60.321   Hemorrhagic otitis externa, right ear
     H60.322   Hemorrhagic otitis externa, left ear
     H60.323   Hemorrhagic otitis externa, bilateral
     H60.329   Hemorrhagic otitis externa, unspecified ear

✓6ᵗʰ H60.33 Swimmer's ear

> **DEF:** Commonly occurs when water gets trapped in the ear after swimming.

     H60.331   Swimmer's ear, right ear
     H60.332   Swimmer's ear, left ear
     H60.333   Swimmer's ear, bilateral
     H60.339   Swimmer's ear, unspecified ear

✓6ᵗʰ H60.39 Other infective otitis externa

     H60.391   Other infective otitis externa, right ear
     H60.392   Other infective otitis externa, left ear
     H60.393   Other infective otitis externa, bilateral
     H60.399   Other infective otitis externa, unspecified ear

✓6ᵗʰ H60.4 Cholesteatoma of external ear

> Keratosis obturans of external ear (canal)
>
> **EXCLUDES 2**   *cholesteatoma of middle ear (H71.-)*
> *recurrent cholesteatoma of postmastoidectomy cavity (H95.0-)*
>
> **DEF:** Cholesteatoma: Noncancerous cyst-like mass of cell debris, including cholesterol and epithelial cells resulting from trauma, repeated or improperly healed infections, and congenital enclosure of epidermal cells.

     H60.40   Cholesteatoma of external ear, unspecified ear
     H60.41   Cholesteatoma of right external ear
     H60.42   Cholesteatoma of left external ear
     H60.43   Cholesteatoma of external ear, bilateral

✓5ᵗʰ H60.5 Acute noninfective otitis externa

✓6ᵗʰ H60.50 Unspecified acute noninfective otitis externa

> Acute otitis externa NOS

     H60.501   Unspecified acute noninfective otitis externa, right ear
     H60.502   Unspecified acute noninfective otitis externa, left ear
     H60.503   Unspecified acute noninfective otitis externa, bilateral
     H60.509   Unspecified acute noninfective otitis externa, unspecified ear

✓6ᵗʰ H60.51 Acute actinic otitis externa

     H60.511   Acute actinic otitis externa, right ear
     H60.512   Acute actinic otitis externa, left ear
     H60.513   Acute actinic otitis externa, bilateral
     H60.519   Acute actinic otitis externa, unspecified ear

✓6ᵗʰ H60.52 Acute chemical otitis externa

     H60.521   Acute chemical otitis externa, right ear
     H60.522   Acute chemical otitis externa, left ear
     H60.523   Acute chemical otitis externa, bilateral
     H60.529   Acute chemical otitis externa, unspecified ear

✓6ᵗʰ H60.53 Acute contact otitis externa

     H60.531   Acute contact otitis externa, right ear
     H60.532   Acute contact otitis externa, left ear
     H60.533   Acute contact otitis externa, bilateral
     H60.539   Acute contact otitis externa, unspecified ear

✓6ᵗʰ H60.54 Acute eczematoid otitis externa

     H60.541   Acute eczematoid otitis externa, right ear
     H60.542   Acute eczematoid otitis externa, left ear
     H60.543   Acute eczematoid otitis externa, bilateral
     H60.549   Acute eczematoid otitis externa, unspecified ear

✓6ᵗʰ H60.55 Acute reactive otitis externa

     H60.551   Acute reactive otitis externa, right ear
     H60.552   Acute reactive otitis externa, left ear
     H60.553   Acute reactive otitis externa, bilateral
     H60.559   Acute reactive otitis externa, unspecified ear

✓6ᵗʰ H60.59 Other noninfective acute otitis externa

     H60.591   Other noninfective acute otitis externa, right ear
     H60.592   Other noninfective acute otitis externa, left ear
     H60.593   Other noninfective acute otitis externa, bilateral
     H60.599   Other noninfective acute otitis externa, unspecified ear

✓5ᵗʰ H60.6 Unspecified chronic otitis externa

     H60.60   Unspecified chronic otitis externa, unspecified ear
     H60.61   Unspecified chronic otitis externa, right ear
     H60.62   Unspecified chronic otitis externa, left ear
     H60.63   Unspecified chronic otitis externa, bilateral

✓5ᵗʰ H60.8 Other otitis externa

✓6ᵗʰ H60.8X Other otitis externa

     H60.8X1   Other otitis externa, right ear
     H60.8X2   Other otitis externa, left ear
     H60.8X3   Other otitis externa, bilateral
     H60.8X9   Other otitis externa, unspecified ear

✓6ᵗʰ H60.9 Unspecified otitis externa

     H60.90   Unspecified otitis externa, unspecified ear
     H60.91   Unspecified otitis externa, right ear

HCC CMS-HCC   **Rx** Rx HCC   **ESR** ESRD HCC   **COM** Commercial HCC   **N** Newborn: 0   **P** Pediatric: 0-17   **M** Maternity: 9-64   **A** Adult: 15-124

648
ICD-10-CM 2023

H60.92　**Unspecified otitis externa, left ear**
H60.93　**Unspecified otitis externa, bilateral**

☑4ᵗʰ **H61**　**Other disorders of external ear**

　☑5ᵗʰ **H61.0**　**Chondritis and perichondritis of external ear**

　　Chondrodermatitis nodularis chronica helicis
　　Perichondritis of auricle
　　Perichondritis of pinna

　　☑6ᵗʰ **H61.00**　**Unspecified perichondritis of external ear**

　　　H61.001　**Unspecified perichondritis of right external ear**
　　　H61.002　**Unspecified perichondritis of left external ear**
　　　H61.003　**Unspecified perichondritis of external ear, bilateral**
　　　H61.009　**Unspecified perichondritis of external ear, unspecified ear**

　　☑6ᵗʰ **H61.01**　**Acute perichondritis of external ear**

　　　H61.011　**Acute perichondritis of right external ear**
　　　H61.012　**Acute perichondritis of left external ear**
　　　H61.013　**Acute perichondritis of external ear, bilateral**
　　　H61.019　**Acute perichondritis of external ear, unspecified ear**

　　☑6ᵗʰ **H61.02**　**Chronic perichondritis of external ear**

　　　H61.021　**Chronic perichondritis of right external ear**
　　　H61.022　**Chronic perichondritis of left external ear**
　　　H61.023　**Chronic perichondritis of external ear, bilateral**
　　　H61.029　**Chronic perichondritis of external ear, unspecified ear**

　　☑6ᵗʰ **H61.03**　**Chondritis of external ear**

　　　Chondritis of auricle
　　　Chondritis of pinna
　　　AHA: 2015,1Q,18
　　　DEF: Infection that has progressed into the cartilage and presents as indurated and edematous skin over the pinna. Vascular compromise occurs with tissue necrosis and deformity.
　　　H61.031　**Chondritis of right external ear**
　　　H61.032　**Chondritis of left external ear**
　　　H61.033　**Chondritis of external ear, bilateral**
　　　H61.039　**Chondritis of external ear, unspecified ear**

　☑5ᵗʰ **H61.1**　**Noninfective disorders of pinna**

　　　EXCLUDES 2　cauliflower ear (M95.1-)
　　　　　　　gouty tophi of ear (M1A.-)

　　☑6ᵗʰ **H61.10**　**Unspecified noninfective disorders of pinna**

　　　Disorder of pinna NOS
　　　H61.101　**Unspecified noninfective disorders of pinna, right ear**
　　　H61.102　**Unspecified noninfective disorders of pinna, left ear**
　　　H61.103　**Unspecified noninfective disorders of pinna, bilateral**
　　　H61.109　**Unspecified noninfective disorders of pinna, unspecified ear**

　　☑6ᵗʰ **H61.11**　**Acquired deformity of pinna**

　　　Acquired deformity of auricle
　　　EXCLUDES 2　cauliflower ear (M95.1-)
　　　H61.111　**Acquired deformity of pinna, right ear**
　　　H61.112　**Acquired deformity of pinna, left ear**
　　　H61.113　**Acquired deformity of pinna, bilateral**
　　　H61.119　**Acquired deformity of pinna, unspecified ear**

　　☑6ᵗʰ **H61.12**　**Hematoma of pinna**

　　　Hematoma of auricle
　　　H61.121　**Hematoma of pinna, right ear**
　　　H61.122　**Hematoma of pinna, left ear**
　　　H61.123　**Hematoma of pinna, bilateral**
　　　H61.129　**Hematoma of pinna, unspecified ear**

　　☑6ᵗʰ **H61.19**　**Other noninfective disorders of pinna**

　　　H61.191　**Noninfective disorders of pinna, right ear**
　　　H61.192　**Noninfective disorders of pinna, left ear**
　　　H61.193　**Noninfective disorders of pinna, bilateral**
　　　H61.199　**Noninfective disorders of pinna, unspecified ear**

☑5ᵗʰ **H61.2**　**Impacted cerumen**

　　Wax in ear
　　H61.20　**Impacted cerumen, unspecified ear**
　　H61.21　**Impacted cerumen, right ear**
　　H61.22　**Impacted cerumen, left ear**
　　H61.23　**Impacted cerumen, bilateral**

☑5ᵗʰ **H61.3**　**Acquired stenosis of external ear canal**

　　Collapse of external ear canal
　　EXCLUDES 1　postprocedural stenosis of external ear canal (H95.81-)

　☑6ᵗʰ **H61.30**　**Acquired stenosis of external ear canal, unspecified**

　　　H61.301　**Acquired stenosis of right external ear canal, unspecified**
　　　H61.302　**Acquired stenosis of left external ear canal, unspecified**
　　　H61.303　**Acquired stenosis of external ear canal, unspecified, bilateral**
　　　H61.309　**Acquired stenosis of external ear canal, unspecified, unspecified ear**

　☑6ᵗʰ **H61.31**　**Acquired stenosis of external ear canal secondary to trauma**

　　　H61.311　**Acquired stenosis of right external ear canal secondary to trauma**
　　　H61.312　**Acquired stenosis of left external ear canal secondary to trauma**
　　　H61.313　**Acquired stenosis of external ear canal secondary to trauma, bilateral**
　　　H61.319　**Acquired stenosis of external ear canal secondary to trauma, unspecified ear**

　☑6ᵗʰ **H61.32**　**Acquired stenosis of external ear canal secondary to inflammation and infection**

　　　DEF: Narrowing of the external ear canal due to chronic inflammation or infection.
　　　H61.321　**Acquired stenosis of right external ear canal secondary to inflammation and infection**
　　　H61.322　**Acquired stenosis of left external ear canal secondary to inflammation and infection**
　　　H61.323　**Acquired stenosis of external ear canal secondary to inflammation and infection, bilateral**
　　　H61.329　**Acquired stenosis of external ear canal secondary to inflammation and infection, unspecified ear**

　☑6ᵗʰ **H61.39**　**Other acquired stenosis of external ear canal**

　　　H61.391　**Other acquired stenosis of right external ear canal**
　　　H61.392　**Other acquired stenosis of left external ear canal**
　　　H61.393　**Other acquired stenosis of external ear canal, bilateral**
　　　H61.399　**Other acquired stenosis of external ear canal, unspecified ear**

☑5ᵗʰ **H61.8**　**Other specified disorders of external ear**

　☑6ᵗʰ **H61.81**　**Exostosis of external canal**

　　　H61.811　**Exostosis of right external canal**
　　　H61.812　**Exostosis of left external canal**
　　　H61.813　**Exostosis of external canal, bilateral**
　　　H61.819　**Exostosis of external canal, unspecified ear**

　☑6ᵗʰ **H61.89**　**Other specified disorders of external ear**

　　　H61.891　**Other specified disorders of right external ear**
　　　H61.892　**Other specified disorders of left external ear**
　　　H61.893　**Other specified disorders of external ear, bilateral**
　　　H61.899　**Other specified disorders of external ear, unspecified ear**

☑5ᵗʰ **H61.9**　**Disorder of external ear, unspecified**

　　H61.90　**Disorder of external ear, unspecified, unspecified ear**
　　H61.91　**Disorder of right external ear, unspecified**
　　H61.92　**Disorder of left external ear, unspecified**
　　H61.93　**Disorder of external ear, unspecified, bilateral**

✅ Additional Character Required　　　✓x7ᵗʰ Placeholder Alert　　　Manifestation　　　Unspecified Dx　　　🄠 QPP　　　UPD Unacceptable PDx

Chapter 8. Diseases of the Ear and Mastoid Process

H62–H65.93

☑4ᵗʰ **H62 Disorders of external ear in diseases classified elsewhere**

☑5ᵗʰ **H62.4 Otitis externa in other diseases classified elsewhere**

Code first underlying disease, such as:
erysipelas (A46)
impetigo (LØ1.Ø)

EXCLUDES 1   otitis externa (in):
candidiasis (B37.84)
herpes viral [herpes simplex] (BØØ.1)
herpes zoster (BØ2.8)

H62.4Ø   *Otitis externa in other diseases classified elsewhere, unspecified ear*

H62.41   *Otitis externa in other diseases classified elsewhere, right ear*

H62.42   *Otitis externa in other diseases classified elsewhere, left ear*

H62.43   *Otitis externa in other diseases classified elsewhere, bilateral*

☑5ᵗʰ **H62.8 Other disorders of external ear in diseases classified elsewhere**

Code first underlying disease, such as:
gout (M1A.-, M1Ø.-)

☑6ᵗʰ **H62.8X Other disorders of external ear in diseases classified elsewhere**

H62.8X1   *Other disorders of right external ear in diseases classified elsewhere*

H62.8X2   *Other disorders of left external ear in diseases classified elsewhere*

H62.8X3   *Other disorders of external ear in diseases classified elsewhere, bilateral*

H62.8X9   *Other disorders of external ear in diseases classified elsewhere, unspecified ear*

Diseases of middle ear and mastoid (H65-H75)

☑4ᵗʰ **H65 Nonsuppurative otitis media**

INCLUDES   nonsuppurative otitis media with myringitis

Use additional code for any associated perforated tympanic membrane (H72.-)

Use additional code, if applicable, to identify:
exposure to environmental tobacco smoke (Z77.22)
exposure to tobacco smoke in the perinatal period (P96.81)
history of tobacco dependence (Z87.891)
infectious agent (B95-B97)
occupational exposure to environmental tobacco smoke (Z57.31)
tobacco dependence (F17.-)
tobacco use (Z72.Ø)

☑5ᵗʰ **H65.Ø Acute serous otitis media**

Acute and subacute secretory otitis

H65.ØØ   **Acute serous otitis media, unspecified ear**

H65.Ø1   **Acute serous otitis media, right ear**

H65.Ø2   **Acute serous otitis media, left ear**

H65.Ø3   **Acute serous otitis media, bilateral**

H65.Ø4   **Acute serous otitis media, recurrent, right ear**

H65.Ø5   **Acute serous otitis media, recurrent, left ear**

H65.Ø6   **Acute serous otitis media, recurrent, bilateral**

H65.Ø7   **Acute serous otitis media, recurrent, unspecified ear**

☑5ᵗʰ **H65.1 Other acute nonsuppurative otitis media**

EXCLUDES 1   otitic barotrauma (T7Ø.Ø)
otitis media (acute) NOS (H66.9)

☑6ᵗʰ **H65.11 Acute and subacute allergic otitis media (mucoid) (sanguinous) (serous)**

H65.111   **Acute and subacute allergic otitis media (mucoid) (sanguinous) (serous), right ear**

H65.112   **Acute and subacute allergic otitis media (mucoid) (sanguinous) (serous), left ear**

H65.113   **Acute and subacute allergic otitis media (mucoid) (sanguinous) (serous), bilateral**

H65.114   **Acute and subacute allergic otitis media (mucoid) (sanguinous) (serous), recurrent, right ear**

H65.115   **Acute and subacute allergic otitis media (mucoid) (sanguinous) (serous), recurrent, left ear**

H65.116   **Acute and subacute allergic otitis media (mucoid) (sanguinous) (serous), recurrent, bilateral**

H65.117   **Acute and subacute allergic otitis media (mucoid) (sanguinous) (serous), recurrent, unspecified ear**

H65.119   **Acute and subacute allergic otitis media (mucoid) (sanguinous) (serous), unspecified ear**

☑6ᵗʰ **H65.19 Other acute nonsuppurative otitis media**

Acute and subacute mucoid otitis media
Acute and subacute nonsuppurative otitis media NOS
Acute and subacute sanguinous otitis media
Acute and subacute seromucinous otitis media

H65.191   **Other acute nonsuppurative otitis media, right ear**

H65.192   **Other acute nonsuppurative otitis media, left ear**

H65.193   **Other acute nonsuppurative otitis media, bilateral**

H65.194   **Other acute nonsuppurative otitis media, recurrent, right ear**

H65.195   **Other acute nonsuppurative otitis media, recurrent, left ear**

H65.196   **Other acute nonsuppurative otitis media, recurrent, bilateral**

H65.197   **Other acute nonsuppurative otitis media recurrent, unspecified ear**

H65.199   **Other acute nonsuppurative otitis media, unspecified ear**

☑5ᵗʰ **H65.2 Chronic serous otitis media**

Chronic tubotympanal catarrh

H65.2Ø   **Chronic serous otitis media, unspecified ear**

H65.21   **Chronic serous otitis media, right ear**

H65.22   **Chronic serous otitis media, left ear**

H65.23   **Chronic serous otitis media, bilateral**

☑5ᵗʰ **H65.3 Chronic mucoid otitis media**

Chronic mucinous otitis media
Chronic secretory otitis media
Chronic transudative otitis media
Glue ear

EXCLUDES 1   adhesive middle ear disease (H74.1)

H65.3Ø   **Chronic mucoid otitis media, unspecified ear**

H65.31   **Chronic mucoid otitis media, right ear**

H65.32   **Chronic mucoid otitis media, left ear**

H65.33   **Chronic mucoid otitis media, bilateral**

☑5ᵗʰ **H65.4 Other chronic nonsuppurative otitis media**

[handwritten: mucoid effusion]

☑6ᵗʰ **H65.41 Chronic allergic otitis media**

H65.411   **Chronic allergic otitis media, right ear**

H65.412   **Chronic allergic otitis media, left ear**

H65.413   **Chronic allergic otitis media, bilateral**

H65.419   **Chronic allergic otitis media, unspecified ear**

☑6ᵗʰ **H65.49 Other chronic nonsuppurative otitis media**

Chronic exudative otitis media
Chronic nonsuppurative otitis media NOS
Chronic otitis media with effusion (nonpurulent)
Chronic seromucinous otitis media

H65.491   **Other chronic nonsuppurative otitis media, right ear**

H65.492   **Other chronic nonsuppurative otitis media, left ear**

H65.493   **Other chronic nonsuppurative otitis media, bilateral**

H65.499   **Other chronic nonsuppurative otitis media, unspecified ear**

☑5ᵗʰ **H65.9 Unspecified nonsuppurative otitis media**

Allergic otitis media NOS
Catarrhal otitis media NOS
Exudative otitis media NOS
Mucoid otitis media NOS
Otitis media with effusion (nonpurulent) NOS
Secretory otitis media NOS
Seromucinous otitis media NOS
Serous otitis media NOS
Transudative otitis media NOS

H65.9Ø   **Unspecified nonsuppurative otitis media, unspecified ear**

H65.91   **Unspecified nonsuppurative otitis media, right ear**

H65.92   **Unspecified nonsuppurative otitis media, left ear**

H65.93   **Unspecified nonsuppurative otitis media, bilateral**

HCC CMS-HCC   **Rx** Rx HCC   **ESR** ESRD HCC   **COM** Commercial HCC   **N** Newborn: 0   **P** Pediatric: 0-17   **M** Maternity: 9-64   **A** Adult: 15-124

650

ICD-10-CM 2023

Chapter 8. Diseases of the Ear and Mastoid Process

✓4ᵗʰ **H66 Suppurative and unspecified otitis media**

     INCLUDES   suppurative and unspecified otitis media with myringitis

     Use additional code to identify:

       exposure to environmental tobacco smoke (Z77.22)

       exposure to tobacco smoke in the perinatal period (P96.81)

       history of tobacco dependence (Z87.891)

       occupational exposure to environmental tobacco smoke (Z57.31)

       tobacco dependence (F17.-)

       tobacco use (Z72.0)

     AHA: 2016,1Q,34

   ✓5ᵗʰ **H66.0** Acute suppurative **otitis media**

     ✓6ᵗʰ **H66.00**   **Acute suppurative otitis media without spontaneous rupture of ear drum**

       H66.001 Acute suppurative otitis media without spontaneous rupture of ear drum, right ear

       H66.002 Acute suppurative otitis media without spontaneous rupture of ear drum, left ear

       H66.003 Acute suppurative otitis media without spontaneous rupture of ear drum, bilateral

       H66.004 Acute suppurative otitis media without spontaneous rupture of ear drum, recurrent, right ear

       H66.005 Acute suppurative otitis media without spontaneous rupture of ear drum, recurrent, left ear

       H66.006 Acute suppurative otitis media without spontaneous rupture of ear drum, recurrent, bilateral

       H66.007 Acute suppurative otitis media without spontaneous rupture of ear drum, recurrent, unspecified ear

       H66.009 Acute suppurative otitis media without spontaneous rupture of ear drum, unspecified ear

     ✓6ᵗʰ **H66.01**   **Acute suppurative otitis media** with spontaneous rupture of ear drum

       DEF: Sudden, severe inflammation of the middle ear, causing pressure that perforates the ear drum tissue.

       H66.011 Acute suppurative otitis media with spontaneous rupture of ear drum, right ear

       H66.012 Acute suppurative otitis media with spontaneous rupture of ear drum, left ear

       H66.013 Acute suppurative otitis media with spontaneous rupture of ear drum, bilateral

       H66.014 Acute suppurative otitis media with spontaneous rupture of ear drum, recurrent, right ear

       H66.015 Acute suppurative otitis media with spontaneous rupture of ear drum, recurrent, left ear

       H66.016 Acute suppurative otitis media with spontaneous rupture of ear drum, recurrent, bilateral

       H66.017 Acute suppurative otitis media with spontaneous rupture of ear drum, recurrent, unspecified ear

       H66.019 Acute suppurative otitis media with spontaneous rupture of ear drum, unspecified ear

   ✓5ᵗʰ **H66.1** Chronic tubotympanic suppurative **otitis media**

     Benign chronic suppurative otitis media

     Chronic tubotympanic disease

     Use additional code for any associated perforated tympanic membrane (H72.-)

     H66.10 Chronic tubotympanic suppurative otitis media, unspecified

     H66.11 Chronic tubotympanic suppurative otitis media, right ear

     H66.12 Chronic tubotympanic suppurative otitis media, left ear

     H66.13 Chronic tubotympanic suppurative otitis media, bilateral

   ✓5ᵗʰ **H66.2** Chronic atticoantral suppurative **otitis media**

     Chronic atticoantral disease

     Use additional code for any associated perforated tympanic membrane (H72.-)

     H66.20 Chronic atticoantral suppurative otitis media, unspecified ear

     H66.21 Chronic atticoantral suppurative otitis media, right ear

     H66.22 Chronic atticoantral suppurative otitis media, left ear

     H66.23 Chronic atticoantral suppurative otitis media, bilateral

   ✓5ᵗʰ **H66.3** Other chronic suppurative otitis media

     Chronic suppurative otitis media NOS

     Use additional code for any associated perforated tympanic membrane (H72.-)

     EXCLUDES 1   tuberculous otitis media (A18.6)

     ✓6ᵗʰ **H66.3X**   Other chronic suppurative otitis media

       H66.3X1 Other chronic suppurative otitis media, right ear

       H66.3X2 Other chronic suppurative otitis media, left ear

       H66.3X3 Other chronic suppurative otitis media, bilateral

       H66.3X9 Other chronic suppurative otitis media, unspecified ear

   ✓5ᵗʰ **H66.4** Suppurative otitis media, unspecified

     Purulent otitis media NOS

     Use additional code for any associated perforated tympanic membrane (H72.-)

     H66.40 Suppurative otitis media, unspecified, unspecified ear

     H66.41 Suppurative otitis media, unspecified, right ear

     H66.42 Suppurative otitis media, unspecified, left ear

     H66.43 Suppurative otitis media, unspecified, bilateral

   ✓5ᵗʰ **H66.9** Otitis media, unspecified

     Otitis media NOS

     Acute otitis media NOS

     Chronic otitis media NOS

     Use additional code for any associated perforated tympanic membrane (H72.-)

     H66.90 Otitis media, unspecified, unspecified ear

     H66.91 Otitis media, unspecified, right ear

     H66.92 Otitis media, unspecified, left ear

     H66.93 Otitis media, unspecified, bilateral

✓4ᵗʰ **H67 Otitis media in diseases classified elsewhere**

     Code first underlying disease, such as:

       plasminogen deficiency (E88.02)

       viral disease NEC (B00-B34)

     Use additional code for any associated perforated tympanic membrane (H72.-)

     EXCLUDES 1   *otitis media in:*

         influenza (J09.X9, J10.83, J11.83)

         measles (B05.3)

         scarlet fever (A38.0)

         tuberculosis (A18.6)

     H67.1 *Otitis media in diseases classified elsewhere, right ear*

     H67.2 *Otitis media in diseases classified elsewhere, left ear*

     H67.3 *Otitis media in diseases classified elsewhere, bilateral*

     H67.9 *Otitis media in diseases classified elsewhere, unspecified ear*

✓4ᵗʰ **H68 Eustachian salpingitis and obstruction**

     DEF: Eustachian tube: Internal channel between the tympanic cavity and the nasopharynx that equalizes internal pressure to the outside pressure and drains mucous production from the middle ear.

   ✓5ᵗʰ **H68.0** Eustachian salpingitis

     ✓6ᵗʰ **H68.00**   Unspecified Eustachian salpingitis

       H68.001 Unspecified Eustachian salpingitis, right ear

       H68.002 Unspecified Eustachian salpingitis, left ear

       H68.003 Unspecified Eustachian salpingitis, bilateral

       H68.009 Unspecified Eustachian salpingitis, unspecified ear

     ✓6ᵗʰ **H68.01**   Acute Eustachian salpingitis

       H68.011 Acute Eustachian salpingitis, right ear

       H68.012 Acute Eustachian salpingitis, left ear

       H68.013 Acute Eustachian salpingitis, bilateral

       H68.019 Acute Eustachian salpingitis, unspecified ear

     ✓6ᵗʰ **H68.02**   Chronic Eustachian salpingitis

       H68.021 Chronic Eustachian salpingitis, right ear

       H68.022 Chronic Eustachian salpingitis, left ear

✔ Additional Character Required   ✓x7ᵗʰ Placeholder Alert   Manifestation   Unspecified Dx   ⚕ QPP   UPD Unacceptable PDx

Chapter 8. Diseases of the Ear and Mastoid Process

H68.023   **Chronic Eustachian salpingitis,** bilateral

H68.029   **Chronic Eustachian salpingitis, unspecified ear**

✓5ᵗʰ **H68.1**   Obstruction **of Eustachian tube**

     Stenosis of Eustachian tube
     Stricture of Eustachian tube

     ✓6ᵗʰ **H68.10**   **Unspecified obstruction of Eustachian tube**

         H68.101   **Unspecified obstruction of Eustachian tube,** right **ear**

         H68.102   **Unspecified obstruction of Eustachian tube,** left **ear**

         H68.103   **Unspecified obstruction of Eustachian tube,** bilateral

         H68.109   **Unspecified obstruction of Eustachian tube, unspecified ear**

     ✓6ᵗʰ **H68.11**   Osseous **obstruction of Eustachian tube**

         H68.111   **Osseous obstruction of Eustachian tube,** right **ear**

         H68.112   **Osseous obstruction of Eustachian tube,** left **ear**

         H68.113   **Osseous obstruction of Eustachian tube,** bilateral

         H68.119   **Osseous obstruction of Eustachian tube, unspecified ear**

     ✓6ᵗʰ **H68.12**   Intrinsic cartilagenous **obstruction of Eustachian tube**

         H68.121   **Intrinsic cartilagenous obstruction of Eustachian tube,** right **ear**

         H68.122   **Intrinsic cartilagenous obstruction of Eustachian tube,** left **ear**

         H68.123   **Intrinsic cartilagenous obstruction of Eustachian tube,** bilateral

         H68.129   **Intrinsic cartilagenous obstruction of Eustachian tube, unspecified ear**

     ✓6ᵗʰ **H68.13**   Extrinsic cartilagenous **obstruction of Eustachian tube**

         Compression of Eustachian tube

         H68.131   **Extrinsic cartilagenous obstruction of Eustachian tube,** right **ear**

         H68.132   **Extrinsic cartilagenous obstruction of Eustachian tube,** left **ear**

         H68.133   **Extrinsic cartilagenous obstruction of Eustachian tube,** bilateral

         H68.139   **Extrinsic cartilagenous obstruction of Eustachian tube, unspecified ear**

✓4ᵗʰ **H69**   **Other and unspecified disorders of Eustachian tube**

     DEF: Eustachian tube: Internal channel between the tympanic cavity and the nasopharynx that equalizes internal pressure to the outside pressure and drains mucous production from the middle ear.

     ✓5ᵗʰ **H69.0**   Patulous **Eustachian tube**

         H69.00   **Patulous Eustachian tube, unspecified ear**

         H69.01   **Patulous Eustachian tube,** right **ear**

         H69.02   **Patulous Eustachian tube,** left **ear**

         H69.03   **Patulous Eustachian tube,** bilateral

     ✓5ᵗʰ **H69.8**   **Other specified disorders of Eustachian tube**

         H69.80   **Other specified disorders of Eustachian tube, unspecified ear**

         H69.81   **Other specified disorders of Eustachian tube,** right **ear**

         H69.82   **Other specified disorders of Eustachian tube,** left **ear**

         H69.83   **Other specified disorders of Eustachian tube,** bilateral

     ✓5ᵗʰ **H69.9**   **Unspecified Eustachian tube disorder**

         H69.90   **Unspecified Eustachian tube disorder, unspecified ear**

         H69.91   **Unspecified Eustachian tube disorder,** right **ear**

         H69.92   **Unspecified Eustachian tube disorder,** left **ear**

         H69.93   **Unspecified Eustachian tube disorder,** bilateral

✓4ᵗʰ **H70**   **Mastoiditis and related conditions**

     ✓5ᵗʰ **H70.0**   Acute **mastoiditis**

         Abscess of mastoid
         Empyema of mastoid

     ✓6ᵗʰ **H70.00**   **Acute mastoiditis** without complications

         H70.001   **Acute mastoiditis without complications,** right **ear**

         H70.002   **Acute mastoiditis without complications,** left **ear**

         H70.003   **Acute mastoiditis without complications,** bilateral

         H70.009   **Acute mastoiditis without complications, unspecified ear**

     ✓6ᵗʰ **H70.01**   Subperiosteal abscess **of mastoid**

         H70.011   **Subperiosteal abscess of mastoid,** right **ear**

         H70.012   **Subperiosteal abscess of mastoid,** left **ear**

         H70.013   **Subperiosteal abscess of mastoid,** bilateral

         H70.019   **Subperiosteal abscess of mastoid, unspecified**

     ✓6ᵗʰ **H70.09**   **Acute mastoiditis with other complications**

         H70.091   **Acute mastoiditis with other complications,** right **ear**

         H70.092   **Acute mastoiditis with other complications,** left **ear**

         H70.093   **Acute mastoiditis with other complications,** bilateral

         H70.099   **Acute mastoiditis with other complications, unspecified ear**

     ✓5ᵗʰ **H70.1**   Chronic **mastoiditis**

         Caries of mastoid
         Fistula of mastoid

         EXCLUDES 1   *tuberculous mastoiditis (A18.03)*

         H70.10   **Chronic mastoiditis, unspecified ear**

         H70.11   **Chronic mastoiditis,** right **ear**

         H70.12   **Chronic mastoiditis,** left **ear**

         H70.13   **Chronic mastoiditis,** bilateral

     ✓5ᵗʰ **H70.2**   Petrositis

         Inflammation of petrous bone

     ✓6ᵗʰ **H70.20**   **Unspecified petrositis**

         H70.201   **Unspecified petrositis,** right **ear**

         H70.202   **Unspecified petrositis,** left **ear**

         H70.203   **Unspecified petrositis,** bilateral

         H70.209   **Unspecified petrositis, unspecified ear**

     ✓6ᵗʰ **H70.21**   Acute **petrositis**

         DEF: Sudden, severe inflammation of the petrous temporal bone behind the ear, associated with a middle ear infection.

         H70.211   **Acute petrositis,** right **ear**

         H70.212   **Acute petrositis,** left **ear**

         H70.213   **Acute petrositis,** bilateral

         H70.219   **Acute petrositis, unspecified ear**

     ✓6ᵗʰ **H70.22**   Chronic **petrositis**

         H70.221   **Chronic petrositis,** right **ear**

         H70.222   **Chronic petrositis,** left **ear**

         H70.223   **Chronic petrositis,** bilateral

         H70.229   **Chronic petrositis, unspecified ear**

     ✓5ᵗʰ **H70.8**   **Other mastoiditis and related conditions**

         EXCLUDES 1   *preauricular sinus and cyst (Q18.1)*

                 sinus, fistula, and cyst of branchial cleft (Q18.0)

     ✓6ᵗʰ **H70.81**   Postauricular fistula

         H70.811   **Postauricular fistula,** right **ear**

         H70.812   **Postauricular fistula,** left **ear**

         H70.813   **Postauricular fistula,** bilateral

         H70.819   **Postauricular fistula, unspecified ear**

     ✓6ᵗʰ **H70.89**   **Other mastoiditis and related conditions**

         H70.891   **Other mastoiditis and related conditions,** right **ear**

         H70.892   **Other mastoiditis and related conditions,** left **ear**

         H70.893   **Other mastoiditis and related conditions,** bilateral

         H70.899   **Other mastoiditis and related conditions, unspecified ear**

     ✓5ᵗʰ **H70.9**   **Unspecified mastoiditis**

         H70.90   **Unspecified mastoiditis, unspecified ear**

         H70.91   **Unspecified mastoiditis,** right **ear**

         H70.92   **Unspecified mastoiditis,** left **ear**

         H70.93   **Unspecified mastoiditis,** bilateral

 HCC CMS-HCC   **Rx** Rx HCC   **ESR** ESRD HCC   **COM** Commercial HCC   **N** Newborn: 0   **P** Pediatric: 0-17   **M** Maternity: 9-64   **A** Adult: 15-124

652   ICD-10-CM 2023

✓4ᵗʰ **H71 Cholesteatoma of middle ear**

     EXCLUDES 2   *cholesteatoma of external ear (H60.4-)*
             recurrent cholesteatoma of postmastoidectomy cavity
                (H95.0-)

AHA: 2021,3Q,8
DEF: Cholesteatoma: Noncancerous cyst-like mass of cell debris, including cholesterol and epithelial cells resulting from trauma, repeated or improperly healed infections, and congenital enclosure of epidermal cells.

Cholesteatoma of Middle Ear

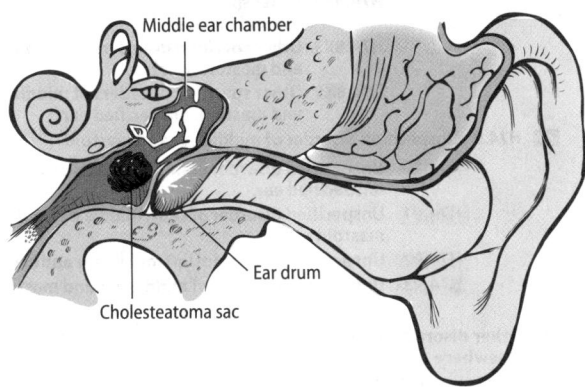

Middle ear chamber

Ear drum

Cholesteatoma sac

✓5ᵗʰ **H71.0 Cholesteatoma of attic**

   H71.00 Cholesteatoma of attic, unspecified ear
   H71.01 Cholesteatoma of attic, right ear
   H71.02 Cholesteatoma of attic, left ear
   H71.03 Cholesteatoma of attic, bilateral

✓5ᵗʰ **H71.1 Cholesteatoma of tympanum**

   H71.10 Cholesteatoma of tympanum, unspecified ear
   H71.11 Cholesteatoma of tympanum, right ear
   H71.12 Cholesteatoma of tympanum, left ear
   H71.13 Cholesteatoma of tympanum, bilateral

✓5ᵗʰ **H71.2 Cholesteatoma of mastoid**

   H71.20 Cholesteatoma of mastoid, unspecified ear
   H71.21 Cholesteatoma of mastoid, right ear
   H71.22 Cholesteatoma of mastoid, left ear
   H71.23 Cholesteatoma of mastoid, bilateral

✓5ᵗʰ **H71.3 Diffuse cholesteatosis**

     AHA: 2021,3Q,8
   H71.30 Diffuse cholesteatosis, unspecified ear
   H71.31 Diffuse cholesteatosis, right ear
   H71.32 Diffuse cholesteatosis, left ear
   H71.33 Diffuse cholesteatosis, bilateral

✓5ᵗʰ **H71.9 Unspecified cholesteatoma**

   H71.90 Unspecified cholesteatoma, unspecified ear
   H71.91 Unspecified cholesteatoma, right ear
   H71.92 Unspecified cholesteatoma, left ear
   H71.93 Unspecified cholesteatoma, bilateral

✓4ᵗʰ **H72 Perforation of tympanic membrane**

     INCLUDES   persistent post-traumatic perforation of ear drum
             postinflammatory perforation of ear drum
   Code first any associated otitis media (H65.-, H66.1-, H66.2-, H66.3-, H66.4-, H66.9-, H67.-)
     EXCLUDES 1   *acute suppurative otitis media with rupture of the tympanic membrane (H66.01-)*
                traumatic rupture of ear drum (S09.2-)

✓5ᵗʰ **H72.0 Central perforation of tympanic membrane**

   H72.00 Central perforation of tympanic membrane, unspecified ear
   H72.01 Central perforation of tympanic membrane, right ear
   H72.02 Central perforation of tympanic membrane, left ear
   H72.03 Central perforation of tympanic membrane, bilateral

✓5ᵗʰ **H72.1 Attic perforation of tympanic membrane**

   Perforation of pars flaccida
   H72.10 Attic perforation of tympanic membrane, unspecified ear
   H72.11 Attic perforation of tympanic membrane, right ear
   H72.12 Attic perforation of tympanic membrane, left ear

   H72.13 Attic perforation of tympanic membrane, bilateral

✓5ᵗʰ **H72.2 Other marginal perforations of tympanic membrane**

   ✓6ᵗʰ **H72.2X Other marginal perforations of tympanic membrane**

     H72.2X1 Other marginal perforations of tympanic membrane, right ear
     H72.2X2 Other marginal perforations of tympanic membrane, left ear
     H72.2X3 Other marginal perforations of tympanic membrane, bilateral
     H72.2X9 Other marginal perforations of tympanic membrane, unspecified ear

✓5ᵗʰ **H72.8 Other perforations of tympanic membrane**

   ✓6ᵗʰ **H72.81 Multiple perforations of tympanic membrane**

     H72.811 Multiple perforations of tympanic membrane, right ear
     H72.812 Multiple perforations of tympanic membrane, left ear
     H72.813 Multiple perforations of tympanic membrane, bilateral
     H72.819 Multiple perforations of tympanic membrane, unspecified ear

   ✓6ᵗʰ **H72.82 Total perforations of tympanic membrane**

     H72.821 Total perforations of tympanic membrane, right ear
     H72.822 Total perforations of tympanic membrane, left ear
     H72.823 Total perforations of tympanic membrane, bilateral
     H72.829 Total perforations of tympanic membrane, unspecified ear

✓5ᵗʰ **H72.9 Unspecified perforation of tympanic membrane**

   H72.90 Unspecified perforation of tympanic membrane, unspecified ear
   H72.91 Unspecified perforation of tympanic membrane, right ear
   H72.92 Unspecified perforation of tympanic membrane, left ear
   H72.93 Unspecified perforation of tympanic membrane, bilateral

✓4ᵗʰ **H73 Other disorders of tympanic membrane**

✓5ᵗʰ **H73.0 Acute myringitis**

     EXCLUDES 1   *acute myringitis with otitis media (H65, H66)*

   ✓6ᵗʰ **H73.00 Unspecified acute myringitis**

     Acute tympanitis NOS
     H73.001 Acute myringitis, right ear
     H73.002 Acute myringitis, left ear
     H73.003 Acute myringitis, bilateral
     H73.009 Acute myringitis, unspecified ear

   ✓6ᵗʰ **H73.01 Bullous myringitis**

     DEF: Bacterial or viral otitis media that is characterized by the appearance of serous or hemorrhagic blebs on the ear drum and sudden onset of severe pain in ear.
     H73.011 Bullous myringitis, right ear
     H73.012 Bullous myringitis, left ear
     H73.013 Bullous myringitis, bilateral
     H73.019 Bullous myringitis, unspecified ear

   ✓6ᵗʰ **H73.09 Other acute myringitis**

     H73.091 Other acute myringitis, right ear
     H73.092 Other acute myringitis, left ear
     H73.093 Other acute myringitis, bilateral
     H73.099 Other acute myringitis, unspecified ear

✓5ᵗʰ **H73.1 Chronic myringitis**

   Chronic tympanitis
     EXCLUDES 1   *chronic myringitis with otitis media (H65, H66)*
   H73.10 Chronic myringitis, unspecified ear
   H73.11 Chronic myringitis, right ear
   H73.12 Chronic myringitis, left ear
   H73.13 Chronic myringitis, bilateral

✓5ᵗʰ **H73.2 Unspecified myringitis**

   H73.20 Unspecified myringitis, unspecified ear
   H73.21 Unspecified myringitis, right ear
   H73.22 Unspecified myringitis, left ear
   H73.23 Unspecified myringitis, bilateral

✓5ᵗʰ **H73.8 Other specified disorders of tympanic membrane**

   ✓6ᵗʰ **H73.81 Atrophic flaccid tympanic membrane**

     H73.811 Atrophic flaccid tympanic membrane, right ear

H73.812   Atrophic flaccid tympanic membrane, left ear
H73.813   Atrophic flaccid tympanic membrane, bilateral
H73.819   Atrophic flaccid tympanic membrane, unspecified ear

✓6ᵗʰ **H73.82 Atrophic nonflaccid tympanic membrane**
H73.821   Atrophic nonflaccid tympanic membrane, right ear
H73.822   Atrophic nonflaccid tympanic membrane, left ear
H73.823   Atrophic nonflaccid tympanic membrane, bilateral
H73.829   Atrophic nonflaccid tympanic membrane, unspecified ear

✓6ᵗʰ **H73.89 Other specified disorders of tympanic membrane**
H73.891   Other specified disorders of tympanic membrane, right ear
H73.892   Other specified disorders of tympanic membrane, left ear
H73.893   Other specified disorders of tympanic membrane, bilateral
H73.899   Other specified disorders of tympanic membrane, unspecified ear

✓5ᵗʰ **H73.9 Unspecified disorder of tympanic membrane**
H73.90   Unspecified disorder of tympanic membrane, unspecified ear
H73.91   Unspecified disorder of tympanic membrane, right ear
H73.92   Unspecified disorder of tympanic membrane, left ear
H73.93   Unspecified disorder of tympanic membrane, bilateral

✓4ᵗʰ **H74 Other disorders of middle ear mastoid**
EXCLUDES 2   mastoiditis (H70.-)

✓5ᵗʰ **H74.0 Tympanosclerosis**
DEF: Calcification of tissue in the ear drum, middle ear bones, and middle ear canal.
H74.01   Tympanosclerosis, right ear
H74.02   Tympanosclerosis, left ear
H74.03   Tympanosclerosis, bilateral
H74.09   Tympanosclerosis, unspecified ear

✓5ᵗʰ **H74.1 Adhesive middle ear disease**
Adhesive otitis
EXCLUDES 1   glue ear (H65.3-)
H74.11   Adhesive right middle ear disease
H74.12   Adhesive left middle ear disease
H74.13   Adhesive middle ear disease, bilateral
H74.19   Adhesive middle ear disease, unspecified ear

✓5ᵗʰ **H74.2 Discontinuity and dislocation of ear ossicles**
H74.20   Discontinuity and dislocation of ear ossicles, unspecified ear
H74.21   Discontinuity and dislocation of right ear ossicles
H74.22   Discontinuity and dislocation of left ear ossicles
H74.23   Discontinuity and dislocation of ear ossicles, bilateral

✓5ᵗʰ **H74.3 Other acquired abnormalities of ear ossicles**
✓6ᵗʰ **H74.31 Ankylosis of ear ossicles**
H74.311   Ankylosis of ear ossicles, right ear
H74.312   Ankylosis of ear ossicles, left ear
H74.313   Ankylosis of ear ossicles, bilateral
H74.319   Ankylosis of ear ossicles, unspecified ear

✓6ᵗʰ **H74.32 Partial loss of ear ossicles**
H74.321   Partial loss of ear ossicles, right ear
H74.322   Partial loss of ear ossicles, left ear
H74.323   Partial loss of ear ossicles, bilateral
H74.329   Partial loss of ear ossicles, unspecified ear

✓6ᵗʰ **H74.39 Other acquired abnormalities of ear ossicles**
H74.391   Other acquired abnormalities of right ear ossicles
H74.392   Other acquired abnormalities of left ear ossicles
H74.393   Other acquired abnormalities of ear ossicles, bilateral
H74.399   Other acquired abnormalities of ear ossicles, unspecified ear

✓5ᵗʰ **H74.4 Polyp of middle ear**
H74.40   Polyp of middle ear, unspecified ear
H74.41   Polyp of right middle ear
H74.42   Polyp of left middle ear
H74.43   Polyp of middle ear, bilateral

✓5ᵗʰ **H74.8 Other specified disorders of middle ear and mastoid**
✓6ᵗʰ **H74.8X Other specified disorders of middle ear and mastoid**
H74.8X1   Other specified disorders of right middle ear and mastoid
H74.8X2   Other specified disorders of left middle ear and mastoid
H74.8X3   Other specified disorders of middle ear and mastoid, bilateral
H74.8X9   Other specified disorders of middle ear and mastoid, unspecified ear

✓5ᵗʰ **H74.9 Unspecified disorder of middle ear and mastoid**
H74.90   Unspecified disorder of middle ear and mastoid, unspecified ear
H74.91   Unspecified disorder of right middle ear and mastoid
H74.92   Unspecified disorder of left middle ear and mastoid
H74.93   Unspecified disorder of middle ear and mastoid, bilateral

✓4ᵗʰ **H75 Other disorders of middle ear and mastoid in diseases classified elsewhere**
Code first underlying disease

✓5ᵗʰ **H75.0 Mastoiditis in infectious and parasitic diseases classified elsewhere**
EXCLUDES 1   mastoiditis (in):
syphilis (A52.77)
tuberculosis (A18.03)
H75.00   Mastoiditis in infectious and parasitic diseases classified elsewhere, unspecified ear
H75.01   Mastoiditis in infectious and parasitic diseases classified elsewhere, right ear
H75.02   Mastoiditis in infectious and parasitic diseases classified elsewhere, left ear
H75.03   Mastoiditis in infectious and parasitic diseases classified elsewhere, bilateral

✓5ᵗʰ **H75.8 Other specified disorders of middle ear and mastoid in diseases classified elsewhere**
H75.80   Other specified disorders of middle ear and mastoid in diseases classified elsewhere, unspecified ear
H75.81   Other specified disorders of right middle ear and mastoid in diseases classified elsewhere
H75.82   Other specified disorders of left middle ear and mastoid in diseases classified elsewhere
H75.83   Other specified disorders of middle ear and mastoid in diseases classified elsewhere, bilateral

Diseases of inner ear (H80-H83)

✓4ᵗʰ **H80 Otosclerosis**
INCLUDES   otospongiosis

✓5ᵗʰ **H80.0 Otosclerosis involving oval window, nonobliterative**
H80.00   Otosclerosis involving oval window, nonobliterative, unspecified ear
H80.01   Otosclerosis involving oval window, nonobliterative, right ear
H80.02   Otosclerosis involving oval window, nonobliterative, left ear
H80.03   Otosclerosis involving oval window, nonobliterative, bilateral

✓5ᵗʰ **H80.1 Otosclerosis involving oval window, obliterative**
H80.10   Otosclerosis involving oval window, obliterative, unspecified ear
H80.11   Otosclerosis involving oval window, obliterative, right ear
H80.12   Otosclerosis involving oval window, obliterative, left ear
H80.13   Otosclerosis involving oval window, obliterative, bilateral

✓5ᵗʰ **H80.2 Cochlear otosclerosis**
Otosclerosis involving otic capsule
Otosclerosis involving round window
H80.20   Cochlear otosclerosis, unspecified ear
H80.21   Cochlear otosclerosis, right ear
H80.22   Cochlear otosclerosis, left ear
H80.23   Cochlear otosclerosis, bilateral

✓5ᵗʰ **H80.8 Other otosclerosis**

    H80.80 Other otosclerosis, unspecified ear

    H80.81 Other otosclerosis, right ear

    H80.82 Other otosclerosis, left ear

    H80.83 Other otosclerosis, bilateral

✓5ᵗʰ **H80.9 Unspecified otosclerosis**

    H80.90 Unspecified otosclerosis, unspecified ear

    H80.91 Unspecified otosclerosis, right ear

    H80.92 Unspecified otosclerosis, left ear

    H80.93 Unspecified otosclerosis, bilateral

✓4ᵗʰ **H81 Disorders of vestibular function**

    EXCLUDES 1   epidemic vertigo (A88.1)

                vertigo NOS (R42)

✓5ᵗʰ **H81.0 Ménière's disease**

    Labyrinthine hydrops

    Ménière's syndrome or vertigo

    DEF: Distended membranous labyrinth of the middle ear from fluctuating pressure of fluid (hydrops) that causes vertigo, tinnitus, pressure, and hearing loss that may last on and off for several hours. Episodes may occur in clusters or may subside for weeks, months, or even years.

    H81.01 Ménière's disease, right ear

    H81.02 Ménière's disease, left ear

    H81.03 Ménière's disease, bilateral

    H81.09 Ménière's disease, unspecified ear

✓5ᵗʰ **H81.1 Benign paroxysmal vertigo**

    H81.10 Benign paroxysmal vertigo, unspecified ear   Q

    H81.11 Benign paroxysmal vertigo, right ear   Q

    H81.12 Benign paroxysmal vertigo, left ear   Q

    H81.13 Benign paroxysmal vertigo, bilateral   Q

✓5ᵗʰ **H81.2 Vestibular neuronitis**

    DEF: Transient benign vertigo caused by inflammation of the vestibular nerve. It is characterized by response to caloric stimulation on one side and nystagmus with rhythmic movement of the eyes. Normal auditory function is present.

    H81.20 Vestibular neuronitis, unspecified ear

    H81.21 Vestibular neuronitis, right ear

    H81.22 Vestibular neuronitis, left ear

    H81.23 Vestibular neuronitis, bilateral

✓5ᵗʰ **H81.3 Other peripheral vertigo**

    ✓6ᵗʰ **H81.31 Aural vertigo**

        H81.311 Aural vertigo, right ear

        H81.312 Aural vertigo, left ear

        H81.313 Aural vertigo, bilateral

        H81.319 Aural vertigo, unspecified ear

    ✓6ᵗʰ **H81.39 Other peripheral vertigo**

        Lermoyez' syndrome

        Otogenic vertigo

        Peripheral vertigo NOS

        H81.391 Other peripheral vertigo, right ear

        H81.392 Other peripheral vertigo, left ear

        H81.393 Other peripheral vertigo, bilateral

        H81.399 Other peripheral vertigo, unspecified ear

    H81.4 Vertigo of central origin

        Central positional nystagmus

✓5ᵗʰ **H81.8 Other disorders of vestibular function**

    ✓6ᵗʰ **H81.8X Other disorders of vestibular function**

        H81.8X1 Other disorders of vestibular function, right ear

        H81.8X2 Other disorders of vestibular function, left ear

        H81.8X3 Other disorders of vestibular function, bilateral

        H81.8X9 Other disorders of vestibular function, unspecified ear

          AHA: 2022,2Q,12

✓5ᵗʰ **H81.9 Unspecified disorder of vestibular function**

    Vertiginous syndrome NOS

    H81.90 Unspecified disorder of vestibular function, unspecified ear

    H81.91 Unspecified disorder of vestibular function, right ear

    H81.92 Unspecified disorder of vestibular function, left ear

    H81.93 Unspecified disorder of vestibular function, bilateral

✓4ᵗʰ **H82 Vertiginous syndromes in diseases classified elsewhere**

    Code first underlying disease

    EXCLUDES 1   epidemic vertigo (A88.1)

    H82.1 Vertiginous syndromes in diseases classified elsewhere, right ear

    H82.2 Vertiginous syndromes in diseases classified elsewhere, left ear

    H82.3 Vertiginous syndromes in diseases classified elsewhere, bilateral

    H82.9 Vertiginous syndromes in diseases classified elsewhere, unspecified ear

✓4ᵗʰ **H83 Other diseases of inner ear**

    ✓5ᵗʰ **H83.0 Labyrinthitis**

        DEF: Inflammation of the inner ear, or labyrinth, characterized by pus, vertigo, dizziness, nausea, and hearing loss.

        H83.01 Labyrinthitis, right ear

        H83.02 Labyrinthitis, left ear

        H83.03 Labyrinthitis, bilateral

        H83.09 Labyrinthitis, unspecified ear

    ✓5ᵗʰ **H83.1 Labyrinthine fistula**

        H83.11 Labyrinthine fistula, right ear

        H83.12 Labyrinthine fistula, left ear

        H83.13 Labyrinthine fistula, bilateral

        H83.19 Labyrinthine fistula, unspecified ear

    ✓5ᵗʰ **H83.2 Labyrinthine dysfunction**

        Labyrinthine hypersensitivity

        Labyrinthine hypofunction

        Labyrinthine loss of function

        DEF: Decreased function of the labyrinth sensors.

        ✓6ᵗʰ **H83.2X Labyrinthine dysfunction**

            H83.2X1 Labyrinthine dysfunction, right ear

            H83.2X2 Labyrinthine dysfunction, left ear

            H83.2X3 Labyrinthine dysfunction, bilateral

            H83.2X9 Labyrinthine dysfunction, unspecified ear

    ✓5ᵗʰ **H83.3 Noise effects on inner ear**

        Acoustic trauma of inner ear

        Noise-induced hearing loss of inner ear

        ✓6ᵗʰ **H83.3X Noise effects on inner ear**

            H83.3X1 Noise effects on right inner ear

            H83.3X2 Noise effects on left inner ear

            H83.3X3 Noise effects on inner ear, bilateral

            H83.3X9 Noise effects on inner ear, unspecified ear

    ✓5ᵗʰ **H83.8 Other specified diseases of inner ear**

        ✓6ᵗʰ **H83.8X Other specified diseases of inner ear**

            H83.8X1 Other specified diseases of right inner ear

            H83.8X2 Other specified diseases of left inner ear

            H83.8X3 Other specified diseases of inner ear, bilateral

            H83.8X9 Other specified diseases of inner ear, unspecified ear

    ✓5ᵗʰ **H83.9 Unspecified disease of inner ear**

        H83.90 Unspecified disease of inner ear, unspecified ear

        H83.91 Unspecified disease of right inner ear

        H83.92 Unspecified disease of left inner ear

        H83.93 Unspecified disease of inner ear, bilateral

Other disorders of ear (H90-H94)

✓4ᵗʰ **H90 Conductive and sensorineural hearing loss**

    EXCLUDES 1   deaf nonspeaking NEC (H91.3)

                deafness NOS (H91.9-)

                hearing loss NOS (H91.9-)

                noise-induced hearing loss (H83.3-)

                ototoxic hearing loss (H91.0-)

                sudden (idiopathic) hearing loss (H91.2-)

    AHA: 2015,2Q,7

    DEF: Conductive hearing loss: Hearing loss due to the inability of soundwaves to move from the outer (external) ear to the inner ear.

    DEF: Sensorineural hearing loss: Hearing loss that occurs from damage to the hair cells of the inner ear or problems with the nerve pathways from the inner ear to the brain.

    H90.0 Conductive hearing loss, bilateral

✓5ᵗʰ **H90.1** Conductive **hearing loss,** unilateral **with unrestricted hearing on the contralateral side**

    H90.11 Conductive hearing loss, unilateral, right ear, with unrestricted hearing on the contralateral side

    H90.12 Conductive hearing loss, unilateral, left ear, with unrestricted hearing on the contralateral side

H90.2 Conductive **hearing loss, unspecified**
    Conductive deafness NOS

H90.3 Sensorineural **hearing loss,** bilateral

✓5ᵗʰ **H90.4** Sensorineural **hearing loss,** unilateral **with unrestricted hearing on the contralateral side**

    H90.41 Sensorineural hearing loss, unilateral, right ear, with unrestricted hearing on the contralateral side

    H90.42 Sensorineural hearing loss, unilateral, left ear, with unrestricted hearing on the contralateral side

H90.5 Unspecified sensorineural **hearing loss**
    Central hearing loss NOS
    Congenital deafness NOS
    Neural hearing loss NOS
    Perceptive hearing loss NOS
    Sensorineural deafness NOS
    Sensory hearing loss NOS
    EXCLUDES 1 *abnormal auditory perception (H93.2-)*
               psychogenic deafness (F44.6)

H90.6 Mixed **conductive and sensorineural hearing loss,** bilateral
    AHA: 2015,2Q,7

✓5ᵗʰ **H90.7** Mixed **conductive and sensorineural hearing loss,** unilateral **with unrestricted hearing on the contralateral side**

    H90.71 Mixed conductive and sensorineural hearing loss, unilateral, right ear, with unrestricted hearing on the contralateral side

    H90.72 Mixed conductive and sensorineural hearing loss, unilateral, left ear, with unrestricted hearing on the contralateral side

H90.8 Mixed **conductive and sensorineural hearing loss, unspecified**

✓5ᵗʰ **H90.A** Conductive and sensorineural hearing loss with restricted hearing on the contralateral side
    AHA: 2016,4Q,23-25

  ✓6ᵗʰ **H90.A1** Conductive hearing loss, unilateral, with restricted hearing on the contralateral side

    H90.A11 Conductive hearing loss, unilateral, right ear with restricted hearing on the contralateral side

    H90.A12 Conductive hearing loss, unilateral, left ear with restricted hearing on the contralateral side

  ✓6ᵗʰ **H90.A2** Sensorineural hearing loss, unilateral, with restricted hearing on the contralateral side

    H90.A21 Sensorineural hearing loss, unilateral, right ear, with restricted hearing on the contralateral side

    H90.A22 Sensorineural hearing loss, unilateral, left ear, with restricted hearing on the contralateral side

  ✓6ᵗʰ **H90.A3** Mixed conductive and sensorineural hearing loss, unilateral with restricted hearing on the contralateral side

    H90.A31 Mixed conductive and sensorineural hearing loss, unilateral, right ear with restricted hearing on the contralateral side

    H90.A32 Mixed conductive and sensorineural hearing, unilateral, left ear with restricted hearing on the contralateral side

✓4ᵗʰ **H91** Other and unspecified hearing loss
    EXCLUDES 1 *abnormal auditory perception (H93.2-)*
           hearing loss as classified in H90.-
           impacted cerumen (H61.2-)
           noise-induced hearing loss (H83.3-)
           psychogenic deafness (F44.6)
           transient ischemic deafness (H93.01-)

✓5ᵗʰ **H91.0** Ototoxic hearing loss
    Code first poisoning due to drug or toxin, if applicable (T36-T65 with fifth or sixth character 1-4 or 6)
    Use additional code for adverse effect, if applicable, to identify drug (T36-T50 with fifth or sixth character 5)

    H91.01 Ototoxic hearing loss, right ear
    H91.02 Ototoxic hearing loss, left ear
    H91.03 Ototoxic hearing loss, bilateral
    H91.09 Ototoxic hearing loss, unspecified ear

✓5ᵗʰ **H91.1** Presbycusis
    Presbyacusia
    H91.10 Presbycusis, unspecified ear
    H91.11 Presbycusis, right ear
    H91.12 Presbycusis, left ear
    H91.13 Presbycusis, bilateral

✓5ᵗʰ **H91.2** Sudden idiopathic hearing loss
    Sudden hearing loss NOS
    H91.20 Sudden idiopathic hearing loss, unspecified ear
    H91.21 Sudden idiopathic hearing loss, right ear
    H91.22 Sudden idiopathic hearing loss, left ear
    H91.23 Sudden idiopathic hearing loss, bilateral

H91.3 Deaf nonspeaking, not elsewhere classified

✓5ᵗʰ **H91.8** Other specified hearing loss

  ✓6ᵗʰ **H91.8X** Other specified hearing loss
    H91.8X1 Other specified hearing loss, right ear
    H91.8X2 Other specified hearing loss, left ear
    H91.8X3 Other specified hearing loss, bilateral
    H91.8X9 Other specified hearing loss, unspecified ear

✓5ᵗʰ **H91.9** Unspecified hearing loss
    Deafness NOS
    High frequency deafness
    Low frequency deafness
    H91.90 Unspecified hearing loss, unspecified ear
    H91.91 Unspecified hearing loss, right ear
    H91.92 Unspecified hearing loss, left ear
    H91.93 Unspecified hearing loss, bilateral

✓4ᵗʰ **H92** Otalgia and effusion of ear

✓5ᵗʰ **H92.0** Otalgia
    H92.01 Otalgia, right ear
    H92.02 Otalgia, left ear
    H92.03 Otalgia, bilateral
    H92.09 Otalgia, unspecified ear

✓5ᵗʰ **H92.1** Otorrhea
    EXCLUDES 1 *leakage of cerebrospinal fluid through ear (G96.0)*
    H92.10 Otorrhea, unspecified ear
    H92.11 Otorrhea, right ear
    H92.12 Otorrhea, left ear
    H92.13 Otorrhea, bilateral

✓5ᵗʰ **H92.2** Otorrhagia
    EXCLUDES 1 *traumatic otorrhagia - code to injury*
    H92.20 Otorrhagia, unspecified ear
    H92.21 Otorrhagia, right ear
    H92.22 Otorrhagia, left ear
    H92.23 Otorrhagia, bilateral

✓4ᵗʰ **H93** Other disorders of ear, not elsewhere classified

✓5ᵗʰ **H93.0** Degenerative and vascular disorders of ear
    EXCLUDES 1 *presbycusis (H91.1)*

  ✓6ᵗʰ **H93.01** Transient ischemic deafness
    H93.011 Transient ischemic deafness, right ear
    H93.012 Transient ischemic deafness, left ear
    H93.013 Transient ischemic deafness, bilateral
    H93.019 Transient ischemic deafness, unspecified ear

  ✓6ᵗʰ **H93.09** Unspecified degenerative and vascular disorders of ear
    H93.091 Unspecified degenerative and vascular disorders of right ear
    H93.092 Unspecified degenerative and vascular disorders of left ear
    H93.093 Unspecified degenerative and vascular disorders of ear, bilateral
    H93.099 Unspecified degenerative and vascular disorders of unspecified ear

✓5ᵗʰ **H93.1** Tinnitus
    H93.11 Tinnitus, right ear
    H93.12 Tinnitus, left ear
    H93.13 Tinnitus, bilateral
    H93.19 Tinnitus, unspecified ear

✓5ᵗʰ **H93.A** Pulsatile tinnitus
    AHA: 2016,4Q,25-26
    H93.A1 Pulsatile tinnitus, right ear
    H93.A2 Pulsatile tinnitus, left ear
    H93.A3 Pulsatile tinnitus, bilateral

HCC CMS-HCC   **Rx** Rx HCC   **ESR** ESRD HCC   **COM** Commercial HCC   **N** Newborn: 0   **P** Pediatric: 0-17   **M** Maternity: 9-64   **A** Adult: 15-124

656   ICD-10-CM 2023

H93.A9   Pulsatile tinnitus, unspecified ear

✓5ᵗʰ **H93.2**   **Other abnormal auditory perceptions**

    EXCLUDES 2   auditory hallucinations (R44.0)

   ✓6ᵗʰ **H93.21**   **Auditory recruitment**

     H93.211   Auditory recruitment, right ear

     H93.212   Auditory recruitment, left ear

     H93.213   Auditory recruitment, bilateral

     H93.219   Auditory recruitment, unspecified ear

   ✓6ᵗʰ **H93.22**   **Diplacusis**

     H93.221   Diplacusis, right ear

     H93.222   Diplacusis, left ear

     H93.223   Diplacusis, bilateral

     H93.229   Diplacusis, unspecified ear

   ✓6ᵗʰ **H93.23**   **Hyperacusis**

     DEF: Exceptionally acute sense of hearing caused by such conditions as Bell's palsy. This term may also refer to painful sensitivity to sounds.

     H93.231   Hyperacusis, right ear

     H93.232   Hyperacusis, left ear

     H93.233   Hyperacusis, bilateral

     H93.239   Hyperacusis, unspecified ear

   ✓6ᵗʰ **H93.24**   **Temporary auditory threshold shift**

     H93.241   Temporary auditory threshold shift, right ear

     H93.242   Temporary auditory threshold shift, left ear

     H93.243   Temporary auditory threshold shift, bilateral

     H93.249   Temporary auditory threshold shift, unspecified ear

   H93.25   **Central auditory processing disorder**

     Congenital auditory imperception

     Word deafness

     EXCLUDES 1   mixed receptive-expressive language disorder (F80.2)

   ✓6ᵗʰ **H93.29**   **Other abnormal auditory perceptions**

     H93.291   Other abnormal auditory perceptions, right ear

     H93.292   Other abnormal auditory perceptions, left ear

     H93.293   Other abnormal auditory perceptions, bilateral

     H93.299   Other abnormal auditory perceptions, unspecified ear

✓5ᵗʰ **H93.3**   **Disorders of acoustic nerve**

    Disorder of 8th cranial nerve

    EXCLUDES 1   acoustic neuroma (D33.3)

               syphilitic acoustic neuritis (A52.15)

   ✓6ᵗʰ **H93.3X**   **Disorders of acoustic nerve**

     H93.3X1   Disorders of right acoustic nerve

     H93.3X2   Disorders of left acoustic nerve

     H93.3X3   Disorders of bilateral acoustic nerves

     H93.3X9   Disorders of unspecified acoustic nerve

✓5ᵗʰ **H93.8**   **Other specified disorders of ear**

   ✓6ᵗʰ **H93.8X**   **Other specified disorders of ear**

     H93.8X1   Other specified disorders of right ear

     H93.8X2   Other specified disorders of left ear

     H93.8X3   Other specified disorders of ear, bilateral

     H93.8X9   Other specified disorders of ear, unspecified ear

✓5ᵗʰ **H93.9**   **Unspecified disorder of ear**

     H93.90   Unspecified disorder of ear, unspecified ear

     H93.91   Unspecified disorder of right ear

     H93.92   Unspecified disorder of left ear

     H93.93   Unspecified disorder of ear, bilateral

✓4ᵗʰ **H94**   **Other disorders of ear in diseases classified elsewhere**

   ✓5ᵗʰ **H94.0**   **Acoustic neuritis in infectious and parasitic diseases classified elsewhere**

     Code first underlying disease, such as:

     parasitic disease (B65-B89)

     EXCLUDES 1   acoustic neuritis (in):

               herpes zoster (B02.29)

               syphilis (A52.15)

     H94.00   *Acoustic neuritis in infectious and parasitic diseases classified elsewhere, unspecified ear*

     H94.01   *Acoustic neuritis in infectious and parasitic diseases classified elsewhere, right ear*

     H94.02   *Acoustic neuritis in infectious and parasitic diseases classified elsewhere, left ear*

     H94.03   *Acoustic neuritis in infectious and parasitic diseases classified elsewhere, bilateral*

   ✓5ᵗʰ **H94.8**   **Other specified disorders of ear in diseases classified elsewhere**

     Code first underlying disease, such as:

     congenital syphilis (A50.0)

     EXCLUDES 1   aural myiasis (B87.4)

               syphilitic labyrinthitis (A52.79)

     H94.80   *Other specified disorders of ear in diseases classified elsewhere, unspecified ear*

     H94.81   *Other specified disorders of right ear in diseases classified elsewhere*

     H94.82   *Other specified disorders of left ear in diseases classified elsewhere*

     H94.83   *Other specified disorders of ear in diseases classified elsewhere, bilateral*

Intraoperative and postprocedural complications and disorders of ear and mastoid process, not elsewhere classified (H95)

✓4ᵗʰ **H95**   **Intraoperative and postprocedural complications and disorders of ear and mastoid process, not elsewhere classified**

    AHA: 2016,4Q,9-10

   ✓6ᵗʰ **H95.0**   **Recurrent cholesteatoma of postmastoidectomy cavity**

     H95.00   Recurrent cholesteatoma of postmastoidectomy cavity, unspecified ear

     H95.01   Recurrent cholesteatoma of postmastoidectomy cavity, right ear

     H95.02   Recurrent cholesteatoma of postmastoidectomy cavity, left ear

     H95.03   Recurrent cholesteatoma of postmastoidectomy cavity, bilateral ears

   ✓5ᵗʰ **H95.1**   **Other disorders of ear and mastoid process following mastoidectomy**

    ✓6ᵗʰ **H95.11**   **Chronic inflammation of postmastoidectomy cavity**

     H95.111   Chronic inflammation of postmastoidectomy cavity, right ear

     H95.112   Chronic inflammation of postmastoidectomy cavity, left ear

     H95.113   Chronic inflammation of postmastoidectomy cavity, bilateral ears

     H95.119   Chronic inflammation of postmastoidectomy cavity, unspecified ear

    ✓6ᵗʰ **H95.12**   **Granulation of postmastoidectomy cavity**

     H95.121   Granulation of postmastoidectomy cavity, right ear

     H95.122   Granulation of postmastoidectomy cavity, left ear

     H95.123   Granulation of postmastoidectomy cavity, bilateral ears

     H95.129   Granulation of postmastoidectomy cavity, unspecified ear

    ✓6ᵗʰ **H95.13**   **Mucosal cyst of postmastoidectomy cavity**

     H95.131   Mucosal cyst of postmastoidectomy cavity, right ear

     H95.132   Mucosal cyst of postmastoidectomy cavity, left ear

     H95.133   Mucosal cyst of postmastoidectomy cavity, bilateral ears

     H95.139   Mucosal cyst of postmastoidectomy cavity, unspecified ear

    ✓6ᵗʰ **H95.19**   **Other disorders following mastoidectomy**

     H95.191   Other disorders following mastoidectomy, right ear

     H95.192   Other disorders following mastoidectomy, left ear

     H95.193   Other disorders following mastoidectomy, bilateral ears

     H95.199   Other disorders following mastoidectomy, unspecified ear

---

☑ Additional Character Required   ✓x7ᵗʰ Placeholder Alert   Manifestation   Unspecified Dx   ◘ QPP   ⦿ Unacceptable PDx

Chapter 8. Diseases of the Ear and Mastoid Process

✓5ᵗʰ **H95.2** Intraoperative hemorrhage and hematoma **of ear and mastoid process complicating a procedure**

> EXCLUDES 1 *intraoperative hemorrhage and hematoma of ear and mastoid process due to accidental puncture or laceration during a procedure (H95.3-)*

H95.21 **Intraoperative hemorrhage and hematoma of ear and mastoid process complicating a** procedure on the ear and mastoid process

H95.22 **Intraoperative hemorrhage and hematoma of ear and mastoid process complicating** other procedure

✓5ᵗʰ **H95.3** Accidental puncture and laceration **of ear and mastoid process during a procedure**

H95.31 **Accidental puncture and laceration of the ear and mastoid process during a** procedure on the ear and mastoid process

H95.32 **Accidental puncture and laceration of the ear and mastoid process during** other procedure

✓5ᵗʰ **H95.4** Postprocedural hemorrhage **of ear and mastoid process following a procedure**

H95.41 **Postprocedural hemorrhage of ear and mastoid process following a** procedure on the ear and mastoid process

H95.42 **Postprocedural hemorrhage of ear and mastoid process following** other procedure

✓5ᵗʰ **H95.5** Postprocedural hematoma and seroma **of ear and mastoid process following a procedure**

H95.51 **Postprocedural** hematoma **of ear and mastoid process following a** procedure on the ear and mastoid process

H95.52 **Postprocedural** hematoma **of ear and mastoid process following** other procedure

H95.53 **Postprocedural** seroma **of ear and mastoid process following a** procedure on the ear and mastoid process

H95.54 **Postprocedural** seroma **of ear and mastoid process following** other procedure

✓5ᵗʰ **H95.8** **Other intraoperative and postprocedural complications and disorders of the ear and mastoid process, not elsewhere classified**

> EXCLUDES 2 *postprocedural complications and disorders following mastoidectomy (H95.0-, H95.1-)*

✓6ᵗʰ **H95.81** Postprocedural stenosis **of external ear canal**

H95.811 **Postprocedural stenosis of** right **external ear canal**

H95.812 **Postprocedural stenosis of** left **external ear canal**

H95.813 **Postprocedural stenosis of external ear canal,** bilateral

H95.819 **Postprocedural stenosis of unspecified external ear canal**

H95.88 **Other intraoperative complications and disorders of the ear and mastoid process, not elsewhere classified**

> Use additional code, if applicable, to further specify disorder

H95.89 **Other postprocedural complications and disorders of the ear and mastoid process, not elsewhere classified**

> Use additional code, if applicable, to further specify disorder

Chapter 9. Diseases of the Circulatory System (I00–I99)

Chapter-specific Guidelines with Coding Examples

The chapter-specific guidelines from the ICD-10-CM Official Guidelines for Coding and Reporting have been provided below. Along with these guidelines are coding examples, contained in the shaded boxes, that have been developed to help illustrate the coding and/or sequencing guidance found in these guidelines.

a. Hypertension

The classification presumes a causal relationship between hypertension and heart involvement and between hypertension and kidney involvement, as the two conditions are linked by the term "with" in the Alphabetic Index. These conditions should be coded as related even in the absence of provider documentation explicitly linking them, unless the documentation clearly states the conditions are unrelated.

For hypertension and conditions not specifically linked by relational terms such as "with," "associated with" or "due to" in the classification, provider documentation must link the conditions in order to code them as related.

1) Hypertension with heart disease

Hypertension with heart conditions classified to I50.- or I51.4-I51.7, I51.89, I51.9, are assigned to a code from category I11, Hypertensive heart disease. Use additional code(s) from category I50, Heart failure, to identify the type(s) of heart failure in those patients with heart failure.

The same heart conditions (I50.-, I51.4-I51.7, I51.89, I51.9) with hypertension are coded separately if the provider has documented they are unrelated to the hypertension. Sequence according to the circumstances of the admission/encounter. *Code separately if not related*

2) Hypertensive chronic kidney disease

Assign codes from category I12, Hypertensive chronic kidney disease, when both hypertension and a condition classifiable to category N18, Chronic kidney disease (CKD), are present. CKD should not be coded as hypertensive if the provider indicates the CKD is not related to the hypertension.

The appropriate code from category N18 should be used as a secondary code with a code from category I12 to identify the stage of chronic kidney disease.

See Section I.C.14. Chronic kidney disease.

If a patient has hypertensive chronic kidney disease and acute renal failure, the acute renal failure should also be coded. Sequence according to the circumstances of the admission/encounter.

> Patient is admitted with stage IV chronic kidney disease (CKD) due to polycystic kidney disease. Patient also is on lisinopril for hypertension.
>
> | | |
> |---|---|
> | **N18.4** | **Chronic kidney disease, stage 4 (severe)** |
> | **Q61.3** | **Polycystic kidney, unspecified** |
> | **I10** | **Essential (primary) hypertension** |
>
> *Explanation:* A combination code describing a relationship between hypertension and CKD is not used because the physician documentation identifies the polycystic kidney disease as the cause for the CKD.

3) Hypertensive heart and chronic kidney disease

Assign codes from combination category I13, Hypertensive heart and chronic kidney disease, when there is hypertension with both heart and kidney involvement. If heart failure is present, assign an additional code from category I50 to identify the type of heart failure.

The appropriate code from category N18, Chronic kidney disease, should be used as a secondary code with a code from category I13 to identify the stage of chronic kidney disease.

See Section I.C.14. Chronic kidney disease.

The codes in category I13, Hypertensive heart and chronic kidney disease, are combination codes that include hypertension, heart disease and chronic kidney disease. The Includes note at I13 specifies that the conditions included at I11 and I12 are included together in I13. If a patient has hypertension, heart disease and chronic kidney disease, then a code from I13 should be used, not individual codes for hypertension, heart disease and chronic kidney disease, or codes from I11 or I12.

For patients with both acute renal failure and chronic kidney disease, the acute renal failure should also be coded. Sequence according to the circumstances of the admission/encounter.

> Hypertensive heart and kidney disease with congestive heart failure and stage 2 chronic kidney disease
>
> | | |
> |---|---|
> | **I13.0** | **Hypertensive heart and chronic kidney disease with heart failure and stage 1 through stage 4 chronic kidney disease, or unspecified chronic kidney disease** |
> | **I50.9** | **Heart failure, unspecified** |
> | **N18.2** | **Chronic kidney disease, stage 2 (mild)** |
>
> *Explanation:* Combination codes in category I13 are used to report conditions classifiable to *both* categories I11 and I12. Do not report conditions classifiable to I11 and I12 separately. Use additional codes to report type of heart failure and stage of CKD.

4) Hypertensive cerebrovascular disease

For hypertensive cerebrovascular disease, first assign the appropriate code from categories I60-I69, followed by the appropriate hypertension code.

> Rupture of cerebral aneurysm caused by malignant hypertension
>
> | | |
> |---|---|
> | **I60.7** | **Nontraumatic subarachnoid hemorrhage from unspecified intracranial artery** |
> | **I10** | **Essential (primary) hypertension** |
>
> *Explanation:* Hypertensive cerebrovascular disease requires two codes: the appropriate I60–I69 code followed by the appropriate hypertension code.

5) Hypertensive retinopathy

Subcategory H35.0, Background retinopathy and retinal vascular changes, should be used along with a code from categories I10-I15, in the Hypertensive diseases section, to include the systemic hypertension. The sequencing is based on the reason for the encounter.

6) Hypertension, secondary

Secondary hypertension is due to an underlying condition. Two codes are required: one to identify the underlying etiology and one from category I15 to identify the hypertension. Sequencing of codes is determined by the reason for admission/encounter.

> Renovascular hypertension due to renal artery atherosclerosis
>
> | | |
> |---|---|
> | **I15.0** | **Renovascular hypertension** |
> | **I70.1** | **Atherosclerosis of renal artery** |
>
> *Explanation:* Secondary hypertension requires two codes: a code to identify the etiology and the appropriate I15 code.

7) Hypertension, transient

Assign code R03.0, Elevated blood pressure reading without diagnosis of hypertension, unless patient has an established diagnosis of hypertension. Assign code O13.-, Gestational [pregnancy-induced] hypertension without significant proteinuria, or O14.-, Pre-eclampsia, for transient hypertension of pregnancy.

8) Hypertension, controlled

This diagnostic statement usually refers to an existing state of hypertension under control by therapy. Assign the appropriate code from categories I10-I15, Hypertensive diseases.

9) Hypertension, uncontrolled

Uncontrolled hypertension may refer to untreated hypertension or hypertension not responding to current therapeutic regimen. In either case, assign the appropriate code from categories I10-I15, Hypertensive diseases.

10) Hypertensive crisis

Assign a code from category I16, Hypertensive crisis, for documented hypertensive urgency, hypertensive emergency or unspecified hypertensive crisis. Code also any identified hypertensive disease (I10-I15). The sequencing is based on the reason for the encounter.

11) Pulmonary hypertension

Pulmonary hypertension is classified to category I27, Other pulmonary heart diseases. For secondary pulmonary hypertension (I27.1, I27.2-), code also any associated conditions or adverse effects of drugs or toxins. The sequencing is based on the reason for the encounter, except for adverse effects of drugs (See Section I.C.19.e.).

b. Atherosclerotic coronary artery disease and angina

ICD-10-CM has combination codes for atherosclerotic heart disease with angina pectoris. The subcategories for these codes are I25.11, Atherosclerotic heart disease of native coronary artery with angina pectoris and I25.7, Atherosclerosis of coronary artery bypass graft(s) and coronary artery of transplanted heart with angina pectoris.

use combination code

☆ do not code angina separately

When using one of these combination codes it is not necessary to use an additional code for angina pectoris. A causal relationship can be assumed in a patient with both atherosclerosis and angina pectoris, unless the documentation indicates the angina is due to something other than the atherosclerosis.

If a patient with coronary artery disease is admitted due to an acute myocardial infarction (AMI), the AMI should be sequenced before the coronary artery disease.

See Section I.C.9. Acute myocardial infarction (AMI)

Patient is being seen for spastic angina pectoris. She also has a documented history of progressive coronary artery disease of the native vessels.

I25.111   Atherosclerotic heart disease of native coronary artery with angina pectoris with documented spasm

Explanation: Report the combination code for atherosclerotic heart disease (coronary artery disease) with angina pectoris. A causal relationship is assumed in a patient with both atherosclerosis and angina pectoris, unless the documentation indicates the angina is due to something other than the atherosclerosis. When using one of these combination codes, it is not necessary to use an additional code for angina pectoris.

---

c. Intraoperative and postprocedural cerebrovascular accident

Medical record documentation should clearly specify the cause- and- effect relationship between the medical intervention and the cerebrovascular accident in order to assign a code for intraoperative or postprocedural cerebrovascular accident.

Proper code assignment depends on whether it was an infarction or hemorrhage and whether it occurred intraoperatively or postoperatively. If it was a cerebral hemorrhage, code assignment depends on the type of procedure performed.

Embolic cerebral infarction of the right middle cerebral artery that occurred during hip replacement surgery. The surgeon documented as due to the surgery.

I97.811   Intraoperative cerebrovascular infarction during other surgery

I63.411   Cerebral infarction due to embolism of right middle cerebral artery

Explanation: Code assignment for intraoperative or postprocedural cerebrovascular accident is based on the provider's documentation of a cause-and-effect relationship between the condition and the procedure. Proper code assignment also depends on whether the cerebrovascular accident was an infarction or hemorrhage, occurred intraoperatively or postoperatively, and the type of procedure performed.

---

d. Sequelae of cerebrovascular disease

1) Category I69, Sequelae of cerebrovascular disease

Category I69 is used to indicate conditions classifiable to categories I60-I67 as the causes of sequela (neurologic deficits), themselves classified elsewhere. These "late effects" include neurologic deficits that persist after initial onset of conditions classifiable to categories I60-I67. The neurologic deficits caused by cerebrovascular disease may be present from the onset or may arise at any time after the onset of the condition classifiable to categories I60-I67.

Codes from category I69, Sequelae of cerebrovascular disease, that specify hemiplegia, hemiparesis and monoplegia identify whether the dominant or nondominant side is affected. Should the affected side be documented, but not specified as dominant or nondominant, and the classification system does not indicate a default, code selection is as follows:

- For ambidextrous patients, the default should be dominant.
- If the left side is affected, the default is non-dominant.
- If the right side is affected, the default is dominant.

2) Codes from category I69 with codes from I60–I67

Codes from category I69 may be assigned on a health care record with codes from I60-I67, if the patient has a current cerebrovascular disease and deficits from an old cerebrovascular disease.

3) Codes from category I69 and personal history of transient ischemic attack (TIA) and cerebral infarction (Z86.73)

Codes from category I69 should not be assigned if the patient does not have neurologic deficits.

See Section I.C.21. 4. History (of) for use of personal history codes

e. Acute myocardial infarction (AMI)

1) Type 1 ST elevation myocardial infarction (STEMI) and non-ST elevation myocardial infarction (NSTEMI)

The ICD-10-CM codes for type 1 acute myocardial infarction (AMI) identify the site, such as anterolateral wall or true posterior wall. Subcategories I21.0-I21.2 and code I21.3 are used for type 1 ST elevation myocardial infarction (STEMI). Code I21.4, Non-ST elevation (NSTEMI) myocardial infarction, is used for type 1 non-ST elevation myocardial infarction (NSTEMI) and nontransmural MIs.

If a type 1 NSTEMI evolves to STEMI, assign the STEMI code. If a type 1 STEMI converts to NSTEMI due to thrombolytic therapy, it is still coded as STEMI.

For encounters occurring while the myocardial infarction is equal to, or less than, four weeks old, including transfers to another acute setting or a postacute setting, and the myocardial infarction meets the definition for "other diagnoses" (see Section III, Reporting Additional Diagnoses), codes from category I21 may continue to be reported. For encounters after the 4-week time frame and the patient is still receiving care related to the myocardial infarction, the appropriate aftercare code should be assigned, rather than a code from category I21. For old or healed myocardial infarctions not requiring further care, code I25.2, Old myocardial infarction, may be assigned.

2) Acute myocardial infarction, unspecified

Code I21.9, Acute myocardial infarction, unspecified, is the default for unspecified acute myocardial infarction or unspecified type. If only type 1 STEMI or transmural MI without the site is documented, assign code I21.3, ST elevation (STEMI) myocardial infarction of unspecified site.

3) AMI documented as nontransmural or subendocardial but site provided

If an AMI is documented as nontransmural or subendocardial, but the site is provided, it is still coded as a subendocardial AMI.

See Section I.C.21.3.for information on coding status post administration of tPA in a different facility within the last 24 hours.

Acute inferior subendocardial myocardial infarction (NSTEMI)

I21.4   Non-ST elevation (NSTEMI) myocardial infarction

Explanation: An AMI documented as subendocardial or nontransmural is coded as such (I21.4, I22.2), even if the site of infarction is specified.

---

4) Subsequent acute myocardial infarction

A code from category I22, Subsequent ST elevation (STEMI) and non-ST elevation (NSTEMI) myocardial infarction, is to be used when a patient who has suffered a type 1 or unspecified AMI has a new AMI within the 4-week time frame of the initial AMI. A code from category I22 must be used in conjunction with a code from category I21. The sequencing of the I22 and I21 codes depends on the circumstances of the encounter.

Do not assign code I22 for subsequent myocardial infarctions other than type 1 or unspecified. For subsequent type 2 AMI assign only code I21.A1. For subsequent type 4 or type 5 AMI, assign only code I21.A9.

If a subsequent myocardial infarction of one type occurs within 4 weeks of a myocardial infarction of a different type, assign the appropriate codes from category I21 to identify each type. Do not assign a code from I22. Codes from category I22 should only be assigned if both the initial and subsequent myocardial infarctions are type 1 or unspecified.

Patient suffered an acute NSTEMI 14 days ago and is now seen for an inferior STEMI.

I22.1   Subsequent ST elevation (STEMI) myocardial infarction of inferior wall

I21.4   Non-ST elevation (NSTEMI) myocardial infarction

Explanation: Both MIs were type 1, and the current MI occurred within the four-week time frame; therefore a code for the current/subsequent STEMI (I22.1) is reported as well as a code for the previous NSTEMI (I21.4).

---

5) Other Types of Myocardial Infarction

The ICD-10-CM provides codes for different types of myocardial infarction. Type 1 myocardial infarctions are assigned to codes I21.0-I21.4.

Type 2 myocardial infarction (myocardial infarction due to demand ischemia or secondary to ischemic imbalance) is assigned to code I21.A1, Myocardial infarction type 2 with the underlying cause coded first. Do not assign code I24.8, Other forms of acute ischemic heart disease, for the demand ischemia. If a type 2 AMI is described as NSTEMI or STEMI, only assign code I21.A1. Codes I21.01-I21.4 should only be assigned for type 1 AMIs.

Acute myocardial infarctions type 3, 4a, 4b, 4c and 5 are assigned to code I21.A9, Other myocardial infarction type.

The "Code also" and "Code first" notes should be followed related to complications, and for coding of postprocedural myocardial infarctions during or following cardiac surgery.

Chapter 9. Diseases of the Circulatory System (I00-I99)

EXCLUDES 2
certain conditions originating in the perinatal period (P04-P96)
certain infectious and parasitic diseases (A00-B99)
complications of pregnancy, childbirth and the puerperium (O00-O9A)
congenital malformations, deformations, and chromosomal abnormalities (Q00-Q99)
endocrine, nutritional and metabolic diseases (E00-E88)
injury, poisoning and certain other consequences of external causes (S00-T88)
neoplasms (C00-D49)
symptoms, signs and abnormal clinical and laboratory findings, not elsewhere classified (R00-R94)
systemic connective tissue disorders (M30-M36)
transient cerebral ischemic attacks and related syndromes (G45.-)

This chapter contains the following blocks:

I00-I02	Acute rheumatic fever
I05-I09	Chronic rheumatic heart diseases
I10-I16	Hypertensive diseases
I20-I25	Ischemic heart diseases
I26-I28	Pulmonary heart disease and diseases of pulmonary circulation
I30-I5A	Other forms of heart disease
I60-I69	Cerebrovascular diseases
I70-I79	Diseases of arteries, arterioles and capillaries
I80-I89	Diseases of veins, lymphatic vessels and lymph nodes, not elsewhere classified
I95-I99	Other and unspecified disorders of the circulatory system

Acute rheumatic fever (I00-I02)

DEF: Rheumatic fever: Inflammatory disease that can follow a throat infection by group A *streptococci*. Complications can involve the joints (arthritis), subcutaneous tissue (nodules), skin (erythema marginatum), heart (carditis), or brain (chorea).

I00 Rheumatic fever without heart involvement
    INCLUDES   arthritis, rheumatic, acute or subacute
    EXCLUDES 1   *rheumatic fever with heart involvement (I01.0-I01.9)*

✓4th I01 Rheumatic fever with heart involvement
    EXCLUDES 1   *chronic diseases of rheumatic origin (I05-I09) unless rheumatic fever is also present or there is evidence of reactivation or activity of the rheumatic process*

    I01.0 Acute rheumatic pericarditis
        Any condition in I00 with pericarditis
        Rheumatic pericarditis (acute)
        EXCLUDES 1   *acute pericarditis not specified as rheumatic (I30.-)*

    I01.1 Acute rheumatic endocarditis
        Any condition in I00 with endocarditis or valvulitis
        Acute rheumatic valvulitis

    I01.2 Acute rheumatic myocarditis
        Any condition in I00 with myocarditis

    I01.8 Other acute rheumatic heart disease
        Any condition in I00 with other or multiple types of heart involvement
        Acute rheumatic pancarditis

    I01.9 Acute rheumatic heart disease, unspecified
        Any condition in I00 with unspecified type of heart involvement
        Rheumatic carditis, acute
        Rheumatic heart disease, active or acute

✓4th I02 Rheumatic chorea
    INCLUDES   Sydenham's chorea
    EXCLUDES 1   *chorea NOS (G25.5)*
              Huntington's chorea (G10)

    I02.0 Rheumatic chorea with heart involvement
        Chorea NOS with heart involvement
        Rheumatic chorea with heart involvement of any type classifiable under I01.-

    I02.9 Rheumatic chorea without heart involvement
        Rheumatic chorea NOS

Chronic rheumatic heart diseases (I05-I09)

✓4th I05 Rheumatic mitral valve diseases
    INCLUDES   conditions classifiable to both I05.0 and I05.2-I05.9, whether specified as rheumatic or not
    EXCLUDES 1   *mitral valve disease specified as nonrheumatic (I34.-)*
              mitral valve disease with aortic and/or tricuspid valve involvement (I08.-)

    I05.0 Rheumatic mitral stenosis
        Mitral (valve) obstruction (rheumatic)

    I05.1 Rheumatic mitral insufficiency
        Rheumatic mitral incompetence
        Rheumatic mitral regurgitation
        EXCLUDES 1   *mitral insufficiency not specified as rheumatic (I34.0)*

    I05.2 Rheumatic mitral stenosis with insufficiency
        Rheumatic mitral stenosis with incompetence or regurgitation

    I05.8 Other rheumatic mitral valve diseases
        Rheumatic mitral (valve) failure

    I05.9 Rheumatic mitral valve disease, unspecified
        Rheumatic mitral (valve) disorder (chronic) NOS

✓4th I06 Rheumatic aortic valve diseases
    EXCLUDES 1   *aortic valve disease not specified as rheumatic (I35.-)*
              aortic valve disease with mitral and/or tricuspid valve involvement (I08.-)

    I06.0 Rheumatic aortic stenosis
        Rheumatic aortic (valve) obstruction

    I06.1 Rheumatic aortic insufficiency
        Rheumatic aortic incompetence
        Rheumatic aortic regurgitation

    I06.2 Rheumatic aortic stenosis with insufficiency
        Rheumatic aortic stenosis with incompetence or regurgitation

    I06.8 Other rheumatic aortic valve diseases

    I06.9 Rheumatic aortic valve disease, unspecified
        Rheumatic aortic (valve) disease NOS

✓4th I07 Rheumatic tricuspid valve diseases
    INCLUDES   rheumatic tricuspid valve diseases specified as rheumatic or unspecified
    EXCLUDES 1   *tricuspid valve disease specified as nonrheumatic (I36.-)*
              tricuspid valve disease with aortic and/or mitral valve involvement (I08.-)

    I07.0 Rheumatic tricuspid stenosis
        Tricuspid (valve) stenosis (rheumatic)

    I07.1 Rheumatic tricuspid insufficiency
        Tricuspid (valve) insufficiency (rheumatic)

    I07.2 Rheumatic tricuspid stenosis and insufficiency

    I07.8 Other rheumatic tricuspid valve diseases

    I07.9 Rheumatic tricuspid valve disease, unspecified
        Rheumatic tricuspid valve disorder NOS

✓4th I08 Multiple valve diseases
    INCLUDES   multiple valve diseases specified as rheumatic or unspecified
    EXCLUDES 1   *endocarditis, valve unspecified (I38)*
              multiple valve disease specified a nonrheumatic (I34.-, I35.-, I36.-, I37.-, I38.-, Q22.-, Q23.-, Q24.8-)
              rheumatic valve disease NOS (I09.1)

    I08.0 Rheumatic disorders of both mitral and aortic valves
        Involvement of both mitral and aortic valves specified as rheumatic or unspecified
        AHA: 2019, 2Q, 5

    I08.1 Rheumatic disorders of both mitral and tricuspid valves

    I08.2 Rheumatic disorders of both aortic and tricuspid valves

    I08.3 Combined rheumatic disorders of mitral, aortic and tricuspid valves

    I08.8 Other rheumatic multiple valve diseases

    I08.9 Rheumatic multiple valve disease, unspecified

✓4th I09 Other rheumatic heart diseases

    I09.0 Rheumatic myocarditis
        EXCLUDES 1   *myocarditis not specified as rheumatic (I51.4)*

    I09.1 Rheumatic diseases of endocardium, valve unspecified
        Rheumatic endocarditis (chronic)
        Rheumatic valvulitis (chronic)
        EXCLUDES 1   *endocarditis, valve unspecified (I38)*

    I09.2 Chronic rheumatic pericarditis
        Adherent pericardium, rheumatic
        Chronic rheumatic mediastinopericarditis
        Chronic rheumatic myopericarditis
        EXCLUDES 1   *chronic pericarditis not specified as rheumatic (I31.-)*

    ✓5th I09.8 Other specified rheumatic heart diseases

        I09.81 Rheumatic heart failure   HCC Rx ESR COM
            Use additional code to identify type of heart failure (I50.-)

        I09.89 Other specified rheumatic heart diseases
            Rheumatic disease of pulmonary valve

Chapter 9. Diseases of the Circulatory System

I09.9   **Rheumatic heart disease, unspecified**
    Rheumatic carditis
      EXCLUDES 1   *rheumatoid carditis (M05.31)*

Hypertensive diseases (I10-I16)

Use additional code to identify:
    exposure to environmental tobacco smoke (Z77.22)
    history of tobacco dependence (Z87.891)
    occupational exposure to environmental tobacco smoke (Z57.31)
    tobacco dependence (F17.-)
    tobacco use (Z72.0)
   EXCLUDES 1   *neonatal hypertension (P29.2)*
            primary pulmonary hypertension (I27.0)
   EXCLUDES 2   *hypertensive disease complicating pregnancy, childbirth and the puerperium (O10-O11, O13-O16)*

I10   **Essential (primary) hypertension**   Rx   Q
    INCLUDES   high blood pressure
          hypertension (arterial) (benign) (essential) (malignant) (primary) (systemic)
     EXCLUDES 1   *hypertensive disease complicating pregnancy, childbirth and the puerperium (O10-O11, O13-O16)*
     EXCLUDES 2   *essential (primary) hypertension involving vessels of brain (I60-I69)*
             essential (primary) hypertension involving vessels of eye (H35.0-)
    AHA: 2022,1Q,36; 2020,1Q,12; 2018,2Q,9; 2016,4Q,27

I11   **Hypertensive heart disease**
    INCLUDES   any condition in I50.- or I51.4-I51.7, I51.89, I51.9 due to hypertension
    AHA: 2018,2Q,9
    TIP: Do not assign a code from this category when provider documentation indicates the heart disease is attributable to another cause.

   I11.0   **Hypertensive heart disease with heart failure**   HCC Rx ESR COM
      Hypertensive heart failure
      Use additional code to identify type of heart failure (I50.-)
      AHA: 2017,1Q,47

   I11.9   **Hypertensive heart disease without heart failure**   Rx
      Hypertensive heart disease NOS

I12   **Hypertensive chronic kidney disease**
    INCLUDES   any condition in N18 and N26 — due to hypertension
          arteriosclerosis of kidney
          arteriosclerotic nephritis (chronic) (interstitial)
          hypertensive nephropathy
          nephrosclerosis
     EXCLUDES 1   *hypertension due to kidney disease (I15.0, I15.1)*
             renovascular hypertension (I15.0)
             secondary hypertension (I15.-)
     EXCLUDES 2   *acute kidney failure (N17.-)*
    AHA: 2019,3Q,3; 2018,4Q,88; 2016,3Q,22
    TIP: Do not assign a code from this category when provider documentation indicates the chronic kidney disease (CKD) is attributable to another cause.

   I12.0   **Hypertensive chronic kidney disease with stage 5 chronic kidney disease or end stage renal disease**   HCC Rx ESR COM
      Use additional code to identify the stage of chronic kidney disease (N18.5, N18.6)

   I12.9   **Hypertensive chronic kidney disease with stage 1 through stage 4 chronic kidney disease, or unspecified chronic kidney disease**   Rx
      Hypertensive chronic kidney disease NOS
      Hypertensive renal disease NOS
      Use additional code to identify the stage of chronic kidney disease (N18.1-N18.4, N18.9)

I13   **Hypertensive heart and chronic kidney disease**
    INCLUDES   any condition in I11.- with any condition in I12.-
          cardiorenal disease
          cardiovascular renal disease
    TIP: Do not assign a code from this category when provider documentation indicates the heart and/or chronic kidney disease is attributable to another cause.

   I13.0   **Hypertensive heart and chronic kidney disease with heart failure and stage 1 through stage 4 chronic kidney disease, or unspecified chronic kidney disease**   HCC Rx ESR COM
      Use additional code to identify type of heart failure (I50.-)
      Use additional code to identify stage of chronic kidney disease (N18.1-N18.4, N18.9)

   I13.1   **Hypertensive heart and chronic kidney disease without heart failure**
     I13.10   **Hypertensive heart and chronic kidney disease without heart failure, with stage 1 through stage 4 chronic kidney disease, or unspecified chronic kidney disease**   Rx
        Hypertensive heart disease and hypertensive chronic kidney disease NOS
        Use additional code to identify the stage of chronic kidney disease (N18.1-N18.4, N18.9)
     I13.11   **Hypertensive heart and chronic kidney disease without heart failure, with stage 5 chronic kidney disease, or end stage renal disease**   HCC Rx ESR COM
        Use additional code to identify the stage of chronic kidney disease (N18.5, N18.6)

   I13.2   **Hypertensive heart and chronic kidney disease with heart failure and with stage 5 chronic kidney disease, or end stage renal disease**   HCC Rx ESR COM
      Use additional code to identify type of heart failure (I50.-)
      Use additional code to identify the stage of chronic kidney disease (N18.5, N18.6)

I15   **Secondary hypertension**
    Code also underlying condition
     EXCLUDES 1   *postprocedural hypertension (I97.3)*
     EXCLUDES 2   *secondary hypertension involving vessels of brain (I60-I69)*
             secondary hypertension involving vessels of eye (H35.0-)

   I15.0   **Renovascular hypertension**   Rx
   I15.1   **Hypertension secondary to other renal disorders**   Rx
      AHA: 2016,3Q,22
   I15.2   **Hypertension secondary to endocrine disorders**   Rx
   I15.8   **Other secondary hypertension**   Rx
   I15.9   **Secondary hypertension, unspecified**   Rx

I16   **Hypertensive crisis**
    Code also any identified hypertensive disease (I10-I15)
    AHA: 2016,4Q,26-28
   I16.0   **Hypertensive urgency**   Rx
   I16.1   **Hypertensive emergency**   Rx
   I16.9   **Hypertensive crisis, unspecified**   Rx

Ischemic heart diseases (I20-I25)

Code also the presence of hypertension (I10-I16)

I20   **Angina pectoris**
    Use additional code to identify:
      exposure to environmental tobacco smoke (Z77.22)
      history of tobacco dependence (Z87.891)
      occupational exposure to environmental tobacco smoke (Z57.31)
      tobacco dependence (F17.-)
      tobacco use (Z72.0)
     EXCLUDES 1   *angina pectoris with atherosclerotic heart disease of native coronary arteries (I25.1-)*
             atherosclerosis of coronary artery bypass graft(s) and coronary artery of transplanted heart with angina pectoris (I25.7-)
             postinfarction angina (I23.7)
    DEF: Chest pain due to reduced blood flow resulting in a lack of oxygen to the heart muscles.

   I20.0   **Unstable angina**   HCC Rx ESR COM
      Accelerated angina
      Crescendo angina
      De novo effort angina
      Intermediate coronary syndrome
      Preinfarction syndrome
      Worsening effort angina

   I20.1   **Angina pectoris with documented spasm**   HCC Rx ESR
      Angiospastic angina
      Prinzmetal angina
      Spasm-induced angina
      Variant angina

   I20.2   **Refractory angina pectoris**

I20.8   **Other forms of angina pectoris** `HCC` `Rx` `ESR`
Angina equivalent
Angina of effort
Coronary slow flow syndrome
Stable angina
Stenocardia
Use additional code(s) for symptoms associated with angina equivalent

I20.9   **Angina pectoris, unspecified** `HCC` `Rx` `ESR`
Angina NOS
Anginal syndrome
Cardiac angina
Ischemic chest pain

✓4ᵗʰ **I21**   **Acute myocardial infarction**
`INCLUDES` cardiac infarction
coronary (artery) embolism
coronary (artery) occlusion
coronary (artery) rupture
coronary (artery) thrombosis
infarction of heart, myocardium, or ventricle
myocardial infarction specified as acute or with a stated duration of 4 weeks (28 days) or less from onset
Use additional code, if applicable, to identify:
exposure to environmental tobacco smoke (Z77.22)
history of tobacco dependence (Z87.891)
occupational exposure to environmental tobacco smoke (Z57.31)
status post administration of tPA (rtPA) in a different facility within the last 24 hours prior to admission to current facility (Z92.82)
tobacco dependence (F17.-)
tobacco use (Z72.0)
`EXCLUDES 2` old myocardial infarction (I25.2)
postmyocardial infarction syndrome (I24.1)
subsequent type 1 myocardial infarction (I22.-)
AHA: 2019,2Q,5; 2018,4Q,68; 2018,3Q,5; 2017,4Q,12-14; 2017,1Q,44-45; 2016,4Q,140; 2015,2Q,16; 2013,1Q,25; 2012,4Q,96,102-103
TIP: When chronic total occlusion and myocardial infarction are documented as being in different vessels, assign code I25.82 Chronic total occlusion of coronary artery, in addition to the myocardial infarction code.

✓5ᵗʰ **I21.0**   **ST elevation (STEMI) myocardial infarction of anterior wall**
Type 1 ST elevation myocardial infarction of anterior wall
DEF: ST elevation myocardial infarction: Complete obstruction of one or more coronary arteries causing decreased blood flow (ischemia) and necrosis of myocardial muscle cells.

I21.01   **ST elevation (STEMI) myocardial infarction involving left main coronary artery** `HCC` `Rx` `ESR` `COM`

I21.02   **ST elevation (STEMI) myocardial infarction involving left anterior descending coronary artery** `HCC` `Rx` `ESR` `COM`
ST elevation (STEMI) myocardial infarction involving diagonal coronary artery
AHA: 2013,1Q,25

I21.09   **ST elevation (STEMI) myocardial infarction involving other coronary artery of anterior wall** `HCC` `Rx` `ESR` `COM`
Acute transmural myocardial infarction of anterior wall
Anteroapical transmural (Q wave) infarction (acute)
Anterolateral transmural (Q wave) infarction (acute)
Anteroseptal transmural (Q wave) infarction (acute)
Transmural (Q wave) infarction (acute) (of) anterior (wall) NOS
AHA: 2012,4Q,102-103

✓5ᵗʰ **I21.1**   **ST elevation (STEMI) myocardial infarction of inferior wall**
Type 1 ST elevation myocardial infarction of inferior wall
DEF: ST elevation myocardial infarction: Complete obstruction of one or more coronary arteries causing decreased blood flow (ischemia) and necrosis of myocardial muscle cells.

I21.11   **ST elevation (STEMI) myocardial infarction involving right coronary artery** `HCC` `Rx` `ESR` `COM`
Inferoposterior transmural (Q wave) infarction (acute)

I21.19   **ST elevation (STEMI) myocardial infarction involving other coronary artery of inferior wall** `HCC` `Rx` `ESR` `COM`
Acute transmural myocardial infarction of inferior wall
Inferolateral transmural (Q wave) infarction (acute)
Transmural (Q wave) infarction (acute) (of) diaphragmatic wall
Transmural (Q wave) infarction (acute) (of) inferior (wall) NOS
`EXCLUDES 2` ST elevation (STEMI) myocardial infarction involving left circumflex coronary artery (I21.21)
AHA: 2012,4Q,96

✓5ᵗʰ **I21.2**   **ST elevation (STEMI) myocardial infarction of other sites**
Type 1 ST elevation myocardial infarction of other sites
DEF: ST elevation myocardial infarction: Complete obstruction of one or more coronary arteries causing decreased blood flow (ischemia) and necrosis of myocardial muscle cells.

I21.21   **ST elevation (STEMI) myocardial infarction involving left circumflex coronary artery** `HCC` `Rx` `ESR` `COM`
ST elevation (STEMI) myocardial infarction involving oblique marginal coronary artery

I21.29   **ST elevation (STEMI) myocardial infarction involving other sites** `HCC` `Rx` `ESR` `COM`
Acute transmural myocardial infarction of other sites
Apical-lateral transmural (Q wave) infarction (acute)
Basal-lateral transmural (Q wave) infarction (acute)
High lateral transmural (Q wave) infarction (acute)
Lateral (wall) NOS transmural (Q wave) infarction (acute)
Posterior (true) transmural (Q wave) infarction (acute)
Posterobasal transmural (Q wave) infarction (acute)
Posterolateral transmural (Q wave) infarction (acute)
Posteroseptal transmural (Q wave) infarction (acute)
Septal transmural (Q wave) infarction (acute) NOS

I21.3   **ST elevation (STEMI) myocardial infarction of unspecified site** `HCC` `Rx` `ESR` `COM`
Acute transmural myocardial infarction of unspecified site
Transmural (Q wave) myocardial infarction NOS
Type 1 ST elevation myocardial infarction of unspecified site
DEF: ST elevation myocardial infarction: Complete obstruction of one or more coronary arteries causing decreased blood flow (ischemia) and necrosis of myocardial muscle cells.

I21.4   **Non-ST elevation (NSTEMI) myocardial infarction** `HCC` `Rx` `ESR` `COM`
Acute subendocardial myocardial infarction
Non-Q wave myocardial infarction NOS
Nontransmural myocardial infarction NOS
Type 1 non-ST elevation myocardial infarction
AHA: 2021,3Q,6; 2019,2Q,33; 2017,1Q,44-45
DEF: Partial obstruction of one or more coronary arteries that causes decreased blood flow (ischemia) and may cause partial thickness necrosis of myocardial muscle cells.

I21.9   **Acute myocardial infarction, unspecified** `HCC` `Rx` `ESR` `COM`
Myocardial infarction (acute) NOS

✓5ᵗʰ **I21.A**   **Other type of myocardial infarction**
AHA: 2019,2Q,5

I21.A1   **Myocardial infarction type 2** `HCC` `Rx` `ESR` `COM`
Myocardial infarction due to demand ischemia
Myocardial infarction secondary to ischemic imbalance
Code first the underlying cause, such as:
anemia (D50.0-D64.9)
chronic obstructive pulmonary disease (J44.-)
paroxysmal tachycardia (I47.0-I47.9)
shock (R57.0-R57.9)
AHA: 2019,4Q,53; 2017,4Q,13-14
DEF: Often referred to as due to demand ischemia, myocardial infarction (MI) type 2 refers to an MI due to ischemia and necrosis resulting from an oxygen imbalance to the heart. This mismatch between oxygen decreased supply and increased demand is caused by conditions other than coronary artery disease such as vasospasm, embolism, anemia, hypertension, hypotension, or arrhythmias.

Chapter 9. Diseases of the Circulatory System *(side margin)*

I21.A9   **Other myocardial infarction type** `HCC` `Rx` `ESR` `COM`

Myocardial infarction associated with revascularization procedure

Myocardial infarction type 3

Myocardial infarction type 4a *[handwritten: related to PCI]*

Myocardial infarction type 4b *[handwritten: stent thrombosis]*

Myocardial infarction type 4c *[handwritten: restenosis ←]*

Myocardial infarction type 5 *[handwritten: → CABG]*

Code first, if applicable, postprocedural myocardial infarction following cardiac surgery (I97.190), or postprocedural myocardial infarction during cardiac surgery (I97.790)

Code also complication, if known and applicable, such as:

(acute) stent occlusion (T82.897-)

(acute) stent stenosis (T82.855-)

(acute) stent thrombosis (T82.867-)

cardiac arrest due to underlying cardiac condition (I46.2)

complication of percutaneous coronary intervention (PCI) (I97.89)

occlusion of coronary artery bypass graft (T82.218-)

AHA: 2021,3Q,6; 2019,2Q,33

✓4ᵗʰ **I22** **Subsequent ST elevation (STEMI) and non-ST elevation (NSTEMI) myocardial infarction**

INCLUDES acute myocardial infarction occurring within four weeks (28 days) of a previous acute myocardial infarction, regardless of site

cardiac infarction

coronary (artery) embolism

coronary (artery) occlusion

coronary (artery) rupture

coronary (artery) thrombosis

infarction of heart, myocardium, or ventricle

recurrent myocardial infarction

reinfarction of myocardium

rupture of heart, myocardium, or ventricle

subsequent type 1 myocardial infarction

Use additional code, if applicable, to identify:

exposure to environmental tobacco smoke (Z77.22)

history of tobacco dependence (Z87.891)

occupational exposure to environmental tobacco smoke (Z57.31)

status post administration of tPA (rtPA) in a different facility within the last 24 hours prior to admission to current facility (Z92.82)

tobacco dependence (F17.-)

tobacco use (Z72.0)

EXCLUDES 1 *subsequent myocardial infarction, type 2 (I21.A1)*

subsequent myocardial infarction of other type (type 3) (type 4) (type 5) (I21.A9)

AHA: 2018,4Q,68; 2018,3Q,5; 2017,4Q,12-13; 2017,2Q,11; 2013,1Q,25; 2012,4Q,97,102-103

DEF: Non-ST elevation myocardial infarction: Partial obstruction of one or more coronary arteries that causes decreased blood flow (ischemia) and may cause partial thickness necrosis of myocardial muscle cells.

DEF: ST elevation myocardial infarction: Complete obstruction of one or more coronary arteries causing decreased blood flow (ischemia) and necrosis of myocardial muscle cells.

TIP: When chronic total occlusion and myocardial infarction are documented as being in different vessels, assign code I25.82 Chronic total occlusion of coronary artery, in addition to the myocardial infarction code.

I22.0 **Subsequent ST elevation (STEMI) myocardial infarction of anterior wall** `HCC` `Rx` `ESR` `COM`

Subsequent acute transmural myocardial infarction of anterior wall

Subsequent transmural (Q wave) infarction (acute)(of) anterior (wall) NOS

Subsequent anteroapical transmural (Q wave) infarction (acute)

Subsequent anterolateral transmural (Q wave) infarction (acute)

Subsequent anteroseptal transmural (Q wave) infarction (acute)

I22.1 **Subsequent ST elevation (STEMI) myocardial infarction of inferior wall** `HCC` `Rx` `ESR` `COM`

Subsequent acute transmural myocardial infarction of inferior wall

Subsequent transmural (Q wave) infarction (acute)(of) diaphragmatic wall

Subsequent transmural (Q wave) infarction (acute)(of) inferior (wall) NOS

Subsequent inferolateral transmural (Q wave) infarction (acute)

Subsequent inferoposterior transmural (Q wave) infarction (acute)

AHA: 2012,4Q,102

I22.2 **Subsequent non-ST elevation (NSTEMI) myocardial infarction** `HCC` `Rx` `ESR` `COM`

Subsequent acute subendocardial myocardial infarction

Subsequent non-Q wave myocardial infarction NOS

Subsequent nontransmural myocardial infarction NOS

I22.8 **Subsequent ST elevation (STEMI) myocardial infarction of other sites** `HCC` `Rx` `ESR` `COM`

Subsequent acute transmural myocardial infarction of other sites

Subsequent apical-lateral transmural (Q wave) myocardial infarction (acute)

Subsequent basal-lateral transmural (Q wave) myocardial infarction (acute)

Subsequent high lateral transmural (Q wave) myocardial infarction (acute)

Subsequent transmural (Q wave) myocardial infarction (acute)(of) lateral (wall) NOS

Subsequent posterior (true) transmural (Q wave) myocardial infarction (acute)

Subsequent posterobasal transmural (Q wave) myocardial infarction (acute)

Subsequent posterolateral transmural (Q wave) myocardial infarction (acute)

Subsequent posteroseptal transmural (Q wave) myocardial infarction (acute)

Subsequent septal NOS transmural (Q wave) myocardial infarction (acute)

I22.9 **Subsequent ST elevation (STEMI) myocardial infarction of unspecified site** `HCC` `Rx` `ESR` `COM`

Subsequent acute myocardial infarction of unspecified site

Subsequent myocardial infarction (acute) NOS

✓4ᵗʰ **I23** **Certain current complications following ST elevation (STEMI) and non-ST elevation (NSTEMI) myocardial infarction (within the 28 day period)**

AHA: 2017,2Q,11

DEF: ST elevation myocardial infarction: Complete obstruction of one or more coronary arteries causing decreased blood flow (ischemia) and necrosis of myocardial muscle cells.

DEF: Non-ST elevation myocardial infarction: Partial obstruction of one or more coronary arteries that causes decreased blood flow (ischemia) and may cause partial thickness necrosis of myocardial muscle cells.

I23.0 **Hemopericardium as current complication following acute myocardial infarction** `HCC` `Rx` `ESR` `COM` `A`

EXCLUDES 1 *hemopericardium not specified as current complication following acute myocardial infarction (I31.2)*

I23.1 **Atrial septal defect as current complication following acute myocardial infarction** `HCC` `Rx` `ESR` `COM` `A`

EXCLUDES 1 *acquired atrial septal defect not specified as current complication following acute myocardial infarction (I51.0)*

I23.2 **Ventricular septal defect as current complication following acute myocardial infarction** `HCC` `Rx` `ESR` `COM` `A`

EXCLUDES 1 *acquired ventricular septal defect not specified as current complication following acute myocardial infarction (I51.0)*

I23.3 **Rupture of cardiac wall without hemopericardium as current complication following acute myocardial infarction** `HCC` `Rx` `ESR` `COM` `A`

I23.4 **Rupture of chordae tendineae as current complication following acute myocardial infarction** `HCC` `Rx` `ESR` `COM`

EXCLUDES 1 *rupture of chordae tendineae not specified as current complication following acute myocardial infarction (I51.1)*

[Handwritten notes at bottom:]
Initial/Acute MI : < 4 weeks (28 days)
Subsequent = within/after 4 weeks of the previous acute MI
Old MI = as having occurred > 4 weeks

`HCC` CMS-HCC   `Rx` Rx HCC   `ESR` ESRD HCC   `COM` Commercial HCC   `N` Newborn: 0   `P` Pediatric: 0-17   `M` Maternity: 9-64   `A` Adult: 15-124

664

ICD-10-CM 2023

I23.5 Rupture of papillary muscle **as current complication following acute myocardial infarction** `HCC` `Rx` `ESR` `COM`
     EXCLUDES 1   *rupture of papillary muscle not specified as current complication following acute myocardial infarction (I51.2)*

I23.6 Thrombosis of atrium, auricular appendage, and ventricle **as current complications following acute myocardial infarction** `HCC` `Rx` `ESR` `COM` `A`
     EXCLUDES 1   *thrombosis of atrium, auricular appendage, and ventricle not specified as current complication following acute myocardial infarction (I51.3)*

I23.7 Postinfarction angina   `HCC` `Rx` `ESR` `COM` `A`
     AHA: 2015,2Q,16
     TIP: When postinfarction angina occurs with atherosclerotic coronary artery disease, code both I23.7 and I25.118 for atherosclerotic disease with other forms of angina pectoris.

I23.8 Other current complications following acute myocardial infarction   `HCC` `Rx` `ESR` `COM` `A`

✓4ᵗʰ **I24 Other acute ischemic heart diseases**
     EXCLUDES 1   *angina pectoris (I20.-)*
               transient myocardial ischemia in newborn (P29.4)
     EXCLUDES 2   *non-ischemic myocardial injury (I5A)*

I24.0 Acute coronary thrombosis not resulting in myocardial infarction   `HCC` `Rx` `ESR` `COM`
     Acute coronary (artery) (vein) embolism not resulting in myocardial infarction
     Acute coronary (artery) (vein) occlusion not resulting in myocardial infarction
     Acute coronary (artery) (vein) thromboembolism not resulting in myocardial infarction
     EXCLUDES 1   *atherosclerotic heart disease (I25.1-)*
     AHA: 2013,1Q,24

I24.1 Dressler's syndrome   `HCC` `Rx` `ESR` `COM`
     Postmyocardial infarction syndrome
     EXCLUDES 1   *postinfarction angina (I23.7)*
     DEF: Fever, leukocytosis, chest pain, evidence of pericarditis, pleurisy, and pneumonia occurring days or weeks after a myocardial infarction.

I24.8 Other forms of acute ischemic heart disease   `HCC` `Rx` `ESR` `COM`
     EXCLUDES 1   *myocardial infarction due to demand ischemia (I21.A1)*
     AHA: 2019,4Q,53; 2017,4Q,13

I24.9 Acute ischemic heart disease, unspecified   `HCC` `Rx` `ESR` `COM`
     EXCLUDES 1   *ischemic heart disease (chronic) NOS (I25.9)*

✓4ᵗʰ **I25 Chronic ischemic heart disease**
     Use additional code to identify:
     chronic total occlusion of coronary artery (I25.82)
     exposure to environmental tobacco smoke (Z77.22)
     history of tobacco dependence (Z87.891)
     occupational exposure to environmental tobacco smoke (Z57.31)
     tobacco dependence (F17.-)
     tobacco use (Z72.0)
     EXCLUDES 2   *non-ischemic myocardial injury (I5A)*

✓5ᵗʰ **I25.1 Atherosclerotic heart disease of native coronary artery**
     Atherosclerotic cardiovascular disease
     Coronary (artery) atheroma
     Coronary (artery) atherosclerosis
     Coronary (artery) disease
     Coronary (artery) sclerosis
     Use additional code, if applicable, to identify:
     coronary atherosclerosis due to calcified coronary lesion (I25.84)
     coronary atherosclerosis due to lipid rich plaque (I25.83)
     EXCLUDES 2   *atheroembolism (I75.-)*
               atherosclerosis of coronary artery bypass graft(s) and transplanted heart (I25.7-)

Atheromas

Atheromas (fatty tissue and/or plaque)   Lumen

I25.10 Atherosclerotic heart disease of native coronary artery **without angina pectoris**   `Rx` `A`
     Atherosclerotic heart disease NOS
     AHA: 2021,3Q,6-7; 2015,2Q,16; 2012,4Q,92

✓6ᵗʰ **I25.11** Atherosclerotic heart disease of native coronary artery **with angina pectoris**

     I25.110 Atherosclerotic heart disease of native coronary artery with **unstable** angina pectoris   `HCC` `Rx` `ESR` `COM` `A`
         EXCLUDES 1   *unstable angina without atherosclerotic heart disease (I20.0)*

     I25.111 Atherosclerotic heart disease of native coronary artery with angina pectoris with **documented spasm**   `HCC` `Rx` `ESR` `A`
         EXCLUDES 1   *angina pectoris with documented spasm without atherosclerotic heart disease (I20.1)*

     I25.112 Atherosclerosic heart disease of native coronary artery with **refractory** angina pectoris

     I25.118 Atherosclerotic heart disease of native coronary artery with other forms of angina pectoris   `HCC` `Rx` `ESR` `A`
         EXCLUDES 1   *other forms of angina pectoris without atherosclerotic heart disease (I20.8)*
         AHA: 2015,2Q,16
         TIP: When postinfarction angina occurs with atherosclerotic coronary artery disease, code both I23.7 and I25.118 for atherosclerotic disease with other forms of angina pectoris.

     I25.119 Atherosclerotic heart disease of native coronary artery with unspecified angina pectoris   `HCC` `Rx` `ESR` `A`
         Atherosclerotic heart disease with angina NOS
         Atherosclerotic heart disease with ischemic chest pain
         EXCLUDES 1   *unspecified angina pectoris without atherosclerotic heart disease (I20.9)*

[Handwritten margin notes:]

former smoker

No previous MI = I21

yes previous MI = I22, I21 (<28 days)

yes previous MI = I21, I25.2 (>28 days)

other reason RFE (head ache) and happen MI at hospital:

No previous MI = 1. RFE
           2. I21

yes. <28 days 1. RFE
           2. I22
           3. I21

yes >28 days: 1. RFE
           2. I21 or I25.2
           3. I22

I25.2   **Old myocardial infarction** `Rx`
Healed myocardial infarction
Past myocardial infarction diagnosed by ECG or other
investigation, but currently presenting no symptoms

I25.3   **Aneurysm of heart** `Rx`
Mural aneurysm
Ventricular aneurysm

√6th **I25.4**   **Coronary artery aneurysm and dissection**

I25.41   **Coronary artery aneurysm** `Rx`
Coronary arteriovenous fistula, acquired
EXCLUDES 1   congenital coronary (artery) aneurysm
(Q24.5)

I25.42   **Coronary artery dissection** `Rx`
DEF: Tear in the intimal arterial wall of a coronary artery
resulting in the sudden intrusion of blood within the
layers of the wall.

I25.5   **Ischemic cardiomyopathy** `Rx`
EXCLUDES 2   coronary atherosclerosis (I25.1-, I25.7-)

I25.6   **Silent myocardial ischemia** `Rx`

√5th **I25.7**   **Atherosclerosis of coronary artery bypass graft(s) and coronary artery of transplanted heart with angina pectoris**
Use additional code, if applicable, to identify:
coronary atherosclerosis due to calcified coronary lesion
(I25.84)
coronary atherosclerosis due to lipid rich plaque (I25.83)
EXCLUDES 1   atherosclerosis of bypass graft(s) of transplanted
heart without angina pectoris (I25.812)
atherosclerosis of coronary artery bypass graft(s)
without angina pectoris (I25.810)
atherosclerosis of native coronary artery of
transplanted heart without angina pectoris
(I25.811)

√6th **I25.70**   **Atherosclerosis of coronary artery bypass graft(s), unspecified, with angina pectoris**

I25.700   **Atherosclerosis of coronary artery bypass graft(s), unspecified, with unstable angina pectoris** `HCC` `Rx` `ESR` `COM` `A`
EXCLUDES 1   unstable angina pectoris
without atherosclerosis of
coronary artery bypass
graft (I20.0)

I25.701   **Atherosclerosis of coronary artery bypass graft(s), unspecified, with angina pectoris with documented spasm** `HCC` `Rx` `ESR` `A`
EXCLUDES 1   angina pectoris with
documented spasm
without atherosclerosis of
coronary artery bypass
graft (I20.1)

I25.702   **Atherosclerosis of coronary artery bypass graft(s), unspecified, with refractory angina pectoris**

I25.708   **Atherosclerosis of coronary artery bypass graft(s), unspecified, with other forms of angina pectoris** `HCC` `Rx` `ESR` `A`
EXCLUDES 1   other forms of angina pectoris
without atherosclerosis of
coronary artery bypass
graft (I20.8)

I25.709   **Atherosclerosis of coronary artery bypass graft(s), unspecified, with unspecified angina pectoris** `HCC` `Rx` `ESR` `A`
EXCLUDES 1   unspecified angina pectoris
without atherosclerosis of
coronary artery bypass
graft (I20.9)

√6th **I25.71**   **Atherosclerosis of autologous vein coronary artery bypass graft(s) with angina pectoris**

I25.710   **Atherosclerosis of autologous vein coronary artery bypass graft(s) with unstable angina pectoris** `HCC` `Rx` `ESR` `COM` `A`
EXCLUDES 1   unstable angina without
atherosclerosis of
autologous vein coronary
artery bypass graft(s)
(I20.0)
EXCLUDES 2   embolism or thrombus of
coronary artery bypass
graft(s) (T82.8-)

I25.711   **Atherosclerosis of autologous vein coronary artery bypass graft(s) with angina pectoris with documented spasm** `HCC` `Rx` `ESR` `A`
EXCLUDES 1   angina pectoris with
documented spasm
without atherosclerosis of
autologous vein coronary
artery bypass graft(s)
(I20.1)

I25.712   **Atherosclerosis of autologous vein coronary artery bypass graft(s) with refractory angina pectoris**

I25.718   **Atherosclerosis of autologous vein coronary artery bypass graft(s) with other forms of angina pectoris** `HCC` `Rx` `ESR` `A`
EXCLUDES 1   other forms of angina pectoris
without atherosclerosis of
autologous vein coronary
artery bypass graft(s)
(I20.8)

I25.719   **Atherosclerosis of autologous vein coronary artery bypass graft(s) with unspecified angina pectoris** `HCC` `Rx` `ESR` `A`
EXCLUDES 1   unspecified angina pectoris
without atherosclerosis of
autologous vein coronary
artery bypass graft(s)
(I20.9)

√6th **I25.72**   **Atherosclerosis of autologous artery coronary artery bypass graft(s) with angina pectoris**
Atherosclerosis of internal mammary artery graft with
angina pectoris

I25.720   **Atherosclerosis of autologous artery coronary artery bypass graft(s) with unstable angina pectoris** `HCC` `Rx` `ESR` `COM` `A`
EXCLUDES 1   unstable angina without
atherosclerosis of
autologous artery
coronary artery bypass
graft(s) (I20.0)

I25.721   **Atherosclerosis of autologous artery coronary artery bypass graft(s) with angina pectoris with documented spasm** `HCC` `Rx` `ESR` `A`
EXCLUDES 1   angina pectoris with
documented spasm
without atherosclerosis of
autologous artery
coronary artery bypass
graft(s) (I20.1)

I25.722   **Atherosclerosis of autologous artery coronary artery bypass graft(s) with refractory angina pectoris**

I25.728   **Atherosclerosis of autologous artery coronary artery bypass graft(s) with other forms of angina pectoris** `HCC` `Rx` `ESR` `A`
EXCLUDES 1   other forms of angina pectoris
without atherosclerosis of
autologous artery
coronary artery bypass
graft(s) (I20.8)

`HCC` CMS-HCC   `Rx` Rx HCC   `ESR` ESRD HCC   `COM` Commercial HCC   `N` Newborn: 0   `P` Pediatric: 0-17   `M` Maternity: 9-64   `A` Adult: 15-124

666

ICD-10-CM 2023

I25.729 **Atherosclerosis of autologous artery coronary artery bypass graft(s) with unspecified angina pectoris** `HCC` `Rx` `ESR` `A`
> *EXCLUDES 1*   unspecified angina pectoris without atherosclerosis of autologous artery coronary artery bypass graft(s) (I20.9)

√6ᵗʰ **I25.73 Atherosclerosis of nonautologous biological coronary artery bypass graft(s) with angina pectoris**

I25.730 **Atherosclerosis of nonautologous biological coronary artery bypass graft(s) with unstable angina pectoris** `HCC` `Rx` `ESR` `COM` `A`
> *EXCLUDES 1*   unstable angina without atherosclerosis of nonautologous biological coronary artery bypass graft(s) (I20.0)

I25.731 **Atherosclerosis of nonautologous biological coronary artery bypass graft(s) with angina pectoris with documented spasm** `HCC` `Rx` `ESR` `A`
> *EXCLUDES 1*   angina pectoris with documented spasm without atherosclerosis of nonautologous biological coronary artery bypass graft(s) (I20.1)

I25.732 **Atherosclerosis of nonautologous biological coronary artery bypass graft(s) with refractory angina pectoris**

I25.738 **Atherosclerosis of nonautologous biological coronary artery bypass graft(s) with other forms of angina pectoris** `HCC` `Rx` `ESR` `A`
> *EXCLUDES 1*   other forms of angina pectoris without atherosclerosis of nonautologous biological coronary artery bypass graft(s) (I20.8)

I25.739 **Atherosclerosis of nonautologous biological coronary artery bypass graft(s) with unspecified angina pectoris** `HCC` `Rx` `ESR` `A`
> *EXCLUDES 1*   unspecified angina pectoris without atherosclerosis of nonautologous biological coronary artery bypass graft(s) (I20.9)

√6ᵗʰ **I25.75 Atherosclerosis of native coronary artery of transplanted heart with angina pectoris**
> *EXCLUDES 1*   atherosclerosis of native coronary artery of transplanted heart without angina pectoris (I25.811)

I25.750 **Atherosclerosis of native coronary artery of transplanted heart with unstable angina** `HCC` `Rx` `ESR` `COM`

I25.751 **Atherosclerosis of native coronary artery of transplanted heart with angina pectoris with documented spasm** `HCC` `Rx` `ESR`

I25.752 **Atherosclerosis of native coronary artery of transplanted heart with refractory angina pectoris**

I25.758 **Atherosclerosis of native coronary artery of transplanted heart with other forms of angina pectoris** `HCC` `Rx` `ESR`

I25.759 **Atherosclerosis of native coronary artery of transplanted heart with unspecified angina pectoris** `HCC` `Rx` `ESR`

√6ᵗʰ **I25.76 Atherosclerosis of bypass graft of coronary artery of transplanted heart with angina pectoris**
> *EXCLUDES 1*   atherosclerosis of bypass graft of coronary artery of transplanted heart without angina pectoris (I25.812)

I25.760 **Atherosclerosis of bypass graft of coronary artery of transplanted heart with unstable angina** `HCC` `Rx` `ESR` `COM` `A`

I25.761 **Atherosclerosis of bypass graft of coronary artery of transplanted heart with angina pectoris with documented spasm** `HCC` `Rx` `ESR` `A`

I25.762 **Atherosclerosis of bypass graft of coronary artery of transplanted heart with refractory angina pectoris**

I25.768 **Atherosclerosis of bypass graft of coronary artery of transplanted heart with other forms of angina pectoris** `HCC` `Rx` `ESR` `A`

I25.769 **Atherosclerosis of bypass graft of coronary artery of transplanted heart with unspecified angina pectoris** `HCC` `Rx` `ESR` `A`

√6ᵗʰ **I25.79 Atherosclerosis of other coronary artery bypass graft(s) with angina pectoris**

I25.790 **Atherosclerosis of other coronary artery bypass graft(s) with unstable angina pectoris** `HCC` `Rx` `ESR` `COM` `A`
> *EXCLUDES 1*   unstable angina without atherosclerosis of other coronary artery bypass graft(s) (I20.0)

I25.791 **Atherosclerosis of other coronary artery bypass graft(s) with angina pectoris with documented spasm** `HCC` `Rx` `ESR` `A`
> *EXCLUDES 1*   angina pectoris with documented spasm without atherosclerosis of other coronary artery bypass graft(s) (I20.1)

I25.792 **Atherosclerosis of other coronary artery bypass graft(s) with refractory angina pectoris**

I25.798 **Atherosclerosis of other coronary artery bypass graft(s) with other forms of angina pectoris** `HCC` `Rx` `ESR` `A`
> *EXCLUDES 1*   other forms of angina pectoris without atherosclerosis of other coronary artery bypass graft(s) (I20.8)

I25.799 **Atherosclerosis of other coronary artery bypass graft(s) with unspecified angina pectoris** `HCC` `Rx` `ESR` `A`
> *EXCLUDES 1*   unspecified angina pectoris without atherosclerosis of other coronary artery bypass graft(s) (I20.9)

√5ᵗʰ **I25.8 Other forms of chronic ischemic heart disease**

√6ᵗʰ **I25.81 Atherosclerosis of other coronary vessels without angina pectoris**
Use additional code, if applicable, to identify:
  coronary atherosclerosis due to calcified coronary lesion (I25.84)
  coronary atherosclerosis due to lipid rich plaque (I25.83)
> *EXCLUDES 2*   atherosclerotic heart disease of native coronary artery without angina pectoris (I25.10)

I25.810 **Atherosclerosis of coronary artery bypass graft(s) without angina pectoris** `Rx` `A`
Atherosclerosis of coronary artery bypass graft NOS
> *EXCLUDES 1*   atherosclerosis of coronary bypass graft(s) with angina pectoris (I25.70-I25.73-, I25.79-)

I25.811 **Atherosclerosis of native coronary artery of transplanted heart without angina pectoris** `Rx`
Atherosclerosis of native coronary artery of transplanted heart NOS
> *EXCLUDES 1*   atherosclerosis of native coronary artery of transplanted heart with angina pectoris (I25.75-)

Chapter 9. Diseases of the Circulatory System

I25.812 Atherosclerosis of bypass graft of coronary artery of transplanted heart without angina pectoris `Rx` `A`

Atherosclerosis of bypass graft of transplanted heart NOS

EXCLUDES 1 atherosclerosis of bypass graft of transplanted heart with angina pectoris (I25.76)

I25.82 Chronic total occlusion of coronary artery `Rx` `UPD`

Complete occlusion of coronary artery

Total occlusion of coronary artery

Code first coronary atherosclerosis (I25.1-, I25.7-, I25.81-)

EXCLUDES 1 acute coronary occlusion with myocardial infarction (I21.0-I21.9, I22.-)

acute coronary occlusion without myocardial infarction (I24.0)

AHA: 2018,3Q,5

DEF: Complete blockage of the coronary artery due to plaque accumulation over an extended period of time, resulting in substantial reduction of blood flow. Symptoms include angina or chest pain.

TIP: Report this code in addition to a code from category I21 or I22 when the chronic total occlusion and the myocardial infarction are documented as being in different vessels.

I25.83 Coronary atherosclerosis due to lipid rich plaque `Rx` `UPD` `A`

Code first coronary atherosclerosis (I25.1-, I25.7-, I25.81-)

I25.84 Coronary atherosclerosis due to calcified coronary lesion `Rx` `UPD`

Coronary atherosclerosis due to severely calcified coronary lesion

Code first coronary atherosclerosis (I25.1-, I25.7-, I25.81-)

I25.89 Other forms of chronic ischemic heart disease `Rx`

I25.9 Chronic ischemic heart disease, unspecified `Rx`

Ischemic heart disease (chronic) NOS

Pulmonary heart disease and diseases of pulmonary circulation (I26-I28)

✓4ᵗʰ I26 **Pulmonary embolism**

INCLUDES pulmonary (acute)(artery)(vein) infarction

pulmonary (acute) (artery)(vein) thromboembolism

pulmonary (acute)(artery)(vein) thrombosis

EXCLUDES 2 chronic pulmonary embolism (I27.82)

personal history of pulmonary embolism (Z86.711)

pulmonary embolism complicating abortion, ectopic or molar pregnancy (O00-O07, O08.2)

pulmonary embolism complicating pregnancy, childbirth and the puerperium (O88.-)

pulmonary embolism due to trauma (T79.0, T79.1)

pulmonary embolism due to complications of surgical and medical care (T80.0, T81.7-, T82.8-)

septic (non-pulmonary) arterial embolism (I76)

✓5ᵗʰ I26.0 **Pulmonary embolism** with acute cor pulmonale

DEF: Cor pulmonale: Heart-lung disease appearing in identifiable forms as chronic or acute. The chronic form of this heart-lung disease is marked by dilation, hypertrophy and failure of the right ventricle due to a disease that has affected the function of the lungs, excluding congenital or left heart diseases and is also called chronic cardiopulmonary disease. The acute form is an overload of the right ventricle from a rapid onset of pulmonary hypertension, usually arising from a pulmonary embolism.

I26.01 Septic pulmonary embolism with acute cor pulmonale `HCC` `Rx` `ESR` `COM` `UPD`

Code first underlying infection

I26.02 Saddle embolus of pulmonary artery with acute cor pulmonale `HCC` `Rx` `ESR` `COM`

I26.09 Other pulmonary embolism with acute cor pulmonale `HCC` `Rx` `ESR` `COM`

Acute cor pulmonale NOS

AHA: 2014,4Q,21

✓5ᵗʰ I26.9 **Pulmonary embolism** without acute cor pulmonale

I26.90 Septic pulmonary embolism without acute cor pulmonale `HCC` `Rx` `ESR` `COM` `UPD`

Code first underlying infection

I26.92 Saddle embolus of pulmonary artery without acute cor pulmonale `HCC` `Rx` `ESR` `COM`

I26.93 Single subsegmental pulmonary embolism without acute cor pulmonale `HCC` `Rx` `ESR` `COM`

Subsegmental pulmonary embolism NOS

AHA: 2021,2Q,9; 2019,4Q,6-7

I26.94 Multiple subsegmental pulmonary emboli without acute cor pulmonale `HCC` `Rx` `ESR` `COM`

AHA: 2022,2Q,13; 2021,2Q,9; 2019,4Q,6-7

I26.99 Other pulmonary embolism without acute cor pulmonale `HCC` `Rx` `ESR` `COM`

Acute pulmonary embolism NOS

Pulmonary embolism NOS

AHA: 2022,2Q,13; 2020,3Q,10-11; 2019,2Q,22

✓4ᵗʰ I27 **Other pulmonary heart diseases**

I27.0 Primary pulmonary hypertension `HCC` `Rx` `ESR` `COM`

Heritable pulmonary arterial hypertension

Idiopathic pulmonary arterial hypertension

Primary group 1 pulmonary hypertension

Primary pulmonary arterial hypertension

EXCLUDES 1 persistent pulmonary hypertension of newborn (P29.30)

pulmonary hypertension NOS (I27.20)

secondary pulmonary arterial hypertension (I27.21)

secondary pulmonary hypertension (I27.29)

DEF: Condition that occurs when pressure within the pulmonary artery is elevated and vascular resistance is observed in the lungs.

I27.1 Kyphoscoliotic heart disease `HCC` `Rx` `ESR` `COM`

✓5ᵗʰ I27.2 **Other** secondary pulmonary hypertension

Code also associated underlying condition

EXCLUDES 1 Eisenmenger's syndrome (I27.83)

AHA: 2017,4Q,14-15; 2014,4Q,21

DEF: Condition that occurs when pressure within the pulmonary artery is elevated and vascular resistance is observed in the lungs.

I27.20 Pulmonary hypertension, unspecified `HCC` `Rx` `ESR` `COM`

Pulmonary hypertension NOS

I27.21 Secondary pulmonary arterial hypertension `HCC` `Rx` `ESR` `COM`

(Associated) (drug-induced) (toxin-induced) pulmonary arterial hypertension NOS

(Associated) (drug-induced) (toxin-induced) (secondary) group 1 pulmonary hypertension

Code also associated conditions if applicable, or adverse effects of drugs or toxins, such as:

adverse effect of appetite depressants (T50.5X5)

congenital heart disease (Q20-Q28)

human immunodeficiency virus [HIV] disease (B20)

polymyositis (M33.2-)

portal hypertension (K76.6)

rheumatoid arthritis (M05.-)

schistosomiasis (B65.-)

Sjögren syndrome (M35.0-)

systemic sclerosis (M34.-)

I27.22 Pulmonary hypertension due to left heart disease `HCC` `Rx` `ESR` `COM`

Group 2 pulmonary hypertension

Code also associated left heart disease, if known, such as:

multiple valve disease (I08.-)

rheumatic aortic valve diseases (I06.-)

rheumatic mitral valve diseases (I05.-)

I27.23 Pulmonary hypertension due to lung diseases and hypoxia `HCC` `Rx` `ESR` `COM`

Group 3 pulmonary hypertension

Code also associated lung disease, if known, such as:

bronchiectasis (J47.-)

cystic fibrosis with pulmonary manifestations (E84.0)

interstitial lung disease (J84.-)

pleural effusion (J90)

sleep apnea (G47.3-)

`HCC` CMS-HCC   `Rx` Rx HCC   `ESR` ESRD HCC   `COM` Commercial HCC   `N` Newborn: 0   `P` Pediatric: 0-17   `M` Maternity: 9-64   `A` Adult: 15-124

668   ICD-10-CM 2023

I27.24 Chronic thromboembolic pulmonary hypertension `HCC` `Rx` `ESR` `COM`
Group 4 pulmonary hypertension
Code also associated pulmonary embolism, if applicable (I26.-, I27.82)

I27.29 Other secondary pulmonary hypertension `HCC` `Rx` `ESR` `COM`
Group 5 pulmonary hypertension
Pulmonary hypertension with unclear multifactorial mechanisms
Pulmonary hypertension due to hematologic disorders
Pulmonary hypertension due to metabolic disorders
Pulmonary hypertension due to other systemic disorders
Code also other associated disorders, if known, such as:
    chronic myeloid leukemia (C92.10-C92.22)
    essential thrombocythemia (D47.3)
    Gaucher disease (E75.22)
    hypertensive chronic kidney disease with end stage renal disease (I12.0, I13.11, I13.2)
    hyperthyroidism (E05.-)
    hypothyroidism (E00-E03)
    polycythemia vera (D45)
    sarcoidosis (D86.-)
AHA: 2016,2Q,8

✓5th **I27.8 Other specified pulmonary heart diseases**

I27.81 Cor pulmonale (chronic) `HCC` `Rx` `ESR` `COM`
Cor pulmonale NOS
EXCLUDES 1   *acute cor pulmonale (I26.0-)*
AHA: 2014,4Q,21
DEF: Heart-lung disease appearing in identifiable forms as chronic or acute. The chronic form of this heart-lung disease is marked by dilation, hypertrophy and failure of the right ventricle due to a disease that has affected the function of the lungs, excluding congenital or left heart diseases and is also called chronic cardiopulmonary disease. The acute form is an overload of the right ventricle from a rapid onset of pulmonary hypertension, usually arising from a pulmonary embolism.

I27.82 Chronic pulmonary embolism `HCC` `Rx` `ESR` `COM`
Use additional code, if applicable, for associated long-term (current) use of anticoagulants (Z79.01)
EXCLUDES 1   *personal history of pulmonary embolism (Z86.711)*
AHA: 2021,2Q,9
DEF: Long-standing condition commonly associated with pulmonary hypertension in which small blood clots travel to the lungs repeatedly over many weeks, months, or years, requiring continuation of established anticoagulant or thrombolytic therapy.

I27.83 Eisenmenger's syndrome `HCC` `Rx` `ESR` `COM`
Eisenmenger's complex
(Irreversible) Eisenmenger's disease
Pulmonary hypertension with right to left shunt related to congenital heart disease
Code also underlying heart defect, if known, such as:
    atrial septal defect ▶(Q21.1-)◀
    Eisenmenger's defect (Q21.8)
    patent ductus arteriosus (Q25.0)
    ventricular septal defect (Q21.0)
DEF: Pulmonary hypertension with congenital communication between two circulations resulting in a right to left shunt. This causes reduced oxygen saturation in the arterial blood, leading to cyanosis and organ damage. Once it develops, this life-threating condition is irreversible.

I27.89 Other specified pulmonary heart diseases `HCC` `Rx` `ESR` `COM`

I27.9 Pulmonary heart disease, unspecified `HCC` `Rx` `ESR` `COM`
Chronic cardiopulmonary disease

✓4th **I28 Other diseases of pulmonary vessels**

I28.0 Arteriovenous fistula of pulmonary vessels `HCC` `Rx` `ESR` `COM`
EXCLUDES 1   *congenital arteriovenous fistula (Q25.72)*

I28.1 Aneurysm of pulmonary artery `HCC` `Rx` `ESR` `COM`
EXCLUDES 1   *congenital aneurysm (Q25.79)*
      congenital arteriovenous aneurysm (Q25.72)

I28.8 Other diseases of pulmonary vessels `HCC` `Rx` `ESR` `COM`
Pulmonary arteritis
Pulmonary endarteritis
Rupture of pulmonary vessels
Stenosis of pulmonary vessels
Stricture of pulmonary vessels

I28.9 Disease of pulmonary vessels, unspecified `HCC` `Rx` `ESR` `COM`

Other forms of heart disease (I30-I5A)

✓4th **I30 Acute pericarditis**
INCLUDES   acute mediastinopericarditis
      acute myopericarditis
      acute pericardial effusion
      acute pleuropericarditis
      acute pneumopericarditis
EXCLUDES 1   *Dressler's syndrome (I24.1)*
      rheumatic pericarditis (acute) (I01.0)
      viral pericarditis due to Coxsakie virus (B33.23)
DEF: Pericarditis: Inflammation affecting the pericardium, the fibroserous membrane that surrounds the heart.

I30.0 Acute nonspecific idiopathic pericarditis `COM`

I30.1 Infective pericarditis `COM`
Pneumococcal pericarditis
Pneumopyopericardium
Purulent pericarditis
Pyopericarditis
Pyopericardium
Pyopneumopericardium
Staphylococcal pericarditis
Streptococcal pericarditis
Suppurative pericarditis
Viral pericarditis
Use additional code (B95-B97) to identify infectious agent

I30.8 Other forms of acute pericarditis `COM`

I30.9 Acute pericarditis, unspecified `COM`

✓4th **I31 Other diseases of pericardium**
EXCLUDES 1   *diseases of pericardium specified as rheumatic (I09.2)*
      postcardiotomy syndrome (I97.0)
      traumatic injury to pericardium (S26.-)

I31.0 Chronic adhesive pericarditis `COM`
Accretio cordis
Adherent pericardium
Adhesive mediastinopericarditis

I31.1 Chronic constrictive pericarditis `COM`
Concretio cordis
Pericardial calcification

I31.2 Hemopericardium, not elsewhere classified `COM`
EXCLUDES 1   *hemopericardium as current complication following acute myocardial infarction (I23.0)*
      ▶*malignant pericardial effusion (I31.31)*◀
DEF: Presence of blood in the pericardial sac (pericardium). It can lead to potentially fatal cardiac tamponade if enough blood enters the pericardial cavity.

▲ ✓5th **I31.3 Pericardial effusion (noninflammatory)**
~~Chylopericardium~~
EXCLUDES 1   *acute pericardial effusion (I30.9)*
AHA: 2019,1Q,16

● **I31.31 Malignant pericardial effusion in diseases classified elsewhere**
Code first underlying neoplasm (C00-D49)

● **I31.39 Other pericardial effusion (noninflammatory)**
Chylopericardium

I31.4 **Cardiac tamponade** `COM` `UPD`
Code first underlying cause
DEF: Life-threatening condition in which fluid or blood accumulates in the space between the muscle of the heart (myocardium) and the outer sac that covers the heart (pericardium), resulting in compression of the heart.

Cardiac Tamponade

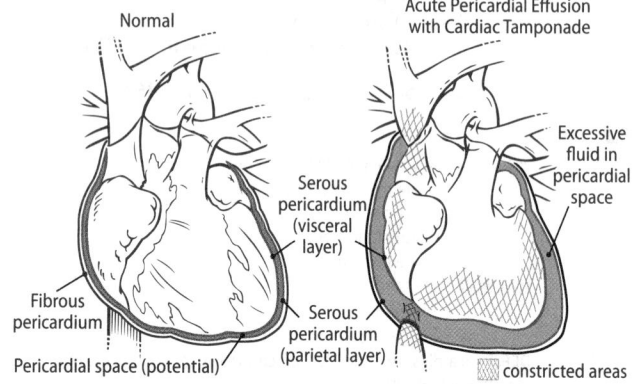

Normal

Acute Pericardial Effusion with Cardiac Tamponade

Excessive fluid in pericardial space

Serous pericardium (visceral layer)

Fibrous pericardium

Serous pericardium (parietal layer)

Pericardial space (potential)

constricted areas

I31.8 **Other specified diseases of pericardium** `COM`
Epicardial plaques
Focal pericardial adhesions

I31.9 **Disease of pericardium, unspecified** `COM`
Pericarditis (chronic) NOS

I32 *Pericarditis in diseases classified elsewhere* `COM`
Code first underlying disease
EXCLUDES 1   *pericarditis (in):*
    coxsackie (virus) (B33.23)
    gonococcal (A54.83)
    meningococcal (A39.53)
    rheumatoid (arthritis) (M05.31)
    syphilitic (A52.06)
    systemic lupus erythematosus (M32.12)
    tuberculosis (A18.84)
DEF: Pericarditis: Inflammation affecting the pericardium, the fibroserous membrane that surrounds the heart.

✓4ᵗʰ **I33** **Acute and subacute endocarditis**
EXCLUDES 1   *acute rheumatic endocarditis (I01.1)*
    endocarditis NOS (I38)
DEF: Endocarditis: Inflammatory disease of the interior lining of the heart chamber and heart valves.

I33.0 **Acute and subacute infective endocarditis** `COM`
Bacterial endocarditis (acute) (subacute)
Infective endocarditis (acute) (subacute) NOS
Endocarditis lenta (acute) (subacute)
Malignant endocarditis (acute) (subacute)
Purulent endocarditis (acute) (subacute)
Septic endocarditis (acute) (subacute)
Ulcerative endocarditis (acute) (subacute)
Vegetative endocarditis (acute) (subacute)
Use additional code (B95-B97) to identify infectious agent

I33.9 **Acute and subacute endocarditis, unspecified** `COM`
Acute endocarditis NOS
Acute myoendocarditis NOS
Acute periendocarditis NOS
Subacute endocarditis NOS
Subacute myoendocarditis NOS
Subacute periendocarditis NOS

✓4ᵗʰ **I34** **Nonrheumatic mitral valve disorders**
EXCLUDES 1   *mitral valve disease (I05.9)*
    mitral valve failure (I05.8)
    mitral valve stenosis (I05.0)
    mitral valve disorder of unspecified cause with diseases of aortic and/or tricuspid valve(s) (I08.-)
    mitral valve disorder of unspecified cause with mitral stenosis or obstruction (I05.0)
    mitral valve disorder specified as congenital (Q23.2, Q23.9)
    mitral valve disorder specified as rheumatic (I05.-)

I34.0 **Nonrheumatic mitral (valve) insufficiency**
Nonrheumatic mitral (valve) incompetence NOS
Nonrheumatic mitral (valve) regurgitation NOS
▶Code also, if applicable:◀
▶nonrheumatic mitral (valve) annulus calcification (I34.81)◀

I34.1 **Nonrheumatic mitral (valve) prolapse**
Floppy nonrheumatic mitral valve syndrome
EXCLUDES 1   *Marfan's syndrome (Q87.4-)*

I34.2 **Nonrheumatic mitral (valve) stenosis**
▶Code also, if applicable:◀
▶nonrheumatic mitral (valve) annulus calcification (I34.81)◀

▲ ✓5ᵗʰ **I34.8** **Other nonrheumatic mitral valve disorders**
●   **I34.81** **Nonrheumatic mitral (valve) annulus calcification**
Nonrheumatic mitral (valve) annular calcification
Mitral (valve) annulus calcification NOS
Code also, if applicable:
  nonrheumatic mitral (valve) insufficiency (I34.0)
  nonrheumatic mitral (valve) stenosis (I34.2)
●   **I34.89** **Other nonrheumatic mitral valve disorders**

I34.9 **Nonrheumatic mitral valve disorder, unspecified**

✓4ᵗʰ **I35** **Nonrheumatic aortic valve disorders**
EXCLUDES 1   *aortic valve disorder of unspecified cause but with diseases of mitral and/or tricuspid valve(s) (I08.-)*
    aortic valve disorder specified as congenital (Q23.0, Q23.1)
    aortic valve disorder specified as rheumatic (I06.-)
    hypertrophic subaortic stenosis (I42.1)

I35.0 **Nonrheumatic aortic (valve) stenosis**
I35.1 **Nonrheumatic aortic (valve) insufficiency**
Nonrheumatic aortic (valve) incompetence NOS
Nonrheumatic aortic (valve) regurgitation NOS
I35.2 **Nonrheumatic aortic (valve) stenosis with insufficiency**
I35.8 **Other nonrheumatic aortic valve disorders**
I35.9 **Nonrheumatic aortic valve disorder, unspecified**

✓4ᵗʰ **I36** **Nonrheumatic tricuspid valve disorders**
EXCLUDES 1   *tricuspid valve disorders of unspecified cause (I07.-)*
    tricuspid valve disorders specified as congenital (Q22.4, Q22.8, Q22.9)
    tricuspid valve disorders specified as rheumatic (I07.-)
    tricuspid valve disorders with aortic and/or mitral valve involvement (I08.-)

I36.0 **Nonrheumatic tricuspid (valve) stenosis**
I36.1 **Nonrheumatic tricuspid (valve) insufficiency**
Nonrheumatic tricuspid (valve) incompetence
Nonrheumatic tricuspid (valve) regurgitation
I36.2 **Nonrheumatic tricuspid (valve) stenosis with insufficiency**
I36.8 **Other nonrheumatic tricuspid valve disorders**
I36.9 **Nonrheumatic tricuspid valve disorder, unspecified**

✓4ᵗʰ **I37** **Nonrheumatic pulmonary valve disorders**
EXCLUDES 1   *pulmonary valve disorder specified as congenital (Q22.1, Q22.2, Q22.3)*
    pulmonary valve disorder specified as rheumatic (I09.89)

I37.0 **Nonrheumatic pulmonary valve stenosis**
I37.1 **Nonrheumatic pulmonary valve insufficiency**
Nonrheumatic pulmonary valve incompetence
Nonrheumatic pulmonary valve regurgitation
I37.2 **Nonrheumatic pulmonary valve stenosis with insufficiency**
I37.8 **Other nonrheumatic pulmonary valve disorders**
I37.9 **Nonrheumatic pulmonary valve disorder, unspecified**

I38 Endocarditis, valve unspecified

INCLUDES   endocarditis (chronic) NOS
valvular incompetence NOS
valvular insufficiency NOS
valvular regurgitation NOS
valvular stenosis NOS
valvulitis (chronic) NOS

EXCLUDES 1   congenital insufficiency of cardiac valve NOS (Q24.8)
congenital stenosis of cardiac valve NOS (Q24.8)
endocardial fibroelastosis (I42.4)
endocarditis specified as rheumatic (I09.1)

DEF: Endocarditis: Inflammatory disease of the interior lining of the heart chamber and heart valves.

I39 *Endocarditis and heart valve disorders in diseases classified elsewhere*

Code first underlying disease, such as:
Q fever (A78)

EXCLUDES 1   endocardial involvement in:
candidiasis (B37.6)
gonococcal infection (A54.83)
Libman-Sacks disease (M32.11)
listerosis (A32.82)
meningococcal infection (A39.51)
rheumatoid arthritis (M05.31)
syphilis (A52.03)
tuberculosis (A18.84)
typhoid fever (A01.02)

DEF: Endocarditis: Inflammatory disease of the interior lining of the heart chamber and heart valves.

☑4ᵗʰ I40 Acute myocarditis

INCLUDES   subacute myocarditis
EXCLUDES 1   acute rheumatic myocarditis (I01.2)
DEF: Myocarditis: Inflammation of the middle layer of the heart, which is composed of muscle tissue.

I40.0 Infective myocarditis   COM
Septic myocarditis
Use additional code (B95-B97) to identify infectious agent

I40.1 Isolated myocarditis   COM
Fiedler's myocarditis
Giant cell myocarditis
Idiopathic myocarditis

I40.8 Other acute myocarditis   COM

I40.9 Acute myocarditis, unspecified   COM

I41 *Myocarditis in diseases classified elsewhere*   COM

Code first underlying disease, such as:
typhus (A75.0-A75.9)

EXCLUDES 1   myocarditis (in):
Chagas' disease (chronic) (B57.2)
acute (B57.0)
coxsackie (virus) infection (B33.22)
diphtheritic (A36.81)
gonococcal (A54.83)
influenzal (J09.X9, J10.82, J11.82)
meningococcal (A39.52)
mumps (B26.82)
rheumatoid arthritis (M05.31)
sarcoid (D86.85)
syphilis (A52.06)
toxoplasmosis (B58.81)
tuberculous (A18.84)

DEF: Myocarditis: Inflammation of the middle layer of the heart, which is composed of muscle tissue.

☑4ᵗʰ I42 Cardiomyopathy

INCLUDES   myocardiopathy
Code first pre-existing cardiomyopathy complicating pregnancy and puerperium (O99.4)
EXCLUDES 2   ischemic cardiomyopathy (I25.5)
peripartum cardiomyopathy (O90.3)
ventricular hypertrophy (I51.7)

I42.0 Dilated cardiomyopathy   HCC Rx ESR COM
Congestive cardiomyopathy

I42.1 Obstructive hypertrophic cardiomyopathy   HCC Rx ESR COM
Hypertrophic subaortic stenosis (idiopathic)
DEF: Cardiomyopathy marked by left ventricle hypertrophy and an enlarged septum that result in obstructed blood flow, arrhythmias, mitral regurgitation, and sudden cardiac death.
TIP: When this condition is described as inherited, assign code Q24.8.

I42.2 Other hypertrophic cardiomyopathy   HCC Rx ESR COM
Nonobstructive hypertrophic cardiomyopathy

I42.3 Endomyocardial (eosinophilic) disease   HCC Rx ESR COM
Endomyocardial (tropical) fibrosis
Löffler's endocarditis

I42.4 Endocardial fibroelastosis   HCC Rx ESR COM
Congenital cardiomyopathy
Elastomyofibrosis

I42.5 Other restrictive cardiomyopathy   HCC Rx ESR COM
Constrictive cardiomyopathy NOS

I42.6 Alcoholic cardiomyopathy   HCC Rx ESR COM
Code also presence of alcoholism (F10.-)

I42.7 Cardiomyopathy due to drug and external agent   HCC Rx ESR COM
Code first poisoning due to drug or toxin, if applicable (T36-T65 with fifth or sixth character 1-4 or 6)
Use additional code for adverse effect, if applicable, to identify drug (T36-T50 with fifth or sixth character 5)
AHA: 2021,3Q,8

I42.8 Other cardiomyopathies   HCC Rx ESR COM

I42.9 Cardiomyopathy, unspecified   HCC Rx ESR COM
Cardiomyopathy (primary) (secondary) NOS

I43 *Cardiomyopathy in diseases classified elsewhere*   HCC Rx ESR COM

Code first underlying disease, such as:
amyloidosis (E85.-)
glycogen storage disease (E74.0)
gout (M10.0-)
thyrotoxicosis (E05.0-E05.9-)

EXCLUDES 1   cardiomyopathy (in):
coxsackie (virus) (B33.24)
diphtheria (A36.81)
sarcoidosis (D86.85)
tuberculosis (A18.84)

☑4ᵗʰ I44 Atrioventricular and left bundle-branch block

I44.0 Atrioventricular block, first degree

I44.1 Atrioventricular block, second degree
Atrioventricular block, type I and II
Möbitz block, type I and II
Second degree block, type I and II
Wenckebach's block

I44.2 Atrioventricular block, complete   HCC ESR COM
Complete heart block NOS
Third degree block
AHA: 2019,2Q,4

☑5ᵗʰ I44.3 Other and unspecified atrioventricular block
Atrioventricular block NOS

I44.30 Unspecified atrioventricular block
I44.39 Other atrioventricular block

I44.4 Left anterior fascicular block
I44.5 Left posterior fascicular block
☑5ᵗʰ I44.6 Other and unspecified fascicular block

I44.60 Unspecified fascicular block
Left bundle-branch hemiblock NOS

I44.69 Other fascicular block

Chapter 9. Diseases of the Circulatory System

I44.7   Left bundle-branch block, unspecified

Conduction Disorders

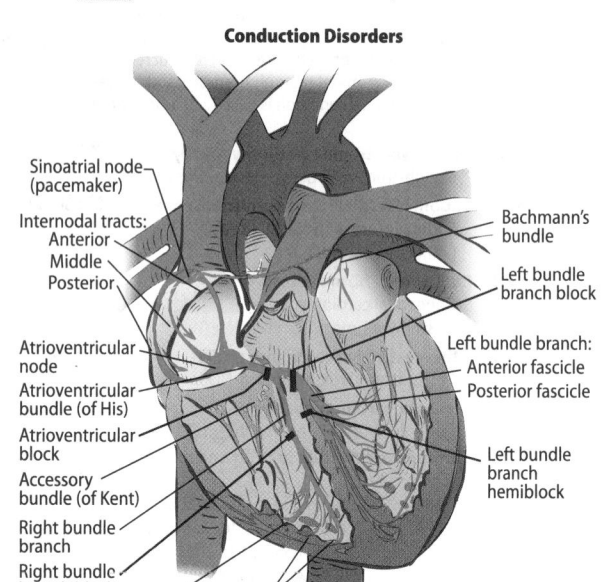

Sinoatrial node (pacemaker)

Internodal tracts:
Anterior
Middle
Posterior

Atrioventricular node
Atrioventricular bundle (of His)
Atrioventricular block
Accessory bundle (of Kent)
Right bundle branch
Right bundle branch block
Moderator band

Bachmann's bundle
Left bundle branch block
Left bundle branch:
Anterior fascicle
Posterior fascicle
Left bundle branch hemiblock
Purkinje fibers

✓4ᵗʰ I45 Other conduction disorders

I45.0   Right fascicular block

✓5ᵗʰ I45.1   Other and unspecified right bundle-branch block

     I45.10   Unspecified right bundle-branch block
               Right bundle-branch block NOS

     I45.19   Other right bundle-branch block

I45.2   Bifascicular block

I45.3   Trifascicular block

I45.4   Nonspecific intraventricular block
     Bundle-branch block NOS

I45.5   Other specified heart block
     Sinoatrial block
     Sinoauricular block
     EXCLUDES 1   heart block NOS (I45.9)

I45.6   Pre-excitation syndrome
     Accelerated atrioventricular conduction
     Accessory atrioventricular conduction
     Anomalous atrioventricular excitation
     Lown-Ganong-Levine syndrome
     Pre-excitation atrioventricular conduction
     Wolff-Parkinson-White syndrome

✓5ᵗʰ I45.8   Other specified conduction disorders

     I45.81   Long QT syndrome
         DEF: Condition characterized by recurrent syncope, malignant arrhythmias, and sudden death. This syndrome has a characteristic prolonged Q-T interval on an electrocardiogram.

     I45.89   Other specified conduction disorders
         Atrioventricular [AV] dissociation
         Interference dissociation
         Isorhythmic dissociation
         Nonparoxysmal AV nodal tachycardia
         AHA: 2013,2Q,31

I45.9   Conduction disorder, unspecified
     Heart block NOS
     Stokes-Adams syndrome

✓4ᵗʰ I46 Cardiac arrest

     EXCLUDES 2   cardiogenic shock (R57.0)
     AHA: 2019,2Q,4-5

I46.2   Cardiac arrest due to underlying cardiac condition   `HCC` `ESR` `COM` `UPD`
     Code first underlying cardiac condition

I46.8   Cardiac arrest due to other underlying condition   `HCC` `ESR` `COM` `UPD`
     Code first underlying condition

I46.9   Cardiac arrest, cause unspecified   `HCC` `ESR` `COM`
     AHA: 2020,3Q,26

✓4ᵗʰ I47 Paroxysmal tachycardia

     Code first tachycardia complicating:
       abortion or ectopic or molar pregnancy (O00-O07, O08.8)
       obstetric surgery and procedures (O75.4)
       EXCLUDES 1   tachycardia NOS (R00.0)
               sinoauricular tachycardia NOS (R00.0)
               sinus [sinusal] tachycardia NOS (R00.0)

I47.0   Re-entry ventricular arrhythmia   `HCC` `ESR` `COM`

I47.1   Supraventricular tachycardia   `HCC` `Rx` `ESR` `COM`
     Atrial (paroxysmal) tachycardia
     Atrioventricular [AV] (paroxysmal) tachycardia
     Atrioventricular re-entrant (nodal) tachycardia [AVNRT] [AVRT]
     Junctional (paroxysmal) tachycardia
     Nodal (paroxysmal) tachycardia

▲   **✓5ᵗʰ I47.2**   Ventricular tachycardia
     AHA: 2021,3Q,11; 2013,3Q,23

●   **I47.20**   Ventricular tachycardia, unspecified

●   **I47.21**   Torsades de pointes
         Code also, if applicable, long QT syndrome (I45.81)
         Use additional code for adverse effect, if applicable, to identify drug (T36-T50 with fifth or sixth character 5)
         DEF: Torsades de pointes (TdP): Accelerated heart rhythm, anywhere between 150 and 300 beats per minute, that initiates in the lower chambers of the heart (ventricles). Most commonly occurs in the setting of inherited or medication-induced long QT syndrome.

●   **I47.29**   Other ventricular tachycardia

I47.9   Paroxysmal tachycardia, unspecified   `HCC` `Rx` `ESR` `COM`
     Bouveret (-Hoffman) syndrome

✓4ᵗʰ I48 Atrial fibrillation and flutter

I48.0   Paroxysmal atrial fibrillation   `HCC` `Rx` `ESR` `COM`
     AHA: 2021,2Q,8; 2018,3Q,6

✓5ᵗʰ I48.1   Persistent atrial fibrillation
     EXCLUDES 1   permanent atrial fibrillation (I48.21)
     AHA: 2021,2Q,8; 2019,4Q,7; 2019,2Q,3; 2018,3Q,6

     I48.11   Longstanding persistent atrial fibrillation   `HCC` `Rx` `ESR` `COM`

     I48.19   Other persistent atrial fibrillation   `HCC` `Rx` `ESR` `COM`
         Chronic persistent atrial fibrillation
         Persistent atrial fibrillation, NOS
         AHA: 2019,4Q,7

✓5ᵗʰ I48.2   Chronic atrial fibrillation
     AHA: 2021,2Q,8; 2019,4Q,7; 2019,2Q,3; 2018,3Q,6

     I48.20   Chronic atrial fibrillation, unspecified   `HCC` `Rx` `ESR` `COM`
         EXCLUDES 1   chronic persistent atrial fibrillation (I48.19)

     I48.21   Permanent atrial fibrillation   `HCC` `Rx` `ESR` `COM`

I48.3   Typical atrial flutter   `HCC` `Rx` `ESR` `COM`
     Type I atrial flutter

I48.4   Atypical atrial flutter   `HCC` `Rx` `ESR` `COM`
     Type II atrial flutter

✓5ᵗʰ I48.9   Unspecified atrial fibrillation and atrial flutter

     I48.91   Unspecified atrial fibrillation   `HCC` `Rx` `ESR` `COM`

     I48.92   Unspecified atrial flutter   `HCC` `Rx` `ESR` `COM`

✓4ᵗʰ I49 Other cardiac arrhythmias

     Code first cardiac arrhythmia complicating:
       abortion or ectopic or molar pregnancy (O00-O07, O08.8)
       obstetric surgery and procedures (O75.4)
       EXCLUDES 1   neonatal dysrhythmia (P29.1-)
               sinoatrial bradycardia (R00.1)
               sinus bradycardia (R00.1)
               vagal bradycardia (R00.1)
       EXCLUDES 2   bradycardia NOS (R00.1)

✓5ᵗʰ I49.0   Ventricular fibrillation and flutter

     I49.01   Ventricular fibrillation   `HCC` `ESR` `COM`
         AHA: 2022,2Q,14

     I49.02   Ventricular flutter   `HCC` `ESR` `COM`

I49.1   Atrial premature depolarization
     Atrial premature beats

I49.2   Junctional premature depolarization   `HCC` `Rx` `ESR` `COM`

`HCC` CMS-HCC   `Rx` Rx HCC   `ESR` ESRD HCC   `COM` Commercial HCC   `N` Newborn: 0   `P` Pediatric: 0-17   `M` Maternity: 9-64   `A` Adult: 15-124

672   ICD-10-CM 2023

I49.3 Ventricular **premature** depolarization
  AHA: 2020,2Q,23

✓5ᵗʰ **I49.4** **Other and unspecified premature depolarization**

  I49.40 **Unspecified premature depolarization**
    Premature beats NOS

  I49.49 **Other premature depolarization**
    Ectopic beats
    Extrasystoles
    Extrasystolic arrhythmias
    Premature contractions

I49.5 **Sick sinus syndrome** HCC ESR COM
  Tachycardia-bradycardia syndrome
  AHA: 2019,1Q,33
  TIP: The presence of a pacemaker controls but does not cure sick sinus syndrome and therefore is considered a reportable chronic condition. When a pacemaker is evaluated by a provider, this code and code Z95.0 Presence of cardiac pacemaker, should be reported, even in the absence of any notable changes or management.

I49.8 **Other specified cardiac arrhythmias**
  Brugada syndrome
  Coronary sinus rhythm disorder
  Ectopic rhythm disorder
  Nodal rhythm disorder

I49.9 **Cardiac arrhythmia, unspecified**
  Arrhythmia (cardiac) NOS

✓4ᵗʰ **I50 Heart failure**
  Code first:
    heart failure complicating abortion or ectopic or molar pregnancy (O00-O07, O08.8)
    heart failure due to hypertension (I11.0)
    heart failure due to hypertension with chronic kidney disease (I13.-)
    heart failure following surgery (I97.13-)
    obstetric surgery and procedures (O75.4)
    rheumatic heart failure (I09.81)
    EXCLUDES 2   cardiac arrest (I46.-)
               neonatal cardiac failure (P29.0)
  AHA: 2018,4Q,67; 2018,2Q,9; 2017,1Q,47; 2014,1Q,25; 2013,2Q,33

  I50.1 Left ventricular **failure, unspecified** HCC Rx ESR COM
    Cardiac asthma
    Edema of lung with heart disease NOS
    Edema of lung with heart failure
    Left heart failure
    Pulmonary edema with heart disease NOS
    Pulmonary edema with heart failure
    EXCLUDES 1   edema of lung without heart disease or heart failure (J81.-)
               pulmonary edema without heart disease or failure (J81.-)

✓5ᵗʰ **I50.2** **Systolic (congestive) heart failure**
    Heart failure with reduced ejection fraction [HFrEF]
    Systolic left ventricular heart failure
    Code also end stage heart failure, if applicable (I50.84)
    EXCLUDES 1   combined systolic (congestive) and diastolic (congestive) heart failure (I50.4-)
    AHA: 2020,3Q,32; 2017,1Q,46; 2016,1Q,10

    I50.20 **Unspecified systolic (congestive) heart failure** HCC Rx ESR COM

    I50.21 **Acute systolic (congestive) heart failure** HCC Rx ESR COM

    I50.22 **Chronic systolic (congestive) heart failure** HCC Rx ESR COM

    I50.23 **Acute on chronic systolic (congestive) heart failure** HCC Rx ESR COM

✓5ᵗʰ **I50.3** **Diastolic (congestive) heart failure**
    Diastolic left ventricular heart failure
    Heart failure with normal ejection fraction
    Heart failure with preserved ejection fraction [HFpEF]
    Code also end stage heart failure, if applicable (I50.84)
    EXCLUDES 1   combined systolic (congestive) and diastolic (congestive) heart failure (I50.4-)
    AHA: 2020,3Q,32; 2017,1Q,46; 2016,1Q,10

    I50.30 **Unspecified diastolic (congestive) heart failure** HCC Rx ESR COM

    I50.31 Acute **diastolic (congestive) heart failure** HCC Rx ESR COM

    I50.32 Chronic **diastolic (congestive) heart failure** HCC Rx ESR COM

    I50.33 Acute on chronic **diastolic (congestive) heart failure** HCC Rx ESR COM

✓5ᵗʰ **I50.4** Combined **systolic (congestive) and diastolic (congestive) heart failure**
    Combined systolic and diastolic left ventricular heart failure
    Heart failure with reduced ejection fraction and diastolic dysfunction
    Code also end stage heart failure, if applicable (I50.84)
    AHA: 2017,1Q,46; 2016,1Q,10

    I50.40 **Unspecified combined systolic (congestive) and diastolic (congestive) heart failure** HCC Rx ESR COM

    I50.41 **Acute combined systolic (congestive) and diastolic (congestive) heart failure** HCC Rx ESR COM

    I50.42 Chronic **combined systolic (congestive) and diastolic (congestive) heart failure** HCC Rx ESR COM

    I50.43 **Acute on chronic combined systolic (congestive) and diastolic (congestive) heart failure** HCC Rx ESR COM

✓5ᵗʰ **I50.8** **Other heart failure**
    AHA: 2017,4Q,15-16

  ✓6ᵗʰ **I50.81** **Right heart failure**
      Right ventricular failure

      I50.810 **Right heart failure, unspecified** HCC Rx ESR COM
        Right heart failure without mention of left heart failure
        Right ventricular failure NOS

      I50.811 **Acute right heart failure** HCC Rx ESR COM
        Acute isolated right heart failure
        Acute (isolated) right ventricular failure

      I50.812 **Chronic right heart failure** HCC Rx ESR COM
        Chronic isolated right heart failure
        Chronic (isolated) right ventricular failure

      I50.813 **Acute on chronic right heart failure** HCC Rx ESR COM
        Acute on chronic isolated right heart failure
        Acute on chronic (isolated) right ventricular failure
        Acute decompensation of chronic (isolated) right ventricular failure
        Acute exacerbation of chronic (isolated) right ventricular failure

      I50.814 **Right heart failure** due to left heart **failure** HCC Rx ESR COM
        Right ventricular failure secondary to left ventricular failure
        Code also the type of left ventricular failure, if known (I50.2-I50.43)
        EXCLUDES 1   right heart failure with but not due to left heart failure (I50.82)

    I50.82 Biventricular **heart failure** HCC Rx ESR COM
      Code also the type of left ventricular failure as systolic, diastolic, or combined, if known (I50.2-I50.43)

    I50.83 **High output heart failure** HCC Rx ESR COM
      DEF: Occurs when the high demand for blood exceeds the capacity of a normally functioning heart to meet the demand.

    I50.84 **End stage heart failure** HCC Rx ESR COM
      Stage D heart failure
      Code also the type of heart failure as systolic, diastolic, or combined, if known (I50.2-I50.43)

    I50.89 **Other heart failure** HCC Rx ESR COM

  I50.9 **Heart failure, unspecified** HCC Rx ESR COM
    Cardiac, heart or myocardial failure NOS
    Congestive heart disease
    Congestive heart failure NOS
    EXCLUDES 2   fluid overload unrelated to congestive heart failure (E87.70)
    AHA: 2017,4Q,15-16; 2017,1Q,45-46; 2014,4Q,21; 2012,4Q,92

Chapter 9. Diseases of the Circulatory System

☑4ᵗʰ I51 Complications and ill-defined descriptions of heart disease

> EXCLUDES 1   *any condition in I51.4-I51.9 due to hypertension (I11.-)*
> *any condition in I51.4-I51.9 due to hypertension and chronic kidney disease (I13.-)*
> *heart disease specified as rheumatic (I00-I09)*

I51.0 Cardiac septal defect, acquired   [A]
Acquired septal atrial defect (old)
Acquired septal auricular defect (old)
Acquired septal ventricular defect (old)

> EXCLUDES 1   *cardiac septal defect as current complication following acute myocardial infarction (I23.1, I23.2)*

DEF: Abnormal communication between opposite heart chambers due to a defect of the septum. It is not present at birth.

I51.1 Rupture of chordae tendineae, not elsewhere classified   HCC Rx ESR COM

> EXCLUDES 1   *rupture of chordae tendineae as current complication following acute myocardial infarction (I23.4)*

I51.2 Rupture of papillary muscle, not elsewhere classified   HCC Rx ESR COM

> EXCLUDES 1   *rupture of papillary muscle as current complication following acute myocardial infarction (I23.5)*

I51.3 Intracardiac thrombosis, not elsewhere classified
Apical thrombosis (old)
Atrial thrombosis (old)
Auricular thrombosis (old)
Mural thrombosis (old)
Ventricular thrombosis (old)

> EXCLUDES 1   *intracardiac thrombosis as current complication following acute myocardial infarction (I23.6)*

AHA: 2013,1Q,24

I51.4 Myocarditis, unspecified   HCC Rx ESR COM
Chronic (interstitial) myocarditis
Myocardial fibrosis
Myocarditis NOS

> EXCLUDES 1   *acute or subacute myocarditis (I40.-)*

AHA: 2018,4Q,67; 2018,2Q,9

I51.5 Myocardial degeneration   HCC Rx ESR COM
Fatty degeneration of heart or myocardium
Myocardial disease
Senile degeneration of heart or myocardium

AHA: 2018,4Q,67; 2018,2Q,9

I51.7 Cardiomegaly
Cardiac dilatation
Cardiac hypertrophy
Ventricular dilatation

AHA: 2018,4Q,67; 2018,2Q,9

☑5ᵗʰ I51.8 Other ill-defined heart diseases
AHA: 2018,2Q,9

I51.81 Takotsubo syndrome
Reversible left ventricular dysfunction following sudden emotional stress
Stress induced cardiomyopathy
Takotsubo cardiomyopathy
Transient left ventricular apical ballooning syndrome

DEF: Complex of symptoms mimicking myocardial infarct in absence of heart disease, with the majority of cases occurring in postmenopausal women. Heart muscles are temporarily weakened, and a sudden, massive surge of adrenalin stuns the heart, greatly reducing the ability to pump blood.

I51.89 Other ill-defined heart diseases
Carditis (acute)(chronic)
Pancarditis (acute)(chronic)

AHA: 2019,2Q,5; 2018,4Q,67

I51.9 Heart disease, unspecified
AHA: 2018,4Q,67; 2018,2Q,9

I52 Other heart disorders in diseases classified elsewhere
Code first underlying disease, such as:
   congenital syphilis (A50.5)
   mucopolysaccharidosis (E76.3)
   schistosomiasis (B65.0-B65.9)

> EXCLUDES 1   *heart disease (in):*
> *gonococcal infection (A54.83)*
> *meningococcal infection (A39.50)*
> *rheumatoid arthritis (M05.31)*
> *syphilis (A52.06)*

I5A Non-ischemic myocardial injury (non-traumatic)
Acute (non-ischemic) myocardial injury
Chronic (non-ischemic) myocardial injury
Unspecified (non-ischemic) myocardial injury
Code first the underlying cause, if known and applicable, such as:
   acute kidney failure (N17.-)
   acute myocarditis (I40.-)
   cardiomyopathy (I42.-)
   chronic kidney disease (CKD) (N18.-)
   heart failure (I50.-)
   hypertensive urgency (I16.0)
   nonrheumatic aortic valve disorders (I35.-)
   paroxysmal tachycardia (I47.-)
   pulmonary embolism (I26.-)
   pulmonary hypertension (I27.0, I27.2-)
   sepsis (A41.-)
   takotsubo syndrome (I51.81)

> EXCLUDES 1   *acute myocardial infarction (I21.-)*
> *injury of heart (S26.-)*

> EXCLUDES 2   *other acute ischemic heart diseases (I24.-)*

AHA: 2021,4Q,14-15

Cerebrovascular diseases (I60-I69)

Use additional code to identify presence of:
   alcohol abuse and dependence (F10.-)
   exposure to environmental tobacco smoke (Z77.22)
   history of tobacco dependence (Z87.891)
   hypertension (I10-I16)
   occupational exposure to environmental tobacco smoke (Z57.31)
   tobacco dependence (F17.-)
   tobacco use (Z72.0)

> EXCLUDES 1   *traumatic intracranial hemorrhage (S06.-)*

AHA: 2014,3Q,5; 2012,4Q,91-92

☑4ᵗʰ I60 Nontraumatic subarachnoid hemorrhage

> EXCLUDES 1   *syphilitic ruptured cerebral aneurysm (A52.05)*
> EXCLUDES 2   *sequelae of subarachnoid hemorrhage (I69.0-)*

☑5ᵗʰ I60.0 Nontraumatic subarachnoid hemorrhage from carotid siphon and bifurcation

I60.00 Nontraumatic subarachnoid hemorrhage from unspecified carotid siphon and bifurcation   HCC ESR COM

I60.01 Nontraumatic subarachnoid hemorrhage from right carotid siphon and bifurcation   HCC ESR COM

I60.02 Nontraumatic subarachnoid hemorrhage from left carotid siphon and bifurcation   HCC ESR COM

☑5ᵗʰ I60.1 Nontraumatic subarachnoid hemorrhage from middle cerebral artery

I60.10 Nontraumatic subarachnoid hemorrhage from unspecified middle cerebral artery   HCC ESR COM

I60.11 Nontraumatic subarachnoid hemorrhage from right middle cerebral artery   HCC ESR COM

I60.12 Nontraumatic subarachnoid hemorrhage from left middle cerebral artery   HCC ESR COM

I60.2 Nontraumatic subarachnoid hemorrhage from anterior communicating artery   HCC ESR COM

☑5ᵗʰ I60.3 Nontraumatic subarachnoid hemorrhage from posterior communicating artery

I60.30 Nontraumatic subarachnoid hemorrhage from unspecified posterior communicating artery   HCC ESR COM

I60.31 Nontraumatic subarachnoid hemorrhage from right posterior communicating artery   HCC ESR COM

I60.32 Nontraumatic subarachnoid hemorrhage from left posterior communicating artery   HCC ESR COM

I60.4 Nontraumatic subarachnoid hemorrhage from basilar artery   HCC ESR COM

✓5ᵗʰ **I60.5** **Nontraumatic subarachnoid hemorrhage from** vertebral artery

     I60.50 **Nontraumatic subarachnoid hemorrhage from unspecified vertebral artery** `HCC` `ESR` `COM`

     I60.51 **Nontraumatic subarachnoid hemorrhage from** right **vertebral artery** `HCC` `ESR` `COM`

     I60.52 **Nontraumatic subarachnoid hemorrhage from** left **vertebral artery** `HCC` `ESR` `COM`

I60.6 **Nontraumatic subarachnoid hemorrhage from other intracranial arteries** `HCC` `ESR` `COM`

I60.7 **Nontraumatic subarachnoid hemorrhage from unspecified intracranial artery** `HCC` `ESR` `COM`

     Ruptured (congenital) berry aneurysm

     Ruptured (congenital) cerebral aneurysm

     Subarachnoid hemorrhage (nontraumatic) from cerebral artery NOS

     Subarachnoid hemorrhage (nontraumatic) from communicating artery NOS

     EXCLUDES 1   berry aneurysm, nonruptured (I67.1)

I60.8 **Other nontraumatic subarachnoid hemorrhage** `HCC` `ESR` `COM`

     Meningeal hemorrhage

     Rupture of cerebral arteriovenous malformation

I60.9 **Nontraumatic subarachnoid hemorrhage, unspecified** `HCC` `ESR` `COM`

✓4ᵗʰ **I61** Nontraumatic intracerebral **hemorrhage**

     EXCLUDES 2   sequelae of intracerebral hemorrhage (I69.1-)

     AHA: 2017,2Q,9-10

I61.0 **Nontraumatic intracerebral hemorrhage in** hemisphere, subcortical `HCC` `ESR` `COM`

     Deep intracerebral hemorrhage (nontraumatic)

     AHA: 2016,4Q,27

I61.1 **Nontraumatic intracerebral hemorrhage in** hemisphere, cortical `HCC` `ESR` `COM`

     Cerebral lobe hemorrhage (nontraumatic)

     Superficial intracerebral hemorrhage (nontraumatic)

I61.2 **Nontraumatic intracerebral hemorrhage in** hemisphere, **unspecified** `HCC` `ESR` `COM`

I61.3 **Nontraumatic intracerebral hemorrhage in** brain stem `HCC` `ESR` `COM`

I61.4 **Nontraumatic intracerebral hemorrhage in** cerebellum `HCC` `ESR` `COM`

I61.5 **Nontraumatic intracerebral hemorrhage,** intraventricular `HCC` `ESR` `COM`

I61.6 **Nontraumatic intracerebral hemorrhage,** multiple localized `HCC` `ESR` `COM`

I61.8 **Other nontraumatic intracerebral hemorrhage** `HCC` `ESR` `COM`

I61.9 **Nontraumatic intracerebral hemorrhage, unspecified** `HCC` `ESR` `COM`

✓4ᵗʰ **I62** Other and unspecified nontraumatic intracranial **hemorrhage**

     EXCLUDES 2   sequelae of intracranial hemorrhage (I69.2)

✓5ᵗʰ **I62.0** **Nontraumatic** subdural **hemorrhage**

     I62.00 **Nontraumatic subdural hemorrhage, unspecified** `HCC` `ESR` `COM`

     I62.01 **Nontraumatic** acute subdural **hemorrhage** `HCC` `ESR` `COM`

     I62.02 **Nontraumatic** subacute subdural **hemorrhage** `HCC` `ESR` `COM`

     I62.03 **Nontraumatic** chronic subdural **hemorrhage** `HCC` `ESR` `COM`

I62.1 **Nontraumatic** extradural **hemorrhage** `HCC` `ESR` `COM`

     Nontraumatic epidural hemorrhage

I62.9 **Nontraumatic intracranial hemorrhage, unspecified** `HCC` `ESR` `COM`

✓4ᵗʰ **I63** Cerebral infarction

     INCLUDES   occlusion and stenosis of cerebral and precerebral arteries, resulting in cerebral infarction

     Use additional code, if applicable, to identify status post administration of tPA (rtPA) in a different facility within the last 24 hours prior to admission to current facility (Z92.82)

     Use additional code, if known, to identify National Institutes of Health Stroke Scale (NIHSS) score (R29.7-)

     EXCLUDES 1   neonatal cerebral infarction (P91.82-)

     EXCLUDES 2   sequelae of cerebral infarction (I69.3-)

     AHA: 2017,2Q,9-10; 2016,4Q,28,61-62; 2015,1Q,25; 2014,1Q,23

     TIP: Weakness on one side of the body documented as secondary to stroke is synonymous with hemiparesis/hemiplegia (G81.-). Weakness of one limb documented as secondary to stroke is synonymous with monoplegia (G83.1-, G83.2-, G83.3-).

✓5ᵗʰ **I63.0** **Cerebral infarction due to** thrombosis of precerebral **arteries**

     I63.00 **Cerebral infarction due to thrombosis of unspecified precerebral artery** `HCC` `ESR` `COM`

     ✓6ᵗʰ **I63.01** **Cerebral infarction due to thrombosis of** vertebral **artery**

         I63.011 **Cerebral infarction due to thrombosis of** right **vertebral artery** `HCC` `ESR` `COM`

         I63.012 **Cerebral infarction due to thrombosis of** left **vertebral artery** `HCC` `ESR` `COM`

         I63.013 **Cerebral infarction due to thrombosis of** bilateral **vertebral arteries** `HCC` `ESR` `COM`

         I63.019 **Cerebral infarction due to thrombosis of unspecified vertebral artery** `HCC` `ESR` `COM`

     I63.02 **Cerebral infarction due to thrombosis of** basilar **artery** `HCC` `ESR` `COM`

     ✓6ᵗʰ **I63.03** **Cerebral infarction due to thrombosis of** carotid **artery**

         I63.031 **Cerebral infarction due to thrombosis of** right **carotid artery** `HCC` `ESR` `COM`

         I63.032 **Cerebral infarction due to thrombosis of** left **carotid artery** `HCC` `ESR` `COM`

         I63.033 **Cerebral infarction due to thrombosis of** bilateral **carotid arteries** `HCC` `ESR` `COM`

         I63.039 **Cerebral infarction due to thrombosis of unspecified carotid artery** `HCC` `ESR` `COM`

     I63.09 **Cerebral infarction due to thrombosis of other precerebral artery** `HCC` `ESR` `COM`

✓5ᵗʰ **I63.1** **Cerebral infarction due to** embolism of precerebral **arteries**

     I63.10 **Cerebral infarction due to embolism of unspecified precerebral artery** `HCC` `ESR` `COM`

     ✓6ᵗʰ **I63.11** **Cerebral infarction due to embolism of** vertebral **artery**

         I63.111 **Cerebral infarction due to embolism of** right **vertebral artery** `HCC` `ESR` `COM`

         I63.112 **Cerebral infarction due to embolism of** left **vertebral artery** `HCC` `ESR` `COM`

         I63.113 **Cerebral infarction due to embolism of** bilateral **vertebral arteries** `HCC` `ESR` `COM`

         I63.119 **Cerebral infarction due to embolism of unspecified vertebral artery** `HCC` `ESR` `COM`

     I63.12 **Cerebral infarction due to embolism of** basilar **artery** `HCC` `ESR` `COM`

     ✓6ᵗʰ **I63.13** **Cerebral infarction due to embolism of** carotid **artery**

         I63.131 **Cerebral infarction due to embolism of** right **carotid artery** `HCC` `ESR` `COM`

         I63.132 **Cerebral infarction due to embolism of** left **carotid artery** `HCC` `ESR` `COM`

         I63.133 **Cerebral infarction due to embolism of** bilateral **carotid arteries** `HCC` `ESR` `COM`

         I63.139 **Cerebral infarction due to embolism of unspecified carotid artery** `HCC` `ESR` `COM`

     I63.19 **Cerebral infarction due to embolism of other precerebral artery** `HCC` `ESR` `COM`

✓5ᵗʰ **I63.2** **Cerebral infarction due to unspecified** occlusion or stenosis of precerebral **arteries**

     AHA: 2020,3Q,27-28

     I63.20 **Cerebral infarction due to unspecified occlusion or stenosis of unspecified precerebral arteries** `HCC` `ESR` `COM`

✅ Additional Character Required   ✓x7ᵗʰ Placeholder Alert   Manifestation   Unspecified Dx   **Q** QPP   **UPD** Unacceptable PDx

√6th **I63.21** Cerebral infarction due to unspecified occlusion or stenosis of vertebral arteries

    I63.211 Cerebral infarction due to unspecified occlusion or stenosis of right vertebral artery `HCC` `ESR` `COM`

    I63.212 Cerebral infarction due to unspecified occlusion or stenosis of left vertebral artery `HCC` `ESR` `COM`

    I63.213 Cerebral infarction due to unspecified occlusion or stenosis of bilateral vertebral arteries `HCC` `ESR` `COM`

    I63.219 Cerebral infarction due to unspecified occlusion or stenosis of unspecified vertebral artery `HCC` `ESR` `COM`

I63.22 Cerebral infarction due to unspecified occlusion or stenosis of basilar artery `HCC` `ESR` `COM`

√6th **I63.23** Cerebral infarction due to unspecified occlusion or stenosis of carotid arteries

    I63.231 Cerebral infarction due to unspecified occlusion or stenosis of right carotid arteries `HCC` `ESR` `COM`

    I63.232 Cerebral infarction due to unspecified occlusion or stenosis of left carotid arteries `HCC` `ESR` `COM`

    I63.233 Cerebral infarction due to unspecified occlusion or stenosis of bilateral carotid arteries `HCC` `ESR` `COM`

    I63.239 Cerebral infarction due to unspecified occlusion or stenosis of unspecified carotid artery `HCC` `ESR` `COM`

I63.29 Cerebral infarction due to unspecified occlusion or stenosis of other precerebral arteries `HCC` `ESR` `COM`

√5th **I63.3** Cerebral infarction due to thrombosis of cerebral arteries

    I63.30 Cerebral infarction due to thrombosis of unspecified cerebral artery `HCC` `ESR` `COM`

√6th **I63.31** Cerebral infarction due to thrombosis of middle cerebral artery

    I63.311 Cerebral infarction due to thrombosis of right middle cerebral artery `HCC` `ESR` `COM`

    I63.312 Cerebral infarction due to thrombosis of left middle cerebral artery `HCC` `ESR` `COM`

    I63.313 Cerebral infarction due to thrombosis of bilateral middle cerebral arteries `HCC` `ESR` `COM`

    I63.319 Cerebral infarction due to thrombosis of unspecified middle cerebral artery `HCC` `ESR` `COM`

√6th **I63.32** Cerebral infarction due to thrombosis of anterior cerebral artery

    I63.321 Cerebral infarction due to thrombosis of right anterior cerebral artery `HCC` `ESR` `COM`

    I63.322 Cerebral infarction due to thrombosis of left anterior cerebral artery `HCC` `ESR` `COM`

    I63.323 Cerebral infarction due to thrombosis of bilateral anterior cerebral arteries `HCC` `ESR` `COM`

    I63.329 Cerebral infarction due to thrombosis of unspecified anterior cerebral artery `HCC` `ESR` `COM`

√6th **I63.33** Cerebral infarction due to thrombosis of posterior cerebral artery

    I63.331 Cerebral infarction due to thrombosis of right posterior cerebral artery `HCC` `ESR` `COM`

    I63.332 Cerebral infarction due to thrombosis of left posterior cerebral artery `HCC` `ESR` `COM`

    I63.333 Cerebral infarction due to thrombosis of bilateral posterior cerebral arteries `HCC` `ESR` `COM`

    I63.339 Cerebral infarction due to thrombosis of unspecified posterior cerebral artery `HCC` `ESR` `COM`

√6th **I63.34** Cerebral infarction due to thrombosis of cerebellar artery

    I63.341 Cerebral infarction due to thrombosis of right cerebellar artery `HCC` `ESR` `COM`

    I63.342 Cerebral infarction due to thrombosis of left cerebellar artery `HCC` `ESR` `COM`

    I63.343 Cerebral infarction due to thrombosis of bilateral cerebellar arteries `HCC` `ESR` `COM`

    I63.349 Cerebral infarction due to thrombosis of unspecified cerebellar artery `HCC` `ESR` `COM`

I63.39 Cerebral infarction due to thrombosis of other cerebral artery `HCC` `ESR` `COM`

√5th **I63.4** Cerebral infarction due to embolism of cerebral arteries

    I63.40 Cerebral infarction due to embolism of unspecified cerebral artery `HCC` `ESR` `COM`

√6th **I63.41** Cerebral infarction due to embolism of middle cerebral artery

    I63.411 Cerebral infarction due to embolism of right middle cerebral artery `HCC` `ESR` `COM`

    I63.412 Cerebral infarction due to embolism of left middle cerebral artery `HCC` `ESR` `COM`

    I63.413 Cerebral infarction due to embolism of bilateral middle cerebral arteries `HCC` `ESR` `COM`

    I63.419 Cerebral infarction due to embolism of unspecified middle cerebral artery `HCC` `ESR` `COM`

√6th **I63.42** Cerebral infarction due to embolism of anterior cerebral artery

    I63.421 Cerebral infarction due to embolism of right anterior cerebral artery `HCC` `ESR` `COM`

    I63.422 Cerebral infarction due to embolism of left anterior cerebral artery `HCC` `ESR` `COM`

    I63.423 Cerebral infarction due to embolism of bilateral anterior cerebral arteries `HCC` `ESR` `COM`

    I63.429 Cerebral infarction due to embolism of unspecified anterior cerebral artery `HCC` `ESR` `COM`

√6th **I63.43** Cerebral infarction due to embolism of posterior cerebral artery

    I63.431 Cerebral infarction due to embolism of right posterior cerebral artery `HCC` `ESR` `COM`

    I63.432 Cerebral infarction due to embolism of left posterior cerebral artery `HCC` `ESR` `COM`

    I63.433 Cerebral infarction due to embolism of bilateral posterior cerebral arteries `HCC` `ESR` `COM`

    I63.439 Cerebral infarction due to embolism of unspecified posterior cerebral artery `HCC` `ESR` `COM`

√6th **I63.44** Cerebral infarction due to embolism of cerebellar artery

    I63.441 Cerebral infarction due to embolism of right cerebellar artery `HCC` `ESR` `COM`

    I63.442 Cerebral infarction due to embolism of left cerebellar artery `HCC` `ESR` `COM`

    I63.443 Cerebral infarction due to embolism of bilateral cerebellar arteries `HCC` `ESR` `COM`

    I63.449 Cerebral infarction due to embolism of unspecified cerebellar artery `HCC` `ESR` `COM`

I63.49 Cerebral infarction due to embolism of other cerebral artery `HCC` `ESR` `COM`

√5th **I63.5** Cerebral infarction due to unspecified occlusion or stenosis of cerebral arteries

    I63.50 Cerebral infarction due to unspecified occlusion or stenosis of unspecified cerebral artery `HCC` `ESR` `COM`

√6th **I63.51** Cerebral infarction due to unspecified occlusion or stenosis of middle cerebral artery

    I63.511 Cerebral infarction due to unspecified occlusion or stenosis of right middle cerebral artery `HCC` `ESR` `COM`

    I63.512 Cerebral infarction due to unspecified occlusion or stenosis of left middle cerebral artery `HCC` `ESR` `COM`

`HCC` CMS-HCC   `Rx` Rx HCC   `ESR` ESRD HCC   `COM` Commercial HCC   N Newborn: 0   P Pediatric: 0-17   M Maternity: 9-64   A Adult: 15-124

676

ICD-10-CM 2023

Chapter 9. Diseases of the Circulatory System

I63.513	Cerebral infarction due to unspecified occlusion or stenosis of bilateral middle cerebral arteries	HCC ESR COM
I63.519	Cerebral infarction due to unspecified occlusion or stenosis of unspecified middle cerebral artery	HCC ESR COM

√6th **I63.52** Cerebral infarction due to unspecified occlusion or stenosis of anterior cerebral artery

I63.521	Cerebral infarction due to unspecified occlusion or stenosis of right anterior cerebral artery	HCC ESR COM
I63.522	Cerebral infarction due to unspecified occlusion or stenosis of left anterior cerebral artery	HCC ESR COM
I63.523	Cerebral infarction due to unspecified occlusion or stenosis of bilateral anterior cerebral arteries	HCC ESR COM
I63.529	Cerebral infarction due to unspecified occlusion or stenosis of unspecified anterior cerebral artery	HCC ESR COM

√6th **I63.53** Cerebral infarction due to unspecified occlusion or stenosis of posterior cerebral artery

I63.531	Cerebral infarction due to unspecified occlusion or stenosis of right posterior cerebral artery	HCC ESR COM
I63.532	Cerebral infarction due to unspecified occlusion or stenosis of left posterior cerebral artery	HCC ESR COM
I63.533	Cerebral infarction due to unspecified occlusion or stenosis of bilateral posterior cerebral arteries	HCC ESR COM
I63.539	Cerebral infarction due to unspecified occlusion or stenosis of unspecified posterior cerebral artery	HCC ESR COM

√6th **I63.54** Cerebral infarction due to unspecified occlusion or stenosis of cerebellar artery

I63.541	Cerebral infarction due to unspecified occlusion or stenosis of right cerebellar artery	HCC ESR COM
I63.542	Cerebral infarction due to unspecified occlusion or stenosis of left cerebellar artery	HCC ESR COM
I63.543	Cerebral infarction due to unspecified occlusion or stenosis of bilateral cerebellar arteries	HCC ESR COM
I63.549	Cerebral infarction due to unspecified occlusion or stenosis of unspecified cerebellar artery	HCC ESR COM

I63.59 Cerebral infarction due to unspecified occlusion or stenosis of other cerebral artery HCC ESR COM

I63.6 Cerebral infarction due to cerebral venous thrombosis, nonpyogenic HCC ESR COM

√5th **I63.8** Other cerebral infarction
    AHA: 2018,4Q,16

I63.81 Other cerebral infarction due to occlusion or stenosis of small artery HCC ESR COM
    Lacunar infarction
    AHA: 2020,3Q,27

I63.89 Other cerebral infarction HCC ESR COM
    AHA: 2022,1Q,25

I63.9 Cerebral infarction, unspecified HCC ESR COM
    Stroke NOS
    EXCLUDES 2 *transient cerebral ischemic attacks and related syndromes (G45.-)*
    AHA: 2020,2Q,29
    TIP: When provider documentation does not identify the location of an infarction, imaging reports can be used to pinpoint the location and lead to a more specific infarction code.

√4th **I65** Occlusion and stenosis of precerebral arteries, not resulting in cerebral infarction
    INCLUDES embolism of precerebral artery
          narrowing of precerebral artery
          obstruction (complete) (partial) of precerebral artery
          thrombosis of precerebral artery
    EXCLUDES 1 *insufficiency, NOS, of precerebral artery (G45.-)*
          insufficiency of precerebral arteries causing cerebral infarction (I63.0-I63.2)
    AHA: 2018,2Q,9

√5th **I65.0** Occlusion and stenosis of vertebral artery

I65.01 Occlusion and stenosis of right vertebral artery

I65.02	Occlusion and stenosis of left vertebral artery	
I65.03	Occlusion and stenosis of bilateral vertebral arteries	
I65.09	Occlusion and stenosis of unspecified vertebral artery	

I65.1 Occlusion and stenosis of basilar artery

√5th **I65.2** Occlusion and stenosis of carotid artery
    AHA: 2021,1Q,4; 2020,3Q,28

I65.21	Occlusion and stenosis of right carotid artery
I65.22	Occlusion and stenosis of left carotid artery
I65.23	Occlusion and stenosis of bilateral carotid arteries
I65.29	Occlusion and stenosis of unspecified carotid artery

I65.8 Occlusion and stenosis of other precerebral arteries

I65.9 Occlusion and stenosis of unspecified precerebral artery
    Occlusion and stenosis of precerebral artery NOS

√4th **I66** Occlusion and stenosis of cerebral arteries, not resulting in cerebral infarction
    INCLUDES embolism of cerebral artery
          narrowing of cerebral artery
          obstruction (complete) (partial) of cerebral artery
          thrombosis of cerebral artery
    EXCLUDES 1 *occlusion and stenosis of cerebral artery causing cerebral infarction (I63.3-I63.5)*

√5th **I66.0** Occlusion and stenosis of middle cerebral artery

I66.01	Occlusion and stenosis of right middle cerebral artery
I66.02	Occlusion and stenosis of left middle cerebral artery
I66.03	Occlusion and stenosis of bilateral middle cerebral arteries
I66.09	Occlusion and stenosis of unspecified middle cerebral artery

√5th **I66.1** Occlusion and stenosis of anterior cerebral artery

I66.11	Occlusion and stenosis of right anterior cerebral artery
I66.12	Occlusion and stenosis of left anterior cerebral artery
I66.13	Occlusion and stenosis of bilateral anterior cerebral arteries
I66.19	Occlusion and stenosis of unspecified anterior cerebral artery

√5th **I66.2** Occlusion and stenosis of posterior cerebral artery

I66.21	Occlusion and stenosis of right posterior cerebral artery
I66.22	Occlusion and stenosis of left posterior cerebral artery
I66.23	Occlusion and stenosis of bilateral posterior cerebral arteries
I66.29	Occlusion and stenosis of unspecified posterior cerebral artery

I66.3 Occlusion and stenosis of cerebellar arteries

I66.8 Occlusion and stenosis of other cerebral arteries
    Occlusion and stenosis of perforating arteries

I66.9 Occlusion and stenosis of unspecified cerebral artery *thrombosis*

√4th **I67** Other cerebrovascular diseases
    EXCLUDES 2 *sequelae of the listed conditions (I69.8)*

I67.0 Dissection of cerebral arteries, nonruptured HCC ESR COM
    EXCLUDES 1 *ruptured cerebral arteries (I60.7)*
    AHA: 2021,3Q,5
    DEF: Dissecting aneurysm: Tear within an arterial wall that allows blood to accumulate between the outer and middle layers, creating a false lumen.

I67.1   Cerebral aneurysm, nonruptured   COM
  Cerebral aneurysm NOS
  Cerebral arteriovenous fistula, acquired
  Internal carotid artery aneurysm, intracranial portion
  Internal carotid artery aneurysm, NOS
  EXCLUDES 1   *congenital cerebral aneurysm, nonruptured (Q28.-)*
               ruptured cerebral aneurysm (I6Ø.7)
  AHA: 2021,3Q,5
  TIP: A diagnosis of dissecting aneurysm should be coded to the dissection code, I67.Ø. The bulging/aneurysm, although present, occurred secondary to the dissection. The dissection represents the most significant problem.

Berry Aneurysm

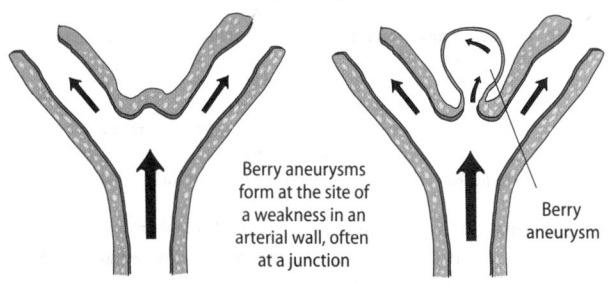

Berry aneurysms form at the site of a weakness in an arterial wall, often at a junction

Berry aneurysm

Anterior communicating artery
40%
34%
Anterior cerebral artery
20%
Internal carotid
4%
Middle cerebral artery
Posterior cerebral artery
Posterior communicating artery
Basilar artery

Common sites of berry aneurysms in the circle of Willis arteries

I67.2   Cerebral atherosclerosis   A
  Atheroma of cerebral and precerebral arteries

I67.3   Progressive vascular leukoencephalopathy   HCC Rx ESR
  Binswanger's disease

I67.4   Hypertensive encephalopathy   Rx
  EXCLUDES 2   *insufficiency, NOS, of precerebral arteries (G45.2)*

I67.5   Moyamoya disease
  DEF: Cerebrovascular ischemia. Vessels occlude and rupture, causing tiny hemorrhages at the base of brain. It affects predominantly Japanese people.

I67.6   Nonpyogenic thrombosis of intracranial venous system
  Nonpyogenic thrombosis of cerebral vein
  Nonpyogenic thrombosis of intracranial venous sinus
  EXCLUDES 1   *nonpyogenic thrombosis of intracranial venous system causing infarction (I63.6)*

I67.7   Cerebral arteritis, not elsewhere classified
  Granulomatous angiitis of the nervous system
  EXCLUDES 1   *allergic granulomatous angiitis (M3Ø.1)*

√5ᵗʰ I67.8   Other specified cerebrovascular diseases

  I67.81   Acute cerebrovascular insufficiency
    Acute cerebrovascular insufficiency unspecified as to location or reversibility

  I67.82   Cerebral ischemia
    Chronic cerebral ischemia

  I67.83   Posterior reversible encephalopathy syndrome
    PRES

  √6ᵗʰ I67.84   Cerebral vasospasm and vasoconstriction

    I67.841   Reversible cerebrovascular vasoconstriction syndrome
      Call-Fleming syndrome
      Code first underlying condition, if applicable, such as eclampsia (O15.ØØ-O15.9)

    I67.848   Other cerebrovascular vasospasm and vasoconstriction

---

√6ᵗʰ I67.85   Hereditary cerebrovascular diseases
  AHA: 2018,4Q,17

  I67.85Ø   Cerebral autosomal dominant arteriopathy with subcortical infarcts and leukoencephalopathy
    CADASIL
    Code also any associated diagnoses, such as:
    epilepsy (G4Ø.-)
    stroke (I63.-)
    vascular dementia (FØ1.-)

  I67.858   Other hereditary cerebrovascular disease

I67.89   Other cerebrovascular disease

I67.9   Cerebrovascular disease, unspecified

√4ᵗʰ I68   Cerebrovascular disorders in diseases classified elsewhere

  I68.Ø   *Cerebral amyloid angiopathy*
    Code first underlying amyloidosis (E85.-)

  I68.2   *Cerebral arteritis in other diseases classified elsewhere*
    Code first underlying disease
    EXCLUDES 1   *cerebral arteritis (in):*
         listerosis (A32.89)
         syphilis (A52.Ø4)
         systemic lupus erythematosus (M32.19)
         tuberculosis (A18.89)

  I68.8   *Other cerebrovascular disorders in diseases classified elsewhere*
    Code first underlying disease
    EXCLUDES 1   *syphilitic cerebral aneurysm (A52.Ø5)*

√4ᵗʰ I69   Sequelae of cerebrovascular disease   *[handwritten: not for traumatic]*

  NOTE   Category I69 is to be used to indicate conditions in I6Ø-I67 as the cause of sequelae. The "sequelae" include conditions specified as such or as residuals which may occur at any time after the onset of the causal condition

  [handwritten: 1. I69 (sequelae) 2. I6Ø-I67]

  EXCLUDES 1   *personal history of cerebral infarction without residual deficit (Z86.73)*
       personal history of prolonged reversible ischemic neurologic deficit (PRIND) (Z86.73)
       personal history of reversible ischemic neurologcial deficit (RIND) (Z86.73)
       sequelae of traumatic intracranial injury (SØ6.-)

  AHA: 2020,2Q,29; 2017,1Q,47; 2016,4Q,28; 2015,1Q,25; 2012,4Q,106
  TIP: Weakness on one side of the body (unilateral weakness) documented as secondary to old cerebrovascular disease is synonymous with hemiparesis/hemiplegia. Weakness of one limb documented as secondary to old cerebrovascular disease is synonymous with monoplegia.
  TIP: For codes describing hemiplegia, hemiparesis, and monoplegia; if the documentation identifies the affected side but not whether it is the dominant or nondominant side, the default is as follows: for ambidextrous patients, the default is dominant; when the left side is affected, the default is nondominant; and when the right side is affected, the default is dominant.

  √5ᵗʰ I69.Ø   Sequelae of nontraumatic subarachnoid hemorrhage

    I69.ØØ   Unspecified sequelae of nontraumatic subarachnoid hemorrhage

    √6ᵗʰ I69.Ø1   Cognitive deficits following nontraumatic subarachnoid hemorrhage

      I69.Ø1Ø   Attention and concentration deficit following nontraumatic subarachnoid hemorrhage

      I69.Ø11   Memory deficit following nontraumatic subarachnoid hemorrhage

      I69.Ø12   Visuospatial deficit and spatial neglect following nontraumatic subarachnoid hemorrhage

      I69.Ø13   Psychomotor deficit following nontraumatic subarachnoid hemorrhage

      I69.Ø14   Frontal lobe and executive function deficit following nontraumatic subarachnoid hemorrhage

      I69.Ø15   Cognitive social or emotional deficit following nontraumatic subarachnoid hemorrhage

      I69.Ø18   Other symptoms and signs involving cognitive functions following nontraumatic subarachnoid hemorrhage

      I69.Ø19   Unspecified symptoms and signs involving cognitive functions following nontraumatic subarachnoid hemorrhage

---

✓6ᵗʰ **I69.02** Speech and language deficits following nontraumatic subarachnoid hemorrhage

I69.020 Aphasia following nontraumatic subarachnoid hemorrhage

I69.021 Dysphasia following nontraumatic subarachnoid hemorrhage

I69.022 Dysarthria following nontraumatic subarachnoid hemorrhage

I69.023 Fluency disorder following nontraumatic subarachnoid hemorrhage
Stuttering following nontraumatic subarachnoid hemorrhage

I69.028 Other speech and language deficits following nontraumatic subarachnoid hemorrhage

✓6ᵗʰ **I69.03** Monoplegia of upper limb following nontraumatic subarachnoid hemorrhage
AHA: 2017,1Q,47

I69.031 Monoplegia of upper limb following nontraumatic subarachnoid hemorrhage affecting right dominant side `HCC` `ESR` `COM`

I69.032 Monoplegia of upper limb following nontraumatic subarachnoid hemorrhage affecting left dominant side `HCC` `ESR` `COM`

I69.033 Monoplegia of upper limb following nontraumatic subarachnoid hemorrhage affecting right non-dominant side `HCC` `ESR` `COM`

I69.034 Monoplegia of upper limb following nontraumatic subarachnoid hemorrhage affecting left non-dominant side `HCC` `ESR` `COM`

I69.039 Monoplegia of upper limb following nontraumatic subarachnoid hemorrhage affecting unspecified side `HCC` `ESR` `COM`

✓6ᵗʰ **I69.04** Monoplegia of lower limb following nontraumatic subarachnoid hemorrhage
AHA: 2017,1Q,47

I69.041 Monoplegia of lower limb following nontraumatic subarachnoid hemorrhage affecting right dominant side `HCC` `ESR` `COM`

I69.042 Monoplegia of lower limb following nontraumatic subarachnoid hemorrhage affecting left dominant side `HCC` `ESR` `COM`

I69.043 Monoplegia of lower limb following nontraumatic subarachnoid hemorrhage affecting right non-dominant side `HCC` `ESR` `COM`

I69.044 Monoplegia of lower limb following nontraumatic subarachnoid hemorrhage affecting left non-dominant side `HCC` `ESR` `COM`

I69.049 Monoplegia of lower limb following nontraumatic subarachnoid hemorrhage affecting unspecified side `HCC` `ESR` `COM`

✓6ᵗʰ **I69.05** Hemiplegia and hemiparesis following nontraumatic subarachnoid hemorrhage
AHA: 2015,1Q,25

I69.051 Hemiplegia and hemiparesis following nontraumatic subarachnoid hemorrhage affecting right dominant side `HCC` `ESR` `COM`

I69.052 Hemiplegia and hemiparesis following nontraumatic subarachnoid hemorrhage affecting left dominant side `HCC` `ESR` `COM`

I69.053 Hemiplegia and hemiparesis following nontraumatic subarachnoid hemorrhage affecting right non-dominant side `HCC` `ESR` `COM`

I69.054 Hemiplegia and hemiparesis following nontraumatic subarachnoid hemorrhage affecting left non-dominant side `HCC` `ESR` `COM`

I69.059 Hemiplegia and hemiparesis following nontraumatic subarachnoid hemorrhage affecting unspecified side `HCC` `ESR` `COM`

✓6ᵗʰ **I69.06** Other paralytic syndrome following nontraumatic subarachnoid hemorrhage
Use additional code to identify type of paralytic syndrome, such as:
locked-in state (G83.5)
quadriplegia (G82.5-)
EXCLUDES 1 hemiplegia/hemiparesis following nontraumatic subarachnoid hemorrhage (I69.05-)
monoplegia of lower limb following nontraumatic subarachnoid hemorrhage (I69.04-)
monoplegia of upper limb following nontraumatic subarachnoid hemorrhage (I69.03-)

I69.061 Other paralytic syndrome following nontraumatic subarachnoid hemorrhage affecting right dominant side `HCC` `ESR` `COM`

I69.062 Other paralytic syndrome following nontraumatic subarachnoid hemorrhage affecting left dominant side `HCC` `ESR` `COM`

I69.063 Other paralytic syndrome following nontraumatic subarachnoid hemorrhage affecting right non-dominant side `HCC` `ESR` `COM`

I69.064 Other paralytic syndrome following nontraumatic subarachnoid hemorrhage affecting left non-dominant side `HCC` `ESR` `COM`

I69.065 Other paralytic syndrome following nontraumatic subarachnoid hemorrhage, bilateral `HCC` `ESR` `COM`

I69.069 Other paralytic syndrome following nontraumatic subarachnoid hemorrhage affecting unspecified side `HCC` `ESR` `COM`

✓6ᵗʰ **I69.09** Other sequelae of nontraumatic subarachnoid hemorrhage

I69.090 Apraxia following nontraumatic subarachnoid hemorrhage

I69.091 Dysphagia following nontraumatic subarachnoid hemorrhage
Use additional code to identify the type of dysphagia, if known
▶(R13.11-R13.19)◀

I69.092 Facial weakness following nontraumatic subarachnoid hemorrhage
Facial droop following nontraumatic subarachnoid hemorrhage

I69.093 Ataxia following nontraumatic subarachnoid hemorrhage

I69.098 Other sequelae following nontraumatic subarachnoid hemorrhage
Alterations of sensation following nontraumatic subarachnoid hemorrhage
Disturbance of vision following nontraumatic subarachnoid hemorrhage
Use additional code to identify the sequelae

✓5ᵗʰ **I69.1** Sequelae of nontraumatic intracerebral hemorrhage

I69.10 Unspecified sequelae of nontraumatic intracerebral hemorrhage

✓6ᵗʰ **I69.11** Cognitive deficits following nontraumatic intracerebral hemorrhage

I69.110 Attention and concentration deficit following nontraumatic intracerebral hemorrhage

I69.111 Memory deficit following nontraumatic intracerebral hemorrhage

I69.112 Visuospatial deficit and spatial neglect following nontraumatic intracerebral hemorrhage

I69.113 Psychomotor deficit following nontraumatic intracerebral hemorrhage

I69.114 Frontal lobe and executive function deficit following nontraumatic intracerebral hemorrhage

Chapter 9. Diseases of the Circulatory System

I69.115 Cognitive social or emotional deficit following nontraumatic intracerebral hemorrhage

I69.118 Other symptoms and signs involving cognitive functions following nontraumatic intracerebral hemorrhage

I69.119 Unspecified symptoms and signs involving cognitive functions following nontraumatic intracerebral hemorrhage

✓6ᵗʰ **I69.12** Speech and language deficits following nontraumatic intracerebral hemorrhage

I69.120 Aphasia following nontraumatic intracerebral hemorrhage

I69.121 Dysphasia following nontraumatic intracerebral hemorrhage

I69.122 Dysarthria following nontraumatic intracerebral hemorrhage

I69.123 Fluency disorder following nontraumatic intracerebral hemorrhage

Stuttering following nontraumatic intracerebral hemorrhage

I69.128 Other speech and language deficits following nontraumatic intracerebral hemorrhage

✓6ᵗʰ **I69.13** Monoplegia of upper limb following nontraumatic intracerebral hemorrhage
AHA: 2017,1Q,47

I69.131 Monoplegia of upper limb following nontraumatic intracerebral hemorrhage affecting right dominant side `HCC` `ESR` `COM`

I69.132 Monoplegia of upper limb following nontraumatic intracerebral hemorrhage affecting left dominant side `HCC` `ESR` `COM`

I69.133 Monoplegia of upper limb following nontraumatic intracerebral hemorrhage affecting right non-dominant side `HCC` `ESR` `COM`

I69.134 Monoplegia of upper limb following nontraumatic intracerebral hemorrhage affecting left non-dominant side `HCC` `ESR` `COM`

I69.139 Monoplegia of upper limb following nontraumatic intracerebral hemorrhage affecting unspecified side `HCC` `ESR` `COM`

✓6ᵗʰ **I69.14** Monoplegia of lower limb following nontraumatic intracerebral hemorrhage
AHA: 2017,1Q,47

I69.141 Monoplegia of lower limb following nontraumatic intracerebral hemorrhage affecting right dominant side `HCC` `ESR` `COM`

I69.142 Monoplegia of lower limb following nontraumatic intracerebral hemorrhage affecting left dominant side `HCC` `ESR` `COM`

I69.143 Monoplegia of lower limb following nontraumatic intracerebral hemorrhage affecting right non-dominant side `HCC` `ESR` `COM`

I69.144 Monoplegia of lower limb following nontraumatic intracerebral hemorrhage affecting left non-dominant side `HCC` `ESR` `COM`

I69.149 Monoplegia of lower limb following nontraumatic intracerebral hemorrhage affecting unspecified side `HCC` `ESR` `COM`

✓6ᵗʰ **I69.15** Hemiplegia and hemiparesis following nontraumatic intracerebral hemorrhage
AHA: 2015,1Q,25

I69.151 Hemiplegia and hemiparesis following nontraumatic intracerebral hemorrhage affecting right dominant side `HCC` `ESR` `COM`

I69.152 Hemiplegia and hemiparesis following nontraumatic intracerebral hemorrhage affecting left dominant side `HCC` `ESR` `COM`

I69.153 Hemiplegia and hemiparesis following nontraumatic intracerebral hemorrhage affecting right non-dominant side `HCC` `ESR` `COM`

I69.154 Hemiplegia and hemiparesis following nontraumatic intracerebral hemorrhage affecting left non-dominant side `HCC` `ESR` `COM`

I69.159 Hemiplegia and hemiparesis following nontraumatic intracerebral hemorrhage affecting unspecified side `HCC` `ESR` `COM`

✓6ᵗʰ **I69.16** Other paralytic syndrome following nontraumatic intracerebral hemorrhage
Use additional code to identify type of paralytic syndrome, such as:
locked-in state (G83.5)
quadriplegia (G82.5-)

EXCLUDES 1 hemiplegia/hemiparesis following nontraumatic intracerebral hemorrhage (I69.15-)
monoplegia of lower limb following nontraumatic intracerebral hemorrhage (I69.14-)
monoplegia of upper limb following nontraumatic intracerebral hemorrhage (I69.13-)

I69.161 Other paralytic syndrome following nontraumatic intracerebral hemorrhage affecting right dominant side `HCC` `ESR` `COM`

I69.162 Other paralytic syndrome following nontraumatic intracerebral hemorrhage affecting left dominant side `HCC` `ESR` `COM`

I69.163 Other paralytic syndrome following nontraumatic intracerebral hemorrhage affecting right non-dominant side `HCC` `ESR` `COM`

I69.164 Other paralytic syndrome following nontraumatic intracerebral hemorrhage affecting left non-dominant side `HCC` `ESR` `COM`

I69.165 Other paralytic syndrome following nontraumatic intracerebral hemorrhage, bilateral `HCC` `ESR` `COM`

I69.169 Other paralytic syndrome following nontraumatic intracerebral hemorrhage affecting unspecified side `HCC` `ESR` `COM`

✓6ᵗʰ **I69.19** Other sequelae of nontraumatic intracerebral hemorrhage

I69.190 Apraxia following nontraumatic intracerebral hemorrhage

I69.191 Dysphagia following nontraumatic intracerebral hemorrhage
Use additional code to identify the type of dysphagia, if known
▶(R13.11-R13.19)◀

I69.192 Facial weakness following nontraumatic intracerebral hemorrhage
Facial droop following nontraumatic intracerebral hemorrhage

I69.193 Ataxia following nontraumatic intracerebral hemorrhage

I69.198 Other sequelae of nontraumatic intracerebral hemorrhage
Alteration of sensations following nontraumatic intracerebral hemorrhage
Disturbance of vision following nontraumatic intracerebral hemorrhage
Use additional code to identify the sequelae

✓5ᵗʰ **I69.2** Sequelae of other nontraumatic intracranial hemorrhage

I69.20 Unspecified sequelae of other nontraumatic intracranial hemorrhage

✓6ᵗʰ **I69.21** Cognitive deficits following other nontraumatic intracranial hemorrhage

I69.210 Attention and concentration deficit following other nontraumatic intracranial hemorrhage

I69.211 Memory deficit following other nontraumatic intracranial hemorrhage

I69.212 Visuospatial deficit and spatial neglect following other nontraumatic intracranial hemorrhage

I69.213   Psychomotor deficit following other nontraumatic intracranial hemorrhage

I69.214   Frontal lobe and executive function deficit following other nontraumatic intracranial hemorrhage

I69.215   Cognitive social or emotional deficit following other nontraumatic intracranial hemorrhage

I69.218   Other symptoms and signs involving cognitive functions following other nontraumatic intracranial hemorrhage

I69.219   Unspecified symptoms and signs involving cognitive functions following other nontraumatic intracranial hemorrhage

✓6ᵗʰ   **I69.22**   Speech and language deficits following other nontraumatic intracranial hemorrhage

I69.220   Aphasia following other nontraumatic intracranial hemorrhage

I69.221   Dysphasia following other nontraumatic intracranial hemorrhage

I69.222   Dysarthria following other nontraumatic intracranial hemorrhage

I69.223   Fluency disorder following other nontraumatic intracranial hemorrhage
Stuttering following other nontraumatic intracranial hemorrhage

I69.228   Other speech and language deficits following other nontraumatic intracranial hemorrhage

✓6ᵗʰ   **I69.23**   Monoplegia of upper limb following other nontraumatic intracranial hemorrhage
AHA: 2017,1Q,47

I69.231   Monoplegia of upper limb following other nontraumatic intracranial hemorrhage affecting right dominant side   HCC ESR COM

I69.232   Monoplegia of upper limb following other nontraumatic intracranial hemorrhage affecting left dominant side   HCC ESR COM

I69.233   Monoplegia of upper limb following other nontraumatic intracranial hemorrhage affecting right non-dominant side   HCC ESR COM

I69.234   Monoplegia of upper limb following other nontraumatic intracranial hemorrhage affecting left non-dominant side   HCC ESR COM

I69.239   Monoplegia of upper limb following other nontraumatic intracranial hemorrhage affecting unspecified side   HCC ESR COM

✓6ᵗʰ   **I69.24**   Monoplegia of lower limb following other nontraumatic intracranial hemorrhage
AHA: 2017,1Q,47

I69.241   Monoplegia of lower limb following other nontraumatic intracranial hemorrhage affecting right dominant side   HCC ESR COM

I69.242   Monoplegia of lower limb following other nontraumatic intracranial hemorrhage affecting left dominant side   HCC ESR COM

I69.243   Monoplegia of lower limb following other nontraumatic intracranial hemorrhage affecting right non-dominant side   HCC ESR COM

I69.244   Monoplegia of lower limb following other nontraumatic intracranial hemorrhage affecting left non-dominant side   HCC ESR COM

I69.249   Monoplegia of lower limb following other nontraumatic intracranial hemorrhage affecting unspecified side   HCC ESR COM

✓6ᵗʰ   **I69.25**   Hemiplegia and hemiparesis following other nontraumatic intracranial hemorrhage
AHA: 2015,1Q,25

I69.251   Hemiplegia and hemiparesis following other nontraumatic intracranial hemorrhage affecting right dominant side   HCC ESR COM

I69.252   Hemiplegia and hemiparesis following other nontraumatic intracranial hemorrhage affecting left dominant side   HCC ESR COM

I69.253   Hemiplegia and hemiparesis following other nontraumatic intracranial hemorrhage affecting right non-dominant side   HCC ESR COM

I69.254   Hemiplegia and hemiparesis following other nontraumatic intracranial hemorrhage affecting left non-dominant side   HCC ESR COM

I69.259   Hemiplegia and hemiparesis following other nontraumatic intracranial hemorrhage affecting unspecified side   HCC ESR COM

✓6ᵗʰ   **I69.26**   Other paralytic syndrome following other nontraumatic intracranial hemorrhage
Use additional code to identify type of paralytic syndrome, such as:
locked-in state (G83.5)
quadriplegia (G82.5-)
EXCLUDES 1   hemiplegia/hemiparesis following other nontraumatic intracranial hemorrhage (I69.25-)
monoplegia of lower limb following other nontraumatic intracranial hemorrhage (I69.24-)
monoplegia of upper limb following other nontraumatic intracranial hemorrhage (I69.23-)

I69.261   Other paralytic syndrome following other nontraumatic intracranial hemorrhage affecting right dominant side   HCC ESR COM

I69.262   Other paralytic syndrome following other nontraumatic intracranial hemorrhage affecting left dominant side   HCC ESR COM

I69.263   Other paralytic syndrome following other nontraumatic intracranial hemorrhage affecting right non-dominant side   HCC ESR COM

I69.264   Other paralytic syndrome following other nontraumatic intracranial hemorrhage affecting left non-dominant side   HCC ESR COM

I69.265   Other paralytic syndrome following other nontraumatic intracranial hemorrhage, bilateral   HCC ESR COM

I69.269   Other paralytic syndrome following other nontraumatic intracranial hemorrhage affecting unspecified side   HCC ESR COM

✓6ᵗʰ   **I69.29**   Other sequelae of other nontraumatic intracranial hemorrhage

I69.290   Apraxia following other nontraumatic intracranial hemorrhage

I69.291   Dysphagia following other nontraumatic intracranial hemorrhage
Use additional code to identify the type of dysphagia, if known
▶(R13.11-R13.19)◀

I69.292   Facial weakness following other nontraumatic intracranial hemorrhage
Facial droop following other nontraumatic intracranial hemorrhage

I69.293   Ataxia following other nontraumatic intracranial hemorrhage

I69.298   Other sequelae of other nontraumatic intracranial hemorrhage
Alteration of sensation following other nontraumatic intracranial hemorrhage
Disturbance of vision following other nontraumatic intracranial hemorrhage
Use additional code to identify the sequelae

☑ Additional Character Required   ✓x7ᵗʰ Placeholder Alert   Manifestation   Unspecified Dx   Q QPP   UPD Unacceptable PDx

Chapter 9. Diseases of the Circulatory System

✓5ᵗʰ **I69.3 Sequelae of** cerebral infarction
Sequelae of stroke NOS
AHA: 2013,4Q,127-128; 2012,4Q,92,94

I69.30 Unspecified sequelae of cerebral infarction

✓6ᵗʰ **I69.31 Cognitive** deficits following cerebral infarction

I69.310 Attention and concentration deficit following cerebral infarction

I69.311 Memory deficit following cerebral infarction

I69.312 Visuospatial deficit and spatial neglect following cerebral infarction

I69.313 Psychomotor deficit following cerebral infarction

I69.314 Frontal lobe and executive function deficit following cerebral infarction

I69.315 Cognitive social or emotional deficit following cerebral infarction

I69.318 Other symptoms and signs involving cognitive functions following cerebral infarction

I69.319 Unspecified symptoms and signs involving cognitive functions following cerebral infarction

✓6ᵗʰ **I69.32 Speech and language deficits** following cerebral infarction

dysphasia

I69.320 Aphasia following cerebral infarction

I69.321 Dysphasia following cerebral infarction
AHA: 2012,4Q,91

I69.322 Dysarthria following cerebral infarction
EXCLUDES 2   transient ischemic attack (TIA) (G45.9)

I69.323 Fluency disorder following cerebral infarction
Stuttering following cerebral infarction

I69.328 Other speech and language deficits following cerebral infarction

✓6ᵗʰ **I69.33 Monoplegia of upper limb** following cerebral infarction
AHA: 2017,1Q,47

I69.331 Monoplegia of upper limb following cerebral infarction affecting right dominant side   HCC ESR COM

I69.332 Monoplegia of upper limb following cerebral infarction affecting left dominant side   HCC ESR COM

I69.333 Monoplegia of upper limb following cerebral infarction affecting right non-dominant side   HCC ESR COM

I69.334 Monoplegia of upper limb following cerebral infarction affecting left non-dominant side   HCC ESR COM

I69.339 Monoplegia of upper limb following cerebral infarction affecting unspecified side   HCC ESR COM

✓6ᵗʰ **I69.34 Monoplegia of lower limb** following cerebral infarction
AHA: 2017,1Q,47

I69.341 Monoplegia of lower limb following cerebral infarction affecting right dominant side   HCC ESR COM

I69.342 Monoplegia of lower limb following cerebral infarction affecting left dominant side   HCC ESR COM

I69.343 Monoplegia of lower limb following cerebral infarction affecting right non-dominant side   HCC ESR COM

I69.344 Monoplegia of lower limb following cerebral infarction affecting left non-dominant side   HCC ESR COM

I69.349 Monoplegia of lower limb following cerebral infarction affecting unspecified side   HCC ESR COM

✓6ᵗʰ **I69.35 Hemiplegia and hemiparesis** following cerebral infarction
AHA: 2015,1Q,25

I69.351 Hemiplegia and hemiparesis following cerebral infarction affecting right dominant side   HCC ESR COM
EXCLUDES 2   transient ischemic attack (TIA) (G45.9)

I69.352 Hemiplegia and hemiparesis following cerebral infarction affecting left dominant side   HCC ESR COM

I69.353 Hemiplegia and hemiparesis following cerebral infarction affecting right non-dominant side   HCC ESR COM

I69.354 Hemiplegia and hemiparesis following cerebral infarction affecting left non-dominant side   HCC ESR COM
AHA: 2012,4Q,91

I69.359 Hemiplegia and hemiparesis following cerebral infarction affecting unspecified side   HCC ESR COM

✓6ᵗʰ **I69.36 Other paralytic syndrome** following cerebral infarction
Use additional code to identify type of paralytic syndrome, such as:
locked-in state (G83.5)
quadriplegia (G82.5-)
EXCLUDES 1   hemiplegia/hemiparesis following cerebral infarction (I69.35-)
monoplegia of lower limb following cerebral infarction (I69.34-)
monoplegia of upper limb following cerebral infarction (I69.33-)

I69.361 Other paralytic syndrome following cerebral infarction affecting right dominant side   HCC ESR COM

I69.362 Other paralytic syndrome following cerebral infarction affecting left dominant side   HCC ESR COM

I69.363 Other paralytic syndrome following cerebral infarction affecting right non-dominant side   HCC ESR COM

I69.364 Other paralytic syndrome following cerebral infarction affecting left non-dominant side   HCC ESR COM

I69.365 Other paralytic syndrome following cerebral infarction, bilateral   HCC ESR COM

I69.369 Other paralytic syndrome following cerebral infarction affecting unspecified side   HCC ESR COM

✓6ᵗʰ **I69.39 Other sequelae of cerebral infarction**

I69.390 Apraxia following cerebral infarction

I69.391 Dysphagia following cerebral infarction
Use additional code to identify the type of dysphagia, if known
▶(R13.11-R13.19)◀

dysphagia

I69.392 Facial weakness following cerebral infarction
Facial droop following cerebral infarction

I69.393 Ataxia following cerebral infarction

I69.398 Other sequelae of cerebral infarction
Alteration of sensation following cerebral infarction
Disturbance of vision following cerebral infarction
Use additional code to identify the sequelae
AHA: 2020,2Q,29

✓5ᵗʰ **I69.8 Sequelae of other** cerebrovascular diseases
EXCLUDES 1   sequelae of traumatic intracranial injury (S06.-)

I69.80 Unspecified sequelae of other cerebrovascular disease

✓6ᵗʰ **I69.81 Cognitive deficits following other cerebrovascular** disease

I69.810 Attention and concentration deficit following other cerebrovascular disease

I69.811 Memory deficit following other cerebrovascular disease

I69.812 Visuospatial deficit and spatial neglect following other cerebrovascular disease

I69.813 Psychomotor deficit following other cerebrovascular disease

I69.814 Frontal lobe and executive function deficit following other cerebrovascular disease

I69.815 Cognitive social or emotional deficit following other cerebrovascular disease

I69.818   Other symptoms and signs involving cognitive functions following other cerebrovascular disease

I69.819   Unspecified symptoms and signs involving cognitive functions following other cerebrovascular disease

✓6ᵗʰ **I69.82**   Speech and language deficits following other cerebrovascular disease

I69.820   Aphasia following other cerebrovascular disease

I69.821   Dysphasia following other cerebrovascular disease

I69.822   Dysarthria following other cerebrovascular disease

I69.823   Fluency disorder following other cerebrovascular disease
Stuttering following other cerebrovascular disease

I69.828   Other speech and language deficits following other cerebrovascular disease
AHA: 2019,3Q,8

✓6ᵗʰ **I69.83**   Monoplegia of upper limb following other cerebrovascular disease
AHA: 2017,1Q,47

I69.831   Monoplegia of upper limb following other cerebrovascular disease affecting right dominant side   HCC ESR COM

I69.832   Monoplegia of upper limb following other cerebrovascular disease affecting left dominant side   HCC ESR COM

I69.833   Monoplegia of upper limb following other cerebrovascular disease affecting right non-dominant side   HCC ESR COM

I69.834   Monoplegia of upper limb following other cerebrovascular disease affecting left non-dominant side   HCC ESR COM

I69.839   Monoplegia of upper limb following other cerebrovascular disease affecting unspecified side   HCC ESR COM

✓6ᵗʰ **I69.84**   Monoplegia of lower limb following other cerebrovascular disease
AHA: 2017,1Q,47

I69.841   Monoplegia of lower limb following other cerebrovascular disease affecting right dominant side   HCC ESR COM

I69.842   Monoplegia of lower limb following other cerebrovascular disease affecting left dominant side   HCC ESR COM

I69.843   Monoplegia of lower limb following other cerebrovascular disease affecting right non-dominant side   HCC ESR COM

I69.844   Monoplegia of lower limb following other cerebrovascular disease affecting left non-dominant side   HCC ESR COM

I69.849   Monoplegia of lower limb following other cerebrovascular disease affecting unspecified side   HCC ESR COM

✓6ᵗʰ **I69.85**   Hemiplegia and hemiparesis following other cerebrovascular disease
AHA: 2015,1Q,25

I69.851   Hemiplegia and hemiparesis following other cerebrovascular disease affecting right dominant side   HCC ESR COM

I69.852   Hemiplegia and hemiparesis following other cerebrovascular disease affecting left dominant side   HCC ESR COM

I69.853   Hemiplegia and hemiparesis following other cerebrovascular disease affecting right non-dominant side   HCC ESR COM

I69.854   Hemiplegia and hemiparesis following other cerebrovascular disease affecting left non-dominant side   HCC ESR COM

I69.859   Hemiplegia and hemiparesis following other cerebrovascular disease affecting unspecified side   HCC ESR COM

✓6ᵗʰ **I69.86**   Other paralytic syndrome following other cerebrovascular disease
Use additional code to identify type of paralytic syndrome, such as:
locked-in state (G83.5)
quadriplegia (G82.5-)
EXCLUDES 1   hemiplegia/hemiparesis following other cerebrovascular disease (I69.85-)
monoplegia of lower limb following other cerebrovascular disease (I69.84-)
monoplegia of upper limb following other cerebrovascular disease (I69.83-)

I69.861   Other paralytic syndrome following other cerebrovascular disease affecting right dominant side   HCC ESR COM

I69.862   Other paralytic syndrome following other cerebrovascular disease affecting left dominant side   HCC ESR COM

I69.863   Other paralytic syndrome following other cerebrovascular disease affecting right non-dominant side   HCC ESR COM

I69.864   Other paralytic syndrome following other cerebrovascular disease affecting left non-dominant side   HCC ESR COM

I69.865   Other paralytic syndrome following other cerebrovascular disease, bilateral   HCC ESR COM

I69.869   Other paralytic syndrome following other cerebrovascular disease affecting unspecified side   HCC ESR COM

✓6ᵗʰ **I69.89**   Other sequelae of other cerebrovascular disease

I69.890   Apraxia following other cerebrovascular disease

I69.891   Dysphagia following other cerebrovascular disease
Use additional code to identify the type of dysphagia, if known
▶(R13.11-R13.19)◀

I69.892   Facial weakness following other cerebrovascular disease
Facial droop following other cerebrovascular disease

I69.893   Ataxia following other cerebrovascular disease

I69.898   Other sequelae of other cerebrovascular disease
Alteration of sensation following other cerebrovascular disease
Disturbance of vision following other cerebrovascular disease
Use additional code to identify the sequelae

✓5ᵗʰ **I69.9**   Sequelae of unspecified cerebrovascular diseases
EXCLUDES 1   sequelae of stroke (I69.3)
sequelae of traumatic intracranial injury (S06.-)

I69.90   Unspecified sequelae of unspecified cerebrovascular disease

✓6ᵗʰ **I69.91**   Cognitive deficits following unspecified cerebrovascular disease

I69.910   Attention and concentration deficit following unspecified cerebrovascular disease

I69.911   Memory deficit following unspecified cerebrovascular disease

I69.912   Visuospatial deficit and spatial neglect following unspecified cerebrovascular disease

I69.913   Psychomotor deficit following unspecified cerebrovascular disease

I69.914   Frontal lobe and executive function deficit following unspecified cerebrovascular disease

I69.915   Cognitive social or emotional deficit following unspecified cerebrovascular disease

I69.918   Other symptoms and signs involving cognitive functions following unspecified cerebrovascular disease

I69.919   Unspecified symptoms and signs involving cognitive functions following unspecified cerebrovascular disease

✓6ᵗʰ I69.92 Speech and language deficits following unspecified cerebrovascular disease

   I69.920 Aphasia following unspecified cerebrovascular disease

   I69.921 Dysphasia following unspecified cerebrovascular disease

   I69.922 Dysarthria following unspecified cerebrovascular disease

   I69.923 Fluency disorder following unspecified cerebrovascular disease

      Stuttering following unspecified cerebrovascular disease

   I69.928 Other speech and language deficits following unspecified cerebrovascular disease

✓6ᵗʰ I69.93 Monoplegia of upper limb following unspecified cerebrovascular disease

   AHA: 2017,1Q,47

   I69.931 Monoplegia of upper limb following unspecified cerebrovascular disease affecting right dominant side HCC ESR COM

   I69.932 Monoplegia of upper limb following unspecified cerebrovascular disease affecting left dominant side HCC ESR COM

   I69.933 Monoplegia of upper limb following unspecified cerebrovascular disease affecting right non-dominant side HCC ESR COM

   I69.934 Monoplegia of upper limb following unspecified cerebrovascular disease affecting left non-dominant side HCC ESR COM

   I69.939 Monoplegia of upper limb following unspecified cerebrovascular disease affecting unspecified side HCC ESR COM

✓6ᵗʰ I69.94 Monoplegia of lower limb following unspecified cerebrovascular disease

   AHA: 2017,1Q,47

   I69.941 Monoplegia of lower limb following unspecified cerebrovascular disease affecting right dominant side HCC ESR COM

   I69.942 Monoplegia of lower limb following unspecified cerebrovascular disease affecting left dominant side HCC ESR COM

   I69.943 Monoplegia of lower limb following unspecified cerebrovascular disease affecting right non-dominant side HCC ESR COM

   I69.944 Monoplegia of lower limb following unspecified cerebrovascular disease affecting left non-dominant side HCC ESR COM

   I69.949 Monoplegia of lower limb following unspecified cerebrovascular disease affecting unspecified side HCC ESR COM

✓6ᵗʰ I69.95 Hemiplegia and hemiparesis following unspecified cerebrovascular disease

   AHA: 2015,1Q,25

   I69.951 Hemiplegia and hemiparesis following unspecified cerebrovascular disease affecting right dominant side HCC ESR COM

   I69.952 Hemiplegia and hemiparesis following unspecified cerebrovascular disease affecting left dominant side HCC ESR COM

   I69.953 Hemiplegia and hemiparesis following unspecified cerebrovascular disease affecting right non-dominant side HCC ESR COM

   I69.954 Hemiplegia and hemiparesis following unspecified cerebrovascular disease affecting left non-dominant side HCC ESR COM

   I69.959 Hemiplegia and hemiparesis following unspecified cerebrovascular disease affecting unspecified side HCC ESR COM

✓6ᵗʰ I69.96 Other paralytic syndrome following unspecified cerebrovascular disease

   Use additional code to identify type of paralytic syndrome, such as:

   locked-in state (G83.5)

   quadriplegia (G82.5-)

   EXCLUDES 1 *hemiplegia/hemiparesis following unspecified cerebrovascular disease (I69.95-)*

      monoplegia of lower limb following unspecified cerebrovascular disease (I69.94-)

      monoplegia of upper limb following unspecified cerebrovascular disease (I69.93-)

   I69.961 Other paralytic syndrome following unspecified cerebrovascular disease affecting right dominant side HCC ESR COM

   I69.962 Other paralytic syndrome following unspecified cerebrovascular disease affecting left dominant side HCC ESR COM

   I69.963 Other paralytic syndrome following unspecified cerebrovascular disease affecting right non-dominant side HCC ESR COM

   I69.964 Other paralytic syndrome following unspecified cerebrovascular disease affecting left non-dominant side HCC ESR COM

   I69.965 Other paralytic syndrome following unspecified cerebrovascular disease, bilateral HCC ESR COM

   I69.969 Other paralytic syndrome following unspecified cerebrovascular disease affecting unspecified side HCC ESR COM

✓6ᵗʰ I69.99 Other sequelae of unspecified cerebrovascular disease

   I69.990 Apraxia following unspecified cerebrovascular disease

   I69.991 Dysphagia following unspecified cerebrovascular disease

      Use additional code to identify the type of dysphagia, if known ▶(R13.11-R13.19)◀

   I69.992 Facial weakness following unspecified cerebrovascular disease

      Facial droop following unspecified cerebrovascular disease

   I69.993 Ataxia following unspecified cerebrovascular disease

   I69.998 Other sequelae following unspecified cerebrovascular disease

      Alteration in sensation following unspecified cerebrovascular disease

      Disturbance of vision following unspecified cerebrovascular disease

      Use additional code to identify the sequelae

Diseases of arteries, arterioles and capillaries (I70-I79)

✓4ᵗʰ I70 Atherosclerosis

     INCLUDES   arterial degeneration
            arteriolosclerosis
            arteriosclerosis
            arteriosclerotic vascular disease
            arteriovascular degeneration
            atheroma
            endarteritis deformans or obliterans
            senile arteritis
            senile endarteritis
            vascular degeneration

     Use additional code to identify:
       exposure to environmental tobacco smoke (Z77.22)
       history of tobacco dependence (Z87.891)
       occupational exposure to environmental tobacco smoke (Z57.31)
       tobacco dependence (F17.-)
       tobacco use (Z72.0)

     EXCLUDES 2   *arteriosclerotic cardiovascular disease (I25.1-)*
            arteriosclerotic heart disease (I25.1-)
            atheroembolism (I75.-)
            cerebral atherosclerosis (I67.2)
            coronary atherosclerosis (I25.1-)
            mesenteric atherosclerosis (K55.1)
            precerebral atherosclerosis (I67.2)
            primary pulmonary atherosclerosis (I27.0)

I70.0 Atherosclerosis of aorta   HCC ESR A

I70.1 Atherosclerosis of renal artery   HCC ESR A
     Goldblatt's kidney
     EXCLUDES 2   *atherosclerosis of renal arterioles (I12.-)*

✓5ᵗʰ I70.2 Atherosclerosis of native arteries of the extremities
     Mönckeberg's (medial) sclerosis
     Use additional code, if applicable, to identify chronic total
       occlusion of artery of extremity (I70.92)
     EXCLUDES 2   *atherosclerosis of bypass graft of extremities*
            (I70.30-I70.79)

     AHA: 2020,4Q,98; 2018,3Q,4; 2018,2Q,7

     ✓6ᵗʰ I70.20 Unspecified atherosclerosis of native arteries of extremities

       I70.201 Unspecified atherosclerosis of native arteries of extremities, right leg   HCC ESR A

       I70.202 Unspecified atherosclerosis of native arteries of extremities, left leg   HCC ESR A

       I70.203 Unspecified atherosclerosis of native arteries of extremities, bilateral legs   HCC ESR A

       I70.208 Unspecified atherosclerosis of native arteries of extremities, other extremity   HCC ESR A

       I70.209 Unspecified atherosclerosis of native arteries of extremities, unspecified extremity   HCC ESR A

     ✓6ᵗʰ I70.21 Atherosclerosis of native arteries of extremities with intermittent claudication

       I70.211 Atherosclerosis of native arteries of extremities with intermittent claudication, right leg   HCC ESR A

       I70.212 Atherosclerosis of native arteries of extremities with intermittent claudication, left leg   HCC ESR A

       I70.213 Atherosclerosis of native arteries of extremities with intermittent claudication, bilateral legs   HCC ESR A

       I70.218 Atherosclerosis of native arteries of extremities with intermittent claudication, other extremity   HCC ESR A

       I70.219 Atherosclerosis of native arteries of extremities with intermittent claudication, unspecified extremity   HCC ESR A

     ✓6ᵗʰ I70.22 Atherosclerosis of native arteries of extremities with rest pain

       INCLUDES   any condition classifiable to I70.21-
           chronic limb-threatening ischemia NOS of native arteries of extremities
           chronic limb-threatening ischemia of native arteries of extremities with rest pain
           critical limb ischemia NOS of native arteries of extremities
           critical limb ischemia of native arteries of extremities with rest pain

       I70.221 Atherosclerosis of native arteries of extremities with rest pain, right leg   HCC ESR A

       I70.222 Atherosclerosis of native arteries of extremities with rest pain, left leg   HCC ESR A

       I70.223 Atherosclerosis of native arteries of extremities with rest pain, bilateral legs   HCC ESR A

       I70.228 Atherosclerosis of native arteries of extremities with rest pain, other extremity   HCC ESR A

       I70.229 Atherosclerosis of native arteries of extremities with rest pain, unspecified extremity   HCC ESR A

     ✓6ᵗʰ I70.23 Atherosclerosis of native arteries of right leg with ulceration

       INCLUDES   any condition classifiable to I70.211 and I70.221
           chronic limb-threatening ischemia of native arteries of right leg with ulceration
           critical limb ischemia of native arteries of right leg with ulceration

       Use additional code to identify severity of ulcer (L97.-)

       I70.231 Atherosclerosis of native arteries of right leg with ulceration of thigh   HCC Rx ESR COM A

       I70.232 Atherosclerosis of native arteries of right leg with ulceration of calf   HCC Rx ESR COM A

       I70.233 Atherosclerosis of native arteries of right leg with ulceration of ankle   HCC Rx ESR COM A

       I70.234 Atherosclerosis of native arteries of right leg with ulceration of heel and midfoot   HCC Rx ESR COM A
           Atherosclerosis of native arteries of right leg with ulceration of plantar surface of midfoot

       I70.235 Atherosclerosis of native arteries of right leg with ulceration of other part of foot   HCC Rx ESR COM A
           Atherosclerosis of native arteries of right leg extremities with ulceration of toe

       I70.238 Atherosclerosis of native arteries of right leg with ulceration of other part of lower leg   HCC Rx ESR COM A

       I70.239 Atherosclerosis of native arteries of right leg with ulceration of unspecified site   HCC Rx ESR COM A

     ✓6ᵗʰ I70.24 Atherosclerosis of native arteries of left leg with ulceration

       INCLUDES   any condition classifiable to I70.212 and I70.222
           chronic limb-threatening ischemia of native arteries of left leg with ulceration
           critical limb ischemia of native arteries of left leg with ulceration

       Use additional code to identify severity of ulcer (L97.-)

       I70.241 Atherosclerosis of native arteries of left leg with ulceration of thigh   HCC Rx ESR COM A

       I70.242 Atherosclerosis of native arteries of left leg with ulceration of calf   HCC Rx ESR COM A

☑ Additional Character Required   ✓x7ᵗʰ Placeholder Alert   Manifestation   Unspecified Dx   Q QPP   UPD Unacceptable PDx

I70.243 Atherosclerosis of native arteries of left leg with ulceration of ankle `HCC` `Rx` `ESR` `COM` `A`

I70.244 Atherosclerosis of native arteries of left leg with ulceration of heel and midfoot `HCC` `Rx` `ESR` `COM` `A`
Atherosclerosis of native arteries of left leg with ulceration of plantar surface of midfoot

I70.245 Atherosclerosis of native arteries of left leg with ulceration of other part of foot `HCC` `Rx` `ESR` `COM` `A`
Atherosclerosis of native arteries of left leg extremities with ulceration of toe

I70.248 Atherosclerosis of native arteries of left leg with ulceration of other part of lower leg `HCC` `Rx` `ESR` `COM` `A`

I70.249 Atherosclerosis of native arteries of left leg with ulceration of unspecified site `HCC` `Rx` `ESR` `COM` `A`

I70.25 Atherosclerosis of native arteries of other extremities with ulceration `HCC` `Rx` `ESR` `COM` `A`
INCLUDES any condition classifiable to I70.218 and I70.228
Use additional code to identify the severity of the ulcer (L98.49-)

✓6ᵗʰ **I70.26** Atherosclerosis of native arteries of extremities with gangrene
INCLUDES any condition classifiable to I70.21-, I70.22-, I70.23-, I70.24-, and I70.25-
chronic limb-threatening ischemia of native arteries of extremities with gangrene
critical limb ischemia of native arteries of extremities with gangrene
Use additional code to identify the severity of any ulcer (L97.-, L98.49-), if applicable

I70.261 Atherosclerosis of native arteries of extremities with gangrene, right leg `HCC` `ESR` `COM` `A`

I70.262 Atherosclerosis of native arteries of extremities with gangrene, left leg `HCC` `ESR` `COM` `A`

I70.263 Atherosclerosis of native arteries of extremities with gangrene, bilateral legs `HCC` `ESR` `COM` `A`

I70.268 Atherosclerosis of native arteries of extremities with gangrene, other extremity `HCC` `ESR` `COM` `A`

I70.269 Atherosclerosis of native arteries of extremities with gangrene, unspecified extremity `HCC` `ESR` `COM` `A`

✓6ᵗʰ **I70.29** Other atherosclerosis of native arteries of extremities

I70.291 Other atherosclerosis of native arteries of extremities, right leg `HCC` `ESR` `A`

I70.292 Other atherosclerosis of native arteries of extremities, left leg `HCC` `ESR` `A`

I70.293 Other atherosclerosis of native arteries of extremities, bilateral legs `HCC` `ESR` `A`

I70.298 Other atherosclerosis of native arteries of extremities, other extremity `HCC` `ESR` `A`

I70.299 Other atherosclerosis of native arteries of extremities, unspecified extremity `HCC` `ESR` `A`

✓5ᵗʰ **I70.3** Atherosclerosis of unspecified type of bypass graft(s) of the extremities
Use additional code, if applicable, to identify chronic total occlusion of artery of extremity (I70.92)
EXCLUDES 1 embolism or thrombus of bypass graft(s) of extremities (T82.8-)
AHA: 2020,4Q,98

✓6ᵗʰ **I70.30** Unspecified atherosclerosis of unspecified type of bypass graft(s) of the extremities

I70.301 Unspecified atherosclerosis of unspecified type of bypass graft(s) of the extremities, right leg `HCC` `ESR` `A`

I70.302 Unspecified atherosclerosis of unspecified type of bypass graft(s) of the extremities, left leg `HCC` `ESR` `A`

I70.303 Unspecified atherosclerosis of unspecified type of bypass graft(s) of the extremities, bilateral legs `HCC` `ESR` `A`

I70.308 Unspecified atherosclerosis of unspecified type of bypass graft(s) of the extremities, other extremity `HCC` `ESR` `A`

I70.309 Unspecified atherosclerosis of unspecified type of bypass graft(s) of the extremities, unspecified extremity `HCC` `ESR` `A`

✓6ᵗʰ **I70.31** Atherosclerosis of unspecified type of bypass graft(s) of the extremities with intermittent claudication

I70.311 Atherosclerosis of unspecified type of bypass graft(s) of the extremities with intermittent claudication, right leg `HCC` `ESR` `A`

I70.312 Atherosclerosis of unspecified type of bypass graft(s) of the extremities with intermittent claudication, left leg `HCC` `ESR` `A`

I70.313 Atherosclerosis of unspecified type of bypass graft(s) of the extremities with intermittent claudication, bilateral legs `HCC` `ESR` `A`

I70.318 Atherosclerosis of unspecified type of bypass graft(s) of the extremities with intermittent claudication, other extremity `HCC` `ESR` `A`

I70.319 Atherosclerosis of unspecified type of bypass graft(s) of the extremities with intermittent claudication, unspecified extremity `HCC` `ESR` `A`

✓6ᵗʰ **I70.32** Atherosclerosis of unspecified type of bypass graft(s) of the extremities with rest pain
INCLUDES any condition classifiable to I70.31-
chronic limb-threatening ischemia NOS of unspecified type of bypass graft(s) of the extremities
▶chronic limb-threatening ischemia of unspecified type of bypass graft(s) of the extremities with rest pain◀
critical limb ischemia NOS of unspecified type of bypass graft(s) of the extremities
critical limb ischemia of unspecified type of bypass graft(s) of the extremities with rest pain

I70.321 Atherosclerosis of unspecified type of bypass graft(s) of the extremities with rest pain, right leg `HCC` `ESR` `A`

I70.322 Atherosclerosis of unspecified type of bypass graft(s) of the extremities with rest pain, left leg `HCC` `ESR` `A`

I70.323 Atherosclerosis of unspecified type of bypass graft(s) of the extremities with rest pain, bilateral legs `HCC` `ESR` `A`

I70.328 Atherosclerosis of unspecified type of bypass graft(s) of the extremities with rest pain, other extremity `HCC` `ESR` `A`

I70.329 Atherosclerosis of unspecified type of bypass graft(s) of the extremities with rest pain, unspecified extremity `HCC` `ESR` `A`

✓6ᵗʰ **I70.33** Atherosclerosis of unspecified type of bypass graft(s) of the right leg with ulceration
INCLUDES any condition classifiable to I70.311 and I70.321
chronic limb-threatening ischemia of unspecified type of bypass graft(s) of the right leg with ulceration
critical limb ischemia of unspecified type of bypass graft(s) of the right leg with ulceration
Use additional code to identify severity of ulcer (L97.-)

I70.331 Atherosclerosis of unspecified type of bypass graft(s) of the right leg with ulceration of thigh `HCC` `Rx` `ESR` `COM` `A`

I70.332 Atherosclerosis of unspecified type of bypass graft(s) of the right leg with ulceration of calf `HCC` `Rx` `ESR` `COM` `A`

I70.333 Atherosclerosis of unspecified type of bypass graft(s) of the right leg with ulceration of ankle `HCC` `Rx` `ESR` `COM` `A`

I70.334 Atherosclerosis of unspecified type of bypass graft(s) of the right leg with ulceration of heel and midfoot `HCC` `Rx` `ESR` `COM` `A`
Atherosclerosis of unspecified type of bypass graft(s) of right leg with ulceration of plantar surface of midfoot

I70.335 Atherosclerosis of unspecified type of bypass graft(s) of the right leg with ulceration of other part of foot `HCC` `Rx` `ESR` `COM` `A`
Atherosclerosis of unspecified type of bypass graft(s) of the right leg with ulceration of toe

I70.338 Atherosclerosis of unspecified type of bypass graft(s) of the right leg with ulceration of other part of lower leg `HCC` `Rx` `ESR` `COM` `A`

I70.339 Atherosclerosis of unspecified type of bypass graft(s) of the right leg with ulceration of unspecified site `HCC` `Rx` `ESR` `COM` `A`

√6ᵗʰ I70.34 Atherosclerosis of unspecified type of bypass graft(s) of the left leg with ulceration
INCLUDES any condition classifiable to I70.312 and I70.322
chronic limb-threatening ischemia of unspecified type of bypass graft(s) of the left leg with ulceration
critical limb ischemia of unspecified type of bypass graft(s) of the left leg with ulceration
Use additional code to identify severity of ulcer (L97.-)

I70.341 Atherosclerosis of unspecified type of bypass graft(s) of the left leg with ulceration of thigh `HCC` `Rx` `ESR` `COM` `A`

I70.342 Atherosclerosis of unspecified type of bypass graft(s) of the left leg with ulceration of calf `HCC` `Rx` `ESR` `COM` `A`

I70.343 Atherosclerosis of unspecified type of bypass graft(s) of the left leg with ulceration of ankle `HCC` `Rx` `ESR` `COM` `A`

I70.344 Atherosclerosis of unspecified type of bypass graft(s) of the left leg with ulceration of heel and midfoot `HCC` `Rx` `ESR` `COM` `A`
Atherosclerosis of unspecified type of bypass graft(s) of left leg with ulceration of plantar surface of midfoot

I70.345 Atherosclerosis of unspecified type of bypass graft(s) of the left leg with ulceration of other part of foot `HCC` `Rx` `ESR` `COM` `A`
Atherosclerosis of unspecified type of bypass graft(s) of the left leg with ulceration of toe

I70.348 Atherosclerosis of unspecified type of bypass graft(s) of the left leg with ulceration of other part of lower leg `HCC` `Rx` `ESR` `COM` `A`

I70.349 Atherosclerosis of unspecified type of bypass graft(s) of the left leg with ulceration of unspecified site `HCC` `Rx` `ESR` `COM` `A`

I70.35 Atherosclerosis of unspecified type of bypass graft(s) of other extremity with ulceration `HCC` `Rx` `ESR` `COM` `A`
INCLUDES any condition classifiable to I70.318 and I70.328
Use additional code to identify severity of ulcer (L98.49-)

√6ᵗʰ I70.36 Atherosclerosis of unspecified type of bypass graft(s) of the extremities with gangrene
INCLUDES any condition classifiable to I70.31-, I70.32-, I70.33-, I70.34-, I70.35
chronic limb-threatening ischemia of unspecified type of bypass graft(s) of the extremities with gangrene
critical limb ischemia of unspecified type of bypass graft(s) of the extremities with gangrene
Use additional code to identify the severity of any ulcer (L97.-, L98.49-), if applicable

I70.361 Atherosclerosis of unspecified type of bypass graft(s) of the extremities with gangrene, right leg `HCC` `ESR` `COM` `A`

I70.362 Atherosclerosis of unspecified type of bypass graft(s) of the extremities with gangrene, left leg `HCC` `ESR` `COM` `A`

I70.363 Atherosclerosis of unspecified type of bypass graft(s) of the extremities with gangrene, bilateral legs `HCC` `ESR` `COM` `A`

I70.368 Atherosclerosis of unspecified type of bypass graft(s) of the extremities with gangrene, other extremity `HCC` `ESR` `COM` `A`

I70.369 Atherosclerosis of unspecified type of bypass graft(s) of the extremities with gangrene, unspecified extremity `HCC` `ESR` `COM` `A`

√6ᵗʰ I70.39 Other atherosclerosis of unspecified type of bypass graft(s) of the extremities

I70.391 Other atherosclerosis of unspecified type of bypass graft(s) of the extremities, right leg `HCC` `ESR` `A`

I70.392 Other atherosclerosis of unspecified type of bypass graft(s) of the extremities, left leg `HCC` `ESR` `A`

I70.393 Other atherosclerosis of unspecified type of bypass graft(s) of the extremities, bilateral legs `HCC` `ESR` `A`

I70.398 Other atherosclerosis of unspecified type of bypass graft(s) of the extremities, other extremity `HCC` `ESR` `A`

I70.399 Other atherosclerosis of unspecified type of bypass graft(s) of the extremities, unspecified extremity `HCC` `ESR` `A`

√5ᵗʰ I70.4 Atherosclerosis of autologous vein bypass graft(s) of the extremities
Use additional code, if applicable, to identify chronic total occlusion of artery of extremity (I70.92)
AHA: 2020,4Q,98

√6ᵗʰ I70.40 Unspecified atherosclerosis of autologous vein bypass graft(s) of the extremities

I70.401 Unspecified atherosclerosis of autologous vein bypass graft(s) of the extremities, right leg `HCC` `ESR` `A`

I70.402 Unspecified atherosclerosis of autologous vein bypass graft(s) of the extremities, left leg `HCC` `ESR` `A`

I70.403 Unspecified atherosclerosis of autologous vein bypass graft(s) of the extremities, bilateral legs `HCC` `ESR` `A`

I70.408 Unspecified atherosclerosis of autologous vein bypass graft(s) of the extremities, other extremity `HCC` `ESR` `A`

I70.409 Unspecified atherosclerosis of autologous vein bypass graft(s) of the extremities, unspecified extremity `HCC` `ESR` `A`

√6ᵗʰ I70.41 Atherosclerosis of autologous vein bypass graft(s) of the extremities with intermittent claudication

I70.411 Atherosclerosis of autologous vein bypass graft(s) of the extremities with intermittent claudication, right leg `HCC` `ESR` `A`

I70.412 Atherosclerosis of autologous vein bypass graft(s) of the extremities with intermittent claudication, left leg `HCC` `ESR` `A`

I70.413 Atherosclerosis of autologous vein bypass graft(s) of the extremities with intermittent claudication, bilateral legs `HCC` `ESR` `A`

Chapter 9. Diseases of the Circulatory System

I70.418 Atherosclerosis of autologous vein bypass graft(s) of the extremities with intermittent claudication, other extremity `HCC` `ESR` `A`

I70.419 Atherosclerosis of autologous vein bypass graft(s) of the extremities with intermittent claudication, unspecified extremity `HCC` `ESR` `A`

✓6th **I70.42 Atherosclerosis of autologous vein bypass graft(s) of the extremities with rest pain**
   `INCLUDES` any condition classifiable to I70.41-
      chronic limb-threatening ischemia NOS of autologous vein bypass graft(s) of the extremities
      chronic limb-threatening ischemia of autologous vein bypass graft(s) of the extremities with rest pain
      critical limb ischemia NOS of autologous vein bypass graft(s) of the extremities
      critical limb ischemia of autologous vein bypass graft(s) of the extremities with rest pain

I70.421 Atherosclerosis of autologous vein bypass graft(s) of the extremities with rest pain, right leg `HCC` `ESR` `A`

I70.422 Atherosclerosis of autologous vein bypass graft(s) of the extremities with rest pain, left leg `HCC` `ESR` `A`

I70.423 Atherosclerosis of autologous vein bypass graft(s) of the extremities with rest pain, bilateral legs `HCC` `ESR` `A`

I70.428 Atherosclerosis of autologous vein bypass graft(s) of the extremities with rest pain, other extremity `HCC` `ESR` `A`

I70.429 Atherosclerosis of autologous vein bypass graft(s) of the extremities with rest pain, unspecified extremity `HCC` `ESR` `A`

✓6th **I70.43 Atherosclerosis of autologous vein bypass graft(s) of the right leg with ulceration**
   `INCLUDES` any condition classifiable to I70.411 and I70.421
      chronic limb-threatening ischemia of autologous vein bypass graft(s) of the right leg with ulceration
      critical limb ischemia of autologous vein bypass graft(s) of the right leg with ulceration
   Use additional code to identify severity of ulcer (L97.-)

I70.431 Atherosclerosis of autologous vein bypass graft(s) of the right leg with ulceration of thigh `HCC` `Rx` `ESR` `COM` `A`

I70.432 Atherosclerosis of autologous vein bypass graft(s) of the right leg with ulceration of calf `HCC` `Rx` `ESR` `COM` `A`

I70.433 Atherosclerosis of autologous vein bypass graft(s) of the right leg with ulceration of ankle `HCC` `Rx` `ESR` `COM` `A`

I70.434 Atherosclerosis of autologous vein bypass graft(s) of the right leg with ulceration of heel and midfoot `HCC` `Rx` `ESR` `COM` `A`
      Atherosclerosis of autologous vein bypass graft(s) of right leg with ulceration of plantar surface of midfoot

I70.435 Atherosclerosis of autologous vein bypass graft(s) of the right leg with ulceration of other part of foot `HCC` `Rx` `ESR` `COM` `A`
      Atherosclerosis of autologous vein bypass graft(s) of right leg with ulceration of toe

I70.438 Atherosclerosis of autologous vein bypass graft(s) of the right leg with ulceration of other part of lower leg `HCC` `Rx` `ESR` `COM` `A`

I70.439 Atherosclerosis of autologous vein bypass graft(s) of the right leg with ulceration of unspecified site `HCC` `Rx` `ESR` `COM` `A`

✓6th **I70.44 Atherosclerosis of autologous vein bypass graft(s) of the left leg with ulceration**
   `INCLUDES` any condition classifiable to I70.412 and I70.422
      chronic limb-threatening ischemia of autologous vein bypass graft(s) of the left leg with ulceration
      critical limb ischemia of autologous vein bypass graft(s) of the left leg with ulceration
   Use additional code to identify severity of ulcer (L97.-)

I70.441 Atherosclerosis of autologous vein bypass graft(s) of the left leg with ulceration of thigh `HCC` `Rx` `ESR` `COM` `A`

I70.442 Atherosclerosis of autologous vein bypass graft(s) of the left leg with ulceration of calf `HCC` `Rx` `ESR` `COM` `A`

I70.443 Atherosclerosis of autologous vein bypass graft(s) of the left leg with ulceration of ankle `HCC` `Rx` `ESR` `COM` `A`

I70.444 Atherosclerosis of autologous vein bypass graft(s) of the left leg with ulceration of heel and midfoot `HCC` `Rx` `ESR` `COM` `A`
      Atherosclerosis of autologous vein bypass graft(s) of left leg with ulceration of plantar surface of midfoot

I70.445 Atherosclerosis of autologous vein bypass graft(s) of the left leg with ulceration of other part of foot `HCC` `Rx` `ESR` `COM` `A`
      Atherosclerosis of autologous vein bypass graft(s) of left leg with ulceration of toe

I70.448 Atherosclerosis of autologous vein bypass graft(s) of the left leg with ulceration of other part of lower leg `HCC` `Rx` `ESR` `COM` `A`

I70.449 Atherosclerosis of autologous vein bypass graft(s) of the left leg with ulceration of unspecified site `HCC` `Rx` `ESR` `COM` `A`

I70.45 Atherosclerosis of autologous vein bypass graft(s) of other extremity with ulceration `HCC` `Rx` `ESR` `COM` `A`
   `INCLUDES` any condition classifiable to I70.418, I70.428, and I70.438
   Use additional code to identify severity of ulcer (L98.49)

✓6th **I70.46 Atherosclerosis of autologous vein bypass graft(s) of the extremities with gangrene**
   `INCLUDES` any condition classifiable to I70.41-, I70.42-, and I70.43-, I70.44-, I70.45
      chronic limb-threatening ischemia of autologous vein bypass graft(s) of the extremities with gangrene
      critical limb ischemia of autologous vein bypass graft(s) of the extremities with gangrene
   Use additional code to identify the severity of any ulcer (L97.-, L98.49-), if applicable

I70.461 Atherosclerosis of autologous vein bypass graft(s) of the extremities with gangrene, right leg `HCC` `ESR` `COM` `A`

I70.462 Atherosclerosis of autologous vein bypass graft(s) of the extremities with gangrene, left leg `HCC` `ESR` `COM` `A`

I70.463 Atherosclerosis of autologous vein bypass graft(s) of the extremities with gangrene, bilateral legs `HCC` `ESR` `COM` `A`

I70.468 Atherosclerosis of autologous vein bypass graft(s) of the extremities with gangrene, other extremity `HCC` `ESR` `COM` `A`

I70.469 Atherosclerosis of autologous vein bypass graft(s) of the extremities with gangrene, unspecified extremity `HCC` `ESR` `COM` `A`

✓6th **I70.49 Other atherosclerosis of autologous vein bypass graft(s) of the extremities**

I70.491 Other atherosclerosis of autologous vein bypass graft(s) of the extremities, right leg `HCC` `ESR` `A`

I70.492 Other atherosclerosis of autologous vein bypass graft(s) of the extremities, left leg `HCC` `ESR` `A`

`HCC` CMS-HCC   `Rx` Rx HCC   `ESR` ESRD HCC   `COM` Commercial HCC   `N` Newborn: 0   `P` Pediatric: 0-17   `M` Maternity: 9-64   `A` Adult: 15-124

688   ICD-10-CM 2023

I70.493 Other atherosclerosis of autologous vein bypass graft(s) of the extremities, bilateral legs   HCC ESR A

I70.498 Other atherosclerosis of autologous vein bypass graft(s) of the extremities, other extremity   HCC ESR A

I70.499 Other atherosclerosis of autologous vein bypass graft(s) of the extremities, unspecified extremity   HCC ESR A

√5th **I70.5** **Atherosclerosis of nonautologous biological bypass graft(s) of the extremities**

Use additional code, if applicable, to identify chronic total occlusion of artery of extremity (I70.92)

AHA: 2020,4Q,98

√6th **I70.50** **Unspecified atherosclerosis of nonautologous biological bypass graft(s) of the extremities**

I70.501 Unspecified atherosclerosis of nonautologous biological bypass graft(s) of the extremities, right leg   HCC ESR A

I70.502 Unspecified atherosclerosis of nonautologous biological bypass graft(s) of the extremities, left leg   HCC ESR A

I70.503 Unspecified atherosclerosis of nonautologous biological bypass graft(s) of the extremities, bilateral legs   HCC ESR A

I70.508 Unspecified atherosclerosis of nonautologous biological bypass graft(s) of the extremities, other extremity   HCC ESR A

I70.509 Unspecified atherosclerosis of nonautologous biological bypass graft(s) of the extremities, unspecified extremity   HCC ESR A

√6th **I70.51** **Atherosclerosis of nonautologous biological bypass graft(s) of the extremities intermittent claudication**

I70.511 Atherosclerosis of nonautologous biological bypass graft(s) of the extremities with intermittent claudication, right leg   HCC ESR A

I70.512 Atherosclerosis of nonautologous biological bypass graft(s) of the extremities with intermittent claudication, left leg   HCC ESR A

I70.513 Atherosclerosis of nonautologous biological bypass graft(s) of the extremities with intermittent claudication, bilateral legs   HCC ESR A

I70.518 Atherosclerosis of nonautologous biological bypass graft(s) of the extremities with intermittent claudication, other extremity   HCC ESR A

I70.519 Atherosclerosis of nonautologous biological bypass graft(s) of the extremities with intermittent claudication, unspecified extremity   HCC ESR A

√6th **I70.52** **Atherosclerosis of nonautologous biological bypass graft(s) of the extremities with rest pain**

INCLUDES   any condition classifiable to I70.51-
chronic limb-threatening ischemia NOS of nonautologous biological bypass graft(s) of the extremities
chronic limb-threatening ischemia of nonautologous biological bypass graft(s) of the extremities with rest pain
critical limb ischemia NOS of nonautologous biological bypass graft(s) of the extremities
critical limb ischemia of nonautologous biological bypass graft(s) of the extremities with rest pain

I70.521 Atherosclerosis of nonautologous biological bypass graft(s) of the extremities with rest pain, right leg   HCC ESR A

I70.522 Atherosclerosis of nonautologous biological bypass graft(s) of the extremities with rest pain, left leg   HCC ESR A

I70.523 Atherosclerosis of nonautologous biological bypass graft(s) of the extremities with rest pain, bilateral legs   HCC ESR A

I70.528 Atherosclerosis of nonautologous biological bypass graft(s) of the extremities with rest pain, other extremity   HCC ESR A

I70.529 Atherosclerosis of nonautologous biological bypass graft(s) of the extremities with rest pain, unspecified extremity   HCC ESR A

√6th **I70.53** **Atherosclerosis of nonautologous biological bypass graft(s) of the right leg with ulceration**

INCLUDES   any condition classifiable to I70.511 and I70.521
chronic limb-threatening ischemia of nonautologous biological bypass graft(s) of the right leg with ulceration
critical limb ischemia of nonautologous biological bypass graft(s) of the right leg with ulceration

Use additional code to identify severity of ulcer (L97.-)

I70.531 Atherosclerosis of nonautologous biological bypass graft(s) of the right leg with ulceration of thigh   HCC Rx ESR COM A

I70.532 Atherosclerosis of nonautologous biological bypass graft(s) of the right leg with ulceration of calf   HCC Rx ESR COM A

I70.533 Atherosclerosis of nonautologous biological bypass graft(s) of the right leg with ulceration of ankle   HCC Rx ESR COM A

I70.534 Atherosclerosis of nonautologous biological bypass graft(s) of the right leg with ulceration of heel and midfoot   HCC Rx ESR COM A

Atherosclerosis of nonautologous biological bypass graft(s) of right leg with ulceration of plantar surface of midfoot

I70.535 Atherosclerosis of nonautologous biological bypass graft(s) of the right leg with ulceration of other part of foot   HCC Rx ESR COM A

Atherosclerosis of nonautologous biological bypass graft(s) of the right leg with ulceration of toe

I70.538 Atherosclerosis of nonautologous biological bypass graft(s) of the right leg with ulceration of other part of lower leg   HCC Rx ESR COM A

I70.539 Atherosclerosis of nonautologous biological bypass graft(s) of the right leg with ulceration of unspecified site   HCC Rx ESR COM A

√6th **I70.54** **Atherosclerosis of nonautologous biological bypass graft(s) of the left leg with ulceration**

INCLUDES   any condition classifiable to I70.512 and I70.522
chronic limb-threatening ischemia of nonautologous biological bypass graft(s) of the left leg with ulceration
critical limb ischemia of nonautologous biological bypass graft(s) of the left leg with ulceration

Use additional code to identify severity of ulcer (L97.-)

I70.541 Atherosclerosis of nonautologous biological bypass graft(s) of the left leg with ulceration of thigh   HCC Rx ESR COM A

I70.542 Atherosclerosis of nonautologous biological bypass graft(s) of the left leg with ulceration of calf   HCC Rx ESR COM A

I70.543   **Atherosclerosis of nonautologous biological bypass graft(s) of the left leg with ulceration of** ankle   `HCC` `Rx` `ESR` `COM` `A`

I70.544   **Atherosclerosis of nonautologous biological bypass graft(s) of the left leg with ulceration of** heel and midfoot   `HCC` `Rx` `ESR` `COM` `A`
     Atherosclerosis of nonautologous biological bypass graft(s) of left leg with ulceration of plantar surface of midfoot

I70.545   **Atherosclerosis of nonautologous biological bypass graft(s) of the left leg with ulceration of other part of** foot   `HCC` `Rx` `ESR` `COM` `A`
     Atherosclerosis of nonautologous biological bypass graft(s) of the left leg with ulceration of toe

I70.548   **Atherosclerosis of nonautologous biological bypass graft(s) of the left leg with ulceration of other part of lower leg**   `HCC` `Rx` `ESR` `COM` `A`

I70.549   **Atherosclerosis of nonautologous biological bypass graft(s) of the left leg with ulceration of unspecified site**   `HCC` `Rx` `ESR` `COM` `A`

I70.55   **Atherosclerosis of nonautologous biological bypass graft(s) of other extremity with** ulceration   `HCC` `Rx` `ESR` `COM` `A`
     `INCLUDES` any condition classifiable to I70.518, I70.528, and I70.538
     Use additional code to identify severity of ulcer (L98.49)

✓6th I70.56   **Atherosclerosis of nonautologous biological bypass graft(s) of the extremities with** gangrene
     `INCLUDES` any condition classifiable to I70.51-, I70.52-, and I70.53-, I70.54-, I70.55
     chronic limb-threatening ischemia of nonautologous biological bypass graft(s) of the extremities with gangrene
     critical limb ischemia of nonautologous biological bypass graft(s) of the extremities with gangrene
     Use additional code to identify the severity of any ulcer (L97.-, L98.49-), if applicable

I70.561   **Atherosclerosis of nonautologous biological bypass graft(s) of the extremities with gangrene,** right leg   `HCC` `ESR` `COM` `A`

I70.562   **Atherosclerosis of nonautologous biological bypass graft(s) of the extremities with gangrene,** left leg   `HCC` `ESR` `COM` `A`

I70.563   **Atherosclerosis of nonautologous biological bypass graft(s) of the extremities with gangrene,** bilateral legs   `HCC` `ESR` `COM` `A`

I70.568   **Atherosclerosis of nonautologous biological bypass graft(s) of the extremities with gangrene, other extremity**   `HCC` `ESR` `COM` `A`

I70.569   **Atherosclerosis of nonautologous biological bypass graft(s) of the extremities with gangrene, unspecified extremity**   `HCC` `ESR` `COM` `A`

✓6th I70.59   **Other atherosclerosis of nonautologous biological bypass graft(s) of the extremities**

I70.591   **Other atherosclerosis of nonautologous biological bypass graft(s) of the extremities,** right leg   `HCC` `ESR` `A`

I70.592   **Other atherosclerosis of nonautologous biological bypass graft(s) of the extremities,** left leg   `HCC` `ESR` `A`

I70.593   **Other atherosclerosis of nonautologous biological bypass graft(s) of the extremities,** bilateral legs   `HCC` `ESR` `A`

I70.598   **Other atherosclerosis of nonautologous biological bypass graft(s) of the extremities, other extremity**   `HCC` `ESR` `A`

I70.599   **Other atherosclerosis of nonautologous biological bypass graft(s) of the extremities, unspecified extremity**   `HCC` `ESR` `A`

✓5th I70.6   **Atherosclerosis of** nonbiological bypass graft(s) of the extremities
     Use additional code, if applicable, to identify chronic total occlusion of artery of extremity (I70.92)
     AHA: 2020,4Q,98

✓6th I70.60   **Unspecified atherosclerosis of nonbiological bypass graft(s) of the extremities**

I70.601   **Unspecified atherosclerosis of nonbiological bypass graft(s) of the extremities,** right leg   `HCC` `ESR` `A`

I70.602   **Unspecified atherosclerosis of nonbiological bypass graft(s) of the extremities,** left leg   `HCC` `ESR` `A`

I70.603   **Unspecified atherosclerosis of nonbiological bypass graft(s) of the extremities,** bilateral legs   `HCC` `ESR` `A`

I70.608   **Unspecified atherosclerosis of nonbiological bypass graft(s) of the extremities, other extremity**   `HCC` `ESR` `A`

I70.609   **Unspecified atherosclerosis of nonbiological bypass graft(s) of the extremities, unspecified extremity**   `HCC` `ESR` `A`

✓6th I70.61   **Atherosclerosis of nonbiological bypass graft(s) of the extremities with** intermittent claudication

I70.611   **Atherosclerosis of nonbiological bypass graft(s) of the extremities with intermittent claudication,** right leg   `HCC` `ESR` `A`

I70.612   **Atherosclerosis of nonbiological bypass graft(s) of the extremities with intermittent claudication,** left leg   `HCC` `ESR` `A`

I70.613   **Atherosclerosis of nonbiological bypass graft(s) of the extremities with intermittent claudication,** bilateral legs   `HCC` `ESR` `A`

I70.618   **Atherosclerosis of nonbiological bypass graft(s) of the extremities with intermittent claudication, other extremity**   `HCC` `ESR` `A`

I70.619   **Atherosclerosis of nonbiological bypass graft(s) of the extremities with intermittent claudication, unspecified extremity**   `HCC` `ESR` `A`

✓6th I70.62   **Atherosclerosis of nonbiological bypass graft(s) of the extremities with** rest pain
     `INCLUDES` any condition classifiable to I70.61-
     chronic limb-threatening ischemia NOS of nonbiological bypass graft(s) of the extremities
     chronic limb-threatening ischemia of nonbiological bypass graft(s) of the extremities with rest pain
     critical limb ischemia NOS of nonbiological bypass graft(s) of the extremities
     critical limb ischemia of nonbiological bypass graft(s) of the extremities with rest pain

I70.621   **Atherosclerosis of nonbiological bypass graft(s) of the extremities with rest pain,** right leg   `HCC` `ESR` `A`

I70.622   **Atherosclerosis of nonbiological bypass graft(s) of the extremities with rest pain,** left leg   `HCC` `ESR` `A`

I70.623   **Atherosclerosis of nonbiological bypass graft(s) of the extremities with rest pain,** bilateral legs   `HCC` `ESR` `A`

I70.628   **Atherosclerosis of nonbiological bypass graft(s) of the extremities with rest pain, other extremity**   `HCC` `ESR` `A`

I70.629   **Atherosclerosis of nonbiological bypass graft(s) of the extremities with rest pain, unspecified extremity**   `HCC` `ESR` `A`

`HCC` CMS-HCC   `Rx` Rx HCC   `ESR` ESRD HCC   `COM` Commercial HCC   `N` Newborn: 0   `P` Pediatric: 0-17   `M` Maternity: 9-64   `A` Adult: 15-124

√6ᵗʰ **I70.63** **Atherosclerosis of nonbiological bypass graft(s) of the right leg with ulceration**
    INCLUDES   any condition classifiable to I70.611 and I70.621
      chronic limb-threatening ischemia of nonbiological bypass graft(s) of the right leg with ulceration
      critical limb ischemia of nonbiological bypass graft(s) of the right leg with ulceration
   Use additional code to identify severity of ulcer (L97.-)

    I70.631 **Atherosclerosis of nonbiological bypass graft(s) of the right leg with ulceration of thigh** HCC Rx ESR COM A

    I70.632 **Atherosclerosis of nonbiological bypass graft(s) of the right leg with ulceration of calf** HCC Rx ESR COM A

    I70.633 **Atherosclerosis of nonbiological bypass graft(s) of the right leg with ulceration of ankle** HCC Rx ESR COM A

    I70.634 **Atherosclerosis of nonbiological bypass graft(s) of the right leg with ulceration of heel and midfoot** HCC Rx ESR COM A
      Atherosclerosis of nonbiological bypass graft(s) of right leg with ulceration of plantar surface of midfoot

    I70.635 **Atherosclerosis of nonbiological bypass graft(s) of the right leg with ulceration of other part of foot** HCC Rx ESR COM A
      Atherosclerosis of nonbiological bypass graft(s) of the right leg with ulceration of toe

    I70.638 **Atherosclerosis of nonbiological bypass graft(s) of the right leg with ulceration of other part of lower leg** HCC Rx ESR COM A

    I70.639 **Atherosclerosis of nonbiological bypass graft(s) of the right leg with ulceration of unspecified site** HCC Rx ESR COM A

√6ᵗʰ **I70.64** **Atherosclerosis of nonbiological bypass graft(s) of the left leg with ulceration**
    INCLUDES   any condition classifiable to I70.612 and I70.622
      chronic limb-threatening ischemia of nonbiological bypass graft(s) of the left leg with ulceration
      critical limb ischemia of nonbiological bypass graft(s) of the left leg with ulceration
   Use additional code to identify severity of ulcer (L97.-)

    I70.641 **Atherosclerosis of nonbiological bypass graft(s) of the left leg with ulceration of thigh** HCC Rx ESR COM A

    I70.642 **Atherosclerosis of nonbiological bypass graft(s) of the left leg with ulceration of calf** HCC Rx ESR COM A

    I70.643 **Atherosclerosis of nonbiological bypass graft(s) of the left leg with ulceration of ankle** HCC Rx ESR COM A

    I70.644 **Atherosclerosis of nonbiological bypass graft(s) of the left leg with ulceration of heel and midfoot** HCC Rx ESR COM A
      Atherosclerosis of nonbiological bypass graft(s) of left leg with ulceration of plantar surface of midfoot

    I70.645 **Atherosclerosis of nonbiological bypass graft(s) of the left leg with ulceration of other part of foot** HCC Rx ESR COM A
      Atherosclerosis of nonbiological bypass graft(s) of the left leg with ulceration of toe

    I70.648 **Atherosclerosis of nonbiological bypass graft(s) of the left leg with ulceration of other part of lower leg** HCC Rx ESR COM A

    I70.649 **Atherosclerosis of nonbiological bypass graft(s) of the left leg with ulceration of unspecified site** HCC Rx ESR COM A

I70.65 **Atherosclerosis of nonbiological bypass graft(s) of other extremity with ulceration** HCC Rx ESR COM
    INCLUDES   any condition classifiable to I70.618 and I70.628
   Use additional code to identify severity of ulcer (L98.49)

√6ᵗʰ **I70.66** **Atherosclerosis of nonbiological bypass graft(s) of the extremities with gangrene**
    INCLUDES   any condition classifiable to I70.61-, I70.62-, I70.63-, I70.64-, I70.65
      chronic limb-threatening ischemia of nonbiological bypass graft(s) of the extremities with gangrene
      critical limb ischemia of nonbiological bypass graft(s) of the extremities with gangrene
   Use additional code to identify the severity of any ulcer (L97.-, L98.49-), if applicable

    I70.661 **Atherosclerosis of nonbiological bypass graft(s) of the extremities with gangrene, right leg** HCC ESR COM A

    I70.662 **Atherosclerosis of nonbiological bypass graft(s) of the extremities with gangrene, left leg** HCC ESR COM A

    I70.663 **Atherosclerosis of nonbiological bypass graft(s) of the extremities with gangrene, bilateral legs** HCC ESR COM A

    I70.668 **Atherosclerosis of nonbiological bypass graft(s) of the extremities with gangrene, other extremity** HCC ESR COM A

    I70.669 **Atherosclerosis of nonbiological bypass graft(s) of the extremities with gangrene, unspecified extremity** HCC ESR COM A

√6ᵗʰ **I70.69** **Other atherosclerosis of nonbiological bypass graft(s) of the extremities**

    I70.691 **Other atherosclerosis of nonbiological bypass graft(s) of the extremities, right leg** HCC ESR

    I70.692 **Other atherosclerosis of nonbiological bypass graft(s) of the extremities, left leg** HCC ESR

    I70.693 **Other atherosclerosis of nonbiological bypass graft(s) of the extremities, bilateral legs** HCC ESR

    I70.698 **Other atherosclerosis of nonbiological bypass graft(s) of the extremities, other extremity** HCC ESR

    I70.699 **Other atherosclerosis of nonbiological bypass graft(s) of the extremities, unspecified extremity** HCC ESR

√5ᵗʰ **I70.7** **Atherosclerosis of other type of bypass graft(s) of the extremities**
   Use additional code, if applicable, to identify chronic total occlusion of artery of extremity (I70.92)
   AHA: 2020,4Q,98

√6ᵗʰ **I70.70** **Unspecified atherosclerosis of other type of bypass graft(s) of the extremities**

    I70.701 **Unspecified atherosclerosis of other type of bypass graft(s) of the extremities, right leg** HCC ESR A

    I70.702 **Unspecified atherosclerosis of other type of bypass graft(s) of the extremities, left leg** HCC ESR A

    I70.703 **Unspecified atherosclerosis of other type of bypass graft(s) of the extremities, bilateral legs** HCC ESR A

    I70.708 **Unspecified atherosclerosis of other type of bypass graft(s) of the extremities, other extremity** HCC ESR A

    I70.709 **Unspecified atherosclerosis of other type of bypass graft(s) of the extremities, unspecified extremity** HCC ESR A

√6ᵗʰ **I70.71** **Atherosclerosis of other type of bypass graft(s) of the extremities with intermittent claudication**

    I70.711 **Atherosclerosis of other type of bypass graft(s) of the extremities with intermittent claudication, right leg** HCC ESR A

Chapter 9. Diseases of the Circulatory System

I70.712–I70.791

I70.712   **Atherosclerosis of other type of bypass graft(s) of the extremities with intermittent claudication, left leg** `HCC` `ESR` `A`

I70.713   **Atherosclerosis of other type of bypass graft(s) of the extremities with intermittent claudication, bilateral legs** `HCC` `ESR` `A`

I70.718   **Atherosclerosis of other type of bypass graft(s) of the extremities with intermittent claudication, other extremity** `HCC` `ESR` `A`

I70.719   **Atherosclerosis of other type of bypass graft(s) of the extremities with intermittent claudication, unspecified extremity** `HCC` `ESR` `A`

√6ᵗʰ **I70.72**   **Atherosclerosis of other type of bypass graft(s) of the extremities with rest pain**
> `INCLUDES`   any condition classifiable to I70.71-
> chronic limb-threatening ischemia NOS of other type of bypass graft(s) of the extremities
> chronic limb-threatening ischemia of other type of bypass graft(s) of the extremities with rest pain
> critical limb ischemia NOS of other type of bypass graft(s) of the extremities
> critical limb ischemia of other type of bypass graft(s) of the extremities with rest pain

I70.721   **Atherosclerosis of other type of bypass graft(s) of the extremities with rest pain, right leg** `HCC` `ESR` `A`

I70.722   **Atherosclerosis of other type of bypass graft(s) of the extremities with rest pain, left leg** `HCC` `ESR` `A`

I70.723   **Atherosclerosis of other type of bypass graft(s) of the extremities with rest pain, bilateral legs** `HCC` `ESR` `A`

I70.728   **Atherosclerosis of other type of bypass graft(s) of the extremities with rest pain, other extremity** `HCC` `ESR` `A`

I70.729   **Atherosclerosis of other type of bypass graft(s) of the extremities with rest pain, unspecified extremity** `HCC` `ESR` `A`

√6ᵗʰ **I70.73**   **Atherosclerosis of other type of bypass graft(s) of the right leg with ulceration**
> `INCLUDES`   any condition classifiable to I70.711 and I70.721
> chronic limb-threatening ischemia of other type of bypass graft(s) of the right leg with ulceration
> critical limb ischemia of other type of bypass graft(s) of the right leg with ulceration
> Use additional code to identify severity of ulcer (L97.-)

I70.731   **Atherosclerosis of other type of bypass graft(s) of the right leg with ulceration of thigh** `HCC` `Rx` `ESR` `COM` `A`

I70.732   **Atherosclerosis of other type of bypass graft(s) of the right leg with ulceration of calf** `HCC` `Rx` `ESR` `COM` `A`

I70.733   **Atherosclerosis of other type of bypass graft(s) of the right leg with ulceration of ankle** `HCC` `Rx` `ESR` `COM` `A`

I70.734   **Atherosclerosis of other type of bypass graft(s) of the right leg with ulceration of heel and midfoot** `HCC` `Rx` `ESR` `COM` `A`
> Atherosclerosis of other type of bypass graft(s) of right leg with ulceration of plantar surface of midfoot

I70.735   **Atherosclerosis of other type of bypass graft(s) of the right leg with ulceration of other part of foot** `HCC` `Rx` `ESR` `COM` `A`
> Atherosclerosis of other type of bypass graft(s) of right leg with ulceration of toe

I70.738   **Atherosclerosis of other type of bypass graft(s) of the right leg with ulceration of other part of lower leg** `HCC` `Rx` `ESR` `COM` `A`

I70.739   **Atherosclerosis of other type of bypass graft(s) of the right leg with ulceration of unspecified site** `HCC` `Rx` `ESR` `COM` `A`

√6ᵗʰ **I70.74**   **Atherosclerosis of other type of bypass graft(s) of the left leg with ulceration**
> `INCLUDES`   any condition classifiable to I70.712 and I70.722
> chronic limb-threatening ischemia of other type of bypass graft(s) of the left leg with ulceration
> critical limb ischemia of other type of bypass graft(s) of the left leg with ulceration
> Use additional code to identify severity of ulcer (L97.-)

I70.741   **Atherosclerosis of other type of bypass graft(s) of the left leg with ulceration of thigh** `HCC` `Rx` `ESR` `COM` `A`

I70.742   **Atherosclerosis of other type of bypass graft(s) of the left leg with ulceration of calf** `HCC` `Rx` `ESR` `COM` `A`

I70.743   **Atherosclerosis of other type of bypass graft(s) of the left leg with ulceration of ankle** `HCC` `Rx` `ESR` `COM` `A`

I70.744   **Atherosclerosis of other type of bypass graft(s) of the left leg with ulceration of heel and midfoot** `HCC` `Rx` `ESR` `COM` `A`
> Atherosclerosis of other type of bypass graft(s) of left leg with ulceration of plantar surface of midfoot

I70.745   **Atherosclerosis of other type of bypass graft(s) of the left leg with ulceration of other part of foot** `HCC` `Rx` `ESR` `COM` `A`
> Atherosclerosis of other type of bypass graft(s) of left leg with ulceration of toe

I70.748   **Atherosclerosis of other type of bypass graft(s) of the left leg with ulceration of other part of lower leg** `HCC` `Rx` `ESR` `COM` `A`

I70.749   **Atherosclerosis of other type of bypass graft(s) of the left leg with ulceration of unspecified site** `HCC` `Rx` `ESR` `COM` `A`

I70.75   **Atherosclerosis of other type of bypass graft(s) of other extremity with ulceration** `HCC` `Rx` `ESR` `COM` `A`
> `INCLUDES`   any condition classifiable to I70.718 and I70.728
> Use additional code to identify severity of ulcer (L98.49)

√6ᵗʰ **I70.76**   **Atherosclerosis of other type of bypass graft(s) of the extremities with gangrene**
> `INCLUDES`   any condition classifiable to I70.71-, I70.72-, I70.73-, I70.74-, I70.75
> chronic limb-threatening ischemia of other type of bypass graft(s) of the extremities with gangrene
> critical limb ischemia of other type of bypass graft(s) of the extremities with gangrene
> Use additional code to identify the severity of any ulcer (L97.-, L98.49-), if applicable

I70.761   **Atherosclerosis of other type of bypass graft(s) of the extremities with gangrene, right leg** `HCC` `ESR` `COM` `A`

I70.762   **Atherosclerosis of other type of bypass graft(s) of the extremities with gangrene, left leg** `HCC` `ESR` `COM` `A`

I70.763   **Atherosclerosis of other type of bypass graft(s) of the extremities with gangrene, bilateral legs** `HCC` `ESR` `COM` `A`

I70.768   **Atherosclerosis of other type of bypass graft(s) of the extremities with gangrene, other extremity** `HCC` `ESR` `COM` `A`

I70.769   **Atherosclerosis of other type of bypass graft(s) of the extremities with gangrene, unspecified extremity** `HCC` `ESR` `COM` `A`

√6ᵗʰ **I70.79**   **Other atherosclerosis of other type of bypass graft(s) of the extremities**

I70.791   **Other atherosclerosis of other type of bypass graft(s) of the extremities, right leg** `HCC` `ESR` `A`

`HCC` CMS-HCC   `Rx` Rx HCC   `ESR` ESRD HCC   `COM` Commercial HCC   `N` Newborn: 0   `P` Pediatric: 0-17   `M` Maternity: 9-64   `A` Adult: 15-124

692

ICD-10-CM 2023

I70.792   Other atherosclerosis of other type of bypass graft(s) of the extremities, left leg   `HCC` `ESR` `A`

I70.793   Other atherosclerosis of other type of bypass graft(s) of the extremities, bilateral legs   `HCC` `ESR` `A`

I70.798   Other atherosclerosis of other type of bypass graft(s) of the extremities, other extremity   `HCC` `ESR` `A`

I70.799   Other atherosclerosis of other type of bypass graft(s) of the extremities, unspecified extremity   `HCC` `ESR` `A`

I70.8   **Atherosclerosis of other arteries**   `A`
> **TIP:** Arteriosclerosis of the iliac arteries is coded here.

✓5ᵗʰ **I70.9**   **Other and unspecified atherosclerosis**

    I70.90   **Unspecified atherosclerosis**   `A`

    I70.91   **Generalized atherosclerosis**   `A`

    I70.92   **Chronic total occlusion of artery of the extremities**   `HCC` `ESR` `UPD` `A`
> Complete occlusion of artery of the extremities
> Total occlusion of artery of the extremities
> Code first atherosclerosis of arteries of the extremities (I70.2-, I70.3-, I70.4-, I70.5-, I70.6-, I70.7-)

✓4ᵗʰ **I71**   **Aortic aneurysm and dissection**

    `EXCLUDES 1`   *aortic ectasia (I77.81-)*
             syphilitic aortic aneurysm (A52.01)
             traumatic aortic aneurysm (S25.09, S35.09)

    ▶Code first, if applicable:◀
    ▶syphilitic aortic aneurysm (A52.01)◀
    ▶traumatic aortic aneurysm (S25.09, S35.09)◀

✓5ᵗʰ **I71.0**   **Dissection of aorta**

    I71.00   **Dissection of unspecified site of aorta**   `HCC` `ESR` `COM`

▲ ✓6ᵗʰ **I71.01**   **Dissection of thoracic aorta**

    ● **I71.010**   **Dissection of ascending aorta**

    ● **I71.011**   **Dissection of aortic arch**

    ● **I71.012**   **Dissection of descending thoracic aorta**

    ● **I71.019**   **Dissection of thoracic aorta, unspecified**

    I71.02   **Dissection of abdominal aorta**   `HCC` `ESR` `COM`

    I71.03   **Dissection of thoracoabdominal aorta**   `HCC` `ESR` `COM`

▲ ✓5ᵗʰ **I71.1**   **Thoracic aortic aneurysm, ruptured**

    I71.10   **Thoracic aortic aneurysm, ruptured, unspecified**

    I71.11   **Aneurysm of the ascending aorta, ruptured**

    I71.12   **Aneurysm of the aortic arch, ruptured**

    I71.13   **Aneurysm of the descending thoracic aorta, ruptured**

▲ ✓5ᵗʰ **I71.2**   **Thoracic aortic aneurysm, without rupture**

    I71.20   **Thoracic aortic aneurysm, without rupture, unspecified**

    I71.21   **Aneurysm of the ascending aorta, without rupture**

    I71.22   **Aneurysm of the aortic arch, without rupture**

    I71.23   **Aneurysm of the descending thoracic aorta, without rupture**

▲ ✓5ᵗʰ **I71.3**   **Abdominal aortic aneurysm, ruptured**

    I71.30   **Abdominal aortic aneurysm, ruptured, unspecified**

    I71.31   **Pararenal abdominal aortic aneurysm, ruptured**

    I71.32   **Juxtarenal abdominal aortic aneurysm, ruptured**

    I71.33   **Infrarenal abdominal aortic aneurysm, ruptured**

▲ ✓5ᵗʰ **I71.4**   **Abdominal aortic aneurysm, without rupture**

    I71.40   **Abdominal aortic aneurysm, without rupture, unspecified**

    I71.41   **Pararenal abdominal aortic aneurysm, without rupture**

    I71.42   **Juxtarenal abdominal aortic aneurysm, without rupture**

    I71.43   **Infrarenal abdominal aortic aneurysm, without rupture**

▲ ✓5ᵗʰ **I71.5**   **Thoracoabdominal aortic aneurysm, ruptured**

    I71.50   **Thoracoabdominal aortic aneurysm, ruptured, unspecified**

    I71.51   **Supraceliac aneurysm of the abdominal aorta, ruptured**

● **I71.52**   **Paravisceral aneurysm of the abdominal aorta, ruptured**

▲ ✓5ᵗʰ **I71.6**   **Thoracoabdominal aortic aneurysm, without rupture**

    ● **I71.60**   **Thoracoabdominal aortic aneurysm, without rupture, unspecified**

    ● **I71.61**   **Supraceliac aneurysm of the abdominal aorta, without rupture**

    ● **I71.62**   **Paravisceral aneurysm of the abdominal aorta, without rupture**

I71.8   **Aortic aneurysm of unspecified site, ruptured**   `HCC` `ESR` `COM`
> Rupture of aorta NOS

I71.9   **Aortic aneurysm of unspecified site, without rupture**   `HCC` `ESR`
> Aneurysm of aorta
> Dilatation of aorta
> Hyaline necrosis of aorta

✓4ᵗʰ **I72**   **Other aneurysm**

    `INCLUDES`   aneurysm (cirsoid) (false) (ruptured)
    `EXCLUDES 2`   *acquired aneurysm (I77.0)*
             aneurysm (of) aorta (I71.-)
             aneurysm (of) arteriovenous NOS (Q27.3-)
             carotid artery dissection (I77.71)
             cerebral (nonruptured) aneurysm (I67.1)
             coronary aneurysm (I25.4)
             coronary artery dissection (I25.42)
             dissection of artery NEC (I77.79)
             dissection of precerebral artery, congenital (nonruptured) (Q28.1)
             heart aneurysm (I25.3)
             iliac artery dissection (I77.72)
             precerebral artery, congential (nonruptured) (Q28.1)
             pulmonary artery aneurysm (I28.1)
             renal artery dissection (I77.73)
             retinal aneurysm (H35.0)
             ruptured cerebral aneurysm (I60.7)
             varicose aneurysm (I77.0)
             vertebral artery dissection (I77.74)
    AHA: 2016,4Q,28-29

I72.0   **Aneurysm of carotid artery**   `HCC` `ESR`
> Aneurysm of common carotid artery
> Aneurysm of external carotid artery
> Aneurysm of internal carotid artery, extracranial portion
>> `EXCLUDES 1`   *aneurysm of internal carotid artery, intracranial portion (I67.1)*
>>   *aneurysm of internal carotid artery NOS (I67.1)*

I72.1   **Aneurysm of artery of upper extremity**   `HCC` `ESR`

I72.2   **Aneurysm of renal artery**   `HCC` `ESR`

I72.3   **Aneurysm of iliac artery**   `HCC` `ESR`

I72.4   **Aneurysm of artery of lower extremity**   `HCC` `ESR`
> **AHA:** 2019,2Q,21

I72.5   **Aneurysm of other precerebral arteries**   `HCC` `ESR`
> Aneurysm of basilar artery (trunk)
>> `EXCLUDES 2`   *aneurysm of carotid artery (I72.0)*
>>   *aneurysm of vertebral artery (I72.6)*
>>   *dissection of carotid artery (I77.71)*
>>   *dissection of other precerebral arteries (I77.75)*
>>   *dissection of vertebral artery (I77.74)*

I72.6   **Aneurysm of vertebral artery**   `HCC` `ESR`
>> `EXCLUDES 2`   *dissection of vertebral artery (I77.74)*

I72.8   **Aneurysm of other specified arteries**   `HCC` `ESR`

Chapter 9. Diseases of the Circulatory System

I72.9   Aneurysm of unspecified site   `HCC` `ESR`

Aneurysm

Outer layer
Layers of muscular and elastic tissue
Inner layer
Aneurysm

✓4th I73   Other peripheral vascular diseases
    EXCLUDES 2   chilblains (T69.1)
          frostbite (T33-T34)
          immersion hand or foot (T69.0-)
          spasm of cerebral artery (G45.9)
    AHA: 2018,4Q,87

✓5th I73.0   Raynaud's syndrome
      Raynaud's disease
      Raynaud's phenomenon (secondary)
      DEF: Constriction of the arteries of the digits caused by cold or by nerve or arterial damage and can be prompted by stress or emotion. Blood cannot reach the skin and soft tissues and the skin turns white with blue mottling.
      I73.00   Raynaud's syndrome without gangrene
      I73.01   Raynaud's syndrome with gangrene   `HCC` `ESR` `COM`

I73.1   Thromboangiitis obliterans [Buerger's disease]   `HCC` `ESR`
      DEF: Inflammatory disease of the extremity blood vessels, mainly the lower blood vessels. This disease is associated with heavy tobacco use. The arteries are more affected than veins. It occurs primarily in young men and leads to tissue ischemia and gangrene.

✓5th I73.8   Other specified peripheral vascular diseases
    EXCLUDES 1   diabetic (peripheral) angiopathy (E08-E13 with .51-.52)
      I73.81   Erythromelalgia   `HCC` `ESR`
      I73.89   Other specified peripheral vascular diseases   `HCC` `ESR`
          Acrocyanosis
          Erythrocyanosis
          Simple acroparesthesia [Schultze's type]
          Vasomotor acroparesthesia [Nothnagel's type]

I73.9   Peripheral vascular disease, unspecified   `HCC` `ESR`
      Intermittent claudication
      Peripheral angiopathy NOS
      Spasm of artery
    EXCLUDES 1   atherosclerosis of the extremities (I70.2-I70.7-)
    AHA: 2018,2Q,7

✓4th I74   Arterial embolism and thrombosis
    `INCLUDES`   embolic infarction
          embolic occlusion
          thrombotic infarction
          thrombotic occlusion
    Code first:
      embolism and thrombosis complicating abortion or ectopic or molar pregnancy (O00-O07, O08.2)
      embolism and thrombosis complicating pregnancy, childbirth and the puerperium (O88.-)
    EXCLUDES 2   atheroembolism (I75.-)
          basilar embolism and thrombosis (I63.0-I63.2, I65.1)
          carotid embolism and thrombosis (I63.0-I63.2, I65.2)
          cerebral embolism and thrombosis (I63.3-I63.5, I66.-)
          coronary embolism and thrombosis (I21-I25)
          mesenteric embolism and thrombosis (K55.0-)
          ophthalmic embolism and thrombosis (H34.-)
          precerebral embolism and thrombosis NOS (I63.0-I63.2, I65.9)
          pulmonary embolism and thrombosis (I26.-)
          renal embolism and thrombosis (N28.0)
          retinal embolism and thrombosis (H34.-)
          septic embolism and thrombosis (I76)
          vertebral embolism and thrombosis (I63.0-I63.2, I65.0)

✓5th I74.0   Embolism and thrombosis of abdominal aorta
      I74.01   Saddle embolus of abdominal aorta   `HCC` `ESR` `COM`
      I74.09   Other arterial embolism and thrombosis of abdominal aorta   `HCC` `ESR` `COM`
          Aortic bifurcation syndrome
          Aortoiliac obstruction
          Leriche's syndrome

✓5th I74.1   Embolism and thrombosis of other and unspecified parts of aorta
      I74.10   Embolism and thrombosis of unspecified parts of aorta   `HCC` `ESR` `COM`
      I74.11   Embolism and thrombosis of thoracic aorta   `HCC` `ESR` `COM`
      I74.19   Embolism and thrombosis of other parts of aorta   `HCC` `ESR` `COM`

I74.2   Embolism and thrombosis of arteries of the upper extremities   `HCC` `ESR` `COM`
I74.3   Embolism and thrombosis of arteries of the lower extremities   `HCC` `ESR` `COM`
I74.4   Embolism and thrombosis of arteries of extremities, unspecified   `HCC` `ESR` `COM`
      Peripheral arterial embolism NOS
I74.5   Embolism and thrombosis of iliac artery   `HCC` `ESR` `COM`
I74.8   Embolism and thrombosis of other arteries   `HCC` `ESR` `COM`
I74.9   Embolism and thrombosis of unspecified artery   `HCC` `ESR` `COM`

✓4th I75   Atheroembolism
    `INCLUDES`   atherothrombotic microembolism
          cholesterol embolism

✓5th I75.0   Atheroembolism of extremities
    ✓6th I75.01   Atheroembolism of upper extremity
        I75.011   Atheroembolism of right upper extremity   `HCC` `ESR` `COM`
        I75.012   Atheroembolism of left upper extremity   `HCC` `ESR` `COM`
        I75.013   Atheroembolism of bilateral upper extremities   `HCC` `ESR` `COM`
        I75.019   Atheroembolism of unspecified upper extremity   `HCC` `ESR` `COM`
    ✓6th I75.02   Atheroembolism of lower extremity
        I75.021   Atheroembolism of right lower extremity   `HCC` `ESR` `COM`
        I75.022   Atheroembolism of left lower extremity   `HCC` `ESR` `COM`
        I75.023   Atheroembolism of bilateral lower extremities   `HCC` `ESR` `COM`
        I75.029   Atheroembolism of unspecified lower extremity   `HCC` `ESR` `COM`

✓5th I75.8   Atheroembolism of other sites
      I75.81   Atheroembolism of kidney   `HCC` `ESR` `COM`
          Use additional code for any associated acute kidney failure and chronic kidney disease (N17.-, N18.-)
      I75.89   Atheroembolism of other site   `HCC` `ESR` `COM`

I76 Septic arterial embolism `HCC` `ESR` `COM` `UPD`
Code first underlying infection, such as:
  infective endocarditis (I33.0)
  lung abscess (J85.-)
Use additional code to identify the site of the embolism (I74.-)
  `EXCLUDES 2`   septic pulmonary embolism (I26.01, I26.90)

✓4th **I77 Other disorders of arteries and arterioles**
  `EXCLUDES 2`   collagen (vascular) diseases (M30-M36)
           hypersensitivity angiitis (M31.0)
           pulmonary artery (I28.-)

I77.0 Arteriovenous fistula, acquired `HCC` `ESR`
Aneurysmal varix
Arteriovenous aneurysm, acquired
  `EXCLUDES 1`   arteriovenous aneurysm NOS (Q27.3-)
           presence of arteriovenous shunt (fistula) for dialysis (Z99.2)
           traumatic - see injury of blood vessel by body region
  `EXCLUDES 2`   cerebral (I67.1)
           coronary (I25.4)
  DEF: Communication between an artery and vein caused by trauma or invasive procedures.

I77.1 Stricture of artery `HCC` `ESR`
Narrowing of artery
AHA: 2021,3Q,12

I77.2 Rupture of artery `HCC` `ESR`
Erosion of artery
Fistula of artery
Ulcer of artery
  `EXCLUDES 1`   traumatic rupture of artery - see injury of blood vessel by body region

I77.3 Arterial fibromuscular dysplasia `HCC` `ESR`
Fibromuscular hyperplasia (of) carotid artery
Fibromuscular hyperplasia (of) renal artery

I77.4 Celiac artery compression syndrome `HCC` `ESR`
AHA: 2021,3Q,12

I77.5 Necrosis of artery `HCC` `ESR`

I77.6 Arteritis, unspecified `HCC` `ESR`
Aortitis NOS
Endarteritis NOS
  `EXCLUDES 1`   arteritis or endarteritis:
           aortic arch (M31.4)
           cerebral NEC (I67.7)
           coronary (I25.89)
           deformans (I70.-)
           giant cell (M31.5, M31.6)
           obliterans (I70.-)
           senile (I70.-)

✓5th **I77.7 Other arterial dissection**
  `EXCLUDES 2`   dissection of aorta (I71.0-)
           dissection of coronary artery (I25.42)
  AHA: 2016,4Q,28-29

  I77.70 Dissection of unspecified artery `HCC` `ESR` `COM`
  I77.71 Dissection of carotid artery `HCC` `ESR` `COM`
  I77.72 Dissection of iliac artery `HCC` `ESR` `COM`
  I77.73 Dissection of renal artery `HCC` `ESR` `COM`
  I77.74 Dissection of vertebral artery `HCC` `ESR` `COM`
    `EXCLUDES 2`   aneurysm of vertebral artery (I72.6)
  I77.75 Dissection of other precerebral arteries `HCC` `ESR` `COM`
    Dissection of basilar artery (trunk)
    `EXCLUDES 2`   aneurysm of carotid artery (I72.0)
            aneurysm of other precerebral arteries (I72.5)
            aneurysm of vertebral artery (I72.6)
            dissection of carotid artery (I77.71)
            dissection of vertebral artery (I77.74)
  I77.76 Dissection of artery of upper extremity `HCC` `ESR` `COM`
  I77.77 Dissection of artery of lower extremity `HCC` `ESR` `COM`
  I77.79 Dissection of other specified artery `HCC` `ESR` `COM`

✓5th **I77.8 Other specified disorders of arteries and arterioles**
✓6th **I77.81 Aortic ectasia**
  Ectasis aorta
  `EXCLUDES 1`   aortic aneurysm and dissection ▶(I71.-)◀
  I77.810 Thoracic aortic ectasia `HCC` `ESR`
  I77.811 Abdominal aortic ectasia `HCC` `ESR`
  I77.812 Thoracoabdominal aortic ectasia `HCC` `ESR`
  I77.819 Aortic ectasia, unspecified site `HCC` `ESR`

  I77.82 Antineutrophilic cytoplasmic antibody [ANCA] vasculitis
  ANCA associated vasculitis
  ANCA positive vasculitis
  `EXCLUDES 2`   eosinophilic granulomatosis with polyangiitis (M30.1)
           granulomatosis with polyangiitis (M31.3-)
           microscopic polyangiitis (M31.7)

  I77.89 Other specified disorders of arteries and arterioles `HCC` `ESR`
  AHA: 2021,1Q,23

  I77.9 Disorder of arteries and arterioles, unspecified `HCC` `ESR`
  AHA: 2021,1Q,4; 2018,2Q,7

✓4th **I78 Diseases of capillaries**

I78.0 Hereditary hemorrhagic telangiectasia `HCC` `ESR`
Rendu-Osler-Weber disease

I78.1 Nevus, non-neoplastic
Araneus nevus
Senile nevus
Spider nevus
Stellar nevus
  `EXCLUDES 1`   nevus NOS (D22.-)
           vascular NOS (Q82.5)
  `EXCLUDES 2`   blue nevus (D22.-)
           flammeus nevus (Q82.5)
           hairy nevus (D22.-)
           melanocytic nevus (D22.-)
           pigmented nevus (D22.-)
           portwine nevus (Q82.5)
           sanguineous nevus (Q82.5)
           strawberry nevus (Q82.5)
           verrucous nevus (Q82.5)
AHA: 2019,1Q,21

I78.8 Other diseases of capillaries

I78.9 Disease of capillaries, unspecified

✓4th **I79 Disorders of arteries, arterioles and capillaries in diseases classified elsewhere**

I79.0 Aneurysm of aorta in diseases classified elsewhere `HCC` `ESR`
Code first underlying disease
  `EXCLUDES 1`   syphilitic aneurysm (A52.01)

I79.1 Aortitis in diseases classified elsewhere `HCC` `ESR`
Code first underlying disease
  `EXCLUDES 1`   syphilitic aortitis (A52.02)

I79.8 Other disorders of arteries, arterioles and capillaries in diseases classified elsewhere `HCC` `ESR`
Code first underlying disease, such as:
  amyloidosis (E85.-)
  `EXCLUDES 1`   diabetic (peripheral) angiopathy (E08-E13 with .51-.52)
           syphilitic endarteritis (A52.09)
           tuberculous endarteritis (A18.89)

Chapter 9. Diseases of the Circulatory System

Diseases of veins, lymphatic vessels and lymph nodes, not elsewhere classified (I8Ø-I89)

✓4ᵗʰ I8Ø Phlebitis and thrombophlebitis

> INCLUDES   endophlebitis
> inflammation, vein
> periphlebitis
> suppurative phlebitis

Code first:
phlebitis and thrombophlebitis complicating abortion, ectopic or molar pregnancy (OØØ-OØ7, OØ8.7)
phlebitis and thrombophlebitis complicating pregnancy, childbirth and the puerperium (O22.-, O87.-)

> EXCLUDES 1   *venous embolism and thrombosis of lower extremities (I82.4-, I82.5-, I82.81-)*

✓5ᵗʰ I8Ø.Ø Phlebitis and thrombophlebitis of superficial vessels of lower extremities

Phlebitis and thrombophlebitis of femoropopliteal vein

- **I8Ø.ØØ**   **Phlebitis and thrombophlebitis of superficial vessels of unspecified lower extremity**
- **I8Ø.Ø1**   **Phlebitis and thrombophlebitis of superficial vessels of** right **lower extremity**
- **I8Ø.Ø2**   **Phlebitis and thrombophlebitis of superficial vessels of** left **lower extremity**
- **I8Ø.Ø3**   **Phlebitis and thrombophlebitis of superficial vessels of lower extremities,** bilateral

✓5ᵗʰ I8Ø.1 Phlebitis and thrombophlebitis of femoral vein

Phlebitis and thrombophlebitis of common femoral vein
Phlebitis and thrombophlebitis of deep femoral vein

- **I8Ø.1Ø**   **Phlebitis and thrombophlebitis of unspecified femoral vein** HCC Rx ESR COM
- **I8Ø.11**   **Phlebitis and thrombophlebitis of** right **femoral vein** HCC Rx ESR COM
- **I8Ø.12**   **Phlebitis and thrombophlebitis of** left **femoral vein** HCC Rx ESR COM
- **I8Ø.13**   **Phlebitis and thrombophlebitis of femoral vein,** bilateral HCC Rx ESR COM

✓5ᵗʰ I8Ø.2 Phlebitis and thrombophlebitis of other and unspecified deep vessels of lower extremities

- **✓6ᵗʰ I8Ø.2Ø**   **Phlebitis and thrombophlebitis of unspecified deep vessels of lower extremities**
  - **I8Ø.2Ø1**   **Phlebitis and thrombophlebitis of unspecified deep vessels of** right **lower extremity** HCC Rx ESR COM
  - **I8Ø.2Ø2**   **Phlebitis and thrombophlebitis of unspecified deep vessels of** left **lower extremity** HCC Rx ESR COM
  - **I8Ø.2Ø3**   **Phlebitis and thrombophlebitis of unspecified deep vessels of lower extremities,** bilateral HCC Rx ESR COM
  - **I8Ø.2Ø9**   **Phlebitis and thrombophlebitis of unspecified deep vessels of unspecified lower extremity** HCC Rx ESR COM
- **✓6ᵗʰ I8Ø.21**   **Phlebitis and thrombophlebitis of** iliac vein

  Phlebitis and thrombophlebitis of common iliac vein
  Phlebitis and thrombophlebitis of external iliac vein
  Phlebitis and thrombophlebitis of internal iliac vein
  - **I8Ø.211**   **Phlebitis and thrombophlebitis of** right **iliac vein** HCC Rx ESR COM
  - **I8Ø.212**   **Phlebitis and thrombophlebitis of** left **iliac vein** HCC Rx ESR COM
  - **I8Ø.213**   **Phlebitis and thrombophlebitis of iliac vein,** bilateral HCC Rx ESR COM
  - **I8Ø.219**   **Phlebitis and thrombophlebitis of unspecified iliac vein** HCC Rx ESR COM
- **✓6ᵗʰ I8Ø.22**   **Phlebitis and thrombophlebitis of** popliteal vein
  - **I8Ø.221**   **Phlebitis and thrombophlebitis of** right **popliteal vein** HCC Rx ESR COM
  - **I8Ø.222**   **Phlebitis and thrombophlebitis of** left **popliteal vein** HCC Rx ESR COM
  - **I8Ø.223**   **Phlebitis and thrombophlebitis of popliteal vein,** bilateral HCC Rx ESR COM
  - **I8Ø.229**   **Phlebitis and thrombophlebitis of unspecified popliteal vein** HCC Rx ESR COM

- **✓6ᵗʰ I8Ø.23**   **Phlebitis and thrombophlebitis of** tibial vein

  Phlebitis and thrombophlebitis of anterior tibial vein
  Phlebitis and thrombophlebitis of posterior tibial vein
  - **I8Ø.231**   **Phlebitis and thrombophlebitis of** right **tibial vein** HCC Rx ESR COM
  - **I8Ø.232**   **Phlebitis and thrombophlebitis of** left **tibial vein** HCC Rx ESR COM
  - **I8Ø.233**   **Phlebitis and thrombophlebitis of tibial vein,** bilateral HCC Rx ESR COM
  - **I8Ø.239**   **Phlebitis and thrombophlebitis of unspecified tibial vein** HCC Rx ESR COM
- **✓6ᵗʰ I8Ø.24**   **Phlebitis and thrombophlebitis of** peroneal vein

  AHA: 2019,4Q,8
  - **I8Ø.241**   **Phlebitis and thrombophlebitis of** right **peroneal vein** HCC Rx ESR COM
  - **I8Ø.242**   **Phlebitis and thrombophlebitis of** left **peroneal vein** HCC Rx ESR COM
  - **I8Ø.243**   **Phlebitis and thrombophlebitis of peroneal vein,** bilateral HCC Rx ESR COM
  - **I8Ø.249**   **Phlebitis and thrombophlebitis of unspecified peroneal vein** HCC Rx ESR COM
- **✓6ᵗʰ I8Ø.25**   **Phlebitis and thrombophlebitis of** calf muscular vein

  Phlebitis and thrombophlebitis of calf muscular vein, NOS
  Phlebitis and thrombophlebitis of gastrocnemial vein
  Phlebitis and thrombophlebitis of soleal vein

  AHA: 2019,4Q,8
  - **I8Ø.251**   **Phlebitis and thrombophlebitis of** right **calf muscular vein** HCC Rx ESR COM
  - **I8Ø.252**   **Phlebitis and thrombophlebitis of** left **calf muscular vein** HCC Rx ESR COM
  - **I8Ø.253**   **Phlebitis and thrombophlebitis of calf muscular vein,** bilateral HCC Rx ESR COM
  - **I8Ø.259**   **Phlebitis and thrombophlebitis of unspecified calf muscular vein** HCC Rx ESR COM
- **✓6ᵗʰ I8Ø.29**   **Phlebitis and thrombophlebitis of other deep vessels of lower extremities**
  - **I8Ø.291**   **Phlebitis and thrombophlebitis of other deep vessels of** right **lower extremity** HCC Rx ESR COM
  - **I8Ø.292**   **Phlebitis and thrombophlebitis of other deep vessels of** left **lower extremity** HCC Rx ESR COM
  - **I8Ø.293**   **Phlebitis and thrombophlebitis of other deep vessels of lower extremity,** bilateral HCC Rx ESR COM
  - **I8Ø.299**   **Phlebitis and thrombophlebitis of other deep vessels of unspecified lower extremity** HCC Rx ESR COM

I8Ø.3   **Phlebitis and thrombophlebitis of lower extremities, unspecified**

I8Ø.8   **Phlebitis and thrombophlebitis of other sites**

I8Ø.9   **Phlebitis and thrombophlebitis of unspecified site**

I81 Portal vein thrombosis

Portal (vein) obstruction

> EXCLUDES 2   *hepatic vein thrombosis (I82.Ø)*
> *phlebitis of portal vein (K75.1)*

AHA: 2019,4Q,68

Chapter 9. Diseases of the Circulatory System

I8Ø–I81

✓4th I82 Other venous embolism and thrombosis

Code first venous embolism and thrombosis complicating:
abortion, ectopic or molar pregnancy (O00-O07, O08.7)
pregnancy, childbirth and the puerperium (O22.-, O87.-)

> *EXCLUDES 2*   *venous embolism and thrombosis (of):*
> *cerebral (I63.6, I67.6)*
> *coronary (I21-I25)*
> *intracranial and intraspinal, septic or NOS (G08)*
> *intracranial, nonpyogenic (I67.6)*
> *intraspinal, nonpyogenic (G95.1)*
> *mesenteric (K55.0-)*
> *portal (I81)*
> *pulmonary (I26.-)*

I82.0 Budd-Chiari syndrome `HCC` `Rx` `ESR` `COM`

Hepatic vein thrombosis
DEF: Thrombosis or other obstruction of the hepatic veins. Symptoms include an enlarged liver, extensive collateral vessels, intractable ascites, and severe portal hypertension.

I82.1 Thrombophlebitis migrans

✓5th I82.2 Embolism and thrombosis of vena cava and other thoracic veins

> **✓6th I82.21 Embolism and thrombosis of superior vena cava**
>
>> **I82.210 Acute embolism and thrombosis of superior vena cava** `HCC` `Rx` `ESR` `COM`
>> Embolism and thrombosis of superior vena cava NOS
>>
>> **I82.211 Chronic embolism and thrombosis of superior vena cava** `HCC` `Rx` `ESR` `COM`
>
> **✓6th I82.22 Embolism and thrombosis of inferior vena cava**
>
>> **I82.220 Acute embolism and thrombosis of inferior vena cava** `HCC` `Rx` `ESR` `COM`
>> Embolism and thrombosis of inferior vena cava NOS
>>
>> **I82.221 Chronic embolism and thrombosis of inferior vena cava** `HCC` `Rx` `ESR` `COM`
>
> **✓6th I82.29 Embolism and thrombosis of other thoracic veins**
> Embolism and thrombosis of brachiocephalic (innominate) vein
>
>> **I82.290 Acute embolism and thrombosis of other thoracic veins** `HCC` `Rx` `ESR` `COM`
>>
>> **I82.291 Chronic embolism and thrombosis of other thoracic veins** `HCC` `Rx` `ESR` `COM`

I82.3 Embolism and thrombosis of renal vein `HCC` `Rx` `ESR` `COM`

✓5th I82.4 Acute embolism and thrombosis of deep veins of lower extremity

> **✓6th I82.40 Acute embolism and thrombosis of unspecified deep veins of lower extremity**
> Deep vein thrombosis NOS
> DVT NOS
>
>> *EXCLUDES 1*   *acute embolism and thrombosis of unspecified deep veins of distal lower extremity (I82.4Z-)*
>> *acute embolism and thrombosis of unspecified deep veins of proximal lower extremity (I82.4Y-)*
>
>> **I82.401 Acute embolism and thrombosis of unspecified deep veins of right lower extremity** `HCC` `Rx` `ESR` `COM`
>>
>> **I82.402 Acute embolism and thrombosis of unspecified deep veins of left lower extremity** `HCC` `Rx` `ESR` `COM`
>>
>> **I82.403 Acute embolism and thrombosis of unspecified deep veins of lower extremity, bilateral** `HCC` `Rx` `ESR` `COM`
>>
>> **I82.409 Acute embolism and thrombosis of unspecified deep veins of unspecified lower extremity** `HCC` `Rx` `ESR` `COM`
>
> **✓6th I82.41 Acute embolism and thrombosis of femoral vein**
> Acute embolism and thrombosis of common femoral vein
> Acute embolism and thrombosis of deep femoral vein
>
>> **I82.411 Acute embolism and thrombosis of right femoral vein** `HCC` `Rx` `ESR` `COM`
>>
>> **I82.412 Acute embolism and thrombosis of left femoral vein** `HCC` `Rx` `ESR` `COM`
>>
>> **I82.413 Acute embolism and thrombosis of femoral vein, bilateral** `HCC` `Rx` `ESR` `COM`

> **I82.419 Acute embolism and thrombosis of unspecified femoral vein** `HCC` `Rx` `ESR` `COM`

> **✓6th I82.42 Acute embolism and thrombosis of iliac vein**
> Acute embolism and thrombosis of common iliac vein
> Acute embolism and thrombosis of external iliac vein
> Acute embolism and thrombosis of internal iliac vein
>
>> **I82.421 Acute embolism and thrombosis of right iliac vein** `HCC` `Rx` `ESR` `COM`
>>
>> **I82.422 Acute embolism and thrombosis of left iliac vein** `HCC` `Rx` `ESR` `COM`
>>
>> **I82.423 Acute embolism and thrombosis of iliac vein, bilateral** `HCC` `Rx` `ESR` `COM`
>>
>> **I82.429 Acute embolism and thrombosis of unspecified iliac vein** `HCC` `Rx` `ESR` `COM`
>
> **✓6th I82.43 Acute embolism and thrombosis of popliteal vein**
>
>> **I82.431 Acute embolism and thrombosis of right popliteal vein** `HCC` `Rx` `ESR` `COM`
>>
>> **I82.432 Acute embolism and thrombosis of left popliteal vein** `HCC` `Rx` `ESR` `COM`
>>
>> **I82.433 Acute embolism and thrombosis of popliteal vein, bilateral** `HCC` `Rx` `ESR` `COM`
>>
>> **I82.439 Acute embolism and thrombosis of unspecified popliteal vein** `HCC` `Rx` `ESR` `COM`
>
> **✓6th I82.44 Acute embolism and thrombosis of tibial vein**
> Acute embolism and thrombosis of anterior tibial vein
> Acute embolism and thrombosis of posterior tibial vein
>
>> **I82.441 Acute embolism and thrombosis of right tibial vein** `HCC` `Rx` `ESR` `COM`
>>
>> **I82.442 Acute embolism and thrombosis of left tibial vein** `HCC` `Rx` `ESR` `COM`
>>
>> **I82.443 Acute embolism and thrombosis of tibial vein, bilateral** `HCC` `Rx` `ESR` `COM`
>>
>> **I82.449 Acute embolism and thrombosis of unspecified tibial vein** `HCC` `Rx` `ESR` `COM`
>
> **✓6th I82.45 Acute embolism and thrombosis of peroneal vein**
> **AHA:** 2019,4Q,8-10
>
>> **I82.451 Acute embolism and thrombosis of right peroneal vein** `HCC` `Rx` `ESR` `COM`
>>
>> **I82.452 Acute embolism and thrombosis of left peroneal vein** `HCC` `Rx` `ESR` `COM`
>>
>> **I82.453 Acute embolism and thrombosis of peroneal vein, bilateral** `HCC` `Rx` `ESR` `COM`
>>
>> **I82.459 Acute embolism and thrombosis of unspecified peroneal vein** `HCC` `Rx` `ESR` `COM`
>
> **✓6th I82.46 Acute embolism and thrombosis of calf muscular vein**
> Acute embolism and thrombosis of calf muscular vein, NOS
> Acute embolism and thrombosis of gastrocnemial vein
> Acute embolism and thrombosis of soleal vein
> **AHA:** 2019,4Q,8-10
>
>> **I82.461 Acute embolism and thrombosis of right calf muscular vein** `HCC` `Rx` `ESR` `COM`
>>
>> **I82.462 Acute embolism and thrombosis of left calf muscular vein** `HCC` `Rx` `ESR` `COM`
>>
>> **I82.463 Acute embolism and thrombosis of calf muscular vein, bilateral** `HCC` `Rx` `ESR` `COM`
>>
>> **I82.469 Acute embolism and thrombosis of unspecified calf muscular vein** `HCC` `Rx` `ESR` `COM`
>
> **✓6th I82.49 Acute embolism and thrombosis of other specified deep vein of lower extremity**
>
>> **I82.491 Acute embolism and thrombosis of other specified deep vein of right lower extremity** `HCC` `Rx` `ESR` `COM`
>>
>> **I82.492 Acute embolism and thrombosis of other specified deep vein of left lower extremity** `HCC` `Rx` `ESR` `COM`
>>
>> **I82.493 Acute embolism and thrombosis of other specified deep vein of lower extremity, bilateral** `HCC` `Rx` `ESR` `COM`
>>
>> **I82.499 Acute embolism and thrombosis of other specified deep vein of unspecified lower extremity** `HCC` `Rx` `ESR` `COM`

☑ Additional Character Required   ✓x7th Placeholder Alert   Manifestation   Unspecified Dx   Q QPP   UPD Unacceptable PDx

√6ᵗʰ **I82.4Y Acute embolism and thrombosis of unspecified deep veins of proximal lower extremity**
Acute embolism and thrombosis of deep vein of thigh NOS
Acute embolism and thrombosis of deep vein of upper leg NOS

I82.4Y1 Acute embolism and thrombosis of unspecified deep veins of right proximal lower extremity HCC Rx ESR COM

I82.4Y2 Acute embolism and thrombosis of unspecified deep veins of left proximal lower extremity HCC Rx ESR COM

I82.4Y3 Acute embolism and thrombosis of unspecified deep veins of proximal lower extremity, bilateral HCC Rx ESR COM

I82.4Y9 Acute embolism and thrombosis of unspecified deep veins of unspecified proximal lower extremity HCC Rx ESR COM

√6ᵗʰ **I82.4Z Acute embolism and thrombosis of unspecified deep veins of distal lower extremity**
Acute embolism and thrombosis of deep vein of calf NOS
Acute embolism and thrombosis of deep vein of lower leg NOS

I82.4Z1 Acute embolism and thrombosis of unspecified deep veins of right distal lower extremity HCC Rx ESR COM

I82.4Z2 Acute embolism and thrombosis of unspecified deep veins of left distal lower extremity HCC Rx ESR COM

I82.4Z3 Acute embolism and thrombosis of unspecified deep veins of distal lower extremity, bilateral HCC Rx ESR COM

I82.4Z9 Acute embolism and thrombosis of unspecified deep veins of unspecified distal lower extremity HCC Rx ESR COM

√5ᵗʰ **I82.5 Chronic embolism and thrombosis of deep veins of lower extremity**
Use additional code, if applicable, for associated long-term (current) use of anticoagulants (Z79.01)
EXCLUDES 1 *personal history of venous embolism and thrombosis (Z86.718)*
AHA: 2020,2Q,20

√6ᵗʰ **I82.50 Chronic embolism and thrombosis of unspecified deep veins of lower extremity**
EXCLUDES 1 *chronic embolism and thrombosis of unspecified deep veins of distal lower extremity (I82.5Z-)*
chronic embolism and thrombosis of unspecified deep veins of proximal lower extremity (I82.5Y-)

I82.501 Chronic embolism and thrombosis of unspecified deep veins of right lower extremity HCC Rx ESR COM

I82.502 Chronic embolism and thrombosis of unspecified deep veins of left lower extremity HCC Rx ESR COM

I82.503 Chronic embolism and thrombosis of unspecified deep veins of lower extremity, bilateral HCC Rx ESR COM

I82.509 Chronic embolism and thrombosis of unspecified deep veins of unspecified lower extremity HCC Rx ESR COM

√6ᵗʰ **I82.51 Chronic embolism and thrombosis of femoral vein**
Chronic embolism and thrombosis of common femoral vein
Chronic embolism and thrombosis of deep femoral vein

I82.511 Chronic embolism and thrombosis of right femoral vein HCC Rx ESR COM

I82.512 Chronic embolism and thrombosis of left femoral vein HCC Rx ESR COM

I82.513 Chronic embolism and thrombosis of femoral vein, bilateral HCC Rx ESR COM

I82.519 Chronic embolism and thrombosis of unspecified femoral vein HCC Rx ESR COM

√6ᵗʰ **I82.52 Chronic embolism and thrombosis of iliac vein**
Chronic embolism and thrombosis of common iliac vein
Chronic embolism and thrombosis of external iliac vein
Chronic embolism and thrombosis of internal iliac vein

I82.521 Chronic embolism and thrombosis of right iliac vein HCC Rx ESR COM

I82.522 Chronic embolism and thrombosis of left iliac vein HCC Rx ESR COM

I82.523 Chronic embolism and thrombosis of iliac vein, bilateral HCC Rx ESR COM

I82.529 Chronic embolism and thrombosis of unspecified iliac vein HCC Rx ESR COM

√6ᵗʰ **I82.53 Chronic embolism and thrombosis of popliteal vein**

I82.531 Chronic embolism and thrombosis of right popliteal vein HCC Rx ESR COM

I82.532 Chronic embolism and thrombosis of left popliteal vein HCC Rx ESR COM

I82.533 Chronic embolism and thrombosis of popliteal vein, bilateral HCC Rx ESR COM

I82.539 Chronic embolism and thrombosis of unspecified popliteal vein HCC Rx ESR COM

√6ᵗʰ **I82.54 Chronic embolism and thrombosis of tibial vein**
Chronic embolism and thrombosis of anterior tibial vein
Chronic embolism and thrombosis of posterior tibial vein

I82.541 Chronic embolism and thrombosis of right tibial vein HCC Rx ESR COM

I82.542 Chronic embolism and thrombosis of left tibial vein HCC Rx ESR COM

I82.543 Chronic embolism and thrombosis of tibial vein, bilateral HCC Rx ESR COM

I82.549 Chronic embolism and thrombosis of unspecified tibial vein HCC Rx ESR COM

√6ᵗʰ **I82.55 Chronic embolism and thrombosis of peroneal vein**
AHA: 2019,4Q,8-10

I82.551 Chronic embolism and thrombosis of right peroneal vein HCC Rx ESR COM

I82.552 Chronic embolism and thrombosis of left peroneal vein HCC Rx ESR COM

I82.553 Chronic embolism and thrombosis of peroneal vein, bilateral HCC Rx ESR COM

I82.559 Chronic embolism and thrombosis of unspecified peroneal vein HCC Rx ESR COM

√6ᵗʰ **I82.56 Chronic embolism and thrombosis of calf muscular vein**
Chronic embolism and thrombosis of calf muscular vein NOS
Chronic embolism and thrombosis of gastrocnemial vein
Chronic embolism and thrombosis of soleal vein
AHA: 2019,4Q,8-10

I82.561 Chronic embolism and thrombosis of right calf muscular vein HCC Rx ESR COM

I82.562 Chronic embolism and thrombosis of left calf muscular vein HCC Rx ESR COM

I82.563 Chronic embolism and thrombosis of calf muscular vein, bilateral HCC Rx ESR COM

I82.569 Chronic embolism and thrombosis of unspecified calf muscular vein HCC Rx ESR COM

√6ᵗʰ **I82.59 Chronic embolism and thrombosis of other specified deep vein of lower extremity**

I82.591 Chronic embolism and thrombosis of other specified deep vein of right lower extremity HCC Rx ESR COM

I82.592 Chronic embolism and thrombosis of other specified deep vein of left lower extremity HCC Rx ESR COM

I82.593 Chronic embolism and thrombosis of other specified deep vein of lower extremity, bilateral HCC Rx ESR COM

I82.599 Chronic embolism and thrombosis of other specified deep vein of unspecified lower extremity HCC Rx ESR COM

√6ᵗʰ **I82.5Y** **Chronic embolism and thrombosis of unspecified deep veins of proximal lower extremity**
Chronic embolism and thrombosis of deep veins of thigh NOS
Chronic embolism and thrombosis of deep veins of upper leg NOS

     I82.5Y1 **Chronic embolism and thrombosis of unspecified deep veins of right proximal lower extremity** HCC Rx ESR COM

     I82.5Y2 **Chronic embolism and thrombosis of unspecified deep veins of left proximal lower extremity** HCC Rx ESR COM

     I82.5Y3 **Chronic embolism and thrombosis of unspecified deep veins of proximal lower extremity, bilateral** HCC Rx ESR COM

     I82.5Y9 **Chronic embolism and thrombosis of unspecified deep veins of unspecified proximal lower extremity** HCC Rx ESR COM

√6ᵗʰ **I82.5Z** **Chronic embolism and thrombosis of unspecified deep veins of distal lower extremity**
Chronic embolism and thrombosis of deep veins of calf NOS
Chronic embolism and thrombosis of deep veins of lower leg NOS

     I82.5Z1 **Chronic embolism and thrombosis of unspecified deep veins of right distal lower extremity** HCC Rx ESR COM

     I82.5Z2 **Chronic embolism and thrombosis of unspecified deep veins of left distal lower extremity** HCC Rx ESR COM

     I82.5Z3 **Chronic embolism and thrombosis of unspecified deep veins of distal lower extremity, bilateral** HCC Rx ESR COM

     I82.5Z9 **Chronic embolism and thrombosis of unspecified deep veins of unspecified distal lower extremity** HCC Rx ESR COM

√5ᵗʰ **I82.6** **Acute embolism and thrombosis of veins of upper extremity**

     √6ᵗʰ **I82.60** **Acute embolism and thrombosis of unspecified veins of upper extremity**

         I82.601 **Acute embolism and thrombosis of unspecified veins of right upper extremity**

         I82.602 **Acute embolism and thrombosis of unspecified veins of left upper extremity**

         I82.603 **Acute embolism and thrombosis of unspecified veins of upper extremity, bilateral**

         I82.609 **Acute embolism and thrombosis of unspecified veins of unspecified upper extremity**

     √6ᵗʰ **I82.61** **Acute embolism and thrombosis of superficial veins of upper extremity**
Acute embolism and thrombosis of antecubital vein
Acute embolism and thrombosis of basilic vein
Acute embolism and thrombosis of cephalic vein

         I82.611 **Acute embolism and thrombosis of superficial veins of right upper extremity**

         I82.612 **Acute embolism and thrombosis of superficial veins of left upper extremity**

         I82.613 **Acute embolism and thrombosis of superficial veins of upper extremity, bilateral**

         I82.619 **Acute embolism and thrombosis of superficial veins of unspecified upper extremity**

     √6ᵗʰ **I82.62** **Acute embolism and thrombosis of deep veins of upper extremity**
Acute embolism and thrombosis of brachial vein
Acute embolism and thrombosis of radial vein
Acute embolism and thrombosis of ulnar vein

         I82.621 **Acute embolism and thrombosis of deep veins of right upper extremity** HCC Rx ESR COM

         I82.622 **Acute embolism and thrombosis of deep veins of left upper extremity** HCC Rx ESR COM

         I82.623 **Acute embolism and thrombosis of deep veins of upper extremity, bilateral** HCC Rx ESR COM

         I82.629 **Acute embolism and thrombosis of deep veins of unspecified upper extremity** HCC Rx ESR COM

√5ᵗʰ **I82.7** **Chronic embolism and thrombosis of veins of upper extremity**
Use additional code, if applicable, for associated long-term (current) use of anticoagulants (Z79.01)
     EXCLUDES 1   *personal history of venous embolism and thrombosis (Z86.718)*

     √6ᵗʰ **I82.70** **Chronic embolism and thrombosis of unspecified veins of upper extremity**

         I82.701 **Chronic embolism and thrombosis of unspecified veins of right upper extremity**

         I82.702 **Chronic embolism and thrombosis of unspecified veins of left upper extremity**

         I82.703 **Chronic embolism and thrombosis of unspecified veins of upper extremity, bilateral**

         I82.709 **Chronic embolism and thrombosis of unspecified veins of unspecified upper extremity**

     √6ᵗʰ **I82.71** **Chronic embolism and thrombosis of superficial veins of upper extremity**
Chronic embolism and thrombosis of antecubital vein
Chronic embolism and thrombosis of basilic vein
Chronic embolism and thrombosis of cephalic vein

         I82.711 **Chronic embolism and thrombosis of superficial veins of right upper extremity**

         I82.712 **Chronic embolism and thrombosis of superficial veins of left upper extremity**

         I82.713 **Chronic embolism and thrombosis of superficial veins of upper extremity, bilateral**

         I82.719 **Chronic embolism and thrombosis of superficial veins of unspecified upper extremity**

     √6ᵗʰ **I82.72** **Chronic embolism and thrombosis of deep veins of upper extremity**
Chronic embolism and thrombosis of brachial vein
Chronic embolism and thrombosis of radial vein
Chronic embolism and thrombosis of ulnar vein

         I82.721 **Chronic embolism and thrombosis of deep veins of right upper extremity** HCC Rx ESR COM

         I82.722 **Chronic embolism and thrombosis of deep veins of left upper extremity** HCC Rx ESR COM

         I82.723 **Chronic embolism and thrombosis of deep veins of upper extremity, bilateral** HCC Rx ESR COM

         I82.729 **Chronic embolism and thrombosis of deep veins of unspecified upper extremity** HCC Rx ESR COM

√5ᵗʰ **I82.A** **Embolism and thrombosis of axillary vein**

     √6ᵗʰ **I82.A1** **Acute embolism and thrombosis of axillary vein**

         I82.A11 **Acute embolism and thrombosis of right axillary vein** HCC Rx ESR COM

         I82.A12 **Acute embolism and thrombosis of left axillary vein** HCC Rx ESR COM

         I82.A13 **Acute embolism and thrombosis of axillary vein, bilateral** HCC Rx ESR COM

         I82.A19 **Acute embolism and thrombosis of unspecified axillary vein** HCC Rx ESR COM

     √6ᵗʰ **I82.A2** **Chronic embolism and thrombosis of axillary vein**

         I82.A21 **Chronic embolism and thrombosis of right axillary vein** HCC Rx ESR COM

         I82.A22 **Chronic embolism and thrombosis of left axillary vein** HCC Rx ESR COM

         I82.A23 **Chronic embolism and thrombosis of axillary vein, bilateral** HCC Rx ESR COM

         I82.A29 **Chronic embolism and thrombosis of unspecified axillary vein** HCC Rx ESR COM

√5ᵗʰ **I82.B** **Embolism and thrombosis of subclavian vein**

     √6ᵗʰ **I82.B1** **Acute embolism and thrombosis of subclavian vein**

         I82.B11 **Acute embolism and thrombosis of right subclavian vein** HCC Rx ESR COM

         I82.B12 **Acute embolism and thrombosis of left subclavian vein** HCC Rx ESR COM

      I82.B13 **Acute embolism and thrombosis of subclavian vein, bilateral** `HCC` `Rx` `ESR` `COM`

      I82.B19 **Acute embolism and thrombosis of unspecified subclavian vein** `HCC` `Rx` `ESR` `COM`

✓6ᵗʰ **I82.B2** **Chronic embolism and thrombosis of subclavian vein**

      I82.B21 **Chronic embolism and thrombosis of right subclavian vein** `HCC` `Rx` `ESR` `COM`

      I82.B22 **Chronic embolism and thrombosis of left subclavian vein** `HCC` `Rx` `ESR` `COM`

      I82.B23 **Chronic embolism and thrombosis of subclavian vein, bilateral** `HCC` `Rx` `ESR` `COM`

      I82.B29 **Chronic embolism and thrombosis of unspecified subclavian vein** `HCC` `Rx` `ESR` `COM`

✓5ᵗʰ **I82.C** **Embolism and thrombosis of internal jugular vein**

✓6ᵗʰ **I82.C1** **Acute embolism and thrombosis of internal jugular vein**

      I82.C11 **Acute embolism and thrombosis of right internal jugular vein** `HCC` `Rx` `ESR` `COM`

      I82.C12 **Acute embolism and thrombosis of left internal jugular vein** `HCC` `Rx` `ESR` `COM`

      I82.C13 **Acute embolism and thrombosis of internal jugular vein, bilateral** `HCC` `Rx` `ESR` `COM`

      I82.C19 **Acute embolism and thrombosis of unspecified internal jugular vein** `HCC` `Rx` `ESR` `COM`

✓6ᵗʰ **I82.C2** **Chronic embolism and thrombosis of internal jugular vein**

      I82.C21 **Chronic embolism and thrombosis of right internal jugular vein** `HCC` `Rx` `ESR` `COM`

      I82.C22 **Chronic embolism and thrombosis of left internal jugular vein** `HCC` `Rx` `ESR` `COM`

      I82.C23 **Chronic embolism and thrombosis of internal jugular vein, bilateral** `HCC` `Rx` `ESR` `COM`

      I82.C29 **Chronic embolism and thrombosis of unspecified internal jugular vein** `HCC` `Rx` `ESR` `COM`

✓5ᵗʰ **I82.8** **Embolism and thrombosis of other specified veins**

Use additional code, if applicable, for associated long-term (current) use of anticoagulants (Z79.01)

✓6ᵗʰ **I82.81** **Embolism and thrombosis of superficial veins of lower extremities**

Embolism and thrombosis of saphenous vein (greater) (lesser)

      I82.811 **Embolism and thrombosis of superficial veins of right lower extremity**

      I82.812 **Embolism and thrombosis of superficial veins of left lower extremity**

      I82.813 **Embolism and thrombosis of superficial veins of lower extremities, bilateral**

      I82.819 **Embolism and thrombosis of superficial veins of unspecified lower extremity**

✓6ᵗʰ **I82.89** **Embolism and thrombosis of other specified veins**

      I82.890 **Acute embolism and thrombosis of other specified veins**

      I82.891 **Chronic embolism and thrombosis of other specified veins**

✓5ᵗʰ **I82.9** **Embolism and thrombosis of unspecified vein**

      I82.90 **Acute embolism and thrombosis of unspecified vein**

Embolism of vein NOS
Thrombosis (vein) NOS

      I82.91 **Chronic embolism and thrombosis of unspecified vein**

✓4ᵗʰ **I83** **Varicose veins of lower extremities**

EXCLUDES 2   *varicose veins complicating pregnancy (O22.0-)*
             varicose veins complicating the puerperium (O87.4)

✓5ᵗʰ **I83.0** **Varicose veins of lower extremities with ulcer**

Use additional code to identify severity of ulcer (L97.-)

✓6ᵗʰ **I83.00** **Varicose veins of unspecified lower extremity with ulcer**

      I83.001 **Varicose veins of unspecified lower extremity with ulcer of thigh** `HCC` `ESR` `COM` `A`

      I83.002 **Varicose veins of unspecified lower extremity with ulcer of calf** `HCC` `ESR` `COM` `A`

      I83.003 **Varicose veins of unspecified lower extremity with ulcer of ankle** `HCC` `ESR` `COM` `A`

      I83.004 **Varicose veins of unspecified lower extremity with ulcer of heel and midfoot** `HCC` `ESR` `COM` `A`

Varicose veins of unspecified lower extremity with ulcer of plantar surface of midfoot

      I83.005 **Varicose veins of unspecified lower extremity with ulcer other part of foot** `HCC` `ESR` `COM` `A`

Varicose veins of unspecified lower extremity with ulcer of toe

      I83.008 **Varicose veins of unspecified lower extremity with ulcer other part of lower leg** `HCC` `ESR` `COM` `A`

      I83.009 **Varicose veins of unspecified lower extremity with ulcer of unspecified site** `HCC` `ESR` `COM` `A`

✓6ᵗʰ **I83.01** **Varicose veins of right lower extremity with ulcer**

      I83.011 **Varicose veins of right lower extremity with ulcer of thigh** `HCC` `ESR` `COM` `A`

      I83.012 **Varicose veins of right lower extremity with ulcer of calf** `HCC` `ESR` `COM` `A`

      I83.013 **Varicose veins of right lower extremity with ulcer of ankle** `HCC` `ESR` `COM` `A`

      I83.014 **Varicose veins of right lower extremity with ulcer of heel and midfoot** `HCC` `ESR` `COM` `A`

Varicose veins of right lower extremity with ulcer of plantar surface of midfoot

      I83.015 **Varicose veins of right lower extremity with ulcer other part of foot** `HCC` `ESR` `COM` `A`

Varicose veins of right lower extremity with ulcer of toe

      I83.018 **Varicose veins of right lower extremity with ulcer other part of lower leg** `HCC` `ESR` `COM` `A`

      I83.019 **Varicose veins of right lower extremity with ulcer of unspecified site** `HCC` `ESR` `COM` `A`

✓6ᵗʰ **I83.02** **Varicose veins of left lower extremity with ulcer**

      I83.021 **Varicose veins of left lower extremity with ulcer of thigh** `HCC` `ESR` `COM` `A`

      I83.022 **Varicose veins of left lower extremity with ulcer of calf** `HCC` `ESR` `COM` `A`

      I83.023 **Varicose veins of left lower extremity with ulcer of ankle** `HCC` `ESR` `COM` `A`

      I83.024 **Varicose veins of left lower extremity with ulcer of heel and midfoot** `HCC` `ESR` `COM` `A`

Varicose veins of left lower extremity with ulcer of plantar surface of midfoot

      I83.025 **Varicose veins of left lower extremity with ulcer other part of foot** `HCC` `ESR` `COM` `A`

Varicose veins of left lower extremity with ulcer of toe

      I83.028 **Varicose veins of left lower extremity with ulcer other part of lower leg** `HCC` `ESR` `COM` `A`

      I83.029 **Varicose veins of left lower extremity with ulcer of unspecified site** `HCC` `ESR` `COM` `A`

✓5ᵗʰ **I83.1** **Varicose veins of lower extremities with inflammation**

      I83.10 **Varicose veins of unspecified lower extremity with inflammation** `A`

      I83.11 **Varicose veins of right lower extremity with inflammation** `A`

      I83.12 **Varicose veins of left lower extremity with inflammation** `A`

√5th **I83.2 Varicose veins of lower extremities with both ulcer and inflammation**
    Use additional code to identify severity of ulcer (L97.-)

√6th **I83.20 Varicose veins of unspecified lower extremity with both ulcer and inflammation**

    I83.201 Varicose veins of unspecified lower extremity with both ulcer of thigh and inflammation HCC ESR COM A

    I83.202 Varicose veins of unspecified lower extremity with both ulcer of calf and inflammation HCC ESR COM A

    I83.203 Varicose veins of unspecified lower extremity with both ulcer of ankle and inflammation HCC ESR COM A

    I83.204 Varicose veins of unspecified lower extremity with both ulcer of heel and midfoot and inflammation HCC ESR COM A
        Varicose veins of unspecified lower extremity with both ulcer of plantar surface of midfoot and inflammation

    I83.205 Varicose veins of unspecified lower extremity with both ulcer of other part of foot and inflammation HCC ESR COM A
        Varicose veins of unspecified lower extremity with both ulcer of toe and inflammation

    I83.208 Varicose veins of unspecified lower extremity with both ulcer of other part of lower extremity and inflammation HCC ESR COM A

    I83.209 Varicose veins of unspecified lower extremity with both ulcer of unspecified site and inflammation HCC ESR COM A

√6th **I83.21 Varicose veins of right lower extremity with both ulcer and inflammation**

    I83.211 Varicose veins of right lower extremity with both ulcer of thigh and inflammation HCC ESR COM A

    I83.212 Varicose veins of right lower extremity with both ulcer of calf and inflammation HCC ESR COM A

    I83.213 Varicose veins of right lower extremity with both ulcer of ankle and inflammation HCC ESR COM A

    I83.214 Varicose veins of right lower extremity with both ulcer of heel and midfoot and inflammation HCC ESR COM A
        Varicose veins of right lower extremity with both ulcer of plantar surface of midfoot and inflammation

    I83.215 Varicose veins of right lower extremity with both ulcer other part of foot and inflammation HCC ESR COM A
        Varicose veins of right lower extremity with both ulcer of toe and inflammation

    I83.218 Varicose veins of right lower extremity with both ulcer of other part of lower extremity and inflammation HCC ESR COM A

    I83.219 Varicose veins of right lower extremity with both ulcer of unspecified site and inflammation HCC ESR COM A

√6th **I83.22 Varicose veins of left lower extremity with both ulcer and inflammation**

    I83.221 Varicose veins of left lower extremity with both ulcer of thigh and inflammation HCC ESR COM A

    I83.222 Varicose veins of left lower extremity with both ulcer of calf and inflammation HCC ESR COM A

    I83.223 Varicose veins of left lower extremity with both ulcer of ankle and inflammation HCC ESR COM A

    I83.224 Varicose veins of left lower extremity with both ulcer of heel and midfoot and inflammation HCC ESR COM A
        Varicose veins of left lower extremity with both ulcer of plantar surface of midfoot and inflammation

    I83.225 Varicose veins of left lower extremity with both ulcer other part of foot and inflammation HCC ESR COM A
        Varicose veins of left lower extremity with both ulcer of toe and inflammation

    I83.228 Varicose veins of left lower extremity with both ulcer of other part of lower extremity and inflammation HCC ESR COM A

    I83.229 Varicose veins of left lower extremity with both ulcer of unspecified site and inflammation HCC ESR COM A

√5th **I83.8 Varicose veins of lower extremities with other complications**

√6th **I83.81 Varicose veins of lower extremities with pain**

    I83.811 Varicose veins of right lower extremity with pain A

    I83.812 Varicose veins of left lower extremity with pain A

    I83.813 Varicose veins of bilateral lower extremities with pain A

    I83.819 Varicose veins of unspecified lower extremity with pain A

√6th **I83.89 Varicose veins of lower extremities with other complications**
    Varicose veins of lower extremities with edema
    Varicose veins of lower extremities with swelling

    I83.891 Varicose veins of right lower extremity with other complications A

    I83.892 Varicose veins of left lower extremity with other complications A

    I83.893 Varicose veins of bilateral lower extremities with other complications A

    I83.899 Varicose veins of unspecified lower extremity with other complications A

√5th **I83.9 Asymptomatic varicose veins of lower extremities**
    Phlebectasia of lower extremities
    Varicose veins of lower extremities
    Varix of lower extremities

    I83.90 Asymptomatic varicose veins of unspecified lower extremity A
        Varicose veins NOS

    I83.91 Asymptomatic varicose veins of right lower extremity A

    I83.92 Asymptomatic varicose veins of left lower extremity A

    I83.93 Asymptomatic varicose veins of bilateral lower extremities A

√4th **I85 Esophageal varices**
    Use additional code to identify:
    alcohol abuse and dependence (F10.-)

√5th **I85.0 Esophageal varices**
    Idiopathic esophageal varices
    Primary esophageal varices

    I85.00 Esophageal varices without bleeding HCC ESR COM
        Esophageal varices NOS

    I85.01 Esophageal varices with bleeding HCC ESR COM

√5th **I85.1 Secondary esophageal varices**

    Esophageal varices secondary to alcoholic liver disease
    Esophageal varices secondary to cirrhosis of liver
    Esophageal varices secondary to schistosomiasis
    Esophageal varices secondary to toxic liver disease
    Code first underlying disease

[handwritten: first code: cirrhosis of liver K74.60]

    I85.10 Secondary esophageal varices without bleeding HCC ESR COM

    I85.11 Secondary esophageal varices with bleeding HCC ESR COM

√4th **I86 Varicose veins of other sites**
    EXCLUDES 1 varicose veins of unspecified site (I83.9-)
    EXCLUDES 2 retinal varices (H35.0-)

    I86.0 Sublingual varices
        DEF: Distended, tortuous veins beneath the tongue.

    I86.1 Scrotal varices ♂
        Varicocele

    I86.2 Pelvic varices

Chapter 9. Diseases of the Circulatory System

186.3 **Vulval varices** ♀

> EXCLUDES 1   *vulval varices complicating childbirth and the puerperium (O87.8)*
> *vulval varices complicating pregnancy (O22.1-)*

[handwritten: varicose vein]

186.4 **Gastric varices**

186.8 **Varicose veins of other specified sites** 🅰
> Varicose ulcer of nasal septum

✓4ᵗʰ **187** **Other disorders of veins**

✓5ᵗʰ **187.0** **Postthrombotic syndrome**
> Chronic venous hypertension due to deep vein thrombosis
> Postphlebitic syndrome
> EXCLUDES 1   *chronic venous hypertension without deep vein thrombosis (187.3-)*

✓6ᵗʰ **187.00** **Postthrombotic syndrome** without complications
> Asymptomatic postthrombotic syndrome

187.001 **Postthrombotic syndrome without complications of** right lower **extremity**

187.002 **Postthrombotic syndrome without complications of** left lower **extremity**

187.003 **Postthrombotic syndrome without complications of** bilateral lower **extremity**

187.009 **Postthrombotic syndrome without complications of unspecified extremity**
> Postthrombotic syndrome NOS

✓6ᵗʰ **187.01** **Postthrombotic syndrome with** ulcer
> Use additional code to specify site and severity of ulcer (L97.-)

187.011 **Postthrombotic syndrome with ulcer of** right lower **extremity** HCC ESR COM

187.012 **Postthrombotic syndrome with ulcer of** left lower **extremity** HCC ESR COM

187.013 **Postthrombotic syndrome with ulcer of** bilateral lower **extremity** HCC ESR COM

187.019 **Postthrombotic syndrome with ulcer of unspecified lower extremity** HCC ESR COM

✓6ᵗʰ **187.02** **Postthrombotic syndrome with** inflammation

187.021 **Postthrombotic syndrome with inflammation of** right lower **extremity**

187.022 **Postthrombotic syndrome with inflammation of** left lower **extremity**

187.023 **Postthrombotic syndrome with inflammation of** bilateral lower **extremity**

187.029 **Postthrombotic syndrome with inflammation of unspecified lower extremity**

✓6ᵗʰ **187.03** **Postthrombotic syndrome with** ulcer and inflammation
> Use additional code to specify site and severity of ulcer (L97.-)

187.031 **Postthrombotic syndrome with ulcer and inflammation of** right lower **extremity** HCC ESR COM

187.032 **Postthrombotic syndrome with ulcer and inflammation of** left lower **extremity** HCC ESR COM

187.033 **Postthrombotic syndrome with ulcer and inflammation of** bilateral lower **extremity** HCC ESR COM

187.039 **Postthrombotic syndrome with ulcer and inflammation of unspecified lower extremity** HCC ESR COM

✓6ᵗʰ **187.09** **Postthrombotic syndrome with other complications**

187.091 **Postthrombotic syndrome with other complications of** right lower **extremity**

187.092 **Postthrombotic syndrome with other complications of** left lower **extremity**

187.093 **Postthrombotic syndrome with other complications of** bilateral lower **extremity**

187.099 **Postthrombotic syndrome with other complications of unspecified lower extremity**

187.1 **Compression of vein**
> Stricture of vein
> Vena cava syndrome (inferior) (superior)
> EXCLUDES 2   *compression of pulmonary vein (I28.8)*

187.2 **Venous insufficiency (chronic) (peripheral)**
> Stasis dermatitis
> EXCLUDES 1   *stasis dermatitis with varicose veins of lower extremities (I83.1-, I83.2-)*
> **DEF:** Insufficient drainage of venous blood in any part of the body that results in edema or dermatosis.

✓5ᵗʰ **187.3** **Chronic venous hypertension (idiopathic)**
> Stasis edema
> EXCLUDES 1   *chronic venous hypertension due to deep vein thrombosis (187.0-)*
> *varicose veins of lower extremities (I83.-)*

✓6ᵗʰ **187.30** **Chronic venous hypertension (idiopathic)** without complications
> Asymptomatic chronic venous hypertension (idiopathic)

187.301 **Chronic venous hypertension (idiopathic) without complications of** right lower **extremity**

187.302 **Chronic venous hypertension (idiopathic) without complications of** left lower **extremity**

187.303 **Chronic venous hypertension (idiopathic) without complications of** bilateral lower **extremity**

187.309 **Chronic venous hypertension (idiopathic) without complications of unspecified lower extremity**
> Chronic venous hypertension NOS

✓6ᵗʰ **187.31** **Chronic venous hypertension (idiopathic) with** ulcer
> Use additional code to specify site and severity of ulcer (L97.-)

187.311 **Chronic venous hypertension (idiopathic) with ulcer of** right lower **extremity** HCC ESR COM

187.312 **Chronic venous hypertension (idiopathic) with ulcer of** left lower **extremity** HCC ESR COM

187.313 **Chronic venous hypertension (idiopathic) with ulcer of** bilateral lower **extremity** HCC ESR COM

187.319 **Chronic venous hypertension (idiopathic) with ulcer of unspecified lower extremity** HCC ESR COM

✓6ᵗʰ **187.32** **Chronic venous hypertension (idiopathic) with** inflammation

187.321 **Chronic venous hypertension (idiopathic) with inflammation of** right lower **extremity**

187.322 **Chronic venous hypertension (idiopathic) with inflammation of** left lower **extremity**

187.323 **Chronic venous hypertension (idiopathic) with inflammation of** bilateral lower **extremity**

187.329 **Chronic venous hypertension (idiopathic) with inflammation of unspecified lower extremity**

✓6ᵗʰ **187.33** **Chronic venous hypertension (idiopathic) with** ulcer and inflammation
> Use additional code to specify site and severity of ulcer (L97.-)

187.331 **Chronic venous hypertension (idiopathic) with ulcer and inflammation of** right lower **extremity** HCC ESR COM

187.332 **Chronic venous hypertension (idiopathic) with ulcer and inflammation of** left lower **extremity** HCC ESR COM

187.333 **Chronic venous hypertension (idiopathic) with ulcer and inflammation of** bilateral lower **extremity** HCC ESR COM

187.339 **Chronic venous hypertension (idiopathic) with ulcer and inflammation of unspecified lower extremity** HCC ESR COM

✓6ᵗʰ **187.39** **Chronic venous hypertension (idiopathic) with other complications**

187.391 **Chronic venous hypertension (idiopathic) with other complications of** right lower **extremity**

187.392 **Chronic venous hypertension (idiopathic) with other complications of** left lower **extremity**

I87.393 Chronic venous hypertension (idiopathic) with other complications of bilateral lower extremity

I87.399 Chronic venous hypertension (idiopathic) with other complications of unspecified lower extremity

I87.8 Other specified disorders of veins
Phlebosclerosis
Venofibrosis

I87.9 Disorder of vein, unspecified

✓4ᵗʰ **I88 Nonspecific lymphadenitis**
EXCLUDES 1   acute lymphadenitis, except mesenteric (L04.-)
enlarged lymph nodes NOS (R59.-)
human immunodeficiency virus [HIV] disease resulting in generalized lymphadenopathy (B20)

I88.0 Nonspecific mesenteric lymphadenitis
Mesenteric lymphadenitis (acute)(chronic)

I88.1 Chronic lymphadenitis, except mesenteric
Adenitis
Lymphadenitis

I88.8 Other nonspecific lymphadenitis

I88.9 Nonspecific lymphadenitis, unspecified
Lymphadenitis NOS

✓4ᵗʰ **I89 Other noninfective disorders of lymphatic vessels and lymph nodes**
EXCLUDES 1   chylocele, tunica vaginalis (nonfilarial) NOS (N50.89)
enlarged lymph nodes NOS (R59.-)
filarial chylocele (B74.-)
hereditary lymphedema (Q82.0)

I89.0 Lymphedema, not elsewhere classified
Elephantiasis (nonfilarial) NOS
Lymphangiectasis
Obliteration, lymphatic vessel
Praecox lymphedema
Secondary lymphedema
EXCLUDES 1   postmastectomy lymphedema (I97.2)

I89.1 Lymphangitis
Chronic lymphangitis
Lymphangitis NOS
Subacute lymphangitis
EXCLUDES 1   acute lymphangitis (L03.-)

I89.8 Other specified noninfective disorders of lymphatic vessels and lymph nodes
Chylocele (nonfilarial)
Chylous ascites
Chylous cyst
Lipomelanotic reticulosis
Lymph node or vessel fistula
Lymph node or vessel infarction
Lymph node or vessel rupture

I89.9 Noninfective disorder of lymphatic vessels and lymph nodes, unspecified
Disease of lymphatic vessels NOS

Other and unspecified disorders of the circulatory system (I95-I99)

✓4ᵗʰ **I95 Hypotension**
EXCLUDES 1   cardiovascular collapse (R57.9) (~R57.9)
maternal hypotension syndrome (O26.5-)
nonspecific low blood pressure reading NOS (R03.1)

I95.0 Idiopathic hypotension

I95.1 Orthostatic hypotension
Hypotension, postural
EXCLUDES 1   neurogenic orthostatic hypotension [Shy-Drager] (G90.3)
orthostatic hypotension due to drugs (I95.2)

I95.2 Hypotension due to drugs
Orthostatic hypotension due to drugs
Use additional code for adverse effect, if applicable, to identify drug (T36-T50 with fifth or sixth character 5)

I95.3 Hypotension of hemodialysis
Intra-dialytic hypotension

✓5ᵗʰ **I95.8 Other hypotension**

I95.81 Postprocedural hypotension

I95.89 Other hypotension
Chronic hypotension

I95.9 Hypotension, unspecified

I96 Gangrene, not elsewhere classified   HCC ESR COM
Gangrenous cellulitis
EXCLUDES 1   gangrene in atherosclerosis of native arteries of the extremities (I70.26)
gangrene in hernia (K40.1, K40.4, K41.1, K41.4, K42.1, K43.1-, K44.1, K45.1, K46.1)
gangrene in other peripheral vascular diseases (I73.-)
gangrene of certain specified sites - see Alphabetical Index
gas gangrene (A48.0)
pyoderma gangrenosum (L88)
EXCLUDES 2   gangrene in diabetes mellitus (E08-E13 with .52)
AHA: 2018,4Q,87; 2018,3Q,3; 2017,3Q,6; 2013,2Q,34

✓4ᵗʰ **I97 Intraoperative and postprocedural complications and disorders of circulatory system, not elsewhere classified**
EXCLUDES 2   postprocedural shock (T81.1-)
AHA: 2021,1Q,13; 2019,2Q,21

I97.0 Postcardiotomy syndrome

✓5ᵗʰ **I97.1 Other postprocedural cardiac functional disturbances**
EXCLUDES 2   acute pulmonary insufficiency following thoracic surgery (J95.1)
intraoperative cardiac functional disturbances (I97.7-)

✓6ᵗʰ **I97.11 Postprocedural cardiac insufficiency**

I97.110 Postprocedural cardiac insufficiency following cardiac surgery

I97.111 Postprocedural cardiac insufficiency following other surgery

✓6ᵗʰ **I97.12 Postprocedural cardiac arrest**

I97.120 Postprocedural cardiac arrest following cardiac surgery

I97.121 Postprocedural cardiac arrest following other surgery

✓6ᵗʰ **I97.13 Postprocedural heart failure**
Use additional code to identify the heart failure (I50.-)

I97.130 Postprocedural heart failure following cardiac surgery

I97.131 Postprocedural heart failure following other surgery

✓6ᵗʰ **I97.19 Other postprocedural cardiac functional disturbances**
Use additional code, if applicable, to further specify disorder

I97.190 Other postprocedural cardiac functional disturbances following cardiac surgery
Use additional code, if applicable, for type 4 or type 5 myocardial infarction, to further specify disorder
AHA: 2019,2Q,33

I97.191 Other postprocedural cardiac functional disturbances following other surgery

I97.2 Postmastectomy lymphedema syndrome   A
Elephantiasis due to mastectomy
Obliteration of lymphatic vessels

I97.3 Postprocedural hypertension

✓5ᵗʰ **I97.4 Intraoperative hemorrhage and hematoma of a circulatory system organ or structure complicating a procedure**
EXCLUDES 1   intraoperative hemorrhage and hematoma of a circulatory system organ or structure due to accidental puncture and laceration during a procedure (I97.5-)
EXCLUDES 2   intraoperative cerebrovascular hemorrhage complicating a procedure (G97.3-)

✓6ᵗʰ **I97.41 Intraoperative hemorrhage and hematoma of a circulatory system organ or structure complicating a circulatory system procedure**

I97.410 Intraoperative hemorrhage and hematoma of a circulatory system organ or structure complicating a cardiac catheterization

I97.411 Intraoperative hemorrhage and hematoma of a circulatory system organ or structure complicating a cardiac bypass

| ✓ Additional Character Required | ✓x7ᵗʰ Placeholder Alert | Manifestation | Unspecified Dx | Q QPP | UPD Unacceptable PDx |

ICD-10-CM 2023   703

Chapter 9. Diseases of the Circulatory System

I97.418   **Intraoperative hemorrhage and hematoma of a circulatory system organ or structure complicating** other circulatory system procedure

I97.42   **Intraoperative hemorrhage and hematoma of a circulatory system organ or structure complicating** other procedure
     AHA: 2020,1Q,19

✓5ᵗʰ   I97.5   Accidental puncture and laceration **of a circulatory system organ or structure during a procedure**
     EXCLUDES 2   *accidental puncture and laceration of brain during a procedure (G97.4-)*

I97.51   **Accidental puncture and laceration of a circulatory system organ or structure during a** circulatory system procedure
     AHA: 2019,2Q,24

I97.52   **Accidental puncture and laceration of a circulatory system organ or structure during** other procedure

✓5ᵗʰ   I97.6   Postprocedural hemorrhage, hematoma and seroma **of a circulatory system organ or structure following a procedure**
     EXCLUDES 2   *postprocedural cerebrovascular hemorrhage complicating a procedure (G97.5-)*
     AHA: 2016,4Q,9-10

✓6ᵗʰ   I97.61   Postprocedural hemorrhage **of a circulatory system organ or structure following a** circulatory system procedure

I97.610   **Postprocedural hemorrhage of a circulatory system organ or structure following a** cardiac catheterization

I97.611   **Postprocedural hemorrhage of a circulatory system organ or structure following** cardiac bypass

I97.618   **Postprocedural hemorrhage of a circulatory system organ or structure following** other circulatory system procedure

✓6ᵗʰ   I97.62   Postprocedural hemorrhage, hematoma and seroma **of a circulatory system organ or structure following** other procedure

I97.620   **Postprocedural** hemorrhage **of a circulatory system organ or structure following other procedure**

I97.621   **Postprocedural** hematoma **of a circulatory system organ or structure following other procedure**

I97.622   **Postprocedural** seroma **of a circulatory system organ or structure following other procedure**

✓6ᵗʰ   I97.63   Postprocedural hematoma **of a circulatory system organ or structure following a** circulatory system procedure

I97.630   **Postprocedural hematoma of a circulatory system organ or structure following a** cardiac catheterization

I97.631   **Postprocedural hematoma of a circulatory system organ or structure following** cardiac bypass

I97.638   **Postprocedural hematoma of a circulatory system organ or structure following** other circulatory system procedure

✓6ᵗʰ   I97.64   Postprocedural seroma **of a circulatory system organ or structure following a circulatory system procedure**

I97.640   **Postprocedural seroma of a circulatory system organ or structure following a** cardiac catheterization

I97.641   **Postprocedural seroma of a circulatory system organ or structure following** cardiac bypass

I97.648   **Postprocedural seroma of a circulatory system organ or structure following** other circulatory system procedure

✓5ᵗʰ   I97.7   Intraoperative **cardiac** functional disturbances
     EXCLUDES 2   *acute pulmonary insufficiency following thoracic surgery (J95.1)*
          postprocedural cardiac functional disturbances (I97.1-)

✓6ᵗʰ   I97.71   Intraoperative cardiac arrest

I97.710   **Intraoperative cardiac arrest during** cardiac surgery

I97.711   **Intraoperative cardiac arrest during** other surgery

✓6ᵗʰ   I97.79   **Other intraoperative cardiac functional disturbances**
     Use additional code, if applicable, to further specify disorder

I97.790   **Other intraoperative cardiac functional disturbances during** cardiac surgery

I97.791   **Other intraoperative cardiac functional disturbances during** other surgery

✓5ᵗʰ   I97.8   **Other intraoperative and postprocedural complications and disorders of the circulatory system, not elsewhere classified**
     Use additional code, if applicable, to further specify disorder

✓6ᵗʰ   I97.81   Intraoperative **cerebrovascular infarction**

I97.810   **Intraoperative cerebrovascular infarction during** cardiac surgery   HCC ESR

I97.811   **Intraoperative cerebrovascular infarction during** other surgery   HCC ESR

✓6ᵗʰ   I97.82   Postprocedural **cerebrovascular infarction**

I97.820   **Postprocedural cerebrovascular infarction following** cardiac surgery   HCC ESR

I97.821   **Postprocedural cerebrovascular infarction following** other surgery   HCC ESR

I97.88   **Other intraoperative complications of the circulatory system, not elsewhere classified**

I97.89   **Other postprocedural complications and disorders of the circulatory system, not elsewhere classified**
     AHA: 2021,3Q,33; 2020,3Q,3-8; 2019,2Q,33

✓4ᵗʰ   **I99   Other and unspecified disorders of circulatory system**

I99.8   **Other disorder of circulatory system**
     AHA: 2020,4Q,98

I99.9   **Unspecified disorder of circulatory system**

Chapter 10. Diseases of the Respiratory System (J00–J99)

Chapter-specific Guidelines with Coding Examples

The chapter-specific guidelines from the ICD-10-CM Official Guidelines for Coding and Reporting have been provided below. Along with these guidelines are coding examples, contained in the shaded boxes, that have been developed to help illustrate the coding and/or sequencing guidance found in these guidelines.

a. Chronic obstructive pulmonary disease [COPD] and asthma

1) Acute exacerbation of chronic obstructive bronchitis and asthma

The codes in categories J44 and J45 distinguish between uncomplicated cases and those in acute exacerbation. An acute exacerbation is a worsening or a decompensation of a chronic condition. An acute exacerbation is not equivalent to an infection superimposed on a chronic condition, though an exacerbation may be triggered by an infection.

> Acute streptococcal bronchitis with acute exacerbation of COPD
>
> | J20.2 | Acute bronchitis due to streptococcus |
> |---|---|
> | J44.0 | Chronic obstructive pulmonary disease with (acute) lower respiratory infection |
> | J44.1 | Chronic obstructive pulmonary disease with (acute) exacerbation |
>
> *Explanation*: ICD-10-CM uses combination codes to create organism-specific classifications for acute bronchitis. Category J44 codes include combination codes with severity components, which differentiate between COPD with acute lower respiratory infection (acute bronchitis), COPD with acute exacerbation, and COPD without mention of a complication (unspecified).
>
> An acute exacerbation is a worsening or a decompensation of a chronic condition. An acute exacerbation is not equivalent to an infection superimposed on a chronic condition, though an exacerbation may be triggered by an infection, as in this example.

> Exacerbation of moderate persistent asthma with status asthmaticus
>
> | J45.42 | Moderate persistent asthma with status asthmaticus |
> |---|---|
>
> *Explanation*: Category J45 Asthma includes severity-specific subcategories and fifth-character codes to distinguish between uncomplicated cases, those in acute exacerbation, and those with status asthmaticus.

b. Acute respiratory failure

1) Acute respiratory failure as principal diagnosis

A code from subcategory J96.0, Acute respiratory failure, or subcategory J96.2, Acute and chronic respiratory failure, may be assigned as a principal diagnosis when it is the condition established after study to be chiefly responsible for occasioning the admission to the hospital, and the selection is supported by the Alphabetic Index and Tabular List. However, chapter-specific coding guidelines (such as obstetrics, poisoning, HIV, newborn) that provide sequencing direction take precedence.

> Acute hypoxic respiratory failure due to exacerbation of chronic obstructive bronchitis
>
> | J96.01 | Acute respiratory failure with hypoxia |
> |---|---|
> | J44.1 | Chronic obstructive pulmonary disease with (acute) exacerbation |
>
> *Explanation*: Category J96 classifies respiratory failure with combination codes that designate the severity and the presence of hypoxia and hypercapnia. Code J96.01 is sequenced as the first-listed diagnosis, as the reason for the encounter. Respiratory failure may be assigned as a principal diagnosis when it is the condition established after study to be chiefly responsible for occasioning the encounter and the selection is supported by the Alphabetic Index and Tabular List.

2) Acute respiratory failure as secondary diagnosis

Respiratory failure may be listed as a secondary diagnosis if it occurs after admission, or if it is present on admission, but does not meet the definition of principal diagnosis.

> Acute respiratory failure due to accidental oxycodone overdose
>
> | T40.2X1A | Poisoning by other opioids, accidental (unintentional), initial encounter |
> |---|---|
> | J96.00 | Acute respiratory failure, unspecified whether with hypoxia or hypercapnia |
>
> *Explanation*: Respiratory failure may be assigned as a principal diagnosis when it is the condition established after study to be chiefly responsible for occasioning the encounter, and the selection is supported by the Alphabetic Index and Tabular List. However, chapter-specific coding guidelines, such as poisoning, that provide sequencing direction take precedence. When coding a poisoning or reaction to the improper use of a medication (e.g., overdose, wrong substance given or taken in error, wrong route of administration), first assign the appropriate code from categories T36–T50. Use additional code(s) for all manifestations of the poisoning. In this instance, the respiratory failure is a manifestation of the poisoning and is sequenced as a secondary diagnosis.

3) Sequencing of acute respiratory failure and another acute condition

When a patient is admitted with respiratory failure and another acute condition, (e.g., myocardial infarction, cerebrovascular accident, aspiration pneumonia), the principal diagnosis will not be the same in every situation. This applies whether the other acute condition is a respiratory or nonrespiratory condition. Selection of the principal diagnosis will be dependent on the circumstances of admission. If both the respiratory failure and the other acute condition are equally responsible for occasioning the admission to the hospital, and there are no chapter-specific sequencing rules, the guideline regarding two or more diagnoses that equally meet the definition for principal diagnosis (*Section II, C.*) may be applied in these situations.

If the documentation is not clear as to whether acute respiratory failure and another condition are equally responsible for occasioning the admission, query the provider for clarification.

> Patient presents with acute pneumococcal pneumonia and acute respiratory failure
>
> | J96.00 | Acute respiratory failure, unspecified whether with hypoxia or hypercapnia |
> |---|---|
> | J13 | Pneumonia due to Streptococcus pneumoniae |
>
> *Explanation*: When a patient is seen for respiratory failure and another acute condition, such as a bacterial pneumonia, the principal or first-listed diagnosis is not the same in every situation. This applies whether the other acute condition is a respiratory or nonrespiratory condition. The principal diagnosis depends on the problem chiefly responsible for the encounter.

c. Influenza due to certain identified influenza viruses

Code only confirmed cases of influenza due to certain identified influenza viruses (category J09), and due to other identified influenza virus (category J10). This is an exception to the hospital inpatient guideline Section II, H. (Uncertain Diagnosis).

In this context, "confirmation" does not require documentation of positive laboratory testing specific for avian or other novel influenza A or other identified influenza virus. However, coding should be based on the provider's diagnostic statement that the patient has avian influenza, or other novel influenza A, for category J09, or has another particular identified strain of influenza, such as H1N1 or H3N2, but not identified as novel or variant, for category J10.

If the provider records "suspected" or "possible" or "probable" avian influenza, or novel influenza, or other identified influenza, then the appropriate influenza code from category J11, Influenza due to unidentified influenza virus, should be assigned. A code from category J09, Influenza due to certain identified influenza viruses, should not be assigned nor should a code from category J10, Influenza due to other identified influenza virus.

Influenza due to avian influenza virus with pneumonia

J09.X1   Influenza due to identified novel influenza A virus with pneumonia

Explanation: Codes in category J09 Influenza due to certain identified influenza viruses should be assigned only for confirmed cases. "Confirmation" does not require positive laboratory testing of a specific influenza virus but does need to be based on the provider's diagnostic statement, which should not include terms such as "possible," "probable," or "suspected."

d. Ventilator associated pneumonia

1) Documentation of ventilator associated pneumonia

As with all procedural or postprocedural complications, code assignment is based on the provider's documentation of the relationship between the condition and the procedure.

Code J95.851, Ventilator associated pneumonia, should be assigned only when the provider has documented ventilator associated pneumonia (VAP). An additional code to identify the organism (e.g., Pseudomonas aeruginosa, code B96.5) should also be assigned. Do not assign an additional code from categories J12-J18 to identify the type of pneumonia.

Code J95.851 should not be assigned for cases where the patient has pneumonia and is on a mechanical ventilator and the provider has not specifically stated that the pneumonia is ventilator-associated pneumonia. If the documentation is unclear as to whether the patient has a pneumonia that is a complication attributable to the mechanical ventilator, query the provider.

2) Ventilator associated pneumonia develops after admission

A patient may be admitted with one type of pneumonia (e.g., code J13, Pneumonia due to Streptococcus pneumonia) and subsequently develop VAP. In this instance, the principal diagnosis would be the appropriate code from categories J12-J18 for the pneumonia diagnosed at the time of admission. Code J95.851, Ventilator associated pneumonia, would be assigned as an additional diagnosis when the provider has also documented the presence of ventilator associated pneumonia.

e. Vaping-related disorders

For patients presenting with condition(s) related to vaping, assign code U07.0, Vaping-related disorder, as the principal diagnosis. For lung injury due to vaping, assign only code U07.0. Assign additional codes for other manifestations, such as acute respiratory failure (subcategory J96.0-) or pneumonitis (code J68.0).

Associated respiratory signs and symptoms due to vaping, such as cough, shortness of breath, etc., are not coded separately, when a definitive diagnosis has been established. However, it would be appropriate to code separately any gastrointestinal symptoms, such as diarrhea and abdominal pain.

See Section I.C.1.g.1.c.i. for Pneumonia confirmed as due to COVID-19

Chapter 10. Diseases of the Respiratory System (J00-J99)

NOTE   When a respiratory condition is described as occurring in more than one site and is not specifically indexed, it should be classified to the lower anatomic site (e.g., tracheobronchitis to bronchitis in J40).

Use additional code, where applicable, to identify:
- exposure to environmental tobacco smoke (Z77.22)
- exposure to tobacco smoke in the perinatal period (P96.81)
- history of tobacco dependence (Z87.891)
- occupational exposure to environmental tobacco smoke (Z57.31)
- tobacco dependence (F17.-)
- tobacco use (Z72.0)

EXCLUDES 2   certain conditions originating in the perinatal period (P04-P96)
certain infectious and parasitic diseases (A00-B99)
complications of pregnancy, childbirth and the puerperium (O00-O9A)
congenital malformations, deformations and chromosomal abnormalities (Q00-Q99)
endocrine, nutritional and metabolic diseases (E00-E88)
injury, poisoning and certain other consequences of external causes (S00-T88)
neoplasms (C00-D49)
smoke inhalation (T59.81-)
symptoms, signs and abnormal clinical and laboratory findings, not elsewhere classified (R00-R94)

This chapter contains the following blocks:
J00-J06	Acute upper respiratory infections
J09-J18	Influenza and pneumonia
J20-J22	Other acute lower respiratory infections
J30-J39	Other diseases of upper respiratory tract
J40-J47	Chronic lower respiratory diseases
J60-J70	Lung diseases due to external agents
J80-J84	Other respiratory diseases principally affecting the interstitium
J85-J86	Suppurative and necrotic conditions of the lower respiratory tract
J90-J94	Other diseases of the pleura
J95	Intraoperative and postprocedural complications and disorders of respiratory system, not elsewhere classified
J96-J99	Other diseases of the respiratory system

Acute upper respiratory infections (J00-J06)

EXCLUDES 1   chronic obstructive pulmonary disease with acute lower respiratory infection (J44.0)

J00   **Acute nasopharyngitis [common cold]**
Acute rhinitis
Coryza (acute)
Infective nasopharyngitis NOS
Infective rhinitis
Nasal catarrh, acute
Nasopharyngitis NOS
   EXCLUDES 1   acute pharyngitis (J02.-)
acute sore throat NOS (J02.9)
influenza virus with other respiratory manifestations (J09.X2, J10.1, J11.1)
pharyngitis NOS (J02.9)
rhinitis NOS (J31.0)
sore throat NOS (J02.9)
   EXCLUDES 2   allergic rhinitis (J30.1-J30.9)
chronic pharyngitis (J31.2)
chronic rhinitis (J31.0)
chronic sore throat (J31.2)
nasopharyngitis, chronic (J31.1)
vasomotor rhinitis (J30.0)

a Cute (handwritten annotation)

✓4ᵗʰ J01   **Acute sinusitis**
   INCLUDES   acute abscess of sinus
acute empyema of sinus
acute infection of sinus
acute inflammation of sinus
acute suppuration of sinus
Use additional code (B95-B97) to identify infectious agent
   EXCLUDES 1   sinusitis NOS (J32.9)
   EXCLUDES 2   chronic sinusitis (J32.0-J32.8)

   ✓5ᵗʰ J01.0   **Acute maxillary sinusitis**
Acute antritis
     J01.00   **Acute maxillary sinusitis, unspecified**
     J01.01   **Acute recurrent maxillary sinusitis**
   ✓5ᵗʰ J01.1   **Acute frontal sinusitis**
     J01.10   **Acute frontal sinusitis, unspecified**
     J01.11   **Acute recurrent frontal sinusitis**

✓5ᵗʰ J01.2   **Acute ethmoidal sinusitis**
   J01.20   **Acute ethmoidal sinusitis, unspecified**
   J01.21   **Acute recurrent ethmoidal sinusitis**
✓5ᵗʰ J01.3   **Acute sphenoidal sinusitis**
   J01.30   **Acute sphenoidal sinusitis, unspecified**
   J01.31   **Acute recurrent sphenoidal sinusitis**
✓5ᵗʰ J01.4   **Acute pansinusitis**
   J01.40   **Acute pansinusitis, unspecified**
   J01.41   **Acute recurrent pansinusitis**
✓5ᵗʰ J01.8   **Other acute sinusitis**
   J01.80   **Other acute sinusitis**
     Acute sinusitis involving more than one sinus but not pansinusitis
   J01.81   **Other acute recurrent sinusitis**
     Acute recurrent sinusitis involving more than one sinus but not pansinusitis
✓5ᵗʰ J01.9   **Acute sinusitis, unspecified**
   J01.90   **Acute sinusitis, unspecified**
   J01.91   **Acute recurrent sinusitis, unspecified**

✓4ᵗʰ J02   **Acute pharyngitis**
   INCLUDES   acute sore throat
   EXCLUDES 1   acute laryngopharyngitis (J06.0)
peritonsillar abscess (J36)
pharyngeal abscess (J39.1)
retropharyngeal abscess (J39.0)
   EXCLUDES 2   chronic pharyngitis (J31.2)

   J02.0   **Streptococcal pharyngitis**
Septic pharyngitis
Streptococcal sore throat
     EXCLUDES 2   scarlet fever (A38.-)
   J02.8   **Acute pharyngitis due to other specified organisms**
Use additional code (B95-B97) to identify infectious agent
     EXCLUDES 1   acute pharyngitis due to coxsackie virus (B08.5)
acute pharyngitis due to gonococcus (A54.5)
acute pharyngitis due to herpes [simplex] virus (B00.2)
acute pharyngitis due to infectious mononucleosis (B27.-)
enteroviral vesicular pharyngitis (B08.5)
   J02.9   **Acute pharyngitis, unspecified**
Gangrenous pharyngitis (acute)
Infective pharyngitis (acute) NOS
Pharyngitis (acute) NOS
Sore throat (acute) NOS
Suppurative pharyngitis (acute)
Ulcerative pharyngitis (acute)
     EXCLUDES 1   influenza virus with other respiratory manifestations (J09.X2, J10.1, J11.1)

✓4ᵗʰ J03   **Acute tonsillitis**
   EXCLUDES 1   acute sore throat (J02.-)
hypertrophy of tonsils (J35.1)
peritonsillar abscess (J36)
sore throat NOS (J02.9)
streptococcal sore throat (J02.0)
   EXCLUDES 2   chronic tonsillitis (J35.0)

   ✓5ᵗʰ J03.0   **Streptococcal tonsillitis**
     J03.00   **Acute streptococcal tonsillitis, unspecified**
     J03.01   **Acute recurrent streptococcal tonsillitis**
   ✓5ᵗʰ J03.8   **Acute tonsillitis due to other specified organisms**
Use additional code (B95-B97) to identify infectious agent
     EXCLUDES 1   diphtheritic tonsillitis (A36.0)
herpesviral pharyngotonsillitis (B00.2)
streptococcal tonsillitis (J03.0)
tuberculous tonsillitis (A15.8)
Vincent's tonsillitis (A69.1)
     J03.80   **Acute tonsillitis due to other specified organisms**
     J03.81   **Acute recurrent tonsillitis due to other specified organisms**

Chapter 10. Diseases of the Respiratory System

✓5ᵗʰ **J03.9 Acute tonsillitis, unspecified**
     Follicular tonsillitis (acute)
     Gangrenous tonsillitis (acute)
     Infective tonsillitis (acute)
     Tonsillitis (acute) NOS
     Ulcerative tonsillitis (acute)
       EXCLUDES 1   *influenza virus with other respiratory manifestations (J09.X2, J10.1, J11.1)*

     J03.90 Acute tonsillitis, unspecified
     J03.91 Acute recurrent tonsillitis, unspecified

✓4ᵗʰ **J04 Acute laryngitis and tracheitis**
     Code also influenza, if present, such as:
       influenza due to identified novel influenza A virus with other respiratory manifestations (J09.X2)
       influenza due to other identified influenza virus with other respiratory manifestations (J10.1)
       influenza due to unidentified influenza virus with other respiratory manifestations (J11.1)
     Use additional code (B95-B97) to identify infectious agent
       EXCLUDES 1   *acute obstructive laryngitis [croup] and epiglottitis (J05.-)*
       EXCLUDES 2   *laryngismus (stridulus) (J38.5)*

     J04.0 Acute laryngitis
       Edematous laryngitis (acute)
       Laryngitis (acute) NOS
       Subglottic laryngitis (acute)
       Suppurative laryngitis (acute)
       Ulcerative laryngitis (acute)
         EXCLUDES 1   *acute obstructive laryngitis (J05.0)*
         EXCLUDES 2   *chronic laryngitis (J37.0)*

✓5ᵗʰ **J04.1 Acute tracheitis**
       Acute viral tracheitis
       Catarrhal tracheitis (acute)
       Tracheitis (acute) NOS
         EXCLUDES 2   *chronic tracheitis (J42)*

     J04.10 Acute tracheitis without obstruction
     J04.11 Acute tracheitis with obstruction
     J04.2 Acute laryngotracheitis
       Laryngotracheitis NOS
       Tracheitis (acute) with laryngitis (acute)
         EXCLUDES 1   *acute obstructive laryngotracheitis (J05.0)*
         EXCLUDES 2   *chronic laryngotracheitis (J37.1)*

✓5ᵗʰ **J04.3 Supraglottitis, unspecified**
     J04.30 Supraglottitis, unspecified, without obstruction
     J04.31 Supraglottitis, unspecified, with obstruction

✓4ᵗʰ **J05 Acute obstructive laryngitis [croup] and epiglottitis** *Won't*

a Cute

Croup

     Code also, influenza, if present, such as:
       influenza due to identified novel influenza A virus with other respiratory manifestations (J09.X2)
       influenza due to other identified influenza virus with other respiratory manifestations (J10.1)
       influenza due to unidentified influenza virus with other respiratory manifestations (J11.1)
     Use additional code (B95-B97) to identify infectious agent
     J05.0 Acute obstructive laryngitis [croup]
       Obstructive laryngitis (acute) NOS
       Obstructive laryngotracheitis NOS
       DEF: Acute laryngeal obstruction due to allergies, foreign bodies, or in the majority of cases a viral infection. Symptoms include a harsh, barking cough, hoarseness, and a persistent, high-pitched respiratory sound (stridor).

✓5ᵗʰ **J05.1 Acute epiglottitis**
       EXCLUDES 2   *epiglottitis, chronic (J37.0)*
     J05.10 Acute epiglottitis without obstruction
       Epiglottitis NOS
     J05.11 Acute epiglottitis with obstruction

✓4ᵗʰ **J06 Acute upper respiratory infections of multiple and unspecified sites**
       EXCLUDES 1   *acute respiratory infection NOS (J22)*
          influenza virus with other respiratory manifestations (J09.X2, J10.1, J11.1)
          streptococcal pharyngitis (J02.0)
     J06.0 Acute laryngopharyngitis

J06.9 Acute upper respiratory infection, unspecified
     Upper respiratory disease, acute
     Upper respiratory infection NOS
     Use additional code (B95-B97) to identify infectious agent, if known, such as:
       respiratory syncytial virus (RSV) (B97.4)
     AHA: 2020,1Q,22

Influenza and pneumonia (J09-J18)

     EXCLUDES 2   *allergic or eosinophilic pneumonia (J82)*
         aspiration pneumonia NOS (J69.0)
         meconium pneumonia (P24.01)
         neonatal aspiration pneumonia (P24.-)
         pneumonia due to solids and liquids (J69.-)
         congenital pneumonia (P23.9)
         lipid pneumonia (J69.1)
         rheumatic pneumonia (I00)
         ventilator associated pneumonia (J95.851)
AHA: 2017,4Q,96
TIP: Hemoptysis (R04.2) is not customarily associated with pneumonia and may be reported separately.

✓4ᵗʰ **J09 Influenza due to certain identified influenza viruses**
       EXCLUDES 1   *influenza A/H1N1 (J10.-)*
          influenza due to other identified influenza virus (J10.-)
          influenza due to unidentified influenza virus (J11.-)
          seasonal influenza due to other identified influenza virus (J10.-)
          seasonal influenza due to unidentified influenza virus (J11.-)

✓5ᵗʰ **J09.X Influenza due to identified novel influenza A virus**
     Avian influenza
     Bird influenza
     Influenza A/H5N1
     Influenza of other animal origin, not bird or swine
     Swine influenza virus (viruses that normally cause infections in pigs)
     AHA: 2016,3Q,10

     J09.X1 Influenza due to identified novel influenza A virus with pneumonia
       Code also, if applicable, associated:
         lung abscess (J85.1)
         other specified type of pneumonia

influenza

     J09.X2 Influenza due to identified novel influenza A virus with other respiratory manifestations
       Influenza due to identified novel influenza A virus NOS
       Influenza due to identified novel influenza A virus with laryngitis
       Influenza due to identified novel influenza A virus with pharyngitis
       Influenza due to identified novel influenza A virus with upper respiratory symptoms
       Use additional code, if applicable, for associated:
         pleural effusion (J91.8)
         sinusitis (J01.-)

     J09.X3 Influenza due to identified novel influenza A virus with gastrointestinal manifestations
       Influenza due to identified novel influenza A virus gastroenteritis
         EXCLUDES 1   *'intestinal flu' [viral gastroenteritis] (A08.-)*

     J09.X9 Influenza due to identified novel influenza A virus with other manifestations
       Influenza due to identified novel influenza A virus with encephalopathy
       Influenza due to identified novel influenza A virus with myocarditis
       Influenza due to identified novel influenza A virus with otitis media
       Use additional code to identify manifestation

☑4ᵗʰ **J10** **Influenza due to** other **identified influenza virus**

INCLUDES   influenza A (non-novel)
influenza B
influenza C

EXCLUDES 1   *influenza due to avian influenza virus (J09.X-)*
influenza due to swine flu (J09.X-)
influenza due to unidentifed influenza virus (J11.-)

☑5ᵗʰ **J10.0** **Influenza due to other identified influenza virus with** pneumonia
Code also associated lung abscess, if applicable (J85.1)

J10.00 **Influenza due to other identified influenza virus with unspecified type of pneumonia**

J10.01 **Influenza due to other identified influenza virus with** the same other identified influenza virus **pneumonia**

J10.08 **Influenza due to other identified influenza virus with other specified pneumonia**
Code also other specified type of pneumonia

J10.1 **Influenza due to other identified influenza virus with** other respiratory manifestations
Influenza due to other identified influenza virus NOS
Influenza due to other identified influenza virus with laryngitis
Influenza due to other identified influenza virus with pharyngitis
Influenza due to other identified influenza virus with upper respiratory symptoms
Use additional code for associated pleural effusion, if applicable (J91.8)
Use additional code for associated sinusitis, if applicable (J01.-)
AHA: 2016,3Q,10-11

J10.2 **Influenza due to other identified influenza virus with** gastrointestinal manifestations
Influenza due to other identified influenza virus gastroenteritis
EXCLUDES 1   *"intestinal flu" [viral gastroenteritis] (A08.-)*

☑5ᵗʰ **J10.8** **Influenza due to other identified influenza virus with other manifestations**

J10.81 **Influenza due to other identified influenza virus with** encephalopathy

J10.82 **Influenza due to other identified influenza virus with** myocarditis

J10.83 **Influenza due to other identified influenza virus with** otitis media
Use additional code for any associated perforated tympanic membrane (H72.-)

J10.89 **Influenza due to other identified influenza virus with other manifestations**
Use additional codes to identify the manifestations

☑4ᵗʰ **J11** **Influenza due to** unidentified **influenza virus**

☑5ᵗʰ **J11.0** **Influenza due to unidentified influenza virus with** pneumonia
Code also associated lung abscess, if applicable (J85.1)
AHA: 2016,3Q,11

J11.00 **Influenza due to unidentified influenza virus with unspecified type of pneumonia**
Influenza with pneumonia NOS

J11.08 **Influenza due to unidentified influenza virus with** specified **pneumonia**
Code also other specified type of pneumonia

J11.1 **Influenza due to unidentified influenza virus with** other respiratory manifestations
Influenza NOS
Influenzal laryngitis NOS
Influenzal pharyngitis NOS
Influenza with upper respiratory symptoms NOS
Use additional code for associated pleural effusion, if applicable (J91.8)
Use additional code for associated sinusitis, if applicable (J01.-)

J11.2 **Influenza due to unidentified influenza virus with** gastrointestinal manifestations
Influenza gastroenteritis NOS
EXCLUDES 1   *"intestinal flu" [viral gastroenteritis] (A08.-)*

☑5ᵗʰ **J11.8** **Influenza due to unidentified influenza virus with other manifestations**

J11.81 **Influenza due to unidentified influenza virus with** encephalopathy
Influenzal encephalopathy NOS

J11.82 **Influenza due to unidentified influenza virus with** myocarditis
Influenzal myocarditis NOS

J11.83 **Influenza due to unidentified influenza virus with** otitis media
Influenzal otitis media NOS
Use additional code for any associated perforated tympanic membrane (H72.-)

J11.89 **Influenza due to unidentified influenza virus with other manifestations**
Use additional codes to identify the manifestations

☑4ᵗʰ **J12** **Viral pneumonia, not elsewhere classified**

INCLUDES   bronchopneumonia due to viruses other than influenza viruses
Code first associated influenza, if applicable (J09.X1, J10.0-, J11.0-)
Code also associated abscess, if applicable (J85.1)

EXCLUDES 1   *aspiration pneumonia due to anesthesia during labor and delivery (O74.0)*
aspiration pneumonia due to anesthesia during pregnancy (O29)
aspiration pneumonia due to anesthesia during puerperium (O89.0)
aspiration pneumonia due to solids and liquids (J69.-)
aspiration pneumonia NOS (J69.0)
congenital pneumonia (P23.0)
congenital rubella pneumonitis (P35.0)
interstitial pneumonia NOS (J84.9)
lipid pneumonia (J69.1)
neonatal aspiration pneumonia (P24.-)
AHA: 2020,2Q,28; 2019,1Q,35; 2018,3Q,24; 2016,3Q,15; 2013,4Q,118

J12.0 Adenoviral **pneumonia**

J12.1 Respiratory syncytial **virus pneumonia**
RSV pneumonia

J12.2 Parainfluenza **virus pneumonia**

J12.3 Human metapneumovirus **pneumonia**

☑5ᵗʰ **J12.8** **Other viral pneumonia**

J12.81 **Pneumonia due to** SARS-associated coronavirus
Severe acute respiratory syndrome NOS
DEF: Inflammation of the lungs with consolidation, caused by the severe adult respiratory syndrome (SARS)-associated coronavirus or SARS-CoV. This pneumonia should not be confused with that caused by SARS-CoV-2 (COVID-19).

J12.82 **Pneumonia due to** coronavirus disease 2019   UPD
Pneumonia due to 2019 novel coronavirus (SARS-CoV-2)
Pneumonia due to COVID-19
Code first COVID-19 (U07.1)
AHA: 2021,1Q,25-30,31-49

J12.89 **Other viral pneumonia**
AHA: 2021,1Q,33-34; 2020,2Q,8,11; 2020,1Q,34-36

J12.9 **Viral pneumonia, unspecified**

J13 **Pneumonia due to** Streptococcus pneumoniae   HCC ESR
Bronchopneumonia due to S. pneumoniae
Code first associated influenza, if applicable (J09.X1, J10.0-, J11.0-)
Code also associated abscess, if applicable (J85.1)
EXCLUDES 1   *congenital pneumonia due to S. pneumoniae (P23.6)*
lobar pneumonia, unspecified organism (J18.1)
pneumonia due to other streptococci (J15.3-J15.4)
AHA: 2020,2Q,28; 2019,1Q,35; 2018,3Q,24; 2016,3Q,15; 2013,4Q,118

J14 **Pneumonia due to** Hemophilus influenzae   HCC ESR
Bronchopneumonia due to H. influenzae
Code first associated influenza, if applicable (J09.X1, J10.0-, J11.0-)
Code also associated abscess, if applicable (J85.1)
EXCLUDES 1   *congenital pneumonia due to H. influenzae (P23.6)*
AHA: 2020,2Q,28; 2019,1Q,35; 2018,3Q,24; 2016,3Q,15; 2013,4Q,118

☑4ᵗʰ **J15** Bacterial **pneumonia, not elsewhere classified**
INCLUDES   Bronchopneumonia due to bacteria other than S. pneumoniae and H. influenzae
Code first associated influenza, if applicable (J09.X1, J10.0-, -J11.0-)
Code also associated abscess, if applicable (J85.1)
EXCLUDES 1   *chlamydial pneumonia (J16.0)*
congenital pneumonia (P23.-)
Legionnaires' disease (A48.1)
spirochetal pneumonia (A69.8)
AHA: 2020,2Q,28; 2019,1Q,35; 2018,3Q,24; 2016,3Q,15; 2013,4Q,118

J15.0 **Pneumonia due to** Klebsiella pneumoniae   HCC ESR COM

J15.1 **Pneumonia due to** Pseudomonas   HCC ESR COM

Chapter 10. Diseases of the Respiratory System

pneumonia

√5ᵗʰ J15.2 Pneumonia due to staphylococcus

    J15.20 Pneumonia due to staphylococcus, unspecified `HCC` `ESR` `COM`

    √6ᵗʰ J15.21 Pneumonia due to Staphylococcus aureus

        J15.211 Pneumonia due to methicillin susceptible Staphylococcus aureus `HCC` `ESR` `COM`
            MSSA pneumonia
            Pneumonia due to Staphylococcus aureus NOS

        J15.212 Pneumonia due to methicillin resistant Staphylococcus aureus `HCC` `ESR` `COM`

    J15.29 Pneumonia due to other staphylococcus `HCC` `ESR` `COM`

J15.3 Pneumonia due to streptococcus, group B `HCC` `ESR`

J15.4 Pneumonia due to other streptococci `HCC` `ESR`
    EXCLUDES 1   pneumonia due to streptococcus, group B (J15.3)
               pneumonia due to Streptococcus pneumoniae (J13)

J15.5 Pneumonia due to Escherichia coli `HCC` `ESR` `COM`

J15.6 Pneumonia due to other Gram-negative bacteria `HCC` `ESR` `COM`
    Pneumonia due to other aerobic Gram-negative bacteria
    Pneumonia due to Serratia marcescens
    AHA: 2020,2Q,28

J15.7 Pneumonia due to Mycoplasma pneumoniae

J15.8 Pneumonia due to other specified bacteria `HCC` `ESR` `COM`

J15.9 Unspecified bacterial pneumonia
    Pneumonia due to gram-positive bacteria

√4ᵗʰ J16 Pneumonia due to other infectious organisms, not elsewhere classified
    Code first associated influenza, if applicable (J09.X1, J10.0-, J11.0-)
    Code also associated abscess, if applicable (J85.1)
    EXCLUDES 1   congenital pneumonia (P23.-)
               ornithosis (A70)
               pneumocystosis (B59)
               pneumonia NOS (J18.9)
    AHA: 2020,2Q,28; 2019,1Q,35; 2018,3Q,24; 2016,3Q,15; 2013,4Q,118

J16.0 Chlamydial pneumonia

J16.8 Pneumonia due to other specified infectious organisms

J17 Pneumonia in diseases classified elsewhere
    Code first underlying disease, such as:
    Q fever (A78)
    rheumatic fever (I00)
    schistosomiasis (B65.0-B65.9)
    EXCLUDES 1   candidial pneumonia (B37.1)
               chlamydial pneumonia (J16.0)
               gonorrheal pneumonia (A54.84)
               histoplasmosis pneumonia (B39.0-B39.2)
               measles pneumonia (B05.2)
               nocardiosis pneumonia (A43.0)
               pneumocystosis (B59)
               pneumonia due to Pneumocystis carinii (B59)
               pneumonia due to Pneumocystis jiroveci (B59)
               pneumonia in actinomycosis (A42.0)
               pneumonia in anthrax (A22.1)
               pneumonia in ascariasis (B77.81)
               pneumonia in aspergillosis (B44.0-B44.1)
               pneumonia in coccidioidomycosis (B38.0-B38.2)
               pneumonia in cytomegalovirus disease (B25.0)
               pneumonia in toxoplasmosis (B58.3)
               rubella pneumonia (B06.81)
               salmonella pneumonia (A02.22)
               spirochetal infection NEC with pneumonia (A69.8)
               tularemia pneumonia (A21.2)
               typhoid fever with pneumonia (A01.03)
               varicella pneumonia (B01.2)
               whooping cough with pneumonia (A37 with fifth character 1)
    AHA: 2020,2Q,28; 2019,1Q,35; 2016,3Q,15; 2013,4Q,118

√4ᵗʰ J18 Pneumonia, unspecified organism
    Code first associated influenza, if applicable (J09.X1, J10.0-, J11.0-)
    EXCLUDES 1   abscess of lung with pneumonia (J85.1)
               aspiration pneumonia due to anesthesia during labor and delivery (O74.0)
               aspiration pneumonia due to anesthesia during pregnancy (O29)
               aspiration pneumonia due to anesthesia during puerperium (O89.0)
               aspiration pneumonia due to solids and liquids (J69.-)
               aspiration pneumonia NOS (J69.0)
               congenital pneumonia (P23.0)
               drug-induced interstitial lung disorder (J70.2-J70.4)
               interstitial pneumonia NOS (J84.9)
               lipid pneumonia (J69.1)
               neonatal aspiration pneumonia (P24.-)
               pneumonitis due to external agents (J67-J70)
               pneumonitis due to fumes and vapors (J68.0)
               usual interstitial pneumonia (J84.178)
    AHA: 2020,2Q,28; 2019,1Q,35; 2016,3Q,15; 2013,4Q,118

J18.0 Bronchopneumonia, unspecified organism
    EXCLUDES 1   hypostatic bronchopneumonia (J18.2)
               lipid pneumonia (J69.1)
    EXCLUDES 2   acute bronchiolitis (J21.-)
               chronic bronchiolitis (J44.9)

J18.1 Lobar pneumonia, unspecified organism `HCC` `ESR`
    AHA: 2019,3Q,37; 2018,3Q,24
    DEF: Lobar pneumonia is characterized by consolidated inflammation confined or localized to only one or a few lobes of the lung. The consolidation affects primarily the alveolar air spaces, unlike bronchopneumonia, which arises from the bronchi or bronchioles and affects a wide area without any localization.
    TIP: Documentation of right upper lobe, left upper lobe, right lower lobe, left lower lobe, or right middle lobe pneumonia alone is not synonymous with "lobar pneumonia," nor should a diagnosis of lobar pneumonia be assumed based on an imaging report that identifies pneumonia in a specific lobe. Assign J18.1 only when the provider specifically documents "lobar pneumonia" without specifying a causal organism.

J18.2 Hypostatic pneumonia, unspecified organism `COM`
    Hypostatic bronchopneumonia
    Passive pneumonia

J18.8 Other pneumonia, unspecified organism

J18.9 Pneumonia, unspecified organism
    AHA: 2020,2Q,28; 2019,3Q,15; 2019,2Q,28; 2014,3Q,4; 2013,4Q,119; 2012,4Q,94

`HCC` CMS-HCC   `Rx` Rx HCC   `ESR` ESRD HCC   `COM` Commercial HCC   `N` Newborn: 0   `P` Pediatric: 0-17   `M` Maternity: 9-64   `A` Adult: 15-124

710   ICD-10-CM 2023

Other acute lower respiratory infections (J20-J22)

EXCLUDES 2　chronic obstructive pulmonary disease with acute lower respiratory infection (J44.0)

✓4ᵗʰ J20　Acute bronchitis

INCLUDES　acute and subacute bronchitis (with) bronchospasm
acute and subacute bronchitis (with) tracheitis
acute and subacute bronchitis (with) tracheobronchitis, acute
acute and subacute fibrinous bronchitis
acute and subacute membranous bronchitis
acute and subacute purulent bronchitis
acute and subacute septic bronchitis

EXCLUDES 1　bronchitis NOS (J40)
tracheobronchitis NOS (J40)

EXCLUDES 2　acute bronchitis with bronchiectasis (J47.0)
acute bronchitis with chronic obstructive asthma (J44.0)
acute bronchitis with chronic obstructive pulmonary disease (J44.0)
allergic bronchitis NOS (J45.909-)
bronchitis due to chemicals, fumes and vapors (J68.0)
chronic bronchitis NOS (J42)
chronic mucopurulent bronchitis (J41.1)
chronic obstructive bronchitis (J44.-)
chronic obstructive tracheobronchitis (J44.-)
chronic simple bronchitis (J41.0)
chronic tracheobronchitis (J42)

AHA: 2019,1Q,35; 2016,3Q,10,16
DEF: Acute inflammation of the main branches of the bronchial tree due to infectious or irritant agents. Symptoms include cough with a varied production of sputum, fever, substernal soreness, and lung rales. Bronchitis usually lasts three to 10 days.

J20.0　Acute bronchitis due to Mycoplasma pneumoniae
J20.1　Acute bronchitis due to Hemophilus influenzae
J20.2　Acute bronchitis due to streptococcus
J20.3　Acute bronchitis due to coxsackievirus
J20.4　Acute bronchitis due to parainfluenza virus
J20.5　Acute bronchitis due to respiratory syncytial virus
　　　　Acute bronchitis due to RSV
J20.6　Acute bronchitis due to rhinovirus
J20.7　Acute bronchitis due to echovirus
J20.8　Acute bronchitis due to other specified organisms
　　　　AHA: 2020,1Q,34-36
　　　　TIP: Assign as a secondary code for a patient with acute bronchitis confirmed as due to COVID-19; assign U07.1 as the principal or first-listed code.
J20.9　Acute bronchitis, unspecified

✓4ᵗʰ J21　Acute bronchiolitis

INCLUDES　acute bronchiolitis with bronchospasm
EXCLUDES 2　respiratory bronchiolitis interstitial lung disease (J84.115)

J21.0　Acute bronchiolitis due to respiratory syncytial virus
　　　　Acute bronchiolitis due to RSV
J21.1　Acute bronchiolitis due to human metapneumovirus
J21.8　Acute bronchiolitis due to other specified organisms
J21.9　Acute bronchiolitis, unspecified
　　　　Bronchiolitis (acute)
　　　　EXCLUDES 1　chronic bronchiolitis (J44.-)

J22　Unspecified acute lower respiratory infection

Acute (lower) respiratory (tract) infection NOS
EXCLUDES 1　upper respiratory infection (acute) (J06.9)
AHA: 2020,1Q,22,34-36
TIP: Assign as a secondary code for a patient with a respiratory infection specified as acute or lower that is documented as being associated with COVID-19; assign U07.1 as the principal or first-listed code. If the respiratory infection documentation does not specify acute or lower, assign J98.8.

Other diseases of upper respiratory tract (J30-J39)

✓4ᵗʰ J30　Vasomotor and allergic rhinitis

INCLUDES　spasmodic rhinorrhea
EXCLUDES 1　allergic rhinitis with asthma (bronchial) (J45.909)
rhinitis NOS (J31.0)

J30.0　Vasomotor rhinitis
　　　　DEF: Noninfectious and nonallergic type of rhinitis for which the cause is often unknown. Symptoms often mimic those of allergic rhinitis with a diagnosis of vasomotor rhinitis typically made after ruling out allergens as the cause.

J30.1　Allergic rhinitis due to pollen
　　　　Allergy NOS due to pollen
　　　　Hay fever
　　　　Pollinosis

J30.2　Other seasonal allergic rhinitis
J30.5　Allergic rhinitis due to food

✓5ᵗʰ J30.8　Other allergic rhinitis
　　　　J30.81　Allergic rhinitis due to animal (cat) (dog) hair and dander
　　　　J30.89　Other allergic rhinitis
　　　　　　　　Perennial allergic rhinitis

J30.9　Allergic rhinitis, unspecified

✓4ᵗʰ J31　Chronic rhinitis, nasopharyngitis and pharyngitis

Use additional code to identify:
exposure to environmental tobacco smoke (Z77.22)
exposure to tobacco smoke in the perinatal period (P96.81)
history of tobacco dependence (Z87.891)
occupational exposure to environmental tobacco smoke (Z57.31)
tobacco dependence (F17.-)
tobacco use (Z72.0)

J31.0　Chronic rhinitis
　　　　Atrophic rhinitis (chronic)
　　　　Granulomatous rhinitis (chronic)
　　　　Hypertrophic rhinitis (chronic)
　　　　Obstructive rhinitis (chronic)
　　　　Ozena
　　　　Purulent rhinitis (chronic)
　　　　Rhinitis (chronic) NOS
　　　　Ulcerative rhinitis (chronic)
　　　　EXCLUDES 1　allergic rhinitis (J30.1-J30.9)
　　　　　　　　　　vasomotor rhinitis (J30.0)
　　　　DEF: Persistent inflammation of the mucous membranes of the nose, characterized by a postnasal drip.

J31.1　Chronic nasopharyngitis
　　　　EXCLUDES 1　acute nasopharyngitis (J00)
　　　　DEF: Persistent inflammation of the mucous membranes extending from the nares to the pharynx. It is characterized by constant irritation in the nasopharynx and postnasal drip.

J31.2　Chronic pharyngitis
　　　　Atrophic pharyngitis (chronic)
　　　　Chronic sore throat
　　　　Granular pharyngitis (chronic)
　　　　Hypertrophic pharyngitis (chronic)
　　　　EXCLUDES 2　acute pharyngitis (J02.9)

✓4ᵗʰ J32　Chronic sinusitis

INCLUDES　sinus abscess
sinus empyema
sinus infection
sinus suppuration
Use additional code to identify:
exposure to environmental tobacco smoke (Z77.22)
exposure to tobacco smoke in the perinatal period (P96.81)
history of tobacco dependence (Z87.891)
infectious agent (B95-B97)
occupational exposure to environmental tobacco smoke (Z57.31)
tobacco dependence (F17.-)
tobacco use (Z72.0)
EXCLUDES 2　acute sinusitis (J01.-)

J32.0　Chronic maxillary sinusitis
　　　　Antritis (chronic)
　　　　Maxillary sinusitis NOS

J32.1　Chronic frontal sinusitis
　　　　Frontal sinusitis NOS

| ✔ Additional Character Required | ✓x7ᵗʰ Placeholder Alert | Manifestation | Unspecified Dx | ◻ QPP | UPD Unacceptable PDx |

ICD-10-CM 2023　　　　　　　　　　　　　　　　　　　　　　　　　　　　　　　　711

J32.2　**Chronic ethmoidal sinusitis**
　　Ethmoidal sinusitis NOS
　　EXCLUDES 1　Woakes' ethmoiditis (J33.1)

J32.3　**Chronic sphenoidal sinusitis**
　　Sphenoidal sinusitis NOS

J32.4　**Chronic pansinusitis**
　　Pansinusitis NOS

J32.8　**Other chronic sinusitis**
　　Sinusitis (chronic) involving more than one sinus but not
　　pansinusitis

J32.9　**Chronic sinusitis, unspecified**
　　Sinusitis (chronic) NOS

✓4ᵗʰ **J33**　**Nasal polyp**
　　Use additional code to identify:
　　　exposure to environmental tobacco smoke (Z77.22)
　　　exposure to tobacco smoke in the perinatal period (P96.81)
　　　history of tobacco dependence (Z87.891)
　　　occupational exposure to environmental tobacco smoke (Z57.31)
　　　tobacco dependence (F17.-)
　　　tobacco use (Z72.0)
　　EXCLUDES 1　adenomatous polyps (D14.0)

J33.0　**Polyp of nasal cavity**
　　Choanal polyp
　　Nasopharyngeal polyp

J33.1　**Polypoid sinus degeneration**
　　Woakes' syndrome or ethmoiditis

J33.8　**Other polyp of sinus**
　　Accessory polyp of sinus
　　Ethmoidal polyp of sinus
　　Maxillary polyp of sinus
　　Sphenoidal polyp of sinus

J33.9　**Nasal polyp, unspecified**

✓4ᵗʰ **J34**　**Other and unspecified disorders of nose and nasal sinuses**
　　EXCLUDES 2　varicose ulcer of nasal septum (I86.8)

J34.0　**Abscess, furuncle and carbuncle of nose**
　　Cellulitis of nose
　　Necrosis of nose
　　Ulceration of nose

J34.1　**Cyst and mucocele of nose and nasal sinus**

J34.2　**Deviated nasal septum**
　　Deflection or deviation of septum (nasal) (acquired)
　　EXCLUDES 1　congenital deviated nasal septum (Q67.4)
　　DEF: Condition in which the nasal septum, a thin wall composed
　　of cartilage and bone that separates the two nostrils, is crooked
　　or displaced from the midline.

J34.3　**Hypertrophy of nasal turbinates**
　　DEF: Overgrowth of bones within the nasal turbinate, which are
　　ridges of bone and soft tissue that project from the sidewalls of
　　the nasal passages. Hypertrophy can cause obstruction of the
　　nasal passages.

✓5ᵗʰ **J34.8**　**Other specified disorders of nose and nasal sinuses**

　　J34.81　**Nasal mucositis (ulcerative)**
　　　　Code also type of associated therapy, such as:
　　　　antineoplastic and immunosuppressive drugs
　　　　　(T45.1X-)
　　　　radiological procedure and radiotherapy (Y84.2)
　　　　EXCLUDES 2　gastrointestinal mucositis (ulcerative)
　　　　　　(K92.81)
　　　　　　mucositis (ulcerative) of vagina and vulva
　　　　　　(N76.81)
　　　　　　oral mucositis (ulcerative) (K12.3-)

　　J34.89　**Other specified disorders of nose and nasal sinuses**
　　　　Perforation of nasal septum NOS
　　　　Rhinolith

J34.9　**Unspecified disorder of nose and nasal sinuses**

✓4ᵗʰ **J35**　**Chronic diseases of tonsils and adenoids**
　　Use additional code to identify:
　　　exposure to environmental tobacco smoke (Z77.22)
　　　exposure to tobacco smoke in the perinatal period (P96.81)
　　　history of tobacco dependence (Z87.891)
　　　occupational exposure to environmental tobacco smoke (Z57.31)
　　　tobacco dependence (F17.-)
　　　tobacco use (Z72.0)

✓5ᵗʰ **J35.0**　**Chronic tonsillitis and adenoiditis**
　　　EXCLUDES 2　acute tonsillitis (J03.-)

　　J35.01　**Chronic tonsillitis**

　　J35.02　**Chronic adenoiditis**

　　J35.03　**Chronic tonsillitis and adenoiditis**

J35.1　**Hypertrophy of tonsils**
　　Enlargement of tonsils
　　EXCLUDES 1　hypertrophy of tonsils with tonsillitis (J35.0-)

J35.2　**Hypertrophy of adenoids**
　　Enlargement of adenoids
　　EXCLUDES 1　hypertrophy of adenoids with adenoiditis (J35.0-)

J35.3　**Hypertrophy of tonsils with hypertrophy of adenoids**
　　EXCLUDES 1　hypertrophy of tonsils and adenoids with tonsillitis
　　　　and adenoiditis (J35.03)

J35.8　**Other chronic diseases of tonsils and adenoids**
　　Adenoid vegetations
　　Amygdalolith
　　Calculus, tonsil
　　Cicatrix of tonsil (and adenoid)
　　Tonsillar tag
　　Ulcer of tonsil

J35.9　**Chronic disease of tonsils and adenoids, unspecified**
　　Disease (chronic) of tonsils and adenoids NOS

J36　**Peritonsillar abscess**
　　INCLUDES　abscess of tonsil
　　　　peritonsillar cellulitis
　　　　quinsy
　　Use additional code (B95-B97) to identify infectious agent
　　EXCLUDES 1　acute tonsillitis (J03.-)
　　　　chronic tonsillitis (J35.0)
　　　　retropharyngeal abscess (J39.0)
　　　　tonsillitis NOS (J03.9-)

✓4ᵗʰ **J37**　**Chronic laryngitis and laryngotracheitis**
　　Use additional code to identify:
　　　exposure to environmental tobacco smoke (Z77.22)
　　　exposure to tobacco smoke in the perinatal period (P96.81)
　　　history of tobacco dependence (Z87.891)
　　　infectious agent (B95-B97)
　　　occupational exposure to environmental tobacco smoke (Z57.31)
　　　tobacco dependence (F17.-)
　　　tobacco use (Z72.0)

J37.0　**Chronic laryngitis**
　　Catarrhal laryngitis
　　Hypertrophic laryngitis
　　Sicca laryngitis
　　EXCLUDES 2　acute laryngitis (J04.0)
　　　　obstructive (acute) laryngitis (J05.0)

J37.1　**Chronic laryngotracheitis**
　　Laryngitis, chronic, with tracheitis (chronic)
　　Tracheitis, chronic, with laryngitis
　　EXCLUDES 1　chronic tracheitis (J42)
　　EXCLUDES 2　acute laryngotracheitis (J04.2)
　　　　acute tracheitis (J04.1)

✓4ᵗʰ **J38**　**Diseases of vocal cords and larynx, not elsewhere classified**
　　Use additional code to identify:
　　　exposure to environmental tobacco smoke (Z77.22)
　　　exposure to tobacco smoke in the perinatal period (P96.81)
　　　history of tobacco dependence (Z87.891)
　　　occupational exposure to environmental tobacco smoke (Z57.31)
　　　tobacco dependence (F17.-)
　　　tobacco use (Z72.0)
　　EXCLUDES 1　congenital laryngeal stridor (P28.89)
　　　　obstructive laryngitis (acute) (J05.0)
　　　　postprocedural subglottic stenosis (J95.5)
　　　　stridor (R06.1)
　　　　ulcerative laryngitis (J04.0)

✓5ᵗʰ **J38.0**　**Paralysis of vocal cords and larynx**
　　Laryngoplegia
　　Paralysis of glottis

　　J38.00　**Paralysis of vocal cords and larynx, unspecified**

　　J38.01　**Paralysis of vocal cords and larynx, unilateral**

　　J38.02　**Paralysis of vocal cords and larynx, bilateral**

J38.1　**Polyp of vocal cord and larynx**
　　EXCLUDES 1　adenomatous polyps (D14.1)

Chapter 10. Diseases of the Respiratory System

J38.2 **Nodules** of vocal cords
     Chorditis (fibrinous)(nodosa)(tuberosa)
     Singer's nodes
     Teacher's nodes

J38.3 **Other diseases of vocal cords**
     Abscess of vocal cords
     Cellulitis of vocal cords
     Granuloma of vocal cords
     Leukokeratosis of vocal cords
     Leukoplakia of vocal cords

J38.4 **Edema** of larynx
     Edema (of) glottis
     Subglottic edema
     Supraglottic edema
     EXCLUDES 1   *acute obstructive laryngitis [croup] (J05.0)*
             edematous laryngitis (J04.0)

J38.5 **Laryngeal** spasm
     Laryngismus (stridulus)

J38.6 **Stenosis** of larynx

J38.7 **Other diseases of larynx**
     Abscess of larynx
     Cellulitis of larynx
     Disease of larynx NOS
     Necrosis of larynx
     Pachyderma of larynx
     Perichondritis of larynx
     Ulcer of larynx

√4ᵗʰ J39 **Other diseases of upper respiratory tract**
     EXCLUDES 1   *acute respiratory infection NOS (J22)*
             acute upper respiratory infection (J06.9)
             upper respiratory inflammation due to chemicals, gases,
                fumes or vapors (J68.2)

J39.0 **Retropharyngeal** and **parapharyngeal** abscess
     Peripharyngeal abscess
     EXCLUDES 1   *peritonsillar abscess (J36)*
     DEF: Purulent infection behind the pharynx and the front of the
     precerebral fascia, characterized by neck stiffness, cervical
     lymphadenopathy, sore throat, fever, and stridor.

J39.1 **Other abscess of pharynx**
     Cellulitis of pharynx
     Nasopharyngeal abscess

J39.2 **Other diseases of pharynx**
     Cyst of pharynx
     Edema of pharynx
     EXCLUDES 2   *chronic pharyngitis (J31.2)*
             ulcerative pharyngitis (J02.9)

J39.3 **Upper respiratory tract hypersensitivity reaction, site unspecified**
     EXCLUDES 1   *hypersensitivity reaction of upper respiratory tract,*
                such as:
                extrinsic allergic alveolitis (J67.9)
                pneumoconiosis (J60-J67.9)

J39.8 **Other specified diseases of upper respiratory tract**

J39.9 **Disease of upper respiratory tract, unspecified**

Chronic lower respiratory diseases (J40-J47)

     EXCLUDES 1   *bronchitis due to chemicals, gases, fumes and vapors (J68.0)*
     EXCLUDES 2   *cystic fibrosis (E84.-)*

J40 **Bronchitis, not specified as acute or chronic**
     Bronchitis NOS
     Bronchitis with tracheitis NOS
     Catarrhal bronchitis
     Tracheobronchitis NOS
     Use additional code to identify:
     exposure to environmental tobacco smoke (Z77.22)
     exposure to tobacco smoke in the perinatal period (P96.81)
     history of tobacco dependence (Z87.891)
     occupational exposure to environmental tobacco smoke (Z57.31)
     tobacco dependence (F17.-)
     tobacco use (Z72.0)
     EXCLUDES 1   *acute bronchitis (J20.-)*
             allergic bronchitis NOS (J45.909-)
             asthmatic bronchitis NOS (J45.9-)
             bronchitis due to chemicals, fumes and vapors (J68.0)
     AHA: 2020,1Q,34-36
     TIP: Assign as a secondary code for a patient with bronchitis of unspecified
     acuity due to COVID-19; assign U07.1 as the principal or first-listed code.

√4ᵗʰ J41 **Simple and mucopurulent chronic bronchitis**
     Use additional code to identify:
     exposure to environmental tobacco smoke (Z77.22)
     exposure to tobacco smoke in the perinatal period (P96.81)
     history of tobacco dependence (Z87.891)
     occupational exposure to environmental tobacco smoke (Z57.31)
     tobacco dependence (F17.-)
     tobacco use (Z72.0)
     EXCLUDES 1   *chronic bronchitis NOS (J42)*
             chronic obstructive bronchitis (J44.-)

     J41.0 **Simple chronic bronchitis**   `HCC` `Rx` `ESR` `COM`

     J41.1 **Mucopurulent chronic bronchitis**   `HCC` `Rx` `ESR` `COM`

     J41.8 **Mixed simple and mucopurulent chronic bronchitis**   `HCC` `Rx` `ESR` `COM`

J42 **Unspecified chronic bronchitis**   `HCC` `Rx` `ESR` `COM`
     Chronic bronchitis NOS
     Chronic tracheitis
     Chronic tracheobronchitis
     Use additional code to identify:
     exposure to environmental tobacco smoke (Z77.22)
     exposure to tobacco smoke in the perinatal period (P96.81)
     history of tobacco dependence (Z87.891)
     occupational exposure to environmental tobacco smoke (Z57.31)
     tobacco dependence (F17.-)
     tobacco use (Z72.0)
     EXCLUDES 1   *chronic asthmatic bronchitis (J44.-)*
             chronic bronchitis with airways obstruction (J44.-)
             chronic emphysematous bronchitis (J44.-)
             chronic obstructive pulmonary disease NOS (J44.9)
             simple and mucopurulent chronic bronchitis (J41.-)

✓4ᵗʰ **J43 Emphysema**

Use additional code to identify:
exposure to environmental tobacco smoke (Z77.22)
history of tobacco dependence (Z87.891)
occupational exposure to environmental tobacco smoke (Z57.31)
tobacco dependence (F17.-)
tobacco use (Z72.0)

EXCLUDES 1   *compensatory emphysema (J98.3)*
emphysema due to inhalation of chemicals, gases, fumes or vapors (J68.4)
emphysema with chronic (obstructive) bronchitis (J44.-)
emphysematous (obstructive) bronchitis (J44.-)
interstitial emphysema (J98.2)
mediastinal emphysema (J98.2)
neonatal interstitial emphysema (P25.0)
surgical (subcutaneous) emphysema (T81.82)

EXCLUDES 2   *traumatic subcutaneous emphysema (T79.7)*

DEF: Pathological condition in which there is destructive enlargement of the air sacs in the lungs resulting in damage and lack of elasticity to the alveolar walls, commonly seen in long-term smokers.

Emphysema

Healthy alveoli — Patent bronchiole — Well-vascularized — Dilated alveoli — Excess mucus

Alveoli w/ Emphysema — Collapsed bronchiole — Broken/fewer capillaries — Enlarged alveoli — Alveolar membranes break down

(margin handwritten notes: chronic (low), chronic)

J43.0   **Unilateral pulmonary emphysema [MacLeod's syndrome]**   HCC Rx ESR COM
Swyer-James syndrome
Unilateral emphysema
Unilateral hyperlucent lung
Unilateral pulmonary artery functional hypoplasia
Unilateral transparency of lung

J43.1   **Panlobular emphysema**   HCC Rx ESR COM
Panacinar emphysema

J43.2   **Centrilobular emphysema**   HCC Rx ESR COM

J43.8   **Other emphysema**   HCC Rx ESR COM

J43.9   **Emphysema, unspecified**   HCC Rx ESR COM
Bullous emphysema (lung)(pulmonary)
Emphysema (lung)(pulmonary) NOS
Emphysematous bleb
Vesicular emphysema (lung)(pulmonary)
AHA: 2019,1Q,34-36; 2017,4Q,97-98

✓4ᵗʰ **J44 Other chronic obstructive pulmonary disease**

INCLUDES   asthma with chronic obstructive pulmonary disease
chronic asthmatic (obstructive) bronchitis
chronic bronchitis with airway obstruction
chronic bronchitis with emphysema
chronic emphysematous bronchitis
chronic obstructive asthma
chronic obstructive bronchitis
chronic obstructive tracheobronchitis

Code also type of asthma, if applicable (J45.-)
Use additional code to identify:
exposure to environmental tobacco smoke (Z77.22)
history of tobacco dependence (Z87.891)
occupational exposure to environmental tobacco smoke (Z57.31)
tobacco dependence (F17.-)
tobacco use (Z72.0)

EXCLUDES 1   *bronchiectasis (J47.-)*
chronic bronchitis NOS (J42)
chronic simple and mucopurulent bronchitis (J41.-)
chronic tracheitis (J42)
chronic tracheobronchitis (J42)
emphysema without chronic bronchitis (J43.-)

AHA: 2019,1Q,34-36; 2017,4Q,97-98; 2017,1Q,25-26; 2016,3Q,15-16; 2013,4Q,109

J44.0   **Chronic obstructive pulmonary disease with (acute) lower respiratory infection**   HCC Rx ESR COM
Code also to identify the infection
AHA: 2019,1Q,35; 2017,4Q,96; 2017,1Q,24-25
TIP: Do not assign when only aspiration pneumonia is present. Aspiration pneumonia is not classified as a respiratory infection.

J44.1   **Chronic obstructive pulmonary disease with (acute) exacerbation**   HCC Rx ESR COM
Decompensated COPD
Decompensated COPD with (acute) exacerbation

EXCLUDES 2   *chronic obstructive pulmonary disease [COPD] with acute bronchitis (J44.0)*
lung diseases due to external agents (J60-J70)

AHA: 2019,1Q,34; 2017,4Q,96; 2017,1Q,26; 2016,1Q,36
TIP: Exacerbation of COPD should not be assumed based upon worsening of a concomitant respiratory disease or when COPD is described as end-stage.
TIP: Assign J43.9 when COPD exacerbation with emphysema is documented.

(margin handwritten note: chronic obstructive asthma → ER)

J44.9   **Chronic obstructive pulmonary disease, unspecified**   HCC Rx ESR COM
Chronic obstructive airway disease NOS
Chronic obstructive lung disease NOS

EXCLUDES 2   *lung diseases due to external agents (J60-J70)*

AHA: 2019,1Q,36; 2017,4Q,96-97; 2016,1Q,36; 2014,4Q,21; 2013,4Q,109

Asthma (handwritten)

chronic low (handwritten, left margin)

☑4ᵗʰ **J45 Asthma**

INCLUDES

- allergic (predominantly) asthma
- allergic bronchitis NOS
- allergic rhinitis with asthma
- atopic asthma
- extrinsic allergic asthma
- hay fever with asthma
- idiosyncratic asthma
- intrinsic nonallergic asthma
- nonallergic asthma

Use additional code to identify:

- eosinophilic asthma (J82.83)
- exposure to environmental tobacco smoke (Z77.22)
- exposure to tobacco smoke in the perinatal period (P96.81)
- history of tobacco dependence (Z87.891)
- occupational exposure to environmental tobacco smoke (Z57.31)
- tobacco dependence (F17.-)
- tobacco use (Z72.0)

EXCLUDES 1
- detergent asthma (J69.8)
- eosinophilic asthma (J82)
- miner's asthma (J60)
- wheezing NOS (R06.2)
- wood asthma (J67.8)

EXCLUDES 2
- asthma with chronic obstructive pulmonary disease (J44.9)
- chronic asthmatic (obstructive) bronchitis (J44.9)
- chronic obstructive asthma (J44.9)

AHA: 2019,1Q,36; 2017,1Q,25-26; 2012,4Q,99

DEF: Status asthmaticus: Severe, intractable episode of asthma that is unresponsive to normal therapeutic measures.

☑5ᵗʰ **J45.2 Mild intermittent asthma**

    J45.20 Mild intermittent asthma, uncomplicated Rx COM
      Mild intermittent asthma NOS

    J45.21 Mild intermittent asthma with (acute) exacerbation Rx COM

    J45.22 Mild intermittent asthma with status asthmaticus Rx COM

☑5ᵗʰ **J45.3 Mild persistent asthma**

    J45.30 Mild persistent asthma, uncomplicated Rx COM
      Mild persistent asthma NOS

    J45.31 Mild persistent asthma with (acute) exacerbation Rx COM
      AHA: 2016,1Q,35

    J45.32 Mild persistent asthma with status asthmaticus Rx COM

☑5ᵗʰ **J45.4 Moderate persistent asthma**

    J45.40 Moderate persistent asthma, uncomplicated Rx COM
      Moderate persistent asthma NOS

    J45.41 Moderate persistent asthma with (acute) exacerbation Rx COM
      AHA: 2017,1Q,26

    J45.42 Moderate persistent asthma with status asthmaticus Rx COM

☑5ᵗʰ **J45.5 Severe persistent asthma**

    J45.50 Severe persistent asthma, uncomplicated Rx COM
      Severe persistent asthma NOS

    J45.51 Severe persistent asthma with (acute) exacerbation Rx COM

    J45.52 Severe persistent asthma with status asthmaticus Rx COM

☑5ᵗʰ **J45.9 Other and unspecified asthma**

    ☑6ᵗʰ **J45.90 Unspecified asthma**
      Asthmatic bronchitis NOS
      Childhood asthma NOS
      Late onset asthma
      AHA: 2017,4Q,96; 2017,1Q,25

reactive airway disease (handwritten) *RAD* →

      J45.901 Unspecified asthma with (acute) exacerbation Rx COM

      J45.902 Unspecified asthma with status asthmaticus Rx COM

if not mentioned complicated asthma or uncomplicated - treat as uncomplicated (handwritten)

    J45.909 Unspecified asthma, uncomplicated Rx COM
      Asthma NOS
      EXCLUDES 2   lung diseases due to external agents (J60-J70)
      AHA: 2017,1Q,25

    ☑6ᵗʰ **J45.99 Other asthma**

      J45.990 Exercise induced bronchospasm Rx COM

      J45.991 Cough variant asthma Rx COM

      J45.998 Other asthma Rx COM

☑4ᵗʰ **J47 Bronchiectasis**

INCLUDES   bronchiolectasis

Use additional code to identify:

- exposure to environmental tobacco smoke (Z77.22)
- exposure to tobacco smoke in the perinatal period (P96.81)
- history of tobacco dependence (Z87.891)
- occupational exposure to environmental tobacco smoke (Z57.31)
- tobacco dependence (F17.-)
- tobacco use (Z72.0)

EXCLUDES 1
- congenital bronchiectasis (Q33.4)
- tuberculous bronchiectasis (current disease) (A15.0)

DEF: Dilation of the bronchi with mucus production and persistent cough due to infection or chronic conditions that causes diminished lung capacity and frequent infections of the lung.

    J47.0 Bronchiectasis with acute lower respiratory infection HCC Rx ESR COM
      Bronchiectasis with acute bronchitis
      Code also to identify infection, if applicable

    J47.1 Bronchiectasis with (acute) exacerbation HCC Rx ESR COM
      AHA: 2021,1Q,23

    J47.9 Bronchiectasis, uncomplicated HCC Rx ESR COM
      Bronchiectasis NOS

Lung diseases due to external agents (J60-J70)

lung (handwritten, left margin)

EXCLUDES 2   asthma (J45.-)
           malignant neoplasm of bronchus and lung (C34.-)

DEF: Pneumoconiosis: Condition caused by inhaling inorganic dust particles, typically associated with occupations that require regular exposure to mineral dusts. A form of interstitial lung disease that contributes to the inflammation of the air sacs, causing the lung tissue to harden.

    J60 Coalworker's pneumoconiosis HCC ESR COM A
      Anthracosilicosis
      Anthracosis
      Black lung disease
      Coalworker's lung
      EXCLUDES 1   coalworker pneumoconiosis with tuberculosis, any type in A15 (J65)

    J61 Pneumoconiosis due to asbestos and other mineral fibers HCC ESR COM A
      Asbestosis
      EXCLUDES 1   pleural plaque with asbestosis (J92.0)
              pneumoconiosis with tuberculosis, any type in A15 (J65)

☑4ᵗʰ **J62 Pneumoconiosis due to dust containing silica**
      INCLUDES   silicotic fibrosis (massive) of lung
      EXCLUDES 1   pneumoconiosis with tuberculosis, any type in A15 (J65)

    J62.0 Pneumoconiosis due to talc dust HCC ESR COM

    J62.8 Pneumoconiosis due to other dust containing silica HCC ESR COM
      Silicosis NOS

☑4ᵗʰ **J63 Pneumoconiosis due to other inorganic dusts**
      EXCLUDES 1   pneumoconiosis with tuberculosis, any type in A15 (J65)

    J63.0 Aluminosis (of lung) HCC ESR COM

    J63.1 Bauxite fibrosis (of lung) HCC ESR COM

    J63.2 Berylliosis HCC ESR COM

    J63.3 Graphite fibrosis (of lung) HCC ESR COM

    J63.4 Siderosis HCC ESR COM
      AHA: 2019,3Q,8

    J63.5 Stannosis HCC ESR COM

    J63.6 Pneumoconiosis due to other specified inorganic dusts HCC ESR COM

    J64 Unspecified pneumoconiosis HCC ESR COM
      EXCLUDES 1   pneumonoconiosis with tuberculosis, any type in A15 (J65)

J65 Pneumoconiosis associated with tuberculosis `HCC` `ESR` `COM`
Any condition in J60-J64 with tuberculosis, any type in A15
Silicotuberculosis

✓4ᵗʰ **J66 Airway disease due to specific** organic dust
EXCLUDES 2 allergic alveolitis (J67.-)
asbestosis (J61)
bagassosis (J67.1)
farmer's lung (J67.0)
hypersensitivity pneumonitis due to organic dust (J67.-)
reactive airways dysfunction syndrome (J68.3)

J66.0 Byssinosis `HCC` `ESR` `COM`
Airway disease due to cotton dust

J66.1 Flax-dressers' disease `HCC` `ESR` `COM`

J66.2 Cannabinosis `HCC` `ESR` `COM`

J66.8 Airway disease due to other specific organic dusts `HCC` `ESR` `COM`

✓4ᵗʰ **J67 Hypersensitivity pneumonitis due to organic dust**
INCLUDES allergic alveolitis and pneumonitis due to inhaled organic dust and particles of fungal, actinomycetic or other origin
EXCLUDES 1 pneumonitis due to inhalation of chemicals, gases, fumes or vapors (J68.0)

J67.0 Farmer's lung `HCC` `ESR` `COM`
Harvester's lung
Haymaker's lung
Moldy hay disease

J67.1 Bagassosis `HCC` `ESR` `COM`
Bagasse disease
Bagasse pneumonitis

J67.2 Bird fancier's lung `HCC` `ESR` `COM`
Budgerigar fancier's disease or lung
Pigeon fancier's disease or lung

J67.3 Suberosis `HCC` `ESR` `COM`
Corkhandler's disease or lung
Corkworker's disease or lung

J67.4 Maltworker's lung `HCC` `ESR` `COM`
Alveolitis due to Aspergillus clavatus

J67.5 Mushroom-worker's lung `HCC` `ESR` `COM`

J67.6 Maple-bark-stripper's lung `HCC` `ESR` `COM`
Alveolitis due to Cryptostroma corticale
Cryptostromosis

J67.7 Air conditioner and humidifier lung `HCC` `ESR` `COM`
Allergic alveolitis due to fungal, thermophilic actinomycetes and other organisms growing in ventilation [air conditioning] systems

J67.8 Hypersensitivity pneumonitis due to other organic dusts `HCC` `ESR` `COM`
Cheese-washer's lung
Coffee-worker's lung
Fish-meal worker's lung
Furrier's lung
Sequoiosis

J67.9 Hypersensitivity pneumonitis due to unspecified organic dust `HCC` `ESR` `COM`
Allergic alveolitis (extrinsic) NOS
Hypersensitivity pneumonitis NOS

✓4ᵗʰ **J68 Respiratory conditions due to inhalation of chemicals, gases, fumes and vapors**
Code first (T51-T65) to identify cause
Use additional code to identify associated respiratory conditions, such as:
acute respiratory failure (J96.0-)

J68.0 Bronchitis and pneumonitis due to chemicals, gases, fumes and vapors `HCC` `ESR` `COM`
Chemical bronchitis (acute)
AHA: 2019,2Q,31

J68.1 Pulmonary edema due to chemicals, gases, fumes and vapors `HCC` `ESR` `COM`
Chemical pulmonary edema (acute) (chronic)
EXCLUDES 1 pulmonary edema (acute) (chronic) NOS (J81.-)

J68.2 Upper respiratory inflammation due to chemicals, gases, fumes and vapors, not elsewhere classified `HCC` `ESR` `COM`

J68.3 Other acute and subacute respiratory conditions due to chemicals, gases, fumes and vapors `HCC` `ESR` `COM`
Reactive airways dysfunction syndrome

J68.4 Chronic respiratory conditions due to chemicals, gases, fumes and vapors `HCC` `ESR` `COM`
Emphysema (diffuse) (chronic) due to inhalation of chemicals, gases, fumes and vapors
Obliterative bronchiolitis (chronic) (subacute) due to inhalation of chemicals, gases, fumes and vapors
Pulmonary fibrosis (chronic) due to inhalation of chemicals, gases, fumes and vapors
EXCLUDES 1 chronic pulmonary edema due to chemicals, gases, fumes and vapors (J68.1)

J68.8 Other respiratory conditions due to chemicals, gases, fumes and vapors `HCC` `ESR` `COM`

J68.9 Unspecified respiratory condition due to chemicals, gases, fumes and vapors `HCC` `ESR` `COM`

✓4ᵗʰ **J69 Pneumonitis due to solids and liquids**
EXCLUDES 1 neonatal aspiration syndromes (P24.-)
postprocedural pneumonitis (J95.4)
AHA: 2017,1Q,24
DEF: Pneumonitis: Noninfectious inflammation of the walls of the alveoli in the lung tissue due to inhalation of food, vomit, oils, essences, or other solids or liquids.

J69.0 Pneumonitis due to inhalation of food and vomit `HCC` `ESR` `COM`
Aspiration pneumonia NOS
Aspiration pneumonia (due to) food (regurgitated)
Aspiration pneumonia (due to) gastric secretions
Aspiration pneumonia (due to) milk
Aspiration pneumonia (due to) vomit
Code also any associated foreign body in respiratory tract (T17.-)
EXCLUDES 1 chemical pneumonitis due to anesthesia (J95.4)
obstetric aspiration pneumonia (O74.0)
AHA: 2020,2Q,11,28; 2019,3Q,17; 2019,2Q,6,31

J69.1 Pneumonitis due to inhalation of oils and essences `HCC` `ESR` `COM`
Exogenous lipoid pneumonia
Lipid pneumonia NOS
Code first (T51-T65) to identify substance
EXCLUDES 1 endogenous lipoid pneumonia (J84.89)

J69.8 Pneumonitis due to inhalation of other solids and liquids `HCC` `ESR` `COM`
Pneumonitis due to aspiration of blood
Pneumonitis due to aspiration of detergent
Code first (T51-T65) to identify substance

✓4ᵗʰ **J70 Respiratory conditions due to other external agents**

J70.0 Acute pulmonary manifestations due to radiation `HCC` `ESR` `COM`
Radiation pneumonitis
Use additional code (W88-W90, X39.0-) to identify the external cause

J70.1 Chronic and other pulmonary manifestations due to radiation `HCC` `ESR` `COM`
Fibrosis of lung following radiation
Use additional code (W88-W90, X39.0-) to identify the external cause

J70.2 Acute drug-induced interstitial lung disorders `HCC` `ESR`
Use additional code for adverse effect, if applicable, to identify drug (T36-T50 with fifth or sixth character 5)
EXCLUDES 1 interstitial pneumonia NOS (J84.9)
lymphoid interstitial pneumonia (J84.2)
AHA: 2019,2Q,28

J70.3 Chronic drug-induced interstitial lung disorders `HCC` `ESR`
Use additional code for adverse effect, if applicable, to identify drug (T36-T50 with fifth or sixth character 5)
EXCLUDES 1 interstitial pneumonia NOS (J84.9)
lymphoid interstitial pneumonia (J84.2)

J70.4 Drug-induced interstitial lung disorders, unspecified `HCC` `ESR`
Use additional code for adverse effect, if applicable, to identify drug (T36-T50 with fifth or sixth character 5)
EXCLUDES 1 interstitial pneumonia NOS (J84.9)
lymphoid interstitial pneumonia (J84.2)
AHA: 2019,2Q,28

J70.5   **Respiratory conditions due to smoke inhalation** `HCC` `ESR`
Code first smoke inhalation (T59.81-)
   EXCLUDES 2   smoke inhalation due to chemicals, gases, fumes and vapors (J68.9)
AHA: 2013,4Q,121

J70.8   **Respiratory conditions due to other specified external agents** `HCC` `ESR`
Code first (T51-T65) to identify the external agent

J70.9   **Respiratory conditions due to unspecified external agent** `HCC` `ESR`
Code first (T51-T65) to identify the external agent

Other respiratory diseases principally affecting the interstitium (J80-J84)

J80   **Acute respiratory distress syndrome** `HCC` `ESR` `COM`
Acute respiratory distress syndrome in adult or child
Adult hyaline membrane disease
   EXCLUDES 1   respiratory distress syndrome in newborn (perinatal) (P22.0)
AHA: 2021,1Q,23; 2020,4Q,96; 2020,1Q,34-36; 2017,1Q,26
DEF: Lung inflammation or injury resulting in a build-up of fluid in the air sacs, preventing the passage of oxygen from the air into the bloodstream.
TIP: Assign as a secondary code for a patient with acute respiratory distress syndrome (ARDS) due to COVID-19; assign code U07.1 as the principal or first-listed code.

✓4ᵗʰ **J81**   **Pulmonary edema**
Use additional code to identify:
exposure to environmental tobacco smoke (Z77.22)
history of tobacco dependence (Z87.891)
occupational exposure to environmental tobacco smoke (Z57.31)
tobacco dependence (F17.-)
tobacco use (Z72.0)
   EXCLUDES 1   chemical (acute) pulmonary edema (J68.1)
hypostatic pneumonia (J18.2)
passive pneumonia (J18.2)
pulmonary edema due to external agents (J60-J70)
pulmonary edema with heart disease NOS (I50.1)
pulmonary edema with heart failure (I50.1)
DEF: Accumulation of fluid in the air sacs of the lungs, making it difficult to breathe.

J81.0   **Acute pulmonary edema** `HCC` `ESR` `COM`
Acute edema of lung
AHA: 2020,3Q,27

J81.1   **Chronic pulmonary edema** `COM`
Pulmonary congestion (chronic) (passive)
Pulmonary edema NOS

✓4ᵗʰ **J82**   **Pulmonary eosinophilia, not elsewhere classified**
   EXCLUDES 2   pulmonary eosinophilia due to aspergillosis (B44.-)
pulmonary eosinophilia due to drugs (J70.2-J70.4)
pulmonary eosinophilia due to specified parasitic infection (B50-B83)
pulmonary eosinophilia due to systemic connective tissue disorders (M30-M36)
pulmonary infiltrate NOS (R91.8)
DEF: Infiltration of eosinophils (white blood cells of the immune system) into the parenchyma of the lungs, resulting in cough, fever, and dyspnea.

✓5ᵗʰ **J82.8**   **Pulmonary eosinophilia, not elsewhere classified**
AHA: 2020,4Q,25-27

J82.81   **Chronic eosinophilic pneumonia** `HCC` `Rx` `ESR` `COM`
Eosinophilic pneumonia, NOS

J82.82   **Acute eosinophilic pneumonia**

J82.83   **Eosinophilic asthma** `Rx` `COM`
Code first asthma, by type, such as:
mild intermittent asthma (J45.2-)
mild persistent asthma (J45.3-)
moderate persistent asthma (J45.4-)
severe persistent asthma (J45.5-)

J82.89   **Other pulmonary eosinophilia, not elsewhere classified** `HCC` `ESR` `COM`
Allergic pneumonia
Löffler's pneumonia
Tropical (pulmonary) eosinophilia NOS

✓4ᵗʰ **J84**   **Other interstitial pulmonary diseases**
   EXCLUDES 1   drug-induced interstitial lung disorders (J70.2-J70.4)
interstitial emphysema (J98.2)
   EXCLUDES 2   lung diseases due to external agents (J60-J70)
DEF: Interstitial: Within the small spaces or gaps occurring in tissue or organs.

✓5ᵗʰ **J84.0**   **Alveolar and parieto-alveolar conditions**

J84.01   **Alveolar proteinosis** `HCC` `Rx` `ESR` `COM`
DEF: Reduced ventilation due to proteinaceous deposits on alveoli. Symptoms include dyspnea, cough, chest pain, weakness, weight loss, and hemoptysis.

J84.02   **Pulmonary alveolar microlithiasis** `HCC` `Rx` `ESR` `COM`

J84.03   **Idiopathic pulmonary hemosiderosis** `HCC` `Rx` `ESR` `COM`
Essential brown induration of lung
Code first underlying disease, such as:
disorders of iron metabolism (E83.1-)
   EXCLUDES 1   acute idiopathic pulmonary hemorrhage in infants [AIPHI] (R04.81)
DEF: Fibrosis of the alveolar walls marked by abnormal accumulation of iron as hemosiderin in the lungs. It primarily affects children and symptoms include anemia, fluid in the lungs, and blood in the sputum. Etiology is unknown.

J84.09   **Other alveolar and parieto-alveolar conditions** `HCC` `Rx` `ESR` `COM`

✓5ᵗʰ **J84.1**   **Other interstitial pulmonary diseases with fibrosis**
   EXCLUDES 1   pulmonary fibrosis (chronic) due to inhalation of chemicals, gases, fumes or vapors (J68.4)
pulmonary fibrosis (chronic) following radiation (J70.1)

J84.10   **Pulmonary fibrosis, unspecified** `HCC` `Rx` `ESR` `COM`
Capillary fibrosis of lung
Cirrhosis of lung (chronic) NOS
Fibrosis of lung (atrophic) (chronic) (confluent) (massive) (perialveolar) (peribronchial) NOS
Induration of lung (chronic) NOS
Postinflammatory pulmonary fibrosis

✓6ᵗʰ **J84.11**   **Idiopathic interstitial pneumonia**
   EXCLUDES 1   lymphoid interstitial pneumonia (J84.2)
pneumocystis pneumonia (B59)

J84.111   **Idiopathic interstitial pneumonia, not otherwise specified** `HCC` `Rx` `ESR` `COM`

J84.112   **Idiopathic pulmonary fibrosis** `HCC` `Rx` `ESR` `COM`
Cryptogenic fibrosing alveolitis
Idiopathic fibrosing alveolitis

J84.113   **Idiopathic non-specific interstitial pneumonitis** `HCC` `Rx` `ESR` `COM`
   EXCLUDES 1   non-specific interstitial pneumonia NOS, or due to known underlying cause (J84.89)

J84.114   **Acute interstitial pneumonitis** `HCC` `Rx` `ESR` `COM`
Hamman-Rich syndrome
   EXCLUDES 1   pneumocystis pneumonia (B59)

J84.115   **Respiratory bronchiolitis interstitial lung disease** `HCC` `Rx` `ESR` `COM`

J84.116   **Cryptogenic organizing pneumonia** `HCC` `Rx` `ESR` `COM`
   EXCLUDES 1   organizing pneumonia NOS, or due to known underlying cause (J84.89)

J84.117   **Desquamative interstitial pneumonia** `HCC` `Rx` `ESR` `COM`

✓6ᵗʰ **J84.17** **Other interstitial pulmonary diseases with fibrosis in diseases classified elsewhere**
AHA: 2020,4Q,27-28

J84.170 *Interstitial lung disease with progressive fibrotic phenotype in diseases classified elsewhere* HCC Rx ESR COM
Progressive fibrotic interstitial lung disease
Code first underlying disease, such as:
lung diseases due to external agents (J60-J70)
rheumatoid arthritis (M05.00-M06.9)
sarcoidosis (D86)
systemic connective tissue disorders (M30-M36)

J84.178 *Other interstitial pulmonary diseases with fibrosis in diseases classified elsewhere* HCC Rx ESR COM
Interstitial pneumonia (nonspecific) (usual) due to collagen vascular disease
Interstitial pneumonia (nonspecific) (usual) in diseases classified elsewhere
Organizing pneumonia due to collagen vascular disease
Organizing pneumonia in diseases classified elsewhere
Code first underlying disease, such as:
progressive systemic sclerosis (M34.0)
rheumatoid arthritis (M05.00-M06.9)
systemic lupus erythematosis (M32.0-M32.9)

J84.2 **Lymphoid interstitial pneumonia** HCC Rx ESR COM
Lymphoid interstitial pneumonitis

✓5ᵗʰ **J84.8** **Other specified interstitial pulmonary diseases**
EXCLUDES 1   exogenous lipoid pneumonia (J69.1)
unspecified lipoid pneumonia (J69.1)

J84.81 **Lymphangioleiomyomatosis** HCC Rx ESR COM
Lymphangiomyomatosis

J84.82 **Adult pulmonary Langerhans cell histiocytosis** HCC Rx ESR COM A
Adult PLCH

J84.83 **Surfactant mutations of the lung** HCC Rx ESR COM
DEF: Genetic disorder resulting in insufficient secretion of a complex mixture of phospholipids and proteins that reduce surface tension in the alveoli following the onset of breathing to facilitate lung expansion in the newborn. It is the leading indication for pediatric lung transplantation.

✓6ᵗʰ **J84.84** **Other interstitial lung diseases of childhood**

J84.841 **Neuroendocrine cell hyperplasia of infancy** HCC Rx ESR COM

J84.842 **Pulmonary interstitial glycogenosis** HCC Rx ESR COM

J84.843 **Alveolar capillary dysplasia with vein misalignment** HCC Rx ESR COM

J84.848 **Other interstitial lung diseases of childhood** HCC Rx ESR COM

J84.89 **Other specified interstitial pulmonary diseases** HCC Rx ESR COM
Endogenous lipoid pneumonia
Interstitial pneumonitis
Non-specific interstitial pneumonitis NOS
Organizing pneumonia NOS
Code first, if applicable:
poisoning due to drug or toxin (T51-T65 with fifth or sixth character to indicate intent), for toxic pneumonopathy
underlying cause of pneumonopathy, if known
Use additional code, for adverse effect, to identify drug (T36-T50 with fifth or sixth character 5), if drug-induced
EXCLUDES 1   *cryptogenic organizing pneumonia (J84.116)*
idiopathic non-specific interstitial pneumonitis (J84.113)
lymphoid interstitial pneumonia (J84.2)
lipoid pneumonia, exogenous or unspecified (J69.1)
AHA: 2021,4Q,106; 2021,1Q,48; 2019,2Q,28

J84.9 **Interstitial pulmonary disease, unspecified** HCC Rx ESR COM
Interstitial pneumonia NOS

Suppurative and necrotic conditions of the lower respiratory tract (J85-J86)

✓4ᵗʰ **J85** **Abscess of lung and mediastinum**
Use additional code (B95-B97) to identify infectious agent

J85.0 **Gangrene and necrosis of lung** HCC ESR COM

J85.1 **Abscess of lung with pneumonia** HCC ESR COM
Code also the type of pneumonia

J85.2 **Abscess of lung without pneumonia** HCC ESR COM
Abscess of lung NOS

J85.3 **Abscess of mediastinum** HCC ESR COM

✓4ᵗʰ **J86** **Pyothorax**
Use additional code (B95-B97) to identify infectious agent
EXCLUDES 1   *abscess of lung (J85.-)*
pyothorax due to tuberculosis (A15.6)
DEF: Collection of pus in the pleural space that is commonly caused by an infection that spreads from the lung, such as bacterial pneumonia or a lung abscess.

J86.0 **Pyothorax with fistula** HCC ESR COM
Bronchocutaneous fistula
Bronchopleural fistula
Hepatopleural fistula
Mediastinal fistula
Pleural fistula
Thoracic fistula
Any condition classifiable to J86.9 with fistula
DEF: Purulent infection of the respiratory cavity, with communication from a cavity to another structure.

J86.9 **Pyothorax without fistula** HCC ESR COM
Abscess of pleura
Abscess of thorax
Empyema (chest) (lung) (pleura)
Fibrinopurulent pleurisy
Purulent pleurisy
Pyopneumothorax
Septic pleurisy
Seropurulent pleurisy
Suppurative pleurisy

Other diseases of the pleura (J90-J94)

J90 **Pleural effusion, not elsewhere classified**
Encysted pleurisy
Pleural effusion NOS
Pleurisy with effusion (exudative) (serous)
EXCLUDES 1   *chylous (pleural) effusion (J94.0)*
malignant pleural effusion (J91.0)
pleurisy NOS (R09.1)
tuberculous pleural effusion (A15.6)
DEF: Collection of lymph and other fluid within the pleural space.

✓4ᵗʰ J91 Pleural effusion in conditions classified elsewhere

> **EXCLUDES 2**   *pleural effusion in heart failure (I50.-)*
> *pleural effusion in systemic lupus erythematosus (M32.13)*

> **DEF:** Collection of lymph and other fluid within the pleural space.

J91.0 Malignant pleural effusion
> Code first underlying neoplasm ▶(C00-D49)◀

J91.8 Pleural effusion in other conditions classified elsewhere
> Code first underlying disease, such as:
> filariasis (B74.0-B74.9)
> influenza (J09.X2, J10.1, J11.1)
> **AHA:** 2015,2Q,15
> **TIP:** Assign this code as a secondary diagnosis to congestive heart failure (I50.-) only if pleural effusion is specifically evaluated or treated.

Pleural Effusion

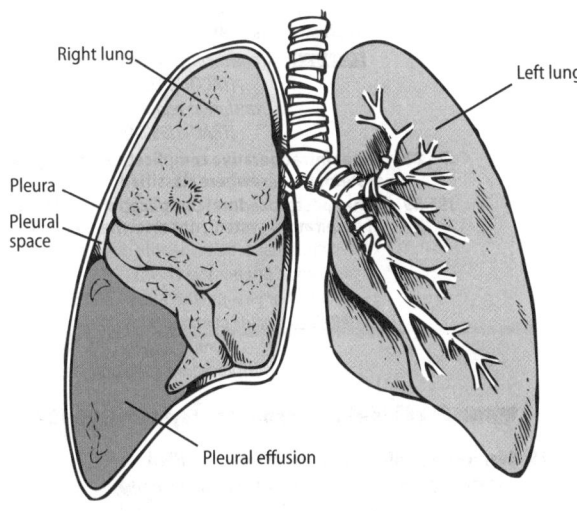

Right lung
Left lung
Pleura
Pleural space
Pleural effusion

✓4ᵗʰ J92 Pleural plaque

> **INCLUDES**   pleural thickening
> **DEF:** Areas of fibrous thickening that form on the parietal or visceral pleura, the membranes that line the ribs and lungs.

J92.0 Pleural plaque with presence of asbestos

J92.9 Pleural plaque without asbestos
> Pleural plaque NOS

✓4ᵗʰ J93 Pneumothorax and air leak

> **EXCLUDES 1**   *congenital or perinatal pneumothorax (P25.1)*
> *postprocedural air leak (J95.812)*
> *postprocedural pneumothorax (J95.811)*
> *pyopneumothorax (J86.-)*
> *traumatic pneumothorax (S27.0)*
> *tuberculous (current disease) pneumothorax (A15.-)*

> **DEF:** Pneumothorax: Lung displacement due to abnormal leakage of air or gas that is trapped in the pleural space formed by the membrane that encloses the lungs and lines the thoracic cavity.

J93.0 Spontaneous tension pneumothorax
> **DEF:** Leaking air from the lung into the lining, causing collapse.

✓5ᵗʰ J93.1 Other spontaneous pneumothorax

> **J93.11 Primary spontaneous pneumothorax**

> **J93.12 Secondary spontaneous pneumothorax**   **UPD**
> Code first underlying condition, such as:
> catamenial pneumothorax due to endometriosis ▶(N80.B-)◀
> cystic fibrosis (E84.-)
> eosinophilic pneumonia (J82)
> lymphangioleiomyomatosis (J84.81)
> malignant neoplasm of bronchus and lung (C34.-)
> Marfan's syndrome (Q87.4)
> pneumonia due to Pneumocystis carinii (B59)
> secondary malignant neoplasm of lung (C78.0-)
> spontaneous rupture of the esophagus (K22.3)

✓5ᵗʰ J93.8 Other pneumothorax and air leak

> **J93.81 Chronic pneumothorax**

> **J93.82 Other air leak**
> Persistent air leak

J93.83 Other pneumothorax
> Acute pneumothorax
> Spontaneous pneumothorax NOS
> **AHA:** 2020,3Q,9-10

J93.9 Pneumothorax, unspecified
> Pneumothorax NOS

✓4ᵗʰ J94 Other pleural conditions

> **EXCLUDES 1**   *pleurisy NOS (R09.1)*
> *traumatic hemopneumothorax (S27.2)*
> *traumatic hemothorax (S27.1)*
> *tuberculous pleural conditions (current disease) (A15.-)*

J94.0 Chylous effusion
> Chyliform effusion
> **DEF:** Fluid within the pleural space due to the leaking of lymph contents into the space, usually as a result of thoracic duct damage or injury or mediastinal lymphoma.

J94.1 Fibrothorax
> **DEF:** Fibrosis within the pleural lining of the lungs commonly seen as a stiff layer surrounding the lung typically attributed to traumatic hemothorax or pleural effusion.

J94.2 Hemothorax
> Hemopneumothorax

J94.8 Other specified pleural conditions
> Hydropneumothorax
> Hydrothorax
> **AHA:** 2021,1Q,48

J94.9 Pleural condition, unspecified

Intraoperative and postprocedural complications and disorders of respiratory system, not elsewhere classified (J95)

✓4ᵗʰ J95 Intraoperative and postprocedural complications and disorders of respiratory system, not elsewhere classified

> **EXCLUDES 2**   *aspiration pneumonia (J69.-)*
> *emphysema (subcutaneous) resulting from a procedure (T81.82)*
> *hypostatic pneumonia (J18.2)*
> *pulmonary manifestations due to radiation (J70.0-J70.1)*

✓5ᵗʰ J95.0 Tracheostomy complications
> **DEF:** Tracheostomy: Formation of a tracheal opening on the neck surface with tube insertion to allow for respiration in cases of obstruction or decreased patency. A tracheostomy may be planned or performed on an emergency basis for temporary or long-term use.

> **J95.00 Unspecified tracheostomy complication**   HCC ESR COM

> **J95.01 Hemorrhage from tracheostomy stoma**   HCC ESR COM

> **J95.02 Infection of tracheostomy stoma**   HCC ESR COM
> Use additional code to identify type of infection, such as:
> cellulitis of neck (L03.221)
> sepsis (A40, A41.-)

> **J95.03 Malfunction of tracheostomy stoma**   HCC ESR COM
> Mechanical complication of tracheostomy stoma
> Obstruction of tracheostomy airway
> Tracheal stenosis due to tracheostomy

> **J95.04 Tracheo-esophageal fistula following tracheostomy**   HCC ESR COM

> **J95.09 Other tracheostomy complication**   HCC ESR COM

J95.1 Acute pulmonary insufficiency following thoracic surgery   HCC ESR
> **EXCLUDES 2**   *functional disturbances following cardiac surgery (I97.0, I97.1-)*

J95.2 Acute pulmonary insufficiency following nonthoracic surgery   HCC ESR
> **EXCLUDES 2**   *functional disturbances following cardiac surgery (I97.0, I97.1-)*

J95.3 Chronic pulmonary insufficiency following surgery   HCC ESR
> **EXCLUDES 2**   *functional disturbances following cardiac surgery (I97.0, I97.1-)*

J95.4 Chemical pneumonitis **due to** anesthesia
  Mendelson's syndrome
  Postprocedural aspiration pneumonia
  Use additional code for adverse effect, if applicable, to identify drug (T41.- with fifth or sixth character 5)
   EXCLUDES 1   *aspiration pneumonia due to anesthesia complicating labor and delivery (O74.0)*
    aspiration pneumonia due to anesthesia complicating pregnancy (O29)
    aspiration pneumonia due to anesthesia complicating the puerperium (O89.01)

J95.5 Postprocedural subglottic stenosis

√5th **J95.6** Intraoperative hemorrhage and hematoma **of a respiratory system organ or structure complicating a procedure**
   EXCLUDES 1   *intraoperative hemorrhage and hematoma of a respiratory system organ or structure due to accidental puncture and laceration during procedure (J95.7-)*

  J95.61 Intraoperative hemorrhage and hematoma of a respiratory system organ or structure complicating a respiratory system procedure

  J95.62 Intraoperative hemorrhage and hematoma of a respiratory system organ or structure complicating other procedure

√5th **J95.7** Accidental puncture and laceration **of a respiratory system organ or structure during a procedure**
   EXCLUDES 2   *postprocedural pneumothorax (J95.811)*

  J95.71 Accidental puncture and laceration of a respiratory system organ or structure during a respiratory system procedure

  J95.72 Accidental puncture and laceration of a respiratory system organ or structure during other procedure

√5th **J95.8** Other intraoperative and postprocedural complications and disorders of respiratory system, not elsewhere classified
  AHA: 2016,4Q,9-10

  √6th **J95.81** Postprocedural pneumothorax and air leak
    J95.811 Postprocedural pneumothorax
      AHA: 2021,1Q,48
    J95.812 Postprocedural air leak

  √6th **J95.82** Postprocedural respiratory failure
    EXCLUDES 1   *respiratory failure in other conditions (J96.-)*
    J95.821 Acute postprocedural respiratory failure   HCC ESR
      Postprocedural respiratory failure NOS
    J95.822 Acute and chronic postprocedural respiratory failure   HCC ESR

  √6th **J95.83** Postprocedural hemorrhage of a respiratory system organ or structure following a procedure
    J95.830 Postprocedural hemorrhage of a respiratory system organ or structure following a respiratory system procedure
    J95.831 Postprocedural hemorrhage of a respiratory system organ or structure following other procedure

  J95.84 Transfusion-related acute lung injury **(TRALI)**
    DEF: Relatively rare, but serious, pulmonary complication of blood transfusion, with acute respiratory distress, noncardiogenic pulmonary edema, cyanosis, hypoxemia, hypotension, fever, and chills.

  √6th **J95.85** Complication of respirator [ventilator]
    J95.850 Mechanical complication of respirator   HCC ESR COM
      EXCLUDES 1   *encounter for respirator [ventilator] dependence during power failure (Z99.12)*
    J95.851 Ventilator associated pneumonia   HCC ESR
      Ventilator associated pneumonitis
      Use additional code to identify the organism, if known (B95.-, B96.-, B97.-)
      EXCLUDES 1   *ventilator lung in newborn (P27.8)*
      AHA: 2020,2Q,17; 2017,1Q,25

  J95.859 Other complication of respirator [ventilator]   HCC ESR COM
    AHA: 2021,1Q,48

√6th **J95.86** Postprocedural hematoma and seroma **of a respiratory system organ or structure following a procedure**
  J95.860 Postprocedural hematoma of a respiratory system organ or structure following a respiratory system procedure
  J95.861 Postprocedural hematoma of a respiratory system organ or structure following other procedure
  J95.862 Postprocedural seroma of a respiratory system organ or structure following a respiratory system procedure
  J95.863 Postprocedural seroma of a respiratory system organ or structure following other procedure

J95.87 Transfusion-associated dyspnea **(TAD)**
   EXCLUDES 1   *transfusion associated circulatory overload (TACO) (E87.71)*
    transfusion-related acute lung injury (TRALI) (J95.84)

J95.88 Other intraoperative complications of respiratory system, not elsewhere classified

J95.89 Other postprocedural complications and disorders of respiratory system, not elsewhere classified
  Use additional code to identify disorder, such as:
  aspiration pneumonia (J69.-)
  bacterial or viral pneumonia (J12-J18)
   EXCLUDES 2   *acute pulmonary insufficiency following thoracic surgery (J95.1)*
    postprocedural subglottic stenosis (J95.5)

Other diseases of the respiratory system (J96-J99)

√4th **J96** Respiratory failure, not elsewhere classified
   EXCLUDES 1   *acute respiratory distress syndrome (J80)*
    cardiorespiratory failure (R09.2)
    newborn respiratory distress syndrome (P22.0)
    postprocedural respiratory failure (J95.82-)
    respiratory arrest (R09.2)
    respiratory arrest of newborn (P28.81)
    respiratory failure of newborn (P28.5)
  AHA: 2021,1Q,27,44-45; 2020,4Q,96

  √5th **J96.0** Acute respiratory failure
    J96.00 Acute respiratory failure, unspecified whether with hypoxia or hypercapnia   HCC ESR COM
      AHA: 2016,3Q,14; 2013,4Q,121
    J96.01 Acute respiratory failure with hypoxia   HCC ESR COM
      AHA: 2020,3Q,12
    J96.02 Acute respiratory failure with hypercapnia   HCC ESR COM
      ▶Acute respiratory acidosis◀

  √5th **J96.1** Chronic respiratory failure
    J96.10 Chronic respiratory failure, unspecified whether with hypoxia or hypercapnia   HCC ESR COM
      AHA: 2016,1Q,38; 2015,1Q,21
    J96.11 Chronic respiratory failure with hypoxia   HCC ESR COM
      AHA: 2013,4Q,129
    J96.12 Chronic respiratory failure with hypercapnia   HCC ESR COM
      ▶Chronic respiratory acidosis◀

  √5th **J96.2** Acute and chronic respiratory failure
    Acute on chronic respiratory failure
    J96.20 Acute and chronic respiratory failure, unspecified whether with hypoxia or hypercapnia   HCC ESR COM
    J96.21 Acute and chronic respiratory failure with hypoxia   HCC ESR COM
    J96.22 Acute and chronic respiratory failure with hypercapnia   HCC ESR COM

  √5th **J96.9** Respiratory failure, unspecified
    J96.90 Respiratory failure, unspecified, unspecified whether with hypoxia or hypercapnia   HCC ESR COM

J96.91	**Respiratory failure, unspecified with hypoxia**	`HCC` `ESR` `COM`
J96.92	**Respiratory failure, unspecified with hypercapnia**	`HCC` `ESR` `COM`

✓4ᵗʰ J98 Other respiratory disorders

Use additional code to identify:
exposure to environmental tobacco smoke (Z77.22)
exposure to tobacco smoke in the perinatal period (P96.81)
history of tobacco dependence (Z87.891)
occupational exposure to environmental tobacco smoke (Z57.31)
tobacco dependence (F17.-)
tobacco use (Z72.Ø)

EXCLUDES 1   *newborn apnea ▶(P28.4-)◀*
            newborn sleep apnea ▶(P28.3-)◀

EXCLUDES 2   *apnea NOS (RØ6.81)*
            sleep apnea (G47.3-)

✓5ᵗʰ J98.Ø Diseases of bronchus, not elsewhere classified

J98.Ø1 Acute bronchospasm

EXCLUDES 1   *acute bronchiolitis with bronchospasm (J21.-)*
          acute bronchitis with bronchospasm (J2Ø.-)
          asthma (J45.-)
          exercise induced bronchospasm (J45.99Ø)

J98.Ø9 Other diseases of bronchus, not elsewhere classified
Broncholithiasis
Calcification of bronchus
Stenosis of bronchus
Tracheobronchial collapse
Tracheobronchial dyskinesia
Ulcer of bronchus

✓5ᵗʰ J98.1 Pulmonary collapse

EXCLUDES 1   *therapeutic collapse of lung status (Z98.3)*

J98.11 Atelectasis

EXCLUDES 1   *newborn atelectasis*
          tuberculous atelectasis (current disease) (A15)

DEF: Collapse of lung tissue affecting part or all of one lung, preventing normal oxygen absorption to healthy tissues.

J98.19 Other pulmonary collapse

J98.2 Interstitial emphysema   `HCC` `Rx` `ESR` `COM`
Mediastinal emphysema

EXCLUDES 1   *emphysema NOS (J43.9)*
          emphysema in newborn (P25.Ø)
          surgical emphysema (subcutaneous) (T81.82)
          traumatic subcutaneous emphysema (T79.7)

J98.3 Compensatory emphysema   `HCC` `Rx` `ESR` `COM`
DEF: Distention of all or part of the lung caused by disease processes or surgical intervention that decreased volume in another part of the lung, causing an overcompensation reaction. Compensatory emphysema occurs in association with pneumonias, pleural effusions, atelectasis, empyema, and pneumothorax.

J98.4 Other disorders of lung
Calcification of lung
Cystic lung disease (acquired)
Lung disease NOS
Pulmolithiasis

EXCLUDES 1   *acute interstitial pneumonitis (J84.114)*
          pulmonary insufficiency following surgery (J95.1-J95.2)

✓5ᵗʰ J98.5 Diseases of mediastinum, not elsewhere classified

EXCLUDES 2   *abscess of mediastinum (J85.3)*

AHA: 2016,4Q,29

J98.51 Mediastinitis
Code first underlying condition, if applicable, such as postoperative mediastinitis (T81.-)

J98.59 Other diseases of mediastinum, not elsewhere classified
Fibrosis of mediastinum
Hernia of mediastinum
Retraction of mediastinum

J98.6 Disorders of diaphragm
Diaphragmatitis
Paralysis of diaphragm
Relaxation of diaphragm

EXCLUDES 1   *congenital malformation of diaphragm NEC (Q79.1)*
          congenital diaphragmatic hernia (Q79.Ø)

EXCLUDES 2   *diaphragmatic hernia (K44.-)*

J98.8 Other specified respiratory disorders
AHA: 2020,1Q,34-36
TIP: Assign as a secondary code for a patient with a respiratory infection that is not further specified but is documented as being associated with COVID-19; assign U07.1 as the principal or first-listed code. If the respiratory infection documentation specifies acute or lower respiratory infection (NOS), assign J22 instead.

J98.9 Respiratory disorder, unspecified
Respiratory disease (chronic) NOS

J99 Respiratory disorders in diseases classified elsewhere   `HCC` `Rx` `ESR` `COM`

Code first underlying disease, such as:
amyloidosis (E85.-)
ankylosing spondylitis (M45)
congenital syphilis (A5Ø.5)
cryoglobulinemia (D89.1)
early congenital syphilis (A5Ø.Ø)
plasminogen deficiency (E88.Ø2)
schistosomiasis (B65.Ø-B65.9)

EXCLUDES 1   *respiratory disorders in:*
          amebiasis (AØ6.5)
          blastomycosis (B4Ø.Ø-B4Ø.2)
          candidiasis (B37.1)
          coccidioidomycosis (B38.Ø-B38.2)
          cystic fibrosis with pulmonary manifestations (E84.Ø)
          dermatomyositis (M33.Ø1, M33.11)
          histoplasmosis (B39.Ø-B39.2)
          late syphilis (A52.72, A52.73)
          polymyositis (M33.21)
          Sjögren syndrome (M35.Ø2)
          systemic lupus erythematosus (M32.13)
          systemic sclerosis (M34.81)
          Wegener's granulomatosis (M31.3Ø-M31.31)

Chapter 11. Diseases of the Digestive System (KØØ–K95)

Chapter-specific Guidelines with Coding Examples
Reserved for future guideline expansion.

Chapter 11. Diseases of the Digestive System (K00-K95)

EXCLUDES 2   *certain conditions originating in the perinatal period (P04-P96)*
certain infectious and parasitic diseases (A00-B99)
complications of pregnancy, childbirth and the puerperium (O00-O9A)
congenital malformations, deformations and chromosomal abnormalities (Q00-Q99)
endocrine, nutritional and metabolic diseases (E00-E88)
injury, poisoning and certain other consequences of external causes (S00-T88)
neoplasms (C00-D49)
symptoms, signs and abnormal clinical and laboratory findings, not elsewhere classified (R00-R94)

This chapter contains the following blocks:

K00-K14   Diseases of oral cavity and salivary glands
K20-K31   Diseases of esophagus, stomach and duodenum
K35-K38   Diseases of appendix
K40-K46   Hernia
K50-K52   Noninfective enteritis and colitis
K55-K64   Other diseases of intestines
K65-K68   Diseases of peritoneum and retroperitoneum
K70-K77   Diseases of liver
K80-K87   Disorders of gallbladder, biliary tract and pancreas
K90-K95   Other diseases of the digestive system

Diseases of oral cavity and salivary glands (K00-K14)

✓4ᵗʰ K00 Disorders of tooth development and eruption

EXCLUDES 2   *embedded and impacted teeth (K01.-)*

K00.0 Anodontia
Hypodontia
Oligodontia
EXCLUDES 1   *acquired absence of teeth (K08.1-)*
DEF: Partial or complete absence of teeth due to a congenital defect involving the tooth bud.

K00.1 Supernumerary teeth
Distomolar
Fourth molar
Mesiodens
Paramolar
Supplementary teeth
EXCLUDES 2   *supernumerary roots (K00.2)*

K00.2 Abnormalities of size and form of teeth
Concrescence of teeth
Fusion of teeth
Gemination of teeth
Dens evaginatus
Dens in dente
Dens invaginatus
Enamel pearls
Macrodontia
Microdontia
Peg-shaped [conical] teeth
Supernumerary roots
Taurodontism
Tuberculum paramolare
EXCLUDES 1   *abnormalities of teeth due to congenital syphilis (A50.5)*
tuberculum Carabelli, which is regarded as a normal variation and should not be coded

K00.3 Mottled teeth
Dental fluorosis
Mottling of enamel
Nonfluoride enamel opacities
EXCLUDES 2   *deposits [accretions] on teeth (K03.6)*

K00.4 Disturbances in tooth formation
Aplasia and hypoplasia of cementum
Dilaceration of tooth
Enamel hypoplasia (neonatal) (postnatal) (prenatal)
Regional odontodysplasia
Turner's tooth
EXCLUDES 1   *Hutchinson's teeth and mulberry molars in congenital syphilis (A50.5)*
EXCLUDES 2   *mottled teeth (K00.3)*

K00.5 Hereditary disturbances in tooth structure, not elsewhere classified
Amelogenesis imperfecta
Dentinogenesis imperfecta
Odontogenesis imperfecta
Dentinal dysplasia
Shell teeth

K00.6 Disturbances in tooth eruption
Dentia praecox
Natal tooth
Neonatal tooth
Premature eruption of tooth
Premature shedding of primary [deciduous] tooth
Prenatal teeth
Retained [persistent] primary tooth
EXCLUDES 2   *embedded and impacted teeth (K01.-)*

K00.7 Teething syndrome

K00.8 Other disorders of tooth development
Color changes during tooth formation
Intrinsic staining of teeth NOS
EXCLUDES 2   *posteruptive color changes (K03.7)*

K00.9 Disorder of tooth development, unspecified
Disorder of odontogenesis NOS

✓4ᵗʰ K01 Embedded and impacted teeth

EXCLUDES 1   *abnormal position of fully erupted teeth (M26.3-)*

K01.0 Embedded teeth

K01.1 Impacted teeth

✓4ᵗʰ K02 Dental caries

INCLUDES   caries of dentine
dental cavities
early childhood caries
pre-eruptive caries
recurrent caries (dentino enamel junction) (enamel) (to the pulp)
tooth decay

Tooth Anatomy

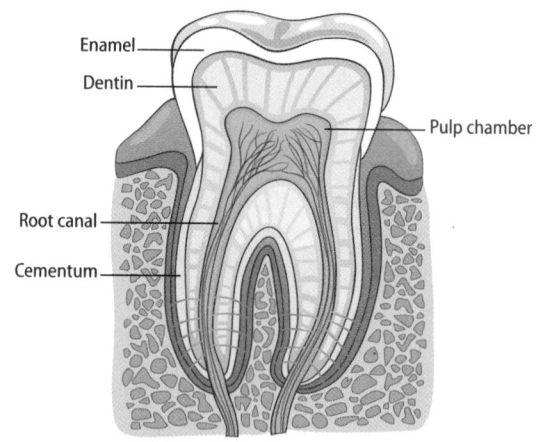

Enamel
Dentin
Pulp chamber
Root canal
Cementum

K02.3 Arrested dental caries
Arrested coronal and root caries

✓5ᵗʰ K02.5 Dental caries on pit and fissure surface
Dental caries on chewing surface of tooth

K02.51 Dental caries on pit and fissure surface limited to enamel
White spot lesions [initial caries] on pit and fissure surface of tooth

K02.52 Dental caries on pit and fissure surface penetrating into dentin
Primary dental caries, cervical origin

K02.53 Dental caries on pit and fissure surface penetrating into pulp

✓5ᵗʰ K02.6 Dental caries on smooth surface

K02.61 Dental caries on smooth surface limited to enamel
White spot lesions [initial caries] on smooth surface of tooth

K02.62 Dental caries on smooth surface penetrating into dentin

K02.63 Dental caries on smooth surface penetrating into pulp

K02.7 **Dental root caries**
K02.9 **Dental caries, unspecified**

✓4ᵗʰ **K03 Other diseases of hard tissues of teeth**
     EXCLUDES 2   *bruxism (F45.8)*
              dental caries (K02.-)
              teeth-grinding NOS (F45.8)

K03.0 **Excessive attrition of teeth**
     Approximal wear of teeth
     Occlusal wear of teeth
     DEF: Attrition: In dentistry, wearing away or erosion of tooth surface from abrasive food or grinding teeth.

K03.1 **Abrasion of teeth**
     Dentifrice abrasion of teeth
     Habitual abrasion of teeth
     Occupational abrasion of teeth
     Ritual abrasion of teeth
     Traditional abrasion of teeth
     Wedge defect NOS

K03.2 **Erosion of teeth**
     Erosion of teeth due to diet
     Erosion of teeth due to drugs and medicaments
     Erosion of teeth due to persistent vomiting
     Erosion of teeth NOS
     Idiopathic erosion of teeth
     Occupational erosion of teeth

K03.3 **Pathological resorption of teeth**
     Internal granuloma of pulp
     Resorption of teeth (external)

K03.4 **Hypercementosis**
     Cementation hyperplasia

K03.5 **Ankylosis of teeth**

K03.6 **Deposits [accretions] on teeth**
     Betel deposits [accretions] on teeth
     Black deposits [accretions] on teeth
     Extrinsic staining of teeth NOS
     Green deposits [accretions] on teeth
     Materia alba deposits [accretions] on teeth
     Orange deposits [accretions] on teeth
     Staining of teeth NOS
     Subgingival dental calculus
     Supragingival dental calculus
     Tobacco deposits [accretions] on teeth

K03.7 **Posteruptive color changes of dental hard tissues**
     EXCLUDES 2   *deposits [accretions] on teeth (K03.6)*

✓5ᵗʰ **K03.8 Other specified diseases of hard tissues of teeth**
     K03.81 **Cracked tooth**
         EXCLUDES 1   *asymptomatic craze lines in enamel - omit code*
                broken or fractured tooth due to trauma (S02.5)
     K03.89 **Other specified diseases of hard tissues of teeth**

K03.9 **Disease of hard tissues of teeth, unspecified**

✓4ᵗʰ **K04 Diseases of pulp and periapical tissues**
     AHA: 2016,4Q,29-30

✓5ᵗʰ **K04.0 Pulpitis**
     Acute pulpitis
     Chronic (hyperplastic) (ulcerative) pulpitis
     K04.01 **Reversible pulpitis**
     K04.02 **Irreversible pulpitis**

K04.1 **Necrosis of pulp**
     Pulpal gangrene

K04.2 **Pulp degeneration**
     Denticles
     Pulpal calcifications
     Pulpal stones

K04.3 **Abnormal hard tissue formation in pulp**
     Secondary or irregular dentine

K04.4 **Acute apical periodontitis of pulpal origin**
     Acute apical periodontitis NOS
     EXCLUDES 1   *acute periodontitis (K05.2-)*
     DEF: Severe inflammation of the area surrounding the tip of a tooth's root that is often secondary to infection or trauma.

K04.5 **Chronic apical periodontitis**
     Apical or periapical granuloma
     Apical periodontitis NOS
     EXCLUDES 1   *chronic periodontitis (K05.3-)*

K04.6 **Periapical abscess with sinus**
     Dental abscess with sinus
     Dentoalveolar abscess with sinus

K04.7 **Periapical abscess without sinus**
     Dental abscess without sinus
     Dentoalveolar abscess without sinus

K04.8 **Radicular cyst**
     Apical (periodontal) cyst
     Periapical cyst
     Residual radicular cyst
     EXCLUDES 2   *lateral periodontal cyst (K09.0)*
     DEF: Most common odontogenic cyst in tissue around the tooth apex due to chronic inflammation of dental pulp.

✓5ᵗʰ **K04.9 Other and unspecified diseases of pulp and periapical tissues**
     K04.90 **Unspecified diseases of pulp and periapical tissues**
     K04.99 **Other diseases of pulp and periapical tissues**

✓4ᵗʰ **K05 Gingivitis and periodontal diseases**
     Use additional code to identify:
     alcohol abuse and dependence (F10.-)
     exposure to environmental tobacco smoke (Z77.22)
     exposure to tobacco smoke in the perinatal period (P96.81)
     history of tobacco dependence (Z87.891)
     occupational exposure to environmental tobacco smoke (Z57.31)
     tobacco dependence (F17.-)
     tobacco use (Z72.0)
     AHA: 2016,4Q,29-30

✓5ᵗʰ **K05.0 Acute gingivitis**
     EXCLUDES 1   *acute necrotizing ulcerative gingivitis (A69.1)*
                herpesviral [herpes simplex] gingivostomatitis (B00.2)
     K05.00 **Acute gingivitis, plaque induced**
         Acute gingivitis NOS
         Plaque induced gingival disease
     K05.01 **Acute gingivitis, non-plaque induced**

✓5ᵗʰ **K05.1 Chronic gingivitis**
     Desquamative gingivitis (chronic)
     Gingivitis (chronic) NOS
     Hyperplastic gingivitis (chronic)
     Pregnancy associated gingivitis
     Simple marginal gingivitis (chronic)
     Ulcerative gingivitis (chronic)
     Code first, if applicable, diseases of the digestive system complicating pregnacy (O99.61-)
     K05.10 **Chronic gingivitis, plaque induced**
         Chronic gingivitis NOS
         Gingivitis NOS
     K05.11 **Chronic gingivitis, non-plaque induced**

✓5ᵗʰ **K05.2 Aggressive periodontitis**
     Acute pericoronitis
     EXCLUDES 1   *acute apical periodontitis (K04.4)*
                periapical abscess (K04.7)
                periapical abscess with sinus (K04.6)
     K05.20 **Aggressive periodontitis, unspecified**
     ✓6ᵗʰ K05.21 **Aggressive periodontitis, localized**
         Periodontal abscess
         K05.211 **Aggressive periodontitis, localized, slight**
         K05.212 **Aggressive periodontitis, localized, moderate**
         K05.213 **Aggressive periodontitis, localized, severe**
         K05.219 **Aggressive periodontitis, localized, unspecified severity**
     ✓6ᵗʰ K05.22 **Aggressive periodontitis, generalized**
         K05.221 **Aggressive periodontitis, generalized, slight**
         K05.222 **Aggressive periodontitis, generalized, moderate**
         K05.223 **Aggressive periodontitis, generalized, severe**
         K05.229 **Aggressive periodontitis, generalized, unspecified severity**

☑ Additional Character Required   ✓x7ᵗʰ Placeholder Alert   Manifestation   Unspecified Dx   🇶 QPP   UPD Unacceptable PDx
ICD-10-CM 2023   725

K02.7–K05.229

Chapter 11. Diseases of the Digestive System

K05.3–K08.3

✓5ᵗʰ **K05.3** **Chronic periodontitis**
Chronic pericoronitis
Complex periodontitis
Periodontitis NOS
Simplex periodontitis
EXCLUDES 1   chronic apical periodontitis (K04.5)

   K05.30 **Chronic periodontitis, unspecified**

✓6ᵗʰ **K05.31** **Chronic periodontitis, localized**

     K05.311 **Chronic periodontitis, localized, slight**
     K05.312 **Chronic periodontitis, localized, moderate**
     K05.313 **Chronic periodontitis, localized, severe**
     K05.319 **Chronic periodontitis, localized, unspecified severity**

✓6ᵗʰ **K05.32** **Chronic periodontitis, generalized**

     K05.321 **Chronic periodontitis, generalized, slight**
     K05.322 **Chronic periodontitis, generalized, moderate**
     K05.323 **Chronic periodontitis, generalized, severe**
     K05.329 **Chronic periodontitis, generalized, unspecified**

K05.4 **Periodontosis**
Juvenile periodontosis

K05.5 **Other periodontal diseases**
Combined periodontic-endodontic lesion
Narrow gingival width (of periodontal soft tissue)
EXCLUDES 2   leukoplakia of gingiva (K13.21)

K05.6 **Periodontal disease, unspecified**

✓4ᵗʰ **K06** **Other disorders of gingiva and edentulous alveolar ridge**
EXCLUDES 2   acute gingivitis (K05.0)
           atrophy of edentulous alveolar ridge (K08.2)
           chronic gingivitis (K05.1)
           gingivitis NOS (K05.1)
AHA: 2016,4Q,29-30

✓5ᵗʰ **K06.0** **Gingival recession**
Gingival recession (postinfective) (postprocedural)
AHA: 2017,4Q,16

✓6ᵗʰ **K06.01** **Gingival recession, localized**

     K06.010 **Localized gingival recession, unspecified**
Localized gingival recession, NOS
     K06.011 **Localized gingival recession, minimal**
     K06.012 **Localized gingival recession, moderate**
     K06.013 **Localized gingival recession, severe**

✓6ᵗʰ **K06.02** **Gingival recession, generalized**

     K06.020 **Generalized gingival recession, unspecified**
Generalized gingival recession, NOS
     K06.021 **Generalized gingival recession, minimal**
     K06.022 **Generalized gingival recession, moderate**
     K06.023 **Generalized gingival recession, severe**

K06.1 **Gingival enlargement**
Gingival fibromatosis

K06.2 **Gingival and edentulous alveolar ridge lesions associated with trauma**
Irritative hyperplasia of edentulous ridge [denture hyperplasia]
Use additional code (Chapter 20) to identify external cause or denture status (Z97.2)

K06.3 **Horizontal alveolar bone loss**

K06.8 **Other specified disorders of gingiva and edentulous alveolar ridge**
Fibrous epulis
Flabby alveolar ridge
Giant cell epulis
Peripheral giant cell granuloma of gingiva
Pyogenic granuloma of gingiva
Vertical ridge deficiency
EXCLUDES 2   gingival cyst (K09.0)

K06.9 **Disorder of gingiva and edentulous alveolar ridge, unspecified**

✓4ᵗʰ **K08** **Other disorders of teeth and supporting structures**
EXCLUDES 2   dentofacial anomalies [including malocclusion] (M26.-)
           disorders of jaw (M27.-)
AHA: 2016,4Q,29-30

K08.0 **Exfoliation of teeth due to systemic causes**
Code also underlying systemic condition

✓5ᵗʰ **K08.1** **Complete loss of teeth**
Acquired loss of teeth, complete
EXCLUDES 1   congenital absence of teeth (K00.0)
           exfoliation of teeth due to systemic causes (K08.0)
           partial loss of teeth (K08.4-)

✓6ᵗʰ **K08.10** **Complete loss of teeth, unspecified cause**

     K08.101 **Complete loss of teeth, unspecified cause, class I**
     K08.102 **Complete loss of teeth, unspecified cause, class II**
     K08.103 **Complete loss of teeth, unspecified cause, class III**
     K08.104 **Complete loss of teeth, unspecified cause, class IV**
     K08.109 **Complete loss of teeth, unspecified cause, unspecified class**
Edentulism NOS

✓6ᵗʰ **K08.11** **Complete loss of teeth due to trauma**

     K08.111 **Complete loss of teeth due to trauma, class I**
     K08.112 **Complete loss of teeth due to trauma, class II**
     K08.113 **Complete loss of teeth due to trauma, class III**
     K08.114 **Complete loss of teeth due to trauma, class IV**
     K08.119 **Complete loss of teeth due to trauma, unspecified class**

✓6ᵗʰ **K08.12** **Complete loss of teeth due to periodontal diseases**

     K08.121 **Complete loss of teeth due to periodontal diseases, class I**
     K08.122 **Complete loss of teeth due to periodontal diseases, class II**
     K08.123 **Complete loss of teeth due to periodontal diseases, class III**
     K08.124 **Complete loss of teeth due to periodontal diseases, class IV**
     K08.129 **Complete loss of teeth due to periodontal diseases, unspecified class**

✓6ᵗʰ **K08.13** **Complete loss of teeth due to caries**

     K08.131 **Complete loss of teeth due to caries, class I**
     K08.132 **Complete loss of teeth due to caries, class II**
     K08.133 **Complete loss of teeth due to caries, class III**
     K08.134 **Complete loss of teeth due to caries, class IV**
     K08.139 **Complete loss of teeth due to caries, unspecified class**

✓6ᵗʰ **K08.19** **Complete loss of teeth due to other specified cause**

     K08.191 **Complete loss of teeth due to other specified cause, class I**
     K08.192 **Complete loss of teeth due to other specified cause, class II**
     K08.193 **Complete loss of teeth due to other specified cause, class III**
     K08.194 **Complete loss of teeth due to other specified cause, class IV**
     K08.199 **Complete loss of teeth due to other specified cause, unspecified class**

✓5ᵗʰ **K08.2** **Atrophy of edentulous alveolar ridge**

   K08.20 **Unspecified atrophy of edentulous alveolar ridge**
Atrophy of the mandible NOS
Atrophy of the maxilla NOS
   K08.21 **Minimal atrophy of the mandible**
Minimal atrophy of the edentulous mandible
   K08.22 **Moderate atrophy of the mandible**
Moderate atrophy of the edentulous mandible
   K08.23 **Severe atrophy of the mandible**
Severe atrophy of the edentulous mandible
   K08.24 **Minimal atrophy of maxilla**
Minimal atrophy of the edentulous maxilla
   K08.25 **Moderate atrophy of the maxilla**
Moderate atrophy of the edentulous maxilla
   K08.26 **Severe atrophy of the maxilla**
Severe atrophy of the edentulous maxilla

K08.3 **Retained dental root**

 CMS-HCC   **Rx** Rx HCC   **ESR** ESRD HCC   **COM** Commercial HCC   **N** Newborn: 0   **P** Pediatric: 0-17   **M** Maternity: 9-64   **A** Adult: 15-124

726

ICD-10-CM 2023

☑5ᵗʰ KØ8.4 Partial loss of teeth
     Acquired loss of teeth, partial
     EXCLUDES 1   *complete loss of teeth (KØ8.1-)*
                congenital absence of teeth (KØØ.Ø)
     EXCLUDES 2   *exfoliation of teeth due to systemic causes (KØ8.Ø)*

   ☑6ᵗʰ KØ8.4Ø Partial loss of teeth, unspecified cause
      KØ8.4Ø1 Partial loss of teeth, unspecified cause, class I
      KØ8.4Ø2 Partial loss of teeth, unspecified cause, class II
      KØ8.4Ø3 Partial loss of teeth, unspecified cause, class III
      KØ8.4Ø4 Partial loss of teeth, unspecified cause, class IV
      KØ8.4Ø9 Partial loss of teeth, unspecified cause, unspecified class
         Tooth extraction status NOS

   ☑6ᵗʰ KØ8.41 Partial loss of teeth due to trauma
      KØ8.411 Partial loss of teeth due to trauma, class I
      KØ8.412 Partial loss of teeth due to trauma, class II
      KØ8.413 Partial loss of teeth due to trauma, class III
      KØ8.414 Partial loss of teeth due to trauma, class IV
      KØ8.419 Partial loss of teeth due to trauma, unspecified class

   ☑6ᵗʰ KØ8.42 Partial loss of teeth due to periodontal diseases
      KØ8.421 Partial loss of teeth due to periodontal diseases, class I
      KØ8.422 Partial loss of teeth due to periodontal diseases, class II
      KØ8.423 Partial loss of teeth due to periodontal diseases, class III
      KØ8.424 Partial loss of teeth due to periodontal diseases, class IV
      KØ8.429 Partial loss of teeth due to periodontal diseases, unspecified class

   ☑6ᵗʰ KØ8.43 Partial loss of teeth due to caries
      KØ8.431 Partial loss of teeth due to caries, class I
      KØ8.432 Partial loss of teeth due to caries, class II
      KØ8.433 Partial loss of teeth due to caries, class III
      KØ8.434 Partial loss of teeth due to caries, class IV
      KØ8.439 Partial loss of teeth due to caries, unspecified class

   ☑6ᵗʰ KØ8.49 Partial loss of teeth due to other specified cause
      KØ8.491 Partial loss of teeth due to other specified cause, class I
      KØ8.492 Partial loss of teeth due to other specified cause, class II
      KØ8.493 Partial loss of teeth due to other specified cause, class III
      KØ8.494 Partial loss of teeth due to other specified cause, class IV
      KØ8.499 Partial loss of teeth due to other specified cause, unspecified class

☑5ᵗʰ KØ8.5 Unsatisfactory restoration of tooth
     Defective bridge, crown, filling
     Defective dental restoration
     EXCLUDES 1   *dental restoration status (Z98.811)*
     EXCLUDES 2   *endosseous dental implant failure (M27.6-)*
                unsatisfactory endodontic treatment (M27.5-)

   KØ8.5Ø Unsatisfactory restoration of tooth, unspecified
      Defective dental restoration NOS
   KØ8.51 Open restoration margins of tooth
      Dental restoration failure of marginal integrity
      Open margin on tooth restoration
      Poor gingival margin to tooth restoration
   KØ8.52 Unrepairable overhanging of dental restorative materials
      Overhanging of tooth restoration
   ☑6ᵗʰ KØ8.53 Fractured dental restorative material
      EXCLUDES 1   *cracked tooth (KØ3.81)*
                traumatic fracture of tooth (SØ2.5)
      KØ8.53Ø Fractured dental restorative material without loss of material
      KØ8.531 Fractured dental restorative material with loss of material

      KØ8.539 Fractured dental restorative material, unspecified
   KØ8.54 Contour of existing restoration of tooth biologically incompatible with oral health
      Dental restoration failure of periodontal anatomical integrity
      Unacceptable contours of existing restoration of tooth
      Unacceptable morphology of existing restoration of tooth
   KØ8.55 Allergy to existing dental restorative material
      Use additional code to identify the specific type of allergy
   KØ8.56 Poor aesthetic of existing restoration of tooth
      Dental restoration aesthetically inadequate or displeasing
   KØ8.59 Other unsatisfactory restoration of tooth
      Other defective dental restoration

☑5ᵗʰ KØ8.8 Other specified disorders of teeth and supporting structures
   KØ8.81 Primary occlusal trauma
   KØ8.82 Secondary occlusal trauma
   KØ8.89 Other specified disorders of teeth and supporting structures
      Enlargement of alveolar ridge NOS
      Insufficient anatomic crown height
      Insufficient clinical crown length
      Irregular alveolar process
      Toothache NOS

KØ8.9 Disorder of teeth and supporting structures, unspecified

☑4ᵗʰ KØ9 Cysts of oral region, not elsewhere classified
     INCLUDES   lesions showing histological features both of aneurysmal cyst and of another fibro-osseous lesion
     EXCLUDES 2   *cysts of jaw (M27.Ø-, M27.4-)*
                radicular cyst (KØ4.8)

   KØ9.Ø Developmental odontogenic cysts
      Dentigerous cyst
      Eruption cyst
      Follicular cyst
      Gingival cyst
      Lateral periodontal cyst
      Primordial cyst
      EXCLUDES 2   *keratocysts (D16.4, D16.5)*
                odontogenic keratocystic tumors (D16.4, D16.5)

   KØ9.1 Developmental (nonodontogenic) cysts of oral region
      Cyst (of) incisive canal
      Cyst (of) palatine of papilla
      Globulomaxillary cyst
      Median palatal cyst
      Nasoalveolar cyst
      Nasolabial cyst
      Nasopalatine duct cyst

   KØ9.8 Other cysts of oral region, not elsewhere classified
      Dermoid cyst
      Epidermoid cyst
      Lymphoepithelial cyst
      Epstein's pearl

KØ9.9 Cyst of oral region, unspecified

☑4ᵗʰ K11 Diseases of salivary glands
     Use additional code to identify:
     alcohol abuse and dependence (F1Ø.-)
     exposure to environmental tobacco smoke (Z77.22)
     exposure to tobacco smoke in the perinatal period (P96.81)
     history of tobacco dependence (Z87.891)
     occupational exposure to environmental tobacco smoke (Z57.31)
     tobacco dependence (F17.-)
     tobacco use (Z72.Ø)

   K11.Ø Atrophy of salivary gland
   K11.1 Hypertrophy of salivary gland
      DEF: Overgrowth of or enlarged salivary gland tissue caused by infection, salivary duct blockage, autoimmune diseases, and benign and malignant tumors.
   ☑5ᵗʰ K11.2 Sialoadenitis
      Parotitis
      EXCLUDES 1   *epidemic parotitis (B26.-)*
                mumps (B26.-)
                uveoparotid fever [Heerfordt] (D86.89)
      DEF: Inflammation of the salivary gland.
     K11.2Ø Sialoadenitis, unspecified

K11.21 **Acute** sialoadenitis
　　EXCLUDES 1　*acute recurrent sialoadenitis (K11.22)*

K11.22 **Acute recurrent** sialoadenitis

K11.23 **Chronic** sialoadenitis

K11.3 **Abscess** of salivary gland

K11.4 **Fistula** of salivary gland
　　EXCLUDES 1　*congenital fistula of salivary gland (Q38.4)*

K11.5 **Sialolithiasis**
Calculus of salivary gland or duct
Stone of salivary gland or duct

K11.6 **Mucocele** of salivary gland
Mucous extravasation cyst of salivary gland
Mucous retention cyst of salivary gland
Ranula

K11.7 **Disturbances of salivary** secretion
Hypoptyalism
Ptyalism
Xerostomia
　　EXCLUDES 2　*dry mouth NOS (R68.2)*

K11.8 **Other diseases of salivary glands**
Benign lymphoepithelial lesion of salivary gland
Mikulicz' disease
Necrotizing sialometaplasia
Sialectasia
Stenosis of salivary duct
Stricture of salivary duct
　　EXCLUDES 1　*Sjögren syndrome (M35.0-)*

K11.9 **Disease of salivary gland, unspecified**
Sialoadenopathy NOS

✓4ᵗʰ **K12** **Stomatitis and related lesions**
Use additional code to identify:
alcohol abuse and dependence (F10.-)
exposure to environmental tobacco smoke (Z77.22)
exposure to tobacco smoke in the perinatal period (P96.81)
history of tobacco dependence (Z87.891)
occupational exposure to environmental tobacco smoke (Z57.31)
tobacco dependence (F17.-)
tobacco use (Z72.0)
　　EXCLUDES 1　*cancrum oris (A69.0)*
　　　　　　　　cheilitis (K13.0)
　　　　　　　　gangrenous stomatitis (A69.0)
　　　　　　　　herpesviral [herpes simplex] gingivostomatitis (B00.2)
　　　　　　　　noma (A69.0)

K12.0 **Recurrent oral aphthae**
Aphthous stomatitis (major) (minor)
Bednar's aphthae
Periadenitis mucosa necrotica recurrens
Recurrent aphthous ulcer
Stomatitis herpetiformis
DEF: Disorder of unknown etiology with small oval or round painful ulcers of the mouth marked by a grayish exudate and a red halo effect.

K12.1 **Other forms of stomatitis**
Stomatitis NOS
Denture stomatitis
Ulcerative stomatitis
Vesicular stomatitis
　　EXCLUDES 1　*acute necrotizing ulcerative stomatitis (A69.1)*
　　　　　　　　Vincent's stomatitis (A69.1)

K12.2 **Cellulitis and abscess of mouth**
Cellulitis of mouth (floor)
Submandibular abscess
　　EXCLUDES 2　*abscess of salivary gland (K11.3)*
　　　　　　　　abscess of tongue (K14.0)
　　　　　　　　periapical abscess (K04.6-K04.7)
　　　　　　　　periodontal abscess (K05.21)
　　　　　　　　peritonsillar abscess (J36)

✓5ᵗʰ **K12.3** **Oral mucositis (ulcerative)**
Mucositis (oral) (oropharyneal)
　　EXCLUDES 2　*gastrointestinal mucositis (ulcerative) (K92.81)*
　　　　　　　　mucositis (ulcerative) of vagina and vulva (N76.81)
　　　　　　　　nasal mucositis (ulcerative) (J34.81)

K12.30 **Oral mucositis (ulcerative), unspecified**

K12.31 **Oral mucositis (ulcerative) due to** antineoplastic therapy
Use additional code for adverse effect, if applicable, to identify antineoplastic and immunosuppressive drugs (T45.1X5)
Use additional code for other antineoplastic therapy, such as:
radiological procedure and radiotherapy (Y84.2)

K12.32 **Oral mucositis (ulcerative) due to other drugs**
Use additional code for adverse effect, if applicable, to identify drug (T36-T50 with fifth or sixth character 5)

K12.33 **Oral mucositis (ulcerative) due to** radiation
Use additional external cause code (W88-W90, X39.0-) to identify cause

K12.39 **Other oral mucositis (ulcerative)**
Viral oral mucositis (ulcerative)

✓4ᵗʰ **K13** **Other diseases of lip and oral mucosa**
INCLUDES　epithelial disturbances of tongue
Use additional code to identify:
alcohol abuse and dependence (F10.-)
exposure to environmental tobacco smoke (Z77.22)
exposure to tobacco smoke in the perinatal period (P96.81)
history of tobacco dependence (Z87.891)
occupational exposure to environmental tobacco smoke (Z57.31)
tobacco dependence (F17.-)
tobacco use (Z72.0)
　　EXCLUDES 2　*certain disorders of gingiva and edentulous alveolar ridge (K05-K06)*
　　　　　　　　cysts of oral region (K09.-)
　　　　　　　　diseases of tongue (K14.-)
　　　　　　　　stomatitis and related lesions (K12.-)

K13.0 **Diseases of lips**
Abscess of lips
Angular cheilitis
Cellulitis of lips
Cheilitis NOS
Cheilodynia
Cheilosis
Exfoliative cheilitis
Fistula of lips
Glandular cheilitis
Hypertrophy of lips
Perlèche NEC
　　EXCLUDES 1　*ariboflavinosis (E53.0)*
　　　　　　　　cheilitis due to radiation-related disorders (L55-L59)
　　　　　　　　congenital fistula of lips (Q38.0)
　　　　　　　　congenital hypertrophy of lips (Q18.6)
　　　　　　　　perlèche due to candidiasis (B37.83)
　　　　　　　　perlèche due to riboflavin deficiency (E53.0)

K13.1 **Cheek and lip biting**

✓5ᵗʰ **K13.2** **Leukoplakia and other disturbances of oral epithelium, including tongue**
　　EXCLUDES 1　*carcinoma in situ of oral epithelium (D00.0-)*
　　　　　　　　hairy leukoplakia (K13.3)
DEF: Leukoplakia: Thickened white patches or lesions appearing on a mucous membrane, such as oral mucosa or tongue.

K13.21 **Leukoplakia of** oral mucosa, including tongue
Leukokeratosis of oral mucosa
Leukoplakia of gingiva, lips, tongue
　　EXCLUDES 1　*hairy leukoplakia (K13.3)*
　　　　　　　　leukokeratosis nicotina palati (K13.24)

K13.22 **Minimal keratinized residual ridge mucosa**
Minimal keratinization of alveolar ridge mucosa

K13.23 **Excessive keratinized residual ridge mucosa**
Excessive keratinization of alveolar ridge mucosa

K13.24 **Leukokeratosis nicotina palati**
Smoker's palate

K13.29 **Other disturbances of oral epithelium, including tongue**
Erythroplakia of mouth or tongue
Focal epithelial hyperplasia of mouth or tongue
Leukoedema of mouth or tongue
Other oral epithelium disturbances

K13.3 **Hairy leukoplakia**

K13.4 Granuloma and granuloma-like lesions of oral mucosa
Eosinophilic granuloma
Granuloma pyogenicum
Verrucous xanthoma

K13.5 Oral submucous fibrosis
Submucous fibrosis of tongue

K13.6 Irritative hyperplasia of oral mucosa
EXCLUDES 2   *irritative hyperplasia of edentulous ridge [denture hyperplasia] (K06.2)*

✓5th **K13.7 Other and unspecified lesions of oral mucosa**

K13.70 Unspecified lesions of oral mucosa

K13.79 Other lesions of oral mucosa
Focal oral mucinosis
AHA: 2022,2Q,7

✓4th **K14 Diseases of tongue**
Use additional code to identify:
alcohol abuse and dependence (F10.-)
exposure to environmental tobacco smoke (Z77.22)
history of tobacco dependence (Z87.891)
occupational exposure to environmental tobacco smoke (Z57.31)
tobacco dependence (F17.-)
tobacco use (Z72.0)
EXCLUDES 2   *erythroplakia (K13.29)*
focal epithelial hyperplasia (K13.29)
leukedema of tongue (K13.29)
leukoplakia of tongue (K13.21)
hairy leukoplakia (K13.3)
macroglossia (congenital) (Q38.2)
submucous fibrosis of tongue (K13.5)

K14.0 Glossitis
Abscess of tongue
Ulceration (traumatic) of tongue
EXCLUDES 1   *atrophic glossitis (K14.4)*
DEF: Inflammation and swelling of the tongue that may be associated with infection, adverse drug reactions, smoking, or injury.

K14.1 Geographic tongue
Benign migratory glossitis
Glossitis areata exfoliativa

K14.2 Median rhomboid glossitis

K14.3 Hypertrophy of tongue papillae
Black hairy tongue
Coated tongue
Hypertrophy of foliate papillae
Lingua villosa nigra

K14.4 Atrophy of tongue papillae
Atrophic glossitis

K14.5 Plicated tongue
Fissured tongue
Furrowed tongue
Scrotal tongue
EXCLUDES 1   *fissured tongue, congenital (Q38.3)*

K14.6 Glossodynia
Glossopyrosis
Painful tongue

K14.8 Other diseases of tongue
Atrophy of tongue
Crenated tongue
Enlargement of tongue
Glossocele
Glossoptosis
Hypertrophy of tongue

K14.9 Disease of tongue, unspecified
Glossopathy NOS

Diseases of esophagus, stomach and duodenum (K20-K31)

EXCLUDES 2   *hiatus hernia (K44.-)*

✓4th **K20 Esophagitis**
Use additional code to identify:
alcohol abuse and dependence (F10.-)
EXCLUDES 1   *erosion of esophagus (K22.1-)*
esophagitis with gastro-esophageal reflux disease (K21.0-)
reflux esophagitis (K21.0-)
ulcerative esophagitis (K22.1-)
EXCLUDES 2   *eosinophilic gastritis or gastroenteritis (K52.81)*

K20.0 Eosinophilic esophagitis
AHA: 2020,4Q,9

✓5th **K20.8 Other esophagitis**
AHA: 2020,4Q,28-29

K20.80 Other esophagitis without bleeding
Abscess of esophagus
Other esophagitis NOS

K20.81 Other esophagitis with bleeding

✓5th **K20.9 Esophagitis, unspecified**
AHA: 2020,4Q,28-29

K20.90 Esophagitis, unspecified without bleeding
Esophagitis NOS

K20.91 Esophagitis, unspecified with bleeding

✓4th **K21 Gastro-esophageal reflux disease**
EXCLUDES 1   *newborn esophageal reflux (P78.83)*

✓5th **K21.0 Gastro-esophageal reflux disease** with esophagitis
AHA: 2020,4Q,28-29

K21.00 Gastro-esophageal reflux disease with esophagitis, without bleeding
Reflux esophagitis

K21.01 Gastro-esophageal reflux disease with esophagitis, with bleeding

K21.9 Gastro-esophageal reflux disease without esophagitis
Esophageal reflux NOS
AHA: 2016,1Q,18

✓4th **K22 Other diseases of esophagus**
EXCLUDES 2   *esophageal varices (I85.-)*

K22.0 Achalasia of cardia
Achalasia NOS
Cardiospasm
EXCLUDES 1   *congenital cardiospasm (Q39.5)*
DEF: Esophageal motility disorder that is caused by absence of the esophageal peristalsis and impaired relaxation of the lower esophageal sphincter. It is characterized by dysphagia, regurgitation, and heartburn.

✓5th **K22.1 Ulcer of esophagus**
Barrett's ulcer
Erosion of esophagus
Fungal ulcer of esophagus
Peptic ulcer of esophagus
Ulcer of esophagus due to ingestion of chemicals
Ulcer of esophagus due to ingestion of drugs and medicaments
Ulcerative esophagitis
Code first poisoning due to drug or toxin, if applicable (T36-T65 with fifth or sixth character 1-4 or 6)
Use additional code for adverse effect, if applicable, to identify drug (T36-T50 with fifth or sixth character 5)
EXCLUDES 1   *Barrett's esophagus (K22.7-)*
AHA: 2018,3Q,22; 2017,3Q,27
TIP: Assign a code for "with bleeding" when an esophageal ulcer and bleeding (hematemesis) are documented. The ICD-10-CM classification assumes the two are related without the provider linking the two conditions. Evidence of bleeding during a procedure is not required.

K22.10 Ulcer of esophagus without bleeding
Ulcer of esophagus NOS

K22.11 Ulcer of esophagus with bleeding
EXCLUDES 2   *bleeding esophageal varices (I85.01, I85.11)*
TIP: For bleeding esophageal ulcers resulting from anticoagulant therapy, assign this code, code D68.32 Hemorrhagic disorder due to extrinsic circulating anticoagulant, and adverse effect code T45.515- with the appropriate seventh character.

Chapter 11. Diseases of the Digestive System *(side margin)*

K22.2 **Esophageal** obstruction
Compression of esophagus
Constriction of esophagus
Stenosis of esophagus
Stricture of esophagus
EXCLUDES 1 congenital stenosis or stricture of esophagus (Q39.3)

K22.3 **Perforation** of esophagus
Rupture of esophagus
EXCLUDES 1 traumatic perforation of (thoracic) esophagus
(S27.8-)

K22.4 **Dyskinesia** of esophagus
Corkscrew esophagus
Diffuse esophageal spasm
Spasm of esophagus
EXCLUDES 1 cardiospasm (K22.0)

K22.5 **Diverticulum** of esophagus, acquired   *epiphrenic*
Esophageal pouch, acquired   *(handwritten: traction)*
EXCLUDES 1 diverticulum of esophagus (congenital) (Q39.6)

K22.6 **Gastro-esophageal** laceration-hemorrhage **syndrome**
Mallory-Weiss syndrome

✓5ᵗʰ K22.7 **Barrett's esophagus**
Barrett's disease
Barrett's syndrome
EXCLUDES 1 Barrett's ulcer (K22.1)
malignant neoplasm of esophagus (C15.-)
DEF: Metaplastic disorder in which specialized columnar epithelial cells replace the normal squamous epithelial cells. Secondary to chronic gastroesophageal reflux damage to the mucosa, this disorder increases the risk of developing adenocarcinoma.

  K22.70 **Barrett's esophagus** without dysplasia **Q**
Barrett's esophagus NOS
  ✓6ᵗʰ K22.71 **Barrett's esophagus** with dysplasia
    K22.710 **Barrett's esophagus with** low grade **dysplasia** **Q**
    K22.711 **Barrett's esophagus with** high grade **dysplasia** **Q**
    K22.719 **Barrett's esophagus with dysplasia, unspecified** **Q**

✓5ᵗʰ K22.8 **Other specified diseases of esophagus**
EXCLUDES 2 esophageal varices (I85.-)
Paterson-Kelly syndrome (D50.1)
AHA: 2021,4Q,15; 2020,1Q,16
  K22.81 **Esophageal polyp**
EXCLUDES 1 benign neoplasm of esophagus (D13.0)
  K22.82 **Esophagogastric junction polyp**
EXCLUDES 1 benign neoplasm of stomach (D13.1)
  K22.89 **Other specified disease of esophagus**
Hemorrhage of esophagus NOS
(handwritten: esophagus Dieulafoy lesion)
K22.9 **Disease of esophagus, unspecified**

K23 **Disorders of esophagus in diseases classified elsewhere**
Code first underlying disease, such as:
congenital syphilis (A50.5)
EXCLUDES 1 late syphilis (A52.79)
megaesophagus due to Chagas' disease (B57.31)
tuberculosis (A18.83)

✓4ᵗʰ K25 **Gastric ulcer**
INCLUDES erosion (acute) of stomach
pylorus ulcer (peptic)
stomach ulcer (peptic)
Use additional code to identify:
alcohol abuse and dependence (F10.-)
EXCLUDES 1 acute gastritis (K29.0-)
peptic ulcer NOS (K27.-)
AHA: 2021,1Q,9,11; 2017,3Q,27
TIP: Assign a code for "with hemorrhage" when a gastric ulcer and GI bleeding are documented. The ICD-10-CM classification assumes the two are related without the provider linking the two conditions. Evidence of bleeding during a procedure is not required.
TIP: For bleeding ulcers resulting from anticoagulant therapy, assign the appropriate "with hemorrhage" ulcer code from this category, code D68.32 Hemorrhagic disorder due to extrinsic circulating anticoagulant, and adverse effect code T45.515- with the appropriate seventh character.
K25.0 **Acute gastric ulcer** with hemorrhage
K25.1 **Acute gastric ulcer** with perforation HCC ESR COM
K25.2 **Acute gastric ulcer** with both hemorrhage and perforation HCC ESR COM

K25.3 **Acute gastric ulcer without hemorrhage or perforation**
K25.4 **Chronic or unspecified gastric ulcer** with hemorrhage
K25.5 **Chronic or unspecified gastric ulcer** with perforation HCC ESR COM
K25.6 **Chronic or unspecified gastric ulcer** with both hemorrhage and perforation HCC ESR COM
K25.7 **Chronic gastric ulcer without hemorrhage or perforation**
K25.9 **Gastric ulcer, unspecified as acute or chronic, without hemorrhage or perforation**

Gastrointestinal Ulcers

Esophagus
Esophageal ulcer
Stomach
Duodenal ulcer
Gastric ulcer
Small intestine

✓4ᵗʰ K26 **Duodenal ulcer**
INCLUDES erosion (acute) of duodenum
duodenum ulcer (peptic)
postpyloric ulcer (peptic)
Use additional code to identify:
alcohol abuse and dependence (F10.-)
EXCLUDES 1 peptic ulcer NOS (K27.-)
AHA: 2017,3Q,27
TIP: Assign a code for "with hemorrhage" when a duodenal ulcer and GI bleeding are documented. The ICD-10-CM classification assumes the two are related without the provider linking the two conditions. Evidence of bleeding during a procedure is not required.
TIP: For bleeding ulcers resulting from anticoagulant therapy, assign the appropriate "with hemorrhage" ulcer code from this category, code D68.32 Hemorrhagic disorder due to extrinsic circulating anticoagulant, and adverse effect code T45.515- with the appropriate seventh character.
K26.0 **Acute duodenal ulcer** with hemorrhage
K26.1 **Acute duodenal ulcer** with perforation HCC ESR COM
K26.2 **Acute duodenal ulcer** with both hemorrhage and perforation HCC ESR COM
K26.3 **Acute duodenal ulcer without hemorrhage or perforation**
K26.4 **Chronic or unspecified duodenal ulcer** with hemorrhage
AHA: 2016,1Q,14
K26.5 **Chronic or unspecified duodenal ulcer** with perforation HCC ESR COM
K26.6 **Chronic or unspecified duodenal ulcer** with both hemorrhage and perforation HCC ESR COM
K26.7 **Chronic duodenal ulcer without hemorrhage or perforation**
K26.9 **Duodenal ulcer, unspecified as acute or chronic, without hemorrhage or perforation**

✓4ᵗʰ K27 **Peptic ulcer, site unspecified**
INCLUDES gastroduodenal ulcer NOS
peptic ulcer NOS
Use additional code to identify:
alcohol abuse and dependence (F10.-)
EXCLUDES 1 peptic ulcer of newborn (P78.82)
AHA: 2017,3Q,27
TIP: Assign a code for "with hemorrhage" when a peptic ulcer and GI bleeding are documented. The ICD-10-CM classification assumes the two are related without the provider linking the two conditions. Evidence of bleeding during a procedure is not required.
TIP: For bleeding ulcers resulting from anticoagulant therapy, assign the appropriate "with hemorrhage" ulcer code from this category, code D68.32 Hemorrhagic disorder due to extrinsic circulating anticoagulant, and adverse effect code T45.515- with the appropriate seventh character.
K27.0 **Acute peptic ulcer, site unspecified,** with hemorrhage
K27.1 **Acute peptic ulcer, site unspecified,** with perforation HCC ESR COM
K27.2 **Acute peptic ulcer, site unspecified,** with both hemorrhage and perforation HCC ESR COM

K27.3 Acute **peptic ulcer, site unspecified, without hemorrhage or perforation**

K27.4 Chronic **or unspecified peptic ulcer, site unspecified, with hemorrhage**

K27.5 Chronic **or unspecified peptic ulcer, site unspecified, with perforation** `HCC` `ESR` `COM`

K27.6 Chronic **or unspecified peptic ulcer, site unspecified, with both hemorrhage and perforation** `HCC` `ESR` `COM`

K27.7 Chronic **peptic ulcer, site unspecified, without hemorrhage or perforation**

K27.9 **Peptic ulcer, site unspecified, unspecified as acute or chronic, without hemorrhage or perforation**

✓4ᵗʰ K28 Gastrojejunal ulcer

    `INCLUDES`   anastomotic ulcer (peptic) or erosion
                    gastrocolic ulcer (peptic) or erosion
                    gastrointestinal ulcer (peptic) or erosion
                    gastrojejunal ulcer (peptic) or erosion
                    jejunal ulcer (peptic) or erosion
                    marginal ulcer (peptic) or erosion
                    stomal ulcer (peptic) or erosion

    Use additional code to identify:
         alcohol abuse and dependence (F10.-)
    `EXCLUDES 1`   *primary ulcer of small intestine (K63.3)*

    AHA: 2017,3Q,27
    TIP: Assign a code for "with hemorrhage" when a gastrojejunal ulcer and GI bleeding are documented. The ICD-10-CM classification assumes the two are related without the provider linking the two conditions. Evidence of bleeding during a procedure is not required.
    TIP: For bleeding ulcers resulting from anticoagulant therapy, assign the appropriate "with hemorrhage" ulcer code from this category, code D68.32 Hemorrhagic disorder due to extrinsic circulating anticoagulant, and adverse effect code T45.515- with the appropriate seventh character.

K28.0 Acute **gastrojejunal ulcer with hemorrhage**

K28.1 Acute **gastrojejunal ulcer with perforation** `HCC` `ESR` `COM`

K28.2 Acute **gastrojejunal ulcer with both hemorrhage and perforation** `HCC` `ESR` `COM`

K28.3 Acute **gastrojejunal ulcer without hemorrhage or perforation**

K28.4 Chronic **or unspecified gastrojejunal ulcer with hemorrhage**

K28.5 Chronic **or unspecified gastrojejunal ulcer with perforation** `HCC` `ESR` `COM`

K28.6 Chronic **or unspecified gastrojejunal ulcer with both hemorrhage and perforation** `HCC` `ESR` `COM`

K28.7 Chronic **gastrojejunal ulcer without hemorrhage or perforation**

K28.9 **Gastrojejunal ulcer, unspecified as acute or chronic, without hemorrhage or perforation**

✓4ᵗʰ K29 Gastritis and duodenitis

    `EXCLUDES 1`   *eosinophilic gastritis or gastroenteritis (K52.81)*
                    Zollinger-Ellison syndrome (E16.4)

    AHA: 2018,3Q,22
    TIP: Assign a code for "with bleeding" when gastritis or duodenitis and GI bleeding are documented. The ICD-10-CM classification assumes the two are related without the provider linking the two conditions. Evidence of bleeding during a procedure is not required.
    TIP: For bleeding ulcers resulting from anticoagulant therapy, assign the appropriate "with hemorrhage" ulcer code from this category, code D68.32 Hemorrhagic disorder due to extrinsic circulating anticoagulant, and adverse effect code T45.515- with the appropriate seventh character.

✓5ᵗʰ K29.0 Acute gastritis

    Use additional code to identify:
         alcohol abuse and dependence (F10.-)
    `EXCLUDES 1`   *erosion (acute) of stomach (K25.-)*

    K29.00 **Acute gastritis** without bleeding
    K29.01 **Acute gastritis** with bleeding

✓5ᵗʰ K29.2 Alcoholic gastritis

    Use additional code to identify:
         alcohol abuse and dependence (F10.-)

    K29.20 **Alcoholic gastritis** without bleeding
    K29.21 **Alcoholic gastritis** with bleeding

✓5ᵗʰ K29.3 Chronic superficial gastritis

    K29.30 **Chronic superficial gastritis** without bleeding
    K29.31 **Chronic superficial gastritis** with bleeding

✓5ᵗʰ K29.4 Chronic atrophic gastritis

    Gastric atrophy

    K29.40 **Chronic atrophic gastritis** without bleeding
    K29.41 **Chronic atrophic gastritis** with bleeding

✓5ᵗʰ K29.5 Unspecified chronic gastritis

    Chronic antral gastritis
    Chronic fundal gastritis

    K29.50 **Unspecified chronic gastritis** without bleeding
    K29.51 **Unspecified chronic gastritis** with bleeding

✓5ᵗʰ K29.6 Other gastritis

    Giant hypertrophic gastritis
    Granulomatous gastritis
    Ménétrier's disease

    K29.60 **Other gastritis** without bleeding
    K29.61 **Other gastritis** with bleeding

✓5ᵗʰ K29.7 Gastritis, unspecified

    K29.70 **Gastritis, unspecified,** without bleeding
    K29.71 **Gastritis, unspecified,** with bleeding

✓5ᵗʰ K29.8 Duodenitis

    K29.80 **Duodenitis** without bleeding
    K29.81 **Duodenitis** with bleeding

✓5ᵗʰ K29.9 Gastroduodenitis, unspecified

    K29.90 **Gastroduodenitis, unspecified,** without bleeding
    K29.91 **Gastroduodenitis, unspecified,** with bleeding

K30 Functional dyspepsia

    Indigestion
    `EXCLUDES 1`   *dyspepsia NOS (R10.13)*
                    heartburn (R12)
                    nervous dyspepsia (F45.8)
                    neurotic dyspepsia (F45.8)
                    psychogenic dyspepsia (F45.8)

✓4ᵗʰ K31 Other diseases of stomach and duodenum

    `INCLUDES`   functional disorders of stomach
    `EXCLUDES 2`   *diabetic gastroparesis (E08.43, E09.43, E10.43, E11.43, E13.43)*
                    diverticulum of duodenum (K57.00-K57.13)

K31.0 Acute dilatation of stomach

    Acute distention of stomach

K31.1 Adult hypertrophic pyloric stenosis   `COM` `A`

    Pyloric stenosis NOS
    `EXCLUDES 1`   *congenital or infantile pyloric stenosis (Q40.0)*

K31.2 Hourglass stricture and stenosis of stomach

    `EXCLUDES 1`   *congenital hourglass stomach (Q40.2)*
                    hourglass contraction of stomach (K31.89)

K31.3 Pylorospasm, not elsewhere classified   `COM`

    `EXCLUDES 1`   *congenital or infantile pylorospasm (Q40.0)*
                    neurotic pylorospasm (F45.8)
                    psychogenic pylorospasm (F45.8)

K31.4 Gastric diverticulum

    `EXCLUDES 1`   *congenital diverticulum of stomach (Q40.2)*

K31.5 Obstruction of duodenum   `COM`

    Constriction of duodenum
    Duodenal ileus (chronic)
    Stenosis of duodenum
    Stricture of duodenum
    Volvulus of duodenum
    `EXCLUDES 1`   *congenital stenosis of duodenum (Q41.0)*

K31.6 Fistula of stomach and duodenum

    Gastrocolic fistula
    Gastrojejunocolic fistula

K31.7 Polyp of stomach and duodenum

    `EXCLUDES 1`   *adenomatous polyp of stomach (D13.1)*
    AHA: 2020,1Q,16

✓5ᵗʰ K31.8 Other specified diseases of stomach and duodenum

✓6ᵗʰ K31.81 Angiodysplasia of stomach and duodenum

    TIP: Assign a code for "with bleeding" when angiodysplasia of the stomach or the duodenum and GI bleeding are documented. The ICD-10-CM classification assumes the two are related without the provider linking the two conditions. Evidence of bleeding during a procedure is not required.

    K31.811 **Angiodysplasia of stomach and duodenum** with bleeding
    K31.819 **Angiodysplasia of stomach and duodenum** without bleeding
           Angiodysplasia of stomach and duodenum NOS

K31.82   Dieulafoy lesion (hemorrhagic) of stomach and duodenum
> EXCLUDES 2   *Dieulafoy lesion of intestine (K63.81)*
> **DEF:** Abnormally large submucosal artery protruding through a defect in the stomach mucosa or intestines that can cause massive and life-threatening hemorrhaging.

K31.83   Achlorhydria
> **DEF:** Absence of hydrochloric acid in gastric secretions due to gastric mucosa atrophy. Achlorhydria is unresponsive to histamines.

K31.84   Gastroparesis
> Gastroparalysis
> Code first underlying disease, if known, such as:
> anorexia nervosa (F50.0-)
> diabetes mellitus (E08.43, E09.43, E10.43, E11.43, E13.43)
> scleroderma (M34.-)
> AHA: 2013,4Q,114

K31.89   Other diseases of stomach and duodenum
> AHA: 2020,1Q,15; 2017,1Q,28

K31.9   Disease of stomach and duodenum, unspecified

✓5ᵗʰ **K31.A   Gastric intestinal** metaplasia
> AHA: 2021,4Q,15-16

K31.A0   Gastric intestinal metaplasia, unspecified
> Gastric intestinal metaplasia indefinite for dysplasia
> Gastric intestinal metaplasia NOS

✓6ᵗʰ **K31.A1   Gastric intestinal metaplasia** without dysplasia

> **K31.A11   Gastric intestinal metaplasia without dysplasia,** involving the antrum
> **K31.A12   Gastric intestinal metaplasia without dysplasia,** involving the body **(corpus)**
> **K31.A13   Gastric intestinal metaplasia without dysplasia,** involving the fundus
> **K31.A14   Gastric intestinal metaplasia without dysplasia,** involving the cardia
> **K31.A15   Gastric intestinal metaplasia without dysplasia,** involving multiple sites
> **K31.A19   Gastric intestinal metaplasia without dysplasia, unspecified site**

✓6ᵗʰ **K31.A2   Gastric intestinal metaplasia** with dysplasia

> **K31.A21   Gastric intestinal metaplasia with** low grade **dysplasia**
> **K31.A22   Gastric intestinal metaplasia with** high grade **dysplasia**
> **K31.A29   Gastric intestinal metaplasia with dysplasia, unspecified**

Diseases of appendix (K35-K38)

✓4ᵗʰ **K35   Acute appendicitis**
> AHA: 2018,4Q,17-18

✓5ᵗʰ **K35.2   Acute appendicitis** with generalized peritonitis
> Appendicitis (acute) with generalized (diffuse) peritonitis following rupture or perforation of appendix

> **K35.20   Acute appendicitis with generalized peritonitis,** without abscess
> (Acute) appendicitis with generalized peritonitis NOS
> **K35.21   Acute appendicitis with generalized peritonitis,** with abscess

✓5ᵗʰ **K35.3   Acute appendicitis** with localized peritonitis

> **K35.30   Acute appendicitis with localized peritonitis,** without perforation or gangrene
> Acute appendicitis with localized peritonitis NOS
> **K35.31   Acute appendicitis with localized peritonitis and gangrene,** without perforation
> ▲ **K35.32   Acute appendicitis with perforation, localized peritonitis, and gangrene,** without abscess
> (Acute) appendicitis with perforation NOS
> Perforated appendix NOS
> Ruptured appendix (with localized peritonitis) NOS
> AHA: 2020,1Q,16
> ▲ **K35.33   Acute appendicitis with perforation, localized peritonitis, and gangrene,** with abscess
> (Acute) appendicitis with (peritoneal) abscess NOS
> Ruptured appendix with localized peritonitis and abscess

✓5ᵗʰ **K35.8   Other and unspecified acute appendicitis**

> **K35.80   Unspecified acute appendicitis**
> Acute appendicitis NOS
> Acute appendicitis without (localized) (generalized) peritonitis
> ✓6ᵗʰ **K35.89   Other acute appendicitis**
> AHA: 2020,1Q,16
> **K35.890   Other acute appendicitis** without perforation or gangrene
> **K35.891   Other acute appendicitis** without perforation, with gangrene
> (Acute) appendicitis with gangrene NOS

K36   Other appendicitis
> Chronic appendicitis
> Recurrent appendicitis

K37   Unspecified appendicitis
> EXCLUDES 1   *unspecified appendicitis with peritonitis (K35.2-, K35.3-)*

✓4ᵗʰ **K38   Other diseases of appendix**

K38.0   Hyperplasia of appendix

K38.1   Appendicular concretions
> Fecalith of appendix
> Stercolith of appendix

K38.2   Diverticulum of appendix

K38.3   Fistula of appendix

K38.8   Other specified diseases of appendix
> Intussusception of appendix

K38.9   Disease of appendix, unspecified

Hernia (K40-K46)

> **NOTE**   Hernia with both gangrene and obstruction is classified to hernia with gangrene.

> **INCLUDES**   acquired hernia
> congenital [except diaphragmatic or hiatus] hernia
> recurrent hernia

AHA: 2021,3Q,30-31

TIP: Do not assign a code for bilateral hernia when the right and left sides have differing pathology. For example, two codes would be assigned for bilateral femoral hernia in which the left side is incarcerated (with obstruction) but the right side is not incarcerated; the code for bilateral would not apply in this case.

✓4ᵗʰ **K40   Inguinal** hernia

> **INCLUDES**   bubonocele
> direct inguinal hernia
> double inguinal hernia
> indirect inguinal hernia
> inguinal hernia NOS
> oblique inguinal hernia
> scrotal hernia
> **DEF:** Within the groin region.

✓5ᵗʰ **K40.0   Bilateral** inguinal hernia, with obstruction, without gangrene
> Inguinal hernia (bilateral) causing obstruction without gangrene
> Incarcerated inguinal hernia (bilateral) without gangrene
> Irreducible inguinal hernia (bilateral) without gangrene
> Strangulated inguinal hernia (bilateral) without gangrene

> **K40.00   Bilateral inguinal hernia, with obstruction, without gangrene,** not specified as recurrent
> Bilateral inguinal hernia, with obstruction, without gangrene NOS
> **K40.01   Bilateral inguinal hernia, with obstruction, without gangrene,** recurrent

✓5ᵗʰ **K40.1   Bilateral** inguinal hernia, with gangrene

> **K40.10   Bilateral inguinal hernia, with gangrene,** not specified as recurrent
> Bilateral inguinal hernia, with gangrene NOS
> **K40.11   Bilateral inguinal hernia, with gangrene,** recurrent

✓5ᵗʰ **K40.2   Bilateral** inguinal hernia, without obstruction or gangrene

> **K40.20   Bilateral inguinal hernia, without obstruction or gangrene,** not specified as recurrent
> Bilateral inguinal hernia NOS
> **K40.21   Bilateral inguinal hernia, without obstruction or gangrene,** recurrent

✓5ʰ **K40.3** Unilateral **inguinal hernia, with obstruction, without gangrene**
Inguinal hernia (unilateral) causing obstruction without gangrene
Incarcerated inguinal hernia (unilateral) without gangrene
Irreducible inguinal hernia (unilateral) without gangrene
Strangulated inguinal hernia (unilateral) without gangrene

     K40.30 Unilateral inguinal hernia, with obstruction, without gangrene, not specified as recurrent
Inguinal hernia, with obstruction NOS
Unilateral inguinal hernia, with obstruction, without gangrene NOS

     K40.31 Unilateral inguinal hernia, with obstruction, without gangrene, recurrent

✓5ʰ **K40.4** Unilateral **inguinal hernia, with gangrene**

     K40.40 Unilateral inguinal hernia, with gangrene, not specified as recurrent
Inguinal hernia with gangrene NOS
Unilateral inguinal hernia with gangrene NOS

     K40.41 Unilateral **inguinal hernia, with gangrene,** recurrent

✓5ʰ **K40.9** Unilateral **inguinal hernia, without obstruction or gangrene**

     K40.90 Unilateral inguinal hernia, without obstruction or gangrene, not specified as recurrent
Inguinal hernia NOS
Unilateral inguinal hernia NOS

     K40.91 Unilateral inguinal hernia, without obstruction or gangrene, recurrent

Hernia Sites

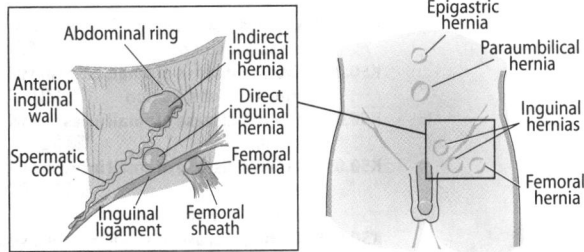

✓4ʰ **K41** Femoral **hernia**

✓5ʰ **K41.0** Bilateral **femoral hernia, with obstruction, without gangrene**
Femoral hernia (bilateral) causing obstruction, without gangrene
Incarcerated femoral hernia (bilateral), without gangrene
Irreducible femoral hernia (bilateral), without gangrene
Strangulated femoral hernia (bilateral), without gangrene

     K41.00 Bilateral femoral hernia, with obstruction, without gangrene, not specified as recurrent
Bilateral femoral hernia, with obstruction, without gangrene NOS

     K41.01 Bilateral femoral hernia, with obstruction, without gangrene, recurrent

✓5ʰ **K41.1** Bilateral **femoral hernia, with gangrene**

     K41.10 Bilateral femoral hernia, with gangrene, not specified as recurrent
Bilateral femoral hernia, with gangrene NOS

     K41.11 Bilateral femoral hernia, with gangrene, recurrent

✓5ʰ **K41.2** Bilateral **femoral hernia, without obstruction or gangrene**

     K41.20 Bilateral femoral hernia, without obstruction or gangrene, not specified as recurrent
Bilateral femoral hernia NOS

     K41.21 Bilateral femoral hernia, without obstruction or gangrene, recurrent

✓5ʰ **K41.3** Unilateral **femoral hernia, with obstruction, without gangrene**
Femoral hernia (unilateral) causing obstruction, without gangrene
Incarcerated femoral hernia (unilateral), without gangrene
Irreducible femoral hernia (unilateral), without gangrene
Strangulated femoral hernia (unilateral), without gangrene

     K41.30 Unilateral femoral hernia, with obstruction, without gangrene, not specified as recurrent
Femoral hernia, with obstruction NOS
Unilateral femoral hernia, with obstruction NOS

     K41.31 Unilateral femoral hernia, with obstruction, without gangrene, recurrent

✓5ʰ **K41.4** Unilateral **femoral hernia, with gangrene**

     K41.40 Unilateral femoral hernia, with gangrene, not specified as recurrent
Femoral hernia, with gangrene NOS
Unilateral femoral hernia, with gangrene NOS

     K41.41 Unilateral **femoral hernia, with gangrene,** recurrent

✓5ʰ **K41.9** Unilateral **femoral hernia, without obstruction or gangrene**

     K41.90 Unilateral femoral hernia, without obstruction or gangrene, not specified as recurrent
Femoral hernia NOS
Unilateral femoral hernia NOS

     K41.91 Unilateral femoral hernia, without obstruction or gangrene, recurrent

✓4ʰ **K42** Umbilical **hernia**

     [INCLUDES] paraumbilical hernia
     EXCLUDES 1 *omphalocele (Q79.2)*

     K42.0 Umbilical hernia **with obstruction, without gangrene**
Umbilical hernia causing obstruction, without gangrene
Incarcerated umbilical hernia, without gangrene
Irreducible umbilical hernia, without gangrene
Strangulated umbilical hernia, without gangrene

     K42.1 Umbilical hernia **with gangrene**
Gangrenous umbilical hernia

     K42.9 Umbilical hernia **without obstruction or gangrene**
Umbilical hernia NOS

✓4ʰ **K43** Ventral **hernia**

     DEF: Condition in which a loop of bowel protrudes through a weakness in the abdominal wall muscles that may occur as a birth defect, past surgical site (incisional), or form at a stomal site (parastomal).

     K43.0 Incisional **hernia with obstruction, without gangrene**
Incisional hernia causing obstruction, without gangrene
Incarcerated incisional hernia, without gangrene
Irreducible incisional hernia, without gangrene
Strangulated incisional hernia, without gangrene

     K43.1 Incisional **hernia with gangrene**
Gangrenous incisional hernia
AHA: 2020,2Q,22

     K43.2 Incisional **hernia without obstruction or gangrene**
Incisional hernia NOS

     K43.3 Parastomal **hernia with obstruction, without gangrene**
Incarcerated parastomal hernia, without gangrene
Irreducible parastomal hernia, without gangrene
Parastomal hernia causing obstruction, without gangrene
Strangulated parastomal hernia, without gangrene

     K43.4 Parastomal **hernia with gangrene**
Gangrenous parastomal hernia

     K43.5 Parastomal **hernia without obstruction or gangrene**
Parastomal hernia NOS

     K43.6 Other and unspecified ventral hernia with obstruction, without gangrene
Epigastric hernia causing obstruction, without gangrene
Hypogastric hernia causing obstruction, without gangrene
Incarcerated epigastric hernia without gangrene
Incarcerated hypogastric hernia without gangrene
Incarcerated midline hernia without gangrene
Incarcerated spigelian hernia without gangrene
Incarcerated subxiphoid hernia without gangrene
Irreducible epigastric hernia without gangrene
Irreducible hypogastric hernia without gangrene
Irreducible midline hernia without gangrene
Irreducible spigelian hernia without gangrene
Irreducible subxiphoid hernia without gangrene
Midline hernia causing obstruction, without gangrene
Spigelian hernia causing obstruction, without gangrene
Strangulated epigastric hernia without gangrene
Strangulated hypogastric hernia without gangrene
Strangulated midline hernia without gangrene
Strangulated spigelian hernia without gangrene
Strangulated subxiphoid hernia without gangrene
Subxiphoid hernia causing obstruction, without gangrene

     K43.7 Other and unspecified ventral hernia **with gangrene**
Any condition listed under K43.6 specified as gangrenous

     K43.9 Ventral hernia **without obstruction or gangrene**
Epigastric hernia
Ventral hernia NOS

☑ Additional Character Required   ✓×7ʰ Placeholder Alert   Manifestation   Unspecified Dx   🄠 QPP   UPD Unacceptable PDx

✓4ᵗʰ **K44 Diaphragmatic hernia**

INCLUDES   hiatus hernia (esophageal) (sliding)
paraesophageal hernia

EXCLUDES 1   *congenital diaphragmatic hernia (Q79.0)*
congenital hiatus hernia (Q40.1)

DEF: Protrusion of an abdominal organ, usually the stomach, through the esophageal opening within the diaphragm and occurring in two types: the sliding hiatal hernia and the paraesophageal hernia.

Hiatal Hernia

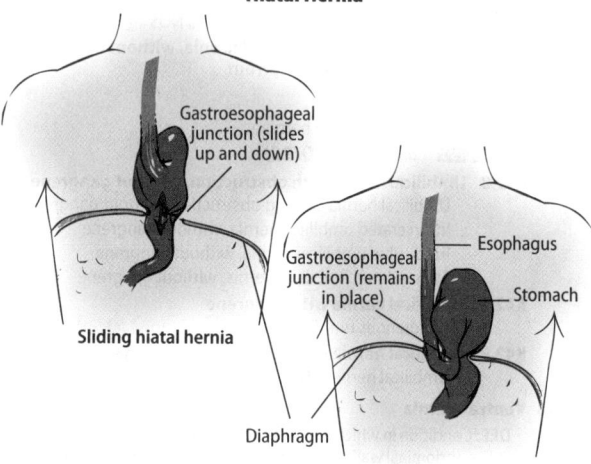

Gastroesophageal junction (slides up and down)

Sliding hiatal hernia

Gastroesophageal junction (remains in place)

Esophagus

Stomach

Diaphragm

Paraesophageal hiatal hernia

K44.0 Diaphragmatic hernia with obstruction, without gangrene
Diaphragmatic hernia causing obstruction
Incarcerated diaphragmatic hernia
Irreducible diaphragmatic hernia
Strangulated diaphragmatic hernia
AHA: 2022,2Q,13

[handwritten: Paraesophageal hernia]

K44.1 Diaphragmatic hernia with gangrene
Gangrenous diaphragmatic hernia

K44.9 Diaphragmatic hernia without obstruction or gangrene
Diaphragmatic hernia NOS

✓4ᵗʰ **K45 Other abdominal hernia**

INCLUDES   abdominal hernia, specified site NEC
lumbar hernia
obturator hernia
pudendal hernia
retroperitoneal hernia
sciatic hernia

K45.0 Other specified abdominal hernia with obstruction, without gangrene
Other specified abdominal hernia causing obstruction
Other specified incarcerated abdominal hernia
Other specified irreducible abdominal hernia
Other specified strangulated abdominal hernia

K45.1 Other specified abdominal hernia with gangrene
Any condition listed under K45 specified as gangrenous

K45.8 Other specified abdominal hernia without obstruction or gangrene

✓4ᵗʰ **K46 Unspecified abdominal hernia**

INCLUDES   enterocele
epiplocele
hernia NOS
interstitial hernia
intestinal hernia
intra-abdominal hernia

EXCLUDES 1   *vaginal enterocele (N81.5)*

K46.0 Unspecified abdominal hernia with obstruction, without gangrene
Unspecified abdominal hernia causing obstruction
Unspecified incarcerated abdominal hernia
Unspecified irreducible abdominal hernia
Unspecified strangulated abdominal hernia

K46.1 Unspecified abdominal hernia with gangrene
Any condition listed under K46 specified as gangrenous

K46.9 Unspecified abdominal hernia without obstruction or gangrene
Abdominal hernia NOS

Noninfective enteritis and colitis (K50-K52)

INCLUDES   noninfective inflammatory bowel disease

EXCLUDES 1   *irritable bowel syndrome (K58.-)*
megacolon (K59.3-)

✓4ᵗʰ **K50 Crohn's disease [regional enteritis]**

INCLUDES   granulomatous enteritis

Use additional code to identify manifestations, such as:
pyoderma gangrenosum (L88)

EXCLUDES 1   *ulcerative colitis (K51.-)*

AHA: 2019,3Q,5; 2012,4Q,104

DEF: Chronic inflammation of the gastrointestinal tract characterized by chronic granulomatous disease, most commonly affecting the intestines and the terminal ileum.

✓5ᵗʰ **K50.0 Crohn's disease of** small intestine
Crohn's disease [regional enteritis] of duodenum
Crohn's disease [regional enteritis] of ileum
Crohn's disease [regional enteritis] of jejunum
Regional ileitis
Terminal ileitis

EXCLUDES 1   *Crohn's disease of both small and large intestine (K50.8-)*

K50.00 Crohn's disease of small intestine without complications   HCC Rx ESR COM

✓6ᵗʰ **K50.01 Crohn's disease of small intestine** with complications

K50.011 Crohn's disease of small intestine with rectal bleeding HCC Rx ESR COM

K50.012 Crohn's disease of small intestine with intestinal obstruction HCC Rx ESR COM

K50.013 Crohn's disease of small intestine with fistula HCC Rx ESR COM

K50.014 Crohn's disease of small intestine with abscess HCC Rx ESR COM
AHA: 2012,4Q,104

K50.018 Crohn's disease of small intestine with other complication HCC Rx ESR COM

K50.019 Crohn's disease of small intestine with unspecified complications HCC Rx ESR COM

✓5ᵗʰ **K50.1 Crohn's disease of** large intestine
Crohn's disease [regional enteritis] of colon
Crohn's disease [regional enteritis] of large bowel
Crohn's disease [regional enteritis] of rectum
Granulomatous colitis
Regional colitis

EXCLUDES 1   *Crohn's disease of both small and large intestine (K50.8)*

K50.10 Crohn's disease of large intestine without complications   HCC Rx ESR COM

✓6ᵗʰ **K50.11 Crohn's disease of large intestine** with complications

K50.111 Crohn's disease of large intestine with rectal bleeding HCC Rx ESR COM

K50.112 Crohn's disease of large intestine with intestinal obstruction HCC Rx ESR COM

K50.113 Crohn's disease of large intestine with fistula HCC Rx ESR COM

K50.114 Crohn's disease of large intestine with abscess HCC Rx ESR COM

K50.118 Crohn's disease of large intestine with other complication HCC Rx ESR COM

K50.119 Crohn's disease of large intestine with unspecified complications HCC Rx ESR COM

✓5ᵗʰ **K50.8 Crohn's disease of** both small and large intestine

K50.80 Crohn's disease of both small and large intestine without complications   HCC Rx ESR COM

✓6ᵗʰ **K50.81 Crohn's disease of both small and large intestine** with complications

K50.811 Crohn's disease of both small and large intestine with rectal bleeding HCC Rx ESR COM

K50.812 Crohn's disease of both small and large intestine with intestinal obstruction `HCC` `Rx` `ESR` `COM`

K50.813 Crohn's disease of both small and large intestine with fistula `HCC` `Rx` `ESR` `COM`

K50.814 Crohn's disease of both small and large intestine with abscess `HCC` `Rx` `ESR` `COM`

K50.818 Crohn's disease of both small and large intestine with other complication `HCC` `Rx` `ESR` `COM`

K50.819 Crohn's disease of both small and large intestine with unspecified complications `HCC` `Rx` `ESR` `COM`

√5th **K50.9 Crohn's disease, unspecified**

K50.90 Crohn's disease, unspecified, without complications `HCC` `Rx` `ESR` `COM`
Crohn's disease NOS
Regional enteritis NOS

√6th **K50.91** Crohn's disease, unspecified, with complications

K50.911 Crohn's disease, unspecified, with rectal bleeding `HCC` `Rx` `ESR` `COM`

K50.912 Crohn's disease, unspecified, with intestinal obstruction `HCC` `Rx` `ESR` `COM`

K50.913 Crohn's disease, unspecified, with fistula `HCC` `Rx` `ESR` `COM`

K50.914 Crohn's disease, unspecified, with abscess `HCC` `Rx` `ESR` `COM`

K50.918 Crohn's disease, unspecified, with other complication `HCC` `Rx` `ESR` `COM`

K50.919 Crohn's disease, unspecified, with unspecified complications `HCC` `Rx` `ESR` `COM`

√4th **K51 Ulcerative colitis**

Use additional code to identify manifestations, such as:
pyoderma gangrenosum (L88)
EXCLUDES 1   *Crohn's disease [regional enteritis] (K50.-)*

√5th **K51.0 Ulcerative (chronic) pancolitis**
Backwash ileitis

K51.00 Ulcerative (chronic) pancolitis without complications `HCC` `Rx` `ESR` `COM`
Ulcerative (chronic) pancolitis NOS

√6th **K51.01** Ulcerative (chronic) pancolitis with complications

K51.011 Ulcerative (chronic) pancolitis with rectal bleeding `HCC` `Rx` `ESR` `COM`

K51.012 Ulcerative (chronic) pancolitis with intestinal obstruction `HCC` `Rx` `ESR` `COM`

K51.013 Ulcerative (chronic) pancolitis with fistula `HCC` `Rx` `ESR` `COM`

K51.014 Ulcerative (chronic) pancolitis with abscess `HCC` `Rx` `ESR` `COM`

K51.018 Ulcerative (chronic) pancolitis with other complication `HCC` `Rx` `ESR` `COM`

K51.019 Ulcerative (chronic) pancolitis with unspecified complications `HCC` `Rx` `ESR` `COM`

√5th **K51.2 Ulcerative (chronic) proctitis**

K51.20 Ulcerative (chronic) proctitis without complications `HCC` `Rx` `ESR` `COM`
Ulcerative (chronic) proctitis NOS

√6th **K51.21** Ulcerative (chronic) proctitis with complications

K51.211 Ulcerative (chronic) proctitis with rectal bleeding `HCC` `Rx` `ESR` `COM`

K51.212 Ulcerative (chronic) proctitis with intestinal obstruction `HCC` `Rx` `ESR` `COM`

K51.213 Ulcerative (chronic) proctitis with fistula `HCC` `Rx` `ESR` `COM`

K51.214 Ulcerative (chronic) proctitis with abscess `HCC` `Rx` `ESR` `COM`

K51.218 Ulcerative (chronic) proctitis with other complication `HCC` `Rx` `ESR` `COM`

K51.219 Ulcerative (chronic) proctitis with unspecified complications `HCC` `Rx` `ESR` `COM`

√5th **K51.3 Ulcerative (chronic) rectosigmoiditis**

K51.30 Ulcerative (chronic) rectosigmoiditis without complications `HCC` `Rx` `ESR` `COM`
Ulcerative (chronic) rectosigmoiditis NOS

√6th **K51.31** Ulcerative (chronic) rectosigmoiditis with complications

K51.311 Ulcerative (chronic) rectosigmoiditis with rectal bleeding `HCC` `Rx` `ESR` `COM`

K51.312 Ulcerative (chronic) rectosigmoiditis with intestinal obstruction `HCC` `Rx` `ESR` `COM`

K51.313 Ulcerative (chronic) rectosigmoiditis with fistula `HCC` `Rx` `ESR` `COM`

K51.314 Ulcerative (chronic) rectosigmoiditis with abscess `HCC` `Rx` `ESR` `COM`

K51.318 Ulcerative (chronic) rectosigmoiditis with other complication `HCC` `Rx` `ESR` `COM`

K51.319 Ulcerative (chronic) rectosigmoiditis with unspecified complications `HCC` `Rx` `ESR` `COM`

√5th **K51.4 Inflammatory polyps of colon**

EXCLUDES 1   *adenomatous polyp of colon (D12.6)*
polyposis of colon (D12.6)
polyps of colon NOS (K63.5)

K51.40 Inflammatory polyps of colon without complications `HCC` `Rx` `ESR` `COM`
Inflammatory polyps of colon NOS

√6th **K51.41** Inflammatory polyps of colon with complications

K51.411 Inflammatory polyps of colon with rectal bleeding `HCC` `Rx` `ESR` `COM`

K51.412 Inflammatory polyps of colon with intestinal obstruction `HCC` `Rx` `ESR` `COM`

K51.413 Inflammatory polyps of colon with fistula `HCC` `Rx` `ESR` `COM`

K51.414 Inflammatory polyps of colon with abscess `HCC` `Rx` `ESR` `COM`

K51.418 Inflammatory polyps of colon with other complication `HCC` `Rx` `ESR` `COM`

K51.419 Inflammatory polyps of colon with unspecified complications `HCC` `Rx` `ESR` `COM`

√5th **K51.5 Left sided colitis**
Left hemicolitis

K51.50 Left sided colitis without complications `HCC` `Rx` `ESR` `COM`
Left sided colitis NOS

√6th **K51.51** Left sided colitis with complications

K51.511 Left sided colitis with rectal bleeding `HCC` `Rx` `ESR` `COM`

K51.512 Left sided colitis with intestinal obstruction `HCC` `Rx` `ESR` `COM`

K51.513 Left sided colitis with fistula `HCC` `Rx` `ESR` `COM`

K51.514 Left sided colitis with abscess `HCC` `Rx` `ESR` `COM`

K51.518 Left sided colitis with other complication `HCC` `Rx` `ESR` `COM`

K51.519 Left sided colitis with unspecified complications `HCC` `Rx` `ESR` `COM`

√5th **K51.8 Other ulcerative colitis**

K51.80 Other ulcerative colitis without complications `HCC` `Rx` `ESR` `COM`

√6th **K51.81** Other ulcerative colitis with complications

K51.811 Other ulcerative colitis with rectal bleeding `HCC` `Rx` `ESR` `COM`

K51.812 Other ulcerative colitis with intestinal obstruction `HCC` `Rx` `ESR` `COM`

K51.813 Other ulcerative colitis with fistula `HCC` `Rx` `ESR` `COM`

K51.814 Other ulcerative colitis with abscess `HCC` `Rx` `ESR` `COM`

K51.818 Other ulcerative colitis with other complication `HCC` `Rx` `ESR` `COM`

K51.819 Other ulcerative colitis with unspecified complications `HCC` `Rx` `ESR` `COM`

√5th **K51.9 Ulcerative colitis, unspecified**

K51.90 Ulcerative colitis, unspecified, without complications `HCC` `Rx` `ESR` `COM`

√6th **K51.91** Ulcerative colitis, unspecified, with complications

K51.911 Ulcerative colitis, unspecified with rectal bleeding `HCC` `Rx` `ESR` `COM`

K51.912 Ulcerative colitis, unspecified with intestinal obstruction `HCC` `Rx` `ESR` `COM`

K51.913 **Ulcerative colitis, unspecified with fistula** `HCC` `Rx` `ESR` `COM`

K51.914 **Ulcerative colitis, unspecified with abscess** `HCC` `Rx` `ESR` `COM`

K51.918 **Ulcerative colitis, unspecified with other complication** `HCC` `Rx` `ESR` `COM`

K51.919 **Ulcerative colitis, unspecified with unspecified complications** `HCC` `Rx` `ESR` `COM`

✓4ᵗʰ **K52** **Other and unspecified noninfective gastroenteritis and colitis**
AHA: 2016,4Q,30-31

K52.0 **Gastroenteritis and colitis due to** radiation

K52.1 **Toxic gastroenteritis and colitis**
Drug-induced gastroenteritis and colitis
Code first (T51-T65) to identify toxic agent
Use additional code for adverse effect, if applicable, to identify drug (T36-T50 with fifth or sixth character 5)
AHA: 2019,1Q,17

✓5ᵗʰ **K52.2** **Allergic and dietetic gastroenteritis and colitis**
Food hypersensitivity gastroenteritis or colitis
Use additional code to identify type of food allergy (Z91.01-, Z91.02-)
EXCLUDES 2 *allergic eosinophilic colitis (K52.82)*
allergic eosinophilic esophagitis (K20.0)
allergic eosinophilic gastritis (K52.81)
allergic eosinophilic gastroenteritis (K52.81)
DEF: True immunoglobulin E (IgE)-mediated allergic reaction of the lining of the stomach, intestines, or colon to food proteins. It causes nausea, vomiting, diarrhea, and abdominal cramping.

K52.21 **Food protein-induced** enterocolitis syndrome
FPIES
Use additional code for hypovolemic shock, if present (R57.1)

K52.22 **Food protein-induced** enteropathy

K52.29 **Other allergic and dietetic gastroenteritis and colitis**
Allergic proctocolitis
Food hypersensitivity gastroenteritis or colitis
Food-induced eosinophilic proctocolitis
Food protein-induced proctocolitis
Immediate gastrointestinal hypersensitivity
Milk protein-induced proctocolitis

K52.3 **Indeterminate colitis**
Colonic inflammatory bowel disease unclassified (IBDU)
EXCLUDES 1 *unspecified colitis (K52.9)*

✓5ᵗʰ **K52.8** **Other specified noninfective gastroenteritis and colitis**

K52.81 **Eosinophilic gastritis or gastroenteritis**
Eosinophilic enteritis
EXCLUDES 2 *eosinophilic esophagitis (K20.0)*
DEF: Disorder involving the accumulation of eosinophil in the lining of the stomach or multiple levels of the gastrointestinal tract, but without a known cause such as connective tissue disease, drug reaction, malignancy, or parasitic infection.

K52.82 **Eosinophilic colitis**
EXCLUDES 2 *allergic proctocolitis (K52.29)*
food-induced eosinophilic proctocolitis (K52.29)
food protein-induced enterocolitis syndrome (FPIES) (K52.21)
food protein-induced proctocolitis (K52.29)
milk protein-induced proctocolitis (K52.29)
DEF: Disorder involving the accumulation of eosinophil in the tissues lining the colon, but without a known cause such as connective tissue disease, drug reaction, malignancy, or parasitic infection. The resultant inflammation may cause extreme abdominal pain, diarrhea, or bloody stool.

✓6ᵗʰ **K52.83** **Microscopic colitis**

K52.831 **Collagenous colitis** `Rx`

K52.832 **Lymphocytic colitis** `Rx`

K52.838 **Other microscopic colitis** `Rx`

K52.839 **Microscopic colitis, unspecified** `Rx`

K52.89 **Other specified noninfective gastroenteritis and colitis**
AHA: 2019,1Q,20

K52.9 **Noninfective gastroenteritis and colitis, unspecified**
Colitis NOS
Enteritis NOS
Gastroenteritis NOS
Ileitis NOS
Jejunitis NOS
Sigmoiditis NOS
EXCLUDES 1 *diarrhea NOS (R19.7)*
functional diarrhea (K59.1)
infectious gastroenteritis and colitis NOS (A09)
neonatal diarrhea (noninfective) (P78.3)
psychogenic diarrhea (F45.8)
AHA: 2021,3Q,3

Other diseases of intestines (K55-K64)

✓4ᵗʰ **K55** **Vascular disorders of intestine**
EXCLUDES 1 *necrotizing enterocolitis of newborn (P77.-)*
AHA: 2016,4Q,32

✓5ᵗʰ **K55.0** **Acute vascular disorders of intestine**
Infarction of appendices epiploicae
Mesenteric (artery) (vein) embolism
Mesenteric (artery) (vein) infarction
Mesenteric (artery) (vein) thrombosis
AHA: 2019,4Q,68

✓6ᵗʰ **K55.01** **Acute (reversible)** ischemia of small intestine

K55.011 **Focal (segmental) acute (reversible) ischemia of small intestine** `HCC` `ESR` `COM`

K55.012 **Diffuse acute (reversible) ischemia of small intestine** `HCC` `ESR` `COM`

K55.019 **Acute (reversible) ischemia of small intestine, extent unspecified** `HCC` `ESR` `COM`

✓6ᵗʰ **K55.02** **Acute infarction of small intestine**
Gangrene of small intestine
Necrosis of small intestine

K55.021 **Focal (segmental) acute infarction of small intestine** `HCC` `ESR` `COM`

K55.022 **Diffuse acute infarction of small intestine** `HCC` `ESR` `COM`

K55.029 **Acute infarction of small intestine, extent unspecified** `HCC` `ESR` `COM`

✓6ᵗʰ **K55.03** **Acute (reversible) ischemia of large intestine**
Acute fulminant ischemic colitis
Subacute ischemic colitis

K55.031 **Focal (segmental) acute (reversible) ischemia of large intestine** `HCC` `ESR` `COM`

K55.032 **Diffuse acute (reversible) ischemia of large intestine** `HCC` `ESR` `COM`

K55.039 **Acute (reversible) ischemia of large intestine, extent unspecified** `HCC` `ESR` `COM`
AHA: 2019,4Q,68

✓6ᵗʰ **K55.04** **Acute infarction of large intestine**
Gangrene of large intestine
Necrosis of large intestine

K55.041 **Focal (segmental) acute infarction of large intestine** `HCC` `ESR` `COM`

K55.042 **Diffuse acute infarction of large intestine** `HCC` `ESR` `COM`

K55.049 **Acute infarction of large intestine, extent unspecified** `HCC` `ESR` `COM`

✓6ᵗʰ **K55.05** **Acute (reversible) ischemia of intestine, part unspecified**

K55.051 **Focal (segmental) acute (reversible) ischemia of intestine, part unspecified** `HCC` `ESR` `COM`

K55.052 **Diffuse acute (reversible) ischemia of intestine, part unspecified** `HCC` `ESR` `COM`

K55.059 **Acute (reversible) ischemia of intestine, part and extent unspecified** `HCC` `ESR` `COM`

√6ᵗʰ **K55.06 Acute infarction of intestine, part unspecified**
Acute intestinal infarction
Gangrene of intestine
Necrosis of intestine

K55.061 Focal (segmental) acute infarction of intestine, part unspecified `HCC` `ESR` `COM`

K55.062 Diffuse acute infarction of intestine, part unspecified `HCC` `ESR` `COM`

K55.069 Acute infarction of intestine, part and extent unspecified `HCC` `ESR` `COM`

K55.1 Chronic vascular disorders of intestine `HCC` `ESR` `COM`
Chronic ischemic colitis
Chronic ischemic enteritis
Chronic ischemic enterocolitis
Ischemic stricture of intestine
Mesenteric atherosclerosis
Mesenteric vascular insufficiency

√5ᵗʰ **K55.2 Angiodysplasia of colon**
AHA: 2018,3Q,21
TIP: Assign a code for "with hemorrhage" when angiodysplasia and GI bleeding are documented. The ICD-10-CM classification assumes the two are related without the provider linking the two conditions. Evidence of bleeding during a procedure is not required.

K55.20 Angiodysplasia of colon without hemorrhage
K55.21 Angiodysplasia of colon with hemorrhage
DEF: Small vascular abnormalities due to fragile blood vessels in the colon, resulting in blood loss from the gastrointestinal (GI) tract.

√5ᵗʰ **K55.3 Necrotizing enterocolitis**
EXCLUDES 1 necrotizing enterocolitis of newborn (P77.-)
EXCLUDES 2 necrotizing enterocolitis due to Clostridium difficile (A04.7-)

K55.30 Necrotizing enterocolitis, unspecified `HCC` `ESR` `COM`
Necrotizing enterocolitis, NOS

K55.31 Stage 1 necrotizing enterocolitis `HCC` `ESR` `COM`
Necrotizing enterocolitis without pneumatosis, without perforation

K55.32 Stage 2 necrotizing enterocolitis `HCC` `ESR` `COM`
Necrotizing enterocolitis with pneumatosis, without perforation

K55.33 Stage 3 necrotizing enterocolitis `HCC` `ESR` `COM`
Necrotizing enterocolitis with perforation
Necrotizing enterocolitis with pneumatosis and perforation

K55.8 Other vascular disorders of intestine `HCC` `ESR` `COM`

K55.9 Vascular disorder of intestine, unspecified `HCC` `ESR` `COM`
Ischemic colitis
Ischemic enteritis
Ischemic enterocolitis

√4ᵗʰ **K56 Paralytic ileus and intestinal obstruction without hernia**
EXCLUDES 1 congenital stricture or stenosis of intestine (Q41-Q42)
cystic fibrosis with meconium ileus (E84.11)
ischemic stricture of intestine (K55.1)
meconium ileus NOS (P76.0)
neonatal intestinal obstructions classifiable to P76.-
obstruction of duodenum (K31.5)
postprocedural intestinal obstruction (K91.3-)
EXCLUDES 2 stenosis of anus or rectum (K62.4)

K56.0 Paralytic ileus `HCC` `ESR` `COM`
Paralysis of bowel
Paralysis of colon
Paralysis of intestine
EXCLUDES 1 gallstone ileus (K56.3)
ileus NOS (K56.7)
obstructive ileus NOS (K56.69-)
DEF: Intestinal obstruction due to paralysis of bowel motility or peristalsis.

K56.1 Intussusception `HCC` `ESR` `COM`
Intussusception or invagination of bowel
Intussusception or invagination of colon
Intussusception or invagination of intestine
Intussusception or invagination of rectum
EXCLUDES 2 intussusception of appendix (K38.8)
DEF: Intestinal obstruction due to prolapse of a bowel section into an adjacent section. It occurs primarily in children and symptoms include acute abdominal pain, vomiting, and passage of blood and mucus from the rectum.

K56.2 Volvulus `HCC` `ESR` `COM`
Strangulation of colon or intestine
Torsion of colon or intestine
Twist of colon or intestine
EXCLUDES 2 volvulus of duodenum (K31.5)
DEF: Twisting, knotting, or entanglement of the bowel on itself that may quickly compromise oxygen supply to the intestinal tissues. A volvulus usually occurs at the sigmoid and ileocecal areas of the intestines.

Volvulus

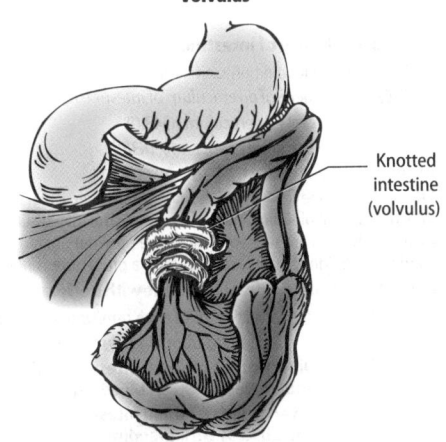

Knotted intestine (volvulus)

K56.3 Gallstone ileus `HCC` `ESR` `COM`
Obstruction of intestine by gallstone

√5ᵗʰ **K56.4 Other impaction of intestine**

K56.41 Fecal impaction `HCC` `ESR` `COM`
EXCLUDES 1 constipation (K59.0-)
incomplete defecation (R15.0)

K56.49 Other impaction of intestine `HCC` `ESR` `COM`

√5ᵗʰ **K56.5 Intestinal adhesions [bands] with obstruction (postinfection)**
Abdominal hernia due to adhesions with obstruction
Peritoneal adhesions [bands] with intestinal obstruction (postinfection)
AHA: 2017,4Q,16-17

K56.50 Intestinal adhesions [bands], unspecified as to partial versus complete obstruction `HCC` `ESR` `COM`
Intestinal adhesions with obstruction NOS

K56.51 Intestinal adhesions [bands], with partial obstruction `HCC` `ESR` `COM`
Intestinal adhesions with incomplete obstruction

K56.52 Intestinal adhesions [bands] with complete obstruction `HCC` `ESR` `COM`

√5ᵗʰ **K56.6 Other and unspecified intestinal obstruction**
AHA: 2017,4Q,16-17; 2017,2Q,12

√6ᵗʰ **K56.60 Unspecified intestinal obstruction**

K56.600 Partial intestinal obstruction, unspecified as to cause `HCC` `ESR` `COM`
Incomplete intestinal obstruction, NOS

K56.601 Complete intestinal obstruction, unspecified as to cause `HCC` `ESR` `COM`

K56.609 Unspecified intestinal obstruction, unspecified as to partial versus complete obstruction `HCC` `ESR` `COM`
Intestinal obstruction NOS

✓6ᵗʰ **K56.69 Other intestinal obstruction**
Enterostenosis NOS
Obstructive ileus NOS
Occlusion of colon or intestine NOS
Stenosis of colon or intestine NOS
Stricture of colon or intestine NOS
> *EXCLUDES 1*   intestinal obstruction due to specified condition - code to condition

    K56.690 Other partial intestinal obstruction `HCC` `ESR` `COM`
         Other incomplete intestinal obstruction

    K56.691 Other complete intestinal obstruction `HCC` `ESR` `COM`

    K56.699 Other intestinal obstruction unspecified as to partial versus complete obstruction `HCC` `ESR` `COM`
         Other intestinal obstruction, NEC

K56.7 Ileus, unspecified `HCC` `ESR` `COM`
> *EXCLUDES 1*   obstructive ileus (K56.69-)
> *EXCLUDES 2*   intestinal obstruction with hernia (K40-K46)

   AHA: 2017,1Q,40

✓4ᵗʰ **K57 Diverticular disease of intestine**
Code also if applicable peritonitis K65.-
> *EXCLUDES 1*   congenital diverticulum of intestine (Q43.8)
>   Meckel's diverticulum (Q43.0)
> *EXCLUDES 2*   diverticulum of appendix (K38.2)

   AHA: 2022,1Q,26-27; 2021,1Q,9,11; 2018,3Q,21
   TIP: Assign a code for "with bleeding" when diverticular disease of the intestine and GI bleeding are documented. The ICD-10-CM classification assumes the two are related without the provider linking the two conditions. Evidence of bleeding during a procedure is not required.

✓5ᵗʰ **K57.0 Diverticulitis of small intestine with perforation and abscess**
> *EXCLUDES 1*   diverticulitis of both small and large intestine with perforation and abscess (K57.4-)

    K57.00 Diverticulitis of small intestine with perforation and abscess without bleeding

    K57.01 Diverticulitis of small intestine with perforation and abscess with bleeding

✓5ᵗʰ **K57.1 Diverticular disease of small intestine without perforation or abscess**
> *EXCLUDES 1*   diverticular disease of both small and large intestine without perforation or abscess (K57.5-)

    K57.10 Diverticulosis of small intestine without perforation or abscess without bleeding
         Diverticular disease of small intestine NOS

    K57.11 Diverticulosis of small intestine without perforation or abscess with bleeding

    K57.12 Diverticulitis of small intestine without perforation or abscess without bleeding

    K57.13 Diverticulitis of small intestine without perforation or abscess with bleeding

✓5ᵗʰ **K57.2 Diverticulitis of large intestine with perforation and abscess**
> *EXCLUDES 1*   diverticulitis of both small and large intestine with perforation and abscess (K57.4-)

    K57.20 Diverticulitis of large intestine with perforation and abscess without bleeding

    K57.21 Diverticulitis of large intestine with perforation and abscess with bleeding

✓5ᵗʰ **K57.3 Diverticular disease of large intestine without perforation or abscess**
> *EXCLUDES 1*   diverticular disease of both small and large intestine without perforation or abscess (K57.5-)

    K57.30 Diverticulosis of large intestine without perforation or abscess without bleeding
         Diverticular disease of colon NOS

    K57.31 Diverticulosis of large intestine without perforation or abscess with bleeding

    K57.32 Diverticulitis of large intestine without perforation or abscess without bleeding

    K57.33 Diverticulitis of large intestine without perforation or abscess with bleeding

✓5ᵗʰ **K57.4 Diverticulitis of both small and large intestine with perforation and abscess**

    K57.40 Diverticulitis of both small and large intestine with perforation and abscess without bleeding

    K57.41 Diverticulitis of both small and large intestine with perforation and abscess with bleeding

✓5ᵗʰ **K57.5 Diverticular disease of both small and large intestine without perforation or abscess**

    K57.50 Diverticulosis of both small and large intestine without perforation or abscess without bleeding
         Diverticular disease of both small and large intestine NOS

    K57.51 Diverticulosis of both small and large intestine without perforation or abscess with bleeding

    K57.52 Diverticulitis of both small and large intestine without perforation or abscess without bleeding

    K57.53 Diverticulitis of both small and large intestine without perforation or abscess with bleeding

✓5ᵗʰ **K57.8 Diverticulitis of intestine, part unspecified, with perforation and abscess**

    K57.80 Diverticulitis of intestine, part unspecified, with perforation and abscess without bleeding

    K57.81 Diverticulitis of intestine, part unspecified, with perforation and abscess with bleeding

✓5ᵗʰ **K57.9 Diverticular disease of intestine, part unspecified, without perforation or abscess**

    K57.90 Diverticulosis of intestine, part unspecified, without perforation or abscess without bleeding
         Diverticular disease of intestine NOS

    K57.91 Diverticulosis of intestine, part unspecified, without perforation or abscess with bleeding

    K57.92 Diverticulitis of intestine, part unspecified, without perforation or abscess without bleeding

    K57.93 Diverticulitis of intestine, part unspecified, without perforation or abscess with bleeding

✓4ᵗʰ **K58 Irritable bowel syndrome**
> *INCLUDES*   irritable colon
>   spastic colon

   AHA: 2016,4Q,32-33

K58.0 Irritable bowel syndrome with diarrhea

K58.1 Irritable bowel syndrome with constipation

K58.2 Mixed irritable bowel syndrome

K58.8 Other irritable bowel syndrome

K58.9 Irritable bowel syndrome without diarrhea
     Irritable bowel syndrome NOS

✓4ᵗʰ **K59 Other functional intestinal disorders**
> *EXCLUDES 1*   change in bowel habit NOS (R19.4)
>   intestinal malabsorption (K90.-)
>   psychogenic intestinal disorders (F45.8)
> *EXCLUDES 2*   functional disorders of stomach (K31.-)

✓5ᵗʰ **K59.0 Constipation**
> *EXCLUDES 1*   fecal impaction (K56.41)
>   incomplete defecation (R15.0)

   AHA: 2016,4Q,33

    K59.00 Constipation, unspecified

    K59.01 Slow transit constipation
         DEF: Delay in the transit of fecal material through the colon secondary to smooth muscle dysfunction or decreased peristaltic contractions along the colon.

    K59.02 Outlet dysfunction constipation

    K59.03 Drug induced constipation
         Use additional code for adverse effect, if applicable, to identify drug (T36-T50 with fifth or sixth character 5)

    K59.04 Chronic idiopathic constipation
         Functional constipation

    K59.09 Other constipation
         Chronic constipation

K59.1 Functional diarrhea
> *EXCLUDES 1*   diarrhea NOS (R19.7)
>   irritable bowel syndrome with diarrhea (K58.0)

K59.2 Neurogenic bowel, not elsewhere classified
     DEF: Disorder of bowel due to a spinal cord lesion because of injury or as a complication of conditions such as multiple sclerosis (MS) or spina bifida. Loss of bowel control is the primary symptom, manifested as constipation or bowel incontinence.

☑5ᵗʰ K59.3 Megacolon, not elsewhere classified
Dilatation of colon
Code first, if applicable (T51-T65) to identify toxic agent
EXCLUDES 1   *congenital megacolon (aganglionic) (Q43.1)*
     megacolon (due to) (in) Chagas' disease (B57.32)
     megacolon (due to) (in) Clostridium difficile (A04.7-)
     megacolon (due to) (in) Hirschsprung's disease
       (Q43.1)
AHA: 2016,4Q,33-34

   K59.31 Toxic megacolon   `HCC` `ESR` `COM`
   K59.39 Other megacolon
     Megacolon NOS

K59.4 Anal spasm
Proctalgia fugax

☑5ᵗʰ K59.8 Other specified functional intestinal disorders
AHA: 2020,4Q,29-30

   K59.81 Ogilvie syndrome
     Acute colonic pseudo-obstruction (ACPO)
   K59.89 Other specified functional intestinal disorders
     Atony of colon
     Pseudo-obstruction (acute) (chronic) of intestine

K59.9 Functional intestinal disorder, unspecified

☑4ᵗʰ K60 Fissure and fistula of anal and rectal regions
EXCLUDES 1   *fissure and fistula of anal and rectal regions with abscess or*
     cellulitis (K61.-)
EXCLUDES 2   *anal sphincter tear (healed) (nontraumatic) (old) (K62.81)*

K60.0 Acute anal fissure
K60.1 Chronic anal fissure
K60.2 Anal fissure, unspecified
K60.3 Anal fistula
K60.4 Rectal fistula
   Fistula of rectum to skin
   EXCLUDES 1   *rectovaginal fistula (N82.3)*
     vesicorectal fistual (N32.1)
K60.5 Anorectal fistula

☑4ᵗʰ K61 Abscess of anal and rectal regions
INCLUDES   abscess of anal and rectal regions
     cellulitis of anal and rectal regions

K61.0 Anal abscess
   Perianal abscess
   EXCLUDES 2   *intrasphincteric abscess (K61.4)*
K61.1 Rectal abscess
   Perirectal abscess
   EXCLUDES 1   *ischiorectal abscess (K61.39)*
   AHA: 2012,4Q,104
K61.2 Anorectal abscess
☑5ᵗʰ K61.3 Ischiorectal abscess
   AHA: 2018,4Q,19
   K61.31 Horseshoe abscess
   K61.39 Other ischiorectal abscess
     Abscess of ischiorectal fossa
     Ischiorectal abscess, NOS
K61.4 Intrasphincteric abscess
   Intersphincteric abscess
K61.5 Supralevator abscess
   AHA: 2018,4Q,19

☑4ᵗʰ K62 Other diseases of anus and rectum
INCLUDES   anal canal
EXCLUDES 2   *colostomy and enterostomy malfunction (K94.0-, K94.1-)*
     fecal incontinence (R15.-)
     hemorrhoids (K64.-)

K62.0 Anal polyp
K62.1 Rectal polyp
   EXCLUDES 1   *adenomatous polyp (D12.8)*
   AHA: 2018,1Q,6
K62.2 Anal prolapse
   Prolapse of anal canal
K62.3 Rectal prolapse
   Prolapse of rectal mucosa
K62.4 Stenosis of anus and rectum
   Stricture of anus (sphincter)
   AHA: 2019,2Q,13

K62.5 Hemorrhage of anus and rectum
   EXCLUDES 1   *gastrointestinal bleeding NOS (K92.2)*
     melena (K92.1)
     neonatal rectal hemorrhage (P54.2)
   AHA: 2019,1Q,21
K62.6 Ulcer of anus and rectum
   Solitary ulcer of anus and rectum
   Stercoral ulcer of anus and rectum
   EXCLUDES 1   *fissure and fistula of anus and rectum (K60.-)*
     ulcerative colitis (K51.-)
K62.7 Radiation proctitis
   Use additional code to identify the type of radiation (W88.-) or
     radiation therapy (Y84.2)
   AHA: 2019,1Q,21
☑5ᵗʰ K62.8 Other specified diseases of anus and rectum
   EXCLUDES 2   *ulcerative proctitis (K51.2)*

   K62.81 Anal sphincter tear (healed) (nontraumatic) (old)
     Tear of anus, nontraumatic
     Use additional code for any associated fecal
       incontinence (R15.-)
     EXCLUDES 2   *anal fissure (K60.-)*
       anal sphincter tear (healed) (old)
         complicating delivery (O34.7-)
       traumatic tear of anal sphincter (S31.831)

   K62.82 Dysplasia of anus
     Anal intraepithelial neoplasia I and II (AIN I and II)
       (histologically confirmed)
     Dysplasia of anus NOS
     Mild and moderate dysplasia of anus (histologically
       confirmed)
     EXCLUDES 1   *abnormal results from anal cytologic*
       examination without histologic
       confirmation (R85.61-)
       anal intraepithelial neoplasia III (D01.3)
       carcinoma in situ of anus (D01.3)
       HGSIL of anus (R85.613)
       severe dysplasia of anus (D01.3)

   K62.89 Other specified diseases of anus and rectum
     Proctitis NOS
     Use additional code for any associated fecal
       incontinence (R15.-)

K62.9 Disease of anus and rectum, unspecified

☑4ᵗʰ K63 Other diseases of intestine
K63.0 Abscess of intestine
   EXCLUDES 1   *abscess of intestine with Crohn's disease (K50.014,*
     K50.114, K50.814, K50.914)
     abscess of intestine with diverticular disease (K57.0,
       K57.2, K57.4, K57.8)
     abscess of intestine with ulcerative colitis (K51.014,
       K51.214, K51.314, K51.414, K51.514, K51.814,
       K51.914)
   EXCLUDES 2   *abscess of anal and rectal regions (K61.-)*
     abscess of appendix (K35.3-)
K63.1 Perforation of intestine (nontraumatic)   `HCC` `ESR` `COM`
   Perforation (nontraumatic) of rectum
   EXCLUDES 1   *perforation (nontraumatic) of duodenum (K26.-)*
     perforation (nontraumatic) of intestine with
       diverticular disease (K57.0, K57.2, K57.4, K57.8)
   EXCLUDES 2   *perforation (nontraumatic) of appendix (K35.2-,*
     K35.3-)
   AHA: 2020,2Q,22
K63.2 Fistula of intestine
   EXCLUDES 1   *fistula of duodenum (K31.6)*
     fistula of intestine with Crohn's disease (K50.013,
       K50.113, K50.813, K50.913)
     fistula of intestine with ulcerative colitis (K51.013,
       K51.213, K51.313, K51.413, K51.513, K51.813,
       K51.913)
   EXCLUDES 2   *fistula of anal and rectal regions (K60.-)*
     fistula of appendix (K38.3)
     intestinal-genital fistula, female (N82.2-N82.4)
     vesicointestinal fistula (N32.1)
   AHA: 2017,3Q,4

Chapter 11. Diseases of the Digestive System

K63.3   Ulcer **of intestine**
Primary ulcer of small intestine
> EXCLUDES 1   *duodenal ulcer (K26.-)*
> *gastrointestinal ulcer (K28.-)*
> *gastrojejunal ulcer (K28.-)*
> *jejunal ulcer (K28.-)*
> *peptic ulcer, site unspecified (K27.-)*
> *ulcer of intestine with perforation (K63.1)*
> *ulcer of anus or rectum (K62.6)*
> *ulcerative colitis (K51.-)*

K63.4   Enteroptosis

K63.5   Polyp **of colon**
> EXCLUDES 1   *adenomatous polyp of colon (D12.-)*
> *inflammatory polyp of colon (K51.4-)*
> *polyposis of colon (D12.6)*

AHA: 2019,1Q,33; 2018,2Q,14; 2017,1Q,15; 2015,2Q,14
TIP: Assign this code when documentation states hyperplastic colon polyp regardless of the site in the colon. Slow-growing, hyperplastic polyps are not precancerous and are classified differently from benign or adenomatous polyps.

✓5ᵗʰ **K63.8**   **Other specified diseases of intestine**

     K63.81   **Dieulafoy lesion of intestine**
> EXCLUDES 2   *Dieulafoy lesion of stomach and duodenum (K31.82)*

         DEF: Abnormally large submucosal artery protruding through a defect in the stomach mucosa or intestines that can cause massive and life-threatening hemorrhaging.

     K63.89   **Other specified diseases of intestine**
         AHA: 2013,2Q,31

K63.9   **Disease of intestine, unspecified**

✓4ᵗʰ **K64**   **Hemorrhoids and perianal venous thrombosis**
> INCLUDES   piles
> EXCLUDES 1   *hemorrhoids complicating childbirth and the puerperium (O87.2)*
> *hemorrhoids complicating pregnancy (O22.4)*

Hemorrhoids

External anal sphincter
External hemorrhoid
Anoderm
Pectinate line
Prolapsing internal hemorrhoid
Internal hemorrhoid
Internal anal sphincter
Perianal vessels

K64.0   First degree **hemorrhoids**
Grade/stage I hemorrhoids
Hemorrhoids (bleeding) without prolapse outside of anal canal

K64.1   Second degree **hemorrhoids**
Grade/stage II hemorrhoids
Hemorrhoids (bleeding) that prolapse with straining, but retract spontaneously

K64.2   Third degree **hemorrhoids**
Grade/stage III hemorrhoids
Hemorrhoids (bleeding) that prolapse with straining and require manual replacement back inside anal canal

K64.3   Fourth degree **hemorrhoids**
Grade/stage IV hemorrhoids
Hemorrhoids (bleeding) with prolapsed tissue that cannot be manually replaced

K64.4   Residual **hemorrhoidal** skin tags
External hemorrhoids, NOS
Skin tags of anus

K64.5   Perianal venous thrombosis
External hemorrhoids with thrombosis
Perianal hematoma
Thrombosed hemorrhoids NOS

K64.8   **Other hemorrhoids**
Internal hemorrhoids, without mention of degree
Prolapsed hemorrhoids, degree not specified

K64.9   **Unspecified hemorrhoids**
Hemorrhoids (bleeding) NOS
Hemorrhoids (bleeding) without mention of degree

Diseases of peritoneum and retroperitoneum (K65-K68)

✓4ᵗʰ **K65**   **Peritonitis**
Use additional code (B95-B97), to identify infectious agent, if known
Code also if applicable diverticular disease of intestine (K57.-)
> EXCLUDES 1   *acute appendicitis with generalized peritonitis (K35.2-)*
> *aseptic peritonitis (T81.6)*
> *benign paroxysmal peritonitis (E85.0)*
> *chemical peritonitis (T81.6)*
> *gonococcal peritonitis (A54.85)*
> *neonatal peritonitis (P78.0-P78.1)*
> *pelvic peritonitis, female (N73.3-N73.5)*
> *periodic familial peritonitis (E85.0)*
> *peritonitis due to talc or other foreign substance (T81.6)*
> *peritonitis in chlamydia (A74.81)*
> *peritonitis in diphtheria (A36.89)*
> *peritonitis in syphilis (late) (A52.74)*
> *peritonitis in tuberculosis (A18.31)*
> *peritonitis with or following abortion or ectopic or molar pregnancy (O00-O07, O08.0)*
> *peritonitis with or following appendicitis (K35.-)*
> *puerperal peritonitis (O85)*
> *retroperitoneal infections (K68.-)*

K65.0   Generalized (acute) **peritonitis**   `HCC` `ESR` `COM`
Pelvic peritonitis (acute), male
Subphrenic peritonitis (acute)
Suppurative peritonitis (acute)

K65.1   **Peritoneal** abscess   `HCC` `ESR` `COM`
Abdominopelvic abscess
Abscess (of) omentum
Abscess (of) peritoneum
Mesenteric abscess
Retrocecal abscess
Subdiaphragmatic abscess
Subhepatic abscess
Subphrenic abscess
AHA: 2022,1Q,26; 2019,1Q,15

K65.2   Spontaneous bacterial **peritonitis**   `HCC` `ESR` `COM`
> EXCLUDES 1   *bacterial peritonitis NOS (K65.9)*

K65.3   **Choleperitonitis**   `HCC` `ESR` `COM`
Peritonitis due to bile
DEF: Inflammation of the peritoneum due to leakage of bile into the peritoneal cavity resulting from rupture of the bile passages or gallbladder.

K65.4   **Sclerosing mesenteritis**   `HCC` `ESR` `COM`
Fat necrosis of peritoneum
(Idiopathic) sclerosing mesenteric fibrosis
Mesenteric lipodystrophy
Mesenteric panniculitis
Retractile mesenteritis

K65.8   **Other peritonitis**   `HCC` `ESR` `COM`
Chronic proliferative peritonitis
Peritonitis due to urine

K65.9   **Peritonitis, unspecified**   `HCC` `ESR` `COM`
Bacterial peritonitis NOS
AHA: 2022,1Q,27; 2013,2Q,31

`HCC` CMS-HCC   `Rx` Rx HCC   `ESR` ESRD HCC   `COM` Commercial HCC   `N` Newborn: 0   `P` Pediatric: 0-17   `M` Maternity: 9-64   `A` Adult: 15-124

740   ICD-10-CM 2023

☑️4ᵗʰ **K66 Other disorders of peritoneum**
> EXCLUDES 2   *ascites (R18.-)*
> *peritoneal effusion (chronic) (R18.8)*

K66.0 Peritoneal adhesions (postprocedural) (postinfection)
Adhesions (of) abdominal (wall)
Adhesions (of) diaphragm
Adhesions (of) intestine
Adhesions (of) male pelvis
Adhesions (of) omentum
Adhesions (of) stomach
Adhesive bands
Mesenteric adhesions
> EXCLUDES 1   *female pelvic adhesions [bands] (N73.6)*
> *peritoneal adhesions with intestinal obstruction (K56.5-)*

K66.1 Hemoperitoneum
> EXCLUDES 1   *traumatic hemoperitoneum (S36.8-)*
> **AHA:** 2022,1Q,22-23

K66.8 Other specified disorders of peritoneum

K66.9 Disorder of peritoneum, unspecified

K67   ***Disorders of peritoneum in infectious diseases classified elsewhere***   HCC ESR COM
Code first underlying disease, such as:
congenital syphilis (A50.0)
helminthiasis (B65.0-B83.9)
> EXCLUDES 1   *peritonitis in chlamydia (A74.81)*
> *peritonitis in diphtheria (A36.89)*
> *peritonitis in gonococcal (A54.85)*
> *peritonitis in syphilis (late) (A52.74)*
> *peritonitis in tuberculosis (A18.31)*

☑️4ᵗʰ **K68 Disorders of retroperitoneum**

☑️5ᵗʰ **K68.1 Retroperitoneal abscess**

K68.11 Postprocedural retroperitoneal abscess
> EXCLUDES 2   *infection following procedure (T81.4-)*

K68.12 Psoas muscle abscess   HCC ESR COM

K68.19 Other retroperitoneal abscess   HCC ESR COM
> **AHA:** 2019,1Q,15
> **TIP:** This code should be used for a diagnosis of internal presacral abscess. If an intra-abdominal abscess is also present, code K65.1 can also be assigned; sequencing depends on the circumstances of admission.

K68.9 Other disorders of retroperitoneum

Diseases of liver (K70-K77)

> EXCLUDES 1   *jaundice NOS (R17)*
> EXCLUDES 2   *hemochromatosis (E83.11-)*
> *Reye's syndrome (G93.7)*
> *viral hepatitis (B15-B19)*
> *Wilson's disease (E83.0)*

☑️4ᵗʰ **K70 Alcoholic liver disease**
Use additional code to identify:
alcohol abuse and dependence (F10.-)

K70.0 Alcoholic fatty liver   A

☑️5ᵗʰ **K70.1 Alcoholic hepatitis**

K70.10 Alcoholic hepatitis without ascites   COM A

K70.11 Alcoholic hepatitis with ascites   COM A

K70.2 Alcoholic fibrosis and sclerosis of liver   A

☑️5ᵗʰ **K70.3 Alcoholic cirrhosis of liver**
Alcoholic cirrhosis NOS

K70.30 Alcoholic cirrhosis of liver without ascites   HCC ESR COM A

Laennec's

K70.31 Alcoholic cirrhosis of liver with ascites   HCC ESR COM A
> **AHA:** 2018,1Q,4

☑️5ᵗʰ **K70.4 Alcoholic hepatic failure**
Acute alcoholic hepatic failure
Alcoholic hepatic failure NOS
Chronic alcoholic hepatic failure
Subacute alcoholic hepatic failure

K70.40 Alcoholic hepatic failure without coma   HCC ESR COM A

K70.41 Alcoholic hepatic failure with coma   HCC ESR COM A

K70.9 Alcoholic liver disease, unspecified   HCC ESR A

☑️4ᵗʰ **K71 Toxic liver disease**
> INCLUDES   drug-induced idiosyncratic (unpredictable) liver disease
> drug-induced toxic (predictable) liver disease
Code first poisoning due to drug or toxin, if applicable (T36-T65 with fifth or sixth character 1-4 or 6)
Use additional code for adverse effect, if applicable, to identify drug (T36-T50 with fifth or sixth character 5)
> EXCLUDES 2   *alcoholic liver disease (K70.-)*
> *Budd-Chiari syndrome (I82.0)*

K71.0 Toxic liver disease with cholestasis
Cholestasis with hepatocyte injury
"Pure" cholestasis

☑️5ᵗʰ **K71.1 Toxic liver disease with hepatic necrosis**
Hepatic failure (acute) (chronic) due to drugs

K71.10 Toxic liver disease with hepatic necrosis, without coma   COM

K71.11 Toxic liver disease with hepatic necrosis, with coma   HCC ESR COM

K71.2 Toxic liver disease with acute hepatitis

K71.3 Toxic liver disease with chronic persistent hepatitis   COM

K71.4 Toxic liver disease with chronic lobular hepatitis   COM

☑️5ᵗʰ **K71.5 Toxic liver disease with chronic active hepatitis**
Toxic liver disease with lupoid hepatitis

K71.50 Toxic liver disease with chronic active hepatitis without ascites   COM

K71.51 Toxic liver disease with chronic active hepatitis with ascites   COM
> **AHA:** 2018,1Q,4

K71.6 Toxic liver disease with hepatitis, not elsewhere classified

K71.7 Toxic liver disease with fibrosis and cirrhosis of liver   COM

K71.8 Toxic liver disease with other disorders of liver
Toxic liver disease with focal nodular hyperplasia
Toxic liver disease with hepatic granulomas
Toxic liver disease with peliosis hepatis
Toxic liver disease with veno-occlusive disease of liver

K71.9 Toxic liver disease, unspecified

☑️4ᵗʰ **K72 Hepatic failure, not elsewhere classified**
> INCLUDES   fulminant hepatitis NEC, with hepatic failure
> ~~hepatic encephalopathy NOS~~
> liver (cell) necrosis with hepatic failure
> malignant hepatitis NEC, with hepatic failure
> yellow liver atrophy or dystrophy
> EXCLUDES 1   *alcoholic hepatic failure (K70.4)*
> *hepatic failure with toxic liver disease (K71.1-)*
> *icterus of newborn (P55-P59)*
> *postprocedural hepatic failure (K91.82)*
> EXCLUDES 2   *hepatic failure complicating abortion or ectopic or molar pregnancy (O00-O07, O08.8)*
> *hepatic failure complicating pregnancy, childbirth and the puerperium (O26.6-)*
> *viral hepatitis with hepatic coma (B15-B19)*

AHA: 2017,1Q,41

☑️5ᵗʰ **K72.0 Acute and subacute hepatic failure**
Acute non-viral hepatitis NOS
AHA: 2015,2Q,17; 2014,2Q,13

K72.00 Acute and subacute hepatic failure without coma   COM
> **AHA:** 2021,1Q,13

K72.01 Acute and subacute hepatic failure with coma   HCC ESR COM

☑️5ᵗʰ **K72.1 Chronic hepatic failure**
End stage liver disease

K72.10 Chronic hepatic failure without coma   HCC ESR COM
> **AHA:** 2021,1Q,13

K72.11 Chronic hepatic failure with coma   HCC ESR COM

☑️5ᵗʰ **K72.9 Hepatic failure, unspecified**

K72.90 Hepatic failure, unspecified without coma   HCC ESR COM
> **AHA:** 2022,1Q,52; 2018,4Q,20; 2016,2Q,35

K72.91 Hepatic failure, unspecified with coma   HCC ESR COM
Hepatic coma NOS

Chapter 11. Diseases of the Digestive System

K73–K76.81

✓4ᵗʰ **K73 Chronic hepatitis, not elsewhere classified**

> *EXCLUDES 1* alcoholic hepatitis (chronic) (K70.1-)
> drug-induced hepatitis (chronic) (K71.-)
> granulomatous hepatitis (chronic) NEC (K75.3)
> reactive, nonspecific hepatitis (chronic) (K75.2)
> viral hepatitis (chronic) (B15-B19)

K73.0 Chronic persistent hepatitis, not elsewhere classified `HCC` `ESR` `COM`

K73.1 Chronic lobular hepatitis, not elsewhere classified `HCC` `ESR` `COM`

K73.2 Chronic active hepatitis, not elsewhere classified `HCC` `ESR` `COM`

K73.8 Other chronic hepatitis, not elsewhere classified `HCC` `ESR` `COM`

K73.9 Chronic hepatitis, unspecified `HCC` `ESR` `COM`

✓4ᵗʰ **K74 Fibrosis and cirrhosis of liver**

> Code also, if applicable, viral hepatitis (acute) (chronic) (B15-B19)
> *EXCLUDES 1* alcoholic cirrhosis (of liver) (K70.3)
> alcoholic fibrosis of liver (K70.2)
> cardiac sclerosis of liver (K76.1)
> cirrhosis (of liver) with toxic liver disease (K71.7)
> congenital cirrhosis (of liver) (P78.81)
> pigmentary cirrhosis (of liver) (E83.110)

✓5ᵗʰ **K74.0 Hepatic fibrosis**

> Code first underlying liver disease, such as:
> nonalcoholic steatohepatitis (NASH) (K75.81)
> **AHA:** 2020,4Q,30-31

K74.00 Hepatic fibrosis, unspecified

K74.01 Hepatic fibrosis, early fibrosis
> Hepatic fibrosis, stage F1 or stage F2

K74.02 Hepatic fibrosis, advanced fibrosis
> Hepatic fibrosis, stage F3
> *EXCLUDES 1* cirrhosis of liver (K74.6-)
> hepatic fibrosis, stage F4 (K74.6-)

K74.1 Hepatic sclerosis

K74.2 Hepatic fibrosis with hepatic sclerosis

K74.3 Primary biliary cirrhosis `HCC` `Rx` `ESR` `COM`
> Chronic nonsuppurative destructive cholangitis
> Primary biliary cholangitis
> *EXCLUDES 2* primary sclerosing cholangitis (K83.01)

K74.4 Secondary biliary cirrhosis `HCC` `ESR` `COM`

K74.5 Biliary cirrhosis, unspecified `HCC` `ESR` `COM`

✓5ᵗʰ **K74.6 Other and unspecified cirrhosis of liver**
> **AHA:** 2020,4Q,30-31

K74.60 Unspecified cirrhosis of liver `HCC` `ESR` `COM`
> Cirrhosis (of liver) NOS
> **AHA:** 2018,1Q,4

K74.69 Other cirrhosis of liver `HCC` `ESR` `COM`
> Cryptogenic cirrhosis (of liver)
> Macronodular cirrhosis (of liver)
> Micronodular cirrhosis (of liver)
> Mixed type cirrhosis (of liver)
> Portal cirrhosis (of liver)
> Postnecrotic cirrhosis (of liver)

✓4ᵗʰ **K75 Other inflammatory liver diseases**

> *EXCLUDES 2* toxic liver disease (K71.-)

K75.0 Abscess of liver `COM`
> Cholangitic hepatic abscess
> Hematogenic hepatic abscess
> Hepatic abscess NOS
> Lymphogenic hepatic abscess
> Pylephlebitic hepatic abscess
> *EXCLUDES 1* amebic liver abscess (A06.4)
> cholangitis without liver abscess (K83.09)
> pylephlebitis without liver abscess (K75.1)
> *EXCLUDES 2* acute or subacute hepatitis NOS (B17.9)
> acute or subacute non-viral hepatitis (K72.0)
> chronic hepatitis NEC (K73.8)

K75.1 Phlebitis of portal vein `COM`
> Pylephlebitis
> *EXCLUDES 1* pylephlebitic liver abscess (K75.0)
> **DEF:** Inflammation of the portal vein or branches due to diverticulitis, perforated appendicitis, or peritonitis. Symptoms include fever, chills, jaundice, sweating, and abscess in various body parts.

K75.2 Nonspecific reactive hepatitis
> *EXCLUDES 1* acute or subacute hepatitis (K72.0-)
> chronic hepatitis NEC (K73.-)
> viral hepatitis (B15-B19)

K75.3 Granulomatous hepatitis, not elsewhere classified
> *EXCLUDES 1* acute or subacute hepatitis (K72.0-)
> chronic hepatitis NEC (K73.-)
> viral hepatitis (B15-B19)

K75.4 Autoimmune hepatitis `HCC` `ESR` `COM`
> Lupoid hepatitis NEC

✓5ᵗʰ **K75.8 Other specified inflammatory liver diseases**

K75.81 Nonalcoholic steatohepatitis (NASH)
> Use additional code, if applicable, hepatic fibrosis (K74.0-)

K75.89 Other specified inflammatory liver diseases

K75.9 Inflammatory liver disease, unspecified
> Hepatitis NOS
> *EXCLUDES 1* acute or subacute hepatitis (K72.0-)
> chronic hepatitis NEC (K73.-)
> viral hepatitis (B15-B19)
> **AHA:** 2015,2Q,17

✓4ᵗʰ **K76 Other diseases of liver**

> *EXCLUDES 2* alcoholic liver disease (K70.-)
> amyloid degeneration of liver (E85.-)
> cystic disease of liver (congenital) (Q44.6)
> hepatic vein thrombosis (I82.0)
> hepatomegaly NOS (R16.0)
> pigmentary cirrhosis (of liver) (E83.110)
> portal vein thrombosis (I81)
> toxic liver disease (K71.-)

K76.0 Fatty (change of) liver, not elsewhere classified
> Nonalcoholic fatty liver disease (NAFLD)
> *EXCLUDES 1* nonalcoholic steatohepatitis (NASH) (K75.81)

K76.1 Chronic passive congestion of liver
> Cardiac cirrhosis
> Cardiac sclerosis

K76.2 Central hemorrhagic necrosis of liver `COM`
> *EXCLUDES 1* liver necrosis with hepatic failure (K72.-)

K76.3 Infarction of liver `COM`

K76.4 Peliosis hepatis
> Hepatic angiomatosis

K76.5 Hepatic veno-occlusive disease
> *EXCLUDES 1* Budd-Chiari syndrome (I82.0)

K76.6 Portal hypertension `HCC` `ESR` `COM`
> Use additional code for any associated complications, such as:
> portal hypertensive gastropathy (K31.89)
> **AHA:** 2020,1Q,15

K76.7 Hepatorenal syndrome `HCC` `ESR` `COM`
> *EXCLUDES 1* hepatorenal syndrome following labor and delivery (O90.4)
> postprocedural hepatorenal syndrome (K91.83)

✓5ᵗʰ **K76.8 Other specified diseases of liver**

K76.81 Hepatopulmonary syndrome `HCC` `ESR` `COM`
> Code first underlying liver disease, such as:
> alcoholic cirrhosis of liver (K70.3-)
> cirrhosis of liver without mention of alcohol (K74.6-)

`HCC` CMS-HCC   `Rx` Rx HCC   `ESR` ESRD HCC   `COM` Commercial HCC   N Newborn: 0   P Pediatric: 0-17   M Maternity: 9-64   A Adult: 15-124

742

ICD-10-CM 2023

●   **K76.82**   Hepatic encephalopathy
         Hepatic encephalopathy, NOS
         Hepatic encephalopathy without coma
         Hepatocerebral intoxication
         Portal-systemic encephalopathy
         Code also underlying liver disease, such as:
            acute and subacute hepatic failure without coma
               (K72.00)
            alcoholic hepatic failure without coma (K70.40)
            chronic hepatic failure without coma (K72.10)
            hepatic failure with toxic liver disease without coma
               (K71.10)
            hepatic failure without coma (K72.90)
            icterus of newborn (P55-P59)
            postprocedural hepatic failure (K91.82)
            viral hepatitis without hepatic coma (B15.9, B16.1,
               B16.9, B17.10, B19.10, B19.20, B19.9)
         EXCLUDES 1   *acute and subacute hepatic failure with*
                coma (K72.01)
             alcoholic hepatic failure with coma
                (K70.41)
             chronic hepatic failure with coma (K72.11)
             hepatic failure with coma (K72.91)

      K76.89   Other specified diseases of liver
         Cyst (simple) of liver
         Focal nodular hyperplasia of liver
         Hepatoptosis

    K76.9   Liver disease, unspecified

K77   *Liver disorders in diseases classified elsewhere*
         Code first underlying disease, such as:
            amyloidosis (E85.-)
            congenital syphilis (A50.0, A50.5)
            congenital toxoplasmosis (P37.1)
            infectious mononucleosis with liver disease ▶(B27.0-B27.9 with fifth
               character 9)◀
            schistosomiasis (B65.0-B65.9)
         EXCLUDES 1   *alcoholic hepatitis (K70.1-)*
             alcoholic liver disease (K70.-)
             cytomegaloviral hepatitis (B25.1)
             herpesviral [herpes simplex] hepatitis (B00.81)
             mumps hepatitis (B26.81)
             sarcoidosis with liver disease (D86.89)
             secondary syphilis with liver disease (A51.45)
             syphilis (late) with liver disease (A52.74)
             toxoplasmosis (acquired) hepatitis (B58.1)
             tuberculosis with liver disease (A18.83)

Disorders of gallbladder, biliary tract and pancreas (K80-K87)

☑4ᵗʰ **K80**   **Cholelithiasis**
      EXCLUDES 1   *retained cholelithiasis following cholecystectomy (K91.86)*
      AHA: 2018,4Q,20
      DEF: Presence or formation of concretions (calculi or "gallstones") in the gallbladder. The stones contain cholesterol, calcium carbonate, or calcium bilirubinate in pure forms or in various combinations.

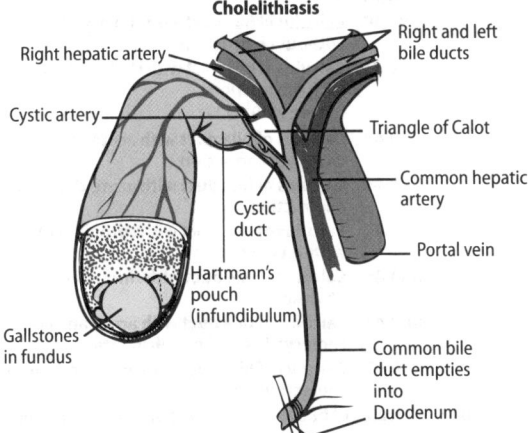

Cholelithiasis

Right hepatic artery — Right and left bile ducts — Cystic artery — Triangle of Calot — Common hepatic artery — Cystic duct — Portal vein — Hartmann's pouch (infundibulum) — Gallstones in fundus — Common bile duct empties into Duodenum

☑5ᵗʰ **K80.0**   **Calculus of** gallbladder **with acute cholecystitis**
         Any condition listed in K80.2 with acute cholecystitis
         Use additional code if applicable for associated gangrene of gallbladder (K82.A1), or perforation of gallbladder (K82.A2)
      K80.00   **Calculus of gallbladder with acute cholecystitis** without obstruction
      K80.01   **Calculus of gallbladder with acute cholecystitis** with obstruction

☑5ᵗʰ **K80.1**   **Calculus of** gallbladder **with other cholecystitis**
         Use additional code if applicable for associated gangrene of gallbladder (K82.A1), or perforation of gallbladder (K82.A2)
      K80.10   **Calculus of gallbladder with** chronic **cholecystitis** without obstruction
         Cholelithiasis with cholecystitis NOS
      K80.11   **Calculus of gallbladder with** chronic **cholecystitis** with obstruction
      K80.12   **Calculus of gallbladder with** acute and chronic **cholecystitis** without obstruction
      K80.13   **Calculus of gallbladder with** acute and chronic **cholecystitis** with obstruction
      K80.18   **Calculus of gallbladder with other cholecystitis** without obstruction
      K80.19   **Calculus of gallbladder with other cholecystitis with** obstruction

☑5ᵗʰ **K80.2**   **Calculus of** gallbladder without cholecystitis
         Cholecystolithiasis without cholecystitis
         Cholelithiasis (without cholecystitis)
         Colic (recurrent) of gallbladder (without cholecystitis)
         Gallstone (impacted) of cystic duct (without cholecystitis)
         Gallstone (impacted) of gallbladder (without cholecystitis)
      K80.20   **Calculus of gallbladder without cholecystitis** without obstruction
      K80.21   **Calculus of gallbladder without cholecystitis** with obstruction

(handwritten annotation: w/o cholecystitis)

☑5ᵗʰ **K80.3**   **Calculus of** bile duct **with cholangitis**
         Any condition listed in K80.5 with cholangitis
         DEF: Cholangitis: Inflammation of the bile ducts.
      K80.30   **Calculus of bile duct with cholangitis, unspecified,** without obstruction
      K80.31   **Calculus of bile duct with cholangitis, unspecified,** with obstruction
      K80.32   **Calculus of bile duct with** acute **cholangitis** without obstruction
      K80.33   **Calculus of bile duct with** acute **cholangitis** with obstruction
      K80.34   **Calculus of bile duct with** chronic **cholangitis** without obstruction
      K80.35   **Calculus of bile duct with** chronic **cholangitis** with obstruction

K80.36 **Calculus of bile duct with** acute and chronic cholangitis without obstruction

K80.37 **Calculus of bile duct with** acute and chronic cholangitis with obstruction

✓5ᵗʰ **K80.4** **Calculus of** bile duct with cholecystitis

Any condition listed in K80.5 with cholecystitis (with cholangitis)
►Code also fistula of bile duct◄ (K83.3)
Use additional code if applicable for associated gangrene of gallbladder (K82.A1), or perforation of gallbladder (K82.A2)
AHA: 2019,1Q,17

K80.40 **Calculus of bile duct with cholecystitis, unspecified, without obstruction**

K80.41 **Calculus of bile duct with cholecystitis, unspecified, with obstruction**
AHA: 2019,1Q,17

K80.42 **Calculus of bile duct with** acute **cholecystitis** without obstruction

K80.43 **Calculus of bile duct with** acute **cholecystitis** with obstruction

K80.44 **Calculus of bile duct with** chronic **cholecystitis** without obstruction

K80.45 **Calculus of bile duct with** chronic **cholecystitis** with obstruction

K80.46 **Calculus of bile duct with** acute and chronic cholecystitis without obstruction

K80.47 **Calculus of bile duct with** acute and chronic cholecystitis with obstruction

✓5ᵗʰ **K80.5** **Calculus of** bile duct without cholangitis or cholecystitis

Choledocholithiasis (without cholangitis or cholecystitis)
Gallstone (impacted) of bile duct NOS (without cholangitis or cholecystitis)
Gallstone (impacted) of common duct (without cholangitis or cholecystitis)
Gallstone (impacted) of hepatic duct (without cholangitis or cholecystitis)
Hepatic cholelithiasis (without cholangitis or cholecystitis)
Hepatic colic (recurrent) (without cholangitis or cholecystitis)
DEF: Cholangitis: Inflammation of the bile ducts.

K80.50 **Calculus of bile duct without cholangitis or cholecystitis** without obstruction

K80.51 **Calculus of bile duct without cholangitis or cholecystitis** with obstruction

✓5ᵗʰ **K80.6** **Calculus of** gallbladder and bile duct with cholecystitis

Use additional code if applicable for associated gangrene of gallbladder (K82.A1), or perforation of gallbladder (K82.A2)

K80.60 **Calculus of gallbladder and bile duct with cholecystitis, unspecified, without obstruction**

K80.61 **Calculus of gallbladder and bile duct with cholecystitis, unspecified, with obstruction**

K80.62 **Calculus of gallbladder and bile duct with** acute cholecystitis without obstruction

K80.63 **Calculus of gallbladder and bile duct with** acute cholecystitis with obstruction

K80.64 **Calculus of gallbladder and bile duct with** chronic cholecystitis without obstruction

K80.65 **Calculus of gallbladder and bile duct with** chronic cholecystitis with obstruction

K80.66 **Calculus of gallbladder and bile duct with** acute and chronic cholecystitis without obstruction

K80.67 **Calculus of gallbladder and bile duct with** acute and chronic cholecystitis with obstruction

✓5ᵗʰ **K80.7** **Calculus of** gallbladder and bile duct without cholecystitis

K80.70 **Calculus of gallbladder and bile duct without cholecystitis** without obstruction

K80.71 **Calculus of gallbladder and bile duct without cholecystitis** with obstruction

✓5ᵗʰ **K80.8** **Other cholelithiasis**

K80.80 **Other cholelithiasis** without obstruction

K80.81 **Other cholelithiasis** with obstruction

✓4ᵗʰ **K81** **Cholecystitis**

Use additional code if applicable for associated gangrene of gallbladder (K82.A1), or perforation of gallbladder (K82.A2)
EXCLUDES 1 *cholecystitis with cholelithiasis (K80.-)*
AHA: 2018,4Q,20

K81.0 **Acute cholecystitis**
Abscess of gallbladder
Angiocholecystitis
Emphysematous (acute) cholecystitis
Empyema of gallbladder
Gangrene of gallbladder
Gangrenous cholecystitis
Suppurative cholecystitis

K81.1 **Chronic cholecystitis**

K81.2 **Acute cholecystitis with chronic cholecystitis**

K81.9 **Cholecystitis, unspecified**

✓4ᵗʰ **K82** **Other diseases of gallbladder**
EXCLUDES 1 *nonvisualization of gallbladder (R93.2)*
postcholecystectomy syndrome (K91.5)

K82.0 **Obstruction of gallbladder**
Occlusion of cystic duct or gallbladder without cholelithiasis
Stenosis of cystic duct or gallbladder without cholelithiasis
Stricture of cystic duct or gallbladder without cholelithiasis
EXCLUDES 1 *obstruction of gallbladder with cholelithiasis (K80.-)*

K82.1 **Hydrops of gallbladder**
Mucocele of gallbladder

K82.2 **Perforation of gallbladder**
Rupture of cystic duct or gallbladder
EXCLUDES 1 *perforation of gallbladder in cholecystitis (K82.A2)*

K82.3 **Fistula of gallbladder**
Cholecystocolic fistula
Cholecystoduodenal fistula

K82.4 **Cholesterolosis of gallbladder**
Strawberry gallbladder
EXCLUDES 1 *cholesterolosis of gallbladder with cholecystitis (K81.-)*
cholesterolosis of gallbladder with cholelithiasis (K80.-)

K82.8 **Other specified diseases of gallbladder**
Adhesions of cystic duct or gallbladder
Atrophy of cystic duct or gallbladder
Cyst of cystic duct or gallbladder
Dyskinesia of cystic duct or gallbladder
Hypertrophy of cystic duct or gallbladder
Nonfunctioning of cystic duct or gallbladder
Ulcer of cystic duct or gallbladder

K82.9 **Disease of gallbladder, unspecified**

✓5ᵗʰ **K82.A** **Disorders of gallbladder in diseases classified elsewhere**
Code first the type of cholecystitis (K81.-), or cholelithiasis with cholecystitis (K80.00-K80.19, K80.40-K80.47, K80.60-K80.67)
AHA: 2018,4Q,19-20

K82.A1 *Gangrene of gallbladder in cholecystitis*

K82.A2 *Perforation of gallbladder in cholecystitis*

✓4ᵗʰ **K83** **Other diseases of biliary tract**
EXCLUDES 1 *postcholecystectomy syndrome (K91.5)*
EXCLUDES 2 *conditions involving the gallbladder (K81-K82)*
conditions involving the cystic duct (K81-K82)

✓5ᵗʰ **K83.0** **Cholangitis**
EXCLUDES 1 *cholangitic liver abscess (K75.0)*
cholangitis with choledocholithiasis (K80.3-, K80.4-)
EXCLUDES 2 *chronic nonsuppurative destructive cholangitis (K74.3)*
primary biliary cholangitis (K74.3)
primary biliary cirrhosis (K74.3)
AHA: 2018,4Q,20

K83.01 **Primary sclerosing cholangitis**

K83.Ø9   **Other cholangitis**
- Ascending cholangitis
- Cholangitis NOS
- Primary cholangitis
- Recurrent cholangitis
- Sclerosing cholangitis
- Secondary cholangitis
- Stenosing cholangitis
- Suppurative cholangitis

K83.1   **Obstruction of bile duct**
- Occlusion of bile duct without cholelithiasis
- Stenosis of bile duct without cholelithiasis
- Stricture of bile duct without cholelithiasis
  - *EXCLUDES 1*   *congenital obstruction of bile duct (Q44.3)*
  - *obstruction of bile duct with cholelithiasis (K8Ø.-)*
- **AHA:** 2016,1Q,18

K83.2   **Perforation of bile duct**
- Rupture of bile duct

K83.3   **Fistula of bile duct**
- Choledochoduodenal fistula
- **AHA:** 2019,1Q,17

K83.4   **Spasm of sphincter of Oddi**

K83.5   **Biliary cyst**

K83.8   **Other specified diseases of biliary tract**
- Adhesions of biliary tract
- Atrophy of biliary tract
- Hypertrophy of biliary tract
- Ulcer of biliary tract

K83.9   **Disease of biliary tract, unspecified**

K85   **Acute pancreatitis**
- *INCLUDES*   acute (recurrent) pancreatitis
  - subacute pancreatitis
- **AHA:** 2016,4Q,34

  K85.Ø   **Idiopathic acute pancreatitis**
- **K85.ØØ**   **Idiopathic acute pancreatitis** without necrosis or infection   COM
- **K85.Ø1**   **Idiopathic acute pancreatitis** with uninfected necrosis   COM
- **K85.Ø2**   **Idiopathic acute pancreatitis** with infected necrosis   COM

  K85.1   **Biliary acute pancreatitis**
- Gallstone pancreatitis
- **K85.1Ø**   **Biliary acute pancreatitis** without necrosis or infection   COM
- **K85.11**   **Biliary acute pancreatitis** with uninfected necrosis   COM
- **K85.12**   **Biliary acute pancreatitis** with infected necrosis   COM

  K85.2   **Alcohol induced acute pancreatitis**
- *EXCLUDES 2*   *alcohol induced chronic pancreatitis (K86.Ø)*
- **K85.2Ø**   **Alcohol induced acute pancreatitis** without necrosis or infection   COM
  - **AHA:** 2020,1Q,9
- **K85.21**   **Alcohol induced acute pancreatitis** with uninfected necrosis   COM
- **K85.22**   **Alcohol induced acute pancreatitis** with infected necrosis   COM

  K85.3   **Drug induced acute pancreatitis**
- Use additional code for adverse effect, if applicable, to identify drug (T36-T5Ø with fifth or sixth character 5)
- Use additional code to identify drug abuse and dependence (F11.- F17.-)
- **K85.3Ø**   **Drug induced acute pancreatitis** without necrosis or infection   COM
- **K85.31**   **Drug induced acute pancreatitis** with uninfected necrosis   COM
- **K85.32**   **Drug induced acute pancreatitis** with infected necrosis   COM

  K85.8   **Other acute pancreatitis**
- **K85.8Ø**   **Other acute pancreatitis** without necrosis or infection   COM
- **K85.81**   **Other acute pancreatitis** with uninfected necrosis   COM
- **K85.82**   **Other acute pancreatitis** with infected necrosis   COM

  K85.9   **Acute pancreatitis, unspecified**
- Pancreatitis NOS
- **K85.9Ø**   **Acute pancreatitis** without necrosis or infection, unspecified   COM
- **K85.91**   **Acute pancreatitis** with uninfected necrosis, unspecified   COM
- **K85.92**   **Acute pancreatitis** with infected necrosis, unspecified   COM

K86   **Other diseases of pancreas**
- *EXCLUDES 2*   *fibrocystic disease of pancreas (E84.-)*
  - *islet cell tumor (of pancreas) (D13.7)*
  - *pancreatic steatorrhea (K9Ø.3)*

  K86.Ø   **Alcohol-induced chronic pancreatitis**   HCC Rx ESR COM
- Use additional code to identify:
  - alcohol abuse and dependence (F1Ø.-)
- Code also exocrine pancreatic insufficiency (K86.81)
- *EXCLUDES 2*   *alcohol induced acute pancreatitis (K85.2-)*

  K86.1   **Other chronic pancreatitis**   HCC Rx ESR COM
- Chronic pancreatitis NOS
- Infectious chronic pancreatitis
- Recurrent chronic pancreatitis
- Relapsing chronic pancreatitis
- Code also exocrine pancreatic insufficiency (K86.81)

  K86.2   **Cyst of pancreas**   Rx

  K86.3   **Pseudocyst of pancreas**   Rx

  K86.8   **Other specified diseases of pancreas**
- **AHA:** 2016,4Q,34-35
- **K86.81**   **Exocrine pancreatic insufficiency**   Rx
- **K86.89**   **Other specified diseases of pancreas**   Rx
  - Aseptic pancreatic necrosis, unrelated to acute pancreatitis
  - Atrophy of pancreas
  - Calculus of pancreas
  - Cirrhosis of pancreas
  - Fibrosis of pancreas
  - Pancreatic fat necrosis, unrelated to acute pancreatitis
  - Pancreatic infantilism
  - Pancreatic necrosis NOS, unrelated to acute pancreatitis

  K86.9   **Disease of pancreas, unspecified**   Rx

K87   *Disorders of gallbladder, biliary tract and pancreas in diseases classified elsewhere*   Rx
- Code first underlying disease
- *EXCLUDES 1*   *cytomegaloviral pancreatitis (B25.2)*
  - *mumps pancreatitis (B26.3)*
  - *syphilitic gallbladder (A52.74)*
  - *syphilitic pancreas (A52.74)*
  - *tuberculosis of gallbladder (A18.83)*
  - *tuberculosis of pancreas (A18.83)*

Other diseases of the digestive system (K9Ø-K95)

K9Ø   **Intestinal malabsorption**
- *EXCLUDES 1*   *intestinal malabsorption following gastrointestinal surgery (K91.2)*
- **AHA:** 2017,4Q,108

  K9Ø.Ø   **Celiac disease**   Rx
- Celiac disease with steatorrhea
- Celiac gluten-sensitive enteropathy
- Nontropical sprue
- Use additional code for associated disorders including:
  - dermatitis herpetiformis (L13.Ø)
  - gluten ataxia (G32.81)
- Code also exocrine pancreatic insufficiency (K86.81)
- **DEF:** Malabsorption syndrome due to gluten consumption. Symptoms include fetid, bulky, frothy, oily stools; a distended abdomen; gas; asthenia; electrolyte depletion; and vitamin B, D, and K deficiency.

  K9Ø.1   **Tropical sprue**   Rx
- Sprue NOS
- Tropical steatorrhea

  K9Ø.2   **Blind loop syndrome, not elsewhere classified**   Rx
- Blind loop syndrome NOS
- *EXCLUDES 1*   *congenital blind loop syndrome (Q43.8)*
  - *postsurgical blind loop syndrome (K91.2)*

  K9Ø.3   **Pancreatic steatorrhea**   Rx

✓5ᵗʰ **K90.4 Other malabsorption due to intolerance**

> *EXCLUDES 2*   celiac gluten-sensitive enteropathy (K90.0)
>
>   lactose intolerance (E73.-)

AHA: 2016,4Q,35-36

   K90.41 Non-celiac gluten sensitivity
     Gluten sensitivity NOS
     Non-celiac gluten sensitive enteropathy

   K90.49 Malabsorption due to intolerance, not elsewhere classified `Rx`
     Malabsorption due to intolerance to carbohydrate
     Malabsorption due to intolerance to fat
     Malabsorption due to intolerance to protein
     Malabsorption due to intolerance to starch

✓5ᵗʰ **K90.8 Other intestinal malabsorption**

   K90.81 Whipple's disease `Rx`

   K90.89 Other intestinal malabsorption `Rx`

K90.9 Intestinal malabsorption, unspecified `Rx`

✓4ᵗʰ **K91 Intraoperative and postprocedural complications and disorders of digestive system, not elsewhere classified**

> *EXCLUDES 2*   complications of artificial opening of digestive system (K94.-)
>
>   complications of bariatric procedures (K95.-)
>
>   gastrojejunal ulcer (K28.-)
>
>   postprocedural (radiation) retroperitoneal abscess (K68.11)
>
>   radiation colitis (K52.0)
>
>   radiation gastroenteritis (K52.0)
>
>   radiation proctitis (K62.7)

AHA: 2016,4Q,9-10

K91.0 Vomiting following gastrointestinal surgery

K91.1 Postgastric surgery syndromes
   Dumping syndrome
   Postgastrectomy syndrome
   Postvagotomy syndrome

K91.2 Postsurgical malabsorption, not elsewhere classified `Rx`
   Postsurgical blind loop syndrome

> *EXCLUDES 1*   malabsorption osteomalacia in adults (M83.2)
>
>   malabsorption osteoporosis, postsurgical (M80.8-, M81.8)

✓5ᵗʰ **K91.3 Postprocedural intestinal obstruction**

AHA: 2017,4Q,16-17; 2017,1Q,40

   K91.30 Postprocedural intestinal obstruction, unspecified as to partial versus complete
     Postprocedural intestinal obstruction NOS

   K91.31 Postprocedural partial intestinal obstruction
     Postprocedural incomplete intestinal obstruction

   K91.32 Postprocedural complete intestinal obstruction

K91.5 Postcholecystectomy syndrome

✓5ᵗʰ **K91.6 Intraoperative hemorrhage and hematoma of a digestive system organ or structure complicating a procedure**

> *EXCLUDES 1*   intraoperative hemorrhage and hematoma of a digestive system organ or structure due to accidental puncture and laceration during a procedure (K91.7-)

   K91.61 Intraoperative hemorrhage and hematoma of a digestive system organ or structure complicating a digestive system procedure
     AHA: 2020,1Q,19

   K91.62 Intraoperative hemorrhage and hematoma of a digestive system organ or structure complicating other procedure

✓5ᵗʰ **K91.7 Accidental puncture and laceration of a digestive system organ or structure during a procedure**

AHA: 2022,1Q,51

   K91.71 Accidental puncture and laceration of a digestive system organ or structure during a digestive system procedure
     AHA: 2021,2Q,11

   K91.72 Accidental puncture and laceration of a digestive system organ or structure during other procedure
     AHA: 2019,2Q,23

✓5ᵗʰ **K91.8 Other intraoperative and postprocedural complications and disorders of digestive system**

   K91.81 Other intraoperative complications of digestive system

   K91.82 Postprocedural hepatic failure

   K91.83 Postprocedural hepatorenal syndrome

✓6ᵗʰ **K91.84 Postprocedural hemorrhage of a digestive system organ or structure following a procedure**

   K91.840 Postprocedural hemorrhage of a digestive system organ or structure following a digestive system procedure
     AHA: 2016,1Q,15

   K91.841 Postprocedural hemorrhage of a digestive system organ or structure following other procedure

✓6ᵗʰ **K91.85 Complications of intestinal pouch**

   K91.850 Pouchitis `HCC` `ESR` `COM`
     Inflammation of internal ileoanal pouch
     DEF: Inflammatory complication of an existing surgically created ileoanal pouch, resulting in multiple GI complaints, including diarrhea, abdominal pain, rectal bleeding, fecal urgency, or incontinence.

   K91.858 Other complications of intestinal pouch `HCC` `ESR` `COM`
     AHA: 2019,2Q,13

K91.86 Retained cholelithiasis following cholecystectomy

✓6ᵗʰ **K91.87 Postprocedural hematoma and seroma of a digestive system organ or structure following a procedure**

   K91.870 Postprocedural hematoma of a digestive system organ or structure following a digestive system procedure
     AHA: 2022,1Q,24

   K91.871 Postprocedural hematoma of a digestive system organ or structure following other procedure

   K91.872 Postprocedural seroma of a digestive system organ or structure following a digestive system procedure

   K91.873 Postprocedural seroma of a digestive system organ or structure following other procedure

K91.89 Other postprocedural complications and disorders of digestive system
   Use additional code, if applicable, to further specify disorder

> *EXCLUDES 2*   postprocedural retroperitoneal abscess (K68.11)

AHA: 2020,2Q,22; 2017,1Q,40

✓4ᵗʰ **K92 Other diseases of digestive system**

> *EXCLUDES 1*   neonatal gastrointestinal hemorrhage (P54.0-P54.3)

K92.0 Hematemesis

K92.1 Melena

> *EXCLUDES 1*   occult blood in feces (R19.5)

K92.2 Gastrointestinal hemorrhage, unspecified
   Gastric hemorrhage NOS
   Intestinal hemorrhage NOS

> *EXCLUDES 1*   acute hemorrhagic gastritis (K29.01)
>
>   hemorrhage of anus and rectum (K62.5)
>
>   angiodysplasia of stomach with hemorrhage (K31.811)
>
>   diverticular disease with hemorrhage (K57.-)
>
>   gastritis and duodenitis with hemorrhage (K29.-)
>
>   peptic ulcer with hemorrhage (K25-K28)

AHA: 2021,1Q,11

✓5ᵗʰ **K92.8 Other specified diseases of the digestive system**

   K92.81 Gastrointestinal mucositis (ulcerative)
     Code also type of associated therapy, such as:
     antineoplastic and immunosuppressive drugs (T45.1X-)
     radiological procedure and radiotherapy (Y84.2)

> *EXCLUDES 2*   mucositis (ulcerative) of vagina and vulva (N76.81)
>
>   nasal mucositis (ulcerative) (J34.81)
>
>   oral mucositis (ulcerative) (K12.3-)

   K92.89 Other specified diseases of the digestive system

K92.9 Disease of digestive system, unspecified

✓4ᵗʰ **K94 Complications of artificial openings of the digestive system**

✓5ᵗʰ **K94.0 Colostomy complications**

   K94.00 Colostomy complication, unspecified `HCC` `ESR` `COM`

   K94.01 Colostomy hemorrhage `HCC` `ESR` `COM`

`HCC` CMS-HCC   `Rx` Rx HCC   `ESR` ESRD HCC   `COM` Commercial HCC   `N` Newborn: 0   `P` Pediatric: 0-17   `M` Maternity: 9-64   `A` Adult: 15-124

    K94.02   **Colostomy** infection   `HCC` `ESR` `COM`
           Use additional code to specify type of infection, such as:
             cellulitis of abdominal wall (L03.311)
             sepsis (A40.-, A41.-)

    K94.03   **Colostomy** malfunction   `HCC` `ESR` `COM`
           Mechanical complication of colostomy

    K94.09   **Other complications of colostomy**   `HCC` `ESR` `COM`

☑5ᵗʰ   **K94.1**   **Enterostomy** complications

    K94.10   **Enterostomy complication, unspecified**   `HCC` `ESR` `COM`

    K94.11   **Enterostomy** hemorrhage   `HCC` `ESR` `COM`

    K94.12   **Enterostomy** infection   `HCC` `ESR` `COM`
           Use additional code to specify type of infection, such as:
             cellulitis of abdominal wall (L03.311)
             sepsis (A40.-, A41.-)

    K94.13   **Enterostomy** malfunction   `HCC` `ESR` `COM`
           Mechanical complication of enterostomy

    K94.19   **Other complications of enterostomy**   `HCC` `ESR` `COM`

☑5ᵗʰ   **K94.2**   **Gastrostomy** complications

    K94.20   **Gastrostomy complication, unspecified**   `HCC` `ESR` `COM`

    K94.21   **Gastrostomy** hemorrhage   `HCC` `ESR` `COM`

    K94.22   **Gastrostomy** infection   `HCC` `ESR` `COM`
           Use additional code to specify type of infection, such as:
             cellulitis of abdominal wall (L03.311)
             sepsis (A40.-, A41.-)

    K94.23   **Gastrostomy** malfunction   `HCC` `ESR` `COM`
           Mechanical complication of gastrostomy
           AHA: 2019,1Q,26

[handwritten note: Clogged tube]

    K94.29   **Other complications of gastrostomy**   `HCC` `ESR` `COM`

☑5ᵗʰ   **K94.3**   **Esophagostomy** complications

    K94.30   **Esophagostomy complications, unspecified**   `HCC` `ESR` `COM`

    K94.31   **Esophagostomy** hemorrhage   `HCC` `ESR` `COM`

    K94.32   **Esophagostomy** infection   `HCC` `ESR` `COM`
           Use additional code to identify the infection

    K94.33   **Esophagostomy** malfunction   `HCC` `ESR` `COM`
           Mechanical complication of esophagostomy

    K94.39   **Other complications of esophagostomy**   `HCC` `ESR` `COM`

☑4ᵗʰ   **K95**   **Complications of bariatric procedures**

   ☑5ᵗʰ   **K95.0**   **Complications of** gastric band procedure

    K95.01   **Infection due to gastric band procedure**
           Use additional code to specify type of infection or organism, such as:
             bacterial and viral infectious agents (B95.-, B96.-)
             cellulitis of abdominal wall (L03.311)
             sepsis (A40.-, A41.-)

    K95.09   **Other complications of gastric band procedure**
           Use additional code, if applicable, to further specify complication

   ☑5ᵗʰ   **K95.8**   **Complications of other bariatric procedure**
         `EXCLUDES 1`   complications of gastric band surgery (K95.0-)

    K95.81   **Infection due to other bariatric procedure**
           Use additional code to specify type of infection or organism, such as:
             bacterial and viral infectious agents (B95.-, B96.-)
             cellulitis of abdominal wall (L03.311)
             sepsis (A40.-, A41.-)

    K95.89   **Other complications of other bariatric procedure**
           Use additional code, if applicable, to further specify complication

---

☑ Additional Character Required   ☑x7ᵗʰ Placeholder Alert   Manifestation   Unspecified Dx   Q QPP   UPD Unacceptable PDx

Chapter 12. Diseases of the Skin and Subcutaneous Tissue (LØØ–L99)

Chapter-specific Guidelines with Coding Examples

The chapter-specific guidelines from the ICD-10-CM Official Guidelines for Coding and Reporting have been provided below. Along with these guidelines are coding examples, contained in the shaded boxes, that have been developed to help illustrate the coding and/or sequencing guidance found in these guidelines.

a. Pressure ulcer stage codes

1) Pressure ulcer stages

Codes in category L89, Pressure ulcer, identify the site and stage of the pressure ulcer.

The ICD-1Ø-CM classifies pressure ulcer stages based on severity, which is designated by stages 1-4, deep tissue pressure injury, unspecified stage, and unstageable.

Assign as many codes from category L89 as needed to identify all the pressure ulcers the patient has, if applicable.

See Section I.B.14. for pressure ulcer stage documentation by clinicians other than patient's provider.

> Stage 3 pressure ulcer left ankle, 6 x 7 cm that invades the fascia; stage 2 pressure ulcer of left hip
>
> **L89.523**   **Pressure ulcer of left ankle, stage 3**
>
> **L89.222**   **Pressure ulcer of left hip, stage 2**
>
> *Explanation:* Patient has a left ankle pressure ulcer documented as stage 3 and a left hip pressure ulcer documented as stage 2. Combination codes from category L89 Pressure ulcer, identify the site of the pressure ulcer as well as the stage. Assign as many codes from category L89 as needed to identify all the pressure ulcers the patient has.

2) Unstageable pressure ulcers

Assignment of the code for unstageable pressure ulcer (L89.--Ø) should be based on the clinical documentation. These codes are used for pressure ulcers whose stage cannot be clinically determined (e.g., the ulcer is covered by eschar or has been treated with a skin or muscle graft). This code should not be confused with the codes for unspecified stage (L89.--9). When there is no documentation regarding the stage of the pressure ulcer, assign the appropriate code for unspecified stage (L89.--9).

> Pressure ulcer of the right lower back documented as unstageable due to the presence of thick eschar covering the ulcer
>
> **L89.13Ø**   **Pressure ulcer of right lower back, unstageable**
>
> *Explanation:* Codes for unstageable pressure ulcers are assigned when the stage cannot be clinically determined (e.g., the ulcer is covered by eschar or has been treated with a skin or muscle graft).

If during an encounter, the stage of an unstageable pressure ulcer is revealed after debridement, assign only the code for the stage revealed following debridement.

3) Documented pressure ulcer stage

Assignment of the pressure ulcer stage code should be guided by clinical documentation of the stage or documentation of the terms found in the Alphabetic Index. For clinical terms describing the stage that are not found in the Alphabetic Index, and there is no documentation of the stage, the provider should be queried.

> Left heel pressure ulcer with partial thickness skin loss involving the dermis
>
> **L89.622**   **Pressure ulcer of left heel, stage 2**
>
> *Explanation:* Code assignment for the pressure ulcer stage should be guided by either the clinical documentation of the stage or the documentation of terms found in the Alphabetic Index. The clinical documentation describing the left heel pressure ulcer "partial thickness skin loss involving the dermis" matches the ICD-10-CM index parenthetical description for stage 2 "(abrasion, blister, partial thickness skin loss involving epidermis and/or dermis)."

4) Patients admitted with pressure ulcers documented as healed

No code is assigned if the documentation states that the pressure ulcer is completely healed at the time of admission.

> Patient receiving follow-up examination of a completely healed pressure ulcer of the foot
>
> **ZØ9**   **Encounter for follow-up examination after completed treatment for conditions other than malignant neoplasm**
>
> **Z87.2**   **Personal history of diseases of the skin and subcutaneous tissue**
>
> *Explanation:* Assign only codes for the reason for the encounter and the personal history of the pressure ulcer. Personal history code Z87.2 includes conditions classifiable to LØØ–L99 such as pressure ulcer. No code is assigned for a pressure ulcer documented as completely healed.

5) Pressure ulcers documented as healing

Pressure ulcers described as healing should be assigned the appropriate pressure ulcer stage code based on the documentation in the medical record. If the documentation does not provide information about the stage of the healing pressure ulcer, assign the appropriate code for unspecified stage.

If the documentation is unclear as to whether the patient has a current (new) pressure ulcer or if the patient is being treated for a healing pressure ulcer, query the provider.

For ulcers that were present on admission but healed at the time of discharge, assign the code for the site and stage of the pressure ulcer at the time of admission.

6) Patient admitted with pressure ulcer evolving into another stage during the admission

If a patient is admitted to an inpatient hospital with a pressure ulcer at one stage and it progresses to a higher stage, two separate codes should be assigned: one code for the site and stage of the ulcer on admission and a second code for the same ulcer site and the highest stage reported during the stay.

7) Pressure-induced deep tissue damage

For pressure-induced deep tissue damage or deep tissue pressure injury, assign only the appropriate code for pressure-induced deep tissue damage (L89.--6).

b. Non-pressure chronic ulcers

1) Patients admitted with non-pressure ulcers documented as healed

No code is assigned if the documentation states that the non-pressure ulcer is completely healed at the time of admission.

2) Non-pressure ulcers documented as healing

Non-pressure ulcers described as healing should be assigned the appropriate non-pressure ulcer code based on the documentation in the medical record. If the documentation does not provide information about the severity of the healing non-pressure ulcer, assign the appropriate code for unspecified severity.

If the documentation is unclear as to whether the patient has a current (new) non-pressure ulcer or if the patient is being treated for a healing non-pressure ulcer, query the provider.

For ulcers that were present on admission but healed at the time of discharge, assign the code for the site and severity of the non-pressure ulcer at the time of admission.

3) Patient admitted with non-pressure ulcer that progresses to another severity level during the admission

If a patient is admitted to an inpatient hospital with a non-pressure ulcer at one severity level and it progresses to a higher severity level, two separate codes should be assigned: one code for the site and severity level of the ulcer on admission and a second code for the same ulcer site and the highest severity level reported during the stay.

See Section I.B.14. for pressure ulcer stage documentation by clinicians other than patient's provider.

Chapter 12. Diseases of the Skin and Subcutaneous Tissue (L00-L99)

EXCLUDES 2
certain conditions originating in the perinatal period (P04-P96)
certain infectious and parasitic diseases (A00-B99)
complications of pregnancy, childbirth and the puerperium (O00-O9A)
congenital malformations, deformations, and chromosomal abnormalities (Q00-Q99)
endocrine, nutritional and metabolic diseases (E00-E88)
lipomelanotic reticulosis (I89.8)
neoplasms (C00-D49)
symptoms, signs and abnormal clinical and laboratory findings, not elsewhere classified (R00-R94)
systemic connective tissue disorders (M30-M36)
viral warts (B07.-)

AHA: 2022,2Q,7

This chapter contains the following blocks:

L00-L08	Infections of the skin and subcutaneous tissue
L10-L14	Bullous disorders
L20-L30	Dermatitis and eczema
L40-L45	Papulosquamous disorders
L49-L54	Urticaria and erythema
L55-L59	Radiation-related disorders of the skin and subcutaneous tissue
L60-L75	Disorders of skin appendages
L76	Intraoperative and postprocedural complications of skin and subcutaneous tissue
L80-L99	Other disorders of the skin and subcutaneous tissue

Infections of the skin and subcutaneous tissue (L00-L8)

Use additional code (B95-B97) to identify infectious agent

EXCLUDES 2
hordeolum (H00.0)
infective dermatitis (L30.3)
local infections of skin classified in Chapter 1
lupus panniculitis (L93.2)
panniculitis NOS (M79.3)
panniculitis of neck and back (M54.0-)
perlèche NOS (K13.0)
perlèche due to candidiasis (B37.0)
perlèche due to riboflavin deficiency (E53.0)
pyogenic granuloma (L98.0)
relapsing panniculitis [Weber-Christian] (M35.6)
viral warts (B07.-)
zoster (B02.-)

L00 Staphylococcal scalded skin syndrome   **COM**
Ritter's disease
Use additional code to identify percentage of skin exfoliation (L49.-)

EXCLUDES 1
bullous impetigo (L01.03)
pemphigus neonatorum (L01.03)
toxic epidermal necrolysis [Lyell] (L51.2)

DEF: Infectious skin disease of children younger than 5 years marked by eruptions ranging from a few localized blisters to widespread, easily ruptured, fine vesicles and bullae affecting almost the entire body. It results in exfoliation of large planes of skin and leaves raw areas.

✓4ᵗʰ L01 Impetigo
EXCLUDES 1 *impetigo herpetiformis (L40.1)*
DEF: Acute, superficial, highly contagious skin infection commonly occurring in children. Skin lesions usually appear on the face and consist of vesicles and bullae that burst and form yellow crusts.

✓5ᵗʰ L01.0 Impetigo
Impetigo contagiosa
Impetigo vulgaris

L01.00 Impetigo, unspecified
Impetigo NOS

L01.01 Non-bullous impetigo

L01.02 Bockhart's impetigo
Impetigo follicularis
Perifolliculitis NOS
Superficial pustular perifolliculitis
DEF: Superficial inflammation of the hair follicles commonly caused by *Staphylococcus aureus* that manifests as rounded, sphere-shaped, pustular eruptions in the areas of the scalp, beard, underarms, extremities, and buttocks.

L01.03 Bullous impetigo
Impetigo neonatorum
Pemphigus neonatorum

L01.09 Other impetigo
Ulcerative impetigo

L01.1 Impetiginization of other dermatoses

✓4ᵗʰ L02 Cutaneous abscess, furuncle and carbuncle
Use additional code to identify organism (B95-B96)

EXCLUDES 2
abscess of anus and rectal regions (K61.-)
abscess of female genital organs (external) (N76.4)
abscess of male genital organs (external) (N48.2, N49.-)

DEF: Carbuncle: Infection of the skin that arises from a collection of interconnected infected boils or furuncles, usually from hair follicles infected by *Staphylococcus*. This condition can produce pus and form drainage cavities.
DEF: Furuncle: Inflamed, painful abscess, cyst, or nodule on the skin caused by bacteria, often *Staphylococcus*, entering along the hair follicle.

✓5ᵗʰ L02.0 Cutaneous abscess, furuncle and carbuncle of face
EXCLUDES 2
abscess of ear, external (H60.0)
abscess of eyelid (H00.0)
abscess of head [any part, except face] (L02.8)
abscess of lacrimal gland (H04.0)
abscess of lacrimal passages (H04.3)
abscess of mouth (K12.2)
abscess of nose (J34.0)
abscess of orbit (H05.0)
submandibular abscess (K12.2)

L02.01 Cutaneous abscess of face
L02.02 Furuncle of face
Boil of face
Folliculitis of face
L02.03 Carbuncle of face

✓5ᵗʰ L02.1 Cutaneous abscess, furuncle and carbuncle of neck
L02.11 Cutaneous abscess of neck
L02.12 Furuncle of neck
Boil of neck
Folliculitis of neck
L02.13 Carbuncle of neck

✓5ᵗʰ L02.2 Cutaneous abscess, furuncle and carbuncle of trunk
EXCLUDES 1
non-newborn omphalitis (L08.82)
omphalitis of newborn (P38.-)
EXCLUDES 2
abscess of breast (N61.1)
abscess of buttocks (L02.3)
abscess of female external genital organs (N76.4)
abscess of hip (L02.4)
abscess of male external genital organs (N48.2, N49.-)

✓6ᵗʰ L02.21 Cutaneous abscess of trunk
L02.211 Cutaneous abscess of abdominal wall
L02.212 Cutaneous abscess of back [any part, except buttock]
L02.213 Cutaneous abscess of chest wall
L02.214 Cutaneous abscess of groin
L02.215 Cutaneous abscess of perineum
L02.216 Cutaneous abscess of umbilicus
L02.219 Cutaneous abscess of trunk, unspecified

✓6ᵗʰ L02.22 Furuncle of trunk
Boil of trunk
Folliculitis of trunk
L02.221 Furuncle of abdominal wall
L02.222 Furuncle of back [any part, except buttock]
L02.223 Furuncle of chest wall
L02.224 Furuncle of groin
L02.225 Furuncle of perineum
L02.226 Furuncle of umbilicus
L02.229 Furuncle of trunk, unspecified

✓6ᵗʰ L02.23 Carbuncle of trunk
L02.231 Carbuncle of abdominal wall
L02.232 Carbuncle of back [any part, except buttock]
L02.233 Carbuncle of chest wall
L02.234 Carbuncle of groin
L02.235 Carbuncle of perineum
L02.236 Carbuncle of umbilicus
L02.239 Carbuncle of trunk, unspecified

✓5ᵗʰ L02.3 Cutaneous abscess, furuncle and carbuncle of buttock
EXCLUDES 1 *pilonidal cyst with abscess (L05.01)*
L02.31 Cutaneous abscess of buttock
Cutaneous abscess of gluteal region

HCC CMS-HCC   **Rx** Rx HCC   **ESR** ESRD HCC   **COM** Commercial HCC   **N** Newborn: 0   **P** Pediatric: 0-17   **M** Maternity: 9-64   **A** Adult: 15-124

750   ICD-10-CM 2023

LØ2.32   Furuncle **of buttock**
    Boil of buttock
    Folliculitis of buttock
    Furuncle of gluteal region

LØ2.33   Carbuncle **of buttock**
    Carbuncle of gluteal region

✓5ᵗʰ **LØ2.4**   **Cutaneous abscess, furuncle and carbuncle of** limb
    EXCLUDES 2   *cutaneous abscess, furuncle and carbuncle of groin (LØ2.214, LØ2.224, LØ2.234)*
         cutaneous abscess, furuncle and carbuncle of hand (LØ2.5-)
         cutaneous abscess, furuncle and carbuncle of foot (LØ2.6-)

   ✓6ᵗʰ **LØ2.41**   **Cutaneous abscess of** limb
      LØ2.411   **Cutaneous abscess of** right axilla
      LØ2.412   **Cutaneous abscess of** left axilla
      LØ2.413   **Cutaneous abscess of** right upper **limb**
      LØ2.414   **Cutaneous abscess of** left upper **limb**
      LØ2.415   **Cutaneous abscess of** right lower **limb**
      LØ2.416   **Cutaneous abscess of** left lower **limb**
      LØ2.419   **Cutaneous abscess of limb, unspecified**

   ✓6ᵗʰ **LØ2.42**   **Furuncle of** limb
      Boil of limb
      Folliculitis of limb
      LØ2.421   **Furuncle of** right axilla
      LØ2.422   **Furuncle of** left axilla
      LØ2.423   **Furuncle of** right upper **limb**
      LØ2.424   **Furuncle of** left upper **limb**
      LØ2.425   **Furuncle of** right lower **limb**
      LØ2.426   **Furuncle of** left lower **limb**
      LØ2.429   **Furuncle of limb, unspecified**

   ✓6ᵗʰ **LØ2.43**   **Carbuncle of** limb
      LØ2.431   **Carbuncle of** right axilla
      LØ2.432   **Carbuncle of** left axilla
      LØ2.433   **Carbuncle of** right upper **limb**
      LØ2.434   **Carbuncle of** left upper **limb**
      LØ2.435   **Carbuncle of** right lower **limb**
      LØ2.436   **Carbuncle of** left lower **limb**
      LØ2.439   **Carbuncle of limb, unspecified**

✓5ᵗʰ **LØ2.5**   **Cutaneous abscess, furuncle and carbuncle of** hand
   ✓6ᵗʰ **LØ2.51**   **Cutaneous abscess of** hand
      LØ2.511   **Cutaneous abscess of** right **hand**
      LØ2.512   **Cutaneous abscess of** left **hand**
      LØ2.519   **Cutaneous abscess of unspecified hand**

   ✓6ᵗʰ **LØ2.52**   **Furuncle hand**
      Boil of hand
      Folliculitis of hand
      LØ2.521   **Furuncle** right **hand**
      LØ2.522   **Furuncle** left **hand**
      LØ2.529   **Furuncle unspecified hand**

   ✓6ᵗʰ **LØ2.53**   **Carbuncle of** hand
      LØ2.531   **Carbuncle of** right **hand**
      LØ2.532   **Carbuncle of** left **hand**
      LØ2.539   **Carbuncle of unspecified hand**

✓5ᵗʰ **LØ2.6**   **Cutaneous abscess, furuncle and carbuncle of** foot
   ✓6ᵗʰ **LØ2.61**   **Cutaneous abscess of** foot
      LØ2.611   **Cutaneous abscess of** right **foot**
      LØ2.612   **Cutaneous abscess of** left **foot**
      LØ2.619   **Cutaneous abscess of unspecified foot**

   ✓6ᵗʰ **LØ2.62**   **Furuncle of** foot
      Boil of foot
      Folliculitis of foot
      LØ2.621   **Furuncle of** right **foot**
      LØ2.622   **Furuncle of** left **foot**
      LØ2.629   **Furuncle of unspecified foot**

   ✓6ᵗʰ **LØ2.63**   **Carbuncle of** foot
      LØ2.631   **Carbuncle of** right **foot**
      LØ2.632   **Carbuncle of** left **foot**
      LØ2.639   **Carbuncle of unspecified foot**

✓5ᵗʰ **LØ2.8**   **Cutaneous abscess, furuncle and carbuncle of other sites**
   ✓6ᵗʰ **LØ2.81**   **Cutaneous abscess of other sites**
      LØ2.811   **Cutaneous abscess of** head [any part, except face]
      LØ2.818   **Cutaneous abscess of other sites**

✓6ᵗʰ **LØ2.82**   **Furuncle of other sites**
    Boil of other sites
    Folliculitis of other sites
    LØ2.821   **Furuncle of** head **[any part, except face]**
    LØ2.828   **Furuncle of other sites**

✓6ᵗʰ **LØ2.83**   **Carbuncle of other sites**
    LØ2.831   **Carbuncle of** head **[any part, except face]**
    LØ2.838   **Carbuncle of other sites**

✓5ᵗʰ **LØ2.9**   **Cutaneous abscess, furuncle and carbuncle, unspecified**
   LØ2.91   **Cutaneous abscess, unspecified**
   LØ2.92   **Furuncle, unspecified**
      Boil NOS
      Furunculosis NOS
   LØ2.93   **Carbuncle, unspecified**

✓4ᵗʰ **LØ3**   **Cellulitis and acute lymphangitis**
   EXCLUDES 2   *cellulitis of anal and rectal region (K61.-)*
         cellulitis of external auditory canal (H6Ø.1)
         cellulitis of eyelid (HØØ.Ø)
         cellulitis of female external genital organs (N76.4)
         cellulitis of lacrimal apparatus (HØ4.3)
         cellulitis of male external genital organs (N48.2, N49.-)
         cellulitis of mouth (K12.2)
         cellulitis of nose (J34.Ø)
         eosinophilic cellulitis [Wells] (L98.3)
         febrile neutrophilic dermatosis [Sweet] (L98.2)
         lymphangitis (chronic) (subacute) (I89.1)

   AHA: 2017,4Q,100
   DEF: Cellulitis: Infection of the skin and subcutaneous tissues, most often caused by *Staphylococcus* or *Streptococcus* bacteria secondary to a cutaneous lesion. Progression of the inflammation may lead to abscess and tissue death, or even systemic infection-like bacteremia.
   DEF: Lymphangitis: Inflammation of the lymph channels most often caused by *Streptococcus*.

✓5ᵗʰ **LØ3.Ø**   **Cellulitis and acute lymphangitis of** finger and toe
    Infection of nail
    Onychia
    Paronychia
    Perionychia

   ✓6ᵗʰ **LØ3.Ø1**   **Cellulitis of** finger
      Felon
      Whitlow
      EXCLUDES 1   *herpetic whitlow (BØØ.89)*
      DEF: Felon: Superficial bacterial skin infection at the tip of the finger.
      LØ3.Ø11   **Cellulitis of** right **finger**
      LØ3.Ø12   **Cellulitis of** left **finger**
      LØ3.Ø19   **Cellulitis of unspecified finger**

   ✓6ᵗʰ **LØ3.Ø2**   **Acute lymphangitis of** finger
      Hangnail with lymphangitis of finger
      LØ3.Ø21   **Acute lymphangitis of** right **finger**
      LØ3.Ø22   **Acute lymphangitis of** left **finger**
      LØ3.Ø29   **Acute lymphangitis of unspecified finger**

   ✓6ᵗʰ **LØ3.Ø3**   **Cellulitis of** toe
      LØ3.Ø31   **Cellulitis of** right **toe**
      LØ3.Ø32   **Cellulitis of** left **toe**
      LØ3.Ø39   **Cellulitis of unspecified toe**

   ✓6ᵗʰ **LØ3.Ø4**   **Acute lymphangitis of** toe
      Hangnail with lymphangitis of toe
      LØ3.Ø41   **Acute lymphangitis of** right **toe**
      LØ3.Ø42   **Acute lymphangitis of** left **toe**
      LØ3.Ø49   **Acute lymphangitis of unspecified toe**

✓5ᵗʰ **LØ3.1**   **Cellulitis and acute lymphangitis of other parts of limb**
   ✓6ᵗʰ **LØ3.11**   **Cellulitis of other parts of limb**
      EXCLUDES 2   *cellulitis of fingers (LØ3.Ø1-)*
         cellulitis of toes (LØ3.Ø3-)
         groin (LØ3.314)
      LØ3.111   **Cellulitis of** right axilla
      LØ3.112   **Cellulitis of** left axilla
      LØ3.113   **Cellulitis of** right upper limb
      LØ3.114   **Cellulitis of** left upper limb
      LØ3.115   **Cellulitis of** right lower limb
      LØ3.116   **Cellulitis of** left lower limb
      LØ3.119   **Cellulitis of unspecified part of limb**

Chapter 12. Diseases of the Skin and Subcutaneous Tissue

L03.12–L05.92

√6ᵗʰ **L03.12**   **Acute lymphangitis** of other parts of limb
> EXCLUDES 2   *acute lymphangitis of fingers (L03.2-)*
> *acute lymphangitis of groin (L03.324)*
> *acute lymphangitis of toes (L03.04-)*

L03.121   **Acute lymphangitis** of **right** axilla
L03.122   **Acute lymphangitis** of **left** axilla
L03.123   **Acute lymphangitis** of **right upper limb**
L03.124   **Acute lymphangitis** of **left upper limb**
L03.125   **Acute lymphangitis** of **right lower limb**
L03.126   **Acute lymphangitis** of **left lower limb**
L03.129   **Acute lymphangitis** of **unspecified part of limb**

√5ᵗʰ **L03.2**   **Cellulitis and acute lymphangitis** of **face and neck**

√6ᵗʰ **L03.21**   **Cellulitis and acute lymphangitis** of **face**

L03.211   **Cellulitis** of **face**
> EXCLUDES 2   *abscess of orbit (H05.01-)*
> *cellulitis of ear (H60.1-)*
> *cellulitis of eyelid (H00.0-)*
> *cellulitis of head (L03.81)*
> *cellulitis of lacrimal apparatus (H04.3)*
> *cellulitis of lip (K13.0)*
> *cellulitis of mouth (K12.2)*
> *cellulitis of nose (internal) (J34.0)*
> *cellulitis of orbit (H05.01-)*
> *cellulitis of scalp (L03.81)*

AHA: 2013,4Q,123

L03.212   **Acute lymphangitis** of **face**
L03.213   **Periorbital cellulitis**
Preseptal cellulitis
AHA: 2016,4Q,36

√6ᵗʰ **L03.22**   **Cellulitis and acute lymphangitis** of **neck**

L03.221   **Cellulitis** of **neck**
L03.222   **Acute lymphangitis** of **neck**

√5ᵗʰ **L03.3**   **Cellulitis and acute lymphangitis** of **trunk**

√6ᵗʰ **L03.31**   **Cellulitis** of **trunk**
> EXCLUDES 2   *cellulitis of anal and rectal regions (K61.-)*
> *cellulitis of breast NOS (N61.0)*
> *cellulitis of female external genital organs (N76.4)*
> *cellulitis of male external genital organs (N48.2, N49.-)*
> *omphalitis of newborn (P38.-)*
> *puerperal cellulitis of breast (O91.2)*

L03.311   **Cellulitis** of **abdominal wall**
> EXCLUDES 2   *cellulitis of umbilicus (L03.316)*
> *cellulitis of groin (L03.314)*

L03.312   **Cellulitis** of **back** [any part except buttock]
L03.313   **Cellulitis** of **chest wall**
L03.314   **Cellulitis** of **groin**
L03.315   **Cellulitis** of **perineum**
L03.316   **Cellulitis** of **umbilicus**
L03.317   **Cellulitis** of **buttock**
L03.319   **Cellulitis** of **trunk, unspecified**

√6ᵗʰ **L03.32**   **Acute lymphangitis** of **trunk**

L03.321   **Acute lymphangitis** of **abdominal wall**
L03.322   **Acute lymphangitis** of **back** [any part except buttock]
L03.323   **Acute lymphangitis** of **chest wall**
L03.324   **Acute lymphangitis** of **groin**
L03.325   **Acute lymphangitis** of **perineum**
L03.326   **Acute lymphangitis** of **umbilicus**
L03.327   **Acute lymphangitis** of **buttock**
L03.329   **Acute lymphangitis** of **trunk, unspecified**

√5ᵗʰ **L03.8**   **Cellulitis and acute lymphangitis** of other sites

√6ᵗʰ **L03.81**   **Cellulitis** of **other sites**

L03.811   **Cellulitis** of **head** [any part, except face]
Cellulitis of scalp
> EXCLUDES 2   *cellulitis of face (L03.211)*

L03.818   **Cellulitis** of other sites

√6ᵗʰ **L03.89**   **Acute lymphangitis** of other sites

L03.891   **Acute lymphangitis** of **head** [any part, except face]

L03.898   **Acute lymphangitis** of other sites

√5ᵗʰ **L03.9**   **Cellulitis and acute lymphangitis, unspecified**

L03.90   **Cellulitis, unspecified**
L03.91   **Acute lymphangitis, unspecified**
> EXCLUDES 1   *lymphangitis NOS (I89.1)*

√4ᵗʰ **L04**   **Acute lymphadenitis**
> INCLUDES   abscess (acute) of lymph nodes, except mesenteric
> acute lymphadenitis, except mesenteric
> EXCLUDES 1   *chronic or subacute lymphadenitis, except mesenteric (I88.1)*
> *enlarged lymph nodes (R59.-)*
> *human immunodeficiency virus [HIV] disease resulting in generalized lymphadenopathy (B20)*
> *lymphadenitis NOS (I88.9)*
> *nonspecific mesenteric lymphadenitis (I88.0)*

DEF: Inflammation or enlargement of the lymph nodes.

L04.0   **Acute lymphadenitis** of **face, head and neck**
L04.1   **Acute lymphadenitis** of **trunk**
L04.2   **Acute lymphadenitis** of **upper limb**
Acute lymphadenitis of axilla
Acute lymphadenitis of shoulder
L04.3   **Acute lymphadenitis** of **lower limb**
Acute lymphadenitis of hip
> EXCLUDES 2   *acute lymphadenitis of groin (L04.1)*

L04.8   **Acute lymphadenitis** of other sites
L04.9   **Acute lymphadenitis, unspecified**

√4ᵗʰ **L05**   **Pilonidal cyst and sinus**
> **DEF:** Pilonidal cyst: Sac or sinus cavity of trapped epithelial tissues in the sacrococcygeal region, usually associated with ingrown hair.
> **DEF:** Pilonidal sinus: Fistula, tract, or channel that extends from an infected area of ingrown hair to another site within the skin or out to the skin surface.

Pilonidal Cyst

- Skin
- Fistula
- Pilonidal cyst
- Fat
- Bone

√5ᵗʰ **L05.0**   **Pilonidal cyst and sinus** with abscess

L05.01   **Pilonidal cyst** with abscess
Pilonidal abscess
Pilonidal dimple with abscess
Postanal dimple with abscess
> EXCLUDES 2   *congenital sacral dimple (Q82.6)*
> *parasacral dimple (Q82.6)*

L05.02   **Pilonidal sinus** with abscess
Coccygeal fistula with abscess
Coccygeal sinus with abscess
Pilonidal fistula with abscess

√5ᵗʰ **L05.9**   **Pilonidal cyst and sinus** without abscess

L05.91   **Pilonidal cyst** without abscess
Pilonidal dimple
Postanal dimple
Pilonidal cyst NOS
> EXCLUDES 2   *congenital sacral dimple (Q82.6)*
> *parasacral dimple (Q82.6)*

L05.92   **Pilonidal sinus** without abscess
Coccygeal fistula
Coccygeal sinus without abscess
Pilonidal fistula

HCC CMS-HCC   **Rx** Rx HCC   **ESR** ESRD HCC   **COM** Commercial HCC   **N** Newborn: 0   **P** Pediatric: 0-17   **M** Maternity: 9-64   **A** Adult: 15-124

752   ICD-10-CM 2023

☑4ᵗʰ **L08 Other local infections of skin and subcutaneous tissue**

L08.0 Pyoderma
Dermatitis gangrenosa
Purulent dermatitis
Septic dermatitis
Suppurative dermatitis
EXCLUDES 1   *pyoderma gangrenosum (L88)*
pyoderma vegetans (L08.81)
DEF: Any superficial skin disease commonly characterized by the discharging of pus not attributed to another condition.

L08.1 Erythrasma
DEF: Chronic, superficial skin infection of brown scaly patches, commonly found in skin folds most prevalent in the overweight or diabetic population.

☑5ᵗʰ **L08.8 Other specified local infections of the skin and subcutaneous tissue**
L08.81 Pyoderma vegetans
EXCLUDES 1   *pyoderma gangrenosum (L88)*
pyoderma NOS (L08.0)
L08.82 Omphalitis not of newborn
EXCLUDES 1   *omphalitis of newborn (P38.-)*
L08.89 Other specified local infections of the skin and subcutaneous tissue
L08.9 Local infection of the skin and subcutaneous tissue, unspecified

Bullous disorders (L10-L14)

EXCLUDES 1   *benign familial pemphigus [Hailey-Hailey] (Q82.8)*
staphylococcal scalded skin syndrome (L00)
toxic epidermal necrolysis [Lyell] (L51.2)

☑4ᵗʰ **L10 Pemphigus**
EXCLUDES 1   *pemphigus neonatorum (L01.03)*

L10.0 Pemphigus vulgaris `Rx` `COM`
L10.1 Pemphigus vegetans `Rx` `COM`
L10.2 Pemphigus foliaceous `Rx` `COM`
L10.3 Brazilian pemphigus [fogo selvagem] `Rx` `COM`
L10.4 Pemphigus erythematosus `Rx` `COM`
Senear-Usher syndrome
L10.5 Drug-induced pemphigus `Rx` `COM`
Use additional code for adverse effect, if applicable, to identify drug (T36-T50 with fifth or sixth character 5)
☑5ᵗʰ **L10.8 Other pemphigus**
L10.81 Paraneoplastic pemphigus `Rx` `COM`
L10.89 Other pemphigus `Rx` `COM`
L10.9 Pemphigus, unspecified `Rx` `COM`

☑4ᵗʰ **L11 Other acantholytic disorders**
L11.0 Acquired keratosis follicularis
EXCLUDES 1   *keratosis follicularis (congenital) [Darier-White] (Q82.8)*
AHA: 2021,3Q,10
L11.1 Transient acantholytic dermatosis [Grover]
L11.8 Other specified acantholytic disorders
L11.9 Acantholytic disorder, unspecified

☑4ᵗʰ **L12 Pemphigoid**
EXCLUDES 1   *herpes gestationis (O26.4-)*
impetigo herpetiformis (L40.1)
L12.0 Bullous pemphigoid `Rx` `COM`
L12.1 Cicatricial pemphigoid `Rx` `COM`
Benign mucous membrane pemphigoid
DEF: Chronic autoimmune disease characterized by subepidermal blistering lesions of the mucosa, including the conjunctiva. It is seen predominantly in the elderly and produces adhesions and scarring.
L12.2 Chronic bullous disease of childhood `Rx` `P`
Juvenile dermatitis herpetiformis
☑5ᵗʰ **L12.3 Acquired epidermolysis bullosa**
EXCLUDES 1   *epidermolysis bullosa (congenital) (Q81.-)*
L12.30 Acquired epidermolysis bullosa, unspecified `HCC` `ESR` `COM`
L12.31 Epidermolysis bullosa due to drug `HCC` `ESR` `COM`
Use additional code for adverse effect, if applicable, to identify drug (T36-T50 with fifth or sixth character 5)
L12.35 Other acquired epidermolysis bullosa `HCC` `ESR` `COM`

L12.8 Other pemphigoid `Rx` `COM`
L12.9 Pemphigoid, unspecified `Rx` `COM`

☑4ᵗʰ **L13 Other bullous disorders**
L13.0 Dermatitis herpetiformis `Rx`
Duhring's disease
Hydroa herpetiformis
EXCLUDES 1   *juvenile dermatitis herpetiformis (L12.2)*
senile dermatitis herpetiformis (L12.0)
DEF: Skin disease to which people are genetically predisposed resulting from an immunological response to gluten. Dermatitis herpetiformis is an extremely pruritic eruption of various lesions that frequently heal, leaving hyperpigmentation or hypopigmentation and occasionally scarring. It is usually associated with asymptomatic gluten-sensitive enteropathy.
L13.1 Subcorneal pustular dermatitis `Rx`
Sneddon-Wilkinson disease
L13.8 Other specified bullous disorders `Rx`
L13.9 Bullous disorder, unspecified `Rx`

L14 Bullous disorders in diseases classified elsewhere `Rx`
Code first underlying disease

Dermatitis and eczema (L20-L30)

`NOTE` In this block the terms dermatitis and eczema are used synonymously and interchangeably.

EXCLUDES 2   *chronic (childhood) granulomatous disease (D71)*
dermatitis gangrenosa (L08.0)
dermatitis herpetiformis (L13.0)
dry skin dermatitis (L85.3)
factitial dermatitis (L98.1)
perioral dermatitis (L71.0)
radiation-related disorders of the skin and subcutaneous tissue (L55-L59)
stasis dermatitis (I87.2)

☑4ᵗʰ **L20 Atopic dermatitis**
L20.0 Besnier's prurigo
☑5ᵗʰ **L20.8 Other atopic dermatitis**
EXCLUDES 2   *circumscribed neurodermatitis (L28.0)*
L20.81 Atopic neurodermatitis
Diffuse neurodermatitis
L20.82 Flexural eczema
L20.83 Infantile (acute) (chronic) eczema `P`
L20.84 Intrinsic (allergic) eczema
L20.89 Other atopic dermatitis
L20.9 Atopic dermatitis, unspecified

☑4ᵗʰ **L21 Seborrheic dermatitis**
EXCLUDES 2   *infective dermatitis (L30.3)*
seborrheic keratosis (L82.-)
L21.0 Seborrhea capitis
Cradle cap
AHA: 2018,1Q,6
TIP: Assign for dandruff in an adult patient.
L21.1 Seborrheic infantile dermatitis `P`
L21.8 Other seborrheic dermatitis
L21.9 Seborrheic dermatitis, unspecified
Seborrhea NOS

L22 Diaper dermatitis
Diaper erythema
Diaper rash
Psoriasiform diaper rash
AHA: 2021,4Q,18

Chapter 12. Diseases of the Skin and Subcutaneous Tissue

L08–L22

✓4ᵗʰ **L23　Allergic contact dermatitis**
- EXCLUDES 1　*allergy NOS (T78.40)*
  contact dermatitis NOS (L25.9)
  dermatitis NOS (L30.9)
- EXCLUDES 2　*dermatitis due to substances taken internally (L27.-)*
  dermatitis of eyelid (H01.1-)
  diaper dermatitis (L22)
  eczema of external ear (H60.5-)
  irritant contact dermatitis (L24.-)
  perioral dermatitis (L71.0)
  radiation-related disorders of the skin and subcutaneous tissue (L55-L59)

L23.0　Allergic contact dermatitis due to metals
　Allergic contact dermatitis due to chromium
　Allergic contact dermatitis due to nickel

L23.1　Allergic contact dermatitis due to adhesives

L23.2　Allergic contact dermatitis due to cosmetics

L23.3　Allergic contact dermatitis due to drugs in contact with skin
　Use additional code for adverse effect, if applicable, to identify drug (T36-T50 with fifth or sixth character 5)
- EXCLUDES 2　*dermatitis due to ingested drugs and medicaments (L27.0-L27.1)*

L23.4　Allergic contact dermatitis due to dyes

L23.5　Allergic contact dermatitis due to other chemical products
　Allergic contact dermatitis due to cement
　Allergic contact dermatitis due to insecticide
　Allergic contact dermatitis due to plastic
　Allergic contact dermatitis due to rubber

L23.6　Allergic contact dermatitis due to food in contact with the skin
- EXCLUDES 2　*dermatitis due to ingested food (L27.2)*

L23.7　Allergic contact dermatitis due to plants, except food
- EXCLUDES 2　*allergy NOS due to pollen (J30.1)*

✓5ᵗʰ **L23.8　Allergic contact dermatitis due to other agents**

　L23.81　Allergic contact dermatitis due to animal (cat) (dog) dander
　　Allergic contact dermatitis due to animal (cat) (dog) hair

　L23.89　Allergic contact dermatitis due to other agents

L23.9　Allergic contact dermatitis, unspecified cause
　Allergic contact eczema NOS

✓4ᵗʰ **L24　Irritant contact dermatitis**
- EXCLUDES 1　*allergy NOS (T78.40)*
  contact dermatitis NOS (L25.9)
  dermatitis NOS (L30.9)
- EXCLUDES 2　*allergic contact dermatitis (L23.-)*
  dermatitis due to substances taken internally (L27.-)
  dermatitis of eyelid (H01.1-)
  diaper dermatitis (L22)
  eczema of external ear (H60.5-)
  perioral dermatitis (L71.0)
  radiation-related disorders of the skin and subcutaneous tissue (L55-L59)

L24.0　Irritant contact dermatitis due to detergents

L24.1　Irritant contact dermatitis due to oils and greases

L24.2　Irritant contact dermatitis due to solvents
　Irritant contact dermatitis due to chlorocompound
　Irritant contact dermatitis due to cyclohexane
　Irritant contact dermatitis due to ester
　Irritant contact dermatitis due to glycol
　Irritant contact dermatitis due to hydrocarbon
　Irritant contact dermatitis due to ketone

L24.3　Irritant contact dermatitis due to cosmetics

L24.4　Irritant contact dermatitis due to drugs in contact with skin
　Use additional code for adverse effect, if applicable, to identify drug (T36-T50 with fifth or sixth character 5)

L24.5　Irritant contact dermatitis due to other chemical products
　Irritant contact dermatitis due to cement
　Irritant contact dermatitis due to insecticide
　Irritant contact dermatitis due to plastic
　Irritant contact dermatitis due to rubber

L24.6　Irritant contact dermatitis due to food in contact with skin
- EXCLUDES 2　*dermatitis due to ingested food (L27.2)*

L24.7　Irritant contact dermatitis due to plants, except food
- EXCLUDES 2　*allergy NOS to pollen (J30.1)*

✓5ᵗʰ **L24.8　Irritant contact dermatitis due to other agents**

　L24.81　Irritant contact dermatitis due to metals
　　Irritant contact dermatitis due to chromium
　　Irritant contact dermatitis due to nickel

　L24.89　Irritant contact dermatitis due to other agents
　　Irritant contact dermatitis due to dyes

L24.9　Irritant contact dermatitis, unspecified cause
　Irritant contact eczema NOS

✓5ᵗʰ **L24.A　Irritant contact dermatitis due to friction or contact with body fluids**
- EXCLUDES 1　*irritant contact dermatitis related to stoma or fistula (L24.B-)*
- EXCLUDES 2　*erythema intertrigo (L30.4)*
- AHA: 2021,4Q,16-18

　L24.A0　Irritant contact dermatitis due to friction or contact with body fluids, unspecified

　L24.A1　Irritant contact dermatitis due to saliva

　L24.A2　Irritant contact dermatitis due to fecal, urinary or dual incontinence
- EXCLUDES 1　*diaper dermatitis (L22)*

　L24.A9　Irritant contact dermatitis due friction or contact with other specified body fluids
　　Irritant contact dermatitis related to endotracheal tube
　　Wound fluids, exudate

✓5ᵗʰ **L24.B　Irritant contact dermatitis related to stoma or fistula**
　Use additional code to identify any artificial opening status (Z93.-), if applicable, for contact dermatitis related to stoma secretions
- AHA: 2021,4Q,16-18

　L24.B0　Irritant contact dermatitis related to unspecified stoma or fistula
　　Irritant contact dermatitis related to fistula NOS
　　Irritant contact dermatitis related to stoma NOS

　L24.B1　Irritant contact dermatitis related to digestive stoma or fistula
　　Irritant contact dermatitis related to gastrostomy
　　Irritant contact dermatitis related to jejunostomy
　　Irritant contact dermatitis related to saliva or spit fistula

　L24.B2　Irritant contact dermatitis related to respiratory stoma or fistula
　　Irritant contact dermatitis related to tracheostomy

　L24.B3　Irritant contact dermatitis related to fecal or urinary stoma or fistula
　　Irritant contact dermatitis related to colostomy
　　Irritant contact dermatitis related to enterocutaneous fistula
　　Irritant contact dermatitis related to ileostomy

✓4ᵗʰ **L25　Unspecified contact dermatitis**
- EXCLUDES 1　*allergic contact dermatitis (L23.-)*
  allergy NOS (T78.40)
  dermatitis NOS (L30.9)
  irritant contact dermatitis (L24.-)
- EXCLUDES 2　*dermatitis due to ingested substances (L27.-)*
  dermatitis of eyelid (H01.1-)
  eczema of external ear (H60.5-)
  perioral dermatitis (L71.0)
  radiation-related disorders of the skin and subcutaneous tissue (L55-L59)

L25.0　Unspecified contact dermatitis due to cosmetics

L25.1　Unspecified contact dermatitis due to drugs in contact with skin
　Use additional code for adverse effect, if applicable, to identify drug (T36-T50 with fifth or sixth character 5)
- EXCLUDES 2　*dermatitis due to ingested drugs and medicaments (L27.0-L27.1)*

L25.2　Unspecified contact dermatitis due to dyes

L25.3　Unspecified contact dermatitis due to other chemical products
　Unspecified contact dermatitis due to cement
　Unspecified contact dermatitis due to insecticide

| HCC CMS-HCC | Rx Rx HCC | ESR ESRD HCC | COM Commercial HCC | N Newborn: 0 | P Pediatric: 0-17 | M Maternity: 9-64 | A Adult: 15-124 |

754

ICD-10-CM 2023

L25.4 Unspecified contact dermatitis due to food in contact with skin
> EXCLUDES 2   dermatitis due to ingested food (L27.2)

L25.5 Unspecified contact dermatitis due to plants, except food
> EXCLUDES 1   nettle rash (L50.9)
> EXCLUDES 2   allergy NOS due to pollen (J30.1)

L25.8 Unspecified contact dermatitis due to other agents

L25.9 Unspecified contact dermatitis, unspecified cause
> Contact dermatitis (occupational) NOS
> Contact eczema (occupational) NOS

L26 Exfoliative dermatitis
> Hebra's pityriasis
> EXCLUDES 1   Ritter's disease (L00)

✓4th **L27** Dermatitis due to substances taken internally
> EXCLUDES 1   allergy NOS (T78.40)
> EXCLUDES 2   adverse food reaction, except dermatitis (T78.0-T78.1)
> contact dermatitis (L23-L25)
> drug photoallergic response (L56.1)
> drug phototoxic response (L56.0)
> urticaria (L50.-)

L27.0 Generalized skin eruption due to drugs and medicaments taken internally
> Use additional code for adverse effect, if applicable, to identify drug (T36-T50 with fifth or sixth character 5)

L27.1 Localized skin eruption due to drugs and medicaments taken internally
> Use additional code for adverse effect, if applicable, to identify drug (T36-T50 with fifth or sixth character 5)

L27.2 Dermatitis due to ingested food
> EXCLUDES 2   dermatitis due to food in contact with skin (L23.6, L24.6, L25.4)

L27.8 Dermatitis due to other substances taken internally

L27.9 Dermatitis due to unspecified substance taken internally

✓4th **L28** Lichen simplex chronicus and prurigo

L28.0 Lichen simplex chronicus
> Circumscribed neurodermatitis
> Lichen NOS

L28.1 Prurigo nodularis

L28.2 Other prurigo
> Prurigo NOS
> Prurigo Hebra
> Prurigo mitis
> Urticaria papulosa

✓4th **L29** Pruritus   *itching*
> EXCLUDES 1   neurotic excoriation (L98.1)
> psychogenic pruritus (F45.8)

L29.0 Pruritus ani

L29.1 Pruritus scroti   ♂

L29.2 Pruritus vulvae   ♀

L29.3 Anogenital pruritus, unspecified

L29.8 Other pruritus

L29.9 Pruritus, unspecified
> Itch NOS

✓4th **L30** Other and unspecified dermatitis
> EXCLUDES 2   contact dermatitis (L23-L25)
> dry skin dermatitis (L85.3)
> small plaque parapsoriasis (L41.3)
> stasis dermatitis (I87.2)

L30.0 Nummular dermatitis

L30.1 Dyshidrosis [pompholyx]

L30.2 Cutaneous autosensitization
> Candidid [levurid]
> Dermatophytid
> Eczematid

L30.3 Infective dermatitis
> Infectious eczematoid dermatitis

L30.4 Erythema intertrigo

L30.5 Pityriasis alba
> AHA: 2018,1Q,6

L30.8 Other specified dermatitis

L30.9 Dermatitis, unspecified
> Eczema NOS

Papulosquamous disorders (L40-L45)

✓4th **L40** Psoriasis
> DEF: Chronic autoimmune condition that speeds up skin cell growth, causing excessive immature skin cells to form raised, rounded erythematous lesions covered by dry, silvery scaling patches. Most commonly found on the scalp, elbows, knees, hands, feet, and genitals, it can also affect the joints with stiffness and swelling.

L40.0 Psoriasis vulgaris   `Rx`
> Nummular psoriasis
> Plaque psoriasis

L40.1 Generalized pustular psoriasis   `Rx`
> Impetigo herpetiformis
> Von Zumbusch's disease

L40.2 Acrodermatitis continua   `Rx`

L40.3 Pustulosis palmaris et plantaris   `Rx`

L40.4 Guttate psoriasis   `Rx`

✓5th **L40.5** Arthropathic psoriasis

L40.50 Arthropathic psoriasis, unspecified   `HCC` `Rx` `ESR` `COM`

L40.51 Distal interphalangeal psoriatic arthropathy   `HCC` `Rx` `ESR` `COM`

L40.52 Psoriatic arthritis mutilans   `HCC` `Rx` `ESR` `COM`

L40.53 Psoriatic spondylitis   `HCC` `Rx` `ESR` `COM`

L40.54 Psoriatic juvenile arthropathy   `HCC` `Rx` `ESR` `COM`

L40.59 Other psoriatic arthropathy   `HCC` `Rx` `ESR` `COM`

L40.8 Other psoriasis   `Rx`
> Flexural psoriasis

L40.9 Psoriasis, unspecified   `Rx`

✓4th **L41** Parapsoriasis
> EXCLUDES 1   poikiloderma vasculare atrophicans (L94.5)

L41.0 Pityriasis lichenoides et varioliformis acuta   `Rx`
> Mucha-Habermann disease

L41.1 Pityriasis lichenoides chronica   `Rx`

L41.3 Small plaque parapsoriasis   `Rx`

L41.4 Large plaque parapsoriasis   `Rx`

L41.5 Retiform parapsoriasis   `Rx`

L41.8 Other parapsoriasis   `Rx`

L41.9 Parapsoriasis, unspecified   `Rx`

L42 Pityriasis rosea

✓4th **L43** Lichen planus
> EXCLUDES 1   lichen planopilaris (L66.1)

L43.0 Hypertrophic lichen planus

L43.1 Bullous lichen planus

L43.2 Lichenoid drug reaction
> Use additional code for adverse effect, if applicable, to identify drug (T36-T50 with fifth or sixth character 5)

L43.3 Subacute (active) lichen planus
> Lichen planus tropicus

L43.8 Other lichen planus

L43.9 Lichen planus, unspecified

✓4th **L44** Other papulosquamous disorders

L44.0 Pityriasis rubra pilaris

L44.1 Lichen nitidus
> DEF: Chronic, inflammatory, asymptomatic skin disorder, characterized by numerous glistening, flat-topped, discrete, skin-colored micropapules, most often on the penis, lower abdomen, inner thighs, wrists, forearms, breasts, and buttocks.

L44.2 Lichen striatus

L44.3 Lichen ruber moniliformis

L44.4 Infantile papular acrodermatitis [Gianotti-Crosti]   `P`

L44.8 Other specified papulosquamous disorders

L44.9 Papulosquamous disorder, unspecified

L45 *Papulosquamous disorders in diseases classified elsewhere*
> Code first underlying disease

| ✓ Additional Character Required | ✓x7th Placeholder Alert | Manifestation | Unspecified Dx | Q QPP | UPD Unacceptable PDx |

ICD-10-CM 2023   755

Chapter 12. Diseases of the Skin and Subcutaneous Tissue

L25.4–L45

Urticaria and erythema (L49-L54)

EXCLUDES 1   Lyme disease (A69.2-)
        rosacea (L71.-)

✓4ᵗʰ **L49   Exfoliation due to erythematous conditions according to extent of body surface involved**
     Code first erythematous condition causing exfoliation, such as:
        Ritter's disease (L00)
        (Staphylococcal) scalded skin syndrome (L00)
        Stevens-Johnson syndrome (L51.1)
        Stevens-Johnson syndrome-toxic epidermal necrolysis overlap
           syndrome (L51.3)
        toxic epidermal necrolysis (L51.2)
    DEF: Exfoliation: Falling or sloughing off skin in layers.

   L49.0   Exfoliation due to erythematous condition involving less than 10 percent of body surface   `UPD`
       Exfoliation due to erythematous condition NOS

   L49.1   Exfoliation due to erythematous condition involving 10-19 percent of body surface   `COM` `UPD`

   L49.2   Exfoliation due to erythematous condition involving 20-29 percent of body surface   `COM` `UPD`

   L49.3   Exfoliation due to erythematous condition involving 30-39 percent of body surface   `COM` `UPD`

   L49.4   Exfoliation due to erythematous condition involving 40-49 percent of body surface   `COM` `UPD`

   L49.5   Exfoliation due to erythematous condition involving 50-59 percent of body surface   `COM` `UPD`

   L49.6   Exfoliation due to erythematous condition involving 60-69 percent of body surface   `COM` `UPD`

   L49.7   Exfoliation due to erythematous condition involving 70-79 percent of body surface   `COM` `UPD`

   L49.8   Exfoliation due to erythematous condition involving 80-89 percent of body surface   `COM` `UPD`

   L49.9   Exfoliation due to erythematous condition involving 90 or more percent of body surface   `COM` `UPD`

✓4ᵗʰ **L50   Urticaria**

     EXCLUDES 1   allergic contact dermatitis (L23.-)
        angioneurotic edema (T78.3)
        giant urticaria (T78.3)
        hereditary angio-edema (D84.1)
        Quincke's edema (T78.3)
        serum urticaria (T80.6-)
        solar urticaria (L56.3)
        urticaria neonatorum (P83.8)
        urticaria papulosa (L28.2)
        urticaria pigmentosa (D47.01)
    DEF: Eruption of itching edema of the skin. **Synonym(s):** hives.

   L50.0   Allergic urticaria
   L50.1   Idiopathic urticaria
   L50.2   Urticaria due to cold and heat
       EXCLUDES 2   familial cold urticaria (M04.2)
   L50.3   Dermatographic urticaria
   L50.4   Vibratory urticaria
   L50.5   Cholinergic urticaria
   L50.6   Contact urticaria
   L50.8   Other urticaria
       Chronic urticaria
       Recurrent periodic urticaria
   L50.9   Urticaria, unspecified

✓4ᵗʰ **L51   Erythema multiforme**
     Use additional code for adverse effect, if applicable, to identify drug
        (T36-T50 with fifth or sixth character 5)
     Use additional code to identify associated manifestations, such as:
        arthropathy associated with dermatological disorders (M14.8-)
        conjunctival edema (H11.42)
        conjunctivitis (H10.22-)
        corneal scars and opacities (H17.-)
        corneal ulcer (H16.0-)
        edema of eyelid (H02.84-)
        inflammation of eyelid (H01.8)
        keratoconjunctivitis sicca (H16.22-)
        mechanical lagophthalmos (H02.22-)
        stomatitis (K12.-)
        symblepharon (H11.23-)
     Use additional code to identify percentage of skin exfoliation (L49.-)
     EXCLUDES 1   staphylococcal scalded skin syndrome (L00)
            Ritter's disease (L00)
    DEF: Acute complex of symptoms with a varied pattern of skin eruptions, such as macular, bullous, papular, nodose, or vesicular lesions on the neck, face, and legs. Erythema (redness of skin and mucous membranes) multiforme (multiple forms) is a hypersensitivity (allergic) reaction that can occur at any age but primarily affects children or young adults.

   L51.0   Nonbullous erythema multiforme
   L51.1   Stevens-Johnson syndrome   `HCC` `ESR` `COM`
   L51.2   Toxic epidermal necrolysis [Lyell]   `HCC` `ESR` `COM`
   L51.3   Stevens-Johnson syndrome-toxic epidermal necrolysis overlap syndrome   `HCC` `ESR` `COM`
       SJS-TEN overlap syndrome
   L51.8   Other erythema multiforme
   L51.9   Erythema multiforme, unspecified
       Erythema iris
       Erythema multiforme major NOS
       Erythema multiforme minor NOS
       Herpes iris

L52   Erythema nodosum
     EXCLUDES 1   tuberculous erythema nodosum (A18.4)
    DEF: Form of panniculitis (inflammation of the fat layer beneath the skin) most often occurring in women. Commonly seen as a hypersensitivity reaction to infections, drugs, sarcoidosis, and specific enteropathies. The acute stage is associated with fever, malaise, and arthralgia. The lesions are pink to blue in color as tender nodules and are found on the front of the legs below the knees.

✓4ᵗʰ **L53   Other erythematous conditions**
     EXCLUDES 1   erythema ab igne (L59.0)
            erythema due to external agents in contact with skin (L23-L25)
            erythema intertrigo (L30.4)

   L53.0   Toxic erythema
       Code first poisoning due to drug or toxin, if applicable (T36-T65 with fifth or sixth character 1-4 or 6)
       Use additional code for adverse effect, if applicable, to identify drug (T36-T50 with fifth or sixth character 5)
       EXCLUDES 1   neonatal erythema toxicum (P83.1)
   L53.1   Erythema annulare centrifugum
   L53.2   Erythema marginatum
   L53.3   Other chronic figurate erythema
   L53.8   Other specified erythematous conditions
   L53.9   Erythematous condition, unspecified
       Erythema NOS
       Erythroderma NOS

L54   Erythema in diseases classified elsewhere
     Code first underlying disease

Radiation-related disorders of the skin and subcutaneous tissue (L55-L59)

✓4ᵗʰ **L55   Sunburn**
   L55.0   Sunburn of first degree
   L55.1   Sunburn of second degree
   L55.2   Sunburn of third degree   `COM`
   L55.9   Sunburn, unspecified

`HCC` CMS-HCC   `Rx` Rx HCC   `ESR` ESRD HCC   `COM` Commercial HCC   `N` Newborn: 0   `P` Pediatric: 0-17   `M` Maternity: 9-64   `A` Adult: 15-124

756   ICD-10-CM 2023

☑4ᵗʰ **L56 Other acute skin changes due to ultraviolet radiation**

Use additional code to identify the source of the ultraviolet radiation (W89, X32)

L56.0 Drug phototoxic response
Use additional code for adverse effect, if applicable, to identify drug (T36-T50 with fifth or sixth character 5)

L56.1 Drug photoallergic response
Use additional code for adverse effect, if applicable, to identify drug (T36-T50 with fifth or sixth character 5)

L56.2 Photocontact dermatitis [berloque dermatitis]

L56.3 Solar urticaria

L56.4 Polymorphous light eruption

L56.5 Disseminated superficial actinic porokeratosis (DSAP)
DEF: Autosomal dominant skin condition occurring in sun-exposed areas of the skin (particularly the arms and legs), characterized by superficial annular, keratotic, brownish-red spots or thickenings with depressed centers and sharp, ridged borders. It may evolve into squamous cell carcinoma.

L56.8 Other specified acute skin changes due to ultraviolet radiation

L56.9 Acute skin change due to ultraviolet radiation, unspecified

☑4ᵗʰ **L57 Skin changes due to chronic exposure to nonionizing radiation**

Use additional code to identify the source of the ultraviolet radiation (W89), or other nonionizing radiation (W90)

L57.0 Actinic keratosis
Keratosis NOS
Senile keratosis
Solar keratosis

L57.1 Actinic reticuloid

L57.2 Cutis rhomboidalis nuchae

L57.3 Poikiloderma of Civatte

L57.4 Cutis laxa senilis
Elastosis senilis

L57.5 Actinic granuloma

L57.8 Other skin changes due to chronic exposure to nonionizing radiation
Farmer's skin
Sailor's skin
Solar dermatitis

L57.9 Skin changes due to chronic exposure to nonionizing radiation, unspecified

☑4ᵗʰ **L58 Radiodermatitis**

Use additional code to identify the source of the radiation (W88, W90)

L58.0 Acute radiodermatitis

L58.1 Chronic radiodermatitis

L58.9 Radiodermatitis, unspecified

☑4ᵗʰ **L59 Other disorders of skin and subcutaneous tissue related to radiation**

L59.0 Erythema ab igne [dermatitis ab igne]

L59.8 Other specified disorders of the skin and subcutaneous tissue related to radiation
AHA: 2017,1Q,33

L59.9 Disorder of the skin and subcutaneous tissue related to radiation, unspecified

Disorders of skin appendages (L60-L75)

EXCLUDES 1   *congenital malformations of integument (Q84.-)*

☑4ᵗʰ **L60 Nail disorders**

EXCLUDES 2   *clubbing of nails (R68.3)*
onychia and paronychia (L03.0-)

Nail Disorders

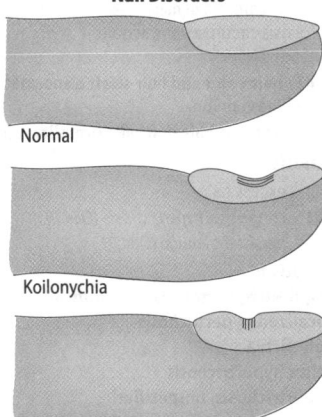

Normal

Koilonychia

Beau's Lines

L60.0 Ingrowing nail

L60.1 Onycholysis

L60.2 Onychogryphosis

L60.3 Nail dystrophy

L60.4 Beau's lines

L60.5 Yellow nail syndrome

L60.8 Other nail disorders

L60.9 Nail disorder, unspecified

L62 Nail disorders in diseases classified elsewhere
Code first underlying disease, such as:
pachydermoperiostosis (M89.4-)

☑4ᵗʰ **L63 Alopecia areata**

L63.0 Alopecia (capitis) totalis

L63.1 Alopecia universalis

L63.2 Ophiasis

L63.8 Other alopecia areata

L63.9 Alopecia areata, unspecified

☑4ᵗʰ **L64 Androgenic alopecia**

INCLUDES   male-pattern baldness

L64.0 Drug-induced androgenic alopecia
Use additional code for adverse effect, if applicable, to identify drug (T36-T50 with fifth or sixth character 5)

L64.8 Other androgenic alopecia

L64.9 Androgenic alopecia, unspecified

☑4ᵗʰ **L65 Other nonscarring hair loss**

Use additional code for adverse effect, if applicable, to identify drug (T36-T50 with fifth or sixth character 5)

EXCLUDES 1   *trichotillomania (F63.3)*

L65.0 Telogen effluvium
DEF: Form of nonscarring alopecia characterized by shedding of hair from premature telogen development in follicles due to stress, including shock, childbirth, surgery, drugs, or weight loss.

L65.1 Anagen effluvium

L65.2 Alopecia mucinosa

L65.8 Other specified nonscarring hair loss

L65.9 Nonscarring hair loss, unspecified
Alopecia NOS

☑4ᵗʰ **L66 Cicatricial alopecia [scarring hair loss]**

L66.0 Pseudopelade

L66.1 Lichen planopilaris
Follicular lichen planus

L66.2 Folliculitis decalvans

L66.3 Perifolliculitis capitis abscedens

L66.4 Folliculitis ulerythematosa reticulata

L66.8 Other cicatricial alopecia
AHA: 2015,1Q,19

L66.9 Cicatricial alopecia, unspecified

Chapter 12. Diseases of the Skin and Subcutaneous Tissue *(side margin)*

L67–L76.22 *(side margin)*

✓4ᵗʰ **L67 Hair color and hair shaft abnormalities**

> EXCLUDES 1   monilethrix (Q84.1)
> pili annulati (Q84.1)
> telogen effluvium (L65.0)

L67.0 Trichorrhexis nodosa

L67.1 Variations in hair color
Canities
Greyness, hair (premature)
Heterochromia of hair
Poliosis circumscripta, acquired
Poliosis NOS

L67.8 Other hair color and hair shaft abnormalities
Fragilitas crinium

L67.9 Hair color and hair shaft abnormality, unspecified

✓4ᵗʰ **L68 Hypertrichosis**

> INCLUDES   excess hair
> EXCLUDES 1   congenital hypertrichosis (Q84.2)
> persistent lanugo (Q84.2)

L68.0 Hirsutism

L68.1 Acquired hypertrichosis lanuginosa

L68.2 Localized hypertrichosis

L68.3 Polytrichia

L68.8 Other hypertrichosis

L68.9 Hypertrichosis, unspecified

✓4ᵗʰ **L70 Acne**

> EXCLUDES 2   acne keloid (L73.0)

L70.0 Acne vulgaris

L70.1 Acne conglobata

L70.2 Acne varioliformis
Acne necrotica miliaris
DEF: Rare form of acne characterized by development of persistent brown papulopustules followed by scar formation. This type of acne usually presents on the brow and temporoparietal part of the scalp.

L70.3 Acne tropica

L70.4 Infantile acne   P

L70.5 Acné excoriée
Acné excoriée des jeunes filles
Picker's acne

L70.8 Other acne

L70.9 Acne, unspecified

✓4ᵗʰ **L71 Rosacea**

> Use additional code for adverse effect, if applicable, to identify drug (T36-T50 with fifth or sixth character 5)

L71.0 Perioral dermatitis

L71.1 Rhinophyma

L71.8 Other rosacea
AHA: 2018,4Q,15

L71.9 Rosacea, unspecified

✓4ᵗʰ **L72 Follicular cysts of skin and subcutaneous tissue**

L72.0 Epidermal cyst

✓5ᵗʰ **L72.1 Pilar and trichodermal cyst**

L72.11 Pilar cyst

L72.12 Trichodermal cyst
Trichilemmal (proliferating) cyst

L72.2 Steatocystoma multiplex

L72.3 Sebaceous cyst

> EXCLUDES 2   pilar cyst (L72.11)
> trichilemmal (proliferating) cyst (L72.12)

L72.8 Other follicular cysts of the skin and subcutaneous tissue

L72.9 Follicular cyst of the skin and subcutaneous tissue, unspecified

✓4ᵗʰ **L73 Other follicular disorders**

L73.0 Acne keloid

L73.1 Pseudofolliculitis barbae

L73.2 Hidradenitis suppurativa — *pus, abscess* (handwritten)

L73.8 Other specified follicular disorders
Sycosis barbae

L73.9 Follicular disorder, unspecified

✓4ᵗʰ **L74 Eccrine sweat disorders**

> EXCLUDES 2   generalized hyperhidrosis (R61)

DEF: Eccrine sweat glands: Glands found in the dermal and hypodermal layer of the skin throughout the body, particularly on the forehead, scalp, axillae, palms, and soles. These glands produce watery and neutral or slightly acidic sweat.

L74.0 Miliaria rubra

L74.1 Miliaria crystallina

L74.2 Miliaria profunda
Miliaria tropicalis

L74.3 Miliaria, unspecified

L74.4 Anhidrosis
Hypohidrosis
DEF: Inability to sweat normally. When the body can't cool itself through perspiration it can lead to heatstroke, a life-threatening condition.

✓5ᵗʰ **L74.5 Focal hyperhidrosis**

✓6ᵗʰ **L74.51 Primary focal hyperhidrosis**

L74.510 Primary focal hyperhidrosis, axilla

L74.511 Primary focal hyperhidrosis, face

L74.512 Primary focal hyperhidrosis, palms

L74.513 Primary focal hyperhidrosis, soles

L74.519 Primary focal hyperhidrosis, unspecified

L74.52 Secondary focal hyperhidrosis
Frey's syndrome

L74.8 Other eccrine sweat disorders

L74.9 Eccrine sweat disorder, unspecified
Sweat gland disorder NOS

✓4ᵗʰ **L75 Apocrine sweat disorders**

> EXCLUDES 1   dyshidrosis (L30.1)
> hidradenitis suppurativa (L73.2)

DEF: Apocrine sweat glands: Found in the axilla, areola, and circumanal region, these glands begin to function in puberty and produce viscid milky secretions in response to external stimuli.

L75.0 Bromhidrosis

L75.1 Chromhidrosis

L75.2 Apocrine miliaria
Fox-Fordyce disease
DEF: Chronic, usually pruritic disease evidenced by small follicular papular eruptions, especially in the axillary and pubic areas. Apocrine miliaria develops from the closure and rupture of the affected apocrine glands' intraepidermal portion of the ducts.

L75.8 Other apocrine sweat disorders

L75.9 Apocrine sweat disorder, unspecified

Intraoperative and postprocedural complications of skin and subcutaneous tissue (L76)

✓4ᵗʰ **L76 Intraoperative and postprocedural complications of skin and subcutaneous tissue**
AHA: 2016,4Q,9-10

✓5ᵗʰ **L76.0 Intraoperative hemorrhage and hematoma of skin and subcutaneous tissue complicating a procedure**

> EXCLUDES 1   intraoperative hemorrhage and hematoma of skin and subcutaneous tissue due to accidental puncture and laceration during a procedure (L76.1-)

L76.01 Intraoperative hemorrhage and hematoma of skin and subcutaneous tissue complicating a dermatologic procedure

L76.02 Intraoperative hemorrhage and hematoma of skin and subcutaneous tissue complicating other procedure

✓5ᵗʰ **L76.1 Accidental puncture and laceration of skin and subcutaneous tissue during a procedure**

L76.11 Accidental puncture and laceration of skin and subcutaneous tissue during a dermatologic procedure

L76.12 Accidental puncture and laceration of skin and subcutaneous tissue during other procedure

✓5ᵗʰ **L76.2 Postprocedural hemorrhage of skin and subcutaneous tissue following a procedure**

L76.21 Postprocedural hemorrhage of skin and subcutaneous tissue following a dermatologic procedure

L76.22 Postprocedural hemorrhage of skin and subcutaneous tissue following other procedure

✓5ᵗʰ **L76.3** Postprocedural hematoma and seroma of skin and subcutaneous tissue following a procedure

     L76.31 Postprocedural hematoma of skin and subcutaneous tissue following a dermatologic procedure

     L76.32 Postprocedural hematoma of skin and subcutaneous tissue following other procedure

     L76.33 Postprocedural seroma of skin and subcutaneous tissue following a dermatologic procedure

     L76.34 Postprocedural seroma of skin and subcutaneous tissue following other procedure

✓5ᵗʰ **L76.8** Other intraoperative and postprocedural complications of skin and subcutaneous tissue

     Use additional code, if applicable, to further specify disorder

     L76.81 Other intraoperative complications of skin and subcutaneous tissue

     L76.82 Other postprocedural complications of skin and subcutaneous tissue

       AHA: 2017,3Q,6

Other disorders of the skin and subcutaneous tissue (L80-L99)

L80 Vitiligo

     EXCLUDES 2   vitiligo of eyelids (H02.73-)

                  vitiligo of vulva (N90.89)

     DEF: Persistent, progressive development of nonpigmented white patches on otherwise normal skin.

✓4ᵗʰ **L81 Other disorders of pigmentation**

     EXCLUDES 1   birthmark NOS (Q82.5)

                  Peutz-Jeghers syndrome ▶(Q85.89)◀

     EXCLUDES 2   nevus - see Alphabetical Index

     L81.0 Postinflammatory hyperpigmentation

     L81.1 Chloasma

     L81.2 Freckles

     L81.3 Café au lait spots

     L81.4 Other melanin hyperpigmentation

       Lentigo

     L81.5 Leukoderma, not elsewhere classified

     L81.6 Other disorders of diminished melanin formation

     L81.7 Pigmented purpuric dermatosis

       Angioma serpiginosum

     L81.8 Other specified disorders of pigmentation

       Iron pigmentation

       Tattoo pigmentation

     L81.9 Disorder of pigmentation, unspecified

✓4ᵗʰ **L82 Seborrheic keratosis**

     INCLUDES   basal cell papilloma

                dermatosis papulosa nigra

                Leser-Trélat disease

     EXCLUDES 2   seborrheic dermatitis (L21.-)

     DEF: Common, benign, noninvasive, lightly pigmented, warty growth composed of basaloid cells that usually appear at middle age as soft, easily crumbling plaques on the face, trunk, and extremities.

     L82.0 Inflamed seborrheic keratosis

       AHA: 2021,3Q,10

     L82.1 Other seborrheic keratosis

       Seborrheic keratosis NOS

L83 Acanthosis nigricans

     Confluent and reticulated papillomatosis

     DEF: Diffuse, velvety hyperplasia of the spinous skin layer of the axilla and other body folds marked by gray, brown, or black pigmentation. In adult form, it is often associated with malignant acanthosis nigricans in a benign, nevoid form relatively generalized.

L84 Corns and callosities

     Callus

     Clavus

✓4ᵗʰ **L85 Other epidermal thickening**

     EXCLUDES 2   hypertrophic disorders of the skin (L91.-)

     L85.0 Acquired ichthyosis

       EXCLUDES 1   congenital ichthyosis (Q80.-)

     L85.1 Acquired keratosis [keratoderma] palmaris et plantaris

       EXCLUDES 1   inherited keratosis palmaris et plantaris (Q82.8)

     L85.2 Keratosis punctata (palmaris et plantaris)

     L85.3 Xerosis cutis

       Dry skin dermatitis

     L85.8 Other specified epidermal thickening

       Cutaneous horn

     L85.9 Epidermal thickening, unspecified

*L86 **Keratoderma in diseases classified elsewhere***

     Code first underlying disease, such as:

     Reiter's disease (M02.3-)

     EXCLUDES 1   gonococcal keratoderma (A54.89)

                gonococcal keratosis (A54.89)

                keratoderma due to vitamin A deficiency (E50.8)

                keratosis due to vitamin A deficiency (E50.8)

                xeroderma due to vitamin A deficiency (E50.8)

✓4ᵗʰ **L87 Transepidermal elimination disorders**

     EXCLUDES 1   granuloma annulare (perforating) (L92.0)

     L87.0 Keratosis follicularis et parafollicularis in cutem penetrans

       Hyperkeratosis follicularis penetrans

       Kyrle disease

     L87.1 Reactive perforating collagenosis

     L87.2 Elastosis perforans serpiginosa

     L87.8 Other transepidermal elimination disorders

     L87.9 Transepidermal elimination disorder, unspecified

L88 Pyoderma gangrenosum   Rx COM

     Phagedenic pyoderma

     EXCLUDES 1   dermatitis gangrenosa (L08.0)

     DEF: Persistent debilitating skin disease characterized by irregular, boggy, blue-red ulcerations, with central healing and undermined edges.

✓4ᵗʰ **L89 Pressure ulcer**

     INCLUDES   bed sore

                decubitus ulcer

                plaster ulcer

                pressure area

                pressure sore

     Code first any associated gangrene (I96)

     EXCLUDES 2   decubitus (trophic) ulcer of cervix (uteri) (N86)

                diabetic ulcers (E08.621, E08.622, E09.621, E09.622, E10.621, E10.622, E11.621, E11.622, E13.621, E13.622)

                non-pressure chronic ulcer of skin (L97.-)

                skin infections (L00-L08)

                varicose ulcer (I83.0, I83.2)

     AHA: 2022,2Q,8; 2021,1Q,24; 2019,4Q,10-11,54; 2018,4Q,69; 2018,3Q,3; 2018,2Q,21; 2017,4Q,109; 2017,1Q,49; 2016,4Q,143

     TIP: The stage of a diagnosed pressure ulcer can be based on documentation from clinicians who are not the patient's provider.

Four Stages of Pressure Ulcer

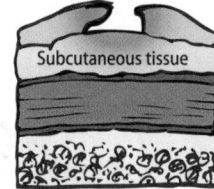

Epidermis — Dermis —

Subcutaneous tissue

Stage 1
Persistent focal edema

Stage 2
Abrasion, blister, partial thickness skin loss involving epidermis and/or dermis

Superficial fascia — Muscle —

Deep fascia — Bone —

Stage 3
Full thickness skin loss involving damage or necrosis of subcutaneous tissue

Stage 4
Necrosis of soft tissues through to underlying muscle, tendon, or bone

✓5ᵗʰ **L89.0** Pressure ulcer of elbow

     ✓6ᵗʰ **L89.00** Pressure ulcer of unspecified elbow

         L89.000 Pressure ulcer of unspecified elbow, unstageable   HCC ESR

Chapter 12. Diseases of the Skin and Subcutaneous Tissue

L89.001 **Pressure ulcer of unspecified elbow, stage 1**
    Healing pressure ulcer of unspecified elbow, stage 1
    Pressure pre-ulcer skin changes limited to persistent focal edema, unspecified elbow

L89.002 **Pressure ulcer of unspecified elbow, stage 2** `HCC` `ESR`
    Healing pressure ulcer of unspecified elbow, stage 2
    Pressure ulcer with abrasion, blister, partial thickness skin loss involving epidermis and/or dermis, unspecified elbow

L89.003 **Pressure ulcer of unspecified elbow, stage 3** `HCC` `ESR`
    Healing pressure ulcer of unspecified elbow, stage 3
    Pressure ulcer with full thickness skin loss involving damage or necrosis of subcutaneous tissue, unspecified elbow

L89.004 **Pressure ulcer of unspecified elbow, stage 4** `HCC` `ESR`
    Healing pressure ulcer of unspecified elbow, stage 4
    Pressure ulcer with necrosis of soft tissues through to underlying muscle, tendon, or bone, unspecified elbow

L89.006 **Pressure-induced deep tissue damage of unspecified elbow**

L89.009 **Pressure ulcer of unspecified elbow, unspecified stage**
    Healing pressure ulcer of elbow NOS
    Healing pressure ulcer of unspecified elbow, unspecified stage

√6ᵗʰ **L89.01** **Pressure ulcer of right elbow**

L89.010 **Pressure ulcer of right elbow, unstageable** `HCC` `ESR`

L89.011 **Pressure ulcer of right elbow, stage 1**
    Healing pressure ulcer of right elbow, stage 1
    Pressure pre-ulcer skin changes limited to persistent focal edema, right elbow

L89.012 **Pressure ulcer of right elbow, stage 2** `HCC` `ESR`
    Healing pressure ulcer of right elbow, stage 2
    Pressure ulcer with abrasion, blister, partial thickness skin loss involving epidermis and/or dermis, right elbow

L89.013 **Pressure ulcer of right elbow, stage 3** `HCC` `ESR`
    Healing pressure ulcer of right elbow, stage 3
    Pressure ulcer with full thickness skin loss involving damage or necrosis of subcutaneous tissue, right elbow

L89.014 **Pressure ulcer of right elbow, stage 4** `HCC` `ESR`
    Healing pressure ulcer of right elbow, stage 4
    Pressure ulcer with necrosis of soft tissues through to underlying muscle, tendon, or bone, right elbow

L89.016 **Pressure-induced deep tissue damage of right elbow**

L89.019 **Pressure ulcer of right elbow, unspecified stage**
    Healing pressure ulcer of right elbow NOS

√6ᵗʰ **L89.02** **Pressure ulcer of left elbow**

L89.020 **Pressure ulcer of left elbow, unstageable** `HCC` `ESR`

L89.021 **Pressure ulcer of left elbow, stage 1**
    Healing pressure ulcer of left elbow, stage 1
    Pressure pre-ulcer skin changes limited to persistent focal edema, left elbow

L89.022 **Pressure ulcer of left elbow, stage 2** `HCC` `ESR`
    Healing pressure ulcer of left elbow, stage 2
    Pressure ulcer with abrasion, blister, partial thickness skin loss involving epidermis and/or dermis, left elbow

L89.023 **Pressure ulcer of left elbow, stage 3** `HCC` `ESR`
    Healing pressure ulcer of left elbow, stage 3
    Pressure ulcer with full thickness skin loss involving damage or necrosis of subcutaneous tissue, left elbow

L89.024 **Pressure ulcer of left elbow, stage 4** `HCC` `ESR`
    Healing pressure ulcer of left elbow, stage 4
    Pressure ulcer with necrosis of soft tissues through to underlying muscle, tendon, or bone, left elbow

L89.026 **Pressure-induced deep tissue damage of left elbow**

L89.029 **Pressure ulcer of left elbow, unspecified stage**
    Healing pressure ulcer of left elbow NOS

√5ᵗʰ **L89.1** **Pressure ulcer of back**

√6ᵗʰ **L89.10** **Pressure ulcer of unspecified part of back**

L89.100 **Pressure ulcer of unspecified part of back, unstageable** `HCC` `ESR`

L89.101 **Pressure ulcer of unspecified part of back, stage 1**
    Healing pressure ulcer of unspecified part of back, stage 1
    Pressure pre-ulcer skin changes limited to persistent focal edema, unspecified part of back

L89.102 **Pressure ulcer of unspecified part of back, stage 2** `HCC` `ESR`
    Healing pressure ulcer of unspecified part of back, stage 2
    Pressure ulcer with abrasion, blister, partial thickness skin loss involving epidermis and/or dermis, unspecified part of back

L89.103 **Pressure ulcer of unspecified part of back, stage 3** `HCC` `ESR`
    Healing pressure ulcer of unspecified part of back, stage 3
    Pressure ulcer with full thickness skin loss involving damage or necrosis of subcutaneous tissue, unspecified part of back

L89.104 **Pressure ulcer of unspecified part of back, stage 4** `HCC` `ESR`
    Healing pressure ulcer of unspecified part of back, stage 4
    Pressure ulcer with necrosis of soft tissues through to underlying muscle, tendon, or bone, unspecified part of back

L89.106 **Pressure-induced deep tissue damage of unspecified part of back**

L89.109 **Pressure ulcer of unspecified part of back, unspecified stage**
    Healing pressure ulcer of unspecified part of back NOS
    Healing pressure ulcer of unspecified part of back, unspecified stage

√6ᵗʰ **L89.11** **Pressure ulcer of right upper back**
    Pressure ulcer of right shoulder blade

L89.110 **Pressure ulcer of right upper back, unstageable** `HCC` `ESR`

L89.111 **Pressure ulcer of right upper back, stage 1**
Healing pressure ulcer of right upper back, stage 1
Pressure pre-ulcer skin changes limited to persistent focal edema, right upper back

L89.112 **Pressure ulcer of right upper back, stage 2** `HCC` `ESR`
Healing pressure ulcer of right upper back, stage 2
Pressure ulcer with abrasion, blister, partial thickness skin loss involving epidermis and/or dermis, right upper back

L89.113 **Pressure ulcer of right upper back, stage 3** `HCC` `ESR`
Healing pressure ulcer of right upper back, stage 3
Pressure ulcer with full thickness skin loss involving damage or necrosis of subcutaneous tissue, right upper back

L89.114 **Pressure ulcer of right upper back, stage 4** `HCC` `ESR`
Healing pressure ulcer of right upper back, stage 4
Pressure ulcer with necrosis of soft tissues through to underlying muscle, tendon, or bone, right upper back

L89.116 **Pressure-induced deep tissue damage of right upper back**

L89.119 **Pressure ulcer of right upper back, unspecified stage**
Healing pressure ulcer of right upper back NOS
Healing pressure ulcer of right upper back, unspecified stage

✓6ᵗʰ L89.12 **Pressure ulcer of left upper back**
Pressure ulcer of left shoulder blade

L89.120 **Pressure ulcer of left upper back, unstageable** `HCC` `ESR`

L89.121 **Pressure ulcer of left upper back, stage 1**
Healing pressure ulcer of left upper back, stage 1
Pressure pre-ulcer skin changes limited to persistent focal edema, left upper back

L89.122 **Pressure ulcer of left upper back, stage 2** `HCC` `ESR`
Healing pressure ulcer of left upper back, stage 2
Pressure ulcer with abrasion, blister, partial thickness skin loss involving epidermis and/or dermis, left upper back

L89.123 **Pressure ulcer of left upper back, stage 3** `HCC` `ESR`
Healing pressure ulcer of left upper back, stage 3
Pressure ulcer with full thickness skin loss involving damage or necrosis of subcutaneous tissue, left upper back

L89.124 **Pressure ulcer of left upper back, stage 4** `HCC` `ESR`
Healing pressure ulcer of left upper back, stage 4
Pressure ulcer with necrosis of soft tissues through to underlying muscle, tendon, or bone, left upper back

L89.126 **Pressure-induced deep tissue damage of left upper back**

L89.129 **Pressure ulcer of left upper back, unspecified stage**
Healing pressure ulcer of left upper back NOS
Healing pressure ulcer of left upper back, unspecified stage

✓6ᵗʰ L89.13 **Pressure ulcer of right lower back**

L89.130 **Pressure ulcer of right lower back, unstageable** `HCC` `ESR`

L89.131 **Pressure ulcer of right lower back, stage 1**
Healing pressure ulcer of right lower back, stage 1
Pressure pre-ulcer skin changes limited to persistent focal edema, right lower back

L89.132 **Pressure ulcer of right lower back, stage 2** `HCC` `ESR`
Healing pressure ulcer of right lower back, stage 2
Pressure ulcer with abrasion, blister, partial thickness skin loss involving epidermis and/or dermis, right lower back

L89.133 **Pressure ulcer of right lower back, stage 3** `HCC` `ESR`
Healing pressure ulcer of right lower back, stage 3
Pressure ulcer with full thickness skin loss involving damage or necrosis of subcutaneous tissue, right lower back

L89.134 **Pressure ulcer of right lower back, stage 4** `HCC` `ESR`
Healing pressure ulcer of right lower back, stage 4
Pressure ulcer with necrosis of soft tissues through to underlying muscle, tendon, or bone, right lower back

L89.136 **Pressure-induced deep tissue damage of right lower back**

L89.139 **Pressure ulcer of right lower back, unspecified stage**
Healing pressure ulcer of right lower back NOS
Healing pressure ulcer of right lower back, unspecified stage

✓6ᵗʰ L89.14 **Pressure ulcer of left lower back**

L89.140 **Pressure ulcer of left lower back, unstageable** `HCC` `ESR`

L89.141 **Pressure ulcer of left lower back, stage 1**
Healing pressure ulcer of left lower back, stage 1
Pressure pre-ulcer skin changes limited to persistent focal edema, left lower back

L89.142 **Pressure ulcer of left lower back, stage 2** `HCC` `ESR`
Healing pressure ulcer of left lower back, stage 2
Pressure ulcer with abrasion, blister, partial thickness skin loss involving epidermis and/or dermis, left lower back

L89.143 **Pressure ulcer of left lower back, stage 3** `HCC` `ESR`
Healing pressure ulcer of left lower back, stage 3
Pressure ulcer with full thickness skin loss involving damage or necrosis of subcutaneous tissue, left lower back

L89.144 **Pressure ulcer of left lower back, stage 4** `HCC` `ESR`
Healing pressure ulcer of left lower back, stage 4
Pressure ulcer with necrosis of soft tissues through to underlying muscle, tendon, or bone, left lower back

L89.146 **Pressure-induced deep tissue damage of left lower back**

L89.149 **Pressure ulcer of left lower back, unspecified stage**
Healing pressure ulcer of left lower back NOS
Healing pressure ulcer of left lower back, unspecified stage

☑ Additional Character Required   ✓x7ᵗʰ Placeholder Alert   **Manifestation**   **Unspecified Dx**   **Q** QPP   **UPD** Unacceptable PDx

√6ᵗʰ **L89.15** **Pressure ulcer of** sacral region
     Pressure ulcer of coccyx
     Pressure ulcer of tailbone
     AHA: 2021,3Q,10

     L89.150 **Pressure ulcer of sacral region,** unstageable   HCC ESR

     L89.151 **Pressure ulcer of sacral region,** stage 1
        Healing pressure ulcer of sacral region, stage 1
        Pressure pre-ulcer skin changes limited to persistent focal edema, sacral region

     L89.152 **Pressure ulcer of sacral region, stage 2**   HCC ESR
        Healing pressure ulcer of sacral region, stage 2
        Pressure ulcer with abrasion, blister, partial thickness skin loss involving epidermis and/or dermis, sacral region

     L89.153 **Pressure ulcer of sacral region, stage 3**   HCC ESR
        Healing pressure ulcer of sacral region, stage 3
        Pressure ulcer with full thickness skin loss involving damage or necrosis of subcutaneous tissue, sacral region

     L89.154 **Pressure ulcer of sacral region, stage 4**   HCC ESR
        Healing pressure ulcer of sacral region, stage 4
        Pressure ulcer with necrosis of soft tissues through to underlying muscle, tendon, or bone, sacral region
        AHA: 2022,2Q,8

     L89.156 **Pressure-induced** deep tissue damage **of sacral region**

     L89.159 **Pressure ulcer of sacral region, unspecified stage**
        Healing pressure ulcer of sacral region NOS
        Healing pressure ulcer of sacral region, unspecified stage

√5ᵗʰ **L89.2** **Pressure ulcer of** hip

     √6ᵗʰ **L89.20** **Pressure ulcer of unspecified hip**

     L89.200 **Pressure ulcer of unspecified hip,** unstageable   HCC ESR

     L89.201 **Pressure ulcer of unspecified hip,** stage 1
        Healing pressure ulcer of unspecified hip back, stage 1
        Pressure pre-ulcer skin changes limited to persistent focal edema, unspecified hip

     L89.202 **Pressure ulcer of unspecified hip,** stage 2   HCC ESR
        Healing pressure ulcer of unspecified hip, stage 2
        Pressure ulcer with abrasion, blister, partial thickness skin loss involving epidermis and/or dermis, unspecified hip

     L89.203 **Pressure ulcer of unspecified hip,** stage 3   HCC ESR
        Healing pressure ulcer of unspecified hip, stage 3
        Pressure ulcer with full thickness skin loss involving damage or necrosis of subcutaneous tissue, unspecified hip

     L89.204 **Pressure ulcer of unspecified hip,** stage 4   HCC ESR
        Healing pressure ulcer of unspecified hip, stage 4
        Pressure ulcer with necrosis of soft tissues through to underlying muscle, tendon, or bone, unspecified hip

     L89.206 **Pressure-induced** deep tissue damage **of unspecified hip**

     L89.209 **Pressure ulcer of unspecified hip, unspecified stage**
        Healing pressure ulcer of unspecified hip NOS
        Healing pressure ulcer of unspecified hip, unspecified stage

√6ᵗʰ **L89.21** **Pressure ulcer of** right **hip**

     L89.210 **Pressure ulcer of right hip,** unstageable   HCC ESR

     L89.211 **Pressure ulcer of right hip,** stage 1
        Healing pressure ulcer of right hip back, stage 1
        Pressure pre-ulcer skin changes limited to persistent focal edema, right hip

     L89.212 **Pressure ulcer of right hip,** stage 2   HCC ESR
        Healing pressure ulcer of right hip, stage 2
        Pressure ulcer with abrasion, blister, partial thickness skin loss involving epidermis and/or dermis, right hip

     L89.213 **Pressure ulcer of right hip,** stage 3   HCC ESR
        Healing pressure ulcer of right hip, stage 3
        Pressure ulcer with full thickness skin loss involving damage or necrosis of subcutaneous tissue, right hip

     L89.214 **Pressure ulcer of right hip,** stage 4   HCC ESR
        Healing pressure ulcer of right hip, stage 4
        Pressure ulcer with necrosis of soft tissues through to underlying muscle, tendon, or bone, right hip

     L89.216 **Pressure-induced** deep tissue damage **of right hip**

     L89.219 **Pressure ulcer of right hip, unspecified stage**
        Healing pressure ulcer of right hip NOS
        Healing pressure ulcer of right hip, unspecified stage

√6ᵗʰ **L89.22** **Pressure ulcer of** left **hip**

     L89.220 **Pressure ulcer of left hip,** unstageable   HCC ESR

     L89.221 **Pressure ulcer of left hip,** stage 1
        Healing pressure ulcer of left hip back, stage 1
        Pressure pre-ulcer skin changes limited to persistent focal edema, left hip

     L89.222 **Pressure ulcer of left hip,** stage 2   HCC ESR
        Healing pressure ulcer of left hip, stage 2
        Pressure ulcer with abrasion, blister, partial thickness skin loss involving epidermis and/or dermis, left hip

     L89.223 **Pressure ulcer of left hip,** stage 3   HCC ESR
        Healing pressure ulcer of left hip, stage 3
        Pressure ulcer with full thickness skin loss involving damage or necrosis of subcutaneous tissue, left hip

     L89.224 **Pressure ulcer of left hip,** stage 4   HCC ESR
        Healing pressure ulcer of left hip, stage 4
        Pressure ulcer with necrosis of soft tissues through to underlying muscle, tendon, or bone, left hip

     L89.226 **Pressure-induced** deep tissue damage **of left hip**

     L89.229 **Pressure ulcer of left hip, unspecified stage**
        Healing pressure ulcer of left hip NOS
        Healing pressure ulcer of left hip, unspecified stage

√5ᵗʰ **L89.3** **Pressure ulcer of** buttock
     AHA: 2021,3Q,10

     √6ᵗʰ **L89.30** **Pressure ulcer of unspecified buttock**

     L89.300 **Pressure ulcer of unspecified buttock,** unstageable   HCC ESR

L89.301 **Pressure ulcer of unspecified buttock, stage 1**
　　　Healing pressure ulcer of unspecified buttock, stage 1
　　　Pressure pre-ulcer skin changes limited to persistent focal edema, unspecified buttock

L89.302 **Pressure ulcer of unspecified buttock, stage 2** `HCC` `ESR`
　　　Healing pressure ulcer of unspecified buttock, stage 2
　　　Pressure ulcer with abrasion, blister, partial thickness skin loss involving epidermis and/or dermis, unspecified buttock

L89.303 **Pressure ulcer of unspecified buttock, stage 3** `HCC` `ESR`
　　　Healing pressure ulcer of unspecified buttock, stage 3
　　　Pressure ulcer with full thickness skin loss involving damage or necrosis of subcutaneous tissue, unspecified buttock

L89.304 **Pressure ulcer of unspecified buttock, stage 4** `HCC` `ESR`
　　　Healing pressure ulcer of unspecified buttock, stage 4
　　　Pressure ulcer with necrosis of soft tissues through to underlying muscle, tendon, or bone, unspecified buttock

L89.306 **Pressure-induced deep tissue damage of unspecified buttock**

L89.309 **Pressure ulcer of unspecified buttock, unspecified stage**
　　　Healing pressure ulcer of unspecified buttock NOS
　　　Healing pressure ulcer of unspecified buttock, unspecified stage

✓6th **L89.31** **Pressure ulcer of right buttock**

L89.310 **Pressure ulcer of right buttock, unstageable** `HCC` `ESR`

L89.311 **Pressure ulcer of right buttock, stage 1**
　　　Healing pressure ulcer of right buttock, stage 1
　　　Pressure pre-ulcer skin changes limited to persistent focal edema, right buttock

L89.312 **Pressure ulcer of right buttock, stage 2** `HCC` `ESR`
　　　Healing pressure ulcer of right buttock, stage 2
　　　Pressure ulcer with abrasion, blister, partial thickness skin loss involving epidermis and/or dermis, right buttock

L89.313 **Pressure ulcer of right buttock, stage 3** `HCC` `ESR`
　　　Healing pressure ulcer of right buttock, stage 3
　　　Pressure ulcer with full thickness skin loss involving damage or necrosis of subcutaneous tissue, right buttock

L89.314 **Pressure ulcer of right buttock, stage 4** `HCC` `ESR`
　　　Healing pressure ulcer of right buttock, stage 4
　　　Pressure ulcer with necrosis of soft tissues through to underlying muscle, tendon, or bone, right buttock

L89.316 **Pressure-induced deep tissue damage of right buttock**

L89.319 **Pressure ulcer of right buttock, unspecified stage**
　　　Healing pressure ulcer of right buttock NOS
　　　Healing pressure ulcer of right buttock, unspecified stage

✓6th **L89.32** **Pressure ulcer of left buttock**

L89.320 **Pressure ulcer of left buttock, unstageable** `HCC` `ESR`

L89.321 **Pressure ulcer of left buttock, stage 1**
　　　Healing pressure ulcer of left buttock, stage 1
　　　Pressure pre-ulcer skin changes limited to persistent focal edema, left buttock

L89.322 **Pressure ulcer of left buttock, stage 2** `HCC` `ESR`
　　　Healing pressure ulcer of left buttock, stage 2
　　　Pressure ulcer with abrasion, blister, partial thickness skin loss involving epidermis and/or dermis, left buttock

L89.323 **Pressure ulcer of left buttock, stage 3** `HCC` `ESR`
　　　Healing pressure ulcer of left buttock, stage 3
　　　Pressure ulcer with full thickness skin loss involving damage or necrosis of subcutaneous tissue, left buttock

L89.324 **Pressure ulcer of left buttock, stage 4** `HCC` `ESR`
　　　Healing pressure ulcer of left buttock, stage 4
　　　Pressure ulcer with necrosis of soft tissues through to underlying muscle, tendon, or bone, left buttock

L89.326 **Pressure-induced deep tissue damage of left buttock**

L89.329 **Pressure ulcer of left buttock, unspecified stage**
　　　Healing pressure ulcer of left buttock NOS
　　　Healing pressure ulcer of left buttock, unspecified stage

✓5th **L89.4** **Pressure ulcer of contiguous site of back, buttock and hip**

L89.40 **Pressure ulcer of contiguous site of back, buttock and hip, unspecified stage**
　　　Healing pressure ulcer of contiguous site of back, buttock and hip NOS
　　　Healing pressure ulcer of contiguous site of back, buttock and hip, unspecified stage

L89.41 **Pressure ulcer of contiguous site of back, buttock and hip, stage 1**
　　　Healing pressure ulcer of contiguous site of back, buttock and hip, stage 1
　　　Pressure pre-ulcer skin changes limited to persistent focal edema, contiguous site of back, buttock and hip

L89.42 **Pressure ulcer of contiguous site of back, buttock and hip, stage 2** `HCC` `ESR`
　　　Healing pressure ulcer of contiguous site of back, buttock and hip, stage 2
　　　Pressure ulcer with abrasion, blister, partial thickness skin loss involving epidermis and/or dermis, contiguous site of back, buttock and hip

L89.43 **Pressure ulcer of contiguous site of back, buttock and hip, stage 3** `HCC` `ESR`
　　　Healing pressure ulcer of contiguous site of back, buttock and hip, stage 3
　　　Pressure ulcer with full thickness skin loss involving damage or necrosis of subcutaneous tissue, contiguous site of back, buttock and hip

L89.44 **Pressure ulcer of contiguous site of back, buttock and hip, stage 4** `HCC` `ESR`
　　　Healing pressure ulcer of contiguous site of back, buttock and hip, stage 4
　　　Pressure ulcer with necrosis of soft tissues through to underlying muscle, tendon, or bone, contiguous site of back, buttock and hip

L89.45 **Pressure ulcer of contiguous site of back, buttock and hip, unstageable** `HCC` `ESR`

L89.46 **Pressure-induced deep tissue damage of contiguous site of back, buttock and hip**

✓5th **L89.5** **Pressure ulcer of ankle**

✓6th **L89.50** **Pressure ulcer of unspecified ankle**

L89.500 **Pressure ulcer of unspecified ankle, unstageable** `HCC` `ESR`

L89.501 **Pressure ulcer of unspecified ankle,** stage 1

     Healing pressure ulcer of unspecified ankle, stage 1

     Pressure pre-ulcer skin changes limited to persistent focal edema, unspecified ankle

L89.502 **Pressure ulcer of unspecified ankle,** stage 2   HCC ESR

     Healing pressure ulcer of unspecified ankle, stage 2

     Pressure ulcer with abrasion, blister, partial thickness skin loss involving epidermis and/or dermis, unspecified ankle

L89.503 **Pressure ulcer of unspecified ankle,** stage 3   HCC ESR

     Healing pressure ulcer of unspecified ankle, stage 3

     Pressure ulcer with full thickness skin loss involving damage or necrosis of subcutaneous tissue, unspecified ankle

L89.504 **Pressure ulcer of unspecified ankle,** stage 4   HCC ESR

     Healing pressure ulcer of unspecified ankle, stage 4

     Pressure ulcer with necrosis of soft tissues through to underlying muscle, tendon, or bone, unspecified ankle

L89.506 **Pressure-induced** deep tissue damage of **unspecified ankle**

L89.509 **Pressure ulcer of unspecified ankle, unspecified stage**

     Healing pressure ulcer of unspecified ankle NOS

     Healing pressure ulcer of unspecified ankle, unspecified stage

√6th **L89.51** **Pressure ulcer of** right **ankle**

L89.510 **Pressure ulcer of right ankle,** unstageable   HCC ESR

L89.511 **Pressure ulcer of right ankle,** stage 1

     Healing pressure ulcer of right ankle, stage 1

     Pressure pre-ulcer skin changes limited to persistent focal edema, right ankle

L89.512 **Pressure ulcer of right ankle,** stage 2   HCC ESR

     Healing pressure ulcer of right ankle, stage 2

     Pressure ulcer with abrasion, blister, partial thickness skin loss involving epidermis and/or dermis, right ankle

L89.513 **Pressure ulcer of right ankle,** stage 3   HCC ESR

     Healing pressure ulcer of right ankle, stage 3

     Pressure ulcer with full thickness skin loss involving damage or necrosis of subcutaneous tissue, right ankle

L89.514 **Pressure ulcer of right ankle,** stage 4   HCC ESR

     Healing pressure ulcer of right ankle, stage 4

     Pressure ulcer with necrosis of soft tissues through to underlying muscle, tendon, or bone, right ankle

L89.516 **Pressure-induced** deep tissue damage of **right ankle**

L89.519 **Pressure ulcer of right ankle, unspecified stage**

     Healing pressure ulcer of right ankle NOS

     Healing pressure ulcer of right ankle, unspecified stage

√6th **L89.52** **Pressure ulcer of** left **ankle**

L89.520 **Pressure ulcer of left ankle,** unstageable   HCC ESR

L89.521 **Pressure ulcer of left ankle,** stage 1

     Healing pressure ulcer of left ankle, stage 1

     Pressure pre-ulcer skin changes limited to persistent focal edema, left ankle

L89.522 **Pressure ulcer of left ankle,** stage 2   HCC ESR

     Healing pressure ulcer of left ankle, stage 2

     Pressure ulcer with abrasion, blister, partial thickness skin loss involving epidermis and/or dermis, left ankle

L89.523 **Pressure ulcer of left ankle,** stage 3   HCC ESR

     Healing pressure ulcer of left ankle, stage 3

     Pressure ulcer with full thickness skin loss involving damage or necrosis of subcutaneous tissue, left ankle

L89.524 **Pressure ulcer of left ankle,** stage 4   HCC ESR

     Healing pressure ulcer of left ankle, stage 4

     Pressure ulcer with necrosis of soft tissues through to underlying muscle, tendon, or bone, left ankle

L89.526 **Pressure-induced** deep tissue damage of **left ankle**

L89.529 **Pressure ulcer of left ankle, unspecified stage**

     Healing pressure ulcer of left ankle NOS

     Healing pressure ulcer of left ankle, unspecified stage

√5th **L89.6** **Pressure ulcer of** heel

√6th **L89.60** **Pressure ulcer of unspecified heel**

L89.600 **Pressure ulcer of unspecified heel,** unstageable   HCC ESR

L89.601 **Pressure ulcer of unspecified heel,** stage 1

     Healing pressure ulcer of unspecified heel, stage 1

     Pressure pre-ulcer skin changes limited to persistent focal edema, unspecified heel

L89.602 **Pressure ulcer of unspecified heel,** stage 2   HCC ESR

     Healing pressure ulcer of unspecified heel, stage 2

     Pressure ulcer with abrasion, blister, partial thickness skin loss involving epidermis and/or dermis, unspecified heel

L89.603 **Pressure ulcer of unspecified heel,** stage 3   HCC ESR

     Healing pressure ulcer of unspecified heel, stage 3

     Pressure ulcer with full thickness skin loss involving damage or necrosis of subcutaneous tissue, unspecified heel

L89.604 **Pressure ulcer of unspecified heel,** stage 4   HCC ESR

     Healing pressure ulcer of unspecified heel, stage 4

     Pressure ulcer with necrosis of soft tissues through to underlying muscle, tendon, or bone, unspecified heel

L89.606 **Pressure-induced** deep tissue damage of **unspecified heel**

L89.609 **Pressure ulcer of unspecified heel, unspecified stage**

     Healing pressure ulcer of unspecified heel NOS

     Healing pressure ulcer of unspecified heel, unspecified stage

√6th **L89.61** **Pressure ulcer of** right **heel**

L89.610 **Pressure ulcer of right heel,** unstageable   HCC ESR

L89.611 **Pressure ulcer of right heel,** stage 1

     Healing pressure ulcer of right heel, stage 1

     Pressure pre-ulcer skin changes limited to persistent focal edema, right heel

L89.612 Pressure ulcer of right heel, stage 2 `HCC` `ESR`
Healing pressure ulcer of right heel, stage 2
Pressure ulcer with abrasion, blister, partial thickness skin loss involving epidermis and/or dermis, right heel

L89.613 Pressure ulcer of right heel, stage 3 `HCC` `ESR`
Healing pressure ulcer of right heel, stage 3
Pressure ulcer with full thickness skin loss involving damage or necrosis of subcutaneous tissue, right heel

L89.614 Pressure ulcer of right heel, stage 4 `HCC` `ESR`
Healing pressure ulcer of right heel, stage 4
Pressure ulcer with necrosis of soft tissues through to underlying muscle, tendon, or bone, right heel

L89.616 Pressure-induced deep tissue damage of right heel

L89.619 Pressure ulcer of right heel, unspecified stage
Healing pressure ulcer of right heel NOS
Healing pressure ulcer of right heel, unspecified stage

√6th **L89.62 Pressure ulcer of left heel**

L89.620 Pressure ulcer of left heel, unstageable `HCC` `ESR`

L89.621 Pressure ulcer of left heel, stage 1
Healing pressure ulcer of left heel, stage 1
Pressure pre-ulcer skin changes limited to persistent focal edema, left heel

L89.622 Pressure ulcer of left heel, stage 2 `HCC` `ESR`
Healing pressure ulcer of left heel, stage 2
Pressure ulcer with abrasion, blister, partial thickness skin loss involving epidermis and/or dermis, left heel

L89.623 Pressure ulcer of left heel, stage 3 `HCC` `ESR`
Healing pressure ulcer of left heel, stage 3
Pressure ulcer with full thickness skin loss involving damage or necrosis of subcutaneous tissue, left heel

L89.624 Pressure ulcer of left heel, stage 4 `HCC` `ESR`
Healing pressure ulcer of left heel, stage 4
Pressure ulcer with necrosis of soft tissues through to underlying muscle, tendon, or bone, left heel

L89.626 Pressure-induced deep tissue damage of left heel

L89.629 Pressure ulcer of left heel, unspecified stage
Healing pressure ulcer of left heel NOS
Healing pressure ulcer of left heel, unspecified stage

√5th **L89.8 Pressure ulcer of other site**

√6th **L89.81 Pressure ulcer of head**
Pressure ulcer of face

L89.810 Pressure ulcer of head, unstageable `HCC` `ESR`

L89.811 Pressure ulcer of head, stage 1
Healing pressure ulcer of head, stage 1
Pressure pre-ulcer skin changes limited to persistent focal edema, head

L89.812 Pressure ulcer of head, stage 2 `HCC` `ESR`
Healing pressure ulcer of head, stage 2
Pressure ulcer with abrasion, blister, partial thickness skin loss involving epidermis and/or dermis, head

L89.813 Pressure ulcer of head, stage 3 `HCC` `ESR`
Healing pressure ulcer of head, stage 3
Pressure ulcer with full thickness skin loss involving damage or necrosis of subcutaneous tissue, head

L89.814 Pressure ulcer of head, stage 4 `HCC` `ESR`
Healing pressure ulcer of head, stage 4
Pressure ulcer with necrosis of soft tissues through to underlying muscle, tendon, or bone, head

L89.816 Pressure-induced deep tissue damage of head

L89.819 Pressure ulcer of head, unspecified stage
Healing pressure ulcer of head NOS
Healing pressure ulcer of head, unspecified stage

√6th **L89.89 Pressure ulcer of other site**

L89.890 Pressure ulcer of other site, unstageable `HCC` `ESR`

L89.891 Pressure ulcer of other site, stage 1
Healing pressure ulcer of other site, stage 1
Pressure pre-ulcer skin changes limited to persistent focal edema, other site

L89.892 Pressure ulcer of other site, stage 2 `HCC` `ESR`
Healing pressure ulcer of other site, stage 2
Pressure ulcer with abrasion, blister, partial thickness skin loss involving epidermis and/or dermis, other site

L89.893 Pressure ulcer of other site, stage 3 `HCC` `ESR`
Healing pressure ulcer of other site, stage 3
Pressure ulcer with full thickness skin loss involving damage or necrosis of subcutaneous tissue, other site

L89.894 Pressure ulcer of other site, stage 4 `HCC` `ESR`
Healing pressure ulcer of other site, stage 4
Pressure ulcer with necrosis of soft tissues through to underlying muscle, tendon, or bone, other site

L89.896 Pressure-induced deep tissue damage of other site

L89.899 Pressure ulcer of other site, unspecified stage
Healing pressure ulcer of other site NOS
Healing pressure ulcer of other site, unspecified stage

√5th **L89.9 Pressure ulcer of unspecified site**

L89.90 Pressure ulcer of unspecified site, unspecified stage
Healing pressure ulcer of unspecified site NOS
Healing pressure ulcer of unspecified site, unspecified stage

L89.91 Pressure ulcer of unspecified site, stage 1
Healing pressure ulcer of unspecified site, stage 1
Pressure pre-ulcer skin changes limited to persistent focal edema, unspecified site

L89.92 Pressure ulcer of unspecified site, stage 2 `HCC` `ESR`
Healing pressure ulcer of unspecified site, stage 2
Pressure ulcer with abrasion, blister, partial thickness skin loss involving epidermis and/or dermis, unspecified site

L89.93 Pressure ulcer of unspecified site, stage 3 `HCC` `ESR`
Healing pressure ulcer of unspecified site, stage 3
Pressure ulcer with full thickness skin loss involving damage or necrosis of subcutaneous tissue, unspecified site

L89.94 Pressure ulcer of unspecified site, stage 4 `HCC` `ESR`
Healing pressure ulcer of unspecified site, stage 4
Pressure ulcer with necrosis of soft tissues through to underlying muscle, tendon, or bone, unspecified site

L89.95 Pressure ulcer of unspecified site, unstageable `HCC` `ESR`

L89.96 Pressure-induced deep tissue damage of unspecified site

Chapter 12. Diseases of the Skin and Subcutaneous Tissue
L90–L97.109

☑4ᵗʰ **L90 Atrophic disorders of skin**

L90.0 Lichen sclerosus et atrophicus
    EXCLUDES 2   *lichen sclerosus of external female genital organs (N90.4)*
           lichen sclerosus of external male genital organs (N48.0)

L90.1 Anetoderma of Schweninger-Buzzi
L90.2 Anetoderma of Jadassohn-Pellizzari
L90.3 Atrophoderma of Pasini and Pierini
L90.4 Acrodermatitis chronica atrophicans
L90.5 Scar conditions and fibrosis of skin
    Adherent scar (skin)
    Cicatrix
    Disfigurement of skin due to scar
    Fibrosis of skin NOS
    Scar NOS
    EXCLUDES 2   *hypertrophic scar (L91.0)*
           keloid scar (L91.0)
    AHA: 2016,2Q,5; 2015,1Q,19

L90.6 Striae atrophicae
L90.8 Other atrophic disorders of skin
L90.9 Atrophic disorder of skin, unspecified

☑4ᵗʰ **L91 Hypertrophic disorders of skin**

L91.0 Hypertrophic scar
    Keloid
    Keloid scar
    EXCLUDES 2   *acne keloid (L73.0)*
           scar NOS (L90.5)
    DEF: Overgrowth of scar tissue due to excess amounts of collagen during connective tissue repair, occurring mainly on the upper trunk and face.

L91.8 Other hypertrophic disorders of the skin
L91.9 Hypertrophic disorder of the skin, unspecified   *Skin tag*

☑4ᵗʰ **L92 Granulomatous disorders of skin and subcutaneous tissue**
    EXCLUDES 2   *actinic granuloma (L57.5)*

L92.0 Granuloma annulare
    Perforating granuloma annulare
L92.1 Necrobiosis lipoidica, not elsewhere classified
    EXCLUDES 1   *necrobiosis lipoidica associated with diabetes mellitus (E08-E13 with .620)*
L92.2 Granuloma faciale [eosinophilic granuloma of skin]
L92.3 Foreign body granuloma of the skin and subcutaneous tissue
    Use additional code to identify the type of retained foreign body (Z18.-)
L92.8 Other granulomatous disorders of the skin and subcutaneous tissue
L92.9 Granulomatous disorder of the skin and subcutaneous tissue, unspecified
    EXCLUDES 2   *umbilical granuloma (P83.81)*
    AHA: 2017,4Q,21-22

☑4ᵗʰ **L93 Lupus erythematosus**
    Use additional code for adverse effect, if applicable, to identify drug (T36-T50 with fifth or sixth character 5)
    EXCLUDES 1   *lupus exedens (A18.4)*
           lupus vulgaris (A18.4)
           scleroderma (M34.-)
           systemic lupus erythematosus (M32.-)
    DEF: Inflammatory, autoimmune skin condition in which the body's autoimmune system attacks healthy tissue of the integumentary system.

L93.0 Discoid lupus erythematosus   Rx
    Lupus erythematosus NOS
L93.1 Subacute cutaneous lupus erythematosus   Rx
L93.2 Other local lupus erythematosus   Rx
    Lupus erythematosus profundus
    Lupus panniculitis

☑4ᵗʰ **L94 Other localized connective tissue disorders**
    EXCLUDES 1   *systemic connective tissue disorders (M30-M36)*

L94.0 Localized scleroderma [morphea]
    Circumscribed scleroderma
L94.1 Linear scleroderma
    En coup de sabre lesion
L94.2 Calcinosis cutis
L94.3 Sclerodactyly
L94.4 Gottron's papules
L94.5 Poikiloderma vasculare atrophicans   Rx

L94.6 Ainhum
L94.8 Other specified localized connective tissue disorders
L94.9 Localized connective tissue disorder, unspecified

☑4ᵗʰ **L95 Vasculitis limited to skin, not elsewhere classified**
    EXCLUDES 1   *angioma serpiginosum (L81.7)*
           Henoch(-Schönlein) purpura (D69.0)
           hypersensitivity angiitis (M31.0)
           lupus panniculitis (L93.2)
           panniculitis NOS (M79.3)
           panniculitis of neck and back (M54.0-)
           polyarteritis nodosa (M30.0)
           relapsing panniculitis (M35.6)
           rheumatoid vasculitis (M05.2)
           serum sickness (T80.6-)
           urticaria (L50.-)
           Wegener's granulomatosis (M31.3-)

L95.0 Livedoid vasculitis
    Atrophie blanche (en plaque)
L95.1 Erythema elevatum diutinum
L95.8 Other vasculitis limited to the skin
L95.9 Vasculitis limited to the skin, unspecified

☑4ᵗʰ **L97 Non-pressure chronic ulcer of lower limb, not elsewhere classified**
    INCLUDES   chronic ulcer of skin of lower limb NOS
           non-healing ulcer of skin
           non-infected sinus of skin
           trophic ulcer NOS
           tropical ulcer NOS
           ulcer of skin of lower limb NOS
    Code first any associated underlying condition, such as:
        any associated gangrene (I96)
        atherosclerosis of the lower extremities (I70.23-, I70.24-, I70.33-, I70.34-, I70.43-, I70.44-, I70.53-, I70.54-, I70.63-, I70.64-, I70.73-, I70.74-)
        chronic venous hypertension (I87.31-, I87.33-)
        diabetic ulcers (E08.621, E08.622, E09.621, E09.622, E10.621, E10.622, E11.621, E11.622, E13.621, E13.622)
        postphlebitic syndrome (I87.01-, I87.03-)
        postthrombotic syndrome (I87.01-, I87.03-)
        varicose ulcer (I83.0-, I83.2-)
    EXCLUDES 2   *pressure ulcer (pressure area) (L89.-)*
           skin infections (L00-L08)
           specific infections classified to A00-B99
    AHA: 2021,1Q,7; 2020,2Q,19; 2018,4Q,69; 2017,4Q,17
    TIP: Assign a code from this category/subcategory for nonpressure ulcers documented as acute.
    TIP: The depth and/or severity of a diagnosed nonpressure ulcer can be determined based on medical record documentation from clinicians who are not the patient's provider.

☑5ᵗʰ **L97.1 Non-pressure chronic ulcer of thigh**

☑6ᵗʰ **L97.10 Non-pressure chronic ulcer of unspecified thigh**

L97.101 Non-pressure chronic ulcer of unspecified thigh limited to breakdown of skin HCC Rx ESR COM
L97.102 Non-pressure chronic ulcer of unspecified thigh with fat layer exposed HCC Rx ESR COM
L97.103 Non-pressure chronic ulcer of unspecified thigh with necrosis of muscle HCC Rx ESR COM
L97.104 Non-pressure chronic ulcer of unspecified thigh with necrosis of bone HCC Rx ESR COM
L97.105 Non-pressure chronic ulcer of unspecified thigh with muscle involvement without evidence of necrosis HCC Rx ESR COM
L97.106 Non-pressure chronic ulcer of unspecified thigh with bone involvement without evidence of necrosis HCC Rx ESR COM
L97.108 Non-pressure chronic ulcer of unspecified thigh with other specified severity HCC Rx ESR COM
L97.109 Non-pressure chronic ulcer of unspecified thigh with unspecified severity HCC Rx ESR COM

√6ᵗʰ **L97.11** Non-pressure chronic ulcer of right thigh

    L97.111 **Non-pressure chronic ulcer of right thigh limited to breakdown of skin** `HCC` `Rx` `ESR` `COM`

    L97.112 **Non-pressure chronic ulcer of right thigh with fat layer exposed** `HCC` `Rx` `ESR` `COM`

    L97.113 **Non-pressure chronic ulcer of right thigh with necrosis of muscle** `HCC` `Rx` `ESR` `COM`

    L97.114 **Non-pressure chronic ulcer of right thigh with necrosis of bone** `HCC` `Rx` `ESR` `COM`

    L97.115 **Non-pressure chronic ulcer of right thigh with muscle involvement without evidence of necrosis** `HCC` `Rx` `ESR` `COM`

    L97.116 **Non-pressure chronic ulcer of right thigh with bone involvement without evidence of necrosis** `HCC` `Rx` `ESR` `COM`

    L97.118 **Non-pressure chronic ulcer of right thigh with other specified severity** `HCC` `Rx` `ESR` `COM`

    L97.119 **Non-pressure chronic ulcer of right thigh with unspecified severity** `HCC` `Rx` `ESR` `COM`

√6ᵗʰ **L97.12** Non-pressure chronic ulcer of left thigh

    L97.121 **Non-pressure chronic ulcer of left thigh limited to breakdown of skin** `HCC` `Rx` `ESR` `COM`

    L97.122 **Non-pressure chronic ulcer of left thigh with fat layer exposed** `HCC` `Rx` `ESR` `COM`

    L97.123 **Non-pressure chronic ulcer of left thigh with necrosis of muscle** `HCC` `Rx` `ESR` `COM`

    L97.124 **Non-pressure chronic ulcer of left thigh with necrosis of bone** `HCC` `Rx` `ESR` `COM`

    L97.125 **Non-pressure chronic ulcer of left thigh with muscle involvement without evidence of necrosis** `HCC` `Rx` `ESR` `COM`

    L97.126 **Non-pressure chronic ulcer of left thigh with bone involvement without evidence of necrosis** `HCC` `Rx` `ESR` `COM`

    L97.128 **Non-pressure chronic ulcer of left thigh with other specified severity** `HCC` `Rx` `ESR` `COM`

    L97.129 **Non-pressure chronic ulcer of left thigh with unspecified severity** `HCC` `Rx` `ESR` `COM`

√5ᵗʰ **L97.2** Non-pressure chronic ulcer of calf

√6ᵗʰ **L97.20** Non-pressure chronic ulcer of unspecified calf

    L97.201 **Non-pressure chronic ulcer of unspecified calf limited to breakdown of skin** `HCC` `Rx` `ESR` `COM`

    L97.202 **Non-pressure chronic ulcer of unspecified calf with fat layer exposed** `HCC` `Rx` `ESR` `COM`

    L97.203 **Non-pressure chronic ulcer of unspecified calf with necrosis of muscle** `HCC` `Rx` `ESR` `COM`

    L97.204 **Non-pressure chronic ulcer of unspecified calf with necrosis of bone** `HCC` `Rx` `ESR` `COM`

    L97.205 **Non-pressure chronic ulcer of unspecified calf with muscle involvement without evidence of necrosis** `HCC` `Rx` `ESR` `COM`

    L97.206 **Non-pressure chronic ulcer of unspecified calf with bone involvement without evidence of necrosis** `HCC` `Rx` `ESR` `COM`

    L97.208 **Non-pressure chronic ulcer of unspecified calf with other specified severity** `HCC` `Rx` `ESR` `COM`

    L97.209 **Non-pressure chronic ulcer of unspecified calf with unspecified severity** `HCC` `Rx` `ESR` `COM`

√6ᵗʰ **L97.21** Non-pressure chronic ulcer of right calf

    L97.211 **Non-pressure chronic ulcer of right calf limited to breakdown of skin** `HCC` `Rx` `ESR` `COM`

    L97.212 **Non-pressure chronic ulcer of right calf with fat layer exposed** `HCC` `Rx` `ESR` `COM`

    L97.213 **Non-pressure chronic ulcer of right calf with necrosis of muscle** `HCC` `Rx` `ESR` `COM`

    L97.214 **Non-pressure chronic ulcer of right calf with necrosis of bone** `HCC` `Rx` `ESR` `COM`

    L97.215 **Non-pressure chronic ulcer of right calf with muscle involvement without evidence of necrosis** `HCC` `Rx` `ESR` `COM`

    L97.216 **Non-pressure chronic ulcer of right calf with bone involvement without evidence of necrosis** `HCC` `Rx` `ESR` `COM`

    L97.218 **Non-pressure chronic ulcer of right calf with other specified severity** `HCC` `Rx` `ESR` `COM`

    L97.219 **Non-pressure chronic ulcer of right calf with unspecified severity** `HCC` `Rx` `ESR` `COM`

√6ᵗʰ **L97.22** Non-pressure chronic ulcer of left calf

    L97.221 **Non-pressure chronic ulcer of left calf limited to breakdown of skin** `HCC` `Rx` `ESR` `COM`

    L97.222 **Non-pressure chronic ulcer of left calf with fat layer exposed** `HCC` `Rx` `ESR` `COM`

    L97.223 **Non-pressure chronic ulcer of left calf with necrosis of muscle** `HCC` `Rx` `ESR` `COM`

    L97.224 **Non-pressure chronic ulcer of left calf with necrosis of bone** `HCC` `Rx` `ESR` `COM`

    L97.225 **Non-pressure chronic ulcer of left calf with muscle involvement without evidence of necrosis** `HCC` `Rx` `ESR` `COM`

    L97.226 **Non-pressure chronic ulcer of left calf with bone involvement without evidence of necrosis** `HCC` `Rx` `ESR` `COM`

    L97.228 **Non-pressure chronic ulcer of left calf with other specified severity** `HCC` `Rx` `ESR` `COM`

    L97.229 **Non-pressure chronic ulcer of left calf with unspecified severity** `HCC` `Rx` `ESR` `COM`

√5ᵗʰ **L97.3** Non-pressure chronic ulcer of ankle

√6ᵗʰ **L97.30** Non-pressure chronic ulcer of unspecified ankle

    L97.301 **Non-pressure chronic ulcer of unspecified ankle limited to breakdown of skin** `HCC` `Rx` `ESR` `COM`

    L97.302 **Non-pressure chronic ulcer of unspecified ankle with fat layer exposed** `HCC` `Rx` `ESR` `COM`

    L97.303 **Non-pressure chronic ulcer of unspecified ankle with necrosis of muscle** `HCC` `Rx` `ESR` `COM`

    L97.304 **Non-pressure chronic ulcer of unspecified ankle with necrosis of bone** `HCC` `Rx` `ESR` `COM`

    L97.305 **Non-pressure chronic ulcer of unspecified ankle with muscle involvement without evidence of necrosis** `HCC` `Rx` `ESR` `COM`

    L97.306 **Non-pressure chronic ulcer of unspecified ankle with bone involvement without evidence of necrosis** `HCC` `Rx` `ESR` `COM`

    L97.308 **Non-pressure chronic ulcer of unspecified ankle with other specified severity** `HCC` `Rx` `ESR` `COM`

    L97.309 **Non-pressure chronic ulcer of unspecified ankle with unspecified severity** `HCC` `Rx` `ESR` `COM`

√6ᵗʰ **L97.31** Non-pressure chronic ulcer of right ankle

    L97.311 **Non-pressure chronic ulcer of right ankle limited to breakdown of skin** `HCC` `Rx` `ESR` `COM`

    L97.312 **Non-pressure chronic ulcer of right ankle with fat layer exposed** `HCC` `Rx` `ESR` `COM`

    L97.313 **Non-pressure chronic ulcer of right ankle with necrosis of muscle** `HCC` `Rx` `ESR` `COM`

    L97.314 **Non-pressure chronic ulcer of right ankle with necrosis of bone** `HCC` `Rx` `ESR` `COM`

    L97.315 **Non-pressure chronic ulcer of right ankle with muscle involvement without evidence of necrosis** `HCC` `Rx` `ESR` `COM`

    L97.316 **Non-pressure chronic ulcer of right ankle with bone involvement without evidence of necrosis** `HCC` `Rx` `ESR` `COM`

    L97.318 **Non-pressure chronic ulcer of right ankle with other specified severity** `HCC` `Rx` `ESR` `COM`

L97.319 Non-pressure chronic ulcer of right ankle with unspecified severity `HCC` `Rx` `ESR` `COM`

✓6ᵗʰ **L97.32 Non-pressure chronic ulcer of left ankle**

L97.321 Non-pressure chronic ulcer of left ankle limited to breakdown of skin `HCC` `Rx` `ESR` `COM`

L97.322 Non-pressure chronic ulcer of left ankle with fat layer exposed `HCC` `Rx` `ESR` `COM`

L97.323 Non-pressure chronic ulcer of left ankle with necrosis of muscle `HCC` `Rx` `ESR` `COM`

L97.324 Non-pressure chronic ulcer of left ankle with necrosis of bone `HCC` `Rx` `ESR` `COM`

L97.325 Non-pressure chronic ulcer of left ankle with muscle involvement without evidence of necrosis `HCC` `Rx` `ESR` `COM`

L97.326 Non-pressure chronic ulcer of left ankle with bone involvement without evidence of necrosis `HCC` `Rx` `ESR` `COM`

L97.328 Non-pressure chronic ulcer of left ankle with other specified severity `HCC` `Rx` `ESR` `COM`

L97.329 Non-pressure chronic ulcer of left ankle with unspecified severity `HCC` `Rx` `ESR` `COM`

✓5ᵗʰ **L97.4 Non-pressure chronic ulcer of heel and midfoot**

Non-pressure chronic ulcer of plantar surface of midfoot

✓6ᵗʰ **L97.40 Non-pressure chronic ulcer of unspecified heel and midfoot**

L97.401 Non-pressure chronic ulcer of unspecified heel and midfoot limited to breakdown of skin `HCC` `Rx` `ESR` `COM`

L97.402 Non-pressure chronic ulcer of unspecified heel and midfoot with fat layer exposed `HCC` `Rx` `ESR` `COM`

L97.403 Non-pressure chronic ulcer of unspecified heel and midfoot with necrosis of muscle `HCC` `Rx` `ESR` `COM`

L97.404 Non-pressure chronic ulcer of unspecified heel and midfoot with necrosis of bone `HCC` `Rx` `ESR` `COM`

L97.405 Non-pressure chronic ulcer of unspecified heel and midfoot with muscle involvement without evidence of necrosis `HCC` `Rx` `ESR` `COM`

L97.406 Non-pressure chronic ulcer of unspecified heel and midfoot with bone involvement without evidence of necrosis `HCC` `Rx` `ESR` `COM`

L97.408 Non-pressure chronic ulcer of unspecified heel and midfoot with other specified severity `HCC` `Rx` `ESR` `COM`

L97.409 Non-pressure chronic ulcer of unspecified heel and midfoot with unspecified severity `HCC` `Rx` `ESR` `COM`

✓6ᵗʰ **L97.41 Non-pressure chronic ulcer of right heel and midfoot**

L97.411 Non-pressure chronic ulcer of right heel and midfoot limited to breakdown of skin `HCC` `Rx` `ESR` `COM`

L97.412 Non-pressure chronic ulcer of right heel and midfoot with fat layer exposed `HCC` `Rx` `ESR` `COM`
AHA: 2020,2Q,19

L97.413 Non-pressure chronic ulcer of right heel and midfoot with necrosis of muscle `HCC` `Rx` `ESR` `COM`

L97.414 Non-pressure chronic ulcer of right heel and midfoot with necrosis of bone `HCC` `Rx` `ESR` `COM`

L97.415 Non-pressure chronic ulcer of right heel and midfoot with muscle involvement without evidence of necrosis `HCC` `Rx` `ESR` `COM`

L97.416 Non-pressure chronic ulcer of right heel and midfoot with bone involvement without evidence of necrosis `HCC` `Rx` `ESR` `COM`

L97.418 Non-pressure chronic ulcer of right heel and midfoot with other specified severity `HCC` `Rx` `ESR` `COM`

L97.419 Non-pressure chronic ulcer of right heel and midfoot with unspecified severity `HCC` `Rx` `ESR` `COM`

✓6ᵗʰ **L97.42 Non-pressure chronic ulcer of left heel and midfoot**

L97.421 Non-pressure chronic ulcer of left heel and midfoot limited to breakdown of skin `HCC` `Rx` `ESR` `COM`
AHA: 2016,1Q,12

L97.422 Non-pressure chronic ulcer of left heel and midfoot with fat layer exposed `HCC` `Rx` `ESR` `COM`
AHA: 2020,2Q,19

L97.423 Non-pressure chronic ulcer of left heel and midfoot with necrosis of muscle `HCC` `Rx` `ESR` `COM`

L97.424 Non-pressure chronic ulcer of left heel and midfoot with necrosis of bone `HCC` `Rx` `ESR` `COM`

L97.425 Non-pressure chronic ulcer of left heel and midfoot with muscle involvement without evidence of necrosis `HCC` `Rx` `ESR` `COM`

L97.426 Non-pressure chronic ulcer of left heel and midfoot with bone involvement without evidence of necrosis `HCC` `Rx` `ESR` `COM`

L97.428 Non-pressure chronic ulcer of left heel and midfoot with other specified severity `HCC` `Rx` `ESR` `COM`

L97.429 Non-pressure chronic ulcer of left heel and midfoot with unspecified severity `HCC` `Rx` `ESR` `COM`

✓5ᵗʰ **L97.5 Non-pressure chronic ulcer of other part of foot**

Non-pressure chronic ulcer of toe

✓6ᵗʰ **L97.50 Non-pressure chronic ulcer of other part of unspecified foot**

L97.501 Non-pressure chronic ulcer of other part of unspecified foot limited to breakdown of skin `HCC` `Rx` `ESR` `COM`

L97.502 Non-pressure chronic ulcer of other part of unspecified foot with fat layer exposed `HCC` `Rx` `ESR` `COM`

L97.503 Non-pressure chronic ulcer of other part of unspecified foot with necrosis of muscle `HCC` `Rx` `ESR` `COM`

L97.504 Non-pressure chronic ulcer of other part of unspecified foot with necrosis of bone `HCC` `Rx` `ESR` `COM`

L97.505 Non-pressure chronic ulcer of other part of unspecified foot with muscle involvement without evidence of necrosis `HCC` `Rx` `ESR` `COM`

L97.506 Non-pressure chronic ulcer of other part of unspecified foot with bone involvement without evidence of necrosis `HCC` `Rx` `ESR` `COM`

L97.508 Non-pressure chronic ulcer of other part of unspecified foot with other specified severity `HCC` `Rx` `ESR` `COM`

L97.509 Non-pressure chronic ulcer of other part of unspecified foot with unspecified severity `HCC` `Rx` `ESR` `COM`

✓6ᵗʰ **L97.51 Non-pressure chronic ulcer of other part of right foot**
AHA: 2020,1Q,12

L97.511 Non-pressure chronic ulcer of other part of right foot limited to breakdown of skin `HCC` `Rx` `ESR` `COM`

L97.512 Non-pressure chronic ulcer of other part of right foot with fat layer exposed `HCC` `Rx` `ESR` `COM`
AHA: 2020,2Q,19

L97.513 Non-pressure chronic ulcer of other part of right foot with necrosis of muscle `HCC` `Rx` `ESR` `COM`

L97.514 Non-pressure chronic ulcer of other part of right foot with necrosis of bone `HCC` `Rx` `ESR` `COM`

L97.515 Non-pressure chronic ulcer of other part of right foot with muscle involvement without evidence of necrosis `HCC` `Rx` `ESR` `COM`

L97.516   Non-pressure chronic ulcer of other part of right foot with bone involvement without evidence of necrosis   HCC Rx ESR COM

L97.518   Non-pressure chronic ulcer of other part of right foot with other specified severity   HCC Rx ESR COM

L97.519   Non-pressure chronic ulcer of other part of right foot with unspecified severity   HCC Rx ESR COM

√6ᵗʰ L97.52   Non-pressure chronic ulcer of other part of left foot

AHA: 2020,1Q,12

L97.521   Non-pressure chronic ulcer of other part of left foot limited to breakdown of skin   HCC Rx ESR COM

L97.522   Non-pressure chronic ulcer of other part of left foot with fat layer exposed   HCC Rx ESR COM

AHA: 2020,2Q,19

L97.523   Non-pressure chronic ulcer of other part of left foot with necrosis of muscle   HCC Rx ESR COM

L97.524   Non-pressure chronic ulcer of other part of left foot with necrosis of bone   HCC Rx ESR COM

L97.525   Non-pressure chronic ulcer of other part of left foot with muscle involvement without evidence of necrosis   HCC Rx ESR COM

L97.526   Non-pressure chronic ulcer of other part of left foot with bone involvement without evidence of necrosis   HCC Rx ESR COM

L97.528   Non-pressure chronic ulcer of other part of left foot with other specified severity   HCC Rx ESR COM

L97.529   Non-pressure chronic ulcer of other part of left foot with unspecified severity   HCC Rx ESR COM

√5ᵗʰ L97.8   Non-pressure chronic ulcer of other part of lower leg

√6ᵗʰ L97.80   Non-pressure chronic ulcer of other part of unspecified lower leg

L97.801   Non-pressure chronic ulcer of other part of unspecified lower leg limited to breakdown of skin   HCC Rx ESR COM

L97.802   Non-pressure chronic ulcer of other part of unspecified lower leg with fat layer exposed   HCC Rx ESR COM

L97.803   Non-pressure chronic ulcer of other part of unspecified lower leg with necrosis of muscle   HCC Rx ESR COM

L97.804   Non-pressure chronic ulcer of other part of unspecified lower leg with necrosis of bone   HCC Rx ESR COM

L97.805   Non-pressure chronic ulcer of other part of unspecified lower leg with muscle involvement without evidence of necrosis   HCC Rx ESR COM

L97.806   Non-pressure chronic ulcer of other part of unspecified lower leg with bone involvement without evidence of necrosis   HCC Rx ESR COM

L97.808   Non-pressure chronic ulcer of other part of unspecified lower leg with other specified severity   HCC Rx ESR COM

L97.809   Non-pressure chronic ulcer of other part of unspecified lower leg with unspecified severity   HCC Rx ESR COM

√6ᵗʰ L97.81   Non-pressure chronic ulcer of other part of right lower leg

L97.811   Non-pressure chronic ulcer of other part of right lower leg limited to breakdown of skin   HCC Rx ESR COM

L97.812   Non-pressure chronic ulcer of other part of right lower leg with fat layer exposed   HCC Rx ESR COM

L97.813   Non-pressure chronic ulcer of other part of right lower leg with necrosis of muscle   HCC Rx ESR COM

L97.814   Non-pressure chronic ulcer of other part of right lower leg with necrosis of bone   HCC Rx ESR COM

L97.815   Non-pressure chronic ulcer of other part of right lower leg with muscle involvement without evidence of necrosis   HCC Rx ESR COM

L97.816   Non-pressure chronic ulcer of other part of right lower leg with bone involvement without evidence of necrosis   HCC Rx ESR COM

L97.818   Non-pressure chronic ulcer of other part of right lower leg with other specified severity   HCC Rx ESR COM

L97.819   Non-pressure chronic ulcer of other part of right lower leg with unspecified severity   HCC Rx ESR COM

√6ᵗʰ L97.82   Non-pressure chronic ulcer of other part of left lower leg

L97.821   Non-pressure chronic ulcer of other part of left lower leg limited to breakdown of skin   HCC Rx ESR COM

L97.822   Non-pressure chronic ulcer of other part of left lower leg with fat layer exposed   HCC Rx ESR COM

L97.823   Non-pressure chronic ulcer of other part of left lower leg with necrosis of muscle   HCC Rx ESR COM

L97.824   Non-pressure chronic ulcer of other part of left lower leg with necrosis of bone   HCC Rx ESR COM

L97.825   Non-pressure chronic ulcer of other part of left lower leg with muscle involvement without evidence of necrosis   HCC Rx ESR COM

L97.826   Non-pressure chronic ulcer of other part of left lower leg with bone involvement without evidence of necrosis   HCC Rx ESR COM

L97.828   Non-pressure chronic ulcer of other part of left lower leg with other specified severity   HCC Rx ESR COM

L97.829   Non-pressure chronic ulcer of other part of left lower leg with unspecified severity   HCC Rx ESR COM

√5ᵗʰ L97.9   Non-pressure chronic ulcer of unspecified part of lower leg

√6ᵗʰ L97.90   Non-pressure chronic ulcer of unspecified part of unspecified lower leg

L97.901   Non-pressure chronic ulcer of unspecified part of unspecified lower leg limited to breakdown of skin   HCC Rx ESR COM

L97.902   Non-pressure chronic ulcer of unspecified part of unspecified lower leg with fat layer exposed   HCC Rx ESR COM

L97.903   Non-pressure chronic ulcer of unspecified part of unspecified lower leg with necrosis of muscle   HCC Rx ESR COM

L97.904   Non-pressure chronic ulcer of unspecified part of unspecified lower leg with necrosis of bone   HCC Rx ESR COM

L97.905   Non-pressure chronic ulcer of unspecified part of unspecified lower leg with muscle involvement without evidence of necrosis   HCC Rx ESR COM

L97.906   Non-pressure chronic ulcer of unspecified part of unspecified lower leg with bone involvement without evidence of necrosis   HCC Rx ESR COM

L97.908   Non-pressure chronic ulcer of unspecified part of unspecified lower leg with other specified severity   HCC Rx ESR COM

L97.909   Non-pressure chronic ulcer of unspecified part of unspecified lower leg with unspecified severity   HCC Rx ESR COM

√6ᵗʰ L97.91   Non-pressure chronic ulcer of unspecified part of right lower leg

L97.911   Non-pressure chronic ulcer of unspecified part of right lower leg limited to breakdown of skin   HCC Rx ESR COM

L97.912   Non-pressure chronic ulcer of unspecified part of right lower leg with fat layer exposed   HCC Rx ESR COM

L97.913   Non-pressure chronic ulcer of unspecified part of right lower leg with necrosis of muscle   HCC Rx ESR COM

✅ Additional Character Required   √x7ᵗʰ Placeholder Alert   Manifestation   Unspecified Dx   Q QPP   UPD Unacceptable PDx

L97.914 Non-pressure chronic ulcer of unspecified part of right lower leg with necrosis of bone `HCC` `Rx` `ESR` `COM`

L97.915 Non-pressure chronic ulcer of unspecified part of right lower leg with muscle involvement without evidence of necrosis `HCC` `Rx` `ESR` `COM`

L97.916 Non-pressure chronic ulcer of unspecified part of right lower leg with bone involvement without evidence of necrosis `HCC` `Rx` `ESR` `COM`

L97.918 Non-pressure chronic ulcer of unspecified part of right lower leg with other specified severity `HCC` `Rx` `ESR` `COM`

L97.919 Non-pressure chronic ulcer of unspecified part of right lower leg with unspecified severity `HCC` `Rx` `ESR` `COM`

✓6ᵗʰ **L97.92** Non-pressure chronic ulcer of unspecified part of left lower leg

L97.921 Non-pressure chronic ulcer of unspecified part of left lower leg limited to breakdown of skin `HCC` `Rx` `ESR` `COM`

L97.922 Non-pressure chronic ulcer of unspecified part of left lower leg with fat layer exposed `HCC` `Rx` `ESR` `COM`

L97.923 Non-pressure chronic ulcer of unspecified part of left lower leg with necrosis of muscle `HCC` `Rx` `ESR` `COM`

L97.924 Non-pressure chronic ulcer of unspecified part of left lower leg with necrosis of bone `HCC` `Rx` `ESR` `COM`

L97.925 Non-pressure chronic ulcer of unspecified part of left lower leg with muscle involvement without evidence of necrosis `HCC` `Rx` `ESR` `COM`

L97.926 Non-pressure chronic ulcer of unspecified part of left lower leg with bone involvement without evidence of necrosis `HCC` `Rx` `ESR` `COM`

L97.928 Non-pressure chronic ulcer of unspecified part of left lower leg with other specified severity `HCC` `Rx` `ESR` `COM`

L97.929 Non-pressure chronic ulcer of unspecified part of left lower leg with unspecified severity `HCC` `Rx` `ESR` `COM`

✓4ᵗʰ **L98** Other disorders of skin and subcutaneous tissue, not elsewhere classified

L98.0 Pyogenic granuloma

EXCLUDES 2   pyogenic granuloma of gingiva (K06.8)
pyogenic granuloma of maxillary alveolar ridge (K04.5)
pyogenic granuloma of oral mucosa (K13.4)

DEF: Solitary polypoid capillary hemangioma often associated with local irritation, trauma, and superimposed inflammation. Located on the skin and gingival or oral mucosa, they bleed easily and may ulcerate and form crusted sores.

L98.1 Factitial dermatitis
Neurotic excoriation
EXCLUDES 1   excoriation (skin-picking) disorder (F42.4)
AHA: 2016,4Q,15
DEF: Self-inflicted skin lesions to satisfy an unconscious psychological or emotional need. Methods used to injure the skin include deep excoriations with a sharp instrument, scarification with a knife, or the application of caustic chemicals and burning, sometimes with a cigarette.

L98.2 Febrile neutrophilic dermatosis [Sweet]

L98.3 Eosinophilic cellulitis [Wells]

✓5ᵗʰ **L98.4** Non-pressure chronic ulcer of skin, not elsewhere classified
Chronic ulcer of skin NOS
Tropical ulcer NOS
Ulcer of skin NOS
EXCLUDES 2   gangrene (I96)
pressure ulcer (pressure area) (L89.-)
skin infections (L00-L08)
specific infections classified to A00-B99
ulcer of lower limb NEC (L97.-)
varicose ulcer (I83.0-I83.93)

AHA: 2017,4Q,17
TIP: The depth and/or severity of a diagnosed nonpressure ulcer can be determined based on medical record documentation from clinicians who are not the patient's provider.
TIP: Assign a code from this category/subcategory for nonpressure ulcers documented as acute.

✓6ᵗʰ **L98.41** Non-pressure chronic ulcer of buttock

L98.411 Non-pressure chronic ulcer of buttock limited to breakdown of skin `HCC` `Rx` `ESR` `COM`

L98.412 Non-pressure chronic ulcer of buttock with fat layer exposed `HCC` `Rx` `ESR` `COM`

L98.413 Non-pressure chronic ulcer of buttock with necrosis of muscle `HCC` `Rx` `ESR` `COM`

L98.414 Non-pressure chronic ulcer of buttock with necrosis of bone `HCC` `Rx` `ESR` `COM`

L98.415 Non-pressure chronic ulcer of buttock with muscle involvement without evidence of necrosis `HCC` `Rx` `ESR` `COM`

L98.416 Non-pressure chronic ulcer of buttock with bone involvement without evidence of necrosis `HCC` `Rx` `ESR` `COM`

L98.418 Non-pressure chronic ulcer of buttock with other specified severity `HCC` `Rx` `ESR` `COM`

L98.419 Non-pressure chronic ulcer of buttock with unspecified severity `HCC` `Rx` `ESR` `COM`

✓6ᵗʰ **L98.42** Non-pressure chronic ulcer of back

DM related ulcer

L98.421 Non-pressure chronic ulcer of back limited to breakdown of skin `HCC` `Rx` `ESR` `COM`

L98.422 Non-pressure chronic ulcer of back with fat layer exposed `HCC` `Rx` `ESR` `COM`

L98.423 Non-pressure chronic ulcer of back with necrosis of muscle `HCC` `Rx` `ESR` `COM`

L98.424 Non-pressure chronic ulcer of back with necrosis of bone `HCC` `Rx` `ESR` `COM`

L98.425 Non-pressure chronic ulcer of back with muscle involvement without evidence of necrosis `HCC` `Rx` `ESR` `COM`

L98.426 Non-pressure chronic ulcer of back with bone involvement without evidence of necrosis `HCC` `Rx` `ESR` `COM`

L98.428 Non-pressure chronic ulcer of back with other specified severity `HCC` `Rx` `ESR` `COM`

L98.429 Non-pressure chronic ulcer of back with unspecified severity `HCC` `Rx` `ESR` `COM`

✓6ᵗʰ **L98.49** Non-pressure chronic ulcer of skin of other sites
Non-pressure chronic ulcer of skin NOS

L98.491 Non-pressure chronic ulcer of skin of other sites limited to breakdown of skin `HCC` `Rx` `ESR` `COM`

L98.492 Non-pressure chronic ulcer of skin of other sites with fat layer exposed `HCC` `Rx` `ESR` `COM`

L98.493 Non-pressure chronic ulcer of skin of other sites with necrosis of muscle `HCC` `Rx` `ESR` `COM`

L98.494 Non-pressure chronic ulcer of skin of other sites with necrosis of bone `HCC` `Rx` `ESR` `COM`

L98.495 Non-pressure chronic ulcer of skin of other sites with muscle involvement without evidence of necrosis `HCC` `Rx` `ESR` `COM`

L98.496 Non-pressure chronic ulcer of skin of other sites with bone involvement without evidence of necrosis `HCC` `Rx` `ESR` `COM`

L98.498   **Non-pressure chronic ulcer of skin of other sites with other specified severity** `HCC` `Rx` `ESR` `COM`

L98.499   **Non-pressure chronic ulcer of skin of other sites with unspecified severity** `HCC` `Rx` `ESR` `COM`

L98.5   **Mucinosis of the skin**
Focal mucinosis
Lichen myxedematosus
Reticular erythematous mucinosis
EXCLUDES 1   *focal oral mucinosis (K13.79)*
      myxedema (E03.9)

L98.6   **Other infiltrative disorders of the skin and subcutaneous tissue**
EXCLUDES 1   *hyalinosis cutis et mucosae (E78.89)*

L98.7   **Excessive and redundant skin and subcutaneous tissue**
Loose or sagging skin, following bariatric surgery weight loss
Loose or sagging skin following dietary weight loss
Loose or sagging skin, NOS
EXCLUDES 2   *acquired excess or redundant skin of eyelid (H02.3-)*
      congenital excess or redundant skin of eyelid (Q10.3)
      skin changes due to chronic exposure to nonionizing radiation (L57.-)

AHA: 2016,4Q,36

L98.8   **Other specified disorders of the skin and subcutaneous tissue**
AHA: 2013,2Q,32

L98.9   **Disorder of the skin and subcutaneous tissue, unspecified**

L99   **Other disorders of skin and subcutaneous tissue in diseases classified elsewhere**
Code first underlying disease, such as:
amyloidosis (E85.-)
EXCLUDES 1   *skin disorders in diabetes (E08-E13 with .62-)*
      skin disorders in gonorrhea (A54.89)
      skin disorders in syphilis (A51.31, A52.79)

AHA: 2021,1Q,39

Chapter 13. Diseases of the Musculoskeletal System and Connective Tissue (M00–M99)

Chapter-specific Guidelines with Coding Examples

The chapter-specific guidelines from the ICD-10-CM Official Guidelines for Coding and Reporting have been provided below. Along with these guidelines are coding examples, contained in the shaded boxes, that have been developed to help illustrate the coding and/or sequencing guidance found in these guidelines.

a. Site and laterality

Most of the codes within Chapter 13 have site and laterality designations. The site represents the bone, joint or the muscle involved. For some conditions where more than one bone, joint or muscle is usually involved, such as osteoarthritis, there is a "multiple sites" code available. For categories where no multiple site code is provided and more than one bone, joint or muscle is involved, multiple codes should be used to indicate the different sites involved.

> Rheumatoid arthritis of multiple sites without rheumatoid factor
>
> **M06.09**   **Rheumatoid arthritis without rheumatoid factor, multiple sites**
>
> *Explanation:* For some conditions where more than one bone, joint or muscle is usually involved, such as osteoarthritis, there is a "multiple sites" code available.

> Adolescent scoliosis in the upper thoracic region and the lumbar vertebrae
>
> **M41.124**   **Adolescent idiopathic scoliosis, thoracic region**
>
> **M41.126**   **Adolescent idiopathic scoliosis, lumbar region**
>
> *Explanation:* For categories without a multiple site code and more than one bone, joint, or muscle is involved, multiple codes should be used to indicate the different sites involved.

1) Bone versus joint

For certain conditions, the bone may be affected at the upper or lower end, (e.g., avascular necrosis of bone, M87, Osteoporosis, M80, M81). Though the portion of the bone affected may be at the joint, the site designation will be the bone, not the joint.

> Idiopathic avascular necrosis of the femoral head of the left hip joint
>
> **M87.052**   **Idiopathic aseptic necrosis of left femur**
>
> *Explanation:* For certain conditions such as avascular necrosis, the bone may be affected at the joint, but the site designation is the bone, not the joint.

b. Acute traumatic versus chronic or recurrent musculoskeletal conditions

Many musculoskeletal conditions are a result of previous injury or trauma to a site, or are recurrent conditions. Bone, joint or muscle conditions that are the result of a healed injury are usually found in chapter 13. Recurrent bone, joint or muscle conditions are also usually found in chapter 13. Any current, acute injury should be coded to the appropriate injury code from chapter 19. Chronic or recurrent conditions should generally be coded with a code from chapter 13. If it is difficult to determine from the documentation in the record which code is best to describe a condition, query the provider.

> Acute traumatic bucket handle tear of right medial meniscus
>
> **S83.211A**   **Bucket-handle tear of medial meniscus, current injury, right knee, initial encounter**
>
> *Explanation:* Any current, acute injury is not coded in chapter 13. It should instead be coded to the appropriate injury code from chapter 19.

> Old bucket handle tear of right medial meniscus
>
> **M23.203**   **Derangement of unspecified medial meniscus due to old tear or injury, right knee**
>
> *Explanation:* Chronic or recurrent conditions should generally be coded with a code from chapter 13.

c. Coding of Pathologic Fractures

7th character A is for use as long as the patient is receiving active treatment for the fracture. Examples of active treatment are: surgical treatment, emergency department encounter, evaluation and continuing treatment by the same or a different physician. While the patient may be seen by a new or different provider over the course of treatment for a pathological fracture, assignment of the 7th character is based on whether the patient is undergoing active treatment and not whether the provider is seeing the patient for the first time.

> Pathologic fracture of left foot, unknown cause, currently under active treatment by a follow-up provider
>
> **M84.475A**   **Pathological fracture, left foot, initial encounter for fracture**
>
> *Explanation:* Seventh character A is for use as long as the patient is receiving active treatment for a pathologic fracture. Examples of active treatment are surgical treatment, emergency department encounter, evaluation, and continuing treatment by the same or a different physician.
>
> The seventh character is based on whether the patient is undergoing active treatment and not whether the provider is seeing the patient for the first time.

7th character D is to be used for encounters after the patient has completed active treatment for the fracture and is receiving routine care for the fracture during the healing or recovery phase. The other 7th characters, listed under each subcategory in the Tabular List, are to be used for subsequent encounters for treatment of problems associated with the healing, such as malunions, nonunions, and sequelae.

Care for complications of surgical treatment for fracture repairs during the healing or recovery phase should be coded with the appropriate complication codes.

See Section I.C.19. Coding of traumatic fractures.

d. Osteoporosis

Osteoporosis is a systemic condition, meaning that all bones of the musculoskeletal system are affected. Therefore, site is not a component of the codes under category M81, Osteoporosis without current pathological fracture. The site codes under category M80, Osteoporosis with current pathological fracture, identify the site of the fracture, not the osteoporosis.

1) Osteoporosis without pathological fracture

Category M81, Osteoporosis without current pathological fracture, is for use for patients with osteoporosis who do not currently have a pathologic fracture due to the osteoporosis, even if they have had a fracture in the past. For patients with a history of osteoporosis fractures, status code Z87.310, Personal history of (healed) osteoporosis fracture, should follow the code from M81.

> Age-related osteoporosis with healed osteoporotic fracture of the lumbar vertebra
>
> **M81.0**   **Age-related osteoporosis without current pathological fracture**
>
> **Z87.310**   **Personal history of (healed) osteoporosis fracture**
>
> *Explanation:* Category M81 is used for patients with osteoporosis who do not currently have a pathologic fracture due to the osteoporosis. To report a previous (healed) fracture, status code Z87.310 Personal history of (healed) osteoporosis fracture, should follow the code from M81.

2) Osteoporosis with current pathological fracture

Category M80, Osteoporosis with current pathological fracture, is for patients who have a current pathologic fracture at the time of an encounter. The codes under M80 identify the site of the fracture. A code from category M80, not a traumatic fracture code, should be used for any patient with known osteoporosis who suffers a fracture, even if the patient had a minor fall or trauma, if that fall or trauma would not usually break a normal, healthy bone.

> Disuse osteoporosis with current fracture of right shoulder sustained lifting a grocery bag, initial encounter
>
> **M80.811A**   **Other osteoporosis with current pathological fracture, right shoulder, initial encounter for fracture**
>
> *Explanation:* A code from category M80, not a traumatic fracture code, should be used for any patient with known osteoporosis who suffers a fracture, even if the patient had a minor fall or trauma, if that fall or trauma would not usually break a normal, healthy bone.

e. Multisystem inflammatory syndrome

See Section I.C.1.g.1.l. for Multisystem Inflammatory Syndrome

Muscle/Tendon Table

ICD-10-CM categorizes certain muscles and tendons in the upper and lower extremities by their action (e.g., extension, flexion), their anatomical location (e.g., posterior, anterior), and/or whether they are intrinsic or extrinsic to a certain anatomical area. The Muscle/Tendon Table is provided at the beginning of chapters 13 and 19 as a resource to help users when code selection depends on one or more of these characteristics. A **TIP** has been placed at those categories and/or subcategories that relate to this table. Please note that this table is not all-inclusive, and proper code assignment should be based on the provider's documentation.

Body Region	Muscle	Extensor Tendon	Flexor Tendon	Other Tendon
Shoulder				
	Deltoid	Posterior deltoid	Anterior deltoid	
	Rotator cuff			
	Infraspinatus			Infraspinatus
	Subscapularis			Subscapularis
	Supraspinatus			Supraspinatus
	Teres minor			Teres minor
	Teres major	Teres major		
Upper arm				
	Anterior muscles			
	Biceps brachii — long head		Biceps brachii — long head	
	Biceps brachii — short head		Biceps brachii — short head	
	Brachialis		Brachialis	
	Coracobrachialis		Coracobrachialis	
	Posterior muscles			
	Triceps brachii	Triceps brachii		
Forearm				
	Anterior muscles			
	Flexors			
	Deep			
	Flexor digitorum profundus		Flexor digitorum profundus	
	Flexor pollicis longus		Flexor pollicis longus	
	Intermediate			
	Flexor digitorum superficialis		Flexor digitorum superficialis	
	Superficial			
	Flexor carpi radialis		Flexor carpi radialis	
	Flexor carpi ulnaris		Flexor carpi ulnaris	
	Palmaris longus		Palmaris longus	
	Pronators			
	Pronator quadratus			Pronator quadratus
	Pronator teres			Pronator teres
	Posterior muscles			
	Extensors			
	Deep			
	Abductor pollicis longus			Abductor pollicis longus
	Extensor indicis	Extensor indicis		
	Extensor pollicis brevis	Extensor pollicis brevis		
	Extensor pollicis longus	Extensor pollicis longus		
	Superficial			
	Brachioradialis			Brachioradialis
	Extensor carpi radialis brevis	Extensor carpi radialis brevis		
	Extensor carpi radialis longus	Extensor carpi radialis longus		
	Extensor carpi ulnaris	Extensor carpi ulnaris		
	Extensor digiti minimi	Extensor digiti minimi		
	Extensor digitorum	Extensor digitorum		
	Anconeus	Anconeus		
	Supinator			Supinator

Body Region	Muscle	Extensor Tendon	Flexor Tendon	Other Tendon
Hand				
Extrinsic — attach to a site in the forearm as well as a site in the hand with action related to hand movement at the wrist				
	Extensor carpi radialis brevis	Extensor carpi radialis brevis		
	Extensor carpi radialis longus	Extensor carpi radialis longus		
	Extensor carpi ulnaris	Extensor carpi ulnaris		
	Flexor carpi radialis		Flexor carpi radialis	
	Flexor carpi ulnaris		Flexor carpi ulnaris	
	Flexor digitorum superficialis		Flexor digitorum superficialis	
	Palmaris longus		Palmaris longus	
Extrinsic — attach to a site in the forearm as well as a site in the hand with action in the hand related to finger movement				
	Adductor pollicis longus			Adductor pollicis longus
	Extensor digiti minimi	Extensor digiti minimi		
	Extensor digitorum	Extensor digitorum		
	Extensor indicis	Extensor indicis		
	Flexor digitorum profundus		Flexor digitorum profundus	
	Flexor digitorum superficialis		Flexor digitorum superficialis	
Extrinsic — attach to a site in the forearm as well as a site in the hand with action in the hand related to thumb movement				
	Extensor pollicis brevis	Extensor pollicis brevis		
	Extensor pollicis longus	Extensor pollicis longus		
	Flexor pollicis longus		Flexor pollicis longus	
Intrinsic — found within the hand only				
	Adductor pollicis			Adductor pollicis
	Dorsal interossei	Dorsal interossei	Dorsal interossei	
	Lumbricals	Lumbricals	Lumbricals	
	Palmaris brevis			Palmaris brevis
	Palmar interossei	Palmar interossei	Palmar interossei	
	Hypothenar muscles			
	Abductor digiti minimi			Abductor digiti minimi
	Flexor digiti minimi brevis		Flexor digiti minimi brevis	
	Opponens digiti minimi		Opponens digiti minimi	
	Thenar muscles			
	Abductor pollicis brevis			Abductor pollicis brevis
	Flexor pollicis brevis		Flexor pollicis brevis	
	Opponens pollicis		Opponens pollicis	
Thigh				
	Anterior muscles			
	Iliopsoas		Iliopsoas	
	Pectineus		Pectineus	
	Quadriceps	Quadriceps		
	Rectus femoris	Rectus femoris — Extends knee	Rectus femoris — Flexes hip	
	Vastus intermedius	Vastus intermedius		
	Vastus lateralis	Vastus lateralis		
	Vastus medialis	Vastus medialis		
	Sartorius		Sartorius	
	Medial muscles			
	Adductor brevis			Adductor brevis
	Adductor longus			Adductor longus
	Adductor magnus			Adductor magnus
	Gracilis			Gracilis
	Obturator externus			Obturator externus
	Posterior muscles			
	Hamstring	Hamstring — Extends hip	Hamstring — Flexes knee	
	Biceps femoris	Biceps femoris	Biceps femoris	
	Semimembranosus	Semimembranosus	Semimembranosus	
	Semitendinosus	Semitendinosus	Semitendinosus	

Body Region	Muscle	Extensor Tendon	Flexor Tendon	Other Tendon
Lower leg				
	Anterior muscles			
	Extensor digitorum longus	Extensor digitorum longus		
	Extensor hallucis longus	Extensor hallucis longus		
	Fibularis (peroneus) tertius	Fibularis (peroneus) tertius		
	Tibialis anterior	Tibialis anterior		Tibialis anterior
	Lateral muscles			
	Fibularis (peroneus) brevis		Fibularis (peroneus) brevis	
	Fibularis (peroneus) longus		Fibularis (peroneus) longus	
	Posterior muscles			
	Deep			
	Flexor digitorum longus		Flexor digitorum longus	
	Flexor hallucis longus		Flexor hallucis longus	
	Popliteus		Popliteus	
	Tibialis posterior		Tibialis posterior	
	Superficial			
	Gastrocnemius		Gastrocnemius	
	Plantaris		Plantaris	
	Soleus		Soleus	
				Calcaneal (Achilles)
Ankle/Foot				
Extrinsic — attach to a site in the lower leg as well as a site in the foot with action related to foot movement at the ankle				
	Plantaris		Plantaris	
	Soleus		Soleus	
	Tibialis anterior	Tibialis anterior		
	Tibialis posterior		Tibialis posterior	
Extrinsic — attach to a site in the lower leg as well as a site in the foot with action in the foot related to toe movement				
	Extensor digitorum longus	Extensor digitorum longus		
	Extensor hallucis longus	Extensor hallucis longus		
	Flexor digitorum longus		Flexor digitorum longus	
	Flexor hallucis longus		Flexor hallucis longus	
Intrinsic — found within the ankle/foot only				
	Dorsal muscles			
	Extensor digitorum brevis	Extensor digitorum brevis		
	Extensor hallucis brevis	Extensor hallucis brevis		
	Plantar muscles			
	Abductor digiti minimi		Abductor digiti minimi	
	Abductor hallucis		Abductor hallucis	
	Dorsal interossei	Dorsal interossei	Dorsal interossei	
	Flexor digiti minimi brevis		Flexor digiti minimi brevis	
	Flexor digitorum brevis		Flexor digitorum brevis	
	Flexor hallucis brevis		Flexor hallucis brevis	
	Lumbricals	Lumbricals	Lumbricals	
	Quadratus plantae		Quadratus plantae	
	Plantar interossei	Plantar interossei	Plantar interossei	

Chapter 13. Diseases of the Musculoskeletal System and Connective Tissue (M00-M99)

NOTE   Use an external cause code following the code for the musculoskeletal condition, if applicable, to identify the cause of the musculoskeletal condition

EXCLUDES 2   *arthropathic psoriasis (L40.5-)*
certain conditions originating in the perinatal period (P04-P96)
certain infectious and parasitic diseases (A00-B99)
compartment syndrome (traumatic) (T79.A-)
complications of pregnancy, childbirth and the puerperium (O00-O9A)
congenital malformations, deformations, and chromosomal abnormalities (Q00-Q99)
endocrine, nutritional and metabolic diseases (E00-E88)
injury, poisoning and certain other consequences of external causes (S00-T88)
neoplasms (C00-D49)
symptoms, signs and abnormal clinical and laboratory findings, not elsewhere classified (R00-R94)

This chapter contains the following blocks:

M00-M02   Infectious arthropathies
M04   Autoinflammatory syndromes
M05-M14   Inflammatory polyarthropathies
M15-M19   Osteoarthritis
M20-M25   Other joint disorders
M26-M27   Dentofacial anomalies [including malocclusion] and other disorders of jaw
M30-M36   Systemic connective tissue disorders
M40-M43   Deforming dorsopathies
M45-M49   Spondylopathies
M50-M54   Other dorsopathies
M60-M63   Disorders of muscles
M65-M67   Disorders of synovium and tendon
M70-M79   Other soft tissue disorders
M80-M85   Disorders of bone density and structure
M86-M90   Other osteopathies
M91-M94   Chondropathies
M95   Other disorders of the musculoskeletal system and connective tissue
M96   Intraoperative and postprocedural complications and disorders of musculoskeletal system, not elsewhere classified
M97   Periprosthetic fracture around internal prosthetic joint
M99   Biomechanical lesions, not elsewhere classified

ARTHROPATHIES (M00-M25)

INCLUDES   disorders affecting predominantly peripheral (limb) joints

Infectious arthropathies (M00-M02)

NOTE   This block comprises arthropathies due to microbiological agents. Distinction is made between the following types of etiological relationship:

a) direct infection of joint, where organisms invade synovial tissue and microbial antigen is present in the joint;

b) indirect infection, which may be of two types: a reactive arthropathy, where microbial infection of the body is established but neither organisms nor antigens can be identified in the joint, and a postinfective arthropathy, where microbial antigen is present but recovery of an organism is inconstant and evidence of local multiplication is lacking.

AHA: 2019,3Q,16

✓4ᵗʰ **M00 Pyogenic arthritis**

    EXCLUDES 2   *infection and inflammatory reaction due to internal joint prosthesis (T84.5-)*

    AHA: 2022,1Q,31
    DEF: Pyogenic: Relating to or involving pus production, often referred to as suppurative or purulent.

    ✓5ᵗʰ **M00.0 Staphylococcal arthritis and polyarthritis**
       Use additional code (B95.61-B95.8) to identify bacterial agent

       M00.00 Staphylococcal arthritis, unspecified joint   HCC ESR COM

       ✓6ᵗʰ **M00.01** Staphylococcal arthritis, shoulder
          M00.011 Staphylococcal arthritis, right shoulder   HCC ESR COM
          M00.012 Staphylococcal arthritis, left shoulder   HCC ESR COM
          M00.019 Staphylococcal arthritis, unspecified shoulder   HCC ESR COM

       ✓6ᵗʰ **M00.02** Staphylococcal arthritis, elbow
          M00.021 Staphylococcal arthritis, right elbow   HCC ESR COM
          M00.022 Staphylococcal arthritis, left elbow   HCC ESR COM

          M00.029 Staphylococcal arthritis, unspecified elbow   HCC ESR COM

       ✓6ᵗʰ **M00.03** Staphylococcal arthritis, wrist
          Staphylococcal arthritis of carpal bones
          M00.031 Staphylococcal arthritis, right wrist   HCC ESR COM
          M00.032 Staphylococcal arthritis, left wrist   HCC ESR COM
          M00.039 Staphylococcal arthritis, unspecified wrist   HCC ESR COM

       ✓6ᵗʰ **M00.04** Staphylococcal arthritis, hand
          Staphylococcal arthritis of metacarpus and phalanges
          M00.041 Staphylococcal arthritis, right hand   HCC ESR COM
          M00.042 Staphylococcal arthritis, left hand   HCC ESR COM
          M00.049 Staphylococcal arthritis, unspecified hand   HCC ESR COM

       ✓6ᵗʰ **M00.05** Staphylococcal arthritis, hip
          M00.051 Staphylococcal arthritis, right hip   HCC ESR COM
          M00.052 Staphylococcal arthritis, left hip   HCC ESR COM
          M00.059 Staphylococcal arthritis, unspecified hip   HCC ESR COM

       ✓6ᵗʰ **M00.06** Staphylococcal arthritis, knee
          M00.061 Staphylococcal arthritis, right knee   HCC ESR COM
          M00.062 Staphylococcal arthritis, left knee   HCC ESR COM
          M00.069 Staphylococcal arthritis, unspecified knee   HCC ESR COM

       ✓6ᵗʰ **M00.07** Staphylococcal arthritis, ankle and foot
          Staphylococcal arthritis, tarsus, metatarsus and phalanges
          M00.071 Staphylococcal arthritis, right ankle and foot   HCC ESR COM
          M00.072 Staphylococcal arthritis, left ankle and foot   HCC ESR COM
          M00.079 Staphylococcal arthritis, unspecified ankle and foot   HCC ESR COM

       M00.08 Staphylococcal arthritis, vertebrae   HCC ESR COM
       M00.09 Staphylococcal polyarthritis   HCC ESR COM

    ✓5ᵗʰ **M00.1 Pneumococcal arthritis and polyarthritis**
       M00.10 Pneumococcal arthritis, unspecified joint   HCC ESR COM

       ✓6ᵗʰ **M00.11** Pneumococcal arthritis, shoulder
          M00.111 Pneumococcal arthritis, right shoulder   HCC ESR COM
          M00.112 Pneumococcal arthritis, left shoulder   HCC ESR COM
          M00.119 Pneumococcal arthritis, unspecified shoulder   HCC ESR COM

       ✓6ᵗʰ **M00.12** Pneumococcal arthritis, elbow
          M00.121 Pneumococcal arthritis, right elbow   HCC ESR COM
          M00.122 Pneumococcal arthritis, left elbow   HCC ESR COM
          M00.129 Pneumococcal arthritis, unspecified elbow   HCC ESR COM

       ✓6ᵗʰ **M00.13** Pneumococcal arthritis, wrist
          Pneumococcal arthritis of carpal bones
          M00.131 Pneumococcal arthritis, right wrist   HCC ESR COM
          M00.132 Pneumococcal arthritis, left wrist   HCC ESR COM
          M00.139 Pneumococcal arthritis, unspecified wrist   HCC ESR COM

       ✓6ᵗʰ **M00.14** Pneumococcal arthritis, hand
          Pneumococcal arthritis of metacarpus and phalanges
          M00.141 Pneumococcal arthritis, right hand   HCC ESR COM
          M00.142 Pneumococcal arthritis, left hand   HCC ESR COM
          M00.149 Pneumococcal arthritis, unspecified hand   HCC ESR COM

Chapter 13. Diseases of the Musculoskeletal System and Connective Tissue

✓6ᵗʰ **M00.15 Pneumococcal arthritis,** hip

   M00.151 Pneumococcal arthritis, right hip `HCC` `ESR` `COM`

   M00.152 Pneumococcal arthritis, left hip `HCC` `ESR` `COM`

   M00.159 Pneumococcal arthritis, unspecified hip `HCC` `ESR` `COM`

✓6ᵗʰ **M00.16 Pneumococcal arthritis,** knee

   M00.161 Pneumococcal arthritis, right knee `HCC` `ESR` `COM`

   M00.162 Pneumococcal arthritis, left knee `HCC` `ESR` `COM`

   M00.169 Pneumococcal arthritis, unspecified knee `HCC` `ESR` `COM`

✓6ᵗʰ **M00.17 Pneumococcal arthritis,** ankle and foot

   Pneumococcal arthritis, tarsus, metatarsus and phalanges

   M00.171 Pneumococcal arthritis, right ankle and foot `HCC` `ESR` `COM`

   M00.172 Pneumococcal arthritis, left ankle and foot `HCC` `ESR` `COM`

   M00.179 Pneumococcal arthritis, unspecified ankle and foot `HCC` `ESR` `COM`

M00.18 Pneumococcal arthritis, vertebrae `HCC` `ESR` `COM`

M00.19 Pneumococcal polyarthritis `HCC` `ESR` `COM`

✓5ᵗʰ **M00.2 Other streptococcal arthritis and polyarthritis**

   Use additional code (B95.0-B95.2, B95.4-B95.5) to identify bacterial agent

   M00.20 Other streptococcal arthritis, unspecified joint `HCC` `ESR` `COM`

✓6ᵗʰ **M00.21 Other streptococcal arthritis,** shoulder

   M00.211 Other streptococcal arthritis, right shoulder `HCC` `ESR` `COM`

   M00.212 Other streptococcal arthritis, left shoulder `HCC` `ESR` `COM`

   M00.219 Other streptococcal arthritis, unspecified shoulder `HCC` `ESR` `COM`

✓6ᵗʰ **M00.22 Other streptococcal arthritis,** elbow

   M00.221 Other streptococcal arthritis, right elbow `HCC` `ESR` `COM`

   M00.222 Other streptococcal arthritis, left elbow `HCC` `ESR` `COM`

   M00.229 Other streptococcal arthritis, unspecified elbow `HCC` `ESR` `COM`

✓6ᵗʰ **M00.23 Other streptococcal arthritis,** wrist

   Other streptococcal arthritis of carpal bones

   M00.231 Other streptococcal arthritis, right wrist `HCC` `ESR` `COM`

   M00.232 Other streptococcal arthritis, left wrist `HCC` `ESR` `COM`

   M00.239 Other streptococcal arthritis, unspecified wrist `HCC` `ESR` `COM`

✓6ᵗʰ **M00.24 Other streptococcal arthritis,** hand

   Other streptococcal arthritis metacarpus and phalanges

   M00.241 Other streptococcal arthritis, right hand `HCC` `ESR` `COM`

   M00.242 Other streptococcal arthritis, left hand `HCC` `ESR` `COM`

   M00.249 Other streptococcal arthritis, unspecified hand `HCC` `ESR` `COM`

✓6ᵗʰ **M00.25 Other streptococcal arthritis,** hip

   M00.251 Other streptococcal arthritis, right hip `HCC` `ESR` `COM`

   M00.252 Other streptococcal arthritis, left hip `HCC` `ESR` `COM`

   M00.259 Other streptococcal arthritis, unspecified hip `HCC` `ESR` `COM`

✓6ᵗʰ **M00.26 Other streptococcal arthritis,** knee

   M00.261 Other streptococcal arthritis, right knee `HCC` `ESR` `COM`

   M00.262 Other streptococcal arthritis, left knee `HCC` `ESR` `COM`

   M00.269 Other streptococcal arthritis, unspecified knee `HCC` `ESR` `COM`

✓6ᵗʰ **M00.27 Other streptococcal arthritis,** ankle and foot

   Other streptococcal arthritis, tarsus, metatarsus and phalanges

   M00.271 Other streptococcal arthritis, right ankle and foot `HCC` `ESR` `COM`

   M00.272 Other streptococcal arthritis, left ankle and foot `HCC` `ESR` `COM`

   M00.279 Other streptococcal arthritis, unspecified ankle and foot `HCC` `ESR` `COM`

M00.28 Other streptococcal arthritis, vertebrae `HCC` `ESR` `COM`

M00.29 Other streptococcal polyarthritis `HCC` `ESR` `COM`

✓5ᵗʰ **M00.8 Arthritis and polyarthritis due to other bacteria**

   Use additional code (B96) to identify bacteria

   M00.80 Arthritis due to other bacteria, unspecified joint `HCC` `ESR` `COM`

✓6ᵗʰ **M00.81 Arthritis due to other bacteria,** shoulder

   M00.811 Arthritis due to other bacteria, right shoulder `HCC` `ESR` `COM`

   M00.812 Arthritis due to other bacteria, left shoulder `HCC` `ESR` `COM`

   M00.819 Arthritis due to other bacteria, unspecified shoulder `HCC` `ESR` `COM`

✓6ᵗʰ **M00.82 Arthritis due to other bacteria,** elbow

   M00.821 Arthritis due to other bacteria, right elbow `HCC` `ESR` `COM`

   M00.822 Arthritis due to other bacteria, left elbow `HCC` `ESR` `COM`

   M00.829 Arthritis due to other bacteria, unspecified elbow `HCC` `ESR` `COM`

✓6ᵗʰ **M00.83 Arthritis due to other bacteria,** wrist

   Arthritis due to other bacteria, carpal bones

   M00.831 Arthritis due to other bacteria, right wrist `HCC` `ESR` `COM`

   M00.832 Arthritis due to other bacteria, left wrist `HCC` `ESR` `COM`

   M00.839 Arthritis due to other bacteria, unspecified wrist `HCC` `ESR` `COM`

✓6ᵗʰ **M00.84 Arthritis due to other bacteria,** hand

   Arthritis due to other bacteria, metacarpus and phalanges

   M00.841 Arthritis due to other bacteria, right hand `HCC` `ESR` `COM`

   M00.842 Arthritis due to other bacteria, left hand `HCC` `ESR` `COM`

   M00.849 Arthritis due to other bacteria, unspecified hand `HCC` `ESR` `COM`

✓6ᵗʰ **M00.85 Arthritis due to other bacteria,** hip

   M00.851 Arthritis due to other bacteria, right hip `HCC` `ESR` `COM`

   M00.852 Arthritis due to other bacteria, left hip `HCC` `ESR` `COM`

   M00.859 Arthritis due to other bacteria, unspecified hip `HCC` `ESR` `COM`

✓6ᵗʰ **M00.86 Arthritis due to other bacteria,** knee

   AHA: 2019,3Q,16

   M00.861 Arthritis due to other bacteria, right knee `HCC` `ESR` `COM`

   M00.862 Arthritis due to other bacteria, left knee `HCC` `ESR` `COM`

   M00.869 Arthritis due to other bacteria, unspecified knee `HCC` `ESR` `COM`

✓6ᵗʰ **M00.87 Arthritis due to other bacteria,** ankle and foot

   Arthritis due to other bacteria, tarsus, metatarsus, and phalanges

   M00.871 Arthritis due to other bacteria, right ankle and foot `HCC` `ESR` `COM`

   M00.872 Arthritis due to other bacteria, left ankle and foot `HCC` `ESR` `COM`

   M00.879 Arthritis due to other bacteria, unspecified ankle and foot `HCC` `ESR` `COM`

M00.88 Arthritis due to other bacteria, vertebrae `HCC` `ESR` `COM`

M00.89 Polyarthritis due to other bacteria `HCC` `ESR` `COM`

`HCC` CMS-HCC   `Rx` Rx HCC   `ESR` ESRD HCC   `COM` Commercial HCC   `N` Newborn: 0   `P` Pediatric: 0-17   `M` Maternity: 9-64   `A` Adult: 15-124

778   ICD-10-CM 2023

M00.9   **Pyogenic arthritis, unspecified**   HCC ESR COM
    Infective arthritis NOS

✓4ᵗʰ **M01**   **Direct infections of joint in infectious and parasitic diseases classified elsewhere**
    Code first underlying disease, such as:
      leprosy [Hansen's disease] (A30.-)
      mycoses (B35-B49)
      O'nyong-nyong fever (A92.1)
      paratyphoid fever (A01.1-A01.4)
    EXCLUDES 1   *arthropathy in Lyme disease (A69.23)*
          gonococcal arthritis (A54.42)
          meningococcal arthritis (A39.83)
          mumps arthritis (B26.85)
          postinfective arthropathy (M02.-)
          postmeningococcal arthritis (A39.84)
          reactive arthritis (M02.3)
          rubella arthritis (B06.82)
          sarcoidosis arthritis (D86.86)
          typhoid fever arthritis (A01.04)
          tuberculosis arthritis (A18.01-A18.02)

✓5ᵗʰ **M01.X**   **Direct infection of joint in infectious and parasitic diseases classified elsewhere**

    M01.X0   *Direct infection of unspecified joint in infectious and parasitic diseases classified elsewhere*   HCC ESR COM

✓6ᵗʰ **M01.X1**   **Direct infection of shoulder joint in infectious and parasitic diseases classified elsewhere**
    M01.X11   *Direct infection of right shoulder in infectious and parasitic diseases classified elsewhere*   HCC ESR COM
    M01.X12   *Direct infection of left shoulder in infectious and parasitic diseases classified elsewhere*   HCC ESR COM
    M01.X19   *Direct infection of unspecified shoulder in infectious and parasitic diseases classified elsewhere*   HCC ESR COM

✓6ᵗʰ **M01.X2**   **Direct infection of elbow in infectious and parasitic diseases classified elsewhere**
    M01.X21   *Direct infection of right elbow in infectious and parasitic diseases classified elsewhere*   HCC ESR COM
    M01.X22   *Direct infection of left elbow in infectious and parasitic diseases classified elsewhere*   HCC ESR COM
    M01.X29   *Direct infection of unspecified elbow in infectious and parasitic diseases classified elsewhere*   HCC ESR COM

✓6ᵗʰ **M01.X3**   **Direct infection of wrist in infectious and parasitic diseases classified elsewhere**
    Direct infection of carpal bones in infectious and parasitic diseases classified elsewhere
    M01.X31   *Direct infection of right wrist in infectious and parasitic diseases classified elsewhere*   HCC ESR COM
    M01.X32   *Direct infection of left wrist in infectious and parasitic diseases classified elsewhere*   HCC ESR COM
    M01.X39   *Direct infection of unspecified wrist in infectious and parasitic diseases classified elsewhere*   HCC ESR COM

✓6ᵗʰ **M01.X4**   **Direct infection of hand in infectious and parasitic diseases classified elsewhere**
    Direct infection of metacarpus and phalanges in infectious and parasitic diseases classified elsewhere
    M01.X41   *Direct infection of right hand in infectious and parasitic diseases classified elsewhere*   HCC ESR COM
    M01.X42   *Direct infection of left hand in infectious and parasitic diseases classified elsewhere*   HCC ESR COM
    M01.X49   *Direct infection of unspecified hand in infectious and parasitic diseases classified elsewhere*   HCC ESR COM

✓6ᵗʰ **M01.X5**   **Direct infection of hip in infectious and parasitic diseases classified elsewhere**
    M01.X51   *Direct infection of right hip in infectious and parasitic diseases classified elsewhere*   HCC ESR COM

    M01.X52   *Direct infection of left hip in infectious and parasitic diseases classified elsewhere*   HCC ESR COM
    M01.X59   *Direct infection of unspecified hip in infectious and parasitic diseases classified elsewhere*   HCC ESR COM

✓6ᵗʰ **M01.X6**   **Direct infection of knee in infectious and parasitic diseases classified elsewhere**
    M01.X61   *Direct infection of right knee in infectious and parasitic diseases classified elsewhere*   HCC ESR COM
    M01.X62   *Direct infection of left knee in infectious and parasitic diseases classified elsewhere*   HCC ESR COM
    M01.X69   *Direct infection of unspecified knee in infectious and parasitic diseases classified elsewhere*   HCC ESR COM

✓6ᵗʰ **M01.X7**   **Direct infection of ankle and foot in infectious and parasitic diseases classified elsewhere**
    Direct infection of tarsus, metatarsus and phalanges in infectious and parasitic diseases classified elsewhere
    M01.X71   *Direct infection of right ankle and foot in infectious and parasitic diseases classified elsewhere*   HCC ESR COM
    M01.X72   *Direct infection of left ankle and foot in infectious and parasitic diseases classified elsewhere*   HCC ESR COM
    M01.X79   *Direct infection of unspecified ankle and foot in infectious and parasitic diseases classified elsewhere*   HCC ESR COM

    M01.X8   *Direct infection of vertebrae in infectious and parasitic diseases classified elsewhere*   HCC ESR COM

    M01.X9   *Direct infection of multiple joints in infectious and parasitic diseases classified elsewhere*   HCC ESR COM

✓4ᵗʰ **M02**   **Postinfective and reactive arthropathies**
    Code first underlying disease, such as:
      congenital syphilis [Clutton's joints] (A50.5)
      enteritis due to Yersinia enterocolitica (A04.6)
      infective endocarditis (I33.0)
      viral hepatitis (B15-B19)
    EXCLUDES 1   *Behçet's disease (M35.2)*
          direct infections of joint in infectious and parasitic diseases classified elsewhere (M01.-)
          mumps arthritis (B26.85)
          postmeningococcal arthritis (A39.84)
          rheumatic fever (I00)
          rubella arthritis (B06.82)
          syphilis arthritis (late) (A52.77)
          tabetic arthropathy [Charcôt's] (A52.16)

✓5ᵗʰ **M02.0**   **Arthropathy following intestinal bypass**

    M02.00   **Arthropathy following intestinal bypass, unspecified site**

✓6ᵗʰ **M02.01**   **Arthropathy following intestinal bypass, shoulder**
    M02.011   **Arthropathy following intestinal bypass, right shoulder**
    M02.012   **Arthropathy following intestinal bypass, left shoulder**
    M02.019   **Arthropathy following intestinal bypass, unspecified shoulder**

✓6ᵗʰ **M02.02**   **Arthropathy following intestinal bypass, elbow**
    M02.021   **Arthropathy following intestinal bypass, right elbow**
    M02.022   **Arthropathy following intestinal bypass, left elbow**
    M02.029   **Arthropathy following intestinal bypass, unspecified elbow**

✓6ᵗʰ **M02.03**   **Arthropathy following intestinal bypass, wrist**
    Arthropathy following intestinal bypass, carpal bones
    M02.031   **Arthropathy following intestinal bypass, right wrist**
    M02.032   **Arthropathy following intestinal bypass, left wrist**
    M02.039   **Arthropathy following intestinal bypass, unspecified wrist**

✓ Additional Character Required   ✓x7ᵗʰ Placeholder Alert   Manifestation   Unspecified Dx   Q QPP   UPD Unacceptable PDx

√6ᵗʰ **M02.04 Arthropathy following intestinal bypass,** hand
  Arthropathy following intestinal bypass, metacarpals and phalanges
  M02.041 Arthropathy following intestinal bypass, right hand
  M02.042 Arthropathy following intestinal bypass, left hand
  M02.049 Arthropathy following intestinal bypass, unspecified hand

√6ᵗʰ **M02.05 Arthropathy following intestinal bypass,** hip
  M02.051 Arthropathy following intestinal bypass, right hip
  M02.052 Arthropathy following intestinal bypass, left hip
  M02.059 Arthropathy following intestinal bypass, unspecified hip

√6ᵗʰ **M02.06 Arthropathy following intestinal bypass,** knee
  M02.061 Arthropathy following intestinal bypass, right knee
  M02.062 Arthropathy following intestinal bypass, left knee
  M02.069 Arthropathy following intestinal bypass, unspecified knee

√6ᵗʰ **M02.07 Arthropathy following intestinal bypass,** ankle and foot
  Arthropathy following intestinal bypass, tarsus, metatarsus and phalanges
  M02.071 Arthropathy following intestinal bypass, right ankle and foot
  M02.072 Arthropathy following intestinal bypass, left ankle and foot
  M02.079 Arthropathy following intestinal bypass, unspecified ankle and foot

M02.08 Arthropathy following intestinal bypass, vertebrae
M02.09 Arthropathy following intestinal bypass, multiple sites

√5ᵗʰ **M02.1** Postdysenteric **arthropathy**
  M02.10 Postdysenteric arthropathy, unspecified site HCC ESR COM
  √6ᵗʰ **M02.11 Postdysenteric arthropathy,** shoulder
    M02.111 Postdysenteric arthropathy, right shoulder HCC ESR COM
    M02.112 Postdysenteric arthropathy, left shoulder HCC ESR COM
    M02.119 Postdysenteric arthropathy, unspecified shoulder HCC ESR COM
  √6ᵗʰ **M02.12 Postdysenteric arthropathy,** elbow
    M02.121 Postdysenteric arthropathy, right elbow HCC ESR COM
    M02.122 Postdysenteric arthropathy, left elbow HCC ESR COM
    M02.129 Postdysenteric arthropathy, unspecified elbow HCC ESR COM
  √6ᵗʰ **M02.13 Postdysenteric arthropathy,** wrist
    Postdysenteric arthropathy, carpal bones
    M02.131 Postdysenteric arthropathy, right wrist HCC ESR COM
    M02.132 Postdysenteric arthropathy, left wrist HCC ESR COM
    M02.139 Postdysenteric arthropathy, unspecified wrist HCC ESR COM
  √6ᵗʰ **M02.14 Postdysenteric arthropathy,** hand
    Postdysenteric arthropathy, metacarpus and phalanges
    M02.141 Postdysenteric arthropathy, right hand HCC ESR COM
    M02.142 Postdysenteric arthropathy, left hand HCC ESR COM
    M02.149 Postdysenteric arthropathy, unspecified hand HCC ESR COM
  √6ᵗʰ **M02.15 Postdysenteric arthropathy,** hip
    M02.151 Postdysenteric arthropathy, right hip HCC ESR COM
    M02.152 Postdysenteric arthropathy, left hip HCC ESR COM
    M02.159 Postdysenteric arthropathy, unspecified hip HCC ESR COM

√6ᵗʰ **M02.16 Postdysenteric arthropathy,** knee
  M02.161 Postdysenteric arthropathy, right knee HCC ESR COM
  M02.162 Postdysenteric arthropathy, left knee HCC ESR COM
  M02.169 Postdysenteric arthropathy, unspecified knee HCC ESR COM
√6ᵗʰ **M02.17 Postdysenteric arthropathy,** ankle and foot
  Postdysenteric arthropathy, tarsus, metatarsus and phalanges
  M02.171 Postdysenteric arthropathy, right ankle and foot HCC ESR COM
  M02.172 Postdysenteric arthropathy, left ankle and foot HCC ESR COM
  M02.179 Postdysenteric arthropathy, unspecified ankle and foot HCC ESR COM
M02.18 Postdysenteric arthropathy, vertebrae HCC ESR COM
M02.19 Postdysenteric arthropathy, multiple sites HCC ESR COM

√5ᵗʰ **M02.2** Postimmunization **arthropathy**
  M02.20 Postimmunization arthropathy, unspecified site
  √6ᵗʰ **M02.21 Postimmunization arthropathy,** shoulder
    M02.211 Postimmunization arthropathy, right shoulder
    M02.212 Postimmunization arthropathy, left shoulder
    M02.219 Postimmunization arthropathy, unspecified shoulder
  √6ᵗʰ **M02.22 Postimmunization arthropathy,** elbow
    M02.221 Postimmunization arthropathy, right elbow
    M02.222 Postimmunization arthropathy, left elbow
    M02.229 Postimmunization arthropathy, unspecified elbow
  √6ᵗʰ **M02.23 Postimmunization arthropathy,** wrist
    Postimmunization arthropathy, carpal bones
    M02.231 Postimmunization arthropathy, right wrist
    M02.232 Postimmunization arthropathy, left wrist
    M02.239 Postimmunization arthropathy, unspecified wrist
  √6ᵗʰ **M02.24 Postimmunization arthropathy,** hand
    Postimmunization arthropathy, metacarpus and phalanges
    M02.241 Postimmunization arthropathy, right hand
    M02.242 Postimmunization arthropathy, left hand
    M02.249 Postimmunization arthropathy, unspecified hand
  √6ᵗʰ **M02.25 Postimmunization arthropathy,** hip
    M02.251 Postimmunization arthropathy, right hip
    M02.252 Postimmunization arthropathy, left hip
    M02.259 Postimmunization arthropathy, unspecified hip
  √6ᵗʰ **M02.26 Postimmunization arthropathy,** knee
    M02.261 Postimmunization arthropathy, right knee
    M02.262 Postimmunization arthropathy, left knee
    M02.269 Postimmunization arthropathy, unspecified knee
  √6ᵗʰ **M02.27 Postimmunization arthropathy,** ankle and foot
    Postimmunization arthropathy, tarsus, metatarsus and phalanges
    M02.271 Postimmunization arthropathy, right ankle and foot
    M02.272 Postimmunization arthropathy, left ankle and foot
    M02.279 Postimmunization arthropathy, unspecified ankle and foot
  M02.28 Postimmunization arthropathy, vertebrae
  M02.29 Postimmunization arthropathy, multiple sites

√5ᵗʰ **M02.3** Reiter's disease
  Reactive arthritis
  DEF: Arthritis, iridocyclitis, and urethritis, sometimes with diarrhea. While symptoms may recur, arthritis is constant.
  M02.30 Reiter's disease, unspecified site HCC Rx ESR COM

√6ᵗʰ **M02.31** Reiter's disease, shoulder

    M02.311 Reiter's disease, right shoulder `HCC` `Rx` `ESR` `COM`

    M02.312 Reiter's disease, left shoulder `HCC` `Rx` `ESR` `COM`

    M02.319 Reiter's disease, unspecified shoulder `HCC` `Rx` `ESR` `COM`

√6ᵗʰ **M02.32** Reiter's disease, elbow

    M02.321 Reiter's disease, right elbow `HCC` `Rx` `ESR` `COM`

    M02.322 Reiter's disease, left elbow `HCC` `Rx` `ESR` `COM`

    M02.329 Reiter's disease, unspecified elbow `HCC` `Rx` `ESR` `COM`

√6ᵗʰ **M02.33** Reiter's disease, wrist

    Reiter's disease, carpal bones

    M02.331 Reiter's disease, right wrist `HCC` `Rx` `ESR` `COM`

    M02.332 Reiter's disease, left wrist `HCC` `Rx` `ESR` `COM`

    M02.339 Reiter's disease, unspecified wrist `HCC` `Rx` `ESR` `COM`

√6ᵗʰ **M02.34** Reiter's disease, hand

    Reiter's disease, metacarpus and phalanges

    M02.341 Reiter's disease, right hand `HCC` `Rx` `ESR` `COM`

    M02.342 Reiter's disease, left hand `HCC` `Rx` `ESR` `COM`

    M02.349 Reiter's disease, unspecified hand `HCC` `Rx` `ESR` `COM`

√6ᵗʰ **M02.35** Reiter's disease, hip

    M02.351 Reiter's disease, right hip `HCC` `Rx` `ESR` `COM`

    M02.352 Reiter's disease, left hip `HCC` `Rx` `ESR` `COM`

    M02.359 Reiter's disease, unspecified hip `HCC` `Rx` `ESR` `COM`

√6ᵗʰ **M02.36** Reiter's disease, knee

    M02.361 Reiter's disease, right knee `HCC` `Rx` `ESR` `COM`

    M02.362 Reiter's disease, left knee `HCC` `Rx` `ESR` `COM`

    M02.369 Reiter's disease, unspecified knee `HCC` `Rx` `ESR` `COM`

√6ᵗʰ **M02.37** Reiter's disease, ankle and foot

    Reiter's disease, tarsus, metatarsus and phalanges

    M02.371 Reiter's disease, right ankle and foot `HCC` `Rx` `ESR` `COM`

    M02.372 Reiter's disease, left ankle and foot `HCC` `Rx` `ESR` `COM`

    M02.379 Reiter's disease, unspecified ankle and foot `HCC` `Rx` `ESR` `COM`

    M02.38 Reiter's disease, vertebrae `HCC` `Rx` `ESR` `COM`

    M02.39 Reiter's disease, multiple sites `HCC` `Rx` `ESR` `COM`

√5ᵗʰ **M02.8** Other reactive arthropathies

    M02.80 *Other reactive arthropathies, unspecified site* `HCC` `ESR` `COM`

√6ᵗʰ **M02.81** Other reactive arthropathies, shoulder

    M02.811 *Other reactive arthropathies, right shoulder* `HCC` `ESR` `COM`

    M02.812 *Other reactive arthropathies, left shoulder* `HCC` `ESR` `COM`

    M02.819 *Other reactive arthropathies, unspecified shoulder* `HCC` `ESR` `COM`

√6ᵗʰ **M02.82** Other reactive arthropathies, elbow

    M02.821 *Other reactive arthropathies, right elbow* `HCC` `ESR` `COM`

    M02.822 *Other reactive arthropathies, left elbow* `HCC` `ESR` `COM`

    M02.829 *Other reactive arthropathies, unspecified elbow* `HCC` `ESR` `COM`

√6ᵗʰ **M02.83** Other reactive arthropathies, wrist

    Other reactive arthropathies, carpal bones

    M02.831 *Other reactive arthropathies, right wrist* `HCC` `ESR` `COM`

    M02.832 *Other reactive arthropathies, left wrist* `HCC` `ESR` `COM`

    M02.839 *Other reactive arthropathies, unspecified wrist* `HCC` `ESR` `COM`

√6ᵗʰ **M02.84** Other reactive arthropathies, hand

    Other reactive arthropathies, metacarpus and phalanges

    M02.841 *Other reactive arthropathies, right hand* `HCC` `ESR` `COM`

    M02.842 *Other reactive arthropathies, left hand* `HCC` `ESR` `COM`

    M02.849 *Other reactive arthropathies, unspecified hand* `HCC` `ESR` `COM`

√6ᵗʰ **M02.85** Other reactive arthropathies, hip

    M02.851 *Other reactive arthropathies, right hip* `HCC` `ESR` `COM`

    M02.852 *Other reactive arthropathies, left hip* `HCC` `ESR` `COM`

    M02.859 *Other reactive arthropathies, unspecified hip* `HCC` `ESR` `COM`

√6ᵗʰ **M02.86** Other reactive arthropathies, knee

    M02.861 *Other reactive arthropathies, right knee* `HCC` `ESR` `COM`

    M02.862 *Other reactive arthropathies, left knee* `HCC` `ESR` `COM`

    M02.869 *Other reactive arthropathies, unspecified knee* `HCC` `ESR` `COM`

√6ᵗʰ **M02.87** Other reactive arthropathies, ankle and foot

    Other reactive arthropathies, tarsus, metatarsus and phalanges

    M02.871 *Other reactive arthropathies, right ankle and foot* `HCC` `ESR` `COM`

    M02.872 *Other reactive arthropathies, left ankle and foot* `HCC` `ESR` `COM`

    M02.879 *Other reactive arthropathies, unspecified ankle and foot* `HCC` `ESR` `COM`

    M02.88 *Other reactive arthropathies, vertebrae* `HCC` `ESR` `COM`

    M02.89 *Other reactive arthropathies, multiple sites* `HCC` `ESR` `COM`

M02.9 Reactive arthropathy, unspecified `HCC` `ESR` `COM`

Autoinflammatory syndromes (M04)

√4ᵗʰ **M04** Autoinflammatory syndromes

    `EXCLUDES 2`   *Crohn's disease (K50.-)*

    AHA: 2016,4Q,37

    M04.1 Periodic fever syndromes `HCC` `Rx` `ESR` `COM`

        Familial Mediterranean fever

        Hyperimmunoglobin D syndrome

        Mevalonate kinase deficiency

        Tumor necrosis factor receptor associated periodic syndrome [TRAPS]

    M04.2 Cryopyrin-associated periodic syndromes `HCC` `Rx` `ESR` `COM`

        Chronic infantile neurological, cutaneous and articular syndrome [CINCA]

        Familial cold autoinflammatory syndrome

        Familial cold urticaria

        Muckle-Wells syndrome

        Neonatal onset multisystemic inflammatory disorder [NOMID]

    M04.8 Other autoinflammatory syndromes `HCC` `Rx` `ESR` `COM`

        Blau syndrome

        Deficiency of interleukin 1 receptor antagonist [DIRA]

        Majeed syndrome

        Periodic fever, aphthous stomatitis, pharyngitis, and adenopathy syndrome [PFAPA]

        Pyogenic arthritis, pyoderma gangrenosum, and acne syndrome [PAPA]

    M04.9 Autoinflammatory syndrome, unspecified `HCC` `Rx` `ESR` `COM`

Inflammatory polyarthropathies (M05-M14)

✓4ᵗʰ **M05 Rheumatoid arthritis with rheumatoid factor**

EXCLUDES 1   *rheumatic fever (I00)*
     juvenile rheumatoid arthritis (M08.-)
     rheumatoid arthritis of spine (M45.-)

AHA: 2020,4Q,31-32

DEF: Rheumatoid arthritis: Autoimmune systemic disease that causes chronic inflammation of the joints and other areas of the body, manifested by inflammatory changes in articular structures and synovial membranes, atrophy, and loss in bone density.

✓5ᵗʰ **M05.0 Felty's syndrome**

   Rheumatoid arthritis with splenoadenomegaly and leukopenia

     M05.00 Felty's syndrome, unspecified site HCC Rx ESR COM

✓6ᵗʰ   **M05.01 Felty's syndrome, shoulder**

     M05.011 Felty's syndrome, right shoulder HCC Rx ESR COM

     M05.012 Felty's syndrome, left shoulder HCC Rx ESR COM

     M05.019 Felty's syndrome, unspecified shoulder HCC Rx ESR COM

✓6ᵗʰ   **M05.02 Felty's syndrome, elbow**

     M05.021 Felty's syndrome, right elbow HCC Rx ESR COM

     M05.022 Felty's syndrome, left elbow HCC Rx ESR COM

     M05.029 Felty's syndrome, unspecified elbow HCC Rx ESR COM

✓6ᵗʰ   **M05.03 Felty's syndrome, wrist**

   Felty's syndrome, carpal bones

     M05.031 Felty's syndrome, right wrist HCC Rx ESR COM

     M05.032 Felty's syndrome, left wrist HCC Rx ESR COM

     M05.039 Felty's syndrome, unspecified wrist HCC Rx ESR COM

✓6ᵗʰ   **M05.04 Felty's syndrome, hand**

   Felty's syndrome, metacarpus and phalanges

     M05.041 Felty's syndrome, right hand HCC Rx ESR COM

     M05.042 Felty's syndrome, left hand HCC Rx ESR COM

     M05.049 Felty's syndrome, unspecified hand HCC Rx ESR COM

✓6ᵗʰ   **M05.05 Felty's syndrome, hip**

     M05.051 Felty's syndrome, right hip HCC Rx ESR COM

     M05.052 Felty's syndrome, left hip HCC Rx ESR COM

     M05.059 Felty's syndrome, unspecified hip HCC Rx ESR COM

✓6ᵗʰ   **M05.06 Felty's syndrome, knee**

     M05.061 Felty's syndrome, right knee HCC Rx ESR COM

     M05.062 Felty's syndrome, left knee HCC Rx ESR COM

     M05.069 Felty's syndrome, unspecified knee HCC Rx ESR COM

✓6ᵗʰ   **M05.07 Felty's syndrome, ankle and foot**

   Felty's syndrome, tarsus, metatarsus and phalanges

     M05.071 Felty's syndrome, right ankle and foot HCC Rx ESR COM

     M05.072 Felty's syndrome, left ankle and foot HCC Rx ESR COM

     M05.079 Felty's syndrome, unspecified ankle and foot HCC Rx ESR COM

     M05.09 Felty's syndrome, multiple sites HCC Rx ESR COM

✓5ᵗʰ **M05.1 Rheumatoid lung disease with rheumatoid arthritis**

     M05.10 Rheumatoid lung disease with rheumatoid arthritis of unspecified site HCC Rx ESR COM

✓6ᵗʰ   **M05.11 Rheumatoid lung disease with rheumatoid arthritis of shoulder**

     M05.111 Rheumatoid lung disease with rheumatoid arthritis of right shoulder HCC Rx ESR COM

     M05.112 Rheumatoid lung disease with rheumatoid arthritis of left shoulder HCC Rx ESR COM

     M05.119 Rheumatoid lung disease with rheumatoid arthritis of unspecified shoulder HCC Rx ESR COM

✓6ᵗʰ   **M05.12 Rheumatoid lung disease with rheumatoid arthritis of elbow**

     M05.121 Rheumatoid lung disease with rheumatoid arthritis of right elbow HCC Rx ESR COM

     M05.122 Rheumatoid lung disease with rheumatoid arthritis of left elbow HCC Rx ESR COM

     M05.129 Rheumatoid lung disease with rheumatoid arthritis of unspecified elbow HCC Rx ESR COM

✓6ᵗʰ   **M05.13 Rheumatoid lung disease with rheumatoid arthritis of wrist**

   Rheumatoid lung disease with rheumatoid arthritis, carpal bones

     M05.131 Rheumatoid lung disease with rheumatoid arthritis of right wrist HCC Rx ESR COM

     M05.132 Rheumatoid lung disease with rheumatoid arthritis of left wrist HCC Rx ESR COM

     M05.139 Rheumatoid lung disease with rheumatoid arthritis of unspecified wrist HCC Rx ESR COM

✓6ᵗʰ   **M05.14 Rheumatoid lung disease with rheumatoid arthritis of hand**

   Rheumatoid lung disease with rheumatoid arthritis, metacarpus and phalanges

     M05.141 Rheumatoid lung disease with rheumatoid arthritis of right hand HCC Rx ESR COM

     M05.142 Rheumatoid lung disease with rheumatoid arthritis of left hand HCC Rx ESR COM

     M05.149 Rheumatoid lung disease with rheumatoid arthritis of unspecified hand HCC Rx ESR COM

✓6ᵗʰ   **M05.15 Rheumatoid lung disease with rheumatoid arthritis of hip**

     M05.151 Rheumatoid lung disease with rheumatoid arthritis of right hip HCC Rx ESR COM

     M05.152 Rheumatoid lung disease with rheumatoid arthritis of left hip HCC Rx ESR COM

     M05.159 Rheumatoid lung disease with rheumatoid arthritis of unspecified hip HCC Rx ESR COM

✓6ᵗʰ   **M05.16 Rheumatoid lung disease with rheumatoid arthritis of knee**

     M05.161 Rheumatoid lung disease with rheumatoid arthritis of right knee HCC Rx ESR COM

     M05.162 Rheumatoid lung disease with rheumatoid arthritis of left knee HCC Rx ESR COM

     M05.169 Rheumatoid lung disease with rheumatoid arthritis of unspecified knee HCC Rx ESR COM

✓6ᵗʰ   **M05.17 Rheumatoid lung disease with rheumatoid arthritis of ankle and foot**

   Rheumatoid lung disease with rheumatoid arthritis, tarsus, metatarsus and phalanges

     M05.171 Rheumatoid lung disease with rheumatoid arthritis of right ankle and foot HCC Rx ESR COM

     M05.172 Rheumatoid lung disease with rheumatoid arthritis of left ankle and foot HCC Rx ESR COM

     M05.179 Rheumatoid lung disease with rheumatoid arthritis of unspecified ankle and foot HCC Rx ESR COM

     M05.19 Rheumatoid lung disease with rheumatoid arthritis of multiple sites HCC Rx ESR COM

√5ᵗʰ **M05.2** **Rheumatoid** vasculitis with rheumatoid arthritis

M05.20 Rheumatoid vasculitis with rheumatoid arthritis of unspecified site `HCC` `Rx` `ESR` `COM`

√6ᵗʰ **M05.21** Rheumatoid vasculitis with rheumatoid arthritis of shoulder

- **M05.211** Rheumatoid vasculitis with rheumatoid arthritis of right shoulder `HCC` `Rx` `ESR` `COM`
- **M05.212** Rheumatoid vasculitis with rheumatoid arthritis of left shoulder `HCC` `Rx` `ESR` `COM`
- **M05.219** Rheumatoid vasculitis with rheumatoid arthritis of unspecified shoulder `HCC` `Rx` `ESR` `COM`

√6ᵗʰ **M05.22** Rheumatoid vasculitis with rheumatoid arthritis of elbow

- **M05.221** Rheumatoid vasculitis with rheumatoid arthritis of right elbow `HCC` `Rx` `ESR` `COM`
- **M05.222** Rheumatoid vasculitis with rheumatoid arthritis of left elbow `HCC` `Rx` `ESR` `COM`
- **M05.229** Rheumatoid vasculitis with rheumatoid arthritis of unspecified elbow `HCC` `Rx` `ESR` `COM`

√6ᵗʰ **M05.23** Rheumatoid vasculitis with rheumatoid arthritis of wrist

Rheumatoid vasculitis with rheumatoid arthritis, carpal bones

- **M05.231** Rheumatoid vasculitis with rheumatoid arthritis of right wrist `HCC` `Rx` `ESR` `COM`
- **M05.232** Rheumatoid vasculitis with rheumatoid arthritis of left wrist `HCC` `Rx` `ESR` `COM`
- **M05.239** Rheumatoid vasculitis with rheumatoid arthritis of unspecified wrist `HCC` `Rx` `ESR` `COM`

√6ᵗʰ **M05.24** Rheumatoid vasculitis with rheumatoid arthritis of hand

Rheumatoid vasculitis with rheumatoid arthritis, metacarpus and phalanges

- **M05.241** Rheumatoid vasculitis with rheumatoid arthritis of right hand `HCC` `Rx` `ESR` `COM`
- **M05.242** Rheumatoid vasculitis with rheumatoid arthritis of left hand `HCC` `Rx` `ESR` `COM`
- **M05.249** Rheumatoid vasculitis with rheumatoid arthritis of unspecified hand `HCC` `Rx` `ESR` `COM`

√6ᵗʰ **M05.25** Rheumatoid vasculitis with rheumatoid arthritis of hip

- **M05.251** Rheumatoid vasculitis with rheumatoid arthritis of right hip `HCC` `Rx` `ESR` `COM`
- **M05.252** Rheumatoid vasculitis with rheumatoid arthritis of left hip `HCC` `Rx` `ESR` `COM`
- **M05.259** Rheumatoid vasculitis with rheumatoid arthritis of unspecified hip `HCC` `Rx` `ESR` `COM`

√6ᵗʰ **M05.26** Rheumatoid vasculitis with rheumatoid arthritis of knee

- **M05.261** Rheumatoid vasculitis with rheumatoid arthritis of right knee `HCC` `Rx` `ESR` `COM`
- **M05.262** Rheumatoid vasculitis with rheumatoid arthritis of left knee `HCC` `Rx` `ESR` `COM`
- **M05.269** Rheumatoid vasculitis with rheumatoid arthritis of unspecified knee `HCC` `Rx` `ESR` `COM`

√6ᵗʰ **M05.27** Rheumatoid vasculitis with rheumatoid arthritis of ankle and foot

Rheumatoid vasculitis with rheumatoid arthritis, tarsus, metatarsus and phalanges

- **M05.271** Rheumatoid vasculitis with rheumatoid arthritis of right ankle and foot `HCC` `Rx` `ESR` `COM`
- **M05.272** Rheumatoid vasculitis with rheumatoid arthritis of left ankle and foot `HCC` `Rx` `ESR` `COM`
- **M05.279** Rheumatoid vasculitis with rheumatoid arthritis of unspecified ankle and foot `HCC` `Rx` `ESR` `COM`

M05.29 Rheumatoid vasculitis with rheumatoid arthritis of multiple sites `HCC` `Rx` `ESR` `COM`

√5ᵗʰ **M05.3** **Rheumatoid** heart disease with rheumatoid arthritis

Rheumatoid carditis
Rheumatoid endocarditis
Rheumatoid myocarditis
Rheumatoid pericarditis

M05.30 Rheumatoid heart disease with rheumatoid arthritis of unspecified site `HCC` `Rx` `ESR` `COM`

√6ᵗʰ **M05.31** Rheumatoid heart disease with rheumatoid arthritis of shoulder

- **M05.311** Rheumatoid heart disease with rheumatoid arthritis of right shoulder `HCC` `Rx` `ESR` `COM`
- **M05.312** Rheumatoid heart disease with rheumatoid arthritis of left shoulder `HCC` `Rx` `ESR` `COM`
- **M05.319** Rheumatoid heart disease with rheumatoid arthritis of unspecified shoulder `HCC` `Rx` `ESR` `COM`

√6ᵗʰ **M05.32** Rheumatoid heart disease with rheumatoid arthritis of elbow

- **M05.321** Rheumatoid heart disease with rheumatoid arthritis of right elbow `HCC` `Rx` `ESR` `COM`
- **M05.322** Rheumatoid heart disease with rheumatoid arthritis of left elbow `HCC` `Rx` `ESR` `COM`
- **M05.329** Rheumatoid heart disease with rheumatoid arthritis of unspecified elbow `HCC` `Rx` `ESR` `COM`

√6ᵗʰ **M05.33** Rheumatoid heart disease with rheumatoid arthritis of wrist

Rheumatoid heart disease with rheumatoid arthritis, carpal bones

- **M05.331** Rheumatoid heart disease with rheumatoid arthritis of right wrist `HCC` `Rx` `ESR` `COM`
- **M05.332** Rheumatoid heart disease with rheumatoid arthritis of left wrist `HCC` `Rx` `ESR` `COM`
- **M05.339** Rheumatoid heart disease with rheumatoid arthritis of unspecified wrist `HCC` `Rx` `ESR` `COM`

√6ᵗʰ **M05.34** Rheumatoid heart disease with rheumatoid arthritis of hand

Rheumatoid heart disease with rheumatoid arthritis, metacarpus and phalanges

- **M05.341** Rheumatoid heart disease with rheumatoid arthritis of right hand `HCC` `Rx` `ESR` `COM`
- **M05.342** Rheumatoid heart disease with rheumatoid arthritis of left hand `HCC` `Rx` `ESR` `COM`
- **M05.349** Rheumatoid heart disease with rheumatoid arthritis of unspecified hand `HCC` `Rx` `ESR` `COM`

√6ᵗʰ **M05.35** Rheumatoid heart disease with rheumatoid arthritis of hip

- **M05.351** Rheumatoid heart disease with rheumatoid arthritis of right hip `HCC` `Rx` `ESR` `COM`
- **M05.352** Rheumatoid heart disease with rheumatoid arthritis of left hip `HCC` `Rx` `ESR` `COM`
- **M05.359** Rheumatoid heart disease with rheumatoid arthritis of unspecified hip `HCC` `Rx` `ESR` `COM`

√6ᵗʰ **M05.36** Rheumatoid heart disease with rheumatoid arthritis of knee

- **M05.361** Rheumatoid heart disease with rheumatoid arthritis of right knee `HCC` `Rx` `ESR` `COM`
- **M05.362** Rheumatoid heart disease with rheumatoid arthritis of left knee `HCC` `Rx` `ESR` `COM`
- **M05.369** Rheumatoid heart disease with rheumatoid arthritis of unspecified knee `HCC` `Rx` `ESR` `COM`

✓6ᵗʰ **M05.37 Rheumatoid heart disease with rheumatoid arthritis of** ankle and foot

     Rheumatoid heart disease with rheumatoid arthritis, tarsus, metatarsus and phalanges

     M05.371 Rheumatoid heart disease with rheumatoid arthritis of right **ankle and foot** `HCC` `Rx` `ESR` `COM`

     M05.372 Rheumatoid heart disease with rheumatoid arthritis of left **ankle and foot** `HCC` `Rx` `ESR` `COM`

     M05.379 Rheumatoid heart disease with rheumatoid arthritis of unspecified ankle and foot `HCC` `Rx` `ESR` `COM`

M05.39 Rheumatoid heart disease with rheumatoid arthritis of multiple sites `HCC` `Rx` `ESR` `COM`

✓5ᵗʰ **M05.4 Rheumatoid** myopathy with rheumatoid arthritis

     M05.40 Rheumatoid myopathy with rheumatoid arthritis of unspecified site `HCC` `Rx` `ESR` `COM`

✓6ᵗʰ **M05.41 Rheumatoid myopathy with rheumatoid arthritis of** shoulder

     M05.411 Rheumatoid myopathy with rheumatoid arthritis of right **shoulder** `HCC` `Rx` `ESR` `COM`

     M05.412 Rheumatoid myopathy with rheumatoid arthritis of left **shoulder** `HCC` `Rx` `ESR` `COM`

     M05.419 Rheumatoid myopathy with rheumatoid arthritis of unspecified shoulder `HCC` `Rx` `ESR` `COM`

✓6ᵗʰ **M05.42 Rheumatoid myopathy with rheumatoid arthritis of** elbow

     M05.421 Rheumatoid myopathy with rheumatoid arthritis of right **elbow** `HCC` `Rx` `ESR` `COM`

     M05.422 Rheumatoid myopathy with rheumatoid arthritis of left **elbow** `HCC` `Rx` `ESR` `COM`

     M05.429 Rheumatoid myopathy with rheumatoid arthritis of unspecified elbow `HCC` `Rx` `ESR` `COM`

✓6ᵗʰ **M05.43 Rheumatoid myopathy with rheumatoid arthritis of** wrist

     Rheumatoid myopathy with rheumatoid arthritis, carpal bones

     M05.431 Rheumatoid myopathy with rheumatoid arthritis of right **wrist** `HCC` `Rx` `ESR` `COM`

     M05.432 Rheumatoid myopathy with rheumatoid arthritis of left **wrist** `HCC` `Rx` `ESR` `COM`

     M05.439 Rheumatoid myopathy with rheumatoid arthritis of unspecified wrist `HCC` `Rx` `ESR` `COM`

✓6ᵗʰ **M05.44 Rheumatoid myopathy with rheumatoid arthritis of** hand

     Rheumatoid myopathy with rheumatoid arthritis, metacarpus and phalanges

     M05.441 Rheumatoid myopathy with rheumatoid arthritis of right **hand** `HCC` `Rx` `ESR` `COM`

     M05.442 Rheumatoid myopathy with rheumatoid arthritis of left **hand** `HCC` `Rx` `ESR` `COM`

     M05.449 Rheumatoid myopathy with rheumatoid arthritis of unspecified hand `HCC` `Rx` `ESR` `COM`

✓6ᵗʰ **M05.45 Rheumatoid myopathy with rheumatoid arthritis of** hip

     M05.451 Rheumatoid myopathy with rheumatoid arthritis of right **hip** `HCC` `Rx` `ESR` `COM`

     M05.452 Rheumatoid myopathy with rheumatoid arthritis of left **hip** `HCC` `Rx` `ESR` `COM`

     M05.459 Rheumatoid myopathy with rheumatoid arthritis of unspecified hip `HCC` `Rx` `ESR` `COM`

✓6ᵗʰ **M05.46 Rheumatoid myopathy with rheumatoid arthritis of** knee

     M05.461 Rheumatoid myopathy with rheumatoid arthritis of right **knee** `HCC` `Rx` `ESR` `COM`

     M05.462 Rheumatoid myopathy with rheumatoid arthritis of left **knee** `HCC` `Rx` `ESR` `COM`

     M05.469 Rheumatoid myopathy with rheumatoid arthritis of unspecified knee `HCC` `Rx` `ESR` `COM`

✓6ᵗʰ **M05.47 Rheumatoid myopathy with rheumatoid arthritis of** ankle and foot

     Rheumatoid myopathy with rheumatoid arthritis, tarsus, metatarsus and phalanges

     M05.471 Rheumatoid myopathy with rheumatoid arthritis of right **ankle and foot** `HCC` `Rx` `ESR` `COM`

     M05.472 Rheumatoid myopathy with rheumatoid arthritis of left **ankle and foot** `HCC` `Rx` `ESR` `COM`

     M05.479 Rheumatoid myopathy with rheumatoid arthritis of unspecified ankle and foot `HCC` `Rx` `ESR` `COM`

M05.49 Rheumatoid myopathy with rheumatoid arthritis of multiple sites `HCC` `Rx` `ESR` `COM`

✓5ᵗʰ **M05.5 Rheumatoid** polyneuropathy with rheumatoid arthritis

     M05.50 Rheumatoid polyneuropathy with rheumatoid arthritis of unspecified site `HCC` `Rx` `ESR` `COM`

✓6ᵗʰ **M05.51 Rheumatoid polyneuropathy with rheumatoid arthritis of** shoulder

     M05.511 Rheumatoid polyneuropathy with rheumatoid arthritis of right **shoulder** `HCC` `Rx` `ESR` `COM`

     M05.512 Rheumatoid polyneuropathy with rheumatoid arthritis of left **shoulder** `HCC` `Rx` `ESR` `COM`

     M05.519 Rheumatoid polyneuropathy with rheumatoid arthritis of unspecified shoulder `HCC` `Rx` `ESR` `COM`

✓6ᵗʰ **M05.52 Rheumatoid polyneuropathy with rheumatoid arthritis of** elbow

     M05.521 Rheumatoid polyneuropathy with rheumatoid arthritis of right **elbow** `HCC` `Rx` `ESR` `COM`

     M05.522 Rheumatoid polyneuropathy with rheumatoid arthritis of left **elbow** `HCC` `Rx` `ESR` `COM`

     M05.529 Rheumatoid polyneuropathy with rheumatoid arthritis of unspecified elbow `HCC` `Rx` `ESR` `COM`

✓6ᵗʰ **M05.53 Rheumatoid polyneuropathy with rheumatoid arthritis of** wrist

     Rheumatoid polyneuropathy with rheumatoid arthritis, carpal bones

     M05.531 Rheumatoid polyneuropathy with rheumatoid arthritis of right **wrist** `HCC` `Rx` `ESR` `COM`

     M05.532 Rheumatoid polyneuropathy with rheumatoid arthritis of left **wrist** `HCC` `Rx` `ESR` `COM`

     M05.539 Rheumatoid polyneuropathy with rheumatoid arthritis of unspecified wrist `HCC` `Rx` `ESR` `COM`

✓6ᵗʰ **M05.54 Rheumatoid polyneuropathy with rheumatoid arthritis of** hand

     Rheumatoid polyneuropathy with rheumatoid arthritis, metacarpus and phalanges

     M05.541 Rheumatoid polyneuropathy with rheumatoid arthritis of right **hand** `HCC` `Rx` `ESR` `COM`

     M05.542 Rheumatoid polyneuropathy with rheumatoid arthritis of left **hand** `HCC` `Rx` `ESR` `COM`

     M05.549 Rheumatoid polyneuropathy with rheumatoid arthritis of unspecified hand `HCC` `Rx` `ESR` `COM`

✓6ᵗʰ **M05.55 Rheumatoid polyneuropathy with rheumatoid arthritis of** hip

     M05.551 Rheumatoid polyneuropathy with rheumatoid arthritis of right **hip** `HCC` `Rx` `ESR` `COM`

     M05.552 Rheumatoid polyneuropathy with rheumatoid arthritis of left **hip** `HCC` `Rx` `ESR` `COM`

     M05.559 Rheumatoid polyneuropathy with rheumatoid arthritis of unspecified hip `HCC` `Rx` `ESR` `COM`

✓6ᵗʰ **M05.56 Rheumatoid polyneuropathy with rheumatoid arthritis of** knee

     M05.561 Rheumatoid polyneuropathy with rheumatoid arthritis of right **knee** `HCC` `Rx` `ESR` `COM`

`HCC` CMS-HCC   `Rx` Rx HCC   `ESR` ESRD HCC   `COM` Commercial HCC   N Newborn: 0   P Pediatric: 0-17   M Maternity: 9-64   A Adult: 15-124

784   ICD-10-CM 2023

M05.562   Rheumatoid polyneuropathy with rheumatoid arthritis of left knee   `HCC` `Rx` `ESR` `COM`

M05.569   Rheumatoid polyneuropathy with rheumatoid arthritis of unspecified knee   `HCC` `Rx` `ESR` `COM`

√6ᵗʰ M05.57   Rheumatoid polyneuropathy with rheumatoid arthritis of ankle and foot

    Rheumatoid polyneuropathy with rheumatoid arthritis, tarsus, metatarsus and phalanges

M05.571   Rheumatoid polyneuropathy with rheumatoid arthritis of right ankle and foot   `HCC` `Rx` `ESR` `COM`

M05.572   Rheumatoid polyneuropathy with rheumatoid arthritis of left ankle and foot   `HCC` `Rx` `ESR` `COM`

M05.579   Rheumatoid polyneuropathy with rheumatoid arthritis of unspecified ankle and foot   `HCC` `Rx` `ESR` `COM`

M05.59   Rheumatoid polyneuropathy with rheumatoid arthritis of multiple sites   `HCC` `Rx` `ESR` `COM`

√5ᵗʰ M05.6   Rheumatoid arthritis with involvement of other organs and systems

M05.60   Rheumatoid arthritis of unspecified site with involvement of other organs and systems   `HCC` `Rx` `ESR` `COM`

√6ᵗʰ M05.61   Rheumatoid arthritis of shoulder with involvement of other organs and systems

M05.611   Rheumatoid arthritis of right shoulder with involvement of other organs and systems   `HCC` `Rx` `ESR` `COM`

M05.612   Rheumatoid arthritis of left shoulder with involvement of other organs and systems   `HCC` `Rx` `ESR` `COM`

M05.619   Rheumatoid arthritis of unspecified shoulder with involvement of other organs and systems   `HCC` `Rx` `ESR` `COM`

√6ᵗʰ M05.62   Rheumatoid arthritis of elbow with involvement of other organs and systems

M05.621   Rheumatoid arthritis of right elbow with involvement of other organs and systems   `HCC` `Rx` `ESR` `COM`

M05.622   Rheumatoid arthritis of left elbow with involvement of other organs and systems   `HCC` `Rx` `ESR` `COM`

M05.629   Rheumatoid arthritis of unspecified elbow with involvement of other organs and systems   `HCC` `Rx` `ESR` `COM`

√6ᵗʰ M05.63   Rheumatoid arthritis of wrist with involvement of other organs and systems

    Rheumatoid arthritis of carpal bones with involvement of other organs and systems

M05.631   Rheumatoid arthritis of right wrist with involvement of other organs and systems   `HCC` `Rx` `ESR` `COM`

M05.632   Rheumatoid arthritis of left wrist with involvement of other organs and systems   `HCC` `Rx` `ESR` `COM`

M05.639   Rheumatoid arthritis of unspecified wrist with involvement of other organs and systems   `HCC` `Rx` `ESR` `COM`

√6ᵗʰ M05.64   Rheumatoid arthritis of hand with involvement of other organs and systems

    Rheumatoid arthritis of metacarpus and phalanges with involvement of other organs and systems

M05.641   Rheumatoid arthritis of right hand with involvement of other organs and systems   `HCC` `Rx` `ESR` `COM`

M05.642   Rheumatoid arthritis of left hand with involvement of other organs and systems   `HCC` `Rx` `ESR` `COM`

M05.649   Rheumatoid arthritis of unspecified hand with involvement of other organs and systems   `HCC` `Rx` `ESR` `COM`

√6ᵗʰ M05.65   Rheumatoid arthritis of hip with involvement of other organs and systems

M05.651   Rheumatoid arthritis of right hip with involvement of other organs and systems   `HCC` `Rx` `ESR` `COM`

M05.652   Rheumatoid arthritis of left hip with involvement of other organs and systems   `HCC` `Rx` `ESR` `COM`

M05.659   Rheumatoid arthritis of unspecified hip with involvement of other organs and systems   `HCC` `Rx` `ESR` `COM`

√6ᵗʰ M05.66   Rheumatoid arthritis of knee with involvement of other organs and systems

M05.661   Rheumatoid arthritis of right knee with involvement of other organs and systems   `HCC` `Rx` `ESR` `COM`

M05.662   Rheumatoid arthritis of left knee with involvement of other organs and systems   `HCC` `Rx` `ESR` `COM`

M05.669   Rheumatoid arthritis of unspecified knee with involvement of other organs and systems   `HCC` `Rx` `ESR` `COM`

√6ᵗʰ M05.67   Rheumatoid arthritis of ankle and foot with involvement of other organs and systems

    Rheumatoid arthritis of tarsus, metatarsus and phalanges with involvement of other organs and systems

M05.671   Rheumatoid arthritis of right ankle and foot with involvement of other organs and systems   `HCC` `Rx` `ESR` `COM`

M05.672   Rheumatoid arthritis of left ankle and foot with involvement of other organs and systems   `HCC` `Rx` `ESR` `COM`

M05.679   Rheumatoid arthritis of unspecified ankle and foot with involvement of other organs and systems   `HCC` `Rx` `ESR` `COM`

M05.69   Rheumatoid arthritis of multiple sites with involvement of other organs and systems   `HCC` `Rx` `ESR` `COM`

√5ᵗʰ M05.7   Rheumatoid arthritis with rheumatoid factor without organ or systems involvement

M05.70   Rheumatoid arthritis with rheumatoid factor of unspecified site without organ or systems involvement   `HCC` `Rx` `ESR` `COM`

√6ᵗʰ M05.71   Rheumatoid arthritis with rheumatoid factor of shoulder without organ or systems involvement

M05.711   Rheumatoid arthritis with rheumatoid factor of right shoulder without organ or systems involvement   `HCC` `Rx` `ESR` `COM`

M05.712   Rheumatoid arthritis with rheumatoid factor of left shoulder without organ or systems involvement   `HCC` `Rx` `ESR` `COM`

M05.719   Rheumatoid arthritis with rheumatoid factor of unspecified shoulder without organ or systems involvement   `HCC` `Rx` `ESR` `COM`

√6ᵗʰ M05.72   Rheumatoid arthritis with rheumatoid factor of elbow without organ or systems involvement

M05.721   Rheumatoid arthritis with rheumatoid factor of right elbow without organ or systems involvement   `HCC` `Rx` `ESR` `COM`

M05.722   Rheumatoid arthritis with rheumatoid factor of left elbow without organ or systems involvement   `HCC` `Rx` `ESR` `COM`

M05.729   Rheumatoid arthritis with rheumatoid factor of unspecified elbow without organ or systems involvement   `HCC` `Rx` `ESR` `COM`

√6ᵗʰ M05.73   Rheumatoid arthritis with rheumatoid factor of wrist without organ or systems involvement

M05.731   Rheumatoid arthritis with rheumatoid factor of right wrist without organ or systems involvement   `HCC` `Rx` `ESR` `COM`

M05.732   Rheumatoid arthritis with rheumatoid factor of left wrist without organ or systems involvement   `HCC` `Rx` `ESR` `COM`

M05.739   Rheumatoid arthritis with rheumatoid factor of unspecified wrist without organ or systems involvement   `HCC` `Rx` `ESR` `COM`

√6ᵗʰ M05.74   Rheumatoid arthritis with rheumatoid factor of hand without organ or systems involvement

M05.741   Rheumatoid arthritis with rheumatoid factor of right hand without organ or systems involvement   `HCC` `Rx` `ESR` `COM`

M05.742   Rheumatoid arthritis with rheumatoid factor of left hand without organ or systems involvement   `HCC` `Rx` `ESR` `COM`

M05.749 Rheumatoid arthritis with rheumatoid factor of unspecified hand without organ or systems involvement `HCC` `Rx` `ESR` `COM`

✓6ᵗʰ **M05.75** Rheumatoid arthritis with rheumatoid factor of hip without organ or systems involvement

M05.751 Rheumatoid arthritis with rheumatoid factor of right hip without organ or systems involvement `HCC` `Rx` `ESR` `COM`

M05.752 Rheumatoid arthritis with rheumatoid factor of left hip without organ or systems involvement `HCC` `Rx` `ESR` `COM`

M05.759 Rheumatoid arthritis with rheumatoid factor of unspecified hip without organ or systems involvement `HCC` `Rx` `ESR` `COM`

✓6ᵗʰ **M05.76** Rheumatoid arthritis with rheumatoid factor of knee without organ or systems involvement

M05.761 Rheumatoid arthritis with rheumatoid factor of right knee without organ or systems involvement `HCC` `Rx` `ESR` `COM`

M05.762 Rheumatoid arthritis with rheumatoid factor of left knee without organ or systems involvement `HCC` `Rx` `ESR` `COM`

M05.769 Rheumatoid arthritis with rheumatoid factor of unspecified knee without organ or systems involvement `HCC` `Rx` `ESR` `COM`

✓6ᵗʰ **M05.77** Rheumatoid arthritis with rheumatoid factor of ankle and foot without organ or systems involvement

M05.771 Rheumatoid arthritis with rheumatoid factor of right ankle and foot without organ or systems involvement `HCC` `Rx` `ESR` `COM`

M05.772 Rheumatoid arthritis with rheumatoid factor of left ankle and foot without organ or systems involvement `HCC` `Rx` `ESR` `COM`

M05.779 Rheumatoid arthritis with rheumatoid factor of unspecified ankle and foot without organ or systems involvement `HCC` `Rx` `ESR` `COM`

M05.79 Rheumatoid arthritis with rheumatoid factor of multiple sites without organ or systems involvement `HCC` `Rx` `ESR` `COM`

M05.7A Rheumatoid arthritis with rheumatoid factor of other specified site without organ or systems involvement `HCC` `Rx` `ESR` `COM`

✓5ᵗʰ **M05.8** Other rheumatoid arthritis with rheumatoid factor

M05.80 Other rheumatoid arthritis with rheumatoid factor of unspecified site `HCC` `Rx` `ESR` `COM`

✓6ᵗʰ **M05.81** Other rheumatoid arthritis with rheumatoid factor of shoulder

M05.811 Other rheumatoid arthritis with rheumatoid factor of right shoulder `HCC` `Rx` `ESR` `COM`

M05.812 Other rheumatoid arthritis with rheumatoid factor of left shoulder `HCC` `Rx` `ESR` `COM`

M05.819 Other rheumatoid arthritis with rheumatoid factor of unspecified shoulder `HCC` `Rx` `ESR` `COM`

✓6ᵗʰ **M05.82** Other rheumatoid arthritis with rheumatoid factor of elbow

M05.821 Other rheumatoid arthritis with rheumatoid factor of right elbow `HCC` `Rx` `ESR` `COM`

M05.822 Other rheumatoid arthritis with rheumatoid factor of left elbow `HCC` `Rx` `ESR` `COM`

M05.829 Other rheumatoid arthritis with rheumatoid factor of unspecified elbow `HCC` `Rx` `ESR` `COM`

✓6ᵗʰ **M05.83** Other rheumatoid arthritis with rheumatoid factor of wrist

M05.831 Other rheumatoid arthritis with rheumatoid factor of right wrist `HCC` `Rx` `ESR` `COM`

M05.832 Other rheumatoid arthritis with rheumatoid factor of left wrist `HCC` `Rx` `ESR` `COM`

M05.839 Other rheumatoid arthritis with rheumatoid factor of unspecified wrist `HCC` `Rx` `ESR` `COM`

✓6ᵗʰ **M05.84** Other rheumatoid arthritis with rheumatoid factor of hand

M05.841 Other rheumatoid arthritis with rheumatoid factor of right hand `HCC` `Rx` `ESR` `COM`

M05.842 Other rheumatoid arthritis with rheumatoid factor of left hand `HCC` `Rx` `ESR` `COM`

M05.849 Other rheumatoid arthritis with rheumatoid factor of unspecified hand `HCC` `Rx` `ESR` `COM`

✓6ᵗʰ **M05.85** Other rheumatoid arthritis with rheumatoid factor of hip

M05.851 Other rheumatoid arthritis with rheumatoid factor of right hip `HCC` `Rx` `ESR` `COM`

M05.852 Other rheumatoid arthritis with rheumatoid factor of left hip `HCC` `Rx` `ESR` `COM`

M05.859 Other rheumatoid arthritis with rheumatoid factor of unspecified hip `HCC` `Rx` `ESR` `COM`

✓6ᵗʰ **M05.86** Other rheumatoid arthritis with rheumatoid factor of knee

M05.861 Other rheumatoid arthritis with rheumatoid factor of right knee `HCC` `Rx` `ESR` `COM`

M05.862 Other rheumatoid arthritis with rheumatoid factor of left knee `HCC` `Rx` `ESR` `COM`

M05.869 Other rheumatoid arthritis with rheumatoid factor of unspecified knee `HCC` `Rx` `ESR` `COM`

✓6ᵗʰ **M05.87** Other rheumatoid arthritis with rheumatoid factor of ankle and foot

M05.871 Other rheumatoid arthritis with rheumatoid factor of right ankle and foot `HCC` `Rx` `ESR` `COM`

M05.872 Other rheumatoid arthritis with rheumatoid factor of left ankle and foot `HCC` `Rx` `ESR` `COM`

M05.879 Other rheumatoid arthritis with rheumatoid factor of unspecified ankle and foot `HCC` `Rx` `ESR` `COM`

M05.89 Other rheumatoid arthritis with rheumatoid factor of multiple sites `HCC` `Rx` `ESR` `COM`

M05.8A Other rheumatoid arthritis with rheumatoid factor of other specified site `HCC` `Rx` `ESR` `COM`

M05.9 Rheumatoid arthritis with rheumatoid factor, unspecified `HCC` `Rx` `ESR` `COM`

✓4ᵗʰ **M06** Other rheumatoid arthritis

AHA: 2020,4Q,31-32

DEF: Rheumatoid arthritis: Autoimmune systemic disease that causes chronic inflammation of the joints and other areas of the body, manifested by inflammatory changes in articular structures and synovial membranes, atrophy, and loss in bone density.

✓5ᵗʰ **M06.0** Rheumatoid arthritis without rheumatoid factor

M06.00 Rheumatoid arthritis without rheumatoid factor, unspecified site `HCC` `Rx` `ESR` `COM`

✓6ᵗʰ **M06.01** Rheumatoid arthritis without rheumatoid factor, shoulder

M06.011 Rheumatoid arthritis without rheumatoid factor, right shoulder `HCC` `Rx` `ESR` `COM`

M06.012 Rheumatoid arthritis without rheumatoid factor, left shoulder `HCC` `Rx` `ESR` `COM`

M06.019 Rheumatoid arthritis without rheumatoid factor, unspecified shoulder `HCC` `Rx` `ESR` `COM`

✓6ᵗʰ **M06.02** Rheumatoid arthritis without rheumatoid factor, elbow

M06.021 Rheumatoid arthritis without rheumatoid factor, right elbow `HCC` `Rx` `ESR` `COM`

M06.022 Rheumatoid arthritis without rheumatoid factor, left elbow `HCC` `Rx` `ESR` `COM`

M06.029 Rheumatoid arthritis without rheumatoid factor, unspecified elbow `HCC` `Rx` `ESR` `COM`

`HCC` CMS-HCC   `Rx` Rx HCC   `ESR` ESRD HCC   `COM` Commercial HCC   N Newborn: 0   P Pediatric: 0-17   M Maternity: 9-64   A Adult: 15-124

786   ICD-10-CM 2023

√6ᵗʰ **M06.03** **Rheumatoid arthritis without rheumatoid factor, wrist**

M06.031 Rheumatoid arthritis without rheumatoid factor, right wrist `HCC` `Rx` `ESR` `COM`

M06.032 Rheumatoid arthritis without rheumatoid factor, left wrist `HCC` `Rx` `ESR` `COM`

M06.039 Rheumatoid arthritis without rheumatoid factor, unspecified wrist `HCC` `Rx` `ESR` `COM`

√6ᵗʰ **M06.04** **Rheumatoid arthritis without rheumatoid factor, hand**

M06.041 Rheumatoid arthritis without rheumatoid factor, right hand `HCC` `Rx` `ESR` `COM`

M06.042 Rheumatoid arthritis without rheumatoid factor, left hand `HCC` `Rx` `ESR` `COM`

M06.049 Rheumatoid arthritis without rheumatoid factor, unspecified hand `HCC` `Rx` `ESR` `COM`

√6ᵗʰ **M06.05** **Rheumatoid arthritis without rheumatoid factor, hip**

M06.051 Rheumatoid arthritis without rheumatoid factor, right hip `HCC` `Rx` `ESR` `COM`

M06.052 Rheumatoid arthritis without rheumatoid factor, left hip `HCC` `Rx` `ESR` `COM`

M06.059 Rheumatoid arthritis without rheumatoid factor, unspecified hip `HCC` `Rx` `ESR` `COM`

√6ᵗʰ **M06.06** **Rheumatoid arthritis without rheumatoid factor, knee**

M06.061 Rheumatoid arthritis without rheumatoid factor, right knee `HCC` `Rx` `ESR` `COM`

M06.062 Rheumatoid arthritis without rheumatoid factor, left knee `HCC` `Rx` `ESR` `COM`

M06.069 Rheumatoid arthritis without rheumatoid factor, unspecified knee `HCC` `Rx` `ESR` `COM`

√6ᵗʰ **M06.07** **Rheumatoid arthritis without rheumatoid factor, ankle and foot**

M06.071 Rheumatoid arthritis without rheumatoid factor, right ankle and foot `HCC` `Rx` `ESR` `COM`

M06.072 Rheumatoid arthritis without rheumatoid factor, left ankle and foot `HCC` `Rx` `ESR` `COM`

M06.079 Rheumatoid arthritis without rheumatoid factor, unspecified ankle and foot `HCC` `Rx` `ESR` `COM`

M06.08 Rheumatoid arthritis without rheumatoid factor, vertebrae `HCC` `Rx` `ESR` `COM`

M06.09 Rheumatoid arthritis without rheumatoid factor, multiple sites `HCC` `Rx` `ESR` `COM`

M06.0A Rheumatoid arthritis without rheumatoid factor, other specified site `HCC` `Rx` `ESR` `COM`

M06.1 **Adult-onset Still's disease** `HCC` `Rx` `ESR` `COM` `A`

> **EXCLUDES 1**   Still's disease NOS (M08.2-)
>
> **DEF:** Type of systemic arthritis characterized by a transient rash and spiking fevers. This condition may resolve or develop into a chronic condition and may affect internal organs, as well as joints. **Synonym(s):** AOSD

√5ᵗʰ **M06.2** **Rheumatoid bursitis**

M06.20 Rheumatoid bursitis, unspecified site `HCC` `Rx` `ESR` `COM`

√6ᵗʰ **M06.21** **Rheumatoid bursitis, shoulder**

M06.211 Rheumatoid bursitis, right shoulder `HCC` `Rx` `ESR` `COM`

M06.212 Rheumatoid bursitis, left shoulder `HCC` `Rx` `ESR` `COM`

M06.219 Rheumatoid bursitis, unspecified shoulder `HCC` `Rx` `ESR` `COM`

√6ᵗʰ **M06.22** **Rheumatoid bursitis, elbow**

M06.221 Rheumatoid bursitis, right elbow `HCC` `Rx` `ESR` `COM`

M06.222 Rheumatoid bursitis, left elbow `HCC` `Rx` `ESR` `COM`

M06.229 Rheumatoid bursitis, unspecified elbow `HCC` `Rx` `ESR` `COM`

√6ᵗʰ **M06.23** **Rheumatoid bursitis, wrist**

M06.231 Rheumatoid bursitis, right wrist `HCC` `Rx` `ESR` `COM`

M06.232 Rheumatoid bursitis, left wrist `HCC` `Rx` `ESR` `COM`

M06.239 Rheumatoid bursitis, unspecified wrist `HCC` `Rx` `ESR` `COM`

√6ᵗʰ **M06.24** **Rheumatoid bursitis, hand**

M06.241 Rheumatoid bursitis, right hand `HCC` `Rx` `ESR` `COM`

M06.242 Rheumatoid bursitis, left hand `HCC` `Rx` `ESR` `COM`

M06.249 Rheumatoid bursitis, unspecified hand `HCC` `Rx` `ESR` `COM`

√6ᵗʰ **M06.25** **Rheumatoid bursitis, hip**

M06.251 Rheumatoid bursitis, right hip `HCC` `Rx` `ESR` `COM`

M06.252 Rheumatoid bursitis, left hip `HCC` `Rx` `ESR` `COM`

M06.259 Rheumatoid bursitis, unspecified hip `HCC` `Rx` `ESR` `COM`

√6ᵗʰ **M06.26** **Rheumatoid bursitis, knee**

M06.261 Rheumatoid bursitis, right knee `HCC` `Rx` `ESR` `COM`

M06.262 Rheumatoid bursitis, left knee `HCC` `Rx` `ESR` `COM`

M06.269 Rheumatoid bursitis, unspecified knee `HCC` `Rx` `ESR` `COM`

√6ᵗʰ **M06.27** **Rheumatoid bursitis, ankle and foot**

M06.271 Rheumatoid bursitis, right ankle and foot `HCC` `Rx` `ESR` `COM`

M06.272 Rheumatoid bursitis, left ankle and foot `HCC` `Rx` `ESR` `COM`

M06.279 Rheumatoid bursitis, unspecified ankle and foot `HCC` `Rx` `ESR` `COM`

M06.28 Rheumatoid bursitis, vertebrae `HCC` `Rx` `ESR` `COM`

M06.29 Rheumatoid bursitis, multiple sites `HCC` `Rx` `ESR` `COM`

√5ᵗʰ **M06.3** **Rheumatoid nodule**

M06.30 Rheumatoid nodule, unspecified site `HCC` `Rx` `ESR` `COM`

√6ᵗʰ **M06.31** **Rheumatoid nodule, shoulder**

M06.311 Rheumatoid nodule, right shoulder `HCC` `Rx` `ESR` `COM`

M06.312 Rheumatoid nodule, left shoulder `HCC` `Rx` `ESR` `COM`

M06.319 Rheumatoid nodule, unspecified shoulder `HCC` `Rx` `ESR` `COM`

√6ᵗʰ **M06.32** **Rheumatoid nodule, elbow**

M06.321 Rheumatoid nodule, right elbow `HCC` `Rx` `ESR` `COM`

M06.322 Rheumatoid nodule, left elbow `HCC` `Rx` `ESR` `COM`

M06.329 Rheumatoid nodule, unspecified elbow `HCC` `Rx` `ESR` `COM`

√6ᵗʰ **M06.33** **Rheumatoid nodule, wrist**

M06.331 Rheumatoid nodule, right wrist `HCC` `Rx` `ESR` `COM`

M06.332 Rheumatoid nodule, left wrist `HCC` `Rx` `ESR` `COM`

M06.339 Rheumatoid nodule, unspecified wrist `HCC` `Rx` `ESR` `COM`

√6ᵗʰ **M06.34** **Rheumatoid nodule, hand**

M06.341 Rheumatoid nodule, right hand `HCC` `Rx` `ESR` `COM`

M06.342 Rheumatoid nodule, left hand `HCC` `Rx` `ESR` `COM`

M06.349 Rheumatoid nodule, unspecified hand `HCC` `Rx` `ESR` `COM`

√6ᵗʰ **M06.35** **Rheumatoid nodule, hip**

M06.351 Rheumatoid nodule, right hip `HCC` `Rx` `ESR` `COM`

M06.352 Rheumatoid nodule, left hip `HCC` `Rx` `ESR` `COM`

M06.359 Rheumatoid nodule, unspecified hip `HCC` `Rx` `ESR` `COM`

√6ᵗʰ **M06.36** **Rheumatoid nodule, knee**

M06.361 Rheumatoid nodule, right knee `HCC` `Rx` `ESR` `COM`

M06.362 Rheumatoid nodule, left knee `HCC` `Rx` `ESR` `COM`

Chapter 13. Diseases of the Musculoskeletal System and Connective Tissue

M06.369–M08.029

        M06.369 Rheumatoid nodule, unspecified knee   `HCC` `Rx` `ESR` `COM`

    ✓6ᵗʰ **M06.37** Rheumatoid nodule, ankle and foot

        M06.371 Rheumatoid nodule, right ankle and foot   `HCC` `Rx` `ESR` `COM`

        M06.372 Rheumatoid nodule, left ankle and foot   `HCC` `Rx` `ESR` `COM`

        M06.379 Rheumatoid nodule, unspecified ankle and foot   `HCC` `Rx` `ESR` `COM`

    M06.38 Rheumatoid nodule, vertebrae   `HCC` `Rx` `ESR` `COM`

    M06.39 Rheumatoid nodule, multiple sites   `HCC` `Rx` `ESR` `COM`

  M06.4 **Inflammatory polyarthropathy**   `HCC` `Rx` `ESR` `COM`
      EXCLUDES 1   polyarthritis NOS (M13.0)

  ✓5ᵗʰ **M06.8** **Other specified rheumatoid arthritis**

    M06.80 Other specified rheumatoid arthritis, unspecified site   `HCC` `Rx` `ESR` `COM`

    ✓6ᵗʰ **M06.81** Other specified rheumatoid arthritis, shoulder

        M06.811 Other specified rheumatoid arthritis, right shoulder   `HCC` `Rx` `ESR` `COM`

        M06.812 Other specified rheumatoid arthritis, left shoulder   `HCC` `Rx` `ESR` `COM`

        M06.819 Other specified rheumatoid arthritis, unspecified shoulder   `HCC` `Rx` `ESR` `COM`

    ✓6ᵗʰ **M06.82** Other specified rheumatoid arthritis, elbow

        M06.821 Other specified rheumatoid arthritis, right elbow   `HCC` `Rx` `ESR` `COM`

        M06.822 Other specified rheumatoid arthritis, left elbow   `HCC` `Rx` `ESR` `COM`

        M06.829 Other specified rheumatoid arthritis, unspecified elbow   `HCC` `Rx` `ESR` `COM`

    ✓6ᵗʰ **M06.83** Other specified rheumatoid arthritis, wrist

        M06.831 Other specified rheumatoid arthritis, right wrist   `HCC` `Rx` `ESR` `COM`

        M06.832 Other specified rheumatoid arthritis, left wrist   `HCC` `Rx` `ESR` `COM`

        M06.839 Other specified rheumatoid arthritis, unspecified wrist   `HCC` `Rx` `ESR` `COM`

    ✓6ᵗʰ **M06.84** Other specified rheumatoid arthritis, hand

        M06.841 Other specified rheumatoid arthritis, right hand   `HCC` `Rx` `ESR` `COM`

        M06.842 Other specified rheumatoid arthritis, left hand   `HCC` `Rx` `ESR` `COM`

        M06.849 Other specified rheumatoid arthritis, unspecified hand   `HCC` `Rx` `ESR` `COM`

    ✓6ᵗʰ **M06.85** Other specified rheumatoid arthritis, hip

        M06.851 Other specified rheumatoid arthritis, right hip   `HCC` `Rx` `ESR` `COM`

        M06.852 Other specified rheumatoid arthritis, left hip   `HCC` `Rx` `ESR` `COM`

        M06.859 Other specified rheumatoid arthritis, unspecified hip   `HCC` `Rx` `ESR` `COM`

    ✓6ᵗʰ **M06.86** Other specified rheumatoid arthritis, knee

        M06.861 Other specified rheumatoid arthritis, right knee   `HCC` `Rx` `ESR` `COM`

        M06.862 Other specified rheumatoid arthritis, left knee   `HCC` `Rx` `ESR` `COM`

        M06.869 Other specified rheumatoid arthritis, unspecified knee   `HCC` `Rx` `ESR` `COM`

    ✓6ᵗʰ **M06.87** Other specified rheumatoid arthritis, ankle and foot

        M06.871 Other specified rheumatoid arthritis, right ankle and foot   `HCC` `Rx` `ESR` `COM`

        M06.872 Other specified rheumatoid arthritis, left ankle and foot   `HCC` `Rx` `ESR` `COM`

        M06.879 Other specified rheumatoid arthritis, unspecified ankle and foot   `HCC` `Rx` `ESR` `COM`

    M06.88 Other specified rheumatoid arthritis, vertebrae   `HCC` `Rx` `ESR` `COM`

    M06.89 Other specified rheumatoid arthritis, multiple sites   `HCC` `Rx` `ESR` `COM`

    M06.8A Other specified rheumatoid arthritis, other specified site   `HCC` `Rx` `ESR` `COM`

  M06.9 **Rheumatoid arthritis, unspecified**   `HCC` `Rx` `ESR` `COM`

✓4ᵗʰ **M07** **Enteropathic arthropathies**
    Code also associated enteropathy, such as:
      regional enteritis [Crohn's disease] (K50.-)
      ulcerative colitis (K51.-)
      EXCLUDES 1   psoriatic arthropathies (L40.5-)

  ✓5ᵗʰ **M07.6** **Enteropathic arthropathies**

    M07.60 Enteropathic arthropathies, unspecified site

    ✓6ᵗʰ **M07.61** Enteropathic arthropathies, shoulder

        M07.611 Enteropathic arthropathies, right shoulder

        M07.612 Enteropathic arthropathies, left shoulder

        M07.619 Enteropathic arthropathies, unspecified shoulder

    ✓6ᵗʰ **M07.62** Enteropathic arthropathies, elbow

        M07.621 Enteropathic arthropathies, right elbow

        M07.622 Enteropathic arthropathies, left elbow

        M07.629 Enteropathic arthropathies, unspecified elbow

    ✓6ᵗʰ **M07.63** Enteropathic arthropathies, wrist

        M07.631 Enteropathic arthropathies, right wrist

        M07.632 Enteropathic arthropathies, left wrist

        M07.639 Enteropathic arthropathies, unspecified wrist

    ✓6ᵗʰ **M07.64** Enteropathic arthropathies, hand

        M07.641 Enteropathic arthropathies, right hand

        M07.642 Enteropathic arthropathies, left hand

        M07.649 Enteropathic arthropathies, unspecified hand

    ✓6ᵗʰ **M07.65** Enteropathic arthropathies, hip

        M07.651 Enteropathic arthropathies, right hip

        M07.652 Enteropathic arthropathies, left hip

        M07.659 Enteropathic arthropathies, unspecified hip

    ✓6ᵗʰ **M07.66** Enteropathic arthropathies, knee

        M07.661 Enteropathic arthropathies, right knee

        M07.662 Enteropathic arthropathies, left knee

        M07.669 Enteropathic arthropathies, unspecified knee

    ✓6ᵗʰ **M07.67** Enteropathic arthropathies, ankle and foot

        M07.671 Enteropathic arthropathies, right ankle and foot

        M07.672 Enteropathic arthropathies, left ankle and foot

        M07.679 Enteropathic arthropathies, unspecified ankle and foot

    M07.68 Enteropathic arthropathies, vertebrae

    M07.69 Enteropathic arthropathies, multiple sites

✓4ᵗʰ **M08** **Juvenile arthritis**
    Code also any associated underlying condition, such as:
      regional enteritis [Crohn's disease] (K50.-)
      ulcerative colitis (K51.-)
      EXCLUDES 1   arthropathy in Whipple's disease (M14.8)
                 Felty's syndrome (M05.0)
                 juvenile dermatomyositis (M33.0-)
                 psoriatic juvenile arthropathy (L40.54)
    AHA: 2020,4Q,31-32

  ✓5ᵗʰ **M08.0** **Unspecified juvenile rheumatoid arthritis**
    Juvenile rheumatoid arthritis with or without rheumatoid factor

    M08.00 Unspecified juvenile rheumatoid arthritis of unspecified site   `HCC` `Rx` `ESR` `COM`

    ✓6ᵗʰ **M08.01** Unspecified juvenile rheumatoid arthritis, shoulder

        M08.011 Unspecified juvenile rheumatoid arthritis, right shoulder   `HCC` `Rx` `ESR` `COM`

        M08.012 Unspecified juvenile rheumatoid arthritis, left shoulder   `HCC` `Rx` `ESR` `COM`

        M08.019 Unspecified juvenile rheumatoid arthritis, unspecified shoulder   `HCC` `Rx` `ESR` `COM`

    ✓6ᵗʰ **M08.02** Unspecified juvenile rheumatoid arthritis of elbow

        M08.021 Unspecified juvenile rheumatoid arthritis, right elbow   `HCC` `Rx` `ESR` `COM`

        M08.022 Unspecified juvenile rheumatoid arthritis, left elbow   `HCC` `Rx` `ESR` `COM`

        M08.029 Unspecified juvenile rheumatoid arthritis, unspecified elbow   `HCC` `Rx` `ESR` `COM`

`HCC` CMS-HCC   `Rx` Rx HCC   `ESR` ESRD HCC   `COM` Commercial HCC   Ⓝ Newborn: 0   Ⓟ Pediatric: 0-17   Ⓜ Maternity: 9-64   Ⓐ Adult: 15-124

788   ICD-10-CM 2023

√6ᵗʰ **M08.03** Unspecified juvenile rheumatoid arthritis, wrist

     M08.031 Unspecified juvenile rheumatoid arthritis, right wrist `HCC` `Rx` `ESR` `COM`

     M08.032 Unspecified juvenile rheumatoid arthritis, left wrist `HCC` `Rx` `ESR` `COM`

     M08.039 Unspecified juvenile rheumatoid arthritis, unspecified wrist `HCC` `Rx` `ESR` `COM`

√6ᵗʰ **M08.04** Unspecified juvenile rheumatoid arthritis, hand

     M08.041 Unspecified juvenile rheumatoid arthritis, right hand `HCC` `Rx` `ESR` `COM`

     M08.042 Unspecified juvenile rheumatoid arthritis, left hand `HCC` `Rx` `ESR` `COM`

     M08.049 Unspecified juvenile rheumatoid arthritis, unspecified hand `HCC` `Rx` `ESR` `COM`

√6ᵗʰ **M08.05** Unspecified juvenile rheumatoid arthritis, hip

     M08.051 Unspecified juvenile rheumatoid arthritis, right hip `HCC` `Rx` `ESR` `COM`

     M08.052 Unspecified juvenile rheumatoid arthritis, left hip `HCC` `Rx` `ESR` `COM`

     M08.059 Unspecified juvenile rheumatoid arthritis, unspecified hip `HCC` `Rx` `ESR` `COM`

√6ᵗʰ **M08.06** Unspecified juvenile rheumatoid arthritis, knee

     M08.061 Unspecified juvenile rheumatoid arthritis, right knee `HCC` `Rx` `ESR` `COM`

     M08.062 Unspecified juvenile rheumatoid arthritis, left knee `HCC` `Rx` `ESR` `COM`

     M08.069 Unspecified juvenile rheumatoid arthritis, unspecified knee `HCC` `Rx` `ESR` `COM`

√6ᵗʰ **M08.07** Unspecified juvenile rheumatoid arthritis, ankle and foot

     M08.071 Unspecified juvenile rheumatoid arthritis, right ankle and foot `HCC` `Rx` `ESR` `COM`

     M08.072 Unspecified juvenile rheumatoid arthritis, left ankle and foot `HCC` `Rx` `ESR` `COM`

     M08.079 Unspecified juvenile rheumatoid arthritis, unspecified ankle and foot `HCC` `Rx` `ESR` `COM`

M08.08 Unspecified juvenile rheumatoid arthritis, vertebrae `HCC` `Rx` `ESR` `COM`

M08.09 Unspecified juvenile rheumatoid arthritis, multiple sites `HCC` `Rx` `ESR` `COM`

M08.0A Unspecified juvenile rheumatoid arthritis, other specified site `HCC` `Rx` `ESR` `COM`

M08.1 Juvenile ankylosing spondylitis

     EXCLUDES 1   ankylosing spondylitis in adults (M45.0-)

√5ᵗʰ **M08.2** Juvenile rheumatoid arthritis with systemic onset

     Still's disease NOS

     EXCLUDES 1   adult-onset Still's disease (M06.1-)

     DEF: Systemic juvenile rheumatoid arthritis characterized by a transient rash and spiking fevers that may affect internal organs, as well as joints.

     M08.20 Juvenile rheumatoid arthritis with systemic onset, unspecified site `HCC` `Rx` `ESR` `COM`

√6ᵗʰ **M08.21** Juvenile rheumatoid arthritis with systemic onset, shoulder

     M08.211 Juvenile rheumatoid arthritis with systemic onset, right shoulder `HCC` `Rx` `ESR` `COM`

     M08.212 Juvenile rheumatoid arthritis with systemic onset, left shoulder `HCC` `Rx` `ESR` `COM`

     M08.219 Juvenile rheumatoid arthritis with systemic onset, unspecified shoulder `HCC` `Rx` `ESR` `COM`

√6ᵗʰ **M08.22** Juvenile rheumatoid arthritis with systemic onset, elbow

     M08.221 Juvenile rheumatoid arthritis with systemic onset, right elbow `HCC` `Rx` `ESR` `COM`

     M08.222 Juvenile rheumatoid arthritis with systemic onset, left elbow `HCC` `Rx` `ESR` `COM`

     M08.229 Juvenile rheumatoid arthritis with systemic onset, unspecified elbow `HCC` `Rx` `ESR` `COM`

√6ᵗʰ **M08.23** Juvenile rheumatoid arthritis with systemic onset, wrist

     M08.231 Juvenile rheumatoid arthritis with systemic onset, right wrist `HCC` `Rx` `ESR` `COM`

     M08.232 Juvenile rheumatoid arthritis with systemic onset, left wrist `HCC` `Rx` `ESR` `COM`

     M08.239 Juvenile rheumatoid arthritis with systemic onset, unspecified wrist `HCC` `Rx` `ESR` `COM`

√6ᵗʰ **M08.24** Juvenile rheumatoid arthritis with systemic onset, hand

     M08.241 Juvenile rheumatoid arthritis with systemic onset, right hand `HCC` `Rx` `ESR` `COM`

     M08.242 Juvenile rheumatoid arthritis with systemic onset, left hand `HCC` `Rx` `ESR` `COM`

     M08.249 Juvenile rheumatoid arthritis with systemic onset, unspecified hand `HCC` `Rx` `ESR` `COM`

√6ᵗʰ **M08.25** Juvenile rheumatoid arthritis with systemic onset, hip

     M08.251 Juvenile rheumatoid arthritis with systemic onset, right hip `HCC` `Rx` `ESR` `COM`

     M08.252 Juvenile rheumatoid arthritis with systemic onset, left hip `HCC` `Rx` `ESR` `COM`

     M08.259 Juvenile rheumatoid arthritis with systemic onset, unspecified hip `HCC` `Rx` `ESR` `COM`

√6ᵗʰ **M08.26** Juvenile rheumatoid arthritis with systemic onset, knee

     M08.261 Juvenile rheumatoid arthritis with systemic onset, right knee `HCC` `Rx` `ESR` `COM`

     M08.262 Juvenile rheumatoid arthritis with systemic onset, left knee `HCC` `Rx` `ESR` `COM`

     M08.269 Juvenile rheumatoid arthritis with systemic onset, unspecified knee `HCC` `Rx` `ESR` `COM`

√6ᵗʰ **M08.27** Juvenile rheumatoid arthritis with systemic onset, ankle and foot

     M08.271 Juvenile rheumatoid arthritis with systemic onset, right ankle and foot `HCC` `Rx` `ESR` `COM`

     M08.272 Juvenile rheumatoid arthritis with systemic onset, left ankle and foot `HCC` `Rx` `ESR` `COM`

     M08.279 Juvenile rheumatoid arthritis with systemic onset, unspecified ankle and foot `HCC` `Rx` `ESR` `COM`

M08.28 Juvenile rheumatoid arthritis with systemic onset, vertebrae `HCC` `Rx` `ESR` `COM`

M08.29 Juvenile rheumatoid arthritis with systemic onset, multiple sites `HCC` `Rx` `ESR` `COM`

M08.2A Juvenile rheumatoid arthritis with systemic onset, other specified site `HCC` `Rx` `ESR` `COM`

M08.3 Juvenile rheumatoid polyarthritis (seronegative) `HCC` `Rx` `ESR` `COM`

√5ᵗʰ **M08.4** Pauciarticular juvenile rheumatoid arthritis

     M08.40 Pauciarticular juvenile rheumatoid arthritis, unspecified site `HCC` `Rx` `ESR` `COM`

√6ᵗʰ **M08.41** Pauciarticular juvenile rheumatoid arthritis, shoulder

     M08.411 Pauciarticular juvenile rheumatoid arthritis, right shoulder `HCC` `Rx` `ESR` `COM`

     M08.412 Pauciarticular juvenile rheumatoid arthritis, left shoulder `HCC` `Rx` `ESR` `COM`

     M08.419 Pauciarticular juvenile rheumatoid arthritis, unspecified shoulder `HCC` `Rx` `ESR` `COM`

√6ᵗʰ **M08.42** Pauciarticular juvenile rheumatoid arthritis, elbow

     M08.421 Pauciarticular juvenile rheumatoid arthritis, right elbow `HCC` `Rx` `ESR` `COM`

     M08.422 Pauciarticular juvenile rheumatoid arthritis, left elbow `HCC` `Rx` `ESR` `COM`

     M08.429 Pauciarticular juvenile rheumatoid arthritis, unspecified elbow `HCC` `Rx` `ESR` `COM`

√6ᵗʰ **M08.43** Pauciarticular juvenile rheumatoid arthritis, wrist

     M08.431 Pauciarticular juvenile rheumatoid arthritis, right wrist `HCC` `Rx` `ESR` `COM`

✔ Additional Character Required   √x7ᵗʰ Placeholder Alert   Manifestation   Unspecified Dx   Q QPP   UPD Unacceptable PDx

Chapter 13. Diseases of the Musculoskeletal System and Connective Tissue

M08.432–M08.979

           M08.432 Pauciarticular juvenile rheumatoid arthritis, left wrist `HCC` `Rx` `ESR` `COM`

           M08.439 Pauciarticular juvenile rheumatoid arthritis, unspecified wrist `HCC` `Rx` `ESR` `COM`

    ✓6ᵗʰ **M08.44** Pauciarticular juvenile rheumatoid arthritis, hand

           M08.441 Pauciarticular juvenile rheumatoid arthritis, right hand `HCC` `Rx` `ESR` `COM`

           M08.442 Pauciarticular juvenile rheumatoid arthritis, left hand `HCC` `Rx` `ESR` `COM`

           M08.449 Pauciarticular juvenile rheumatoid arthritis, unspecified hand `HCC` `Rx` `ESR` `COM`

    ✓6ᵗʰ **M08.45** Pauciarticular juvenile rheumatoid arthritis, hip

           M08.451 Pauciarticular juvenile rheumatoid arthritis, right hip `HCC` `Rx` `ESR` `COM`

           M08.452 Pauciarticular juvenile rheumatoid arthritis, left hip `HCC` `Rx` `ESR` `COM`

           M08.459 Pauciarticular juvenile rheumatoid arthritis, unspecified hip `HCC` `Rx` `ESR` `COM`

    ✓6ᵗʰ **M08.46** Pauciarticular juvenile rheumatoid arthritis, knee

           M08.461 Pauciarticular juvenile rheumatoid arthritis, right knee `HCC` `Rx` `ESR` `COM`

           M08.462 Pauciarticular juvenile rheumatoid arthritis, left knee `HCC` `Rx` `ESR` `COM`

           M08.469 Pauciarticular juvenile rheumatoid arthritis, unspecified knee `HCC` `Rx` `ESR` `COM`

    ✓6ᵗʰ **M08.47** Pauciarticular juvenile rheumatoid arthritis, ankle and foot

           M08.471 Pauciarticular juvenile rheumatoid arthritis, right ankle and foot `HCC` `Rx` `ESR` `COM`

           M08.472 Pauciarticular juvenile rheumatoid arthritis, left ankle and foot `HCC` `Rx` `ESR` `COM`

           M08.479 Pauciarticular juvenile rheumatoid arthritis, unspecified ankle and foot `HCC` `Rx` `ESR` `COM`

    M08.48 Pauciarticular juvenile rheumatoid arthritis, vertebrae `HCC` `Rx` `ESR` `COM`

    M08.4A Pauciarticular juvenile rheumatoid arthritis, other specified site `HCC` `Rx` `ESR` `COM`

✓5ᵗʰ **M08.8** Other juvenile arthritis

    M08.80 Other juvenile arthritis, unspecified site `HCC` `Rx` `ESR` `COM`

    ✓6ᵗʰ **M08.81** Other juvenile arthritis, shoulder

           M08.811 Other juvenile arthritis, right shoulder `HCC` `Rx` `ESR` `COM`

           M08.812 Other juvenile arthritis, left shoulder `HCC` `Rx` `ESR` `COM`

           M08.819 Other juvenile arthritis, unspecified shoulder `HCC` `Rx` `ESR` `COM`

    ✓6ᵗʰ **M08.82** Other juvenile arthritis, elbow

           M08.821 Other juvenile arthritis, right elbow `HCC` `Rx` `ESR` `COM`

           M08.822 Other juvenile arthritis, left elbow `HCC` `Rx` `ESR` `COM`

           M08.829 Other juvenile arthritis, unspecified elbow `HCC` `Rx` `ESR` `COM`

    ✓6ᵗʰ **M08.83** Other juvenile arthritis, wrist

           M08.831 Other juvenile arthritis, right wrist `HCC` `Rx` `ESR` `COM`

           M08.832 Other juvenile arthritis, left wrist `HCC` `Rx` `ESR` `COM`

           M08.839 Other juvenile arthritis, unspecified wrist `HCC` `Rx` `ESR` `COM`

    ✓6ᵗʰ **M08.84** Other juvenile arthritis, hand

           M08.841 Other juvenile arthritis, right hand `HCC` `Rx` `ESR` `COM`

           M08.842 Other juvenile arthritis, left hand `HCC` `Rx` `ESR` `COM`

           M08.849 Other juvenile arthritis, unspecified hand `HCC` `Rx` `ESR` `COM`

    ✓6ᵗʰ **M08.85** Other juvenile arthritis, hip

           M08.851 Other juvenile arthritis, right hip `HCC` `Rx` `ESR` `COM`

           M08.852 Other juvenile arthritis, left hip `HCC` `Rx` `ESR` `COM`

           M08.859 Other juvenile arthritis, unspecified hip `HCC` `Rx` `ESR` `COM`

    ✓6ᵗʰ **M08.86** Other juvenile arthritis, knee

           M08.861 Other juvenile arthritis, right knee `HCC` `Rx` `ESR` `COM`

           M08.862 Other juvenile arthritis, left knee `HCC` `Rx` `ESR` `COM`

           M08.869 Other juvenile arthritis, unspecified knee `HCC` `Rx` `ESR` `COM`

    ✓6ᵗʰ **M08.87** Other juvenile arthritis, ankle and foot

           M08.871 Other juvenile arthritis, right ankle and foot `HCC` `Rx` `ESR` `COM`

           M08.872 Other juvenile arthritis, left ankle and foot `HCC` `Rx` `ESR` `COM`

           M08.879 Other juvenile arthritis, unspecified ankle and foot `HCC` `Rx` `ESR` `COM`

    M08.88 Other juvenile arthritis, other specified site `HCC` `Rx` `ESR` `COM`

        Other juvenile arthritis, vertebrae

    M08.89 Other juvenile arthritis, multiple sites `HCC` `Rx` `ESR` `COM`

✓5ᵗʰ **M08.9** Juvenile arthritis, unspecified

      EXCLUDES 1   *juvenile rheumatoid arthritis, unspecified (M08.0-)*

    M08.90 Juvenile arthritis, unspecified, unspecified site `HCC` `Rx` `ESR` `COM`

    ✓6ᵗʰ **M08.91** Juvenile arthritis, unspecified, shoulder

           M08.911 Juvenile arthritis, unspecified, right shoulder `HCC` `Rx` `ESR` `COM`

           M08.912 Juvenile arthritis, unspecified, left shoulder `HCC` `Rx` `ESR` `COM`

           M08.919 Juvenile arthritis, unspecified, unspecified shoulder `HCC` `Rx` `ESR` `COM`

    ✓6ᵗʰ **M08.92** Juvenile arthritis, unspecified, elbow

           M08.921 Juvenile arthritis, unspecified, right elbow `HCC` `Rx` `ESR` `COM`

           M08.922 Juvenile arthritis, unspecified, left elbow `HCC` `Rx` `ESR` `COM`

           M08.929 Juvenile arthritis, unspecified, unspecified elbow `HCC` `Rx` `ESR` `COM`

    ✓6ᵗʰ **M08.93** Juvenile arthritis, unspecified, wrist

           M08.931 Juvenile arthritis, unspecified, right wrist `HCC` `Rx` `ESR` `COM`

           M08.932 Juvenile arthritis, unspecified, left wrist `HCC` `Rx` `ESR` `COM`

           M08.939 Juvenile arthritis, unspecified, unspecified wrist `HCC` `Rx` `ESR` `COM`

    ✓6ᵗʰ **M08.94** Juvenile arthritis, unspecified, hand

           M08.941 Juvenile arthritis, unspecified, right hand `HCC` `Rx` `ESR` `COM`

           M08.942 Juvenile arthritis, unspecified, left hand `HCC` `Rx` `ESR` `COM`

           M08.949 Juvenile arthritis, unspecified, unspecified hand `HCC` `Rx` `ESR` `COM`

    ✓6ᵗʰ **M08.95** Juvenile arthritis, unspecified, hip

           M08.951 Juvenile arthritis, unspecified, right hip `HCC` `Rx` `ESR` `COM`

           M08.952 Juvenile arthritis, unspecified, left hip `HCC` `Rx` `ESR` `COM`

           M08.959 Juvenile arthritis, unspecified, unspecified hip `HCC` `Rx` `ESR` `COM`

    ✓6ᵗʰ **M08.96** Juvenile arthritis, unspecified, knee

           M08.961 Juvenile arthritis, unspecified, right knee `HCC` `Rx` `ESR` `COM`

           M08.962 Juvenile arthritis, unspecified, left knee `HCC` `Rx` `ESR` `COM`

           M08.969 Juvenile arthritis, unspecified, unspecified knee `HCC` `Rx` `ESR` `COM`

    ✓6ᵗʰ **M08.97** Juvenile arthritis, unspecified, ankle and foot

           M08.971 Juvenile arthritis, unspecified, right ankle and foot `HCC` `Rx` `ESR` `COM`

           M08.972 Juvenile arthritis, unspecified, left ankle and foot `HCC` `Rx` `ESR` `COM`

           M08.979 Juvenile arthritis, unspecified, unspecified ankle and foot `HCC` `Rx` `ESR` `COM`

`HCC` CMS-HCC   `Rx` Rx HCC   `ESR` ESRD HCC   `COM` Commercial HCC   N Newborn: 0   P Pediatric: 0-17   M Maternity: 9-64   A Adult: 15-124

790   ICD-10-CM 2023

M08.98   **Juvenile arthritis, unspecified,** vertebrae   `HCC` `Rx` `ESR` `COM`

M08.99   **Juvenile arthritis, unspecified, multiple** sites   `HCC` `Rx` `ESR` `COM`

M08.9A   **Juvenile arthritis, unspecified, other specified** site   `HCC` `Rx` `ESR` `COM`

✓4ᵗʰ **M1A**   **Chronic gout**

Use additional code to identify:
autonomic neuropathy in diseases classified elsewhere (G99.Ø)
calculus of urinary tract in diseases classified elsewhere (N22)
cardiomyopathy in diseases classified elsewhere (I43)
disorders of external ear in diseases classified elsewhere (H61.1-, H62.8-)
disorders of iris and ciliary body in diseases classified elsewhere (H22)
glomerular disorders in diseases classified elsewhere (NØ8)

EXCLUDES 1   gout NOS (M1Ø.-)

EXCLUDES 2   acute gout (M1Ø.-)

> The appropriate 7th character is to be added to each code from category M1A.
> Ø   without tophus (tophi)
> 1   with tophus (tophi)

✓5ᵗʰ **M1A.Ø**   **Idiopathic chronic gout**

Chronic gouty bursitis
Primary chronic gout

✓x7ᵗʰ   **M1A.ØØ**   **Idiopathic chronic gout, unspecified site**

✓6ᵗʰ   **M1A.Ø1**   **Idiopathic chronic gout, shoulder**

    ✓7ᵗʰ   **M1A.Ø11**   **Idiopathic chronic gout, right shoulder**

    ✓7ᵗʰ   **M1A.Ø12**   **Idiopathic chronic gout, left shoulder**

    ✓7ᵗʰ   **M1A.Ø19**   **Idiopathic chronic gout, unspecified shoulder**

✓6ᵗʰ   **M1A.Ø2**   **Idiopathic chronic gout, elbow**

    ✓7ᵗʰ   **M1A.Ø21**   **Idiopathic chronic gout, right elbow**

    ✓7ᵗʰ   **M1A.Ø22**   **Idiopathic chronic gout, left elbow**

    ✓7ᵗʰ   **M1A.Ø29**   **Idiopathic chronic gout, unspecified elbow**

✓6ᵗʰ   **M1A.Ø3**   **Idiopathic chronic gout, wrist**

    ✓7ᵗʰ   **M1A.Ø31**   **Idiopathic chronic gout, right wrist**

    ✓7ᵗʰ   **M1A.Ø32**   **Idiopathic chronic gout, left wrist**

    ✓7ᵗʰ   **M1A.Ø39**   **Idiopathic chronic gout, unspecified wrist**

✓6ᵗʰ   **M1A.Ø4**   **Idiopathic chronic gout, hand**

    ✓7ᵗʰ   **M1A.Ø41**   **Idiopathic chronic gout, right hand**

    ✓7ᵗʰ   **M1A.Ø42**   **Idiopathic chronic gout, left hand**

    ✓7ᵗʰ   **M1A.Ø49**   **Idiopathic chronic gout, unspecified hand**

✓6ᵗʰ   **M1A.Ø5**   **Idiopathic chronic gout, hip**

    ✓7ᵗʰ   **M1A.Ø51**   **Idiopathic chronic gout, right hip**

    ✓7ᵗʰ   **M1A.Ø52**   **Idiopathic chronic gout, left hip**

    ✓7ᵗʰ   **M1A.Ø59**   **Idiopathic chronic gout, unspecified hip**

✓6ᵗʰ   **M1A.Ø6**   **Idiopathic chronic gout, knee**

    ✓7ᵗʰ   **M1A.Ø61**   **Idiopathic chronic gout, right knee**

    ✓7ᵗʰ   **M1A.Ø62**   **Idiopathic chronic gout, left knee**

    ✓7ᵗʰ   **M1A.Ø69**   **Idiopathic chronic gout, unspecified knee**

✓6ᵗʰ   **M1A.Ø7**   **Idiopathic chronic gout, ankle and foot**

    ✓7ᵗʰ   **M1A.Ø71**   **Idiopathic chronic gout, right ankle and foot**

    ✓7ᵗʰ   **M1A.Ø72**   **Idiopathic chronic gout, left ankle and foot**

    ✓7ᵗʰ   **M1A.Ø79**   **Idiopathic chronic gout, unspecified ankle and foot**

✓x7ᵗʰ   **M1A.Ø8**   **Idiopathic chronic gout, vertebrae**

✓x7ᵗʰ   **M1A.Ø9**   **Idiopathic chronic gout, multiple sites**

✓5ᵗʰ **M1A.1**   **Lead-induced chronic gout**

Code first toxic effects of lead and its compounds (T56.Ø-)

✓x7ᵗʰ   **M1A.1Ø**   **Lead-induced chronic gout, unspecified site**

✓6ᵗʰ   **M1A.11**   **Lead-induced chronic gout, shoulder**

    ✓7ᵗʰ   **M1A.111**   **Lead-induced chronic gout, right shoulder**

    ✓7ᵗʰ   **M1A.112**   **Lead-induced chronic gout, left shoulder**

    ✓7ᵗʰ   **M1A.119**   **Lead-induced chronic gout, unspecified shoulder**

✓6ᵗʰ   **M1A.12**   **Lead-induced chronic gout, elbow**

    ✓7ᵗʰ   **M1A.121**   **Lead-induced chronic gout, right elbow**

    ✓7ᵗʰ   **M1A.122**   **Lead-induced chronic gout, left elbow**

    ✓7ᵗʰ   **M1A.129**   **Lead-induced chronic gout, unspecified elbow**

✓6ᵗʰ   **M1A.13**   **Lead-induced chronic gout, wrist**

    ✓7ᵗʰ   **M1A.131**   **Lead-induced chronic gout, right wrist**

    ✓7ᵗʰ   **M1A.132**   **Lead-induced chronic gout, left wrist**

    ✓7ᵗʰ   **M1A.139**   **Lead-induced chronic gout, unspecified wrist**

✓6ᵗʰ   **M1A.14**   **Lead-induced chronic gout, hand**

    ✓7ᵗʰ   **M1A.141**   **Lead-induced chronic gout, right hand**

    ✓7ᵗʰ   **M1A.142**   **Lead-induced chronic gout, left hand**

    ✓7ᵗʰ   **M1A.149**   **Lead-induced chronic gout, unspecified hand**

✓6ᵗʰ   **M1A.15**   **Lead-induced chronic gout, hip**

    ✓7ᵗʰ   **M1A.151**   **Lead-induced chronic gout, right hip**

    ✓7ᵗʰ   **M1A.152**   **Lead-induced chronic gout, left hip**

    ✓7ᵗʰ   **M1A.159**   **Lead-induced chronic gout, unspecified hip**

✓6ᵗʰ   **M1A.16**   **Lead-induced chronic gout, knee**

    ✓7ᵗʰ   **M1A.161**   **Lead-induced chronic gout, right knee**

    ✓7ᵗʰ   **M1A.162**   **Lead-induced chronic gout, left knee**

    ✓7ᵗʰ   **M1A.169**   **Lead-induced chronic gout, unspecified knee**

✓6ᵗʰ   **M1A.17**   **Lead-induced chronic gout, ankle and foot**

    ✓7ᵗʰ   **M1A.171**   **Lead-induced chronic gout, right ankle and foot**

    ✓7ᵗʰ   **M1A.172**   **Lead-induced chronic gout, left ankle and foot**

    ✓7ᵗʰ   **M1A.179**   **Lead-induced chronic gout, unspecified ankle and foot**

✓x7ᵗʰ   **M1A.18**   **Lead-induced chronic gout, vertebrae**

✓x7ᵗʰ   **M1A.19**   **Lead-induced chronic gout, multiple sites**

✓5ᵗʰ **M1A.2**   **Drug-induced chronic gout**

Use additional code for adverse effect, if applicable, to identify drug (T36-T5Ø with fifth or sixth character 5)

✓x7ᵗʰ   **M1A.2Ø**   **Drug-induced chronic gout, unspecified site**

✓6ᵗʰ   **M1A.21**   **Drug-induced chronic gout, shoulder**

    ✓7ᵗʰ   **M1A.211**   **Drug-induced chronic gout, right shoulder**

    ✓7ᵗʰ   **M1A.212**   **Drug-induced chronic gout, left shoulder**

    ✓7ᵗʰ   **M1A.219**   **Drug-induced chronic gout, unspecified shoulder**

✓6ᵗʰ   **M1A.22**   **Drug-induced chronic gout, elbow**

    ✓7ᵗʰ   **M1A.221**   **Drug-induced chronic gout, right elbow**

    ✓7ᵗʰ   **M1A.222**   **Drug-induced chronic gout, left elbow**

    ✓7ᵗʰ   **M1A.229**   **Drug-induced chronic gout, unspecified elbow**

✓6ᵗʰ   **M1A.23**   **Drug-induced chronic gout, wrist**

    ✓7ᵗʰ   **M1A.231**   **Drug-induced chronic gout, right wrist**

    ✓7ᵗʰ   **M1A.232**   **Drug-induced chronic gout, left wrist**

    ✓7ᵗʰ   **M1A.239**   **Drug-induced chronic gout, unspecified wrist**

✓6ᵗʰ   **M1A.24**   **Drug-induced chronic gout, hand**

    ✓7ᵗʰ   **M1A.241**   **Drug-induced chronic gout, right hand**

    ✓7ᵗʰ   **M1A.242**   **Drug-induced chronic gout, left hand**

    ✓7ᵗʰ   **M1A.249**   **Drug-induced chronic gout, unspecified hand**

✓6ᵗʰ   **M1A.25**   **Drug-induced chronic gout, hip**

    ✓7ᵗʰ   **M1A.251**   **Drug-induced chronic gout, right hip**

    ✓7ᵗʰ   **M1A.252**   **Drug-induced chronic gout, left hip**

    ✓7ᵗʰ   **M1A.259**   **Drug-induced chronic gout, unspecified hip**

✓6ᵗʰ   **M1A.26**   **Drug-induced chronic gout, knee**

    ✓7ᵗʰ   **M1A.261**   **Drug-induced chronic gout, right knee**

    ✓7ᵗʰ   **M1A.262**   **Drug-induced chronic gout, left knee**

    ✓7ᵗʰ   **M1A.269**   **Drug-induced chronic gout, unspecified knee**

✓6ᵗʰ   **M1A.27**   **Drug-induced chronic gout, ankle and foot**

    ✓7ᵗʰ   **M1A.271**   **Drug-induced chronic gout, right ankle and foot**

    ✓7ᵗʰ   **M1A.272**   **Drug-induced chronic gout, left ankle and foot**

☑ Additional Character Required   ✓x7ᵗʰ Placeholder Alert   Manifestation   Unspecified Dx   Q QPP   UPD Unacceptable PDx

√7ᵗʰ **M1A.279** Drug-induced chronic gout, unspecified ankle and foot

√x7ᵗʰ **M1A.28** Drug-induced chronic gout, vertebrae

√x7ᵗʰ **M1A.29** Drug-induced chronic gout, multiple sites

√5ᵗʰ **M1A.3** Chronic gout due to renal impairment

Code first associated renal disease

√x7ᵗʰ **M1A.30** Chronic gout due to renal impairment, unspecified site

√6ᵗʰ **M1A.31** Chronic gout due to renal impairment, shoulder

√7ᵗʰ **M1A.311** Chronic gout due to renal impairment, right shoulder

√7ᵗʰ **M1A.312** Chronic gout due to renal impairment, left shoulder

√7ᵗʰ **M1A.319** Chronic gout due to renal impairment, unspecified shoulder

√6ᵗʰ **M1A.32** Chronic gout due to renal impairment, elbow

√7ᵗʰ **M1A.321** Chronic gout due to renal impairment, right elbow

√7ᵗʰ **M1A.322** Chronic gout due to renal impairment, left elbow

√7ᵗʰ **M1A.329** Chronic gout due to renal impairment, unspecified elbow

√6ᵗʰ **M1A.33** Chronic gout due to renal impairment, wrist

√7ᵗʰ **M1A.331** Chronic gout due to renal impairment, right wrist

√7ᵗʰ **M1A.332** Chronic gout due to renal impairment, left wrist

√7ᵗʰ **M1A.339** Chronic gout due to renal impairment, unspecified wrist

√6ᵗʰ **M1A.34** Chronic gout due to renal impairment, hand

√7ᵗʰ **M1A.341** Chronic gout due to renal impairment, right hand

√7ᵗʰ **M1A.342** Chronic gout due to renal impairment, left hand

√7ᵗʰ **M1A.349** Chronic gout due to renal impairment, unspecified hand

√6ᵗʰ **M1A.35** Chronic gout due to renal impairment, hip

√7ᵗʰ **M1A.351** Chronic gout due to renal impairment, right hip

√7ᵗʰ **M1A.352** Chronic gout due to renal impairment, left hip

√7ᵗʰ **M1A.359** Chronic gout due to renal impairment, unspecified hip

√6ᵗʰ **M1A.36** Chronic gout due to renal impairment, knee

√7ᵗʰ **M1A.361** Chronic gout due to renal impairment, right knee

√7ᵗʰ **M1A.362** Chronic gout due to renal impairment, left knee

√7ᵗʰ **M1A.369** Chronic gout due to renal impairment, unspecified knee

√6ᵗʰ **M1A.37** Chronic gout due to renal impairment, ankle and foot

√7ᵗʰ **M1A.371** Chronic gout due to renal impairment, right ankle and foot

√7ᵗʰ **M1A.372** Chronic gout due to renal impairment, left ankle and foot

√7ᵗʰ **M1A.379** Chronic gout due to renal impairment, unspecified ankle and foot

√x7ᵗʰ **M1A.38** Chronic gout due to renal impairment, vertebrae

√x7ᵗʰ **M1A.39** Chronic gout due to renal impairment, multiple sites

√5ᵗʰ **M1A.4** Other secondary chronic gout

Code first associated condition

√x7ᵗʰ **M1A.40** Other secondary chronic gout, unspecified site

√6ᵗʰ **M1A.41** Other secondary chronic gout, shoulder

√7ᵗʰ **M1A.411** Other secondary chronic gout, right shoulder

√7ᵗʰ **M1A.412** Other secondary chronic gout, left shoulder

√7ᵗʰ **M1A.419** Other secondary chronic gout, unspecified shoulder

√6ᵗʰ **M1A.42** Other secondary chronic gout, elbow

√7ᵗʰ **M1A.421** Other secondary chronic gout, right elbow

√7ᵗʰ **M1A.422** Other secondary chronic gout, left elbow

√7ᵗʰ **M1A.429** Other secondary chronic gout, unspecified elbow

√6ᵗʰ **M1A.43** Other secondary chronic gout, wrist

√7ᵗʰ **M1A.431** Other secondary chronic gout, right wrist

√7ᵗʰ **M1A.432** Other secondary chronic gout, left wrist

√7ᵗʰ **M1A.439** Other secondary chronic gout, unspecified wrist

√6ᵗʰ **M1A.44** Other secondary chronic gout, hand

√7ᵗʰ **M1A.441** Other secondary chronic gout, right hand

√7ᵗʰ **M1A.442** Other secondary chronic gout, left hand

√7ᵗʰ **M1A.449** Other secondary chronic gout, unspecified hand

√6ᵗʰ **M1A.45** Other secondary chronic gout, hip

√7ᵗʰ **M1A.451** Other secondary chronic gout, right hip

√7ᵗʰ **M1A.452** Other secondary chronic gout, left hip

√7ᵗʰ **M1A.459** Other secondary chronic gout, unspecified hip

√6ᵗʰ **M1A.46** Other secondary chronic gout, knee

√7ᵗʰ **M1A.461** Other secondary chronic gout, right knee

√7ᵗʰ **M1A.462** Other secondary chronic gout, left knee

√7ᵗʰ **M1A.469** Other secondary chronic gout, unspecified knee

√6ᵗʰ **M1A.47** Other secondary chronic gout, ankle and foot

√7ᵗʰ **M1A.471** Other secondary chronic gout, right ankle and foot

√7ᵗʰ **M1A.472** Other secondary chronic gout, left ankle and foot

√7ᵗʰ **M1A.479** Other secondary chronic gout, unspecified ankle and foot

√x7ᵗʰ **M1A.48** Other secondary chronic gout, vertebrae

√x7ᵗʰ **M1A.49** Other secondary chronic gout, multiple sites

√x7ᵗʰ **M1A.9** Chronic gout, unspecified

√4ᵗʰ **M10** Gout

Acute gout

Gout attack

Gout flare

Podagra

Use additional code to identify:

autonomic neuropathy in diseases classified elsewhere (G99.0)

calculus of urinary tract in diseases classified elsewhere (N22)

cardiomyopathy in diseases classified elsewhere (I43)

disorders of external ear in diseases classified elsewhere (H61.1-, H62.8-)

disorders of iris and ciliary body in diseases classified elsewhere (H22)

glomerular disorders in diseases classified elsewhere (N08)

EXCLUDES 2   chronic gout (M1A.-)

DEF: Purine and pyrimidine metabolic disorders, manifested by hyperuricemia and recurrent acute inflammatory arthritis. Monosodium urate or monohydrate crystals may be deposited in and around the joints, leading to joint destruction and severe crippling.

√5ᵗʰ **M10.0** Idiopathic gout

Gouty bursitis

Primary gout

M10.00 Idiopathic gout, unspecified site

√6ᵗʰ **M10.01** Idiopathic gout, shoulder

M10.011 Idiopathic gout, right shoulder

M10.012 Idiopathic gout, left shoulder

M10.019 Idiopathic gout, unspecified shoulder

√6ᵗʰ **M10.02** Idiopathic gout, elbow

M10.021 Idiopathic gout, right elbow

M10.022 Idiopathic gout, left elbow

M10.029 Idiopathic gout, unspecified elbow

√6ᵗʰ **M10.03** Idiopathic gout, wrist

M10.031 Idiopathic gout, right wrist

M10.032 Idiopathic gout, left wrist

M10.039 Idiopathic gout, unspecified wrist

√6ᵗʰ **M10.04** Idiopathic gout, hand

M10.041 Idiopathic gout, right hand

M10.042 Idiopathic gout, left hand

M10.049 Idiopathic gout, unspecified hand

√6ᵗʰ **M10.05** Idiopathic gout, hip

M10.051 Idiopathic gout, right hip

M10.052 Idiopathic gout, left hip

M10.059 Idiopathic gout, unspecified hip

√6ᵗʰ **M10.06** Idiopathic gout, knee

M10.061 Idiopathic gout, right knee

HCC CMS-HCC **Rx** Rx HCC **ESR** ESRD HCC **COM** Commercial HCC   **N** Newborn: 0 **P** Pediatric: 0-17 **M** Maternity: 9-64 **A** Adult: 15-124

792   ICD-10-CM 2023

M10.062 Idiopathic gout, left knee
M10.069 Idiopathic gout, unspecified knee
√6ᵗʰ M10.07 Idiopathic gout, ankle and foot
M10.071 Idiopathic gout, right ankle and foot
M10.072 Idiopathic gout, left ankle and foot
M10.079 Idiopathic gout, unspecified ankle and foot
M10.08 Idiopathic gout, vertebrae
M10.09 Idiopathic gout, multiple sites
√5ᵗʰ M10.1 Lead-induced gout
Code first toxic effects of lead and its compounds (T56.0-)
M10.10 Lead-induced gout, unspecified site
√6ᵗʰ M10.11 Lead-induced gout, shoulder
M10.111 Lead-induced gout, right shoulder
M10.112 Lead-induced gout, left shoulder
M10.119 Lead-induced gout, unspecified shoulder
√6ᵗʰ M10.12 Lead-induced gout, elbow
M10.121 Lead-induced gout, right elbow
M10.122 Lead-induced gout, left elbow
M10.129 Lead-induced gout, unspecified elbow
√6ᵗʰ M10.13 Lead-induced gout, wrist
M10.131 Lead-induced gout, right wrist
M10.132 Lead-induced gout, left wrist
M10.139 Lead-induced gout, unspecified wrist
√6ᵗʰ M10.14 Lead-induced gout, hand
M10.141 Lead-induced gout, right hand
M10.142 Lead-induced gout, left hand
M10.149 Lead-induced gout, unspecified hand
√6ᵗʰ M10.15 Lead-induced gout, hip
M10.151 Lead-induced gout, right hip
M10.152 Lead-induced gout, left hip
M10.159 Lead-induced gout, unspecified hip
√6ᵗʰ M10.16 Lead-induced gout, knee
M10.161 Lead-induced gout, right knee
M10.162 Lead-induced gout, left knee
M10.169 Lead-induced gout, unspecified knee
√6ᵗʰ M10.17 Lead-induced gout, ankle and foot
M10.171 Lead-induced gout, right ankle and foot
M10.172 Lead-induced gout, left ankle and foot
M10.179 Lead-induced gout, unspecified ankle and foot
M10.18 Lead-induced gout, vertebrae
M10.19 Lead-induced gout, multiple sites
√5ᵗʰ M10.2 Drug-induced gout
Use additional code for adverse effect, if applicable, to identify drug (T36-T50 with fifth or sixth character 5)
M10.20 Drug-induced gout, unspecified site
√6ᵗʰ M10.21 Drug-induced gout, shoulder
M10.211 Drug-induced gout, right shoulder
M10.212 Drug-induced gout, left shoulder
M10.219 Drug-induced gout, unspecified shoulder
√6ᵗʰ M10.22 Drug-induced gout, elbow
M10.221 Drug-induced gout, right elbow
M10.222 Drug-induced gout, left elbow
M10.229 Drug-induced gout, unspecified elbow
√6ᵗʰ M10.23 Drug-induced gout, wrist
M10.231 Drug-induced gout, right wrist
M10.232 Drug-induced gout, left wrist
M10.239 Drug-induced gout, unspecified wrist
√6ᵗʰ M10.24 Drug-induced gout, hand
M10.241 Drug-induced gout, right hand
M10.242 Drug-induced gout, left hand
M10.249 Drug-induced gout, unspecified hand
√6ᵗʰ M10.25 Drug-induced gout, hip
M10.251 Drug-induced gout, right hip
M10.252 Drug-induced gout, left hip
M10.259 Drug-induced gout, unspecified hip
√6ᵗʰ M10.26 Drug-induced gout, knee
M10.261 Drug-induced gout, right knee
M10.262 Drug-induced gout, left knee
M10.269 Drug-induced gout, unspecified knee
√6ᵗʰ M10.27 Drug-induced gout, ankle and foot
M10.271 Drug-induced gout, right ankle and foot
M10.272 Drug-induced gout, left ankle and foot

M10.279 Drug-induced gout, unspecified ankle and foot
M10.28 Drug-induced gout, vertebrae
M10.29 Drug-induced gout, multiple sites
√5ᵗʰ M10.3 Gout due to renal impairment
Code first associated renal disease
M10.30 Gout due to renal impairment, unspecified site
√6ᵗʰ M10.31 Gout due to renal impairment, shoulder
M10.311 Gout due to renal impairment, right shoulder
M10.312 Gout due to renal impairment, left shoulder
M10.319 Gout due to renal impairment, unspecified shoulder
√6ᵗʰ M10.32 Gout due to renal impairment, elbow
M10.321 Gout due to renal impairment, right elbow
M10.322 Gout due to renal impairment, left elbow
M10.329 Gout due to renal impairment, unspecified elbow
√6ᵗʰ M10.33 Gout due to renal impairment, wrist
M10.331 Gout due to renal impairment, right wrist
M10.332 Gout due to renal impairment, left wrist
M10.339 Gout due to renal impairment, unspecified wrist
√6ᵗʰ M10.34 Gout due to renal impairment, hand
M10.341 Gout due to renal impairment, right hand
M10.342 Gout due to renal impairment, left hand
M10.349 Gout due to renal impairment, unspecified hand
√6ᵗʰ M10.35 Gout due to renal impairment, hip
M10.351 Gout due to renal impairment, right hip
M10.352 Gout due to renal impairment, left hip
M10.359 Gout due to renal impairment, unspecified hip
√6ᵗʰ M10.36 Gout due to renal impairment, knee
M10.361 Gout due to renal impairment, right knee
M10.362 Gout due to renal impairment, left knee
M10.369 Gout due to renal impairment, unspecified knee
√6ᵗʰ M10.37 Gout due to renal impairment, ankle and foot
M10.371 Gout due to renal impairment, right ankle and foot
M10.372 Gout due to renal impairment, left ankle and foot
M10.379 Gout due to renal impairment, unspecified ankle and foot
M10.38 Gout due to renal impairment, vertebrae
M10.39 Gout due to renal impairment, multiple sites
√5ᵗʰ M10.4 Other secondary gout
Code first associated condition
M10.40 Other secondary gout, unspecified site
√6ᵗʰ M10.41 Other secondary gout, shoulder
M10.411 Other secondary gout, right shoulder
M10.412 Other secondary gout, left shoulder
M10.419 Other secondary gout, unspecified shoulder
√6ᵗʰ M10.42 Other secondary gout, elbow
M10.421 Other secondary gout, right elbow
M10.422 Other secondary gout, left elbow
M10.429 Other secondary gout, unspecified elbow
√6ᵗʰ M10.43 Other secondary gout, wrist
M10.431 Other secondary gout, right wrist
M10.432 Other secondary gout, left wrist
M10.439 Other secondary gout, unspecified wrist
√6ᵗʰ M10.44 Other secondary gout, hand
M10.441 Other secondary gout, right hand
M10.442 Other secondary gout, left hand
M10.449 Other secondary gout, unspecified hand
√6ᵗʰ M10.45 Other secondary gout, hip
M10.451 Other secondary gout, right hip
M10.452 Other secondary gout, left hip
M10.459 Other secondary gout, unspecified hip
√6ᵗʰ M10.46 Other secondary gout, knee
M10.461 Other secondary gout, right knee
M10.462 Other secondary gout, left knee
M10.469 Other secondary gout, unspecified knee

✓6ᵗʰ **M10.47** **Other secondary gout,** ankle and foot

    M10.471 Other secondary gout, right ankle and foot
    M10.472 Other secondary gout, left ankle and foot
    M10.479 Other secondary gout, unspecified ankle and foot

M10.48 **Other secondary gout,** vertebrae
M10.49 **Other secondary gout,** multiple sites

M10.9 **Gout, unspecified**
    Gout NOS

✓4ᵗʰ **M11** **Other crystal arthropathies**

✓5ᵗʰ **M11.0** **Hydroxyapatite deposition disease**

    DEF: Disease caused by deposits of calcium phosphate crystals in the soft tissues close to the joint (especially tendons) or in the joints. These calcifications can be mono or polyarticular and can cause destruction of the joint involved.

    M11.00 **Hydroxyapatite deposition disease, unspecified site**

✓6ᵗʰ **M11.01** **Hydroxyapatite deposition disease,** shoulder

    M11.011 Hydroxyapatite deposition disease, right shoulder
    M11.012 Hydroxyapatite deposition disease, left shoulder
    M11.019 Hydroxyapatite deposition disease, unspecified shoulder

✓6ᵗʰ **M11.02** **Hydroxyapatite deposition disease,** elbow

    M11.021 Hydroxyapatite deposition disease, right elbow
    M11.022 Hydroxyapatite deposition disease, left elbow
    M11.029 Hydroxyapatite deposition disease, unspecified elbow

✓6ᵗʰ **M11.03** **Hydroxyapatite deposition disease,** wrist

    M11.031 Hydroxyapatite deposition disease, right wrist
    M11.032 Hydroxyapatite deposition disease, left wrist
    M11.039 Hydroxyapatite deposition disease, unspecified wrist

✓6ᵗʰ **M11.04** **Hydroxyapatite deposition disease,** hand

    M11.041 Hydroxyapatite deposition disease, right hand
    M11.042 Hydroxyapatite deposition disease, left hand
    M11.049 Hydroxyapatite deposition disease, unspecified hand

✓6ᵗʰ **M11.05** **Hydroxyapatite deposition disease,** hip

    M11.051 Hydroxyapatite deposition disease, right hip
    M11.052 Hydroxyapatite deposition disease, left hip
    M11.059 Hydroxyapatite deposition disease, unspecified hip

✓6ᵗʰ **M11.06** **Hydroxyapatite deposition disease,** knee

    M11.061 Hydroxyapatite deposition disease, right knee
    M11.062 Hydroxyapatite deposition disease, left knee
    M11.069 Hydroxyapatite deposition disease, unspecified knee

✓6ᵗʰ **M11.07** **Hydroxyapatite deposition disease,** ankle and foot

    M11.071 Hydroxyapatite deposition disease, right ankle and foot
    M11.072 Hydroxyapatite deposition disease, left ankle and foot
    M11.079 Hydroxyapatite deposition disease, unspecified ankle and foot

M11.08 **Hydroxyapatite deposition disease,** vertebrae
M11.09 **Hydroxyapatite deposition disease,** multiple sites

✓5ᵗʰ **M11.1** **Familial chondrocalcinosis**

    M11.10 **Familial chondrocalcinosis, unspecified site**

✓6ᵗʰ **M11.11** **Familial chondrocalcinosis,** shoulder

    M11.111 Familial chondrocalcinosis, right shoulder
    M11.112 Familial chondrocalcinosis, left shoulder
    M11.119 Familial chondrocalcinosis, unspecified shoulder

✓6ᵗʰ **M11.12** **Familial chondrocalcinosis,** elbow

    M11.121 Familial chondrocalcinosis, right elbow
    M11.122 Familial chondrocalcinosis, left elbow

    M11.129 Familial chondrocalcinosis, unspecified elbow

✓6ᵗʰ **M11.13** **Familial chondrocalcinosis,** wrist

    M11.131 Familial chondrocalcinosis, right wrist
    M11.132 Familial chondrocalcinosis, left wrist
    M11.139 Familial chondrocalcinosis, unspecified wrist

✓6ᵗʰ **M11.14** **Familial chondrocalcinosis,** hand

    M11.141 Familial chondrocalcinosis, right hand
    M11.142 Familial chondrocalcinosis, left hand
    M11.149 Familial chondrocalcinosis, unspecified hand

✓6ᵗʰ **M11.15** **Familial chondrocalcinosis,** hip

    M11.151 Familial chondrocalcinosis, right hip
    M11.152 Familial chondrocalcinosis, left hip
    M11.159 Familial chondrocalcinosis, unspecified hip

✓6ᵗʰ **M11.16** **Familial chondrocalcinosis,** knee

    M11.161 Familial chondrocalcinosis, right knee
    M11.162 Familial chondrocalcinosis, left knee
    M11.169 Familial chondrocalcinosis, unspecified knee

✓6ᵗʰ **M11.17** **Familial chondrocalcinosis,** ankle and foot

    M11.171 Familial chondrocalcinosis, right ankle and foot
    M11.172 Familial chondrocalcinosis, left ankle and foot
    M11.179 Familial chondrocalcinosis, unspecified ankle and foot

M11.18 **Familial chondrocalcinosis,** vertebrae
M11.19 **Familial chondrocalcinosis,** multiple sites

✓5ᵗʰ **M11.2** **Other chondrocalcinosis**

    Chondrocalcinosis NOS
    AHA: 2018,3Q,20
    TIP: Pseudogout is captured with codes in this subcategory.

    M11.20 **Other chondrocalcinosis, unspecified site**

✓6ᵗʰ **M11.21** **Other chondrocalcinosis,** shoulder

    M11.211 Other chondrocalcinosis, right shoulder
    M11.212 Other chondrocalcinosis, left shoulder
    M11.219 Other chondrocalcinosis, unspecified shoulder

✓6ᵗʰ **M11.22** **Other chondrocalcinosis,** elbow

    M11.221 Other chondrocalcinosis, right elbow
    M11.222 Other chondrocalcinosis, left elbow
    M11.229 Other chondrocalcinosis, unspecified elbow

✓6ᵗʰ **M11.23** **Other chondrocalcinosis,** wrist

    M11.231 Other chondrocalcinosis, right wrist
    M11.232 Other chondrocalcinosis, left wrist
    M11.239 Other chondrocalcinosis, unspecified wrist

✓6ᵗʰ **M11.24** **Other chondrocalcinosis,** hand

    M11.241 Other chondrocalcinosis, right hand
    M11.242 Other chondrocalcinosis, left hand
    M11.249 Other chondrocalcinosis, unspecified hand

✓6ᵗʰ **M11.25** **Other chondrocalcinosis,** hip

    M11.251 Other chondrocalcinosis, right hip
    M11.252 Other chondrocalcinosis, left hip
    M11.259 Other chondrocalcinosis, unspecified hip

✓6ᵗʰ **M11.26** **Other chondrocalcinosis,** knee

    M11.261 Other chondrocalcinosis, right knee
    M11.262 Other chondrocalcinosis, left knee
    M11.269 Other chondrocalcinosis, unspecified knee

✓6ᵗʰ **M11.27** **Other chondrocalcinosis,** ankle and foot

    M11.271 Other chondrocalcinosis, right ankle and foot
    M11.272 Other chondrocalcinosis, left ankle and foot
    M11.279 Other chondrocalcinosis, unspecified ankle and foot

M11.28 **Other chondrocalcinosis,** vertebrae
M11.29 **Other chondrocalcinosis,** multiple sites

✓5ᵗʰ **M11.8** **Other specified crystal arthropathies**

    M11.80 **Other specified crystal arthropathies, unspecified site**

√6ᵗʰ **M11.81** Other specified crystal arthropathies, shoulder

     M11.811 Other specified crystal arthropathies, right shoulder

     M11.812 Other specified crystal arthropathies, left shoulder

     M11.819 Other specified crystal arthropathies, unspecified shoulder

√6ᵗʰ **M11.82** Other specified crystal arthropathies, elbow

     M11.821 Other specified crystal arthropathies, right elbow

     M11.822 Other specified crystal arthropathies, left elbow

     M11.829 Other specified crystal arthropathies, unspecified elbow

√6ᵗʰ **M11.83** Other specified crystal arthropathies, wrist

     M11.831 Other specified crystal arthropathies, right wrist

     M11.832 Other specified crystal arthropathies, left wrist

     M11.839 Other specified crystal arthropathies, unspecified wrist

√6ᵗʰ **M11.84** Other specified crystal arthropathies, hand

     M11.841 Other specified crystal arthropathies, right hand

     M11.842 Other specified crystal arthropathies, left hand

     M11.849 Other specified crystal arthropathies, unspecified hand

√6ᵗʰ **M11.85** Other specified crystal arthropathies, hip

     M11.851 Other specified crystal arthropathies, right hip

     M11.852 Other specified crystal arthropathies, left hip

     M11.859 Other specified crystal arthropathies, unspecified hip

√6ᵗʰ **M11.86** Other specified crystal arthropathies, knee

     M11.861 Other specified crystal arthropathies, right knee

     M11.862 Other specified crystal arthropathies, left knee

     M11.869 Other specified crystal arthropathies, unspecified knee

√6ᵗʰ **M11.87** Other specified crystal arthropathies, ankle and foot

     M11.871 Other specified crystal arthropathies, right ankle and foot

     M11.872 Other specified crystal arthropathies, left ankle and foot

     M11.879 Other specified crystal arthropathies, unspecified ankle and foot

     M11.88 Other specified crystal arthropathies, vertebrae

     M11.89 Other specified crystal arthropathies, multiple sites

M11.9 Crystal arthropathy, unspecified

√4ᵗʰ **M12** **Other and unspecified arthropathy**

     EXCLUDES 1   arthrosis (M15-M19)

              cricoarytenoid arthropathy (J38.7)

√5ᵗʰ **M12.0** Chronic postrheumatic arthropathy [Jaccoud]

     M12.00 Chronic postrheumatic arthropathy [Jaccoud], unspecified site   HCC Rx ESR COM

√6ᵗʰ **M12.01** Chronic postrheumatic arthropathy [Jaccoud], shoulder

     M12.011 Chronic postrheumatic arthropathy [Jaccoud], right shoulder   HCC Rx ESR COM

     M12.012 Chronic postrheumatic arthropathy [Jaccoud], left shoulder   HCC Rx ESR COM

     M12.019 Chronic postrheumatic arthropathy [Jaccoud], unspecified shoulder   HCC Rx ESR COM

√6ᵗʰ **M12.02** Chronic postrheumatic arthropathy [Jaccoud], elbow

     M12.021 Chronic postrheumatic arthropathy [Jaccoud], right elbow   HCC Rx ESR COM

     M12.022 Chronic postrheumatic arthropathy [Jaccoud], left elbow   HCC Rx ESR COM

     M12.029 Chronic postrheumatic arthropathy [Jaccoud], unspecified elbow   HCC Rx ESR COM

√6ᵗʰ **M12.03** Chronic postrheumatic arthropathy [Jaccoud], wrist

     M12.031 Chronic postrheumatic arthropathy [Jaccoud], right wrist   HCC Rx ESR COM

     M12.032 Chronic postrheumatic arthropathy [Jaccoud], left wrist   HCC Rx ESR COM

     M12.039 Chronic postrheumatic arthropathy [Jaccoud], unspecified wrist   HCC Rx ESR COM

√6ᵗʰ **M12.04** Chronic postrheumatic arthropathy [Jaccoud], hand

     M12.041 Chronic postrheumatic arthropathy [Jaccoud], right hand   HCC Rx ESR COM

     M12.042 Chronic postrheumatic arthropathy [Jaccoud], left hand   HCC Rx ESR COM

     M12.049 Chronic postrheumatic arthropathy [Jaccoud], unspecified hand   HCC Rx ESR COM

√6ᵗʰ **M12.05** Chronic postrheumatic arthropathy [Jaccoud], hip

     M12.051 Chronic postrheumatic arthropathy [Jaccoud], right hip   HCC Rx ESR COM

     M12.052 Chronic postrheumatic arthropathy [Jaccoud], left hip   HCC Rx ESR COM

     M12.059 Chronic postrheumatic arthropathy [Jaccoud], unspecified hip   HCC Rx ESR COM

√6ᵗʰ **M12.06** Chronic postrheumatic arthropathy [Jaccoud], knee

     M12.061 Chronic postrheumatic arthropathy [Jaccoud], right knee   HCC Rx ESR COM

     M12.062 Chronic postrheumatic arthropathy [Jaccoud], left knee   HCC Rx ESR COM

     M12.069 Chronic postrheumatic arthropathy [Jaccoud], unspecified knee   HCC Rx ESR COM

√6ᵗʰ **M12.07** Chronic postrheumatic arthropathy [Jaccoud], ankle and foot

     M12.071 Chronic postrheumatic arthropathy [Jaccoud], right ankle and foot   HCC Rx ESR COM

     M12.072 Chronic postrheumatic arthropathy [Jaccoud], left ankle and foot   HCC Rx ESR COM

     M12.079 Chronic postrheumatic arthropathy [Jaccoud], unspecified ankle and foot   HCC Rx ESR COM

     M12.08 Chronic postrheumatic arthropathy [Jaccoud], other specified site   HCC Rx ESR COM

         Chronic postrheumatic arthropathy [Jaccoud], vertebrae

     M12.09 Chronic postrheumatic arthropathy [Jaccoud], multiple sites   HCC Rx ESR COM

√5ᵗʰ **M12.1** Kaschin-Beck disease

     Osteochondroarthrosis deformans endemica

     M12.10 Kaschin-Beck disease, unspecified site

√6ᵗʰ **M12.11** Kaschin-Beck disease, shoulder

     M12.111 Kaschin-Beck disease, right shoulder

     M12.112 Kaschin-Beck disease, left shoulder

     M12.119 Kaschin-Beck disease, unspecified shoulder

√6ᵗʰ **M12.12** Kaschin-Beck disease, elbow

     M12.121 Kaschin-Beck disease, right elbow

     M12.122 Kaschin-Beck disease, left elbow

     M12.129 Kaschin-Beck disease, unspecified elbow

√6ᵗʰ **M12.13** Kaschin-Beck disease, wrist

     M12.131 Kaschin-Beck disease, right wrist

     M12.132 Kaschin-Beck disease, left wrist

     M12.139 Kaschin-Beck disease, unspecified wrist

√6ᵗʰ **M12.14** Kaschin-Beck disease, hand

     M12.141 Kaschin-Beck disease, right hand

     M12.142 Kaschin-Beck disease, left hand

     M12.149 Kaschin-Beck disease, unspecified hand

√6ᵗʰ **M12.15** Kaschin-Beck disease, hip

     M12.151 Kaschin-Beck disease, right hip

     M12.152 Kaschin-Beck disease, left hip

     M12.159 Kaschin-Beck disease, unspecified hip

√6ᵗʰ **M12.16** Kaschin-Beck disease, knee

     M12.161 Kaschin-Beck disease, right knee

     M12.162 Kaschin-Beck disease, left knee

     M12.169 Kaschin-Beck disease, unspecified knee

✓6ᵗʰ **M12.17 Kaschin-Beck disease, ankle and foot**

    M12.171 Kaschin-Beck disease, right ankle and foot

    M12.172 Kaschin-Beck disease, left ankle and foot

    M12.179 Kaschin-Beck disease, unspecified ankle and foot

M12.18 Kaschin-Beck disease, vertebrae

M12.19 Kaschin-Beck disease, multiple sites

✓5ᵗʰ **M12.2 Villonodular synovitis (pigmented)**

    M12.20 Villonodular synovitis (pigmented), unspecified site

✓6ᵗʰ **M12.21 Villonodular synovitis (pigmented), shoulder**

    M12.211 Villonodular synovitis (pigmented), right shoulder

    M12.212 Villonodular synovitis (pigmented), left shoulder

    M12.219 Villonodular synovitis (pigmented), unspecified shoulder

✓6ᵗʰ **M12.22 Villonodular synovitis (pigmented), elbow**

    M12.221 Villonodular synovitis (pigmented), right elbow

    M12.222 Villonodular synovitis (pigmented), left elbow

    M12.229 Villonodular synovitis (pigmented), unspecified elbow

✓6ᵗʰ **M12.23 Villonodular synovitis (pigmented), wrist**

    M12.231 Villonodular synovitis (pigmented), right wrist

    M12.232 Villonodular synovitis (pigmented), left wrist

    M12.239 Villonodular synovitis (pigmented), unspecified wrist

✓6ᵗʰ **M12.24 Villonodular synovitis (pigmented), hand**

    M12.241 Villonodular synovitis (pigmented), right hand

    M12.242 Villonodular synovitis (pigmented), left hand

    M12.249 Villonodular synovitis (pigmented), unspecified hand

✓6ᵗʰ **M12.25 Villonodular synovitis (pigmented), hip**

    M12.251 Villonodular synovitis (pigmented), right hip

    M12.252 Villonodular synovitis (pigmented), left hip

    M12.259 Villonodular synovitis (pigmented), unspecified hip

✓6ᵗʰ **M12.26 Villonodular synovitis (pigmented), knee**

    M12.261 Villonodular synovitis (pigmented), right knee

    M12.262 Villonodular synovitis (pigmented), left knee

    M12.269 Villonodular synovitis (pigmented), unspecified knee

✓6ᵗʰ **M12.27 Villonodular synovitis (pigmented), ankle and foot**

    M12.271 Villonodular synovitis (pigmented), right ankle and foot

    M12.272 Villonodular synovitis (pigmented), left ankle and foot

    M12.279 Villonodular synovitis (pigmented), unspecified ankle and foot

M12.28 Villonodular synovitis (pigmented), other specified site

    Villonodular synovitis (pigmented), vertebrae

M12.29 Villonodular synovitis (pigmented), multiple sites

✓5ᵗʰ **M12.3 Palindromic rheumatism**

    DEF: Sudden and recurring attacks of moderate to severe joint pain and swelling generally occurring in the hands or feet of unknown etiology. After the attack subsides, the joints appear normal again.

    M12.30 Palindromic rheumatism, unspecified site

✓6ᵗʰ **M12.31 Palindromic rheumatism, shoulder**

    M12.311 Palindromic rheumatism, right shoulder

    M12.312 Palindromic rheumatism, left shoulder

    M12.319 Palindromic rheumatism, unspecified shoulder

✓6ᵗʰ **M12.32 Palindromic rheumatism, elbow**

    M12.321 Palindromic rheumatism, right elbow

    M12.322 Palindromic rheumatism, left elbow

    M12.329 Palindromic rheumatism, unspecified elbow

✓6ᵗʰ **M12.33 Palindromic rheumatism, wrist**

    M12.331 Palindromic rheumatism, right wrist

    M12.332 Palindromic rheumatism, left wrist

    M12.339 Palindromic rheumatism, unspecified wrist

✓6ᵗʰ **M12.34 Palindromic rheumatism, hand**

    M12.341 Palindromic rheumatism, right hand

    M12.342 Palindromic rheumatism, left hand

    M12.349 Palindromic rheumatism, unspecified hand

✓6ᵗʰ **M12.35 Palindromic rheumatism, hip**

    M12.351 Palindromic rheumatism, right hip

    M12.352 Palindromic rheumatism, left hip

    M12.359 Palindromic rheumatism, unspecified hip

✓6ᵗʰ **M12.36 Palindromic rheumatism, knee**

    M12.361 Palindromic rheumatism, right knee

    M12.362 Palindromic rheumatism, left knee

    M12.369 Palindromic rheumatism, unspecified knee

✓6ᵗʰ **M12.37 Palindromic rheumatism, ankle and foot**

    M12.371 Palindromic rheumatism, right ankle and foot

    M12.372 Palindromic rheumatism, left ankle and foot

    M12.379 Palindromic rheumatism, unspecified ankle and foot

M12.38 Palindromic rheumatism, other specified site

    Palindromic rheumatism, vertebrae

M12.39 Palindromic rheumatism, multiple sites

✓5ᵗʰ **M12.4 Intermittent hydrarthrosis**

    M12.40 Intermittent hydrarthrosis, unspecified site

✓6ᵗʰ **M12.41 Intermittent hydrarthrosis, shoulder**

    M12.411 Intermittent hydrarthrosis, right shoulder

    M12.412 Intermittent hydrarthrosis, left shoulder

    M12.419 Intermittent hydrarthrosis, unspecified shoulder

✓6ᵗʰ **M12.42 Intermittent hydrarthrosis, elbow**

    M12.421 Intermittent hydrarthrosis, right elbow

    M12.422 Intermittent hydrarthrosis, left elbow

    M12.429 Intermittent hydrarthrosis, unspecified elbow

✓6ᵗʰ **M12.43 Intermittent hydrarthrosis, wrist**

    M12.431 Intermittent hydrarthrosis, right wrist

    M12.432 Intermittent hydrarthrosis, left wrist

    M12.439 Intermittent hydrarthrosis, unspecified wrist

✓6ᵗʰ **M12.44 Intermittent hydrarthrosis, hand**

    M12.441 Intermittent hydrarthrosis, right hand

    M12.442 Intermittent hydrarthrosis, left hand

    M12.449 Intermittent hydrarthrosis, unspecified hand

✓6ᵗʰ **M12.45 Intermittent hydrarthrosis, hip**

    M12.451 Intermittent hydrarthrosis, right hip

    M12.452 Intermittent hydrarthrosis, left hip

    M12.459 Intermittent hydrarthrosis, unspecified hip

✓6ᵗʰ **M12.46 Intermittent hydrarthrosis, knee**

    M12.461 Intermittent hydrarthrosis, right knee

    M12.462 Intermittent hydrarthrosis, left knee

    M12.469 Intermittent hydrarthrosis, unspecified knee

✓6ᵗʰ **M12.47 Intermittent hydrarthrosis, ankle and foot**

    M12.471 Intermittent hydrarthrosis, right ankle and foot

    M12.472 Intermittent hydrarthrosis, left ankle and foot

    M12.479 Intermittent hydrarthrosis, unspecified ankle and foot

M12.48 Intermittent hydrarthrosis, other site

M12.49 Intermittent hydrarthrosis, multiple sites

√5ᵗʰ M12.5 Traumatic arthropathy

> **EXCLUDES 1**   current injury-see Alphabetic Index
> post-traumatic osteoarthritis of first carpometacarpal joint (M18.2-M18.3)
> post-traumatic osteoarthritis of hip (M16.4-M16.5)
> post-traumatic osteoarthritis of knee (M17.2-M17.3)
> post-traumatic osteoarthritis NOS (M19.1-)
> post-traumatic osteoarthritis of other single joints (M19.1-)

AHA: 2015,1Q,17

M12.50 Traumatic arthropathy, unspecified site

√6ᵗʰ **M12.51** Traumatic arthropathy, shoulder
- M12.511 Traumatic arthropathy, right shoulder
- M12.512 Traumatic arthropathy, left shoulder
- M12.519 Traumatic arthropathy, unspecified shoulder

√6ᵗʰ **M12.52** Traumatic arthropathy, elbow
- M12.521 Traumatic arthropathy, right elbow
- M12.522 Traumatic arthropathy, left elbow
- M12.529 Traumatic arthropathy, unspecified elbow

√6ᵗʰ **M12.53** Traumatic arthropathy, wrist
- M12.531 Traumatic arthropathy, right wrist
- M12.532 Traumatic arthropathy, left wrist
- M12.539 Traumatic arthropathy, unspecified wrist

√6ᵗʰ **M12.54** Traumatic arthropathy, hand
- M12.541 Traumatic arthropathy, right hand
- M12.542 Traumatic arthropathy, left hand
- M12.549 Traumatic arthropathy, unspecified hand

√6ᵗʰ **M12.55** Traumatic arthropathy, hip
- M12.551 Traumatic arthropathy, right hip
- M12.552 Traumatic arthropathy, left hip
- M12.559 Traumatic arthropathy, unspecified hip

√6ᵗʰ **M12.56** Traumatic arthropathy, knee
- M12.561 Traumatic arthropathy, right knee
- M12.562 Traumatic arthropathy, left knee
- M12.569 Traumatic arthropathy, unspecified knee

√6ᵗʰ **M12.57** Traumatic arthropathy, ankle and foot
- M12.571 Traumatic arthropathy, right ankle and foot
- M12.572 Traumatic arthropathy, left ankle and foot
- M12.579 Traumatic arthropathy, unspecified ankle and foot

M12.58 Traumatic arthropathy, other specified site
    Traumatic arthropathy, vertebrae

M12.59 Traumatic arthropathy, multiple sites

√5ᵗʰ M12.8 Other specific arthropathies, not elsewhere classified
    Transient arthropathy

M12.80 Other specific arthropathies, not elsewhere classified, unspecified site

√6ᵗʰ **M12.81** Other specific arthropathies, not elsewhere classified, shoulder
- M12.811 Other specific arthropathies, not elsewhere classified, right shoulder
- M12.812 Other specific arthropathies, not elsewhere classified, left shoulder
- M12.819 Other specific arthropathies, not elsewhere classified, unspecified shoulder

√6ᵗʰ **M12.82** Other specific arthropathies, not elsewhere classified, elbow
- M12.821 Other specific arthropathies, not elsewhere classified, right elbow
- M12.822 Other specific arthropathies, not elsewhere classified, left elbow
- M12.829 Other specific arthropathies, not elsewhere classified, unspecified elbow

√6ᵗʰ **M12.83** Other specific arthropathies, not elsewhere classified, wrist
- M12.831 Other specific arthropathies, not elsewhere classified, right wrist
- M12.832 Other specific arthropathies, not elsewhere classified, left wrist
- M12.839 Other specific arthropathies, not elsewhere classified, unspecified wrist

√6ᵗʰ **M12.84** Other specific arthropathies, not elsewhere classified, hand
- M12.841 Other specific arthropathies, not elsewhere classified, right hand
- M12.842 Other specific arthropathies, not elsewhere classified, left hand
- M12.849 Other specific arthropathies, not elsewhere classified, unspecified hand

√6ᵗʰ **M12.85** Other specific arthropathies, not elsewhere classified, hip
- M12.851 Other specific arthropathies, not elsewhere classified, right hip
- M12.852 Other specific arthropathies, not elsewhere classified, left hip
- M12.859 Other specific arthropathies, not elsewhere classified, unspecified hip

√6ᵗʰ **M12.86** Other specific arthropathies, not elsewhere classified, knee
- M12.861 Other specific arthropathies, not elsewhere classified, right knee
- M12.862 Other specific arthropathies, not elsewhere classified, left knee
- M12.869 Other specific arthropathies, not elsewhere classified, unspecified knee

√6ᵗʰ **M12.87** Other specific arthropathies, not elsewhere classified, ankle and foot
- M12.871 Other specific arthropathies, not elsewhere classified, right ankle and foot
- M12.872 Other specific arthropathies, not elsewhere classified, left ankle and foot
- M12.879 Other specific arthropathies, not elsewhere classified, unspecified ankle and foot

M12.88 Other specific arthropathies, not elsewhere classified, other specified site
    Other specific arthropathies, not elsewhere classified, vertebrae

M12.89 Other specific arthropathies, not elsewhere classified, multiple sites

M12.9 Arthropathy, unspecified

√4ᵗʰ M13 Other arthritis

> **EXCLUDES 1**   arthrosis (M15-M19)
> osteoarthritis (M15-M19)

M13.0 Polyarthritis, unspecified

√5ᵗʰ M13.1 Monoarthritis, not elsewhere classified

M13.10 Monoarthritis, not elsewhere classified, unspecified site

√6ᵗʰ **M13.11** Monoarthritis, not elsewhere classified, shoulder
- M13.111 Monoarthritis, not elsewhere classified, right shoulder
- M13.112 Monoarthritis, not elsewhere classified, left shoulder
- M13.119 Monoarthritis, not elsewhere classified, unspecified shoulder

√6ᵗʰ **M13.12** Monoarthritis, not elsewhere classified, elbow
- M13.121 Monoarthritis, not elsewhere classified, right elbow
- M13.122 Monoarthritis, not elsewhere classified, left elbow
- M13.129 Monoarthritis, not elsewhere classified, unspecified elbow

√6ᵗʰ **M13.13** Monoarthritis, not elsewhere classified, wrist
- M13.131 Monoarthritis, not elsewhere classified, right wrist
- M13.132 Monoarthritis, not elsewhere classified, left wrist
- M13.139 Monoarthritis, not elsewhere classified, unspecified wrist

√6ᵗʰ **M13.14** Monoarthritis, not elsewhere classified, hand
- M13.141 Monoarthritis, not elsewhere classified, right hand
- M13.142 Monoarthritis, not elsewhere classified, left hand
- M13.149 Monoarthritis, not elsewhere classified, unspecified hand

√6ᵗʰ **M13.15** Monoarthritis, not elsewhere classified, hip
- M13.151 Monoarthritis, not elsewhere classified, right hip
- M13.152 Monoarthritis, not elsewhere classified, left hip

Chapter 13. Diseases of the Musculoskeletal System and Connective Tissue

M13.159 Monoarthritis, not elsewhere classified, unspecified hip

✓6th M13.16 **Monoarthritis, not elsewhere classified,** knee

M13.161 Monoarthritis, not elsewhere classified, right knee

M13.162 Monoarthritis, not elsewhere classified, left knee

M13.169 Monoarthritis, not elsewhere classified, unspecified knee

✓6th M13.17 **Monoarthritis, not elsewhere classified,** ankle and foot

M13.171 Monoarthritis, not elsewhere classified, right ankle and foot

M13.172 Monoarthritis, not elsewhere classified, left ankle and foot

M13.179 Monoarthritis, not elsewhere classified, unspecified ankle and foot

✓5th M13.8 **Other specified arthritis**

Allergic arthritis

EXCLUDES 1 osteoarthritis (M15-M19)

M13.80 **Other specified arthritis, unspecified site**

✓6th M13.81 **Other specified arthritis,** shoulder

M13.811 Other specified arthritis, right shoulder
M13.812 Other specified arthritis, left shoulder
M13.819 Other specified arthritis, unspecified shoulder

✓6th M13.82 **Other specified arthritis,** elbow

M13.821 Other specified arthritis, right elbow
M13.822 Other specified arthritis, left elbow
M13.829 Other specified arthritis, unspecified elbow

✓6th M13.83 **Other specified arthritis,** wrist

M13.831 Other specified arthritis, right wrist
M13.832 Other specified arthritis, left wrist
M13.839 Other specified arthritis, unspecified wrist

✓6th M13.84 **Other specified arthritis,** hand

M13.841 Other specified arthritis, right hand
M13.842 Other specified arthritis, left hand
M13.849 Other specified arthritis, unspecified hand

✓6th M13.85 **Other specified arthritis,** hip

M13.851 Other specified arthritis, right hip
M13.852 Other specified arthritis, left hip
M13.859 Other specified arthritis, unspecified hip

✓6th M13.86 **Other specified arthritis,** knee

M13.861 Other specified arthritis, right knee
M13.862 Other specified arthritis, left knee
M13.869 Other specified arthritis, unspecified knee

✓6th M13.87 **Other specified arthritis,** ankle and foot

M13.871 Other specified arthritis, right ankle and foot
M13.872 Other specified arthritis, left ankle and foot
M13.879 Other specified arthritis, unspecified ankle and foot

M13.88 **Other specified arthritis, other site**
M13.89 **Other specified arthritis,** multiple sites

✓4th M14 **Arthropathies in other diseases classified elsewhere**

EXCLUDES 1 arthropathy in:
diabetes mellitus (E08-E13 with .61-)
hematological disorders (M36.2-M36.3)
hypersensitivity reactions (M36.4)
neoplastic disease (M36.1)
neurosyphillis (A52.16)
sarcoidosis (D86.86)
enteropathic arthropathies (M07.-)
juvenile psoriatic arthropathy (L40.54)
lipoid dermatoarthritis (E78.81)

✓5th M14.6 **Charcôt's joint**

Neuropathic arthropathy

EXCLUDES 1 Charcôt's joint in diabetes mellitus (E08-E13 with .610)
Charcôt's joint in tabes dorsalis (A52.16)

DEF: Progressive neurologic arthropathy in which chronic degeneration of joints in the weight-bearing areas with peripheral hypertrophy occurs as a complication of a neuropathy disorder. Supporting structures relax from a loss of sensation resulting in chronic joint instability.

M14.60 **Charcôt's joint, unspecified site**

✓6th M14.61 **Charcôt's joint,** shoulder

M14.611 Charcôt's joint, right shoulder
M14.612 Charcôt's joint, left shoulder
M14.619 Charcôt's joint, unspecified shoulder

✓6th M14.62 **Charcôt's joint,** elbow

M14.621 Charcôt's joint, right elbow
M14.622 Charcôt's joint, left elbow
M14.629 Charcôt's joint, unspecified elbow

✓6th M14.63 **Charcôt's joint,** wrist

M14.631 Charcôt's joint, right wrist
M14.632 Charcôt's joint, left wrist
M14.639 Charcôt's joint, unspecified wrist

✓6th M14.64 **Charcôt's joint,** hand

M14.641 Charcôt's joint, right hand
M14.642 Charcôt's joint, left hand
M14.649 Charcôt's joint, unspecified hand

✓6th M14.65 **Charcôt's joint,** hip

M14.651 Charcôt's joint, right hip
M14.652 Charcôt's joint, left hip
M14.659 Charcôt's joint, unspecified hip

✓6th M14.66 **Charcôt's joint,** knee

M14.661 Charcôt's joint, right knee
M14.662 Charcôt's joint, left knee
M14.669 Charcôt's joint, unspecified knee

✓6th M14.67 **Charcôt's joint,** ankle and foot

M14.671 Charcôt's joint, right ankle and foot
M14.672 Charcôt's joint, left ankle and foot
M14.679 Charcôt's joint, unspecified ankle and foot

M14.68 **Charcôt's joint,** vertebrae
M14.69 **Charcôt's joint,** multiple sites

✓5th M14.8 **Arthropathies in other specified diseases classified elsewhere**

Code first underlying disease, such as:
amyloidosis (E85.-)
erythema multiforme (L51.-)
erythema nodosum (L52)
hemochromatosis (E83.11-)
hyperparathyroidism (E21.-)
hypothyroidism (E00-E03)
sickle-cell disorders (D57.-)
thyrotoxicosis [hyperthyroidism] (E05.-)
Whipple's disease (K90.81)

M14.80 *Arthropathies in other specified diseases classified elsewhere, unspecified site*

✓6th M14.81 **Arthropathies in other specified diseases classified elsewhere,** shoulder

M14.811 *Arthropathies in other specified diseases classified elsewhere, right shoulder*
M14.812 *Arthropathies in other specified diseases classified elsewhere, left shoulder*
M14.819 *Arthropathies in other specified diseases classified elsewhere, unspecified shoulder*

[handwritten: degenerative joint disease (DJD)]

M14.82 Arthropathies in other specified diseases classified elsewhere, **elbow**
- **M14.821** Arthropathies in other specified diseases classified elsewhere, *right* **elbow**
- **M14.822** Arthropathies in other specified diseases classified elsewhere, *left* **elbow**
- **M14.829** Arthropathies in other specified diseases classified elsewhere, *unspecified* **elbow**

M14.83 Arthropathies in other specified diseases classified elsewhere, **wrist**
- **M14.831** Arthropathies in other specified diseases classified elsewhere, *right* **wrist**
- **M14.832** Arthropathies in other specified diseases classified elsewhere, *left* **wrist**
- **M14.839** Arthropathies in other specified diseases classified elsewhere, *unspecified* **wrist**

M14.84 Arthropathies in other specified diseases classified elsewhere, **hand**
- **M14.841** Arthropathies in other specified diseases classified elsewhere, *right* **hand**
- **M14.842** Arthropathies in other specified diseases classified elsewhere, *left* **hand**
- **M14.849** Arthropathies in other specified diseases classified elsewhere, *unspecified* **hand**

M14.85 Arthropathies in other specified diseases classified elsewhere, **hip**
- **M14.851** Arthropathies in other specified diseases classified elsewhere, *right* **hip**
- **M14.852** Arthropathies in other specified diseases classified elsewhere, *left* **hip**
- **M14.859** Arthropathies in other specified diseases classified elsewhere, *unspecified* **hip**

M14.86 Arthropathies in other specified diseases classified elsewhere, **knee**
- **M14.861** Arthropathies in other specified diseases classified elsewhere, *right* **knee**
- **M14.862** Arthropathies in other specified diseases classified elsewhere, *left* **knee**
- **M14.869** Arthropathies in other specified diseases classified elsewhere, *unspecified* **knee**

M14.87 Arthropathies in other specified diseases classified elsewhere, **ankle and foot**
- **M14.871** Arthropathies in other specified diseases classified elsewhere, *right* **ankle and foot**
- **M14.872** Arthropathies in other specified diseases classified elsewhere, *left* **ankle and foot**
- **M14.879** Arthropathies in other specified diseases classified elsewhere, *unspecified* **ankle and foot**

M14.88 Arthropathies in other specified diseases classified elsewhere, *vertebrae*

M14.89 Arthropathies in other specified diseases classified elsewhere, *multiple sites*

[handwritten margin note: osteoarthritis || OJD / degenerative joint disease]

Osteoarthritis (M15-M19)

EXCLUDES 2   osteoarthritis of spine (M47.-)
AHA: 2020,2Q,14; 2016,4Q,147
TIP: Assign a primary osteoarthritis code when the site of the osteoarthritis is documented but the type of osteoarthritis — primary, secondary, generalized, or post-traumatic — is not documented. Primary is considered the default.

M15 Polyosteoarthritis
INCLUDES   arthritis of multiple sites
EXCLUDES 1   bilateral involvement of single joint (M16-M19)

- **M15.0** Primary generalized (osteo)arthritis
- **M15.1** Heberden's nodes (with arthropathy)
  - Interphalangeal distal osteoarthritis
- **M15.2** Bouchard's nodes (with arthropathy)
  - Juxtaphalangeal distal osteoarthritis
- **M15.3** Secondary multiple arthritis
  - Post-traumatic polyosteoarthritis
- **M15.4** Erosive (osteo)arthritis
- **M15.8** Other polyosteoarthritis
- **M15.9** Polyosteoarthritis, unspecified
  - Generalized osteoarthritis NOS

M16 Osteoarthritis of hip
AHA: 2016,4Q,146

- **M16.0** Bilateral primary osteoarthritis of hip
  - **AHA:** 2018,2Q,15

M16.1 Unilateral primary **osteoarthritis of hip**
  - Primary osteoarthritis of hip NOS
  - **AHA:** 2018,2Q,15
  - **M16.10** Unilateral primary osteoarthritis, unspecified hip
  - **M16.11** Unilateral primary osteoarthritis, right hip
  - **M16.12** Unilateral primary osteoarthritis, left hip

- **M16.2** Bilateral **osteoarthritis resulting from hip dysplasia**

M16.3 Unilateral **osteoarthritis resulting from hip dysplasia**
  - Dysplastic osteoarthritis of hip NOS
  - **M16.30** Unilateral osteoarthritis resulting from hip dysplasia, unspecified hip
  - **M16.31** Unilateral osteoarthritis resulting from hip dysplasia, right hip
  - **M16.32** Unilateral osteoarthritis resulting from hip dysplasia, left hip

- **M16.4** Bilateral post-traumatic **osteoarthritis of hip**

M16.5 Unilateral post-traumatic **osteoarthritis of hip**
  - Post-traumatic osteoarthritis of hip NOS
  - **M16.50** Unilateral post-traumatic osteoarthritis, unspecified hip
  - **M16.51** Unilateral post-traumatic osteoarthritis, right hip
  - **M16.52** Unilateral post-traumatic osteoarthritis, left hip

- **M16.6** Other bilateral secondary **osteoarthritis of hip**
- **M16.7** Other unilateral secondary **osteoarthritis of hip**
  - Secondary osteoarthritis of hip NOS
- **M16.9** Osteoarthritis of hip, unspecified

M17 Osteoarthritis of knee
AHA: 2016,4Q,146-147

- **M17.0** Bilateral primary **osteoarthritis of knee**
  - **AHA:** 2018,2Q,15

M17.1 Unilateral primary **osteoarthritis of knee**
  - Primary osteoarthritis of knee NOS
  - **AHA:** 2018,2Q,15
  - **M17.10** Unilateral primary osteoarthritis, unspecified knee
  - **M17.11** Unilateral primary osteoarthritis, right knee
  - **M17.12** Unilateral primary osteoarthritis, left knee

- **M17.2** Bilateral post-traumatic **osteoarthritis of knee**

M17.3 Unilateral post-traumatic **osteoarthritis of knee**
  - Post-traumatic osteoarthritis of knee NOS
  - **M17.30** Unilateral post-traumatic osteoarthritis, unspecified knee
  - **M17.31** Unilateral post-traumatic osteoarthritis, right knee
  - **M17.32** Unilateral post-traumatic osteoarthritis, left knee

- **M17.4** Other bilateral secondary **osteoarthritis of knee**
- **M17.5** Other unilateral secondary **osteoarthritis of knee**
  - Secondary osteoarthritis of knee NOS
- **M17.9** Osteoarthritis of knee, unspecified

[handwritten: primary is specified, both knee]

M18 Osteoarthritis of first carpometacarpal joint

- **M18.0** Bilateral primary **osteoarthritis of first carpometacarpal joints**

M18.1 Unilateral primary **osteoarthritis of first carpometacarpal joint**
  - Primary osteoarthritis of first carpometacarpal joint NOS
  - **M18.10** Unilateral primary osteoarthritis of first carpometacarpal joint, unspecified hand
  - **M18.11** Unilateral primary osteoarthritis of first carpometacarpal joint, right hand
  - **M18.12** Unilateral primary osteoarthritis of first carpometacarpal joint, left hand

- **M18.2** Bilateral post-traumatic **osteoarthritis of first carpometacarpal joints**

M18.3 Unilateral post-traumatic **osteoarthritis of first carpometacarpal joint**
  - Post-traumatic osteoarthritis of first carpometacarpal joint NOS
  - **M18.30** Unilateral post-traumatic osteoarthritis of first carpometacarpal joint, unspecified hand
  - **M18.31** Unilateral post-traumatic osteoarthritis of first carpometacarpal joint, right hand
  - **M18.32** Unilateral post-traumatic osteoarthritis of first carpometacarpal joint, left hand

- **M18.4** Other bilateral secondary **osteoarthritis of first carpometacarpal joints**

M18.5 Other unilateral secondary **osteoarthritis of first carpometacarpal joint**
  - Secondary osteoarthritis of first carpometacarpal joint NOS
  - **M18.50** Other unilateral secondary osteoarthritis of first carpometacarpal joint, unspecified hand

M18.51 Other unilateral secondary osteoarthritis of first carpometacarpal joint, right hand

M18.52 Other unilateral secondary osteoarthritis of first carpometacarpal joint, left hand

M18.9 Osteoarthritis of first carpometacarpal joint, unspecified

✓4ᵗʰ **M19** Other and unspecified osteoarthritis

EXCLUDES 1   polyarthritis (M15.-)

EXCLUDES 2   arthrosis of spine (M47.-)

hallux rigidus (M20.2)

osteoarthritis of spine (M47.-)

AHA: 2020,4Q,31-32

✓5ᵗʰ **M19.0** Primary osteoarthritis of other joints

AHA: 2018,2Q,15; 2016,4Q,145

✓6ᵗʰ **M19.01** Primary osteoarthritis, shoulder

M19.011 Primary osteoarthritis, right shoulder

M19.012 Primary osteoarthritis, left shoulder

M19.019 Primary osteoarthritis, unspecified shoulder

✓6ᵗʰ **M19.02** Primary osteoarthritis, elbow

M19.021 Primary osteoarthritis, right elbow

M19.022 Primary osteoarthritis, left elbow

M19.029 Primary osteoarthritis, unspecified elbow

✓6ᵗʰ **M19.03** Primary osteoarthritis, wrist

M19.031 Primary osteoarthritis, right wrist

M19.032 Primary osteoarthritis, left wrist

M19.039 Primary osteoarthritis, unspecified wrist

✓6ᵗʰ **M19.04** Primary osteoarthritis, hand

EXCLUDES 2   primary osteoarthritis of first carpometacarpal joint (M18.0-, M18.1-)

M19.041 Primary osteoarthritis, right hand

M19.042 Primary osteoarthritis, left hand

M19.049 Primary osteoarthritis, unspecified hand

✓6ᵗʰ **M19.07** Primary osteoarthritis ankle and foot

M19.071 Primary osteoarthritis, right ankle and foot

M19.072 Primary osteoarthritis, left ankle and foot

M19.079 Primary osteoarthritis, unspecified ankle and foot

M19.09 Primary osteoarthritis, other specified site

✓5ᵗʰ **M19.1** Post-traumatic osteoarthritis of other joints

✓6ᵗʰ **M19.11** Post-traumatic osteoarthritis, shoulder

M19.111 Post-traumatic osteoarthritis, right shoulder

M19.112 Post-traumatic osteoarthritis, left shoulder

M19.119 Post-traumatic osteoarthritis, unspecified shoulder

✓6ᵗʰ **M19.12** Post-traumatic osteoarthritis, elbow

M19.121 Post-traumatic osteoarthritis, right elbow

M19.122 Post-traumatic osteoarthritis, left elbow

M19.129 Post-traumatic osteoarthritis, unspecified elbow

✓6ᵗʰ **M19.13** Post-traumatic osteoarthritis, wrist

M19.131 Post-traumatic osteoarthritis, right wrist

M19.132 Post-traumatic osteoarthritis, left wrist

M19.139 Post-traumatic osteoarthritis, unspecified wrist

✓6ᵗʰ **M19.14** Post-traumatic osteoarthritis, hand

EXCLUDES 2   post-traumatic osteoarthritis of first carpometacarpal joint (M18.2-, M18.3-)

M19.141 Post-traumatic osteoarthritis, right hand

M19.142 Post-traumatic osteoarthritis, left hand

M19.149 Post-traumatic osteoarthritis, unspecified hand

✓6ᵗʰ **M19.17** Post-traumatic osteoarthritis, ankle and foot

M19.171 Post-traumatic osteoarthritis, right ankle and foot

M19.172 Post-traumatic osteoarthritis, left ankle and foot

M19.179 Post-traumatic osteoarthritis, unspecified ankle and foot

M19.19 Post-traumatic osteoarthritis, other specified site

✓5ᵗʰ **M19.2** Secondary osteoarthritis of other joints

✓6ᵗʰ **M19.21** Secondary osteoarthritis, shoulder

M19.211 Secondary osteoarthritis, right shoulder

M19.212 Secondary osteoarthritis, left shoulder

M19.219 Secondary osteoarthritis, unspecified shoulder

✓6ᵗʰ **M19.22** Secondary osteoarthritis, elbow

M19.221 Secondary osteoarthritis, right elbow

M19.222 Secondary osteoarthritis, left elbow

M19.229 Secondary osteoarthritis, unspecified elbow

✓6ᵗʰ **M19.23** Secondary osteoarthritis, wrist

M19.231 Secondary osteoarthritis, right wrist

M19.232 Secondary osteoarthritis, left wrist

M19.239 Secondary osteoarthritis, unspecified wrist

✓6ᵗʰ **M19.24** Secondary osteoarthritis, hand

M19.241 Secondary osteoarthritis, right hand

M19.242 Secondary osteoarthritis, left hand

M19.249 Secondary osteoarthritis, unspecified hand

✓6ᵗʰ **M19.27** Secondary osteoarthritis, ankle and foot

M19.271 Secondary osteoarthritis, right ankle and foot

M19.272 Secondary osteoarthritis, left ankle and foot

M19.279 Secondary osteoarthritis, unspecified ankle and foot

M19.29 Secondary osteoarthritis, other specified site

✓5ᵗʰ **M19.9** Osteoarthritis, unspecified site

TIP: Assign M19.90 when neither the site nor the type of osteoarthritis — primary, secondary, or post-traumatic — is documented.

M19.90 Unspecified osteoarthritis, unspecified site

Arthrosis NOS

Arthritis NOS

Osteoarthritis NOS

AHA: 2016,4Q,145-147

M19.91 Primary osteoarthritis, unspecified site

Primary osteoarthritis NOS

M19.92 Post-traumatic osteoarthritis, unspecified site

Post-traumatic osteoarthritis NOS

M19.93 Secondary osteoarthritis, unspecified site

Secondary osteoarthritis NOS

Other joint disorders (M20-M25)

EXCLUDES 2   joints of the spine (M40-M54)

✓4ᵗʰ **M20** Acquired deformities of fingers and toes

EXCLUDES 1   acquired absence of fingers and toes (Z89.-)

congenital absence of fingers and toes (Q71.3-, Q72.3-)

congenital deformities and malformations of fingers and toes (Q66.-, Q68-Q70, Q74.-)

✓5ᵗʰ **M20.0** Deformity of finger(s)

EXCLUDES 1   clubbing of fingers (R68.3)

palmar fascial fibromatosis [Dupuytren] (M72.0)

trigger finger (M65.3)

✓6ᵗʰ **M20.00** Unspecified deformity of finger(s)

M20.001 Unspecified deformity of right finger(s)

M20.002 Unspecified deformity of left finger(s)

M20.009 Unspecified deformity of unspecified finger(s)

✓6ᵗʰ **M20.01** Mallet finger

M20.011 Mallet finger of right finger(s)

M20.012 Mallet finger of left finger(s)

M20.019 Mallet finger of unspecified finger(s)

✓6ᵗʰ **M20.02** Boutonnière deformity

DEF: Deformity of the finger caused by flexion of the proximal interphalangeal joint and hyperextension of the distal joint. The deformity results from rheumatoid arthritis, osteoarthritis, or injury.

M20.021 Boutonnière deformity of right finger(s)

M20.022 Boutonnière deformity of left finger(s)

M20.029 Boutonnière deformity of unspecified finger(s)

√6ᵗʰ **M20.03** Swan-neck **deformity**

> **DEF:** Flexed distal and hyperextended proximal interphalangeal joint most commonly caused by rheumatoid arthritis.

     M20.031 Swan-neck deformity of right **finger(s)**
     M20.032 Swan-neck deformity of left **finger(s)**
     M20.039 Swan-neck deformity of unspecified **finger(s)**

√6ᵗʰ **M20.09** Other deformity of **finger(s)**

     M20.091 Other deformity of right **finger(s)**
     M20.092 Other deformity of left **finger(s)**
     M20.099 Other deformity of **finger(s), unspecified finger(s)**

√5ᵗʰ **M20.1** Hallux valgus (acquired)

> EXCLUDES 2   bunion (M21.6-)
> **AHA:** 2016,4Q,38
> **DEF:** Deformity in which the great toe deviates toward the other toes and may even be positioned over or under the second toe.

Hallux Valgus

Hallux valgus —

Medial eminence of metatarsal bone —

Right foot

     M20.10 Hallux valgus (acquired), unspecified **foot**
     M20.11 Hallux valgus (acquired), right **foot**
     M20.12 Hallux valgus (acquired), left **foot**

√5ᵗʰ **M20.2** Hallux rigidus

     M20.20 Hallux rigidus, unspecified **foot**
     M20.21 Hallux rigidus, right **foot**
     M20.22 Hallux rigidus, left **foot**

√5ᵗʰ **M20.3** Hallux varus (acquired)

> **DEF:** Deformity in which the great toe deviates away from the other toes.

     M20.30 Hallux varus (acquired), unspecified **foot**
     M20.31 Hallux varus (acquired), right **foot**
     M20.32 Hallux varus (acquired), left **foot**

√5ᵗʰ **M20.4** Other hammer toe(s) (acquired)

     M20.40 Other hammer toe(s) (acquired), unspecified **foot**
     M20.41 Other hammer toe(s) (acquired), right **foot**
     M20.42 Other hammer toe(s) (acquired), left **foot**

√5ᵗʰ **M20.5** Other deformities of toe(s) (acquired)

   √6ᵗʰ **M20.5X** Other deformities of **toe(s) (acquired)**

     M20.5X1 Other deformities of toe(s) (acquired), right **foot**
     M20.5X2 Other deformities of toe(s) (acquired), left **foot**
     M20.5X9 Other deformities of toe(s) (acquired), unspecified **foot**

√5ᵗʰ **M20.6** Acquired deformities of **toe(s), unspecified**

     M20.60 Acquired deformities of toe(s), unspecified, unspecified **foot**
     M20.61 Acquired deformities of toe(s), unspecified, right **foot**
     M20.62 Acquired deformities of toe(s), unspecified, left **foot**

√4ᵗʰ **M21** Other acquired deformities of limbs

> EXCLUDES 1   acquired absence of limb (Z89.-)
>   congenital absence of limbs (Q71-Q73)
>   congenital deformities and malformations of limbs (Q65-Q66, Q68-Q74)
> EXCLUDES 2   acquired deformities of fingers or toes (M20.-)
>   coxa plana (M91.2)

√5ᵗʰ **M21.0** Valgus **deformity, not elsewhere classified**

> EXCLUDES 1   metatarsus valgus (Q66.6)
>   talipes calcaneovalgus (Q66.4-)

     M21.00 Valgus deformity, not elsewhere classified, unspecified site

√6ᵗʰ **M21.02** Valgus deformity, not elsewhere classified, elbow

> Cubitus valgus

     M21.021 Valgus deformity, not elsewhere classified, right **elbow**
     M21.022 Valgus deformity, not elsewhere classified, left **elbow**
     M21.029 Valgus deformity, not elsewhere classified, unspecified **elbow**

√6ᵗʰ **M21.05** Valgus deformity, not elsewhere classified, hip

     M21.051 Valgus deformity, not elsewhere classified, right **hip**
     M21.052 Valgus deformity, not elsewhere classified, left **hip**
     M21.059 Valgus deformity, not elsewhere classified, unspecified **hip**

√6ᵗʰ **M21.06** Valgus deformity, not elsewhere classified, knee

> Genu valgum
> Knock knee
> **DEF:** Genu valga/valgum: Condition in which the thighs slant inward, causing the knees to be angled abnormally close together, leaving the space between the ankles wider than normal.

Genu Valga (knock-knee)

     M21.061 Valgus deformity, not elsewhere classified, right **knee**
     M21.062 Valgus deformity, not elsewhere classified, left **knee**
     M21.069 Valgus deformity, not elsewhere classified, unspecified **knee**

√6ᵗʰ **M21.07** Valgus deformity, not elsewhere classified, ankle

     M21.071 Valgus deformity, not elsewhere classified, right **ankle**
     M21.072 Valgus deformity, not elsewhere classified, left **ankle**
     M21.079 Valgus deformity, not elsewhere classified, unspecified **ankle**

√5ᵗʰ **M21.1** Varus **deformity, not elsewhere classified**

> EXCLUDES 1   metatarsus varus (Q66.22-)
>   tibia vara (M92.51-)

     M21.10 Varus deformity, not elsewhere classified, unspecified site

✔6ᵗʰ **M21.12** **Varus deformity, not elsewhere classified,** elbow

    Cubitus varus, elbow

    M21.121 **Varus deformity, not elsewhere classified, right elbow**

    M21.122 **Varus deformity, not elsewhere classified, left elbow**

    M21.129 **Varus deformity, not elsewhere classified, unspecified elbow**

✔6ᵗʰ **M21.15** **Varus deformity, not elsewhere classified,** hip

    M21.151 **Varus deformity, not elsewhere classified, right hip**

    M21.152 **Varus deformity, not elsewhere classified, left hip**

    M21.159 **Varus deformity, not elsewhere classified, unspecified**

✔6ᵗʰ **M21.16** **Varus deformity, not elsewhere classified,** knee

    Bow leg

    Genu varum

    DEF: Genu varus/varum: Condition in which the thighs and/or legs are bowed in an outward curve with an abnormally increased space between the knees.

Genu Varus (bowleg)

    M21.161 **Varus deformity, not elsewhere classified, right knee**

    M21.162 **Varus deformity, not elsewhere classified, left knee**

    M21.169 **Varus deformity, not elsewhere classified, unspecified knee**

✔6ᵗʰ **M21.17** **Varus deformity, not elsewhere classified,** ankle

    M21.171 **Varus deformity, not elsewhere classified, right ankle**

    M21.172 **Varus deformity, not elsewhere classified, left ankle**

    M21.179 **Varus deformity, not elsewhere classified, unspecified ankle**

✔5ᵗʰ **M21.2** **Flexion deformity**

    M21.20 **Flexion deformity, unspecified site**

  ✔6ᵗʰ **M21.21** **Flexion deformity,** shoulder

    M21.211 **Flexion deformity, right shoulder**

    M21.212 **Flexion deformity, left shoulder**

    M21.219 **Flexion deformity, unspecified shoulder**

  ✔6ᵗʰ **M21.22** **Flexion deformity,** elbow

    M21.221 **Flexion deformity, right elbow**

    M21.222 **Flexion deformity, left elbow**

    M21.229 **Flexion deformity, unspecified elbow**

  ✔6ᵗʰ **M21.23** **Flexion deformity,** wrist

    M21.231 **Flexion deformity, right wrist**

    M21.232 **Flexion deformity, left wrist**

    M21.239 **Flexion deformity, unspecified wrist**

  ✔6ᵗʰ **M21.24** **Flexion deformity,** finger joints

    M21.241 **Flexion deformity, right finger joints**

    M21.242 **Flexion deformity, left finger joints**

    M21.249 **Flexion deformity, unspecified finger joints**

✔6ᵗʰ **M21.25** **Flexion deformity,** hip

    M21.251 **Flexion deformity, right hip**

    M21.252 **Flexion deformity, left hip**

    M21.259 **Flexion deformity, unspecified hip**

✔6ᵗʰ **M21.26** **Flexion deformity,** knee

    M21.261 **Flexion deformity, right knee**

    M21.262 **Flexion deformity, left knee**

    M21.269 **Flexion deformity, unspecified knee**

✔6ᵗʰ **M21.27** **Flexion deformity,** ankle and toes

    M21.271 **Flexion deformity, right ankle and toes**

    M21.272 **Flexion deformity, left ankle and toes**

    M21.279 **Flexion deformity, unspecified ankle and toes**

✔5ᵗʰ **M21.3** **Wrist or foot drop (acquired)**

  ✔6ᵗʰ **M21.33** **Wrist drop (acquired)**

    M21.331 **Wrist drop, right wrist**

    M21.332 **Wrist drop, left wrist**

    M21.339 **Wrist drop, unspecified wrist**

  ✔6ᵗʰ **M21.37** **Foot drop (acquired)**

    M21.371 **Foot drop, right foot**

    M21.372 **Foot drop, left foot**

    M21.379 **Foot drop, unspecified foot**

✔5ᵗʰ **M21.4** **Flat foot [pes planus] (acquired)**

    EXCLUDES 1 *congenital pes planus (Q66.5-)*

    M21.40 **Flat foot [pes planus] (acquired), unspecified foot**

    M21.41 **Flat foot [pes planus] (acquired), right foot**

    M21.42 **Flat foot [pes planus] (acquired), left foot**

✔5ᵗʰ **M21.5** **Acquired** clawhand, clubhand, clawfoot and clubfoot

    EXCLUDES 1 *clubfoot, not specified as acquired (Q66.89)*

  ✔6ᵗʰ **M21.51** **Acquired** clawhand

    M21.511 **Acquired clawhand, right hand**

    M21.512 **Acquired clawhand, left hand**

    M21.519 **Acquired clawhand, unspecified hand**

  ✔6ᵗʰ **M21.52** **Acquired** clubhand

    M21.521 **Acquired clubhand, right hand**

    M21.522 **Acquired clubhand, left hand**

    M21.529 **Acquired clubhand, unspecified hand**

  ✔6ᵗʰ **M21.53** **Acquired** clawfoot

    DEF: High foot arch with hyperextended toes at the metatarsophalangeal joint and flexed toes at the distal joints.

    M21.531 **Acquired clawfoot, right foot**

    M21.532 **Acquired clawfoot, left foot**

    M21.539 **Acquired clawfoot, unspecified foot**

  ✔6ᵗʰ **M21.54** **Acquired** clubfoot

    DEF: Acquired anomaly of the foot with the heel elevated and rotated outward and the toes pointing inward.

    M21.541 **Acquired clubfoot, right foot**

    M21.542 **Acquired clubfoot, left foot**

    M21.549 **Acquired clubfoot, unspecified foot**

✔5ᵗʰ **M21.6** **Other acquired deformities of foot**

    EXCLUDES 2 *deformities of toe (acquired) (M20.1-M20.6-)*

    AHA: 2016,4Q,38

  ✔6ᵗʰ **M21.61** **Bunion**

    M21.611 **Bunion of right foot**

    M21.612 **Bunion of left foot**

    M21.619 **Bunion of unspecified foot**

  ✔6ᵗʰ **M21.62** **Bunionette**

    M21.621 **Bunionette of right foot**

    M21.622 **Bunionette of left foot**

    M21.629 **Bunionette of unspecified foot**

  ✔6ᵗʰ **M21.6X** **Other acquired deformities of** foot

    M21.6X1 **Other acquired deformities of right foot**

    M21.6X2 **Other acquired deformities of left foot**

    M21.6X9 **Other acquired deformities of unspecified foot**

✔5ᵗʰ **M21.7** **Unequal limb length (acquired)**

    NOTE The site used should correspond to the shorter limb

    M21.70 **Unequal limb length (acquired), unspecified site**

  ✔6ᵗʰ **M21.72** **Unequal limb length (acquired),** humerus

    M21.721 **Unequal limb length (acquired), right humerus**

           M21.722 Unequal limb length (acquired), left humerus

           M21.729 Unequal limb length (acquired), unspecified humerus

√6ᵗʰ **M21.73** Unequal limb length (acquired), ulna and radius

           M21.731 Unequal limb length (acquired), right ulna

           M21.732 Unequal limb length (acquired), left ulna

           M21.733 Unequal limb length (acquired), right radius

           M21.734 Unequal limb length (acquired), left radius

           M21.739 Unequal limb length (acquired), unspecified ulna and radius

√6ᵗʰ **M21.75** Unequal limb length (acquired), femur

           M21.751 Unequal limb length (acquired), right femur

           M21.752 Unequal limb length (acquired), left femur

           M21.759 Unequal limb length (acquired), unspecified femur

√6ᵗʰ **M21.76** Unequal limb length (acquired), tibia and fibula

           M21.761 Unequal limb length (acquired), right tibia

           M21.762 Unequal limb length (acquired), left tibia

           M21.763 Unequal limb length (acquired), right fibula

           M21.764 Unequal limb length (acquired), left fibula

           M21.769 Unequal limb length (acquired), unspecified tibia and fibula

√5ᵗʰ **M21.8** Other specified acquired deformities of limbs

        EXCLUDES 2   coxa plana (M91.2)

      M21.80 Other specified acquired deformities of unspecified limb

√6ᵗʰ **M21.82** Other specified acquired deformities of upper arm

           M21.821 Other specified acquired deformities of right upper arm

           M21.822 Other specified acquired deformities of left upper arm

           M21.829 Other specified acquired deformities of unspecified upper arm

√6ᵗʰ **M21.83** Other specified acquired deformities of forearm

           M21.831 Other specified acquired deformities of right forearm

           M21.832 Other specified acquired deformities of left forearm

           M21.839 Other specified acquired deformities of unspecified forearm

√6ᵗʰ **M21.85** Other specified acquired deformities of thigh

           M21.851 Other specified acquired deformities of right thigh

           M21.852 Other specified acquired deformities of left thigh

           M21.859 Other specified acquired deformities of unspecified thigh

√6ᵗʰ **M21.86** Other specified acquired deformities of lower leg

           M21.861 Other specified acquired deformities of right lower leg

           M21.862 Other specified acquired deformities of left lower leg

           M21.869 Other specified acquired deformities of unspecified lower leg

√5ᵗʰ **M21.9** Unspecified acquired deformity of limb and hand

      M21.90 Unspecified acquired deformity of unspecified limb

√6ᵗʰ **M21.92** Unspecified acquired deformity of upper arm

           M21.921 Unspecified acquired deformity of right upper arm

           M21.922 Unspecified acquired deformity of left upper arm

           M21.929 Unspecified acquired deformity of unspecified upper arm

√6ᵗʰ **M21.93** Unspecified acquired deformity of forearm

           M21.931 Unspecified acquired deformity of right forearm

           M21.932 Unspecified acquired deformity of left forearm

           M21.939 Unspecified acquired deformity of unspecified forearm

√6ᵗʰ **M21.94** Unspecified acquired deformity of hand

           M21.941 Unspecified acquired deformity of hand, right hand

           M21.942 Unspecified acquired deformity of hand, left hand

           M21.949 Unspecified acquired deformity of hand, unspecified hand

√6ᵗʰ **M21.95** Unspecified acquired deformity of thigh

           M21.951 Unspecified acquired deformity of right thigh

           M21.952 Unspecified acquired deformity of left thigh

           M21.959 Unspecified acquired deformity of unspecified thigh

√6ᵗʰ **M21.96** Unspecified acquired deformity of lower leg

           M21.961 Unspecified acquired deformity of right lower leg

           M21.962 Unspecified acquired deformity of left lower leg

           M21.969 Unspecified acquired deformity of unspecified lower leg

√4ᵗʰ **M22 Disorder of patella**

        EXCLUDES 2   traumatic dislocation of patella (S83.0-)

√5ᵗʰ **M22.0** Recurrent dislocation of patella

      M22.00 Recurrent dislocation of patella, unspecified knee

      M22.01 Recurrent dislocation of patella, right knee

      M22.02 Recurrent dislocation of patella, left knee

√5ᵗʰ **M22.1** Recurrent subluxation of patella

        Incomplete dislocation of patella

      M22.10 Recurrent subluxation of patella, unspecified knee

      M22.11 Recurrent subluxation of patella, right knee

      M22.12 Recurrent subluxation of patella, left knee

√5ᵗʰ **M22.2** Patellofemoral disorders

    √6ᵗʰ **M22.2X** Patellofemoral disorders

        M22.2X1 Patellofemoral disorders, right knee

        M22.2X2 Patellofemoral disorders, left knee

        M22.2X9 Patellofemoral disorders, unspecified knee

√5ᵗʰ **M22.3** Other derangements of patella

    √6ᵗʰ **M22.3X** Other derangements of patella

        M22.3X1 Other derangements of patella, right knee

        M22.3X2 Other derangements of patella, left knee

        M22.3X9 Other derangements of patella, unspecified knee

√5ᵗʰ **M22.4** Chondromalacia patellae

      M22.40 Chondromalacia patellae, unspecified knee

      M22.41 Chondromalacia patellae, right knee

      M22.42 Chondromalacia patellae, left knee

√5ᵗʰ **M22.8** Other disorders of patella

    √6ᵗʰ **M22.8X** Other disorders of patella

        M22.8X1 Other disorders of patella, right knee

        M22.8X2 Other disorders of patella, left knee

        M22.8X9 Other disorders of patella, unspecified knee

√5ᵗʰ **M22.9** Unspecified disorder of patella

      M22.90 Unspecified disorder of patella, unspecified knee

      M22.91 Unspecified disorder of patella, right knee

      M22.92 Unspecified disorder of patella, left knee

√4ᵗʰ **M23 Internal derangement of knee**

        EXCLUDES 1   ankylosis (M24.66)

                 deformity of knee (M21.-)

                 osteochondritis dissecans (M93.2)

        EXCLUDES 2   current injury - see injury of knee and lower leg (S80-S89)

                 recurrent dislocation or subluxation of joints (M24.4)

                 recurrent dislocation or subluxation of patella (M22.0-M22.1)

√5ᵗʰ **M23.0** Cystic meniscus

    √6ᵗʰ **M23.00** Cystic meniscus, unspecified meniscus

        Cystic meniscus, unspecified lateral meniscus

        Cystic meniscus, unspecified medial meniscus

        M23.000 Cystic meniscus, unspecified lateral meniscus, right knee

        M23.001 Cystic meniscus, unspecified lateral meniscus, left knee

M23.002 Cystic meniscus, unspecified lateral meniscus, unspecified knee

M23.003 Cystic meniscus, unspecified medial meniscus, right knee

M23.004 Cystic meniscus, unspecified medial meniscus, left knee

M23.005 Cystic meniscus, unspecified medial meniscus, unspecified knee

M23.006 Cystic meniscus, unspecified meniscus, right knee

M23.007 Cystic meniscus, unspecified meniscus, left knee

M23.009 Cystic meniscus, unspecified meniscus, unspecified knee

√6th **M23.01** Cystic meniscus, anterior horn of medial meniscus

M23.011 Cystic meniscus, anterior horn of medial meniscus, right knee

M23.012 Cystic meniscus, anterior horn of medial meniscus, left knee

M23.019 Cystic meniscus, anterior horn of medial meniscus, unspecified knee

√6th **M23.02** Cystic meniscus, posterior horn of medial meniscus

M23.021 Cystic meniscus, posterior horn of medial meniscus, right knee

M23.022 Cystic meniscus, posterior horn of medial meniscus, left knee

M23.029 Cystic meniscus, posterior horn of medial meniscus, unspecified knee

√6th **M23.03** Cystic meniscus, other medial meniscus

M23.031 Cystic meniscus, other medial meniscus, right knee

M23.032 Cystic meniscus, other medial meniscus, left knee

M23.039 Cystic meniscus, other medial meniscus, unspecified knee

√6th **M23.04** Cystic meniscus, anterior horn of lateral meniscus

M23.041 Cystic meniscus, anterior horn of lateral meniscus, right knee

M23.042 Cystic meniscus, anterior horn of lateral meniscus, left knee

M23.049 Cystic meniscus, anterior horn of lateral meniscus, unspecified knee

√6th **M23.05** Cystic meniscus, posterior horn of lateral meniscus

M23.051 Cystic meniscus, posterior horn of lateral meniscus, right knee

M23.052 Cystic meniscus, posterior horn of lateral meniscus, left knee

M23.059 Cystic meniscus, posterior horn of lateral meniscus, unspecified knee

√6th **M23.06** Cystic meniscus, other lateral meniscus

M23.061 Cystic meniscus, other lateral meniscus, right knee

M23.062 Cystic meniscus, other lateral meniscus, left knee

M23.069 Cystic meniscus, other lateral meniscus, unspecified knee

√5th **M23.2** Derangement of meniscus due to old tear or injury

Old bucket-handle tear

AHA: 2019,2Q,26

Derangement of Meniscus

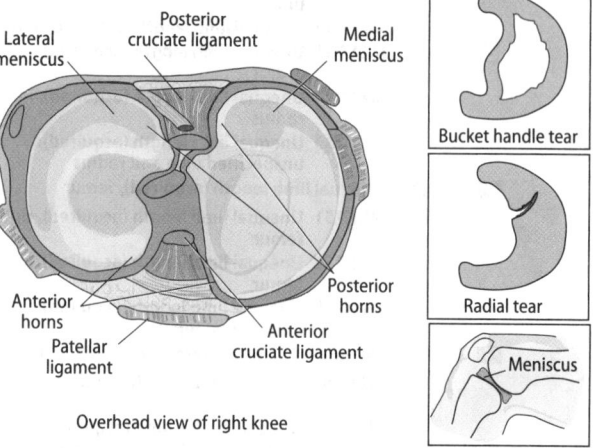

Overhead view of right knee

√6th **M23.20** Derangement of unspecified meniscus due to old tear or injury

Derangement of unspecified lateral meniscus due to old tear or injury

Derangement of unspecified medial meniscus due to old tear or injury

M23.200 Derangement of unspecified lateral meniscus due to old tear or injury, right knee

M23.201 Derangement of unspecified lateral meniscus due to old tear or injury, left knee

M23.202 Derangement of unspecified lateral meniscus due to old tear or injury, unspecified knee

M23.203 Derangement of unspecified medial meniscus due to old tear or injury, right knee

M23.204 Derangement of unspecified medial meniscus due to old tear or injury, left knee

M23.205 Derangement of unspecified medial meniscus due to old tear or injury, unspecified knee

M23.206 Derangement of unspecified meniscus due to old tear or injury, right knee

M23.207 Derangement of unspecified meniscus due to old tear or injury, left knee

M23.209 Derangement of unspecified meniscus due to old tear or injury, unspecified knee

√6th **M23.21** Derangement of anterior horn of medial meniscus due to old tear or injury

M23.211 Derangement of anterior horn of medial meniscus due to old tear or injury, right knee

M23.212 Derangement of anterior horn of medial meniscus due to old tear or injury, left knee

M23.219 Derangement of anterior horn of medial meniscus due to old tear or injury, unspecified knee

√6th **M23.22** Derangement of posterior horn of medial meniscus due to old tear or injury

M23.221 Derangement of posterior horn of medial meniscus due to old tear or injury, right knee

M23.222 Derangement of posterior horn of medial meniscus due to old tear or injury, left knee

M23.229 Derangement of posterior horn of medial meniscus due to old tear or injury, unspecified knee

√6th **M23.23** Derangement of other medial meniscus due to old tear or injury

M23.231 Derangement of other medial meniscus due to old tear or injury, right knee

M23.232 Derangement of other medial meniscus due to old tear or injury, left knee

M23.239 Derangement of other medial meniscus due to old tear or injury, unspecified knee

✓6ᵗʰ **M23.24** Derangement of anterior horn of lateral meniscus due to old tear or injury

M23.241 Derangement of anterior horn of lateral meniscus due to old tear or injury, right knee

M23.242 Derangement of anterior horn of lateral meniscus due to old tear or injury, left knee

M23.249 Derangement of anterior horn of lateral meniscus due to old tear or injury, unspecified knee

✓6ᵗʰ **M23.25** Derangement of posterior horn of lateral meniscus due to old tear or injury

M23.251 Derangement of posterior horn of lateral meniscus due to old tear or injury, right knee

M23.252 Derangement of posterior horn of lateral meniscus due to old tear or injury, left knee

M23.259 Derangement of posterior horn of lateral meniscus due to old tear or injury, unspecified knee

✓6ᵗʰ **M23.26** Derangement of other lateral meniscus due to old tear or injury

M23.261 Derangement of other lateral meniscus due to old tear or injury, right knee

M23.262 Derangement of other lateral meniscus due to old tear or injury, left knee

M23.269 Derangement of other lateral meniscus due to old tear or injury, unspecified knee

✓5ᵗʰ **M23.3** Other meniscus derangements

Degenerate meniscus
Detached meniscus
Retained meniscus

✓6ᵗʰ **M23.30** Other meniscus derangements, unspecified meniscus

Other meniscus derangements, unspecified lateral meniscus
Other meniscus derangements, unspecified medial meniscus

M23.300 Other meniscus derangements, unspecified lateral meniscus, right knee

M23.301 Other meniscus derangements, unspecified lateral meniscus, left knee

M23.302 Other meniscus derangements, unspecified lateral meniscus, unspecified knee

M23.303 Other meniscus derangements, unspecified medial meniscus, right knee

M23.304 Other meniscus derangements, unspecified medial meniscus, left knee

M23.305 Other meniscus derangements, unspecified medial meniscus, unspecified knee

M23.306 Other meniscus derangements, unspecified meniscus, right knee

M23.307 Other meniscus derangements, unspecified meniscus, left knee

M23.309 Other meniscus derangements, unspecified meniscus, unspecified knee

✓6ᵗʰ **M23.31** Other meniscus derangements, anterior horn of medial meniscus

M23.311 Other meniscus derangements, anterior horn of medial meniscus, right knee

M23.312 Other meniscus derangements, anterior horn of medial meniscus, left knee

M23.319 Other meniscus derangements, anterior horn of medial meniscus, unspecified knee

✓6ᵗʰ **M23.32** Other meniscus derangements, posterior horn of medial meniscus

M23.321 Other meniscus derangements, posterior horn of medial meniscus, right knee

M23.322 Other meniscus derangements, posterior horn of medial meniscus, left knee

M23.329 Other meniscus derangements, posterior horn of medial meniscus, unspecified knee

✓6ᵗʰ **M23.33** Other meniscus derangements, other medial meniscus

M23.331 Other meniscus derangements, other medial meniscus, right knee

M23.332 Other meniscus derangements, other medial meniscus, left knee

M23.339 Other meniscus derangements, other medial meniscus, unspecified knee

✓6ᵗʰ **M23.34** Other meniscus derangements, anterior horn of lateral meniscus

M23.341 Other meniscus derangements, anterior horn of lateral meniscus, right knee

M23.342 Other meniscus derangements, anterior horn of lateral meniscus, left knee

M23.349 Other meniscus derangements, anterior horn of lateral meniscus, unspecified knee

✓6ᵗʰ **M23.35** Other meniscus derangements, posterior horn of lateral meniscus

M23.351 Other meniscus derangements, posterior horn of lateral meniscus, right knee

M23.352 Other meniscus derangements, posterior horn of lateral meniscus, left knee

M23.359 Other meniscus derangements, posterior horn of lateral meniscus, unspecified knee

✓6ᵗʰ **M23.36** Other meniscus derangements, other lateral meniscus

M23.361 Other meniscus derangements, other lateral meniscus, right knee

M23.362 Other meniscus derangements, other lateral meniscus, left knee

M23.369 Other meniscus derangements, other lateral meniscus, unspecified knee

✓5ᵗʰ **M23.4** Loose body in knee

M23.40 Loose body in knee, unspecified knee
M23.41 Loose body in knee, right knee
M23.42 Loose body in knee, left knee

✓5ᵗʰ **M23.5** Chronic instability of knee

M23.50 Chronic instability of knee, unspecified knee
M23.51 Chronic instability of knee, right knee
M23.52 Chronic instability of knee, left knee

✓5ᵗʰ **M23.6** Other spontaneous disruption of ligament(s) of knee

✓6ᵗʰ **M23.60** Other spontaneous disruption of unspecified ligament of knee

M23.601 Other spontaneous disruption of unspecified ligament of right knee
M23.602 Other spontaneous disruption of unspecified ligament of left knee
M23.609 Other spontaneous disruption of unspecified ligament of unspecified knee

✓6ᵗʰ **M23.61** Other spontaneous disruption of anterior cruciate ligament of knee

M23.611 Other spontaneous disruption of anterior cruciate ligament of right knee
M23.612 Other spontaneous disruption of anterior cruciate ligament of left knee
M23.619 Other spontaneous disruption of anterior cruciate ligament of unspecified knee

✓6ᵗʰ **M23.62** Other spontaneous disruption of posterior cruciate ligament of knee

M23.621 Other spontaneous disruption of posterior cruciate ligament of right knee
M23.622 Other spontaneous disruption of posterior cruciate ligament of left knee
M23.629 Other spontaneous disruption of posterior cruciate ligament of unspecified knee

✓6ᵗʰ **M23.63** Other spontaneous disruption of medial collateral ligament of knee

M23.631 Other spontaneous disruption of medial collateral ligament of right knee
M23.632 Other spontaneous disruption of medial collateral ligament of left knee
M23.639 Other spontaneous disruption of medial collateral ligament of unspecified knee

✓6ᵗʰ **M23.64** Other spontaneous disruption of lateral collateral ligament of knee

M23.641 Other spontaneous disruption of lateral collateral ligament of right knee
M23.642 Other spontaneous disruption of lateral collateral ligament of left knee

M23.649 Other spontaneous disruption of lateral collateral ligament of unspecified knee

✓6ᵗʰ M23.67 Other spontaneous disruption of capsular ligament of knee

M23.671 Other spontaneous disruption of capsular ligament of right knee

M23.672 Other spontaneous disruption of capsular ligament of left knee

M23.679 Other spontaneous disruption of capsular ligament of unspecified knee

✓5ᵗʰ M23.8 Other internal derangements of knee
Laxity of ligament of knee
Snapping knee

✓6ᵗʰ M23.8X Other internal derangements of knee

M23.8X1 Other internal derangements of right knee

M23.8X2 Other internal derangements of left knee

M23.8X9 Other internal derangements of unspecified knee

✓5ᵗʰ M23.9 Unspecified internal derangement of knee

M23.90 Unspecified internal derangement of unspecified knee

M23.91 Unspecified internal derangement of right knee

M23.92 Unspecified internal derangement of left knee

✓4ᵗʰ M24 Other specific joint derangements

EXCLUDES 1 current injury - see injury of joint by body region

EXCLUDES 2 ganglion (M67.4)
snapping knee (M23.8-)
temporomandibular joint disorders (M26.6-)

AHA: 2020,4Q,31-32

✓5ᵗʰ M24.0 Loose body in joint

EXCLUDES 2 loose body in knee (M23.4)

M24.00 Loose body in unspecified joint

✓6ᵗʰ M24.01 Loose body in shoulder

M24.011 Loose body in right shoulder
M24.012 Loose body in left shoulder
M24.019 Loose body in unspecified shoulder

✓6ᵗʰ M24.02 Loose body in elbow

M24.021 Loose body in right elbow
M24.022 Loose body in left elbow
M24.029 Loose body in unspecified elbow

✓6ᵗʰ M24.03 Loose body in wrist

M24.031 Loose body in right wrist
M24.032 Loose body in left wrist
M24.039 Loose body in unspecified wrist

✓6ᵗʰ M24.04 Loose body in finger joints

M24.041 Loose body in right finger joint(s)
M24.042 Loose body in left finger joint(s)
M24.049 Loose body in unspecified finger joint(s)

✓6ᵗʰ M24.05 Loose body in hip

M24.051 Loose body in right hip
M24.052 Loose body in left hip
M24.059 Loose body in unspecified hip

✓6ᵗʰ M24.07 Loose body in ankle and toe joints

M24.071 Loose body in right ankle
M24.072 Loose body in left ankle
M24.073 Loose body in unspecified ankle
M24.074 Loose body in right toe joint(s)
M24.075 Loose body in left toe joint(s)
M24.076 Loose body in unspecified toe joints

M24.08 Loose body, other site

✓5ᵗʰ M24.1 Other articular cartilage disorders

EXCLUDES 2 chondrocalcinosis (M11.1, M11.2-)
internal derangement of knee (M23.-)
metastatic calcification (E83.5)
ochronosis (E70.2)

M24.10 Other articular cartilage disorders, unspecified site

✓6ᵗʰ M24.11 Other articular cartilage disorders, shoulder

M24.111 Other articular cartilage disorders, right shoulder

M24.112 Other articular cartilage disorders, left shoulder

M24.119 Other articular cartilage disorders, unspecified shoulder

✓6ᵗʰ M24.12 Other articular cartilage disorders, elbow

M24.121 Other articular cartilage disorders, right elbow

M24.122 Other articular cartilage disorders, left elbow

M24.129 Other articular cartilage disorders, unspecified elbow

✓6ᵗʰ M24.13 Other articular cartilage disorders, wrist

M24.131 Other articular cartilage disorders, right wrist

M24.132 Other articular cartilage disorders, left wrist

M24.139 Other articular cartilage disorders, unspecified wrist

✓6ᵗʰ M24.14 Other articular cartilage disorders, hand

M24.141 Other articular cartilage disorders, right hand

M24.142 Other articular cartilage disorders, left hand

M24.149 Other articular cartilage disorders, unspecified hand

✓6ᵗʰ M24.15 Other articular cartilage disorders, hip

M24.151 Other articular cartilage disorders, right hip

M24.152 Other articular cartilage disorders, left hip

M24.159 Other articular cartilage disorders, unspecified hip

✓6ᵗʰ M24.17 Other articular cartilage disorders, ankle and foot

M24.171 Other articular cartilage disorders, right ankle

M24.172 Other articular cartilage disorders, left ankle

M24.173 Other articular cartilage disorders, unspecified ankle

M24.174 Other articular cartilage disorders, right foot

M24.175 Other articular cartilage disorders, left foot

M24.176 Other articular cartilage disorders, unspecified foot

M24.19 Other articular cartilage disorders, other specified site

✓5ᵗʰ M24.2 Disorder of ligament
Instability secondary to old ligament injury
Ligamentous laxity NOS

EXCLUDES 1 familial ligamentous laxity (M35.7)

EXCLUDES 2 internal derangement of knee (M23.5-M23.8X9)

M24.20 Disorder of ligament, unspecified site

✓6ᵗʰ M24.21 Disorder of ligament, shoulder

M24.211 Disorder of ligament, right shoulder
M24.212 Disorder of ligament, left shoulder
M24.219 Disorder of ligament, unspecified shoulder

✓6ᵗʰ M24.22 Disorder of ligament, elbow

M24.221 Disorder of ligament, right elbow
M24.222 Disorder of ligament, left elbow
M24.229 Disorder of ligament, unspecified elbow

✓6ᵗʰ M24.23 Disorder of ligament, wrist

M24.231 Disorder of ligament, right wrist
M24.232 Disorder of ligament, left wrist
M24.239 Disorder of ligament, unspecified wrist

✓6ᵗʰ M24.24 Disorder of ligament, hand

M24.241 Disorder of ligament, right hand
M24.242 Disorder of ligament, left hand
M24.249 Disorder of ligament, unspecified hand

✓6ᵗʰ M24.25 Disorder of ligament, hip

M24.251 Disorder of ligament, right hip
M24.252 Disorder of ligament, left hip
M24.259 Disorder of ligament, unspecified hip

✓6ᵗʰ M24.27 Disorder of ligament, ankle and foot

M24.271 Disorder of ligament, right ankle
M24.272 Disorder of ligament, left ankle
M24.273 Disorder of ligament, unspecified ankle
M24.274 Disorder of ligament, right foot
M24.275 Disorder of ligament, left foot
M24.276 Disorder of ligament, unspecified foot

M24.28 Disorder of ligament, vertebrae

M24.29   Disorder of ligament, other specified site

√5ᵗʰ **M24.3**   **Pathological dislocation of joint, not elsewhere classified**

> **EXCLUDES 1**   *congenital dislocation or displacement of joint - see congenital malformations and deformations of the musculoskeletal system (Q65-Q79)*
> *current injury - see injury of joints and ligaments by body region*
> *recurrent dislocation of joint (M24.4-)*

M24.30   Pathological dislocation of unspecified joint, not elsewhere classified

√6ᵗʰ **M24.31**   Pathological dislocation of shoulder, not elsewhere classified
- M24.311   Pathological dislocation of right shoulder, not elsewhere classified
- M24.312   Pathological dislocation of left shoulder, not elsewhere classified
- **M24.319**   Pathological dislocation of unspecified shoulder, not elsewhere classified

√6ᵗʰ **M24.32**   Pathological dislocation of elbow, not elsewhere classified
- M24.321   Pathological dislocation of right elbow, not elsewhere classified
- M24.322   Pathological dislocation of left elbow, not elsewhere classified
- **M24.329**   Pathological dislocation of unspecified elbow, not elsewhere classified

√6ᵗʰ **M24.33**   Pathological dislocation of wrist, not elsewhere classified
- M24.331   Pathological dislocation of right wrist, not elsewhere classified
- M24.332   Pathological dislocation of left wrist, not elsewhere classified
- **M24.339**   Pathological dislocation of unspecified wrist, not elsewhere classified

√6ᵗʰ **M24.34**   Pathological dislocation of hand, not elsewhere classified
- M24.341   Pathological dislocation of right hand, not elsewhere classified
- M24.342   Pathological dislocation of left hand, not elsewhere classified
- **M24.349**   Pathological dislocation of unspecified hand, not elsewhere classified

√6ᵗʰ **M24.35**   Pathological dislocation of hip, not elsewhere classified
> AHA: 2022,1Q,32
- M24.351   Pathological dislocation of right hip, not elsewhere classified
- M24.352   Pathological dislocation of left hip, not elsewhere classified
- **M24.359**   Pathological dislocation of unspecified hip, not elsewhere classified

√6ᵗʰ **M24.36**   Pathological dislocation of knee, not elsewhere classified
- M24.361   Pathological dislocation of right knee, not elsewhere classified
- M24.362   Pathological dislocation of left knee, not elsewhere classified
- **M24.369**   Pathological dislocation of unspecified knee, not elsewhere classified

√6ᵗʰ **M24.37**   Pathological dislocation of ankle and foot, not elsewhere classified
- M24.371   Pathological dislocation of right ankle, not elsewhere classified
- M24.372   Pathological dislocation of left ankle, not elsewhere classified
- **M24.373**   Pathological dislocation of unspecified ankle, not elsewhere classified
- M24.374   Pathological dislocation of right foot, not elsewhere classified
- M24.375   Pathological dislocation of left foot, not elsewhere classified
- **M24.376**   Pathological dislocation of unspecified foot, not elsewhere classified

M24.39   Pathological dislocation of other specified joint, not elsewhere classified

√5ᵗʰ **M24.4**   **Recurrent dislocation of joint**
> Recurrent subluxation of joint
> **EXCLUDES 2**   *recurrent dislocation of patella (M22.0-M22.1)*
> *recurrent vertebral dislocation (M43.3-, M43.4, M43.5-)*

M24.40   **Recurrent dislocation, unspecified joint**

√6ᵗʰ **M24.41**   Recurrent dislocation, shoulder
- M24.411   Recurrent dislocation, right shoulder
- M24.412   Recurrent dislocation, left shoulder
- **M24.419**   Recurrent dislocation, unspecified shoulder

√6ᵗʰ **M24.42**   Recurrent dislocation, elbow
- M24.421   Recurrent dislocation, right elbow
- M24.422   Recurrent dislocation, left elbow
- **M24.429**   Recurrent dislocation, unspecified elbow

√6ᵗʰ **M24.43**   Recurrent dislocation, wrist
- M24.431   Recurrent dislocation, right wrist
- M24.432   Recurrent dislocation, left wrist
- **M24.439**   Recurrent dislocation, unspecified wrist

√6ᵗʰ **M24.44**   Recurrent dislocation, hand and finger(s)
- M24.441   Recurrent dislocation, right hand
- M24.442   Recurrent dislocation, left hand
- **M24.443**   Recurrent dislocation, unspecified hand
- M24.444   Recurrent dislocation, right finger
- M24.445   Recurrent dislocation, left finger
- **M24.446**   Recurrent dislocation, unspecified finger

√6ᵗʰ **M24.45**   Recurrent dislocation, hip
- M24.451   Recurrent dislocation, right hip
- M24.452   Recurrent dislocation, left hip
- **M24.459**   Recurrent dislocation, unspecified hip

√6ᵗʰ **M24.46**   Recurrent dislocation, knee
- M24.461   Recurrent dislocation, right knee
- M24.462   Recurrent dislocation, left knee
- **M24.469**   Recurrent dislocation, unspecified knee

√6ᵗʰ **M24.47**   Recurrent dislocation, ankle, foot and toes
- M24.471   Recurrent dislocation, right ankle
- M24.472   Recurrent dislocation, left ankle
- **M24.473**   Recurrent dislocation, unspecified ankle
- M24.474   Recurrent dislocation, right foot
- M24.475   Recurrent dislocation, left foot
- **M24.476**   Recurrent dislocation, unspecified foot
- M24.477   Recurrent dislocation, right toe(s)
- M24.478   Recurrent dislocation, left toe(s)
- **M24.479**   Recurrent dislocation, unspecified toe(s)

M24.49   Recurrent dislocation, other specified joint

√5ᵗʰ **M24.5**   **Contracture of joint**
> **EXCLUDES 1**   *contracture of muscle without contracture of joint (M62.4-)*
> *contracture of tendon (sheath) without contracture of joint (M62.4-)*
> *Dupuytren's contracture (M72.0)*
> **EXCLUDES 2**   *acquired deformities of limbs (M20-M21)*
> AHA: 2016,2Q,6

M24.50   Contracture, unspecified joint

√6ᵗʰ **M24.51**   Contracture, shoulder
- M24.511   Contracture, right shoulder
- M24.512   Contracture, left shoulder
- **M24.519**   Contracture, unspecified shoulder

√6ᵗʰ **M24.52**   Contracture, elbow
- M24.521   Contracture, right elbow
- M24.522   Contracture, left elbow
- **M24.529**   Contracture, unspecified elbow

√6ᵗʰ **M24.53**   Contracture, wrist
- M24.531   Contracture, right wrist
- M24.532   Contracture, left wrist
- **M24.539**   Contracture, unspecified wrist

√6ᵗʰ **M24.54**   Contracture, hand
- M24.541   Contracture, right hand
- M24.542   Contracture, left hand
- **M24.549**   Contracture, unspecified hand

√6ᵗʰ **M24.55**   Contracture, hip
- M24.551   Contracture, right hip
- M24.552   Contracture, left hip
- **M24.559**   Contracture, unspecified hip

√6ᵗʰ **M24.56**   Contracture, knee
- M24.561   Contracture, right knee
- M24.562   Contracture, left knee
- **M24.569**   Contracture, unspecified knee

√6ᵗʰ **M24.57**   Contracture, ankle and foot
- M24.571   Contracture, right ankle
- M24.572   Contracture, left ankle

M24.573   **Contracture, unspecified ankle**
M24.574   **Contracture,** right foot
M24.575   **Contracture,** left foot
M24.576   **Contracture, unspecified foot**
M24.59   **Contracture, other specified joint**

√5ᵗʰ **M24.6   Ankylosis of joint**

> EXCLUDES 1   *stiffness of joint without ankylosis (M25.6-)*
> EXCLUDES 2   *spine (M43.2-)*

DEF: Ankylosis: Abnormal union or fusion of bones in a joint, which is normally moveable.

M24.60   Ankylosis, unspecified joint

√6ᵗʰ **M24.61   Ankylosis,** shoulder
M24.611   **Ankylosis,** right shoulder
M24.612   **Ankylosis,** left shoulder
M24.619   **Ankylosis, unspecified shoulder**

√6ᵗʰ **M24.62   Ankylosis,** elbow
M24.621   **Ankylosis,** right elbow
M24.622   **Ankylosis,** left elbow
M24.629   **Ankylosis, unspecified elbow**

√6ᵗʰ **M24.63   Ankylosis,** wrist
M24.631   **Ankylosis,** right wrist
M24.632   **Ankylosis,** left wrist
M24.639   **Ankylosis, unspecified wrist**

√6ᵗʰ **M24.64   Ankylosis,** hand
M24.641   **Ankylosis,** right hand
M24.642   **Ankylosis,** left hand
M24.649   **Ankylosis, unspecified hand**

√6ᵗʰ **M24.65   Ankylosis,** hip
M24.651   **Ankylosis,** right hip
M24.652   **Ankylosis,** left hip
M24.659   **Ankylosis, unspecified hip**

√6ᵗʰ **M24.66   Ankylosis,** knee
M24.661   **Ankylosis,** right knee
M24.662   **Ankylosis,** left knee
M24.669   **Ankylosis, unspecified knee**

√6ᵗʰ **M24.67   Ankylosis,** ankle and foot
M24.671   **Ankylosis,** right ankle
M24.672   **Ankylosis,** left ankle
M24.673   **Ankylosis, unspecified ankle**
M24.674   **Ankylosis,** right foot
M24.675   **Ankylosis,** left foot
M24.676   **Ankylosis, unspecified foot**
M24.69   **Ankylosis, other specified joint**

M24.7   Protrusio acetabuli

DEF: Intrapelvic protrusion of the acetabulum characterized by the sinking of the floor of the acetabulum, causing the femoral head to protrude. It limits hip movement and is of unknown etiology. **Synonym(s):** *Otto's pelvis.*

√5ᵗʰ **M24.8   Other specific joint derangements, not elsewhere classified**

> EXCLUDES 2   *iliotibial band syndrome (M76.3)*

M24.80   Other specific joint derangements of unspecified joint, not elsewhere classified

√6ᵗʰ **M24.81   Other specific joint derangements of** shoulder, **not elsewhere classified**
M24.811   **Other specific joint derangements of** right shoulder, not elsewhere classified
M24.812   **Other specific joint derangements of** left shoulder, not elsewhere classified
M24.819   **Other specific joint derangements of unspecified shoulder, not elsewhere classified**

√6ᵗʰ **M24.82   Other specific joint derangements of** elbow, **not elsewhere classified**
M24.821   **Other specific joint derangements of** right elbow, not elsewhere classified
M24.822   **Other specific joint derangements of** left elbow, not elsewhere classified
M24.829   **Other specific joint derangements of unspecified elbow, not elsewhere classified**

√6ᵗʰ **M24.83   Other specific joint derangements of** wrist, **not elsewhere classified**
M24.831   **Other specific joint derangements of** right wrist, not elsewhere classified
M24.832   **Other specific joint derangements of** left wrist, not elsewhere classified
M24.839   **Other specific joint derangements of unspecified wrist, not elsewhere classified**

√6ᵗʰ **M24.84   Other specific joint derangements of** hand, **not elsewhere classified**
M24.841   **Other specific joint derangements of** right hand, not elsewhere classified
M24.842   **Other specific joint derangements of** left hand, not elsewhere classified
M24.849   **Other specific joint derangements of unspecified hand, not elsewhere classified**

√6ᵗʰ **M24.85   Other specific joint derangements of** hip, **not elsewhere classified**
Irritable hip
M24.851   **Other specific joint derangements of** right hip, not elsewhere classified
M24.852   **Other specific joint derangements of** left hip, not elsewhere classified
M24.859   **Other specific joint derangements of unspecified hip, not elsewhere classified**

√6ᵗʰ **M24.87   Other specific joint derangements of** ankle and foot, **not elsewhere classified**
M24.871   **Other specific joint derangements of** right ankle, not elsewhere classified
M24.872   **Other specific joint derangements of** left ankle, not elsewhere classified
M24.873   **Other specific joint derangements of unspecified ankle, not elsewhere classified**
M24.874   **Other specific joint derangements of** right foot, not elsewhere classified
M24.875   **Other specific joint derangements of** left foot, not elsewhere classified
M24.876   **Other specific joint derangements of unspecified foot, not elsewhere classified**
M24.89   **Other specific joint derangement of other specified joint, not elsewhere classified**

M24.9   Joint derangement, unspecified

√4ᵗʰ **M25   Other joint disorder, not elsewhere classified**

> EXCLUDES 2   *abnormality of gait and mobility (R26.-)*
> *acquired deformities of limb (M20-M21)*
> *calcification of bursa (M71.4-)*
> *calcification of shoulder (joint) (M75.3)*
> *calcification of tendon (M65.2-)*
> *difficulty in walking (R26.2)*
> *temporomandibular joint disorder (M26.6-)*

AHA: 2020,4Q,31-32

√5ᵗʰ **M25.0   Hemarthrosis**

> EXCLUDES 1   *current injury - see injury of joint by body region*
> *hemophilic arthropathy (M36.2)*

M25.00   Hemarthrosis, unspecified joint

√6ᵗʰ **M25.01   Hemarthrosis,** shoulder
M25.011   **Hemarthrosis,** right shoulder
M25.012   **Hemarthrosis,** left shoulder
M25.019   **Hemarthrosis, unspecified shoulder**

√6ᵗʰ **M25.02   Hemarthrosis,** elbow
M25.021   **Hemarthrosis,** right elbow
M25.022   **Hemarthrosis,** left elbow
M25.029   **Hemarthrosis, unspecified elbow**

√6ᵗʰ **M25.03   Hemarthrosis,** wrist
M25.031   **Hemarthrosis,** right wrist
M25.032   **Hemarthrosis,** left wrist
M25.039   **Hemarthrosis, unspecified wrist**

√6ᵗʰ **M25.04   Hemarthrosis,** hand
M25.041   **Hemarthrosis,** right hand
M25.042   **Hemarthrosis,** left hand
M25.049   **Hemarthrosis, unspecified hand**

√6ᵗʰ **M25.05   Hemarthrosis,** hip
M25.051   **Hemarthrosis,** right hip
M25.052   **Hemarthrosis,** left hip
M25.059   **Hemarthrosis, unspecified hip**

√6ᵗʰ **M25.06   Hemarthrosis,** knee
M25.061   **Hemarthrosis,** right knee
M25.062   **Hemarthrosis,** left knee
M25.069   **Hemarthrosis, unspecified knee**

√6ᵗʰ **M25.07   Hemarthrosis,** ankle and foot
M25.071   **Hemarthrosis,** right ankle
M25.072   **Hemarthrosis,** left ankle
M25.073   **Hemarthrosis, unspecified ankle**
M25.074   **Hemarthrosis,** right foot

      M25.Ø75 Hemarthrosis, left foot
      M25.Ø76 Hemarthrosis, unspecified foot
   M25.Ø8 Hemarthrosis, other specified site
      Hemarthrosis, vertebrae

✓5ᵗʰ M25.1 **Fistula of joint**

   M25.10 Fistula, unspecified joint
✓6ᵗʰ M25.11 Fistula, shoulder

      M25.111 Fistula, right shoulder
      M25.112 Fistula, left shoulder
      M25.119 Fistula, unspecified shoulder
✓6ᵗʰ M25.12 Fistula, elbow

      M25.121 Fistula, right elbow
      M25.122 Fistula, left elbow
      M25.129 Fistula, unspecified elbow
✓6ᵗʰ M25.13 Fistula, wrist

      M25.131 Fistula, right wrist
      M25.132 Fistula, left wrist
      M25.139 Fistula, unspecified wrist
✓6ᵗʰ M25.14 Fistula, hand

      M25.141 Fistula, right hand
      M25.142 Fistula, left hand
      M25.149 Fistula, unspecified hand
✓6ᵗʰ M25.15 Fistula, hip

      M25.151 Fistula, right hip
      M25.152 Fistula, left hip
      M25.159 Fistula, unspecified hip
✓6ᵗʰ M25.16 Fistula, knee

      M25.161 Fistula, right knee
      M25.162 Fistula, left knee
      M25.169 Fistula, unspecified knee
✓6ᵗʰ M25.17 Fistula, ankle and foot

      M25.171 Fistula, right ankle
      M25.172 Fistula, left ankle
      M25.173 Fistula, unspecified ankle
      M25.174 Fistula, right foot
      M25.175 Fistula, left foot
      M25.176 Fistula, unspecified foot
   M25.18 Fistula, other specified site
      Fistula, vertebrae

✓5ᵗʰ M25.2 **Flail joint**
      DEF: Hinged joint that exhibits an abnormal or excessive degree of range and mobility.
   M25.20 Flail joint, unspecified joint
✓6ᵗʰ M25.21 Flail joint, shoulder

      M25.211 Flail joint, right shoulder
      M25.212 Flail joint, left shoulder
      M25.219 Flail joint, unspecified shoulder
✓6ᵗʰ M25.22 Flail joint, elbow

      M25.221 Flail joint, right elbow
      M25.222 Flail joint, left elbow
      M25.229 Flail joint, unspecified elbow
✓6ᵗʰ M25.23 Flail joint, wrist

      M25.231 Flail joint, right wrist
      M25.232 Flail joint, left wrist
      M25.239 Flail joint, unspecified wrist
✓6ᵗʰ M25.24 Flail joint, hand

      M25.241 Flail joint, right hand
      M25.242 Flail joint, left hand
      M25.249 Flail joint, unspecified hand
✓6ᵗʰ M25.25 Flail joint, hip

      M25.251 Flail joint, right hip
      M25.252 Flail joint, left hip
      M25.259 Flail joint, unspecified hip
✓6ᵗʰ M25.26 Flail joint, knee

      M25.261 Flail joint, right knee
      M25.262 Flail joint, left knee
      M25.269 Flail joint, unspecified knee
✓6ᵗʰ M25.27 Flail joint, ankle and foot

      M25.271 Flail joint, right ankle and foot
      M25.272 Flail joint, left ankle and foot
      M25.279 Flail joint, unspecified ankle and foot
   M25.28 Flail joint, other site

✓5ᵗʰ M25.3 **Other instability of joint**
     EXCLUDES 1 *instability of joint secondary to old ligament injury (M24.2-)*
           instability of joint secondary to removal of joint prosthesis (M96.8-)
     EXCLUDES 2 *spinal instabilities (M53.2-)*
   M25.30 Other instability, unspecified joint
✓6ᵗʰ M25.31 Other instability, shoulder

      M25.311 Other instability, right shoulder
      M25.312 Other instability, left shoulder
      M25.319 Other instability, unspecified shoulder
✓6ᵗʰ M25.32 Other instability, elbow

      M25.321 Other instability, right elbow
      M25.322 Other instability, left elbow
      M25.329 Other instability, unspecified elbow
✓6ᵗʰ M25.33 Other instability, wrist

      M25.331 Other instability, right wrist
      M25.332 Other instability, left wrist
      M25.339 Other instability, unspecified wrist
✓6ᵗʰ M25.34 Other instability, hand

      M25.341 Other instability, right hand
      M25.342 Other instability, left hand
      M25.349 Other instability, unspecified hand
✓6ᵗʰ M25.35 Other instability, hip

      M25.351 Other instability, right hip
      M25.352 Other instability, left hip
      M25.359 Other instability, unspecified hip
✓6ᵗʰ M25.36 Other instability, knee

      M25.361 Other instability, right knee
      M25.362 Other instability, left knee
      M25.369 Other instability, unspecified knee
✓6ᵗʰ M25.37 Other instability, ankle and foot

      M25.371 Other instability, right ankle
      M25.372 Other instability, left ankle
      M25.373 Other instability, unspecified ankle
      M25.374 Other instability, right foot
      M25.375 Other instability, left foot
      M25.376 Other instability, unspecified foot
   M25.39 Other instability, other specified joint

✓5ᵗʰ M25.4 **Effusion of joint**
     EXCLUDES 1 *hydrarthrosis in yaws (A66.6)*
           intermittent hydrarthrosis (M12.4-)
           other infective (teno)synovitis (M65.1-)
   M25.40 Effusion, unspecified joint
✓6ᵗʰ M25.41 Effusion, shoulder

      M25.411 Effusion, right shoulder
      M25.412 Effusion, left shoulder
      M25.419 Effusion, unspecified shoulder
✓6ᵗʰ M25.42 Effusion, elbow

      M25.421 Effusion, right elbow
      M25.422 Effusion, left elbow
      M25.429 Effusion, unspecified elbow
✓6ᵗʰ M25.43 Effusion, wrist

      M25.431 Effusion, right wrist
      M25.432 Effusion, left wrist
      M25.439 Effusion, unspecified wrist
✓6ᵗʰ M25.44 Effusion, hand

      M25.441 Effusion, right hand
      M25.442 Effusion, left hand
      M25.449 Effusion, unspecified hand
✓6ᵗʰ M25.45 Effusion, hip

      M25.451 Effusion, right hip
      M25.452 Effusion, left hip
      M25.459 Effusion, unspecified hip
✓6ᵗʰ M25.46 Effusion, knee

      M25.461 Effusion, right knee
      M25.462 Effusion, left knee
      M25.469 Effusion, unspecified knee
✓6ᵗʰ M25.47 Effusion, ankle and foot

      M25.471 Effusion, right ankle
      M25.472 Effusion, left ankle
      M25.473 Effusion, unspecified ankle
      M25.474 Effusion, right foot
      M25.475 Effusion, left foot
      M25.476 Effusion, unspecified foot

M25.48   **Effusion, other site**

✓5ᵗʰ M25.5 **Pain in joint**

　　EXCLUDES 2　*pain in hand (M79.64-)*
　　　　　　　pain in fingers (M79.64-)
　　　　　　　pain in foot (M79.67-)
　　　　　　　pain in limb (M79.6-)
　　　　　　　pain in toes (M79.67-)

M25.50   **Pain in unspecified joint**

✓6ᵗʰ M25.51 **Pain in shoulder**

M25.511   **Pain in right shoulder**
M25.512   **Pain in left shoulder**
M25.519   **Pain in unspecified shoulder**

✓6ᵗʰ M25.52 **Pain in elbow**

M25.521   **Pain in right elbow**
M25.522   **Pain in left elbow**
M25.529   **Pain in unspecified elbow**

✓6ᵗʰ M25.53 **Pain in wrist**

M25.531   **Pain in right wrist**
M25.532   **Pain in left wrist**
M25.539   **Pain in unspecified wrist**

✓6ᵗʰ M25.54 **Pain in joints of hand**

AHA: 2016,4Q,38

M25.541   **Pain in joints of right hand**
M25.542   **Pain in joints of left hand**
M25.549   **Pain in joints of unspecified hand**
　　　　　　Pain in joints of hand NOS

✓6ᵗʰ M25.55 **Pain in hip**

M25.551   **Pain in right hip**
M25.552   **Pain in left hip**
M25.559   **Pain in unspecified hip**

✓6ᵗʰ M25.56 **Pain in knee**

M25.561   **Pain in right knee**
M25.562   **Pain in left knee**
M25.569   **Pain in unspecified knee**

✓6ᵗʰ M25.57 **Pain in ankle and joints of foot**

M25.571   **Pain in right ankle and joints of right foot**
M25.572   **Pain in left ankle and joints of left foot**
M25.579   **Pain in unspecified ankle and joints of unspecified foot**

M25.59   **Pain in other specified joint**

✓5ᵗʰ M25.6 **Stiffness of joint, not elsewhere classified**

　　EXCLUDES 1　*ankylosis of joint (M24.6-)*
　　　　　　　contracture of joint (M24.5-)

M25.60   **Stiffness of unspecified joint, not elsewhere classified**

✓6ᵗʰ M25.61 **Stiffness of shoulder, not elsewhere classified**

M25.611   **Stiffness of right shoulder, not elsewhere classified**
M25.612   **Stiffness of left shoulder, not elsewhere classified**
M25.619   **Stiffness of unspecified shoulder, not elsewhere classified**

✓6ᵗʰ M25.62 **Stiffness of elbow, not elsewhere classified**

M25.621   **Stiffness of right elbow, not elsewhere classified**
M25.622   **Stiffness of left elbow, not elsewhere classified**
M25.629   **Stiffness of unspecified elbow, not elsewhere classified**

✓6ᵗʰ M25.63 **Stiffness of wrist, not elsewhere classified**

M25.631   **Stiffness of right wrist, not elsewhere classified**
M25.632   **Stiffness of left wrist, not elsewhere classified**
M25.639   **Stiffness of unspecified wrist, not elsewhere classified**

✓6ᵗʰ M25.64 **Stiffness of hand, not elsewhere classified**

M25.641   **Stiffness of right hand, not elsewhere classified**
M25.642   **Stiffness of left hand, not elsewhere classified**
M25.649   **Stiffness of unspecified hand, not elsewhere classified**

✓6ᵗʰ M25.65 **Stiffness of hip, not elsewhere classified**

M25.651   **Stiffness of right hip, not elsewhere classified**

M25.652   **Stiffness of left hip, not elsewhere classified**
M25.659   **Stiffness of unspecified hip, not elsewhere classified**

✓6ᵗʰ M25.66 **Stiffness of knee, not elsewhere classified**

M25.661   **Stiffness of right knee, not elsewhere classified**
M25.662   **Stiffness of left knee, not elsewhere classified**
M25.669   **Stiffness of unspecified knee, not elsewhere classified**

✓6ᵗʰ M25.67 **Stiffness of ankle and foot, not elsewhere classified**

M25.671   **Stiffness of right ankle, not elsewhere classified**
M25.672   **Stiffness of left ankle, not elsewhere classified**
M25.673   **Stiffness of unspecified ankle, not elsewhere classified**
M25.674   **Stiffness of right foot, not elsewhere classified**
M25.675   **Stiffness of left foot, not elsewhere classified**
M25.676   **Stiffness of unspecified foot, not elsewhere classified**

M25.69   **Stiffness of other specified joint, not elsewhere classified**

✓5ᵗʰ M25.7 **Osteophyte**

M25.70   **Osteophyte, unspecified joint**

✓6ᵗʰ M25.71 **Osteophyte, shoulder**

M25.711   **Osteophyte, right shoulder**
M25.712   **Osteophyte, left shoulder**
M25.719   **Osteophyte, unspecified shoulder**

✓6ᵗʰ M25.72 **Osteophyte, elbow**

M25.721   **Osteophyte, right elbow**
M25.722   **Osteophyte, left elbow**
M25.729   **Osteophyte, unspecified elbow**

✓6ᵗʰ M25.73 **Osteophyte, wrist**

M25.731   **Osteophyte, right wrist**
M25.732   **Osteophyte, left wrist**
M25.739   **Osteophyte, unspecified wrist**

✓6ᵗʰ M25.74 **Osteophyte, hand**

M25.741   **Osteophyte, right hand**
M25.742   **Osteophyte, left hand**
M25.749   **Osteophyte, unspecified hand**

✓6ᵗʰ M25.75 **Osteophyte, hip**

M25.751   **Osteophyte, right hip**
M25.752   **Osteophyte, left hip**
M25.759   **Osteophyte, unspecified hip**

✓6ᵗʰ M25.76 **Osteophyte, knee**

M25.761   **Osteophyte, right knee**
M25.762   **Osteophyte, left knee**
M25.769   **Osteophyte, unspecified knee**

✓6ᵗʰ M25.77 **Osteophyte, ankle and foot**

M25.771   **Osteophyte, right ankle**
M25.772   **Osteophyte, left ankle**
M25.773   **Osteophyte, unspecified ankle**
M25.774   **Osteophyte, right foot**
M25.775   **Osteophyte, left foot**
M25.776   **Osteophyte, unspecified foot**

M25.78   **Osteophyte, vertebrae**

✓5ᵗʰ M25.8 **Other specified joint disorders**

M25.80   **Other specified joint disorders, unspecified joint**

✓6ᵗʰ M25.81 **Other specified joint disorders, shoulder**

M25.811   **Other specified joint disorders, right shoulder**
M25.812   **Other specified joint disorders, left shoulder**
M25.819   **Other specified joint disorders, unspecified shoulder**

✓6ᵗʰ M25.82 **Other specified joint disorders, elbow**

M25.821   **Other specified joint disorders, right elbow**
M25.822   **Other specified joint disorders, left elbow**
M25.829   **Other specified joint disorders, unspecified elbow**

✓6ᵗʰ M25.83 **Other specified joint disorders, wrist**

M25.831   **Other specified joint disorders, right wrist**

M25.832   Other specified joint disorders, left wrist
M25.839   Other specified joint disorders, unspecified wrist

√6ᵗʰ   M25.84   Other specified joint disorders, hand

M25.841   Other specified joint disorders, right hand
M25.842   Other specified joint disorders, left hand
M25.849   Other specified joint disorders, unspecified hand

√6ᵗʰ   M25.85   Other specified joint disorders, hip
     AHA: 2014,4Q,25

M25.851   Other specified joint disorders, right hip
M25.852   Other specified joint disorders, left hip
M25.859   Other specified joint disorders, unspecified hip

√6ᵗʰ   M25.86   Other specified joint disorders, knee

M25.861   Other specified joint disorders, right knee
M25.862   Other specified joint disorders, left knee
M25.869   Other specified joint disorders, unspecified knee

√6ᵗʰ   M25.87   Other specified joint disorders, ankle and foot

M25.871   Other specified joint disorders, right ankle and foot
M25.872   Other specified joint disorders, left ankle and foot
M25.879   Other specified joint disorders, unspecified ankle and foot

M25.9   Joint disorder, unspecified

Dentofacial anomalies [including malocclusion] and other disorders of jaw (M26-M27)

EXCLUDES 1   *hemifacial atrophy or hypertrophy (Q67.4)*
          unilateral condylar hyperplasia or hypoplasia (M27.8)

√4ᵗʰ   **M26   Dentofacial anomalies [including malocclusion]**

√5ᵗʰ   M26.0   Major anomalies of jaw size

     EXCLUDES 1   *acromegaly (E22.0)*
               Robin's syndrome (Q87.0)

M26.00   Unspecified anomaly of jaw size
M26.01   Maxillary hyperplasia
M26.02   Maxillary hypoplasia
     AHA: 2014,3Q,23
M26.03   Mandibular hyperplasia
M26.04   Mandibular hypoplasia
M26.05   Macrogenia
M26.06   Microgenia
M26.07   Excessive tuberosity of jaw
     Entire maxillary tuberosity
M26.09   Other specified anomalies of jaw size

√5ᵗʰ   M26.1   Anomalies of jaw-cranial base relationship

M26.10   Unspecified anomaly of jaw-cranial base relationship
M26.11   Maxillary asymmetry
M26.12   Other jaw asymmetry
M26.19   Other specified anomalies of jaw-cranial base relationship
     AHA: 2020,1Q,21

√5ᵗʰ   M26.2   Anomalies of dental arch relationship

M26.20   Unspecified anomaly of dental arch relationship
√6ᵗʰ   M26.21   Malocclusion, Angle's class

M26.211   Malocclusion, Angle's class I
     Neutro-occlusion
M26.212   Malocclusion, Angle's class II
     Disto-occlusion Division I
     Disto-occlusion Division II
M26.213   Malocclusion, Angle's class III
     Mesio-occlusion
M26.219   Malocclusion, Angle's class, unspecified

√6ᵗʰ   M26.22   Open occlusal relationship

M26.220   Open anterior occlusal relationship
     Anterior open bite
M26.221   Open posterior occlusal relationship
     Posterior open bite

M26.23   Excessive horizontal overlap
     Excessive horizontal overjet
M26.24   Reverse articulation
     Crossbite (anterior) (posterior)
M26.25   Anomalies of interarch distance

M26.29   Other anomalies of dental arch relationship
     Midline deviation of dental arch
     Overbite (excessive) deep
     Overbite (excessive) horizontal
     Overbite (excessive) vertical
     Posterior lingual occlusion of mandibular teeth

√5ᵗʰ   M26.3   Anomalies of tooth position of fully erupted tooth or teeth

     EXCLUDES 2   *embedded and impacted teeth (K01.-)*

M26.30   Unspecified anomaly of tooth position of fully erupted tooth or teeth
     Abnormal spacing of fully erupted tooth or teeth NOS
     Displacement of fully erupted tooth or teeth NOS
     Transposition of fully erupted tooth or teeth NOS

M26.31   Crowding of fully erupted teeth
M26.32   Excessive spacing of fully erupted teeth
     Diastema of fully erupted tooth or teeth NOS
M26.33   Horizontal displacement of fully erupted tooth or teeth
     Tipped tooth or teeth
     Tipping of fully erupted tooth
M26.34   Vertical displacement of fully erupted tooth or teeth
     Extruded tooth
     Infraeruption of tooth or teeth
     Supraeruption of tooth or teeth
M26.35   Rotation of fully erupted tooth or teeth
M26.36   Insufficient interocclusal distance of fully erupted teeth (ridge)
     Lack of adequate intermaxillary vertical dimension of fully erupted teeth
M26.37   Excessive interocclusal distance of fully erupted teeth
     Excessive intermaxillary vertical dimension of fully erupted teeth
     Loss of occlusal vertical dimension of fully erupted teeth
M26.39   Other anomalies of tooth position of fully erupted tooth or teeth

M26.4   Malocclusion, unspecified

√5ᵗʰ   M26.5   Dentofacial functional abnormalities

     EXCLUDES 1   *bruxism (F45.8)*
               teeth-grinding NOS (F45.8)

M26.50   Dentofacial functional abnormalities, unspecified
M26.51   Abnormal jaw closure
M26.52   Limited mandibular range of motion
M26.53   Deviation in opening and closing of the mandible
M26.54   Insufficient anterior guidance
     Insufficient anterior occlusal guidance
M26.55   Centric occlusion maximum intercuspation discrepancy
     EXCLUDES 1   *centric occlusion NOS (M26.59)*
M26.56   Non-working side interference
     Balancing side interference
M26.57   Lack of posterior occlusal support
M26.59   Other dentofacial functional abnormalities
     Centric occlusion (of teeth) NOS
     Malocclusion due to abnormal swallowing
     Malocclusion due to mouth breathing
     Malocclusion due to tongue, lip or finger habits

[handwritten notes:]
A. initial encounter
D. subsequent encounter for fracture with routine healing.
G: delayed healing
K: healing with no union
P: healing with mal union

✓ Additional Character Required   √x7ᵗʰ Placeholder Alert   Manifestation   Unspecified Dx   Q QPP   UPD Unacceptable PDx

√5ᵗʰ **M26.6 Temporomandibular joint disorders**

     EXCLUDES 2   *current temporomandibular joint dislocation (S03.0)*
                   current temporomandibular joint sprain (S03.4)

     AHA: 2016,4Q,38-39

Temporomandibular Joint

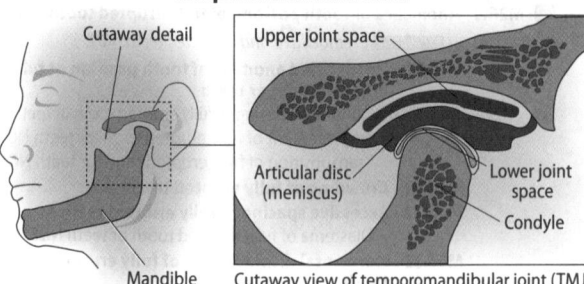

Cutaway detail

Upper joint space

Articular disc (meniscus)

Lower joint space

Condyle

Mandible   Cutaway view of temporomandibular joint (TMJ)

√6ᵗʰ **M26.60 Temporomandibular joint disorder, unspecified**

     M26.601 Right temporomandibular joint disorder, unspecified

     M26.602 Left temporomandibular joint disorder, unspecified

     M26.603 Bilateral temporomandibular joint disorder, unspecified

     M26.609 Unspecified temporomandibular joint disorder, unspecified side

         Temporomandibular joint disorder NOS

√6ᵗʰ **M26.61 Adhesions and ankylosis of temporomandibular joint**

     M26.611 Adhesions and ankylosis of right temporomandibular joint

     M26.612 Adhesions and ankylosis of left temporomandibular joint

     M26.613 Adhesions and ankylosis of bilateral temporomandibular joint

     M26.619 Adhesions and ankylosis of temporomandibular joint, unspecified side

√6ᵗʰ **M26.62 Arthralgia of temporomandibular joint**

     M26.621 Arthralgia of right temporomandibular joint

     M26.622 Arthralgia of left temporomandibular joint

     M26.623 Arthralgia of bilateral temporomandibular joint

     M26.629 Arthralgia of temporomandibular joint, unspecified side

√6ᵗʰ **M26.63 Articular disc disorder of temporomandibular joint**

     M26.631 Articular disc disorder of right temporomandibular joint

     M26.632 Articular disc disorder of left temporomandibular joint

     M26.633 Articular disc disorder of bilateral temporomandibular joint

     M26.639 Articular disc disorder of temporomandibular joint, unspecified side

√6ᵗʰ **M26.64 Arthritis of temporomandibular joint**

     AHA: 2020,4Q,32

     M26.641 Arthritis of right temporomandibular joint

     M26.642 Arthritis of left temporomandibular joint

     M26.643 Arthritis of bilateral temporomandibular joint

     M26.649 Arthritis of unspecified temporomandibular joint

√6ᵗʰ **M26.65 Arthropathy of temporomandibular joint**

     AHA: 2020,4Q,32

     M26.651 Arthropathy of right temporomandibular joint

     M26.652 Arthropathy of left temporomandibular joint

     M26.653 Arthropathy of bilateral temporomandibular joint

     M26.659 Arthropathy of unspecified temporomandibular joint

     M26.69 Other specified disorders of temporomandibular joint

√5ᵗʰ **M26.7 Dental alveolar anomalies**

     M26.70 Unspecified alveolar anomaly

     M26.71 Alveolar maxillary hyperplasia

     M26.72 Alveolar mandibular hyperplasia

     M26.73 Alveolar maxillary hypoplasia

     M26.74 Alveolar mandibular hypoplasia

     M26.79 Other specified alveolar anomalies

√5ᵗʰ **M26.8 Other dentofacial anomalies**

     M26.81 Anterior soft tissue impingement

         Anterior soft tissue impingement on teeth

     M26.82 Posterior soft tissue impingement

         Posterior soft tissue impingement on teeth

     M26.89 Other dentofacial anomalies

M26.9 Dentofacial anomaly, unspecified

√4ᵗʰ **M27 Other diseases of jaws**

     M27.0 Developmental disorders of jaws

         Latent bone cyst of jaw

         Stafne's cyst

         Torus mandibularis

         Torus palatinus

     M27.1 Giant cell granuloma, central

         Giant cell granuloma NOS

         EXCLUDES 1   *peripheral giant cell granuloma (K06.8)*

     M27.2 Inflammatory conditions of jaws

         Osteitis of jaw(s)

         Osteomyelitis (neonatal) jaw(s)

         Osteoradionecrosis jaw(s)

         Periostitis jaw(s)

         Sequestrum of jaw bone

         Use additional code (W88-W90, X39.0) to identify radiation, if radiation-induced

         EXCLUDES 2   *osteonecrosis of jaw due to drug (M87.180)*

     M27.3 Alveolitis of jaws

         Alveolar osteitis

         Dry socket

√5ᵗʰ **M27.4 Other and unspecified cysts of jaw**

         EXCLUDES 1   *cysts of oral region (K09.-)*
                  latent bone cyst of jaw (M27.0)
                  Stafne's cyst (M27.0)

     M27.40 Unspecified cyst of jaw

         Cyst of jaw NOS

     M27.49 Other cysts of jaw

         Aneurysmal cyst of jaw

         Hemorrhagic cyst of jaw

         Traumatic cyst of jaw

√5ᵗʰ **M27.5 Periradicular pathology associated with previous endodontic treatment**

     M27.51 Perforation of root canal space due to endodontic treatment

     M27.52 Endodontic overfill

     M27.53 Endodontic underfill

     M27.59 Other periradicular pathology associated with previous endodontic treatment

√5ᵗʰ **M27.6 Endosseous dental implant failure**

     M27.61 Osseointegration failure of dental implant

         Hemorrhagic complications of dental implant placement

         Iatrogenic osseointegration failure of dental implant

         Osseointegration failure of dental implant due to complications of systemic disease

         Osseointegration failure of dental implant due to poor bone quality

         Pre-integration failure of dental implant NOS

         Pre-osseointegration failure of dental implant

HCC CMS-HCC   **Rx** Rx HCC   **ESR** ESRD HCC   **COM** Commercial HCC   **N** Newborn: 0   **P** Pediatric: 0-17   **M** Maternity: 9-64   **A** Adult: 15-124

812   ICD-10-CM 2023

M27.62 **Post-osseointegration biological failure of dental implant**
Failure of dental implant due to lack of attached gingiva
Failure of dental implant due to occlusal trauma (caused by poor prosthetic design)
Failure of dental implant due to parafunctional habits
Failure of dental implant due to periodontal infection (peri-implantitis)
Failure of dental implant due to poor oral hygiene
Iatrogenic post-osseointegration failure of dental implant
Post-osseointegration failure of dental implant due to complications of systemic disease

M27.63 **Post-osseointegration mechanical failure of dental implant**
Failure of dental prosthesis causing loss of dental implant
Fracture of dental implant
> EXCLUDES 2   *cracked tooth (KØ3.81)*
> *fractured dental restorative material with loss of material (KØ8.531)*
> *fractured dental restorative material without loss of material (KØ8.53Ø)*
> *fractured tooth (SØ2.5)*

M27.69 **Other endosseous dental implant failure**
Dental implant failure NOS

M27.8 **Other specified diseases of jaws**
Cherubism
Exostosis
Fibrous dysplasia
Unilateral condylar hyperplasia
Unilateral condylar hypoplasia
> EXCLUDES 1   *jaw pain (R68.84)*

M27.9 **Disease of jaws, unspecified**

Systemic connective tissue disorders (M3Ø-M36)

> INCLUDES   autoimmune disease NOS
> collagen (vascular) disease NOS
> systemic autoimmune disease
> systemic collagen (vascular) disease
> EXCLUDES 1   *autoimmune disease, single organ or single cell-type-code to relevant condition category*

☑4ᵗʰ **M3Ø Polyarteritis nodosa and related conditions**
> EXCLUDES 1   *microscopic polyarteritis (M31.7)*

M3Ø.Ø **Polyarteritis nodosa** `HCC` `Rx` `ESR` `COM`

M3Ø.1 **Polyarteritis with lung involvement [Churg-Strauss]** `HCC` `Rx` `ESR` `COM`
Allergic granulomatous angiitis
Eosinophilic granulomatosis with polyangiitis [EGPA]
AHA: 2021,1Q,23

M3Ø.2 **Juvenile polyarteritis** `HCC` `Rx` `ESR` `COM`

M3Ø.3 **Mucocutaneous lymph node syndrome [Kawasaki]** `HCC` `Rx` `ESR` `COM`

M3Ø.8 **Other conditions related to polyarteritis nodosa** `HCC` `Rx` `ESR` `COM`
Polyangiitis overlap syndrome

☑4ᵗʰ **M31 Other necrotizing vasculopathies**

M31.Ø **Hypersensitivity angiitis** `HCC` `Rx` `ESR` `COM`
Goodpasture's syndrome

☑6ᵗʰ M31.1 **Thrombotic microangiopathy**
AHA: 2021,4Q,19
M31.1Ø **Thrombotic microangiopathy, unspecified** `HCC` `Rx` `ESR` `COM`

M31.11 **Hematopoietic stem cell transplantation-associated thrombotic microangiopathy [HSCT-TMA]** `HCC` `Rx` `ESR` `COM`
Transplant-associated thrombotic microangiopathy [TA-TMA]
Code first if applicable:
complications of bone marrow transplant (T86.Ø-)
complications of stem cell transplant (T86.5)
Use additional code to identify specific organ dysfunction, such as:
acute kidney failure (N17.-)
acute respiratory distress syndrome (J8Ø)
capillary leak syndrome (I78.8)
diffuse alveolar hemorrhage (RØ4.89)
encephalopathy (metabolic) (septic) (G93.41)
fluid overload, unspecified (E87.7Ø)
graft versus host disease (D89.81-)
hemolytic uremic syndrome ▶(D59.3-)◀
hepatic failure (K72.-)
hepatic veno-occlusive disease (K76.5)
idiopathic interstitial pneumonia (J84.11-)
sinusoidal obstruction syndrome (K76.5)

M31.19 **Other thrombotic microangiopathy** `HCC` `Rx` `ESR` `COM`
Thrombotic thrombocytopenic purpura

M31.2 **Lethal midline granuloma** `HCC` `Rx` `ESR` `COM`

☑5ᵗʰ M31.3 **Wegener's granulomatosis**
Granulomatosis with polyangiitis
Necrotizing respiratory granulomatosis
AHA: 2021,1Q,23

M31.3Ø **Wegener's granulomatosis without renal involvement** `HCC` `Rx` `ESR` `COM`
Wegener's granulomatosis NOS
AHA: 2021,2Q,10

M31.31 **Wegener's granulomatosis with renal involvement** `HCC` `Rx` `ESR` `COM`

M31.4 **Aortic arch syndrome [Takayasu]** `HCC` `Rx` `ESR` `COM`

M31.5 **Giant cell arteritis with polymyalgia rheumatica** `HCC` `Rx` `ESR` `COM`

M31.6 **Other giant cell arteritis** `HCC` `Rx` `ESR` `COM`

M31.7 **Microscopic polyangiitis** `HCC` `Rx` `ESR` `COM`
Microscopic polyarteritis
> EXCLUDES 1   *polyarteritis nodosa (M3Ø.Ø)*
AHA: 2021,1Q,23

M31.8 **Other specified necrotizing vasculopathies** `HCC` `ESR`
Hypocomplementemic vasculitis
Septic vasculitis

M31.9 **Necrotizing vasculopathy, unspecified** `HCC` `ESR`

☑4ᵗʰ **M32 Systemic lupus erythematosus (SLE)**
> EXCLUDES 1   *lupus erythematosus (discoid) (NOS) (L93.Ø)*
AHA: 2020,4Q,11; 2018,3Q,14
TIP: There is no default code for "lupus NOS." Query the provider for the specific type of lupus in order to assign the appropriate code.

M32.Ø **Drug-induced systemic lupus erythematosus** `HCC` `Rx` `ESR` `COM`
Use additional code for adverse effect, if applicable, to identify drug (T36-T5Ø with fifth or sixth character 5)

☑5ᵗʰ M32.1 **Systemic lupus erythematosus with organ or system involvement**

M32.1Ø **Systemic lupus erythematosus, organ or system involvement unspecified** `HCC` `Rx` `ESR` `COM`

M32.11 **Endocarditis in systemic lupus erythematosus** `HCC` `Rx` `ESR` `COM`
Libman-Sacks disease

M32.12 **Pericarditis in systemic lupus erythematosus** `HCC` `Rx` `ESR` `COM`
Lupus pericarditis

M32.13 **Lung involvement in systemic lupus erythematosus** `HCC` `Rx` `ESR` `COM`
Pleural effusion due to systemic lupus erythematosus

M32.14 **Glomerular disease in systemic lupus erythematosus** `HCC` `Rx` `ESR` `COM`
Lupus renal disease NOS
AHA: 2013,4Q,125

M32.15 **Tubulo-interstitial nephropathy in systemic lupus erythematosus** `HCC` `Rx` `ESR` `COM`

Chapter 13. Diseases of the Musculoskeletal System and Connective Tissue

M32.19   **Other organ or system involvement in systemic lupus erythematosus** `HCC` `Rx` `ESR` `COM`

M32.8   Other forms of systemic lupus erythematosus `HCC` `Rx` `ESR` `COM`

M32.9   Systemic lupus erythematosus, unspecified `HCC` `Rx` `ESR` `COM`
SLE NOS
Systemic lupus erythematosus NOS
Systemic lupus erythematosus without organ involvement

✓4ᵗʰ **M33   Dermatopolymyositis**
AHA: 2017,4Q,18

✓5ᵗʰ **M33.0   Juvenile dermatomyositis**

M33.00   Juvenile dermatomyositis, organ involvement unspecified `HCC` `Rx` `ESR` `COM`

M33.01   Juvenile dermatomyositis with respiratory involvement `HCC` `Rx` `ESR` `COM`

M33.02   Juvenile dermatomyositis with myopathy `HCC` `Rx` `ESR` `COM`

M33.03   Juvenile dermatomyositis without myopathy `HCC` `Rx` `ESR` `COM`

M33.09   Juvenile dermatomyositis with other organ involvement `HCC` `Rx` `ESR` `COM`

✓5ᵗʰ **M33.1   Other dermatomyositis**
Adult dermatomyositis

M33.10   Other dermatomyositis, organ involvement unspecified `HCC` `Rx` `ESR` `COM`

M33.11   Other dermatomyositis with respiratory involvement `HCC` `Rx` `ESR` `COM`

M33.12   Other dermatomyositis with myopathy `HCC` `Rx` `ESR` `COM`

M33.13   Other dermatomyositis without myopathy `HCC` `Rx` `ESR` `COM`
Dermatomyositis NOS

M33.19   Other dermatomyositis with other organ involvement `HCC` `Rx` `ESR` `COM`

✓5ᵗʰ **M33.2   Polymyositis**

M33.20   Polymyositis, organ involvement unspecified `HCC` `Rx` `ESR` `COM`

M33.21   Polymyositis with respiratory involvement `HCC` `Rx` `ESR` `COM`

M33.22   Polymyositis with myopathy `HCC` `Rx` `ESR` `COM`

M33.29   Polymyositis with other organ involvement `HCC` `Rx` `ESR` `COM`

✓5ᵗʰ **M33.9   Dermatopolymyositis, unspecified**

M33.90   Dermatopolymyositis, unspecified, organ involvement unspecified `HCC` `Rx` `ESR` `COM`

M33.91   Dermatopolymyositis, unspecified with respiratory involvement `HCC` `Rx` `ESR` `COM`

M33.92   Dermatopolymyositis, unspecified with myopathy `HCC` `Rx` `ESR` `COM`

M33.93   Dermatopolymyositis, unspecified without myopathy `HCC` `Rx` `ESR` `COM`

M33.99   Dermatopolymyositis, unspecified with other organ involvement `HCC` `Rx` `ESR` `COM`

✓4ᵗʰ **M34   Systemic sclerosis [scleroderma]**
EXCLUDES 1   *circumscribed scleroderma (L94.0)*
neonatal scleroderma (P83.88)

M34.0   Progressive systemic sclerosis `HCC` `Rx` `ESR` `COM`

M34.1   CR(E)ST syndrome `HCC` `Rx` `ESR` `COM`
Combination of calcinosis, Raynaud's phenomenon, esophageal dysfunction, sclerodactyly, telangiectasia

M34.2   Systemic sclerosis induced by drug and chemical `HCC` `Rx` `ESR` `COM`
Code first poisoning due to drug or toxin, if applicable (T36-T65 with fifth or sixth character 1-4 or 6)
Use additional code for adverse effect, if applicable, to identify drug (T36-T50 with fifth or sixth character 5)

✓5ᵗʰ **M34.8   Other forms of systemic sclerosis**

M34.81   Systemic sclerosis with lung involvement `HCC` `Rx` `ESR` `COM`
Code also if applicable:
other interstitial pulmonary diseases (J84.89)
secondary pulmonary arterial hypertension (I27.21)

M34.82   Systemic sclerosis with myopathy `HCC` `Rx` `ESR` `COM`

M34.83   Systemic sclerosis with polyneuropathy `HCC` `Rx` `ESR` `COM`

M34.89   Other systemic sclerosis `HCC` `Rx` `ESR` `COM`

M34.9   Systemic sclerosis, unspecified `HCC` `Rx` `ESR` `COM`

✓4ᵗʰ **M35   Other systemic involvement of connective tissue**
EXCLUDES 1   *reactive perforating collagenosis (L87.1)*

✓5ᵗʰ **M35.0   Sjögren syndrome**
Sicca syndrome
Use additional code to identify associated manifestations
EXCLUDES 1   *dry mouth, unspecified (R68.2)*
AHA: 2021,4Q,20
DEF: Autoimmune disease associated with keratoconjunctivitis, laryngopharyngitis, rhinitis, dry mouth, enlarged parotid gland, and chronic polyarthritis.

M35.00   Sjögren syndrome, unspecified `HCC` `Rx` `ESR` `COM`

M35.01   Sjögren syndrome with keratoconjunctivitis `HCC` `Rx` `ESR` `COM`

M35.02   Sjögren syndrome with lung involvement `HCC` `Rx` `ESR` `COM`

M35.03   Sjögren syndrome with myopathy `HCC` `Rx` `ESR` `COM`

M35.04   Sjögren syndrome with tubulo-interstitial nephropathy `HCC` `Rx` `ESR` `COM`
Renal tubular acidosis in sicca syndrome

M35.05   Sjögren syndrome with inflammatory arthritis `HCC` `Rx` `ESR` `COM`

M35.06   Sjögren syndrome with peripheral nervous system involvement `HCC` `Rx` `ESR` `COM`

M35.07   Sjögren syndrome with central nervous system involvement `HCC` `Rx` `ESR` `COM`

M35.08   Sjögren syndrome with gastrointestinal involvement `HCC` `Rx` `ESR` `COM`

M35.0A   Sjögren syndrome with glomerular disease `HCC` `Rx` `ESR` `COM`

M35.0B   Sjögren syndrome with vasculitis `HCC` `Rx` `ESR` `COM`

M35.0C   Sjögren syndrome with dental involvement `HCC` `Rx` `ESR` `COM`

M35.09   Sjögren syndrome with other organ involvement `HCC` `Rx` `ESR` `COM`

M35.1   Other overlap syndromes `HCC` `Rx` `ESR` `COM`
Mixed connective tissue disease
EXCLUDES 1   *polyangiitis overlap syndrome (M30.8)*

M35.2   Behçet's disease `HCC` `Rx` `ESR` `COM`

M35.3   Polymyalgia rheumatica `HCC` `ESR` `COM`
EXCLUDES 1   *polymyalgia rheumatica with giant cell arteritis (M31.5)*

M35.4   Diffuse (eosinophilic) fasciitis

M35.5   Multifocal fibrosclerosis `HCC` `Rx` `ESR` `COM`

M35.6   Relapsing panniculitis [Weber-Christian]
EXCLUDES 1   *lupus panniculitis (L93.2)*
panniculitis NOS (M79.3-)

M35.7   Hypermobility syndrome
Familial ligamentous laxity
EXCLUDES 1   *ligamentous laxity, NOS (M24.2-)*
EXCLUDES 2   *Ehlers-Danlos syndromes (Q79.6-)*

`HCC` CMS-HCC   `Rx` Rx HCC   `ESR` ESRD HCC   `COM` Commercial HCC   `N` Newborn: 0   `P` Pediatric: 0-17   `M` Maternity: 9-64   `A` Adult: 15-124

814   ICD-10-CM 2023

✓5ᵗʰ **M35.8 Other specified systemic involvement of connective tissue**
AHA: 2021,1Q,36; 2020,3Q,13-14

M35.81 Multisystem inflammatory syndrome `HCC` `ESR` `COM`
MIS-A
MIS-C
Multisystem inflammatory syndrome in adults
Multisystem inflammatory syndrome in children
Pediatric inflammatory multisystem syndrome
PIMS
Code first, if applicable, COVID-19 (U07.1)
Code also any associated complications such as:
  acute hepatic failure (K72.0-)
  acute kidney failure (N17.-)
  acute myocarditis (I40.-)
  acute respiratory distress syndrome (J80)
  cardiac arrhythmia (I47-I49.-)
  pneumonia due to COVID-19 (J12.82)
  severe sepsis (R65.2-)
  viral cardiomyopathy (B33.24)
  viral pericarditis (B33.23)
Use additional code, if applicable, for:
  exposure to COVID-19 or SARS-CoV-2 infection (Z20.822)
  personal history of COVID-19 (Z86.16)
  post COVID-19 condition (U09.9)
AHA: 2021,4Q,102; 2021,1Q,29,36,41
DEF: Hyperinflammatory condition that seems to be largely associated with past or present coronavirus disease 2019 (COVID-19) infection. Predominantly occurring in children, with less frequent occurrences in adults, symptoms often include fever, laboratory evidence of inflammation, and evidence of clinically severe illness requiring hospitalization with multisystem (two or more) organ involvement. *Synonym(s): MIS, MIS-C.*

M35.89 Other specified systemic involvement of connective tissue `HCC` `Rx` `ESR` `COM`

M35.9 Systemic involvement of connective tissue, unspecified `HCC` `Rx` `ESR` `COM`
Autoimmune disease (systemic) NOS
Collagen (vascular) disease NOS

✓4ᵗʰ **M36 Systemic disorders of connective tissue in diseases classified elsewhere**
EXCLUDES 2 *arthropathies in diseases classified elsewhere (M14.-)*

M36.0 Dermato(poly)myositis in neoplastic disease `HCC` `Rx` `ESR` `COM`
Code first underlying neoplasm (C00-D49)

M36.1 Arthropathy in neoplastic disease
Code first underlying neoplasm, such as:
  leukemia (C91-C95)
  malignant histiocytosis (C96.A)
  multiple myeloma (C90.0)

M36.2 Hemophilic arthropathy
Hemarthrosis in hemophilic arthropathy
Code first underlying disease, such as:
  factor VIII deficiency (D66)
    with vascular defect ▶(D68.0-)◀
  factor IX deficiency (D67)
  hemophilia (classical) (D66)
  hemophilia B (D67)
  hemophilia C (D68.1)

M36.3 Arthropathy in other blood disorders

M36.4 Arthropathy in hypersensitivity reactions classified elsewhere
Code first underlying disease, such as:
  Henoch (-Schönlein) purpura (D69.0)
  serum sickness (T80.6-)

M36.8 Systemic disorders of connective tissue in other diseases classified elsewhere `HCC` `Rx` `ESR` `COM`
Code first underlying disease, such as:
  alkaptonuria (E70.2)
  hypogammaglobulinemia (D80.-)
  ochronosis (E70.2)

DORSOPATHIES (M40-M54)

Deforming dorsopathies (M40-M43)

✓4ᵗʰ **M40 Kyphosis and lordosis**
Code first underlying disease
EXCLUDES 1 *congenital kyphosis and lordosis (Q76.4)*
  kyphoscoliosis (M41.-)
  postprocedural kyphosis and lordosis (M96.-)

Kyphosis and Lordosis

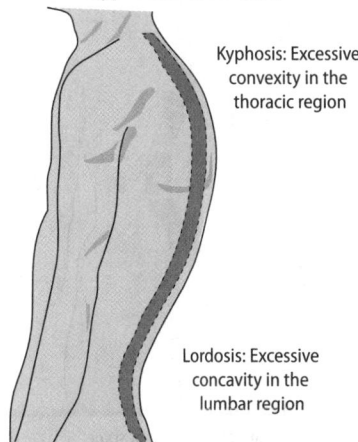

Kyphosis: Excessive convexity in the thoracic region

Lordosis: Excessive concavity in the lumbar region

✓5ᵗʰ **M40.0 Postural kyphosis**
EXCLUDES 1 *osteochondrosis of spine (M42.-)*
M40.00 Postural kyphosis, site unspecified
M40.03 Postural kyphosis, cervicothoracic region
M40.04 Postural kyphosis, thoracic region
M40.05 Postural kyphosis, thoracolumbar region

✓5ᵗʰ **M40.1 Other secondary kyphosis**
M40.10 Other secondary kyphosis, site unspecified `UPD`
M40.12 Other secondary kyphosis, cervical region `UPD`
M40.13 Other secondary kyphosis, cervicothoracic region `UPD`
M40.14 Other secondary kyphosis, thoracic region `UPD`
M40.15 Other secondary kyphosis, thoracolumbar region `UPD`

✓5ᵗʰ **M40.2 Other and unspecified kyphosis**
✓6ᵗʰ **M40.20 Unspecified kyphosis**
M40.202 Unspecified kyphosis, cervical region
M40.203 Unspecified kyphosis, cervicothoracic region
M40.204 Unspecified kyphosis, thoracic region
M40.205 Unspecified kyphosis, thoracolumbar region
M40.209 Unspecified kyphosis, site unspecified
✓6ᵗʰ **M40.29 Other kyphosis**
M40.292 Other kyphosis, cervical region
M40.293 Other kyphosis, cervicothoracic region
M40.294 Other kyphosis, thoracic region
M40.295 Other kyphosis, thoracolumbar region
M40.299 Other kyphosis, site unspecified

✓5ᵗʰ **M40.3 Flatback syndrome**
M40.30 Flatback syndrome, site unspecified
M40.35 Flatback syndrome, thoracolumbar region
M40.36 Flatback syndrome, lumbar region
M40.37 Flatback syndrome, lumbosacral region

✓5ᵗʰ **M40.4 Postural lordosis**
Acquired lordosis
M40.40 Postural lordosis, site unspecified
M40.45 Postural lordosis, thoracolumbar region
M40.46 Postural lordosis, lumbar region
M40.47 Postural lordosis, lumbosacral region

✓5ᵗʰ **M40.5 Lordosis, unspecified**
M40.50 Lordosis, unspecified, site unspecified
M40.55 Lordosis, unspecified, thoracolumbar region
M40.56 Lordosis, unspecified, lumbar region
M40.57 Lordosis, unspecified, lumbosacral region

Chapter 13. Diseases of the Musculoskeletal System and Connective Tissue

✓4th **M41 Scoliosis**

     INCLUDES   kyphoscoliosis

     EXCLUDES 1   *congenital scoliosis due to bony malformation (Q76.3)*

                  congenital scoliosis NOS (Q67.5)

                  kyphoscoliotic heart disease (I27.1)

                  postural congenital scoliosis (Q67.5)

     EXCLUDES 2   *postprocedural scoliosis (M96.-)*

     AHA: 2022,1Q,30

Scoliosis

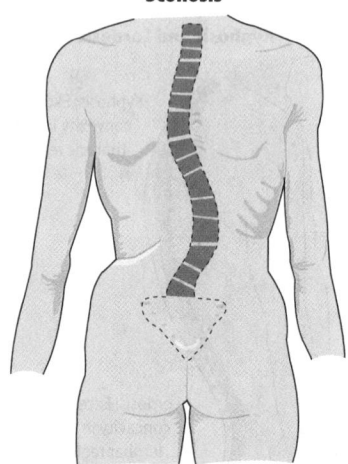

Lateral curvature of spine

✓5th **M41.0 Infantile idiopathic scoliosis**

     AHA: 2014,4Q,26

     M41.00 Infantile idiopathic scoliosis, site unspecified

     M41.02 Infantile idiopathic scoliosis, cervical region

     M41.03 Infantile idiopathic scoliosis, cervicothoracic region

     M41.04 Infantile idiopathic scoliosis, thoracic region

     M41.05 Infantile idiopathic scoliosis, thoracolumbar region

     M41.06 Infantile idiopathic scoliosis, lumbar region

     M41.07 Infantile idiopathic scoliosis, lumbosacral region

     M41.08 Infantile idiopathic scoliosis, sacral and sacrococcygeal region

✓5th **M41.1 Juvenile and adolescent idiopathic scoliosis**

     ✓6th **M41.11 Juvenile idiopathic scoliosis**

         AHA: 2014,4Q,28

         M41.112 Juvenile idiopathic scoliosis, cervical region

         M41.113 Juvenile idiopathic scoliosis, cervicothoracic region

         M41.114 Juvenile idiopathic scoliosis, thoracic region

         M41.115 Juvenile idiopathic scoliosis, thoracolumbar region

         M41.116 Juvenile idiopathic scoliosis, lumbar region

         M41.117 Juvenile idiopathic scoliosis, lumbosacral region

         M41.119 Juvenile idiopathic scoliosis, site unspecified

     ✓6th **M41.12 Adolescent scoliosis**

         M41.122 Adolescent idiopathic scoliosis, cervical region

         M41.123 Adolescent idiopathic scoliosis, cervicothoracic region

         M41.124 Adolescent idiopathic scoliosis, thoracic region

         M41.125 Adolescent idiopathic scoliosis, thoracolumbar region

         M41.126 Adolescent idiopathic scoliosis, lumbar region

         M41.127 Adolescent idiopathic scoliosis, lumbosacral region

         M41.129 Adolescent idiopathic scoliosis, site unspecified

✓5th **M41.2 Other idiopathic scoliosis**

     M41.20 Other idiopathic scoliosis, site unspecified

     M41.22 Other idiopathic scoliosis, cervical region

     M41.23 Other idiopathic scoliosis, cervicothoracic region

     M41.24 Other idiopathic scoliosis, thoracic region

     M41.25 Other idiopathic scoliosis, thoracolumbar region

     M41.26 Other idiopathic scoliosis, lumbar region

     M41.27 Other idiopathic scoliosis, lumbosacral region

✓5th **M41.3 Thoracogenic scoliosis**

     M41.30 Thoracogenic scoliosis, site unspecified

     M41.34 Thoracogenic scoliosis, thoracic region

     M41.35 Thoracogenic scoliosis, thoracolumbar region

✓5th **M41.4 Neuromuscular scoliosis**

     Scoliosis secondary to cerebral palsy, Friedreich's ataxia, poliomyelitis and other neuromuscular disorders

     Code also underlying condition

     AHA: 2014,4Q,27

     M41.40 Neuromuscular scoliosis, site unspecified

     M41.41 Neuromuscular scoliosis, occipito-atlanto-axial region

     M41.42 Neuromuscular scoliosis, cervical region

     M41.43 Neuromuscular scoliosis, cervicothoracic region

     M41.44 Neuromuscular scoliosis, thoracic region

     M41.45 Neuromuscular scoliosis, thoracolumbar region

     M41.46 Neuromuscular scoliosis, lumbar region

     M41.47 Neuromuscular scoliosis, lumbosacral region

✓5th **M41.5 Other secondary scoliosis**

     Code first underlying disease

     AHA: 2019,1Q,19

     M41.50 Other secondary scoliosis, site unspecified `UPD`

     M41.52 Other secondary scoliosis, cervical region `UPD`

     M41.53 Other secondary scoliosis, cervicothoracic region `UPD`

     M41.54 Other secondary scoliosis, thoracic region `UPD`

     M41.55 Other secondary scoliosis, thoracolumbar region `UPD`

     M41.56 Other secondary scoliosis, lumbar region `UPD`

     M41.57 Other secondary scoliosis, lumbosacral region `UPD`

✓5th **M41.8 Other forms of scoliosis**

     AHA: 2022,1Q,30

     M41.80 Other forms of scoliosis, site unspecified

     M41.82 Other forms of scoliosis, cervical region

     M41.83 Other forms of scoliosis, cervicothoracic region

     M41.84 Other forms of scoliosis, thoracic region

     M41.85 Other forms of scoliosis, thoracolumbar region

     M41.86 Other forms of scoliosis, lumbar region

     M41.87 Other forms of scoliosis, lumbosacral region

     M41.9 Scoliosis, unspecified

     AHA: 2022,1Q,30

✓4th **M42 Spinal osteochondrosis**

     ✓5th **M42.0 Juvenile osteochondrosis of spine**

         Calvé's disease

         Scheuermann's disease

         EXCLUDES 1   *postural kyphosis (M40.0)*

         M42.00 Juvenile osteochondrosis of spine, site unspecified `COM`

         M42.01 Juvenile osteochondrosis of spine, occipito-atlanto-axial region `COM`

         M42.02 Juvenile osteochondrosis of spine, cervical region `COM`

         M42.03 Juvenile osteochondrosis of spine, cervicothoracic region `COM`

         M42.04 Juvenile osteochondrosis of spine, thoracic region `COM`

         M42.05 Juvenile osteochondrosis of spine, thoracolumbar region `COM`

         M42.06 Juvenile osteochondrosis of spine, lumbar region `COM`

         M42.07 Juvenile osteochondrosis of spine, lumbosacral region `COM`

         M42.08 Juvenile osteochondrosis of spine, sacral and sacrococcygeal region `COM`

         M42.09 Juvenile osteochondrosis of spine, multiple sites in spine `COM`

     ✓5th **M42.1 Adult osteochondrosis of spine**

         M42.10 Adult osteochondrosis of spine, site unspecified `A`

         M42.11 Adult osteochondrosis of spine, occipito-atlanto-axial region `A`

HCC CMS-HCC   **Rx** Rx HCC   **ESR** ESRD HCC   **COM** Commercial HCC   **N** Newborn: 0   **P** Pediatric: 0-17   **M** Maternity: 9-64   **A** Adult: 15-124

816   ICD-10-CM 2023

M42.12 **Adult osteochondrosis of spine,** cervical region   A

M42.13 **Adult osteochondrosis of spine,** cervicothoracic region   A

M42.14 **Adult osteochondrosis of spine,** thoracic region   A

M42.15 **Adult osteochondrosis of spine,** thoracolumbar region   A

M42.16 **Adult osteochondrosis of spine,** lumbar region   A

M42.17 **Adult osteochondrosis of spine,** lumbosacral region   A

M42.18 **Adult osteochondrosis of** spine, sacral and sacrococcygeal **region**   A

M42.19 **Adult osteochondrosis of spine,** multiple sites in spine   A

M42.9 **Spinal osteochondrosis, unspecified**

✓4ᵗʰ **M43 Other deforming dorsopathies**

    EXCLUDES 1   *congenital spondylolysis and spondylolisthesis (Q76.2)*
hemivertebra (Q76.3-Q76.4)
Klippel-Feil syndrome (Q76.1)
lumbarization and sacralization (Q76.4)
platyspondylisis (Q76.4)
spina bifida occulta (Q76.0)
spinal curvature in osteoporosis (M80.-)
spinal curvature in Paget's disease of bone [osteitis deformans] (M88.-)

✓5ᵗʰ **M43.0 Spondylolysis**

    EXCLUDES 1   *congenital spondylolysis (Q76.2)*
spondylolisthesis (M43.1)

M43.00 **Spondylolysis, site unspecified**

M43.01 **Spondylolysis,** occipito-atlanto-axial **region**

M43.02 **Spondylolysis,** cervical **region**

M43.03 **Spondylolysis,** cervicothoracic **region**

M43.04 **Spondylolysis,** thoracic **region**

M43.05 **Spondylolysis,** thoracolumbar **region**

M43.06 **Spondylolysis,** lumbar **region**

M43.07 **Spondylolysis,** lumbosacral **region**

M43.08 **Spondylolysis,** sacral and sacrococcygeal **region**

M43.09 **Spondylolysis,** multiple sites in spine

✓5ᵗʰ **M43.1 Spondylolisthesis**

    EXCLUDES 1   *acute traumatic of lumbosacral region (S33.1)*
acute traumatic of sites other than lumbosacral - code to Fracture, vertebra, by region
congenital spondylolisthesis (Q76.2)

AHA: 2020,2Q,21; 2018,3Q,18
TIP: Code also any associated radiculopathy (M54.1-) and/or myelopathy (G99.2).

M43.10 **Spondylolisthesis, site unspecified**

M43.11 **Spondylolisthesis,** occipito-atlanto-axial **region**

M43.12 **Spondylolisthesis,** cervical **region**

M43.13 **Spondylolisthesis,** cervicothoracic **region**

M43.14 **Spondylolisthesis,** thoracic **region**

M43.15 **Spondylolisthesis,** thoracolumbar **region**

M43.16 **Spondylolisthesis,** lumbar **region**

M43.17 **Spondylolisthesis,** lumbosacral **region**

M43.18 **Spondylolisthesis,** sacral and sacrococcygeal **region**

M43.19 **Spondylolisthesis,** multiple sites in spine

✓5ᵗʰ **M43.2 Fusion of spine**

Ankylosis of spinal joint

    EXCLUDES 1   *ankylosing spondylitis (M45.0-)*
congenital fusion of spine (Q76.4)

    EXCLUDES 2   *arthrodesis status (Z98.1)*
pseudoarthrosis after fusion or arthrodesis (M96.0)

M43.20 **Fusion of spine, site unspecified**

M43.21 **Fusion of spine,** occipito-atlanto-axial **region**

M43.22 **Fusion of spine,** cervical **region**

M43.23 **Fusion of spine,** cervicothoracic **region**

M43.24 **Fusion of spine,** thoracic **region**

M43.25 **Fusion of spine,** thoracolumbar **region**

M43.26 **Fusion of spine,** lumbar **region**

M43.27 **Fusion of spine,** lumbosacral **region**

M43.28 **Fusion of spine,** sacral and sacrococcygeal **region**

M43.3 **Recurrent atlantoaxial dislocation with myelopathy**

M43.4 **Other recurrent atlantoaxial dislocation**

✓5ᵗʰ **M43.5 Other recurrent vertebral dislocation**

    EXCLUDES 1   *biomechanical lesions NEC (M99.-)*

✓6ᵗʰ **M43.5X Other recurrent vertebral dislocation**

M43.5X2 **Other recurrent vertebral dislocation,** cervical **region**

M43.5X3 **Other recurrent vertebral dislocation,** cervicothoracic **region**

M43.5X4 **Other recurrent vertebral dislocation,** thoracic **region**

M43.5X5 **Other recurrent vertebral dislocation,** thoracolumbar **region**

M43.5X6 **Other recurrent vertebral dislocation,** lumbar **region**

M43.5X7 **Other recurrent vertebral dislocation,** lumbosacral **region**

M43.5X8 **Other recurrent vertebral dislocation,** sacral and sacrococcygeal **region**

M43.5X9 **Other recurrent vertebral dislocation, site unspecified**

M43.6 **Torticollis**

    EXCLUDES 1   *congenital (sternomastoid) torticollis (Q68.0)*
current injury - see Injury, of spine, by body region
ocular torticollis (R29.891)
psychogenic torticollis (F45.8)
spasmodic torticollis (G24.3)
torticollis due to birth injury (P15.2)

DEF: Twisted, unnatural position of the neck due to contracted cervical muscles that pull the head to one side.

✓5ᵗʰ **M43.8 Other specified deforming dorsopathies**

    EXCLUDES 2   *kyphosis and lordosis (M40.-)*
scoliosis (M41.-)

✓6ᵗʰ **M43.8X Other specified deforming dorsopathies**

M43.8X1 **Other specified deforming dorsopathies,** occipito-atlanto-axial **region**

M43.8X2 **Other specified deforming dorsopathies,** cervical **region**

M43.8X3 **Other specified deforming dorsopathies,** cervicothoracic **region**

M43.8X4 **Other specified deforming dorsopathies,** thoracic **region**

M43.8X5 **Other specified deforming dorsopathies,** thoracolumbar **region**

M43.8X6 **Other specified deforming dorsopathies,** lumbar **region**

M43.8X7 **Other specified deforming dorsopathies,** lumbosacral **region**

M43.8X8 **Other specified deforming dorsopathies,** sacral and sacrococcygeal **region**

M43.8X9 **Other specified deforming dorsopathies, site unspecified**

M43.9 **Deforming dorsopathy, unspecified**

Curvature of spine NOS

Spondylopathies (M45-M49)

✓4ᵗʰ **M45 Ankylosing spondylitis**

Rheumatoid arthritis of spine

    EXCLUDES 1   *arthropathy in Reiter's disease (M02.3-)*
juvenile (ankylosing) spondylitis (M08.1)

    EXCLUDES 2   *Behçet's disease (M35.2)*

M45.0 **Ankylosing spondylitis of** multiple sites in spine   HCC Rx ESR COM

M45.1 **Ankylosing spondylitis of** occipito-atlanto-axial region   HCC Rx ESR COM

M45.2 **Ankylosing spondylitis of** cervical region   HCC Rx ESR COM

M45.3 **Ankylosing spondylitis of** cervicothoracic region   HCC Rx ESR COM

M45.4 **Ankylosing spondylitis of** thoracic region   HCC Rx ESR COM

M45.5 **Ankylosing spondylitis of** thoracolumbar region   HCC Rx ESR COM

M45.6 **Ankylosing spondylitis** lumbar region   HCC Rx ESR COM

M45.7 **Ankylosing spondylitis of** lumbosacral region   HCC Rx ESR COM

M45.8 **Ankylosing spondylitis** sacral and sacrococcygeal region   HCC Rx ESR COM

M45.9 **Ankylosing spondylitis of** unspecified sites in spine   HCC Rx ESR COM

Chapter 13. Diseases of the Musculoskeletal System and Connective Tissue

✓5ᵗʰ **M45.A Non-radiographic axial spondyloarthritis**
    AHA: 2021,4Q,21-22

M45.A0 Non-radiographic axial spondyloarthritis of unspecified sites in spine `HCC` `Rx` `ESR` `COM`

M45.A1 Non-radiographic axial spondyloarthritis of occipito-atlanto-axial region `HCC` `Rx` `ESR` `COM`

M45.A2 Non-radiographic axial spondyloarthritis of cervical region `HCC` `Rx` `ESR` `COM`

M45.A3 Non-radiographic axial spondyloarthritis of cervicothoracic region `HCC` `Rx` `ESR` `COM`

M45.A4 Non-radiographic axial spondyloarthritis of thoracic region `HCC` `Rx` `ESR` `COM`

M45.A5 Non-radiographic axial spondyloarthritis of thoracolumbar region `HCC` `Rx` `ESR` `COM`

M45.A6 Non-radiographic axial spondyloarthritis of lumbar region `HCC` `Rx` `ESR` `COM`

M45.A7 Non-radiographic axial spondyloarthritis of lumbosacral region `HCC` `Rx` `ESR` `COM`

M45.A8 Non-radiographic axial spondyloarthritis of sacral and sacrococcygeal region `HCC` `Rx` `ESR` `COM`

M45.AB Non-radiographic axial spondyloarthritis of multiple sites in spine `HCC` `Rx` `ESR` `COM`

✓4ᵗʰ **M46 Other inflammatory spondylopathies**

✓5ᵗʰ **M46.0 Spinal enthesopathy**
    Disorder of ligamentous or muscular attachments of spine

M46.00 Spinal enthesopathy, site unspecified `HCC` `ESR`

M46.01 Spinal enthesopathy, occipito-atlanto-axial region `HCC` `ESR`

M46.02 Spinal enthesopathy, cervical region `HCC` `ESR`

M46.03 Spinal enthesopathy, cervicothoracic region `HCC` `ESR`

M46.04 Spinal enthesopathy, thoracic region `HCC` `ESR`

M46.05 Spinal enthesopathy, thoracolumbar region `HCC` `ESR`

M46.06 Spinal enthesopathy, lumbar region `HCC` `ESR`

M46.07 Spinal enthesopathy, lumbosacral region `HCC` `ESR`

M46.08 Spinal enthesopathy, sacral and sacrococcygeal region `HCC` `ESR`

M46.09 Spinal enthesopathy, multiple sites in spine `HCC` `ESR`

M46.1 Sacroiliitis, not elsewhere classified `HCC` `ESR`
    AHA: 2020,2Q,14
    DEF: Inflammation of the sacroiliac joint (situated at the juncture of the sacrum and hip). Symptoms include pain in the buttocks or lower back that can extend down one or both legs.

✓5ᵗʰ **M46.2 Osteomyelitis of vertebra**

M46.20 Osteomyelitis of vertebra, site unspecified `HCC` `ESR` `COM`

M46.21 Osteomyelitis of vertebra, occipito-atlanto-axial region `HCC` `ESR` `COM`

M46.22 Osteomyelitis of vertebra, cervical region `HCC` `ESR` `COM`

M46.23 Osteomyelitis of vertebra, cervicothoracic region `HCC` `ESR` `COM`

M46.24 Osteomyelitis of vertebra, thoracic region `HCC` `ESR` `COM`

M46.25 Osteomyelitis of vertebra, thoracolumbar region `HCC` `ESR` `COM`

M46.26 Osteomyelitis of vertebra, lumbar region `HCC` `ESR` `COM`

M46.27 Osteomyelitis of vertebra, lumbosacral region `HCC` `ESR` `COM`

M46.28 Osteomyelitis of vertebra, sacral and sacrococcygeal region `HCC` `ESR` `COM`

✓5ᵗʰ **M46.3 Infection of intervertebral disc (pyogenic)**
    Use additional code (B95-B97) to identify infectious agent

M46.30 Infection of intervertebral disc (pyogenic), site unspecified `HCC` `ESR` `COM`

M46.31 Infection of intervertebral disc (pyogenic), occipito-atlanto-axial region `HCC` `ESR` `COM`

M46.32 Infection of intervertebral disc (pyogenic), cervical region `HCC` `ESR` `COM`

M46.33 Infection of intervertebral disc (pyogenic), cervicothoracic region `HCC` `ESR` `COM`

M46.34 Infection of intervertebral disc (pyogenic), thoracic region `HCC` `ESR` `COM`

M46.35 Infection of intervertebral disc (pyogenic), thoracolumbar region `HCC` `ESR` `COM`

M46.36 Infection of intervertebral disc (pyogenic), lumbar region `HCC` `ESR` `COM`

M46.37 Infection of intervertebral disc (pyogenic), lumbosacral region `HCC` `ESR` `COM`

M46.38 Infection of intervertebral disc (pyogenic), sacral and sacrococcygeal region `HCC` `ESR` `COM`

M46.39 Infection of intervertebral disc (pyogenic), multiple sites in spine `HCC` `ESR` `COM`

✓5ᵗʰ **M46.4 Discitis, unspecified**

M46.40 Discitis, unspecified, site unspecified

M46.41 Discitis, unspecified, occipito-atlanto-axial region

M46.42 Discitis, unspecified, cervical region

M46.43 Discitis, unspecified, cervicothoracic region

M46.44 Discitis, unspecified, thoracic region

M46.45 Discitis, unspecified, thoracolumbar region

M46.46 Discitis, unspecified, lumbar region

M46.47 Discitis, unspecified, lumbosacral region

M46.48 Discitis, unspecified, sacral and sacrococcygeal region

M46.49 Discitis, unspecified, multiple sites in spine

✓5ᵗʰ **M46.5 Other infective spondylopathies**

M46.50 Other infective spondylopathies, site unspecified `HCC` `ESR`

M46.51 Other infective spondylopathies, occipito-atlanto-axial region `HCC` `ESR`

M46.52 Other infective spondylopathies, cervical region `HCC` `ESR`

M46.53 Other infective spondylopathies, cervicothoracic region `HCC` `ESR`

M46.54 Other infective spondylopathies, thoracic region `HCC` `ESR`

M46.55 Other infective spondylopathies, thoracolumbar region `HCC` `ESR`

M46.56 Other infective spondylopathies, lumbar region `HCC` `ESR`

M46.57 Other infective spondylopathies, lumbosacral region `HCC` `ESR`

M46.58 Other infective spondylopathies, sacral and sacrococcygeal region `HCC` `ESR`

M46.59 Other infective spondylopathies, multiple sites in spine `HCC` `ESR`

✓5ᵗʰ **M46.8 Other specified inflammatory spondylopathies**

M46.80 Other specified inflammatory spondylopathies, site unspecified `HCC` `ESR`

M46.81 Other specified inflammatory spondylopathies, occipito-atlanto-axial region `HCC` `ESR`

M46.82 Other specified inflammatory spondylopathies, cervical region `HCC` `ESR`

M46.83 Other specified inflammatory spondylopathies, cervicothoracic region `HCC` `ESR`

M46.84 Other specified inflammatory spondylopathies, thoracic region `HCC` `ESR`

M46.85 Other specified inflammatory spondylopathies, thoracolumbar region `HCC` `ESR`

M46.86 Other specified inflammatory spondylopathies, lumbar region `HCC` `ESR`

M46.87 Other specified inflammatory spondylopathies, lumbosacral region `HCC` `ESR`

M46.88 Other specified inflammatory spondylopathies, sacral and sacrococcygeal region `HCC` `ESR`

M46.89 Other specified inflammatory spondylopathies, multiple sites in spine `HCC` `ESR`

✓5ᵗʰ **M46.9 Unspecified inflammatory spondylopathy**

M46.90 Unspecified inflammatory spondylopathy, site unspecified `HCC` `ESR`

M46.91 Unspecified inflammatory spondylopathy, occipito-atlanto-axial region `HCC` `ESR`

M46.92 Unspecified inflammatory spondylopathy, cervical region `HCC` `ESR`
    AHA: 2019,3Q,10

M46.93 Unspecified inflammatory spondylopathy, cervicothoracic region `HCC` `ESR`

M46.94 Unspecified inflammatory spondylopathy, thoracic region `HCC` `ESR`

M46.95 Unspecified inflammatory spondylopathy, thoracolumbar region `HCC` `ESR`

`HCC` CMS-HCC   `Rx` Rx HCC   `ESR` ESRD HCC   `COM` Commercial HCC   N Newborn: 0   P Pediatric: 0-17   M Maternity: 9-64   A Adult: 15-124

818   ICD-10-CM 2023

M46.96 Unspecified inflammatory spondylopathy, lumbar region `HCC` `ESR`

M46.97 Unspecified inflammatory spondylopathy, lumbosacral region `HCC` `ESR`

M46.98 Unspecified inflammatory spondylopathy, sacral and sacrococcygeal region `HCC` `ESR`

M46.99 Unspecified inflammatory spondylopathy, multiple sites in spine `HCC` `ESR`

`✓4ᵗʰ` **M47   Spondylosis**

> INCLUDES   arthrosis or osteoarthritis of spine
> degeneration of facet joints
> **AHA:** 2020,1Q,17; 2019,3Q,10-11; 2016,4Q,147

`✓5ᵗʰ` **M47.0   Anterior spinal and vertebral artery compression syndromes**

     `✓6ᵗʰ` **M47.01   Anterior spinal artery compression syndromes**

         M47.011   Anterior spinal artery compression syndromes, occipito-atlanto-axial region

         M47.012   Anterior spinal artery compression syndromes, cervical region

         M47.013   Anterior spinal artery compression syndromes, cervicothoracic region

         M47.014   Anterior spinal artery compression syndromes, thoracic region

         M47.015   Anterior spinal artery compression syndromes, thoracolumbar region

         M47.016   Anterior spinal artery compression syndromes, lumbar region

         M47.019   Anterior spinal artery compression syndromes, site unspecified

     `✓6ᵗʰ` **M47.02   Vertebral artery compression syndromes**

         M47.021   Vertebral artery compression syndromes, occipito-atlanto-axial region

         M47.022   Vertebral artery compression syndromes, cervical region

         M47.029   Vertebral artery compression syndromes, site unspecified

`✓5ᵗʰ` **M47.1   Other spondylosis with myelopathy**

> Spondylogenic compression of spinal cord
> EXCLUDES 1   vertebral subluxation (M43.3-M43.5X9)
> **AHA:** 2020,1Q,17

     M47.10   Other spondylosis with myelopathy, site unspecified

     M47.11   Other spondylosis with myelopathy, occipito-atlanto-axial region

     M47.12   Other spondylosis with myelopathy, cervical region

     M47.13   Other spondylosis with myelopathy, cervicothoracic region

     M47.14   Other spondylosis with myelopathy, thoracic region

     M47.15   Other spondylosis with myelopathy, thoracolumbar region

     M47.16   Other spondylosis with myelopathy, lumbar region

`✓5ᵗʰ` **M47.2   Other spondylosis with radiculopathy**

> **AHA:** 2020,1Q,17

     M47.20   Other spondylosis with radiculopathy, site unspecified

     M47.21   Other spondylosis with radiculopathy, occipito-atlanto-axial region

     M47.22   Other spondylosis with radiculopathy, cervical region

     M47.23   Other spondylosis with radiculopathy, cervicothoracic region

     M47.24   Other spondylosis with radiculopathy, thoracic region

     M47.25   Other spondylosis with radiculopathy, thoracolumbar region

     M47.26   Other spondylosis with radiculopathy, lumbar region

     M47.27   Other spondylosis with radiculopathy, lumbosacral region

     M47.28   Other spondylosis with radiculopathy, sacral and sacrococcygeal region

`✓5ᵗʰ` **M47.8   Other spondylosis**

     `✓6ᵗʰ` **M47.81   Spondylosis without myelopathy or radiculopathy**

         AHA: 2019,3Q,10-11; 2018,2Q,14

         M47.811   Spondylosis without myelopathy or radiculopathy, occipito-atlanto-axial region

         M47.812   Spondylosis without myelopathy or radiculopathy, cervical region

M47.813   Spondylosis without myelopathy or radiculopathy, cervicothoracic region

M47.814   Spondylosis without myelopathy or radiculopathy, thoracic region

M47.815   Spondylosis without myelopathy or radiculopathy, thoracolumbar region

M47.816   Spondylosis without myelopathy or radiculopathy, lumbar region

M47.817   Spondylosis without myelopathy or radiculopathy, lumbosacral region

M47.818   Spondylosis without myelopathy or radiculopathy, sacral and sacrococcygeal region

M47.819   Spondylosis without myelopathy or radiculopathy, site unspecified

     `✓6ᵗʰ` **M47.89   Other spondylosis**

         M47.891   Other spondylosis, occipito-atlanto-axial region

         M47.892   Other spondylosis, cervical region

         M47.893   Other spondylosis, cervicothoracic region

         M47.894   Other spondylosis, thoracic region

         M47.895   Other spondylosis, thoracolumbar region

         M47.896   Other spondylosis, lumbar region

         M47.897   Other spondylosis, lumbosacral region

         M47.898   Other spondylosis, sacral and sacrococcygeal region

         M47.899   Other spondylosis, site unspecified

M47.9   Spondylosis, unspecified

`✓4ᵗʰ` **M48   Other spondylopathies**

`✓5ᵗʰ` **M48.0   Spinal stenosis**

> Caudal stenosis
> **AHA:** 2020,1Q,17; 2018,3Q,18-19
> **TIP:** Code also any associated radiculopathy (M54.1-) and/or myelopathy (G99.2).

     M48.00   Spinal stenosis, site unspecified

     M48.01   Spinal stenosis, occipito-atlanto-axial region

     M48.02   Spinal stenosis, cervical region

     M48.03   Spinal stenosis, cervicothoracic region

     M48.04   Spinal stenosis, thoracic region

     M48.05   Spinal stenosis, thoracolumbar region

     `✓6ᵗʰ` **M48.06   Spinal stenosis, lumbar region**

         AHA: 2018,3Q,19; 2017,4Q,18-19

         M48.061   Spinal stenosis, lumbar region without neurogenic claudication
             Spinal stenosis, lumbar region NOS

         M48.062   Spinal stenosis, lumbar region with neurogenic claudication

     M48.07   Spinal stenosis, lumbosacral region

     M48.08   Spinal stenosis, sacral and sacrococcygeal region

`✓5ᵗʰ` **M48.1   Ankylosing hyperostosis [Forestier]**

> Diffuse idiopathic skeletal hyperostosis [DISH]

     M48.10   Ankylosing hyperostosis [Forestier], site unspecified

     M48.11   Ankylosing hyperostosis [Forestier], occipito-atlanto-axial region

     M48.12   Ankylosing hyperostosis [Forestier], cervical region

     M48.13   Ankylosing hyperostosis [Forestier], cervicothoracic region

     M48.14   Ankylosing hyperostosis [Forestier], thoracic region

     M48.15   Ankylosing hyperostosis [Forestier], thoracolumbar region

     M48.16   Ankylosing hyperostosis [Forestier], lumbar region

     M48.17   Ankylosing hyperostosis [Forestier], lumbosacral region

     M48.18   Ankylosing hyperostosis [Forestier], sacral and sacrococcygeal region

     M48.19   Ankylosing hyperostosis [Forestier], multiple sites in spine

`✓5ᵗʰ` **M48.2   Kissing spine**

     M48.20   Kissing spine, site unspecified

     M48.21   Kissing spine, occipito-atlanto-axial region

     M48.22   Kissing spine, cervical region

     M48.23   Kissing spine, cervicothoracic region

     M48.24   Kissing spine, thoracic region

     M48.25   Kissing spine, thoracolumbar region

     M48.26   Kissing spine, lumbar region

     M48.27   Kissing spine, lumbosacral region

Chapter 13. Diseases of the Musculoskeletal System and Connective Tissue

✓5ᵗʰ **M48.3 Traumatic spondylopathy**

     M48.30 Traumatic spondylopathy, site unspecified

     M48.31 Traumatic spondylopathy, occipito-atlanto-axial region

     M48.32 Traumatic spondylopathy, cervical region

     M48.33 Traumatic spondylopathy, cervicothoracic region

     M48.34 Traumatic spondylopathy, thoracic region

     M48.35 Traumatic spondylopathy, thoracolumbar region

     M48.36 Traumatic spondylopathy, lumbar region

     M48.37 Traumatic spondylopathy, lumbosacral region

     M48.38 Traumatic spondylopathy, sacral and sacrococcygeal region

✓5ᵗʰ **M48.4 Fatigue fracture of vertebra**

     Stress fracture of vertebra

     EXCLUDES 1   *pathological fracture NOS (M84.4-)*

         pathological fracture of vertebra due to neoplasm (M84.58)

         pathological fracture of vertebra due to osteoporosis (M80.-)

         pathological fracture of vertebra due to other diagnosis (M84.68)

         traumatic fracture of vertebrae (S12.0-S12.3-, S22.0-, S32.0-)

> The appropriate 7th character is to be added to each code from subcategory M48.4.
> A   initial encounter for fracture
> D   subsequent encounter for fracture with routine healing
> G   subsequent encounter for fracture with delayed healing
> S   sequela of fracture

     ✓x7ᵗʰ **M48.40** Fatigue fracture of vertebra, site unspecified Q

     ✓x7ᵗʰ **M48.41** Fatigue fracture of vertebra, occipito-atlanto-axial region Q

     ✓x7ᵗʰ **M48.42** Fatigue fracture of vertebra, cervical region Q

     ✓x7ᵗʰ **M48.43** Fatigue fracture of vertebra, cervicothoracic region Q

     ✓x7ᵗʰ **M48.44** Fatigue fracture of vertebra, thoracic region Q

     ✓x7ᵗʰ **M48.45** Fatigue fracture of vertebra, thoracolumbar region Q

     ✓x7ᵗʰ **M48.46** Fatigue fracture of vertebra, lumbar region Q

     ✓x7ᵗʰ **M48.47** Fatigue fracture of vertebra, lumbosacral region Q

     ✓x7ᵗʰ **M48.48** Fatigue fracture of vertebra, sacral and sacrococcygeal region Q

✓5ᵗʰ **M48.5 Collapsed vertebra, not elsewhere classified**

     Collapsed vertebra NOS

     Compression fracture of vertebra NOS

     Wedging of vertebra NOS

     EXCLUDES 1   *current injury - see Injury of spine, by body region*

         fatigue fracture of vertebra (M48.4)

         pathological fracture NOS (M84.4-)

         pathological fracture of vertebra due to neoplasm (M84.58)

         pathological fracture of vertebra due to osteoporosis (M80.-)

         pathological fracture of vertebra due to other diagnosis (M84.68)

         stress fracture of vertebra (M48.4-)

         traumatic fracture of vertebra (S12.-, S22.-, S32.-)

> The appropriate 7th character is to be added to each code from subcategory M48.5.
> A   initial encounter for fracture
> D   subsequent encounter for fracture with routine healing
> G   subsequent encounter for fracture with delayed healing
> S   sequela of fracture

     ¹ ✓x7ᵗʰ **M48.50** Collapsed vertebra, not elsewhere classified, site unspecified HCC Rx ESR COM

     ¹ ✓x7ᵗʰ **M48.51** Collapsed vertebra, not elsewhere classified, occipito-atlanto-axial region HCC Rx ESR COM

     ¹ ✓x7ᵗʰ **M48.52** Collapsed vertebra, not elsewhere classified, cervical region HCC Rx ESR COM

     ¹ ✓x7ᵗʰ **M48.53** Collapsed vertebra, not elsewhere classified, cervicothoracic region HCC Rx ESR COM

     ¹ ✓x7ᵗʰ **M48.54** Collapsed vertebra, not elsewhere classified, thoracic region HCC Rx ESR COM

     ¹ ✓x7ᵗʰ **M48.55** Collapsed vertebra, not elsewhere classified, thoracolumbar region HCC Rx ESR COM

     ¹ ✓x7ᵗʰ **M48.56** Collapsed vertebra, not elsewhere classified, lumbar region HCC Rx ESR COM

     ¹ ✓x7ᵗʰ **M48.57** Collapsed vertebra, not elsewhere classified, lumbosacral region HCC Rx ESR COM

     ¹ ✓x7ᵗʰ **M48.58** Collapsed vertebra, not elsewhere classified, sacral and sacrococcygeal region HCC Rx ESR COM

✓5ᵗʰ **M48.8 Other specified spondylopathies**

     Ossification of posterior longitudinal ligament

     ✓6ᵗʰ **M48.8X** Other specified spondylopathies

         M48.8X1 Other specified spondylopathies, occipito-atlanto-axial region HCC Rx ESR COM

         M48.8X2 Other specified spondylopathies, cervical region HCC Rx ESR COM

         M48.8X3 Other specified spondylopathies, cervicothoracic region HCC Rx ESR COM

         M48.8X4 Other specified spondylopathies, thoracic region HCC Rx ESR COM

         M48.8X5 Other specified spondylopathies, thoracolumbar region HCC Rx ESR COM

         M48.8X6 Other specified spondylopathies, lumbar region HCC Rx ESR COM

         M48.8X7 Other specified spondylopathies, lumbosacral region HCC Rx ESR COM

         M48.8X8 Other specified spondylopathies, sacral and sacrococcygeal region HCC Rx ESR COM

         M48.8X9 Other specified spondylopathies, site unspecified HCC Rx ESR COM

     M48.9 Spondylopathy, unspecified

✓4ᵗʰ **M49 Spondylopathies in diseases classified elsewhere**

     INCLUDES   curvature of spine in diseases classified elsewhere

         deformity of spine in diseases classified elsewhere

         kyphosis in diseases classified elsewhere

         scoliosis in diseases classified elsewhere

         spondylopathy in diseases classified elsewhere

     Code first underlying disease, such as:

         brucellosis (A23.-)

         Charcôt-Marie-Tooth disease (G60.0)

         enterobacterial infections (A01-A04)

         osteitis fibrosa cystica (E21.0)

     EXCLUDES 1   *curvature of spine in tuberculosis [Pott's] (A18.01)*

         enteropathic arthropathies (M07.-)

         gonococcal spondylitis (A54.41)

         neuropathic spondylopathy in syringomyelia (G95.0)

         neuropathic spondylopathy in tabes dorsalis (A52.11)

         neuropathic [tabes dorsalis] spondylitis (A52.11)

         nonsyphilitic neuropathic spondylopathy NEC (G98.0)

         spondylitis in syphilis (acquired) (A52.77)

         tuberculous spondylitis (A18.01)

         typhoid fever spondylitis (A01.05)

     ✓5ᵗʰ **M49.8 Spondylopathy in diseases classified elsewhere**

         M49.80 *Spondylopathy in diseases classified elsewhere, site unspecified* HCC ESR

         M49.81 *Spondylopathy in diseases classified elsewhere, occipito-atlanto-axial region* HCC ESR

         M49.82 *Spondylopathy in diseases classified elsewhere, cervical region* HCC ESR

         M49.83 *Spondylopathy in diseases classified elsewhere, cervicothoracic region* HCC ESR

         M49.84 *Spondylopathy in diseases classified elsewhere, thoracic region* HCC ESR

         M49.85 *Spondylopathy in diseases classified elsewhere, thoracolumbar region* HCC ESR

         M49.86 *Spondylopathy in diseases classified elsewhere, lumbar region* HCC ESR

         M49.87 *Spondylopathy in diseases classified elsewhere, lumbosacral region* HCC ESR

         M49.88 *Spondylopathy in diseases classified elsewhere, sacral and sacrococcygeal region* HCC ESR

         M49.89 *Spondylopathy in diseases classified elsewhere, multiple sites in spine* HCC ESR

Other dorsopathies (M50-M54)

EXCLUDES 1   current injury - see injury of spine by body region
discitis NOS (M46.4-)

✓4ᵗʰ M50 Cervical disc disorders

> **NOTE**   ~~Code to the most superior level of disorder~~
>
> **INCLUDES**   cervicothoracic disc disorders
> cervicothoracic disc disorders with cervicalgia
>
> AHA: 2016,4Q,39-40; 2016,1Q,17

✓5ᵗʰ M50.0 Cervical disc disorder with myelopathy

> AHA: 2018,3Q,19

> **M50.00** Cervical disc disorder with myelopathy, unspecified cervical region

> **M50.01** Cervical disc disorder with myelopathy, high cervical region
> C2-C3 disc disorder with myelopathy
> C3-C4 disc disorder with myelopathy

> **✓6ᵗʰ M50.02** Cervical disc disorder with myelopathy, mid-cervical region
> > **M50.020** Cervical disc disorder with myelopathy, mid-cervical region, unspecified level
> > **M50.021** Cervical disc disorder at C4-C5 level with myelopathy
> > C4-C5 disc disorder with myelopathy
> > **M50.022** Cervical disc disorder at C5-C6 level with myelopathy
> > C5-C6 disc disorder with myelopathy
> > **M50.023** Cervical disc disorder at C6-C7 level with myelopathy
> > C6-C7 disc disorder with myelopathy

> **M50.03** Cervical disc disorder with myelopathy, cervicothoracic region
> C7-T1 disc disorder with myelopathy

✓5ᵗʰ M50.1 Cervical disc disorder with radiculopathy

> **EXCLUDES 2**   brachial radiculitis NOS (M54.13)

> AHA: 2018,3Q,19

> **M50.10** Cervical disc disorder with radiculopathy, unspecified cervical region

> **M50.11** Cervical disc disorder with radiculopathy, high cervical region
> C2-C3 disc disorder with radiculopathy
> C3 radiculopathy due to disc disorder
> C3-C4 disc disorder with radiculopathy
> C4 radiculopathy due to disc disorder

> **✓6ᵗʰ M50.12** Cervical disc disorder with radiculopathy, mid-cervical region
> > **M50.120** Mid-cervical disc disorder, unspecified level
> > **M50.121** Cervical disc disorder at C4-C5 level with radiculopathy
> > C4-C5 disc disorder with radiculopathy
> > C5 radiculopathy due to disc disorder
> > **M50.122** Cervical disc disorder at C5-C6 level with radiculopathy
> > C5-C6 disc disorder with radiculopathy
> > C6 radiculopathy due to disc disorder
> > **M50.123** Cervical disc disorder at C6-C7 level with radiculopathy
> > C6-C7 disc disorder with radiculopathy
> > C7 radiculopathy due to disc disorder

> **M50.13** Cervical disc disorder with radiculopathy, cervicothoracic region
> C7-T1 disc disorder with radiculopathy
> C8 radiculopathy due to disc disorder

✓6ᵗʰ M50.2 Other cervical disc displacement

> **M50.20** Other cervical disc displacement, unspecified cervical region

> **M50.21** Other cervical disc displacement, high cervical region
> Other C2-C3 cervical disc displacement
> Other C3-C4 cervical disc displacement

> **✓6ᵗʰ M50.22** Other cervical disc displacement, mid-cervical region
> > **M50.220** Other cervical disc displacement, mid-cervical region, unspecified level
> > **M50.221** Other cervical disc displacement at C4-C5 level
> > Other C4-C5 cervical disc displacement
> > **M50.222** Other cervical disc displacement at C5-C6 level
> > Other C5-C6 cervical disc displacement
> > **M50.223** Other cervical disc displacement at C6-C7 level
> > Other C6-C7 cervical disc displacement

> **M50.23** Other cervical disc displacement, cervicothoracic region
> Other C7-T1 cervical disc displacement

✓5ᵗʰ M50.3 Other cervical disc degeneration

> **M50.30** Other cervical disc degeneration, unspecified cervical region

> **M50.31** Other cervical disc degeneration, high cervical region
> Other C2-C3 cervical disc degeneration
> Other C3-C4 cervical disc degeneration

> **✓6ᵗʰ M50.32** Other cervical disc degeneration, mid-cervical region
> > **M50.320** Other cervical disc degeneration, mid-cervical region, unspecified level
> > **M50.321** Other cervical disc degeneration at C4-C5 level
> > Other C4-C5 cervical disc degeneration
> > **M50.322** Other cervical disc degeneration at C5-C6 level
> > Other C5-C6 cervical disc degeneration
> > **M50.323** Other cervical disc degeneration at C6-C7 level
> > Other C6-C7 cervical disc degeneration

> **M50.33** Other cervical disc degeneration, cervicothoracic region
> Other C7-T1 cervical disc degeneration

✓6ᵗʰ M50.8 Other cervical disc disorders

> **M50.80** Other cervical disc disorders, unspecified cervical region

> **M50.81** Other cervical disc disorders, high cervical region
> Other C2-C3 cervical disc disorders
> Other C3-C4 cervical disc disorders

> **✓6ᵗʰ M50.82** Other cervical disc disorders, mid-cervical region
> > **M50.820** Other cervical disc disorders, mid-cervical region, unspecified level
> > **M50.821** Other cervical disc disorders at C4-C5 level
> > Other C4-C5 cervical disc disorders
> > **M50.822** Other cervical disc disorders at C5-C6 level
> > Other C5-C6 cervical disc disorders
> > **M50.823** Other cervical disc disorders at C6-C7 level
> > Other C6-C7 cervical disc disorders

> **M50.83** Other cervical disc disorders, cervicothoracic region
> Other C7-T1 cervical disc disorders

✓5ᵗʰ M50.9 Cervical disc disorder, unspecified

> **M50.90** Cervical disc disorder, unspecified, unspecified cervical region

> **M50.91** Cervical disc disorder, unspecified, high cervical region
> C2-C3 cervical disc disorder, unspecified
> C3-C4 cervical disc disorder, unspecified

> **✓6ᵗʰ M50.92** Cervical disc disorder, unspecified, mid-cervical region
> > **M50.920** Unspecified cervical disc disorder, mid-cervical region, unspecified level
> > **M50.921** Unspecified cervical disc disorder at C4-C5 level
> > Unspecified C4-C5 cervical disc disorder
> > **M50.922** Unspecified cervical disc disorder at C5-C6 level
> > Unspecified C5-C6 cervical disc disorder
> > **M50.923** Unspecified cervical disc disorder at C6-C7 level
> > Unspecified C6-C7 cervical disc disorder

> **M50.93** Cervical disc disorder, unspecified, cervicothoracic region
> C7-T1 cervical disc disorder, unspecified

✓ Additional Character Required   ✓×7ᵗʰ Placeholder Alert   Manifestation   Unspecified Dx   Q QPP   UPD Unacceptable PDx

✓4ᵗʰ **M51 Thoracic, thoracolumbar, and lumbosacral intervertebral disc disorders**
> EXCLUDES 2   *cervical and cervicothoracic disc disorders (M50.-)*
> *sacral and sacrococcygeal disorders (M53.3)*

✓5ᵗʰ **M51.0 Thoracic, thoracolumbar and lumbosacral intervertebral disc disorders with myelopathy**
- **M51.04** Intervertebral disc disorders with myelopathy, **thoracic region**
- **M51.05** Intervertebral disc disorders with myelopathy, **thoracolumbar region**
- **M51.06** Intervertebral disc disorders with myelopathy, **lumbar region**

✓5ᵗʰ **M51.1 Thoracic, thoracolumbar and lumbosacral intervertebral disc disorders with radiculopathy**
> Sciatica due to intervertebral disc disorder
> EXCLUDES 1   *lumbar radiculitis NOS (M54.16)*
> *sciatica NOS (M54.3)*
> **AHA:** 2018,3Q,18
- **M51.14** Intervertebral disc disorders with radiculopathy, **thoracic region**
- **M51.15** Intervertebral disc disorders with radiculopathy, **thoracolumbar region**
- **M51.16** Intervertebral disc disorders with radiculopathy, **lumbar region**
- **M51.17** Intervertebral disc disorders with radiculopathy, **lumbosacral region**

✓5ᵗʰ **M51.2 Other thoracic, thoracolumbar and lumbosacral intervertebral disc displacement**
> Lumbago due to displacement of intervertebral disc
> **AHA:** 2022,1Q,26

Displacement Intervertebral Disc

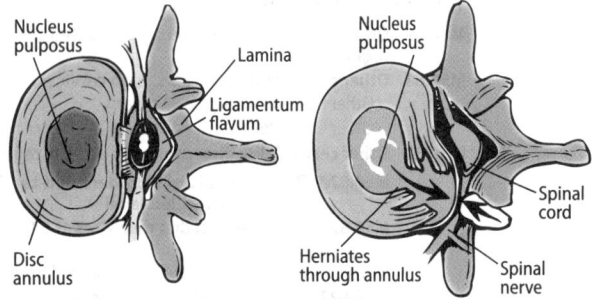

Normal Top View   Herniated Top View

- **M51.24** Other intervertebral disc displacement, **thoracic region**
- **M51.25** Other intervertebral disc displacement, **thoracolumbar region**
- **M51.26** Other intervertebral disc displacement, **lumbar region**
- **M51.27** Other intervertebral disc displacement, **lumbosacral region**

✓5ᵗʰ **M51.3 Other thoracic, thoracolumbar and lumbosacral intervertebral disc degeneration**
> **AHA:** 2022,1Q,26; 2018,2Q,15; 2013,3Q,22
- **M51.34** Other intervertebral disc degeneration, **thoracic region**
- **M51.35** Other intervertebral disc degeneration, **thoracolumbar region**
- **M51.36** Other intervertebral disc degeneration, **lumbar region**
- **M51.37** Other intervertebral disc degeneration, **lumbosacral region**

✓5ᵗʰ **M51.4 Schmorl's nodes**
> **DEF:** Irregular bone defect in the margin of the vertebral body that causes herniation into the end plate of the vertebral body.
- **M51.44** Schmorl's nodes, **thoracic region**
- **M51.45** Schmorl's nodes, **thoracolumbar region**
- **M51.46** Schmorl's nodes, **lumbar region**
- **M51.47** Schmorl's nodes, **lumbosacral region**

✓6ᵗʰ **M51.8 Other thoracic, thoracolumbar and lumbosacral intervertebral disc disorders**
- **M51.84** Other intervertebral disc disorders, **thoracic region**
- **M51.85** Other intervertebral disc disorders, **thoracolumbar region**
- **M51.86** Other intervertebral disc disorders, **lumbar region**
- **M51.87** Other intervertebral disc disorders, **lumbosacral region**

M51.9 Unspecified thoracic, thoracolumbar and lumbosacral intervertebral disc disorder

✓6ᵗʰ **M51.A Other lumbar and lumbosacral annulus fibrosus disc defects**
- **M51.A0** Intervertebral annulus fibrosus defect, **lumbar region, unspecified size**
  > Code first, if applicable, lumbar disc herniation (M51.06, M51.16, M51.26)
- **M51.A1** Intervertebral annulus fibrosus defect, **small, lumbar region**
  > Code first, if applicable, lumbar disc herniation (M51.06, M51.16, M51.26)
- **M51.A2** Intervertebral annulus fibrosus defect, **large, lumbar region**
  > Code first, if applicable, lumbar disc herniation (M51.06, M51.16, M51.26)
- **M51.A3** Intervertebral annulus fibrosus defect, **lumbosacral region, unspecified size**
  > Code first, if applicable, lumbosacral disc herniation (M51.17, M51.27)
- **M51.A4** Intervertebral annulus fibrosus defect, **small, lumbosacral region**
  > Code first, if applicable, lumbosacral disc herniation (M51.17, M51.27)
- **M51.A5** Intervertebral annulus fibrosus defect, **large, lumbosacral region**
  > Code first, if applicable, lumbosacral disc herniation (M51.17, M51.27)

✓4ᵗʰ **M53 Other and unspecified dorsopathies, not elsewhere classified**

M53.0 Cervicocranial syndrome
> Posterior cervical sympathetic syndrome

M53.1 Cervicobrachial syndrome
> EXCLUDES 2   *cervical disc disorder (M50.-)*
> *thoracic outlet syndrome (G54.0)*

✓5ᵗʰ **M53.2 Spinal instabilities**
✓6ᵗʰ **M53.2X Spinal instabilities**
- **M53.2X1** Spinal instabilities, **occipito-atlanto-axial region**
- **M53.2X2** Spinal instabilities, **cervical region**
- **M53.2X3** Spinal instabilities, **cervicothoracic region**
- **M53.2X4** Spinal instabilities, **thoracic region**
- **M53.2X5** Spinal instabilities, **thoracolumbar region**
- **M53.2X6** Spinal instabilities, **lumbar region**
- **M53.2X7** Spinal instabilities, **lumbosacral region**
- **M53.2X8** Spinal instabilities, **sacral and sacrococcygeal region**
- **M53.2X9** Spinal instabilities, **site unspecified**

M53.3 Sacrococcygeal disorders, not elsewhere classified
> Coccygodynia

✓5ᵗʰ **M53.8 Other specified dorsopathies**
- **M53.80** Other specified dorsopathies, **site unspecified**
- **M53.81** Other specified dorsopathies, **occipito-atlanto-axial region**
- **M53.82** Other specified dorsopathies, **cervical region**
- **M53.83** Other specified dorsopathies, **cervicothoracic region**
- **M53.84** Other specified dorsopathies, **thoracic region**
- **M53.85** Other specified dorsopathies, **thoracolumbar region**
- **M53.86** Other specified dorsopathies, **lumbar region**
- **M53.87** Other specified dorsopathies, **lumbosacral region**
- **M53.88** Other specified dorsopathies, **sacral and sacrococcygeal region**

M53.9 Dorsopathy, unspecified

✓4ᵗʰ **M54 Dorsalgia**
> EXCLUDES 1   *psychogenic dorsalgia (F45.41)*

✓5ᵗʰ **M54.0 Panniculitis affecting regions of neck and back**
> EXCLUDES 1   *lupus panniculitis (L93.2)*
> *panniculitis NOS (M79.3)*
> *relapsing [Weber-Christian] panniculitis (M35.6)*
- **M54.00** Panniculitis affecting regions of neck and back, **site unspecified**
- **M54.01** Panniculitis affecting regions of neck and back, **occipito-atlanto-axial region**
- **M54.02** Panniculitis affecting regions of neck and back, **cervical region**

HCC CMS-HCC   **Rx** Rx HCC   **ESR** ESRD HCC   **COM** Commercial HCC   **N** Newborn: 0   **P** Pediatric: 0-17   **M** Maternity: 9-64   **A** Adult: 15-124

822   ICD-10-CM 2023

M54.03 **Panniculitis affecting regions of neck and back, cervicothoracic region**

M54.04 **Panniculitis affecting regions of neck and back, thoracic region**

M54.05 **Panniculitis affecting regions of neck and back, thoracolumbar region**

M54.06 **Panniculitis affecting regions of neck and back, lumbar region**

M54.07 **Panniculitis affecting regions of neck and back, lumbosacral region**

M54.08 **Panniculitis affecting regions of neck and back, sacral and sacrococcygeal region**

M54.09 **Panniculitis affecting regions, neck and back, multiple sites in spine**

√5ᵗʰ M54.1 **Radiculopathy**

Brachial neuritis or radiculitis NOS
Lumbar neuritis or radiculitis NOS
Lumbosacral neuritis or radiculitis NOS
Thoracic neuritis or radiculitis NOS
Radiculitis NOS

EXCLUDES 1   *neuralgia and neuritis NOS (M79.2)*
radiculopathy with cervical disc disorder (M50.1)
radiculopathy with lumbar and other intervertebral disc disorder (M51.1-)
radiculopathy with spondylosis (M47.2-)

AHA: 2018,3Q,18

TIP: A code from this subcategory can be used in addition to a spondylolisthesis code (M43.1-) or a spinal stenosis code (M48.0-) when either condition is documented as the cause of the radiculopathy.

M54.10 **Radiculopathy, site unspecified**

M54.11 **Radiculopathy, occipito-atlanto-axial region**

M54.12 **Radiculopathy, cervical region**

M54.13 **Radiculopathy, cervicothoracic region**

M54.14 **Radiculopathy, thoracic region**

M54.15 **Radiculopathy, thoracolumbar region**

M54.16 **Radiculopathy, lumbar region**

M54.17 **Radiculopathy, lumbosacral region**

M54.18 **Radiculopathy, sacral and sacrococcygeal region**

M54.2 **Cervicalgia**

EXCLUDES 1   *cervicalgia due to intervertebral cervical disc disorder (M50.-)*

√5ᵗʰ M54.3 **Sciatica**

EXCLUDES 1   *lesion of sciatic nerve (G57.0)*
sciatica due to intervertebral disc disorder (M51.1-)
sciatica with lumbago (M54.4-)

M54.30 **Sciatica, unspecified side**

M54.31 **Sciatica, right side**

M54.32 **Sciatica, left side**

√5ᵗʰ M54.4 **Lumbago with sciatica**

EXCLUDES 1   *lumbago with sciatica due to intervertebral disc disorder (M51.1-)*

AHA: 2016,2Q,7

M54.40 **Lumbago with sciatica, unspecified side**

M54.41 **Lumbago with sciatica, right side**

M54.42 **Lumbago with sciatica, left side**

√5ᵗʰ M54.5 **Low back pain**

EXCLUDES 1   *low back strain (S39.012)*
lumbago due to intervertebral disc displacement (M51.2-)
lumbago with sciatica (M54.4-)

AHA: 2021,4Q,22

M54.50 **Low back pain, unspecified**
Loin pain
Lumbago NOS

M54.51 **Vertebrogenic low back pain**
Low back vertebral endplate pain

M54.59 **Other low back pain**

M54.6 **Pain in thoracic spine**

EXCLUDES 1   *pain in thoracic spine due to intervertebral disc disorder (M51.-)*

√5ᵗʰ M54.8 **Other dorsalgia**

EXCLUDES 1   *dorsalgia in thoracic region (M54.6)*
low back pain (M54.5-)

M54.81 **Occipital neuralgia**

M54.89 **Other dorsalgia**

M54.9 **Dorsalgia, unspecified**
Backache NOS
Back pain NOS

SOFT TISSUE DISORDERS (M60-M79)

Disorders of muscles (M60-M63)

EXCLUDES 1   *dermatopolymyositis (M33.-)*
~~*muscular dystrophies and myopathies (G71-G72)*~~
myopathy in amyloidosis (E85.-)
myopathy in polyarteritis nodosa (M30.0)
myopathy in rheumatoid arthritis (M05.32)
myopathy in scleroderma (M34.-)
myopathy in Sjögren's syndrome (M35.03)
myopathy in systemic lupus erythematosus (M32.-)

EXCLUDES 2 ▶*muscular dystrophies and myopathies (G71-G72)*◀

√4ᵗʰ M60 **Myositis**

EXCLUDES 2   *inclusion body myositis [IBM] (G72.41)*

√5ᵗʰ M60.0 **Infective myositis**
Tropical pyomyositis
Use additional code (B95-B97) to identify infectious agent

√6ᵗʰ M60.00 **Infective myositis, unspecified site**

M60.000 **Infective myositis, unspecified right arm**
Infective myositis, right upper limb NOS

M60.001 **Infective myositis, unspecified left arm**
Infective myositis, left upper limb NOS

M60.002 **Infective myositis, unspecified arm**
Infective myositis, upper limb NOS

M60.003 **Infective myositis, unspecified right leg**
Infective myositis, right lower limb NOS

M60.004 **Infective myositis, unspecified left leg**
Infective myositis, left lower limb NOS

M60.005 **Infective myositis, unspecified leg**
Infective myositis, lower limb NOS

M60.009 **Infective myositis, unspecified site**

√6ᵗʰ M60.01 **Infective myositis, shoulder**

M60.011 **Infective myositis, right shoulder**

M60.012 **Infective myositis, left shoulder**

M60.019 **Infective myositis, unspecified shoulder**

√6ᵗʰ M60.02 **Infective myositis, upper arm**

M60.021 **Infective myositis, right upper arm**

M60.022 **Infective myositis, left upper arm**

M60.029 **Infective myositis, unspecified upper arm**

√6ᵗʰ M60.03 **Infective myositis, forearm**

M60.031 **Infective myositis, right forearm**

M60.032 **Infective myositis, left forearm**

M60.039 **Infective myositis, unspecified forearm**

√6ᵗʰ M60.04 **Infective myositis, hand and fingers**

M60.041 **Infective myositis, right hand**

M60.042 **Infective myositis, left hand**

M60.043 **Infective myositis, unspecified hand**

M60.044 **Infective myositis, right finger(s)**

M60.045 **Infective myositis, left finger(s)**

M60.046 **Infective myositis, unspecified finger(s)**

√6ᵗʰ M60.05 **Infective myositis, thigh**

M60.051 **Infective myositis, right thigh**

M60.052 **Infective myositis, left thigh**

M60.059 **Infective myositis, unspecified thigh**

√6ᵗʰ M60.06 **Infective myositis, lower leg**

M60.061 **Infective myositis, right lower leg**

M60.062 **Infective myositis, left lower leg**

M60.069 **Infective myositis, unspecified lower leg**

√6ᵗʰ M60.07 **Infective myositis, ankle, foot and toes**

M60.070 **Infective myositis, right ankle**

M60.071 **Infective myositis, left ankle**

M60.072 **Infective myositis, unspecified ankle**

M60.073 **Infective myositis, right foot**

M60.074 **Infective myositis, left foot**

M60.075 **Infective myositis, unspecified foot**

M60.076 **Infective myositis, right toe(s)**

M60.077 **Infective myositis, left toe(s)**

M60.078 **Infective myositis, unspecified toe(s)**

M60.08 **Infective myositis, other site**

M60.09 **Infective myositis, multiple sites**

√5ᵗʰ M60.1 **Interstitial myositis**

M60.10 **Interstitial myositis of unspecified site**

✓6ᵗʰ **M60.11 Interstitial myositis, shoulder**

     M60.111 Interstitial myositis, right shoulder
     M60.112 Interstitial myositis, left shoulder
     M60.119 Interstitial myositis, unspecified shoulder

✓6ᵗʰ **M60.12 Interstitial myositis, upper arm**

     M60.121 Interstitial myositis, right upper arm
     M60.122 Interstitial myositis, left upper arm
     M60.129 Interstitial myositis, unspecified upper arm

✓6ᵗʰ **M60.13 Interstitial myositis, forearm**

     M60.131 Interstitial myositis, right forearm
     M60.132 Interstitial myositis, left forearm
     M60.139 Interstitial myositis, unspecified forearm

✓6ᵗʰ **M60.14 Interstitial myositis, hand**

     M60.141 Interstitial myositis, right hand
     M60.142 Interstitial myositis, left hand
     M60.149 Interstitial myositis, unspecified hand

✓6ᵗʰ **M60.15 Interstitial myositis, thigh**

     M60.151 Interstitial myositis, right thigh
     M60.152 Interstitial myositis, left thigh
     M60.159 Interstitial myositis, unspecified thigh

✓6ᵗʰ **M60.16 Interstitial myositis, lower leg**

     M60.161 Interstitial myositis, right lower leg
     M60.162 Interstitial myositis, left lower leg
     M60.169 Interstitial myositis, unspecified lower leg

✓6ᵗʰ **M60.17 Interstitial myositis, ankle and foot**

     M60.171 Interstitial myositis, right ankle and foot
     M60.172 Interstitial myositis, left ankle and foot
     M60.179 Interstitial myositis, unspecified ankle and foot

     M60.18 Interstitial myositis, other site
     M60.19 Interstitial myositis, multiple sites

✓5ᵗʰ **M60.2 Foreign body granuloma of soft tissue, not elsewhere classified**

     Use additional code to identify the type of retained foreign body (Z18.-)

     EXCLUDES 1   *foreign body granuloma of skin and subcutaneous tissue (L92.3)*

     M60.20 Foreign body granuloma of soft tissue, not elsewhere classified, unspecified site

✓6ᵗʰ **M60.21 Foreign body granuloma of soft tissue, not elsewhere classified, shoulder**

     M60.211 Foreign body granuloma of soft tissue, not elsewhere classified, right shoulder
     M60.212 Foreign body granuloma of soft tissue, not elsewhere classified, left shoulder
     M60.219 Foreign body granuloma of soft tissue, not elsewhere classified, unspecified shoulder

✓6ᵗʰ **M60.22 Foreign body granuloma of soft tissue, not elsewhere classified, upper arm**

     M60.221 Foreign body granuloma of soft tissue, not elsewhere classified, right upper arm
     M60.222 Foreign body granuloma of soft tissue, not elsewhere classified, left upper arm
     M60.229 Foreign body granuloma of soft tissue, not elsewhere classified, unspecified upper arm

✓6ᵗʰ **M60.23 Foreign body granuloma of soft tissue, not elsewhere classified, forearm**

     M60.231 Foreign body granuloma of soft tissue, not elsewhere classified, right forearm
     M60.232 Foreign body granuloma of soft tissue, not elsewhere classified, left forearm
     M60.239 Foreign body granuloma of soft tissue, not elsewhere classified, unspecified forearm

✓6ᵗʰ **M60.24 Foreign body granuloma of soft tissue, not elsewhere classified, hand**

     M60.241 Foreign body granuloma of soft tissue, not elsewhere classified, right hand
     M60.242 Foreign body granuloma of soft tissue, not elsewhere classified, left hand
     M60.249 Foreign body granuloma of soft tissue, not elsewhere classified, unspecified hand

✓6ᵗʰ **M60.25 Foreign body granuloma of soft tissue, not elsewhere classified, thigh**

     M60.251 Foreign body granuloma of soft tissue, not elsewhere classified, right thigh
     M60.252 Foreign body granuloma of soft tissue, not elsewhere classified, left thigh
     M60.259 Foreign body granuloma of soft tissue, not elsewhere classified, unspecified thigh

✓6ᵗʰ **M60.26 Foreign body granuloma of soft tissue, not elsewhere classified, lower leg**

     M60.261 Foreign body granuloma of soft tissue, not elsewhere classified, right lower leg
     M60.262 Foreign body granuloma of soft tissue, not elsewhere classified, left lower leg
     M60.269 Foreign body granuloma of soft tissue, not elsewhere classified, unspecified lower leg

✓6ᵗʰ **M60.27 Foreign body granuloma of soft tissue, not elsewhere classified, ankle and foot**

     M60.271 Foreign body granuloma of soft tissue, not elsewhere classified, right ankle and foot
     M60.272 Foreign body granuloma of soft tissue, not elsewhere classified, left ankle and foot
     M60.279 Foreign body granuloma of soft tissue, not elsewhere classified, unspecified ankle and foot

     M60.28 Foreign body granuloma of soft tissue, not elsewhere classified, other site

✓5ᵗʰ **M60.8 Other myositis**

     M60.80 Other myositis, unspecified site

✓6ᵗʰ **M60.81 Other myositis shoulder**

     M60.811 Other myositis, right shoulder
     M60.812 Other myositis, left shoulder
     M60.819 Other myositis, unspecified shoulder

✓6ᵗʰ **M60.82 Other myositis, upper arm**

     M60.821 Other myositis, right upper arm
     M60.822 Other myositis, left upper arm
     M60.829 Other myositis, unspecified upper arm

✓6ᵗʰ **M60.83 Other myositis, forearm**

     M60.831 Other myositis, right forearm
     M60.832 Other myositis, left forearm
     M60.839 Other myositis, unspecified forearm

✓6ᵗʰ **M60.84 Other myositis, hand**

     M60.841 Other myositis, right hand
     M60.842 Other myositis, left hand
     M60.849 Other myositis, unspecified hand

✓6ᵗʰ **M60.85 Other myositis, thigh**

     M60.851 Other myositis, right thigh
     M60.852 Other myositis, left thigh
     M60.859 Other myositis, unspecified thigh

✓6ᵗʰ **M60.86 Other myositis, lower leg**

     M60.861 Other myositis, right lower leg
     M60.862 Other myositis, left lower leg
     M60.869 Other myositis, unspecified lower leg

✓6ᵗʰ **M60.87 Other myositis, ankle and foot**

     M60.871 Other myositis, right ankle and foot
     M60.872 Other myositis, left ankle and foot
     M60.879 Other myositis, unspecified ankle and foot

     M60.88 Other myositis, other site
     M60.89 Other myositis, multiple sites

     M60.9 Myositis, unspecified

✓4ᵗʰ **M61 Calcification and ossification of muscle**

✓5ᵗʰ **M61.0 Myositis ossificans traumatica**

     M61.00 Myositis ossificans traumatica, unspecified site

✓6ᵗʰ **M61.01 Myositis ossificans traumatica, shoulder**

     M61.011 Myositis ossificans traumatica, right shoulder
     M61.012 Myositis ossificans traumatica, left shoulder
     M61.019 Myositis ossificans traumatica, unspecified shoulder

✓6ᵗʰ **M61.02 Myositis ossificans traumatica, upper arm**

     M61.021 Myositis ossificans traumatica, right upper arm

M61.022   Myositis ossificans traumatica, left upper arm

M61.029   Myositis ossificans traumatica, unspecified upper arm

√6ᵗʰ   **M61.03**   Myositis ossificans traumatica, forearm

     M61.031   Myositis ossificans traumatica, right forearm

     M61.032   Myositis ossificans traumatica, left forearm

     M61.039   Myositis ossificans traumatica, unspecified forearm

√6ᵗʰ   **M61.04**   Myositis ossificans traumatica, hand

     M61.041   Myositis ossificans traumatica, right hand

     M61.042   Myositis ossificans traumatica, left hand

     M61.049   Myositis ossificans traumatica, unspecified hand

√6ᵗʰ   **M61.05**   Myositis ossificans traumatica, thigh

     M61.051   Myositis ossificans traumatica, right thigh

     M61.052   Myositis ossificans traumatica, left thigh

     M61.059   Myositis ossificans traumatica, unspecified thigh

√6ᵗʰ   **M61.06**   Myositis ossificans traumatica, lower leg

     M61.061   Myositis ossificans traumatica, right lower leg

     M61.062   Myositis ossificans traumatica, left lower leg

     M61.069   Myositis ossificans traumatica, unspecified lower leg

√6ᵗʰ   **M61.07**   Myositis ossificans traumatica, ankle and foot

     M61.071   Myositis ossificans traumatica, right ankle and foot

     M61.072   Myositis ossificans traumatica, left ankle and foot

     M61.079   Myositis ossificans traumatica, unspecified ankle and foot

     M61.08   Myositis ossificans traumatica, other site

     M61.09   Myositis ossificans traumatica, multiple sites

√5ᵗʰ   **M61.1**   **Myositis ossificans progressiva**

     Fibrodysplasia ossificans progressiva

     M61.10   Myositis ossificans progressiva, unspecified site

√6ᵗʰ   **M61.11**   Myositis ossificans progressiva, shoulder

     M61.111   Myositis ossificans progressiva, right shoulder

     M61.112   Myositis ossificans progressiva, left shoulder

     M61.119   Myositis ossificans progressiva, unspecified shoulder

√6ᵗʰ   **M61.12**   Myositis ossificans progressiva, upper arm

     M61.121   Myositis ossificans progressiva, right upper arm

     M61.122   Myositis ossificans progressiva, left upper arm

     M61.129   Myositis ossificans progressiva, unspecified arm

√6ᵗʰ   **M61.13**   Myositis ossificans progressiva, forearm

     M61.131   Myositis ossificans progressiva, right forearm

     M61.132   Myositis ossificans progressiva, left forearm

     M61.139   Myositis ossificans progressiva, unspecified forearm

√6ᵗʰ   **M61.14**   Myositis ossificans progressiva, hand and finger(s)

     M61.141   Myositis ossificans progressiva, right hand

     M61.142   Myositis ossificans progressiva, left hand

     M61.143   Myositis ossificans progressiva, unspecified hand

     M61.144   Myositis ossificans progressiva, right finger(s)

     M61.145   Myositis ossificans progressiva, left finger(s)

     M61.146   Myositis ossificans progressiva, unspecified finger(s)

√6ᵗʰ   **M61.15**   Myositis ossificans progressiva, thigh

     M61.151   Myositis ossificans progressiva, right thigh

     M61.152   Myositis ossificans progressiva, left thigh

     M61.159   Myositis ossificans progressiva, unspecified thigh

√6ᵗʰ   **M61.16**   Myositis ossificans progressiva, lower leg

     M61.161   Myositis ossificans progressiva, right lower leg

     M61.162   Myositis ossificans progressiva, left lower leg

     M61.169   Myositis ossificans progressiva, unspecified lower leg

√6ᵗʰ   **M61.17**   Myositis ossificans progressiva, ankle, foot and toe(s)

     M61.171   Myositis ossificans progressiva, right ankle

     M61.172   Myositis ossificans progressiva, left ankle

     M61.173   Myositis ossificans progressiva, unspecified ankle

     M61.174   Myositis ossificans progressiva, right foot

     M61.175   Myositis ossificans progressiva, left foot

     M61.176   Myositis ossificans progressiva, unspecified foot

     M61.177   Myositis ossificans progressiva, right toe(s)

     M61.178   Myositis ossificans progressiva, left toe(s)

     M61.179   Myositis ossificans progressiva, unspecified toe(s)

     M61.18   Myositis ossificans progressiva, other site

     M61.19   Myositis ossificans progressiva, multiple sites

√5ᵗʰ   **M61.2**   **Paralytic calcification and ossification of muscle**

     Myositis ossificans associated with quadriplegia or paraplegia

     M61.20   Paralytic calcification and ossification of muscle, unspecified site

√6ᵗʰ   **M61.21**   Paralytic calcification and ossification of muscle, shoulder

     M61.211   Paralytic calcification and ossification of muscle, right shoulder

     M61.212   Paralytic calcification and ossification of muscle, left shoulder

     M61.219   Paralytic calcification and ossification of muscle, unspecified shoulder

√6ᵗʰ   **M61.22**   Paralytic calcification and ossification of muscle, upper arm

     M61.221   Paralytic calcification and ossification of muscle, right upper arm

     M61.222   Paralytic calcification and ossification of muscle, left upper arm

     M61.229   Paralytic calcification and ossification of muscle, unspecified upper arm

√6ᵗʰ   **M61.23**   Paralytic calcification and ossification of muscle, forearm

     M61.231   Paralytic calcification and ossification of muscle, right forearm

     M61.232   Paralytic calcification and ossification of muscle, left forearm

     M61.239   Paralytic calcification and ossification of muscle, unspecified forearm

√6ᵗʰ   **M61.24**   Paralytic calcification and ossification of muscle, hand

     M61.241   Paralytic calcification and ossification of muscle, right hand

     M61.242   Paralytic calcification and ossification of muscle, left hand

     M61.249   Paralytic calcification and ossification of muscle, unspecified hand

√6ᵗʰ   **M61.25**   Paralytic calcification and ossification of muscle, thigh

     M61.251   Paralytic calcification and ossification of muscle, right thigh

     M61.252   Paralytic calcification and ossification of muscle, left thigh

     M61.259   Paralytic calcification and ossification of muscle, unspecified thigh

√6ᵗʰ   **M61.26**   Paralytic calcification and ossification of muscle, lower leg

     M61.261   Paralytic calcification and ossification of muscle, right lower leg

     M61.262   Paralytic calcification and ossification of muscle, left lower leg

     M61.269   Paralytic calcification and ossification of muscle, unspecified lower leg

√6ᵗʰ   **M61.27**   Paralytic calcification and ossification of muscle, ankle and foot

     M61.271   Paralytic calcification and ossification of muscle, right ankle and foot

---

☑ Additional Character Required   √x7ᵗʰ Placeholder Alert   Manifestation   Unspecified Dx   Q QPP   UPD Unacceptable PDx

M61.272   **Paralytic calcification and ossification of muscle, left ankle and foot**

M61.279   **Paralytic calcification and ossification of muscle, unspecified ankle and foot**

M61.28   **Paralytic calcification and ossification of muscle, other site**

M61.29   **Paralytic calcification and ossification of muscle, multiple sites**

✓5ᵗʰ M61.3   **Calcification and ossification of muscles associated with burns**

Myositis ossificans associated with burns

M61.30   **Calcification and ossification of muscles associated with burns, unspecified site**

✓6ᵗʰ M61.31   **Calcification and ossification of muscles associated with burns, shoulder**

    M61.311   **Calcification and ossification of muscles associated with burns, right shoulder**

    M61.312   **Calcification and ossification of muscles associated with burns, left shoulder**

    M61.319   **Calcification and ossification of muscles associated with burns, unspecified shoulder**

✓6ᵗʰ M61.32   **Calcification and ossification of muscles associated with burns, upper arm**

    M61.321   **Calcification and ossification of muscles associated with burns, right upper arm**

    M61.322   **Calcification and ossification of muscles associated with burns, left upper arm**

    M61.329   **Calcification and ossification of muscles associated with burns, unspecified upper arm**

✓6ᵗʰ M61.33   **Calcification and ossification of muscles associated with burns, forearm**

    M61.331   **Calcification and ossification of muscles associated with burns, right forearm**

    M61.332   **Calcification and ossification of muscles associated with burns, left forearm**

    M61.339   **Calcification and ossification of muscles associated with burns, unspecified forearm**

✓6ᵗʰ M61.34   **Calcification and ossification of muscles associated with burns, hand**

    M61.341   **Calcification and ossification of muscles associated with burns, right hand**

    M61.342   **Calcification and ossification of muscles associated with burns, left hand**

    M61.349   **Calcification and ossification of muscles associated with burns, unspecified hand**

✓6ᵗʰ M61.35   **Calcification and ossification of muscles associated with burns, thigh**

    M61.351   **Calcification and ossification of muscles associated with burns, right thigh**

    M61.352   **Calcification and ossification of muscles associated with burns, left thigh**

    M61.359   **Calcification and ossification of muscles associated with burns, unspecified thigh**

✓6ᵗʰ M61.36   **Calcification and ossification of muscles associated with burns, lower leg**

    M61.361   **Calcification and ossification of muscles associated with burns, right lower leg**

    M61.362   **Calcification and ossification of muscles associated with burns, left lower leg**

    M61.369   **Calcification and ossification of muscles associated with burns, unspecified lower leg**

✓6ᵗʰ M61.37   **Calcification and ossification of muscles associated with burns, ankle and foot**

    M61.371   **Calcification and ossification of muscles associated with burns, right ankle and foot**

    M61.372   **Calcification and ossification of muscles associated with burns, left ankle and foot**

    M61.379   **Calcification and ossification of muscles associated with burns, unspecified ankle and foot**

M61.38   **Calcification and ossification of muscles associated with burns, other site**

M61.39   **Calcification and ossification of muscles associated with burns, multiple sites**

✓5ᵗʰ M61.4   **Other calcification of muscle**

    EXCLUDES 1   calcific tendinitis NOS (M65.2-)

               calcific tendinitis of shoulder (M75.3)

M61.40   **Other calcification of muscle, unspecified site**

✓6ᵗʰ M61.41   **Other calcification of muscle, shoulder**

    M61.411   **Other calcification of muscle, right shoulder**

    M61.412   **Other calcification of muscle, left shoulder**

    M61.419   **Other calcification of muscle, unspecified shoulder**

✓6ᵗʰ M61.42   **Other calcification of muscle, upper arm**

    M61.421   **Other calcification of muscle, right upper arm**

    M61.422   **Other calcification of muscle, left upper arm**

    M61.429   **Other calcification of muscle, unspecified upper arm**

✓6ᵗʰ M61.43   **Other calcification of muscle, forearm**

    M61.431   **Other calcification of muscle, right forearm**

    M61.432   **Other calcification of muscle, left forearm**

    M61.439   **Other calcification of muscle, unspecified forearm**

✓6ᵗʰ M61.44   **Other calcification of muscle, hand**

    M61.441   **Other calcification of muscle, right hand**

    M61.442   **Other calcification of muscle, left hand**

    M61.449   **Other calcification of muscle, unspecified hand**

✓6ᵗʰ M61.45   **Other calcification of muscle, thigh**

    M61.451   **Other calcification of muscle, right thigh**

    M61.452   **Other calcification of muscle, left thigh**

    M61.459   **Other calcification of muscle, unspecified thigh**

✓6ᵗʰ M61.46   **Other calcification of muscle, lower leg**

    M61.461   **Other calcification of muscle, right lower leg**

    M61.462   **Other calcification of muscle, left lower leg**

    M61.469   **Other calcification of muscle, unspecified lower leg**

✓6ᵗʰ M61.47   **Other calcification of muscle, ankle and foot**

    M61.471   **Other calcification of muscle, right ankle and foot**

    M61.472   **Other calcification of muscle, left ankle and foot**

    M61.479   **Other calcification of muscle, unspecified ankle and foot**

M61.48   **Other calcification of muscle, other site**

M61.49   **Other calcification of muscle, multiple sites**

✓5ᵗʰ M61.5   **Other ossification of muscle**

M61.50   **Other ossification of muscle, unspecified site**

✓6ᵗʰ M61.51   **Other ossification of muscle, shoulder**

    M61.511   **Other ossification of muscle, right shoulder**

    M61.512   **Other ossification of muscle, left shoulder**

    M61.519   **Other ossification of muscle, unspecified shoulder**

✓6ᵗʰ M61.52   **Other ossification of muscle, upper arm**

    M61.521   **Other ossification of muscle, right upper arm**

    M61.522   **Other ossification of muscle, left upper arm**

    M61.529   **Other ossification of muscle, unspecified upper arm**

✓6ᵗʰ M61.53   **Other ossification of muscle, forearm**

    M61.531   **Other ossification of muscle, right forearm**

    M61.532   **Other ossification of muscle, left forearm**

    M61.539   **Other ossification of muscle, unspecified forearm**

✓6ᵗʰ M61.54   **Other ossification of muscle, hand**

    M61.541   **Other ossification of muscle, right hand**

    M61.542   **Other ossification of muscle, left hand**

    M61.549   **Other ossification of muscle, unspecified hand**

✓6ᵗʰ M61.55   **Other ossification of muscle, thigh**

    M61.551   **Other ossification of muscle, right thigh**

    M61.552   **Other ossification of muscle, left thigh**

    M61.559   **Other ossification of muscle, unspecified thigh**

✓6ᵗʰ **M61.56** Other ossification of muscle, lower leg

    M61.561 Other ossification of muscle, right lower leg

    M61.562 Other ossification of muscle, left lower leg

    M61.569 Other ossification of muscle, unspecified lower leg

✓6ᵗʰ **M61.57** Other ossification of muscle, ankle and foot

    M61.571 Other ossification of muscle, right ankle and foot

    M61.572 Other ossification of muscle, left ankle and foot

    M61.579 Other ossification of muscle, unspecified ankle and foot

  M61.58 Other ossification of muscle, other site

  M61.59 Other ossification of muscle, multiple sites

M61.9 Calcification and ossification of muscle, unspecified

✓4ᵗʰ **M62 Other disorders of muscle**

  EXCLUDES 1   alcoholic myopathy (G72.1)

           cramp and spasm (R25.2)

           drug-induced myopathy (G72.0)

           myalgia (M79.1-)

           stiff-man syndrome (G25.82)

  EXCLUDES 2   nontraumatic hematoma of muscle (M79.81)

✓5ᵗʰ **M62.0 Separation of muscle (nontraumatic)**

    Diastasis of muscle

    EXCLUDES 1   diastasis recti complicating pregnancy, labor and delivery (O71.8)

              traumatic separation of muscle - see strain of muscle by body region

  M62.00 Separation of muscle (nontraumatic), unspecified site

✓6ᵗʰ **M62.01** Separation of muscle (nontraumatic), shoulder

    M62.011 Separation of muscle (nontraumatic), right shoulder

    M62.012 Separation of muscle (nontraumatic), left shoulder

    M62.019 Separation of muscle (nontraumatic), unspecified shoulder

✓6ᵗʰ **M62.02** Separation of muscle (nontraumatic), upper arm

    M62.021 Separation of muscle (nontraumatic), right upper arm

    M62.022 Separation of muscle (nontraumatic), left upper arm

    M62.029 Separation of muscle (nontraumatic), unspecified upper arm

✓6ᵗʰ **M62.03** Separation of muscle (nontraumatic), forearm

    M62.031 Separation of muscle (nontraumatic), right forearm

    M62.032 Separation of muscle (nontraumatic), left forearm

    M62.039 Separation of muscle (nontraumatic), unspecified forearm

✓6ᵗʰ **M62.04** Separation of muscle (nontraumatic), hand

    M62.041 Separation of muscle (nontraumatic), right hand

    M62.042 Separation of muscle (nontraumatic), left hand

    M62.049 Separation of muscle (nontraumatic), unspecified hand

✓6ᵗʰ **M62.05** Separation of muscle (nontraumatic), thigh

    M62.051 Separation of muscle (nontraumatic), right thigh

    M62.052 Separation of muscle (nontraumatic), left thigh

    M62.059 Separation of muscle (nontraumatic), unspecified thigh

✓6ᵗʰ **M62.06** Separation of muscle (nontraumatic), lower leg

    M62.061 Separation of muscle (nontraumatic), right lower leg

    M62.062 Separation of muscle (nontraumatic), left lower leg

    M62.069 Separation of muscle (nontraumatic), unspecified lower leg

✓6ᵗʰ **M62.07** Separation of muscle (nontraumatic), ankle and foot

    M62.071 Separation of muscle (nontraumatic), right ankle and foot

    M62.072 Separation of muscle (nontraumatic), left ankle and foot

    M62.079 Separation of muscle (nontraumatic), unspecified ankle and foot

  M62.08 Separation of muscle (nontraumatic), other site

✓5ᵗʰ **M62.1 Other rupture of muscle (nontraumatic)**

    EXCLUDES 1   traumatic rupture of muscle - see strain of muscle by body region

    EXCLUDES 2   rupture of tendon (M66.-)

  M62.10 Other rupture of muscle (nontraumatic), unspecified site

✓6ᵗʰ **M62.11** Other rupture of muscle (nontraumatic), shoulder

    M62.111 Other rupture of muscle (nontraumatic), right shoulder

    M62.112 Other rupture of muscle (nontraumatic), left shoulder

    M62.119 Other rupture of muscle (nontraumatic), unspecified shoulder

✓6ᵗʰ **M62.12** Other rupture of muscle (nontraumatic), upper arm

    M62.121 Other rupture of muscle (nontraumatic), right upper arm

    M62.122 Other rupture of muscle (nontraumatic), left upper arm

    M62.129 Other rupture of muscle (nontraumatic), unspecified upper arm

✓6ᵗʰ **M62.13** Other rupture of muscle (nontraumatic), forearm

    M62.131 Other rupture of muscle (nontraumatic), right forearm

    M62.132 Other rupture of muscle (nontraumatic), left forearm

    M62.139 Other rupture of muscle (nontraumatic), unspecified forearm

✓6ᵗʰ **M62.14** Other rupture of muscle (nontraumatic), hand

    M62.141 Other rupture of muscle (nontraumatic), right hand

    M62.142 Other rupture of muscle (nontraumatic), left hand

    M62.149 Other rupture of muscle (nontraumatic), unspecified hand

✓6ᵗʰ **M62.15** Other rupture of muscle (nontraumatic), thigh

    M62.151 Other rupture of muscle (nontraumatic), right thigh

    M62.152 Other rupture of muscle (nontraumatic), left thigh

    M62.159 Other rupture of muscle (nontraumatic), unspecified thigh

✓6ᵗʰ **M62.16** Other rupture of muscle (nontraumatic), lower leg

    M62.161 Other rupture of muscle (nontraumatic), right lower leg

    M62.162 Other rupture of muscle (nontraumatic), left lower leg

    M62.169 Other rupture of muscle (nontraumatic), unspecified lower leg

✓6ᵗʰ **M62.17** Other rupture of muscle (nontraumatic), ankle and foot

    M62.171 Other rupture of muscle (nontraumatic), right ankle and foot

    M62.172 Other rupture of muscle (nontraumatic), left ankle and foot

    M62.179 Other rupture of muscle (nontraumatic), unspecified ankle and foot

  M62.18 Other rupture of muscle (nontraumatic), other site

✓5ᵗʰ **M62.2 Nontraumatic ischemic infarction of muscle**

    EXCLUDES 1   compartment syndrome (traumatic) (T79.A-)

              nontraumatic compartment syndrome (M79.A-)

              rhabdomyolysis (M62.82)

              traumatic ischemia of muscle (T79.6)

              Volkmann's ischemic contracture (T79.6)

  M62.20 Nontraumatic ischemic infarction of muscle, unspecified site

✓6ᵗʰ **M62.21** Nontraumatic ischemic infarction of muscle, shoulder

    M62.211 Nontraumatic ischemic infarction of muscle, right shoulder

    M62.212 Nontraumatic ischemic infarction of muscle, left shoulder

    M62.219 Nontraumatic ischemic infarction of muscle, unspecified shoulder

✓6ᵗʰ **M62.22 Nontraumatic ischemic infarction of muscle, upper arm**
    M62.221 Nontraumatic ischemic infarction of muscle, right upper arm
    M62.222 Nontraumatic ischemic infarction of muscle, left upper arm
    M62.229 Nontraumatic ischemic infarction of muscle, unspecified upper arm

✓6ᵗʰ **M62.23 Nontraumatic ischemic infarction of muscle, forearm**
    M62.231 Nontraumatic ischemic infarction of muscle, right forearm
    M62.232 Nontraumatic ischemic infarction of muscle, left forearm
    M62.239 Nontraumatic ischemic infarction of muscle, unspecified forearm

✓6ᵗʰ **M62.24 Nontraumatic ischemic infarction of muscle, hand**
    M62.241 Nontraumatic ischemic infarction of muscle, right hand
    M62.242 Nontraumatic ischemic infarction of muscle, left hand
    M62.249 Nontraumatic ischemic infarction of muscle, unspecified hand

✓6ᵗʰ **M62.25 Nontraumatic ischemic infarction of muscle, thigh**
    M62.251 Nontraumatic ischemic infarction of muscle, right thigh
    M62.252 Nontraumatic ischemic infarction of muscle, left thigh
    M62.259 Nontraumatic ischemic infarction of muscle, unspecified thigh

✓6ᵗʰ **M62.26 Nontraumatic ischemic infarction of muscle, lower leg**
    M62.261 Nontraumatic ischemic infarction of muscle, right lower leg
    M62.262 Nontraumatic ischemic infarction of muscle, left lower leg
    M62.269 Nontraumatic ischemic infarction of muscle, unspecified lower leg

✓6ᵗʰ **M62.27 Nontraumatic ischemic infarction of muscle, ankle and foot**
    M62.271 Nontraumatic ischemic infarction of muscle, right ankle and foot
    M62.272 Nontraumatic ischemic infarction of muscle, left ankle and foot
    M62.279 Nontraumatic ischemic infarction of muscle, unspecified ankle and foot

M62.28 Nontraumatic ischemic infarction of muscle, other site

M62.3 Immobility syndrome (paraplegic)

✓5ᵗʰ **M62.4 Contracture of muscle**
  Contracture of tendon (sheath)
  EXCLUDES 1 contracture of joint (M24.5-)
  M62.40 Contracture of muscle, unspecified site

✓6ᵗʰ **M62.41 Contracture of muscle, shoulder**
    M62.411 Contracture of muscle, right shoulder
    M62.412 Contracture of muscle, left shoulder
    M62.419 Contracture of muscle, unspecified shoulder

✓6ᵗʰ **M62.42 Contracture of muscle, upper arm**
    M62.421 Contracture of muscle, right upper arm
    M62.422 Contracture of muscle, left upper arm
    M62.429 Contracture of muscle, unspecified upper arm

✓6ᵗʰ **M62.43 Contracture of muscle, forearm**
    M62.431 Contracture of muscle, right forearm
    M62.432 Contracture of muscle, left forearm
    M62.439 Contracture of muscle, unspecified forearm

✓6ᵗʰ **M62.44 Contracture of muscle, hand**
    M62.441 Contracture of muscle, right hand
    M62.442 Contracture of muscle, left hand
    M62.449 Contracture of muscle, unspecified hand

✓6ᵗʰ **M62.45 Contracture of muscle, thigh**
    M62.451 Contracture of muscle, right thigh
    M62.452 Contracture of muscle, left thigh
    M62.459 Contracture of muscle, unspecified thigh

✓6ᵗʰ **M62.46 Contracture of muscle, lower leg**
    M62.461 Contracture of muscle, right lower leg
    M62.462 Contracture of muscle, left lower leg

    M62.469 Contracture of muscle, unspecified lower leg

✓6ᵗʰ **M62.47 Contracture of muscle, ankle and foot**
    M62.471 Contracture of muscle, right ankle and foot
    M62.472 Contracture of muscle, left ankle and foot
    M62.479 Contracture of muscle, unspecified ankle and foot

M62.48 Contracture of muscle, other site
M62.49 Contracture of muscle, multiple sites

✓6ᵗʰ **M62.5 Muscle wasting and atrophy, not elsewhere classified**
  Disuse atrophy NEC
  EXCLUDES 1 neuralgic amyotrophy (G54.5)
    progressive muscular atrophy (G12.21)
    sarcopenia (M62.84)
  EXCLUDES 2 pelvic muscle wasting (N81.84)

M62.50 Muscle wasting and atrophy, not elsewhere classified, unspecified site

✓6ᵗʰ **M62.51 Muscle wasting and atrophy, not elsewhere classified, shoulder**
    M62.511 Muscle wasting and atrophy, not elsewhere classified, right shoulder
    M62.512 Muscle wasting and atrophy, not elsewhere classified, left shoulder
    M62.519 Muscle wasting and atrophy, not elsewhere classified, unspecified shoulder

✓6ᵗʰ **M62.52 Muscle wasting and atrophy, not elsewhere classified, upper arm**
    M62.521 Muscle wasting and atrophy, not elsewhere classified, right upper arm
    M62.522 Muscle wasting and atrophy, not elsewhere classified, left upper arm
    M62.529 Muscle wasting and atrophy, not elsewhere classified, unspecified upper arm

✓6ᵗʰ **M62.53 Muscle wasting and atrophy, not elsewhere classified, forearm**
    M62.531 Muscle wasting and atrophy, not elsewhere classified, right forearm
    M62.532 Muscle wasting and atrophy, not elsewhere classified, left forearm
    M62.539 Muscle wasting and atrophy, not elsewhere classified, unspecified forearm

✓6ᵗʰ **M62.54 Muscle wasting and atrophy, not elsewhere classified, hand**
    M62.541 Muscle wasting and atrophy, not elsewhere classified, right hand
    M62.542 Muscle wasting and atrophy, not elsewhere classified, left hand
    M62.549 Muscle wasting and atrophy, not elsewhere classified, unspecified hand

✓6ᵗʰ **M62.55 Muscle wasting and atrophy, not elsewhere classified, thigh**
    M62.551 Muscle wasting and atrophy, not elsewhere classified, right thigh
    M62.552 Muscle wasting and atrophy, not elsewhere classified, left thigh
    M62.559 Muscle wasting and atrophy, not elsewhere classified, unspecified thigh

✓6ᵗʰ **M62.56 Muscle wasting and atrophy, not elsewhere classified, lower leg**
    M62.561 Muscle wasting and atrophy, not elsewhere classified, right lower leg
    M62.562 Muscle wasting and atrophy, not elsewhere classified, left lower leg
    M62.569 Muscle wasting and atrophy, not elsewhere classified, unspecified lower leg

✓6ᵗʰ **M62.57 Muscle wasting and atrophy, not elsewhere classified, ankle and foot**
    M62.571 Muscle wasting and atrophy, not elsewhere classified, right ankle and foot
    M62.572 Muscle wasting and atrophy, not elsewhere classified, left ankle and foot
    M62.579 Muscle wasting and atrophy, not elsewhere classified, unspecified ankle and foot

M62.58 Muscle wasting and atrophy, not elsewhere classified, other site
M62.59 Muscle wasting and atrophy, not elsewhere classified, multiple sites

- ✓6ᵗʰ **M62.5A** **Muscle wasting and atrophy, not elsewhere classified,** back
- **M62.5A0** **Muscle wasting and atrophy, not elsewhere classified, back,** cervical
- **M62.5A1** **Muscle wasting and atrophy, not elsewhere classified, back,** thoracic
- **M62.5A2** **Muscle wasting and atrophy, not elsewhere classified, back,** lumbosacral
- **M62.5A9** **Muscle wasting and atrophy, not elsewhere classified, back, unspecified level**

✓5ᵗʰ **M62.8** **Other specified disorders of muscle**
> EXCLUDES 2   nontraumatic hematoma of muscle (M79.81)

    M62.81 **Muscle weakness (generalized)**
> EXCLUDES 1   muscle weakness in sarcopenia (M62.84)

    M62.82 **Rhabdomyolysis**
> EXCLUDES 1   traumatic rhabdomyolysis (T79.6)

     AHA: 2019,2Q,12
     DEF: Rapid disintegration or destruction of skeletal muscle caused by direct or indirect injury, resulting in the excretion of muscle protein myoglobin into the urine.

    ✓6ᵗʰ **M62.83** **Muscle spasm**
     M62.830 **Muscle spasm of** back
     M62.831 **Muscle spasm of** calf
       Charley-horse
     M62.838 **Other muscle spasm**

    M62.84 **Sarcopenia**
     Age-related sarcopenia
     Code first underlying disease, if applicable, such as:
       disorders of myoneural junction and muscle disease in diseases classified elsewhere (G73.-)
       other and unspecified myopathies (G72.-)
       primary disorders of muscles (G71.-)
     AHA: 2016,4Q,41

    M62.89 **Other specified disorders of muscle**
     Muscle (sheath) hernia

    M62.9 **Disorder of muscle, unspecified**

✓4ᵗʰ **M63** **Disorders of muscle in diseases classified elsewhere**
    Code first underlying disease, such as:
     leprosy (A30.-)
     neoplasm (C49.-, C79.89, D21.-, D48.1)
     schistosomiasis (B65.-)
     trichinellosis (B75)
> EXCLUDES 1   myopathy in cysticercosis (B69.81)
> myopathy in endocrine diseases (G73.7)
> myopathy in metabolic diseases (G73.7)
> myopathy in sarcoidosis (D86.87)
> myopathy in secondary syphilis (A51.49)
> myopathy in syphilis (late) (A52.78)
> myopathy in toxoplasmosis (B58.82)
> myopathy in tuberculosis (A18.09)

✓5ᵗʰ **M63.8** **Disorders of muscle in diseases classified elsewhere**
    M63.80 *Disorders of muscle in diseases classified elsewhere, unspecified site*
    ✓6ᵗʰ **M63.81** **Disorders of muscle in diseases classified elsewhere,** shoulder
     M63.811 *Disorders of muscle in diseases classified elsewhere, right shoulder*
     M63.812 *Disorders of muscle in diseases classified elsewhere, left shoulder*
     M63.819 *Disorders of muscle in diseases classified elsewhere, unspecified shoulder*
    ✓6ᵗʰ **M63.82** **Disorders of muscle in diseases classified elsewhere,** upper arm
     M63.821 *Disorders of muscle in diseases classified elsewhere, right upper arm*
     M63.822 *Disorders of muscle in diseases classified elsewhere, left upper arm*
     M63.829 *Disorders of muscle in diseases classified elsewhere, unspecified upper arm*
    ✓6ᵗʰ **M63.83** **Disorders of muscle in diseases classified elsewhere,** forearm
     M63.831 *Disorders of muscle in diseases classified elsewhere, right forearm*
     M63.832 *Disorders of muscle in diseases classified elsewhere, left forearm*
     M63.839 *Disorders of muscle in diseases classified elsewhere, unspecified forearm*

    ✓6ᵗʰ **M63.84** **Disorders of muscle in diseases classified elsewhere,** hand
     M63.841 *Disorders of muscle in diseases classified elsewhere, right hand*
     M63.842 *Disorders of muscle in diseases classified elsewhere, left hand*
     M63.849 *Disorders of muscle in diseases classified elsewhere, unspecified hand*
    ✓6ᵗʰ **M63.85** **Disorders of muscle in diseases classified elsewhere,** thigh
     M63.851 *Disorders of muscle in diseases classified elsewhere, right thigh*
     M63.852 *Disorders of muscle in diseases classified elsewhere, left thigh*
     M63.859 *Disorders of muscle in diseases classified elsewhere, unspecified thigh*
    ✓6ᵗʰ **M63.86** **Disorders of muscle in diseases classified elsewhere,** lower leg
     M63.861 *Disorders of muscle in diseases classified elsewhere, right lower leg*
     M63.862 *Disorders of muscle in diseases classified elsewhere, left lower leg*
     M63.869 *Disorders of muscle in diseases classified elsewhere, unspecified lower leg*
    ✓6ᵗʰ **M63.87** **Disorders of muscle in diseases classified elsewhere,** ankle and foot
     M63.871 *Disorders of muscle in diseases classified elsewhere, right ankle and foot*
     M63.872 *Disorders of muscle in diseases classified elsewhere, left ankle and foot*
     M63.879 *Disorders of muscle in diseases classified elsewhere, unspecified ankle and foot*
    M63.88 *Disorders of muscle in diseases classified elsewhere, other site*
    M63.89 *Disorders of muscle in diseases classified elsewhere, multiple sites*

Disorders of synovium and tendon (M65-M67)

✓4ᵗʰ **M65** **Synovitis and tenosynovitis**
> EXCLUDES 1   chronic crepitant synovitis of hand and wrist (M70.0-)
> current injury - see injury of ligament or tendon by body region
> soft tissue disorders related to use, overuse and pressure (M70.-)

✓5ᵗʰ **M65.0** **Abscess of tendon sheath**
    Use additional code (B95-B96) to identify bacterial agent.
    M65.00 **Abscess of tendon sheath, unspecified site**
    ✓6ᵗʰ **M65.01** **Abscess of tendon sheath,** shoulder
     M65.011 **Abscess of tendon sheath,** right shoulder
     M65.012 **Abscess of tendon sheath,** left shoulder
     M65.019 **Abscess of tendon sheath, unspecified shoulder**
    ✓6ᵗʰ **M65.02** **Abscess of tendon sheath,** upper arm
     M65.021 **Abscess of tendon sheath,** right upper arm
     M65.022 **Abscess of tendon sheath,** left upper arm
     M65.029 **Abscess of tendon sheath, unspecified upper arm**
    ✓6ᵗʰ **M65.03** **Abscess of tendon sheath,** forearm
     M65.031 **Abscess of tendon sheath,** right forearm
     M65.032 **Abscess of tendon sheath,** left forearm
     M65.039 **Abscess of tendon sheath, unspecified forearm**
    ✓6ᵗʰ **M65.04** **Abscess of tendon sheath,** hand
     M65.041 **Abscess of tendon sheath,** right hand
     M65.042 **Abscess of tendon sheath,** left hand
     M65.049 **Abscess of tendon sheath, unspecified hand**
    ✓6ᵗʰ **M65.05** **Abscess of tendon sheath,** thigh
     M65.051 **Abscess of tendon sheath,** right thigh
     M65.052 **Abscess of tendon sheath,** left thigh
     M65.059 **Abscess of tendon sheath, unspecified thigh**
    ✓6ᵗʰ **M65.06** **Abscess of tendon sheath,** lower leg
     M65.061 **Abscess of tendon sheath,** right lower leg
     M65.062 **Abscess of tendon sheath,** left lower leg
     M65.069 **Abscess of tendon sheath, unspecified lower leg**

✓6ᵗʰ **M65.Ø7** Abscess of tendon sheath, ankle and foot
- **M65.Ø71** Abscess of tendon sheath, right ankle and foot
- **M65.Ø72** Abscess of tendon sheath, left ankle and foot
- **M65.Ø79** Abscess of tendon sheath, unspecified ankle and foot

M65.Ø8 Abscess of tendon sheath, other site

✓5ᵗʰ **M65.1** Other infective (teno)synovitis
- **M65.1Ø** Other infective (teno)synovitis, unspecified site
- ✓6ᵗʰ **M65.11** Other infective (teno)synovitis, shoulder
  - **M65.111** Other infective (teno)synovitis, right shoulder
  - **M65.112** Other infective (teno)synovitis, left shoulder
  - **M65.119** Other infective (teno)synovitis, unspecified shoulder
- ✓6ᵗʰ **M65.12** Other infective (teno)synovitis, elbow
  - **M65.121** Other infective (teno)synovitis, right elbow
  - **M65.122** Other infective (teno)synovitis, left elbow
  - **M65.129** Other infective (teno)synovitis, unspecified elbow
- ✓6ᵗʰ **M65.13** Other infective (teno)synovitis, wrist
  - **M65.131** Other infective (teno)synovitis, right wrist
  - **M65.132** Other infective (teno)synovitis, left wrist
  - **M65.139** Other infective (teno)synovitis, unspecified wrist
- ✓6ᵗʰ **M65.14** Other infective (teno)synovitis, hand
  - **M65.141** Other infective (teno)synovitis, right hand
  - **M65.142** Other infective (teno)synovitis, left hand
  - **M65.149** Other infective (teno)synovitis, unspecified hand
- ✓6ᵗʰ **M65.15** Other infective (teno)synovitis, hip
  - **M65.151** Other infective (teno)synovitis, right hip
  - **M65.152** Other infective (teno)synovitis, left hip
  - **M65.159** Other infective (teno)synovitis, unspecified hip
- ✓6ᵗʰ **M65.16** Other infective (teno)synovitis, knee
  - **M65.161** Other infective (teno)synovitis, right knee
  - **M65.162** Other infective (teno)synovitis, left knee
  - **M65.169** Other infective (teno)synovitis, unspecified knee
- ✓6ᵗʰ **M65.17** Other infective (teno)synovitis, ankle and foot
  - **M65.171** Other infective (teno)synovitis, right ankle and foot
  - **M65.172** Other infective (teno)synovitis, left ankle and foot
  - **M65.179** Other infective (teno)synovitis, unspecified ankle and foot

M65.18 Other infective (teno)synovitis, other site

M65.19 Other infective (teno)synovitis, multiple sites

✓5ᵗʰ **M65.2** Calcific tendinitis
- **EXCLUDES 1** tendinitis as classified in M75-M77
  calcified tendinitis of shoulder (M75.3)
- **M65.2Ø** Calcific tendinitis, unspecified site
- ✓6ᵗʰ **M65.22** Calcific tendinitis, upper arm
  - **M65.221** Calcific tendinitis, right upper arm
  - **M65.222** Calcific tendinitis, left upper arm
  - **M65.229** Calcific tendinitis, unspecified upper arm
- ✓6ᵗʰ **M65.23** Calcific tendinitis, forearm
  - **M65.231** Calcific tendinitis, right forearm
  - **M65.232** Calcific tendinitis, left forearm
  - **M65.239** Calcific tendinitis, unspecified forearm
- ✓6ᵗʰ **M65.24** Calcific tendinitis, hand
  - **M65.241** Calcific tendinitis, right hand
  - **M65.242** Calcific tendinitis, left hand
  - **M65.249** Calcific tendinitis, unspecified hand
- ✓6ᵗʰ **M65.25** Calcific tendinitis, thigh
  - **M65.251** Calcific tendinitis, right thigh
  - **M65.252** Calcific tendinitis, left thigh
  - **M65.259** Calcific tendinitis, unspecified thigh
- ✓6ᵗʰ **M65.26** Calcific tendinitis, lower leg
  - **M65.261** Calcific tendinitis, right lower leg
  - **M65.262** Calcific tendinitis, left lower leg
  - **M65.269** Calcific tendinitis, unspecified lower leg

✓6ᵗʰ **M65.27** Calcific tendinitis, ankle and foot
- **M65.271** Calcific tendinitis, right ankle and foot
- **M65.272** Calcific tendinitis, left ankle and foot
- **M65.279** Calcific tendinitis, unspecified ankle and foot

M65.28 Calcific tendinitis, other site

M65.29 Calcific tendinitis, multiple sites

✓6ᵗʰ **M65.3** Trigger finger
- Nodular tendinous disease
- **M65.3Ø** Trigger finger, unspecified finger
- ✓6ᵗʰ **M65.31** Trigger thumb
  - **M65.311** Trigger thumb, right thumb
  - **M65.312** Trigger thumb, left thumb
  - **M65.319** Trigger thumb, unspecified thumb
- ✓6ᵗʰ **M65.32** Trigger finger, index finger
  - **M65.321** Trigger finger, right index finger
  - **M65.322** Trigger finger, left index finger
  - **M65.329** Trigger finger, unspecified index finger
- ✓6ᵗʰ **M65.33** Trigger finger, middle finger
  - **M65.331** Trigger finger, right middle finger
  - **M65.332** Trigger finger, left middle finger
  - **M65.339** Trigger finger, unspecified middle finger
- ✓6ᵗʰ **M65.34** Trigger finger, ring finger
  - **M65.341** Trigger finger, right ring finger
  - **M65.342** Trigger finger, left ring finger
  - **M65.349** Trigger finger, unspecified ring finger
- ✓6ᵗʰ **M65.35** Trigger finger, little finger
  - **M65.351** Trigger finger, right little finger
  - **M65.352** Trigger finger, left little finger
  - **M65.359** Trigger finger, unspecified little finger

M65.4 Radial styloid tenosynovitis [de Quervain]

✓5ᵗʰ **M65.8** Other synovitis and tenosynovitis
- **M65.8Ø** Other synovitis and tenosynovitis, unspecified site
- ✓6ᵗʰ **M65.81** Other synovitis and tenosynovitis, shoulder
  - **M65.811** Other synovitis and tenosynovitis, right shoulder
  - **M65.812** Other synovitis and tenosynovitis, left shoulder
  - **M65.819** Other synovitis and tenosynovitis, unspecified shoulder
- ✓6ᵗʰ **M65.82** Other synovitis and tenosynovitis, upper arm
  - **M65.821** Other synovitis and tenosynovitis, right upper arm
  - **M65.822** Other synovitis and tenosynovitis, left upper arm
  - **M65.829** Other synovitis and tenosynovitis, unspecified upper arm
- ✓6ᵗʰ **M65.83** Other synovitis and tenosynovitis, forearm
  - **M65.831** Other synovitis and tenosynovitis, right forearm
  - **M65.832** Other synovitis and tenosynovitis, left forearm
  - **M65.839** Other synovitis and tenosynovitis, unspecified forearm
- ✓6ᵗʰ **M65.84** Other synovitis and tenosynovitis, hand
  - **M65.841** Other synovitis and tenosynovitis, right hand
  - **M65.842** Other synovitis and tenosynovitis, left hand
  - **M65.849** Other synovitis and tenosynovitis, unspecified hand
- ✓6ᵗʰ **M65.85** Other synovitis and tenosynovitis, thigh
  - **M65.851** Other synovitis and tenosynovitis, right thigh
  - **M65.852** Other synovitis and tenosynovitis, left thigh
  - **M65.859** Other synovitis and tenosynovitis, unspecified thigh
- ✓6ᵗʰ **M65.86** Other synovitis and tenosynovitis, lower leg
  - **M65.861** Other synovitis and tenosynovitis, right lower leg
  - **M65.862** Other synovitis and tenosynovitis, left lower leg
  - **M65.869** Other synovitis and tenosynovitis, unspecified lower leg
- ✓6ᵗʰ **M65.87** Other synovitis and tenosynovitis, ankle and foot
  - **M65.871** Other synovitis and tenosynovitis, right ankle and foot

M65.872 **Other synovitis and tenosynovitis,** left **ankle and foot**
M65.879 **Other synovitis and tenosynovitis, unspecified ankle and foot**
M65.88 **Other synovitis and tenosynovitis, other site**
M65.89 **Other synovitis and tenosynovitis,** multiple sites
M65.9 Synovitis and tenosynovitis, unspecified

✅4ᵗʰ **M66 Spontaneous rupture of synovium and tendon**

INCLUDES   rupture that occurs when a normal force is applied to tissues that are inferred to have less than normal strength

EXCLUDES 2   rotator cuff syndrome (M75.1-)
rupture where an abnormal force is applied to normal tissue - see injury of tendon by body region

M66.0 Rupture of popliteal cyst
✅5ᵗʰ **M66.1 Rupture of** synovium
Rupture of synovial cyst
EXCLUDES 2   rupture of popliteal cyst (M66.0)
M66.10 **Rupture of synovium, unspecified joint**
✅6ᵗʰ M66.11 **Rupture of synovium,** shoulder
M66.111 **Rupture of synovium,** right **shoulder**
M66.112 **Rupture of synovium,** left **shoulder**
M66.119 **Rupture of synovium, unspecified shoulder**
✅6ᵗʰ M66.12 **Rupture of synovium,** elbow
M66.121 **Rupture of synovium,** right **elbow**
M66.122 **Rupture of synovium,** left **elbow**
M66.129 **Rupture of synovium, unspecified elbow**
✅6ᵗʰ M66.13 **Rupture of synovium,** wrist
M66.131 **Rupture of synovium,** right **wrist**
M66.132 **Rupture of synovium,** left **wrist**
M66.139 **Rupture of synovium, unspecified wrist**
✅6ᵗʰ M66.14 **Rupture of synovium,** hand and fingers
M66.141 **Rupture of synovium,** right **hand**
M66.142 **Rupture of synovium,** left **hand**
M66.143 **Rupture of synovium, unspecified hand**
M66.144 **Rupture of synovium,** right **finger(s)**
M66.145 **Rupture of synovium,** left **finger(s)**
M66.146 **Rupture of synovium, unspecified finger(s)**
✅6ᵗʰ M66.15 **Rupture of synovium,** hip
M66.151 **Rupture of synovium,** right **hip**
M66.152 **Rupture of synovium,** left **hip**
M66.159 **Rupture of synovium, unspecified hip**
✅6ᵗʰ M66.17 **Rupture of synovium,** ankle, foot and toes
M66.171 **Rupture of synovium,** right **ankle**
M66.172 **Rupture of synovium,** left **ankle**
M66.173 **Rupture of synovium, unspecified ankle**
M66.174 **Rupture of synovium,** right **foot**
M66.175 **Rupture of synovium,** left **foot**
M66.176 **Rupture of synovium, unspecified foot**
M66.177 **Rupture of synovium,** right **toe(s)**
M66.178 **Rupture of synovium,** left **toe(s)**
M66.179 **Rupture of synovium, unspecified toe(s)**
M66.18 **Rupture of synovium, other site**
✅5ᵗʰ **M66.2 Spontaneous rupture of** extensor tendons
TIP: Refer to the Muscle/Tendon table at the beginning of this chapter.
M66.20 **Spontaneous rupture of extensor tendons, unspecified site**
✅6ᵗʰ M66.21 **Spontaneous rupture of extensor tendons,** shoulder
M66.211 **Spontaneous rupture of extensor tendons,** right **shoulder**
M66.212 **Spontaneous rupture of extensor tendons,** left **shoulder**
M66.219 **Spontaneous rupture of extensor tendons, unspecified shoulder**
✅6ᵗʰ M66.22 **Spontaneous rupture of extensor tendons,** upper arm
M66.221 **Spontaneous rupture of extensor tendons,** right **upper arm**
M66.222 **Spontaneous rupture of extensor tendons,** left **upper arm**
M66.229 **Spontaneous rupture of extensor tendons, unspecified upper arm**

✅6ᵗʰ M66.23 **Spontaneous rupture of extensor tendons,** forearm
M66.231 **Spontaneous rupture of extensor tendons,** right **forearm**
M66.232 **Spontaneous rupture of extensor tendons,** left **forearm**
M66.239 **Spontaneous rupture of extensor tendons, unspecified forearm**
✅6ᵗʰ M66.24 **Spontaneous rupture of extensor tendons,** hand
M66.241 **Spontaneous rupture of extensor tendons,** right **hand**
M66.242 **Spontaneous rupture of extensor tendons,** left **hand**
M66.249 **Spontaneous rupture of extensor tendons, unspecified hand**
✅6ᵗʰ M66.25 **Spontaneous rupture of extensor tendons,** thigh
M66.251 **Spontaneous rupture of extensor tendons,** right **thigh**
M66.252 **Spontaneous rupture of extensor tendons,** left **thigh**
M66.259 **Spontaneous rupture of extensor tendons, unspecified thigh**
✅6ᵗʰ M66.26 **Spontaneous rupture of extensor tendons,** lower leg
M66.261 **Spontaneous rupture of extensor tendons,** right **lower leg**
M66.262 **Spontaneous rupture of extensor tendons,** left **lower leg**
M66.269 **Spontaneous rupture of extensor tendons, unspecified lower leg**
✅6ᵗʰ M66.27 **Spontaneous rupture of extensor tendons,** ankle and foot
M66.271 **Spontaneous rupture of extensor tendons,** right **ankle and foot**
M66.272 **Spontaneous rupture of extensor tendons,** left **ankle and foot**
M66.279 **Spontaneous rupture of extensor tendons, unspecified ankle and foot**
M66.28 **Spontaneous rupture of extensor tendons, other site**
M66.29 **Spontaneous rupture of extensor tendons,** multiple sites
✅5ᵗʰ **M66.3 Spontaneous rupture of** flexor tendons
TIP: Refer to the Muscle/Tendon table at the beginning of this chapter.
M66.30 **Spontaneous rupture of flexor tendons, unspecified site**
✅6ᵗʰ M66.31 **Spontaneous rupture of flexor tendons,** shoulder
M66.311 **Spontaneous rupture of flexor tendons,** right **shoulder**
M66.312 **Spontaneous rupture of flexor tendons,** left **shoulder**
M66.319 **Spontaneous rupture of flexor tendons, unspecified shoulder**
✅6ᵗʰ M66.32 **Spontaneous rupture of flexor tendons,** upper arm
M66.321 **Spontaneous rupture of flexor tendons,** right **upper arm**
M66.322 **Spontaneous rupture of flexor tendons,** left **upper arm**
M66.329 **Spontaneous rupture of flexor tendons, unspecified upper arm**
✅6ᵗʰ M66.33 **Spontaneous rupture of flexor tendons,** forearm
M66.331 **Spontaneous rupture of flexor tendons,** right **forearm**
M66.332 **Spontaneous rupture of flexor tendons,** left **forearm**
M66.339 **Spontaneous rupture of flexor tendons, unspecified forearm**
✅6ᵗʰ M66.34 **Spontaneous rupture of flexor tendons,** hand
M66.341 **Spontaneous rupture of flexor tendons,** right **hand**
M66.342 **Spontaneous rupture of flexor tendons,** left **hand**
M66.349 **Spontaneous rupture of flexor tendons, unspecified hand**
✅6ᵗʰ M66.35 **Spontaneous rupture of flexor tendons,** thigh
M66.351 **Spontaneous rupture of flexor tendons,** right **thigh**
M66.352 **Spontaneous rupture of flexor tendons,** left **thigh**
M66.359 **Spontaneous rupture of flexor tendons, unspecified thigh**

✓6ᵗʰ **M66.36** Spontaneous rupture of flexor tendons, lower leg
    M66.361 Spontaneous rupture of flexor tendons, right lower leg
    M66.362 Spontaneous rupture of flexor tendons, left lower leg
    M66.369 Spontaneous rupture of flexor tendons, unspecified lower leg

✓6ᵗʰ **M66.37** Spontaneous rupture of flexor tendons, ankle and foot
    M66.371 Spontaneous rupture of flexor tendons, right ankle and foot
    M66.372 Spontaneous rupture of flexor tendons, left ankle and foot
    M66.379 Spontaneous rupture of flexor tendons, unspecified ankle and foot

M66.38 Spontaneous rupture of flexor tendons, other site
M66.39 Spontaneous rupture of flexor tendons, multiple sites

✓5ᵗʰ **M66.8** Spontaneous rupture of other tendons
    TIP: Refer to the Muscle/Tendon table at the beginning of this chapter.
    M66.80 Spontaneous rupture of other tendons, unspecified site

✓6ᵗʰ **M66.81** Spontaneous rupture of other tendons, shoulder
    M66.811 Spontaneous rupture of other tendons, right shoulder
    M66.812 Spontaneous rupture of other tendons, left shoulder
    M66.819 Spontaneous rupture of other tendons, unspecified shoulder

✓6ᵗʰ **M66.82** Spontaneous rupture of other tendons, upper arm
    M66.821 Spontaneous rupture of other tendons, right upper arm
    M66.822 Spontaneous rupture of other tendons, left upper arm
    M66.829 Spontaneous rupture of other tendons, unspecified upper arm

✓6ᵗʰ **M66.83** Spontaneous rupture of other tendons, forearm
    M66.831 Spontaneous rupture of other tendons, right forearm
    M66.832 Spontaneous rupture of other tendons, left forearm
    M66.839 Spontaneous rupture of other tendons, unspecified forearm

✓6ᵗʰ **M66.84** Spontaneous rupture of other tendons, hand
    M66.841 Spontaneous rupture of other tendons, right hand
    M66.842 Spontaneous rupture of other tendons, left hand
    M66.849 Spontaneous rupture of other tendons, unspecified hand

✓6ᵗʰ **M66.85** Spontaneous rupture of other tendons, thigh
    M66.851 Spontaneous rupture of other tendons, right thigh
    M66.852 Spontaneous rupture of other tendons, left thigh
    M66.859 Spontaneous rupture of other tendons, unspecified thigh

✓6ᵗʰ **M66.86** Spontaneous rupture of other tendons, lower leg
    M66.861 Spontaneous rupture of other tendons, right lower leg
    M66.862 Spontaneous rupture of other tendons, left lower leg
    M66.869 Spontaneous rupture of other tendons, unspecified lower leg

✓6ᵗʰ **M66.87** Spontaneous rupture of other tendons, ankle and foot
    M66.871 Spontaneous rupture of other tendons, right ankle and foot
    M66.872 Spontaneous rupture of other tendons, left ankle and foot
    M66.879 Spontaneous rupture of other tendons, unspecified ankle and foot

M66.88 Spontaneous rupture of other tendons, other sites
M66.89 Spontaneous rupture of other tendons, multiple sites

M66.9 Spontaneous rupture of unspecified tendon
    Rupture at musculotendinous junction, nontraumatic

✓4ᵗʰ **M67** Other disorders of synovium and tendon
    EXCLUDES 1 palmar fascial fibromatosis [Dupuytren] (M72.0)
       tendinitis NOS (M77.9-)
       xanthomatosis localized to tendons (E78.2)

✓5ᵗʰ **M67.0** Short Achilles tendon (acquired)
    M67.00 Short Achilles tendon (acquired), unspecified ankle
    M67.01 Short Achilles tendon (acquired), right ankle
    M67.02 Short Achilles tendon (acquired), left ankle

✓5ᵗʰ **M67.2** Synovial hypertrophy, not elsewhere classified
    EXCLUDES 1 villonodular synovitis (pigmented) (M12.2-)
    M67.20 Synovial hypertrophy, not elsewhere classified, unspecified site

✓6ᵗʰ **M67.21** Synovial hypertrophy, not elsewhere classified, shoulder
    M67.211 Synovial hypertrophy, not elsewhere classified, right shoulder
    M67.212 Synovial hypertrophy, not elsewhere classified, left shoulder
    M67.219 Synovial hypertrophy, not elsewhere classified, unspecified shoulder

✓6ᵗʰ **M67.22** Synovial hypertrophy, not elsewhere classified, upper arm
    M67.221 Synovial hypertrophy, not elsewhere classified, right upper arm
    M67.222 Synovial hypertrophy, not elsewhere classified, left upper arm
    M67.229 Synovial hypertrophy, not elsewhere classified, unspecified upper arm

✓6ᵗʰ **M67.23** Synovial hypertrophy, not elsewhere classified, forearm
    M67.231 Synovial hypertrophy, not elsewhere classified, right forearm
    M67.232 Synovial hypertrophy, not elsewhere classified, left forearm
    M67.239 Synovial hypertrophy, not elsewhere classified, unspecified forearm

✓6ᵗʰ **M67.24** Synovial hypertrophy, not elsewhere classified, hand
    M67.241 Synovial hypertrophy, not elsewhere classified, right hand
    M67.242 Synovial hypertrophy, not elsewhere classified, left hand
    M67.249 Synovial hypertrophy, not elsewhere classified, unspecified hand

✓6ᵗʰ **M67.25** Synovial hypertrophy, not elsewhere classified, thigh
    M67.251 Synovial hypertrophy, not elsewhere classified, right thigh
    M67.252 Synovial hypertrophy, not elsewhere classified, left thigh
    M67.259 Synovial hypertrophy, not elsewhere classified, unspecified thigh

✓6ᵗʰ **M67.26** Synovial hypertrophy, not elsewhere classified, lower leg
    M67.261 Synovial hypertrophy, not elsewhere classified, right lower leg
    M67.262 Synovial hypertrophy, not elsewhere classified, left lower leg
    M67.269 Synovial hypertrophy, not elsewhere classified, unspecified lower leg

✓6ᵗʰ **M67.27** Synovial hypertrophy, not elsewhere classified, ankle and foot
    M67.271 Synovial hypertrophy, not elsewhere classified, right ankle and foot
    M67.272 Synovial hypertrophy, not elsewhere classified, left ankle and foot
    M67.279 Synovial hypertrophy, not elsewhere classified, unspecified ankle and foot

M67.28 Synovial hypertrophy, not elsewhere classified, other site
M67.29 Synovial hypertrophy, not elsewhere classified, multiple sites

✓5ᵗʰ **M67.3** Transient synovitis
    Toxic synovitis
    EXCLUDES 1 palindromic rheumatism (M12.3-)
    M67.30 Transient synovitis, unspecified site

✓6ᵗʰ **M67.31** Transient synovitis, shoulder
    M67.311 Transient synovitis, right shoulder
    M67.312 Transient synovitis, left shoulder
    M67.319 Transient synovitis, unspecified shoulder

✓6ᵗʰ **M67.32** **Transient synovitis,** elbow

    M67.321 **Transient synovitis,** right **elbow**
    M67.322 **Transient synovitis,** left **elbow**
    M67.329 **Transient synovitis, unspecified elbow**

✓6ᵗʰ **M67.33** **Transient synovitis,** wrist

    M67.331 **Transient synovitis,** right **wrist**
    M67.332 **Transient synovitis,** left **wrist**
    M67.339 **Transient synovitis, unspecified wrist**

✓6ᵗʰ **M67.34** **Transient synovitis,** hand

    M67.341 **Transient synovitis,** right **hand**
    M67.342 **Transient synovitis,** left **hand**
    M67.349 **Transient synovitis, unspecified hand**

✓6ᵗʰ **M67.35** **Transient synovitis,** hip

    M67.351 **Transient synovitis,** right **hip**
    M67.352 **Transient synovitis,** left **hip**
    M67.359 **Transient synovitis, unspecified hip**

✓6ᵗʰ **M67.36** **Transient synovitis,** knee

    M67.361 **Transient synovitis,** right **knee**
    M67.362 **Transient synovitis,** left **knee**
    M67.369 **Transient synovitis, unspecified knee**

✓6ᵗʰ **M67.37** **Transient synovitis,** ankle and foot

    M67.371 **Transient synovitis,** right **ankle and foot**
    M67.372 **Transient synovitis,** left **ankle and foot**
    M67.379 **Transient synovitis, unspecified ankle and foot**

    M67.38 **Transient synovitis, other site**
    M67.39 **Transient synovitis,** multiple sites

✓5ᵗʰ **M67.4** **Ganglion**

    Ganglion of joint or tendon (sheath)

    EXCLUDES 1   ganglion in yaws (A66.6)
    EXCLUDES 2   cyst of bursa (M71.2-M71.3)
            cyst of synovium (M71.2-M71.3)

    DEF: Fluid-filled, benign cyst appearing on a tendon sheath or aponeurosis, frequently connecting to an underlying joint.

    M67.40 **Ganglion, unspecified site**

✓6ᵗʰ **M67.41** **Ganglion,** shoulder

    M67.411 **Ganglion,** right **shoulder**
    M67.412 **Ganglion,** left **shoulder**
    M67.419 **Ganglion, unspecified shoulder**

✓6ᵗʰ **M67.42** **Ganglion,** elbow

    M67.421 **Ganglion,** right **elbow**
    M67.422 **Ganglion,** left **elbow**
    M67.429 **Ganglion, unspecified elbow**

✓6ᵗʰ **M67.43** **Ganglion,** wrist

Ganglion of Wrist

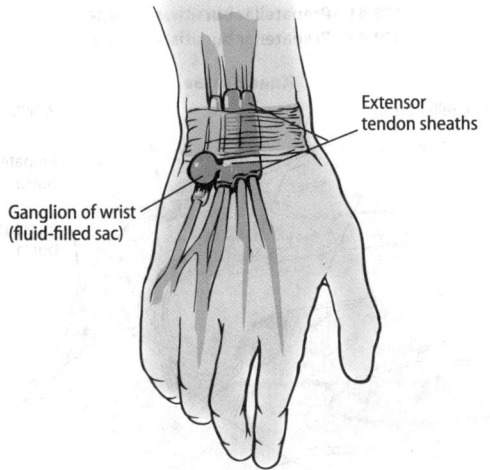

Extensor tendon sheaths

Ganglion of wrist (fluid-filled sac)

    M67.431 **Ganglion,** right **wrist**
    M67.432 **Ganglion,** left **wrist**
    M67.439 **Ganglion, unspecified wrist**

✓6ᵗʰ **M67.44** **Ganglion,** hand

    M67.441 **Ganglion,** right **hand**
    M67.442 **Ganglion,** left **hand**
    M67.449 **Ganglion, unspecified hand**

✓6ᵗʰ **M67.45** **Ganglion,** hip

    M67.451 **Ganglion, right hip**

    M67.452 **Ganglion, left hip**
    M67.459 **Ganglion, unspecified hip**

✓6ᵗʰ **M67.46** **Ganglion,** knee

    M67.461 **Ganglion,** right **knee**
    M67.462 **Ganglion,** left **knee**
    M67.469 **Ganglion, unspecified knee**

✓6ᵗʰ **M67.47** **Ganglion,** ankle and foot

    M67.471 **Ganglion,** right **ankle and foot**
    M67.472 **Ganglion,** left **ankle and foot**
    M67.479 **Ganglion, unspecified ankle and foot**

    M67.48 **Ganglion, other site**
    M67.49 **Ganglion,** multiple sites

✓5ᵗʰ **M67.5** **Plica syndrome**

    Plica knee

    M67.50 **Plica syndrome, unspecified knee**
    M67.51 **Plica syndrome,** right **knee**
    M67.52 **Plica syndrome,** left **knee**

✓5ᵗʰ **M67.8** **Other specified disorders of synovium and tendon**

    M67.80 **Other specified disorders of synovium and tendon, unspecified site**

✓6ᵗʰ **M67.81** **Other specified disorders of synovium and tendon,** shoulder

    M67.811 **Other specified disorders of synovium,** right **shoulder**
    M67.812 **Other specified disorders of synovium,** left **shoulder**
    M67.813 **Other specified disorders of tendon,** right **shoulder**
    M67.814 **Other specified disorders of tendon,** left **shoulder**
    M67.819 **Other specified disorders of synovium and tendon, unspecified shoulder**

✓6ᵗʰ **M67.82** **Other specified disorders of synovium and tendon,** elbow

    M67.821 **Other specified disorders of synovium,** right **elbow**
    M67.822 **Other specified disorders of synovium,** left **elbow**
    M67.823 **Other specified disorders of tendon,** right **elbow**
    M67.824 **Other specified disorders of tendon,** left **elbow**
    M67.829 **Other specified disorders of synovium and tendon, unspecified elbow**

✓6ᵗʰ **M67.83** **Other specified disorders of synovium and tendon,** wrist

    M67.831 **Other specified disorders of synovium,** right **wrist**
    M67.832 **Other specified disorders of synovium,** left **wrist**
    M67.833 **Other specified disorders of tendon,** right **wrist**
    M67.834 **Other specified disorders of tendon,** left **wrist**
    M67.839 **Other specified disorders of synovium and tendon, unspecified wrist**

✓6ᵗʰ **M67.84** **Other specified disorders of synovium and tendon,** hand

    M67.841 **Other specified disorders of synovium,** right **hand**
    M67.842 **Other specified disorders of synovium,** left **hand**
    M67.843 **Other specified disorders of tendon,** right **hand**
    M67.844 **Other specified disorders of tendon,** left **hand**
    M67.849 **Other specified disorders of synovium and tendon, unspecified hand**

✓6ᵗʰ **M67.85** **Other specified disorders of synovium and tendon,** hip

    M67.851 **Other specified disorders of synovium,** right **hip**
    M67.852 **Other specified disorders of synovium,** left **hip**
    M67.853 **Other specified disorders of tendon,** right **hip**
    M67.854 **Other specified disorders of tendon,** left **hip**
    M67.859 **Other specified disorders of synovium and tendon, unspecified hip**

Chapter 13. Diseases of the Musculoskeletal System and Connective Tissue

M67.86–M70.52

✓6ᵗʰ **M67.86** Other specified disorders of synovium and tendon, knee

     M67.861 Other specified disorders of synovium, right knee

     M67.862 Other specified disorders of synovium, left knee

     M67.863 Other specified disorders of tendon, right knee

     M67.864 Other specified disorders of tendon, left knee

     M67.869 Other specified disorders of synovium and tendon, unspecified knee

✓6ᵗʰ **M67.87** Other specified disorders of synovium and tendon, ankle and foot

     M67.871 Other specified disorders of synovium, right ankle and foot

     M67.872 Other specified disorders of synovium, left ankle and foot

     M67.873 Other specified disorders of tendon, right ankle and foot

     M67.874 Other specified disorders of tendon, left ankle and foot

     M67.879 Other specified disorders of synovium and tendon, unspecified ankle and foot

   M67.88 Other specified disorders of synovium and tendon, other site

   M67.89 Other specified disorders of synovium and tendon, multiple sites

✓5ᵗʰ **M67.9** Unspecified disorder of synovium and tendon

   M67.90 Unspecified disorder of synovium and tendon, unspecified site

✓6ᵗʰ **M67.91** Unspecified disorder of synovium and tendon, shoulder

     M67.911 Unspecified disorder of synovium and tendon, right shoulder

     M67.912 Unspecified disorder of synovium and tendon, left shoulder

     M67.919 Unspecified disorder of synovium and tendon, unspecified shoulder

✓6ᵗʰ **M67.92** Unspecified disorder of synovium and tendon, upper arm

     M67.921 Unspecified disorder of synovium and tendon, right upper arm

     M67.922 Unspecified disorder of synovium and tendon, left upper arm

     M67.929 Unspecified disorder of synovium and tendon, unspecified upper arm

✓6ᵗʰ **M67.93** Unspecified disorder of synovium and tendon, forearm

     M67.931 Unspecified disorder of synovium and tendon, right forearm

     M67.932 Unspecified disorder of synovium and tendon, left forearm

     M67.939 Unspecified disorder of synovium and tendon, unspecified forearm

✓6ᵗʰ **M67.94** Unspecified disorder of synovium and tendon, hand

     M67.941 Unspecified disorder of synovium and tendon, right hand

     M67.942 Unspecified disorder of synovium and tendon, left hand

     M67.949 Unspecified disorder of synovium and tendon, unspecified hand

✓6ᵗʰ **M67.95** Unspecified disorder of synovium and tendon, thigh

     M67.951 Unspecified disorder of synovium and tendon, right thigh

     M67.952 Unspecified disorder of synovium and tendon, left thigh

     M67.959 Unspecified disorder of synovium and tendon, unspecified thigh

✓6ᵗʰ **M67.96** Unspecified disorder of synovium and tendon, lower leg

     M67.961 Unspecified disorder of synovium and tendon, right lower leg

     M67.962 Unspecified disorder of synovium and tendon, left lower leg

     M67.969 Unspecified disorder of synovium and tendon, unspecified lower leg

✓6ᵗʰ **M67.97** Unspecified disorder of synovium and tendon, ankle and foot

     M67.971 Unspecified disorder of synovium and tendon, right ankle and foot

     M67.972 Unspecified disorder of synovium and tendon, left ankle and foot

     M67.979 Unspecified disorder of synovium and tendon, unspecified ankle and foot

   M67.98 Unspecified disorder of synovium and tendon, other site

   M67.99 Unspecified disorder of synovium and tendon, multiple sites

Other soft tissue disorders (M70-M79)

✓4ᵗʰ **M70** Soft tissue disorders related to use, overuse and pressure

   INCLUDES   soft tissue disorders of occupational origin

   Use additional external cause code to identify activity causing disorder (Y93.-)

   EXCLUDES 1   bursitis NOS (M71.9-)

   EXCLUDES 2   bursitis of shoulder (M75.5)

                    enthesopathies (M76-M77)

                    pressure ulcer (pressure area) (L89.-)

✓5ᵗʰ **M70.0** Crepitant synovitis (acute) (chronic) of hand and wrist

   ✓6ᵗʰ **M70.03** Crepitant synovitis (acute) (chronic), wrist

     M70.031 Crepitant synovitis (acute) (chronic), right wrist

     M70.032 Crepitant synovitis (acute) (chronic), left wrist

     M70.039 Crepitant synovitis (acute) (chronic), unspecified wrist

   ✓6ᵗʰ **M70.04** Crepitant synovitis (acute) (chronic), hand

     M70.041 Crepitant synovitis (acute) (chronic), right hand

     M70.042 Crepitant synovitis (acute) (chronic), left hand

     M70.049 Crepitant synovitis (acute) (chronic), unspecified hand

✓5ᵗʰ **M70.1** Bursitis of hand

   M70.10 Bursitis, unspecified hand

   M70.11 Bursitis, right hand

   M70.12 Bursitis, left hand

✓5ᵗʰ **M70.2** Olecranon bursitis

   M70.20 Olecranon bursitis, unspecified elbow

   M70.21 Olecranon bursitis, right elbow

   M70.22 Olecranon bursitis, left elbow

✓5ᵗʰ **M70.3** Other bursitis of elbow

   M70.30 Other bursitis of elbow, unspecified elbow

   M70.31 Other bursitis of elbow, right elbow

   M70.32 Other bursitis of elbow, left elbow

✓5ᵗʰ **M70.4** Prepatellar bursitis

   M70.40 Prepatellar bursitis, unspecified knee

   M70.41 Prepatellar bursitis, right knee

   M70.42 Prepatellar bursitis, left knee

Knee Bursae

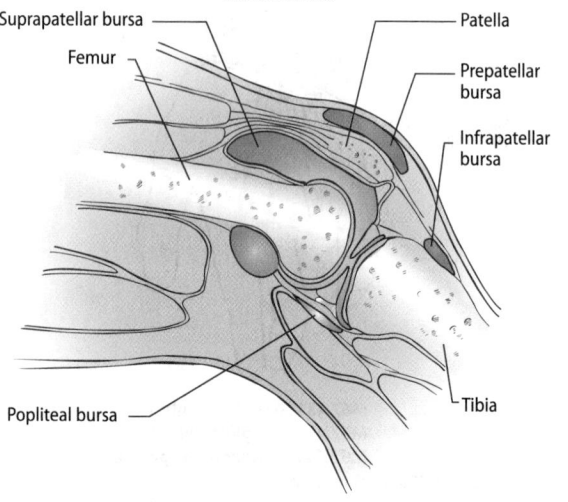

Suprapatellar bursa — Femur — Patella — Prepatellar bursa — Infrapatellar bursa — Popliteal bursa — Tibia

✓5ᵗʰ **M70.5** Other bursitis of knee

   M70.50 Other bursitis of knee, unspecified knee

   M70.51 Other bursitis of knee, right knee

   M70.52 Other bursitis of knee, left knee

HCC CMS-HCC   **Rx** Rx HCC   **ESR** ESRD HCC   **COM** Commercial HCC   **N** Newborn: 0   **P** Pediatric: 0-17   **M** Maternity: 9-64   **A** Adult: 15-124

834   ICD-10-CM 2023

✓5ᵗʰ **M70.6** Trochanteric bursitis
Trochanteric tendinitis
- **M70.60** Trochanteric bursitis, unspecified hip
- **M70.61** Trochanteric bursitis, right hip
- **M70.62** Trochanteric bursitis, left hip

✓5ᵗʰ **M70.7** Other bursitis of hip
Ischial bursitis
- **M70.70** Other bursitis of hip, unspecified hip
- **M70.71** Other bursitis of hip, right hip
- **M70.72** Other bursitis of hip, left hip

✓5ᵗʰ **M70.8** Other soft tissue disorders related to use, overuse and pressure
- **M70.80** Other soft tissue disorders related to use, overuse and pressure of unspecified site
- ✓6ᵗʰ **M70.81** Other soft tissue disorders related to use, overuse and pressure of shoulder
  - M70.811 Other soft tissue disorders related to use, overuse and pressure, right shoulder
  - M70.812 Other soft tissue disorders related to use, overuse and pressure, left shoulder
  - **M70.819** Other soft tissue disorders related to use, overuse and pressure, unspecified shoulder
- ✓6ᵗʰ **M70.82** Other soft tissue disorders related to use, overuse and pressure of upper arm
  - M70.821 Other soft tissue disorders related to use, overuse and pressure, right upper arm
  - M70.822 Other soft tissue disorders related to use, overuse and pressure, left upper arm
  - **M70.829** Other soft tissue disorders related to use, overuse and pressure, unspecified upper arms
- ✓6ᵗʰ **M70.83** Other soft tissue disorders related to use, overuse and pressure of forearm
  - M70.831 Other soft tissue disorders related to use, overuse and pressure, right forearm
  - M70.832 Other soft tissue disorders related to use, overuse and pressure, left forearm
  - **M70.839** Other soft tissue disorders related to use, overuse and pressure, unspecified forearm
- ✓6ᵗʰ **M70.84** Other soft tissue disorders related to use, overuse and pressure of hand
  - M70.841 Other soft tissue disorders related to use, overuse and pressure, right hand
  - M70.842 Other soft tissue disorders related to use, overuse and pressure, left hand
  - **M70.849** Other soft tissue disorders related to use, overuse and pressure, unspecified hand
- ✓6ᵗʰ **M70.85** Other soft tissue disorders related to use, overuse and pressure of thigh
  - M70.851 Other soft tissue disorders related to use, overuse and pressure, right thigh
  - M70.852 Other soft tissue disorders related to use, overuse and pressure, left thigh
  - **M70.859** Other soft tissue disorders related to use, overuse and pressure, unspecified thigh
- ✓6ᵗʰ **M70.86** Other soft tissue disorders related to use, overuse and pressure lower leg
  - M70.861 Other soft tissue disorders related to use, overuse and pressure, right lower leg
  - M70.862 Other soft tissue disorders related to use, overuse and pressure, left lower leg
  - **M70.869** Other soft tissue disorders related to use, overuse and pressure, unspecified leg
- ✓6ᵗʰ **M70.87** Other soft tissue disorders related to use, overuse and pressure of ankle and foot
  - M70.871 Other soft tissue disorders related to use, overuse and pressure, right ankle and foot
  - M70.872 Other soft tissue disorders related to use, overuse and pressure, left ankle and foot
  - **M70.879** Other soft tissue disorders related to use, overuse and pressure, unspecified ankle and foot
- **M70.88** Other soft tissue disorders related to use, overuse and pressure other site
- **M70.89** Other soft tissue disorders related to use, overuse and pressure multiple sites

✓5ᵗʰ **M70.9** Unspecified soft tissue disorder related to use, overuse and pressure
- **M70.90** Unspecified soft tissue disorder related to use, overuse and pressure of unspecified site
- ✓6ᵗʰ **M70.91** Unspecified soft tissue disorder related to use, overuse and pressure of shoulder
  - **M70.911** Unspecified soft tissue disorder related to use, overuse and pressure, right shoulder
  - **M70.912** Unspecified soft tissue disorder related to use, overuse and pressure, left shoulder
  - **M70.919** Unspecified soft tissue disorder related to use, overuse and pressure, unspecified shoulder
- ✓6ᵗʰ **M70.92** Unspecified soft tissue disorder related to use, overuse and pressure of upper arm
  - **M70.921** Unspecified soft tissue disorder related to use, overuse and pressure, right upper arm
  - **M70.922** Unspecified soft tissue disorder related to use, overuse and pressure, left upper arm
  - **M70.929** Unspecified soft tissue disorder related to use, overuse and pressure, unspecified upper arm
- ✓6ᵗʰ **M70.93** Unspecified soft tissue disorder related to use, overuse and pressure of forearm
  - **M70.931** Unspecified soft tissue disorder related to use, overuse and pressure, right forearm
  - **M70.932** Unspecified soft tissue disorder related to use, overuse and pressure, left forearm
  - **M70.939** Unspecified soft tissue disorder related to use, overuse and pressure, unspecified forearm
- ✓6ᵗʰ **M70.94** Unspecified soft tissue disorder related to use, overuse and pressure of hand
  - **M70.941** Unspecified soft tissue disorder related to use, overuse and pressure, right hand
  - **M70.942** Unspecified soft tissue disorder related to use, overuse and pressure, left hand
  - **M70.949** Unspecified soft tissue disorder related to use, overuse and pressure, unspecified hand
- ✓6ᵗʰ **M70.95** Unspecified soft tissue disorder related to use, overuse and pressure of thigh
  - **M70.951** Unspecified soft tissue disorder related to use, overuse and pressure, right thigh
  - **M70.952** Unspecified soft tissue disorder related to use, overuse and pressure, left thigh
  - **M70.959** Unspecified soft tissue disorder related to use, overuse and pressure, unspecified thigh
- ✓6ᵗʰ **M70.96** Unspecified soft tissue disorder related to use, overuse and pressure lower leg
  - **M70.961** Unspecified soft tissue disorder related to use, overuse and pressure, right lower leg
  - **M70.962** Unspecified soft tissue disorder related to use, overuse and pressure, left lower leg
  - **M70.969** Unspecified soft tissue disorder related to use, overuse and pressure, unspecified lower leg
- ✓6ᵗʰ **M70.97** Unspecified soft tissue disorder related to use, overuse and pressure of ankle and foot
  - **M70.971** Unspecified soft tissue disorder related to use, overuse and pressure, right ankle and foot
  - **M70.972** Unspecified soft tissue disorder related to use, overuse and pressure, left ankle and foot
  - **M70.979** Unspecified soft tissue disorder related to use, overuse and pressure, unspecified ankle and foot
- **M70.98** Unspecified soft tissue disorder related to use, overuse and pressure other
- **M70.99** Unspecified soft tissue disorder related to use, overuse and pressure multiple sites

Chapter 13. Diseases of the Musculoskeletal System and Connective Tissue

✓4th **M71 Other bursopathies**

> EXCLUDES 1   bunion (M20.1)
> bursitis related to use, overuse or pressure (M70.-)
> enthesopathies (M76-M77)

✓5th **M71.0 Abscess of bursa**

> Use additional code (B95.-, B96.-) to identify causative organism

    M71.00 Abscess of bursa, unspecified site

✓6th **M71.01 Abscess of bursa, shoulder**

     M71.011 Abscess of bursa, right shoulder
     M71.012 Abscess of bursa, left shoulder
     M71.019 Abscess of bursa, unspecified shoulder

✓6th **M71.02 Abscess of bursa, elbow**

     M71.021 Abscess of bursa, right elbow
     M71.022 Abscess of bursa, left elbow
     M71.029 Abscess of bursa, unspecified elbow

✓6th **M71.03 Abscess of bursa, wrist**

     M71.031 Abscess of bursa, right wrist
     M71.032 Abscess of bursa, left wrist
     M71.039 Abscess of bursa, unspecified wrist

✓6th **M71.04 Abscess of bursa, hand**

     M71.041 Abscess of bursa, right hand
     M71.042 Abscess of bursa, left hand
     M71.049 Abscess of bursa, unspecified hand

✓6th **M71.05 Abscess of bursa, hip**

     M71.051 Abscess of bursa, right hip
     M71.052 Abscess of bursa, left hip
     M71.059 Abscess of bursa, unspecified hip

✓6th **M71.06 Abscess of bursa, knee**

     M71.061 Abscess of bursa, right knee
     M71.062 Abscess of bursa, left knee
     M71.069 Abscess of bursa, unspecified knee

✓6th **M71.07 Abscess of bursa, ankle and foot**

     M71.071 Abscess of bursa, right ankle and foot
     M71.072 Abscess of bursa, left ankle and foot
     M71.079 Abscess of bursa, unspecified ankle and foot

    M71.08 Abscess of bursa, other site

    M71.09 Abscess of bursa, multiple sites

✓5th **M71.1 Other infective bursitis**

> Use additional code (B95.-, B96.-) to identify causative organism

    M71.10 Other infective bursitis, unspecified site

✓6th **M71.11 Other infective bursitis, shoulder**

     M71.111 Other infective bursitis, right shoulder
     M71.112 Other infective bursitis, left shoulder
     M71.119 Other infective bursitis, unspecified shoulder

✓6th **M71.12 Other infective bursitis, elbow**

     M71.121 Other infective bursitis, right elbow
     M71.122 Other infective bursitis, left elbow
     M71.129 Other infective bursitis, unspecified elbow

✓6th **M71.13 Other infective bursitis, wrist**

     M71.131 Other infective bursitis, right wrist
     M71.132 Other infective bursitis, left wrist
     M71.139 Other infective bursitis, unspecified wrist

✓6th **M71.14 Other infective bursitis, hand**

     M71.141 Other infective bursitis, right hand
     M71.142 Other infective bursitis, left hand
     M71.149 Other infective bursitis, unspecified hand

✓6th **M71.15 Other infective bursitis, hip**

     M71.151 Other infective bursitis, right hip
     M71.152 Other infective bursitis, left hip
     M71.159 Other infective bursitis, unspecified hip

✓6th **M71.16 Other infective bursitis, knee**

     M71.161 Other infective bursitis, right knee
     M71.162 Other infective bursitis, left knee
     M71.169 Other infective bursitis, unspecified knee

✓6th **M71.17 Other infective bursitis, ankle and foot**

     M71.171 Other infective bursitis, right ankle and foot
     M71.172 Other infective bursitis, left ankle and foot
     M71.179 Other infective bursitis, unspecified ankle and foot

    M71.18 Other infective bursitis, other site

    M71.19 Other infective bursitis, multiple sites

✓5th **M71.2 Synovial cyst of popliteal space [Baker]**

> EXCLUDES 1   synovial cyst of popliteal space with rupture (M66.0)

DEF: Sac filled with clear synovial fluid in adults, usually secondary to disease inside the joint, located on the back of the knee in the popliteal fossa area. In children, the cyst usually represents a ganglion of one of the tendons in the knee.

Baker's Cyst

Baker's cyst connected to knee joint synovial cavity

    M71.20 Synovial cyst of popliteal space [Baker], unspecified knee

    M71.21 Synovial cyst of popliteal space [Baker], right knee

    M71.22 Synovial cyst of popliteal space [Baker], left knee

✓5th **M71.3 Other bursal cyst**

> Synovial cyst NOS
> EXCLUDES 1   synovial cyst with rupture (M66.1-)

    M71.30 Other bursal cyst, unspecified site

✓6th **M71.31 Other bursal cyst, shoulder**

     M71.311 Other bursal cyst, right shoulder
     M71.312 Other bursal cyst, left shoulder
     M71.319 Other bursal cyst, unspecified shoulder

✓6th **M71.32 Other bursal cyst, elbow**

     M71.321 Other bursal cyst, right elbow
     M71.322 Other bursal cyst, left elbow
     M71.329 Other bursal cyst, unspecified elbow

✓6th **M71.33 Other bursal cyst, wrist**

     M71.331 Other bursal cyst, right wrist
     M71.332 Other bursal cyst, left wrist
     M71.339 Other bursal cyst, unspecified wrist

✓6th **M71.34 Other bursal cyst, hand**

     M71.341 Other bursal cyst, right hand
     M71.342 Other bursal cyst, left hand
     M71.349 Other bursal cyst, unspecified hand

✓6th **M71.35 Other bursal cyst, hip**

     M71.351 Other bursal cyst, right hip
     M71.352 Other bursal cyst, left hip
     M71.359 Other bursal cyst, unspecified hip

✓6th **M71.37 Other bursal cyst, ankle and foot**

     M71.371 Other bursal cyst, right ankle and foot
     M71.372 Other bursal cyst, left ankle and foot
     M71.379 Other bursal cyst, unspecified ankle and foot

    M71.38 Other bursal cyst, other site

    M71.39 Other bursal cyst, multiple sites

✓5th **M71.4 Calcium deposit in bursa**

> EXCLUDES 2   calcium deposit in bursa of shoulder (M75.3)

    M71.40 Calcium deposit in bursa, unspecified site

✓6th **M71.42 Calcium deposit in bursa, elbow**

     M71.421 Calcium deposit in bursa, right elbow
     M71.422 Calcium deposit in bursa, left elbow
     M71.429 Calcium deposit in bursa, unspecified elbow

✓6th **M71.43 Calcium deposit in bursa, wrist**

     M71.431 Calcium deposit in bursa, right wrist
     M71.432 Calcium deposit in bursa, left wrist

M71.439 Calcium deposit in bursa, unspecified wrist

✓6ᵗʰ M71.44 **Calcium deposit in bursa, hand**
  M71.441 Calcium deposit in bursa, right hand
  M71.442 Calcium deposit in bursa, left hand
  M71.449 Calcium deposit in bursa, unspecified hand

✓6ᵗʰ M71.45 **Calcium deposit in bursa, hip**
  M71.451 Calcium deposit in bursa, right hip
  M71.452 Calcium deposit in bursa, left hip
  M71.459 Calcium deposit in bursa, unspecified hip

✓6ᵗʰ M71.46 **Calcium deposit in bursa, knee**
  M71.461 Calcium deposit in bursa, right knee
  M71.462 Calcium deposit in bursa, left knee
  M71.469 Calcium deposit in bursa, unspecified knee

✓6ᵗʰ M71.47 **Calcium deposit in bursa, ankle and foot**
  M71.471 Calcium deposit in bursa, right ankle and foot
  M71.472 Calcium deposit in bursa, left ankle and foot
  M71.479 Calcium deposit in bursa, unspecified ankle and foot

M71.48 Calcium deposit in bursa, other site
M71.49 Calcium deposit in bursa, multiple sites

✓5ᵗʰ M71.5 **Other bursitis, not elsewhere classified**
  EXCLUDES 1 bursitis NOS (M71.9-)
  EXCLUDES 2 bursitis of shoulder (M75.5)
              bursitis of tibial collateral [Pellegrini-Stieda] (M76.4-)

M71.50 Other bursitis, not elsewhere classified, unspecified site

✓6ᵗʰ M71.52 **Other bursitis, not elsewhere classified, elbow**
  M71.521 Other bursitis, not elsewhere classified, right elbow
  M71.522 Other bursitis, not elsewhere classified, left elbow
  M71.529 Other bursitis, not elsewhere classified, unspecified elbow

✓6ᵗʰ M71.53 **Other bursitis, not elsewhere classified, wrist**
  M71.531 Other bursitis, not elsewhere classified, right wrist
  M71.532 Other bursitis, not elsewhere classified, left wrist
  M71.539 Other bursitis, not elsewhere classified, unspecified wrist

✓6ᵗʰ M71.54 **Other bursitis, not elsewhere classified, hand**
  M71.541 Other bursitis, not elsewhere classified, right hand
  M71.542 Other bursitis, not elsewhere classified, left hand
  M71.549 Other bursitis, not elsewhere classified, unspecified hand

✓6ᵗʰ M71.55 **Other bursitis, not elsewhere classified, hip**
  M71.551 Other bursitis, not elsewhere classified, right hip
  M71.552 Other bursitis, not elsewhere classified, left hip
  M71.559 Other bursitis, not elsewhere classified, unspecified hip

✓6ᵗʰ M71.56 **Other bursitis, not elsewhere classified, knee**
  M71.561 Other bursitis, not elsewhere classified, right knee
  M71.562 Other bursitis, not elsewhere classified, left knee
  M71.569 Other bursitis, not elsewhere classified, unspecified knee

✓6ᵗʰ M71.57 **Other bursitis, not elsewhere classified, ankle and foot**
  M71.571 Other bursitis, not elsewhere classified, right ankle and foot
  M71.572 Other bursitis, not elsewhere classified, left ankle and foot
  M71.579 Other bursitis, not elsewhere classified, unspecified ankle and foot

M71.58 Other bursitis, not elsewhere classified, other site

✓5ᵗʰ M71.8 **Other specified bursopathies**
M71.80 Other specified bursopathies, unspecified site

✓6ᵗʰ M71.81 **Other specified bursopathies, shoulder**
  M71.811 Other specified bursopathies, right shoulder
  M71.812 Other specified bursopathies, left shoulder
  M71.819 Other specified bursopathies, unspecified shoulder

✓6ᵗʰ M71.82 **Other specified bursopathies, elbow**
  M71.821 Other specified bursopathies, right elbow
  M71.822 Other specified bursopathies, left elbow
  M71.829 Other specified bursopathies, unspecified elbow

✓6ᵗʰ M71.83 **Other specified bursopathies, wrist**
  M71.831 Other specified bursopathies, right wrist
  M71.832 Other specified bursopathies, left wrist
  M71.839 Other specified bursopathies, unspecified wrist

✓6ᵗʰ M71.84 **Other specified bursopathies, hand**
  M71.841 Other specified bursopathies, right hand
  M71.842 Other specified bursopathies, left hand
  M71.849 Other specified bursopathies, unspecified hand

✓6ᵗʰ M71.85 **Other specified bursopathies, hip**
  M71.851 Other specified bursopathies, right hip
  M71.852 Other specified bursopathies, left hip
  M71.859 Other specified bursopathies, unspecified hip

✓6ᵗʰ M71.86 **Other specified bursopathies, knee**
  M71.861 Other specified bursopathies, right knee
  M71.862 Other specified bursopathies, left knee
  M71.869 Other specified bursopathies, unspecified knee

✓6ᵗʰ M71.87 **Other specified bursopathies, ankle and foot**
  M71.871 Other specified bursopathies, right ankle and foot
  M71.872 Other specified bursopathies, left ankle and foot
  M71.879 Other specified bursopathies, unspecified ankle and foot

M71.88 Other specified bursopathies, other site
M71.89 Other specified bursopathies, multiple sites

M71.9 **Bursopathy, unspecified**
  Bursitis NOS

✓4ᵗʰ **M72 Fibroblastic disorders**
  EXCLUDES 2 retroperitoneal fibromatosis (D48.3)

M72.0 **Palmar fascial fibromatosis [Dupuytren]**   [A]
  DEF: Dupuytren's contracture: Flexion deformity of a finger, due to shortened, thickened fibrosing of palmar fascia. The cause is unknown, but it is associated with long-standing epilepsy.

M72.1 **Knuckle pads**

M72.2 **Plantar fascial fibromatosis**
  Plantar fasciitis
  DEF: Rapid-growing and multiplanar nodular swellings and pain in the foot that is not associated with contractures.

M72.4 **Pseudosarcomatous fibromatosis**
  Nodular fasciitis

M72.6 **Necrotizing fasciitis**   HCC ESR COM
  Use additional code (B95.-, B96.-) to identify causative organism

M72.8 **Other fibroblastic disorders**
  Abscess of fascia
  Fasciitis NEC
  Other infective fasciitis
  Use additional code to (B95.-, B96.-) identify causative organism
  EXCLUDES 1 diffuse (eosinophilic) fasciitis (M35.4)
              necrotizing fasciitis (M72.6)
              nodular fasciitis (M72.4)
              perirenal fasciitis NOS (N13.5)
              perirenal fasciitis with infection (N13.6)
              plantar fasciitis (M72.2)

M72.9 **Fibroblastic disorder, unspecified**
  Fasciitis NOS
  Fibromatosis NOS

Chapter 13. Diseases of the Musculoskeletal System and Connective Tissue

M75–M77.32

☑4ᵗʰ **M75 Shoulder lesions**

    EXCLUDES 2   shoulder-hand syndrome (M89.0-)

  ☑5ᵗʰ **M75.0 Adhesive capsulitis of shoulder**

    Frozen shoulder

    Periarthritis of shoulder

    AHA: 2015,2Q,23

    M75.00   **Adhesive capsulitis of unspecified shoulder**

    M75.01   **Adhesive capsulitis of** right **shoulder**

    M75.02   **Adhesive capsulitis of** left **shoulder**

  ☑5ᵗʰ **M75.1 Rotator cuff tear or rupture, not specified as traumatic**

    Rotator cuff syndrome

    Supraspinatus syndrome

    Supraspinatus tear or rupture, not specified as traumatic

    EXCLUDES 1   tear of rotator cuff, traumatic (S46.01-)

    ☑6ᵗʰ **M75.10**   **Unspecified rotator cuff tear or rupture, not specified as traumatic**

      M75.100   **Unspecified rotator cuff tear or rupture of unspecified shoulder, not specified as traumatic**

      M75.101   **Unspecified rotator cuff tear or rupture of** right **shoulder, not specified as traumatic**

      M75.102   **Unspecified rotator cuff tear or rupture of** left **shoulder, not specified as traumatic**

    ☑6ᵗʰ **M75.11**   **Incomplete rotator cuff tear or rupture not specified as traumatic**

      M75.110   **Incomplete rotator cuff tear or rupture of unspecified shoulder, not specified as traumatic**

      M75.111   **Incomplete rotator cuff tear or rupture of** right **shoulder, not specified as traumatic**

      M75.112   **Incomplete rotator cuff tear or rupture of** left **shoulder, not specified as traumatic**

    ☑6ᵗʰ **M75.12**   **Complete rotator cuff tear or rupture not specified as traumatic**

      M75.120   **Complete rotator cuff tear or rupture of unspecified shoulder, not specified as traumatic**

      M75.121   **Complete rotator cuff tear or rupture of** right **shoulder, not specified as traumatic**

      M75.122   **Complete rotator cuff tear or rupture of** left **shoulder, not specified as traumatic**

  ☑5ᵗʰ **M75.2** Bicipital **tendinitis**

    M75.20   **Bicipital tendinitis, unspecified shoulder**

    M75.21   **Bicipital tendinitis,** right **shoulder**

    M75.22   **Bicipital tendinitis,** left **shoulder**

  ☑5ᵗʰ **M75.3** Calcific **tendinitis of shoulder**

    Calcified bursa of shoulder

    M75.30   **Calcific tendinitis of unspecified shoulder**

    M75.31   **Calcific tendinitis of** right **shoulder**

    M75.32   **Calcific tendinitis of** left **shoulder**

  ☑5ᵗʰ **M75.4** Impingement syndrome **of shoulder**

    M75.40   **Impingement syndrome of unspecified shoulder**

    M75.41   **Impingement syndrome of** right **shoulder**

    M75.42   **Impingement syndrome of** left **shoulder**

  ☑5ᵗʰ **M75.5 Bursitis of shoulder**

    M75.50   **Bursitis of unspecified shoulder**

    M75.51   **Bursitis of** right **shoulder**

    M75.52   **Bursitis of** left **shoulder**

  ☑5ᵗʰ **M75.8 Other shoulder lesions**

    M75.80   **Other shoulder lesions, unspecified shoulder**

    M75.81   **Other shoulder lesions,** right **shoulder**

    M75.82   **Other shoulder lesions,** left **shoulder**

  ☑5ᵗʰ **M75.9 Shoulder lesion, unspecified**

    M75.90   **Shoulder lesion, unspecified, unspecified shoulder**

    M75.91   **Shoulder lesion, unspecified,** right **shoulder**

    M75.92   **Shoulder lesion, unspecified,** left **shoulder**

☑4ᵗʰ **M76 Enthesopathies, lower limb, excluding foot**

    EXCLUDES 2   bursitis due to use, overuse and pressure (M70.-)

                  enthesopathies of ankle and foot (M77.5-)

  ☑5ᵗʰ **M76.0** Gluteal **tendinitis**

    M76.00   **Gluteal tendinitis, unspecified hip**

    M76.01   **Gluteal tendinitis,** right **hip**

    M76.02   **Gluteal tendinitis,** left **hip**

☑5ᵗʰ **M76.1** Psoas **tendinitis**

    M76.10   **Psoas tendinitis, unspecified hip**

    M76.11   **Psoas tendinitis,** right **hip**

    M76.12   **Psoas tendinitis,** left **hip**

☑5ᵗʰ **M76.2 Iliac crest spur**

    M76.20   **Iliac crest spur, unspecified hip**

    M76.21   **Iliac crest spur,** right **hip**

    M76.22   **Iliac crest spur,** left **hip**

☑5ᵗʰ **M76.3 Iliotibial band syndrome**

    M76.30   **Iliotibial band syndrome, unspecified leg**

    M76.31   **Iliotibial band syndrome,** right **leg**

    M76.32   **Iliotibial band syndrome,** left **leg**

☑5ᵗʰ **M76.4 Tibial collateral bursitis [Pellegrini-Stieda]**

    M76.40   **Tibial collateral bursitis [Pellegrini-Stieda], unspecified leg**

    M76.41   **Tibial collateral bursitis [Pellegrini-Stieda],** right **leg**

    M76.42   **Tibial collateral bursitis [Pellegrini-Stieda],** left **leg**

☑5ᵗʰ **M76.5** Patellar **tendinitis**

    M76.50   **Patellar tendinitis, unspecified knee**

    M76.51   **Patellar tendinitis,** right **knee**

    M76.52   **Patellar tendinitis,** left **knee**

☑5ᵗʰ **M76.6** Achilles **tendinitis**

    Achilles bursitis

    M76.60   **Achilles tendinitis, unspecified leg**

    M76.61   **Achilles tendinitis,** right **leg**

    M76.62   **Achilles tendinitis,** left **leg**

☑5ᵗʰ **M76.7** Peroneal **tendinitis**

    M76.70   **Peroneal tendinitis, unspecified leg**

    M76.71   **Peroneal tendinitis,** right **leg**

    M76.72   **Peroneal tendinitis,** left **leg**

☑5ᵗʰ **M76.8 Other specified enthesopathies of lower limb, excluding foot**

    ☑6ᵗʰ **M76.81** Anterior tibial syndrome

      M76.811   **Anterior tibial syndrome,** right **leg**

      M76.812   **Anterior tibial syndrome,** left **leg**

      M76.819   **Anterior tibial syndrome, unspecified leg**

    ☑6ᵗʰ **M76.82** Posterior tibial tendinitis

      M76.821   **Posterior tibial tendinitis,** right **leg**

      M76.822   **Posterior tibial tendinitis,** left **leg**

      M76.829   **Posterior tibial tendinitis, unspecified leg**

    ☑6ᵗʰ **M76.89** **Other specified enthesopathies of** lower limb, excluding foot

      M76.891   **Other specified enthesopathies of** right **lower limb, excluding foot**

      M76.892   **Other specified enthesopathies of** left **lower limb, excluding foot**

      M76.899   **Other specified enthesopathies of unspecified lower limb, excluding foot**

  M76.9   **Unspecified enthesopathy, lower limb, excluding foot**

☑4ᵗʰ **M77 Other enthesopathies**

    EXCLUDES 1   bursitis NOS (M71.9-)

    EXCLUDES 2   bursitis due to use, overuse and pressure (M70.-)

                  osteophyte (M25.7)

                  spinal enthesopathy (M46.0-)

  ☑5ᵗʰ **M77.0** Medial **epicondylitis**

    M77.00   **Medial epicondylitis, unspecified elbow**

    M77.01   **Medial epicondylitis,** right **elbow**

    M77.02   **Medial epicondylitis,** left **elbow**

  ☑5ᵗʰ **M77.1** Lateral **epicondylitis**

    Tennis elbow

    M77.10   **Lateral epicondylitis, unspecified elbow**

    M77.11   **Lateral epicondylitis,** right **elbow**

    M77.12   **Lateral epicondylitis,** left **elbow**

  ☑5ᵗʰ **M77.2 Periarthritis of wrist**

    M77.20   **Periarthritis, unspecified wrist**

    M77.21   **Periarthritis,** right **wrist**

    M77.22   **Periarthritis,** left **wrist**

  ☑5ᵗʰ **M77.3 Calcaneal spur**

    DEF: Overgrowth of calcaneus bone on the underside of the heel that causes pain on walking. Calcaneal spur is due to a chronic avulsion injury of the plantar fascia from the calcaneus.

    M77.30   **Calcaneal spur, unspecified foot**

    M77.31   **Calcaneal spur,** right **foot**

    M77.32   **Calcaneal spur,** left **foot**

☑5ᵗʰ **M77.4 Metatarsalgia**
     EXCLUDES 1   *Morton's metatarsalgia (G57.6)*
     M77.40 Metatarsalgia, unspecified foot
     M77.41 Metatarsalgia, right foot
     M77.42 Metatarsalgia, left foot

☑5ᵗʰ **M77.5 Other enthesopathy of foot and ankle**
     M77.50 Other enthesopathy of unspecified foot and ankle
     M77.51 Other enthesopathy of right foot and ankle
     M77.52 Other enthesopathy of left foot and ankle

M77.8 Other enthesopathies, not elsewhere classified

M77.9 Enthesopathy, unspecified
     Bone spur NOS
     Capsulitis NOS
     Periarthritis NOS
     Tendinitis NOS

☑4ᵗʰ **M79 Other and unspecified soft tissue disorders, not elsewhere classified**
     EXCLUDES 1   *psychogenic rheumatism (F45.8)*
                soft tissue pain, psychogenic (F45.41)

M79.0 Rheumatism, unspecified
     EXCLUDES 1   *fibromyalgia (M79.7)*
                palindromic rheumatism (M12.3-)

☑5ᵗʰ **M79.1 Myalgia**
     Myofascial pain syndrome
     EXCLUDES 1   *fibromyalgia (M79.7)*
                myositis (M60.-)
     AHA: 2018,4Q,21
     M79.10 Myalgia, unspecified site
     M79.11 Myalgia of mastication muscle
     M79.12 Myalgia of auxiliary muscles, head and neck
     M79.18 Myalgia, other site

M79.2 Neuralgia and neuritis, unspecified
     EXCLUDES 1   *brachial radiculitis NOS (M54.1)*
                lumbosacral radiculitis NOS (M54.1)
                mononeuropathies (G56-G58)
                radiculitis NOS (M54.1)
                sciatica (M54.3-M54.4)
     TIP: Assign for documented neuropathic pain.

M79.3 Panniculitis, unspecified
     EXCLUDES 1   *lupus panniculitis (L93.2)*
                neck and back panniculitis (M54.0-)
                relapsing [Weber-Christian] panniculitis (M35.6)

M79.4 Hypertrophy of (infrapatellar) fat pad

M79.5 Residual foreign body in soft tissue
     EXCLUDES 1   *foreign body granuloma of skin and subcutaneous tissue (L92.3)*
                foreign body granuloma of soft tissue (M60.2-)

☑5ᵗʰ **M79.6 Pain in limb, hand, foot, fingers and toes**
     EXCLUDES 2   *pain in joint (M25.5-)*
     ☑6ᵗʰ **M79.60 Pain in limb, unspecified**
         M79.601 Pain in right arm
              Pain in right upper limb NOS
         M79.602 Pain in left arm
              Pain in left upper limb NOS
         M79.603 Pain in arm, unspecified
              Pain in upper limb NOS
         M79.604 Pain in right leg
              Pain in right lower limb NOS
         M79.605 Pain in left leg
              Pain in left lower limb NOS
         M79.606 Pain in leg, unspecified
              Pain in lower limb NOS
         M79.609 Pain in unspecified limb
              Pain in limb NOS
     ☑6ᵗʰ **M79.62 Pain in upper arm**
         Pain in axillary region
         M79.621 Pain in right upper arm
         M79.622 Pain in left upper arm
         M79.629 Pain in unspecified upper arm
     ☑6ᵗʰ **M79.63 Pain in forearm**
         M79.631 Pain in right forearm
         M79.632 Pain in left forearm
         M79.639 Pain in unspecified forearm
     ☑6ᵗʰ **M79.64 Pain in hand and fingers**
         M79.641 Pain in right hand

         M79.642 Pain in left hand
         M79.643 Pain in unspecified hand
         M79.644 Pain in right finger(s)
         M79.645 Pain in left finger(s)
         M79.646 Pain in unspecified finger(s)
     ☑6ᵗʰ **M79.65 Pain in thigh**
         M79.651 Pain in right thigh
         M79.652 Pain in left thigh
         M79.659 Pain in unspecified thigh
     ☑6ᵗʰ **M79.66 Pain in lower leg**
         M79.661 Pain in right lower leg
         M79.662 Pain in left lower leg
         M79.669 Pain in unspecified lower leg
     ☑6ᵗʰ **M79.67 Pain in foot and toes**
         M79.671 Pain in right foot
         M79.672 Pain in left foot
         M79.673 Pain in unspecified foot
         M79.674 Pain in right toe(s)
         M79.675 Pain in left toe(s)
         M79.676 Pain in unspecified toe(s)

M79.7 Fibromyalgia
     Fibromyositis
     Fibrositis
     Myofibrositis

☑5ᵗʰ **M79.A Nontraumatic compartment syndrome**
     Code first, if applicable, associated postprocedural complication
     EXCLUDES 1   *compartment syndrome NOS (T79.A-)*
                fibromyalgia (M79.7)
                nontraumatic ischemic infarction of muscle (M62.2-)
                traumatic compartment syndrome (T79.A-)
     ☑6ᵗʰ **M79.A1 Nontraumatic compartment syndrome of upper extremity**
         Nontraumatic compartment syndrome of shoulder, arm, forearm, wrist, hand, and fingers
         M79.A11 Nontraumatic compartment syndrome of right upper extremity
         M79.A12 Nontraumatic compartment syndrome of left upper extremity
         M79.A19 Nontraumatic compartment syndrome of unspecified upper extremity
     ☑6ᵗʰ **M79.A2 Nontraumatic compartment syndrome of lower extremity**
         Nontraumatic compartment syndrome of hip, buttock, thigh, leg, foot, and toes
         M79.A21 Nontraumatic compartment syndrome of right lower extremity
         M79.A22 Nontraumatic compartment syndrome of left lower extremity
         M79.A29 Nontraumatic compartment syndrome of unspecified lower extremity
     M79.A3 Nontraumatic compartment syndrome of abdomen
     M79.A9 Nontraumatic compartment syndrome of other sites

☑5ᵗʰ **M79.8 Other specified soft tissue disorders**
     M79.81 Nontraumatic hematoma of soft tissue
         Nontraumatic hematoma of muscle
         Nontraumatic seroma of muscle and soft tissue
     M79.89 Other specified soft tissue disorders
         Polyalgia

M79.9 Soft tissue disorder, unspecified

☑ Additional Character Required   ☑x7ᵗʰ Placeholder Alert   Manifestation   Unspecified Dx   Q QPP   UPD Unacceptable PDx

Chapter 13. Diseases of the Musculoskeletal System and Connective Tissue

OSTEOPATHIES AND CHONDROPATHIES (M80-M94)

Disorders of bone density and structure (M80-M85)

✓4ᵗʰ **M80 Osteoporosis** with current pathological fracture

> **INCLUDES**   osteoporosis with current fragility fracture
>
> Use additional code to identify major osseous defect, if applicable (M89.7-)
>
> **EXCLUDES 1**   collapsed vertebra NOS (M48.5)
> pathological fracture NOS (M84.4)
> wedging of vertebra NOS (M48.5)
>
> **EXCLUDES 2**   personal history of (healed) osteoporosis fracture (Z87.310)
>
> **AHA:** 2018,2Q,12
>
> **TIP:** The site codes in this category identify the site of the fracture, not the site of the osteoporosis.

> The appropriate 7th character is to be added to each code from category M80:
> A   initial encounter for fracture
> D   subsequent encounter for fracture with routine healing
> G   subsequent encounter for fracture with delayed healing
> K   subsequent encounter for fracture with nonunion
> P   subsequent encounter for fracture with malunion
> S   sequela

✓5ᵗʰ **M80.0 Age-related** osteoporosis with current pathological fracture

> Involutional osteoporosis with current pathological fracture
> Osteoporosis NOS with current pathological fracture
> Postmenopausal osteoporosis with current pathological fracture
> Senile osteoporosis with current pathological fracture

     ✓x7ᵗʰ **M80.00 Age-related osteoporosis with current pathological fracture, unspecified site**   Rx Q A

     ✓6ᵗʰ **M80.01 Age-related osteoporosis with current pathological fracture, shoulder**

         ✓7ᵗʰ **M80.011 Age-related osteoporosis with current pathological fracture, right shoulder**   Rx Q A

         ✓7ᵗʰ **M80.012 Age-related osteoporosis with current pathological fracture, left shoulder**   Rx Q A

         ✓7ᵗʰ **M80.019 Age-related osteoporosis with current pathological fracture, unspecified shoulder**   Rx Q A

     ✓6ᵗʰ **M80.02 Age-related osteoporosis with current pathological fracture, humerus**

         ✓7ᵗʰ **M80.021 Age-related osteoporosis with current pathological fracture, right humerus**   Rx Q A

pathological

         ✓7ᵗʰ **M80.022 Age-related osteoporosis with current pathological fracture, left humerus**   Rx Q A

         ✓7ᵗʰ **M80.029 Age-related osteoporosis with current pathological fracture, unspecified humerus**   Rx Q A

     ✓6ᵗʰ **M80.03 Age-related osteoporosis with current pathological fracture, forearm**
> Age-related osteoporosis with current pathological fracture of wrist

         ✓7ᵗʰ **M80.031 Age-related osteoporosis with current pathological fracture, right forearm**   Rx Q A

         ✓7ᵗʰ **M80.032 Age-related osteoporosis with current pathological fracture, left forearm**   Rx Q A

         ✓7ᵗʰ **M80.039 Age-related osteoporosis with current pathological fracture, unspecified forearm**   Rx Q A

     ✓6ᵗʰ **M80.04 Age-related osteoporosis with current pathological fracture, hand**

         ✓7ᵗʰ **M80.041 Age-related osteoporosis with current pathological fracture, right hand**   Rx Q A

         ✓7ᵗʰ **M80.042 Age-related osteoporosis with current pathological fracture, left hand**   Rx Q A

         ✓7ᵗʰ **M80.049 Age-related osteoporosis with current pathological fracture, unspecified hand**   Rx Q A

     ✓6ᵗʰ **M80.05 Age-related osteoporosis with current pathological fracture, femur**
> Age-related osteoporosis with current pathological fracture of hip

         1 ✓7ᵗʰ **M80.051 Age-related osteoporosis with current pathological fracture, right femur**   HCC Rx ESR COM Q A

         1 ✓7ᵗʰ **M80.052 Age-related osteoporosis with current pathological fracture, left femur**   HCC Rx ESR COM Q A

         1 ✓7ᵗʰ **M80.059 Age-related osteoporosis with current pathological fracture, unspecified femur**   HCC Rx ESR COM Q A

     ✓6ᵗʰ **M80.06 Age-related osteoporosis with current pathological fracture, lower leg**

         ✓7ᵗʰ **M80.061 Age-related osteoporosis with current pathological fracture, right lower leg**   Rx Q A

         ✓7ᵗʰ **M80.062 Age-related osteoporosis with current pathological fracture, left lower leg**   Rx Q A

         ✓7ᵗʰ **M80.069 Age-related osteoporosis with current pathological fracture, unspecified lower leg**   Rx Q A

     ✓6ᵗʰ **M80.07 Age-related osteoporosis with current pathological fracture, ankle and foot**

         ✓7ᵗʰ **M80.071 Age-related osteoporosis with current pathological fracture, right ankle and foot**   Rx Q A

         ✓7ᵗʰ **M80.072 Age-related osteoporosis with current pathological fracture, left ankle and foot**   Rx Q A

         ✓7ᵗʰ **M80.079 Age-related osteoporosis with current pathological fracture, unspecified ankle and foot**   Rx Q A

     1 ✓x7ᵗʰ **M80.08 Age-related osteoporosis with current pathological fracture, vertebra(e)**   HCC Rx ESR COM Q A

     ✓x7ᵗʰ **M80.0A Age-related osteoporosis with current pathological fracture, other site**   Rx Q A
> **AHA:** 2020,4Q,32-33

✓5ᵗʰ **M80.8 Other osteoporosis with current pathological fracture**

> Drug-induced osteoporosis with current pathological fracture
> Idiopathic osteoporosis with current pathological fracture
> Osteoporosis of disuse with current pathological fracture
> Postoophorectomy osteoporosis with current pathological fracture
> Postsurgical malabsorption osteoporosis with current pathological fracture
> Post-traumatic osteoporosis with current pathological fracture
> Use additional code for adverse effect, if applicable, to identify drug (T36-T50 with fifth or sixth character 5)

     ✓x7ᵗʰ **M80.80 Other osteoporosis with current pathological fracture, unspecified site**   Rx Q

     ✓6ᵗʰ **M80.81 Other osteoporosis with pathological fracture, shoulder**

         ✓7ᵗʰ **M80.811 Other osteoporosis with current pathological fracture, right shoulder**   Rx Q

         ✓7ᵗʰ **M80.812 Other osteoporosis with current pathological fracture, left shoulder**   Rx Q

         ✓7ᵗʰ **M80.819 Other osteoporosis with current pathological fracture, unspecified shoulder**   Rx Q

     ✓6ᵗʰ **M80.82 Other osteoporosis with current pathological fracture, humerus**

         ✓7ᵗʰ **M80.821 Other osteoporosis with current pathological fracture, right humerus**   Rx Q

         ✓7ᵗʰ **M80.822 Other osteoporosis with current pathological fracture, left humerus**   Rx Q

         ✓7ᵗʰ **M80.829 Other osteoporosis with current pathological fracture, unspecified humerus**   Rx Q

✓6ᵗʰ **M80.83** **Other osteoporosis with current pathological fracture,** forearm

Other osteoporosis with current pathological fracture of wrist

     ✓7ᵗʰ **M80.831** **Other osteoporosis with current pathological fracture,** right forearm   Rx Q

     ✓7ᵗʰ **M80.832** **Other osteoporosis with current pathological fracture,** left forearm   Rx Q

     ✓7ᵗʰ **M80.839** **Other osteoporosis with current pathological fracture, unspecified forearm**   Rx Q

✓6ᵗʰ **M80.84** **Other osteoporosis with current pathological fracture,** hand

     ✓7ᵗʰ **M80.841** **Other osteoporosis with current pathological fracture,** right hand   Rx Q

     ✓7ᵗʰ **M80.842** **Other osteoporosis with current pathological fracture,** left hand   Rx Q

     ✓7ᵗʰ **M80.849** **Other osteoporosis with current pathological fracture, unspecified hand**   Rx Q

✓6ᵗʰ **M80.85** **Other osteoporosis with current pathological fracture,** femur

Other osteoporosis with current pathological fracture of hip

     ¹ ✓7ᵗʰ **M80.851** **Other osteoporosis with current pathological fracture,** right femur   HCC Rx ESR COM Q

     ¹ ✓7ᵗʰ **M80.852** **Other osteoporosis with current pathological fracture,** left femur   HCC Rx ESR COM Q

     ¹ ✓7ᵗʰ **M80.859** **Other osteoporosis with current pathological fracture, unspecified femur**   HCC Rx ESR COM Q

✓6ᵗʰ **M80.86** **Other osteoporosis with current pathological fracture,** lower leg

     ✓7ᵗʰ **M80.861** **Other osteoporosis with current pathological fracture,** right lower leg   Rx Q

     ✓7ᵗʰ **M80.862** **Other osteoporosis with current pathological fracture,** left lower leg   Rx Q

     ✓7ᵗʰ **M80.869** **Other osteoporosis with current pathological fracture, unspecified lower leg**   Rx Q

✓6ᵗʰ **M80.87** **Other osteoporosis with current pathological fracture,** ankle and foot

     ✓7ᵗʰ **M80.871** **Other osteoporosis with current pathological fracture,** right ankle and foot   Rx Q

     ✓7ᵗʰ **M80.872** **Other osteoporosis with current pathological fracture,** left ankle and foot   Rx Q

     ✓7ᵗʰ **M80.879** **Other osteoporosis with current pathological fracture, unspecified ankle and foot**   Rx Q

¹ ✓x7ᵗʰ **M80.88** **Other osteoporosis with current pathological fracture,** vertebra(e)   HCC Rx ESR COM Q

✓x7ᵗʰ **M80.8A** **Other osteoporosis with current pathological fracture, other site**   Rx Q

AHA: 2020,4Q,32

✓4ᵗʰ **M81 Osteoporosis** without current pathological fracture

Use additional code to identify:

major osseous defect, if applicable (M89.7-)

personal history of (healed) osteoporosis fracture, if applicable (Z87.310)

     EXCLUDES 1   *osteoporosis with current pathological fracture (M80.-)*

     Sudeck's atrophy (M89.0)

M81.0 Age-related **osteoporosis without current pathological fracture**   Rx Q A

Involutional osteoporosis without current pathological fracture

Osteoporosis NOS

Postmenopausal osteoporosis without current pathological fracture

Senile osteoporosis without current pathological fracture

M81.6 Localized **osteoporosis [Lequesne]**   Rx Q

     EXCLUDES 1   *Sudeck's atrophy (M89.0)*

M81.8 **Other osteoporosis without current pathological fracture**   Rx Q

Drug-induced osteoporosis without current pathological fracture

Idiopathic osteoporosis without current pathological fracture

Osteoporosis of disuse without current pathological fracture

Postoophorectomy osteoporosis without current pathological fracture

Postsurgical malabsorption osteoporosis without current pathological fracture

Post-traumatic osteoporosis without current pathological fracture

Use additional code for adverse effect, if applicable, to identify drug (T36-T50 with fifth or sixth character 5)

✓4ᵗʰ **M83 Adult osteomalacia**

     EXCLUDES 1   *infantile and juvenile osteomalacia (E55.0)*

     renal osteodystrophy (N25.0)

     rickets (active) (E55.0)

     rickets (active) sequelae (E64.3)

     vitamin D-resistant osteomalacia (E83.3)

     vitamin D-resistant rickets (active) (E83.3)

M83.0 Puerperal **osteomalacia**   Rx M ♀

M83.1 Senile **osteomalacia**   Rx A

M83.2 **Adult osteomalacia** due to malabsorption   Rx A

Postsurgical malabsorption osteomalacia in adults

M83.3 **Adult osteomalacia** due to malnutrition   Rx A

M83.4 Aluminum bone disease   Rx

M83.5 **Other** drug-induced **osteomalacia in adults**   Rx A

Use additional code for adverse effect, if applicable, to identify drug (T36-T50 with fifth or sixth character 5)

M83.8 **Other adult osteomalacia**   Rx A

M83.9 **Adult osteomalacia, unspecified**   Rx A

✓4ᵗʰ **M84 Disorder of continuity of bone**

     EXCLUDES 2   *traumatic fracture of bone-see fracture, by site*

✓5ᵗʰ **M84.3 Stress fracture**

Fatigue fracture

March fracture

Stress fracture NOS

Stress reaction

Use additional external cause code(s) to identify the cause of the stress fracture

     EXCLUDES 1   *pathological fracture due to osteoporosis (M80.-)*

     pathological fracture NOS (M84.4.-)

     traumatic fracture (S12.-, S22.-, S32.-, S42.-, S52.-, S62.-, S72.-, S82.-, S92.-)

     EXCLUDES 2   *personal history of (healed) stress (fatigue) fracture (Z87.312)*

     stress fracture of vertebra (M48.4-)

> The appropriate 7th character is to be added to each code from subcategory M84.3.
> A   initial encounter for fracture
> D   subsequent encounter for fracture with routine healing
> G   subsequent encounter for fracture with delayed healing
> K   subsequent encounter for fracture with nonunion
> P   subsequent encounter for fracture with malunion
> S   sequela

✓x7ᵗʰ **M84.30** **Stress fracture, unspecified site**

✓6ᵗʰ **M84.31** **Stress fracture,** shoulder

     ✓7ᵗʰ **M84.311** **Stress fracture, right shoulder**   Q

     ✓7ᵗʰ **M84.312** **Stress fracture, left shoulder**   Q

     ✓7ᵗʰ **M84.319** **Stress fracture, unspecified shoulder**   Q

✓6ᵗʰ **M84.32** **Stress fracture,** humerus

     ✓7ᵗʰ **M84.321** **Stress fracture, right humerus**   Q

     ✓7ᵗʰ **M84.322** **Stress fracture, left humerus**   Q

     ✓7ᵗʰ **M84.329** **Stress fracture, unspecified humerus**   Q

✓6ᵗʰ **M84.33** **Stress fracture,** ulna and radius

     ✓7ᵗʰ **M84.331** **Stress fracture, right ulna**   Q

     ✓7ᵗʰ **M84.332** **Stress fracture, left ulna**   Q

     ✓7ᵗʰ **M84.333** **Stress fracture, right radius**   Q

     ✓7ᵗʰ **M84.334** **Stress fracture, left radius**   Q

√7ᵗʰ **M84.339** Stress fracture, unspecified ulna and radius ▫

√6ᵗʰ **M84.34** Stress fracture, hand and fingers

　√7ᵗʰ **M84.341** Stress fracture, right hand ▫
　√7ᵗʰ **M84.342** Stress fracture, left hand ▫
　√7ᵗʰ **M84.343** Stress fracture, unspecified hand ▫
　√7ᵗʰ **M84.344** Stress fracture, right finger(s)
　√7ᵗʰ **M84.345** Stress fracture, left finger(s)
　√7ᵗʰ **M84.346** Stress fracture, unspecified finger(s)

√6ᵗʰ **M84.35** Stress fracture, pelvis and femur

　　Stress fracture, hip

　√7ᵗʰ **M84.350** Stress fracture, pelvis ▫
　√7ᵗʰ **M84.351** Stress fracture, right femur ▫
　√7ᵗʰ **M84.352** Stress fracture, left femur ▫
　√7ᵗʰ **M84.353** Stress fracture, unspecified femur ▫
　√7ᵗʰ **M84.359** Stress fracture, hip, unspecified ▫

√6ᵗʰ **M84.36** Stress fracture, tibia and fibula

　√7ᵗʰ **M84.361** Stress fracture, right tibia ▫
　√7ᵗʰ **M84.362** Stress fracture, left tibia ▫
　√7ᵗʰ **M84.363** Stress fracture, right fibula ▫
　√7ᵗʰ **M84.364** Stress fracture, left fibula ▫
　√7ᵗʰ **M84.369** Stress fracture, unspecified tibia and fibula ▫

√6ᵗʰ **M84.37** Stress fracture, ankle, foot and toes

　√7ᵗʰ **M84.371** Stress fracture, right ankle ▫
　√7ᵗʰ **M84.372** Stress fracture, left ankle ▫
　√7ᵗʰ **M84.373** Stress fracture, unspecified ankle ▫
　√7ᵗʰ **M84.374** Stress fracture, right foot ▫
　√7ᵗʰ **M84.375** Stress fracture, left foot ▫
　√7ᵗʰ **M84.376** Stress fracture, unspecified foot ▫
　√7ᵗʰ **M84.377** Stress fracture, right toe(s)
　√7ᵗʰ **M84.378** Stress fracture, left toe(s)
　√7ᵗʰ **M84.379** Stress fracture, unspecified toe(s)

√x7ᵗʰ **M84.38** Stress fracture, other site ▫

　　EXCLUDES 2　stress fracture of vertebra (M48.4-)

√5ᵗʰ **M84.4** Pathological fracture, not elsewhere classified

　　Chronic fracture
　　Pathological fracture NOS

　　EXCLUDES 1　collapsed vertebra NEC (M48.5)
　　　　pathological fracture in neoplastic disease (M84.5-)
　　　　pathological fracture in osteoporosis (M80.-)
　　　　pathological fracture in other disease (M84.6-)
　　　　stress fracture (M84.3-)
　　　　traumatic fracture (S12.-, S22.-, S32.-, S42.-, S52.-, S62.-, S72.-, S82.-, S92.-)

　　EXCLUDES 2　personal history of (healed) pathological fracture (Z87.311)

The appropriate 7th character is to be added to each code from subcategory M84.4.
A　initial encounter for fracture
D　subsequent encounter for fracture with routine healing
G　subsequent encounter for fracture with delayed healing
K　subsequent encounter for fracture with nonunion
P　subsequent encounter for fracture with malunion
S　sequela

√x7ᵗʰ **M84.40** Pathological fracture, unspecified site `Rx`

√6ᵗʰ **M84.41** Pathological fracture, shoulder

　√7ᵗʰ **M84.411** Pathological fracture, right shoulder `Rx`
　√7ᵗʰ **M84.412** Pathological fracture, left shoulder `Rx`
　√7ᵗʰ **M84.419** Pathological fracture, unspecified shoulder `Rx`

√6ᵗʰ **M84.42** Pathological fracture, humerus

　√7ᵗʰ **M84.421** Pathological fracture, right humerus `Rx`
　√7ᵗʰ **M84.422** Pathological fracture, left humerus `Rx`
　√7ᵗʰ **M84.429** Pathological fracture, unspecified humerus `Rx`

√6ᵗʰ **M84.43** Pathological fracture, ulna and radius

　√7ᵗʰ **M84.431** Pathological fracture, right ulna `Rx`

　√7ᵗʰ **M84.432** Pathological fracture, left ulna `Rx`
　√7ᵗʰ **M84.433** Pathological fracture, right radius `Rx`
　√7ᵗʰ **M84.434** Pathological fracture, left radius `Rx`
　√7ᵗʰ **M84.439** Pathological fracture, unspecified ulna and radius `Rx`

√6ᵗʰ **M84.44** Pathological fracture, hand and fingers

　√7ᵗʰ **M84.441** Pathological fracture, right hand `Rx`
　√7ᵗʰ **M84.442** Pathological fracture, left hand `Rx`
　√7ᵗʰ **M84.443** Pathological fracture, unspecified hand `Rx`
　√7ᵗʰ **M84.444** Pathological fracture, right finger(s) `Rx`
　√7ᵗʰ **M84.445** Pathological fracture, left finger(s) `Rx`
　√7ᵗʰ **M84.446** Pathological fracture, unspecified finger(s) `Rx`

√6ᵗʰ **M84.45** Pathological fracture, femur and pelvis

　　AHA: 2016,4Q,43

　¹ √7ᵗʰ **M84.451** Pathological fracture, right femur `HCC` `Rx` `ESR` `COM`
　¹ √7ᵗʰ **M84.452** Pathological fracture, left femur `HCC` `Rx` `ESR` `COM`
　¹ √7ᵗʰ **M84.453** Pathological fracture, unspecified femur `HCC` `Rx` `ESR` `COM`
　√7ᵗʰ **M84.454** Pathological fracture, pelvis `Rx`
　¹ √7ᵗʰ **M84.459** Pathological fracture, hip, unspecified `HCC` `Rx` `ESR` `COM`

√6ᵗʰ **M84.46** Pathological fracture, tibia and fibula

　√7ᵗʰ **M84.461** Pathological fracture, right tibia `Rx`
　√7ᵗʰ **M84.462** Pathological fracture, left tibia `Rx`
　√7ᵗʰ **M84.463** Pathological fracture, right fibula `Rx`
　√7ᵗʰ **M84.464** Pathological fracture, left fibula `Rx`
　√7ᵗʰ **M84.469** Pathological fracture, unspecified tibia and fibula `Rx`

√6ᵗʰ **M84.47** Pathological fracture, ankle, foot and toes

　√7ᵗʰ **M84.471** Pathological fracture, right ankle `Rx`
　√7ᵗʰ **M84.472** Pathological fracture, left ankle `Rx`
　√7ᵗʰ **M84.473** Pathological fracture, unspecified ankle `Rx`
　√7ᵗʰ **M84.474** Pathological fracture, right foot `Rx`
　√7ᵗʰ **M84.475** Pathological fracture, left foot `Rx`
　√7ᵗʰ **M84.476** Pathological fracture, unspecified foot `Rx`
　√7ᵗʰ **M84.477** Pathological fracture, right toe(s) `Rx`
　√7ᵗʰ **M84.478** Pathological fracture, left toe(s) `Rx`
　√7ᵗʰ **M84.479** Pathological fracture, unspecified toe(s) `Rx`

√x7ᵗʰ **M84.48** Pathological fracture, other site `Rx`

√5ᵗʰ **M84.5** Pathological fracture in neoplastic disease

　　Code also underlying neoplasm

The appropriate 7th character is to be added to each code from subcategory M84.5.
A　initial encounter for fracture
D　subsequent encounter for fracture with routine healing
G　subsequent encounter for fracture with delayed healing
K　subsequent encounter for fracture with nonunion
P　subsequent encounter for fracture with malunion
S　sequela

√x7ᵗʰ **M84.50** Pathological fracture in neoplastic disease, unspecified site `Rx`

√6ᵗʰ **M84.51** Pathological fracture in neoplastic disease, shoulder

　√7ᵗʰ **M84.511** Pathological fracture in neoplastic disease, right shoulder `Rx`
　√7ᵗʰ **M84.512** Pathological fracture in neoplastic disease, left shoulder `Rx`
　√7ᵗʰ **M84.519** Pathological fracture in neoplastic disease, unspecified shoulder `Rx`

√6ᵗʰ **M84.52** Pathological fracture in neoplastic disease, humerus

　√7ᵗʰ **M84.521** Pathological fracture in neoplastic disease, right humerus `Rx`
　√7ᵗʰ **M84.522** Pathological fracture in neoplastic disease, left humerus `Rx`

√7ᵗʰ **M84.529** Pathological fracture in neoplastic disease, unspecified humerus   Rx

√6ᵗʰ **M84.53** Pathological fracture in neoplastic disease, ulna and radius

    √7ᵗʰ **M84.531** Pathological fracture in neoplastic disease, right ulna   Rx

    √7ᵗʰ **M84.532** Pathological fracture in neoplastic disease, left ulna   Rx

    √7ᵗʰ **M84.533** Pathological fracture in neoplastic disease, right radius   Rx

    √7ᵗʰ **M84.534** Pathological fracture in neoplastic disease, left radius   Rx

    √7ᵗʰ **M84.539** Pathological fracture in neoplastic disease, unspecified ulna and radius   Rx

√6ᵗʰ **M84.54** Pathological fracture in neoplastic disease, hand

    √7ᵗʰ **M84.541** Pathological fracture in neoplastic disease, right hand   Rx

    √7ᵗʰ **M84.542** Pathological fracture in neoplastic disease, left hand   Rx

    √7ᵗʰ **M84.549** Pathological fracture in neoplastic disease, unspecified hand   Rx

√6ᵗʰ **M84.55** Pathological fracture in neoplastic disease, pelvis and femur

    √7ᵗʰ **M84.550** Pathological fracture in neoplastic disease, pelvis   Rx

    ¹ √7ᵗʰ **M84.551** Pathological fracture in neoplastic disease, right femur   HCC Rx ESR COM

    ¹ √7ᵗʰ **M84.552** Pathological fracture in neoplastic disease, left femur   HCC Rx ESR COM

    ¹ √7ᵗʰ **M84.553** Pathological fracture in neoplastic disease, unspecified femur   HCC Rx ESR COM

    ¹ √7ᵗʰ **M84.559** Pathological fracture in neoplastic disease, hip, unspecified   HCC Rx ESR COM

√6ᵗʰ **M84.56** Pathological fracture in neoplastic disease, tibia and fibula

    √7ᵗʰ **M84.561** Pathological fracture in neoplastic disease, right tibia   Rx

    √7ᵗʰ **M84.562** Pathological fracture in neoplastic disease, left tibia   Rx

    √7ᵗʰ **M84.563** Pathological fracture in neoplastic disease, right fibula   Rx

    √7ᵗʰ **M84.564** Pathological fracture in neoplastic disease, left fibula   Rx

    √7ᵗʰ **M84.569** Pathological fracture in neoplastic disease, unspecified tibia and fibula   Rx

√6ᵗʰ **M84.57** Pathological fracture in neoplastic disease, ankle and foot

    √7ᵗʰ **M84.571** Pathological fracture in neoplastic disease, right ankle   Rx

    √7ᵗʰ **M84.572** Pathological fracture in neoplastic disease, left ankle   Rx

    √7ᵗʰ **M84.573** Pathological fracture in neoplastic disease, unspecified ankle   Rx

    √7ᵗʰ **M84.574** Pathological fracture in neoplastic disease, right foot   Rx

    √7ᵗʰ **M84.575** Pathological fracture in neoplastic disease, left foot   Rx

    √7ᵗʰ **M84.576** Pathological fracture in neoplastic disease, unspecified foot   Rx

√x7ᵗʰ **M84.58** Pathological fracture in neoplastic disease, other specified site   Rx

    Pathological fracture in neoplastic disease, vertebrae

√6ᵗʰ **M84.6** Pathological fracture in other disease

Code also underlying condition

EXCLUDES 1   *pathological fracture in osteoporosis (M80.-)*

The appropriate 7th character is to be added to each code from subcategory M84.6.
A   initial encounter for fracture
D   subsequent encounter for fracture with routine healing
G   subsequent encounter for fracture with delayed healing
K   subsequent encounter for fracture with nonunion
P   subsequent encounter for fracture with malunion
S   sequela

√x7ᵗʰ **M84.60** Pathological fracture in other disease, unspecified site   Rx

√6ᵗʰ **M84.61** Pathological fracture in other disease, shoulder

    √7ᵗʰ **M84.611** Pathological fracture in other disease, right shoulder   Rx

    √7ᵗʰ **M84.612** Pathological fracture in other disease, left shoulder   Rx

    √7ᵗʰ **M84.619** Pathological fracture in other disease, unspecified shoulder   Rx

√6ᵗʰ **M84.62** Pathological fracture in other disease, humerus

    √7ᵗʰ **M84.621** Pathological fracture in other disease, right humerus   Rx

    √7ᵗʰ **M84.622** Pathological fracture in other disease, left humerus   Rx

    √7ᵗʰ **M84.629** Pathological fracture in other disease, unspecified humerus   Rx

√6ᵗʰ **M84.63** Pathological fracture in other disease, ulna and radius

    √7ᵗʰ **M84.631** Pathological fracture in other disease, right ulna   Rx

    √7ᵗʰ **M84.632** Pathological fracture in other disease, left ulna   Rx

    √7ᵗʰ **M84.633** Pathological fracture in other disease, right radius   Rx

    √7ᵗʰ **M84.634** Pathological fracture in other disease, left radius   Rx

    √7ᵗʰ **M84.639** Pathological fracture in other disease, unspecified ulna and radius   Rx

√6ᵗʰ **M84.64** Pathological fracture in other disease, hand

    √7ᵗʰ **M84.641** Pathological fracture in other disease, right hand   Rx

    √7ᵗʰ **M84.642** Pathological fracture in other disease, left hand   Rx

    √7ᵗʰ **M84.649** Pathological fracture in other disease, unspecified hand   Rx

√6ᵗʰ **M84.65** Pathological fracture in other disease, pelvis and femur

    √7ᵗʰ **M84.650** Pathological fracture in other disease, pelvis   Rx

    ¹ √7ᵗʰ **M84.651** Pathological fracture in other disease, right femur   HCC Rx ESR COM

    ¹ √7ᵗʰ **M84.652** Pathological fracture in other disease, left femur   HCC Rx ESR COM

    ¹ √7ᵗʰ **M84.653** Pathological fracture in other disease, unspecified femur   HCC Rx ESR COM

    ¹ √7ᵗʰ **M84.659** Pathological fracture in other disease, hip, unspecified   HCC Rx ESR COM

√6ᵗʰ **M84.66** Pathological fracture in other disease, tibia and fibula

    √7ᵗʰ **M84.661** Pathological fracture in other disease, right tibia   Rx

    √7ᵗʰ **M84.662** Pathological fracture in other disease, left tibia   Rx

    √7ᵗʰ **M84.663** Pathological fracture in other disease, right fibula   Rx

    √7ᵗʰ **M84.664** Pathological fracture in other disease, left fibula   Rx

    √7ᵗʰ **M84.669** Pathological fracture in other disease, unspecified tibia and fibula   Rx

√6ᵗʰ **M84.67** Pathological fracture in other disease, ankle and foot

    √7ᵗʰ **M84.671** Pathological fracture in other disease, right ankle   Rx

    √7ᵗʰ **M84.672** Pathological fracture in other disease, left ankle   Rx

    √7ᵗʰ **M84.673** Pathological fracture in other disease, unspecified ankle   Rx

    √7ᵗʰ **M84.674** Pathological fracture in other disease, right foot   Rx

    √7ᵗʰ **M84.675** Pathological fracture in other disease, left foot   Rx

    √7ᵗʰ **M84.676** Pathological fracture in other disease, unspecified foot   Rx

√x7ᵗʰ **M84.68** Pathological fracture in other disease, other site   Rx

☑5ᵗʰ **M84.7 Nontraumatic fracture, not elsewhere classified**

☑6ᵗʰ **M84.75 Atypical femoral fracture**

AHA: 2016,4Q,41-42

> The appropriate 7th character is to be added to each code from M84.75.
> A initial encounter for fracture
> D subsequent encounter for fracture with routine healing
> G subsequent encounter for fracture with delayed healing
> K subsequent encounter for fracture with nonunion
> P subsequent encounter for fracture with malunion
> S sequela

☑7ᵗʰ **M84.75Ø Atypical femoral fracture, unspecified** ◨
☑7ᵗʰ **M84.751 Incomplete atypical femoral fracture, right leg** ◨
☑7ᵗʰ **M84.752 Incomplete atypical femoral fracture, left leg** ◨
☑7ᵗʰ **M84.753 Incomplete atypical femoral fracture, unspecified leg** ◨
¹ ☑7ᵗʰ **M84.754 Complete transverse atypical femoral fracture, right leg** HCC ESR COM ◨
¹ ☑7ᵗʰ **M84.755 Complete transverse atypical femoral fracture, left leg** HCC ESR COM ◨
¹ ☑7ᵗʰ **M84.756 Complete transverse atypical femoral fracture, unspecified leg** HCC ESR COM ◨
¹ ☑7ᵗʰ **M84.757 Complete oblique atypical femoral fracture, right leg** HCC ESR COM ◨
¹ ☑7ᵗʰ **M84.758 Complete oblique atypical femoral fracture, left leg** HCC ESR COM
¹ ☑7ᵗʰ **M84.759 Complete oblique atypical femoral fracture, unspecified leg** HCC ESR COM ◨

☑5ᵗʰ **M84.8 Other disorders of continuity of bone**

M84.8Ø Other disorders of continuity of bone, unspecified site
☑6ᵗʰ **M84.81 Other disorders of continuity of bone, shoulder**
M84.811 Other disorders of continuity of bone, right shoulder
M84.812 Other disorders of continuity of bone, left shoulder
M84.819 Other disorders of continuity of bone, unspecified shoulder
☑6ᵗʰ **M84.82 Other disorders of continuity of bone, humerus**
M84.821 Other disorders of continuity of bone, right humerus
M84.822 Other disorders of continuity of bone, left humerus
M84.829 Other disorders of continuity of bone, unspecified humerus
☑6ᵗʰ **M84.83 Other disorders of continuity of bone, ulna and radius**
M84.831 Other disorders of continuity of bone, right ulna
M84.832 Other disorders of continuity of bone, left ulna
M84.833 Other disorders of continuity of bone, right radius
M84.834 Other disorders of continuity of bone, left radius
M84.839 Other disorders of continuity of bone, unspecified ulna and radius
☑6ᵗʰ **M84.84 Other disorders of continuity of bone, hand**
M84.841 Other disorders of continuity of bone, right hand
M84.842 Other disorders of continuity of bone, left hand
M84.849 Other disorders of continuity of bone, unspecified hand
☑6ᵗʰ **M84.85 Other disorders of continuity of bone, pelvic region and thigh**
M84.851 Other disorders of continuity of bone, right pelvic region and thigh
M84.852 Other disorders of continuity of bone, left pelvic region and thigh
M84.859 Other disorders of continuity of bone, unspecified pelvic region and thigh
☑6ᵗʰ **M84.86 Other disorders of continuity of bone, tibia and fibula**
M84.861 Other disorders of continuity of bone, right tibia
M84.862 Other disorders of continuity of bone, left tibia
M84.863 Other disorders of continuity of bone, right fibula
M84.864 Other disorders of continuity of bone, left fibula
M84.869 Other disorders of continuity of bone, unspecified tibia and fibula
☑6ᵗʰ **M84.87 Other disorders of continuity of bone, ankle and foot**
M84.871 Other disorders of continuity of bone, right ankle and foot
M84.872 Other disorders of continuity of bone, left ankle and foot
M84.879 Other disorders of continuity of bone, unspecified ankle and foot
M84.88 Other disorders of continuity of bone, other site
M84.9 Disorder of continuity of bone, unspecified

☑4ᵗʰ **M85 Other disorders of bone density and structure**

EXCLUDES 1 osteogenesis imperfecta (Q78.Ø)
osteopetrosis (Q78.2)
osteopoikilosis (Q78.8)
polyostotic fibrous dysplasia (Q78.1)

☑5ᵗʰ **M85.Ø Fibrous dysplasia (monostotic)**

EXCLUDES 2 fibrous dysplasia of jaw (M27.8)

M85.ØØ Fibrous dysplasia (monostotic), unspecified site
☑6ᵗʰ **M85.Ø1 Fibrous dysplasia (monostotic), shoulder**
M85.Ø11 Fibrous dysplasia (monostotic), right shoulder
M85.Ø12 Fibrous dysplasia (monostotic), left shoulder
M85.Ø19 Fibrous dysplasia (monostotic), unspecified shoulder
☑6ᵗʰ **M85.Ø2 Fibrous dysplasia (monostotic), upper arm**
M85.Ø21 Fibrous dysplasia (monostotic), right upper arm
M85.Ø22 Fibrous dysplasia (monostotic), left upper arm
M85.Ø29 Fibrous dysplasia (monostotic), unspecified upper arm
☑6ᵗʰ **M85.Ø3 Fibrous dysplasia (monostotic), forearm**
M85.Ø31 Fibrous dysplasia (monostotic), right forearm
M85.Ø32 Fibrous dysplasia (monostotic), left forearm
M85.Ø39 Fibrous dysplasia (monostotic), unspecified forearm
☑6ᵗʰ **M85.Ø4 Fibrous dysplasia (monostotic), hand**
M85.Ø41 Fibrous dysplasia (monostotic), right hand
M85.Ø42 Fibrous dysplasia (monostotic), left hand
M85.Ø49 Fibrous dysplasia (monostotic), unspecified hand
☑6ᵗʰ **M85.Ø5 Fibrous dysplasia (monostotic), thigh**
M85.Ø51 Fibrous dysplasia (monostotic), right thigh
M85.Ø52 Fibrous dysplasia (monostotic), left thigh
M85.Ø59 Fibrous dysplasia (monostotic), unspecified thigh
☑6ᵗʰ **M85.Ø6 Fibrous dysplasia (monostotic), lower leg**
M85.Ø61 Fibrous dysplasia (monostotic), right lower leg
M85.Ø62 Fibrous dysplasia (monostotic), left lower leg
M85.Ø69 Fibrous dysplasia (monostotic), unspecified lower leg
☑6ᵗʰ **M85.Ø7 Fibrous dysplasia (monostotic), ankle and foot**
M85.Ø71 Fibrous dysplasia (monostotic), right ankle and foot
M85.Ø72 Fibrous dysplasia (monostotic), left ankle and foot
M85.Ø79 Fibrous dysplasia (monostotic), unspecified ankle and foot

M85.08   Fibrous dysplasia (monostotic), other site
M85.09   Fibrous dysplasia (monostotic), multiple sites

✓5ᵗʰ M85.1   **Skeletal fluorosis**

M85.10   Skeletal fluorosis, unspecified site

✓6ᵗʰ M85.11   Skeletal fluorosis, shoulder

M85.111   Skeletal fluorosis, right shoulder
M85.112   Skeletal fluorosis, left shoulder
M85.119   Skeletal fluorosis, unspecified shoulder

✓6ᵗʰ M85.12   Skeletal fluorosis, upper arm

M85.121   Skeletal fluorosis, right upper arm
M85.122   Skeletal fluorosis, left upper arm
M85.129   Skeletal fluorosis, unspecified upper arm

✓6ᵗʰ M85.13   Skeletal fluorosis, forearm

M85.131   Skeletal fluorosis, right forearm
M85.132   Skeletal fluorosis, left forearm
M85.139   Skeletal fluorosis, unspecified forearm

✓6ᵗʰ M85.14   Skeletal fluorosis, hand

M85.141   Skeletal fluorosis, right hand
M85.142   Skeletal fluorosis, left hand
M85.149   Skeletal fluorosis, unspecified hand

✓6ᵗʰ M85.15   Skeletal fluorosis, thigh

M85.151   Skeletal fluorosis, right thigh
M85.152   Skeletal fluorosis, left thigh
M85.159   Skeletal fluorosis, unspecified thigh

✓6ᵗʰ M85.16   Skeletal fluorosis, lower leg

M85.161   Skeletal fluorosis, right lower leg
M85.162   Skeletal fluorosis, left lower leg
M85.169   Skeletal fluorosis, unspecified lower leg

✓6ᵗʰ M85.17   Skeletal fluorosis, ankle and foot

M85.171   Skeletal fluorosis, right ankle and foot
M85.172   Skeletal fluorosis, left ankle and foot
M85.179   Skeletal fluorosis, unspecified ankle and foot

M85.18   Skeletal fluorosis, other site
M85.19   Skeletal fluorosis, multiple sites

M85.2   **Hyperostosis of skull**
DEF: Abnormal bone growth on the inner aspect of the cranial bones.

✓5ᵗʰ M85.3   **Osteitis condensans**

M85.30   Osteitis condensans, unspecified site

✓6ᵗʰ M85.31   Osteitis condensans, shoulder

M85.311   Osteitis condensans, right shoulder
M85.312   Osteitis condensans, left shoulder
M85.319   Osteitis condensans, unspecified shoulder

✓6ᵗʰ M85.32   Osteitis condensans, upper arm

M85.321   Osteitis condensans, right upper arm
M85.322   Osteitis condensans, left upper arm
M85.329   Osteitis condensans, unspecified upper arm

✓6ᵗʰ M85.33   Osteitis condensans, forearm

M85.331   Osteitis condensans, right forearm
M85.332   Osteitis condensans, left forearm
M85.339   Osteitis condensans, unspecified forearm

✓6ᵗʰ M85.34   Osteitis condensans, hand

M85.341   Osteitis condensans, right hand
M85.342   Osteitis condensans, left hand
M85.349   Osteitis condensans, unspecified hand

✓6ᵗʰ M85.35   Osteitis condensans, thigh

M85.351   Osteitis condensans, right thigh
M85.352   Osteitis condensans, left thigh
M85.359   Osteitis condensans, unspecified thigh

✓6ᵗʰ M85.36   Osteitis condensans, lower leg

M85.361   Osteitis condensans, right lower leg
M85.362   Osteitis condensans, left lower leg
M85.369   Osteitis condensans, unspecified lower leg

✓6ᵗʰ M85.37   Osteitis condensans, ankle and foot

M85.371   Osteitis condensans, right ankle and foot
M85.372   Osteitis condensans, left ankle and foot
M85.379   Osteitis condensans, unspecified ankle and foot

M85.38   Osteitis condensans, other site
M85.39   Osteitis condensans, multiple sites

✓5ᵗʰ M85.4   **Solitary bone cyst**
EXCLUDES 2   solitary cyst of jaw (M27.4)

M85.40   Solitary bone cyst, unspecified site

✓6ᵗʰ M85.41   Solitary bone cyst, shoulder

M85.411   Solitary bone cyst, right shoulder
M85.412   Solitary bone cyst, left shoulder
M85.419   Solitary bone cyst, unspecified shoulder

✓6ᵗʰ M85.42   Solitary bone cyst, humerus

M85.421   Solitary bone cyst, right humerus
M85.422   Solitary bone cyst, left humerus
M85.429   Solitary bone cyst, unspecified humerus

✓6ᵗʰ M85.43   Solitary bone cyst, ulna and radius

M85.431   Solitary bone cyst, right ulna and radius
M85.432   Solitary bone cyst, left ulna and radius
M85.439   Solitary bone cyst, unspecified ulna and radius

✓6ᵗʰ M85.44   Solitary bone cyst, hand

M85.441   Solitary bone cyst, right hand
M85.442   Solitary bone cyst, left hand
M85.449   Solitary bone cyst, unspecified hand

✓6ᵗʰ M85.45   Solitary bone cyst, pelvis

M85.451   Solitary bone cyst, right pelvis
M85.452   Solitary bone cyst, left pelvis
M85.459   Solitary bone cyst, unspecified pelvis

✓6ᵗʰ M85.46   Solitary bone cyst, tibia and fibula

M85.461   Solitary bone cyst, right tibia and fibula
M85.462   Solitary bone cyst, left tibia and fibula
M85.469   Solitary bone cyst, unspecified tibia and fibula

✓6ᵗʰ M85.47   Solitary bone cyst, ankle and foot

M85.471   Solitary bone cyst, right ankle and foot
M85.472   Solitary bone cyst, left ankle and foot
M85.479   Solitary bone cyst, unspecified ankle and foot

M85.48   Solitary bone cyst, other site

✓5ᵗʰ M85.5   **Aneurysmal bone cyst**
EXCLUDES 2   aneurysmal cyst of jaw (M27.4)
DEF: Solitary bone lesion that bulges into the periosteum and is marked by a calcified rim.

M85.50   Aneurysmal bone cyst, unspecified site

✓6ᵗʰ M85.51   Aneurysmal bone cyst, shoulder

M85.511   Aneurysmal bone cyst, right shoulder
M85.512   Aneurysmal bone cyst, left shoulder
M85.519   Aneurysmal bone cyst, unspecified shoulder

✓6ᵗʰ M85.52   Aneurysmal bone cyst, upper arm

M85.521   Aneurysmal bone cyst, right upper arm
M85.522   Aneurysmal bone cyst, left upper arm
M85.529   Aneurysmal bone cyst, unspecified upper arm

✓6ᵗʰ M85.53   Aneurysmal bone cyst, forearm

M85.531   Aneurysmal bone cyst, right forearm
M85.532   Aneurysmal bone cyst, left forearm
M85.539   Aneurysmal bone cyst, unspecified forearm

✓6ᵗʰ M85.54   Aneurysmal bone cyst, hand

M85.541   Aneurysmal bone cyst, right hand
M85.542   Aneurysmal bone cyst, left hand
M85.549   Aneurysmal bone cyst, unspecified hand

✓6ᵗʰ M85.55   Aneurysmal bone cyst, thigh

M85.551   Aneurysmal bone cyst, right thigh
M85.552   Aneurysmal bone cyst, left thigh
M85.559   Aneurysmal bone cyst, unspecified thigh

✓6ᵗʰ M85.56   Aneurysmal bone cyst, lower leg

M85.561   Aneurysmal bone cyst, right lower leg
M85.562   Aneurysmal bone cyst, left lower leg
M85.569   Aneurysmal bone cyst, unspecified lower leg

✓6ᵗʰ M85.57   Aneurysmal bone cyst, ankle and foot

M85.571   Aneurysmal bone cyst, right ankle and foot
M85.572   Aneurysmal bone cyst, left ankle and foot
M85.579   Aneurysmal bone cyst, unspecified ankle and foot

M85.58   Aneurysmal bone cyst, other site
M85.59   Aneurysmal bone cyst, multiple sites

Chapter 13. Diseases of the Musculoskeletal System and Connective Tissue

M85.6–M86.049

✓5ᵗʰ **M85.6 Other cyst of bone**

> EXCLUDES 1   cyst of jaw NEC (M27.4)
> osteitis fibrosa cystica generalisata [von Recklinghausen's disease of bone] (E21.0)

     M85.60 Other cyst of bone, unspecified site

✓6ᵗʰ   **M85.61 Other cyst of bone, shoulder**

     M85.611 Other cyst of bone, right shoulder
     M85.612 Other cyst of bone, left shoulder
     M85.619 Other cyst of bone, unspecified shoulder

✓6ᵗʰ   **M85.62 Other cyst of bone, upper arm**

     M85.621 Other cyst of bone, right upper arm
     M85.622 Other cyst of bone, left upper arm
     M85.629 Other cyst of bone, unspecified upper arm

✓6ᵗʰ   **M85.63 Other cyst of bone, forearm**

     M85.631 Other cyst of bone, right forearm
     M85.632 Other cyst of bone, left forearm
     M85.639 Other cyst of bone, unspecified forearm

✓6ᵗʰ   **M85.64 Other cyst of bone, hand**

     M85.641 Other cyst of bone, right hand
     M85.642 Other cyst of bone, left hand
     M85.649 Other cyst of bone, unspecified hand

✓6ᵗʰ   **M85.65 Other cyst of bone, thigh**

     M85.651 Other cyst of bone, right thigh
     M85.652 Other cyst of bone, left thigh
     M85.659 Other cyst of bone, unspecified thigh

✓6ᵗʰ   **M85.66 Other cyst of bone, lower leg**

     M85.661 Other cyst of bone, right lower leg
     M85.662 Other cyst of bone, left lower leg
     M85.669 Other cyst of bone, unspecified lower leg

✓6ᵗʰ   **M85.67 Other cyst of bone, ankle and foot**

     M85.671 Other cyst of bone, right ankle and foot
     M85.672 Other cyst of bone, left ankle and foot
     M85.679 Other cyst of bone, unspecified ankle and foot

     M85.68 Other cyst of bone, other site
     M85.69 Other cyst of bone, multiple sites

✓5ᵗʰ **M85.8 Other specified disorders of bone density and structure**

     Hyperostosis of bones, except skull
     Osteosclerosis, acquired

> EXCLUDES 1   diffuse idiopathic skeletal hyperostosis [DISH] (M48.1)
> osteosclerosis congenita (Q77.4)
> osteosclerosis fragilitas (generalista) (Q78.2)
> osteosclerosis myelofibrosis (D75.81)

     M85.80 Other specified disorders of bone density and structure, unspecified site

✓6ᵗʰ   **M85.81 Other specified disorders of bone density and structure, shoulder**

     M85.811 Other specified disorders of bone density and structure, right shoulder
     M85.812 Other specified disorders of bone density and structure, left shoulder
     M85.819 Other specified disorders of bone density and structure, unspecified shoulder

✓6ᵗʰ   **M85.82 Other specified disorders of bone density and structure, upper arm**

     M85.821 Other specified disorders of bone density and structure, right upper arm
     M85.822 Other specified disorders of bone density and structure, left upper arm
     M85.829 Other specified disorders of bone density and structure, unspecified upper arm

✓6ᵗʰ   **M85.83 Other specified disorders of bone density and structure, forearm**

     M85.831 Other specified disorders of bone density and structure, right forearm
     M85.832 Other specified disorders of bone density and structure, left forearm
     M85.839 Other specified disorders of bone density and structure, unspecified forearm

✓6ᵗʰ   **M85.84 Other specified disorders of bone density and structure, hand**

     M85.841 Other specified disorders of bone density and structure, right hand
     M85.842 Other specified disorders of bone density and structure, left hand
     M85.849 Other specified disorders of bone density and structure, unspecified hand

✓6ᵗʰ   **M85.85 Other specified disorders of bone density and structure, thigh**

     M85.851 Other specified disorders of bone density and structure, right thigh
     M85.852 Other specified disorders of bone density and structure, left thigh
     M85.859 Other specified disorders of bone density and structure, unspecified thigh

✓6ᵗʰ   **M85.86 Other specified disorders of bone density and structure, lower leg**

     M85.861 Other specified disorders of bone density and structure, right lower leg
     M85.862 Other specified disorders of bone density and structure, left lower leg
     M85.869 Other specified disorders of bone density and structure, unspecified lower leg

✓6ᵗʰ   **M85.87 Other specified disorders of bone density and structure, ankle and foot**

     M85.871 Other specified disorders of bone density and structure, right ankle and foot
     M85.872 Other specified disorders of bone density and structure, left ankle and foot
     M85.879 Other specified disorders of bone density and structure, unspecified ankle and foot

     M85.88 Other specified disorders of bone density and structure, other site
     M85.89 Other specified disorders of bone density and structure, multiple sites

M85.9 Disorder of bone density and structure, unspecified

     AHA: 2021,3Q,11

Other osteopathies (M86-M90)

> EXCLUDES 1   postprocedural osteopathies (M96.-)

✓4ᵗʰ **M86 Osteomyelitis**

     Use additional code (B95-B97) to identify infectious agent
     Use additional code to identify major osseous defect, if applicable (M89.7-)

> EXCLUDES 1   osteomyelitis due to:
> echinococcus (B67.2)
> gonococcus (A54.43)
> salmonella (A02.24)

> EXCLUDES 2   ostemyelitis of:
> orbit (H05.0-)
> petrous bone (H70.2-)
> vertebra (M46.2-)

✓5ᵗʰ **M86.0 Acute hematogenous osteomyelitis**

     M86.00 Acute hematogenous osteomyelitis, unspecified site   HCC ESR COM

✓6ᵗʰ   **M86.01 Acute hematogenous osteomyelitis, shoulder**

     M86.011 Acute hematogenous osteomyelitis, right shoulder   HCC ESR COM
     M86.012 Acute hematogenous osteomyelitis, left shoulder   HCC ESR COM
     M86.019 Acute hematogenous osteomyelitis, unspecified shoulder   HCC ESR COM

✓6ᵗʰ   **M86.02 Acute hematogenous osteomyelitis, humerus**

     M86.021 Acute hematogenous osteomyelitis, right humerus   HCC ESR COM
     M86.022 Acute hematogenous osteomyelitis, left humerus   HCC ESR COM
     M86.029 Acute hematogenous osteomyelitis, unspecified humerus   HCC ESR COM

✓6ᵗʰ   **M86.03 Acute hematogenous osteomyelitis, radius and ulna**

     M86.031 Acute hematogenous osteomyelitis, right radius and ulna   HCC ESR COM
     M86.032 Acute hematogenous osteomyelitis, left radius and ulna   HCC ESR COM
     M86.039 Acute hematogenous osteomyelitis, unspecified radius and ulna   HCC ESR COM

✓6ᵗʰ   **M86.04 Acute hematogenous osteomyelitis, hand**

     M86.041 Acute hematogenous osteomyelitis, right hand   HCC ESR COM
     M86.042 Acute hematogenous osteomyelitis, left hand   HCC ESR COM
     M86.049 Acute hematogenous osteomyelitis, unspecified hand   HCC ESR COM

✓6th **M86.05** Acute hematogenous osteomyelitis, femur

     M86.051 Acute hematogenous osteomyelitis, right femur `HCC` `ESR` `COM`

     M86.052 Acute hematogenous osteomyelitis, left femur `HCC` `ESR` `COM`

     M86.059 Acute hematogenous osteomyelitis, unspecified femur `HCC` `ESR` `COM`

✓6th **M86.06** Acute hematogenous osteomyelitis, tibia and fibula

     M86.061 Acute hematogenous osteomyelitis, right tibia and fibula `HCC` `ESR` `COM`

     M86.062 Acute hematogenous osteomyelitis, left tibia and fibula `HCC` `ESR` `COM`

     M86.069 Acute hematogenous osteomyelitis, unspecified tibia and fibula `HCC` `ESR` `COM`

✓6th **M86.07** Acute hematogenous osteomyelitis, ankle and foot

     M86.071 Acute hematogenous osteomyelitis, right ankle and foot `HCC` `ESR` `COM`

     M86.072 Acute hematogenous osteomyelitis, left ankle and foot `HCC` `ESR` `COM`

     M86.079 Acute hematogenous osteomyelitis, unspecified ankle and foot `HCC` `ESR` `COM`

   M86.08 Acute hematogenous osteomyelitis, other sites `HCC` `ESR` `COM`

   M86.09 Acute hematogenous osteomyelitis, multiple sites `HCC` `ESR` `COM`

✓5th **M86.1** Other acute osteomyelitis

   M86.10 Other acute osteomyelitis, unspecified site `HCC` `ESR` `COM`

✓6th **M86.11** Other acute osteomyelitis, shoulder

     M86.111 Other acute osteomyelitis, right shoulder `HCC` `ESR` `COM`

     M86.112 Other acute osteomyelitis, left shoulder `HCC` `ESR` `COM`

     M86.119 Other acute osteomyelitis, unspecified shoulder `HCC` `ESR` `COM`

✓6th **M86.12** Other acute osteomyelitis, humerus

     M86.121 Other acute osteomyelitis, right humerus `HCC` `ESR` `COM`

     M86.122 Other acute osteomyelitis, left humerus `HCC` `ESR` `COM`

     M86.129 Other acute osteomyelitis, unspecified humerus `HCC` `ESR` `COM`

✓6th **M86.13** Other acute osteomyelitis, radius and ulna

     M86.131 Other acute osteomyelitis, right radius and ulna `HCC` `ESR` `COM`

     M86.132 Other acute osteomyelitis, left radius and ulna `HCC` `ESR` `COM`

     M86.139 Other acute osteomyelitis, unspecified radius and ulna `HCC` `ESR` `COM`

✓6th **M86.14** Other acute osteomyelitis, hand

     M86.141 Other acute osteomyelitis, right hand `HCC` `ESR` `COM`

     M86.142 Other acute osteomyelitis, left hand `HCC` `ESR` `COM`

     M86.149 Other acute osteomyelitis, unspecified hand `HCC` `ESR` `COM`

✓6th **M86.15** Other acute osteomyelitis, femur

     M86.151 Other acute osteomyelitis, right femur `HCC` `ESR` `COM`

     M86.152 Other acute osteomyelitis, left femur `HCC` `ESR` `COM`

     M86.159 Other acute osteomyelitis, unspecified femur `HCC` `ESR` `COM`

✓6th **M86.16** Other acute osteomyelitis, tibia and fibula

     M86.161 Other acute osteomyelitis, right tibia and fibula `HCC` `ESR` `COM`

     M86.162 Other acute osteomyelitis, left tibia and fibula `HCC` `ESR` `COM`

     M86.169 Other acute osteomyelitis, unspecified tibia and fibula `HCC` `ESR` `COM`

✓6th **M86.17** Other acute osteomyelitis, ankle and foot

     AHA: 2020,1Q,12

     M86.171 Other acute osteomyelitis, right ankle and foot `HCC` `ESR` `COM`

     M86.172 Other acute osteomyelitis, left ankle and foot `HCC` `ESR` `COM`

     M86.179 Other acute osteomyelitis, unspecified ankle and foot `HCC` `ESR` `COM`

   M86.18 Other acute osteomyelitis, other site `HCC` `ESR` `COM`

   M86.19 Other acute osteomyelitis, multiple sites `HCC` `ESR` `COM`

✓5th **M86.2** Subacute osteomyelitis

   M86.20 Subacute osteomyelitis, unspecified site `HCC` `ESR` `COM`

✓6th **M86.21** Subacute osteomyelitis, shoulder

     M86.211 Subacute osteomyelitis, right shoulder `HCC` `ESR` `COM`

     M86.212 Subacute osteomyelitis, left shoulder `HCC` `ESR` `COM`

     M86.219 Subacute osteomyelitis, unspecified shoulder `HCC` `ESR` `COM`

✓6th **M86.22** Subacute osteomyelitis, humerus

     M86.221 Subacute osteomyelitis, right humerus `HCC` `ESR` `COM`

     M86.222 Subacute osteomyelitis, left humerus `HCC` `ESR` `COM`

     M86.229 Subacute osteomyelitis, unspecified humerus `HCC` `ESR` `COM`

✓6th **M86.23** Subacute osteomyelitis, radius and ulna

     M86.231 Subacute osteomyelitis, right radius and ulna `HCC` `ESR` `COM`

     M86.232 Subacute osteomyelitis, left radius and ulna `HCC` `ESR` `COM`

     M86.239 Subacute osteomyelitis, unspecified radius and ulna `HCC` `ESR` `COM`

✓6th **M86.24** Subacute osteomyelitis, hand

     M86.241 Subacute osteomyelitis, right hand `HCC` `ESR` `COM`

     M86.242 Subacute osteomyelitis, left hand `HCC` `ESR` `COM`

     M86.249 Subacute osteomyelitis, unspecified hand `HCC` `ESR` `COM`

✓6th **M86.25** Subacute osteomyelitis, femur

     M86.251 Subacute osteomyelitis, right femur `HCC` `ESR` `COM`

     M86.252 Subacute osteomyelitis, left femur `HCC` `ESR` `COM`

     M86.259 Subacute osteomyelitis, unspecified femur `HCC` `ESR` `COM`

✓6th **M86.26** Subacute osteomyelitis, tibia and fibula

     M86.261 Subacute osteomyelitis, right tibia and fibula `HCC` `ESR` `COM`

     M86.262 Subacute osteomyelitis, left tibia and fibula `HCC` `ESR` `COM`

     M86.269 Subacute osteomyelitis, unspecified tibia and fibula `HCC` `ESR` `COM`

✓6th **M86.27** Subacute osteomyelitis, ankle and foot

     M86.271 Subacute osteomyelitis, right ankle and foot `HCC` `ESR` `COM`

     M86.272 Subacute osteomyelitis, left ankle and foot `HCC` `ESR` `COM`

     M86.279 Subacute osteomyelitis, unspecified ankle and foot `HCC` `ESR` `COM`

   M86.28 Subacute osteomyelitis, other site `HCC` `ESR` `COM`

   M86.29 Subacute osteomyelitis, multiple sites `HCC` `ESR` `COM`

✓5th **M86.3** Chronic multifocal osteomyelitis

   M86.30 Chronic multifocal osteomyelitis, unspecified site `HCC` `ESR` `COM`

✓6th **M86.31** Chronic multifocal osteomyelitis, shoulder

     M86.311 Chronic multifocal osteomyelitis, right shoulder `HCC` `ESR` `COM`

     M86.312 Chronic multifocal osteomyelitis, left shoulder `HCC` `ESR` `COM`

     M86.319 Chronic multifocal osteomyelitis, unspecified shoulder `HCC` `ESR` `COM`

✓6th **M86.32** Chronic multifocal osteomyelitis, humerus

     M86.321 Chronic multifocal osteomyelitis, right humerus `HCC` `ESR` `COM`

     M86.322 Chronic multifocal osteomyelitis, left humerus `HCC` `ESR` `COM`

✓ Additional Character Required   ✓x7th Placeholder Alert   Manifestation   Unspecified Dx   Ⓠ QPP   `UPD` Unacceptable PDx

Chapter 13. Diseases of the Musculoskeletal System and Connective Tissue

M86.329 Chronic multifocal osteomyelitis, unspecified humerus HCC ESR COM

✓6ᵗʰ M86.33 Chronic multifocal osteomyelitis, radius and ulna

M86.331 Chronic multifocal osteomyelitis, right radius and ulna HCC ESR COM

M86.332 Chronic multifocal osteomyelitis, left radius and ulna HCC ESR COM

M86.339 Chronic multifocal osteomyelitis, unspecified radius and ulna HCC ESR COM

✓6ᵗʰ M86.34 Chronic multifocal osteomyelitis, hand

M86.341 Chronic multifocal osteomyelitis, right hand HCC ESR COM

M86.342 Chronic multifocal osteomyelitis, left hand HCC ESR COM

M86.349 Chronic multifocal osteomyelitis, unspecified hand HCC ESR COM

✓6ᵗʰ M86.35 Chronic multifocal osteomyelitis, femur

M86.351 Chronic multifocal osteomyelitis, right femur HCC ESR COM

M86.352 Chronic multifocal osteomyelitis, left femur HCC ESR COM

M86.359 Chronic multifocal osteomyelitis, unspecified femur HCC ESR COM

✓6ᵗʰ M86.36 Chronic multifocal osteomyelitis, tibia and fibula

M86.361 Chronic multifocal osteomyelitis, right tibia and fibula HCC ESR COM

M86.362 Chronic multifocal osteomyelitis, left tibia and fibula HCC ESR COM

M86.369 Chronic multifocal osteomyelitis, unspecified tibia and fibula HCC ESR COM

✓6ᵗʰ M86.37 Chronic multifocal osteomyelitis, ankle and foot

M86.371 Chronic multifocal osteomyelitis, right ankle and foot HCC ESR COM

M86.372 Chronic multifocal osteomyelitis, left ankle and foot HCC ESR COM

M86.379 Chronic multifocal osteomyelitis, unspecified ankle and foot HCC ESR COM

M86.38 Chronic multifocal osteomyelitis, other site HCC ESR COM

M86.39 Chronic multifocal osteomyelitis, multiple sites HCC ESR COM

✓5ᵗʰ M86.4 Chronic osteomyelitis with draining sinus

M86.40 Chronic osteomyelitis with draining sinus, unspecified site HCC ESR COM

✓6ᵗʰ M86.41 Chronic osteomyelitis with draining sinus, shoulder

M86.411 Chronic osteomyelitis with draining sinus, right shoulder HCC ESR COM

M86.412 Chronic osteomyelitis with draining sinus, left shoulder HCC ESR COM

M86.419 Chronic osteomyelitis with draining sinus, unspecified shoulder HCC ESR COM

✓6ᵗʰ M86.42 Chronic osteomyelitis with draining sinus, humerus

M86.421 Chronic osteomyelitis with draining sinus, right humerus HCC ESR COM

M86.422 Chronic osteomyelitis with draining sinus, left humerus HCC ESR COM

M86.429 Chronic osteomyelitis with draining sinus, unspecified humerus HCC ESR COM

✓6ᵗʰ M86.43 Chronic osteomyelitis with draining sinus, radius and ulna

M86.431 Chronic osteomyelitis with draining sinus, right radius and ulna HCC ESR COM

M86.432 Chronic osteomyelitis with draining sinus, left radius and ulna HCC ESR COM

M86.439 Chronic osteomyelitis with draining sinus, unspecified radius and ulna HCC ESR COM

✓6ᵗʰ M86.44 Chronic osteomyelitis with draining sinus, hand

M86.441 Chronic osteomyelitis with draining sinus, right hand HCC ESR COM

M86.442 Chronic osteomyelitis with draining sinus, left hand HCC ESR COM

M86.449 Chronic osteomyelitis with draining sinus, unspecified hand HCC ESR COM

✓6ᵗʰ M86.45 Chronic osteomyelitis with draining sinus, femur

M86.451 Chronic osteomyelitis with draining sinus, right femur HCC ESR COM

M86.452 Chronic osteomyelitis with draining sinus, left femur HCC ESR COM

M86.459 Chronic osteomyelitis with draining sinus, unspecified femur HCC ESR COM

✓6ᵗʰ M86.46 Chronic osteomyelitis with draining sinus, tibia and fibula

M86.461 Chronic osteomyelitis with draining sinus, right tibia and fibula HCC ESR COM

M86.462 Chronic osteomyelitis with draining sinus, left tibia and fibula HCC ESR COM

M86.469 Chronic osteomyelitis with draining sinus, unspecified tibia and fibula HCC ESR COM

✓6ᵗʰ M86.47 Chronic osteomyelitis with draining sinus, ankle and foot

M86.471 Chronic osteomyelitis with draining sinus, right ankle and foot HCC ESR COM

M86.472 Chronic osteomyelitis with draining sinus, left ankle and foot HCC ESR COM

M86.479 Chronic osteomyelitis with draining sinus, unspecified ankle and foot HCC ESR COM

M86.48 Chronic osteomyelitis with draining sinus, other site HCC ESR COM

M86.49 Chronic osteomyelitis with draining sinus, multiple sites HCC ESR COM

✓5ᵗʰ M86.5 Other chronic hematogenous osteomyelitis

M86.50 Other chronic hematogenous osteomyelitis, unspecified site HCC ESR COM

✓6ᵗʰ M86.51 Other chronic hematogenous osteomyelitis, shoulder

M86.511 Other chronic hematogenous osteomyelitis, right shoulder HCC ESR COM

M86.512 Other chronic hematogenous osteomyelitis, left shoulder HCC ESR COM

M86.519 Other chronic hematogenous osteomyelitis, unspecified shoulder HCC ESR COM

✓6ᵗʰ M86.52 Other chronic hematogenous osteomyelitis, humerus

M86.521 Other chronic hematogenous osteomyelitis, right humerus HCC ESR COM

M86.522 Other chronic hematogenous osteomyelitis, left humerus HCC ESR COM

M86.529 Other chronic hematogenous osteomyelitis, unspecified humerus HCC ESR COM

✓6ᵗʰ M86.53 Other chronic hematogenous osteomyelitis, radius and ulna

M86.531 Other chronic hematogenous osteomyelitis, right radius and ulna HCC ESR COM

M86.532 Other chronic hematogenous osteomyelitis, left radius and ulna HCC ESR COM

M86.539 Other chronic hematogenous osteomyelitis, unspecified radius and ulna HCC ESR COM

✓6ᵗʰ M86.54 Other chronic hematogenous osteomyelitis, hand

M86.541 Other chronic hematogenous osteomyelitis, right hand HCC ESR COM

M86.542 Other chronic hematogenous osteomyelitis, left hand HCC ESR COM

M86.549 Other chronic hematogenous osteomyelitis, unspecified hand HCC ESR COM

✓6ᵗʰ M86.55 Other chronic hematogenous osteomyelitis, femur

M86.551 Other chronic hematogenous osteomyelitis, right femur HCC ESR COM

M86.552 Other chronic hematogenous osteomyelitis, left femur HCC ESR COM

M86.559 Other chronic hematogenous osteomyelitis, unspecified femur HCC ESR COM

√6ᵗʰ **M86.56 Other chronic hematogenous osteomyelitis,** tibia and fibula

    M86.561 Other chronic hematogenous osteomyelitis, right **tibia and fibula** `HCC` `ESR` `COM`

    M86.562 Other chronic hematogenous osteomyelitis, left **tibia and fibula** `HCC` `ESR` `COM`

    M86.569 Other chronic hematogenous osteomyelitis, unspecified tibia and fibula `HCC` `ESR` `COM`

√6ᵗʰ **M86.57 Other chronic hematogenous osteomyelitis,** ankle and foot

    M86.571 Other chronic hematogenous osteomyelitis, right **ankle and foot** `HCC` `ESR` `COM`

    M86.572 Other chronic hematogenous osteomyelitis, left **ankle and foot** `HCC` `ESR` `COM`

    M86.579 Other chronic hematogenous osteomyelitis, unspecified ankle and foot `HCC` `ESR` `COM`

M86.58 Other chronic hematogenous osteomyelitis, other site `HCC` `ESR` `COM`

M86.59 Other chronic hematogenous osteomyelitis, multiple sites `HCC` `ESR` `COM`

√5ᵗʰ **M86.6 Other** chronic osteomyelitis

    M86.60 Other chronic osteomyelitis, unspecified site `HCC` `ESR` `COM`

√6ᵗʰ **M86.61 Other chronic osteomyelitis,** shoulder

    M86.611 Other chronic osteomyelitis, right **shoulder** `HCC` `ESR` `COM`

    M86.612 Other chronic osteomyelitis, left **shoulder** `HCC` `ESR` `COM`

    M86.619 Other chronic osteomyelitis, unspecified shoulder `HCC` `ESR` `COM`

√6ᵗʰ **M86.62 Other chronic osteomyelitis,** humerus

    M86.621 Other chronic osteomyelitis, right **humerus** `HCC` `ESR` `COM`

    M86.622 Other chronic osteomyelitis, left **humerus** `HCC` `ESR` `COM`

    M86.629 Other chronic osteomyelitis, unspecified humerus `HCC` `ESR` `COM`

√6ᵗʰ **M86.63 Other chronic osteomyelitis,** radius and ulna

    M86.631 Other chronic osteomyelitis, right **radius and ulna** `HCC` `ESR` `COM`

    M86.632 Other chronic osteomyelitis, left **radius and ulna** `HCC` `ESR` `COM`

    M86.639 Other chronic osteomyelitis, unspecified radius and ulna `HCC` `ESR` `COM`

√6ᵗʰ **M86.64 Other chronic osteomyelitis,** hand

    M86.641 Other chronic osteomyelitis, right **hand** `HCC` `ESR` `COM`

    M86.642 Other chronic osteomyelitis, left **hand** `HCC` `ESR` `COM`

    M86.649 Other chronic osteomyelitis, unspecified hand `HCC` `ESR` `COM`

√6ᵗʰ **M86.65 Other chronic osteomyelitis,** thigh

    M86.651 Other chronic osteomyelitis, right **thigh** `HCC` `ESR` `COM`

    M86.652 Other chronic osteomyelitis, left **thigh** `HCC` `ESR` `COM`

    M86.659 Other chronic osteomyelitis, unspecified thigh `HCC` `ESR` `COM`

√6ᵗʰ **M86.66 Other chronic osteomyelitis,** tibia and fibula

    M86.661 Other chronic osteomyelitis, right **tibia and fibula** `HCC` `ESR` `COM`

    M86.662 Other chronic osteomyelitis, left **tibia and fibula** `HCC` `ESR` `COM`

    M86.669 Other chronic osteomyelitis, unspecified tibia and fibula `HCC` `ESR` `COM`

√6ᵗʰ **M86.67 Other chronic osteomyelitis,** ankle and foot

    M86.671 Other chronic osteomyelitis, right **ankle and foot** `HCC` `ESR` `COM`

        AHA: 2016,1Q,13

    M86.672 Other chronic osteomyelitis, left **ankle and foot** `HCC` `ESR` `COM`

    M86.679 Other chronic osteomyelitis, unspecified ankle and foot `HCC` `ESR` `COM`

M86.68 Other chronic osteomyelitis, other site `HCC` `ESR` `COM`

M86.69 Other chronic osteomyelitis, multiple sites `HCC` `ESR` `COM`

√5ᵗʰ **M86.8 Other osteomyelitis**

    Brodie's abscess

    AHA: 2022,1Q,31

    √6ᵗʰ **M86.8X Other osteomyelitis**

        M86.8X0 Other osteomyelitis, multiple sites `HCC` `ESR` `COM`

        M86.8X1 Other osteomyelitis, shoulder `HCC` `ESR` `COM`

        M86.8X2 Other osteomyelitis, upper arm `HCC` `ESR` `COM`

        M86.8X3 Other osteomyelitis, forearm `HCC` `ESR` `COM`

        M86.8X4 Other osteomyelitis, hand `HCC` `ESR` `COM`

        M86.8X5 Other osteomyelitis, thigh `HCC` `ESR` `COM`

        M86.8X6 Other osteomyelitis, lower leg `HCC` `ESR` `COM`

        M86.8X7 Other osteomyelitis, ankle and foot `HCC` `ESR` `COM`

        M86.8X8 Other osteomyelitis, other site `HCC` `ESR` `COM`

        M86.8X9 Other osteomyelitis, unspecified sites `HCC` `ESR` `COM`

M86.9 Osteomyelitis, unspecified `HCC` `ESR` `COM`

    Infection of bone NOS

    Periostitis without osteomyelitis

√4ᵗʰ **M87 Osteonecrosis**

    `INCLUDES`   avascular necrosis of bone

    Use additional code to identify major osseous defect, if applicable (M89.7-)

    `EXCLUDES 1`   juvenile osteonecrosis (M91-M92)

               osteochondropathies (M90-M93)

√5ᵗʰ **M87.0** Idiopathic aseptic **necrosis of bone**

    M87.00 Idiopathic aseptic necrosis of unspecified bone `HCC` `Rx` `ESR` `COM`

    √6ᵗʰ **M87.01 Idiopathic aseptic necrosis of** shoulder

        Idiopathic aseptic necrosis of clavicle and scapula

        M87.011 Idiopathic aseptic necrosis of right **shoulder** `HCC` `Rx` `ESR` `COM`

        M87.012 Idiopathic aseptic necrosis of left **shoulder** `HCC` `Rx` `ESR` `COM`

        M87.019 Idiopathic aseptic necrosis of unspecified shoulder `HCC` `Rx` `ESR` `COM`

    √6ᵗʰ **M87.02 Idiopathic aseptic necrosis of** humerus

        M87.021 Idiopathic aseptic necrosis of right **humerus** `HCC` `Rx` `ESR` `COM`

        M87.022 Idiopathic aseptic necrosis of left **humerus** `HCC` `Rx` `ESR` `COM`

        M87.029 Idiopathic aseptic necrosis of unspecified humerus `HCC` `Rx` `ESR` `COM`

    √6ᵗʰ **M87.03 Idiopathic aseptic necrosis of** radius, ulna and carpus

        M87.031 Idiopathic aseptic necrosis of right **radius** `HCC` `Rx` `ESR` `COM`

        M87.032 Idiopathic aseptic necrosis of left **radius** `HCC` `Rx` `ESR` `COM`

        M87.033 Idiopathic aseptic necrosis of unspecified radius `HCC` `Rx` `ESR` `COM`

        M87.034 Idiopathic aseptic necrosis of right **ulna** `HCC` `Rx` `ESR` `COM`

        M87.035 Idiopathic aseptic necrosis of left **ulna** `HCC` `Rx` `ESR` `COM`

        M87.036 Idiopathic aseptic necrosis of unspecified ulna `HCC` `Rx` `ESR` `COM`

        M87.037 Idiopathic aseptic necrosis of right **carpus** `HCC` `Rx` `ESR` `COM`

        M87.038 Idiopathic aseptic necrosis of left **carpus** `HCC` `Rx` `ESR` `COM`

        M87.039 Idiopathic aseptic necrosis of unspecified carpus `HCC` `Rx` `ESR` `COM`

√6ᵗʰ **M87.04** **Idiopathic aseptic necrosis of** hand and fingers

Idiopathic aseptic necrosis of metacarpals and phalanges of hands

M87.041 **Idiopathic aseptic necrosis of** right hand `HCC` `Rx` `ESR` `COM`

M87.042 **Idiopathic aseptic necrosis of** left hand `HCC` `Rx` `ESR` `COM`

M87.043 **Idiopathic aseptic necrosis of unspecified hand** `HCC` `Rx` `ESR` `COM`

M87.044 **Idiopathic aseptic necrosis of** right finger(s) `HCC` `Rx` `ESR` `COM`

M87.045 **Idiopathic aseptic necrosis of** left finger(s) `HCC` `Rx` `ESR` `COM`

M87.046 **Idiopathic aseptic necrosis of unspecified finger(s)** `HCC` `Rx` `ESR` `COM`

√6ᵗʰ **M87.05** **Idiopathic aseptic necrosis of** pelvis and femur

M87.050 **Idiopathic aseptic necrosis of** pelvis `HCC` `Rx` `ESR` `COM`

M87.051 **Idiopathic aseptic necrosis of** right femur `HCC` `Rx` `ESR` `COM`

M87.052 **Idiopathic aseptic necrosis of** left femur `HCC` `Rx` `ESR` `COM`

M87.059 **Idiopathic aseptic necrosis of unspecified femur** `HCC` `Rx` `ESR` `COM`

√6ᵗʰ **M87.06** **Idiopathic aseptic necrosis of** tibia and fibula

M87.061 **Idiopathic aseptic necrosis of** right tibia `HCC` `Rx` `ESR` `COM`

M87.062 **Idiopathic aseptic necrosis of** left tibia `HCC` `Rx` `ESR` `COM`

M87.063 **Idiopathic aseptic necrosis of unspecified tibia** `HCC` `Rx` `ESR` `COM`

M87.064 **Idiopathic aseptic necrosis of** right fibula `HCC` `Rx` `ESR` `COM`

M87.065 **Idiopathic aseptic necrosis of** left fibula `HCC` `Rx` `ESR` `COM`

M87.066 **Idiopathic aseptic necrosis of unspecified fibula** `HCC` `Rx` `ESR` `COM`

√6ᵗʰ **M87.07** **Idiopathic aseptic necrosis of** ankle, foot and toes

Idiopathic aseptic necrosis of metatarsus, tarsus, and phalanges of toes

M87.071 **Idiopathic aseptic necrosis of** right ankle `HCC` `Rx` `ESR` `COM`

M87.072 **Idiopathic aseptic necrosis of** left ankle `HCC` `Rx` `ESR` `COM`

M87.073 **Idiopathic aseptic necrosis of unspecified ankle** `HCC` `Rx` `ESR` `COM`

M87.074 **Idiopathic aseptic necrosis of** right foot `HCC` `Rx` `ESR` `COM`

M87.075 **Idiopathic aseptic necrosis of** left foot `HCC` `Rx` `ESR` `COM`

M87.076 **Idiopathic aseptic necrosis of unspecified foot** `HCC` `Rx` `ESR` `COM`

M87.077 **Idiopathic aseptic necrosis of** right toe(s) `HCC` `Rx` `ESR` `COM`

M87.078 **Idiopathic aseptic necrosis of** left toe(s) `HCC` `Rx` `ESR` `COM`

M87.079 **Idiopathic aseptic necrosis of unspecified toe(s)** `HCC` `Rx` `ESR` `COM`

M87.08 **Idiopathic aseptic necrosis of bone, other site** `HCC` `Rx` `ESR` `COM`

M87.09 **Idiopathic aseptic necrosis of bone,** multiple sites `HCC` `Rx` `ESR` `COM`

√5ᵗʰ **M87.1** **Osteonecrosis** due to drugs

Use additional code for adverse effect, if applicable, to identify drug (T36-T50 with fifth or sixth character 5)

M87.10 **Osteonecrosis due to drugs, unspecified bone** `HCC` `Rx` `ESR` `COM`

√6ᵗʰ **M87.11** **Osteonecrosis due to drugs,** shoulder

M87.111 **Osteonecrosis due to drugs,** right shoulder `HCC` `Rx` `ESR` `COM`

M87.112 **Osteonecrosis due to drugs,** left shoulder `HCC` `Rx` `ESR` `COM`

M87.119 **Osteonecrosis due to drugs, unspecified shoulder** `HCC` `Rx` `ESR` `COM`

√6ᵗʰ **M87.12** **Osteonecrosis due to drugs,** humerus

M87.121 **Osteonecrosis due to drugs,** right humerus `HCC` `Rx` `ESR` `COM`

M87.122 **Osteonecrosis due to drugs,** left humerus `HCC` `Rx` `ESR` `COM`

M87.129 **Osteonecrosis due to drugs, unspecified humerus** `HCC` `Rx` `ESR` `COM`

√6ᵗʰ **M87.13** **Osteonecrosis due to drugs of** radius, ulna and carpus

M87.131 **Osteonecrosis due to drugs of** right radius `HCC` `Rx` `ESR` `COM`

M87.132 **Osteonecrosis due to drugs of** left radius `HCC` `Rx` `ESR` `COM`

M87.133 **Osteonecrosis due to drugs of unspecified radius** `HCC` `Rx` `ESR` `COM`

M87.134 **Osteonecrosis due to drugs of** right ulna `HCC` `Rx` `ESR` `COM`

M87.135 **Osteonecrosis due to drugs of** left ulna `HCC` `Rx` `ESR` `COM`

M87.136 **Osteonecrosis due to drugs of unspecified ulna** `HCC` `Rx` `ESR` `COM`

M87.137 **Osteonecrosis due to drugs of** right carpus `HCC` `Rx` `ESR` `COM`

M87.138 **Osteonecrosis due to drugs of** left carpus `HCC` `Rx` `ESR` `COM`

M87.139 **Osteonecrosis due to drugs of unspecified carpus** `HCC` `Rx` `ESR` `COM`

√6ᵗʰ **M87.14** **Osteonecrosis due to drugs,** hand and fingers

M87.141 **Osteonecrosis due to drugs,** right hand `HCC` `Rx` `ESR` `COM`

M87.142 **Osteonecrosis due to drugs,** left hand `HCC` `Rx` `ESR` `COM`

M87.143 **Osteonecrosis due to drugs, unspecified hand** `HCC` `Rx` `ESR` `COM`

M87.144 **Osteonecrosis due to drugs,** right finger(s) `HCC` `Rx` `ESR` `COM`

M87.145 **Osteonecrosis due to drugs,** left finger(s) `HCC` `Rx` `ESR` `COM`

M87.146 **Osteonecrosis due to drugs, unspecified finger(s)** `HCC` `Rx` `ESR` `COM`

√6ᵗʰ **M87.15** **Osteonecrosis due to drugs,** pelvis and femur

M87.150 **Osteonecrosis due to drugs,** pelvis `HCC` `Rx` `ESR` `COM`

M87.151 **Osteonecrosis due to drugs,** right femur `HCC` `Rx` `ESR` `COM`

M87.152 **Osteonecrosis due to drugs,** left femur `HCC` `Rx` `ESR` `COM`

M87.159 **Osteonecrosis due to drugs, unspecified femur** `HCC` `Rx` `ESR` `COM`

√6ᵗʰ **M87.16** **Osteonecrosis due to drugs,** tibia and fibula

M87.161 **Osteonecrosis due to drugs,** right tibia `HCC` `Rx` `ESR` `COM`

M87.162 **Osteonecrosis due to drugs,** left tibia `HCC` `Rx` `ESR` `COM`

M87.163 **Osteonecrosis due to drugs, unspecified tibia** `HCC` `Rx` `ESR` `COM`

M87.164 **Osteonecrosis due to drugs,** right fibula `HCC` `Rx` `ESR` `COM`

M87.165 **Osteonecrosis due to drugs,** left fibula `HCC` `Rx` `ESR` `COM`

M87.166 **Osteonecrosis due to drugs, unspecified fibula** `HCC` `Rx` `ESR` `COM`

√6ᵗʰ **M87.17** **Osteonecrosis due to drugs,** ankle, foot and toes

M87.171 **Osteonecrosis due to drugs,** right ankle `HCC` `Rx` `ESR` `COM`

M87.172 **Osteonecrosis due to drugs,** left ankle `HCC` `Rx` `ESR` `COM`

M87.173 **Osteonecrosis due to drugs, unspecified ankle** `HCC` `Rx` `ESR` `COM`

M87.174 **Osteonecrosis due to drugs,** right foot `HCC` `Rx` `ESR` `COM`

M87.175 **Osteonecrosis due to drugs,** left foot `HCC` `Rx` `ESR` `COM`

M87.176 **Osteonecrosis due to drugs, unspecified foot** `HCC` `Rx` `ESR` `COM`

M87.177 **Osteonecrosis due to drugs,** right toe(s) `HCC` `Rx` `ESR` `COM`

M87.178 **Osteonecrosis due to drugs,** left toe(s) `HCC` `Rx` `ESR` `COM`

M87.179 **Osteonecrosis due to drugs, unspecified toe(s)** `HCC` `Rx` `ESR` `COM`

`HCC` CMS-HCC   `Rx` Rx HCC   `ESR` ESRD HCC   `COM` Commercial HCC   N Newborn: 0   P Pediatric: 0-17   M Maternity: 9-64   A Adult: 15-124

✓6ᵗʰ **M87.18** **Osteonecrosis due to drugs, other site**

     M87.180 **Osteonecrosis due to drugs, jaw** `HCC` `Rx` `ESR` `COM`

     M87.188 **Osteonecrosis due to drugs, other site** `HCC` `Rx` `ESR` `COM`

   M87.19 **Osteonecrosis due to drugs, multiple sites**

✓5ᵗʰ **M87.2** **Osteonecrosis** due to previous trauma

   M87.20 **Osteonecrosis due to previous trauma, unspecified bone** `HCC` `Rx` `ESR` `COM`

✓6ᵗʰ **M87.21** **Osteonecrosis due to previous trauma, shoulder**

     M87.211 **Osteonecrosis due to previous trauma, right shoulder** `HCC` `Rx` `ESR` `COM`

     M87.212 **Osteonecrosis due to previous trauma, left shoulder** `HCC` `Rx` `ESR` `COM`

     M87.219 **Osteonecrosis due to previous trauma, unspecified shoulder** `HCC` `Rx` `ESR` `COM`

✓6ᵗʰ **M87.22** **Osteonecrosis due to previous trauma, humerus**

     M87.221 **Osteonecrosis due to previous trauma, right humerus** `HCC` `Rx` `ESR` `COM`

     M87.222 **Osteonecrosis due to previous trauma, left humerus** `HCC` `Rx` `ESR` `COM`

     M87.229 **Osteonecrosis due to previous trauma, unspecified humerus** `HCC` `Rx` `ESR` `COM`

✓6ᵗʰ **M87.23** **Osteonecrosis due to previous trauma of radius, ulna and carpus**

     M87.231 **Osteonecrosis due to previous trauma of right radius** `HCC` `Rx` `ESR` `COM`

     M87.232 **Osteonecrosis due to previous trauma of left radius** `HCC` `Rx` `ESR` `COM`

     M87.233 **Osteonecrosis due to previous trauma of unspecified radius** `HCC` `Rx` `ESR` `COM`

     M87.234 **Osteonecrosis due to previous trauma of right ulna** `HCC` `Rx` `ESR` `COM`

     M87.235 **Osteonecrosis due to previous trauma of left ulna** `HCC` `Rx` `ESR` `COM`

     M87.236 **Osteonecrosis due to previous trauma of unspecified ulna** `HCC` `Rx` `ESR` `COM`

     M87.237 **Osteonecrosis due to previous trauma of right carpus** `HCC` `Rx` `ESR` `COM`

     M87.238 **Osteonecrosis due to previous trauma of left carpus** `HCC` `Rx` `ESR` `COM`

     M87.239 **Osteonecrosis due to previous trauma of unspecified carpus** `HCC` `Rx` `ESR` `COM`

✓6ᵗʰ **M87.24** **Osteonecrosis due to previous trauma, hand and fingers**

     M87.241 **Osteonecrosis due to previous trauma, right hand** `HCC` `Rx` `ESR` `COM`

     M87.242 **Osteonecrosis due to previous trauma, left hand** `HCC` `Rx` `ESR` `COM`

     M87.243 **Osteonecrosis due to previous trauma, unspecified hand** `HCC` `Rx` `ESR` `COM`

     M87.244 **Osteonecrosis due to previous trauma, right finger(s)** `HCC` `Rx` `ESR` `COM`

     M87.245 **Osteonecrosis due to previous trauma, left finger(s)** `HCC` `Rx` `ESR` `COM`

     M87.246 **Osteonecrosis due to previous trauma, unspecified finger(s)** `HCC` `Rx` `ESR` `COM`

✓6ᵗʰ **M87.25** **Osteonecrosis due to previous trauma, pelvis and femur**

     M87.250 **Osteonecrosis due to previous trauma, pelvis** `HCC` `Rx` `ESR` `COM`

     M87.251 **Osteonecrosis due to previous trauma, right femur** `HCC` `Rx` `ESR` `COM`

     M87.252 **Osteonecrosis due to previous trauma, left femur** `HCC` `Rx` `ESR` `COM`

     M87.256 **Osteonecrosis due to previous trauma, unspecified femur** `HCC` `Rx` `ESR` `COM`

✓6ᵗʰ **M87.26** **Osteonecrosis due to previous trauma, tibia and fibula**

     M87.261 **Osteonecrosis due to previous trauma, right tibia** `HCC` `Rx` `ESR` `COM`

     M87.262 **Osteonecrosis due to previous trauma, left tibia** `HCC` `Rx` `ESR` `COM`

     M87.263 **Osteonecrosis due to previous trauma, unspecified tibia** `HCC` `Rx` `ESR` `COM`

     M87.264 **Osteonecrosis due to previous trauma, right fibula** `HCC` `Rx` `ESR` `COM`

     M87.265 **Osteonecrosis due to previous trauma, left fibula** `HCC` `Rx` `ESR` `COM`

     M87.266 **Osteonecrosis due to previous trauma, unspecified fibula** `HCC` `Rx` `ESR` `COM`

✓6ᵗʰ **M87.27** **Osteonecrosis due to previous trauma, ankle, foot and toes**

     M87.271 **Osteonecrosis due to previous trauma, right ankle** `HCC` `Rx` `ESR` `COM`

     M87.272 **Osteonecrosis due to previous trauma, left ankle** `HCC` `Rx` `ESR` `COM`

     M87.273 **Osteonecrosis due to previous trauma, unspecified ankle** `HCC` `Rx` `ESR` `COM`

     M87.274 **Osteonecrosis due to previous trauma, right foot** `HCC` `Rx` `ESR` `COM`

     M87.275 **Osteonecrosis due to previous trauma, left foot** `HCC` `Rx` `ESR` `COM`

     M87.276 **Osteonecrosis due to previous trauma, unspecified foot** `HCC` `Rx` `ESR` `COM`

     M87.277 **Osteonecrosis due to previous trauma, right toe(s)** `HCC` `Rx` `ESR` `COM`

     M87.278 **Osteonecrosis due to previous trauma, left toe(s)** `HCC` `Rx` `ESR` `COM`

     M87.279 **Osteonecrosis due to previous trauma, unspecified toe(s)** `HCC` `Rx` `ESR` `COM`

   M87.28 **Osteonecrosis due to previous trauma, other site** `HCC` `Rx` `ESR` `COM`

   M87.29 **Osteonecrosis due to previous trauma, multiple sites** `HCC` `Rx` `ESR` `COM`

✓5ᵗʰ **M87.3** **Other** secondary osteonecrosis

   M87.30 **Other secondary osteonecrosis, unspecified bone** `HCC` `Rx` `ESR` `COM`

✓6ᵗʰ **M87.31** **Other secondary osteonecrosis, shoulder**

     M87.311 **Other secondary osteonecrosis, right shoulder** `HCC` `Rx` `ESR` `COM`

     M87.312 **Other secondary osteonecrosis, left shoulder** `HCC` `Rx` `ESR` `COM`

     M87.319 **Other secondary osteonecrosis, unspecified shoulder** `HCC` `Rx` `ESR` `COM`

✓6ᵗʰ **M87.32** **Other secondary osteonecrosis, humerus**

     M87.321 **Other secondary osteonecrosis, right humerus** `HCC` `Rx` `ESR` `COM`

     M87.322 **Other secondary osteonecrosis, left humerus** `HCC` `Rx` `ESR` `COM`

     M87.329 **Other secondary osteonecrosis, unspecified humerus** `HCC` `Rx` `ESR` `COM`

✓6ᵗʰ **M87.33** **Other secondary osteonecrosis of radius, ulna and carpus**

     M87.331 **Other secondary osteonecrosis of right radius** `HCC` `Rx` `ESR` `COM`

     M87.332 **Other secondary osteonecrosis of left radius** `HCC` `Rx` `ESR` `COM`

     M87.333 **Other secondary osteonecrosis of unspecified radius** `HCC` `Rx` `ESR` `COM`

     M87.334 **Other secondary osteonecrosis of right ulna** `HCC` `Rx` `ESR` `COM`

     M87.335 **Other secondary osteonecrosis of left ulna** `HCC` `Rx` `ESR` `COM`

     M87.336 **Other secondary osteonecrosis of unspecified ulna** `HCC` `Rx` `ESR` `COM`

     M87.337 **Other secondary osteonecrosis of right carpus** `HCC` `Rx` `ESR` `COM`

     M87.338 **Other secondary osteonecrosis of left carpus** `HCC` `Rx` `ESR` `COM`

     M87.339 **Other secondary osteonecrosis of unspecified carpus** `HCC` `Rx` `ESR` `COM`

✓6ᵗʰ **M87.34** **Other secondary osteonecrosis, hand and fingers**

     M87.341 **Other secondary osteonecrosis, right hand** `HCC` `Rx` `ESR` `COM`

     M87.342 **Other secondary osteonecrosis, left hand** `HCC` `Rx` `ESR` `COM`

     M87.343 **Other secondary osteonecrosis, unspecified hand** `HCC` `Rx` `ESR` `COM`

     M87.344 **Other secondary osteonecrosis, right finger(s)** `HCC` `Rx` `ESR` `COM`

     M87.345 **Other secondary osteonecrosis, left finger(s)** `HCC` `Rx` `ESR` `COM`

     M87.346 **Other secondary osteonecrosis, unspecified finger(s)** `HCC` `Rx` `ESR` `COM`

☑ Additional Character Required   ✓x7ᵗʰ Placeholder Alert   Manifestation   Unspecified Dx   Q QPP   UPD Unacceptable PDx

✓6ᵗʰ **M87.35** Other secondary osteonecrosis, pelvis and femur

　　M87.350 Other secondary osteonecrosis, pelvis `HCC` `Rx` `ESR` `COM`

　　M87.351 Other secondary osteonecrosis, right femur `HCC` `Rx` `ESR` `COM`

　　M87.352 Other secondary osteonecrosis, left femur `HCC` `Rx` `ESR` `COM`

　　M87.353 Other secondary osteonecrosis, unspecified femur `HCC` `Rx` `ESR` `COM`

✓6ᵗʰ **M87.36** Other secondary osteonecrosis, tibia and fibula

　　M87.361 Other secondary osteonecrosis, right tibia `HCC` `Rx` `ESR` `COM`

　　M87.362 Other secondary osteonecrosis, left tibia `HCC` `Rx` `ESR` `COM`

　　M87.363 Other secondary osteonecrosis, unspecified tibia `HCC` `Rx` `ESR` `COM`

　　M87.364 Other secondary osteonecrosis, right fibula `HCC` `Rx` `ESR` `COM`

　　M87.365 Other secondary osteonecrosis, left fibula `HCC` `Rx` `ESR` `COM`

　　M87.366 Other secondary osteonecrosis, unspecified fibula `HCC` `Rx` `ESR` `COM`

✓6ᵗʰ **M87.37** Other secondary osteonecrosis, ankle and foot

　　M87.371 Other secondary osteonecrosis, right ankle `HCC` `Rx` `ESR` `COM`

　　M87.372 Other secondary osteonecrosis, left ankle `HCC` `Rx` `ESR` `COM`

　　M87.373 Other secondary osteonecrosis, unspecified ankle `HCC` `Rx` `ESR` `COM`

　　M87.374 Other secondary osteonecrosis, right foot `HCC` `Rx` `ESR` `COM`

　　M87.375 Other secondary osteonecrosis, left foot `HCC` `Rx` `ESR` `COM`

　　M87.376 Other secondary osteonecrosis, unspecified foot `HCC` `Rx` `ESR` `COM`

　　M87.377 Other secondary osteonecrosis, right toe(s) `HCC` `Rx` `ESR` `COM`

　　M87.378 Other secondary osteonecrosis, left toe(s) `HCC` `Rx` `ESR` `COM`

　　M87.379 Other secondary osteonecrosis, unspecified toe(s) `HCC` `Rx` `ESR` `COM`

　M87.38 Other secondary osteonecrosis, other site `HCC` `Rx` `ESR` `COM`

　M87.39 Other secondary osteonecrosis, multiple sites `HCC` `Rx` `ESR` `COM`

✓5ᵗʰ **M87.8** Other osteonecrosis

　M87.80 Other osteonecrosis, unspecified bone `HCC` `Rx` `ESR` `COM`

✓6ᵗʰ **M87.81** Other osteonecrosis, shoulder

　　M87.811 Other osteonecrosis, right shoulder `HCC` `Rx` `ESR` `COM`

　　M87.812 Other osteonecrosis, left shoulder `HCC` `Rx` `ESR` `COM`

　　M87.819 Other osteonecrosis, unspecified shoulder `HCC` `Rx` `ESR` `COM`

✓6ᵗʰ **M87.82** Other osteonecrosis, humerus

　　M87.821 Other osteonecrosis, right humerus `HCC` `Rx` `ESR` `COM`

　　M87.822 Other osteonecrosis, left humerus `HCC` `Rx` `ESR` `COM`

　　M87.829 Other osteonecrosis, unspecified humerus `HCC` `Rx` `ESR` `COM`

✓6ᵗʰ **M87.83** Other osteonecrosis of radius, ulna and carpus

　　M87.831 Other osteonecrosis of right radius `HCC` `Rx` `ESR` `COM`

　　M87.832 Other osteonecrosis of left radius `HCC` `Rx` `ESR` `COM`

　　M87.833 Other osteonecrosis of unspecified radius `HCC` `Rx` `ESR` `COM`

　　M87.834 Other osteonecrosis of right ulna `HCC` `Rx` `ESR` `COM`

　　M87.835 Other osteonecrosis of left ulna `HCC` `Rx` `ESR` `COM`

　　M87.836 Other osteonecrosis of unspecified ulna `HCC` `Rx` `ESR` `COM`

　　M87.837 Other osteonecrosis of right carpus `HCC` `Rx` `ESR` `COM`

　　M87.838 Other osteonecrosis of left carpus `HCC` `Rx` `ESR` `COM`

　　M87.839 Other osteonecrosis of unspecified carpus `HCC` `Rx` `ESR` `COM`

✓6ᵗʰ **M87.84** Other osteonecrosis, hand and fingers

　　M87.841 Other osteonecrosis, right hand `HCC` `Rx` `ESR` `COM`

　　M87.842 Other osteonecrosis, left hand `HCC` `Rx` `ESR` `COM`

　　M87.843 Other osteonecrosis, unspecified hand `HCC` `Rx` `ESR` `COM`

　　M87.844 Other osteonecrosis, right finger(s) `HCC` `Rx` `ESR` `COM`

　　M87.845 Other osteonecrosis, left finger(s) `HCC` `Rx` `ESR` `COM`

　　M87.849 Other osteonecrosis, unspecified finger(s) `HCC` `Rx` `ESR` `COM`

✓6ᵗʰ **M87.85** Other osteonecrosis, pelvis and femur

　　M87.850 Other osteonecrosis, pelvis `HCC` `Rx` `ESR` `COM`

　　M87.851 Other osteonecrosis, right femur `HCC` `Rx` `ESR` `COM`

　　M87.852 Other osteonecrosis, left femur `HCC` `Rx` `ESR` `COM`

　　M87.859 Other osteonecrosis, unspecified femur `HCC` `Rx` `ESR` `COM`

✓6ᵗʰ **M87.86** Other osteonecrosis, tibia and fibula

　　M87.861 Other osteonecrosis, right tibia `HCC` `Rx` `ESR` `COM`

　　M87.862 Other osteonecrosis, left tibia `HCC` `Rx` `ESR` `COM`

　　M87.863 Other osteonecrosis, unspecified tibia `HCC` `Rx` `ESR` `COM`

　　M87.864 Other osteonecrosis, right fibula `HCC` `Rx` `ESR` `COM`

　　M87.865 Other osteonecrosis, left fibula `HCC` `Rx` `ESR` `COM`

　　M87.869 Other osteonecrosis, unspecified fibula `HCC` `Rx` `ESR` `COM`

✓6ᵗʰ **M87.87** Other osteonecrosis, ankle, foot and toes

　　M87.871 Other osteonecrosis, right ankle `HCC` `Rx` `ESR` `COM`

　　M87.872 Other osteonecrosis, left ankle `HCC` `Rx` `ESR` `COM`

　　M87.873 Other osteonecrosis, unspecified ankle `HCC` `Rx` `ESR` `COM`

　　M87.874 Other osteonecrosis, right foot `HCC` `Rx` `ESR` `COM`

　　M87.875 Other osteonecrosis, left foot `HCC` `Rx` `ESR` `COM`

　　M87.876 Other osteonecrosis, unspecified foot `HCC` `Rx` `ESR` `COM`

　　M87.877 Other osteonecrosis, right toe(s) `HCC` `Rx` `ESR` `COM`

　　M87.878 Other osteonecrosis, left toe(s) `HCC` `Rx` `ESR` `COM`

　　M87.879 Other osteonecrosis, unspecified toe(s) `HCC` `Rx` `ESR` `COM`

　M87.88 Other osteonecrosis, other site `HCC` `Rx` `ESR` `COM`

　M87.89 Other osteonecrosis, multiple sites `HCC` `Rx` `ESR` `COM`

M87.9 Osteonecrosis, unspecified `HCC` `Rx` `ESR` `COM`
　Necrosis of bone NOS

✓4ᵗʰ **M88** Osteitis deformans [Paget's disease of bone]

　EXCLUDES 1　osteitis deformans in neoplastic disease (M90.6)

　DEF: Bone disease characterized by numerous cycles of bone resorption by the body. Resorption is followed by accelerated repair attempts, causing bone deformities and bowing, with associated fractures and pain.

M88.0 Osteitis deformans of skull

M88.1 Osteitis deformans of vertebrae

✓5ᵗʰ **M88.8** Osteitis deformans of other bones

✓6ᵗʰ **M88.81** Osteitis deformans of shoulder

　　M88.811 Osteitis deformans of right shoulder

　　M88.812 Osteitis deformans of left shoulder

　　M88.819 Osteitis deformans of unspecified shoulder

`HCC` CMS-HCC　　`Rx` Rx HCC　　`ESR` ESRD HCC　　`COM` Commercial HCC　　N Newborn: 0　　P Pediatric: 0-17　　M Maternity: 9-64　　A Adult: 15-124

852　　　M87.35–M88.819　　　ICD-10-CM 2023

√6ᵗʰ **M88.82 Osteitis deformans of** upper arm

     M88.821 Osteitis deformans of right **upper arm**

     M88.822 Osteitis deformans of left **upper arm**

     M88.829 Osteitis deformans of unspecified upper arm

√6ᵗʰ **M88.83 Osteitis deformans of** forearm

     M88.831 Osteitis deformans of right **forearm**

     M88.832 Osteitis deformans of left **forearm**

     M88.839 Osteitis deformans of unspecified forearm

√6ᵗʰ **M88.84 Osteitis deformans of** hand

     M88.841 Osteitis deformans of right **hand**

     M88.842 Osteitis deformans of left **hand**

     M88.849 Osteitis deformans of unspecified hand

√6ᵗʰ **M88.85 Osteitis deformans of** thigh

     M88.851 Osteitis deformans of right **thigh**

     M88.852 Osteitis deformans of left **thigh**

     M88.859 Osteitis deformans of unspecified thigh

√6ᵗʰ **M88.86 Osteitis deformans of** lower leg

     M88.861 Osteitis deformans of right **lower leg**

     M88.862 Osteitis deformans of left **lower leg**

     M88.869 Osteitis deformans of unspecified lower leg

√6ᵗʰ **M88.87 Osteitis deformans of** ankle and foot

     M88.871 Osteitis deformans of right **ankle and foot**

     M88.872 Osteitis deformans of left **ankle and foot**

     M88.879 Osteitis deformans of unspecified ankle and foot

   M88.88 Osteitis deformans of other bones

     EXCLUDES 2   *osteitis deformans of skull (M88.0)*

                 osteitis deformans of vertebrae (M88.1)

   M88.89 Osteitis deformans of multiple sites

  M88.9 Osteitis deformans of unspecified bone

√4ᵗʰ **M89 Other disorders of bone**

√5ᵗʰ **M89.0 Algoneurodystrophy**

     Shoulder-hand syndrome

     Sudeck's atrophy

     EXCLUDES 1   *causalgia, lower limb (G57.7-)*

                 causalgia, upper limb (G56.4-)

                 complex regional pain syndrome II, lower limb (G57.7-)

                 complex regional pain syndrome II, upper limb (G56.4-)

                 reflex sympathetic dystrophy (G90.5-)

     M89.00 Algoneurodystrophy, unspecified site

√6ᵗʰ **M89.01 Algoneurodystrophy,** shoulder

     M89.011 Algoneurodystrophy, right **shoulder**

     M89.012 Algoneurodystrophy, left **shoulder**

     M89.019 Algoneurodystrophy, unspecified shoulder

√6ᵗʰ **M89.02 Algoneurodystrophy,** upper arm

     M89.021 Algoneurodystrophy, right **upper arm**

     M89.022 Algoneurodystrophy, left **upper arm**

     M89.029 Algoneurodystrophy, unspecified upper arm

√6ᵗʰ **M89.03 Algoneurodystrophy,** forearm

     M89.031 Algoneurodystrophy, right **forearm**

     M89.032 Algoneurodystrophy, left **forearm**

     M89.039 Algoneurodystrophy, unspecified forearm

√6ᵗʰ **M89.04 Algoneurodystrophy,** hand

     M89.041 Algoneurodystrophy, right **hand**

     M89.042 Algoneurodystrophy, left **hand**

     M89.049 Algoneurodystrophy, unspecified hand

√6ᵗʰ **M89.05 Algoneurodystrophy,** thigh

     M89.051 Algoneurodystrophy, right **thigh**

     M89.052 Algoneurodystrophy, left **thigh**

     M89.059 Algoneurodystrophy, unspecified thigh

√6ᵗʰ **M89.06 Algoneurodystrophy,** lower leg

     M89.061 Algoneurodystrophy, right **lower leg**

     M89.062 Algoneurodystrophy, left **lower leg**

     M89.069 Algoneurodystrophy, unspecified lower leg

√6ᵗʰ **M89.07 Algoneurodystrophy,** ankle and foot

     M89.071 Algoneurodystrophy, right **ankle and foot**

     M89.072 Algoneurodystrophy, left **ankle and foot**

     M89.079 Algoneurodystrophy, unspecified ankle and foot

   M89.08 Algoneurodystrophy, other site

   M89.09 Algoneurodystrophy, multiple sites

√5ᵗʰ **M89.1 Physeal arrest**

     Arrest of growth plate

     Epiphyseal arrest

     Growth plate arrest

√6ᵗʰ **M89.12 Physeal arrest,** humerus

     M89.121 Complete physeal arrest, right proximal **humerus**

     M89.122 Complete physeal arrest, left proximal **humerus**

     M89.123 Partial physeal arrest, right proximal **humerus**

     M89.124 Partial physeal arrest, left proximal **humerus**

     M89.125 Complete physeal arrest, right distal **humerus**

     M89.126 Complete physeal arrest, left distal **humerus**

     M89.127 Partial physeal arrest, right distal **humerus**

     M89.128 Partial physeal arrest, left distal **humerus**

     M89.129 Physeal arrest, humerus, unspecified

√6ᵗʰ **M89.13 Physeal arrest,** forearm

     M89.131 Complete physeal arrest, right distal **radius**

     M89.132 Complete physeal arrest, left distal **radius**

     M89.133 Partial physeal arrest, right distal **radius**

     M89.134 Partial physeal arrest, left distal **radius**

     M89.138 Other physeal arrest of forearm

     M89.139 Physeal arrest, forearm, unspecified

√6ᵗʰ **M89.15 Physeal arrest,** femur

     M89.151 Complete physeal arrest, right proximal **femur**

     M89.152 Complete physeal arrest, left proximal **femur**

     M89.153 Partial physeal arrest, right proximal **femur**

     M89.154 Partial physeal arrest, left proximal **femur**

     M89.155 Complete physeal arrest, right distal **femur**

     M89.156 Complete physeal arrest, left distal **femur**

     M89.157 Partial physeal arrest, right distal **femur**

     M89.158 Partial physeal arrest, left distal **femur**

     M89.159 Physeal arrest, femur, unspecified

√6ᵗʰ **M89.16 Physeal arrest,** lower leg

     M89.160 Complete physeal arrest, right proximal **tibia**

     M89.161 Complete physeal arrest, left proximal **tibia**

     M89.162 Partial physeal arrest, right proximal **tibia**

     M89.163 Partial physeal arrest, left proximal **tibia**

     M89.164 Complete physeal arrest, right distal **tibia**

     M89.165 Complete physeal arrest, left distal **tibia**

     M89.166 Partial physeal arrest, right distal **tibia**

     M89.167 Partial physeal arrest, left distal **tibia**

     M89.168 Other physeal arrest of lower leg

     M89.169 Physeal arrest, lower leg, unspecified

   M89.18 Physeal arrest, other site

√5ᵗʰ **M89.2 Other disorders of bone development and growth**

     M89.20 Other disorders of bone development and growth, unspecified site

√6ᵗʰ **M89.21 Other disorders of bone development and growth,** shoulder

     M89.211 Other disorders of bone development and growth, right **shoulder**

     M89.212 Other disorders of bone development and growth, left **shoulder**

     M89.219 Other disorders of bone development and growth, unspecified shoulder

√6ᵗʰ **M89.22 Other disorders of bone development and growth,** humerus

     M89.221 Other disorders of bone development and growth, right **humerus**

     M89.222 Other disorders of bone development and growth, left **humerus**

     M89.229 Other disorders of bone development and growth, unspecified humerus

---

☑ Additional Character Required   √x7ᵗʰ Placeholder Alert   Manifestation   Unspecified Dx   ◘ QPP   UPD Unacceptable PDx

✓6ᵗʰ **M89.23** **Other disorders of bone development and growth, ulna and radius**
  M89.231 Other disorders of bone development and growth, right ulna
  M89.232 Other disorders of bone development and growth, left ulna
  M89.233 Other disorders of bone development and growth, right radius
  M89.234 Other disorders of bone development and growth, left radius
  M89.239 Other disorders of bone development and growth, unspecified ulna and radius
✓6ᵗʰ **M89.24** **Other disorders of bone development and growth, hand**
  M89.241 Other disorders of bone development and growth, right hand
  M89.242 Other disorders of bone development and growth, left hand
  M89.249 Other disorders of bone development and growth, unspecified hand
✓6ᵗʰ **M89.25** **Other disorders of bone development and growth, femur**
  M89.251 Other disorders of bone development and growth, right femur
  M89.252 Other disorders of bone development and growth, left femur
  M89.259 Other disorders of bone development and growth, unspecified femur
✓6ᵗʰ **M89.26** **Other disorders of bone development and growth, tibia and fibula**
  M89.261 Other disorders of bone development and growth, right tibia
  M89.262 Other disorders of bone development and growth, left tibia
  M89.263 Other disorders of bone development and growth, right fibula
  M89.264 Other disorders of bone development and growth, left fibula
  M89.269 Other disorders of bone development and growth, unspecified lower leg
✓6ᵗʰ **M89.27** **Other disorders of bone development and growth, ankle and foot**
  M89.271 Other disorders of bone development and growth, right ankle and foot
  M89.272 Other disorders of bone development and growth, left ankle and foot
  M89.279 Other disorders of bone development and growth, unspecified ankle and foot
  M89.28 Other disorders of bone development and growth, other site
  M89.29 Other disorders of bone development and growth, multiple sites
✓5ᵗʰ **M89.3** **Hypertrophy of bone**
  M89.30 Hypertrophy of bone, unspecified site
✓6ᵗʰ **M89.31** Hypertrophy of bone, shoulder
  M89.311 Hypertrophy of bone, right shoulder
  M89.312 Hypertrophy of bone, left shoulder
  M89.319 Hypertrophy of bone, unspecified shoulder
✓6ᵗʰ **M89.32** Hypertrophy of bone, humerus
  M89.321 Hypertrophy of bone, right humerus
  M89.322 Hypertrophy of bone, left humerus
  M89.329 Hypertrophy of bone, unspecified humerus
✓6ᵗʰ **M89.33** Hypertrophy of bone, ulna and radius
  M89.331 Hypertrophy of bone, right ulna
  M89.332 Hypertrophy of bone, left ulna
  M89.333 Hypertrophy of bone, right radius
  M89.334 Hypertrophy of bone, left radius
  M89.339 Hypertrophy of bone, unspecified ulna and radius
✓6ᵗʰ **M89.34** Hypertrophy of bone, hand
  M89.341 Hypertrophy of bone, right hand
  M89.342 Hypertrophy of bone, left hand
  M89.349 Hypertrophy of bone, unspecified hand
✓6ᵗʰ **M89.35** Hypertrophy of bone, femur
  M89.351 Hypertrophy of bone, right femur
  M89.352 Hypertrophy of bone, left femur
  M89.359 Hypertrophy of bone, unspecified femur

✓6ᵗʰ **M89.36** Hypertrophy of bone, tibia and fibula
  M89.361 Hypertrophy of bone, right tibia
  M89.362 Hypertrophy of bone, left tibia
  M89.363 Hypertrophy of bone, right fibula
  M89.364 Hypertrophy of bone, left fibula
  M89.369 Hypertrophy of bone, unspecified tibia and fibula
✓6ᵗʰ **M89.37** Hypertrophy of bone, ankle and foot
  M89.371 Hypertrophy of bone, right ankle and foot
  M89.372 Hypertrophy of bone, left ankle and foot
  M89.379 Hypertrophy of bone, unspecified ankle and foot
  M89.38 Hypertrophy of bone, other site
  M89.39 Hypertrophy of bone, multiple sites
✓5ᵗʰ **M89.4** **Other hypertrophic osteoarthropathy**
  Marie-Bamberger disease
  Pachydermoperiostosis
  M89.40 Other hypertrophic osteoarthropathy, unspecified site
✓6ᵗʰ **M89.41** Other hypertrophic osteoarthropathy, shoulder
  M89.411 Other hypertrophic osteoarthropathy, right shoulder
  M89.412 Other hypertrophic osteoarthropathy, left shoulder
  M89.419 Other hypertrophic osteoarthropathy, unspecified shoulder
✓6ᵗʰ **M89.42** Other hypertrophic osteoarthropathy, upper arm
  M89.421 Other hypertrophic osteoarthropathy, right upper arm
  M89.422 Other hypertrophic osteoarthropathy, left upper arm
  M89.429 Other hypertrophic osteoarthropathy, unspecified upper arm
✓6ᵗʰ **M89.43** Other hypertrophic osteoarthropathy, forearm
  M89.431 Other hypertrophic osteoarthropathy, right forearm
  M89.432 Other hypertrophic osteoarthropathy, left forearm
  M89.439 Other hypertrophic osteoarthropathy, unspecified forearm
✓6ᵗʰ **M89.44** Other hypertrophic osteoarthropathy, hand
  M89.441 Other hypertrophic osteoarthropathy, right hand
  M89.442 Other hypertrophic osteoarthropathy, left hand
  M89.449 Other hypertrophic osteoarthropathy, unspecified hand
✓6ᵗʰ **M89.45** Other hypertrophic osteoarthropathy, thigh
  M89.451 Other hypertrophic osteoarthropathy, right thigh
  M89.452 Other hypertrophic osteoarthropathy, left thigh
  M89.459 Other hypertrophic osteoarthropathy, unspecified thigh
✓6ᵗʰ **M89.46** Other hypertrophic osteoarthropathy, lower leg
  M89.461 Other hypertrophic osteoarthropathy, right lower leg
  M89.462 Other hypertrophic osteoarthropathy, left lower leg
  M89.469 Other hypertrophic osteoarthropathy, unspecified lower leg
✓6ᵗʰ **M89.47** Other hypertrophic osteoarthropathy, ankle and foot
  M89.471 Other hypertrophic osteoarthropathy, right ankle and foot
  M89.472 Other hypertrophic osteoarthropathy, left ankle and foot
  M89.479 Other hypertrophic osteoarthropathy, unspecified ankle and foot
  M89.48 Other hypertrophic osteoarthropathy, other site
  M89.49 Other hypertrophic osteoarthropathy, multiple sites
✓5ᵗʰ **M89.5** **Osteolysis**
  Use additional code to identify major osseous defect, if applicable (M89.7-)
  EXCLUDES 2 periprosthetic osteolysis of internal prosthetic joint (T84.05-)
  M89.50 Osteolysis, unspecified site

√6ᵗʰ **M89.51 Osteolysis, shoulder**

     M89.511 Osteolysis, right shoulder
     M89.512 Osteolysis, left shoulder
     M89.519 Osteolysis, unspecified shoulder

√6ᵗʰ **M89.52 Osteolysis, upper arm**

     M89.521 Osteolysis, right upper arm
     M89.522 Osteolysis, left upper arm
     M89.529 Osteolysis, unspecified upper arm

√6ᵗʰ **M89.53 Osteolysis, forearm**

     M89.531 Osteolysis, right forearm
     M89.532 Osteolysis, left forearm
     M89.539 Osteolysis, unspecified forearm

√6ᵗʰ **M89.54 Osteolysis, hand**

     M89.541 Osteolysis, right hand
     M89.542 Osteolysis, left hand
     M89.549 Osteolysis, unspecified hand

√6ᵗʰ **M89.55 Osteolysis, thigh**

     M89.551 Osteolysis, right thigh
     M89.552 Osteolysis, left thigh
     M89.559 Osteolysis, unspecified thigh

√6ᵗʰ **M89.56 Osteolysis, lower leg**

     M89.561 Osteolysis, right lower leg
     M89.562 Osteolysis, left lower leg
     M89.569 Osteolysis, unspecified lower leg

√6ᵗʰ **M89.57 Osteolysis, ankle and foot**

     M89.571 Osteolysis, right ankle and foot
     M89.572 Osteolysis, left ankle and foot
     M89.579 Osteolysis, unspecified ankle and foot

     M89.58 Osteolysis, other site
     M89.59 Osteolysis, multiple sites

√5ᵗʰ **M89.6 Osteopathy after poliomyelitis**

     Use additional code (B91) to identify previous poliomyelitis
     EXCLUDES 1   postpolio syndrome (G14)

     M89.60 Osteopathy after poliomyelitis, unspecified site HCC ESR COM

√6ᵗʰ **M89.61 Osteopathy after poliomyelitis, shoulder**

     M89.611 Osteopathy after poliomyelitis, right shoulder HCC ESR COM
     M89.612 Osteopathy after poliomyelitis, left shoulder HCC ESR COM
     M89.619 Osteopathy after poliomyelitis, unspecified shoulder HCC ESR COM

√6ᵗʰ **M89.62 Osteopathy after poliomyelitis, upper arm**

     M89.621 Osteopathy after poliomyelitis, right upper arm HCC ESR COM
     M89.622 Osteopathy after poliomyelitis, left upper arm HCC ESR COM
     M89.629 Osteopathy after poliomyelitis, unspecified upper arm HCC ESR COM

√6ᵗʰ **M89.63 Osteopathy after poliomyelitis, forearm**

     M89.631 Osteopathy after poliomyelitis, right forearm HCC ESR COM
     M89.632 Osteopathy after poliomyelitis, left forearm HCC ESR COM
     M89.639 Osteopathy after poliomyelitis, unspecified forearm HCC ESR COM

√6ᵗʰ **M89.64 Osteopathy after poliomyelitis, hand**

     M89.641 Osteopathy after poliomyelitis, right hand HCC ESR COM
     M89.642 Osteopathy after poliomyelitis, left hand HCC ESR COM
     M89.649 Osteopathy after poliomyelitis, unspecified hand HCC ESR COM

√6ᵗʰ **M89.65 Osteopathy after poliomyelitis, thigh**

     M89.651 Osteopathy after poliomyelitis, right thigh HCC ESR COM
     M89.652 Osteopathy after poliomyelitis, left thigh HCC ESR COM
     M89.659 Osteopathy after poliomyelitis, unspecified thigh HCC ESR COM

√6ᵗʰ **M89.66 Osteopathy after poliomyelitis, lower leg**

     M89.661 Osteopathy after poliomyelitis, right lower leg HCC ESR COM
     M89.662 Osteopathy after poliomyelitis, left lower leg HCC ESR COM

     M89.669 Osteopathy after poliomyelitis, unspecified lower leg HCC ESR COM

√6ᵗʰ **M89.67 Osteopathy after poliomyelitis, ankle and foot**

     M89.671 Osteopathy after poliomyelitis, right ankle and foot HCC ESR COM
     M89.672 Osteopathy after poliomyelitis, left ankle and foot HCC ESR COM
     M89.679 Osteopathy after poliomyelitis, unspecified ankle and foot HCC ESR COM

     M89.68 Osteopathy after poliomyelitis, other site HCC ESR COM
     M89.69 Osteopathy after poliomyelitis, multiple sites HCC ESR COM

√5ᵗʰ **M89.7 Major osseous defect**

     Code first underlying disease, if known, such as:
     aseptic necrosis of bone (M87.-)
     malignant neoplasm of bone (C40.-)
     osteolysis (M89.5)
     osteomyelitis (M86.-)
     osteonecrosis (M87.-)
     osteoporosis (M80.-, M81.-)
     periprosthetic osteolysis (T84.05-)

     M89.70 Major osseous defect, unspecified site

√6ᵗʰ **M89.71 Major osseous defect, shoulder region**

     Major osseous defect clavicle or scapula

     M89.711 Major osseous defect, right shoulder region
     M89.712 Major osseous defect, left shoulder region
     M89.719 Major osseous defect, unspecified shoulder region

√6ᵗʰ **M89.72 Major osseous defect, humerus**

     M89.721 Major osseous defect, right humerus
     M89.722 Major osseous defect, left humerus
     M89.729 Major osseous defect, unspecified humerus

√6ᵗʰ **M89.73 Major osseous defect, forearm**

     Major osseous defect of radius and ulna

     M89.731 Major osseous defect, right forearm
     M89.732 Major osseous defect, left forearm
     M89.739 Major osseous defect, unspecified forearm

√6ᵗʰ **M89.74 Major osseous defect, hand**

     Major osseous defect of carpus, fingers, metacarpus

     M89.741 Major osseous defect, right hand
     M89.742 Major osseous defect, left hand
     M89.749 Major osseous defect, unspecified hand

√6ᵗʰ **M89.75 Major osseous defect, pelvic region and thigh**

     Major osseous defect of femur and pelvis

     M89.751 Major osseous defect, right pelvic region and thigh
     M89.752 Major osseous defect, left pelvic region and thigh
     M89.759 Major osseous defect, unspecified pelvic region and thigh

√6ᵗʰ **M89.76 Major osseous defect, lower leg**

     Major osseous defect of fibula and tibia

     M89.761 Major osseous defect, right lower leg
     M89.762 Major osseous defect, left lower leg
     M89.769 Major osseous defect, unspecified lower leg

√6ᵗʰ **M89.77 Major osseous defect, ankle and foot**

     Major osseous defect of metatarsus, tarsus, toes

     M89.771 Major osseous defect, right ankle and foot
     M89.772 Major osseous defect, left ankle and foot
     M89.779 Major osseous defect, unspecified ankle and foot

     M89.78 Major osseous defect, other site
     M89.79 Major osseous defect, multiple sites

√5ᵗʰ **M89.8 Other specified disorders of bone**

     Infantile cortical hyperostoses
     Post-traumatic subperiosteal ossification
     AHA: 2022,2Q,10

√6ᵗʰ **M89.8X Other specified disorders of bone**

     M89.8X0 Other specified disorders of bone, multiple sites

M89.8X1 Other specified disorders of bone, shoulder

M89.8X2 Other specified disorders of bone, upper arm

M89.8X3 Other specified disorders of bone, forearm
AHA: 2019,3Q,9

M89.8X4 Other specified disorders of bone, hand

M89.8X5 Other specified disorders of bone, thigh

M89.8X6 Other specified disorders of bone, lower leg

M89.8X7 Other specified disorders of bone, ankle and foot

M89.8X8 Other specified disorders of bone, other site

M89.8X9 Other specified disorders of bone, unspecified site

M89.9 Disorder of bone, unspecified

✓4th **M90** Osteopathies in diseases classified elsewhere

EXCLUDES 1   osteochondritis, osteomyelitis, and osteopathy (in):
cryptococcosis (B45.3)
diabetes mellitus (E08-E13 with .69-)
gonococcal (A54.43)
neurogenic syphilis (A52.11)
renal osteodystrophy (N25.0)
salmonellosis (A02.24)
secondary syphilis (A51.46)
syphilis (late) (A52.77)

✓5th **M90.5** Osteonecrosis in diseases classified elsewhere

Code first underlying disease, such as:
caisson disease (T70.3)
hemoglobinopathy (D50-D64)

M90.50 Osteonecrosis in diseases classified elsewhere, unspecified site   HCC Rx ESR COM

✓6th **M90.51** Osteonecrosis in diseases classified elsewhere, shoulder

M90.511 Osteonecrosis in diseases classified elsewhere, right shoulder   HCC Rx ESR COM

M90.512 Osteonecrosis in diseases classified elsewhere, left shoulder   HCC Rx ESR COM

M90.519 Osteonecrosis in diseases classified elsewhere, unspecified shoulder   HCC Rx ESR COM

✓6th **M90.52** Osteonecrosis in diseases classified elsewhere, upper arm

M90.521 Osteonecrosis in diseases classified elsewhere, right upper arm   HCC Rx ESR COM

M90.522 Osteonecrosis in diseases classified elsewhere, left upper arm   HCC Rx ESR COM

M90.529 Osteonecrosis in diseases classified elsewhere, unspecified upper arm   HCC Rx ESR COM

✓6th **M90.53** Osteonecrosis in diseases classified elsewhere, forearm

M90.531 Osteonecrosis in diseases classified elsewhere, right forearm   HCC Rx ESR COM

M90.532 Osteonecrosis in diseases classified elsewhere, left forearm   HCC Rx ESR COM

M90.539 Osteonecrosis in diseases classified elsewhere, unspecified forearm   HCC Rx ESR COM

✓6th **M90.54** Osteonecrosis in diseases classified elsewhere, hand

M90.541 Osteonecrosis in diseases classified elsewhere, right hand   HCC Rx ESR COM

M90.542 Osteonecrosis in diseases classified elsewhere, left hand   HCC Rx ESR COM

M90.549 Osteonecrosis in diseases classified elsewhere, unspecified hand   HCC Rx ESR COM

✓6th **M90.55** Osteonecrosis in diseases classified elsewhere, thigh

M90.551 Osteonecrosis in diseases classified elsewhere, right thigh   HCC Rx ESR COM

M90.552 Osteonecrosis in diseases classified elsewhere, left thigh   HCC Rx ESR COM

M90.559 Osteonecrosis in diseases classified elsewhere, unspecified thigh   HCC Rx ESR COM

✓6th **M90.56** Osteonecrosis in diseases classified elsewhere, lower leg

M90.561 Osteonecrosis in diseases classified elsewhere, right lower leg   HCC Rx ESR COM

M90.562 Osteonecrosis in diseases classified elsewhere, left lower leg   HCC Rx ESR COM

M90.569 Osteonecrosis in diseases classified elsewhere, unspecified lower leg   HCC Rx ESR COM

✓6th **M90.57** Osteonecrosis in diseases classified elsewhere, ankle and foot

M90.571 Osteonecrosis in diseases classified elsewhere, right ankle and foot   HCC Rx ESR COM

M90.572 Osteonecrosis in diseases classified elsewhere, left ankle and foot   HCC Rx ESR COM

M90.579 Osteonecrosis in diseases classified elsewhere, unspecified ankle and foot   HCC Rx ESR COM

M90.58 Osteonecrosis in diseases classified elsewhere, other site   HCC Rx ESR COM

M90.59 Osteonecrosis in diseases classified elsewhere, multiple sites   HCC Rx ESR COM

✓5th **M90.6** Osteitis deformans in neoplastic diseases

Osteitis deformans in malignant neoplasm of bone
Code first the neoplasm (C40.-, C41.-)

EXCLUDES 1   osteitis deformans [Paget's disease of bone] (M88.-)

M90.60 Osteitis deformans in neoplastic diseases, unspecified site

✓6th **M90.61** Osteitis deformans in neoplastic diseases, shoulder

M90.611 Osteitis deformans in neoplastic diseases, right shoulder

M90.612 Osteitis deformans in neoplastic diseases, left shoulder

M90.619 Osteitis deformans in neoplastic diseases, unspecified shoulder

✓6th **M90.62** Osteitis deformans in neoplastic diseases, upper arm

M90.621 Osteitis deformans in neoplastic diseases, right upper arm

M90.622 Osteitis deformans in neoplastic diseases, left upper arm

M90.629 Osteitis deformans in neoplastic diseases, unspecified upper arm

✓6th **M90.63** Osteitis deformans in neoplastic diseases, forearm

M90.631 Osteitis deformans in neoplastic diseases, right forearm

M90.632 Osteitis deformans in neoplastic diseases, left forearm

M90.639 Osteitis deformans in neoplastic diseases, unspecified forearm

✓6th **M90.64** Osteitis deformans in neoplastic diseases, hand

M90.641 Osteitis deformans in neoplastic diseases, right hand

M90.642 Osteitis deformans in neoplastic diseases, left hand

M90.649 Osteitis deformans in neoplastic diseases, unspecified hand

✓6th **M90.65** Osteitis deformans in neoplastic diseases, thigh

M90.651 Osteitis deformans in neoplastic diseases, right thigh

M90.652 Osteitis deformans in neoplastic diseases, left thigh

M90.659 Osteitis deformans in neoplastic diseases, unspecified thigh

✓6th **M90.66** Osteitis deformans in neoplastic diseases, lower leg

M90.661 Osteitis deformans in neoplastic diseases, right lower leg

M90.662 Osteitis deformans in neoplastic diseases, left lower leg

M90.669 Osteitis deformans in neoplastic diseases, unspecified lower leg

✓6ᵗʰ **M90.67** **Osteitis deformans in neoplastic diseases,** ankle and foot
- *M90.671* *Osteitis deformans in neoplastic diseases, right ankle and foot*
- *M90.672* *Osteitis deformans in neoplastic diseases, left ankle and foot*
- *M90.679* *Osteitis deformans in neoplastic diseases, unspecified ankle and foot*
- *M90.68* *Osteitis deformans in neoplastic diseases, other site*
- *M90.69* *Osteitis deformans in neoplastic diseases, multiple sites*

✓5ᵗʰ **M90.8** **Osteopathy in diseases classified elsewhere**
Code first underlying disease, such as:
rickets (E55.0)
vitamin-D-resistant rickets (E83.3)
- *M90.80* *Osteopathy in diseases classified elsewhere, unspecified site*

✓6ᵗʰ **M90.81** **Osteopathy in diseases classified elsewhere,** shoulder
- *M90.811* *Osteopathy in diseases classified elsewhere, right shoulder*
- *M90.812* *Osteopathy in diseases classified elsewhere, left shoulder*
- *M90.819* *Osteopathy in diseases classified elsewhere, unspecified shoulder*

✓6ᵗʰ **M90.82** **Osteopathy in diseases classified elsewhere,** upper arm
- *M90.821* *Osteopathy in diseases classified elsewhere, right upper arm*
- *M90.822* *Osteopathy in diseases classified elsewhere, left upper arm*
- *M90.829* *Osteopathy in diseases classified elsewhere, unspecified upper arm*

✓6ᵗʰ **M90.83** **Osteopathy in diseases classified elsewhere,** forearm
- *M90.831* *Osteopathy in diseases classified elsewhere, right forearm*
- *M90.832* *Osteopathy in diseases classified elsewhere, left forearm*
- *M90.839* *Osteopathy in diseases classified elsewhere, unspecified forearm*

✓6ᵗʰ **M90.84** **Osteopathy in diseases classified elsewhere,** hand
- *M90.841* *Osteopathy in diseases classified elsewhere, right hand*
- *M90.842* *Osteopathy in diseases classified elsewhere, left hand*
- *M90.849* *Osteopathy in diseases classified elsewhere, unspecified hand*

✓6ᵗʰ **M90.85** **Osteopathy in diseases classified elsewhere,** thigh
- *M90.851* *Osteopathy in diseases classified elsewhere, right thigh*
- *M90.852* *Osteopathy in diseases classified elsewhere, left thigh*
- *M90.859* *Osteopathy in diseases classified elsewhere, unspecified thigh*

✓6ᵗʰ **M90.86** **Osteopathy in diseases classified elsewhere,** lower leg
- *M90.861* *Osteopathy in diseases classified elsewhere, right lower leg*
- *M90.862* *Osteopathy in diseases classified elsewhere, left lower leg*
- *M90.869* *Osteopathy in diseases classified elsewhere, unspecified lower leg*

✓6ᵗʰ **M90.87** **Osteopathy in diseases classified elsewhere,** ankle and foot
- *M90.871* *Osteopathy in diseases classified elsewhere, right ankle and foot*
- *M90.872* *Osteopathy in diseases classified elsewhere, left ankle and foot*
- *M90.879* *Osteopathy in diseases classified elsewhere, unspecified ankle and foot*
- *M90.88* *Osteopathy in diseases classified elsewhere, other site*
- *M90.89* *Osteopathy in diseases classified elsewhere, multiple sites*

Chondropathies (M91-M94)

EXCLUDES 1   postprocedural chondropathies (M96.-)

✓4ᵗʰ **M91** **Juvenile osteochondrosis of** hip and pelvis
EXCLUDES 1   slipped upper femoral epiphysis (nontraumatic) ▶(M93.0-)◀

M91.0 **Juvenile osteochondrosis of** pelvis   COM
Osteochondrosis (juvenile) of acetabulum
Osteochondrosis (juvenile) of iliac crest [Buchanan]
Osteochondrosis (juvenile) of ischiopubic synchondrosis [van Neck]
Osteochondrosis (juvenile) of symphysis pubis [Pierson]

✓5ᵗʰ **M91.1** **Juvenile osteochondrosis of** head of femur [Legg-Calvé-Perthes]
- **M91.10** **Juvenile osteochondrosis of head of femur [Legg-Calvé-Perthes], unspecified leg**   COM
- **M91.11** **Juvenile osteochondrosis of head of femur [Legg-Calvé-Perthes],** right leg   COM
- **M91.12** **Juvenile osteochondrosis of head of femur [Legg-Calvé-Perthes],** left leg   COM

✓5ᵗʰ **M91.2** **Coxa plana**
Hip deformity due to previous juvenile osteochondrosis
- **M91.20** **Coxa plana, unspecified hip**   COM
- **M91.21** **Coxa plana,** right hip   COM
- **M91.22** **Coxa plana,** left hip   COM

✓5ᵗʰ **M91.3** **Pseudocoxalgia**
- **M91.30** **Pseudocoxalgia, unspecified hip**   COM
- **M91.31** **Pseudocoxalgia,** right hip   COM
- **M91.32** **Pseudocoxalgia,** left hip   COM

✓5ᵗʰ **M91.4** **Coxa magna**
- **M91.40** **Coxa magna, unspecified hip**   COM
- **M91.41** **Coxa magna,** right hip   COM
- **M91.42** **Coxa magna,** left hip   COM

✓5ᵗʰ **M91.8** **Other juvenile osteochondrosis of hip and pelvis**
Juvenile osteochondrosis after reduction of congenital dislocation of hip
- **M91.80** **Other juvenile osteochondrosis of hip and pelvis, unspecified leg**   COM
- **M91.81** **Other juvenile osteochondrosis of hip and pelvis,** right leg   COM
- **M91.82** **Other juvenile osteochondrosis of hip and pelvis,** left leg   COM

✓5ᵗʰ **M91.9** **Juvenile osteochondrosis of hip and pelvis, unspecified**
- **M91.90** **Juvenile osteochondrosis of hip and pelvis, unspecified, unspecified leg**   COM
- **M91.91** **Juvenile osteochondrosis of hip and pelvis, unspecified,** right leg   COM
- **M91.92** **Juvenile osteochondrosis of hip and pelvis, unspecified,** left leg   COM

✓4ᵗʰ **M92** **Other juvenile osteochondrosis**
✓5ᵗʰ **M92.0** **Juvenile osteochondrosis of** humerus
Osteochondrosis (juvenile) of capitulum of humerus [Panner]
Osteochondrosis (juvenile) of head of humerus [Haas]
- **M92.00** **Juvenile osteochondrosis of humerus, unspecified arm**
- **M92.01** **Juvenile osteochondrosis of humerus,** right arm
- **M92.02** **Juvenile osteochondrosis of humerus,** left arm

✓5ᵗʰ **M92.1** **Juvenile osteochondrosis of** radius and ulna
Osteochondrosis (juvenile) of lower ulna [Burns]
Osteochondrosis (juvenile) of radial head [Brailsford]
- **M92.10** **Juvenile osteochondrosis of radius and ulna, unspecified arm**
- **M92.11** **Juvenile osteochondrosis of radius and ulna,** right arm
- **M92.12** **Juvenile osteochondrosis of radius and ulna,** left arm

✓5ᵗʰ **M92.2** **Juvenile osteochondrosis, hand**
✓6ᵗʰ **M92.20** **Unspecified juvenile osteochondrosis,** hand
- **M92.201** **Unspecified juvenile osteochondrosis, right hand**
- **M92.202** **Unspecified juvenile osteochondrosis, left hand**
- **M92.209** **Unspecified juvenile osteochondrosis, unspecified hand**

M92.21 Osteochondrosis (juvenile) of carpal lunate [Kienböck]
  M92.211 Osteochondrosis (juvenile) of carpal lunate [Kienböck], right hand
  M92.212 Osteochondrosis (juvenile) of carpal lunate [Kienböck], left hand
  M92.219 Osteochondrosis (juvenile) of carpal lunate [Kienböck], unspecified hand

M92.22 Osteochondrosis (juvenile) of metacarpal heads [Mauclaire]
  M92.221 Osteochondrosis (juvenile) of metacarpal heads [Mauclaire], right hand
  M92.222 Osteochondrosis (juvenile) of metacarpal heads [Mauclaire], left hand
  M92.229 Osteochondrosis (juvenile) of metacarpal heads [Mauclaire], unspecified hand

M92.29 Other juvenile osteochondrosis, hand
  M92.291 Other juvenile osteochondrosis, right hand
  M92.292 Other juvenile osteochondrosis, left hand
  M92.299 Other juvenile osteochondrosis, unspecified hand

M92.3 Other juvenile osteochondrosis, upper limb
  M92.30 Other juvenile osteochondrosis, unspecified upper limb
  M92.31 Other juvenile osteochondrosis, right upper limb
  M92.32 Other juvenile osteochondrosis, left upper limb

M92.4 Juvenile osteochondrosis of patella
Osteochondrosis (juvenile) of primary patellar center [Köhler]
Osteochondrosis (juvenile) of secondary patellar centre [Sinding Larsen]
  M92.40 Juvenile osteochondrosis of patella, unspecified knee
  M92.41 Juvenile osteochondrosis of patella, right knee
  M92.42 Juvenile osteochondrosis of patella, left knee

M92.5 Juvenile osteochondrosis of tibia and fibula
AHA: 2020,4Q,33-34
  M92.50 Unspecified juvenile osteochondrosis of tibia and fibula
    M92.501 Unspecified juvenile osteochondrosis, right leg
    M92.502 Unspecified juvenile osteochondrosis, left leg
    M92.503 Unspecified juvenile osteochondrosis, bilateral leg
    M92.509 Unspecified juvenile osteochondrosis, unspecified leg
  M92.51 Juvenile osteochondrosis of proximal tibia
Blount disease
Tibia vara
    M92.511 Juvenile osteochondrosis of proximal tibia, right leg
    M92.512 Juvenile osteochondrosis of proximal tibia, left leg
    M92.513 Juvenile osteochondrosis of proximal tibia, bilateral
    M92.519 Juvenile osteochondrosis of proximal tibia, unspecified leg
  M92.52 Juvenile osteochondrosis of tibia tubercle
Osgood-Schlatter disease
    M92.521 Juvenile osteochondrosis of tibia tubercle, right leg
    M92.522 Juvenile osteochondrosis of tibia tubercle, left leg
    M92.523 Juvenile osteochondrosis of tibia tubercle, bilateral
    M92.529 Juvenile osteochondrosis of tibia tubercle, unspecified leg
  M92.59 Other juvenile osteochondrosis of tibia and fibula
    M92.591 Other juvenile osteochondrosis of tibia and fibula, right leg
    M92.592 Other juvenile osteochondrosis of tibia and fibula, left leg
    M92.593 Other juvenile osteochondrosis of tibia and fibula, bilateral
    M92.599 Other juvenile osteochondrosis of tibia and fibula, unspecified leg

M92.6 Juvenile osteochondrosis of tarsus
Osteochondrosis (juvenile) of calcaneum [Sever]
Osteochondrosis (juvenile) of os tibiale externum [Haglund]
Osteochondrosis (juvenile) of talus [Diaz]
Osteochondrosis (juvenile) of tarsal navicular [Köhler]
  M92.60 Juvenile osteochondrosis of tarsus, unspecified ankle
  M92.61 Juvenile osteochondrosis of tarsus, right ankle
  M92.62 Juvenile osteochondrosis of tarsus, left ankle

M92.7 Juvenile osteochondrosis of metatarsus
Osteochondrosis (juvenile) of fifth metatarsus [Iselin]
Osteochondrosis (juvenile) of second metatarsus [Freiberg]
  M92.70 Juvenile osteochondrosis of metatarsus, unspecified foot
  M92.71 Juvenile osteochondrosis of metatarsus, right foot
  M92.72 Juvenile osteochondrosis of metatarsus, left foot

M92.8 Other specified juvenile osteochondrosis
Calcaneal apophysitis
DEF: Calcaneal apophysitis: Inflammation of the calcaneus at the point of Achilles tendon insertion usually occurring in boys ages 8 to 14. Pain, tenderness, and localized swelling are present.

M92.9 Juvenile osteochondrosis, unspecified
Juvenile apophysitis NOS
Juvenile epiphysitis NOS
Juvenile osteochondritis NOS
Juvenile osteochondrosis NOS

M93 Other osteochondropathies
EXCLUDES 2   osteochondrosis of spine (M42.-)

M93.0 Slipped upper femoral epiphysis (nontraumatic)
▶Slipped capital femoral epiphysis (SCFE)◀
▶Slipped upper femoral epiphysis (SUFE)◀
Use additional code for associated chondrolysis (M94.3)
  M93.00 Unspecified slipped upper femoral epiphysis (nontraumatic)
    M93.001 Unspecified slipped upper femoral epiphysis (nontraumatic), right hip
    M93.002 Unspecified slipped upper femoral epiphysis (nontraumatic), left hip
    M93.003 Unspecified slipped upper femoral epiphysis (nontraumatic), unspecified hip
    M93.004 Unspecified slipped upper femoral epiphysis (nontraumatic), bilateral hips
  M93.01 Acute slipped upper femoral epiphysis, stable (nontraumatic)
    M93.011 Acute slipped upper femoral epiphysis, stable (nontraumatic), right hip
    M93.012 Acute slipped upper femoral epiphysis, stable (nontraumatic), left hip
    M93.013 Acute slipped upper femoral epiphysis, stable (nontraumatic), unspecified hip
    M93.014 Acute slipped upper femoral epiphysis, stable (nontraumatic), bilateral hips
  M93.02 Chronic slipped upper femoral epiphysis, stable (nontraumatic)
    M93.021 Chronic slipped upper femoral epiphysis, stable (nontraumatic), right hip
    M93.022 Chronic slipped upper femoral epiphysis, stable (nontraumatic), left hip
    M93.023 Chronic slipped upper femoral epiphysis, stable (nontraumatic), unspecified hip
    M93.024 Chronic slipped upper femoral epiphysis, stable (nontraumatic), bilateral hips
  M93.03 Acute on chronic slipped upper femoral epiphysis, stable (nontraumatic)
    M93.031 Acute on chronic slipped upper femoral epiphysis, stable (nontraumatic), right hip
    M93.032 Acute on chronic slipped upper femoral epiphysis, stable (nontraumatic), left hip
    M93.033 Acute on chronic slipped upper femoral epiphysis, stable (nontraumatic), unspecified hip
    M93.034 Acute on chronic slipped upper femoral epiphysis, stable (nontraumatic), bilateral hips

- ✓6ᵗʰ **M93.04** Acute slipped upper femoral epiphysis, unstable (nontraumatic)
- **M93.041** Acute slipped upper femoral epiphysis, unstable (nontraumatic), right hip
- **M93.042** Acute slipped upper femoral epiphysis, unstable (nontraumatic), left hip
- **M93.043** Acute slipped upper femoral epiphysis, unstable (nontraumatic), unspecified hip
- **M93.044** Acute slipped upper femoral epiphysis, unstable (nontraumatic), bilateral hips
- ✓6ᵗʰ **M93.05** Acute on chronic slipped upper femoral epiphysis, unstable (nontraumatic)
- **M93.051** Acute on chronic slipped upper femoral epiphysis, unstable (nontraumatic), right hip
- **M93.052** Acute on chronic slipped upper femoral epiphysis, unstable (nontraumatic), left hip
- **M93.053** Acute on chronic slipped upper femoral epiphysis, unstable (nontraumatic), unspecified hip
- **M93.054** Acute on chronic slipped upper femoral epiphysis, unstable (nontraumatic), bilateral hips
- ✓6ᵗʰ **M93.06** Acute slipped upper femoral epiphysis, unspecified stability (nontraumatic)
- **M93.061** Acute slipped upper femoral epiphysis, unspecified stability (nontraumatic), right hip
- **M93.062** Acute slipped upper femoral epiphysis, unspecified stability (nontraumatic), left hip
- **M93.063** Acute slipped upper femoral epiphysis, unspecified stability (nontraumatic), unspecified hip
- **M93.064** Acute slipped upper femoral epiphysis, unspecified stability (nontraumatic), bilateral hips
- ✓6ᵗʰ **M93.07** Acute on chronic slipped upper femoral epiphysis, unspecified stability (nontraumatic)
- **M93.071** Acute on chronic slipped upper femoral epiphysis, unspecified stability (nontraumatic), right hip
- **M93.072** Acute on chronic slipped upper femoral epiphysis, unspecified stability (nontraumatic), left hip
- **M93.073** Acute on chronic slipped upper femoral epiphysis, unspecified stability (nontraumatic), unspecified hip
- **M93.074** Acute on chronic slipped upper femoral epiphysis, unspecified stability (nontraumatic), bilateral hips

M93.1 Kienböck's disease of adults   A
     Adult osteochondrosis of carpal lunates

✓5ᵗʰ **M93.2** Osteochondritis dissecans
     DEF: Avascular necrosis caused by lack of blood flow to the bone and cartilage of a joint causing the bone to die. This can result in splinters or pieces of cartilage breaking off in the joint.

M93.20 Osteochondritis dissecans of unspecified site

✓6ᵗʰ **M93.21** Osteochondritis dissecans of shoulder
     M93.211 Osteochondritis dissecans, right shoulder
     M93.212 Osteochondritis dissecans, left shoulder
     M93.219 Osteochondritis dissecans, unspecified shoulder

✓6ᵗʰ **M93.22** Osteochondritis dissecans of elbow
     M93.221 Osteochondritis dissecans, right elbow
     M93.222 Osteochondritis dissecans, left elbow
     M93.229 Osteochondritis dissecans, unspecified elbow

✓6ᵗʰ **M93.23** Osteochondritis dissecans of wrist
     M93.231 Osteochondritis dissecans, right wrist
     M93.232 Osteochondritis dissecans, left wrist
     M93.239 Osteochondritis dissecans, unspecified wrist

✓6ᵗʰ **M93.24** Osteochondritis dissecans of joints of hand
     M93.241 Osteochondritis dissecans, joints of right hand
     M93.242 Osteochondritis dissecans, joints of left hand
     M93.249 Osteochondritis dissecans, joints of unspecified hand

✓6ᵗʰ **M93.25** Osteochondritis dissecans of hip
     M93.251 Osteochondritis dissecans, right hip
     M93.252 Osteochondritis dissecans, left hip
     M93.259 Osteochondritis dissecans, unspecified hip

✓6ᵗʰ **M93.26** Osteochondritis dissecans knee
     M93.261 Osteochondritis dissecans, right knee
     M93.262 Osteochondritis dissecans, left knee
     M93.269 Osteochondritis dissecans, unspecified knee

✓6ᵗʰ **M93.27** Osteochondritis dissecans of ankle and joints of foot
     M93.271 Osteochondritis dissecans, right ankle and joints of right foot
     M93.272 Osteochondritis dissecans, left ankle and joints of left foot
     M93.279 Osteochondritis dissecans, unspecified ankle and joints of foot

M93.28 Osteochondritis dissecans other site
M93.29 Osteochondritis dissecans multiple sites

✓5ᵗʰ **M93.8** Other specified osteochondropathies

M93.80 Other specified osteochondropathies of unspecified site

✓6ᵗʰ **M93.81** Other specified osteochondropathies of shoulder
     M93.811 Other specified osteochondropathies, right shoulder
     M93.812 Other specified osteochondropathies, left shoulder
     M93.819 Other specified osteochondropathies, unspecified shoulder

✓6ᵗʰ **M93.82** Other specified osteochondropathies of upper arm
     M93.821 Other specified osteochondropathies, right upper arm
     M93.822 Other specified osteochondropathies, left upper arm
     M93.829 Other specified osteochondropathies, unspecified upper arm

✓6ᵗʰ **M93.83** Other specified osteochondropathies of forearm
     M93.831 Other specified osteochondropathies, right forearm
     M93.832 Other specified osteochondropathies, left forearm
     M93.839 Other specified osteochondropathies, unspecified forearm

✓6ᵗʰ **M93.84** Other specified osteochondropathies of hand
     M93.841 Other specified osteochondropathies, right hand
     M93.842 Other specified osteochondropathies, left hand
     M93.849 Other specified osteochondropathies, unspecified hand

✓6ᵗʰ **M93.85** Other specified osteochondropathies of thigh
     M93.851 Other specified osteochondropathies, right thigh
     M93.852 Other specified osteochondropathies, left thigh
     M93.859 Other specified osteochondropathies, unspecified thigh

✓6ᵗʰ **M93.86** Other specified osteochondropathies lower leg
     M93.861 Other specified osteochondropathies, right lower leg
     M93.862 Other specified osteochondropathies, left lower leg
     M93.869 Other specified osteochondropathies, unspecified lower leg

✓6ᵗʰ **M93.87** Other specified osteochondropathies of ankle and foot
     M93.871 Other specified osteochondropathies, right ankle and foot
     M93.872 Other specified osteochondropathies, left ankle and foot
     M93.879 Other specified osteochondropathies, unspecified ankle and foot

M93.88 Other specified osteochondropathies other site
M93.89 Other specified osteochondropathies multiple sites

✔ Additional Character Required   ✓x7ᵗʰ Placeholder Alert   Manifestation   Unspecified Dx   Q QPP   UPD Unacceptable PDx

✓5ᵗʰ **M93.9 Osteochondropathy, unspecified**
    Apophysitis NOS
    Epiphysitis NOS
    Osteochondritis NOS
    Osteochondrosis NOS
    M93.90 Osteochondropathy, unspecified of unspecified site
    ✓6ᵗʰ **M93.91 Osteochondropathy, unspecified of shoulder**
        M93.911 Osteochondropathy, unspecified, right shoulder
        M93.912 Osteochondropathy, unspecified, left shoulder
        M93.919 Osteochondropathy, unspecified, unspecified shoulder
    ✓6ᵗʰ **M93.92 Osteochondropathy, unspecified of upper arm**
        M93.921 Osteochondropathy, unspecified, right upper arm
        M93.922 Osteochondropathy, unspecified, left upper arm
        M93.929 Osteochondropathy, unspecified, unspecified upper arm
    ✓6ᵗʰ **M93.93 Osteochondropathy, unspecified of forearm**
        M93.931 Osteochondropathy, unspecified, right forearm
        M93.932 Osteochondropathy, unspecified, left forearm
        M93.939 Osteochondropathy, unspecified, unspecified forearm
    ✓6ᵗʰ **M93.94 Osteochondropathy, unspecified of hand**
        M93.941 Osteochondropathy, unspecified, right hand
        M93.942 Osteochondropathy, unspecified, left hand
        M93.949 Osteochondropathy, unspecified, unspecified hand
    ✓6ᵗʰ **M93.95 Osteochondropathy, unspecified of thigh**
        M93.951 Osteochondropathy, unspecified, right thigh
        M93.952 Osteochondropathy, unspecified, left thigh
        M93.959 Osteochondropathy, unspecified, unspecified thigh
    ✓6ᵗʰ **M93.96 Osteochondropathy, unspecified lower leg**
        M93.961 Osteochondropathy, unspecified, right lower leg
        M93.962 Osteochondropathy, unspecified, left lower leg
        M93.969 Osteochondropathy, unspecified, unspecified lower leg
    ✓6ᵗʰ **M93.97 Osteochondropathy, unspecified of ankle and foot**
        M93.971 Osteochondropathy, unspecified, right ankle and foot
        M93.972 Osteochondropathy, unspecified, left ankle and foot
        M93.979 Osteochondropathy, unspecified, unspecified ankle and foot
    M93.98 Osteochondropathy, unspecified other site
    M93.99 Osteochondropathy, unspecified multiple sites

✓4ᵗʰ **M94 Other disorders of cartilage**
    M94.0 Chondrocostal junction syndrome [Tietze]
        Costochondritis
    M94.1 Relapsing polychondritis
    ✓5ᵗʰ **M94.2 Chondromalacia**
        EXCLUDES 1 chondromalacia patellae (M22.4)
        M94.20 Chondromalacia, unspecified site
    ✓6ᵗʰ **M94.21 Chondromalacia, shoulder**
        M94.211 Chondromalacia, right shoulder
        M94.212 Chondromalacia, left shoulder
        M94.219 Chondromalacia, unspecified shoulder
    ✓6ᵗʰ **M94.22 Chondromalacia, elbow**
        M94.221 Chondromalacia, right elbow
        M94.222 Chondromalacia, left elbow
        M94.229 Chondromalacia, unspecified elbow
    ✓6ᵗʰ **M94.23 Chondromalacia, wrist**
        M94.231 Chondromalacia, right wrist
        M94.232 Chondromalacia, left wrist
        M94.239 Chondromalacia, unspecified wrist

✓6ᵗʰ **M94.24 Chondromalacia, joints of hand**
    M94.241 Chondromalacia, joints of right hand
    M94.242 Chondromalacia, joints of left hand
    M94.249 Chondromalacia, joints of unspecified hand
✓6ᵗʰ **M94.25 Chondromalacia, hip**
    M94.251 Chondromalacia, right hip
    M94.252 Chondromalacia, left hip
    M94.259 Chondromalacia, unspecified hip
✓6ᵗʰ **M94.26 Chondromalacia, knee**
    M94.261 Chondromalacia, right knee
    M94.262 Chondromalacia, left knee
    M94.269 Chondromalacia, unspecified knee
✓6ᵗʰ **M94.27 Chondromalacia, ankle and joints of foot**
    M94.271 Chondromalacia, right ankle and joints of right foot
    M94.272 Chondromalacia, left ankle and joints of left foot
    M94.279 Chondromalacia, unspecified ankle and joints of foot
    M94.28 Chondromalacia, other site
    M94.29 Chondromalacia, multiple sites
✓5ᵗʰ **M94.3 Chondrolysis**
    Code first any associated slipped upper femoral epiphysis (nontraumatic) (M93.0-)
    ✓6ᵗʰ **M94.35 Chondrolysis, hip**
        M94.351 Chondrolysis, right hip
        M94.352 Chondrolysis, left hip
        M94.359 Chondrolysis, unspecified hip
✓5ᵗʰ **M94.8 Other specified disorders of cartilage**
    ✓6ᵗʰ **M94.8X Other specified disorders of cartilage**
        M94.8X0 Other specified disorders of cartilage, multiple sites
        M94.8X1 Other specified disorders of cartilage, shoulder
        M94.8X2 Other specified disorders of cartilage, upper arm
        M94.8X3 Other specified disorders of cartilage, forearm
        M94.8X4 Other specified disorders of cartilage, hand
        M94.8X5 Other specified disorders of cartilage, thigh
        M94.8X6 Other specified disorders of cartilage, lower leg
        M94.8X7 Other specified disorders of cartilage, ankle and foot
        M94.8X8 Other specified disorders of cartilage, other site
        M94.8X9 Other specified disorders of cartilage, unspecified sites
    M94.9 Disorder of cartilage, unspecified

Other disorders of the musculoskeletal system and connective tissue (M95)

✓4ᵗʰ **M95 Other acquired deformities of musculoskeletal system and connective tissue**
    EXCLUDES 2 *acquired absence of limbs and organs (Z89-Z90)*
        acquired deformities of limbs (M20-M21)
        congenital malformations and deformations of the musculoskeletal system (Q65-Q79)
        deforming dorsopathies (M40-M43)
        dentofacial anomalies [including malocclusion] (M26.-)
        postprocedural musculoskeletal disorders (M96.-)
    M95.0 Acquired deformity of nose
        EXCLUDES 2 *deviated nasal septum (J34.2)*
    ✓5ᵗʰ **M95.1 Cauliflower ear**
        EXCLUDES 2 *other acquired deformities of ear (H61.1)*
        DEF: Acquired deformity of the external ear due to injury or subsequent perichondritis.
        M95.10 Cauliflower ear, unspecified ear
        M95.11 Cauliflower ear, right ear
        M95.12 Cauliflower ear, left ear
    M95.2 Other acquired deformity of head
        AHA: 2022,1Q,34
    M95.3 Acquired deformity of neck

M95.4 Acquired deformity of chest and rib
    AHA: 2022,2Q,14; 2014,4Q,26-27

M95.5 Acquired deformity of pelvis
    EXCLUDES 1   maternal care for known or suspected disproportion (O33.-)

M95.8 Other specified acquired deformities of musculoskeletal system

M95.9 Acquired deformity of musculoskeletal system, unspecified

Intraoperative and postprocedural complications and disorders of musculoskeletal system, not elsewhere classified (M96)

✓4ᵗʰ **M96 Intraoperative and postprocedural complications and disorders of musculoskeletal system, not elsewhere classified**
    EXCLUDES 2   arthropathy following intestinal bypass (M02.0-)
       complications of internal orthopedic prosthetic devices, implants and grafts (T84.-)
       disorders associated with osteoporosis (M80)
       periprosthetic fracture around internal prosthetic joint (M97.-)
       presence of functional implants and other devices (Z96-Z97)

M96.0 Pseudarthrosis after fusion or arthrodesis

M96.1 Postlaminectomy syndrome, not elsewhere classified

M96.2 Postradiation kyphosis

M96.3 Postlaminectomy kyphosis

M96.4 Postsurgical lordosis

M96.5 Postradiation scoliosis

✓5ᵗʰ **M96.6 Fracture of bone following insertion of orthopedic implant, joint prosthesis, or bone plate**
    Intraoperative fracture of bone during insertion of orthopedic implant, joint prosthesis, or bone plate
    EXCLUDES 2   complication of internal orthopedic devices, implants or grafts (T84.-)

   ✓6ᵗʰ **M96.62 Fracture of** humerus **following insertion of orthopedic implant, joint prosthesis, or bone plate**
      M96.621 Fracture of humerus following insertion of orthopedic implant, joint prosthesis, or bone plate, right **arm** `HCC` `ESR`
      M96.622 Fracture of humerus following insertion of orthopedic implant, joint prosthesis, or bone plate, left **arm** `HCC` `ESR`
      M96.629 Fracture of humerus following insertion of orthopedic implant, joint prosthesis, or bone plate, unspecified arm `HCC` `ESR`

   ✓6ᵗʰ **M96.63 Fracture of** radius or ulna **following insertion of orthopedic implant, joint prosthesis, or bone plate**
      M96.631 Fracture of radius or ulna following insertion of orthopedic implant, joint prosthesis, or bone plate, right **arm** `HCC` `ESR`
      M96.632 Fracture of radius or ulna following insertion of orthopedic implant, joint prosthesis, or bone plate, left **arm** `HCC` `ESR`
      M96.639 Fracture of radius or ulna following insertion of orthopedic implant, joint prosthesis, or bone plate, unspecified arm `HCC` `ESR`

   M96.65 Fracture of pelvis **following insertion of orthopedic implant, joint prosthesis, or bone plate** `HCC` `ESR`

   ✓6ᵗʰ **M96.66 Fracture of** femur **following insertion of orthopedic implant, joint prosthesis, or bone plate**
      M96.661 Fracture of femur following insertion of orthopedic implant, joint prosthesis, or bone plate, right **leg** `HCC` `ESR`
      M96.662 Fracture of femur following insertion of orthopedic implant, joint prosthesis, or bone plate, left **leg** `HCC` `ESR`
      M96.669 Fracture of femur following insertion of orthopedic implant, joint prosthesis, or bone plate, unspecified leg `HCC` `ESR`

   ✓6ᵗʰ **M96.67 Fracture of** tibia or fibula **following insertion of orthopedic implant, joint prosthesis, or bone plate**
      M96.671 Fracture of tibia or fibula following insertion of orthopedic implant, joint prosthesis, or bone plate, right **leg** `HCC` `ESR`

      M96.672 Fracture of tibia or fibula following insertion of orthopedic implant, joint prosthesis, or bone plate, left **leg** `HCC` `ESR`
      M96.679 Fracture of tibia or fibula following insertion of orthopedic implant, joint prosthesis, or bone plate, unspecified leg `HCC` `ESR`

   M96.69 Fracture of other bone following insertion of orthopedic implant, joint prosthesis, or bone plate `HCC` `ESR`

✓5ᵗʰ **M96.8 Other intraoperative and postprocedural complications and disorders of musculoskeletal system, not elsewhere classified**
    AHA: 2016,4Q,9-10

   ✓6ᵗʰ **M96.81 Intraoperative hemorrhage and hematoma of a musculoskeletal structure complicating a procedure**
      EXCLUDES 1   intraoperative hemorrhage and hematoma of a musculoskeletal structure due to accidental puncture and laceration during a procedure (M96.82-)
      M96.810 Intraoperative hemorrhage and hematoma of a musculoskeletal structure complicating a musculoskeletal system procedure
      M96.811 Intraoperative hemorrhage and hematoma of a musculoskeletal structure complicating other procedure

   ✓6ᵗʰ **M96.82 Accidental puncture and laceration of a musculoskeletal structure during a procedure**
      M96.820 Accidental puncture and laceration of a musculoskeletal structure during a musculoskeletal system procedure
      M96.821 Accidental puncture and laceration of a musculoskeletal structure during other procedure

   ✓6ᵗʰ **M96.83 Postprocedural hemorrhage of a musculoskeletal structure following a procedure**
      M96.830 Postprocedural hemorrhage of a musculoskeletal structure following a musculoskeletal system procedure
      M96.831 Postprocedural hemorrhage of a musculoskeletal structure following other procedure

   ✓6ᵗʰ **M96.84 Postprocedural hematoma and seroma of a musculoskeletal structure following a procedure**
      M96.840 Postprocedural hematoma **of a musculoskeletal structure following a** musculoskeletal system procedure
      M96.841 Postprocedural hematoma **of a musculoskeletal structure following** other procedure
       AHA: 2016,4Q,10
      M96.842 Postprocedural seroma **of a musculoskeletal structure following a** musculoskeletal system procedure
      M96.843 Postprocedural seroma **of a musculoskeletal structure following** other procedure
       AHA: 2018,3Q,6

   M96.89 Other intraoperative and postprocedural complications and disorders of the musculoskeletal system
      Instability of joint secondary to removal of joint prosthesis
      Use additional code, if applicable, to further specify disorder
      AHA: 2022,2Q,14; 2021,1Q,5

● ✓5ᵗʰ **M96.A Fracture of ribs, sternum and thorax** associated with compression of the chest and cardiopulmonary resuscitation

●   **M96.A1 Fracture of sternum associated with chest compression and cardiopulmonary resuscitation**
      Fracture of xiphoid process associated with chest compression and cardiopulmonary resuscitation

●   **M96.A2 Fracture of one rib associated with chest compression and cardiopulmonary resuscitation**

●   **M96.A3 Multiple fractures of ribs associated with chest compression and cardiopulmonary resuscitation**

●   **M96.A4 Flail chest associated with chest compression and cardiopulmonary resuscitation**

●   **M96.A9 Other fracture associated with chest compression and cardiopulmonary resuscitation**

 Additional Character Required   ✓x7ᵗʰ Placeholder Alert   Manifestation   Unspecified Dx   Q QPP   UPD Unacceptable PDx

Chapter 13. Diseases of the Musculoskeletal System and Connective Tissue

Periprosthetic fractures around internal prosthetic joint (M97)

☑4ᵗʰ **M97 Periprosthetic fracture around internal prosthetic joint**

EXCLUDES 2   *breakage (fracture) of prosthetic joint (T84.01-)*
fracture of bone following insertion of orthopedic implant, joint prosthesis or bone plate (M96.6-)

AHA: 2016,4Q,42-43

> The appropriate 7th character is to be added to each code from category M97.
> A   initial encounter
> D   subsequent encounter
> S   sequela

☑5ᵗʰ **M97.0 Periprosthetic fracture around internal prosthetic** hip **joint**
    AHA: 2018,1Q,21; 2016,4Q,42

¹ ✓x7ᵗʰ **M97.01 Periprosthetic fracture around internal prosthetic** right **hip joint**   HCC ESR Q

¹ ✓x7ᵗʰ **M97.02 Periprosthetic fracture around internal prosthetic** left **hip joint**   HCC ESR Q

☑5ᵗʰ **M97.1 Periprosthetic fracture around internal prosthetic** knee **joint**

✓x7ᵗʰ **M97.11 Periprosthetic fracture around internal prosthetic** right **knee joint**   Q

✓x7ᵗʰ **M97.12 Periprosthetic fracture around internal prosthetic** left **knee joint**   Q

☑5ᵗʰ **M97.2 Periprosthetic fracture around internal prosthetic** ankle **joint**

✓x7ᵗʰ **M97.21 Periprosthetic fracture around internal prosthetic** right **ankle joint**   Q

✓x7ᵗʰ **M97.22 Periprosthetic fracture around internal prosthetic** left **ankle joint**   Q

☑5ᵗʰ **M97.3 Periprosthetic fracture around internal prosthetic** shoulder **joint**

✓x7ᵗʰ **M97.31 Periprosthetic fracture around internal prosthetic** right **shoulder joint**   Q

✓x7ᵗʰ **M97.32 Periprosthetic fracture around internal prosthetic** left **shoulder joint**   Q

☑5ᵗʰ **M97.4 Periprosthetic fracture around internal prosthetic** elbow **joint**

✓x7ᵗʰ **M97.41 Periprosthetic fracture around internal prosthetic** right **elbow joint**   Q

✓x7ᵗʰ **M97.42 Periprosthetic fracture around internal prosthetic** left **elbow joint**   Q

✓x7ᵗʰ **M97.8 Periprosthetic fracture around other internal prosthetic joint**
Periprosthetic fracture around internal prosthetic finger joint
Periprosthetic fracture around internal prosthetic spinal joint
Periprosthetic fracture around internal prosthetic toe joint
Periprosthetic fracture around internal prosthetic wrist joint
Use additional code to identify the joint (Z96.6-)

✓x7ᵗʰ **M97.9 Periprosthetic fracture around unspecified internal prosthetic joint**

Biomechanical lesions, not elsewhere classified (M99)

☑4ᵗʰ **M99 Biomechanical lesions, not elsewhere classified**

NOTE   This category should not be used if the condition can be classified elsewhere.

DEF: Biomechanical lesion: Term used by osteopathic and chiropractic physicians to describe musculoskeletal conditions treated that are not more appropriately classified elsewhere.

☑5ᵗʰ **M99.0 Segmental and somatic dysfunction**

M99.00 Segmental and somatic dysfunction of head **region**
M99.01 Segmental and somatic dysfunction of cervical **region**
M99.02 Segmental and somatic dysfunction of thoracic **region**
M99.03 Segmental and somatic dysfunction of lumbar **region**
M99.04 Segmental and somatic dysfunction of sacral **region**
M99.05 Segmental and somatic dysfunction of pelvic **region**
M99.06 Segmental and somatic dysfunction of lower **extremity**
M99.07 Segmental and somatic dysfunction of upper **extremity**
M99.08 Segmental and somatic dysfunction of rib cage
M99.09 Segmental and somatic dysfunction of abdomen and other **regions**

☑5ᵗʰ **M99.1 Subluxation complex (vertebral)**

M99.10 Subluxation complex (vertebral) of head **region**

M99.11 Subluxation complex (vertebral) of cervical **region**
M99.12 Subluxation complex (vertebral) of thoracic **region**
M99.13 Subluxation complex (vertebral) of lumbar **region**
M99.14 Subluxation complex (vertebral) of sacral **region**
M99.15 Subluxation complex (vertebral) of pelvic **region**
M99.16 Subluxation complex (vertebral) of lower extremity
M99.17 Subluxation complex (vertebral) of upper extremity
M99.18 Subluxation complex (vertebral) of rib cage
M99.19 Subluxation complex (vertebral) of abdomen and other **regions**

☑5ᵗʰ **M99.2 Subluxation stenosis of neural canal**

M99.20 Subluxation stenosis of neural canal of head **region**
M99.21 Subluxation stenosis of neural canal of cervical **region**
M99.22 Subluxation stenosis of neural canal of thoracic **region**
M99.23 Subluxation stenosis of neural canal of lumbar **region**
M99.24 Subluxation stenosis of neural canal of sacral **region**
M99.25 Subluxation stenosis of neural canal of pelvic **region**
M99.26 Subluxation stenosis of neural canal of lower extremity
M99.27 Subluxation stenosis of neural canal of upper extremity
M99.28 Subluxation stenosis of neural canal of rib cage
M99.29 Subluxation stenosis of neural canal of abdomen and other **regions**

☑6ᵗʰ **M99.3 Osseous stenosis of neural canal**

M99.30 Osseous stenosis of neural canal of head **region**
M99.31 Osseous stenosis of neural canal of cervical **region**
M99.32 Osseous stenosis of neural canal of thoracic **region**
M99.33 Osseous stenosis of neural canal of lumbar **region**
M99.34 Osseous stenosis of neural canal of sacral **region**
M99.35 Osseous stenosis of neural canal of pelvic **region**
M99.36 Osseous stenosis of neural canal of lower extremity
M99.37 Osseous stenosis of neural canal of upper extremity
M99.38 Osseous stenosis of neural canal of rib cage
M99.39 Osseous stenosis of neural canal of abdomen and other **regions**

☑5ᵗʰ **M99.4 Connective tissue stenosis of neural canal**

M99.40 Connective tissue stenosis of neural canal of head **region**
M99.41 Connective tissue stenosis of neural canal of cervical **region**
M99.42 Connective tissue stenosis of neural canal of thoracic **region**
M99.43 Connective tissue stenosis of neural canal of lumbar **region**
M99.44 Connective tissue stenosis of neural canal of sacral **region**
M99.45 Connective tissue stenosis of neural canal of pelvic **region**
M99.46 Connective tissue stenosis of neural canal of lower extremity
M99.47 Connective tissue stenosis of neural canal of upper extremity
M99.48 Connective tissue stenosis of neural canal of rib cage
M99.49 Connective tissue stenosis of neural canal of abdomen and other **regions**

☑5ᵗʰ **M99.5 Intervertebral disc stenosis of neural canal**

M99.50 Intervertebral disc stenosis of neural canal of head **region**
M99.51 Intervertebral disc stenosis of neural canal of cervical **region**
M99.52 Intervertebral disc stenosis of neural canal of thoracic **region**
M99.53 Intervertebral disc stenosis of neural canal of lumbar **region**
M99.54 Intervertebral disc stenosis of neural canal of sacral **region**
M99.55 Intervertebral disc stenosis of neural canal of pelvic **region**
M99.56 Intervertebral disc stenosis of neural canal of lower extremity
M99.57 Intervertebral disc stenosis of neural canal of upper extremity
M99.58 Intervertebral disc stenosis of neural canal of rib cage

M99.59   Intervertebral disc stenosis of neural canal of abdomen and other regions

✓5ᵗʰ **M99.6**   **Osseous and subluxation stenosis of intervertebral foramina**

M99.60   Osseous and subluxation stenosis of intervertebral foramina of head region

M99.61   Osseous and subluxation stenosis of intervertebral foramina of cervical region

M99.62   Osseous and subluxation stenosis of intervertebral foramina of thoracic region

M99.63   Osseous and subluxation stenosis of intervertebral foramina of lumbar region

M99.64   Osseous and subluxation stenosis of intervertebral foramina of sacral region

M99.65   Osseous and subluxation stenosis of intervertebral foramina of pelvic region

M99.66   Osseous and subluxation stenosis of intervertebral foramina of lower extremity

M99.67   Osseous and subluxation stenosis of intervertebral foramina of upper extremity

M99.68   Osseous and subluxation stenosis of intervertebral foramina of rib cage

M99.69   Osseous and subluxation stenosis of intervertebral foramina of abdomen and other regions

✓5ᵗʰ **M99.7**   **Connective tissue and disc stenosis of intervertebral foramina**

M99.70   Connective tissue and disc stenosis of intervertebral foramina of head region

M99.71   Connective tissue and disc stenosis of intervertebral foramina of cervical region

M99.72   Connective tissue and disc stenosis of intervertebral foramina of thoracic region

M99.73   Connective tissue and disc stenosis of intervertebral foramina of lumbar region

M99.74   Connective tissue and disc stenosis of intervertebral foramina of sacral region

M99.75   Connective tissue and disc stenosis of intervertebral foramina of pelvic region

M99.76   Connective tissue and disc stenosis of intervertebral foramina of lower extremity

M99.77   Connective tissue and disc stenosis of intervertebral foramina of upper extremity

M99.78   Connective tissue and disc stenosis of intervertebral foramina of rib cage

M99.79   Connective tissue and disc stenosis of intervertebral foramina of abdomen and other regions

✓5ᵗʰ **M99.8**   **Other biomechanical lesions**

M99.80   Other biomechanical lesions of head region

M99.81   Other biomechanical lesions of cervical region

M99.82   Other biomechanical lesions of thoracic region

M99.83   Other biomechanical lesions of lumbar region

M99.84   Other biomechanical lesions of sacral region

M99.85   Other biomechanical lesions of pelvic region

M99.86   Other biomechanical lesions of lower extremity

M99.87   Other biomechanical lesions of upper extremity

M99.88   Other biomechanical lesions of rib cage

M99.89   Other biomechanical lesions of abdomen and other regions

M99.9   **Biomechanical lesion, unspecified**

Chapter 14. Diseases of Genitourinary System (N00–N99)

Chapter-specific Guidelines with Coding Examples

The chapter-specific guidelines from the ICD-10-CM Official Guidelines for Coding and Reporting have been provided below. Along with these guidelines are coding examples, contained in the shaded boxes, that have been developed to help illustrate the coding and/or sequencing guidance found in these guidelines.

a. Chronic kidney disease

1) Stages of chronic kidney disease (CKD)

The ICD-10-CM classifies CKD based on severity. The severity of CKD is designated by stages 1-5. Stage 2, code N18.2, equates to mild CKD; stage 3, codes N18.30-N18.32, equate to moderate CKD; and stage 4, code N18.4, equates to severe CKD. Code N18.6, End stage renal disease (ESRD), is assigned when the provider has documented end-stage renal disease (ESRD).

If both a stage of CKD and ESRD are documented, assign code N18.6 only.

Stage 5 chronic kidney disease with ESRD requiring chronic dialysis

N18.6   **End stage renal disease**

Z99.2   **Dependence on renal dialysis**

Explanation: The diagnostic statement indicates the patient has chronic kidney disease, documented both as stage 5 and as ESRD requiring chronic dialysis. Code N18.6 End stage renal disease (ESRD), is assigned when the provider has documented end-stage-renal disease (ESRD). If both a stage of CKD and ESRD are documented, assign code N18.6 only.

---

2) Chronic kidney disease and kidney transplant status

Patients who have undergone kidney transplant may still have some form of chronic kidney disease (CKD) because the kidney transplant may not fully restore kidney function. Therefore, the presence of CKD alone does not constitute a transplant complication. Assign the appropriate N18 code for the patient's stage of CKD and code Z94.0, Kidney transplant status. If a transplant complication such as failure or rejection or other transplant complication is documented, see section I.C.19.g for information on coding complications of a kidney transplant. If the documentation is unclear as to whether the patient has a complication of the transplant, query the provider.

Patient with residual chronic kidney disease stage 1 after kidney transplant

N18.1   **Chronic kidney disease, stage 1**

Z94.0   **Kidney transplant status**

Explanation: Patients who have undergone kidney transplant may still have some form of chronic kidney disease (CKD) because the kidney transplant may not fully restore kidney function. The presence of CKD alone does not constitute a transplant complication. Assign the appropriate N18 code for the patient's stage of CKD and code Z94.0 Kidney transplant status.

---

3) Chronic kidney disease with other conditions

Patients with CKD may also suffer from other serious conditions, most commonly diabetes mellitus and hypertension. The sequencing of the CKD code in relationship to codes for other contributing conditions is based on the conventions in the Tabular List.

See I.C.9. Hypertensive chronic kidney disease.

See I.C.19. Chronic kidney disease and kidney transplant complications.

Type 1 diabetic chronic kidney disease, stage 2

E10.22   **Type 1 diabetes mellitus with diabetic chronic kidney disease**

N18.2   **Chronic kidney disease, stage 2 (mild)**

Explanation: Patients with CKD may also suffer from other serious conditions such as diabetes mellitus. The sequencing of the CKD code in relationship to codes for other contributing conditions is based on the conventions in the Tabular List. Diabetic CKD code E10.22 includes an instructional note to "Use additional code to identify stage of chronic kidney disease (N18.1–N18.6)," thus providing sequencing direction.

Chapter 14. Diseases of the Genitourinary System (N00-N99)

EXCLUDES 2   certain conditions originating in the perinatal period (P04-P96)
certain infectious and parasitic diseases (A00-B99)
complications of pregnancy, childbirth and the puerperium (O00-O9A)
congenital malformations, deformations and chromosomal abnormalities (Q00-Q99)
endocrine, nutritional and metabolic diseases (E00-E88)
injury, poisoning and certain other consequences of external causes (S00-T88)
neoplasms (C00-D49)
symptoms, signs and abnormal clinical and laboratory findings, not elsewhere classified (R00-R94)

This chapter contains the following blocks:
N00-N08   Glomerular diseases
N10-N16   Renal tubulo-interstitial diseases
N17-N19   Acute kidney failure and chronic kidney disease
N20-N23   Urolithiasis
N25-N29   Other disorders of kidney and ureter
N30-N39   Other diseases of the urinary system
N40-N53   Diseases of male genital organs
N60-N65   Disorders of breast
N70-N77   Inflammatory diseases of female pelvic organs
N80-N98   Noninflammatory disorders of female genital tract
N99   Intraoperative and postprocedural complications and disorders of genitourinary system, not elsewhere classified

Glomerular diseases (N00-N08)

Code also any associated kidney failure (N17-N19).
EXCLUDES 1   hypertensive chronic kidney disease (I12.-)
AHA: 2020,4Q,34-35
DEF: Glomeruli: Clusters of microscopic blood vessels located within the kidneys containing small pores through which waste products are filtered from the blood and urine is formed.
DEF: Glomerulonephritis: Disease of the kidney with diffuse inflammation of the capillary loops of the glomeruli.

✓4ᵗʰ N00 Acute nephritic syndrome
INCLUDES   acute glomerular disease
acute glomerulonephritis
acute nephritis
EXCLUDES 1   acute tubulo-interstitial nephritis (N10)
nephritic syndrome NOS (N05.-)
AHA: 2021,1Q,23
N00.0   Acute nephritic syndrome with minor glomerular abnormality
Acute nephritic syndrome with minimal change lesion
N00.1   Acute nephritic syndrome with focal and segmental glomerular lesions
Acute nephritic syndrome with focal and segmental hyalinosis
Acute nephritic syndrome with focal and segmental sclerosis
Acute nephritic syndrome with focal glomerulonephritis
N00.2   Acute nephritic syndrome with diffuse membranous glomerulonephritis
N00.3   Acute nephritic syndrome with diffuse mesangial proliferative glomerulonephritis
N00.4   Acute nephritic syndrome with diffuse endocapillary proliferative glomerulonephritis
N00.5   Acute nephritic syndrome with diffuse mesangiocapillary glomerulonephritis
Acute nephritic syndrome with membranoproliferative glomerulonephritis, types 1 and 3, or NOS
EXCLUDES 1   acute nephritic syndrome with C3 glomerulonephritis (N00.A)
acute nephritic syndrome with C3 glomerulopathy (N00.A)
N00.6   Acute nephritic syndrome with dense deposit disease
Acute nephritic syndrome with C3 glomerulopathy with dense deposit disease
Acute nephritic syndrome with membranoproliferative glomerulonephritis, type 2
N00.7   Acute nephritic syndrome with diffuse crescentic glomerulonephritis
Acute nephritic syndrome with extracapillary glomerulonephritis
N00.8   Acute nephritic syndrome with other morphologic changes
Acute nephritic syndrome with proliferative glomerulonephritis NOS
N00.9   Acute nephritic syndrome with unspecified morphologic changes

N00.A   Acute nephritic syndrome with C3 glomerulonephritis
Acute nephritic syndrome with C3 glomerulopathy, NOS
EXCLUDES 1   acute nephritic syndrome (with C3 glomerulopathy) with dense deposit disease (N00.6)

✓4ᵗʰ N01 Rapidly progressive nephritic syndrome
INCLUDES   rapidly progressive glomerular disease
rapidly progressive glomerulonephritis
rapidly progressive nephritis
EXCLUDES 1   nephritic syndrome NOS (N05.-)
AHA: 2021,1Q,23
N01.0   Rapidly progressive nephritic syndrome with minor glomerular abnormality
Rapidly progressive nephritic syndrome with minimal change lesion
N01.1   Rapidly progressive nephritic syndrome with focal and segmental glomerular lesions
Rapidly progressive nephritic syndrome with focal and segmental hyalinosis
Rapidly progressive nephritic syndrome with focal and segmental sclerosis
Rapidly progressive nephritic syndrome with focal glomerulonephritis
N01.2   Rapidly progressive nephritic syndrome with diffuse membranous glomerulonephritis
N01.3   Rapidly progressive nephritic syndrome with diffuse mesangial proliferative glomerulonephritis
N01.4   Rapidly progressive nephritic syndrome with diffuse endocapillary proliferative glomerulonephritis
N01.5   Rapidly progressive nephritic syndrome with diffuse mesangiocapillary glomerulonephritis
Rapidly progressive nephritic syndrome with membranoproliferative glomerulonephritis, types 1 and 3, or NOS
EXCLUDES 1   rapidly progressive nephritic syndrome with C3 glomerulonephritis (N01.A)
rapidly progressive nephritic syndrome with C3 glomerulopathy (N01.A)
N01.6   Rapidly progressive nephritic syndrome with dense deposit disease
Rapidly progressive nephritic syndrome with C3 glomerulopathy with dense deposit disease
Rapidly progressive nephritic syndrome with membranoproliferative glomerulonephritis, type 2
N01.7   Rapidly progressive nephritic syndrome with diffuse crescentic glomerulonephritis
Rapidly progressive nephritic syndrome with extracapillary glomerulonephritis
N01.8   Rapidly progressive nephritic syndrome with other morphologic changes
Rapidly progressive nephritic syndrome with proliferative glomerulonephritis NOS
N01.9   Rapidly progressive nephritic syndrome with unspecified morphologic changes
N01.A   Rapidly progressive nephritic syndrome with C3 glomerulonephritis
Rapidly progressive nephritic syndrome with C3 glomerulopathy, NOS
EXCLUDES 1   rapidly progressive nephritic syndrome (with C3 glomerulopathy) with dense deposit disease (N01.6)

✓4ᵗʰ N02 Recurrent and persistent hematuria
EXCLUDES 1   acute cystitis with hematuria (N30.01)
hematuria NOS (R31.9)
hematuria not associated with specified morphologic lesions (R31.-)
N02.0   Recurrent and persistent hematuria with minor glomerular abnormality
Recurrent and persistent hematuria with minimal change lesion
N02.1   Recurrent and persistent hematuria with focal and segmental glomerular lesions
Recurrent and persistent hematuria with focal and segmental hyalinosis
Recurrent and persistent hematuria with focal and segmental sclerosis
Recurrent and persistent hematuria with focal glomerulonephritis
N02.2   Recurrent and persistent hematuria with diffuse membranous glomerulonephritis

NØ2.3 **Recurrent and persistent hematuria with** diffuse mesangial proliferative glomerulonephritis

NØ2.4 **Recurrent and persistent hematuria with** diffuse endocapillary proliferative glomerulonephritis

NØ2.5 **Recurrent and persistent hematuria with** diffuse mesangiocapillary glomerulonephritis

    Recurrent and persistent hematuria with membranoproliferative glomerulonephritis, types 1 and 3, or NOS

    EXCLUDES 1   *recurrent and persistent hematuria with C3 glomerulonephritis (NØ2.A)*

    recurrent and persistent hematuria with C3 glomerulopathy (NØ2.A)

NØ2.6 **Recurrent and persistent hematuria with** dense deposit disease

    Recurrent and persistent hematuria with C3 glomerulopathy with dense deposit disease

    Recurrent and persistent hematuria with membranoproliferative glomerulonephritis, type 2

NØ2.7 **Recurrent and persistent hematuria with** diffuse crescentic glomerulonephritis

    Recurrent and persistent hematuria with extracapillary glomerulonephritis

NØ2.8 **Recurrent and persistent hematuria with other morphologic changes**

    Recurrent and persistent hematuria with proliferative glomerulonephritis NOS

NØ2.9 **Recurrent and persistent hematuria with unspecified morphologic changes**

    AHA: 2017,2Q,5

NØ2.A **Recurrent and persistent hematuria with** C3 glomerulonephritis

    Recurrent and persistent hematuria with C3 glomerulopathy

    EXCLUDES 1   *recurrent and persistent hematuria (with C3 glomerulopathy) with dense deposit disease (NØ2.6)*

✓4ᵗʰ **NØ3** Chronic **nephritic syndrome**

    INCLUDES   chronic glomerular disease

    chronic glomerulonephritis

    chronic nephritis

    EXCLUDES 1   *chronic tubulo-interstitial nephritis (N11.-)*

    diffuse sclerosing glomerulonephritis (NØ5.8-)

    nephritic syndrome NOS (NØ5.-)

    AHA: 2021,1Q,23

    DEF: Slow, progressive type of nephritis characterized by inflammation of the capillary loops in the glomeruli of the kidney, which leads to renal failure.

NØ3.Ø **Chronic nephritic syndrome with** minor glomerular abnormality

    Chronic nephritic syndrome with minimal change lesion

NØ3.1 **Chronic nephritic syndrome with** focal and segmental glomerular lesions

    Chronic nephritic syndrome with focal and segmental hyalinosis

    Chronic nephritic syndrome with focal and segmental sclerosis

    Chronic nephritic syndrome with focal glomerulonephritis

NØ3.2 **Chronic nephritic syndrome with** diffuse membranous glomerulonephritis

NØ3.3 **Chronic nephritic syndrome with** diffuse mesangial proliferative glomerulonephritis

NØ3.4 **Chronic nephritic syndrome with** diffuse endocapillary proliferative glomerulonephritis

NØ3.5 **Chronic nephritic syndrome with diffuse** mesangiocapillary glomerulonephritis

    Chronic nephritic syndrome with membranoproliferative glomerulonephritis, types 1 and 3, or NOS

    EXCLUDES 1   *chronic nephritic syndrome with C3 glomerulonephritis (NØ3.A)*

    chronic nephritic syndrome with C3 glomerulopathy (NØ3.A)

NØ3.6 **Chronic nephritic syndrome with** dense deposit disease

    Chronic nephritic syndrome with C3 glomerulopathy with dense deposit disease

    Chronic nephritic syndrome with membranoproliferative glomerulonephritis, type 2

NØ3.7 **Chronic nephritic syndrome with** diffuse crescentic glomerulonephritis

    Chronic nephritic syndrome with extracapillary glomerulonephritis

NØ3.8 **Chronic nephritic syndrome with other morphologic changes**

    Chronic nephritic syndrome with proliferative glomerulonephritis NOS

NØ3.9 **Chronic nephritic syndrome with unspecified morphologic changes**

NØ3.A **Chronic nephritic syndrome with** C3 glomerulonephritis

    Chronic nephritic syndrome with C3 glomerulopathy

    EXCLUDES 1   *chronic nephritic syndrome (with C3 glomerulopathy) with dense deposit disease (NØ3.6)*

✓4ᵗʰ **NØ4** **Nephrotic syndrome**

    INCLUDES   congenital nephrotic syndrome

    lipoid nephrosis

NØ4.Ø **Nephrotic syndrome with** minor glomerular abnormality

    Nephrotic syndrome with minimal change lesion

NØ4.1 **Nephrotic syndrome with** focal and segmental glomerular lesions

    Nephrotic syndrome with focal and segmental hyalinosis

    Nephrotic syndrome with focal and segmental sclerosis

    Nephrotic syndrome with focal glomerulonephritis

NØ4.2 **Nephrotic syndrome with** diffuse membranous glomerulonephritis

NØ4.3 **Nephrotic syndrome with** diffuse mesangial proliferative glomerulonephritis

NØ4.4 **Nephrotic syndrome with** diffuse endocapillary proliferative glomerulonephritis

NØ4.5 **Nephrotic syndrome with** diffuse mesangiocapillary glomerulonephritis

    Nephrotic syndrome with membranoproliferative glomerulonephritis, types 1 and 3, or NOS

    EXCLUDES 1   *nephrotic syndrome with C3 glomerulonephritis (NØ4.A)*

    nephrotic syndrome with C3 glomerulopathy (NØ4.A)

NØ4.6 **Nephrotic syndrome with** dense deposit disease

    Nephrotic syndrome with C3 glomerulopathy with dense deposit disease

    Nephrotic syndrome with membranoproliferative glomerulonephritis, type 2

NØ4.7 **Nephrotic syndrome with** diffuse crescentic glomerulonephritis

    Nephrotic syndrome with extracapillary glomerulonephritis

NØ4.8 **Nephrotic syndrome with other morphologic changes**

    Nephrotic syndrome with proliferative glomerulonephritis NOS

NØ4.9 **Nephrotic syndrome with unspecified morphologic changes**

NØ4.A **Nephrotic syndrome with** C3 glomerulonephritis

    Nephrotic syndrome with C3 glomerulopathy

    EXCLUDES 1   *nephrotic syndrome (with C3 glomerulopathy) with dense deposit disease (NØ4.6)*

✓4ᵗʰ **NØ5** **Unspecified nephritic syndrome**

    INCLUDES   glomerular disease NOS

    glomerulonephritis NOS

    nephritis NOS

    nephropathy NOS and renal disease NOS with morphological lesion specified in .Ø-.8

    EXCLUDES 1   *nephropathy NOS with no stated morphological lesion (N28.9)*

    renal disease NOS with no stated morphological lesion (N28.9)

    tubulo-interstitial nephritis NOS (N12)

NØ5.Ø **Unspecified nephritic syndrome with** minor glomerular abnormality

    Unspecified nephritic syndrome with minimal change lesion

NØ5.1 **Unspecified nephritic syndrome with** focal and segmental glomerular lesions

    Unspecified nephritic syndrome with focal and segmental hyalinosis

    Unspecified nephritic syndrome with focal and segmental sclerosis

    Unspecified nephritic syndrome with focal glomerulonephritis

NØ5.2 **Unspecified nephritic syndrome with** diffuse membranous glomerulonephritis

NØ5.3 **Unspecified nephritic syndrome with** diffuse mesangial proliferative glomerulonephritis

NØ5.4 **Unspecified nephritic syndrome with** diffuse endocapillary proliferative glomerulonephritis

N05.5 **Unspecified nephritic syndrome with** diffuse mesangiocapillary glomerulonephritis

Unspecified nephritic syndrome with membranoproliferative glomerulonephritis, types 1 and 3, or NOS

> *EXCLUDES 1*   *unspecified nephritic syndrome with C3 glomerulonephritis (N05.A)*
> *unspecified nephritic syndrome with C3 glomerulopathy (N05.A)*

N05.6 **Unspecified nephritic syndrome with** dense deposit disease

Unspecified nephritic syndrome with C3 glomerulopathy with dense deposit disease

Unspecified nephritic syndrome with membranoproliferative glomerulonephritis, type 2

N05.7 **Unspecified nephritic syndrome with** diffuse crescentic glomerulonephritis

Unspecified nephritic syndrome with extracapillary glomerulonephritis

N05.8 **Unspecified nephritic syndrome with other morphologic changes**

Unspecified nephritic syndrome with proliferative glomerulonephritis NOS

N05.9 **Unspecified nephritic syndrome with unspecified morphologic changes**

N05.A **Unspecified nephritic syndrome with** C3 glomerulonephritis

Unspecified nephritic syndrome with C3 glomerulopathy

> *EXCLUDES 1*   *unspecified nephritic syndrome (with C3 glomerulopathy) with dense deposit disease (N05.6)*

☑4ᵗʰ N06 **Isolated proteinuria with specified morphological lesion**

> *EXCLUDES 1*   *proteinuria not associated with specific morphologic lesions (R80.0)*

N06.0 **Isolated proteinuria with** minor glomerular abnormality

Isolated proteinuria with minimal change lesion

N06.1 **Isolated proteinuria with** focal and segmental glomerular lesions

Isolated proteinuria with focal and segmental hyalinosis
Isolated proteinuria with focal and segmental sclerosis
Isolated proteinuria with focal glomerulonephritis

N06.2 **Isolated proteinuria with** diffuse membranous glomerulonephritis

N06.3 **Isolated proteinuria with** diffuse mesangial proliferative glomerulonephritis

N06.4 **Isolated proteinuria with** diffuse endocapillary proliferative glomerulonephritis

N06.5 **Isolated proteinuria with** diffuse mesangiocapillary glomerulonephritis

Isolated proteinuria with membranoproliferative glomerulonephritis, types 1 and 3, or NOS

> *EXCLUDES 1*   *isolated proteinuria with C3 glomerulonephritis (N06.A)*
> *isolated proteinuria with C3 glomerulopathy (N06.A)*

N06.6 **Isolated proteinuria with** dense deposit disease

Isolated proteinuria with C3 glomerulopathy with dense deposit disease

Isolated proteinuria with membranoproliferative glomerulonephritis, type 2

N06.7 **Isolated proteinuria with** diffuse crescentic glomerulonephritis

Isolated proteinuria with extracapillary glomerulonephritis

N06.8 **Isolated proteinuria with other morphologic lesion**

Isolated proteinuria with proliferative glomerulonephritis NOS

N06.9 **Isolated proteinuria with unspecified morphologic lesion**

N06.A **Isolated proteinuria with** C3 glomerulonephritis

Isolated proteinuria with C3 glomerulopathy

> *EXCLUDES 1*   *isolated proteinuria (with C3 glomerulopathy) with dense deposit disease (N06.6)*

☑4ᵗʰ N07 **Hereditary nephropathy, not elsewhere classified**

> *EXCLUDES 2*   *Alport's syndrome (Q87.81-)*
> *hereditary amyloid nephropathy (E85.-)*
> *nail patella syndrome (Q87.2)*
> *non-neuropathic heredofamilial amyloidosis (E85.-)*

N07.0 **Hereditary nephropathy, not elsewhere classified with** minor glomerular abnormality

Hereditary nephropathy, not elsewhere classified with minimal change lesion

N07.1 **Hereditary nephropathy, not elsewhere classified with** focal and segmental glomerular lesions

Hereditary nephropathy, not elsewhere classified with focal and segmental hyalinosis

Hereditary nephropathy, not elsewhere classified with focal and segmental sclerosis

Hereditary nephropathy, not elsewhere classified with focal glomerulonephritis

N07.2 **Hereditary nephropathy, not elsewhere classified with diffuse membranous glomerulonephritis**

N07.3 **Hereditary nephropathy, not elsewhere classified with diffuse mesangial proliferative glomerulonephritis**

N07.4 **Hereditary nephropathy, not elsewhere classified with diffuse endocapillary proliferative glomerulonephritis**

N07.5 **Hereditary nephropathy, not elsewhere classified with diffuse mesangiocapillary glomerulonephritis**

Hereditary nephropathy, not elsewhere classified with membranoproliferative glomerulonephritis, types 1 and 3, or NOS

> *EXCLUDES 1*   *hereditary nephropathy, not elsewhere classified with C3 glomerulonephritis (N07.A)*
> *hereditary nephropathy, not elsewhere classified with C3 glomerulopathy (N07.A)*

N07.6 **Hereditary nephropathy, not elsewhere classified with** dense deposit disease

Hereditary nephropathy, not elsewhere classified with C3 glomerulopathy with dense deposit disease

Hereditary nephropathy, not elsewhere classified with membranoproliferative glomerulonephritis, type 2

N07.7 **Hereditary nephropathy, not elsewhere classified with diffuse crescentic glomerulonephritis**

Hereditary nephropathy, not elsewhere classified with extracapillary glomerulonephritis

N07.8 **Hereditary nephropathy, not elsewhere classified with other morphologic lesions**

Hereditary nephropathy, not elsewhere classified with proliferative glomerulonephritis NOS

N07.9 **Hereditary nephropathy, not elsewhere classified with unspecified morphologic lesions**

N07.A **Hereditary nephropathy, not elsewhere classified with** C3 glomerulonephritis

Hereditary nephropathy, not elsewhere classified with C3 glomerulopathy

> *EXCLUDES 1*   *hereditary nephropathy, not elsewhere classified (with C3 glomerulopathy) with dense deposit disease (N07.6)*

N08 *Glomerular disorders in diseases classified elsewhere*

Glomerulonephritis
Nephritis
Nephropathy
Code first underlying disease, such as:
   amyloidosis (E85.-)
   congenital syphilis (A50.5)
   cryoglobulinemia (D89.1)
   disseminated intravascular coagulation (D65)
   gout (M1A.-, M10.-)
   microscopic polyangiitis (M31.7)
   multiple myeloma (C90.0-)
   sepsis (A40.0-A41.9)
   sickle-cell disease (D57.0-D57.8)

> *EXCLUDES 1*   *glomerulonephritis, nephritis and nephropathy (in):*
>   *antiglomerular basement membrane disease (M31.0)*
>   *diabetes (E08-E13 with .21)*
>   *gonococcal (A54.21)*
>   *Goodpasture's syndrome (M31.0)*
>   *hemolytic-uremic syndrome ▶(D59.3-)◀*
>   *lupus (M32.14)*
>   *mumps (B26.83)*
>   *syphilis (A52.75)*
>   *systemic lupus erythematosus (M32.14)*
>   *Wegener's granulomatosis (M31.31)*
> *pyelonephritis in diseases classified elsewhere (N16)*
> *renal tubulo-interstitial disorders classified elsewhere (N16)*

HCC CMS-HCC   **Rx** Rx HCC   **ESR** ESRD HCC   **COM** Commercial HCC   **N** Newborn: 0   **P** Pediatric: 0-17   **M** Maternity: 9-64   **A** Adult: 15-124

868

ICD-10-CM 2023

Renal tubulo-interstitial diseases (N10-N16)

INCLUDES   pyelonephritis
EXCLUDES 1   *pyeloureteritis cystica (N28.85)*

N10   Acute **pyelonephritis**
Acute infectious interstitial nephritis
Acute pyelitis
Acute tubulo-interstitial nephritis
Hemoglobin nephrosis
Myoglobin nephrosis
Use additional code (B95-B97), to identify infectious agent
AHA: 2020,3Q,25; 2019,3Q,13

✓4ᵗʰ N11   Chronic **tubulo-interstitial nephritis**
INCLUDES   chronic infectious interstitial nephritis
chronic pyelitis
chronic pyelonephritis
Use additional code (B95-B97), to identify infectious agent

N11.0   Nonobstructive reflux-associated **chronic pyelonephritis**
Pyelonephritis (chronic) associated with (vesicoureteral) reflux
EXCLUDES 1   *vesicoureteral reflux NOS (N13.70)*

N11.1   Chronic obstructive **pyelonephritis**
Pyelonephritis (chronic) associated with anomaly of pelviureteric junction
Pyelonephritis (chronic) associated with anomaly of pyeloureteric junction
Pyelonephritis (chronic) associated with crossing of vessel
Pyelonephritis (chronic) associated with kinking of ureter
Pyelonephritis (chronic) associated with obstruction of ureter
Pyelonephritis (chronic) associated with stricture of pelviureteric junction
Pyelonephritis (chronic) associated with stricture of ureter
EXCLUDES 1   *calculous pyelonephritis (N20.9)*
           obstructive uropathy (N13.-)

N11.8   Other chronic tubulo-interstitial nephritis
Nonobstructive chronic pyelonephritis NOS

N11.9   Chronic tubulo-interstitial nephritis, unspecified
Chronic interstitial nephritis NOS
Chronic pyelitis NOS
Chronic pyelonephritis NOS

N12   **Tubulo-interstitial nephritis,** not specified as acute or chronic
Interstitial nephritis NOS
Pyelitis NOS
Pyelonephritis NOS
EXCLUDES 1   *calculous pyelonephritis (N20.9)*

✓4ᵗʰ N13   Obstructive and reflux uropathy
EXCLUDES 2   *calculus of kidney and ureter without hydronephrosis (N20.-)*
      congenital obstructive defects of renal pelvis and ureter (Q62.0-Q62.3)
      hydronephrosis with ureteropelvic junction obstruction (Q62.11)
      obstructive pyelonephritis (N11.1)
DEF: Hydronephrosis: Distension of the kidney caused by an accumulation of urine that cannot flow out due to an obstruction that may be caused by conditions such as kidney stones or vesicoureteral reflux.

N13.0   Hydronephrosis with ureteropelvic junction obstruction
Hydronephrosis due to acquired occlusion of ureteropelvic junction
EXCLUDES 2   *hydronephrosis with ureteropelvic junction obstruction due to calculus (N13.2)*
AHA: 2016,4Q,43

Hydronephrosis/UPJ Obstruction

Hydronephrosis
Ureteropelvic junction obstruction
Kidney
Ureters
Bladder

N13.1   Hydronephrosis with ureteral stricture, not elsewhere classified
EXCLUDES 1   *hydronephrosis with ureteral stricture with infection (N13.6)*

N13.2   Hydronephrosis with renal and ureteral calculous obstruction
EXCLUDES 1   *hydronephrosis with renal and ureteral calculous obstruction with infection (N13.6)*

✓5ᵗʰ N13.3   Other and unspecified hydronephrosis
EXCLUDES 1   *hydronephrosis with infection (N13.6)*

N13.30   Unspecified hydronephrosis
N13.39   Other hydronephrosis

N13.4   Hydroureter
EXCLUDES 1   *congenital hydroureter (Q62.3-)*
      hydroureter with infection (N13.6)
      vesicoureteral-reflux with hydroureter (N13.73-)
DEF: Abnormal enlargement or distension of the ureter with water or urine caused by an obstruction.

N13.5   Crossing vessel and stricture of ureter without hydronephrosis
Kinking and stricture of ureter without hydronephrosis
EXCLUDES 1   *crossing vessel and stricture of ureter without hydronephrosis with infection (N13.6)*

N13.6   Pyonephrosis
Conditions in N13.0-N13.5 with infection
Obstructive uropathy with infection
Use additional code (B95-B97), to identify infectious agent
AHA: 2018,2Q,21

☑ Additional Character Required   ✓x7ᵗʰ Placeholder Alert   Manifestation   Unspecified Dx   ◘ QPP   UPD Unacceptable PDx

Chapter 14. Diseases of the Genitourinary System

☑5ᵗʰ **N13.7   Vesicoureteral-reflux**

> **EXCLUDES 1**   *reflux-associated pyelonephritis (N11.0)*
>
> **DEF:** Urine passage from the bladder flows backward up into the ureter and kidneys that can lead to bacterial infection and an increase in hydrostatic pressure, causing kidney damage.

Vesicoureteral Reflux

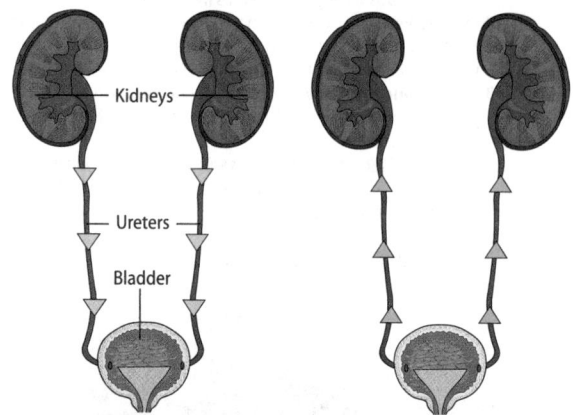

Kidneys

Ureters

Bladder

Normal flow of urine   Urine flowing the wrong way (VUR)

> **N13.70   Vesicoureteral-reflux, unspecified**
> Vesicoureteral-reflux NOS
>
> **N13.71   Vesicoureteral-reflux without reflux nephropathy**
>
> ☑6ᵗʰ **N13.72   Vesicoureteral-reflux with reflux nephropathy without hydroureter**
>> **N13.721   Vesicoureteral-reflux with reflux nephropathy without hydroureter, unilateral**
>> **N13.722   Vesicoureteral-reflux with reflux nephropathy without hydroureter, bilateral**
>> **N13.729   Vesicoureteral-reflux with reflux nephropathy without hydroureter, unspecified**
>
> ☑6ᵗʰ **N13.73   Vesicoureteral-reflux with reflux nephropathy with hydroureter**
>> **N13.731   Vesicoureteral-reflux with reflux nephropathy with hydroureter, unilateral**
>> **N13.732   Vesicoureteral-reflux with reflux nephropathy with hydroureter, bilateral**
>> **N13.739   Vesicoureteral-reflux with reflux nephropathy with hydroureter, unspecified**

N13.8   Other obstructive and reflux uropathy
> Urinary tract obstruction due to specified cause
> Code first, if applicable, any causal condition, such as:
> enlarged prostate (N40.1)

N13.9   Obstructive and reflux uropathy, unspecified
> Urinary tract obstruction NOS

☑4ᵗʰ **N14   Drug- and heavy-metal-induced tubulo-interstitial and tubular conditions**

> Code first poisoning due to drug or toxin, if applicable (T36-T65 with fifth or sixth character 1-4 or 6)
> Use additional code for adverse effect, if applicable, to identify drug (T36-T50 with fifth or sixth character 5)

N14.0   Analgesic nephropathy

▲ ☑5ᵗʰ **N14.1   Nephropathy induced by other drugs, medicaments and biological substances**
> AHA: 2021,3Q,9-10

●   **N14.11   Contrast-induced nephropathy**
>> Contrast medium, radiography nephropathy
>> **EXCLUDES 2**   *acute kidney failure (N17.-)*

●   **N14.19   Nephropathy induced by other drugs, medicaments and biological substances**

N14.2   Nephropathy induced by unspecified drug, medicament or biological substance

N14.3   Nephropathy induced by heavy metals

N14.4   Toxic nephropathy, not elsewhere classified

☑4ᵗʰ **N15   Other renal tubulo-interstitial diseases**

N15.0   Balkan nephropathy
> Balkan endemic nephropathy

N15.1   Renal and perinephric abscess

N15.8   Other specified renal tubulo-interstitial diseases

N15.9   Renal tubulo-interstitial disease, unspecified
> Infection of kidney NOS
> **EXCLUDES 1**   *urinary tract infection NOS (N39.0)*

N16   Renal tubulo-interstitial disorders in diseases classified elsewhere
> Pyelonephritis
> Tubulo-interstitial nephritis
> Code first underlying disease, such as:
> brucellosis (A23.0-A23.9)
> cryoglobulinemia (D89.1)
> glycogen storage disease (E74.0)
> leukemia (C91-C95)
> lymphoma (C81.0-C85.9, C96.0-C96.9)
> multiple myeloma (C90.0-)
> sepsis (A40.0-A41.9)
> Wilson's disease (E83.0)
>
> **EXCLUDES 1**   *diphtheritic pyelonephritis and tubulo-interstitial nephritis (A36.84)*
> *pyelonephritis and tubulo-interstitial nephritis in candidiasis (B37.49)*
> *pyelonephritis and tubulo-interstitial nephritis in cystinosis (E72.04)*
> *pyelonephritis and tubulo-interstitial nephritis in salmonella infection (A02.25)*
> *pyelonephritis and tubulo-interstitial nephritis in sarcoidosis (D86.84)*
> *pyelonephritis and tubulo-interstitial nephritis in Sjögren syndrome (M35.04)*
> *pyelonephritis and tubulo-interstitial nephritis in systemic lupus erythematosus (M32.15)*
> *pyelonephritis and tubulo-interstitial nephritis in toxoplasmosis (B58.83)*
> *renal tubular degeneration in diabetes (E08-E13 with .29)*
> *syphilitic pyelonephritis and tubulo-interstitial nephritis (A52.75)*

Acute kidney failure and chronic kidney disease (N17-N19)

> **EXCLUDES 2**   *congenital renal failure (P96.0)*
> *drug- and heavy-metal-induced tubulo-interstitial and tubular conditions (N14.-)*
> *extrarenal uremia (R39.2)*
> *hemolytic-uremic syndrome ▶(D59.3-)◄*
> *hepatorenal syndrome (K76.7)*
> *postpartum hepatorenal syndrome (O90.4)*
> *posttraumatic renal failure (T79.5)*
> *prerenal uremia (R39.2)*
> *renal failure complicating abortion or ectopic or molar pregnancy (O00-O07, O08.4)*
> *renal failure following labor and delivery (O90.4)*
> *renal failure postprocedural (N99.0)*

☑4ᵗʰ **N17   Acute kidney failure**

> Code also associated underlying condition
> **EXCLUDES 1**   *posttraumatic renal failure (T79.5)*
> **AHA:** 2020,3Q,22; 2019,2Q,7; 2019,1Q,12; 2013,4Q,124

N17.0   Acute kidney failure with tubular necrosis   HCC ESR
> Acute tubular necrosis
> Renal tubular necrosis
> Tubular necrosis NOS
> **AHA:** 2021,3Q,10

N17.1   Acute kidney failure with acute cortical necrosis   HCC ESR
> Acute cortical necrosis
> Cortical necrosis NOS
> Renal cortical necrosis

N17.2   Acute kidney failure with medullary necrosis   HCC ESR
> Medullary [papillary] necrosis NOS
> Acute medullary [papillary] necrosis
> Renal medullary [papillary] necrosis

N17.8   Other acute kidney failure   HCC ESR

N17.9   Acute kidney failure, unspecified   HCC ESR
> Acute kidney injury (nontraumatic)
> **EXCLUDES 2**   *traumatic kidney injury (S37.0-)*

☑4ᵗʰ **N18** Chronic **kidney disease (CKD)**

> Code first any associated:
> > diabetic chronic kidney disease (E08.22, E09.22, E10.22, E11.22, E13.22)
> > hypertensive chronic kidney disease (I12.-, I13.-)
> Use additional code to identify kidney transplant status, if applicable, (Z94.0)
> **AHA:** 2019,3Q,3; 2018,4Q,88; 2013,1Q,24
> **TIP:** CKD/ESRD occurring in an individual with a history of kidney transplant should not be assumed to be a transplant complication unless specifically indicated as such by provider documentation.

N18.1 Chronic kidney disease, stage 1

N18.2 Chronic kidney disease, stage 2 **(mild)**

☑5ᵗʰ **N18.3** Chronic kidney disease, stage 3 (moderate)

> **AHA:** 2020,4Q,35

> **N18.30** Chronic kidney disease, stage 3 unspecified   HCC ESR
>
> **N18.31** Chronic kidney disease, stage 3a   HCC ESR
>
> **N18.32** Chronic kidney disease, stage 3b   HCC ESR

N18.4 Chronic kidney disease, stage 4 (severe)   HCC Rx ESR COM

N18.5 Chronic kidney disease, stage 5   HCC Rx ESR COM

> *EXCLUDES 1*   chronic kidney disease, stage 5 requiring chronic dialysis (N18.6)
> **DEF:** End-stage renal disease (ESRD) with a GFR value of 15 ml/min or less not yet requiring chronic dialysis.
> **TIP:** When both ESRD and CKD 5 are documented, code only for ESRD.

N18.6 End stage **renal disease**   HCC Rx ESR COM

> *stage 5* *need dialysis*
> Chronic kidney disease requiring chronic dialysis
> Use additional code to identify dialysis status (Z99.2)
> **AHA:** 2016,3Q,22; 2016,1Q,12; 2013,4Q,124-125
> **TIP:** When both ESRD and CKD 5 are documented, code only for ESRD.

N18.9 Chronic **kidney disease, unspecified** *nephropathy*

> *CKD*
> Chronic renal disease
> Chronic renal failure NOS
> Chronic renal insufficiency
> Chronic uremia NOS
> Diffuse sclerosing glomerulonephritis NOS

N19 **Unspecified kidney failure**

> Uremia NOS
> *EXCLUDES 1*   acute kidney failure (N17.-)
> > chronic kidney disease (N18.-)
> > chronic uremia (N18.9)
> > extrarenal uremia (R39.2)
> > prerenal uremia (R39.2)
> > renal insufficiency (acute) (N28.9)
> > uremia of newborn (P96.0)

Urolithiasis (N20-N23)

> **AHA:** 2017,1Q,5; 2015,2Q,8
> **TIP:** Codes from this code block can be assigned based on the diagnosis listed in a radiology report when authenticated by a radiologist and available at the time of code assignment.

☑4ᵗʰ **N20** **Calculus of** kidney and ureter

> Calculous pyelonephritis
> *EXCLUDES 1*   nephrocalcinosis (E83.5)
> > that with hydronephrosis (N13.2)
> **AHA:** 2019,3Q,13

N20.0 **Calculus of** kidney

> Nephrolithiasis NOS
> Renal calculus
> Renal stone
> Staghorn calculus
> Stone in kidney
> **AHA:** 2019,3Q,13

N20.1 **Calculus of** ureter

> Calculus of the ureteropelvic junction
> Ureteric stone
> **AHA:** 2016,3Q,22

N20.2 **Calculus of** kidney with calculus of ureter

N20.9 **Urinary calculus, unspecified**

☑4ᵗʰ **N21** **Calculus of** lower urinary tract

> *INCLUDES*   calculus of lower urinary tract with cystitis and urethritis

N21.0 **Calculus in** bladder

> Calculus in diverticulum of bladder
> Urinary bladder stone
> *EXCLUDES 2*   staghorn calculus (N20.0)

N21.1 **Calculus in** urethra

> *EXCLUDES 2*   calculus of prostate (N42.0)

N21.8 **Other lower urinary tract calculus**

N21.9 **Calculus of lower urinary tract, unspecified**

> *EXCLUDES 1*   calculus of urinary tract NOS (N20.9)

N22 *Calculus of urinary tract in diseases classified elsewhere*

> Code first underlying disease, such as:
> > gout (M1A.-, M10.-)
> > schistosomiasis (B65.0-B65.9)

N23 **Unspecified renal colic**

Other disorders of kidney and ureter (N25-N29)

> *EXCLUDES 2*   disorders of kidney and ureter with urolithiasis (N20-N23)

☑4ᵗʰ **N25** **Disorders resulting from impaired renal tubular function**

N25.0 **Renal osteodystrophy**   Rx

> Azotemic osteodystrophy
> Phosphate-losing tubular disorders
> Renal rickets
> Renal short stature
> *EXCLUDES 2*   metabolic disorders classifiable to E70-E88
> **DEF:** Various bone diseases occurring when kidney function is impaired or fails. Abnormal levels of phosphorous and calcium can lead to osteomalacia, osteoporosis, or osteosclerosis.

N25.1 **Nephrogenic diabetes insipidus**   HCC Rx ESR COM

> *EXCLUDES 1*   diabetes insipidus NOS (E23.2)
> **DEF:** Type of diabetes due to the inability of renal tubules to reabsorb water back into the body. It is not responsive to vasopressin (antidiuretic hormone) and it is characterized by excessive thirst and excessive urine production. It may develop into chronic renal insufficiency.

☑5ᵗʰ **N25.8** **Other disorders resulting from impaired renal tubular function**

> **N25.81** **Secondary hyperparathyroidism of renal origin**   HCC Rx ESR COM
> > *EXCLUDES 1*   secondary hyperparathyroidism, non-renal (E21.1)
> > *EXCLUDES 2*   metabolic disorders classifiable to E70-E88
> > **DEF:** Parathyroid dysfunction caused by chronic renal failure. Phosphate clearance and vitamin D production is impaired resulting in lowered calcium blood levels and an excessive production of parathyroid hormone.
>
> **N25.89** **Other disorders resulting from impaired renal tubular function**
> > Hypokalemic nephropathy
> > Lightwood-Albright syndrome
> > Renal tubular acidosis NOS

N25.9 **Disorder resulting from impaired renal tubular function, unspecified**

☑4ᵗʰ **N26** **Unspecified contracted kidney**

> *EXCLUDES 1*   contracted kidney due to hypertension (I12.-)
> > diffuse sclerosing glomerulonephritis (N05.8.-)
> > hypertensive nephrosclerosis (arteriolar) (arteriosclerotic) (I12.-)
> > small kidney of unknown cause (N27.-)

N26.1 **Atrophy of kidney (terminal)**

N26.2 **Page kidney**   Rx

N26.9 **Renal sclerosis, unspecified**

☑4ᵗʰ **N27** **Small kidney of unknown cause**

> *INCLUDES*   oligonephronia

N27.0 **Small kidney, unilateral**

N27.1 **Small kidney, bilateral**

N27.9 **Small kidney, unspecified**

Chapter 14. Diseases of the Genitourinary System

✓4ᵗʰ **N28 Other disorders of kidney and ureter, not elsewhere classified**

N28.0 Ischemia and infarction of kidney   `HCC` `ESR` `COM`
Renal artery embolism
Renal artery obstruction
Renal artery occlusion
Renal artery thrombosis
Renal infarct
EXCLUDES 1   atherosclerosis of renal artery (extrarenal part) (I70.1)
congenital stenosis of renal artery (Q27.1)
Goldblatt's kidney (I70.1)

N28.1 Cyst of kidney, acquired
Cyst (multiple) (solitary) of kidney (acquired)
EXCLUDES 1   cystic kidney disease (congenital) (Q61.-)

✓5ᵗʰ **N28.8 Other specified disorders of kidney and ureter**
EXCLUDES 1   hydroureter (N13.4)
ureteric stricture with hydronephrosis (N13.1)
ureteric stricture without hydronephrosis (N13.5)

N28.81 Hypertrophy of kidney
N28.82 Megaloureter
N28.83 Nephroptosis
N28.84 Pyelitis cystica
N28.85 Pyeloureteritis cystica
N28.86 Ureteritis cystica
N28.89 Other specified disorders of kidney and ureter

N28.9 Disorder of kidney and ureter, unspecified
Nephropathy NOS
Renal disease (acute) NOS
Renal insufficiency (acute)
EXCLUDES 1   chronic renal insufficiency (N18.9)
unspecified nephritic syndrome (N05.-)
AHA: 2016,1Q,13

N29 Other disorders of kidney and ureter in diseases classified elsewhere
Code first underlying disease, such as:
amyloidosis (E85.-)
nephrocalcinosis (E83.5)
schistosomiasis (B65.0-B65.9)
EXCLUDES 1   disorders of kidney and ureter in:
cystinosis (E72.0)
gonorrhea (A54.21)
syphilis (A52.75)
tuberculosis (A18.11)

Other diseases of the urinary system (N30-N39)

EXCLUDES 2   urinary infection (complicating):
abortion or ectopic or molar pregnancy (O00-O07, O08.8)
pregnancy, childbirth and the puerperium (O23.-, O75.3, O86.2-)

✓4ᵗʰ **N30 Cystitis**
Use additional code to identify infectious agent (B95-B97)
EXCLUDES 1   prostatocystitis (N41.3)
AHA: 2017,1Q,6
DEF: Inflammation of the urinary bladder. Symptoms include dysuria, frequency of urination, urgency, and hematuria.

✓5ᵗʰ **N30.0 Acute cystitis**
EXCLUDES 1   irradiation cystitis (N30.4-)
trigonitis (N30.3-)

N30.00 Acute cystitis without hematuria
N30.01 Acute cystitis with hematuria

✓5ᵗʰ **N30.1 Interstitial cystitis (chronic)**
N30.10 Interstitial cystitis (chronic) without hematuria
N30.11 Interstitial cystitis (chronic) with hematuria

✓5ᵗʰ **N30.2 Other chronic cystitis**
N30.20 Other chronic cystitis without hematuria
N30.21 Other chronic cystitis with hematuria

✓5ᵗʰ **N30.3 Trigonitis**
Urethrotrigonitis
N30.30 Trigonitis without hematuria
N30.31 Trigonitis with hematuria

✓5ᵗʰ **N30.4 Irradiation cystitis**
N30.40 Irradiation cystitis without hematuria
N30.41 Irradiation cystitis with hematuria

✓5ᵗʰ **N30.8 Other cystitis**
Abscess of bladder   *bladder infectn*
N30.80 Other cystitis without hematuria
N30.81 Other cystitis with hematuria

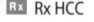

✓5ᵗʰ **N30.9 Cystitis, unspecified**   *E coli*
N30.90 Cystitis, unspecified without hematuria
N30.91 Cystitis, unspecified with hematuria

✓4ᵗʰ **N31 Neuromuscular dysfunction of bladder, not elsewhere classified**
Use additional code to identify any associated urinary incontinence (N39.3-N39.4-)
EXCLUDES 1   cord bladder NOS (G95.89)
neurogenic bladder due to cauda equina syndrome (G83.4)
neuromuscular dysfunction due to spinal cord lesion (G95.89)

N31.0 Uninhibited neuropathic bladder, not elsewhere classified
N31.1 Reflex neuropathic bladder, not elsewhere classified
N31.2 Flaccid neuropathic bladder, not elsewhere classified
Atonic (motor) (sensory) neuropathic bladder
Autonomous neuropathic bladder
Nonreflex neuropathic bladder

N31.8 Other neuromuscular dysfunction of bladder
N31.9 Neuromuscular dysfunction of bladder, unspecified
Neurogenic bladder dysfunction NOS

✓4ᵗʰ **N32 Other disorders of bladder**
EXCLUDES 2   calculus of bladder (N21.0)
cystocele (N81.1-)
hernia or prolapse of bladder, female (N81.1-)

N32.0 Bladder-neck obstruction
Bladder-neck stenosis (acquired)
EXCLUDES 1   congenital bladder-neck obstruction (Q64.3-)
DEF: Bladder outlet and vesicourethral obstruction that occurs as a consequence of benign prostatic hypertrophy or prostatic cancer. It may also occur in either sex due to strictures, radiation, cystoscopy, catheterization, injury, infection, blood clots, bladder cancer, impaction, or other disease that compresses the bladder neck.

N32.1 Vesicointestinal fistula
Vesicorectal fistula

N32.2 Vesical fistula, not elsewhere classified
EXCLUDES 1   fistula between bladder and female genital tract (N82.0-N82.1)

N32.3 Diverticulum of bladder
EXCLUDES 1   congenital diverticulum of bladder (Q64.6)
diverticulitis of bladder (N30.8-)

✓5ᵗʰ **N32.8 Other specified disorders of bladder**
N32.81 Overactive bladder
Detrusor muscle hyperactivity
EXCLUDES 1   frequent urination due to specified bladder condition — code to condition
DEF: Sudden involuntary contractions of the muscular wall of the bladder that results in a sudden, strong urge to urinate.

N32.89 Other specified disorders of bladder
Bladder hemorrhage
Bladder hypertrophy
Calcified bladder
Contracted bladder

N32.9 Bladder disorder, unspecified   *bladder lesion*

N33 Bladder disorders in diseases classified elsewhere
Code first underlying disease, such as:
schistosomiasis (B65.0-B65.9)
EXCLUDES 1   bladder disorder in syphilis (A52.76)
bladder disorder in tuberculosis (A18.12)
candidal cystitis (B37.41)
chlamydial cystitis (A56.01)
cystitis in gonorrhea (A54.01)
cystitis in neurogenic bladder (N31.-)
diphtheritic cystitis (A36.85)
neurogenic bladder (N31.-)
syphilitic cystitis (A52.76)
trichomonal cystitis (A59.03)

☑4ᵗʰ **N34 Urethritis and urethral syndrome**

Use additional code (B95-B97), to identify infectious agent

EXCLUDES 2   *Reiter's disease (M02.3-)*

urethritis in diseases with a predominantly sexual mode of transmission (A50-A64)

urethrotrigonitis (N30.3-)

AHA: 2017,1Q,6

N34.0 Urethral abscess

Abscess (of) Cowper's gland

Abscess (of) Littré's gland

Abscess (of) urethral (gland)

Periurethral abscess

EXCLUDES 1   *urethral caruncle (N36.2)*

N34.1 Nonspecific urethritis

Nongonococcal urethritis

Nonvenereal urethritis

N34.2 Other urethritis

Meatitis, urethral

Postmenopausal urethritis

Ulcer of urethra (meatus)

Urethritis NOS

N34.3 Urethral syndrome, unspecified

☑4ᵗʰ **N35 Urethral stricture**

EXCLUDES 1   *congenital urethral stricture (Q64.3-)*

postprocedural urethral stricture (N99.1-)

AHA: 2018,4Q,21-22

☑5ᵗʰ **N35.0 Post-traumatic urethral stricture**

Urethral stricture due to injury

EXCLUDES 1   *postprocedural urethral stricture (N99.1-)*

  ☑6ᵗʰ **N35.01 Post-traumatic urethral stricture, male**

N35.010 **Post-traumatic urethral stricture, male, meatal** ♂

N35.011 **Post-traumatic bulbous urethral stricture** ♂

N35.012 **Post-traumatic membranous urethral stricture** ♂

N35.013 **Post-traumatic anterior urethral stricture** ♂

N35.014 **Post-traumatic urethral stricture, male, unspecified** ♂

N35.016 **Post-traumatic urethral stricture, male, overlapping sites** ♂

  ☑6ᵗʰ **N35.02 Post-traumatic urethral stricture, female**

N35.021 **Urethral stricture due to childbirth** ♀

N35.028 **Other post-traumatic urethral stricture, female** ♀

☑5ᵗʰ **N35.1 Postinfective urethral stricture, not elsewhere classified**

EXCLUDES 1   *gonococcal urethral stricture (A54.01)*

syphilitic urethral stricture (A52.76)

urethral stricture associated with schistosomiasis (B65.-, N29)

  ☑6ᵗʰ **N35.11 Postinfective urethral stricture, not elsewhere classified, male**

N35.111 **Postinfective urethral stricture, not elsewhere classified, male, meatal** ♂

N35.112 **Postinfective bulbous urethral stricture, not elsewhere classified, male** ♂

N35.113 **Postinfective membranous urethral stricture, not elsewhere classified, male** ♂

N35.114 **Postinfective anterior urethral stricture, not elsewhere classified, male** ♂

N35.116 **Postinfective urethral stricture, not elsewhere classified, male, overlapping sites** ♂

N35.119 **Postinfective urethral stricture, not elsewhere classified, male, unspecified** ♂

N35.12 **Postinfective urethral stricture, not elsewhere classified, female** ♀

☑5ᵗʰ **N35.8 Other urethral stricture**

EXCLUDES 1   *postprocedural urethral stricture (N99.1-)*

  ☑6ᵗʰ **N35.81 Other urethral stricture, male**

N35.811 **Other urethral stricture, male, meatal** ♂

N35.812 **Other urethral bulbous stricture, male** ♂

N35.813 **Other membranous urethral stricture, male** ♂

N35.814 **Other anterior urethral stricture, male** ♂

N35.816 **Other urethral stricture, male, overlapping sites** ♂

N35.819 **Other urethral stricture, male, unspecified site** ♂

N35.82 **Other urethral stricture, female** ♀

☑5ᵗʰ **N35.9 Urethral stricture, unspecified**

  ☑6ᵗʰ **N35.91 Urethral stricture, unspecified, male**

N35.911 **Unspecified urethral stricture, male, meatal** ♂

N35.912 **Unspecified bulbous urethral stricture, male** ♂

N35.913 **Unspecified membranous urethral stricture, male** ♂

N35.914 **Unspecified anterior urethral stricture, male** ♂

N35.916 **Unspecified urethral stricture, male, overlapping sites** ♂

N35.919 **Unspecified urethral stricture, male, unspecified site** ♂

Pinhole meatus NOS

Urethral stricture NOS

N35.92 **Unspecified urethral stricture, female** ♀

☑4ᵗʰ **N36 Other disorders of urethra**

N36.0 Urethral fistula

Urethroperineal fistula

Urethrorectal fistula

Urinary fistula NOS

EXCLUDES 1   *urethroscrotal fistula (N50.89)*

urethrovaginal fistula (N82.1)

urethrovesicovaginal fistula (N82.1)

N36.1 Urethral diverticulum

N36.2 Urethral caruncle

☑5ᵗʰ **N36.4 Urethral functional and muscular disorders**

Use additional code to identify associated urinary stress incontinence (N39.3)

N36.41 Hypermobility of urethra

N36.42 Intrinsic sphincter deficiency (ISD)

N36.43 Combined hypermobility of urethra and intrinsic sphincter deficiency

N36.44 Muscular disorders of urethra

Bladder sphincter dyssynergy

N36.5 Urethral false passage

N36.8 Other specified disorders of urethra

EXCLUDES 1   *congenital urethrocele (Q64.7)*

female urethrocele (N81.0)

AHA: 2022,2Q,7

N36.9 Urethral disorder, unspecified

N37 Urethral disorders in diseases classified elsewhere

Code first underlying disease

EXCLUDES 1   *urethritis (in):*

candidal infection (B37.41)

chlamydial (A56.01)

gonorrhea (A54.01)

syphilis (A52.76)

trichomonal infection (A59.03)

tuberculosis (A18.13)

☑ Additional Character Required   ☑x7ᵗʰ Placeholder Alert   Manifestation   Unspecified Dx   ◐ QPP   UPD Unacceptable PDx

Chapter 14. Diseases of the Genitourinary System

N39–N42.9

✓4ᵗʰ **N39 Other disorders of urinary system**

    EXCLUDES 2   hematuria NOS (R31.-)

         recurrent or persistent hematuria (N02.-)

         recurrent or persistent hematuria with specified

           morphological lesion (N02.-)

         proteinuria NOS (R80.-)

  N39.0 Urinary tract infection, site not specified

       Use additional code (B95-B97), to identify infectious agent

      EXCLUDES 1   candidiasis of urinary tract (B37.4-)

          neonatal urinary tract infection (P39.3)

          pyuria (R82.81)

          urinary tract infection of specified site, such as:

           cystitis (N30.-)

           urethritis (N34.-)

       AHA: 2019,3Q,17; 2018,2Q,21,22; 2018,1Q,16; 2017,1Q,6; 2012,4Q,94

  N39.3 Stress incontinence (female) (male) ~~SUI~~

       Code also any associated overactive bladder (N32.81)

      EXCLUDES 1   mixed incontinence (N39.46)

✓5ᵗʰ **N39.4 Other specified urinary incontinence**

       Code also any associated overactive bladder (N32.81)

      EXCLUDES 1   enuresis NOS (R32)

          functional urinary incontinence (R39.81)

          urinary incontinence associated with cognitive

           impairment (R39.81)

          urinary incontinence NOS (R32)

          urinary incontinence of nonorganic origin (F98.0)

urge   **N39.41 Urge incontinence**

         EXCLUDES 1   mixed incontinence (N39.46)

mix   **N39.42 Incontinence without sensory awareness**

         Insensible (urinary) incontinence

     N39.43 Post-void dribbling

     N39.44 Nocturnal enuresis

        EXCLUDES 2   nocturnal polyuria (R35.81)

     N39.45 Continuous leakage

     N39.46 Mixed incontinence

         Urge and stress incontinence

  ✓6ᵗʰ **N39.49 Other specified urinary incontinence**

         AHA: 2016,4Q,44

uncontrollable   **N39.490 Overflow incontinence**

drug   **N39.491 Coital incontinence**

         N39.492 Postural (urinary) incontinence

         N39.498 Other specified urinary incontinence

            Reflex incontinence

            Total incontinence

  N39.8 Other specified disorders of urinary system

  N39.9 Disorder of urinary system, unspecified

Diseases of male genital organs (N40-N53)

✓4ᵗʰ **N40 Benign prostatic hyperplasia**

    INCLUDES   adenofibromatous hypertrophy of prostate

          benign hypertrophy of the prostate

          benign prostatic hypertrophy

          BPH

          enlarged prostate

          nodular prostate

          polyp of prostate

    EXCLUDES 1   benign neoplasms of prostate (adenoma, benign)

           (fibroadenoma) (fibroma) (myoma) (D29.1)

    EXCLUDES 2   malignant neoplasm of prostate (C61)

    DEF: Enlargement of the prostate gland due to an abnormal proliferation of fibrostromal tissue in the paraurethral glands. This condition causes impingement of the urethra resulting in obstructed urinary flow.

  N40.0 Benign prostatic hyperplasia without lower urinary tract symptoms   🅰 ♂

       Enlarged prostate NOS

       Enlarged prostate without LUTS

  N40.1 Benign prostatic hyperplasia with lower urinary tract symptoms   🅰 ♂

       Enlarged prostate with LUTS

       Use additional code for associated symptoms, when specified:

         incomplete bladder emptying (R39.14)

         nocturia (R35.1)

         straining on urination (R39.16)

         urinary frequency (R35.0)

         urinary hesitancy (R39.11)

         urinary incontinence (N39.4-)

         urinary obstruction (N13.8)

         urinary retention (R33.8)

         urinary urgency (R39.15)

         weak urinary stream (R39.12)

       AHA: 2018,4Q,55

  N40.2 Nodular prostate without lower urinary tract symptoms   🅰 ♂

       Nodular prostate without LUTS

  N40.3 Nodular prostate with lower urinary tract symptoms   🅰 ♂

       Use additional code for associated symptoms, when specified:

         incomplete bladder emptying (R39.14)

         nocturia (R35.1)

         straining on urination (R39.16)

         urinary frequency (R35.0)

         urinary hesitancy (R39.11)

         urinary incontinence (N39.4-)

         urinary obstruction (N13.8)

         urinary retention (R33.8)

         urinary urgency (R39.15)

         weak urinary stream (R39.12)

✓4ᵗʰ **N41 Inflammatory diseases of prostate**

       Use additional code (B95-B97), to identify infectious agent

  N41.0 Acute prostatitis   🅰 ♂

  N41.1 Chronic prostatitis   🅰 ♂

  N41.2 Abscess of prostate   🅰 ♂

  N41.3 Prostatocystitis   🅰 ♂

  N41.4 Granulomatous prostatitis   🅰 ♂

  N41.8 Other inflammatory diseases of prostate   🅰 ♂

  N41.9 Inflammatory disease of prostate, unspecified   🅰 ♂

       Prostatitis NOS

✓4ᵗʰ **N42 Other and unspecified disorders of prostate**

  N42.0 Calculus of prostate   🅰 ♂

       Prostatic stone

       DEF: Formation of a small, solid stone often composed of calcium carbonate or calcium phosphate in the prostate gland.

  N42.1 Congestion and hemorrhage of prostate   🅰 ♂

      EXCLUDES 1   enlarged prostate (N40.-)

          hematuria (R31.-)

          hyperplasia of prostate (N40.-)

          inflammatory diseases of prostate (N41.-)

  ✓5ᵗʰ **N42.3 Dysplasia of prostate**

       AHA: 2016,4Q,44

    N42.30 Unspecified dysplasia of prostate   ♂

    N42.31 Prostatic intraepithelial neoplasia   ♂

       PIN

       Prostatic intraepithelial neoplasia I (PIN I)

       Prostatic intraepithelial neoplasia II (PIN II)

      EXCLUDES 1   prostatic intraepithelial neoplasia III (PIN III) (D07.5)

       DEF: Abnormality of shape and size of the intraepithelial tissues of the prostate. It is a premalignant condition characterized by stalks and absence of a basilar cell layer.

    N42.32 Atypical small acinar proliferation of prostate   ♂

    N42.39 Other dysplasia of prostate   ♂

  ✓5ᵗʰ **N42.8 Other specified disorders of prostate**

    N42.81 Prostatodynia syndrome   🅰 ♂

       Painful prostate syndrome

    N42.82 Prostatosis syndrome   🅰 ♂

    N42.83 Cyst of prostate   🅰 ♂

    N42.89 Other specified disorders of prostate   🅰 ♂

  N42.9 Disorder of prostate, unspecified   🅰 ♂

Chapter 14. Diseases of the Genitourinary System

✓4ᵗʰ **N43 Hydrocele and spermatocele**

    INCLUDES   hydrocele of spermatic cord, testis or tunica vaginalis

    EXCLUDES 1   congenital hydrocele (P83.5)

    DEF: Hydrocele: Serous fluid that collects in the tunica vaginalis of the scrotum along the spermatic cord in males.

  N43.0 Encysted hydrocele

  N43.1 Infected hydrocele   *Swelling is not infectious* ♂

    Use additional code (B95-B97), to identify infectious agent

  N43.2 Other hydrocele   ♂

Hydrocele

Testicle
Scrotum

Normal   Noncommunicating hydrocele   Communicating hydrocele   Hydrocele of the cord

  N43.3 Hydrocele, unspecified   *no pain · only swelling.* ♂

✓5ᵗʰ **N43.4 Spermatocele of epididymis**

    Spermatic cyst

    DEF: Spermatocele: Noncancerous accumulation of fluid and dead sperm cells normally located at the head of the epididymis that exhibits itself as a hard, smooth scrotal mass and do not normally require treatment unless they become enlarged or cause pain.

    N43.40 Spermatocele of epididymis, unspecified   ♂

    N43.41 Spermatocele of epididymis, single   ♂

    N43.42 Spermatocele of epididymis, multiple   ♂

✓4ᵗʰ **N44 Noninflammatory disorders of testis**

✓5ᵗʰ **N44.0 Torsion of testis**

    N44.00 Torsion of testis, unspecified   ♂

    N44.01 Extravaginal torsion of spermatic cord   ♂

      DEF: Torsion of the spermatic cord just below the tunica vaginalis attachments.

    N44.02 Intravaginal torsion of spermatic cord   ♂

      Torsion of spermatic cord NOS

    N44.03 Torsion of appendix testis   ♂

    N44.04 Torsion of appendix epididymis   ♂

  N44.1 Cyst of tunica albuginea testis   ♂

  N44.2 Benign cyst of testis   ♂

  N44.8 Other noninflammatory disorders of the testis   ♂

✓4ᵗʰ **N45 Orchitis and epididymitis**

    Use additional code (B95-B97), to identify infectious agent

  N45.1 Epididymitis   ♂

  N45.2 Orchitis   ♂

  N45.3 Epididymo-orchitis   ♂

  N45.4 Abscess of epididymis or testis   ♂

✓4ᵗʰ **N46 Male infertility**

    EXCLUDES 1   vasectomy status (Z98.52)

✓5ᵗʰ **N46.0 Azoospermia**

    Absolute male infertility

    Male infertility due to germinal (cell) aplasia

    Male infertility due to spermatogenic arrest (complete)

    DEF: Failure of the development of sperm or the absence of sperm in semen.

    N46.01 Organic azoospermia   A ♂

      Azoospermia NOS

  ✓6ᵗʰ **N46.02 Azoospermia due to extratesticular causes**   ♂

      Code also associated cause

      N46.021 Azoospermia due to drug therapy   A ♂

      N46.022 Azoospermia due to infection   A ♂

      N46.023 Azoospermia due to obstruction of efferent ducts   A ♂

      N46.024 Azoospermia due to radiation   A ♂

      N46.025 Azoospermia due to systemic disease   A ♂

      N46.029 Azoospermia due to other extratesticular causes   A ♂

✓5ᵗʰ **N46.1 Oligospermia**

    Male infertility due to germinal cell desquamation

    Male infertility due to hypospermatogenesis

    Male infertility due to incomplete spermatogenic arrest

    DEF: Insufficient production of sperm in semen.

    N46.11 Organic oligospermia   A ♂

      Oligospermia NOS

  ✓6ᵗʰ **N46.12 Oligospermia due to extratesticular causes**   ♂

      Code also associated cause

      N46.121 Oligospermia due to drug therapy   A ♂

      N46.122 Oligospermia due to infection   A ♂

      N46.123 Oligospermia due to obstruction of efferent ducts   A ♂

      N46.124 Oligospermia due to radiation   A ♂

      N46.125 Oligospermia due to systemic disease   A ♂

      N46.129 Oligospermia due to other extratesticular causes   A ♂

  N46.8 Other male infertility   A ♂

  N46.9 Male infertility, unspecified   A ♂

✓4ᵗʰ **N47 Disorders of prepuce**

  N47.0 Adherent prepuce, newborn   N ♂

  N47.1 Phimosis   ♂

    DEF: Condition in which the foreskin is contracted and cannot be drawn back behind the glans penis.

  N47.2 Paraphimosis   ♂

  N47.3 Deficient foreskin   ♂

  N47.4 Benign cyst of prepuce   ♂

  N47.5 Adhesions of prepuce and glans penis   ♂

  N47.6 Balanoposthitis   ♂

    Use additional code (B95-B97), to identify infectious agent

    EXCLUDES 1   balanitis (N48.1)

  N47.7 Other inflammatory diseases of prepuce   ♂

    Use additional code (B95-B97), to identify infectious agent

  N47.8 Other disorders of prepuce   ♂

✓4ᵗʰ **N48 Other disorders of penis**

  N48.0 Leukoplakia of penis   ♂

    Balanitis xerotica obliterans

    Kraurosis of penis

    Lichen sclerosus of external male genital organs

    EXCLUDES 1   carcinoma in situ of penis (D07.4)

  N48.1 Balanitis   ♂

    Use additional code (B95-B97), to identify infectious agent

    EXCLUDES 1   amebic balanitis (A06.8)

         balanitis xerotica obliterans (N48.0)

         candidal balanitis (B37.42)

         gonococcal balanitis (A54.23)

         herpesviral [herpes simplex] balanitis (A60.01)

    DEF: Inflammation of the glans penis, most often affecting uncircumcised males.

✓5ᵗʰ **N48.2 Other inflammatory disorders of penis**

    Use additional code (B95-B97), to identify infectious agent

    EXCLUDES 1   balanitis (N48.1)

         balanitis xerotica obliterans (N48.0)

         balanoposthitis (N47.6)

    N48.21 Abscess of corpus cavernosum and penis   ♂

    N48.22 Cellulitis of corpus cavernosum and penis   ♂

    N48.29 Other inflammatory disorders of penis   ♂

✓5ᵗʰ **N48.3 Priapism**

    Painful erection

    Code first underlying cause

    N48.30 Priapism, unspecified   ♂

    N48.31 Priapism due to trauma   ♂

    N48.32 Priapism due to disease classified elsewhere   ♂

    N48.33 Priapism, drug-induced   ♂

    N48.39 Other priapism   ♂

  N48.5 Ulcer of penis   ♂

Chapter 14. Diseases of the Genitourinary System

N48.6   **Induration penis plastica**   ♂
- Peyronie's disease
- Plastic induration of penis

☑5ᵗʰ **N48.8**   **Other specified disorders of penis**

    N48.81   **Thrombosis of superficial vein of penis**   ♂

    N48.82   **Acquired torsion of penis**   ♂
- Acquired torsion of penis NOS
  - EXCLUDES 1   *congenital torsion of penis (Q55.63)*

    N48.83   **Acquired buried penis**   ♂
- EXCLUDES 1   *congenital hidden penis (Q55.64)*

    N48.89   **Other specified disorders of penis**   ♂

N48.9   **Disorder of penis, unspecified**   ♂

☑4ᵗʰ **N49**   **Inflammatory disorders of male genital organs, not elsewhere classified**
- Use additional code (B95-B97), to identify infectious agent
  - EXCLUDES 1   *inflammation of penis (N48.1, N48.2-)*
  -                *orchitis and epididymitis (N45.-)*

N49.0   **Inflammatory disorders of seminal vesicle**   ♂
- Vesiculitis NOS

N49.1   **Inflammatory disorders of spermatic cord, tunica vaginalis and vas deferens**   ♂
- Vasitis

N49.2   **Inflammatory disorders of scrotum**   ♂

N49.3   **Fournier gangrene**   ♂
- AHA: 2020,2Q,18

N49.8   **Inflammatory disorders of other specified male genital organs**   ♂
- Inflammation of multiple sites in male genital organs

N49.9   **Inflammatory disorder of unspecified male genital organ**   ♂
- Abscess of unspecified male genital organ
- Boil of unspecified male genital organ
- Carbuncle of unspecified male genital organ
- Cellulitis of unspecified male genital organ

☑4ᵗʰ **N50**   **Other and unspecified disorders of male genital organs**
- EXCLUDES 2   *torsion of testis (N44.0-)*

N50.0   **Atrophy of testis**   ♂

N50.1   **Vascular disorders of male genital organs**   ♂
- Hematocele, NOS, of male genital organs
- Hemorrhage of male genital organs
- Thrombosis of male genital organs

N50.3   **Cyst of epididymis**   ♂

☑5ᵗʰ **N50.8**   **Other specified disorders of male genital organs**
- AHA: 2016,4Q,45

    ☑6ᵗʰ **N50.81**   **Testicular pain**

       N50.811   **Right testicular pain**   ♂

       N50.812   **Left testicular pain**   ♂

       N50.819   **Testicular pain, unspecified**   ♂

    N50.82   **Scrotal pain**   ♂

    N50.89   **Other specified disorders of the male genital organs**   ♂
- Atrophy of scrotum, seminal vesicle, spermatic cord, tunica vaginalis and vas deferens
- Chylocele, tunica vaginalis (nonfilarial) NOS
- Edema of scrotum, seminal vesicle, spermatic cord, tunica vaginalis and vas deferens
- Hypertrophy of scrotum, seminal vesicle, spermatic cord, tunica vaginalis and vas deferens
- Stricture of spermatic cord, tunica vaginalis, and vas deferens
- Ulcer of scrotum, seminal vesicle, spermatic cord, testis, tunica vaginalis and vas deferens
- Urethroscrotal fistula

N50.9   **Disorder of male genital organs, unspecified**   ♂

N51   ***Disorders of male genital organs in diseases classified elsewhere***   ♂
- Code first underlying disease, such as:
  - filariasis (B74.0-B74.9)
  - EXCLUDES 1   *amebic balanitis (A06.8)*
  -                *candidal balanitis (B37.42)*
  -                *gonococcal balanitis (A54.23)*
  -                *gonococcal prostatitis (A54.22)*
  -                *herpesviral [herpes simplex] balanitis (A60.01)*
  -                *trichomonal prostatitis (A59.02)*
  -                *tuberculous prostatitis (A18.14)*

☑4ᵗʰ **N52**   **Male erectile dysfunction**
- EXCLUDES 1   *psychogenic impotence (F52.21)*

☑5ᵗʰ **N52.0**   **Vasculogenic erectile dysfunction**

    N52.01   **Erectile dysfunction due to arterial insufficiency**   A ♂

    N52.02   **Corporo-venous occlusive erectile dysfunction**   A ♂

    N52.03   **Combined arterial insufficiency and corporo-venous occlusive erectile dysfunction**   A ♂

N52.1   ***Erectile dysfunction due to diseases classified elsewhere***   A ♂
- Code first underlying disease

N52.2   **Drug-induced erectile dysfunction**   A ♂

☑5ᵗʰ **N52.3**   **Postprocedural erectile dysfunction**
- AHA: 2016,4Q,45

    N52.31   **Erectile dysfunction following radical prostatectomy**   A ♂

    N52.32   **Erectile dysfunction following radical cystectomy**   A ♂

    N52.33   **Erectile dysfunction following urethral surgery**   A ♂

    N52.34   **Erectile dysfunction following simple prostatectomy**   A ♂

    N52.35   **Erectile dysfunction following radiation therapy**   A ♂

    N52.36   **Erectile dysfunction following interstitial seed therapy**   A ♂

    N52.37   **Erectile dysfunction following prostate ablative therapy**   A ♂
- Erectile dysfunction following cryotherapy
- Erectile dysfunction following other prostate ablative therapies
- Erectile dysfunction following ultrasound ablative therapies

    N52.39   **Other and unspecified postprocedural erectile dysfunction**   A ♂

N52.8   **Other male erectile dysfunction**   A ♂

N52.9   **Male erectile dysfunction, unspecified**   A ♂
- Impotence NOS

☑4ᵗʰ **N53**   **Other male sexual dysfunction**
- EXCLUDES 1   *psychogenic sexual dysfunction (F52.-)*

☑5ᵗʰ **N53.1**   **Ejaculatory dysfunction**
- EXCLUDES 1   *premature ejaculation (F52.4)*

    N53.11   **Retarded ejaculation**   ♂

    N53.12   **Painful ejaculation**   ♂

    N53.13   **Anejaculatory orgasm**   ♂

    N53.14   **Retrograde ejaculation**   ♂
- DEF: Form of male sexual dysfunction in which the semen enters the bladder instead of going out through the urethra during ejaculation.

    N53.19   **Other ejaculatory dysfunction**   ♂
- Ejaculatory dysfunction NOS

N53.8   **Other male sexual dysfunction**   ♂

N53.9   **Unspecified male sexual dysfunction**   ♂

Disorders of breast (N60-N65)

EXCLUDES 1   *disorders of breast associated with childbirth (O91-O92)*

☑4ᵗʰ **N60**   **Benign mammary dysplasia**
- INCLUDES   fibrocystic mastopathy

☑5ᵗʰ **N60.0**   **Solitary cyst of breast**
- Cyst of breast

    N60.01   **Solitary cyst of right breast**

    N60.02   **Solitary cyst of left breast**

    N60.09   **Solitary cyst of unspecified breast**

✓5ᵗʰ **N60.1** **Diffuse cystic mastopathy**

Cystic breast
Fibrocystic disease of breast
    EXCLUDES 1   *diffuse cystic mastopathy with epithelial proliferation (N60.3-)*

   N60.11 **Diffuse cystic mastopathy of right breast**   A
   N60.12 **Diffuse cystic mastopathy of left breast**   A
   N60.19 **Diffuse cystic mastopathy of unspecified breast**   A

✓5ᵗʰ **N60.2** **Fibroadenosis of breast**

Adenofibrosis of breast
    EXCLUDES 2   *fibroadenoma of breast (D24.-)*

   N60.21 **Fibroadenosis of right breast**
   N60.22 **Fibroadenosis of left breast**
   N60.29 **Fibroadenosis of unspecified breast**

✓5ᵗʰ **N60.3** **Fibrosclerosis of breast**

Cystic mastopathy with epithelial proliferation
   N60.31 **Fibrosclerosis of right breast**
   N60.32 **Fibrosclerosis of left breast**
   N60.39 **Fibrosclerosis of unspecified breast**

✓5ᵗʰ **N60.4** **Mammary duct ectasia**

   N60.41 **Mammary duct ectasia of right breast**
   N60.42 **Mammary duct ectasia of left breast**
   N60.49 **Mammary duct ectasia of unspecified breast**

✓5ᵗʰ **N60.8** **Other benign mammary dysplasias**

   N60.81 **Other benign mammary dysplasias of right breast**
   N60.82 **Other benign mammary dysplasias of left breast**
   N60.89 **Other benign mammary dysplasias of unspecified breast**

✓5ᵗʰ **N60.9** **Unspecified benign mammary dysplasia**

   N60.91 **Unspecified benign mammary dysplasia of right breast**
   N60.92 **Unspecified benign mammary dysplasia of left breast**
   N60.99 **Unspecified benign mammary dysplasia of unspecified breast**

✓4ᵗʰ **N61** **Inflammatory disorders of breast**

    EXCLUDES 1   *inflammatory carcinoma of breast (C50.9)*
       inflammatory disorder of breast associated with childbirth (O91.-)
       neonatal infective mastitis (P39.0)
       thrombophlebitis of breast [Mondor's disease] (I80.8)

   N61.0 **Mastitis without abscess**
     Infective mastitis (acute) (nonpuerperal) (subacute)
     Mastitis (acute) (nonpuerperal) (subacute) NOS
     Cellulitis (acute) (nonpuerperal) (subacute) of breast NOS
     Cellulitis (acute) (nonpuerperal) (subacute) of nipple NOS

   N61.1 **Abscess of the breast and nipple**
     Abscess (acute) (chronic) (nonpuerperal) of areola
     Abscess (acute) (chronic) (nonpuerperal) of breast
     Carbuncle of breast
     Mastitis with abscess

✓5ᵗʰ   **N61.2** **Granulomatous mastitis**
     AHA: 2020,4Q,35
   N61.20 **Granulomatous mastitis, unspecified breast**
   N61.21 **Granulomatous mastitis, right breast**
   N61.22 **Granulomatous mastitis, left breast**
   N61.23 **Granulomatous mastitis, bilateral breast**

N62 **Hypertrophy of breast**
     Gynecomastia
     Hypertrophy of breast NOS
     Massive pubertal hypertrophy of breast
    EXCLUDES 1   *breast engorgement of newborn (P83.4)*
       disproportion of reconstructed breast (N65.1)

✓4ᵗʰ **N63** **Unspecified lump in breast**
     Nodule(s) NOS in breast
     AHA: 2019,4Q,12; 2017,4Q,19
   N63.0 **Unspecified lump in unspecified breast**
✓5ᵗʰ   **N63.1** **Unspecified lump in the right breast**
   N63.10 **Unspecified lump in the right breast, unspecified quadrant**
   N63.11 **Unspecified lump in the right breast, upper outer quadrant**
   N63.12 **Unspecified lump in the right breast, upper inner quadrant**
   N63.13 **Unspecified lump in the right breast, lower outer quadrant**
   N63.14 **Unspecified lump in the right breast, lower inner quadrant**
   N63.15 **Unspecified lump in the right breast, overlapping quadrants**
✓5ᵗʰ   **N63.2** **Unspecified lump in the left breast**
   N63.20 **Unspecified lump in the left breast, unspecified quadrant**
   N63.21 **Unspecified lump in the left breast, upper outer quadrant**
   N63.22 **Unspecified lump in the left breast, upper inner quadrant**
   N63.23 **Unspecified lump in the left breast, lower outer quadrant**
   N63.24 **Unspecified lump in the left breast, lower inner quadrant**
   N63.25 **Unspecified lump in the left breast, overlapping quadrants**
✓5ᵗʰ   **N63.3** **Unspecified lump in axillary tail**
   N63.31 **Unspecified lump in axillary tail of the right breast**
   N63.32 **Unspecified lump in axillary tail of the left breast**
✓5ᵗʰ   **N63.4** **Unspecified lump in breast, subareolar**
   N63.41 **Unspecified lump in right breast, subareolar**
   N63.42 **Unspecified lump in left breast, subareolar**

✓4ᵗʰ **N64** **Other disorders of breast**
    EXCLUDES 2   *mechanical complication of breast prosthesis and implant (T85.4-)*
   N64.0 **Fissure and fistula of nipple**
   N64.1 **Fat necrosis of breast**
     Fat necrosis (segmental) of breast
     Code first breast necrosis due to breast graft (T85.898)
   N64.2 **Atrophy of breast**
   N64.3 **Galactorrhea not associated with childbirth**
   N64.4 **Mastodynia**
✓5ᵗʰ   **N64.5** **Other signs and symptoms in breast**
    EXCLUDES 2   *abnormal findings on diagnostic imaging of breast (R92.-)*
   N64.51 **Induration of breast**
   N64.52 **Nipple discharge**
    EXCLUDES 1   *abnormal findings in nipple discharge (R89.-)*
   N64.53 **Retraction of nipple**
   N64.59 **Other signs and symptoms in breast**
✓5ᵗʰ   **N64.8** **Other specified disorders of breast**
   N64.81 **Ptosis of breast**   A
    EXCLUDES 1   *ptosis of native breast in relation to reconstructed breast (N65.1)*
   N64.82 **Hypoplasia of breast**   A
     Micromastia
    EXCLUDES 1   *congenital absence of breast (Q83.0)*
       hypoplasia of native breast in relation to reconstructed breast (N65.1)
   N64.89 **Other specified disorders of breast**
     Galactocele
     Subinvolution of breast (postlactational)
     AHA: 2019,1Q,32; 2018,1Q,3
   N64.9 **Disorder of breast, unspecified**

✓4ᵗʰ **N65** **Deformity and disproportion of reconstructed breast**
   N65.0 **Deformity of reconstructed breast**   A
     Contour irregularity in reconstructed breast
     Excess tissue in reconstructed breast
     Misshapen reconstructed breast
   N65.1 **Disproportion of reconstructed breast**   A
     Breast asymmetry between native breast and reconstructed breast
     Disproportion between native breast and reconstructed breast

Inflammatory diseases of female pelvic organs (N70-N77)

EXCLUDES 1   *inflammatory diseases of female pelvic organs complicating:*
abortion or ectopic or molar pregnancy (O00-O07, O08.0)
pregnancy, childbirth and the puerperium (O23.-, O75.3, O85, O86.-)

✓4ᵗʰ **N70 Salpingitis and oophoritis**

    INCLUDES   abscess (of) fallopian tube
          abscess (of) ovary
          pyosalpinx
          salpingo-oophoritis
          tubo-ovarian abscess
          tubo-ovarian inflammatory disease

    Use additional code (B95-B97), to identify infectious agent
      EXCLUDES 1   *gonococcal infection (A54.24)*
                tuberculous infection (A18.17)

   ✓5ᵗʰ **N70.0 Acute salpingitis and oophoritis**

      N70.01 Acute salpingitis ♀
      N70.02 Acute oophoritis ♀
      N70.03 Acute salpingitis and oophoritis ♀

   ✓5ᵗʰ **N70.1 Chronic salpingitis and oophoritis**

      Hydrosalpinx
      N70.11 Chronic salpingitis ♀
      N70.12 Chronic oophoritis ♀
      N70.13 Chronic salpingitis and oophoritis ♀

   ✓5ᵗʰ **N70.9 Salpingitis and oophoritis, unspecified**

      N70.91 Salpingitis, unspecified ♀
      N70.92 Oophoritis, unspecified ♀
      N70.93 Salpingitis and oophoritis, unspecified ♀

✓4ᵗʰ **N71 Inflammatory disease of uterus, except cervix**

    INCLUDES   endo (myo) metritis
          metritis
          myometritis
          pyometra
          uterine abscess

    Use additional code (B95-B97), to identify infectious agent
      EXCLUDES 1   *hyperplastic endometritis (N85.0-)*
                infection of uterus following delivery (O85, O86.-)

   N71.0 Acute inflammatory disease of uterus ♀
   N71.1 Chronic inflammatory disease of uterus ♀
   N71.9 Inflammatory disease of uterus, unspecified ♀

N72 Inflammatory disease of cervix uteri ♀

    INCLUDES   cervicitis (with or without erosion or ectropion)
          endocervicitis (with or without erosion or ectropion)
          exocervicitis (with or without erosion or ectropion)

    Use additional code (B95-B97), to identify infectious agent
      EXCLUDES 1   *erosion and ectropion of cervix without cervicitis (N86)*

✓4ᵗʰ **N73 Other female pelvic inflammatory diseases**

    Use additional code (B95-B97), to identify infectious agent

   N73.0 Acute parametritis and pelvic cellulitis ♀
      Abscess of broad ligament
      Abscess of parametrium
      Pelvic cellulitis, female
      DEF: Parametritis: Inflammation of the parametrium.

   N73.1 Chronic parametritis and pelvic cellulitis ♀
      Any condition in N73.0 specified as chronic
      EXCLUDES 1   *tuberculous parametritis and pelvic cellultis (A18.17)*

   N73.2 Unspecified parametritis and pelvic cellulitis ♀
      Any condition in N73.0 unspecified whether acute or chronic

   N73.3 Female acute pelvic peritonitis ♀
   N73.4 Female chronic pelvic peritonitis ♀
      EXCLUDES 1   *tuberculous pelvic (female) peritonitis (A18.17)*

   N73.5 Female pelvic peritonitis, unspecified ♀
   N73.6 Female pelvic peritoneal adhesions (postinfective) ♀
      EXCLUDES 2   *postprocedural pelvic peritoneal adhesions (N99.4)*
      AHA: 2014,1Q,6

   N73.8 Other specified female pelvic inflammatory diseases ♀
   N73.9 Female pelvic inflammatory disease, unspecified ♀
      Female pelvic infection or inflammation NOS

N74 ***Female pelvic inflammatory disorders in diseases classified elsewhere*** ♀

    Code first underlying disease
      EXCLUDES 1   *chlamydial cervicitis (A56.02)*
                chlamydial pelvic inflammatory disease (A56.11)
                gonococcal cervicitis (A54.03)
                gonococcal pelvic inflammatory disease (A54.24)
                herpesviral [herpes simplex] cervicitis (A60.03)
                herpesviral [herpes simplex] pelvic inflammatory disease (A60.09)
                syphilitic cervicitis (A52.76)
                syphilitic pelvic inflammatory disease (A52.76)
                trichomonal cervicitis (A59.09)
                tuberculous cervicitis (A18.16)
                tuberculous pelvic inflammatory disease (A18.17)

✓4ᵗʰ **N75 Diseases of Bartholin's gland**

    DEF: Bartholin's gland: Mucous-producing gland found in the vestibular bulbs on either side of the vaginal orifice and connected to the mucosal membrane at the opening by a duct.

   N75.0 Cyst of Bartholin's gland ♀
   N75.1 Abscess of Bartholin's gland ♀
   N75.8 Other diseases of Bartholin's gland ♀
      Bartholinitis
   N75.9 Disease of Bartholin's gland, unspecified ♀

✓4ᵗʰ **N76 Other inflammation of vagina and vulva**

    Use additional code (B95-B97), to identify infectious agent
      EXCLUDES 2   *senile (atrophic) vaginitis (N95.2)*
                vulvar vestibulitis (N94.810)

   N76.0 Acute vaginitis ♀
      Acute vulvovaginitis
      Vaginitis NOS
      Vulvovaginitis NOS

   N76.1 Subacute and chronic vaginitis ♀
      Chronic vulvovaginitis
      Subacute vulvovaginitis

   N76.2 Acute vulvitis ♀
      Vulvitis NOS

   N76.3 Subacute and chronic vulvitis ♀
   N76.4 Abscess of vulva ♀
      Furuncle of vulva

   N76.5 Ulceration of vagina ♀
   N76.6 Ulceration of vulva ♀

   ✓5ᵗʰ **N76.8 Other specified inflammation of vagina and vulva**

      N76.81 Mucositis (ulcerative) of vagina and vulva ♀
         Code also type of associated therapy, such as:
           antineoplastic and immunosuppressive drugs (T45.1X-)
           radiological procedure and radiotherapy (Y84.2)
         EXCLUDES 2   *gastrointestinal mucositis (ulcerative) (K92.81)*
                   nasal mucositis (ulcerative) (J34.81)
                   oral mucositis (ulcerative) (K12.3-)

      N76.82 Fournier disease of vagina and vulva
         Fournier gangrene of vagina and vulva
         Code also, if applicable, diabetes mellitus (E08-E13 with .9)
         EXCLUDES 1   *gangrene in diabetes mellitus (E08-E13 with .52)*

      N76.89 Other specified inflammation of vagina and vulva ♀

✓4ᵗʰ **N77 Vulvovaginal ulceration and inflammation in diseases classified elsewhere**

   N77.0 ***Ulceration of vulva in diseases classified elsewhere*** ♀
      Code first underlying disease, such as:
      Behçet's disease (M35.2)
      EXCLUDES 1   *ulceration of vulva in gonococcal infection (A54.02)*
                ulceration of vulva in herpesviral [herpes simplex] infection (A60.04)
                ulceration of vulva in syphilis (A51.0)
                ulceration of vulva in tuberculosis (A18.18)

N80 – 98   *noninflammatory female*

N77.1   *Vaginitis, vulvitis and vulvovaginitis in diseases classified elsewhere* ♀
     Code first underlying disease, such as:
       pinworm (B80)
       EXCLUDES 1   candidal vulvovaginitis ▶(B37.3-)◀
               chlamydial vulvovaginitis (A56.02)
               gonococcal vulvovaginitis (A54.02)
               herpesviral [herpes simplex] vulvovaginitis (A60.04)
               trichomonal vulvovaginitis (A59.01)
               tuberculous vulvovaginitis (A18.18)
               vulvovaginitis in early syphilis (A51.0)
               vulvovaginitis in late syphilis (A52.76)

Noninflammatory disorders of female genital tract (N80-N98)

✓4ᵗʰ N80 Endometriosis
     DEF: Aberrant uterine mucosal tissue appearing in areas of the pelvic cavity outside of its normal location, lining the uterus, and inflaming surrounding tissues often resulting in infertility or spontaneous abortion.

▲   **✓5ᵗʰ N80.0 Endometriosis of** *uterus*
     ~~Adenomyosis~~
     ▶Endometriosis of the cervix◀
       EXCLUDES 1   stromal endometriosis (D39.0)
-    **N80.00**   **Endometriosis of the uterus, unspecified**
-    **N80.01**   **Superficial endometriosis of the uterus**
-    **N80.02**   **Deep endometriosis of the uterus**
         Deep retrocervical endometriosis
-    **N80.03**   **Adenomyosis of the uterus**
         Adenomyosis NOS

▲   **✓5ᵗʰ N80.1 Endometriosis of** *ovary*
-    **✓6ᵗʰ N80.10 Endometriosis of ovary, unspecified depth**

• **ovaries**
• **= bilateral**

       N80.101   **Endometriosis of** right **ovary, unspecified depth**
       N80.102   **Endometriosis of** left **ovary, unspecified depth**
       N80.103   **Endometriosis of** bilateral **ovaries, unspecified depth**
       N80.109   **Endometriosis of ovary, unspecified side, unspecified depth**
           Endometriosis of ovary NOS
-    **✓6ᵗʰ N80.11 Superficial endometriosis of the ovary**
-      **N80.111**   **Superficial endometriosis of** right **ovary**
-      **N80.112**   **Superficial endometriosis of** left **ovary**
-      **N80.113**   **Superficial endometriosis of** bilateral **ovaries**
-      **N80.119**   **Superficial endometriosis of ovary, unspecified ovary**
-    **✓6ᵗʰ N80.12 Deep endometriosis of ovary**
         Deep ovarian endometriosis
         Endometrioma
-      **N80.121**   **Deep endometriosis of** right **ovary**
-      **N80.122**   **Deep endometriosis of** left **ovary**
-      **N80.123**   **Deep endometriosis of** bilateral **ovaries**
-      **N80.129**   **Deep endometriosis of ovary, unspecified ovary**

▲   **✓5ᵗʰ N80.2 Endometriosis of** *fallopian tube*
-    **✓6ᵗʰ N80.20 Endometriosis of fallopian tube, unspecified depth**
       N80.201   **Endometriosis of** right **fallopian tube, unspecified depth**
       N80.202   **Endometriosis of** left **fallopian tube, unspecified depth**
       N80.203   **Endometriosis of** bilateral **fallopian tubes, unspecified depth**
       N80.209   **Endometriosis of unspecified fallopian tube, unspecified depth**
          Endometriosis fallopian tube NOS
-    **✓6ᵗʰ N80.21 Superficial endometriosis of fallopian tube**
-      **N80.211**   **Superficial endometriosis of** right **fallopian tube**
-      **N80.212**   **Superficial endometriosis of** left **fallopian tube**
-      **N80.213**   **Superficial endometriosis of** bilateral **fallopian tubes**
-      **N80.219**   **Superficial endometriosis of unspecified fallopian tube**

-    **✓6ᵗʰ N80.22 Deep endometriosis of the fallopian tube**
         Deep endometriosis involving muscular wall of fallopian tube
-      **N80.221**   **Deep endometriosis of** right **fallopian tube**
-      **N80.222**   **Deep endometriosis of** left **fallopian tube**
-      **N80.223**   **Deep endometriosis of** bilateral **fallopian tubes**
-      **N80.229**   **Deep endometriosis of unspecified fallopian tube**

▲   **✓5ᵗʰ N80.3 Endometriosis of** *pelvic peritoneum*
     N80.30   **Endometriosis of pelvic peritoneum, unspecified**
         Endometriosis of the retroperitoneum NOS
-    **✓6ᵗʰ N80.31 Endometriosis of the** anterior cul-de-sac
-      **N80.311**   **Superficial endometriosis of the anterior cul-de-sac**
-      **N80.312**   **Deep endometriosis of the anterior cul-de-sac**
-      **N80.319**   **Endometriosis of the anterior cul-de-sac, unspecified depth**
           Endometriosis of the anterior cul-de-sac NOS
-    **✓6ᵗʰ N80.32 Endometriosis of the** posterior cul-de-sac
-      **N80.321**   **Superficial endometriosis of the posterior cul-de-sac**
-      **N80.322**   **Deep endometriosis of the posterior cul-de-sac**
-      **N80.329**   **Endometriosis of the posterior cul-de-sac, unspecified depth**
           Endometriosis of the posterior cul-de-sac NOS
-    **✓6ᵗʰ N80.33 Superficial endometriosis of the** pelvic sidewall
-      **N80.331**   **Superficial endometriosis of the** right **pelvic sidewall**
-      **N80.332**   **Superficial endometriosis of the** left **pelvic sidewall**
-      **N80.333**   **Superficial endometriosis of** bilateral **pelvic sidewall**
-      **N80.339**   **Superficial endometriosis of pelvic sidewall, unspecified side**
-    **✓6ᵗʰ N80.34 Deep endometriosis of the** pelvic sidewall
-      **N80.341**   **Deep endometriosis of the** right **pelvic sidewall**
-      **N80.342**   **Deep endometriosis of the** left **pelvic sidewall**
-      **N80.343**   **Deep endometriosis of the** bilateral **pelvic sidewall**
-      **N80.349**   **Deep endometriosis of the pelvic sidewall, unspecified side**
-    **✓6ᵗʰ N80.35 Endometriosis of the pelvic sidewall, unspecified depth**
-      **N80.351**   **Endometriosis of the** right **pelvic sidewall, unspecified depth**
-      **N80.352**   **Endometriosis of the** left **pelvic sidewall, unspecified depth**
-      **N80.353**   **Endometriosis of** bilateral **pelvic sidewall, unspecified depth**
-      **N80.359**   **Endometriosis of pelvic sidewall, unspecified side, unspecified depth**
           Endometriosis of the pelvic sidewall NOS
-    **✓6ᵗʰ N80.36 Superficial endometriosis of the** pelvic brim
-      **N80.361**   **Superficial endometriosis of the** right **pelvic brim**
-      **N80.362**   **Superficial endometriosis of the** left **pelvic brim**
-      **N80.363**   **Superficial endometriosis of** bilateral **pelvic brim**
-      **N80.369**   **Superficial endometriosis of the pelvic brim, unspecified side**
-    **✓6ᵗʰ N80.37 Deep endometriosis of the** pelvic brim
-      **N80.371**   **Deep endometriosis of the** right **pelvic brim**
-      **N80.372**   **Deep endometriosis of the** left **pelvic brim**
-      **N80.373**   **Deep endometriosis of** bilateral **pelvic brim**
-      **N80.379**   **Deep endometriosis of the pelvic brim, unspecified side**
-    **✓6ᵗʰ N80.38 Endometriosis of the pelvic brim, unspecified depth**
-      **N80.381**   **Endometriosis of the** right **pelvic brim, unspecified depth**

female noninflammatory

Chapter 14. Diseases of the Genitourinary System

N80.382 Endometriosis of the left pelvic brim, unspecified depth

N80.383 Endometriosis of bilateral pelvic brim, unspecified depth

N80.389 Endometriosis of the pelvic brim, unspecified side, unspecified depth
> Endometriosis of the pelvic brim NOS

✓6th **N80.3A** Superficial endometriosis of the uterosacral ligament(s)

    N80.3A1 Superficial endometriosis of the right uterosacral ligament

    N80.3A2 Superficial endometriosis of the left uterosacral ligament

    N80.3A3 Superficial endometriosis of the bilateral uterosacral ligament(s)

    N80.3A9 Superficial endometriosis of the uterosacral ligament(s), unspecified side

✓6th **N80.3B** Deep endometriosis of the uterosacral ligament(s)

    N80.3B1 Deep endometriosis of the right uterosacral ligament

    N80.3B2 Deep endometriosis of the left uterosacral ligament

    N80.3B3 Deep endometriosis of bilateral uterosacral ligament(s)

    N80.3B9 Deep endometriosis of the uterosacral ligament(s), unspecified side

✓6th **N80.3C** Endometriosis of the uterosacral ligament(s), unspecified depth

    N80.3C1 Endometriosis of the right uterosacral ligament, unspecified depth

    N80.3C2 Endometriosis of the left uterosacral ligament, unspecified depth

    N80.3C3 Endometriosis of bilateral uterosacral ligament(s), unspecified depth

    N80.3C9 Endometriosis of the uterosacral ligament(s), unspecified side, unspecified depth
> Endometriosis of the uterosacral ligament(s) NOS

✓6th **N80.39** Endometriosis of other pelvic peritoneum

    N80.391 Superficial endometriosis of the pelvic peritoneum, other specified sites

    N80.392 Deep endometriosis of the pelvic peritoneum, other specified sites

    N80.399 Endometriosis of the pelvic peritoneum, other specified sites, unspecified depth

▲ ✓5th **N80.4** Endometriosis of rectovaginal septum and vagina

    N80.40 Endometriosis of rectovaginal septum, unspecified involvement of vagina
> Endometriosis of the rectovaginal septum, NOS

    N80.41 Endometriosis of rectovaginal septum without involvement of vagina

    N80.42 Endometriosis of rectovaginal septum with involvement of vagina

▲ ✓5th **N80.5** Endometriosis of intestine

    N80.50 Endometriosis of intestine, unspecified

✓6th **N80.51** Endometriosis of the rectum

    N80.511 Superficial endometriosis of the rectum

    N80.512 Deep endometriosis of the rectum
> Deep endometriosis of the rectum, multifocal

    N80.519 Endometriosis of the rectum, unspecified depth
> Endometriosis of the rectum NOS

✓6th **N80.52** Endometriosis of the sigmoid colon

    N80.521 Superficial endometriosis of the sigmoid colon

    N80.522 Deep endometriosis of the sigmoid colon

    N80.529 Endometriosis of the sigmoid colon, unspecified depth
> Endometriosis of the sigmoid colon NOS

✓6th **N80.53** Endometriosis of the cecum

    N80.531 Superficial endometriosis of the cecum

    N80.532 Deep endometriosis of the cecum

    N80.539 Endometriosis of the cecum, unspecified depth
> Endometriosis of the cecum NOS

✓6th **N80.54** Endometriosis of the appendix

    N80.541 Superficial endometriosis of the appendix

    N80.542 Deep endometriosis of the appendix

    N80.549 Endometriosis of the appendix, unspecified depth
> Endometriosis of the appendix NOS

✓6th **N80.55** Endometriosis of other parts of the colon
> Endometriosis of descending colon
> Endometriosis of transverse colon

    N80.551 Superficial endometriosis of other parts of the colon

    N80.552 Deep endometriosis of other parts of the colon

    N80.559 Endometriosis of other parts of the colon, unspecified depth
> Endometriosis of colon NOS

✓6th **N80.56** Endometriosis of the small intestine

    N80.561 Superficial endometriosis of the small intestine

    N80.562 Deep endometriosis of the small intestine
> Deep endometriosis of the small intestine, multifocal

    N80.569 Endometriosis of the small intestine, unspecified depth
> Endometriosis of the small intestine NOS

N80.6 Endometriosis in cutaneous scar   ♀

✓5th **N80.A** Endometriosis of bladder and ureters

    N80.A0 Endometriosis of bladder, unspecified depth
> Endometriosis of bladder NOS

    N80.A1 Superficial endometriosis of bladder

    N80.A2 Deep endometriosis of bladder

✓6th **N80.A4** Superficial endometriosis of ureter
> Extrinsic endometriosis of ureter
> Code also, if applicable, obstructive and reflux uropathy (N13.-)

    N80.A41 Superficial endometriosis of right ureter

    N80.A42 Superficial endometriosis of left ureter

    N80.A43 Superficial endometriosis of bilateral ureters

    N80.A49 Superficial endometriosis of unspecified ureter

✓6th **N80.A5** Deep endometriosis of ureter
> Intrinsic endometriosis of ureter
> Code also, if applicable, obstructive and reflux uropathy (N13.-)

    N80.A51 Deep endometriosis of right ureter

    N80.A52 Deep endometriosis of left ureter

    N80.A53 Deep endometriosis of bilateral ureters

    N80.A59 Deep endometriosis of unspecified ureter

✓6th **N80.A6** Endometriosis of ureter, unspecified depth
> Code also, if applicable, obstructive and reflux uropathy (N13.-)

    N80.A61 Endometriosis of right ureter, unspecified depth

    N80.A62 Endometriosis of left ureter, unspecified depth

    N80.A63 Endometriosis of bilateral ureters, unspecified depth

    N80.A69 Endometriosis of unspecified ureter, unspecified depth

✓5th **N80.B** Endometriosis of cardiothoracic space
> Endometriosis of thorax
> Code also, if applicable:
> catamenial hemothorax (J94.2)
> catamenial pneumothorax (J93.12)

    N80.B1 Endometriosis of pleura

    N80.B2 Endometriosis of lung

✓6th **N80.B3** Endometriosis of diaphragm

    N80.B31 Superficial endometriosis of diaphragm

    N80.B32 Deep endometriosis of diaphragm

    N80.B39 Endometriosis of diaphragm, unspecified depth
> Endometriosis of the diaphragm NOS

    N80.B4 Endometriosis of the pericardial space

    N80.B5 Endometriosis of the mediastinal space

    N80.B6 Endometriosis of cardiothoracic space

HCC CMS-HCC   **Rx** Rx HCC   **ESR** ESRD HCC   **COM** Commercial HCC   **N** Newborn: 0   **P** Pediatric: 0-17   **M** Maternity: 9-64   **A** Adult: 15-124

880

ICD-10-CM 2023

[handwritten: urethral vaginal vault (Rectal slings) — Female non inflammatory]

- ✓5ᵗʰ **N80.C** **Endometriosis of the** abdomen
- **N80.C0** **Endometriosis of the abdomen, unspecified**
  Endometriosis of the abdomen NOS
- ✓6ᵗʰ **N80.C1** **Endometriosis of the** anterior **abdominal wall**
  - **N80.C10** **Endometriosis of the anterior abdominal wall,** subcutaneous tissue
  - **N80.C11** **Endometriosis of the anterior abdominal wall,** fascia and muscular layers
  - **N80.C19** **Endometriosis of the anterior abdominal wall, unspecified depth**
    Endometriosis of the anterior abdominal wall NOS
- **N80.C2** **Endometriosis of the** umbilicus
- **N80.C3** **Endometriosis of the** inguinal canal
- **N80.C4** **Endometriosis of** extra-pelvic abdominal peritoneum
- **N80.C9** **Endometriosis of other site of abdomen**
- ✓5ᵗʰ **N80.D** **Endometriosis of the** pelvic nerves
  Endometriosis of the nerves of the retroperitoneum
  - **N80.D0** **Endometriosis of the pelvic nerves, unspecified**
    Endometriosis of nerve of the retroperitoneum, NOS
  - **N80.D1** **Endometriosis of the** sacral splanchnic nerves
    Endometriosis of the pelvic splanchnic nerves
  - **N80.D2** **Endometriosis of the** sacral nerve roots
  - **N80.D3** **Endometriosis of the** obturator nerve
  - **N80.D4** **Endometriosis of the** sciatic nerve
  - **N80.D5** **Endometriosis of the** pudendal nerve
  - **N80.D6** **Endometriosis of the** femoral nerve
  - **N80.D9** **Endometriosis of other pelvic nerve**
    Endometriosis of the other nerves of the retroperitoneum
- **N80.8** **Other endometriosis** ♀
  ▶Endometriosis of other site◀
- **N80.9** **Endometriosis, unspecified** ♀
- ✓4ᵗʰ **N81** **Female genital prolapse**
  EXCLUDES 1   genital prolapse complicating pregnancy, labor or delivery (O34.5-)
  prolapse and hernia of ovary and fallopian tube (N83.4-)
  prolapse of vaginal vault after hysterectomy (N99.3)

Types of Pelvic Organ Prolapse

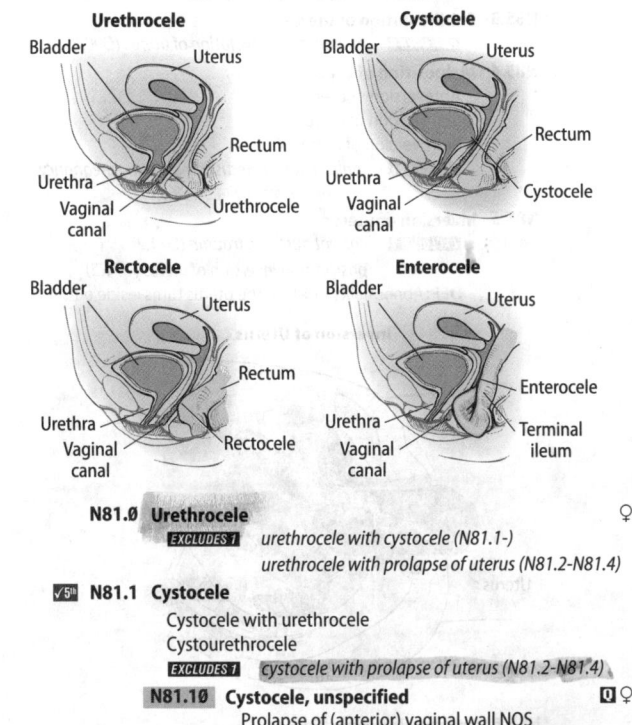

Urethrocele — Bladder, Uterus, Rectum, Urethra, Vaginal canal, Urethrocele
Cystocele — Bladder, Uterus, Rectum, Urethra, Vaginal canal, Cystocele
Rectocele — Bladder, Uterus, Rectum, Urethra, Vaginal canal, Rectocele
Enterocele — Bladder, Uterus, Enterocele, Urethra, Vaginal canal, Terminal ileum

- **N81.0** **Urethrocele** ♀
  EXCLUDES 1   urethrocele with cystocele (N81.1-)
  urethrocele with prolapse of uterus (N81.2-N81.4)
- ✓5ᵗʰ **N81.1** **Cystocele**
  Cystocele with urethrocele
  Cystourethrocele
  EXCLUDES 1   cystocele with prolapse of uterus (N81.2-N81.4)
  - **N81.10** **Cystocele, unspecified** ⓠ♀
    Prolapse of (anterior) vaginal wall NOS
  - **N81.11** **Cystocele, midline** ⓠ♀

[handwritten: ↓ cant be with N81.2 – N81.4]

- **N81.12** **Cystocele,** lateral ⓠ♀
  Paravaginal cystocele
  DEF: Detachment of the lateral support connections of the vagina at the arcus tendineus fasciae pelvis (ATFP) that results in bladder drop. The bladder herniates into the vagina laterally.
- **N81.2** **Incomplete** uterovaginal prolapse ⓠ♀ *[handwritten: +rectocele]*
  First degree uterine prolapse *[handwritten: second degree cystocele]*
  Prolapse of cervix NOS
  Second degree uterine prolapse
  EXCLUDES 1   cervical stump prolapse (N81.85)
- **N81.3** **Complete** uterovaginal prolapse ⓠ♀ *[handwritten: (uterine prolapse)]*
  Procidentia (uteri) NOS
  Third degree uterine prolapse
- **N81.4** **Uterovaginal prolapse, unspecified** ⓠ♀ *[handwritten: +rectocele]*
  Prolapse of uterus NOS *[handwritten: cystocele + uterine prolapse]*
- **N81.5** **Vaginal enterocele**
  EXCLUDES 1   enterocele with prolapse of uterus (N81.2-N81.4)
- **N81.6** **Rectocele**
  Prolapse of posterior vaginal wall
  Use additional code for any associated fecal incontinence, if applicable (R15.-)
  EXCLUDES 2   perineocele (N81.81)
  rectal prolapse (K62.3)
  rectocele with prolapse of uterus (N81.2-N81.4)
- ✓5ᵗʰ **N81.8** **Other female genital prolapse**
  - **N81.81** **Perineocele** ♀
  - **N81.82** **Incompetence or weakening of** pubocervical tissue ♀
  - **N81.83** **Incompetence or weakening of** rectovaginal tissue ♀
  - **N81.84** **Pelvic muscle wasting** ♀
    Disuse atrophy of pelvic muscles and anal sphincter
  - **N81.85** **Cervical stump prolapse** ♀
  - **N81.89** **Other female genital prolapse** ⓠ♀
    Deficient perineum
    Old laceration of muscles of pelvic floor
  - **N81.9** **Female genital prolapse, unspecified** ⓠ♀
- ✓4ᵗʰ **N82** **Fistulae involving female genital tract**
  EXCLUDES 1   vesicointestinal fistulae (N32.1)
  - **N82.0** **Vesicovaginal fistula** ♀ *[handwritten: vesico = bladder]*
  - **N82.1** **Other female urinary-genital tract fistulae** ♀
    Cervicovesical fistula
    Ureterovaginal fistula
    Urethrovaginal fistula *[handwritten: urethra]*
    Uteroureteric fistula
    Uterovesical fistula
    AHA: 2017,3Q,3
  - **N82.2** **Fistula of vagina to** small **intestine** ♀
  - **N82.3** **Fistula of vagina to** large **intestine** ♀
    Rectovaginal fistula *[handwritten: recto]*
  - **N82.4** **Other female intestinal-genital tract fistulae** ♀
    Intestinouterine fistula
  - **N82.5** **Female** genital tract-skin **fistulae** ♀
    Uterus to abdominal wall fistula
    Vaginoperineal fistula
  - **N82.8** **Other female genital tract fistulae** ♀
  - **N82.9** **Female genital tract fistula, unspecified** ♀
- ✓4ᵗʰ **N83** **Noninflammatory disorders of ovary, fallopian tube and broad ligament**
  EXCLUDES 2   hydrosalpinx (N70.1-)
  AHA: 2016,4Q,46
  - ✓5ᵗʰ **N83.0** **Follicular cyst of ovary**
    Cyst of graafian follicle
    Hemorrhagic follicular cyst (of ovary)
    - **N83.00** **Follicular cyst of ovary, unspecified side** ♀
    - **N83.01** **Follicular cyst of** right **ovary** ♀
    - **N83.02** **Follicular cyst of** left **ovary** ♀
  - ✓5ᵗʰ **N83.1** **Corpus luteum cyst**
    Hemorrhagic corpus luteum cyst
    AHA: 2022,1Q,23
    - **N83.10** **Corpus luteum cyst of ovary, unspecified side** ♀
    - **N83.11** **Corpus luteum cyst of** right **ovary** ♀
    - **N83.12** **Corpus luteum cyst of** left **ovary** ♀

[handwritten notes in margin: "Stage II vaginal vault prolapse exclude N81.)" ; "(prolapse uterine complete)" ; "N81.2" "+ N81.6 can be..." ; "same"]

√5ᵗʰ **N83.2** **Other and unspecified ovarian cysts**
- EXCLUDES 1   *developmental ovarian cyst (Q50.1)*
  - *neoplastic ovarian cyst (D27.-)*
  - *polycystic ovarian syndrome (E28.2)*
  - *Stein-Leventhal syndrome (E28.2)*
- **AHA:** 2022,1Q,23

√6ᵗʰ **N83.20** **Unspecified ovarian cysts**
- **N83.201** Unspecified ovarian cyst, right side ♀
- **N83.202** Unspecified ovarian cyst, left side ♀
- **N83.209** Unspecified ovarian cyst, unspecified side ♀
  - Ovarian cyst, NOS

√6ᵗʰ **N83.29** **Other ovarian cysts**
- Retention cyst of ovary
- Simple cyst of ovary
- **N83.291** Other ovarian cyst, right side ♀
- **N83.292** Other ovarian cyst, left side ♀
- **N83.299** Other ovarian cyst, unspecified side ♀

√5ᵗʰ **N83.3** **Acquired atrophy of ovary and fallopian tube**

√6ᵗʰ **N83.31** **Acquired atrophy of ovary**
- **N83.311** Acquired atrophy of right ovary ♀
- **N83.312** Acquired atrophy of left ovary ♀
- **N83.319** Acquired atrophy of ovary, unspecified side ♀
  - Acquired atrophy of ovary, NOS

√6ᵗʰ **N83.32** **Acquired atrophy of fallopian tube**
- **N83.321** Acquired atrophy of right fallopian tube ♀
- **N83.322** Acquired atrophy of left fallopian tube ♀
- **N83.329** Acquired atrophy of fallopian tube, unspecified side ♀
  - Acquired atrophy of fallopian tube, NOS

√6ᵗʰ **N83.33** **Acquired atrophy of ovary and fallopian tube**
- **N83.331** Acquired atrophy of right ovary and fallopian tube ♀
- **N83.332** Acquired atrophy of left ovary and fallopian tube ♀
- **N83.339** Acquired atrophy of ovary and fallopian tube, unspecified side ♀
  - Acquired atrophy of ovary and fallopian tube, NOS

√5ᵗʰ **N83.4** **Prolapse and hernia of ovary and fallopian tube**
- **N83.40** Prolapse and hernia of ovary and fallopian tube, unspecified side ♀
  - Prolapse and hernia of ovary and fallopian tube, NOS
- **N83.41** Prolapse and hernia of right ovary and fallopian tube ♀
- **N83.42** Prolapse and hernia of left ovary and fallopian tube ♀

√5ᵗʰ **N83.5** **Torsion of ovary, ovarian pedicle and fallopian tube**
- Torsion of accessory tube

√6ᵗʰ **N83.51** **Torsion of ovary and ovarian pedicle**
- **N83.511** Torsion of right ovary and ovarian pedicle ♀
- **N83.512** Torsion of left ovary and ovarian pedicle ♀
- **N83.519** Torsion of ovary and ovarian pedicle, unspecified side ♀
  - Torsion of ovary and ovarian pedicle, NOS

√6ᵗʰ **N83.52** **Torsion of fallopian tube**
- Torsion of hydatid of Morgagni
- **N83.521** Torsion of right fallopian tube ♀
- **N83.522** Torsion of left fallopian tube ♀
- **N83.529** Torsion of fallopian tube, unspecified side ♀
  - Torsion of fallopian tube, NOS

N83.53 Torsion of ovary, ovarian pedicle and fallopian tube ♀

N83.6 **Hematosalpinx**
- EXCLUDES 1   *hematosalpinx (with) (in):*
  - *hematocolpos (N89.7)*
  - *hematometra (N85.7)*
  - *tubal pregnancy (O00.1-)*

N83.7 **Hematoma of broad ligament** ♀

N83.8 **Other noninflammatory disorders of ovary, fallopian tube and broad ligament** ♀
- Broad ligament laceration syndrome [Allen-Masters]

N83.9 **Noninflammatory disorder of ovary, fallopian tube and broad ligament, unspecified** ♀

√4ᵗʰ **N84** **Polyp of female genital tract**
- EXCLUDES 1   *adenomatous polyp (D28.-)*
  - *placental polyp (O90.89)*

N84.0 **Polyp of corpus uteri** ♀
- Polyp of endometrium
- Polyp of uterus NOS
- EXCLUDES 1   *polypoid endometrial hyperplasia (N85.0-)*

N84.1 **Polyp of cervix uteri** ♀
- Mucous polyp of cervix

N84.2 **Polyp of vagina** ♀

N84.3 **Polyp of vulva** ♀
- Polyp of labia

N84.8 **Polyp of other parts of female genital tract** ♀

N84.9 **Polyp of female genital tract, unspecified** ♀

√4ᵗʰ **N85** **Other noninflammatory disorders of uterus, except cervix**
- EXCLUDES 1   *endometriosis (N80.-)*
  - *inflammatory diseases of uterus (N71.-)*
  - *noninflammatory disorders of cervix, except malposition (N86-N88)*
  - *polyp of corpus uteri (N84.0)*
  - *uterine prolapse (N81.-)*

√5ᵗʰ **N85.0** **Endometrial hyperplasia**

N85.00 **Endometrial hyperplasia, unspecified** ♀
- Hyperplasia (adenomatous) (cystic) (glandular) of endometrium
- Hyperplastic endometritis

N85.01 **Benign endometrial hyperplasia** ♀
- Endometrial hyperplasia (complex) (simple) without atypia

N85.02 **Endometrial intraepithelial neoplasia [EIN]** ♀
- Endometrial hyperplasia with atypia
- EXCLUDES 1   *malignant neoplasm of endometrium (with endometrial intraepithelial neoplasia [EIN]) (C54.1)*

N85.2 **Hypertrophy of uterus** ♀
- Bulky or enlarged uterus
- EXCLUDES 1   *puerperal hypertrophy of uterus (O90.89)*

N85.3 **Subinvolution of uterus** ♀
- EXCLUDES 1   *puerperal subinvolution of uterus (O90.89)*

N85.4 **Malposition of uterus** ♀
- Anteversion of uterus
- Retroflexion of uterus
- Retroversion of uterus
- EXCLUDES 1   *malposition of uterus complicating pregnancy, labor or delivery (O34.5-, O65.5)*

N85.5 **Inversion of uterus** ♀
- EXCLUDES 1   *current obstetric trauma (O71.2)*
  - *postpartum inversion of uterus (O71.2)*
- **DEF:** Abnormality in which the uterus turns inside out.

Inversion of Uterus

Uterus

N85.6 **Intrauterine synechiae** ♀

| HCC CMS-HCC | Rx Rx HCC | ESRD ESRD HCC | COM Commercial HCC | N Newborn: 0 | P Pediatric: 0-17 | M Maternity: 9-64 | A Adult: 15-124 |

882

ICD-10-CM 2023

N85.7 Hematometra ♀
Hematosalpinx with hematometra
EXCLUDES 1   hematometra with hematocolpos (N89.7)
DEF: Accumulation of blood within the uterus.

N85.8 Other specified noninflammatory disorders of uterus ♀ *Atrophic*
Atrophy of uterus, acquired
Fibrosis of uterus NOS

N85.9 Noninflammatory disorder of uterus, unspecified ♀
Disorder of uterus NOS

● **N85.A Isthmocele**
Isthmocele (non-pregnant state)
Code also any associated conditions such as:
abnormal uterine and vaginal bleeding, unspecified (N93.9)
female infertility of uterine origin (N97.2)
pelvic and perineal pain (R10.2)
EXCLUDES 1   maternal care for cesarean scar defect (isthmocele)
(O34.22)

N86 Erosion and ectropion of cervix uteri ♀
Decubitus (trophic) ulcer of cervix
Eversion of cervix
EXCLUDES 1   erosion and ectropion of cervix with cervicitis (N72)

✓4ᵗʰ N87 Dysplasia of cervix uteri
EXCLUDES 1   abnormal results from cervical cytologic examination without
histologic confirmation (R87.61-)
carcinoma in situ of cervix uteri (D06.-)
cervical intraepithelial neoplasia III [CIN III] (D06.-)
HGSIL of cervix (R87.613)
severe dysplasia of cervix uteri (D06.-)

N87.0 Mild cervical dysplasia
Cervical intraepithelial neoplasia I [CIN I]

CIN I

N87.1 Moderate cervical dysplasia ♀
Cervical intraepithelial neoplasia II [CIN II]

CIN II

N87.9 Dysplasia of cervix uteri, unspecified ♀
Anaplasia of cervix
Cervical atypism
Cervical dysplasia NOS

Severe dysplasia D06-

✓4ᵗʰ N88 Other noninflammatory disorders of cervix uteri
EXCLUDES 2   inflammatory disease of cervix (N72)
polyp of cervix (N84.1)

N88.0 Leukoplakia of cervix uteri ♀

N88.1 Old laceration of cervix uteri ♀
Adhesions of cervix
EXCLUDES 1   current obstetric trauma (O71.3)

N88.2 Stricture and stenosis of cervix uteri ♀
EXCLUDES 1   stricture and stenosis of cervix uteri complicating
labor (O65.5)

N88.3 Incompetence of cervix uteri ♀
Investigation and management of (suspected) cervical
incompetence in a nonpregnant woman
EXCLUDES 1   cervical incompetence complicating pregnancy
(O34.3-)
DEF: Inadequate functioning of the cervix marked by abnormal
widening during pregnancy and causing premature birth or
miscarriage.

N88.4 Hypertrophic elongation of cervix uteri ♀

N88.8 Other specified noninflammatory disorders of cervix uteri ♀
EXCLUDES 1   current obstetric trauma (O71.3)

N88.9 Noninflammatory disorder of cervix uteri, unspecified ♀

✓4ᵗʰ N89 Other noninflammatory disorders of vagina
EXCLUDES 1   abnormal results from vaginal cytologic examination without
histologic confirmation (R87.62-)
carcinoma in situ of vagina (D07.2)
HGSIL of vagina (R87.623)
inflammation of vagina (N76.-)
senile (atrophic) vaginitis (N95.2)
severe dysplasia of vagina (D07.2)
trichomonal leukorrhea (A59.00)
vaginal intraepithelial neoplasia [VAIN], grade III (D07.2)

N89.0 Mild vaginal dysplasia
Vaginal intraepithelial neoplasia [VAIN], grade I

D07- III stem

N89.1 Moderate vaginal dysplasia ♀
Vaginal intraepithelial neoplasia [VAIN], grade II

Vagina

N89.3 Dysplasia of vagina, unspecified ♀

N89.4 Leukoplakia of vagina ♀   *Vagina*

N89.5 Stricture and atresia of vagina ♀
Vaginal adhesions
Vaginal stenosis
EXCLUDES 1   congenital atresia or stricture (Q52.4)
postprocedural adhesions of vagina (N99.2)

N89.6 Tight hymenal ring ♀
Rigid hymen
Tight introitus
EXCLUDES 1   imperforate hymen (Q52.3)

N89.7 Hematocolpos ♀
Hematocolpos with hematometra or hematosalpinx
AHA: 2016,4Q,58

N89.8 Other specified noninflammatory disorders of vagina ♀
Leukorrhea NOS
Old vaginal laceration   *Hematoma of vagina*
Pessary ulcer of vagina   *(non obstetrical)*
EXCLUDES 1   current obstetric trauma (O70.-, O71.4, O71.7-O71.8)
old laceration involving muscles of pelvic floor
(N81.8)

N89.9 Noninflammatory disorder of vagina, unspecified ♀

✓4ᵗʰ N90 Other noninflammatory disorders of vulva and perineum
EXCLUDES 1   anogenital (venereal) warts (A63.0)
carcinoma in situ of vulva (D07.1)
condyloma acuminatum (A63.0)
current obstetric trauma (O70.-, O71.7-O71.8)
inflammation of vulva (N76.-)
severe dysplasia of vulva (D07.1)
vulvar intraepithelial neoplasm III [VIN III] (D07.1)

N90.0 Mild vulvar dysplasia ♀
Vulvar intraepithelial neoplasia [VIN], grade I

N90.1 Moderate vulvar dysplasia ♀
Vulvar intraepithelial neoplasia [VIN], grade II

N90.3 Dysplasia of vulva, unspecified ♀

N90.4 Leukoplakia of vulva ♀   *vulva*
Dystrophy of vulva
Kraurosis of vulva
Lichen sclerosus of external female genital organs

N90.5 Atrophy of vulva ♀
Stenosis of vulva

✓5ᵗʰ N90.6 Hypertrophy of vulva
AHA: 2016,4Q,46

N90.60 Unspecified hypertrophy of vulva ♀
Unspecified hypertrophy of labia

N90.61 Childhood asymmetric labium majus enlargement
CALME

N90.69 Other specified hypertrophy of vulva ♀
Other specified hypertrophy of labia

N90.7 Vulvar cyst ♀

✓5ᵗʰ N90.8 Other specified noninflammatory disorders of vulva and perineum

✓6ᵗʰ N90.81 Female genital mutilation status
Female genital cutting status

N90.810 Female genital mutilation status, unspecified ♀
Female genital cutting status, unspecified
Female genital mutilation status NOS

N90.811 Female genital mutilation Type I status ♀
Clitorectomy status
Female genital cutting Type I status

N90.812 Female genital mutilation Type II status ♀
Clitorectomy with excision of labia minora status
Female genital cutting Type II status

N90.813 Female genital mutilation Type III status ♀
Female genital cutting Type III status
Infibulation status

Chapter 14. Diseases of the Genitourinary System

N90.818   **Other female genital mutilation status** ♀
Female genital cutting Type IV status
Female genital mutilation Type IV status
Other female genital cutting status

N90.89   **Other specified noninflammatory disorders of vulva and perineum** *(non obstetric)*
Hematoma vulva lesion
Adhesions of vulva
Hypertrophy of clitoris

N90.9   **Noninflammatory disorder of vulva and perineum, unspecified** ♀

✓4ᵗʰ **N91**   **Absent, scanty and rare menstruation**
   EXCLUDES 1   *ovarian dysfunction (E28.-)*   *>16y*

N91.0   **Primary amenorrhea** ♀
N91.1   **Secondary amenorrhea** *stop >3m*   *or >6m if irregular* ♀
N91.2   **Amenorrhea, unspecified** *regular* ♀
N91.3   **Primary oligomenorrhea** ♀
N91.4   **Secondary oligomenorrhea** ♀
N91.5   **Oligomenorrhea, unspecified** ♀
Hypomenorrhea NOS

✓4ᵗʰ **N92**   **Excessive, frequent and irregular menstruation**
   EXCLUDES 1   *postmenopausal bleeding (N95.0)*
     precocious puberty (menstruation) (E30.1)

N92.0   **Excessive and frequent menstruation** with regular cycle ♀
heavy prolonged period
Heavy periods NOS
Menorrhagia NOS   *N84O if Polyps*
Polymenorrhea

N92.1   **Excessive and frequent menstruation** with irregular cycle ♀
Metrorrhagia
Irregular intermenstrual bleeding
Irregular, shortened intervals between menstrual bleeding
Menometrorrhagia   *intermenstrual (irregular)*
Metrorrhagia

N92.2   **Excessive menstruation at puberty** P ♀
Excessive bleeding associated with onset of menstrual periods
Pubertal menorrhagia
Puberty bleeding

N92.3   **Ovulation bleeding** ♀
Regular intermenstrual bleeding

N92.4   **Excessive bleeding in the premenopausal period** ♀
Climacteric menorrhagia or metrorrhagia
Menopausal menorrhagia or metrorrhagia
Perimenopausal bleeding
Perimenopausal menorrhagia or metrorrhagia
Preclimacteric menorrhagia or metrorrhagia
Premenopausal menorrhagia or metrorrhagia

N92.5   **Other specified irregular menstruation** ♀
N92.6   **Irregular menstruation, unspecified** ♀
Irregular bleeding NOS
Irregular periods NOS
   EXCLUDES 1   *irregular menstruation with:*
     lengthened intervals or scanty bleeding (N91.3-N91.5)
     shortened intervals or excessive bleeding (N92.1)

✓4ᵗʰ **N93**   **Other abnormal uterine and vaginal bleeding**
   EXCLUDES 1   *neonatal vaginal hemorrhage (P54.6)*
     precocious puberty (menstruation) (E30.1)
     pseudomenses (P54.6)

N93.0   **Postcoital and contact bleeding** ♀
N93.1   **Pre-pubertal vaginal bleeding** ♀
AHA: 2016,4Q,47
N93.8   **Other specified abnormal uterine and vaginal bleeding** ♀
Dysfunctional or functional uterine or vaginal bleeding NOS
N93.9   **Abnormal uterine and vaginal bleeding, unspecified** ♀

✓4ᵗʰ **N94**   **Pain and other conditions associated with female genital organs and menstrual cycle**
N94.0   **Mittelschmerz** ♀
DEF: One-sided, lower abdominal pain occurring between menstrual periods that is associated with ovulation.
✓5ᵗʰ **N94.1**   **Dyspareunia** *pain in sex*
   EXCLUDES 1   *psychogenic dyspareunia (F52.6)*
AHA: 2016,4Q,47
N94.10   **Unspecified dyspareunia** ♀
N94.11   **Superficial (introital) dyspareunia** ♀

N94.12   **Deep dyspareunia** ♀
N94.19   **Other specified dyspareunia** ♀
N94.2   **Vaginismus** ♀
   EXCLUDES 1   *psychogenic vaginismus (F52.5)*
DEF: Spontaneous contractions of the muscles surrounding the vagina, causing it to constrict or close.
N94.3   **Premenstrual tension syndrome**
Code also associated menstrual migraine (G43.82-, G43.83-)
   EXCLUDES 1   *premenstrual dysphoric disorder (F32.81)*
N94.4   **Primary dysmenorrhea** ♀
N94.5   **Secondary dysmenorrhea** ♀
N94.6   **Dysmenorrhea, unspecified** ♀
   EXCLUDES 1   *psychogenic dysmenorrhea (F45.8)*

✓5ᵗʰ **N94.8**   **Other specified conditions associated with female genital organs and menstrual cycle**
✓6ᵗʰ **N94.81**   **Vulvodynia**
N94.810   **Vulvar vestibulitis** ♀
N94.818   **Other vulvodynia** ♀
N94.819   **Vulvodynia, unspecified** ♀
Vulvodynia NOS
N94.89   **Other specified conditions associated with female genital organs and menstrual cycle** ♀
abdominal pain
DEF: Hydrocele: Serous fluid that collects in the canal of Nuck in females.
N94.9   **Unspecified condition associated with female genital organs and menstrual cycle** ♀

✓4ᵗʰ **N95**   **Menopausal and other perimenopausal disorders**
Menopausal and other perimenopausal disorders due to naturally occurring (age-related) menopause and perimenopause
   EXCLUDES 1   *excessive bleeding in the premenopausal period (N92.4)*
     menopausal and perimenopausal disorders due to artificial or premature menopause (E89.4-, E28.31-)
     premature menopause (E28.31-)
   EXCLUDES 2   *postmenopausal osteoporosis (M81.0-)*
     postmenopausal osteoporosis with current pathological fracture (M80.0-)
     postmenopausal urethritis (N34.2)
N95.0   **Postmenopausal bleeding** ♀
N95.1   **Menopausal and female climacteric states** ♀
Symptoms such as flushing, sleeplessness, headache, lack of concentration, associated with natural (age-related) menopause
Use additional code for associated symptoms
   EXCLUDES 1   *asymptomatic menopausal state (Z78.0)*
     symptoms associated with artificial menopause (E89.41)
     symptoms associated with premature menopause (E28.310)
N95.2   **Postmenopausal atrophic vaginitis** ♀
Senile (atrophic) vaginitis
N95.8   **Other specified menopausal and perimenopausal disorders** ♀
N95.9   **Unspecified menopausal and perimenopausal disorder** ♀

N96   **Recurrent pregnancy loss** ♀
Investigation or care in a nonpregnant woman with history of recurrent pregnancy loss
   EXCLUDES 1   *recurrent pregnancy loss with current pregnancy (O26.2-)*

✓4ᵗʰ **N97**   **Female infertility**
   INCLUDES   inability to achieve a pregnancy
     sterility, female NOS
   EXCLUDES 2   *female infertility associated with:*
     hypopituitarism (E23.0)
     Stein-Leventhal syndrome (E28.2)
     incompetence of cervix uteri (N88.3)
DEF: Infertility: Inability to conceive for at least one year with regular intercourse.
DEF: Primary infertility: Infertility occurring in patients who have never conceived.
DEF: Secondary infertility: Infertility occurring in patients who have previously conceived.
N97.0   **Female infertility** associated with anovulation ♀
AHA: 2022,2Q,16

| HCC CMS-HCC | Rx Rx HCC | ESR ESRD HCC | COM Commercial HCC | N Newborn: 0 | P Pediatric: 0-17 | M Maternity: 9-64 | A Adult: 15-124 |

N97.1 Female infertility of tubal origin ♀
Female infertility associated with congenital anomaly of tube
Female infertility due to tubal block
Female infertility due to tubal occlusion
Female infertility due to tubal stenosis

N97.2 Female infertility of uterine origin ♀
Female infertility associated with congenital anomaly of uterus
Female infertility due to nonimplantation of ovum

N97.8 Female infertility of other origin ♀
AHA: 2022,2Q,15

N97.9 Female infertility, unspecified ♀

✓4ᵗʰ **N98 Complications associated with artificial fertilization**

N98.Ø Infection associated with artificial insemination ♀

N98.1 Hyperstimulation of ovaries ♀
Hyperstimulation of ovaries NOS
Hyperstimulation of ovaries associated with induced ovulation

N98.2 Complications of attempted introduction of fertilized ovum following in vitro fertilization ♀

N98.3 Complications of attempted introduction of embryo in embryo transfer ♀

N98.8 Other complications associated with artificial fertilization ♀

N98.9 Complication associated with artificial fertilization, unspecified ♀

Intraoperative and postprocedural complications and disorders of genitourinary system, not elsewhere classified (N99)

✓4ᵗʰ **N99 Intraoperative and postprocedural complications and disorders of genitourinary system, not elsewhere classified**
EXCLUDES 2   irradiation cystitis (N3Ø.4-)
postoophorectomy osteoporosis with current pathological fracture (M8Ø.8-)
postoophorectomy osteoporosis without current pathological fracture (M81.8)

N99.Ø Postprocedural (acute) (chronic) kidney failure
Use additional code to type of kidney disease

✓5ᵗʰ **N99.1** Postprocedural urethral stricture
Postcatheterization urethral stricture

✓6ᵗʰ **N99.11** Postprocedural urethral stricture, male
AHA: 2016,4Q,47-48

N99.11Ø Postprocedural urethral stricture, male, meatal ♂

N99.111 Postprocedural bulbous urethral stricture, male ♂

N99.112 Postprocedural membranous urethral stricture, male ♂

N99.113 Postprocedural anterior bulbous urethral stricture, male ♂

N99.114 Postprocedural urethral stricture, male, unspecified ♂

N99.115 Postprocedural fossa navicularis urethral stricture ♂

N99.116 Postprocedural urethral stricture, male, overlapping sites ♂

N99.12 Postprocedural urethral stricture, female ♀

N99.2 Postprocedural adhesions of vagina ♀

N99.3 Prolapse of vaginal vault after hysterectomy ♀

N99.4 Postprocedural pelvic peritoneal adhesions
EXCLUDES 2   pelvic peritoneal adhesions NOS (N73.6)
postinfective pelvic peritoneal adhesions (N73.6)

✓5ᵗʰ **N99.5** Complications of stoma of urinary tract
EXCLUDES 2   mechanical complication of urinary catheter (T83.Ø-)
AHA: 2016,4Q,48

✓6ᵗʰ **N99.51** Complication of cystostomy
N99.51Ø Cystostomy hemorrhage `HCC` `ESR`
N99.511 Cystostomy infection `HCC` `ESR`
N99.512 Cystostomy malfunction `HCC` `ESR`
N99.518 Other cystostomy complication `HCC` `ESR`

✓6ᵗʰ **N99.52** Complication of incontinent external stoma of urinary tract
N99.52Ø Hemorrhage of incontinent external stoma of urinary tract `HCC` `ESR`
N99.521 Infection of incontinent external stoma of urinary tract `HCC` `ESR`

N99.522 Malfunction of incontinent external stoma of urinary tract `HCC` `ESR`

N99.523 Herniation of incontinent stoma of urinary tract `HCC` `ESR`

N99.524 Stenosis of incontinent stoma of urinary tract `HCC` `ESR`

N99.528 Other complication of incontinent external stoma of urinary tract `HCC` `ESR`

✓6ᵗʰ **N99.53** Complication of continent stoma of urinary tract
N99.53Ø Hemorrhage of continent stoma of urinary tract `HCC` `ESR`
N99.531 Infection of continent stoma of urinary tract `HCC` `ESR`
N99.532 Malfunction of continent stoma of urinary tract `HCC` `ESR`
N99.533 Herniation of continent stoma of urinary tract `HCC` `ESR`
N99.534 Stenosis of continent stoma of urinary tract `HCC` `ESR`
N99.538 Other complication of continent stoma of urinary tract `HCC` `ESR`

✓5ᵗʰ **N99.6** Intraoperative hemorrhage and hematoma of a genitourinary system organ or structure complicating a procedure
EXCLUDES 1   intraoperative hemorrhage and hematoma of a genitourinary system organ or structure due to accidental puncture or laceration during a procedure (N99.7-)

N99.61 Intraoperative hemorrhage and hematoma of a genitourinary system organ or structure complicating a genitourinary system procedure

N99.62 Intraoperative hemorrhage and hematoma of a genitourinary system organ or structure complicating other procedure

✓5ᵗʰ **N99.7** Accidental puncture and laceration of a genitourinary system organ or structure during a procedure
N99.71 Accidental puncture and laceration of a genitourinary system organ or structure during a genitourinary system procedure
N99.72 Accidental puncture and laceration of a genitourinary system organ or structure during other procedure

✓5ᵗʰ **N99.8** Other intraoperative and postprocedural complications and disorders of genitourinary system
AHA: 2016,4Q,9-10
N99.81 Other intraoperative complications of genitourinary system

✓6ᵗʰ **N99.82** Postprocedural hemorrhage of a genitourinary system organ or structure following a procedure
N99.82Ø Postprocedural hemorrhage of a genitourinary system organ or structure following a genitourinary system procedure
N99.821 Postprocedural hemorrhage of a genitourinary system organ or structure following other procedure

N99.83 Residual ovary syndrome ♀

✓6ᵗʰ **N99.84** Postprocedural hematoma and seroma of a genitourinary system organ or structure following a procedure
N99.84Ø Postprocedural hematoma of a genitourinary system organ or structure following a genitourinary system procedure
N99.841 Postprocedural hematoma of a genitourinary system organ or structure following other procedure
N99.842 Postprocedural seroma of a genitourinary system organ or structure following a genitourinary system procedure
N99.843 Postprocedural seroma of a genitourinary system organ or structure following other procedure

N99.85 Post endometrial ablation syndrome ♀
AHA: 2019,4Q,12

N99.89 Other postprocedural complications and disorders of genitourinary system

Chapter 15. Pregnancy, Childbirth, and the Puerperium (O00–O9A)

Chapter-specific Guidelines with Coding Examples

The chapter-specific guidelines from the ICD-10-CM Official Guidelines for Coding and Reporting have been provided below. Along with these guidelines are coding examples, contained in the shaded boxes, that have been developed to help illustrate the coding and/or sequencing guidance found in these guidelines.

a. General rules for obstetric cases

1) Codes from Chapter 15 and sequencing priority

Obstetric cases require codes from chapter 15, codes in the range O00–O9A, Pregnancy, Childbirth, and the Puerperium. Chapter 15 codes have sequencing priority over codes from other chapters. Additional codes from other chapters may be used in conjunction with chapter 15 codes to further specify conditions. Should the provider document that the pregnancy is incidental to the encounter, then code Z33.1, Pregnant state, incidental, should be used in place of any chapter 15 codes. It is the provider's responsibility to state that the condition being treated is not affecting the pregnancy.

> Bladder abscess in pregnant patient at 25 weeks' gestation
>
> **O23.12**   **Infections of bladder in pregnancy, second trimester**
>
> **N30.80**   **Other cystitis without hematuria**
>
> **Z3A.25**   **25 weeks gestation of pregnancy**
>
> *Explanation:* The documentation does not indicate that the pregnancy is incidental or in any way unaffected by the bladder abscess; therefore, an obstetrics code should be sequenced first. An additional code was provided to identify the specific bladder condition as this information is not called out specifically in the obstetrics code.

2) Chapter 15 codes used only on the maternal record

Chapter 15 codes are to be used only on the maternal record, never on the record of the newborn.

3) Final character for trimester

The majority of codes in Chapter 15 have a final character indicating the trimester of pregnancy. The timeframes for the trimesters are indicated at the beginning of the chapter. If trimester is not a component of a code, it is because the condition always occurs in a specific trimester, or the concept of trimester of pregnancy is not applicable. Certain codes have characters for only certain trimesters because the condition does not occur in all trimesters, but it may occur in more than just one. Assignment of the final character for trimester should be based on the provider's documentation of the trimester (or number of weeks) for the current admission/encounter. This applies to the assignment of trimester for pre-existing conditions as well as those that develop during or are due to the pregnancy. The provider's documentation of the number of weeks may be used to assign the appropriate code identifying the trimester.

> Pregnant patient at 21 weeks' gestation admitted with excessive vomiting
>
> **O21.2**   **Late vomiting of pregnancy**
>
> **Z3A.21**   **21 weeks gestation of pregnancy**
>
> *Explanation:* Category O21 classifies vomiting in pregnancy. Although code selection is based on whether the vomiting is before or after 20 completed weeks, these codes are not further classified by trimester. If vomiting only in the second trimester was documented, the provider should be queried for the specific week of gestation, as this will affect code selection.

Whenever delivery occurs during the current admission, and there is an "in childbirth" option for the obstetric complication being coded, the "in childbirth" code should be assigned. When the classification does not provide an obstetric code with an "in childbirth" option, it is appropriate to assign a code describing the current trimester.

4) Selection of trimester for inpatient admissions that encompass more than one trimester

In instances when a patient is admitted to a hospital for complications of pregnancy during one trimester and remains in the hospital into a subsequent trimester, the trimester character for the antepartum complication code should be assigned on the basis of the trimester when the complication developed, not the trimester of the discharge. If the condition developed prior to the current admission/encounter or

represents a pre-existing condition, the trimester character for the trimester at the time of the admission/encounter should be assigned.

5) Unspecified trimester

Each category that includes codes for trimester has a code for "unspecified trimester." The "unspecified trimester" code should rarely be used, such as when the documentation in the record is insufficient to determine the trimester and it is not possible to obtain clarification.

6) 7th character for fetus identification

Where applicable, a 7th character is to be assigned for certain categories (O31, O32, O33.3 - O33.6, O35, O36, O40, O41, O60.1, O60.2, O64, and O69) to identify the fetus for which the complication code applies.

Assign 7th character "0":

- For single gestations.
- When the documentation in the record is insufficient to determine the fetus affected and it is not possible to obtain clarification.
- When it is not possible to clinically determine which fetus is affected.

> Maternal patient with twin gestations is seen after ultrasound identifies fetus B to be in breech presentation
>
> **O32.1XX2**   **Maternal care for breech presentation, fetus 2**
>
> *Explanation:* The documentation indicates that although there are two fetuses, only one fetus is determined to be in breech presentation. Whether fetus 2 or fetus B is used, the coder can assign the seventh character of 2 to identify the second fetus as the one in breech.

7) Completed weeks of gestation

In ICD-10-CM, "completed" weeks of gestation refers to full weeks. For example, if the provider documents gestation at 39 weeks and 6 days, the code for 39 weeks of gestation should be assigned, as the patient has not yet reached 40 completed weeks.

b. Selection of OB principal or first-listed diagnosis

1) Routine outpatient prenatal visits

For routine outpatient prenatal visits when no complications are present, a code from category Z34, Encounter for supervision of normal pregnancy, should be used as the first-listed diagnosis. These codes should not be used in conjunction with chapter 15 codes.

2) Supervision of high-risk pregnancy

Codes from category O09, Supervision of high-risk pregnancy, are intended for use only during the prenatal period. For complications during the labor or delivery episode as a result of a high-risk pregnancy, assign the applicable complication codes from Chapter 15. If there are no complications during the labor or delivery episode, assign code O80, Encounter for full-term uncomplicated delivery.

For routine prenatal outpatient visits for patients with high-risk pregnancies, a code from category O09, Supervision of high-risk pregnancy, should be used as the first-listed diagnosis. Secondary chapter 15 codes may be used in conjunction with these codes if appropriate.

> 36-year-old seen in labor with second child at 39 weeks' gestation, delivered a healthy baby, delivery complicated by tear of fourchette that was repaired
>
> **O70.0**   **First degree perineal laceration during delivery**
>
> **Z3A.39**   **39 weeks gestation of pregnancy**
>
> **Z37.0**   **Single live birth**
>
> Explanation: Although this patient is over 35 and having her second child (elderly multigravida), do not append a code from subcategory O09.52-. A code describing the tear of the fourchette, which complicated the delivery, should be used in addition to the applicable Z codes.

3) Episodes when no delivery occurs

In episodes when no delivery occurs, the principal diagnosis should correspond to the principal complication of the pregnancy which necessitated the encounter. Should more than one complication exist, all of which are treated or monitored, any of the complication codes may be sequenced first.

4) When a delivery occurs

When an obstetric patient is admitted and delivers during that admission, the condition that prompted the admission should be sequenced as the principal diagnosis. If multiple conditions prompted the admission, sequence the one most related to the delivery as the principal diagnosis. A code for any complication of the delivery should be assigned as an additional diagnosis. In cases of cesarean delivery, if the patient was admitted with a condition that resulted in the performance of a cesarean procedure, that condition should be selected as the principal diagnosis. If the reason for the admission was unrelated to the condition resulting in the cesarean delivery, the condition related to the reason for the admission should be selected as the principal diagnosis.

Maternal patient with diet-controlled gestational diabetes was seen at 38 weeks' gestation in obstructed labor due to footling presentation; cesarean performed for the malpresentation

O64.8XX0	Obstructed labor due to other malposition and malpresentation, not applicable or unspecified
O24.420	Gestational diabetes mellitus in childbirth, diet controlled
Z3A.38	38 weeks gestation of pregnancy
Z37.0	Single live birth

Explanation: The obstructed labor necessitated the cesarean procedure.

5) Outcome of delivery

A code from category Z37, Outcome of delivery, should be included on every maternal record when a delivery has occurred. These codes are not to be used on subsequent records or on the newborn record.

c. Pre-existing conditions versus conditions due to the pregnancy

Certain categories in Chapter 15 distinguish between conditions of the mother that existed prior to pregnancy (pre-existing) and those that are a direct result of pregnancy. When assigning codes from Chapter 15, it is important to assess if a condition was pre-existing prior to pregnancy or developed during or due to the pregnancy in order to assign the correct code.

Categories that do not distinguish between pre-existing and pregnancy-related conditions may be used for either. It is acceptable to use codes specifically for the puerperium with codes complicating pregnancy and childbirth if a condition arises postpartum during the delivery encounter.

Type 2 diabetic patient presents at 19 weeks gestation for glucose check. Patient has been taking oral metformin for several years and currently is experiencing no diabetic complications.

O24.112	Pre-existing type 2 diabetes mellitus, in pregnancy, second trimester
E11.9	Type 2 diabetes mellitus without complications
Z79.84	Long term (current) use of oral hypoglycemic drugs

Explanation: The documentation states that the patient has been on a diabetic medication (oral metformin) for several years, indicating the patient was diabetic prior to becoming pregnant. Reporting pre-existing Type 2 diabetes in a pregnant patient requires two codes to capture the condition, a code from category O24 and a code from category E11. A note at E11 indicates that the code for long-term use of oral hypoglycemic drugs should also be reported.

d. Pre-existing hypertension in pregnancy

Category O10, Pre-existing hypertension complicating pregnancy, childbirth and the puerperium, includes codes for hypertensive heart and hypertensive chronic kidney disease. When assigning one of the O10 codes that includes hypertensive heart disease or hypertensive chronic kidney disease, it is necessary to add a secondary code from the appropriate hypertension category to specify the type of heart failure or chronic kidney disease.

See Section I.C.9. Hypertension.

e. Fetal conditions affecting the management of the mother

1) Codes from categories O35 and O36

Codes from categories O35, Maternal care for known or suspected fetal abnormality and damage, and O36, Maternal care for other fetal problems, are assigned only when the fetal condition is actually responsible for modifying the management of the mother, i.e., by requiring diagnostic studies, additional observation, special care, or termination of pregnancy. The fact that the fetal condition exists does not justify assigning a code from this series to the mother's record.

A patient with twin gestation is seen for spotting 15 weeks into her pregnancy; the doctors also suspect fetal hydrocephalus. Patient is instructed to return in one week for additional diagnostic testing, sooner if the problem worsens.

O35.00X0	Maternal care for (suspected) central nervous system malformation or damage in fetus, unspecified, not applicable or unspecified
O26.852	Spotting complicating pregnancy, second trimester
Z3A.15	15 weeks gestation of pregnancy

Explanation: Whether the fetal hydrocephalus was suspected or confirmed, an additional code is warranted for this condition since documentation indicates the patient is to return sooner than her routine visit for further testing.

2) In utero surgery

In cases when surgery is performed on the fetus, a diagnosis code from category O35, Maternal care for known or suspected fetal abnormality and damage, should be assigned identifying the fetal condition. Assign the appropriate procedure code for the procedure performed.

No code from Chapter 16, the perinatal codes, should be used on the mother's record to identify fetal conditions. Surgery performed in utero on a fetus is still to be coded as an obstetric encounter.

f. HIV infection in pregnancy, childbirth and the puerperium

During pregnancy, childbirth or the puerperium, a patient admitted because of an HIV-related illness should receive a principal diagnosis from subcategory O98.7-, Human immunodeficiency [HIV] disease complicating pregnancy, childbirth and the puerperium, followed by the code(s) for the HIV-related illness(es).

Patients with asymptomatic HIV infection status admitted during pregnancy, childbirth, or the puerperium should receive codes of O98.7- and Z21, Asymptomatic human immunodeficiency virus [HIV] infection status.

A previously asymptomatic HIV patient who is 13 weeks pregnant is evaluated for HIV-related candidal bronchitis

O98.711	Human immunodeficiency virus [HIV] disease complicating pregnancy, first trimester
B20	Human immunodeficiency virus [HIV] disease
B37.1	Pulmonary candidiasis
Z3A.13	13 weeks gestation of pregnancy

Explanation: Because candidal bronchitis is an AIDS-related condition, this patient is now considered to have HIV disease. An obstetrics code indicating that HIV is complicating the pregnancy is coded first, followed by B20 for HIV disease as well as a code for the candidal bronchitis.

g. Diabetes mellitus in pregnancy

Diabetes mellitus is a significant complicating factor in pregnancy. Pregnant patients who are diabetic should be assigned a code from category O24, Diabetes mellitus in pregnancy, childbirth, and the puerperium, first, followed by the appropriate diabetes code(s) (E08-E13) from Chapter 4.

h. Long term use of insulin and oral hypoglycemics

See section I.C.4.a.3 for information on the long term-use of insulin and oral hypoglycemics.

i. Gestational (pregnancy induced) diabetes

Gestational (pregnancy induced) diabetes can occur during the second and third trimester of pregnancy in patients who were not diabetic prior to pregnancy. Gestational diabetes can cause complications in the pregnancy similar to those of pre-existing diabetes mellitus. It also puts the patient at greater risk of developing diabetes after the pregnancy.

Codes for gestational diabetes are in subcategory O24.4, Gestational diabetes mellitus. No other code from category O24, Diabetes mellitus in pregnancy, childbirth, and the puerperium, should be used with a code from O24.4.

The codes under subcategory O24.4 include diet controlled, insulin controlled, and controlled by oral hypoglycemic drugs. If a patient with gestational diabetes is treated with both diet and insulin, only the code for insulin-controlled is required. If a patient with gestational diabetes is treated with both diet and oral hypoglycemic medications, only the code for "controlled by oral hypoglycemic drugs" is required. Codes Z79.4, Long-term (current) use of insulin, Z79.84, Long-term (current) use of oral hypoglycemic drugs, **and Z79.85, Long-term (current) use of injectable non-insulin antidiabetic drugs,** should not be assigned with codes from subcategory O24.4.

An abnormal glucose tolerance in pregnancy is assigned a code from subcategory O99.81, Abnormal glucose complicating pregnancy, childbirth, and the puerperium.

j. Sepsis and septic shock complicating abortion, pregnancy, childbirth and the puerperium

When assigning a chapter 15 code for sepsis complicating abortion, pregnancy, childbirth, and the puerperium, a code for the specific type of infection should be assigned as an additional diagnosis. If severe sepsis is present, a code from subcategory R65.2, Severe sepsis, and code(s) for associated organ dysfunction(s) should also be assigned as additional diagnoses.

Patient is seen several days after a miscarriage with sepsis; cultures return MSSA	
O03.87	**Sepsis following complete or unspecified spontaneous abortion**
B95.61	**Methicillin susceptible Staphylococcus aureus infection as the cause of diseases classified elsewhere**

Explanation: The type of infection that caused this patient to become septic was methicillin susceptible *Staphylococcus aureus* (MSSA), which as a secondary code helps capture all aspects related to this patient's septic condition.

k. Puerperal sepsis

Code O85, Puerperal sepsis, should be assigned with a secondary code to identify the causal organism (e.g., for a bacterial infection, assign a code from category B95-B96, Bacterial infections in conditions classified elsewhere). A code from category A40, Streptococcal sepsis, or A41, Other sepsis, should not be used for puerperal sepsis. If applicable, use additional codes to identify severe sepsis (R65.2-) and any associated acute organ dysfunction.

Code O85 should not be assigned for sepsis following an obstetrical procedure (See Section I.C.1.d.5.b., Sepsis due to a postprocedural infection).

l. Alcohol, tobacco and drug use during pregnancy, childbirth and the puerperium

1) Alcohol use during pregnancy, childbirth and the puerperium

Codes under subcategory O99.31, Alcohol use complicating pregnancy, childbirth, and the puerperium, should be assigned for any pregnancy case when a patient uses alcohol during the pregnancy or postpartum. A secondary code from category F10, Alcohol related disorders, should also be assigned to identify manifestations of the alcohol use.

2) Tobacco use during pregnancy, childbirth and the puerperium

Codes under subcategory O99.33, Smoking (tobacco) complicating pregnancy, childbirth, and the puerperium, should be assigned for any pregnancy case when a patient uses any type of tobacco product during the pregnancy or postpartum.

A secondary code from category F17, Nicotine dependence, should also be assigned to identify the type of nicotine dependence.

3) Drug use during pregnancy, childbirth and the puerperium

Codes under subcategory O99.32, Drug use complicating pregnancy, childbirth, and the puerperium, should be assigned for any pregnancy case when a patient uses drugs during the pregnancy or postpartum. This can involve illegal drugs, or inappropriate use or abuse of prescription drugs. Secondary code(s) from categories F11-F16 and F18-F19 should also be assigned to identify manifestations of the drug use.

m. Poisoning, toxic effects, adverse effects and underdosing in a pregnant patient

A code from subcategory O9A.2, Injury, poisoning and certain other consequences of external causes complicating pregnancy, childbirth, and the puerperium, should be sequenced first, followed by the appropriate injury, poisoning, toxic effect, adverse effect or underdosing code, and then the additional code(s) that specifies the condition caused by the poisoning, toxic effect, adverse effect or underdosing.

See Section I.C.19. Adverse effects, poisoning, underdosing and toxic effects.

Patient treated for accidental carbon monoxide poisoning from a gas heating implement; the patient is 18 weeks' pregnant	
O9A.212	**Injury, poisoning and certain other consequences of external causes complicating pregnancy, second trimester**
T58.11XA	**Toxic effect of carbon monoxide from utility gas, accidental (unintentional), initial encounter**
Z3A.18	**18 weeks gestation of pregnancy**

Explanation: Although the carbon monoxide poisoning is the reason for the encounter, a code from the obstetrics chapter must be sequenced first. Chapter 15 codes have sequencing priority over codes from other chapters.

n. Normal delivery, code O80

1) Encounter for full term uncomplicated delivery

Code O80 should be assigned when a patient is admitted for a full-term normal delivery and delivers a single, healthy infant without any complications antepartum, during the delivery, or postpartum during the delivery episode. Code O80 is always a principal diagnosis. It is not to be used if any other code from chapter 15 is needed to describe a current complication of the antenatal, delivery, or postnatal period. Additional codes from other chapters may be used with code O80 if they are not related to or are in any way complicating the pregnancy.

2) Uncomplicated delivery with resolved antepartum complication

Code O80 may be used if the patient had a complication at some point during the pregnancy, but the complication is not present at the time of the admission for delivery.

Patient presents in labor at 39 weeks' gestation and delivers a healthy newborn; patient had abnormal glucose levels in her first trimester, which have since resolved	
O80	**Encounter for full-term uncomplicated delivery**
Z37.0	**Single live birth**

Explanation: The abnormal glucose levels during the first trimester cannot be coded if they are not affecting the patient's current trimester. Without additional complications associated with the pregnancy, fetus, or mother, code O80 is appropriate.

3) Outcome of delivery for O80

Z37.0, Single live birth, is the only outcome of delivery code appropriate for use with O80.

o. The peripartum and postpartum periods

1) Peripartum and postpartum periods

The postpartum period begins immediately after delivery and continues for six weeks following delivery. The peripartum period is defined as the last month of pregnancy to five months postpartum.

2) Peripartum and postpartum complication

A postpartum complication is any complication occurring within the six-week period.

3) Pregnancy-related complications after 6-week period

Chapter 15 codes may also be used to describe pregnancy-related complications after the peripartum or postpartum period if the provider documents that a condition is pregnancy related.

Patient referred for varicose veins. She had a baby boy three months ago; the varicose veins started to appear one month ago. The doctor attributes the patient's pregnancy as the cause of the varicose veins, which continue to be painful and bother the patient. She is seeking surgical relief.	
O87.4	**Varicose veins of the lower extremity in the puerperium**

Explanation: Although the varicose veins occurred several months after the delivery of the newborn, the doctor attributed the varicose veins to pregnancy and therefore a code from chapter 15 is appropriate.

4) Admission for routine postpartum care following delivery outside hospital

When the mother delivers outside the hospital prior to admission and is admitted for routine postpartum care and no complications are noted, code Z39.0, Encounter for care and examination of mother immediately after delivery, should be assigned as the principal diagnosis.

5) Pregnancy associated cardiomyopathy

Pregnancy associated cardiomyopathy, code O90.3, is unique in that it may be diagnosed in the third trimester of pregnancy but may continue to progress months after delivery. For this reason, it is referred to as peripartum cardiomyopathy. Code O90.3 is only for use when the cardiomyopathy develops as a result of pregnancy in a patient who did not have pre-existing heart disease.

p. Code O94, Sequelae of complication of pregnancy, childbirth, and the puerperium

1) Code O94

Code O94, Sequelae of complication of pregnancy, childbirth, and the puerperium, is for use in those cases when an initial complication of a pregnancy develops a sequela or sequelae requiring care or treatment at a future date.

2) After the initial postpartum period

This code may be used at any time after the initial postpartum period.

3) Sequencing of code O94

This code, like all sequela codes, is to be sequenced following the code describing the sequelae of the complication.

q. Termination of pregnancy and spontaneous abortions

1) Abortion with Liveborn Fetus

When an attempted termination of pregnancy results in a liveborn fetus, assign code Z33.2, Encounter for elective termination of pregnancy and a code from category Z37, Outcome of Delivery.

2) Retained Products of Conception following an abortion

Subsequent encounters for retained products of conception following a spontaneous abortion or elective termination of pregnancy, without complications are assigned O03.4, Incomplete spontaneous abortion without complication, or code O07.4, Failed attempted termination of pregnancy without complication. This advice is appropriate even when the patient was discharged previously with a discharge diagnosis of complete abortion. If the patient has a specific complication associated with the spontaneous abortion or elective termination of pregnancy in addition to retained products of conception, assign the appropriate complication code (e.g., O03.-, O04.-, O07.-) instead of code O03.4 or O07.4.

Patient was seen two days ago for complete spontaneous abortion but returns today for urinary tract infection (UTI) with ultrasound showing retained products of conception

O03.38   Urinary tract infection following incomplete spontaneous abortion

Explanation: Although the diagnosis from the patient's previous stay indicated that the patient had a complete abortion, it is now determined that there were actually retained products of conception (POC). An abortion with retained POC is considered incomplete and in this case resulted in the patient developing a UTI.

3) Complications leading to abortion

Codes from Chapter 15 may be used as additional codes to identify any documented complications of the pregnancy in conjunction with codes in categories in O04, O07 and O08.

4) Hemorrhage following elective abortion

For hemorrhage post elective abortion, assign code O04.6, Delayed or excessive hemorrhage following (induced) termination of pregnancy. Do not assign code O72.1, Other immediate postpartum hemorrhage, as this code should not be assigned for post abortion conditions. Do not assign code Z33.2, Encounter for elective termination of pregnancy, when the patient experiences a complication post elective abortion.

r. Abuse in a pregnant patient

For suspected or confirmed cases of abuse of a pregnant patient, a code(s) from subcategories O9A.3, Physical abuse complicating pregnancy, childbirth, and the puerperium, O9A.4, Sexual abuse complicating pregnancy, childbirth, and the puerperium, and O9A.5, Psychological abuse complicating pregnancy, childbirth, and the puerperium, should be sequenced first, followed by the appropriate codes (if applicable) to identify any associated current injury due to physical abuse, sexual abuse, and the perpetrator of abuse.

See Section I.C.19. Adult and child abuse, neglect and other maltreatment.

s. COVID-19 infection in pregnancy, childbirth, and the puerperium

During pregnancy, childbirth or the puerperium, when COVID-19 is the reason for admission/encounter, code O98.5-, Other viral diseases complicating pregnancy, childbirth and the puerperium, should be sequenced as the principal/first-listed diagnosis, and code U07.1, COVID-19, and the appropriate codes for associated manifestation(s) should be assigned as additional diagnoses. Codes from Chapter 15 always take sequencing priority.

If the reason for admission/encounter is unrelated to COVID-19 but the patient tests positive for COVID-19 during the admission/encounter, the appropriate code for the reason for admission/encounter should be sequenced as the principal/first-listed diagnosis, and codes O98.5-and U07.1, as well as the appropriate codes for associated COVID-19 manifestations, should be assigned as additional diagnoses.

Chapter 15. Pregnancy, Childbirth and the Puerperium (O00-O9A)

NOTE   CODES FROM THIS CHAPTER ARE FOR USE ONLY ON MATERNAL RECORDS, NEVER ON NEWBORN RECORDS

Codes from this chapter are for use for conditions related to or aggravated by the pregnancy, childbirth, or by the puerperium (maternal causes or obstetric causes)

NOTE   Trimesters are counted from the first day of the last menstrual period. They are defined as follows:

1st trimester- less than 14 weeks 0 days

2nd trimester- 14 weeks 0 days to less than 28 weeks 0 days

3rd trimester- 28 weeks 0 days until delivery

Use additional code from category Z3A, Weeks of gestation, to identify the specific week of the pregnancy, if known.

EXCLUDES 1   supervision of normal pregnancy (Z34.-)

EXCLUDES 2   mental and behavioral disorders associated with the puerperium (F53.-)
obstetrical tetanus (A34)
postpartum necrosis of pituitary gland (E23.0)
puerperal osteomalacia (M83.0)

AHA: 2016,1Q,3-5; 2014,3Q,17

This chapter contains the following blocks:

O00-O08   Pregnancy with abortive outcome
O09   Supervision of high risk pregnancy
O10-O16   Edema, proteinuria and hypertensive disorders in pregnancy, childbirth and the puerperium
O20-O29   Other maternal disorders predominantly related to pregnancy
O30-O48   Maternal care related to the fetus and amniotic cavity and possible delivery problems
O60-O77   Complications of labor and delivery
O80-O82   Encounter for delivery
O85-O92   Complications predominantly related to the puerperium
O94-O9A   Other obstetric conditions, not elsewhere classified

Pregnancy with abortive outcome (O00-O08)

EXCLUDES 1   continuing pregnancy in multiple gestation after abortion of one fetus or more (O31.1-, O31.3-)

TIP: Do not assign a code from category Z3A with codes in this code block.

O00 Ectopic pregnancy

INCLUDES   ruptured ectopic pregnancy

Use additional code from category O08 to identify any associated complication

AHA: 2016,4Q,48-50; 2014,3Q,17

DEF: Implantation of a fertilized egg outside the uterus, usually in the fallopian tube or abdomen that requires emergency treatment.

O00.0 Abdominal pregnancy

EXCLUDES 1   maternal care for viable fetus in abdominal pregnancy (O36.7-)

O00.00 Abdominal pregnancy without intrauterine pregnancy COM M ♀
Abdominal pregnancy NOS

O00.01 Abdominal pregnancy with intrauterine pregnancy COM M ♀

O00.1 Tubal pregnancy   *Z33.1 Preg stat incidental*
Fallopian pregnancy
Rupture of (fallopian) tube due to pregnancy
Tubal abortion
AHA: 2017,4Q,20

O00.10 Tubal pregnancy without intrauterine pregnancy
Tubal pregnancy NOS

O00.101 Right tubal pregnancy without intrauterine pregnancy COM M ♀

O00.102 Left tubal pregnancy without intrauterine pregnancy COM M ♀

O00.109 Unspecified tubal pregnancy without intrauterine pregnancy COM M ♀

O00.11 Tubal pregnancy with intrauterine pregnancy

O00.111 Right tubal pregnancy with intrauterine pregnancy COM M ♀

O00.112 Left tubal pregnancy with intrauterine pregnancy COM M ♀

O00.119 Unspecified tubal pregnancy with intrauterine pregnancy COM M ♀

O00.2 Ovarian pregnancy
AHA: 2017,4Q,20

O00.20 Ovarian pregnancy without intrauterine pregnancy
Ovarian pregnancy NOS

O00.201 Right ovarian pregnancy without intrauterine pregnancy COM M ♀

O00.202 Left ovarian pregnancy without intrauterine pregnancy COM M ♀

O00.209 Unspecified ovarian pregnancy without intrauterine pregnancy COM M ♀

O00.21 Ovarian pregnancy with intrauterine pregnancy

O00.211 Right ovarian pregnancy with intrauterine pregnancy COM M ♀

O00.212 Left ovarian pregnancy with intrauterine pregnancy COM M ♀

O00.219 Unspecified ovarian pregnancy with intrauterine pregnancy COM M ♀

O00.8 Other ectopic pregnancy
Cervical pregnancy
Cornual pregnancy
Intraligamentous pregnancy
Mural pregnancy

O00.80 Other ectopic pregnancy without intrauterine pregnancy COM M ♀
Other ectopic pregnancy NOS

O00.81 Other ectopic pregnancy with intrauterine pregnancy COM M ♀

O00.9 Ectopic pregnancy, unspecified

O00.90 Unspecified ectopic pregnancy without intrauterine pregnancy COM M ♀
Ectopic pregnancy NOS

O00.91 Unspecified ectopic pregnancy with intrauterine pregnancy COM M ♀

O01 Hydatidiform mole   *molar pregnancy*
Use additional code from category O08 to identify any associated complication   *trophoblastic neoplasm*

EXCLUDES 1   chorioadenoma (destruens) (D39.2)   *PSTT*
malignant hydatidiform mole (D39.2)   *placental-site-trophoblastic*

AHA: 2014,3Q,17   *tumor*

DEF: Abnormal product of pregnancy, marked by a mass of cysts resembling a bunch of grapes due to chorionic villi proliferation and dissolution. It must be surgically removed.

O01.0 Classical hydatidiform mole COM M ♀   *chorioadenoma*
Complete hydatidiform mole

O01.1 Incomplete and partial hydatidiform mole COM M ♀

O01.9 Hydatidiform mole, unspecified COM M ♀
Trophoblastic disease NOS
Vesicular mole NOS

O02 Other abnormal products of conception   *carneous mole*
Use additional code from category O08 to identify any associated complication

EXCLUDES 1   papyraceous fetus (O31.0-)

AHA: 2014,3Q,17   *empty*

O02.0 Blighted ovum and nonhydatidiform mole COM M ♀
Carneous mole
Fleshy mole
Intrauterine mole NOS
Molar pregnancy NEC
Pathological ovum

O02.1 Missed abortion COM M ♀
Early fetal death, before completion of 20 weeks of gestation, with retention of dead fetus

EXCLUDES 1   failed induced abortion (O07.-)
fetal death (intrauterine) (late) (O36.4)
missed abortion with blighted ovum (O02.0)
missed abortion with hydatidiform mole (O01.-)
missed abortion with nonhydatidiform (O02.0)
missed abortion with other abnormal products of conception (O02.8-)
missed delivery (O36.4)
stillbirth (P95)

AHA: 2022,2Q,3; 2019,3Q,11

Z3A... week of pregnancy do not report with abortion code.

✓5ᵗʰ **O02.8 Other specified abnormal products of conception**

    EXCLUDES 1   *abnormal products of conception with blighted ovum (O02.0)*

          abnormal products of conception with hydatidiform mole (O01.-)

          abnormal products of conception with nonhydatidiform mole (O02.0)

O02.81 Inappropriate change in quantitative human chorionic gonadotropin (hCG) in early pregnancy   COM M ♀

    Biochemical pregnancy

    Chemical pregnancy

    Inappropriate level of quantitative human chorionic gonadotropin (hCG) for gestational age in early pregnancy

O02.89 Other abnormal products of conception   COM M ♀

O02.9 Abnormal product of conception, unspecified   COM M ♀

✓4ᵗʰ **O03 Spontaneous abortion**

    NOTE   Incomplete abortion includes retained products of conception following spontaneous abortion

    INCLUDES   miscarriage

O03.0 Genital tract and pelvic infection following incomplete spontaneous abortion   COM M ♀

    Endometritis following incomplete spontaneous abortion

    Oophoritis following incomplete spontaneous abortion

    Parametritis following incomplete spontaneous abortion

    Pelvic peritonitis following incomplete spontaneous abortion

    Salpingitis following incomplete spontaneous abortion

    Salpingo-oophoritis following incomplete spontaneous abortion

    EXCLUDES 1   *sepsis following incomplete spontaneous abortion (O03.37)*

          urinary tract infection following incomplete spontaneous abortion (O03.38)

O03.1 Delayed or excessive hemorrhage following incomplete spontaneous abortion   COM M ♀

    Afibrinogenemia following incomplete spontaneous abortion

    Defibrination syndrome following incomplete spontaneous abortion

    Hemolysis following incomplete spontaneous abortion

    Intravascular coagulation following incomplete spontaneous abortion

    AHA: 2022,1Q,19

O03.2 Embolism following incomplete spontaneous abortion   COM M ♀

    Air embolism following incomplete spontaneous abortion

    Amniotic fluid embolism following incomplete spontaneous abortion

    Blood-clot embolism following incomplete spontaneous abortion

    Embolism NOS following incomplete spontaneous abortion

    Fat embolism following incomplete spontaneous abortion

    Pulmonary embolism following incomplete spontaneous abortion

    Pyemic embolism following incomplete spontaneous abortion

    Septic or septicopyemic embolism following incomplete spontaneous abortion

    Soap embolism following incomplete spontaneous abortion

✓5ᵗʰ **O03.3 Other and unspecified complications following incomplete spontaneous abortion**

O03.30 Unspecified complication following incomplete spontaneous abortion   COM M ♀

O03.31 Shock following incomplete spontaneous abortion   COM M ♀

    Circulatory collapse following incomplete spontaneous abortion

    Shock (postprocedural) following incomplete spontaneous abortion

    EXCLUDES 1   *shock due to infection following incomplete spontaneous abortion (O03.37)*

O03.32 Renal failure following incomplete spontaneous abortion   COM M ♀

    Kidney failure (acute) following incomplete spontaneous abortion

    Oliguria following incomplete spontaneous abortion

    Renal shutdown following incomplete spontaneous abortion

    Renal tubular necrosis following incomplete spontaneous abortion

    Uremia following incomplete spontaneous abortion

O03.33 Metabolic disorder following incomplete spontaneous abortion   COM M ♀

O03.34 Damage to pelvic organs following incomplete spontaneous abortion   COM M ♀

    Laceration, perforation, tear or chemical damage of bladder following incomplete spontaneous abortion

    Laceration, perforation, tear or chemical damage of bowel following incomplete spontaneous abortion

    Laceration, perforation, tear or chemical damage of broad ligament following incomplete spontaneous abortion

    Laceration, perforation, tear or chemical damage of cervix following incomplete spontaneous abortion

    Laceration, perforation, tear or chemical damage of periurethral tissue following incomplete spontaneous abortion

    Laceration, perforation, tear or chemical damage of uterus following incomplete spontaneous abortion

    Laceration, perforation, tear or chemical damage of vagina following incomplete spontaneous abortion

O03.35 Other venous complications following incomplete spontaneous abortion   COM M ♀

O03.36 Cardiac arrest following incomplete spontaneous abortion   COM M ♀

O03.37 Sepsis following incomplete spontaneous abortion   COM M ♀

    Use additional code to identify infectious agent (B95-B97)

    Use additional code to identify severe sepsis, if applicable (R65.2-)

    EXCLUDES 1   *septic or septicopyemic embolism following incomplete spontaneous abortion (O03.2)*

O03.38 Urinary tract infection following incomplete spontaneous abortion   COM M ♀

    Cystitis following incomplete spontaneous abortion

O03.39 Incomplete spontaneous abortion with other complications   COM M ♀

O03.4 Incomplete spontaneous abortion without complication   COM M ♀

O03.5 Genital tract and pelvic infection following complete or unspecified spontaneous abortion   COM M ♀

    Endometritis following complete or unspecified spontaneous abortion

    Oophoritis following complete or unspecified spontaneous abortion

    Parametritis following complete or unspecified spontaneous abortion

    Pelvic peritonitis following complete or unspecified spontaneous abortion

    Salpingitis following complete or unspecified spontaneous abortion

    Salpingo-oophoritis following complete or unspecified spontaneous abortion

    EXCLUDES 1   *sepsis following complete or unspecified spontaneous abortion (O03.87)*

          urinary tract infection following complete or unspecified spontaneous abortion (O03.88)

OØ3.6 Delayed or excessive hemorrhage following complete or unspecified spontaneous abortion ᴄᴏᴍ Ⓜ ♀

   Afibrinogenemia following complete or unspecified spontaneous abortion

   Defibrination syndrome following complete or unspecified spontaneous abortion

   Hemolysis following complete or unspecified spontaneous abortion

   Intravascular coagulation following complete or unspecified spontaneous abortion

   AHA: 2022,1Q,19

OØ3.7 Embolism following complete or unspecified spontaneous abortion ᴄᴏᴍ Ⓜ ♀

   Air embolism following complete or unspecified spontaneous abortion

   Amniotic fluid embolism following complete or unspecified spontaneous abortion

   Blood-clot embolism following complete or unspecified spontaneous abortion

   Embolism NOS following complete or unspecified spontaneous abortion

   Fat embolism following complete or unspecified spontaneous abortion

   Pulmonary embolism following complete or unspecified spontaneous abortion

   Pyemic embolism following complete or unspecified spontaneous abortion

   Septic or septicopyemic embolism following complete or unspecified spontaneous abortion

   Soap embolism following complete or unspecified spontaneous abortion

✓5ᵗʰ **OØ3.8 Other and unspecified complications following complete or unspecified spontaneous abortion**

   OØ3.80 Unspecified complication following complete or unspecified spontaneous abortion ᴄᴏᴍ Ⓜ ♀

   OØ3.81 Shock following complete or unspecified spontaneous abortion ᴄᴏᴍ Ⓜ ♀

      Circulatory collapse following complete or unspecified spontaneous abortion

      Shock (postprocedural) following complete or unspecified spontaneous abortion

      ᴇxᴄʟᴜᴅᴇs 1   *shock due to infection following complete or unspecified spontaneous abortion (OØ3.87)*

   OØ3.82 Renal failure following complete or unspecified spontaneous abortion ᴄᴏᴍ Ⓜ ♀

      Kidney failure (acute) following complete or unspecified spontaneous abortion

      Oliguria following complete or unspecified spontaneous abortion

      Renal shutdown following complete or unspecified spontaneous abortion

      Renal tubular necrosis following complete or unspecified spontaneous abortion

      Uremia following complete or unspecified spontaneous abortion

   OØ3.83 Metabolic disorder following complete or unspecified spontaneous abortion ᴄᴏᴍ Ⓜ ♀

OØ3.84 Damage to pelvic organs following complete or unspecified spontaneous abortion ᴄᴏᴍ Ⓜ ♀

   Laceration, perforation, tear or chemical damage of bladder following complete or unspecified spontaneous abortion

   Laceration, perforation, tear or chemical damage of bowel following complete or unspecified spontaneous abortion

   Laceration, perforation, tear or chemical damage of broad ligament following complete or unspecified spontaneous abortion

   Laceration, perforation, tear or chemical damage of cervix following complete or unspecified spontaneous abortion

   Laceration, perforation, tear or chemical damage of periurethral tissue following complete or unspecified spontaneous abortion

   Laceration, perforation, tear or chemical damage of uterus following complete or unspecified spontaneous abortion

   Laceration, perforation, tear or chemical damage of vagina following complete or unspecified spontaneous abortion

OØ3.85 Other venous complications following complete or unspecified spontaneous abortion ᴄᴏᴍ Ⓜ ♀

OØ3.86 Cardiac arrest following complete or unspecified spontaneous abortion ᴄᴏᴍ Ⓜ ♀

OØ3.87 Sepsis following complete or unspecified spontaneous abortion ᴄᴏᴍ Ⓜ ♀

miscarriage

   Use additional code to identify infectious agent (B95-B97)

   Use additional code to identify severe sepsis, if applicable (R65.2-)

   ᴇxᴄʟᴜᴅᴇs 1   *septic or septicopyemic embolism following complete or unspecified spontaneous abortion (OØ3.7)*

OØ3.88 Urinary tract infection following complete or unspecified spontaneous abortion ᴄᴏᴍ Ⓜ ♀

   Cystitis following complete or unspecified spontaneous abortion

OØ3.89 Complete or unspecified spontaneous abortion with other complications ᴄᴏᴍ Ⓜ ♀

OØ3.9 Complete or unspecified spontaneous abortion without complication ᴄᴏᴍ Ⓜ ♀

elective or therapeutic

   Miscarriage NOS

   Spontaneous abortion NOS

✓4ᵗʰ **OØ4 Complications following (induced) termination of pregnancy**

   ɪɴᴄʟᴜᴅᴇs   complications following (induced) termination of pregnancy

   ᴇxᴄʟᴜᴅᴇs 1   *encounter for elective termination of pregnancy, uncomplicated (Z33.2)*

      failed attempted termination of pregnancy (OØ7.-)

OØ4.5 Genital tract and pelvic infection following (induced) termination of pregnancy Ⓜ ♀

   Endometritis following (induced) termination of pregnancy

   Oophoritis following (induced) termination of pregnancy

   Parametritis following (induced) termination of pregnancy

   Pelvic peritonitis following (induced) termination of pregnancy

   Salpingitis following (induced) termination of pregnancy

   Salpingo-oophoritis following (induced) termination of pregnancy

   ᴇxᴄʟᴜᴅᴇs 1   *sepsis following (induced) termination of pregnancy (OØ4.87)*

      urinary tract infection following (induced) termination of pregnancy (OØ4.88)

OØ4.6 Delayed or excessive hemorrhage following (induced) termination of pregnancy Ⓜ ♀

after induced abortion

   Afibrinogenemia following (induced) termination of pregnancy

   Defibrination syndrome following (induced) termination of pregnancy

   Hemolysis following (induced) termination of pregnancy

   Intravascular coagulation following (induced) termination of pregnancy

   AHA: 2019,3Q,11

 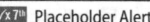

[handwritten: Not abcd]   *[handwritten: Abortion]*

O04.7   Embolism following (induced) termination of pregnancy   Ⓜ ♀

Air embolism following (induced) termination of pregnancy
Amniotic fluid embolism following (induced) termination of pregnancy
Blood-clot embolism following (induced) termination of pregnancy
Embolism NOS following (induced) termination of pregnancy
Fat embolism following (induced) termination of pregnancy
Pulmonary embolism following (induced) termination of pregnancy
Pyemic embolism following (induced) termination of pregnancy
Septic or septicopyemic embolism following (induced) termination of pregnancy
Soap embolism following (induced) termination of pregnancy

✓5ᵗʰ **O04.8   (Induced) termination of pregnancy with other and unspecified complications**

O04.80   (Induced) termination of pregnancy with unspecified complications   Ⓜ ♀

O04.81   Shock following (induced) termination of pregnancy   Ⓜ ♀

Circulatory collapse following (induced) termination of pregnancy
Shock (postprocedural) following (induced) termination of pregnancy

EXCLUDES 1   *shock due to infection following (induced) termination of pregnancy (O04.87)*

O04.82   Renal failure following (induced) termination of pregnancy   Ⓜ ♀

Kidney failure (acute) following (induced) termination of pregnancy
Oliguria following (induced) termination of pregnancy
Renal shutdown following (induced) termination of pregnancy
Renal tubular necrosis following (induced) termination of pregnancy
Uremia following (induced) termination of pregnancy

O04.83   Metabolic disorder following (induced) termination of pregnancy   Ⓜ ♀

O04.84   Damage to pelvic organs following (induced) termination of pregnancy   Ⓜ ♀

Laceration, perforation, tear or chemical damage of bladder following (induced) termination of pregnancy
Laceration, perforation, tear or chemical damage of bowel following (induced) termination of pregnancy
Laceration, perforation, tear or chemical damage of broad ligament following (induced) termination of pregnancy
Laceration, perforation, tear or chemical damage of cervix following (induced) termination of pregnancy
Laceration, perforation, tear or chemical damage of periurethral tissue following (induced) termination of pregnancy
Laceration, perforation, tear or chemical damage of uterus following (induced) termination of pregnancy
Laceration, perforation, tear or chemical damage of vagina following (induced) termination of pregnancy

O04.85   Other venous complications following (induced) termination of pregnancy   Ⓜ ♀

O04.86   Cardiac arrest following (induced) termination of pregnancy   Ⓜ ♀

O04.87   Sepsis following (induced) termination of pregnancy   Ⓜ ♀

Use additional code to identify infectious agent (B95-B97)
Use additional code to identify severe sepsis, if applicable (R65.2-)

EXCLUDES 1   *septic or septicopyemic embolism following (induced) termination of pregnancy (O04.7)*

O04.88   Urinary tract infection following (induced) termination of pregnancy   Ⓜ ♀

Cystitis following (induced) termination of pregnancy

O04.89   (Induced) termination of pregnancy with other complications   Ⓜ ♀

✓4ᵗʰ **O07   Failed attempted termination of pregnancy**

INCLUDES   failure of attempted induction of termination of pregnancy
incomplete elective abortion

EXCLUDES 1   *incomplete spontaneous abortion (O03.0-)*

O07.0   Genital tract and pelvic infection following failed attempted termination of pregnancy   Ⓜ ♀

[handwritten: Retained product of Conception]

Endometritis following failed attempted termination of pregnancy
Oophoritis following failed attempted termination of pregnancy
Parametritis following failed attempted termination of pregnancy
Pelvic peritonitis following failed attempted termination of pregnancy
Salpingitis following failed attempted termination of pregnancy
Salpingo-oophoritis following failed attempted termination of pregnancy

EXCLUDES 1   *sepsis following failed attempted termination of pregnancy (O07.37)*
urinary tract infection following failed attempted termination of pregnancy (O07.38)

O07.1   Delayed or excessive hemorrhage following failed attempted termination of pregnancy   Ⓜ ♀

Afibrinogenemia following failed attempted termination of pregnancy
Defibrination syndrome following failed attempted termination of pregnancy
Hemolysis following failed attempted termination of pregnancy
Intravascular coagulation following failed attempted termination of pregnancy

O07.2   Embolism following failed attempted termination of pregnancy   Ⓜ ♀

Air embolism following failed attempted termination of pregnancy
Amniotic fluid embolism following failed attempted termination of pregnancy
Blood-clot embolism following failed attempted termination of pregnancy
Embolism NOS following failed attempted termination of pregnancy
Fat embolism following failed attempted termination of pregnancy
Pulmonary embolism following failed attempted termination of pregnancy
Pyemic embolism following failed attempted termination of pregnancy
Septic or septicopyemic embolism following failed attempted termination of pregnancy
Soap embolism following failed attempted termination of pregnancy

✓5ᵗʰ **O07.3   Failed attempted termination of pregnancy with other and unspecified complications**

O07.30   Failed attempted termination of pregnancy with unspecified complications   Ⓜ ♀

O07.31   Shock following failed attempted termination of pregnancy   Ⓜ ♀

Circulatory collapse following failed attempted termination of pregnancy
Shock (postprocedural) following failed attempted termination of pregnancy

EXCLUDES 1   *shock due to infection following failed attempted termination of pregnancy (O07.37)*

O07.32   Renal failure following failed attempted termination of pregnancy   Ⓜ ♀

Kidney failure (acute) following failed attempted termination of pregnancy
Oliguria following failed attempted termination of pregnancy
Renal shutdown following failed attempted termination of pregnancy
Renal tubular necrosis following failed attempted termination of pregnancy
Uremia following failed attempted termination of pregnancy

O07.33   Metabolic disorder following failed attempted termination of pregnancy   Ⓜ ♀

O07.34 Damage to pelvic organs **following failed attempted termination of pregnancy**   M ♀
Laceration, perforation, tear or chemical damage of bladder following failed attempted termination of pregnancy
Laceration, perforation, tear or chemical damage of bowel following failed attempted termination of pregnancy
Laceration, perforation, tear or chemical damage of broad ligament following failed attempted termination of pregnancy
Laceration, perforation, tear or chemical damage of cervix following failed attempted termination of pregnancy
Laceration, perforation, tear or chemical damage of periurethral tissue following failed attempted termination of pregnancy
Laceration, perforation, tear or chemical damage of uterus following failed attempted termination of pregnancy
Laceration, perforation, tear or chemical damage of vagina following failed attempted termination of pregnancy

O07.35 Other venous complications **following failed attempted termination of pregnancy**   M ♀

O07.36 Cardiac arrest **following failed attempted termination of pregnancy**   M ♀

O07.37 Sepsis **following failed attempted termination of pregnancy**   M ♀
Use additional code (B95-B97), to identify infectious agent
Use additional code (R65.2-) to identify severe sepsis, if applicable
> *EXCLUDES 1*   *septic or septicopyemic embolism following failed attempted termination of pregnancy (O07.2)*

O07.38 Urinary tract infection **following failed attempted termination of pregnancy**   M ♀
Cystitis following failed attempted termination of pregnancy

O07.39 Failed attempted termination of pregnancy with **other complications**   M ♀

O07.4 Failed attempted termination of pregnancy without complication   M ♀

√4ᵗʰ **O08** Complications following ectopic and molar **pregnancy**
This category is for use with categories O00-O02 to identify any associated complications

O08.0 Genital tract and pelvic infection **following ectopic and molar pregnancy**   COM ♀
Endometritis following ectopic and molar pregnancy
Oophoritis following ectopic and molar pregnancy
Parametritis following ectopic and molar pregnancy
Pelvic peritonitis following ectopic and molar pregnancy
Salpingitis following ectopic and molar pregnancy
Salpingo-oophoritis following ectopic and molar pregnancy
> *EXCLUDES 1*   *sepsis following ectopic and molar pregnancy (O08.82)*
> *urinary tract infection (O08.83)*

O08.1 Delayed or excessive hemorrhage **following ectopic and molar pregnancy**   COM M ♀
Afibrinogenemia following ectopic and molar pregnancy
Defibrination syndrome following ectopic and molar pregnancy
Hemolysis following ectopic and molar pregnancy
Intravascular coagulation following ectopic and molar pregnancy
> *EXCLUDES 1*   *delayed or excessive hemorrhage due to incomplete abortion (O03.1)*

O08.2 Embolism **following ectopic and molar pregnancy**   COM M ♀
Air embolism following ectopic and molar pregnancy
Amniotic fluid embolism following ectopic and molar pregnancy
Blood-clot embolism following ectopic and molar pregnancy
Embolism NOS following ectopic and molar pregnancy
Fat embolism following ectopic and molar pregnancy
Pulmonary embolism following ectopic and molar pregnancy
Pyemic embolism following ectopic and molar pregnancy
Septic or septicopyemic embolism following ectopic and molar pregnancy
Soap embolism following ectopic and molar pregnancy

O08.3 Shock **following ectopic and molar pregnancy**   COM M ♀
Circulatory collapse following ectopic and molar pregnancy
Shock (postprocedural) following ectopic and molar pregnancy
> *EXCLUDES 1*   *shock due to infection following ectopic and molar pregnancy (O08.82)*

O08.4 Renal failure **following ectopic and molar pregnancy**   COM M ♀
Kidney failure (acute) following ectopic and molar pregnancy
Oliguria following ectopic and molar pregnancy
Renal shutdown following ectopic and molar pregnancy
Renal tubular necrosis following ectopic and molar pregnancy
Uremia following ectopic and molar pregnancy

O08.5 Metabolic disorders **following an ectopic and molar pregnancy**   COM M ♀

O08.6 Damage to pelvic organs and tissues **following an ectopic and molar pregnancy**   COM M ♀
Laceration, perforation, tear or chemical damage of bladder following an ectopic and molar pregnancy
Laceration, perforation, tear or chemical damage of bowel following an ectopic and molar pregnancy
Laceration, perforation, tear or chemical damage of broad ligament following an ectopic and molar pregnancy
Laceration, perforation, tear or chemical damage of cervix following an ectopic and molar pregnancy
Laceration, perforation, tear or chemical damage of periurethral tissue following an ectopic and molar pregnancy
Laceration, perforation, tear or chemical damage of uterus following an ectopic and molar pregnancy
Laceration, perforation, tear or chemical damage of vagina following an ectopic and molar pregnancy

O08.7 Other venous complications following an ectopic and molar pregnancy   COM M ♀

√5ᵗʰ **O08.8** Other complications following an ectopic and molar pregnancy

O08.81 Cardiac arrest **following an ectopic and molar pregnancy**   COM M ♀

O08.82 Sepsis **following an ectopic and molar pregnancy**   COM M ♀
Use additional code (B95-B97), to identify infectious agent
Use additional code (R65.2-) to identify severe sepsis, if applicable
> *EXCLUDES 1*   *septic or septicopyemic embolism following ectopic and molar pregnancy (O08.2)*

O08.83 Urinary tract infection **following an ectopic and molar pregnancy**   COM M ♀
Cystitis following an ectopic and molar pregnancy

O08.89 Other complications following an ectopic and molar pregnancy   COM M ♀

O08.9 Unspecified complication following an ectopic and molar pregnancy   COM M ♀

Supervision of high risk pregnancy (O09)

√4ᵗʰ **O09** Supervision of high risk **pregnancy**
AHA: 2019,3Q,5; 2016,4Q,48-50,150

√5ᵗʰ **O09.0** Supervision of pregnancy with history of infertility

O09.00 Supervision of pregnancy with history of infertility, unspecified trimester   COM M ♀

O09.01 Supervision of pregnancy with history of infertility, first trimester   COM M ♀

O09.02 Supervision of pregnancy with history of infertility, second trimester   COM M ♀

O09.03 Supervision of pregnancy with history of infertility, third trimester   COM M ♀

Chapter 15. Pregnancy, Childbirth and the Puerperium

O09.1–O09.822

✓5ᵗʰ **O09.1**   Supervision of pregnancy with history of ectopic pregnancy

O09.10   Supervision of pregnancy with history of ectopic pregnancy, unspecified trimester   COM M ♀

O09.11   Supervision of pregnancy with history of ectopic pregnancy, first trimester   COM M ♀

O09.12   Supervision of pregnancy with history of ectopic pregnancy, second trimester   COM M ♀

O09.13   Supervision of pregnancy with history of ectopic pregnancy, third trimester   COM M ♀

✓5ᵗʰ **O09.A**   Supervision of pregnancy with history of molar pregnancy

DEF: Molar pregnancy: Trophoblastic neoplasm that mimics pregnancy by proliferating from a pathologic ovum and resulting only in a mass of cysts resembling grapes, 80 percent of which are benign, but require surgical removal.

O09.A0   Supervision of pregnancy with history of molar pregnancy, unspecified trimester   COM M ♀

O09.A1   Supervision of pregnancy with history of molar pregnancy, first trimester   COM M ♀

O09.A2   Supervision of pregnancy with history of molar pregnancy, second trimester   COM M ♀

O09.A3   Supervision of pregnancy with history of molar pregnancy, third trimester   COM M ♀

✓5ᵗʰ **O09.2**   Supervision of pregnancy with other poor reproductive or obstetric history

EXCLUDES 2   *pregnancy care for patient with history of recurrent pregnancy loss (O26.2-)*

✓6ᵗʰ **O09.21**   Supervision of pregnancy with history of pre-term labor

O09.211   Supervision of pregnancy with history of pre-term labor, first trimester   COM M ♀

O09.212   Supervision of pregnancy with history of pre-term labor, second trimester   COM M ♀

O09.213   Supervision of pregnancy with history of pre-term labor, third trimester   COM M ♀

O09.219   Supervision of pregnancy with history of pre-term labor, unspecified trimester   COM M ♀

✓6ᵗʰ **O09.29**   Supervision of pregnancy with other poor reproductive or obstetric history

Supervision of pregnancy with history of neonatal death

Supervision of pregnancy with history of stillbirth

still birth

O09.291   Supervision of pregnancy with other poor reproductive or obstetric history, first trimester   COM M ♀

O09.292   Supervision of pregnancy with other poor reproductive or obstetric history, second trimester   COM M ♀

O09.293   Supervision of pregnancy with other poor reproductive or obstetric history, third trimester   COM M ♀

O09.299   Supervision of pregnancy with other poor reproductive or obstetric history, unspecified trimester   COM M ♀

✓5ᵗʰ **O09.3**   Supervision of pregnancy with insufficient antenatal care

Supervision of concealed pregnancy

Supervision of hidden pregnancy

O09.30   Supervision of pregnancy with insufficient antenatal care, unspecified trimester   COM M ♀

O09.31   Supervision of pregnancy with insufficient antenatal care, first trimester   COM M ♀

O09.32   Supervision of pregnancy with insufficient antenatal care, second trimester   COM M ♀

O09.33   Supervision of pregnancy with insufficient antenatal care, third trimester   COM M ♀

✓5ᵗʰ **O09.4**   Supervision of pregnancy with grand multiparity

O09.40   Supervision of pregnancy with grand multiparity, unspecified trimester   COM M ♀

O09.41   Supervision of pregnancy with grand multiparity, first trimester   COM M ♀

O09.42   Supervision of pregnancy with grand multiparity, second trimester   COM M ♀

O09.43   Supervision of pregnancy with grand multiparity, third trimester   COM M ♀

✓5ᵗʰ **O09.5**   Supervision of elderly primigravida and multigravida

Pregnancy for a female 35 years and older at expected date of delivery

>35 at expected date Elderly

✓6ᵗʰ **O09.51**   Supervision of elderly primigravida

O09.511   Supervision of elderly primigravida, first trimester   COM M ♀

O09.512   Supervision of elderly primigravida, second trimester   COM M ♀

O09.513   Supervision of elderly primigravida, third trimester   COM M ♀

O09.519   Supervision of elderly primigravida, unspecified trimester   COM M ♀

✓6ᵗʰ **O09.52**   Supervision of elderly multigravida

O09.521   Supervision of elderly multigravida, first trimester   COM M ♀

O09.522   Supervision of elderly multigravida, second trimester   COM M ♀

O09.523   Supervision of elderly multigravida, third trimester   COM M ♀

O09.529   Supervision of elderly multigravida, unspecified trimester   COM M ♀

✓5ᵗʰ **O09.6**   Supervision of young primigravida and multigravida

Supervision of pregnancy for a female less than 16 years old at expected date of delivery

<16 not use with delivery use antepartum

✓6ᵗʰ **O09.61**   Supervision of young primigravida

O09.611   Supervision of young primigravida, first trimester   COM M ♀

O09.612   Supervision of young primigravida, second trimester   COM M ♀

O09.613   Supervision of young primigravida, third trimester   COM M ♀

O09.619   Supervision of young primigravida, unspecified trimester   COM M ♀

✓6ᵗʰ **O09.62**   Supervision of young multigravida

O09.621   Supervision of young multigravida, first trimester   COM M ♀

O09.622   Supervision of young multigravida, second trimester   COM M ♀

O09.623   Supervision of young multigravida, third trimester   COM M ♀

O09.629   Supervision of young multigravida, unspecified trimester   COM M ♀

✓5ᵗʰ **O09.7**   Supervision of high risk pregnancy due to social problems

O09.70   Supervision of high risk pregnancy due to social problems, unspecified trimester   COM M ♀

O09.71   Supervision of high risk pregnancy due to social problems, first trimester   COM M ♀

O09.72   Supervision of high risk pregnancy due to social problems, second trimester   COM M ♀

O09.73   Supervision of high risk pregnancy due to social problems, third trimester   COM M ♀

✓5ᵗʰ **O09.8**   Supervision of other high risk pregnancies

✓6ᵗʰ **O09.81**   Supervision of pregnancy resulting from assisted reproductive technology

Supervision of pregnancy resulting from in-vitro fertilization

EXCLUDES 2   *gestational carrier status (Z33.3)*

ART assisted reproductive Technology

O09.811   Supervision of pregnancy resulting from assisted reproductive technology, first trimester   COM M ♀

O09.812   Supervision of pregnancy resulting from assisted reproductive technology, second trimester   COM M ♀

O09.813   Supervision of pregnancy resulting from assisted reproductive technology, third trimester   COM M ♀

O09.819   Supervision of pregnancy resulting from assisted reproductive technology, unspecified trimester   COM M ♀

✓6ᵗʰ **O09.82**   Supervision of pregnancy with history of in utero procedure during previous pregnancy

O09.821   Supervision of pregnancy with history of in utero procedure during previous pregnancy, first trimester   COM M ♀

O09.822   Supervision of pregnancy with history of in utero procedure during previous pregnancy, second trimester   COM M ♀

O09.823   **Supervision of pregnancy with history of in utero procedure during previous pregnancy, third trimester** COM M ♀

O09.829   **Supervision of pregnancy with history of in utero procedure during previous pregnancy, unspecified trimester** COM ♀

> EXCLUDES 1   supervision of pregnancy affected by in utero procedure during current pregnancy (O35.7)

✓6ᵗʰ   O09.89   **Supervision of other high risk pregnancies**

O09.891   **Supervision of other high risk pregnancies, first trimester** COM M ♀

O09.892   **Supervision of other high risk pregnancies, second trimester** COM M ♀

O09.893   **Supervision of other high risk pregnancies, third trimester** COM M ♀

O09.899   **Supervision of other high risk pregnancies, unspecified trimester** COM M ♀

✓5ᵗʰ   O09.9   **Supervision of high risk pregnancy, unspecified**

O09.90   **Supervision of high risk pregnancy, unspecified, unspecified trimester** COM M ♀

O09.91   **Supervision of high risk pregnancy, unspecified, first trimester** COM M ♀

O09.92   **Supervision of high risk pregnancy, unspecified, second trimester** COM M ♀

O09.93   **Supervision of high risk pregnancy, unspecified, third trimester** COM M ♀

Edema, proteinuria and hypertensive disorders in pregnancy, childbirth and the puerperium (O10-O16)

AHA: 2016,4Q,50

✓4ᵗʰ   O10   **Pre-existing hypertension complicating pregnancy, childbirth and the puerperium**

> INCLUDES   pre-existing hypertension with pre-existing proteinuria complicating pregnancy, childbirth and the puerperium

> EXCLUDES 2   pre-existing hypertension with superimposed pre-eclampsia complicating pregnancy, childbirth and the puerperium (O11.-)

✓5ᵗʰ   O10.0   **Pre-existing essential hypertension complicating pregnancy, childbirth and the puerperium**

> Any condition in I10 specified as a reason for obstetric care during pregnancy, childbirth or the puerperium

✓6ᵗʰ   O10.01   **Pre-existing essential hypertension complicating pregnancy**

O10.011   **Pre-existing essential hypertension complicating pregnancy, first trimester** COM M ♀

O10.012   **Pre-existing essential hypertension complicating pregnancy, second trimester** COM M ♀

O10.013   **Pre-existing essential hypertension complicating pregnancy, third trimester** COM M ♀

O10.019   **Pre-existing essential hypertension complicating pregnancy, unspecified trimester** COM M ♀

O10.02   **Pre-existing essential hypertension complicating childbirth** COM M ♀

O10.03   **Pre-existing essential hypertension complicating the puerperium** COM M ♀

✓5ᵗʰ   O10.1   **Pre-existing hypertensive heart disease complicating pregnancy, childbirth and the puerperium**

> Any condition in I11 specified as a reason for obstetric care during pregnancy, childbirth or the puerperium
> Use additional code from I11 to identify the type of hypertensive heart disease

✓6ᵗʰ   O10.11   **Pre-existing hypertensive heart disease complicating pregnancy**

O10.111   **Pre-existing hypertensive heart disease complicating pregnancy, first trimester** COM M ♀

O10.112   **Pre-existing hypertensive heart disease complicating pregnancy, second trimester** COM M ♀

O10.113   **Pre-existing hypertensive heart disease complicating pregnancy, third trimester** COM M ♀

O10.119   **Pre-existing hypertensive heart disease complicating pregnancy, unspecified trimester** COM M ♀

O10.12   **Pre-existing hypertensive heart disease complicating childbirth** COM M ♀

O10.13   **Pre-existing hypertensive heart disease complicating the puerperium** COM M ♀

✓5ᵗʰ   O10.2   **Pre-existing hypertensive chronic kidney disease complicating pregnancy, childbirth and the puerperium**

> Any condition in I12 specified as a reason for obstetric care during pregnancy, childbirth or the puerperium
> Use additional code from I12 to identify the type of hypertensive chronic kidney disease

✓6ᵗʰ   O10.21   **Pre-existing hypertensive chronic kidney disease complicating pregnancy**

O10.211   **Pre-existing hypertensive chronic kidney disease complicating pregnancy, first trimester** COM M ♀

O10.212   **Pre-existing hypertensive chronic kidney disease complicating pregnancy, second trimester** COM M ♀

O10.213   **Pre-existing hypertensive chronic kidney disease complicating pregnancy, third trimester** COM M ♀

O10.219   **Pre-existing hypertensive chronic kidney disease complicating pregnancy, unspecified trimester** COM M ♀

O10.22   **Pre-existing hypertensive chronic kidney disease complicating childbirth** COM M ♀

O10.23   **Pre-existing hypertensive chronic kidney disease complicating the puerperium** COM M ♀

✓5ᵗʰ   O10.3   **Pre-existing hypertensive heart and chronic kidney disease complicating pregnancy, childbirth and the puerperium**

> Any condition in I13 specified as a reason for obstetric care during pregnancy, childbirth or the puerperium
> Use additional code from I13 to identify the type of hypertensive heart and chronic kidney disease

✓6ᵗʰ   O10.31   **Pre-existing hypertensive heart and chronic kidney disease complicating pregnancy**

O10.311   **Pre-existing hypertensive heart and chronic kidney disease complicating pregnancy, first trimester** COM M ♀

O10.312   **Pre-existing hypertensive heart and chronic kidney disease complicating pregnancy, second trimester** COM M ♀

O10.313   **Pre-existing hypertensive heart and chronic kidney disease complicating pregnancy, third trimester** COM M ♀

O10.319   **Pre-existing hypertensive heart and chronic kidney disease complicating pregnancy, unspecified trimester** COM M ♀

O10.32   **Pre-existing hypertensive heart and chronic kidney disease complicating childbirth** COM M ♀

O10.33   **Pre-existing hypertensive heart and chronic kidney disease complicating the puerperium** COM M ♀

✓5ᵗʰ   O10.4   **Pre-existing secondary hypertension complicating pregnancy, childbirth and the puerperium**

> Any condition in I15 specified as a reason for obstetric care during pregnancy, childbirth or the puerperium
> Use additional code from I15 to identify the type of secondary hypertension

✓6ᵗʰ   O10.41   **Pre-existing secondary hypertension complicating pregnancy**

O10.411   **Pre-existing secondary hypertension complicating pregnancy, first trimester** COM M ♀

O10.412   **Pre-existing secondary hypertension complicating pregnancy, second trimester** COM M ♀

O10.413   **Pre-existing secondary hypertension complicating pregnancy, third trimester** COM M ♀

O10.419   **Pre-existing secondary hypertension complicating pregnancy, unspecified trimester** COM M ♀

O10.42   **Pre-existing secondary hypertension complicating childbirth** COM M ♀

Chapter 15. Pregnancy, Childbirth and the Puerperium

O10.43 **Pre-existing secondary hypertension complicating the** puerperium   COM M ♀

✓5th O10.9 **Unspecified pre-existing hypertension complicating pregnancy, childbirth and the puerperium**

✓6th O10.91 **Unspecified pre-existing hypertension complicating** pregnancy

CHTN

O10.911 **Unspecified pre-existing hypertension complicating pregnancy, first** trimester   COM M ♀

O10.912 **Unspecified pre-existing hypertension complicating pregnancy, second** trimester   COM M ♀

O10.913 **Unspecified pre-existing hypertension complicating pregnancy, third** trimester   COM M ♀

O10.919 **Unspecified pre-existing hypertension complicating pregnancy, unspecified** trimester   COM M ♀

O10.92 **Unspecified pre-existing hypertension complicating** childbirth   COM M ♀

O10.93 **Unspecified pre-existing hypertension complicating the** puerperium   COM M ♀

✓4th O11 **Pre-existing hypertension with pre-eclampsia**

INCLUDES   conditions in O10 complicated by pre-eclampsia
pre-eclampsia superimposed pre-existing in hypertension
Use additional code from O10 to identify the type of hypertension
DEF: Complication of pregnancy manifesting in the development of borderline hypertension, protein in the urine, and unresponsive swelling between the 20th week of pregnancy and the end of the first week following birth in mild to moderate cases. Severe preeclampsia presents with hypertension, associated with marked swelling, proteinuria, abdominal pain, and/or visual changes.

Hypertension

O11.1 **Pre-existing hypertension with pre-eclampsia, first** trimester   COM M ♀

O11.2 **Pre-existing hypertension with pre-eclampsia, second** trimester   COM M ♀

O11.3 **Pre-existing hypertension with pre-eclampsia, third** trimester   COM M ♀

O11.4 **Pre-existing hypertension with pre-eclampsia, complicating** childbirth   COM M ♀

O11.5 **Pre-existing hypertension with pre-eclampsia, complicating the** puerperium   COM M ♀

O11.9 **Pre-existing hypertension with pre-eclampsia, unspecified** trimester   COM M ♀

✓4th O12 **Gestational [pregnancy-induced] edema and proteinuria without hypertension**

✓5th O12.0 **Gestational** edema

O12.00 **Gestational edema, unspecified** trimester   COM M ♀

O12.01 **Gestational edema, first trimester**   COM M ♀

O12.02 **Gestational edema, second trimester**   COM M ♀

O12.03 **Gestational edema, third trimester**   COM M ♀

edema

O12.04 **Gestational edema, complicating** childbirth   COM M ♀

O12.05 **Gestational edema, complicating the** puerperium   COM M ♀

✓5th O12.1 **Gestational** proteinuria

O12.10 **Gestational proteinuria, unspecified** trimester   COM M ♀

O12.11 **Gestational proteinuria, first trimester**   COM M ♀

O12.12 **Gestational proteinuria, second** trimester   COM M ♀

O12.13 **Gestational proteinuria, third trimester**   COM M ♀

O12.14 **Gestational proteinuria, complicating** childbirth   COM M ♀

O12.15 **Gestational proteinuria, complicating the** puerperium   COM M ♀

✓5th O12.2 **Gestational** edema with proteinuria

O12.20 **Gestational edema with proteinuria, unspecified** trimester   COM M ♀

O12.21 **Gestational edema with proteinuria, first** trimester   COM M ♀

O12.22 **Gestational edema with proteinuria, second** trimester   COM M ♀

O12.23 **Gestational edema with proteinuria, third** trimester   COM M ♀

O12.24 **Gestational edema with proteinuria, complicating** childbirth   COM M ♀

O12.25 **Gestational edema with proteinuria, complicating the** puerperium   COM M ♀

✓4th O13 **Gestational [pregnancy-induced] hypertension without significant proteinuria**

Gestational H

INCLUDES   gestational hypertension NOS
transient hypertension of pregnancy
AHA: 2016,1Q,5

O13.1 **Gestational [pregnancy-induced] hypertension without significant proteinuria, first trimester**   COM M ♀

O13.2 **Gestational [pregnancy-induced] hypertension without significant proteinuria, second trimester**   COM M ♀

GHTN

O13.3 **Gestational [pregnancy-induced] hypertension without significant proteinuria, third trimester**   COM M ♀

O13.4 **Gestational [pregnancy-induced] hypertension without significant proteinuria, complicating** childbirth   COM M ♀

O13.5 **Gestational [pregnancy-induced] hypertension without significant proteinuria, complicating the** puerperium   COM M ♀

O13.9 **Gestational [pregnancy-induced] hypertension without significant proteinuria, unspecified trimester**   COM M ♀

✓4th O14 **Pre-eclampsia**

EXCLUDES 1   pre-existing hypertension with pre-eclampsia (O11)
DEF: Complication of pregnancy manifesting in the development of borderline hypertension, protein in the urine, and unresponsive swelling between the 20th week of pregnancy and the end of the first week following birth in mild to moderate cases. Severe preeclampsia presents with hypertension, associated with marked swelling, proteinuria, abdominal pain, and/or visual changes.

✓5th O14.0 **Mild to moderate pre-eclampsia**

AHA: 2019,3Q,12; 2019,2Q,8

O14.00 **Mild to moderate pre-eclampsia, unspecified** trimester   COM M ♀

O14.02 **Mild to moderate pre-eclampsia, second** trimester   COM M ♀

O14.03 **Mild to moderate pre-eclampsia, third** trimester   COM M ♀

O14.04 **Mild to moderate pre-eclampsia, complicating** childbirth   COM M ♀
AHA: 2019,2Q,8

O14.05 **Mild to moderate pre-eclampsia, complicating the** puerperium   COM M ♀

✓5th O14.1 **Severe pre-eclampsia**

EXCLUDES 1   HELLP syndrome (O14.2-)
AHA: 2019,3Q,12

Severe

O14.10 **Severe pre-eclampsia, unspecified** trimester   COM M ♀

O14.12 **Severe pre-eclampsia, second trimester**   COM M ♀

O14.13 **Severe pre-eclampsia, third trimester**   COM M ♀

O14.14 **Severe pre-eclampsia complicating** childbirth   COM M ♀

O14.15 **Severe pre-eclampsia, complicating the** puerperium   COM M ♀

✓5th O14.2 **HELLP syndrome**

Severe pre-eclampsia with hemolysis, elevated liver enzymes and low platelet count (HELLP)
AHA: 2019,3Q,12

O14.20 **HELLP syndrome (HELLP), unspecified** trimester   COM M ♀

O14.22 **HELLP syndrome (HELLP), second** trimester   COM M ♀

O14.23 **HELLP syndrome (HELLP), third** trimester   COM M ♀

O14.24 **HELLP syndrome, complicating** childbirth   COM M ♀

O14.25 **HELLP syndrome, complicating the** puerperium   COM M ♀

✓5th O14.9 **Unspecified pre-eclampsia**

O14.90 **Unspecified pre-eclampsia, unspecified** trimester   COM M ♀

O14.92 **Unspecified pre-eclampsia, second** trimester   COM M ♀

O14.93 **Unspecified pre-eclampsia, third** trimester   COM M ♀

O14.94 **Unspecified pre-eclampsia, complicating** childbirth   COM M ♀

O14.95 **Unspecified pre-eclampsia, complicating the** puerperium   COM M ♀

O15 Eclampsia

INCLUDES convulsions following conditions in O10-O14 and O16
DEF: Tetany and toxemia producing seizure activity or coma in a pregnant patient who most often has presented with prior preeclampsia (i.e., hypertension, albuminuria, and edema).

O15.0 Eclampsia complicating pregnancy

- **O15.00** Eclampsia complicating pregnancy, unspecified trimester COM M ♀
- **O15.02** Eclampsia complicating pregnancy, second trimester COM M ♀
- **O15.03** Eclampsia complicating pregnancy, third trimester COM M ♀

O15.1 Eclampsia complicating labor COM M ♀

O15.2 Eclampsia complicating the puerperium COM M ♀

O15.9 Eclampsia, unspecified as to time period COM M ♀
Eclampsia NOS

O16 Unspecified maternal hypertension

- **O16.1** Unspecified maternal hypertension, first trimester COM M ♀
- **O16.2** Unspecified maternal hypertension, second trimester COM M ♀
- **O16.3** Unspecified maternal hypertension, third trimester COM M ♀
- **O16.4** Unspecified maternal hypertension, complicating childbirth COM M ♀
- **O16.5** Unspecified maternal hypertension, complicating the puerperium COM M ♀
- **O16.9** Unspecified maternal hypertension, unspecified trimester COM M ♀

Other maternal disorders predominantly related to pregnancy (O20-O29)

EXCLUDES 2 maternal care related to the fetus and amniotic cavity and possible delivery problems (O30-O48)
maternal diseases classifiable elsewhere but complicating pregnancy, labor and delivery, and the puerperium (O98-O99)

O20 Hemorrhage in early pregnancy

INCLUDES hemorrhage before completion of 20 weeks gestation
EXCLUDES 1 pregnancy with abortive outcome (O00-O08)

<20W

O20.0 Threatened abortion COM M ♀
Hemorrhage specified as due to threatened abortion
DEF: Bloody discharge during pregnancy. The cervix may be dilated and pregnancy threatened, but the pregnancy is not terminated.

O20.8 Other hemorrhage in early pregnancy COM M ♀

O20.9 Hemorrhage in early pregnancy, unspecified COM M ♀

O21 Excessive vomiting in pregnancy

<20W or >20W

O21.0 Mild hyperemesis gravidarum COM M ♀
Hyperemesis gravidarum, mild or unspecified, starting before the end of the 20th week of gestation

O21.1 Hyperemesis gravidarum with metabolic disturbance COM M ♀
Hyperemesis gravidarum, starting before the end of the 20th week of gestation, with metabolic disturbance such as carbohydrate depletion
Hyperemesis gravidarum, starting before the end of the 20th week of gestation, with metabolic disturbance such as dehydration
Hyperemesis gravidarum, starting before the end of the 20th week of gestation, with metabolic disturbance such as electrolyte imbalance

O21.2 Late vomiting of pregnancy COM M ♀
Excessive vomiting starting after 20 completed weeks of gestation

>20W

O21.8 Other vomiting complicating pregnancy COM M ♀
Vomiting due to diseases classified elsewhere, complicating pregnancy
Use additional code, to identify cause

O21.9 Vomiting of pregnancy, unspecified COM M ♀

O22 Venous complications and hemorrhoids in pregnancy

EXCLUDES 1 venous complications of:
abortion NOS (O03.9)
ectopic or molar pregnancy (O08.7)
failed attempted abortion (O07.35)
induced abortion (O04.85)
spontaneous abortion (O03.89)
EXCLUDES 2 obstetric pulmonary embolism (O88.-)
venous complications and hemorrhoids of childbirth and the puerperium (O87.-)

O22.0 Varicose veins of lower extremity in pregnancy
Varicose veins NOS in pregnancy
DEF: Distended, tortuous veins of the lower extremities associated with pregnancy.
- **O22.00** Varicose veins of lower extremity in pregnancy, unspecified trimester COM M ♀
- **O22.01** Varicose veins of lower extremity in pregnancy, first trimester COM M ♀
- **O22.02** Varicose veins of lower extremity in pregnancy, second trimester COM M ♀
- **O22.03** Varicose veins of lower extremity in pregnancy, third trimester COM M ♀

O22.1 Genital varices in pregnancy *varicose vein*
Perineal varices in pregnancy
Vaginal varices in pregnancy
Vulval varices in pregnancy
- **O22.10** Genital varices in pregnancy, unspecified trimester COM M ♀
- **O22.11** Genital varices in pregnancy, first trimester COM M ♀
- **O22.12** Genital varices in pregnancy, second trimester COM M ♀
- **O22.13** Genital varices in pregnancy, third trimester COM M ♀

O22.2 Superficial thrombophlebitis in pregnancy
Phlebitis in pregnancy NOS
Thrombophlebitis of legs in pregnancy
Thrombosis in pregnancy NOS
Use additional code to identify the superficial thrombophlebitis (I80.0-)
- **O22.20** Superficial thrombophlebitis in pregnancy, unspecified trimester COM M ♀
- **O22.21** Superficial thrombophlebitis in pregnancy, first trimester COM M ♀
- **O22.22** Superficial thrombophlebitis in pregnancy, second trimester COM M ♀
- **O22.23** Superficial thrombophlebitis in pregnancy, third trimester COM M ♀

O22.3 Deep phlebothrombosis in pregnancy
Deep vein thrombosis, antepartum
Use additional code to identify the deep vein thrombosis (I82.4-, I82.5-, I82.62-, I82.72-)
Use additional code, if applicable, for associated long-term (current) use of anticoagulants (Z79.01)

I82.- thrombosis

- **O22.30** Deep phlebothrombosis in pregnancy, unspecified trimester COM M ♀
- **O22.31** Deep phlebothrombosis in pregnancy, first trimester COM M ♀
- **O22.32** Deep phlebothrombosis in pregnancy, second trimester COM M ♀
- **O22.33** Deep phlebothrombosis in pregnancy, third trimester COM M ♀

O22.4 Hemorrhoids in pregnancy
- **O22.40** Hemorrhoids in pregnancy, unspecified trimester COM M ♀
- **O22.41** Hemorrhoids in pregnancy, first trimester COM M ♀
- **O22.42** Hemorrhoids in pregnancy, second trimester COM M ♀
- **O22.43** Hemorrhoids in pregnancy, third trimester COM M ♀

O22.5 Cerebral venous thrombosis in pregnancy
Cerebrovenous sinus thrombosis in pregnancy
- **O22.50** Cerebral venous thrombosis in pregnancy, unspecified trimester COM M ♀
- **O22.51** Cerebral venous thrombosis in pregnancy, first trimester COM M ♀

Chapter 15. Pregnancy, Childbirth and the Puerperium — *O22.52–O24.03*

       O22.52   **Cerebral venous thrombosis in pregnancy, second trimester**   COM M ♀

       O22.53   **Cerebral venous thrombosis in pregnancy, third trimester**   COM M ♀

✓5ᵗʰ **O22.8   Other venous complications in pregnancy**

   ✓6ᵗʰ **O22.8X   Other venous complications in pregnancy**

       O22.8X1   **Other venous complications in pregnancy, first trimester**   COM M ♀

       O22.8X2   **Other venous complications in pregnancy, second trimester**   COM M ♀

       O22.8X3   **Other venous complications in pregnancy, third trimester**   COM M ♀

       O22.8X9   **Other venous complications in pregnancy, unspecified trimester**   COM M ♀

✓5ᵗʰ **O22.9   Venous complication in pregnancy, unspecified**

       Gestational phlebitis NOS
       Gestational phlebopathy NOS
       Gestational thrombosis NOS

       O22.90   **Venous complication in pregnancy, unspecified, unspecified trimester**   COM M ♀

       O22.91   **Venous complication in pregnancy, unspecified, first trimester**   COM M ♀

       O22.92   **Venous complication in pregnancy, unspecified, second trimester**   COM M ♀

       O22.93   **Venous complication in pregnancy, unspecified, third trimester**   COM M ♀

✓4ᵗʰ **O23   Infections of genitourinary tract in pregnancy**

     Use additional code to identify organism (B95.-, B96.-)

     EXCLUDES 2   *gonococcal infections complicating pregnancy, childbirth and the puerperium (O98.2)*

       infections with a predominantly sexual mode of transmission NOS complicating pregnancy, childbirth and the puerperium (O98.3)

       syphilis complicating pregnancy, childbirth and the puerperium (O98.1)

       tuberculosis of genitourinary system complicating pregnancy, childbirth and the puerperium (O98.0)

       venereal disease NOS complicating pregnancy, childbirth and the puerperium (O98.3)

     AHA: 2018,2Q,20

✓5ᵗʰ **O23.0   Infections of kidney in pregnancy**

     Pyelonephritis in pregnancy

       O23.00   **Infections of kidney in pregnancy, unspecified trimester**   COM M ♀

       O23.01   **Infections of kidney in pregnancy, first trimester**   COM M ♀

       O23.02   **Infections of kidney in pregnancy, second trimester**   COM M ♀

       O23.03   **Infections of kidney in pregnancy, third trimester**   COM M ♀

✓5ᵗʰ **O23.1   Infections of bladder in pregnancy**

       O23.10   **Infections of bladder in pregnancy, unspecified trimester**   COM M ♀

       O23.11   **Infections of bladder in pregnancy, first trimester**   COM M ♀

       O23.12   **Infections of bladder in pregnancy, second trimester**   COM M ♀

       O23.13   **Infections of bladder in pregnancy, third trimester**   COM M ♀

✓5ᵗʰ **O23.2   Infections of urethra in pregnancy**

       O23.20   **Infections of urethra in pregnancy, unspecified trimester**   COM M ♀

       O23.21   **Infections of urethra in pregnancy, first trimester**   COM M ♀

       O23.22   **Infections of urethra in pregnancy, second trimester**   COM M ♀

       O23.23   **Infections of urethra in pregnancy, third trimester**   COM M ♀

✓5ᵗʰ **O23.3   Infections of other parts of urinary tract in pregnancy**

       O23.30   **Infections of other parts of urinary tract in pregnancy, unspecified trimester**   COM M ♀

       O23.31   **Infections of other parts of urinary tract in pregnancy, first trimester**   COM M ♀

       O23.32   **Infections of other parts of urinary tract in pregnancy, second trimester**   COM M ♀

       O23.33   **Infections of other parts of urinary tract in pregnancy, third trimester**   COM M ♀

✓5ᵗʰ **O23.4   Unspecified infection of urinary tract in pregnancy**

       O23.40   **Unspecified infection of urinary tract in pregnancy, unspecified trimester**   COM M ♀

       O23.41   **Unspecified infection of urinary tract in pregnancy, first trimester**   COM M ♀

       O23.42   **Unspecified infection of urinary tract in pregnancy, second trimester**   COM M ♀

       O23.43   **Unspecified infection of urinary tract in pregnancy, third trimester**   COM M ♀

✓5ᵗʰ **O23.5   Infections of the genital tract in pregnancy**

   ✓6ᵗʰ **O23.51   Infection of cervix in pregnancy**

       O23.511   **Infections of cervix in pregnancy, first trimester**   COM M ♀

       O23.512   **Infections of cervix in pregnancy, second trimester**   COM M ♀

       O23.513   **Infections of cervix in pregnancy, third trimester**   COM M ♀

       O23.519   **Infections of cervix in pregnancy, unspecified trimester**   COM M ♀

   ✓6ᵗʰ **O23.52   Salpingo-oophoritis in pregnancy**

     Oophoritis in pregnancy
     Salpingitis in pregnancy

       O23.521   **Salpingo-oophoritis in pregnancy, first trimester**   COM M ♀

       O23.522   **Salpingo-oophoritis in pregnancy, second trimester**   COM M ♀

       O23.523   **Salpingo-oophoritis in pregnancy, third trimester**   COM M ♀

       O23.529   **Salpingo-oophoritis in pregnancy, unspecified trimester**   COM M ♀

   ✓6ᵗʰ **O23.59   Infection of other part of genital tract in pregnancy**

     AHA: 2022,1Q,20

       O23.591   **Infection of other part of genital tract in pregnancy, first trimester**   COM M ♀

       O23.592   **Infection of other part of genital tract in pregnancy, second trimester**   COM M ♀

       O23.593   **Infection of other part of genital tract in pregnancy, third trimester**   COM M ♀

       O23.599   **Infection of other part of genital tract in pregnancy, unspecified trimester**   COM M ♀

✓5ᵗʰ **O23.9   Unspecified genitourinary tract infection in pregnancy**

     Genitourinary tract infection in pregnancy NOS

       O23.90   **Unspecified genitourinary tract infection in pregnancy, unspecified trimester**   COM M ♀

       O23.91   **Unspecified genitourinary tract infection in pregnancy, first trimester**   COM M ♀

       O23.92   **Unspecified genitourinary tract infection in pregnancy, second trimester**   COM M ♀

       O23.93   **Unspecified genitourinary tract infection in pregnancy, third trimester**   COM M ♀

✓4ᵗʰ **O24   Diabetes mellitus in pregnancy, childbirth and the puerperium**

   ✓5ᵗʰ **O24.0   Pre-existing type 1 diabetes mellitus, in pregnancy, childbirth and the puerperium**

     Juvenile onset diabetes mellitus, in pregnancy, childbirth and the puerperium

     Ketosis-prone diabetes mellitus in pregnancy, childbirth and the puerperium

     Use additional code from category E10 to further identify any manifestations

   ✓6ᵗʰ **O24.01   Pre-existing type 1 diabetes mellitus, in pregnancy**

       O24.011   **Pre-existing type 1 diabetes mellitus, in pregnancy, first trimester**   COM 0 M ♀

       O24.012   **Pre-existing type 1 diabetes mellitus, in pregnancy, second trimester**   COM 0 M ♀

       O24.013   **Pre-existing type 1 diabetes mellitus, in pregnancy, third trimester**   COM 0 M ♀

       O24.019   **Pre-existing type 1 diabetes mellitus, in pregnancy, unspecified trimester**   COM 0 M ♀

       O24.02   **Pre-existing type 1 diabetes mellitus, in childbirth**   COM 0 M ♀

       O24.03   **Pre-existing type 1 diabetes mellitus, in the puerperium**   COM 0 M ♀

HCC CMS-HCC   Rx Rx HCC   ESR ESRD HCC   COM Commercial HCC   N Newborn: 0   P Pediatric: 0-17   M Maternity: 9-64   A Adult: 15-124

(handwritten top margin: "Maternal Disorder O24.1–O26.10")

(handwritten top left: "Maternal Disorder")

✓5ᵗʰ O24.1 Pre-existing type 2 diabetes mellitus, in pregnancy, childbirth and the puerperium
Insulin-resistant diabetes mellitus in pregnancy, childbirth and the puerperium
Use additional code (for):
from category E11 to further identify any manifestations
long-term (current) use of insulin (Z79.4)

✓6ᵗʰ O24.11 Pre-existing type 2 diabetes mellitus, in pregnancy
O24.111 Pre-existing type 2 diabetes mellitus, in pregnancy, first trimester COM Q M ♀
O24.112 Pre-existing type 2 diabetes mellitus, in pregnancy, second trimester COM Q M ♀
O24.113 Pre-existing type 2 diabetes mellitus, in pregnancy, third trimester COM Q M ♀
O24.119 Pre-existing type 2 diabetes mellitus, in pregnancy, unspecified trimester COM Q M ♀

(handwritten: "E 11.9 type 2 DM no complicati")

O24.12 Pre-existing type 2 diabetes mellitus, in childbirth COM Q M ♀
O24.13 Pre-existing type 2 diabetes mellitus, in the puerperium COM Q M ♀

✓5ᵗʰ O24.3 Unspecified pre-existing diabetes mellitus in pregnancy, childbirth and the puerperium
Use additional code (for):
from category E11 to further identify any manifestation
long-term (current) use of insulin (Z79.4)

(handwritten: "unspecified DM")

✓6ᵗʰ O24.31 Unspecified pre-existing diabetes mellitus in pregnancy
O24.311 Unspecified pre-existing diabetes mellitus in pregnancy, first trimester COM Q M ♀
O24.312 Unspecified pre-existing diabetes mellitus in pregnancy, second trimester COM Q M ♀
O24.313 Unspecified pre-existing diabetes mellitus in pregnancy, third trimester COM Q M ♀
O24.319 Unspecified pre-existing diabetes mellitus in pregnancy, unspecified trimester COM Q M ♀

O24.32 Unspecified pre-existing diabetes mellitus in childbirth COM Q M ♀
O24.33 Unspecified pre-existing diabetes mellitus in the puerperium COM Q M ♀

✓5ᵗʰ O24.4 Gestational diabetes mellitus
Diabetes mellitus arising in pregnancy
Gestational diabetes mellitus NOS
AHA: 2020,3Q,30; 2016,4Q,50; 2015,4Q,34

(handwritten: "Ø Z79.4 Z79.84 Z79.85")

✓6ᵗʰ O24.41 Gestational diabetes mellitus in pregnancy

(handwritten: "5th digit 1 A₁ GDM → pregnancy")
(handwritten: "A₂ GDM (insulin)")

O24.410 Gestational diabetes mellitus in pregnancy, diet controlled COM M ♀
O24.414 Gestational diabetes mellitus in pregnancy, insulin controlled COM M ♀
O24.415 Gestational diabetes mellitus in pregnancy, controlled by oral hypoglycemic drugs COM M ♀
Gestational diabetes mellitus in pregnancy, controlled by oral antidiabetic drugs
O24.419 Gestational diabetes mellitus in pregnancy, unspecified control COM M ♀

✓6ᵗʰ O24.42 Gestational diabetes mellitus in childbirth
AHA: 2016,1Q,5

(handwritten: "A₁ GDM")
(handwritten: "5th digit 2 – childbirth")

O24.420 Gestational diabetes mellitus in childbirth, diet controlled COM M ♀
O24.424 Gestational diabetes mellitus in childbirth, insulin controlled COM M ♀
O24.425 Gestational diabetes mellitus in childbirth, controlled by oral hypoglycemic drugs COM M ♀
Gestational diabetes mellitus in childbirth, controlled by oral antidiabetic drugs
O24.429 Gestational diabetes mellitus in childbirth, unspecified control COM M ♀

✓6ᵗʰ O24.43 Gestational diabetes mellitus in the puerperium
O24.430 Gestational diabetes mellitus in the puerperium, diet controlled COM M ♀

O24.434 Gestational diabetes mellitus in the puerperium, insulin controlled COM M ♀
O24.435 Gestational diabetes mellitus in puerperium, controlled by oral hypoglycemic drugs COM M ♀
Gestational diabetes mellitus in puerperium, controlled by oral antidiabetic drugs
O24.439 Gestational diabetes mellitus in the puerperium, unspecified control COM M ♀

(handwritten: "5th digit 3 — puerperium")

✓5ᵗʰ O24.8 Other pre-existing diabetes mellitus in pregnancy, childbirth, and the puerperium
Use additional code (for):
from categories E08, E09 and E13 to further identify any manifestation
long-term (current) use of insulin (Z79.4)

✓6ᵗʰ O24.81 Other pre-existing diabetes mellitus in pregnancy
O24.811 Other pre-existing diabetes mellitus in pregnancy, first trimester COM Q M ♀
O24.812 Other pre-existing diabetes mellitus in pregnancy, second trimester COM Q M ♀
O24.813 Other pre-existing diabetes mellitus in pregnancy, third trimester COM Q M ♀
O24.819 Other pre-existing diabetes mellitus in pregnancy, unspecified trimester COM Q M ♀

O24.82 Other pre-existing diabetes mellitus in childbirth COM Q M ♀
O24.83 Other pre-existing diabetes mellitus in the puerperium COM Q M ♀

✓5ᵗʰ O24.9 Unspecified diabetes mellitus in pregnancy, childbirth and the puerperium
Use additional code for long-term (current) use of insulin (Z79.4)

✓6ᵗʰ O24.91 Unspecified diabetes mellitus in pregnancy
O24.911 Unspecified diabetes mellitus in pregnancy, first trimester COM M ♀
O24.912 Unspecified diabetes mellitus in pregnancy, second trimester COM M ♀
O24.913 Unspecified diabetes mellitus in pregnancy, third trimester COM M ♀
O24.919 Unspecified diabetes mellitus in pregnancy, unspecified trimester COM M ♀

O24.92 Unspecified diabetes mellitus in childbirth COM M ♀
O24.93 Unspecified diabetes mellitus in the puerperium COM M ♀

✓4ᵗʰ O25 Malnutrition in pregnancy, childbirth and the puerperium

✓5ᵗʰ O25.1 Malnutrition in pregnancy
O25.10 Malnutrition in pregnancy, unspecified trimester COM M ♀
O25.11 Malnutrition in pregnancy, first trimester COM M ♀
O25.12 Malnutrition in pregnancy, second trimester COM M ♀
O25.13 Malnutrition in pregnancy, third trimester COM M ♀

O25.2 Malnutrition in childbirth COM M ♀
O25.3 Malnutrition in the puerperium COM M ♀

✓4ᵗʰ O26 Maternal care for other conditions predominantly related to pregnancy

✓5ᵗʰ O26.0 Excessive weight gain in pregnancy
EXCLUDES 2 gestational edema (O12.0, O12.2)
O26.00 Excessive weight gain in pregnancy, unspecified trimester COM M ♀
O26.01 Excessive weight gain in pregnancy, first trimester COM M ♀
O26.02 Excessive weight gain in pregnancy, second trimester COM M ♀
O26.03 Excessive weight gain in pregnancy, third trimester COM M ♀

✓5ᵗʰ O26.1 Low weight gain in pregnancy
O26.10 Low weight gain in pregnancy, unspecified trimester COM M ♀

Maternal Disorder (handwritten)

Chapter 15. Pregnancy, Childbirth and the Puerperium (vertical sidebar)

O26.11 Low weight gain in pregnancy, first trimester   COM M ♀

O26.12 Low weight gain in pregnancy, second trimester   COM M ♀

O26.13 Low weight gain in pregnancy, third trimester   COM M ♀

✓5ᵗʰ **O26.2** Pregnancy care for patient with recurrent pregnancy loss

O26.20 Pregnancy care for patient with recurrent pregnancy loss, unspecified trimester   COM M ♀

O26.21 Pregnancy care for patient with recurrent pregnancy loss, first trimester   COM M ♀

O26.22 Pregnancy care for patient with recurrent pregnancy loss, second trimester   COM M ♀

O26.23 Pregnancy care for patient with recurrent pregnancy loss, third trimester   COM M ♀

✓5ᵗʰ **O26.3** Retained intrauterine contraceptive device in pregnancy

O26.30 Retained intrauterine contraceptive device in pregnancy, unspecified trimester   COM M ♀

O26.31 Retained intrauterine contraceptive device in pregnancy, first trimester   COM M ♀

O26.32 Retained intrauterine contraceptive device in pregnancy, second trimester   COM M ♀

O26.33 Retained intrauterine contraceptive device in pregnancy, third trimester   COM M ♀

✓5ᵗʰ **O26.4** Herpes gestationis

DEF: Rare skin disorder of unknown origin that appears on the abdomen in the second and third trimester as intensely itchy blisters that spread to other sites.

O26.40 Herpes gestationis, unspecified trimester   COM M ♀

O26.41 Herpes gestationis, first trimester   COM M ♀

O26.42 Herpes gestationis, second trimester   COM M ♀

O26.43 Herpes gestationis, third trimester   COM M ♀

✓5ᵗʰ **O26.5** Maternal hypotension syndrome

Supine hypotensive syndrome

O26.50 Maternal hypotension syndrome, unspecified trimester   COM M ♀

O26.51 Maternal hypotension syndrome, first trimester   COM M ♀

O26.52 Maternal hypotension syndrome, second trimester   COM M ♀

O26.53 Maternal hypotension syndrome, third trimester   COM M ♀

✓5ᵗʰ **O26.6** Liver and biliary tract disorders in pregnancy, childbirth and the puerperium

Use additional code to identify the specific disorder

EXCLUDES 2   hepatorenal syndrome following labor and delivery (O90.4)

✓6ᵗʰ **O26.61** Liver and biliary tract disorders in pregnancy

O26.611 Liver and biliary tract disorders in pregnancy, first trimester   COM M ♀

O26.612 Liver and biliary tract disorders in pregnancy, second trimester   COM M ♀

O26.613 Liver and biliary tract disorders in pregnancy, third trimester   COM M ♀

O26.619 Liver and biliary tract disorders in pregnancy, unspecified trimester   COM M ♀

O26.62 Liver and biliary tract disorders in childbirth   COM M ♀

O26.63 Liver and biliary tract disorders in the puerperium   COM M ♀

✓5ᵗʰ **O26.7** Subluxation of symphysis (pubis) in pregnancy, childbirth and the puerperium

EXCLUDES 1   traumatic separation of symphysis (pubis) during childbirth (O71.6)

✓6ᵗʰ **O26.71** Subluxation of symphysis (pubis) in pregnancy

O26.711 Subluxation of symphysis (pubis) in pregnancy, first trimester   COM M ♀

O26.712 Subluxation of symphysis (pubis) in pregnancy, second trimester   COM M ♀

O26.713 Subluxation of symphysis (pubis) in pregnancy, third trimester   COM M ♀

O26.719 Subluxation of symphysis (pubis) in pregnancy, unspecified trimester   COM M ♀

O26.72 Subluxation of symphysis (pubis) in childbirth   COM M ♀

O26.73 Subluxation of symphysis (pubis) in the puerperium   COM M ♀

✓5ᵗʰ **O26.8** Other specified pregnancy related conditions

✓6ᵗʰ **O26.81** Pregnancy related exhaustion and fatigue

O26.811 Pregnancy related exhaustion and fatigue, first trimester   COM M ♀

O26.812 Pregnancy related exhaustion and fatigue, second trimester   COM M ♀

O26.813 Pregnancy related exhaustion and fatigue, third trimester   COM M ♀

O26.819 Pregnancy related exhaustion and fatigue, unspecified trimester   COM M ♀

✓6ᵗʰ **O26.82** Pregnancy related peripheral neuritis

O26.821 Pregnancy related peripheral neuritis, first trimester   COM M ♀

O26.822 Pregnancy related peripheral neuritis, second trimester   COM M ♀

O26.823 Pregnancy related peripheral neuritis, third trimester   COM M ♀

O26.829 Pregnancy related peripheral neuritis, unspecified trimester   COM M ♀

✓6ᵗʰ **O26.83** Pregnancy related renal disease

Use additional code to identify the specific disorder

O26.831 Pregnancy related renal disease, first trimester   COM M ♀

O26.832 Pregnancy related renal disease, second trimester   COM M ♀

O26.833 Pregnancy related renal disease, third trimester   COM M ♀

O26.839 Pregnancy related renal disease, unspecified trimester   COM M ♀

✓6ᵗʰ **O26.84** Uterine size-date discrepancy complicating pregnancy

EXCLUDES 1   encounter for suspected problem with fetal growth ruled out (Z03.74)

O26.841 Uterine size-date discrepancy, first trimester   COM M ♀

O26.842 Uterine size-date discrepancy, second trimester   COM M ♀

O26.843 Uterine size-date discrepancy, third trimester   COM M ♀

O26.849 Uterine size-date discrepancy, unspecified trimester   COM M ♀

✓6ᵗʰ **O26.85** Spotting complicating pregnancy

O26.851 Spotting complicating pregnancy, first trimester   COM M ♀

O26.852 Spotting complicating pregnancy, second trimester   COM M ♀

O26.853 Spotting complicating pregnancy, third trimester   COM M ♀

O26.859 Spotting complicating pregnancy, unspecified trimester   COM M ♀

O26.86 Pruritic urticarial papules and plaques of pregnancy (PUPPP)   COM M ♀

Polymorphic eruption of pregnancy

✓6ᵗʰ **O26.87** Cervical shortening

EXCLUDES 1   encounter for suspected cervical shortening ruled out (Z03.75)

DEF: Cervix that has shortened to less than 25 mm before the 24th week of pregnancy. A shortened cervix is a warning sign for impending premature delivery and is treated by cervical cerclage placement or progesterone.

O26.872 Cervical shortening, second trimester   COM M ♀

O26.873 Cervical shortening, third trimester   COM M ♀

O26.879 Cervical shortening, unspecified trimester   COM M ♀

✓6ᵗʰ **O26.89** Other specified pregnancy related conditions

AHA: 2015,3Q,40

O26.891 Other specified pregnancy related conditions, first trimester   COM M ♀

O26.892 Other specified pregnancy related conditions, second trimester   COM M ♀

O26.893 Other specified pregnancy related conditions, third trimester   COM M ♀

(handwritten margin notes: "Spotting", "back pain")

[handwritten: Maternal Disorders]

O26.899 Other specified pregnancy related conditions, unspecified trimester   COM M ♀

✓5th **O26.9** Pregnancy related conditions, unspecified

O26.90 Pregnancy related conditions, unspecified, unspecified trimester   COM M ♀

O26.91 Pregnancy related conditions, unspecified, first trimester   COM M ♀

O26.92 Pregnancy related conditions, unspecified, second trimester   COM M ♀

[handwritten: RH⁻]

O26.93 Pregnancy related conditions, unspecified, third trimester   COM M ♀

✓4th **O28** **Abnormal findings on antenatal screening of mother**

> EXCLUDES 1   *diagnostic findings classified elsewhere - see Alphabetical Index*

O28.0 Abnormal hematological finding on antenatal screening of mother   M ♀

O28.1 Abnormal biochemical finding on antenatal screening of mother   M ♀

O28.2 Abnormal cytological finding on antenatal screening of mother   M ♀

O28.3 Abnormal ultrasonic finding on antenatal screening of mother   M ♀

O28.4 Abnormal radiological finding on antenatal screening of mother   M ♀

O28.5 Abnormal chromosomal and genetic finding on antenatal screening of mother   M ♀

O28.8 Other abnormal findings on antenatal screening of mother   M ♀

O28.9 Unspecified abnormal findings on antenatal screening of mother   M ♀

✓4th **O29** **Complications of anesthesia during pregnancy**

> INCLUDES   maternal complications arising from the administration of a general, regional or local anesthetic, analgesic or other sedation during pregnancy
>
> Use additional code, if necessary, to identify the complication
>
> EXCLUDES 2   *complications of anesthesia during labor and delivery (O74.-)*
> *complications of anesthesia during the puerperium (O89.-)*

✓5th **O29.0** Pulmonary complications of anesthesia during pregnancy

✓6th **O29.01** Aspiration pneumonitis due to anesthesia during pregnancy

> Inhalation of stomach contents or secretions NOS due to anesthesia during pregnancy
> Mendelson's syndrome due to anesthesia during pregnancy

O29.011 Aspiration pneumonitis due to anesthesia during pregnancy, first trimester   COM M ♀

O29.012 Aspiration pneumonitis due to anesthesia during pregnancy, second trimester   COM M ♀

O29.013 Aspiration pneumonitis due to anesthesia during pregnancy, third trimester   COM M ♀

O29.019 Aspiration pneumonitis due to anesthesia during pregnancy, unspecified trimester   COM M ♀

✓6th **O29.02** Pressure collapse of lung due to anesthesia during pregnancy

O29.021 Pressure collapse of lung due to anesthesia during pregnancy, first trimester   COM M ♀

O29.022 Pressure collapse of lung due to anesthesia during pregnancy, second trimester   COM M ♀

O29.023 Pressure collapse of lung due to anesthesia during pregnancy, third trimester   COM M ♀

O29.029 Pressure collapse of lung due to anesthesia during pregnancy, unspecified trimester   COM M ♀

✓6th **O29.09** Other pulmonary complications of anesthesia during pregnancy

O29.091 Other pulmonary complications of anesthesia during pregnancy, first trimester   COM M ♀

O29.092 Other pulmonary complications of anesthesia during pregnancy, second trimester   COM M ♀

O29.093 Other pulmonary complications of anesthesia during pregnancy, third trimester   COM M ♀

O29.099 Other pulmonary complications of anesthesia during pregnancy, unspecified trimester   COM M ♀

✓5th **O29.1** Cardiac complications of anesthesia during pregnancy

✓6th **O29.11** Cardiac arrest due to anesthesia during pregnancy

O29.111 Cardiac arrest due to anesthesia during pregnancy, first trimester   COM M ♀

O29.112 Cardiac arrest due to anesthesia during pregnancy, second trimester   COM M ♀

O29.113 Cardiac arrest due to anesthesia during pregnancy, third trimester   COM M ♀

O29.119 Cardiac arrest due to anesthesia during pregnancy, unspecified trimester   COM M ♀

✓6th **O29.12** Cardiac failure due to anesthesia during pregnancy

O29.121 Cardiac failure due to anesthesia during pregnancy, first trimester   COM M ♀

O29.122 Cardiac failure due to anesthesia during pregnancy, second trimester   COM M ♀

O29.123 Cardiac failure due to anesthesia during pregnancy, third trimester   COM M ♀

O29.129 Cardiac failure due to anesthesia during pregnancy, unspecified trimester   COM M ♀

✓6th **O29.19** Other cardiac complications of anesthesia during pregnancy

O29.191 Other cardiac complications of anesthesia during pregnancy, first trimester   COM M ♀

O29.192 Other cardiac complications of anesthesia during pregnancy, second trimester   COM M ♀

O29.193 Other cardiac complications of anesthesia during pregnancy, third trimester   COM M ♀

O29.199 Other cardiac complications of anesthesia during pregnancy, unspecified trimester   COM M ♀

✓5th **O29.2** Central nervous system complications of anesthesia during pregnancy

✓6th **O29.21** Cerebral anoxia due to anesthesia during pregnancy

O29.211 Cerebral anoxia due to anesthesia during pregnancy, first trimester   COM M ♀

O29.212 Cerebral anoxia due to anesthesia during pregnancy, second trimester   COM M ♀

O29.213 Cerebral anoxia due to anesthesia during pregnancy, third trimester   COM M ♀

O29.219 Cerebral anoxia due to anesthesia during pregnancy, unspecified trimester   COM M ♀

✓6th **O29.29** Other central nervous system complications of anesthesia during pregnancy

O29.291 Other central nervous system complications of anesthesia during pregnancy, first trimester   COM M ♀

O29.292 Other central nervous system complications of anesthesia during pregnancy, second trimester   COM M ♀

O29.293 Other central nervous system complications of anesthesia during pregnancy, third trimester   COM M ♀

O29.299 Other central nervous system complications of anesthesia during pregnancy, unspecified trimester   COM M ♀

✓5th **O29.3** Toxic reaction to local anesthesia during pregnancy

✓6th **O29.3X** Toxic reaction to local anesthesia during pregnancy

O29.3X1 Toxic reaction to local anesthesia during pregnancy, first trimester   COM M ♀

O29.3X2 Toxic reaction to local anesthesia during pregnancy, second trimester   COM M ♀

O29.3X3 Toxic reaction to local anesthesia during pregnancy, third trimester   COM M ♀

O29.3X9 Toxic reaction to local anesthesia during pregnancy, unspecified trimester   COM M ♀

Chapter 15. Pregnancy, Childbirth and the Puerperium

✓5ᵗʰ **O29.4** Spinal and epidural anesthesia induced headache **during pregnancy**

    O29.40 Spinal and epidural anesthesia induced headache during pregnancy, unspecified trimester COM M ♀

    O29.41 Spinal and epidural anesthesia induced headache during pregnancy, first trimester COM M ♀

    O29.42 Spinal and epidural anesthesia induced headache during pregnancy, second trimester COM M ♀

    O29.43 Spinal and epidural anesthesia induced headache during pregnancy, third trimester COM M ♀

✓5ᵗʰ **O29.5** Other complications of spinal and epidural anesthesia **during pregnancy**

  ✓6ᵗʰ **O29.5X** Other complications of spinal and epidural anesthesia during pregnancy

    O29.5X1 Other complications of spinal and epidural anesthesia during pregnancy, first trimester COM M ♀

    O29.5X2 Other complications of spinal and epidural anesthesia during pregnancy, second trimester COM M ♀

    O29.5X3 Other complications of spinal and epidural anesthesia during pregnancy, third trimester COM M ♀

    O29.5X9 Other complications of spinal and epidural anesthesia during pregnancy, unspecified trimester COM M ♀

✓5ᵗʰ **O29.6** Failed or difficult intubation **for anesthesia during pregnancy**

    O29.60 Failed or difficult intubation for anesthesia during pregnancy, unspecified trimester COM M ♀

    O29.61 Failed or difficult intubation for anesthesia during pregnancy, first trimester COM M ♀

    O29.62 Failed or difficult intubation for anesthesia during pregnancy, second trimester COM M ♀

    O29.63 Failed or difficult intubation for anesthesia during pregnancy, third trimester COM M ♀

✓5ᵗʰ **O29.8** Other complications of anesthesia during pregnancy

  ✓6ᵗʰ **O29.8X** Other complications of anesthesia during pregnancy

    O29.8X1 Other complications of anesthesia during pregnancy, first trimester COM M ♀

    O29.8X2 Other complications of anesthesia during pregnancy, second trimester COM M ♀

    O29.8X3 Other complications of anesthesia during pregnancy, third trimester COM M ♀

    O29.8X9 Other complications of anesthesia during pregnancy, unspecified trimester COM M ♀

✓5ᵗʰ **O29.9** Unspecified complication of anesthesia during pregnancy

    O29.90 Unspecified complication of anesthesia during pregnancy, unspecified trimester COM M ♀

    O29.91 Unspecified complication of anesthesia during pregnancy, first trimester COM M ♀

    O29.92 Unspecified complication of anesthesia during pregnancy, second trimester COM M ♀

    O29.93 Unspecified complication of anesthesia during pregnancy, third trimester COM M ♀

Maternal care related to the fetus and amniotic cavity and possible delivery problems (O30-O48)

✓4ᵗʰ **O30** **Multiple gestation**

  Code also any complications specific to multiple gestation

  AHA: 2016,4Q,51

✓5ᵗʰ **O30.0** Twin **pregnancy**

  ✓6ᵗʰ **O30.00** Twin pregnancy, unspecified number of placenta and unspecified number of amniotic sacs

    O30.001 Twin pregnancy, unspecified number of placenta and unspecified number of amniotic sacs, first trimester COM M ♀

    O30.002 Twin pregnancy, unspecified number of placenta and unspecified number of amniotic sacs, second trimester COM M ♀

    O30.003 Twin pregnancy, unspecified number of placenta and unspecified number of amniotic sacs, third trimester COM M ♀

    O30.009 Twin pregnancy, unspecified number of placenta and unspecified number of amniotic sacs, unspecified trimester COM M ♀

  ✓6ᵗʰ **O30.01** Twin pregnancy, monochorionic/monoamniotic

    Twin pregnancy, one placenta, one amniotic sac

    EXCLUDES 1 conjoined twins (O30.02-)

    O30.011 Twin pregnancy, monochorionic/monoamniotic, first trimester COM M ♀

    O30.012 Twin pregnancy, monochorionic/monoamniotic, second trimester COM M ♀

    O30.013 Twin pregnancy, monochorionic/monoamniotic, third trimester COM M ♀

    O30.019 Twin pregnancy, monochorionic/monoamniotic, unspecified trimester COM M ♀

  ✓6ᵗʰ **O30.02** Conjoined twin pregnancy

    O30.021 Conjoined twin pregnancy, first trimester COM M ♀

    O30.022 Conjoined twin pregnancy, second trimester COM M ♀

    O30.023 Conjoined twin pregnancy, third trimester COM M ♀

    O30.029 Conjoined twin pregnancy, unspecified trimester COM M ♀

  ✓6ᵗʰ **O30.03** Twin pregnancy, monochorionic/diamniotic

    Twin pregnancy, one placenta, two amniotic sacs

    O30.031 Twin pregnancy, monochorionic/diamniotic, first trimester COM M ♀

    O30.032 Twin pregnancy, monochorionic/diamniotic, second trimester COM M ♀

    O30.033 Twin pregnancy, monochorionic/diamniotic, third trimester COM M ♀

    O30.039 Twin pregnancy, monochorionic/diamniotic, unspecified trimester COM M ♀

  ✓6ᵗʰ **O30.04** Twin pregnancy, dichorionic/diamniotic

    Twin pregnancy, two placentae, two amniotic sacs

    O30.041 Twin pregnancy, dichorionic/diamniotic, first trimester COM M ♀

    O30.042 Twin pregnancy, dichorionic/diamniotic, second trimester COM M ♀

    O30.043 Twin pregnancy, dichorionic/diamniotic, third trimester COM M ♀

    O30.049 Twin pregnancy, dichorionic/diamniotic, unspecified trimester COM M ♀

  ✓6ᵗʰ **O30.09** Twin pregnancy, unable to determine number of placenta and number of amniotic sacs

    O30.091 Twin pregnancy, unable to determine number of placenta and number of amniotic sacs, first trimester COM M ♀

    O30.092 Twin pregnancy, unable to determine number of placenta and number of amniotic sacs, second trimester COM M ♀

    O30.093 Twin pregnancy, unable to determine number of placenta and number of amniotic sacs, third trimester COM M ♀

    O30.099 Twin pregnancy, unable to determine number of placenta and number of amniotic sacs, unspecified trimester COM M ♀

✓5ᵗʰ **O30.1** Triplet **pregnancy**

  ✓6ᵗʰ **O30.10** Triplet pregnancy, unspecified number of placenta and unspecified number of amniotic sacs

    AHA: 2016,2Q,8

    O30.101 Triplet pregnancy, unspecified number of placenta and unspecified number of amniotic sacs, first trimester COM M ♀

    O30.102 Triplet pregnancy, unspecified number of placenta and unspecified number of amniotic sacs, second trimester COM M ♀

O30.103   Triplet pregnancy, unspecified number of placenta and unspecified number of amniotic sacs, third trimester   COM M ♀

O30.109   Triplet pregnancy, unspecified number of placenta and unspecified number of amniotic sacs, unspecified trimester   COM M ♀

✓6ᵗʰ O30.11   Triplet pregnancy with two or more monochorionic fetuses

O30.111   Triplet pregnancy with two or more monochorionic fetuses, first trimester   COM M ♀

O30.112   Triplet pregnancy with two or more monochorionic fetuses, second trimester   COM M ♀

O30.113   Triplet pregnancy with two or more monochorionic fetuses, third trimester   COM M ♀

O30.119   Triplet pregnancy with two or more monochorionic fetuses, unspecified trimester   COM M ♀

✓6ᵗʰ O30.12   Triplet pregnancy with two or more monoamniotic fetuses

O30.121   Triplet pregnancy with two or more monoamniotic fetuses, first trimester   COM M ♀

O30.122   Triplet pregnancy with two or more monoamniotic fetuses, second trimester   COM M ♀

O30.123   Triplet pregnancy with two or more monoamniotic fetuses, third trimester   COM M ♀

O30.129   Triplet pregnancy with two or more monoamniotic fetuses, unspecified trimester   COM M ♀

✓6ᵗʰ O30.13   Triplet pregnancy, trichorionic/triamniotic
AHA: 2018,4Q,22

O30.131   Triplet pregnancy, trichorionic/triamniotic, first trimester   COM M ♀

O30.132   Triplet pregnancy, trichorionic/triamniotic, second trimester   COM M ♀

O30.133   Triplet pregnancy, trichorionic/triamniotic, third trimester   COM M ♀

O30.139   Triplet pregnancy, trichorionic/triamniotic, unspecified trimester   COM M ♀

✓6ᵗʰ O30.19   Triplet pregnancy, unable to determine number of placenta and number of amniotic sacs

O30.191   Triplet pregnancy, unable to determine number of placenta and number of amniotic sacs, first trimester   COM M ♀

O30.192   Triplet pregnancy, unable to determine number of placenta and number of amniotic sacs, second trimester   COM M ♀

O30.193   Triplet pregnancy, unable to determine number of placenta and number of amniotic sacs, third trimester   COM M ♀

O30.199   Triplet pregnancy, unable to determine number of placenta and number of amniotic sacs, unspecified trimester   COM M ♀

✓5ᵗʰ O30.2   Quadruplet pregnancy

✓6ᵗʰ O30.20   Quadruplet pregnancy, unspecified number of placenta and unspecified number of amniotic sacs

O30.201   Quadruplet pregnancy, unspecified number of placenta and unspecified number of amniotic sacs, first trimester   COM M ♀

O30.202   Quadruplet pregnancy, unspecified number of placenta and unspecified number of amniotic sacs, second trimester   COM M ♀

O30.203   Quadruplet pregnancy, unspecified number of placenta and unspecified number of amniotic sacs, third trimester   COM M ♀

O30.209   Quadruplet pregnancy, unspecified number of placenta and unspecified number of amniotic sacs, unspecified trimester   COM M ♀

✓6ᵗʰ O30.21   Quadruplet pregnancy with two or more monochorionic fetuses

O30.211   Quadruplet pregnancy with two or more monochorionic fetuses, first trimester   COM M ♀

O30.212   Quadruplet pregnancy with two or more monochorionic fetuses, second trimester   COM M ♀

O30.213   Quadruplet pregnancy with two or more monochorionic fetuses, third trimester   COM M ♀

O30.219   Quadruplet pregnancy with two or more monochorionic fetuses, unspecified trimester   COM M ♀

✓6ᵗʰ O30.22   Quadruplet pregnancy with two or more monoamniotic fetuses

O30.221   Quadruplet pregnancy with two or more monoamniotic fetuses, first trimester   COM M ♀

O30.222   Quadruplet pregnancy with two or more monoamniotic fetuses, second trimester   COM M ♀

O30.223   Quadruplet pregnancy with two or more monoamniotic fetuses, third trimester   COM M ♀

O30.229   Quadruplet pregnancy with two or more monoamniotic fetuses, unspecified trimester   COM M ♀

✓6ᵗʰ O30.23   Quadruplet pregnancy, quadrachorionic/quadra-amniotic
AHA: 2018,4Q,22

O30.231   Quadruplet pregnancy, quadrachorionic/quadra-amniotic, first trimester   COM M ♀

O30.232   Quadruplet pregnancy, quadrachorionic/quadra-amniotic, second trimester   COM M ♀

O30.233   Quadruplet pregnancy, quadrachorionic/quadra-amniotic, third trimester   COM M ♀

O30.239   Quadruplet pregnancy, quadrachorionic/quadra-amniotic, unspecified trimester   COM M ♀

✓6ᵗʰ O30.29   Quadruplet pregnancy, unable to determine number of placenta and number of amniotic sacs

O30.291   Quadruplet pregnancy, unable to determine number of placenta and number of amniotic sacs, first trimester   COM M ♀

O30.292   Quadruplet pregnancy, unable to determine number of placenta and number of amniotic sacs, second trimester   COM M ♀

O30.293   Quadruplet pregnancy, unable to determine number of placenta and number of amniotic sacs, third trimester   COM M ♀

O30.299   Quadruplet pregnancy, unable to determine number of placenta and number of amniotic sacs, unspecified trimester   COM M ♀

✓5ᵗʰ O30.8   Other specified multiple gestation
Multiple gestation pregnancy greater then quadruplets

✓6ᵗʰ O30.80   Other specified multiple gestation, unspecified number of placenta and unspecified number of amniotic sacs

O30.801   Other specified multiple gestation, unspecified number of placenta and unspecified number of amniotic sacs, first trimester   COM M ♀

O30.802   Other specified multiple gestation, unspecified number of placenta and unspecified number of amniotic sacs, second trimester   COM M ♀

O30.803   Other specified multiple gestation, unspecified number of placenta and unspecified number of amniotic sacs, third trimester   COM M ♀

Chapter 15. Pregnancy, Childbirth and the Puerperium

O30.809   Other specified multiple gestation, unspecified number of placenta and unspecified number of amniotic sacs, unspecified trimester   COM M ♀

√6ᵗʰ **O30.81**   Other specified multiple gestation with two or more monochorionic fetuses

O30.811   Other specified multiple gestation with two or more monochorionic fetuses, first trimester   COM M ♀

O30.812   Other specified multiple gestation with two or more monochorionic fetuses, second trimester   COM M ♀

O30.813   Other specified multiple gestation with two or more monochorionic fetuses, third trimester   COM M ♀

O30.819   Other specified multiple gestation with two or more monochorionic fetuses, unspecified trimester   COM M ♀

√6ᵗʰ **O30.82**   Other specified multiple gestation with two or more monoamniotic fetuses

O30.821   Other specified multiple gestation with two or more monoamniotic fetuses, first trimester   COM M ♀

O30.822   Other specified multiple gestation with two or more monoamniotic fetuses, second trimester   COM M ♀

O30.823   Other specified multiple gestation with two or more monoamniotic fetuses, third trimester   COM M ♀

O30.829   Other specified multiple gestation with two or more monoamniotic fetuses, unspecified trimester   COM M ♀

√6ᵗʰ **O30.83**   Other specified multiple gestation, number of chorions and amnions are both equal to the number of fetuses

Pentachorionic, penta-amniotic pregnancy (quintuplets)
Hexachorionic, hexa-amniotic pregnancy (sextuplets)
Heptachorionic, hepta-amniotic pregnancy (septuplets)

AHA: 2018,4Q,22

O30.831   Other specified multiple gestation, number of chorions and amnions are both equal to the number of fetuses, first trimester   COM M ♀

O30.832   Other specified multiple gestation, number of chorions and amnions are both equal to the number of fetuses, second trimester   COM M ♀

O30.833   Other specified multiple gestation, number of chorions and amnions are both equal to the number of fetuses, third trimester   COM M ♀

O30.839   Other specified multiple gestation, number of chorions and amnions are both equal to the number of fetuses, unspecified trimester   COM M ♀

√6ᵗʰ **O30.89**   Other specified multiple gestation, unable to determine number of placenta and number of amniotic sacs

O30.891   Other specified multiple gestation, unable to determine number of placenta and number of amniotic sacs, first trimester   COM M ♀

O30.892   Other specified multiple gestation, unable to determine number of placenta and number of amniotic sacs, second trimester   COM M ♀

O30.893   Other specified multiple gestation, unable to determine number of placenta and number of amniotic sacs, third trimester   COM M ♀

O30.899   Other specified multiple gestation, unable to determine number of placenta and number of amniotic sacs, unspecified trimester   COM M ♀

√5ᵗʰ **O30.9**   Multiple gestation, unspecified

Multiple pregnancy NOS

O30.90   Multiple gestation, unspecified, unspecified trimester   COM M ♀

O30.91   Multiple gestation, unspecified, first trimester   COM M ♀

O30.92   Multiple gestation, unspecified, second trimester   COM M ♀

O30.93   Multiple gestation, unspecified, third trimester   COM M ♀

√4ᵗʰ **O31**   **Complications specific to multiple gestation**

EXCLUDES 2   delayed delivery of second twin, triplet, etc. (O63.2)
malpresentation of one fetus or more (O32.9)
placental transfusion syndromes (O43.0-)

AHA: 2012,4Q,107

One of the following 7th characters is to be assigned to each code under category O31. 7th character 0 is for single gestations and multiple gestations where the fetus is unspecified. 7th characters 1 through 9 are for cases of multiple gestations to identify the fetus for which the code applies. The appropriate code from category O30, Multiple gestation, must also be assigned when assigning a code from category O31 that has a 7th character of 1 through 9.

0   not applicable or unspecified
1   fetus 1
2   fetus 2
3   fetus 3
4   fetus 4
5   fetus 5
9   other fetus

√5ᵗʰ **O31.0**   Papyraceous fetus

Fetus compressus
DEF: Fetus that has died, but remains in utero for weeks before delivery, becoming compacted and mummified in appearance, with skin resembling parchment. Occurs most commonly in multigestational pregnancies. *Synonym(s): paper doll fetus.*

√x 7ᵗʰ **O31.00**   Papyraceous fetus, unspecified trimester   COM M ♀

√x 7ᵗʰ **O31.01**   Papyraceous fetus, first trimester   COM M ♀

√x 7ᵗʰ **O31.02**   Papyraceous fetus, second trimester   COM M ♀

√x 7ᵗʰ **O31.03**   Papyraceous fetus, third trimester   COM M ♀

√5ᵗʰ **O31.1**   Continuing pregnancy after spontaneous abortion of one fetus or more

√x 7ᵗʰ **O31.10**   Continuing pregnancy after spontaneous abortion of one fetus or more, unspecified trimester   COM M ♀

√x 7ᵗʰ **O31.11**   Continuing pregnancy after spontaneous abortion of one fetus or more, first trimester   COM M ♀

√x 7ᵗʰ **O31.12**   Continuing pregnancy after spontaneous abortion of one fetus or more, second trimester   COM M ♀

√x 7ᵗʰ **O31.13**   Continuing pregnancy after spontaneous abortion of one fetus or more, third trimester   COM M ♀

√5ᵗʰ **O31.2**   Continuing pregnancy after intrauterine death of one fetus or more

√x 7ᵗʰ **O31.20**   Continuing pregnancy after intrauterine death of one fetus or more, unspecified trimester   COM M ♀

√x 7ᵗʰ **O31.21**   Continuing pregnancy after intrauterine death of one fetus or more, first trimester   COM M ♀

√x 7ᵗʰ **O31.22**   Continuing pregnancy after intrauterine death of one fetus or more, second trimester   COM M ♀

√x 7ᵗʰ **O31.23**   Continuing pregnancy after intrauterine death of one fetus or more, third trimester   COM M ♀

√5ᵗʰ **O31.3**   Continuing pregnancy after elective fetal reduction of one fetus or more

Continuing pregnancy after selective termination of one fetus or more

√x 7ᵗʰ **O31.30**   Continuing pregnancy after elective fetal reduction of one fetus or more, unspecified trimester   COM M ♀

√x 7ᵗʰ **O31.31**   Continuing pregnancy after elective fetal reduction of one fetus or more, first trimester   COM M ♀

√x 7ᵗʰ **O31.32**   Continuing pregnancy after elective fetal reduction of one fetus or more, second trimester   COM M ♀

√x 7ᵗʰ **O31.33**   Continuing pregnancy after elective fetal reduction of one fetus or more, third trimester   COM M ♀

√5ᵗʰ **O31.8**   Other complications specific to multiple gestation   COM

√6ᵗʰ **O31.8X**   Other complications specific to multiple gestation

√7ᵗʰ **O31.8X1**   Other complications specific to multiple gestation, first trimester   M ♀

√7ᵗʰ **O31.8X2**   Other complications specific to multiple gestation, second trimester   M ♀

√7ᵗʰ **O31.8X3**   Other complications specific to multiple gestation, third trimester   M ♀

HCC CMS-HCC   Rx Rx HCC   ESR ESRD HCC   COM Commercial HCC   N Newborn: 0   P Pediatric: 0-17   M Maternity: 9-64   A Adult: 15-124

[handwritten top margin: Fetus Abnormality]

[handwritten right margin, vertical:] Chapter 15. Pregnancy, Childbirth and the Puerperium

√7ᵗʰ O31.8X9 Other complications specific to multiple gestation, unspecified trimester M ♀

√4ᵗʰ O32 Maternal care for malpresentation of fetus

[handwritten left margin: before onset of labor]

INCLUDES the listed conditions as a reason for observation, hospitalization or other obstetric care of the mother, or for cesarean delivery before onset of labor

EXCLUDES 1 malpresentation of fetus with obstructed labor (O64.-)

AHA: 2012,4Q,107

One of the following 7th characters is to be assigned to each code under category O32. 7th character Ø is for single gestations and multiple gestations where the fetus is unspecified. 7th characters 1 through 9 are for cases of multiple gestations to identify the fetus for which the code applies. The appropriate code from category O3Ø, Multiple gestation, must also be assigned when assigning a code from category O32 that has a 7th character of 1 through 9.

[handwritten left margin: Single gestation ←]

Ø not applicable or unspecified
1 fetus 1
2 fetus 2
3 fetus 3
4 fetus 4
5 fetus 5
9 other fetus

Fetal Malpresentation

Breech
Mother's pelvis

Shoulder (arm prolapse)

Compound (extremity together with head)

Face (mentum)

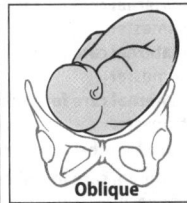
Oblique

√x7ᵗʰ O32.Ø Maternal care for unstable lie COM M ♀

√x7ᵗʰ O32.1 Maternal care for breech presentation COM M ♀
Maternal care for buttocks presentation
Maternal care for complete breech
Maternal care for frank breech
EXCLUDES 1 footling presentation (O32.8)
incomplete breech (O32.8)
DEF: Fetus presentation in a longitudinal lie with the buttocks or feet closest to birth canal that may require external cephalic version or cesarean delivery.

[handwritten left margin: breech for fetus B O32.1XX2]

√x7ᵗʰ O32.2 Maternal care for transverse and oblique lie COM M ♀
Maternal care for oblique presentation
Maternal care for transverse presentation

√x7ᵗʰ O32.3 Maternal care for face, brow and chin presentation COM M ♀

√x7ᵗʰ O32.4 Maternal care for high head at term COM M ♀
Maternal care for failure of head to enter pelvic brim

√x7ᵗʰ O32.6 Maternal care for compound presentation COM M ♀

√x7ᵗʰ O32.8 Maternal care for other malpresentation of fetus COM M ♀
Maternal care for footling presentation
Maternal care for incomplete breech

[handwritten left margin: footling]

√x7ᵗʰ O32.9 Maternal care for malpresentation of fetus, unspecified COM M ♀

√4ᵗʰ O33 Maternal care for disproportion

[handwritten left margin: before onset of labor]

INCLUDES the listed conditions as a reason for observation, hospitalization or other obstetric care of the mother, or for cesarean delivery before onset of labor
EXCLUDES 1 disproportion with obstructed labor (O65-O66)

O33.Ø Maternal care for disproportion due to deformity of maternal pelvic bones COM M ♀
Maternal care for disproportion due to pelvic deformity causing disproportion NOS

O33.1 Maternal care for disproportion due to generally contracted pelvis COM M ♀
Maternal care for disproportion due to contracted pelvis NOS causing disproportion

O33.2 Maternal care for disproportion due to inlet contraction of pelvis COM M ♀
Maternal care for disproportion due to inlet contraction (pelvis) causing disproportion

√x7ᵗʰ O33.3 Maternal care for disproportion due to outlet contraction of pelvis COM M ♀
Maternal care for disproportion due to mid-cavity contraction (pelvis)
Maternal care for disproportion due to outlet contraction (pelvis)

One of the following 7th characters is to be assigned to code O33.3. 7th character Ø is for single gestations and multiple gestations where the fetus is unspecified. 7th characters 1 through 9 are for cases of multiple gestations to identify the fetus for which the code applies. The appropriate code from category O3Ø, Multiple gestation, must also be assigned when assigning code O33.3 with a 7th character of 1 through 9.

[handwritten: Single gestation]

Ø not applicable or unspecified
1 fetus 1
2 fetus 2
3 fetus 3
4 fetus 4
5 fetus 5
9 other fetus

√x7ᵗʰ O33.4 Maternal care for disproportion of mixed maternal and fetal origin COM M ♀

One of the following 7th characters is to be assigned to code O33.4. 7th character Ø is for single gestations and multiple gestations where the fetus is unspecified. 7th characters 1 through 9 are for cases of multiple gestations to identify the fetus for which the code applies. The appropriate code from category O3Ø, Multiple gestation, must also be assigned when assigning code O33.4 with a 7th character of 1 through 9.
Ø not applicable or unspecified
1 fetus 1
2 fetus 2
3 fetus 3
4 fetus 4
5 fetus 5
9 other fetus

√x7ᵗʰ O33.5 Maternal care for disproportion due to unusually large fetus COM M ♀

[handwritten: Macrosomia]

Maternal care for disproportion due to disproportion of fetal origin with normally formed fetus
Maternal care for disproportion due to fetal disproportion NOS

One of the following 7th characters is to be assigned to code O33.5. 7th character Ø is for single gestations and multiple gestations where the fetus is unspecified. 7th characters 1 through 9 are for cases of multiple gestations to identify the fetus for which the code applies. The appropriate code from category O3Ø, Multiple gestation, must also be assigned when assigning code O33.5 with a 7th character of 1 through 9.
Ø not applicable or unspecified
1 fetus 1
2 fetus 2
3 fetus 3
4 fetus 4
5 fetus 5
9 other fetus

*[right margin, vertical: O31.8X9–O33.5]*

Chapter 15. Pregnancy, Childbirth and the Puerperium *(vertical sidebar)*

✓x7ᵗʰ **O33.6 Maternal care for disproportion due to hydrocephalic fetus** COM M ♀

> One of the following 7th characters is to be assigned to code O33.6. 7th character Ø is for single gestations and multiple gestations where the fetus is unspecified. 7th characters 1 through 9 are for cases of multiple gestations to identify the fetus for which the code applies. The appropriate code from category O30, Multiple gestation, must also be assigned when assigning code O33.6 with a 7th character of 1 through 9.
> Ø   not applicable or unspecified
> 1   fetus 1
> 2   fetus 2
> 3   fetus 3
> 4   fetus 4
> 5   fetus 5
> 9   other fetus

✓x7ᵗʰ **O33.7 Maternal care for disproportion due to other fetal deformities** COM M ♀

> Maternal care for disproportion due to fetal ascites
> Maternal care for disproportion due to fetal hydrops
> Maternal care for disproportion due to fetal meningomyelocele
> Maternal care for disproportion due to fetal sacral teratoma
> Maternal care for disproportion due to fetal tumor
> EXCLUDES 1   obstructed labor due to other fetal deformities (O66.3)

> AHA: 2016,4Q,51

> One of the following 7th characters is to be assigned to code O33.7. 7th character Ø is for single gestations and multiple gestations where the fetus is unspecified. 7th characters 1 through 9 are for cases of multiple gestations to identify the fetus for which the code applies. The appropriate code from category O30, Multiple gestation, must also be assigned when assigning code O33.7 with a 7th character of 1 through 9.
> Ø   not applicable or unspecified
> 1   fetus 1
> 2   fetus 2
> 3   fetus 3
> 4   fetus 4
> 5   fetus 5
> 9   other fetus

O33.8 Maternal care for disproportion of other origin COM M ♀

O33.9 Maternal care for disproportion, unspecified COM M ♀

> Maternal care for disproportion due to cephalopelvic disproportion NOS
> Maternal care for disproportion due to fetopelvic disproportion NOS

✓4ᵗʰ **O34 Maternal care for abnormality of pelvic organs**

> INCLUDES   the listed conditions as a reason for hospitalization or other obstetric care of the mother, or for cesarean delivery before onset of labor
> Code first any associated obstructed labor (O65.5)
> Use additional code for specific condition

✓5ᵗʰ **O34.0 Maternal care for congenital malformation of uterus** *(handwritten: Double Q51.3 Q51.4)*

> Maternal care for double uterus
> Maternal care for uterus bicornis *(handwritten: Bicornate)*

O34.00 Maternal care for unspecified congenital malformation of uterus, unspecified trimester COM M ♀ *(handwritten: Septate Q51.28)*

O34.01 Maternal care for unspecified congenital malformation of uterus, first trimester COM M ♀

O34.02 Maternal care for unspecified congenital malformation of uterus, second trimester COM M ♀

O34.03 Maternal care for unspecified congenital malformation of uterus, third trimester COM M ♀

✓5ᵗʰ **O34.1 Maternal care for benign tumor of corpus uteri** *(handwritten: fibroids D25.9)*

> EXCLUDES 2   maternal care for benign tumor of cervix (O34.4-)
> maternal care for malignant neoplasm of uterus (O9A.1-)

O34.10 Maternal care for benign tumor of corpus uteri, unspecified trimester COM M ♀

O34.11 Maternal care for benign tumor of corpus uteri, first trimester COM M ♀

O34.12 Maternal care for benign tumor of corpus uteri, second trimester COM M ♀

O34.13 Maternal care for benign tumor of corpus uteri, third trimester COM M ♀

✓5ᵗʰ **O34.2 Maternal care due to uterine scar from previous surgery**

> AHA: 2020,4Q,36; 2016,4Q,76

✓6ᵗʰ **O34.21 Maternal care for scar from previous cesarean delivery** *(handwritten: after previous c-section)*

> AHA: 2018,3Q,23; 2016,4Q,51-52 *(handwritten: (LT))*

O34.211 Maternal care for low transverse scar from previous cesarean delivery COM M ♀

O34.212 Maternal care for vertical scar from previous cesarean delivery COM M ♀ *(handwritten: classical c-section →)*

> Maternal care for classical scar from previous cesarean delivery

O34.218 Maternal care for other type scar from previous cesarean delivery COM M ♀

> Mid-transverse T incision

O34.219 Maternal care for unspecified type scar from previous cesarean delivery COM M ♀ *(handwritten: VBAC)*

O34.22 Maternal care for cesarean scar defect (isthmocele) COM M ♀ *(handwritten: cesarean history)*

O34.29 Maternal care due to uterine scar from other previous surgery COM M ♀

> Maternal care due to uterine scar from other transmural uterine incision

✓5ᵗʰ **O34.3 Maternal care for cervical incompetence** *(handwritten: cerclage)*

> Maternal care for cerclage with or without cervical incompetence
> Maternal care for Shirodkar suture with or without cervical incompetence
> DEF: Inadequate functioning of the cervix marked by abnormal widening during pregnancy and causing premature birth or miscarriage.

O34.30 Maternal care for cervical incompetence, unspecified trimester COM M ♀

O34.31 Maternal care for cervical incompetence, first trimester COM M ♀

O34.32 Maternal care for cervical incompetence, second trimester COM M ♀

O34.33 Maternal care for cervical incompetence, third trimester COM M ♀

✓5ᵗʰ **O34.4 Maternal care for other abnormalities of cervix**

O34.40 Maternal care for other abnormalities of cervix, unspecified trimester COM M ♀

O34.41 Maternal care for other abnormalities of cervix, first trimester COM M ♀

O34.42 Maternal care for other abnormalities of cervix, second trimester COM M ♀

O34.43 Maternal care for other abnormalities of cervix, third trimester COM M ♀

✓5ᵗʰ **O34.5 Maternal care for other abnormalities of gravid uterus**

✓6ᵗʰ **O34.51 Maternal care for incarceration of gravid uterus**

O34.511 Maternal care for incarceration of gravid uterus, first trimester COM M ♀

O34.512 Maternal care for incarceration of gravid uterus, second trimester COM M ♀

O34.513 Maternal care for incarceration of gravid uterus, third trimester COM M ♀

O34.519 Maternal care for incarceration of gravid uterus, unspecified trimester COM M ♀

✓6ᵗʰ **O34.52 Maternal care for prolapse of gravid uterus**

O34.521 Maternal care for prolapse of gravid uterus, first trimester COM M ♀

O34.522 Maternal care for prolapse of gravid uterus, second trimester COM M ♀

O34.523 Maternal care for prolapse of gravid uterus, third trimester COM M ♀

O34.529 Maternal care for prolapse of gravid uterus, unspecified trimester COM M ♀

✓6ᵗʰ **O34.53 Maternal care for retroversion of gravid uterus**

O34.531 Maternal care for retroversion of gravid uterus, first trimester COM M ♀

O34.532 Maternal care for retroversion of gravid uterus, second trimester COM M ♀

O34.533 Maternal care for retroversion of gravid uterus, third trimester COM M ♀

O34.539 Maternal care for retroversion of gravid uterus, unspecified trimester COM M ♀

| HCC CMS-HCC | Rx Rx HCC | ESR ESRD HCC | COM Commercial HCC | N Newborn: 0 | P Pediatric: 0-17 | M Maternity: 9-64 | A Adult: 15-124 |

908
O33.6–O34.539 *(sidebar)*
ICD-10-CM 2023

(handwritten top-left: "Maternal Abnormality")
(handwritten top-right: "Fetus abnormality")

(handwritten left margin: "IUGR" "SGA" small for dates Z03.74)

O34.59 Maternal care for other abnormalities of gravid uterus

    O34.591 Maternal care for other abnormalities of gravid uterus, **first trimester** COM M ♀

    O34.592 Maternal care for other abnormalities of gravid uterus, **second trimester** COM M ♀

    O34.593 Maternal care for other abnormalities of gravid uterus, **third trimester** COM M ♀

    O34.599 Maternal care for other abnormalities of gravid uterus, **unspecified** COM M ♀

O34.6 Maternal care for abnormality of vagina

    EXCLUDES 2   maternal care for vaginal varices in pregnancy (O22.1-)

    O34.60 Maternal care for abnormality of vagina, **unspecified trimester** COM M ♀

    O34.61 Maternal care for abnormality of vagina, **first trimester** COM M ♀

    O34.62 Maternal care for abnormality of vagina, **second trimester** COM M ♀

    O34.63 Maternal care for abnormality of vagina, **third trimester** COM M ♀

O34.7 Maternal care for abnormality of vulva and perineum

    EXCLUDES 2   maternal care for perineal and vulval varices in pregnancy (O22.1-)

    O34.70 Maternal care for abnormality of vulva and perineum, **unspecified trimester** COM M ♀

    O34.71 Maternal care for abnormality of vulva and perineum, **first trimester** COM M ♀

    O34.72 Maternal care for abnormality of vulva and perineum, **second trimester** COM M ♀

    O34.73 Maternal care for abnormality of vulva and perineum, **third trimester** COM M ♀

O34.8 Maternal care for other abnormalities of pelvic organs

(handwritten left margin: "ovarian cyst")

    O34.80 Maternal care for other abnormalities of pelvic organs, **unspecified trimester** COM M ♀

    O34.81 Maternal care for other abnormalities of pelvic organs, **first trimester** COM M ♀

    O34.82 Maternal care for other abnormalities of pelvic organs, **second trimester** COM M ♀

    O34.83 Maternal care for other abnormalities of pelvic organs, **third trimester** COM M ♀

O34.9 Maternal care for abnormality of pelvic organ, unspecified

    O34.90 Maternal care for abnormality of pelvic organ, unspecified, **unspecified trimester** COM ♀

    O34.91 Maternal care for abnormality of pelvic organ, unspecified, **first trimester** COM M ♀

    O34.92 Maternal care for abnormality of pelvic organ, unspecified, **second trimester** COM M ♀

    O34.93 Maternal care for abnormality of pelvic organ, unspecified, **third trimester** COM M ♀

O35 Maternal care for known or suspected fetal abnormality and damage

    INCLUDES   the listed conditions in the fetus as a reason for hospitalization or other obstetric care to the mother, or for termination of pregnancy

    Code also any associated maternal condition

    EXCLUDES 1   encounter for suspected maternal and fetal conditions ruled out (Z03.7-)

    One of the following 7th characters is to be assigned to each code under category O35. 7th character 0 is for single gestations and multiple gestations where the fetus is unspecified. 7th characters 1 through 9 are for cases of multiple gestations to identify the fetus for which the code applies. The appropriate code from category O30, Multiple gestation, must also be assigned when assigning a code from category O35 that has a 7th character of 1 through 9.

    0   not applicable or unspecified
    1   fetus 1
    2   fetus 2
    3   fetus 3
    4   fetus 4
    5   fetus 5
    9   other fetus

  O35.0 Maternal care for (suspected) central nervous system malformation in fetus

    Maternal care for fetal anencephaly
    Maternal care for fetal hydrocephalus
    Maternal care for fetal spina bifida

    EXCLUDES 2   chromosomal abnormality in fetus ▶(O35.1-)◀

(handwritten: "hydrocephalus" "anencephalic")

    O35.00 Maternal care for (suspected) central nervous system malformation or damage in fetus, **unspecified**

    O35.01 Maternal care for (suspected) central nervous system malformation or damage in fetus, **agenesis of the corpus callosum**

    O35.02 Maternal care for (suspected) central nervous system malformation or damage in fetus, **anencephaly**

    O35.03 Maternal care for (suspected) central nervous system malformation or damage in fetus, **choroid plexus cysts**

    O35.04 Maternal care for (suspected) central nervous system malformation or damage in fetus, **encephalocele**

    O35.05 Maternal care for (suspected) central nervous system malformation or damage in fetus, **holoprosencephaly**

    O35.06 Maternal care for (suspected) central nervous system malformation or damage in fetus, **hydrocephaly**
        Maternal care for fetal hydrocephalus

    O35.07 Maternal care for (suspected) central nervous system malformation or damage in fetus, **microcephaly**

    O35.08 Maternal care for (suspected) central nervous system malformation or damage in fetus, **spina bifida**

    O35.09 Maternal care for (suspected) other central nervous system malformation or damage in fetus

  O35.1 Maternal care for (suspected) chromosomal abnormality in fetus

(handwritten: "second fetus")

    O35.10 Maternal care for (suspected) chromosomal abnormality in fetus, **unspecified**

    O35.11 Maternal care for (suspected) chromosomal abnormality in fetus, **Trisomy 13**

    O35.12 Maternal care for (suspected) chromosomal abnormality in fetus, **Trisomy 18**

(handwritten: "O35.13X2" ←)

    O35.13 Maternal care for (suspected) chromosomal abnormality in fetus, **Trisomy 21**

    O35.14 Maternal care for (suspected) chromosomal abnormality in fetus, **Turner Syndrome**

    O35.15 Maternal care for (suspected) chromosomal abnormality in fetus, **sex chromosome abnormality**

    O35.19 Maternal care for (suspected) chromosomal abnormality in fetus, **other chromosomal abnormality**

  O35.A Maternal care for other (suspected) fetal abnormality and damage, **fetal facial anomalies**

  O35.B Maternal care for other (suspected) fetal abnormality and damage, **fetal cardiac anomalies**

  O35.C Maternal care for other (suspected) fetal abnormality and damage, **fetal pulmonary anomalies**

- ● ✓x7ᵗʰ **O35.D** **Maternal care for other (suspected) fetal abnormality and damage,** fetal gastrointestinal anomalies
- ● ✓x7ᵗʰ **O35.E** **Maternal care for other (suspected) fetal abnormality and damage,** fetal genitourinary anomalies
- ● ✓x7ᵗʰ **O35.F** **Maternal care for other (suspected) fetal abnormality and damage,** fetal musculoskeletal anomalies of trunk
  - EXCLUDES 2   *maternal care for other (suspected) fetal abnormality and damage, fetal lower extremities anomalies (O35.H)*
  - *maternal care for other (suspected) fetal abnormality and damage, fetal upper extremities anomalies (O35.G)*
- ● ✓x7ᵗʰ **O35.G** **Maternal care for other (suspected) fetal abnormality and damage,** fetal upper extremities anomalies
- ● ✓x7ᵗʰ **O35.H** **Maternal care for other (suspected) fetal abnormality and damage,** fetal lower extremities anomalies
- ✓x7ᵗʰ **O35.2** **Maternal care for (suspected)** hereditary disease in fetus   COM Ⓜ ♀
  - EXCLUDES 2   *chromosomal abnormality in fetus ▶(O35.1-)◀*
- ✓x7ᵗʰ **O35.3** **Maternal care for (suspected)** damage to fetus from viral disease in mother   COM Ⓜ ♀
  - Maternal care for damage to fetus from maternal cytomegalovirus infection
  - Maternal care for damage to fetus from maternal rubella
- ✓x7ᵗʰ **O35.4** **Maternal care for (suspected)** damage to fetus from alcohol   COM Ⓜ ♀
- ✓x7ᵗʰ **O35.5** **Maternal care for (suspected)** damage to fetus by drugs   COM Ⓜ ♀
  - Maternal care for damage to fetus from drug addiction
- ✓x7ᵗʰ **O35.6** **Maternal care for (suspected)** damage to fetus by radiation   COM Ⓜ ♀
- ✓x7ᵗʰ **O35.7** **Maternal care for (suspected)** damage to fetus by other medical procedures   COM Ⓜ ♀
  - Maternal care for damage to fetus by amniocentesis
  - Maternal care for damage to fetus by biopsy procedures
  - Maternal care for damage to fetus by hematological investigation
  - Maternal care for damage to fetus by intrauterine contraceptive device
  - Maternal care for damage to fetus by intrauterine surgery
- ✓x7ᵗʰ **O35.8** **Maternal care for other (suspected) fetal abnormality and damage**   COM Ⓜ ♀
  - Maternal care for damage to fetus from maternal listeriosis
  - Maternal care for damage to fetus from maternal toxoplasmosis
- ✓x7ᵗʰ **O35.9** **Maternal care for (suspected) fetal abnormality and damage, unspecified**   COM Ⓜ ♀
- ✓4ᵗʰ **O36** **Maternal care for other fetal problems**
  - INCLUDES   the listed conditions in the fetus as a reason for hospitalization or other obstetric care of the mother, or for termination of pregnancy
  - EXCLUDES 1   *encounter for suspected maternal and fetal conditions ruled out (Z03.7-)*
  - *placental transfusion syndromes (O43.0-)*
  - EXCLUDES 2   *labor and delivery complicated by fetal stress (O77.-)*
  - **AHA:** 2015,3Q,40

  One of the following 7th characters is to be assigned to each code under category O36. 7th character Ø is for single gestations and multiple gestations where the fetus is unspecified. 7th characters 1 through 9 are for cases of multiple gestations to identify the fetus for which the code applies. The appropriate code from category O30, Multiple gestation, must also be assigned when assigning a code from category O36 that has a 7th character of 1 through 9.
  - Ø   not applicable or unspecified
  - 1   fetus 1
  - 2   fetus 2
  - 3   fetus 3
  - 4   fetus 4
  - 5   fetus 5
  - 9   other fetus

- ✓5ᵗʰ **O36.Ø** **Maternal care for rhesus isoimmunization**
  - Maternal care for Rh incompatibility (with hydrops fetalis)
  - ✓6ᵗʰ **O36.01** **Maternal care for** anti-D [Rh] antibodies
    - **AHA:** 2014,4Q,17
    - ✓7ᵗʰ **O36.011** **Maternal care for anti-D [Rh] antibodies, first trimester**   COM Ⓜ ♀
    - ✓7ᵗʰ **O36.012** **Maternal care for anti-D [Rh] antibodies, second trimester**   COM Ⓜ ♀
    - ✓7ᵗʰ **O36.013** **Maternal care for anti-D [Rh] antibodies, third trimester**   COM Ⓜ ♀
    - ✓7ᵗʰ **O36.019** **Maternal care for anti-D [Rh] antibodies, unspecified trimester**   COM Ⓜ ♀
  - ✓6ᵗʰ **O36.09** **Maternal care for other rhesus isoimmunization**
    - ✓7ᵗʰ **O36.091** **Maternal care for other rhesus isoimmunization, first trimester**   COM Ⓜ ♀
    - ✓7ᵗʰ **O36.092** **Maternal care for other rhesus isoimmunization, second trimester**   COM Ⓜ ♀
    - ✓7ᵗʰ **O36.093** **Maternal care for other rhesus isoimmunization, third trimester**   COM Ⓜ ♀
    - ✓7ᵗʰ **O36.099** **Maternal care for other rhesus isoimmunization, unspecified trimester**   COM Ⓜ ♀
- ✓5ᵗʰ **O36.1** **Maternal care for other isoimmunization**
  - Maternal care for ABO isoimmunization

  not for RH-
  - ✓6ᵗʰ **O36.11** **Maternal care for** Anti-A sensitization
    - Maternal care for isoimmunization NOS (with hydrops fetalis)
    - ✓7ᵗʰ **O36.111** **Maternal care for Anti-A sensitization, first trimester**   COM Ⓜ ♀
    - ✓7ᵗʰ **O36.112** **Maternal care for Anti-A sensitization, second trimester**   COM Ⓜ ♀
    - ✓7ᵗʰ **O36.113** **Maternal care for Anti-A sensitization, third trimester**   COM Ⓜ ♀
    - ✓7ᵗʰ **O36.119** **Maternal care for Anti-A sensitization, unspecified trimester**   COM Ⓜ ♀
  - ✓6ᵗʰ **O36.19** **Maternal care for other isoimmunization**
    - Maternal care for Anti-B sensitization
    - ✓7ᵗʰ **O36.191** **Maternal care for other isoimmunization, first trimester**   COM Ⓜ ♀
    - ✓7ᵗʰ **O36.192** **Maternal care for other isoimmunization, second trimester**   COM Ⓜ ♀
    - ✓7ᵗʰ **O36.193** **Maternal care for other isoimmunization, third trimester**   COM Ⓜ ♀
    - ✓7ᵗʰ **O36.199** **Maternal care for other isoimmunization, unspecified trimester**   COM Ⓜ ♀
- ✓5ᵗʰ **O36.2** **Maternal care for hydrops fetalis**
  - Maternal care for hydrops fetalis NOS
  - Maternal care for hydrops fetalis not associated with isoimmunization
  - EXCLUDES 1   *hydrops fetalis associated with ABO isoimmunization (O36.1-)*
  - *hydrops fetalis associated with rhesus isoimmunization (O36.0-)*
  - **DEF:** Hydrops fetalis: Abnormal fluid buildup in at least two of the following fetal organ spaces: the skin (edema), abdomen (ascites), around the heart (pericardia effusion), and around the lung (pleural effusion). Fluid accumulation may also occur in the mother as polyhydramnios and edema of the placenta.
  - ✓x7ᵗʰ **O36.20** **Maternal care for hydrops fetalis, unspecified trimester**   COM Ⓜ ♀
  - ✓x7ᵗʰ **O36.21** **Maternal care for hydrops fetalis, first trimester**   COM Ⓜ ♀
  - ✓x7ᵗʰ **O36.22** **Maternal care for hydrops fetalis, second trimester**   COM Ⓜ ♀
  - ✓x7ᵗʰ **O36.23** **Maternal care for hydrops fetalis, third trimester**   COM Ⓜ ♀
- ✓x7ᵗʰ **O36.4** **Maternal care for intrauterine death**   COM Ⓜ ♀

  Fetal demise missed abortion
  - Maternal care for intrauterine fetal death NOS
  - Maternal care for intrauterine fetal death after completion of 20 weeks of gestation
  - Maternal care for late fetal death
  - Maternal care for missed delivery
  - EXCLUDES 1   *missed abortion (O02.1)*
  - *stillbirth (P95)*
  - **AHA:** 2022,2Q,3
- ✓5ᵗʰ **O36.5** **Maternal care for known or suspected poor fetal growth**
  - ✓6ᵗʰ **O36.51** **Maternal care for known or suspected placental insufficiency**
    - ✓7ᵗʰ **O36.511** **Maternal care for known or suspected placental insufficiency, first trimester**   COM Ⓜ ♀

√7ᵗʰ **O36.512 Maternal care for known or suspected placental insufficiency, second trimester** COM M ♀

√7ᵗʰ **O36.513 Maternal care for known or suspected placental insufficiency, third trimester** COM M ♀

√7ᵗʰ **O36.519 Maternal care for known or suspected placental insufficiency, unspecified trimester** COM M ♀

√6ᵗʰ **O36.59 Maternal care for other known or suspected poor fetal growth**
Maternal care for known or suspected light-for-dates NOS
Maternal care for known or suspected small-for-dates NOS

√7ᵗʰ **O36.591 Maternal care for other known or suspected poor fetal growth, first trimester** COM M ♀

√7ᵗʰ **O36.592 Maternal care for other known or suspected poor fetal growth, second trimester** COM M ♀

√7ᵗʰ **O36.593 Maternal care for other known or suspected poor fetal growth, third trimester** COM M ♀

√7ᵗʰ **O36.599 Maternal care for other known or suspected poor fetal growth, unspecified** COM M ♀

√5ᵗʰ **O36.6 Maternal care for excessive fetal growth**
Maternal care for known or suspected large-for-dates

√x7ᵗʰ **O36.60 Maternal care for excessive fetal growth, unspecified trimester** COM M ♀

√x7ᵗʰ **O36.61 Maternal care for excessive fetal growth, first trimester** COM M ♀

√x7ᵗʰ **O36.62 Maternal care for excessive fetal growth, second trimester** COM M ♀

√x7ᵗʰ **O36.63 Maternal care for excessive fetal growth, third trimester** COM M ♀

√5ᵗʰ **O36.7 Maternal care for viable fetus in abdominal pregnancy**

√x7ᵗʰ **O36.70 Maternal care for viable fetus in abdominal pregnancy, unspecified trimester** COM M ♀

√x7ᵗʰ **O36.71 Maternal care for viable fetus in abdominal pregnancy, first trimester** COM M ♀

√x7ᵗʰ **O36.72 Maternal care for viable fetus in abdominal pregnancy, second trimester** COM M ♀

√x7ᵗʰ **O36.73 Maternal care for viable fetus in abdominal pregnancy, third trimester** COM ♀

√5ᵗʰ **O36.8 Maternal care for other specified fetal problems**

√x7ᵗʰ **O36.80 Pregnancy with inconclusive fetal viability** COM M ♀
Encounter to determine fetal viability of pregnancy
AHA: 2019,2Q,29

√6ᵗʰ **O36.81 Decreased fetal movements**

√7ᵗʰ **O36.812 Decreased fetal movements, second trimester** COM M ♀

√7ᵗʰ **O36.813 Decreased fetal movements, third trimester** COM M ♀

√7ᵗʰ **O36.819 Decreased fetal movements, unspecified trimester** COM M ♀

√6ᵗʰ **O36.82 Fetal anemia and thrombocytopenia**

√7ᵗʰ **O36.821 Fetal anemia and thrombocytopenia, first trimester** COM M ♀

√7ᵗʰ **O36.822 Fetal anemia and thrombocytopenia, second trimester** COM M ♀

√7ᵗʰ **O36.823 Fetal anemia and thrombocytopenia, third trimester** COM M ♀

√7ᵗʰ **O36.829 Fetal anemia and thrombocytopenia, unspecified trimester** COM M ♀

√6ᵗʰ **O36.83 Maternal care for abnormalities of the fetal heart rate or rhythm**
Maternal care for depressed fetal heart rate tones
Maternal care for fetal bradycardia
Maternal care for fetal heart rate abnormal variability
Maternal care for fetal heart rate decelerations
Maternal care for fetal heart rate irregularity
Maternal care for fetal tachycardia
Maternal care for non-reassuring fetal heart rate or rhythm
AHA: 2017,4Q,20
TIP: Assign for documented fetal tachycardia, bradycardia, decelerations, or loss of variability detected during antenatal testing.

√7ᵗʰ **O36.831 Maternal care for abnormalities of the fetal heart rate or rhythm, first trimester** COM M ♀

√7ᵗʰ **O36.832 Maternal care for abnormalities of the fetal heart rate or rhythm, second trimester** COM M ♀

√7ᵗʰ **O36.833 Maternal care for abnormalities of the fetal heart rate or rhythm, third trimester** COM M ♀

√7ᵗʰ **O36.839 Maternal care for abnormalities of the fetal heart rate or rhythm, unspecified trimester** COM M ♀

√6ᵗʰ **O36.89 Maternal care for other specified fetal problems**

√7ᵗʰ **O36.891 Maternal care for other specified fetal problems, first trimester** COM M ♀

√7ᵗʰ **O36.892 Maternal care for other specified fetal problems, second trimester** COM M ♀

√7ᵗʰ **O36.893 Maternal care for other specified fetal problems, third trimester** COM M ♀

√7ᵗʰ **O36.899 Maternal care for other specified fetal problems, unspecified trimester** COM M ♀

√5ᵗʰ **O36.9 Maternal care for fetal problem, unspecified**

√x7ᵗʰ **O36.90 Maternal care for fetal problem, unspecified, unspecified trimester** COM M ♀

√x7ᵗʰ **O36.91 Maternal care for fetal problem, unspecified, first trimester** COM M ♀

√x7ᵗʰ **O36.92 Maternal care for fetal problem, unspecified, second trimester** COM M ♀

√x7ᵗʰ **O36.93 Maternal care for fetal problem, unspecified, third trimester** COM M ♀

√4ᵗʰ **O40 Polyhydramnios**
INCLUDES hydramnios
EXCLUDES 1 encounter for suspected maternal and fetal conditions ruled out (Z03.7-)
AHA: 2016,1Q,4
DEF: Excess amniotic fluid surrounding the fetus, typically defined as a total fluid volume of greater than 24 cm.

One of the following 7th characters is to be assigned to each code under category O40. 7th character 0 is for single gestations and multiple gestations where the fetus is unspecified. 7th characters 1 through 9 are for cases of multiple gestations to identify the fetus for which the code applies. The appropriate code from category O30, Multiple gestation, must also be assigned when assigning a code from category O40 that has a 7th character of 1 through 9.
0 not applicable or unspecified
1 fetus 1
2 fetus 2
3 fetus 3
4 fetus 4
5 fetus 5
9 other fetus

√x7ᵗʰ **O40.1 Polyhydramnios, first trimester** COM M ♀

√x7ᵗʰ **O40.2 Polyhydramnios, second trimester** COM M ♀

√x7ᵗʰ **O40.3 Polyhydramnios, third trimester** COM M ♀

√x7ᵗʰ **O40.9 Polyhydramnios, unspecified trimester** COM M ♀

✓4ᵗʰ **O41 Other disorders of amniotic fluid and membranes**

> **EXCLUDES 1** encounter for suspected maternal and fetal conditions ruled out (Z03.7-)

> One of the following 7th characters is to be assigned to each code under category O41. 7th character Ø is for single gestations and multiple gestations where the fetus is unspecified. 7th characters 1 through 9 are for cases of multiple gestations to identify the fetus for which the code applies. The appropriate code from category O3Ø, Multiple gestation, must also be assigned when assigning a code from category O41 that has a 7th character of 1 through 9.
> Ø not applicable or unspecified
> 1 fetus 1
> 2 fetus 2
> 3 fetus 3
> 4 fetus 4
> 5 fetus 5
> 9 other fetus

✓5ᵗʰ **O41.Ø Oligohydramnios**   *less fluid*

> Oligohydramnios without rupture of membranes
> **DEF:** Low amniotic fluid, occurring most frequently in the last trimester.

  ✓x7ᵗʰ **O41.ØØ Oligohydramnios,** unspecified trimester COM M ♀

  ✓x7ᵗʰ **O41.Ø1 Oligohydramnios,** first trimester COM M ♀

  ✓x7ᵗʰ **O41.Ø2 Oligohydramnios,** second trimester COM M ♀

  ✓x7ᵗʰ **O41.Ø3 Oligohydramnios,** third trimester COM M ♀

✓5ᵗʰ **O41.1 Infection of amniotic sac and membranes**

  ✓6ᵗʰ **O41.1Ø Infection of amniotic sac and membranes, unspecified**

    ✓7ᵗʰ **O41.1Ø1 Infection of amniotic sac and membranes, unspecified,** first trimester COM M ♀

    ✓7ᵗʰ **O41.1Ø2 Infection of amniotic sac and membranes, unspecified,** second trimester COM M ♀

    ✓7ᵗʰ **O41.1Ø3 Infection of amniotic sac and membranes, unspecified,** third trimester COM M ♀

    ✓7ᵗʰ **O41.1Ø9 Infection of amniotic sac and membranes, unspecified, unspecified trimester** COM M ♀

  ✓6ᵗʰ **O41.12 Chorioamnionitis**

    AHA: 2019,2Q,34

    ✓7ᵗʰ **O41.121 Chorioamnionitis,** first trimester COM M ♀

    ✓7ᵗʰ **O41.122 Chorioamnionitis,** second trimester COM M ♀

    ✓7ᵗʰ **O41.123 Chorioamnionitis,** third trimester COM M ♀

    ✓7ᵗʰ **O41.129 Chorioamnionitis, unspecified** trimester COM M ♀

  ✓6ᵗʰ **O41.14 Placentitis**

    ✓7ᵗʰ **O41.141 Placentitis,** first trimester COM M ♀

    ✓7ᵗʰ **O41.142 Placentitis,** second trimester COM M ♀

    ✓7ᵗʰ **O41.143 Placentitis,** third trimester COM M ♀

    ✓7ᵗʰ **O41.149 Placentitis, unspecified** trimester COM M ♀

✓5ᵗʰ **O41.8 Other specified disorders of amniotic fluid and membranes**

  ✓6ᵗʰ **O41.8X Other specified disorders of amniotic fluid and membranes**

    ✓7ᵗʰ **O41.8X1 Other specified disorders of amniotic fluid and membranes,** first trimester COM M ♀

    ✓7ᵗʰ **O41.8X2 Other specified disorders of amniotic fluid and membranes,** second trimester COM M ♀

    ✓7ᵗʰ **O41.8X3 Other specified disorders of amniotic fluid and membranes,** third trimester COM M ♀

    ✓7ᵗʰ **O41.8X9 Other specified disorders of amniotic fluid and membranes, unspecified** trimester COM M ♀

✓5ᵗʰ **O41.9 Disorder of amniotic fluid and membranes, unspecified**

  ✓x7ᵗʰ **O41.9Ø Disorder of amniotic fluid and membranes, unspecified,** unspecified trimester COM M ♀

  ✓x7ᵗʰ **O41.91 Disorder of amniotic fluid and membranes, unspecified,** first trimester COM M ♀

  ✓x7ᵗʰ **O41.92 Disorder of amniotic fluid and membranes, unspecified,** second trimester COM M ♀

✓x7ᵗʰ **O41.93 Disorder of amniotic fluid and membranes, unspecified,** third trimester COM M ♀

✓4ᵗʰ **O42 Premature rupture of membranes**

  AHA: 2016,1Q,3

  ✓5ᵗʰ **O42.Ø Premature rupture of membranes, onset of labor within 24 hours of rupture**

    O42.ØØ Premature rupture of membranes, onset of labor within 24 hours of rupture, unspecified weeks of gestation COM M ♀

    ✓6ᵗʰ **O42.Ø1 Preterm premature rupture of membranes, onset of labor within 24 hours of rupture**

      Premature rupture of membranes before 37 completed weeks of gestation

O60.1 preterm labor w <24h

      O42.Ø11 Preterm premature rupture of membranes, onset of labor within 24 hours of rupture, first trimester COM M ♀

      O42.Ø12 Preterm premature rupture of membranes, onset of labor within 24 hours of rupture, second trimester COM M ♀

      O42.Ø13 Preterm premature rupture of membranes, onset of labor within 24 hours of rupture, third trimester COM M ♀

      O42.Ø19 Preterm premature rupture of membranes, onset of labor within 24 hours of rupture, unspecified trimester COM M ♀

ROM

    O42.Ø2 Full-term premature rupture of membranes, onset of labor within 24 hours of rupture COM M ♀

      Premature rupture of membranes at or after 37 completed weeks of gestation, onset of labor within 24 hours of rupture

  ✓5ᵗʰ **O42.1 Premature rupture of membranes, onset of labor more than 24 hours following rupture**

    AHA: 2016,1Q,5

PROM

    O42.1Ø Premature rupture of membranes, onset of labor more than 24 hours following rupture, unspecified weeks of gestation COM M ♀

    ✓6ᵗʰ **O42.11 Preterm premature rupture of membranes, onset of labor more than 24 hours following rupture**

      Premature rupture of membranes before 37 completed weeks of gestation

>24h

      O42.111 Preterm premature rupture of membranes, onset of labor more than 24 hours following rupture, first trimester COM M ♀

      O42.112 Preterm premature rupture of membranes, onset of labor more than 24 hours following rupture, second trimester COM M ♀

      O42.113 Preterm premature rupture of membranes, onset of labor more than 24 hours following rupture, third trimester COM M ♀

      O42.119 Preterm premature rupture of membranes, onset of labor more than 24 hours following rupture, unspecified trimester COM M ♀

    O42.12 Full-term premature rupture of membranes, onset of labor more than 24 hours following rupture COM M ♀

      Premature rupture of membranes at or after 37 completed weeks of gestation, onset of labor more than 24 hours following rupture

  ✓5ᵗʰ **O42.9 Premature rupture of membranes, unspecified as to length of time between rupture and onset of labor**

    O42.9Ø Premature rupture of membranes, unspecified as to length of time between rupture and onset of labor, unspecified weeks of gestation COM M ♀

    ✓6ᵗʰ **O42.91 Preterm premature rupture of membranes, unspecified as to length of time between rupture and onset of labor**

      Premature rupture of membranes before 37 completed weeks of gestation

PPROM

      O42.911 Preterm premature rupture of membranes, unspecified as to length of time between rupture and onset of labor, first trimester COM M ♀

Chapter 15. Pregnancy, Childbirth and the Puerperium

handwritten: unspecific length time.

O42.912 Preterm premature rupture of membranes, unspecified as to length of time between rupture and onset of labor, second trimester ᴄᴏᴍ Ⓜ ♀

O42.913 Preterm premature rupture of membranes, unspecified as to length of time between rupture and onset of labor, third trimester ᴄᴏᴍ Ⓜ ♀

O42.919 Preterm premature rupture of membranes, unspecified as to length of time between rupture and onset of labor, unspecified trimester ᴄᴏᴍ Ⓜ ♀

O42.92 Full-term premature rupture of membranes, unspecified as to length of time between rupture and onset of labor ᴄᴏᴍ Ⓜ ♀
Premature rupture of membranes at or after 37 completed weeks of gestation, unspecified as to length of time between rupture and onset of labor

✓4ᵗʰ **O43** Placental disorders
  EXCLUDES 2 maternal care for poor fetal growth due to placental insufficiency (O36.5-)
   placenta previa (O44.-)
   placental polyp (O90.89)
   placentitis (O41.14-)
   premature separation of placenta [abruptio placentae] (O45.-)

✓5ᵗʰ **O43.0** Placental transfusion syndromes

  ✓6ᵗʰ **O43.01** Fetomaternal placental transfusion syndrome
   Maternofetal placental transfusion syndrome

    O43.011 Fetomaternal placental transfusion syndrome, first trimester ᴄᴏᴍ Ⓜ ♀

    O43.012 Fetomaternal placental transfusion syndrome, second trimester ᴄᴏᴍ Ⓜ ♀

    O43.013 Fetomaternal placental transfusion syndrome, third trimester ᴄᴏᴍ Ⓜ ♀

    O43.019 Fetomaternal placental transfusion syndrome, unspecified trimester ᴄᴏᴍ Ⓜ ♀

  ✓6ᵗʰ **O43.02** Fetus-to-fetus placental transfusion syndrome
   DEF: Condition in which an imbalance in amniotic fluid occurs due to uneven blood flow between twins sharing a placenta.

Twin to Twin Transfusion Syndrome (TTTS)

Healthy twins   Twins with TTTS

    O43.021 Fetus-to-fetus placental transfusion syndrome, first trimester ᴄᴏᴍ Ⓜ ♀

    O43.022 Fetus-to-fetus placental transfusion syndrome, second trimester ᴄᴏᴍ Ⓜ ♀

    O43.023 Fetus-to-fetus placental transfusion syndrome, third trimester ᴄᴏᴍ Ⓜ ♀

    O43.029 Fetus-to-fetus placental transfusion syndrome, unspecified trimester ᴄᴏᴍ Ⓜ ♀

✓5ᵗʰ **O43.1** Malformation of placenta

  ✓6ᵗʰ **O43.10** Malformation of placenta, unspecified
   Abnormal placenta NOS

    O43.101 Malformation of placenta, unspecified, first trimester ᴄᴏᴍ Ⓜ ♀

    O43.102 Malformation of placenta, unspecified, second trimester ᴄᴏᴍ Ⓜ ♀

    O43.103 Malformation of placenta, unspecified, third trimester ᴄᴏᴍ Ⓜ ♀

    O43.109 Malformation of placenta, unspecified, unspecified trimester ᴄᴏᴍ Ⓜ ♀

  ✓6ᵗʰ **O43.11** Circumvallate placenta

    O43.111 Circumvallate placenta, first trimester ᴄᴏᴍ Ⓜ ♀

    O43.112 Circumvallate placenta, second trimester ᴄᴏᴍ Ⓜ ♀

    O43.113 Circumvallate placenta, third trimester ᴄᴏᴍ Ⓜ ♀

    O43.119 Circumvallate placenta, unspecified trimester ᴄᴏᴍ Ⓜ ♀

  ✓6ᵗʰ **O43.12** Velamentous insertion of umbilical cord

    O43.121 Velamentous insertion of umbilical cord, first trimester ᴄᴏᴍ Ⓜ ♀

    O43.122 Velamentous insertion of umbilical cord, second trimester ᴄᴏᴍ Ⓜ ♀

    O43.123 Velamentous insertion of umbilical cord, third trimester ᴄᴏᴍ Ⓜ ♀

    O43.129 Velamentous insertion of umbilical cord, unspecified trimester ᴄᴏᴍ Ⓜ ♀

  ✓6ᵗʰ **O43.19** Other malformation of placenta

handwritten: eccentric marginal core.

    O43.191 Other malformation of placenta, first trimester ᴄᴏᴍ Ⓜ ♀

    O43.192 Other malformation of placenta, second trimester ᴄᴏᴍ Ⓜ ♀

    O43.193 Other malformation of placenta, third trimester ᴄᴏᴍ Ⓜ ♀

    O43.199 Other malformation of placenta, unspecified trimester ᴄᴏᴍ Ⓜ ♀

✓5ᵗʰ **O43.2** Morbidly adherent placenta
   Code also associated third stage postpartum hemorrhage, if applicable (O72.0)
   EXCLUDES 1 retained placenta (O73.-)

  ✓6ᵗʰ **O43.21** Placenta accreta
   DEF: Condition where the placenta adheres too deeply to the uterine wall; often associated with placenta previa.

    O43.211 Placenta accreta, first trimester ᴄᴏᴍ Ⓜ ♀

    O43.212 Placenta accreta, second trimester ᴄᴏᴍ Ⓜ ♀

    O43.213 Placenta accreta, third trimester ᴄᴏᴍ Ⓜ ♀

    O43.219 Placenta accreta, unspecified trimester ᴄᴏᴍ Ⓜ ♀

  ✓6ᵗʰ **O43.22** Placenta increta
   AHA: 2022,1Q,20
   DEF: Condition where the placenta adheres too deeply to the uterine wall and penetrates the muscle; often associated with placenta previa.

    O43.221 Placenta increta, first trimester ᴄᴏᴍ Ⓜ ♀

    O43.222 Placenta increta, second trimester ᴄᴏᴍ Ⓜ ♀

    O43.223 Placenta increta, third trimester ᴄᴏᴍ Ⓜ ♀

    O43.229 Placenta increta, unspecified trimester ᴄᴏᴍ Ⓜ ♀

  ✓6ᵗʰ **O43.23** Placenta percreta
   DEF: Condition where the placenta attaches through the uterine muscle and may invade other organs, resulting in antenatal complications, premature delivery, retention of all or a portion of the placenta, or postpartum bleeding.

    O43.231 Placenta percreta, first trimester ᴄᴏᴍ Ⓜ ♀

    O43.232 Placenta percreta, second trimester ᴄᴏᴍ Ⓜ ♀

    O43.233 Placenta percreta, third trimester ᴄᴏᴍ Ⓜ ♀

    O43.239 Placenta percreta, unspecified trimester ᴄᴏᴍ Ⓜ ♀

✓5ᵗʰ **O43.8** Other placental disorders

  ✓6ᵗʰ **O43.81** Placental infarction

    O43.811 Placental infarction, first trimester ᴄᴏᴍ Ⓜ ♀

    O43.812 Placental infarction, second trimester ᴄᴏᴍ Ⓜ ♀

✓ Additional Character Required   ✓x7ᵗʰ Placeholder Alert   Manifestation   Unspecified Dx   Ⓠ QPP   ᴜᴘᴅ Unacceptable PDx
ICD-10-CM 2023   913

O42.912–O43.812

O43.813 **Placental infarction**, third trimester COM M ♀

O43.819 **Placental infarction, unspecified** trimester COM M ♀

✓6ᵗʰ O43.89 **Other placental disorders**
Placental dysfunction

O43.891 **Other placental disorders**, first trimester COM M ♀

O43.892 **Other placental disorders**, second trimester COM M ♀

O43.893 **Other placental disorders**, third trimester COM M ♀

O43.899 **Other placental disorders, unspecified** trimester COM M ♀

✓5ᵗʰ O43.9 **Unspecified placental disorder**

O43.90 **Unspecified placental disorder, unspecified** trimester COM M ♀

O43.91 **Unspecified placental disorder**, first trimester COM M ♀

O43.92 **Unspecified placental disorder**, second trimester COM M ♀

O43.93 **Unspecified placental disorder**, third trimester COM M ♀

✓4ᵗʰ **O44 Placenta previa**
AHA: 2016,4Q,52-53
DEF: Placenta implanted in the lower segment of the uterus, which commonly causes hemorrhage in the last trimester of pregnancy.

✓5ᵗʰ O44.0 **Complete placenta previa NOS or** without hemorrhage
Placenta previa NOS

O44.00 **Complete placenta previa NOS or without hemorrhage, unspecified trimester** COM M ♀

O44.01 **Complete placenta previa NOS or without hemorrhage, first trimester** COM M ♀

O44.02 **Complete placenta previa NOS or without hemorrhage, second trimester** COM M ♀

O44.03 **Complete placenta previa NOS or without hemorrhage, third trimester** COM M ♀

✓5ᵗʰ O44.1 **Complete placenta previa** with hemorrhage

EXCLUDES 1   *labor and delivery complicated by hemorrhage from vasa previa (O69.4)*

not specified is complete

O44.10 **Complete placenta previa with hemorrhage, unspecified trimester** COM M ♀

O44.11 **Complete placenta previa with hemorrhage**, first trimester COM M ♀

O44.12 **Complete placenta previa with hemorrhage**, second trimester COM M ♀

O44.13 **Complete placenta previa with hemorrhage**, third trimester COM M ♀

✓5ᵗʰ O44.2 **Partial placenta previa** without hemorrhage
Marginal placenta previa, NOS or without hemorrhage

O44.20 **Partial placenta previa NOS or without hemorrhage, unspecified trimester** COM M ♀

O44.21 **Partial placenta previa NOS or without hemorrhage, first trimester** COM M ♀

O44.22 **Partial placenta previa NOS or without hemorrhage, second trimester** COM M ♀

O44.23 **Partial placenta previa NOS or without hemorrhage, third trimester** COM M ♀

✓5ᵗʰ O44.3 **Partial placenta previa** with hemorrhage
Marginal placenta previa with hemorrhage

O44.30 **Partial placenta previa with hemorrhage, unspecified trimester** COM M ♀

O44.31 **Partial placenta previa with hemorrhage**, first trimester COM M ♀

O44.32 **Partial placenta previa with hemorrhage**, second trimester COM M ♀

O44.33 **Partial placenta previa with hemorrhage**, third trimester COM M ♀

✓5ᵗʰ O44.4 **Low lying placenta NOS or** without hemorrhage
Low implantation of placenta NOS or without hemorrhage

O44.40 **Low lying placenta NOS or without hemorrhage, unspecified trimester** COM M ♀

O44.41 **Low lying placenta NOS or without hemorrhage**, first trimester COM M ♀

O44.42 **Low lying placenta NOS or without hemorrhage**, second trimester COM M ♀

O44.43 **Low lying placenta NOS or without hemorrhage,** third trimester COM M ♀

✓5ᵗʰ O44.5 **Low lying placenta** with hemorrhage
Low implantation of placenta with hemorrhage

O44.50 **Low lying placenta with hemorrhage, unspecified** trimester COM M ♀

O44.51 **Low lying placenta with hemorrhage**, first trimester COM M ♀

O44.52 **Low lying placenta with hemorrhage**, second trimester COM M ♀

O44.53 **Low lying placenta with hemorrhage**, third trimester COM M ♀

✓4ᵗʰ **O45 Premature separation of placenta [abruptio placentae]**

✓5ᵗʰ O45.0 **Premature separation of placenta** with coagulation defect

✓6ᵗʰ O45.00 **Premature separation of placenta with coagulation defect, unspecified**

O45.001 **Premature separation of placenta with coagulation defect, unspecified,** first trimester COM M ♀

O45.002 **Premature separation of placenta with coagulation defect, unspecified,** second trimester COM M ♀

O45.003 **Premature separation of placenta with coagulation defect, unspecified,** third trimester COM M ♀

O45.009 **Premature separation of placenta with coagulation defect, unspecified, unspecified trimester** COM M ♀

✓6ᵗʰ O45.01 **Premature separation of placenta** with afibrinogenemia
Premature separation of placenta with hypofibrinogenemia

O45.011 **Premature separation of placenta with afibrinogenemia,** first trimester COM M ♀

O45.012 **Premature separation of placenta with afibrinogenemia,** second trimester COM M ♀

O45.013 **Premature separation of placenta with afibrinogenemia,** third trimester COM M ♀

O45.019 **Premature separation of placenta with afibrinogenemia, unspecified** trimester COM M ♀

✓6ᵗʰ O45.02 **Premature separation of placenta** with disseminated intravascular coagulation

O45.021 **Premature separation of placenta with disseminated intravascular coagulation,** first trimester COM M ♀

O45.022 **Premature separation of placenta with disseminated intravascular coagulation,** second trimester COM M ♀

O45.023 **Premature separation of placenta with disseminated intravascular coagulation,** third trimester COM M ♀

O45.029 **Premature separation of placenta with disseminated intravascular coagulation, unspecified trimester** COM M ♀

✓6ᵗʰ O45.09 **Premature separation of placenta with other coagulation defect**

O45.091 **Premature separation of placenta with other coagulation defect,** first trimester COM M ♀

O45.092 **Premature separation of placenta with other coagulation defect,** second trimester COM M ♀

O45.093 **Premature separation of placenta with other coagulation defect,** third trimester COM M ♀

O45.099 **Premature separation of placenta with other coagulation defect, unspecified** trimester COM M ♀

✓5ᵗʰ O45.8 **Other premature separation of placenta**

✓6ᵗʰ O45.8X **Other premature separation of placenta**

O45.8X1 **Other premature separation of placenta,** first trimester COM M ♀

O45.8X2 **Other premature separation of placenta,** second trimester COM M ♀

O45.8X3 **Other premature separation of placenta,** third trimester COM M ♀

[handwritten margin: placenta] *[handwritten: Delivery Problem]*

O45.8X9 Other premature separation of placenta, unspecified trimester ⬛COM M ♀

✓5th **O45.9** Premature separation of placenta, unspecified
  Abruptio placentae NOS

[handwritten margin: placental Abruption]

  O45.90 Premature separation of placenta, unspecified, unspecified trimester ⬛COM M ♀
  O45.91 Premature separation of placenta, unspecified, first trimester ⬛COM M ♀
  O45.92 Premature separation of placenta, unspecified, second trimester ⬛COM M ♀
  O45.93 Premature separation of placenta, unspecified, third trimester ⬛COM M ♀

✓4th **O46** Antepartum hemorrhage, not elsewhere classified

[handwritten margin: antepartum Hemorrhage]

  EXCLUDES 1 hemorrhage in early pregnancy (O20.-)
    intrapartum hemorrhage NEC (O67.-)
    placenta previa (O44.-)
    premature separation of placenta [abruptio placentae] (O45.-)
  DEF: Uterine hemorrhage prior to delivery that is not related to placenta previa or abruptio placentae.

✓5th **O46.0** Antepartum hemorrhage with coagulation defect

  ✓6th **O46.00** Antepartum hemorrhage with coagulation defect, unspecified
    O46.001 Antepartum hemorrhage with coagulation defect, unspecified, first trimester ⬛COM M ♀
    O46.002 Antepartum hemorrhage with coagulation defect, unspecified, second trimester ⬛COM M ♀
    O46.003 Antepartum hemorrhage with coagulation defect, unspecified, third trimester ⬛COM M ♀
    O46.009 Antepartum hemorrhage with coagulation defect, unspecified, unspecified trimester ⬛COM M ♀

  ✓6th **O46.01** Antepartum hemorrhage with afibrinogenemia
    Antepartum hemorrhage with hypofibrinogenemia
    O46.011 Antepartum hemorrhage with afibrinogenemia, first trimester ⬛COM M ♀
    O46.012 Antepartum hemorrhage with afibrinogenemia, second trimester ⬛COM M ♀
    O46.013 Antepartum hemorrhage with afibrinogenemia, third trimester ⬛COM M ♀
    O46.019 Antepartum hemorrhage with afibrinogenemia, unspecified trimester ⬛COM M ♀

  ✓6th **O46.02** Antepartum hemorrhage with disseminated intravascular coagulation
    O46.021 Antepartum hemorrhage with disseminated intravascular coagulation, first trimester ⬛COM M ♀
    O46.022 Antepartum hemorrhage with disseminated intravascular coagulation, second trimester ⬛COM M ♀
    O46.023 Antepartum hemorrhage with disseminated intravascular coagulation, third trimester ⬛COM M ♀
    O46.029 Antepartum hemorrhage with disseminated intravascular coagulation, unspecified trimester ⬛COM M ♀

  ✓6th **O46.09** Antepartum hemorrhage with other coagulation defect
    O46.091 Antepartum hemorrhage with other coagulation defect, first trimester ⬛COM M ♀
    O46.092 Antepartum hemorrhage with other coagulation defect, second trimester ⬛COM M ♀
    O46.093 Antepartum hemorrhage with other coagulation defect, third trimester ⬛COM M ♀
    O46.099 Antepartum hemorrhage with other coagulation defect, unspecified trimester ⬛COM M ♀

✓5th **O46.8** Other antepartum hemorrhage
  ✓6th **O46.8X** Other antepartum hemorrhage
    O46.8X1 Other antepartum hemorrhage, first trimester ⬛COM M ♀
    O46.8X2 Other antepartum hemorrhage, second trimester ⬛COM M ♀
    O46.8X3 Other antepartum hemorrhage, third trimester ⬛COM M ♀
    O46.8X9 Other antepartum hemorrhage, unspecified trimester ⬛COM M ♀

✓5th **O46.9** Antepartum hemorrhage, unspecified
    O46.90 Antepartum hemorrhage, unspecified, unspecified trimester ⬛COM M ♀
    O46.91 Antepartum hemorrhage, unspecified, first trimester ⬛COM M ♀
    O46.92 Antepartum hemorrhage, unspecified, second trimester ⬛COM M ♀
    O46.93 Antepartum hemorrhage, unspecified, third trimester ⬛COM M ♀

✓4th **O47** False labor
  INCLUDES Braxton Hicks contractions
    threatened labor
  EXCLUDES 1 preterm labor (O60.-)
  AHA: 2021,1Q,10

[handwritten margin: False labor]

✓5th **O47.0** False labor before 37 completed weeks of gestation
    O47.00 False labor before 37 completed weeks of gestation, unspecified trimester ⬛COM ♀
    O47.02 False labor before 37 completed weeks of gestation, second trimester ⬛COM ♀
    O47.03 False labor before 37 completed weeks of gestation, third trimester ⬛COM ♀
  O47.1 False labor at or after 37 completed weeks of gestation *[handwritten: back home]* ⬛COM ♀
  O47.9 False labor, unspecified ⬛COM ♀

✓4th **O48** Late pregnancy
  AHA: 2022,2Q,3 *[handwritten: ≥ 40 +1 days]*
  O48.0 Post-term pregnancy ⬛COM M ♀
    Pregnancy over 40 completed weeks to 42 completed weeks gestation
  O48.1 Prolonged pregnancy ⬛COM M ♀
    Pregnancy which has advanced beyond 42 completed weeks gestation
    AHA: 2016,1Q,5

Complications of labor and delivery (O60-O77)

✓4th **O60** Preterm labor
  INCLUDES onset (spontaneous) of labor before 37 completed weeks of gestation
  EXCLUDES 1 false labor (O47.0-)
    threatened labor NOS (O47.0-)

✓5th **O60.0** Preterm labor without delivery
    O60.00 Preterm labor without delivery, unspecified trimester ⬛COM M ♀
    O60.02 Preterm labor without delivery, second trimester ⬛COM M ♀
    O60.03 Preterm labor without delivery, third trimester ⬛COM M ♀

✓5th **O60.1** Preterm labor with preterm delivery
    AHA: 2016,2Q,10

[handwritten margin: pre-term labor w/ delivery]

One of the following 7th characters is to be assigned to each code under subcategory O60.1. 7th character 0 is for single gestations and multiple gestations where the fetus is unspecified. 7th characters 1 through 9 are for cases of multiple gestations to identify the fetus for which the code applies. The appropriate code from category O30, Multiple gestation, must also be assigned when assigning a code from subcategory O60.1 that has a 7th character of 1 through 9.
  0   not applicable or unspecified *[handwritten: A]*
  1   fetus 1 *[handwritten: A]*
  2   fetus 2 *[handwritten: B]*
  3   fetus 3 *[handwritten: C]*
  4   fetus 4 *[handwritten: D]*
  5   fetus 5 *[handwritten: E]*
  9   other fetus

  ✓x7th **O60.10** Preterm labor with preterm delivery, unspecified trimester ⬛COM M ♀
    Preterm labor with delivery NOS
  ✓x7th **O60.12** Preterm labor second trimester with preterm delivery second trimester ⬛COM M ♀

☑ Additional Character Required   ✓x7th Placeholder Alert   Manifestation   Unspecified Dx   Q QPP   UPD Unacceptable PDx

[handwritten bottom: during premature labor happen acute renal failure]

labor complication (handwritten)

Delivery problem (handwritten, top)

Chapter 15. Pregnancy, Childbirth and the Puerperium (side vertical text)

√x7th **O60.13** **Preterm labor** second trimester **with preterm delivery** third trimester   COM M ♀

√x7th **O60.14** **Preterm labor** third trimester **with preterm delivery** third trimester   COM M ♀

√5th **O60.2** **Term delivery with preterm labor**

Arrested Dialation (handwritten)
failure to progress (handwritten)

One of the following 7th characters is to be assigned to each code under subcategory O60.2. 7th character Ø is for single gestations and multiple gestations where the fetus is unspecified. 7th characters 1 through 9 are for cases of multiple gestations to identify the fetus for which the code applies. The appropriate code from category O30, Multiple gestation, must also be assigned when assigning a code from subcategory O60.2 that has a 7th character of 1 through 9.

Ø   not applicable or unspecified
1   fetus 1
2   fetus 2
3   fetus 3
4   fetus 4
5   fetus 5
9   other fetus

√x7th **O60.20** **Term delivery with preterm labor, unspecified trimester**   COM M ♀

√x7th **O60.22** **Term delivery with preterm labor,** second trimester   COM M ♀

√x7th **O60.23** **Term delivery with preterm labor,** third trimester   COM M ♀

√4th **O61** **Failed induction of labor**

O61.0 **Failed** medical **induction of labor**   COM M ♀
   Failed induction (of labor) by oxytocin
   Failed induction (of labor) by prostaglandins

O61.1 **Failed** instrumental **induction of labor**   COM M ♀
   Failed mechanical induction (of labor)
   Failed surgical induction (of labor)

O61.8 **Other failed induction of labor**   COM M ♀

O61.9 **Failed induction of labor, unspecified**   COM M ♀

√4th **O62** **Abnormalities of forces of labor**

no aducate contraction (handwritten)
latent phase (handwritten)
not aducate dilation (handwritten)

DEF: Uterine inertia: Weak or poorly coordinated contractions of the uterus during labor.

O47.1 for labor hall "senthone" (handwritten, left margin)

O62.0 **Primary inadequate contractions**   COM M ♀
   Failure of cervical dilatation
   Primary hypotonic uterine dysfunction
   Uterine inertia during latent phase of labor

<4cm process labor (handwritten)

O62.1 **Secondary uterine inertia**   COM M ♀
   Arrested active phase of labor
   Secondary hypotonic uterine dysfunction

>4cm (handwritten)

O62.2 **Other uterine inertia**   COM M ♀
   Atony of uterus without hemorrhage
   Atony of uterus NOS
   Desultory labor
   Hypotonic uterine dysfunction NOS
   Irregular labor
   Poor contractions
   Slow slope active phase of labor
   Uterine inertia NOS

   EXCLUDES 1   atony of uterus with hemorrhage (postpartum) (O72.1)
     postpartum atony of uterus without hemorrhage (O75.89)

   DEF: Uterine atony: Failure of the uterine muscles to contract after the fetus and placenta are delivered.

Qwik (handwritten)

O62.3 **Precipitate labor** *Rapid delivery* (handwritten)   COM M ♀
   DEF: Rapid labor with delivery occurring in three hours or less from the onset of contractions.

O62.4 **Hypertonic, incoordinate, and prolonged uterine contractions**   COM M ♀
   Cervical spasm
   Contraction ring dystocia
   Dyscoordinate labor
   Hour-glass contraction of uterus
   Hypertonic uterine dysfunction
   Incoordinate uterine action
   Tetanic contractions
   Uterine dystocia NOS
   Uterine spasm
   EXCLUDES 1   dystocia (fetal) (maternal) NOS (O66.9)

O62.8 **Other abnormalities of forces of labor**   COM M ♀

O62.9 **Abnormality of forces of labor, unspecified**   COM M ♀

√4th **O63** **Long labor**

active phase (handwritten)

O63.0 **Prolonged first stage** (of labor) *10-14h* (handwritten)   COM M ♀
O63.1 **Prolonged second stage** (of labor) *1-4h (3h push)* (handwritten)   COM M ♀
O63.2 **Delayed delivery of second twin, triplet, etc.**   COM M ♀
O63.9 **Long labor, unspecified**   COM M ♀
   Prolonged labor NOS

√4th **O64** **Obstructed labor due to malposition and malpresentation of fetus**

One of the following 7th characters is to be assigned to each code under category O64. 7th character Ø is for single gestations and multiple gestations where the fetus is unspecified. 7th characters 1 through 9 are for cases of multiple gestations to identify the fetus for which the code applies. The appropriate code from category O30, Multiple gestation, must also be assigned when assigning a code from category O64 that has a 7th character of 1 through 9.

Ø   not applicable or unspecified
1   fetus 1
2   fetus 2
3   fetus 3
4   fetus 4
5   fetus 5
9   other fetus

Fetal Malposition

Breech — Mother's pelvis
Shoulder (arm prolapse)
Compound (extremity together with head)
Face (mentum)
Oblique

obstructive labor (handwritten)

√x7th **O64.0** **Obstructed labor due to** incomplete rotation of fetal head   COM M ♀
   Deep transverse arrest
   Obstructed labor due to persistent occipitoiliac (position)
   Obstructed labor due to persistent occipitoposterior (position)
   Obstructed labor due to persistent occipitosacral (position)
   Obstructed labor due to persistent occipitotransverse (position)

√x7th **O64.1** **Obstructed labor due to** breech presentation   COM M ♀
   Obstructed labor due to buttocks presentation
   Obstructed labor due to complete breech presentation
   Obstructed labor due to frank breech presentation

√x7th **O64.2** **Obstructed labor due to** face presentation   COM M ♀
   Obstructed labor due to chin presentation

√x7th **O64.3** **Obstructed labor due to** brow presentation   COM M ♀

√x7th **O64.4** **Obstructed labor due to** shoulder presentation   COM M ♀
   Prolapsed arm
   EXCLUDES 1   impacted shoulders (O66.0)
     shoulder dystocia (O66.0)

√x7th **O64.5** **Obstructed labor due to** compound presentation   COM M ♀

√x7th **O64.8** **Obstructed labor due to** other malposition and malpresentation   COM M ♀
   Obstructed labor due to footling presentation
   Obstructed labor due to incomplete breech presentation

√x7th **O64.9** **Obstructed labor due to malposition and malpresentation, unspecified**   COM M ♀

√4th **O65** **Obstructed labor due to maternal pelvic abnormality**

O65.0 **Obstructed labor due to** deformed pelvis   COM M ♀
O65.1 **Obstructed labor due to** generally contracted pelvis   COM M ♀
O65.2 **Obstructed labor due to** pelvic inlet contraction   COM M ♀
O65.3 **Obstructed labor due to** pelvic outlet and mid-cavity contraction   COM M ♀

(handwritten bottom margin, illegible)

O65.4 Obstructed labor due to fetopelvic disproportion, unspecified COM M ♀
> EXCLUDES 1 dystocia due to abnormality of fetus (O66.2-O66.3)

O65.5 Obstructed labor due to abnormality of maternal pelvic organs COM M ♀
> Obstructed labor due to conditions listed in O34.-
> Use additional code to identify abnormality of pelvic organs O34.-

O65.8 Obstructed labor due to other maternal pelvic abnormalities COM M ♀

O65.9 Obstructed labor due to maternal pelvic abnormality, unspecified COM M ♀

✓4ᵗʰ **O66 Other obstructed labor**   *too big*

O66.0 Obstructed labor due to shoulder dystocia COM M ♀
> Impacted shoulders
> **DEF:** Obstructed labor due to impacted fetal shoulders. It is an emergency condition that may require cesarean section, forceps delivery, vacuum extraction, or symphysiotomy.

O66.1 Obstructed labor due to locked twins COM M ♀

O66.2 Obstructed labor due to unusually large fetus COM M ♀

O66.3 Obstructed labor due to other abnormalities of fetus COM M ♀
> Dystocia due to fetal ascites
> Dystocia due to fetal hydrops
> Dystocia due to fetal meningomyelocele
> Dystocia due to fetal sacral teratoma
> Dystocia due to fetal tumor
> Dystocia due to hydrocephalic fetus
> Use additional code to identify cause of obstruction

✓5ᵗʰ **O66.4 Failed trial of labor**

> **O66.40 Failed trial of labor, unspecified** COM M ♀
> **O66.41 Failed attempted vaginal birth after previous cesarean delivery** COM M ♀
>> Code first rupture of uterus, if applicable (O71.0-, O71.1)

O66.5 Attempted application of vacuum extractor and forceps COM M ♀
> Attempted application of vacuum or forceps, with subsequent delivery by forceps or cesarean delivery

O66.6 Obstructed labor due to other multiple fetuses COM M ♀

O66.8 Other specified obstructed labor COM M ♀
> Use additional code to identify cause of obstruction

O66.9 Obstructed labor, unspecified COM M ♀
> Dystocia NOS
> Fetal dystocia NOS
> Maternal dystocia NOS

59618
59620
59622

✓4ᵗʰ **O67 Labor and delivery complicated by intrapartum hemorrhage, not elsewhere classified**
> EXCLUDES 1 antepartum hemorrhage NEC (O46.-)
> placenta previa (O44.-)
> premature separation of placenta [abruptio placentae] (O45.-)
> EXCLUDES 2 postpartum hemorrhage (O72.-)

Hemorrhage
intrapartum

O67.0 Intrapartum hemorrhage with coagulation defect COM M ♀
> Intrapartum hemorrhage (excessive) associated with afibrinogenemia
> Intrapartum hemorrhage (excessive) associated with disseminated intravascular coagulation
> Intrapartum hemorrhage (excessive) associated with hyperfibrinolysis
> Intrapartum hemorrhage (excessive) associated with hypofibrinogenemia

O67.8 Other intrapartum hemorrhage COM M ♀
> Excessive intrapartum hemorrhage

O67.9 Intrapartum hemorrhage, unspecified COM M ♀

if antepartum hemorrhage O46.

O68 Labor and delivery complicated by abnormality of fetal acid-base balance COM M ♀
> Fetal acidemia complicating labor and delivery
> Fetal acidosis complicating labor and delivery
> Fetal alkalosis complicating labor and delivery
> Fetal metabolic acidemia complicating labor and delivery
> EXCLUDES 1 fetal stress NOS (O77.9)
>> labor and delivery complicated by electrocardiographic evidence of fetal stress (O77.8)
>> labor and delivery complicated by ultrasonic evidence of fetal stress (O77.8)
> EXCLUDES 2 abnormality in fetal heart rate or rhythm (O76)
>> labor and delivery complicated by meconium in amniotic fluid (O77.0)

acid
base
balance

✓4ᵗʰ **O69 Labor and delivery complicated by umbilical cord complications**
> **AHA:** 2016,1Q,5

> One of the following 7th characters is to be assigned to each code under category O69. 7th character Ø is for single gestations and multiple gestations where the fetus is unspecified. 7th characters 1 through 9 are for cases of multiple gestations to identify the fetus for which the code applies. The appropriate code from category O30, Multiple gestation, must also be assigned when assigning a code from category O69 that has a 7th character of 1 through 9.
> Ø   not applicable or unspecified
> 1   fetus 1
> 2   fetus 2
> 3   fetus 3
> 4   fetus 4
> 5   fetus 5
> 9   other fetus

✓x7ᵗʰ **O69.0 Labor and delivery complicated by prolapse of cord** COM M ♀
> **DEF:** Abnormal presentation of the fetus marked by a protruding umbilical cord during labor. It can cause fetal death.

✓x7ᵗʰ **O69.1 Labor and delivery complicated by cord around neck, with compression** COM M ♀   *Tight*
> EXCLUDES 1 labor and delivery complicated by cord around neck, without compression (O69.81)

✓x7ᵗʰ **O69.2 Labor and delivery complicated by other cord entanglement, with compression** COM M ♀
> Labor and delivery complicated by compression of cord NOS
> Labor and delivery complicated by entanglement of cords of twins in monoamniotic sac   *Knot*
> Labor and delivery complicated by knot in cord
> EXCLUDES 1 labor and delivery complicated by other cord entanglement, without compression (O69.82)

✓x7ᵗʰ **O69.3 Labor and delivery complicated by short cord** COM M ♀

✓x7ᵗʰ **O69.4 Labor and delivery complicated by vasa previa** COM M ♀
> Labor and delivery complicated by hemorrhage from vasa previa

✓x7ᵗʰ **O69.5 Labor and delivery complicated by vascular lesion of cord** COM M ♀
> Labor and delivery complicated by cord bruising
> Labor and delivery complicated by cord hematoma
> Labor and delivery complicated by thrombosis of umbilical vessels

✓5ᵗʰ **O69.8 Labor and delivery complicated by other cord complications**

> ✓x7ᵗʰ **O69.81 Labor and delivery complicated by cord around neck, without compression** COM M ♀
>> **AHA:** 2016,1Q,5
> ✓x7ᵗʰ **O69.82 Labor and delivery complicated by other cord entanglement, without compression** COM M ♀   *truncal*
> ✓x7ᵗʰ **O69.89 Labor and delivery complicated by other cord complications** COM M ♀

✓x7ᵗʰ **O69.9 Labor and delivery complicated by cord complication, unspecified** COM M ♀

2 vessel cord.

[handwritten margin note: tear of forchette]

✓4ᵗʰ **O70 Perineal laceration during delivery**

   INCLUDES episiotomy extended by laceration
   EXCLUDES 1 obstetric high vaginal laceration alone (O71.4)
   AHA: 2016,2Q,34; 2016,1Q,3-4,5

O70.0 First degree perineal laceration during delivery COM M ♀
[handwritten: clitoral]
   Perineal laceration, rupture or tear involving fourchette during delivery
   Perineal laceration, rupture or tear involving labia during delivery
   Perineal laceration, rupture or tear involving skin during delivery
   Perineal laceration, rupture or tear involving vagina during delivery
   Perineal laceration, rupture or tear involving vulva during delivery
   Slight perineal laceration, rupture or tear during delivery

O70.1 Second degree perineal laceration during delivery COM M ♀
   Perineal laceration, rupture or tear during delivery as in O70.0, also involving pelvic floor
   Perineal laceration, rupture or tear during delivery as in O70.0, also involving perineal muscles
   Perineal laceration, rupture or tear during delivery as in O70.0, also involving vaginal muscles
   EXCLUDES 1 perineal laceration involving anal sphincter (O70.2)

✓5ᵗʰ **O70.2 Third degree perineal laceration during delivery**

[handwritten margin note: includes episiotomy extended]

   Perineal laceration, rupture or tear during delivery as in O70.1, also involving anal sphincter
   Perineal laceration, rupture or tear during delivery as in O70.1, also involving rectovaginal septum
   Perineal laceration, rupture or tear during delivery as in O70.1, also involving sphincter NOS
   EXCLUDES 1 anal sphincter tear during delivery without third degree perineal laceration (O70.4)
     perineal laceration involving anal or rectal mucosa (O70.3)
   AHA: 2016,4Q,53-54

   O70.20 Third degree perineal laceration during delivery, unspecified COM M ♀
   O70.21 Third degree perineal laceration during delivery, IIIa COM M ♀
     Third degree perineal laceration during delivery with less than 50% of external anal sphincter (EAS) thickness torn
   O70.22 Third degree perineal laceration during delivery, IIIb COM M ♀
     Third degree perineal laceration during delivery with more than 50% external anal sphincter (EAS) thickness torn
   O70.23 Third degree perineal laceration during delivery, IIIc COM M ♀
     Third degree perineal laceration during delivery with both external anal sphincter (EAS) and internal anal sphincter (IAS) torn

O70.3 Fourth degree perineal laceration during delivery COM M ♀
   Perineal laceration, rupture or tear during delivery as in O70.2, also involving anal mucosa
   Perineal laceration, rupture or tear during delivery as in O70.2, also involving rectal mucosa

O70.4 Anal sphincter tear complicating delivery, not associated with third degree laceration COM M ♀
   EXCLUDES 1 anal sphincter tear with third degree perineal laceration (O70.2)

O70.9 Perineal laceration during delivery, unspecified COM M ♀

✓4ᵗʰ **O71 Other obstetric trauma**
   INCLUDES obstetric damage from instruments

✓5ᵗʰ **O71.0 Rupture of uterus (spontaneous) before onset of labor**
   EXCLUDES 1 disruption of (current) cesarean delivery wound (O90.0)
     laceration of uterus, NEC (O71.81)

   O71.00 Rupture of uterus before onset of labor, unspecified trimester COM M ♀
   O71.02 Rupture of uterus before onset of labor, second trimester COM M ♀
   O71.03 Rupture of uterus before onset of labor, third trimester COM M ♀

O71.1 Rupture of uterus during labor COM M ♀
   Rupture of uterus not stated as occurring before onset of labor
   EXCLUDES 1 disruption of cesarean delivery wound (O90.0)
     laceration of uterus, NEC (O71.81)

O71.2 Postpartum inversion of uterus COM M ♀

O71.3 Obstetric laceration of cervix COM M ♀
   Annular detachment of cervix

O71.4 Obstetric high vaginal laceration alone COM M ♀
   Laceration of vaginal wall without perineal laceration
   EXCLUDES 1 obstetric high vaginal laceration with perineal laceration (O70.-)
   AHA: 2016,1Q,5

O71.5 Other obstetric injury to pelvic organs COM M ♀
   Obstetric injury to bladder
   Obstetric injury to urethra
   EXCLUDES 2 obstetric periurethral trauma (O71.82)
   AHA: 2014,4Q,18

O71.6 Obstetric damage to pelvic joints and ligaments COM M ♀
   Obstetric avulsion of inner symphyseal cartilage
   Obstetric damage to coccyx
   Obstetric traumatic separation of symphysis (pubis)

O71.7 Obstetric hematoma of pelvis COM M ♀
   Obstetric hematoma of perineum
   Obstetric hematoma of vagina
   Obstetric hematoma of vulva

✓5ᵗʰ **O71.8 Other specified obstetric trauma**

   O71.81 Laceration of uterus, not elsewhere classified COM M ♀
   O71.82 Other specified trauma to perineum and vulva COM M ♀
     Obstetric periurethral trauma
     AHA: 2016,1Q,4; 2014,4Q,18
   O71.89 Other specified obstetric trauma COM M ♀

O71.9 Obstetric trauma, unspecified COM M ♀

✓4ᵗʰ **O72 Postpartum hemorrhage**
   INCLUDES hemorrhage after delivery of fetus or infant

[handwritten: placenta over 5'-15']

O72.0 Third-stage hemorrhage COM M ♀
   Hemorrhage associated with retained, trapped or adherent placenta
   Retained placenta NOS
   Code also type of adherent placenta (O43.2-)
   AHA: 2019,3Q,11

O72.1 Other immediate postpartum hemorrhage COM M ♀
   Hemorrhage following delivery of placenta
   Postpartum hemorrhage (atonic) NOS
   Uterine atony with hemorrhage
   EXCLUDES 1 uterine atony NOS (O62.2)
     uterine atony without hemorrhage (O62.2)
     postpartum atony of uterus without hemorrhage (O75.89)

[handwritten: not after abortion]

   AHA: 2016,1Q,4
   DEF: Uterine atony: Failure of the uterine muscles to contract after the fetus and placenta are delivered.

O72.2 Delayed and secondary postpartum hemorrhage COM M ♀
   Hemorrhage associated with retained portions of placenta or membranes after the first 24 hours following delivery of placenta
   Retained products of conception NOS, following delivery

O72.3 Postpartum coagulation defects COM M ♀
   Postpartum afibrinogenemia
   Postpartum fibrinolysis

✓4ᵗʰ **O73 Retained placenta and membranes, without hemorrhage**

[handwritten: placenta over 5'-15]

   EXCLUDES 1 placenta accreta (O43.21-)
     placenta increta (O43.22-)
     placenta percreta (O43.23-)
   DEF: Postpartum condition resulting from failure to expel placental membrane tissues due to failed contractions of the uterine wall.

O73.0 Retained placenta without hemorrhage COM M ♀
   Adherent placenta, without hemorrhage
   Trapped placenta without hemorrhage

O73.1 Retained portions of placenta and membranes, without hemorrhage COM M ♀

[handwritten: Portions]

   Retained products of conception following delivery, without hemorrhage

ICD-10-CM 2023 *labor complication* Chapter 15. Pregnancy, Childbirth and the Puerperium *normal vaginal delivery? documented?* O74–O85

Chapter 15. Pregnancy, Childbirth and the Puerperium

O74–O85

✓4th O74 Complications of anesthesia during labor and delivery

INCLUDES maternal complications arising from the administration of a general, regional or local anesthetic, analgesic or other sedation during labor and delivery

Use additional code, if applicable, to identify specific complication

anesthesia

O74.0 Aspiration pneumonitis due to anesthesia during labor and delivery COM M ♀
Inhalation of stomach contents or secretions NOS due to anesthesia during labor and delivery
Mendelson's syndrome due to anesthesia during labor and delivery

O74.1 Other pulmonary complications of anesthesia during labor and delivery COM M ♀

O74.2 Cardiac complications of anesthesia during labor and delivery COM M ♀

O74.3 Central nervous system complications of anesthesia during labor and delivery COM M ♀

O74.4 Toxic reaction to local anesthesia during labor and delivery COM M ♀

O74.5 Spinal and epidural anesthesia-induced headache during labor and delivery COM M ♀

O74.6 Other complications of spinal and epidural anesthesia during labor and delivery COM M ♀

O74.7 Failed or difficult intubation for anesthesia during labor and delivery COM M ♀

O74.8 Other complications of anesthesia during labor and delivery COM M ♀

O74.9 Complication of anesthesia during labor and delivery, unspecified COM M ♀

✓4th O75 Other complications of labor and delivery, not elsewhere classified

EXCLUDES 2 puerperal (postpartum) infection (O86.-)
puerperal (postpartum) sepsis (O85)

O75.0 Maternal distress during labor and delivery COM M ♀

O75.1 Shock during or following labor and delivery COM M ♀
Obstetric shock following labor and delivery

O75.2 Pyrexia during labor, not elsewhere classified COM M ♀

O75.3 Other infection during labor COM M ♀
Sepsis during labor
Use additional code (B95-B97), to identify infectious agent

O75.4 Other complications of obstetric surgery and procedures COM M ♀
Cardiac arrest following obstetric surgery or procedures
Cardiac failure following obstetric surgery or procedures
Cerebral anoxia following obstetric surgery or procedures
Pulmonary edema following obstetric surgery or procedures
Use additional code to identify specific complication
EXCLUDES 2 complications of anesthesia during labor and delivery (O74.-)
disruption of obstetrical (surgical) wound (O90.0-O90.1)
hematoma of obstetrical (surgical) wound (O90.2)
infection of obstetrical (surgical) wound (O86.0-)

O75.5 Delayed delivery after artificial rupture of membranes COM M ♀

✓5th O75.8 Other specified complications of labor and delivery

O75.81 Maternal exhaustion complicating labor and delivery COM M ♀

O75.82 Onset (spontaneous) of labor after 37 completed weeks of gestation but before 39 completed weeks gestation, with delivery by (planned) cesarean section COM ♀
Delivery by (planned) cesarean section occurring after 37 completed weeks of gestation but before 39 completed weeks gestation due to (spontaneous) onset of labor
Code first to specify reason for planned cesarean section such as:
cephalopelvic disproportion (normally formed fetus) (O33.9)
previous cesarean delivery (O34.21)
AHA: 2022,2Q,3

O75.89 Other specified complications of labor and delivery COM M ♀ *uterine atony w/o hemo*

O75.9 Complication of labor and delivery, unspecified COM M ♀

O76 Abnormality in fetal heart rate and rhythm complicating labor and delivery COM M ♀

Fetal ♡ tb
Depressed fetal heart rate tones complicating labor and delivery
Fetal bradycardia complicating labor and delivery
Fetal heart rate decelerations complicating labor and delivery
Fetal heart rate irregularity complicating labor and delivery
Fetal heart rate abnormal variability complicating labor and delivery
Fetal tachycardia complicating labor and delivery
Non-reassuring fetal heart rate or rhythm complicating labor and delivery *EHR tracing*
EXCLUDES 1 fetal stress NOS (O77.9)
labor and delivery complicated by electrocardiographic evidence of fetal stress (O77.8)
labor and delivery complicated by ultrasonic evidence of fetal stress (O77.8)
EXCLUDES 2 fetal metabolic acidemia (O68)
other fetal stress (O77.0-O77.1)
AHA: 2013,4Q,118

Fetal stress

✓4th O77 Other fetal stress complicating labor and delivery *(MSAF)*

O77.0 Labor and delivery complicated by meconium in amniotic fluid COM M ♀
AHA: 2022,2Q,16; 2013,4Q,117-118

O77.1 Fetal stress in labor or delivery due to drug administration COM M ♀

O77.8 Labor and delivery complicated by other evidence of fetal stress COM M ♀
Labor and delivery complicated by electrocardiographic evidence of fetal stress
Labor and delivery complicated by ultrasonic evidence of fetal stress
EXCLUDES 1 abnormality of fetal acid-base balance (O68)
abnormality in fetal heart rate or rhythm (O76)
fetal metabolic acidemia (O68)

Fetal stress

O77.9 Labor and delivery complicated by fetal stress, unspecified COM M ♀
EXCLUDES 1 abnormality of fetal acid-base balance (O68)
abnormality in fetal heart rate or rhythm (O76)
fetal metabolic acidemia (O68)

Encounter for delivery (O80-O82)

O80 Encounter for full-term uncomplicated delivery COM M ♀

NOTE Delivery requiring minimal or no assistance, with or without episiotomy, without fetal manipulation [e.g., rotation version] or instrumentation [forceps] of a spontaneous, cephalic, vaginal, full-term, single, live-born infant. This code is for use as a single diagnosis code and is not to be used with any other code from chapter 15.
Use additional code to indicate outcome of delivery (Z37.0)
AHA: 2016,4Q,150; 2014,2Q,9

normal delivery single add Z37.0 only

O82 Encounter for cesarean delivery without indication COM M ♀

C-section not documented reason
Use additional code to indicate outcome of delivery (Z37.0) → *fetus abnormal mother condition complication*

Complications predominantly related to the puerperium (O85-O92)

EXCLUDES 2 mental and behavioral disorders associated with the puerperium (F53.-)
obstetrical tetanus (A34)
puerperal osteomalacia (M83.0)

O85 Puerperal sepsis COM M ♀

add B95-B96. No A40 or A41
Postpartum sepsis
Puerperal peritonitis
Puerperal pyemia
Use additional code (B95-B97), to identify infectious agent
Use additional code (R65.2-) to identify severe sepsis, if applicable
EXCLUDES 1 fever of unknown origin following delivery (O86.4)
genital tract infection following delivery (O86.1-)
obstetric pyemic and septic embolism (O88.3-)
puerperal septic thrombophlebitis (O86.81)
urinary tract infection following delivery (O86.2-)
EXCLUDES 2 sepsis during labor (O75.3)
AHA: 2022,2Q,5; 2020,2Q,32; 2019,2Q,39; 2018,4Q,23

Can't use for post procedural infection only for puerperal.

☑4ᵗʰ **O86 Other puerperal infections**
Use additional code (B95-B97), to identify infectious agent
EXCLUDES 2   infection during labor (O75.3)
    obstetrical tetanus (A34)

☑5ᵗʰ **O86.0 Infection of** obstetric surgical wound
Infected cesarean delivery wound following delivery
Infected perineal repair following delivery
EXCLUDES 1   complications of procedures, not elsewhere classified
    (T81.4-)
    postprocedural fever NOS (R50.82)
    postprocedural retroperitoneal abscess (K68.11)
AHA: 2020,2Q,32; 2018,4Q,22-23,62

O86.00 Infection of obstetric surgical wound, unspecified COM M ♀

O86.01 Infection of obstetric surgical wound, superficial incisional site COM M ♀
Subcutaneous abscess following an obstetrical procedure
Stitch abscess following an obstetrical procedure

O86.02 Infection of obstetric surgical wound, deep incisional site COM M ♀
Intramuscular abscess following an obstetrical procedure
Sub-fascial abscess following an obstetrical procedure
AHA: 2020,2Q,32

O86.03 Infection of obstetric surgical wound, organ and space site COM M ♀
Intraabdominal abscess following an obstetrical procedure
Subphrenic abscess following an obstetrical procedure

O86.04 Sepsis following an obstetrical procedure COM ♀
Use additional code to identify the sepsis
AHA: 2020,2Q,32; 2019,2Q,39

O86.09 Infection of obstetric surgical wound, other surgical site COM M ♀

☑5ᵗʰ **O86.1 Other infection of** genital tract following delivery
O86.11 Cervicitis following delivery COM M ♀
O86.12 Endometritis following delivery COM M ♀
O86.13 Vaginitis following delivery COM M ♀
O86.19 Other infection of genital tract following delivery COM M ♀

☑5ᵗʰ **O86.2 Urinary tract infection following delivery**
O86.20 Urinary tract infection following delivery, unspecified COM M ♀
Puerperal urinary tract infection NOS
AHA: 2022,2Q,5
O86.21 Infection of kidney following delivery COM M ♀
O86.22 Infection of bladder following delivery COM M ♀
Infection of urethra following delivery
O86.29 Other urinary tract infection following delivery COM M ♀

O86.4 Pyrexia of unknown origin following delivery COM M ♀
Puerperal infection NOS following delivery
Puerperal pyrexia NOS following delivery
EXCLUDES 2   pyrexia during labor (O75.2)
DEF: Fever of unknown origin experienced by the mother after childbirth.

☑5ᵗʰ **O86.8 Other specified puerperal infections**
O86.81 Puerperal septic thrombophlebitis COM M ♀
O86.89 Other specified puerperal infections COM M ♀

☑4ᵗʰ **O87 Venous complications and hemorrhoids in the puerperium**
INCLUDES venous complications in labor, delivery and the puerperium
EXCLUDES 2   obstetric embolism (O88.-)
    puerperal septic thrombophlebitis (O86.81)
    venous complications in pregnancy (O22.-)

O87.0 Superficial thrombophlebitis in the puerperium COM M ♀
Puerperal phlebitis NOS
Puerperal thrombosis NOS

O87.1 Deep phlebothrombosis in the puerperium COM M ♀
Deep vein thrombosis, postpartum
Pelvic thrombophlebitis, postpartum
Use additional code to identify the deep vein thrombosis (I82.4-, I82.5-, I82.62-, I82.72-)
Use additional code, if applicable, for associated long-term (current) use of anticoagulants (Z79.01)

O87.2 Hemorrhoids in the puerperium COM M ♀
O87.3 Cerebral venous thrombosis in the puerperium COM M ♀
Cerebrovenous sinus thrombosis in the puerperium
O87.4 Varicose veins of lower extremity in the puerperium COM M ♀ *varicositis*
O87.8 Other venous complications in the puerperium COM M ♀
Genital varices in the puerperium
O87.9 Venous complication in the puerperium, unspecified COM M ♀
Puerperal phlebopathy NOS

☑4ᵗʰ **O88 Obstetric embolism**
EXCLUDES 1   embolism complicating abortion NOS (O03.2)
    embolism complicating ectopic or molar pregnancy (O08.2)
    embolism complicating failed attempted abortion (O07.2)
    embolism complicating induced abortion (O04.7)
    embolism complicating spontaneous abortion (O03.2, O03.7)

☑5ᵗʰ **O88.0 Obstetric** air embolism
DEF: Sudden blocking of the pulmonary artery or right ventricle with air or nitrogen bubbles.
☑6ᵗʰ **O88.01 Obstetric air embolism in** pregnancy
O88.011 Air embolism in pregnancy, first trimester COM M ♀
O88.012 Air embolism in pregnancy, second trimester COM M ♀
O88.013 Air embolism in pregnancy, third trimester COM M ♀
O88.019 Air embolism in pregnancy, unspecified trimester COM M ♀
O88.02 Air embolism in childbirth COM M ♀
O88.03 Air embolism in the puerperium COM M ♀

☑5ᵗʰ **O88.1 Amniotic fluid embolism**
Anaphylactoid syndrome in pregnancy
☑6ᵗʰ **O88.11 Amniotic fluid embolism in** pregnancy
O88.111 Amniotic fluid embolism in pregnancy, first trimester COM M ♀
O88.112 Amniotic fluid embolism in pregnancy, second trimester COM M ♀
O88.113 Amniotic fluid embolism in pregnancy, third trimester COM M ♀
O88.119 Amniotic fluid embolism in pregnancy, unspecified trimester COM M ♀
O88.12 Amniotic fluid embolism in childbirth COM M ♀
O88.13 Amniotic fluid embolism in the puerperium COM M ♀

☑5ᵗʰ **O88.2 Obstetric** thromboembolism
☑6ᵗʰ **O88.21 Thromboembolism in** pregnancy
Obstetric (pulmonary) embolism NOS
O88.211 Thromboembolism in pregnancy, first trimester COM M ♀
O88.212 Thromboembolism in pregnancy, second trimester COM M ♀
O88.213 Thromboembolism in pregnancy, third trimester COM M ♀
O88.219 Thromboembolism in pregnancy, unspecified trimester COM M ♀
O88.22 Thromboembolism in childbirth COM M ♀
O88.23 Thromboembolism in the puerperium COM M ♀
Puerperal (pulmonary) embolism NOS

☑5ᵗʰ **O88.3 Obstetric** pyemic and septic embolism
☑6ᵗʰ **O88.31 Pyemic and septic embolism in** pregnancy
O88.311 Pyemic and septic embolism in pregnancy, first trimester COM M ♀
O88.312 Pyemic and septic embolism in pregnancy, second trimester COM M ♀
O88.313 Pyemic and septic embolism in pregnancy, third trimester COM M ♀
O88.319 Pyemic and septic embolism in pregnancy, unspecified trimester COM M ♀

puerperium (handwritten)

O88.32 **Pyemic and septic embolism in childbirth** `COM` `M` ♀

O88.33 **Pyemic and septic embolism in the puerperium** `COM` `M` ♀

√5ᵗʰ O88.8 **Other obstetric embolism**
Obstetric fat embolism

√6ᵗʰ O88.81 **Other embolism in** pregnancy

O88.811 **Other embolism in pregnancy, first trimester** `COM` `M` ♀

O88.812 **Other embolism in pregnancy, second trimester** `COM` `M` ♀

O88.813 **Other embolism in pregnancy, third trimester** `COM` `M` ♀

O88.819 **Other embolism in pregnancy, unspecified trimester** `COM` `M` ♀

O88.82 **Other embolism in** childbirth `COM` `M` ♀

O88.83 **Other embolism in the** puerperium `COM` `M` ♀

√4ᵗʰ O89 **Complications of anesthesia during the puerperium**

`INCLUDES` maternal complications arising from the administration of a general, regional or local anesthetic, analgesic or other sedation during the puerperium

Use additional code, if applicable, to identify specific complication

√5ᵗʰ O89.0 **Pulmonary complications of anesthesia during the puerperium**

O89.01 **Aspiration pneumonitis due to anesthesia during the puerperium** `COM` `M` ♀
Inhalation of stomach contents or secretions NOS due to anesthesia during the puerperium
Mendelson's syndrome due to anesthesia during the puerperium

O89.09 **Other pulmonary complications of anesthesia during the puerperium** `COM` `M` ♀

O89.1 **Cardiac complications of anesthesia during the puerperium** `COM` `M` ♀

O89.2 **Central nervous system complications of anesthesia during the puerperium** `COM` `M` ♀

O89.3 **Toxic reaction to local anesthesia during the puerperium** `COM` `M` ♀

O89.4 **Spinal and epidural anesthesia-induced headache during the puerperium** `COM` `M` ♀

O89.5 **Other complications of spinal and epidural anesthesia during the puerperium** `COM` `M` ♀

O89.6 **Failed or difficult intubation for anesthesia during the puerperium** `COM` `M` ♀

O89.8 **Other complications of anesthesia during the puerperium** `COM` `M` ♀

O89.9 **Complication of anesthesia during the puerperium, unspecified** `COM` `M` ♀

√4ᵗʰ O90 **Complications of the puerperium, not elsewhere classified**

O90.0 **Disruption of cesarean delivery wound** `COM` `M` ♀
Dehiscence of cesarean delivery wound
`EXCLUDES 1` rupture of uterus (spontaneous) before onset of labor (O71.0-)
rupture of uterus during labor (O71.1)

(handwritten: open cesarean wound after 1 year + O94)

O90.1 **Disruption of perineal obstetric wound** `COM` `M` ♀
Disruption of wound of episiotomy
Disruption of wound of perineal laceration
Secondary perineal tear

O90.2 **Hematoma of obstetric wound** `COM` `M` ♀

O90.3 **Peripartum cardiomyopathy** `COM` `M` ♀
Conditions in I42- arising during pregnancy and the puerperium
`EXCLUDES 1` pre-existing heart disease complicating pregnancy and the puerperium (O99.4-)
DEF: Any structural or functional abnormality of the ventricular myocardium. It is a noninflammatory disease of obscure or unknown etiology with onset during the postpartum period.

(handwritten: start 3rd semester; continue 1 month after birth; did not have pre-existing heart disease)

O90.4 **Postpartum acute kidney failure** `COM` `M` ♀
Hepatorenal syndrome following labor and delivery

(handwritten: follow delivery)

O90.5 **Postpartum thyroiditis** `COM` `M` ♀

O90.6 **Postpartum mood disturbance** `COM` `Q` `M` ♀
Postpartum blues
Postpartum dysphoria
Postpartum sadness
`EXCLUDES 1` postpartum depression (F53.0)
puerperal psychosis (F53.1)

√5ᵗʰ O90.8 **Other complications of the puerperium, not elsewhere classified**

O90.81 **Anemia of the puerperium** `COM` `M` ♀
Postpartum anemia NOS
`EXCLUDES 1` pre-existing anemia complicating the puerperium (O99.03)
AHA: 2019,3Q,11

O90.89 **Other complications of the puerperium, not elsewhere classified** `COM` `M` ♀
Placental polyp

O90.9 **Complication of the puerperium, unspecified** `COM` `M` ♀

√4ᵗʰ O91 **Infections of breast associated with pregnancy, the puerperium and lactation**
Use additional code to identify infection

√5ᵗʰ O91.0 **Infection of nipple associated with pregnancy, the puerperium and lactation**

√6ᵗʰ O91.01 **Infection of nipple associated with** pregnancy
Gestational abscess of nipple

O91.011 **Infection of nipple associated with pregnancy, first trimester** `COM` `M` ♀

O91.012 **Infection of nipple associated with pregnancy, second trimester** `COM` `M` ♀

O91.013 **Infection of nipple associated with pregnancy, third trimester** `COM` `M` ♀

O91.019 **Infection of nipple associated with pregnancy, unspecified trimester** `COM` `M` ♀

O91.02 **Infection of nipple associated with the puerperium** `M` ♀
Puerperal abscess of nipple

O91.03 **Infection of nipple associated with** lactation `M` ♀
Abscess of nipple associated with lactation

√5ᵗʰ O91.1 **Abscess of breast associated with pregnancy, the puerperium and lactation**

√6ᵗʰ O91.11 **Abscess of breast associated with** pregnancy
Gestational mammary abscess
Gestational purulent mastitis
Gestational subareolar abscess

O91.111 **Abscess of breast associated with pregnancy, first trimester** `COM` `M` ♀

O91.112 **Abscess of breast associated with pregnancy, second trimester** `COM` `M` ♀

O91.113 **Abscess of breast associated with pregnancy, third trimester** `COM` `M` ♀

O91.119 **Abscess of breast associated with pregnancy, unspecified trimester** `COM` `M` ♀

O91.12 **Abscess of breast associated with the puerperium** `M` ♀
Puerperal mammary abscess
Puerperal purulent mastitis
Puerperal subareolar abscess

O91.13 **Abscess of breast associated with** lactation `M` ♀
Mammary abscess associated with lactation
Purulent mastitis associated with lactation
Subareolar abscess associated with lactation

√5ᵗʰ O91.2 **Nonpurulent mastitis associated with pregnancy, the puerperium and lactation**

√6ᵗʰ O91.21 **Nonpurulent mastitis associated with** pregnancy
Gestational interstitial mastitis
Gestational lymphangitis of breast
Gestational mastitis NOS
Gestational parenchymatous mastitis

O91.211 **Nonpurulent mastitis associated with pregnancy, first trimester** `COM` `M` ♀

O91.212 **Nonpurulent mastitis associated with pregnancy, second trimester** `COM` `M` ♀

O91.213 **Nonpurulent mastitis associated with pregnancy, third trimester** `COM` `M` ♀

O91.219 **Nonpurulent mastitis associated with pregnancy, unspecified trimester** `COM` `M` ♀

(handwritten: peripartum: last month pregnancy to 5 months after delivery)

| ✔ Additional Character Required | ✔x7ᵗʰ Placeholder Alert | Manifestation | Unspecified Dx | `Q` QPP | `UPD` Unacceptable PDx |

ICD-10-CM 2023   921

[handwritten margin notes: "puerperium", "if found at follow up visit code 091.22 first ② Z39.2"]

091.22 Nonpurulent mastitis associated with the puerperium M ♀
Puerperal interstitial mastitis
Puerperal lymphangitis of breast
Puerperal mastitis NOS
Puerperal parenchymatous mastitis

091.23 Nonpurulent mastitis associated with lactation M ♀
Interstitial mastitis associated with lactation
Lymphangitis of breast associated with lactation
Mastitis NOS associated with lactation
Parenchymatous mastitis associated with lactation

☑4ᵗʰ **092 Other disorders of breast and disorders of lactation associated with pregnancy and the puerperium**

☑5ᵗʰ **092.0 Retracted nipple associated with pregnancy, the puerperium, and lactation**

☑6ᵗʰ **092.01 Retracted nipple associated with pregnancy**

092.011 Retracted nipple associated with pregnancy, first trimester COM M ♀

092.012 Retracted nipple associated with pregnancy, second trimester COM M ♀

092.013 Retracted nipple associated with pregnancy, third trimester COM M ♀

092.019 Retracted nipple associated with pregnancy, unspecified trimester COM M ♀

092.02 Retracted nipple associated with the puerperium M ♀

092.03 Retracted nipple associated with lactation M ♀

☑5ᵗʰ **092.1 Cracked nipple associated with pregnancy, the puerperium, and lactation**
Fissure of nipple, gestational or puerperal

☑6ᵗʰ **092.11 Cracked nipple associated with pregnancy**

092.111 Cracked nipple associated with pregnancy, first trimester COM M ♀

092.112 Cracked nipple associated with pregnancy, second trimester COM M ♀

092.113 Cracked nipple associated with pregnancy, third trimester COM M ♀

092.119 Cracked nipple associated with pregnancy, unspecified trimester COM M ♀

092.12 Cracked nipple associated with the puerperium M ♀

092.13 Cracked nipple associated with lactation M ♀

☑5ᵗʰ **092.2 Other and unspecified disorders of breast associated with pregnancy and the puerperium**

092.20 Unspecified disorder of breast associated with pregnancy and the puerperium M ♀

092.29 Other disorders of breast associated with pregnancy and the puerperium M ♀

092.3 Agalactia M ♀
Primary agalactia
EXCLUDES 1   elective agalactia (092.5)
secondary agalactia (092.5)
therapeutic agalactia (092.5)
DEF: Absence of milk secretion in a female after delivery.

092.4 Hypogalactia M ♀

092.5 Suppressed lactation M ♀
Elective agalactia
Secondary agalactia
Therapeutic agalactia
EXCLUDES 1   primary agalactia (092.3)

092.6 Galactorrhea M ♀
DEF: Excessive or persistent milk secretion by the breast that may occur in the absence of nursing.

☑5ᵗʰ **092.7 Other and unspecified disorders of lactation**

092.70 Unspecified disorders of lactation M ♀

092.79 Other disorders of lactation M ♀
Puerperal galactocele

Other obstetric conditions, not elsewhere classified (094-09A)

094 Sequelae of complication of pregnancy, childbirth, and the puerperium UPD M ♀

NOTE   This category is to be used to indicate conditions in 000-077.-, 085-094 and 098-09A.- as the cause of late effects. The sequelae include conditions specified as such, or as late effects, which may occur at any time after the puerperium

Code first condition resulting from (sequela) of complication of pregnancy, childbirth, and the puerperium

[handwritten margin notes: "① Condition", "② sequelae 094"]

☑4ᵗʰ **098 Maternal infectious and parasitic diseases classifiable elsewhere but complicating pregnancy, childbirth and the puerperium**

INCLUDES   the listed conditions when complicating the pregnant state, when aggravated by the pregnancy, or as a reason for obstetric care

Use additional code (Chapter 1), to identify specific infectious or parasitic disease

EXCLUDES 2   herpes gestationis (026.4-)
infectious carrier state (099.82-, 099.83-)
obstetrical tetanus (A34)
puerperal infection (086.-)
puerperal sepsis (085)
when the reason for maternal care is that the disease is known or suspected to have affected the fetus (035-036)

☑5ᵗʰ **098.0 Tuberculosis complicating pregnancy, childbirth and the puerperium**
Conditions in A15-A19

☑6ᵗʰ **098.01 Tuberculosis complicating pregnancy**

098.011 Tuberculosis complicating pregnancy, first trimester COM M ♀

098.012 Tuberculosis complicating pregnancy, second trimester COM M ♀

098.013 Tuberculosis complicating pregnancy, third trimester COM M ♀

098.019 Tuberculosis complicating pregnancy, unspecified trimester COM M ♀

098.02 Tuberculosis complicating childbirth COM M ♀

098.03 Tuberculosis complicating the puerperium COM M ♀

☑5ᵗʰ **098.1 Syphilis complicating pregnancy, childbirth and the puerperium**
Conditions in A50-A53

☑6ᵗʰ **098.11 Syphilis complicating pregnancy**

098.111 Syphilis complicating pregnancy, first trimester COM M ♀

098.112 Syphilis complicating pregnancy, second trimester COM M ♀

098.113 Syphilis complicating pregnancy, third trimester UPD M ♀

098.119 Syphilis complicating pregnancy, unspecified trimester COM M ♀

098.12 Syphilis complicating childbirth COM M ♀

098.13 Syphilis complicating the puerperium COM M ♀

☑5ᵗʰ **098.2 Gonorrhea complicating pregnancy, childbirth and the puerperium**
Conditions in A54.-

☑6ᵗʰ **098.21 Gonorrhea complicating pregnancy**

098.211 Gonorrhea complicating pregnancy, first trimester COM M ♀

098.212 Gonorrhea complicating pregnancy, second trimester COM M ♀

098.213 Gonorrhea complicating pregnancy, third trimester COM M ♀

098.219 Gonorrhea complicating pregnancy, unspecified trimester COM M ♀

098.22 Gonorrhea complicating childbirth COM M ♀

098.23 Gonorrhea complicating the puerperium COM M ♀

✓5ᵗʰ O98.3 Other infections with a predominantly sexual mode of transmission complicating pregnancy, childbirth and the puerperium
  Conditions in A55-A64
  AHA: 2020,1Q,20

  ✓6ᵗʰ O98.31 Other infections with a predominantly sexual mode of transmission complicating pregnancy
    O98.311 Other infections with a predominantly sexual mode of transmission complicating pregnancy, first trimester COM M ♀
    O98.312 Other infections with a predominantly sexual mode of transmission complicating pregnancy, second trimester COM M ♀
    O98.313 Other infections with a predominantly sexual mode of transmission complicating pregnancy, third trimester COM M ♀
    O98.319 Other infections with a predominantly sexual mode of transmission complicating pregnancy, unspecified trimester COM M ♀
  O98.32 Other infections with a predominantly sexual mode of transmission complicating childbirth COM M ♀
  O98.33 Other infections with a predominantly sexual mode of transmission complicating the puerperium COM M ♀

✓5ᵗʰ O98.4 Viral hepatitis complicating pregnancy, childbirth and the puerperium
  Conditions in B15-B19

  ✓6ᵗʰ O98.41 Viral hepatitis complicating pregnancy
    O98.411 Viral hepatitis complicating pregnancy, first trimester COM M ♀
    O98.412 Viral hepatitis complicating pregnancy, second trimester COM M ♀
    O98.413 Viral hepatitis complicating pregnancy, third trimester COM M ♀
    O98.419 Viral hepatitis complicating pregnancy, unspecified trimester COM M ♀
  O98.42 Viral hepatitis complicating childbirth COM M ♀
  O98.43 Viral hepatitis complicating the puerperium COM M ♀

✓5ᵗʰ O98.5 Other viral diseases complicating pregnancy, childbirth and the puerperium
  Conditions in A80-B09, B25-B34, R87.81-, R87.82-
  EXCLUDES 1 human immunodeficiency virus [HIV] disease complicating pregnancy, childbirth and the puerperium (O98.7-)
  TIP: Assign a code from this subcategory as the principal or first-listed diagnosis for a patient admitted/presenting during pregnancy, childbirth, or the puerperium because of COVID-19; assign U07.1 and codes for associated manifestations as secondary codes.

  ✓6ᵗʰ O98.51 Other viral diseases complicating pregnancy
    O98.511 Other viral diseases complicating pregnancy, first trimester COM M ♀
    O98.512 Other viral diseases complicating pregnancy, second trimester COM M ♀
    O98.513 Other viral diseases complicating pregnancy, third trimester COM M ♀
    O98.519 Other viral diseases complicating pregnancy, unspecified trimester COM M ♀
  O98.52 Other viral diseases complicating childbirth COM M ♀
  O98.53 Other viral diseases complicating the puerperium COM M ♀

✓5ᵗʰ O98.6 Protozoal diseases complicating pregnancy, childbirth and the puerperium
  Conditions in B50-B64

  ✓6ᵗʰ O98.61 Protozoal diseases complicating pregnancy
    O98.611 Protozoal diseases complicating pregnancy, first trimester COM M ♀
    O98.612 Protozoal diseases complicating pregnancy, second trimester COM M ♀
    O98.613 Protozoal diseases complicating pregnancy, third trimester COM M ♀
    O98.619 Protozoal diseases complicating pregnancy, unspecified trimester COM M ♀

O98.62 Protozoal diseases complicating childbirth COM M ♀
O98.63 Protozoal diseases complicating the puerperium COM M ♀

✓5ᵗʰ O98.7 Human immunodeficiency virus [HIV] disease complicating pregnancy, childbirth and the puerperium
  Use additional code to identify the type of HIV disease:
  acquired immune deficiency syndrome (AIDS) (B20)
  asymptomatic HIV status (Z21)
  HIV positive NOS (Z21)
  symptomatic HIV disease (B20)

  ✓6ᵗʰ O98.71 Human immunodeficiency virus [HIV] disease complicating pregnancy
    O98.711 Human immunodeficiency virus [HIV] disease complicating pregnancy, first trimester COM M ♀
    O98.712 Human immunodeficiency virus [HIV] disease complicating pregnancy, second trimester COM M ♀
    O98.713 Human immunodeficiency virus [HIV] disease complicating pregnancy, third trimester COM M ♀
    O98.719 Human immunodeficiency virus [HIV] disease complicating pregnancy, unspecified trimester COM M ♀
  O98.72 Human immunodeficiency virus [HIV] disease complicating childbirth COM M ♀
  O98.73 Human immunodeficiency virus [HIV] disease complicating the puerperium COM M ♀

✓5ᵗʰ O98.8 Other maternal infectious and parasitic diseases complicating pregnancy, childbirth and the puerperium
  AHA: 2020,1Q,10

  ✓6ᵗʰ O98.81 Other maternal infectious and parasitic diseases complicating pregnancy
    O98.811 Other maternal infectious and parasitic diseases complicating pregnancy, first trimester COM M ♀
    O98.812 Other maternal infectious and parasitic diseases complicating pregnancy, second trimester COM M ♀
    O98.813 Other maternal infectious and parasitic diseases complicating pregnancy, third trimester COM M ♀
    O98.819 Other maternal infectious and parasitic diseases complicating pregnancy, unspecified trimester COM M ♀
  O98.82 Other maternal infectious and parasitic diseases complicating childbirth COM M ♀
  O98.83 Other maternal infectious and parasitic diseases complicating the puerperium COM M ♀
    AHA: 2022,2Q,5

✓5ᵗʰ O98.9 Unspecified maternal infectious and parasitic disease complicating pregnancy, childbirth and the puerperium

  ✓6ᵗʰ O98.91 Unspecified maternal infectious and parasitic disease complicating pregnancy
    O98.911 Unspecified maternal infectious and parasitic disease complicating pregnancy, first trimester COM M ♀
    O98.912 Unspecified maternal infectious and parasitic disease complicating pregnancy, second trimester COM M ♀
    O98.913 Unspecified maternal infectious and parasitic disease complicating pregnancy, third trimester COM M ♀
    O98.919 Unspecified maternal infectious and parasitic disease complicating pregnancy, unspecified trimester COM M ♀
  O98.92 Unspecified maternal infectious and parasitic disease complicating childbirth COM M ♀
  O98.93 Unspecified maternal infectious and parasitic disease complicating the puerperium COM M ♀

Chapter 15. Pregnancy, Childbirth and the Puerperium

O99–O99.325

√4ᵗʰ O99 Other maternal diseases classifiable elsewhere but complicating pregnancy, childbirth and the puerperium
- INCLUDES   conditions which complicate the pregnant state, are aggravated by the pregnancy or are a main reason for obstetric care
- Use additional code to identify specific condition
- EXCLUDES 2   when the reason for maternal care is that the condition is known or suspected to have affected the fetus (O35-O36)

√5ᵗʰ O99.0 Anemia complicating pregnancy, childbirth and the puerperium
- Conditions in D50-D64
- EXCLUDES 1   anemia arising in the puerperium (O90.81)
  - postpartum anemia NOS (O90.81)
- AHA: 2019,3Q,11

     √6ᵗʰ O99.01 Anemia complicating pregnancy
- AHA: 2016,1Q,4
  - **O99.011 Anemia complicating pregnancy, first trimester** COM M ♀
  - **O99.012 Anemia complicating pregnancy, second trimester** COM M ♀
  - **O99.013 Anemia complicating pregnancy, third trimester** COM M ♀
  - **O99.019 Anemia complicating pregnancy, unspecified trimester** COM M ♀

     O99.02 Anemia complicating childbirth COM M ♀

     O99.03 Anemia complicating the puerperium COM M ♀
- EXCLUDES 1   postpartum anemia not pre-existing prior to delivery (O90.81)

√5ᵗʰ O99.1 Other diseases of the blood and blood-forming organs and certain disorders involving the immune mechanism complicating pregnancy, childbirth and the puerperium
- Conditions in D65-D89
- EXCLUDES 1   hemorrhage with coagulation defects (O45.-, O46.0-, O67.0, O72.3)

     √6ᵗʰ O99.11 Other diseases of the blood and blood-forming organs and certain disorders involving the immune mechanism complicating pregnancy
- **O99.111 Other diseases of the blood and blood-forming organs and certain disorders involving the immune mechanism complicating pregnancy, first trimester** COM M ♀
- **O99.112 Other diseases of the blood and blood-forming organs and certain disorders involving the immune mechanism complicating pregnancy, second trimester** COM M ♀
- **O99.113 Other diseases of the blood and blood-forming organs and certain disorders involving the immune mechanism complicating pregnancy, third trimester** COM M ♀
- **O99.119 Other diseases of the blood and blood-forming organs and certain disorders involving the immune mechanism complicating pregnancy, unspecified trimester** COM M ♀

     O99.12 Other diseases of the blood and blood-forming organs and certain disorders involving the immune mechanism complicating childbirth COM M ♀

     O99.13 Other diseases of the blood and blood-forming organs and certain disorders involving the immune mechanism complicating the puerperium COM M ♀

√5ᵗʰ O99.2 Endocrine, nutritional and metabolic diseases complicating pregnancy, childbirth and the puerperium
- Conditions in E00-E89
- EXCLUDES 2   diabetes mellitus (O24.-)
  - malnutrition (O25.-)
  - postpartum thyroiditis (O90.5)

     √6ᵗʰ O99.21 Obesity complicating pregnancy, childbirth, and the puerperium
- Use additional code to identify the type of obesity (E66.-)
- AHA: 2021,2Q,10; 2018,4Q,80
- TIP: Do not assign a BMI code (Z68.-) for obese or overweight patients who are pregnant.
  - **O99.210 Obesity complicating pregnancy, unspecified trimester** COM M ♀
  - **O99.211 Obesity complicating pregnancy, first trimester** COM M ♀
  - **O99.212 Obesity complicating pregnancy, second trimester** COM M ♀
  - **O99.213 Obesity complicating pregnancy, third trimester** COM M ♀
  - **O99.214 Obesity complicating childbirth** COM M ♀
  - **O99.215 Obesity complicating the puerperium** COM M ♀

     √6ᵗʰ O99.28 Other endocrine, nutritional and metabolic diseases complicating pregnancy, childbirth and the puerperium
- AHA: 2021,1Q,8
  - **O99.280 Endocrine, nutritional and metabolic diseases complicating pregnancy, unspecified trimester** COM ♀
  - **O99.281 Endocrine, nutritional and metabolic diseases complicating pregnancy, first trimester** COM M ♀
  - **O99.282 Endocrine, nutritional and metabolic diseases complicating pregnancy, second trimester** COM M ♀
  - **O99.283 Endocrine, nutritional and metabolic diseases complicating pregnancy, third trimester** COM M ♀
  - **O99.284 Endocrine, nutritional and metabolic diseases complicating childbirth** COM M ♀
  - **O99.285 Endocrine, nutritional and metabolic diseases complicating the puerperium** COM M ♀

√5ᵗʰ O99.3 Mental disorders and diseases of the nervous system complicating pregnancy, childbirth and the puerperium

     √6ᵗʰ O99.31 Alcohol use complicating pregnancy, childbirth, and the puerperium
- Use additional code(s) from F10 to identify manifestations of the alcohol use
  - **O99.310 Alcohol use complicating pregnancy, unspecified trimester** COM M ♀
  - **O99.311 Alcohol use complicating pregnancy, first trimester** COM M ♀
  - **O99.312 Alcohol use complicating pregnancy, second trimester** COM M ♀
  - **O99.313 Alcohol use complicating pregnancy, third trimester** COM M ♀
  - **O99.314 Alcohol use complicating childbirth** COM M ♀
  - **O99.315 Alcohol use complicating the puerperium** COM M ♀

     √6ᵗʰ O99.32 Drug use complicating pregnancy, childbirth, and the puerperium
- Use additional code(s) from F11-F16 and F18-F19 to identify manifestations of the drug use
- AHA: 2018,4Q,69-70; 2018,2Q,10
- TIP: When drug use is documented during pregnancy, assign first a code from this subcategory followed by an additional code from F11-F16 and F18-F19 identifying the specific drug use even if not documented as associated with a physical, mental, or behavioral disorder. According to chapter 15 guidelines, it is the provider's responsibility to state that the condition being treated is *not* affecting the pregnancy.
  - **O99.320 Drug use complicating pregnancy, unspecified trimester** COM M ♀
  - **O99.321 Drug use complicating pregnancy, first trimester** COM M ♀
  - **O99.322 Drug use complicating pregnancy, second trimester** COM M ♀
  - **O99.323 Drug use complicating pregnancy, third trimester** COM M ♀
  - **O99.324 Drug use complicating childbirth** COM M ♀
  - **O99.325 Drug use complicating the puerperium** COM M ♀

Handwritten annotations: "F10 alcohol related disorder"; "Drug Use"; "Drug Dependence F11.20"; "weed F12.90"; "Cannabis F12.20"

✓6ᵗʰ **O99.33 Tobacco use disorder complicating pregnancy, childbirth, and the puerperium**
Smoking complicating pregnancy, childbirth, and the puerperium
Use additional code from category F17 to identify type of tobacco nicotine dependence

O99.330 Smoking (tobacco) complicating pregnancy, unspecified trimester COM M ♀

O99.331 Smoking (tobacco) complicating pregnancy, first trimester COM M ♀

O99.332 Smoking (tobacco) complicating pregnancy, second trimester COM M ♀

O99.333 Smoking (tobacco) complicating pregnancy, third trimester COM M ♀

O99.334 Smoking (tobacco) complicating childbirth COM M ♀

O99.335 Smoking (tobacco) complicating the puerperium COM M ♀

✓6ᵗʰ **O99.34 Other mental disorders complicating pregnancy, childbirth, and the puerperium**
Conditions in F01-F09, F20-F52 and F54-F99
EXCLUDES 2   postpartum mood disturbance (O90.6)
postnatal psychosis (F53.1)
puerperal psychosis (F53.1)

O99.340 Other mental disorders complicating pregnancy, unspecified trimester COM Q M ♀

O99.341 Other mental disorders complicating pregnancy, first trimester COM Q M ♀

O99.342 Other mental disorders complicating pregnancy, second trimester COM Q M ♀

O99.343 Other mental disorders complicating pregnancy, third trimester COM Q M ♀

O99.344 Other mental disorders complicating childbirth COM Q M ♀

O99.345 Other mental disorders complicating the puerperium COM Q M ♀
AHA: 2018,4Q,8

✓6ᵗʰ **O99.35 Diseases of the nervous system complicating pregnancy, childbirth, and the puerperium**
Conditions in G00-G99
EXCLUDES 2   pregnancy related peripheral neuritis (O26.8-)

O99.350 Diseases of the nervous system complicating pregnancy, unspecified trimester COM M ♀

O99.351 Diseases of the nervous system complicating pregnancy, first trimester COM M ♀

O99.352 Diseases of the nervous system complicating pregnancy, second trimester COM M ♀

O99.353 Diseases of the nervous system complicating pregnancy, third trimester COM M ♀

O99.354 Diseases of the nervous system complicating childbirth COM M ♀

O99.355 Diseases of the nervous system complicating the puerperium COM M ♀

✓5ᵗʰ **O99.4 Diseases of the circulatory system complicating pregnancy, childbirth and the puerperium**
Conditions in I00-I99
EXCLUDES 1   peripartum cardiomyopathy (O90.3)
EXCLUDES 2   hypertensive disorders (O10-O16)
obstetric embolism (O88.-)
venous complications and cerebrovenous sinus thrombosis in labor, childbirth and the puerperium (O87.-)
venous complications and cerebrovenous sinus thrombosis in pregnancy (O22.-)
AHA: 2016,2Q,8

✓6ᵗʰ **O99.41 Diseases of the circulatory system complicating pregnancy**

O99.411 Diseases of the circulatory system complicating pregnancy, first trimester COM M ♀

O99.412 Diseases of the circulatory system complicating pregnancy, second trimester COM M ♀

O99.413 Diseases of the circulatory system complicating pregnancy, third trimester COM M ♀

O99.419 Diseases of the circulatory system complicating pregnancy, unspecified trimester COM M ♀

O99.42 Diseases of the circulatory system complicating childbirth COM M ♀

O99.43 Diseases of the circulatory system complicating the puerperium COM M ♀

✓5ᵗʰ **O99.5 Diseases of the respiratory system complicating pregnancy, childbirth and the puerperium**
Conditions in J00-J99

✓6ᵗʰ **O99.51 Diseases of the respiratory system complicating pregnancy**

O99.511 Diseases of the respiratory system complicating pregnancy, first trimester COM M ♀

O99.512 Diseases of the respiratory system complicating pregnancy, second trimester COM M ♀

O99.513 Diseases of the respiratory system complicating pregnancy, third trimester COM M ♀

O99.519 Diseases of the respiratory system complicating pregnancy, unspecified trimester COM M ♀

O99.52 Diseases of the respiratory system complicating childbirth COM M ♀

O99.53 Diseases of the respiratory system complicating the puerperium COM M ♀

✓5ᵗʰ **O99.6 Diseases of the digestive system complicating pregnancy, childbirth and the puerperium**
Conditions in K00-K93
EXCLUDES 2   hemorrhoids in pregnancy (O22.4-)
liver and biliary tract disorders in pregnancy, childbirth and the puerperium (O26.6-)

✓6ᵗʰ **O99.61 Diseases of the digestive system complicating pregnancy**
AHA: 2016,1Q,4

O99.611 Diseases of the digestive system complicating pregnancy, first trimester COM M ♀

O99.612 Diseases of the digestive system complicating pregnancy, second trimester COM M ♀

O99.613 Diseases of the digestive system complicating pregnancy, third trimester COM M ♀

O99.619 Diseases of the digestive system complicating pregnancy, unspecified trimester COM M ♀

O99.62 Diseases of the digestive system complicating childbirth COM M ♀

O99.63 Diseases of the digestive system complicating the puerperium COM M ♀

✓5ᵗʰ **O99.7 Diseases of the skin and subcutaneous tissue complicating pregnancy, childbirth and the puerperium**
Conditions in L00-L99
EXCLUDES 2   herpes gestationis (O26.4)
pruritic urticarial papules and plaques of pregnancy (PUPPP) (O26.86)

✓6ᵗʰ **O99.71 Diseases of the skin and subcutaneous tissue complicating pregnancy**

O99.711 Diseases of the skin and subcutaneous tissue complicating pregnancy, first trimester COM M ♀

O99.712 Diseases of the skin and subcutaneous tissue complicating pregnancy, second trimester COM M ♀

O99.713 Diseases of the skin and subcutaneous tissue complicating pregnancy, third trimester COM M ♀

O99.719 Diseases of the skin and subcutaneous tissue complicating pregnancy, unspecified trimester COM M ♀

O99.72 Diseases of the skin and subcutaneous tissue complicating childbirth COM M ♀

O99.73 Diseases of the skin and subcutaneous tissue complicating the puerperium COM M ♀

✓5ᵗʰ **O99.8 Other specified diseases and conditions complicating pregnancy, childbirth and the puerperium**
Conditions in D00-D48, H00-H95, M00-N99, and Q00-Q99
Use additional code to identify condition
EXCLUDES 2   genitourinary infections in pregnancy (O23.-)
infection of genitourinary tract following delivery (O86.1-O86.4)
malignant neoplasm complicating pregnancy, childbirth and the puerperium (O9A.1-)
maternal care for known or suspected abnormality of maternal pelvic organs (O34.-)
postpartum acute kidney failure (O90.4)
traumatic injuries in pregnancy (O9A.2-)

✓6ᵗʰ **O99.81 Abnormal glucose complicating pregnancy, childbirth and the puerperium**
EXCLUDES 1   gestational diabetes (O24.4-)

O99.810 Abnormal glucose complicating pregnancy COM M ♀
O99.814 Abnormal glucose complicating childbirth COM M ♀
O99.815 Abnormal glucose complicating the puerperium COM M ♀

✓6ᵗʰ **O99.82 Streptococcus B carrier state complicating pregnancy, childbirth and the puerperium**
EXCLUDES 1   carrier of streptococcus group B (GBS) in a nonpregnant woman (Z22.330)
DEF: *Streptococcus* group B colonization: Bacteria normally found in the vagina or lower intestine of many healthy adult women that may infect the fetus during childbirth, causing mental or physical handicaps or death. Women who test positive for *Streptococcus* group B during pregnancy are considered a "colonized" status and are treated with IV antibiotics at the time of delivery and may also be treated with oral antibiotics during the pregnancy.

O99.820 Streptococcus B carrier state complicating pregnancy COM M ♀
O99.824 Streptococcus B carrier state complicating childbirth COM M ♀
AHA: 2019,2Q,8
O99.825 Streptococcus B carrier state complicating the puerperium COM M ♀

✓6ᵗʰ **O99.83 Other infection carrier state complicating pregnancy, childbirth and the puerperium**
Use additional code to identify the carrier state (Z22.-)
O99.830 Other infection carrier state complicating pregnancy COM M ♀
O99.834 Other infection carrier state complicating childbirth COM M ♀
O99.835 Other infection carrier state complicating the puerperium COM M ♀

✓6ᵗʰ **O99.84 Bariatric surgery status complicating pregnancy, childbirth and the puerperium**
Gastric banding status complicating pregnancy, childbirth and the puerperium
Gastric bypass status for obesity complicating pregnancy, childbirth and the puerperium
Obesity surgery status complicating pregnancy, childbirth and the puerperium
O99.840 Bariatric surgery status complicating pregnancy, unspecified trimester COM M ♀
O99.841 Bariatric surgery status complicating pregnancy, first trimester COM M ♀
O99.842 Bariatric surgery status complicating pregnancy, second trimester COM M ♀
O99.843 Bariatric surgery status complicating pregnancy, third trimester COM M ♀
O99.844 Bariatric surgery status complicating childbirth COM M ♀
O99.845 Bariatric surgery status complicating the puerperium COM M ♀

✓6ᵗʰ **O99.89 Other specified diseases and conditions complicating pregnancy, childbirth and the puerperium**
AHA: 2020,4Q,36-37
O99.891 Other specified diseases and conditions complicating pregnancy COM M ♀

O99.892 Other specified diseases and conditions complicating childbirth COM M ♀
O99.893 Other specified diseases and conditions complicating puerperium COM M ♀

✓4ᵗʰ **O9A Maternal malignant neoplasms, traumatic injuries and abuse classifiable elsewhere but complicating pregnancy, childbirth and the puerperium**

✓5ᵗʰ **O9A.1 Malignant neoplasm complicating pregnancy, childbirth and the puerperium**
Conditions in C00-C96
Use additional code to identify neoplasm
EXCLUDES 2   maternal care for benign tumor of corpus uteri (O34.1-)
maternal care for benign tumor of cervix (O34.4-)
AHA: 2015,3Q,19

✓6ᵗʰ **O9A.11 Malignant neoplasm complicating pregnancy**
O9A.111 Malignant neoplasm complicating pregnancy, first trimester COM M ♀
O9A.112 Malignant neoplasm complicating pregnancy, second trimester COM M ♀
O9A.113 Malignant neoplasm complicating pregnancy, third trimester COM M ♀
O9A.119 Malignant neoplasm complicating pregnancy, unspecified trimester COM M ♀

O9A.12 Malignant neoplasm complicating childbirth COM M ♀
O9A.13 Malignant neoplasm complicating the puerperium COM M ♀

✓5ᵗʰ **O9A.2 Injury, poisoning and certain other consequences of external causes complicating pregnancy, childbirth and the puerperium**
Conditions in S00-T88, except T74 and T76
Use additional code(s) to identify the injury or poisoning
EXCLUDES 2   physical, sexual and psychological abuse complicating pregnancy, childbirth and the puerperium (O9A.3-, O9A.4-, O9A.5-)

✓6ᵗʰ **O9A.21 Injury, poisoning and certain other consequences of external causes complicating pregnancy**
O9A.211 Injury, poisoning and certain other consequences of external causes complicating pregnancy, first trimester COM M ♀
O9A.212 Injury, poisoning and certain other consequences of external causes complicating pregnancy, second trimester COM M ♀
O9A.213 Injury, poisoning and certain other consequences of external causes complicating pregnancy, third trimester COM M ♀
O9A.219 Injury, poisoning and certain other consequences of external causes complicating pregnancy, unspecified trimester COM M ♀

O9A.22 Injury, poisoning and certain other consequences of external causes complicating childbirth COM M ♀
O9A.23 Injury, poisoning and certain other consequences of external causes complicating the puerperium COM M ♀

✓5ᵗʰ **O9A.3 Physical abuse complicating pregnancy, childbirth and the puerperium**
Conditions in T74.11 or T76.11
Use additional code (if applicable):
to identify any associated current injury due to physical abuse
to identify the perpetrator of abuse (Y07.-)
EXCLUDES 2   sexual abuse complicating pregnancy, childbirth and the puerperium (O9A.4)

✓6ᵗʰ **O9A.31 Physical abuse complicating pregnancy**
O9A.311 Physical abuse complicating pregnancy, first trimester COM M ♀
O9A.312 Physical abuse complicating pregnancy, second trimester COM M ♀
O9A.313 Physical abuse complicating pregnancy, third trimester COM M ♀
O9A.319 Physical abuse complicating pregnancy, unspecified trimester COM M ♀

O9A.32 Physical abuse complicating childbirth COM M ♀

O9A.33   **Physical abuse complicating the puerperium**   `COM` `M` ♀

✓5ᵗʰ **O9A.4**   Sexual abuse **complicating pregnancy, childbirth and the puerperium**

    Conditions in T74.21 or T76.21

    Use additional code (if applicable):

      to identify any associated current injury due to sexual abuse

      to identify the perpetrator of abuse (Y07.-)

✓6ᵗʰ **O9A.41**   **Sexual abuse complicating** pregnancy

    O9A.411   **Sexual abuse complicating pregnancy, first trimester**   `COM` `M` ♀

    O9A.412   **Sexual abuse complicating pregnancy, second trimester**   `COM` `M` ♀

    O9A.413   **Sexual abuse complicating pregnancy, third trimester**   `COM` `M` ♀

    O9A.419   **Sexual abuse complicating pregnancy, unspecified trimester**   `COM` `M` ♀

O9A.42   **Sexual abuse complicating** childbirth   `COM` `M` ♀

O9A.43   **Sexual abuse complicating the puerperium**   `COM` `M` ♀

✓5ᵗʰ **O9A.5**   Psychological abuse **complicating pregnancy, childbirth and the puerperium**

    Conditions in T74.31 or T76.31

    Use additional code to identify the perpetrator of abuse (Y07.-)

✓6ᵗʰ **O9A.51**   **Psychological abuse complicating** pregnancy

    O9A.511   **Psychological abuse complicating pregnancy,** first trimester   `COM` `M` ♀

    O9A.512   **Psychological abuse complicating pregnancy,** second trimester   `COM` `M` ♀

    O9A.513   **Psychological abuse complicating pregnancy,** third trimester   `COM` `M` ♀

    O9A.519   **Psychological abuse complicating pregnancy, unspecified trimester**   `COM` `M` ♀

O9A.52   **Psychological abuse complicating** childbirth   `COM` `M` ♀

O9A.53   **Psychological abuse complicating the puerperium**   `COM` `M` ♀

☑ Additional Character Required   ✓x7ᵗʰ Placeholder Alert   Manifestation   Unspecified Dx   ◑ QPP   UPD Unacceptable PDx

Chapter 16. Certain Conditions Originating in the Perinatal Period (P00–P96)

Chapter-specific Guidelines with Coding Examples

The chapter-specific guidelines from the ICD-10-CM Official Guidelines for Coding and Reporting have been provided below. Along with these guidelines are coding examples, contained in the shaded boxes, that have been developed to help illustrate the coding and/or sequencing guidance found in these guidelines.

For coding and reporting purposes the perinatal period is defined as before birth through the 28th day following birth. The following guidelines are provided for reporting purposes

a. General perinatal rules

1) Use of Chapter 16 codes

Codes in this chapter are <u>never</u> for use on the maternal record. Codes from Chapter 15, the obstetric chapter, are never permitted on the newborn record. Chapter 16 codes may be used throughout the life of the patient if the condition is still present.

2) Principal diagnosis for birth record

When coding the birth episode in a newborn record, assign a code from category Z38, Liveborn infants according to place of birth and type of delivery, as the principal diagnosis. A code from category Z38 is assigned only once, to a newborn at the time of birth. If a newborn is transferred to another institution, a code from category Z38 should not be used at the receiving hospital.

A code from category Z38 is used only on the newborn record, not on the mother's record.

3) Use of codes from other chapters with codes from Chapter 16

Codes from other chapters may be used with codes from chapter 16 if the codes from the other chapters provide more specific detail. Codes for signs and symptoms may be assigned when a definitive diagnosis has not been established. If the reason for the encounter is a perinatal condition, the code from chapter 16 should be sequenced first.

4) Use of Chapter 16 codes after the perinatal period

Should a condition originate in the perinatal period, and continue throughout the life of the patient, the perinatal code should continue to be used regardless of the patient's age.

> A 7-year-old patient with history of birth injury that resulted in Erb's palsy is seen for subscapularis release
>
> **P14.0**   **Erb's paralysis due to birth injury**
>
> *Explanation:* Although in this instance Erb's palsy is specifically related to a birth injury, it has not resolved and continues to be a health concern. A perinatal code is appropriate even though this patient is beyond the perinatal period.

5) Birth process or community acquired conditions

If a newborn has a condition that may be either due to the birth process or community acquired and the documentation does not indicate which it is, the default is due to the birth process and the code from Chapter 16 should be used. If the condition is community-acquired, a code from Chapter 16 should not be assigned.

For COVID-19 infection in a newborn, see guideline I.C.16.h.

6) Code all clinically significant conditions

All clinically significant conditions noted on routine newborn examination should be coded. A condition is clinically significant if it requires:

clinical evaluation; or

therapeutic treatment; or

diagnostic procedures; or

extended length of hospital stay; or

increased nursing care and/or monitoring; or

has implications for future health care needs

Note: The perinatal guidelines listed above are the same as the general coding guidelines for "additional diagnoses", except for the final point regarding implications for future health care needs. Codes should be assigned for conditions that have been specified by the provider as having implications for future health care needs.

b. Observation and evaluation of newborns for suspected conditions not found

1) Use of Z05 codes

Assign a code from category Z05, Observation and evaluation of newborn for suspected **diseases and** conditions ruled out, to identify those instances when a healthy newborn is evaluated for a suspected condition/**disease** that is determined after study not to be present. Do not use a code from category Z05 when the patient **is documented to have** signs or symptoms of a suspected problem; in such cases code the sign or symptom.

2) Z05 on other than the birth record

A code from category Z05 may also be assigned as a principal or first-listed code for readmissions or encounters when the code from category Z38 code no longer applies. Codes from category Z05 are for use only for healthy newborns and infants for which no condition after study is found to be present.

3) Z05 on a birth record

A code from category Z05 is to be used as a secondary code after the code from category Z38, Liveborn infants according to place of birth and type of delivery.

> Newborn delivered via vaginal delivery; previous ultrasounds showed what appeared to be an abnormality of the right kidney. Kidney function tests were performed and ultrasounds taken and any genitourinary conditions ruled out.
>
> **Z38.00**   **Single liveborn infant, delivered vaginally**
>
> **Z05.6**   **Observation and evaluation of newborn for suspected genitourinary condition ruled out**
>
> *Explanation:* The newborn had no signs or symptoms of kidney or other genitourinary condition but was evaluated after delivery due to the abnormal prenatal ultrasound findings. A Z code describing the type and place of birth should be coded first, followed by a Z05 category code for the work performed to rule out a suspected genitourinary condition.

c. Coding additional perinatal diagnoses

1) Assigning codes for conditions that require treatment

Assign codes for conditions that require treatment or further investigation, prolong the length of stay, or require resource utilization.

2) Codes for conditions specified as having implications for future health care needs

Assign codes for conditions that have been specified by the provider as having implications for future health care needs.

Note: This guideline should not be used for adult patients.

> An abnormal noise was heard in the left hip of a post-term newborn during a physical examination. The pediatrician would like to follow the patient after discharge as a hip click can be an early sign of hip dysplasia. The newborn was delivered via cesarean at 41 weeks.
>
> **Z38.01**   **Single liveborn infant, delivered by cesarean**
>
> **P08.21**   **Post-term newborn**
>
> **R29.4**   **Clicking hip**
>
> *Explanation:* The abnormal hip noise or click is appended as a secondary diagnosis not only because it is an abnormal finding upon examination, but also due to its potential to be part of a bigger health issue. The hip dysplasia has not yet been diagnosed and does not warrant a code at this time.

d. Prematurity and fetal growth retardation

Providers utilize different criteria in determining prematurity. A code for prematurity should not be assigned unless it is documented. Assignment of codes in categories P05, Disorders of newborn related to slow fetal growth and fetal malnutrition, and P07, Disorders of newborn related to short gestation and low birth weight, not elsewhere classified, should be based on the recorded birth weight and estimated gestational age.

When both birth weight and gestational age are available, two codes from category P07 should be assigned, with the code for birth weight sequenced before the code for gestational age.

e. Low birth weight and immaturity status

Codes from category P07, Disorders of newborn related to short gestation and low birth weight, not elsewhere classified, are for use for a child or adult who was premature or had a low birth weight as a newborn and this is affecting the patient's current health status.

See Section I.C.21. Factors influencing health status and contact with health services, Status.

> A 35-year-old patient, who weighed 659 grams at birth, is seen for heart disease documented as being a consequence of the low birth weight
>
> **I51.9**   **Heart disease, unspecified**
>
> **P07.02**   **Extremely low birth weight newborn, 500–749 grams**
>
> *Explanation:* A code from subcategories P07.0- and P07.1- is appropriate, regardless of the age of the patient, as long as the documentation provides a clear link between the patient's current illness and the low birth weight.

f. Bacterial sepsis of newborn

Category P36, Bacterial sepsis of newborn, includes congenital sepsis. If a perinate is documented as having sepsis without documentation of congenital or community acquired, the default is congenital and a code from category P36 should be assigned. If the P36 code includes the causal organism, an additional code from category B95, Streptococcus, Staphylococcus, and Enterococcus as the cause of diseases classified elsewhere, or B96, Other bacterial agents as the cause of diseases classified elsewhere, should not be assigned. If the P36 code does not include the causal organism, assign an additional code from category B96. If applicable, use additional codes to identify severe sepsis (R65.2-) and any associated acute organ dysfunction.

> A full-term infant develops severe sepsis 24 hours after discharge from the hospital and is readmitted; cultures identified *E. coli* as the infective agent
>
> **P36.4**   **Sepsis of newborn due to Escherichia coli**
>
> **R65.20**   **Severe sepsis without septic shock**
>
> *Explanation:* Even though this newborn was discharged and could have acquired *E. coli* from his/her external environment, due to the lack of documentation specifying specifically how this pathogen was acquired, the default is to code the *E. coli* sepsis as congenital. A code from chapter 1, "Certain Infectious and Parasitic Diseases," is not required because the perinatal sepsis code identifies both the sepsis and the bacteria causing the sepsis.

g. Stillbirth

Code P95, Stillbirth, is only for use in institutions that maintain separate records for stillbirths. No other code should be used with P95. Code P95 should not be used on the mother's record.

h. COVID-19 infection in newborn

For a newborn that tests positive for COVID-19, assign code U07.1, COVID-19, and the appropriate codes for associated manifestation(s) in neonates/newborns in the absence of documentation indicating a specific type of transmission. For a newborn that tests positive for COVID-19 and the provider documents the condition was contracted in utero or during the birth process, assign codes P35.8, Other congenital viral diseases, and U07.1, COVID-19. When coding the birth episode in a newborn record, the appropriate code from category Z38, Liveborn infants according to place of birth and type of delivery, should be assigned as the principal diagnosis.

Chapter 16. Certain Conditions Originating in the Perinatal Period

Chapter 16. Certain Conditions Originating in the Perinatal Period (P00-P96)

NOTE Codes from this chapter are for use on newborn records only, never on maternal records

INCLUDES conditions that have their origin in the fetal or perinatal period (before birth through the first 28 days after birth) even if morbidity occurs later

EXCLUDES 2 congenital malformations, deformations and chromosomal abnormalities (Q00-Q99)

endocrine, nutritional and metabolic diseases (E00-E88)

injury, poisoning and certain other consequences of external causes (S00-T88)

neoplasms (C00-D49)

tetanus neonatorum (A33)

This chapter contains the following blocks:

P00-P04   Newborn affected by maternal factors and by complications of pregnancy, labor, and delivery
P05-P08   Disorders of newborn related to length of gestation and fetal growth
P09   Abnormal findings on neonatal screening
P10-P15   Birth trauma
P19-P29   Respiratory and cardiovascular disorders specific to the perinatal period
P35-P39   Infections specific to the perinatal period
P50-P61   Hemorrhagic and hematological disorders of newborn
P70-P74   Transitory endocrine and metabolic disorders specific to newborn
P76-P78   Digestive system disorders of newborn
P80-P83   Conditions involving the integument and temperature regulation of newborn
P84   Other problems with newborn
P90-P96   Other disorders originating in the perinatal period

Newborn affected by maternal factors and by complications of pregnancy, labor, and delivery (P00-P04)

NOTE These codes are for use when the listed maternal conditions are specified as the cause of confirmed morbidity or potential morbidity which have their origin in the perinatal period (before birth through the first 28 days after birth).

AHA: 2016,4Q,54-55

✓4ᵗʰ P00 Newborn affected by maternal conditions that may be unrelated to present pregnancy

Code first any current condition in newborn

EXCLUDES 2 encounter for observation of newborn for suspected diseases and conditions ruled out (Z05.-)

newborn affected by maternal complications of pregnancy (P01.-)

newborn affected by maternal endocrine and metabolic disorders (P70-P74)

newborn affected by noxious substances transmitted via placenta or breast milk (P04.-)

P00.0 Newborn affected by maternal hypertensive disorders

Newborn affected by maternal conditions classifiable to O10-O11, O13-O16

P00.1 Newborn affected by maternal renal and urinary tract diseases

Newborn affected by maternal conditions classifiable to N00-N39

P00.2 Newborn affected by maternal infectious and parasitic diseases

Newborn affected by maternal infectious disease classifiable to A00-B99, J09 and J10

EXCLUDES 1 maternal genital tract or other localized infections (P00.8)

EXCLUDES 2 infections specific to the perinatal period (P35-P39)

newborn affected by (positive) maternal group B streptococcus (GBS) colonization (P00.82)

AHA: 2019,2Q,10; 2015,3Q,20

P00.3 Newborn affected by other maternal circulatory and respiratory diseases

Newborn affected by maternal conditions classifiable to I00-I99, J00-J99, Q20-Q34 and not included in P00.0, P00.2

P00.4 Newborn affected by maternal nutritional disorders

Newborn affected by maternal disorders classifiable to E40-E64

Maternal malnutrition NOS

P00.5 Newborn affected by maternal injury

Newborn affected by maternal conditions classifiable to O9A.2-

P00.6 Newborn affected by surgical procedure on mother

Newborn affected by amniocentesis

EXCLUDES 1 Cesarean delivery for present delivery (P03.4)

damage to placenta from amniocentesis, Cesarean delivery or surgical induction (P02.1)

previous surgery to uterus or pelvic organs (P03.89)

EXCLUDES 2 newborn affected by complication of (fetal) intrauterine procedure (P96.5)

P00.7 Newborn affected by other medical procedures on mother, not elsewhere classified

Newborn affected by radiation to mother

EXCLUDES 1 damage to placenta from amniocentesis, cesarean delivery or surgical induction (P02.1)

newborn affected by other complications of labor and delivery (P03.-)

✓5ᵗʰ P00.8 Newborn affected by other maternal conditions

P00.81 Newborn affected by periodontal disease in mother

P00.82 Newborn affected by (positive) maternal group B streptococcus (GBS) colonization

Contact with positive maternal group B streptococcus

AHA: 2021,4Q,23

P00.89 Newborn affected by other maternal conditions

Newborn affected by conditions classifiable to T80-T88

Newborn affected by maternal genital tract or other localized infections

Newborn affected by maternal systemic lupus erythematosus

Use additional code to identify infectious agent, if known

EXCLUDES 2 newborn affected by positive maternal group B streptococcus (GBS) colonization (P00.82)

AHA: 2019,2Q,9

P00.9 Newborn affected by unspecified maternal condition

✓4ᵗʰ P01 Newborn affected by maternal complications of pregnancy

Code first any current condition in newborn

EXCLUDES 2 encounter for observation of newborn for suspected diseases and conditions ruled out (Z05.-)

P01.0 Newborn affected by incompetent cervix

P01.1 Newborn affected by premature rupture of membranes

P01.2 Newborn affected by oligohydramnios

EXCLUDES 1 oligohydramnios due to premature rupture of membranes (P01.1)

DEF: Low amniotic fluid level, resulting in underdeveloped organs in the fetus.

P01.3 Newborn affected by polyhydramnios

Newborn affected by hydramnios

DEF: Excess amniotic fluid surrounding the fetus, typically defined as a total fluid volume of greater than 24 cm.

P01.4 Newborn affected by ectopic pregnancy

Newborn affected by abdominal pregnancy

P01.5 Newborn affected by multiple pregnancy

Newborn affected by triplet (pregnancy)

Newborn affected by twin (pregnancy)

P01.6 Newborn affected by maternal death

P01.7 Newborn affected by malpresentation before labor

Newborn affected by breech presentation before labor

Newborn affected by external version before labor

Newborn affected by face presentation before labor

Newborn affected by transverse lie before labor

Newborn affected by unstable lie before labor

P01.8 Newborn affected by other maternal complications of pregnancy

P01.9 Newborn affected by maternal complication of pregnancy, unspecified

✓4ᵗʰ P02 Newborn affected by complications of placenta, cord and membranes

Code first any current condition in newborn

EXCLUDES 2 encounter for observation of newborn for suspected diseases and conditions ruled out (Z05.-)

P02.0 Newborn affected by placenta previa

DEF: Placenta developed in the lower segment of the uterus that can cause hemorrhaging leading to preterm delivery.

Chapter 16. Certain Conditions Originating in the Perinatal Period

P02.1   **Newborn affected by other forms of placental** separation and hemorrhage
Newborn affected by abruptio placenta
Newborn affected by accidental hemorrhage
Newborn affected by antepartum hemorrhage
Newborn affected by damage to placenta from amniocentesis, cesarean delivery or surgical induction
Newborn affected by maternal blood loss
Newborn affected by premature separation of placenta

✓5th **P02.2**   **Newborn affected by other and unspecified** morphological and functional abnormalities **of placenta**

    P02.20   **Newborn affected by unspecified morphological and functional abnormalities of placenta**

    P02.29   **Newborn affected by other morphological and functional abnormalities of placenta**
Newborn affected by placental dysfunction
Newborn affected by placental infarction
Newborn affected by placental insufficiency

P02.3   **Newborn affected by** placental transfusion syndromes
Newborn affected by placental and cord abnormalities resulting in twin-to-twin or other transplacental transfusion

P02.4   **Newborn affected by** prolapsed cord

P02.5   **Newborn affected by other compression of umbilical cord**
Newborn affected by umbilical cord (tightly) around neck
Newborn affected by entanglement of umbilical cord
Newborn affected by knot in umbilical cord
AHA: 2022,1Q,22

✓5th **P02.6**   **Newborn affected by other and unspecified** conditions of umbilical cord

    P02.60   **Newborn affected by unspecified conditions of umbilical cord**

    P02.69   **Newborn affected by other conditions of umbilical cord**
Newborn affected by short umbilical cord
Newborn affected by vasa previa
    EXCLUDES 1   *newborn affected by single umbilical artery (Q27.0)*

✓5th **P02.7**   **Newborn affected by** chorioamnionitis
AHA: 2018,4Q,23-24
DEF: Inflammation of the fetal membranes due to maternal infection characterized by fetal tachycardia, respiratory distress, apnea, weak cries, and poor sucking.

    P02.70   **Newborn affected by** fetal inflammatory response syndrome   HCC ESR COM
Newborn affected by FIRS

    P02.78   **Newborn affected by other conditions from chorioamnionitis**
Newborn affected by amnionitis
Newborn affected by membranitis
Newborn affected by placentitis

P02.8   **Newborn affected by other abnormalities of membranes**

P02.9   **Newborn affected by abnormality of membranes, unspecified**

✓4th **P03**   **Newborn affected by other complications of** labor and delivery
Code first any current condition in newborn
    EXCLUDES 2   *encounter for observation of newborn for suspected diseases and conditions ruled out (Z05.-)*

P03.0   **Newborn affected by** breech delivery and extraction

P03.1   **Newborn affected by other** malpresentation, malposition and disproportion **during labor and delivery**
Newborn affected by contracted pelvis
Newborn affected by conditions classifiable to O64-O66
Newborn affected by persistent occipitoposterior
Newborn affected by transverse lie

P03.2   **Newborn affected by** forceps delivery

Forceps Assisted Birth

Forceps extractor

P03.3   **Newborn affected by delivery by** vacuum extractor [ventouse]

Vacuum Assisted Birth

Vacuum extractor

P03.4   **Newborn affected by** Cesarean delivery

P03.5   **Newborn affected by** precipitate delivery
Newborn affected by rapid second stage

P03.6   **Newborn affected by** abnormal uterine contractions
Newborn affected by conditions classifiable to O62.-, except O62.3
Newborn affected by hypertonic labor
Newborn affected by uterine inertia

✓5th **P03.8**   **Newborn affected by other specified complications of labor and delivery**

    ✓6th **P03.81**   **Newborn affected by** abnormality in fetal (intrauterine) heart rate or rhythm
    EXCLUDES 1   *neonatal cardiac dysrhythmia (P29.1-)*

       P03.810   **Newborn affected by abnormality in fetal (intrauterine) heart rate or rhythm** before the onset of labor

       P03.811   **Newborn affected by abnormality in fetal (intrauterine) heart rate or rhythm** during labor

       P03.819   **Newborn affected by abnormality in fetal (intrauterine) heart rate or rhythm, unspecified as to time of onset**

    P03.82   Meconium passage **during delivery**
    EXCLUDES 1   *meconium aspiration (P24.00, P24.01)*
meconium staining (P96.83)
DEF: Fetal intestinal activity that increases in response to a fetomaternal distressed state during delivery. The anal sphincter relaxes and meconium is passed into the amniotic fluid.

    P03.89   **Newborn affected by other specified complications of labor and delivery**
Newborn affected by abnormality of maternal soft tissues
Newborn affected by conditions classifiable to O60-O75 and by procedures used in labor and delivery not included in P02.- and P03.0-P03.6
Newborn affected by induction of labor

P03.9   **Newborn affected by complication of labor and delivery, unspecified**

✓4th **P04**   **Newborn affected by** noxious substances transmitted via placenta or breast milk
    INCLUDES   nonteratogenic effects of substances transmitted via placenta
Code first any current condition in newborn, if applicable
    EXCLUDES 2   *congenital malformations (Q00-Q99)*
encounter for observation of newborn for suspected diseases and conditions ruled out (Z05.-)
neonatal jaundice from excessive hemolysis due to drugs or toxins transmitted from mother (P58.4)
newborn in contact with and (suspected) exposures hazardous to health not transmitted via placenta or breast milk (Z77.-)

P04.0   **Newborn affected by maternal** anesthesia and analgesia **in pregnancy, labor and delivery**   COM
Newborn affected by reactions and intoxications from maternal opiates and tranquilizers administered for procedures during pregnancy or labor and delivery
    EXCLUDES 2   *newborn affected by other maternal medication (P04.1-)*

√5th **P04.1 Newborn affected by other maternal medication**

Code first withdrawal symptoms from maternal use of drugs of addiction, if applicable (P96.1)

    EXCLUDES 1   *dysmorphism due to warfarin (Q86.2)*

               fetal hydantoin syndrome (Q86.1)

    EXCLUDES 2   *maternal anesthesia and analgesia in pregnancy, labor and delivery (P04.0)*

               maternal use of drugs of addiction (P04.4-)

    AHA: 2018,4Q,24-25

    P04.11 Newborn affected by maternal antineoplastic chemotherapy COM

    P04.12 Newborn affected by maternal cytotoxic drugs COM

    P04.13 Newborn affected by maternal use of anticonvulsants COM

    P04.14 Newborn affected by maternal use of opiates COM

    P04.15 Newborn affected by maternal use of antidepressants COM

    P04.16 Newborn affected by maternal use of amphetamines COM

    P04.17 Newborn affected by maternal use of sedative-hypnotics COM

    P04.1A Newborn affected by maternal use of anxiolytics COM

    P04.18 Newborn affected by other maternal medication COM

    P04.19 Newborn affected by maternal use of unspecified medication COM

P04.2 Newborn affected by maternal use of tobacco COM

Newborn affected by exposure in utero to tobacco smoke

    EXCLUDES 2   *newborn exposure to environmental tobacco smoke (P96.81)*

P04.3 Newborn affected by maternal use of alcohol COM

    EXCLUDES 1   *fetal alcohol syndrome (Q86.0)*

√5th **P04.4 Newborn affected by maternal use of** drugs of addiction

    AHA: 2018,4Q,25

    P04.40 Newborn affected by maternal use of unspecified drugs of addiction COM

    P04.41 Newborn affected by maternal use of cocaine COM

    P04.42 Newborn affected by maternal use of hallucinogens COM

        EXCLUDES 2   *newborn affected by other maternal medication (P04.1-)*

    P04.49 Newborn affected by maternal use of other drugs of addiction

        EXCLUDES 2   *newborn affected by maternal anesthesia and analgesia (P04.0)*

                   withdrawal symptoms from maternal use of drugs of addiction (P96.1)

P04.5 Newborn affected by maternal use of nutritional chemical substances COM

P04.6 Newborn affected by maternal exposure to environmental chemical substances COM

√5th **P04.8 Newborn affected by other maternal** noxious substances

    AHA: 2018,4Q,25

    P04.81 Newborn affected by maternal use of cannabis COM

    P04.89 Newborn affected by other maternal noxious substances COM

P04.9 Newborn affected by maternal noxious substance, unspecified COM

Disorders of newborn related to length of gestation and fetal growth (P05-P08)

√4th **P05 Disorders of newborn related to slow fetal growth and fetal malnutrition**

    AHA: 2016,4Q,55-56

√5th **P05.0 Newborn light for gestational age**

Newborn light-for-dates

Weight below but length above 10th percentile for gestational age

    P05.00 Newborn light for gestational age, unspecified weight COM

    P05.01 Newborn light for gestational age, less than 500 grams COM

    P05.02 Newborn light for gestational age, 500-749 grams COM

    P05.03 Newborn light for gestational age, 750-999 grams COM

    P05.04 Newborn light for gestational age, 1000-1249 grams COM

    P05.05 Newborn light for gestational age, 1250-1499 grams COM

    P05.06 Newborn light for gestational age, 1500-1749 grams COM

    P05.07 Newborn light for gestational age, 1750-1999 grams COM

    P05.08 Newborn light for gestational age, 2000-2499 grams COM

    P05.09 Newborn light for gestational age, 2500 grams and over COM

        Newborn light for gestational age, other

√5th **P05.1 Newborn small for gestational age**

Newborn small-and-light-for-dates

Newborn small-for-dates

Weight and length below 10th percentile for gestational age

    P05.10 Newborn small for gestational age, unspecified weight COM

    P05.11 Newborn small for gestational age, less than 500 grams COM

    P05.12 Newborn small for gestational age, 500-749 grams COM

    P05.13 Newborn small for gestational age, 750-999 grams COM

    P05.14 Newborn small for gestational age, 1000-1249 grams COM

    P05.15 Newborn small for gestational age, 1250-1499 grams COM

    P05.16 Newborn small for gestational age, 1500-1749 grams COM

    P05.17 Newborn small for gestational age, 1750-1999 grams COM

    P05.18 Newborn small for gestational age, 2000-2499 grams COM

    P05.19 Newborn small for gestational age, other COM

        Newborn small for gestational age, 2500 grams and over

P05.2 Newborn affected by fetal (intrauterine) malnutrition **not light or small for gestational age** COM

Infant, not light or small for gestational age, showing signs of fetal malnutrition, such as dry, peeling skin and loss of subcutaneous tissue

    EXCLUDES 1   *newborn affected by fetal malnutrition with light for gestational age (P05.0-)*

               newborn affected by fetal malnutrition with small for gestational age (P05.1-)

P05.9 Newborn affected by slow intrauterine growth, unspecified COM

Newborn affected by fetal growth retardation NOS

√4th **P07 Disorders of newborn related to short gestation and low birth weight, not elsewhere classified**

    NOTE   When both birth weight and gestational age of the newborn are available, both should be coded with birth weight sequenced before gestational age

    INCLUDES   the listed conditions, without further specification, as the cause of morbidity or additional care, in newborn

√5th **P07.0 Extremely low birth weight newborn**

Newborn birth weight 999 g. or less

    EXCLUDES 1   *low birth weight due to slow fetal growth and fetal malnutrition (P05.-)*

    P07.00 Extremely low birth weight newborn, unspecified weight COM

    P07.01 Extremely low birth weight newborn, less than 500 grams COM

    P07.02 Extremely low birth weight newborn, 500-749 grams COM

    P07.03 Extremely low birth weight newborn, 750-999 grams COM

Chapter 16. Certain Conditions Originating in the Perinatal Period *(side margin)*

✓5ᵗʰ **P07.1** **Other low birth weight newborn**   *61b = 2729* (handwritten)
Newborn birth weight 1000-2499 g.
> **EXCLUDES 1** *low birth weight due to slow fetal growth and fetal malnutrition (P05.-)*

P07.10 **Other low birth weight newborn, unspecified weight** `COM`

P07.14 **Other low birth weight newborn, 1000-1249 grams** `COM`

P07.15 **Other low birth weight newborn, 1250-1499 grams** `COM`

P07.16 **Other low birth weight newborn, 1500-1749 grams** `COM`

P07.17 **Other low birth weight newborn, 1750-1999 grams** `COM`

P07.18 **Other low birth weight newborn, 2000-2499 grams** `COM`

✓5ᵗʰ **P07.2** **Extreme immaturity of newborn**
Less than 28 completed weeks (less than 196 completed days) of gestation.

P07.20 **Extreme immaturity of newborn, unspecified weeks of gestation** `COM`
Gestational age less than 28 completed weeks NOS

P07.21 **Extreme immaturity of newborn, gestational age less than 23 completed weeks** `COM`
Extreme immaturity of newborn, gestational age less than 23 weeks, 0 days

P07.22 **Extreme immaturity of newborn, gestational age 23 completed weeks** `COM`
Extreme immaturity of newborn, gestational age 23 weeks, 0 days through 23 weeks, 6 days

P07.23 **Extreme immaturity of newborn, gestational age 24 completed weeks** `COM`
Extreme immaturity of newborn, gestational age 24 weeks, 0 days through 24 weeks, 6 days

P07.24 **Extreme immaturity of newborn, gestational age 25 completed weeks** `COM`
Extreme immaturity of newborn, gestational age 25 weeks, 0 days through 25 weeks, 6 days

P07.25 **Extreme immaturity of newborn, gestational age 26 completed weeks** `COM`
Extreme immaturity of newborn, gestational age 26 weeks, 0 days through 26 weeks, 6 days

P07.26 **Extreme immaturity of newborn, gestational age 27 completed weeks** `COM`
Extreme immaturity of newborn, gestational age 27 weeks, 0 days through 27 weeks, 6 days

✓5ᵗʰ **P07.3** **Preterm [premature] newborn [other]**
28 completed weeks or more but less than 37 completed weeks (196 completed days but less than 259 completed days) of gestation
Prematurity NOS
AHA: 2017,3Q,26

P07.30 **Preterm newborn, unspecified weeks of gestation** `COM`

P07.31 **Preterm newborn, gestational age 28 completed weeks** `COM`
Preterm newborn, gestational age 28 weeks, 0 days through 28 weeks, 6 days

P07.32 **Preterm newborn, gestational age 29 completed weeks** `COM`
Preterm newborn, gestational age 29 weeks, 0 days through 29 weeks, 6 days

P07.33 **Preterm newborn, gestational age 30 completed weeks** `COM`
Preterm newborn, gestational age 30 weeks, 0 days through 30 weeks, 6 days

P07.34 **Preterm newborn, gestational age 31 completed weeks** `COM`
Preterm newborn, gestational age 31 weeks, 0 days through 31 weeks, 6 days

P07.35 **Preterm newborn, gestational age 32 completed weeks** `COM`
Preterm newborn, gestational age 32 weeks, 0 days through 32 weeks, 6 days

P07.36 **Preterm newborn, gestational age 33 completed weeks** `COM`
Preterm newborn, gestational age 33 weeks, 0 days through 33 weeks, 6 days

P07.37 **Preterm newborn, gestational age 34 completed weeks** `COM`
Preterm newborn, gestational age 34 weeks, 0 days through 34 weeks, 6 days

P07.38 **Preterm newborn, gestational age 35 completed weeks** `COM`
Preterm newborn, gestational age 35 weeks, 0 days through 35 weeks, 6 days

P07.39 **Preterm newborn, gestational age 36 completed weeks** `COM`
Preterm newborn, gestational age 36 weeks, 0 days through 36 weeks, 6 days

✓4ᵗʰ **P08** **Disorders of newborn related to long gestation and high birth weight**
> **NOTE** When both birth weight and gestational age of the newborn are available, priority of assignment should be given to birth weight
> **INCLUDES** the listed conditions, without further specification, as causes of morbidity or additional care, in newborn

P08.0 **Exceptionally large newborn baby** `COM`
Usually implies a birth weight of 4500 g. or more
> **EXCLUDES 1** *syndrome of infant of diabetic mother (P70.1)*
> *syndrome of infant of mother with gestational diabetes (P70.0)*

P08.1 **Other heavy for gestational age newborn** `COM`
Other newborn heavy- or large-for-dates regardless of period of gestation
Usually implies a birth weight of 4000 g. to 4499 g.
> **EXCLUDES 1** *newborn with a birth weight of 4500 or more (P08.0)*
> *syndrome of infant of diabetic mother (P70.1)*
> *syndrome of infant of mother with gestational diabetes (P70.0)*

✓5ᵗʰ **P08.2** **Late newborn, not heavy for gestational age**
AHA: 2014,1Q,14

P08.21 **Post-term newborn** `COM`
Newborn with gestation period over 40 completed weeks to 42 completed weeks

P08.22 **Prolonged gestation of newborn** `COM`
Newborn with gestation period over 42 completed weeks (294 days or more), not heavy- or large-for-dates.
Postmaturity NOS

Abnormal findings on neonatal screening (P09)

✓4ᵗʰ **P09** **Abnormal findings on neonatal screening**
> **INCLUDES** abnormal findings on state mandated newborn screens
> failed newborn screening
> **EXCLUDES 2** *nonspecific serologic evidence of human immunodeficiency virus [HIV] (R75)*
AHA: 2021,4Q,24

P09.1 **Abnormal findings on neonatal screening for inborn errors of metabolism**

P09.2 **Abnormal findings on neonatal screening for congenital endocrine disease**
Abnormal findings on neonatal screening for congenital adrenal hyperplasia
Abnormal findings on neonatal screening for hypothyroidism screen

P09.3 **Abnormal findings on neonatal screening for congenital hematologic disorders**
Abnormal findings for hemoglobinothies screen
Abnormal findings on red cell membrane defects screen
Abnormal findings on sickle cell screen

P09.4 **Abnormal findings on neonatal screening for cystic fibrosis**

P09.5 **Abnormal findings on neonatal screening for critical congenital heart disease**
Neonatal congenital heart disease screening failure

P09.6 **Abnormal findings on neonatal screening for neonatal hearing loss**
> **EXCLUDES 2** *encounter for hearing examination following failed hearing screening (Z01.110)*

P09.8 **Other abnormal findings on neonatal screening**

`HCC` CMS-HCC	`Rx` Rx HCC	`ESR` ESRD HCC	`COM` Commercial HCC	`N` Newborn: 0	`P` Pediatric: 0-17	`M` Maternity: 9-64	`A` Adult: 15-124

P09.9 **Abnormal findings on neonatal screening, unspecified**

Birth trauma (P10-P15)

☑4ᵗʰ **P10 Intracranial laceration and hemorrhage** due to birth injury
> EXCLUDES 1   intracranial hemorrhage of newborn NOS (P52.9)
> intracranial hemorrhage of newborn due to anoxia or hypoxia (P52.-)
> nontraumatic intracranial hemorrhage of newborn (P52.-)

P10.0 **Subdural** hemorrhage due to birth injury   COM
> Subdural hematoma (localized) due to birth injury
> EXCLUDES 1   subdural hemorrhage accompanying tentorial tear (P10.4)

P10.1 **Cerebral** hemorrhage due to birth injury   COM

P10.2 **Intraventricular** hemorrhage due to birth injury   COM

P10.3 **Subarachnoid** hemorrhage due to birth injury   COM

P10.4 **Tentorial tear** due to birth injury   COM

P10.8 **Other intracranial lacerations and hemorrhages** due to birth injury   COM

P10.9 **Unspecified intracranial laceration and hemorrhage** due to birth injury   COM

☑4ᵗʰ **P11 Other birth injuries to** central nervous system

P11.0 **Cerebral edema** due to birth injury   COM

P11.1 **Other specified brain damage** due to birth injury   COM

P11.2 **Unspecified brain damage** due to birth injury   COM

P11.3 **Birth injury to** facial nerve
> Facial palsy due to birth injury

P11.4 **Birth injury to other cranial nerves**

P11.5 **Birth injury to** spine and spinal cord   COM
> Fracture of spine due to birth injury

P11.9 **Birth injury to central nervous system, unspecified**

☑4ᵗʰ **P12 Birth injury to** scalp

Birth Injuries to Scalp

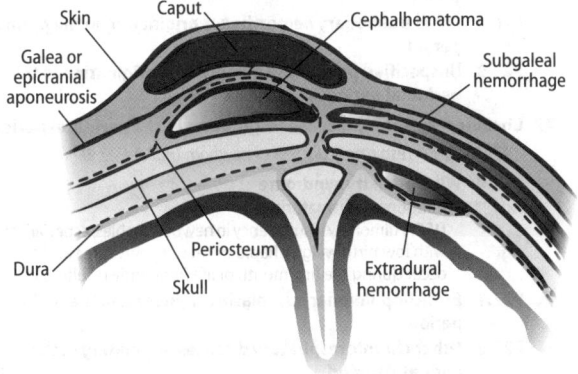

P12.0 **Cephalhematoma** due to birth injury
> **DEF:** Condition that occurs in a neonate when blood vessels between the skull and periosteum rupture and blood collects in the subperiosteal space (below the periosteum). It is typically caused by prolonged labor or trauma due to instrument-assisted delivery (e.g., forceps, vacuum extraction), although in rare circumstances, it may indicate a linear skull fracture with intracranial hemorrhage.

P12.1 **Chignon (from vacuum extraction)** due to birth injury
> **DEF:** Artificial swelling of the scalp that occurs when a collection of interstitial fluid and blood forms in the area of the scalp where the suction cup was applied during a vacuum-assisted delivery.

P12.2 **Epicranial subaponeurotic hemorrhage** due to birth injury
> Subgaleal hemorrhage

P12.3 **Bruising of scalp** due to birth injury

P12.4 **Injury of scalp of newborn** due to monitoring equipment
> Sampling incision of scalp of newborn
> Scalp clip (electrode) injury of newborn

☑5ᵗʰ P12.8 **Other birth injuries to scalp**

P12.81 **Caput succedaneum**
> **DEF:** Swelling of the scalp as a result of pressure being exerted on the head from the vaginal walls, uterus, or instrumentation used in assisting a delivery (e.g., vacuum).

P12.89 **Other birth injuries to scalp**

P12.9 **Birth injury to scalp, unspecified**

☑4ᵗʰ **P13 Birth injury to** skeleton
> EXCLUDES 2   birth injury to spine (P11.5)

P13.0 **Fracture of skull** due to birth injury

P13.1 **Other birth injuries to skull**
> EXCLUDES 1   cephalhematoma (P12.0)

P13.2 **Birth injury to** femur

P13.3 **Birth injury to other long bones**

P13.4 **Fracture of clavicle** due to birth injury

P13.8 **Birth injuries to other parts of skeleton**

P13.9 **Birth injury to skeleton, unspecified**

☑4ᵗʰ **P14 Birth injury to** peripheral nervous system

P14.0 **Erb's paralysis** due to birth injury
> **DEF:** Erb's paralysis: Most common type of brachial plexus (peripheral nerve) injury in a neonate that involves nerve damage at the level of C5-C6. *Synonym(s): Erb's palsy*

P14.1 **Klumpke's paralysis** due to birth injury

P14.2 **Phrenic nerve paralysis** due to birth injury

P14.3 **Other brachial plexus birth injuries**

P14.8 **Birth injuries to other parts of peripheral nervous system**

P14.9 **Birth injury to peripheral nervous system, unspecified**

☑4ᵗʰ **P15 Other birth injuries**

P15.0 **Birth injury to** liver
> Rupture of liver due to birth injury

P15.1 **Birth injury to** spleen
> Rupture of spleen due to birth injury

P15.2 **Sternomastoid** injury due to birth injury

P15.3 **Birth injury to** eye
> Subconjunctival hemorrhage due to birth injury
> Traumatic glaucoma due to birth injury

P15.4 **Birth injury to** face
> Facial congestion due to birth injury

P15.5 **Birth injury to** external genitalia

P15.6 **Subcutaneous fat necrosis** due to birth injury

P15.8 **Other specified birth injuries**

P15.9 **Birth injury, unspecified**

Respiratory and cardiovascular disorders specific to the perinatal period (P19-P29)

☑4ᵗʰ **P19 Metabolic acidemia in newborn**
> INCLUDES   metabolic acidemia in newborn

P19.0 **Metabolic acidemia in newborn first noted** before onset of labor

P19.1 **Metabolic acidemia in newborn first noted** during labor

P19.2 **Metabolic acidemia noted** at birth

P19.9 **Metabolic acidemia, unspecified**

☑4ᵗʰ **P22 Respiratory distress of newborn**
> **AHA:** 2019,2Q,29

P22.0 **Respiratory distress syndrome of newborn**   COM
> Cardiorespiratory distress syndrome of newborn
> Hyaline membrane disease
> Idiopathic respiratory distress syndrome [IRDS or RDS] of newborn
> Pulmonary hypoperfusion syndrome
> Respiratory distress syndrome, type I
> EXCLUDES 2   respiratory arrest of newborn (P28.81)
> respiratory failure of newborn NOS (P28.5)
> **AHA:** 2019,2Q,29
> **DEF:** Severe chest contractions upon air intake and expiratory grunting. The infant appears blue due to oxygen deficiency and has a rapid respiratory rate, formerly called hyaline membrane disease.

P22.1 **Transient tachypnea of newborn**
> Idiopathic tachypnea of newborn
> Respiratory distress syndrome, type II
> Wet lung syndrome
> **DEF:** Rapid, labored breathing of a newborn. It is a short-term problem that begins after birth and lasts about three days.

P22.8 **Other respiratory distress of newborn**
> EXCLUDES 1   respiratory arrest of newborn (P28.81)
> respiratory failure of newborn NOS (P28.5)

P22.9 **Respiratory distress of newborn, unspecified**
> EXCLUDES 1   respiratory arrest of newborn (P28.81)
> respiratory failure of newborn NOS (P28.5)

Chapter 16. Certain Conditions Originating in the Perinatal Period *(side margin)*

P23–P28.2 *(side margin)*

✓4ᵗʰ **P23 Congenital pneumonia**

> INCLUDES   infective pneumonia acquired in utero or during birth
>
> EXCLUDES 1 *neonatal pneumonia resulting from aspiration (P24.-)*

P23.0 Congenital pneumonia due to viral agent COM
Use additional code (B97) to identify organism
> EXCLUDES 1 *congenital rubella pneumonitis (P35.0)*

P23.1 Congenital pneumonia due to Chlamydia COM

P23.2 Congenital pneumonia due to staphylococcus COM

P23.3 Congenital pneumonia due to streptococcus, group B COM

P23.4 Congenital pneumonia due to Escherichia coli COM

P23.5 Congenital pneumonia due to Pseudomonas COM

P23.6 Congenital pneumonia due to other bacterial agents COM
Congenital pneumonia due to Hemophilus influenzae
Congenital pneumonia due to Klebsiella pneumoniae
Congenital pneumonia due to Mycoplasma
Congenital pneumonia due to Streptococcus, except group B
Use additional code (B95-B96) to identify organism

P23.8 Congenital pneumonia due to other organisms COM

P23.9 Congenital pneumonia, unspecified COM

✓4ᵗʰ **P24 Neonatal aspiration**

> INCLUDES   aspiration in utero and during delivery

✓5ᵗʰ **P24.0 Meconium aspiration**

> EXCLUDES 1 *meconium passage (without aspiration) during delivery (P03.82)*
> *meconium staining (P96.83)*

> DEF: Meconium in the trachea or seen on chest x-ray after birth.

P24.00 Meconium aspiration without respiratory symptoms
Meconium aspiration NOS

P24.01 Meconium aspiration with respiratory symptoms COM
Meconium aspiration pneumonia
Meconium aspiration pneumonitis
Meconium aspiration syndrome NOS
Use additional code to identify any secondary pulmonary hypertension, if applicable (I27.2-)
> DEF: Aspiration of fetal intestinal material during or prior to delivery. It is usually a complication of placental insufficiency, causing pneumonitis and bronchial obstruction (inflammatory reaction of lungs).

✓5ᵗʰ **P24.1 Neonatal aspiration of (clear) amniotic fluid and mucus**
Neonatal aspiration of liquor (amnii)

P24.10 Neonatal aspiration of (clear) amniotic fluid and mucus without respiratory symptoms
Neonatal aspiration of amniotic fluid and mucus NOS

P24.11 Neonatal aspiration of (clear) amniotic fluid and mucus with respiratory symptoms COM
Neonatal aspiration of amniotic fluid and mucus with pneumonia
Neonatal aspiration of amniotic fluid and mucus with pneumonitis
Use additional code to identify any secondary pulmonary hypertension, if applicable (I27.2-)

✓5ᵗʰ **P24.2 Neonatal aspiration of blood**

P24.20 Neonatal aspiration of blood without respiratory symptoms
Neonatal aspiration of blood NOS

P24.21 Neonatal aspiration of blood with respiratory symptoms COM
Neonatal aspiration of blood with pneumonia
Neonatal aspiration of blood with pneumonitis
Use additional code to identify any secondary pulmonary hypertension, if applicable (I27.2-)

✓5ᵗʰ **P24.3 Neonatal aspiration of milk and regurgitated food**
Neonatal aspiration of stomach contents

P24.30 Neonatal aspiration of milk and regurgitated food without respiratory symptoms
Neonatal aspiration of milk and regurgitated food NOS

P24.31 Neonatal aspiration of milk and regurgitated food with respiratory symptoms COM
Neonatal aspiration of milk and regurgitated food with pneumonia
Neonatal aspiration of milk and regurgitated food with pneumonitis
Use additional code to identify any secondary pulmonary hypertension, if applicable (I27.2-)

✓5ᵗʰ **P24.8 Other neonatal aspiration**

P24.80 Other neonatal aspiration without respiratory symptoms
Neonatal aspiration NEC

P24.81 Other neonatal aspiration with respiratory symptoms COM
Neonatal aspiration pneumonia NEC
Neonatal aspiration with pneumonitis NEC
Neonatal aspiration with pneumonia NOS
Neonatal aspiration with pneumonitis NOS
Use additional code to identify any secondary pulmonary hypertension, if applicable (I27.2-)

P24.9 Neonatal aspiration, unspecified

✓4ᵗʰ **P25 Interstitial emphysema and related conditions originating in the perinatal period**

P25.0 Interstitial emphysema originating in the perinatal period

P25.1 Pneumothorax originating in the perinatal period

P25.2 Pneumomediastinum originating in the perinatal period

P25.3 Pneumopericardium originating in the perinatal period

P25.8 Other conditions related to interstitial emphysema originating in the perinatal period

✓4ᵗʰ **P26 Pulmonary hemorrhage originating in the perinatal period**

> EXCLUDES 1 *acute idiopathic hemorrhage in infants over 28 days old (R04.81)*

P26.0 Tracheobronchial hemorrhage originating in the perinatal period COM

P26.1 Massive pulmonary hemorrhage originating in the perinatal period COM

P26.8 Other pulmonary hemorrhages originating in the perinatal period COM

P26.9 Unspecified pulmonary hemorrhage originating in the perinatal period COM

✓4ᵗʰ **P27 Chronic respiratory disease originating in the perinatal period**

> EXCLUDES 2 *respiratory distress of newborn (P22.0-P22.9)*

P27.0 Wilson-Mikity syndrome COM
Pulmonary dysmaturity
> DEF: Pulmonary insufficiency in newborn babies, especially those with low birth weight. Rapid onset of hypercapnia and cyanosis occur during the first month of life frequently resulting in death.

P27.1 Bronchopulmonary dysplasia originating in the perinatal period COM

P27.8 Other chronic respiratory diseases originating in the perinatal period COM
Congenital pulmonary fibrosis
Ventilator lung in newborn

P27.9 Unspecified chronic respiratory disease originating in the perinatal period COM

✓4ᵗʰ **P28 Other respiratory conditions originating in the perinatal period**

> ▶Code also, if applicable, congenital malformations of the respiratory system (Q30-Q34)◀
>
> EXCLUDES 1 *congenital malformations of the respiratory system (Q30-Q34)*

P28.0 Primary atelectasis of newborn COM
Primary failure to expand terminal respiratory units
Pulmonary hypoplasia associated with short gestation
Pulmonary immaturity NOS

✓5ᵗʰ **P28.1 Other and unspecified atelectasis of newborn**

P28.10 Unspecified atelectasis of newborn COM
Atelectasis of newborn NOS

P28.11 Resorption atelectasis without respiratory distress syndrome COM
> EXCLUDES 1 *resorption atelectasis with respiratory distress syndrome (P22.0)*

P28.19 Other atelectasis of newborn COM
Partial atelectasis of newborn
Secondary atelectasis of newborn

P28.2 Cyanotic attacks of newborn
> EXCLUDES 1 *apnea of newborn ▶(P28.3- - P28.4-)◀*

▲ ✓5ᵗʰ **P28.3 Primary sleep apnea of newborn**
~~Central sleep apnea of newborn~~
~~Obstructive sleep apnea of newborn~~
Sleep apnea of newborn NOS
EXCLUDES 2 ▶*other apnea of newborn (P28.4-)*◀
DEF: Unexplained cessation of breathing when a neonate makes no respiratory effort for 20 seconds or longer or when a neonate's breathing cessation is accompanied by cyanosis, bradycardia, or hypotonia.

● **P28.30 Primary sleep apnea of newborn, unspecified**
Transient oxygen desaturation spells of newborn during sleep

● **P28.31 Primary central sleep apnea of newborn**

● **P28.32 Primary obstructive sleep apnea of newborn**

● **P28.33 Primary mixed sleep apnea of newborn**

● **P28.39 Other primary sleep apnea of newborn**

▲ ✓5ᵗʰ **P28.4 Other apnea of newborn**
~~Apnea of prematurity~~
~~Obstructive apnea of newborn~~
EXCLUDES 1 *obstructive sleep apnea of newborn (P28.3)*
EXCLUDES 2 ▶*primary sleep apnea of newborn (P28.3-)*◀

● **P28.40 Unspecified apnea of newborn**
Apnea of newborn, NOS
Transient oxygen desaturation spells of newborn

● **P28.41 Central neonatal apnea of newborn**

● **P28.42 Obstructive apnea of newborn**

● **P28.43 Mixed neonatal apnea of newborn**

● **P28.49 Other apnea of newborn**
Apnea of prematurity

P28.5 Respiratory failure of newborn COM
EXCLUDES 1 *respiratory arrest of newborn (P28.81)*
respiratory distress of newborn (P22.0-)
AHA: 2019,2Q,29

✓5ᵗʰ **P28.8 Other specified respiratory conditions of newborn**

P28.81 Respiratory arrest of newborn COM
P28.89 Other specified respiratory conditions of newborn
Congenital laryngeal stridor
Sniffles in newborn
Snuffles in newborn
EXCLUDES 1 *early congenital syphilitic rhinitis (A50.05)*

P28.9 Respiratory condition of newborn, unspecified
Respiratory depression in newborn

✓4ᵗʰ **P29 Cardiovascular disorders originating in the perinatal period**
EXCLUDES 2 *congenital malformations of the circulatory system (Q20-Q28)*

P29.0 Neonatal cardiac failure COM

✓5ᵗʰ **P29.1 Neonatal cardiac dysrhythmia**
P29.11 Neonatal tachycardia
P29.12 Neonatal bradycardia

P29.2 Neonatal hypertension

✓5ᵗʰ **P29.3 Persistent fetal circulation**
AHA: 2017,4Q,20-21

P29.30 Pulmonary hypertension of newborn COM
Persistent pulmonary hypertension of newborn
DEF: Condition that occurs when pressure within the pulmonary artery is elevated and vascular resistance is observed in the lungs.

P29.38 Other persistent fetal circulation COM
Delayed closure of ductus arteriosus

P29.4 Transient myocardial ischemia in newborn

✓5ᵗʰ **P29.8 Other cardiovascular disorders originating in the perinatal period**
P29.81 Cardiac arrest of newborn COM
P29.89 Other cardiovascular disorders originating in the perinatal period
AHA: 2014,4Q,23

P29.9 Cardiovascular disorder originating in the perinatal period, unspecified

Infections specific to the perinatal period (P35-P39)

Infections acquired in utero, during birth via the umbilicus, or during the first 28 days after birth
EXCLUDES 2 *asymptomatic human immunodeficiency virus [HIV] infection status (Z21)*
congenital gonococcal infection (A54.-)
congenital pneumonia (P23.-)
congenital syphilis (A50.-)
human immunodeficiency virus [HIV] disease (B20)
infant botulism (A48.51)
infectious diseases not specific to the perinatal period (A00-B99, J09, J10.-)
intestinal infectious disease (A00-A09)
laboratory evidence of human immunodeficiency virus [HIV] (R75)
tetanus neonatorum (A33)

✓4ᵗʰ **P35 Congenital viral diseases**
INCLUDES infections acquired in utero or during birth

P35.0 Congenital rubella syndrome
Congenital rubella pneumonitis

P35.1 Congenital cytomegalovirus infection COM

P35.2 Congenital herpesviral [herpes simplex] infection

P35.3 Congenital viral hepatitis

P35.4 Congenital Zika virus disease
Use additional code to identify manifestations of congenital Zika virus disease
AHA: 2018,4Q,25-26

P35.8 Other congenital viral diseases
Congenital varicella [chickenpox]
AHA: 2020,2Q,13

P35.9 Congenital viral disease, unspecified

✓4ᵗʰ **P36 Bacterial sepsis of newborn**
INCLUDES congenital sepsis
Use additional code(s), if applicable, to identify severe sepsis (R65.2-) and associated acute organ dysfunction(s)

P36.0 Sepsis of newborn due to streptococcus, group B HCC ESR COM

✓5ᵗʰ **P36.1 Sepsis of newborn due to other and unspecified streptococci**
P36.10 Sepsis of newborn due to unspecified streptococci HCC ESR COM
P36.19 Sepsis of newborn due to other streptococci HCC ESR COM

P36.2 Sepsis of newborn due to Staphylococcus aureus HCC ESR COM

✓5ᵗʰ **P36.3 Sepsis of newborn due to other and unspecified staphylococci**
P36.30 Sepsis of newborn due to unspecified staphylococci HCC ESR COM
P36.39 Sepsis of newborn due to other staphylococci HCC ESR COM

P36.4 Sepsis of newborn due to Escherichia coli HCC ESR COM

P36.5 Sepsis of newborn due to anaerobes HCC ESR COM

P36.8 Other bacterial sepsis of newborn HCC ESR COM
Use additional code from category B96 to identify organism

P36.9 Bacterial sepsis of newborn, unspecified HCC ESR COM

✓4ᵗʰ **P37 Other congenital infectious and parasitic diseases**
EXCLUDES 2 *congenital syphilis (A50.-)*
infectious neonatal diarrhea (A00-A09)
necrotizing enterocolitis in newborn (P77.-)
noninfectious neonatal diarrhea (P78.3)
ophthalmia neonatorum due to gonococcus (A54.31)
tetanus neonatorum (A33)

P37.0 Congenital tuberculosis

P37.1 Congenital toxoplasmosis
Hydrocephalus due to congenital toxoplasmosis

P37.2 Neonatal (disseminated) listeriosis

P37.3 Congenital falciparum malaria

P37.4 Other congenital malaria

P37.5 Neonatal candidiasis

P37.8 Other specified congenital infectious and parasitic diseases

P37.9 Congenital infectious or parasitic disease, unspecified

Chapter 16. Certain Conditions Originating in the Perinatal Period

P38–P56.99

✓4ᵗʰ **P38 Omphalitis of newborn**

> EXCLUDES 1   omphalitis not of newborn (L08.82)
> tetanus omphalitis (A33)
> umbilical hemorrhage of newborn (P51.-)

DEF: Omphalitis: Infection and inflammation of the umbilical stump, often due to bacteria that can spread beyond the umbilical stump to the fascia, muscle, or even the umbilical vessels.

P38.1 Omphalitis with mild hemorrhage

P38.9 Omphalitis without hemorrhage
Omphalitis of newborn NOS

✓4ᵗʰ **P39 Other infections specific to the perinatal period**
Use additional code to identify organism or specific infection

P39.0 Neonatal infective mastitis
> EXCLUDES 1   breast engorgement of newborn (P83.4)
> noninfective mastitis of newborn (P83.4)

P39.1 Neonatal conjunctivitis and dacryocystitis
Neonatal chlamydial conjunctivitis
Ophthalmia neonatorum NOS
> EXCLUDES 1   gonococcal conjunctivitis (A54.31)

P39.2 Intra-amniotic infection affecting newborn, not elsewhere classified

P39.3 Neonatal urinary tract infection

P39.4 Neonatal skin infection
Neonatal pyoderma
> EXCLUDES 1   pemphigus neonatorum (L00)
> staphylococcal scalded skin syndrome (L00)

P39.8 Other specified infections specific to the perinatal period

P39.9 Infection specific to the perinatal period, unspecified

Hemorrhagic and hematological disorders of newborn (P50-P61)

> EXCLUDES 1   congenital stenosis and stricture of bile ducts (Q44.3)
> Crigler-Najjar syndrome (E80.5)
> Dubin-Johnson syndrome (E80.6)
> Gilbert syndrome (E80.4)
> hereditary hemolytic anemias (D55-D58)

✓4ᵗʰ **P50 Newborn affected by intrauterine (fetal) blood loss**
> EXCLUDES 1   congenital anemia from intrauterine (fetal) blood loss (P61.3)

P50.0 Newborn affected by intrauterine (fetal) blood loss from vasa previa

P50.1 Newborn affected by intrauterine (fetal) blood loss from ruptured cord

P50.2 Newborn affected by intrauterine (fetal) blood loss from placenta

P50.3 Newborn affected by hemorrhage into co-twin

P50.4 Newborn affected by hemorrhage into maternal circulation

P50.5 Newborn affected by intrauterine (fetal) blood loss from cut end of co-twin's cord

P50.8 Newborn affected by other intrauterine (fetal) blood loss

P50.9 Newborn affected by intrauterine (fetal) blood loss, unspecified
Newborn affected by fetal hemorrhage NOS

✓4ᵗʰ **P51 Umbilical hemorrhage of newborn**
> EXCLUDES 1   omphalitis with mild hemorrhage (P38.1)
> umbilical hemorrhage from cut end of co-twins cord (P50.5)

P51.0 Massive umbilical hemorrhage of newborn

P51.8 Other umbilical hemorrhages of newborn
Slipped umbilical ligature NOS

P51.9 Umbilical hemorrhage of newborn, unspecified

✓4ᵗʰ **P52 Intracranial nontraumatic hemorrhage of newborn**
> INCLUDES   intracranial hemorrhage due to anoxia or hypoxia
> EXCLUDES 1   intracranial hemorrhage due to birth injury (P10.-)
> intracranial hemorrhage due to other injury (S06.-)

P52.0 Intraventricular (nontraumatic) hemorrhage, grade 1, of newborn COM
Subependymal hemorrhage (without intraventricular extension)
Bleeding into germinal matrix

P52.1 Intraventricular (nontraumatic) hemorrhage, grade 2, of newborn COM
Subependymal hemorrhage with intraventricular extension
Bleeding into ventricle

✓5ᵗʰ **P52.2 Intraventricular (nontraumatic) hemorrhage, grade 3 and grade 4, of newborn**

P52.21 Intraventricular (nontraumatic) hemorrhage, grade 3, of newborn COM
Subependymal hemorrhage with intraventricular extension with enlargement of ventricle

P52.22 Intraventricular (nontraumatic) hemorrhage, grade 4, of newborn COM
Bleeding into cerebral cortex
Subependymal hemorrhage with intracerebral extension

P52.3 Unspecified intraventricular (nontraumatic) hemorrhage of newborn COM

P52.4 Intracerebral (nontraumatic) hemorrhage of newborn COM

P52.5 Subarachnoid (nontraumatic) hemorrhage of newborn COM

P52.6 Cerebellar (nontraumatic) and posterior fossa hemorrhage of newborn COM

P52.8 Other intracranial (nontraumatic) hemorrhages of newborn COM

P52.9 Intracranial (nontraumatic) hemorrhage of newborn, unspecified COM

P53 Hemorrhagic disease of newborn COM
Vitamin K deficiency of newborn

✓4ᵗʰ **P54 Other neonatal hemorrhages**
> EXCLUDES 1   newborn affected by (intrauterine) blood loss (P50.-)
> pulmonary hemorrhage originating in the perinatal period (P26.-)

P54.0 Neonatal hematemesis
> EXCLUDES 1   neonatal hematemesis due to swallowed maternal blood (P78.2)

P54.1 Neonatal melena
> EXCLUDES 1   neonatal melena due to swallowed maternal blood (P78.2)

P54.2 Neonatal rectal hemorrhage

P54.3 Other neonatal gastrointestinal hemorrhage

P54.4 Neonatal adrenal hemorrhage

P54.5 Neonatal cutaneous hemorrhage
Neonatal bruising
Neonatal ecchymoses
Neonatal petechiae
Neonatal superficial hematomata
> EXCLUDES 2   bruising of scalp due to birth injury (P12.3)
> cephalhematoma due to birth injury (P12.0)

P54.6 Neonatal vaginal hemorrhage ♀
Neonatal pseudomenses

P54.8 Other specified neonatal hemorrhages

P54.9 Neonatal hemorrhage, unspecified

✓4ᵗʰ **P55 Hemolytic disease of newborn**

P55.0 Rh isoimmunization of newborn COM
DEF: Incompatible Rh fetal-maternal blood grouping that prematurely destroys red blood cells. Symptoms include jaundice, asphyxia, pulmonary hypertension, edema, respiratory distress, kernicterus, and coagulopathies. It is detected by a Coombs test.
TIP: A positive Coombs test without documentation of associated Rh isoimmunization should be coded to R79.89 Other specified abnormal findings of blood chemistry.

P55.1 ABO isoimmunization of newborn COM
AHA: 2015,3Q,20

P55.8 Other hemolytic diseases of newborn COM
AHA: 2018,3Q,24

P55.9 Hemolytic disease of newborn, unspecified COM

✓4ᵗʰ **P56 Hydrops fetalis due to hemolytic disease**
> EXCLUDES 1   hydrops fetalis NOS (P83.2)

P56.0 Hydrops fetalis due to isoimmunization COM

✓5ᵗʰ **P56.9 Hydrops fetalis due to other and unspecified hemolytic disease**

P56.90 Hydrops fetalis due to unspecified hemolytic disease COM

P56.99 Hydrops fetalis due to other hemolytic disease COM

☑4ᵗʰ **P57 Kernicterus**

    P57.0 Kernicterus due to isoimmunization `COM`
        DEF: Complication of erythroblastosis fetalis associated with severe neural symptoms, high blood bilirubin levels, and nerve cell destruction. It results in bilirubin-pigmented gray matter of the central nervous system.

    P57.8 Other specified kernicterus `COM`
        EXCLUDES 1   *Crigler-Najjar syndrome (E80.5)*

    P57.9 Kernicterus, unspecified `COM`

☑4ᵗʰ **P58 Neonatal jaundice due to other excessive hemolysis**
    EXCLUDES 1   *jaundice due to isoimmunization (P55-P57)*

    P58.0 Neonatal jaundice due to bruising

    P58.1 Neonatal jaundice due to bleeding

    P58.2 Neonatal jaundice due to infection

    P58.3 Neonatal jaundice due to polycythemia

☑5ᵗʰ **P58.4 Neonatal jaundice due to drugs or toxins transmitted from mother or given to newborn**
        Code first poisoning due to drug or toxin, if applicable (T36-T65 with fifth or sixth character 1-4 or 6)
        Use additional code for adverse effect, if applicable, to identify drug (T36-T50 with fifth or sixth character 5)

        P58.41 Neonatal jaundice due to drugs or toxins transmitted from mother

        P58.42 Neonatal jaundice due to drugs or toxins given to newborn

    P58.5 Neonatal jaundice due to swallowed maternal blood

    P58.8 Neonatal jaundice due to other specified excessive hemolysis

    P58.9 Neonatal jaundice due to excessive hemolysis, unspecified

☑4ᵗʰ **P59 Neonatal jaundice from other and unspecified causes**
    EXCLUDES 1   *jaundice due to inborn errors of metabolism (E70-E88)*
               kernicterus (P57.-)

    P59.0 Neonatal jaundice associated with preterm delivery
        Hyperbilirubinemia of prematurity
        Jaundice due to delayed conjugation associated with preterm delivery

    P59.1 Inspissated bile syndrome `COM`
        DEF: Biliary obstruction in newborn resulting from obstruction of outflow tract.

☑5ᵗʰ **P59.2 Neonatal jaundice from other and unspecified hepatocellular damage**
        EXCLUDES 1   *congenital viral hepatitis (P35.3)*

        P59.20 Neonatal jaundice from unspecified hepatocellular damage `COM`

        P59.29 Neonatal jaundice from other hepatocellular damage `COM`
            Neonatal giant cell hepatitis
            Neonatal (idiopathic) hepatitis

    P59.3 Neonatal jaundice from breast milk inhibitor

    P59.8 Neonatal jaundice from other specified causes

    P59.9 Neonatal jaundice, unspecified
        Neonatal physiological jaundice (intense)(prolonged) NOS
        AHA: 2015,3Q,20

  P60 Disseminated intravascular coagulation of newborn `COM`
    Defibrination syndrome of newborn

☑4ᵗʰ **P61 Other perinatal hematological disorders**
    EXCLUDES 1   *transient hypogammaglobulinemia of infancy (D80.7)*

    P61.0 Transient neonatal thrombocytopenia `COM`
        Neonatal thrombocytopenia due to exchange transfusion
        Neonatal thrombocytopenia due to idiopathic maternal thrombocytopenia
        Neonatal thrombocytopenia due to isoimmunization
        DEF: Temporary decrease in blood platelets of a newborn that is secondary to placental insufficiency.

    P61.1 Polycythemia neonatorum
        DEF: Abnormal increase of total red blood cells of a newborn that results in hyperviscosity, which slows the flow of blood through small blood vessels.

    P61.2 Anemia of prematurity

    P61.3 Congenital anemia from fetal blood loss

    P61.4 Other congenital anemias, not elsewhere classified
        Congenital anemia NOS

    P61.5 Transient neonatal neutropenia `COM`
        EXCLUDES 1   *congenital neutropenia (nontransient) (D70.0)*
        DEF: Low blood neutrophil counts of newborn that occurs due to maternal hypertension, sepsis, twin-twin transfusion, alloimmunization, and hemolytic disease.

    P61.6 Other transient neonatal disorders of coagulation `COM`

    P61.8 Other specified perinatal hematological disorders

    P61.9 Perinatal hematological disorder, unspecified

Transitory endocrine and metabolic disorders specific to newborn (P70-P74)

  INCLUDES   transitory endocrine and metabolic disturbances caused by the infant's response to maternal endocrine and metabolic factors, or its adjustment to extrauterine environment

  AHA: 2018,2Q,6

☑4ᵗʰ **P70 Transitory disorders of carbohydrate metabolism specific to newborn**

    P70.0 Syndrome of infant of mother with gestational diabetes
        Newborn (with hypoglycemia) affected by maternal gestational diabetes
        EXCLUDES 1   *newborn (with hypoglycemia) affected by maternal (pre-existing) diabetes mellitus (P70.1)*
               syndrome of infant of a diabetic mother (P70.1)

    P70.1 Syndrome of infant of a diabetic mother
        Newborn (with hypoglycemia) affected by maternal (pre-existing) diabetes mellitus
        EXCLUDES 1   *newborn (with hypoglycemia) affected by maternal gestational diabetes (P70.0)*
               syndrome of infant of mother with gestational diabetes (P70.0)

    P70.2 Neonatal diabetes mellitus

    P70.3 Iatrogenic neonatal hypoglycemia

    P70.4 Other neonatal hypoglycemia
        Transitory neonatal hypoglycemia

    P70.8 Other transitory disorders of carbohydrate metabolism of newborn

    P70.9 Transitory disorder of carbohydrate metabolism of newborn, unspecified

☑4ᵗʰ **P71 Transitory neonatal disorders of calcium and magnesium metabolism**

    P71.0 Cow's milk hypocalcemia in newborn

    P71.1 Other neonatal hypocalcemia
        EXCLUDES 1   *neonatal hypoparathyroidism (P71.4)*

    P71.2 Neonatal hypomagnesemia

    P71.3 Neonatal tetany without calcium or magnesium deficiency
        Neonatal tetany NOS

    P71.4 Transitory neonatal hypoparathyroidism

    P71.8 Other transitory neonatal disorders of calcium and magnesium metabolism
        AHA: 2016,4Q,54

    P71.9 Transitory neonatal disorder of calcium and magnesium metabolism, unspecified

☑4ᵗʰ **P72 Other transitory neonatal endocrine disorders**
    EXCLUDES 1   *congenital hypothyroidism with or without goiter (E03.0-E03.1)*
               dyshormogenetic goiter (E07.1)
               Pendred's syndrome (E07.1)

    P72.0 Neonatal goiter, not elsewhere classified
        Transitory congenital goiter with normal functioning

    P72.1 Transitory neonatal hyperthyroidism
        Neonatal thyrotoxicosis

    P72.2 Other transitory neonatal disorders of thyroid function, not elsewhere classified
        Transitory neonatal hypothyroidism

    P72.8 Other specified transitory neonatal endocrine disorders

    P72.9 Transitory neonatal endocrine disorder, unspecified

☑4ᵗʰ **P74 Other transitory neonatal electrolyte and metabolic disturbances**
    AHA: 2018,4Q,26-27

    P74.0 Late metabolic acidosis of newborn
        EXCLUDES 1   *(fetal) metabolic acidosis of newborn (P19)*

    P74.1 Dehydration of newborn

☑5ᵗʰ **P74.2 Disturbances of sodium balance of newborn**

        P74.21 Hypernatremia of newborn
        P74.22 Hyponatremia of newborn

☑5ᵗʰ **P74.3 Disturbances of potassium balance of newborn**

        P74.31 Hyperkalemia of newborn

P74.32　Hypokalemia of newborn

✓5ᵗʰ **P74.4　Other transitory electrolyte disturbances of newborn**

　　P74.41　Alkalosis of newborn
　　　　Hyperbicarbonatemia

✓6ᵗʰ **P74.42　Disturbances of chlorine balance of newborn**

　　　　P74.421　Hyperchloremia of newborn
　　　　　　Hyperchloremic metabolic acidosis
　　　　　　EXCLUDES 2　*late metabolic acidosis of the newborn (P74.0)*

　　　　P74.422　Hypochloremia of newborn

　　　　P74.49　Other transitory electrolyte disturbance of newborn

P74.5　Transitory tyrosinemia of newborn

P74.6　Transitory hyperammonemia of newborn

P74.8　Other transitory metabolic disturbances of newborn
　　Amino-acid metabolic disorders described as transitory

P74.9　Transitory metabolic disturbance of newborn, unspecified

Digestive system disorders of newborn (P76-P78)

✓4ᵗʰ **P76　Other intestinal obstruction of newborn**

P76.0　Meconium plug syndrome
　　Meconium ileus NOS
　　EXCLUDES 1　*meconium ileus in cystic fibrosis (E84.11)*
　　DEF: Meconium obstruction of a newborn's intestines, resulting from unusually thick or hard meconium.

P76.1　Transitory ileus of newborn
　　EXCLUDES 1　*Hirschsprung's disease (Q43.1)*

P76.2　Intestinal obstruction due to inspissated milk

P76.8　Other specified intestinal obstruction of newborn
　　EXCLUDES 1　*intestinal obstruction classifiable to K56.-*

P76.9　Intestinal obstruction of newborn, unspecified

✓4ᵗʰ **P77　Necrotizing enterocolitis of newborn**
　　DEF: Serious intestinal infection and inflammation in preterm infants. Severity is measured by stages and may progress to life-threatening perforation or peritonitis. Resection surgical treatment may be necessary.

P77.1　Stage 1 necrotizing enterocolitis in newborn　COM
　　Necrotizing enterocolitis without pneumatosis, without perforation
　　DEF: Broad-spectrum symptoms with nonspecific signs, including feeding intolerance, abdominal distention, bradycardia, and metabolic abnormalities.

P77.2　Stage 2 necrotizing enterocolitis in newborn　COM
　　Necrotizing enterocolitis with pneumatosis, without perforation
　　DEF: Radiographic confirmation of necrotizing enterocolitis showing intestinal dilatation, fixed loops of bowels, pneumatosis intestinalis, metabolic acidosis, and thrombocytopenia.

P77.3　Stage 3 necrotizing enterocolitis in newborn　COM
　　Necrotizing enterocolitis with perforation
　　Necrotizing enterocolitis with pneumatosis and perforation
　　DEF: Advanced stage in which an infant demonstrates signs of bowel perforation, septic shock, metabolic acidosis, ascites, disseminated intravascular coagulopathy, and neutropenia.

P77.9　Necrotizing enterocolitis in newborn, unspecified　COM
　　Necrotizing enterocolitis in newborn, NOS

✓4ᵗʰ **P78　Other perinatal digestive system disorders**
　　EXCLUDES 1　*cystic fibrosis (E84.0-E84.9)*
　　　　neonatal gastrointestinal hemorrhages (P54.0-P54.3)

P78.0　Perinatal intestinal perforation　COM
　　Meconium peritonitis

P78.1　Other neonatal peritonitis
　　Neonatal peritonitis NOS

P78.2　Neonatal hematemesis and melena due to swallowed maternal blood

P78.3　Noninfective neonatal diarrhea
　　Neonatal diarrhea NOS

✓5ᵗʰ **P78.8　Other specified perinatal digestive system disorders**

　　P78.81　Congenital cirrhosis (of liver)
　　P78.82　Peptic ulcer of newborn
　　P78.83　Newborn esophageal reflux
　　　　Neonatal esophageal reflux

P78.84　Gestational alloimmune liver disease　COM
　　GALD
　　Neonatal hemochromatosis
　　EXCLUDES 1　*hemochromatosis (E83.11-)*
　　AHA: 2017,4Q,21
　　DEF: Severe hepatic injury with onset during fetal development with manifestations beginning during fetal life. It is due to maternal antibodies to fetal hepatic cells (hepatocytes) that cross the placenta into the fetal circulation, causing hepatic cell necrosis.

P78.89　Other specified perinatal digestive system disorders

P78.9　Perinatal digestive system disorder, unspecified

Conditions involving the integument and temperature regulation of newborn (P80-P83)

✓4ᵗʰ **P80　Hypothermia of newborn**
　　DEF: Decrease in newborn body temperature due to their larger ratio of surface area to body weight, thin skin with blood vessels close to the surface, and a limited amount of subcutaneous fat.

P80.0　Cold injury syndrome
　　Severe and usually chronic hypothermia associated with a pink flushed appearance, edema and neurological and biochemical abnormalities.
　　EXCLUDES 1　*mild hypothermia of newborn (P80.8)*

P80.8　Other hypothermia of newborn
　　Mild hypothermia of newborn

P80.9　Hypothermia of newborn, unspecified

✓4ᵗʰ **P81　Other disturbances of temperature regulation of newborn**

P81.0　Environmental hyperthermia of newborn

P81.8　Other specified disturbances of temperature regulation of newborn

P81.9　Disturbance of temperature regulation of newborn, unspecified
　　Fever of newborn NOS

✓4ᵗʰ **P83　Other conditions of integument specific to newborn**
　　EXCLUDES 1　*congenital malformations of skin and integument (Q80-Q84)*
　　　　hydrops fetalis due to hemolytic disease (P56.-)
　　　　neonatal skin infection (P39.4)
　　　　staphylococcal scalded skin syndrome (L00)
　　EXCLUDES 2　*cradle cap (L21.0)*
　　　　diaper [napkin] dermatitis (L22)

P83.0　Sclerema neonatorum
　　DEF: Diffuse, rapidly progressing white, waxy, nonpitting hardening of tissue, usually of legs and feet that is life-threatening. It is found in preterm or debilitated infants. Etiology is unknown.

P83.1　Neonatal erythema toxicum

P83.2　Hydrops fetalis not due to hemolytic disease
　　Hydrops fetalis NOS
　　DEF: Severe, life-threatening problem of a newborn characterized by severe edema of the entire body. It is unrelated to immune response.

✓5ᵗʰ **P83.3　Other and unspecified edema specific to newborn**

　　P83.30　Unspecified edema specific to newborn
　　P83.39　Other edema specific to newborn

P83.4　Breast engorgement of newborn
　　Noninfective mastitis of newborn

P83.5　Congenital hydrocele　♂
　　DEF: Hydrocele: Serous fluid that collects in the tunica vaginalis of the scrotum along the spermatic cord in males.

P83.6　Umbilical polyp of newborn

✓5ᵗʰ **P83.8　Other specified conditions of integument specific to newborn**
　　AHA: 2017,4Q,21-22

　　P83.81　Umbilical granuloma
　　　　EXCLUDES 2　*granulomatous disorder of the skin and subcutaneous tissue, unspecified (L92.9)*

　　P83.88　Other specified conditions of integument specific to newborn
　　　　Bronze baby syndrome
　　　　Neonatal scleroderma
　　　　Urticaria neonatorum

P83.9　Condition of the integument specific to newborn, unspecified

Other problems with newborn (P84)

P84 Other problems with newborn
Acidemia of newborn
Acidosis of newborn
Anoxia of newborn NOS
Asphyxia of newborn NOS
Hypercapnia of newborn
Hypoxemia of newborn
Hypoxia of newborn NOS
Mixed metabolic and respiratory acidosis of newborn
>EXCLUDES 1   *intracranial hemorrhage due to anoxia or hypoxia (P52.-)*
>*hypoxic ischemic encephalopathy [HIE] (P91.6-)*
>*late metabolic acidosis of newborn (P74.0)*

Other disorders originating in the perinatal period (P90-P96)

P90 Convulsions of newborn   `COM`
>EXCLUDES 1   *benign myoclonic epilepsy in infancy (G40.3-)*
>*benign neonatal convulsions (familial) (G40.3-)*

☑4ᵗʰ **P91 Other disturbances of cerebral status of newborn**

   P91.0 Neonatal cerebral ischemia   `COM`
>EXCLUDES 1   *neonatal cerebral infarction (P91.82-)*

   P91.1 Acquired periventricular cysts of newborn   `COM`

   P91.2 Neonatal cerebral leukomalacia   `COM`
     Periventricular leukomalacia

   P91.3 Neonatal cerebral irritability   `COM`

   P91.4 Neonatal cerebral depression   `COM`

   P91.5 Neonatal coma   `COM`

☑5ᵗʰ   **P91.6 Hypoxic ischemic encephalopathy [HIE]**
>EXCLUDES 1   *neonatal cerebral depression (P91.4)*
>*neonatal cerebral irritability (P91.3)*
>*neonatal coma (P91.5)*

     AHA: 2017,4Q,22

     P91.60 Hypoxic ischemic encephalopathy [HIE], unspecified   `COM`

     P91.61 Mild hypoxic ischemic encephalopathy [HIE]   `COM`

     P91.62 Moderate hypoxic ischemic encephalopathy [HIE]   `COM`

     P91.63 Severe hypoxic ischemic encephalopathy [HIE]   `COM`

☑5ᵗʰ   **P91.8 Other specified disturbances of cerebral status of newborn**
     AHA: 2017,4Q,22

     ☑6ᵗʰ   **P91.81 Neonatal encephalopathy**

       P91.811 Neonatal encephalopathy in diseases classified elsewhere   `COM`
         Code first underlying condition, if known, such as:
           congenital cirrhosis (of liver) (P78.81)
           intracranial nontraumatic hemorrhage of newborn (P52.-)
           kernicterus (P57.-)

       P91.819 Neonatal encephalopathy, unspecified   `COM`

     ☑6ᵗʰ   **P91.82 Neonatal cerebral infarction**
       Neonatal stroke
       Perinatal arterial ischemic stroke
       Perinatal cerebral infarction
>EXCLUDES 1   *cerebral infarction (I63.-)*
>EXCLUDES 2   *intracranial hemorrhage of newborn (P52.-)*

       AHA: 2020,4Q,37-38

       P91.821 Neonatal cerebral infarction, right side of brain   `HCC` `ESR` `COM`

       P91.822 Neonatal cerebral infarction, left side of brain   `HCC` `ESR` `COM`

       P91.823 Neonatal cerebral infarction, bilateral   `HCC` `ESR` `COM`

       P91.829 Neonatal cerebral infarction, unspecified side   `HCC` `ESR` `COM`

     P91.88 Other specified disturbances of cerebral status of newborn   `COM`

   P91.9 Disturbance of cerebral status of newborn, unspecified   `COM`

☑4ᵗʰ **P92 Feeding problems of newborn**
>EXCLUDES 1   *eating disorders (F50.-)*
>EXCLUDES 2   *feeding problems in child over 28 days old (R63.3)*

   AHA: 2016,3Q,19

   ☑5ᵗʰ   **P92.0 Vomiting of newborn**
>EXCLUDES 1   *vomiting of child over 28 days old (R11.-)*

     P92.01 Bilious vomiting of newborn
>EXCLUDES 1   *bilious vomiting in child over 28 days old (R11.14)*

     P92.09 Other vomiting of newborn
>EXCLUDES 1   *regurgitation of food in newborn (P92.1)*

   P92.1 Regurgitation and rumination of newborn

   P92.2 Slow feeding of newborn

   P92.3 Underfeeding of newborn

   P92.4 Overfeeding of newborn

   P92.5 Neonatal difficulty in feeding at breast
     AHA: 2017,1Q,28

   P92.6 Failure to thrive in newborn
>EXCLUDES 1   *failure to thrive in child over 28 days old (R62.51)*

   P92.8 Other feeding problems of newborn

   P92.9 Feeding problem of newborn, unspecified

☑4ᵗʰ **P93 Reactions and intoxications due to drugs administered to newborn**
>INCLUDES   reactions and intoxications due to drugs administered to fetus affecting newborn
>EXCLUDES 1   *jaundice due to drugs or toxins transmitted from mother or given to newborn (P58.4-)*
>*reactions and intoxications from maternal opiates, tranquilizers and other medication (P04.0-P04.1, P04.4-)*
>*withdrawal symptoms from maternal use of drugs of addiction (P96.1)*
>*withdrawal symptoms from therapeutic use of drugs in newborn (P96.2)*

   P93.0 Grey baby syndrome   `COM`
     Grey syndrome from chloramphenicol administration in newborn

   P93.8 Other reactions and intoxications due to drugs administered to newborn   `COM`
     Use additional code for adverse effect, if applicable, to identify drug (T36-T50 with fifth or sixth character 5)

☑4ᵗʰ **P94 Disorders of muscle tone of newborn**

   P94.0 Transient neonatal myasthenia gravis
>EXCLUDES 1   *myasthenia gravis (G70.0)*

   P94.1 Congenital hypertonia

   P94.2 Congenital hypotonia
     Floppy baby syndrome, unspecified

   P94.8 Other disorders of muscle tone of newborn

   P94.9 Disorder of muscle tone of newborn, unspecified

P95 Stillbirth
Deadborn fetus NOS
Fetal death of unspecified cause
Stillbirth NOS
>EXCLUDES 1   *maternal care for intrauterine death (O36.4)*
>*missed abortion (O02.1)*
>*outcome of delivery, stillbirth (Z37.1, Z37.3, Z37.4, Z37.7)*

☑4ᵗʰ **P96 Other conditions originating in the perinatal period**

   P96.0 Congenital renal failure
     Uremia of newborn

   P96.1 Neonatal withdrawal symptoms from maternal use of drugs of addiction   `COM`
     Drug withdrawal syndrome in infant of dependent mother
     Neonatal abstinence syndrome
>EXCLUDES 1   *reactions and intoxications from maternal opiates and tranquilizers administered during labor and delivery (P04.0)*

     AHA: 2018,4Q,24-25

   P96.2 Withdrawal symptoms from therapeutic use of drugs in newborn   `COM`

   P96.3 Wide cranial sutures of newborn
     Neonatal craniotabes

   P96.5 Complication to newborn due to (fetal) intrauterine procedure
>EXCLUDES 2   *newborn affected by amniocentesis (P00.6)*

☑ Additional Character Required   ☑x7ᵗʰ Placeholder Alert   Manifestation   Unspecified Dx   Ⓠ QPP   UPD Unacceptable PDx

✓5ᵗʰ **P96.8　Other specified conditions originating in the perinatal period**

P96.81　Exposure to (parental) (environmental) tobacco smoke in the perinatal period

EXCLUDES 2　*newborn affected by in utero exposure to tobacco (P04.2)*

exposure to environmental tobacco smoke after the perinatal period (Z77.22)

P96.82　Delayed separation of umbilical cord

P96.83　Meconium staining

EXCLUDES 1　*meconium aspiration (P24.00, P24.01)*

meconium passage during delivery (P03.82)

DEF: Meconium passed in utero causing discoloration on the fetal skin and nails or on the umbilicus. This staining may be incidental or may be an indicator of significant fetal stress that could affect outcomes.

P96.89　Other specified conditions originating in the perinatal period

Use additional code to specify condition

P96.9　Condition originating in the perinatal period, unspecified

Congenital debility NOS

Chapter 17. Congenital Malformations, Deformations, and Chromosomal Abnormalities (Q00–Q99)

Chapter-specific Guidelines with Coding Examples

The chapter-specific guidelines from the ICD-10-CM Official Guidelines for Coding and Reporting have been provided below. Along with these guidelines are coding examples, contained in the shaded boxes, that have been developed to help illustrate the coding and/or sequencing guidance found in these guidelines.

Assign an appropriate code(s) from categories Q00-Q99, Congenital malformations, deformations, and chromosomal abnormalities when a malformation/deformation or chromosomal abnormality is documented. A malformation/deformation/or chromosomal abnormality may be the principal/first-listed diagnosis on a record or a secondary diagnosis.

When a malformation/deformation/or chromosomal abnormality does not have a unique code assignment, assign additional code(s) for any manifestations that may be present.

When the code assignment specifically identifies the malformation/deformation/or chromosomal abnormality, manifestations that are an inherent component of the anomaly should not be coded separately. Additional codes should be assigned for manifestations that are not an inherent component.

8-day-old infant with tetralogy of Fallot and pulmonary stenosis

Q21.3   **Tetralogy of Fallot**

Explanation: Pulmonary stenosis is inherent in the disease process of tetralogy of Fallot. When the code assignment specifically identifies the malformation/deformation/or chromosomal abnormality, manifestations that are inherent components of the anomaly should not be coded separately.

7-month-old infant with Down syndrome and common atrioventricular canal

Q90.9   **Down syndrome, unspecified**

Q21.23   **Complete atrioventricular septal defect**

Explanation: While a common atrioventricular canal is often associated with patients with Down syndrome, this manifestation is not an inherent component and may be reported separately. When the code assignment specifically identifies the anomaly, manifestations that are inherent components of the condition should not be coded separately. Additional codes should be assigned for manifestations that are not inherent components.

Codes from Chapter 17 may be used throughout the life of the patient. If a congenital malformation or deformity has been corrected, a personal history code should be used to identify the history of the malformation or deformity. Although present at birth, a malformation/deformation/or chromosomal abnormality may not be identified until later in life. Whenever the condition is diagnosed by the provider, it is appropriate to assign a code from codes Q00-Q99. For the birth admission, the appropriate code from category Z38, Liveborn infants, according to place of birth and type of delivery, should be sequenced as the principal diagnosis, followed by any congenital anomaly codes, Q00- Q99.

Three-year-old with history of corrected ventricular septal defect

Z87.74   **Personal history of (corrected) congenital malformations of heart and circulatory system**

Explanation: If a congenital malformation or deformity has been corrected, a personal history code should be used to identify the history of the malformation or deformity.

Forty-year-old man with headaches diagnosed with congenital arteriovenous malformation of cerebral vessels by brain scan

Q28.2   **Arteriovenous malformation of cerebral vessels**

Explanation: Although present at birth, malformations may not be identified until later in life. Whenever a congenital condition is diagnosed by the physician, it is appropriate to assign a code from the range Q00–Q99.

Chapter 17. Congenital Malformations, Deformations and Chromosomal Abnormalities (Q00–Q99)

NOTE   Codes from this chapter are not for use on maternal records

EXCLUDES 2   *inborn errors of metabolism (E70–E88)*

This chapter contains the following blocks:

Q00–Q07   Congenital malformations of the nervous system
Q10–Q18   Congenital malformations of eye, ear, face and neck
Q20–Q28   Congenital malformations of the circulatory system
Q30–Q34   Congenital malformations of the respiratory system
Q35–Q37   Cleft lip and cleft palate
Q38–Q45   Other congenital malformations of the digestive system
Q50–Q56   Congenital malformations of genital organs
Q60–Q64   Congenital malformations of the urinary system
Q65–Q79   Congenital malformations and deformations of the musculoskeletal system
Q80–Q89   Other congenital malformations
Q90–Q99   Chromosomal abnormalities, not elsewhere classified

Congenital malformations of the nervous system (Q00–Q07)

☑4ᵗʰ **Q00   Anencephaly and similar malformations**

Q00.0   Anencephaly   HCC Rx ESR COM
Acephaly
Acrania
Amyelencephaly
Hemianencephaly
Hemicephaly

Q00.1   Craniorachischisis   HCC Rx ESR COM

Q00.2   Iniencephaly   HCC Rx ESR COM

☑4ᵗʰ **Q01   Encephalocele**

INCLUDES   Arnold-Chiari syndrome, type III
encephalocystocele
encephalomyelocele
hydroencephalocele
hydromeningocele, cranial
meningocele, cerebral
meningoencephalocele

EXCLUDES 1   *Meckel-Gruber syndrome (Q61.9)*

DEF: Congenital protrusion of brain tissue through a defect in the skull.

Q01.0   Frontal encephalocele   HCC Rx ESR COM

Q01.1   Nasofrontal encephalocele   HCC Rx ESR COM

Q01.2   Occipital encephalocele   HCC Rx ESR COM

Q01.8   Encephalocele of other sites   HCC Rx ESR COM

Q01.9   Encephalocele, unspecified   HCC Rx ESR COM

Q02   Microcephaly   HCC Rx ESR COM
INCLUDES   hydromicrocephaly
micrencephalon
Code first, if applicable, congenital Zika virus disease
EXCLUDES 1   *Meckel-Gruber syndrome (Q61.9)*
AHA: 2018,4Q,26
DEF: Congenital disorder in which the head circumference is more than two standard deviations below the mean for age, sex, race, and gestation and associated with a decreased life expectancy.

☑4ᵗʰ **Q03   Congenital hydrocephalus**

INCLUDES   hydrocephalus in newborn

EXCLUDES 1   *Arnold-Chiari syndrome, type II (Q07.0-)*
acquired hydrocephalus (G91.-)
hydrocephalus due to congenital toxoplasmosis (P37.1)
hydrocephalus with spina bifida (Q05.0-Q05.4)

DEF: Hydrocephalus: Abnormal buildup of cerebrospinal fluid in the brain causing dilation of the ventricles.

Congenital Hydrocephalus

Normal ventricles   Hydrocephalic ventricles

Q03.0   Malformations of aqueduct of Sylvius   HCC Rx ESR COM
Anomaly of aqueduct of Sylvius
Obstruction of aqueduct of Sylvius, congenital
Stenosis of aqueduct of Sylvius

Q03.1   Atresia of foramina of Magendie and Luschka   HCC Rx ESR COM
Dandy-Walker syndrome

Q03.8   Other congenital hydrocephalus   HCC Rx ESR COM

Q03.9   Congenital hydrocephalus, unspecified   HCC Rx ESR COM

☑4ᵗʰ **Q04   Other congenital malformations of brain**

EXCLUDES 1   *cyclopia (Q87.0)*
macrocephaly (Q75.3)

Q04.0   Congenital malformations of corpus callosum   HCC Rx ESR COM
Agenesis of corpus callosum

Q04.1   Arhinencephaly   HCC Rx ESR COM

Q04.2   Holoprosencephaly   HCC Rx ESR COM

Q04.3   Other reduction deformities of brain   HCC Rx ESR COM
Absence of part of brain
Agenesis of part of brain
Agyria
Aplasia of part of brain
Hydranencephaly
Hypoplasia of part of brain
Lissencephaly
Microgyria
Pachygyria
EXCLUDES 1   *congenital malformations of corpus callosum (Q04.0)*

Q04.4   Septo-optic dysplasia of brain   HCC Rx ESR COM

Q04.5   Megalencephaly   HCC Rx ESR COM

Q04.6   Congenital cerebral cysts   HCC Rx ESR COM
Porencephaly
Schizencephaly
EXCLUDES 1   *acquired porencephalic cyst (G93.0)*

Q04.8   Other specified congenital malformations of brain   HCC Rx ESR COM
Arnold-Chiari syndrome, type IV
Macrogyria

Q04.9   Congenital malformation of brain, unspecified   HCC Rx ESR COM
Congenital anomaly NOS of brain
Congenital deformity NOS of brain
Congenital disease or lesion NOS of brain
Multiple anomalies NOS of brain, congenital

☑4ᵗʰ **Q05 Spina bifida**

INCLUDES
hydromeningocele (spinal)
meningocele (spinal)
meningomyelocele
myelocele
myelomeningocele
rachischisis
spina bifida (aperta)(cystica)
syringomyelocele

Use additional code for any associated paraplegia (paraparesis) (G82.2-)

EXCLUDES 1   *Arnold-Chiari syndrome, type II (Q07.0-)*
spina bifida occulta (Q76.0)

DEF: Lack of closure in the vertebral column with protrusion of the spinal cord through the defect, often in the lumbosacral area. This condition can be recognized by the presence of alpha-fetoproteins in the amniotic fluid.

Spina Bifida

Spina bifida occulta   Meningocele   Myelomeningocele

Q05.0 **Cervical spina bifida** with hydrocephalus   HCC Rx ESR COM

Q05.1 **Thoracic spina bifida** with hydrocephalus   HCC Rx ESR COM
Dorsal spina bifida with hydrocephalus
Thoracolumbar spina bifida with hydrocephalus

Q05.2 **Lumbar spina bifida** with hydrocephalus   HCC Rx ESR COM
Lumbosacral spina bifida with hydrocephalus

Q05.3 **Sacral spina bifida** with hydrocephalus   HCC Rx ESR COM

Q05.4 **Unspecified spina bifida with hydrocephalus**   HCC Rx ESR COM

Q05.5 **Cervical spina bifida** without hydrocephalus   HCC Rx ESR COM

Q05.6 **Thoracic spina bifida** without hydrocephalus   HCC Rx ESR COM
Dorsal spina bifida NOS
Thoracolumbar spina bifida NOS

Q05.7 **Lumbar spina bifida** without hydrocephalus   HCC Rx ESR COM
Lumbosacral spina bifida NOS

Q05.8 **Sacral spina bifida** without hydrocephalus   HCC Rx ESR COM

Q05.9 **Spina bifida, unspecified**   HCC Rx ESR COM

☑4ᵗʰ **Q06 Other congenital malformations of spinal cord**

Q06.0 **Amyelia**   HCC Rx ESR COM

Q06.1 **Hypoplasia and dysplasia of spinal cord**   HCC Rx ESR COM
Atelomyelia
Myelatelia
Myelodysplasia of spinal cord

Q06.2 **Diastematomyelia**   HCC Rx ESR COM
DEF: Rare congenital anomaly often associated with spina bifida. The spinal cord is separated into longitudinal halves by a bony, cartilaginous or fibrous septum, each half surrounded by a dural sac.

Q06.3 **Other congenital cauda equina malformations**   HCC Rx ESR COM

Q06.4 **Hydromyelia**   HCC Rx ESR COM
Hydrorachis

Q06.8 **Other specified congenital malformations of spinal cord**   HCC Rx ESR COM

Q06.9 **Congenital malformation of spinal cord, unspecified**   HCC Rx ESR COM
Congenital anomaly NOS of spinal cord
Congenital deformity NOS of spinal cord
Congenital disease or lesion NOS of spinal cord

☑4ᵗʰ **Q07 Other congenital malformations of nervous system**

EXCLUDES 2   *congenital central alveolar hypoventilation syndrome (G47.35)*
familial dysautonomia [Riley-Day] (G90.1)
neurofibromatosis (nonmalignant) (Q85.0-)

☑5ᵗʰ **Q07.0 Arnold-Chiari syndrome**
Arnold-Chiari syndrome, type II
EXCLUDES 1   *Arnold-Chiari syndrome, type III (Q01.-)*
Arnold-Chiari syndrome, type IV (Q04.8)
DEF: Congenital malformation of the brain in which the cerebellum protrudes through the foramen magnum into the spinal canal.

Q07.00 **Arnold-Chiari syndrome** without spina bifida or hydrocephalus   HCC Rx ESR COM

Q07.01 **Arnold-Chiari syndrome** with spina bifida   HCC Rx ESR COM

Q07.02 **Arnold-Chiari syndrome** with hydrocephalus   HCC Rx ESR COM

Q07.03 **Arnold-Chiari syndrome** with spina bifida and hydrocephalus   HCC Rx ESR COM

Q07.8 **Other specified congenital malformations of nervous system**   HCC Rx ESR COM
Agenesis of nerve
Displacement of brachial plexus
Jaw-winking syndrome
Marcus Gunn's syndrome

Q07.9 **Congenital malformation of nervous system, unspecified**   HCC Rx ESR COM
Congenital anomaly NOS of nervous system
Congenital deformity NOS of nervous system
Congenital disease or lesion NOS of nervous system

Congenital malformations of eye, ear, face and neck (Q10-Q18)

EXCLUDES 2   *cleft lip and cleft palate (Q35-Q37)*
congenital malformation of cervical spine (Q05.0, Q05.5, Q67.5, Q76.0-Q76.4)
congenital malformation of larynx (Q31.-)
congenital malformation of lip NEC (Q38.0)
congenital malformation of nose (Q30.-)
congenital malformation of parathyroid gland (Q89.2)
congenital malformation of thyroid gland (Q89.2)

☑4ᵗʰ **Q10 Congenital malformations of eyelid, lacrimal apparatus and orbit**

EXCLUDES 1   *cryptophthalmos NOS (Q11.2)*
cryptophthalmos syndrome (Q87.0)

Q10.0 **Congenital ptosis**
DEF: Congenital drooping of the eyelid. Ptosis is mostly idiopathic, but may occur genetically.

Q10.1 **Congenital ectropion**

Q10.2 **Congenital entropion**

Q10.3 **Other congenital malformations of eyelid**
Ablepharon
Blepharophimosis, congenital
Coloboma of eyelid
Congenital absence or agenesis of cilia
Congenital absence or agenesis of eyelid
Congenital accessory eyelid
Congenital accessory eye muscle
Congenital malformation of eyelid NOS

Q10.4 **Absence and agenesis of lacrimal apparatus**
Congenital absence of punctum lacrimale

Q10.5 **Congenital stenosis and stricture of lacrimal duct**

Q10.6 **Other congenital malformations of lacrimal apparatus**
Congenital malformation of lacrimal apparatus NOS

Q10.7 **Congenital malformation of orbit**

☑4ᵗʰ **Q11 Anophthalmos, microphthalmos and macrophthalmos**

Q11.0 **Cystic eyeball**

Q11.1 **Other anophthalmos**
Anophthalmos NOS
Agenesis of eye
Aplasia of eye

Q11.2 **Microphthalmos**
Cryptophthalmos NOS
Dysplasia of eye
Hypoplasia of eye
Rudimentary eye
EXCLUDES 1   *cryptophthalmos syndrome (Q87.0)*

Q11.3 Macrophthalmos
> *EXCLUDES 1*   macrophthalmos in congenital glaucoma (Q15.0)

✓4ᵗʰ Q12 Congenital lens malformations

Q12.0 Congenital cataract

Q12.1 Congenital displaced lens

Q12.2 Coloboma of lens

Coloboma of Lens

Coloboma

Q12.3 Congenital aphakia

Q12.4 Spherophakia

Q12.8 Other congenital lens malformations
Microphakia

Q12.9 Congenital lens malformation, unspecified

✓4ᵗʰ Q13 Congenital malformations of anterior segment of eye

Q13.0 Coloboma of iris
Coloboma NOS
DEF: Defective or absent section of ocular tissue that may present as mild cupping or a small pit in the ocular disc due to extensive defects in the iris, ciliary body, choroids, and retina.

Q13.1 Absence of iris
Aniridia
Use additional code for associated glaucoma (H42)
DEF: Incompletely formed or absent iris. It affects both eyes and is a dominant trait.

Q13.2 Other congenital malformations of iris
Anisocoria, congenital
Atresia of pupil
Congenital malformation of iris NOS
Corectopia

Q13.3 Congenital corneal opacity

Q13.4 Other congenital corneal malformations
Congenital malformation of cornea NOS
Microcornea
Peter's anomaly

Q13.5 Blue sclera

✓5ᵗʰ Q13.8 Other congenital malformations of anterior segment of eye

Q13.81 Rieger's anomaly
Use additional code for associated glaucoma (H42)

Q13.89 Other congenital malformations of anterior segment of eye

Q13.9 Congenital malformation of anterior segment of eye, unspecified

✓4ᵗʰ Q14 Congenital malformations of posterior segment of eye
> *EXCLUDES 2*   optic nerve hypoplasia (H47.03-)

Q14.0 Congenital malformation of vitreous humor
Congenital vitreous opacity

Q14.1 Congenital malformation of retina
Congenital retinal aneurysm

Q14.2 Congenital malformation of optic disc
Coloboma of optic disc

Q14.3 Congenital malformation of choroid

Q14.8 Other congenital malformations of posterior segment of eye
Coloboma of the fundus

Q14.9 Congenital malformation of posterior segment of eye, unspecified

✓4ᵗʰ Q15 Other congenital malformations of eye
> *EXCLUDES 1*   congenital nystagmus (H55.01)
> ocular albinism (E70.31-)
> optic nerve hypoplasia (H47.03-)
> retinitis pigmentosa (H35.52)

Q15.0 Congenital glaucoma
Axenfeld's anomaly
Buphthalmos
Glaucoma of childhood
Glaucoma of newborn
Hydrophthalmos
Keratoglobus, congenital, with glaucoma
Macrocornea with glaucoma
Macrophthalmos in congenital glaucoma
Megalocornea with glaucoma

Q15.8 Other specified congenital malformations of eye

Q15.9 Congenital malformation of eye, unspecified
Congenital anomaly of eye
Congenital deformity of eye

✓4ᵗʰ Q16 Congenital malformations of ear causing impairment of hearing
> *EXCLUDES 1*   congenital deafness (H90.-)

Q16.0 Congenital absence of (ear) auricle

Q16.1 Congenital absence, atresia and stricture of auditory canal (external)
Congenital atresia or stricture of osseous meatus

Q16.2 Absence of eustachian tube

Q16.3 Congenital malformation of ear ossicles
Congenital fusion of ear ossicles

Q16.4 Other congenital malformations of middle ear
Congenital malformation of middle ear NOS

Q16.5 Congenital malformation of inner ear
Congenital anomaly of membranous labyrinth
Congenital anomaly of organ of Corti

Q16.9 Congenital malformation of ear causing impairment of hearing, unspecified
Congenital absence of ear NOS

✓4ᵗʰ Q17 Other congenital malformations of ear
> *EXCLUDES 1*   congenital malformations of ear with impairment of hearing (Q16.0-Q16.9)
> preauricular sinus (Q18.1)

Q17.0 Accessory auricle
Accessory tragus
Polyotia
Preauricular appendage or tag
Supernumerary ear
Supernumerary lobule

Q17.1 Macrotia
DEF: Birth defect characterized by abnormal enlargement of the pinna of the ear.

Q17.2 Microtia

Q17.3 Other misshapen ear
Pointed ear

Q17.4 Misplaced ear
Low-set ears
> *EXCLUDES 1*   cervical auricle (Q18.2)

Q17.5 Prominent ear
Bat ear

Q17.8 Other specified congenital malformations of ear
Congenital absence of lobe of ear

Q17.9 Congenital malformation of ear, unspecified
Congenital anomaly of ear NOS

✓4ᵗʰ Q18 Other congenital malformations of face and neck
> *EXCLUDES 1*   cleft lip and cleft palate (Q35-Q37)
> conditions classified to Q67.0-Q67.4
> congenital malformations of skull and face bones (Q75.-)
> cyclopia (Q87.0)
> dentofacial anomalies [including malocclusion] (M26.-)
> malformation syndromes affecting facial appearance (Q87.0)
> persistent thyroglossal duct (Q89.2)

Q18.0 Sinus, fistula and cyst of branchial cleft
Branchial vestige

Q18.1 Preauricular sinus and cyst
Fistula of auricle, congenital
Cervicoaural fistula

Q18.2 Other branchial cleft malformations
Branchial cleft malformation NOS
Cervical auricle
Otocephaly

Q18.3 Webbing of neck
Pterygium colli
DEF: Congenital malformation characterized by a thick, triangular skinfold that stretches from the lateral side of the neck across the shoulder. It is associated with genetic conditions such as Turner's and Noonan's syndromes.

Q18.4 Macrostomia
DEF: Rare congenital craniofacial bilateral or unilateral anomaly of the mouth due to malformed maxillary and mandibular processes. It results in an abnormally large mouth extending toward the ear.

Q18.5 Microstomia

Q18.6 Macrocheilia
Hypertrophy of lip, congenital

Q18.7 Microcheilia

Q18.8 Other specified congenital malformations of face and neck
Medial cyst of face and neck
Medial fistula of face and neck
Medial sinus of face and neck

Q18.9 Congenital malformation of face and neck, unspecified
Congenital anomaly NOS of face and neck

Congenital malformations of the circulatory system (Q20-Q28)

✓4ᵗʰ Q20 Congenital malformations of cardiac chambers and connections
EXCLUDES 1 dextrocardia with situs inversus (Q89.3)
mirror-image atrial arrangement with situs inversus (Q89.3)

Q20.0 Common arterial trunk Rx COM
Persistent truncus arteriosus
EXCLUDES 1 aortic septal defect (Q21.4)

Q20.1 Double outlet right ventricle Rx COM
Taussig-Bing syndrome

Q20.2 Double outlet left ventricle Rx COM

Q20.3 Discordant ventriculoarterial connection Rx COM
Dextrotransposition of aorta
Transposition of great vessels (complete)

Q20.4 Double inlet ventricle Rx COM
Common ventricle
Cor triloculare biatriatum
Single ventricle

Q20.5 Discordant atrioventricular connection Rx COM
Corrected transposition
Levotransposition
Ventricular inversion

Q20.6 Isomerism of atrial appendages COM
Isomerism of atrial appendages with asplenia or polysplenia

Q20.8 Other congenital malformations of cardiac chambers and connections Rx COM
Cor binoculare

Q20.9 Congenital malformation of cardiac chambers and connections, unspecified COM

✓4ᵗʰ Q21 Congenital malformations of cardiac septa
EXCLUDES 1 acquired cardiac septal defect (I51.0)

Q21.0 Ventricular septal defect Rx COM
Roger's disease

Ventricular Septal Defect

✓5ᵗʰ Q21.1 Atrial septal defect
~~Coronary sinus defect~~
~~Patent or persistent foramen ovale~~
~~Patent or persistent ostium secundum defect (type II)~~
~~Patent or persistent sinus venosus defect~~
EXCLUDES 2 ▶ostium primum atrial septal defect (type I) (Q21.20)◀

Atrial Septal Defect

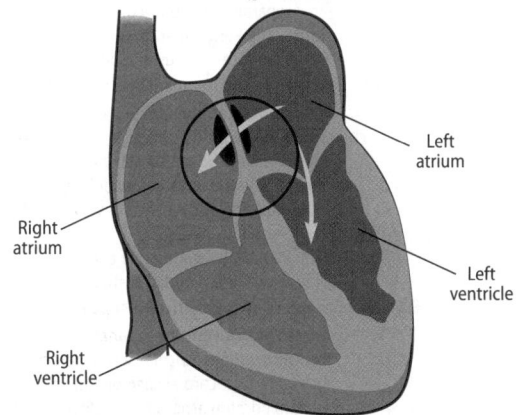

Left atrium

Right atrium

Left ventricle

Right ventricle

Q21.10 Atrial septal defect, unspecified

Q21.11 Secundum atrial septal defect
Fenestrated atrial septum
Patent or persistent ostium secundum defect (type II)

Q21.12 Patent foramen ovale
Persistent foramen ovale

Q21.13 Coronary sinus atrial septal defect
Coronary sinus defect
Unroofed coronary sinus

Q21.14 Superior sinus venosus atrial septal defect
Superior vena cava type atrial septal defect

Q21.15 Inferior sinus venosus atrial septal defect
Inferior vena cava type atrial septal defect

Q21.16 Sinus venosus atrial septal defect, unspecified
Sinus venosus defect, NOS

Q21.19 Other specified atrial septal defect
Common atrium
Other specified atrial septal abnormality

Chapter 17. Congenital Malformations, Deformations and Chromosomal Abnormalities

Q21.2–Q25.0

▲ ✔5ᵗʰ **Q21.2** **Atrioventricular septal defect**
► Atrioventricular canal defect ◄
~~Common atrioventricular canal~~
Endocardial cushion defect
Ostium primum atrial septal defect (type I)

Atrioventricular Septal Defect

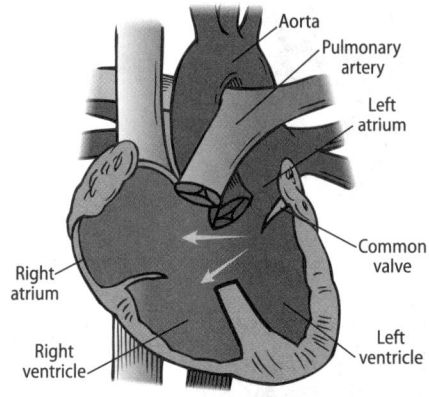

Aorta
Pulmonary artery
Left atrium
Common valve
Right atrium
Left ventricle
Right ventricle

- **Q21.20** **Atrioventricular septal defect, unspecified as to partial or complete**
Atrioventricular canal, NOS
Endocardial cushion defect NOS
Ostium primum atrial septal defect (type I) NOS

- **Q21.21** **Partial atrioventricular septal defect**
Incomplete atrioventricular canal
Incomplete atrioventricular septal defect
Incomplete endocardial cushion defect
Ostium primum atrial septal defect (type I) with separate atrioventricular valves
Partial atrioventricular canal
Partial endocardial cushion defect

- **Q21.22** **Transitional atrioventricular septal defect**
Intermediate atrioventricular canal
Intermediate atrioventricular septal defect
Intermediate endocardial cushion defect
Ostium primum atrial septal defect (type I) with separate atrioventricular valves and a small or restrictive inlet VSD
Transitional atrioventricular canal
Transitional endocardial cushion defect

- **Q21.23** **Complete atrioventricular septal defect**
Common atrioventricular canal
Common atrioventricular septal defect
Common endocardial cushion defect
Ostium primum atrial septal defect (type I) with common atrioventricular valve and a moderate or larger inlet VSD

Q21.3 **Tetralogy of Fallot**   Rx COM
Ventricular septal defect with pulmonary stenosis or atresia, dextroposition of aorta and hypertrophy of right ventricle.
AHA: 2014,3Q,16

Q21.4 **Aortopulmonary septal defect**   COM
Aortic septal defect
Aortopulmonary window

Q21.8 **Other congenital malformations of cardiac septa**   COM
Eisenmenger's defect
Pentalogy of Fallot
Code also, if applicable:
Eisenmenger's complex (I27.83)
Eisenmenger's syndrome (I27.83)

Q21.9 **Congenital malformation of cardiac septum, unspecified**   COM
Septal (heart) defect NOS

✔4ᵗʰ **Q22** **Congenital malformations of pulmonary and tricuspid valves**

Q22.0 **Pulmonary valve atresia**   Rx COM

Q22.1 **Congenital pulmonary valve stenosis**   COM

Q22.2 **Congenital pulmonary valve insufficiency**   COM
Congenital pulmonary valve regurgitation

Q22.3 **Other congenital malformations of pulmonary valve**   COM
Congenital malformation of pulmonary valve NOS
Supernumerary cusps of pulmonary valve

Q22.4 **Congenital tricuspid stenosis**   COM   *atresia* [handwritten]   *fontan procedure* [handwritten]
Congenital tricuspid atresia

Q22.5 **Ebstein's anomaly**   COM
DEF: Malformation of the tricuspid valve characterized by septal and posterior leaflets attaching to the wall of the right ventricle. Ebstein's anomaly causes the right ventricle to fuse with the atrium into a large right atrium and a small ventricle and leads to heart failure and abnormal cardiac rhythm.

Q22.6 **Hypoplastic right heart syndrome**   COM

Q22.8 **Other congenital malformations of tricuspid valve**   COM

Q22.9 **Congenital malformation of tricuspid valve, unspecified**   COM

✔4ᵗʰ **Q23** **Congenital malformations of aortic and mitral valves**

Q23.0 **Congenital stenosis of aortic valve**   COM
Congenital aortic atresia
Congenital aortic stenosis NOS
EXCLUDES 1   *congenital stenosis of aortic valve in hypoplastic left heart syndrome (Q23.4)*
congenital subaortic stenosis (Q24.4)
supravalvular aortic stenosis (congenital) (Q25.3)

Q23.1 **Congenital insufficiency of aortic valve**   COM
Bicuspid aortic valve
Congenital aortic insufficiency

Q23.2 **Congenital mitral stenosis**   COM
Congenital mitral atresia

Q23.3 **Congenital mitral insufficiency**   COM

Q23.4 **Hypoplastic left heart syndrome**   Rx COM

Q23.8 **Other congenital malformations of aortic and mitral valves**   COM

Q23.9 **Congenital malformation of aortic and mitral valves, unspecified**   COM

✔4ᵗʰ **Q24** **Other congenital malformations of heart**
EXCLUDES 1   *endocardial fibroelastosis (I42.4)*

Q24.0 **Dextrocardia**   COM
EXCLUDES 1   *dextrocardia with situs inversus (Q89.3)*
isomerism of atrial appendages (with asplenia or polysplenia) (Q20.6)
mirror-image atrial arrangement with situs inversus (Q89.3)
DEF: Congenital condition in which the heart is located on the right side of the chest rather than in its normal position on the left.

Q24.1 **Levocardia**   COM

Q24.2 **Cor triatriatum**   COM

Q24.3 **Pulmonary infundibular stenosis**   COM
Subvalvular pulmonic stenosis

Q24.4 **Congenital subaortic stenosis**   COM
DEF: Congenital heart defect characterized by stenosis of the left ventricular outflow tract due to a fibrous tissue ring or septal hypertrophy below the aortic valve.

Q24.5 **Malformation of coronary vessels**   Rx COM
Congenital coronary (artery) aneurysm

Q24.6 **Congenital heart block**   COM

Q24.8 **Other specified congenital malformations of heart**   COM
Congenital diverticulum of left ventricle
Congenital malformation of myocardium
Congenital malformation of pericardium
Malposition of heart
Uhl's disease

Q24.9 **Congenital malformation of heart, unspecified**   COM
Congenital anomaly of heart
Congenital disease of heart

✔4ᵗʰ **Q25** **Congenital malformations of great arteries**

Q25.0 **Patent ductus arteriosus**   Rx COM
Patent ductus Botallo
Persistent ductus arteriosus
DEF: Condition in which the normal channel between the pulmonary artery and the aorta fails to close at birth, causing arterial blood to recirculate in the lungs and inhibiting the blood supply to the aorta. *Synonym(s): PDA.*

Q25.1 Coarctation of aorta `COM`
Coarctation of aorta (preductal) (postductal)
Stenosis of aorta
AHA: 2016,4Q,56-57

√5ᵗʰ **Q25.2 Atresia of aorta**
AHA: 2016,4Q,56-57

Q25.21 Interruption of aortic arch `COM`
Atresia of aortic arch

Q25.29 Other atresia of aorta `COM`
Atresia of aorta

Q25.3 Supravalvular aortic stenosis `COM`
EXCLUDES 1   *congenital aortic stenosis NOS (Q23.0)*
congenital stenosis of aortic valve (Q23.0)

√5ᵗʰ **Q25.4 Other congenital malformations of aorta**
EXCLUDES 1   *hypoplasia of aorta in hypoplastic left heart syndrome (Q23.4)*
AHA: 2016,4Q,57

Q25.40 Congenital malformation of aorta unspecified `COM`

Q25.41 Absence and aplasia of aorta `COM`

Q25.42 Hypoplasia of aorta `COM`

Q25.43 Congenital aneurysm of aorta `COM`
Congenital aneurysm of aortic root
Congenital aneurysm of aortic sinus

Q25.44 Congenital dilation of aorta `COM`

Q25.45 Double aortic arch `COM`
Vascular ring of aorta

Aortic Arch Anomalies

Esophagus
Trachea
Aortic arch

Normal aortic arch

Double aortic arch   Right aortic arch

Q25.46 Tortuous aortic arch `COM`
Persistent convolutions of aortic arch

Q25.47 Right aortic arch `COM`
Persistent right aortic arch

Q25.48 Anomalous origin of subclavian artery `COM`

Q25.49 Other congenital malformations of aorta `COM`
Aortic arch
Bovine arch

Q25.5 Atresia of pulmonary artery `Rx` `COM`

Q25.6 Stenosis of pulmonary artery `COM`
Supravalvular pulmonary stenosis

√5ᵗʰ **Q25.7 Other congenital malformations of pulmonary artery**

Q25.71 Coarctation of pulmonary artery `Rx` `COM`

Q25.72 Congenital pulmonary arteriovenous malformation `COM`
Congenital pulmonary arteriovenous aneurysm

Q25.79 Other congenital malformations of pulmonary artery `COM`
Aberrant pulmonary artery
Agenesis of pulmonary artery
Congenital aneurysm of pulmonary artery
Congenital anomaly of pulmonary artery
Hypoplasia of pulmonary artery

Q25.8 Other congenital malformations of other great arteries `COM`

Q25.9 Congenital malformation of great arteries, unspecified `COM`

√4ᵗʰ **Q26 Congenital malformations of great veins**

Q26.0 Congenital stenosis of vena cava `Rx` `COM`
Congenital stenosis of vena cava (inferior)(superior)

Q26.1 Persistent left superior vena cava `Rx` `COM`

Q26.2 Total anomalous pulmonary venous connection `Rx` `COM`
Total anomalous pulmonary venous return [TAPVR], subdiaphragmatic
Total anomalous pulmonary venous return [TAPVR], supradiaphragmatic

Q26.3 Partial anomalous pulmonary venous connection `Rx` `COM`
Partial anomalous pulmonary venous return

Q26.4 Anomalous pulmonary venous connection, unspecified `Rx` `COM`

Q26.5 Anomalous portal venous connection `COM`

Q26.6 Portal vein-hepatic artery fistula `COM`

Q26.8 Other congenital malformations of great veins `Rx` `COM`
Absence of vena cava (inferior) (superior)
Azygos continuation of inferior vena cava
Persistent left posterior cardinal vein
Scimitar syndrome

Q26.9 Congenital malformation of great vein, unspecified `Rx` `COM`
Congenital anomaly of vena cava (inferior) (superior) NOS

√4ᵗʰ **Q27 Other congenital malformations of peripheral vascular system**
EXCLUDES 2   *anomalies of cerebral and precerebral vessels (Q28.0-Q28.3)*
anomalies of coronary vessels (Q24.5)
anomalies of pulmonary artery (Q25.5-Q25.7)
congenital retinal aneurysm (Q14.1)
hemangioma and lymphangioma (D18.-)

Q27.0 Congenital absence and hypoplasia of umbilical artery `COM`
Single umbilical artery

Q27.1 Congenital renal artery stenosis `COM`

Q27.2 Other congenital malformations of renal artery `COM`
Congenital malformation of renal artery NOS
Multiple renal arteries

√5ᵗʰ **Q27.3 Arteriovenous malformation (peripheral)**
Arteriovenous aneurysm
EXCLUDES 1   *acquired arteriovenous aneurysm (I77.0)*
EXCLUDES 2   *arteriovenous malformation of cerebral vessels (Q28.2)*
arteriovenous malformation of precerebral vessels (Q28.0)
DEF: Arteriovenous malformation: Connecting passage between an artery and a vein.

Q27.30 Arteriovenous malformation, site unspecified `COM`

Q27.31 Arteriovenous malformation of vessel of upper limb `COM`

Q27.32 Arteriovenous malformation of vessel of lower limb `COM`

Q27.33 Arteriovenous malformation of digestive system vessel `COM`
AHA: 2018,3Q,21

Q27.34 Arteriovenous malformation of renal vessel `COM`

Q27.39 Arteriovenous malformation, other site `COM`

Q27.4 Congenital phlebectasia `COM`

☑ Additional Character Required   √x7ᵗʰ Placeholder Alert   Manifestation   Unspecified Dx   🅠 QPP   `UPD` Unacceptable PDx

Chapter 17. Congenital Malformations, Deformations and Chromosomal Abnormalities

Q27.8 Other specified congenital malformations of peripheral vascular system `COM`
- Absence of peripheral vascular system
- Atresia of peripheral vascular system
- Congenital aneurysm (peripheral)
- Congenital stricture, artery
- Congenital varix
  - *EXCLUDES 1*   *arteriovenous malformation (Q27.3-)*

Q27.9 Congenital malformation of peripheral vascular system, unspecified `COM`
- Anomaly of artery or vein NOS

✓4ᵗʰ **Q28 Other congenital malformations of circulatory system**
- *EXCLUDES 1*   *congenital aneurysm NOS (Q27.8)*
  - *congenital coronary aneurysm (Q24.5)*
  - *ruptured cerebral arteriovenous malformation (I60.8)*
  - *ruptured malformation of precerebral vessels (I72.0)*
- *EXCLUDES 2*   *congenital peripheral aneurysm (Q27.8)*
  - *congenital pulmonary aneurysm (Q25.79)*
  - *congenital retinal aneurysm (Q14.1)*

Q28.0 Arteriovenous malformation of precerebral vessels `COM`
- Congenital arteriovenous precerebral aneurysm (nonruptured)

Q28.1 Other malformations of precerebral vessels `COM`
- Congenital malformation of precerebral vessels NOS
- Congenital precerebral aneurysm (nonruptured)

Q28.2 Arteriovenous malformation of cerebral vessels `COM`
- Arteriovenous malformation of brain NOS
- Congenital arteriovenous cerebral aneurysm (nonruptured)

Q28.3 Other malformations of cerebral vessels `COM`
- Congenital cerebral aneurysm (nonruptured)
- Congenital malformation of cerebral vessels NOS
- Developmental venous anomaly

Q28.8 Other specified congenital malformations of circulatory system `COM`
- Congenital aneurysm, specified site NEC
- Spinal vessel anomaly

Q28.9 Congenital malformation of circulatory system, unspecified `COM`

Congenital malformations of the respiratory system (Q30-Q34)

✓4ᵗʰ **Q30 Congenital malformations of nose**
- *EXCLUDES 1*   *congenital deviation of nasal septum (Q67.4)*

Q30.0 Choanal atresia
- Atresia of nares (anterior) (posterior)
- Congenital stenosis of nares (anterior) (posterior)

Q30.1 Agenesis and underdevelopment of nose
- Congenital absent of nose

Q30.2 Fissured, notched and cleft nose

Q30.3 Congenital perforated nasal septum

Q30.8 Other congenital malformations of nose
- Accessory nose
- Congenital anomaly of nasal sinus wall
- **AHA:** 2022,2Q,17

Q30.9 Congenital malformation of nose, unspecified

✓4ᵗʰ **Q31 Congenital malformations of larynx**
- *EXCLUDES 1*   *congenital laryngeal stridor NOS (P28.89)*

Q31.0 Web of larynx
- Glottic web of larynx
- Subglottic web of larynx
- Web of larynx NOS
- **DEF:** Congenital malformation of the larynx marked by thin, translucent, or thick fibrotic membrane-like structure between the vocal folds. It is characterized by shortness of breath and stridor.

Q31.1 Congenital subglottic stenosis

Q31.2 Laryngeal hypoplasia

Q31.3 Laryngocele

Q31.5 Congenital laryngomalacia

Q31.8 Other congenital malformations of larynx
- Absence of larynx
- Agenesis of larynx
- Atresia of larynx
- Congenital cleft thyroid cartilage
- Congenital fissure of epiglottis
- Congenital stenosis of larynx NEC
- Posterior cleft of cricoid cartilage

Q31.9 Congenital malformation of larynx, unspecified

✓4ᵗʰ **Q32 Congenital malformations of trachea and bronchus**
- *EXCLUDES 1*   *congenital bronchiectasis (Q33.4)*

Q32.0 Congenital tracheomalacia

Q32.1 Other congenital malformations of trachea
- Atresia of trachea
- Congenital anomaly of tracheal cartilage
- Congenital dilatation of trachea
- Congenital malformation of trachea
- Congenital stenosis of trachea
- Congenital tracheocele

Q32.2 Congenital bronchomalacia

Q32.3 Congenital stenosis of bronchus

Q32.4 Other congenital malformations of bronchus
- Absence of bronchus
- Agenesis of bronchus
- Atresia of bronchus
- Congenital diverticulum of bronchus
- Congenital malformation of bronchus NOS

✓4ᵗʰ **Q33 Congenital malformations of lung**

Q33.0 Congenital cystic lung
- Congenital cystic lung disease
- Congenital honeycomb lung
- Congenital polycystic lung disease
  - *EXCLUDES 1*   *cystic fibrosis (E84.0)*
    - *cystic lung disease, acquired or unspecified (J98.4)*

Q33.1 Accessory lobe of lung
- Azygos lobe (fissured), lung

Q33.2 Sequestration of lung

Q33.3 Agenesis of lung
- Congenital absence of lung (lobe)

Q33.4 Congenital bronchiectasis

Q33.5 Ectopic tissue in lung

Q33.6 Congenital hypoplasia and dysplasia of lung
- *EXCLUDES 1*   *pulmonary hypoplasia associated with short gestation (P28.0)*

Q33.8 Other congenital malformations of lung

Q33.9 Congenital malformation of lung, unspecified

✓4ᵗʰ **Q34 Other congenital malformations of respiratory system**
- *EXCLUDES 2*   *congenital central alveolar hypoventilation syndrome (G47.35)*

Q34.0 Anomaly of pleura

Q34.1 Congenital cyst of mediastinum

Q34.8 Other specified congenital malformations of respiratory system
- Atresia of nasopharynx

Q34.9 Congenital malformation of respiratory system, unspecified
- Congenital absence of respiratory system
- Congenital anomaly of respiratory system NOS

`HCC` CMS-HCC   `Rx` Rx HCC   `ESR` ESRD HCC   `COM` Commercial HCC   `N` Newborn: 0   `P` Pediatric: 0-17   `M` Maternity: 9-64   `A` Adult: 15-124

950   ICD-10-CM 2023

Cleft lip and cleft palate (Q35-Q37)

Use additional code to identify associated malformation of the nose (Q30.2)

EXCLUDES 2   Robin's syndrome (Q87.0)

✓4ᵗʰ Q35 Cleft palate

INCLUDES   fissure of palate
palatoschisis

EXCLUDES 1   cleft palate with cleft lip (Q37.-)

DEF: Congenital fissure or defect of the roof of the mouth opening to the nasal cavity due to failure of embryonic cells to fuse completely.

Cleft Palate

Cleft in soft palate   Cleft in hard and soft palate

Hard palate

Soft palate

Cleft   Cleft

Q35.1 **Cleft hard palate**   COM
Q35.3 **Cleft soft palate**   COM
Q35.5 **Cleft hard palate with cleft soft palate**   COM
Q35.7 **Cleft uvula**   COM
Q35.9 **Cleft palate, unspecified**   COM
      Cleft palate NOS

✓4ᵗʰ Q36 Cleft lip

INCLUDES   cheiloschisis
congenital fissure of lip
harelip
labium leporinum

EXCLUDES 1   cleft lip with cleft palate (Q37.-)

DEF: Congenital fissure or opening in the upper lip due to failure of embryonic cells to fuse completely.

Cleft Lip

Unilateral incomplete   Unilateral complete   Bilateral complete

Q36.0 **Cleft lip, bilateral**   COM
Q36.1 **Cleft lip, median**   COM
Q36.9 **Cleft lip, unilateral**   COM
      Cleft lip NOS

✓4ᵗʰ Q37 Cleft palate with cleft lip

INCLUDES   cheilopalatoschisis

Q37.0 **Cleft hard palate with bilateral cleft lip**   COM
Q37.1 **Cleft hard palate with unilateral cleft lip**   COM
      Cleft hard palate with cleft lip NOS
Q37.2 **Cleft soft palate with bilateral cleft lip**   COM
Q37.3 **Cleft soft palate with unilateral cleft lip**   COM
      Cleft soft palate with cleft lip NOS
Q37.4 **Cleft hard and soft palate with bilateral cleft lip**   COM
Q37.5 **Cleft hard and soft palate with unilateral cleft lip**   COM
      Cleft hard and soft palate with cleft lip NOS
Q37.8 **Unspecified cleft palate with bilateral cleft lip**   COM
Q37.9 **Unspecified cleft palate with unilateral cleft lip**   COM
      Cleft palate with cleft lip NOS

Other congenital malformations of the digestive system (Q38-Q45)

✓4ᵗʰ Q38 Other congenital malformations of tongue, mouth and pharynx

EXCLUDES 1   dentofacial anomalies (M26.-)
macrostomia (Q18.4)
microstomia (Q18.5)

Q38.0 **Congenital malformations of lips, not elsewhere classified**
      Congenital fistula of lip
      Congenital malformation of lip NOS
      Van der Woude's syndrome

      EXCLUDES 1   cleft lip (Q36.-)
               cleft lip with cleft palate (Q37.-)
               macrocheilia (Q18.6)
               microcheilia (Q18.7)

Q38.1 **Ankyloglossia**
      Tongue tie

Q38.2 **Macroglossia**
      Congenital hypertrophy of tongue

Q38.3 **Other congenital malformations of tongue**
      Aglossia
      Bifid tongue
      Congenital adhesion of tongue
      Congenital fissure of tongue
      Congenital malformation of tongue NOS
      Double tongue
      Hypoglossia
      Hypoplasia of tongue
      Microglossia

Q38.4 **Congenital malformations of salivary glands and ducts**
      Atresia of salivary glands and ducts
      Congenital absence of salivary glands and ducts
      Congenital accessory salivary glands and ducts
      Congenital fistula of salivary gland

Q38.5 **Congenital malformations of palate, not elsewhere classified**
      Congenital absence of uvula
      Congenital malformation of palate NOS
      Congenital high arched palate

      EXCLUDES 1   cleft palate (Q35.-)
               cleft palate with cleft lip (Q37.-)

Q38.6 **Other congenital malformations of mouth**
      Congenital malformation of mouth NOS

Q38.7 **Congenital pharyngeal pouch**
      Congenital diverticulum of pharynx

      EXCLUDES 1   pharyngeal pouch syndrome (D82.1)

Q38.8 **Other congenital malformations of pharynx**
      Congenital malformation of pharynx NOS
      Imperforate pharynx

✓4ᵗʰ Q39 Congenital malformations of esophagus

Q39.0 **Atresia of esophagus without fistula**   COM
      Atresia of esophagus NOS

Q39.1 **Atresia of esophagus with tracheo-esophageal fistula**   COM
      Atresia of esophagus with broncho-esophageal fistula

Q39.2 **Congenital tracheo-esophageal fistula without atresia**   COM
      Congenital tracheo-esophageal fistula NOS

Q39.3 **Congenital stenosis and stricture of esophagus**   COM
Q39.4 **Esophageal web**   COM
Q39.5 **Congenital dilatation of esophagus**
      Congenital cardiospasm
Q39.6 **Congenital diverticulum of esophagus**
      Congenital esophageal pouch
Q39.8 **Other congenital malformations of esophagus**
      Congenital absence of esophagus
      Congenital displacement of esophagus
      Congenital duplication of esophagus
Q39.9 **Congenital malformation of esophagus, unspecified**

✓4ᵗʰ Q40 Other congenital malformations of upper alimentary tract

Q40.0 **Congenital hypertrophic pyloric stenosis**   COM
      Congenital or infantile constriction
      Congenital or infantile hypertrophy
      Congenital or infantile spasm
      Congenital or infantile stenosis
      Congenital or infantile stricture

Chapter 17. Congenital Malformations, Deformations and Chromosomal Abnormalities

Q40.1   Congenital hiatus hernia
Congenital displacement of cardia through esophageal hiatus
EXCLUDES 1   *congenital diaphragmatic hernia (Q79.0)*

Q40.2   Other specified congenital malformations of stomach
Congenital displacement of stomach
Congenital diverticulum of stomach
Congenital hourglass stomach
Congenital duplication of stomach
Megalogastria
Microgastria

Q40.3   Congenital malformation of stomach, unspecified

Q40.8   Other specified congenital malformations of upper alimentary tract

Q40.9   Congenital malformation of upper alimentary tract, unspecified
Congenital anomaly of upper alimentary tract
Congenital deformity of upper alimentary tract

✓4th Q41   Congenital absence, atresia and stenosis of small intestine
INCLUDES   congenital obstruction, occlusion or stricture of small intestine or intestine NOS
EXCLUDES 1   *cystic fibrosis with intestinal manifestation (E84.11)*
meconium ileus NOS (without cystic fibrosis) (P76.0)

Q41.0   Congenital absence, atresia and stenosis of duodenum COM

Q41.1   Congenital absence, atresia and stenosis of jejunum COM
Apple peel syndrome
Imperforate jejunum

Q41.2   Congenital absence, atresia and stenosis of ileum COM

Q41.8   Congenital absence, atresia and stenosis of other specified parts of small intestine COM

Q41.9   Congenital absence, atresia and stenosis of small intestine, part unspecified COM
Congenital absence, atresia and stenosis of intestine NOS

✓4th Q42   Congenital absence, atresia and stenosis of large intestine
INCLUDES   congenital obstruction, occlusion and stricture of large intestine

Q42.0   Congenital absence, atresia and stenosis of rectum with fistula COM

Q42.1   Congenital absence, atresia and stenosis of rectum without fistula COM
Imperforate rectum

Q42.2   Congenital absence, atresia and stenosis of anus with fistula COM

Q42.3   Congenital absence, atresia and stenosis of anus without fistula COM
Imperforate anus

Q42.8   Congenital absence, atresia and stenosis of other parts of large intestine COM

Q42.9   Congenital absence, atresia and stenosis of large intestine, part unspecified COM

✓4th Q43   Other congenital malformations of intestine

Q43.0   Meckel's diverticulum (displaced) (hypertrophic)
Persistent omphalomesenteric duct
Persistent vitelline duct
DEF: Congenital, abnormal remnant of embryonic digestive system development that leaves a sacculation or outpouching from the wall of the small intestine near the terminal part of the ileum made of acid-secreting tissue as in the stomach.

Q43.1   Hirschsprung's disease COM
Aganglionosis
Congenital (aganglionic) megacolon
DEF: Congenital enlargement or dilation of the colon, with the absence of nerve cells in a segment of colon distally that causes the inability to defecate.

Q43.2   Other congenital functional disorders of colon COM
Congenital dilatation of colon

Q43.3   Congenital malformations of intestinal fixation COM
Congenital omental, anomalous adhesions [bands]
Congenital peritoneal adhesions [bands]
Incomplete rotation of cecum and colon
Insufficient rotation of cecum and colon
Jackson's membrane
Malrotation of colon
Rotation failure of cecum and colon
Universal mesentery

Q43.4   Duplication of intestine

Q43.5   Ectopic anus

Q43.6   Congenital fistula of rectum and anus
EXCLUDES 1   *congenital fistula of anus with absence, atresia and stenosis (Q42.2)*
congenital fistula of rectum with absence, atresia and stenosis (Q42.0)
congenital rectovaginal fistula (Q52.2)
congenital urethrorectal fistula (Q64.73)
pilonidal fistula or sinus (L05.-)

Q43.7   Persistent cloaca
Cloaca NOS

Q43.8   Other specified congenital malformations of intestine
Congenital blind loop syndrome
Congenital diverticulitis, colon
Congenital diverticulum, intestine
Dolichocolon
Megaloappendix
Megaloduodenum
Microcolon
Transposition of appendix
Transposition of colon
Transposition of intestine
AHA: 2013,2Q,31

Q43.9   Congenital malformation of intestine, unspecified

✓4th Q44   Congenital malformations of gallbladder, bile ducts and liver

Q44.0   Agenesis, aplasia and hypoplasia of gallbladder
Congenital absence of gallbladder

Q44.1   Other congenital malformations of gallbladder
Congenital malformation of gallbladder NOS
Intrahepatic gallbladder

Q44.2   Atresia of bile ducts

Q44.3   Congenital stenosis and stricture of bile ducts

Q44.4   Choledochal cyst

Q44.5   Other congenital malformations of bile ducts
Accessory hepatic duct
Biliary duct duplication
Congenital malformation of bile duct NOS
Cystic duct duplication

Q44.6   Cystic disease of liver
Fibrocystic disease of liver

Q44.7   Other congenital malformations of liver
Accessory liver
Alagille's syndrome
Congenital absence of liver
Congenital hepatomegaly
Congenital malformation of liver NOS

✓4th Q45   Other congenital malformations of digestive system
EXCLUDES 2   *congenital diaphragmatic hernia (Q79.0)*
congenital hiatus hernia (Q40.1)

Q45.0   Agenesis, aplasia and hypoplasia of pancreas
Congenital absence of pancreas

Q45.1   Annular pancreas

Q45.2   Congenital pancreatic cyst

Q45.3   Other congenital malformations of pancreas and pancreatic duct
Accessory pancreas
Congenital malformation of pancreas or pancreatic duct NOS
EXCLUDES 1   *congenital diabetes mellitus (E10.-)*
cystic fibrosis (E84.0-E84.9)
fibrocystic disease of pancreas (E84.-)
neonatal diabetes mellitus (P70.2)

Q45.8   Other specified congenital malformations of digestive system
Absence (complete) (partial) of alimentary tract NOS
Duplication of digestive system
Malposition, congenital of digestive system

Q45.9   Congenital malformation of digestive system, unspecified
Congenital anomaly of digestive system
Congenital deformity of digestive system

Congenital malformations of genital organs (Q50-Q56)

> EXCLUDES 1   androgen insensitivity syndrome (E34.5-)
> syndromes associated with anomalies in the number and form of chromosomes (Q90-Q99)

✓4th Q50 Congenital malformations of ovaries, fallopian tubes and broad ligaments

- **✓5th Q50.0 Congenital absence of ovary**
  > EXCLUDES 1   Turner's syndrome (Q96.-)
  - **Q50.01 Congenital absence of ovary, unilateral** ♀
  - **Q50.02 Congenital absence of ovary, bilateral** ♀
- **Q50.1 Developmental ovarian cyst** ♀
- **Q50.2 Congenital torsion of ovary** ♀
- **✓5th Q50.3 Other congenital malformations of ovary**
  - **Q50.31 Accessory ovary** ♀
  - **Q50.32 Ovarian streak** ♀
    46, XX with streak gonads
  - **Q50.39 Other congenital malformation of ovary** ♀
    Congenital malformation of ovary NOS
- **Q50.4 Embryonic cyst of fallopian tube** ♀
  Fimbrial cyst
- **Q50.5 Embryonic cyst of broad ligament** ♀
  Epoophoron cyst
  Parovarian cyst
- **Q50.6 Other congenital malformations of fallopian tube and broad ligament** ♀
  Absence of fallopian tube and broad ligament
  Accessory fallopian tube and broad ligament
  Atresia of fallopian tube and broad ligament
  Congenital malformation of fallopian tube or broad ligament NOS

✓4th Q51 Congenital malformations of uterus and cervix

- **Q51.0 Agenesis and aplasia of uterus** ♀
  Congenital absence of uterus
- **✓5th Q51.1 Doubling of uterus with doubling of cervix and vagina**
  - **Q51.10 Doubling of uterus with doubling of cervix and vagina without obstruction** ♀
    Doubling of uterus with doubling of cervix and vagina NOS
  - **Q51.11 Doubling of uterus with doubling of cervix and vagina with obstruction** ♀
- **✓5th Q51.2 Other doubling of uterus**
  Doubling of uterus NOS
  Septate uterus
  AHA: 2018,4Q,27
  - **Q51.21 Complete doubling of uterus** ♀
    Complete septate uterus
  - **Q51.22 Partial doubling of uterus** ♀
    Partial septate uterus
  - **Q51.28 Other and unspecified doubling of uterus** ♀
    Septate uterus NOS
- **Q51.3 Bicornate uterus** ♀
  Bicornate uterus, complete or partial
- **Q51.4 Unicornate uterus** ♀
  Unicornate uterus with or without a separate uterine horn
  Uterus with only one functioning horn
- **Q51.5 Agenesis and aplasia of cervix** ♀
  Congenital absence of cervix
- **Q51.6 Embryonic cyst of cervix** ♀
- **Q51.7 Congenital fistulae between uterus and digestive and urinary tracts** ♀
- **✓5th Q51.8 Other congenital malformations of uterus and cervix**
  - **✓6th Q51.81 Other congenital malformations of uterus**
    - **Q51.810 Arcuate uterus** ♀
      Arcuatus uterus
    - **Q51.811 Hypoplasia of uterus** ♀
    - **Q51.818 Other congenital malformations of uterus** ♀
      Müllerian anomaly of uterus NEC
  - **✓6th Q51.82 Other congenital malformations of cervix**
    - **Q51.820 Cervical duplication** ♀
    - **Q51.821 Hypoplasia of cervix** ♀
    - **Q51.828 Other congenital malformations of cervix** ♀

- **Q51.9 Congenital malformation of uterus and cervix, unspecified** ♀

✓4th Q52 Other congenital malformations of female genitalia

- **Q52.0 Congenital absence of vagina** ♀
  Vaginal agenesis, total or partial
- **✓5th Q52.1 Doubling of vagina**
  > EXCLUDES 1   doubling of vagina with doubling of uterus and cervix (Q51.1-)
  - **Q52.10 Doubling of vagina, unspecified** ♀
    Septate vagina NOS
  - **Q52.11 Transverse vaginal septum** ♀
  - **✓6th Q52.12 Longitudinal vaginal septum**
    AHA: 2016,4Q,58-59
    - **Q52.120 Longitudinal vaginal septum, nonobstructing** ♀
    - **Q52.121 Longitudinal vaginal septum, obstructing, right side** ♀
    - **Q52.122 Longitudinal vaginal septum, obstructing, left side** ♀
    - **Q52.123 Longitudinal vaginal septum, microperforate, right side** ♀
    - **Q52.124 Longitudinal vaginal septum, microperforate, left side** ♀
    - **Q52.129 Other and unspecified longitudinal vaginal septum** ♀
- **Q52.2 Congenital rectovaginal fistula** ♀
  > EXCLUDES 1   cloaca (Q43.7)
- **Q52.3 Imperforate hymen** ♀
  DEF: Obstructive anomaly of vagina, characterized by complete closure of the membranous fold around the external opening of the vagina, obstructing the vaginal introitus.
- **Q52.4 Other congenital malformations of vagina** ♀
  Canal of Nuck cyst, congenital
  Congenital malformation of vagina NOS
  Embryonic vaginal cyst
  Gartner's duct cyst
  AHA: 2022,2Q,15
- **Q52.5 Fusion of labia** ♀
- **Q52.6 Congenital malformation of clitoris** ♀
- **✓5th Q52.7 Other and unspecified congenital malformations of vulva**
  - **Q52.70 Unspecified congenital malformations of vulva** ♀
    Congenital malformation of vulva NOS
  - **Q52.71 Congenital absence of vulva** ♀
  - **Q52.79 Other congenital malformations of vulva** ♀
    Congenital cyst of vulva
- **Q52.8 Other specified congenital malformations of female genitalia** ♀
- **Q52.9 Congenital malformation of female genitalia, unspecified** ♀

✓4th Q53 Undescended and ectopic testicle

- **✓5th Q53.0 Ectopic testis**
  - **Q53.00 Ectopic testis, unspecified** ♂
  - **Q53.01 Ectopic testis, unilateral** ♂
  - **Q53.02 Ectopic testes, bilateral** ♂
- **✓5th Q53.1 Undescended testicle, unilateral**
  AHA: 2017,4Q,22-23
  - **Q53.10 Unspecified undescended testicle, unilateral** ♂
  - **✓6th Q53.11 Abdominal testis, unilateral**
    - **Q53.111 Unilateral intraabdominal testis** ♂
    - **Q53.112 Unilateral inguinal testis** ♂
  - **Q53.12 Ectopic perineal testis, unilateral** ♂
  - **Q53.13 Unilateral high scrotal testis** ♂
- **✓5th Q53.2 Undescended testicle, bilateral**
  AHA: 2017,4Q,22-23
  - **Q53.20 Undescended testicle, unspecified, bilateral** ♂
  - **✓6th Q53.21 Abdominal testis, bilateral**
    - **Q53.211 Bilateral intraabdominal testes** ♂
    - **Q53.212 Bilateral inguinal testes** ♂
  - **Q53.22 Ectopic perineal testis, bilateral** ♂
  - **Q53.23 Bilateral high scrotal testes** ♂
- **Q53.9 Undescended testicle, unspecified** ♂
  Cryptorchism NOS

☑ Additional Character Required   ✓x7th Placeholder Alert   Manifestation   Unspecified Dx   Q QPP   UPD Unacceptable PDx

Chapter 17. Congenital Malformations, Deformations and Chromosomal Abnormalities

Q54–Q61.9

☑4ᵗʰ **Q54 Hypospadias**

> EXCLUDES 1   epispadias (Q64.0)
>
> **DEF:** Abnormal opening of the urethra on the ventral (underside) surface of the penis.

Hypospadias

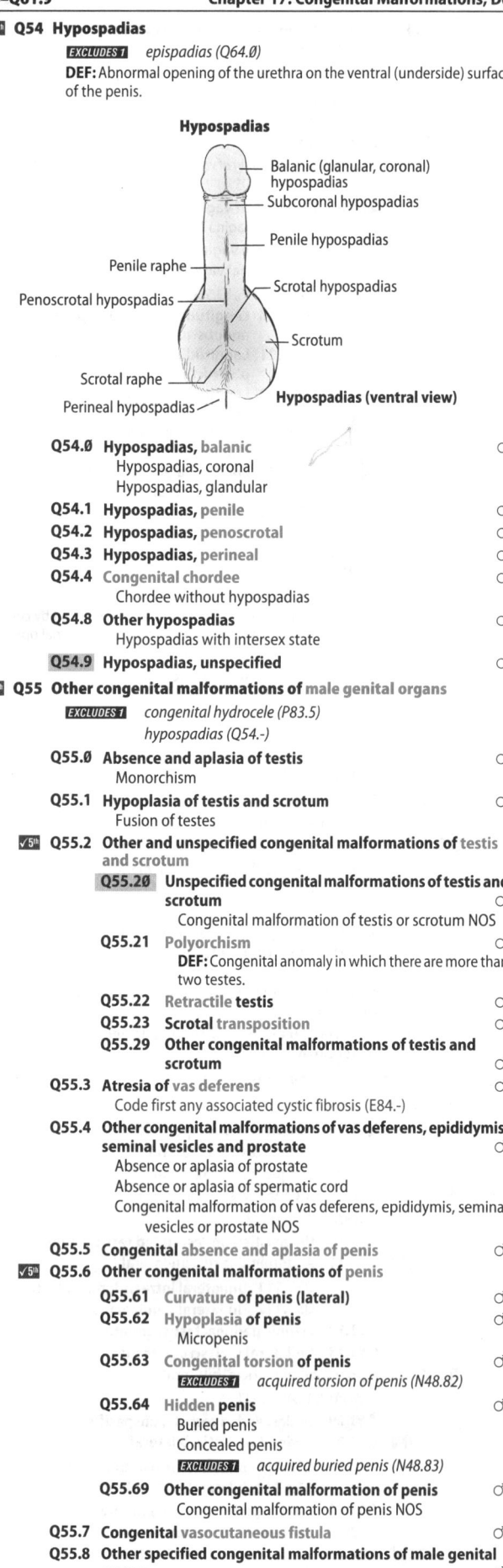

- Balanic (glanular, coronal) hypospadias
- Subcoronal hypospadias
- Penile hypospadias
- Penile raphe
- Scrotal hypospadias
- Penoscrotal hypospadias
- Scrotum
- Scrotal raphe
- Perineal hypospadias

Hypospadias (ventral view)

Q54.0   **Hypospadias,** balanic   ♂
     Hypospadias, coronal
     Hypospadias, glandular

Q54.1   **Hypospadias,** penile   ♂

Q54.2   **Hypospadias,** penoscrotal   ♂

Q54.3   **Hypospadias,** perineal   ♂

Q54.4   **Congenital chordee**   ♂
     Chordee without hypospadias

Q54.8   **Other hypospadias**   ♂
     Hypospadias with intersex state

Q54.9   **Hypospadias, unspecified**   ♂

☑4ᵗʰ **Q55 Other congenital malformations of** male genital organs

> EXCLUDES 1   congenital hydrocele (P83.5)
>
>   hypospadias (Q54.-)

Q55.0   **Absence and aplasia of testis**   ♂
     Monorchism

Q55.1   **Hypoplasia of testis and scrotum**   ♂
     Fusion of testes

☑5ᵗʰ Q55.2   **Other and unspecified congenital malformations of** testis and scrotum

     Q55.20   **Unspecified congenital malformations of testis and scrotum**   ♂
         Congenital malformation of testis or scrotum NOS

     Q55.21   **Polyorchism**   ♂
         DEF: Congenital anomaly in which there are more than two testes.

     Q55.22   **Retractile testis**   ♂

     Q55.23   **Scrotal** transposition   ♂

     Q55.29   **Other congenital malformations of testis and scrotum**   ♂

Q55.3   **Atresia of** vas deferens   ♂
     Code first any associated cystic fibrosis (E84.-)

Q55.4   **Other congenital malformations of vas deferens, epididymis, seminal vesicles and prostate**   ♂
     Absence or aplasia of prostate
     Absence or aplasia of spermatic cord
     Congenital malformation of vas deferens, epididymis, seminal vesicles or prostate NOS

Q55.5   **Congenital** absence and aplasia of penis   ♂

☑5ᵗʰ Q55.6   **Other congenital malformations of** penis

     Q55.61   **Curvature of penis (lateral)**   ♂

     Q55.62   **Hypoplasia of penis**   ♂
         Micropenis

     Q55.63   **Congenital torsion of penis**   ♂
         EXCLUDES 1   acquired torsion of penis (N48.82)

     Q55.64   **Hidden penis**   ♂
         Buried penis
         Concealed penis
         EXCLUDES 1   acquired buried penis (N48.83)

     Q55.69   **Other congenital malformation of penis**   ♂
         Congenital malformation of penis NOS

Q55.7   **Congenital** vasocutaneous fistula   ♂

Q55.8   **Other specified congenital malformations of male genital organs**   ♂

Q55.9   **Congenital malformation of male genital organ, unspecified**   ♂
     Congenital anomaly of male genital organ
     Congenital deformity of male genital organ

☑4ᵗʰ **Q56 Indeterminate sex and pseudohermaphroditism**

> EXCLUDES 1   46, XX true hermaphrodite (Q99.1)
>
>   androgen insensitivity syndrome (E34.5-)
>
>   chimera 46, XX/46, XY true hermaphrodite (Q99.0)
>
>   female pseudohermaphroditism with adrenocortical disorder (E25.)
>
>   pseudohermaphroditism with specified chromosomal anomaly (Q96-Q99)
>
>   pure gonadal dysgenesis (Q99.1)
>
> **DEF:** Indeterminate sex: External genitalia that is nondescript, lacking the physical appearance specific to either sex.
>
> **DEF:** Pseudohermaphroditism: Presence of gonads of one sex and external genitalia of another sex.

Q56.0   **Hermaphroditism,** not elsewhere classified
     Ovotestis

Q56.1   **Male pseudohermaphroditism, not elsewhere classified**   ♂
     46, XY with streak gonads
     Male pseudohermaphroditism NOS

Q56.2   **Female pseudohermaphroditism, not elsewhere classified**   ♀
     Female pseudohermaphroditism NOS

Q56.3   **Pseudohermaphroditism, unspecified**

Q56.4   **Indeterminate sex, unspecified**
     Ambiguous genitalia

Congenital malformations of the urinary system (Q60-Q64)

☑4ᵗʰ **Q60 Renal agenesis and other** reduction defects of kidney

> INCLUDES   congenital absence of kidney
>
>   congenital atrophy of kidney
>
>   infantile atrophy of kidney

Q60.0   **Renal** agenesis, unilateral

Q60.1   **Renal** agenesis, bilateral

Q60.2   **Renal** agenesis, unspecified

Q60.3   **Renal** hypoplasia, unilateral

Q60.4   **Renal** hypoplasia, bilateral

Q60.5   **Renal** hypoplasia, unspecified

Q60.6   **Potter's syndrome**

☑4ᵗʰ **Q61 Cystic kidney disease**

> EXCLUDES 1   acquired cyst of kidney (N28.1)
>
>   Potter's syndrome (Q60.6)

☑5ᵗʰ Q61.0   **Congenital renal** cyst

     Q61.00   **Congenital renal cyst, unspecified**
         Cyst of kidney NOS (congenital)

     Q61.01   **Congenital single renal cyst**

     Q61.02   **Congenital multiple renal cysts**

☑5ᵗʰ Q61.1   **Polycystic kidney, infantile type**
     Polycystic kidney, autosomal recessive

     Q61.11   **Cystic dilatation of collecting ducts**   COM

     Q61.19   **Other polycystic kidney, infantile type**   COM

Q61.2   **Polycystic kidney, adult type**
     Polycystic kidney, autosomal dominant

Q61.3   **Polycystic kidney, unspecified**
     AHA: 2016,3Q,22

Q61.4   **Renal** dysplasia
     Multicystic dysplastic kidney
     Multicystic kidney (development)
     Multicystic kidney disease
     Multicystic renal dysplasia
     EXCLUDES 1   polycystic kidney disease (Q61.11-Q61.3)

Q61.5   **Medullary cystic** kidney
     Nephronophthisis
     Sponge kidney NOS
     DEF: Sponge kidney: Dilated collecting tubules that are usually asymptomatic. Calcinosis in tubules may cause renal insufficiency.

Q61.8   **Other cystic kidney diseases**
     Fibrocystic kidney
     Fibrocystic renal degeneration or disease

Q61.9   **Cystic kidney disease, unspecified**
     Meckel-Gruber syndrome

✓4th **Q62** **Congenital obstructive defects of** renal pelvis **and congenital malformations of** ureter

   Q62.0 **Congenital** hydronephrosis

✓5th **Q62.1** **Congenital** occlusion of ureter

     Atresia and stenosis of ureter

     Q62.10 **Congenital occlusion of ureter, unspecified**

     Q62.11 **Congenital occlusion of** ureteropelvic junction

     Q62.12 **Congenital occlusion of** ureterovesical orifice

   Q62.2 **Congenital** megaureter

     Congenital dilatation of ureter

✓5th **Q62.3** **Other obstructive defects of renal pelvis and ureter**

     Q62.31 **Congenital** ureterocele, orthotopic

     Q62.32 **Cecoureterocele**

       Ectopic ureterocele

     Q62.39 **Other obstructive defects of renal pelvis and ureter**

       Ureteropelvic junction obstruction NOS

   Q62.4 **Agenesis of** ureter

     Congenital absence ureter

   Q62.5 **Duplication of** ureter

     Accessory ureter

     Double ureter

✓5th **Q62.6** **Malposition of** ureter

     Q62.60 **Malposition of ureter, unspecified**

     Q62.61 **Deviation of** ureter

     Q62.62 **Displacement of** ureter

     Q62.63 **Anomalous implantation of** ureter

       Ectopia of ureter

       Ectopic ureter

     Q62.69 **Other malposition of ureter**

   Q62.7 **Congenital** vesico-uretero-renal reflux

   Q62.8 **Other congenital malformations of ureter**

     Anomaly of ureter NOS

✓4th **Q63** **Other congenital malformations of** kidney

   EXCLUDES 1   *congenital nephrotic syndrome (N04.-)*

   Q63.0 **Accessory** kidney

   Q63.1 **Lobulated, fused and horseshoe** kidney

   Q63.2 **Ectopic** kidney

     Congenital displaced kidney

     Malrotation of kidney

   Q63.3 **Hyperplastic and giant** kidney

     Compensatory hypertrophy of kidney

   Q63.8 **Other specified congenital malformations of kidney**

     Congenital renal calculi

   Q63.9 **Congenital malformation of kidney, unspecified**

✓4th **Q64** **Other congenital malformations of** urinary system

   Q64.0 **Epispadias**

     EXCLUDES 1   *hypospadias (Q54.-)*

Epispadias

Normal external urethral orifice —

— Glans penis

Foreskin (retracted) —

Epispadias —

Epispadias (dorsal view)

✓5th **Q64.1** **Exstrophy of** urinary bladder

     Q64.10 **Exstrophy of urinary bladder, unspecified** `COM`

       Ectopia vesicae

     Q64.11 **Supravesical fissure of urinary bladder** `COM`

     Q64.12 **Cloacal exstrophy of urinary bladder** `COM`

     Q64.19 **Other exstrophy of urinary bladder** `COM`

       Extroversion of bladder

   Q64.2 **Congenital** posterior urethral valves

✓5th **Q64.3** **Other atresia and stenosis of** urethra and bladder neck

     Q64.31 **Congenital** bladder neck obstruction

       Congenital obstruction of vesicourethral orifice

     Q64.32 **Congenital** stricture of urethra

     Q64.33 **Congenital** stricture of urinary meatus

     Q64.39 **Other atresia and stenosis of urethra and bladder neck**

       Atresia and stenosis of urethra and bladder neck NOS

   Q64.4 **Malformation of** urachus

     Cyst of urachus

     Patent urachus

     Prolapse of urachus

   Q64.5 **Congenital** absence of bladder and urethra

   Q64.6 **Congenital** diverticulum of bladder

✓5th **Q64.7** **Other and unspecified congenital malformations of bladder and urethra**

     EXCLUDES 1   *congenital prolapse of bladder (mucosa) (Q79.4)*

     Q64.70 **Unspecified congenital malformation of bladder and urethra**

       Malformation of bladder or urethra NOS

     Q64.71 **Congenital** prolapse of urethra

     Q64.72 **Congenital** prolapse of urinary meatus

     Q64.73 **Congenital** urethrorectal fistula

     Q64.74 **Double urethra**

     Q64.75 **Double urinary meatus**

     Q64.79 **Other congenital malformations of bladder and urethra**

   Q64.8 **Other specified congenital malformations of urinary system**

   Q64.9 **Congenital malformation of urinary system, unspecified**

     Congenital anomaly NOS of urinary system

     Congenital deformity NOS of urinary system

Congenital malformations and deformations of the musculoskeletal system (Q65-Q79)

✓4th **Q65** **Congenital deformities of** hip

   EXCLUDES 1   *clicking hip (R29.4)*

✓5th **Q65.0** **Congenital** dislocation of hip, unilateral

     Q65.00 **Congenital dislocation of unspecified hip, unilateral** `COM`

     Q65.01 **Congenital dislocation of** right **hip, unilateral** `COM`

     Q65.02 **Congenital dislocation of left hip, unilateral** `COM`

   Q65.1 **Congenital** dislocation of hip, bilateral `COM`

   Q65.2 **Congenital dislocation of hip, unspecified** `COM`

✓5th **Q65.3** **Congenital** partial dislocation of hip, unilateral

     Q65.30 **Congenital partial dislocation of unspecified hip, unilateral** `COM`

     Q65.31 **Congenital partial dislocation of** right **hip, unilateral** `COM`

     Q65.32 **Congenital partial dislocation of** left **hip, unilateral** `COM`

   Q65.4 **Congenital** partial dislocation of hip, bilateral `COM`

   Q65.5 **Congenital partial dislocation of hip, unspecified** `COM`

   Q65.6 **Congenital** unstable hip `COM`

     Congenital dislocatable hip

✓5th **Q65.8** **Other congenital deformities of hip**

     Q65.81 **Congenital** coxa valga `COM`

     Q65.82 **Congenital** coxa vara `COM`

     Q65.89 **Other specified congenital deformities of hip** `COM`

       Anteversion of femoral neck

       Congenital acetabular dysplasia

   Q65.9 **Congenital deformity of hip, unspecified** `COM`

✓4th **Q66** **Congenital deformities of** feet

   EXCLUDES 1   *reduction defects of feet (Q72.-)*

          valgus deformities (acquired) (M21.0-)

          varus deformities (acquired) (M21.1-)

   AHA: 2019,4Q,13

✓5th **Q66.0** **Congenital** talipes equinovarus

     Q66.00 **Congenital talipes equinovarus, unspecified foot**

     Q66.01 **Congenital talipes equinovarus,** right **foot**

     Q66.02 **Congenital talipes equinovarus,** left **foot**

✓5th **Q66.1** **Congenital** talipes calcaneovarus

     Q66.10 **Congenital talipes calcaneovarus, unspecified foot**

     Q66.11 **Congenital talipes calcaneovarus,** right **foot**

     Q66.12 **Congenital talipes calcaneovarus,** left **foot**

✓ Additional Character Required   ✓x7th Placeholder Alert   Manifestation   Unspecified Dx   Q QPP   UPD Unacceptable PDx

✓5ᵗʰ **Q66.2 Congenital metatarsus (primus) varus**
   AHA: 2016,4Q,59
   ✓6ᵗʰ **Q66.21 Congenital metatarsus primus varus**
      Q66.211 Congenital metatarsus primus varus, right foot
      Q66.212 Congenital metatarsus primus varus, left foot
      Q66.219 Congenital metatarsus primus varus, unspecified foot
   ✓6ᵗʰ **Q66.22 Congenital metatarsus adductus**
      Congenital metatarsus varus
      Q66.221 Congenital metatarsus adductus, right foot
      Q66.222 Congenital metatarsus adductus, left foot
      Q66.229 Congenital metatarsus adductus, unspecified foot

✓5ᵗʰ **Q66.3 Other congenital varus deformities of feet**
   Hallux varus, congenital
      Q66.30 Other congenital varus deformities of feet, unspecified foot
      Q66.31 Other congenital varus deformities of feet, right foot
      Q66.32 Other congenital varus deformities of feet, left foot

✓5ᵗʰ **Q66.4 Congenital talipes calcaneovalgus**
      Q66.40 Congenital talipes calcaneovalgus, unspecified foot
      Q66.41 Congenital talipes calcaneovalgus, right foot
      Q66.42 Congenital talipes calcaneovalgus, left foot

✓5ᵗʰ **Q66.5 Congenital pes planus**
   Congenital flat foot
   Congenital rigid flat foot
   Congenital spastic (everted) flat foot
   EXCLUDES 1 pes planus, acquired (M21.4)
      Q66.50 Congenital pes planus, unspecified foot
      Q66.51 Congenital pes planus, right foot
      Q66.52 Congenital pes planus, left foot

Q66.6 Other congenital valgus deformities of feet
   Congenital metatarsus valgus

✓5ᵗʰ **Q66.7 Congenital pes cavus**
      Q66.70 Congenital pes cavus, unspecified foot
      Q66.71 Congenital pes cavus, right foot
      Q66.72 Congenital pes cavus, left foot

✓5ᵗʰ **Q66.8 Other congenital deformities of feet**
      Q66.80 Congenital vertical talus deformity, unspecified foot
      Q66.81 Congenital vertical talus deformity, right foot
      Q66.82 Congenital vertical talus deformity, left foot
      Q66.89 Other specified congenital deformities of feet
         Congenital asymmetric talipes
         Congenital clubfoot NOS
         Congenital talipes NOS
         Congenital tarsal coalition
         Hammer toe, congenital
         DEF: Clubfoot: Congenital anomaly of the foot with the heel elevated and rotated outward and the toes pointing inward.

✓5ᵗʰ **Q66.9 Congenital deformity of feet, unspecified**
      Q66.90 Congenital deformity of feet, unspecified, unspecified foot
      Q66.91 Congenital deformity of feet, unspecified, right foot
      Q66.92 Congenital deformity of feet, unspecified, left foot

✓4ᵗʰ **Q67 Congenital musculoskeletal deformities of head, face, spine and chest**
   EXCLUDES 1 congenital malformation syndromes classified to Q87.-
               Potter's syndrome (Q60.6)
   Q67.0 Congenital facial asymmetry
   Q67.1 Congenital compression facies
   Q67.2 Dolichocephaly
   Q67.3 Plagiocephaly

Q67.4 Other congenital deformities of skull, face and jaw
   Congenital depressions in skull
   Congenital hemifacial atrophy or hypertrophy
   Deviation of nasal septum, congenital
   Squashed or bent nose, congenital
   EXCLUDES 1 dentofacial anomalies [including malocclusion] (M26.-)
               syphilitic saddle nose (A50.5)
   DEF: Deviated septum: Condition in which the nasal septum, a thin wall composed of cartilage and bone that separates the two nostrils, is crooked or displaced from the midline.

Q67.5 Congenital deformity of spine
   Congenital postural scoliosis
   Congenital scoliosis NOS
   EXCLUDES 1 infantile idiopathic scoliosis (M41.0)
               scoliosis due to congenital bony malformation (Q76.3)
   AHA: 2014,4Q,26

Q67.6 Pectus excavatum
   Congenital funnel chest

Q67.7 Pectus carinatum
   Congenital pigeon chest

Q67.8 Other congenital deformities of chest
   Congenital deformity of chest wall NOS

✓4ᵗʰ **Q68 Other congenital musculoskeletal deformities**
   EXCLUDES 1 reduction defects of limb(s) (Q71-Q73)
   EXCLUDES 2 congenital myotonic chondrodystrophy (G71.13)

   Q68.0 Congenital deformity of sternocleidomastoid muscle
      Congenital contracture of sternocleidomastoid (muscle)
      Congenital (sternomastoid) torticollis
      Sternomastoid tumor (congenital)

   Q68.1 Congenital deformity of finger(s) and hand
      Congenital clubfinger
      Spade-like hand (congenital)

   Q68.2 Congenital deformity of knee
      Congenital dislocation of knee
      Congenital genu recurvatum

   Q68.3 Congenital bowing of femur
      EXCLUDES 1 anteversion of femur (neck) (Q65.89)

   Q68.4 Congenital bowing of tibia and fibula

   Q68.5 Congenital bowing of long bones of leg, unspecified

   Q68.6 Discoid meniscus

   Q68.8 Other specified congenital musculoskeletal deformities
      Congenital deformity of clavicle
      Congenital deformity of elbow
      Congenital deformity of forearm
      Congenital deformity of scapula
      Congenital deformity of wrist
      Congenital dislocation of elbow
      Congenital dislocation of shoulder
      Congenital dislocation of wrist

✓4ᵗʰ **Q69 Polydactyly**
   Q69.0 Accessory finger(s)
   Q69.1 Accessory thumb(s)
   Q69.2 Accessory toe(s)
      Accessory hallux
   Q69.9 Polydactyly, unspecified
      Supernumerary digit(s) NOS

✓4ᵗʰ **Q70 Syndactyly**
   ✓5ᵗʰ **Q70.0 Fused fingers**
      Complex syndactyly of fingers with synostosis
         Q70.00 Fused fingers, unspecified hand
         Q70.01 Fused fingers, right hand
         Q70.02 Fused fingers, left hand
         Q70.03 Fused fingers, bilateral
   ✓5ᵗʰ **Q70.1 Webbed fingers**
      Simple syndactyly of fingers without synostosis
         Q70.10 Webbed fingers, unspecified hand
         Q70.11 Webbed fingers, right hand
         Q70.12 Webbed fingers, left hand
         Q70.13 Webbed fingers, bilateral
   ✓5ᵗʰ **Q70.2 Fused toes**
      Complex syndactyly of toes with synostosis
         Q70.20 Fused toes, unspecified foot
         Q70.21 Fused toes, right foot

Q70.22   **Fused toes,** left **foot**

Q70.23   **Fused toes,** bilateral

√5ᵗʰ **Q70.3**   Webbed toes

     Simple syndactyly of toes without synostosis

     Q70.30   **Webbed toes, unspecified foot**

     Q70.31   **Webbed toes,** right **foot**

     Q70.32   **Webbed toes,** left **foot**

     Q70.33   **Webbed toes,** bilateral

Q70.4   Polysyndactyly, unspecified

     EXCLUDES 1   specified syndactyly of hand and feet - code to specified conditions (Q70.0-Q70.3-)

Q70.9   Syndactyly, unspecified

     Symphalangy NOS

√4ᵗʰ **Q71**   **Reduction defects of** upper limb

√5ᵗʰ **Q71.0**   Congenital complete absence **of upper limb**

     Q71.00   **Congenital complete absence of unspecified upper limb**

     Q71.01   **Congenital complete absence of** right **upper limb**

     Q71.02   **Congenital complete absence of** left **upper limb**

     Q71.03   **Congenital complete absence of upper limb,** bilateral

√5ᵗʰ **Q71.1**   Congenital absence of upper arm and forearm with hand present

     Q71.10   **Congenital absence of unspecified upper arm and forearm with hand present**

     Q71.11   **Congenital absence of** right **upper arm and forearm with hand present**

     Q71.12   **Congenital absence of** left **upper arm and forearm with hand present**

     Q71.13   **Congenital absence of upper arm and forearm with hand present,** bilateral

√5ᵗʰ **Q71.2**   Congenital absence of both forearm and hand

     Q71.20   **Congenital absence of both forearm and hand, unspecified upper limb**

     Q71.21   **Congenital absence of both forearm and hand,** right **upper limb**

     Q71.22   **Congenital absence of both forearm and hand,** left **upper limb**

     Q71.23   **Congenital absence of both forearm and hand,** bilateral

√5ᵗʰ **Q71.3**   Congenital absence of hand and finger

     Q71.30   **Congenital absence of unspecified hand and finger**

     Q71.31   **Congenital absence of** right **hand and finger**

     Q71.32   **Congenital absence of** left **hand and finger**

     Q71.33   **Congenital absence of hand and finger,** bilateral

√5ᵗʰ **Q71.4**   Longitudinal reduction defect of radius

     Clubhand (congenital)

     Radial clubhand

     Q71.40   **Longitudinal reduction defect of unspecified radius**

     Q71.41   **Longitudinal reduction defect of** right **radius**

     Q71.42   **Longitudinal reduction defect of** left **radius**

     Q71.43   **Longitudinal reduction defect of radius,** bilateral

√5ᵗʰ **Q71.5**   Longitudinal reduction defect of ulna

     Q71.50   **Longitudinal reduction defect of unspecified ulna**

     Q71.51   **Longitudinal reduction defect of** right **ulna**

     Q71.52   **Longitudinal reduction defect of** left **ulna**

     Q71.53   **Longitudinal reduction defect of ulna,** bilateral

√5ᵗʰ **Q71.6**   Lobster-claw hand

     Q71.60   **Lobster-claw hand, unspecified hand**

     Q71.61   **Lobster-claw** right **hand**

     Q71.62   **Lobster-claw** left **hand**

     Q71.63   **Lobster-claw hand,** bilateral

√5ᵗʰ **Q71.8**   Other reduction defects of upper limb

     √6ᵗʰ **Q71.81**   **Congenital** shortening **of upper limb**

         Q71.811   **Congenital shortening of** right **upper limb**

         Q71.812   **Congenital shortening of** left **upper limb**

         Q71.813   **Congenital shortening of upper limb, bilateral**

         Q71.819   **Congenital shortening of unspecified upper limb**

     √6ᵗʰ **Q71.89**   **Other reduction defects of upper limb**

         Q71.891   **Other reduction defects of** right **upper limb**

         Q71.892   **Other reduction defects of** left **upper limb**

         Q71.893   **Other reduction defects of upper limb, bilateral**

     Q71.899   **Other reduction defects of unspecified upper limb**

√5ᵗʰ **Q71.9**   Unspecified reduction defect of upper limb

     Q71.90   **Unspecified reduction defect of unspecified upper limb**

     Q71.91   **Unspecified reduction defect of** right **upper limb**

     Q71.92   **Unspecified reduction defect of** left **upper limb**

     Q71.93   **Unspecified reduction defect of upper limb, bilateral**

√4ᵗʰ **Q72**   **Reduction defects of** lower limb

√5ᵗʰ **Q72.0**   Congenital complete absence **of lower limb**

     Q72.00   **Congenital complete absence of unspecified lower limb**

     Q72.01   **Congenital complete absence of** right **lower limb**

     Q72.02   **Congenital complete absence of** left **lower limb**

     Q72.03   **Congenital complete absence of lower limb, bilateral**

√5ᵗʰ **Q72.1**   Congenital absence of thigh and lower leg with foot present

     Q72.10   **Congenital absence of unspecified thigh and lower leg with foot present**

     Q72.11   **Congenital absence of** right **thigh and lower leg with foot present**

     Q72.12   **Congenital absence of** left **thigh and lower leg with foot present**

     Q72.13   **Congenital absence of thigh and lower leg with foot present,** bilateral

√5ᵗʰ **Q72.2**   Congenital absence of both lower leg and foot

     Q72.20   **Congenital absence of both lower leg and foot, unspecified lower limb**

     Q72.21   **Congenital absence of both lower leg and foot,** right **lower limb**

     Q72.22   **Congenital absence of both lower leg and foot,** left **lower limb**

     Q72.23   **Congenital absence of both lower leg and foot, bilateral**

√5ᵗʰ **Q72.3**   Congenital absence of foot and toe(s)

     Q72.30   **Congenital absence of unspecified foot and toe(s)**

     Q72.31   **Congenital absence of** right **foot and toe(s)**

     Q72.32   **Congenital absence of** left **foot and toe(s)**

     Q72.33   **Congenital absence of foot and toe(s),** bilateral

√5ᵗʰ **Q72.4**   Longitudinal reduction defect of femur

     Proximal femoral focal deficiency

     Q72.40   **Longitudinal reduction defect of unspecified femur**

     Q72.41   **Longitudinal reduction defect of** right **femur**

     Q72.42   **Longitudinal reduction defect of** left **femur**

     Q72.43   **Longitudinal reduction defect of femur,** bilateral

√5ᵗʰ **Q72.5**   Longitudinal reduction defect of tibia

     Q72.50   **Longitudinal reduction defect of unspecified tibia**

     Q72.51   **Longitudinal reduction defect of** right **tibia**

     Q72.52   **Longitudinal reduction defect of** left **tibia**

     Q72.53   **Longitudinal reduction defect of tibia,** bilateral

√5ᵗʰ **Q72.6**   Longitudinal reduction defect of fibula

     Q72.60   **Longitudinal reduction defect of unspecified fibula**

     Q72.61   **Longitudinal reduction defect of** right **fibula**

     Q72.62   **Longitudinal reduction defect of** left **fibula**

     Q72.63   **Longitudinal reduction defect of fibula,** bilateral

√5ᵗʰ **Q72.7**   Split foot

     Q72.70   **Split foot, unspecified lower limb**

     Q72.71   **Split foot,** right **lower limb**

     Q72.72   **Split foot,** left **lower limb**

     Q72.73   **Split foot,** bilateral

√5ᵗʰ **Q72.8**   Other reduction defects of lower limb

     √6ᵗʰ **Q72.81**   **Congenital** shortening **of lower limb**

         Q72.811   **Congenital shortening of** right **lower limb**

         Q72.812   **Congenital shortening of** left **lower limb**

         Q72.813   **Congenital shortening of lower limb, bilateral**

         Q72.819   **Congenital shortening of unspecified lower limb**

     √6ᵗʰ **Q72.89**   **Other reduction defects of lower limb**

         Q72.891   **Other reduction defects of** right **lower limb**

         Q72.892   **Other reduction defects of** left **lower limb**

         Q72.893   **Other reduction defects of lower limb, bilateral**

✔️ Additional Character Required   √x7ᵗʰ Placeholder Alert   Manifestation   Unspecified Dx   Q QPP   UPD Unacceptable PDx

Q72.899 Other reduction defects of unspecified lower limb

✓5ᵗʰ **Q72.9 Unspecified reduction defect of lower limb**

Q72.90 Unspecified reduction defect of unspecified lower limb

Q72.91 Unspecified reduction defect of right lower limb

Q72.92 Unspecified reduction defect of left lower limb

Q72.93 Unspecified reduction defect of lower limb, bilateral

✓4ᵗʰ **Q73 Reduction defects of unspecified limb**

Q73.0 Congenital absence of unspecified limb(s)
Amelia NOS

Q73.1 Phocomelia, unspecified limb(s)
Phocomelia NOS

Q73.8 Other reduction defects of unspecified limb(s)
Longitudinal reduction deformity of unspecified limb(s)
Ectromelia of limb NOS
Hemimelia of limb NOS
Reduction defect of limb NOS

✓4ᵗʰ **Q74 Other congenital malformations of limb(s)**
EXCLUDES 1   *polydactyly (Q69.-)*
    reduction defect of limb (Q71-Q73)
    syndactyly (Q70.-)

Q74.0 Other congenital malformations of upper limb(s), including shoulder girdle
Accessory carpal bones
Cleidocranial dysostosis
Congenital pseudarthrosis of clavicle
Macrodactylia (fingers)
Madelung's deformity
Radioulnar synostosis
Sprengel's deformity
Triphalangeal thumb

Q74.1 Congenital malformation of knee
Congenital absence of patella
Congenital dislocation of patella
Congenital genu valgum
Congenital genu varum
Rudimentary patella
EXCLUDES 1   *congenital dislocation of knee (Q68.2)*
    congenital genu recurvatum (Q68.2)
    nail patella syndrome (Q87.2)

Q74.2 Other congenital malformations of lower limb(s), including pelvic girdle
Congenital fusion of sacroiliac joint
Congenital malformation of ankle joint
Congenital malformation of sacroiliac joint
EXCLUDES 1   *anteversion of femur (neck) (Q65.89)*

Q74.3 Arthrogryposis multiplex congenita

Q74.8 Other specified congenital malformations of limb(s)

Q74.9 Unspecified congenital malformation of limb(s)
Congenital anomaly of limb(s) NOS

✓4ᵗʰ **Q75 Other congenital malformations of skull and face bones**
EXCLUDES 1   *congenital malformation of face NOS (Q18.-)*
    congenital malformation syndromes classified to Q87.-
    dentofacial anomalies [including malocclusion] (M26.-)
    musculoskeletal deformities of head and face (Q67.0-Q67.4)
    skull defects associated with congenital anomalies of brain such as:
        anencephaly (Q00.0)
        encephalocele (Q01.-)
        hydrocephalus (Q03.-)
        microcephaly (Q02)

Q75.0 Craniosynostosis
Acrocephaly
Imperfect fusion of skull
Oxycephaly
Trigonocephaly
DEF: Congenital condition in which one or more of the cranial sutures fuse prematurely, creating a deformed or aberrant head shape.

Q75.1 Craniofacial dysostosis
Crouzon's disease

Q75.2 Hypertelorism

Q75.3 Macrocephaly

Q75.4 Mandibulofacial dysostosis
Franceschetti syndrome
Treacher Collins syndrome

Q75.5 Oculomandibular dysostosis

Q75.8 Other specified congenital malformations of skull and face bones
Absence of skull bone, congenital
Congenital deformity of forehead
Platybasia

Q75.9 Congenital malformation of skull and face bones, unspecified
Congenital anomaly of face bones NOS
Congenital anomaly of skull NOS

✓4ᵗʰ **Q76 Congenital malformations of spine and bony thorax**
EXCLUDES 1   *congenital musculoskeletal deformities of spine and chest (Q67.5-Q67.8)*

Q76.0 Spina bifida occulta
EXCLUDES 1   *meningocele (spinal) (Q05.-)*
    spina bifida (aperta) (cystica) (Q05.-)

Q76.1 Klippel-Feil syndrome
Cervical fusion syndrome

Q76.2 Congenital spondylolisthesis
Congenital spondylolysis
EXCLUDES 1   *spondylolisthesis (acquired) (M43.1-)*
    spondylolysis (acquired) (M43.0-)

Q76.3 Congenital scoliosis due to congenital bony malformation
Hemivertebra fusion or failure of segmentation with scoliosis

✓5ᵗʰ **Q76.4 Other congenital malformations of spine, not associated with scoliosis**

✓6ᵗʰ **Q76.41 Congenital kyphosis**

Q76.411 Congenital kyphosis, occipito-atlanto-axial region

Q76.412 Congenital kyphosis, cervical region

Q76.413 Congenital kyphosis, cervicothoracic region

Q76.414 Congenital kyphosis, thoracic region

Q76.415 Congenital kyphosis, thoracolumbar region

Q76.419 Congenital kyphosis, unspecified region

✓6ᵗʰ **Q76.42 Congenital lordosis**

Q76.425 Congenital lordosis, thoracolumbar region

Q76.426 Congenital lordosis, lumbar region

Q76.427 Congenital lordosis, lumbosacral region

Q76.428 Congenital lordosis, sacral and sacrococcygeal region

Q76.429 Congenital lordosis, unspecified region

Q76.49 Other congenital malformations of spine, not associated with scoliosis
Congenital absence of vertebra NOS
Congenital fusion of spine NOS
Congenital malformation of lumbosacral (joint) (region) NOS
Congenital malformation of spine NOS
Hemivertebra NOS
Malformation of spine NOS
Platyspondylisis NOS
Supernumerary vertebra NOS

Q76.5 Cervical rib
Supernumerary rib in cervical region

Q76.6 Other congenital malformations of ribs
Accessory rib
Congenital absence of rib
Congenital fusion of ribs
Congenital malformation of ribs NOS
EXCLUDES 1   *short rib syndrome (Q77.2)*

Q76.7 Congenital malformation of sternum
Congenital absence of sternum
Sternum bifidum

Q76.8 Other congenital malformations of bony thorax

Q76.9 Congenital malformation of bony thorax, unspecified

✓4ᵗʰ **Q77 Osteochondrodysplasia with defects of growth of tubular bones and spine**
EXCLUDES 1   *mucopolysaccharidosis (E76.0-E76.3)*
EXCLUDES 2   *congenital myotonic chondrodystrophy (G71.13)*

Q77.0 Achondrogenesis   COM
Hypochondrogenesis

Q77.1 Thanatophoric short stature   COM

Q77.2 Short rib syndrome `COM`
Asphyxiating thoracic dysplasia [Jeune]

Q77.3 Chondrodysplasia punctata `COM`
EXCLUDES 1   *Rhizomelic chondrodysplasia punctata (E71.43)*

Q77.4 Achondroplasia `COM`
Hypochondroplasia
Osteosclerosis congenita

Q77.5 Diastrophic dysplasia `COM`

Q77.6 Chondroectodermal dysplasia `COM`
Ellis-van Creveld syndrome

Q77.7 Spondyloepiphyseal dysplasia `COM`

Q77.8 Other osteochondrodysplasia with defects of growth of tubular bones and spine `COM`

Q77.9 Osteochondrodysplasia with defects of growth of tubular bones and spine, unspecified `COM`

☑4ᵗʰ **Q78 Other osteochondrodysplasias**
EXCLUDES 2   *congenital myotonic chondrodystrophy (G71.13)*

Q78.0 Osteogenesis imperfecta `COM`
Fragilitas ossium
Osteopsathyrosis

Q78.1 Polyostotic fibrous dysplasia `COM`
Albright(-McCune)(-Sternberg) syndrome

Q78.2 Osteopetrosis `COM`
Albers-Schönberg syndrome
Osteosclerosis NOS
DEF: Rare congenital condition in which the bones are excessively dense, resulting from a discrepancy in the formation and breakdown of bone.

Q78.3 Progressive diaphyseal dysplasia `COM`
Camurati-Engelmann syndrome

Q78.4 Enchondromatosis `COM`
Maffucci's syndrome
Ollier's disease

Q78.5 Metaphyseal dysplasia `COM`
Pyle's syndrome

Q78.6 Multiple congenital exostoses `COM`
Diaphyseal aclasis

Q78.8 Other specified osteochondrodysplasias `COM`
Osteopoikilosis

Q78.9 Osteochondrodysplasia, unspecified `COM`
Chondrodystrophy NOS
Osteodystrophy NOS

☑4ᵗʰ **Q79 Congenital malformations of musculoskeletal system, not elsewhere classified**
EXCLUDES 2   *congenital (sternomastoid) torticollis (Q68.0)*

Q79.0 Congenital diaphragmatic hernia `COM`
EXCLUDES 1   *congenital hiatus hernia (Q40.1)*

Q79.1 Other congenital malformations of diaphragm `COM`
Absence of diaphragm
Congenital malformation of diaphragm NOS
Eventration of diaphragm

Q79.2 Exomphalos `COM`
Omphalocele
EXCLUDES 1   *umbilical hernia (K42.-)*

Q79.3 Gastroschisis `COM`

Gastroschisis

Rectus abdominus m.
Herniated small bowel (gastroschisis)
Umbilicus
skin
distal
proximal
Defect

Q79.4 Prune belly syndrome `COM`
Congenital prolapse of bladder mucosa
Eagle-Barrett syndrome

☑5ᵗʰ **Q79.5 Other congenital malformations of abdominal wall**
EXCLUDES 1   *umbilical hernia (K42.-)*

Q79.51 Congenital hernia of bladder `COM`
Q79.59 Other congenital malformations of abdominal wall

☑5ᵗʰ **Q79.6 Ehlers-Danlos syndromes**
AHA: 2019,4Q,13-14
DEF: Connective tissue disorder that causes hyperextended skin and joints and results in fragile blood vessels with bleeding, poor wound healing, and subcutaneous pseudotumors.

Q79.60 Ehlers-Danlos syndrome, unspecified `Rx` `COM`
Q79.61 Classical Ehlers-Danlos syndrome `Rx` `COM`
Classical EDS (cEDS)
Q79.62 Hypermobile Ehlers-Danlos syndrome `Rx` `COM`
Hypermobile EDS (hEDS)
Q79.63 Vascular Ehlers-Danlos syndrome `Rx` `COM`
Vascular EDS (vEDS)
Q79.69 Other Ehlers-Danlos syndromes `Rx` `COM`

Q79.8 Other congenital malformations of musculoskeletal system
Absence of muscle
Absence of tendon
Accessory muscle
Amyotrophia congenita
Congenital constricting bands
Congenital shortening of tendon
Poland syndrome

Q79.9 Congenital malformation of musculoskeletal system, unspecified
Congenital anomaly of musculoskeletal system NOS
Congenital deformity of musculoskeletal system NOS

Other congenital malformations (Q80-Q89)

☑4ᵗʰ **Q80 Congenital ichthyosis**
EXCLUDES 1   *Refsum's disease (G60.1)*
DEF: Excessive production of skin cells resulting in red, dry, scaly skin.

Q80.0 Ichthyosis vulgaris
Q80.1 X-linked ichthyosis
Q80.2 Lamellar ichthyosis
Collodion baby
Q80.3 Congenital bullous ichthyosiform erythroderma
Q80.4 Harlequin fetus
Q80.8 Other congenital ichthyosis
Q80.9 Congenital ichthyosis, unspecified

☑4ᵗʰ **Q81 Epidermolysis bullosa**
Q81.0 Epidermolysis bullosa simplex `COM`
EXCLUDES 1   *Cockayne's syndrome (Q87.19)*
Q81.1 Epidermolysis bullosa letalis `COM`
Herlitz' syndrome
Q81.2 Epidermolysis bullosa dystrophica `COM`
Q81.8 Other epidermolysis bullosa `COM`
Q81.9 Epidermolysis bullosa, unspecified `COM`

☑4ᵗʰ **Q82 Other congenital malformations of skin**
EXCLUDES 1   *acrodermatitis enteropathica (E83.2)*
            congenital erythropoietic porphyria (E80.0)
            pilonidal cyst or sinus (L05.-)
            Sturge-Weber (-Dimitri) syndrome ▶(Q85.89)◀

Q82.0 Hereditary lymphedema
Q82.1 Xeroderma pigmentosum
Q82.2 Congenital cutaneous mastocytosis
Congenital diffuse cutaneous mastocytosis
Congenital maculopapular cutaneous mastocytosis
Congenital urticaria pigmentosa
EXCLUDES 1   *cutaneous mastocytosis NOS (D47.01)*
            diffuse cutaneous mastocytosis (with onset after newborn period) (D47.01)
            malignant mastocytosis (C96.2-)
            systemic mastocytosis (D47.02)
            urticaria pigmentosa (non-congenital) (with onset after newborn period) (D47.01)
AHA: 2017,4Q,5

Q82.3 Incontinentia pigmenti
Q82.4 Ectodermal dysplasia (anhidrotic)
EXCLUDES 1   *Ellis-van Creveld syndrome (Q77.6)*

Q82.5 Congenital non-neoplastic nevus
Birthmark NOS
Flammeus Nevus
Portwine Nevus
Sanguineous Nevus
Strawberry Nevus
Vascular Nevus NOS
Verrucous Nevus
EXCLUDES 2   *araneus nevus (I78.1)*
Café au lait spots (L81.3)
lentigo (L81.4)
melanocytic nevus (D22.-)
nevus NOS (D22.-)
pigmented nevus (D22.-)
spider nevus (I78.1)
stellar nevus (I78.1)

Q82.6 Congenital sacral dimple
Parasacral dimple
EXCLUDES 2   *pilonidal cyst with abscess (L05.01)*
pilonidal cyst without abscess (L05.91)
AHA: 2016,4Q,60

Q82.8 Other specified congenital malformations of skin
Abnormal palmar creases
Accessory skin tags
Benign familial pemphigus [Hailey-Hailey]
Congenital poikiloderma
Cutis laxa (hyperelastica)
Dermatoglyphic anomalies
Inherited keratosis palmaris et plantaris
Keratosis follicularis [Darier-White]
EXCLUDES 1   *Ehlers-Danlos syndromes (Q79.6-)*
AHA: 2021,3Q,10; 2016,1Q,17

Q82.9 Congenital malformation of skin, unspecified

✓4ᵗʰ **Q83 Congenital malformations of breast**
EXCLUDES 2   *absence of pectoral muscle (Q79.8)*
hypoplasia of breast (N64.82)
micromastia (N64.82)

Q83.0 Congenital absence of breast with absent nipple

Q83.1 Accessory breast
Supernumerary breast

Q83.2 Absent nipple

Q83.3 Accessory nipple
Supernumerary nipple

Q83.8 Other congenital malformations of breast

Q83.9 Congenital malformation of breast, unspecified

✓4ᵗʰ **Q84 Other congenital malformations of integument**

Q84.0 Congenital alopecia
Congenital atrichosis

Q84.1 Congenital morphological disturbances of hair, not elsewhere classified
Beaded hair
Monilethrix
Pili annulati
EXCLUDES 1   *Menkes' kinky hair syndrome (E83.0)*

Q84.2 Other congenital malformations of hair
Congenital hypertrichosis
Congenital malformation of hair NOS
Persistent lanugo

Q84.3 Anonychia
EXCLUDES 1   *nail patella syndrome (Q87.2)*

Q84.4 Congenital leukonychia

Q84.5 Enlarged and hypertrophic nails
Congenital onychauxis
Pachyonychia

Q84.6 Other congenital malformations of nails
Congenital clubnail
Congenital koilonychia
Congenital malformation of nail NOS

Q84.8 Other specified congenital malformations of integument
Aplasia cutis congenita

Q84.9 Congenital malformation of integument, unspecified
Congenital anomaly of integument NOS
Congenital deformity of integument NOS

✓4ᵗʰ **Q85 Phakomatoses, not elsewhere classified**
EXCLUDES 1   *ataxia telangiectasia [Louis-Bar] (G11.3)*
familial dysautonomia [Riley-Day] (G90.1)

✓6ᵗʰ **Q85.0 Neurofibromatosis (nonmalignant)**

Q85.00 Neurofibromatosis, unspecified   HCC ESR COM

Q85.01 Neurofibromatosis, type 1   HCC ESR COM
Von Recklinghausen disease

Q85.02 Neurofibromatosis, type 2   HCC ESR COM
Acoustic neurofibromatosis
DEF: Inherited condition with cutaneous lesions, benign tumors of peripheral nerves, and bilateral 8th nerve masses.

Q85.03 Schwannomatosis   HCC ESR COM
DEF: Genetic mutation (SMARCB1/INI1) causing multiple benign tumors along the nerve pathways, except on the 8th cranial (vestibular) nerve.

Q85.09 Other neurofibromatosis   HCC ESR COM

Q85.1 Tuberous sclerosis   HCC Rx ESR COM
Bourneville's disease
Epiloia

▲ ✓5ᵗʰ **Q85.8 Other phakomatoses, not elsewhere classified**
~~Peutz-Jeghers Syndrome~~
~~Sturge-Weber(-Dimitri) syndrome~~
~~von Hippel-Lindau syndrome~~
EXCLUDES 1   *Meckel-Gruber syndrome (Q61.9)*
AHA: 2021,3Q,12

● **Q85.81 PTEN tumor syndrome**
PHTS
PTEN hamartoma tumor syndrome
PTEN related Cowden syndrome
Code also, if applicable, genetic susceptibility to malignant neoplasm (Z15.0-)

● **Q85.82 Other Cowden syndrome**

● **Q85.83 Von Hippel-Lindau syndrome**
Code also manifestations

● **Q85.89 Other phakomatoses, not elsewhere classified**
Peutz-Jeghers syndrome
Sturge-Weber(-Dimitri) syndrome

Q85.9 Phakomatosis, unspecified   HCC Rx ESR COM
Hamartosis NOS

✓4ᵗʰ **Q86 Congenital malformation syndromes due to known exogenous causes, not elsewhere classified**
EXCLUDES 2   *iodine-deficiency-related hypothyroidism (E00-E02)*
nonteratogenic effects of substances transmitted via placenta or breast milk (P04.-)

Q86.0 Fetal alcohol syndrome (dysmorphic)   COM

Q86.1 Fetal hydantoin syndrome   COM
Meadow's syndrome

Q86.2 Dysmorphism due to warfarin   COM

Q86.8 Other congenital malformation syndromes due to known exogenous causes   COM

✓4ᵗʰ **Q87 Other specified congenital malformation syndromes affecting multiple systems**
Use additional code(s) to identify all associated manifestations

Q87.0 Congenital malformation syndromes predominantly affecting facial appearance
Acrocephalopolysyndactyly
Acrocephalosyndactyly [Apert]
Cryptophthalmos syndrome
Cyclopia
Goldenhar syndrome
Moebius syndrome
Oro-facial-digital syndrome
Robin syndrome
Whistling face

✓5ᵗʰ **Q87.1 Congenital malformation syndromes predominantly associated with short stature**
EXCLUDES 1   *Ellis-van Creveld syndrome (Q77.6)*
Smith-Lemli-Opitz syndrome (E78.72)
AHA: 2019,4Q,14-15

Q87.11 Prader-Willi syndrome   Rx COM

Q87.19 Other congenital malformation syndromes predominantly associated with short stature `COM`
> Aarskog syndrome
> Cockayne syndrome
> De Lange syndrome
> Dubowitz syndrome
> Noonan syndrome
> Robinow-Silverman-Smith syndrome
> Russell-Silver syndrome
> Seckel syndrome

Q87.2 Congenital malformation syndromes predominantly involving limbs `COM`
> Holt-Oram syndrome
> Klippel-Trenaunay-Weber syndrome
> Nail patella syndrome
> Rubinstein-Taybi syndrome
> Sirenomelia syndrome
> Thrombocytopenia with absent radius [TAR] syndrome
> VATER syndrome

Q87.3 Congenital malformation syndromes involving early overgrowth `COM`
> Beckwith-Wiedemann syndrome
> Sotos syndrome
> Weaver syndrome

✓5ᵗʰ **Q87.4 Marfan's syndrome**
> **DEF:** Disorder that affects the connective tissue of multiple systems, including disproportionally long or abnormal bone structure and eye and cardiovascular complications.

  Q87.40 Marfan's syndrome, unspecified `Rx` `COM`

✓6ᵗʰ **Q87.41 Marfan's syndrome with cardiovascular manifestations**
  Q87.410 Marfan's syndrome with aortic dilation `Rx` `COM`
  Q87.418 Marfan's syndrome with other cardiovascular manifestations `Rx` `COM`

  Q87.42 Marfan's syndrome with ocular manifestations `Rx` `COM`
  Q87.43 Marfan's syndrome with skeletal manifestation `Rx` `COM`

Q87.5 Other congenital malformation syndromes with other skeletal changes `COM`

✓5ᵗʰ **Q87.8 Other specified congenital malformation syndromes, not elsewhere classified**
  EXCLUDES 1 Zellweger syndrome (E71.510)

  Q87.81 Alport syndrome `COM`
  > Use additional code to identify stage of chronic kidney disease (N18.1-N18.6)

  Q87.82 Arterial tortuosity syndrome `Rx` `COM`
  > **AHA:** 2016,4Q,60-61

  Q87.89 Other specified congenital malformation syndromes, not elsewhere classified `COM`
  > Laurence-Moon (-Bardet)-Biedl syndrome

✓4ᵗʰ **Q89 Other congenital malformations, not elsewhere classified**

✓5ᵗʰ **Q89.0 Congenital absence and malformations of spleen**
  EXCLUDES 1 isomerism of atrial appendages (with asplenia or polysplenia) (Q20.6)

  Q89.01 Asplenia (congenital)
  Q89.09 Congenital malformations of spleen
  > Congenital splenomegaly

Q89.1 Congenital malformations of adrenal gland
  EXCLUDES 1 adrenogenital disorders (E25.-)
  >   congenital adrenal hyperplasia (E25.0)

Q89.2 Congenital malformations of other endocrine glands
> Congenital malformation of parathyroid or thyroid gland
> Persistent thyroglossal duct
> Thyroglossal cyst
  EXCLUDES 1 congenital goiter (E03.0)
  >   congenital hypothyroidism (E03.1)

Q89.3 Situs inversus `COM`
> Dextrocardia with situs inversus
> Mirror-image atrial arrangement with situs inversus
> Situs inversus or transversus abdominalis
> Situs inversus or transversus thoracis
> Transposition of abdominal viscera
> Transposition of thoracic viscera
  EXCLUDES 1 dextrocardia NOS (Q24.0)
> **DEF:** Congenital anomaly in which the internal thoracic and abdominal organs are transposed laterally and found on the opposite side from the normal position.

Q89.4 Conjoined twins `COM`
> Craniopagus
> Dicephaly
> Pygopagus
> Thoracopagus

Q89.7 Multiple congenital malformations, not elsewhere classified
> Multiple congenital anomalies NOS
> Multiple congenital deformities NOS
  EXCLUDES 1 congenital malformation syndromes affecting multiple systems (Q87.-)

Q89.8 Other specified congenital malformations `COM`
> Use additional code(s) to identify all associated manifestations
> **AHA:** 2021,3Q,12

Q89.9 Congenital malformation, unspecified
> Congenital anomaly NOS
> Congenital deformity NOS

Chromosomal abnormalities, not elsewhere classified (Q90-Q99)

EXCLUDES 2 mitochondrial metabolic disorders (E88.4-)

✓4ᵗʰ **Q90 Down syndrome**
> Use additional code(s) to identify any associated physical conditions and degree of intellectual disabilities (F70-F79)

  Q90.0 Trisomy 21, nonmosaicism (meiotic nondisjunction) `COM`
  Q90.1 Trisomy 21, mosaicism (mitotic nondisjunction) `COM`
  Q90.2 Trisomy 21, translocation `COM`
  Q90.9 Down syndrome, unspecified `COM`
  > Trisomy 21 NOS

✓4ᵗʰ **Q91 Trisomy 18 and Trisomy 13**
  Q91.0 Trisomy 18, nonmosaicism (meiotic nondisjunction) `Rx` `COM`
  Q91.1 Trisomy 18, mosaicism (mitotic nondisjunction) `Rx` `COM`
  Q91.2 Trisomy 18, translocation `Rx` `COM`
  Q91.3 Trisomy 18, unspecified `Rx` `COM`
  Q91.4 Trisomy 13, nonmosaicism (meiotic nondisjunction) `Rx` `COM`
  Q91.5 Trisomy 13, mosaicism (mitotic nondisjunction) `Rx` `COM`
  Q91.6 Trisomy 13, translocation `Rx` `COM`
  Q91.7 Trisomy 13, unspecified `Rx` `COM`

✓4ᵗʰ **Q92 Other trisomies and partial trisomies of the autosomes, not elsewhere classified**
  INCLUDES unbalanced translocations and insertions
  EXCLUDES 1 trisomies of chromosomes 13, 18, 21 (Q90-Q91)

  Q92.0 Whole chromosome trisomy, nonmosaicism (meiotic nondisjunction) `Rx` `COM`
  Q92.1 Whole chromosome trisomy, mosaicism (mitotic nondisjunction) `Rx` `COM`
  Q92.2 Partial trisomy `Rx` `COM`
  > Less than whole arm duplicated
  > Whole arm or more duplicated
  EXCLUDES 1 partial trisomy due to unbalanced translocation (Q92.5)

  Q92.5 Duplications with other complex rearrangements `Rx` `COM`
  > Partial trisomy due to unbalanced translocations
  > Code also any associated deletions due to unbalanced translocations, inversions and insertions (Q93.7)

✓5ᵗʰ **Q92.6 Marker chromosomes**
  > Trisomies due to dicentrics
  > Trisomies due to extra rings
  > Trisomies due to isochromosomes
  > Individual with marker heterochromatin

  Q92.61 Marker chromosomes in normal individual `Rx` `COM`

Q92.62 **Marker chromosomes in** abnormal **individual** `Rx` `COM`

Q92.7 **Triploidy and polyploidy** `Rx` `COM`

Q92.8 **Other specified trisomies and partial trisomies of autosomes** `Rx` `COM`
    Duplications identified by fluorescence in situ hybridization (FISH)
    Duplications identified by in situ hybridization (ISH)
    Duplications seen only at prometaphase

Q92.9 **Trisomy and partial trisomy of autosomes, unspecified** `Rx` `COM`

✓4ᵗʰ **Q93** **Monosomies and deletions from the autosomes, not elsewhere classified**

Q93.0 **Whole** chromosome monosomy, nonmosaicism **(meiotic nondisjunction)** `Rx` `COM`

Q93.1 **Whole chromosome monosomy,** mosaicism **(mitotic nondisjunction)** `Rx` `COM`

Q93.2 **Chromosome** replaced with ring**, dicentric or isochromosome** `Rx` `COM`

Q93.3 **Deletion of short arm of chromosome** 4 `Rx` `COM`
    Wolff-Hirschorn syndrome

Q93.4 **Deletion of short arm of chromosome** 5 `Rx` `COM`
    Cri-du-chat syndrome

✓5ᵗʰ **Q93.5** **Other deletions of** part of a chromosome
    AHA: 2018,4Q,28

    Q93.51 **Angelman syndrome** `Rx` `COM`

    Q93.59 **Other deletions of part of a chromosome** `Rx` `COM`

Q93.7 **Deletions with other complex rearrangements** `Rx` `COM`
    Deletions due to unbalanced translocations, inversions and insertions
    Code also any associated duplications due to unbalanced translocations, inversions and insertions (Q92.5)

✓5ᵗʰ **Q93.8** **Other deletions from the autosomes**

    Q93.81 **Velo-cardio-facial syndrome** `Rx` `COM`
        Deletion 22q11.2
        AHA: 2019,3Q,14
        DEF: Microdeletion syndrome affecting multiple organs characterized by a cleft palate, heart defects, an elongated face with almond-shaped eyes, wide nose, small ears, weak immune system, weak musculature, hypothyroidism, short stature, and scoliosis. The deletion occurs at q11.2 on the long arm of the chromosome 22.

    Q93.82 **Williams syndrome** `Rx` `COM`
        AHA: 2018,4Q,28-29

    Q93.88 **Other microdeletions** `Rx` `COM`
        Miller-Dieker syndrome
        Smith-Magenis syndrome

    Q93.89 **Other deletions from the autosomes** `Rx` `COM`
        Deletions identified by fluorescence in situ hybridization (FISH)
        Deletions identified by in situ hybridization (ISH)
        Deletions seen only at prometaphase

Q93.9 **Deletion from autosomes, unspecified** `Rx` `COM`

✓4ᵗʰ **Q95** **Balanced rearrangements and structural markers, not elsewhere classified**
    INCLUDES Robertsonian and balanced reciprocal translocations and insertions

Q95.0 **Balanced translocation and insertion in normal individual**

Q95.1 **Chromosome inversion in normal individual**

Q95.2 **Balanced autosomal rearrangement in abnormal individual** `Rx` `COM`

Q95.3 **Balanced sex/autosomal rearrangement in abnormal individual** `Rx` `COM`

Q95.5 **Individual with autosomal fragile site**

Q95.8 **Other balanced rearrangements and structural markers**

Q95.9 **Balanced rearrangement and structural marker, unspecified**

✓4ᵗʰ **Q96** **Turner's syndrome**
    EXCLUDES 1 Noonan syndrome (Q87.19)

Q96.0 **Karyotype 45, X** `COM` ♀

Q96.1 **Karyotype 46, X iso (Xq)** `COM` ♀
    Karyotype 46, isochromosome Xq

Q96.2 **Karyotype 46, X with abnormal sex chromosome, except iso (Xq)** `COM` ♀
    Karyotype 46, X with abnormal sex chromosome, except isochromosome Xq

Q96.3 **Mosaicism, 45, X/46, XX or XY** `COM` ♀

Q96.4 **Mosaicism, 45, X/other cell line(s) with abnormal sex chromosome** `COM` ♀

Q96.8 **Other variants of Turner's syndrome** `COM` ♀

Q96.9 **Turner's syndrome, unspecified** `COM` ♀

✓4ᵗʰ **Q97** **Other sex chromosome abnormalities, female phenotype, not elsewhere classified**
    EXCLUDES 1 Turner's syndrome (Q96.-)

Q97.0 **Karyotype 47, XXX** `COM` ♀

Q97.1 **Female with more than three X chromosomes** `COM` ♀

Q97.2 **Mosaicism, lines with various numbers of X chromosomes** `COM` ♀

Q97.3 **Female with 46, XY karyotype** `COM` ♀

Q97.8 **Other specified sex chromosome abnormalities, female phenotype** `COM` ♀

Q97.9 **Sex chromosome abnormality, female phenotype, unspecified** `COM` ♀

✓4ᵗʰ **Q98** **Other sex chromosome abnormalities, male phenotype, not elsewhere classified**

Q98.0 **Klinefelter syndrome karyotype 47, XXY** `COM` ♂

Q98.1 **Klinefelter syndrome, male with more than two X chromosomes** `COM` ♂

Q98.3 **Other male with 46, XX karyotype** `COM` ♂

Q98.4 **Klinefelter syndrome, unspecified** `COM` ♂

Q98.5 **Karyotype 47, XYY** `COM`

Q98.6 **Male with structurally abnormal sex chromosome** `COM` ♂

Q98.7 **Male with sex chromosome mosaicism** `COM` ♂

Q98.8 **Other specified sex chromosome abnormalities, male phenotype** `COM` ♂

Q98.9 **Sex chromosome abnormality, male phenotype, unspecified** `COM` ♂

✓4ᵗʰ **Q99** **Other chromosome abnormalities, not elsewhere classified**

Q99.0 **Chimera 46, XX/46, XY** `COM`
    Chimera 46, XX/46, XY true hermaphrodite

Q99.1 **46, XX true hermaphrodite** `COM`
    46, XX with streak gonads
    46, XY with streak gonads
    Pure gonadal dysgenesis

Q99.2 **Fragile X chromosome** `Rx` `COM`
    Fragile X syndrome

Q99.8 **Other specified chromosome abnormalities** `COM`

Q99.9 **Chromosomal abnormality, unspecified** `COM`

`HCC` CMS-HCC   `Rx` Rx HCC   `ESR` ESRD HCC   `COM` Commercial HCC   N Newborn: 0   P Pediatric: 0-17   M Maternity: 9-64   A Adult: 15-124

962   ICD-10-CM 2023

Chapter 18. Symptoms, Signs and Abnormal Clinical and Laboratory Findings (R00–R99)

Chapter-specific Guidelines with Coding Examples

The chapter-specific guidelines from the ICD-10-CM Official Guidelines for Coding and Reporting have been provided below. Along with these guidelines are coding examples, contained in the shaded boxes, that have been developed to help illustrate the coding and/or sequencing guidance found in these guidelines.

Chapter 18 includes symptoms, signs, abnormal results of clinical or other investigative procedures, and ill-defined conditions regarding which no diagnosis classifiable elsewhere is recorded. Signs and symptoms that point to a specific diagnosis have been assigned to a category in other chapters of the classification.

a. Use of symptom codes

Codes that describe symptoms and signs are acceptable for reporting purposes when a related definitive diagnosis has not been established (confirmed) by the provider.

> Tenderness and localized pain in the right upper quadrant; based on presentation, probable gallstones
>
> **R10.11   Right upper quadrant pain**
>
> **R10.811   Right upper quadrant abdominal tenderness**
>
> *Explanation:* Codes that describe symptoms such as abdominal pain are acceptable for reporting purposes when the provider has not established (confirmed) a definitive diagnosis.

b. Use of a symptom code with a definitive diagnosis code

Codes for signs and symptoms may be reported in addition to a related definitive diagnosis when the sign or symptom is not routinely associated with that diagnosis, such as the various signs and symptoms associated with complex syndromes. The definitive diagnosis code should be sequenced before the symptom code.

Signs or symptoms that are associated routinely with a disease process should not be assigned as additional codes, unless otherwise instructed by the classification.

> Pneumonia with hemoptysis
>
> **J18.9   Pneumonia, unspecified organism**
>
> **R04.2   Hemoptysis**
>
> *Explanation:* Codes for signs and symptoms may be reported in addition to a related definitive diagnosis when the sign or symptom is not routinely associated with that diagnosis.

> Abdominal pain due to acute appendicitis
>
> **K35.80   Unspecified acute appendicitis**
>
> *Explanation:* Codes for signs or symptoms routinely associated with a disease process should not be assigned unless the classification instructs otherwise.

c. Combination codes that include symptoms

ICD-10-CM contains a number of combination codes that identify both the definitive diagnosis and common symptoms of that diagnosis. When using one of these combination codes, an additional code should not be assigned for the symptom.

> IBS with diarrhea
>
> **K58.0   Irritable bowel syndrome with diarrhea**
>
> *Explanation:* When a combination code identifies both the definitive diagnosis and the symptom, an additional code should not be assigned for the symptom.

d. Repeated falls

Code R29.6, Repeated falls, is for use for encounters when a patient has recently fallen and the reason for the fall is being investigated.

Code Z91.81, History of falling, is for use when a patient has fallen in the past and is at risk for future falls. When appropriate, both codes R29.6 and Z91.81 may be assigned together.

e. Coma

Code R40.20, Unspecified coma, may be assigned in conjunction with codes for any medical condition.

Do not report codes for unspecified coma, individual or total Glasgow coma scale scores for a patient with a medically induced coma or a sedated patient.

1) Coma scale

The coma scale codes (R40.21- to R40.24-) can be used in conjunction with traumatic brain injury codes. These codes are primarily for use by trauma registries, but they may be used in any setting where this information is collected. The coma scale codes should be sequenced after the diagnosis code(s).

These codes, one from each subcategory, are needed to complete the scale. The 7th character indicates when the scale was recorded. The 7th character should match for all three codes.

At a minimum, report the initial score documented on presentation at your facility. This may be a score from the emergency medicine technician (EMT) or in the emergency department. If desired, a facility may choose to capture multiple coma scale scores.

Assign code R40.24-, Glasgow coma scale, total score, when only the total score is documented in the medical record and not the individual score(s).

If multiple coma scores are captured within the first 24 hours after hospital admission, assign only the code for the score at the time of admission. ICD-10-CM does not classify coma scores that are reported after admission but less than 24 hours later.

See Section I.B.14. for coma scale documentation by clinicians other than patient's provider

> 36-year-old man found down after unknown injury with skull fracture and with concussion and loss of consciousness of unknown duration. Upon hospital admission, the patient was evaluated with the following Glasgow coma scores:
>
> Eye-opening response—3: eyes open to speech
>
> Verbal response—3: random speech with no conversational exchange
>
> Motor response—4: pulls limb away from painful stimulus
>
> **S02.0XXA   Fracture of vault of skull, initial encounter for closed fracture**
>
> **S06.0X9A   Concussion with loss of consciousness of unspecified duration, initial encounter**
>
> **R40.2133   Coma scale, eyes open, to sound, at hospital admission**
>
> **R40.2233   Coma scale, best verbal response, inappropriate words, at hospital admission**
>
> **R40.2343   Coma scale, best motor response, flexion withdrawal, at hospital admission**
>
> *Explanation:* When individual scores for the Glasgow coma scale are documented, one code from each category is needed to complete the scale. The seventh character indicates when the scale was recorded and should match for all three codes. Assign a code from subcategory R40.24- Glasgow coma scale, total score, when only the total and not the individual score(s) is documented.

f. Functional quadriplegia

GUIDELINE HAS BEEN DELETED EFFECTIVE OCTOBER 1, 2017

g. SIRS due to non-infectious process

The systemic inflammatory response syndrome (SIRS) can develop as a result of certain non-infectious disease processes, such as trauma, malignant neoplasm, or pancreatitis. When SIRS is documented with a noninfectious condition, and no subsequent infection is documented, the code for the underlying condition, such as an injury, should be assigned, followed by code R65.10, Systemic inflammatory response syndrome (SIRS) of non-infectious origin without acute organ dysfunction, or code R65.11, Systemic inflammatory response syndrome (SIRS) of non-infectious origin with acute organ dysfunction. If an associated acute organ dysfunction is documented, the appropriate code(s) for the specific type of organ dysfunction(s) should be assigned in addition to code R65.11. If acute organ dysfunction is documented, but it cannot be determined if the acute organ dysfunction is associated with SIRS or due to another condition (e.g., directly due to the trauma), the provider should be queried.

Systemic inflammatory response syndrome (SIRS) due to acute gallstone pancreatitis

K85.1Ø	**Biliary acute pancreatitis without necrosis or infection**
R65.1Ø	**Systemic inflammatory response syndrome [SIRS] of non-infectious origin without acute organ dysfunction**

Explanation: When SIRS is documented with a non-infectious condition without subsequent infection documented, the code for the underlying condition such as pancreatitis should be assigned followed by the appropriate code for SIRS of noninfectious origin, either with or without associated organ dysfunction.

---

h. Death NOS

Code R99, Ill-defined and unknown cause of mortality, is only for use in the very limited circumstance when a patient who has already died is brought into an emergency department or other healthcare facility and is pronounced dead upon arrival. It does not represent the discharge disposition of death.

i. NIHSS stroke scale

The NIH stroke scale (NIHSS) codes (R29.7- -) can be used in conjunction with acute stroke codes (I63) to identify the patient's neurological status and the severity of the stroke. The stroke scale codes should be sequenced after the acute stroke diagnosis code(s).

At a minimum, report the initial score documented. If desired, a facility may choose to capture multiple stroke scale scores.

See Section I.B.14. for NIHSS stroke scale documentation by clinicians other than patient's provider

Chapter 18. Symptoms, Signs and Abnormal Clinical and Laboratory Findings, Not Elsewhere Classified (R00-R99)

NOTE This chapter includes symptoms, signs, abnormal results of clinical or other investigative procedures, and ill-defined conditions regarding which no diagnosis classifiable elsewhere is recorded.

Signs and symptoms that point rather definitely to a given diagnosis have been assigned to a category in other chapters of the classification. In general, categories in this chapter include the less well-defined conditions and symptoms that, without the necessary study of the case to establish a final diagnosis, point perhaps equally to two or more diseases or to two or more systems of the body. Practically all categories in the chapter could be designated 'not otherwise specified', 'unknown etiology' or 'transient'. The Alphabetical Index should be consulted to determine which symptoms and signs are to be allocated here and which to other chapters. The residual subcategories, numbered .8, are generally provided for other relevant symptoms that cannot be allocated elsewhere in the classification.

The conditions and signs or symptoms included in categories R00-R94 consist of:

(a) cases for which no more specific diagnosis can be made even after all the facts bearing on the case have been investigated;

(b) signs or symptoms existing at the time of initial encounter that proved to be transient and whose causes could not be determined;

(c) provisional diagnosis in a patient who failed to return for further investigation or care;

(d) cases referred elsewhere for investigation or treatment before the diagnosis was made;

(e) cases in which a more precise diagnosis was not available for any other reason;

(f) certain symptoms, for which supplementary information is provided, that represent important problems in medical care in their own right.

EXCLUDES 2 *abnormal findings on antenatal screening of mother (O28.-)*
certain conditions originating in the perinatal period (P04-P96)
signs and symptoms classified in the body system chapters
signs and symptoms of breast (N63, N64.5)

AHA: 2017,1Q,6,7

This chapter contains the following blocks:

R00-R09	Symptoms and signs involving the circulatory and respiratory systems
R10-R19	Symptoms and signs involving the digestive system and abdomen
R20-R23	Symptoms and signs involving the skin and subcutaneous tissue
R25-R29	Symptoms and signs involving the nervous and musculoskeletal systems
R30-R39	Symptoms and signs involving the genitourinary system
R40-R46	Symptoms and signs involving cognition, perception, emotional state and behavior
R47-R49	Symptoms and signs involving speech and voice
R50-R69	General symptoms and signs
R70-R79	Abnormal findings on examination of blood, without diagnosis
R80-R82	Abnormal findings on examination of urine, without diagnosis
R83-R89	Abnormal findings on examination of other body fluids, substances and tissues, without diagnosis
R90-R94	Abnormal findings on diagnostic imaging and in function studies, without diagnosis
R97	Abnormal tumor markers
R99	Ill-defined and unknown cause of mortality

Symptoms and signs involving the circulatory and respiratory systems (R00-R09)

☑4ᵗʰ **R00 Abnormalities of heart beat**

     EXCLUDES 1 *abnormalities originating in the perinatal period (P29.1-)*
     EXCLUDES 2 *specified arrhythmias (I47-I49)*

     R00.0 Tachycardia, unspecified
       Rapid heart beat
       Sinoauricular tachycardia NOS
       Sinus [sinusal] tachycardia NOS
       EXCLUDES 1 *neonatal tachycardia (P29.11)*
           paroxysmal tachycardia (I47.-)
       DEF: Excessively rapid heart rate of more than 100 beats per minute.

R00.1 Bradycardia, unspecified
   Sinoatrial bradycardia
   Sinus bradycardia
   Slow heart beat
   Vagal bradycardia
   Use additional code for adverse effect, if applicable, to identify drug (T36-T50 with fifth or sixth character 5)
   EXCLUDES 1 *neonatal bradycardia (P29.12)*
   AHA: 2020,2Q,23
   DEF: Slowed heartbeat, usually defined as a rate fewer than 60 beats per minute. Heart rhythm may be slow as a result of a congenital defect or an acquired problem.

R00.2 Palpitations
   Awareness of heart beat

R00.8 Other abnormalities of heart beat

R00.9 Unspecified abnormalities of heart beat

☑4ᵗʰ **R01 Cardiac murmurs and other cardiac sounds**

   EXCLUDES 1 *cardiac murmurs and sounds originating in the perinatal period (P29.8)*

   R01.0 Benign and innocent cardiac murmurs
     Functional cardiac murmur

   R01.1 Cardiac murmur, unspecified
     Cardiac bruit NOS
     Heart murmur NOS
     Systolic murmur NOS

   R01.2 Other cardiac sounds
     Cardiac dullness, increased or decreased
     Precordial friction

☑4ᵗʰ **R03 Abnormal blood-pressure reading, without diagnosis**

   R03.0 Elevated blood-pressure reading, without diagnosis of hypertension
     NOTE This category is to be used to record an episode of elevated blood pressure in a patient in whom no formal diagnosis of hypertension has been made, or as an isolated incidental finding.

   R03.1 Nonspecific low blood-pressure reading
     EXCLUDES 1 *hypotension (I95.-)*
         maternal hypotension syndrome (O26.5-)
         neurogenic orthostatic hypotension (G90.3)

☑4ᵗʰ **R04 Hemorrhage from respiratory passages**

   R04.0 Epistaxis
     Hemorrhage from nose
     Nosebleed

   R04.1 Hemorrhage from throat
     EXCLUDES 2 *hemoptysis (R04.2)*

   R04.2 Hemoptysis
     Blood-stained sputum
     Cough with hemorrhage
     AHA: 2013,4Q,118

☑5ᵗʰ **R04.8 Hemorrhage from other sites in respiratory passages**

     R04.81 Acute idiopathic pulmonary hemorrhage in infants Ⓟ
       AIPHI
       Acute idiopathic hemorrhage in infants over 28 days old
       EXCLUDES 1 *perinatal pulmonary hemorrhage (P26.-)*
          ▶*von Willebrand disease (D68.0-)*◀

     R04.89 Hemorrhage from other sites in respiratory passages
       Pulmonary hemorrhage NOS

   R04.9 Hemorrhage from respiratory passages, unspecified

☑4ᵗʰ **R05 Cough**

   EXCLUDES 1 *paroxysmal cough due to Bordetella pertussis (A37.0-)*
         smoker's cough (J41.0)
   EXCLUDES 2 *cough with hemorrhage (R04.2)*
   AHA: 2021,4Q,24-25; 2016,2Q,33

   R05.1 Acute cough

   R05.2 Subacute cough

   R05.3 Chronic cough
     Persistent cough
     Refractory cough
     Unexplained cough

   R05.4 Cough syncope UPD
     Code first syncope and collapse (R55)

   R05.8 Other specified cough

Chapter 18. Symptoms, Signs and Abnormal Clinical and Laboratory Findings

R05.9–R09.89

R05.9   **Cough, unspecified**

✓4ᵗʰ **R06**   **Abnormalities of breathing**

> EXCLUDES 1   acute respiratory distress syndrome (J80)
> respiratory arrest (R09.2)
> respiratory arrest of newborn (P28.81)
> respiratory distress syndrome of newborn (P22.-)
> respiratory failure (J96.-)
> respiratory failure of newborn (P28.5)

✓5ᵗʰ **R06.0**   **Dyspnea**

> EXCLUDES 1   tachypnea NOS (R06.82)
> transient tachypnea of newborn (P22.1)

    R06.00   **Dyspnea, unspecified**
       AHA: 2017,1Q,26

    R06.01   **Orthopnea**

    R06.02   **Shortness of breath**

    R06.03   **Acute respiratory distress**
       AHA: 2017,4Q,23

    R06.09   **Other forms of dyspnea**

   R06.1   **Stridor**

> EXCLUDES 1   congenital laryngeal stridor (P28.89)
> laryngismus (stridulus) (J38.5)

    DEF: Certain type of wheezing described as a loud, constant, musical sound produced when breathing with an obstructed airway, like the inspiratory sound heard when laryngeal or esophageal obstruction is present.

   R06.2   **Wheezing**

> EXCLUDES 1   asthma (J45.-)

    AHA: 2016,2Q,33
    DEF: High-pitched whistling sound during breathing due to stenosis of the respiratory passageway. Wheezing is associated with asthma, sleep apnea, bronchiectasis, bronchiolitis, COPD, and pleural effusion.

   R06.3   **Periodic breathing**
      Cheyne-Stokes breathing

   R06.4   **Hyperventilation**

> EXCLUDES 1   psychogenic hyperventilation (F45.8)

   R06.5   **Mouth breathing**

> EXCLUDES 2   dry mouth NOS (R68.2)

   R06.6   **Hiccough**

> EXCLUDES 1   psychogenic hiccough (F45.8)

   R06.7   **Sneezing**

✓5ᵗʰ **R06.8**   **Other abnormalities of breathing**

    R06.81   **Apnea, not elsewhere classified**
       Apnea NOS

> EXCLUDES 1   apnea (of) newborn ▶(P28.4-)◀
> sleep apnea (G47.3-)
> sleep apnea of newborn (primary) ▶(P28.3-)◀

    R06.82   **Tachypnea, not elsewhere classified**
       Tachypnea NOS

> EXCLUDES 1   transitory tachypnea of newborn (P22.1)

    R06.83   **Snoring**

    R06.89   **Other abnormalities of breathing**
       Breath-holding (spells)
       Sighing

   R06.9   **Unspecified abnormalities of breathing**

✓4ᵗʰ **R07**   **Pain in throat and chest**

> EXCLUDES 1   epidemic myalgia (B33.0)
> EXCLUDES 2   jaw pain R68.84
> pain in breast (N64.4)

   R07.0   **Pain in throat**   *not sore throat*

> EXCLUDES 1   chronic sore throat (J31.2)
> sore throat (acute) NOS (J02.9)
> EXCLUDES 2   dysphagia (R13.1-)
> pain in neck (M54.2)

   R07.1   **Chest pain on breathing**
      Painful respiration

   R07.2   **Precordial pain**
    DEF: Pain felt in the anterior (front) chest wall over the region of the heart. This type of pain is generally felt slightly to the left of the sternum, but may also extend into the surrounding chest wall region.

✓5ᵗʰ **R07.8**   **Other chest pain**

    R07.81   **Pleurodynia**
       Pleurodynia NOS

> EXCLUDES 1   epidemic pleurodynia (B33.0)

    R07.82   **Intercostal pain**

    R07.89   **Other chest pain**
       Anterior chest-wall pain NOS
       AHA: 2021,1Q,42

   R07.9   **Chest pain, unspecified**

✓4ᵗʰ **R09**   **Other symptoms and signs involving the circulatory and respiratory system**

> EXCLUDES 1   acute respiratory distress syndrome (J80)
> respiratory arrest of newborn (P28.81)
> respiratory distress syndrome of newborn (P22.0)
> respiratory failure (J96.-)
> respiratory failure of newborn (P28.5)

✓5ᵗʰ **R09.0**   **Asphyxia and hypoxemia**

> EXCLUDES 1   asphyxia due to carbon monoxide (T58.-)
> asphyxia due to foreign body in respiratory tract (T17.-)
> birth (intrauterine) asphyxia (P84)
> hyperventilation (R06.4)
> traumatic asphyxia (T71.-)
> EXCLUDES 2   hypercapnia (R06.89)

    R09.01   **Asphyxia**
    DEF: Interference of oxygen intake due to obstruction or injury of airways resulting in a lack of oxygen perfusion to the tissues or excessive carbon dioxide in the blood. Can cause unconsciousness or death.

    R09.02   **Hypoxemia**
       AHA: 2019,3Q,15
    DEF: Insufficient oxygen in the arterial blood resulting in inadequate delivery of oxygen to the body tissues.

   R09.1   **Pleurisy**

> EXCLUDES 1   pleurisy with effusion (J90)

   R09.2   **Respiratory arrest**   HCC ESR COM
      Cardiorespiratory failure

> EXCLUDES 1   cardiac arrest (I46.-)
> respiratory arrest of newborn (P28.81)
> respiratory distress of newborn (P22.0)
> respiratory failure (J96.-)
> respiratory failure of newborn (P28.5)
> respiratory insufficiency (R06.89)
> respiratory insufficiency of newborn (P28.5)

   R09.3   **Abnormal sputum**
      Abnormal amount of sputum
      Abnormal color of sputum
      Abnormal odor of sputum
      Excessive sputum

> EXCLUDES 1   blood-stained sputum (R04.2)

✓5ᵗʰ **R09.8**   **Other specified symptoms and signs involving the circulatory and respiratory systems**

    R09.81   **Nasal congestion**

    R09.82   **Postnasal drip**

    R09.89   **Other specified symptoms and signs involving the circulatory and respiratory systems**
       Abnormal chest percussion
       Bruit (arterial)
       Chest tympany
       Choking sensation
       Feeling of foreign body in throat
       Friction sounds in chest
       Rales
       Weak pulse

> EXCLUDES 2   foreign body in throat (T17.2-)
> wheezing (R06.2)

       AHA: 2021,1Q,42

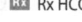

Symptoms and signs involving the digestive system and abdomen (R10-R19)

EXCLUDES 2 *congenital or infantile pylorospasm (Q40.0)*
gastrointestinal hemorrhage (K92.0-K92.2)
intestinal obstruction (K56.-)
newborn gastrointestinal hemorrhage (P54.0-P54.3)
newborn intestinal obstruction (P76.-)
pylorospasm (K31.3)
signs and symptoms involving the urinary system (R30-R39)
symptoms referable to female genital organs (N94.-)
symptoms referable to male genital organs (N48-N50)

✓4th **R10 Abdominal and pelvic pain**

EXCLUDES 1 *renal colic (N23)*
EXCLUDES 2 *dorsalgia (M54.-)*
flatulence and related conditions (R14.-)

R10.0 Acute abdomen
Severe abdominal pain (generalized) (with abdominal rigidity)
EXCLUDES 1 *abdominal rigidity NOS (R19.3)*
generalized abdominal pain NOS (R10.84)
localized abdominal pain (R10.1-R10.3-)

✓5th **R10.1 Pain localized to upper abdomen**

R10.10 Upper abdominal pain, unspecified
R10.11 Right upper quadrant pain
R10.12 Left upper quadrant pain
R10.13 Epigastric pain
Dyspepsia
EXCLUDES 1 *functional dyspepsia (K30)*

Abdominal Pain

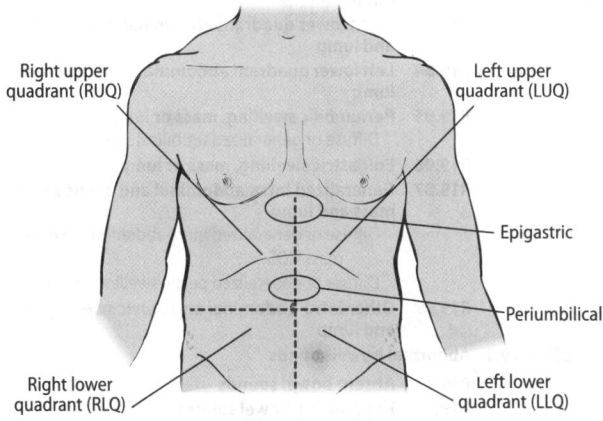

Right upper quadrant (RUQ)
Left upper quadrant (LUQ)
Epigastric
Periumbilical
Right lower quadrant (RLQ)
Left lower quadrant (LLQ)

R10.2 Pelvic and perineal pain
EXCLUDES 1 *vulvodynia (N94.81)*

✓5th **R10.3 Pain localized to other parts of lower abdomen**

R10.30 Lower abdominal pain, unspecified
R10.31 Right lower quadrant pain
R10.32 Left lower quadrant pain
R10.33 Periumbilical pain

✓5th **R10.8 Other abdominal pain**

✓6th **R10.81 Abdominal tenderness**
Abdominal tenderness NOS
R10.811 Right upper quadrant abdominal tenderness
R10.812 Left upper quadrant abdominal tenderness
R10.813 Right lower quadrant abdominal tenderness
R10.814 Left lower quadrant abdominal tenderness
R10.815 Periumbilic abdominal tenderness
R10.816 Epigastric abdominal tenderness
R10.817 Generalized abdominal tenderness
R10.819 Abdominal tenderness, unspecified site

✓6th **R10.82 Rebound abdominal tenderness**
R10.821 Right upper quadrant rebound abdominal tenderness
R10.822 Left upper quadrant rebound abdominal tenderness
R10.823 Right lower quadrant rebound abdominal tenderness

R10.824 Left lower quadrant rebound abdominal tenderness
R10.825 Periumbilic rebound abdominal tenderness
R10.826 Epigastric rebound abdominal tenderness
R10.827 Generalized rebound abdominal tenderness
R10.829 Rebound abdominal tenderness, unspecified site

R10.83 Colic P
Colic NOS
Infantile colic
EXCLUDES 1 *colic in adult and child over 12 months old (R10.84)*
DEF: Inconsolable crying in an otherwise well-fed and healthy infant for more than three hours a day, three days a week, for more than three weeks.

R10.84 Generalized abdominal pain
EXCLUDES 1 *generalized abdominal pain associated with acute abdomen (R10.0)*

R10.9 Unspecified abdominal pain

✓4th **R11 Nausea and vomiting**
EXCLUDES 1 *cyclical vomiting associated with migraine (G43.A-)*
excessive vomiting in pregnancy (O21.-)
hematemesis (K92.0)
neonatal hematemesis (P54.0)
newborn vomiting (P92.0-)
psychogenic vomiting (F50.89)
vomiting associated with bulimia nervosa (F50.2)
vomiting following gastrointestinal surgery (K91.0)
AHA: 2017, 1Q, 28

R11.0 Nausea   *HCli have not Confirmed Pregnancy*
Nausea NOS
Nausea without vomiting

✓5th **R11.1 Vomiting**

R11.10 Vomiting, unspecified
Vomiting NOS
R11.11 Vomiting without nausea
R11.12 Projectile vomiting
R11.13 Vomiting of fecal matter
R11.14 Bilious vomiting
Bilious emesis
R11.15 Cyclical vomiting syndrome unrelated to migraine
Cyclic vomiting syndrome NOS
Persistent vomiting
EXCLUDES 1 *cyclical vomiting in migraine (G43.A-)*
EXCLUDES 2 *bulimia nervosa (F50.2)*
diabetes mellitus due to underlying condition (E08.-)
AHA: 2019, 4Q, 15

R11.2 Nausea with vomiting, unspecified
Persistent nausea with vomiting NOS
AHA: 2020, 1Q, 8

R12 Heartburn
EXCLUDES 1 *dyspepsia NOS (R10.13)*
functional dyspepsia (K30)

✓4th **R13 Aphagia and dysphagia**

R13.0 Aphagia
Inability to swallow
EXCLUDES 1 *psychogenic aphagia (F50.9)*

Chapter 18. Symptoms, Signs and Abnormal Clinical and Laboratory Findings

R10–R13.0

Chapter 18. Symptoms, Signs and Abnormal Clinical and Laboratory Findings

R13.1–R19.4

√5ᵗʰ **R13.1 Dysphagia**

Code first, if applicable, dysphagia following cerebrovascular disease (I69. with final characters -91)

EXCLUDES 1   *psychogenic dysphagia (F45.8)*

Swallowing Function

Oral phase

Oropharyngeal phase

Pharyngeal phase

Pharyngoesophageal phase

R13.10 Dysphagia, unspecified
Difficulty in swallowing NOS

R13.11 Dysphagia, oral phase

R13.12 Dysphagia, oropharyngeal phase

R13.13 Dysphagia, pharyngeal phase

R13.14 Dysphagia, pharyngoesophageal phase

R13.19 Other dysphagia
Cervical dysphagia
Neurogenic dysphagia

√4ᵗʰ **R14 Flatulence and related conditions**

EXCLUDES 1   *psychogenic aerophagy (F45.8)*

R14.0 Abdominal distension (gaseous)
Bloating
Tympanites (abdominal) (intestinal)

R14.1 Gas pain

R14.2 Eructation

R14.3 Flatulence

√4ᵗʰ **R15 Fecal incontinence**

INCLUDES   encopresis NOS

EXCLUDES 1   *fecal incontinence of nonorganic origin (F98.1)*

R15.0 Incomplete defecation

EXCLUDES 1   *constipation (K59.0-)*
fecal impaction (K56.41)

R15.1 Fecal smearing
Fecal soiling

R15.2 Fecal urgency

R15.9 Full incontinence of feces
Fecal incontinence NOS

√4ᵗʰ **R16 Hepatomegaly and splenomegaly, not elsewhere classified**

R16.0 Hepatomegaly, not elsewhere classified
Hepatomegaly NOS

R16.1 Splenomegaly, not elsewhere classified
Splenomegaly NOS

R16.2 Hepatomegaly with splenomegaly, not elsewhere classified
Hepatosplenomegaly NOS

R17 Unspecified jaundice

EXCLUDES 1   *neonatal jaundice (P55, P57-P59)*

√4ᵗʰ **R18 Ascites**

INCLUDES   fluid in peritoneal cavity

EXCLUDES 1   *ascites in alcoholic cirrhosis (K70.31)*
ascites in alcoholic hepatitis (K70.11)
ascites in toxic liver disease with chronic active hepatitis (K71.51)

DEF: Abnormal accumulation of free fluid in the abdominal cavity, causing distention and tightness in addition to shortness of breath as the fluid accumulates. Ascites is usually an underlying disorder and can be a manifestation of any number of diseases.

R18.0 Malignant ascites   UPD
Code first malignancy, such as:
malignant neoplasm of ovary (C56.-)
secondary malignant neoplasm of retroperitoneum and peritoneum (C78.6)

R18.8 Other ascites
Ascites NOS
Peritoneal effusion (chronic)
AHA: 2018,1Q,4

√4ᵗʰ **R19 Other symptoms and signs involving the digestive system and abdomen**

EXCLUDES 1   *acute abdomen (R10.0)*

√5ᵗʰ **R19.0 Intra-abdominal and pelvic swelling, mass and lump**

EXCLUDES 1   *abdominal distension (gaseous) (R14.-)*
ascites (R18.-)

R19.00 Intra-abdominal and pelvic swelling, mass and lump, unspecified site

R19.01 Right upper quadrant abdominal swelling, mass and lump

R19.02 Left upper quadrant abdominal swelling, mass and lump

R19.03 Right lower quadrant abdominal swelling, mass and lump

R19.04 Left lower quadrant abdominal swelling, mass and lump

R19.05 Periumbilic swelling, mass or lump
Diffuse or generalized umbilical swelling or mass

R19.06 Epigastric swelling, mass or lump

R19.07 Generalized intra-abdominal and pelvic swelling, mass and lump
Diffuse or generalized intra-abdominal swelling or mass NOS
Diffuse or generalized pelvic swelling or mass NOS

R19.09 Other intra-abdominal and pelvic swelling, mass and lump

√5ᵗʰ **R19.1 Abnormal bowel sounds**

R19.11 Absent bowel sounds

R19.12 Hyperactive bowel sounds

R19.15 Other abnormal bowel sounds
Abnormal bowel sounds NOS

R19.2 Visible peristalsis
Hyperperistalsis
DEF: Visible movements of muscular attempts to move food through the digestive tract due to pyloric obstruction, stomach obstruction, or intestinal obstruction.

√5ᵗʰ **R19.3 Abdominal rigidity**

EXCLUDES 1   *abdominal rigidity with severe abdominal pain (R10.0)*

R19.30 Abdominal rigidity, unspecified site

R19.31 Right upper quadrant abdominal rigidity

R19.32 Left upper quadrant abdominal rigidity

R19.33 Right lower quadrant abdominal rigidity

R19.34 Left lower quadrant abdominal rigidity

R19.35 Periumbilic abdominal rigidity

R19.36 Epigastric abdominal rigidity

R19.37 Generalized abdominal rigidity

R19.4 Change in bowel habit

EXCLUDES 1   *constipation (K59.0-)*
functional diarrhea (K59.1)

Image labels (Swallowing Function diagrams):
Oral phase: Bolus, Soft palate, Palatine tonsil
Oropharyngeal phase: Pharynx, Oral cavity, Bolus, Trachea
Pharyngeal phase: Tongue, Bolus, Epiglottis, Esophagus
Pharyngoesophageal phase: Bolus, Epiglottis, Trachea

R19.5 **Other fecal abnormalities**
Abnormal stool color
Bulky stools
Mucus in stools
Occult blood in feces
Occult blood in stools
EXCLUDES 1   *melena (K92.1)*
           neonatal melena (P54.1)
AHA: 2021,1Q,9; 2019,1Q,32

R19.6 **Halitosis**

R19.7 **Diarrhea, unspecified**
Diarrhea NOS
EXCLUDES 1   *functional diarrhea (K59.1)*
           neonatal diarrhea (P78.3)
           psychogenic diarrhea (F45.8)
AHA: 2021,3Q,3

R19.8 **Other specified symptoms and signs involving the digestive system and abdomen**

Symptoms and signs involving the skin and subcutaneous tissue (R20-R23)

EXCLUDES 2   *symptoms relating to breast (N64.4-N64.5)*

✓4ᵗʰ **R20** **Disturbances of skin sensation**
EXCLUDES 1   *dissociative anesthesia and sensory loss (F44.6)*
           psychogenic disturbances (F45.8)

R20.0 **Anesthesia of skin**
R20.1 **Hypoesthesia of skin**
R20.2 **Paresthesia of skin**
Formication
Pins and needles
Tingling skin
EXCLUDES 1   *acroparesthesia (I73.8)*
R20.3 **Hyperesthesia**
R20.8 **Other disturbances of skin sensation**
R20.9 **Unspecified disturbances of skin sensation**

R21 **Rash and other nonspecific skin eruption**
INCLUDES   rash NOS
EXCLUDES 1   *specified type of rash - code to condition*
           vesicular eruption (R23.8)

✓4ᵗʰ **R22** **Localized swelling, mass and lump of skin and subcutaneous tissue**
INCLUDES   subcutaneous nodules (localized)(superficial)
EXCLUDES 1   *abnormal findings on diagnostic imaging (R90-R93)*
           edema (R60.-)
           enlarged lymph nodes (R59.-)
           localized adiposity (E65)
           swelling of joint (M25.4-)

R22.0 **Localized swelling, mass and lump, head**
R22.1 **Localized swelling, mass and lump, neck**
R22.2 **Localized swelling, mass and lump, trunk**
EXCLUDES 1   *intra-abdominal or pelvic mass and lump (R19.0-)*
           intra-abdominal or pelvic swelling (R19.0-)
EXCLUDES 2   *breast mass and lump (N63)*

✓5ᵗʰ **R22.3** **Localized swelling, mass and lump, upper limb**
     R22.30 **Localized swelling, mass and lump, unspecified upper limb**
     R22.31 **Localized swelling, mass and lump, right upper limb**
     R22.32 **Localized swelling, mass and lump, left upper limb**
     R22.33 **Localized swelling, mass and lump, upper limb, bilateral**

✓5ᵗʰ **R22.4** **Localized swelling, mass and lump, lower limb**
     R22.40 **Localized swelling, mass and lump, unspecified lower limb**
     R22.41 **Localized swelling, mass and lump, right lower limb**
     R22.42 **Localized swelling, mass and lump, left lower limb**
     R22.43 **Localized swelling, mass and lump, lower limb, bilateral**
R22.9 **Localized swelling, mass and lump, unspecified**

✓4ᵗʰ **R23** **Other skin changes**
R23.0 **Cyanosis**
EXCLUDES 1   *acrocyanosis (I73.8)*
           cyanotic attacks of newborn (P28.2)
DEF: Bluish or purplish discoloration of the skin due to an inadequate oxygen blood level.

R23.1 **Pallor**
Clammy skin
R23.2 **Flushing**
Excessive blushing
Code first, if applicable, menopausal and female climacteric states (N95.1)
R23.3 **Spontaneous ecchymoses**
Petechiae
EXCLUDES 1   *ecchymoses of newborn (P54.5)*
           purpura (D69.-)
R23.4 **Changes in skin texture**
Desquamation of skin
Induration of skin
Scaling of skin
EXCLUDES 1   *epidermal thickening NOS (L85.9)*
R23.8 **Other skin changes**
R23.9 **Unspecified skin changes**

Symptoms and signs involving the nervous and musculoskeletal systems (R25-R29)

✓4ᵗʰ **R25** **Abnormal involuntary movements**
EXCLUDES 1   *specific movement disorders (G20-G26)*
           stereotyped movement disorders (F98.4)
           tic disorders (F95.-)

R25.0 **Abnormal head movements**
R25.1 **Tremor, unspecified**
EXCLUDES 1   *chorea NOS (G25.5)*
           essential tremor (G25.0)
           hysterical tremor (F44.4)
           intention tremor (G25.2)
R25.2 **Cramp and spasm**
EXCLUDES 2   *carpopedal spasm (R29.0)*
           charley-horse (M62.831)
           infantile spasms (G40.4-)
           muscle spasm of back (M62.830)
           muscle spasm of calf (M62.831)
R25.3 **Fasciculation**
Twitching NOS
R25.8 **Other abnormal involuntary movements**
R25.9 **Unspecified abnormal involuntary movements**

✓4ᵗʰ **R26** **Abnormalities of gait and mobility**
EXCLUDES 1   *ataxia NOS (R27.0)*
           hereditary ataxia (G11.-)
           locomotor (syphilitic) ataxia (A52.11)
           immobility syndrome (paraplegic) (M62.3)

R26.0 **Ataxic gait**
Staggering gait
AHA: 2022,2Q,12
R26.1 **Paralytic gait**
Spastic gait
R26.2 **Difficulty in walking, not elsewhere classified**
EXCLUDES 1   *falling (R29.6)*
           unsteadiness on feet (R26.81)
AHA: 2016,2Q,7

✓5ᵗʰ **R26.8** **Other abnormalities of gait and mobility**
     R26.81 **Unsteadiness on feet**
     R26.89 **Other abnormalities of gait and mobility**
           AHA: 2020,2Q,29
R26.9 **Unspecified abnormalities of gait and mobility**

✓4ᵗʰ **R27** **Other lack of coordination**
EXCLUDES 1   *ataxic gait (R26.0)*
           hereditary ataxia (G11.-)
           vertigo NOS (R42)
R27.0 **Ataxia, unspecified**
EXCLUDES 1   *ataxia following cerebrovascular disease (I69. with final characters -93)*
R27.8 **Other lack of coordination**
R27.9 **Unspecified lack of coordination**

✓4ᵗʰ **R29 Other symptoms and signs involving the nervous and musculoskeletal systems**

R29.0 Tetany
Carpopedal spasm
> EXCLUDES 1 *hysterical tetany (F44.5)*
> *neonatal tetany (P71.3)*
> *parathyroid tetany (E20.9)*
> *post-thyroidectomy tetany (E89.2)*
DEF: Calcium or other mineral imbalance causing voluntary muscles such as hands, feet, or larynx to spasm rhythmically.

R29.1 Meningismus

R29.2 Abnormal reflex
> EXCLUDES 2 *abnormal pupillary reflex (H57.0)*
> *hyperactive gag reflex (J39.2)*
> *vasovagal reaction or syncope (R55)*

R29.3 Abnormal posture

R29.4 Clicking hip
> EXCLUDES 1 *congenital deformities of hip (Q65.-)*

R29.5 Transient paralysis
Code first any associated spinal cord injury (S14.0, S14.1-, S24.0, S24.1-, S34.0-, S34.1-)
> EXCLUDES 1 *transient ischemic attack (G45.9)*

R29.6 Repeated falls
Falling
Tendency to fall
> EXCLUDES 2 *at risk for falling (Z91.81)*
> *history of falling (Z91.81)*
AHA: 2016,2Q,6
TIP: Code in addition to Parkinson's disease (G20), when documented.

✓5ᵗʰ **R29.7 National Institutes of Health Stroke Scale (NIHSS) score**
Code first the type of cerebral infarction (I63.-)
AHA: 2016,4Q,61-62
TIP: Codes from this subcategory may be assigned based on medical record documentation from clinicians who are not the patient's provider.

✓6ᵗʰ **R29.70 NIHSS score 0-9**
R29.700	NIHSS score 0	UPD
R29.701	NIHSS score 1	UPD
R29.702	NIHSS score 2	UPD
R29.703	NIHSS score 3	UPD
R29.704	NIHSS score 4	UPD
R29.705	NIHSS score 5	UPD
R29.706	NIHSS score 6	UPD
R29.707	NIHSS score 7	UPD
R29.708	NIHSS score 8	UPD
R29.709	NIHSS score 9	UPD

✓6ᵗʰ **R29.71 NIHSS score 10-19**
R29.710	NIHSS score 10	UPD
R29.711	NIHSS score 11	UPD
R29.712	NIHSS score 12	UPD
R29.713	NIHSS score 13	UPD
R29.714	NIHSS score 14	UPD
R29.715	NIHSS score 15	UPD
R29.716	NIHSS score 16	UPD
R29.717	NIHSS score 17	UPD
R29.718	NIHSS score 18	UPD
R29.719	NIHSS score 19	UPD

✓6ᵗʰ **R29.72 NIHSS score 20-29**
R29.720	NIHSS score 20	UPD
R29.721	NIHSS score 21	UPD
R29.722	NIHSS score 22	UPD
R29.723	NIHSS score 23	UPD
R29.724	NIHSS score 24	UPD
R29.725	NIHSS score 25	UPD
R29.726	NIHSS score 26	UPD
R29.727	NIHSS score 27	UPD
R29.728	NIHSS score 28	UPD
R29.729	NIHSS score 29	UPD

✓6ᵗʰ **R29.73 NIHSS score 30-39**
R29.730	NIHSS score 30	UPD
R29.731	NIHSS score 31	UPD
R29.732	NIHSS score 32	UPD
R29.733	NIHSS score 33	UPD
R29.734	NIHSS score 34	UPD
R29.735	NIHSS score 35	UPD
R29.736	NIHSS score 36	UPD
R29.737	NIHSS score 37	UPD
R29.738	NIHSS score 38	UPD
R29.739	NIHSS score 39	UPD

✓6ᵗʰ **R29.74 NIHSS score 40-42**
R29.740	NIHSS score 40	UPD
R29.741	NIHSS score 41	UPD
R29.742	NIHSS score 42	UPD

✓5ᵗʰ **R29.8 Other symptoms and signs involving the nervous and musculoskeletal systems**

✓6ᵗʰ **R29.81 Other symptoms and signs involving the nervous system**

R29.810 Facial weakness
Facial droop
> EXCLUDES 1 *Bell's palsy (G51.0)*
> *facial weakness following cerebrovascular disease (I69. with final characters -92)*

R29.818 Other symptoms and signs involving the nervous system

✓6ᵗʰ **R29.89 Other symptoms and signs involving the musculoskeletal system**
> EXCLUDES 2 *pain in limb (M79.6-)*

R29.890 Loss of height
> EXCLUDES 1 *osteoporosis (M80-M81)*

R29.891 Ocular torticollis
> EXCLUDES 1 *congenital (sternomastoid) torticollis Q68.0*
> *psychogenic torticollis (F45.8)*
> *spasmodic torticollis (G24.3)*
> *torticollis due to birth injury (P15.8)*
> *torticollis NOS M43.6*
DEF: Abnormal head posture as a result of a contracted state of cervical muscles to correct a visual disturbance, either double vision or a visual field defect.

R29.898 Other symptoms and signs involving the musculoskeletal system

✓5ᵗʰ **R29.9 Unspecified symptoms and signs involving the nervous and musculoskeletal systems**

R29.90 Unspecified symptoms and signs involving the nervous system

R29.91 Unspecified symptoms and signs involving the musculoskeletal system

Symptoms and signs involving the genitourinary system (R30-R39)

✓4ᵗʰ **R30 Pain associated with micturition**
> EXCLUDES 1 *psychogenic pain associated with micturition (F45.8)*

R30.0 Dysuria
Strangury

R30.1 Vesical tenesmus
DEF: Feeling of a full bladder even when there is little or no urine in the bladder.

R30.9 Painful micturition, unspecified
Painful urination NOS

✓4ᵗʰ **R31 Hematuria**
> EXCLUDES 1 *hematuria included with underlying conditions, such as:*
> *acute cystitis with hematuria (N30.01)*
> *recurrent and persistent hematuria in glomerular diseases (N02.-)*
AHA: 2017,1Q,17

R31.0 Gross hematuria

R31.1 Benign essential microscopic hematuria

✓5ᵗʰ **R31.2 Other microscopic hematuria**
AHA: 2016,4Q,62

R31.21 Asymptomatic microscopic hematuria
AMH

R31.29 Other microscopic hematuria

R31.9 Hematuria, unspecified

R32 Unspecified urinary incontinence
Enuresis NOS
> EXCLUDES 1   *functional urinary incontinence (R39.81)*
> *nonorganic enuresis (F98.0)*
> *stress incontinence and other specified urinary incontinence (N39.3-N39.4-)*
> *urinary incontinence associated with cognitive impairment (R39.81)*

✓4th **R33 Retention of urine**
> EXCLUDES 1   *psychogenic retention of urine (F45.8)*

R33.0 Drug induced retention of urine
Use additional code for adverse effect, if applicable, to identify drug (T36-T50 with fifth or sixth character 5)

R33.8 Other retention of urine
Code first, if applicable, any causal condition, such as:
enlarged prostate (N40.1)
AHA: 2018,4Q,55

R33.9 Retention of urine, unspecified

R34 Anuria and oliguria
> EXCLUDES 1   *anuria and oliguria complicating abortion or ectopic or molar pregnancy (O00-O07, O08.4)*
> *anuria and oliguria complicating pregnancy (O26.83-)*
> *anuria and oliguria complicating the puerperium (O90.4)*

✓4th **R35 Polyuria**
Code first, if applicable, any causal condition, such as:
enlarged prostate (N40.1)
> EXCLUDES 1   *psychogenic polyuria (F45.8)*

R35.0 Frequency of micturition   *urinary frequency urgency.*
R35.1 Nocturia
✓5th **R35.8 Other polyuria**
AHA: 2021,4Q,26
R35.81 Nocturnal polyuria
> EXCLUDES 2   *nocturnal enuresis (N39.44)*

R35.89 Other polyuria
Polyuria NOS

✓4th **R36 Urethral discharge**
R36.0 Urethral discharge without blood
R36.1 Hematospermia ♂
R36.9 Urethral discharge, unspecified
Penile discharge NOS
Urethrorrhea

R37 Sexual dysfunction, unspecified

✓4th **R39 Other and unspecified symptoms and signs involving the genitourinary system**
R39.0 Extravasation of urine
✓5th **R39.1 Other difficulties with micturition**
Code first, if applicable, any causal condition, such as:
enlarged prostate (N40.1)
R39.11 Hesitancy of micturition
R39.12 Poor urinary stream
Weak urinary steam
R39.13 Splitting of urinary stream
R39.14 Feeling of incomplete bladder emptying
R39.15 Urgency of urination
> EXCLUDES 1   *urge incontinence (N39.41, N39.46)*

R39.16 Straining to void
✓6th **R39.19 Other difficulties with micturition**
AHA: 2016,4Q,63
R39.191 Need to immediately re-void
R39.192 Position dependent micturition
R39.198 Other difficulties with micturition
R39.2 Extrarenal uremia
Prerenal uremia
> EXCLUDES 1   *uremia NOS (N19)*

✓5th **R39.8 Other symptoms and signs involving the genitourinary system**
AHA: 2017,4Q,22-23
R39.81 Functional urinary incontinence
Urinary incontinence due to cognitive impairment, or severe physical disability or immobility
> EXCLUDES 1   *stress incontinence and other specified urinary incontinence (N39.3-N39.4-)*
> *urinary incontinence NOS (R32)*

physically disable or mentally

R39.82 Chronic bladder pain
AHA: 2016,4Q,64
R39.83 Unilateral non-palpable testicle ♂
R39.84 Bilateral non-palpable testicles ♂
R39.89 Other symptoms and signs involving the genitourinary system
R39.9 Unspecified symptoms and signs involving the genitourinary system

Symptoms and signs involving cognition, perception, emotional state and behavior (R40-R46)

> EXCLUDES 2   *symptoms and signs constituting part of a pattern of mental disorder (F01-F99)*

✓4th **R40 Somnolence, stupor and coma**
> EXCLUDES 1   *neonatal coma (P91.5)*
> *somnolence, stupor and coma in diabetes (E08-E13)*
> *somnolence, stupor and coma in hepatic failure (K72.-)*
> *somnolence, stupor and coma in hypoglycemia (nondiabetic) (E15)*

R40.0 Somnolence
Drowsiness
> EXCLUDES 1   *coma (R40.2-)*

R40.1 Stupor
Catatonic stupor
Semicoma
> EXCLUDES 1   *catatonic schizophrenia (F20.2)*
> *coma (R40.2-)*
> *depressive stupor (F31-F33)*
> *dissociative stupor (F44.2)*
> *manic stupor (F30.2)*

✓5th **R40.2 Coma**
Code first any associated:
fracture of skull (S02.-)
intracranial injury (S06.-)

> NOTE   One code from each subcategory, R40.21-R40.23, is required to complete the coma scale

AHA: 2020,3Q,46; 2019,2Q,12; 2018,4Q,70; 2017,4Q,23-25,95; 2015,2Q,17; 2014,1Q,19
TIP: Codes for individual (R40.21-, R40.22-, R40.23-) or total (R40.24-) coma scale scores may be assigned based on medical record documentation from clinicians who are not the patient's provider.
TIP: It is not appropriate to assign individual (R40.21-, R40.22-, R40.23-) or total (R40.24-) coma scale score codes for patients who are sedated or in medically induced comas.

R40.20 Unspecified coma   HCC ESR COM
Coma NOS
Unconsciousness NOS
AHA: 2021,4Q,112-113; 2021,2Q,5
✓6th **R40.21 Coma scale, eyes open**

> The following appropriate 7th character is to be added to subcategory R40.21-, R40.22-, R40.23-, and R40.24-.
> 0   unspecified time
> 1   in the field [EMT or ambulance]
> 2   at arrival to emergency department
> 3   at hospital admission
> 4   24 hours or more after hospital admission

✓7th **R40.211 Coma scale, eyes open, never**   HCC ESR COM UPD
Coma scale eye opening score of 1
✓7th **R40.212 Coma scale, eyes open, to pain**   HCC ESR COM UPD
Coma scale eye opening score of 2
✓7th **R40.213 Coma scale, eyes open, to sound**   UPD
Coma scale eye opening score of 3
✓7th **R40.214 Coma scale, eyes open, spontaneous**   UPD
Coma scale eye opening score of 4
✓6th **R40.22 Coma scale, best verbal response**
✓7th **R40.221 Coma scale, best verbal response, none**   HCC ESR COM UPD
Coma scale verbal score of 1

☑ Additional Character Required   ✓x7th Placeholder Alert   Manifestation   Unspecified Dx   Q QPP   UPD Unacceptable PDx

Chapter 18. Symptoms, Signs and Abnormal Clinical and Laboratory Findings

R40.222–R43.2

√7th **R40.222** **Coma scale, best verbal response, incomprehensible words** `HCC` `ESR` `COM` `UPD`
     Coma scale verbal score of 2
     Incomprehensible sounds (2-5 years of age)
     Moans/grunts to pain; restless (< 2 years old)

√7th **R40.223** **Coma scale, best verbal response, inappropriate words** `UPD`
     Coma scale verbal score of 3
     Inappropriate crying or screaming (< 2 years of age)
     Screaming (2-5 years of age)

√7th **R40.224** **Coma scale, best verbal response, confused conversation** `UPD`
     Coma scale verbal score of 4
     Inappropriate words (2-5 years of age)
     Irritable cries (< 2 years of age)

√7th **R40.225** **Coma scale, best verbal response, oriented** `UPD`
     Coma scale verbal score of 5
     Cooing or babbling or crying appropriately (< 2 years of age)
     Uses appropriate words (2-5 years of age)

√6th **R40.23** **Coma scale, best motor response**

√7th **R40.231** **Coma scale, best motor response, none** `HCC` `ESR` `COM` `UPD`
     Coma scale motor score of 1

√7th **R40.232** **Coma scale, best motor response, extension** `HCC` `ESR` `COM` `UPD`
     Abnormal extensor posturing to pain or noxious stimuli (< 2 years of age)
     Coma scale motor score of 2
     Extensor posturing to pain or noxious stimuli (2-5 years of age)

√7th **R40.233** **Coma scale, best motor response, abnormal flexion** `UPD`
     Abnormal flexure posturing to pain or noxious stimuli (2-5 years of age)
     Coma scale motor score of 3
     Flexion/decorticate posturing (< 2 years of age)

√7th **R40.234** **Coma scale, best motor response, flexion withdrawal** `HCC` `ESR` `COM` `UPD`
     Coma scale motor score of 4
     Withdraws from pain or noxious stimuli (2-5 years of age)

√7th **R40.235** **Coma scale, best motor response, localizes pain** `UPD`
     Coma scale motor score of 5
     Localizes pain (2-5 years of age)
     Withdraws to touch (< 2 years of age)

√7th **R40.236** **Coma scale, best motor response, obeys commands** `UPD`
     Coma scale motor score of 6
     Normal or spontaneous movement (< 2 years of age)
     Obeys commands (2-5 years of age)

√6th **R40.24** **Glasgow coma scale, total score**

     NOTE   Assign a code from subcategory R40.24, when only the total coma score is documented

     AHA: 2021,2Q,4; 2016,4Q,64-65

√7th **R40.241** **Glasgow coma scale score 13-15** `UPD`

√7th **R40.242** **Glasgow coma scale score 9-12** `UPD`

√7th **R40.243** **Glasgow coma scale score 3-8** `HCC` `ESR` `COM` `UPD`

√7th **R40.244** **Other coma, without documented Glasgow coma scale score, or with partial score reported** `HCC` `ESR` `COM` `UPD`

R40.3 **Persistent vegetative state** `HCC` `ESR` `COM`
     DEF: Persistent wakefulness without consciousness due to a nonfunctioning cerebral cortex.

R40.4 **Transient alteration of awareness**
     AHA: 2020,2Q,24

√4th **R41** **Other symptoms and signs involving cognitive functions and awareness**
     EXCLUDES 1   dissociative [conversion] disorders (F44.-)
         mild cognitive impairment, so stated (G31.84)

R41.0 **Disorientation, unspecified**
     Confusion NOS
     Delirium NOS
     AHA: 2022,2Q,11; 2019,2Q,34

R41.1 **Anterograde amnesia**

R41.2 **Retrograde amnesia**

R41.3 **Other amnesia**
     Amnesia NOS
     Memory loss NOS
     EXCLUDES 1   amnestic disorder due to known physiologic condition (F04)
         amnestic syndrome due to psychoactive substance use (F10-F19 with 5th character .6)
         mild memory disturbance due to known physiological condition (F06.8)
         transient global amnesia (G45.4)

R41.4 **Neurologic neglect syndrome**
     Asomatognosia
     Hemi-akinesia
     Hemi-inattention
     Hemispatial neglect
     Left-sided neglect
     Sensory neglect
     Visuospatial neglect
     EXCLUDES 1   visuospatial deficit (R41.842)

√5th **R41.8** **Other symptoms and signs involving cognitive functions and awareness**

R41.81 **Age-related cognitive decline** `A`
     Senility NOS

R41.82 **Altered mental status, unspecified**
     Change in mental status NOS
     EXCLUDES 1   altered level of consciousness (R40.-)
         altered mental status due to known condition - code to condition delirium NOS (R41.0)
     AHA: 2012,4Q,97

R41.83 **Borderline intellectual functioning**
     IQ level 71 to 84
     EXCLUDES 1   intellectual disabilities (F70-F79)

√6th **R41.84** **Other specified cognitive deficit**
     EXCLUDES 1   cognitive deficits as sequelae of cerebrovascular disease (I69.01-, I69.11-, I69.21-, I69.31-, I69.81-, I69.91-)

R41.840 **Attention and concentration deficit**
     EXCLUDES 1   attention-deficit hyperactivity disorders (F90.-)

R41.841 **Cognitive communication deficit**

R41.842 **Visuospatial deficit**

R41.843 **Psychomotor deficit**

R41.844 **Frontal lobe and executive function deficit**

R41.89 **Other symptoms and signs involving cognitive functions and awareness**
     Anosognosia

R41.9 **Unspecified symptoms and signs involving cognitive functions and awareness**
     Unspecified neurocognitive disorder

R42 **Dizziness and giddiness** `O`
     Light-headedness
     Vertigo NOS
     EXCLUDES 1   vertiginous syndromes (H81.-)
         vertigo from infrasound (T75.23)

√4th **R43** **Disturbances of smell and taste**

R43.0 **Anosmia**
     DEF: Permanent or transient absence of smell that may be congenital or acquired.

R43.1 **Parosmia**
     DEF: Abnormal perception of smell usually triggered by environmental odors.

R43.2 **Parageusia**
     DEF: Abnormal perception of taste.

`HCC` CMS-HCC   `Rx` Rx HCC   `ESR` ESRD HCC   `COM` Commercial HCC   `N` Newborn: 0   `P` Pediatric: 0-17   `M` Maternity: 9-64   `A` Adult: 15-124

972   ICD-10-CM 2023

R43.8   **Other disturbances of smell and taste**
Mixed disturbance of smell and taste

R43.9   **Unspecified disturbances of smell and taste**

✓4ᵗʰ **R44**   **Other symptoms and signs involving general sensations and perceptions**

> EXCLUDES 1   alcoholic hallucinations (F10.151, F10.251, F10.951)
> hallucinations in drug psychosis (F11-F19 with fifth to sixth characters 51)
> hallucinations in mood disorders with psychotic symptoms (F30.2, F31.5, F32.3, F33.3)
> hallucinations in schizophrenia, schizotypal and delusional disorders (F20-F29)

> EXCLUDES 2   disturbances of skin sensation (R20.-)

R44.0   **Auditory hallucinations**

R44.1   **Visual hallucinations**

R44.2   **Other hallucinations**

R44.3   **Hallucinations, unspecified**
AHA: 2022,2Q,11

R44.8   **Other symptoms and signs involving general sensations and perceptions**

R44.9   **Unspecified symptoms and signs involving general sensations and perceptions**

✓4ᵗʰ **R45**   **Symptoms and signs involving emotional state**

R45.0   **Nervousness**
Nervous tension

R45.1   **Restlessness and agitation**

R45.2   **Unhappiness**

R45.3   **Demoralization and apathy**
> EXCLUDES 1   anhedonia (R45.84)

R45.4   **Irritability and anger**

R45.5   **Hostility**

R45.6   **Violent behavior**

R45.7   **State of emotional shock and stress, unspecified**

✓5ᵗʰ **R45.8**   **Other symptoms and signs involving emotional state**

     R45.81   **Low self-esteem**

     R45.82   **Worries**

     R45.83   **Excessive crying of child, adolescent or adult**
> EXCLUDES 1   excessive crying of infant (baby) R68.11

     R45.84   **Anhedonia**

   ✓6ᵗʰ **R45.85**   **Homicidal and suicidal ideations**
> EXCLUDES 1   suicide attempt (T14.91)

       R45.850   **Homicidal ideations**

       R45.851   **Suicidal ideations**
AHA: 2022,1Q,29
DEF: Thoughts of committing suicide but no actual attempt of suicide has been made.

     R45.86   **Emotional lability**

     R45.87   **Impulsiveness**

     R45.88   **Nonsuicidal self-harm**   HCC Rx ESR COM
Nonsuicidal self-injury
Nonsuicidal self-mutilation
Self-inflicted injury without suicidal intent
Code also injury, if known
AHA: 2021,4Q,26-27

     R45.89   **Other symptoms and signs involving emotional state**

✓4ᵗʰ **R46**   **Symptoms and signs involving appearance and behavior**

> EXCLUDES 1   appearance and behavior in schizophrenia, schizotypal and delusional disorders (F20-F29)
> mental and behavioral disorders (F01-F99)

R46.0   **Very low level of personal hygiene**

R46.1   **Bizarre personal appearance**

R46.2   **Strange and inexplicable behavior**

R46.3   **Overactivity**

R46.4   **Slowness and poor responsiveness**
> EXCLUDES 1   stupor (R40.1)

R46.5   **Suspiciousness and marked evasiveness**

R46.6   **Undue concern and preoccupation with stressful events**

R46.7   **Verbosity and circumstantial detail obscuring reason for contact**

✓5ᵗʰ **R46.8**   **Other symptoms and signs involving appearance and behavior**

     R46.81   **Obsessive-compulsive behavior**
> EXCLUDES 1   obsessive-compulsive disorder (F42.-)

R46.89   **Other symptoms and signs involving appearance and behavior**

Symptoms and signs involving speech and voice (R47-R49)

✓4ᵗʰ **R47**   **Speech disturbances, not elsewhere classified**

> EXCLUDES 1   autism (F84.0)
> cluttering (F80.81)
> specific developmental disorders of speech and language (F80.-)
> stuttering (F80.81)

✓5ᵗʰ **R47.0**   **Dysphasia and aphasia**

     R47.01   **Aphasia**
> EXCLUDES 1   aphasia following cerebrovascular disease (I69. with final characters -20)
> progressive isolated aphasia (G31.01)

     R47.02   **Dysphasia**
> EXCLUDES 1   dysphasia following cerebrovascular disease (I69. with final characters -21)

R47.1   **Dysarthria and anarthria**
> EXCLUDES 1   dysarthria following cerebrovascular disease (I69. with final characters -22)

✓5ᵗʰ **R47.8**   **Other speech disturbances**
> EXCLUDES 1   dysarthria following cerebrovascular disease (I69. with final characters -28)

     R47.81   **Slurred speech**

     R47.82   *Fluency disorder in conditions classified elsewhere*
Stuttering in conditions classified elsewhere
Code first underlying disease or condition, such as:
Parkinson's disease (G20)
> EXCLUDES 1   adult onset fluency disorder (F98.5)
> childhood onset fluency disorder (F80.81)
> fluency disorder (stuttering) following cerebrovascular disease (I69. with final characters -23)

     R47.89   **Other speech disturbances**

R47.9   **Unspecified speech disturbances**

✓4ᵗʰ **R48**   **Dyslexia and other symbolic dysfunctions, not elsewhere classified**

> EXCLUDES 1   specific developmental disorders of scholastic skills (F81.-)

R48.0   **Dyslexia and alexia**

R48.1   **Agnosia**
Astereognosia (astereognosis)
Autotopagnosia
> EXCLUDES 1   visual object agnosia (R48.3)
DEF: Inability to recognize common things such as faces, objects, smells, or voices.

R48.2   **Apraxia**
> EXCLUDES 1   apraxia following cerebrovascular disease (I69. with final characters -90)

R48.3   **Visual agnosia**
Prosopagnosia
Simultanagnosia (asimultagnosia)

R48.8   **Other symbolic dysfunctions**
Acalculia
Agraphia
AHA: 2017,1Q,27

R48.9   **Unspecified symbolic dysfunctions**

✓4ᵗʰ **R49**   **Voice and resonance disorders**

> EXCLUDES 1   psychogenic voice and resonance disorders (F44.4)

R49.0   **Dysphonia**
Hoarseness

R49.1   **Aphonia**
Loss of voice

✓5ᵗʰ **R49.2**   **Hypernasality and hyponasality**

     R49.21   **Hypernasality**

     R49.22   **Hyponasality**

R49.8   **Other voice and resonance disorders**

R49.9   **Unspecified voice and resonance disorder**
Change in voice NOS
Resonance disorder NOS

Chapter 18. Symptoms, Signs and Abnormal Clinical and Laboratory Findings

General symptoms and signs (R50-R69)

✓4th R50 Fever of other and unknown origin

> EXCLUDES 1   chills without fever (R68.83)
> febrile convulsions (R56.0-)
> fever of unknown origin during labor (O75.2)
> fever of unknown origin in newborn (P81.9)
> hypothermia due to illness (R68.0)
> malignant hyperthermia due to anesthesia (T88.3)
> puerperal pyrexia NOS (O86.4)

R50.2 Drug induced fever
Use additional code for adverse effect, if applicable, to identify drug (T36-T50 with fifth or sixth character 5)
> EXCLUDES 1   postvaccination (postimmunization) fever (R50.83)

✓5th R50.8 Other specified fever

R50.81 *Fever presenting with conditions classified elsewhere*
Code first underlying condition when associated fever is present, such as with:
leukemia (C91-C95)
neutropenia (D70.-)
sickle-cell disease (D57.-)
AHA: 2020,3Q,22; 2014,4Q,22

R50.82 Postprocedural fever
> EXCLUDES 1   postprocedural infection (T81.4-)
> posttransfusion fever (R50.84)
> postvaccination (postimmunization) fever (R50.83)

R50.83 Postvaccination fever
Postimmunization fever

R50.84 Febrile nonhemolytic transfusion reaction
FNHTR
Posttransfusion fever

R50.9 Fever, unspecified
Fever NOS
Fever of unknown origin [FUO]
Fever with chills
Fever with rigors
Hyperpyrexia NOS
Persistent fever
Pyrexia NOS

✓4th R51 Headache

> EXCLUDES 2   atypical face pain (G50.1)
> migraine and other headache syndromes (G43-G44)
> trigeminal neuralgia (G50.0)

AHA: 2020,4Q,38-39

R51.0 Headache with orthostatic component, not elsewhere classified
Headache with positional component, not elsewhere classified

R51.9 Headache, unspecified
Facial pain NOS

R52 Pain, unspecified
Acute pain NOS
Generalized pain NOS
Pain NOS

> EXCLUDES 1   acute and chronic pain, not elsewhere classified (G89.-)
> localized pain, unspecified type - code to pain by site, such as:
> abdomen pain (R10.-)
> back pain (M54.9)
> breast pain (N64.4)
> chest pain (R07.1-R07.9)
> ear pain (H92.0-)
> eye pain (H57.1)
> headache (R51.9)
> joint pain (M25.5-)
> limb pain (M79.6-)
> lumbar region pain (M54.5-)
> pelvic and perineal pain (R10.2)
> renal colic (N23)
> shoulder pain (M25.51-)
> spine pain (M54.-)
> throat pain (R07.0)
> tongue pain (K14.6)
> tooth pain (K08.8)
> pain disorders exclusively related to psychological factors (F45.41)

✓4th R53 Malaise and fatigue

R53.0 Neoplastic (malignant) related fatigue
Code first associated neoplasm

R53.1 Weakness
Asthenia NOS
> EXCLUDES 1   age-related weakness (R54)
> muscle weakness (generalized) (M62.81)
> sarcopenia (M62.84)
> senile asthenia (R54)

AHA: 2017,1Q,7; 2015,1Q,25

R53.2 Functional quadriplegia   HCC ESR COM
Complete immobility due to severe physical disability or frailty
> EXCLUDES 1   frailty NOS (R54)
> hysterical paralysis (F44.4)
> immobility syndrome (M62.3)
> neurologic quadriplegia (G82.5-)
> quadriplegia (G82.50)

AHA: 2016,2Q,6
DEF: Inability to move due to a nonphysiological condition, such as dementia. The patient has no mental ability to move independently.

✓5th R53.8 Other malaise and fatigue

> EXCLUDES 1   combat exhaustion and fatigue (F43.0)
> congenital debility (P96.9)
> exhaustion and fatigue due to excessive exertion (T73.3)
> exhaustion and fatigue due to exposure (T73.2)
> exhaustion and fatigue due to heat (T67.-)
> exhaustion and fatigue due to pregnancy (O26.8-)
> exhaustion and fatigue due to recurrent depressive episode (F33)
> exhaustion and fatigue due to senile debility (R54)

R53.81 Other malaise
Chronic debility
Debility NOS
General physical deterioration
Malaise NOS
Nervous debility
> EXCLUDES 1   age-related physical debility (R54)
AHA: 2021,1Q,43

R53.82 Chronic fatigue, unspecified
~~Chronic fatigue syndrome NOS~~
> EXCLUDES 1   ►chronic fatigue syndrome (G93.32)◄
> ►myalgic encephalomyelitis (G93.32)◄
> ►post infection and related fatigue syndromes (G93.39)◄
> postviral fatigue syndrome ►(G93.31)◄

R53.83   **Other fatigue**
     Fatigue NOS
     Lack of energy
     Lethargy
     Tiredness
     EXCLUDES 2   exhaustion and fatigue due to depressive
             episode (F32.-)

R54   **Age-related physical debility**   [A]
     Frailty
     Old age
     Senescence
     Senile asthenia
     Senile debility
     EXCLUDES 1   age-related cognitive decline (R41.81)
             sarcopenia (M62.84)
             senile psychosis (F03)
             senility NOS (R41.81)

R55   **Syncope and collapse**
     Blackout
     Fainting
     Vasovagal attack
     EXCLUDES 1   cardiogenic shock (R57.0)
             carotid sinus syncope (G90.01)
             heat syncope (T67.1)
             neurocirculatory asthenia (F45.8)
             neurogenic orthostatic hypotension (G90.3)
             orthostatic hypotension (I95.1)
             postprocedural shock (T81.1-)
             psychogenic syncope (F48.8)
             shock NOS (R57.9)
             shock complicating or following abortion or ectopic or molar
                 pregnancy (O00-O07, O08.3)
             shock complicating or following labor and delivery (O75.1)
             Stokes-Adams attack (I45.9)
             unconsciousness NOS (R40.2-)

✓4ᵗʰ R56   **Convulsions, not elsewhere classified**
     EXCLUDES 1   dissociative convulsions and seizures (F44.5)
             epileptic convulsions and seizures (G40.-)
             newborn convulsions and seizures (P90)

   ✓5ᵗʰ R56.0   **Febrile convulsions**

     R56.00   **Simple febrile convulsions**   HCC ESR COM
         Febrile convulsion NOS
         Febrile seizure NOS

     R56.01   **Complex febrile convulsions**   HCC ESR COM
         Atypical febrile seizure
         Complex febrile seizure
         Complicated febrile seizure
         EXCLUDES 1   status epilepticus (G40.901)

   R56.1   **Post traumatic seizures**   HCC ESR COM
     EXCLUDES 1   post traumatic epilepsy (G40.-)

   R56.9   **Unspecified convulsions**   HCC ESR COM
     Convulsion disorder
     Fit NOS
     Recurrent convulsions
     Seizure(s) (convulsive) NOS
     AHA: 2021,1Q,3; 2019,1Q,19

✓4ᵗʰ R57   **Shock, not elsewhere classified**
     EXCLUDES 1   anaphylactic shock NOS (T78.2)
             anaphylactic reaction or shock due to adverse food reaction
                 (T78.0-)
             anaphylactic shock due to adverse effect of correct drug or
                 medicament properly administered (T88.6)
             anaphylactic shock due to serum (T80.5-)
             electric shock (T75.4)
             obstetric shock (O75.1)
             postprocedural shock (T81.1-)
             psychic shock (F43.0)
             shock complicating or following ectopic or molar pregnancy
                 (O00-O07, O08.3)
             shock due to anesthesia (T88.2)
             shock due to lightning (T75.01)
             toxic shock syndrome (A48.3)
             traumatic shock (T79.4)

   R57.0   **Cardiogenic shock**   HCC ESR COM
     EXCLUDES 2   septic shock (R65.21)
     AHA: 2020,3Q,26
     DEF: Associated with myocardial infarction, cardiac tamponade,
     and massive pulmonary embolism. Symptoms include mental
     confusion, reduced blood pressure, tachycardia, pallor, and cold,
     clammy skin.

   R57.1   **Hypovolemic shock**   HCC ESR COM
     AHA: 2019,2Q,7

   R57.8   **Other shock**   HCC ESR COM

   R57.9   **Shock, unspecified**   HCC ESR COM
     Failure of peripheral circulation NOS

R58   **Hemorrhage, not elsewhere classified**
     Hemorrhage NOS
     EXCLUDES 1   hemorrhage included with underlying conditions, such as:
             acute duodenal ulcer with hemorrhage (K26.0)
             acute gastritis with bleeding (K29.01)
             ulcerative enterocolitis with rectal bleeding (K51.01)

✓4ᵗʰ R59   **Enlarged lymph nodes**
     INCLUDES   swollen glands
     EXCLUDES 1   acute lymphadenitis (L04.-)
             chronic lymphadenitis (I88.1)
             lymphadenitis NOS (I88.9)
             mesenteric (acute) (chronic) lymphadenitis (I88.0)

   R59.0   **Localized enlarged lymph nodes**

   R59.1   **Generalized enlarged lymph nodes**
     Lymphadenopathy NOS

   R59.9   **Enlarged lymph nodes, unspecified**

✓4ᵗʰ R60   **Edema, not elsewhere classified**
     EXCLUDES 1   angioneurotic edema (T78.3)
             ascites (R18.-)
             cerebral edema (G93.6)
             cerebral edema due to birth injury (P11.0)
             edema of larynx (J38.4)
             edema of nasopharynx (J39.2)
             edema of pharynx (J39.2)
             gestational edema (O12.0-)
             hereditary edema (Q82.0)
             hydrops fetalis NOS (P83.2)
             hydrothorax (J94.8)
             newborn edema (P83.3)
             pulmonary edema (J81.-)

   R60.0   **Localized edema**

   R60.1   **Generalized edema**
     EXCLUDES 2   nutritional edema (E40-E46)

   R60.9   **Edema, unspecified**
     Fluid retention NOS

R61   **Generalized hyperhidrosis**
     Excessive sweating
     Night sweats
     Secondary hyperhidrosis
     Code first, if applicable, menopausal and female climacteric states
     (N95.1)
     EXCLUDES 1   focal (primary) (secondary) hyperhidrosis (L74.5-)
             Frey's syndrome (L74.52)
             localized (primary) (secondary) hyperhidrosis (L74.5-)

Chapter 18. Symptoms, Signs and Abnormal Clinical and Laboratory Findings

R53.83–R61

Chapter 18. Symptoms, Signs and Abnormal Clinical and Laboratory Findings

☑4ᵗʰ **R62 Lack of expected normal physiological development in childhood and adults**

     EXCLUDES 1   *delayed puberty (E30.0)*
                  gonadal dysgenesis (Q99.1)
                  hypopituitarism (E23.0)

R62.0 Delayed milestone in childhood   P
     Delayed attainment of expected physiological developmental stage
     Late talker
     Late walker

☑5ᵗʰ **R62.5 Other and unspecified lack of expected normal physiological development in childhood**
     EXCLUDES 1   *HIV disease resulting in failure to thrive (B20)*
                  physical retardation due to malnutrition (E45)

     R62.50 Unspecified lack of expected normal physiological development in childhood
         Infantilism NOS

     R62.51 Failure to thrive (child)   P
         Failure to gain weight
         EXCLUDES 1   *failure to thrive in child under 28 days old (P92.6)*
         AHA: 2018,4Q,82
         DEF: Organic failure to thrive (FTT): Acute or chronic illness that interferes with nutritional intake, absorption, metabolism excretion, and energy requirements.
         DEF: Nonorganic failure to thrive (FTT): Symptom of neglect or abuse.

     R62.52 Short stature (child)
         Lack of growth
         Physical retardation
         Short stature NOS
         EXCLUDES 1   *short stature due to endocrine disorder ▶(E34.3-)◀*

     R62.59 Other lack of expected normal physiological development in childhood

R62.7 Adult failure to thrive   A

☑4ᵗʰ **R63 Symptoms and signs concerning food and fluid intake**
     EXCLUDES 1   *bulimia NOS (F50.2)*

R63.0 Anorexia
     Loss of appetite
     EXCLUDES 1   *anorexia nervosa (F50.0-)*
                  loss of appetite of nonorganic origin (F50.89)
     AHA: 2018,4Q,82
     TIP: Assign an additional code from category Z68 when BMI is documented. BMI can be based on documentation from clinicians who are not the patient's provider.

R63.1 Polydipsia
     Excessive thirst

R63.2 Polyphagia
     Excessive eating
     Hyperalimentation NOS

☑5ᵗʰ **R63.3 Feeding difficulties**
     EXCLUDES 2   *eating disorders (F50.-)*
                  feeding problems of newborn (P92.-)
                  infant feeding disorder of nonorganic origin (F98.2-)
     AHA: 2021,4Q,27-28; 2017,1Q,28; 2016,3Q,19

     R63.30 Feeding difficulties, unspecified

     R63.31 Pediatric feeding disorder, acute   P
         Pediatric feeding dysfunction, acute
         Code also, if applicable, associated conditions such as:
            aspiration pneumonia (J69.0)
            dysphagia (R13.1-)
            gastro-esophageal reflux disease (K21.-)
            malnutrition (E40-E46)

     R63.32 Pediatric feeding disorder, chronic   P
         Pediatric feeding dysfunction, chronic
         Code also, if applicable, associated conditions such as:
            aspiration pneumonia (J69.0)
            dysphagia (R13.1-)
            gastro-esophageal reflux disease (K21.-)
            malnutrition (E40-E46)

     R63.39 Other feeding difficulties
         Feeding problem (elderly) (infant) NOS
         Picky eater

R63.4 Abnormal weight loss
     AHA: 2018,4Q,82
     TIP: Assign an additional code from category Z68 when BMI is documented. BMI can be based on documentation from clinicians who are not the patient's provider.

R63.5 Abnormal weight gain
     EXCLUDES 1   *excessive weight gain in pregnancy (O26.0-)*
                  obesity (E66.-)
     AHA: 2018,4Q,82
     TIP: Assign an additional code from category Z68 when BMI is documented. BMI can be based on documentation from clinicians who are not the patient's provider.

R63.6 Underweight
     Use additional code to identify body mass index (BMI), if known (Z68.-)
     EXCLUDES 1   *abnormal weight loss (R63.4)*
                  anorexia nervosa (F50.0-)
                  malnutrition (E40-E46)
     AHA: 2018,4Q,82

R63.8 Other symptoms and signs concerning food and fluid intake

R64 Cachexia   HCC ESR COM
     Wasting syndrome
     Code first underlying condition, if known
     EXCLUDES 1   *abnormal weight loss (R63.4)*
                  nutritional marasmus (E41)
     AHA: 2018,4Q,82; 2017,3Q,24
     TIP: Assign code E43 when emaciated or emaciation is documented in relation to malnutrition.

☑4ᵗʰ **R65 Symptoms and signs specifically associated with systemic inflammation and infection**
     AHA: 2019,2Q,38
     TIP: When documentation states SIRS with an infection, assign only a code for the infection. ICD-10-CM does not offer a code for SIRS due to infectious process. If sepsis is suspected, query the provider.

☑5ᵗʰ **R65.1 Systemic inflammatory response syndrome [SIRS] of non-infectious origin**
     Code first underlying condition, such as:
         heatstroke (T67.0-)
         injury and trauma (S00-T88)
     EXCLUDES 1   *sepsis - code to infection*
                  severe sepsis (R65.2)

     R65.10 Systemic inflammatory response syndrome [SIRS] of non-infectious origin without acute organ dysfunction   HCC ESR COM UPD
         Systemic inflammatory response syndrome (SIRS) NOS
         AHA: 2019,2Q,24

     R65.11 Systemic inflammatory response syndrome [SIRS] of non-infectious origin with acute organ dysfunction   HCC ESR COM UPD
         Use additional code to identify specific acute organ dysfunction, such as:
         acute kidney failure (N17.-)
         acute respiratory failure (J96.0-)
         critical illness myopathy (G72.81)
         critical illness polyneuropathy (G62.81)
         disseminated intravascular coagulopathy [DIC] (D65)
         encephalopathy (metabolic) (septic) (G93.41)
         hepatic failure (K72.0-)

(handwritten, left margin) underlying systematic condition first code

✓5ᵗʰ R65.2 Severe sepsis *(handwritten: never be principal diagnosis)*

Infection with associated acute organ dysfunction

Sepsis with acute organ dysfunction

Sepsis with multiple organ dysfunction

Systemic inflammatory response syndrome due to infectious process with acute organ dysfunction

Code first underlying infection, such as:

infection following a procedure (T81.4-)

infections following infusion, transfusion and therapeutic injection (T80.2-)

puerperal sepsis (O85)

sepsis following complete or unspecified spontaneous abortion (O03.87)

sepsis following ectopic and molar pregnancy (O08.82)

sepsis following incomplete spontaneous abortion (O03.37)

sepsis following (induced) termination of pregnancy (O04.87)

sepsis NOS (A41.9)

Use additional code to identify specific acute organ dysfunction, such as:

acute kidney failure (N17.-)

acute respiratory failure (J96.0-)

critical illness myopathy (G72.81)

critical illness polyneuropathy (G62.81)

disseminated intravascular coagulopathy [DIC] (D65)

encephalopathy (metabolic) (septic) (G93.41)

hepatic failure (K72.0-)

AHA: 2020,2Q,17; 2018,4Q,62-63; 2017,4Q,98-99; 2016,3Q,8

R65.20 Severe sepsis without septic shock `HCC` `ESR` `COM` `UPD`

Severe sepsis NOS

AHA: 2020,2Q,17; 2016,3Q,14; 2013,4Q,119

R65.21 Severe sepsis with septic shock `HCC` `ESR` `COM` `UPD`

AHA: 2018,4Q,63

✓4ᵗʰ R68 Other general symptoms and signs

R68.0 Hypothermia, not associated with low environmental temperature

EXCLUDES 1   *hypothermia NOS (accidental) (T68)*

hypothermia due to anesthesia (T88.51)

hypothermia due to low environmental temperature (T68)

newborn hypothermia (P80.-)

✓5ᵗʰ R68.1 Nonspecific symptoms peculiar to infancy

EXCLUDES 1   *colic, infantile (R10.83)*

neonatal cerebral irritability (P91.3)

teething syndrome (K00.7)

R68.11 Excessive crying of infant (baby) `P`

EXCLUDES 1   *excessive crying of child, adolescent, or adult (R45.83)*

R68.12 Fussy infant (baby) `P`

Irritable infant

R68.13 Apparent life threatening event in infant (ALTE) `P`

Apparent life threatening event in newborn

Brief resolved unexplained event (BRUE)

Code first confirmed diagnosis, if known

Use additional code(s) for associated signs and symptoms if no confirmed diagnosis established, or if signs and symptoms are not associated routinely with confirmed diagnosis, or provide additional information for cause of ALTE

R68.19 Other nonspecific symptoms peculiar to infancy `P`

R68.2 Dry mouth, unspecified

EXCLUDES 1   *dry mouth due to dehydration (E86.0)*

dry mouth due to Sjögren syndrome (M35.0-)

salivary gland hyposecretion (K11.7)

R68.3 Clubbing of fingers

Clubbing of nails

EXCLUDES 1   *congenital clubfinger (Q68.1)*

DEF: Enlarged soft tissue of the distal fingers that usually occurs in heart and lung diseases.

✓5ᵗʰ R68.8 Other general symptoms and signs

R68.81 Early satiety

DEF: Premature feeling of being full after eating only a small amount of food. The mechanism of satiety is multifactorial.

R68.82 Decreased libido `A`

Decreased sexual desire

R68.83 Chills (without fever)

Chills NOS

EXCLUDES 1   *chills with fever (R50.9)*

R68.84 Jaw pain

Mandibular pain

Maxilla pain

EXCLUDES 1   *temporomandibular joint arthralgia (M26.62-)*

R68.89 Other general symptoms and signs

R69 Illness, unspecified

Unknown and unspecified cases of morbidity

Abnormal findings on examination of blood, without diagnosis (R70-R79)

EXCLUDES 2   *abnormal findings on antenatal screening of mother (O28.-)*

abnormalities of lipids (E78.-)

abnormalities of platelets and thrombocytes (D69.-)

abnormalities of white blood cells classified elsewhere (D70-D72)

coagulation hemorrhagic disorders (D65-D68)

diagnostic abnormal findings classified elsewhere - see Alphabetical Index

hemorrhagic and hematological disorders of newborn (P50-P61)

✓4ᵗʰ R70 Elevated erythrocyte sedimentation rate and abnormality of plasma viscosity

R70.0 Elevated erythrocyte sedimentation rate

R70.1 Abnormal plasma viscosity

✓4ᵗʰ R71 Abnormality of red blood cells

EXCLUDES 1   *anemias (D50-D64)*

anemia of premature infant (P61.2)

benign (familial) polycythemia (D75.0)

congenital anemias (P61.2-P61.4)

newborn anemia due to isoimmunization (P55.-)

polycythemia neonatorum (P61.1)

polycythemia NOS (D75.1)

polycythemia vera (D45)

secondary polycythemia (D75.1)

R71.0 Precipitous drop in hematocrit

Drop (precipitous) in hemoglobin

Drop in hematocrit

R71.8 Other abnormality of red blood cells

Abnormal red-cell morphology NOS

Abnormal red-cell volume NOS

Anisocytosis

Poikilocytosis

✓4ᵗʰ R73 Elevated blood glucose level

EXCLUDES 1   *diabetes mellitus (E08-E13)*

diabetes mellitus in pregnancy, childbirth and the puerperium (O24.-)

neonatal disorders (P70.0-P70.2)

postsurgical hypoinsulinemia (E89.1)

✓5ᵗʰ R73.0 Abnormal glucose

EXCLUDES 1   *abnormal glucose in pregnancy (O99.81-)*

diabetes mellitus (E08-E13)

dysmetabolic syndrome X (E88.81)

gestational diabetes (O24.4-)

glycosuria (R81)

hypoglycemia (E16.2)

R73.01 Impaired fasting glucose

Elevated fasting glucose

R73.02 Impaired glucose tolerance (oral)

Elevated glucose tolerance

R73.03 Prediabetes *(handwritten: borderline)*

Latent diabetes

AHA: 2016,4Q,65

R73.09 Other abnormal glucose

Abnormal glucose NOS

Abnormal non-fasting glucose tolerance

R73.9 Hyperglycemia, unspecified

✓4ᵗʰ **R74 Abnormal serum enzyme levels**

✓5ᵗʰ **R74.0 Nonspecific elevation of levels of transaminase and lactic acid dehydrogenase [LDH]**
AHA: 2020,4Q,39

R74.01 Elevation of levels of liver transaminase levels
Elevation of levels of alanine transaminase (ALT)
Elevation of levels of aspartate transaminase (AST)

R74.02 Elevation of levels of lactic acid dehydrogenase [LDH]

R74.8 Abnormal levels of other serum enzymes
Abnormal level of acid phosphatase
Abnormal level of alkaline phosphatase
Abnormal level of amylase
Abnormal level of lipase [triacylglycerol lipase]
AHA: 2019,2Q,6

R74.9 Abnormal serum enzyme level, unspecified

R75 Inconclusive laboratory evidence of human immunodeficiency virus [HIV]
Nonconclusive HIV-test finding in infants
EXCLUDES 1   asymptomatic human immunodeficiency virus [HIV] infection status (Z21)
human immunodeficiency virus [HIV] disease (B20)

✓4ᵗʰ **R76 Other abnormal immunological findings in serum**

R76.0 Raised antibody titer
EXCLUDES 1   isoimmunization in pregnancy (O36.0-O36.1)
isoimmunization affecting newborn (P55.-)
AHA: 2021,1Q,6

✓5ᵗʰ **R76.1 Nonspecific reaction to test for tuberculosis**

R76.11 Nonspecific reaction to tuberculin skin test without active tuberculosis
Abnormal result of Mantoux test
PPD positive
Tuberculin (skin test) positive
Tuberculin (skin test) reactor
EXCLUDES 1   nonspecific reaction to cell mediated immunity measurement of gamma interferon antigen response without active tuberculosis (R76.12)

R76.12 Nonspecific reaction to cell mediated immunity measurement of gamma interferon antigen response without active tuberculosis
Nonspecific reaction to QuantiFERON-TB test (QFT) without active tuberculosis
EXCLUDES 1   nonspecific reaction to tuberculin skin test without active tuberculosis (R76.11)
positive tuberculin skin test (R76.11)

R76.8 Other specified abnormal immunological findings in serum
Raised level of immunoglobulins NOS
AHA: 2021,1Q,6

R76.9 Abnormal immunological finding in serum, unspecified

✓4ᵗʰ **R77 Other abnormalities of plasma proteins**
EXCLUDES 1   disorders of plasma-protein metabolism (E88.0-)

R77.0 Abnormality of albumin

R77.1 Abnormality of globulin
Hyperglobulinemia NOS

R77.2 Abnormality of alphafetoprotein

R77.8 Other specified abnormalities of plasma proteins

R77.9 Abnormality of plasma protein, unspecified
AHA: 2019,2Q,6

✓4ᵗʰ **R78 Findings of drugs and other substances, not normally found in blood**
Use additional code to identify the any retained foreign body, if applicable (Z18.-)
EXCLUDES 1   mental or behavioral disorders due to psychoactive substance use (F10-F19)

R78.0 Finding of alcohol in blood
Use additional external cause code (Y90.-), for detail regarding alcohol level

R78.1 Finding of opiate drug in blood

R78.2 Finding of cocaine in blood

R78.3 Finding of hallucinogen in blood

R78.4 Finding of other drugs of addictive potential in blood

R78.5 Finding of other psychotropic drug in blood

R78.6 Finding of steroid agent in blood

✓5ᵗʰ **R78.7 Finding of abnormal level of heavy metals in blood**

R78.71 Abnormal lead level in blood
EXCLUDES 1   lead poisoning (T56.0-)

R78.79 Finding of abnormal level of heavy metals in blood

✓5ᵗʰ **R78.8 Finding of other specified substances, not normally found in blood**

R78.81 Bacteremia
EXCLUDES 1   sepsis — code to specified infection
DEF: Laboratory finding of bacteria in the blood in the absence of two or more signs of sepsis. Transient in nature, it can progress to septicemia with a severe infectious process.

R78.89 Finding of other specified substances, not normally found in blood
Finding of abnormal level of lithium in blood

R78.9 Finding of unspecified substance, not normally found in blood

✓4ᵗʰ **R79 Other abnormal findings of blood chemistry**
Use additional code to identify any retained foreign body, if applicable (Z18.-)
EXCLUDES 1   asymptomatic hyperuricemia (E79.0)
hyperglycemia NOS (R73.9)
hypoglycemia NOS (E16.2)
neonatal hypoglycemia (P70.3-P70.4)
specific findings indicating disorder of amino-acid metabolism (E70-E72)
specific findings indicating disorder of carbohydrate metabolism (E73-E74)
specific findings indicating disorder of lipid metabolism (E75.-)

R79.0 Abnormal level of blood mineral
Abnormal blood level of cobalt
Abnormal blood level of copper
Abnormal blood level of iron
Abnormal blood level of magnesium
Abnormal blood level of mineral NEC
Abnormal blood level of zinc
EXCLUDES 1   abnormal level of lithium (R78.89)
disorders of mineral metabolism (E83.-)
neonatal hypomagnesemia (P71.2)
nutritional mineral deficiency (E58-E61)

R79.1 Abnormal coagulation profile
Abnormal or prolonged bleeding time
Abnormal or prolonged coagulation time
Abnormal or prolonged partial thromboplastin time [PTT]
Abnormal or prolonged prothrombin time [PT]
▶Low von Willebrand factor◀
EXCLUDES 1   coagulation defects (D68.-)
EXCLUDES 2   abnormality of fluid, electrolyte or acid-base balance (E86-E87)

✓5ᵗʰ **R79.8 Other specified abnormal findings of blood chemistry**

R79.81 Abnormal blood-gas level

R79.82 Elevated C-reactive protein [CRP]

R79.83 Abnormal findings of blood amino-acid level
Homocysteinemia
EXCLUDES 1   disorders of amino-acid metabolism (E70-E72)
AHA: 2021,4Q,28

R79.89 Other specified abnormal findings of blood chemistry
AHA: 2019,2Q,6
TIP: Assign for positive Coombs test when not further clarified in the documentation.

R79.9 Abnormal finding of blood chemistry, unspecified

Abnormal findings on examination of urine, without diagnosis (R80-R82)

EXCLUDES 1   *abnormal findings on antenatal screening of mother (O28.-)*
diagnostic abnormal findings classified elsewhere - see Alphabetical Index
specific findings indicating disorder of amino-acid metabolism (E70-E72)
specific findings indicating disorder of carbohydrate metabolism (E73-E74)

✓4ᵗʰ **R80 Proteinuria**

  EXCLUDES 1   *gestational proteinuria (O12.1-)*

  R80.0 Isolated proteinuria
    Idiopathic proteinuria
    EXCLUDES 1   *isolated proteinuria with specific morphological lesion (N06.-)*

  R80.1 Persistent proteinuria, unspecified
  R80.2 Orthostatic proteinuria, unspecified
    Postural proteinuria
  R80.3 Bence Jones proteinuria
  R80.8 Other proteinuria
  R80.9 Proteinuria, unspecified
    Albuminuria NOS

R81 Glycosuria
  EXCLUDES 1   *renal glycosuria (E74.818)*

✓4ᵗʰ **R82 Other and unspecified abnormal findings in urine**

  INCLUDES   chromoabnormalities in urine
  Use additional code to identify any retained foreign body, if applicable (Z18.-)
  EXCLUDES 2   *hematuria (R31.-)*

  R82.0 Chyluria
    EXCLUDES 1   *filarial chyluria (B74.-)*

  R82.1 Myoglobinuria
  R82.2 Biliuria
  R82.3 Hemoglobinuria
    EXCLUDES 1   *hemoglobinuria due to hemolysis from external causes NEC (D59.6)*
      hemoglobinuria due to paroxysmal nocturnal [Marchiafava-Micheli] (D59.5)
    DEF: Free hemoglobin in blood due to rapid hemolysis of red blood cells. Causes include burns, crushed injury, sickle cell anemia, thalassemia, parasitic infections, or kidney infections.

  R82.4 Acetonuria
    Ketonuria
    DEF: Excessive excretion of acetone in urine that commonly occurs in diabetic acidosis.

  R82.5 Elevated urine levels of drugs, medicaments and biological substances
    Elevated urine levels of catecholamines
    Elevated urine levels of indoleacetic acid
    Elevated urine levels of 17-ketosteroids
    Elevated urine levels of steroids

  R82.6 Abnormal urine levels of substances chiefly nonmedicinal as to source
    Abnormal urine level of heavy metals

✓5ᵗʰ   **R82.7 Abnormal findings on microbiological examination of urine**
    EXCLUDES 1   *colonization status (Z22.-)*
    AHA: 2016,4Q,65
    R82.71 Bacteriuria
    R82.79 Other abnormal findings on microbiological examination of urine
      Positive culture findings of urine

✓5ᵗʰ   **R82.8 Abnormal findings on cytological and histological examination of urine**
    AHA: 2019,4Q,16
    R82.81 Pyuria
      Sterile pyuria
    R82.89 Other abnormal findings on cytological and histological examination of urine

✓5ᵗʰ   **R82.9 Other and unspecified abnormal findings in urine**
    R82.90 Unspecified abnormal findings in urine

  R82.91 Other chromoabnormalities of urine
    Chromoconversion (dipstick)
    Idiopathic dipstick converts positive for blood with no cellular forms in sediment
    EXCLUDES 1   *hemoglobinuria (R82.3)*
      myoglobinuria (R82.1)

✓6ᵗʰ   **R82.99 Other abnormal findings in urine**
    AHA: 2018,4Q,29-30
    R82.991 Hypocitraturia
    R82.992 Hyperoxaluria
      EXCLUDES 1   *primary hyperoxaluria (E72.53)*
    R82.993 Hyperuricosuria
    R82.994 Hypercalciuria
      Idiopathic hypercalciuria
    R82.998 Other abnormal findings in urine
      Cells and casts in urine
      Crystalluria
      Melanuria

Abnormal findings on examination of other body fluids, substances and tissues, without diagnosis (R83-R89)

EXCLUDES 1   *abnormal findings on antenatal screening of mother (O28.-)*
diagnostic abnormal findings classified elsewhere - see Alphabetical Index

EXCLUDES 2   *abnormal findings on examination of blood, without diagnosis (R70-R79)*
abnormal findings on examination of urine, without diagnosis (R80-R82)
abnormal tumor markers (R97.-)

✓4ᵗʰ **R83 Abnormal findings in cerebrospinal fluid**

  R83.0 Abnormal level of enzymes in cerebrospinal fluid
  R83.1 Abnormal level of hormones in cerebrospinal fluid
  R83.2 Abnormal level of other drugs, medicaments and biological substances in cerebrospinal fluid
  R83.3 Abnormal level of substances chiefly nonmedicinal as to source in cerebrospinal fluid
  R83.4 Abnormal immunological findings in cerebrospinal fluid
  R83.5 Abnormal microbiological findings in cerebrospinal fluid
    Positive culture findings in cerebrospinal fluid
    EXCLUDES 1   *colonization status (Z22.-)*
  R83.6 Abnormal cytological findings in cerebrospinal fluid
  R83.8 Other abnormal findings in cerebrospinal fluid
    Abnormal chromosomal findings in cerebrospinal fluid
  R83.9 Unspecified abnormal finding in cerebrospinal fluid

✓4ᵗʰ **R84 Abnormal findings in specimens from respiratory organs and thorax**

  INCLUDES   abnormal findings in bronchial washings
    abnormal findings in nasal secretions
    abnormal findings in pleural fluid
    abnormal findings in sputum
    abnormal findings in throat scrapings
  EXCLUDES 1   *blood-stained sputum (R04.2)*

  R84.0 Abnormal level of enzymes in specimens from respiratory organs and thorax
  R84.1 Abnormal level of hormones in specimens from respiratory organs and thorax
  R84.2 Abnormal level of other drugs, medicaments and biological substances in specimens from respiratory organs and thorax
  R84.3 Abnormal level of substances chiefly nonmedicinal as to source in specimens from respiratory organs and thorax
  R84.4 Abnormal immunological findings in specimens from respiratory organs and thorax
  R84.5 Abnormal microbiological findings in specimens from respiratory organs and thorax
    Positive culture findings in specimens from respiratory organs and thorax
    EXCLUDES 1   *colonization status (Z22.-)*
  R84.6 Abnormal cytological findings in specimens from respiratory organs and thorax
  R84.7 Abnormal histological findings in specimens from respiratory organs and thorax
  R84.8 Other abnormal findings in specimens from respiratory organs and thorax
    Abnormal chromosomal findings in specimens from respiratory organs and thorax
  R84.9 Unspecified abnormal finding in specimens from respiratory organs and thorax

Chapter 18. Symptoms, Signs and Abnormal Clinical and Laboratory Findings

R85–R87.5

✓4ᵗʰ **R85 Abnormal findings in specimens from** digestive organs and abdominal cavity

     INCLUDES   abnormal findings in peritoneal fluid
              abnormal findings in saliva

     EXCLUDES 1   *cloudy peritoneal dialysis effluent (R88.0)*
              fecal abnormalities (R19.5)

R85.0 Abnormal level of enzymes **in specimens from digestive organs and abdominal cavity**

R85.1 Abnormal level of hormones **in specimens from digestive organs and abdominal cavity**

R85.2 Abnormal level of other drugs, medicaments and biological substances in specimens from digestive organs and abdominal cavity

R85.3 Abnormal level of substances chiefly nonmedicinal **as to source in specimens from digestive organs and abdominal cavity**

R85.4 Abnormal immunological **findings in specimens from digestive organs and abdominal cavity**

R85.5 Abnormal microbiological **findings in specimens from digestive organs and abdominal cavity**

     Positive culture findings in specimens from digestive organs and abdominal cavity
     EXCLUDES 1   *colonization status (Z22.-)*

✓5ᵗʰ **R85.6 Abnormal** cytological **findings in specimens from digestive organs and abdominal cavity**

     ✓6ᵗʰ **R85.61 Abnormal cytologic smear of** anus

         EXCLUDES 1   *abnormal cytological findings in specimens from other digestive organs and abdominal cavity (R85.69)*
              anal intraepithelial neoplasia I [AIN I] (K62.82)
              anal intraepithelial neoplasia II [AIN II] (K62.82)
              anal intraepithelial neoplasia III [AIN III] (D01.3)
              carcinoma in situ of anus (histologically confirmed) (D01.3)
              dysplasia (mild) (moderate) of anus (histologically confirmed) (K62.82)
              severe dysplasia of anus (histologically confirmed) (D01.3)

         EXCLUDES 2   *anal high risk human papillomavirus (HPV) DNA test positive (R85.81)*
              anal low risk human papillomavirus (HPV) DNA test positive (R85.82)

         R85.610 Atypical squamous cells of undetermined significance **on cytologic smear of anus [ASC-US]**

         R85.611 Atypical squamous cells cannot exclude high grade **squamous intraepithelial lesion on cytologic smear of anus [ASC-H]**

         R85.612 Low grade squamous intraepithelial **lesion on cytologic smear of anus [LGSIL]**

         R85.613 High grade squamous intraepithelial **lesion on cytologic smear of anus [HGSIL]**

         R85.614 Cytologic evidence of malignancy **on smear of anus**

         R85.615 Unsatisfactory cytologic smear of anus
              Inadequate sample of cytologic smear of anus

         R85.616 Satisfactory anal smear but lacking transformation zone

         R85.618 Other abnormal cytological findings on specimens from anus

         R85.619 Unspecified abnormal cytological findings in specimens from anus
              Abnormal anal cytology NOS
              Atypical glandular cells of anus NOS

     R85.69 Abnormal cytological findings in specimens from other digestive organs and abdominal cavity

R85.7 Abnormal histological **findings in specimens from digestive organs and abdominal cavity**

✓5ᵗʰ **R85.8 Other abnormal findings in specimens from digestive organs and abdominal cavity**

     R85.81 Anal high risk human papillomavirus **[HPV] DNA test positive**
         EXCLUDES 1   *anogenital warts due to human papillomavirus (HPV) (A63.0)*
              condyloma acuminatum (A63.0)

     R85.82 Anal low risk human papillomavirus **[HPV] DNA test positive**
         Use additional code for associated human papillomavirus (B97.7)

     R85.89 Other abnormal findings in specimens from digestive organs and abdominal cavity
         Abnormal chromosomal findings in specimens from digestive organs and abdominal cavity

R85.9 Unspecified abnormal finding in specimens from digestive organs and abdominal cavity

✓4ᵗʰ **R86 Abnormal findings in specimens from** male genital organs

     INCLUDES   abnormal findings in prostatic secretions
              abnormal findings in semen, seminal fluid
              abnormal spermatozoa

     EXCLUDES 1   *azoospermia (N46.0-)*
              oligospermia (N46.1-)

R86.0 Abnormal level of enzymes **in specimens from male genital organs** ♂

R86.1 Abnormal level of hormones **in specimens from male genital organs** ♂

R86.2 Abnormal level of other drugs, medicaments and biological substances in specimens from male genital organs ♂

R86.3 Abnormal level of substances chiefly nonmedicinal **as to source in specimens from male genital organs** ♂

R86.4 Abnormal immunological **findings in specimens from male genital organs** ♂

R86.5 Abnormal microbiological **findings in specimens from male genital organs** ♂
     Positive culture findings in specimens from male genital organs
     EXCLUDES 1   *colonization status (Z22.-)*

R86.6 Abnormal cytological **findings in specimens from male genital organs** ♂

R86.7 Abnormal histological **findings in specimens from male genital organs** ♂

R86.8 Other abnormal findings in specimens from male genital organs ♂
     Abnormal chromosomal findings in specimens from male genital organs

R86.9 Unspecified abnormal finding in specimens from male genital organs ♂

✓4ᵗʰ **R87 Abnormal findings in specimens from** female genital organs

     INCLUDES   abnormal findings in secretion and smears from cervix uteri
              abnormal findings in secretion and smears from vagina
              abnormal findings in secretion and smears from vulva

R87.0 Abnormal level of enzymes **in specimens from female genital organs** ♀

R87.1 Abnormal level of hormones **in specimens from female genital organs** ♀

R87.2 Abnormal level of other drugs, medicaments and biological substances in specimens from female genital organs ♀

R87.3 Abnormal level of substances chiefly nonmedicinal **as to source in specimens from female genital organs** ♀

R87.4 Abnormal immunological **findings in specimens from female genital organs** ♀

R87.5 Abnormal microbiological **findings in specimens from female genital organs** ♀
     Positive culture findings in specimens from female genital organs
     EXCLUDES 1   *colonization status (Z22.-)*

[handwritten margin note: abnormal pap smear]

☑5ᵗʰ R87.6 Abnormal cytological findings in specimens from female genital organs

[handwritten margin note: can't be together]

☑6ᵗʰ R87.61 Abnormal cytological findings in specimens from cervix uteri

EXCLUDES 1   abnormal cytological findings in specimens from other female genital organs (R87.69)
abnormal cytological findings in specimens from vagina (R87.62-)
carcinoma in situ of cervix uteri (histologically confirmed) (D06.-)
cervical intraepithelial neoplasia I [CIN I] (N87.0)
cervical intraepithelial neoplasia II [CIN II] (N87.1)
cervical intraepithelial neoplasia III [CIN III] (D06.-)
dysplasia (mild) (moderate) of cervix uteri (histologically confirmed) (N87.-)
severe dysplasia of cervix uteri (histologically confirmed) (D06.-)

EXCLUDES 2   cervical high risk human papillomavirus (HPV) DNA test positive (R87.810)
cervical low risk human papillomavirus (HPV) DNA test positive (R87.820)

[handwritten: (ASC-US)] R87.610 Atypical squamous cells of undetermined significance on cytologic smear of cervix [ASC-US] ♀

R87.611 Atypical squamous cells cannot exclude high grade squamous intraepithelial lesion on cytologic smear of cervix [ASC-H] ♀

R87.612 Low grade squamous intraepithelial lesion on cytologic smear of cervix [LGSIL] ♀

R87.613 High grade squamous intraepithelial lesion on cytologic smear of cervix [HGSIL] ♀

R87.614 Cytologic evidence of malignancy on smear of cervix ♀

R87.615 Unsatisfactory cytologic smear of cervix ♀
Inadequate sample of cytologic smear of cervix

R87.616 Satisfactory cervical smear but lacking transformation zone ♀

R87.618 Other abnormal cytological findings on specimens from cervix uteri ♀

R87.619 Unspecified abnormal cytological findings in specimens from cervix uteri ♀
Abnormal cervical cytology NOS
Abnormal Papanicolaou smear of cervix NOS
Abnormal thin preparation smear of cervix NOS
Atypical endocervical cells of cervix NOS
Atypical endometrial cells of cervix NOS
Atypical glandular cells of cervix NOS

[handwritten note: pap smear: atypical glandular cells]

☑6ᵗʰ R87.62 Abnormal cytological findings in specimens from vagina
Use additional code to identify acquired absence of uterus and cervix, if applicable (Z90.71-)

EXCLUDES 1   abnormal cytological findings in specimens from cervix uteri (R87.61-)
abnormal cytological findings in specimens from other female genital organs (R87.69)
carcinoma in situ of vagina (histologically confirmed) (D07.2)
dysplasia (mild) (moderate) of vagina (histologically confirmed) (N89.-)
severe dysplasia of vagina (histologically confirmed) (D07.2)
vaginal intraepithelial neoplasia I [VAIN I] (N89.0)
vaginal intraepithelial neoplasia II [VAIN II] (N89.1)
vaginal intraepithelial neoplasia III [VAIN III] (D07.2)

EXCLUDES 2   vaginal high risk human papillomavirus (HPV) DNA test positive (R87.811)
vaginal low risk human papillomavirus (HPV) DNA test positive (R87.821)

R87.620 Atypical squamous cells of undetermined significance on cytologic smear of vagina [ASC-US] ♀

R87.621 Atypical squamous cells cannot exclude high grade squamous intraepithelial lesion on cytologic smear of vagina [ASC-H] ♀

R87.622 Low grade squamous intraepithelial lesion on cytologic smear of vagina [LGSIL] ♀

R87.623 High grade squamous intraepithelial lesion on cytologic smear of vagina [HGSIL] ♀

R87.624 Cytologic evidence of malignancy on smear of vagina ♀

R87.625 Unsatisfactory cytologic smear of vagina ♀
Inadequate sample of cytologic smear of vagina

R87.628 Other abnormal cytological findings on specimens from vagina ♀

R87.629 Unspecified abnormal cytological findings in specimens from vagina ♀
Abnormal Papanicolaou smear of vagina NOS
Abnormal thin preparation smear of vagina NOS
Abnormal vaginal cytology NOS
Atypical endocervical cells of vagina NOS
Atypical endometrial cells of vagina NOS
Atypical glandular cells of vagina NOS

R87.69 Abnormal cytological findings in specimens from other female genital organs ♀
Abnormal cytological findings in specimens from female genital organs NOS

EXCLUDES 1   dysplasia of vulva (histologically confirmed) (N90.0-N90.3)

[handwritten note: cervical cancer history for 2 years not use "C" code. use Z85 (history of malignant neoplasm)]

Chapter 18. Symptoms, Signs and Abnormal Clinical and Laboratory Findings

R87.7   **Abnormal histological findings in specimens from female genital organs** ♀
> EXCLUDES 1   *carcinoma in situ (histologically confirmed) of female genital organs (D06-D07.3)*
> *cervical intraepithelial neoplasia I [CIN I] (N87.0)*
> *cervical intraepithelial neoplasia II [CIN II] (N87.1)*
> *cervical intraepithelial neoplasia III [CIN III] (D06.-)*
> *dysplasia (mild) (moderate) of cervix uteri (histologically confirmed) (N87.-)*
> *dysplasia (mild) (moderate) of vagina (histologically confirmed) (N89.-)*
> *severe dysplasia of cervix uteri (histologically confirmed) (D06.-)*
> *severe dysplasia of vagina (histologically confirmed) (D07.2)*
> *vaginal intraepithelial neoplasia I [VAIN I] (N89.0)*
> *vaginal intraepithelial neoplasia II [VAIN II] (N89.1)*
> *vaginal intraepithelial neoplasia III [VAIN III] (D07.2)*

√5ᵗʰ R87.8   **Other abnormal findings in specimens from female genital organs**

   √6ᵗʰ R87.81   High risk human papillomavirus [HPV] DNA test positive from female genital organs
> EXCLUDES 1   *anogenital warts due to human papillomavirus (HPV) (A63.0)*
> *condyloma acuminatum (A63.0)*

     R87.810   Cervical high risk human papillomavirus [HPV] DNA test positive ♀

     R87.811   Vaginal high risk human papillomavirus [HPV] DNA test positive ♀

   √6ᵗʰ R87.82   Low risk human papillomavirus [HPV] DNA test positive from female genital organs
> Use additional code for associated human papillomavirus (B97.7)

     R87.820   Cervical low risk human papillomavirus [HPV] DNA test positive ♀

     R87.821   Vaginal low risk human papillomavirus [HPV] DNA test positive ♀

   R87.89   Other abnormal findings in specimens from female genital organs ♀
> Abnormal chromosomal findings in specimens from female genital organs

   R87.9   Unspecified abnormal finding in specimens from female genital organs ♀

√4ᵗʰ R88   **Abnormal findings in other body fluids and substances**

   R88.0   Cloudy (hemodialysis) (peritoneal) dialysis effluent

   R88.8   Abnormal findings in other body fluids and substances

√4ᵗʰ R89   **Abnormal findings in specimens from other organs, systems and tissues**
> INCLUDES   abnormal findings in nipple discharge
> abnormal findings in synovial fluid
> abnormal findings in wound secretions

   R89.0   Abnormal level of enzymes in specimens from other organs, systems and tissues

   R89.1   Abnormal level of hormones in specimens from other organs, systems and tissues

   R89.2   Abnormal level of other drugs, medicaments and biological substances in specimens from other organs, systems and tissues

   R89.3   Abnormal level of substances chiefly nonmedicinal as to source in specimens from other organs, systems and tissues

   R89.4   Abnormal immunological findings in specimens from other organs, systems and tissues

   R89.5   Abnormal microbiological findings in specimens from other organs, systems and tissues
> Positive culture findings in specimens from other organs, systems and tissues
> EXCLUDES 1   *colonization status (Z22.-)*

   R89.6   Abnormal cytological findings in specimens from other organs, systems and tissues

   R89.7   Abnormal histological findings in specimens from other organs, systems and tissues

   R89.8   Other abnormal findings in specimens from other organs, systems and tissues
> Abnormal chromosomal findings in specimens from other organs, systems and tissues

   R89.9   Unspecified abnormal finding in specimens from other organs, systems and tissues

Abnormal findings on diagnostic imaging and in function studies, without diagnosis (R90-R94)

> INCLUDES   nonspecific abnormal findings on diagnostic imaging by computerized axial tomography [CAT scan]
> nonspecific abnormal findings on diagnostic imaging by magnetic resonance imaging [MRI][NMR]
> nonspecific abnormal findings on diagnostic imaging by positron emission tomography [PET scan]
> nonspecific abnormal findings on diagnostic imaging by thermography
> nonspecific abnormal findings on diagnostic imaging by ultrasound [echogram]
> nonspecific abnormal findings on diagnostic imaging by X-ray examination
> EXCLUDES 1   *abnormal findings on antenatal screening of mother (O28.-)*
> *diagnostic abnormal findings classified elsewhere - see Alphabetical Index*

√4ᵗʰ R90   **Abnormal findings on diagnostic imaging of central nervous system**

   R90.0   Intracranial space-occupying lesion found on diagnostic imaging of central nervous system

   √5ᵗʰ R90.8   Other abnormal findings on diagnostic imaging of central nervous system

     R90.81   Abnormal echoencephalogram

     R90.82   White matter disease, unspecified

     R90.89   Other abnormal findings on diagnostic imaging of central nervous system
> Other cerebrovascular abnormality found on diagnostic imaging of central nervous system

√4ᵗʰ R91   **Abnormal findings on diagnostic imaging of lung**

   R91.1   Solitary pulmonary nodule
> Coin lesion lung
> Solitary pulmonary nodule, subsegmental branch of the bronchial tree

   R91.8   Other nonspecific abnormal finding of lung field
> Lung mass NOS found on diagnostic imaging of lung
> Pulmonary infiltrate NOS
> Shadow, lung

√4ᵗʰ R92   **Abnormal and inconclusive findings on diagnostic imaging of breast**

   R92.0   Mammographic microcalcification found on diagnostic imaging of breast
> EXCLUDES 2   *mammographic calcification (calculus) found on diagnostic imaging of breast (R92.1)*
> DEF: Calcium and cellular debris deposits in the breast that cannot be felt but can be detected on a mammogram. The deposits can be a sign of cancer, benign conditions, or changes in the breast tissue as a result of inflammation, injury, or an obstructed duct.

   R92.1   Mammographic calcification found on diagnostic imaging of breast
> Mammographic calculus found on diagnostic imaging of breast

   R92.2   Inconclusive mammogram
> Dense breasts NOS
> Inconclusive mammogram NEC
> Inconclusive mammography due to dense breasts
> Inconclusive mammography NEC
> AHA: 2015,1Q,24

   R92.8   Other abnormal and inconclusive findings on diagnostic imaging of breast

√4ᵗʰ R93   **Abnormal findings on diagnostic imaging of other body structures**

   R93.0   Abnormal findings on diagnostic imaging of skull and head, not elsewhere classified
> EXCLUDES 1   *intracranial space-occupying lesion found on diagnostic imaging (R90.0)*

   R93.1   Abnormal findings on diagnostic imaging of heart and coronary circulation
> Abnormal echocardiogram NOS
> Abnormal heart shadow

   R93.2   Abnormal findings on diagnostic imaging of liver and biliary tract
> Nonvisualization of gallbladder

   R93.3   Abnormal findings on diagnostic imaging of other parts of digestive tract

✓5ᵗʰ R93.4 Abnormal findings on diagnostic imaging of urinary organs
    EXCLUDES 2   hypertrophy of kidney (N28.81)
    AHA: 2016,4Q,66

R93.41 Abnormal radiologic findings on diagnostic imaging of renal pelvis, ureter, or bladder
    Filling defect of bladder found on diagnostic imaging
    Filling defect of renal pelvis found on diagnostic imaging
    Filling defect of ureter found on diagnostic imaging

✓6ᵗʰ R93.42 Abnormal radiologic findings on diagnostic imaging of kidney
    R93.421 Abnormal radiologic findings on diagnostic imaging of right **kidney**
    R93.422 Abnormal radiologic findings on diagnostic imaging of left **kidney**
    R93.429 Abnormal radiologic findings on diagnostic imaging of unspecified kidney

R93.49 Abnormal radiologic findings on diagnostic imaging of other urinary organs

R93.5 Abnormal findings on diagnostic imaging of other abdominal regions, including retroperitoneum

R93.6 Abnormal findings on diagnostic imaging of limbs
    EXCLUDES 2   abnormal finding in skin and subcutaneous tissue (R93.8-)
    AHA: 2020,1Q,14

R93.7 Abnormal findings on diagnostic imaging of other parts of musculoskeletal system
    EXCLUDES 2   abnormal findings on diagnostic imaging of skull (R93.0)

✓5ᵗʰ R93.8 Abnormal findings on diagnostic imaging of other specified body structures
    AHA: 2018,4Q,30

✓6ᵗʰ R93.81 Abnormal radiologic findings on diagnostic imaging of testis
    R93.811 Abnormal radiologic findings on diagnostic imaging of right **testicle** ♂
    R93.812 Abnormal radiologic findings on diagnostic imaging of left **testicle** ♂
    R93.813 Abnormal radiologic findings on diagnostic imaging of testicles, bilateral ♂
    R93.819 Abnormal radiologic findings on diagnostic imaging of unspecified testicle ♂

R93.89 Abnormal findings on diagnostic imaging of other specified body structures
    Abnormal finding by radioisotope localization of placenta
    Abnormal radiological finding in skin and subcutaneous tissue
    Mediastinal shift

[handwritten: thickened endometrium]

R93.9 Diagnostic imaging inconclusive due to excess body fat **of patient**

✓4ᵗʰ R94 Abnormal results of function studies
    INCLUDES   abnormal results of radionuclide [radioisotope] uptake studies
    abnormal results of scintigraphy

✓5ᵗʰ R94.0 Abnormal results of function studies of central nervous system
    R94.01 Abnormal electroencephalogram [EEG]
    R94.02 Abnormal brain scan
    R94.09 Abnormal results of other function studies of central nervous system

✓5ᵗʰ R94.1 Abnormal results of function studies of peripheral nervous system and special senses
    ✓6ᵗʰ R94.11 Abnormal results of function studies of eye
    R94.110 Abnormal electro-oculogram [EOG]
    R94.111 Abnormal electroretinogram [ERG]
    Abnormal retinal function study
    R94.112 Abnormal visually evoked potential [VEP]
    R94.113 Abnormal oculomotor **study**
    R94.118 Abnormal results of other function studies of eye
    ✓6ᵗʰ R94.12 Abnormal results of function studies of ear and other special senses
    AHA: 2016,3Q,17
    R94.120 Abnormal auditory **function study**
    R94.121 Abnormal vestibular **function study**
    R94.128 Abnormal results of other function studies of ear and other special senses

✓6ᵗʰ R94.13 Abnormal results of function studies of peripheral nervous system
    R94.130 Abnormal response to nerve stimulation, unspecified
    R94.131 Abnormal electromyogram [EMG]
    EXCLUDES 1   electromyogram of eye (R94.113)
    R94.138 Abnormal results of other function studies of peripheral nervous system

R94.2 Abnormal results of pulmonary function **studies**
    Reduced ventilatory capacity
    Reduced vital capacity

✓5ᵗʰ R94.3 Abnormal results of cardiovascular function **studies**
    R94.30 Abnormal result of cardiovascular function study, unspecified
    R94.31 Abnormal electrocardiogram [ECG] [EKG]
    EXCLUDES 1   long QT syndrome (I45.81)
    R94.39 Abnormal result of other cardiovascular function study
    Abnormal electrophysiological intracardiac studies
    Abnormal phonocardiogram
    Abnormal vectorcardiogram

R94.4 Abnormal results of kidney function **studies**
    Abnormal renal function test

R94.5 Abnormal results of liver function **studies**

R94.6 Abnormal results of thyroid function **studies**

R94.7 Abnormal results of other endocrine function studies
    EXCLUDES 2   abnormal glucose (R73.0-)

R94.8 Abnormal results of function studies of other organs and systems
    Abnormal basal metabolic rate [BMR]
    Abnormal bladder function test
    Abnormal splenic function test

Abnormal tumor markers (R97)

✓4ᵗʰ R97 Abnormal tumor markers
    Elevated tumor associated antigens [TAA]
    Elevated tumor specific antigens [TSA]

R97.0 Elevated carcinoembryonic antigen [CEA]

R97.1 Elevated cancer antigen 125 [CA 125]

✓5ᵗʰ R97.2 Elevated prostate specific antigen [PSA]
    AHA: 2016,4Q,66
    R97.20 Elevated prostate specific antigen [PSA] A ♂
    R97.21 Rising PSA following treatment for malignant neoplasm of prostate A ♂

R97.8 Other abnormal tumor markers

Ill-defined and unknown cause of mortality (R99)

R99 Ill-defined and unknown cause of mortality
    Death (unexplained) NOS
    Unspecified cause of mortality

Chapter 19. Injury, Poisoning, and Certain Other Consequences of External Causes (S00–T88)

Chapter-specific Guidelines with Coding Examples

The chapter-specific guidelines from the ICD-10-CM Official Guidelines for Coding and Reporting have been provided below. Along with these guidelines are coding examples, contained in the shaded boxes, that have been developed to help illustrate the coding and/or sequencing guidance found in these guidelines.

a. Application of 7th characters in Chapter 19

Most categories in chapter 19 have a 7th character requirement for each applicable code. Most categories in this chapter have three 7th character values (with the exception of fractures): A, initial encounter, D, subsequent encounter and S, sequela. Categories for traumatic fractures have additional 7th character values. While the patient may be seen by a new or different provider over the course of treatment for an injury, assignment of the 7th character is based on whether the patient is undergoing active treatment and not whether the provider is seeing the patient for the first time.

For complication codes, active treatment refers to treatment for the condition described by the code, even though it may be related to an earlier precipitating problem. For example, code T84.50XA, Infection and inflammatory reaction due to unspecified internal joint prosthesis, initial encounter, is used when active treatment is provided for the infection, even though the condition relates to the prosthetic device, implant or graft that was placed at a previous encounter.

7th character "A", initial encounter is used for each encounter where the patient is receiving active treatment for the condition.

> Patient evaluated after fall from a skateboard onto the sidewalk, x-rays identify a nondisplaced fracture to the distal pole of the right scaphoid bone. The patient is placed in a cast.
>
> **S62.014A   Nondisplaced fracture of distal pole of navicular [scaphoid] bone of right wrist, initial encounter for closed fracture**
>
> **V00.131A   Fall from skateboard, initial encounter**
>
> **Y93.51   Activity, roller skating (inline) and skateboarding**
>
> **Y92.480   Sidewalk as the place of occurrence of the external cause**
>
> **Y99.8   Other external cause status**
>
> *Explanation:* This fracture would be coded with a seventh character A for initial encounter because the patient received x-rays to identify the site of the fracture and treatment was rendered; this would be considered active treatment.

7th character "D" subsequent encounter is used for encounters after the patient has completed active treatment of the condition and is receiving routine care for the condition during the healing or recovery phase.

> Patient seen in follow-up after fall from a skateboard onto the sidewalk resulted in casting of the right arm. X-rays are taken to evaluate how well the nondisplaced fracture to the distal pole of the right scaphoid bone is healing. The physician feels the fracture is healing appropriately; no adjustments to the cast are made.
>
> **S62.014D   Nondisplaced fracture of distal pole of navicular [scaphoid] bone of right wrist, subsequent encounter for fracture with routine healing**
>
> **V00.131D   Fall from skateboard, subsequent encounter**
>
> *Explanation:* This fracture would be coded with a seventh character D for subsequent encounter, whether the same physician who provided the initial cast application or a different physician is now seeing the patient. Although the patient received x-rays, the intent of the x-rays was to assess how the fracture was healing. There was no active treatment rendered and the visit is therefore considered a subsequent encounter.

The aftercare Z codes should not be used for aftercare for conditions such as injuries or poisonings, where 7th characters are provided to identify subsequent care. For example, for aftercare of an injury, assign the acute injury code with the 7th character "D" (subsequent encounter).

7th character "S", sequela, is for use for complications or conditions that arise as a direct result of a condition, such as scar formation after a burn. The scars are sequelae of the burn. When using 7th character "S", it is necessary to use both the injury code that precipitated the sequela and the code for the sequela itself. The "S" is added only to the injury code, not the sequela code. The 7th character "S" identifies the injury responsible for the sequela. The specific type of sequela (e.g. scar) is sequenced first, followed by the injury code.

See Section I.B.10. Sequelae, (Late Effects)

> Patient with a history of a nondisplaced fracture to the distal pole of the right scaphoid bone due to a fall from a skateboard is seen for evaluation of arthritis to the right wrist that has developed as a consequence of the traumatic fracture.
>
> **M12.531   Traumatic arthropathy, right wrist**
>
> **S62.014S   Nondisplaced fracture of distal pole of navicular [scaphoid] bone of right wrist, sequela**
>
> **V00.131S   Fall from skateboard, sequela**
>
> *Explanation:* The code identifying the specific sequela condition (traumatic arthritis) should be coded first followed by the injury that instigated the development of the sequela (fracture). The scaphoid fracture injury code is given a 7th character S for sequela to represent its role as the inciting injury. The fracture has healed and is not being managed or treated on this admit and therefore is not applicable as a first listed or principal diagnosis. However, it is directly related to the development of the arthritis and should be appended as a secondary code to signify this cause and effect relationship.

b. Coding of injuries

When coding injuries, assign separate codes for each injury unless a combination code is provided, in which case the combination code is assigned. Codes from category T07, Unspecified multiple injuries should not be assigned in the inpatient setting unless information for a more specific code is not available. Traumatic injury codes (S00-T14.9) are not to be used for normal, healing surgical wounds or to identify complications of surgical wounds.

> 11-year-old girl fell from her horse, resulting in a laceration to her right forearm with several large pieces of wooden fragments embedded in the wound as well as abrasions to her right ear; in addition, her right shoulder was dislocated.
>
> **S43.004A   Unspecified dislocation of right shoulder joint, initial encounter**
>
> **S51.821A   Laceration with foreign body of right forearm, initial encounter**
>
> **S00.411A   Abrasion of right ear, initial encounter**
>
> **V80.010A   Animal-rider injured by fall from or being thrown from horse in noncollision accident, initial encounter**
>
> **Y93.52   Activity, horseback riding**
>
> *Explanation:* Each separate injury should be reported. The patient's injury to the forearm is reported with one combination code that captures both the laceration and the foreign body.

The code for the most serious injury, as determined by the provider and the focus of treatment, is sequenced first.

1) Superficial injuries

Superficial injuries such as abrasions or contusions are not coded when associated with more severe injuries of the same site.

2) Primary injury with damage to nerves/blood vessels

When a primary injury results in minor damage to peripheral nerves or blood vessels, the primary injury is sequenced first with additional code(s) for injuries to nerves and spinal cord (such as category S04), and/or injury to blood vessels (such as category S15). When the primary injury is to the blood vessels or nerves, that injury should be sequenced first.

3) Iatrogenic injuries

Injury codes from Chapter 19 should not be assigned for injuries that occur during, or as a result of, a medical intervention. Assign the appropriate complication code(s).

c. Coding of traumatic fractures

The principles of multiple coding of injuries should be followed in coding fractures. Fractures of specified sites are coded individually by site in accordance with both the provisions within categories S02, S12, S22, S32, S42, S49, S52, S59, S62, S72, S79, S82, S89, S92 and the level of detail furnished by medical record content.

A fracture not indicated as open or closed should be coded to closed. A fracture not indicated whether displaced or not displaced should be coded to displaced.

More specific guidelines are as follows:

1) Initial vs. subsequent encounter for fractures

Traumatic fractures are coded using the appropriate 7th character for initial encounter (A, B, C) for each encounter where the patient is receiving active treatment for the fracture. The appropriate 7th character for initial encounter should also be assigned for a patient who delayed seeking treatment for the fracture or nonunion.

Fractures are coded using the appropriate 7th character for subsequent care for encounters after the patient has completed active treatment of the fracture and is receiving routine care for the fracture during the healing or recovery phase.

Care for complications of surgical treatment for fracture repairs during the healing or recovery phase should be coded with the appropriate complication codes.

Care of complications of fractures, such as malunion and nonunion, should be reported with the appropriate 7th character for subsequent care with nonunion (K, M, N,) or subsequent care with malunion (P, Q, R).

Malunion/nonunion: The appropriate 7th character for initial encounter should also be assigned for a patient who delayed seeking treatment for the fracture or nonunion.

Female patient fell during a forest hiking excursion almost six months ago and until recently did not feel she needed to seek medical attention for her left ankle pain; x-rays show nonunion of lateral malleolus and surgery has been scheduled

S82.62XA	Displaced fracture of lateral malleolus of left fibula, initial encounter for closed fracture
W01.0XXA	Fall on same level from slipping, tripping and stumbling without subsequent striking against object, initial encounter
Y92.821	Forest as place of occurrence of the external cause
Y93.01	Activity, walking, marching and hiking
Y99.8	Other external cause status

Explanation: A seventh character of A is used for the lateral malleolus nonunion fracture to signify that the fracture is receiving active treatment. The delayed care for the fracture has resulted in a nonunion, but capturing the nonunion in the seventh character is trumped by the provision of active care.

The open fracture designations in the assignment of the 7th character for fractures of the forearm, femur and lower leg, including ankle are based on the Gustilo open fracture classification. When the Gustilo classification type is not specified for an open fracture, the 7th character for open fracture type I or II should be assigned (B, E, H, M, Q).

A code from category M80, not a traumatic fracture code, should be used for any patient with known osteoporosis who suffers a fracture, even if the patient had a minor fall or trauma, if that fall or trauma would not usually break a normal, healthy bone.

See Section I.C.13. Osteoporosis.

The aftercare Z codes should not be used for aftercare for traumatic fractures. For aftercare of a traumatic fracture, assign the acute fracture code with the appropriate 7th character.

2) Multiple fractures sequencing

Multiple fractures are sequenced in accordance with the severity of the fracture.

3) Physeal fractures

For physeal fractures, assign only the code identifying the type of physeal fracture. Do not assign a separate code to identify the specific bone that is fractured.

d. Coding of burns and corrosions

The ICD-10-CM makes a distinction between burns and corrosions. The burn codes are for thermal burns, except sunburns, that come from a heat source, such as a fire or hot appliance. The burn codes are also for burns resulting from electricity and radiation. Corrosions are burns due to chemicals. The guidelines are the same for burns and corrosions.

Current burns (T20-T25) are classified by depth, extent and by agent (X code). Burns are classified by depth as first degree (erythema), second degree (blistering), and third degree (full-thickness involvement). Burns of the eye and internal organs (T26-T28) are classified by site, but not by degree.

1) Sequencing of burn and related condition codes

Sequence first the code that reflects the highest degree of burn when more than one burn is present.

a. When the reason for the admission or encounter is for treatment of external multiple burns, sequence first the code that reflects the burn of the highest degree.

b. When a patient has both internal and external burns, the circumstances of admission govern the selection of the principal diagnosis or first-listed diagnosis.

c. When a patient is admitted for burn injuries and other related conditions such as smoke inhalation and/or respiratory failure, the circumstances of admission govern the selection of the principal or first-listed diagnosis.

Patient referred for minor first-degree burns to multiple sites of her right and left hands as well as severe smoke inhalation. While she was sleeping at home, a candle on her dresser lit the bedroom curtains on fire.

T59.811A	Toxic effect of smoke, accidental (unintentional), initial encounter
J70.5	Respiratory conditions due to smoke inhalation
T23.191A	Burn of first degree of multiple sites of right wrist and hand, initial encounter
T23.192A	Burn of first degree of multiple sites of left wrist and hand, initial encounter
X08.8XXA	Exposure to other specified smoke, fire and flames, initial encounter
Y99.8	Other external cause status
Y92.003	Bedroom of unspecified non-institutional (private) residence as the place of occurrence of the external cause
Y93.84	Activity, sleeping

Explanation: Based on the documentation, the inhalation injury is more severe than the first-degree burns and is sequenced first. The burns to the hands are appended as secondary diagnoses.

---

2) Burns of the same anatomic site

Classify burns of the same anatomic site and on the same side but of different degrees to the subcategory identifying the highest degree recorded in the diagnosis (e.g., for second and third degree burns of right thigh, assign only code T24.311-).

3) Non-healing burns

Non-healing burns are coded as acute burns.

Necrosis of burned skin should be coded as a non-healed burn.

4) Infected burn

For any documented infected burn site, use an additional code for the infection.

5) Assign separate codes for each burn site

When coding burns, assign separate codes for each burn site. Category T30, Burn and corrosion, body region unspecified is extremely vague and should rarely be used.

Codes for burns of "multiple sites" should only be assigned when the medical record documentation does not specify the individual sites.

6) Burns and corrosions classified according to extent of body surface involved

Assign codes from category T31, Burns classified according to extent of body surface involved, or T32, Corrosions classified according to extent of body surface involved, for acute burns or corrosions when the site of the burn or corrosion is not specified or when there is a need for additional data. It is advisable to use category T31 as additional coding when needed to provide data for evaluating burn mortality, such as that needed by burn units. It is also advisable to use category T31 as an additional code for reporting purposes when there is mention of a third- degree burn involving 20 percent or more of the body surface. Codes from categories T31 and T32 should not be used for sequelae of burns or corrosions.

Categories T31 and T32 are based on the classic "rule of nines" in estimating body surface involved: head and neck are assigned nine percent, each arm nine percent, each leg 18 percent, the anterior trunk 18 percent, posterior trunk 18 percent, and genitalia one percent. Providers may change these percentage assignments where necessary to accommodate infants and children who have proportionally larger heads than adults, and patients who have large buttocks, thighs, or abdomen that involve burns.

Patient seen for dressing change after he accidentally spilled acetic acid on himself two days ago. The second-degree burns to his right thigh, covering about 3 percent of his body surface, are healing appropriately.

T54.2X1D	Toxic effect of corrosive acids and acid-like substances, accidental (unintentional), subsequent encounter
T24.611D	Corrosion of second degree of right thigh, subsequent encounter
T32.0	Corrosions involving less than 10% of body surface

Explanation: Code T32.0 provides additional information as to how much of the patient's body was affected by the corrosive substance.

7) Encounters for treatment of sequela of burns

Encounters for the treatment of the late effects of burns or corrosions (i.e., scars or joint contractures) should be coded with a burn or corrosion code with the 7th character "S" for sequela.

8) Sequelae with a late effect code and current burn

When appropriate, both a code for a current burn or corrosion with 7th character "A" or "D" and a burn or corrosion code with 7th character "S" may be assigned on the same record (when both a current burn and sequelae of an old burn exist). Burns and corrosions do not heal at the same rate and a current healing wound may still exist with sequela of a healed burn or corrosion.

See Section I.B.10. Sequela (Late Effects)

Female patient seen for second-degree burn to the left ear; she also has significant scarring on her left elbow from a third-degree burn from childhood

T20.212A	Burn of second degree of left ear [any part, except ear drum], initial encounter
L90.5	Scar conditions and fibrosis of skin
T22.322S	Burn of third degree of left elbow, sequela

Explanation: The patient is being seen for management of a current second-degree burn, which is reflected in the code by appending the seventh character of A, indicating active treatment or management of this burn. The elbow scarring is a sequela of a previous third-degree burn. The sequela condition precedes the original burn injury, which is appended with a seventh character of S.

9) Use of an external cause code with burns and corrosions

An external cause code should be used with burns and corrosions to identify the source and intent of the burn, as well as the place where it occurred.

e. Adverse effects, poisoning, underdosing and toxic effects

Codes in categories T36-T65 are combination codes that include the substance that was taken as well as the intent. No additional external cause code is required for poisonings, toxic effects, adverse effects and underdosing codes.

1) Do not code directly from the Table of Drugs

Do not code directly from the Table of Drugs and Chemicals. Always refer back to the Tabular List.

2) Use as many codes as necessary to describe

Use as many codes as necessary to describe completely all drugs, medicinal or biological substances.

3) If the same code would describe the causative agent

If the same code would describe the causative agent for more than one adverse reaction, poisoning, toxic effect or underdosing, assign the code only once.

4) If two or more drugs, medicinal or biological substances

If two or more drugs, medicinal or biological substances are taken, code each individually unless a combination code is listed in the Table of Drugs and Chemicals.

If multiple unspecified drugs, medicinal or biological substances were taken, assign the appropriate code from subcategory T50.91, Poisoning by, adverse effect of and underdosing of multiple unspecified drugs, medicaments and biological substances.

5) The occurrence of drug toxicity is classified in ICD-10-CM as follows:

(a) Adverse effect

When coding an adverse effect of a drug that has been correctly prescribed and properly administered, assign the appropriate code for the nature of the adverse effect followed by the appropriate code for the adverse effect of the drug (T36-T50). The code for the drug should have a 5th or 6th character "5" (for example T36.0X5-) Examples of the nature of an adverse effect are tachycardia, delirium, gastrointestinal hemorrhaging, vomiting, hypokalemia, hepatitis, renal failure, or respiratory failure.

(b) Poisoning

When coding a poisoning or reaction to the improper use of a medication (e.g., overdose, wrong substance given or taken in error, wrong route of administration), first assign the appropriate code from categories T36-T50. The poisoning codes have an associated intent as their 5th or 6th character (accidental, intentional self-harm, assault and undetermined). If the intent of the poisoning is unknown or unspecified, code the intent as accidental intent. The undetermined intent is only for use if the documentation in the record specifies that the intent cannot be determined. Use additional code(s) for all manifestations of poisonings.

If there is also a diagnosis of abuse or dependence of the substance, the abuse or dependence is assigned as an additional code.

Examples of poisoning include:

(i)   Error was made in drug prescription
Errors made in drug prescription or in the administration of the drug by provider, nurse, patient, or other person.

(ii   Overdose of a drug intentionally taken
If an overdose of a drug was intentionally taken or administered and resulted in drug toxicity, it would be coded as a poisoning.

(iii)   Nonprescribed drug taken with correctly prescribed and properly administered drug
If a nonprescribed drug or medicinal agent was taken in combination with a correctly prescribed and properly administered drug, any drug toxicity or other reaction resulting from the interaction of the two drugs would be classified as a poisoning.

(iv)   Interaction of drug(s) and alcohol
When a reaction results from the interaction of a drug(s) and alcohol, this would be classified as poisoning.
See Section I.C.4. if poisoning is the result of insulin pump malfunctions.

(c) Underdosing

Underdosing refers to taking less of a medication than is prescribed by a provider or a manufacturer's instruction. Discontinuing the use of a prescribed medication on the patient's own initiative (not directed by the patient's provider) is also classified as an underdosing. For underdosing, assign the code from categories T36-T50 (fifth or sixth character "6"). **Documentation of a change in the patient's condition is not required in order to assign an underdosing code. Documentation that the patient is taking less of a medication than is prescribed or discontinued the prescribed medication is sufficient for code assignment.**

Codes for underdosing should never be assigned as principal or first-listed codes. If a patient has a relapse or exacerbation of the medical condition for which the drug is prescribed because of the reduction in dose, then the medical condition itself should be coded.

Noncompliance (Z91.12-, Z91.13- and Z91.14-) or complication of care (Y63.6-Y63.9) codes are to be used with an underdosing code to indicate intent, if known.

Patient referred for atrial fibrillation with history of chronic atrial fibrillation for which she is prescribed amiodarone. Financial concerns have left the patient unable to pay for her prescriptions and she has been skipping her amiodarone dose every other day to offset the cost.

I48.20	Chronic atrial fibrillation, unspecified
T46.2X6A	Underdosing of other antidysrhythmic drugs, initial encounter
Z91.120	Patient's intentional underdosing of medication regimen due to financial hardship

Explanation: By skipping her amiodarone pill every other day, the patient's atrial fibrillation returned. The condition for which the drug was being taken is reported first, followed by an underdosing code to show that the patient was not adhering to her prescription regiment. The Z code helps elaborate on the patient's social and/or economic circumstances that led to the patient taking less then what she was prescribed.

(d) Toxic effects

When a harmful substance is ingested or comes in contact with a person, this is classified as a toxic effect. The toxic effect codes are in categories T51-T65.

Toxic effect codes have an associated intent: accidental, intentional self-harm, assault and undetermined.

f. Adult and child abuse, neglect and other maltreatment

Sequence first the appropriate code from categories T74, Adult and child abuse, neglect and other maltreatment, confirmed, or T76, Adult and child abuse, neglect and other maltreatment, suspected, for abuse, neglect and other maltreatment, followed by any accompanying mental health or injury code(s).

If the documentation in the medical record states abuse or neglect, it is coded as confirmed (T74.-). It is coded as suspected if it is documented as suspected (T76.-).

For cases of confirmed abuse or neglect an external cause code from the assault section (X92-Y09) should be added to identify the cause of any physical injuries. A perpetrator code (Y07) should be added when the perpetrator of the abuse is known. For suspected cases of abuse or neglect, do not report external cause or perpetrator code.

If a suspected case of abuse, neglect or mistreatment is ruled out during an encounter code Z04.71, Encounter for examination and observation following alleged physical adult abuse, ruled out, or code Z04.72, Encounter for examination and observation following alleged child physical abuse, ruled out, should be used, not a code from T76.

If a suspected case of alleged rape or sexual abuse is ruled out during an encounter code Z04.41, Encounter for examination and observation following alleged adult rape or code Z04.42, Encounter for examination and observation following alleged child rape, should be used, not a code from T76.

If a suspected case of forced sexual exploitation or forced labor exploitation is ruled out during an encounter, code Z04.81, Encounter for examination and observation of victim following forced sexual exploitation, or code Z04.82, Encounter for examination and observation of victim following forced labor exploitation, should be used, not a code from T76.

See Section I.C.15. Abuse in a pregnant patient.

g. Complications of care

1) General guidelines for complications of care

(a) Documentation of complications of care

See Section I.B.16. for information on documentation of complications of care.

2) Pain due to medical devices

Pain associated with devices, implants or grafts left in a surgical site (for example painful hip prosthesis) is assigned to the appropriate code(s) found in Chapter 19, Injury, poisoning, and certain other consequences of external causes. Specific codes for pain due to medical devices are found in the T code section of the ICD-10-CM. Use additional code(s) from category G89 to identify acute or chronic pain due to presence of the device, implant or graft (G89.18 or G89.28).

Chronic left breast pain secondary to breast implant	
T85.848A	Pain due to other internal prosthetic devices, implants and grafts, initial encounter
N64.4	Mastodynia
G89.28	Other chronic postprocedural pain

Explanation: As the pain is a complication related to the breast implant, the complication code is sequenced first. The T code does not describe the site or type of pain, so additional codes may be appended to indicate that the patient is experiencing chronic pain in the breast.

3) Transplant complications

(a) Transplant complications other than kidney

Codes under category T86, Complications of transplanted organs and tissues, are for use for both complications and rejection of transplanted organs. A transplant complication code is only assigned if the complication affects the function of the transplanted organ. Two codes are required to fully describe a transplant complication: the appropriate code from category T86 and a secondary code that identifies the complication.

Pre-existing conditions or conditions that develop after the transplant are not coded as complications unless they affect the function of the transplanted organs.

See I.C.21. for transplant organ removal status

See I.C.2. for malignant neoplasm associated with transplanted organ.

(b) Kidney transplant complications

Patients who have undergone kidney transplant may still have some form of chronic kidney disease (CKD) because the kidney transplant may not fully restore kidney function. Code T86.1- should be assigned for documented complications of a kidney transplant, such as transplant failure or rejection or other transplant complication. Code T86.1- should not be assigned for post kidney transplant patients who have chronic kidney (CKD) unless a transplant complication such as transplant failure or rejection is documented. If the documentation is unclear as to whether the patient has a complication of the transplant, query the provider.

Conditions that affect the function of the transplanted kidney, other than CKD, should be assigned a code from subcategory T86.1, Complications of transplanted organ, Kidney, and a secondary code that identifies the complication.

For patients with CKD following a kidney transplant, but who do not have a complication such as failure or rejection, *see section I.C.14. Chronic kidney disease and kidney transplant status.*

Patient seen for chronic kidney disease stage 2; history of successful kidney transplant with no complications identified	
N18.2	Chronic kidney disease, stage 2 (mild)
Z94.0	Kidney transplant status

Explanation: This patient's stage 2 CKD is not indicated as being due to the transplanted kidney but instead is just the residual disease the patient had prior to the transplant.

4) Complication codes that include the external cause

As with certain other T codes, some of the complications of care codes have the external cause included in the code. The code includes the nature of the complication as well as the type of procedure that caused the complication. No external cause code indicating the type of procedure is necessary for these codes.

5) Complications of care codes within the body system chapters

Intraoperative and postprocedural complication codes are found within the body system chapters with codes specific to the organs and structures of that body system. These codes should be sequenced first, followed by a code(s) for the specific complication, if applicable.

Postprocedural ischemic infarction of the left middle cerebral artery due to cardiac surgery	
I97.820	Postprocedural cerebrovascular infarction following cardiac surgery
I63.512	Cerebral infarction due to unspecified occlusion or stenosis of left middle cerebral artery

Explanation: The infarction was caused by the cardiac procedure and is coded as a postprocedural complication. The postprocedural cerebrovascular infarction is the first-listed diagnosis, followed by the code for the infarction itself.

Complication codes from the body system chapters should be assigned for intraoperative and postprocedural complications (e.g., the appropriate complication code from chapter 9 would be assigned for a vascular intraoperative or postprocedural complication) unless the complication is specifically indexed to a T code in chapter 19.

Muscle/Tendon Table

ICD-10-CM categorizes certain muscles and tendons in the upper and lower extremities by their action (e.g., extension, flexion), their anatomical location (e.g., posterior, anterior), and/or whether they are intrinsic or extrinsic to a certain anatomical area. The Muscle/Tendon Table is provided at the beginning of chapters 13 and 19 as a resource to help users when code selection depends on one or more of these characteristics. A **TIP** has been placed at those categories and/or subcategories that relate to this table. Please note that this table is not all-inclusive, and proper code assignment should be based on the provider's documentation.

Body Region	Muscle	Extensor Tendon	Flexor Tendon	Other Tendon
Shoulder				
	Deltoid	Posterior deltoid	Anterior deltoid	
	Rotator cuff			
	Infraspinatus			Infraspinatus
	Subscapularis			Subscapularis
	Supraspinatus			Supraspinatus
	Teres minor			Teres minor
	Teres major	Teres major		
Upper arm				
	Anterior muscles			
	Biceps brachii — long head		Biceps brachii — long head	
	Biceps brachii — short head		Biceps brachii — short head	
	Brachialis		Brachialis	
	Coracobrachialis		Coracobrachialis	
	Posterior muscles			
	Triceps brachii	Triceps brachii		
Forearm				
	Anterior muscles			
	Flexors			
	Deep			
	Flexor digitorum profundus		Flexor digitorum profundus	
	Flexor pollicis longus		Flexor pollicis longus	
	Intermediate			
	Flexor digitorum superficialis		Flexor digitorum superficialis	
	Superficial			
	Flexor carpi radialis		Flexor carpi radialis	
	Flexor carpi ulnaris		Flexor carpi ulnaris	
	Palmaris longus		Palmaris longus	
	Pronators			
	Pronator quadratus			Pronator quadratus
	Pronator teres			Pronator teres
	Posterior muscles			
	Extensors			
	Deep			
	Abductor pollicis longus			Abductor pollicis longus
	Extensor indicis	Extensor indicis		
	Extensor pollicis brevis	Extensor pollicis brevis		
	Extensor pollicis longus	Extensor pollicis longus		
	Superficial			
	Brachioradialis			Brachioradialis
	Extensor carpi radialis brevis	Extensor carpi radialis brevis		
	Extensor carpi radialis longus	Extensor carpi radialis longus		
	Extensor carpi ulnaris	Extensor carpi ulnaris		
	Extensor digiti minimi	Extensor digiti minimi		
	Extensor digitorum	Extensor digitorum		
	Anconeus	Anconeus		
	Supinator			Supinator

Body Region	Muscle	Extensor Tendon	Flexor Tendon	Other Tendon
Hand				
Extrinsic — attach to a site in the forearm as well as a site in the hand with action related to hand movement at the wrist				
	Extensor carpi radialis brevis	Extensor carpi radialis brevis		
	Extensor carpi radialis longus	Extensor carpi radialis longus		
	Extensor carpi ulnaris	Extensor carpi ulnaris		
	Flexor carpi radialis		Flexor carpi radialis	
	Flexor carpi ulnaris		Flexor carpi ulnaris	
	Flexor digitorum superficialis		Flexor digitorum superficialis	
	Palmaris longus		Palmaris longus	
Extrinsic — attach to a site in the forearm as well as a site in the hand with action in the hand related to finger movement				
	Adductor pollicis longus			Adductor pollicis longus
	Extensor digiti minimi	Extensor digiti minimi		
	Extensor digitorum	Extensor digitorum		
	Extensor indicis	Extensor indicis		
	Flexor digitorum profundus		Flexor digitorum profundus	
	Flexor digitorum superficialis		Flexor digitorum superficialis	
Extrinsic — attach to a site in the forearm as well as a site in the hand with action in the hand related to thumb movement				
	Extensor pollicis brevis	Extensor pollicis brevis		
	Extensor pollicis longus	Extensor pollicis longus		
	Flexor pollicis longus		Flexor pollicis longus	
Intrinsic — found within the hand only				
	Adductor pollicis			Adductor pollicis
	Dorsal interossei	Dorsal interossei	Dorsal interossei	
	Lumbricals	Lumbricals	Lumbricals	
	Palmaris brevis			Palmaris brevis
	Palmar interossei	Palmar interossei	Palmar interossei	
	Hypothenar muscles			
	Abductor digiti minimi			Abductor digiti minimi
	Flexor digiti minimi brevis		Flexor digiti minimi brevis	
	Opponens digiti minimi		Opponens digiti minimi	
	Thenar muscles			
	Abductor pollicis brevis			Abductor pollicis brevis
	Flexor pollicis brevis		Flexor pollicis brevis	
	Opponens pollicis		Opponens pollicis	
Thigh				
	Anterior muscles			
	Iliopsoas		Iliopsoas	
	Pectineus		Pectineus	
	Quadriceps	Quadriceps		
	Rectus femoris	Rectus femoris — Extends knee	Rectus femoris — Flexes hip	
	Vastus intermedius	Vastus intermedius		
	Vastus lateralis	Vastus lateralis		
	Vastus medialis	Vastus medialis		
	Sartorius		Sartorius	
	Medial muscles			
	Adductor brevis			Adductor brevis
	Adductor longus			Adductor longus
	Adductor magnus			Adductor magnus
	Gracilis			Gracilis
	Obturator externus			Obturator externus
	Posterior muscles			
	Hamstring	Hamstring — Extends hip	Hamstring — Flexes knee	
	Biceps femoris	Biceps femoris	Biceps femoris	
	Semimembranosus	Semimembranosus	Semimembranosus	
	Semitendinosus	Semitendinosus	Semitendinosus	

Body Region	Muscle	Extensor Tendon	Flexor Tendon	Other Tendon
Lower leg				
	Anterior muscles			
	Extensor digitorum longus	Extensor digitorum longus		
	Extensor hallucis longus	Extensor hallucis longus		
	Fibularis (peroneus) tertius	Fibularis (peroneus) tertius		
	Tibialis anterior	Tibialis anterior		Tibialis anterior
	Lateral muscles			
	Fibularis (peroneus) brevis		Fibularis (peroneus) brevis	
	Fibularis (peroneus) longus		Fibularis (peroneus) longus	
	Posterior muscles			
	Deep			
	Flexor digitorum longus		Flexor digitorum longus	
	Flexor hallucis longus		Flexor hallucis longus	
	Popliteus		Popliteus	
	Tibialis posterior		Tibialis posterior	
	Superficial			
	Gastrocnemius		Gastrocnemius	
	Plantaris		Plantaris	
	Soleus		Soleus	
				Calcaneal (Achilles)
Ankle/Foot				
Extrinsic — attach to a site in the lower leg as well as a site in the foot with action related to foot movement at the ankle				
	Plantaris		Plantaris	
	Soleus		Soleus	
	Tibialis anterior	Tibialis anterior		
	Tibialis posterior		Tibialis posterior	
Extrinsic — attach to a site in the lower leg as well as a site in the foot with action in the foot related to toe movement				
	Extensor digitorum longus	Extensor digitorum longus		
	Extensor hallucis longus	Extensor hallucis longus		
	Flexor digitorum longus		Flexor digitorum longus	
	Flexor hallucis longus		Flexor hallucis longus	
Intrinsic — found within the ankle/foot only				
	Dorsal muscles			
	Extensor digitorum brevis	Extensor digitorum brevis		
	Extensor hallucis brevis	Extensor hallucis brevis		
	Plantar muscles			
	Abductor digiti minimi		Abductor digiti minimi	
	Abductor hallucis		Abductor hallucis	
	Dorsal interossei	Dorsal interossei	Dorsal interossei	
	Flexor digiti minimi brevis		Flexor digiti minimi brevis	
	Flexor digitorum brevis		Flexor digitorum brevis	
	Flexor hallucis brevis		Flexor hallucis brevis	
	Lumbricals	Lumbricals	Lumbricals	
	Quadratus plantae		Quadratus plantae	
	Plantar interossei	Plantar interossei	Plantar interossei	

Chapter 19. Injury, Poisoning and Certain Other Consequences of External Causes (S00-T88)

NOTE Use secondary code(s) from Chapter 20, External causes of morbidity, to indicate cause of injury. Codes within the T section that include the external cause do not require an additional external cause code.

Use additional code to identify any retained foreign body, if applicable (Z18.-)

EXCLUDES 1 *birth trauma (P10-P15)*
obstetric trauma (O70-O71)

NOTE The chapter uses the S-section for coding different types of injuries related to single body regions and the T-section to cover injuries to unspecified body regions as well as poisoning and certain other consequences of external causes.

AHA: 2016,2Q,3-7; 2015,4Q,35-38; 2015,3Q,37-39,40; 2015,2Q,6; 2015,1Q,3-21

TIP: The specific site of an injury can be determined from the radiology report when authenticated by a radiologist and available at the time of code assignment.

This chapter contains the following blocks:

S00-S09	Injuries to the head
S10-S19	Injuries to the neck
S20-S29	Injuries to the thorax
S30-S39	Injuries to the abdomen, lower back, lumbar spine, pelvis and external genitals
S40-S49	Injuries to the shoulder and upper arm
S50-S59	Injuries to the elbow and forearm
S60-S69	Injuries to the wrist, hand and fingers
S70-S79	Injuries to the hip and thigh
S80-S89	Injuries to the knee and lower leg
S90-S99	Injuries to the ankle and foot
T07	Injuries involving multiple body regions
T14	Injury of unspecified body region
T15-T19	Effects of foreign body entering through natural orifice
T20-T25	Burns and corrosions of external body surface, specified by site
T26-T28	Burns and corrosions confined to eye and internal organs
T30-T32	Burns and corrosions of multiple and unspecified body regions
T33-T34	Frostbite
T36-T50	Poisoning by, adverse effect of and underdosing of drugs, medicaments and biological substances
T51-T65	Toxic effects of substances chiefly nonmedicinal as to source
T66-T78	Other and unspecified effects of external causes
T79	Certain early complications of trauma
T80-T88	Complications of surgical and medical care, not elsewhere classified

Injuries to the head (S00-S09)

INCLUDES injuries of ear
injuries of eye
injuries of face [any part]
injuries of gum
injuries of jaw
injuries of oral cavity
injuries of palate
injuries of periocular area
injuries of scalp
injuries of temporomandibular joint area
injuries of tongue
injuries of tooth

Code also for any associated infection

EXCLUDES 2 *burns and corrosions (T20-T32)*
effects of foreign body in ear (T16)
effects of foreign body in larynx (T17.3)
effects of foreign body in mouth NOS (T18.0)
effects of foreign body in nose (T17.0-T17.1)
effects of foreign body in pharynx (T17.2)
effects of foreign body on external eye (T15.-)
frostbite (T33-T34)
insect bite or sting, venomous (T63.4)

✓4th **S00** **Superficial injury of head**

EXCLUDES 1 *diffuse cerebral contusion (S06.2-)*
focal cerebral contusion (S06.3-)
injury of eye and orbit (S05.-)
open wound of head (S01.-)

Head

The appropriate 7th character is to be added to each code from category S00.
A   initial encounter
D   subsequent encounter
S   sequela

✓5th **S00.0** **Superficial injury of scalp**

   ✓x7th **S00.00** Unspecified superficial injury of scalp

   ✓x7th **S00.01** Abrasion of scalp

   ✓x7th **S00.02** Blister (nonthermal) of scalp

   ✓x7th **S00.03** Contusion of scalp　　　🅾
     Bruise of scalp
     Hematoma of scalp

   ✓x7th **S00.04** External constriction of part of scalp

   ✓x7th **S00.05** Superficial foreign body of scalp
     Splinter in the scalp

   ✓x7th **S00.06** Insect bite (nonvenomous) of scalp

   ✓x7th **S00.07** Other superficial bite of scalp
     EXCLUDES 1 *open bite of scalp (S01.05)*

✓5th **S00.1** **Contusion of eyelid and periocular area**
   Black eye
   EXCLUDES 2 *contusion of eyeball and orbital tissues (S05.1-)*

   ✓x7th **S00.10** Contusion of unspecified eyelid and periocular area

   ✓x7th **S00.11** Contusion of right eyelid and periocular area

   ✓x7th **S00.12** Contusion of left eyelid and periocular area

✓5th **S00.2** **Other and unspecified superficial injuries of eyelid and periocular area**
   EXCLUDES 2 *superficial injury of conjunctiva and cornea (S05.0-)*

   ✓6th **S00.20** Unspecified superficial injury of eyelid and periocular area

     ✓7th **S00.201** Unspecified superficial injury of right eyelid and periocular area

     ✓7th **S00.202** Unspecified superficial injury of left eyelid and periocular area

     ✓7th **S00.209** Unspecified superficial injury of unspecified eyelid and periocular area

   ✓6th **S00.21** Abrasion of eyelid and periocular area

     ✓7th **S00.211** Abrasion of right eyelid and periocular area

     ✓7th **S00.212** Abrasion of left eyelid and periocular area

     ✓7th **S00.219** Abrasion of unspecified eyelid and periocular area

   ✓6th **S00.22** Blister (nonthermal) of eyelid and periocular area

     ✓7th **S00.221** Blister (nonthermal) of right eyelid and periocular area

     ✓7th **S00.222** Blister (nonthermal) of left eyelid and periocular area

     ✓7th **S00.229** Blister (nonthermal) of unspecified eyelid and periocular area

   ✓6th **S00.24** External constriction of eyelid and periocular area

     ✓7th **S00.241** External constriction of right eyelid and periocular area

     ✓7th **S00.242** External constriction of left eyelid and periocular area

     ✓7th **S00.249** External constriction of unspecified eyelid and periocular area

   ✓6th **S00.25** Superficial foreign body of eyelid and periocular area
     Splinter of eyelid and periocular area
     EXCLUDES 2 *retained foreign body in eyelid (H02.81-)*

     ✓7th **S00.251** Superficial foreign body of right eyelid and periocular area

     ✓7th **S00.252** Superficial foreign body of left eyelid and periocular area

     ✓7th **S00.259** Superficial foreign body of unspecified eyelid and periocular area

   ✓6th **S00.26** Insect bite (nonvenomous) of eyelid and periocular area

     ✓7th **S00.261** Insect bite (nonvenomous) of right eyelid and periocular area

     ✓7th **S00.262** Insect bite (nonvenomous) of left eyelid and periocular area

     ✓7th **S00.269** Insect bite (nonvenomous) of unspecified eyelid and periocular area

   ✓6th **S00.27** Other superficial bite of eyelid and periocular area
     EXCLUDES 1 *open bite of eyelid and periocular area (S01.15)*

     ✓7th **S00.271** Other superficial bite of right eyelid and periocular area

     ✓7th **S00.272** Other superficial bite of left eyelid and periocular area

     ✓7th **S00.279** Other superficial bite of unspecified eyelid and periocular area

✓5th **S00.3** **Superficial injury of nose**

   ✓x7th **S00.30** Unspecified superficial injury of nose

   ✓x7th **S00.31** Abrasion of nose

   ✓x7th **S00.32** Blister (nonthermal) of nose

√x 7ᵗʰ **S00.33** **Contusion** of nose   **Q**
Bruise of nose
Hematoma of nose

√x 7ᵗʰ **S00.34** **External constriction** of nose

√x 7ᵗʰ **S00.35** **Superficial foreign body** of nose
Splinter in the nose

√x 7ᵗʰ **S00.36** **Insect bite (nonvenomous)** of nose

√x 7ᵗʰ **S00.37** **Other superficial bite** of nose
EXCLUDES 1   open bite of nose (S01.25)

√5ᵗʰ **S00.4 Superficial injury of ear**

√6ᵗʰ **S00.40** **Unspecified superficial injury of ear**

√7ᵗʰ **S00.401** Unspecified superficial injury of **right** ear

√7ᵗʰ **S00.402** Unspecified superficial injury of **left** ear

√7ᵗʰ **S00.409** Unspecified superficial injury of unspecified ear

√6ᵗʰ **S00.41** **Abrasion** of ear

√7ᵗʰ **S00.411** Abrasion of **right** ear

√7ᵗʰ **S00.412** Abrasion of **left** ear

√7ᵗʰ **S00.419** Abrasion of unspecified ear

√6ᵗʰ **S00.42** **Blister (nonthermal)** of ear

√7ᵗʰ **S00.421** Blister (nonthermal) of **right** ear

√7ᵗʰ **S00.422** Blister (nonthermal) of **left** ear

√7ᵗʰ **S00.429** Blister (nonthermal) of unspecified ear

√6ᵗʰ **S00.43** **Contusion** of ear
Bruise of ear
Hematoma of ear

√7ᵗʰ **S00.431** Contusion of **right** ear   **Q**

√7ᵗʰ **S00.432** Contusion of **left** ear   **Q**

√7ᵗʰ **S00.439** Contusion of unspecified ear   **Q**

√6ᵗʰ **S00.44** **External constriction** of ear

√7ᵗʰ **S00.441** External constriction of **right** ear

√7ᵗʰ **S00.442** External constriction of **left** ear

√7ᵗʰ **S00.449** External constriction of unspecified ear

√6ᵗʰ **S00.45** **Superficial foreign body** of ear
Splinter in the ear

√7ᵗʰ **S00.451** Superficial foreign body of **right** ear

√7ᵗʰ **S00.452** Superficial foreign body of **left** ear

√7ᵗʰ **S00.459** Superficial foreign body of unspecified ear

√6ᵗʰ **S00.46** **Insect bite (nonvenomous)** of ear

√7ᵗʰ **S00.461** Insect bite (nonvenomous) of **right** ear

√7ᵗʰ **S00.462** Insect bite (nonvenomous) of **left** ear

√7ᵗʰ **S00.469** Insect bite (nonvenomous) of unspecified ear

√6ᵗʰ **S00.47** **Other superficial bite** of ear
EXCLUDES 1   open bite of ear (S01.35)

√7ᵗʰ **S00.471** Other superficial bite of **right** ear

√7ᵗʰ **S00.472** Other superficial bite of **left** ear

√7ᵗʰ **S00.479** Other superficial bite of unspecified ear

√5ᵗʰ **S00.5 Superficial injury of lip and oral cavity**

√6ᵗʰ **S00.50** **Unspecified superficial injury of lip and oral cavity**

√7ᵗʰ **S00.501** Unspecified superficial injury of **lip**

√7ᵗʰ **S00.502** Unspecified superficial injury of **oral cavity**

√6ᵗʰ **S00.51** **Abrasion of lip and oral cavity**

√7ᵗʰ **S00.511** Abrasion of **lip**

√7ᵗʰ **S00.512** Abrasion of **oral cavity**

√6ᵗʰ **S00.52** **Blister (nonthermal) of lip and oral cavity**

√7ᵗʰ **S00.521** Blister (nonthermal) of **lip**

√7ᵗʰ **S00.522** Blister (nonthermal) of **oral cavity**

√6ᵗʰ **S00.53** **Contusion of lip and oral cavity**

√7ᵗʰ **S00.531** **Contusion** of **lip**   **Q**
Bruise of lip
Hematoma of lip

√7ᵗʰ **S00.532** **Contusion** of **oral cavity**   **Q**
Bruise of oral cavity
Hematoma of oral cavity

√6ᵗʰ **S00.54** **External constriction of lip and oral cavity**

√7ᵗʰ **S00.541** **External constriction** of **lip**

√7ᵗʰ **S00.542** **External constriction** of **oral cavity**

√6ᵗʰ **S00.55** **Superficial foreign body of lip and oral cavity**

√7ᵗʰ **S00.551** **Superficial foreign body** of **lip**
Splinter of lip and oral cavity

√7ᵗʰ **S00.552** **Superficial foreign body** of **oral cavity**
Splinter of lip and oral cavity

√6ᵗʰ **S00.56** **Insect bite (nonvenomous)** of lip and oral cavity

√7ᵗʰ **S00.561** Insect bite (nonvenomous) of **lip**

√7ᵗʰ **S00.562** Insect bite (nonvenomous) of **oral cavity**

√6ᵗʰ **S00.57** **Other superficial bite** of lip and oral cavity

√7ᵗʰ **S00.571** Other superficial bite of **lip**
EXCLUDES 1   open bite of lip (S01.551)

√7ᵗʰ **S00.572** Other superficial bite of **oral cavity**
EXCLUDES 1   open bite of oral cavity (S01.552)

√5ᵗʰ **S00.8 Superficial injury of other parts of head**
Superficial injuries of face [any part]

√x 7ᵗʰ **S00.80** **Unspecified superficial injury of other part of head**

√x 7ᵗʰ **S00.81** **Abrasion** of other part of head

√x 7ᵗʰ **S00.82** **Blister (nonthermal)** of other part of head

√x 7ᵗʰ **S00.83** **Contusion** of other part of head   **Q**
Bruise of other part of head
Hematoma of other part of head

√x 7ᵗʰ **S00.84** **External constriction** of other part of head

√x 7ᵗʰ **S00.85** **Superficial foreign body** of other part of head
Splinter in other part of head

√x 7ᵗʰ **S00.86** **Insect bite (nonvenomous)** of other part of head

√x 7ᵗʰ **S00.87** **Other superficial bite** of other part of head
EXCLUDES 1   open bite of other part of head (S01.85)

√5ᵗʰ **S00.9 Superficial injury of unspecified part of head**

√x 7ᵗʰ **S00.90** **Unspecified superficial injury of unspecified part of head**

√x 7ᵗʰ **S00.91** **Abrasion** of unspecified part of head

√x 7ᵗʰ **S00.92** **Blister (nonthermal)** of unspecified part of head

√x 7ᵗʰ **S00.93** **Contusion** of unspecified part of head   **Q**
Bruise of head
Hematoma of head

√x 7ᵗʰ **S00.94** **External constriction** of unspecified part of head

√x 7ᵗʰ **S00.95** **Superficial foreign body** of unspecified part of head
Splinter of head

√x 7ᵗʰ **S00.96** **Insect bite (nonvenomous)** of unspecified part of head

√x 7ᵗʰ **S00.97** **Other superficial bite** of unspecified part of head
EXCLUDES 1   open bite of head (S01.95)

√4ᵗʰ **S01 Open wound of head**
Code also any associated:
injury of cranial nerve (S04.-)
injury of muscle and tendon of head (S09.1-)
intracranial injury (S06.-)
wound infection
EXCLUDES 1   open skull fracture (S02.- with 7th character B)
EXCLUDES 2   injury of eye and orbit (S05.-)
traumatic amputation of part of head (S08.-)

The appropriate 7th character is to be added to each code from category S01.
A   initial encounter
D   subsequent encounter
S   sequela

√5ᵗʰ **S01.0 Open wound of scalp**
EXCLUDES 1   avulsion of scalp (S08.0-)

√x 7ᵗʰ **S01.00** **Unspecified open wound of scalp**

√x 7ᵗʰ **S01.01** **Laceration without foreign body** of scalp

√x 7ᵗʰ **S01.02** **Laceration with foreign body** of scalp

√x 7ᵗʰ **S01.03** **Puncture wound without foreign body** of scalp

√x 7ᵗʰ **S01.04** **Puncture wound with foreign body** of scalp

√x 7ᵗʰ **S01.05** **Open bite** of scalp
Bite of scalp NOS
EXCLUDES 1   superficial bite of scalp (S00.06, S00.07-)

✓5ᵗʰ **S01.1** **Open wound of** eyelid and periocular area

     Open wound of eyelid and periocular area with or without involvement of lacrimal passages

     ✓6ᵗʰ **S01.10** **Unspecified open wound of eyelid and periocular area**

         ✓7ᵗʰ **S01.101** **Unspecified open wound of** right **eyelid and periocular area**

         ✓7ᵗʰ **S01.102** **Unspecified open wound of** left **eyelid and periocular area**

         ✓7ᵗʰ **S01.109** **Unspecified open wound of unspecified eyelid and periocular area**

     ✓6ᵗʰ **S01.11** Laceration without foreign body of eyelid and periocular area

         ✓7ᵗʰ **S01.111** **Laceration without foreign body of** right **eyelid and periocular area**

         ✓7ᵗʰ **S01.112** **Laceration without foreign body of** left **eyelid and periocular area**

         ✓7ᵗʰ **S01.119** **Laceration without foreign body of unspecified eyelid and periocular area**

     ✓6ᵗʰ **S01.12** Laceration with foreign body of eyelid and periocular area

         ✓7ᵗʰ **S01.121** **Laceration with foreign body of** right **eyelid and periocular area**

         ✓7ᵗʰ **S01.122** **Laceration with foreign body of** left **eyelid and periocular area**

         ✓7ᵗʰ **S01.129** **Laceration with foreign body of unspecified eyelid and periocular area**

     ✓6ᵗʰ **S01.13** Puncture wound without foreign body of eyelid and periocular area

         ✓7ᵗʰ **S01.131** **Puncture wound without foreign body of** right **eyelid and periocular area**

         ✓7ᵗʰ **S01.132** **Puncture wound without foreign body of** left **eyelid and periocular area**

         ✓7ᵗʰ **S01.139** **Puncture wound without foreign body of unspecified eyelid and periocular area**

     ✓6ᵗʰ **S01.14** Puncture wound with foreign body of eyelid and periocular area

         ✓7ᵗʰ **S01.141** **Puncture wound with foreign body of** right **eyelid and periocular area**

         ✓7ᵗʰ **S01.142** **Puncture wound with foreign body of** left **eyelid and periocular area**

         ✓7ᵗʰ **S01.149** **Puncture wound with foreign body of unspecified eyelid and periocular area**

     ✓6ᵗʰ **S01.15** Open bite of eyelid and periocular area

         Bite of eyelid and periocular area NOS

             EXCLUDES 1   *superficial bite of eyelid and periocular area (S00.26, S00.27)*

         ✓7ᵗʰ **S01.151** **Open bite of** right **eyelid and periocular area**

         ✓7ᵗʰ **S01.152** **Open bite of** left **eyelid and periocular area**

         ✓7ᵗʰ **S01.159** **Open bite of unspecified eyelid and periocular area**

✓5ᵗʰ **S01.2** **Open wound of** nose

     ✓x7ᵗʰ **S01.20** **Unspecified open wound of nose**

     ✓x7ᵗʰ **S01.21** Laceration without foreign body **of nose**

     ✓x7ᵗʰ **S01.22** Laceration with foreign body **of nose**

     ✓x7ᵗʰ **S01.23** Puncture wound without foreign body **of nose**

     ✓x7ᵗʰ **S01.24** Puncture wound with foreign body **of nose**

     ✓x7ᵗʰ **S01.25** Open bite **of nose**

         Bite of nose NOS

             EXCLUDES 1   *superficial bite of nose (S00.36, S00.37)*

✓5ᵗʰ **S01.3** **Open wound of** ear

     ✓6ᵗʰ **S01.30** **Unspecified open wound of ear**

         ✓7ᵗʰ **S01.301** **Unspecified open wound of** right **ear**

         ✓7ᵗʰ **S01.302** **Unspecified open wound of** left **ear**

         ✓7ᵗʰ **S01.309** **Unspecified open wound of unspecified ear**

     ✓6ᵗʰ **S01.31** Laceration without foreign body **of ear**

         ✓7ᵗʰ **S01.311** **Laceration without foreign body of** right **ear**

         ✓7ᵗʰ **S01.312** **Laceration without foreign body of** left **ear**

         ✓7ᵗʰ **S01.319** **Laceration without foreign body of unspecified ear**

     ✓6ᵗʰ **S01.32** Laceration with foreign body **of ear**

         ✓7ᵗʰ **S01.321** **Laceration with foreign body of** right **ear**

         ✓7ᵗʰ **S01.322** **Laceration with foreign body of** left **ear**

         ✓7ᵗʰ **S01.329** **Laceration with foreign body of unspecified ear**

     ✓6ᵗʰ **S01.33** Puncture wound without foreign body **of ear**

         ✓7ᵗʰ **S01.331** **Puncture wound without foreign body of** right **ear**

         ✓7ᵗʰ **S01.332** **Puncture wound without foreign body of** left **ear**

         ✓7ᵗʰ **S01.339** **Puncture wound without foreign body of unspecified ear**

     ✓6ᵗʰ **S01.34** Puncture wound with foreign body **of ear**

         ✓7ᵗʰ **S01.341** **Puncture wound with foreign body of** right **ear**

         ✓7ᵗʰ **S01.342** **Puncture wound with foreign body of** left **ear**

         ✓7ᵗʰ **S01.349** **Puncture wound with foreign body of unspecified ear**

     ✓6ᵗʰ **S01.35** Open bite **of ear**

         Bite of ear NOS

             EXCLUDES 1   *superficial bite of ear (S00.46, S00.47)*

         ✓7ᵗʰ **S01.351** **Open bite of** right **ear**

         ✓7ᵗʰ **S01.352** **Open bite of** left **ear**

         ✓7ᵗʰ **S01.359** **Open bite of unspecified ear**

✓5ᵗʰ **S01.4** **Open wound of** cheek and temporomandibular area

     ✓6ᵗʰ **S01.40** **Unspecified open wound of cheek and temporomandibular area**

         ✓7ᵗʰ **S01.401** **Unspecified open wound of** right **cheek and temporomandibular area**

         ✓7ᵗʰ **S01.402** **Unspecified open wound of** left **cheek and temporomandibular area**

         ✓7ᵗʰ **S01.409** **Unspecified open wound of unspecified cheek and temporomandibular area**

     ✓6ᵗʰ **S01.41** Laceration without foreign body of cheek and temporomandibular area

         ✓7ᵗʰ **S01.411** **Laceration without foreign body of** right **cheek and temporomandibular area**

         ✓7ᵗʰ **S01.412** **Laceration without foreign body of** left **cheek and temporomandibular area**

         ✓7ᵗʰ **S01.419** **Laceration without foreign body of unspecified cheek and temporomandibular area**

     ✓6ᵗʰ **S01.42** Laceration with foreign body of cheek and temporomandibular area

         ✓7ᵗʰ **S01.421** **Laceration with foreign body of** right **cheek and temporomandibular area**

         ✓7ᵗʰ **S01.422** **Laceration with foreign body of** left **cheek and temporomandibular area**

         ✓7ᵗʰ **S01.429** **Laceration with foreign body of unspecified cheek and temporomandibular area**

     ✓6ᵗʰ **S01.43** Puncture wound without foreign body of cheek and temporomandibular area

         ✓7ᵗʰ **S01.431** **Puncture wound without foreign body of** right **cheek and temporomandibular area**

         ✓7ᵗʰ **S01.432** **Puncture wound without foreign body of** left **cheek and temporomandibular area**

         ✓7ᵗʰ **S01.439** **Puncture wound without foreign body of unspecified cheek and temporomandibular area**

     ✓6ᵗʰ **S01.44** Puncture wound with foreign body of cheek and temporomandibular area

         ✓7ᵗʰ **S01.441** **Puncture wound with foreign body of** right **cheek and temporomandibular area**

         ✓7ᵗʰ **S01.442** **Puncture wound with foreign body of** left **cheek and temporomandibular area**

         ✓7ᵗʰ **S01.449** **Puncture wound with foreign body of unspecified cheek and temporomandibular area**

     ✓6ᵗʰ **S01.45** Open bite of cheek and temporomandibular area

         Bite of cheek and temporomandibular area NOS

             EXCLUDES 2   *superficial bite of cheek and temporomandibular area (S00.86, S00.87)*

         ✓7ᵗʰ **S01.451** **Open bite of** right **cheek and temporomandibular area**

         ✓7ᵗʰ **S01.452** **Open bite of** left **cheek and temporomandibular area**

         ✓7ᵗʰ **S01.459** **Open bite of unspecified cheek and temporomandibular area**

HCC CMS-HCC   **Rx** Rx HCC   **ESR** ESRD HCC   **COM** Commercial HCC   **N** Newborn: 0   **P** Pediatric: 0-17   **M** Maternity: 9-64   **A** Adult: 15-124

994

ICD-10-CM 2023

√5ᵗʰ **S01.5 Open wound of lip and oral cavity**
EXCLUDES 2   tooth dislocation (S03.2)
tooth fracture (S02.5)
√6ᵗʰ **S01.50 Unspecified open wound of lip and oral cavity**
√7ᵗʰ **S01.501 Unspecified open wound of lip**
√7ᵗʰ **S01.502 Unspecified open wound of oral cavity**
√6ᵗʰ **S01.51 Laceration of lip and oral cavity without foreign body**
√7ᵗʰ **S01.511 Laceration without foreign body of lip**
√7ᵗʰ **S01.512 Laceration without foreign body of oral cavity**
√6ᵗʰ **S01.52 Laceration of lip and oral cavity with foreign body**
√7ᵗʰ **S01.521 Laceration with foreign body of lip**
√7ᵗʰ **S01.522 Laceration with foreign body of oral cavity**
√6ᵗʰ **S01.53 Puncture wound of lip and oral cavity without foreign body**
√7ᵗʰ **S01.531 Puncture wound without foreign body of lip**
√7ᵗʰ **S01.532 Puncture wound without foreign body of oral cavity**
√6ᵗʰ **S01.54 Puncture wound of lip and oral cavity with foreign body**
√7ᵗʰ **S01.541 Puncture wound with foreign body of lip**
√7ᵗʰ **S01.542 Puncture wound with foreign body of oral cavity**
√6ᵗʰ **S01.55 Open bite of lip and oral cavity**
√7ᵗʰ **S01.551 Open bite of lip**
Bite of lip NOS
EXCLUDES 1   superficial bite of lip (S00.571)
√7ᵗʰ **S01.552 Open bite of oral cavity**
Bite of oral cavity NOS
EXCLUDES 1   superficial bite of oral cavity (S00.572)
√5ᵗʰ **S01.8 Open wound of other parts of head**
√x7ᵗʰ **S01.80 Unspecified open wound of other part of head**
√x7ᵗʰ **S01.81 Laceration without foreign body of other part of head**
√x7ᵗʰ **S01.82 Laceration with foreign body of other part of head**
√x7ᵗʰ **S01.83 Puncture wound without foreign body of other part of head**
√x7ᵗʰ **S01.84 Puncture wound with foreign body of other part of head**
√x7ᵗʰ **S01.85 Open bite of other part of head**
Bite of other part of head NOS
EXCLUDES 1   superficial bite of other part of head (S00.87)
√5ᵗʰ **S01.9 Open wound of unspecified part of head**
√x7ᵗʰ **S01.90 Unspecified open wound of unspecified part of head**
√x7ᵗʰ **S01.91 Laceration without foreign body of unspecified part of head**
√x7ᵗʰ **S01.92 Laceration with foreign body of unspecified part of head**
√x7ᵗʰ **S01.93 Puncture wound without foreign body of unspecified part of head**
√x7ᵗʰ **S01.94 Puncture wound with foreign body of unspecified part of head**
√x7ᵗʰ **S01.95 Open bite of unspecified part of head**
Bite of head NOS
EXCLUDES 1   superficial bite of head NOS (S00.97)

√4ᵗʰ **S02 Fracture of skull and facial bones**
NOTE   A fracture not indicated as open or closed should be coded to closed.
Code also any associated intracranial injury (S06.-)
AHA: 2021,1Q,6; 2017,1Q,42; 2016,4Q,66-67
The appropriate 7th character is to be added to each code from category S02.
A   initial encounter for closed fracture
B   initial encounter for open fracture
D   subsequent encounter for fracture with routine healing
G   subsequent encounter for fracture with delayed healing
K   subsequent encounter for fracture with nonunion
S   sequela
√x7ᵗʰ **S02.0 Fracture of vault of skull** HCC ESR
Fracture of frontal bone
Fracture of parietal bone
√5ᵗʰ **S02.1 Fracture of base of skull**
EXCLUDES 2   lateral orbital wall (S02.84-)
medial orbital wall (S02.83-)
orbital floor (S02.3-)
AHA: 2019,4Q,16-17
√6ᵗʰ **S02.10 Unspecified fracture of base of skull**
√7ᵗʰ **S02.101 Fracture of base of skull, right side** HCC ESR
√7ᵗʰ **S02.102 Fracture of base of skull, left side** HCC ESR
√7ᵗʰ **S02.109 Fracture of base of skull, unspecified side** HCC ESR
√6ᵗʰ **S02.11 Fracture of occiput**
√7ᵗʰ **S02.110 Type I occipital condyle fracture, unspecified side** HCC ESR
√7ᵗʰ **S02.111 Type II occipital condyle fracture, unspecified side** HCC ESR
√7ᵗʰ **S02.112 Type III occipital condyle fracture, unspecified side** HCC ESR
√7ᵗʰ **S02.113 Unspecified occipital condyle fracture** HCC ESR
√7ᵗʰ **S02.118 Other fracture of occiput, unspecified side** HCC ESR
√7ᵗʰ **S02.119 Unspecified fracture of occiput** HCC ESR
√7ᵗʰ **S02.11A Type I occipital condyle fracture, right side** HCC ESR
√7ᵗʰ **S02.11B Type I occipital condyle fracture, left side** HCC ESR
√7ᵗʰ **S02.11C Type II occipital condyle fracture, right side** HCC ESR
√7ᵗʰ **S02.11D Type II occipital condyle fracture, left side** HCC ESR
√7ᵗʰ **S02.11E Type III occipital condyle fracture, right side** HCC ESR
√7ᵗʰ **S02.11F Type III occipital condyle fracture, left side** HCC ESR
√7ᵗʰ **S02.11G Other fracture of occiput, right side** HCC ESR
√7ᵗʰ **S02.11H Other fracture of occiput, left side** HCC ESR
√6ᵗʰ **S02.12 Fracture of orbital roof**
AHA: 2019,4Q,16-17
√7ᵗʰ **S02.121 Fracture of orbital roof, right side** HCC ESR
√7ᵗʰ **S02.122 Fracture of orbital roof, left side** HCC ESR
√7ᵗʰ **S02.129 Fracture of orbital roof, unspecified side** HCC ESR
√x7ᵗʰ **S02.19 Other fracture of base of skull**
Fracture of anterior fossa of base of skull
Fracture of ethmoid sinus
Fracture of frontal sinus
Fracture of middle fossa of base of skull
Fracture of posterior fossa of base of skull
Fracture of sphenoid
Fracture of temporal bone
√x7ᵗʰ **S02.2 Fracture of nasal bones**

☑ Additional Character Required   √x7ᵗʰ Placeholder Alert   Manifestation   Unspecified Dx   ⓠ QPP   UPD Unacceptable PDx

✓5th **S02.3** **Fracture of orbital floor**

Fracture of inferior orbital wall

EXCLUDES 1 *orbit NOS (S02.85)*

EXCLUDES 2 *lateral orbital wall (S02.84-)*
medial orbital wall (S02.83-)
orbital roof (S02.1-)

2 ✓x7th **S02.30** **Fracture of orbital floor, unspecified side** HCC ESR

2 ✓x7th **S02.31** **Fracture of orbital floor, right side** HCC ESR

2 ✓x7th **S02.32** **Fracture of orbital floor, left side** HCC ESR

✓5th **S02.4** **Fracture of malar, maxillary and zygoma bones**

Fracture of superior maxilla

Fracture of upper jaw (bone)

Fracture of zygomatic process of temporal bone

✓6th **S02.40** **Fracture of malar, maxillary and zygoma bones, unspecified**

2 ✓7th **S02.400** **Malar fracture, unspecified side** HCC ESR

2 ✓7th **S02.401** **Maxillary fracture, unspecified side** HCC ESR

2 ✓7th **S02.402** **Zygomatic fracture, unspecified side** HCC ESR

2 ✓7th **S02.40A** **Malar fracture, right side** HCC ESR

2 ✓7th **S02.40B** **Malar fracture, left side** HCC ESR

2 ✓7th **S02.40C** **Maxillary fracture, right side** HCC ESR

2 ✓7th **S02.40D** **Maxillary fracture, left side** HCC ESR

2 ✓7th **S02.40E** **Zygomatic fracture, right side** HCC ESR

2 ✓7th **S02.40F** **Zygomatic fracture, left side** HCC ESR

✓6th **S02.41** **LeFort fracture**

DEF: Named for Rene Le Fort, these fractures describe different combinations of multiple fractures that occur from significant force to the midface. A common denominator in all three types of LeFort fractures is fracture of the pterygoid processes, which are two bony plates resembling wings that extend downward from the sphenoid bone.

LeFort Fracture Types

Frontal bone
Type III
Nasal bone
Orbital floor
Type II
Type I
Maxilla
Zygomatic bone (malar) and arch

2 ✓7th **S02.411** **LeFort I fracture** HCC ESR

2 ✓7th **S02.412** **LeFort II fracture** HCC ESR

2 ✓7th **S02.413** **LeFort III fracture** HCC ESR

2 ✓x7th **S02.42** **Fracture of alveolus of maxilla** HCC ESR

✓x7th **S02.5** **Fracture of tooth (traumatic)**

Broken tooth

EXCLUDES 1 *cracked tooth (nontraumatic) (K03.81)*

✓5th **S02.6** **Fracture of mandible**

Fracture of lower jaw (bone)

✓6th **S02.60** **Fracture of mandible, unspecified**

2 ✓7th **S02.600** **Fracture of unspecified part of body of mandible, unspecified side** HCC ESR

2 ✓7th **S02.601** **Fracture of unspecified part of body of right mandible** HCC ESR

2 ✓7th **S02.602** **Fracture of unspecified part of body of left mandible** HCC ESR

2 ✓7th **S02.609** **Fracture of mandible, unspecified** HCC ESR

✓6th **S02.61** **Fracture of condylar process of mandible**

2 ✓7th **S02.610** **Fracture of condylar process of mandible, unspecified side** HCC ESR

2 ✓7th **S02.611** **Fracture of condylar process of right mandible** HCC ESR

2 ✓7th **S02.612** **Fracture of condylar process of left mandible** HCC ESR

✓6th **S02.62** **Fracture of subcondylar process of mandible**

2 ✓7th **S02.620** **Fracture of subcondylar process of mandible, unspecified side** HCC ESR

2 ✓7th **S02.621** **Fracture of subcondylar process of right mandible** HCC ESR

2 ✓7th **S02.622** **Fracture of subcondylar process of left mandible** HCC ESR

✓6th **S02.63** **Fracture of coronoid process of mandible**

2 ✓7th **S02.630** **Fracture of coronoid process of mandible, unspecified side** HCC ESR

2 ✓7th **S02.631** **Fracture of coronoid process of right mandible** HCC ESR

2 ✓7th **S02.632** **Fracture of coronoid process of left mandible** HCC ESR

✓6th **S02.64** **Fracture of ramus of mandible**

2 ✓7th **S02.640** **Fracture of ramus of mandible, unspecified side** HCC ESR

2 ✓7th **S02.641** **Fracture of ramus of right mandible** HCC ESR

2 ✓7th **S02.642** **Fracture of ramus of left mandible** HCC ESR

✓6th **S02.65** **Fracture of angle of mandible**

2 ✓7th **S02.650** **Fracture of angle of mandible, unspecified side** HCC ESR

2 ✓7th **S02.651** **Fracture of angle of right mandible** HCC ESR

2 ✓7th **S02.652** **Fracture of angle of left mandible** HCC ESR

2 ✓x7th **S02.66** **Fracture of symphysis of mandible** HCC ESR

✓6th **S02.67** **Fracture of alveolus of mandible**

2 ✓7th **S02.670** **Fracture of alveolus of mandible, unspecified side** HCC ESR

2 ✓7th **S02.671** **Fracture of alveolus of right mandible** HCC ESR

2 ✓7th **S02.672** **Fracture of alveolus of left mandible** HCC ESR

2 ✓x7th **S02.69** **Fracture of mandible of other specified site** HCC ESR

✓5th **S02.8** **Fractures of other specified skull and facial bones**

Fracture of palate

EXCLUDES 2 *fracture of orbital floor (S02.3-)*
fracture of orbital roof (S02.12-)

2 ✓x7th **S02.80** **Fracture of other specified skull and facial bones, unspecified side** HCC ESR

2 ✓x7th **S02.81** **Fracture of other specified skull and facial bones, right side** HCC ESR

2 ✓x7th **S02.82** **Fracture of other specified skull and facial bones, left side** HCC ESR

✓6th **S02.83** **Fracture of medial orbital wall**

EXCLUDES 2 *orbital floor (S02.3-)*
orbital roof (S02.12-)

AHA: 2019,4Q,16-17

2 ✓7th **S02.831** **Fracture of medial orbital wall, right side** HCC ESR

2 ✓7th **S02.832** **Fracture of medial orbital wall, left side** HCC ESR

2 ✓7th **S02.839** **Fracture of medial orbital wall, unspecified side** HCC ESR

✓6th **S02.84** **Fracture of lateral orbital wall**

EXCLUDES 2 *orbital floor (S02.3-)*
orbital roof (S02.12-)

AHA: 2019,4Q,16-17

2 ✓7th **S02.841** **Fracture of lateral orbital wall, right side** HCC ESR

2 ✓7th **S02.842** **Fracture of lateral orbital wall, left side** HCC ESR

2 ✓7th **S02.849** **Fracture of lateral orbital wall, unspecified side** HCC ESR

2 √x7ᵗʰ S02.85 Fracture of orbit, unspecified HCC ESR
Fracture of orbit NOS
Fracture of orbit wall NOS
EXCLUDES 1   lateral orbital wall (S02.84-)
   medial orbital wall (S02.83-)
   orbital floor (S02.3-)
   orbital roof (S02.12-)

√5ᵗʰ S02.9 Fracture of unspecified skull and facial bones

2 √x7ᵗʰ S02.91 Unspecified fracture of skull HCC ESR
AHA: 2020,2Q,24

2 √x7ᵗʰ S02.92 Unspecified fracture of facial bones HCC ESR

√4ᵗʰ S03 Dislocation and sprain of joints and ligaments of head
INCLUDES   avulsion of joint (capsule) or ligament of head
laceration of cartilage, joint (capsule) or ligament of head
sprain of cartilage, joint (capsule) or ligament of head
traumatic hemarthrosis of joint or ligament of head
traumatic rupture of joint or ligament of head
traumatic subluxation of joint or ligament of head
traumatic tear of joint or ligament of head
Code also any associated open wound
EXCLUDES 2   strain of muscle or tendon of head (S09.1)

The appropriate 7th character is to be added to each code from category S03.
A   initial encounter
D   subsequent encounter
S   sequela

√5ᵗʰ S03.0 Dislocation of jaw
Dislocation of jaw (cartilage) (meniscus)
Dislocation of mandible
Dislocation of temporomandibular (joint)
AHA: 2016,4Q,67

√x7ᵗʰ S03.00 Dislocation of jaw, unspecified side
√x7ᵗʰ S03.01 Dislocation of jaw, right side
√x7ᵗʰ S03.02 Dislocation of jaw, left side
√x7ᵗʰ S03.03 Dislocation of jaw, bilateral

√x7ᵗʰ S03.1 Dislocation of septal cartilage of nose
√x7ᵗʰ S03.2 Dislocation of tooth

√5ᵗʰ S03.4 Sprain of jaw
Sprain of temporomandibular (joint) (ligament)
AHA: 2016,4Q,67

√x7ᵗʰ S03.40 Sprain of jaw, unspecified side
√x7ᵗʰ S03.41 Sprain of jaw, right side
√x7ᵗʰ S03.42 Sprain of jaw, left side
√x7ᵗʰ S03.43 Sprain of jaw, bilateral

√x7ᵗʰ S03.8 Sprain of joints and ligaments of other parts of head
√x7ᵗʰ S03.9 Sprain of joints and ligaments of unspecified parts of head

√4ᵗʰ S04 Injury of cranial nerve
The selection of side should be based on the side of the body being affected
Code first any associated intracranial injury (S06.-)
Code also any associated:
open wound of head (S01.-)
skull fracture (S02.-)

The appropriate 7th character is to be added to each code from category S04.
A   initial encounter
D   subsequent encounter
S   sequela

√5ᵗʰ S04.0 Injury of optic nerve and pathways
Use additional code to identify any visual field defect or blindness (H53.4-, H54.-)

√6ᵗʰ S04.01 Injury of optic nerve
Injury of 2nd cranial nerve
√7ᵗʰ S04.011 Injury of optic nerve, right eye
√7ᵗʰ S04.012 Injury of optic nerve, left eye
√7ᵗʰ S04.019 Injury of optic nerve, unspecified eye
Injury of optic nerve NOS

√x7ᵗʰ S04.02 Injury of optic chiasm

√6ᵗʰ S04.03 Injury of optic tract and pathways
Injury of optic radiation
√7ᵗʰ S04.031 Injury of optic tract and pathways, right side
√7ᵗʰ S04.032 Injury of optic tract and pathways, left side
√7ᵗʰ S04.039 Injury of optic tract and pathways, unspecified side
Injury of optic tract and pathways NOS

√6ᵗʰ S04.04 Injury of visual cortex
√7ᵗʰ S04.041 Injury of visual cortex, right side
√7ᵗʰ S04.042 Injury of visual cortex, left side
√7ᵗʰ S04.049 Injury of visual cortex, unspecified side
Injury of visual cortex NOS

√5ᵗʰ S04.1 Injury of oculomotor nerve
Injury of 3rd cranial nerve
√x7ᵗʰ S04.10 Injury of oculomotor nerve, unspecified side
√x7ᵗʰ S04.11 Injury of oculomotor nerve, right side
√x7ᵗʰ S04.12 Injury of oculomotor nerve, left side

√5ᵗʰ S04.2 Injury of trochlear nerve
Injury of 4th cranial nerve
√x7ᵗʰ S04.20 Injury of trochlear nerve, unspecified side
√x7ᵗʰ S04.21 Injury of trochlear nerve, right side
√x7ᵗʰ S04.22 Injury of trochlear nerve, left side

√5ᵗʰ S04.3 Injury of trigeminal nerve
Injury of 5th cranial nerve
√x7ᵗʰ S04.30 Injury of trigeminal nerve, unspecified side
√x7ᵗʰ S04.31 Injury of trigeminal nerve, right side
√x7ᵗʰ S04.32 Injury of trigeminal nerve, left side

√5ᵗʰ S04.4 Injury of abducent nerve
Injury of 6th cranial nerve
√x7ᵗʰ S04.40 Injury of abducent nerve, unspecified side
√x7ᵗʰ S04.41 Injury of abducent nerve, right side
√x7ᵗʰ S04.42 Injury of abducent nerve, left side

√5ᵗʰ S04.5 Injury of facial nerve
Injury of 7th cranial nerve
√x7ᵗʰ S04.50 Injury of facial nerve, unspecified side
√x7ᵗʰ S04.51 Injury of facial nerve, right side
√x7ᵗʰ S04.52 Injury of facial nerve, left side

√5ᵗʰ S04.6 Injury of acoustic nerve
Injury of auditory nerve
Injury of 8th cranial nerve
√x7ᵗʰ S04.60 Injury of acoustic nerve, unspecified side
√x7ᵗʰ S04.61 Injury of acoustic nerve, right side
√x7ᵗʰ S04.62 Injury of acoustic nerve, left side

√5ᵗʰ S04.7 Injury of accessory nerve
Injury of 11th cranial nerve
√x7ᵗʰ S04.70 Injury of accessory nerve, unspecified side
√x7ᵗʰ S04.71 Injury of accessory nerve, right side
√x7ᵗʰ S04.72 Injury of accessory nerve, left side

√5ᵗʰ S04.8 Injury of other cranial nerves
√6ᵗʰ S04.81 Injury of olfactory [1st] nerve
√7ᵗʰ S04.811 Injury of olfactory [1st] nerve, right side
√7ᵗʰ S04.812 Injury of olfactory [1st] nerve, left side
√7ᵗʰ S04.819 Injury of olfactory [1st] nerve, unspecified side

√6ᵗʰ S04.89 Injury of other cranial nerves
Injury of vagus [10th] nerve
√7ᵗʰ S04.891 Injury of other cranial nerves, right side
√7ᵗʰ S04.892 Injury of other cranial nerves, left side
√7ᵗʰ S04.899 Injury of other cranial nerves, unspecified side

√x7ᵗʰ S04.9 Injury of unspecified cranial nerve

√4ᵗʰ **S05 Injury of eye and orbit**

     INCLUDES   open wound of eye and orbit

     EXCLUDES 2   *2nd cranial [optic] nerve injury (S04.0-)*
           3rd cranial [oculomotor] nerve injury (S04.1-)
           open wound of eyelid and periocular area (S01.1-)
           orbital bone fracture (S02.1-, S02.3-, S02.8-)
           superficial injury of eyelid (S00.1-S00.2)

> The appropriate 7th character is to be added to each code from category S05.
> A   initial encounter
> D   subsequent encounter
> S   sequela

√5ᵗʰ **S05.0 Injury of conjunctiva and corneal abrasion** without foreign body

     EXCLUDES 1   *foreign body in conjunctival sac (T15.1)*
           foreign body in cornea (T15.0)

   √x7ᵗʰ **S05.00 Injury of conjunctiva and corneal abrasion without foreign body, unspecified eye**

   √x7ᵗʰ **S05.01 Injury of conjunctiva and corneal abrasion without foreign body, right eye**

   √x7ᵗʰ **S05.02 Injury of conjunctiva and corneal abrasion without foreign body, left eye**

√5ᵗʰ **S05.1 Contusion of eyeball and orbital tissues**

     Traumatic hyphema

     EXCLUDES 2   *black eye NOS (S00.1)*
           contusion of eyelid and periocular area (S00.1)

   √x7ᵗʰ **S05.10 Contusion of eyeball and orbital tissues, unspecified eye**

   √x7ᵗʰ **S05.11 Contusion of eyeball and orbital tissues, right eye**

   √x7ᵗʰ **S05.12 Contusion of eyeball and orbital tissues, left eye**

√5ᵗʰ **S05.2 Ocular laceration and rupture** with prolapse or loss of intraocular tissue

   √x7ᵗʰ **S05.20 Ocular laceration and rupture with prolapse or loss of intraocular tissue, unspecified eye**

   √x7ᵗʰ **S05.21 Ocular laceration and rupture with prolapse or loss of intraocular tissue, right eye**

   √x7ᵗʰ **S05.22 Ocular laceration and rupture with prolapse or loss of intraocular tissue, left eye**

√5ᵗʰ **S05.3 Ocular laceration** without prolapse or loss of intraocular tissue

     Laceration of eye NOS

     AHA: 2022,1Q,33

     DEF: Tear in ocular tissue without displacing structures that is due to blunt trauma. It is characterized by pain, redness, and decreased vision.

   √x7ᵗʰ **S05.30 Ocular laceration without prolapse or loss of intraocular tissue, unspecified eye**

   √x7ᵗʰ **S05.31 Ocular laceration without prolapse or loss of intraocular tissue, right eye**

   √x7ᵗʰ **S05.32 Ocular laceration without prolapse or loss of intraocular tissue, left eye**

√5ᵗʰ **S05.4 Penetrating wound of orbit** with or without foreign body

     EXCLUDES 2   *retained (old) foreign body following penetrating wound in orbit (H05.5-)*

   √x7ᵗʰ **S05.40 Penetrating wound of orbit with or without foreign body, unspecified eye**

   √x7ᵗʰ **S05.41 Penetrating wound of orbit with or without foreign body, right eye**

   √x7ᵗʰ **S05.42 Penetrating wound of orbit with or without foreign body, left eye**

√5ᵗʰ **S05.5 Penetrating wound with foreign body of eyeball**

     EXCLUDES 2   *retained (old) intraocular foreign body (H44.6-, H44.7)*

   √x7ᵗʰ **S05.50 Penetrating wound with foreign body of unspecified eyeball**

   √x7ᵗʰ **S05.51 Penetrating wound with foreign body of right eyeball**

   √x7ᵗʰ **S05.52 Penetrating wound with foreign body of left eyeball**

√5ᵗʰ **S05.6 Penetrating wound without foreign body of eyeball**

     Ocular penetration NOS

   √x7ᵗʰ **S05.60 Penetrating wound without foreign body of unspecified eyeball**

   √x7ᵗʰ **S05.61 Penetrating wound without foreign body of right eyeball**

   √x7ᵗʰ **S05.62 Penetrating wound without foreign body of left eyeball**

√5ᵗʰ **S05.7 Avulsion of eye**

     Traumatic enucleation

   √x7ᵗʰ **S05.70 Avulsion of unspecified eye**

   √x7ᵗʰ **S05.71 Avulsion of right eye**

   √x7ᵗʰ **S05.72 Avulsion of left eye**

√5ᵗʰ **S05.8 Other injuries of eye and orbit**

     Lacrimal duct injury

   √6ᵗʰ **S05.8X Other injuries of eye and orbit**

     √7ᵗʰ **S05.8X1 Other injuries of right eye and orbit**

     √7ᵗʰ **S05.8X2 Other injuries of left eye and orbit**

     √7ᵗʰ **S05.8X9 Other injuries of unspecified eye and orbit**

√5ᵗʰ **S05.9 Unspecified injury of eye and orbit**

     Injury of eye NOS

   √x7ᵗʰ **S05.90 Unspecified injury of unspecified eye and orbit**

   √x7ᵗʰ **S05.91 Unspecified injury of right eye and orbit**

   √x7ᵗʰ **S05.92 Unspecified injury of left eye and orbit**

√4ᵗʰ **S06 Intracranial injury**

     NOTE   7th characters D and S do not apply to codes in category S06 with 6th character 7 – death due to brain injury prior to regaining consciousness, or 8 – death due to other cause prior to regaining consciousness.

     INCLUDES   traumatic brain injury

     Code also any associated:
       open wound of head (S01.-)
       skull fracture (S02.-)

     ▶Use additional code, if applicable, to identify mild neurocognitive disorders due to known physiological condition (F06.7-)◀

     EXCLUDES 1   *head injury NOS (S09.90)*

     AHA: 2017,4Q,25; 2017,1Q,42; 2015,3Q,37

     TIP: Do not assign Z87.820 Personal history of traumatic brain injury, when residual conditions persist after an intracranial injury. The codes for the residual conditions should be first listed, followed by a code from category S06 using seventh character S to identify sequela.

> The appropriate 7th character is to be added to each code from category S06.
> A   initial encounter
> D   subsequent encounter
> S   sequela

√5ᵗʰ **S06.0 Concussion**

     Commotio cerebri

     EXCLUDES 1   ▶*concussion with other intracranial injuries classified in subcategories S06.1- to S06.6-, and S06.81- to S06.89-, code to specified intracranial injury*◀

     AHA: 2016,4Q,67-68

   √6ᵗʰ **S06.0X Concussion**

     ³ √7ᵗʰ **S06.0X0 Concussion without loss of consciousness** HCC ESR Q

     ³ √7ᵗʰ **S06.0X1 Concussion with loss of consciousness of 30 minutes or less** HCC ESR Q
          ▶Concussion with brief loss of consciousness◀

     √7ᵗʰ **S06.0XA Concussion with loss of consciousness status unknown**
          Concussion NOS

     ³ √7ᵗʰ **S06.0X9 Concussion with loss of consciousness of unspecified duration** HCC ESR Q
          ~~Concussion NOS~~

√5ᵗʰ **S06.1 Traumatic cerebral edema**

     Diffuse traumatic cerebral edema
     Focal traumatic cerebral edema
     AHA: 2019,3Q,35; 2015,1Q,12-13

   √6ᵗʰ **S06.1X Traumatic cerebral edema**

     ² √7ᵗʰ **S06.1X0 Traumatic cerebral edema without loss of consciousness** HCC ESR Q

     ² √7ᵗʰ **S06.1X1 Traumatic cerebral edema with loss of consciousness of 30 minutes or less** HCC ESR Q
          ▶Traumatic cerebral edema with brief loss of consciousness◀

     ² √7ᵗʰ **S06.1X2 Traumatic cerebral edema with loss of consciousness of 31 minutes to 59 minutes** HCC ESR Q

Head

² √7ᵗʰ **S06.1X3 Traumatic cerebral edema with loss of consciousness of** 1 hour to 5 hours 59 minutes   HCC ESR COM Q

² √7ᵗʰ **S06.1X4 Traumatic cerebral edema with loss of consciousness of** 6 hours to 24 hours   HCC ESR COM Q

² √7ᵗʰ **S06.1X5 Traumatic cerebral edema with loss of consciousness** greater than 24 hours with return to pre-existing conscious level   HCC ESR COM

² √7ᵗʰ **S06.1X6 Traumatic cerebral edema with loss of consciousness** greater than 24 hours without return to pre-existing conscious level with patient surviving   HCC ESR COM

√7ᵗʰ **S06.1X7 Traumatic cerebral edema with loss of consciousness of** any duration with death due to brain injury prior to regaining consciousness

√7ᵗʰ **S06.1X8 Traumatic cerebral edema with loss of consciousness of** any duration with death due to **other** cause prior to regaining consciousness

√7ᵗʰ **S06.1XA Traumatic cerebral edema with loss of consciousness** status unknown
Traumatic cerebral edema NOS

² √7ᵗʰ **S06.1X9 Traumatic cerebral edema with loss of consciousness of unspecified duration**   HCC ESR Q
~~Traumatic cerebral edema NOS~~

√5ᵗʰ **S06.2 Diffuse traumatic brain injury**
Diffuse axonal brain injury
Use additional code, if applicable, for traumatic brain compression or herniation (S06.A-)
EXCLUDES 1   traumatic diffuse cerebral edema (S06.1X-)
AHA: 2020,3Q,46

√6ᵗʰ **S06.2X Diffuse traumatic brain injury**

² √7ᵗʰ **S06.2X0 Diffuse traumatic brain injury** without loss of consciousness   HCC ESR Q

² √7ᵗʰ **S06.2X1 Diffuse traumatic brain injury with loss of consciousness of** 30 minutes or less   HCC ESR Q
▶Diffuse traumatic brain injury with brief loss of consciousness◀

² √7ᵗʰ **S06.2X2 Diffuse traumatic brain injury with loss of consciousness of** 31 minutes to 59 minutes   HCC ESR Q

² √7ᵗʰ **S06.2X3 Diffuse traumatic brain injury with loss of consciousness of** 1 hour to 5 hours 59 minutes   HCC ESR COM Q

² √7ᵗʰ **S06.2X4 Diffuse traumatic brain injury with loss of consciousness of** 6 hours to 24 hours   HCC ESR COM Q

² √7ᵗʰ **S06.2X5 Diffuse traumatic brain injury with loss of consciousness** greater than 24 hours with return to pre-existing conscious levels   HCC ESR COM

² √7ᵗʰ **S06.2X6 Diffuse traumatic brain injury with loss of consciousness** greater than 24 hours without return to pre-existing conscious level with patient surviving   HCC ESR COM

√7ᵗʰ **S06.2X7 Diffuse traumatic brain injury with loss of consciousness of** any duration with death due to brain injury prior to regaining consciousness

√7ᵗʰ **S06.2X8 Diffuse traumatic brain injury with loss of consciousness of** any duration with death due to **other** cause prior to regaining consciousness

√7ᵗʰ **S06.2XA Diffuse traumatic brain injury with loss of consciousness** status unknown
Diffuse traumatic brain injury NOS

² √7ᵗʰ **S06.2X9 Diffuse traumatic brain injury with loss of consciousness of unspecified duration**   HCC ESR Q
~~Diffuse traumatic brain injury NOS~~

√5ᵗʰ **S06.3 Focal traumatic brain injury**
Use additional code, if applicable, for traumatic brain compression or herniation (S06.A-)
EXCLUDES 1   any condition classifiable to S06.4-S06.6
EXCLUDES 2   focal cerebral edema (S06.1)
AHA: 2020,3Q,46; 2019,3Q,35; 2015,1Q,12-13

√6ᵗʰ **S06.30 Unspecified focal traumatic brain injury**

² √7ᵗʰ **S06.300 Unspecified focal traumatic brain injury** without loss of consciousness   HCC ESR Q

² √7ᵗʰ **S06.301 Unspecified focal traumatic brain injury with loss of consciousness of** 30 minutes or less   HCC ESR Q
▶Unspecified focal traumatic brain injury with brief loss of consciousness◀

² √7ᵗʰ **S06.302 Unspecified focal traumatic brain injury with loss of consciousness of** 31 minutes to 59 minutes   HCC ESR Q

² √7ᵗʰ **S06.303 Unspecified focal traumatic brain injury with loss of consciousness of** 1 hour to 5 hours 59 minutes   HCC ESR COM Q

² √7ᵗʰ **S06.304 Unspecified focal traumatic brain injury with loss of consciousness of** 6 hours to 24 hours   HCC ESR COM Q

² √7ᵗʰ **S06.305 Unspecified focal traumatic brain injury with loss of consciousness** greater than 24 hours with return to pre-existing conscious level   HCC ESR COM

² √7ᵗʰ **S06.306 Unspecified focal traumatic brain injury with loss of consciousness** greater than 24 hours without return to pre-existing conscious level with patient surviving   HCC ESR COM

√7ᵗʰ **S06.307 Unspecified focal traumatic brain injury with loss of consciousness of** any duration with death due to brain injury prior to regaining consciousness

√7ᵗʰ **S06.308 Unspecified focal traumatic brain injury with loss of consciousness of** any duration with death due to **other** cause prior to regaining consciousness

√7ᵗʰ **S06.30A Unspecified focal traumatic brain injury with loss of consciousness** status unknown
Unspecified focal traumatic brain injury NOS

² √7ᵗʰ **S06.309 Unspecified focal traumatic brain injury with loss of consciousness of unspecified duration**   HCC ESR Q
~~Unspecified focal traumatic brain injury NOS~~

√6ᵗʰ **S06.31 Contusion and laceration of** right cerebrum

² √7ᵗʰ **S06.310 Contusion and laceration of right cerebrum** without loss of consciousness   HCC ESR

² √7ᵗʰ **S06.311 Contusion and laceration of right cerebrum with loss of consciousness of** 30 minutes or less   HCC ESR
▶Contusion and laceration of right cerebrum with brief loss of consciousness◀

² √7ᵗʰ **S06.312 Contusion and laceration of right cerebrum with loss of consciousness of** 31 minutes to 59 minutes   HCC ESR

² √7ᵗʰ **S06.313 Contusion and laceration of right cerebrum with loss of consciousness of** 1 hour to 5 hours 59 minutes   HCC ESR COM

² √7ᵗʰ **S06.314 Contusion and laceration of right cerebrum with loss of consciousness of** 6 hours to 24 hours   HCC ESR COM

² √7ᵗʰ **S06.315 Contusion and laceration of right cerebrum with loss of consciousness** greater than 24 hours with return to pre-existing conscious level   HCC ESR COM

² √7ᵗʰ **S06.316 Contusion and laceration of right cerebrum with loss of consciousness** greater than 24 hours without return to pre-existing conscious level with patient surviving   HCC ESR COM

Chapter 19. Injury, Poisoning and Certain Other Consequences of External Causes

✓7ᵗʰ **S06.317 Contusion and laceration of right cerebrum with loss of consciousness of** any duration with death due to brain injury prior to regaining consciousness

✓7ᵗʰ **S06.318 Contusion and laceration of right cerebrum with loss of consciousness of** any duration with death due to **other** cause prior to regaining consciousness

✓7ᵗʰ **S06.31A Contusion and laceration of right cerebrum with loss of consciousness** status unknown
>> Contusion and laceration of right cerebrum NOS

2 ✓7ᵗʰ **S06.319 Contusion and laceration of right cerebrum with loss of consciousness of** unspecified duration   HCC ESR
>> ~~Contusion and laceration of right cerebrum NOS~~

✓6ᵗʰ **S06.32 Contusion and laceration of** left cerebrum

2 ✓7ᵗʰ **S06.320 Contusion and laceration of left cerebrum** without loss of consciousness   HCC ESR

2 ✓7ᵗʰ **S06.321 Contusion and laceration of left cerebrum with loss of consciousness of** 30 minutes or less   HCC ESR
>> ▶Contusion and laceration of left cerebrum with brief loss of consciousness◀

2 ✓7ᵗʰ **S06.322 Contusion and laceration of left cerebrum with loss of consciousness of** 31 minutes to 59 minutes   HCC ESR

2 ✓7ᵗʰ **S06.323 Contusion and laceration of left cerebrum with loss of consciousness of** 1 hour to 5 hours 59 minutes   HCC ESR COM

2 ✓7ᵗʰ **S06.324 Contusion and laceration of left cerebrum with loss of consciousness of** 6 hours to 24 hours   HCC ESR COM

2 ✓7ᵗʰ **S06.325 Contusion and laceration of left cerebrum with loss of consciousness** greater than 24 hours with return to pre-existing conscious level   HCC ESR COM

2 ✓7ᵗʰ **S06.326 Contusion and laceration of left cerebrum with loss of consciousness** greater than 24 hours without return to pre-existing conscious level with patient surviving   HCC ESR COM

✓7ᵗʰ **S06.327 Contusion and laceration of left cerebrum with loss of consciousness of** any duration with death due to brain injury prior to regaining consciousness

✓7ᵗʰ **S06.328 Contusion and laceration of left cerebrum with loss of consciousness of** any duration with death due to **other** cause prior to regaining consciousness

✓7ᵗʰ **S06.32A Contusion and laceration of left cerebrum with loss of consciousness** status unknown
>> Contusion and laceration of left cerebrum NOS

2 ✓7ᵗʰ **S06.329 Contusion and laceration of left cerebrum with loss of consciousness of** unspecified duration   HCC ESR
>> ~~Contusion and laceration of left cerebrum NOS~~

✓6ᵗʰ **S06.33 Contusion and laceration of cerebrum, unspecified**

2 ✓7ᵗʰ **S06.330 Contusion and laceration of cerebrum, unspecified,** without loss of consciousness   HCC ESR

2 ✓7ᵗʰ **S06.331 Contusion and laceration of cerebrum, unspecified, with loss of consciousness of** 30 minutes or less   HCC ESR
>> ▶Contusion and laceration of cerebrum, unspecified, with brief loss of consciousness◀

2 ✓7ᵗʰ **S06.332 Contusion and laceration of cerebrum, unspecified, with loss of consciousness of** 31 minutes to 59 minutes   HCC ESR

2 ✓7ᵗʰ **S06.333 Contusion and laceration of cerebrum, unspecified, with loss of consciousness of** 1 hour to 5 hours 59 minutes   HCC ESR COM

2 ✓7ᵗʰ **S06.334 Contusion and laceration of cerebrum, unspecified, with loss of consciousness of** 6 hours to 24 hours   HCC ESR COM

2 ✓7ᵗʰ **S06.335 Contusion and laceration of cerebrum, unspecified, with loss of consciousness** greater than 24 hours with return to pre-existing conscious level   HCC ESR COM

2 ✓7ᵗʰ **S06.336 Contusion and laceration of cerebrum, unspecified, with loss of consciousness** greater than 24 hours without return to pre-existing conscious level with patient surviving   HCC ESR COM

✓7ᵗʰ **S06.337 Contusion and laceration of cerebrum, unspecified, with loss of consciousness of** any duration with death due to brain injury prior to regaining consciousness

✓7ᵗʰ **S06.338 Contusion and laceration of cerebrum, unspecified, with loss of consciousness of** any duration with death due to **other** cause prior to regaining consciousness

✓7ᵗʰ **S06.33A Contusion and laceration of cerebrum, unspecified, with loss of consciousness** status unknown
>> Contusion and laceration of cerebrum NOS

2 ✓7ᵗʰ **S06.339 Contusion and laceration of cerebrum, unspecified, with loss of consciousness of** unspecified duration   HCC ESR
>> ~~Contusion and laceration of cerebrum NOS~~

✓6ᵗʰ **S06.34 Traumatic hemorrhage of** right cerebrum
> Traumatic intracerebral hemorrhage and hematoma of right cerebrum

2 ✓7ᵗʰ **S06.340 Traumatic hemorrhage of right cerebrum** without loss of consciousness   HCC ESR Q

2 ✓7ᵗʰ **S06.341 Traumatic hemorrhage of right cerebrum with loss of consciousness of** 30 minutes or less   HCC ESR Q
>> ▶Traumatic hemorrhage of right cerebrum with loss of consciousness◀

2 ✓7ᵗʰ **S06.342 Traumatic hemorrhage of right cerebrum with loss of consciousness of** 31 minutes to 59 minutes   HCC ESR Q

2 ✓7ᵗʰ **S06.343 Traumatic hemorrhage of right cerebrum with loss of consciousness of** 1 hours to 5 hours 59 minutes   HCC ESR COM Q

2 ✓7ᵗʰ **S06.344 Traumatic hemorrhage of right cerebrum with loss of consciousness of** 6 hours to 24 hours   HCC ESR COM Q

2 ✓7ᵗʰ **S06.345 Traumatic hemorrhage of right cerebrum with loss of consciousness** greater than 24 hours with return to pre-existing conscious level   HCC ESR COM

2 ✓7ᵗʰ **S06.346 Traumatic hemorrhage of right cerebrum with loss of consciousness** greater than 24 hours without return to pre-existing conscious level with patient surviving   HCC ESR COM

✓7ᵗʰ **S06.347 Traumatic hemorrhage of right cerebrum with loss of consciousness of** any duration with death due to brain injury prior to regaining consciousness

✓7ᵗʰ **S06.348 Traumatic hemorrhage of right cerebrum with loss of consciousness of** any duration with death due to **other** cause prior to regaining consciousness

✓7ᵗʰ **S06.34A Traumatic hemorrhage of right cerebrum with loss of consciousness** status unknown
>> Traumatic hemorrhage of right cerebrum NOS

2 ✓7ᵗʰ **S06.349 Traumatic hemorrhage of right cerebrum with loss of consciousness of** unspecified duration   HCC ESR Q
>> ~~Traumatic hemorrhage of right cerebrum NOS~~

✓6ᵗʰ **S06.35 Traumatic hemorrhage of** left cerebrum
> Traumatic intracerebral hemorrhage and hematoma of left cerebrum

2 ✓7ᵗʰ **S06.350 Traumatic hemorrhage of left cerebrum** without loss of consciousness   HCC ESR Q

Head

2 √7ᵗʰ **S06.351 Traumatic hemorrhage of left cerebrum with loss of consciousness of** 30 minutes or less   HCC ESR Q
▶Traumatic hemorrhage of left cerebrum with brief loss of consciousness◀

2 √7ᵗʰ **S06.352 Traumatic hemorrhage of left cerebrum with loss of consciousness of** 31 minutes to 59 minutes   HCC ESR Q

2 √7ᵗʰ **S06.353 Traumatic hemorrhage of left cerebrum with loss of consciousness of** 1 hours to 5 hours 59 minutes   HCC ESR COM Q

2 √7ᵗʰ **S06.354 Traumatic hemorrhage of left cerebrum with loss of consciousness of** 6 hours to 24 hours   HCC ESR COM Q

2 √7ᵗʰ **S06.355 Traumatic hemorrhage of left cerebrum with loss of consciousness** greater than 24 hours with return to pre-existing conscious level   HCC ESR COM

2 √7ᵗʰ **S06.356 Traumatic hemorrhage of left cerebrum with loss of consciousness** greater than 24 hours without return to pre-existing conscious level with patient surviving   HCC ESR COM

√7ᵗʰ **S06.357 Traumatic hemorrhage of left cerebrum with loss of consciousness of** any duration with death due to brain injury prior to regaining consciousness

√7ᵗʰ **S06.358 Traumatic hemorrhage of left cerebrum with loss of consciousness of** any duration with death due to **other** cause prior to regaining consciousness

√7ᵗʰ **S06.35A Traumatic hemorrhage of left cerebrum with loss of consciousness** status unknown
Traumatic hemorrhage of left cerebrum NOS

2 √7ᵗʰ **S06.359 Traumatic hemorrhage of left cerebrum with loss of consciousness of unspecified duration**   HCC ESR Q
Traumatic hemorrhage of left cerebrum NOS

√6ᵗʰ **S06.36 Traumatic hemorrhage of cerebrum, unspecified**
Traumatic intracerebral hemorrhage and hematoma, unspecified

2 √7ᵗʰ **S06.360 Traumatic hemorrhage of cerebrum, unspecified,** without loss of consciousness   HCC ESR Q

2 √7ᵗʰ **S06.361 Traumatic hemorrhage of cerebrum, unspecified, with loss of consciousness of** 30 minutes or less   HCC ESR Q
▶Traumatic hemorrhage of cerebrum, unspecified, with brief loss of consciousness◀

2 √7ᵗʰ **S06.362 Traumatic hemorrhage of cerebrum, unspecified, with loss of consciousness of** 31 minutes to 59 minutes   HCC ESR Q

2 √7ᵗʰ **S06.363 Traumatic hemorrhage of cerebrum, unspecified, with loss of consciousness of** 1 hours to 5 hours 59 minutes   HCC ESR COM Q

2 √7ᵗʰ **S06.364 Traumatic hemorrhage of cerebrum, unspecified, with loss of consciousness of** 6 hours to 24 hours   HCC ESR COM Q

2 √7ᵗʰ **S06.365 Traumatic hemorrhage of cerebrum, unspecified, with loss of consciousness** greater than 24 hours with return to pre-existing conscious level   HCC ESR COM

2 √7ᵗʰ **S06.366 Traumatic hemorrhage of cerebrum, unspecified, with loss of consciousness** greater than 24 hours without return to pre-existing conscious level with patient surviving   HCC ESR COM

√7ᵗʰ **S06.367 Traumatic hemorrhage of cerebrum, unspecified, with loss of consciousness of** any duration with death due to brain injury prior to regaining consciousness

√7ᵗʰ **S06.368 Traumatic hemorrhage of cerebrum, unspecified, with loss of consciousness of** any duration with death due to **other** cause prior to regaining consciousness

√7ᵗʰ **S06.36A Traumatic hemorrhage of cerebrum, unspecified, with loss of consciousness** status unknown
Traumatic hemorrhage of cerebrum NOS

2 √7ᵗʰ **S06.369 Traumatic hemorrhage of cerebrum, unspecified, with loss of consciousness of unspecified duration**   HCC ESR Q
Traumatic hemorrhage of cerebrum NOS

√6ᵗʰ **S06.37 Contusion, laceration, and hemorrhage of cerebellum**

2 √7ᵗʰ **S06.370 Contusion, laceration, and hemorrhage of cerebellum** without loss of consciousness   HCC ESR

2 √7ᵗʰ **S06.371 Contusion, laceration, and hemorrhage of cerebellum with loss of consciousness of** 30 minutes or less   HCC ESR
▶Contusion, laceration, and hemorrhage of cerebellum with brief loss of consciousness◀

2 √7ᵗʰ **S06.372 Contusion, laceration, and hemorrhage of cerebellum with loss of consciousness of** 31 minutes to 59 minutes   HCC ESR

2 √7ᵗʰ **S06.373 Contusion, laceration, and hemorrhage of cerebellum with loss of consciousness of** 1 hour to 5 hours 59 minutes   HCC ESR COM

2 √7ᵗʰ **S06.374 Contusion, laceration, and hemorrhage of cerebellum with loss of consciousness of** 6 hours to 24 hours   HCC ESR COM

2 √7ᵗʰ **S06.375 Contusion, laceration, and hemorrhage of cerebellum with loss of consciousness** greater than 24 hours with return to pre-existing conscious level   HCC ESR COM

2 √7ᵗʰ **S06.376 Contusion, laceration, and hemorrhage of cerebellum with loss of consciousness** greater than 24 hours without return to pre-existing conscious level with patient surviving   HCC ESR COM

√7ᵗʰ **S06.377 Contusion, laceration, and hemorrhage of cerebellum with loss of consciousness of** any duration with death due to brain injury prior to regaining consciousness

√7ᵗʰ **S06.378 Contusion, laceration, and hemorrhage of cerebellum with loss of consciousness of** any duration with death due to **other** cause prior to regaining consciousness

√7ᵗʰ **S06.37A Contusion, laceration, and hemorrhage of cerebellum with loss of consciousness** status unknown
Contusion, laceration, and hemorrhage of cerebellum NOS

2 √7ᵗʰ **S06.379 Contusion, laceration, and hemorrhage of cerebellum with loss of consciousness of unspecified duration**   HCC ESR
Contusion, laceration, and hemorrhage of cerebellum NOS

√6ᵗʰ **S06.38 Contusion, laceration, and hemorrhage of brainstem**

2 √7ᵗʰ **S06.380 Contusion, laceration, and hemorrhage of brainstem** without loss of consciousness   HCC ESR

2 √7ᵗʰ **S06.381 Contusion, laceration, and hemorrhage of brainstem with loss of consciousness of** 30 minutes or less   HCC ESR
▶Contusion, laceration, and hemorrhage of brainstem with brief loss of consciousness◀

2 √7ᵗʰ **S06.382 Contusion, laceration, and hemorrhage of brainstem with loss of consciousness of** 31 minutes to 59 minutes   HCC ESR

2 √7ᵗʰ **S06.383 Contusion, laceration, and hemorrhage of brainstem with loss of consciousness of** 1 hour to 5 hours 59 minutes   HCC ESR COM

2 √7ᵗʰ **S06.384 Contusion, laceration, and hemorrhage of brainstem with loss of consciousness of** 6 hours to 24 hours   HCC ESR COM

2 √7ᵗʰ **S06.385 Contusion, laceration, and hemorrhage of brainstem with loss of consciousness** greater than 24 hours with return to pre-existing conscious level   HCC ESR COM

Head

² ✓7ᵗʰ **S06.386** **Contusion, laceration, and hemorrhage of brainstem with loss of consciousness** greater than 24 hours without return to pre-existing conscious level with patient surviving `HCC` `ESR` `COM`

✓7ᵗʰ **S06.387** **Contusion, laceration, and hemorrhage of brainstem with loss of consciousness** of any duration with death due to brain injury prior to regaining consciousness

✓7ᵗʰ **S06.388** **Contusion, laceration, and hemorrhage of brainstem with loss of consciousness** of any duration with death due to **other** cause prior to regaining consciousness

✓7ᵗʰ **S06.38A** **Contusion, laceration, and hemorrhage of brainstem with loss of consciousness** status unknown
Contusion, laceration, and hemorrhage of brainstem NOS

² ✓7ᵗʰ **S06.389** **Contusion, laceration, and hemorrhage of brainstem with loss of consciousness** of unspecified duration `HCC` `ESR`
~~Contusion, laceration, and hemorrhage of brainstem NOS~~

✓5ᵗʰ **S06.4** **Epidural** **hemorrhage**
Extradural hemorrhage NOS
Extradural hemorrhage (traumatic)
DEF: Epidural space: Space between the endosteum of the cranium (skull) and the dura mater, the outermost layer of a three-layer membrane that covers the brain.

✓6ᵗʰ **S06.4X** **Epidural hemorrhage**

² ✓7ᵗʰ **S06.4X0** **Epidural hemorrhage** without loss of consciousness `HCC` `ESR` `Q`

² ✓7ᵗʰ **S06.4X1** **Epidural hemorrhage with loss of consciousness of** 30 minutes or less `HCC` `ESR` `Q`
▶Epidural hemorrhage with brief loss of consciousness◀

² ✓7ᵗʰ **S06.4X2** **Epidural hemorrhage with loss of consciousness of** 31 minutes to 59 minutes `HCC` `ESR` `Q`

² ✓7ᵗʰ **S06.4X3** **Epidural hemorrhage with loss of consciousness of** 1 hour to 5 hours 59 minutes `HCC` `ESR` `COM` `Q`

² ✓7ᵗʰ **S06.4X4** **Epidural hemorrhage with loss of consciousness of** 6 hours to 24 hours `HCC` `ESR` `COM` `Q`

² ✓7ᵗʰ **S06.4X5** **Epidural hemorrhage with loss of consciousness** greater than 24 hours with return to pre-existing conscious level `HCC` `ESR` `COM`

² ✓7ᵗʰ **S06.4X6** **Epidural hemorrhage with loss of consciousness** greater than 24 hours without return to pre-existing conscious level with patient surviving `HCC` `ESR` `COM`

✓7ᵗʰ **S06.4X7** **Epidural hemorrhage with loss of consciousness of** any duration with death due to brain injury prior to regaining consciousness

✓7ᵗʰ **S06.4X8** **Epidural hemorrhage with loss of consciousness of** any duration with death due to **other** causes prior to regaining consciousness

✓7ᵗʰ **S06.4XA** **Epidural hemorrhage with loss of consciousness** status unknown
Epidural hemorrhage NOS

² ✓7ᵗʰ **S06.4X9** **Epidural hemorrhage with loss of consciousness of unspecified duration** `HCC` `ESR` `Q`
~~Epidural hemorrhage NOS~~

✓5ᵗʰ **S06.5** **Traumatic** **subdural** **hemorrhage**
Use additional code, if applicable, for traumatic brain compression or herniation (S06.A-)
AHA: 2021,2Q,5; 2021,1Q,4
DEF: Subdural: Potential space between the dura mater and arachnoid membrane around the brain.

✓6ᵗʰ **S06.5X** **Traumatic subdural hemorrhage**

² ✓7ᵗʰ **S06.5X0** **Traumatic subdural hemorrhage** without loss of consciousness `HCC` `ESR` `Q`

² ✓7ᵗʰ **S06.5X1** **Traumatic subdural hemorrhage with loss of consciousness of** 30 minutes or less `HCC` `ESR` `Q`
▶Traumatic subdural hemorrhage with brief loss of consciousness◀

² ✓7ᵗʰ **S06.5X2** **Traumatic subdural hemorrhage with loss of consciousness of** 31 minutes to 59 minutes `HCC` `ESR` `Q`

² ✓7ᵗʰ **S06.5X3** **Traumatic subdural hemorrhage with loss of consciousness of** 1 hour to 5 hours 59 minutes `HCC` `ESR` `COM` `Q`

² ✓7ᵗʰ **S06.5X4** **Traumatic subdural hemorrhage with loss of consciousness of** 6 hours to 24 hours `HCC` `ESR` `COM` `Q`

² ✓7ᵗʰ **S06.5X5** **Traumatic subdural hemorrhage with loss of consciousness** greater than 24 hours with return to pre-existing conscious level `HCC` `ESR` `COM`

² ✓7ᵗʰ **S06.5X6** **Traumatic subdural hemorrhage with loss of consciousness** greater than 24 hours without return to pre-existing conscious level with patient surviving `HCC` `ESR` `COM`

✓7ᵗʰ **S06.5X7** **Traumatic subdural hemorrhage with loss of consciousness of** any duration with death due to brain injury before regaining consciousness

✓7ᵗʰ **S06.5X8** **Traumatic subdural hemorrhage with loss of consciousness of** any duration with death due to **other** cause before regaining consciousness

✓7ᵗʰ **S06.5XA** **Traumatic subdural hemorrhage with loss of consciousness** status unknown
Traumatic subdural hemorrhage NOS

² ✓7ᵗʰ **S06.5X9** **Traumatic subdural hemorrhage with loss of consciousness of unspecified duration** `HCC` `ESR` `Q`
~~Traumatic subdural hemorrhage NOS~~

✓5ᵗʰ **S06.6** **Traumatic** **subarachnoid** **hemorrhage**
Use additional code, if applicable, for traumatic brain compression or herniation (S06.A-)
AHA: 2021,2Q,5; 2021,1Q,4
DEF: Subarachnoid: Space located between the arachnoid membrane and the pia mater that contains cerebrospinal fluid.

✓6ᵗʰ **S06.6X** **Traumatic subarachnoid hemorrhage**

² ✓7ᵗʰ **S06.6X0** **Traumatic subarachnoid hemorrhage** without loss of consciousness `HCC` `ESR` `Q`

² ✓7ᵗʰ **S06.6X1** **Traumatic subarachnoid hemorrhage with loss of consciousness of** 30 minutes or less `HCC` `ESR` `Q`
▶Traumatic subarachnoid hemorrhage with brief loss of consciousness◀

² ✓7ᵗʰ **S06.6X2** **Traumatic subarachnoid hemorrhage with loss of consciousness of** 31 minutes to 59 minutes `HCC` `ESR` `Q`

² ✓7ᵗʰ **S06.6X3** **Traumatic subarachnoid hemorrhage with loss of consciousness of** 1 hour to 5 hours 59 minutes `HCC` `ESR` `COM` `Q`

² ✓7ᵗʰ **S06.6X4** **Traumatic subarachnoid hemorrhage with loss of consciousness of** 6 hours to 24 hours `HCC` `ESR` `COM` `Q`

² ✓7ᵗʰ **S06.6X5** **Traumatic subarachnoid hemorrhage with loss of consciousness** greater than 24 hours with return to pre-existing conscious level `HCC` `ESR` `COM`

² ✓7ᵗʰ **S06.6X6** **Traumatic subarachnoid hemorrhage with loss of consciousness** greater than 24 hours without return to pre-existing conscious level with patient surviving `HCC` `ESR` `COM`

✓7ᵗʰ **S06.6X7** **Traumatic subarachnoid hemorrhage with loss of consciousness of** any duration with death due to brain injury prior to regaining consciousness

✓7ᵗʰ **S06.6X8** **Traumatic subarachnoid hemorrhage with loss of consciousness of** any duration with death due to **other** cause prior to regaining consciousness

(handwritten note in left margin: "Head")

√7ᵗʰ **S06.6XA** **Traumatic subarachnoid hemorrhage with loss of consciousness** status unknown
> Traumatic subarachnoid hemorrhage NOS

² √7ᵗʰ **S06.6X9** **Traumatic subarachnoid hemorrhage with loss of consciousness of unspecified duration** HCC ESR Q
> ~~Traumatic subarachnoid hemorrhage NOS~~

√5ᵗʰ **S06.8** **Other specified intracranial injuries**

√6ᵗʰ **S06.81** **Injury of right internal carotid artery, intracranial portion, not elsewhere classified**

² √7ᵗʰ **S06.810** **Injury of right internal carotid artery, intracranial portion, not elsewhere classified** without loss of consciousness HCC ESR Q

² √7ᵗʰ **S06.811** **Injury of right internal carotid artery, intracranial portion, not elsewhere classified with loss of consciousness of** 30 minutes or less HCC ESR Q
> ▶Injury of right internal carotid artery, intracranial portion, not elsewhere classified with brief loss of consciousness◀

² √7ᵗʰ **S06.812** **Injury of right internal carotid artery, intracranial portion, not elsewhere classified with loss of consciousness of** 31 minutes to 59 minutes HCC ESR Q

² √7ᵗʰ **S06.813** **Injury of right internal carotid artery, intracranial portion, not elsewhere classified with loss of consciousness of** 1 hour to 5 hours 59 minutes HCC ESR COM Q

² √7ᵗʰ **S06.814** **Injury of right internal carotid artery, intracranial portion, not elsewhere classified with loss of consciousness of** 6 hours to 24 hours HCC ESR COM Q

² √7ᵗʰ **S06.815** **Injury of right internal carotid artery, intracranial portion, not elsewhere classified with loss of consciousness** greater than 24 hours with return to pre-existing conscious level HCC ESR COM

² √7ᵗʰ **S06.816** **Injury of right internal carotid artery, intracranial portion, not elsewhere classified with loss of consciousness** greater than 24 hours without return to pre-existing conscious level with patient surviving HCC ESR COM

√7ᵗʰ **S06.817** **Injury of right internal carotid artery, intracranial portion, not elsewhere classified with loss of consciousness of** any duration with death due to brain injury prior to regaining consciousness

√7ᵗʰ **S06.818** **Injury of right internal carotid artery, intracranial portion, not elsewhere classified with loss of consciousness of** any duration with death due to other cause prior to regaining consciousness

√7ᵗʰ **S06.81A** **Injury of right internal carotid artery, intracranial portion, not elsewhere classified with loss of consciousness** status unknown
> Injury of right internal carotid artery, intracranial portion, not elsewhere classified NOS

² √7ᵗʰ **S06.819** **Injury of right internal carotid artery, intracranial portion, not elsewhere classified with loss of consciousness of** unspecified duration HCC ESR Q
> ~~Injury of right internal carotid artery, intracranial portion, not elsewhere classified NOS~~

√6ᵗʰ **S06.82** **Injury of left internal carotid artery, intracranial portion, not elsewhere classified**

² √7ᵗʰ **S06.820** **Injury of left internal carotid artery, intracranial portion, not elsewhere classified** without loss of consciousness HCC ESR Q

² √7ᵗʰ **S06.821** **Injury of left internal carotid artery, intracranial portion, not elsewhere classified with loss of consciousness of** 30 minutes or less HCC ESR Q
> ▶Injury of left internal carotid artery, intracranial portion, not elsewhere classified with brief loss of consciousness◀

² √7ᵗʰ **S06.822** **Injury of left internal carotid artery, intracranial portion, not elsewhere classified with loss of consciousness of** 31 minutes to 59 minutes HCC ESR Q

² √7ᵗʰ **S06.823** **Injury of left internal carotid artery, intracranial portion, not elsewhere classified with loss of consciousness of** 1 hour to 5 hours 59 minutes HCC ESR COM Q

² √7ᵗʰ **S06.824** **Injury of left internal carotid artery, intracranial portion, not elsewhere classified with loss of consciousness of** 6 hours to 24 hours HCC ESR COM Q

² √7ᵗʰ **S06.825** **Injury of left internal carotid artery, intracranial portion, not elsewhere classified with loss of consciousness** greater than 24 hours with return to pre-existing conscious level HCC ESR COM

² √7ᵗʰ **S06.826** **Injury of left internal carotid artery, intracranial portion, not elsewhere classified with loss of consciousness** greater than 24 hours without return to pre-existing conscious level with patient surviving HCC ESR COM

√7ᵗʰ **S06.827** **Injury of left internal carotid artery, intracranial portion, not elsewhere classified with loss of consciousness of** any duration with death due to brain injury prior to regaining consciousness

√7ᵗʰ **S06.828** **Injury of left internal carotid artery, intracranial portion, not elsewhere classified with loss of consciousness of** any duration with death due to other cause prior to regaining consciousness

√7ᵗʰ **S06.82A** **Injury of left internal carotid artery, intracranial portion, not elsewhere classified with loss of consciousness** status unknown
> Injury of left internal carotid artery, intracranial portion, not elsewhere classified NOS

² √7ᵗʰ **S06.829** **Injury of left internal carotid artery, intracranial portion, not elsewhere classified with loss of consciousness of** unspecified duration HCC ESR Q
> ~~Injury of left internal carotid artery, intracranial portion, not elsewhere classified NOS~~

√6ᵗʰ **S06.8A** **Primary blast injury of brain, not elsewhere classified**
> Code also, if applicable, focal traumatic brain injury (S06.3-)
>
> EXCLUDES 2   traumatic cerebral edema (S06.1)

√7ᵗʰ **S06.8A0** **Primary blast injury of brain, not elsewhere classified** without loss of consciousness

√7ᵗʰ **S06.8A1** **Primary blast injury of brain, not elsewhere classified with loss of consciousness of** 30 minutes or less
> Primary blast injury of brain, not elsewhere classified with brief loss of consciousness

√7ᵗʰ **S06.8A2** **Primary blast injury of brain, not elsewhere classified with loss of consciousness of** 31 minutes to 59 minutes

√7ᵗʰ **S06.8A3** **Primary blast injury of brain, not elsewhere classified with loss of consciousness of** 1 hour to 5 hours 59 minutes

√7ᵗʰ **S06.8A4** **Primary blast injury of brain, not elsewhere classified with loss of consciousness of** 6 hours to 24 hours

Head

- ✓7th **S06.8A5** **Primary blast injury of brain, not elsewhere classified with loss of consciousness** greater than 24 hours with return to pre-existing conscious level
- ✓7th **S06.8A6** **Primary blast injury of brain, not elsewhere classified with loss of consciousness** greater than 24 hours without return to pre-existing conscious level with patient surviving
- ✓7th **S06.8A7** **Primary blast injury of brain, not elsewhere classified with loss of consciousness of** any duration with death due to brain injury prior to regaining consciousness
- ✓7th **S06.8A8** **Primary blast injury of brain, not elsewhere classified with loss of consciousness of** any duration with death due to other cause prior to regaining consciousness
- ✓7th **S06.8AA** **Primary blast injury of brain, not elsewhere classified with loss of consciousness** status unknown
  Primary blast injury of brain NOS
- ✓7th **S06.8A9** **Primary blast injury of brain, not elsewhere classified with loss of consciousness of unspecified duration**

✓6th **S06.89** **Other specified intracranial injury**
  EXCLUDES 1   concussion (S06.0X-)

- 2 ✓7th **S06.890** **Other specified intracranial injury** without loss of consciousness   HCC ESR Q
- 2 ✓7th **S06.891** **Other specified intracranial injury with loss of consciousness of** 30 minutes or less   HCC ESR Q
  ▶Other specified intracranial injury with brief loss of consciousness◀
- 2 ✓7th **S06.892** **Other specified intracranial injury with loss of consciousness of** 31 minutes to 59 minutes   HCC ESR Q
- 2 ✓7th **S06.893** **Other specified intracranial injury with loss of consciousness of** 1 hour to 5 hours 59 minutes   HCC ESR COM Q
- 2 ✓7th **S06.894** **Other specified intracranial injury with loss of consciousness of** 6 hours to 24 hours   HCC ESR COM Q
- 2 ✓7th **S06.895** **Other specified intracranial injury with loss of consciousness** greater than 24 hours with return to pre-existing conscious level   HCC ESR COM
- 2 ✓7th **S06.896** **Other specified intracranial injury with loss of consciousness** greater than 24 hours without return to pre-existing conscious level with patient surviving   HCC ESR COM
- ✓7th **S06.897** **Other specified intracranial injury with loss of consciousness of** any duration with death due to brain injury prior to regaining consciousness
- ✓7th **S06.898** **Other specified intracranial injury with loss of consciousness of** any duration with death due to other cause prior to regaining consciousness
- ✓7th **S06.89A** **Other specified intracranial injury with loss of consciousness** status unknown
- 2 ✓7th **S06.899** **Other specified intracranial injury with loss of consciousness of unspecified duration**   HCC ESR Q

✓5th **S06.9** **Unspecified intracranial injury**
  Brain injury NOS
  Head injury NOS with loss of consciousness
  Traumatic brain injury NOS
  EXCLUDES 1   conditions classifiable to S06.0- to S06.8- code to specified intracranial injury
  head injury NOS (S09.90)
  AHA: 2020,3Q,46; 2020,2Q,31

✓6th **S06.9X** **Unspecified intracranial injury**
- 2 ✓7th **S06.9X0** **Unspecified intracranial injury** without loss of consciousness   HCC ESR Q

- 2 ✓7th **S06.9X1** **Unspecified intracranial injury with loss of consciousness of** 30 minutes or less   HCC ESR Q
  ▶Unspecified intracranial injury with brief loss of consciousness◀
- 2 ✓7th **S06.9X2** **Unspecified intracranial injury with loss of consciousness of** 31 minutes to 59 minutes   HCC ESR Q
- 2 ✓7th **S06.9X3** **Unspecified intracranial injury with loss of consciousness of** 1 hour to 5 hours 59 minutes   HCC ESR COM Q
- 2 ✓7th **S06.9X4** **Unspecified intracranial injury with loss of consciousness of** 6 hours to 24 hours   HCC ESR COM Q
- 2 ✓7th **S06.9X5** **Unspecified intracranial injury with loss of consciousness** greater than 24 hours with return to pre-existing conscious level   HCC ESR COM
- 2 ✓7th **S06.9X6** **Unspecified intracranial injury with loss of consciousness** greater than 24 hours without return to pre-existing conscious level with patient surviving   HCC ESR COM
- ✓7th **S06.9X7** **Unspecified intracranial injury with loss of consciousness of** any duration with death due to brain injury prior to regaining consciousness
- ✓7th **S06.9X8** **Unspecified intracranial injury with loss of consciousness of** any duration with death due to other cause prior to regaining consciousness
- ✓7th **S06.9XA** **Unspecified intracranial injury with loss of consciousness** status unknown
- 2 ✓7th **S06.9X9** **Unspecified intracranial injury with loss of consciousness of unspecified duration**   HCC ESR Q

✓5th **S06.A** **Traumatic brain compression and herniation**
  Traumatic cerebral compression
  Code first the underlying traumatic brain injury, such as:
    diffuse traumatic brain injury (S06.2-)
    focal traumatic brain injury (S06.3-)
    traumatic subdural hemorrhage (S06.5-)
    traumatic subarachnoid hemorrhage (S06.6-)
  AHA: 2021,4Q,29

✓x7th **S06.A0** **Traumatic brain compression** without herniation   HCC ESR UPD
  Traumatic brain compression NOS
  Traumatic cerebral compression NOS

✓x7th **S06.A1** **Traumatic brain compression** with herniation   HCC ESR UPD
  Traumatic brain herniation
  Traumatic brainstem compression with herniation
  Traumatic cerebellar compression with herniation
  Traumatic cerebral compression with herniation

✓4th **S07** **Crushing injury of head**
  Use additional code for all associated injuries, such as:
    intracranial injuries (S06.-)
    skull fractures (S02.-)

  The appropriate 7th character is to be added to each code from category S07.
  A   initial encounter
  D   subsequent encounter
  S   sequela

✓x7th **S07.0** **Crushing injury of** face

✓x7th **S07.1** **Crushing injury of** skull

✓x7th **S07.8** **Crushing injury of** other parts of head

✓x7th **S07.9** **Crushing injury of head**, part unspecified

✓4th **S08** **Avulsion and traumatic amputation of part of head**
  An amputation not identified as partial or complete should be coded to complete

  The appropriate 7th character is to be added to each code from category S08.
  A   initial encounter
  D   subsequent encounter
  S   sequela

✓x7th **S08.0** **Avulsion of** scalp

√5ᵗʰ **S08.1 Traumatic amputation of** ear

  √6ᵗʰ **S08.11 Complete traumatic amputation of ear**

    √7ᵗʰ **S08.111 Complete traumatic amputation of** right ear

    √7ᵗʰ **S08.112 Complete traumatic amputation of** left ear

    √7ᵗʰ **S08.119 Complete traumatic amputation of unspecified ear**

  √6ᵗʰ **S08.12 Partial traumatic amputation of ear**

    √7ᵗʰ **S08.121 Partial traumatic amputation of** right ear

    √7ᵗʰ **S08.122 Partial traumatic amputation of** left ear

    √7ᵗʰ **S08.129 Partial traumatic amputation of unspecified ear**

√5ᵗʰ **S08.8 Traumatic amputation of other parts of head**

  √6ᵗʰ **S08.81 Traumatic amputation of** nose

    √7ᵗʰ **S08.811 Complete traumatic amputation of nose**

    √7ᵗʰ **S08.812 Partial traumatic amputation of nose**

  √x7ᵗʰ **S08.89 Traumatic amputation of other parts of head**

√4ᵗʰ **S09 Other and unspecified injuries of head**

> The appropriate 7th character is to be added to each code from category S09.
> A   initial encounter
> D   subsequent encounter
> S   sequela

√x7ᵗʰ **S09.0 Injury of** blood vessels **of head, not elsewhere classified**

    EXCLUDES 1 *injury of cerebral blood vessels (S06.-)*
                injury of precerebral blood vessels (S15.-)

√5ᵗʰ **S09.1 Injury of** muscle and tendon **of head**

   Code also any associated open wound (S01.-)
     EXCLUDES 2 *sprain to joints and ligament of head (S03.9)*

  √x7ᵗʰ **S09.10 Unspecified injury of muscle and tendon of head**
     Injury of muscle and tendon of head NOS

  √x7ᵗʰ **S09.11 Strain of muscle and tendon of head** ▢

  √x7ᵗʰ **S09.12 Laceration of muscle and tendon of head**

  √x7ᵗʰ **S09.19 Other specified injury of muscle and tendon of head** ▢

√5ᵗʰ **S09.2 Traumatic rupture of** ear drum

    EXCLUDES 1 *traumatic rupture of ear drum due to blast injury (S09.31-)*

  √x7ᵗʰ **S09.20 Traumatic rupture of unspecified ear drum**

  √x7ᵗʰ **S09.21 Traumatic rupture of** right **ear drum**

  √x7ᵗʰ **S09.22 Traumatic rupture of** left **ear drum**

√5ᵗʰ **S09.3 Other specified and unspecified injury of middle and inner ear**

    EXCLUDES 1 *injury to ear NOS (S09.91-)*
    EXCLUDES 2 *injury to external ear (S00.4-, S01.3-, S08.1-)*

  √6ᵗʰ **S09.30 Unspecified injury of** middle and inner ear

    √7ᵗʰ **S09.301 Unspecified injury of** right **middle and inner ear**

    √7ᵗʰ **S09.302 Unspecified injury of** left **middle and inner ear**

    √7ᵗʰ **S09.309 Unspecified injury of unspecified middle and inner ear**

  √6ᵗʰ **S09.31 Primary** blast injury **of ear**
     Blast injury of ear NOS

    √7ᵗʰ **S09.311 Primary blast injury of** right **ear**

    √7ᵗʰ **S09.312 Primary blast injury of** left **ear**

    √7ᵗʰ **S09.313 Primary blast injury of ear,** bilateral

    √7ᵗʰ **S09.319 Primary blast injury of unspecified ear**

  √6ᵗʰ **S09.39 Other specified injury of middle and inner ear**
     Secondary blast injury to ear

    √7ᵗʰ **S09.391 Other specified injury of** right **middle and inner ear**

    √7ᵗʰ **S09.392 Other specified injury of** left **middle and inner ear**

    √7ᵗʰ **S09.399 Other specified injury of unspecified middle and inner ear**

√x7ᵗʰ **S09.8 Other specified injuries of head** ▢

√5ᵗʰ **S09.9 Unspecified injury of face and head**

  √x7ᵗʰ **S09.90 Unspecified injury of** head
     Head injury NOS

     EXCLUDES 1 *brain injury NOS (S06.9-)*
             head injury NOS with loss of consciousness (S06.9-)
             intracranial injury NOS (S06.9-)

  √x7ᵗʰ **S09.91 Unspecified injury of** ear
     Injury of ear NOS

  √x7ᵗʰ **S09.92 Unspecified injury of** nose
     Injury of nose NOS

  √x7ᵗʰ **S09.93 Unspecified injury of** face
     Injury of face NOS
     AHA: 2019,2Q,23

Injuries to the neck (S10-S19)

INCLUDES   injuries of nape
               injuries of supraclavicular region
               injuries of throat

EXCLUDES 2 *burns and corrosions (T20-T32)*
           effects of foreign body in esophagus (T18.1)
           effects of foreign body in larynx (T17.3)
           effects of foreign body in pharynx (T17.2)
           effects of foreign body in trachea (T17.4)
           frostbite (T33-T34)
           insect bite or sting, venomous (T63.4)

√4ᵗʰ **S10 Superficial injury of neck**

> The appropriate 7th character is to be added to each code from category S10.
> A   initial encounter
> D   subsequent encounter
> S   sequela

√x7ᵗʰ **S10.0 Contusion of throat**

    Contusion of cervical esophagus
    Contusion of larynx
    Contusion of pharynx
    Contusion of trachea

√5ᵗʰ **S10.1 Other and unspecified superficial injuries of throat**

  √x7ᵗʰ **S10.10 Unspecified superficial injuries of throat**

  √x7ᵗʰ **S10.11 Abrasion of throat**

  √x7ᵗʰ **S10.12 Blister (nonthermal) of throat**

  √x7ᵗʰ **S10.14 External constriction of part of throat**

  √x7ᵗʰ **S10.15 Superficial foreign body of throat**
     Splinter in the throat

  √x7ᵗʰ **S10.16 Insect bite (nonvenomous) of throat**

  √x7ᵗʰ **S10.17 Other superficial bite of throat**
     EXCLUDES 1 *open bite of throat (S11.85)*

√5ᵗʰ **S10.8 Superficial injury of other specified parts of neck**

  √x7ᵗʰ **S10.80 Unspecified superficial injury of other specified part of neck**

  √x7ᵗʰ **S10.81 Abrasion of other specified part of neck**

  √x7ᵗʰ **S10.82 Blister (nonthermal) of other specified part of neck**

  √x7ᵗʰ **S10.83 Contusion of other specified part of neck**

  √x7ᵗʰ **S10.84 External constriction of other specified part of neck**

  √x7ᵗʰ **S10.85 Superficial foreign body of other specified part of neck**
     Splinter in other specified part of neck

  √x7ᵗʰ **S10.86 Insect bite of other specified part of neck**

  √x7ᵗʰ **S10.87 Other superficial bite of other specified part of neck**
     EXCLUDES 1 *open bite of other specified parts of neck (S11.85)*

√5ᵗʰ **S10.9 Superficial injury of unspecified part of neck**

  √x7ᵗʰ **S10.90 Unspecified superficial injury of unspecified part of neck**

  √x7ᵗʰ **S10.91 Abrasion of unspecified part of neck**

  √x7ᵗʰ **S10.92 Blister (nonthermal) of unspecified part of neck**

  √x7ᵗʰ **S10.93 Contusion of unspecified part of neck**

  √x7ᵗʰ **S10.94 External constriction of unspecified part of neck**

  √x7ᵗʰ **S10.95 Superficial foreign body of unspecified part of neck**

  √x7ᵗʰ **S10.96 Insect bite of unspecified part of neck**

  √x7ᵗʰ **S10.97 Other superficial bite of unspecified part of neck**

Chapter 19. Injury, Poisoning and Certain Other Consequences of External Causes

☑️4th **S11 Open wound of neck**

Code also any associated:
  spinal cord injury (S14.0, S14.1-)
  wound infection
  EXCLUDES 2   open fracture of vertebra (S12.- with 7th character B)

> The appropriate 7th character is to be added to each code from category S11.
> A   initial encounter
> D   subsequent encounter
> S   sequela

☑️5th **S11.0 Open wound of larynx and trachea**

☑️6th **S11.01   Open wound of larynx**
  EXCLUDES 2   open wound of vocal cord (S11.03)

☑️7th **S11.011 Laceration without foreign body of larynx**
☑️7th **S11.012 Laceration with foreign body of larynx**
☑️7th **S11.013 Puncture wound without foreign body of larynx**
☑️7th **S11.014 Puncture wound with foreign body of larynx**
☑️7th **S11.015 Open bite of larynx**
  Bite of larynx NOS
☑️7th **S11.019 Unspecified open wound of larynx**

☑️6th **S11.02   Open wound of trachea**
  Open wound of cervical trachea
  Open wound of trachea NOS
  EXCLUDES 2   open wound of thoracic trachea (S27.5-)

☑️7th **S11.021 Laceration without foreign body of trachea**
☑️7th **S11.022 Laceration with foreign body of trachea**
☑️7th **S11.023 Puncture wound without foreign body of trachea**
☑️7th **S11.024 Puncture wound with foreign body of trachea**
☑️7th **S11.025 Open bite of trachea**
  Bite of trachea NOS
☑️7th **S11.029 Unspecified open wound of trachea**

☑️6th **S11.03   Open wound of vocal cord**

☑️7th **S11.031 Laceration without foreign body of vocal cord**
☑️7th **S11.032 Laceration with foreign body of vocal cord**
☑️7th **S11.033 Puncture wound without foreign body of vocal cord**
☑️7th **S11.034 Puncture wound with foreign body of vocal cord**
☑️7th **S11.035 Open bite of vocal cord**
  Bite of vocal cord NOS
☑️7th **S11.039 Unspecified open wound of vocal cord**

☑️5th **S11.1 Open wound of thyroid gland**

☑x7th **S11.10   Unspecified open wound of thyroid gland**
☑x7th **S11.11   Laceration without foreign body of thyroid gland**
☑x7th **S11.12   Laceration with foreign body of thyroid gland**
☑x7th **S11.13   Puncture wound without foreign body of thyroid gland**
☑x7th **S11.14   Puncture wound with foreign body of thyroid gland**
☑x7th **S11.15   Open bite of thyroid gland**
  Bite of thyroid gland NOS

☑️5th **S11.2 Open wound of pharynx and cervical esophagus**
  EXCLUDES 1   open wound of esophagus NOS (S27.8-)

☑x7th **S11.20   Unspecified open wound of pharynx and cervical esophagus**
☑x7th **S11.21   Laceration without foreign body of pharynx and cervical esophagus**
☑x7th **S11.22   Laceration with foreign body of pharynx and cervical esophagus**
☑x7th **S11.23   Puncture wound without foreign body of pharynx and cervical esophagus**
☑x7th **S11.24   Puncture wound with foreign body of pharynx and cervical esophagus**
☑x7th **S11.25   Open bite of pharynx and cervical esophagus**
  Bite of pharynx and cervical esophagus NOS

☑️5th **S11.8 Open wound of other specified parts of neck**

☑x7th **S11.80   Unspecified open wound of other specified part of neck**

☑x7th **S11.81   Laceration without foreign body of other specified part of neck**
☑x7th **S11.82   Laceration with foreign body of other specified part of neck**
☑x7th **S11.83   Puncture wound without foreign body of other specified part of neck**
☑x7th **S11.84   Puncture wound with foreign body of other specified part of neck**
☑x7th **S11.85   Open bite of other specified part of neck**
  Bite of other specified part of neck NOS
  EXCLUDES 1   superficial bite of other specified part of neck (S10.87)
☑x7th **S11.89   Other open wound of other specified part of neck**

☑️5th **S11.9 Open wound of unspecified part of neck**

☑x7th **S11.90   Unspecified open wound of unspecified part of neck**
☑x7th **S11.91   Laceration without foreign body of unspecified part of neck**
☑x7th **S11.92   Laceration with foreign body of unspecified part of neck**
☑x7th **S11.93   Puncture wound without foreign body of unspecified part of neck**
☑x7th **S11.94   Puncture wound with foreign body of unspecified part of neck**
☑x7th **S11.95   Open bite of unspecified part of neck**
  Bite of neck NOS
  EXCLUDES 1   superficial bite of neck (S10.97)

☑️4th **S12 Fracture of cervical vertebra and other parts of neck**

> **NOTE**   A fracture not indicated as displaced or nondisplaced should be coded to displaced.
> A fracture not indicated as open or closed should be coded to closed.

INCLUDES   fracture of cervical neural arch
  fracture of cervical spine
  fracture of cervical spinous process
  fracture of cervical transverse process
  fracture of cervical vertebral arch
  fracture of neck

Code first any associated cervical spinal cord injury (S14.0, S14.1-)
AHA: 2021,1Q,6; 2018,2Q,12; 2015,3Q,37-39

> The appropriate 7th character is to be added to all codes from subcategories S12.0-S12.6.
> A   initial encounter for closed fracture
> B   initial encounter for open fracture
> D   subsequent encounter for fracture with routine healing
> G   subsequent encounter for fracture with delayed healing
> K   subsequent encounter for fracture with nonunion
> S   sequela

☑️5th **S12.0 Fracture of first cervical vertebra**
  Atlas

☑️6th **S12.00   Unspecified fracture of first cervical vertebra**
  [1] ☑️7th **S12.000 Unspecified displaced fracture of first cervical vertebra** HCC ESR COM Q
  [1] ☑️7th **S12.001 Unspecified nondisplaced fracture of first cervical vertebra** HCC ESR COM Q
[1] ☑x7th **S12.01   Stable burst fracture of first cervical vertebra** HCC ESR COM Q
[1] ☑x7th **S12.02   Unstable burst fracture of first cervical vertebra** HCC ESR COM Q
☑️6th **S12.03   Posterior arch fracture of first cervical vertebra**
  [1] ☑️7th **S12.030 Displaced posterior arch fracture of first cervical vertebra** HCC ESR COM Q
  [1] ☑️7th **S12.031 Nondisplaced posterior arch fracture of first cervical vertebra** HCC ESR COM Q
☑️6th **S12.04   Lateral mass fracture of first cervical vertebra**
  [1] ☑️7th **S12.040 Displaced lateral mass fracture of first cervical vertebra** HCC ESR COM Q
  [1] ☑️7th **S12.041 Nondisplaced lateral mass fracture of first cervical vertebra** HCC ESR COM Q
☑️6th **S12.09   Other fracture of first cervical vertebra**
  [1] ☑️7th **S12.090 Other displaced fracture of first cervical vertebra** HCC ESR COM Q
  [1] ☑️7th **S12.091 Other nondisplaced fracture of first cervical vertebra** HCC ESR COM Q

√5ᵗʰ **S12.1** **Fracture of** second **cervical vertebra**
Axis

√6ᵗʰ **S12.10** **Unspecified fracture of second cervical vertebra**

¹ √7ᵗʰ **S12.100** **Unspecified** displaced **fracture of second cervical vertebra** `HCC` `ESR` `COM` `Q`

¹ √7ᵗʰ **S12.101** **Unspecified** nondisplaced **fracture of second cervical vertebra** `HCC` `ESR` `COM` `Q`

√6ᵗʰ **S12.11** **Type II** dens **fracture**

¹ √7ᵗʰ **S12.110** Anterior displaced **Type II dens fracture** `HCC` `ESR` `COM` `Q`

¹ √7ᵗʰ **S12.111** Posterior displaced **Type II dens fracture** `HCC` `ESR` `COM` `Q`

¹ √7ᵗʰ **S12.112** Nondisplaced **Type II dens fracture** `HCC` `ESR` `COM` `Q`

√6ᵗʰ **S12.12** **Other dens fracture**

¹ √7ᵗʰ **S12.120** **Other** displaced **dens fracture** `HCC` `ESR` `COM` `Q`

¹ √7ᵗʰ **S12.121** **Other** nondisplaced **dens fracture** `HCC` `ESR` `COM` `Q`

√6ᵗʰ **S12.13** **Unspecified traumatic** spondylolisthesis **of second cervical vertebra**

¹ √7ᵗʰ **S12.130** **Unspecified traumatic** displaced **spondylolisthesis of second cervical vertebra** `HCC` `ESR` `COM` `Q`

¹ √7ᵗʰ **S12.131** **Unspecified traumatic** nondisplaced **spondylolisthesis of second cervical vertebra** `HCC` `ESR` `COM` `Q`

¹ √x7ᵗʰ **S12.14** Type III **traumatic** spondylolisthesis **of second cervical vertebra** `HCC` `ESR` `COM` `Q`

√6ᵗʰ **S12.15** **Other traumatic** spondylolisthesis **of second cervical vertebra**

¹ √7ᵗʰ **S12.150** **Other traumatic** displaced **spondylolisthesis of second cervical vertebra** `HCC` `ESR` `COM` `Q`

¹ √7ᵗʰ **S12.151** **Other traumatic** nondisplaced **spondylolisthesis of second cervical vertebra** `HCC` `ESR` `COM` `Q`

√6ᵗʰ **S12.19** **Other fracture of second cervical vertebra**

¹ √7ᵗʰ **S12.190** **Other** displaced **fracture of second cervical vertebra** `HCC` `ESR` `COM` `Q`

¹ √7ᵗʰ **S12.191** **Other** nondisplaced **fracture of second cervical vertebra** `HCC` `ESR` `COM` `Q`

√5ᵗʰ **S12.2** **Fracture of** third **cervical vertebra**

√6ᵗʰ **S12.20** **Unspecified fracture of third cervical vertebra**

¹ √7ᵗʰ **S12.200** **Unspecified** displaced **fracture of third cervical vertebra** `HCC` `ESR` `COM` `Q`

¹ √7ᵗʰ **S12.201** **Unspecified** nondisplaced **fracture of third cervical vertebra** `HCC` `ESR` `COM` `Q`

√6ᵗʰ **S12.23** **Unspecified traumatic** spondylolisthesis **of third cervical vertebra**

¹ √7ᵗʰ **S12.230** **Unspecified traumatic** displaced **spondylolisthesis of third cervical vertebra** `HCC` `ESR` `COM` `Q`

¹ √7ᵗʰ **S12.231** **Unspecified traumatic** nondisplaced **spondylolisthesis of third cervical vertebra** `HCC` `ESR` `COM` `Q`

¹ √x7ᵗʰ **S12.24** Type III **traumatic** spondylolisthesis **of third cervical vertebra**

√6ᵗʰ **S12.25** **Other traumatic spondylolisthesis of third cervical vertebra**

¹ √7ᵗʰ **S12.250** **Other traumatic** displaced **spondylolisthesis of third cervical vertebra**

¹ √7ᵗʰ **S12.251** **Other traumatic** nondisplaced **spondylolisthesis of third cervical vertebra** `HCC` `ESR` `COM` `Q`

√6ᵗʰ **S12.29** **Other fracture of third cervical vertebra**

¹ √7ᵗʰ **S12.290** **Other** displaced **fracture of third cervical vertebra** `HCC` `ESR` `COM` `Q`

¹ √7ᵗʰ **S12.291** **Other** nondisplaced **fracture of third cervical vertebra**

√5ᵗʰ **S12.3** **Fracture of** fourth **cervical vertebra**

√6ᵗʰ **S12.30** **Unspecified fracture of fourth cervical vertebra**

¹ √7ᵗʰ **S12.300** **Unspecified** displaced **fracture of fourth cervical vertebra** `HCC` `ESR` `COM` `Q`

¹ √7ᵗʰ **S12.301** **Unspecified** nondisplaced **fracture of fourth cervical vertebra** `HCC` `ESR` `COM` `Q`

√6ᵗʰ **S12.33** **Unspecified traumatic spondylolisthesis of fourth cervical vertebra**

¹ √7ᵗʰ **S12.330** **Unspecified traumatic** displaced **spondylolisthesis of fourth cervical vertebra** `HCC` `ESR` `COM` `Q`

¹ √7ᵗʰ **S12.331** **Unspecified traumatic** nondisplaced **spondylolisthesis of fourth cervical vertebra** `HCC` `ESR` `COM` `Q`

¹ √x7ᵗʰ **S12.34** **Type III** traumatic spondylolisthesis **of fourth cervical vertebra** `HCC` `ESR` `COM` `Q`

√6ᵗʰ **S12.35** **Other traumatic** spondylolisthesis **of fourth cervical vertebra**

¹ √7ᵗʰ **S12.350** **Other traumatic** displaced **spondylolisthesis of fourth cervical vertebra** `HCC` `ESR` `COM` `Q`

¹ √7ᵗʰ **S12.351** **Other traumatic** nondisplaced **spondylolisthesis of fourth cervical vertebra**

√6ᵗʰ **S12.39** **Other fracture of fourth cervical vertebra**

¹ √7ᵗʰ **S12.390** **Other** displaced **fracture of fourth cervical vertebra** `HCC` `ESR` `COM` `Q`

¹ √7ᵗʰ **S12.391** **Other** nondisplaced **fracture of fourth cervical vertebra** `HCC` `ESR` `COM` `Q`

√5ᵗʰ **S12.4** **Fracture of** fifth **cervical vertebra**

√6ᵗʰ **S12.40** **Unspecified fracture of fifth cervical vertebra**

¹ √7ᵗʰ **S12.400** **Unspecified** displaced **fracture of fifth cervical vertebra** `HCC` `ESR` `COM` `Q`

¹ √7ᵗʰ **S12.401** **Unspecified** nondisplaced **fracture of fifth cervical vertebra** `HCC` `ESR` `COM` `Q`

√6ᵗʰ **S12.43** **Unspecified traumatic** spondylolisthesis **of fifth cervical vertebra**

¹ √7ᵗʰ **S12.430** **Unspecified traumatic** displaced **spondylolisthesis of fifth cervical vertebra** `HCC` `ESR` `COM` `Q`

¹ √7ᵗʰ **S12.431** **Unspecified traumatic** nondisplaced **spondylolisthesis of fifth cervical vertebra** `HCC` `ESR` `COM` `Q`

¹ √x7ᵗʰ **S12.44** **Type III** traumatic spondylolisthesis **of fifth cervical vertebra** `HCC` `ESR` `COM` `Q`

√6ᵗʰ **S12.45** **Other traumatic** spondylolisthesis **of fifth cervical vertebra**

¹ √7ᵗʰ **S12.450** **Other traumatic** displaced **spondylolisthesis of fifth cervical vertebra** `HCC` `ESR` `COM` `Q`

¹ √7ᵗʰ **S12.451** **Other traumatic** nondisplaced **spondylolisthesis of fifth cervical vertebra** `HCC` `ESR` `COM` `Q`

√6ᵗʰ **S12.49** **Other fracture of fifth cervical vertebra**

¹ √7ᵗʰ **S12.490** **Other** displaced **fracture of fifth cervical vertebra** `HCC` `ESR` `COM` `Q`

¹ √7ᵗʰ **S12.491** **Other** nondisplaced **fracture of fifth cervical vertebra** `HCC` `ESR` `COM` `Q`

√5ᵗʰ **S12.5** **Fracture of** sixth **cervical vertebra**

√6ᵗʰ **S12.50** **Unspecified fracture of sixth cervical vertebra**

¹ √7ᵗʰ **S12.500** **Unspecified** displaced **fracture of sixth cervical vertebra** `HCC` `ESR` `COM` `Q`

¹ √7ᵗʰ **S12.501** **Unspecified** nondisplaced **fracture of sixth cervical vertebra** `HCC` `ESR` `COM` `Q`

√6ᵗʰ **S12.53** **Unspecified traumatic** spondylolisthesis **of sixth cervical vertebra**

¹ √7ᵗʰ **S12.530** **Unspecified traumatic** displaced **spondylolisthesis of sixth cervical vertebra** `HCC` `ESR` `COM` `Q`

¹ √7ᵗʰ **S12.531** **Unspecified traumatic** nondisplaced **spondylolisthesis of sixth cervical vertebra** `HCC` `ESR` `COM` `Q`

¹ √x7ᵗʰ **S12.54** **Type III** traumatic spondylolisthesis **of sixth cervical vertebra** `HCC` `ESR` `COM` `Q`

√6ᵗʰ **S12.55** **Other traumatic** spondylolisthesis **of sixth cervical vertebra**

¹ √7ᵗʰ **S12.550** **Other traumatic** displaced **spondylolisthesis of sixth cervical vertebra** `HCC` `ESR` `COM` `Q`

¹ √7ᵗʰ **S12.551** **Other traumatic** nondisplaced **spondylolisthesis of sixth cervical vertebra** `HCC` `ESR` `COM` `Q`

√6ᵗʰ **S12.59** **Other fracture of sixth cervical vertebra**

¹ √7ᵗʰ **S12.590** **Other** displaced **fracture of sixth cervical vertebra** `HCC` `ESR` `COM` `Q`

---

¹ ✓7ᵗʰ **S12.591** Other nondisplaced fracture of sixth cervical vertebra `HCC` `ESR` `COM` `Q`

✓5ᵗʰ **S12.6 Fracture of seventh cervical vertebra**

  ✓6ᵗʰ **S12.60 Unspecified fracture of seventh cervical vertebra**

    ¹ ✓7ᵗʰ **S12.600** Unspecified displaced fracture of seventh cervical vertebra `HCC` `ESR` `COM` `Q`

    ¹ ✓7ᵗʰ **S12.601** Unspecified nondisplaced fracture of seventh cervical vertebra `HCC` `ESR` `COM` `Q`

  ✓6ᵗʰ **S12.63 Unspecified traumatic spondylolisthesis of seventh cervical vertebra**

    ¹ ✓7ᵗʰ **S12.630** Unspecified traumatic displaced spondylolisthesis of seventh cervical vertebra `HCC` `ESR` `COM` `Q`

    ¹ ✓7ᵗʰ **S12.631** Unspecified traumatic nondisplaced spondylolisthesis of seventh cervical vertebra `HCC` `ESR` `COM` `Q`

  ¹ ✓x7ᵗʰ **S12.64 Type III traumatic spondylolisthesis of seventh cervical vertebra** `HCC` `ESR` `COM` `Q`

  ✓6ᵗʰ **S12.65 Other traumatic spondylolisthesis of seventh cervical vertebra**

    ¹ ✓7ᵗʰ **S12.650** Other traumatic displaced spondylolisthesis of seventh cervical vertebra `HCC` `ESR` `COM` `Q`

    ¹ ✓7ᵗʰ **S12.651** Other traumatic nondisplaced spondylolisthesis of seventh cervical vertebra `HCC` `ESR` `COM` `Q`

  ✓6ᵗʰ **S12.69 Other fracture of seventh cervical vertebra**

    ¹ ✓7ᵗʰ **S12.690** Other displaced fracture of seventh cervical vertebra `HCC` `ESR` `COM` `Q`

    ¹ ✓7ᵗʰ **S12.691** Other nondisplaced fracture of seventh cervical vertebra `HCC` `ESR` `COM` `Q`

¹ ✓x7ᵗʰ **S12.8 Fracture of other parts of neck** `HCC` `ESR` `COM` `Q`

  Hyoid bone
  Larynx
  Thyroid cartilage
  Trachea

> The appropriate 7th character is to be added to code S12.8.
> A initial encounter
> D subsequent encounter
> S sequela

¹ ✓x7ᵗʰ **S12.9 Fracture of neck, unspecified** `HCC` `ESR` `COM` `Q`

  Fracture of neck NOS
  Fracture of cervical spine NOS
  Fracture of cervical vertebra NOS

> The appropriate 7th character is to be added to code S12.9.
> A initial encounter
> D subsequent encounter
> S sequela

✓4ᵗʰ **S13 Dislocation and sprain of joints and ligaments at neck level**

  INCLUDES avulsion of joint or ligament at neck level
    laceration of cartilage, joint or ligament at neck level
    sprain of cartilage, joint or ligament at neck level
    traumatic hemarthrosis of joint or ligament at neck level
    traumatic rupture of joint or ligament at neck level
    traumatic subluxation of joint or ligament at neck level
    traumatic tear of joint or ligament at neck level

  Code also any associated open wound
  EXCLUDES 2 *strain of muscle or tendon at neck level (S16.1)*

> The appropriate 7th character is to be added to each code from category S13.
> A initial encounter
> D subsequent encounter
> S sequela

  ✓x7ᵗʰ **S13.0 Traumatic rupture of cervical intervertebral disc**

    EXCLUDES 1 *rupture or displacement (nontraumatic) of cervical intervertebral disc NOS (M50.-)*

  ✓5ᵗʰ **S13.1 Subluxation and dislocation of cervical vertebrae**

    Code also any associated:
      open wound of neck (S11.-)
      spinal cord injury (S14.1-)
    EXCLUDES 2 *fracture of cervical vertebrae (S12.0-S12.3-)*

    ✓6ᵗʰ **S13.10 Subluxation and dislocation of unspecified cervical vertebrae**

      ✓7ᵗʰ **S13.100** Subluxation of unspecified cervical vertebra

      ✓7ᵗʰ **S13.101** Dislocation of unspecified cervical vertebra

    ✓6ᵗʰ **S13.11 Subluxation and dislocation of C0/C1 cervical vertebrae**

      Subluxation and dislocation of atlantooccipital joint
      Subluxation and dislocation of atloidooccipital joint
      Subluxation and dislocation of occipitoatloid joint

      ✓7ᵗʰ **S13.110** Subluxation of C0/C1 cervical vertebrae

      ✓7ᵗʰ **S13.111** Dislocation of C0/C1 cervical vertebrae

    ✓6ᵗʰ **S13.12 Subluxation and dislocation of C1/C2 cervical vertebrae**

      Subluxation and dislocation of atlantoaxial joint

      ✓7ᵗʰ **S13.120** Subluxation of C1/C2 cervical vertebrae

      ✓7ᵗʰ **S13.121** Dislocation of C1/C2 cervical vertebrae

    ✓6ᵗʰ **S13.13 Subluxation and dislocation of C2/C3 cervical vertebrae**

      ✓7ᵗʰ **S13.130** Subluxation of C2/C3 cervical vertebrae

      ✓7ᵗʰ **S13.131** Dislocation of C2/C3 cervical vertebrae

    ✓6ᵗʰ **S13.14 Subluxation and dislocation of C3/C4 cervical vertebrae**

      ✓7ᵗʰ **S13.140** Subluxation of C3/C4 cervical vertebrae

      ✓7ᵗʰ **S13.141** Dislocation of C3/C4 cervical vertebrae

    ✓6ᵗʰ **S13.15 Subluxation and dislocation of C4/C5 cervical vertebrae**

      ✓7ᵗʰ **S13.150** Subluxation of C4/C5 cervical vertebrae

      ✓7ᵗʰ **S13.151** Dislocation of C4/C5 cervical vertebrae

    ✓6ᵗʰ **S13.16 Subluxation and dislocation of C5/C6 cervical vertebrae**

      ✓7ᵗʰ **S13.160** Subluxation of C5/C6 cervical vertebrae

      ✓7ᵗʰ **S13.161** Dislocation of C5/C6 cervical vertebrae

    ✓6ᵗʰ **S13.17 Subluxation and dislocation of C6/C7 cervical vertebrae**

      ✓7ᵗʰ **S13.170** Subluxation of C6/C7 cervical vertebrae

      ✓7ᵗʰ **S13.171** Dislocation of C6/C7 cervical vertebrae

    ✓6ᵗʰ **S13.18 Subluxation and dislocation of C7/T1 cervical vertebrae**

      ✓7ᵗʰ **S13.180** Subluxation of C7/T1 cervical vertebrae

      ✓7ᵗʰ **S13.181** Dislocation of C7/T1 cervical vertebrae

  ✓5ᵗʰ **S13.2 Dislocation of other and unspecified parts of neck**

    ✓x7ᵗʰ **S13.20 Dislocation of unspecified parts of neck**

    ✓x7ᵗʰ **S13.29 Dislocation of other parts of neck**

  ✓x7ᵗʰ **S13.4 Sprain of ligaments of cervical spine**

    Sprain of anterior longitudinal (ligament), cervical
    Sprain of atlanto-axial (joints)
    Sprain of atlanto-occipital (joints)
    Whiplash injury of cervical spine

  ✓x7ᵗʰ **S13.5 Sprain of thyroid region**

    Sprain of cricoarytenoid (joint) (ligament)
    Sprain of cricothyroid (joint) (ligament)
    Sprain of thyroid cartilage

  ✓x7ᵗʰ **S13.8 Sprain of joints and ligaments of other parts of neck**

  ✓x7ᵗʰ **S13.9 Sprain of joints and ligaments of unspecified parts of neck**

✓4ᵗʰ **S14 Injury of nerves and spinal cord at neck level**

  NOTE Code to highest level of cervical cord injury

  Code also any associated:
    fracture of cervical vertebra (S12.0- — S12.6.-)
    open wound of neck (S11.-)
    transient paralysis (R29.5)

> The appropriate 7th character is to be added to each code from category S14.
> A initial encounter
> D subsequent encounter
> S sequela

  ✓x7ᵗʰ **S14.0 Concussion and edema of cervical spinal cord** `HCC` `ESR` `COM`

  ✓5ᵗʰ **S14.1 Other and unspecified injuries of cervical spinal cord**

    ✓6ᵗʰ **S14.10 Unspecified injury of cervical spinal cord**

      ✓7ᵗʰ **S14.101** Unspecified injury at C1 level of cervical spinal cord `HCC` `ESR` `COM`

      ✓7ᵗʰ **S14.102** Unspecified injury at C2 level of cervical spinal cord `HCC` `ESR` `COM`

      ✓7ᵗʰ **S14.103** Unspecified injury at C3 level of cervical spinal cord `HCC` `ESR` `COM`

√7ᵗʰ **S14.104 Unspecified injury at** C4 **level of cervical spinal cord** HCC ESR COM

√7ᵗʰ **S14.105 Unspecified injury at** C5 **level of cervical spinal cord** HCC ESR COM

√7ᵗʰ **S14.106 Unspecified injury at** C6 **level of cervical spinal cord** HCC ESR COM

√7ᵗʰ **S14.107 Unspecified injury at** C7 **level of cervical spinal cord** HCC ESR COM

√7ᵗʰ **S14.108 Unspecified injury at** C8 **level of cervical spinal cord** HCC ESR COM

√7ᵗʰ **S14.109 Unspecified injury at unspecified level of cervical spinal cord** HCC ESR COM
Injury of cervical spinal cord NOS

√6ᵗʰ **S14.11 Complete lesion of cervical spinal cord**

√7ᵗʰ **S14.111 Complete lesion at** C1 **level of cervical spinal cord** HCC ESR COM

√7ᵗʰ **S14.112 Complete lesion at** C2 **level of cervical spinal cord** HCC ESR COM

√7ᵗʰ **S14.113 Complete lesion at** C3 **level of cervical spinal cord** HCC ESR COM

√7ᵗʰ **S14.114 Complete lesion at** C4 **level of cervical spinal cord** HCC ESR COM

√7ᵗʰ **S14.115 Complete lesion at** C5 **level of cervical spinal cord** HCC ESR COM

√7ᵗʰ **S14.116 Complete lesion at** C6 **level of cervical spinal cord** HCC ESR COM

√7ᵗʰ **S14.117 Complete lesion at** C7 **level of cervical spinal cord** HCC ESR COM

√7ᵗʰ **S14.118 Complete lesion at** C8 **level of cervical spinal cord** HCC ESR COM

√7ᵗʰ **S14.119 Complete lesion at unspecified level of cervical spinal cord** HCC ESR COM

√6ᵗʰ **S14.12 Central cord syndrome of cervical spinal cord**

√7ᵗʰ **S14.121 Central cord syndrome at** C1 **level of cervical spinal cord** HCC ESR COM

√7ᵗʰ **S14.122 Central cord syndrome at** C2 **level of cervical spinal cord** HCC ESR COM

√7ᵗʰ **S14.123 Central cord syndrome at** C3 **level of cervical spinal cord** HCC ESR COM

√7ᵗʰ **S14.124 Central cord syndrome at** C4 **level of cervical spinal cord** HCC ESR COM

√7ᵗʰ **S14.125 Central cord syndrome at** C5 **level of cervical spinal cord** HCC ESR COM

√7ᵗʰ **S14.126 Central cord syndrome at** C6 **level of cervical spinal cord** HCC ESR COM

√7ᵗʰ **S14.127 Central cord syndrome at** C7 **level of cervical spinal cord** HCC ESR COM

√7ᵗʰ **S14.128 Central cord syndrome at** C8 **level of cervical spinal cord** HCC ESR COM

√7ᵗʰ **S14.129 Central cord syndrome at unspecified level of cervical spinal cord** HCC ESR COM

√6ᵗʰ **S14.13 Anterior cord syndrome of cervical spinal cord**

√7ᵗʰ **S14.131 Anterior cord syndrome at** C1 **level of cervical spinal cord** HCC ESR COM

√7ᵗʰ **S14.132 Anterior cord syndrome at** C2 **level of cervical spinal cord** HCC ESR COM

√7ᵗʰ **S14.133 Anterior cord syndrome at** C3 **level of cervical spinal cord** HCC ESR COM

√7ᵗʰ **S14.134 Anterior cord syndrome at** C4 **level of cervical spinal cord** HCC ESR COM

√7ᵗʰ **S14.135 Anterior cord syndrome at** C5 **level of cervical spinal cord** HCC ESR COM

√7ᵗʰ **S14.136 Anterior cord syndrome at** C6 **level of cervical spinal cord** HCC ESR COM

√7ᵗʰ **S14.137 Anterior cord syndrome at** C7 **level of cervical spinal cord** HCC ESR COM

√7ᵗʰ **S14.138 Anterior cord syndrome at** C8 **level of cervical spinal cord** HCC ESR COM

√7ᵗʰ **S14.139 Anterior cord syndrome at unspecified level of cervical spinal cord** HCC ESR COM

√6ᵗʰ **S14.14 Brown-Séquard syndrome of cervical spinal cord**

√7ᵗʰ **S14.141 Brown-Séquard syndrome at** C1 **level of cervical spinal cord** HCC ESR COM

√7ᵗʰ **S14.142 Brown-Séquard syndrome at** C2 **level of cervical spinal cord** HCC ESR COM

√7ᵗʰ **S14.143 Brown-Séquard syndrome at** C3 **level of cervical spinal cord** HCC ESR COM

√7ᵗʰ **S14.144 Brown-Séquard syndrome at** C4 **level of cervical spinal cord** HCC ESR COM

√7ᵗʰ **S14.145 Brown-Séquard syndrome at** C5 **level of cervical spinal cord** HCC ESR COM

√7ᵗʰ **S14.146 Brown-Séquard syndrome at** C6 **level of cervical spinal cord** HCC ESR COM

√7ᵗʰ **S14.147 Brown-Séquard syndrome at** C7 **level of cervical spinal cord** HCC ESR COM

√7ᵗʰ **S14.148 Brown-Séquard syndrome at** C8 **level of cervical spinal cord** HCC ESR COM

√7ᵗʰ **S14.149 Brown-Séquard syndrome at unspecified level of cervical spinal cord** HCC ESR COM

√6ᵗʰ **S14.15 Other incomplete lesions of cervical spinal cord**
Incomplete lesion of cervical spinal cord NOS
Posterior cord syndrome of cervical spinal cord

√7ᵗʰ **S14.151 Other incomplete lesion at** C1 **level of cervical spinal cord** HCC ESR COM

√7ᵗʰ **S14.152 Other incomplete lesion at** C2 **level of cervical spinal cord** HCC ESR COM

√7ᵗʰ **S14.153 Other incomplete lesion at** C3 **level of cervical spinal cord** HCC ESR COM

√7ᵗʰ **S14.154 Other incomplete lesion at** C4 **level of cervical spinal cord** HCC ESR COM

√7ᵗʰ **S14.155 Other incomplete lesion at** C5 **level of cervical spinal cord** HCC ESR COM

√7ᵗʰ **S14.156 Other incomplete lesion at** C6 **level of cervical spinal cord** HCC ESR COM

√7ᵗʰ **S14.157 Other incomplete lesion at** C7 **level of cervical spinal cord** HCC ESR COM

√7ᵗʰ **S14.158 Other incomplete lesion at** C8 **level of cervical spinal cord** HCC ESR COM

√7ᵗʰ **S14.159 Other incomplete lesion at unspecified level of cervical spinal cord** HCC ESR COM

√x7ᵗʰ **S14.2 Injury of** nerve root of cervical spine

√x7ᵗʰ **S14.3 Injury of** brachial plexus

√x7ᵗʰ **S14.4 Injury of** peripheral nerves of neck

√x7ᵗʰ **S14.5 Injury of** cervical sympathetic nerves

√x7ᵗʰ **S14.8 Injury of other specified nerves of neck**

√x7ᵗʰ **S14.9 Injury of unspecified nerves of neck**

√4ᵗʰ **S15 Injury of blood vessels at neck level**
Code also any associated open wound (S11.-)

The appropriate 7th character is to be added to each code from category S15.
A initial encounter
D subsequent encounter
S sequela

√5ᵗʰ **S15.0 Injury of** carotid artery **of neck**
Injury of carotid artery (common) (external) (internal, extracranial portion)
Injury of carotid artery NOS

EXCLUDES 1   *injury of internal carotid artery, intracranial portion (S06.8)*

√6ᵗʰ **S15.00 Unspecified injury of carotid artery**

√7ᵗʰ **S15.001 Unspecified injury of** right **carotid artery**

√7ᵗʰ **S15.002 Unspecified injury of** left **carotid artery**

√7ᵗʰ **S15.009 Unspecified injury of unspecified carotid artery**

√6ᵗʰ **S15.01 Minor laceration of carotid artery**
Incomplete transection of carotid artery
Laceration of carotid artery NOS
Superficial laceration of carotid artery

√7ᵗʰ **S15.011 Minor laceration of** right **carotid artery**

√7ᵗʰ **S15.012 Minor laceration of** left **carotid artery**

√7ᵗʰ **S15.019 Minor laceration of unspecified carotid artery**

√6ᵗʰ **S15.02 Major laceration of carotid artery**
Complete transection of carotid artery
Traumatic rupture of carotid artery

√7ᵗʰ **S15.021 Major laceration of** right **carotid artery**

√7ᵗʰ **S15.022 Major laceration of** left **carotid artery**

√7ᵗʰ **S15.029 Major laceration of unspecified carotid artery**

√6ᵗʰ **S15.09**   Other specified injury of carotid artery

√7ᵗʰ   **S15.091**   Other specified injury of right carotid artery

√7ᵗʰ   **S15.092**   Other specified injury of left carotid artery

√7ᵗʰ   **S15.099**   Other specified injury of unspecified carotid artery

√5ᵗʰ **S15.1**   Injury of vertebral artery

√6ᵗʰ   **S15.10**   Unspecified injury of vertebral artery

√7ᵗʰ   **S15.101**   Unspecified injury of right vertebral artery

√7ᵗʰ   **S15.102**   Unspecified injury of left vertebral artery

√7ᵗʰ   **S15.109**   Unspecified injury of unspecified vertebral artery

√6ᵗʰ   **S15.11**   Minor laceration of vertebral artery

Incomplete transection of vertebral artery

Laceration of vertebral artery NOS

Superficial laceration of vertebral artery

√7ᵗʰ   **S15.111**   Minor laceration of right vertebral artery

√7ᵗʰ   **S15.112**   Minor laceration of left vertebral artery

√7ᵗʰ   **S15.119**   Minor laceration of unspecified vertebral artery

√6ᵗʰ   **S15.12**   Major laceration of vertebral artery

Complete transection of vertebral artery

Traumatic rupture of vertebral artery

√7ᵗʰ   **S15.121**   Major laceration of right vertebral artery

√7ᵗʰ   **S15.122**   Major laceration of left vertebral artery

√7ᵗʰ   **S15.129**   Major laceration of unspecified vertebral artery

√6ᵗʰ   **S15.19**   Other specified injury of vertebral artery

√7ᵗʰ   **S15.191**   Other specified injury of right vertebral artery

√7ᵗʰ   **S15.192**   Other specified injury of left vertebral artery

√7ᵗʰ   **S15.199**   Other specified injury of unspecified vertebral artery

√5ᵗʰ **S15.2**   Injury of external jugular vein

√6ᵗʰ   **S15.20**   Unspecified injury of external jugular vein

√7ᵗʰ   **S15.201**   Unspecified injury of right external jugular vein

√7ᵗʰ   **S15.202**   Unspecified injury of left external jugular vein

√7ᵗʰ   **S15.209**   Unspecified injury of unspecified external jugular vein

√6ᵗʰ   **S15.21**   Minor laceration of external jugular vein

Incomplete transection of external jugular vein

Laceration of external jugular vein NOS

Superficial laceration of external jugular vein

√7ᵗʰ   **S15.211**   Minor laceration of right external jugular vein

√7ᵗʰ   **S15.212**   Minor laceration of left external jugular vein

√7ᵗʰ   **S15.219**   Minor laceration of unspecified external jugular vein

√6ᵗʰ   **S15.22**   Major laceration of external jugular vein

Complete transection of external jugular vein

Traumatic rupture of external jugular vein

√7ᵗʰ   **S15.221**   Major laceration of right external jugular vein

√7ᵗʰ   **S15.222**   Major laceration of left external jugular vein

√7ᵗʰ   **S15.229**   Major laceration of unspecified external jugular vein

√6ᵗʰ   **S15.29**   Other specified injury of external jugular vein

√7ᵗʰ   **S15.291**   Other specified injury of right external jugular vein

√7ᵗʰ   **S15.292**   Other specified injury of left external jugular vein

√7ᵗʰ   **S15.299**   Other specified injury of unspecified external jugular vein

√5ᵗʰ **S15.3**   Injury of internal jugular vein

√6ᵗʰ   **S15.30**   Unspecified injury of internal jugular vein

√7ᵗʰ   **S15.301**   Unspecified injury of right internal jugular vein

√7ᵗʰ   **S15.302**   Unspecified injury of left internal jugular vein

√7ᵗʰ   **S15.309**   Unspecified injury of unspecified internal jugular vein

√6ᵗʰ   **S15.31**   Minor laceration of internal jugular vein

Incomplete transection of internal jugular vein

Laceration of internal jugular vein NOS

Superficial laceration of internal jugular vein

√7ᵗʰ   **S15.311**   Minor laceration of right internal jugular vein

√7ᵗʰ   **S15.312**   Minor laceration of left internal jugular vein

√7ᵗʰ   **S15.319**   Minor laceration of unspecified internal jugular vein

√6ᵗʰ   **S15.32**   Major laceration of internal jugular vein

Complete transection of internal jugular vein

Traumatic rupture of internal jugular vein

√7ᵗʰ   **S15.321**   Major laceration of right internal jugular vein

√7ᵗʰ   **S15.322**   Major laceration of left internal jugular vein

√7ᵗʰ   **S15.329**   Major laceration of unspecified internal jugular vein

√6ᵗʰ   **S15.39**   Other specified injury of internal jugular vein

√7ᵗʰ   **S15.391**   Other specified injury of right internal jugular vein

√7ᵗʰ   **S15.392**   Other specified injury of left internal jugular vein

√7ᵗʰ   **S15.399**   Other specified injury of unspecified internal jugular vein

√x7ᵗʰ **S15.8**   Injury of other specified blood vessels at neck level

√x7ᵗʰ **S15.9**   Injury of unspecified blood vessel at neck level

√4ᵗʰ **S16**   **Injury of muscle, fascia and tendon at neck level**

Code also any associated open wound (S11.-)

EXCLUDES 2   sprain of joint or ligament at neck level (S13.9)

The appropriate 7th character is to be added to each code from category S16.
A   initial encounter
D   subsequent encounter
S   sequela

√x7ᵗʰ **S16.1**   Strain of muscle, fascia and tendon at neck level

√x7ᵗʰ **S16.2**   Laceration of muscle, fascia and tendon at neck level

√x7ᵗʰ **S16.8**   Other specified injury of muscle, fascia and tendon at neck level

√x7ᵗʰ **S16.9**   Unspecified injury of muscle, fascia and tendon at neck level

√4ᵗʰ **S17**   **Crushing injury of neck**

Use additional code for all associated injuries, such as:
injury of blood vessels (S15.-)
open wound of neck (S11.-)
spinal cord injury (S14.0, S14.1-)
vertebral fracture (S12.0- — S12.3-)

The appropriate 7th character is to be added to each code from category S17.
A   initial encounter
D   subsequent encounter
S   sequela

√x7ᵗʰ **S17.0**   Crushing injury of larynx and trachea

√x7ᵗʰ **S17.8**   Crushing injury of other specified parts of neck

√x7ᵗʰ **S17.9**   Crushing injury of neck, part unspecified

√4ᵗʰ **S19**   **Other specified and unspecified injuries of neck**

The appropriate 7th character is to be added to each code from category S19.
A   initial encounter
D   subsequent encounter
S   sequela

√5ᵗʰ **S19.8**   Other specified injuries of neck

√x7ᵗʰ   **S19.80**   Other specified injuries of unspecified part of neck

√x7ᵗʰ   **S19.81**   Other specified injuries of larynx

√x7ᵗʰ   **S19.82**   Other specified injuries of cervical trachea

EXCLUDES 2   other specified injury of thoracic trachea (S27.5-)

√x7ᵗʰ   **S19.83**   Other specified injuries of vocal cord

√x7ᵗʰ   **S19.84**   Other specified injuries of thyroid gland

√x7ᵗʰ   **S19.85**   Other specified injuries of pharynx and cervical esophagus

AHA: 2022,1Q,27

HCC CMS-HCC   **Rx** Rx HCC   **ESR** ESRD HCC   **COM** Commercial HCC   **N** Newborn: 0   **P** Pediatric: 0-17   **M** Maternity: 9-64   **A** Adult: 15-124

1010

ICD-10-CM 2023

√x7ᵗʰ **S19.89** Other specified injuries of other specified part of neck

√x7ᵗʰ **S19.9** Unspecified injury of neck

Injuries to the thorax (S20-S29)

INCLUDES	injuries of breast
	injuries of chest (wall)
	injuries of interscapular area

EXCLUDES 2
burns and corrosions (T20-T32)
effects of foreign body in bronchus (T17.5)
effects of foreign body in esophagus (T18.1)
effects of foreign body in lung (T17.8)
effects of foreign body in trachea (T17.4)
frostbite (T33-T34)
injuries of axilla
injuries of clavicle
injuries of scapular region
injuries of shoulder
insect bite or sting, venomous (T63.4)

Neck

√4ᵗʰ **S20** Superficial injury of thorax

AHA: 2020,4Q,39

The appropriate 7th character is to be added to each code from category S20.
A   initial encounter
D   subsequent encounter
S   sequela

√5ᵗʰ **S20.0** Contusion of breast
- √x7ᵗʰ **S20.00** Contusion of breast, unspecified breast
- √x7ᵗʰ **S20.01** Contusion of right breast
- √x7ᵗʰ **S20.02** Contusion of left breast

√5ᵗʰ **S20.1** Other and unspecified superficial injuries of breast
- √6ᵗʰ **S20.10** Unspecified superficial injuries of breast
  - √7ᵗʰ **S20.101** Unspecified superficial injuries of breast, right breast
  - √7ᵗʰ **S20.102** Unspecified superficial injuries of breast, left breast
  - √7ᵗʰ **S20.109** Unspecified superficial injuries of breast, unspecified breast
- √6ᵗʰ **S20.11** Abrasion of breast
  - √7ᵗʰ **S20.111** Abrasion of breast, right breast
  - √7ᵗʰ **S20.112** Abrasion of breast, left breast
  - √7ᵗʰ **S20.119** Abrasion of breast, unspecified breast
- √6ᵗʰ **S20.12** Blister (nonthermal) of breast
  - √7ᵗʰ **S20.121** Blister (nonthermal) of breast, right breast
  - √7ᵗʰ **S20.122** Blister (nonthermal) of breast, left breast
  - √7ᵗʰ **S20.129** Blister (nonthermal) of breast, unspecified breast
- √6ᵗʰ **S20.14** External constriction of part of breast
  - √7ᵗʰ **S20.141** External constriction of part of breast, right breast
  - √7ᵗʰ **S20.142** External constriction of part of breast, left breast
  - √7ᵗʰ **S20.149** External constriction of part of breast, unspecified breast
- √6ᵗʰ **S20.15** Superficial foreign body of breast
  Splinter in the breast
  - √7ᵗʰ **S20.151** Superficial foreign body of breast, right breast
  - √7ᵗʰ **S20.152** Superficial foreign body of breast, left breast
  - √7ᵗʰ **S20.159** Superficial foreign body of breast, unspecified breast
- √6ᵗʰ **S20.16** Insect bite (nonvenomous) of breast
  - √7ᵗʰ **S20.161** Insect bite (nonvenomous) of breast, right breast
  - √7ᵗʰ **S20.162** Insect bite (nonvenomous) of breast, left breast
  - √7ᵗʰ **S20.169** Insect bite (nonvenomous) of breast, unspecified breast
- √6ᵗʰ **S20.17** Other superficial bite of breast
  - EXCLUDES 1 open bite of breast (S21.05-)
  - √7ᵗʰ **S20.171** Other superficial bite of breast, right breast
  - √7ᵗʰ **S20.172** Other superficial bite of breast, left breast

√7ᵗʰ **S20.179** Other superficial bite of breast, unspecified breast

√5ᵗʰ **S20.2** Contusion of thorax
- √x7ᵗʰ **S20.20** Contusion of thorax, unspecified
- √6ᵗʰ **S20.21** Contusion of front wall of thorax
  - √7ᵗʰ **S20.211** Contusion of right front wall of thorax
  - √7ᵗʰ **S20.212** Contusion of left front wall of thorax
  - √7ᵗʰ **S20.213** Contusion of bilateral front wall of thorax
  - √7ᵗʰ **S20.214** Contusion of middle front wall of thorax
  - √7ᵗʰ **S20.219** Contusion of unspecified front wall of thorax
- √6ᵗʰ **S20.22** Contusion of back wall of thorax
  - √7ᵗʰ **S20.221** Contusion of right back wall of thorax
  - √7ᵗʰ **S20.222** Contusion of left back wall of thorax
  - √7ᵗʰ **S20.223** Contusion of bilateral back wall of thorax
  - √7ᵗʰ **S20.224** Contusion of middle back wall of thorax
  - √7ᵗʰ **S20.229** Contusion of unspecified back wall of thorax

√5ᵗʰ **S20.3** Other and unspecified superficial injuries of front wall of thorax
- √6ᵗʰ **S20.30** Unspecified superficial injuries of front wall of thorax
  - √7ᵗʰ **S20.301** Unspecified superficial injuries of right front wall of thorax
  - √7ᵗʰ **S20.302** Unspecified superficial injuries of left front wall of thorax
  - √7ᵗʰ **S20.303** Unspecified superficial injuries of bilateral front wall of thorax
  - √7ᵗʰ **S20.304** Unspecified superficial injuries of middle front wall of thorax
  - √7ᵗʰ **S20.309** Unspecified superficial injuries of unspecified front wall of thorax
- √6ᵗʰ **S20.31** Abrasion of front wall of thorax
  - √7ᵗʰ **S20.311** Abrasion of right front wall of thorax
  - √7ᵗʰ **S20.312** Abrasion of left front wall of thorax
  - √7ᵗʰ **S20.313** Abrasion of bilateral front wall of thorax
  - √7ᵗʰ **S20.314** Abrasion of middle front wall of thorax
  - √7ᵗʰ **S20.319** Abrasion of unspecified front wall of thorax
- √6ᵗʰ **S20.32** Blister (nonthermal) of front wall of thorax
  - √7ᵗʰ **S20.321** Blister (nonthermal) of right front wall of thorax
  - √7ᵗʰ **S20.322** Blister (nonthermal) of left front wall of thorax
  - √7ᵗʰ **S20.323** Blister (nonthermal) of bilateral front wall of thorax
  - √7ᵗʰ **S20.324** Blister (nonthermal) of middle front wall of thorax
  - √7ᵗʰ **S20.329** Blister (nonthermal) of unspecified front wall of thorax
- √6ᵗʰ **S20.34** External constriction of front wall of thorax
  - √7ᵗʰ **S20.341** External constriction of right front wall of thorax
  - √7ᵗʰ **S20.342** External constriction of left front wall of thorax
  - √7ᵗʰ **S20.343** External constriction of bilateral front wall of thorax
  - √7ᵗʰ **S20.344** External constriction of middle front wall of thorax
  - √7ᵗʰ **S20.349** External constriction of unspecified front wall of thorax
- √6ᵗʰ **S20.35** Superficial foreign body of front wall of thorax
  Splinter in front wall of thorax
  - √7ᵗʰ **S20.351** Superficial foreign body of right front wall of thorax
  - √7ᵗʰ **S20.352** Superficial foreign body of left front wall of thorax
  - √7ᵗʰ **S20.353** Superficial foreign body of bilateral front wall of thorax
  - √7ᵗʰ **S20.354** Superficial foreign body of middle front wall of thorax
  - √7ᵗʰ **S20.359** Superficial foreign body of unspecified front wall of thorax
- √6ᵗʰ **S20.36** Insect bite (nonvenomous) of front wall of thorax
  - √7ᵗʰ **S20.361** Insect bite (nonvenomous) of right front wall of thorax

Neck

✔ Additional Character Required   √x7ᵗʰ Placeholder Alert   Manifestation   Unspecified Dx   ◘ QPP   UPD Unacceptable PDx
ICD-10-CM 2023   **1011**

Chapter 19. Injury, Poisoning and Certain Other Consequences of External Causes

S19.89-S20.361

√7ᵗʰ **S20.362** Insect bite (nonvenomous) of left front wall of thorax

√7ᵗʰ **S20.363** Insect bite (nonvenomous) of bilateral front wall of thorax

√7ᵗʰ **S20.364** Insect bite (nonvenomous) of middle front wall of thorax

√7ᵗʰ **S20.369** Insect bite (nonvenomous) of unspecified front wall of thorax

√6ᵗʰ **S20.37** Other superficial bite of front wall of thorax
> EXCLUDES 1　　open bite of front wall of thorax (S21.15)

√7ᵗʰ **S20.371** Other superficial bite of right front wall of thorax

√7ᵗʰ **S20.372** Other superficial bite of left front wall of thorax

√7ᵗʰ **S20.373** Other superficial bite of bilateral front wall of thorax

√7ᵗʰ **S20.374** Other superficial bite of middle front wall of thorax

√7ᵗʰ **S20.379** Other superficial bite of unspecified front wall of thorax

√5ᵗʰ **S20.4** Other and unspecified superficial injuries of back wall of thorax

√6ᵗʰ **S20.40** Unspecified superficial injuries of back wall of thorax

√7ᵗʰ **S20.401** Unspecified superficial injuries of right back wall of thorax

√7ᵗʰ **S20.402** Unspecified superficial injuries of left back wall of thorax

√7ᵗʰ **S20.409** Unspecified superficial injuries of unspecified back wall of thorax

√6ᵗʰ **S20.41** Abrasion of back wall of thorax

√7ᵗʰ **S20.411** Abrasion of right back wall of thorax

√7ᵗʰ **S20.412** Abrasion of left back wall of thorax

√7ᵗʰ **S20.419** Abrasion of unspecified back wall of thorax

√6ᵗʰ **S20.42** Blister (nonthermal) of back wall of thorax

√7ᵗʰ **S20.421** Blister (nonthermal) of right back wall of thorax

√7ᵗʰ **S20.422** Blister (nonthermal) of left back wall of thorax

√7ᵗʰ **S20.429** Blister (nonthermal) of unspecified back wall of thorax

√6ᵗʰ **S20.44** External constriction of back wall of thorax

√7ᵗʰ **S20.441** External constriction of right back wall of thorax

√7ᵗʰ **S20.442** External constriction of left back wall of thorax

√7ᵗʰ **S20.449** External constriction of unspecified back wall of thorax

√6ᵗʰ **S20.45** Superficial foreign body of back wall of thorax
> Splinter of back wall of thorax

√7ᵗʰ **S20.451** Superficial foreign body of right back wall of thorax

√7ᵗʰ **S20.452** Superficial foreign body of left back wall of thorax

√7ᵗʰ **S20.459** Superficial foreign body of unspecified back wall of thorax

√6ᵗʰ **S20.46** Insect bite (nonvenomous) of back wall of thorax

√7ᵗʰ **S20.461** Insect bite (nonvenomous) of right back wall of thorax

√7ᵗʰ **S20.462** Insect bite (nonvenomous) of left back wall of thorax

√7ᵗʰ **S20.469** Insect bite (nonvenomous) of unspecified back wall of thorax

√6ᵗʰ **S20.47** Other superficial bite of back wall of thorax
> EXCLUDES 1　　open bite of back wall of thorax (S21.25)

√7ᵗʰ **S20.471** Other superficial bite of right back wall of thorax

√7ᵗʰ **S20.472** Other superficial bite of left back wall of thorax

√7ᵗʰ **S20.479** Other superficial bite of unspecified back wall of thorax

√5ᵗʰ **S20.9** Superficial injury of unspecified parts of thorax
> EXCLUDES 1　　contusion of thorax NOS (S20.20)

√x7ᵗʰ **S20.90** Unspecified superficial injury of unspecified parts of thorax
> Superficial injury of thoracic wall NOS

√x7ᵗʰ **S20.91** Abrasion of unspecified parts of thorax

√x7ᵗʰ **S20.92** Blister (nonthermal) of unspecified parts of thorax

√x7ᵗʰ **S20.94** External constriction of unspecified parts of thorax

√x7ᵗʰ **S20.95** Superficial foreign body of unspecified parts of thorax
> Splinter in thorax NOS

√x7ᵗʰ **S20.96** Insect bite (nonvenomous) of unspecified parts of thorax

√x7ᵗʰ **S20.97** Other superficial bite of unspecified parts of thorax
> EXCLUDES 1　　open bite of thorax NOS (S21.95)

√4ᵗʰ **S21** Open wound of thorax
> Code also any associated injury, such as:
> injury of heart (S26.-)
> injury of intrathoracic organs (S27.-)
> rib fracture (S22.3-, S22.4-)
> spinal cord injury (S24.0-, S24.1-)
> traumatic hemopneumothorax (S27.3)
> traumatic hemothorax (S27.1)
> traumatic pneumothorax (S27.0)
> wound infection
> EXCLUDES 1　　traumatic amputation (partial) of thorax (S28.1)

> The appropriate 7th character is to be added to each code from category S21.
> A　initial encounter
> D　subsequent encounter
> S　sequela

√5ᵗʰ **S21.0** Open wound of breast

√6ᵗʰ **S21.00** Unspecified open wound of breast

√7ᵗʰ **S21.001** Unspecified open wound of right breast

√7ᵗʰ **S21.002** Unspecified open wound of left breast

√7ᵗʰ **S21.009** Unspecified open wound of unspecified breast

√6ᵗʰ **S21.01** Laceration without foreign body of breast

√7ᵗʰ **S21.011** Laceration without foreign body of right breast

√7ᵗʰ **S21.012** Laceration without foreign body of left breast

√7ᵗʰ **S21.019** Laceration without foreign body of unspecified breast

√6ᵗʰ **S21.02** Laceration with foreign body of breast

√7ᵗʰ **S21.021** Laceration with foreign body of right breast

√7ᵗʰ **S21.022** Laceration with foreign body of left breast

√7ᵗʰ **S21.029** Laceration with foreign body of unspecified breast

√6ᵗʰ **S21.03** Puncture wound without foreign body of breast

√7ᵗʰ **S21.031** Puncture wound without foreign body of right breast

√7ᵗʰ **S21.032** Puncture wound without foreign body of left breast

√7ᵗʰ **S21.039** Puncture wound without foreign body of unspecified breast

√6ᵗʰ **S21.04** Puncture wound with foreign body of breast

√7ᵗʰ **S21.041** Puncture wound with foreign body of right breast

√7ᵗʰ **S21.042** Puncture wound with foreign body of left breast

√7ᵗʰ **S21.049** Puncture wound with foreign body of unspecified breast

√6ᵗʰ **S21.05** Open bite of breast
> Bite of breast NOS
> EXCLUDES 1　　superficial bite of breast (S20.17)

√7ᵗʰ **S21.051** Open bite of right breast

√7ᵗʰ **S21.052** Open bite of left breast

√7ᵗʰ **S21.059** Open bite of unspecified breast

√5ᵗʰ **S21.1** Open wound of front wall of thorax without penetration into thoracic cavity
> Open wound of chest without penetration into thoracic cavity

√6ᵗʰ **S21.10** Unspecified open wound of front wall of thorax without penetration into thoracic cavity

√7ᵗʰ **S21.101** Unspecified open wound of right front wall of thorax without penetration into thoracic cavity

√7ᵗʰ **S21.102** Unspecified open wound of left front wall of thorax without penetration into thoracic cavity

√7ᵗʰ **S21.109** Unspecified open wound of unspecified front wall of thorax without penetration into thoracic cavity

√6ᵗʰ **S21.11** Laceration without foreign body of front wall of thorax without penetration into thoracic cavity

√7ᵗʰ **S21.111** Laceration without foreign body of right front wall of thorax without penetration into thoracic cavity

√7ᵗʰ **S21.112** Laceration without foreign body of left front wall of thorax without penetration into thoracic cavity

√7ᵗʰ **S21.119** Laceration without foreign body of unspecified front wall of thorax without penetration into thoracic cavity

√6ᵗʰ **S21.12** Laceration with foreign body of front wall of thorax without penetration into thoracic cavity

√7ᵗʰ **S21.121** Laceration with foreign body of right front wall of thorax without penetration into thoracic cavity

√7ᵗʰ **S21.122** Laceration with foreign body of left front wall of thorax without penetration into thoracic cavity

√7ᵗʰ **S21.129** Laceration with foreign body of unspecified front wall of thorax without penetration into thoracic cavity

√6ᵗʰ **S21.13** Puncture wound without foreign body of front wall of thorax without penetration into thoracic cavity

√7ᵗʰ **S21.131** Puncture wound without foreign body of right front wall of thorax without penetration into thoracic cavity

√7ᵗʰ **S21.132** Puncture wound without foreign body of left front wall of thorax without penetration into thoracic cavity

√7ᵗʰ **S21.139** Puncture wound without foreign body of unspecified front wall of thorax without penetration into thoracic cavity

√6ᵗʰ **S21.14** Puncture wound with foreign body of front wall of thorax without penetration into thoracic cavity

√7ᵗʰ **S21.141** Puncture wound with foreign body of right front wall of thorax without penetration into thoracic cavity

√7ᵗʰ **S21.142** Puncture wound with foreign body of left front wall of thorax without penetration into thoracic cavity

√7ᵗʰ **S21.149** Puncture wound with foreign body of unspecified front wall of thorax without penetration into thoracic cavity

√6ᵗʰ **S21.15** Open bite of front wall of thorax without penetration into thoracic cavity

Bite of front wall of thorax NOS

EXCLUDES 1 superficial bite of front wall of thorax (S20.37)

√7ᵗʰ **S21.151** Open bite of right front wall of thorax without penetration into thoracic cavity

√7ᵗʰ **S21.152** Open bite of left front wall of thorax without penetration into thoracic cavity

√7ᵗʰ **S21.159** Open bite of unspecified front wall of thorax without penetration into thoracic cavity

√5ᵗʰ **S21.2** Open wound of back wall of thorax without penetration into thoracic cavity

√6ᵗʰ **S21.20** Unspecified open wound of back wall of thorax without penetration into thoracic cavity

√7ᵗʰ **S21.201** Unspecified open wound of right back wall of thorax without penetration into thoracic cavity

√7ᵗʰ **S21.202** Unspecified open wound of left back wall of thorax without penetration into thoracic cavity

√7ᵗʰ **S21.209** Unspecified open wound of unspecified back wall of thorax without penetration into thoracic cavity

√6ᵗʰ **S21.21** Laceration without foreign body of back wall of thorax without penetration into thoracic cavity

√7ᵗʰ **S21.211** Laceration without foreign body of right back wall of thorax without penetration into thoracic cavity

√7ᵗʰ **S21.212** Laceration without foreign body of left back wall of thorax without penetration into thoracic cavity

√7ᵗʰ **S21.219** Laceration without foreign body of unspecified back wall of thorax without penetration into thoracic cavity

√6ᵗʰ **S21.22** Laceration with foreign body of back wall of thorax without penetration into thoracic cavity

√7ᵗʰ **S21.221** Laceration with foreign body of right back wall of thorax without penetration into thoracic cavity

√7ᵗʰ **S21.222** Laceration with foreign body of left back wall of thorax without penetration into thoracic cavity

√7ᵗʰ **S21.229** Laceration with foreign body of unspecified back wall of thorax without penetration into thoracic cavity

√6ᵗʰ **S21.23** Puncture wound without foreign body of back wall of thorax without penetration into thoracic cavity

√7ᵗʰ **S21.231** Puncture wound without foreign body of right back wall of thorax without penetration into thoracic cavity

√7ᵗʰ **S21.232** Puncture wound without foreign body of left back wall of thorax without penetration into thoracic cavity

√7ᵗʰ **S21.239** Puncture wound without foreign body of unspecified back wall of thorax without penetration into thoracic cavity

√6ᵗʰ **S21.24** Puncture wound with foreign body of back wall of thorax without penetration into thoracic cavity

√7ᵗʰ **S21.241** Puncture wound with foreign body of right back wall of thorax without penetration into thoracic cavity

√7ᵗʰ **S21.242** Puncture wound with foreign body of left back wall of thorax without penetration into thoracic cavity

√7ᵗʰ **S21.249** Puncture wound with foreign body of unspecified back wall of thorax without penetration into thoracic cavity

√6ᵗʰ **S21.25** Open bite of back wall of thorax without penetration into thoracic cavity

Bite of back wall of thorax NOS

EXCLUDES 1 superficial bite of back wall of thorax (S20.47)

√7ᵗʰ **S21.251** Open bite of right back wall of thorax without penetration into thoracic cavity

√7ᵗʰ **S21.252** Open bite of left back wall of thorax without penetration into thoracic cavity

√7ᵗʰ **S21.259** Open bite of unspecified back wall of thorax without penetration into thoracic cavity

√5ᵗʰ **S21.3** Open wound of front wall of thorax with penetration into thoracic cavity

Open wound of chest with penetration into thoracic cavity

√6ᵗʰ **S21.30** Unspecified open wound of front wall of thorax with penetration into thoracic cavity

√7ᵗʰ **S21.301** Unspecified open wound of right front wall of thorax with penetration into thoracic cavity

√7ᵗʰ **S21.302** Unspecified open wound of left front wall of thorax with penetration into thoracic cavity

√7ᵗʰ **S21.309** Unspecified open wound of unspecified front wall of thorax with penetration into thoracic cavity

√6ᵗʰ **S21.31** Laceration without foreign body of front wall of thorax with penetration into thoracic cavity

√7ᵗʰ **S21.311** Laceration without foreign body of right front wall of thorax with penetration into thoracic cavity

√7ᵗʰ **S21.312** Laceration without foreign body of left front wall of thorax with penetration into thoracic cavity

√7ᵗʰ **S21.319** Laceration without foreign body of unspecified front wall of thorax with penetration into thoracic cavity

√6ᵗʰ **S21.32** Laceration with foreign body of front wall of thorax with penetration into thoracic cavity

√7ᵗʰ **S21.321** Laceration with foreign body of right front wall of thorax with penetration into thoracic cavity

√7ᵗʰ **S21.322** Laceration with foreign body of left front wall of thorax with penetration into thoracic cavity

√7ᵗʰ **S21.329** Laceration with foreign body of unspecified front wall of thorax with penetration into thoracic cavity

√6ᵗʰ **S21.33** Puncture wound without foreign body of front wall of thorax with penetration into thoracic cavity

√7ᵗʰ **S21.331** Puncture wound without foreign body of right front wall of thorax with penetration into thoracic cavity

√7ᵗʰ **S21.332** Puncture wound without foreign body of left front wall of thorax with penetration into thoracic cavity

√7ᵗʰ **S21.339** Puncture wound without foreign body of unspecified front wall of thorax with penetration into thoracic cavity

√6ᵗʰ **S21.34** Puncture wound with foreign body of front wall of thorax with penetration into thoracic cavity

√7ᵗʰ **S21.341** Puncture wound with foreign body of right front wall of thorax with penetration into thoracic cavity

√7ᵗʰ **S21.342** Puncture wound with foreign body of left front wall of thorax with penetration into thoracic cavity

√7ᵗʰ **S21.349** Puncture wound with foreign body of unspecified front wall of thorax with penetration into thoracic cavity

√6ᵗʰ **S21.35** Open bite of front wall of thorax with penetration into thoracic cavity

EXCLUDES 1   superficial bite of front wall of thorax (S20.37)

√7ᵗʰ **S21.351** Open bite of right front wall of thorax with penetration into thoracic cavity

√7ᵗʰ **S21.352** Open bite of left front wall of thorax with penetration into thoracic cavity

√7ᵗʰ **S21.359** Open bite of unspecified front wall of thorax with penetration into thoracic cavity

√5ᵗʰ **S21.4** Open wound of back wall of thorax with penetration into thoracic cavity

√6ᵗʰ **S21.40** Unspecified open wound of back wall of thorax with penetration into thoracic cavity

√7ᵗʰ **S21.401** Unspecified open wound of right back wall of thorax with penetration into thoracic cavity

√7ᵗʰ **S21.402** Unspecified open wound of left back wall of thorax with penetration into thoracic cavity

√7ᵗʰ **S21.409** Unspecified open wound of unspecified back wall of thorax with penetration into thoracic cavity

√6ᵗʰ **S21.41** Laceration without foreign body of back wall of thorax with penetration into thoracic cavity

√7ᵗʰ **S21.411** Laceration without foreign body of right back wall of thorax with penetration into thoracic cavity

√7ᵗʰ **S21.412** Laceration without foreign body of left back wall of thorax with penetration into thoracic cavity

√7ᵗʰ **S21.419** Laceration without foreign body of unspecified back wall of thorax with penetration into thoracic cavity

√6ᵗʰ **S21.42** Laceration with foreign body of back wall of thorax with penetration into thoracic cavity

√7ᵗʰ **S21.421** Laceration with foreign body of right back wall of thorax with penetration into thoracic cavity

√7ᵗʰ **S21.422** Laceration with foreign body of left back wall of thorax with penetration into thoracic cavity

√7ᵗʰ **S21.429** Laceration with foreign body of unspecified back wall of thorax with penetration into thoracic cavity

√6ᵗʰ **S21.43** Puncture wound without foreign body of back wall of thorax with penetration into thoracic cavity

√7ᵗʰ **S21.431** Puncture wound without foreign body of right back wall of thorax with penetration into thoracic cavity

√7ᵗʰ **S21.432** Puncture wound without foreign body of left back wall of thorax with penetration into thoracic cavity

√7ᵗʰ **S21.439** Puncture wound without foreign body of unspecified back wall of thorax with penetration into thoracic cavity

√6ᵗʰ **S21.44** Puncture wound with foreign body of back wall of thorax with penetration into thoracic cavity

√7ᵗʰ **S21.441** Puncture wound with foreign body of right back wall of thorax with penetration into thoracic cavity

√7ᵗʰ **S21.442** Puncture wound with foreign body of left back wall of thorax with penetration into thoracic cavity

√7ᵗʰ **S21.449** Puncture wound with foreign body of unspecified back wall of thorax with penetration into thoracic cavity

√6ᵗʰ **S21.45** Open bite of back wall of thorax with penetration into thoracic cavity

Bite of back wall of thorax NOS

EXCLUDES 1   superficial bite of back wall of thorax (S20.47)

√7ᵗʰ **S21.451** Open bite of right back wall of thorax with penetration into thoracic cavity

√7ᵗʰ **S21.452** Open bite of left back wall of thorax with penetration into thoracic cavity

√7ᵗʰ **S21.459** Open bite of unspecified back wall of thorax with penetration into thoracic cavity

√5ᵗʰ **S21.9** Open wound of unspecified part of thorax

Open wound of thoracic wall NOS

√x7ᵗʰ **S21.90** Unspecified open wound of unspecified part of thorax

√x7ᵗʰ **S21.91** Laceration without foreign body of unspecified part of thorax

√x7ᵗʰ **S21.92** Laceration with foreign body of unspecified part of thorax

√x7ᵗʰ **S21.93** Puncture wound without foreign body of unspecified part of thorax

√x7ᵗʰ **S21.94** Puncture wound with foreign body of unspecified part of thorax

√x7ᵗʰ **S21.95** Open bite of unspecified part of thorax

EXCLUDES 1   superficial bite of thorax (S20.97)

√4ᵗʰ **S22** Fracture of rib(s), sternum and thoracic spine

NOTE   A fracture not indicated as displaced or nondisplaced should be coded to displaced

A fracture not indicated as open or closed should be coded to closed

INCLUDES   fracture of thoracic neural arch
fracture of thoracic spinous process
fracture of thoracic transverse process
fracture of thoracic vertebra
fracture of thoracic vertebral arch

Code first any associated:
injury of intrathoracic organ (S27.-)
spinal cord injury (S24.0-, S24.1-)

EXCLUDES 1   transection of thorax (S28.1)

EXCLUDES 2   fracture of clavicle (S42.0-)
fracture of scapula (S42.1-)

AHA: 2021,1Q,6; 2018,2Q,12; 2015,3Q,37-39

The appropriate 7th character is to be added to each code from category S22.
A   initial encounter for closed fracture
B   initial encounter for open fracture
D   subsequent encounter for fracture with routine healing
G   subsequent encounter for fracture with delayed healing
K   subsequent encounter for fracture with nonunion
S   sequela

√5ᵗʰ **S22.0** Fracture of thoracic vertebra

√6ᵗʰ **S22.00** Fracture of unspecified thoracic vertebra

¹ √7ᵗʰ **S22.000** Wedge compression fracture of unspecified thoracic vertebra   HCC ESR COM Q

¹ √7ᵗʰ **S22.001** Stable burst fracture of unspecified thoracic vertebra   HCC ESR COM Q

¹ √7ᵗʰ **S22.002** Unstable burst fracture of unspecified thoracic vertebra   HCC ESR COM Q

¹ √7ᵗʰ **S22.008** Other fracture of unspecified thoracic vertebra   HCC ESR COM Q

¹ √7ᵗʰ **S22.009** Unspecified fracture of unspecified thoracic vertebra   HCC ESR COM Q

√6ᵗʰ **S22.01** Fracture of first thoracic vertebra

¹ √7ᵗʰ **S22.010** Wedge compression fracture of first thoracic vertebra   HCC ESR COM Q

¹ √7ᵗʰ **S22.011** Stable burst fracture of first thoracic vertebra   HCC ESR COM Q

¹ √7ᵗʰ **S22.012** Unstable burst fracture of first thoracic vertebra   HCC ESR COM Q

¹ ✓7ᵗʰ **S22.018** Other fracture of first thoracic vertebra   `HCC` `ESR` `COM` `Q`

¹ ✓7ᵗʰ **S22.019** Unspecified fracture of first thoracic vertebra   `HCC` `ESR` `COM` `Q`

✓6ᵗʰ **S22.02** Fracture of second thoracic vertebra

¹ ✓7ᵗʰ **S22.020** Wedge compression fracture of second thoracic vertebra   `HCC` `ESR` `COM` `Q`

¹ ✓7ᵗʰ **S22.021** Stable burst fracture of second thoracic vertebra   `HCC` `ESR` `COM` `Q`

¹ ✓7ᵗʰ **S22.022** Unstable burst fracture of second thoracic vertebra   `HCC` `ESR` `COM` `Q`

¹ ✓7ᵗʰ **S22.028** Other fracture of second thoracic vertebra   `HCC` `ESR` `COM` `Q`

¹ ✓7ᵗʰ **S22.029** Unspecified fracture of second thoracic vertebra   `HCC` `ESR` `COM` `Q`

✓6ᵗʰ **S22.03** Fracture of third thoracic vertebra

¹ ✓7ᵗʰ **S22.030** Wedge compression fracture of third thoracic vertebra   `HCC` `ESR` `COM` `Q`

¹ ✓7ᵗʰ **S22.031** Stable burst fracture of third thoracic vertebra   `HCC` `ESR` `COM` `Q`

¹ ✓7ᵗʰ **S22.032** Unstable burst fracture of third thoracic vertebra   `HCC` `ESR` `COM` `Q`

¹ ✓7ᵗʰ **S22.038** Other fracture of third thoracic vertebra   `HCC` `ESR` `COM` `Q`

¹ ✓7ᵗʰ **S22.039** Unspecified fracture of third thoracic vertebra   `HCC` `ESR` `COM` `Q`

✓6ᵗʰ **S22.04** Fracture of fourth thoracic vertebra

¹ ✓7ᵗʰ **S22.040** Wedge compression fracture of fourth thoracic vertebra   `HCC` `ESR` `COM` `Q`

¹ ✓7ᵗʰ **S22.041** Stable burst fracture of fourth thoracic vertebra   `HCC` `ESR` `COM` `Q`

¹ ✓7ᵗʰ **S22.042** Unstable burst fracture of fourth thoracic vertebra   `HCC` `ESR` `COM` `Q`

¹ ✓7ᵗʰ **S22.048** Other fracture of fourth thoracic vertebra   `HCC` `ESR` `COM` `Q`

¹ ✓7ᵗʰ **S22.049** Unspecified fracture of fourth thoracic vertebra   `HCC` `ESR` `COM` `Q`

✓6ᵗʰ **S22.05** Fracture of T5-T6 vertebra

¹ ✓7ᵗʰ **S22.050** Wedge compression fracture of T5-T6 vertebra   `HCC` `ESR` `COM` `Q`

¹ ✓7ᵗʰ **S22.051** Stable burst fracture of T5-T6 vertebra   `HCC` `ESR` `COM` `Q`

¹ ✓7ᵗʰ **S22.052** Unstable burst fracture of T5-T6 vertebra   `HCC` `ESR` `COM` `Q`

¹ ✓7ᵗʰ **S22.058** Other fracture of T5-T6 vertebra   `HCC` `ESR` `COM` `Q`

¹ ✓7ᵗʰ **S22.059** Unspecified fracture of T5-T6 vertebra   `HCC` `ESR` `COM` `Q`

✓6ᵗʰ **S22.06** Fracture of T7-T8 vertebra

¹ ✓7ᵗʰ **S22.060** Wedge compression fracture of T7-T8 vertebra   `HCC` `ESR` `COM` `Q`

¹ ✓7ᵗʰ **S22.061** Stable burst fracture of T7-T8 vertebra   `HCC` `ESR` `COM` `Q`

¹ ✓7ᵗʰ **S22.062** Unstable burst fracture of T7-T8 vertebra   `HCC` `ESR` `COM` `Q`

¹ ✓7ᵗʰ **S22.068** Other fracture of T7-T8 thoracic vertebra   `HCC` `ESR` `COM` `Q`

¹ ✓7ᵗʰ **S22.069** Unspecified fracture of T7-T8 vertebra   `HCC` `ESR` `COM` `Q`

✓6ᵗʰ **S22.07** Fracture of T9-T10 vertebra

¹ ✓7ᵗʰ **S22.070** Wedge compression fracture of T9-T10 vertebra   `HCC` `ESR` `COM` `Q`

¹ ✓7ᵗʰ **S22.071** Stable burst fracture of T9-T10 vertebra   `HCC` `ESR` `COM` `Q`

¹ ✓7ᵗʰ **S22.072** Unstable burst fracture of T9-T10 vertebra   `HCC` `ESR` `COM` `Q`

¹ ✓7ᵗʰ **S22.078** Other fracture of T9-T10 vertebra   `HCC` `ESR` `COM` `Q`

¹ ✓7ᵗʰ **S22.079** Unspecified fracture of T9-T10 vertebra   `HCC` `ESR` `COM` `Q`

✓6ᵗʰ **S22.08** Fracture of T11-T12 vertebra

¹ ✓7ᵗʰ **S22.080** Wedge compression fracture of T11-T12 vertebra   `HCC` `ESR` `COM` `Q`

¹ ✓7ᵗʰ **S22.081** Stable burst fracture of T11-T12 vertebra   `HCC` `ESR` `COM` `Q`

¹ ✓7ᵗʰ **S22.082** Unstable burst fracture of T11-T12 vertebra   `HCC` `ESR` `COM` `Q`

¹ ✓7ᵗʰ **S22.088** Other fracture of T11-T12 vertebra   `HCC` `ESR` `COM` `Q`

¹ ✓7ᵗʰ **S22.089** Unspecified fracture of T11-T12 vertebra   `HCC` `ESR` `COM` `Q`

✓5ᵗʰ **S22.2** Fracture of sternum

DEF: Break in flat bone (breast bone) in the anterior thorax caused by blunt trauma to the anterior chest.

✓x7ᵗʰ **S22.20** Unspecified fracture of sternum   `Q`

✓x7ᵗʰ **S22.21** Fracture of manubrium   `Q`

✓x7ᵗʰ **S22.22** Fracture of body of sternum   `Q`

✓x7ᵗʰ **S22.23** Sternal manubrial dissociation   `Q`

✓x7ᵗʰ **S22.24** Fracture of xiphoid process   `Q`

✓5ᵗʰ **S22.3** Fracture of one rib

AHA: 2021,1Q,5

✓x7ᵗʰ **S22.31** Fracture of one rib, right side   `Q`

✓x7ᵗʰ **S22.32** Fracture of one rib, left side   `Q`

✓x7ᵗʰ **S22.39** Fracture of one rib, unspecified side   `Q`

✓5ᵗʰ **S22.4** Multiple fractures of ribs

Fractures of two or more ribs

EXCLUDES 1 flail chest (S22.5-)

AHA: 2021,1Q,5

✓x7ᵗʰ **S22.41** Multiple fractures of ribs, right side   `Q`

✓x7ᵗʰ **S22.42** Multiple fractures of ribs, left side   `Q`

✓x7ᵗʰ **S22.43** Multiple fractures of ribs, bilateral   `Q`

✓x7ᵗʰ **S22.49** Multiple fractures of ribs, unspecified side   `Q`

✓x7ᵗʰ **S22.5** Flail chest   `Q`

✓x7ᵗʰ **S22.9** Fracture of bony thorax, part unspecified   `Q`

✓4ᵗʰ **S23** Dislocation and sprain of joints and ligaments of thorax

INCLUDES avulsion of joint or ligament of thorax
laceration of cartilage, joint or ligament of thorax
sprain of cartilage, joint or ligament of thorax
traumatic hemarthrosis of joint or ligament of thorax
traumatic rupture of joint or ligament of thorax
traumatic subluxation of joint or ligament of thorax
traumatic tear of joint or ligament of thorax

Code also any associated open wound

EXCLUDES 2 dislocation, sprain of sternoclavicular joint (S43.2, S43.6)
strain of muscle or tendon of thorax (S29.01-)

The appropriate 7th character is to be added to each code from category S23.
A   initial encounter
D   subsequent encounter
S   sequela

✓x7ᵗʰ **S23.0** Traumatic rupture of thoracic intervertebral disc

EXCLUDES 1 rupture or displacement (nontraumatic) of thoracic intervertebral disc NOS (M51.- with fifth character 4)

✓5ᵗʰ **S23.1** Subluxation and dislocation of thoracic vertebra

Code also any associated:
open wound of thorax (S21.-)
spinal cord injury (S24.0-, S24.1-)

EXCLUDES 2 fracture of thoracic vertebrae (S22.0-)

✓6ᵗʰ **S23.10** Subluxation and dislocation of unspecified thoracic vertebra

✓7ᵗʰ **S23.100** Subluxation of unspecified thoracic vertebra

✓7ᵗʰ **S23.101** Dislocation of unspecified thoracic vertebra

✓6ᵗʰ **S23.11** Subluxation and dislocation of T1/T2 thoracic vertebra

✓7ᵗʰ **S23.110** Subluxation of T1/T2 thoracic vertebra

✓7ᵗʰ **S23.111** Dislocation of T1/T2 thoracic vertebra

✓6ᵗʰ **S23.12** Subluxation and dislocation of T2/T3-T3/T4 thoracic vertebra

✓7ᵗʰ **S23.120** Subluxation of T2/T3 thoracic vertebra

✓7ᵗʰ **S23.121** Dislocation of T2/T3 thoracic vertebra

✓7ᵗʰ **S23.122** Subluxation of T3/T4 thoracic vertebra

✓7ᵗʰ **S23.123** Dislocation of T3/T4 thoracic vertebra

✓6ᵗʰ **S23.13** Subluxation and dislocation of T4/T5-T5/T6 thoracic vertebra

✓7ᵗʰ **S23.130** Subluxation of T4/T5 thoracic vertebra

✓7ᵗʰ **S23.131** Dislocation of T4/T5 thoracic vertebra

☑7ᵗʰ **S23.132** Subluxation of T5/T6 thoracic vertebra
☑7ᵗʰ **S23.133** Dislocation of T5/T6 thoracic vertebra

☑6ᵗʰ **S23.14** **Subluxation and dislocation of** T6/T7-T7/T8 **thoracic vertebra**
    ☑7ᵗʰ **S23.14Ø** Subluxation of T6/T7 thoracic vertebra
    ☑7ᵗʰ **S23.141** Dislocation of T6/T7 thoracic vertebra
    ☑7ᵗʰ **S23.142** Subluxation of T7/T8 thoracic vertebra
    ☑7ᵗʰ **S23.143** Dislocation of T7/T8 thoracic vertebra

☑6ᵗʰ **S23.15** **Subluxation and dislocation of** T8/T9-T9/T1Ø **thoracic vertebra**
    ☑7ᵗʰ **S23.15Ø** Subluxation of T8/T9 thoracic vertebra
    ☑7ᵗʰ **S23.151** Dislocation of T8/T9 thoracic vertebra
    ☑7ᵗʰ **S23.152** Subluxation of T9/T1Ø thoracic vertebra
    ☑7ᵗʰ **S23.153** Dislocation of T9/T1Ø thoracic vertebra

☑6ᵗʰ **S23.16** **Subluxation and dislocation of** T1Ø/T11-T11/T12 **thoracic vertebra**
    ☑7ᵗʰ **S23.16Ø** Subluxation of T1Ø/T11 thoracic vertebra
    ☑7ᵗʰ **S23.161** Dislocation of T1Ø/T11 thoracic vertebra
    ☑7ᵗʰ **S23.162** Subluxation of T11/T12 thoracic vertebra
    ☑7ᵗʰ **S23.163** Dislocation of T11/T12 thoracic vertebra

☑6ᵗʰ **S23.17** **Subluxation and dislocation of** T12/L1 **thoracic vertebra**
    ☑7ᵗʰ **S23.17Ø** Subluxation of T12/L1 thoracic vertebra
    ☑7ᵗʰ **S23.171** Dislocation of T12/L1 thoracic vertebra

☑5ᵗʰ **S23.2** **Dislocation of other and unspecified parts of thorax**
    ☑x7ᵗʰ **S23.2Ø** **Dislocation of unspecified part of thorax**
    ☑x7ᵗʰ **S23.29** **Dislocation of other parts of thorax**

☑x7ᵗʰ **S23.3** **Sprain of ligaments of thoracic spine**

☑5ᵗʰ **S23.4** **Sprain of ribs and sternum**
    ☑x7ᵗʰ **S23.41** **Sprain of ribs**
    ☑6ᵗʰ **S23.42** **Sprain of sternum**
        ☑7ᵗʰ **S23.42Ø** **Sprain of sternoclavicular (joint) (ligament)**
        ☑7ᵗʰ **S23.421** **Sprain of chondrosternal joint**
        ☑7ᵗʰ **S23.428** **Other sprain of sternum**
        ☑7ᵗʰ **S23.429** **Unspecified sprain of sternum**

☑x7ᵗʰ **S23.8** **Sprain of other specified parts of thorax**

☑x7ᵗʰ **S23.9** **Sprain of unspecified parts of thorax**

☑4ᵗʰ **S24** **Injury of nerves and spinal cord at thorax level**

> **NOTE**   Code to highest level of thoracic spinal cord injury.
> Injuries to the spinal cord (S24.Ø and S24.1) refer to the cord level and not bone level injury, and can affect nerve roots at and below the level given.

Code also any associated:
    fracture of thoracic vertebra (S22.Ø-)
    open wound of thorax (S21.-)
    transient paralysis (R29.5)
EXCLUDES 2   injury of brachial plexus (S14.3)

> The appropriate 7th character is to be added to each code from category S24.
> A   initial encounter
> D   subsequent encounter
> S   sequela

☑x7ᵗʰ **S24.Ø** **Concussion and edema of thoracic spinal cord** HCC ESR COM

☑5ᵗʰ **S24.1** **Other and unspecified injuries of thoracic spinal cord**
    ☑6ᵗʰ **S24.1Ø** **Unspecified injury of thoracic spinal cord**
        ☑7ᵗʰ **S24.1Ø1** **Unspecified injury at** T1 **level of thoracic spinal cord** HCC ESR COM
        ☑7ᵗʰ **S24.1Ø2** **Unspecified injury at** T2-T6 **level of thoracic spinal cord** HCC ESR COM
        ☑7ᵗʰ **S24.1Ø3** **Unspecified injury at** T7-T1Ø **level of thoracic spinal cord** HCC ESR COM
        ☑7ᵗʰ **S24.1Ø4** **Unspecified injury at** T11-T12 **level of thoracic spinal cord** HCC ESR COM
        ☑7ᵗʰ **S24.1Ø9** **Unspecified injury at unspecified level of thoracic spinal cord** HCC ESR COM
             Injury of thoracic spinal cord NOS

    ☑6ᵗʰ **S24.11** Complete lesion **of thoracic spinal cord**
        ☑7ᵗʰ **S24.111** **Complete lesion at** T1 **level of thoracic spinal cord** HCC ESR COM

        ☑7ᵗʰ **S24.112** **Complete lesion at** T2-T6 **level of thoracic spinal cord** HCC ESR COM
        ☑7ᵗʰ **S24.113** **Complete lesion at** T7-T1Ø **level of thoracic spinal cord** HCC ESR COM
        ☑7ᵗʰ **S24.114** **Complete lesion at** T11-T12 **level of thoracic spinal cord** HCC ESR COM
        ☑7ᵗʰ **S24.119** **Complete lesion at unspecified level of thoracic spinal cord** HCC ESR COM

    ☑6ᵗʰ **S24.13** Anterior cord syndrome **of thoracic spinal cord**
        ☑7ᵗʰ **S24.131** **Anterior cord syndrome at** T1 **level of thoracic spinal cord** HCC ESR COM
        ☑7ᵗʰ **S24.132** **Anterior cord syndrome at** T2-T6 **level of thoracic spinal cord** HCC ESR COM
        ☑7ᵗʰ **S24.133** **Anterior cord syndrome at** T7-T1Ø **level of thoracic spinal cord** HCC ESR COM
        ☑7ᵗʰ **S24.134** **Anterior cord syndrome at** T11-T12 **level of thoracic spinal cord** HCC ESR COM
        ☑7ᵗʰ **S24.139** **Anterior cord syndrome at unspecified level of thoracic spinal cord** HCC ESR COM

    ☑6ᵗʰ **S24.14** Brown-Séquard syndrome **of thoracic spinal cord**
        ☑7ᵗʰ **S24.141** **Brown-Séquard syndrome at** T1 **level of thoracic spinal cord** HCC ESR COM
        ☑7ᵗʰ **S24.142** **Brown-Séquard syndrome at** T2-T6 **level of thoracic spinal cord** HCC ESR COM
        ☑7ᵗʰ **S24.143** **Brown-Séquard syndrome at** T7-T1Ø **level of thoracic spinal cord** HCC ESR COM
        ☑7ᵗʰ **S24.144** **Brown-Séquard syndrome at** T11-T12 **level of thoracic spinal cord** HCC ESR COM
        ☑7ᵗʰ **S24.149** **Brown-Séquard syndrome at unspecified level of thoracic spinal cord** HCC ESR COM

    ☑6ᵗʰ **S24.15** **Other** incomplete lesions **of thoracic spinal cord**
         Incomplete lesion of thoracic spinal cord NOS
         Posterior cord syndrome of thoracic spinal cord
        ☑7ᵗʰ **S24.151** **Other incomplete lesion at** T1 **level of thoracic spinal cord** HCC ESR COM
        ☑7ᵗʰ **S24.152** **Other incomplete lesion at** T2-T6 **level of thoracic spinal cord** HCC ESR COM
        ☑7ᵗʰ **S24.153** **Other incomplete lesion at** T7-T1Ø **level of thoracic spinal cord** HCC ESR COM
        ☑7ᵗʰ **S24.154** **Other incomplete lesion at** T11-T12 **level of thoracic spinal cord** HCC ESR COM
        ☑7ᵗʰ **S24.159** **Other incomplete lesion at unspecified level of thoracic spinal cord** HCC ESR COM

☑x7ᵗʰ **S24.2** **Injury of nerve root of thoracic spine**

☑x7ᵗʰ **S24.3** **Injury of peripheral nerves of thorax**

☑x7ᵗʰ **S24.4** **Injury of thoracic sympathetic nervous system**
     Injury of cardiac plexus
     Injury of esophageal plexus
     Injury of pulmonary plexus
     Injury of stellate ganglion
     Injury of thoracic sympathetic ganglion

☑x7ᵗʰ **S24.8** **Injury of other specified nerves of thorax**

☑x7ᵗʰ **S24.9** **Injury of unspecified nerve of thorax**

☑4ᵗʰ **S25** **Injury of blood vessels of thorax**
     Code also any associated open wound (S21.-)

> The appropriate 7th character is to be added to each code from category S25.
> A   initial encounter
> D   subsequent encounter
> S   sequela

☑5ᵗʰ **S25.Ø** **Injury of** thoracic aorta
     Injury of aorta NOS
    ☑x7ᵗʰ **S25.ØØ** **Unspecified injury of thoracic aorta**
    ☑x7ᵗʰ **S25.Ø1** Minor laceration **of thoracic aorta**
         Incomplete transection of thoracic aorta
         Laceration of thoracic aorta NOS
         Superficial laceration of thoracic aorta
    ☑x7ᵗʰ **S25.Ø2** Major laceration **of thoracic aorta**
         Complete transection of thoracic aorta
         Traumatic rupture of thoracic aorta
    ☑x7ᵗʰ **S25.Ø9** **Other specified injury of thoracic aorta**

√5ᵗʰ **S25.1** Injury of innominate or subclavian artery

  √6ᵗʰ **S25.10** Unspecified injury of innominate or subclavian artery

    √7ᵗʰ **S25.101** Unspecified injury of right innominate or subclavian artery

    √7ᵗʰ **S25.102** Unspecified injury of left innominate or subclavian artery

    √7ᵗʰ **S25.109** Unspecified injury of unspecified innominate or subclavian artery

  √6ᵗʰ **S25.11** Minor laceration of innominate or subclavian artery

    Incomplete transection of innominate or subclavian artery

    Laceration of innominate or subclavian artery NOS

    Superficial laceration of innominate or subclavian artery

    √7ᵗʰ **S25.111** Minor laceration of right innominate or subclavian artery

    √7ᵗʰ **S25.112** Minor laceration of left innominate or subclavian artery

    √7ᵗʰ **S25.119** Minor laceration of unspecified innominate or subclavian artery

  √6ᵗʰ **S25.12** Major laceration of innominate or subclavian artery

    Complete transection of innominate or subclavian artery

    Traumatic rupture of innominate or subclavian artery

    √7ᵗʰ **S25.121** Major laceration of right innominate or subclavian artery

    √7ᵗʰ **S25.122** Major laceration of left innominate or subclavian artery

    √7ᵗʰ **S25.129** Major laceration of unspecified innominate or subclavian artery

  √6ᵗʰ **S25.19** Other specified injury of innominate or subclavian artery

    √7ᵗʰ **S25.191** Other specified injury of right innominate or subclavian artery

    √7ᵗʰ **S25.192** Other specified injury of left innominate or subclavian artery

    √7ᵗʰ **S25.199** Other specified injury of unspecified innominate or subclavian artery

√5ᵗʰ **S25.2** Injury of superior vena cava

  Injury of vena cava NOS

  √x7ᵗʰ **S25.20** Unspecified injury of superior vena cava

  √x7ᵗʰ **S25.21** Minor laceration of superior vena cava

    Incomplete transection of superior vena cava

    Laceration of superior vena cava NOS

    Superficial laceration of superior vena cava

  √x7ᵗʰ **S25.22** Major laceration of superior vena cava

    Complete transection of superior vena cava

    Traumatic rupture of superior vena cava

  √x7ᵗʰ **S25.29** Other specified injury of superior vena cava

√5ᵗʰ **S25.3** Injury of innominate or subclavian vein

  √6ᵗʰ **S25.30** Unspecified injury of innominate or subclavian vein

    √7ᵗʰ **S25.301** Unspecified injury of right innominate or subclavian vein

    √7ᵗʰ **S25.302** Unspecified injury of left innominate or subclavian vein

    √7ᵗʰ **S25.309** Unspecified injury of unspecified innominate or subclavian vein

  √6ᵗʰ **S25.31** Minor laceration of innominate or subclavian vein

    Incomplete transection of innominate or subclavian vein

    Laceration of innominate or subclavian vein NOS

    Superficial laceration of innominate or subclavian vein

    √7ᵗʰ **S25.311** Minor laceration of right innominate or subclavian vein

    √7ᵗʰ **S25.312** Minor laceration of left innominate or subclavian vein

    √7ᵗʰ **S25.319** Minor laceration of unspecified innominate or subclavian vein

  √6ᵗʰ **S25.32** Major laceration of innominate or subclavian vein

    Complete transection of innominate or subclavian vein

    Traumatic rupture of innominate or subclavian vein

    √7ᵗʰ **S25.321** Major laceration of right innominate or subclavian vein

    √7ᵗʰ **S25.322** Major laceration of left innominate or subclavian vein

    √7ᵗʰ **S25.329** Major laceration of unspecified innominate or subclavian vein

  √6ᵗʰ **S25.39** Other specified injury of innominate or subclavian vein

    √7ᵗʰ **S25.391** Other specified injury of right innominate or subclavian vein

    √7ᵗʰ **S25.392** Other specified injury of left innominate or subclavian vein

    √7ᵗʰ **S25.399** Other specified injury of unspecified innominate or subclavian vein

√5ᵗʰ **S25.4** Injury of pulmonary blood vessels

  √6ᵗʰ **S25.40** Unspecified injury of pulmonary blood vessels

    √7ᵗʰ **S25.401** Unspecified injury of right pulmonary blood vessels

    √7ᵗʰ **S25.402** Unspecified injury of left pulmonary blood vessels

    √7ᵗʰ **S25.409** Unspecified injury of unspecified pulmonary blood vessels

  √6ᵗʰ **S25.41** Minor laceration of pulmonary blood vessels

    Incomplete transection of pulmonary blood vessels

    Laceration of pulmonary blood vessels NOS

    Superficial laceration of pulmonary blood vessels

    √7ᵗʰ **S25.411** Minor laceration of right pulmonary blood vessels

    √7ᵗʰ **S25.412** Minor laceration of left pulmonary blood vessels

    √7ᵗʰ **S25.419** Minor laceration of unspecified pulmonary blood vessels

  √6ᵗʰ **S25.42** Major laceration of pulmonary blood vessels

    Complete transection of pulmonary blood vessels

    Traumatic rupture of pulmonary blood vessels

    √7ᵗʰ **S25.421** Major laceration of right pulmonary blood vessels

    √7ᵗʰ **S25.422** Major laceration of left pulmonary blood vessels

    √7ᵗʰ **S25.429** Major laceration of unspecified pulmonary blood vessels

  √6ᵗʰ **S25.49** Other specified injury of pulmonary blood vessels

    √7ᵗʰ **S25.491** Other specified injury of right pulmonary blood vessels

    √7ᵗʰ **S25.492** Other specified injury of left pulmonary blood vessels

    √7ᵗʰ **S25.499** Other specified injury of unspecified pulmonary blood vessels

√5ᵗʰ **S25.5** Injury of intercostal blood vessels

  √6ᵗʰ **S25.50** Unspecified injury of intercostal blood vessels

    √7ᵗʰ **S25.501** Unspecified injury of intercostal blood vessels, right side

    √7ᵗʰ **S25.502** Unspecified injury of intercostal blood vessels, left side

    √7ᵗʰ **S25.509** Unspecified injury of intercostal blood vessels, unspecified side

  √6ᵗʰ **S25.51** Laceration of intercostal blood vessels

    √7ᵗʰ **S25.511** Laceration of intercostal blood vessels, right side

    √7ᵗʰ **S25.512** Laceration of intercostal blood vessels, left side

    √7ᵗʰ **S25.519** Laceration of intercostal blood vessels, unspecified side

  √6ᵗʰ **S25.59** Other specified injury of intercostal blood vessels

    √7ᵗʰ **S25.591** Other specified injury of intercostal blood vessels, right side

    √7ᵗʰ **S25.592** Other specified injury of intercostal blood vessels, left side

    √7ᵗʰ **S25.599** Other specified injury of intercostal blood vessels, unspecified side

√5ᵗʰ **S25.8** Injury of other blood vessels of thorax

  Injury of azygos vein

  Injury of mammary artery or vein

  √6ᵗʰ **S25.80** Unspecified injury of other blood vessels of thorax

    √7ᵗʰ **S25.801** Unspecified injury of other blood vessels of thorax, right side

    √7ᵗʰ **S25.802** Unspecified injury of other blood vessels of thorax, left side

    √7ᵗʰ **S25.809** Unspecified injury of other blood vessels of thorax, unspecified side

  √6ᵗʰ **S25.81** Laceration of other blood vessels of thorax

    √7ᵗʰ **S25.811** Laceration of other blood vessels of thorax, right side

---

☑7ᵗʰ **S25.812 Laceration of other blood vessels of thorax, left side**

☑7ᵗʰ **S25.819 Laceration of other blood vessels of thorax, unspecified side**

☑6ᵗʰ **S25.89 Other specified injury of other blood vessels of thorax**

☑7ᵗʰ **S25.891 Other specified injury of other blood vessels of thorax, right side**

☑7ᵗʰ **S25.892 Other specified injury of other blood vessels of thorax, left side**

☑7ᵗʰ **S25.899 Other specified injury of other blood vessels of thorax, unspecified side**

☑5ᵗʰ **S25.9 Injury of unspecified blood vessel of thorax**

☑x7ᵗʰ **S25.90 Unspecified injury of unspecified blood vessel of thorax**

☑x7ᵗʰ **S25.91 Laceration of unspecified blood vessel of thorax**

☑x7ᵗʰ **S25.99 Other specified injury of unspecified blood vessel of thorax**

☑4ᵗʰ **S26 Injury of heart**

Code also any associated:
open wound of thorax (S21.-)
traumatic hemopneumothorax (S27.2)
traumatic hemothorax (S27.1)
traumatic pneumothorax (S27.0)

The appropriate 7th character is to be added to each code from category S26.
A   initial encounter
D   subsequent encounter
S   sequela

☑5ᵗʰ **S26.0 Injury of heart with hemopericardium**

☑x7ᵗʰ **S26.00 Unspecified injury of heart with hemopericardium**

☑x7ᵗʰ **S26.01 Contusion of heart with hemopericardium**

☑6ᵗʰ **S26.02 Laceration of heart with hemopericardium**

☑7ᵗʰ **S26.020 Mild laceration of heart with hemopericardium**
Laceration of heart without penetration of heart chamber

☑7ᵗʰ **S26.021 Moderate laceration of heart with hemopericardium**
Laceration of heart with penetration of heart chamber

☑7ᵗʰ **S26.022 Major laceration of heart with hemopericardium**
Laceration of heart with penetration of multiple heart chambers

☑x7ᵗʰ **S26.09 Other injury of heart with hemopericardium**

☑5ᵗʰ **S26.1 Injury of heart without hemopericardium**

☑x7ᵗʰ **S26.10 Unspecified injury of heart without hemopericardium**

☑x7ᵗʰ **S26.11 Contusion of heart without hemopericardium**

☑x7ᵗʰ **S26.12 Laceration of heart without hemopericardium**

☑x7ᵗʰ **S26.19 Other injury of heart without hemopericardium**

☑5ᵗʰ **S26.9 Injury of heart, unspecified with or without hemopericardium**

☑x7ᵗʰ **S26.90 Unspecified injury of heart, unspecified with or without hemopericardium**

☑x7ᵗʰ **S26.91 Contusion of heart, unspecified with or without hemopericardium**
DEF: Bruising within the heart muscle, with no mention of an open wound, usually caused by blunt chest trauma in motor vehicle accidents, falling from great heights, or receiving CPR.

☑x7ᵗʰ **S26.92 Laceration of heart, unspecified with or without hemopericardium**
Laceration of heart NOS
AHA: 2019,2Q,24

☑x7ᵗʰ **S26.99 Other injury of heart, unspecified with or without hemopericardium**

☑4ᵗʰ **S27 Injury of other and unspecified intrathoracic organs**

Code also any associated open wound of thorax (S21.-)

EXCLUDES 2   injury of cervical esophagus (S10-S19)
injury of trachea (cervical) (S10-S19)

The appropriate 7th character is to be added to each code from category S27.
A   initial encounter
D   subsequent encounter
S   sequela

☑x7ᵗʰ **S27.0 Traumatic pneumothorax**
EXCLUDES 1   spontaneous pneumothorax (J93.-)

☑x7ᵗʰ **S27.1 Traumatic hemothorax**

☑x7ᵗʰ **S27.2 Traumatic hemopneumothorax**

☑5ᵗʰ **S27.3 Other and unspecified injuries of lung**

☑6ᵗʰ **S27.30 Unspecified injury of lung**

☑7ᵗʰ **S27.301 Unspecified injury of lung, unilateral**

☑7ᵗʰ **S27.302 Unspecified injury of lung, bilateral**

☑7ᵗʰ **S27.309 Unspecified injury of lung, unspecified**

☑6ᵗʰ **S27.31 Primary blast injury of lung**
Blast injury of lung NOS

☑7ᵗʰ **S27.311 Primary blast injury of lung, unilateral**

☑7ᵗʰ **S27.312 Primary blast injury of lung, bilateral**

☑7ᵗʰ **S27.319 Primary blast injury of lung, unspecified**

☑6ᵗʰ **S27.32 Contusion of lung**
DEF: Bruising of the lung without mention of an open wound.

☑7ᵗʰ **S27.321 Contusion of lung, unilateral**

☑7ᵗʰ **S27.322 Contusion of lung, bilateral**

☑7ᵗʰ **S27.329 Contusion of lung, unspecified**

☑6ᵗʰ **S27.33 Laceration of lung**

☑7ᵗʰ **S27.331 Laceration of lung, unilateral**

☑7ᵗʰ **S27.332 Laceration of lung, bilateral**

☑7ᵗʰ **S27.339 Laceration of lung, unspecified**

☑6ᵗʰ **S27.39 Other injuries of lung**
Secondary blast injury of lung

☑7ᵗʰ **S27.391 Other injuries of lung, unilateral**

☑7ᵗʰ **S27.392 Other injuries of lung, bilateral**

☑7ᵗʰ **S27.399 Other injuries of lung, unspecified**

☑5ᵗʰ **S27.4 Injury of bronchus**

☑6ᵗʰ **S27.40 Unspecified injury of bronchus**

☑7ᵗʰ **S27.401 Unspecified injury of bronchus, unilateral**

☑7ᵗʰ **S27.402 Unspecified injury of bronchus, bilateral**

☑7ᵗʰ **S27.409 Unspecified injury of bronchus, unspecified**

☑6ᵗʰ **S27.41 Primary blast injury of bronchus**
Blast injury of bronchus NOS

☑7ᵗʰ **S27.411 Primary blast injury of bronchus, unilateral**

☑7ᵗʰ **S27.412 Primary blast injury of bronchus, bilateral**

☑7ᵗʰ **S27.419 Primary blast injury of bronchus, unspecified**

☑6ᵗʰ **S27.42 Contusion of bronchus**

☑7ᵗʰ **S27.421 Contusion of bronchus, unilateral**

☑7ᵗʰ **S27.422 Contusion of bronchus, bilateral**

☑7ᵗʰ **S27.429 Contusion of bronchus, unspecified**

☑6ᵗʰ **S27.43 Laceration of bronchus**

☑7ᵗʰ **S27.431 Laceration of bronchus, unilateral**

☑7ᵗʰ **S27.432 Laceration of bronchus, bilateral**

☑7ᵗʰ **S27.439 Laceration of bronchus, unspecified**

☑6ᵗʰ **S27.49 Other injury of bronchus**
Secondary blast injury of bronchus

☑7ᵗʰ **S27.491 Other injury of bronchus, unilateral**

☑7ᵗʰ **S27.492 Other injury of bronchus, bilateral**

☑7ᵗʰ **S27.499 Other injury of bronchus, unspecified**

☑5ᵗʰ **S27.5 Injury of thoracic trachea**

☑x7ᵗʰ **S27.50 Unspecified injury of thoracic trachea**

☑x7ᵗʰ **S27.51 Primary blast injury of thoracic trachea**
Blast injury of thoracic trachea NOS

☑x7ᵗʰ **S27.52 Contusion of thoracic trachea**

√x7ᵗʰ **S27.53** Laceration of thoracic trachea

√x7ᵗʰ **S27.59** Other injury of thoracic trachea

     Secondary blast injury of thoracic trachea

√5ᵗʰ **S27.6** Injury of pleura

   √x7ᵗʰ **S27.60** Unspecified injury of pleura

   √x7ᵗʰ **S27.63** Laceration of pleura

   √x7ᵗʰ **S27.69** Other injury of pleura

√5ᵗʰ **S27.8** Injury of other specified intrathoracic organs

   √6ᵗʰ **S27.80** Injury of diaphragm

     √7ᵗʰ **S27.802** Contusion of diaphragm

     √7ᵗʰ **S27.803** Laceration of diaphragm

     √7ᵗʰ **S27.808** Other injury of diaphragm

     √7ᵗʰ **S27.809** Unspecified injury of diaphragm

   √6ᵗʰ **S27.81** Injury of esophagus (thoracic part)

     √7ᵗʰ **S27.812** Contusion of esophagus (thoracic part)

     √7ᵗʰ **S27.813** Laceration of esophagus (thoracic part)

     √7ᵗʰ **S27.818** Other injury of esophagus (thoracic part)

     √7ᵗʰ **S27.819** Unspecified injury of esophagus (thoracic part)

   √6ᵗʰ **S27.89** Injury of other specified intrathoracic organs

     Injury of lymphatic thoracic duct

     Injury of thymus gland

     √7ᵗʰ **S27.892** Contusion of other specified intrathoracic organs

     √7ᵗʰ **S27.893** Laceration of other specified intrathoracic organs

     √7ᵗʰ **S27.898** Other injury of other specified intrathoracic organs

     √7ᵗʰ **S27.899** Unspecified injury of other specified intrathoracic organs

√x7ᵗʰ **S27.9** Injury of unspecified intrathoracic organ

√4ᵗʰ **S28** **Crushing injury of thorax, and traumatic amputation of part of thorax**

   The appropriate 7th character is to be added to each code from category S28.
   A   initial encounter
   D   subsequent encounter
   S   sequela

√x7ᵗʰ **S28.0** Crushed chest

   Use additional code for all associated injuries
   EXCLUDES 1   flail chest (S22.5)

√x7ᵗʰ **S28.1** Traumatic amputation (partial) of part of thorax, except breast

√5ᵗʰ **S28.2** Traumatic amputation of breast

   √6ᵗʰ **S28.21** Complete traumatic amputation of breast

     Traumatic amputation of breast NOS

     √7ᵗʰ **S28.211** Complete traumatic amputation of right breast

     √7ᵗʰ **S28.212** Complete traumatic amputation of left breast

     √7ᵗʰ **S28.219** Complete traumatic amputation of unspecified breast

   √6ᵗʰ **S28.22** Partial traumatic amputation of breast

     √7ᵗʰ **S28.221** Partial traumatic amputation of right breast

     √7ᵗʰ **S28.222** Partial traumatic amputation of left breast

     √7ᵗʰ **S28.229** Partial traumatic amputation of unspecified breast

√4ᵗʰ **S29** **Other and unspecified injuries of thorax**

   Code also any associated open wound (S21.-)

   The appropriate 7th character is to be added to each code from category S29.
   A   initial encounter
   D   subsequent encounter
   S   sequela

√5ᵗʰ **S29.0** Injury of muscle and tendon at thorax level

   √6ᵗʰ **S29.00** Unspecified injury of muscle and tendon of thorax

     √7ᵗʰ **S29.001** Unspecified injury of muscle and tendon of front wall of thorax

     √7ᵗʰ **S29.002** Unspecified injury of muscle and tendon of back wall of thorax

     √7ᵗʰ **S29.009** Unspecified injury of muscle and tendon of unspecified wall of thorax

   √6ᵗʰ **S29.01** Strain of muscle and tendon of thorax

     √7ᵗʰ **S29.011** Strain of muscle and tendon of front wall of thorax

     √7ᵗʰ **S29.012** Strain of muscle and tendon of back wall of thorax

     √7ᵗʰ **S29.019** Strain of muscle and tendon of unspecified wall of thorax

   √6ᵗʰ **S29.02** Laceration of muscle and tendon of thorax

     √7ᵗʰ **S29.021** Laceration of muscle and tendon of front wall of thorax

     √7ᵗʰ **S29.022** Laceration of muscle and tendon of back wall of thorax

     √7ᵗʰ **S29.029** Laceration of muscle and tendon of unspecified wall of thorax

   √6ᵗʰ **S29.09** Other injury of muscle and tendon of thorax

     √7ᵗʰ **S29.091** Other injury of muscle and tendon of front wall of thorax

     √7ᵗʰ **S29.092** Other injury of muscle and tendon of back wall of thorax

     √7ᵗʰ **S29.099** Other injury of muscle and tendon of unspecified wall of thorax

√x7ᵗʰ **S29.8** Other specified injuries of thorax

√x7ᵗʰ **S29.9** Unspecified injury of thorax

Injuries to the abdomen, lower back, lumbar spine, pelvis and external genitals (S30-S39)

INCLUDES   injuries to the abdominal wall
     injuries to the anus
     injuries to the buttock
     injuries to the external genitalia
     injuries to the flank
     injuries to the groin

EXCLUDES 2   burns and corrosions (T20-T32)
     effects of foreign body in anus and rectum (T18.5)
     effects of foreign body in genitourinary tract (T19.-)
     effects of foreign body in stomach, small intestine and colon (T18.2-T18.4)
     frostbite (T33-T34)
     insect bite or sting, venomous (T63.4)

√4ᵗʰ **S30** **Superficial injury of abdomen, lower back, pelvis and external genitals**

   EXCLUDES 2   superficial injury of hip (S70.-)

   The appropriate 7th character is to be added to each code from category S30.
   A   initial encounter
   D   subsequent encounter
   S   sequela

√x7ᵗʰ **S30.0** Contusion of lower back and pelvis

   Contusion of buttock

√x7ᵗʰ **S30.1** Contusion of abdominal wall

   Contusion of flank

   Contusion of groin

√5ᵗʰ **S30.2** Contusion of external genital organs

   √6ᵗʰ **S30.20** Contusion of unspecified external genital organ

     √7ᵗʰ **S30.201** Contusion of unspecified external genital organ, male ♂

     √7ᵗʰ **S30.202** Contusion of unspecified external genital organ, female ♀

   √x7ᵗʰ **S30.21** Contusion of penis

   √x7ᵗʰ **S30.22** Contusion of scrotum and testes ♂

   √x7ᵗʰ **S30.23** Contusion of vagina and vulva ♀

√x7ᵗʰ **S30.3** Contusion of anus

√5ᵗʰ **S30.8** Other superficial injuries of abdomen, lower back, pelvis and external genitals

   √6ᵗʰ **S30.81** Abrasion of abdomen, lower back, pelvis and external genitals

     √7ᵗʰ **S30.810** Abrasion of lower back and pelvis

     √7ᵗʰ **S30.811** Abrasion of abdominal wall

     √7ᵗʰ **S30.812** Abrasion of penis ♂

     √7ᵗʰ **S30.813** Abrasion of scrotum and testes ♂

     √7ᵗʰ **S30.814** Abrasion of vagina and vulva ♀

     √7ᵗʰ **S30.815** Abrasion of unspecified external genital organs, male ♂

√7ᵗʰ **S30.816** **Abrasion of unspecified** external genital organs, female ♀

√7ᵗʰ **S30.817** **Abrasion of** anus

√6ᵗʰ **S30.82** Blister (nonthermal) of **abdomen, lower back, pelvis and external genitals**

√7ᵗʰ **S30.820** **Blister (nonthermal) of** lower back and pelvis

√7ᵗʰ **S30.821** **Blister (nonthermal) of** abdominal wall

√7ᵗʰ **S30.822** **Blister (nonthermal) of** penis ♂

√7ᵗʰ **S30.823** **Blister (nonthermal) of** scrotum and testes ♂

√7ᵗʰ **S30.824** **Blister (nonthermal) of** vagina and vulva ♀

√7ᵗʰ **S30.825** **Blister (nonthermal) of unspecified external genital organs, male** ♂

√7ᵗʰ **S30.826** **Blister (nonthermal) of unspecified external genital organs, female** ♀

√7ᵗʰ **S30.827** **Blister (nonthermal) of** anus

√6ᵗʰ **S30.84** External constriction of **abdomen, lower back, pelvis and external genitals**

√7ᵗʰ **S30.840** **External constriction of** lower back and pelvis

√7ᵗʰ **S30.841** **External constriction of** abdominal wall

√7ᵗʰ **S30.842** **External constriction of** penis ♂

Hair tourniquet syndrome of penis
Use additional cause code to identify the constricting item (W49.0-)

√7ᵗʰ **S30.843** **External constriction of** scrotum and testes ♂

√7ᵗʰ **S30.844** **External constriction of** vagina and vulva ♀

√7ᵗʰ **S30.845** **External constriction of unspecified external genital organs, male** ♂

√7ᵗʰ **S30.846** **External constriction of unspecified external genital organs, female** ♀

√6ᵗʰ **S30.85** Superficial foreign body of **abdomen, lower back, pelvis and external genitals**

Splinter in the abdomen, lower back, pelvis and external genitals

√7ᵗʰ **S30.850** **Superficial foreign body of** lower back and pelvis

√7ᵗʰ **S30.851** **Superficial foreign body of** abdominal wall

√7ᵗʰ **S30.852** **Superficial foreign body of** penis ♂

√7ᵗʰ **S30.853** **Superficial foreign body of** scrotum and testes ♂

√7ᵗʰ **S30.854** **Superficial foreign body of** vagina and vulva ♀

√7ᵗʰ **S30.855** **Superficial foreign body of unspecified external genital organs, male** ♂

√7ᵗʰ **S30.856** **Superficial foreign body of unspecified external genital organs, female** ♀

√7ᵗʰ **S30.857** **Superficial foreign body of** anus

√6ᵗʰ **S30.86** Insect bite (nonvenomous) of **abdomen, lower back, pelvis and external genitals**

√7ᵗʰ **S30.860** **Insect bite (nonvenomous) of** lower back and pelvis

√7ᵗʰ **S30.861** **Insect bite (nonvenomous) of** abdominal wall

√7ᵗʰ **S30.862** **Insect bite (nonvenomous) of** penis ♂

√7ᵗʰ **S30.863** **Insect bite (nonvenomous) of** scrotum and testes ♂

√7ᵗʰ **S30.864** **Insect bite (nonvenomous) of** vagina and vulva ♀

√7ᵗʰ **S30.865** **Insect bite (nonvenomous) of unspecified external genital organs, male** ♂

√7ᵗʰ **S30.866** **Insect bite (nonvenomous) of unspecified external genital organs, female** ♀

√7ᵗʰ **S30.867** **Insect bite (nonvenomous) of** anus

√6ᵗʰ **S30.87** Other superficial bite of **abdomen, lower back, pelvis and external genitals**

EXCLUDES 1 open bite of abdomen, lower back, pelvis and external genitals (S31.05, S31.15, S31.25, S31.35, S31.45, S31.55)

√7ᵗʰ **S30.870** **Other superficial bite of** lower back and pelvis

√7ᵗʰ **S30.871** **Other superficial bite of** abdominal wall

√7ᵗʰ **S30.872** **Other superficial bite of** penis ♂

√7ᵗʰ **S30.873** **Other superficial bite of** scrotum and testes ♂

√7ᵗʰ **S30.874** **Other superficial bite of** vagina and vulva ♀

√7ᵗʰ **S30.875** **Other superficial bite of unspecified external genital organs, male** ♂

√7ᵗʰ **S30.876** **Other superficial bite of unspecified external genital organs, female** ♀

√7ᵗʰ **S30.877** **Other superficial bite of** anus

√5ᵗʰ **S30.9** Unspecified superficial injury of abdomen, **lower back, pelvis and external genitals**

√x7ᵗʰ **S30.91** **Unspecified superficial injury of** lower back and pelvis

√x7ᵗʰ **S30.92** **Unspecified superficial injury of** abdominal wall

√x7ᵗʰ **S30.93** **Unspecified superficial injury of** penis ♂

√x7ᵗʰ **S30.94** **Unspecified superficial injury of** scrotum and testes ♂

√x7ᵗʰ **S30.95** **Unspecified superficial injury of** vagina and vulva ♀

√x7ᵗʰ **S30.96** **Unspecified superficial injury of unspecified external genital organs, male** ♂

√x7ᵗʰ **S30.97** **Unspecified superficial injury of unspecified external genital organs, female** ♀

√x7ᵗʰ **S30.98** **Unspecified superficial injury of** anus

√4ᵗʰ **S31** Open wound of abdomen, **lower back, pelvis and external genitals**

Code also any associated:
spinal cord injury (S24.0, S24.1-, S34.0-, S34.1-)
wound infection

EXCLUDES 1 traumatic amputation of part of abdomen, lower back and pelvis (S38.2-, S38.3)

EXCLUDES 2 open wound of hip (S71.00-S71.02)
open fracture of pelvis (S32.1- - S32.9 with 7th character B)

The appropriate 7th character is to be added to each code from category S31.
A   initial encounter
D   subsequent encounter
S   sequela

√5ᵗʰ **S31.0** Open wound of lower back and pelvis

√6ᵗʰ **S31.00** Unspecified open wound of lower back and pelvis

√7ᵗʰ **S31.000** Unspecified open wound of lower back and pelvis **without penetration into retroperitoneum**

Unspecified open wound of lower back and pelvis NOS

√7ᵗʰ **S31.001** Unspecified open wound of lower back and pelvis **with penetration into retroperitoneum**

√6ᵗʰ **S31.01** Laceration without foreign body **of lower back and pelvis**

√7ᵗʰ **S31.010** **Laceration without foreign body of lower back and pelvis** without penetration into retroperitoneum

Laceration without foreign body of lower back and pelvis NOS

√7ᵗʰ **S31.011** **Laceration without foreign body of lower back and pelvis** with penetration into retroperitoneum

√6ᵗʰ **S31.02** Laceration with foreign body **of lower back and pelvis**

√7ᵗʰ **S31.020** **Laceration with foreign body of lower back and pelvis** without penetration into retroperitoneum

Laceration with foreign body of lower back and pelvis NOS

√7ᵗʰ **S31.021** **Laceration with foreign body of lower back and pelvis** with penetration into retroperitoneum

√6ᵗʰ **S31.03** Puncture wound without foreign body **of lower back and pelvis**

√7ᵗʰ **S31.030** **Puncture wound without foreign body of lower back and pelvis** without penetration into retroperitoneum

Puncture wound without foreign body of lower back and pelvis NOS

√7ᵗʰ **S31.031** **Puncture wound without foreign body of lower back and pelvis** with penetration into retroperitoneum

√6ᵗʰ **S31.04** Puncture wound with foreign body of lower back and pelvis

√7ᵗʰ **S31.040** Puncture wound with foreign body of lower back and pelvis without penetration into retroperitoneum

Puncture wound with foreign body of lower back and pelvis NOS

√7ᵗʰ **S31.041** Puncture wound with foreign body of lower back and pelvis with penetration into retroperitoneum

√6ᵗʰ **S31.05** Open bite of lower back and pelvis

Bite of lower back and pelvis NOS

EXCLUDES 1   superficial bite of lower back and pelvis (S30.860, S30.870)

√7ᵗʰ **S31.050** Open bite of lower back and pelvis without penetration into retroperitoneum

Open bite of lower back and pelvis NOS

√7ᵗʰ **S31.051** Open bite of lower back and pelvis with penetration into retroperitoneum

√5ᵗʰ **S31.1** Open wound of abdominal wall without penetration into peritoneal cavity

Open wound of abdominal wall NOS

EXCLUDES 2   open wound of abdominal wall with penetration into peritoneal cavity (S31.6-)

√6ᵗʰ **S31.10** Unspecified open wound of abdominal wall without penetration into peritoneal cavity

√7ᵗʰ **S31.100** Unspecified open wound of abdominal wall, right upper quadrant without penetration into peritoneal cavity

√7ᵗʰ **S31.101** Unspecified open wound of abdominal wall, left upper quadrant without penetration into peritoneal cavity

√7ᵗʰ **S31.102** Unspecified open wound of abdominal wall, epigastric region without penetration into peritoneal cavity

√7ᵗʰ **S31.103** Unspecified open wound of abdominal wall, right lower quadrant without penetration into peritoneal cavity

√7ᵗʰ **S31.104** Unspecified open wound of abdominal wall, left lower quadrant without penetration into peritoneal cavity

√7ᵗʰ **S31.105** Unspecified open wound of abdominal wall, periumbilic region without penetration into peritoneal cavity

√7ᵗʰ **S31.109** Unspecified open wound of abdominal wall, unspecified quadrant without penetration into peritoneal cavity

Unspecified open wound of abdominal wall NOS

√6ᵗʰ **S31.11** Laceration without foreign body of abdominal wall without penetration into peritoneal cavity

√7ᵗʰ **S31.110** Laceration without foreign body of abdominal wall, right upper quadrant without penetration into peritoneal cavity

√7ᵗʰ **S31.111** Laceration without foreign body of abdominal wall, left upper quadrant without penetration into peritoneal cavity

√7ᵗʰ **S31.112** Laceration without foreign body of abdominal wall, epigastric region without penetration into peritoneal cavity

√7ᵗʰ **S31.113** Laceration without foreign body of abdominal wall, right lower quadrant without penetration into peritoneal cavity

√7ᵗʰ **S31.114** Laceration without foreign body of abdominal wall, left lower quadrant without penetration into peritoneal cavity

√7ᵗʰ **S31.115** Laceration without foreign body of abdominal wall, periumbilic region without penetration into peritoneal cavity

√7ᵗʰ **S31.119** Laceration without foreign body of abdominal wall, unspecified quadrant without penetration into peritoneal cavity

√6ᵗʰ **S31.12** Laceration with foreign body of abdominal wall without penetration into peritoneal cavity

√7ᵗʰ **S31.120** Laceration of abdominal wall with foreign body, right upper quadrant without penetration into peritoneal cavity

√7ᵗʰ **S31.121** Laceration of abdominal wall with foreign body, left upper quadrant without penetration into peritoneal cavity

√7ᵗʰ **S31.122** Laceration of abdominal wall with foreign body, epigastric region without penetration into peritoneal cavity

√7ᵗʰ **S31.123** Laceration of abdominal wall with foreign body, right lower quadrant without penetration into peritoneal cavity

√7ᵗʰ **S31.124** Laceration of abdominal wall with foreign body, left lower quadrant without penetration into peritoneal cavity

√7ᵗʰ **S31.125** Laceration of abdominal wall with foreign body, periumbilic region without penetration into peritoneal cavity

√7ᵗʰ **S31.129** Laceration of abdominal wall with foreign body, unspecified quadrant without penetration into peritoneal cavity

√6ᵗʰ **S31.13** Puncture wound of abdominal wall without foreign body without penetration into peritoneal cavity

√7ᵗʰ **S31.130** Puncture wound of abdominal wall without foreign body, right upper quadrant without penetration into peritoneal cavity

√7ᵗʰ **S31.131** Puncture wound of abdominal wall without foreign body, left upper quadrant without penetration into peritoneal cavity

√7ᵗʰ **S31.132** Puncture wound of abdominal wall without foreign body, epigastric region without penetration into peritoneal cavity

√7ᵗʰ **S31.133** Puncture wound of abdominal wall without foreign body, right lower quadrant without penetration into peritoneal cavity

√7ᵗʰ **S31.134** Puncture wound of abdominal wall without foreign body, left lower quadrant without penetration into peritoneal cavity

√7ᵗʰ **S31.135** Puncture wound of abdominal wall without foreign body, periumbilic region without penetration into peritoneal cavity

√7ᵗʰ **S31.139** Puncture wound of abdominal wall without foreign body, unspecified quadrant without penetration into peritoneal cavity

√6ᵗʰ **S31.14** Puncture wound of abdominal wall with foreign body without penetration into peritoneal cavity

√7ᵗʰ **S31.140** Puncture wound of abdominal wall with foreign body, right upper quadrant without penetration into peritoneal cavity

√7ᵗʰ **S31.141** Puncture wound of abdominal wall with foreign body, left upper quadrant without penetration into peritoneal cavity

√7ᵗʰ **S31.142** Puncture wound of abdominal wall with foreign body, epigastric region without penetration into peritoneal cavity

√7ᵗʰ **S31.143** Puncture wound of abdominal wall with foreign body, right lower quadrant without penetration into peritoneal cavity

√7ᵗʰ **S31.144** Puncture wound of abdominal wall with foreign body, left lower quadrant without penetration into peritoneal cavity

√7ᵗʰ **S31.145** Puncture wound of abdominal wall with foreign body, periumbilic region without penetration into peritoneal cavity

√7ᵗʰ **S31.149** Puncture wound of abdominal wall with foreign body, unspecified quadrant without penetration into peritoneal cavity

√6ᵗʰ **S31.15** Open bite of abdominal wall without penetration into peritoneal cavity

Bite of abdominal wall NOS

EXCLUDES 1   superficial bite of abdominal wall (S30.871)

√7ᵗʰ **S31.150** Open bite of abdominal wall, right upper quadrant without penetration into peritoneal cavity

---

√7ᵗʰ **S31.151 Open bite of abdominal wall,** left upper quadrant **without penetration into peritoneal cavity**

√7ᵗʰ **S31.152 Open bite of abdominal wall,** epigastric region **without penetration into peritoneal cavity**

√7ᵗʰ **S31.153 Open bite of abdominal wall,** right lower quadrant **without penetration into peritoneal cavity**

√7ᵗʰ **S31.154 Open bite of abdominal wall,** left lower quadrant **without penetration into peritoneal cavity**

√7ᵗʰ **S31.155 Open bite of abdominal wall,** periumbilic region **without penetration into peritoneal cavity**

√7ᵗʰ **S31.159 Open bite of abdominal wall, unspecified quadrant without penetration into peritoneal cavity**

√5ᵗʰ **S31.2 Open wound of** penis

√x7ᵗʰ **S31.20 Unspecified open wound of penis** ♂

√x7ᵗʰ **S31.21 Laceration without foreign body of penis** ♂

√x7ᵗʰ **S31.22 Laceration with foreign body of penis** ♂

√x7ᵗʰ **S31.23 Puncture wound without foreign body of penis** ♂

√x7ᵗʰ **S31.24 Puncture wound with foreign body of penis** ♂

√x7ᵗʰ **S31.25 Open bite of penis** ♂

Bite of penis NOS

EXCLUDES 1   *superficial bite of penis (S30.862, S30.872)*

√5ᵗʰ **S31.3 Open wound of** scrotum and testes

√x7ᵗʰ **S31.30 Unspecified open wound of scrotum and testes** ♂

√x7ᵗʰ **S31.31 Laceration without foreign body of scrotum and testes** ♂

√x7ᵗʰ **S31.32 Laceration with foreign body of scrotum and testes** ♂

√x7ᵗʰ **S31.33 Puncture wound without foreign body of scrotum and testes** ♂

√x7ᵗʰ **S31.34 Puncture wound with foreign body of scrotum and testes** ♂

√x7ᵗʰ **S31.35 Open bite of scrotum and testes** ♂

Bite of scrotum and testes NOS

EXCLUDES 1   *superficial bite of scrotum and testes (S30.863, S30.873)*

√5ᵗʰ **S31.4 Open wound of** vagina and vulva

EXCLUDES 1   *injury to vagina and vulva during delivery (O70.-, O71.4)*

√x7ᵗʰ **S31.40 Unspecified open wound of vagina and vulva** ♀

√x7ᵗʰ **S31.41 Laceration without foreign body of vagina and vulva** ♀

√x7ᵗʰ **S31.42 Laceration with foreign body of vagina and vulva** ♀

√x7ᵗʰ **S31.43 Puncture wound without foreign body of vagina and vulva** ♀

√x7ᵗʰ **S31.44 Puncture wound with foreign body of vagina and vulva** ♀

√x7ᵗʰ **S31.45 Open bite of vagina and vulva** ♀

Bite of vagina and vulva NOS

EXCLUDES 1   *superficial bite of vagina and vulva (S30.864, S30.874)*

√5ᵗʰ **S31.5 Open wound of unspecified external genital organs**

EXCLUDES 1   *traumatic amputation of external genital organs (S38.21, S38.22)*

√6ᵗʰ **S31.50 Unspecified open wound of unspecified external genital organs**

√7ᵗʰ **S31.501 Unspecified open wound of unspecified external genital organs,** male ♂

√7ᵗʰ **S31.502 Unspecified open wound of unspecified external genital organs,** female ♀

√6ᵗʰ **S31.51 Laceration without foreign body of unspecified external genital organs**

√7ᵗʰ **S31.511 Laceration without foreign body of unspecified external genital organs,** male ♂

√7ᵗʰ **S31.512 Laceration without foreign body of unspecified external genital organs,** female ♀

√6ᵗʰ **S31.52 Laceration with foreign body of unspecified external genital organs**

√7ᵗʰ **S31.521 Laceration with foreign body of unspecified external genital organs,** male ♂

√7ᵗʰ **S31.522 Laceration with foreign body of unspecified external genital organs,** female ♀

√6ᵗʰ **S31.53 Puncture wound without foreign body of unspecified external genital organs**

√7ᵗʰ **S31.531 Puncture wound without foreign body of unspecified external genital organs,** male ♂

√7ᵗʰ **S31.532 Puncture wound without foreign body of unspecified external genital organs,** female ♀

√6ᵗʰ **S31.54 Puncture wound with foreign body of unspecified external genital organs**

√7ᵗʰ **S31.541 Puncture wound with foreign body of unspecified external genital organs,** male ♂

√7ᵗʰ **S31.542 Puncture wound with foreign body of unspecified external genital organs,** female ♀

√6ᵗʰ **S31.55 Open bite of unspecified external genital organs**

Bite of unspecified external genital organs NOS

EXCLUDES 1   *superficial bite of unspecified external genital organs (S30.865, S30.866, S30.875, S30.876)*

√7ᵗʰ **S31.551 Open bite of unspecified external genital organs,** male ♂

√7ᵗʰ **S31.552 Open bite of unspecified external genital organs,** female ♀

√5ᵗʰ **S31.6 Open wound of** abdominal wall with penetration into peritoneal cavity

√6ᵗʰ **S31.60 Unspecified open wound of abdominal wall with penetration into peritoneal cavity**

√7ᵗʰ **S31.600 Unspecified open wound of abdominal wall,** right upper quadrant **with penetration into peritoneal cavity**

√7ᵗʰ **S31.601 Unspecified open wound of abdominal wall,** left upper quadrant **with penetration into peritoneal cavity**

√7ᵗʰ **S31.602 Unspecified open wound of abdominal wall,** epigastric region **with penetration into peritoneal cavity**

√7ᵗʰ **S31.603 Unspecified open wound of abdominal wall,** right lower quadrant **with penetration into peritoneal cavity**

√7ᵗʰ **S31.604 Unspecified open wound of abdominal wall,** left lower quadrant **with penetration into peritoneal cavity**

√7ᵗʰ **S31.605 Unspecified open wound of abdominal wall,** periumbilic region **with penetration into peritoneal cavity**

√7ᵗʰ **S31.609 Unspecified open wound of abdominal wall, unspecified quadrant with penetration into peritoneal cavity**

√6ᵗʰ **S31.61 Laceration without foreign body of abdominal wall with penetration into peritoneal cavity**

√7ᵗʰ **S31.610 Laceration without foreign body of abdominal wall,** right upper quadrant **with penetration into peritoneal cavity**

√7ᵗʰ **S31.611 Laceration without foreign body of abdominal wall,** left upper quadrant **with penetration into peritoneal cavity**

√7ᵗʰ **S31.612 Laceration without foreign body of abdominal wall,** epigastric region **with penetration into peritoneal cavity**

√7ᵗʰ **S31.613 Laceration without foreign body of abdominal wall,** right lower quadrant **with penetration into peritoneal cavity**

√7ᵗʰ **S31.614 Laceration without foreign body of abdominal wall,** left lower quadrant **with penetration into peritoneal cavity**

√7ᵗʰ **S31.615 Laceration without foreign body of abdominal wall,** periumbilic region **with penetration into peritoneal cavity**

√7ᵗʰ **S31.619 Laceration without foreign body of abdominal wall, unspecified quadrant with penetration into peritoneal cavity**

√6ᵗʰ **S31.62** Laceration with foreign body of abdominal wall with penetration into peritoneal cavity

   √7ᵗʰ **S31.620** **Laceration with foreign body of abdominal wall, right upper quadrant with penetration into peritoneal cavity**

   √7ᵗʰ **S31.621** **Laceration with foreign body of abdominal wall, left upper quadrant with penetration into peritoneal cavity**

   √7ᵗʰ **S31.622** **Laceration with foreign body of abdominal wall, epigastric region with penetration into peritoneal cavity**

   √7ᵗʰ **S31.623** **Laceration with foreign body of abdominal wall, right lower quadrant with penetration into peritoneal cavity**

   √7ᵗʰ **S31.624** **Laceration with foreign body of abdominal wall, left lower quadrant with penetration into peritoneal cavity**

   √7ᵗʰ **S31.625** **Laceration with foreign body of abdominal wall, periumbilic region with penetration into peritoneal cavity**

   √7ᵗʰ **S31.629** **Laceration with foreign body of abdominal wall, unspecified quadrant with penetration into peritoneal cavity**

√6ᵗʰ **S31.63** Puncture wound without foreign body of abdominal wall with penetration into peritoneal cavity

   √7ᵗʰ **S31.630** **Puncture wound without foreign body of abdominal wall, right upper quadrant with penetration into peritoneal cavity**

   √7ᵗʰ **S31.631** **Puncture wound without foreign body of abdominal wall, left upper quadrant with penetration into peritoneal cavity**

   √7ᵗʰ **S31.632** **Puncture wound without foreign body of abdominal wall, epigastric region with penetration into peritoneal cavity**

   √7ᵗʰ **S31.633** **Puncture wound without foreign body of abdominal wall, right lower quadrant with penetration into peritoneal cavity**

   √7ᵗʰ **S31.634** **Puncture wound without foreign body of abdominal wall, left lower quadrant with penetration into peritoneal cavity**

   √7ᵗʰ **S31.635** **Puncture wound without foreign body of abdominal wall, periumbilic region with penetration into peritoneal cavity**

   √7ᵗʰ **S31.639** **Puncture wound without foreign body of abdominal wall, unspecified quadrant with penetration into peritoneal cavity**

√6ᵗʰ **S31.64** Puncture wound with foreign body of abdominal wall with penetration into peritoneal cavity

   √7ᵗʰ **S31.640** **Puncture wound with foreign body of abdominal wall, right upper quadrant with penetration into peritoneal cavity**

   √7ᵗʰ **S31.641** **Puncture wound with foreign body of abdominal wall, left upper quadrant with penetration into peritoneal cavity**

   √7ᵗʰ **S31.642** **Puncture wound with foreign body of abdominal wall, epigastric region with penetration into peritoneal cavity**

   √7ᵗʰ **S31.643** **Puncture wound with foreign body of abdominal wall, right lower quadrant with penetration into peritoneal cavity**

   √7ᵗʰ **S31.644** **Puncture wound with foreign body of abdominal wall, left lower quadrant with penetration into peritoneal cavity**

   √7ᵗʰ **S31.645** **Puncture wound with foreign body of abdominal wall, periumbilic region with penetration into peritoneal cavity**

   √7ᵗʰ **S31.649** **Puncture wound with foreign body of abdominal wall, unspecified quadrant with penetration into peritoneal cavity**

√6ᵗʰ **S31.65** Open bite of abdominal wall with penetration into peritoneal cavity

   EXCLUDES 1   *superficial bite of abdominal wall (S30.861, S30.871)*

   √7ᵗʰ **S31.650** **Open bite of abdominal wall, right upper quadrant with penetration into peritoneal cavity**

   √7ᵗʰ **S31.651** **Open bite of abdominal wall, left upper quadrant with penetration into peritoneal cavity**

   √7ᵗʰ **S31.652** **Open bite of abdominal wall, epigastric region with penetration into peritoneal cavity**

   √7ᵗʰ **S31.653** **Open bite of abdominal wall, right lower quadrant with penetration into peritoneal cavity**

   √7ᵗʰ **S31.654** **Open bite of abdominal wall, left lower quadrant with penetration into peritoneal cavity**

   √7ᵗʰ **S31.655** **Open bite of abdominal wall, periumbilic region with penetration into peritoneal cavity**

   √7ᵗʰ **S31.659** **Open bite of abdominal wall, unspecified quadrant with penetration into peritoneal cavity**

√5ᵗʰ **S31.8** **Open wound of other parts of abdomen, lower back and pelvis**

√6ᵗʰ **S31.80** **Open wound of unspecified buttock**

   √7ᵗʰ **S31.801** **Laceration without foreign body of unspecified buttock**

   √7ᵗʰ **S31.802** **Laceration with foreign body of unspecified buttock**

   √7ᵗʰ **S31.803** **Puncture wound without foreign body of unspecified buttock**

   √7ᵗʰ **S31.804** **Puncture wound with foreign body of unspecified buttock**

   √7ᵗʰ **S31.805** **Open bite of unspecified buttock**

       Bite of buttock NOS

       EXCLUDES 1   *superficial bite of buttock (S30.870)*

   √7ᵗʰ **S31.809** **Unspecified open wound of unspecified buttock**

√6ᵗʰ **S31.81** **Open wound of right buttock**

   √7ᵗʰ **S31.811** **Laceration without foreign body of right buttock**

   √7ᵗʰ **S31.812** **Laceration with foreign body of right buttock**

   √7ᵗʰ **S31.813** **Puncture wound without foreign body of right buttock**

   √7ᵗʰ **S31.814** **Puncture wound with foreign body of right buttock**

   √7ᵗʰ **S31.815** **Open bite of right buttock**

       Bite of right buttock NOS

       EXCLUDES 1   *superficial bite of buttock (S30.870)*

   √7ᵗʰ **S31.819** **Unspecified open wound of right buttock**

√6ᵗʰ **S31.82** **Open wound of left buttock**

   √7ᵗʰ **S31.821** **Laceration without foreign body of left buttock**

   √7ᵗʰ **S31.822** **Laceration with foreign body of left buttock**

   √7ᵗʰ **S31.823** **Puncture wound without foreign body of left buttock**

   √7ᵗʰ **S31.824** **Puncture wound with foreign body of left buttock**

   √7ᵗʰ **S31.825** **Open bite of left buttock**

       Bite of left buttock NOS

       EXCLUDES 1   *superficial bite of buttock (S30.870)*

   √7ᵗʰ **S31.829** **Unspecified open wound of left buttock**

√6ᵗʰ **S31.83** **Open wound of anus**

   √7ᵗʰ **S31.831** **Laceration without foreign body of anus**

   √7ᵗʰ **S31.832** **Laceration with foreign body of anus**

   √7ᵗʰ **S31.833** **Puncture wound without foreign body of anus**

   √7ᵗʰ **S31.834** **Puncture wound with foreign body of anus**

   √7ᵗʰ **S31.835** **Open bite of anus**

       Bite of anus NOS

       EXCLUDES 1   *superficial bite of anus (S30.877)*

   √7ᵗʰ **S31.839** **Unspecified open wound of anus**

Chapter 19. Injury, Poisoning and Certain Other Consequences of External Causes *(side margin)*

✓4ᵗʰ **S32 Fracture of lumbar spine and pelvis**

> **NOTE**   A fracture not indicated as displaced or nondisplaced should be coded to displaced.
>
> A fracture not indicated as opened or closed should be coded to closed.

> **INCLUDES**   fracture of lumbosacral neural arch
> fracture of lumbosacral spinous process
> fracture of lumbosacral transverse process
> fracture of lumbosacral vertebra
> fracture of lumbosacral vertebral arch

Code first any associated spinal cord and spinal nerve injury (S34.-)

EXCLUDES 1   transection of abdomen (S38.3)

EXCLUDES 2   fracture of hip NOS (S72.0-)

AHA: 2021,1Q,6; 2018,2Q,12; 2015,3Q,37-39; 2012,4Q,93

> The appropriate 7th character is to be added to each code from category S32.
> A   initial encounter for closed fracture
> B   initial encounter for open fracture
> D   subsequent encounter for fracture with routine healing
> G   subsequent encounter for fracture with delayed healing
> K   subsequent encounter for fracture with nonunion
> S   sequela

✓5ᵗʰ **S32.0 Fracture of lumbar vertebra**
    Fracture of lumbar spine NOS

   ✓6ᵗʰ **S32.00 Fracture of unspecified lumbar vertebra**

     1 ✓7ᵗʰ **S32.000** Wedge compression fracture of unspecified lumbar vertebra   HCC ESR COM Q

     1 ✓7ᵗʰ **S32.001** Stable burst fracture of unspecified lumbar vertebra   HCC ESR COM Q

     1 ✓7ᵗʰ **S32.002** Unstable burst fracture of unspecified lumbar vertebra   HCC ESR COM Q

     1 ✓7ᵗʰ **S32.008** Other fracture of unspecified lumbar vertebra   HCC ESR COM Q

     1 ✓7ᵗʰ **S32.009** Unspecified fracture of unspecified lumbar vertebra   HCC ESR COM Q

   ✓6ᵗʰ **S32.01 Fracture of first lumbar vertebra**

     1 ✓7ᵗʰ **S32.010** Wedge compression fracture of first lumbar vertebra   HCC ESR COM Q

     1 ✓7ᵗʰ **S32.011** Stable burst fracture of first lumbar vertebra   HCC ESR COM Q

     1 ✓7ᵗʰ **S32.012** Unstable burst fracture of first lumbar vertebra   HCC ESR COM Q

     1 ✓7ᵗʰ **S32.018** Other fracture of first lumbar vertebra   HCC ESR COM Q

     1 ✓7ᵗʰ **S32.019** Unspecified fracture of first lumbar vertebra   HCC ESR COM Q

   ✓6ᵗʰ **S32.02 Fracture of second lumbar vertebra**

     1 ✓7ᵗʰ **S32.020** Wedge compression fracture of second lumbar vertebra   HCC ESR COM Q

     1 ✓7ᵗʰ **S32.021** Stable burst fracture of second lumbar vertebra   HCC ESR COM Q

     1 ✓7ᵗʰ **S32.022** Unstable burst fracture of second lumbar vertebra   HCC ESR COM Q

     1 ✓7ᵗʰ **S32.028** Other fracture of second lumbar vertebra   HCC ESR COM Q

     1 ✓7ᵗʰ **S32.029** Unspecified fracture of second lumbar vertebra   HCC ESR COM Q

   ✓6ᵗʰ **S32.03 Fracture of third lumbar vertebra**

     1 ✓7ᵗʰ **S32.030** Wedge compression fracture of third lumbar vertebra   HCC ESR COM Q

     1 ✓7ᵗʰ **S32.031** Stable burst fracture of third lumbar vertebra   HCC ESR COM Q

     1 ✓7ᵗʰ **S32.032** Unstable burst fracture of third lumbar vertebra   HCC ESR COM Q

     1 ✓7ᵗʰ **S32.038** Other fracture of third lumbar vertebra   HCC ESR COM Q

     1 ✓7ᵗʰ **S32.039** Unspecified fracture of third lumbar vertebra   HCC ESR COM Q

   ✓6ᵗʰ **S32.04 Fracture of fourth lumbar vertebra**

     1 ✓7ᵗʰ **S32.040** Wedge compression fracture of fourth lumbar vertebra   HCC ESR COM Q

     1 ✓7ᵗʰ **S32.041** Stable burst fracture of fourth lumbar vertebra   HCC ESR COM Q

     1 ✓7ᵗʰ **S32.042** Unstable burst fracture of fourth lumbar vertebra

     1 ✓7ᵗʰ **S32.048** Other fracture of fourth lumbar vertebra   HCC ESR COM Q

     1 ✓7ᵗʰ **S32.049** Unspecified fracture of fourth lumbar vertebra   HCC ESR COM Q

   ✓6ᵗʰ **S32.05 Fracture of fifth lumbar vertebra**

     1 ✓7ᵗʰ **S32.050** Wedge compression fracture of fifth lumbar vertebra   HCC ESR COM Q

     1 ✓7ᵗʰ **S32.051** Stable burst fracture of fifth lumbar vertebra   HCC ESR COM Q

     1 ✓7ᵗʰ **S32.052** Unstable burst fracture of fifth lumbar vertebra   HCC ESR COM Q

     1 ✓7ᵗʰ **S32.058** Other fracture of fifth lumbar vertebra   HCC ESR COM Q

     1 ✓7ᵗʰ **S32.059** Unspecified fracture of fifth lumbar vertebra   HCC ESR COM Q

✓5ᵗʰ **S32.1 Fracture of sacrum**

> **NOTE**   For vertical fractures, code to most medial fracture extension
>
> Use two codes if both a vertical and transverse fracture are present

Code also any associated fracture of pelvic ring (S32.8-)

   1 ✓x7ᵗʰ **S32.10 Unspecified fracture of sacrum**   HCC ESR COM Q

   ✓6ᵗʰ **S32.11 Zone I fracture of sacrum**
     Vertical sacral ala fracture of sacrum

Vertical Sacral Fracture Zones

     1 ✓7ᵗʰ **S32.110** Nondisplaced Zone I fracture of sacrum   HCC ESR COM Q

     1 ✓7ᵗʰ **S32.111** Minimally displaced Zone I fracture of sacrum   HCC ESR COM Q

     1 ✓7ᵗʰ **S32.112** Severely displaced Zone I fracture of sacrum   HCC ESR COM Q

     1 ✓7ᵗʰ **S32.119** Unspecified Zone I fracture of sacrum   HCC ESR COM Q

   ✓6ᵗʰ **S32.12 Zone II fracture of sacrum**
     Vertical foraminal region fracture of sacrum

     1 ✓7ᵗʰ **S32.120** Nondisplaced Zone II fracture of sacrum   HCC ESR COM Q

     1 ✓7ᵗʰ **S32.121** Minimally displaced Zone II fracture of sacrum   HCC ESR COM Q

     1 ✓7ᵗʰ **S32.122** Severely displaced Zone II fracture of sacrum   HCC ESR COM Q

     1 ✓7ᵗʰ **S32.129** Unspecified Zone II fracture of sacrum   HCC ESR COM Q

   ✓6ᵗʰ **S32.13 Zone III fracture of sacrum**
     Vertical fracture into spinal canal region of sacrum

     1 ✓7ᵗʰ **S32.130** Nondisplaced Zone III fracture of sacrum   HCC ESR COM Q

     1 ✓7ᵗʰ **S32.131** Minimally displaced Zone III fracture of sacrum   HCC ESR COM Q

     1 ✓7ᵗʰ **S32.132** Severely displaced Zone III fracture of sacrum   HCC ESR COM Q

¹ √x7ᵗʰ **S32.139** Unspecified Zone III fracture of sacrum HCC ESR COM Q

Transverse Sacral Fracture Types

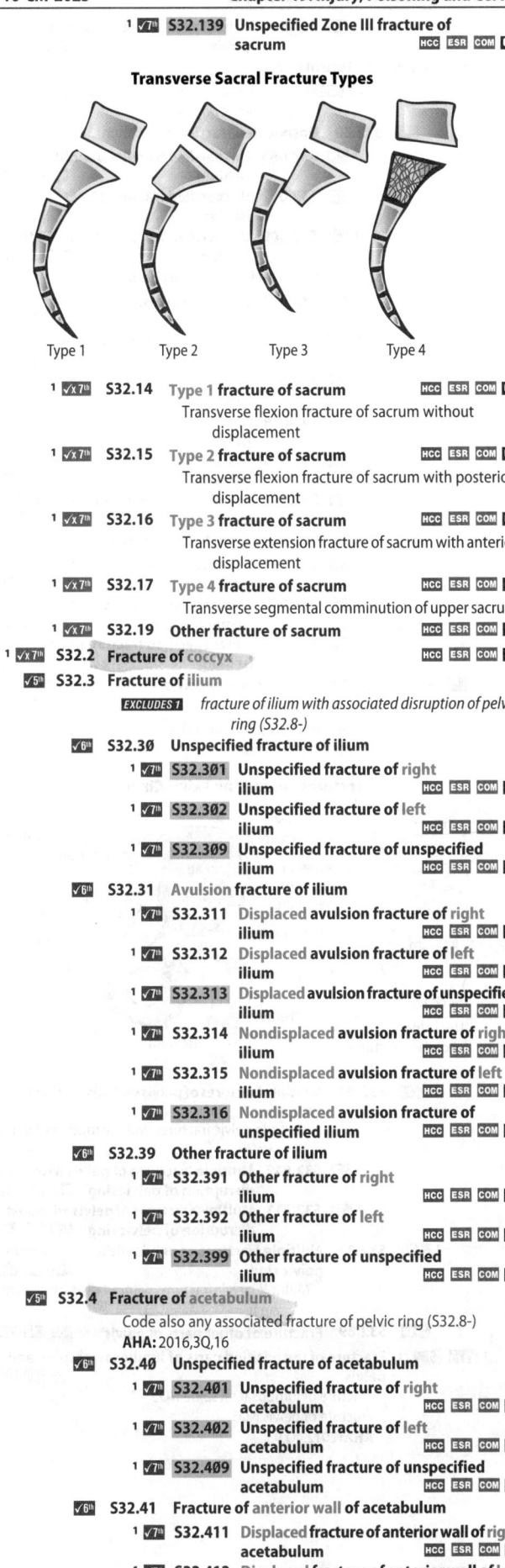

Type 1   Type 2   Type 3   Type 4

¹ √x7ᵗʰ **S32.14** Type 1 fracture of sacrum HCC ESR COM Q
Transverse flexion fracture of sacrum without displacement

¹ √x7ᵗʰ **S32.15** Type 2 fracture of sacrum HCC ESR COM Q
Transverse flexion fracture of sacrum with posterior displacement

¹ √x7ᵗʰ **S32.16** Type 3 fracture of sacrum HCC ESR COM Q
Transverse extension fracture of sacrum with anterior displacement

¹ √x7ᵗʰ **S32.17** Type 4 fracture of sacrum HCC ESR COM Q
Transverse segmental comminution of upper sacrum

¹ √x7ᵗʰ **S32.19** Other fracture of sacrum HCC ESR COM Q

¹ √x7ᵗʰ **S32.2** Fracture of coccyx HCC ESR COM Q

√5ᵗʰ **S32.3** Fracture of ilium

EXCLUDES 1 fracture of ilium with associated disruption of pelvic ring (S32.8-)

√6ᵗʰ **S32.30** Unspecified fracture of ilium

¹ √7ᵗʰ **S32.301** Unspecified fracture of right ilium HCC ESR COM Q

¹ √7ᵗʰ **S32.302** Unspecified fracture of left ilium HCC ESR COM Q

¹ √7ᵗʰ **S32.309** Unspecified fracture of unspecified ilium HCC ESR COM Q

√6ᵗʰ **S32.31** Avulsion fracture of ilium

¹ √7ᵗʰ **S32.311** Displaced avulsion fracture of right ilium HCC ESR COM Q

¹ √7ᵗʰ **S32.312** Displaced avulsion fracture of left ilium HCC ESR COM Q

¹ √7ᵗʰ **S32.313** Displaced avulsion fracture of unspecified ilium HCC ESR COM Q

¹ √7ᵗʰ **S32.314** Nondisplaced avulsion fracture of right ilium HCC ESR COM Q

¹ √7ᵗʰ **S32.315** Nondisplaced avulsion fracture of left ilium HCC ESR COM Q

¹ √7ᵗʰ **S32.316** Nondisplaced avulsion fracture of unspecified ilium HCC ESR COM Q

√6ᵗʰ **S32.39** Other fracture of ilium

¹ √7ᵗʰ **S32.391** Other fracture of right ilium HCC ESR COM Q

¹ √7ᵗʰ **S32.392** Other fracture of left ilium HCC ESR COM Q

¹ √7ᵗʰ **S32.399** Other fracture of unspecified ilium HCC ESR COM Q

√5ᵗʰ **S32.4** Fracture of acetabulum

Code also any associated fracture of pelvic ring (S32.8-)
AHA: 2016,3Q,16

√6ᵗʰ **S32.40** Unspecified fracture of acetabulum

¹ √7ᵗʰ **S32.401** Unspecified fracture of right acetabulum HCC ESR COM Q

¹ √7ᵗʰ **S32.402** Unspecified fracture of left acetabulum HCC ESR COM Q

¹ √7ᵗʰ **S32.409** Unspecified fracture of unspecified acetabulum HCC ESR COM Q

√6ᵗʰ **S32.41** Fracture of anterior wall of acetabulum

¹ √7ᵗʰ **S32.411** Displaced fracture of anterior wall of right acetabulum HCC ESR COM Q

¹ √7ᵗʰ **S32.412** Displaced fracture of anterior wall of left acetabulum

¹ √7ᵗʰ **S32.413** Displaced fracture of anterior wall of unspecified acetabulum HCC ESR COM Q

¹ √7ᵗʰ **S32.414** Nondisplaced fracture of anterior wall of right acetabulum HCC ESR COM Q

¹ √7ᵗʰ **S32.415** Nondisplaced fracture of anterior wall of left acetabulum HCC ESR COM Q

¹ √7ᵗʰ **S32.416** Nondisplaced fracture of anterior wall of unspecified acetabulum HCC ESR COM Q

√6ᵗʰ **S32.42** Fracture of posterior wall of acetabulum

¹ √7ᵗʰ **S32.421** Displaced fracture of posterior wall of right acetabulum HCC ESR COM Q

¹ √7ᵗʰ **S32.422** Displaced fracture of posterior wall of left acetabulum HCC ESR COM Q

¹ √7ᵗʰ **S32.423** Displaced fracture of posterior wall of unspecified acetabulum HCC ESR COM Q

¹ √7ᵗʰ **S32.424** Nondisplaced fracture of posterior wall of right acetabulum HCC ESR COM Q

¹ √7ᵗʰ **S32.425** Nondisplaced fracture of posterior wall of left acetabulum HCC ESR COM Q

¹ √7ᵗʰ **S32.426** Nondisplaced fracture of posterior wall of unspecified acetabulum HCC ESR COM Q

√6ᵗʰ **S32.43** Fracture of anterior column [iliopubic] of acetabulum

¹ √7ᵗʰ **S32.431** Displaced fracture of anterior column [iliopubic] of right acetabulum HCC ESR COM Q

¹ √7ᵗʰ **S32.432** Displaced fracture of anterior column [iliopubic] of left acetabulum HCC ESR COM Q

¹ √7ᵗʰ **S32.433** Displaced fracture of anterior column [iliopubic] of unspecified acetabulum HCC ESR COM Q

¹ √7ᵗʰ **S32.434** Nondisplaced fracture of anterior column [iliopubic] of right acetabulum HCC ESR COM Q

¹ √7ᵗʰ **S32.435** Nondisplaced fracture of anterior column [iliopubic] of left acetabulum HCC ESR COM Q

¹ √7ᵗʰ **S32.436** Nondisplaced fracture of anterior column [iliopubic] of unspecified acetabulum HCC ESR COM Q

√6ᵗʰ **S32.44** Fracture of posterior column [ilioischial] of acetabulum

¹ √7ᵗʰ **S32.441** Displaced fracture of posterior column [ilioischial] of right acetabulum HCC ESR COM Q

¹ √7ᵗʰ **S32.442** Displaced fracture of posterior column [ilioischial] of left acetabulum HCC ESR COM Q

¹ √7ᵗʰ **S32.443** Displaced fracture of posterior column [ilioischial] of unspecified acetabulum HCC ESR COM Q

¹ √7ᵗʰ **S32.444** Nondisplaced fracture of posterior column [ilioischial] of right acetabulum HCC ESR COM Q

¹ √7ᵗʰ **S32.445** Nondisplaced fracture of posterior column [ilioischial] of left acetabulum HCC ESR COM Q

¹ √7ᵗʰ **S32.446** Nondisplaced fracture of posterior column [ilioischial] of unspecified acetabulum HCC ESR COM Q

√6ᵗʰ **S32.45** Transverse fracture of acetabulum

¹ √7ᵗʰ **S32.451** Displaced transverse fracture of right acetabulum HCC ESR COM Q

¹ √7ᵗʰ **S32.452** Displaced transverse fracture of left acetabulum HCC ESR COM Q

¹ √7ᵗʰ **S32.453** Displaced transverse fracture of unspecified acetabulum HCC ESR COM Q

¹ √7ᵗʰ **S32.454** Nondisplaced transverse fracture of right acetabulum HCC ESR COM Q

¹ √7ᵗʰ **S32.455** Nondisplaced transverse fracture of left acetabulum HCC ESR COM Q

¹ √7ᵗʰ **S32.456** Nondisplaced transverse fracture of unspecified acetabulum HCC ESR COM Q

√6ᵗʰ **S32.46** Associated transverse-posterior fracture of acetabulum

¹ √7ᵗʰ **S32.461** Displaced associated transverse-posterior fracture of right acetabulum   HCC ESR COM Q

¹ √7ᵗʰ **S32.462** Displaced associated transverse-posterior fracture of left acetabulum   HCC ESR COM Q

¹ √7ᵗʰ **S32.463** Displaced associated transverse-posterior fracture of unspecified acetabulum   HCC ESR COM Q

¹ √7ᵗʰ **S32.464** Nondisplaced associated transverse-posterior fracture of right acetabulum   HCC ESR COM Q

¹ √7ᵗʰ **S32.465** Nondisplaced associated transverse-posterior fracture of left acetabulum   HCC ESR COM Q

¹ √7ᵗʰ **S32.466** Nondisplaced associated transverse-posterior fracture of unspecified acetabulum   HCC ESR COM Q

√6ᵗʰ **S32.47** Fracture of medial wall of acetabulum

¹ √7ᵗʰ **S32.471** Displaced fracture of medial wall of right acetabulum   HCC ESR COM Q

¹ √7ᵗʰ **S32.472** Displaced fracture of medial wall of left acetabulum   HCC ESR COM Q

¹ √7ᵗʰ **S32.473** Displaced fracture of medial wall of unspecified acetabulum   HCC ESR COM Q

¹ √7ᵗʰ **S32.474** Nondisplaced fracture of medial wall of right acetabulum   HCC ESR COM Q

¹ √7ᵗʰ **S32.475** Nondisplaced fracture of medial wall of left acetabulum   HCC ESR COM Q

¹ √7ᵗʰ **S32.476** Nondisplaced fracture of medial wall of unspecified acetabulum   HCC ESR COM Q

√6ᵗʰ **S32.48** Dome fracture of acetabulum

¹ √7ᵗʰ **S32.481** Displaced dome fracture of right acetabulum   HCC ESR COM Q

¹ √7ᵗʰ **S32.482** Displaced dome fracture of left acetabulum   HCC ESR COM Q

¹ √7ᵗʰ **S32.483** Displaced dome fracture of unspecified acetabulum   HCC ESR COM Q

¹ √7ᵗʰ **S32.484** Nondisplaced dome fracture of right acetabulum   HCC ESR COM Q

¹ √7ᵗʰ **S32.485** Nondisplaced dome fracture of left acetabulum   HCC ESR COM Q

¹ √7ᵗʰ **S32.486** Nondisplaced dome fracture of unspecified acetabulum   HCC ESR COM Q

√6ᵗʰ **S32.49** Other specified fracture of acetabulum

¹ √7ᵗʰ **S32.491** Other specified fracture of right acetabulum   HCC ESR COM Q

¹ √7ᵗʰ **S32.492** Other specified fracture of left acetabulum   HCC ESR COM Q

¹ √7ᵗʰ **S32.499** Other specified fracture of unspecified acetabulum   HCC ESR COM Q

√5ᵗʰ **S32.5** Fracture of pubis

EXCLUDES 1   *fracture of pubis with associated disruption of pelvic ring (S32.8-)*

√6ᵗʰ **S32.50** Unspecified fracture of pubis

¹ √7ᵗʰ **S32.501** Unspecified fracture of right pubis   HCC ESR COM Q

¹ √7ᵗʰ **S32.502** Unspecified fracture of left pubis   HCC ESR COM Q

¹ √7ᵗʰ **S32.509** Unspecified fracture of unspecified pubis   HCC ESR COM Q

√6ᵗʰ **S32.51** Fracture of superior rim of pubis

¹ √7ᵗʰ **S32.511** Fracture of superior rim of right pubis   HCC ESR COM Q

¹ √7ᵗʰ **S32.512** Fracture of superior rim of left pubis   HCC ESR COM Q

¹ √7ᵗʰ **S32.519** Fracture of superior rim of unspecified pubis   HCC ESR COM Q

√6ᵗʰ **S32.59** Other specified fracture of pubis

¹ √7ᵗʰ **S32.591** Other specified fracture of right pubis   HCC ESR COM Q

¹ √7ᵗʰ **S32.592** Other specified fracture of left pubis   HCC ESR COM Q

¹ √7ᵗʰ **S32.599** Other specified fracture of unspecified pubis   HCC ESR COM Q

√5ᵗʰ **S32.6** Fracture of ischium

EXCLUDES 1   *fracture of ischium with associated disruption of pelvic ring (S32.8-)*

√6ᵗʰ **S32.60** Unspecified fracture of ischium

¹ √7ᵗʰ **S32.601** Unspecified fracture of right ischium   HCC ESR COM Q

¹ √7ᵗʰ **S32.602** Unspecified fracture of left ischium   HCC ESR COM Q

¹ √7ᵗʰ **S32.609** Unspecified fracture of unspecified ischium   HCC ESR COM Q

√6ᵗʰ **S32.61** Avulsion fracture of ischium

¹ √7ᵗʰ **S32.611** Displaced avulsion fracture of right ischium   HCC ESR COM Q

¹ √7ᵗʰ **S32.612** Displaced avulsion fracture of left ischium   HCC ESR COM Q

¹ √7ᵗʰ **S32.613** Displaced avulsion fracture of unspecified ischium   HCC ESR COM Q

¹ √7ᵗʰ **S32.614** Nondisplaced avulsion fracture of right ischium   HCC ESR COM Q

¹ √7ᵗʰ **S32.615** Nondisplaced avulsion fracture of left ischium   HCC ESR COM Q

¹ √7ᵗʰ **S32.616** Nondisplaced avulsion fracture of unspecified ischium   HCC ESR COM Q

√6ᵗʰ **S32.69** Other specified fracture of ischium

¹ √7ᵗʰ **S32.691** Other specified fracture of right ischium   HCC ESR COM Q

¹ √7ᵗʰ **S32.692** Other specified fracture of left ischium   HCC ESR COM Q

¹ √7ᵗʰ **S32.699** Other specified fracture of unspecified ischium   HCC ESR COM Q

√5ᵗʰ **S32.8** Fracture of other parts of pelvis

Code also any associated:
    fracture of acetabulum (S32.4-)
    sacral fracture (S32.1-)

Fractures Disrupting Pelvic Circle

Pelvic circle — Stable

Unstable (two-place fracture)

Pelvic Bones

Iliac crest; Anterior superior iliac spine; Ischial spine; Acetabulum; Femur; Ilium; L5; Sacrum; Coccyx; Pubis; Ischium; Pubic symphysis

√6ᵗʰ **S32.81** Multiple fractures of pelvis with disruption of pelvic ring

Multiple pelvic fractures with disruption of pelvic circle

¹ √7ᵗʰ **S32.810** Multiple fractures of pelvis with stable disruption of pelvic ring   HCC ESR COM Q

¹ √7ᵗʰ **S32.811** Multiple fractures of pelvis with unstable disruption of pelvic ring   HCC ESR COM Q

¹ √x7ᵗʰ **S32.82** Multiple fractures of pelvis without disruption of pelvic ring   HCC ESR COM Q

Multiple pelvic fractures without disruption of pelvic circle

¹ √x7ᵗʰ **S32.89** Fracture of other parts of pelvis   HCC ESR COM Q

¹ √x7ᵗʰ **S32.9** Fracture of unspecified parts of lumbosacral spine and pelvis   HCC ESR COM Q

Fracture of lumbosacral spine NOS
Fracture of pelvis NOS
AHA: 2012,4Q,93

☑4ᵗʰ **S33 Dislocation and sprain of joints and ligaments of lumbar spine and pelvis**

INCLUDES   avulsion of joint or ligament of lumbar spine and pelvis

laceration of cartilage, joint or ligament of lumbar spine and pelvis

sprain of cartilage, joint or ligament of lumbar spine and pelvis

traumatic hemarthrosis of joint or ligament of lumbar spine and pelvis

traumatic rupture of joint or ligament of lumbar spine and pelvis

traumatic subluxation of joint or ligament of lumbar spine and pelvis

traumatic tear of joint or ligament of lumbar spine and pelvis

Code also any associated open wound

EXCLUDES 1   nontraumatic rupture or displacement of lumbar intervertebral disc NOS (M51.-)

obstetric damage to pelvic joints and ligaments (O71.6)

EXCLUDES 2   dislocation and sprain of joints and ligaments of hip (S73.-)

strain of muscle of lower back and pelvis (S39.01-)

The appropriate 7th character is to be added to each code from category S33.
A   initial encounter
D   subsequent encounter
S   sequela

☑x7ᵗʰ **S33.0 Traumatic rupture of lumbar intervertebral disc**

EXCLUDES 1   rupture or displacement (nontraumatic) of lumbar intervertebral disc NOS (M51.- with fifth character 6)

☑5ᵗʰ **S33.1 Subluxation and dislocation of** lumbar vertebra

Code also any associated:
open wound of abdomen, lower back and pelvis (S31)
spinal cord injury (S24.0, S24.1-, S34.0-, S34.1-)

EXCLUDES 2   fracture of lumbar vertebrae (S32.0-)

☑6ᵗʰ **S33.10 Subluxation and dislocation of unspecified lumbar vertebra**

☑7ᵗʰ **S33.100** Subluxation of unspecified lumbar vertebra

☑7ᵗʰ **S33.101** Dislocation of unspecified lumbar vertebra

☑6ᵗʰ **S33.11 Subluxation and dislocation of** L1/L2 **lumbar vertebra**

☑7ᵗʰ **S33.110** Subluxation of L1/L2 lumbar vertebra

☑7ᵗʰ **S33.111** Dislocation of L1/L2 lumbar vertebra

☑6ᵗʰ **S33.12 Subluxation and dislocation of** L2/L3 **lumbar vertebra**

☑7ᵗʰ **S33.120** Subluxation of L2/L3 lumbar vertebra

☑7ᵗʰ **S33.121** Dislocation of L2/L3 lumbar vertebra

☑6ᵗʰ **S33.13 Subluxation and dislocation of** L3/L4 **lumbar vertebra**

☑7ᵗʰ **S33.130** Subluxation of L3/L4 lumbar vertebra

☑7ᵗʰ **S33.131** Dislocation of L3/L4 lumbar vertebra

☑6ᵗʰ **S33.14 Subluxation and dislocation of** L4/L5 **lumbar vertebra**

☑7ᵗʰ **S33.140** Subluxation of L4/L5 lumbar vertebra

☑7ᵗʰ **S33.141** Dislocation of L4/L5 lumbar vertebra

☑x7ᵗʰ **S33.2 Dislocation of** sacroiliac and sacrococcygeal **joint**

☑5ᵗʰ **S33.3 Dislocation of other and unspecified parts of lumbar spine and pelvis**

☑x7ᵗʰ **S33.30** Dislocation of unspecified parts of lumbar spine and pelvis

☑x7ᵗʰ **S33.39** Dislocation of other parts of lumbar spine and pelvis

☑x7ᵗʰ **S33.4 Traumatic rupture of** symphysis pubis

☑x7ᵗʰ **S33.5 Sprain of ligaments of** lumbar spine

☑x7ᵗʰ **S33.6 Sprain of** sacroiliac joint

☑x7ᵗʰ **S33.8 Sprain of other parts of lumbar spine and pelvis**

☑x7ᵗʰ **S33.9 Sprain of unspecified parts of lumbar spine and pelvis**

☑4ᵗʰ **S34 Injury of lumbar and sacral spinal cord and nerves at abdomen, lower back and pelvis level**

NOTE   Code to highest level of lumbar cord injury.

Injuries to the spinal cord (S34.0 and S34.1) refer to the cord level and not bone level injury, and can affect nerve roots at and below the level given.

Code also any associated:
fracture of vertebra (S22.0-, S32.0-)
open wound of abdomen, lower back and pelvis (S31.-)
transient paralysis (R29.5)

The appropriate 7th character is to be added to each code from category S34.
A   initial encounter
D   subsequent encounter
S   sequela

☑5ᵗʰ **S34.0 Concussion and edema** of lumbar and sacral spinal cord

☑x7ᵗʰ **S34.01 Concussion and edema of** lumbar **spinal cord** HCC ESR COM

☑x7ᵗʰ **S34.02 Concussion and edema of** sacral **spinal cord** HCC ESR COM

Concussion and edema of conus medullaris

☑5ᵗʰ **S34.1 Other and unspecified injury of lumbar and sacral spinal cord**

☑6ᵗʰ **S34.10 Unspecified injury to lumbar spinal cord**

☑7ᵗʰ **S34.101 Unspecified injury to** L1 level **of lumbar spinal cord** HCC ESR COM

Unspecified injury to lumbar spinal cord level 1

☑7ᵗʰ **S34.102 Unspecified injury to** L2 level **of lumbar spinal cord** HCC ESR COM

Unspecified injury to lumbar spinal cord level 2

☑7ᵗʰ **S34.103 Unspecified injury to** L3 level **of lumbar spinal cord** HCC ESR COM

Unspecified injury to lumbar spinal cord level 3

☑7ᵗʰ **S34.104 Unspecified injury to** L4 level **of lumbar spinal cord** HCC ESR COM

Unspecified injury to lumbar spinal cord level 4

☑7ᵗʰ **S34.105 Unspecified injury to** L5 level **of lumbar spinal cord** HCC ESR COM

Unspecified injury to lumbar spinal cord level 5

☑7ᵗʰ **S34.109 Unspecified injury to unspecified level of lumbar spinal cord** HCC ESR COM

☑6ᵗʰ **S34.11 Complete lesion** of lumbar spinal cord

☑7ᵗʰ **S34.111 Complete lesion of** L1 level **of lumbar spinal cord** HCC ESR COM

Complete lesion of lumbar spinal cord level 1

☑7ᵗʰ **S34.112 Complete lesion of** L2 level **of lumbar spinal cord** HCC ESR COM

Complete lesion of lumbar spinal cord level 2

☑7ᵗʰ **S34.113 Complete lesion of** L3 level **of lumbar spinal cord** HCC ESR COM

Complete lesion of lumbar spinal cord level 3

☑7ᵗʰ **S34.114 Complete lesion of** L4 level **of lumbar spinal cord** HCC ESR COM

Complete lesion of lumbar spinal cord level 4

☑7ᵗʰ **S34.115 Complete lesion of** L5 level **of lumbar spinal cord** HCC ESR COM

Complete lesion of lumbar spinal cord level 5

☑7ᵗʰ **S34.119 Complete lesion of unspecified level of lumbar spinal cord** HCC ESR COM

☑6ᵗʰ **S34.12 Incomplete lesion** of lumbar spinal cord

☑7ᵗʰ **S34.121 Incomplete lesion of** L1 level **of lumbar spinal cord** HCC ESR COM

Incomplete lesion of lumbar spinal cord level 1

√7ᵗʰ **S34.122 Incomplete lesion of** L2 level **of lumbar spinal cord** HCC ESR COM
     Incomplete lesion of lumbar spinal cord level 2

√7ᵗʰ **S34.123 Incomplete lesion of** L3 level **of lumbar spinal cord** HCC ESR COM
     Incomplete lesion of lumbar spinal cord level 3

√7ᵗʰ **S34.124 Incomplete lesion of** L4 level **of lumbar spinal cord** HCC ESR COM
     Incomplete lesion of lumbar spinal cord level 4

√7ᵗʰ **S34.125 Incomplete lesion of** L5 level **of lumbar spinal cord** HCC ESR COM
     Incomplete lesion of lumbar spinal cord level 5

√7ᵗʰ **S34.129 Incomplete lesion of unspecified level of lumbar spinal cord** HCC ESR COM

√6ᵗʰ **S34.13 Other and unspecified injury to sacral spinal cord**
     Other injury to conus medullaris

√7ᵗʰ **S34.131 Complete lesion of sacral spinal cord** HCC ESR COM
     Complete lesion of conus medullaris

√7ᵗʰ **S34.132 Incomplete lesion of sacral spinal cord** HCC ESR COM
     Incomplete lesion of conus medullaris

√7ᵗʰ **S34.139 Unspecified injury to sacral spinal cord** HCC ESR COM
     Unspecified injury of conus medullaris

√5ᵗʰ **S34.2 Injury of nerve root of lumbar and sacral spine**

√x 7ᵗʰ **S34.21 Injury of nerve root of** lumbar spine

√x 7ᵗʰ **S34.22 Injury of nerve root of** sacral spine

¹ √x 7ᵗʰ **S34.3 Injury of cauda equina** HCC ESR COM

√x 7ᵗʰ **S34.4 Injury of lumbosacral plexus**

√x 7ᵗʰ **S34.5 Injury of lumbar, sacral and pelvic sympathetic nerves**
     Injury of celiac ganglion or plexus
     Injury of hypogastric plexus
     Injury of mesenteric plexus (inferior) (superior)
     Injury of splanchnic nerve

√x 7ᵗʰ **S34.6 Injury of peripheral nerve(s) at abdomen, lower back and pelvis level**

√x 7ᵗʰ **S34.8 Injury of other nerves at abdomen, lower back and pelvis level**

√x 7ᵗʰ **S34.9 Injury of unspecified nerves at abdomen, lower back and pelvis level**

√4ᵗʰ **S35 Injury of blood vessels at abdomen, lower back and pelvis level**
Code also any associated open wound (S31.-)

> The appropriate 7th character is to be added to each code from category S35.
> A   initial encounter
> D   subsequent encounter
> S   sequela

√5ᵗʰ **S35.0 Injury of** abdominal aorta
     EXCLUDES 1   injury of aorta NOS (S25.0)

√x 7ᵗʰ **S35.00 Unspecified injury of abdominal aorta**

√x 7ᵗʰ **S35.01 Minor laceration of abdominal aorta**
     Incomplete transection of abdominal aorta
     Laceration of abdominal aorta NOS
     Superficial laceration of abdominal aorta

√x 7ᵗʰ **S35.02 Major laceration of abdominal aorta**
     Complete transection of abdominal aorta
     Traumatic rupture of abdominal aorta

√x 7ᵗʰ **S35.09 Other injury of abdominal aorta**

√5ᵗʰ **S35.1 Injury of** inferior vena cava
     Injury of hepatic vein
     EXCLUDES 1   injury of vena cava NOS (S25.2)

√x 7ᵗʰ **S35.10 Unspecified injury of inferior vena cava**

√x 7ᵗʰ **S35.11 Minor laceration of inferior vena cava**
     Incomplete transection of inferior vena cava
     Laceration of inferior vena cava NOS
     Superficial laceration of inferior vena cava

√x 7ᵗʰ **S35.12 Major laceration of inferior vena cava**
     Complete transection of inferior vena cava
     Traumatic rupture of inferior vena cava

√x 7ᵗʰ **S35.19 Other injury of inferior vena cava**

√5ᵗʰ **S35.2 Injury of celiac or mesenteric artery and branches**

√6ᵗʰ **S35.21 Injury of** celiac artery

√7ᵗʰ **S35.211 Minor laceration of celiac artery**
     Incomplete transection of celiac artery
     Laceration of celiac artery NOS
     Superficial laceration of celiac artery

√7ᵗʰ **S35.212 Major laceration of celiac artery**
     Complete transection of celiac artery
     Traumatic rupture of celiac artery

√7ᵗʰ **S35.218 Other injury of celiac artery**

√7ᵗʰ **S35.219 Unspecified injury of celiac artery**

√6ᵗʰ **S35.22 Injury of** superior mesenteric artery

√7ᵗʰ **S35.221 Minor laceration of superior mesenteric artery**
     Incomplete transection of superior mesenteric artery
     Laceration of superior mesenteric artery NOS
     Superficial laceration of superior mesenteric artery

√7ᵗʰ **S35.222 Major laceration of superior mesenteric artery**
     Complete transection of superior mesenteric artery
     Traumatic rupture of superior mesenteric artery

√7ᵗʰ **S35.228 Other injury of superior mesenteric artery**

√7ᵗʰ **S35.229 Unspecified injury of superior mesenteric artery**

√6ᵗʰ **S35.23 Injury of** inferior mesenteric artery

√7ᵗʰ **S35.231 Minor laceration of inferior mesenteric artery**
     Incomplete transection of inferior mesenteric artery
     Laceration of inferior mesenteric artery NOS
     Superficial laceration of inferior mesenteric artery

√7ᵗʰ **S35.232 Major laceration of inferior mesenteric artery**
     Complete transection of inferior mesenteric artery
     Traumatic rupture of inferior mesenteric artery

√7ᵗʰ **S35.238 Other injury of inferior mesenteric artery**

√7ᵗʰ **S35.239 Unspecified injury of inferior mesenteric artery**

√6ᵗʰ **S35.29 Injury of** branches of celiac and mesenteric artery
     Injury of gastric artery
     Injury of gastroduodenal artery
     Injury of hepatic artery
     Injury of splenic artery

√7ᵗʰ **S35.291 Minor laceration of branches of celiac and mesenteric artery**
     Incomplete transection of branches of celiac and mesenteric artery
     Laceration of branches of celiac and mesenteric artery NOS
     Superficial laceration of branches of celiac and mesenteric artery

√7ᵗʰ **S35.292 Major laceration of branches of celiac and mesenteric artery**
     Complete transection of branches of celiac and mesenteric artery
     Traumatic rupture of branches of celiac and mesenteric artery

√7ᵗʰ **S35.298 Other injury of branches of celiac and mesenteric artery**

√7ᵗʰ **S35.299 Unspecified injury of branches of celiac and mesenteric artery**

√5ᵗʰ **S35.3 Injury of portal or splenic vein and branches**

  √6ᵗʰ **S35.31 Injury of portal vein**

    √7ᵗʰ **S35.311 Laceration of portal vein**

    √7ᵗʰ **S35.318 Other specified injury of portal vein**

    √7ᵗʰ **S35.319 Unspecified injury of portal vein**

  √6ᵗʰ **S35.32 Injury of splenic vein**

    √7ᵗʰ **S35.321 Laceration of splenic vein**

    √7ᵗʰ **S35.328 Other specified injury of splenic vein**

    √7ᵗʰ **S35.329 Unspecified injury of splenic vein**

  √6ᵗʰ **S35.33 Injury of superior mesenteric vein**

    √7ᵗʰ **S35.331 Laceration of superior mesenteric vein**

    √7ᵗʰ **S35.338 Other specified injury of superior mesenteric vein**

    √7ᵗʰ **S35.339 Unspecified injury of superior mesenteric vein**

  √6ᵗʰ **S35.34 Injury of inferior mesenteric vein**

    √7ᵗʰ **S35.341 Laceration of inferior mesenteric vein**

    √7ᵗʰ **S35.348 Other specified injury of inferior mesenteric vein**

    √7ᵗʰ **S35.349 Unspecified injury of inferior mesenteric vein**

√5ᵗʰ **S35.4 Injury of renal blood vessels**

  √6ᵗʰ **S35.40 Unspecified injury of renal blood vessel**

    √7ᵗʰ **S35.401 Unspecified injury of right renal artery**

    √7ᵗʰ **S35.402 Unspecified injury of left renal artery**

    √7ᵗʰ **S35.403 Unspecified injury of unspecified renal artery**

    √7ᵗʰ **S35.404 Unspecified injury of right renal vein**

    √7ᵗʰ **S35.405 Unspecified injury of left renal vein**

    √7ᵗʰ **S35.406 Unspecified injury of unspecified renal vein**

  √6ᵗʰ **S35.41 Laceration of renal blood vessel**

    √7ᵗʰ **S35.411 Laceration of right renal artery**

    √7ᵗʰ **S35.412 Laceration of left renal artery**

    √7ᵗʰ **S35.413 Laceration of unspecified renal artery**

    √7ᵗʰ **S35.414 Laceration of right renal vein**

    √7ᵗʰ **S35.415 Laceration of left renal vein**

    √7ᵗʰ **S35.416 Laceration of unspecified renal vein**

  √6ᵗʰ **S35.49 Other specified injury of renal blood vessel**

    √7ᵗʰ **S35.491 Other specified injury of right renal artery**

    √7ᵗʰ **S35.492 Other specified injury of left renal artery**

    √7ᵗʰ **S35.493 Other specified injury of unspecified renal artery**

    √7ᵗʰ **S35.494 Other specified injury of right renal vein**

    √7ᵗʰ **S35.495 Other specified injury of left renal vein**

    √7ᵗʰ **S35.496 Other specified injury of unspecified renal vein**

√5ᵗʰ **S35.5 Injury of iliac blood vessels**

  √x7ᵗʰ **S35.50 Injury of unspecified iliac blood vessel(s)**

  √6ᵗʰ **S35.51 Injury of iliac artery or vein**

    Injury of hypogastric artery or vein

    √7ᵗʰ **S35.511 Injury of right iliac artery**

    √7ᵗʰ **S35.512 Injury of left iliac artery**

    √7ᵗʰ **S35.513 Injury of unspecified iliac artery**

    √7ᵗʰ **S35.514 Injury of right iliac vein**

    √7ᵗʰ **S35.515 Injury of left iliac vein**

    √7ᵗʰ **S35.516 Injury of unspecified iliac vein**

  √6ᵗʰ **S35.53 Injury of uterine artery or vein**

    √7ᵗʰ **S35.531 Injury of right uterine artery** ♀

    √7ᵗʰ **S35.532 Injury of left uterine artery** ♀

    √7ᵗʰ **S35.533 Injury of unspecified uterine artery** ♀

    √7ᵗʰ **S35.534 Injury of right uterine vein** ♀

    √7ᵗʰ **S35.535 Injury of left uterine vein** ♀

    √7ᵗʰ **S35.536 Injury of unspecified uterine vein** ♀

  √x7ᵗʰ **S35.59 Injury of other iliac blood vessels**

√5ᵗʰ **S35.8 Injury of other blood vessels at abdomen, lower back and pelvis level**

  Injury of ovarian artery or vein

  √6ᵗʰ **S35.8X Injury of other blood vessels at abdomen, lower back and pelvis level**

    √7ᵗʰ **S35.8X1 Laceration of other blood vessels at abdomen, lower back and pelvis level**

    √7ᵗʰ **S35.8X8 Other specified injury of other blood vessels at abdomen, lower back and pelvis level**

    √7ᵗʰ **S35.8X9 Unspecified injury of other blood vessels at abdomen, lower back and pelvis level**

√5ᵗʰ **S35.9 Injury of unspecified blood vessel at abdomen, lower back and pelvis level**

  √x7ᵗʰ **S35.90 Unspecified injury of unspecified blood vessel at abdomen, lower back and pelvis level**

  √x7ᵗʰ **S35.91 Laceration of unspecified blood vessel at abdomen, lower back and pelvis level**

  √x7ᵗʰ **S35.99 Other specified injury of unspecified blood vessel at abdomen, lower back and pelvis level**

√4ᵗʰ **S36 Injury of intra-abdominal organs**

  Code also any associated open wound (S31.-)

  The appropriate 7th character is to be added to each code from category S36.
  A   initial encounter
  D   subsequent encounter
  S   sequela

√5ᵗʰ **S36.0 Injury of spleen**

  AHA: 2015,2Q,36; 2015,1Q,10

  √x7ᵗʰ **S36.00 Unspecified injury of spleen**

  √6ᵗʰ **S36.02 Contusion of spleen**

    √7ᵗʰ **S36.020 Minor contusion of spleen**

      Contusion of spleen less than 2 cm

    √7ᵗʰ **S36.021 Major contusion of spleen**

      Contusion of spleen greater than 2 cm

    √7ᵗʰ **S36.029 Unspecified contusion of spleen**

  √6ᵗʰ **S36.03 Laceration of spleen**

    √7ᵗʰ **S36.030 Superficial (capsular) laceration of spleen**

      Laceration of spleen less than 1 cm
      Minor laceration of spleen

    √7ᵗʰ **S36.031 Moderate laceration of spleen**

      Laceration of spleen 1 to 3 cm

    √7ᵗʰ **S36.032 Major laceration of spleen**

      Avulsion of spleen
      Laceration of spleen greater than 3 cm
      Massive laceration of spleen
      Multiple moderate lacerations of spleen
      Stellate laceration of spleen

    √7ᵗʰ **S36.039 Unspecified laceration of spleen**

  √x7ᵗʰ **S36.09 Other injury of spleen**

√5ᵗʰ **S36.1 Injury of liver and gallbladder and bile duct**

  √6ᵗʰ **S36.11 Injury of liver**

    √7ᵗʰ **S36.112 Contusion of liver**

    √7ᵗʰ **S36.113 Laceration of liver, unspecified degree**

    √7ᵗʰ **S36.114 Minor laceration of liver**

      Laceration involving capsule only, or, without significant involvement of hepatic parenchyma [i.e., less than 1 cm deep]

    √7ᵗʰ **S36.115 Moderate laceration of liver**

      Laceration involving parenchyma but without major disruption of parenchyma [i.e., less than 10 cm long and less than 3 cm deep]

    √7ᵗʰ **S36.116 Major laceration of liver**

      Laceration with significant disruption of hepatic parenchyma [i.e., greater than 10 cm long and 3 cm deep]
      Multiple moderate lacerations, with or without hematoma
      Stellate laceration of liver

    √7ᵗʰ **S36.118 Other injury of liver**

    √7ᵗʰ **S36.119 Unspecified injury of liver**

Chapter 19. Injury, Poisoning and Certain Other Consequences of External Causes

S36.12–S36.69

√6ᵗʰ **S36.12**   Injury of gallbladder
- √7ᵗʰ **S36.122**   Contusion of gallbladder
- √7ᵗʰ **S36.123**   Laceration of gallbladder
- √7ᵗʰ **S36.128**   Other injury of gallbladder
- √7ᵗʰ **S36.129**   Unspecified injury of gallbladder

√x7ᵗʰ **S36.13**   Injury of bile duct

√5ᵗʰ **S36.2**   Injury of pancreas

√6ᵗʰ **S36.20**   Unspecified injury of pancreas
- √7ᵗʰ **S36.200**   Unspecified injury of head of pancreas
- √7ᵗʰ **S36.201**   Unspecified injury of body of pancreas
- √7ᵗʰ **S36.202**   Unspecified injury of tail of pancreas
- √7ᵗʰ **S36.209**   Unspecified injury of unspecified part of pancreas

√6ᵗʰ **S36.22**   Contusion of pancreas
- √7ᵗʰ **S36.220**   Contusion of head of pancreas
- √7ᵗʰ **S36.221**   Contusion of body of pancreas
- √7ᵗʰ **S36.222**   Contusion of tail of pancreas
- √7ᵗʰ **S36.229**   Contusion of unspecified part of pancreas

√6ᵗʰ **S36.23**   Laceration of pancreas, unspecified degree
- √7ᵗʰ **S36.230**   Laceration of head of pancreas, unspecified degree
- √7ᵗʰ **S36.231**   Laceration of body of pancreas, unspecified degree
- √7ᵗʰ **S36.232**   Laceration of tail of pancreas, unspecified degree
- √7ᵗʰ **S36.239**   Laceration of unspecified part of pancreas, unspecified degree

√6ᵗʰ **S36.24**   Minor laceration of pancreas
- √7ᵗʰ **S36.240**   Minor laceration of head of pancreas
- √7ᵗʰ **S36.241**   Minor laceration of body of pancreas
- √7ᵗʰ **S36.242**   Minor laceration of tail of pancreas
- √7ᵗʰ **S36.249**   Minor laceration of unspecified part of pancreas

√6ᵗʰ **S36.25**   Moderate laceration of pancreas
- √7ᵗʰ **S36.250**   Moderate laceration of head of pancreas
- √7ᵗʰ **S36.251**   Moderate laceration of body of pancreas
- √7ᵗʰ **S36.252**   Moderate laceration of tail of pancreas
- √7ᵗʰ **S36.259**   Moderate laceration of unspecified part of pancreas

√6ᵗʰ **S36.26**   Major laceration of pancreas
- √7ᵗʰ **S36.260**   Major laceration of head of pancreas
- √7ᵗʰ **S36.261**   Major laceration of body of pancreas
- √7ᵗʰ **S36.262**   Major laceration of tail of pancreas
- √7ᵗʰ **S36.269**   Major laceration of unspecified part of pancreas

√6ᵗʰ **S36.29**   Other injury of pancreas
- √7ᵗʰ **S36.290**   Other injury of head of pancreas
- √7ᵗʰ **S36.291**   Other injury of body of pancreas
- √7ᵗʰ **S36.292**   Other injury of tail of pancreas
- √7ᵗʰ **S36.299**   Other injury of unspecified part of pancreas

√5ᵗʰ **S36.3**   Injury of stomach

√x7ᵗʰ **S36.30**   Unspecified injury of stomach

√x7ᵗʰ **S36.32**   Contusion of stomach

√x7ᵗʰ **S36.33**   Laceration of stomach

√x7ᵗʰ **S36.39**   Other injury of stomach

√5ᵗʰ **S36.4**   Injury of small intestine

√6ᵗʰ **S36.40**   Unspecified injury of small intestine
- √7ᵗʰ **S36.400**   Unspecified injury of duodenum
- √7ᵗʰ **S36.408**   Unspecified injury of other part of small intestine
- √7ᵗʰ **S36.409**   Unspecified injury of unspecified part of small intestine

√6ᵗʰ **S36.41**   Primary blast injury of small intestine
    Blast injury of small intestine NOS
- √7ᵗʰ **S36.410**   Primary blast injury of duodenum
- √7ᵗʰ **S36.418**   Primary blast injury of other part of small intestine
- √7ᵗʰ **S36.419**   Primary blast injury of unspecified part of small intestine

√6ᵗʰ **S36.42**   Contusion of small intestine
- √7ᵗʰ **S36.420**   Contusion of duodenum
- √7ᵗʰ **S36.428**   Contusion of other part of small intestine
- √7ᵗʰ **S36.429**   Contusion of unspecified part of small intestine

√6ᵗʰ **S36.43**   Laceration of small intestine
- √7ᵗʰ **S36.430**   Laceration of duodenum
- √7ᵗʰ **S36.438**   Laceration of other part of small intestine
- √7ᵗʰ **S36.439**   Laceration of unspecified part of small intestine

√6ᵗʰ **S36.49**   Other injury of small intestine
- √7ᵗʰ **S36.490**   Other injury of duodenum
- √7ᵗʰ **S36.498**   Other injury of other part of small intestine
- √7ᵗʰ **S36.499**   Other injury of unspecified part of small intestine

√5ᵗʰ **S36.5**   Injury of colon
    EXCLUDES 2   injury of rectum (S36.6-)

√6ᵗʰ **S36.50**   Unspecified injury of colon
- √7ᵗʰ **S36.500**   Unspecified injury of ascending [right] colon
- √7ᵗʰ **S36.501**   Unspecified injury of transverse colon
- √7ᵗʰ **S36.502**   Unspecified injury of descending [left] colon
- √7ᵗʰ **S36.503**   Unspecified injury of sigmoid colon
- √7ᵗʰ **S36.508**   Unspecified injury of other part of colon
- √7ᵗʰ **S36.509**   Unspecified injury of unspecified part of colon

√6ᵗʰ **S36.51**   Primary blast injury of colon
    Blast injury of colon NOS
- √7ᵗʰ **S36.510**   Primary blast injury of ascending [right] colon
- √7ᵗʰ **S36.511**   Primary blast injury of transverse colon
- √7ᵗʰ **S36.512**   Primary blast injury of descending [left] colon
- √7ᵗʰ **S36.513**   Primary blast injury of sigmoid colon
- √7ᵗʰ **S36.518**   Primary blast injury of other part of colon
- √7ᵗʰ **S36.519**   Primary blast injury of unspecified part of colon

√6ᵗʰ **S36.52**   Contusion of colon
- √7ᵗʰ **S36.520**   Contusion of ascending [right] colon
- √7ᵗʰ **S36.521**   Contusion of transverse colon
- √7ᵗʰ **S36.522**   Contusion of descending [left] colon
- √7ᵗʰ **S36.523**   Contusion of sigmoid colon
- √7ᵗʰ **S36.528**   Contusion of other part of colon
- √7ᵗʰ **S36.529**   Contusion of unspecified part of colon

√6ᵗʰ **S36.53**   Laceration of colon
- √7ᵗʰ **S36.530**   Laceration of ascending [right] colon
- √7ᵗʰ **S36.531**   Laceration of transverse colon
- √7ᵗʰ **S36.532**   Laceration of descending [left] colon
- √7ᵗʰ **S36.533**   Laceration of sigmoid colon
- √7ᵗʰ **S36.538**   Laceration of other part of colon
- √7ᵗʰ **S36.539**   Laceration of unspecified part of colon

√6ᵗʰ **S36.59**   Other injury of colon
    Secondary blast injury of colon
- √7ᵗʰ **S36.590**   Other injury of ascending [right] colon
- √7ᵗʰ **S36.591**   Other injury of transverse colon
- √7ᵗʰ **S36.592**   Other injury of descending [left] colon
- √7ᵗʰ **S36.593**   Other injury of sigmoid colon
- √7ᵗʰ **S36.598**   Other injury of other part of colon
- √7ᵗʰ **S36.599**   Other injury of unspecified part of colon

√5ᵗʰ **S36.6**   Injury of rectum

√x7ᵗʰ **S36.60**   Unspecified injury of rectum

√x7ᵗʰ **S36.61**   Primary blast injury of rectum
    Blast injury of rectum NOS

√x7ᵗʰ **S36.62**   Contusion of rectum

√x7ᵗʰ **S36.63**   Laceration of rectum

√x7ᵗʰ **S36.69**   Other injury of rectum
    Secondary blast injury of rectum

HCC CMS-HCC   **Rx** Rx HCC   **ESR** ESRD HCC   **COM** Commercial HCC   **N** Newborn: 0   **P** Pediatric: 0-17   **M** Maternity: 9-64   **A** Adult: 15-124

1030   ICD-10-CM 2023

✓5ᵗʰ **S36.8** Injury of other intra-abdominal organs

   ✓x7ᵗʰ **S36.81** Injury of peritoneum

   ✓6ᵗʰ **S36.89** Injury of other intra-abdominal organs

       Injury of retroperitoneum

      ✓7ᵗʰ **S36.892** Contusion of other intra-abdominal organs

      ✓7ᵗʰ **S36.893** Laceration of other intra-abdominal organs

      ✓7ᵗʰ **S36.898** Other injury of other intra-abdominal organs

      ✓7ᵗʰ **S36.899** Unspecified injury of other intra-abdominal organs

✓5ᵗʰ **S36.9** Injury of unspecified intra-abdominal organ

   ✓7ᵗʰ **S36.90** Unspecified injury of unspecified intra-abdominal organ

   ✓x7ᵗʰ **S36.92** Contusion of unspecified intra-abdominal organ

   ✓x7ᵗʰ **S36.93** Laceration of unspecified intra-abdominal organ

   ✓x7ᵗʰ **S36.99** Other injury of unspecified intra-abdominal organ

✓4ᵗʰ **S37** Injury of urinary and pelvic organs

       Code also any associated open wound (S31.-)

       EXCLUDES 1 obstetric trauma to pelvic organs (O71.-)

       EXCLUDES 2 injury of peritoneum (S36.81)

               injury of retroperitoneum (S36.89-)

       The appropriate 7th character is to be added to each code from category S37.

       A   initial encounter

       D   subsequent encounter

       S   sequela

  ✓5ᵗʰ **S37.0** Injury of kidney

       EXCLUDES 2 acute kidney injury (nontraumatic) (N17.9)

   ✓6ᵗʰ **S37.00** Unspecified injury of kidney

      ✓7ᵗʰ **S37.001** Unspecified injury of right kidney

      ✓7ᵗʰ **S37.002** Unspecified injury of left kidney

      ✓7ᵗʰ **S37.009** Unspecified injury of unspecified kidney

   ✓6ᵗʰ **S37.01** Minor contusion of kidney

       Contusion of kidney less than 2 cm

       Contusion of kidney NOS

      ✓7ᵗʰ **S37.011** Minor contusion of right kidney

      ✓7ᵗʰ **S37.012** Minor contusion of left kidney

      ✓7ᵗʰ **S37.019** Minor contusion of unspecified kidney

   ✓6ᵗʰ **S37.02** Major contusion of kidney

       Contusion of kidney greater than 2 cm

      ✓7ᵗʰ **S37.021** Major contusion of right kidney

      ✓7ᵗʰ **S37.022** Major contusion of left kidney

      ✓7ᵗʰ **S37.029** Major contusion of unspecified kidney

   ✓6ᵗʰ **S37.03** Laceration of kidney, unspecified degree

      ✓7ᵗʰ **S37.031** Laceration of right kidney, unspecified degree

      ✓7ᵗʰ **S37.032** Laceration of left kidney, unspecified degree

      ✓7ᵗʰ **S37.039** Laceration of unspecified kidney, unspecified degree

   ✓6ᵗʰ **S37.04** Minor laceration of kidney

       Laceration of kidney less than 1 cm

      ✓7ᵗʰ **S37.041** Minor laceration of right kidney

      ✓7ᵗʰ **S37.042** Minor laceration of left kidney

      ✓7ᵗʰ **S37.049** Minor laceration of unspecified kidney

   ✓6ᵗʰ **S37.05** Moderate laceration of kidney

       Laceration of kidney 1 to 3 cm

      ✓7ᵗʰ **S37.051** Moderate laceration of right kidney

      ✓7ᵗʰ **S37.052** Moderate laceration of left kidney

      ✓7ᵗʰ **S37.059** Moderate laceration of unspecified kidney

   ✓6ᵗʰ **S37.06** Major laceration of kidney

       Avulsion of kidney

       Laceration of kidney greater than 3 cm

       Massive laceration of kidney

       Multiple moderate lacerations of kidney

       Stellate laceration of kidney

      ✓7ᵗʰ **S37.061** Major laceration of right kidney

      ✓7ᵗʰ **S37.062** Major laceration of left kidney

      ✓7ᵗʰ **S37.069** Major laceration of unspecified kidney

   ✓6ᵗʰ **S37.09** Other injury of kidney

      ✓7ᵗʰ **S37.091** Other injury of right kidney

      ✓7ᵗʰ **S37.092** Other injury of left kidney

      ✓7ᵗʰ **S37.099** Other injury of unspecified kidney

  ✓5ᵗʰ **S37.1** Injury of ureter

   ✓x7ᵗʰ **S37.10** Unspecified injury of ureter

   ✓x7ᵗʰ **S37.12** Contusion of ureter

   ✓x7ᵗʰ **S37.13** Laceration of ureter

   ✓x7ᵗʰ **S37.19** Other injury of ureter

  ✓5ᵗʰ **S37.2** Injury of bladder *(bladder)*

   ✓x7ᵗʰ **S37.20** Unspecified injury of bladder

   ✓x7ᵗʰ **S37.22** Contusion of bladder

   ✓x7ᵗʰ **S37.23** Laceration of bladder

   ✓x7ᵗʰ **S37.29** Other injury of bladder

  ✓5ᵗʰ **S37.3** Injury of urethra

   ✓x7ᵗʰ **S37.30** Unspecified injury of urethra

   ✓x7ᵗʰ **S37.32** Contusion of urethra

   ✓x7ᵗʰ **S37.33** Laceration of urethra

   ✓x7ᵗʰ **S37.39** Other injury of urethra

  ✓5ᵗʰ **S37.4** Injury of ovary

   ✓6ᵗʰ **S37.40** Unspecified injury of ovary

      ✓7ᵗʰ **S37.401** Unspecified injury of ovary, unilateral ♀

      ✓7ᵗʰ **S37.402** Unspecified injury of ovary, bilateral ♀

      ✓7ᵗʰ **S37.409** Unspecified injury of ovary, unspecified ♀

   ✓6ᵗʰ **S37.42** Contusion of ovary

      ✓7ᵗʰ **S37.421** Contusion of ovary, unilateral ♀

      ✓7ᵗʰ **S37.422** Contusion of ovary, bilateral ♀

      ✓7ᵗʰ **S37.429** Contusion of ovary, unspecified ♀

   ✓6ᵗʰ **S37.43** Laceration of ovary

      ✓7ᵗʰ **S37.431** Laceration of ovary, unilateral ♀

      ✓7ᵗʰ **S37.432** Laceration of ovary, bilateral ♀

      ✓7ᵗʰ **S37.439** Laceration of ovary, unspecified ♀

   ✓6ᵗʰ **S37.49** Other injury of ovary

      ✓7ᵗʰ **S37.491** Other injury of ovary, unilateral ♀

      ✓7ᵗʰ **S37.492** Other injury of ovary, bilateral ♀

      ✓7ᵗʰ **S37.499** Other injury of ovary, unspecified ♀

  ✓5ᵗʰ **S37.5** Injury of fallopian tube

   ✓6ᵗʰ **S37.50** Unspecified injury of fallopian tube

      ✓7ᵗʰ **S37.501** Unspecified injury of fallopian tube, unilateral ♀

      ✓7ᵗʰ **S37.502** Unspecified injury of fallopian tube, bilateral ♀

      ✓7ᵗʰ **S37.509** Unspecified injury of fallopian tube, unspecified ♀

   ✓6ᵗʰ **S37.51** Primary blast injury of fallopian tube

       Blast injury of fallopian tube NOS

      ✓7ᵗʰ **S37.511** Primary blast injury of fallopian tube, unilateral ♀

      ✓7ᵗʰ **S37.512** Primary blast injury of fallopian tube, bilateral ♀

      ✓7ᵗʰ **S37.519** Primary blast injury of fallopian tube, unspecified ♀

   ✓6ᵗʰ **S37.52** Contusion of fallopian tube

      ✓7ᵗʰ **S37.521** Contusion of fallopian tube, unilateral ♀

      ✓7ᵗʰ **S37.522** Contusion of fallopian tube, bilateral ♀

      ✓7ᵗʰ **S37.529** Contusion of fallopian tube, unspecified ♀

   ✓6ᵗʰ **S37.53** Laceration of fallopian tube

      ✓7ᵗʰ **S37.531** Laceration of fallopian tube, unilateral ♀

      ✓7ᵗʰ **S37.532** Laceration of fallopian tube, bilateral ♀

      ✓7ᵗʰ **S37.539** Laceration of fallopian tube, unspecified ♀

✅ Additional Character Required   ✓x7ᵗʰ Placeholder Alert   Manifestation   Unspecified Dx   **Q** QPP   **UPD** Unacceptable PDx

Chapter 19. Injury, Poisoning and Certain Other Consequences of External Causes

S37.59–S39.91

☑6ᵗʰ **S37.59** **Other injury of fallopian tube**
    Secondary blast injury of fallopian tube

    ☑7ᵗʰ **S37.591** **Other injury of fallopian tube, unilateral** ♀

    ☑7ᵗʰ **S37.592** **Other injury of fallopian tube, bilateral** ♀

    ☑7ᵗʰ **S37.599** **Other injury of fallopian tube, unspecified** ♀

☑5ᵗʰ **S37.6** **Injury of uterus**
    EXCLUDES 1   *injury to gravid uterus (O9A.2-)*
        injury to uterus during delivery (O71.-)

  ☑✗7ᵗʰ **S37.60** **Unspecified injury of uterus** ♀

  ☑✗7ᵗʰ **S37.62** **Contusion of uterus** ♀

  ☑✗7ᵗʰ **S37.63** **Laceration of uterus** ♀

  ☑✗7ᵗʰ **S37.69** **Other injury of uterus** ♀

☑5ᵗʰ **S37.8** **Injury of other urinary and pelvic organs**

  ☑6ᵗʰ **S37.81** **Injury of adrenal gland**

    ☑7ᵗʰ **S37.812** **Contusion of adrenal gland**

    ☑7ᵗʰ **S37.813** **Laceration of adrenal gland**

    ☑7ᵗʰ **S37.818** **Other injury of adrenal gland**

    ☑7ᵗʰ **S37.819** **Unspecified injury of adrenal gland**

  ☑6ᵗʰ **S37.82** **Injury of prostate**

    ☑7ᵗʰ **S37.822** **Contusion of prostate** ♂

    ☑7ᵗʰ **S37.823** **Laceration of prostate** ♂

    ☑7ᵗʰ **S37.828** **Other injury of prostate** ♂

    ☑7ᵗʰ **S37.829** **Unspecified injury of prostate** ♂

  ☑6ᵗʰ **S37.89** **Injury of other urinary and pelvic organ**

    ☑7ᵗʰ **S37.892** **Contusion of other urinary and pelvic organ**

    ☑7ᵗʰ **S37.893** **Laceration of other urinary and pelvic organ**

    ☑7ᵗʰ **S37.898** **Other injury of other urinary and pelvic organ**

    ☑7ᵗʰ **S37.899** **Unspecified injury of other urinary and pelvic organ**

☑5ᵗʰ **S37.9** **Injury of unspecified urinary and pelvic organ**

  ☑✗7ᵗʰ **S37.90** **Unspecified injury of unspecified urinary and pelvic organ**

  ☑✗7ᵗʰ **S37.92** **Contusion of unspecified urinary and pelvic organ**

  ☑✗7ᵗʰ **S37.93** **Laceration of unspecified urinary and pelvic organ**

  ☑✗7ᵗʰ **S37.99** **Other injury of unspecified urinary and pelvic organ**

☑4ᵗʰ **S38** **Crushing injury and traumatic amputation of abdomen, lower back, pelvis and external genitals**

  NOTE   An amputation not identified as partial or complete should be coded to complete

The appropriate 7th character is to be added to each code from category S38.
A   initial encounter
D   subsequent encounter
S   sequela

☑5ᵗʰ **S38.0** **Crushing injury of external genital organs**
    Use additional code for any associated injuries

  ☑6ᵗʰ **S38.00** **Crushing injury of unspecified external genital organs**

    ☑7ᵗʰ **S38.001** **Crushing injury of unspecified external genital organs, male** ♂

    ☑7ᵗʰ **S38.002** **Crushing injury of unspecified external genital organs, female** ♀

  ☑✗7ᵗʰ **S38.01** **Crushing injury of penis** ♂

  ☑✗7ᵗʰ **S38.02** **Crushing injury of scrotum and testis** ♂

  ☑✗7ᵗʰ **S38.03** **Crushing injury of vulva** ♀

☑✗7ᵗʰ **S38.1** **Crushing injury of abdomen, lower back, and pelvis**
    Use additional code for all associated injuries, such as:
    fracture of thoracic or lumbar spine and pelvis (S22.0-, S32.-)
    injury to intra-abdominal organs (S36.-)
    injury to urinary and pelvic organs (S37.-)
    open wound of abdominal wall (S31.-)
    spinal cord injury (S34.0, S34.1-)
    EXCLUDES 2   *crushing injury of external genital organs (S38.0-)*

☑5ᵗʰ **S38.2** **Traumatic amputation of external genital organs**

  ☑6ᵗʰ **S38.21** **Traumatic amputation of female external genital organs**
    Traumatic amputation of clitoris
    Traumatic amputation of labium (majus) (minus)
    Traumatic amputation of vulva

    ☑7ᵗʰ **S38.211** **Complete traumatic amputation of female external genital organs** ♀

    ☑7ᵗʰ **S38.212** **Partial traumatic amputation of female external genital organs** ♀

  ☑6ᵗʰ **S38.22** **Traumatic amputation of penis**

    ☑7ᵗʰ **S38.221** **Complete traumatic amputation of penis** ♂

    ☑7ᵗʰ **S38.222** **Partial traumatic amputation of penis** ♂

  ☑6ᵗʰ **S38.23** **Traumatic amputation of scrotum and testis**

    ☑7ᵗʰ **S38.231** **Complete traumatic amputation of scrotum and testis** ♂

    ☑7ᵗʰ **S38.232** **Partial traumatic amputation of scrotum and testis** ♂

☑✗7ᵗʰ **S38.3** **Transection (partial) of abdomen**

☑4ᵗʰ **S39** **Other and unspecified injuries of abdomen, lower back, pelvis and external genitals**
    Code also any associated open wound (S31.-)
    EXCLUDES 2   *sprain of joints and ligaments of lumbar spine and pelvis (S33.-)*

The appropriate 7th character is to be added to each code from category S39.
A   initial encounter
D   subsequent encounter
S   sequela

☑5ᵗʰ **S39.0** **Injury of muscle, fascia and tendon of abdomen, lower back and pelvis**

  ☑6ᵗʰ **S39.00** **Unspecified injury of muscle, fascia and tendon of abdomen, lower back and pelvis**

    ☑7ᵗʰ **S39.001** **Unspecified injury of muscle, fascia and tendon of abdomen**

    ☑7ᵗʰ **S39.002** **Unspecified injury of muscle, fascia and tendon of lower back**

    ☑7ᵗʰ **S39.003** **Unspecified injury of muscle, fascia and tendon of pelvis**

  ☑6ᵗʰ **S39.01** **Strain of muscle, fascia and tendon of abdomen, lower back and pelvis**

    ☑7ᵗʰ **S39.011** **Strain of muscle, fascia and tendon of abdomen**

    ☑7ᵗʰ **S39.012** **Strain of muscle, fascia and tendon of lower back**

    ☑7ᵗʰ **S39.013** **Strain of muscle, fascia and tendon of pelvis**

  ☑6ᵗʰ **S39.02** **Laceration of muscle, fascia and tendon of abdomen, lower back and pelvis**

    ☑7ᵗʰ **S39.021** **Laceration of muscle, fascia and tendon of abdomen**

    ☑7ᵗʰ **S39.022** **Laceration of muscle, fascia and tendon of lower back**

    ☑7ᵗʰ **S39.023** **Laceration of muscle, fascia and tendon of pelvis**

  ☑6ᵗʰ **S39.09** **Other injury of muscle, fascia and tendon of abdomen, lower back and pelvis**

    ☑7ᵗʰ **S39.091** **Other injury of muscle, fascia and tendon of abdomen**

    ☑7ᵗʰ **S39.092** **Other injury of muscle, fascia and tendon of lower back**

    ☑7ᵗʰ **S39.093** **Other injury of muscle, fascia and tendon of pelvis**

☑5ᵗʰ **S39.8** **Other specified injuries of abdomen, lower back, pelvis and external genitals**

  ☑✗7ᵗʰ **S39.81** **Other specified injuries of abdomen**

  ☑✗7ᵗʰ **S39.82** **Other specified injuries of lower back**

  ☑✗7ᵗʰ **S39.83** **Other specified injuries of pelvis**

  ☑6ᵗʰ **S39.84** **Other specified injuries of external genitals**

    ☑7ᵗʰ **S39.840** **Fracture of corpus cavernosum penis** ♂

    ☑7ᵗʰ **S39.848** **Other specified injuries of external genitals**

☑5ᵗʰ **S39.9** **Unspecified injury of abdomen, lower back, pelvis and external genitals**

  ☑✗7ᵗʰ **S39.91** **Unspecified injury of abdomen**

√x7ᵗʰ   **S39.92**   Unspecified injury of lower back

√x7ᵗʰ   **S39.93**   Unspecified injury of pelvis

√x7ᵗʰ   **S39.94**   Unspecified injury of external genitals

Injuries to the shoulder and upper arm (S40-S49)

INCLUDES   injuries of axilla
     injuries of scapular region
EXCLUDES 2   burns and corrosions (T20-T32)
     frostbite (T33-T34)
     injuries of elbow (S50-S59)
     insect bite or sting, venomous (T63.4)

√4ᵗʰ   **S40**   **Superficial injury of shoulder and upper arm**

> The appropriate 7th character is to be added to each code from category S40.
> A   initial encounter
> D   subsequent encounter
> S   sequela

√5ᵗʰ   **S40.0**   Contusion of shoulder and upper arm

√6ᵗʰ   **S40.01**   Contusion of shoulder

     √7ᵗʰ   **S40.011**   Contusion of right shoulder

     √7ᵗʰ   **S40.012**   Contusion of left shoulder

     √7ᵗʰ   **S40.019**   Contusion of unspecified shoulder

√6ᵗʰ   **S40.02**   Contusion of upper arm

     √7ᵗʰ   **S40.021**   Contusion of right upper arm

     √7ᵗʰ   **S40.022**   Contusion of left upper arm

     √7ᵗʰ   **S40.029**   Contusion of unspecified upper arm

√5ᵗʰ   **S40.2**   Other superficial injuries of shoulder

√6ᵗʰ   **S40.21**   Abrasion of shoulder

     √7ᵗʰ   **S40.211**   Abrasion of right shoulder

     √7ᵗʰ   **S40.212**   Abrasion of left shoulder

     √7ᵗʰ   **S40.219**   Abrasion of unspecified shoulder

√6ᵗʰ   **S40.22**   Blister (nonthermal) of shoulder

     √7ᵗʰ   **S40.221**   Blister (nonthermal) of right shoulder

     √7ᵗʰ   **S40.222**   Blister (nonthermal) of left shoulder

     √7ᵗʰ   **S40.229**   Blister (nonthermal) of unspecified shoulder

√6ᵗʰ   **S40.24**   External constriction of shoulder

     √7ᵗʰ   **S40.241**   External constriction of right shoulder

     √7ᵗʰ   **S40.242**   External constriction of left shoulder

     √7ᵗʰ   **S40.249**   External constriction of unspecified shoulder

√6ᵗʰ   **S40.25**   Superficial foreign body of shoulder
     Splinter in the shoulder

     √7ᵗʰ   **S40.251**   Superficial foreign body of right shoulder

     √7ᵗʰ   **S40.252**   Superficial foreign body of left shoulder

     √7ᵗʰ   **S40.259**   Superficial foreign body of unspecified shoulder

√6ᵗʰ   **S40.26**   Insect bite (nonvenomous) of shoulder

     √7ᵗʰ   **S40.261**   Insect bite (nonvenomous) of right shoulder

     √7ᵗʰ   **S40.262**   Insect bite (nonvenomous) of left shoulder

     √7ᵗʰ   **S40.269**   Insect bite (nonvenomous) of unspecified shoulder

√6ᵗʰ   **S40.27**   Other superficial bite of shoulder
     EXCLUDES 1   open bite of shoulder (S41.05)

     √7ᵗʰ   **S40.271**   Other superficial bite of right shoulder

     √7ᵗʰ   **S40.272**   Other superficial bite of left shoulder

     √7ᵗʰ   **S40.279**   Other superficial bite of unspecified shoulder

√5ᵗʰ   **S40.8**   Other superficial injuries of upper arm

√6ᵗʰ   **S40.81**   Abrasion of upper arm

     √7ᵗʰ   **S40.811**   Abrasion of right upper arm

     √7ᵗʰ   **S40.812**   Abrasion of left upper arm

     √7ᵗʰ   **S40.819**   Abrasion of unspecified upper arm

√6ᵗʰ   **S40.82**   Blister (nonthermal) of upper arm

     √7ᵗʰ   **S40.821**   Blister (nonthermal) of right upper arm

     √7ᵗʰ   **S40.822**   Blister (nonthermal) of left upper arm

     √7ᵗʰ   **S40.829**   Blister (nonthermal) of unspecified upper arm

√6ᵗʰ   **S40.84**   External constriction of upper arm

     √7ᵗʰ   **S40.841**   External constriction of right upper arm

     √7ᵗʰ   **S40.842**   External constriction of left upper arm

     √7ᵗʰ   **S40.849**   External constriction of unspecified upper arm

√6ᵗʰ   **S40.85**   Superficial foreign body of upper arm
     Splinter in the upper arm

     √7ᵗʰ   **S40.851**   Superficial foreign body of right upper arm

     √7ᵗʰ   **S40.852**   Superficial foreign body of left upper arm

     √7ᵗʰ   **S40.859**   Superficial foreign body of unspecified upper arm

√6ᵗʰ   **S40.86**   Insect bite (nonvenomous) of upper arm

     √7ᵗʰ   **S40.861**   Insect bite (nonvenomous) of right upper arm

     √7ᵗʰ   **S40.862**   Insect bite (nonvenomous) of left upper arm

     √7ᵗʰ   **S40.869**   Insect bite (nonvenomous) of unspecified upper arm

√6ᵗʰ   **S40.87**   Other superficial bite of upper arm
     EXCLUDES 1   open bite of upper arm (S41.14)
     EXCLUDES 2   other superficial bite of shoulder (S40.27-)

     √7ᵗʰ   **S40.871**   Other superficial bite of right upper arm

     √7ᵗʰ   **S40.872**   Other superficial bite of left upper arm

     √7ᵗʰ   **S40.879**   Other superficial bite of unspecified upper arm

√5ᵗʰ   **S40.9**   Unspecified superficial injury of shoulder and upper arm

√6ᵗʰ   **S40.91**   Unspecified superficial injury of shoulder

     √7ᵗʰ   **S40.911**   Unspecified superficial injury of right shoulder

     √7ᵗʰ   **S40.912**   Unspecified superficial injury of left shoulder

     √7ᵗʰ   **S40.919**   Unspecified superficial injury of unspecified shoulder

√6ᵗʰ   **S40.92**   Unspecified superficial injury of upper arm

     √7ᵗʰ   **S40.921**   Unspecified superficial injury of right upper arm

     √7ᵗʰ   **S40.922**   Unspecified superficial injury of left upper arm

     √7ᵗʰ   **S40.929**   Unspecified superficial injury of unspecified upper arm

√4ᵗʰ   **S41**   **Open wound of shoulder and upper arm**

> Code also any associated wound infection
> EXCLUDES 1   traumatic amputation of shoulder and upper arm (S48.-)
> EXCLUDES 2   open fracture of shoulder and upper arm (S42.- with 7th character B or C)

> The appropriate 7th character is to be added to each code from category S41.
> A   initial encounter
> D   subsequent encounter
> S   sequela

√5ᵗʰ   **S41.0**   Open wound of shoulder

√6ᵗʰ   **S41.00**   Unspecified open wound of shoulder

     √7ᵗʰ   **S41.001**   Unspecified open wound of right shoulder

     √7ᵗʰ   **S41.002**   Unspecified open wound of left shoulder

     √7ᵗʰ   **S41.009**   Unspecified open wound of unspecified shoulder

√6ᵗʰ   **S41.01**   Laceration without foreign body of shoulder

     √7ᵗʰ   **S41.011**   Laceration without foreign body of right shoulder

     √7ᵗʰ   **S41.012**   Laceration without foreign body of left shoulder

     √7ᵗʰ   **S41.019**   Laceration without foreign body of unspecified shoulder

√6ᵗʰ   **S41.02**   Laceration with foreign body of shoulder

     √7ᵗʰ   **S41.021**   Laceration with foreign body of right shoulder

     √7ᵗʰ   **S41.022**   Laceration with foreign body of left shoulder

     √7ᵗʰ   **S41.029**   Laceration with foreign body of unspecified shoulder

√6ᵗʰ   **S41.03**   Puncture wound without foreign body of shoulder

     √7ᵗʰ   **S41.031**   Puncture wound without foreign body of right shoulder

---

✓ Additional Character Required   √x7ᵗʰ Placeholder Alert   Manifestation   Unspecified Dx   Q QPP   UPD Unacceptable PDx

√7ᵗʰ **S41.032** **Puncture wound without foreign body of** left **shoulder**

√7ᵗʰ **S41.039** **Puncture wound without foreign body of unspecified shoulder**

√6ᵗʰ **S41.04** Puncture wound with foreign body **of shoulder**

√7ᵗʰ **S41.041** **Puncture wound with foreign body of** right **shoulder**

√7ᵗʰ **S41.042** **Puncture wound with foreign body of** left **shoulder**

√7ᵗʰ **S41.049** **Puncture wound with foreign body of unspecified shoulder**

√6ᵗʰ **S41.05** Open bite **of shoulder**

Bite of shoulder NOS

EXCLUDES 1   *superficial bite of shoulder (S40.27)*

√7ᵗʰ **S41.051** **Open bite of** right **shoulder**

√7ᵗʰ **S41.052** **Open bite of** left **shoulder**

√7ᵗʰ **S41.059** **Open bite of unspecified shoulder**

√5ᵗʰ **S41.1** **Open wound of** upper arm

√6ᵗʰ **S41.10** **Unspecified open wound of upper arm**

AHA: 2016,3Q,24

√7ᵗʰ **S41.101** **Unspecified open wound of** right **upper arm**

√7ᵗʰ **S41.102** **Unspecified open wound of** left **upper arm**

√7ᵗʰ **S41.109** **Unspecified open wound of unspecified upper arm**

√6ᵗʰ **S41.11** Laceration without foreign body **of upper arm**

√7ᵗʰ **S41.111** **Laceration without foreign body of** right **upper arm**

√7ᵗʰ **S41.112** **Laceration without foreign body of** left **upper arm**

√7ᵗʰ **S41.119** **Laceration without foreign body of unspecified upper arm**

√6ᵗʰ **S41.12** Laceration with foreign body **of upper arm**

√7ᵗʰ **S41.121** **Laceration with foreign body of** right **upper arm**

√7ᵗʰ **S41.122** **Laceration with foreign body of** left **upper arm**

√7ᵗʰ **S41.129** **Laceration with foreign body of unspecified upper arm**

√6ᵗʰ **S41.13** Puncture wound without foreign body **of upper arm**

AHA: 2016,3Q,24

√7ᵗʰ **S41.131** **Puncture wound without foreign body of** right **upper arm**

√7ᵗʰ **S41.132** **Puncture wound without foreign body of** left **upper arm**

√7ᵗʰ **S41.139** **Puncture wound without foreign body of unspecified upper arm**

√6ᵗʰ **S41.14** Puncture wound with foreign body **of upper arm**

AHA: 2016,3Q,24

√7ᵗʰ **S41.141** **Puncture wound with foreign body of** right **upper arm**

√7ᵗʰ **S41.142** **Puncture wound with foreign body of** left **upper arm**

√7ᵗʰ **S41.149** **Puncture wound with foreign body of unspecified upper arm**

√6ᵗʰ **S41.15** Open bite **of upper arm**

Bite of upper arm NOS

EXCLUDES 1   *superficial bite of upper arm (S40.87)*

√7ᵗʰ **S41.151** **Open bite of** right **upper arm**

√7ᵗʰ **S41.152** **Open bite of** left **upper arm**

√7ᵗʰ **S41.159** **Open bite of unspecified upper arm**

√4ᵗʰ **S42** **Fracture of shoulder and upper arm**

NOTE   A fracture not indicated as displaced or nondisplaced should be coded to displaced

A fracture not indicated as open or closed should be coded to closed

EXCLUDES 1   *traumatic amputation of shoulder and upper arm (S48.-)*

AHA: 2018,2Q,12; 2015,3Q,37-39

DEF: Diaphysis: Central shaft of a long bone.

DEF: Epiphysis: Proximal and distal rounded ends of a long bone, communicates with the joint.

DEF: Metaphysis: Section of a long bone located between the epiphysis and diaphysis at the proximal and distal ends.

DEF: Physis (growth plate): Narrow zone of cartilaginous tissue between the epiphysis and metaphysis at each end of a long bone. In childhood, proliferation of cells in this zone lengthens the bone. As the bone matures, this area thins, ossification eventually fusing into solid bone and growth stops. *Synonym(s): Epiphyseal plate.*

> The appropriate 7th character is to be added to all codes from category S42 [unless otherwise indicated].
> A   initial encounter for closed fracture
> B   initial encounter for open fracture
> D   subsequent encounter for fracture with routine healing
> G   subsequent encounter for fracture with delayed healing
> K   subsequent encounter for fracture with nonunion
> P   subsequent encounter for fracture with malunion
> S   sequela

√5ᵗʰ **S42.0** **Fracture of** clavicle

√6ᵗʰ **S42.00** **Fracture of unspecified part of clavicle**

√7ᵗʰ **S42.001** **Fracture of unspecified part of** right **clavicle** ▢

√7ᵗʰ **S42.002** **Fracture of unspecified part of** left **clavicle** ▢

√7ᵗʰ **S42.009** **Fracture of unspecified part of unspecified clavicle** ▢

AHA: 2012,4Q,93

√6ᵗʰ **S42.01** **Fracture of** sternal end **of clavicle**

√7ᵗʰ **S42.011** **Anterior displaced fracture of sternal end of** right **clavicle** ▢

√7ᵗʰ **S42.012** **Anterior displaced fracture of sternal end of** left **clavicle** ▢

√7ᵗʰ **S42.013** **Anterior displaced fracture of sternal end of unspecified clavicle** ▢

Displaced fracture of sternal end of clavicle NOS

√7ᵗʰ **S42.014** **Posterior displaced fracture of sternal end of** right **clavicle** ▢

√7ᵗʰ **S42.015** **Posterior displaced fracture of sternal end of** left **clavicle** ▢

√7ᵗʰ **S42.016** **Posterior displaced fracture of sternal end of unspecified clavicle** ▢

√7ᵗʰ **S42.017** **Nondisplaced fracture of sternal end of** right **clavicle** ▢

√7ᵗʰ **S42.018** **Nondisplaced fracture of sternal end of** left **clavicle** ▢

√7ᵗʰ **S42.019** **Nondisplaced fracture of sternal end of unspecified clavicle** ▢

√6ᵗʰ **S42.02** **Fracture of** shaft **of clavicle**

√7ᵗʰ **S42.021** **Displaced fracture of shaft of** right **clavicle** ▢

√7ᵗʰ **S42.022** **Displaced fracture of shaft of** left **clavicle** ▢

√7ᵗʰ **S42.023** **Displaced fracture of shaft of unspecified clavicle** ▢

√7ᵗʰ **S42.024** **Nondisplaced fracture of shaft of** right **clavicle** ▢

√7ᵗʰ **S42.025** **Nondisplaced fracture of shaft of** left **clavicle** ▢

√7ᵗʰ **S42.026** **Nondisplaced fracture of shaft of unspecified clavicle** ▢

√6ᵗʰ **S42.03** **Fracture of** lateral end **of clavicle**

Fracture of acromial end of clavicle

√7ᵗʰ **S42.031** **Displaced fracture of lateral end of** right **clavicle** ▢

√7ᵗʰ **S42.032** **Displaced fracture of lateral end of** left **clavicle** ▢

√7ᵗʰ **S42.033** **Displaced fracture of lateral end of unspecified clavicle** ▢

HCC CMS-HCC   **Rx** Rx HCC   **ESR** ESRD HCC   **COM** Commercial HCC   **N** Newborn: 0   **P** Pediatric: 0-17   **M** Maternity: 9-64   **A** Adult: 15-124

1034   ICD-10-CM 2023

√7ᵗʰ **S42.034** Nondisplaced **fracture of lateral end of** right **clavicle** Q

√7ᵗʰ **S42.035** Nondisplaced **fracture of lateral end of** left **clavicle** Q

√7ᵗʰ **S42.036** Nondisplaced **fracture of lateral end of unspecified clavicle** Q

√5ᵗʰ **S42.1** **Fracture of** scapula

√6ᵗʰ **S42.10** **Fracture of unspecified part of scapula**

√7ᵗʰ **S42.101** **Fracture of unspecified part of scapula,** right **shoulder** Q

√7ᵗʰ **S42.102** **Fracture of unspecified part of scapula,** left **shoulder** Q

√7ᵗʰ **S42.109** **Fracture of unspecified part of scapula, unspecified shoulder** Q

√6ᵗʰ **S42.11** **Fracture of** body **of scapula**

√7ᵗʰ **S42.111** Displaced **fracture of body of scapula,** right **shoulder** Q

√7ᵗʰ **S42.112** Displaced **fracture of body of scapula,** left **shoulder** Q

√7ᵗʰ **S42.113** Displaced **fracture of body of scapula, unspecified shoulder** Q

√7ᵗʰ **S42.114** Nondisplaced **fracture of body of scapula,** right **shoulder** Q

√7ᵗʰ **S42.115** Nondisplaced **fracture of body of scapula,** left **shoulder** Q

√7ᵗʰ **S42.116** Nondisplaced **fracture of body of scapula, unspecified shoulder** Q

√6ᵗʰ **S42.12** **Fracture of** acromial process

√7ᵗʰ **S42.121** Displaced **fracture of acromial process,** right **shoulder** Q

√7ᵗʰ **S42.122** Displaced **fracture of acromial process,** left **shoulder** Q

√7ᵗʰ **S42.123** Displaced **fracture of acromial process, unspecified shoulder** Q

√7ᵗʰ **S42.124** Nondisplaced **fracture of acromial process,** right **shoulder** Q

√7ᵗʰ **S42.125** Nondisplaced **fracture of acromial process,** left **shoulder** Q

√7ᵗʰ **S42.126** Nondisplaced **fracture of acromial process, unspecified shoulder** Q

√6ᵗʰ **S42.13** **Fracture of** coracoid process

√7ᵗʰ **S42.131** Displaced **fracture of coracoid process,** right **shoulder** Q

√7ᵗʰ **S42.132** Displaced **fracture of coracoid process,** left **shoulder** Q

√7ᵗʰ **S42.133** Displaced **fracture of coracoid process, unspecified shoulder** Q

√7ᵗʰ **S42.134** Nondisplaced **fracture of coracoid process,** right **shoulder** Q

√7ᵗʰ **S42.135** Nondisplaced **fracture of coracoid process,** left **shoulder** Q

√7ᵗʰ **S42.136** Nondisplaced **fracture of coracoid process, unspecified shoulder** Q

√6ᵗʰ **S42.14** **Fracture of** glenoid cavity **of scapula**

√7ᵗʰ **S42.141** Displaced **fracture of glenoid cavity of scapula,** right **shoulder** Q

√7ᵗʰ **S42.142** Displaced **fracture of glenoid cavity of scapula,** left **shoulder** Q

√7ᵗʰ **S42.143** Displaced **fracture of glenoid cavity of scapula, unspecified shoulder** Q

√7ᵗʰ **S42.144** Nondisplaced **fracture of glenoid cavity of scapula,** right **shoulder** Q

√7ᵗʰ **S42.145** Nondisplaced **fracture of glenoid cavity of scapula,** left **shoulder** Q

√7ᵗʰ **S42.146** Nondisplaced **fracture of glenoid cavity of scapula, unspecified shoulder** Q

√6ᵗʰ **S42.15** **Fracture of** neck **of scapula**

√7ᵗʰ **S42.151** Displaced **fracture of neck of scapula,** right **shoulder** Q

√7ᵗʰ **S42.152** Displaced **fracture of neck of scapula,** left **shoulder** Q

√7ᵗʰ **S42.153** Displaced **fracture of neck of scapula, unspecified shoulder** Q

√7ᵗʰ **S42.154** Nondisplaced **fracture of neck of scapula,** right **shoulder** Q

√7ᵗʰ **S42.155** Nondisplaced **fracture of neck of scapula,** left **shoulder** Q

√7ᵗʰ **S42.156** Nondisplaced **fracture of neck of scapula, unspecified shoulder** Q

√6ᵗʰ **S42.19** **Fracture of other part of scapula**

√7ᵗʰ **S42.191** **Fracture of other part of scapula,** right **shoulder** Q

√7ᵗʰ **S42.192** **Fracture of other part of scapula,** left **shoulder** Q

√7ᵗʰ **S42.199** **Fracture of other part of scapula, unspecified shoulder** Q

√5ᵗʰ **S42.2** **Fracture of** upper end of humerus

Fracture of proximal end of humerus

EXCLUDES 2   *fracture of shaft of humerus (S42.3-)*

physeal fracture of upper end of humerus (S49.0-)

√6ᵗʰ **S42.20** **Unspecified fracture of upper end of humerus**

√7ᵗʰ **S42.201** **Unspecified fracture of upper end of** right **humerus** Q

√7ᵗʰ **S42.202** **Unspecified fracture of upper end of** left **humerus** Q

√7ᵗʰ **S42.209** **Unspecified fracture of upper end of unspecified humerus** Q

√6ᵗʰ **S42.21** **Unspecified fracture of** surgical neck **of humerus**

Fracture of neck of humerus NOS

√7ᵗʰ **S42.211** **Unspecified** displaced **fracture of surgical neck of** right **humerus** Q

√7ᵗʰ **S42.212** **Unspecified** displaced **fracture of surgical neck of** left **humerus** Q

√7ᵗʰ **S42.213** **Unspecified** displaced **fracture of surgical neck of unspecified humerus** Q

√7ᵗʰ **S42.214** **Unspecified** nondisplaced **fracture of surgical neck of** right **humerus** Q

√7ᵗʰ **S42.215** **Unspecified** nondisplaced **fracture of surgical neck of** left **humerus** Q

√7ᵗʰ **S42.216** **Unspecified** nondisplaced **fracture of surgical neck of unspecified humerus** Q

√6ᵗʰ **S42.22** **2-part** fracture of surgical neck **of humerus**

√7ᵗʰ **S42.221** **2-part** displaced **fracture of surgical neck of** right **humerus** Q

√7ᵗʰ **S42.222** **2-part** displaced **fracture of surgical neck of** left **humerus** Q

√7ᵗʰ **S42.223** **2-part** displaced **fracture of surgical neck of unspecified humerus** Q

√7ᵗʰ **S42.224** **2-part** nondisplaced **fracture of surgical neck of** right **humerus** Q

√7ᵗʰ **S42.225** **2-part** nondisplaced **fracture of surgical neck of** left **humerus** Q

√7ᵗʰ **S42.226** **2-part** nondisplaced **fracture of surgical neck of unspecified humerus** Q

√6ᵗʰ **S42.23** **3-part** fracture of surgical neck **of humerus**

√7ᵗʰ **S42.231** **3-part fracture of surgical neck of** right **humerus** Q

√7ᵗʰ **S42.232** **3-part fracture of surgical neck of** left **humerus** Q

√7ᵗʰ **S42.239** **3-part fracture of surgical neck of unspecified humerus** Q

√6ᵗʰ **S42.24** **4-part** fracture of surgical neck **of humerus**

√7ᵗʰ **S42.241** **4-part fracture of surgical neck of** right **humerus** Q

√7ᵗʰ **S42.242** **4-part fracture of surgical neck of** left **humerus** Q

√7ᵗʰ **S42.249** **4-part fracture of surgical neck of unspecified humerus** Q

√6ᵗʰ **S42.25** **Fracture of** greater tuberosity **of humerus**

√7ᵗʰ **S42.251** Displaced **fracture of greater tuberosity of** right **humerus** Q

√7ᵗʰ **S42.252** Displaced **fracture of greater tuberosity of** left **humerus** Q

√7ᵗʰ **S42.253** Displaced **fracture of greater tuberosity of unspecified humerus** Q

√7ᵗʰ **S42.254** Nondisplaced **fracture of greater tuberosity of** right **humerus** Q

√7ᵗʰ **S42.255** Nondisplaced **fracture of greater tuberosity of** left **humerus** Q

√7ᵗʰ **S42.256** Nondisplaced **fracture of greater tuberosity of unspecified humerus** Q

√6ᵗʰ **S42.26** **Fracture of** lesser tuberosity **of humerus**

√7ᵗʰ **S42.261** Displaced **fracture of lesser tuberosity of** right **humerus** Q

√7ᵗʰ **S42.262** Displaced **fracture of lesser tuberosity of** left **humerus** Q

Chapter 19. Injury, Poisoning and Certain Other Consequences of External Causes

√7ᵗʰ **S42.263** Displaced **fracture of lesser tuberosity of unspecified humerus** Ø

√7ᵗʰ **S42.264** Nondisplaced **fracture of lesser tuberosity of** right **humerus** Ø

√7ᵗʰ **S42.265** Nondisplaced **fracture of lesser tuberosity of** left **humerus** Ø

√7ᵗʰ **S42.266** Nondisplaced **fracture of lesser tuberosity of unspecified humerus** Ø

√6ᵗʰ **S42.27** Torus **fracture of upper end of humerus**

The appropriate 7th character is to be added to all codes in subcategory S42.27
A   initial encounter for closed fracture
D   subsequent encounter for fracture with routine healing
G   subsequent encounter for fracture with delayed healing
K   subsequent encounter for fracture with nonunion
P   subsequent encounter for fracture with malunion
S   sequela

√7ᵗʰ **S42.271** Torus **fracture of upper end of** right **humerus** Ø

√7ᵗʰ **S42.272** Torus **fracture of upper end of** left **humerus** Ø

√7ᵗʰ **S42.279** Torus **fracture of upper end of unspecified humerus** Ø

√6ᵗʰ **S42.29** Other **fracture of upper end of humerus**

Fracture of anatomical neck of humerus
Fracture of articular head of humerus
AHA: 2019,1Q,18

√7ᵗʰ **S42.291** Other displaced **fracture of upper end of** right **humerus** Ø

√7ᵗʰ **S42.292** Other displaced **fracture of upper end of** left **humerus** Ø

√7ᵗʰ **S42.293** Other displaced **fracture of upper end of unspecified humerus** Ø

√7ᵗʰ **S42.294** Other nondisplaced **fracture of upper end of** right **humerus** Ø

√7ᵗʰ **S42.295** Other nondisplaced **fracture of upper end of** left **humerus** Ø

√7ᵗʰ **S42.296** Other nondisplaced **fracture of upper end of unspecified humerus** Ø

√5ᵗʰ **S42.3** Fracture of shaft **of humerus**

Fracture of humerus NOS
Fracture of upper arm NOS
EXCLUDES 2   physeal fractures of upper end of humerus (S49.0-)
     physeal fractures of lower end of humerus (S49.1-)

√6ᵗʰ **S42.30** Unspecified **fracture of shaft of humerus**

√7ᵗʰ **S42.301** Unspecified **fracture of shaft of humerus,** right arm Ø

√7ᵗʰ **S42.302** Unspecified **fracture of shaft of humerus,** left **arm** Ø

√7ᵗʰ **S42.309** Unspecified **fracture of shaft of humerus, unspecified arm** Ø

√6ᵗʰ **S42.31** Greenstick **fracture of shaft of humerus**

The appropriate 7th character is to be added to all codes in subcategory S42.31
A   initial encounter for closed fracture
D   subsequent encounter for fracture with routine healing
G   subsequent encounter for fracture with delayed healing
K   subsequent encounter for fracture with nonunion
P   subsequent encounter for fracture with malunion
S   sequela

√7ᵗʰ **S42.311** Greenstick **fracture of shaft of humerus,** right **arm** Ø

√7ᵗʰ **S42.312** Greenstick **fracture of shaft of humerus,** left **arm** Ø

√7ᵗʰ **S42.319** Greenstick **fracture of shaft of humerus, unspecified arm** Ø

√6ᵗʰ **S42.32** Transverse **fracture of shaft of humerus**

√7ᵗʰ **S42.321** Displaced **transverse fracture of shaft of humerus,** right **arm** Ø

√7ᵗʰ **S42.322** Displaced **transverse fracture of shaft of humerus,** left **arm** Ø

√7ᵗʰ **S42.323** Displaced **transverse fracture of shaft of humerus, unspecified arm** Ø

√7ᵗʰ **S42.324** Nondisplaced **transverse fracture of shaft of humerus,** right **arm** Ø

√7ᵗʰ **S42.325** Nondisplaced **transverse fracture of shaft of humerus,** left **arm** Ø

√7ᵗʰ **S42.326** Nondisplaced **transverse fracture of shaft of humerus, unspecified arm** Ø

√6ᵗʰ **S42.33** Oblique **fracture of shaft of humerus**

√7ᵗʰ **S42.331** Displaced **oblique fracture of shaft of humerus,** right **arm** Ø

√7ᵗʰ **S42.332** Displaced **oblique fracture of shaft of humerus,** left **arm** Ø

√7ᵗʰ **S42.333** Displaced **oblique fracture of shaft of humerus, unspecified arm** Ø

√7ᵗʰ **S42.334** Nondisplaced **oblique fracture of shaft of humerus,** right **arm** Ø

√7ᵗʰ **S42.335** Nondisplaced **oblique fracture of shaft of humerus,** left **arm** Ø

√7ᵗʰ **S42.336** Nondisplaced **oblique fracture of shaft of humerus, unspecified arm** Ø

√6ᵗʰ **S42.34** Spiral **fracture of shaft of humerus**

√7ᵗʰ **S42.341** Displaced **spiral fracture of shaft of humerus,** right **arm** Ø

√7ᵗʰ **S42.342** Displaced **spiral fracture of shaft of humerus,** left **arm** Ø

√7ᵗʰ **S42.343** Displaced **spiral fracture of shaft of humerus, unspecified arm** Ø

√7ᵗʰ **S42.344** Nondisplaced **spiral fracture of shaft of humerus,** right **arm** Ø

√7ᵗʰ **S42.345** Nondisplaced **spiral fracture of shaft of humerus,** left **arm** Ø

√7ᵗʰ **S42.346** Nondisplaced **spiral fracture of shaft of humerus, unspecified arm** Ø

√6ᵗʰ **S42.35** Comminuted **fracture of shaft of humerus**

√7ᵗʰ **S42.351** Displaced **comminuted fracture of shaft of humerus,** right **arm** Ø

√7ᵗʰ **S42.352** Displaced **comminuted fracture of shaft of humerus,** left **arm** Ø

√7ᵗʰ **S42.353** Displaced **comminuted fracture of shaft of humerus, unspecified arm** Ø

√7ᵗʰ **S42.354** Nondisplaced **comminuted fracture of shaft of humerus,** right **arm** Ø

√7ᵗʰ **S42.355** Nondisplaced **comminuted fracture of shaft of humerus,** left **arm** Ø

√7ᵗʰ **S42.356** Nondisplaced **comminuted fracture of shaft of humerus, unspecified arm** Ø

√6ᵗʰ **S42.36** Segmental **fracture of shaft of humerus**

√7ᵗʰ **S42.361** Displaced **segmental fracture of shaft of humerus,** right **arm** Ø

√7ᵗʰ **S42.362** Displaced **segmental fracture of shaft of humerus,** left **arm** Ø

√7ᵗʰ **S42.363** Displaced **segmental fracture of shaft of humerus, unspecified arm** Ø

√7ᵗʰ **S42.364** Nondisplaced **segmental fracture of shaft of humerus,** right **arm** Ø

√7ᵗʰ **S42.365** Nondisplaced **segmental fracture of shaft of humerus,** left **arm** Ø

√7ᵗʰ **S42.366** Nondisplaced **segmental fracture of shaft of humerus, unspecified arm** Ø

√6ᵗʰ **S42.39** Other **fracture of shaft of humerus**

√7ᵗʰ **S42.391** Other **fracture of shaft of** right **humerus** Ø

√7ᵗʰ **S42.392** Other **fracture of shaft of** left **humerus** Ø

√7ᵗʰ **S42.399** Other **fracture of shaft of unspecified humerus** Ø

√5ᵗʰ **S42.4** Fracture of lower end **of humerus**

Fracture of distal end of humerus
EXCLUDES 2   fracture of shaft of humerus (S42.3-)
     physeal fracture of lower end of humerus (S49.1-)

√6ᵗʰ **S42.40** Unspecified **fracture of lower end of humerus**

Fracture of elbow NOS

√7ᵗʰ **S42.401** Unspecified **fracture of lower end of** right **humerus** Ø

√7ᵗʰ **S42.402** Unspecified **fracture of lower end of** left **humerus** Ø

√7ᵗʰ S42.409 Unspecified fracture of lower end of unspecified humerus ◘

√6ᵗʰ S42.41 Simple supracondylar fracture without intercondylar fracture of humerus

√7ᵗʰ S42.411 Displaced simple supracondylar fracture without intercondylar fracture of right humerus ◘

√7ᵗʰ S42.412 Displaced simple supracondylar fracture without intercondylar fracture of left humerus ◘

√7ᵗʰ S42.413 Displaced simple supracondylar fracture without intercondylar fracture of unspecified humerus ◘

√7ᵗʰ S42.414 Nondisplaced simple supracondylar fracture without intercondylar fracture of right humerus ◘

√7ᵗʰ S42.415 Nondisplaced simple supracondylar fracture without intercondylar fracture of left humerus ◘

√7ᵗʰ S42.416 Nondisplaced simple supracondylar fracture without intercondylar fracture of unspecified humerus ◘

√6ᵗʰ S42.42 Comminuted supracondylar fracture without intercondylar fracture of humerus

√7ᵗʰ S42.421 Displaced comminuted supracondylar fracture without intercondylar fracture of right humerus ◘

√7ᵗʰ S42.422 Displaced comminuted supracondylar fracture without intercondylar fracture of left humerus ◘

√7ᵗʰ S42.423 Displaced comminuted supracondylar fracture without intercondylar fracture of unspecified humerus ◘

√7ᵗʰ S42.424 Nondisplaced comminuted supracondylar fracture without intercondylar fracture of right humerus ◘

√7ᵗʰ S42.425 Nondisplaced comminuted supracondylar fracture without intercondylar fracture of left humerus ◘

√7ᵗʰ S42.426 Nondisplaced comminuted supracondylar fracture without intercondylar fracture of unspecified humerus ◘

√6ᵗʰ S42.43 Fracture (avulsion) of lateral epicondyle of humerus

√7ᵗʰ S42.431 Displaced fracture (avulsion) of lateral epicondyle of right humerus ◘

√7ᵗʰ S42.432 Displaced fracture (avulsion) of lateral epicondyle of left humerus ◘

√7ᵗʰ S42.433 Displaced fracture (avulsion) of lateral epicondyle of unspecified humerus ◘

√7ᵗʰ S42.434 Nondisplaced fracture (avulsion) of lateral epicondyle of right humerus ◘

√7ᵗʰ S42.435 Nondisplaced fracture (avulsion) of lateral epicondyle of left humerus ◘

√7ᵗʰ S42.436 Nondisplaced fracture (avulsion) of lateral epicondyle of unspecified humerus ◘

√6ᵗʰ S42.44 Fracture (avulsion) of medial epicondyle of humerus

√7ᵗʰ S42.441 Displaced fracture (avulsion) of medial epicondyle of right humerus ◘

√7ᵗʰ S42.442 Displaced fracture (avulsion) of medial epicondyle of left humerus ◘

√7ᵗʰ S42.443 Displaced fracture (avulsion) of medial epicondyle of unspecified humerus ◘

√7ᵗʰ S42.444 Nondisplaced fracture (avulsion) of medial epicondyle of right humerus ◘

√7ᵗʰ S42.445 Nondisplaced fracture (avulsion) of medial epicondyle of left humerus ◘

√7ᵗʰ S42.446 Nondisplaced fracture (avulsion) of medial epicondyle of unspecified humerus ◘

√7ᵗʰ S42.447 Incarcerated fracture (avulsion) of medial epicondyle of right humerus ◘

√7ᵗʰ S42.448 Incarcerated fracture (avulsion) of medial epicondyle of left humerus ◘

√7ᵗʰ S42.449 Incarcerated fracture (avulsion) of medial epicondyle of unspecified humerus ◘

√6ᵗʰ S42.45 Fracture of lateral condyle of humerus

Fracture of capitellum of humerus

√7ᵗʰ S42.451 Displaced fracture of lateral condyle of right humerus ◘

√7ᵗʰ S42.452 Displaced fracture of lateral condyle of left humerus ◘

√7ᵗʰ S42.453 Displaced fracture of lateral condyle of unspecified humerus ◘

√7ᵗʰ S42.454 Nondisplaced fracture of lateral condyle of right humerus ◘

√7ᵗʰ S42.455 Nondisplaced fracture of lateral condyle of left humerus ◘

√7ᵗʰ S42.456 Nondisplaced fracture of lateral condyle of unspecified humerus ◘

√6ᵗʰ S42.46 Fracture of medial condyle of humerus

Trochlea fracture of humerus

√7ᵗʰ S42.461 Displaced fracture of medial condyle of right humerus ◘

√7ᵗʰ S42.462 Displaced fracture of medial condyle of left humerus ◘

√7ᵗʰ S42.463 Displaced fracture of medial condyle of unspecified humerus ◘

√7ᵗʰ S42.464 Nondisplaced fracture of medial condyle of right humerus ◘

√7ᵗʰ S42.465 Nondisplaced fracture of medial condyle of left humerus ◘

√7ᵗʰ S42.466 Nondisplaced fracture of medial condyle of unspecified humerus ◘

√6ᵗʰ S42.47 Transcondylar fracture of humerus

√7ᵗʰ S42.471 Displaced transcondylar fracture of right humerus ◘

√7ᵗʰ S42.472 Displaced transcondylar fracture of left humerus ◘

√7ᵗʰ S42.473 Displaced transcondylar fracture of unspecified humerus ◘

√7ᵗʰ S42.474 Nondisplaced transcondylar fracture of right humerus ◘

√7ᵗʰ S42.475 Nondisplaced transcondylar fracture of left humerus ◘

√7ᵗʰ S42.476 Nondisplaced transcondylar fracture of unspecified humerus ◘

√6ᵗʰ S42.48 Torus fracture of lower end of humerus

> The appropriate 7th character is to be added to all codes in subcategory S42.48.
> A   initial encounter for closed fracture
> D   subsequent encounter for fracture with routine healing
> G   subsequent encounter for fracture with delayed healing
> K   subsequent encounter for fracture with nonunion
> P   subsequent encounter for fracture with malunion
> S   sequela

√7ᵗʰ S42.481 Torus fracture of lower end of right humerus ◘

√7ᵗʰ S42.482 Torus fracture of lower end of left humerus ◘

√7ᵗʰ S42.489 Torus fracture of lower end of unspecified humerus ◘

√6ᵗʰ S42.49 Other fracture of lower end of humerus

√7ᵗʰ S42.491 Other displaced fracture of lower end of right humerus ◘

√7ᵗʰ S42.492 Other displaced fracture of lower end of left humerus ◘

√7ᵗʰ S42.493 Other displaced fracture of lower end of unspecified humerus ◘

√7ᵗʰ S42.494 Other nondisplaced fracture of lower end of right humerus ◘

√7ᵗʰ S42.495 Other nondisplaced fracture of lower end of left humerus ◘

√7ᵗʰ S42.496 Other nondisplaced fracture of lower end of unspecified humerus ◘

√5ᵗʰ S42.9 Fracture of shoulder girdle, part unspecified

Fracture of shoulder NOS

√x7ᵗʰ S42.90 Fracture of unspecified shoulder girdle, part unspecified ◘

√x7ᵗʰ S42.91 Fracture of right shoulder girdle, part unspecified ◘

√x7ᵗʰ S42.92 Fracture of left shoulder girdle, part unspecified ◘

✓4ᵗʰ **S43 Dislocation and sprain of joints and ligaments of shoulder girdle**

INCLUDES avulsion of joint or ligament of shoulder girdle
laceration of cartilage, joint or ligament of shoulder girdle
sprain of cartilage, joint or ligament of shoulder girdle
traumatic hemarthrosis of joint or ligament of shoulder girdle
traumatic rupture of joint or ligament of shoulder girdle
traumatic subluxation of joint or ligament of shoulder girdle
traumatic tear of joint or ligament of shoulder girdle

Code also any associated open wound

EXCLUDES 2 *strain of muscle, fascia and tendon of shoulder and upper arm (S46.-)*

> The appropriate 7th character is to be added to each code from category S43.
> A　initial encounter
> D　subsequent encounter
> S　sequela

✓5ᵗʰ **S43.0 Subluxation and dislocation of shoulder joint**

Dislocation of glenohumeral joint
Subluxation of glenohumeral joint

✓6ᵗʰ **S43.00 Unspecified subluxation and dislocation of shoulder joint**

Dislocation of humerus NOS
Subluxation of humerus NOS

✓7ᵗʰ **S43.001 Unspecified subluxation of right shoulder joint**

✓7ᵗʰ **S43.002 Unspecified subluxation of left shoulder joint**

✓7ᵗʰ **S43.003 Unspecified subluxation of unspecified shoulder joint**

✓7ᵗʰ **S43.004 Unspecified dislocation of right shoulder joint**

✓7ᵗʰ **S43.005 Unspecified dislocation of left shoulder joint**

✓7ᵗʰ **S43.006 Unspecified dislocation of unspecified shoulder joint**

✓6ᵗʰ **S43.01 Anterior subluxation and dislocation of humerus**

✓7ᵗʰ **S43.011 Anterior subluxation of right humerus**

✓7ᵗʰ **S43.012 Anterior subluxation of left humerus**

✓7ᵗʰ **S43.013 Anterior subluxation of unspecified humerus**

✓7ᵗʰ **S43.014 Anterior dislocation of right humerus**

✓7ᵗʰ **S43.015 Anterior dislocation of left humerus**

✓7ᵗʰ **S43.016 Anterior dislocation of unspecified humerus**

✓6ᵗʰ **S43.02 Posterior subluxation and dislocation of humerus**

✓7ᵗʰ **S43.021 Posterior subluxation of right humerus**

✓7ᵗʰ **S43.022 Posterior subluxation of left humerus**

✓7ᵗʰ **S43.023 Posterior subluxation of unspecified humerus**

✓7ᵗʰ **S43.024 Posterior dislocation of right humerus**

✓7ᵗʰ **S43.025 Posterior dislocation of left humerus**

✓7ᵗʰ **S43.026 Posterior dislocation of unspecified humerus**

✓6ᵗʰ **S43.03 Inferior subluxation and dislocation of humerus**

✓7ᵗʰ **S43.031 Inferior subluxation of right humerus**

✓7ᵗʰ **S43.032 Inferior subluxation of left humerus**

✓7ᵗʰ **S43.033 Inferior subluxation of unspecified humerus**

✓7ᵗʰ **S43.034 Inferior dislocation of right humerus**

✓7ᵗʰ **S43.035 Inferior dislocation of left humerus**

✓7ᵗʰ **S43.036 Inferior dislocation of unspecified humerus**

✓6ᵗʰ **S43.08 Other subluxation and dislocation of shoulder joint**

✓7ᵗʰ **S43.081 Other subluxation of right shoulder joint**

✓7ᵗʰ **S43.082 Other subluxation of left shoulder joint**

✓7ᵗʰ **S43.083 Other subluxation of unspecified shoulder joint**

✓7ᵗʰ **S43.084 Other dislocation of right shoulder joint**

✓7ᵗʰ **S43.085 Other dislocation of left shoulder joint**

✓7ᵗʰ **S43.086 Other dislocation of unspecified shoulder joint**

✓5ᵗʰ **S43.1 Subluxation and dislocation of acromioclavicular joint**

✓6ᵗʰ **S43.10 Unspecified dislocation of acromioclavicular joint**

✓7ᵗʰ **S43.101 Unspecified dislocation of right acromioclavicular joint**

✓7ᵗʰ **S43.102 Unspecified dislocation of left acromioclavicular joint**

✓7ᵗʰ **S43.109 Unspecified dislocation of unspecified acromioclavicular joint**

✓6ᵗʰ **S43.11 Subluxation of acromioclavicular joint**

✓7ᵗʰ **S43.111 Subluxation of right acromioclavicular joint**

✓7ᵗʰ **S43.112 Subluxation of left acromioclavicular joint**

✓7ᵗʰ **S43.119 Subluxation of unspecified acromioclavicular joint**

✓6ᵗʰ **S43.12 Dislocation of acromioclavicular joint, 100%-200% displacement**

✓7ᵗʰ **S43.121 Dislocation of right acromioclavicular joint, 100%-200% displacement**

✓7ᵗʰ **S43.122 Dislocation of left acromioclavicular joint, 100%-200% displacement**

✓7ᵗʰ **S43.129 Dislocation of unspecified acromioclavicular joint, 100%-200% displacement**

✓6ᵗʰ **S43.13 Dislocation of acromioclavicular joint, greater than 200% displacement**

✓7ᵗʰ **S43.131 Dislocation of right acromioclavicular joint, greater than 200% displacement**

✓7ᵗʰ **S43.132 Dislocation of left acromioclavicular joint, greater than 200% displacement**

✓7ᵗʰ **S43.139 Dislocation of unspecified acromioclavicular joint, greater than 200% displacement**

✓6ᵗʰ **S43.14 Inferior dislocation of acromioclavicular joint**

✓7ᵗʰ **S43.141 Inferior dislocation of right acromioclavicular joint**

✓7ᵗʰ **S43.142 Inferior dislocation of left acromioclavicular joint**

✓7ᵗʰ **S43.149 Inferior dislocation of unspecified acromioclavicular joint**

✓6ᵗʰ **S43.15 Posterior dislocation of acromioclavicular joint**

✓7ᵗʰ **S43.151 Posterior dislocation of right acromioclavicular joint**

✓7ᵗʰ **S43.152 Posterior dislocation of left acromioclavicular joint**

✓7ᵗʰ **S43.159 Posterior dislocation of unspecified acromioclavicular joint**

✓5ᵗʰ **S43.2 Subluxation and dislocation of sternoclavicular joint**

✓6ᵗʰ **S43.20 Unspecified subluxation and dislocation of sternoclavicular joint**

✓7ᵗʰ **S43.201 Unspecified subluxation of right sternoclavicular joint**

✓7ᵗʰ **S43.202 Unspecified subluxation of left sternoclavicular joint**

✓7ᵗʰ **S43.203 Unspecified subluxation of unspecified sternoclavicular joint**

✓7ᵗʰ **S43.204 Unspecified dislocation of right sternoclavicular joint**

✓7ᵗʰ **S43.205 Unspecified dislocation of left sternoclavicular joint**

✓7ᵗʰ **S43.206 Unspecified dislocation of unspecified sternoclavicular joint**

✓6ᵗʰ **S43.21 Anterior subluxation and dislocation of sternoclavicular joint**

✓7ᵗʰ **S43.211 Anterior subluxation of right sternoclavicular joint**

✓7ᵗʰ **S43.212 Anterior subluxation of left sternoclavicular joint**

✓7ᵗʰ **S43.213 Anterior subluxation of unspecified sternoclavicular joint**

✓7ᵗʰ **S43.214 Anterior dislocation of right sternoclavicular joint**

✓7ᵗʰ **S43.215 Anterior dislocation of left sternoclavicular joint**

✓7ᵗʰ **S43.216 Anterior dislocation of unspecified sternoclavicular joint**

✓6ᵗʰ **S43.22 Posterior subluxation and dislocation of sternoclavicular joint**

✓7ᵗʰ **S43.221 Posterior subluxation of right sternoclavicular joint**

✓7ᵗʰ **S43.222 Posterior subluxation of left sternoclavicular joint**

√7ᵗʰ **S43.223** Posterior subluxation of unspecified sternoclavicular joint

√7ᵗʰ **S43.224** Posterior dislocation of right sternoclavicular joint

√7ᵗʰ **S43.225** Posterior dislocation of left sternoclavicular joint

√7ᵗʰ **S43.226** Posterior dislocation of unspecified sternoclavicular joint

√5ᵗʰ **S43.3** Subluxation and dislocation of other and unspecified parts of shoulder girdle

√6ᵗʰ **S43.30** Subluxation and dislocation of unspecified parts of shoulder girdle

     Dislocation of shoulder girdle NOS
     Subluxation of shoulder girdle NOS

√7ᵗʰ **S43.301** Subluxation of unspecified parts of right shoulder girdle

√7ᵗʰ **S43.302** Subluxation of unspecified parts of left shoulder girdle

√7ᵗʰ **S43.303** Subluxation of unspecified parts of unspecified shoulder girdle

√7ᵗʰ **S43.304** Dislocation of unspecified parts of right shoulder girdle

√7ᵗʰ **S43.305** Dislocation of unspecified parts of left shoulder girdle

√7ᵗʰ **S43.306** Dislocation of unspecified parts of unspecified shoulder girdle

√6ᵗʰ **S43.31** Subluxation and dislocation of scapula

√7ᵗʰ **S43.311** Subluxation of right scapula

√7ᵗʰ **S43.312** Subluxation of left scapula

√7ᵗʰ **S43.313** Subluxation of unspecified scapula

√7ᵗʰ **S43.314** Dislocation of right scapula

√7ᵗʰ **S43.315** Dislocation of left scapula

√7ᵗʰ **S43.316** Dislocation of unspecified scapula

√6ᵗʰ **S43.39** Subluxation and dislocation of other parts of shoulder girdle

√7ᵗʰ **S43.391** Subluxation of other parts of right shoulder girdle

√7ᵗʰ **S43.392** Subluxation of other parts of left shoulder girdle

√7ᵗʰ **S43.393** Subluxation of other parts of unspecified shoulder girdle

√7ᵗʰ **S43.394** Dislocation of other parts of right shoulder girdle

√7ᵗʰ **S43.395** Dislocation of other parts of left shoulder girdle

√7ᵗʰ **S43.396** Dislocation of other parts of unspecified shoulder girdle

√5ᵗʰ **S43.4** Sprain of shoulder joint

√6ᵗʰ **S43.40** Unspecified sprain of shoulder joint

√7ᵗʰ **S43.401** Unspecified sprain of right shoulder joint

√7ᵗʰ **S43.402** Unspecified sprain of left shoulder joint

√7ᵗʰ **S43.409** Unspecified sprain of unspecified shoulder joint

√6ᵗʰ **S43.41** Sprain of coracohumeral (ligament)

√7ᵗʰ **S43.411** Sprain of right coracohumeral (ligament)

√7ᵗʰ **S43.412** Sprain of left coracohumeral (ligament)

√7ᵗʰ **S43.419** Sprain of unspecified coracohumeral (ligament)

√6ᵗʰ **S43.42** Sprain of rotator cuff capsule

     EXCLUDES 1   rotator cuff syndrome (complete) (incomplete), not specified as traumatic (M75.1-)
     EXCLUDES 2   injury of tendon of rotator cuff (S46.0-)

√7ᵗʰ **S43.421** Sprain of right rotator cuff capsule

√7ᵗʰ **S43.422** Sprain of left rotator cuff capsule

√7ᵗʰ **S43.429** Sprain of unspecified rotator cuff capsule

√6ᵗʰ **S43.43** Superior glenoid labrum lesion

     SLAP lesion
     AHA: 2019,2Q,26
     DEF: Detachment injury of the superior aspect of the glenoid labrum, which is the ring of fibrocartilage attached to the rim of the glenoid cavity of the scapula.

√7ᵗʰ **S43.431** Superior glenoid labrum lesion of right shoulder

√7ᵗʰ **S43.432** Superior glenoid labrum lesion of left shoulder

√7ᵗʰ **S43.439** Superior glenoid labrum lesion of unspecified shoulder

√6ᵗʰ **S43.49** Other sprain of shoulder joint

√7ᵗʰ **S43.491** Other sprain of right shoulder joint

√7ᵗʰ **S43.492** Other sprain of left shoulder joint

√7ᵗʰ **S43.499** Other sprain of unspecified shoulder joint

√5ᵗʰ **S43.5** Sprain of acromioclavicular joint

     Sprain of acromioclavicular ligament

√x7ᵗʰ **S43.50** Sprain of unspecified acromioclavicular joint

√x7ᵗʰ **S43.51** Sprain of right acromioclavicular joint

√x7ᵗʰ **S43.52** Sprain of left acromioclavicular joint

√5ᵗʰ **S43.6** Sprain of sternoclavicular joint

√x7ᵗʰ **S43.60** Sprain of unspecified sternoclavicular joint

√x7ᵗʰ **S43.61** Sprain of right sternoclavicular joint

√x7ᵗʰ **S43.62** Sprain of left sternoclavicular joint

√5ᵗʰ **S43.8** Sprain of other specified parts of shoulder girdle

√x7ᵗʰ **S43.80** Sprain of other specified parts of unspecified shoulder girdle

√x7ᵗʰ **S43.81** Sprain of other specified parts of right shoulder girdle

√x7ᵗʰ **S43.82** Sprain of other specified parts of left shoulder girdle

√5ᵗʰ **S43.9** Sprain of unspecified parts of shoulder girdle

√x7ᵗʰ **S43.90** Sprain of unspecified parts of unspecified shoulder girdle

     Sprain of shoulder girdle NOS

√x7ᵗʰ **S43.91** Sprain of unspecified parts of right shoulder girdle

√x7ᵗʰ **S43.92** Sprain of unspecified parts of left shoulder girdle

√4ᵗʰ **S44** **Injury of nerves at shoulder and upper arm level**

     Code also any associated open wound (S41.-)
     EXCLUDES 2   injury of brachial plexus (S14.3-)

     The appropriate 7th character is to be added to each code from category S44.
     A   initial encounter
     D   subsequent encounter
     S   sequela

√5ᵗʰ **S44.0** Injury of ulnar nerve at upper arm level

     EXCLUDES 1   ulnar nerve NOS (S54.0)

√x7ᵗʰ **S44.00** Injury of ulnar nerve at upper arm level, unspecified arm

√x7ᵗʰ **S44.01** Injury of ulnar nerve at upper arm level, right arm

√x7ᵗʰ **S44.02** Injury of ulnar nerve at upper arm level, left arm

√5ᵗʰ **S44.1** Injury of median nerve at upper arm level

     EXCLUDES 1   median nerve NOS (S54.1)

√x7ᵗʰ **S44.10** Injury of median nerve at upper arm level, unspecified arm

√x7ᵗʰ **S44.11** Injury of median nerve at upper arm level, right arm

√x7ᵗʰ **S44.12** Injury of median nerve at upper arm level, left arm

√5ᵗʰ **S44.2** Injury of radial nerve at upper arm level

     EXCLUDES 1   radial nerve NOS (S54.2)

√x7ᵗʰ **S44.20** Injury of radial nerve at upper arm level, unspecified arm

√x7ᵗʰ **S44.21** Injury of radial nerve at upper arm level, right arm

√x7ᵗʰ **S44.22** Injury of radial nerve at upper arm level, left arm

√5ᵗʰ **S44.3** Injury of axillary nerve

√x7ᵗʰ **S44.30** Injury of axillary nerve, unspecified arm

√x7ᵗʰ **S44.31** Injury of axillary nerve, right arm

√x7ᵗʰ **S44.32** Injury of axillary nerve, left arm

√5ᵗʰ **S44.4** Injury of musculocutaneous nerve

√x7ᵗʰ **S44.40** Injury of musculocutaneous nerve, unspecified arm

√x7ᵗʰ **S44.41** Injury of musculocutaneous nerve, right arm

√x7ᵗʰ **S44.42** Injury of musculocutaneous nerve, left arm

√5ᵗʰ **S44.5** Injury of cutaneous sensory nerve at shoulder and upper arm level

√x7ᵗʰ **S44.50** Injury of cutaneous sensory nerve at shoulder and upper arm level, unspecified arm

√x7ᵗʰ **S44.51** Injury of cutaneous sensory nerve at shoulder and upper arm level, right arm

√x7ᵗʰ **S44.52** Injury of cutaneous sensory nerve at shoulder and upper arm level, left arm

Chapter 19. Injury, Poisoning and Certain Other Consequences of External Causes

S44.8–S45.901

- ✓5ᵗʰ **S44.8** Injury of other nerves at shoulder and upper arm level
  - ✓6ᵗʰ **S44.8X** Injury of other nerves at shoulder and upper arm level
    - ✓7ᵗʰ **S44.8X1** Injury of other nerves at shoulder and upper arm level, right arm
    - ✓7ᵗʰ **S44.8X2** Injury of other nerves at shoulder and upper arm level, left arm
    - ✓7ᵗʰ **S44.8X9** Injury of other nerves at shoulder and upper arm level, unspecified arm
- ✓5ᵗʰ **S44.9** Injury of unspecified nerve at shoulder and upper arm level
  - ✓x7ᵗʰ **S44.90** Injury of unspecified nerve at shoulder and upper arm level, unspecified arm
  - ✓x7ᵗʰ **S44.91** Injury of unspecified nerve at shoulder and upper arm level, right arm
  - ✓x7ᵗʰ **S44.92** Injury of unspecified nerve at shoulder and upper arm level, left arm

- ✓4ᵗʰ **S45** **Injury of blood vessels at shoulder and upper arm level**

  Code also any associated open wound (S41.-)

  EXCLUDES 2   injury of subclavian artery (S25.1)
  injury of subclavian vein (S25.3)

  > The appropriate 7th character is to be added to each code from category S45.
  > A   initial encounter
  > D   subsequent encounter
  > S   sequela

  - ✓5ᵗʰ **S45.0** Injury of axillary artery
    - ✓6ᵗʰ **S45.00** Unspecified injury of axillary artery
      - ✓7ᵗʰ **S45.001** Unspecified injury of axillary artery, right side
      - ✓7ᵗʰ **S45.002** Unspecified injury of axillary artery, left side
      - ✓7ᵗʰ **S45.009** Unspecified injury of axillary artery, unspecified side
    - ✓6ᵗʰ **S45.01** Laceration of axillary artery
      - ✓7ᵗʰ **S45.011** Laceration of axillary artery, right side
      - ✓7ᵗʰ **S45.012** Laceration of axillary artery, left side
      - ✓7ᵗʰ **S45.019** Laceration of axillary artery, unspecified side
    - ✓6ᵗʰ **S45.09** Other specified injury of axillary artery
      - ✓7ᵗʰ **S45.091** Other specified injury of axillary artery, right side
      - ✓7ᵗʰ **S45.092** Other specified injury of axillary artery, left side
      - ✓7ᵗʰ **S45.099** Other specified injury of axillary artery, unspecified side
  - ✓5ᵗʰ **S45.1** Injury of brachial artery
    - ✓6ᵗʰ **S45.10** Unspecified injury of brachial artery
      - ✓7ᵗʰ **S45.101** Unspecified injury of brachial artery, right side
      - ✓7ᵗʰ **S45.102** Unspecified injury of brachial artery, left side
      - ✓7ᵗʰ **S45.109** Unspecified injury of brachial artery, unspecified side
    - ✓6ᵗʰ **S45.11** Laceration of brachial artery
      - ✓7ᵗʰ **S45.111** Laceration of brachial artery, right side
      - ✓7ᵗʰ **S45.112** Laceration of brachial artery, left side
      - ✓7ᵗʰ **S45.119** Laceration of brachial artery, unspecified side
    - ✓6ᵗʰ **S45.19** Other specified injury of brachial artery
      - ✓7ᵗʰ **S45.191** Other specified injury of brachial artery, right side
      - ✓7ᵗʰ **S45.192** Other specified injury of brachial artery, left side
      - ✓7ᵗʰ **S45.199** Other specified injury of brachial artery, unspecified side
  - ✓5ᵗʰ **S45.2** Injury of axillary or brachial vein
    - ✓6ᵗʰ **S45.20** Unspecified injury of axillary or brachial vein
      - ✓7ᵗʰ **S45.201** Unspecified injury of axillary or brachial vein, right side
      - ✓7ᵗʰ **S45.202** Unspecified injury of axillary or brachial vein, left side
      - ✓7ᵗʰ **S45.209** Unspecified injury of axillary or brachial vein, unspecified side
    - ✓6ᵗʰ **S45.21** Laceration of axillary or brachial vein
      - ✓7ᵗʰ **S45.211** Laceration of axillary or brachial vein, right side
      - ✓7ᵗʰ **S45.212** Laceration of axillary or brachial vein, left side
      - ✓7ᵗʰ **S45.219** Laceration of axillary or brachial vein, unspecified side
    - ✓6ᵗʰ **S45.29** Other specified injury of axillary or brachial vein
      - ✓7ᵗʰ **S45.291** Other specified injury of axillary or brachial vein, right side
      - ✓7ᵗʰ **S45.292** Other specified injury of axillary or brachial vein, left side
      - ✓7ᵗʰ **S45.299** Other specified injury of axillary or brachial vein, unspecified side
  - ✓5ᵗʰ **S45.3** Injury of superficial vein at shoulder and upper arm level
    - ✓6ᵗʰ **S45.30** Unspecified injury of superficial vein at shoulder and upper arm level
      - ✓7ᵗʰ **S45.301** Unspecified injury of superficial vein at shoulder and upper arm level, right arm
      - ✓7ᵗʰ **S45.302** Unspecified injury of superficial vein at shoulder and upper arm level, left arm
      - ✓7ᵗʰ **S45.309** Unspecified injury of superficial vein at shoulder and upper arm level, unspecified arm
    - ✓6ᵗʰ **S45.31** Laceration of superficial vein at shoulder and upper arm level
      - ✓7ᵗʰ **S45.311** Laceration of superficial vein at shoulder and upper arm level, right arm
      - ✓7ᵗʰ **S45.312** Laceration of superficial vein at shoulder and upper arm level, left arm
      - ✓7ᵗʰ **S45.319** Laceration of superficial vein at shoulder and upper arm level, unspecified arm
    - ✓6ᵗʰ **S45.39** Other specified injury of superficial vein at shoulder and upper arm level
      - ✓7ᵗʰ **S45.391** Other specified injury of superficial vein at shoulder and upper arm level, right arm
      - ✓7ᵗʰ **S45.392** Other specified injury of superficial vein at shoulder and upper arm level, left arm
      - ✓7ᵗʰ **S45.399** Other specified injury of superficial vein at shoulder and upper arm level, unspecified arm
  - ✓5ᵗʰ **S45.8** Injury of other specified blood vessels at shoulder and upper arm level
    - ✓6ᵗʰ **S45.80** Unspecified injury of other specified blood vessels at shoulder and upper arm level
      - ✓7ᵗʰ **S45.801** Unspecified injury of other specified blood vessels at shoulder and upper arm level, right arm
      - ✓7ᵗʰ **S45.802** Unspecified injury of other specified blood vessels at shoulder and upper arm level, left arm
      - ✓7ᵗʰ **S45.809** Unspecified injury of other specified blood vessels at shoulder and upper arm level, unspecified arm
    - ✓6ᵗʰ **S45.81** Laceration of other specified blood vessels at shoulder and upper arm level
      - ✓7ᵗʰ **S45.811** Laceration of other specified blood vessels at shoulder and upper arm level, right arm
      - ✓7ᵗʰ **S45.812** Laceration of other specified blood vessels at shoulder and upper arm level, left arm
      - ✓7ᵗʰ **S45.819** Laceration of other specified blood vessels at shoulder and upper arm level, unspecified arm
    - ✓6ᵗʰ **S45.89** Other specified injury of other specified blood vessels at shoulder and upper arm level
      - ✓7ᵗʰ **S45.891** Other specified injury of other specified blood vessels at shoulder and upper arm level, right arm
      - ✓7ᵗʰ **S45.892** Other specified injury of other specified blood vessels at shoulder and upper arm level, left arm
      - ✓7ᵗʰ **S45.899** Other specified injury of other specified blood vessels at shoulder and upper arm level, unspecified arm
  - ✓5ᵗʰ **S45.9** Injury of unspecified blood vessel at shoulder and upper arm level
    - ✓6ᵗʰ **S45.90** Unspecified injury of unspecified blood vessel at shoulder and upper arm level
      - ✓7ᵗʰ **S45.901** Unspecified injury of unspecified blood vessel at shoulder and upper arm level, right arm

HCC CMS-HCC   **Rx** Rx HCC   **ESR** ESRD HCC   **COM** Commercial HCC   **N** Newborn: 0   **P** Pediatric: 0-17   **M** Maternity: 9-64   **A** Adult: 15-124

1040

ICD-10-CM 2023

✓7ᵗʰ **S45.902** Unspecified injury of unspecified blood vessel at shoulder and upper arm level, left arm

✓7ᵗʰ **S45.909** Unspecified injury of unspecified blood vessel at shoulder and upper arm level, unspecified arm

✓6ᵗʰ **S45.91** Laceration of unspecified blood vessel at shoulder and upper arm level

✓7ᵗʰ **S45.911** Laceration of unspecified blood vessel at shoulder and upper arm level, right arm

✓7ᵗʰ **S45.912** Laceration of unspecified blood vessel at shoulder and upper arm level, left arm

✓7ᵗʰ **S45.919** Laceration of unspecified blood vessel at shoulder and upper arm level, unspecified arm

✓6ᵗʰ **S45.99** Other specified injury of unspecified blood vessel at shoulder and upper arm level

✓7ᵗʰ **S45.991** Other specified injury of unspecified blood vessel at shoulder and upper arm level, right arm

✓7ᵗʰ **S45.992** Other specified injury of unspecified blood vessel at shoulder and upper arm level, left arm

✓7ᵗʰ **S45.999** Other specified injury of unspecified blood vessel at shoulder and upper arm level, unspecified arm

✓4ᵗʰ **S46** Injury of muscle, fascia and tendon at shoulder and upper arm level

Code also any associated open wound (S41.-)

EXCLUDES 2 injury of muscle, fascia and tendon at elbow (S56.-)
sprain of joints and ligaments of shoulder girdle (S43.9)

TIP: Refer to the Muscle/Tendon table at the beginning of this chapter.

The appropriate 7th character is to be added to each code from category S46.
A initial encounter
D subsequent encounter
S sequela

✓5ᵗʰ **S46.0** Injury of muscle(s) and tendon(s) of the rotator cuff of shoulder

✓6ᵗʰ **S46.00** Unspecified injury of muscle(s) and tendon(s) of the rotator cuff of shoulder

✓7ᵗʰ **S46.001** Unspecified injury of muscle(s) and tendon(s) of the rotator cuff of right shoulder

✓7ᵗʰ **S46.002** Unspecified injury of muscle(s) and tendon(s) of the rotator cuff of left shoulder

✓7ᵗʰ **S46.009** Unspecified injury of muscle(s) and tendon(s) of the rotator cuff of unspecified shoulder

✓6ᵗʰ **S46.01** Strain of muscle(s) and tendon(s) of the rotator cuff of shoulder

✓7ᵗʰ **S46.011** Strain of muscle(s) and tendon(s) of the rotator cuff of right shoulder

✓7ᵗʰ **S46.012** Strain of muscle(s) and tendon(s) of the rotator cuff of left shoulder

✓7ᵗʰ **S46.019** Strain of muscle(s) and tendon(s) of the rotator cuff of unspecified shoulder

✓6ᵗʰ **S46.02** Laceration of muscle(s) and tendon(s) of the rotator cuff of shoulder

✓7ᵗʰ **S46.021** Laceration of muscle(s) and tendon(s) of the rotator cuff of right shoulder

✓7ᵗʰ **S46.022** Laceration of muscle(s) and tendon(s) of the rotator cuff of left shoulder

✓7ᵗʰ **S46.029** Laceration of muscle(s) and tendon(s) of the rotator cuff of unspecified shoulder

✓6ᵗʰ **S46.09** Other injury of muscle(s) and tendon(s) of the rotator cuff of shoulder

✓7ᵗʰ **S46.091** Other injury of muscle(s) and tendon(s) of the rotator cuff of right shoulder

✓7ᵗʰ **S46.092** Other injury of muscle(s) and tendon(s) of the rotator cuff of left shoulder

✓7ᵗʰ **S46.099** Other injury of muscle(s) and tendon(s) of the rotator cuff of unspecified shoulder

✓5ᵗʰ **S46.1** Injury of muscle, fascia and tendon of long head of biceps

✓6ᵗʰ **S46.10** Unspecified injury of muscle, fascia and tendon of long head of biceps

✓7ᵗʰ **S46.101** Unspecified injury of muscle, fascia and tendon of long head of biceps, right arm

✓7ᵗʰ **S46.102** Unspecified injury of muscle, fascia and tendon of long head of biceps, left arm

✓7ᵗʰ **S46.109** Unspecified injury of muscle, fascia and tendon of long head of biceps, unspecified arm

✓6ᵗʰ **S46.11** Strain of muscle, fascia and tendon of long head of biceps

AHA: 2020,1Q,38; 2019,2Q,27

✓7ᵗʰ **S46.111** Strain of muscle, fascia and tendon of long head of biceps, right arm

✓7ᵗʰ **S46.112** Strain of muscle, fascia and tendon of long head of biceps, left arm

✓7ᵗʰ **S46.119** Strain of muscle, fascia and tendon of long head of biceps, unspecified arm

✓6ᵗʰ **S46.12** Laceration of muscle, fascia and tendon of long head of biceps

✓7ᵗʰ **S46.121** Laceration of muscle, fascia and tendon of long head of biceps, right arm

✓7ᵗʰ **S46.122** Laceration of muscle, fascia and tendon of long head of biceps, left arm

✓7ᵗʰ **S46.129** Laceration of muscle, fascia and tendon of long head of biceps, unspecified arm

✓6ᵗʰ **S46.19** Other injury of muscle, fascia and tendon of long head of biceps

✓7ᵗʰ **S46.191** Other injury of muscle, fascia and tendon of long head of biceps, right arm

✓7ᵗʰ **S46.192** Other injury of muscle, fascia and tendon of long head of biceps, left arm

✓7ᵗʰ **S46.199** Other injury of muscle, fascia and tendon of long head of biceps, unspecified arm

✓5ᵗʰ **S46.2** Injury of muscle, fascia and tendon of other parts of biceps

✓6ᵗʰ **S46.20** Unspecified injury of muscle, fascia and tendon of other parts of biceps

✓7ᵗʰ **S46.201** Unspecified injury of muscle, fascia and tendon of other parts of biceps, right arm

✓7ᵗʰ **S46.202** Unspecified injury of muscle, fascia and tendon of other parts of biceps, left arm

✓7ᵗʰ **S46.209** Unspecified injury of muscle, fascia and tendon of other parts of biceps, unspecified arm

✓6ᵗʰ **S46.21** Strain of muscle, fascia and tendon of other parts of biceps

✓7ᵗʰ **S46.211** Strain of muscle, fascia and tendon of other parts of biceps, right arm

✓7ᵗʰ **S46.212** Strain of muscle, fascia and tendon of other parts of biceps, left arm

✓7ᵗʰ **S46.219** Strain of muscle, fascia and tendon of other parts of biceps, unspecified arm

✓6ᵗʰ **S46.22** Laceration of muscle, fascia and tendon of other parts of biceps

✓7ᵗʰ **S46.221** Laceration of muscle, fascia and tendon of other parts of biceps, right arm

✓7ᵗʰ **S46.222** Laceration of muscle, fascia and tendon of other parts of biceps, left arm

✓7ᵗʰ **S46.229** Laceration of muscle, fascia and tendon of other parts of biceps, unspecified arm

✓6ᵗʰ **S46.29** Other injury of muscle, fascia and tendon of other parts of biceps

✓7ᵗʰ **S46.291** Other injury of muscle, fascia and tendon of other parts of biceps, right arm

✓7ᵗʰ **S46.292** Other injury of muscle, fascia and tendon of other parts of biceps, left arm

✓7ᵗʰ **S46.299** Other injury of muscle, fascia and tendon of other parts of biceps, unspecified arm

✓5ᵗʰ **S46.3** Injury of muscle, fascia and tendon of triceps

✓6ᵗʰ **S46.30** Unspecified injury of muscle, fascia and tendon of triceps

✓7ᵗʰ **S46.301** Unspecified injury of muscle, fascia and tendon of triceps, right arm

✓7ᵗʰ **S46.302** Unspecified injury of muscle, fascia and tendon of triceps, left arm

✓7ᵗʰ **S46.309** Unspecified injury of muscle, fascia and tendon of triceps, unspecified arm

✓6ᵗʰ **S46.31** Strain of muscle, fascia and tendon of triceps

✓7ᵗʰ **S46.311** Strain of muscle, fascia and tendon of triceps, right arm

✓7ᵗʰ **S46.312** Strain of muscle, fascia and tendon of triceps, left arm

✓7ᵗʰ **S46.319** Strain of muscle, fascia and tendon of triceps, unspecified arm

✓6ᵗʰ **S46.32** Laceration of muscle, fascia and tendon of triceps

✓7ᵗʰ **S46.321** Laceration of muscle, fascia and tendon of triceps, right arm

√7th **S46.322** Laceration of muscle, fascia and tendon of triceps, left arm

√7th **S46.329** Laceration of muscle, fascia and tendon of triceps, unspecified arm

√6th **S46.39** Other injury of muscle, fascia and tendon of triceps

√7th **S46.391** Other injury of muscle, fascia and tendon of triceps, right arm

√7th **S46.392** Other injury of muscle, fascia and tendon of triceps, left arm

√7th **S46.399** Other injury of muscle, fascia and tendon of triceps, unspecified arm

√5th **S46.8** Injury of other muscles, fascia and tendons at shoulder and upper arm level

√6th **S46.80** Unspecified injury of other muscles, fascia and tendons at shoulder and upper arm level

√7th **S46.801** Unspecified injury of other muscles, fascia and tendons at shoulder and upper arm level, right arm

√7th **S46.802** Unspecified injury of other muscles, fascia and tendons at shoulder and upper arm level, left arm

√7th **S46.809** Unspecified injury of other muscles, fascia and tendons at shoulder and upper arm level, unspecified arm

√6th **S46.81** Strain of other muscles, fascia and tendons at shoulder and upper arm level

√7th **S46.811** Strain of other muscles, fascia and tendons at shoulder and upper arm level, right arm

√7th **S46.812** Strain of other muscles, fascia and tendons at shoulder and upper arm level, left arm

√7th **S46.819** Strain of other muscles, fascia and tendons at shoulder and upper arm level, unspecified arm

√6th **S46.82** Laceration of other muscles, fascia and tendons at shoulder and upper arm level

√7th **S46.821** Laceration of other muscles, fascia and tendons at shoulder and upper arm level, right arm

√7th **S46.822** Laceration of other muscles, fascia and tendons at shoulder and upper arm level, left arm

√7th **S46.829** Laceration of other muscles, fascia and tendons at shoulder and upper arm level, unspecified arm

√6th **S46.89** Other injury of other muscles, fascia and tendons at shoulder and upper arm level

√7th **S46.891** Other injury of other muscles, fascia and tendons at shoulder and upper arm level, right arm

√7th **S46.892** Other injury of other muscles, fascia and tendons at shoulder and upper arm level, left arm

√7th **S46.899** Other injury of other muscles, fascia and tendons at shoulder and upper arm level, unspecified arm

√5th **S46.9** Injury of unspecified muscle, fascia and tendon at shoulder and upper arm level

√6th **S46.90** Unspecified injury of unspecified muscle, fascia and tendon at shoulder and upper arm level

√7th **S46.901** Unspecified injury of unspecified muscle, fascia and tendon at shoulder and upper arm level, right arm

√7th **S46.902** Unspecified injury of unspecified muscle, fascia and tendon at shoulder and upper arm level, left arm

√7th **S46.909** Unspecified injury of unspecified muscle, fascia and tendon at shoulder and upper arm level, unspecified arm

√6th **S46.91** Strain of unspecified muscle, fascia and tendon at shoulder and upper arm level

√7th **S46.911** Strain of unspecified muscle, fascia and tendon at shoulder and upper arm level, right arm

√7th **S46.912** Strain of unspecified muscle, fascia and tendon at shoulder and upper arm level, left arm

√7th **S46.919** Strain of unspecified muscle, fascia and tendon at shoulder and upper arm level, unspecified arm

√6th **S46.92** Laceration of unspecified muscle, fascia and tendon at shoulder and upper arm level

√7th **S46.921** Laceration of unspecified muscle, fascia and tendon at shoulder and upper arm level, right arm

√7th **S46.922** Laceration of unspecified muscle, fascia and tendon at shoulder and upper arm level, left arm

√7th **S46.929** Laceration of unspecified muscle, fascia and tendon at shoulder and upper arm level, unspecified arm

√6th **S46.99** Other injury of unspecified muscle, fascia and tendon at shoulder and upper arm level

√7th **S46.991** Other injury of unspecified muscle, fascia and tendon at shoulder and upper arm level, right arm

√7th **S46.992** Other injury of unspecified muscle, fascia and tendon at shoulder and upper arm level, left arm

√7th **S46.999** Other injury of unspecified muscle, fascia and tendon at shoulder and upper arm level, unspecified arm

√4th **S47** **Crushing injury of shoulder and upper arm**

Use additional code for all associated injuries

EXCLUDES 2　crushing injury of elbow (S57.0-)

The appropriate 7th character is to be added to each code from category S47.
A　initial encounter
D　subsequent encounter
S　sequela

√x7th **S47.1** Crushing injury of right shoulder and upper arm

√x7th **S47.2** Crushing injury of left shoulder and upper arm

√x7th **S47.9** Crushing injury of shoulder and upper arm, unspecified arm

√4th **S48** **Traumatic amputation of shoulder and upper arm**

An amputation not identified as partial or complete should be coded to complete

EXCLUDES 1　traumatic amputation at elbow level (S58.0)

The appropriate 7th character is to be added to each code from category S48.
A　initial encounter
D　subsequent encounter
S　sequela

√5th **S48.0** Traumatic amputation at shoulder joint

√6th **S48.01** Complete traumatic amputation at shoulder joint

² √7th **S48.011** Complete traumatic amputation at right shoulder joint　HCC ESR COM

² √7th **S48.012** Complete traumatic amputation at left shoulder joint　HCC ESR COM

² √7th **S48.019** Complete traumatic amputation at unspecified shoulder joint　HCC ESR COM

√6th **S48.02** Partial traumatic amputation at shoulder joint

² √7th **S48.021** Partial traumatic amputation at right shoulder joint　HCC ESR COM

² √7th **S48.022** Partial traumatic amputation at left shoulder joint　HCC ESR COM

² √7th **S48.029** Partial traumatic amputation at unspecified shoulder joint　HCC ESR COM

√5th **S48.1** Traumatic amputation at level between shoulder and elbow

√6th **S48.11** Complete traumatic amputation at level between shoulder and elbow

² √7th **S48.111** Complete traumatic amputation at level between right shoulder and elbow　HCC ESR COM

² √7th **S48.112** Complete traumatic amputation at level between left shoulder and elbow　HCC ESR COM

² √7th **S48.119** Complete traumatic amputation at level between unspecified shoulder and elbow　HCC ESR COM

√6th **S48.12** Partial traumatic amputation at level between shoulder and elbow

² √7th **S48.121** Partial traumatic amputation at level between right shoulder and elbow　HCC ESR COM

² √7th **S48.122** Partial traumatic amputation at level between left shoulder and elbow　HCC ESR COM

² ✓7ᵗʰ **S48.129** Partial traumatic amputation at level between unspecified shoulder and elbow   `HCC` `ESR` `COM`

✓5ᵗʰ **S48.9** Traumatic amputation of shoulder and upper arm, level unspecified

  ✓6ᵗʰ **S48.91** Complete traumatic amputation of shoulder and upper arm, level unspecified

    ² ✓7ᵗʰ **S48.911** Complete traumatic amputation of right shoulder and upper arm, level unspecified   `HCC` `ESR` `COM`

    ² ✓7ᵗʰ **S48.912** Complete traumatic amputation of left shoulder and upper arm, level unspecified   `HCC` `ESR` `COM`

    ² ✓7ᵗʰ **S48.919** Complete traumatic amputation of unspecified shoulder and upper arm, level unspecified   `HCC` `ESR` `COM`

  ✓6ᵗʰ **S48.92** Partial traumatic amputation of shoulder and upper arm, level unspecified

    ² ✓7ᵗʰ **S48.921** Partial traumatic amputation of right shoulder and upper arm, level unspecified   `HCC` `ESR` `COM`

    ² ✓7ᵗʰ **S48.922** Partial traumatic amputation of left shoulder and upper arm, level unspecified   `HCC` `ESR` `COM`

    ² ✓7ᵗʰ **S48.929** Partial traumatic amputation of unspecified shoulder and upper arm, level unspecified   `HCC` `ESR` `COM`

✓4ᵗʰ **S49** Other and unspecified injuries of shoulder and upper arm

  AHA: 2018,2Q,12; 2018,1Q,3

> The appropriate 7th character is to be added to each code from subcategories S49.0 and S49.1.
> A   initial encounter for closed fracture
> D   subsequent encounter for fracture with routine healing
> G   subsequent encounter for fracture with delayed healing
> K   subsequent encounter for fracture with nonunion
> P   subsequent encounter for fracture with malunion
> S   sequela

✓5ᵗʰ **S49.0** Physeal fracture of upper end of humerus

  AHA: 2019,4Q,56

  ✓6ᵗʰ **S49.00** Unspecified physeal fracture of upper end of humerus

    ✓7ᵗʰ **S49.001** Unspecified physeal fracture of upper end of humerus, right arm   `Q`

    ✓7ᵗʰ **S49.002** Unspecified physeal fracture of upper end of humerus, left arm   `Q`

    ✓7ᵗʰ **S49.009** Unspecified physeal fracture of upper end of humerus, unspecified arm   `Q`

  ✓6ᵗʰ **S49.01** Salter-Harris Type I physeal fracture of upper end of humerus

    ✓7ᵗʰ **S49.011** Salter-Harris Type I physeal fracture of upper end of humerus, right arm   `Q`

    ✓7ᵗʰ **S49.012** Salter-Harris Type I physeal fracture of upper end of humerus, left arm   `Q`

    ✓7ᵗʰ **S49.019** Salter-Harris Type I physeal fracture of upper end of humerus, unspecified arm   `Q`

  ✓6ᵗʰ **S49.02** Salter-Harris Type II physeal fracture of upper end of humerus

    ✓7ᵗʰ **S49.021** Salter-Harris Type II physeal fracture of upper end of humerus, right arm   `Q`

    ✓7ᵗʰ **S49.022** Salter-Harris Type II physeal fracture of upper end of humerus, left arm   `Q`

    ✓7ᵗʰ **S49.029** Salter-Harris Type II physeal fracture of upper end of humerus, unspecified arm   `Q`

  ✓6ᵗʰ **S49.03** Salter-Harris Type III physeal fracture of upper end of humerus

    ✓7ᵗʰ **S49.031** Salter-Harris Type III physeal fracture of upper end of humerus, right arm   `Q`

    ✓7ᵗʰ **S49.032** Salter-Harris Type III physeal fracture of upper end of humerus, left arm   `Q`

    ✓7ᵗʰ **S49.039** Salter-Harris Type III physeal fracture of upper end of humerus, unspecified arm   `Q`

  ✓6ᵗʰ **S49.04** Salter-Harris Type IV physeal fracture of upper end of humerus

    ✓7ᵗʰ **S49.041** Salter-Harris Type IV physeal fracture of upper end of humerus, right arm   `Q`

    ✓7ᵗʰ **S49.042** Salter-Harris Type IV physeal fracture of upper end of humerus, left arm   `Q`

    ✓7ᵗʰ **S49.049** Salter-Harris Type IV physeal fracture of upper end of humerus, unspecified arm   `Q`

  ✓6ᵗʰ **S49.09** Other physeal fracture of upper end of humerus

    ✓7ᵗʰ **S49.091** Other physeal fracture of upper end of humerus, right arm   `Q`

    ✓7ᵗʰ **S49.092** Other physeal fracture of upper end of humerus, left arm   `Q`

    ✓7ᵗʰ **S49.099** Other physeal fracture of upper end of humerus, unspecified arm   `Q`

✓5ᵗʰ **S49.1** Physeal fracture of lower end of humerus

  AHA: 2019,4Q,56

  ✓6ᵗʰ **S49.10** Unspecified physeal fracture of lower end of humerus

    ✓7ᵗʰ **S49.101** Unspecified physeal fracture of lower end of humerus, right arm   `Q`

    ✓7ᵗʰ **S49.102** Unspecified physeal fracture of lower end of humerus, left arm   `Q`

    ✓7ᵗʰ **S49.109** Unspecified physeal fracture of lower end of humerus, unspecified arm   `Q`

  ✓6ᵗʰ **S49.11** Salter-Harris Type I physeal fracture of lower end of humerus

    ✓7ᵗʰ **S49.111** Salter-Harris Type I physeal fracture of lower end of humerus, right arm   `Q`

    ✓7ᵗʰ **S49.112** Salter-Harris Type I physeal fracture of lower end of humerus, left arm   `Q`

    ✓7ᵗʰ **S49.119** Salter-Harris Type I physeal fracture of lower end of humerus, unspecified arm   `Q`

  ✓6ᵗʰ **S49.12** Salter-Harris Type II physeal fracture of lower end of humerus

    ✓7ᵗʰ **S49.121** Salter-Harris Type II physeal fracture of lower end of humerus, right arm   `Q`

    ✓7ᵗʰ **S49.122** Salter-Harris Type II physeal fracture of lower end of humerus, left arm   `Q`

    ✓7ᵗʰ **S49.129** Salter-Harris Type II physeal fracture of lower end of humerus, unspecified arm   `Q`

  ✓6ᵗʰ **S49.13** Salter-Harris Type III physeal fracture of lower end of humerus

    ✓7ᵗʰ **S49.131** Salter-Harris Type III physeal fracture of lower end of humerus, right arm   `Q`

    ✓7ᵗʰ **S49.132** Salter-Harris Type III physeal fracture of lower end of humerus, left arm   `Q`

    ✓7ᵗʰ **S49.139** Salter-Harris Type III physeal fracture of lower end of humerus, unspecified arm   `Q`

  ✓6ᵗʰ **S49.14** Salter-Harris Type IV physeal fracture of lower end of humerus

    ✓7ᵗʰ **S49.141** Salter-Harris Type IV physeal fracture of lower end of humerus, right arm   `Q`

    ✓7ᵗʰ **S49.142** Salter-Harris Type IV physeal fracture of lower end of humerus, left arm   `Q`

    ✓7ᵗʰ **S49.149** Salter-Harris Type IV physeal fracture of lower end of humerus, unspecified arm   `Q`

  ✓6ᵗʰ **S49.19** Other physeal fracture of lower end of humerus

    ✓7ᵗʰ **S49.191** Other physeal fracture of lower end of humerus, right arm   `Q`

    ✓7ᵗʰ **S49.192** Other physeal fracture of lower end of humerus, left arm   `Q`

    ✓7ᵗʰ **S49.199** Other physeal fracture of lower end of humerus, unspecified arm   `Q`

✓5ᵗʰ **S49.8** Other specified injuries of shoulder and upper arm

> The appropriate 7th character is to be added to each code in subcategory S49.8.
> A   initial encounter
> D   subsequent encounter
> S   sequela

  ✓×7ᵗʰ **S49.80** Other specified injuries of shoulder and upper arm, unspecified arm

  ✓×7ᵗʰ **S49.81** Other specified injuries of right shoulder and upper arm

  ✓×7ᵗʰ **S49.82** Other specified injuries of left shoulder and upper arm

☑5ᵗʰ S49.9 Unspecified injury of shoulder and upper arm

The appropriate 7th character is to be added to each code in subcategory S49.9.
A   initial encounter
D   subsequent encounter
S   sequela

☑x7ᵗʰ **S49.90** Unspecified injury of shoulder and upper arm, unspecified arm
☑x7ᵗʰ **S49.91** Unspecified injury of right shoulder and upper arm
☑x7ᵗʰ **S49.92** Unspecified injury of left shoulder and upper arm

Injuries to the elbow and forearm (S50-S59)

EXCLUDES 2   burns and corrosions (T20-T32)
frostbite (T33-T34)
injuries of wrist and hand (S60-S69)
insect bite or sting, venomous (T63.4)

☑4ᵗʰ S50 Superficial injury of elbow and forearm

EXCLUDES 2   superficial injury of wrist and hand (S60.-)

The appropriate 7th character is to be added to each code from category S50.
A   initial encounter
D   subsequent encounter
S   sequela

☑5ᵗʰ S50.0 Contusion of elbow
☑x7ᵗʰ **S50.00** Contusion of unspecified elbow
☑x7ᵗʰ **S50.01** Contusion of right elbow
☑x7ᵗʰ **S50.02** Contusion of left elbow

☑5ᵗʰ S50.1 Contusion of forearm
☑x7ᵗʰ **S50.10** Contusion of unspecified forearm
☑x7ᵗʰ **S50.11** Contusion of right forearm
☑x7ᵗʰ **S50.12** Contusion of left forearm

☑5ᵗʰ S50.3 Other superficial injuries of elbow
☑6ᵗʰ **S50.31** Abrasion of elbow
☑7ᵗʰ **S50.311** Abrasion of right elbow
☑7ᵗʰ **S50.312** Abrasion of left elbow
☑7ᵗʰ **S50.319** Abrasion of unspecified elbow
☑6ᵗʰ **S50.32** Blister (nonthermal) of elbow
☑7ᵗʰ **S50.321** Blister (nonthermal) of right elbow
☑7ᵗʰ **S50.322** Blister (nonthermal) of left elbow
☑7ᵗʰ **S50.329** Blister (nonthermal) of unspecified elbow
☑6ᵗʰ **S50.34** External constriction of elbow
☑7ᵗʰ **S50.341** External constriction of right elbow
☑7ᵗʰ **S50.342** External constriction of left elbow
☑7ᵗʰ **S50.349** External constriction of unspecified elbow
☑6ᵗʰ **S50.35** Superficial foreign body of elbow
Splinter in the elbow
☑7ᵗʰ **S50.351** Superficial foreign body of right elbow
☑7ᵗʰ **S50.352** Superficial foreign body of left elbow
☑7ᵗʰ **S50.359** Superficial foreign body of unspecified elbow
☑6ᵗʰ **S50.36** Insect bite (nonvenomous) of elbow
☑7ᵗʰ **S50.361** Insect bite (nonvenomous) of right elbow
☑7ᵗʰ **S50.362** Insect bite (nonvenomous) of left elbow
☑7ᵗʰ **S50.369** Insect bite (nonvenomous) of unspecified elbow
☑6ᵗʰ **S50.37** Other superficial bite of elbow
EXCLUDES 1   open bite of elbow (S51.05)
☑7ᵗʰ **S50.371** Other superficial bite of right elbow
☑7ᵗʰ **S50.372** Other superficial bite of left elbow
☑7ᵗʰ **S50.379** Other superficial bite of unspecified elbow

☑5ᵗʰ S50.8 Other superficial injuries of forearm
☑6ᵗʰ **S50.81** Abrasion of forearm
☑7ᵗʰ **S50.811** Abrasion of right forearm
☑7ᵗʰ **S50.812** Abrasion of left forearm
☑7ᵗʰ **S50.819** Abrasion of unspecified forearm
☑6ᵗʰ **S50.82** Blister (nonthermal) of forearm
☑7ᵗʰ **S50.821** Blister (nonthermal) of right forearm

☑7ᵗʰ **S50.822** Blister (nonthermal) of left forearm
☑7ᵗʰ **S50.829** Blister (nonthermal) of unspecified forearm
☑6ᵗʰ **S50.84** External constriction of forearm
☑7ᵗʰ **S50.841** External constriction of right forearm
☑7ᵗʰ **S50.842** External constriction of left forearm
☑7ᵗʰ **S50.849** External constriction of unspecified forearm
☑6ᵗʰ **S50.85** Superficial foreign body of forearm
Splinter in the forearm
☑7ᵗʰ **S50.851** Superficial foreign body of right forearm
☑7ᵗʰ **S50.852** Superficial foreign body of left forearm
☑7ᵗʰ **S50.859** Superficial foreign body of unspecified forearm
☑6ᵗʰ **S50.86** Insect bite (nonvenomous) of forearm
☑7ᵗʰ **S50.861** Insect bite (nonvenomous) of right forearm
☑7ᵗʰ **S50.862** Insect bite (nonvenomous) of left forearm
☑7ᵗʰ **S50.869** Insect bite (nonvenomous) of unspecified forearm
☑6ᵗʰ **S50.87** Other superficial bite of forearm
EXCLUDES 1   open bite of forearm (S51.85)
☑7ᵗʰ **S50.871** Other superficial bite of right forearm
☑7ᵗʰ **S50.872** Other superficial bite of left forearm
☑7ᵗʰ **S50.879** Other superficial bite of unspecified forearm

☑5ᵗʰ S50.9 Unspecified superficial injury of elbow and forearm
☑6ᵗʰ **S50.90** Unspecified superficial injury of elbow
☑7ᵗʰ **S50.901** Unspecified superficial injury of right elbow
☑7ᵗʰ **S50.902** Unspecified superficial injury of left elbow
☑7ᵗʰ **S50.909** Unspecified superficial injury of unspecified elbow
☑6ᵗʰ **S50.91** Unspecified superficial injury of forearm
☑7ᵗʰ **S50.911** Unspecified superficial injury of right forearm
☑7ᵗʰ **S50.912** Unspecified superficial injury of left forearm
☑7ᵗʰ **S50.919** Unspecified superficial injury of unspecified forearm

☑4ᵗʰ S51 Open wound of elbow and forearm
Code also any associated wound infection
EXCLUDES 1   open fracture of elbow and forearm (S52.- with open fracture 7th character)
traumatic amputation of elbow and forearm (S58.-)
EXCLUDES 2   open wound of wrist and hand (S61.-)

The appropriate 7th character is to be added to each code from category S51.
A   initial encounter
D   subsequent encounter
S   sequela

☑5ᵗʰ S51.0 Open wound of elbow
☑6ᵗʰ **S51.00** Unspecified open wound of elbow
☑7ᵗʰ **S51.001** Unspecified open wound of right elbow
AHA: 2012,4Q,108
☑7ᵗʰ **S51.002** Unspecified open wound of left elbow
☑7ᵗʰ **S51.009** Unspecified open wound of unspecified elbow
Open wound of elbow NOS
☑6ᵗʰ **S51.01** Laceration without foreign body of elbow
☑7ᵗʰ **S51.011** Laceration without foreign body of right elbow
☑7ᵗʰ **S51.012** Laceration without foreign body of left elbow
☑7ᵗʰ **S51.019** Laceration without foreign body of unspecified elbow
☑6ᵗʰ **S51.02** Laceration with foreign body of elbow
☑7ᵗʰ **S51.021** Laceration with foreign body of right elbow
☑7ᵗʰ **S51.022** Laceration with foreign body of left elbow
☑7ᵗʰ **S51.029** Laceration with foreign body of unspecified elbow

☑6ᵗʰ **S51.Ø3** Puncture wound without foreign body **of elbow**

     ☑7ᵗʰ **S51.Ø31** Puncture wound without foreign body of right **elbow**

     ☑7ᵗʰ **S51.Ø32** Puncture wound without foreign body of left **elbow**

     ☑7ᵗʰ **S51.Ø39** Puncture wound without foreign body of unspecified **elbow**

☑6ᵗʰ **S51.Ø4** Puncture wound with foreign body **of elbow**

     ☑7ᵗʰ **S51.Ø41** Puncture wound with foreign body of right **elbow**

     ☑7ᵗʰ **S51.Ø42** Puncture wound with foreign body of left **elbow**

     ☑7ᵗʰ **S51.Ø49** Puncture wound with foreign body of unspecified **elbow**

☑6ᵗʰ **S51.Ø5** Open bite **of elbow**

     Bite of elbow NOS

        EXCLUDES 1   superficial bite of elbow (S5Ø.36, S5Ø.37)

     ☑7ᵗʰ **S51.Ø51** Open bite, right **elbow**

     ☑7ᵗʰ **S51.Ø52** Open bite, left **elbow**

     ☑7ᵗʰ **S51.Ø59** Open bite, unspecified **elbow**

☑5ᵗʰ **S51.8** **Open wound of** forearm

     EXCLUDES 2   open wound of elbow (S51.Ø-)

☑6ᵗʰ **S51.8Ø** **Unspecified open wound of forearm**

     AHA: 2016,3Q,24

     ☑7ᵗʰ **S51.8Ø1** Unspecified open wound of right **forearm**

     ☑7ᵗʰ **S51.8Ø2** Unspecified open wound of left **forearm**

     ☑7ᵗʰ **S51.8Ø9** Unspecified open wound of unspecified **forearm**

        Open wound of forearm NOS

☑6ᵗʰ **S51.81** Laceration without foreign body **of forearm**

     ☑7ᵗʰ **S51.811** Laceration without foreign body of right **forearm**

     ☑7ᵗʰ **S51.812** Laceration without foreign body of left **forearm**

     ☑7ᵗʰ **S51.819** Laceration without foreign body of unspecified **forearm**

☑6ᵗʰ **S51.82** Laceration with foreign body **of forearm**

     ☑7ᵗʰ **S51.821** Laceration with foreign body of right **forearm**

     ☑7ᵗʰ **S51.822** Laceration with foreign body of left **forearm**

     ☑7ᵗʰ **S51.829** Laceration with foreign body of unspecified **forearm**

☑6ᵗʰ **S51.83** Puncture wound without foreign body **of forearm**

     AHA: 2016,3Q,24

     ☑7ᵗʰ **S51.831** Puncture wound without foreign body of right **forearm**

     ☑7ᵗʰ **S51.832** Puncture wound without foreign body of left **forearm**

     ☑7ᵗʰ **S51.839** Puncture wound without foreign body of unspecified **forearm**

☑6ᵗʰ **S51.84** Puncture wound with foreign body **of forearm**

     AHA: 2016,3Q,24

     ☑7ᵗʰ **S51.841** Puncture wound with foreign body of right **forearm**

     ☑7ᵗʰ **S51.842** Puncture wound with foreign body of left **forearm**

     ☑7ᵗʰ **S51.849** Puncture wound with foreign body of unspecified **forearm**

☑6ᵗʰ **S51.85** Open bite **of forearm**

     Bite of forearm NOS

        EXCLUDES 1   superficial bite of forearm (S5Ø.86, S5Ø.87)

     ☑7ᵗʰ **S51.851** Open bite of right **forearm**

     ☑7ᵗʰ **S51.852** Open bite of left **forearm**

     ☑7ᵗʰ **S51.859** Open bite of unspecified **forearm**

☑4ᵗʰ **S52** **Fracture of forearm**

     NOTE   A fracture not indicated as displaced or nondisplaced should be coded to displaced.

        A fracture not indicated as open or closed should be coded to closed.

        The open fracture designations are based on the Gustilo open fracture classification.

     EXCLUDES 1   traumatic amputation of forearm (S58.-)

     EXCLUDES 2   fracture at wrist and hand level (S62.-)

     AHA: 2018,2Q,12; 2016,1Q,33; 2015,3Q,37-39

     DEF: Diaphysis: Central shaft of a long bone.

     DEF: Epiphysis: Proximal and distal rounded ends of a long bone, communicates with the joint.

     DEF: Metaphysis: Section of a long bone located between the epiphysis and diaphysis at the proximal and distal ends.

     DEF: Physis (growth plate): Narrow zone of cartilaginous tissue between the epiphysis and metaphysis at each end of a long bone. In childhood, proliferation of cells in this zone lengthens the bone. As the bone matures, this area thins, ossification eventually fusing into solid bone and growth stops. **Synonym(s):** Epiphyseal plate.

The appropriate 7th character is to be added to all codes from category S52 [unless otherwise indicated].

A   initial encounter for closed fracture

B   initial encounter for open fracture type I or II

     initial encounter for open fracture NOS

C   initial encounter for open fracture type IIIA, IIIB, or IIIC

D   subsequent encounter for closed fracture with routine healing

E   subsequent encounter for open fracture type I or II with routine healing

F   subsequent encounter for open fracture type IIIA, IIIB, or IIIC with routine healing

G   subsequent encounter for closed fracture with delayed healing

H   subsequent encounter for open fracture type I or II with delayed healing

J   subsequent encounter for open fracture type IIIA, IIIB, or IIIC with delayed healing

K   subsequent encounter for closed fracture with nonunion

M   subsequent encounter for open fracture type I or II with nonunion

N   subsequent encounter for open fracture type IIIA, IIIB, or IIIC with nonunion

P   subsequent encounter for closed fracture with malunion

Q   subsequent encounter for open fracture type I or II with malunion

R   subsequent encounter for open fracture type IIIA, IIIB, or IIIC with malunion

S   sequela

☑5ᵗʰ **S52.Ø** **Fracture of** upper end of ulna

     Fracture of proximal end of ulna

     EXCLUDES 2   fracture of elbow NOS (S42.4Ø-)

          fractures of shaft of ulna (S52.2-)

     ☑6ᵗʰ **S52.ØØ** **Unspecified fracture of upper end of ulna**

        ☑7ᵗʰ **S52.ØØ1** Unspecified fracture of upper end of right **ulna** 🆀

        ☑7ᵗʰ **S52.ØØ2** Unspecified fracture of upper end of left **ulna** 🆀

        ☑7ᵗʰ **S52.ØØ9** Unspecified fracture of upper end of unspecified **ulna** 🆀

     ☑6ᵗʰ **S52.Ø1** Torus **fracture of upper end of ulna**

The appropriate 7th character is to be added to all codes in subcategory S52.Ø1

A   initial encounter for closed fracture

D   subsequent encounter for fracture with routine healing

G   subsequent encounter for fracture with delayed healing

K   subsequent encounter for fracture with nonunion

P   subsequent encounter for fracture with malunion

S   sequela

        ☑7ᵗʰ **S52.Ø11** Torus fracture of upper end of right **ulna** 🆀

        ☑7ᵗʰ **S52.Ø12** Torus fracture of upper end of left **ulna** 🆀

        ☑7ᵗʰ **S52.Ø19** Torus fracture of upper end of unspecified **ulna** 🆀

✓6ᵗʰ **S52.02 Fracture of** olecranon process without intraarticular extension **of ulna**

✓7ᵗʰ **S52.021** Displaced **fracture of olecranon process without intraarticular extension of** right **ulna** ▢

✓7ᵗʰ **S52.022** Displaced **fracture of olecranon process without intraarticular extension of** left **ulna** ▢

✓7ᵗʰ **S52.023** Displaced **fracture of olecranon process without intraarticular extension of unspecified ulna** ▢

✓7ᵗʰ **S52.024** Nondisplaced **fracture of olecranon process without intraarticular extension of** right **ulna** ▢

✓7ᵗʰ **S52.025** Nondisplaced **fracture of olecranon process without intraarticular extension of** left **ulna** ▢

✓7ᵗʰ **S52.026** Nondisplaced **fracture of olecranon process without intraarticular extension of unspecified ulna** ▢

✓6ᵗʰ **S52.03 Fracture of** olecranon process with intraarticular extension **of ulna**

✓7ᵗʰ **S52.031** Displaced **fracture of olecranon process with intraarticular extension of** right **ulna** ▢

✓7ᵗʰ **S52.032** Displaced **fracture of olecranon process with intraarticular extension of** left **ulna** ▢

✓7ᵗʰ **S52.033** Displaced **fracture of olecranon process with intraarticular extension of unspecified ulna** ▢

✓7ᵗʰ **S52.034** Nondisplaced **fracture of olecranon process with intraarticular extension of** right **ulna** ▢

✓7ᵗʰ **S52.035** Nondisplaced **fracture of olecranon process with intraarticular extension of** left **ulna** ▢

✓7ᵗʰ **S52.036** Nondisplaced **fracture of olecranon process with intraarticular extension of unspecified ulna** ▢

✓6ᵗʰ **S52.04 Fracture of** coronoid process **of ulna**

✓7ᵗʰ **S52.041** Displaced **fracture of coronoid process of** right **ulna** ▢

✓7ᵗʰ **S52.042** Displaced **fracture of coronoid process of** left **ulna** ▢

✓7ᵗʰ **S52.043** Displaced **fracture of coronoid process of unspecified ulna** ▢

✓7ᵗʰ **S52.044** Nondisplaced **fracture of coronoid process of** right **ulna** ▢

✓7ᵗʰ **S52.045** Nondisplaced **fracture of coronoid process of** left **ulna** ▢

✓7ᵗʰ **S52.046** Nondisplaced **fracture of coronoid process of unspecified ulna** ▢

✓6ᵗʰ **S52.09 Other fracture of upper end of ulna**

✓7ᵗʰ **S52.091** Other **fracture of upper end of** right **ulna** ▢

✓7ᵗʰ **S52.092** Other **fracture of upper end of** left **ulna** ▢

✓7ᵗʰ **S52.099** Other **fracture of upper end of unspecified ulna** ▢

✓5ᵗʰ **S52.1 Fracture of** upper end of radius

Fracture of proximal end of radius

EXCLUDES 2 *physeal fractures of upper end of radius (S59.2-)*
fracture of shaft of radius (S52.3-)

✓6ᵗʰ **S52.10 Unspecified fracture of upper end of radius**

✓7ᵗʰ **S52.101** Unspecified **fracture of upper end of** right **radius** ▢

✓7ᵗʰ **S52.102** Unspecified **fracture of upper end of** left **radius** ▢

✓7ᵗʰ **S52.109** Unspecified **fracture of upper end of unspecified radius** ▢

✓6ᵗʰ **S52.11 Torus fracture of upper end of radius**

The appropriate 7th character is to be added to all codes in subcategory S52.11
A initial encounter for closed fracture
D subsequent encounter for fracture with routine healing
G subsequent encounter for fracture with delayed healing
K subsequent encounter for fracture with nonunion
P subsequent encounter for fracture with malunion
S sequela

✓7ᵗʰ **S52.111 Torus fracture of upper end of** right **radius** ▢

✓7ᵗʰ **S52.112 Torus fracture of upper end of** left **radius** ▢

✓7ᵗʰ **S52.119 Torus fracture of upper end of unspecified radius** ▢

✓6ᵗʰ **S52.12 Fracture of** head of radius

✓7ᵗʰ **S52.121** Displaced **fracture of head of** right **radius** ▢

✓7ᵗʰ **S52.122** Displaced **fracture of head of** left **radius** ▢

✓7ᵗʰ **S52.123** Displaced **fracture of head of unspecified radius** ▢

✓7ᵗʰ **S52.124** Nondisplaced **fracture of head of** right **radius** ▢

✓7ᵗʰ **S52.125** Nondisplaced **fracture of head of** left **radius** ▢

✓7ᵗʰ **S52.126** Nondisplaced **fracture of head of unspecified radius** ▢

✓6ᵗʰ **S52.13 Fracture of** neck of radius

✓7ᵗʰ **S52.131** Displaced **fracture of neck of** right **radius** ▢

✓7ᵗʰ **S52.132** Displaced **fracture of neck of** left **radius** ▢

✓7ᵗʰ **S52.133** Displaced **fracture of neck of unspecified radius** ▢

✓7ᵗʰ **S52.134** Nondisplaced **fracture of neck of** right **radius** ▢

✓7ᵗʰ **S52.135** Nondisplaced **fracture of neck of** left **radius** ▢

✓7ᵗʰ **S52.136** Nondisplaced **fracture of neck of unspecified radius** ▢

✓6ᵗʰ **S52.18 Other fracture of upper end of radius**

✓7ᵗʰ **S52.181** Other **fracture of upper end of** right **radius** ▢

✓7ᵗʰ **S52.182** Other **fracture of upper end of** left **radius** ▢

✓7ᵗʰ **S52.189** Other **fracture of upper end of unspecified radius** ▢

✓5ᵗʰ **S52.2 Fracture of** shaft of ulna

✓6ᵗʰ **S52.20 Unspecified fracture of shaft of ulna**

Fracture of ulna NOS

✓7ᵗʰ **S52.201** Unspecified **fracture of shaft of** right **ulna** ▢

✓7ᵗʰ **S52.202** Unspecified **fracture of shaft of** left **ulna** ▢

✓7ᵗʰ **S52.209** Unspecified **fracture of shaft of unspecified ulna** ▢

✓6ᵗʰ **S52.21 Greenstick fracture of shaft of ulna**

The appropriate 7th character is to be added to all codes in subcategory S52.21
A initial encounter for closed fracture
D subsequent encounter for fracture with routine healing
G subsequent encounter for fracture with delayed healing
K subsequent encounter for fracture with nonunion
P subsequent encounter for fracture with malunion
S sequela

✓7ᵗʰ **S52.211 Greenstick fracture of shaft of** right **ulna** ▢

✓7ᵗʰ **S52.212 Greenstick fracture of shaft of** left **ulna** ▢

HCC CMS-HCC   **Rx** Rx HCC   **ESR** ESRD HCC   **COM** Commercial HCC   **N** Newborn: 0   **P** Pediatric: 0-17   **M** Maternity: 9-64   **A** Adult: 15-124

1046   ICD-10-CM 2023

√7ᵗʰ **S52.219** Greenstick fracture of shaft of unspecified ulna 🅀

√6ᵗʰ **S52.22** Transverse fracture of shaft of ulna

√7ᵗʰ **S52.221** Displaced transverse fracture of shaft of right ulna 🅀

√7ᵗʰ **S52.222** Displaced transverse fracture of shaft of left ulna 🅀

√7ᵗʰ **S52.223** Displaced transverse fracture of shaft of unspecified ulna 🅀

√7ᵗʰ **S52.224** Nondisplaced transverse fracture of shaft of right ulna 🅀

√7ᵗʰ **S52.225** Nondisplaced transverse fracture of shaft of left ulna 🅀

√7ᵗʰ **S52.226** Nondisplaced transverse fracture of shaft of unspecified ulna 🅀

√6ᵗʰ **S52.23** Oblique fracture of shaft of ulna

√7ᵗʰ **S52.231** Displaced oblique fracture of shaft of right ulna 🅀

√7ᵗʰ **S52.232** Displaced oblique fracture of shaft of left ulna 🅀

√7ᵗʰ **S52.233** Displaced oblique fracture of shaft of unspecified ulna 🅀

√7ᵗʰ **S52.234** Nondisplaced oblique fracture of shaft of right ulna 🅀

√7ᵗʰ **S52.235** Nondisplaced oblique fracture of shaft of left ulna 🅀

√7ᵗʰ **S52.236** Nondisplaced oblique fracture of shaft of unspecified ulna 🅀

√6ᵗʰ **S52.24** Spiral fracture of shaft of ulna

√7ᵗʰ **S52.241** Displaced spiral fracture of shaft of ulna, right arm 🅀

√7ᵗʰ **S52.242** Displaced spiral fracture of shaft of ulna, left arm 🅀

√7ᵗʰ **S52.243** Displaced spiral fracture of shaft of ulna, unspecified arm 🅀

√7ᵗʰ **S52.244** Nondisplaced spiral fracture of shaft of ulna, right arm 🅀

√7ᵗʰ **S52.245** Nondisplaced spiral fracture of shaft of ulna, left arm 🅀

√7ᵗʰ **S52.246** Nondisplaced spiral fracture of shaft of ulna, unspecified arm 🅀

√6ᵗʰ **S52.25** Comminuted fracture of shaft of ulna

√7ᵗʰ **S52.251** Displaced comminuted fracture of shaft of ulna, right arm 🅀

√7ᵗʰ **S52.252** Displaced comminuted fracture of shaft of ulna, left arm 🅀

√7ᵗʰ **S52.253** Displaced comminuted fracture of shaft of ulna, unspecified arm 🅀

√7ᵗʰ **S52.254** Nondisplaced comminuted fracture of shaft of ulna, right arm 🅀

√7ᵗʰ **S52.255** Nondisplaced comminuted fracture of shaft of ulna, left arm 🅀

√7ᵗʰ **S52.256** Nondisplaced comminuted fracture of shaft of ulna, unspecified arm 🅀

√6ᵗʰ **S52.26** Segmental fracture of shaft of ulna

√7ᵗʰ **S52.261** Displaced segmental fracture of shaft of ulna, right arm 🅀

√7ᵗʰ **S52.262** Displaced segmental fracture of shaft of ulna, left arm 🅀

√7ᵗʰ **S52.263** Displaced segmental fracture of shaft of ulna, unspecified arm 🅀

√7ᵗʰ **S52.264** Nondisplaced segmental fracture of shaft of ulna, right arm 🅀

√7ᵗʰ **S52.265** Nondisplaced segmental fracture of shaft of ulna, left arm 🅀

√7ᵗʰ **S52.266** Nondisplaced segmental fracture of shaft of ulna, unspecified arm 🅀

√6ᵗʰ **S52.27** Monteggia's fracture of ulna

Fracture of upper shaft of ulna with dislocation of radial head

√7ᵗʰ **S52.271** Monteggia's fracture of right ulna 🅀

√7ᵗʰ **S52.272** Monteggia's fracture of left ulna 🅀

√7ᵗʰ **S52.279** Monteggia's fracture of unspecified ulna 🅀

√6ᵗʰ **S52.28** Bent bone of ulna

√7ᵗʰ **S52.281** Bent bone of right ulna 🅀

√7ᵗʰ **S52.282** Bent bone of left ulna 🅀

√7ᵗʰ **S52.283** Bent bone of unspecified ulna 🅀

√6ᵗʰ **S52.29** Other fracture of shaft of ulna

√7ᵗʰ **S52.291** Other fracture of shaft of right ulna 🅀

√7ᵗʰ **S52.292** Other fracture of shaft of left ulna 🅀

√7ᵗʰ **S52.299** Other fracture of shaft of unspecified ulna 🅀

√5ᵗʰ **S52.3** **Fracture of** shaft of radius

√6ᵗʰ **S52.30** Unspecified fracture of shaft of radius

√7ᵗʰ **S52.301** Unspecified fracture of shaft of right radius 🅀

√7ᵗʰ **S52.302** Unspecified fracture of shaft of left radius 🅀

√7ᵗʰ **S52.309** Unspecified fracture of shaft of unspecified radius 🅀

√6ᵗʰ **S52.31** Greenstick fracture of shaft of radius

> The appropriate 7th character is to be added to all codes in subcategory S52.31.
> A   initial encounter for closed fracture
> D   subsequent encounter for fracture with routine healing
> G   subsequent encounter for fracture with delayed healing
> K   subsequent encounter for fracture with nonunion
> P   subsequent encounter for fracture with malunion
> S   sequela

√7ᵗʰ **S52.311** Greenstick fracture of shaft of radius, right arm 🅀

√7ᵗʰ **S52.312** Greenstick fracture of shaft of radius, left arm 🅀

√7ᵗʰ **S52.319** Greenstick fracture of shaft of radius, unspecified arm 🅀

√6ᵗʰ **S52.32** Transverse fracture of shaft of radius

√7ᵗʰ **S52.321** Displaced transverse fracture of shaft of right radius 🅀

√7ᵗʰ **S52.322** Displaced transverse fracture of shaft of left radius 🅀

√7ᵗʰ **S52.323** Displaced transverse fracture of shaft of unspecified radius 🅀

√7ᵗʰ **S52.324** Nondisplaced transverse fracture of shaft of right radius 🅀

√7ᵗʰ **S52.325** Nondisplaced transverse fracture of shaft of left radius 🅀

√7ᵗʰ **S52.326** Nondisplaced transverse fracture of shaft of unspecified radius 🅀

√6ᵗʰ **S52.33** Oblique fracture of shaft of radius

√7ᵗʰ **S52.331** Displaced oblique fracture of shaft of right radius 🅀

√7ᵗʰ **S52.332** Displaced oblique fracture of shaft of left radius 🅀

√7ᵗʰ **S52.333** Displaced oblique fracture of shaft of unspecified radius 🅀

√7ᵗʰ **S52.334** Nondisplaced oblique fracture of shaft of right radius 🅀

√7ᵗʰ **S52.335** Nondisplaced oblique fracture of shaft of left radius 🅀

√7ᵗʰ **S52.336** Nondisplaced oblique fracture of shaft of unspecified radius 🅀

√6ᵗʰ **S52.34** Spiral fracture of shaft of radius

√7ᵗʰ **S52.341** Displaced spiral fracture of shaft of radius, right arm 🅀

√7ᵗʰ **S52.342** Displaced spiral fracture of shaft of radius, left arm 🅀

√7ᵗʰ **S52.343** Displaced spiral fracture of shaft of radius, unspecified arm 🅀

√7ᵗʰ **S52.344** Nondisplaced spiral fracture of shaft of radius, right arm 🅀

√7ᵗʰ **S52.345** Nondisplaced spiral fracture of shaft of radius, left arm 🅀

√7ᵗʰ **S52.346** Nondisplaced spiral fracture of shaft of radius, unspecified arm 🅀

√6ᵗʰ **S52.35** Comminuted fracture of shaft of radius

√7ᵗʰ **S52.351** Displaced comminuted fracture of shaft of radius, right arm 🅀

√7ᵗʰ **S52.352** Displaced comminuted fracture of shaft of radius, left arm 🅀

√7ᵗʰ **S52.353** Displaced comminuted fracture of shaft of radius, unspecified arm 🅀

☑️ Additional Character Required   √x7ᵗʰ Placeholder Alert   Manifestation   Unspecified Dx   🅀 QPP   UPD Unacceptable PDx

√6ᵗʰ **S52.354** Nondisplaced **comminuted fracture of shaft of radius, right arm** ⚪

√7ᵗʰ **S52.355** Nondisplaced **comminuted fracture of shaft of radius, left arm** ⚪

√7ᵗʰ **S52.356** Nondisplaced **comminuted fracture of shaft of radius, unspecified arm** ⚪

√6ᵗʰ **S52.36** Segmental **fracture of shaft of radius**

√7ᵗʰ **S52.361** Displaced **segmental fracture of shaft of radius, right arm** ⚪

√7ᵗʰ **S52.362** Displaced **segmental fracture of shaft of radius, left arm** ⚪

√7ᵗʰ **S52.363** Displaced **segmental fracture of shaft of radius, unspecified arm** ⚪

√7ᵗʰ **S52.364** Nondisplaced **segmental fracture of shaft of radius, right arm** ⚪

√7ᵗʰ **S52.365** Nondisplaced **segmental fracture of shaft of radius, left arm** ⚪

√7ᵗʰ **S52.366** Nondisplaced **segmental fracture of shaft of radius, unspecified arm** ⚪

√6ᵗʰ **S52.37** Galeazzi's **fracture**

Fracture of lower shaft of radius with radioulnar joint dislocation

√7ᵗʰ **S52.371** Galeazzi's **fracture of** right **radius** ⚪

√7ᵗʰ **S52.372** Galeazzi's **fracture of** left **radius** ⚪

√7ᵗʰ **S52.379** Galeazzi's **fracture of unspecified radius** ⚪

√6ᵗʰ **S52.38** Bent bone **of radius**

√7ᵗʰ **S52.381** Bent bone **of** right **radius** ⚪

√7ᵗʰ **S52.382** Bent bone **of** left **radius** ⚪

√7ᵗʰ **S52.389** Bent bone **of unspecified radius** ⚪

√6ᵗʰ **S52.39** Other fracture of shaft of radius

√7ᵗʰ **S52.391** Other fracture of shaft of radius, right arm ⚪

√7ᵗʰ **S52.392** Other fracture of shaft of radius, left arm ⚪

√7ᵗʰ **S52.399** Other fracture of shaft of radius, unspecified arm ⚪

√5ᵗʰ **S52.5** **Fracture of** lower end of radius

Fracture of distal end of radius

EXCLUDES 2   physeal fractures of lower end of radius (S59.2-)

DEF: Fracture of the distal end of the radius above the wrist, most commonly caused by a fall onto an outstretched hand.

√6ᵗʰ **S52.50** Unspecified fracture of the lower end of radius

√7ᵗʰ **S52.501** Unspecified fracture of the lower end of right radius ⚪

√7ᵗʰ **S52.502** Unspecified fracture of the lower end of left radius ⚪

√7ᵗʰ **S52.509** Unspecified fracture of the lower end of unspecified radius ⚪

√6ᵗʰ **S52.51** Fracture of **radial styloid process**

√7ᵗʰ **S52.511** Displaced **fracture of** right **radial styloid process** ⚪

√7ᵗʰ **S52.512** Displaced **fracture of** left **radial styloid process** ⚪

√7ᵗʰ **S52.513** Displaced **fracture of unspecified radial styloid process** ⚪

√7ᵗʰ **S52.514** Nondisplaced **fracture of** right **radial styloid process** ⚪

√7ᵗʰ **S52.515** Nondisplaced **fracture of** left **radial styloid process** ⚪

√7ᵗʰ **S52.516** Nondisplaced **fracture of unspecified radial styloid process** ⚪

√6ᵗʰ **S52.52** Torus **fracture of lower end of radius**

The appropriate 7th character is to be added to all codes in subcategory S52.52.
A   initial encounter for closed fracture
D   subsequent encounter for fracture with routine healing
G   subsequent encounter for fracture with delayed healing
K   subsequent encounter for fracture with nonunion
P   subsequent encounter for fracture with malunion
S   sequela

√7ᵗʰ **S52.521** Torus **fracture of lower end of** right **radius** ⚪

√7ᵗʰ **S52.522** Torus **fracture of lower end of** left **radius** ⚪

√7ᵗʰ **S52.529** Torus **fracture of lower end of unspecified radius** ⚪

√6ᵗʰ **S52.53** Colles' **fracture**

AHA: 2016,2Q,4

DEF: Fracture of the radius at the wrist in which the distal fragment is pushed posteriorly. The dorsal angulation of the fragment results in the wrist cocking up.

√7ᵗʰ **S52.531** Colles' **fracture of** right **radius** ⚪

√7ᵗʰ **S52.532** Colles' **fracture of** left **radius** ⚪

√7ᵗʰ **S52.539** Colles' **fracture of unspecified radius** ⚪

√6ᵗʰ **S52.54** Smith's **fracture**

√7ᵗʰ **S52.541** Smith's **fracture of** right **radius** ⚪

√7ᵗʰ **S52.542** Smith's **fracture of** left **radius** ⚪

√7ᵗʰ **S52.549** Smith's **fracture of unspecified radius** ⚪

√6ᵗʰ **S52.55** Other extraarticular **fracture of lower end of radius**

√7ᵗʰ **S52.551** Other extraarticular **fracture of lower end of** right **radius** ⚪

√7ᵗʰ **S52.552** Other extraarticular **fracture of lower end of** left **radius** ⚪

√7ᵗʰ **S52.559** Other extraarticular **fracture of lower end of unspecified radius** ⚪

√6ᵗʰ **S52.56** Barton's **fracture**

√7ᵗʰ **S52.561** Barton's **fracture of** right **radius** ⚪

√7ᵗʰ **S52.562** Barton's **fracture of** left **radius** ⚪

√7ᵗʰ **S52.569** Barton's **fracture of unspecified radius** ⚪

√6ᵗʰ **S52.57** Other intraarticular **fracture of lower end of radius**

√7ᵗʰ **S52.571** Other intraarticular **fracture of lower end of** right **radius** ⚪

√7ᵗʰ **S52.572** Other intraarticular **fracture of lower end of** left **radius** ⚪

√7ᵗʰ **S52.579** Other intraarticular **fracture of lower end of unspecified radius** ⚪

√6ᵗʰ **S52.59** Other fractures of lower end of radius

AHA: 2019,3Q,9

√7ᵗʰ **S52.591** Other fractures of lower end of right radius ⚪

√7ᵗʰ **S52.592** Other fractures of lower end of left radius ⚪

√7ᵗʰ **S52.599** Other fractures of lower end of unspecified radius ⚪

√5ᵗʰ **S52.6** **Fracture of** lower end of ulna

√6ᵗʰ **S52.60** Unspecified fracture of lower end of ulna

√7ᵗʰ **S52.601** Unspecified fracture of lower end of right ulna ⚪

√7ᵗʰ **S52.602** Unspecified fracture of lower end of left ulna ⚪

√7ᵗʰ **S52.609** Unspecified fracture of lower end of unspecified ulna ⚪

√6ᵗʰ **S52.61** Fracture of ulna styloid process

√7ᵗʰ **S52.611** Displaced **fracture of** right **ulna styloid process** ⚪

√7ᵗʰ **S52.612** Displaced **fracture of** left **ulna styloid process** ⚪

√7ᵗʰ **S52.613** Displaced **fracture of unspecified ulna styloid process** ⚪

√7ᵗʰ **S52.614** Nondisplaced **fracture of** right **ulna styloid process** ⚪

√7ᵗʰ **S52.615** Nondisplaced **fracture of** left **ulna styloid process** ⚪

√7ᵗʰ **S52.616** Nondisplaced **fracture of unspecified ulna styloid process** ⚪

HCC CMS-HCC   **Rx** Rx HCC   **ESR** ESRD HCC   **COM** Commercial HCC   **N** Newborn: 0   **P** Pediatric: 0-17   **M** Maternity: 9-64   **A** Adult: 15-124

ICD-10-CM 2023

√6ᵗʰ **S52.62** Torus fracture of lower end of ulna

> The appropriate 7th character is to be added to all codes in subcategory S52.62.
> A initial encounter for closed fracture
> D subsequent encounter for fracture with routine healing
> G subsequent encounter for fracture with delayed healing
> K subsequent encounter for fracture with nonunion
> P subsequent encounter for fracture with malunion
> S sequela

     √7ᵗʰ **S52.621** Torus fracture of lower end of right ulna   Q

     √7ᵗʰ **S52.622** Torus fracture of lower end of left ulna   Q

     √7ᵗʰ **S52.629** Torus fracture of lower end of unspecified ulna   Q

√6ᵗʰ **S52.69** Other fracture of lower end of ulna

     AHA: 2019,3Q,9

     √7ᵗʰ **S52.691** Other fracture of lower end of right ulna   Q

     √7ᵗʰ **S52.692** Other fracture of lower end of left ulna   Q

     √7ᵗʰ **S52.699** Other fracture of lower end of unspecified ulna   Q

√5ᵗʰ **S52.9** Unspecified fracture of forearm

     √x7ᵗʰ **S52.90** Unspecified fracture of unspecified forearm   Q

     √x7ᵗʰ **S52.91** Unspecified fracture of right forearm   Q

     √x7ᵗʰ **S52.92** Unspecified fracture of left forearm   Q

√4ᵗʰ **S53** Dislocation and sprain of joints and ligaments of elbow

     INCLUDES   avulsion of joint or ligament of elbow
                laceration of cartilage, joint or ligament of elbow
                sprain of cartilage, joint or ligament of elbow
                traumatic hemarthrosis of joint or ligament of elbow
                traumatic rupture of joint or ligament of elbow
                traumatic subluxation of joint or ligament of elbow
                traumatic tear of joint or ligament of elbow

     Code also any associated open wound

     EXCLUDES 2   strain of muscle, fascia and tendon at forearm level (S56.-)

> The appropriate 7th character is to be added to each code from category S53.
> A initial encounter
> D subsequent encounter
> S sequela

√5ᵗʰ **S53.0** Subluxation and dislocation of radial head

     Dislocation of radiohumeral joint
     Subluxation of radiohumeral joint

     EXCLUDES 1   Monteggia's fracture-dislocation (S52.27-)

     √6ᵗʰ **S53.00** Unspecified subluxation and dislocation of radial head

         √7ᵗʰ **S53.001** Unspecified subluxation of right radial head

         √7ᵗʰ **S53.002** Unspecified subluxation of left radial head

         √7ᵗʰ **S53.003** Unspecified subluxation of unspecified radial head

         √7ᵗʰ **S53.004** Unspecified dislocation of right radial head

         √7ᵗʰ **S53.005** Unspecified dislocation of left radial head

         √7ᵗʰ **S53.006** Unspecified dislocation of unspecified radial head

     √6ᵗʰ **S53.01** Anterior subluxation and dislocation of radial head

         Anteriomedial subluxation and dislocation of radial head

         √7ᵗʰ **S53.011** Anterior subluxation of right radial head

         √7ᵗʰ **S53.012** Anterior subluxation of left radial head

         √7ᵗʰ **S53.013** Anterior subluxation of unspecified radial head

         √7ᵗʰ **S53.014** Anterior dislocation of right radial head

         √7ᵗʰ **S53.015** Anterior dislocation of left radial head

         √7ᵗʰ **S53.016** Anterior dislocation of unspecified radial head

√6ᵗʰ **S53.02** Posterior subluxation and dislocation of radial head

     Posteriolateral subluxation and dislocation of radial head

     √7ᵗʰ **S53.021** Posterior subluxation of right radial head

     √7ᵗʰ **S53.022** Posterior subluxation of left radial head

     √7ᵗʰ **S53.023** Posterior subluxation of unspecified radial head

     √7ᵗʰ **S53.024** Posterior dislocation of right radial head

     √7ᵗʰ **S53.025** Posterior dislocation of left radial head

     √7ᵗʰ **S53.026** Posterior dislocation of unspecified radial head

√6ᵗʰ **S53.03** Nursemaid's elbow

     √7ᵗʰ **S53.031** Nursemaid's elbow, right elbow

     √7ᵗʰ **S53.032** Nursemaid's elbow, left elbow

     √7ᵗʰ **S53.033** Nursemaid's elbow, unspecified elbow

√6ᵗʰ **S53.09** Other subluxation and dislocation of radial head

     √7ᵗʰ **S53.091** Other subluxation of right radial head

     √7ᵗʰ **S53.092** Other subluxation of left radial head

     √7ᵗʰ **S53.093** Other subluxation of unspecified radial head

     √7ᵗʰ **S53.094** Other dislocation of right radial head

     √7ᵗʰ **S53.095** Other dislocation of left radial head

     √7ᵗʰ **S53.096** Other dislocation of unspecified radial head

√5ᵗʰ **S53.1** Subluxation and dislocation of ulnohumeral joint

     Subluxation and dislocation of elbow NOS

     EXCLUDES 1   dislocation of radial head alone (S53.0-)

     √6ᵗʰ **S53.10** Unspecified subluxation and dislocation of ulnohumeral joint

         √7ᵗʰ **S53.101** Unspecified subluxation of right ulnohumeral joint

         √7ᵗʰ **S53.102** Unspecified subluxation of left ulnohumeral joint

         √7ᵗʰ **S53.103** Unspecified subluxation of unspecified ulnohumeral joint

         √7ᵗʰ **S53.104** Unspecified dislocation of right ulnohumeral joint

         √7ᵗʰ **S53.105** Unspecified dislocation of left ulnohumeral joint

         √7ᵗʰ **S53.106** Unspecified dislocation of unspecified ulnohumeral joint

     √6ᵗʰ **S53.11** Anterior subluxation and dislocation of ulnohumeral joint

         √7ᵗʰ **S53.111** Anterior subluxation of right ulnohumeral joint

         √7ᵗʰ **S53.112** Anterior subluxation of left ulnohumeral joint

         √7ᵗʰ **S53.113** Anterior subluxation of unspecified ulnohumeral joint

         √7ᵗʰ **S53.114** Anterior dislocation of right ulnohumeral joint

             AHA: 2012,4Q,108

         √7ᵗʰ **S53.115** Anterior dislocation of left ulnohumeral joint

         √7ᵗʰ **S53.116** Anterior dislocation of unspecified ulnohumeral joint

     √6ᵗʰ **S53.12** Posterior subluxation and dislocation of ulnohumeral joint

         √7ᵗʰ **S53.121** Posterior subluxation of right ulnohumeral joint

         √7ᵗʰ **S53.122** Posterior subluxation of left ulnohumeral joint

         √7ᵗʰ **S53.123** Posterior subluxation of unspecified ulnohumeral joint

         √7ᵗʰ **S53.124** Posterior dislocation of right ulnohumeral joint

         √7ᵗʰ **S53.125** Posterior dislocation of left ulnohumeral joint

         √7ᵗʰ **S53.126** Posterior dislocation of unspecified ulnohumeral joint

     √6ᵗʰ **S53.13** Medial subluxation and dislocation of ulnohumeral joint

         √7ᵗʰ **S53.131** Medial subluxation of right ulnohumeral joint

         √7ᵗʰ **S53.132** Medial subluxation of left ulnohumeral joint

         √7ᵗʰ **S53.133** Medial subluxation of unspecified ulnohumeral joint

Chapter 19. Injury, Poisoning and Certain Other Consequences of External Causes

√7ᵗʰ **S53.134** Medial dislocation of right ulnohumeral joint

√7ᵗʰ **S53.135** Medial dislocation of left ulnohumeral joint

√7ᵗʰ **S53.136** Medial dislocation of unspecified ulnohumeral joint

√6ᵗʰ **S53.14** Lateral subluxation and dislocation of ulnohumeral joint

√7ᵗʰ **S53.141** Lateral subluxation of right ulnohumeral joint

√7ᵗʰ **S53.142** Lateral subluxation of left ulnohumeral joint

√7ᵗʰ **S53.143** Lateral subluxation of unspecified ulnohumeral joint

√7ᵗʰ **S53.144** Lateral dislocation of right ulnohumeral joint

√7ᵗʰ **S53.145** Lateral dislocation of left ulnohumeral joint

√7ᵗʰ **S53.146** Lateral dislocation of unspecified ulnohumeral joint

√6ᵗʰ **S53.19** Other subluxation and dislocation of ulnohumeral joint

√7ᵗʰ **S53.191** Other subluxation of right ulnohumeral joint

√7ᵗʰ **S53.192** Other subluxation of left ulnohumeral joint

√7ᵗʰ **S53.193** Other subluxation of unspecified ulnohumeral joint

√7ᵗʰ **S53.194** Other dislocation of right ulnohumeral joint

√7ᵗʰ **S53.195** Other dislocation of left ulnohumeral joint

√7ᵗʰ **S53.196** Other dislocation of unspecified ulnohumeral joint

√5ᵗʰ **S53.2** Traumatic rupture of radial collateral ligament

EXCLUDES 1   sprain of radial collateral ligament NOS (S53.43-)

√x7ᵗʰ **S53.20** Traumatic rupture of unspecified radial collateral ligament

√x7ᵗʰ **S53.21** Traumatic rupture of right radial collateral ligament

√x7ᵗʰ **S53.22** Traumatic rupture of left radial collateral ligament

√5ᵗʰ **S53.3** Traumatic rupture of ulnar collateral ligament

EXCLUDES 1   sprain of ulnar collateral ligament (S53.44-)

√x7ᵗʰ **S53.30** Traumatic rupture of unspecified ulnar collateral ligament

√x7ᵗʰ **S53.31** Traumatic rupture of right ulnar collateral ligament

√x7ᵗʰ **S53.32** Traumatic rupture of left ulnar collateral ligament

√5ᵗʰ **S53.4** Sprain of elbow

EXCLUDES 2   traumatic rupture of radial collateral ligament (S53.2-)

traumatic rupture of ulnar collateral ligament (S53.3-)

√6ᵗʰ **S53.40** Unspecified sprain of elbow

√7ᵗʰ **S53.401** Unspecified sprain of right elbow

√7ᵗʰ **S53.402** Unspecified sprain of left elbow

√7ᵗʰ **S53.409** Unspecified sprain of unspecified elbow

Sprain of elbow NOS

√6ᵗʰ **S53.41** Radiohumeral (joint) sprain

√7ᵗʰ **S53.411** Radiohumeral (joint) sprain of right elbow

√7ᵗʰ **S53.412** Radiohumeral (joint) sprain of left elbow

√7ᵗʰ **S53.419** Radiohumeral (joint) sprain of unspecified elbow

√6ᵗʰ **S53.42** Ulnohumeral (joint) sprain

√7ᵗʰ **S53.421** Ulnohumeral (joint) sprain of right elbow

√7ᵗʰ **S53.422** Ulnohumeral (joint) sprain of left elbow

√7ᵗʰ **S53.429** Ulnohumeral (joint) sprain of unspecified elbow

√6ᵗʰ **S53.43** Radial collateral ligament sprain

√7ᵗʰ **S53.431** Radial collateral ligament sprain of right elbow

√7ᵗʰ **S53.432** Radial collateral ligament sprain of left elbow

√7ᵗʰ **S53.439** Radial collateral ligament sprain of unspecified elbow

√6ᵗʰ **S53.44** Ulnar collateral ligament sprain

√7ᵗʰ **S53.441** Ulnar collateral ligament sprain of right elbow

√7ᵗʰ **S53.442** Ulnar collateral ligament sprain of left elbow

√7ᵗʰ **S53.449** Ulnar collateral ligament sprain of unspecified elbow

√6ᵗʰ **S53.49** Other sprain of elbow

√7ᵗʰ **S53.491** Other sprain of right elbow

√7ᵗʰ **S53.492** Other sprain of left elbow

√7ᵗʰ **S53.499** Other sprain of unspecified elbow

√4ᵗʰ **S54** Injury of nerves at forearm level

Code also any associated open wound (S51.-)

EXCLUDES 2   injury of nerves at wrist and hand level (S64.-)

The appropriate 7th character is to be added to each code from category S54.

A   initial encounter

D   subsequent encounter

S   sequela

√5ᵗʰ **S54.0** Injury of ulnar nerve at forearm level

Injury of ulnar nerve NOS

√x7ᵗʰ **S54.00** Injury of ulnar nerve at forearm level, unspecified arm

√x7ᵗʰ **S54.01** Injury of ulnar nerve at forearm level, right arm

√x7ᵗʰ **S54.02** Injury of ulnar nerve at forearm level, left arm

√5ᵗʰ **S54.1** Injury of median nerve at forearm level

Injury of median nerve NOS

√x7ᵗʰ **S54.10** Injury of median nerve at forearm level, unspecified arm

√x7ᵗʰ **S54.11** Injury of median nerve at forearm level, right arm

√x7ᵗʰ **S54.12** Injury of median nerve at forearm level, left arm

√5ᵗʰ **S54.2** Injury of radial nerve at forearm level

Injury of radial nerve NOS

√x7ᵗʰ **S54.20** Injury of radial nerve at forearm level, unspecified arm

√x7ᵗʰ **S54.21** Injury of radial nerve at forearm level, right arm

√x7ᵗʰ **S54.22** Injury of radial nerve at forearm level, left arm

√5ᵗʰ **S54.3** Injury of cutaneous sensory nerve at forearm level

√x7ᵗʰ **S54.30** Injury of cutaneous sensory nerve at forearm level, unspecified arm

√x7ᵗʰ **S54.31** Injury of cutaneous sensory nerve at forearm level, right arm

√x7ᵗʰ **S54.32** Injury of cutaneous sensory nerve at forearm level, left arm

√5ᵗʰ **S54.8** Injury of other nerves at forearm level

√6ᵗʰ **S54.8X** Injury of other nerves at forearm level

√7ᵗʰ **S54.8X1** Injury of other nerves at forearm level, right arm

√7ᵗʰ **S54.8X2** Injury of other nerves at forearm level, left arm

√7ᵗʰ **S54.8X9** Injury of other nerves at forearm level, unspecified arm

√5ᵗʰ **S54.9** Injury of unspecified nerve at forearm level

√x7ᵗʰ **S54.90** Injury of unspecified nerve at forearm level, unspecified arm

√x7ᵗʰ **S54.91** Injury of unspecified nerve at forearm level, right arm

√x7ᵗʰ **S54.92** Injury of unspecified nerve at forearm level, left arm

√4ᵗʰ **S55** Injury of blood vessels at forearm level

Code also any associated open wound (S51.-)

EXCLUDES 2   injury of blood vessels at wrist and hand level (S65.-)

injury of brachial vessels (S45.1-S45.2)

The appropriate 7th character is to be added to each code from category S55.

A   initial encounter

D   subsequent encounter

S   sequela

√5ᵗʰ **S55.0** Injury of ulnar artery at forearm level

√6ᵗʰ **S55.00** Unspecified injury of ulnar artery at forearm level

√7ᵗʰ **S55.001** Unspecified injury of ulnar artery at forearm level, right arm

√7ᵗʰ **S55.002** Unspecified injury of ulnar artery at forearm level, left arm

√7ᵗʰ **S55.009** Unspecified injury of ulnar artery at forearm level, unspecified arm

HCC CMS-HCC   **Rx** Rx HCC   **ESR** ESRD HCC   **COM** Commercial HCC   **N** Newborn: 0   **P** Pediatric: 0-17   **M** Maternity: 9-64   **A** Adult: 15-124

1050

ICD-10-CM 2023

√6ᵗʰ **S55.01** Laceration of ulnar artery at forearm level

√7ᵗʰ **S55.011** Laceration of ulnar artery at forearm level, right arm

√7ᵗʰ **S55.012** Laceration of ulnar artery at forearm level, left arm

√7ᵗʰ **S55.019** Laceration of ulnar artery at forearm level, unspecified arm

√6ᵗʰ **S55.09** Other specified injury of ulnar artery at forearm level

√7ᵗʰ **S55.091** Other specified injury of ulnar artery at forearm level, right arm

√7ᵗʰ **S55.092** Other specified injury of ulnar artery at forearm level, left arm

√7ᵗʰ **S55.099** Other specified injury of ulnar artery at forearm level, unspecified arm

√5ᵗʰ **S55.1** Injury of radial artery at forearm level

√6ᵗʰ **S55.10** Unspecified injury of radial artery at forearm level

√7ᵗʰ **S55.101** Unspecified injury of radial artery at forearm level, right arm

√7ᵗʰ **S55.102** Unspecified injury of radial artery at forearm level, left arm

√7ᵗʰ **S55.109** Unspecified injury of radial artery at forearm level, unspecified arm

√6ᵗʰ **S55.11** Laceration of radial artery at forearm level

√7ᵗʰ **S55.111** Laceration of radial artery at forearm level, right arm

√7ᵗʰ **S55.112** Laceration of radial artery at forearm level, left arm

√7ᵗʰ **S55.119** Laceration of radial artery at forearm level, unspecified arm

√6ᵗʰ **S55.19** Other specified injury of radial artery at forearm level

√7ᵗʰ **S55.191** Other specified injury of radial artery at forearm level, right arm

√7ᵗʰ **S55.192** Other specified injury of radial artery at forearm level, left arm

√7ᵗʰ **S55.199** Other specified injury of radial artery at forearm level, unspecified arm

√5ᵗʰ **S55.2** Injury of vein at forearm level

√6ᵗʰ **S55.20** Unspecified injury of vein at forearm level

√7ᵗʰ **S55.201** Unspecified injury of vein at forearm level, right arm

√7ᵗʰ **S55.202** Unspecified injury of vein at forearm level, left arm

√7ᵗʰ **S55.209** Unspecified injury of vein at forearm level, unspecified arm

√6ᵗʰ **S55.21** Laceration of vein at forearm level

√7ᵗʰ **S55.211** Laceration of vein at forearm level, right arm

√7ᵗʰ **S55.212** Laceration of vein at forearm level, left arm

√7ᵗʰ **S55.219** Laceration of vein at forearm level, unspecified arm

√6ᵗʰ **S55.29** Other specified injury of vein at forearm level

√7ᵗʰ **S55.291** Other specified injury of vein at forearm level, right arm

√7ᵗʰ **S55.292** Other specified injury of vein at forearm level, left arm

√7ᵗʰ **S55.299** Other specified injury of vein at forearm level, unspecified arm

√5ᵗʰ **S55.8** Injury of other blood vessels at forearm level

√6ᵗʰ **S55.80** Unspecified injury of other blood vessels at forearm level

√7ᵗʰ **S55.801** Unspecified injury of other blood vessels at forearm level, right arm

√7ᵗʰ **S55.802** Unspecified injury of other blood vessels at forearm level, left arm

√7ᵗʰ **S55.809** Unspecified injury of other blood vessels at forearm level, unspecified arm

√6ᵗʰ **S55.81** Laceration of other blood vessels at forearm level

√7ᵗʰ **S55.811** Laceration of other blood vessels at forearm level, right arm

√7ᵗʰ **S55.812** Laceration of other blood vessels at forearm level, left arm

√7ᵗʰ **S55.819** Laceration of other blood vessels at forearm level, unspecified arm

√6ᵗʰ **S55.89** Other specified injury of other blood vessels at forearm level

√7ᵗʰ **S55.891** Other specified injury of other blood vessels at forearm level, right arm

√7ᵗʰ **S55.892** Other specified injury of other blood vessels at forearm level, left arm

√7ᵗʰ **S55.899** Other specified injury of other blood vessels at forearm level, unspecified arm

√5ᵗʰ **S55.9** Injury of unspecified blood vessel at forearm level

√6ᵗʰ **S55.90** Unspecified injury of unspecified blood vessel at forearm level

√7ᵗʰ **S55.901** Unspecified injury of unspecified blood vessel at forearm level, right arm

√7ᵗʰ **S55.902** Unspecified injury of unspecified blood vessel at forearm level, left arm

√7ᵗʰ **S55.909** Unspecified injury of unspecified blood vessel at forearm level, unspecified arm

√6ᵗʰ **S55.91** Laceration of unspecified blood vessel at forearm level

√7ᵗʰ **S55.911** Laceration of unspecified blood vessel at forearm level, right arm

√7ᵗʰ **S55.912** Laceration of unspecified blood vessel at forearm level, left arm

√7ᵗʰ **S55.919** Laceration of unspecified blood vessel at forearm level, unspecified arm

√6ᵗʰ **S55.99** Other specified injury of unspecified blood vessel at forearm level

√7ᵗʰ **S55.991** Other specified injury of unspecified blood vessel at forearm level, right arm

√7ᵗʰ **S55.992** Other specified injury of unspecified blood vessel at forearm level, left arm

√7ᵗʰ **S55.999** Other specified injury of unspecified blood vessel at forearm level, unspecified arm

√4ᵗʰ **S56** **Injury of muscle, fascia and tendon at forearm level**

Code also any associated open wound (S51.-)

EXCLUDES 2   *injury of muscle, fascia and tendon at or below wrist (S66.-)*
           sprain of joints and ligaments of elbow (S53.4-)

TIP: Refer to the Muscle/Tendon table at the beginning of this chapter

The appropriate 7th character is to be added to each code from category S56.
A   initial encounter
D   subsequent encounter
S   sequela

√5ᵗʰ **S56.0** Injury of flexor muscle, fascia and tendon of thumb at forearm level

√6ᵗʰ **S56.00** Unspecified injury of flexor muscle, fascia and tendon of thumb at forearm level

√7ᵗʰ **S56.001** Unspecified injury of flexor muscle, fascia and tendon of right thumb at forearm level

√7ᵗʰ **S56.002** Unspecified injury of flexor muscle, fascia and tendon of left thumb at forearm level

√7ᵗʰ **S56.009** Unspecified injury of flexor muscle, fascia and tendon of unspecified thumb at forearm level

√6ᵗʰ **S56.01** Strain of flexor muscle, fascia and tendon of thumb at forearm level

√7ᵗʰ **S56.011** Strain of flexor muscle, fascia and tendon of right thumb at forearm level

√7ᵗʰ **S56.012** Strain of flexor muscle, fascia and tendon of left thumb at forearm level

√7ᵗʰ **S56.019** Strain of flexor muscle, fascia and tendon of unspecified thumb at forearm level

√6ᵗʰ **S56.02** Laceration of flexor muscle, fascia and tendon of thumb at forearm level

√7ᵗʰ **S56.021** Laceration of flexor muscle, fascia and tendon of right thumb at forearm level

√7ᵗʰ **S56.022** Laceration of flexor muscle, fascia and tendon of left thumb at forearm level

√7ᵗʰ **S56.029** Laceration of flexor muscle, fascia and tendon of unspecified thumb at forearm level

√6ᵗʰ **S56.09** Other injury of flexor muscle, fascia and tendon of thumb at forearm level

√7ᵗʰ **S56.091** Other injury of flexor muscle, fascia and tendon of right thumb at forearm level

√7ᵗʰ **S56.092** Other injury of flexor muscle, fascia and tendon of left thumb at forearm level

√7ᵗʰ **S56.099** Other injury of flexor muscle, fascia and tendon of unspecified thumb at forearm level

---

☑ Additional Character Required   √x7ᵗʰ Placeholder Alert   Manifestation   Unspecified Dx   ℚ QPP   UPD Unacceptable PDx

√5ᵗʰ **S56.1** Injury of flexor muscle, fascia and tendon of other and unspecified finger at forearm level

√6ᵗʰ **S56.10** Unspecified injury of flexor muscle, fascia and tendon of other and unspecified finger at forearm level

√7ᵗʰ **S56.101** Unspecified injury of flexor muscle, fascia and tendon of right index finger at forearm level

√7ᵗʰ **S56.102** Unspecified injury of flexor muscle, fascia and tendon of left index finger at forearm level

√7ᵗʰ **S56.103** Unspecified injury of flexor muscle, fascia and tendon of right middle finger at forearm level

√7ᵗʰ **S56.104** Unspecified injury of flexor muscle, fascia and tendon of left middle finger at forearm level

√7ᵗʰ **S56.105** Unspecified injury of flexor muscle, fascia and tendon of right ring finger at forearm level

√7ᵗʰ **S56.106** Unspecified injury of flexor muscle, fascia and tendon of left ring finger at forearm level

√7ᵗʰ **S56.107** Unspecified injury of flexor muscle, fascia and tendon of right little finger at forearm level

√7ᵗʰ **S56.108** Unspecified injury of flexor muscle, fascia and tendon of left little finger at forearm level

√7ᵗʰ **S56.109** Unspecified injury of flexor muscle, fascia and tendon of unspecified finger at forearm level

√6ᵗʰ **S56.11** Strain of flexor muscle, fascia and tendon of other and unspecified finger at forearm level

√7ᵗʰ **S56.111** Strain of flexor muscle, fascia and tendon of right index finger at forearm level

√7ᵗʰ **S56.112** Strain of flexor muscle, fascia and tendon of left index finger at forearm level

√7ᵗʰ **S56.113** Strain of flexor muscle, fascia and tendon of right middle finger at forearm level

√7ᵗʰ **S56.114** Strain of flexor muscle, fascia and tendon of left middle finger at forearm level

√7ᵗʰ **S56.115** Strain of flexor muscle, fascia and tendon of right ring finger at forearm level

√7ᵗʰ **S56.116** Strain of flexor muscle, fascia and tendon of left ring finger at forearm level

√7ᵗʰ **S56.117** Strain of flexor muscle, fascia and tendon of right little finger at forearm level

√7ᵗʰ **S56.118** Strain of flexor muscle, fascia and tendon of left little finger at forearm level

√7ᵗʰ **S56.119** Strain of flexor muscle, fascia and tendon of finger of unspecified finger at forearm level

√6ᵗʰ **S56.12** Laceration of flexor muscle, fascia and tendon of other and unspecified finger at forearm level

√7ᵗʰ **S56.121** Laceration of flexor muscle, fascia and tendon of right index finger at forearm level

√7ᵗʰ **S56.122** Laceration of flexor muscle, fascia and tendon of left index finger at forearm level

√7ᵗʰ **S56.123** Laceration of flexor muscle, fascia and tendon of right middle finger at forearm level

√7ᵗʰ **S56.124** Laceration of flexor muscle, fascia and tendon of left middle finger at forearm level

√7ᵗʰ **S56.125** Laceration of flexor muscle, fascia and tendon of right ring finger at forearm level

√7ᵗʰ **S56.126** Laceration of flexor muscle, fascia and tendon of left ring finger at forearm level

√7ᵗʰ **S56.127** Laceration of flexor muscle, fascia and tendon of right little finger at forearm level

√7ᵗʰ **S56.128** Laceration of flexor muscle, fascia and tendon of left little finger at forearm level

√7ᵗʰ **S56.129** Laceration of flexor muscle, fascia and tendon of unspecified finger at forearm level

√6ᵗʰ **S56.19** Other injury of flexor muscle, fascia and tendon of other and unspecified finger at forearm level

√7ᵗʰ **S56.191** Other injury of flexor muscle, fascia and tendon of right index finger at forearm level

√7ᵗʰ **S56.192** Other injury of flexor muscle, fascia and tendon of left index finger at forearm level

√7ᵗʰ **S56.193** Other injury of flexor muscle, fascia and tendon of right middle finger at forearm level

√7ᵗʰ **S56.194** Other injury of flexor muscle, fascia and tendon of left middle finger at forearm level

√7ᵗʰ **S56.195** Other injury of flexor muscle, fascia and tendon of right ring finger at forearm level

√7ᵗʰ **S56.196** Other injury of flexor muscle, fascia and tendon of left ring finger at forearm level

√7ᵗʰ **S56.197** Other injury of flexor muscle, fascia and tendon of right little finger at forearm level

√7ᵗʰ **S56.198** Other injury of flexor muscle, fascia and tendon of left little finger at forearm level

√7ᵗʰ **S56.199** Other injury of flexor muscle, fascia and tendon of unspecified finger at forearm level

√5ᵗʰ **S56.2** Injury of other flexor muscle, fascia and tendon at forearm level

√6ᵗʰ **S56.20** Unspecified injury of other flexor muscle, fascia and tendon at forearm level

√7ᵗʰ **S56.201** Unspecified injury of other flexor muscle, fascia and tendon at forearm level, right arm

√7ᵗʰ **S56.202** Unspecified injury of other flexor muscle, fascia and tendon at forearm level, left arm

√7ᵗʰ **S56.209** Unspecified injury of other flexor muscle, fascia and tendon at forearm level, unspecified arm

√6ᵗʰ **S56.21** Strain of other flexor muscle, fascia and tendon at forearm level

√7ᵗʰ **S56.211** Strain of other flexor muscle, fascia and tendon at forearm level, right arm

√7ᵗʰ **S56.212** Strain of other flexor muscle, fascia and tendon at forearm level, left arm

√7ᵗʰ **S56.219** Strain of other flexor muscle, fascia and tendon at forearm level, unspecified arm

√6ᵗʰ **S56.22** Laceration of other flexor muscle, fascia and tendon at forearm level

√7ᵗʰ **S56.221** Laceration of other flexor muscle, fascia and tendon at forearm level, right arm

√7ᵗʰ **S56.222** Laceration of other flexor muscle, fascia and tendon at forearm level, left arm

√7ᵗʰ **S56.229** Laceration of other flexor muscle, fascia and tendon at forearm level, unspecified arm

√6ᵗʰ **S56.29** Other injury of other flexor muscle, fascia and tendon at forearm level

√7ᵗʰ **S56.291** Other injury of other flexor muscle, fascia and tendon at forearm level, right arm

√7ᵗʰ **S56.292** Other injury of other flexor muscle, fascia and tendon at forearm level, left arm

√7ᵗʰ **S56.299** Other injury of other flexor muscle, fascia and tendon at forearm level, unspecified arm

√5ᵗʰ **S56.3** Injury of extensor or abductor muscles, fascia and tendons of thumb at forearm level

√6ᵗʰ **S56.30** Unspecified injury of extensor or abductor muscles, fascia and tendons of thumb at forearm level

√7ᵗʰ **S56.301** Unspecified injury of extensor or abductor muscles, fascia and tendons of right thumb at forearm level

√7ᵗʰ **S56.302** Unspecified injury of extensor or abductor muscles, fascia and tendons of left thumb at forearm level

√7ᵗʰ **S56.309** Unspecified injury of extensor or abductor muscles, fascia and tendons of unspecified thumb at forearm level

√6ᵗʰ **S56.31** Strain of extensor or abductor muscles, fascia and tendons of thumb at forearm level

√7ᵗʰ **S56.311** Strain of extensor or abductor muscles, fascia and tendons of right thumb at forearm level

√7ᵗʰ **S56.312** Strain of extensor or abductor muscles, fascia and tendons of left thumb at forearm level

✓7ᵗʰ **S56.319** Strain of extensor or abductor muscles, fascia and tendons of unspecified thumb at forearm level

✓6ᵗʰ **S56.32** Laceration of extensor or abductor muscles, fascia and tendons of thumb at forearm level

  ✓7ᵗʰ **S56.321** Laceration of extensor or abductor muscles, fascia and tendons of right thumb at forearm level

  ✓7ᵗʰ **S56.322** Laceration of extensor or abductor muscles, fascia and tendons of left thumb at forearm level

  ✓7ᵗʰ **S56.329** Laceration of extensor or abductor muscles, fascia and tendons of unspecified thumb at forearm level

✓6ᵗʰ **S56.39** Other injury of extensor or abductor muscles, fascia and tendons of thumb at forearm level

  ✓7ᵗʰ **S56.391** Other injury of extensor or abductor muscles, fascia and tendons of right thumb at forearm level

  ✓7ᵗʰ **S56.392** Other injury of extensor or abductor muscles, fascia and tendons of left thumb at forearm level

  ✓7ᵗʰ **S56.399** Other injury of extensor or abductor muscles, fascia and tendons of unspecified thumb at forearm level

✓5ᵗʰ **S56.4** Injury of extensor muscle, fascia and tendon of other and unspecified finger at forearm level

✓6ᵗʰ **S56.40** Unspecified injury of extensor muscle, fascia and tendon of other and unspecified finger at forearm level

  ✓7ᵗʰ **S56.401** Unspecified injury of extensor muscle, fascia and tendon of right index finger at forearm level

  ✓7ᵗʰ **S56.402** Unspecified injury of extensor muscle, fascia and tendon of left index finger at forearm level

  ✓7ᵗʰ **S56.403** Unspecified injury of extensor muscle, fascia and tendon of right middle finger at forearm level

  ✓7ᵗʰ **S56.404** Unspecified injury of extensor muscle, fascia and tendon of left middle finger at forearm level

  ✓7ᵗʰ **S56.405** Unspecified injury of extensor muscle, fascia and tendon of right ring finger at forearm level

  ✓7ᵗʰ **S56.406** Unspecified injury of extensor muscle, fascia and tendon of left ring finger at forearm level

  ✓7ᵗʰ **S56.407** Unspecified injury of extensor muscle, fascia and tendon of right little finger at forearm level

  ✓7ᵗʰ **S56.408** Unspecified injury of extensor muscle, fascia and tendon of left little finger at forearm level

  ✓7ᵗʰ **S56.409** Unspecified injury of extensor muscle, fascia and tendon of unspecified finger at forearm level

✓6ᵗʰ **S56.41** Strain of extensor muscle, fascia and tendon of other and unspecified finger at forearm level

  ✓7ᵗʰ **S56.411** Strain of extensor muscle, fascia and tendon of right index finger at forearm level

  ✓7ᵗʰ **S56.412** Strain of extensor muscle, fascia and tendon of left index finger at forearm level

  ✓7ᵗʰ **S56.413** Strain of extensor muscle, fascia and tendon of right middle finger at forearm level

  ✓7ᵗʰ **S56.414** Strain of extensor muscle, fascia and tendon of left middle finger at forearm level

  ✓7ᵗʰ **S56.415** Strain of extensor muscle, fascia and tendon of right ring finger at forearm level

  ✓7ᵗʰ **S56.416** Strain of extensor muscle, fascia and tendon of left ring finger at forearm level

  ✓7ᵗʰ **S56.417** Strain of extensor muscle, fascia and tendon of right little finger at forearm level

  ✓7ᵗʰ **S56.418** Strain of extensor muscle, fascia and tendon of left little finger at forearm level

  ✓7ᵗʰ **S56.419** Strain of extensor muscle, fascia and tendon of finger, unspecified finger at forearm level

✓6ᵗʰ **S56.42** Laceration of extensor muscle, fascia and tendon of other and unspecified finger at forearm level

  ✓7ᵗʰ **S56.421** Laceration of extensor muscle, fascia and tendon of right index finger at forearm level

  ✓7ᵗʰ **S56.422** Laceration of extensor muscle, fascia and tendon of left index finger at forearm level

  ✓7ᵗʰ **S56.423** Laceration of extensor muscle, fascia and tendon of right middle finger at forearm level

  ✓7ᵗʰ **S56.424** Laceration of extensor muscle, fascia and tendon of left middle finger at forearm level

  ✓7ᵗʰ **S56.425** Laceration of extensor muscle, fascia and tendon of right ring finger at forearm level

  ✓7ᵗʰ **S56.426** Laceration of extensor muscle, fascia and tendon of left ring finger at forearm level

  ✓7ᵗʰ **S56.427** Laceration of extensor muscle, fascia and tendon of right little finger at forearm level

  ✓7ᵗʰ **S56.428** Laceration of extensor muscle, fascia and tendon of left little finger at forearm level

  ✓7ᵗʰ **S56.429** Laceration of extensor muscle, fascia and tendon of unspecified finger at forearm level

✓6ᵗʰ **S56.49** Other injury of extensor muscle, fascia and tendon of other and unspecified finger at forearm level

  ✓7ᵗʰ **S56.491** Other injury of extensor muscle, fascia and tendon of right index finger at forearm level

  ✓7ᵗʰ **S56.492** Other injury of extensor muscle, fascia and tendon of left index finger at forearm level

  ✓7ᵗʰ **S56.493** Other injury of extensor muscle, fascia and tendon of right middle finger at forearm level

  ✓7ᵗʰ **S56.494** Other injury of extensor muscle, fascia and tendon of left middle finger at forearm level

  ✓7ᵗʰ **S56.495** Other injury of extensor muscle, fascia and tendon of right ring finger at forearm level

  ✓7ᵗʰ **S56.496** Other injury of extensor muscle, fascia and tendon of left ring finger at forearm level

  ✓7ᵗʰ **S56.497** Other injury of extensor muscle, fascia and tendon of right little finger at forearm level

  ✓7ᵗʰ **S56.498** Other injury of extensor muscle, fascia and tendon of left little finger at forearm level

  ✓7ᵗʰ **S56.499** Other injury of extensor muscle, fascia and tendon of unspecified finger at forearm level

✓5ᵗʰ **S56.5** Injury of other extensor muscle, fascia and tendon at forearm level

✓6ᵗʰ **S56.50** Unspecified injury of other extensor muscle, fascia and tendon at forearm level

  ✓7ᵗʰ **S56.501** Unspecified injury of other extensor muscle, fascia and tendon at forearm level, right arm

  ✓7ᵗʰ **S56.502** Unspecified injury of other extensor muscle, fascia and tendon at forearm level, left arm

  ✓7ᵗʰ **S56.509** Unspecified injury of other extensor muscle, fascia and tendon at forearm level, unspecified arm

✓6ᵗʰ **S56.51** Strain of other extensor muscle, fascia and tendon at forearm level

  ✓7ᵗʰ **S56.511** Strain of other extensor muscle, fascia and tendon at forearm level, right arm

  ✓7ᵗʰ **S56.512** Strain of other extensor muscle, fascia and tendon at forearm level, left arm

  ✓7ᵗʰ **S56.519** Strain of other extensor muscle, fascia and tendon at forearm level, unspecified arm

✓6ᵗʰ **S56.52** Laceration of other extensor muscle, fascia and tendon at forearm level

  ✓7ᵗʰ **S56.521** Laceration of other extensor muscle, fascia and tendon at forearm level, right arm

---

√7ᵗʰ **S56.522** Laceration of other extensor muscle, fascia and tendon at forearm level, left arm

√7ᵗʰ **S56.529** Laceration of other extensor muscle, fascia and tendon at forearm level, unspecified arm

√6ᵗʰ **S56.59** Other injury of other extensor muscle, fascia and tendon at forearm level

√7ᵗʰ **S56.591** Other injury of other extensor muscle, fascia and tendon at forearm level, right arm

√7ᵗʰ **S56.592** Other injury of other extensor muscle, fascia and tendon at forearm level, left arm

√7ᵗʰ **S56.599** Other injury of other extensor muscle, fascia and tendon at forearm level, unspecified arm

√5ᵗʰ **S56.8** Injury of other muscles, fascia and tendons at forearm level

√6ᵗʰ **S56.80** Unspecified injury of other muscles, fascia and tendons at forearm level

√7ᵗʰ **S56.801** Unspecified injury of other muscles, fascia and tendons at forearm level, right arm

√7ᵗʰ **S56.802** Unspecified injury of other muscles, fascia and tendons at forearm level, left arm

√7ᵗʰ **S56.809** Unspecified injury of other muscles, fascia and tendons at forearm level, unspecified arm

√6ᵗʰ **S56.81** Strain of other muscles, fascia and tendons at forearm level

√7ᵗʰ **S56.811** Strain of other muscles, fascia and tendons at forearm level, right arm

√7ᵗʰ **S56.812** Strain of other muscles, fascia and tendons at forearm level, left arm

√7ᵗʰ **S56.819** Strain of other muscles, fascia and tendons at forearm level, unspecified arm

√6ᵗʰ **S56.82** Laceration of other muscles, fascia and tendons at forearm level

√7ᵗʰ **S56.821** Laceration of other muscles, fascia and tendons at forearm level, right arm

√7ᵗʰ **S56.822** Laceration of other muscles, fascia and tendons at forearm level, left arm

√7ᵗʰ **S56.829** Laceration of other muscles, fascia and tendons at forearm level, unspecified arm

√6ᵗʰ **S56.89** Other injury of other muscles, fascia and tendons at forearm level

√7ᵗʰ **S56.891** Other injury of other muscles, fascia and tendons at forearm level, right arm

√7ᵗʰ **S56.892** Other injury of other muscles, fascia and tendons at forearm level, left arm

√7ᵗʰ **S56.899** Other injury of other muscles, fascia and tendons at forearm level, unspecified arm

√5ᵗʰ **S56.9** Injury of unspecified muscles, fascia and tendons at forearm level

√6ᵗʰ **S56.90** Unspecified injury of unspecified muscles, fascia and tendons at forearm level

√7ᵗʰ **S56.901** Unspecified injury of unspecified muscles, fascia and tendons at forearm level, right arm

√7ᵗʰ **S56.902** Unspecified injury of unspecified muscles, fascia and tendons at forearm level, left arm

√7ᵗʰ **S56.909** Unspecified injury of unspecified muscles, fascia and tendons at forearm level, unspecified arm

√6ᵗʰ **S56.91** Strain of unspecified muscles, fascia and tendons at forearm level

√7ᵗʰ **S56.911** Strain of unspecified muscles, fascia and tendons at forearm level, right arm

√7ᵗʰ **S56.912** Strain of unspecified muscles, fascia and tendons at forearm level, left arm

√7ᵗʰ **S56.919** Strain of unspecified muscles, fascia and tendons at forearm level, unspecified arm

√6ᵗʰ **S56.92** Laceration of unspecified muscles, fascia and tendons at forearm level

√7ᵗʰ **S56.921** Laceration of unspecified muscles, fascia and tendons at forearm level, right arm

√7ᵗʰ **S56.922** Laceration of unspecified muscles, fascia and tendons at forearm level, left arm

√7ᵗʰ **S56.929** Laceration of unspecified muscles, fascia and tendons at forearm level, unspecified arm

√6ᵗʰ **S56.99** Other injury of unspecified muscles, fascia and tendons at forearm level

√7ᵗʰ **S56.991** Other injury of unspecified muscles, fascia and tendons at forearm level, right arm

√7ᵗʰ **S56.992** Other injury of unspecified muscles, fascia and tendons at forearm level, left arm

√7ᵗʰ **S56.999** Other injury of unspecified muscles, fascia and tendons at forearm level, unspecified arm

√4ᵗʰ **S57** Crushing injury of elbow and forearm

Use additional code(s) for all associated injuries

EXCLUDES 2   crushing injury of wrist and hand (S67.-)

The appropriate 7th character is to be added to each code from category S57.
A   initial encounter
D   subsequent encounter
S   sequela

√5ᵗʰ **S57.0** Crushing injury of elbow

√x7ᵗʰ **S57.00** Crushing injury of unspecified elbow

√x7ᵗʰ **S57.01** Crushing injury of right elbow

√x7ᵗʰ **S57.02** Crushing injury of left elbow

√5ᵗʰ **S57.8** Crushing injury of forearm

√x7ᵗʰ **S57.80** Crushing injury of unspecified forearm

√x7ᵗʰ **S57.81** Crushing injury of right forearm

√x7ᵗʰ **S57.82** Crushing injury of left forearm

√4ᵗʰ **S58** Traumatic amputation of elbow and forearm

An amputation not identified as partial or complete should be coded to complete

EXCLUDES 1   traumatic amputation of wrist and hand (S68.-)

The appropriate 7th character is to be added to each code from category S58.
A   initial encounter
D   subsequent encounter
S   sequela

√5ᵗʰ **S58.0** Traumatic amputation at elbow level

√6ᵗʰ **S58.01** Complete traumatic amputation at elbow level

² √7ᵗʰ **S58.011** Complete traumatic amputation at elbow level, right arm   HCC ESR COM

² √7ᵗʰ **S58.012** Complete traumatic amputation at elbow level, left arm   HCC ESR COM

² √7ᵗʰ **S58.019** Complete traumatic amputation at elbow level, unspecified arm   HCC ESR COM

√6ᵗʰ **S58.02** Partial traumatic amputation at elbow level

² √7ᵗʰ **S58.021** Partial traumatic amputation at elbow level, right arm   HCC ESR COM

² √7ᵗʰ **S58.022** Partial traumatic amputation at elbow level, left arm   HCC ESR COM

² √7ᵗʰ **S58.029** Partial traumatic amputation at elbow level, unspecified arm   HCC ESR COM

√5ᵗʰ **S58.1** Traumatic amputation at level between elbow and wrist

√6ᵗʰ **S58.11** Complete traumatic amputation at level between elbow and wrist

² √7ᵗʰ **S58.111** Complete traumatic amputation at level between elbow and wrist, right arm   HCC ESR COM

² √7ᵗʰ **S58.112** Complete traumatic amputation at level between elbow and wrist, left arm   HCC ESR COM

² √7ᵗʰ **S58.119** Complete traumatic amputation at level between elbow and wrist, unspecified arm   HCC ESR COM

√6ᵗʰ **S58.12** Partial traumatic amputation at level between elbow and wrist

² √7ᵗʰ **S58.121** Partial traumatic amputation at level between elbow and wrist, right arm   HCC ESR COM

² √7ᵗʰ **S58.122** Partial traumatic amputation at level between elbow and wrist, left arm   HCC ESR COM

² √7ᵗʰ **S58.129** Partial traumatic amputation at level between elbow and wrist, unspecified arm   HCC ESR COM

√5ᵗʰ **S58.9** **Traumatic amputation of** forearm, level unspecified

> EXCLUDES 1   *traumatic amputation of wrist (S68.-)*

√6ᵗʰ **S58.91** **Complete traumatic amputation of forearm, level unspecified**

2 √7ᵗʰ **S58.911** Complete traumatic amputation of right forearm, level unspecified   HCC ESR COM

2 √7ᵗʰ **S58.912** Complete traumatic amputation of left forearm, level unspecified   HCC ESR COM

2 √7ᵗʰ **S58.919** Complete traumatic amputation of unspecified forearm, level unspecified   HCC ESR COM

√6ᵗʰ **S58.92** **Partial traumatic amputation of forearm, level unspecified**

2 √7ᵗʰ **S58.921** Partial traumatic amputation of right forearm, level unspecified   HCC ESR COM

2 √7ᵗʰ **S58.922** Partial traumatic amputation of left forearm, level unspecified   HCC ESR COM

2 √7ᵗʰ **S58.929** Partial traumatic amputation of unspecified forearm, level unspecified   HCC ESR COM

√4ᵗʰ **S59** **Other and unspecified injuries of elbow and forearm**

> EXCLUDES 2   *other and unspecified injuries of wrist and hand (S69.-)*

AHA: 2018,2Q,12; 2018,1Q,3; 2015,3Q,37-39

> The appropriate 7th character is to be added to each code from subcategories S59.0, S59.1, and S59.2.
> A   initial encounter for closed fracture
> D   subsequent encounter for fracture with routine healing
> G   subsequent encounter for fracture with delayed healing
> K   subsequent encounter for fracture with nonunion
> P   subsequent encounter for fracture with malunion
> S   sequela

√5ᵗʰ **S59.0** **Physeal fracture of** lower end of ulna

AHA: 2019,4Q,56

√6ᵗʰ **S59.00** **Unspecified physeal fracture of lower end of ulna**

√7ᵗʰ **S59.001** Unspecified physeal fracture of lower end of ulna, right arm   Q

√7ᵗʰ **S59.002** Unspecified physeal fracture of lower end of ulna, left arm   Q

√7ᵗʰ **S59.009** Unspecified physeal fracture of lower end of ulna, unspecified arm   Q

√6ᵗʰ **S59.01** **Salter-Harris Type I physeal fracture of lower end of ulna**

√7ᵗʰ **S59.011** Salter-Harris Type I physeal fracture of lower end of ulna, right arm   Q

√7ᵗʰ **S59.012** Salter-Harris Type I physeal fracture of lower end of ulna, left arm   Q

√7ᵗʰ **S59.019** Salter-Harris Type I physeal fracture of lower end of ulna, unspecified arm   Q

√6ᵗʰ **S59.02** **Salter-Harris Type II physeal fracture of lower end of ulna**

√7ᵗʰ **S59.021** Salter-Harris Type II physeal fracture of lower end of ulna, right arm   Q

√7ᵗʰ **S59.022** Salter-Harris Type II physeal fracture of lower end of ulna, left arm   Q

√7ᵗʰ **S59.029** Salter-Harris Type II physeal fracture of lower end of ulna, unspecified arm   Q

√6ᵗʰ **S59.03** **Salter-Harris Type III physeal fracture of lower end of ulna**

√7ᵗʰ **S59.031** Salter-Harris Type III physeal fracture of lower end of ulna, right arm   Q

√7ᵗʰ **S59.032** Salter-Harris Type III physeal fracture of lower end of ulna, left arm   Q

√7ᵗʰ **S59.039** Salter-Harris Type III physeal fracture of lower end of ulna, unspecified arm   Q

√6ᵗʰ **S59.04** **Salter-Harris Type IV physeal fracture of lower end of ulna**

√7ᵗʰ **S59.041** Salter-Harris Type IV physeal fracture of lower end of ulna, right arm   Q

√7ᵗʰ **S59.042** Salter-Harris Type IV physeal fracture of lower end of ulna, left arm   Q

√7ᵗʰ **S59.049** Salter-Harris Type IV physeal fracture of lower end of ulna, unspecified arm   Q

√6ᵗʰ **S59.09** **Other physeal fracture of lower end of ulna**

√7ᵗʰ **S59.091** Other physeal fracture of lower end of ulna, right arm   Q

√7ᵗʰ **S59.092** Other physeal fracture of lower end of ulna, left arm   Q

√7ᵗʰ **S59.099** Other physeal fracture of lower end of ulna, unspecified arm   Q

√5ᵗʰ **S59.1** **Physeal fracture of** upper end of radius

AHA: 2019,4Q,56

√6ᵗʰ **S59.10** **Unspecified physeal fracture of upper end of radius**

√7ᵗʰ **S59.101** Unspecified physeal fracture of upper end of radius, right arm   Q

√7ᵗʰ **S59.102** Unspecified physeal fracture of upper end of radius, left arm   Q

√7ᵗʰ **S59.109** Unspecified physeal fracture of upper end of radius, unspecified arm   Q

√6ᵗʰ **S59.11** **Salter-Harris Type I physeal fracture of upper end of radius**

√7ᵗʰ **S59.111** Salter-Harris Type I physeal fracture of upper end of radius, right arm   Q

√7ᵗʰ **S59.112** Salter-Harris Type I physeal fracture of upper end of radius, left arm   Q

√7ᵗʰ **S59.119** Salter-Harris Type I physeal fracture of upper end of radius, unspecified arm   Q

√6ᵗʰ **S59.12** **Salter-Harris Type II physeal fracture of upper end of radius**

√7ᵗʰ **S59.121** Salter-Harris Type II physeal fracture of upper end of radius, right arm   Q

√7ᵗʰ **S59.122** Salter-Harris Type II physeal fracture of upper end of radius, left arm   Q

√7ᵗʰ **S59.129** Salter-Harris Type II physeal fracture of upper end of radius, unspecified arm   Q

√6ᵗʰ **S59.13** **Salter-Harris Type III physeal fracture of upper end of radius**

√7ᵗʰ **S59.131** Salter-Harris Type III physeal fracture of upper end of radius, right arm   Q

√7ᵗʰ **S59.132** Salter-Harris Type III physeal fracture of upper end of radius, left arm   Q

√7ᵗʰ **S59.139** Salter-Harris Type III physeal fracture of upper end of radius, unspecified arm   Q

√6ᵗʰ **S59.14** **Salter-Harris Type IV physeal fracture of upper end of radius**

√7ᵗʰ **S59.141** Salter-Harris Type IV physeal fracture of upper end of radius, right arm   Q

√7ᵗʰ **S59.142** Salter-Harris Type IV physeal fracture of upper end of radius, left arm   Q

√7ᵗʰ **S59.149** Salter-Harris Type IV physeal fracture of upper end of radius, unspecified arm   Q

√6ᵗʰ **S59.19** **Other physeal fracture of upper end of radius**

√7ᵗʰ **S59.191** Other physeal fracture of upper end of radius, right arm   Q

√7ᵗʰ **S59.192** Other physeal fracture of upper end of radius, left arm   Q

√7ᵗʰ **S59.199** Other physeal fracture of upper end of radius, unspecified arm   Q

√5ᵗʰ **S59.2** **Physeal fracture of** lower end of radius

AHA: 2019,4Q,56

√6ᵗʰ **S59.20** **Unspecified physeal fracture of lower end of radius**

√7ᵗʰ **S59.201** Unspecified physeal fracture of lower end of radius, right arm   Q

√7ᵗʰ **S59.202** Unspecified physeal fracture of lower end of radius, left arm   Q

√7ᵗʰ **S59.209** Unspecified physeal fracture of lower end of radius, unspecified arm   Q

√6ᵗʰ **S59.21** **Salter-Harris Type I physeal fracture of lower end of radius**

√7ᵗʰ **S59.211** Salter-Harris Type I physeal fracture of lower end of radius, right arm   Q

√7ᵗʰ **S59.212** Salter-Harris Type I physeal fracture of lower end of radius, left arm   Q

√7ᵗʰ **S59.219** Salter-Harris Type I physeal fracture of lower end of radius, unspecified arm   Q

√6ᵗʰ **S59.22** **Salter-Harris Type II physeal fracture of lower end of radius**

√7ᵗʰ **S59.221** Salter-Harris Type II physeal fracture of lower end of radius, right arm   Q

√7ᵗʰ **S59.222** Salter-Harris Type II physeal fracture of lower end of radius, left arm   Q

√7ᵗʰ **S59.229** Salter-Harris Type II physeal fracture of lower end of radius, unspecified arm   Q

Chapter 19. Injury, Poisoning and Certain Other Consequences of External Causes

√6ᵗʰ **S59.23** Salter-Harris Type III physeal fracture of lower end of radius

     √7ᵗʰ **S59.231** Salter-Harris Type III physeal fracture of lower end of radius, right arm ▢

     √7ᵗʰ **S59.232** Salter-Harris Type III physeal fracture of lower end of radius, left arm ▢

     √7ᵗʰ **S59.239** Salter-Harris Type III physeal fracture of lower end of radius, unspecified arm ▢

√6ᵗʰ **S59.24** Salter-Harris Type IV physeal fracture of lower end of radius

     √7ᵗʰ **S59.241** Salter-Harris Type IV physeal fracture of lower end of radius, right arm ▢

     √7ᵗʰ **S59.242** Salter-Harris Type IV physeal fracture of lower end of radius, left arm ▢

     √7ᵗʰ **S59.249** Salter-Harris Type IV physeal fracture of lower end of radius, unspecified arm ▢

√6ᵗʰ **S59.29** Other physeal fracture of lower end of radius

     √7ᵗʰ **S59.291** Other physeal fracture of lower end of radius, right arm ▢

     √7ᵗʰ **S59.292** Other physeal fracture of lower end of radius, left arm ▢

     √7ᵗʰ **S59.299** Other physeal fracture of lower end of radius, unspecified arm ▢

√5ᵗʰ **S59.8 Other specified injuries of elbow and forearm**

> The appropriate 7th character is to be added to each code in subcategory S59.8.
> A   initial encounter
> D   subsequent encounter
> S   sequela

√6ᵗʰ **S59.80** Other specified injuries of elbow

     √7ᵗʰ **S59.801** Other specified injuries of right elbow

     √7ᵗʰ **S59.802** Other specified injuries of left elbow

     √7ᵗʰ **S59.809** Other specified injuries of unspecified elbow

√6ᵗʰ **S59.81** Other specified injuries of forearm

     √7ᵗʰ **S59.811** Other specified injuries right forearm

     √7ᵗʰ **S59.812** Other specified injuries left forearm

     √7ᵗʰ **S59.819** Other specified injuries unspecified forearm

√5ᵗʰ **S59.9 Unspecified injury of elbow and forearm**

> The appropriate 7th character is to be added to each code in subcategory S59.9.
> A   initial encounter
> D   subsequent encounter
> S   sequela

√6ᵗʰ **S59.90** Unspecified injury of elbow

     √7ᵗʰ **S59.901** Unspecified injury of right elbow

     √7ᵗʰ **S59.902** Unspecified injury of left elbow

     √7ᵗʰ **S59.909** Unspecified injury of unspecified elbow

√6ᵗʰ **S59.91** Unspecified injury of forearm

     √7ᵗʰ **S59.911** Unspecified injury of right forearm

     √7ᵗʰ **S59.912** Unspecified injury of left forearm

     √7ᵗʰ **S59.919** Unspecified injury of unspecified forearm

Injuries to the wrist, hand and fingers (S60-S69)

EXCLUDES 2   burns and corrosions (T20-T32)
         frostbite (T33-T34)
         insect bite or sting, venomous (T63.4)

√4ᵗʰ **S60 Superficial injury of wrist, hand and fingers**

> The appropriate 7th character is to be added to each code from category S60.
> A   initial encounter
> D   subsequent encounter
> S   sequela

√5ᵗʰ **S60.0 Contusion of finger without damage to nail**

     EXCLUDES 1   contusion involving nail (matrix) (S60.1)

     √x7ᵗʰ **S60.00** Contusion of unspecified finger without damage to nail

         Contusion of finger(s) NOS

     √6ᵗʰ **S60.01** Contusion of thumb without damage to nail

         √7ᵗʰ **S60.011** Contusion of right thumb without damage to nail

         √7ᵗʰ **S60.012** Contusion of left thumb without damage to nail

         √7ᵗʰ **S60.019** Contusion of unspecified thumb without damage to nail

     √6ᵗʰ **S60.02** Contusion of index finger without damage to nail

         √7ᵗʰ **S60.021** Contusion of right index finger without damage to nail

         √7ᵗʰ **S60.022** Contusion of left index finger without damage to nail

         √7ᵗʰ **S60.029** Contusion of unspecified index finger without damage to nail

     √6ᵗʰ **S60.03** Contusion of middle finger without damage to nail

         √7ᵗʰ **S60.031** Contusion of right middle finger without damage to nail

         √7ᵗʰ **S60.032** Contusion of left middle finger without damage to nail

         √7ᵗʰ **S60.039** Contusion of unspecified middle finger without damage to nail

     √6ᵗʰ **S60.04** Contusion of ring finger without damage to nail

         √7ᵗʰ **S60.041** Contusion of right ring finger without damage to nail

         √7ᵗʰ **S60.042** Contusion of left ring finger without damage to nail

         √7ᵗʰ **S60.049** Contusion of unspecified ring finger without damage to nail

     √6ᵗʰ **S60.05** Contusion of little finger without damage to nail

         √7ᵗʰ **S60.051** Contusion of right little finger without damage to nail

         √7ᵗʰ **S60.052** Contusion of left little finger without damage to nail

         √7ᵗʰ **S60.059** Contusion of unspecified little finger without damage to nail

√5ᵗʰ **S60.1 Contusion of finger with damage to nail**

     √x7ᵗʰ **S60.10** Contusion of unspecified finger with damage to nail

     √6ᵗʰ **S60.11** Contusion of thumb with damage to nail

         √7ᵗʰ **S60.111** Contusion of right thumb with damage to nail

         √7ᵗʰ **S60.112** Contusion of left thumb with damage to nail

         √7ᵗʰ **S60.119** Contusion of unspecified thumb with damage to nail

     √6ᵗʰ **S60.12** Contusion of index finger with damage to nail

         √7ᵗʰ **S60.121** Contusion of right index finger with damage to nail

         √7ᵗʰ **S60.122** Contusion of left index finger with damage to nail

         √7ᵗʰ **S60.129** Contusion of unspecified index finger with damage to nail

     √6ᵗʰ **S60.13** Contusion of middle finger with damage to nail

         √7ᵗʰ **S60.131** Contusion of right middle finger with damage to nail

         √7ᵗʰ **S60.132** Contusion of left middle finger with damage to nail

         √7ᵗʰ **S60.139** Contusion of unspecified middle finger with damage to nail

     √6ᵗʰ **S60.14** Contusion of ring finger with damage to nail

         √7ᵗʰ **S60.141** Contusion of right ring finger with damage to nail

         √7ᵗʰ **S60.142** Contusion of left ring finger with damage to nail

         √7ᵗʰ **S60.149** Contusion of unspecified ring finger with damage to nail

     √6ᵗʰ **S60.15** Contusion of little finger with damage to nail

         √7ᵗʰ **S60.151** Contusion of right little finger with damage to nail

         √7ᵗʰ **S60.152** Contusion of left little finger with damage to nail

         √7ᵗʰ **S60.159** Contusion of unspecified little finger with damage to nail

√5ᵗʰ **S60.2 Contusion of wrist and hand**

     EXCLUDES 2   contusion of fingers (S60.0-, S60.1-)

     √6ᵗʰ **S60.21** Contusion of wrist

         √7ᵗʰ **S60.211** Contusion of right wrist

         √7ᵗʰ **S60.212** Contusion of left wrist

         √7ᵗʰ **S60.219** Contusion of unspecified wrist

     √6ᵗʰ **S60.22** Contusion of hand

         √7ᵗʰ **S60.221** Contusion of right hand

√7ᵗʰ **S60.222** Contusion of left hand
√7ᵗʰ **S60.229** Contusion of unspecified hand

√5ᵗʰ **S60.3** Other superficial injuries of thumb

√6ᵗʰ **S60.31** Abrasion of thumb
√7ᵗʰ **S60.311** Abrasion of right thumb
√7ᵗʰ **S60.312** Abrasion of left thumb
√7ᵗʰ **S60.319** Abrasion of unspecified thumb

√6ᵗʰ **S60.32** Blister (nonthermal) of thumb
√7ᵗʰ **S60.321** Blister (nonthermal) of right thumb
√7ᵗʰ **S60.322** Blister (nonthermal) of left thumb
√7ᵗʰ **S60.329** Blister (nonthermal) of unspecified thumb

√6ᵗʰ **S60.34** External constriction of thumb
Hair tourniquet syndrome of thumb
Use additional cause code to identify the constricting item (W49.0-)
√7ᵗʰ **S60.341** External constriction of right thumb
√7ᵗʰ **S60.342** External constriction of left thumb
√7ᵗʰ **S60.349** External constriction of unspecified thumb

√6ᵗʰ **S60.35** Superficial foreign body of thumb
Splinter in the thumb
√7ᵗʰ **S60.351** Superficial foreign body of right thumb
√7ᵗʰ **S60.352** Superficial foreign body of left thumb
√7ᵗʰ **S60.359** Superficial foreign body of unspecified thumb

√6ᵗʰ **S60.36** Insect bite (nonvenomous) of thumb
√7ᵗʰ **S60.361** Insect bite (nonvenomous) of right thumb
√7ᵗʰ **S60.362** Insect bite (nonvenomous) of left thumb
√7ᵗʰ **S60.369** Insect bite (nonvenomous) of unspecified thumb

√6ᵗʰ **S60.37** Other superficial bite of thumb
EXCLUDES 1   open bite of thumb (S61.05-, S61.15-)
√7ᵗʰ **S60.371** Other superficial bite of right thumb
√7ᵗʰ **S60.372** Other superficial bite of left thumb
√7ᵗʰ **S60.379** Other superficial bite of unspecified thumb

√6ᵗʰ **S60.39** Other superficial injuries of thumb
√7ᵗʰ **S60.391** Other superficial injuries of right thumb
√7ᵗʰ **S60.392** Other superficial injuries of left thumb
√7ᵗʰ **S60.399** Other superficial injuries of unspecified thumb

√5ᵗʰ **S60.4** Other superficial injuries of other fingers

√6ᵗʰ **S60.41** Abrasion of fingers
√7ᵗʰ **S60.410** Abrasion of right index finger
√7ᵗʰ **S60.411** Abrasion of left index finger
√7ᵗʰ **S60.412** Abrasion of right middle finger
√7ᵗʰ **S60.413** Abrasion of left middle finger
√7ᵗʰ **S60.414** Abrasion of right ring finger
√7ᵗʰ **S60.415** Abrasion of left ring finger
√7ᵗʰ **S60.416** Abrasion of right little finger
√7ᵗʰ **S60.417** Abrasion of left little finger
√7ᵗʰ **S60.418** Abrasion of other finger
Abrasion of specified finger with unspecified laterality
√7ᵗʰ **S60.419** Abrasion of unspecified finger

√6ᵗʰ **S60.42** Blister (nonthermal) of fingers
√7ᵗʰ **S60.420** Blister (nonthermal) of right index finger
√7ᵗʰ **S60.421** Blister (nonthermal) of left index finger
√7ᵗʰ **S60.422** Blister (nonthermal) of right middle finger
√7ᵗʰ **S60.423** Blister (nonthermal) of left middle finger
√7ᵗʰ **S60.424** Blister (nonthermal) of right ring finger
√7ᵗʰ **S60.425** Blister (nonthermal) of left ring finger
√7ᵗʰ **S60.426** Blister (nonthermal) of right little finger
√7ᵗʰ **S60.427** Blister (nonthermal) of left little finger
√7ᵗʰ **S60.428** Blister (nonthermal) of other finger
Blister (nonthermal) of specified finger with unspecified laterality
√7ᵗʰ **S60.429** Blister (nonthermal) of unspecified finger

√6ᵗʰ **S60.44** External constriction of fingers
Hair tourniquet syndrome of finger
Use additional cause code to identify the constricting item (W49.0-)
√7ᵗʰ **S60.440** External constriction of right index finger
√7ᵗʰ **S60.441** External constriction of left index finger
√7ᵗʰ **S60.442** External constriction of right middle finger
√7ᵗʰ **S60.443** External constriction of left middle finger
√7ᵗʰ **S60.444** External constriction of right ring finger
√7ᵗʰ **S60.445** External constriction of left ring finger
√7ᵗʰ **S60.446** External constriction of right little finger
√7ᵗʰ **S60.447** External constriction of left little finger
√7ᵗʰ **S60.448** External constriction of other finger
External constriction of specified finger with unspecified laterality
√7ᵗʰ **S60.449** External constriction of unspecified finger

√6ᵗʰ **S60.45** Superficial foreign body of fingers
Splinter in the finger(s)
√7ᵗʰ **S60.450** Superficial foreign body of right index finger
√7ᵗʰ **S60.451** Superficial foreign body of left index finger
√7ᵗʰ **S60.452** Superficial foreign body of right middle finger
√7ᵗʰ **S60.453** Superficial foreign body of left middle finger
√7ᵗʰ **S60.454** Superficial foreign body of right ring finger
√7ᵗʰ **S60.455** Superficial foreign body of left ring finger
√7ᵗʰ **S60.456** Superficial foreign body of right little finger
√7ᵗʰ **S60.457** Superficial foreign body of left little finger
√7ᵗʰ **S60.458** Superficial foreign body of other finger
Superficial foreign body of specified finger with unspecified laterality
√7ᵗʰ **S60.459** Superficial foreign body of unspecified finger

√6ᵗʰ **S60.46** Insect bite (nonvenomous) of fingers
√7ᵗʰ **S60.460** Insect bite (nonvenomous) of right index finger
√7ᵗʰ **S60.461** Insect bite (nonvenomous) of left index finger
√7ᵗʰ **S60.462** Insect bite (nonvenomous) of right middle finger
√7ᵗʰ **S60.463** Insect bite (nonvenomous) of left middle finger
√7ᵗʰ **S60.464** Insect bite (nonvenomous) of right ring finger
√7ᵗʰ **S60.465** Insect bite (nonvenomous) of left ring finger
√7ᵗʰ **S60.466** Insect bite (nonvenomous) of right little finger
√7ᵗʰ **S60.467** Insect bite (nonvenomous) of left little finger
√7ᵗʰ **S60.468** Insect bite (nonvenomous) of other finger
Insect bite (nonvenomous) of specified finger with unspecified laterality
√7ᵗʰ **S60.469** Insect bite (nonvenomous) of unspecified finger

√6ᵗʰ **S60.47** Other superficial bite of fingers
EXCLUDES 1   open bite of fingers (S61.25-, S61.35-)
√7ᵗʰ **S60.470** Other superficial bite of right index finger
√7ᵗʰ **S60.471** Other superficial bite of left index finger
√7ᵗʰ **S60.472** Other superficial bite of right middle finger
√7ᵗʰ **S60.473** Other superficial bite of left middle finger
√7ᵗʰ **S60.474** Other superficial bite of right ring finger
√7ᵗʰ **S60.475** Other superficial bite of left ring finger
√7ᵗʰ **S60.476** Other superficial bite of right little finger
√7ᵗʰ **S60.477** Other superficial bite of left little finger
√7ᵗʰ **S60.478** Other superficial bite of other finger
Other superficial bite of specified finger with unspecified laterality

---

☑ Additional Character Required   √x7ᵗʰ Placeholder Alert   Manifestation   Unspecified Dx   Q QPP   UPD Unacceptable PDx

√7ᵗʰ **S60.479** Other superficial bite of unspecified finger

√5ᵗʰ **S60.5** Other superficial injuries of hand

     EXCLUDES 2   superficial injuries of fingers (S60.3-, S60.4-)

√6ᵗʰ **S60.51** Abrasion of hand
- √7ᵗʰ **S60.511** Abrasion of right hand
- √7ᵗʰ **S60.512** Abrasion of left hand
- √7ᵗʰ **S60.519** Abrasion of unspecified hand

√6ᵗʰ **S60.52** Blister (nonthermal) of hand
- √7ᵗʰ **S60.521** Blister (nonthermal) of right hand
- √7ᵗʰ **S60.522** Blister (nonthermal) of left hand
- √7ᵗʰ **S60.529** Blister (nonthermal) of unspecified hand

√6ᵗʰ **S60.54** External constriction of hand
- √7ᵗʰ **S60.541** External constriction of right hand
- √7ᵗʰ **S60.542** External constriction of left hand
- √7ᵗʰ **S60.549** External constriction of unspecified hand

√6ᵗʰ **S60.55** Superficial foreign body of hand

    Splinter in the hand
- √7ᵗʰ **S60.551** Superficial foreign body of right hand
- √7ᵗʰ **S60.552** Superficial foreign body of left hand
- √7ᵗʰ **S60.559** Superficial foreign body of unspecified hand

√6ᵗʰ **S60.56** Insect bite (nonvenomous) of hand
- √7ᵗʰ **S60.561** Insect bite (nonvenomous) of right hand
- √7ᵗʰ **S60.562** Insect bite (nonvenomous) of left hand
- √7ᵗʰ **S60.569** Insect bite (nonvenomous) of unspecified hand

√6ᵗʰ **S60.57** Other superficial bite of hand

     EXCLUDES 1   open bite of hand (S61.45-)
- √7ᵗʰ **S60.571** Other superficial bite of hand of right hand
- √7ᵗʰ **S60.572** Other superficial bite of hand of left hand
- √7ᵗʰ **S60.579** Other superficial bite of hand of unspecified hand

√5ᵗʰ **S60.8** Other superficial injuries of wrist

√6ᵗʰ **S60.81** Abrasion of wrist
- √7ᵗʰ **S60.811** Abrasion of right wrist
- √7ᵗʰ **S60.812** Abrasion of left wrist
- √7ᵗʰ **S60.819** Abrasion of unspecified wrist

√6ᵗʰ **S60.82** Blister (nonthermal) of wrist
- √7ᵗʰ **S60.821** Blister (nonthermal) of right wrist
- √7ᵗʰ **S60.822** Blister (nonthermal) of left wrist
- √7ᵗʰ **S60.829** Blister (nonthermal) of unspecified wrist

√6ᵗʰ **S60.84** External constriction of wrist
- √7ᵗʰ **S60.841** External constriction of right wrist
- √7ᵗʰ **S60.842** External constriction of left wrist
- √7ᵗʰ **S60.849** External constriction of unspecified wrist

√6ᵗʰ **S60.85** Superficial foreign body of wrist

    Splinter in the wrist
- √7ᵗʰ **S60.851** Superficial foreign body of right wrist
- √7ᵗʰ **S60.852** Superficial foreign body of left wrist
- √7ᵗʰ **S60.859** Superficial foreign body of unspecified wrist

√6ᵗʰ **S60.86** Insect bite (nonvenomous) of wrist
- √7ᵗʰ **S60.861** Insect bite (nonvenomous) of right wrist
- √7ᵗʰ **S60.862** Insect bite (nonvenomous) of left wrist
- √7ᵗʰ **S60.869** Insect bite (nonvenomous) of unspecified wrist

√6ᵗʰ **S60.87** Other superficial bite of wrist

     EXCLUDES 1   open bite of wrist (S61.55)
- √7ᵗʰ **S60.871** Other superficial bite of right wrist
- √7ᵗʰ **S60.872** Other superficial bite of left wrist
- √7ᵗʰ **S60.879** Other superficial bite of unspecified wrist

√6ᵗʰ **S60.9** Unspecified superficial injury of wrist, hand and fingers

√6ᵗʰ **S60.91** Unspecified superficial injury of wrist
- √7ᵗʰ **S60.911** Unspecified superficial injury of right wrist
- √7ᵗʰ **S60.912** Unspecified superficial injury of left wrist
- √7ᵗʰ **S60.919** Unspecified superficial injury of unspecified wrist

√6ᵗʰ **S60.92** Unspecified superficial injury of hand
- √7ᵗʰ **S60.921** Unspecified superficial injury of right hand
- √7ᵗʰ **S60.922** Unspecified superficial injury of left hand
- √7ᵗʰ **S60.929** Unspecified superficial injury of unspecified hand

√6ᵗʰ **S60.93** Unspecified superficial injury of thumb
- √7ᵗʰ **S60.931** Unspecified superficial injury of right thumb
- √7ᵗʰ **S60.932** Unspecified superficial injury of left thumb
- √7ᵗʰ **S60.939** Unspecified superficial injury of unspecified thumb

√6ᵗʰ **S60.94** Unspecified superficial injury of other fingers
- √7ᵗʰ **S60.940** Unspecified superficial injury of right index finger
- √7ᵗʰ **S60.941** Unspecified superficial injury of left index finger
- √7ᵗʰ **S60.942** Unspecified superficial injury of right middle finger
- √7ᵗʰ **S60.943** Unspecified superficial injury of left middle finger
- √7ᵗʰ **S60.944** Unspecified superficial injury of right ring finger
- √7ᵗʰ **S60.945** Unspecified superficial injury of left ring finger
- √7ᵗʰ **S60.946** Unspecified superficial injury of right little finger
- √7ᵗʰ **S60.947** Unspecified superficial injury of left little finger
- √7ᵗʰ **S60.948** Unspecified superficial injury of other finger

    Unspecified superficial injury of specified finger with unspecified laterality
- √7ᵗʰ **S60.949** Unspecified superficial injury of unspecified finger

√4ᵗʰ **S61** Open wound of wrist, hand and fingers

    Code also any associated wound infection

     EXCLUDES 1   open fracture of wrist, hand and finger (S62.- with 7th character B)

                  traumatic amputation of wrist and hand (S68.-)

> The appropriate 7th character is to be added to each code from category S61.
> A   initial encounter
> D   subsequent encounter
> S   sequela

√5ᵗʰ **S61.0** Open wound of thumb without damage to nail

     EXCLUDES 1   open wound of thumb with damage to nail (S61.1-)

√6ᵗʰ **S61.00** Unspecified open wound of thumb without damage to nail
- √7ᵗʰ **S61.001** Unspecified open wound of right thumb without damage to nail
- √7ᵗʰ **S61.002** Unspecified open wound of left thumb without damage to nail
- √7ᵗʰ **S61.009** Unspecified open wound of unspecified thumb without damage to nail

√6ᵗʰ **S61.01** Laceration without foreign body of thumb without damage to nail
- √7ᵗʰ **S61.011** Laceration without foreign body of right thumb without damage to nail
- √7ᵗʰ **S61.012** Laceration without foreign body of left thumb without damage to nail
- √7ᵗʰ **S61.019** Laceration without foreign body of unspecified thumb without damage to nail

√6ᵗʰ **S61.02** Laceration with foreign body of thumb without damage to nail
- √7ᵗʰ **S61.021** Laceration with foreign body of right thumb without damage to nail
- √7ᵗʰ **S61.022** Laceration with foreign body of left thumb without damage to nail
- √7ᵗʰ **S61.029** Laceration with foreign body of unspecified thumb without damage to nail

√6ᵗʰ **S61.03** Puncture wound without foreign body of thumb without damage to nail
- √7ᵗʰ **S61.031** Puncture wound without foreign body of right thumb without damage to nail
- √7ᵗʰ **S61.032** Puncture wound without foreign body of left thumb without damage to nail

√7ᵗʰ **S61.039** Puncture wound without foreign body of unspecified thumb without damage to nail

√6ᵗʰ **S61.04** Puncture wound with foreign body of thumb without damage to nail

√7ᵗʰ **S61.041** Puncture wound with foreign body of right thumb without damage to nail

√7ᵗʰ **S61.042** Puncture wound with foreign body of left thumb without damage to nail

√7ᵗʰ **S61.049** Puncture wound with foreign body of unspecified thumb without damage to nail

√6ᵗʰ **S61.05** Open bite of thumb without damage to nail

Bite of thumb NOS

EXCLUDES 1   superficial bite of thumb (S60.36-, S60.37-)

√7ᵗʰ **S61.051** Open bite of right thumb without damage to nail

√7ᵗʰ **S61.052** Open bite of left thumb without damage to nail

√7ᵗʰ **S61.059** Open bite of unspecified thumb without damage to nail

√5ᵗʰ **S61.1** Open wound of thumb with damage to nail

√6ᵗʰ **S61.10** Unspecified open wound of thumb with damage to nail

√7ᵗʰ **S61.101** Unspecified open wound of right thumb with damage to nail

√7ᵗʰ **S61.102** Unspecified open wound of left thumb with damage to nail

√7ᵗʰ **S61.109** Unspecified open wound of unspecified thumb with damage to nail

√6ᵗʰ **S61.11** Laceration without foreign body of thumb with damage to nail

√7ᵗʰ **S61.111** Laceration without foreign body of right thumb with damage to nail

√7ᵗʰ **S61.112** Laceration without foreign body of left thumb with damage to nail

√7ᵗʰ **S61.119** Laceration without foreign body of unspecified thumb with damage to nail

√6ᵗʰ **S61.12** Laceration with foreign body of thumb with damage to nail

√7ᵗʰ **S61.121** Laceration with foreign body of right thumb with damage to nail

√7ᵗʰ **S61.122** Laceration with foreign body of left thumb with damage to nail

√7ᵗʰ **S61.129** Laceration with foreign body of unspecified thumb with damage to nail

√6ᵗʰ **S61.13** Puncture wound without foreign body of thumb with damage to nail

√7ᵗʰ **S61.131** Puncture wound without foreign body of right thumb with damage to nail

√7ᵗʰ **S61.132** Puncture wound without foreign body of left thumb with damage to nail

√7ᵗʰ **S61.139** Puncture wound without foreign body of unspecified thumb with damage to nail

√6ᵗʰ **S61.14** Puncture wound with foreign body of thumb with damage to nail

√7ᵗʰ **S61.141** Puncture wound with foreign body of right thumb with damage to nail

√7ᵗʰ **S61.142** Puncture wound with foreign body of left thumb with damage to nail

√7ᵗʰ **S61.149** Puncture wound with foreign body of unspecified thumb with damage to nail

√6ᵗʰ **S61.15** Open bite of thumb with damage to nail

Bite of thumb with damage to nail NOS

EXCLUDES 1   superficial bite of thumb (S60.36-, S60.37-)

√7ᵗʰ **S61.151** Open bite of right thumb with damage to nail

√7ᵗʰ **S61.152** Open bite of left thumb with damage to nail

√7ᵗʰ **S61.159** Open bite of unspecified thumb with damage to nail

√5ᵗʰ **S61.2** Open wound of other finger without damage to nail

EXCLUDES 1   open wound of finger involving nail (matrix) (S61.3-)

EXCLUDES 2   open wound of thumb without damage to nail (S61.0-)

√6ᵗʰ **S61.20** Unspecified open wound of other finger without damage to nail

√7ᵗʰ **S61.200** Unspecified open wound of right index finger without damage to nail

√7ᵗʰ **S61.201** Unspecified open wound of left index finger without damage to nail

√7ᵗʰ **S61.202** Unspecified open wound of right middle finger without damage to nail

√7ᵗʰ **S61.203** Unspecified open wound of left middle finger without damage to nail

√7ᵗʰ **S61.204** Unspecified open wound of right ring finger without damage to nail

√7ᵗʰ **S61.205** Unspecified open wound of left ring finger without damage to nail

√7ᵗʰ **S61.206** Unspecified open wound of right little finger without damage to nail

√7ᵗʰ **S61.207** Unspecified open wound of left little finger without damage to nail

√7ᵗʰ **S61.208** Unspecified open wound of other finger without damage to nail

Unspecified open wound of specified finger with unspecified laterality without damage to nail

√7ᵗʰ **S61.209** Unspecified open wound of unspecified finger without damage to nail

√6ᵗʰ **S61.21** Laceration without foreign body of finger without damage to nail

√7ᵗʰ **S61.210** Laceration without foreign body of right index finger without damage to nail

√7ᵗʰ **S61.211** Laceration without foreign body of left index finger without damage to nail

√7ᵗʰ **S61.212** Laceration without foreign body of right middle finger without damage to nail

√7ᵗʰ **S61.213** Laceration without foreign body of left middle finger without damage to nail

√7ᵗʰ **S61.214** Laceration without foreign body of right ring finger without damage to nail

√7ᵗʰ **S61.215** Laceration without foreign body of left ring finger without damage to nail

√7ᵗʰ **S61.216** Laceration without foreign body of right little finger without damage to nail

√7ᵗʰ **S61.217** Laceration without foreign body of left little finger without damage to nail

√7ᵗʰ **S61.218** Laceration without foreign body of other finger without damage to nail

Laceration without foreign body of specified finger with unspecified laterality without damage to nail

√7ᵗʰ **S61.219** Laceration without foreign body of unspecified finger without damage to nail

√6ᵗʰ **S61.22** Laceration with foreign body of finger without damage to nail

√7ᵗʰ **S61.220** Laceration with foreign body of right index finger without damage to nail

√7ᵗʰ **S61.221** Laceration with foreign body of left index finger without damage to nail

√7ᵗʰ **S61.222** Laceration with foreign body of right middle finger without damage to nail

√7ᵗʰ **S61.223** Laceration with foreign body of left middle finger without damage to nail

√7ᵗʰ **S61.224** Laceration with foreign body of right ring finger without damage to nail

√7ᵗʰ **S61.225** Laceration with foreign body of left ring finger without damage to nail

√7ᵗʰ **S61.226** Laceration with foreign body of right little finger without damage to nail

√7ᵗʰ **S61.227** Laceration with foreign body of left little finger without damage to nail

√7ᵗʰ **S61.228** Laceration with foreign body of other finger without damage to nail

Laceration with foreign body of specified finger with unspecified laterality without damage to nail

√7ᵗʰ **S61.229** Laceration with foreign body of unspecified finger without damage to nail

√6ᵗʰ **S61.23** Puncture wound without foreign body of finger without damage to nail

√7ᵗʰ **S61.230** Puncture wound without foreign body of right index finger without damage to nail

√7ᵗʰ **S61.231** Puncture wound without foreign body of left index finger without damage to nail

√7ᵗʰ **S61.232** Puncture wound without foreign body of right middle finger without damage to nail

√7ᵗʰ **S61.233** Puncture wound without foreign body of left middle finger without damage to nail

Chapter 19. Injury, Poisoning and Certain Other Consequences of External Causes

√7ᵗʰ **S61.234** **Puncture wound without foreign body of** right ring **finger without damage to nail**

√7ᵗʰ **S61.235** **Puncture wound without foreign body of** left ring **finger without damage to nail**

√7ᵗʰ **S61.236** **Puncture wound without foreign body of** right little **finger without damage to nail**

√7ᵗʰ **S61.237** **Puncture wound without foreign body of** left little **finger without damage to nail**

√7ᵗʰ **S61.238** **Puncture wound without foreign body of other finger without damage to nail**

Puncture wound without foreign body of specified finger with unspecified laterality without damage to nail

√7ᵗʰ **S61.239** **Puncture wound without foreign body of unspecified finger without damage to nail**

√6ᵗʰ **S61.24** **Puncture wound with foreign body** of finger without damage to nail

√7ᵗʰ **S61.240** **Puncture wound with foreign body of** right index **finger without damage to nail**

√7ᵗʰ **S61.241** **Puncture wound with foreign body of** left index **finger without damage to nail**

√7ᵗʰ **S61.242** **Puncture wound with foreign body of** right middle **finger without damage to nail**

√7ᵗʰ **S61.243** **Puncture wound with foreign body of** left middle **finger without damage to nail**

√7ᵗʰ **S61.244** **Puncture wound with foreign body of** right ring **finger without damage to nail**

√7ᵗʰ **S61.245** **Puncture wound with foreign body of** left ring **finger without damage to nail**

√7ᵗʰ **S61.246** **Puncture wound with foreign body of** right little **finger without damage to nail**

√7ᵗʰ **S61.247** **Puncture wound with foreign body of** left little **finger without damage to nail**

√7ᵗʰ **S61.248** **Puncture wound with foreign body of other finger without damage to nail**

Puncture wound with foreign body of specified finger with unspecified laterality without damage to nail

√7ᵗʰ **S61.249** **Puncture wound with foreign body of unspecified finger without damage to nail**

√6ᵗʰ **S61.25** **Open bite** of finger without damage to nail

Bite of finger without damage to nail NOS

EXCLUDES 1   superficial bite of finger (S60.46-, S60.47-)

√7ᵗʰ **S61.250** **Open bite of** right index **finger without damage to nail**

√7ᵗʰ **S61.251** **Open bite of** left index **finger without damage to nail**

√7ᵗʰ **S61.252** **Open bite of** right middle **finger without damage to nail**

√7ᵗʰ **S61.253** **Open bite of** left middle **finger without damage to nail**

√7ᵗʰ **S61.254** **Open bite of** right ring **finger without damage to nail**

√7ᵗʰ **S61.255** **Open bite of** left ring **finger without damage to nail**

√7ᵗʰ **S61.256** **Open bite of** right little **finger without damage to nail**

√7ᵗʰ **S61.257** **Open bite of** left little **finger without damage to nail**

√7ᵗʰ **S61.258** **Open bite of other finger without damage to nail**

Open bite of specified finger with unspecified laterality without damage to nail

√7ᵗʰ **S61.259** **Open bite of unspecified finger without damage to nail**

√5ᵗʰ **S61.3** **Open wound of other** finger with damage to nail

√6ᵗʰ **S61.30** **Unspecified open wound of finger with damage to nail**

√7ᵗʰ **S61.300** **Unspecified open wound of** right index **finger with damage to nail**

√7ᵗʰ **S61.301** **Unspecified open wound of** left index **finger with damage to nail**

√7ᵗʰ **S61.302** **Unspecified open wound of** right middle **finger with damage to nail**

√7ᵗʰ **S61.303** **Unspecified open wound of** left middle **finger with damage to nail**

√7ᵗʰ **S61.304** **Unspecified open wound of** right ring **finger with damage to nail**

√7ᵗʰ **S61.305** **Unspecified open wound of** left ring **finger with damage to nail**

√7ᵗʰ **S61.306** **Unspecified open wound of** right little **finger with damage to nail**

√7ᵗʰ **S61.307** **Unspecified open wound of** left little **finger with damage to nail**

√7ᵗʰ **S61.308** **Unspecified open wound of other finger with damage to nail**

Unspecified open wound of specified finger with unspecified laterality with damage to nail

√7ᵗʰ **S61.309** **Unspecified open wound of unspecified finger with damage to nail**

√6ᵗʰ **S61.31** **Laceration without foreign body** of finger with damage to nail

√7ᵗʰ **S61.310** **Laceration without foreign body of** right index **finger with damage to nail**

√7ᵗʰ **S61.311** **Laceration without foreign body of** left index **finger with damage to nail**

√7ᵗʰ **S61.312** **Laceration without foreign body of** right middle **finger with damage to nail**

√7ᵗʰ **S61.313** **Laceration without foreign body of** left middle **finger with damage to nail**

√7ᵗʰ **S61.314** **Laceration without foreign body of** right ring **finger with damage to nail**

√7ᵗʰ **S61.315** **Laceration without foreign body of** left ring **finger with damage to nail**

√7ᵗʰ **S61.316** **Laceration without foreign body of** right little **finger with damage to nail**

√7ᵗʰ **S61.317** **Laceration without foreign body of** left little **finger with damage to nail**

√7ᵗʰ **S61.318** **Laceration without foreign body of other finger with damage to nail**

Laceration without foreign body of specified finger with unspecified laterality with damage to nail

√7ᵗʰ **S61.319** **Laceration without foreign body of unspecified finger with damage to nail**

√6ᵗʰ **S61.32** **Laceration with foreign body** of finger with damage to nail

√7ᵗʰ **S61.320** **Laceration with foreign body of** right index **finger with damage to nail**

√7ᵗʰ **S61.321** **Laceration with foreign body of** left index **finger with damage to nail**

√7ᵗʰ **S61.322** **Laceration with foreign body of** right middle **finger with damage to nail**

√7ᵗʰ **S61.323** **Laceration with foreign body of** left middle **finger with damage to nail**

√7ᵗʰ **S61.324** **Laceration with foreign body of** right ring **finger with damage to nail**

√7ᵗʰ **S61.325** **Laceration with foreign body of** left ring **finger with damage to nail**

√7ᵗʰ **S61.326** **Laceration with foreign body of** right little **finger with damage to nail**

√7ᵗʰ **S61.327** **Laceration with foreign body of** left little **finger with damage to nail**

√7ᵗʰ **S61.328** **Laceration with foreign body of other finger with damage to nail**

Laceration with foreign body of specified finger with unspecified laterality with damage to nail

√7ᵗʰ **S61.329** **Laceration with foreign body of unspecified finger with damage to nail**

√6ᵗʰ **S61.33** **Puncture wound without foreign body** of finger with damage to nail

√7ᵗʰ **S61.330** **Puncture wound without foreign body of** right index **finger with damage to nail**

√7ᵗʰ **S61.331** **Puncture wound without foreign body of** left index **finger with damage to nail**

√7ᵗʰ **S61.332** **Puncture wound without foreign body of** right middle **finger with damage to nail**

√7ᵗʰ **S61.333** **Puncture wound without foreign body of** left middle **finger with damage to nail**

√7ᵗʰ **S61.334** **Puncture wound without foreign body of** right ring **finger with damage to nail**

√7ᵗʰ **S61.335** **Puncture wound without foreign body of** left ring **finger with damage to nail**

√7ᵗʰ **S61.336** **Puncture wound without foreign body of** right little **finger with damage to nail**

√7ᵗʰ **S61.337** **Puncture wound without foreign body of** left little **finger with damage to nail**

√7ᵗʰ **S61.338 Puncture wound without foreign body of other finger with damage to nail**
    Puncture wound without foreign body of specified finger with unspecified laterality with damage to nail

√7ᵗʰ **S61.339 Puncture wound without foreign body of unspecified finger with damage to nail**

√6ᵗʰ **S61.34 Puncture wound with foreign body of finger with damage to nail**

√7ᵗʰ **S61.340 Puncture wound with foreign body of right index finger with damage to nail**

√7ᵗʰ **S61.341 Puncture wound with foreign body of left index finger with damage to nail**

√7ᵗʰ **S61.342 Puncture wound with foreign body of right middle finger with damage to nail**

√7ᵗʰ **S61.343 Puncture wound with foreign body of left middle finger with damage to nail**

√7ᵗʰ **S61.344 Puncture wound with foreign body of right ring finger with damage to nail**

√7ᵗʰ **S61.345 Puncture wound with foreign body of left ring finger with damage to nail**

√7ᵗʰ **S61.346 Puncture wound with foreign body of right little finger with damage to nail**

√7ᵗʰ **S61.347 Puncture wound with foreign body of left little finger with damage to nail**

√7ᵗʰ **S61.348 Puncture wound with foreign body of other finger with damage to nail**
    Puncture wound with foreign body of specified finger with unspecified laterality with damage to nail

√7ᵗʰ **S61.349 Puncture wound with foreign body of unspecified finger with damage to nail**

√6ᵗʰ **S61.35 Open bite of finger with damage to nail**
    Bite of finger with damage to nail NOS
    EXCLUDES 1   superficial bite of finger (S60.46-, S60.47-)

√7ᵗʰ **S61.350 Open bite of right index finger with damage to nail**

√7ᵗʰ **S61.351 Open bite of left index finger with damage to nail**

√7ᵗʰ **S61.352 Open bite of right middle finger with damage to nail**

√7ᵗʰ **S61.353 Open bite of left middle finger with damage to nail**

√7ᵗʰ **S61.354 Open bite of right ring finger with damage to nail**

√7ᵗʰ **S61.355 Open bite of left ring finger with damage to nail**

√7ᵗʰ **S61.356 Open bite of right little finger with damage to nail**

√7ᵗʰ **S61.357 Open bite of left little finger with damage to nail**

√7ᵗʰ **S61.358 Open bite of other finger with damage to nail**
    Open bite of specified finger with unspecified laterality with damage to nail

√7ᵗʰ **S61.359 Open bite of unspecified finger with damage to nail**

√5ᵗʰ **S61.4 Open wound of hand**

√6ᵗʰ **S61.40 Unspecified open wound of hand**

√7ᵗʰ **S61.401 Unspecified open wound of right hand**

√7ᵗʰ **S61.402 Unspecified open wound of left hand**

√7ᵗʰ **S61.409 Unspecified open wound of unspecified hand**

√6ᵗʰ **S61.41 Laceration without foreign body of hand**

√7ᵗʰ **S61.411 Laceration without foreign body of right hand**

√7ᵗʰ **S61.412 Laceration without foreign body of left hand**

√7ᵗʰ **S61.419 Laceration without foreign body of unspecified hand**

√6ᵗʰ **S61.42 Laceration with foreign body of hand**

√7ᵗʰ **S61.421 Laceration with foreign body of right hand**

√7ᵗʰ **S61.422 Laceration with foreign body of left hand**

√7ᵗʰ **S61.429 Laceration with foreign body of unspecified hand**

√6ᵗʰ **S61.43 Puncture wound without foreign body of hand**

√7ᵗʰ **S61.431 Puncture wound without foreign body of right hand**

√7ᵗʰ **S61.432 Puncture wound without foreign body of left hand**

√7ᵗʰ **S61.439 Puncture wound without foreign body of unspecified hand**

√6ᵗʰ **S61.44 Puncture wound with foreign body of hand**

√7ᵗʰ **S61.441 Puncture wound with foreign body of right hand**

√7ᵗʰ **S61.442 Puncture wound with foreign body of left hand**

√7ᵗʰ **S61.449 Puncture wound with foreign body of unspecified hand**

√6ᵗʰ **S61.45 Open bite of hand**
    Bite of hand NOS
    EXCLUDES 1   superficial bite of hand (S60.56-, S60.57-)

√7ᵗʰ **S61.451 Open bite of right hand**

√7ᵗʰ **S61.452 Open bite of left hand**

√7ᵗʰ **S61.459 Open bite of unspecified hand**

√5ᵗʰ **S61.5 Open wound of wrist**

√6ᵗʰ **S61.50 Unspecified open wound of wrist**

√7ᵗʰ **S61.501 Unspecified open wound of right wrist**

√7ᵗʰ **S61.502 Unspecified open wound of left wrist**

√7ᵗʰ **S61.509 Unspecified open wound of unspecified wrist**

√6ᵗʰ **S61.51 Laceration without foreign body of wrist**

√7ᵗʰ **S61.511 Laceration without foreign body of right wrist**

√7ᵗʰ **S61.512 Laceration without foreign body of left wrist**

√7ᵗʰ **S61.519 Laceration without foreign body of unspecified wrist**

√6ᵗʰ **S61.52 Laceration with foreign body of wrist**

√7ᵗʰ **S61.521 Laceration with foreign body of right wrist**

√7ᵗʰ **S61.522 Laceration with foreign body of left wrist**

√7ᵗʰ **S61.529 Laceration with foreign body of unspecified wrist**

√6ᵗʰ **S61.53 Puncture wound without foreign body of wrist**

√7ᵗʰ **S61.531 Puncture wound without foreign body of right wrist**

√7ᵗʰ **S61.532 Puncture wound without foreign body of left wrist**

√7ᵗʰ **S61.539 Puncture wound without foreign body of unspecified wrist**

√6ᵗʰ **S61.54 Puncture wound with foreign body of wrist**

√7ᵗʰ **S61.541 Puncture wound with foreign body of right wrist**

√7ᵗʰ **S61.542 Puncture wound with foreign body of left wrist**

√7ᵗʰ **S61.549 Puncture wound with foreign body of unspecified wrist**

√6ᵗʰ **S61.55 Open bite of wrist**
    Bite of wrist NOS
    EXCLUDES 1   superficial bite of wrist (S60.86-, S60.87-)

√7ᵗʰ **S61.551 Open bite of right wrist**

√7ᵗʰ **S61.552 Open bite of left wrist**

√7ᵗʰ **S61.559 Open bite of unspecified wrist**

☑ Additional Character Required   √x7ᵗʰ Placeholder Alert   Manifestation   Unspecified Dx   ◘ QPP   UPD Unacceptable PDx

Chapter 19. Injury, Poisoning and Certain Other Consequences of External Causes

S62–S62.146

✓4ᵗʰ **S62** **Fracture at wrist and hand level**

> **NOTE** A fracture not indicated as displaced or nondisplaced should be coded to displaced
>
> A fracture not indicated as open or closed should be coded to closed

> **EXCLUDES 1** traumatic amputation of wrist and hand (S68.-)
>
> **EXCLUDES 2** fracture of distal parts of ulna and radius (S52.-)

AHA: 2018,2Q,12; 2015,3Q,37-39

> The appropriate 7th character is to be added to each code from category S62.
> A   initial encounter for closed fracture
> B   initial encounter for open fracture
> D   subsequent encounter for fracture with routine healing
> G   subsequent encounter for fracture with delayed healing
> K   subsequent encounter for fracture with nonunion
> P   subsequent encounter for fracture with malunion
> S   sequela

✓5ᵗʰ **S62.0** **Fracture of navicular [scaphoid] bone of wrist**

    ✓6ᵗʰ **S62.00** **Unspecified fracture of navicular [scaphoid] bone of wrist**

       ✓7ᵗʰ **S62.001** **Unspecified fracture of navicular [scaphoid] bone of right wrist**   Q

       ✓7ᵗʰ **S62.002** **Unspecified fracture of navicular [scaphoid] bone of left wrist**   Q

         AHA: 2012,4Q,106

       ✓7ᵗʰ **S62.009** **Unspecified fracture of navicular [scaphoid] bone of unspecified wrist**   Q

    ✓6ᵗʰ **S62.01** **Fracture of distal pole of navicular [scaphoid] bone of wrist**

         Fracture of volar tuberosity of navicular [scaphoid] bone of wrist

       ✓7ᵗʰ **S62.011** **Displaced fracture of distal pole of navicular [scaphoid] bone of right wrist**   Q

       ✓7ᵗʰ **S62.012** **Displaced fracture of distal pole of navicular [scaphoid] bone of left wrist**   Q

       ✓7ᵗʰ **S62.013** **Displaced fracture of distal pole of navicular [scaphoid] bone of unspecified wrist**   Q

       ✓7ᵗʰ **S62.014** **Nondisplaced fracture of distal pole of navicular [scaphoid] bone of right wrist**   Q

       ✓7ᵗʰ **S62.015** **Nondisplaced fracture of distal pole of navicular [scaphoid] bone of left wrist**   Q

       ✓7ᵗʰ **S62.016** **Nondisplaced fracture of distal pole of navicular [scaphoid] bone of unspecified wrist**   Q

    ✓6ᵗʰ **S62.02** **Fracture of middle third of navicular [scaphoid] bone of wrist**

       ✓7ᵗʰ **S62.021** **Displaced fracture of middle third of navicular [scaphoid] bone of right wrist**   Q

       ✓7ᵗʰ **S62.022** **Displaced fracture of middle third of navicular [scaphoid] bone of left wrist**   Q

       ✓7ᵗʰ **S62.023** **Displaced fracture of middle third of navicular [scaphoid] bone of unspecified wrist**   Q

       ✓7ᵗʰ **S62.024** **Nondisplaced fracture of middle third of navicular [scaphoid] bone of right wrist**   Q

       ✓7ᵗʰ **S62.025** **Nondisplaced fracture of middle third of navicular [scaphoid] bone of left wrist**   Q

       ✓7ᵗʰ **S62.026** **Nondisplaced fracture of middle third of navicular [scaphoid] bone of unspecified wrist**   Q

    ✓6ᵗʰ **S62.03** **Fracture of proximal third of navicular [scaphoid] bone of wrist**

       ✓7ᵗʰ **S62.031** **Displaced fracture of proximal third of navicular [scaphoid] bone of right wrist**   Q

       ✓7ᵗʰ **S62.032** **Displaced fracture of proximal third of navicular [scaphoid] bone of left wrist**   Q

       ✓7ᵗʰ **S62.033** **Displaced fracture of proximal third of navicular [scaphoid] bone of unspecified wrist**   Q

       ✓7ᵗʰ **S62.034** **Nondisplaced fracture of proximal third of navicular [scaphoid] bone of right wrist**   Q

       ✓7ᵗʰ **S62.035** **Nondisplaced fracture of proximal third of navicular [scaphoid] bone of left wrist**   Q

       ✓7ᵗʰ **S62.036** **Nondisplaced fracture of proximal third of navicular [scaphoid] bone of unspecified wrist**   Q

✓5ᵗʰ **S62.1** **Fracture of other and unspecified carpal bone(s)**

> **EXCLUDES 2** fracture of scaphoid of wrist (S62.0-)

    ✓6ᵗʰ **S62.10** **Fracture of unspecified carpal bone**

         Fracture of wrist NOS

       ✓7ᵗʰ **S62.101** **Fracture of unspecified carpal bone, right wrist**   Q

       ✓7ᵗʰ **S62.102** **Fracture of unspecified carpal bone, left wrist**   Q

         AHA: 2012,4Q,95

       ✓7ᵗʰ **S62.109** **Fracture of unspecified carpal bone, unspecified wrist**   Q

    ✓6ᵗʰ **S62.11** **Fracture of triquetrum [cuneiform] bone of wrist**

       ✓7ᵗʰ **S62.111** **Displaced fracture of triquetrum [cuneiform] bone, right wrist**   Q

       ✓7ᵗʰ **S62.112** **Displaced fracture of triquetrum [cuneiform] bone, left wrist**   Q

       ✓7ᵗʰ **S62.113** **Displaced fracture of triquetrum [cuneiform] bone, unspecified wrist**   Q

       ✓7ᵗʰ **S62.114** **Nondisplaced fracture of triquetrum [cuneiform] bone, right wrist**   Q

       ✓7ᵗʰ **S62.115** **Nondisplaced fracture of triquetrum [cuneiform] bone, left wrist**   Q

       ✓7ᵗʰ **S62.116** **Nondisplaced fracture of triquetrum [cuneiform] bone, unspecified wrist**   Q

    ✓6ᵗʰ **S62.12** **Fracture of lunate [semilunar]**

       ✓7ᵗʰ **S62.121** **Displaced fracture of lunate [semilunar], right wrist**   Q

       ✓7ᵗʰ **S62.122** **Displaced fracture of lunate [semilunar], left wrist**   Q

       ✓7ᵗʰ **S62.123** **Displaced fracture of lunate [semilunar], unspecified wrist**   Q

       ✓7ᵗʰ **S62.124** **Nondisplaced fracture of lunate [semilunar], right wrist**   Q

       ✓7ᵗʰ **S62.125** **Nondisplaced fracture of lunate [semilunar], left wrist**   Q

       ✓7ᵗʰ **S62.126** **Nondisplaced fracture of lunate [semilunar], unspecified wrist**   Q

    ✓6ᵗʰ **S62.13** **Fracture of capitate [os magnum] bone**

       ✓7ᵗʰ **S62.131** **Displaced fracture of capitate [os magnum] bone, right wrist**   Q

       ✓7ᵗʰ **S62.132** **Displaced fracture of capitate [os magnum] bone, left wrist**   Q

       ✓7ᵗʰ **S62.133** **Displaced fracture of capitate [os magnum] bone, unspecified wrist**   Q

       ✓7ᵗʰ **S62.134** **Nondisplaced fracture of capitate [os magnum] bone, right wrist**   Q

       ✓7ᵗʰ **S62.135** **Nondisplaced fracture of capitate [os magnum] bone, left wrist**   Q

       ✓7ᵗʰ **S62.136** **Nondisplaced fracture of capitate [os magnum] bone, unspecified wrist**   Q

    ✓6ᵗʰ **S62.14** **Fracture of body of hamate [unciform] bone**

         Fracture of hamate [unciform] bone NOS

       ✓7ᵗʰ **S62.141** **Displaced fracture of body of hamate [unciform] bone, right wrist**   Q

       ✓7ᵗʰ **S62.142** **Displaced fracture of body of hamate [unciform] bone, left wrist**   Q

       ✓7ᵗʰ **S62.143** **Displaced fracture of body of hamate [unciform] bone, unspecified wrist**   Q

       ✓7ᵗʰ **S62.144** **Nondisplaced fracture of body of hamate [unciform] bone, right wrist**   Q

       ✓7ᵗʰ **S62.145** **Nondisplaced fracture of body of hamate [unciform] bone, left wrist**   Q

       ✓7ᵗʰ **S62.146** **Nondisplaced fracture of body of hamate [unciform] bone, unspecified wrist**   Q

HCC CMS-HCC   **Rx** Rx HCC   **ESR** ESRD HCC   **COM** Commercial HCC   **N** Newborn: 0   **P** Pediatric: 0-17   **M** Maternity: 9-64   **A** Adult: 15-124

1062   ICD-10-CM 2023

☑6ᵗʰ **S62.15** **Fracture of** hook process of hamate [unciform] **bone**
Fracture of unciform process of hamate [unciform] bone

☑7ᵗʰ **S62.151** Displaced **fracture of hook process of hamate [unciform] bone,** right **wrist** ⓠ

☑7ᵗʰ **S62.152** Displaced **fracture of hook process of hamate [unciform] bone,** left **wrist** ⓠ

☑7ᵗʰ **S62.153** Displaced **fracture of hook process of hamate [unciform] bone, unspecified wrist** ⓠ

☑7ᵗʰ **S62.154** Nondisplaced **fracture of hook process of hamate [unciform] bone,** right **wrist** ⓠ

☑7ᵗʰ **S62.155** Nondisplaced **fracture of hook process of hamate [unciform] bone,** left **wrist** ⓠ

☑7ᵗʰ **S62.156** Nondisplaced **fracture of hook process of hamate [unciform] bone, unspecified wrist** ⓠ

☑6ᵗʰ **S62.16** **Fracture of** pisiform

☑7ᵗʰ **S62.161** Displaced **fracture of pisiform,** right **wrist** ⓠ

☑7ᵗʰ **S62.162** Displaced **fracture of pisiform,** left **wrist** ⓠ

☑7ᵗʰ **S62.163** Displaced **fracture of pisiform, unspecified wrist** ⓠ

☑7ᵗʰ **S62.164** Nondisplaced **fracture of pisiform,** right **wrist** ⓠ

☑7ᵗʰ **S62.165** Nondisplaced **fracture of pisiform,** left **wrist** ⓠ

☑7ᵗʰ **S62.166** Nondisplaced **fracture of pisiform, unspecified wrist** ⓠ

☑6ᵗʰ **S62.17** **Fracture of** trapezium [larger multangular]

☑7ᵗʰ **S62.171** Displaced **fracture of trapezium [larger multangular],** right **wrist** ⓠ

☑7ᵗʰ **S62.172** Displaced **fracture of trapezium [larger multangular],** left **wrist** ⓠ

☑7ᵗʰ **S62.173** Displaced **fracture of trapezium [larger multangular], unspecified wrist** ⓠ

☑7ᵗʰ **S62.174** Nondisplaced **fracture of trapezium [larger multangular],** right **wrist** ⓠ

☑7ᵗʰ **S62.175** Nondisplaced **fracture of trapezium [larger multangular],** left **wrist** ⓠ

☑7ᵗʰ **S62.176** Nondisplaced **fracture of trapezium [larger multangular], unspecified wrist** ⓠ

☑6ᵗʰ **S62.18** **Fracture of** trapezoid [smaller multangular]

☑7ᵗʰ **S62.181** Displaced **fracture of trapezoid [smaller multangular],** right **wrist** ⓠ

☑7ᵗʰ **S62.182** Displaced **fracture of trapezoid [smaller multangular],** left **wrist** ⓠ

☑7ᵗʰ **S62.183** Displaced **fracture of trapezoid [smaller multangular], unspecified wrist** ⓠ

☑7ᵗʰ **S62.184** Nondisplaced **fracture of trapezoid [smaller multangular],** right **wrist** ⓠ

☑7ᵗʰ **S62.185** Nondisplaced **fracture of trapezoid [smaller multangular],** left **wrist** ⓠ

☑7ᵗʰ **S62.186** Nondisplaced **fracture of trapezoid [smaller multangular], unspecified wrist** ⓠ

☑5ᵗʰ **S62.2** **Fracture of** first metacarpal **bone**

☑6ᵗʰ **S62.20** **Unspecified fracture of first metacarpal bone**

☑7ᵗʰ **S62.201** **Unspecified fracture of first metacarpal bone,** right **hand** ⓠ

☑7ᵗʰ **S62.202** **Unspecified fracture of first metacarpal bone,** left **hand** ⓠ

☑7ᵗʰ **S62.209** **Unspecified fracture of first metacarpal bone, unspecified hand** ⓠ

☑6ᵗʰ **S62.21** Bennett's **fracture**
DEF: Intra-articular, two-part fracture at the base of the first metacarpal bone (thumb) on the ulnar side at the carpometacarpal (CMC) joint.

☑7ᵗʰ **S62.211** **Bennett's fracture,** right **hand** ⓠ

☑7ᵗʰ **S62.212** **Bennett's fracture,** left **hand** ⓠ

☑7ᵗʰ **S62.213** **Bennett's fracture, unspecified hand** ⓠ

☑6ᵗʰ **S62.22** Rolando's **fracture**
DEF: Comminuted, three part intra-articular fracture at the base of the thumb metacarpal.

☑7ᵗʰ **S62.221** Displaced **Rolando's fracture,** right **hand** ⓠ

☑7ᵗʰ **S62.222** Displaced **Rolando's fracture,** left **hand** ⓠ

☑7ᵗʰ **S62.223** Displaced **Rolando's fracture, unspecified hand** ⓠ

☑7ᵗʰ **S62.224** Nondisplaced **Rolando's fracture,** right **hand** ⓠ

☑7ᵗʰ **S62.225** Nondisplaced **Rolando's fracture,** left **hand** ⓠ

☑7ᵗʰ **S62.226** Nondisplaced **Rolando's fracture, unspecified hand** ⓠ

☑6ᵗʰ **S62.23** **Other fracture of** base of first metacarpal bone

☑7ᵗʰ **S62.231** **Other** displaced **fracture of base of first metacarpal bone,** right **hand** ⓠ

☑7ᵗʰ **S62.232** **Other** displaced **fracture of base of first metacarpal bone,** left **hand** ⓠ

☑7ᵗʰ **S62.233** **Other** displaced **fracture of base of first metacarpal bone, unspecified hand** ⓠ

☑7ᵗʰ **S62.234** **Other** nondisplaced **fracture of base of first metacarpal bone,** right **hand** ⓠ

☑7ᵗʰ **S62.235** **Other** nondisplaced **fracture of base of first metacarpal bone,** left **hand** ⓠ

☑7ᵗʰ **S62.236** **Other** nondisplaced **fracture of base of first metacarpal bone, unspecified hand** ⓠ

☑6ᵗʰ **S62.24** **Fracture of** shaft of first metacarpal bone

☑7ᵗʰ **S62.241** Displaced **fracture of shaft of first metacarpal bone,** right **hand** ⓠ

☑7ᵗʰ **S62.242** Displaced **fracture of shaft of first metacarpal bone,** left **hand** ⓠ

☑7ᵗʰ **S62.243** Displaced **fracture of shaft of first metacarpal bone, unspecified hand** ⓠ

☑7ᵗʰ **S62.244** Nondisplaced **fracture of shaft of first metacarpal bone,** right **hand** ⓠ

☑7ᵗʰ **S62.245** Nondisplaced **fracture of shaft of first metacarpal bone,** left **hand** ⓠ

☑7ᵗʰ **S62.246** Nondisplaced **fracture of shaft of first metacarpal bone, unspecified hand** ⓠ

☑6ᵗʰ **S62.25** **Fracture of** neck of first metacarpal bone

☑7ᵗʰ **S62.251** Displaced **fracture of neck of first metacarpal bone,** right **hand** ⓠ

☑7ᵗʰ **S62.252** Displaced **fracture of neck of first metacarpal bone,** left **hand** ⓠ

☑7ᵗʰ **S62.253** Displaced **fracture of neck of first metacarpal bone, unspecified hand** ⓠ

☑7ᵗʰ **S62.254** Nondisplaced **fracture of neck of first metacarpal bone,** right **hand** ⓠ

☑7ᵗʰ **S62.255** Nondisplaced **fracture of neck of first metacarpal bone,** left **hand** ⓠ

☑7ᵗʰ **S62.256** Nondisplaced **fracture of neck of first metacarpal bone, unspecified hand** ⓠ

☑6ᵗʰ **S62.29** **Other fracture of first metacarpal bone**

☑7ᵗʰ **S62.291** **Other fracture of first metacarpal bone,** right **hand** ⓠ

☑7ᵗʰ **S62.292** **Other fracture of first metacarpal bone,** left **hand** ⓠ

☑7ᵗʰ **S62.299** **Other fracture of first metacarpal bone, unspecified hand** ⓠ

☑5ᵗʰ **S62.3** **Fracture of other and unspecified metacarpal bone**
EXCLUDES 2   *fracture of first metacarpal bone (S62.2-)*

☑6ᵗʰ **S62.30** **Unspecified fracture of other metacarpal bone**

☑7ᵗʰ **S62.300** **Unspecified fracture of** second **metacarpal bone,** right **hand** ⓠ

☑7ᵗʰ **S62.301** **Unspecified fracture of** second **metacarpal bone,** left **hand** ⓠ

☑7ᵗʰ **S62.302** **Unspecified fracture of** third **metacarpal bone,** right **hand** ⓠ

☑7ᵗʰ **S62.303** **Unspecified fracture of** third **metacarpal bone,** left **hand** ⓠ

☑7ᵗʰ **S62.304** **Unspecified fracture of** fourth **metacarpal bone,** right **hand** ⓠ

☑7ᵗʰ **S62.305** **Unspecified fracture of** fourth **metacarpal bone,** left **hand** ⓠ

☑7ᵗʰ **S62.306** **Unspecified fracture of** fifth **metacarpal bone,** right **hand** ⓠ

☑7ᵗʰ **S62.307** **Unspecified fracture of** fifth **metacarpal bone,** left **hand** ⓠ

Chapter 19. Injury, Poisoning and Certain Other Consequences of External Causes

S62.308–S62.391

√7ᵗʰ **S62.308** **Unspecified fracture of other metacarpal bone** Ⓠ
Unspecified fracture of specified metacarpal bone with unspecified laterality

√7ᵗʰ **S62.309** **Unspecified fracture of unspecified metacarpal bone** Ⓠ

√6ᵗʰ **S62.31** Displaced fracture of base of other metacarpal bone

√7ᵗʰ **S62.310** **Displaced fracture of base of second metacarpal bone, right hand** Ⓠ

√7ᵗʰ **S62.311** **Displaced fracture of base of second metacarpal bone, left hand** Ⓠ

√7ᵗʰ **S62.312** **Displaced fracture of base of third metacarpal bone, right hand** Ⓠ

√7ᵗʰ **S62.313** **Displaced fracture of base of third metacarpal bone, left hand** Ⓠ

√7ᵗʰ **S62.314** **Displaced fracture of base of fourth metacarpal bone, right hand** Ⓠ

√7ᵗʰ **S62.315** **Displaced fracture of base of fourth metacarpal bone, left hand** Ⓠ

√7ᵗʰ **S62.316** **Displaced fracture of base of fifth metacarpal bone, right hand** Ⓠ

√7ᵗʰ **S62.317** **Displaced fracture of base of fifth metacarpal bone, left hand** Ⓠ

√7ᵗʰ **S62.318** **Displaced fracture of base of other metacarpal bone** Ⓠ
Displaced fracture of base of specified metacarpal bone with unspecified laterality

√7ᵗʰ **S62.319** **Displaced fracture of base of unspecified metacarpal bone** Ⓠ

√6ᵗʰ **S62.32** Displaced fracture of shaft of other metacarpal bone

√7ᵗʰ **S62.320** **Displaced fracture of shaft of second metacarpal bone, right hand** Ⓠ

√7ᵗʰ **S62.321** **Displaced fracture of shaft of second metacarpal bone, left hand** Ⓠ

√7ᵗʰ **S62.322** **Displaced fracture of shaft of third metacarpal bone, right hand** Ⓠ

√7ᵗʰ **S62.323** **Displaced fracture of shaft of third metacarpal bone, left hand** Ⓠ

√7ᵗʰ **S62.324** **Displaced fracture of shaft of fourth metacarpal bone, right hand** Ⓠ

√7ᵗʰ **S62.325** **Displaced fracture of shaft of fourth metacarpal bone, left hand** Ⓠ

√7ᵗʰ **S62.326** **Displaced fracture of shaft of fifth metacarpal bone, right hand** Ⓠ

√7ᵗʰ **S62.327** **Displaced fracture of shaft of fifth metacarpal bone, left hand** Ⓠ

√7ᵗʰ **S62.328** **Displaced fracture of shaft of other metacarpal bone** Ⓠ
Displaced fracture of shaft of specified metacarpal bone with unspecified laterality

√7ᵗʰ **S62.329** **Displaced fracture of shaft of unspecified metacarpal bone** Ⓠ

√6ᵗʰ **S62.33** Displaced fracture of neck of other metacarpal bone

√7ᵗʰ **S62.330** **Displaced fracture of neck of second metacarpal bone, right hand** Ⓠ

√7ᵗʰ **S62.331** **Displaced fracture of neck of second metacarpal bone, left hand** Ⓠ

√7ᵗʰ **S62.332** **Displaced fracture of neck of third metacarpal bone, right hand** Ⓠ

√7ᵗʰ **S62.333** **Displaced fracture of neck of third metacarpal bone, left hand** Ⓠ

√7ᵗʰ **S62.334** **Displaced fracture of neck of fourth metacarpal bone, right hand** Ⓠ

√7ᵗʰ **S62.335** **Displaced fracture of neck of fourth metacarpal bone, left hand** Ⓠ

√7ᵗʰ **S62.336** **Displaced fracture of neck of fifth metacarpal bone, right hand** Ⓠ

√7ᵗʰ **S62.337** **Displaced fracture of neck of fifth metacarpal bone, left hand** Ⓠ

√7ᵗʰ **S62.338** **Displaced fracture of neck of other metacarpal bone** Ⓠ
Displaced fracture of neck of specified metacarpal bone with unspecified laterality

√7ᵗʰ **S62.339** **Displaced fracture of neck of unspecified metacarpal bone** Ⓠ

√6ᵗʰ **S62.34** Nondisplaced fracture of base of other metacarpal bone

√7ᵗʰ **S62.340** **Nondisplaced fracture of base of second metacarpal bone, right hand** Ⓠ

√7ᵗʰ **S62.341** **Nondisplaced fracture of base of second metacarpal bone, left hand** Ⓠ

√7ᵗʰ **S62.342** **Nondisplaced fracture of base of third metacarpal bone, right hand** Ⓠ

√7ᵗʰ **S62.343** **Nondisplaced fracture of base of third metacarpal bone, left hand** Ⓠ

√7ᵗʰ **S62.344** **Nondisplaced fracture of base of fourth metacarpal bone, right hand** Ⓠ

√7ᵗʰ **S62.345** **Nondisplaced fracture of base of fourth metacarpal bone, left hand** Ⓠ

√7ᵗʰ **S62.346** **Nondisplaced fracture of base of fifth metacarpal bone, right hand** Ⓠ

√7ᵗʰ **S62.347** **Nondisplaced fracture of base of fifth metacarpal bone, left hand** Ⓠ

√7ᵗʰ **S62.348** **Nondisplaced fracture of base of other metacarpal bone** Ⓠ
Nondisplaced fracture of base of specified metacarpal bone with unspecified laterality

√7ᵗʰ **S62.349** **Nondisplaced fracture of base of unspecified metacarpal bone** Ⓠ

√6ᵗʰ **S62.35** Nondisplaced fracture of shaft of other metacarpal bone

√7ᵗʰ **S62.350** **Nondisplaced fracture of shaft of second metacarpal bone, right hand** Ⓠ

√7ᵗʰ **S62.351** **Nondisplaced fracture of shaft of second metacarpal bone, left hand** Ⓠ

√7ᵗʰ **S62.352** **Nondisplaced fracture of shaft of third metacarpal bone, right hand** Ⓠ

√7ᵗʰ **S62.353** **Nondisplaced fracture of shaft of third metacarpal bone, left hand** Ⓠ

√7ᵗʰ **S62.354** **Nondisplaced fracture of shaft of fourth metacarpal bone, right hand** Ⓠ

√7ᵗʰ **S62.355** **Nondisplaced fracture of shaft of fourth metacarpal bone, left hand** Ⓠ

√7ᵗʰ **S62.356** **Nondisplaced fracture of shaft of fifth metacarpal bone, right hand** Ⓠ

√7ᵗʰ **S62.357** **Nondisplaced fracture of shaft of fifth metacarpal bone, left hand** Ⓠ

√7ᵗʰ **S62.358** **Nondisplaced fracture of shaft of other metacarpal bone** Ⓠ
Nondisplaced fracture of shaft of specified metacarpal bone with unspecified laterality

√7ᵗʰ **S62.359** **Nondisplaced fracture of shaft of unspecified metacarpal bone** Ⓠ

√6ᵗʰ **S62.36** Nondisplaced fracture of neck of other metacarpal bone

√7ᵗʰ **S62.360** **Nondisplaced fracture of neck of second metacarpal bone, right hand** Ⓠ

√7ᵗʰ **S62.361** **Nondisplaced fracture of neck of second metacarpal bone, left hand** Ⓠ

√7ᵗʰ **S62.362** **Nondisplaced fracture of neck of third metacarpal bone, right hand** Ⓠ

√7ᵗʰ **S62.363** **Nondisplaced fracture of neck of third metacarpal bone, left hand** Ⓠ

√7ᵗʰ **S62.364** **Nondisplaced fracture of neck of fourth metacarpal bone, right hand** Ⓠ

√7ᵗʰ **S62.365** **Nondisplaced fracture of neck of fourth metacarpal bone, left hand** Ⓠ

√7ᵗʰ **S62.366** **Nondisplaced fracture of neck of fifth metacarpal bone, right hand** Ⓠ

√7ᵗʰ **S62.367** **Nondisplaced fracture of neck of fifth metacarpal bone, left hand** Ⓠ

√7ᵗʰ **S62.368** **Nondisplaced fracture of neck of other metacarpal bone** Ⓠ
Nondisplaced fracture of neck of specified metacarpal bone with unspecified laterality

√7ᵗʰ **S62.369** **Nondisplaced fracture of neck of unspecified metacarpal bone** Ⓠ

√6ᵗʰ **S62.39** Other fracture of other metacarpal bone

√7ᵗʰ **S62.390** **Other fracture of second metacarpal bone, right hand** Ⓠ

√7ᵗʰ **S62.391** **Other fracture of second metacarpal bone, left hand** Ⓠ

| HCC CMS-HCC | Rx Rx HCC | ESR ESRD HCC | COM Commercial HCC | N Newborn: 0 | P Pediatric: 0-17 | M Maternity: 9-64 | A Adult: 15-124 |

1064

ICD-10-CM 2023

√7ᵗʰ **S62.392** Other fracture of third metacarpal bone, right hand   ◘

√7ᵗʰ **S62.393** Other fracture of third metacarpal bone, left hand   ◘

√7ᵗʰ **S62.394** Other fracture of fourth metacarpal bone, right hand   ◘

√7ᵗʰ **S62.395** Other fracture of fourth metacarpal bone, left hand   ◘

√7ᵗʰ **S62.396** Other fracture of fifth metacarpal bone, right hand   ◘

√7ᵗʰ **S62.397** Other fracture of fifth metacarpal bone, left hand   ◘

√7ᵗʰ **S62.398** Other fracture of other metacarpal bone   ◘
> Other fracture of specified metacarpal bone with unspecified laterality

√7ᵗʰ **S62.399** Other fracture of unspecified metacarpal bone   ◘

√5ᵗʰ **S62.5** Fracture of thumb

  √6ᵗʰ **S62.50** Fracture of unspecified phalanx of thumb

    √7ᵗʰ **S62.501** Fracture of unspecified phalanx of right thumb

    √7ᵗʰ **S62.502** Fracture of unspecified phalanx of left thumb

    √7ᵗʰ **S62.509** Fracture of unspecified phalanx of unspecified thumb

  √6ᵗʰ **S62.51** Fracture of proximal phalanx of thumb

    √7ᵗʰ **S62.511** Displaced fracture of proximal phalanx of right thumb

    √7ᵗʰ **S62.512** Displaced fracture of proximal phalanx of left thumb

    √7ᵗʰ **S62.513** Displaced fracture of proximal phalanx of unspecified thumb

    √7ᵗʰ **S62.514** Nondisplaced fracture of proximal phalanx of right thumb

    √7ᵗʰ **S62.515** Nondisplaced fracture of proximal phalanx of left thumb

    √7ᵗʰ **S62.516** Nondisplaced fracture of proximal phalanx of unspecified thumb

  √6ᵗʰ **S62.52** Fracture of distal phalanx of thumb

    √7ᵗʰ **S62.521** Displaced fracture of distal phalanx of right thumb

    √7ᵗʰ **S62.522** Displaced fracture of distal phalanx of left thumb

    √7ᵗʰ **S62.523** Displaced fracture of distal phalanx of unspecified thumb

    √7ᵗʰ **S62.524** Nondisplaced fracture of distal phalanx of right thumb

    √7ᵗʰ **S62.525** Nondisplaced fracture of distal phalanx of left thumb

    √7ᵗʰ **S62.526** Nondisplaced fracture of distal phalanx of unspecified thumb

√5ᵗʰ **S62.6** Fracture of other and unspecified finger(s)
> **EXCLUDES 2**   fracture of thumb (S62.5-)

  √6ᵗʰ **S62.60** Fracture of unspecified phalanx of finger

    √7ᵗʰ **S62.600** Fracture of unspecified phalanx of right index finger

    √7ᵗʰ **S62.601** Fracture of unspecified phalanx of left index finger

    √7ᵗʰ **S62.602** Fracture of unspecified phalanx of right middle finger

    √7ᵗʰ **S62.603** Fracture of unspecified phalanx of left middle finger

    √7ᵗʰ **S62.604** Fracture of unspecified phalanx of right ring finger

    √7ᵗʰ **S62.605** Fracture of unspecified phalanx of left ring finger

    √7ᵗʰ **S62.606** Fracture of unspecified phalanx of right little finger

    √7ᵗʰ **S62.607** Fracture of unspecified phalanx of left little finger

    √7ᵗʰ **S62.608** Fracture of unspecified phalanx of other finger
> Fracture of unspecified phalanx of specified finger with unspecified laterality

    √7ᵗʰ **S62.609** Fracture of unspecified phalanx of unspecified finger

√6ᵗʰ **S62.61** Displaced fracture of proximal phalanx of finger

    √7ᵗʰ **S62.610** Displaced fracture of proximal phalanx of right index finger

    √7ᵗʰ **S62.611** Displaced fracture of proximal phalanx of left index finger

    √7ᵗʰ **S62.612** Displaced fracture of proximal phalanx of right middle finger

    √7ᵗʰ **S62.613** Displaced fracture of proximal phalanx of left middle finger

    √7ᵗʰ **S62.614** Displaced fracture of proximal phalanx of right ring finger

    √7ᵗʰ **S62.615** Displaced fracture of proximal phalanx of left ring finger

    √7ᵗʰ **S62.616** Displaced fracture of proximal phalanx of right little finger

    √7ᵗʰ **S62.617** Displaced fracture of proximal phalanx of left little finger

    √7ᵗʰ **S62.618** Displaced fracture of proximal phalanx of other finger
> Displaced fracture of proximal phalanx of specified finger with unspecified laterality

    √7ᵗʰ **S62.619** Displaced fracture of proximal phalanx of unspecified finger

√6ᵗʰ **S62.62** Displaced fracture of middle phalanx of finger

    √7ᵗʰ **S62.620** Displaced fracture of middle phalanx of right index finger

    √7ᵗʰ **S62.621** Displaced fracture of middle phalanx of left index finger

    √7ᵗʰ **S62.622** Displaced fracture of middle phalanx of right middle finger

    √7ᵗʰ **S62.623** Displaced fracture of middle phalanx of left middle finger

    √7ᵗʰ **S62.624** Displaced fracture of middle phalanx of right ring finger

    √7ᵗʰ **S62.625** Displaced fracture of middle phalanx of left ring finger

    √7ᵗʰ **S62.626** Displaced fracture of middle phalanx of right little finger

    √7ᵗʰ **S62.627** Displaced fracture of middle phalanx of left little finger

    √7ᵗʰ **S62.628** Displaced fracture of middle phalanx of other finger
> Displaced fracture of middle phalanx of specified finger with unspecified laterality

    √7ᵗʰ **S62.629** Displaced fracture of middle phalanx of unspecified finger

√6ᵗʰ **S62.63** Displaced fracture of distal phalanx of finger

    √7ᵗʰ **S62.630** Displaced fracture of distal phalanx of right index finger

    √7ᵗʰ **S62.631** Displaced fracture of distal phalanx of left index finger

    √7ᵗʰ **S62.632** Displaced fracture of distal phalanx of right middle finger

    √7ᵗʰ **S62.633** Displaced fracture of distal phalanx of left middle finger

    √7ᵗʰ **S62.634** Displaced fracture of distal phalanx of right ring finger

    √7ᵗʰ **S62.635** Displaced fracture of distal phalanx of left ring finger

    √7ᵗʰ **S62.636** Displaced fracture of distal phalanx of right little finger

    √7ᵗʰ **S62.637** Displaced fracture of distal phalanx of left little finger

    √7ᵗʰ **S62.638** Displaced fracture of distal phalanx of other finger
> Displaced fracture of distal phalanx of specified finger with unspecified laterality

    √7ᵗʰ **S62.639** Displaced fracture of distal phalanx of unspecified finger

√6ᵗʰ **S62.64** Nondisplaced fracture of proximal phalanx of finger

    √7ᵗʰ **S62.640** Nondisplaced fracture of proximal phalanx of right index finger

    √7ᵗʰ **S62.641** Nondisplaced fracture of proximal phalanx of left index finger

    √7ᵗʰ **S62.642** Nondisplaced fracture of proximal phalanx of right middle finger

    √7ᵗʰ **S62.643** Nondisplaced fracture of proximal phalanx of left middle finger

√7ᵗʰ **S62.644** **Nondisplaced fracture of proximal phalanx of right ring finger**

√7ᵗʰ **S62.645** **Nondisplaced fracture of proximal phalanx of left ring finger**

√7ᵗʰ **S62.646** **Nondisplaced fracture of proximal phalanx of right little finger**

√7ᵗʰ **S62.647** **Nondisplaced fracture of proximal phalanx of left little finger**

√7ᵗʰ **S62.648** **Nondisplaced fracture of proximal phalanx of other finger**
Nondisplaced fracture of proximal phalanx of specified finger with unspecified laterality

√7ᵗʰ **S62.649** **Nondisplaced fracture of proximal phalanx of unspecified finger**

√6ᵗʰ **S62.65** **Nondisplaced fracture of middle phalanx of finger**

√7ᵗʰ **S62.650** **Nondisplaced fracture of middle phalanx of right index finger**

√7ᵗʰ **S62.651** **Nondisplaced fracture of middle phalanx of left index finger**

√7ᵗʰ **S62.652** **Nondisplaced fracture of middle phalanx of right middle finger**

√7ᵗʰ **S62.653** **Nondisplaced fracture of middle phalanx of left middle finger**

√7ᵗʰ **S62.654** **Nondisplaced fracture of middle phalanx of right ring finger**

√7ᵗʰ **S62.655** **Nondisplaced fracture of middle phalanx of left ring finger**

√7ᵗʰ **S62.656** **Nondisplaced fracture of middle phalanx of right little finger**

√7ᵗʰ **S62.657** **Nondisplaced fracture of middle phalanx of left little finger**

√7ᵗʰ **S62.658** **Nondisplaced fracture of middle phalanx of other finger**
Nondisplaced fracture of middle phalanx of specified finger with unspecified laterality

√7ᵗʰ **S62.659** **Nondisplaced fracture of middle phalanx of unspecified finger**

√6ᵗʰ **S62.66** **Nondisplaced fracture of distal phalanx of finger**

√7ᵗʰ **S62.660** **Nondisplaced fracture of distal phalanx of right index finger**

√7ᵗʰ **S62.661** **Nondisplaced fracture of distal phalanx of left index finger**

√7ᵗʰ **S62.662** **Nondisplaced fracture of distal phalanx of right middle finger**

√7ᵗʰ **S62.663** **Nondisplaced fracture of distal phalanx of left middle finger**

√7ᵗʰ **S62.664** **Nondisplaced fracture of distal phalanx of right ring finger**

√7ᵗʰ **S62.665** **Nondisplaced fracture of distal phalanx of left ring finger**

√7ᵗʰ **S62.666** **Nondisplaced fracture of distal phalanx of right little finger**

√7ᵗʰ **S62.667** **Nondisplaced fracture of distal phalanx of left little finger**

√7ᵗʰ **S62.668** **Nondisplaced fracture of distal phalanx of other finger**
Nondisplaced fracture of distal phalanx of specified finger with unspecified laterality

√7ᵗʰ **S62.669** **Nondisplaced fracture of distal phalanx of unspecified finger**

√5ᵗʰ **S62.9** **Unspecified fracture of wrist and hand**

√x7ᵗʰ **S62.90** **Unspecified fracture of unspecified wrist and hand** ▯

√x7ᵗʰ **S62.91** **Unspecified fracture of right wrist and hand** ▯

√x7ᵗʰ **S62.92** **Unspecified fracture of left wrist and hand** ▯

√4ᵗʰ **S63** **Dislocation and sprain of joints and ligaments at wrist and hand level**

INCLUDES   avulsion of joint or ligament at wrist and hand level
laceration of cartilage, joint or ligament at wrist and hand level
sprain of cartilage, joint or ligament at wrist and hand level
traumatic hemarthrosis of joint or ligament at wrist and hand level
traumatic rupture of joint or ligament at wrist and hand level
traumatic subluxation of joint or ligament at wrist and hand level
traumatic tear of joint or ligament at wrist and hand level

Code also any associated open wound

EXCLUDES 2   *strain of muscle, fascia and tendon of wrist and hand (S66.-)*

The appropriate 7th character is to be added to each code from category S63.
A   initial encounter
D   subsequent encounter
S   sequela

√5ᵗʰ **S63.0** **Subluxation and dislocation of wrist and hand joints**

√6ᵗʰ **S63.00** **Unspecified subluxation and dislocation of wrist and hand**
Dislocation of carpal bone NOS
Dislocation of distal end of radius NOS
Subluxation of carpal bone NOS
Subluxation of distal end of radius NOS

√7ᵗʰ **S63.001** **Unspecified subluxation of right wrist and hand**

√7ᵗʰ **S63.002** **Unspecified subluxation of left wrist and hand**

√7ᵗʰ **S63.003** **Unspecified subluxation of unspecified wrist and hand**

√7ᵗʰ **S63.004** **Unspecified dislocation of right wrist and hand**

√7ᵗʰ **S63.005** **Unspecified dislocation of left wrist and hand**

√7ᵗʰ **S63.006** **Unspecified dislocation of unspecified wrist and hand**

√6ᵗʰ **S63.01** **Subluxation and dislocation of distal radioulnar joint**

√7ᵗʰ **S63.011** **Subluxation of distal radioulnar joint of right wrist**

√7ᵗʰ **S63.012** **Subluxation of distal radioulnar joint of left wrist**

√7ᵗʰ **S63.013** **Subluxation of distal radioulnar joint of unspecified wrist**

√7ᵗʰ **S63.014** **Dislocation of distal radioulnar joint of right wrist**

√7ᵗʰ **S63.015** **Dislocation of distal radioulnar joint of left wrist**

√7ᵗʰ **S63.016** **Dislocation of distal radioulnar joint of unspecified wrist**

√6ᵗʰ **S63.02** **Subluxation and dislocation of radiocarpal joint**

√7ᵗʰ **S63.021** **Subluxation of radiocarpal joint of right wrist**

√7ᵗʰ **S63.022** **Subluxation of radiocarpal joint of left wrist**

√7ᵗʰ **S63.023** **Subluxation of radiocarpal joint of unspecified wrist**

√7ᵗʰ **S63.024** **Dislocation of radiocarpal joint of right wrist**

√7ᵗʰ **S63.025** **Dislocation of radiocarpal joint of left wrist**

√7ᵗʰ **S63.026** **Dislocation of radiocarpal joint of unspecified wrist**

√6ᵗʰ **S63.03** **Subluxation and dislocation of midcarpal joint**

√7ᵗʰ **S63.031** **Subluxation of midcarpal joint of right wrist**

√7ᵗʰ **S63.032** **Subluxation of midcarpal joint of left wrist**

√7ᵗʰ **S63.033** **Subluxation of midcarpal joint of unspecified wrist**

√7ᵗʰ **S63.034** **Dislocation of midcarpal joint of right wrist**

√7ᵗʰ **S63.035** **Dislocation of midcarpal joint of left wrist**

√7ᵗʰ **S63.036** **Dislocation of midcarpal joint of unspecified wrist**

☑6ᵗʰ **S63.04 Subluxation and dislocation of carpometacarpal joint of thumb**
> EXCLUDES 2   *interphalangeal subluxation and dislocation of thumb (S63.1-)*

- ☑7ᵗʰ **S63.041** Subluxation of carpometacarpal joint of right thumb
- ☑7ᵗʰ **S63.042** Subluxation of carpometacarpal joint of left thumb
- ☑7ᵗʰ **S63.043** Subluxation of carpometacarpal joint of unspecified thumb
- ☑7ᵗʰ **S63.044** Dislocation of carpometacarpal joint of right thumb
- ☑7ᵗʰ **S63.045** Dislocation of carpometacarpal joint of left thumb
- ☑7ᵗʰ **S63.046** Dislocation of carpometacarpal joint of unspecified thumb

☑6ᵗʰ **S63.05 Subluxation and dislocation of other carpometacarpal joint**
> EXCLUDES 2   *subluxation and dislocation of carpometacarpal joint of thumb (S63.04-)*

- ☑7ᵗʰ **S63.051** Subluxation of other carpometacarpal joint of right hand
- ☑7ᵗʰ **S63.052** Subluxation of other carpometacarpal joint of left hand
- ☑7ᵗʰ **S63.053** Subluxation of other carpometacarpal joint of unspecified hand
- ☑7ᵗʰ **S63.054** Dislocation of other carpometacarpal joint of right hand
- ☑7ᵗʰ **S63.055** Dislocation of other carpometacarpal joint of left hand
- ☑7ᵗʰ **S63.056** Dislocation of other carpometacarpal joint of unspecified hand

☑6ᵗʰ **S63.06 Subluxation and dislocation of metacarpal (bone), proximal end**

- ☑7ᵗʰ **S63.061** Subluxation of metacarpal (bone), proximal end of right hand
- ☑7ᵗʰ **S63.062** Subluxation of metacarpal (bone), proximal end of left hand
- ☑7ᵗʰ **S63.063** Subluxation of metacarpal (bone), proximal end of unspecified hand
- ☑7ᵗʰ **S63.064** Dislocation of metacarpal (bone), proximal end of right hand
- ☑7ᵗʰ **S63.065** Dislocation of metacarpal (bone), proximal end of left hand
- ☑7ᵗʰ **S63.066** Dislocation of metacarpal (bone), proximal end of unspecified hand

☑6ᵗʰ **S63.07 Subluxation and dislocation of distal end of ulna**

- ☑7ᵗʰ **S63.071** Subluxation of distal end of right ulna
- ☑7ᵗʰ **S63.072** Subluxation of distal end of left ulna
- ☑7ᵗʰ **S63.073** Subluxation of distal end of unspecified ulna
- ☑7ᵗʰ **S63.074** Dislocation of distal end of right ulna
- ☑7ᵗʰ **S63.075** Dislocation of distal end of left ulna
- ☑7ᵗʰ **S63.076** Dislocation of distal end of unspecified ulna

☑6ᵗʰ **S63.09 Other subluxation and dislocation of wrist and hand**

- ☑7ᵗʰ **S63.091** Other subluxation of right wrist and hand
- ☑7ᵗʰ **S63.092** Other subluxation of left wrist and hand
- ☑7ᵗʰ **S63.093** Other subluxation of unspecified wrist and hand
- ☑7ᵗʰ **S63.094** Other dislocation of right wrist and hand
- ☑7ᵗʰ **S63.095** Other dislocation of left wrist and hand
- ☑7ᵗʰ **S63.096** Other dislocation of unspecified wrist and hand

☑5ᵗʰ **S63.1 Subluxation and dislocation of thumb**

☑6ᵗʰ **S63.10 Unspecified subluxation and dislocation of thumb**

- ☑7ᵗʰ **S63.101** Unspecified subluxation of right thumb
- ☑7ᵗʰ **S63.102** Unspecified subluxation of left thumb
- ☑7ᵗʰ **S63.103** Unspecified subluxation of unspecified thumb
- ☑7ᵗʰ **S63.104** Unspecified dislocation of right thumb
- ☑7ᵗʰ **S63.105** Unspecified dislocation of left thumb
- ☑7ᵗʰ **S63.106** Unspecified dislocation of unspecified thumb

☑6ᵗʰ **S63.11 Subluxation and dislocation of metacarpophalangeal joint of thumb**

- ☑7ᵗʰ **S63.111** Subluxation of metacarpophalangeal joint of right thumb
- ☑7ᵗʰ **S63.112** Subluxation of metacarpophalangeal joint of left thumb
- ☑7ᵗʰ **S63.113** Subluxation of metacarpophalangeal joint of unspecified thumb
- ☑7ᵗʰ **S63.114** Dislocation of metacarpophalangeal joint of right thumb
- ☑7ᵗʰ **S63.115** Dislocation of metacarpophalangeal joint of left thumb
- ☑7ᵗʰ **S63.116** Dislocation of metacarpophalangeal joint of unspecified thumb

☑6ᵗʰ **S63.12 Subluxation and dislocation of interphalangeal joint of thumb**

- ☑7ᵗʰ **S63.121** Subluxation of interphalangeal joint of right thumb
- ☑7ᵗʰ **S63.122** Subluxation of interphalangeal joint of left thumb
- ☑7ᵗʰ **S63.123** Subluxation of interphalangeal joint of unspecified thumb
- ☑7ᵗʰ **S63.124** Dislocation of interphalangeal joint of right thumb
- ☑7ᵗʰ **S63.125** Dislocation of interphalangeal joint of left thumb
- ☑7ᵗʰ **S63.126** Dislocation of interphalangeal joint of unspecified thumb

☑5ᵗʰ **S63.2 Subluxation and dislocation of other finger(s)**
> EXCLUDES 2   *subluxation and dislocation of thumb (S63.1-)*

☑6ᵗʰ **S63.20 Unspecified subluxation of other finger**

- ☑7ᵗʰ **S63.200** Unspecified subluxation of right index finger
- ☑7ᵗʰ **S63.201** Unspecified subluxation of left index finger
- ☑7ᵗʰ **S63.202** Unspecified subluxation of right middle finger
- ☑7ᵗʰ **S63.203** Unspecified subluxation of left middle finger
- ☑7ᵗʰ **S63.204** Unspecified subluxation of right ring finger
- ☑7ᵗʰ **S63.205** Unspecified subluxation of left ring finger
- ☑7ᵗʰ **S63.206** Unspecified subluxation of right little finger
- ☑7ᵗʰ **S63.207** Unspecified subluxation of left little finger
- ☑7ᵗʰ **S63.208** Unspecified subluxation of other finger
  > Unspecified subluxation of specified finger with unspecified laterality
- ☑7ᵗʰ **S63.209** Unspecified subluxation of unspecified finger

☑6ᵗʰ **S63.21 Subluxation of metacarpophalangeal joint of finger**

- ☑7ᵗʰ **S63.210** Subluxation of metacarpophalangeal joint of right index finger
- ☑7ᵗʰ **S63.211** Subluxation of metacarpophalangeal joint of left index finger
- ☑7ᵗʰ **S63.212** Subluxation of metacarpophalangeal joint of right middle finger
- ☑7ᵗʰ **S63.213** Subluxation of metacarpophalangeal joint of left middle finger
- ☑7ᵗʰ **S63.214** Subluxation of metacarpophalangeal joint of right ring finger
- ☑7ᵗʰ **S63.215** Subluxation of metacarpophalangeal joint of left ring finger
- ☑7ᵗʰ **S63.216** Subluxation of metacarpophalangeal joint of right little finger
- ☑7ᵗʰ **S63.217** Subluxation of metacarpophalangeal joint of left little finger
- ☑7ᵗʰ **S63.218** Subluxation of metacarpophalangeal joint of other finger
  > Subluxation of metacarpophalangeal joint of specified finger with unspecified laterality
- ☑7ᵗʰ **S63.219** Subluxation of metacarpophalangeal joint of unspecified finger

☑6ᵗʰ **S63.22 Subluxation of unspecified interphalangeal joint of finger**

- ☑7ᵗʰ **S63.220** Subluxation of unspecified interphalangeal joint of right index finger
- ☑7ᵗʰ **S63.221** Subluxation of unspecified interphalangeal joint of left index finger
- ☑7ᵗʰ **S63.222** Subluxation of unspecified interphalangeal joint of right middle finger
- ☑7ᵗʰ **S63.223** Subluxation of unspecified interphalangeal joint of left middle finger

√7th **S63.224** Subluxation of unspecified interphalangeal joint of right ring finger
√7th **S63.225** Subluxation of unspecified interphalangeal joint of left ring finger
√7th **S63.226** Subluxation of unspecified interphalangeal joint of right little finger
√7th **S63.227** Subluxation of unspecified interphalangeal joint of left little finger
√7th **S63.228** Subluxation of unspecified interphalangeal joint of other finger
  Subluxation of unspecified interphalangeal joint of specified finger with unspecified laterality
√7th **S63.229** Subluxation of unspecified interphalangeal joint of unspecified finger

√6th **S63.23** Subluxation of proximal interphalangeal joint of finger
√7th **S63.230** Subluxation of proximal interphalangeal joint of right index finger
√7th **S63.231** Subluxation of proximal interphalangeal joint of left index finger
√7th **S63.232** Subluxation of proximal interphalangeal joint of right middle finger
√7th **S63.233** Subluxation of proximal interphalangeal joint of left middle finger
√7th **S63.234** Subluxation of proximal interphalangeal joint of right ring finger
√7th **S63.235** Subluxation of proximal interphalangeal joint of left ring finger
√7th **S63.236** Subluxation of proximal interphalangeal joint of right little finger
√7th **S63.237** Subluxation of proximal interphalangeal joint of left little finger
√7th **S63.238** Subluxation of proximal interphalangeal joint of other finger
  Subluxation of proximal interphalangeal joint of specified finger with unspecified laterality
√7th **S63.239** Subluxation of proximal interphalangeal joint of unspecified finger

√6th **S63.24** Subluxation of distal interphalangeal joint of finger
√7th **S63.240** Subluxation of distal interphalangeal joint of right index finger
√7th **S63.241** Subluxation of distal interphalangeal joint of left index finger
√7th **S63.242** Subluxation of distal interphalangeal joint of right middle finger
√7th **S63.243** Subluxation of distal interphalangeal joint of left middle finger
√7th **S63.244** Subluxation of distal interphalangeal joint of right ring finger
√7th **S63.245** Subluxation of distal interphalangeal joint of left ring finger
√7th **S63.246** Subluxation of distal interphalangeal joint of right little finger
√7th **S63.247** Subluxation of distal interphalangeal joint of left little finger
√7th **S63.248** Subluxation of distal interphalangeal joint of other finger
  Subluxation of distal interphalangeal joint of specified finger with unspecified laterality
√7th **S63.249** Subluxation of distal interphalangeal joint of unspecified finger

√6th **S63.25** Unspecified dislocation of other finger
√7th **S63.250** Unspecified dislocation of right index finger
√7th **S63.251** Unspecified dislocation of left index finger
√7th **S63.252** Unspecified dislocation of right middle finger
√7th **S63.253** Unspecified dislocation of left middle finger
√7th **S63.254** Unspecified dislocation of right ring finger
√7th **S63.255** Unspecified dislocation of left ring finger
√7th **S63.256** Unspecified dislocation of right little finger
√7th **S63.257** Unspecified dislocation of left little finger

√7th **S63.258** Unspecified dislocation of other finger
  Unspecified dislocation of specified finger with unspecified laterality
√7th **S63.259** Unspecified dislocation of unspecified finger
  Unspecified dislocation of unspecified finger with unspecified laterality

√6th **S63.26** Dislocation of metacarpophalangeal joint of finger
√7th **S63.260** Dislocation of metacarpophalangeal joint of right index finger
√7th **S63.261** Dislocation of metacarpophalangeal joint of left index finger
√7th **S63.262** Dislocation of metacarpophalangeal joint of right middle finger
√7th **S63.263** Dislocation of metacarpophalangeal joint of left middle finger
√7th **S63.264** Dislocation of metacarpophalangeal joint of right ring finger
√7th **S63.265** Dislocation of metacarpophalangeal joint of left ring finger
√7th **S63.266** Dislocation of metacarpophalangeal joint of right little finger
√7th **S63.267** Dislocation of metacarpophalangeal joint of left little finger
√7th **S63.268** Dislocation of metacarpophalangeal joint of other finger
  Dislocation of metacarpophalangeal joint of specified finger with unspecified laterality
√7th **S63.269** Dislocation of metacarpophalangeal joint of unspecified finger

√6th **S63.27** Dislocation of unspecified interphalangeal joint of finger
√7th **S63.270** Dislocation of unspecified interphalangeal joint of right index finger
√7th **S63.271** Dislocation of unspecified interphalangeal joint of left index finger
√7th **S63.272** Dislocation of unspecified interphalangeal joint of right middle finger
√7th **S63.273** Dislocation of unspecified interphalangeal joint of left middle finger
√7th **S63.274** Dislocation of unspecified interphalangeal joint of right ring finger
√7th **S63.275** Dislocation of unspecified interphalangeal joint of left ring finger
√7th **S63.276** Dislocation of unspecified interphalangeal joint of right little finger
√7th **S63.277** Dislocation of unspecified interphalangeal joint of left little finger
√7th **S63.278** Dislocation of unspecified interphalangeal joint of other finger
  Dislocation of unspecified interphalangeal joint of specified finger with unspecified laterality
√7th **S63.279** Dislocation of unspecified interphalangeal joint of unspecified finger
  Dislocation of unspecified interphalangeal joint of unspecified finger without specified laterality

√6th **S63.28** Dislocation of proximal interphalangeal joint of finger
√7th **S63.280** Dislocation of proximal interphalangeal joint of right index finger
√7th **S63.281** Dislocation of proximal interphalangeal joint of left index finger
√7th **S63.282** Dislocation of proximal interphalangeal joint of right middle finger
√7th **S63.283** Dislocation of proximal interphalangeal joint of left middle finger
√7th **S63.284** Dislocation of proximal interphalangeal joint of right ring finger
√7th **S63.285** Dislocation of proximal interphalangeal joint of left ring finger
√7th **S63.286** Dislocation of proximal interphalangeal joint of right little finger
√7th **S63.287** Dislocation of proximal interphalangeal joint of left little finger

√7ᵗʰ **S63.288 Dislocation of proximal interphalangeal joint of other finger**
Dislocation of proximal interphalangeal joint of specified finger with unspecified laterality

√7ᵗʰ **S63.289 Dislocation of proximal interphalangeal joint of unspecified finger**

√6ᵗʰ **S63.29 Dislocation of distal interphalangeal joint of finger**

√7ᵗʰ **S63.290 Dislocation of distal interphalangeal joint of right index finger**

√7ᵗʰ **S63.291 Dislocation of distal interphalangeal joint of left index finger**

√7ᵗʰ **S63.292 Dislocation of distal interphalangeal joint of right middle finger**

√7ᵗʰ **S63.293 Dislocation of distal interphalangeal joint of left middle finger**

√7ᵗʰ **S63.294 Dislocation of distal interphalangeal joint of right ring finger**

√7ᵗʰ **S63.295 Dislocation of distal interphalangeal joint of left ring finger**

√7ᵗʰ **S63.296 Dislocation of distal interphalangeal joint of right little finger**

√7ᵗʰ **S63.297 Dislocation of distal interphalangeal joint of left little finger**

√7ᵗʰ **S63.298 Dislocation of distal interphalangeal joint of other finger**
Dislocation of distal interphalangeal joint of specified finger with unspecified laterality

√7ᵗʰ **S63.299 Dislocation of distal interphalangeal joint of unspecified finger**

√5ᵗʰ **S63.3 Traumatic rupture of ligament of wrist**

√6ᵗʰ **S63.30 Traumatic rupture of unspecified ligament of wrist**

√7ᵗʰ **S63.301 Traumatic rupture of unspecified ligament of right wrist**

√7ᵗʰ **S63.302 Traumatic rupture of unspecified ligament of left wrist**

√7ᵗʰ **S63.309 Traumatic rupture of unspecified ligament of unspecified wrist**

√6ᵗʰ **S63.31 Traumatic rupture of collateral ligament of wrist**

√7ᵗʰ **S63.311 Traumatic rupture of collateral ligament of right wrist**

√7ᵗʰ **S63.312 Traumatic rupture of collateral ligament of left wrist**

√7ᵗʰ **S63.319 Traumatic rupture of collateral ligament of unspecified wrist**

√6ᵗʰ **S63.32 Traumatic rupture of radiocarpal ligament**

√7ᵗʰ **S63.321 Traumatic rupture of right radiocarpal ligament**

√7ᵗʰ **S63.322 Traumatic rupture of left radiocarpal ligament**

√7ᵗʰ **S63.329 Traumatic rupture of unspecified radiocarpal ligament**

√6ᵗʰ **S63.33 Traumatic rupture of ulnocarpal (palmar) ligament**

√7ᵗʰ **S63.331 Traumatic rupture of right ulnocarpal (palmar) ligament**

√7ᵗʰ **S63.332 Traumatic rupture of left ulnocarpal (palmar) ligament**

√7ᵗʰ **S63.339 Traumatic rupture of unspecified ulnocarpal (palmar) ligament**

√6ᵗʰ **S63.39 Traumatic rupture of other ligament of wrist**

√7ᵗʰ **S63.391 Traumatic rupture of other ligament of right wrist**

√7ᵗʰ **S63.392 Traumatic rupture of other ligament of left wrist**

√7ᵗʰ **S63.399 Traumatic rupture of other ligament of unspecified wrist**

√5ᵗʰ **S63.4 Traumatic rupture of ligament of finger at metacarpophalangeal and interphalangeal joint(s)**

√6ᵗʰ **S63.40 Traumatic rupture of unspecified ligament of finger at metacarpophalangeal and interphalangeal joint**

√7ᵗʰ **S63.400 Traumatic rupture of unspecified ligament of right index finger at metacarpophalangeal and interphalangeal joint**

√7ᵗʰ **S63.401 Traumatic rupture of unspecified ligament of left index finger at metacarpophalangeal and interphalangeal joint**

√7ᵗʰ **S63.402 Traumatic rupture of unspecified ligament of right middle finger at metacarpophalangeal and interphalangeal joint**

√7ᵗʰ **S63.403 Traumatic rupture of unspecified ligament of left middle finger at metacarpophalangeal and interphalangeal joint**

√7ᵗʰ **S63.404 Traumatic rupture of unspecified ligament of right ring finger at metacarpophalangeal and interphalangeal joint**

√7ᵗʰ **S63.405 Traumatic rupture of unspecified ligament of left ring finger at metacarpophalangeal and interphalangeal joint**

√7ᵗʰ **S63.406 Traumatic rupture of unspecified ligament of right little finger at metacarpophalangeal and interphalangeal joint**

√7ᵗʰ **S63.407 Traumatic rupture of unspecified ligament of left little finger at metacarpophalangeal and interphalangeal joint**

√7ᵗʰ **S63.408 Traumatic rupture of unspecified ligament of other finger at metacarpophalangeal and interphalangeal joint**
Traumatic rupture of unspecified ligament of specified finger with unspecified laterality at metacarpophalangeal and interphalangeal joint

√7ᵗʰ **S63.409 Traumatic rupture of unspecified ligament of unspecified finger at metacarpophalangeal and interphalangeal joint**

√6ᵗʰ **S63.41 Traumatic rupture of collateral ligament of finger at metacarpophalangeal and interphalangeal joint**

√7ᵗʰ **S63.410 Traumatic rupture of collateral ligament of right index finger at metacarpophalangeal and interphalangeal joint**

√7ᵗʰ **S63.411 Traumatic rupture of collateral ligament of left index finger at metacarpophalangeal and interphalangeal joint**

√7ᵗʰ **S63.412 Traumatic rupture of collateral ligament of right middle finger at metacarpophalangeal and interphalangeal joint**

√7ᵗʰ **S63.413 Traumatic rupture of collateral ligament of left middle finger at metacarpophalangeal and interphalangeal joint**

√7ᵗʰ **S63.414 Traumatic rupture of collateral ligament of right ring finger at metacarpophalangeal and interphalangeal joint**

√7ᵗʰ **S63.415 Traumatic rupture of collateral ligament of left ring finger at metacarpophalangeal and interphalangeal joint**

√7ᵗʰ **S63.416 Traumatic rupture of collateral ligament of right little finger at metacarpophalangeal and interphalangeal joint**

√7ᵗʰ **S63.417 Traumatic rupture of collateral ligament of left little finger at metacarpophalangeal and interphalangeal joint**

√7ᵗʰ **S63.418 Traumatic rupture of collateral ligament of other finger at metacarpophalangeal and interphalangeal joint**
Traumatic rupture of collateral ligament of specified finger with unspecified laterality at metacarpophalangeal and interphalangeal joint

√7ᵗʰ **S63.419 Traumatic rupture of collateral ligament of unspecified finger at metacarpophalangeal and interphalangeal joint**

√6ᵗʰ **S63.42** **Traumatic rupture of** palmar ligament **of finger at metacarpophalangeal and interphalangeal joint**

  √7ᵗʰ **S63.420** Traumatic rupture of palmar ligament of right index finger at metacarpophalangeal and interphalangeal joint

  √7ᵗʰ **S63.421** Traumatic rupture of palmar ligament of left index finger at metacarpophalangeal and interphalangeal joint

  √7ᵗʰ **S63.422** Traumatic rupture of palmar ligament of right middle finger at metacarpophalangeal and interphalangeal joint

  √7ᵗʰ **S63.423** Traumatic rupture of palmar ligament of left middle finger at metacarpophalangeal and interphalangeal joint

  √7ᵗʰ **S63.424** Traumatic rupture of palmar ligament of right ring finger at metacarpophalangeal and interphalangeal joint

  √7ᵗʰ **S63.425** Traumatic rupture of palmar ligament of left ring finger at metacarpophalangeal and interphalangeal joint

  √7ᵗʰ **S63.426** Traumatic rupture of palmar ligament of right little finger at metacarpophalangeal and interphalangeal joint

  √7ᵗʰ **S63.427** Traumatic rupture of palmar ligament of left little finger at metacarpophalangeal and interphalangeal joint

  √7ᵗʰ **S63.428** Traumatic rupture of palmar ligament of other finger at metacarpophalangeal and interphalangeal joint
    Traumatic rupture of palmar ligament of specified finger with unspecified laterality at metacarpophalangeal and interphalangeal joint

  √7ᵗʰ **S63.429** Traumatic rupture of palmar ligament of unspecified finger at metacarpophalangeal and interphalangeal joint

√6ᵗʰ **S63.43** **Traumatic rupture of** volar plate **of finger at metacarpophalangeal and interphalangeal joint**

  √7ᵗʰ **S63.430** Traumatic rupture of volar plate of right index finger at metacarpophalangeal and interphalangeal joint

  √7ᵗʰ **S63.431** Traumatic rupture of volar plate of left index finger at metacarpophalangeal and interphalangeal joint

  √7ᵗʰ **S63.432** Traumatic rupture of volar plate of right middle finger at metacarpophalangeal and interphalangeal joint

  √7ᵗʰ **S63.433** Traumatic rupture of volar plate of left middle finger at metacarpophalangeal and interphalangeal joint

  √7ᵗʰ **S63.434** Traumatic rupture of volar plate of right ring finger at metacarpophalangeal and interphalangeal joint

  √7ᵗʰ **S63.435** Traumatic rupture of volar plate of left ring finger at metacarpophalangeal and interphalangeal joint

  √7ᵗʰ **S63.436** Traumatic rupture of volar plate of right little finger at metacarpophalangeal and interphalangeal joint

  √7ᵗʰ **S63.437** Traumatic rupture of volar plate of left little finger at metacarpophalangeal and interphalangeal joint

  √7ᵗʰ **S63.438** Traumatic rupture of volar plate of other finger at metacarpophalangeal and interphalangeal joint
    Traumatic rupture of volar plate of specified finger with unspecified laterality at metacarpophalangeal and interphalangeal joint

  √7ᵗʰ **S63.439** Traumatic rupture of volar plate of unspecified finger at metacarpophalangeal and interphalangeal joint

√6ᵗʰ **S63.49** **Traumatic rupture of other ligament of finger at metacarpophalangeal and interphalangeal joint**

  √7ᵗʰ **S63.490** Traumatic rupture of other ligament of right index finger at metacarpophalangeal and interphalangeal joint

  √7ᵗʰ **S63.491** Traumatic rupture of other ligament of left index finger at metacarpophalangeal and interphalangeal joint

  √7ᵗʰ **S63.492** Traumatic rupture of other ligament of right middle finger at metacarpophalangeal and interphalangeal joint

  √7ᵗʰ **S63.493** Traumatic rupture of other ligament of left middle finger at metacarpophalangeal and interphalangeal joint

  √7ᵗʰ **S63.494** Traumatic rupture of other ligament of right ring finger at metacarpophalangeal and interphalangeal joint

  √7ᵗʰ **S63.495** Traumatic rupture of other ligament of left ring finger at metacarpophalangeal and interphalangeal joint

  √7ᵗʰ **S63.496** Traumatic rupture of other ligament of right little finger at metacarpophalangeal and interphalangeal joint

  √7ᵗʰ **S63.497** Traumatic rupture of other ligament of left little finger at metacarpophalangeal and interphalangeal joint

  √7ᵗʰ **S63.498** Traumatic rupture of other ligament of other finger at metacarpophalangeal and interphalangeal joint
    Traumatic rupture of ligament of specified finger with unspecified laterality at metacarpophalangeal and interphalangeal joint

  √7ᵗʰ **S63.499** Traumatic rupture of other ligament of unspecified finger at metacarpophalangeal and interphalangeal joint

√5ᵗʰ **S63.5** **Other and unspecified** sprain of wrist

  √6ᵗʰ **S63.50** **Unspecified sprain of wrist**

    √7ᵗʰ **S63.501** Unspecified sprain of right wrist

    √7ᵗʰ **S63.502** Unspecified sprain of left wrist

    √7ᵗʰ **S63.509** Unspecified sprain of unspecified wrist

  √6ᵗʰ **S63.51** **Sprain of** carpal **(joint)**

    √7ᵗʰ **S63.511** Sprain of carpal joint of right wrist

    √7ᵗʰ **S63.512** Sprain of carpal joint of left wrist

    √7ᵗʰ **S63.519** Sprain of carpal joint of unspecified wrist

  √6ᵗʰ **S63.52** **Sprain of** radiocarpal **joint**
    EXCLUDES 1 *traumatic rupture of radiocarpal ligament (S63.32-)*

    √7ᵗʰ **S63.521** Sprain of radiocarpal joint of right wrist

    √7ᵗʰ **S63.522** Sprain of radiocarpal joint of left wrist

    √7ᵗʰ **S63.529** Sprain of radiocarpal joint of unspecified wrist

  √6ᵗʰ **S63.59** **Other specified sprain of wrist**

    √7ᵗʰ **S63.591** Other specified sprain of right wrist

    √7ᵗʰ **S63.592** Other specified sprain of left wrist

    √7ᵗʰ **S63.599** Other specified sprain of unspecified wrist

√5ᵗʰ **S63.6** **Other and unspecified sprain of finger(s)**
  EXCLUDES 1 *traumatic rupture of ligament of finger at metacarpophalangeal and interphalangeal joint(s) (S63.4-)*

  √6ᵗʰ **S63.60** **Unspecified sprain of** thumb

    √7ᵗʰ **S63.601** Unspecified sprain of right thumb

    √7ᵗʰ **S63.602** Unspecified sprain of left thumb

    √7ᵗʰ **S63.609** Unspecified sprain of unspecified thumb

  √6ᵗʰ **S63.61** **Unspecified sprain of other and unspecified** finger(s)

    √7ᵗʰ **S63.610** Unspecified sprain of right index finger

    √7ᵗʰ **S63.611** Unspecified sprain of left index finger

    √7ᵗʰ **S63.612** Unspecified sprain of right middle finger

    √7ᵗʰ **S63.613** Unspecified sprain of left middle finger

    √7ᵗʰ **S63.614** Unspecified sprain of right ring finger

    √7ᵗʰ **S63.615** Unspecified sprain of left ring finger

    √7ᵗʰ **S63.616** Unspecified sprain of right little finger

    √7ᵗʰ **S63.617** Unspecified sprain of left little finger

---

√7ᵗʰ **S63.618** Unspecified sprain of other finger
Unspecified sprain of specified finger with unspecified laterality

√7ᵗʰ **S63.619** Unspecified sprain of unspecified finger

√6ᵗʰ **S63.62** Sprain of interphalangeal joint of thumb

√7ᵗʰ **S63.621** Sprain of interphalangeal joint of right thumb

√7ᵗʰ **S63.622** Sprain of interphalangeal joint of left thumb

√7ᵗʰ **S63.629** Sprain of interphalangeal joint of unspecified thumb

√6ᵗʰ **S63.63** Sprain of interphalangeal joint of other and unspecified finger(s)

√7ᵗʰ **S63.630** Sprain of interphalangeal joint of right index finger

√7ᵗʰ **S63.631** Sprain of interphalangeal joint of left index finger

√7ᵗʰ **S63.632** Sprain of interphalangeal joint of right middle finger

√7ᵗʰ **S63.633** Sprain of interphalangeal joint of left middle finger

√7ᵗʰ **S63.634** Sprain of interphalangeal joint of right ring finger

√7ᵗʰ **S63.635** Sprain of interphalangeal joint of left ring finger

√7ᵗʰ **S63.636** Sprain of interphalangeal joint of right little finger

√7ᵗʰ **S63.637** Sprain of interphalangeal joint of left little finger

√7ᵗʰ **S63.638** Sprain of interphalangeal joint of other finger

√7ᵗʰ **S63.639** Sprain of interphalangeal joint of unspecified finger

√6ᵗʰ **S63.64** Sprain of metacarpophalangeal joint of thumb

√7ᵗʰ **S63.641** Sprain of metacarpophalangeal joint of right thumb

√7ᵗʰ **S63.642** Sprain of metacarpophalangeal joint of left thumb

√7ᵗʰ **S63.649** Sprain of metacarpophalangeal joint of unspecified thumb

√6ᵗʰ **S63.65** Sprain of metacarpophalangeal joint of other and unspecified finger(s)

√7ᵗʰ **S63.650** Sprain of metacarpophalangeal joint of right index finger

√7ᵗʰ **S63.651** Sprain of metacarpophalangeal joint of left index finger

√7ᵗʰ **S63.652** Sprain of metacarpophalangeal joint of right middle finger

√7ᵗʰ **S63.653** Sprain of metacarpophalangeal joint of left middle finger

√7ᵗʰ **S63.654** Sprain of metacarpophalangeal joint of right ring finger

√7ᵗʰ **S63.655** Sprain of metacarpophalangeal joint of left ring finger

√7ᵗʰ **S63.656** Sprain of metacarpophalangeal joint of right little finger

√7ᵗʰ **S63.657** Sprain of metacarpophalangeal joint of left little finger

√7ᵗʰ **S63.658** Sprain of metacarpophalangeal joint of other finger
Sprain of metacarpophalangeal joint of specified finger with unspecified laterality

√7ᵗʰ **S63.659** Sprain of metacarpophalangeal joint of unspecified finger

√6ᵗʰ **S63.68** Other sprain of thumb

√7ᵗʰ **S63.681** Other sprain of right thumb

√7ᵗʰ **S63.682** Other sprain of left thumb

√7ᵗʰ **S63.689** Other sprain of unspecified thumb

√6ᵗʰ **S63.69** Other sprain of other and unspecified finger(s)

√7ᵗʰ **S63.690** Other sprain of right index finger

√7ᵗʰ **S63.691** Other sprain of left index finger

√7ᵗʰ **S63.692** Other sprain of right middle finger

√7ᵗʰ **S63.693** Other sprain of left middle finger

√7ᵗʰ **S63.694** Other sprain of right ring finger

√7ᵗʰ **S63.695** Other sprain of left ring finger

√7ᵗʰ **S63.696** Other sprain of right little finger

√7ᵗʰ **S63.697** Other sprain of left little finger

√7ᵗʰ **S63.698** Other sprain of other finger
Other sprain of specified finger with unspecified laterality

√7ᵗʰ **S63.699** Other sprain of unspecified finger

√5ᵗʰ **S63.8** Sprain of other part of wrist and hand

√6ᵗʰ **S63.8X** Sprain of other part of wrist and hand

√7ᵗʰ **S63.8X1** Sprain of other part of right wrist and hand

√7ᵗʰ **S63.8X2** Sprain of other part of left wrist and hand

√7ᵗʰ **S63.8X9** Sprain of other part of unspecified wrist and hand

√5ᵗʰ **S63.9** Sprain of unspecified part of wrist and hand

√x7ᵗʰ **S63.90** Sprain of unspecified part of unspecified wrist and hand

√x7ᵗʰ **S63.91** Sprain of unspecified part of right wrist and hand

√x7ᵗʰ **S63.92** Sprain of unspecified part of left wrist and hand

√4ᵗʰ **S64** **Injury of nerves at wrist and hand level**
Code also any associated open wound (S61.-)

The appropriate 7th character is to be added to each code from category S64.
A   initial encounter
D   subsequent encounter
S   sequela

√5ᵗʰ **S64.0** Injury of ulnar nerve at wrist and hand level

√x7ᵗʰ **S64.00** Injury of ulnar nerve at wrist and hand level of unspecified arm

√x7ᵗʰ **S64.01** Injury of ulnar nerve at wrist and hand level of right arm

√x7ᵗʰ **S64.02** Injury of ulnar nerve at wrist and hand level of left arm

√5ᵗʰ **S64.1** Injury of median nerve at wrist and hand level

√x7ᵗʰ **S64.10** Injury of median nerve at wrist and hand level of unspecified arm

√x7ᵗʰ **S64.11** Injury of median nerve at wrist and hand level of right arm

√x7ᵗʰ **S64.12** Injury of median nerve at wrist and hand level of left arm

√5ᵗʰ **S64.2** Injury of radial nerve at wrist and hand level

√x7ᵗʰ **S64.20** Injury of radial nerve at wrist and hand level of unspecified arm

√x7ᵗʰ **S64.21** Injury of radial nerve at wrist and hand level of right arm

√x7ᵗʰ **S64.22** Injury of radial nerve at wrist and hand level of left arm

√5ᵗʰ **S64.3** Injury of digital nerve of thumb

√x7ᵗʰ **S64.30** Injury of digital nerve of unspecified thumb

√x7ᵗʰ **S64.31** Injury of digital nerve of right thumb

√x7ᵗʰ **S64.32** Injury of digital nerve of left thumb

√5ᵗʰ **S64.4** Injury of digital nerve of other and unspecified finger

√x7ᵗʰ **S64.40** Injury of digital nerve of unspecified finger

√6ᵗʰ **S64.49** Injury of digital nerve of other finger

√7ᵗʰ **S64.490** Injury of digital nerve of right index finger

√7ᵗʰ **S64.491** Injury of digital nerve of left index finger

√7ᵗʰ **S64.492** Injury of digital nerve of right middle finger

√7ᵗʰ **S64.493** Injury of digital nerve of left middle finger

√7ᵗʰ **S64.494** Injury of digital nerve of right ring finger

√7ᵗʰ **S64.495** Injury of digital nerve of left ring finger

√7ᵗʰ **S64.496** Injury of digital nerve of right little finger

√7ᵗʰ **S64.497** Injury of digital nerve of left little finger

√7ᵗʰ **S64.498** Injury of digital nerve of other finger
Injury of digital nerve of specified finger with unspecified laterality

√5ᵗʰ **S64.8** Injury of other nerves at wrist and hand level

√6ᵗʰ **S64.8X** Injury of other nerves at wrist and hand level

√7ᵗʰ **S64.8X1** Injury of other nerves at wrist and hand level of right arm

√7ᵗʰ **S64.8X2** Injury of other nerves at wrist and hand level of left arm

√7ᵗʰ **S64.8X9** Injury of other nerves at wrist and hand level of unspecified arm

√5ᵗʰ **S64.9** Injury of unspecified nerve at wrist and hand level

√x7ᵗʰ **S64.90** Injury of unspecified nerve at wrist and hand level of unspecified arm

√x7ᵗʰ **S64.91** Injury of unspecified nerve at wrist and hand level of right arm

√x7ᵗʰ **S64.92** Injury of unspecified nerve at wrist and hand level of left arm

√4ᵗʰ **S65** **Injury of blood vessels at wrist and hand level**

Code also any associated open wound (S61.-)

> The appropriate 7th character is to be added to each code from category S65.
> A   initial encounter
> D   subsequent encounter
> S   sequela

√5ᵗʰ **S65.0** Injury of ulnar artery at wrist and hand level

√6ᵗʰ **S65.00** Unspecified injury of ulnar artery at wrist and hand level

√7ᵗʰ **S65.001** Unspecified injury of ulnar artery at wrist and hand level of right arm

√7ᵗʰ **S65.002** Unspecified injury of ulnar artery at wrist and hand level of left arm

√7ᵗʰ **S65.009** Unspecified injury of ulnar artery at wrist and hand level of unspecified arm

√6ᵗʰ **S65.01** Laceration of ulnar artery at wrist and hand level

√7ᵗʰ **S65.011** Laceration of ulnar artery at wrist and hand level of right arm

√7ᵗʰ **S65.012** Laceration of ulnar artery at wrist and hand level of left arm

√7ᵗʰ **S65.019** Laceration of ulnar artery at wrist and hand level of unspecified arm

√6ᵗʰ **S65.09** Other specified injury of ulnar artery at wrist and hand level

√7ᵗʰ **S65.091** Other specified injury of ulnar artery at wrist and hand level of right arm

√7ᵗʰ **S65.092** Other specified injury of ulnar artery at wrist and hand level of left arm

√7ᵗʰ **S65.099** Other specified injury of ulnar artery at wrist and hand level of unspecified arm

√5ᵗʰ **S65.1** Injury of radial artery at wrist and hand level

√6ᵗʰ **S65.10** Unspecified injury of radial artery at wrist and hand level

√7ᵗʰ **S65.101** Unspecified injury of radial artery at wrist and hand level of right arm

√7ᵗʰ **S65.102** Unspecified injury of radial artery at wrist and hand level of left arm

√7ᵗʰ **S65.109** Unspecified injury of radial artery at wrist and hand level of unspecified arm

√6ᵗʰ **S65.11** Laceration of radial artery at wrist and hand level

√7ᵗʰ **S65.111** Laceration of radial artery at wrist and hand level of right arm

√7ᵗʰ **S65.112** Laceration of radial artery at wrist and hand level of left arm

√7ᵗʰ **S65.119** Laceration of radial artery at wrist and hand level of unspecified arm

√6ᵗʰ **S65.19** Other specified injury of radial artery at wrist and hand level

√7ᵗʰ **S65.191** Other specified injury of radial artery at wrist and hand level of right arm

√7ᵗʰ **S65.192** Other specified injury of radial artery at wrist and hand level of left arm

√7ᵗʰ **S65.199** Other specified injury of radial artery at wrist and hand level of unspecified arm

√5ᵗʰ **S65.2** Injury of superficial palmar arch

√6ᵗʰ **S65.20** Unspecified injury of superficial palmar arch

√7ᵗʰ **S65.201** Unspecified injury of superficial palmar arch of right hand

√7ᵗʰ **S65.202** Unspecified injury of superficial palmar arch of left hand

√7ᵗʰ **S65.209** Unspecified injury of superficial palmar arch of unspecified hand

√6ᵗʰ **S65.21** Laceration of superficial palmar arch

√7ᵗʰ **S65.211** Laceration of superficial palmar arch of right hand

√7ᵗʰ **S65.212** Laceration of superficial palmar arch of left hand

√7ᵗʰ **S65.219** Laceration of superficial palmar arch of unspecified hand

√6ᵗʰ **S65.29** Other specified injury of superficial palmar arch

√7ᵗʰ **S65.291** Other specified injury of superficial palmar arch of right hand

√7ᵗʰ **S65.292** Other specified injury of superficial palmar arch of left hand

√7ᵗʰ **S65.299** Other specified injury of superficial palmar arch of unspecified hand

√5ᵗʰ **S65.3** Injury of deep palmar arch

√6ᵗʰ **S65.30** Unspecified injury of deep palmar arch

√7ᵗʰ **S65.301** Unspecified injury of deep palmar arch of right hand

√7ᵗʰ **S65.302** Unspecified injury of deep palmar arch of left hand

√7ᵗʰ **S65.309** Unspecified injury of deep palmar arch of unspecified hand

√6ᵗʰ **S65.31** Laceration of deep palmar arch

√7ᵗʰ **S65.311** Laceration of deep palmar arch of right hand

√7ᵗʰ **S65.312** Laceration of deep palmar arch of left hand

√7ᵗʰ **S65.319** Laceration of deep palmar arch of unspecified hand

√6ᵗʰ **S65.39** Other specified injury of deep palmar arch

√7ᵗʰ **S65.391** Other specified injury of deep palmar arch of right hand

√7ᵗʰ **S65.392** Other specified injury of deep palmar arch of left hand

√7ᵗʰ **S65.399** Other specified injury of deep palmar arch of unspecified hand

√5ᵗʰ **S65.4** Injury of blood vessel of thumb

√6ᵗʰ **S65.40** Unspecified injury of blood vessel of thumb

√7ᵗʰ **S65.401** Unspecified injury of blood vessel of right thumb

√7ᵗʰ **S65.402** Unspecified injury of blood vessel of left thumb

√7ᵗʰ **S65.409** Unspecified injury of blood vessel of unspecified thumb

√6ᵗʰ **S65.41** Laceration of blood vessel of thumb

√7ᵗʰ **S65.411** Laceration of blood vessel of right thumb

√7ᵗʰ **S65.412** Laceration of blood vessel of left thumb

√7ᵗʰ **S65.419** Laceration of blood vessel of unspecified thumb

√6ᵗʰ **S65.49** Other specified injury of blood vessel of thumb

√7ᵗʰ **S65.491** Other specified injury of blood vessel of right thumb

√7ᵗʰ **S65.492** Other specified injury of blood vessel of left thumb

√7ᵗʰ **S65.499** Other specified injury of blood vessel of unspecified thumb

√5ᵗʰ **S65.5** Injury of blood vessel of other and unspecified finger

√6ᵗʰ **S65.50** Unspecified injury of blood vessel of other and unspecified finger

√7ᵗʰ **S65.500** Unspecified injury of blood vessel of right index finger

√7ᵗʰ **S65.501** Unspecified injury of blood vessel of left index finger

√7ᵗʰ **S65.502** Unspecified injury of blood vessel of right middle finger

√7ᵗʰ **S65.503** Unspecified injury of blood vessel of left middle finger

√7ᵗʰ **S65.504** Unspecified injury of blood vessel of right ring finger

√7ᵗʰ **S65.505** Unspecified injury of blood vessel of left ring finger

√7ᵗʰ **S65.506** Unspecified injury of blood vessel of right little finger

√7ᵗʰ **S65.507** Unspecified injury of blood vessel of left little finger

√7ᵗʰ **S65.508** Unspecified injury of blood vessel of other finger

Unspecified injury of blood vessel of specified finger with unspecified laterality

√7ᵗʰ **S65.509** Unspecified injury of blood vessel of unspecified finger

√6ᵗʰ **S65.51** Laceration of blood vessel of other and unspecified finger

√7ᵗʰ **S65.510** Laceration of blood vessel of right index finger

√7ᵗʰ **S65.511** **Laceration of blood vessel of** left index finger

√7ᵗʰ **S65.512** **Laceration of blood vessel of** right middle finger

√7ᵗʰ **S65.513** **Laceration of blood vessel of** left middle finger

√7ᵗʰ **S65.514** **Laceration of blood vessel of** right ring finger

√7ᵗʰ **S65.515** **Laceration of blood vessel of** left ring finger

√7ᵗʰ **S65.516** **Laceration of blood vessel of** right little finger

√7ᵗʰ **S65.517** **Laceration of blood vessel of** left little finger

√7ᵗʰ **S65.518** **Laceration of blood vessel of other finger**

Laceration of blood vessel of specified finger with unspecified laterality

√7ᵗʰ **S65.519** **Laceration of blood vessel of unspecified finger**

√6ᵗʰ **S65.59** **Other specified injury of blood vessel of other and unspecified finger**

√7ᵗʰ **S65.590** **Other specified injury of blood vessel of** right index **finger**

√7ᵗʰ **S65.591** **Other specified injury of blood vessel of** left index **finger**

√7ᵗʰ **S65.592** **Other specified injury of blood vessel of** right middle **finger**

√7ᵗʰ **S65.593** **Other specified injury of blood vessel of** left middle **finger**

√7ᵗʰ **S65.594** **Other specified injury of blood vessel of** right ring **finger**

√7ᵗʰ **S65.595** **Other specified injury of blood vessel of** left ring **finger**

√7ᵗʰ **S65.596** **Other specified injury of blood vessel of** right little **finger**

√7ᵗʰ **S65.597** **Other specified injury of blood vessel of** left little **finger**

√7ᵗʰ **S65.598** **Other specified injury of blood vessel of other finger**

Other specified injury of blood vessel of specified finger with unspecified laterality

√7ᵗʰ **S65.599** **Other specified injury of blood vessel of unspecified finger**

√5ᵗʰ **S65.8** **Injury of other blood vessels at** wrist and hand level

√6ᵗʰ **S65.80** **Unspecified injury of other blood vessels at wrist and hand level**

√7ᵗʰ **S65.801** **Unspecified injury of other blood vessels at wrist and hand level of right arm**

√7ᵗʰ **S65.802** **Unspecified injury of other blood vessels at wrist and hand level of left arm**

√7ᵗʰ **S65.809** **Unspecified injury of other blood vessels at wrist and hand level of unspecified arm**

√6ᵗʰ **S65.81** **Laceration of other blood vessels at wrist and hand level**

√7ᵗʰ **S65.811** **Laceration of other blood vessels at wrist and hand level of** right **arm**

√7ᵗʰ **S65.812** **Laceration of other blood vessels at wrist and hand level of** left **arm**

√7ᵗʰ **S65.819** **Laceration of other blood vessels at wrist and hand level of unspecified arm**

√6ᵗʰ **S65.89** **Other specified injury of other blood vessels at wrist and hand level**

√7ᵗʰ **S65.891** **Other specified injury of other blood vessels at wrist and hand level of** right **arm**

√7ᵗʰ **S65.892** **Other specified injury of other blood vessels at wrist and hand level of** left **arm**

√7ᵗʰ **S65.899** **Other specified injury of other blood vessels at wrist and hand level of unspecified arm**

√5ᵗʰ **S65.9** **Injury of unspecified blood vessel at** wrist and hand level

√6ᵗʰ **S65.90** **Unspecified injury of unspecified blood vessel at wrist and hand level**

√7ᵗʰ **S65.901** **Unspecified injury of unspecified blood vessel at wrist and hand level of** right **arm**

√7ᵗʰ **S65.902** **Unspecified injury of unspecified blood vessel at wrist and hand level of** left **arm**

√7ᵗʰ **S65.909** **Unspecified injury of unspecified blood vessel at wrist and hand level of unspecified arm**

√6ᵗʰ **S65.91** **Laceration** of unspecified blood vessel at wrist and hand level

√7ᵗʰ **S65.911** **Laceration of unspecified blood vessel at wrist and hand level of** right **arm**

√7ᵗʰ **S65.912** **Laceration of unspecified blood vessel at wrist and hand level of** left **arm**

√7ᵗʰ **S65.919** **Laceration of unspecified blood vessel at wrist and hand level of unspecified arm**

√6ᵗʰ **S65.99** **Other specified injury of unspecified blood vessel at wrist and hand level**

√7ᵗʰ **S65.991** **Other specified injury of unspecified blood vessel at wrist and hand of** right **arm**

√7ᵗʰ **S65.992** **Other specified injury of unspecified blood vessel at wrist and hand of** left **arm**

√7ᵗʰ **S65.999** **Other specified injury of unspecified blood vessel at wrist and hand of unspecified arm**

√4ᵗʰ **S66** **Injury of muscle, fascia and tendon at wrist and hand level**

Code also any associated open wound (S61.-)

EXCLUDES 2   *sprain of joints and ligaments of wrist and hand (S63.-)*

TIP: Refer to the Muscle/Tendon table at the beginning of this chapter.

The appropriate 7th character is to be added to each code from category S66.
A   initial encounter
D   subsequent encounter
S   sequela

√5ᵗʰ **S66.0** **Injury of** long flexor **muscle, fascia and tendon of** thumb **at wrist and hand level**

√6ᵗʰ **S66.00** **Unspecified injury of long flexor muscle, fascia and tendon of thumb at wrist and hand level**

√7ᵗʰ **S66.001** **Unspecified injury of long flexor muscle, fascia and tendon of** right **thumb at wrist and hand level**

√7ᵗʰ **S66.002** **Unspecified injury of long flexor muscle, fascia and tendon of** left **thumb at wrist and hand level**

√7ᵗʰ **S66.009** **Unspecified injury of long flexor muscle, fascia and tendon of unspecified thumb at wrist and hand level**

√6ᵗʰ **S66.01** **Strain of long flexor muscle, fascia and tendon of thumb at wrist and hand level**

√7ᵗʰ **S66.011** **Strain of long flexor muscle, fascia and tendon of** right **thumb at wrist and hand level**

√7ᵗʰ **S66.012** **Strain of long flexor muscle, fascia and tendon of** left **thumb at wrist and hand level**

√7ᵗʰ **S66.019** **Strain of long flexor muscle, fascia and tendon of unspecified thumb at wrist and hand level**

√6ᵗʰ **S66.02** **Laceration** of long flexor muscle, fascia and tendon of thumb at wrist and hand level

√7ᵗʰ **S66.021** **Laceration of long flexor muscle, fascia and tendon of** right **thumb at wrist and hand level**

√7ᵗʰ **S66.022** **Laceration of long flexor muscle, fascia and tendon of** left **thumb at wrist and hand level**

√7ᵗʰ **S66.029** **Laceration of long flexor muscle, fascia and tendon of unspecified thumb at wrist and hand level**

√6ᵗʰ **S66.09** **Other specified injury of long flexor muscle, fascia and tendon of thumb at wrist and hand level**

√7ᵗʰ **S66.091** **Other specified injury of long flexor muscle, fascia and tendon of** right **thumb at wrist and hand level**

√7ᵗʰ **S66.092** **Other specified injury of long flexor muscle, fascia and tendon of** left **thumb at wrist and hand level**

√7ᵗʰ **S66.099** **Other specified injury of long flexor muscle, fascia and tendon of unspecified thumb at wrist and hand level**

√5ᵗʰ **S66.1** **Injury of** flexor **muscle, fascia and tendon of other and unspecified** finger **at wrist and hand level**

EXCLUDES 2   *injury of long flexor muscle, fascia and tendon of thumb at wrist and hand level (S66.0-)*

√6ᵗʰ **S66.10** **Unspecified injury of flexor muscle, fascia and tendon of other and unspecified finger at wrist and hand level**

√7ᵗʰ **S66.100** **Unspecified injury of flexor muscle, fascia and tendon of** right index **finger at wrist and hand level**

√7ᵗʰ S66.101 Unspecified injury of flexor muscle, fascia and tendon of left index finger at wrist and hand level

√7ᵗʰ S66.102 Unspecified injury of flexor muscle, fascia and tendon of right middle finger at wrist and hand level

√7ᵗʰ S66.103 Unspecified injury of flexor muscle, fascia and tendon of left middle finger at wrist and hand level

√7ᵗʰ S66.104 Unspecified injury of flexor muscle, fascia and tendon of right ring finger at wrist and hand level

√7ᵗʰ S66.105 Unspecified injury of flexor muscle, fascia and tendon of left ring finger at wrist and hand level

√7ᵗʰ S66.106 Unspecified injury of flexor muscle, fascia and tendon of right little finger at wrist and hand level

√7ᵗʰ S66.107 Unspecified injury of flexor muscle, fascia and tendon of left little finger at wrist and hand level

√7ᵗʰ S66.108 Unspecified injury of flexor muscle, fascia and tendon of other finger at wrist and hand level

Unspecified injury of flexor muscle, fascia and tendon of specified finger with unspecified laterality at wrist and hand level

√7ᵗʰ S66.109 Unspecified injury of flexor muscle, fascia and tendon of unspecified finger at wrist and hand level

√6ᵗʰ S66.11 Strain of flexor muscle, fascia and tendon of other and unspecified finger at wrist and hand level

√7ᵗʰ S66.110 Strain of flexor muscle, fascia and tendon of right index finger at wrist and hand level

√7ᵗʰ S66.111 Strain of flexor muscle, fascia and tendon of left index finger at wrist and hand level

√7ᵗʰ S66.112 Strain of flexor muscle, fascia and tendon of right middle finger at wrist and hand level

√7ᵗʰ S66.113 Strain of flexor muscle, fascia and tendon of left middle finger at wrist and hand level

√7ᵗʰ S66.114 Strain of flexor muscle, fascia and tendon of right ring finger at wrist and hand level

√7ᵗʰ S66.115 Strain of flexor muscle, fascia and tendon of left ring finger at wrist and hand level

√7ᵗʰ S66.116 Strain of flexor muscle, fascia and tendon of right little finger at wrist and hand level

√7ᵗʰ S66.117 Strain of flexor muscle, fascia and tendon of left little finger at wrist and hand level

√7ᵗʰ S66.118 Strain of flexor muscle, fascia and tendon of other finger at wrist and hand level

Strain of flexor muscle, fascia and tendon of specified finger with unspecified laterality at wrist and hand level

√7ᵗʰ S66.119 Strain of flexor muscle, fascia and tendon of unspecified finger at wrist and hand level

√6ᵗʰ S66.12 Laceration of flexor muscle, fascia and tendon of other and unspecified finger at wrist and hand level

√7ᵗʰ S66.120 Laceration of flexor muscle, fascia and tendon of right index finger at wrist and hand level

√7ᵗʰ S66.121 Laceration of flexor muscle, fascia and tendon of left index finger at wrist and hand level

√7ᵗʰ S66.122 Laceration of flexor muscle, fascia and tendon of right middle finger at wrist and hand level

√7ᵗʰ S66.123 Laceration of flexor muscle, fascia and tendon of left middle finger at wrist and hand level

√7ᵗʰ S66.124 Laceration of flexor muscle, fascia and tendon of right ring finger at wrist and hand level

√7ᵗʰ S66.125 Laceration of flexor muscle, fascia and tendon of left ring finger at wrist and hand level

√7ᵗʰ S66.126 Laceration of flexor muscle, fascia and tendon of right little finger at wrist and hand level

√7ᵗʰ S66.127 Laceration of flexor muscle, fascia and tendon of left little finger at wrist and hand level

√7ᵗʰ S66.128 Laceration of flexor muscle, fascia and tendon of other finger at wrist and hand level

Laceration of flexor muscle, fascia and tendon of specified finger with unspecified laterality at wrist and hand level

√7ᵗʰ S66.129 Laceration of flexor muscle, fascia and tendon of unspecified finger at wrist and hand level

√6ᵗʰ S66.19 Other injury of flexor muscle, fascia and tendon of other and unspecified finger at wrist and hand level

√7ᵗʰ S66.190 Other injury of flexor muscle, fascia and tendon of right index finger at wrist and hand level

√7ᵗʰ S66.191 Other injury of flexor muscle, fascia and tendon of left index finger at wrist and hand level

√7ᵗʰ S66.192 Other injury of flexor muscle, fascia and tendon of right middle finger at wrist and hand level

√7ᵗʰ S66.193 Other injury of flexor muscle, fascia and tendon of left middle finger at wrist and hand level

√7ᵗʰ S66.194 Other injury of flexor muscle, fascia and tendon of right ring finger at wrist and hand level

√7ᵗʰ S66.195 Other injury of flexor muscle, fascia and tendon of left ring finger at wrist and hand level

√7ᵗʰ S66.196 Other injury of flexor muscle, fascia and tendon of right little finger at wrist and hand level

√7ᵗʰ S66.197 Other injury of flexor muscle, fascia and tendon of left little finger at wrist and hand level

√7ᵗʰ S66.198 Other injury of flexor muscle, fascia and tendon of other finger at wrist and hand level

Other injury of flexor muscle, fascia and tendon of specified finger with unspecified laterality at wrist and hand level

√7ᵗʰ S66.199 Other injury of flexor muscle, fascia and tendon of unspecified finger at wrist and hand level

√5ᵗʰ S66.2 Injury of extensor muscle, fascia and tendon of thumb at wrist and hand level

√6ᵗʰ S66.20 Unspecified injury of extensor muscle, fascia and tendon of thumb at wrist and hand level

√7ᵗʰ S66.201 Unspecified injury of extensor muscle, fascia and tendon of right thumb at wrist and hand level

√7ᵗʰ S66.202 Unspecified injury of extensor muscle, fascia and tendon of left thumb at wrist and hand level

√7ᵗʰ S66.209 Unspecified injury of extensor muscle, fascia and tendon of unspecified thumb at wrist and hand level

√6ᵗʰ S66.21 Strain of extensor muscle, fascia and tendon of thumb at wrist and hand level

√7ᵗʰ S66.211 Strain of extensor muscle, fascia and tendon of right thumb at wrist and hand level

√7ᵗʰ S66.212 Strain of extensor muscle, fascia and tendon of left thumb at wrist and hand level

√7ᵗʰ S66.219 Strain of extensor muscle, fascia and tendon of unspecified thumb at wrist and hand level

√6ᵗʰ S66.22 Laceration of extensor muscle, fascia and tendon of thumb at wrist and hand level

√7ᵗʰ S66.221 Laceration of extensor muscle, fascia and tendon of right thumb at wrist and hand level

√7ᵗʰ S66.222 Laceration of extensor muscle, fascia and tendon of left thumb at wrist and hand level

√7ᵗʰ S66.229 Laceration of extensor muscle, fascia and tendon of unspecified thumb at wrist and hand level

√6ᵗʰ **S66.29** **Other specified injury of extensor muscle, fascia and tendon of thumb at wrist and hand level**

√7ᵗʰ **S66.291** Other specified injury of extensor muscle, fascia and tendon of right thumb at wrist and hand level

√7ᵗʰ **S66.292** Other specified injury of extensor muscle, fascia and tendon of left thumb at wrist and hand level

√7ᵗʰ **S66.299** Other specified injury of extensor muscle, fascia and tendon of unspecified thumb at wrist and hand level

√6ᵗʰ **S66.3** Injury of extensor muscle, fascia and tendon of other and unspecified finger at wrist and hand level

EXCLUDES 2   injury of extensor muscle, fascia and tendon of thumb at wrist and hand level (S66.2-)

√6ᵗʰ **S66.30** **Unspecified injury of extensor muscle, fascia and tendon of other and unspecified finger at wrist and hand level**

√7ᵗʰ **S66.300** Unspecified injury of extensor muscle, fascia and tendon of right index finger at wrist and hand level

√7ᵗʰ **S66.301** Unspecified injury of extensor muscle, fascia and tendon of left index finger at wrist and hand level

√7ᵗʰ **S66.302** Unspecified injury of extensor muscle, fascia and tendon of right middle finger at wrist and hand level

√7ᵗʰ **S66.303** Unspecified injury of extensor muscle, fascia and tendon of left middle finger at wrist and hand level

√7ᵗʰ **S66.304** Unspecified injury of extensor muscle, fascia and tendon of right ring finger at wrist and hand level

√7ᵗʰ **S66.305** Unspecified injury of extensor muscle, fascia and tendon of left ring finger at wrist and hand level

√7ᵗʰ **S66.306** Unspecified injury of extensor muscle, fascia and tendon of right little finger at wrist and hand level

√7ᵗʰ **S66.307** Unspecified injury of extensor muscle, fascia and tendon of left little finger at wrist and hand level

√7ᵗʰ **S66.308** Unspecified injury of extensor muscle, fascia and tendon of other finger at wrist and hand level

Unspecified injury of extensor muscle, fascia and tendon of specified finger with unspecified laterality at wrist and hand level

√7ᵗʰ **S66.309** Unspecified injury of extensor muscle, fascia and tendon of unspecified finger at wrist and hand level

√6ᵗʰ **S66.31** Strain of extensor muscle, fascia and tendon of other and unspecified finger at wrist and hand level

√7ᵗʰ **S66.310** Strain of extensor muscle, fascia and tendon of right index finger at wrist and hand level

√7ᵗʰ **S66.311** Strain of extensor muscle, fascia and tendon of left index finger at wrist and hand level

√7ᵗʰ **S66.312** Strain of extensor muscle, fascia and tendon of right middle finger at wrist and hand level

√7ᵗʰ **S66.313** Strain of extensor muscle, fascia and tendon of left middle finger at wrist and hand level

√7ᵗʰ **S66.314** Strain of extensor muscle, fascia and tendon of right ring finger at wrist and hand level

√7ᵗʰ **S66.315** Strain of extensor muscle, fascia and tendon of left ring finger at wrist and hand level

√7ᵗʰ **S66.316** Strain of extensor muscle, fascia and tendon of right little finger at wrist and hand level

√7ᵗʰ **S66.317** Strain of extensor muscle, fascia and tendon of left little finger at wrist and hand level

√7ᵗʰ **S66.318** Strain of extensor muscle, fascia and tendon of other finger at wrist and hand level

Strain of extensor muscle, fascia and tendon of specified finger with unspecified laterality at wrist and hand level

√7ᵗʰ **S66.319** Strain of extensor muscle, fascia and tendon of unspecified finger at wrist and hand level

√6ᵗʰ **S66.32** Laceration of extensor muscle, fascia and tendon of other and unspecified finger at wrist and hand level

√7ᵗʰ **S66.320** Laceration of extensor muscle, fascia and tendon of right index finger at wrist and hand level

√7ᵗʰ **S66.321** Laceration of extensor muscle, fascia and tendon of left index finger at wrist and hand level

√7ᵗʰ **S66.322** Laceration of extensor muscle, fascia and tendon of right middle finger at wrist and hand level

√7ᵗʰ **S66.323** Laceration of extensor muscle, fascia and tendon of left middle finger at wrist and hand level

√7ᵗʰ **S66.324** Laceration of extensor muscle, fascia and tendon of right ring finger at wrist and hand level

√7ᵗʰ **S66.325** Laceration of extensor muscle, fascia and tendon of left ring finger at wrist and hand level

√7ᵗʰ **S66.326** Laceration of extensor muscle, fascia and tendon of right little finger at wrist and hand level

√7ᵗʰ **S66.327** Laceration of extensor muscle, fascia and tendon of left little finger at wrist and hand level

√7ᵗʰ **S66.328** Laceration of extensor muscle, fascia and tendon of other finger at wrist and hand level

Laceration of extensor muscle, fascia and tendon of specified finger with unspecified laterality at wrist and hand level

√7ᵗʰ **S66.329** Laceration of extensor muscle, fascia and tendon of unspecified finger at wrist and hand level

√6ᵗʰ **S66.39** Other injury of extensor muscle, fascia and tendon of other and unspecified finger at wrist and hand level

√7ᵗʰ **S66.390** Other injury of extensor muscle, fascia and tendon of right index finger at wrist and hand level

√7ᵗʰ **S66.391** Other injury of extensor muscle, fascia and tendon of left index finger at wrist and hand level

√7ᵗʰ **S66.392** Other injury of extensor muscle, fascia and tendon of right middle finger at wrist and hand level

√7ᵗʰ **S66.393** Other injury of extensor muscle, fascia and tendon of left middle finger at wrist and hand level

√7ᵗʰ **S66.394** Other injury of extensor muscle, fascia and tendon of right ring finger at wrist and hand level

√7ᵗʰ **S66.395** Other injury of extensor muscle, fascia and tendon of left ring finger at wrist and hand level

√7ᵗʰ **S66.396** Other injury of extensor muscle, fascia and tendon of right little finger at wrist and hand level

√7ᵗʰ **S66.397** Other injury of extensor muscle, fascia and tendon of left little finger at wrist and hand level

√7ᵗʰ **S66.398** Other injury of extensor muscle, fascia and tendon of other finger at wrist and hand level

Other injury of extensor muscle, fascia and tendon of specified finger with unspecified laterality at wrist and hand level

√7ᵗʰ **S66.399** Other injury of extensor muscle, fascia and tendon of unspecified finger at wrist and hand level

√5ᵗʰ **S66.4 Injury of** intrinsic **muscle, fascia and tendon of** thumb **at wrist and hand level**

√6ᵗʰ **S66.40 Unspecified injury of intrinsic muscle, fascia and tendon of thumb at wrist and hand level**

√7ᵗʰ **S66.401 Unspecified injury of intrinsic muscle, fascia and tendon of** right **thumb at wrist and hand level**

√7ᵗʰ **S66.402 Unspecified injury of intrinsic muscle, fascia and tendon of** left **thumb at wrist and hand level**

√7ᵗʰ **S66.409 Unspecified injury of intrinsic muscle, fascia and tendon of unspecified thumb at wrist and hand level**

√6ᵗʰ **S66.41** Strain **of intrinsic muscle, fascia and tendon of thumb at wrist and hand level**

√7ᵗʰ **S66.411 Strain of intrinsic muscle, fascia and tendon of** right **thumb at wrist and hand level**

√7ᵗʰ **S66.412 Strain of intrinsic muscle, fascia and tendon of** left **thumb at wrist and hand level**

√7ᵗʰ **S66.419 Strain of intrinsic muscle, fascia and tendon of unspecified thumb at wrist and hand level**

√6ᵗʰ **S66.42** Laceration **of intrinsic muscle, fascia and tendon of thumb at wrist and hand level**

√7ᵗʰ **S66.421 Laceration of intrinsic muscle, fascia and tendon of** right **thumb at wrist and hand level**

√7ᵗʰ **S66.422 Laceration of intrinsic muscle, fascia and tendon of** left **thumb at wrist and hand level**

√7ᵗʰ **S66.429 Laceration of intrinsic muscle, fascia and tendon of unspecified thumb at wrist and hand level**

√6ᵗʰ **S66.49 Other specified injury of intrinsic muscle, fascia and tendon of thumb at wrist and hand level**

√7ᵗʰ **S66.491 Other specified injury of intrinsic muscle, fascia and tendon of** right **thumb at wrist and hand level**

√7ᵗʰ **S66.492 Other specified injury of intrinsic muscle, fascia and tendon of** left **thumb at wrist and hand level**

√7ᵗʰ **S66.499 Other specified injury of intrinsic muscle, fascia and tendon of unspecified thumb at wrist and hand level**

√5ᵗʰ **S66.5 Injury of** intrinsic **muscle, fascia and tendon of other and unspecified** finger **at wrist and hand level**

> EXCLUDES 2 *injury of intrinsic muscle, fascia and tendon of thumb at wrist and hand level (S66.4-)*

√6ᵗʰ **S66.50 Unspecified injury of intrinsic muscle, fascia and tendon of other and unspecified finger at wrist and hand level**

√7ᵗʰ **S66.500 Unspecified injury of intrinsic muscle, fascia and tendon of** right index **finger at wrist and hand level**

√7ᵗʰ **S66.501 Unspecified injury of intrinsic muscle, fascia and tendon of** left index **finger at wrist and hand level**

√7ᵗʰ **S66.502 Unspecified injury of intrinsic muscle, fascia and tendon of** right middle **finger at wrist and hand level**

√7ᵗʰ **S66.503 Unspecified injury of intrinsic muscle, fascia and tendon of** left middle **finger at wrist and hand level**

√7ᵗʰ **S66.504 Unspecified injury of intrinsic muscle, fascia and tendon of** right ring **finger at wrist and hand level**

√7ᵗʰ **S66.505 Unspecified injury of intrinsic muscle, fascia and tendon of** left ring **finger at wrist and hand level**

√7ᵗʰ **S66.506 Unspecified injury of intrinsic muscle, fascia and tendon of** right little **finger at wrist and hand level**

√7ᵗʰ **S66.507 Unspecified injury of intrinsic muscle, fascia and tendon of** left little **finger at wrist and hand level**

√7ᵗʰ **S66.508 Unspecified injury of intrinsic muscle, fascia and tendon of other finger at wrist and hand level**

Unspecified injury of intrinsic muscle, fascia and tendon of specified finger with unspecified laterality at wrist and hand level

√7ᵗʰ **S66.509 Unspecified injury of intrinsic muscle, fascia and tendon of unspecified finger at wrist and hand level**

√6ᵗʰ **S66.51** Strain **of intrinsic muscle, fascia and tendon of other and unspecified finger at wrist and hand level**

√7ᵗʰ **S66.510 Strain of intrinsic muscle, fascia and tendon of** right index **finger at wrist and hand level**

√7ᵗʰ **S66.511 Strain of intrinsic muscle, fascia and tendon of** left index **finger at wrist and hand level**

√7ᵗʰ **S66.512 Strain of intrinsic muscle, fascia and tendon of** right middle **finger at wrist and hand level**

√7ᵗʰ **S66.513 Strain of intrinsic muscle, fascia and tendon of** left middle **finger at wrist and hand level**

√7ᵗʰ **S66.514 Strain of intrinsic muscle, fascia and tendon of** right ring **finger at wrist and hand level**

√7ᵗʰ **S66.515 Strain of intrinsic muscle, fascia and tendon of** left ring **finger at wrist and hand level**

√7ᵗʰ **S66.516 Strain of intrinsic muscle, fascia and tendon of** right little **finger at wrist and hand level**

√7ᵗʰ **S66.517 Strain of intrinsic muscle, fascia and tendon of** left little **finger at wrist and hand level**

√7ᵗʰ **S66.518 Strain of intrinsic muscle, fascia and tendon of other finger at wrist and hand level**

Strain of intrinsic muscle, fascia and tendon of specified finger with unspecified laterality at wrist and hand level

√7ᵗʰ **S66.519 Strain of intrinsic muscle, fascia and tendon of unspecified finger at wrist and hand level**

√6ᵗʰ **S66.52** Laceration **of intrinsic muscle, fascia and tendon of other and unspecified finger at wrist and hand level**

√7ᵗʰ **S66.520 Laceration of intrinsic muscle, fascia and tendon of** right index **finger at wrist and hand level**

√7ᵗʰ **S66.521 Laceration of intrinsic muscle, fascia and tendon of** left index **finger at wrist and hand level**

√7ᵗʰ **S66.522 Laceration of intrinsic muscle, fascia and tendon of** right middle **finger at wrist and hand level**

√7ᵗʰ **S66.523 Laceration of intrinsic muscle, fascia and tendon of** left middle **finger at wrist and hand level**

√7ᵗʰ **S66.524 Laceration of intrinsic muscle, fascia and tendon of** right ring **finger at wrist and hand level**

√7ᵗʰ **S66.525 Laceration of intrinsic muscle, fascia and tendon of** left ring **finger at wrist and hand level**

√7ᵗʰ **S66.526 Laceration of intrinsic muscle, fascia and tendon of** right little **finger at wrist and hand level**

√7ᵗʰ **S66.527 Laceration of intrinsic muscle, fascia and tendon of** left little **finger at wrist and hand level**

√7ᵗʰ **S66.528 Laceration of intrinsic muscle, fascia and tendon of other finger at wrist and hand level**

Laceration of intrinsic muscle, fascia and tendon of specified finger with unspecified laterality at wrist and hand level

√7ᵗʰ **S66.529 Laceration of intrinsic muscle, fascia and tendon of unspecified finger at wrist and hand level**

✓6th **S66.59** Other injury of intrinsic muscle, fascia and tendon of other and unspecified finger at wrist and hand level

     ✓7th **S66.590** Other injury of intrinsic muscle, fascia and tendon of right index finger at wrist and hand level

     ✓7th **S66.591** Other injury of intrinsic muscle, fascia and tendon of left index finger at wrist and hand level

     ✓7th **S66.592** Other injury of intrinsic muscle, fascia and tendon of right middle finger at wrist and hand level

     ✓7th **S66.593** Other injury of intrinsic muscle, fascia and tendon of left middle finger at wrist and hand level

     ✓7th **S66.594** Other injury of intrinsic muscle, fascia and tendon of right ring finger at wrist and hand level

     ✓7th **S66.595** Other injury of intrinsic muscle, fascia and tendon of left ring finger at wrist and hand level

     ✓7th **S66.596** Other injury of intrinsic muscle, fascia and tendon of right little finger at wrist and hand level

     ✓7th **S66.597** Other injury of intrinsic muscle, fascia and tendon of left little finger at wrist and hand level

     ✓7th **S66.598** Other injury of intrinsic muscle, fascia and tendon of other finger at wrist and hand level

         Other injury of intrinsic muscle, fascia and tendon of specified finger with unspecified laterality at wrist and hand level

     ✓7th **S66.599** Other injury of intrinsic muscle, fascia and tendon of unspecified finger at wrist and hand level

✓5th **S66.8** Injury of other specified muscles, fascia and tendons at wrist and hand level

     ✓6th **S66.80** Unspecified injury of other specified muscles, fascia and tendons at wrist and hand level

         ✓7th **S66.801** Unspecified injury of other specified muscles, fascia and tendons at wrist and hand level, right hand

         ✓7th **S66.802** Unspecified injury of other specified muscles, fascia and tendons at wrist and hand level, left hand

         ✓7th **S66.809** Unspecified injury of other specified muscles, fascia and tendons at wrist and hand level, unspecified hand

     ✓6th **S66.81** Strain of other specified muscles, fascia and tendons at wrist and hand level

         ✓7th **S66.811** Strain of other specified muscles, fascia and tendons at wrist and hand level, right hand

         ✓7th **S66.812** Strain of other specified muscles, fascia and tendons at wrist and hand level, left hand

         ✓7th **S66.819** Strain of other specified muscles, fascia and tendons at wrist and hand level, unspecified hand

     ✓6th **S66.82** Laceration of other specified muscles, fascia and tendons at wrist and hand level

         ✓7th **S66.821** Laceration of other specified muscles, fascia and tendons at wrist and hand level, right hand

         ✓7th **S66.822** Laceration of other specified muscles, fascia and tendons at wrist and hand level, left hand

         ✓7th **S66.829** Laceration of other specified muscles, fascia and tendons at wrist and hand level, unspecified hand

     ✓6th **S66.89** Other injury of other specified muscles, fascia and tendons at wrist and hand level

         ✓7th **S66.891** Other injury of other specified muscles, fascia and tendons at wrist and hand level, right hand

         ✓7th **S66.892** Other injury of other specified muscles, fascia and tendons at wrist and hand level, left hand

         ✓7th **S66.899** Other injury of other specified muscles, fascia and tendons at wrist and hand level, unspecified hand

✓5th **S66.9** Injury of unspecified muscle, fascia and tendon at wrist and hand level

     ✓6th **S66.90** Unspecified injury of unspecified muscle, fascia and tendon at wrist and hand level

         ✓7th **S66.901** Unspecified injury of unspecified muscle, fascia and tendon at wrist and hand level, right hand

         ✓7th **S66.902** Unspecified injury of unspecified muscle, fascia and tendon at wrist and hand level, left hand

         ✓7th **S66.909** Unspecified injury of unspecified muscle, fascia and tendon at wrist and hand level, unspecified hand

     ✓6th **S66.91** Strain of unspecified muscle, fascia and tendon at wrist and hand level

         ✓7th **S66.911** Strain of unspecified muscle, fascia and tendon at wrist and hand level, right hand

         ✓7th **S66.912** Strain of unspecified muscle, fascia and tendon at wrist and hand level, left hand

         ✓7th **S66.919** Strain of unspecified muscle, fascia and tendon at wrist and hand level, unspecified hand

     ✓6th **S66.92** Laceration of unspecified muscle, fascia and tendon at wrist and hand level

         ✓7th **S66.921** Laceration of unspecified muscle, fascia and tendon at wrist and hand level, right hand

         ✓7th **S66.922** Laceration of unspecified muscle, fascia and tendon at wrist and hand level, left hand

         ✓7th **S66.929** Laceration of unspecified muscle, fascia and tendon at wrist and hand level, unspecified hand

     ✓6th **S66.99** Other injury of unspecified muscle, fascia and tendon at wrist and hand level

         ✓7th **S66.991** Other injury of unspecified muscle, fascia and tendon at wrist and hand level, right hand

         ✓7th **S66.992** Other injury of unspecified muscle, fascia and tendon at wrist and hand level, left hand

         ✓7th **S66.999** Other injury of unspecified muscle, fascia and tendon at wrist and hand level, unspecified hand

✓4th **S67** Crushing injury of wrist, hand and fingers

     Use additional code for all associated injuries, such as:
         fracture of wrist and hand (S62.-)
         open wound of wrist and hand (S61.-)

     The appropriate 7th character is to be added to each code from category S67.
     A   initial encounter
     D   subsequent encounter
     S   sequela

     ✓5th **S67.0** Crushing injury of thumb

         ✓x7th **S67.00** Crushing injury of unspecified thumb

         ✓x7th **S67.01** Crushing injury of right thumb

         ✓x7th **S67.02** Crushing injury of left thumb

     ✓5th **S67.1** Crushing injury of other and unspecified finger(s)

         EXCLUDES 2   crushing injury of thumb (S67.0-)

         ✓x7th **S67.10** Crushing injury of unspecified finger(s)

         ✓6th **S67.19** Crushing injury of other finger(s)

             ✓7th **S67.190** Crushing injury of right index finger

             ✓7th **S67.191** Crushing injury of left index finger

             ✓7th **S67.192** Crushing injury of right middle finger

             ✓7th **S67.193** Crushing injury of left middle finger

             ✓7th **S67.194** Crushing injury of right ring finger

             ✓7th **S67.195** Crushing injury of left ring finger

             ✓7th **S67.196** Crushing injury of right little finger

             ✓7th **S67.197** Crushing injury of left little finger

             ✓7th **S67.198** Crushing injury of other finger

                 Crushing injury of specified finger with unspecified laterality

     ✓5th **S67.2** Crushing injury of hand

         EXCLUDES 2   crushing injury of fingers (S67.1-)
                    crushing injury of thumb (S67.0-)

         ✓x7th **S67.20** Crushing injury of unspecified hand

√x7ᵗʰ **S67.21** Crushing injury of right hand

√x7ᵗʰ **S67.22** Crushing injury of left hand

√5ᵗʰ **S67.3** **Crushing injury of** wrist

√x7ᵗʰ **S67.30** Crushing injury of unspecified wrist

√x7ᵗʰ **S67.31** Crushing injury of right wrist

√x7ᵗʰ **S67.32** Crushing injury of left wrist

√5ᵗʰ **S67.4** **Crushing injury of** wrist and hand

> EXCLUDES 1 *crushing injury of hand alone (S67.2-)*
> *crushing injury of wrist alone (S67.3-)*
> EXCLUDES 2 *crushing injury of fingers (S67.1-)*
> *crushing injury of thumb (S67.0-)*

√x7ᵗʰ **S67.40** Crushing injury of unspecified wrist and hand

√x7ᵗʰ **S67.41** Crushing injury of right wrist and hand

√x7ᵗʰ **S67.42** Crushing injury of left wrist and hand

√5ᵗʰ **S67.9** **Crushing injury of unspecified part(s) of wrist, hand and fingers**

√x7ᵗʰ **S67.90** Crushing injury of unspecified part(s) of unspecified wrist, hand and fingers

√x7ᵗʰ **S67.91** Crushing injury of unspecified part(s) of right wrist, hand and fingers

√x7ᵗʰ **S67.92** Crushing injury of unspecified part(s) of left wrist, hand and fingers

√4ᵗʰ **S68** **Traumatic amputation of wrist, hand and fingers**

An amputation not identified as partial or complete should be coded to complete.

> The appropriate 7th character is to be added to each code from category S68.
> A initial encounter
> D subsequent encounter
> S sequela

√5ᵗʰ **S68.0** **Traumatic** metacarpophalangeal **amputation of** thumb

Traumatic amputation of thumb NOS

√6ᵗʰ **S68.01** **Complete** traumatic metacarpophalangeal amputation of thumb

³ √7ᵗʰ **S68.011** Complete traumatic metacarpophalangeal amputation of right thumb HCC ESR

³ √7ᵗʰ **S68.012** Complete traumatic metacarpophalangeal amputation of left thumb HCC ESR

³ √7ᵗʰ **S68.019** Complete traumatic metacarpophalangeal amputation of unspecified thumb HCC ESR

√6ᵗʰ **S68.02** **Partial** traumatic metacarpophalangeal amputation of thumb

³ √7ᵗʰ **S68.021** Partial traumatic metacarpophalangeal amputation of right thumb HCC ESR

³ √7ᵗʰ **S68.022** Partial traumatic metacarpophalangeal amputation of left thumb HCC ESR

³ √7ᵗʰ **S68.029** Partial traumatic metacarpophalangeal amputation of unspecified thumb HCC ESR

√5ᵗʰ **S68.1** **Traumatic** metacarpophalangeal **amputation of other and unspecified** finger

Traumatic amputation of finger NOS

> EXCLUDES 2 *traumatic metacarpophalangeal amputation of thumb (S68.0-)*

√6ᵗʰ **S68.11** **Complete** traumatic metacarpophalangeal amputation of other and unspecified finger

³ √7ᵗʰ **S68.110** Complete traumatic metacarpophalangeal amputation of right index finger HCC ESR

³ √7ᵗʰ **S68.111** Complete traumatic metacarpophalangeal amputation of left index finger HCC ESR

³ √7ᵗʰ **S68.112** Complete traumatic metacarpophalangeal amputation of right middle finger HCC ESR

³ √7ᵗʰ **S68.113** Complete traumatic metacarpophalangeal amputation of left middle finger HCC ESR

³ √7ᵗʰ **S68.114** Complete traumatic metacarpophalangeal amputation of right ring finger HCC ESR

³ √7ᵗʰ **S68.115** Complete traumatic metacarpophalangeal amputation of left ring finger HCC ESR

³ √7ᵗʰ **S68.116** Complete traumatic metacarpophalangeal amputation of right little finger HCC ESR

³ √7ᵗʰ **S68.117** Complete traumatic metacarpophalangeal amputation of left little finger HCC ESR

³ √7ᵗʰ **S68.118** Complete traumatic metacarpophalangeal amputation of other finger HCC ESR

Complete traumatic metacarpophalangeal amputation of specified finger with unspecified laterality

³ √7ᵗʰ **S68.119** Complete traumatic metacarpophalangeal amputation of unspecified finger HCC ESR

√6ᵗʰ **S68.12** **Partial** traumatic metacarpophalangeal amputation of other and unspecified finger

³ √7ᵗʰ **S68.120** Partial traumatic metacarpophalangeal amputation of right index finger HCC ESR

³ √7ᵗʰ **S68.121** Partial traumatic metacarpophalangeal amputation of left index finger HCC ESR

³ √7ᵗʰ **S68.122** Partial traumatic metacarpophalangeal amputation of right middle finger HCC ESR

³ √7ᵗʰ **S68.123** Partial traumatic metacarpophalangeal amputation of left middle finger HCC ESR

³ √7ᵗʰ **S68.124** Partial traumatic metacarpophalangeal amputation of right ring finger HCC ESR

³ √7ᵗʰ **S68.125** Partial traumatic metacarpophalangeal amputation of left ring finger HCC ESR

³ √7ᵗʰ **S68.126** Partial traumatic metacarpophalangeal amputation of right little finger HCC ESR

³ √7ᵗʰ **S68.127** Partial traumatic metacarpophalangeal amputation of left little finger HCC ESR

³ √7ᵗʰ **S68.128** Partial traumatic metacarpophalangeal amputation of other finger HCC ESR

Partial traumatic metacarpophalangeal amputation of specified finger with unspecified laterality

³ √7ᵗʰ **S68.129** Partial traumatic metacarpophalangeal amputation of unspecified finger HCC ESR

√5ᵗʰ **S68.4** **Traumatic amputation of** hand at wrist level

Traumatic amputation of hand NOS
Traumatic amputation of wrist

√6ᵗʰ **S68.41** **Complete** traumatic amputation of hand at wrist level

² √7ᵗʰ **S68.411** Complete traumatic amputation of right hand at wrist level HCC ESR COM

² √7ᵗʰ **S68.412** Complete traumatic amputation of left hand at wrist level HCC ESR COM

² √7ᵗʰ **S68.419** Complete traumatic amputation of unspecified hand at wrist level HCC ESR COM

√6ᵗʰ **S68.42** **Partial** traumatic amputation of hand at wrist level

² √7ᵗʰ **S68.421** Partial traumatic amputation of right hand at wrist level HCC ESR COM

² √7ᵗʰ **S68.422** Partial traumatic amputation of left hand at wrist level HCC ESR COM

² √7ᵗʰ **S68.429** Partial traumatic amputation of unspecified hand at wrist level HCC ESR COM

√6ᵗʰ **S68.5** **Traumatic** transphalangeal **amputation of** thumb

Traumatic interphalangeal joint amputation of thumb

√6ᵗʰ **S68.51** **Complete** traumatic transphalangeal amputation of thumb

³ √7ᵗʰ **S68.511** Complete traumatic transphalangeal amputation of right thumb HCC ESR

³ √7ᵗʰ **S68.512** Complete traumatic transphalangeal amputation of left thumb HCC ESR

³ √7ᵗʰ **S68.519** Complete traumatic transphalangeal amputation of unspecified thumb HCC ESR

HCC CMS-HCC　　Rx Rx HCC　　ESR ESRD HCC　　COM Commercial HCC　　N Newborn: 0　　P Pediatric: 0-17　　M Maternity: 9-64　　A Adult: 15-124

☑6ᵗʰ **S68.52** Partial traumatic transphalangeal amputation of thumb

   ³ ☑7ᵗʰ **S68.521** Partial traumatic transphalangeal amputation of right thumb   HCC ESR

   ³ ☑7ᵗʰ **S68.522** Partial traumatic transphalangeal amputation of left thumb   HCC ESR

   ³ ☑7ᵗʰ **S68.529** Partial traumatic transphalangeal amputation of unspecified thumb   HCC ESR

☑5ᵗʰ **S68.6** Traumatic transphalangeal amputation of other and unspecified finger

  ☑6ᵗʰ **S68.61** Complete traumatic transphalangeal amputation of other and unspecified finger(s)

   ³ ☑7ᵗʰ **S68.610** Complete traumatic transphalangeal amputation of right index finger   HCC ESR

   ³ ☑7ᵗʰ **S68.611** Complete traumatic transphalangeal amputation of left index finger   HCC ESR

   ³ ☑7ᵗʰ **S68.612** Complete traumatic transphalangeal amputation of right middle finger   HCC ESR

   ³ ☑7ᵗʰ **S68.613** Complete traumatic transphalangeal amputation of left middle finger   HCC ESR

   ³ ☑7ᵗʰ **S68.614** Complete traumatic transphalangeal amputation of right ring finger   HCC ESR

   ³ ☑7ᵗʰ **S68.615** Complete traumatic transphalangeal amputation of left ring finger   HCC ESR

   ³ ☑7ᵗʰ **S68.616** Complete traumatic transphalangeal amputation of right little finger   HCC ESR

   ³ ☑7ᵗʰ **S68.617** Complete traumatic transphalangeal amputation of left little finger   HCC ESR

   ³ ☑7ᵗʰ **S68.618** Complete traumatic transphalangeal amputation of other finger   HCC ESR

     Complete traumatic transphalangeal amputation of specified finger with unspecified laterality

   ³ ☑7ᵗʰ **S68.619** Complete traumatic transphalangeal amputation of unspecified finger   HCC ESR

  ☑6ᵗʰ **S68.62** Partial traumatic transphalangeal amputation of other and unspecified finger

   ³ ☑7ᵗʰ **S68.620** Partial traumatic transphalangeal amputation of right index finger   HCC ESR

   ³ ☑7ᵗʰ **S68.621** Partial traumatic transphalangeal amputation of left index finger   HCC ESR

   ³ ☑7ᵗʰ **S68.622** Partial traumatic transphalangeal amputation of right middle finger   HCC ESR

   ³ ☑7ᵗʰ **S68.623** Partial traumatic transphalangeal amputation of left middle finger   HCC ESR

   ³ ☑7ᵗʰ **S68.624** Partial traumatic transphalangeal amputation of right ring finger   HCC ESR

   ³ ☑7ᵗʰ **S68.625** Partial traumatic transphalangeal amputation of left ring finger   HCC ESR

   ³ ☑7ᵗʰ **S68.626** Partial traumatic transphalangeal amputation of right little finger   HCC ESR

   ³ ☑7ᵗʰ **S68.627** Partial traumatic transphalangeal amputation of left little finger   HCC ESR

   ³ ☑7ᵗʰ **S68.628** Partial traumatic transphalangeal amputation of other finger   HCC ESR

     Partial traumatic transphalangeal amputation of specified finger with unspecified laterality

   ³ ☑7ᵗʰ **S68.629** Partial traumatic transphalangeal amputation of unspecified finger   HCC ESR

☑5ᵗʰ **S68.7** Traumatic transmetacarpal amputation of hand

  ☑6ᵗʰ **S68.71** Complete traumatic transmetacarpal amputation of hand

   ² ☑7ᵗʰ **S68.711** Complete traumatic transmetacarpal amputation of right hand   HCC ESR COM

   ² ☑7ᵗʰ **S68.712** Complete traumatic transmetacarpal amputation of left hand   HCC ESR COM

   ² ☑7ᵗʰ **S68.719** Complete traumatic transmetacarpal amputation of unspecified hand   HCC ESR COM

  ☑6ᵗʰ **S68.72** Partial traumatic transmetacarpal amputation of hand

   ² ☑7ᵗʰ **S68.721** Partial traumatic transmetacarpal amputation of right hand   HCC ESR COM

   ² ☑7ᵗʰ **S68.722** Partial traumatic transmetacarpal amputation of left hand   HCC ESR COM

   ² ☑7ᵗʰ **S68.729** Partial traumatic transmetacarpal amputation of unspecified hand   HCC ESR COM

☑4ᵗʰ **S69** Other and unspecified injuries of wrist, hand and finger(s)

  The appropriate 7th character is to be added to each code from category S69.
  A initial encounter
  D subsequent encounter
  S sequela

  ☑5ᵗʰ **S69.8** Other specified injuries of wrist, hand and finger(s)

   ☑x7ᵗʰ **S69.80** Other specified injuries of unspecified wrist, hand and finger(s)

   ☑x7ᵗʰ **S69.81** Other specified injuries of right wrist, hand and finger(s)

   ☑x7ᵗʰ **S69.82** Other specified injuries of left wrist, hand and finger(s)

  ☑5ᵗʰ **S69.9** Unspecified injury of wrist, hand and finger(s)

   ☑x7ᵗʰ **S69.90** Unspecified injury of unspecified wrist, hand and finger(s)

   ☑x7ᵗʰ **S69.91** Unspecified injury of right wrist, hand and finger(s)

   ☑x7ᵗʰ **S69.92** Unspecified injury of left wrist, hand and finger(s)

Injuries to the hip and thigh (S70-S79)

EXCLUDES 2   *burns and corrosions (T20-T32)*
          frostbite (T33-T34)
          snake bite (T63.0-)
          venomous insect bite or sting (T63.4-)

☑4ᵗʰ **S70** Superficial injury of hip and thigh

  The appropriate 7th character is to be added to each code from category S70.
  A initial encounter
  D subsequent encounter
  S sequela

  ☑5ᵗʰ **S70.0** Contusion of hip

   ☑x7ᵗʰ **S70.00** Contusion of unspecified hip

   ☑x7ᵗʰ **S70.01** Contusion of right hip

   ☑x7ᵗʰ **S70.02** Contusion of left hip

  ☑5ᵗʰ **S70.1** Contusion of thigh

   ☑x7ᵗʰ **S70.10** Contusion of unspecified thigh

   ☑x7ᵗʰ **S70.11** Contusion of right thigh

   ☑x7ᵗʰ **S70.12** Contusion of left thigh

  ☑5ᵗʰ **S70.2** Other superficial injuries of hip

   ☑6ᵗʰ **S70.21** Abrasion of hip

    ☑7ᵗʰ **S70.211** Abrasion, right hip

    ☑7ᵗʰ **S70.212** Abrasion, left hip

    ☑7ᵗʰ **S70.219** Abrasion, unspecified hip

   ☑6ᵗʰ **S70.22** Blister (nonthermal) of hip

    ☑7ᵗʰ **S70.221** Blister (nonthermal), right hip

    ☑7ᵗʰ **S70.222** Blister (nonthermal), left hip

    ☑7ᵗʰ **S70.229** Blister (nonthermal), unspecified hip

   ☑6ᵗʰ **S70.24** External constriction of hip

    ☑7ᵗʰ **S70.241** External constriction, right hip

    ☑7ᵗʰ **S70.242** External constriction, left hip

    ☑7ᵗʰ **S70.249** External constriction, unspecified hip

   ☑6ᵗʰ **S70.25** Superficial foreign body of hip

     Splinter in the hip

    ☑7ᵗʰ **S70.251** Superficial foreign body, right hip

    ☑7ᵗʰ **S70.252** Superficial foreign body, left hip

    ☑7ᵗʰ **S70.259** Superficial foreign body, unspecified hip

---

☑ Additional Character Required   ☑x7ᵗʰ Placeholder Alert   Manifestation   Unspecified Dx   🇶 QPP   UPD Unacceptable PDx

✓6ᵗʰ **S70.26** Insect bite (nonvenomous) of hip
     ✓7ᵗʰ **S70.261** Insect bite (nonvenomous), right hip
     ✓7ᵗʰ **S70.262** Insect bite (nonvenomous), left hip
     ✓7ᵗʰ **S70.269** Insect bite (nonvenomous), unspecified hip

✓6ᵗʰ **S70.27** Other superficial bite of hip
     EXCLUDES 1   open bite of hip (S71.05-)
     ✓7ᵗʰ **S70.271** Other superficial bite of hip, right hip
     ✓7ᵗʰ **S70.272** Other superficial bite of hip, left hip
     ✓7ᵗʰ **S70.279** Other superficial bite of hip, unspecified hip

✓5ᵗʰ **S70.3** Other superficial injuries of thigh
     ✓6ᵗʰ **S70.31** Abrasion of thigh
         ✓7ᵗʰ **S70.311** Abrasion, right thigh
         ✓7ᵗʰ **S70.312** Abrasion, left thigh
         ✓7ᵗʰ **S70.319** Abrasion, unspecified thigh

     ✓6ᵗʰ **S70.32** Blister (nonthermal) of thigh
         ✓7ᵗʰ **S70.321** Blister (nonthermal), right thigh
         ✓7ᵗʰ **S70.322** Blister (nonthermal), left thigh
         ✓7ᵗʰ **S70.329** Blister (nonthermal), unspecified thigh

     ✓6ᵗʰ **S70.34** External constriction of thigh
         ✓7ᵗʰ **S70.341** External constriction, right thigh
         ✓7ᵗʰ **S70.342** External constriction, left thigh
         ✓7ᵗʰ **S70.349** External constriction, unspecified thigh

     ✓6ᵗʰ **S70.35** Superficial foreign body of thigh
         Splinter in the thigh
         ✓7ᵗʰ **S70.351** Superficial foreign body, right thigh
         ✓7ᵗʰ **S70.352** Superficial foreign body, left thigh
         ✓7ᵗʰ **S70.359** Superficial foreign body, unspecified thigh

     ✓6ᵗʰ **S70.36** Insect bite (nonvenomous) of thigh
         ✓7ᵗʰ **S70.361** Insect bite (nonvenomous), right thigh
         ✓7ᵗʰ **S70.362** Insect bite (nonvenomous), left thigh
         ✓7ᵗʰ **S70.369** Insect bite (nonvenomous), unspecified thigh

     ✓6ᵗʰ **S70.37** Other superficial bite of thigh
         EXCLUDES 1   open bite of thigh (S71.15)
         ✓7ᵗʰ **S70.371** Other superficial bite of right thigh
         ✓7ᵗʰ **S70.372** Other superficial bite of left thigh
         ✓7ᵗʰ **S70.379** Other superficial bite of unspecified thigh

✓5ᵗʰ **S70.9** Unspecified superficial injury of hip and thigh
     ✓6ᵗʰ **S70.91** Unspecified superficial injury of hip
         ✓7ᵗʰ **S70.911** Unspecified superficial injury of right hip
         ✓7ᵗʰ **S70.912** Unspecified superficial injury of left hip
         ✓7ᵗʰ **S70.919** Unspecified superficial injury of unspecified hip

     ✓6ᵗʰ **S70.92** Unspecified superficial injury of thigh
         ✓7ᵗʰ **S70.921** Unspecified superficial injury of right thigh
         ✓7ᵗʰ **S70.922** Unspecified superficial injury of left thigh
         ✓7ᵗʰ **S70.929** Unspecified superficial injury of unspecified thigh

✓4ᵗʰ **S71** Open wound of hip and thigh
     Code also any associated wound infection
     EXCLUDES 1   open fracture of hip and thigh (S72.-)
         traumatic amputation of hip and thigh (S78.-)
     EXCLUDES 2   bite of venomous animal (T63.-)
         open wound of ankle, foot and toes (S91.-)
         open wound of knee and lower leg (S81.-)

     The appropriate 7th character is to be added to each code from category S71.
     A   initial encounter
     D   subsequent encounter
     S   sequela

     ✓5ᵗʰ **S71.0** Open wound of hip
         ✓6ᵗʰ **S71.00** Unspecified open wound of hip
             ✓7ᵗʰ **S71.001** Unspecified open wound, right hip
             ✓7ᵗʰ **S71.002** Unspecified open wound, left hip
             ✓7ᵗʰ **S71.009** Unspecified open wound, unspecified hip

         ✓6ᵗʰ **S71.01** Laceration without foreign body of hip
             ✓7ᵗʰ **S71.011** Laceration without foreign body, right hip
             ✓7ᵗʰ **S71.012** Laceration without foreign body, left hip
             ✓7ᵗʰ **S71.019** Laceration without foreign body, unspecified hip

         ✓6ᵗʰ **S71.02** Laceration with foreign body of hip
             ✓7ᵗʰ **S71.021** Laceration with foreign body, right hip
             ✓7ᵗʰ **S71.022** Laceration with foreign body, left hip
             ✓7ᵗʰ **S71.029** Laceration with foreign body, unspecified hip

         ✓6ᵗʰ **S71.03** Puncture wound without foreign body of hip
             ✓7ᵗʰ **S71.031** Puncture wound without foreign body, right hip
             ✓7ᵗʰ **S71.032** Puncture wound without foreign body, left hip
             ✓7ᵗʰ **S71.039** Puncture wound without foreign body, unspecified hip

         ✓6ᵗʰ **S71.04** Puncture wound with foreign body of hip
             ✓7ᵗʰ **S71.041** Puncture wound with foreign body, right hip
             ✓7ᵗʰ **S71.042** Puncture wound with foreign body, left hip
             ✓7ᵗʰ **S71.049** Puncture wound with foreign body, unspecified hip

         ✓6ᵗʰ **S71.05** Open bite of hip
             Bite of hip NOS
             EXCLUDES 1   superficial bite of hip (S70.26, S70.27)
             ✓7ᵗʰ **S71.051** Open bite, right hip
             ✓7ᵗʰ **S71.052** Open bite, left hip
             ✓7ᵗʰ **S71.059** Open bite, unspecified hip

     ✓5ᵗʰ **S71.1** Open wound of thigh
         ✓6ᵗʰ **S71.10** Unspecified open wound of thigh
             AHA: 2016,3Q,24
             ✓7ᵗʰ **S71.101** Unspecified open wound, right thigh
             ✓7ᵗʰ **S71.102** Unspecified open wound, left thigh
             ✓7ᵗʰ **S71.109** Unspecified open wound, unspecified thigh

         ✓6ᵗʰ **S71.11** Laceration without foreign body of thigh
             ✓7ᵗʰ **S71.111** Laceration without foreign body, right thigh
             ✓7ᵗʰ **S71.112** Laceration without foreign body, left thigh
             ✓7ᵗʰ **S71.119** Laceration without foreign body, unspecified thigh

         ✓6ᵗʰ **S71.12** Laceration with foreign body of thigh
             ✓7ᵗʰ **S71.121** Laceration with foreign body, right thigh
             ✓7ᵗʰ **S71.122** Laceration with foreign body, left thigh
             ✓7ᵗʰ **S71.129** Laceration with foreign body, unspecified thigh

         ✓6ᵗʰ **S71.13** Puncture wound without foreign body of thigh
             AHA: 2016,3Q,24
             ✓7ᵗʰ **S71.131** Puncture wound without foreign body, right thigh
             ✓7ᵗʰ **S71.132** Puncture wound without foreign body, left thigh
             ✓7ᵗʰ **S71.139** Puncture wound without foreign body, unspecified thigh

         ✓6ᵗʰ **S71.14** Puncture wound with foreign body of thigh
             AHA: 2016,3Q,24
             ✓7ᵗʰ **S71.141** Puncture wound with foreign body, right thigh
             ✓7ᵗʰ **S71.142** Puncture wound with foreign body, left thigh
             ✓7ᵗʰ **S71.149** Puncture wound with foreign body, unspecified thigh

         ✓6ᵗʰ **S71.15** Open bite of thigh
             Bite of thigh NOS
             EXCLUDES 1   superficial bite of thigh (S70.37-)
             ✓7ᵗʰ **S71.151** Open bite, right thigh
             ✓7ᵗʰ **S71.152** Open bite, left thigh
             ✓7ᵗʰ **S71.159** Open bite, unspecified thigh

☑4ᵗʰ **S72 Fracture of femur**

> **NOTE** A fracture not indicated as displaced or nondisplaced should be coded to displaced.
>
> A fracture not indicated as open or closed should be coded to closed.
>
> The open fracture designations are based on the Gustilo open fracture classification.

EXCLUDES 1   traumatic amputation of hip and thigh (S78.-)
EXCLUDES 2   fracture of lower leg and ankle (S82.-)
           fracture of foot (S92.-)
           periprosthetic fracture of prosthetic implant of hip (M97.0-)

AHA: 2018,2Q,12; 2016,1Q,33; 2015,3Q,37-39; 2015,1Q,17; 2013,4Q,128
DEF: Diaphysis: Central shaft of a long bone.
DEF: Epiphysis: Proximal and distal rounded ends of a long bone communicates with the joint.
DEF: Metaphysis: Section of a long bone located between the epiphysis and diaphysis at the proximal and distal ends.
DEF: Physis (growth plate): Narrow zone of cartilaginous tissue between the epiphysis and metaphysis at each end of a long bone. In childhood, proliferation of cells in this zone lengthens the bone. As the bone matures, this area thins, ossification eventually fusing into solid bone and growth stops. *Synonym(s):* Epiphyseal plate.

The appropriate 7th character is to be added to all codes from category S72 [unless otherwise indicated].
A   initial encounter for closed fracture
B   initial encounter for open fracture type I or II
     initial encounter for open fracture NOS
C   initial encounter for open fracture type IIIA, IIIB, or IIIC
D   subsequent encounter for closed fracture with routine healing
E   subsequent encounter for open fracture type I or II with routine healing
F   subsequent encounter for open fracture type IIIA, IIIB, or IIIC with routine healing
G   subsequent encounter for closed fracture with delayed healing
H   subsequent encounter for open fracture type I or II with delayed healing
J   subsequent encounter for open fracture type IIIA, IIIB, or IIIC with delayed healing
K   subsequent encounter for closed fracture with nonunion
M   subsequent encounter for open fracture type I or II with nonunion
N   subsequent encounter for open fracture type IIIA, IIIB, or IIIC with nonunion
P   subsequent encounter for closed fracture with malunion
Q   subsequent encounter for open fracture type I or II with malunion
R   subsequent encounter for open fracture type IIIA, IIIB, or IIIC with malunion
S   sequela

☑5ᵗʰ **S72.0 Fracture of head and neck of femur**

     EXCLUDES 2   physeal fracture of upper end of femur (S79.0-)

     AHA: 2016,3Q,16

☑6ᵗʰ **S72.00 Fracture of unspecified part of neck of femur**

     Fracture of hip NOS
     Fracture of neck of femur NOS

     ¹ ☑7ᵗʰ **S72.001 Fracture of unspecified part of neck of right femur** HCC ESR COM Q

     ¹ ☑7ᵗʰ **S72.002 Fracture of unspecified part of neck of left femur** HCC ESR COM Q

     ¹ ☑7ᵗʰ **S72.009 Fracture of unspecified part of neck of unspecified femur** HCC ESR COM Q

☑6ᵗʰ **S72.01 Unspecified intracapsular fracture of femur**

     Subcapital fracture of femur

     ¹ ☑7ᵗʰ **S72.011 Unspecified intracapsular fracture of right femur** HCC ESR COM Q

     ¹ ☑7ᵗʰ **S72.012 Unspecified intracapsular fracture of left femur** HCC ESR COM Q

     ¹ ☑7ᵗʰ **S72.019 Unspecified intracapsular fracture of unspecified femur** HCC ESR COM Q

☑6ᵗʰ **S72.02 Fracture of epiphysis (separation) (upper) of femur**

     Transepiphyseal fracture of femur

     EXCLUDES 1   capital femoral epiphyseal fracture (pediatric) of femur (S79.01-)
               Salter-Harris Type I physeal fracture of upper end of femur (S79.01-)

     ¹ ☑7ᵗʰ **S72.021 Displaced fracture of epiphysis (separation) (upper) of right femur** HCC ESR COM Q

     ¹ ☑7ᵗʰ **S72.022 Displaced fracture of epiphysis (separation) (upper) of left femur** HCC ESR COM Q

     ¹ ☑7ᵗʰ **S72.023 Displaced fracture of epiphysis (separation) (upper) of unspecified femur** HCC ESR COM Q

     ¹ ☑7ᵗʰ **S72.024 Nondisplaced fracture of epiphysis (separation) (upper) of right femur** HCC ESR COM Q

     ¹ ☑7ᵗʰ **S72.025 Nondisplaced fracture of epiphysis (separation) (upper) of left femur** HCC ESR COM Q

     ¹ ☑7ᵗʰ **S72.026 Nondisplaced fracture of epiphysis (separation) (upper) of unspecified femur** HCC ESR COM Q

☑6ᵗʰ **S72.03 Midcervical fracture of femur**

     Transcervical fracture of femur NOS

     ¹ ☑7ᵗʰ **S72.031 Displaced midcervical fracture of right femur** HCC ESR COM Q

     ¹ ☑7ᵗʰ **S72.032 Displaced midcervical fracture of left femur** HCC ESR COM Q

     ¹ ☑7ᵗʰ **S72.033 Displaced midcervical fracture of unspecified femur** HCC ESR COM Q

     ¹ ☑7ᵗʰ **S72.034 Nondisplaced midcervical fracture of right femur** HCC ESR COM Q

     ¹ ☑7ᵗʰ **S72.035 Nondisplaced midcervical fracture of left femur** HCC ESR COM Q

     ¹ ☑7ᵗʰ **S72.036 Nondisplaced midcervical fracture of unspecified femur** HCC ESR COM Q

☑6ᵗʰ **S72.04 Fracture of base of neck of femur**

     Cervicotrochanteric fracture of femur

     ¹ ☑7ᵗʰ **S72.041 Displaced fracture of base of neck of right femur** HCC ESR COM Q

     ¹ ☑7ᵗʰ **S72.042 Displaced fracture of base of neck of left femur** HCC ESR COM Q

     ¹ ☑7ᵗʰ **S72.043 Displaced fracture of base of neck of unspecified femur** HCC ESR COM Q

     ¹ ☑7ᵗʰ **S72.044 Nondisplaced fracture of base of neck of right femur** HCC ESR COM Q

     ¹ ☑7ᵗʰ **S72.045 Nondisplaced fracture of base of neck of left femur** HCC ESR COM Q

     ¹ ☑7ᵗʰ **S72.046 Nondisplaced fracture of base of neck of unspecified femur** HCC ESR COM Q

☑6ᵗʰ **S72.05 Unspecified fracture of head of femur**

     Fracture of head of femur NOS

     ¹ ☑7ᵗʰ **S72.051 Unspecified fracture of head of right femur** HCC ESR COM Q

     ¹ ☑7ᵗʰ **S72.052 Unspecified fracture of head of left femur** HCC ESR COM Q

     ¹ ☑7ᵗʰ **S72.059 Unspecified fracture of head of unspecified femur** HCC ESR COM Q

☑6ᵗʰ **S72.06 Articular fracture of head of femur**

     ¹ ☑7ᵗʰ **S72.061 Displaced articular fracture of head of right femur** HCC ESR COM Q

     ¹ ☑7ᵗʰ **S72.062 Displaced articular fracture of head of left femur** HCC ESR COM Q

     ¹ ☑7ᵗʰ **S72.063 Displaced articular fracture of head of unspecified femur** HCC ESR COM Q

     ¹ ☑7ᵗʰ **S72.064 Nondisplaced articular fracture of head of right femur** HCC ESR COM Q

     ¹ ☑7ᵗʰ **S72.065 Nondisplaced articular fracture of head of left femur** HCC ESR COM Q

     ¹ ☑7ᵗʰ **S72.066 Nondisplaced articular fracture of head of unspecified femur** HCC ESR COM Q

☑6ᵗʰ **S72.09 Other fracture of head and neck of femur**

     ¹ ☑7ᵗʰ **S72.091 Other fracture of head and neck of right femur** HCC ESR COM Q

     ¹ ☑7ᵗʰ **S72.092 Other fracture of head and neck of left femur** HCC ESR COM Q

     ¹ ☑7ᵗʰ **S72.099 Other fracture of head and neck of unspecified femur** HCC ESR COM Q

☑5ᵗʰ **S72.1 Pertrochanteric fracture**

     AHA: 2016,3Q,16

☑6ᵗʰ **S72.10 Unspecified trochanteric fracture of femur**

     Fracture of trochanter NOS

     ¹ ☑7ᵗʰ **S72.101 Unspecified trochanteric fracture of right femur** HCC ESR COM Q

     ¹ ☑7ᵗʰ **S72.102 Unspecified trochanteric fracture of left femur** HCC ESR COM Q

¹ √7ᵗʰ **S72.109** Unspecified trochanteric fracture of unspecified femur `HCC` `ESR` `COM` `Q`

√6ᵗʰ **S72.11** Fracture of greater trochanter of femur

¹ √7ᵗʰ **S72.111** Displaced fracture of greater trochanter of right femur `HCC` `ESR` `COM` `Q`

¹ √7ᵗʰ **S72.112** Displaced fracture of greater trochanter of left femur `HCC` `ESR` `COM` `Q`

¹ √7ᵗʰ **S72.113** Displaced fracture of greater trochanter of unspecified femur `HCC` `ESR` `COM` `Q`

¹ √7ᵗʰ **S72.114** Nondisplaced fracture of greater trochanter of right femur `HCC` `ESR` `COM` `Q`

¹ √7ᵗʰ **S72.115** Nondisplaced fracture of greater trochanter of left femur `HCC` `ESR` `COM` `Q`

¹ √7ᵗʰ **S72.116** Nondisplaced fracture of greater trochanter of unspecified femur `HCC` `ESR` `COM` `Q`

√6ᵗʰ **S72.12** Fracture of lesser trochanter of femur

¹ √7ᵗʰ **S72.121** Displaced fracture of lesser trochanter of right femur `HCC` `ESR` `COM` `Q`

¹ √7ᵗʰ **S72.122** Displaced fracture of lesser trochanter of left femur `HCC` `ESR` `COM` `Q`

¹ √7ᵗʰ **S72.123** Displaced fracture of lesser trochanter of unspecified femur `HCC` `ESR` `COM` `Q`

¹ √7ᵗʰ **S72.124** Nondisplaced fracture of lesser trochanter of right femur `HCC` `ESR` `COM` `Q`

¹ √7ᵗʰ **S72.125** Nondisplaced fracture of lesser trochanter of left femur `HCC` `ESR` `COM` `Q`

¹ √7ᵗʰ **S72.126** Nondisplaced fracture of lesser trochanter of unspecified femur `HCC` `ESR` `COM` `Q`

√6ᵗʰ **S72.13** Apophyseal fracture of femur

EXCLUDES 1 chronic (nontraumatic) slipped upper femoral epiphysis (M93.0-)

¹ √7ᵗʰ **S72.131** Displaced apophyseal fracture of right femur `HCC` `ESR` `COM` `Q`

¹ √7ᵗʰ **S72.132** Displaced apophyseal fracture of left femur `HCC` `ESR` `COM` `Q`

¹ √7ᵗʰ **S72.133** Displaced apophyseal fracture of unspecified femur `HCC` `ESR` `COM` `Q`

¹ √7ᵗʰ **S72.134** Nondisplaced apophyseal fracture of right femur `HCC` `ESR` `COM` `Q`

¹ √7ᵗʰ **S72.135** Nondisplaced apophyseal fracture of left femur `HCC` `ESR` `COM` `Q`

¹ √7ᵗʰ **S72.136** Nondisplaced apophyseal fracture of unspecified femur `HCC` `ESR` `COM` `Q`

√6ᵗʰ **S72.14** Intertrochanteric fracture of femur

¹ √7ᵗʰ **S72.141** Displaced intertrochanteric fracture of right femur `HCC` `ESR` `COM` `Q`

¹ √7ᵗʰ **S72.142** Displaced intertrochanteric fracture of left femur `HCC` `ESR` `COM` `Q`

¹ √7ᵗʰ **S72.143** Displaced intertrochanteric fracture of unspecified femur `HCC` `ESR` `COM` `Q`

¹ √7ᵗʰ **S72.144** Nondisplaced intertrochanteric fracture of right femur `HCC` `ESR` `COM` `Q`

¹ √7ᵗʰ **S72.145** Nondisplaced intertrochanteric fracture of left femur `HCC` `ESR` `COM` `Q`

¹ √7ᵗʰ **S72.146** Nondisplaced intertrochanteric fracture of unspecified femur `HCC` `ESR` `COM` `Q`

√5ᵗʰ **S72.2** Subtrochanteric fracture of femur

¹ √x7ᵗʰ **S72.21** Displaced subtrochanteric fracture of right femur `HCC` `ESR` `COM` `Q`

¹ √x7ᵗʰ **S72.22** Displaced subtrochanteric fracture of left femur `HCC` `ESR` `COM` `Q`

¹ √x7ᵗʰ **S72.23** Displaced subtrochanteric fracture of unspecified femur `HCC` `ESR` `COM` `Q`

¹ √x7ᵗʰ **S72.24** Nondisplaced subtrochanteric fracture of right femur `HCC` `ESR` `COM` `Q`

¹ √x7ᵗʰ **S72.25** Nondisplaced subtrochanteric fracture of left femur `HCC` `ESR` `COM` `Q`

¹ √x7ᵗʰ **S72.26** Nondisplaced subtrochanteric fracture of unspecified femur `HCC` `ESR` `COM` `Q`

√5ᵗʰ **S72.3** Fracture of shaft of femur

√6ᵗʰ **S72.30** Unspecified fracture of shaft of femur

¹ √7ᵗʰ **S72.301** Unspecified fracture of shaft of right femur `HCC` `ESR` `Q`

¹ √7ᵗʰ **S72.302** Unspecified fracture of shaft of left femur `HCC` `ESR` `Q`

¹ √7ᵗʰ **S72.309** Unspecified fracture of shaft of unspecified femur `HCC` `ESR` `Q`

√6ᵗʰ **S72.32** Transverse fracture of shaft of femur

¹ √7ᵗʰ **S72.321** Displaced transverse fracture of shaft of right femur `HCC` `ESR` `Q`

¹ √7ᵗʰ **S72.322** Displaced transverse fracture of shaft of left femur `HCC` `ESR` `Q`

¹ √7ᵗʰ **S72.323** Displaced transverse fracture of shaft of unspecified femur `HCC` `ESR` `Q`

¹ √7ᵗʰ **S72.324** Nondisplaced transverse fracture of shaft of right femur `HCC` `ESR` `Q`

¹ √7ᵗʰ **S72.325** Nondisplaced transverse fracture of shaft of left femur `HCC` `ESR` `Q`

¹ √7ᵗʰ **S72.326** Nondisplaced transverse fracture of shaft of unspecified femur `HCC` `ESR` `Q`

√6ᵗʰ **S72.33** Oblique fracture of shaft of femur

¹ √7ᵗʰ **S72.331** Displaced oblique fracture of shaft of right femur `HCC` `ESR` `Q`

¹ √7ᵗʰ **S72.332** Displaced oblique fracture of shaft of left femur `HCC` `ESR` `Q`

¹ √7ᵗʰ **S72.333** Displaced oblique fracture of shaft of unspecified femur `HCC` `ESR` `Q`

¹ √7ᵗʰ **S72.334** Nondisplaced oblique fracture of shaft of right femur `HCC` `ESR` `Q`

¹ √7ᵗʰ **S72.335** Nondisplaced oblique fracture of shaft of left femur `HCC` `ESR` `Q`

¹ √7ᵗʰ **S72.336** Nondisplaced oblique fracture of shaft of unspecified femur `HCC` `ESR` `Q`

√6ᵗʰ **S72.34** Spiral fracture of shaft of femur

¹ √7ᵗʰ **S72.341** Displaced spiral fracture of shaft of right femur `HCC` `ESR` `Q`

¹ √7ᵗʰ **S72.342** Displaced spiral fracture of shaft of left femur `HCC` `ESR` `Q`

¹ √7ᵗʰ **S72.343** Displaced spiral fracture of shaft of unspecified femur `HCC` `ESR` `Q`

¹ √7ᵗʰ **S72.344** Nondisplaced spiral fracture of shaft of right femur `HCC` `ESR` `Q`

¹ √7ᵗʰ **S72.345** Nondisplaced spiral fracture of shaft of left femur `HCC` `ESR` `Q`

¹ √7ᵗʰ **S72.346** Nondisplaced spiral fracture of shaft of unspecified femur `HCC` `ESR` `Q`

√6ᵗʰ **S72.35** Comminuted fracture of shaft of femur

¹ √7ᵗʰ **S72.351** Displaced comminuted fracture of shaft of right femur `HCC` `ESR` `Q`

¹ √7ᵗʰ **S72.352** Displaced comminuted fracture of shaft of left femur `HCC` `ESR` `Q`

¹ √7ᵗʰ **S72.353** Displaced comminuted fracture of shaft of unspecified femur `HCC` `ESR` `Q`

¹ √7ᵗʰ **S72.354** Nondisplaced comminuted fracture of shaft of right femur `HCC` `ESR` `Q`

¹ √7ᵗʰ **S72.355** Nondisplaced comminuted fracture of shaft of left femur `HCC` `ESR` `Q`

¹ √7ᵗʰ **S72.356** Nondisplaced comminuted fracture of shaft of unspecified femur `HCC` `ESR` `Q`

√6ᵗʰ **S72.36** Segmental fracture of shaft of femur

¹ √7ᵗʰ **S72.361** Displaced segmental fracture of shaft of right femur `HCC` `ESR` `Q`

¹ √7ᵗʰ **S72.362** Displaced segmental fracture of shaft of left femur `HCC` `ESR` `Q`

¹ √7ᵗʰ **S72.363** Displaced segmental fracture of shaft of unspecified femur `HCC` `ESR` `Q`

¹ √7ᵗʰ **S72.364** Nondisplaced segmental fracture of shaft of right femur `HCC` `ESR` `Q`

¹ √7ᵗʰ **S72.365** Nondisplaced segmental fracture of shaft of left femur `HCC` `ESR` `Q`

¹ √7ᵗʰ **S72.366** Nondisplaced segmental fracture of shaft of unspecified femur `HCC` `ESR` `Q`

√6ᵗʰ **S72.39** Other fracture of shaft of femur

¹ √7ᵗʰ **S72.391** Other fracture of shaft of right femur `HCC` `ESR` `Q`

¹ √7ᵗʰ **S72.392** Other fracture of shaft of left femur `HCC` `ESR` `Q`

¹ √7ᵗʰ **S72.399** Other fracture of shaft of unspecified femur `HCC` `ESR` `Q`

`HCC` CMS-HCC   `Rx` Rx HCC   `ESR` ESRD HCC   `COM` Commercial HCC   `N` Newborn: 0   `P` Pediatric: 0-17   `M` Maternity: 9-64   `A` Adult: 15-124

1082   ICD-10-CM 2023

√5ᵗʰ **S72.4 Fracture of lower end of femur**
Fracture of distal end of femur
> EXCLUDES 2   fracture of shaft of femur (S72.3-)
> physeal fracture of lower end of femur (S79.1-)

AHA: 2016,4Q,42

√6ᵗʰ **S72.40 Unspecified fracture of lower end of femur**
AHA: 2018,1Q,21; 2016,4Q,42

¹ √7ᵗʰ **S72.401 Unspecified fracture of lower end of right femur** HCC ESR Q

¹ √7ᵗʰ **S72.402 Unspecified fracture of lower end of left femur** HCC ESR Q

¹ √7ᵗʰ **S72.409 Unspecified fracture of lower end of unspecified femur** HCC ESR Q

√6ᵗʰ **S72.41 Unspecified condyle fracture of lower end of femur**
Condyle fracture of femur NOS

¹ √7ᵗʰ **S72.411 Displaced unspecified condyle fracture of lower end of right femur** HCC ESR Q

¹ √7ᵗʰ **S72.412 Displaced unspecified condyle fracture of lower end of left femur** HCC ESR Q

¹ √7ᵗʰ **S72.413 Displaced unspecified condyle fracture of lower end of unspecified femur** HCC ESR Q

¹ √7ᵗʰ **S72.414 Nondisplaced unspecified condyle fracture of lower end of right femur** HCC ESR Q

¹ √7ᵗʰ **S72.415 Nondisplaced unspecified condyle fracture of lower end of left femur** HCC ESR Q

¹ √7ᵗʰ **S72.416 Nondisplaced unspecified condyle fracture of lower end of unspecified femur** HCC ESR Q

√6ᵗʰ **S72.42 Fracture of lateral condyle of femur**

¹ √7ᵗʰ **S72.421 Displaced fracture of lateral condyle of right femur** HCC ESR Q

¹ √7ᵗʰ **S72.422 Displaced fracture of lateral condyle of left femur** HCC ESR Q

¹ √7ᵗʰ **S72.423 Displaced fracture of lateral condyle of unspecified femur** HCC ESR Q

¹ √7ᵗʰ **S72.424 Nondisplaced fracture of lateral condyle of right femur** HCC ESR Q

¹ √7ᵗʰ **S72.425 Nondisplaced fracture of lateral condyle of left femur** HCC ESR Q

¹ √7ᵗʰ **S72.426 Nondisplaced fracture of lateral condyle of unspecified femur** HCC ESR Q

√6ᵗʰ **S72.43 Fracture of medial condyle of femur**

¹ √7ᵗʰ **S72.431 Displaced fracture of medial condyle of right femur** HCC ESR Q

¹ √7ᵗʰ **S72.432 Displaced fracture of medial condyle of left femur** HCC ESR Q

¹ √7ᵗʰ **S72.433 Displaced fracture of medial condyle of unspecified femur** HCC ESR Q

¹ √7ᵗʰ **S72.434 Nondisplaced fracture of medial condyle of right femur** HCC ESR Q

¹ √7ᵗʰ **S72.435 Nondisplaced fracture of medial condyle of left femur** HCC ESR Q

¹ √7ᵗʰ **S72.436 Nondisplaced fracture of medial condyle of unspecified femur** HCC ESR Q

√6ᵗʰ **S72.44 Fracture of lower epiphysis (separation) of femur**
> EXCLUDES 1   Salter-Harris Type I physeal fracture of lower end of femur (S79.11-)

¹ √7ᵗʰ **S72.441 Displaced fracture of lower epiphysis (separation) of right femur** HCC ESR Q

¹ √7ᵗʰ **S72.442 Displaced fracture of lower epiphysis (separation) of left femur** HCC ESR Q

¹ √7ᵗʰ **S72.443 Displaced fracture of lower epiphysis (separation) of unspecified femur** HCC ESR Q

¹ √7ᵗʰ **S72.444 Nondisplaced fracture of lower epiphysis (separation) of right femur** HCC ESR Q

¹ √7ᵗʰ **S72.445 Nondisplaced fracture of lower epiphysis (separation) of left femur** HCC ESR Q

¹ √7ᵗʰ **S72.446 Nondisplaced fracture of lower epiphysis (separation) of unspecified femur** HCC ESR Q

√6ᵗʰ **S72.45 Supracondylar fracture without intracondylar extension of lower end of femur**
Supracondylar fracture of lower end of femur NOS
> EXCLUDES 1   supracondylar fracture with intracondylar extension of lower end of femur (S72.46-)

¹ √7ᵗʰ **S72.451 Displaced supracondylar fracture without intracondylar extension of lower end of right femur** HCC ESR Q

¹ √7ᵗʰ **S72.452 Displaced supracondylar fracture without intracondylar extension of lower end of left femur** HCC ESR Q

¹ √7ᵗʰ **S72.453 Displaced supracondylar fracture without intracondylar extension of lower end of unspecified femur** HCC ESR Q

¹ √7ᵗʰ **S72.454 Nondisplaced supracondylar fracture without intracondylar extension of lower end of right femur** HCC ESR Q

¹ √7ᵗʰ **S72.455 Nondisplaced supracondylar fracture without intracondylar extension of lower end of left femur** HCC ESR Q

¹ √7ᵗʰ **S72.456 Nondisplaced supracondylar fracture without intracondylar extension of lower end of unspecified femur** HCC ESR Q

√6ᵗʰ **S72.46 Supracondylar fracture with intracondylar extension of lower end of femur**
> EXCLUDES 1   supracondylar fracture without intracondylar extension of lower end of femur (S72.45-)

¹ √7ᵗʰ **S72.461 Displaced supracondylar fracture with intracondylar extension of lower end of right femur** HCC ESR Q

¹ √7ᵗʰ **S72.462 Displaced supracondylar fracture with intracondylar extension of lower end of left femur** HCC ESR Q

¹ √7ᵗʰ **S72.463 Displaced supracondylar fracture with intracondylar extension of lower end of unspecified femur** HCC ESR Q

¹ √7ᵗʰ **S72.464 Nondisplaced supracondylar fracture with intracondylar extension of lower end of right femur** HCC ESR Q

¹ √7ᵗʰ **S72.465 Nondisplaced supracondylar fracture with intracondylar extension of lower end of left femur** HCC ESR Q

¹ √7ᵗʰ **S72.466 Nondisplaced supracondylar fracture with intracondylar extension of lower end of unspecified femur** HCC ESR Q

√6ᵗʰ **S72.47 Torus fracture of lower end of femur**

> The appropriate 7th character is to be added to all codes in subcategory S72.47.
> A   initial encounter for closed fracture
> D   subsequent encounter for fracture with routine healing
> G   subsequent encounter for fracture with delayed healing
> K   subsequent encounter for fracture with nonunion
> P   subsequent encounter for fracture with malunion
> S   sequela

¹ √7ᵗʰ **S72.471 Torus fracture of lower end of right femur** HCC ESR Q

¹ √7ᵗʰ **S72.472 Torus fracture of lower end of left femur** HCC ESR Q

¹ √7ᵗʰ **S72.479 Torus fracture of lower end of unspecified femur** HCC ESR Q

√6ᵗʰ **S72.49 Other fracture of lower end of femur**

¹ √7ᵗʰ **S72.491 Other fracture of lower end of right femur** HCC ESR Q

¹ √7ᵗʰ **S72.492 Other fracture of lower end of left femur** HCC ESR Q

¹ √7ᵗʰ **S72.499 Other fracture of lower end of unspecified femur** HCC ESR Q

√5ᵗʰ **S72.8 Other fracture of femur**

√6ᵗʰ **S72.8X Other fracture of femur**

¹ √7ᵗʰ **S72.8X1 Other fracture of right femur** HCC ESR Q

¹ √7ᵗʰ **S72.8X2 Other fracture of left femur** HCC ESR Q

☑ Additional Character Required   √x7ᵗʰ Placeholder Alert   Manifestation   Unspecified Dx   Q QPP   UPD Unacceptable PDx

¹ √7ᵗʰ **S72.8X9** Other fracture of unspecified femur   `HCC` `ESR` `Q`

√5ᵗʰ **S72.9** **Unspecified fracture of femur**
 Fracture of thigh NOS
 Fracture of upper leg NOS
 `EXCLUDES 1`   fracture of hip NOS (S72.00-, S72.01-)

¹ √x 7ᵗʰ **S72.90** **Unspecified fracture of unspecified femur**   `HCC` `ESR` `Q`
 AHA: 2012,4Q,93

¹ √x 7ᵗʰ **S72.91** **Unspecified fracture of right femur**   `HCC` `ESR` `Q`

¹ √x 7ᵗʰ **S72.92** **Unspecified fracture of left femur**   `HCC` `ESR` `Q`

√4ᵗʰ **S73** **Dislocation and sprain of joint and ligaments of hip**
 `INCLUDES`   avulsion of joint or ligament of hip
 laceration of cartilage, joint or ligament of hip
 sprain of cartilage, joint or ligament of hip
 traumatic hemarthrosis of joint or ligament of hip
 traumatic rupture of joint or ligament of hip
 traumatic subluxation of joint or ligament of hip
 traumatic tear of joint or ligament of hip
 Code also any associated open wound
 `EXCLUDES 2`   strain of muscle, fascia and tendon of hip and thigh (S76.-)

 The appropriate 7th character is to be added to each code from category S73.
 A   initial encounter
 D   subsequent encounter
 S   sequela

√5ᵗʰ **S73.0** **Subluxation and dislocation of hip**
 `EXCLUDES 2`   dislocation and subluxation of hip prosthesis (T84.020, T84.021)

√6ᵗʰ **S73.00** **Unspecified subluxation and dislocation of hip**
 Dislocation of hip NOS
 Subluxation of hip NOS

¹ √7ᵗʰ **S73.001** Unspecified subluxation of right hip   `HCC` `ESR`

¹ √7ᵗʰ **S73.002** Unspecified subluxation of left hip   `HCC` `ESR`

¹ √7ᵗʰ **S73.003** Unspecified subluxation of unspecified hip   `HCC` `ESR`

¹ √7ᵗʰ **S73.004** Unspecified dislocation of right hip   `HCC` `ESR`

¹ √7ᵗʰ **S73.005** Unspecified dislocation of left hip   `HCC` `ESR`

¹ √7ᵗʰ **S73.006** Unspecified dislocation of unspecified hip   `HCC` `ESR`

√6ᵗʰ **S73.01** **Posterior subluxation and dislocation of hip**

¹ √7ᵗʰ **S73.011** Posterior subluxation of right hip   `HCC` `ESR`

¹ √7ᵗʰ **S73.012** Posterior subluxation of left hip   `HCC` `ESR`

¹ √7ᵗʰ **S73.013** Posterior subluxation of unspecified hip   `HCC` `ESR`

¹ √7ᵗʰ **S73.014** Posterior dislocation of right hip   `HCC` `ESR`

¹ √7ᵗʰ **S73.015** Posterior dislocation of left hip   `HCC` `ESR`

¹ √7ᵗʰ **S73.016** Posterior dislocation of unspecified hip   `HCC` `ESR`

√6ᵗʰ **S73.02** **Obturator subluxation and dislocation of hip**

¹ √7ᵗʰ **S73.021** Obturator subluxation of right hip   `HCC` `ESR`

¹ √7ᵗʰ **S73.022** Obturator subluxation of left hip   `HCC` `ESR`

¹ √7ᵗʰ **S73.023** Obturator subluxation of unspecified hip   `HCC` `ESR`

¹ √7ᵗʰ **S73.024** Obturator dislocation of right hip   `HCC` `ESR`

¹ √7ᵗʰ **S73.025** Obturator dislocation of left hip   `HCC` `ESR`

¹ √7ᵗʰ **S73.026** Obturator dislocation of unspecified hip   `HCC` `ESR`

√6ᵗʰ **S73.03** **Other anterior subluxation and dislocation of hip**

¹ √7ᵗʰ **S73.031** Other anterior subluxation of right hip   `HCC` `ESR`

¹ √7ᵗʰ **S73.032** Other anterior subluxation of left hip   `HCC` `ESR`

¹ √7ᵗʰ **S73.033** Other anterior subluxation of unspecified hip   `HCC` `ESR`

¹ √7ᵗʰ **S73.034** Other anterior dislocation of right hip   `HCC` `ESR`

¹ √7ᵗʰ **S73.035** Other anterior dislocation of left hip   `HCC` `ESR`

¹ √7ᵗʰ **S73.036** Other anterior dislocation of unspecified hip   `HCC` `ESR`

√6ᵗʰ **S73.04** **Central subluxation and dislocation of hip**

¹ √7ᵗʰ **S73.041** Central subluxation of right hip   `HCC` `ESR`

¹ √7ᵗʰ **S73.042** Central subluxation of left hip   `HCC` `ESR`

¹ √7ᵗʰ **S73.043** Central subluxation of unspecified hip   `HCC` `ESR`

¹ √7ᵗʰ **S73.044** Central dislocation of right hip   `HCC` `ESR`

¹ √7ᵗʰ **S73.045** Central dislocation of left hip   `HCC` `ESR`

¹ √7ᵗʰ **S73.046** Central dislocation of unspecified hip   `HCC` `ESR`

√5ᵗʰ **S73.1** **Sprain of hip**
 AHA: 2014,4Q,25

√6ᵗʰ **S73.10** **Unspecified sprain of hip**

√7ᵗʰ **S73.101** Unspecified sprain of right hip

√7ᵗʰ **S73.102** Unspecified sprain of left hip

√7ᵗʰ **S73.109** Unspecified sprain of unspecified hip

√6ᵗʰ **S73.11** **Iliofemoral ligament sprain of hip**

√7ᵗʰ **S73.111** Iliofemoral ligament sprain of right hip

√7ᵗʰ **S73.112** Iliofemoral ligament sprain of left hip

√7ᵗʰ **S73.119** Iliofemoral ligament sprain of unspecified hip

√6ᵗʰ **S73.12** **Ischiocapsular (ligament) sprain of hip**

√7ᵗʰ **S73.121** Ischiocapsular ligament sprain of right hip

√7ᵗʰ **S73.122** Ischiocapsular ligament sprain of left hip

√7ᵗʰ **S73.129** Ischiocapsular ligament sprain of unspecified hip

√6ᵗʰ **S73.19** **Other sprain of hip**

√7ᵗʰ **S73.191** Other sprain of right hip

√7ᵗʰ **S73.192** Other sprain of left hip

√7ᵗʰ **S73.199** Other sprain of unspecified hip

√4ᵗʰ **S74** **Injury of nerves at hip and thigh level**
 Code also any associated open wound (S71.-)
 `EXCLUDES 2`   injury of nerves at ankle and foot level (S94.-)
 injury of nerves at lower leg level (S84.-)

 The appropriate 7th character is to be added to each code from category S74.
 A   initial encounter
 D   subsequent encounter
 S   sequela

√5ᵗʰ **S74.0** **Injury of sciatic nerve at hip and thigh level**

√x 7ᵗʰ **S74.00** Injury of sciatic nerve at hip and thigh level, unspecified leg

√x 7ᵗʰ **S74.01** Injury of sciatic nerve at hip and thigh level, right leg

√x 7ᵗʰ **S74.02** Injury of sciatic nerve at hip and thigh level, left leg

√5ᵗʰ **S74.1** **Injury of femoral nerve at hip and thigh level**

√x 7ᵗʰ **S74.10** Injury of femoral nerve at hip and thigh level, unspecified leg

√x 7ᵗʰ **S74.11** Injury of femoral nerve at hip and thigh level, right leg

√x 7ᵗʰ **S74.12** Injury of femoral nerve at hip and thigh level, left leg

√5ᵗʰ **S74.2** **Injury of cutaneous sensory nerve at hip and thigh level**

√x 7ᵗʰ **S74.20** Injury of cutaneous sensory nerve at hip and thigh level, unspecified leg

√x 7ᵗʰ **S74.21** Injury of cutaneous sensory nerve at hip and thigh level, right leg

√x 7ᵗʰ **S74.22** Injury of cutaneous sensory nerve at hip and thigh level, left leg

√5ᵗʰ **S74.8** **Injury of other nerves at hip and thigh level**

√6ᵗʰ **S74.8X** **Injury of other nerves at hip and thigh level**

√7ᵗʰ **S74.8X1** Injury of other nerves at hip and thigh level, right leg

Femur

Nerve

Thigh

   ✓7ᵗʰ **S74.8X2** Injury of other nerves at hip and thigh level, left leg

   ✓7ᵗʰ **S74.8X9** Injury of other nerves at hip and thigh level, unspecified leg

✓5ᵗʰ **S74.9** Injury of unspecified nerve at hip and thigh level

   ✓ₓ7ᵗʰ **S74.90** Injury of unspecified nerve at hip and thigh level, unspecified leg

   ✓ₓ7ᵗʰ **S74.91** Injury of unspecified nerve at hip and thigh level, right leg

   ✓ₓ7ᵗʰ **S74.92** Injury of unspecified nerve at hip and thigh level, left leg

✓4ᵗʰ **S75** Injury of blood vessels at hip and thigh level

Code also any associated open wound (S71.-)

EXCLUDES 2   injury of blood vessels at lower leg level (S85.-)

        injury of popliteal artery (S85.0)

The appropriate 7th character is to be added to each code from category S75.
A   initial encounter
D   subsequent encounter
S   sequela

✓5ᵗʰ **S75.0** Injury of femoral artery

   ✓6ᵗʰ **S75.00** Unspecified injury of femoral artery

      ✓7ᵗʰ **S75.001** Unspecified injury of femoral artery, right leg

      ✓7ᵗʰ **S75.002** Unspecified injury of femoral artery, left leg

      ✓7ᵗʰ **S75.009** Unspecified injury of femoral artery, unspecified leg

   ✓6ᵗʰ **S75.01** Minor laceration of femoral artery

       Incomplete transection of femoral artery
       Laceration of femoral artery NOS
       Superficial laceration of femoral artery

      ✓7ᵗʰ **S75.011** Minor laceration of femoral artery, right leg

      ✓7ᵗʰ **S75.012** Minor laceration of femoral artery, left leg

      ✓7ᵗʰ **S75.019** Minor laceration of femoral artery, unspecified leg

   ✓6ᵗʰ **S75.02** Major laceration of femoral artery

       Complete transection of femoral artery
       Traumatic rupture of femoral artery

      ✓7ᵗʰ **S75.021** Major laceration of femoral artery, right leg

      ✓7ᵗʰ **S75.022** Major laceration of femoral artery, left leg

      ✓7ᵗʰ **S75.029** Major laceration of femoral artery, unspecified leg

   ✓6ᵗʰ **S75.09** Other specified injury of femoral artery

      ✓7ᵗʰ **S75.091** Other specified injury of femoral artery, right leg

      ✓7ᵗʰ **S75.092** Other specified injury of femoral artery, left leg

      ✓7ᵗʰ **S75.099** Other specified injury of femoral artery, unspecified leg

✓5ᵗʰ **S75.1** Injury of femoral vein at hip and thigh level

   ✓6ᵗʰ **S75.10** Unspecified injury of femoral vein at hip and thigh level

      ✓7ᵗʰ **S75.101** Unspecified injury of femoral vein at hip and thigh level, right leg

      ✓7ᵗʰ **S75.102** Unspecified injury of femoral vein at hip and thigh level, left leg

      ✓7ᵗʰ **S75.109** Unspecified injury of femoral vein at hip and thigh level, unspecified leg

   ✓6ᵗʰ **S75.11** Minor laceration of femoral vein at hip and thigh level

       Incomplete transection of femoral vein at hip and thigh level
       Laceration of femoral vein at hip and thigh level NOS
       Superficial laceration of femoral vein at hip and thigh level

      ✓7ᵗʰ **S75.111** Minor laceration of femoral vein at hip and thigh level, right leg

      ✓7ᵗʰ **S75.112** Minor laceration of femoral vein at hip and thigh level, left leg

      ✓7ᵗʰ **S75.119** Minor laceration of femoral vein at hip and thigh level, unspecified leg

   ✓6ᵗʰ **S75.12** Major laceration of femoral vein at hip and thigh level

       Complete transection of femoral vein at hip and thigh level
       Traumatic rupture of femoral vein at hip and thigh level

      ✓7ᵗʰ **S75.121** Major laceration of femoral vein at hip and thigh level, right leg

      ✓7ᵗʰ **S75.122** Major laceration of femoral vein at hip and thigh level, left leg

      ✓7ᵗʰ **S75.129** Major laceration of femoral vein at hip and thigh level, unspecified leg

   ✓6ᵗʰ **S75.19** Other specified injury of femoral vein at hip and thigh level

      ✓7ᵗʰ **S75.191** Other specified injury of femoral vein at hip and thigh level, right leg

      ✓7ᵗʰ **S75.192** Other specified injury of femoral vein at hip and thigh level, left leg

      ✓7ᵗʰ **S75.199** Other specified injury of femoral vein at hip and thigh level, unspecified leg

✓5ᵗʰ **S75.2** Injury of greater saphenous vein at hip and thigh level

EXCLUDES 1   greater saphenous vein NOS (S85.3)

   ✓6ᵗʰ **S75.20** Unspecified injury of greater saphenous vein at hip and thigh level

      ✓7ᵗʰ **S75.201** Unspecified injury of greater saphenous vein at hip and thigh level, right leg

      ✓7ᵗʰ **S75.202** Unspecified injury of greater saphenous vein at hip and thigh level, left leg

      ✓7ᵗʰ **S75.209** Unspecified injury of greater saphenous vein at hip and thigh level, unspecified leg

   ✓6ᵗʰ **S75.21** Minor laceration of greater saphenous vein at hip and thigh level

       Incomplete transection of greater saphenous vein at hip and thigh level
       Laceration of greater saphenous vein at hip and thigh level NOS
       Superficial laceration of greater saphenous vein at hip and thigh level

      ✓7ᵗʰ **S75.211** Minor laceration of greater saphenous vein at hip and thigh level, right leg

      ✓7ᵗʰ **S75.212** Minor laceration of greater saphenous vein at hip and thigh level, left leg

      ✓7ᵗʰ **S75.219** Minor laceration of greater saphenous vein at hip and thigh level, unspecified leg

   ✓6ᵗʰ **S75.22** Major laceration of greater saphenous vein at hip and thigh level

       Complete transection of greater saphenous vein at hip and thigh level
       Traumatic rupture of greater saphenous vein at hip and thigh level

      ✓7ᵗʰ **S75.221** Major laceration of greater saphenous vein at hip and thigh level, right leg

      ✓7ᵗʰ **S75.222** Major laceration of greater saphenous vein at hip and thigh level, left leg

      ✓7ᵗʰ **S75.229** Major laceration of greater saphenous vein at hip and thigh level, unspecified leg

   ✓6ᵗʰ **S75.29** Other specified injury of greater saphenous vein at hip and thigh level

      ✓7ᵗʰ **S75.291** Other specified injury of greater saphenous vein at hip and thigh level, right leg

      ✓7ᵗʰ **S75.292** Other specified injury of greater saphenous vein at hip and thigh level, left leg

      ✓7ᵗʰ **S75.299** Other specified injury of greater saphenous vein at hip and thigh level, unspecified leg

✓5ᵗʰ **S75.8** Injury of other blood vessels at hip and thigh level

   ✓6ᵗʰ **S75.80** Unspecified injury of other blood vessels at hip and thigh level

      ✓7ᵗʰ **S75.801** Unspecified injury of other blood vessels at hip and thigh level, right leg

      ✓7ᵗʰ **S75.802** Unspecified injury of other blood vessels at hip and thigh level, left leg

      ✓7ᵗʰ **S75.809** Unspecified injury of other blood vessels at hip and thigh level, unspecified leg

Chapter 19. Injury, Poisoning and Certain Other Consequences of External Causes

✓6ᵗʰ **S75.81** Laceration of other blood vessels at hip and thigh level
- ✓7ᵗʰ **S75.811** Laceration of other blood vessels at hip and thigh level, right leg
- ✓7ᵗʰ **S75.812** Laceration of other blood vessels at hip and thigh level, left leg
- ✓7ᵗʰ **S75.819** Laceration of other blood vessels at hip and thigh level, unspecified leg

✓6ᵗʰ **S75.89** Other specified injury of other blood vessels at hip and thigh level
- ✓7ᵗʰ **S75.891** Other specified injury of other blood vessels at hip and thigh level, right leg
- ✓7ᵗʰ **S75.892** Other specified injury of other blood vessels at hip and thigh level, left leg
- ✓7ᵗʰ **S75.899** Other specified injury of other blood vessels at hip and thigh level, unspecified leg

✓5ᵗʰ **S75.9** Injury of unspecified blood vessel at hip and thigh level

✓6ᵗʰ **S75.90** Unspecified injury of unspecified blood vessel at hip and thigh level
- ✓7ᵗʰ **S75.901** Unspecified injury of unspecified blood vessel at hip and thigh level, right leg
- ✓7ᵗʰ **S75.902** Unspecified injury of unspecified blood vessel at hip and thigh level, left leg
- ✓7ᵗʰ **S75.909** Unspecified injury of unspecified blood vessel at hip and thigh level, unspecified leg

✓6ᵗʰ **S75.91** Laceration of unspecified blood vessel at hip and thigh level
- ✓7ᵗʰ **S75.911** Laceration of unspecified blood vessel at hip and thigh level, right leg
- ✓7ᵗʰ **S75.912** Laceration of unspecified blood vessel at hip and thigh level, left leg
- ✓7ᵗʰ **S75.919** Laceration of unspecified blood vessel at hip and thigh level, unspecified leg

✓6ᵗʰ **S75.99** Other specified injury of unspecified blood vessel at hip and thigh level
- ✓7ᵗʰ **S75.991** Other specified injury of unspecified blood vessel at hip and thigh level, right leg
- ✓7ᵗʰ **S75.992** Other specified injury of unspecified blood vessel at hip and thigh level, left leg
- ✓7ᵗʰ **S75.999** Other specified injury of unspecified blood vessel at hip and thigh level, unspecified leg

✓4ᵗʰ **S76 Injury of muscle, fascia and tendon at hip and thigh level**

Code also any associated open wound (S71.-)

EXCLUDES 2   injury of muscle, fascia and tendon at lower leg level (S86)
sprain of joint and ligament of hip (S73.1)

TIP: Refer to the Muscle/Tendon table at the beginning of this chapter.

The appropriate 7th character is to be added to each code from category S76.
A   initial encounter
D   subsequent encounter
S   sequela

✓5ᵗʰ **S76.0** Injury of muscle, fascia and tendon of hip

✓6ᵗʰ **S76.00** Unspecified injury of muscle, fascia and tendon of hip
- ✓7ᵗʰ **S76.001** Unspecified injury of muscle, fascia and tendon of right hip
- ✓7ᵗʰ **S76.002** Unspecified injury of muscle, fascia and tendon of left hip
- ✓7ᵗʰ **S76.009** Unspecified injury of muscle, fascia and tendon of unspecified hip

✓6ᵗʰ **S76.01** Strain of muscle, fascia and tendon of hip
- ✓7ᵗʰ **S76.011** Strain of muscle, fascia and tendon of right hip
- ✓7ᵗʰ **S76.012** Strain of muscle, fascia and tendon of left hip
- ✓7ᵗʰ **S76.019** Strain of muscle, fascia and tendon of unspecified hip

✓6ᵗʰ **S76.02** Laceration of muscle, fascia and tendon of hip
- ✓7ᵗʰ **S76.021** Laceration of muscle, fascia and tendon of right hip
- ✓7ᵗʰ **S76.022** Laceration of muscle, fascia and tendon of left hip
- ✓7ᵗʰ **S76.029** Laceration of muscle, fascia and tendon of unspecified hip

✓6ᵗʰ **S76.09** Other specified injury of muscle, fascia and tendon of hip
- ✓7ᵗʰ **S76.091** Other specified injury of muscle, fascia and tendon of right hip
- ✓7ᵗʰ **S76.092** Other specified injury of muscle, fascia and tendon of left hip
- ✓7ᵗʰ **S76.099** Other specified injury of muscle, fascia and tendon of unspecified hip

✓5ᵗʰ **S76.1** Injury of quadriceps muscle, fascia and tendon

Injury of patellar ligament (tendon)

✓6ᵗʰ **S76.10** Unspecified injury of quadriceps muscle, fascia and tendon
- ✓7ᵗʰ **S76.101** Unspecified injury of right quadriceps muscle, fascia and tendon
- ✓7ᵗʰ **S76.102** Unspecified injury of left quadriceps muscle, fascia and tendon
- ✓7ᵗʰ **S76.109** Unspecified injury of unspecified quadriceps muscle, fascia and tendon

✓6ᵗʰ **S76.11** Strain of quadriceps muscle, fascia and tendon
- ✓7ᵗʰ **S76.111** Strain of right quadriceps muscle, fascia and tendon
- ✓7ᵗʰ **S76.112** Strain of left quadriceps muscle, fascia and tendon
- ✓7ᵗʰ **S76.119** Strain of unspecified quadriceps muscle, fascia and tendon

✓6ᵗʰ **S76.12** Laceration of quadriceps muscle, fascia and tendon
- ✓7ᵗʰ **S76.121** Laceration of right quadriceps muscle, fascia and tendon
- ✓7ᵗʰ **S76.122** Laceration of left quadriceps muscle, fascia and tendon
- ✓7ᵗʰ **S76.129** Laceration of unspecified quadriceps muscle, fascia and tendon

✓6ᵗʰ **S76.19** Other specified injury of quadriceps muscle, fascia and tendon
- ✓7ᵗʰ **S76.191** Other specified injury of right quadriceps muscle, fascia and tendon
- ✓7ᵗʰ **S76.192** Other specified injury of left quadriceps muscle, fascia and tendon
- ✓7ᵗʰ **S76.199** Other specified injury of unspecified quadriceps muscle, fascia and tendon

✓5ᵗʰ **S76.2** Injury of adductor muscle, fascia and tendon of thigh

✓6ᵗʰ **S76.20** Unspecified injury of adductor muscle, fascia and tendon of thigh
- ✓7ᵗʰ **S76.201** Unspecified injury of adductor muscle, fascia and tendon of right thigh
- ✓7ᵗʰ **S76.202** Unspecified injury of adductor muscle, fascia and tendon of left thigh
- ✓7ᵗʰ **S76.209** Unspecified injury of adductor muscle, fascia and tendon of unspecified thigh

✓6ᵗʰ **S76.21** Strain of adductor muscle, fascia and tendon of thigh
- ✓7ᵗʰ **S76.211** Strain of adductor muscle, fascia and tendon of right thigh
- ✓7ᵗʰ **S76.212** Strain of adductor muscle, fascia and tendon of left thigh
- ✓7ᵗʰ **S76.219** Strain of adductor muscle, fascia and tendon of unspecified thigh

✓6ᵗʰ **S76.22** Laceration of adductor muscle, fascia and tendon of thigh
- ✓7ᵗʰ **S76.221** Laceration of adductor muscle, fascia and tendon of right thigh
- ✓7ᵗʰ **S76.222** Laceration of adductor muscle, fascia and tendon of left thigh
- ✓7ᵗʰ **S76.229** Laceration of adductor muscle, fascia and tendon of unspecified thigh

✓6ᵗʰ **S76.29** Other injury of adductor muscle, fascia and tendon of thigh
- ✓7ᵗʰ **S76.291** Other injury of adductor muscle, fascia and tendon of right thigh
- ✓7ᵗʰ **S76.292** Other injury of adductor muscle, fascia and tendon of left thigh
- ✓7ᵗʰ **S76.299** Other injury of adductor muscle, fascia and tendon of unspecified thigh

✓5ᵗʰ **S76.3** Injury of muscle, fascia and tendon of the posterior muscle group at thigh level

✓6ᵗʰ **S76.30** Unspecified injury of muscle, fascia and tendon of the posterior muscle group at thigh level
- ✓7ᵗʰ **S76.301** Unspecified injury of muscle, fascia and tendon of the posterior muscle group at thigh level, right thigh

---

√7ᵗʰ **S76.302** Unspecified injury of muscle, fascia and tendon of the posterior muscle group at thigh level, left thigh

√7ᵗʰ **S76.309** Unspecified injury of muscle, fascia and tendon of the posterior muscle group at thigh level, unspecified thigh

√6ᵗʰ **S76.31** Strain of muscle, fascia and tendon of the posterior muscle group at thigh level

√7ᵗʰ **S76.311** Strain of muscle, fascia and tendon of the posterior muscle group at thigh level, right thigh

√7ᵗʰ **S76.312** Strain of muscle, fascia and tendon of the posterior muscle group at thigh level, left thigh

√7ᵗʰ **S76.319** Strain of muscle, fascia and tendon of the posterior muscle group at thigh level, unspecified thigh

√6ᵗʰ **S76.32** Laceration of muscle, fascia and tendon of the posterior muscle group at thigh level

√7ᵗʰ **S76.321** Laceration of muscle, fascia and tendon of the posterior muscle group at thigh level, right thigh

√7ᵗʰ **S76.322** Laceration of muscle, fascia and tendon of the posterior muscle group at thigh level, left thigh

√7ᵗʰ **S76.329** Laceration of muscle, fascia and tendon of the posterior muscle group at thigh level, unspecified thigh

√6ᵗʰ **S76.39** Other specified injury of muscle, fascia and tendon of the posterior muscle group at thigh level

√7ᵗʰ **S76.391** Other specified injury of muscle, fascia and tendon of the posterior muscle group at thigh level, right thigh

√7ᵗʰ **S76.392** Other specified injury of muscle, fascia and tendon of the posterior muscle group at thigh level, left thigh

√7ᵗʰ **S76.399** Other specified injury of muscle, fascia and tendon of the posterior muscle group at thigh level, unspecified thigh

√5ᵗʰ **S76.8** Injury of other specified muscles, fascia and tendons at thigh level

√6ᵗʰ **S76.80** Unspecified injury of other specified muscles, fascia and tendons at thigh level

√7ᵗʰ **S76.801** Unspecified injury of other specified muscles, fascia and tendons at thigh level, right thigh

√7ᵗʰ **S76.802** Unspecified injury of other specified muscles, fascia and tendons at thigh level, left thigh

√7ᵗʰ **S76.809** Unspecified injury of other specified muscles, fascia and tendons at thigh level, unspecified thigh

√6ᵗʰ **S76.81** Strain of other specified muscles, fascia and tendons at thigh level

√7ᵗʰ **S76.811** Strain of other specified muscles, fascia and tendons at thigh level, right thigh

√7ᵗʰ **S76.812** Strain of other specified muscles, fascia and tendons at thigh level, left thigh

√7ᵗʰ **S76.819** Strain of other specified muscles, fascia and tendons at thigh level, unspecified thigh

√6ᵗʰ **S76.82** Laceration of other specified muscles, fascia and tendons at thigh level

√7ᵗʰ **S76.821** Laceration of other specified muscles, fascia and tendons at thigh level, right thigh

√7ᵗʰ **S76.822** Laceration of other specified muscles, fascia and tendons at thigh level, left thigh

√7ᵗʰ **S76.829** Laceration of other specified muscles, fascia and tendons at thigh level, unspecified thigh

√6ᵗʰ **S76.89** Other injury of other specified muscles, fascia and tendons at thigh level

√7ᵗʰ **S76.891** Other injury of other specified muscles, fascia and tendons at thigh level, right thigh

√7ᵗʰ **S76.892** Other injury of other specified muscles, fascia and tendons at thigh level, left thigh

√7ᵗʰ **S76.899** Other injury of other specified muscles, fascia and tendons at thigh level, unspecified thigh

√5ᵗʰ **S76.9** Injury of unspecified muscles, fascia and tendons at thigh level

√6ᵗʰ **S76.90** Unspecified injury of unspecified muscles, fascia and tendons at thigh level

√7ᵗʰ **S76.901** Unspecified injury of unspecified muscles, fascia and tendons at thigh level, right thigh

√7ᵗʰ **S76.902** Unspecified injury of unspecified muscles, fascia and tendons at thigh level, left thigh

√7ᵗʰ **S76.909** Unspecified injury of unspecified muscles, fascia and tendons at thigh level, unspecified thigh

√6ᵗʰ **S76.91** Strain of unspecified muscles, fascia and tendons at thigh level

√7ᵗʰ **S76.911** Strain of unspecified muscles, fascia and tendons at thigh level, right thigh

√7ᵗʰ **S76.912** Strain of unspecified muscles, fascia and tendons at thigh level, left thigh

√7ᵗʰ **S76.919** Strain of unspecified muscles, fascia and tendons at thigh level, unspecified thigh

√6ᵗʰ **S76.92** Laceration of unspecified muscles, fascia and tendons at thigh level

√7ᵗʰ **S76.921** Laceration of unspecified muscles, fascia and tendons at thigh level, right thigh

√7ᵗʰ **S76.922** Laceration of unspecified muscles, fascia and tendons at thigh level, left thigh

√7ᵗʰ **S76.929** Laceration of unspecified muscles, fascia and tendons at thigh level, unspecified thigh

√6ᵗʰ **S76.99** Other specified injury of unspecified muscles, fascia and tendons at thigh level

√7ᵗʰ **S76.991** Other specified injury of unspecified muscles, fascia and tendons at thigh level, right thigh

√7ᵗʰ **S76.992** Other specified injury of unspecified muscles, fascia and tendons at thigh level, left thigh

√7ᵗʰ **S76.999** Other specified injury of unspecified muscles, fascia and tendons at thigh level, unspecified thigh

√4ᵗʰ **S77** Crushing injury of hip and thigh

Use additional code(s) for all associated injuries

EXCLUDES 2　crushing injury of ankle and foot (S97.-)
　　　　　　crushing injury of lower leg (S87.-)

The appropriate 7th character is to be added to each code from category S77.
A initial encounter
D subsequent encounter
S sequela

√5ᵗʰ **S77.0** Crushing injury of hip

√x7ᵗʰ **S77.00** Crushing injury of unspecified hip

√x7ᵗʰ **S77.01** Crushing injury of right hip

√x7ᵗʰ **S77.02** Crushing injury of left hip

√5ᵗʰ **S77.1** Crushing injury of thigh

√x7ᵗʰ **S77.10** Crushing injury of unspecified thigh

√x7ᵗʰ **S77.11** Crushing injury of right thigh

√x7ᵗʰ **S77.12** Crushing injury of left thigh

√5ᵗʰ **S77.2** Crushing injury of hip with thigh

√x7ᵗʰ **S77.20** Crushing injury of unspecified hip with thigh

√x7ᵗʰ **S77.21** Crushing injury of right hip with thigh

√x7ᵗʰ **S77.22** Crushing injury of left hip with thigh

√4ᵗʰ **S78** Traumatic amputation of hip and thigh

An amputation not identified as partial or complete should be coded to complete

EXCLUDES 1　traumatic amputation of knee (S88.0-)

The appropriate 7th character is to be added to each code from category S78.
A initial encounter
D subsequent encounter
S sequela

√5ᵗʰ **S78.0** Traumatic amputation at hip joint

√6ᵗʰ **S78.01** Complete traumatic amputation at hip joint

√7ᵗʰ **S78.011** Complete traumatic amputation at right hip joint　HCC ESR COM

✓7ᵗʰ **S78.012 Complete traumatic amputation at left hip joint** HCC ESR COM

✓7ᵗʰ **S78.019 Complete traumatic amputation at unspecified hip joint** HCC ESR COM

✓6ᵗʰ **S78.02 Partial traumatic amputation at hip joint**

✓7ᵗʰ **S78.021 Partial traumatic amputation at right hip joint** HCC ESR COM

✓7ᵗʰ **S78.022 Partial traumatic amputation at left hip joint** HCC ESR COM

✓7ᵗʰ **S78.029 Partial traumatic amputation at unspecified hip joint** HCC ESR COM

✓5ᵗʰ **S78.1 Traumatic amputation at level between hip and knee**

EXCLUDES 1　traumatic amputation of knee (S88.0-)

Amputation

✓6ᵗʰ **S78.11 Complete traumatic amputation at level between hip and knee**

✓7ᵗʰ **S78.111 Complete traumatic amputation at level between right hip and knee** HCC ESR COM

✓7ᵗʰ **S78.112 Complete traumatic amputation at level between left hip and knee** HCC ESR COM

✓7ᵗʰ **S78.119 Complete traumatic amputation at level between unspecified hip and knee** HCC ESR COM

✓6ᵗʰ **S78.12 Partial traumatic amputation at level between hip and knee**

✓7ᵗʰ **S78.121 Partial traumatic amputation at level between right hip and knee** HCC ESR COM

✓7ᵗʰ **S78.122 Partial traumatic amputation at level between left hip and knee** HCC ESR COM

✓7ᵗʰ **S78.129 Partial traumatic amputation at level between unspecified hip and knee** HCC ESR COM

✓5ᵗʰ **S78.9 Traumatic amputation of hip and thigh, level unspecified**

✓6ᵗʰ **S78.91 Complete traumatic amputation of hip and thigh, level unspecified**

✓7ᵗʰ **S78.911 Complete traumatic amputation of right hip and thigh, level unspecified** HCC ESR COM

✓7ᵗʰ **S78.912 Complete traumatic amputation of left hip and thigh, level unspecified** HCC ESR COM

✓7ᵗʰ **S78.919 Complete traumatic amputation of unspecified hip and thigh, level unspecified** HCC ESR COM

✓6ᵗʰ **S78.92 Partial traumatic amputation of hip and thigh, level unspecified**

✓7ᵗʰ **S78.921 Partial traumatic amputation of right hip and thigh, level unspecified** HCC ESR COM

✓7ᵗʰ **S78.922 Partial traumatic amputation of left hip and thigh, level unspecified** HCC ESR COM

✓7ᵗʰ **S78.929 Partial traumatic amputation of unspecified hip and thigh, level unspecified** HCC ESR COM

✓4ᵗʰ **S79 Other and unspecified injuries of hip and thigh**

NOTE　A fracture not indicated as open or closed should be coded to closed

AHA: 2018,2Q,12; 2018,1Q,3; 2015,3Q,37-39

The appropriate 7th character is to be added to each code from subcategories S79.0 and S79.1.
A initial encounter for closed fracture
D subsequent encounter for fracture with routine healing
G subsequent encounter for fracture with delayed healing
K subsequent encounter for fracture with nonunion
P subsequent encounter for fracture with malunion
S sequela

✓5ᵗʰ **S79.0 Physeal fracture of upper end of femur**

EXCLUDES 1　apophyseal fracture of upper end of femur (S72.13-)
nontraumatic slipped upper femoral epiphysis (M93.0-)

AHA: 2019,4Q,56

✓6ᵗʰ **S79.00 Unspecified physeal fracture of upper end of femur**

1 ✓7ᵗʰ **S79.001 Unspecified physeal fracture of upper end of right femur** HCC ESR COM Q

1 ✓7ᵗʰ **S79.002 Unspecified physeal fracture of upper end of left femur** HCC ESR COM Q

1 ✓7ᵗʰ **S79.009 Unspecified physeal fracture of upper end of unspecified femur** HCC ESR COM Q

✓6ᵗʰ **S79.01 Salter-Harris Type I physeal fracture of upper end of femur**

Acute on chronic slipped capital femoral epiphysis (traumatic)
Acute slipped capital femoral epiphysis (traumatic)
Capital femoral epiphyseal fracture

EXCLUDES 1　chronic slipped upper femoral epiphysis (nontraumatic) (M93.02-)

1 ✓7ᵗʰ **S79.011 Salter-Harris Type I physeal fracture of upper end of right femur** HCC ESR COM Q

1 ✓7ᵗʰ **S79.012 Salter-Harris Type I physeal fracture of upper end of left femur** HCC ESR COM Q

1 ✓7ᵗʰ **S79.019 Salter-Harris Type I physeal fracture of upper end of unspecified femur** HCC ESR COM Q

✓6ᵗʰ **S79.09 Other physeal fracture of upper end of femur**

1 ✓7ᵗʰ **S79.091 Other physeal fracture of upper end of right femur** HCC ESR COM Q

1 ✓7ᵗʰ **S79.092 Other physeal fracture of upper end of left femur** HCC ESR COM Q

1 ✓7ᵗʰ **S79.099 Other physeal fracture of upper end of unspecified femur** HCC ESR COM Q

✓5ᵗʰ **S79.1 Physeal fracture of lower end of femur**

AHA: 2019,4Q,56

✓6ᵗʰ **S79.10 Unspecified physeal fracture of lower end of femur**

1 ✓7ᵗʰ **S79.101 Unspecified physeal fracture of lower end of right femur** HCC ESR Q

1 ✓7ᵗʰ **S79.102 Unspecified physeal fracture of lower end of left femur** HCC ESR Q

1 ✓7ᵗʰ **S79.109 Unspecified physeal fracture of lower end of unspecified femur** HCC ESR Q

✓6ᵗʰ **S79.11 Salter-Harris Type I physeal fracture of lower end of femur**

1 ✓7ᵗʰ **S79.111 Salter-Harris Type I physeal fracture of lower end of right femur** HCC ESR Q

1 ✓7ᵗʰ **S79.112 Salter-Harris Type I physeal fracture of lower end of left femur** HCC ESR Q

1 ✓7ᵗʰ **S79.119 Salter-Harris Type I physeal fracture of lower end of unspecified femur** HCC ESR Q

✓6ᵗʰ **S79.12 Salter-Harris Type II physeal fracture of lower end of femur**

1 ✓7ᵗʰ **S79.121 Salter-Harris Type II physeal fracture of lower end of right femur** HCC ESR Q

1 ✓7ᵗʰ **S79.122 Salter-Harris Type II physeal fracture of lower end of left femur** HCC ESR Q

1 ✓7ᵗʰ **S79.129 Salter-Harris Type II physeal fracture of lower end of unspecified femur** HCC ESR Q

✓6ᵗʰ **S79.13 Salter-Harris Type III physeal fracture of lower end of femur**

1 ✓7ᵗʰ **S79.131 Salter-Harris Type III physeal fracture of lower end of right femur** HCC ESR Q

1 ✓7ᵗʰ **S79.132 Salter-Harris Type III physeal fracture of lower end of left femur** HCC ESR Q

1 ✓7ᵗʰ **S79.139 Salter-Harris Type III physeal fracture of lower end of unspecified femur** HCC ESR Q

✓6ᵗʰ **S79.14 Salter-Harris Type IV physeal fracture of lower end of femur**

1 ✓7ᵗʰ **S79.141 Salter-Harris Type IV physeal fracture of lower end of right femur** HCC ESR Q

1 ✓7ᵗʰ **S79.142 Salter-Harris Type IV physeal fracture of lower end of left femur** HCC ESR Q

1 ✓7ᵗʰ **S79.149 Salter-Harris Type IV physeal fracture of lower end of unspecified femur** HCC ESR Q

✓6ᵗʰ **S79.19 Other physeal fracture of lower end of femur**

1 ✓7ᵗʰ **S79.191 Other physeal fracture of lower end of right femur** HCC ESR Q

1 ✓7ᵗʰ **S79.192 Other physeal fracture of lower end of left femur** HCC ESR Q

1 ✓7ᵗʰ **S79.199 Other physeal fracture of lower end of unspecified femur** HCC ESR Q

✓5ᵗʰ **S79.8 Other specified injuries of hip and thigh**

The appropriate 7th character is to be added to each code in subcategory S79.8.
A   initial encounter
D   subsequent encounter
S   sequela

✓6ᵗʰ **S79.81   Other specified injuries of hip**
    ✓7ᵗʰ **S79.811 Other specified injuries of right hip**
    ✓7ᵗʰ **S79.812 Other specified injuries of left hip**
    ✓7ᵗʰ **S79.819 Other specified injuries of unspecified hip**

✓6ᵗʰ **S79.82   Other specified injuries of thigh**
    ✓7ᵗʰ **S79.821 Other specified injuries of right thigh**
    ✓7ᵗʰ **S79.822 Other specified injuries of left thigh**
    ✓7ᵗʰ **S79.829 Other specified injuries of unspecified thigh**

✓5ᵗʰ **S79.9 Unspecified injury of hip and thigh**

The appropriate 7th character is to be added to each code in subcategory S79.9.
A   initial encounter
D   subsequent encounter
S   sequela

✓6ᵗʰ **S79.91   Unspecified injury of hip**
    ✓7ᵗʰ **S79.911 Unspecified injury of right hip**
    ✓7ᵗʰ **S79.912 Unspecified injury of left hip**
    ✓7ᵗʰ **S79.919 Unspecified injury of unspecified hip**

✓6ᵗʰ **S79.92   Unspecified injury of thigh**
    ✓7ᵗʰ **S79.921 Unspecified injury of right thigh**
    ✓7ᵗʰ **S79.922 Unspecified injury of left thigh**
    ✓7ᵗʰ **S79.929 Unspecified injury of unspecified thigh**

Injuries to the knee and lower leg (S80-S89)

EXCLUDES 2   burns and corrosions (T20-T32)
    frostbite (T33-T34)
    injuries of ankle and foot, except fracture of ankle and malleolus (S90-S99)
    insect bite or sting, venomous (T63.4)

✓4ᵗʰ **S80 Superficial injury of knee and lower leg**
EXCLUDES 2   superficial injury of ankle and foot (S90.-)

The appropriate 7th character is to be added to each code from category S80.
A   initial encounter
D   subsequent encounter
S   sequela

✓5ᵗʰ **S80.0 Contusion of knee**
  ✓x7ᵗʰ **S80.00 Contusion of unspecified knee**
  ✓x7ᵗʰ **S80.01 Contusion of right knee**
  ✓x7ᵗʰ **S80.02 Contusion of left knee**

✓5ᵗʰ **S80.1 Contusion of lower leg**
  ✓x7ᵗʰ **S80.10 Contusion of unspecified lower leg**
  ✓x7ᵗʰ **S80.11 Contusion of right lower leg**
  ✓x7ᵗʰ **S80.12 Contusion of left lower leg**

✓5ᵗʰ **S80.2 Other superficial injuries of knee**
  ✓6ᵗʰ **S80.21   Abrasion of knee**
    ✓7ᵗʰ **S80.211 Abrasion, right knee**
    ✓7ᵗʰ **S80.212 Abrasion, left knee**
    ✓7ᵗʰ **S80.219 Abrasion, unspecified knee**

  ✓6ᵗʰ **S80.22   Blister (nonthermal) of knee**
    ✓7ᵗʰ **S80.221 Blister (nonthermal), right knee**
    ✓7ᵗʰ **S80.222 Blister (nonthermal), left knee**
    ✓7ᵗʰ **S80.229 Blister (nonthermal), unspecified knee**

  ✓6ᵗʰ **S80.24   External constriction of knee**
    ✓7ᵗʰ **S80.241 External constriction, right knee**
    ✓7ᵗʰ **S80.242 External constriction, left knee**
    ✓7ᵗʰ **S80.249 External constriction, unspecified knee**

  ✓6ᵗʰ **S80.25   Superficial foreign body of knee**
    Splinter in the knee
    ✓7ᵗʰ **S80.251 Superficial foreign body, right knee**
    ✓7ᵗʰ **S80.252 Superficial foreign body, left knee**

    ✓7ᵗʰ **S80.259 Superficial foreign body, unspecified knee**

  ✓6ᵗʰ **S80.26   Insect bite (nonvenomous) of knee**
    ✓7ᵗʰ **S80.261 Insect bite (nonvenomous), right knee**
    ✓7ᵗʰ **S80.262 Insect bite (nonvenomous), left knee**
    ✓7ᵗʰ **S80.269 Insect bite (nonvenomous), unspecified knee**

  ✓6ᵗʰ **S80.27   Other superficial bite of knee**
    EXCLUDES 1   open bite of knee (S81.05-)
    ✓7ᵗʰ **S80.271 Other superficial bite of right knee**
    ✓7ᵗʰ **S80.272 Other superficial bite of left knee**
    ✓7ᵗʰ **S80.279 Other superficial bite of unspecified knee**

✓5ᵗʰ **S80.8 Other superficial injuries of lower leg**
  ✓6ᵗʰ **S80.81   Abrasion of lower leg**
    ✓7ᵗʰ **S80.811 Abrasion, right lower leg**
    ✓7ᵗʰ **S80.812 Abrasion, left lower leg**
    ✓7ᵗʰ **S80.819 Abrasion, unspecified lower leg**

  ✓6ᵗʰ **S80.82   Blister (nonthermal) of lower leg**
    ✓7ᵗʰ **S80.821 Blister (nonthermal), right lower leg**
    ✓7ᵗʰ **S80.822 Blister (nonthermal), left lower leg**
    ✓7ᵗʰ **S80.829 Blister (nonthermal), unspecified lower leg**

  ✓6ᵗʰ **S80.84   External constriction of lower leg**
    ✓7ᵗʰ **S80.841 External constriction, right lower leg**
    ✓7ᵗʰ **S80.842 External constriction, left lower leg**
    ✓7ᵗʰ **S80.849 External constriction, unspecified leg**

  ✓6ᵗʰ **S80.85   Superficial foreign body of lower leg**
    Splinter in the lower leg
    ✓7ᵗʰ **S80.851 Superficial foreign body, right lower leg**
    ✓7ᵗʰ **S80.852 Superficial foreign body, left lower leg**
    ✓7ᵗʰ **S80.859 Superficial foreign body, unspecified lower leg**

  ✓6ᵗʰ **S80.86   Insect bite (nonvenomous) of lower leg**
    ✓7ᵗʰ **S80.861 Insect bite (nonvenomous), right lower leg**
    ✓7ᵗʰ **S80.862 Insect bite (nonvenomous), left lower leg**
    ✓7ᵗʰ **S80.869 Insect bite (nonvenomous), unspecified lower leg**

  ✓6ᵗʰ **S80.87   Other superficial bite of lower leg**
    EXCLUDES 1   open bite of lower leg (S81.85-)
    ✓7ᵗʰ **S80.871 Other superficial bite, right lower leg**
    ✓7ᵗʰ **S80.872 Other superficial bite, left lower leg**
    ✓7ᵗʰ **S80.879 Other superficial bite, unspecified lower leg**

✓5ᵗʰ **S80.9 Unspecified superficial injury of knee and lower leg**
  ✓6ᵗʰ **S80.91   Unspecified superficial injury of knee**
    ✓7ᵗʰ **S80.911 Unspecified superficial injury of right knee**
    ✓7ᵗʰ **S80.912 Unspecified superficial injury of left knee**
    ✓7ᵗʰ **S80.919 Unspecified superficial injury of unspecified knee**

  ✓6ᵗʰ **S80.92   Unspecified superficial injury of lower leg**
    ✓7ᵗʰ **S80.921 Unspecified superficial injury of right lower leg**
    ✓7ᵗʰ **S80.922 Unspecified superficial injury of left lower leg**
    ✓7ᵗʰ **S80.929 Unspecified superficial injury of unspecified lower leg**

✓4ᵗʰ **S81 Open wound of knee and lower leg**
Code also any associated wound infection
EXCLUDES 1   open fracture of knee and lower leg (S82.-)
    traumatic amputation of lower leg (S88.-)
EXCLUDES 2   open wound of ankle and foot (S91.-)

The appropriate 7th character is to be added to each code from category S81.
A   initial encounter
D   subsequent encounter
S   sequela

✓5ᵗʰ **S81.0 Open wound of knee**
  ✓6ᵗʰ **S81.00   Unspecified open wound of knee**
    ✓7ᵗʰ **S81.001 Unspecified open wound, right knee**

☑ Additional Character Required   ✓x7ᵗʰ Placeholder Alert   Manifestation   Unspecified Dx   Q QPP   UPD Unacceptable PDx

Chapter 19. Injury, Poisoning and Certain Other Consequences of External Causes

√7ᵗʰ **S81.002** Unspecified open wound, left knee

√7ᵗʰ **S81.009** Unspecified open wound, unspecified knee

√6ᵗʰ **S81.01** Laceration without foreign body of knee

√7ᵗʰ **S81.011** Laceration without foreign body, right knee

√7ᵗʰ **S81.012** Laceration without foreign body, left knee

√7ᵗʰ **S81.019** Laceration without foreign body, unspecified knee

√6ᵗʰ **S81.02** Laceration with foreign body of knee

√7ᵗʰ **S81.021** Laceration with foreign body, right knee

√7ᵗʰ **S81.022** Laceration with foreign body, left knee

√7ᵗʰ **S81.029** Laceration with foreign body, unspecified knee

√6ᵗʰ **S81.03** Puncture wound without foreign body of knee

√7ᵗʰ **S81.031** Puncture wound without foreign body, right knee

√7ᵗʰ **S81.032** Puncture wound without foreign body, left knee

√7ᵗʰ **S81.039** Puncture wound without foreign body, unspecified knee

√6ᵗʰ **S81.04** Puncture wound with foreign body of knee

√7ᵗʰ **S81.041** Puncture wound with foreign body, right knee

√7ᵗʰ **S81.042** Puncture wound with foreign body, left knee

√7ᵗʰ **S81.049** Puncture wound with foreign body, unspecified knee

√6ᵗʰ **S81.05** Open bite of knee

Bite of knee NOS

EXCLUDES 1   superficial bite of knee (S80.27-)

√7ᵗʰ **S81.051** Open bite, right knee

√7ᵗʰ **S81.052** Open bite, left knee

√7ᵗʰ **S81.059** Open bite, unspecified knee

√5ᵗʰ **S81.8** Open wound of lower leg

√6ᵗʰ **S81.80** Unspecified open wound of lower leg

AHA: 2016,3Q,24

√7ᵗʰ **S81.801** Unspecified open wound, right lower leg

√7ᵗʰ **S81.802** Unspecified open wound, left lower leg

√7ᵗʰ **S81.809** Unspecified open wound, unspecified lower leg

√6ᵗʰ **S81.81** Laceration without foreign body of lower leg

√7ᵗʰ **S81.811** Laceration without foreign body, right lower leg

√7ᵗʰ **S81.812** Laceration without foreign body, left lower leg

√7ᵗʰ **S81.819** Laceration without foreign body, unspecified lower leg

√6ᵗʰ **S81.82** Laceration with foreign body of lower leg

√7ᵗʰ **S81.821** Laceration with foreign body, right lower leg

√7ᵗʰ **S81.822** Laceration with foreign body, left lower leg

√7ᵗʰ **S81.829** Laceration with foreign body, unspecified lower leg

√6ᵗʰ **S81.83** Puncture wound without foreign body of lower leg

AHA: 2016,3Q,24

√7ᵗʰ **S81.831** Puncture wound without foreign body, right lower leg

√7ᵗʰ **S81.832** Puncture wound without foreign body, left lower leg

√7ᵗʰ **S81.839** Puncture wound without foreign body, unspecified lower leg

√6ᵗʰ **S81.84** Puncture wound with foreign body of lower leg

AHA: 2016,3Q,24

√7ᵗʰ **S81.841** Puncture wound with foreign body, right lower leg

√7ᵗʰ **S81.842** Puncture wound with foreign body, left lower leg

√7ᵗʰ **S81.849** Puncture wound with foreign body, unspecified lower leg

√6ᵗʰ **S81.85** Open bite of lower leg

Bite of lower leg NOS

EXCLUDES 1   superficial bite of lower leg (S80.86-, S80.87-)

√7ᵗʰ **S81.851** Open bite, right lower leg

√7ᵗʰ **S81.852** Open bite, left lower leg

√7ᵗʰ **S81.859** Open bite, unspecified lower leg

√4ᵗʰ **S82** Fracture of lower leg, including ankle

NOTE   A fracture not indicated as displaced or nondisplaced should be coded to displaced

A fracture not indicated as open or closed should be coded to closed

The open fracture designations are based on the Gustilo open fracture classification.

INCLUDES   fracture of malleolus

EXCLUDES 1   traumatic amputation of lower leg (S88.-)

EXCLUDES 2   fracture of foot, except ankle (S92.-)

periprosthetic fracture around internal prosthetic implant of knee joint (M97.1-)

AHA: 2018,2Q,12; 2016,1Q,33; 2015,3Q,37-39

DEF: Diaphysis: Central shaft of a long bone.

DEF: Epiphysis: Proximal and distal rounded ends of a long bone, communicates with the joint.

DEF: Metaphysis: Section of a long bone located between the epiphysis and diaphysis at the proximal and distal ends.

DEF: Physis (growth plate): Narrow zone of cartilaginous tissue between the epiphysis and metaphysis at each end of a long bone. In childhood, proliferation of cells in this zone lengthens the bone. As the bone matures, this area thins, ossification eventually fusing into solid bone and growth stops. **Synonym(s):** Epiphyseal plate.

The appropriate 7th character is to be added to all codes from category S82 [unless otherwise indicated].

A   initial encounter for closed fracture

B   initial encounter for open fracture type I or II
    initial encounter for open fracture NOS

C   initial encounter for open fracture type IIIA, IIIB, or IIIC

D   subsequent encounter for closed fracture with routine healing

E   subsequent encounter for open fracture type I or II with routine healing

F   subsequent encounter for open fracture type IIIA, IIIB, or IIIC with routine healing

G   subsequent encounter for closed fracture with delayed healing

H   subsequent encounter for open fracture type I or II with delayed healing

J   subsequent encounter for open fracture type IIIA, IIIB, or IIIC with delayed healing

K   subsequent encounter for closed fracture with nonunion

M   subsequent encounter for open fracture type I or II with nonunion

N   subsequent encounter for open fracture type IIIA, IIIB, or IIIC with nonunion

P   subsequent encounter for closed fracture with malunion

Q   subsequent encounter for open fracture type I or II with malunion

R   subsequent encounter for open fracture type IIIA, IIIB, or IIIC with malunion

S   sequela

√5ᵗʰ **S82.0** Fracture of patella

Knee cap

√6ᵗʰ **S82.00** Unspecified fracture of patella

√7ᵗʰ **S82.001** Unspecified fracture of right patella ◨

√7ᵗʰ **S82.002** Unspecified fracture of left patella ◨

√7ᵗʰ **S82.009** Unspecified fracture of unspecified patella ◨

√6ᵗʰ **S82.01** Osteochondral fracture of patella

√7ᵗʰ **S82.011** Displaced osteochondral fracture of right patella ◨

√7ᵗʰ **S82.012** Displaced osteochondral fracture of left patella ◨

√7ᵗʰ **S82.013** Displaced osteochondral fracture of unspecified patella ◨

√7ᵗʰ **S82.014** Nondisplaced osteochondral fracture of right patella ◨

√7ᵗʰ **S82.015** Nondisplaced osteochondral fracture of left patella ◨

√7ᵗʰ **S82.016** Nondisplaced osteochondral fracture of unspecified patella ◨

√6ᵗʰ **S82.02** Longitudinal fracture of patella

√7ᵗʰ **S82.021** Displaced longitudinal fracture of right patella ◨

√7ᵗʰ **S82.022** Displaced longitudinal fracture of left patella ◨

√7th **S82.023** Displaced **longitudinal** fracture of unspecified **patella** ◘

√7th **S82.024** Nondisplaced **longitudinal** fracture of right **patella** ◘

√7th **S82.025** Nondisplaced **longitudinal fracture of** left **patella** ◘

√7th **S82.026** Nondisplaced **longitudinal** fracture of unspecified **patella** ◘

√6th **S82.03** Transverse **fracture of patella**

√7th **S82.031** Displaced **transverse** fracture of right **patella** ◘

√7th **S82.032** Displaced **transverse** fracture of left **patella** ◘

√7th **S82.033** Displaced **transverse** fracture of unspecified **patella** ◘

√7th **S82.034** Nondisplaced **transverse** fracture of right **patella** ◘

√7th **S82.035** Nondisplaced **transverse** fracture of left **patella** ◘

√7th **S82.036** Nondisplaced **transverse** fracture of unspecified **patella** ◘

√6th **S82.04** Comminuted **fracture of patella**

√7th **S82.041** Displaced **comminuted** fracture of right **patella** ◘

√7th **S82.042** Displaced **comminuted** fracture of left **patella** ◘

√7th **S82.043** Displaced **comminuted** fracture of unspecified **patella** ◘

√7th **S82.044** Nondisplaced **comminuted** fracture of right **patella** ◘

√7th **S82.045** Nondisplaced **comminuted** fracture of left **patella** ◘

√7th **S82.046** Nondisplaced **comminuted** fracture of unspecified **patella** ◘

√6th **S82.09** Other fracture of patella

√7th **S82.091** Other fracture of right **patella** ◘

√7th **S82.092** Other fracture of left **patella** ◘

√7th **S82.099** Other fracture of unspecified **patella** ◘

√5th **S82.1** Fracture of upper end of tibia

Fracture of proximal end of tibia

EXCLUDES 2 fracture of shaft of tibia (S82.2-)

physeal fracture of upper end of tibia (S89.0-)

√6th **S82.10** Unspecified fracture of upper end of tibia

√7th **S82.101** Unspecified fracture of upper end of right **tibia** ◘

√7th **S82.102** Unspecified fracture of upper end of left **tibia** ◘

√7th **S82.109** Unspecified fracture of upper end of unspecified **tibia** ◘

√6th **S82.11** Fracture of tibial spine

√7th **S82.111** Displaced fracture of right **tibial spine** ◘

√7th **S82.112** Displaced fracture of left **tibial spine** ◘

√7th **S82.113** Displaced fracture of unspecified **tibial spine** ◘

√7th **S82.114** Nondisplaced fracture of right **tibial spine** ◘

√7th **S82.115** Nondisplaced fracture of left **tibial spine** ◘

√7th **S82.116** Nondisplaced fracture of unspecified **tibial spine** ◘

√6th **S82.12** Fracture of lateral condyle of tibia

√7th **S82.121** Displaced fracture of lateral condyle of right **tibia** ◘

√7th **S82.122** Displaced fracture of lateral condyle of left **tibia** ◘

√7th **S82.123** Displaced fracture of lateral condyle of unspecified **tibia** ◘

√7th **S82.124** Nondisplaced fracture of lateral condyle of right **tibia** ◘

√7th **S82.125** Nondisplaced fracture of lateral condyle of left **tibia** ◘

√7th **S82.126** Nondisplaced fracture of lateral condyle of unspecified **tibia** ◘

√6th **S82.13** Fracture of medial condyle of tibia

√7th **S82.131** Displaced **fracture of medial condyle of** right **tibia** ◘

√7th **S82.132** Displaced **fracture of medial condyle of** left **tibia** ◘

√7th **S82.133** Displaced **fracture of medial condyle of** unspecified **tibia** ◘

√7th **S82.134** Nondisplaced **fracture of medial condyle** of right **tibia** ◘

√7th **S82.135** Nondisplaced **fracture of medial condyle** of left **tibia** ◘

√7th **S82.136** Nondisplaced **fracture of medial condyle** of unspecified **tibia** ◘

√6th **S82.14** Bicondylar **fracture of tibia**

Fracture of tibial plateau NOS

√7th **S82.141** Displaced **bicondylar** fracture of right **tibia** ◘

√7th **S82.142** Displaced **bicondylar** fracture of left **tibia** ◘

√7th **S82.143** Displaced **bicondylar** fracture of unspecified **tibia** ◘

√7th **S82.144** Nondisplaced **bicondylar** fracture of right **tibia** ◘

√7th **S82.145** Nondisplaced **bicondylar** fracture of left **tibia** ◘

√7th **S82.146** Nondisplaced **bicondylar** fracture of unspecified **tibia** ◘

√6th **S82.15** Fracture of tibial tuberosity

√7th **S82.151** Displaced **fracture of right tibial tuberosity** ◘

√7th **S82.152** Displaced **fracture of left tibial tuberosity** ◘

√7th **S82.153** Displaced **fracture of unspecified tibial tuberosity** ◘

√7th **S82.154** Nondisplaced **fracture of right tibial tuberosity** ◘

√7th **S82.155** Nondisplaced **fracture of left tibial tuberosity** ◘

√7th **S82.156** Nondisplaced **fracture of unspecified tibial tuberosity** ◘

√6th **S82.16** Torus **fracture of upper end of tibia**

The appropriate 7th character is to be added to all codes in subcategory S82.16.

A   initial encounter for closed fracture

D   subsequent encounter for fracture with routine healing

G   subsequent encounter for fracture with delayed healing

K   subsequent encounter for fracture with nonunion

P   subsequent encounter for fracture with malunion

S   sequela

√7th **S82.161** Torus fracture of upper end of right **tibia** ◘

√7th **S82.162** Torus fracture of upper end of left **tibia** ◘

√7th **S82.169** Torus fracture of upper end of unspecified **tibia** ◘

√6th **S82.19** Other fracture of upper end of tibia

√7th **S82.191** Other fracture of upper end of right **tibia** ◘

√7th **S82.192** Other fracture of upper end of left **tibia** ◘

√7th **S82.199** Other fracture of upper end of unspecified **tibia** ◘

√5th **S82.2** Fracture of shaft of tibia

√6th **S82.20** Unspecified fracture of shaft of tibia

Fracture of tibia NOS

√7th **S82.201** Unspecified fracture of shaft of right **tibia** ◘

√7th **S82.202** Unspecified fracture of shaft of left **tibia** ◘

√7th **S82.209** Unspecified fracture of shaft of unspecified **tibia** ◘

√6th **S82.22** Transverse fracture of shaft of tibia

√7th **S82.221** Displaced transverse fracture of shaft of right **tibia** ◘

√7ᵗʰ **S82.222** Displaced transverse fracture of shaft of left tibia ⬚

√7ᵗʰ **S82.223** Displaced transverse fracture of shaft of unspecified tibia ⬚

√7ᵗʰ S82.224 Nondisplaced transverse fracture of shaft of right tibia ⬚

√7ᵗʰ S82.225 Nondisplaced transverse fracture of shaft of left tibia ⬚

√7ᵗʰ **S82.226** Nondisplaced transverse fracture of shaft of unspecified tibia ⬚

√6ᵗʰ **S82.23** Oblique fracture of shaft of tibia

√7ᵗʰ S82.231 Displaced oblique fracture of shaft of right tibia ⬚

√7ᵗʰ S82.232 Displaced oblique fracture of shaft of left tibia ⬚

√7ᵗʰ **S82.233** Displaced oblique fracture of shaft of unspecified tibia ⬚

√7ᵗʰ S82.234 Nondisplaced oblique fracture of shaft of right tibia ⬚

√7ᵗʰ S82.235 Nondisplaced oblique fracture of shaft of left tibia ⬚

√7ᵗʰ **S82.236** Nondisplaced oblique fracture of shaft of unspecified tibia ⬚

√6ᵗʰ **S82.24** Spiral fracture of shaft of tibia
Toddler fracture

√7ᵗʰ S82.241 Displaced spiral fracture of shaft of right tibia ⬚

√7ᵗʰ S82.242 Displaced spiral fracture of shaft of left tibia ⬚

√7ᵗʰ **S82.243** Displaced spiral fracture of shaft of unspecified tibia ⬚

√7ᵗʰ S82.244 Nondisplaced spiral fracture of shaft of right tibia ⬚

√7ᵗʰ S82.245 Nondisplaced spiral fracture of shaft of left tibia ⬚

√7ᵗʰ **S82.246** Nondisplaced spiral fracture of shaft of unspecified tibia ⬚

√6ᵗʰ **S82.25** Comminuted fracture of shaft of tibia

√7ᵗʰ S82.251 Displaced comminuted fracture of shaft of right tibia ⬚

√7ᵗʰ S82.252 Displaced comminuted fracture of shaft of left tibia ⬚

√7ᵗʰ **S82.253** Displaced comminuted fracture of shaft of unspecified tibia ⬚

√7ᵗʰ S82.254 Nondisplaced comminuted fracture of shaft of right tibia ⬚

√7ᵗʰ S82.255 Nondisplaced comminuted fracture of shaft of left tibia ⬚

√7ᵗʰ **S82.256** Nondisplaced comminuted fracture of shaft of unspecified tibia ⬚

√6ᵗʰ **S82.26** Segmental fracture of shaft of tibia

√7ᵗʰ S82.261 Displaced segmental fracture of shaft of right tibia ⬚

√7ᵗʰ S82.262 Displaced segmental fracture of shaft of left tibia ⬚

√7ᵗʰ **S82.263** Displaced segmental fracture of shaft of unspecified tibia ⬚

√7ᵗʰ S82.264 Nondisplaced segmental fracture of shaft of right tibia ⬚

√7ᵗʰ S82.265 Nondisplaced segmental fracture of shaft of left tibia ⬚

√7ᵗʰ **S82.266** Nondisplaced segmental fracture of shaft of unspecified tibia ⬚

√6ᵗʰ **S82.29** Other fracture of shaft of tibia

√7ᵗʰ S82.291 Other fracture of shaft of right tibia ⬚

√7ᵗʰ S82.292 Other fracture of shaft of left tibia ⬚

√7ᵗʰ **S82.299** Other fracture of shaft of unspecified tibia ⬚

√5ᵗʰ **S82.3** Fracture of lower end of tibia

EXCLUDES 1   bimalleolar fracture of lower leg (S82.84-)
fracture of medial malleolus alone (S82.5-)
Maisonneuve's fracture (S82.86-)
pilon fracture of distal tibia (S82.87-)
trimalleolar fractures of lower leg (S82.85-)

√6ᵗʰ **S82.30** Unspecified fracture of lower end of tibia

√7ᵗʰ **S82.301** Unspecified fracture of lower end of right tibia ⬚

√7ᵗʰ **S82.302** Unspecified fracture of lower end of left tibia ⬚

√7ᵗʰ S82.309 Unspecified fracture of lower end of unspecified tibia ⬚

√6ᵗʰ S82.31 Torus fracture of lower end of tibia

> The appropriate 7th character is to be added to all codes in subcategory S82.31.
> A   initial encounter for closed fracture
> D   subsequent encounter for fracture with routine healing
> G   subsequent encounter for fracture with delayed healing
> K   subsequent encounter for fracture with nonunion
> P   subsequent encounter for fracture with malunion
> S   sequela

√7ᵗʰ S82.311 Torus fracture of lower end of right tibia ⬚

√7ᵗʰ S82.312 Torus fracture of lower end of left tibia ⬚

√7ᵗʰ **S82.319** Torus fracture of lower end of unspecified tibia ⬚

√6ᵗʰ **S82.39** Other fracture of lower end of tibia
AHA: 2015,1Q,25

√7ᵗʰ S82.391 Other fracture of lower end of right tibia ⬚

√7ᵗʰ S82.392 Other fracture of lower end of left tibia ⬚

√7ᵗʰ **S82.399** Other fracture of lower end of unspecified tibia ⬚

√5ᵗʰ **S82.4** Fracture of shaft of fibula

EXCLUDES 2   fracture of lateral malleolus alone (S82.6-)

√6ᵗʰ **S82.40** Unspecified fracture of shaft of fibula

√7ᵗʰ **S82.401** Unspecified fracture of shaft of right fibula ⬚

√7ᵗʰ **S82.402** Unspecified fracture of shaft of left fibula ⬚

√7ᵗʰ **S82.409** Unspecified fracture of shaft of unspecified fibula ⬚

√6ᵗʰ **S82.42** Transverse fracture of shaft of fibula

√7ᵗʰ S82.421 Displaced transverse fracture of shaft of right fibula ⬚

√7ᵗʰ S82.422 Displaced transverse fracture of shaft of left fibula ⬚

√7ᵗʰ **S82.423** Displaced transverse fracture of shaft of unspecified fibula ⬚

√7ᵗʰ S82.424 Nondisplaced transverse fracture of shaft of right fibula ⬚

√7ᵗʰ S82.425 Nondisplaced transverse fracture of shaft of left fibula ⬚

√7ᵗʰ **S82.426** Nondisplaced transverse fracture of shaft of unspecified fibula ⬚

√6ᵗʰ **S82.43** Oblique fracture of shaft of fibula

√7ᵗʰ S82.431 Displaced oblique fracture of shaft of right fibula ⬚

√7ᵗʰ S82.432 Displaced oblique fracture of shaft of left fibula ⬚

√7ᵗʰ **S82.433** Displaced oblique fracture of shaft of unspecified fibula ⬚

√7ᵗʰ S82.434 Nondisplaced oblique fracture of shaft of right fibula ⬚

√7ᵗʰ S82.435 Nondisplaced oblique fracture of shaft of left fibula ⬚

√7ᵗʰ **S82.436** Nondisplaced oblique fracture of shaft of unspecified fibula ⬚

√6ᵗʰ **S82.44** Spiral fracture of shaft of fibula

√7ᵗʰ S82.441 Displaced spiral fracture of shaft of right fibula ⬚

√7ᵗʰ S82.442 Displaced spiral fracture of shaft of left fibula ⬚

√7ᵗʰ **S82.443** Displaced spiral fracture of shaft of unspecified fibula ⬚

√7ᵗʰ S82.444 Nondisplaced spiral fracture of shaft of right fibula ⬚

√7ᵗʰ S82.445 Nondisplaced spiral fracture of shaft of left fibula ⬚

HCC CMS-HCC   **Rx** Rx HCC   **ESR** ESRD HCC   **OOM** Commercial HCC   **N** Newborn: 0   **P** Pediatric: 0-17   **M** Maternity: 9-64   **A** Adult: 15-124

1092   ICD-10-CM 2023

√7ᵗʰ **S82.446** Nondisplaced **spiral fracture of shaft of** unspecified **fibula** 🅠

√6ᵗʰ **S82.45** Comminuted **fracture of shaft of fibula**

  √7ᵗʰ **S82.451** Displaced **comminuted fracture of shaft of** right **fibula** 🅠

  √7ᵗʰ **S82.452** Displaced **comminuted fracture of shaft of** left **fibula** 🅠

  √7ᵗʰ **S82.453** Displaced **comminuted fracture of shaft of** unspecified **fibula** 🅠

  √7ᵗʰ **S82.454** Nondisplaced **comminuted fracture of shaft of** right **fibula** 🅠

  √7ᵗʰ **S82.455** Nondisplaced **comminuted fracture of shaft of** left **fibula** 🅠

  √7ᵗʰ **S82.456** Nondisplaced **comminuted fracture of shaft of** unspecified **fibula** 🅠

√6ᵗʰ **S82.46** Segmental **fracture of shaft of fibula**

  √7ᵗʰ **S82.461** Displaced **segmental fracture of shaft of** right **fibula** 🅠

  √7ᵗʰ **S82.462** Displaced **segmental fracture of shaft of** left **fibula** 🅠

  √7ᵗʰ **S82.463** Displaced **segmental fracture of shaft of** unspecified **fibula** 🅠

  √7ᵗʰ **S82.464** Nondisplaced **segmental fracture of shaft of** right **fibula** 🅠

  √7ᵗʰ **S82.465** Nondisplaced **segmental fracture of shaft of** left **fibula** 🅠

  √7ᵗʰ **S82.466** Nondisplaced **segmental fracture of shaft of** unspecified **fibula** 🅠

√6ᵗʰ **S82.49** Other **fracture of shaft of fibula**

  √7ᵗʰ **S82.491** Other **fracture of shaft of** right **fibula** 🅠

  √7ᵗʰ **S82.492** Other **fracture of shaft of** left **fibula** 🅠

  √7ᵗʰ **S82.499** Other **fracture of shaft of** unspecified **fibula** 🅠

fibula

√5ᵗʰ **S82.5** Fracture of medial malleolus

   EXCLUDES 1   pilon fracture of distal tibia (S82.87-)
              Salter-Harris type III of lower end of tibia (S89.13-)
              Salter-Harris type IV of lower end of tibia (S89.14-)

  √x7ᵗʰ **S82.51** Displaced **fracture of medial malleolus of** right **tibia** 🅠

  √x7ᵗʰ **S82.52** Displaced **fracture of medial malleolus of** left **tibia** 🅠

  √x7ᵗʰ **S82.53** Displaced **fracture of medial malleolus of** unspecified **tibia** 🅠

  √x7ᵗʰ **S82.54** Nondisplaced **fracture of medial malleolus of** right **tibia** 🅠

  √x7ᵗʰ **S82.55** Nondisplaced **fracture of medial malleolus of** left **tibia** 🅠

  √x7ᵗʰ **S82.56** Nondisplaced **fracture of medial malleolus of** unspecified **tibia** 🅠

√5ᵗʰ **S82.6** Fracture of lateral malleolus

   EXCLUDES 1   pilon fracture of distal tibia (S82.87-)

  √x7ᵗʰ **S82.61** Displaced **fracture of lateral malleolus of** right **fibula** 🅠

  √x7ᵗʰ **S82.62** Displaced **fracture of lateral malleolus of** left **fibula** 🅠

  √x7ᵗʰ **S82.63** Displaced **fracture of lateral malleolus of** unspecified **fibula** 🅠

  √x7ᵗʰ **S82.64** Nondisplaced **fracture of lateral malleolus of** right **fibula** 🅠

  √x7ᵗʰ **S82.65** Nondisplaced **fracture of lateral malleolus of** left **fibula** 🅠

  √x7ᵗʰ **S82.66** Nondisplaced **fracture of lateral malleolus of** unspecified **fibula** 🅠

√5ᵗʰ **S82.8** Other fractures of lower leg

  √6ᵗʰ **S82.81** Torus **fracture of upper end of fibula**

> The appropriate 7th character is to be added to all codes in subcategory S82.81
> A   initial encounter for closed fracture
> D   subsequent encounter for fracture with routine healing
> G   subsequent encounter for fracture with delayed healing
> K   subsequent encounter for fracture with nonunion
> P   subsequent encounter for fracture with malunion
> S   sequela

  √7ᵗʰ **S82.811** Torus fracture of upper end of right fibula 🅠

  √7ᵗʰ **S82.812** Torus fracture of upper end of left fibula 🅠

  √7ᵗʰ **S82.819** Torus fracture of upper end of unspecified fibula 🅠

√6ᵗʰ **S82.82** Torus **fracture of lower end of fibula**

> The appropriate 7th character is to be added to all codes in subcategory S82.82.
> A   initial encounter for closed fracture
> D   subsequent encounter for fracture with routine healing
> G   subsequent encounter for fracture with delayed healing
> K   subsequent encounter for fracture with nonunion
> P   subsequent encounter for fracture with malunion
> S   sequela

fibula

  √7ᵗʰ **S82.821** Torus fracture of lower end of right fibula 🅠

  √7ᵗʰ **S82.822** Torus fracture of lower end of left fibula 🅠

  √7ᵗʰ **S82.829** Torus fracture of lower end of unspecified fibula 🅠

  √6ᵗʰ **S82.83** Other fracture of upper and lower end of fibula
       AHA: 2015,1Q,25

  √7ᵗʰ **S82.831** Other fracture of upper and lower end of right fibula 🅠

  √7ᵗʰ **S82.832** Other fracture of upper and lower end of left fibula 🅠

  √7ᵗʰ **S82.839** Other fracture of upper and lower end of unspecified fibula 🅠

  √6ᵗʰ **S82.84** Bimalleolar **fracture of lower leg**

Right Bimalleolar Fracture

  √7ᵗʰ **S82.841** Displaced **bimalleolar fracture of** right **lower leg** 🅠

√7th **S82.842** Displaced **bimalleolar fracture of left lower leg** ◘

√7th **S82.843** Displaced **bimalleolar fracture of unspecified lower leg** ◘

√7th **S82.844** Nondisplaced **bimalleolar fracture of right lower leg** ◘

√7th **S82.845** Nondisplaced **bimalleolar fracture of left lower leg** ◘

√7th **S82.846** Nondisplaced **bimalleolar fracture of unspecified lower leg** ◘

√6th **S82.85** Trimalleolar **fracture of lower leg**

√7th **S82.851** Displaced **trimalleolar fracture of right lower leg** ◘

√7th **S82.852** Displaced **trimalleolar fracture of left lower leg** ◘

√7th **S82.853** Displaced **trimalleolar fracture of unspecified lower leg** ◘

√7th **S82.854** Nondisplaced **trimalleolar fracture of right lower leg** ◘

√7th **S82.855** Nondisplaced **trimalleolar fracture of left lower leg** ◘

√7th **S82.856** Nondisplaced **trimalleolar fracture of unspecified lower leg** ◘

√6th **S82.86** Maisonneuve's **fracture**

√7th **S82.861** Displaced **Maisonneuve's fracture of right leg** ◘

√7th **S82.862** Displaced **Maisonneuve's fracture of left leg** ◘

√7th **S82.863** Displaced **Maisonneuve's fracture of unspecified leg** ◘

√7th **S82.864** Nondisplaced **Maisonneuve's fracture of right leg** ◘

√7th **S82.865** Nondisplaced **Maisonneuve's fracture of left leg** ◘

√7th **S82.866** Nondisplaced **Maisonneuve's fracture of unspecified leg** ◘

√6th **S82.87** Pilon **fracture of tibia**

√7th **S82.871** Displaced **pilon fracture of right tibia** ◘

√7th **S82.872** Displaced **pilon fracture of left tibia** ◘

√7th **S82.873** Displaced **pilon fracture of unspecified tibia** ◘

√7th **S82.874** Nondisplaced **pilon fracture of right tibia** ◘

√7th **S82.875** Nondisplaced **pilon fracture of left tibia** ◘

√7th **S82.876** Nondisplaced **pilon fracture of unspecified tibia** ◘

√6th **S82.89** Other fractures of lower leg

Fracture of ankle NOS

√7th **S82.891** Other fracture of **right lower leg** ◘

√7th **S82.892** Other fracture of **left lower leg** ◘

√7th **S82.899** Other fracture of unspecified lower leg ◘

√5th **S82.9** Unspecified fracture of lower leg

√x7th **S82.90** Unspecified fracture of unspecified lower leg ◘

√x7th **S82.91** Unspecified fracture of **right lower leg** ◘

√x7th **S82.92** Unspecified fracture of **left lower leg** ◘

S82.92XS

√4th **S83** **Dislocation and sprain of joints and ligaments of knee**

INCLUDES   avulsion of joint or ligament of knee

laceration of cartilage, joint or ligament of knee

sprain of cartilage, joint or ligament of knee

traumatic hemarthrosis of joint or ligament of knee

traumatic rupture of joint or ligament of knee

traumatic subluxation of joint or ligament of knee

traumatic tear of joint or ligament of knee

Code also any associated open wound

EXCLUDES 2   derangement of patella (M22.0-M22.3)

injury of patellar ligament (tendon) (S76.1-)

internal derangement of knee (M23.-)

old dislocation of knee (M24.36)

pathological dislocation of knee (M24.36)

recurrent dislocation of knee (M22.0)

strain of muscle, fascia and tendon of lower leg (S86.-)

The appropriate 7th character is to be added to each code from category S83.

A   initial encounter

D   subsequent encounter

S   sequela

√5th **S83.0** **Subluxation and dislocation of patella**

√6th **S83.00** **Unspecified subluxation and dislocation of patella**

√7th **S83.001** Unspecified **subluxation of right patella**

√7th **S83.002** Unspecified **subluxation of left patella**

√7th **S83.003** Unspecified **subluxation of unspecified patella**

√7th **S83.004** Unspecified **dislocation of right patella**

√7th **S83.005** Unspecified **dislocation of left patella**

√7th **S83.006** Unspecified **dislocation of unspecified patella**

√6th **S83.01** **Lateral subluxation and dislocation of patella**

√7th **S83.011** Lateral **subluxation of right patella**

√7th **S83.012** Lateral **subluxation of left patella**

√7th **S83.013** Lateral **subluxation of unspecified patella**

√7th **S83.014** Lateral **dislocation of right patella**

√7th **S83.015** Lateral **dislocation of left patella**

√7th **S83.016** Lateral **dislocation of unspecified patella**

√6th **S83.09** **Other subluxation and dislocation of patella**

√7th **S83.091** Other **subluxation of right patella**

√7th **S83.092** Other **subluxation of left patella**

√7th **S83.093** Other **subluxation of unspecified patella**

√7th **S83.094** Other **dislocation of right patella**

√7th **S83.095** Other **dislocation of left patella**

√7th **S83.096** Other **dislocation of unspecified patella**

√5th **S83.1** **Subluxation and dislocation of knee**

EXCLUDES 2   instability of knee prosthesis (T84.022, T84.023)

√6th **S83.10** **Unspecified subluxation and dislocation of knee**

√7th **S83.101** Unspecified **subluxation of right knee**

√7th **S83.102** Unspecified **subluxation of left knee**

√7th **S83.103** Unspecified **subluxation of unspecified knee**

√7th **S83.104** Unspecified **dislocation of right knee**

√7th **S83.105** Unspecified **dislocation of left knee**

√7th **S83.106** Unspecified **dislocation of unspecified knee**

√6th **S83.11** **Anterior subluxation and dislocation of proximal end of tibia**

Posterior subluxation and dislocation of distal end of femur

√7th **S83.111** Anterior **subluxation of proximal end of tibia, right knee**

√7th **S83.112** Anterior **subluxation of proximal end of tibia, left knee**

√7th **S83.113** Anterior **subluxation of proximal end of tibia, unspecified knee**

√7th **S83.114** Anterior **dislocation of proximal end of tibia, right knee**

√7th **S83.115** Anterior **dislocation of proximal end of tibia, left knee**

√7th **S83.116** Anterior **dislocation of proximal end of tibia, unspecified knee**

✓6ᵗʰ **S83.12** Posterior subluxation and dislocation of proximal end of tibia

Anterior dislocation of distal end of femur

     ✓7ᵗʰ **S83.121** Posterior subluxation of proximal end of tibia, right knee

     ✓7ᵗʰ **S83.122** Posterior subluxation of proximal end of tibia, left knee

     ✓7ᵗʰ **S83.123** Posterior subluxation of proximal end of tibia, unspecified knee

     ✓7ᵗʰ **S83.124** Posterior dislocation of proximal end of tibia, right knee

     ✓7ᵗʰ **S83.125** Posterior dislocation of proximal end of tibia, left knee

     ✓7ᵗʰ **S83.126** Posterior dislocation of proximal end of tibia, unspecified knee

✓6ᵗʰ **S83.13** Medial subluxation and dislocation of proximal end of tibia

     ✓7ᵗʰ **S83.131** Medial subluxation of proximal end of tibia, right knee

     ✓7ᵗʰ **S83.132** Medial subluxation of proximal end of tibia, left knee

     ✓7ᵗʰ **S83.133** Medial subluxation of proximal end of tibia, unspecified knee

     ✓7ᵗʰ **S83.134** Medial dislocation of proximal end of tibia, right knee

     ✓7ᵗʰ **S83.135** Medial dislocation of proximal end of tibia, left knee

     ✓7ᵗʰ **S83.136** Medial dislocation of proximal end of tibia, unspecified knee

✓6ᵗʰ **S83.14** Lateral subluxation and dislocation of proximal end of tibia

     ✓7ᵗʰ **S83.141** Lateral subluxation of proximal end of tibia, right knee

     ✓7ᵗʰ **S83.142** Lateral subluxation of proximal end of tibia, left knee

     ✓7ᵗʰ **S83.143** Lateral subluxation of proximal end of tibia, unspecified knee

     ✓7ᵗʰ **S83.144** Lateral dislocation of proximal end of tibia, right knee

     ✓7ᵗʰ **S83.145** Lateral dislocation of proximal end of tibia, left knee

     ✓7ᵗʰ **S83.146** Lateral dislocation of proximal end of tibia, unspecified knee

✓6ᵗʰ **S83.19** Other subluxation and dislocation of knee

     ✓7ᵗʰ **S83.191** Other subluxation of right knee

     ✓7ᵗʰ **S83.192** Other subluxation of left knee

     ✓7ᵗʰ **S83.193** Other subluxation of unspecified knee

     ✓7ᵗʰ **S83.194** Other dislocation of right knee

     ✓7ᵗʰ **S83.195** Other dislocation of left knee

     ✓7ᵗʰ **S83.196** Other dislocation of unspecified knee

✓5ᵗʰ **S83.2** Tear of meniscus, current injury

     EXCLUDES 1   old bucket-handle tear (M23.2)

     AHA: 2019,2Q,26

✓6ᵗʰ **S83.20** Tear of unspecified meniscus, current injury

     Tear of meniscus of knee NOS

     ✓7ᵗʰ **S83.200** Bucket-handle tear of unspecified meniscus, current injury, right knee

     ✓7ᵗʰ **S83.201** Bucket-handle tear of unspecified meniscus, current injury, left knee

     ✓7ᵗʰ **S83.202** Bucket-handle tear of unspecified meniscus, current injury, unspecified knee

     ✓7ᵗʰ **S83.203** Other tear of unspecified meniscus, current injury, right knee

     ✓7ᵗʰ **S83.204** Other tear of unspecified meniscus, current injury, left knee

     ✓7ᵗʰ **S83.205** Other tear of unspecified meniscus, current injury, unspecified knee

     ✓7ᵗʰ **S83.206** Unspecified tear of unspecified meniscus, current injury, right knee

     ✓7ᵗʰ **S83.207** Unspecified tear of unspecified meniscus, current injury, left knee

     ✓7ᵗʰ **S83.209** Unspecified tear of unspecified meniscus, current injury, unspecified knee

✓6ᵗʰ **S83.21** Bucket-handle tear of medial meniscus, current injury

     ✓7ᵗʰ **S83.211** Bucket-handle tear of medial meniscus, current injury, right knee

     ✓7ᵗʰ **S83.212** Bucket-handle tear of medial meniscus, current injury, left knee

     ✓7ᵗʰ **S83.219** Bucket-handle tear of medial meniscus, current injury, unspecified knee

✓6ᵗʰ **S83.22** Peripheral tear of medial meniscus, current injury

     ✓7ᵗʰ **S83.221** Peripheral tear of medial meniscus, current injury, right knee

     ✓7ᵗʰ **S83.222** Peripheral tear of medial meniscus, current injury, left knee

     ✓7ᵗʰ **S83.229** Peripheral tear of medial meniscus, current injury, unspecified knee

✓6ᵗʰ **S83.23** Complex tear of medial meniscus, current injury

     ✓7ᵗʰ **S83.231** Complex tear of medial meniscus, current injury, right knee

     ✓7ᵗʰ **S83.232** Complex tear of medial meniscus, current injury, left knee

     ✓7ᵗʰ **S83.239** Complex tear of medial meniscus, current injury, unspecified knee

✓6ᵗʰ **S83.24** Other tear of medial meniscus, current injury

     ✓7ᵗʰ **S83.241** Other tear of medial meniscus, current injury, right knee

     ✓7ᵗʰ **S83.242** Other tear of medial meniscus, current injury, left knee

     ✓7ᵗʰ **S83.249** Other tear of medial meniscus, current injury, unspecified knee

✓6ᵗʰ **S83.25** Bucket-handle tear of lateral meniscus, current injury

     ✓7ᵗʰ **S83.251** Bucket-handle tear of lateral meniscus, current injury, right knee

     ✓7ᵗʰ **S83.252** Bucket-handle tear of lateral meniscus, current injury, left knee

     ✓7ᵗʰ **S83.259** Bucket-handle tear of lateral meniscus, current injury, unspecified knee

✓6ᵗʰ **S83.26** Peripheral tear of lateral meniscus, current injury

     ✓7ᵗʰ **S83.261** Peripheral tear of lateral meniscus, current injury, right knee

     ✓7ᵗʰ **S83.262** Peripheral tear of lateral meniscus, current injury, left knee

     ✓7ᵗʰ **S83.269** Peripheral tear of lateral meniscus, current injury, unspecified knee

✓6ᵗʰ **S83.27** Complex tear of lateral meniscus, current injury

     ✓7ᵗʰ **S83.271** Complex tear of lateral meniscus, current injury, right knee

     ✓7ᵗʰ **S83.272** Complex tear of lateral meniscus, current injury, left knee

     ✓7ᵗʰ **S83.279** Complex tear of lateral meniscus, current injury, unspecified knee

✓6ᵗʰ **S83.28** Other tear of lateral meniscus, current injury

     ✓7ᵗʰ **S83.281** Other tear of lateral meniscus, current injury, right knee

     ✓7ᵗʰ **S83.282** Other tear of lateral meniscus, current injury, left knee

     ✓7ᵗʰ **S83.289** Other tear of lateral meniscus, current injury, unspecified knee

✓5ᵗʰ **S83.3** Tear of articular cartilage of knee, current

     ✓x7ᵗʰ **S83.30** Tear of articular cartilage of unspecified knee, current

     ✓x7ᵗʰ **S83.31** Tear of articular cartilage of right knee, current

     ✓x7ᵗʰ **S83.32** Tear of articular cartilage of left knee, current

✓5ᵗʰ **S83.4** Sprain of collateral ligament of knee

     ✓6ᵗʰ **S83.40** Sprain of unspecified collateral ligament of knee

         ✓7ᵗʰ **S83.401** Sprain of unspecified collateral ligament of right knee

         ✓7ᵗʰ **S83.402** Sprain of unspecified collateral ligament of left knee

         ✓7ᵗʰ **S83.409** Sprain of unspecified collateral ligament of unspecified knee

     ✓6ᵗʰ **S83.41** Sprain of medial collateral ligament of knee

         Sprain of tibial collateral ligament

         ✓7ᵗʰ **S83.411** Sprain of medial collateral ligament of right knee

         ✓7ᵗʰ **S83.412** Sprain of medial collateral ligament of left knee

         ✓7ᵗʰ **S83.419** Sprain of medial collateral ligament of unspecified knee

     ✓6ᵗʰ **S83.42** Sprain of lateral collateral ligament of knee

         Sprain of fibular collateral ligament

         ✓7ᵗʰ **S83.421** Sprain of lateral collateral ligament of right knee

         ✓7ᵗʰ **S83.422** Sprain of lateral collateral ligament of left knee

✓7ᵗʰ **S83.429** Sprain of lateral collateral ligament of unspecified knee

✓5ᵗʰ **S83.5** Sprain of cruciate ligament of knee

    AHA: 2016,2Q,3

  ✓6ᵗʰ **S83.50** Sprain of unspecified cruciate ligament of knee

    ✓7ᵗʰ **S83.501** Sprain of unspecified cruciate ligament of right knee

    ✓7ᵗʰ **S83.502** Sprain of unspecified cruciate ligament of left knee

    ✓7ᵗʰ **S83.509** Sprain of unspecified cruciate ligament of unspecified knee

  ✓6ᵗʰ **S83.51** Sprain of anterior cruciate ligament of knee

    ✓7ᵗʰ **S83.511** Sprain of anterior cruciate ligament of right knee

    ✓7ᵗʰ **S83.512** Sprain of anterior cruciate ligament of left knee

    ✓7ᵗʰ **S83.519** Sprain of anterior cruciate ligament of unspecified knee

  ✓6ᵗʰ **S83.52** Sprain of posterior cruciate ligament of knee

    ✓7ᵗʰ **S83.521** Sprain of posterior cruciate ligament of right knee

    ✓7ᵗʰ **S83.522** Sprain of posterior cruciate ligament of left knee

    ✓7ᵗʰ **S83.529** Sprain of posterior cruciate ligament of unspecified knee

✓5ᵗʰ **S83.6** Sprain of the superior tibiofibular joint and ligament

  ✓x7ᵗʰ **S83.60** Sprain of the superior tibiofibular joint and ligament, unspecified knee

  ✓x7ᵗʰ **S83.61** Sprain of the superior tibiofibular joint and ligament, right knee

  ✓x7ᵗʰ **S83.62** Sprain of the superior tibiofibular joint and ligament, left knee

✓5ᵗʰ **S83.8** Sprain of other specified parts of knee

  ✓6ᵗʰ **S83.8X** Sprain of other specified parts of knee

    ✓7ᵗʰ **S83.8X1** Sprain of other specified parts of right knee

    ✓7ᵗʰ **S83.8X2** Sprain of other specified parts of left knee

    ✓7ᵗʰ **S83.8X9** Sprain of other specified parts of unspecified knee

✓5ᵗʰ **S83.9** Sprain of unspecified site of knee

  ✓x7ᵗʰ **S83.90** Sprain of unspecified site of unspecified knee

  ✓x7ᵗʰ **S83.91** Sprain of unspecified site of right knee

  ✓x7ᵗʰ **S83.92** Sprain of unspecified site of left knee

✓4ᵗʰ **S84** Injury of nerves at lower leg level

  Code also any associated open wound (S81.-)

  EXCLUDES 2   injury of nerves at ankle and foot level (S94.-)

  The appropriate 7th character is to be added to each code from category S84.

  A   initial encounter

  D   subsequent encounter

  S   sequela

Nerve

✓5ᵗʰ **S84.0** Injury of tibial nerve at lower leg level

  ✓x7ᵗʰ **S84.00** Injury of tibial nerve at lower leg level, unspecified leg

  ✓x7ᵗʰ **S84.01** Injury of tibial nerve at lower leg level, right leg

  ✓x7ᵗʰ **S84.02** Injury of tibial nerve at lower leg level, left leg

✓5ᵗʰ **S84.1** Injury of peroneal nerve at lower leg level

  ✓x7ᵗʰ **S84.10** Injury of peroneal nerve at lower leg level, unspecified leg

  ✓x7ᵗʰ **S84.11** Injury of peroneal nerve at lower leg level, right leg

  ✓x7ᵗʰ **S84.12** Injury of peroneal nerve at lower leg level, left leg

✓5ᵗʰ **S84.2** Injury of cutaneous sensory nerve at lower leg level

  ✓x7ᵗʰ **S84.20** Injury of cutaneous sensory nerve at lower leg level, unspecified leg

  ✓x7ᵗʰ **S84.21** Injury of cutaneous sensory nerve at lower leg level, right leg

  ✓x7ᵗʰ **S84.22** Injury of cutaneous sensory nerve at lower leg level, left leg

✓5ᵗʰ **S84.8** Injury of other nerves at lower leg level

  ✓6ᵗʰ **S84.80** Injury of other nerves at lower leg level

    ✓7ᵗʰ **S84.801** Injury of other nerves at lower leg level, right leg

    ✓7ᵗʰ **S84.802** Injury of other nerves at lower leg level, left leg

    ✓7ᵗʰ **S84.809** Injury of other nerves at lower leg level, unspecified leg

✓5ᵗʰ **S84.9** Injury of unspecified nerve at lower leg level

  ✓x7ᵗʰ **S84.90** Injury of unspecified nerve at lower leg level, unspecified leg

  ✓x7ᵗʰ **S84.91** Injury of unspecified nerve at lower leg level, right leg

  ✓x7ᵗʰ **S84.92** Injury of unspecified nerve at lower leg level, left leg

✓4ᵗʰ **S85** Injury of blood vessels at lower leg level

  Code also any associated open wound (S81.-)

  EXCLUDES 2   injury of blood vessels at ankle and foot level (S95.-)

  The appropriate 7th character is to be added to each code from category S85.

  A   initial encounter

  D   subsequent encounter

  S   sequela

✓5ᵗʰ **S85.0** Injury of popliteal artery

  ✓6ᵗʰ **S85.00** Unspecified injury of popliteal artery

    ✓7ᵗʰ **S85.001** Unspecified injury of popliteal artery, right leg

    ✓7ᵗʰ **S85.002** Unspecified injury of popliteal artery, left leg

    ✓7ᵗʰ **S85.009** Unspecified injury of popliteal artery, unspecified leg

  ✓6ᵗʰ **S85.01** Laceration of popliteal artery

    ✓7ᵗʰ **S85.011** Laceration of popliteal artery, right leg

    ✓7ᵗʰ **S85.012** Laceration of popliteal artery, left leg

    ✓7ᵗʰ **S85.019** Laceration of popliteal artery, unspecified leg

  ✓6ᵗʰ **S85.09** Other specified injury of popliteal artery

    ✓7ᵗʰ **S85.091** Other specified injury of popliteal artery, right leg

    ✓7ᵗʰ **S85.092** Other specified injury of popliteal artery, left leg

    ✓7ᵗʰ **S85.099** Other specified injury of popliteal artery, unspecified leg

✓5ᵗʰ **S85.1** Injury of tibial artery

  ✓6ᵗʰ **S85.10** Unspecified injury of unspecified tibial artery

    Injury of tibial artery NOS

    ✓7ᵗʰ **S85.101** Unspecified injury of unspecified tibial artery, right leg

    ✓7ᵗʰ **S85.102** Unspecified injury of unspecified tibial artery, left leg

    ✓7ᵗʰ **S85.109** Unspecified injury of unspecified tibial artery, unspecified leg

  ✓6ᵗʰ **S85.11** Laceration of unspecified tibial artery

    ✓7ᵗʰ **S85.111** Laceration of unspecified tibial artery, right leg

    ✓7ᵗʰ **S85.112** Laceration of unspecified tibial artery, left leg

    ✓7ᵗʰ **S85.119** Laceration of unspecified tibial artery, unspecified leg

  ✓6ᵗʰ **S85.12** Other specified injury of unspecified tibial artery

    ✓7ᵗʰ **S85.121** Other specified injury of unspecified tibial artery, right leg

    ✓7ᵗʰ **S85.122** Other specified injury of unspecified tibial artery, left leg

    ✓7ᵗʰ **S85.129** Other specified injury of unspecified tibial artery, unspecified leg

  ✓6ᵗʰ **S85.13** Unspecified injury of anterior tibial artery

    ✓7ᵗʰ **S85.131** Unspecified injury of anterior tibial artery, right leg

    ✓7ᵗʰ **S85.132** Unspecified injury of anterior tibial artery, left leg

    ✓7ᵗʰ **S85.139** Unspecified injury of anterior tibial artery, unspecified leg

  ✓6ᵗʰ **S85.14** Laceration of anterior tibial artery

    ✓7ᵗʰ **S85.141** Laceration of anterior tibial artery, right leg

    ✓7ᵗʰ **S85.142** Laceration of anterior tibial artery, left leg

    ✓7ᵗʰ **S85.149** Laceration of anterior tibial artery, unspecified leg

  ✓6ᵗʰ **S85.15** Other specified injury of anterior tibial artery

    ✓7ᵗʰ **S85.151** Other specified injury of anterior tibial artery, right leg

Tibial

Artery

✓7th **S85.152** Other specified injury of anterior tibial artery, **left leg**

✓7th **S85.159** Other specified injury of anterior tibial artery, unspecified leg

✓6th **S85.16** Unspecified injury of posterior tibial artery

✓7th **S85.161** Unspecified injury of posterior tibial artery, **right leg**

✓7th **S85.162** Unspecified injury of posterior tibial artery, **left leg**

✓7th **S85.169** Unspecified injury of posterior tibial artery, unspecified leg

✓6th **S85.17** Laceration of posterior tibial artery

✓7th **S85.171** Laceration of posterior tibial artery, **right leg**

✓7th **S85.172** Laceration of posterior tibial artery, **left leg**

✓7th **S85.179** Laceration of posterior tibial artery, unspecified leg

✓6th **S85.18** Other specified injury of posterior tibial artery

✓7th **S85.181** Other specified injury of posterior tibial artery, **right leg**

✓7th **S85.182** Other specified injury of posterior tibial artery, **left leg**

✓7th **S85.189** Other specified injury of posterior tibial artery, unspecified leg

✓5th **S85.2** Injury of peroneal artery

✓6th **S85.20** Unspecified injury of peroneal artery

✓7th **S85.201** Unspecified injury of peroneal artery, **right leg**

✓7th **S85.202** Unspecified injury of peroneal artery, **left leg**

✓7th **S85.209** Unspecified injury of peroneal artery, unspecified leg

✓6th **S85.21** Laceration of peroneal artery

✓7th **S85.211** Laceration of peroneal artery, **right leg**

✓7th **S85.212** Laceration of peroneal artery, **left leg**

✓7th **S85.219** Laceration of peroneal artery, unspecified leg

✓6th **S85.29** Other specified injury of peroneal artery

✓7th **S85.291** Other specified injury of peroneal artery, **right leg**

✓7th **S85.292** Other specified injury of peroneal artery, **left leg**

✓7th **S85.299** Other specified injury of peroneal artery, unspecified leg

✓5th **S85.3** Injury of greater saphenous vein at lower leg level

Injury of greater saphenous vein NOS
Injury of saphenous vein NOS

✓6th **S85.30** Unspecified injury of greater saphenous vein at lower leg level

✓7th **S85.301** Unspecified injury of greater saphenous vein at lower leg level, **right leg**

✓7th **S85.302** Unspecified injury of greater saphenous vein at lower leg level, **left leg**

✓7th **S85.309** Unspecified injury of greater saphenous vein at lower leg level, unspecified leg

✓6th **S85.31** Laceration of greater saphenous vein at lower leg level

✓7th **S85.311** Laceration of greater saphenous vein at lower leg level, **right leg**

✓7th **S85.312** Laceration of greater saphenous vein at lower leg level, **left leg**

✓7th **S85.319** Laceration of greater saphenous vein at lower leg level, unspecified leg

✓6th **S85.39** Other specified injury of greater saphenous vein at lower leg level

✓7th **S85.391** Other specified injury of greater saphenous vein at lower leg level, **right leg**

✓7th **S85.392** Other specified injury of greater saphenous vein at lower leg level, **left leg**

✓7th **S85.399** Other specified injury of greater saphenous vein at lower leg level, unspecified leg

✓5th **S85.4** Injury of lesser saphenous vein at lower leg level

✓6th **S85.40** Unspecified injury of lesser saphenous vein at lower leg level

✓7th **S85.401** Unspecified injury of lesser saphenous vein at lower leg level, **right leg**

✓7th **S85.402** Unspecified injury of lesser saphenous vein at lower leg level, **left leg**

✓7th **S85.409** Unspecified injury of lesser saphenous vein at lower leg level, unspecified leg

✓6th **S85.41** Laceration of lesser saphenous vein at lower leg level

✓7th **S85.411** Laceration of lesser saphenous vein at lower leg level, **right leg**

✓7th **S85.412** Laceration of lesser saphenous vein at lower leg level, **left leg**

✓7th **S85.419** Laceration of lesser saphenous vein at lower leg level, unspecified leg

✓6th **S85.49** Other specified injury of lesser saphenous vein at lower leg level

✓7th **S85.491** Other specified injury of lesser saphenous vein at lower leg level, **right leg**

✓7th **S85.492** Other specified injury of lesser saphenous vein at lower leg level, **left leg**

✓7th **S85.499** Other specified injury of lesser saphenous vein at lower leg level, unspecified leg

✓5th **S85.5** Injury of popliteal vein

✓6th **S85.50** Unspecified injury of popliteal vein

✓7th **S85.501** Unspecified injury of popliteal vein, **right leg**

✓7th **S85.502** Unspecified injury of popliteal vein, **left leg**

✓7th **S85.509** Unspecified injury of popliteal vein, unspecified leg

✓6th **S85.51** Laceration of popliteal vein

✓7th **S85.511** Laceration of popliteal vein, **right leg**

✓7th **S85.512** Laceration of popliteal vein, **left leg**

✓7th **S85.519** Laceration of popliteal vein, unspecified leg

✓6th **S85.59** Other specified injury of popliteal vein

✓7th **S85.591** Other specified injury of popliteal vein, **right leg**

✓7th **S85.592** Other specified injury of popliteal vein, **left leg**

✓7th **S85.599** Other specified injury of popliteal vein, unspecified leg

✓5th **S85.8** Injury of other blood vessels at lower leg level

✓6th **S85.80** Unspecified injury of other blood vessels at lower leg level

✓7th **S85.801** Unspecified injury of other blood vessels at lower leg level, **right leg**

✓7th **S85.802** Unspecified injury of other blood vessels at lower leg level, **left leg**

✓7th **S85.809** Unspecified injury of other blood vessels at lower leg level, unspecified leg

✓6th **S85.81** Laceration of other blood vessels at lower leg level

✓7th **S85.811** Laceration of other blood vessels at lower leg level, **right leg**

✓7th **S85.812** Laceration of other blood vessels at lower leg level, **left leg**

✓7th **S85.819** Laceration of other blood vessels at lower leg level, unspecified leg

✓6th **S85.89** Other specified injury of other blood vessels at lower leg level

✓7th **S85.891** Other specified injury of other blood vessels at lower leg level, **right leg**

✓7th **S85.892** Other specified injury of other blood vessels at lower leg level, **left leg**

✓7th **S85.899** Other specified injury of other blood vessels at lower leg level, unspecified leg

✓5th **S85.9** Injury of unspecified blood vessel at lower leg level

✓6th **S85.90** Unspecified injury of unspecified blood vessel at lower leg level

✓7th **S85.901** Unspecified injury of unspecified blood vessel at lower leg level, **right leg**

✓7th **S85.902** Unspecified injury of unspecified blood vessel at lower leg level, **left leg**

✓7th **S85.909** Unspecified injury of unspecified blood vessel at lower leg level, unspecified leg

✓6th **S85.91** Laceration of unspecified blood vessel at lower leg level

✓7th **S85.911** Laceration of unspecified blood vessel at lower leg level, **right leg**

✓7th **S85.912** Laceration of unspecified blood vessel at lower leg level, **left leg**

✓7th **S85.919** Laceration of unspecified blood vessel at lower leg level, unspecified leg

✓6ᵗʰ S85.99 Other specified injury of unspecified blood vessel at lower leg level
- **✓7ᵗʰ S85.991** Other specified injury of unspecified blood vessel at lower leg level, **right** leg
- **✓7ᵗʰ S85.992** Other specified injury of unspecified blood vessel at lower leg level, **left** leg
- **✓7ᵗʰ S85.999** Other specified injury of unspecified blood vessel at lower leg level, unspecified leg

✓4ᵗʰ S86 Injury of muscle, fascia and tendon at lower leg level

Code also any associated open wound (S81.-)

EXCLUDES 2   injury of muscle, fascia and tendon at ankle (S96.-)
injury of patellar ligament (tendon) (S76.1-)
sprain of joints and ligaments of knee (S83.-)

TIP: Refer to the Muscle/Tendon table at the beginning of this chapter.

The appropriate 7th character is to be added to each code from category S86.
A   initial encounter
D   subsequent encounter
S   sequela

✓5ᵗʰ S86.0 Injury of Achilles tendon
- **✓6ᵗʰ S86.00 Unspecified injury of Achilles tendon**
  - **✓7ᵗʰ S86.001** Unspecified injury of **right** Achilles tendon
  - **✓7ᵗʰ S86.002** Unspecified injury of **left** Achilles tendon
  - **✓7ᵗʰ S86.009** Unspecified injury of unspecified Achilles tendon
- **✓6ᵗʰ S86.01 Strain of Achilles tendon**
  - **✓7ᵗʰ S86.011** Strain of **right** Achilles tendon
  - **✓7ᵗʰ S86.012** Strain of **left** Achilles tendon
  - **✓7ᵗʰ S86.019** Strain of unspecified Achilles tendon
- **✓6ᵗʰ S86.02 Laceration of Achilles tendon**
  - **✓7ᵗʰ S86.021** Laceration of **right** Achilles tendon
  - **✓7ᵗʰ S86.022** Laceration of **left** Achilles tendon
  - **✓7ᵗʰ S86.029** Laceration of unspecified Achilles tendon
- **✓6ᵗʰ S86.09 Other specified injury of Achilles tendon**
  - **✓7ᵗʰ S86.091** Other specified injury of **right** Achilles tendon
  - **✓7ᵗʰ S86.092** Other specified injury of **left** Achilles tendon
  - **✓7ᵗʰ S86.099** Other specified injury of unspecified Achilles tendon

✓5ᵗʰ S86.1 Injury of other muscle(s) and tendon(s) of posterior muscle group at lower leg level
- **✓6ᵗʰ S86.10 Unspecified injury of other muscle(s) and tendon(s) of posterior muscle group at lower leg level**
  - **✓7ᵗʰ S86.101** Unspecified injury of other muscle(s) and tendon(s) of posterior muscle group at lower leg level, **right** leg
  - **✓7ᵗʰ S86.102** Unspecified injury of other muscle(s) and tendon(s) of posterior muscle group at lower leg level, **left** leg
  - **✓7ᵗʰ S86.109** Unspecified injury of other muscle(s) and tendon(s) of posterior muscle group at lower leg level, unspecified leg
- **✓6ᵗʰ S86.11 Strain of other muscle(s) and tendon(s) of posterior muscle group at lower leg level**
  - **✓7ᵗʰ S86.111** Strain of other muscle(s) and tendon(s) of posterior muscle group at lower leg level, **right** leg
  - **✓7ᵗʰ S86.112** Strain of other muscle(s) and tendon(s) of posterior muscle group at lower leg level, **left** leg
  - **✓7ᵗʰ S86.119** Strain of other muscle(s) and tendon(s) of posterior muscle group at lower leg level, unspecified leg
- **✓6ᵗʰ S86.12 Laceration of other muscle(s) and tendon(s) of posterior muscle group at lower leg level**
  - **✓7ᵗʰ S86.121** Laceration of other muscle(s) and tendon(s) of posterior muscle group at lower leg level, **right** leg
  - **✓7ᵗʰ S86.122** Laceration of other muscle(s) and tendon(s) of posterior muscle group at lower leg level, **left** leg
  - **✓7ᵗʰ S86.129** Laceration of other muscle(s) and tendon(s) of posterior muscle group at lower leg level, unspecified leg

✓6ᵗʰ S86.19 Other injury of other muscle(s) and tendon(s) of posterior muscle group at lower leg level
- **✓7ᵗʰ S86.191** Other injury of other muscle(s) and tendon(s) of posterior muscle group at lower leg level, **right** leg
- **✓7ᵗʰ S86.192** Other injury of other muscle(s) and tendon(s) of posterior muscle group at lower leg level, **left** leg
- **✓7ᵗʰ S86.199** Other injury of other muscle(s) and tendon(s) of posterior muscle group at lower leg level, unspecified leg

✓5ᵗʰ S86.2 Injury of muscle(s) and tendon(s) of anterior muscle group at lower leg level
- **✓6ᵗʰ S86.20 Unspecified injury of muscle(s) and tendon(s) of anterior muscle group at lower leg level**
  - **✓7ᵗʰ S86.201** Unspecified injury of muscle(s) and tendon(s) of anterior muscle group at lower leg level, **right** leg
  - **✓7ᵗʰ S86.202** Unspecified injury of muscle(s) and tendon(s) of anterior muscle group at lower leg level, **left** leg
  - **✓7ᵗʰ S86.209** Unspecified injury of muscle(s) and tendon(s) of anterior muscle group at lower leg level, unspecified leg
- **✓6ᵗʰ S86.21 Strain of muscle(s) and tendon(s) of anterior muscle group at lower leg level**
  - **S86.211** Strain of muscle(s) and tendon(s) of anterior muscle group at lower leg level, **right** leg
  - **✓7ᵗʰ S86.212** Strain of muscle(s) and tendon(s) of anterior muscle group at lower leg level, **left** leg
  - **✓7ᵗʰ S86.219** Strain of muscle(s) and tendon(s) of anterior muscle group at lower leg level, unspecified leg
- **✓6ᵗʰ S86.22 Laceration of muscle(s) and tendon(s) of anterior muscle group at lower leg level**
  - **✓7ᵗʰ S86.221** Laceration of muscle(s) and tendon(s) of anterior muscle group at lower leg level, **right** leg
  - **✓7ᵗʰ S86.222** Laceration of muscle(s) and tendon(s) of anterior muscle group at lower leg level, **left** leg
  - **✓7ᵗʰ S86.229** Laceration of muscle(s) and tendon(s) of anterior muscle group at lower leg level, unspecified leg
- **✓6ᵗʰ S86.29 Other injury of muscle(s) and tendon(s) of anterior muscle group at lower leg level**
  - **✓7ᵗʰ S86.291** Other injury of muscle(s) and tendon(s) of anterior muscle group at lower leg level, **right** leg
  - **✓7ᵗʰ S86.292** Other injury of muscle(s) and tendon(s) of anterior muscle group at lower leg level, **left** leg
  - **✓7ᵗʰ S86.299** Other injury of muscle(s) and tendon(s) of anterior muscle group at lower leg level, unspecified leg

✓5ᵗʰ S86.3 Injury of muscle(s) and tendon(s) of peroneal muscle group at lower leg level
- **✓6ᵗʰ S86.30 Unspecified injury of muscle(s) and tendon(s) of peroneal muscle group at lower leg level**
  - **✓7ᵗʰ S86.301** Unspecified injury of muscle(s) and tendon(s) of peroneal muscle group at lower leg level, **right** leg
  - **✓7ᵗʰ S86.302** Unspecified injury of muscle(s) and tendon(s) of peroneal muscle group at lower leg level, **left** leg
  - **✓7ᵗʰ S86.309** Unspecified injury of muscle(s) and tendon(s) of peroneal muscle group at lower leg level, unspecified leg
- **✓6ᵗʰ S86.31 Strain of muscle(s) and tendon(s) of peroneal muscle group at lower leg level**
  - **✓7ᵗʰ S86.311** Strain of muscle(s) and tendon(s) of peroneal muscle group at lower leg level, **right** leg
  - **✓7ᵗʰ S86.312** Strain of muscle(s) and tendon(s) of peroneal muscle group at lower leg level, **left** leg
  - **✓7ᵗʰ S86.319** Strain of muscle(s) and tendon(s) of peroneal muscle group at lower leg level, unspecified leg

√6ᵗʰ **S86.32** Laceration of muscle(s) and tendon(s) of peroneal muscle group at lower leg level
- √7ᵗʰ **S86.321** Laceration of muscle(s) and tendon(s) of peroneal muscle group at lower leg level, right leg
- √7ᵗʰ **S86.322** Laceration of muscle(s) and tendon(s) of peroneal muscle group at lower leg level, left leg
- √7ᵗʰ **S86.329** Laceration of muscle(s) and tendon(s) of peroneal muscle group at lower leg level, unspecified leg

√6ᵗʰ **S86.39** Other injury of muscle(s) and tendon(s) of peroneal muscle group at lower leg level
- √7ᵗʰ **S86.391** Other injury of muscle(s) and tendon(s) of peroneal muscle group at lower leg level, right leg
- √7ᵗʰ **S86.392** Other injury of muscle(s) and tendon(s) of peroneal muscle group at lower leg level, left leg
- √7ᵗʰ **S86.399** Other injury of muscle(s) and tendon(s) of peroneal muscle group at lower leg level, unspecified leg

√5ᵗʰ **S86.8** Injury of other muscles and tendons at lower leg level

√6ᵗʰ **S86.80** Unspecified injury of other muscles and tendons at lower leg level
- √7ᵗʰ **S86.801** Unspecified injury of other muscle(s) and tendon(s) at lower leg level, right leg
- √7ᵗʰ **S86.802** Unspecified injury of other muscle(s) and tendon(s) at lower leg level, left leg
- √7ᵗʰ **S86.809** Unspecified injury of other muscle(s) and tendon(s) at lower leg level, unspecified leg

√6ᵗʰ **S86.81** Strain of other muscles and tendons at lower leg level
- √7ᵗʰ **S86.811** Strain of other muscle(s) and tendon(s) at lower leg level, right leg
- √7ᵗʰ **S86.812** Strain of other muscle(s) and tendon(s) at lower leg level, left leg
- √7ᵗʰ **S86.819** Strain of other muscle(s) and tendon(s) at lower leg level, unspecified leg

√6ᵗʰ **S86.82** Laceration of other muscles and tendons at lower leg level
- √7ᵗʰ **S86.821** Laceration of other muscle(s) and tendon(s) at lower leg level, right leg
- √7ᵗʰ **S86.822** Laceration of other muscle(s) and tendon(s) at lower leg level, left leg
- √7ᵗʰ **S86.829** Laceration of other muscle(s) and tendon(s) at lower leg level, unspecified leg

√6ᵗʰ **S86.89** Other injury of other muscles and tendons at lower leg level
- √7ᵗʰ **S86.891** Other injury of other muscle(s) and tendon(s) at lower leg level, right leg
- √7ᵗʰ **S86.892** Other injury of other muscle(s) and tendon(s) at lower leg level, left leg
- √7ᵗʰ **S86.899** Other injury of other muscle(s) and tendon(s) at lower leg level, unspecified leg

√5ᵗʰ **S86.9** Injury of unspecified muscle and tendon at lower leg level

√6ᵗʰ **S86.90** Unspecified injury of unspecified muscle and tendon at lower leg level
- √7ᵗʰ **S86.901** Unspecified injury of unspecified muscle(s) and tendon(s) at lower leg level, right leg
- √7ᵗʰ **S86.902** Unspecified injury of unspecified muscle(s) and tendon(s) at lower leg level, left leg
- √7ᵗʰ **S86.909** Unspecified injury of unspecified muscle(s) and tendon(s) at lower leg level, unspecified leg

√6ᵗʰ **S86.91** Strain of unspecified muscle and tendon at lower leg level
- √7ᵗʰ **S86.911** Strain of unspecified muscle(s) and tendon(s) at lower leg level, right leg
- √7ᵗʰ **S86.912** Strain of unspecified muscle(s) and tendon(s) at lower leg level, left leg
- √7ᵗʰ **S86.919** Strain of unspecified muscle(s) and tendon(s) at lower leg level, unspecified leg

√6ᵗʰ **S86.92** Laceration of unspecified muscle and tendon at lower leg level
- √7ᵗʰ **S86.921** Laceration of unspecified muscle(s) and tendon(s) at lower leg level, right leg

- √7ᵗʰ **S86.922** Laceration of unspecified muscle(s) and tendon(s) at lower leg level, left leg
- √7ᵗʰ **S86.929** Laceration of unspecified muscle(s) and tendon(s) at lower leg level, unspecified leg

√6ᵗʰ **S86.99** Other injury of unspecified muscle and tendon at lower leg level
- √7ᵗʰ **S86.991** Other injury of unspecified muscle(s) and tendon(s) at lower leg level, right leg
- √7ᵗʰ **S86.992** Other injury of unspecified muscle(s) and tendon(s) at lower leg level, left leg
- √7ᵗʰ **S86.999** Other injury of unspecified muscle(s) and tendon(s) at lower leg level, unspecified leg

√4ᵗʰ **S87** Crushing injury of lower leg

Use additional code(s) for all associated injuries
EXCLUDES 2   crushing injury of ankle and foot (S97.-)

The appropriate 7th character is to be added to each code from category S87.
- A   initial encounter
- D   subsequent encounter
- S   sequela

√5ᵗʰ **S87.0** Crushing injury of knee
- √x7ᵗʰ **S87.00** Crushing injury of unspecified knee
- √x7ᵗʰ **S87.01** Crushing injury of right knee
- √x7ᵗʰ **S87.02** Crushing injury of left knee

√5ᵗʰ **S87.8** Crushing injury of lower leg
- √x7ᵗʰ **S87.80** Crushing injury of unspecified lower leg
- √x7ᵗʰ **S87.81** Crushing injury of right lower leg
- √x7ᵗʰ **S87.82** Crushing injury of left lower leg

√4ᵗʰ **S88** Traumatic amputation of lower leg

An amputation not identified as partial or complete should be coded to complete
EXCLUDES 1   traumatic amputation of ankle and foot (S98.-)

The appropriate 7th character is to be added to each code from category S88.
- A   initial encounter
- D   subsequent encounter
- S   sequela

√5ᵗʰ **S88.0** Traumatic amputation at knee level

√6ᵗʰ **S88.01** Complete traumatic amputation at knee level
- √7ᵗʰ **S88.011** Complete traumatic amputation at knee level, right lower leg   HCC ESR COM
- √7ᵗʰ **S88.012** Complete traumatic amputation at knee level, left lower leg   HCC ESR COM
- √7ᵗʰ **S88.019** Complete traumatic amputation at knee level, unspecified lower leg   HCC ESR COM

√6ᵗʰ **S88.02** Partial traumatic amputation at knee level
- √7ᵗʰ **S88.021** Partial traumatic amputation at knee level, right lower leg   HCC ESR COM
- √7ᵗʰ **S88.022** Partial traumatic amputation at knee level, left lower leg   HCC ESR COM
- √7ᵗʰ **S88.029** Partial traumatic amputation at knee level, unspecified lower leg   HCC ESR COM

√5ᵗʰ **S88.1** Traumatic amputation at level between knee and ankle

√6ᵗʰ **S88.11** Complete traumatic amputation at level between knee and ankle
- √7ᵗʰ **S88.111** Complete traumatic amputation at level between knee and ankle, right lower leg   HCC ESR COM
- √7ᵗʰ **S88.112** Complete traumatic amputation at level between knee and ankle, left lower leg   HCC ESR COM
- √7ᵗʰ **S88.119** Complete traumatic amputation at level between knee and ankle, unspecified lower leg   HCC ESR COM

√6ᵗʰ **S88.12** Partial traumatic amputation at level between knee and ankle
- √7ᵗʰ **S88.121** Partial traumatic amputation at level between knee and ankle, right lower leg   HCC ESR COM
- √7ᵗʰ **S88.122** Partial traumatic amputation at level between knee and ankle, left lower leg   HCC ESR COM

Chapter 19. Injury, Poisoning and Certain Other Consequences of External Causes

S88.129–S89.221

✓7ᵗʰ **S88.129** Partial traumatic amputation at level between knee and ankle, unspecified lower leg   HCC ESR COM

✓5ᵗʰ **S88.9** Traumatic amputation of lower leg, level unspecified

  ✓6ᵗʰ **S88.91** Complete traumatic amputation of lower leg, level unspecified

    ✓7ᵗʰ **S88.911** Complete traumatic amputation of right lower leg, level unspecified   HCC ESR COM

    ✓7ᵗʰ **S88.912** Complete traumatic amputation of left lower leg, level unspecified   HCC ESR COM

    ✓7ᵗʰ **S88.919** Complete traumatic amputation of unspecified lower leg, level unspecified   HCC ESR COM

  ✓6ᵗʰ **S88.92** Partial traumatic amputation of lower leg, level unspecified

    ✓7ᵗʰ **S88.921** Partial traumatic amputation of right lower leg, level unspecified   HCC ESR COM

    ✓7ᵗʰ **S88.922** Partial traumatic amputation of left lower leg, level unspecified   HCC ESR COM

    ✓7ᵗʰ **S88.929** Partial traumatic amputation of unspecified lower leg, level unspecified   HCC ESR COM

✓4ᵗʰ **S89** Other and unspecified injuries of lower leg

> **NOTE**   A fracture not indicated as open or closed should be coded to closed.

> **EXCLUDES 2**   *other and unspecified injuries of ankle and foot (S99.-)*

AHA: 2018,2Q,12; 2018,1Q,3; 2015,3Q,37-39

The appropriate 7th character is to be added to each code from subcategories S89.Ø, S89.1, S89.2, and S89.3.
- A   initial encounter for closed fracture
- D   subsequent encounter for fracture with routine healing
- G   subsequent encounter for fracture with delayed healing
- K   subsequent encounter for fracture with nonunion
- P   subsequent encounter for fracture with malunion
- S   sequela

✓5ᵗʰ **S89.Ø** Physeal fracture of upper end of tibia

AHA: 2019,4Q,56

  ✓6ᵗʰ **S89.ØØ** Unspecified physeal fracture of upper end of tibia

    ✓7ᵗʰ **S89.ØØ1** Unspecified physeal fracture of upper end of right tibia   Q

    ✓7ᵗʰ **S89.ØØ2** Unspecified physeal fracture of upper end of left tibia   Q

    ✓7ᵗʰ **S89.ØØ9** Unspecified physeal fracture of upper end of unspecified tibia   Q

  ✓6ᵗʰ **S89.Ø1** Salter-Harris Type I physeal fracture of upper end of tibia

    ✓7ᵗʰ **S89.Ø11** Salter-Harris Type I physeal fracture of upper end of right tibia   Q

    ✓7ᵗʰ **S89.Ø12** Salter-Harris Type I physeal fracture of upper end of left tibia   Q

    ✓7ᵗʰ **S89.Ø19** Salter-Harris Type I physeal fracture of upper end of unspecified tibia   Q

  ✓6ᵗʰ **S89.Ø2** Salter-Harris Type II physeal fracture of upper end of tibia

    ✓7ᵗʰ **S89.Ø21** Salter-Harris Type II physeal fracture of upper end of right tibia   Q

    ✓7ᵗʰ **S89.Ø22** Salter-Harris Type II physeal fracture of upper end of left tibia   Q

    ✓7ᵗʰ **S89.Ø29** Salter-Harris Type II physeal fracture of upper end of unspecified tibia   Q

  ✓6ᵗʰ **S89.Ø3** Salter-Harris Type III physeal fracture of upper end of tibia

    ✓7ᵗʰ **S89.Ø31** Salter-Harris Type III physeal fracture of upper end of right tibia   Q

    ✓7ᵗʰ **S89.Ø32** Salter-Harris Type III physeal fracture of upper end of left tibia   Q

    ✓7ᵗʰ **S89.Ø39** Salter-Harris Type III physeal fracture of upper end of unspecified tibia   Q

  ✓6ᵗʰ **S89.Ø4** Salter-Harris Type IV physeal fracture of upper end of tibia

    ✓7ᵗʰ **S89.Ø41** Salter-Harris Type IV physeal fracture of upper end of right tibia   Q

    ✓7ᵗʰ **S89.Ø42** Salter-Harris Type IV physeal fracture of upper end of left tibia   Q

    ✓7ᵗʰ **S89.Ø49** Salter-Harris Type IV physeal fracture of upper end of unspecified tibia   Q

✓6ᵗʰ **S89.Ø9** Other physeal fracture of upper end of tibia

    ✓7ᵗʰ **S89.Ø91** Other physeal fracture of upper end of right tibia   Q

    ✓7ᵗʰ **S89.Ø92** Other physeal fracture of upper end of left tibia   Q

    ✓7ᵗʰ **S89.Ø99** Other physeal fracture of upper end of unspecified tibia   Q

✓5ᵗʰ **S89.1** Physeal fracture of lower end of tibia

AHA: 2019,4Q,56

  ✓6ᵗʰ **S89.1Ø** Unspecified physeal fracture of lower end of tibia

    ✓7ᵗʰ **S89.1Ø1** Unspecified physeal fracture of lower end of right tibia   Q

    ✓7ᵗʰ **S89.1Ø2** Unspecified physeal fracture of lower end of left tibia   Q

    ✓7ᵗʰ **S89.1Ø9** Unspecified physeal fracture of lower end of unspecified tibia   Q

  ✓6ᵗʰ **S89.11** Salter-Harris Type I physeal fracture of lower end of tibia

    ✓7ᵗʰ **S89.111** Salter-Harris Type I physeal fracture of lower end of right tibia   Q

    ✓7ᵗʰ **S89.112** Salter-Harris Type I physeal fracture of lower end of left tibia   Q

    ✓7ᵗʰ **S89.119** Salter-Harris Type I physeal fracture of lower end of unspecified tibia   Q

  ✓6ᵗʰ **S89.12** Salter-Harris Type II physeal fracture of lower end of tibia

    ✓7ᵗʰ **S89.121** Salter-Harris Type II physeal fracture of lower end of right tibia   Q

    ✓7ᵗʰ **S89.122** Salter-Harris Type II physeal fracture of lower end of left tibia   Q

    ✓7ᵗʰ **S89.129** Salter-Harris Type II physeal fracture of lower end of unspecified tibia   Q

  ✓6ᵗʰ **S89.13** Salter-Harris Type III physeal fracture of lower end of tibia

> **EXCLUDES 1**   *fracture of medial malleolus (adult) (S82.5-)*

    ✓7ᵗʰ **S89.131** Salter-Harris Type III physeal fracture of lower end of right tibia   Q

    ✓7ᵗʰ **S89.132** Salter-Harris Type III physeal fracture of lower end of left tibia   Q

    ✓7ᵗʰ **S89.139** Salter-Harris Type III physeal fracture of lower end of unspecified tibia   Q

  ✓6ᵗʰ **S89.14** Salter-Harris Type IV physeal fracture of lower end of tibia

> **EXCLUDES 1**   *fracture of medial malleolus (adult) (S82.5-)*

    ✓7ᵗʰ **S89.141** Salter-Harris Type IV physeal fracture of lower end of right tibia   Q

    ✓7ᵗʰ **S89.142** Salter-Harris Type IV physeal fracture of lower end of left tibia   Q

    ✓7ᵗʰ **S89.149** Salter-Harris Type IV physeal fracture of lower end of unspecified tibia   Q

  ✓6ᵗʰ **S89.19** Other physeal fracture of lower end of tibia

    ✓7ᵗʰ **S89.191** Other physeal fracture of lower end of right tibia   Q

    ✓7ᵗʰ **S89.192** Other physeal fracture of lower end of left tibia   Q

    ✓7ᵗʰ **S89.199** Other physeal fracture of lower end of unspecified tibia   Q

✓5ᵗʰ **S89.2** Physeal fracture of upper end of fibula

AHA: 2019,4Q,56

  ✓6ᵗʰ **S89.2Ø** Unspecified physeal fracture of upper end of fibula

    ✓7ᵗʰ **S89.2Ø1** Unspecified physeal fracture of upper end of right fibula   Q

    ✓7ᵗʰ **S89.2Ø2** Unspecified physeal fracture of upper end of left fibula   Q

    ✓7ᵗʰ **S89.2Ø9** Unspecified physeal fracture of upper end of unspecified fibula   Q

  ✓6ᵗʰ **S89.21** Salter-Harris Type I physeal fracture of upper end of fibula

    ✓7ᵗʰ **S89.211** Salter-Harris Type I physeal fracture of upper end of right fibula   Q

    ✓7ᵗʰ **S89.212** Salter-Harris Type I physeal fracture of upper end of left fibula   Q

    ✓7ᵗʰ **S89.219** Salter-Harris Type I physeal fracture of upper end of unspecified fibula   Q

  ✓6ᵗʰ **S89.22** Salter-Harris Type II physeal fracture of upper end of fibula

    ✓7ᵗʰ **S89.221** Salter-Harris Type II physeal fracture of upper end of right fibula   Q

√7ᵗʰ **S89.222** Salter-Harris Type II physeal fracture of upper end of **left** fibula ◳

√7ᵗʰ **S89.229** Salter-Harris Type II physeal fracture of upper end of unspecified fibula ◳

√6ᵗʰ **S89.29** Other physeal fracture of upper end of fibula

√7ᵗʰ **S89.291** Other physeal fracture of upper end of **right** fibula ◳

√7ᵗʰ **S89.292** Other physeal fracture of upper end of **left** fibula ◳

√7ᵗʰ **S89.299** Other physeal fracture of upper end of unspecified fibula ◳

√5ᵗʰ **S89.3** **Physeal fracture of lower end of fibula**

AHA: 2019,4Q,56

√6ᵗʰ **S89.30** Unspecified physeal fracture of lower end of fibula

√7ᵗʰ **S89.301** Unspecified physeal fracture of lower end of **right** fibula ◳

√7ᵗʰ **S89.302** Unspecified physeal fracture of lower end of **left** fibula ◳

√7ᵗʰ **S89.309** Unspecified physeal fracture of lower end of unspecified fibula ◳

√6ᵗʰ **S89.31** Salter-Harris Type I physeal fracture of lower end of fibula

√7ᵗʰ **S89.311** Salter-Harris Type I physeal fracture of lower end of **right** fibula ◳

√7ᵗʰ **S89.312** Salter-Harris Type I physeal fracture of lower end of **left** fibula ◳

√7ᵗʰ **S89.319** Salter-Harris Type I physeal fracture of lower end of unspecified fibula ◳

√6ᵗʰ **S89.32** Salter-Harris Type II physeal fracture of lower end of fibula

√7ᵗʰ **S89.321** Salter-Harris Type II physeal fracture of lower end of **right** fibula ◳

√7ᵗʰ **S89.322** Salter-Harris Type II physeal fracture of lower end of **left** fibula ◳

√7ᵗʰ **S89.329** Salter-Harris Type II physeal fracture of lower end of unspecified fibula ◳

√6ᵗʰ **S89.39** Other physeal fracture of lower end of fibula

√7ᵗʰ **S89.391** Other physeal fracture of lower end of **right** fibula ◳

√7ᵗʰ **S89.392** Other physeal fracture of lower end of **left** fibula ◳

√7ᵗʰ **S89.399** Other physeal fracture of lower end of unspecified fibula ◳

√5ᵗʰ **S89.8** Other specified injuries of lower leg

The appropriate 7th character is to be added to each code in subcategory S89.8.
A initial encounter
D subsequent encounter
S sequela

√x7ᵗʰ **S89.80** Other specified injuries of unspecified lower leg

√x7ᵗʰ **S89.81** Other specified injuries of **right** lower leg

√x7ᵗʰ **S89.82** Other specified injuries of **left** lower leg

√5ᵗʰ **S89.9** Unspecified injury of lower leg

The appropriate 7th character is to be added to each code in subcategory S89.9.
A initial encounter
D subsequent encounter
S sequela

√x7ᵗʰ **S89.90** Unspecified injury of unspecified lower leg

√x7ᵗʰ **S89.91** Unspecified injury of **right** lower leg

√x7ᵗʰ **S89.92** Unspecified injury of **left** lower leg

Injuries to the ankle and foot (S90-S99)

EXCLUDES 2 burns and corrosions (T20-T32)
fracture of ankle and malleolus (S82.-)
frostbite (T33-T34)
insect bite or sting, venomous (T63.4)

√4ᵗʰ **S90** **Superficial injury of ankle, foot and toes**

The appropriate 7th character is to be added to each code from category S90.
A initial encounter
D subsequent encounter
S sequela

√5ᵗʰ **S90.0** Contusion of ankle

√x7ᵗʰ **S90.00** Contusion of unspecified ankle

√x7ᵗʰ **S90.01** Contusion of **right** ankle

√x7ᵗʰ **S90.02** Contusion of **left** ankle

√5ᵗʰ **S90.1** Contusion of toe without damage to nail

√6ᵗʰ **S90.11** Contusion of **great** toe without damage to nail

√7ᵗʰ **S90.111** Contusion of **right** great toe without damage to nail

√7ᵗʰ **S90.112** Contusion of **left** great toe without damage to nail

√7ᵗʰ **S90.119** Contusion of unspecified great toe without damage to nail

√6ᵗʰ **S90.12** Contusion of **lesser** toe without damage to nail

√7ᵗʰ **S90.121** Contusion of **right** lesser toe(s) without damage to nail

√7ᵗʰ **S90.122** Contusion of **left** lesser toe(s) without damage to nail

√7ᵗʰ **S90.129** Contusion of unspecified lesser toe(s) without damage to nail
Contusion of toe NOS

√5ᵗʰ **S90.2** Contusion of toe with damage to nail

√6ᵗʰ **S90.21** Contusion of **great** toe with damage to nail

√7ᵗʰ **S90.211** Contusion of **right** great toe with damage to nail

√7ᵗʰ **S90.212** Contusion of **left** great toe with damage to nail

√7ᵗʰ **S90.219** Contusion of unspecified great toe with damage to nail

√6ᵗʰ **S90.22** Contusion of **lesser** toe with damage to nail

√7ᵗʰ **S90.221** Contusion of **right** lesser toe(s) with damage to nail

√7ᵗʰ **S90.222** Contusion of **left** lesser toe(s) with damage to nail

√7ᵗʰ **S90.229** Contusion of unspecified lesser toe(s) with damage to nail

√5ᵗʰ **S90.3** Contusion of foot

EXCLUDES 2 contusion of toes (S90.1-, S90.2-)

√x7ᵗʰ **S90.30** Contusion of unspecified foot
Contusion of foot NOS

√x7ᵗʰ **S90.31** Contusion of **right** foot

√x7ᵗʰ **S90.32** Contusion of **left** foot

√5ᵗʰ **S90.4** Other superficial injuries of toe

√6ᵗʰ **S90.41** Abrasion of toe

√7ᵗʰ **S90.411** Abrasion, **right** great toe

√7ᵗʰ **S90.412** Abrasion, **left** great toe

√7ᵗʰ **S90.413** Abrasion, unspecified great toe

√7ᵗʰ **S90.414** Abrasion, **right** lesser toe(s)

√7ᵗʰ **S90.415** Abrasion, **left** lesser toe(s)

√7ᵗʰ **S90.416** Abrasion, unspecified lesser toe(s)

√6ᵗʰ **S90.42** Blister (nonthermal) of toe

√7ᵗʰ **S90.421** Blister (nonthermal), **right** great toe

√7ᵗʰ **S90.422** Blister (nonthermal), **left** great toe

√7ᵗʰ **S90.423** Blister (nonthermal), unspecified great toe

√7ᵗʰ **S90.424** Blister (nonthermal), **right** lesser toe(s)

√7ᵗʰ **S90.425** Blister (nonthermal), **left** lesser toe(s)

√7ᵗʰ **S90.426** Blister (nonthermal), unspecified lesser toe(s)

√6ᵗʰ **S90.44** External constriction of toe
Hair tourniquet syndrome of toe

√7ᵗʰ **S90.441** External constriction, **right** great toe

√7ᵗʰ **S90.442** External constriction, **left** great toe

√7ᵗʰ **S90.443** External constriction, unspecified great toe

√7ᵗʰ **S90.444** External constriction, **right** lesser toe(s)

√7ᵗʰ **S90.445** External constriction, **left** lesser toe(s)

√7ᵗʰ **S90.446** External constriction, unspecified lesser toe(s)

√6ᵗʰ **S90.45** Superficial foreign body of toe
Splinter in the toe

√7ᵗʰ **S90.451** Superficial foreign body, **right** great toe

√7ᵗʰ **S90.452** Superficial foreign body, **left** great toe

√7ᵗʰ **S90.453** Superficial foreign body, unspecified great toe

√7ᵗʰ **S90.454** Superficial foreign body, **right** lesser toe(s)

√7ᵗʰ **S90.455** Superficial foreign body, left lesser toe(s)

√7ᵗʰ **S90.456** Superficial foreign body, unspecified lesser toe(s)

√6ᵗʰ **S90.46** Insect bite (nonvenomous) of toe

√7ᵗʰ **S90.461** Insect bite (nonvenomous), right great toe

√7ᵗʰ **S90.462** Insect bite (nonvenomous), left great toe

√7ᵗʰ **S90.463** Insect bite (nonvenomous), unspecified great toe

√7ᵗʰ **S90.464** Insect bite (nonvenomous), right lesser toe(s)

√7ᵗʰ **S90.465** Insect bite (nonvenomous), left lesser toe(s)

√7ᵗʰ **S90.466** Insect bite (nonvenomous), unspecified lesser toe(s)

√6ᵗʰ **S90.47** Other superficial bite of toe

     EXCLUDES 1   open bite of toe (S91.15-, S91.25-)

√7ᵗʰ **S90.471** Other superficial bite of right great toe

√7ᵗʰ **S90.472** Other superficial bite of left great toe

√7ᵗʰ **S90.473** Other superficial bite of unspecified great toe

√7ᵗʰ **S90.474** Other superficial bite of right lesser toe(s)

√7ᵗʰ **S90.475** Other superficial bite of left lesser toe(s)

√7ᵗʰ **S90.476** Other superficial bite of unspecified lesser toe(s)

√5ᵗʰ **S90.5** Other superficial injuries of ankle

√6ᵗʰ **S90.51** Abrasion of ankle

√7ᵗʰ **S90.511** Abrasion, right ankle

√7ᵗʰ **S90.512** Abrasion, left ankle

√7ᵗʰ **S90.519** Abrasion, unspecified ankle

√6ᵗʰ **S90.52** Blister (nonthermal) of ankle

√7ᵗʰ **S90.521** Blister (nonthermal), right ankle

√7ᵗʰ **S90.522** Blister (nonthermal), left ankle

√7ᵗʰ **S90.529** Blister (nonthermal), unspecified ankle

√6ᵗʰ **S90.54** External constriction of ankle

√7ᵗʰ **S90.541** External constriction, right ankle

√7ᵗʰ **S90.542** External constriction, left ankle

√7ᵗʰ **S90.549** External constriction, unspecified ankle

√6ᵗʰ **S90.55** Superficial foreign body of ankle

     Splinter in the ankle

√7ᵗʰ **S90.551** Superficial foreign body, right ankle

√7ᵗʰ **S90.552** Superficial foreign body, left ankle

√7ᵗʰ **S90.559** Superficial foreign body, unspecified ankle

√6ᵗʰ **S90.56** Insect bite (nonvenomous) of ankle

√7ᵗʰ **S90.561** Insect bite (nonvenomous), right ankle

√7ᵗʰ **S90.562** Insect bite (nonvenomous), left ankle

√7ᵗʰ **S90.569** Insect bite (nonvenomous), unspecified ankle

√6ᵗʰ **S90.57** Other superficial bite of ankle

     EXCLUDES 1   open bite of ankle (S91.05-)

√7ᵗʰ **S90.571** Other superficial bite of ankle, right ankle

√7ᵗʰ **S90.572** Other superficial bite of ankle, left ankle

√7ᵗʰ **S90.579** Other superficial bite of ankle, unspecified ankle

√5ᵗʰ **S90.8** Other superficial injuries of foot

√6ᵗʰ **S90.81** Abrasion of foot

√7ᵗʰ **S90.811** Abrasion, right foot

√7ᵗʰ **S90.812** Abrasion, left foot

√7ᵗʰ **S90.819** Abrasion, unspecified foot

√6ᵗʰ **S90.82** Blister (nonthermal) of foot

√7ᵗʰ **S90.821** Blister (nonthermal), right foot

√7ᵗʰ **S90.822** Blister (nonthermal), left foot

√7ᵗʰ **S90.829** Blister (nonthermal), unspecified foot

√6ᵗʰ **S90.84** External constriction of foot

√7ᵗʰ **S90.841** External constriction, right foot

√7ᵗʰ **S90.842** External constriction, left foot

√7ᵗʰ **S90.849** External constriction, unspecified foot

√6ᵗʰ **S90.85** Superficial foreign body of foot

     Splinter in the foot

√7ᵗʰ **S90.851** Superficial foreign body, right foot

√7ᵗʰ **S90.852** Superficial foreign body, left foot

√7ᵗʰ **S90.859** Superficial foreign body, unspecified foot

√6ᵗʰ **S90.86** Insect bite (nonvenomous) of foot

√7ᵗʰ **S90.861** Insect bite (nonvenomous), right foot

√7ᵗʰ **S90.862** Insect bite (nonvenomous), left foot

√7ᵗʰ **S90.869** Insect bite (nonvenomous), unspecified foot

√6ᵗʰ **S90.87** Other superficial bite of foot

     EXCLUDES 1   open bite of foot (S91.35-)

√7ᵗʰ **S90.871** Other superficial bite of right foot

√7ᵗʰ **S90.872** Other superficial bite of left foot

√7ᵗʰ **S90.879** Other superficial bite of unspecified foot

√5ᵗʰ **S90.9** Unspecified superficial injury of ankle, foot and toe

√6ᵗʰ **S90.91** Unspecified superficial injury of ankle

√7ᵗʰ **S90.911** Unspecified superficial injury of right ankle

√7ᵗʰ **S90.912** Unspecified superficial injury of left ankle

√7ᵗʰ **S90.919** Unspecified superficial injury of unspecified ankle

√6ᵗʰ **S90.92** Unspecified superficial injury of foot

√7ᵗʰ **S90.921** Unspecified superficial injury of right foot

√7ᵗʰ **S90.922** Unspecified superficial injury of left foot

√7ᵗʰ **S90.929** Unspecified superficial injury of unspecified foot

√6ᵗʰ **S90.93** Unspecified superficial injury of toes

√7ᵗʰ **S90.931** Unspecified superficial injury of right great toe

√7ᵗʰ **S90.932** Unspecified superficial injury of left great toe

√7ᵗʰ **S90.933** Unspecified superficial injury of unspecified great toe

√7ᵗʰ **S90.934** Unspecified superficial injury of right lesser toe(s)

√7ᵗʰ **S90.935** Unspecified superficial injury of left lesser toe(s)

√7ᵗʰ **S90.936** Unspecified superficial injury of unspecified lesser toe(s)

√4ᵗʰ **S91** Open wound of ankle, foot and toes

     Code also any associated wound infection

     EXCLUDES 1   open fracture of ankle, foot and toes (S92.- with 7th character B)

                   traumatic amputation of ankle and foot (S98.-)

     AHA: 2021,1Q,7

The appropriate 7th character is to be added to each code from category S91.
A   initial encounter
D   subsequent encounter
S   sequela

√5ᵗʰ **S91.0** Open wound of ankle

√6ᵗʰ **S91.00** Unspecified open wound of ankle

√7ᵗʰ **S91.001** Unspecified open wound, right ankle

√7ᵗʰ **S91.002** Unspecified open wound, left ankle

√7ᵗʰ **S91.009** Unspecified open wound, unspecified ankle

√6ᵗʰ **S91.01** Laceration without foreign body of ankle

√7ᵗʰ **S91.011** Laceration without foreign body, right ankle

√7ᵗʰ **S91.012** Laceration without foreign body, left ankle

√7ᵗʰ **S91.019** Laceration without foreign body, unspecified ankle

√6ᵗʰ **S91.02** Laceration with foreign body of ankle

√7ᵗʰ **S91.021** Laceration with foreign body, right ankle

√7ᵗʰ **S91.022** Laceration with foreign body, left ankle

√7ᵗʰ **S91.029** Laceration with foreign body, unspecified ankle

√6ᵗʰ **S91.03** Puncture wound without foreign body of ankle

√7ᵗʰ **S91.031** Puncture wound without foreign body, right ankle

√7ᵗʰ **S91.032** Puncture wound without foreign body, left ankle

√7ᵗʰ **S91.039** Puncture wound without foreign body, unspecified ankle

√6ᵗʰ **S91.04** Puncture wound with foreign body of ankle

    √7ᵗʰ **S91.041** Puncture wound with foreign body, right ankle

    √7ᵗʰ **S91.042** Puncture wound with foreign body, left ankle

    √7ᵗʰ **S91.049** Puncture wound with foreign body, unspecified ankle

√6ᵗʰ **S91.05** Open bite of ankle

    EXCLUDES 1   superficial bite of ankle (S90.56-, S90.57-)

    √7ᵗʰ **S91.051** Open bite, right ankle

    √7ᵗʰ **S91.052** Open bite, left ankle

    √7ᵗʰ **S91.059** Open bite, unspecified ankle

√5ᵗʰ **S91.1** Open wound of toe without damage to nail

√6ᵗʰ **S91.10** Unspecified open wound of toe without damage to nail

    √7ᵗʰ **S91.101** Unspecified open wound of right great toe without damage to nail

    √7ᵗʰ **S91.102** Unspecified open wound of left great toe without damage to nail

    √7ᵗʰ **S91.103** Unspecified open wound of unspecified great toe without damage to nail

    √7ᵗʰ **S91.104** Unspecified open wound of right lesser toe(s) without damage to nail

    √7ᵗʰ **S91.105** Unspecified open wound of left lesser toe(s) without damage to nail

    √7ᵗʰ **S91.106** Unspecified open wound of unspecified lesser toe(s) without damage to nail

    √7ᵗʰ **S91.109** Unspecified open wound of unspecified toe(s) without damage to nail

√6ᵗʰ **S91.11** Laceration without foreign body of toe without damage to nail

    √7ᵗʰ **S91.111** Laceration without foreign body of right great toe without damage to nail

    √7ᵗʰ **S91.112** Laceration without foreign body of left great toe without damage to nail

    √7ᵗʰ **S91.113** Laceration without foreign body of unspecified great toe without damage to nail

    √7ᵗʰ **S91.114** Laceration without foreign body of right lesser toe(s) without damage to nail

    √7ᵗʰ **S91.115** Laceration without foreign body of left lesser toe(s) without damage to nail

    √7ᵗʰ **S91.116** Laceration without foreign body of unspecified lesser toe(s) without damage to nail

    √7ᵗʰ **S91.119** Laceration without foreign body of unspecified toe without damage to nail

√6ᵗʰ **S91.12** Laceration with foreign body of toe without damage to nail

    √7ᵗʰ **S91.121** Laceration with foreign body of right great toe without damage to nail

    √7ᵗʰ **S91.122** Laceration with foreign body of left great toe without damage to nail

    √7ᵗʰ **S91.123** Laceration with foreign body of unspecified great toe without damage to nail

    √7ᵗʰ **S91.124** Laceration with foreign body of right lesser toe(s) without damage to nail

    √7ᵗʰ **S91.125** Laceration with foreign body of left lesser toe(s) without damage to nail

    √7ᵗʰ **S91.126** Laceration with foreign body of unspecified lesser toe(s) without damage to nail

    √7ᵗʰ **S91.129** Laceration with foreign body of unspecified toe(s) without damage to nail

√6ᵗʰ **S91.13** Puncture wound without foreign body of toe without damage to nail

    √7ᵗʰ **S91.131** Puncture wound without foreign body of right great toe without damage to nail

    √7ᵗʰ **S91.132** Puncture wound without foreign body of left great toe without damage to nail

    √7ᵗʰ **S91.133** Puncture wound without foreign body of unspecified great toe without damage to nail

    √7ᵗʰ **S91.134** Puncture wound without foreign body of right lesser toe(s) without damage to nail

    √7ᵗʰ **S91.135** Puncture wound without foreign body of left lesser toe(s) without damage to nail

    √7ᵗʰ **S91.136** Puncture wound without foreign body of unspecified lesser toe(s) without damage to nail

    √7ᵗʰ **S91.139** Puncture wound without foreign body of unspecified toe(s) without damage to nail

√6ᵗʰ **S91.14** Puncture wound with foreign body of toe without damage to nail

    √7ᵗʰ **S91.141** Puncture wound with foreign body of right great toe without damage to nail

    √7ᵗʰ **S91.142** Puncture wound with foreign body of left great toe without damage to nail

    √7ᵗʰ **S91.143** Puncture wound with foreign body of unspecified great toe without damage to nail

    √7ᵗʰ **S91.144** Puncture wound with foreign body of right lesser toe(s) without damage to nail

    √7ᵗʰ **S91.145** Puncture wound with foreign body of left lesser toe(s) without damage to nail

    √7ᵗʰ **S91.146** Puncture wound with foreign body of unspecified lesser toe(s) without damage to nail

    √7ᵗʰ **S91.149** Puncture wound with foreign body of unspecified toe(s) without damage to nail

√6ᵗʰ **S91.15** Open bite of toe without damage to nail

    Bite of toe NOS

    EXCLUDES 1   superficial bite of toe (S90.46-, S90.47-)

    √7ᵗʰ **S91.151** Open bite of right great toe without damage to nail

    √7ᵗʰ **S91.152** Open bite of left great toe without damage to nail

    √7ᵗʰ **S91.153** Open bite of unspecified great toe without damage to nail

    √7ᵗʰ **S91.154** Open bite of right lesser toe(s) without damage to nail

    √7ᵗʰ **S91.155** Open bite of left lesser toe(s) without damage to nail

    √7ᵗʰ **S91.156** Open bite of unspecified lesser toe(s) without damage to nail

    √7ᵗʰ **S91.159** Open bite of unspecified toe(s) without damage to nail

√5ᵗʰ **S91.2** Open wound of toe with damage to nail

√6ᵗʰ **S91.20** Unspecified open wound of toe with damage to nail

    √7ᵗʰ **S91.201** Unspecified open wound of right great toe with damage to nail

    √7ᵗʰ **S91.202** Unspecified open wound of left great toe with damage to nail

    √7ᵗʰ **S91.203** Unspecified open wound of unspecified great toe with damage to nail

    √7ᵗʰ **S91.204** Unspecified open wound of right lesser toe(s) with damage to nail

    √7ᵗʰ **S91.205** Unspecified open wound of left lesser toe(s) with damage to nail

    √7ᵗʰ **S91.206** Unspecified open wound of unspecified lesser toe(s) with damage to nail

    √7ᵗʰ **S91.209** Unspecified open wound of unspecified toe(s) with damage to nail

√6ᵗʰ **S91.21** Laceration without foreign body of toe with damage to nail

    √7ᵗʰ **S91.211** Laceration without foreign body of right great toe with damage to nail

    √7ᵗʰ **S91.212** Laceration without foreign body of left great toe with damage to nail

    √7ᵗʰ **S91.213** Laceration without foreign body of unspecified great toe with damage to nail

    √7ᵗʰ **S91.214** Laceration without foreign body of right lesser toe(s) with damage to nail

    √7ᵗʰ **S91.215** Laceration without foreign body of left lesser toe(s) with damage to nail

    √7ᵗʰ **S91.216** Laceration without foreign body of unspecified lesser toe(s) with damage to nail

    √7ᵗʰ **S91.219** Laceration without foreign body of unspecified toe(s) with damage to nail

√6ᵗʰ **S91.22** Laceration with foreign body of toe with damage to nail

    √7ᵗʰ **S91.221** Laceration with foreign body of right great toe with damage to nail

    √7ᵗʰ **S91.222** Laceration with foreign body of left great toe with damage to nail

    √7ᵗʰ **S91.223** Laceration with foreign body of unspecified great toe with damage to nail

    √7ᵗʰ **S91.224** Laceration with foreign body of right lesser toe(s) with damage to nail

    √7ᵗʰ **S91.225** Laceration with foreign body of left lesser toe(s) with damage to nail

√7ᵗʰ **S91.226** Laceration with foreign body of unspecified lesser toe(s) with damage to nail

√7ᵗʰ **S91.229** Laceration with foreign body of unspecified toe(s) with damage to nail

√6ᵗʰ **S91.23** Puncture wound without foreign body of toe with damage to nail

√7ᵗʰ **S91.231** Puncture wound without foreign body of right great toe with damage to nail

√7ᵗʰ **S91.232** Puncture wound without foreign body of left great toe with damage to nail

√7ᵗʰ **S91.233** Puncture wound without foreign body of unspecified great toe with damage to nail

√7ᵗʰ **S91.234** Puncture wound without foreign body of right lesser toe(s) with damage to nail

√7ᵗʰ **S91.235** Puncture wound without foreign body of left lesser toe(s) with damage to nail

√7ᵗʰ **S91.236** Puncture wound without foreign body of unspecified lesser toe(s) with damage to nail

√7ᵗʰ **S91.239** Puncture wound without foreign body of unspecified toe(s) with damage to nail

√6ᵗʰ **S91.24** Puncture wound with foreign body of toe with damage to nail

√7ᵗʰ **S91.241** Puncture wound with foreign body of right great toe with damage to nail

√7ᵗʰ **S91.242** Puncture wound with foreign body of left great toe with damage to nail

√7ᵗʰ **S91.243** Puncture wound with foreign body of unspecified great toe with damage to nail

√7ᵗʰ **S91.244** Puncture wound with foreign body of right lesser toe(s) with damage to nail

√7ᵗʰ **S91.245** Puncture wound with foreign body of left lesser toe(s) with damage to nail

√7ᵗʰ **S91.246** Puncture wound with foreign body of unspecified lesser toe(s) with damage to nail

√7ᵗʰ **S91.249** Puncture wound with foreign body of unspecified toe(s) with damage to nail

√6ᵗʰ **S91.25** Open bite of toe with damage to nail

Bite of toe with damage to nail NOS

EXCLUDES 1   superficial bite of toe (S90.46-, S90.47-)

√7ᵗʰ **S91.251** Open bite of right great toe with damage to nail

√7ᵗʰ **S91.252** Open bite of left great toe with damage to nail

√7ᵗʰ **S91.253** Open bite of unspecified great toe with damage to nail

√7ᵗʰ **S91.254** Open bite of right lesser toe(s) with damage to nail

√7ᵗʰ **S91.255** Open bite of left lesser toe(s) with damage to nail

√7ᵗʰ **S91.256** Open bite of unspecified lesser toe(s) with damage to nail

√7ᵗʰ **S91.259** Open bite of unspecified toe(s) with damage to nail

√5ᵗʰ **S91.3** Open wound of foot

√6ᵗʰ **S91.30** Unspecified open wound of foot

√7ᵗʰ **S91.301** Unspecified open wound, right foot

√7ᵗʰ **S91.302** Unspecified open wound, left foot

√7ᵗʰ **S91.309** Unspecified open wound, unspecified foot

√6ᵗʰ **S91.31** Laceration without foreign body of foot

√7ᵗʰ **S91.311** Laceration without foreign body, right foot

√7ᵗʰ **S91.312** Laceration without foreign body, left foot

√7ᵗʰ **S91.319** Laceration without foreign body, unspecified foot

√6ᵗʰ **S91.32** Laceration with foreign body of foot

√7ᵗʰ **S91.321** Laceration with foreign body, right foot

√7ᵗʰ **S91.322** Laceration with foreign body, left foot

√7ᵗʰ **S91.329** Laceration with foreign body, unspecified foot

√6ᵗʰ **S91.33** Puncture wound without foreign body of foot

√7ᵗʰ **S91.331** Puncture wound without foreign body, right foot

√7ᵗʰ **S91.332** Puncture wound without foreign body, left foot

√7ᵗʰ **S91.339** Puncture wound without foreign body, unspecified foot

√6ᵗʰ **S91.34** Puncture wound with foreign body of foot

√7ᵗʰ **S91.341** Puncture wound with foreign body, right foot

√7ᵗʰ **S91.342** Puncture wound with foreign body, left foot

√7ᵗʰ **S91.349** Puncture wound with foreign body, unspecified foot

√6ᵗʰ **S91.35** Open bite of foot

EXCLUDES 1   superficial bite of foot (S90.86-, S90.87-)

√7ᵗʰ **S91.351** Open bite, right foot

√7ᵗʰ **S91.352** Open bite, left foot

√7ᵗʰ **S91.359** Open bite, unspecified foot

√4ᵗʰ **S92 Fracture of foot and toe, except ankle**

NOTE A fracture not indicated as displaced or nondisplaced should be coded to displaced

A fracture not indicated as open or closed should be coded to closed.

EXCLUDES 2   fracture of ankle (S82.-)
fracture of malleolus (S82.-)
traumatic amputation of ankle and foot (S98.-)

AHA: 2018,2Q,12; 2015,3Q,37-39

The appropriate 7th character is to be added to each code from category S92.
A   initial encounter for closed fracture
B   initial encounter for open fracture
D   subsequent encounter for fracture with routine healing
G   subsequent encounter for fracture with delayed healing
K   subsequent encounter for fracture with nonunion
P   subsequent encounter for fracture with malunion
S   sequela

√5ᵗʰ **S92.0** Fracture of calcaneus

Heel bone
Os calcis
EXCLUDES 2   physeal fracture of calcaneus (S99.0-)

√6ᵗʰ **S92.00** Unspecified fracture of calcaneus

√7ᵗʰ **S92.001** Unspecified fracture of right calcaneus   Q

√7ᵗʰ **S92.002** Unspecified fracture of left calcaneus   Q

√7ᵗʰ **S92.009** Unspecified fracture of unspecified calcaneus   Q

√6ᵗʰ **S92.01** Fracture of body of calcaneus

√7ᵗʰ **S92.011** Displaced fracture of body of right calcaneus   Q

√7ᵗʰ **S92.012** Displaced fracture of body of left calcaneus   Q

√7ᵗʰ **S92.013** Displaced fracture of body of unspecified calcaneus   Q

√7ᵗʰ **S92.014** Nondisplaced fracture of body of right calcaneus   Q

√7ᵗʰ **S92.015** Nondisplaced fracture of body of left calcaneus   Q

√7ᵗʰ **S92.016** Nondisplaced fracture of body of unspecified calcaneus   Q

√6ᵗʰ **S92.02** Fracture of anterior process of calcaneus

√7ᵗʰ **S92.021** Displaced fracture of anterior process of right calcaneus   Q

√7ᵗʰ **S92.022** Displaced fracture of anterior process of left calcaneus   Q

√7ᵗʰ **S92.023** Displaced fracture of anterior process of unspecified calcaneus   Q

√7ᵗʰ **S92.024** Nondisplaced fracture of anterior process of right calcaneus   Q

√7ᵗʰ **S92.025** Nondisplaced fracture of anterior process of left calcaneus   Q

√7ᵗʰ **S92.026** Nondisplaced fracture of anterior process of unspecified calcaneus   Q

√6ᵗʰ **S92.03** Avulsion fracture of tuberosity of calcaneus

√7ᵗʰ **S92.031** Displaced avulsion fracture of tuberosity of right calcaneus   Q

√7ᵗʰ **S92.032** Displaced avulsion fracture of tuberosity of left calcaneus   Q

√7ᵗʰ **S92.033** Displaced avulsion fracture of tuberosity of unspecified calcaneus   Q

√7ᵗʰ **S92.034** Nondisplaced avulsion fracture of tuberosity of right calcaneus   Q

√7ᵗʰ **S92.035** Nondisplaced avulsion fracture of tuberosity of left calcaneus Q

√7ᵗʰ **S92.036** Nondisplaced avulsion fracture of tuberosity of unspecified calcaneus Q

√6ᵗʰ **S92.04** Other fracture of tuberosity of calcaneus

√7ᵗʰ **S92.041** Displaced other fracture of tuberosity of right calcaneus Q

√7ᵗʰ **S92.042** Displaced other fracture of tuberosity of left calcaneus Q

√7ᵗʰ **S92.043** Displaced other fracture of tuberosity of unspecified calcaneus Q

√7ᵗʰ **S92.044** Nondisplaced other fracture of tuberosity of right calcaneus Q

√7ᵗʰ **S92.045** Nondisplaced other fracture of tuberosity of left calcaneus Q

√7ᵗʰ **S92.046** Nondisplaced other fracture of tuberosity of unspecified calcaneus Q

√6ᵗʰ **S92.05** Other extraarticular fracture of calcaneus

√7ᵗʰ **S92.051** Displaced other extraarticular fracture of right calcaneus Q

√7ᵗʰ **S92.052** Displaced other extraarticular fracture of left calcaneus Q

√7ᵗʰ **S92.053** Displaced other extraarticular fracture of unspecified calcaneus Q

√7ᵗʰ **S92.054** Nondisplaced other extraarticular fracture of right calcaneus Q

√7ᵗʰ **S92.055** Nondisplaced other extraarticular fracture of left calcaneus Q

√7ᵗʰ **S92.056** Nondisplaced other extraarticular fracture of unspecified calcaneus Q

√6ᵗʰ **S92.06** Intraarticular fracture of calcaneus

√7ᵗʰ **S92.061** Displaced intraarticular fracture of right calcaneus Q

√7ᵗʰ **S92.062** Displaced intraarticular fracture of left calcaneus Q

√7ᵗʰ **S92.063** Displaced intraarticular fracture of unspecified calcaneus Q

√7ᵗʰ **S92.064** Nondisplaced intraarticular fracture of right calcaneus Q

√7ᵗʰ **S92.065** Nondisplaced intraarticular fracture of left calcaneus Q

√7ᵗʰ **S92.066** Nondisplaced intraarticular fracture of unspecified calcaneus Q

√5ᵗʰ **S92.1** Fracture of talus
Astragalus

√6ᵗʰ **S92.10** Unspecified fracture of talus

√7ᵗʰ **S92.101** Unspecified fracture of right talus Q

√7ᵗʰ **S92.102** Unspecified fracture of left talus Q

√7ᵗʰ **S92.109** Unspecified fracture of unspecified talus Q

√6ᵗʰ **S92.11** Fracture of neck of talus

√7ᵗʰ **S92.111** Displaced fracture of neck of right talus Q

√7ᵗʰ **S92.112** Displaced fracture of neck of left talus Q

√7ᵗʰ **S92.113** Displaced fracture of neck of unspecified talus Q

√7ᵗʰ **S92.114** Nondisplaced fracture of neck of right talus Q

√7ᵗʰ **S92.115** Nondisplaced fracture of neck of left talus Q

√7ᵗʰ **S92.116** Nondisplaced fracture of neck of unspecified talus Q

√6ᵗʰ **S92.12** Fracture of body of talus

√7ᵗʰ **S92.121** Displaced fracture of body of right talus Q

√7ᵗʰ **S92.122** Displaced fracture of body of left talus Q

√7ᵗʰ **S92.123** Displaced fracture of body of unspecified talus Q

√7ᵗʰ **S92.124** Nondisplaced fracture of body of right talus Q

√7ᵗʰ **S92.125** Nondisplaced fracture of body of left talus Q

√7ᵗʰ **S92.126** Nondisplaced fracture of body of unspecified talus Q

√6ᵗʰ **S92.13** Fracture of posterior process of talus

√7ᵗʰ **S92.131** Displaced fracture of posterior process of right talus

√7ᵗʰ **S92.132** Displaced fracture of posterior process of left talus Q

√7ᵗʰ **S92.133** Displaced fracture of posterior process of unspecified talus Q

√7ᵗʰ **S92.134** Nondisplaced fracture of posterior process of right talus Q

√7ᵗʰ **S92.135** Nondisplaced fracture of posterior process of left talus Q

√7ᵗʰ **S92.136** Nondisplaced fracture of posterior process of unspecified talus Q

√6ᵗʰ **S92.14** Dome fracture of talus

EXCLUDES 1   osteochondritis dissecans (M93.2)

√7ᵗʰ **S92.141** Displaced dome fracture of right talus Q

√7ᵗʰ **S92.142** Displaced dome fracture of left talus Q

√7ᵗʰ **S92.143** Displaced dome fracture of unspecified talus Q

√7ᵗʰ **S92.144** Nondisplaced dome fracture of right talus Q

√7ᵗʰ **S92.145** Nondisplaced dome fracture of left talus Q

√7ᵗʰ **S92.146** Nondisplaced dome fracture of unspecified talus Q

√6ᵗʰ **S92.15** Avulsion fracture (chip fracture) of talus

√7ᵗʰ **S92.151** Displaced avulsion fracture (chip fracture) of right talus Q

√7ᵗʰ **S92.152** Displaced avulsion fracture (chip fracture) of left talus Q

√7ᵗʰ **S92.153** Displaced avulsion fracture (chip fracture) of unspecified talus Q

√7ᵗʰ **S92.154** Nondisplaced avulsion fracture (chip fracture) of right talus Q

√7ᵗʰ **S92.155** Nondisplaced avulsion fracture (chip fracture) of left talus Q

√7ᵗʰ **S92.156** Nondisplaced avulsion fracture (chip fracture) of unspecified talus Q

√6ᵗʰ **S92.19** Other fracture of talus

√7ᵗʰ **S92.191** Other fracture of right talus Q

√7ᵗʰ **S92.192** Other fracture of left talus Q

√7ᵗʰ **S92.199** Other fracture of unspecified talus Q

√5ᵗʰ **S92.2** Fracture of other and unspecified tarsal bone(s)

√6ᵗʰ **S92.20** Fracture of unspecified tarsal bone(s)

√7ᵗʰ **S92.201** Fracture of unspecified tarsal bone(s) of right foot Q

√7ᵗʰ **S92.202** Fracture of unspecified tarsal bone(s) of left foot Q

√7ᵗʰ **S92.209** Fracture of unspecified tarsal bone(s) of unspecified foot Q

√6ᵗʰ **S92.21** Fracture of cuboid bone

√7ᵗʰ **S92.211** Displaced fracture of cuboid bone of right foot Q

√7ᵗʰ **S92.212** Displaced fracture of cuboid bone of left foot Q

√7ᵗʰ **S92.213** Displaced fracture of cuboid bone of unspecified foot Q

√7ᵗʰ **S92.214** Nondisplaced fracture of cuboid bone of right foot Q

√7ᵗʰ **S92.215** Nondisplaced fracture of cuboid bone of left foot Q

√7ᵗʰ **S92.216** Nondisplaced fracture of cuboid bone of unspecified foot Q

√6ᵗʰ **S92.22** Fracture of lateral cuneiform

√7ᵗʰ **S92.221** Displaced fracture of lateral cuneiform of right foot Q

√7ᵗʰ **S92.222** Displaced fracture of lateral cuneiform of left foot Q

√7ᵗʰ **S92.223** Displaced fracture of lateral cuneiform of unspecified foot Q

√7ᵗʰ **S92.224** Nondisplaced fracture of lateral cuneiform of right foot Q

√7ᵗʰ **S92.225** Nondisplaced fracture of lateral cuneiform of left foot Q

√7ᵗʰ **S92.226** Nondisplaced fracture of lateral cuneiform of unspecified foot Q

√6ᵗʰ **S92.23** Fracture of intermediate cuneiform

√7ᵗʰ **S92.231** Displaced fracture of intermediate cuneiform of right foot Q

☑ Additional Character Required   √x7ᵗʰ Placeholder Alert   Manifestation   Unspecified Dx   Q QPP   UPD Unacceptable PDx

☑7th **S92.232** Displaced fracture of intermediate cuneiform of left foot ▢

☑7th **S92.233** Displaced fracture of intermediate cuneiform of unspecified foot ▢

☑7th **S92.234** Nondisplaced fracture of intermediate cuneiform of right foot ▢

☑7th **S92.235** Nondisplaced fracture of intermediate cuneiform of left foot ▢

☑7th **S92.236** Nondisplaced fracture of intermediate cuneiform of unspecified foot ▢

☑6th **S92.24** Fracture of medial cuneiform

☑7th **S92.241** Displaced fracture of medial cuneiform of right foot ▢

☑7th **S92.242** Displaced fracture of medial cuneiform of left foot ▢

☑7th **S92.243** Displaced fracture of medial cuneiform of unspecified foot ▢

☑7th **S92.244** Nondisplaced fracture of medial cuneiform of right foot ▢

☑7th **S92.245** Nondisplaced fracture of medial cuneiform of left foot ▢

☑7th **S92.246** Nondisplaced fracture of medial cuneiform of unspecified foot ▢

☑6th **S92.25** Fracture of navicular [scaphoid] of foot

☑7th **S92.251** Displaced fracture of navicular [scaphoid] of right foot ▢

☑7th **S92.252** Displaced fracture of navicular [scaphoid] of left foot ▢

☑7th **S92.253** Displaced fracture of navicular [scaphoid] of unspecified foot ▢

☑7th **S92.254** Nondisplaced fracture of navicular [scaphoid] of right foot ▢

☑7th **S92.255** Nondisplaced fracture of navicular [scaphoid] of left foot ▢

☑7th **S92.256** Nondisplaced fracture of navicular [scaphoid] of unspecified foot ▢

☑5th **S92.3** Fracture of metatarsal bone(s)

> **EXCLUDES 2** physeal fracture of metatarsal (S99.1-)

AHA: 2018,1Q,3

☑6th **S92.30** Fracture of unspecified metatarsal bone(s)

☑7th **S92.301** Fracture of unspecified metatarsal bone(s), right foot ▢

☑7th **S92.302** Fracture of unspecified metatarsal bone(s), left foot ▢

☑7th **S92.309** Fracture of unspecified metatarsal bone(s), unspecified foot ▢

☑6th **S92.31** Fracture of first metatarsal bone

☑7th **S92.311** Displaced fracture of first metatarsal bone, right foot ▢

☑7th **S92.312** Displaced fracture of first metatarsal bone, left foot ▢

☑7th **S92.313** Displaced fracture of first metatarsal bone, unspecified foot ▢

☑7th **S92.314** Nondisplaced fracture of first metatarsal bone, right foot ▢

☑7th **S92.315** Nondisplaced fracture of first metatarsal bone, left foot ▢

☑7th **S92.316** Nondisplaced fracture of first metatarsal bone, unspecified foot ▢

☑6th **S92.32** Fracture of second metatarsal bone

☑7th **S92.321** Displaced fracture of second metatarsal bone, right foot ▢

☑7th **S92.322** Displaced fracture of second metatarsal bone, left foot ▢

☑7th **S92.323** Displaced fracture of second metatarsal bone, unspecified foot ▢

☑7th **S92.324** Nondisplaced fracture of second metatarsal bone, right foot ▢

☑7th **S92.325** Nondisplaced fracture of second metatarsal bone, left foot ▢

☑7th **S92.326** Nondisplaced fracture of second metatarsal bone, unspecified foot ▢

☑6th **S92.33** Fracture of third metatarsal bone

☑7th **S92.331** Displaced fracture of third metatarsal bone, right foot ▢

☑7th **S92.332** Displaced fracture of third metatarsal bone, left foot ▢

☑7th **S92.333** Displaced fracture of third metatarsal bone, unspecified foot ▢

☑7th **S92.334** Nondisplaced fracture of third metatarsal bone, right foot ▢

☑7th **S92.335** Nondisplaced fracture of third metatarsal bone, left foot ▢

☑7th **S92.336** Nondisplaced fracture of third metatarsal bone, unspecified foot ▢

☑6th **S92.34** Fracture of fourth metatarsal bone

☑7th **S92.341** Displaced fracture of fourth metatarsal bone, right foot ▢

☑7th **S92.342** Displaced fracture of fourth metatarsal bone, left foot ▢

☑7th **S92.343** Displaced fracture of fourth metatarsal bone, unspecified foot ▢

☑7th **S92.344** Nondisplaced fracture of fourth metatarsal bone, right foot ▢

☑7th **S92.345** Nondisplaced fracture of fourth metatarsal bone, left foot ▢

☑7th **S92.346** Nondisplaced fracture of fourth metatarsal bone, unspecified foot ▢

☑6th **S92.35** Fracture of fifth metatarsal bone

☑7th **S92.351** Displaced fracture of fifth metatarsal bone, right foot ▢

☑7th **S92.352** Displaced fracture of fifth metatarsal bone, left foot ▢

☑7th **S92.353** Displaced fracture of fifth metatarsal bone, unspecified foot ▢

☑7th **S92.354** Nondisplaced fracture of fifth metatarsal bone, right foot ▢

☑7th **S92.355** Nondisplaced fracture of fifth metatarsal bone, left foot ▢

☑7th **S92.356** Nondisplaced fracture of fifth metatarsal bone, unspecified foot ▢

☑5th **S92.4** Fracture of great toe

> **EXCLUDES 2** physeal fracture of phalanx of toe (S99.2-)

☑6th **S92.40** Unspecified fracture of great toe

☑7th **S92.401** Displaced unspecified fracture of right great toe

☑7th **S92.402** Displaced unspecified fracture of left great toe

☑7th **S92.403** Displaced unspecified fracture of unspecified great toe

☑7th **S92.404** Nondisplaced unspecified fracture of right great toe

☑7th **S92.405** Nondisplaced unspecified fracture of left great toe

☑7th **S92.406** Nondisplaced unspecified fracture of unspecified great toe

☑6th **S92.41** Fracture of proximal phalanx of great toe

☑7th **S92.411** Displaced fracture of proximal phalanx of right great toe

☑7th **S92.412** Displaced fracture of proximal phalanx of left great toe

☑7th **S92.413** Displaced fracture of proximal phalanx of unspecified great toe

☑7th **S92.414** Nondisplaced fracture of proximal phalanx of right great toe

☑7th **S92.415** Nondisplaced fracture of proximal phalanx of left great toe

☑7th **S92.416** Nondisplaced fracture of proximal phalanx of unspecified great toe

☑6th **S92.42** Fracture of distal phalanx of great toe

☑7th **S92.421** Displaced fracture of distal phalanx of right great toe

☑7th **S92.422** Displaced fracture of distal phalanx of left great toe

☑7th **S92.423** Displaced fracture of distal phalanx of unspecified great toe

☑7th **S92.424** Nondisplaced fracture of distal phalanx of right great toe

☑7th **S92.425** Nondisplaced fracture of distal phalanx of left great toe

☑7th **S92.426** Nondisplaced fracture of distal phalanx of unspecified great toe

☑6th **S92.49** Other fracture of great toe

☑7th **S92.491** Other fracture of right great toe

☑7th **S92.492** Other fracture of left great toe

☑7th **S92.499** Other fracture of unspecified great toe

HCC CMS-HCC **Rx** Rx HCC **ESR** ESRD HCC **COM** Commercial HCC **N** Newborn: 0 **P** Pediatric: 0-17 **M** Maternity: 9-64 **A** Adult: 15-124

1106 ICD-10-CM 2023

☑5ᵗʰ **S92.5**   Fracture of **lesser** toe(s)

    EXCLUDES 2   *physeal fracture of phalanx of toe (S99.2-)*

   ☑6ᵗʰ **S92.50**   Unspecified fracture of lesser toe(s)

     ☑7ᵗʰ **S92.501**   Displaced unspecified fracture of right lesser toe(s)

     ☑7ᵗʰ **S92.502**   Displaced unspecified fracture of left lesser toe(s)

     ☑7ᵗʰ **S92.503**   Displaced unspecified fracture of unspecified lesser toe(s)

     ☑7ᵗʰ **S92.504**   Nondisplaced unspecified fracture of right lesser toe(s)

     ☑7ᵗʰ **S92.505**   Nondisplaced unspecified fracture of left lesser toe(s)

     ☑7ᵗʰ **S92.506**   Nondisplaced unspecified fracture of unspecified lesser toe(s)

   ☑6ᵗʰ **S92.51**   Fracture of proximal phalanx of lesser toe(s)

     ☑7ᵗʰ **S92.511**   Displaced fracture of proximal phalanx of right lesser toe(s)

     ☑7ᵗʰ **S92.512**   Displaced fracture of proximal phalanx of left lesser toe(s)

     ☑7ᵗʰ **S92.513**   Displaced fracture of proximal phalanx of unspecified lesser toe(s)

     ☑7ᵗʰ **S92.514**   Nondisplaced fracture of proximal phalanx of right lesser toe(s)

     ☑7ᵗʰ **S92.515**   Nondisplaced fracture of proximal phalanx of left lesser toe(s)

     ☑7ᵗʰ **S92.516**   Nondisplaced fracture of proximal phalanx of unspecified lesser toe(s)

   ☑6ᵗʰ **S92.52**   Fracture of middle phalanx of lesser toe(s)

     ☑7ᵗʰ **S92.521**   Displaced fracture of middle phalanx of right lesser toe(s)

     ☑7ᵗʰ **S92.522**   Displaced fracture of middle phalanx of left lesser toe(s)

     ☑7ᵗʰ **S92.523**   Displaced fracture of middle phalanx of unspecified lesser toe(s)

     ☑7ᵗʰ **S92.524**   Nondisplaced fracture of middle phalanx of right lesser toe(s)

     ☑7ᵗʰ **S92.525**   Nondisplaced fracture of middle phalanx of left lesser toe(s)

     ☑7ᵗʰ **S92.526**   Nondisplaced fracture of middle phalanx of unspecified lesser toe(s)

   ☑6ᵗʰ **S92.53**   Fracture of distal phalanx of lesser toe(s)

     ☑7ᵗʰ **S92.531**   Displaced fracture of distal phalanx of right lesser toe(s)

     ☑7ᵗʰ **S92.532**   Displaced fracture of distal phalanx of left lesser toe(s)

     ☑7ᵗʰ **S92.533**   Displaced fracture of distal phalanx of unspecified lesser toe(s)

     ☑7ᵗʰ **S92.534**   Nondisplaced fracture of distal phalanx of right lesser toe(s)

     ☑7ᵗʰ **S92.535**   Nondisplaced fracture of distal phalanx of left lesser toe(s)

     ☑7ᵗʰ **S92.536**   Nondisplaced fracture of distal phalanx of unspecified lesser toe(s)

   ☑6ᵗʰ **S92.59**   Other fracture of lesser toe(s)

     ☑7ᵗʰ **S92.591**   Other fracture of right lesser toe(s)

     ☑7ᵗʰ **S92.592**   Other fracture of left lesser toe(s)

     ☑7ᵗʰ **S92.599**   Other fracture of unspecified lesser toe(s)

☑5ᵗʰ **S92.8**   Other fracture of foot, except ankle

   ☑6ᵗʰ **S92.81**   Other fracture of foot

     Sesamoid fracture of foot

     AHA: 2016,4Q,68

     ☑7ᵗʰ **S92.811**   Other fracture of right foot   🄌

     ☑7ᵗʰ **S92.812**   Other fracture of left foot   🄌

     ☑7ᵗʰ **S92.819**   Other fracture of unspecified foot   🄌

☑5ᵗʰ **S92.9**   Unspecified fracture of foot and toe

   ☑6ᵗʰ **S92.90**   Unspecified fracture of foot

     ☑7ᵗʰ **S92.901**   Unspecified fracture of right foot   🄌

     ☑7ᵗʰ **S92.902**   Unspecified fracture of left foot   🄌

     ☑7ᵗʰ **S92.909**   Unspecified fracture of unspecified foot   🄌

   ☑6ᵗʰ **S92.91**   Unspecified fracture of toe

     ☑7ᵗʰ **S92.911**   Unspecified fracture of right toe(s)

     ☑7ᵗʰ **S92.912**   Unspecified fracture of left toe(s)

     ☑7ᵗʰ **S92.919**   Unspecified fracture of unspecified toe(s)

☑4ᵗʰ **S93**   Dislocation and sprain of joints and ligaments at ankle, foot and toe level

   INCLUDES   avulsion of joint or ligament of ankle, foot and toe

     laceration of cartilage, joint or ligament of ankle, foot and toe

     sprain of cartilage, joint or ligament of ankle, foot and toe

     traumatic hemarthrosis of joint or ligament of ankle, foot and toe

     traumatic rupture of joint or ligament of ankle, foot and toe

     traumatic subluxation of joint or ligament of ankle, foot and toe

     traumatic tear of joint or ligament of ankle, foot and toe

Code also any associated open wound

   EXCLUDES 2   *strain of muscle and tendon of ankle and foot (S96.-)*

> The appropriate 7th character is to be added to each code from category S93.
> A   initial encounter
> D   subsequent encounter
> S   sequela

   ☑5ᵗʰ **S93.0**   Subluxation and dislocation of ankle joint

     Subluxation and dislocation of astragalus

     Subluxation and dislocation of fibula, lower end

     Subluxation and dislocation of talus

     Subluxation and dislocation of tibia, lower end

     ✓x7ᵗʰ **S93.01**   Subluxation of right ankle joint

     ✓x7ᵗʰ **S93.02**   Subluxation of left ankle joint

     ✓x7ᵗʰ **S93.03**   Subluxation of unspecified ankle joint

     ✓x7ᵗʰ **S93.04**   Dislocation of right ankle joint

     ✓x7ᵗʰ **S93.05**   Dislocation of left ankle joint

     ✓x7ᵗʰ **S93.06**   Dislocation of unspecified ankle joint

   ☑5ᵗʰ **S93.1**   Subluxation and dislocation of toe

     ☑6ᵗʰ **S93.10**   Unspecified subluxation and dislocation of toe

      Dislocation of toe NOS

      Subluxation of toe NOS

      ☑7ᵗʰ **S93.101**   Unspecified subluxation of right toe(s)

      ☑7ᵗʰ **S93.102**   Unspecified subluxation of left toe(s)

      ☑7ᵗʰ **S93.103**   Unspecified subluxation of unspecified toe(s)

      ☑7ᵗʰ **S93.104**   Unspecified dislocation of right toe(s)

      ☑7ᵗʰ **S93.105**   Unspecified dislocation of left toe(s)

      ☑7ᵗʰ **S93.106**   Unspecified dislocation of unspecified toe(s)

     ☑6ᵗʰ **S93.11**   Dislocation of interphalangeal joint

      ☑7ᵗʰ **S93.111**   Dislocation of interphalangeal joint of right great toe

      ☑7ᵗʰ **S93.112**   Dislocation of interphalangeal joint of left great toe

      ☑7ᵗʰ **S93.113**   Dislocation of interphalangeal joint of unspecified great toe

      ☑7ᵗʰ **S93.114**   Dislocation of interphalangeal joint of right lesser toe(s)

      ☑7ᵗʰ **S93.115**   Dislocation of interphalangeal joint of left lesser toe(s)

      ☑7ᵗʰ **S93.116**   Dislocation of interphalangeal joint of unspecified lesser toe(s)

      ☑7ᵗʰ **S93.119**   Dislocation of interphalangeal joint of unspecified toe(s)

     ☑6ᵗʰ **S93.12**   Dislocation of metatarsophalangeal joint

      ☑7ᵗʰ **S93.121**   Dislocation of metatarsophalangeal joint of right great toe

      ☑7ᵗʰ **S93.122**   Dislocation of metatarsophalangeal joint of left great toe

      ☑7ᵗʰ **S93.123**   Dislocation of metatarsophalangeal joint of unspecified great toe

      ☑7ᵗʰ **S93.124**   Dislocation of metatarsophalangeal joint of right lesser toe(s)

      ☑7ᵗʰ **S93.125**   Dislocation of metatarsophalangeal joint of left lesser toe(s)

      ☑7ᵗʰ **S93.126**   Dislocation of metatarsophalangeal joint of unspecified lesser toe(s)

      ☑7ᵗʰ **S93.129**   Dislocation of metatarsophalangeal joint of unspecified toe(s)

     ☑6ᵗʰ **S93.13**   Subluxation of interphalangeal joint

      ☑7ᵗʰ **S93.131**   Subluxation of interphalangeal joint of right great toe

---

Chapter 19. Injury, Poisoning and Certain Other Consequences of External Causes

S93.132–S93.602

(margin handwritten notes: "Subluxation", "foot", "Sprain", "Toe")

✓7th **S93.132** Subluxation of interphalangeal joint of left great toe

✓7th **S93.133** Subluxation of interphalangeal joint of unspecified great toe

✓7th **S93.134** Subluxation of interphalangeal joint of right lesser toe(s)

✓7th **S93.135** Subluxation of interphalangeal joint of left lesser toe(s)

✓7th **S93.136** Subluxation of interphalangeal joint of unspecified lesser toe(s)

✓7th **S93.139** Subluxation of interphalangeal joint of unspecified toe(s)

✓6th **S93.14** Subluxation of metatarsophalangeal joint

✓7th **S93.141** Subluxation of metatarsophalangeal joint of right great toe

✓7th **S93.142** Subluxation of metatarsophalangeal joint of left great toe

✓7th **S93.143** Subluxation of metatarsophalangeal joint of unspecified great toe

✓7th **S93.144** Subluxation of metatarsophalangeal joint of right lesser toe(s)

✓7th **S93.145** Subluxation of metatarsophalangeal joint of left lesser toe(s)

✓7th **S93.146** Subluxation of metatarsophalangeal joint of unspecified lesser toe(s)

✓7th **S93.149** Subluxation of metatarsophalangeal joint of unspecified toe(s)

✓5th **S93.3** Subluxation and dislocation of foot

EXCLUDES 2 dislocation of toe (S93.1-)

✓6th **S93.30** Unspecified subluxation and dislocation of foot

Dislocation of foot NOS
Subluxation of foot NOS

✓7th **S93.301** Unspecified subluxation of right foot

✓7th **S93.302** Unspecified subluxation of left foot

✓7th **S93.303** Unspecified subluxation of unspecified foot

✓7th **S93.304** Unspecified dislocation of right foot

✓7th **S93.305** Unspecified dislocation of left foot

✓7th **S93.306** Unspecified dislocation of unspecified foot

✓6th **S93.31** Subluxation and dislocation of tarsal joint

✓7th **S93.311** Subluxation of tarsal joint of right foot

✓7th **S93.312** Subluxation of tarsal joint of left foot

✓7th **S93.313** Subluxation of tarsal joint of unspecified foot

✓7th **S93.314** Dislocation of tarsal joint of right foot

✓7th **S93.315** Dislocation of tarsal joint of left foot

✓7th **S93.316** Dislocation of tarsal joint of unspecified foot

✓6th **S93.32** Subluxation and dislocation of tarsometatarsal joint

✓7th **S93.321** Subluxation of tarsometatarsal joint of right foot

✓7th **S93.322** Subluxation of tarsometatarsal joint of left foot

✓7th **S93.323** Subluxation of tarsometatarsal joint of unspecified foot

✓7th **S93.324** Dislocation of tarsometatarsal joint of right foot

✓7th **S93.325** Dislocation of tarsometatarsal joint of left foot

✓7th **S93.326** Dislocation of tarsometatarsal joint of unspecified foot

✓6th **S93.33** Other subluxation and dislocation of foot

✓7th **S93.331** Other subluxation of right foot

✓7th **S93.332** Other subluxation of left foot

✓7th **S93.333** Other subluxation of unspecified foot

✓7th **S93.334** Other dislocation of right foot

✓7th **S93.335** Other dislocation of left foot

✓7th **S93.336** Other dislocation of unspecified foot

✓5th **S93.4** Sprain of ankle

EXCLUDES 2 injury of Achilles tendon (S86.0-)

✓6th **S93.40** Sprain of unspecified ligament of ankle

Sprain of ankle NOS
Sprained ankle NOS

✓7th **S93.401** Sprain of unspecified ligament of right ankle

✓7th **S93.402** Sprain of unspecified ligament of left ankle

✓7th **S93.409** Sprain of unspecified ligament of unspecified ankle

✓6th **S93.41** Sprain of calcaneofibular ligament

✓7th **S93.411** Sprain of calcaneofibular ligament of right ankle

✓7th **S93.412** Sprain of calcaneofibular ligament of left ankle

✓7th **S93.419** Sprain of calcaneofibular ligament of unspecified ankle

✓6th **S93.42** Sprain of deltoid ligament

✓7th **S93.421** Sprain of deltoid ligament of right ankle

✓7th **S93.422** Sprain of deltoid ligament of left ankle

✓7th **S93.429** Sprain of deltoid ligament of unspecified ankle

✓6th **S93.43** Sprain of tibiofibular ligament

✓7th **S93.431** Sprain of tibiofibular ligament of right ankle

✓7th **S93.432** Sprain of tibiofibular ligament of left ankle

✓7th **S93.439** Sprain of tibiofibular ligament of unspecified ankle

✓6th **S93.49** Sprain of other ligament of ankle

Sprain of internal collateral ligament
Sprain of talofibular ligament

✓7th **S93.491** Sprain of other ligament of right ankle

✓7th **S93.492** Sprain of other ligament of left ankle

✓7th **S93.499** Sprain of other ligament of unspecified ankle

✓5th **S93.5** Sprain of toe

✓6th **S93.50** Unspecified sprain of toe

✓7th **S93.501** Unspecified sprain of right great toe

✓7th **S93.502** Unspecified sprain of left great toe

✓7th **S93.503** Unspecified sprain of unspecified great toe

✓7th **S93.504** Unspecified sprain of right lesser toe(s)

✓7th **S93.505** Unspecified sprain of left lesser toe(s)

✓7th **S93.506** Unspecified sprain of unspecified lesser toe(s)

✓7th **S93.509** Unspecified sprain of unspecified toe(s)

✓6th **S93.51** Sprain of interphalangeal joint of toe

✓7th **S93.511** Sprain of interphalangeal joint of right great toe

✓7th **S93.512** Sprain of interphalangeal joint of left great toe

✓7th **S93.513** Sprain of interphalangeal joint of unspecified great toe

✓7th **S93.514** Sprain of interphalangeal joint of right lesser toe(s)

✓7th **S93.515** Sprain of interphalangeal joint of left lesser toe(s)

✓7th **S93.516** Sprain of interphalangeal joint of unspecified lesser toe(s)

✓7th **S93.519** Sprain of interphalangeal joint of unspecified toe(s)

✓6th **S93.52** Sprain of metatarsophalangeal joint of toe

✓7th **S93.521** Sprain of metatarsophalangeal joint of right great toe

✓7th **S93.522** Sprain of metatarsophalangeal joint of left great toe

✓7th **S93.523** Sprain of metatarsophalangeal joint of unspecified great toe

✓7th **S93.524** Sprain of metatarsophalangeal joint of right lesser toe(s)

✓7th **S93.525** Sprain of metatarsophalangeal joint of left lesser toe(s)

✓7th **S93.526** Sprain of metatarsophalangeal joint of unspecified lesser toe(s)

✓7th **S93.529** Sprain of metatarsophalangeal joint of unspecified toe(s)

✓5th **S93.6** Sprain of foot

EXCLUDES 2 sprain of metatarsophalangeal joint of toe (S93.52-)
sprain of toe (S93.5-)

✓6th **S93.60** Unspecified sprain of foot

✓7th **S93.601** Unspecified sprain of right foot

✓7th **S93.602** Unspecified sprain of left foot

HCC CMS-HCC   **Rx** Rx HCC   **ESR** ESRD HCC   **COM** Commercial HCC   **N** Newborn: 0   **P** Pediatric: 0-17   **M** Maternity: 9-64   **A** Adult: 15-124

1108   ICD-10-CM 2023

    ☑7ᵗʰ **S93.609** Unspecified sprain of unspecified foot

☑6ᵗʰ **S93.61 Sprain of tarsal ligament of foot**
    ☑7ᵗʰ **S93.611** Sprain of tarsal ligament of right foot
    ☑7ᵗʰ **S93.612** Sprain of tarsal ligament of left foot
    ☑7ᵗʰ **S93.619** Sprain of tarsal ligament of unspecified foot

☑6ᵗʰ **S93.62 Sprain of tarsometatarsal ligament of foot**
    ☑7ᵗʰ **S93.621** Sprain of tarsometatarsal ligament of right foot
    ☑7ᵗʰ **S93.622** Sprain of tarsometatarsal ligament of left foot
    ☑7ᵗʰ **S93.629** Sprain of tarsometatarsal ligament of unspecified foot

☑6ᵗʰ **S93.69 Other sprain of foot**
    ☑7ᵗʰ **S93.691** Other sprain of right foot
    ☑7ᵗʰ **S93.692** Other sprain of left foot
    ☑7ᵗʰ **S93.699** Other sprain of unspecified foot

☑4ᵗʰ **S94 Injury of nerves at ankle and foot level**
Code also any associated open wound (S91.-)

The appropriate 7th character is to be added to each code from category S94.
A   initial encounter
D   subsequent encounter
S   sequela

☑5ᵗʰ **S94.0 Injury of lateral plantar nerve**
    ☑x7ᵗʰ **S94.00** Injury of lateral plantar nerve, unspecified leg
    ☑x7ᵗʰ **S94.01** Injury of lateral plantar nerve, right leg
    ☑x7ᵗʰ **S94.02** Injury of lateral plantar nerve, left leg

☑5ᵗʰ **S94.1 Injury of medial plantar nerve**
    ☑x7ᵗʰ **S94.10** Injury of medial plantar nerve, unspecified leg
    ☑x7ᵗʰ **S94.11** Injury of medial plantar nerve, right leg
    ☑x7ᵗʰ **S94.12** Injury of medial plantar nerve, left leg

☑5ᵗʰ **S94.2 Injury of deep peroneal nerve at ankle and foot level**
Injury of terminal, lateral branch of deep peroneal nerve
    ☑x7ᵗʰ **S94.20** Injury of deep peroneal nerve at ankle and foot level, unspecified leg
    ☑x7ᵗʰ **S94.21** Injury of deep peroneal nerve at ankle and foot level, right leg
    ☑x7ᵗʰ **S94.22** Injury of deep peroneal nerve at ankle and foot level, left leg

☑5ᵗʰ **S94.3 Injury of cutaneous sensory nerve at ankle and foot level**
    ☑x7ᵗʰ **S94.30** Injury of cutaneous sensory nerve at ankle and foot level, unspecified leg
    ☑x7ᵗʰ **S94.31** Injury of cutaneous sensory nerve at ankle and foot level, right leg
    ☑x7ᵗʰ **S94.32** Injury of cutaneous sensory nerve at ankle and foot level, left leg

☑5ᵗʰ **S94.8 Injury of other nerves at ankle and foot level**
    ☑6ᵗʰ **S94.8X** Injury of other nerves at ankle and foot level
        ☑7ᵗʰ **S94.8X1** Injury of other nerves at ankle and foot level, right leg
        ☑7ᵗʰ **S94.8X2** Injury of other nerves at ankle and foot level, left leg
        ☑7ᵗʰ **S94.8X9** Injury of other nerves at ankle and foot level, unspecified leg

☑5ᵗʰ **S94.9 Injury of unspecified nerve at ankle and foot level**
    ☑x7ᵗʰ **S94.90** Injury of unspecified nerve at ankle and foot level, unspecified leg
    ☑x7ᵗʰ **S94.91** Injury of unspecified nerve at ankle and foot level, right leg
    ☑x7ᵗʰ **S94.92** Injury of unspecified nerve at ankle and foot level, left leg

☑4ᵗʰ **S95 Injury of blood vessels at ankle and foot level**
Code also any associated open wound (S91.-)
EXCLUDES 2   injury of posterior tibial artery and vein (S85.1-, S85.8-)

The appropriate 7th character is to be added to each code from category S95.
A   initial encounter
D   subsequent encounter
S   sequela

☑5ᵗʰ **S95.0 Injury of dorsal artery of foot**
    ☑6ᵗʰ **S95.00** Unspecified injury of dorsal artery of foot
        ☑7ᵗʰ **S95.001** Unspecified injury of dorsal artery of right foot
        ☑7ᵗʰ **S95.002** Unspecified injury of dorsal artery of left foot
        ☑7ᵗʰ **S95.009** Unspecified injury of dorsal artery of unspecified foot

    ☑6ᵗʰ **S95.01** Laceration of dorsal artery of foot
        ☑7ᵗʰ **S95.011** Laceration of dorsal artery of right foot
        ☑7ᵗʰ **S95.012** Laceration of dorsal artery of left foot
        ☑7ᵗʰ **S95.019** Laceration of dorsal artery of unspecified foot

    ☑6ᵗʰ **S95.09** Other specified injury of dorsal artery of foot
        ☑7ᵗʰ **S95.091** Other specified injury of dorsal artery of right foot
        ☑7ᵗʰ **S95.092** Other specified injury of dorsal artery of left foot
        ☑7ᵗʰ **S95.099** Other specified injury of dorsal artery of unspecified foot

☑5ᵗʰ **S95.1 Injury of plantar artery of foot**
    ☑6ᵗʰ **S95.10** Unspecified injury of plantar artery of foot
        ☑7ᵗʰ **S95.101** Unspecified injury of plantar artery of right foot
        ☑7ᵗʰ **S95.102** Unspecified injury of plantar artery of left foot
        ☑7ᵗʰ **S95.109** Unspecified injury of plantar artery of unspecified foot

    ☑6ᵗʰ **S95.11** Laceration of plantar artery of foot
        ☑7ᵗʰ **S95.111** Laceration of plantar artery of right foot
        ☑7ᵗʰ **S95.112** Laceration of plantar artery of left foot
        ☑7ᵗʰ **S95.119** Laceration of plantar artery of unspecified foot

    ☑6ᵗʰ **S95.19** Other specified injury of plantar artery of foot
        ☑7ᵗʰ **S95.191** Other specified injury of plantar artery of right foot
        ☑7ᵗʰ **S95.192** Other specified injury of plantar artery of left foot
        ☑7ᵗʰ **S95.199** Other specified injury of plantar artery of unspecified foot

☑5ᵗʰ **S95.2 Injury of dorsal vein of foot**
    ☑6ᵗʰ **S95.20** Unspecified injury of dorsal vein of foot
        ☑7ᵗʰ **S95.201** Unspecified injury of dorsal vein of right foot
        ☑7ᵗʰ **S95.202** Unspecified injury of dorsal vein of left foot
        ☑7ᵗʰ **S95.209** Unspecified injury of dorsal vein of unspecified foot

    ☑6ᵗʰ **S95.21** Laceration of dorsal vein of foot
        ☑7ᵗʰ **S95.211** Laceration of dorsal vein of right foot
        ☑7ᵗʰ **S95.212** Laceration of dorsal vein of left foot
        ☑7ᵗʰ **S95.219** Laceration of dorsal vein of unspecified foot

    ☑6ᵗʰ **S95.29** Other specified injury of dorsal vein of foot
        ☑7ᵗʰ **S95.291** Other specified injury of dorsal vein of right foot
        ☑7ᵗʰ **S95.292** Other specified injury of dorsal vein of left foot
        ☑7ᵗʰ **S95.299** Other specified injury of dorsal vein of unspecified foot

☑5ᵗʰ **S95.8 Injury of other blood vessels at ankle and foot level**
    ☑6ᵗʰ **S95.80** Unspecified injury of other blood vessels at ankle and foot level
        ☑7ᵗʰ **S95.801** Unspecified injury of other blood vessels at ankle and foot level, right leg
        ☑7ᵗʰ **S95.802** Unspecified injury of other blood vessels at ankle and foot level, left leg
        ☑7ᵗʰ **S95.809** Unspecified injury of other blood vessels at ankle and foot level, unspecified leg

√6ᵗʰ **S95.81** Laceration of other blood vessels at ankle and foot level
- √7ᵗʰ **S95.811** Laceration of other blood vessels at ankle and foot level, right leg
- √7ᵗʰ **S95.812** Laceration of other blood vessels at ankle and foot level, left leg
- √7ᵗʰ **S95.819** Laceration of other blood vessels at ankle and foot level, unspecified leg

√6ᵗʰ **S95.89** Other specified injury of other blood vessels at ankle and foot level
- √7ᵗʰ **S95.891** Other specified injury of other blood vessels at ankle and foot level, right leg
- √7ᵗʰ **S95.892** Other specified injury of other blood vessels at ankle and foot level, left leg
- √7ᵗʰ **S95.899** Other specified injury of other blood vessels at ankle and foot level, unspecified leg

√5ᵗʰ **S95.9** Injury of unspecified blood vessel at ankle and foot level

√6ᵗʰ **S95.90** Unspecified injury of unspecified blood vessel at ankle and foot level
- √7ᵗʰ **S95.901** Unspecified injury of unspecified blood vessel at ankle and foot level, right leg
- √7ᵗʰ **S95.902** Unspecified injury of unspecified blood vessel at ankle and foot level, left leg
- √7ᵗʰ **S95.909** Unspecified injury of unspecified blood vessel at ankle and foot level, unspecified leg

√6ᵗʰ **S95.91** Laceration of unspecified blood vessel at ankle and foot level
- √7ᵗʰ **S95.911** Laceration of unspecified blood vessel at ankle and foot level, right leg
- √7ᵗʰ **S95.912** Laceration of unspecified blood vessel at ankle and foot level, left leg
- √7ᵗʰ **S95.919** Laceration of unspecified blood vessel at ankle and foot level, unspecified leg

√6ᵗʰ **S95.99** Other specified injury of unspecified blood vessel at ankle and foot level
- √7ᵗʰ **S95.991** Other specified injury of unspecified blood vessel at ankle and foot level, right leg
- √7ᵗʰ **S95.992** Other specified injury of unspecified blood vessel at ankle and foot level, left leg
- √7ᵗʰ **S95.999** Other specified injury of unspecified blood vessel at ankle and foot level, unspecified leg

√4ᵗʰ **S96** Injury of muscle and tendon at ankle and foot level

     Code also any associated open wound (S91.-)

     EXCLUDES 2   injury of Achilles tendon (S86.0-)

         sprain of joints and ligaments of ankle and foot (S93.-)

     TIP: Refer to the Muscle/Tendon table at the beginning of this chapter.

     The appropriate 7th character is to be added to each code from category S96.
- A   initial encounter
- D   subsequent encounter
- S   sequela

√5ᵗʰ **S96.0** Injury of muscle and tendon of long flexor muscle of toe at ankle and foot level

√6ᵗʰ **S96.00** Unspecified injury of muscle and tendon of long flexor muscle of toe at ankle and foot level
- √7ᵗʰ **S96.001** Unspecified injury of muscle and tendon of long flexor muscle of toe at ankle and foot level, right foot
- √7ᵗʰ **S96.002** Unspecified injury of muscle and tendon of long flexor muscle of toe at ankle and foot level, left foot
- √7ᵗʰ **S96.009** Unspecified injury of muscle and tendon of long flexor muscle of toe at ankle and foot level, unspecified foot

√6ᵗʰ **S96.01** Strain of muscle and tendon of long flexor muscle of toe at ankle and foot level
- √7ᵗʰ **S96.011** Strain of muscle and tendon of long flexor muscle of toe at ankle and foot level, right foot
- √7ᵗʰ **S96.012** Strain of muscle and tendon of long flexor muscle of toe at ankle and foot level, left foot
- √7ᵗʰ **S96.019** Strain of muscle and tendon of long flexor muscle of toe at ankle and foot level, unspecified foot

√6ᵗʰ **S96.02** Laceration of muscle and tendon of long flexor muscle of toe at ankle and foot level
- √7ᵗʰ **S96.021** Laceration of muscle and tendon of long flexor muscle of toe at ankle and foot level, right foot
- √7ᵗʰ **S96.022** Laceration of muscle and tendon of long flexor muscle of toe at ankle and foot level, left foot
- √7ᵗʰ **S96.029** Laceration of muscle and tendon of long flexor muscle of toe at ankle and foot level, unspecified foot

√6ᵗʰ **S96.09** Other injury of muscle and tendon of long flexor muscle of toe at ankle and foot level
- √7ᵗʰ **S96.091** Other injury of muscle and tendon of long flexor muscle of toe at ankle and foot level, right foot
- √7ᵗʰ **S96.092** Other injury of muscle and tendon of long flexor muscle of toe at ankle and foot level, left foot
- √7ᵗʰ **S96.099** Other injury of muscle and tendon of long flexor muscle of toe at ankle and foot level, unspecified foot

√5ᵗʰ **S96.1** Injury of muscle and tendon of long extensor muscle of toe at ankle and foot level

√6ᵗʰ **S96.10** Unspecified injury of muscle and tendon of long extensor muscle of toe at ankle and foot level
- √7ᵗʰ **S96.101** Unspecified injury of muscle and tendon of long extensor muscle of toe at ankle and foot level, right foot
- √7ᵗʰ **S96.102** Unspecified injury of muscle and tendon of long extensor muscle of toe at ankle and foot level, left foot
- √7ᵗʰ **S96.109** Unspecified injury of muscle and tendon of long extensor muscle of toe at ankle and foot level, unspecified foot

√6ᵗʰ **S96.11** Strain of muscle and tendon of long extensor muscle of toe at ankle and foot level
- √7ᵗʰ **S96.111** Strain of muscle and tendon of long extensor muscle of toe at ankle and foot level, right foot
- √7ᵗʰ **S96.112** Strain of muscle and tendon of long extensor muscle of toe at ankle and foot level, left foot
- √7ᵗʰ **S96.119** Strain of muscle and tendon of long extensor muscle of toe at ankle and foot level, unspecified foot

√6ᵗʰ **S96.12** Laceration of muscle and tendon of long extensor muscle of toe at ankle and foot level
- √7ᵗʰ **S96.121** Laceration of muscle and tendon of long extensor muscle of toe at ankle and foot level, right foot
- √7ᵗʰ **S96.122** Laceration of muscle and tendon of long extensor muscle of toe at ankle and foot level, left foot
- √7ᵗʰ **S96.129** Laceration of muscle and tendon of long extensor muscle of toe at ankle and foot level, unspecified foot

√6ᵗʰ **S96.19** Other specified injury of muscle and tendon of long extensor muscle of toe at ankle and foot level
- √7ᵗʰ **S96.191** Other specified injury of muscle and tendon of long extensor muscle of toe at ankle and foot level, right foot
- √7ᵗʰ **S96.192** Other specified injury of muscle and tendon of long extensor muscle of toe at ankle and foot level, left foot
- √7ᵗʰ **S96.199** Other specified injury of muscle and tendon of long extensor muscle of toe at ankle and foot level, unspecified foot

√5ᵗʰ **S96.2** Injury of intrinsic muscle and tendon at ankle and foot level

√6ᵗʰ **S96.20** Unspecified injury of intrinsic muscle and tendon at ankle and foot level
- √7ᵗʰ **S96.201** Unspecified injury of intrinsic muscle and tendon at ankle and foot level, right foot
- √7ᵗʰ **S96.202** Unspecified injury of intrinsic muscle and tendon at ankle and foot level, left foot
- √7ᵗʰ **S96.209** Unspecified injury of intrinsic muscle and tendon at ankle and foot level, unspecified foot

√6ᵗʰ **S96.21** Strain of intrinsic muscle and tendon at ankle and foot level
- √7ᵗʰ **S96.211** Strain of intrinsic muscle and tendon at ankle and foot level, right foot
- √7ᵗʰ **S96.212** Strain of intrinsic muscle and tendon at ankle and foot level, left foot

HCC CMS-HCC   **Rx** Rx HCC   **ESH** ESRD HCC   **COM** Commercial HCC   **N** Newborn: 0   **P** Pediatric: 0-17   **M** Maternity: 9-64   **A** Adult: 15-124

1110   ICD-10-CM 2023

√7ᵗʰ **S96.219** Strain of intrinsic muscle and tendon at ankle and foot level, unspecified foot

√6ᵗʰ **S96.22** Laceration of intrinsic muscle and tendon at ankle and foot level

    √7ᵗʰ **S96.221** Laceration of intrinsic muscle and tendon at ankle and foot level, right foot

    √7ᵗʰ **S96.222** Laceration of intrinsic muscle and tendon at ankle and foot level, left foot

    √7ᵗʰ **S96.229** Laceration of intrinsic muscle and tendon at ankle and foot level, unspecified foot

√6ᵗʰ **S96.29** Other specified injury of intrinsic muscle and tendon at ankle and foot level

    √7ᵗʰ **S96.291** Other specified injury of intrinsic muscle and tendon at ankle and foot level, right foot

    √7ᵗʰ **S96.292** Other specified injury of intrinsic muscle and tendon at ankle and foot level, left foot

    √7ᵗʰ **S96.299** Other specified injury of intrinsic muscle and tendon at ankle and foot level, unspecified foot

√5ᵗʰ **S96.8** Injury of other specified muscles and tendons at ankle and foot level

√6ᵗʰ **S96.80** Unspecified injury of other specified muscles and tendons at ankle and foot level

    √7ᵗʰ **S96.801** Unspecified injury of other specified muscles and tendons at ankle and foot level, right foot

    √7ᵗʰ **S96.802** Unspecified injury of other specified muscles and tendons at ankle and foot level, left foot

    √7ᵗʰ **S96.809** Unspecified injury of other specified muscles and tendons at ankle and foot level, unspecified foot

√6ᵗʰ **S96.81** Strain of other specified muscles and tendons at ankle and foot level

    √7ᵗʰ **S96.811** Strain of other specified muscles and tendons at ankle and foot level, right foot

    √7ᵗʰ **S96.812** Strain of other specified muscles and tendons at ankle and foot level, left foot

    √7ᵗʰ **S96.819** Strain of other specified muscles and tendons at ankle and foot level, unspecified foot

√6ᵗʰ **S96.82** Laceration of other specified muscles and tendons at ankle and foot level

    √7ᵗʰ **S96.821** Laceration of other specified muscles and tendons at ankle and foot level, right foot

    √7ᵗʰ **S96.822** Laceration of other specified muscles and tendons at ankle and foot level, left foot

    √7ᵗʰ **S96.829** Laceration of other specified muscles and tendons at ankle and foot level, unspecified foot

√6ᵗʰ **S96.89** Other specified injury of other specified muscles and tendons at ankle and foot level

    √7ᵗʰ **S96.891** Other specified injury of other specified muscles and tendons at ankle and foot level, right foot

    √7ᵗʰ **S96.892** Other specified injury of other specified muscles and tendons at ankle and foot level, left foot

    √7ᵗʰ **S96.899** Other specified injury of other specified muscles and tendons at ankle and foot level, unspecified foot

√5ᵗʰ **S96.9** Injury of unspecified muscle and tendon at ankle and foot level

√6ᵗʰ **S96.90** Unspecified injury of unspecified muscle and tendon at ankle and foot level

    √7ᵗʰ **S96.901** Unspecified injury of unspecified muscle and tendon at ankle and foot level, right foot

    √7ᵗʰ **S96.902** Unspecified injury of unspecified muscle and tendon at ankle and foot level, left foot

    √7ᵗʰ **S96.909** Unspecified injury of unspecified muscle and tendon at ankle and foot level, unspecified foot

√6ᵗʰ **S96.91** Strain of unspecified muscle and tendon at ankle and foot level

    √7ᵗʰ **S96.911** Strain of unspecified muscle and tendon at ankle and foot level, right foot

    √7ᵗʰ **S96.912** Strain of unspecified muscle and tendon at ankle and foot level, left foot

    √7ᵗʰ **S96.919** Strain of unspecified muscle and tendon at ankle and foot level, unspecified foot

√6ᵗʰ **S96.92** Laceration of unspecified muscle and tendon at ankle and foot level

    √7ᵗʰ **S96.921** Laceration of unspecified muscle and tendon at ankle and foot level, right foot

    √7ᵗʰ **S96.922** Laceration of unspecified muscle and tendon at ankle and foot level, left foot

    √7ᵗʰ **S96.929** Laceration of unspecified muscle and tendon at ankle and foot level, unspecified foot

√6ᵗʰ **S96.99** Other specified injury of unspecified muscle and tendon at ankle and foot level

    √7ᵗʰ **S96.991** Other specified injury of unspecified muscle and tendon at ankle and foot level, right foot

    √7ᵗʰ **S96.992** Other specified injury of unspecified muscle and tendon at ankle and foot level, left foot

    √7ᵗʰ **S96.999** Other specified injury of unspecified muscle and tendon at ankle and foot level, unspecified foot

√4ᵗʰ **S97** Crushing injury of ankle and foot

Use additional code(s) for all associated injuries

The appropriate 7th character is to be added to each code from category S97.
A   initial encounter
D   subsequent encounter
S   sequela

√5ᵗʰ **S97.0** Crushing injury of ankle

    √x7ᵗʰ **S97.00** Crushing injury of unspecified ankle

    √x7ᵗʰ **S97.01** Crushing injury of right ankle

    √x7ᵗʰ **S97.02** Crushing injury of left ankle

√5ᵗʰ **S97.1** Crushing injury of toe

√6ᵗʰ **S97.10** Crushing injury of unspecified toe(s)

    √7ᵗʰ **S97.101** Crushing injury of unspecified right toe(s)

    √7ᵗʰ **S97.102** Crushing injury of unspecified left toe(s)

    √7ᵗʰ **S97.109** Crushing injury of unspecified toe(s)

      Crushing injury of toe NOS

√6ᵗʰ **S97.11** Crushing injury of great toe

    √7ᵗʰ **S97.111** Crushing injury of right great toe

    √7ᵗʰ **S97.112** Crushing injury of left great toe

    √7ᵗʰ **S97.119** Crushing injury of unspecified great toe

√6ᵗʰ **S97.12** Crushing injury of lesser toe(s)

    √7ᵗʰ **S97.121** Crushing injury of right lesser toe(s)

    √7ᵗʰ **S97.122** Crushing injury of left lesser toe(s)

    √7ᵗʰ **S97.129** Crushing injury of unspecified lesser toe(s)

√5ᵗʰ **S97.8** Crushing injury of foot

    √x7ᵗʰ **S97.80** Crushing injury of unspecified foot

      Crushing injury of foot NOS

    √x7ᵗʰ **S97.81** Crushing injury of right foot

    √x7ᵗʰ **S97.82** Crushing injury of left foot

√4ᵗʰ **S98** Traumatic amputation of ankle and foot

An amputation not identified as partial or complete should be coded to complete

The appropriate 7th character is to be added to each code from category S98.
A   initial encounter
D   subsequent encounter
S   sequela

√5ᵗʰ **S98.0** Traumatic amputation of foot at ankle level

√6ᵗʰ **S98.01** Complete traumatic amputation of foot at ankle level

    √7ᵗʰ **S98.011** Complete traumatic amputation of right foot at ankle level   HCC ESR COM

    √7ᵗʰ **S98.012** Complete traumatic amputation of left foot at ankle level   HCC ESR COM

    √7ᵗʰ **S98.019** Complete traumatic amputation of unspecified foot at ankle level   HCC ESR COM

√6ᵗʰ **S98.02** Partial traumatic amputation of foot at ankle level

    √7ᵗʰ **S98.021** Partial traumatic amputation of right foot at ankle level   HCC ESR COM

    √7ᵗʰ **S98.022** Partial traumatic amputation of left foot at ankle level   HCC ESR COM

√7ᵗʰ **S98.029** Partial traumatic amputation of unspecified foot at ankle level   HCC ESR COM

√5ᵗʰ **S98.1** Traumatic amputation of one toe

√6ᵗʰ **S98.11** Complete traumatic amputation of great toe

√7ᵗʰ **S98.111** Complete traumatic amputation of right great toe   HCC ESR

√7ᵗʰ **S98.112** Complete traumatic amputation of left great toe   HCC ESR

√7ᵗʰ **S98.119** Complete traumatic amputation of unspecified great toe   HCC ESR

√6ᵗʰ **S98.12** Partial traumatic amputation of great toe

√7ᵗʰ **S98.121** Partial traumatic amputation of right great toe   HCC ESR

√7ᵗʰ **S98.122** Partial traumatic amputation of left great toe   HCC ESR

√7ᵗʰ **S98.129** Partial traumatic amputation of unspecified great toe   HCC ESR

√6ᵗʰ **S98.13** Complete traumatic amputation of one lesser toe
Traumatic amputation of toe NOS

√7ᵗʰ **S98.131** Complete traumatic amputation of one right lesser toe   HCC ESR

√7ᵗʰ **S98.132** Complete traumatic amputation of one left lesser toe   HCC ESR

√7ᵗʰ **S98.139** Complete traumatic amputation of one unspecified lesser toe   HCC ESR

√6ᵗʰ **S98.14** Partial traumatic amputation of one lesser toe

√7ᵗʰ **S98.141** Partial traumatic amputation of one right lesser toe   HCC ESR

√7ᵗʰ **S98.142** Partial traumatic amputation of one left lesser toe   HCC ESR

√7ᵗʰ **S98.149** Partial traumatic amputation of one unspecified lesser toe   HCC ESR

√5ᵗʰ **S98.2** Traumatic amputation of two or more lesser toes

√6ᵗʰ **S98.21** Complete traumatic amputation of two or more lesser toes

√7ᵗʰ **S98.211** Complete traumatic amputation of two or more right lesser toes   HCC ESR

√7ᵗʰ **S98.212** Complete traumatic amputation of two or more left lesser toes   HCC ESR

√7ᵗʰ **S98.219** Complete traumatic amputation of two or more unspecified lesser toes   HCC ESR

√6ᵗʰ **S98.22** Partial traumatic amputation of two or more lesser toes

√7ᵗʰ **S98.221** Partial traumatic amputation of two or more right lesser toes   HCC ESR

√7ᵗʰ **S98.222** Partial traumatic amputation of two or more left lesser toes   HCC ESR

√7ᵗʰ **S98.229** Partial traumatic amputation of two or more unspecified lesser toes   HCC ESR

√5ᵗʰ **S98.3** Traumatic amputation of midfoot

√6ᵗʰ **S98.31** Complete traumatic amputation of midfoot

√7ᵗʰ **S98.311** Complete traumatic amputation of right midfoot   HCC ESR COM

√7ᵗʰ **S98.312** Complete traumatic amputation of left midfoot   HCC ESR COM

√7ᵗʰ **S98.319** Complete traumatic amputation of unspecified midfoot   HCC ESR COM

√6ᵗʰ **S98.32** Partial traumatic amputation of midfoot

√7ᵗʰ **S98.321** Partial traumatic amputation of right midfoot   HCC ESR COM

√7ᵗʰ **S98.322** Partial traumatic amputation of left midfoot   HCC ESR COM

√7ᵗʰ **S98.329** Partial traumatic amputation of unspecified midfoot   HCC ESR COM

√5ᵗʰ **S98.9** Traumatic amputation of foot, level unspecified

√6ᵗʰ **S98.91** Complete traumatic amputation of foot, level unspecified

√7ᵗʰ **S98.911** Complete traumatic amputation of right foot, level unspecified   HCC ESR COM

√7ᵗʰ **S98.912** Complete traumatic amputation of left foot, level unspecified   HCC ESR COM

√7ᵗʰ **S98.919** Complete traumatic amputation of unspecified foot, level unspecified   HCC ESR COM

√6ᵗʰ **S98.92** Partial traumatic amputation of foot, level unspecified

√7ᵗʰ **S98.921** Partial traumatic amputation of right foot, level unspecified   HCC ESR COM

√7ᵗʰ **S98.922** Partial traumatic amputation of left foot, level unspecified   HCC ESR COM

√7ᵗʰ **S98.929** Partial traumatic amputation of unspecified foot, level unspecified   HCC ESR COM

√4ᵗʰ **S99** Other and unspecified injuries of ankle and foot
AHA: 2018,2Q,12; 2018,1Q,3; 2016,4Q,68-69

√5ᵗʰ **S99.0** Physeal fracture of calcaneus
AHA: 2019,4Q,56

> The appropriate 7th character is to be added to each code from subcategory S99.0.
> A   initial encounter for closed fracture
> B   initial encounter for open fracture
> D   subsequent encounter for fracture with routine healing
> G   subsequent encounter for fracture with delayed healing
> K   subsequent encounter for fracture with nonunion
> P   subsequent encounter for fracture with malunion
> S   sequela

√6ᵗʰ **S99.00** Unspecified physeal fracture of calcaneus

√7ᵗʰ **S99.001** Unspecified physeal fracture of right calcaneus   Q

√7ᵗʰ **S99.002** Unspecified physeal fracture of left calcaneus   Q

√7ᵗʰ **S99.009** Unspecified physeal fracture of unspecified calcaneus   Q

√6ᵗʰ **S99.01** Salter-Harris Type I physeal fracture of calcaneus

√7ᵗʰ **S99.011** Salter-Harris Type I physeal fracture of right calcaneus   Q

√7ᵗʰ **S99.012** Salter-Harris Type I physeal fracture of left calcaneus   Q

√7ᵗʰ **S99.019** Salter-Harris Type I physeal fracture of unspecified calcaneus   Q

√6ᵗʰ **S99.02** Salter-Harris Type II physeal fracture of calcaneus

√7ᵗʰ **S99.021** Salter-Harris Type II physeal fracture of right calcaneus   Q

√7ᵗʰ **S99.022** Salter-Harris Type II physeal fracture of left calcaneus   Q

√7ᵗʰ **S99.029** Salter-Harris Type II physeal fracture of unspecified calcaneus   Q

√6ᵗʰ **S99.03** Salter-Harris Type III physeal fracture of calcaneus

√7ᵗʰ **S99.031** Salter-Harris Type III physeal fracture of right calcaneus   Q

√7ᵗʰ **S99.032** Salter-Harris Type III physeal fracture of left calcaneus   Q

√7ᵗʰ **S99.039** Salter-Harris Type III physeal fracture of unspecified calcaneus   Q

√6ᵗʰ **S99.04** Salter-Harris Type IV physeal fracture of calcaneus

√7ᵗʰ **S99.041** Salter-Harris Type IV physeal fracture of right calcaneus   Q

√7ᵗʰ **S99.042** Salter-Harris Type IV physeal fracture of left calcaneus   Q

√7ᵗʰ **S99.049** Salter-Harris Type IV physeal fracture of unspecified calcaneus   Q

√6ᵗʰ **S99.09** Other physeal fracture of calcaneus

√7ᵗʰ **S99.091** Other physeal fracture of right calcaneus   Q

√7ᵗʰ **S99.092** Other physeal fracture of left calcaneus   Q

√7ᵗʰ **S99.099** Other physeal fracture of unspecified calcaneus   Q

√5ᵗʰ **S99.1** **Physeal fracture of metatarsal**

     AHA: 2019,4Q,56

The appropriate 7th character is to be added to each code from subcategory S99.1
A   initial encounter for closed fracture
B   initial encounter for open fracture
D   subsequent encounter for fracture with routine healing
G   subsequent encounter for fracture with delayed healing
K   subsequent encounter for fracture with nonunion
P   subsequent encounter for fracture with malunion
S   sequela

√6ᵗʰ **S99.10** **Unspecified physeal fracture of metatarsal**

     √7ᵗʰ **S99.101** Unspecified physeal fracture of right metatarsal   🄠

     √7ᵗʰ **S99.102** Unspecified physeal fracture of left metatarsal   🄠

     √7ᵗʰ **S99.109** Unspecified physeal fracture of unspecified metatarsal   🄠

√6ᵗʰ **S99.11** Salter-Harris Type I physeal fracture of metatarsal

     √7ᵗʰ **S99.111** Salter-Harris Type I physeal fracture of right metatarsal   🄠

     √7ᵗʰ **S99.112** Salter-Harris Type I physeal fracture of left metatarsal   🄠

     √7ᵗʰ **S99.119** Salter-Harris Type I physeal fracture of unspecified metatarsal   🄠

√6ᵗʰ **S99.12** Salter-Harris Type II physeal fracture of metatarsal

     √7ᵗʰ **S99.121** Salter-Harris Type II physeal fracture of right metatarsal   🄠

     √7ᵗʰ **S99.122** Salter-Harris Type II physeal fracture of left metatarsal   🄠

     √7ᵗʰ **S99.129** Salter-Harris Type II physeal fracture of unspecified metatarsal   🄠

√6ᵗʰ **S99.13** Salter-Harris Type III physeal fracture of metatarsal

     √7ᵗʰ **S99.131** Salter-Harris Type III physeal fracture of right metatarsal   🄠

     √7ᵗʰ **S99.132** Salter-Harris Type III physeal fracture of left metatarsal   🄠

     √7ᵗʰ **S99.139** Salter-Harris Type III physeal fracture of unspecified metatarsal   🄠

√6ᵗʰ **S99.14** Salter-Harris Type IV physeal fracture of metatarsal

     √7ᵗʰ **S99.141** Salter-Harris Type IV physeal fracture of right metatarsal   🄠

     √7ᵗʰ **S99.142** Salter-Harris Type IV physeal fracture of left metatarsal   🄠

     √7ᵗʰ **S99.149** Salter-Harris Type IV physeal fracture of unspecified metatarsal   🄠

√6ᵗʰ **S99.19** Other physeal fracture of metatarsal

     √7ᵗʰ **S99.191** Other physeal fracture of right metatarsal   🄠

     √7ᵗʰ **S99.192** Other physeal fracture of left metatarsal   🄠

     √7ᵗʰ **S99.199** Other physeal fracture of unspecified metatarsal   🄠

√5ᵗʰ **S99.2** **Physeal fracture of phalanx of toe**

     AHA: 2019,4Q,56

The appropriate 7th character is to be added to each code from subcategories S99.2.
A   initial encounter for closed fracture
B   initial encounter for open fracture
D   subsequent encounter for fracture with routine healing
G   subsequent encounter for fracture with delayed healing
K   subsequent encounter for fracture with nonunion
P   subsequent encounter for fracture with malunion
S   sequela

√6ᵗʰ **S99.20** **Unspecified physeal fracture of phalanx of toe**

     √7ᵗʰ **S99.201** Unspecified physeal fracture of phalanx of right toe

     √7ᵗʰ **S99.202** Unspecified physeal fracture of phalanx of left toe

     √7ᵗʰ **S99.209** Unspecified physeal fracture of phalanx of unspecified toe

√6ᵗʰ **S99.21** Salter-Harris Type I physeal fracture of phalanx of toe

     √7ᵗʰ **S99.211** Salter-Harris Type I physeal fracture of phalanx of right toe

     √7ᵗʰ **S99.212** Salter-Harris Type I physeal fracture of phalanx of left toe

     √7ᵗʰ **S99.219** Salter-Harris Type I physeal fracture of phalanx of unspecified toe

√6ᵗʰ **S99.22** Salter-Harris Type II physeal fracture of phalanx of toe

     √7ᵗʰ **S99.221** Salter-Harris Type II physeal fracture of phalanx of right toe

     √7ᵗʰ **S99.222** Salter-Harris Type II physeal fracture of phalanx of left toe

     √7ᵗʰ **S99.229** Salter-Harris Type II physeal fracture of phalanx of unspecified toe

√6ᵗʰ **S99.23** Salter-Harris Type III physeal fracture of phalanx of toe

     √7ᵗʰ **S99.231** Salter-Harris Type III physeal fracture of phalanx of right toe

     √7ᵗʰ **S99.232** Salter-Harris Type III physeal fracture of phalanx of left toe

     √7ᵗʰ **S99.239** Salter-Harris Type III physeal fracture of phalanx of unspecified toe

√6ᵗʰ **S99.24** Salter-Harris Type IV physeal fracture of phalanx of toe

     √7ᵗʰ **S99.241** Salter-Harris Type IV physeal fracture of phalanx of right toe

     √7ᵗʰ **S99.242** Salter-Harris Type IV physeal fracture of phalanx of left toe

     √7ᵗʰ **S99.249** Salter-Harris Type IV physeal fracture of phalanx of unspecified toe

√6ᵗʰ **S99.29** Other physeal fracture of phalanx of toe

     √7ᵗʰ **S99.291** Other physeal fracture of phalanx of right toe

     √7ᵗʰ **S99.292** Other physeal fracture of phalanx of left toe

     √7ᵗʰ **S99.299** Other physeal fracture of phalanx of unspecified toe

√5ᵗʰ **S99.8** Other specified injuries of ankle and foot

The appropriate 7th character is to be added to each code from subcategory S99.8.
A   initial encounter
D   subsequent encounter
S   sequela

√6ᵗʰ **S99.81** Other specified injuries of ankle

     √7ᵗʰ **S99.811** Other specified injuries of right ankle

     √7ᵗʰ **S99.812** Other specified injuries of left ankle

     √7ᵗʰ **S99.819** Other specified injuries of unspecified ankle

√6ᵗʰ **S99.82** Other specified injuries of foot

     √7ᵗʰ **S99.821** Other specified injuries of right foot

     √7ᵗʰ **S99.822** Other specified injuries of left foot

     √7ᵗʰ **S99.829** Other specified injuries of unspecified foot

√5ᵗʰ **S99.9** Unspecified injury of ankle and foot

The appropriate 7th character is to be added to each code from subcategory S99.9.
A   initial encounter
D   subsequent encounter
S   sequela

√6ᵗʰ **S99.91** **Unspecified injury of ankle**

     √7ᵗʰ **S99.911** Unspecified injury of right ankle

     √7ᵗʰ **S99.912** Unspecified injury of left ankle

     √7ᵗʰ **S99.919** Unspecified injury of unspecified ankle

√6ᵗʰ **S99.92** Unspecified injury of foot

     √7ᵗʰ **S99.921** Unspecified injury of right foot

     √7ᵗʰ **S99.922** Unspecified injury of left foot

     √7ᵗʰ **S99.929** Unspecified injury of unspecified foot

INJURY, POISONING AND CERTAIN OTHER CONSEQUENCES OF EXTERNAL CAUSES (T07-T88)

Injuries involving multiple body regions (T07)

EXCLUDES 1   burns and corrosions (T20-T32)
frostbite (T33-T34)
insect bite or sting, venomous (T63.4)
sunburn (L55.-)

✓x7ᵗʰ **T07**   **Unspecified multiple injuries**
     EXCLUDES 1   injury NOS (T14.90)
     AHA: 2017,4Q,26

> The appropriate 7th character is to be added to code T07.
> A   initial encounter
> D   subsequent encounter
> S   sequela

Injury of unspecified body region (T14)

✓4ᵗʰ **T14**   **Injury of unspecified body region**
     EXCLUDES 1   multiple unspecified injuries (T07)
     AHA: 2017,4Q,26

> The appropriate 7th character is to be added to each code from category T14.
> A   initial encounter
> D   subsequent encounter
> S   sequela

✓x7ᵗʰ **T14.8**   **Other injury of unspecified body region**
     Abrasion NOS
     Contusion NOS
     Crush injury NOS
     Fracture NOS
     Skin injury NOS
     Vascular injury NOS
     Wound NOS

✓5ᵗʰ **T14.9**   **Unspecified injury**
     ✓x7ᵗʰ **T14.90**   **Injury, unspecified**
         Injury NOS
     ✓x7ᵗʰ **T14.91**   **Suicide attempt**   HCC Rx ESR COM
         Attempted suicide NOS

Effects of foreign body entering through natural orifice (T15-T19)

EXCLUDES 2   foreign body accidentally left in operation wound (T81.5-)
foreign body in penetrating wound - see open wound by body region
residual foreign body in soft tissue (M79.5)
splinter, without open wound - see superficial injury by body region

✓4ᵗʰ **T15**   **Foreign body on external eye**
     EXCLUDES 2   foreign body in penetrating wound of orbit and eye ball (S05.4-, S05.5-)
         open wound of eyelid and periocular area (S01.1-)
         retained foreign body in eyelid (H02.8-)
         retained (old) foreign body in penetrating wound of orbit and eye ball (H05.5-, H44.6-, H44.7-)
         superficial foreign body of eyelid and periocular area (S00.25-)

> The appropriate 7th character is to be added to each code from category T15.
> A   initial encounter
> D   subsequent encounter
> S   sequela

✓5ᵗʰ **T15.0**   **Foreign body in cornea**
     ✓x7ᵗʰ **T15.00**   **Foreign body in cornea, unspecified eye**
     ✓x7ᵗʰ **T15.01**   **Foreign body in cornea, right eye**
     ✓x7ᵗʰ **T15.02**   **Foreign body in cornea, left eye**

✓5ᵗʰ **T15.1**   **Foreign body in conjunctival sac**
     ✓x7ᵗʰ **T15.10**   **Foreign body in conjunctival sac, unspecified eye**
     ✓x7ᵗʰ **T15.11**   **Foreign body in conjunctival sac, right eye**
     ✓x7ᵗʰ **T15.12**   **Foreign body in conjunctival sac, left eye**

✓5ᵗʰ **T15.8**   **Foreign body in other and multiple parts of external eye**
     Foreign body in lacrimal punctum
     ✓x7ᵗʰ **T15.80**   **Foreign body in other and multiple parts of external eye, unspecified eye**

✓x7ᵗʰ **T15.81**   **Foreign body in other and multiple parts of external eye, right eye**
✓x7ᵗʰ **T15.82**   **Foreign body in other and multiple parts of external eye, left eye**

✓5ᵗʰ **T15.9**   **Foreign body on external eye, part unspecified**
     ✓x7ᵗʰ **T15.90**   **Foreign body on external eye, part unspecified, unspecified eye**
     ✓x7ᵗʰ **T15.91**   **Foreign body on external eye, part unspecified, right eye**
     ✓x7ᵗʰ **T15.92**   **Foreign body on external eye, part unspecified, left eye**

✓4ᵗʰ **T16**   **Foreign body in ear**
     INCLUDES   foreign body in auditory canal

> The appropriate 7th character is to be added to each code from category T16.
> A   initial encounter
> D   subsequent encounter
> S   sequela

✓x7ᵗʰ **T16.1**   **Foreign body in right ear**
✓x7ᵗʰ **T16.2**   **Foreign body in left ear**
✓x7ᵗʰ **T16.9**   **Foreign body in ear, unspecified ear**

✓4ᵗʰ **T17**   **Foreign body in respiratory tract**

> The appropriate 7th character is to be added to each code from category T17.
> A   initial encounter
> D   subsequent encounter
> S   sequela

✓x7ᵗʰ **T17.0**   **Foreign body in nasal sinus**
✓x7ᵗʰ **T17.1**   **Foreign body in nostril**
     Foreign body in nose NOS

✓5ᵗʰ **T17.2**   **Foreign body in pharynx**
     Foreign body in nasopharynx
     Foreign body in throat NOS
     ✓6ᵗʰ **T17.20**   **Unspecified foreign body in pharynx**
         ✓7ᵗʰ **T17.200**   **Unspecified foreign body in pharynx causing asphyxiation**
         ✓7ᵗʰ **T17.208**   **Unspecified foreign body in pharynx causing other injury**
     ✓6ᵗʰ **T17.21**   **Gastric contents in pharynx**
         Aspiration of gastric contents into pharynx
         Vomitus in pharynx
         ✓7ᵗʰ **T17.210**   **Gastric contents in pharynx causing asphyxiation**
         ✓7ᵗʰ **T17.218**   **Gastric contents in pharynx causing other injury**
     ✓6ᵗʰ **T17.22**   **Food in pharynx**
         Bones in pharynx
         Seeds in pharynx
         ✓7ᵗʰ **T17.220**   **Food in pharynx causing asphyxiation**
         ✓7ᵗʰ **T17.228**   **Food in pharynx causing other injury**
     ✓6ᵗʰ **T17.29**   **Other foreign object in pharynx**
         ✓7ᵗʰ **T17.290**   **Other foreign object in pharynx causing asphyxiation**
         ✓7ᵗʰ **T17.298**   **Other foreign object in pharynx causing other injury**

✓5ᵗʰ **T17.3**   **Foreign body in larynx**
     ✓6ᵗʰ **T17.30**   **Unspecified foreign body in larynx**
         ✓7ᵗʰ **T17.300**   **Unspecified foreign body in larynx causing asphyxiation**
         ✓7ᵗʰ **T17.308**   **Unspecified foreign body in larynx causing other injury**
     ✓6ᵗʰ **T17.31**   **Gastric contents in larynx**
         Aspiration of gastric contents into larynx
         Vomitus in larynx
         ✓7ᵗʰ **T17.310**   **Gastric contents in larynx causing asphyxiation**
         ✓7ᵗʰ **T17.318**   **Gastric contents in larynx causing other injury**
     ✓6ᵗʰ **T17.32**   **Food in larynx**
         Bones in larynx
         Seeds in larynx
         ✓7ᵗʰ **T17.320**   **Food in larynx causing asphyxiation**
         ✓7ᵗʰ **T17.328**   **Food in larynx causing other injury**

√6ᵗʰ **T17.39** **Other foreign object in larynx**

√7ᵗʰ **T17.390** **Other foreign object in larynx** causing asphyxiation

√7ᵗʰ **T17.398** **Other foreign object in larynx** causing other injury

√5ᵗʰ **T17.4** **Foreign body in** trachea

√6ᵗʰ **T17.40** **Unspecified foreign body in trachea**

√7ᵗʰ **T17.400** **Unspecified foreign body in trachea** causing asphyxiation

√7ᵗʰ **T17.408** **Unspecified foreign body in trachea** causing other injury

√6ᵗʰ **T17.41** **Gastric contents in trachea**

Aspiration of gastric contents into trachea
Vomitus in trachea

√7ᵗʰ **T17.410** **Gastric contents in trachea** causing asphyxiation

√7ᵗʰ **T17.418** **Gastric contents in trachea** causing other injury

√6ᵗʰ **T17.42** **Food in trachea**

Bones in trachea
Seeds in trachea

√7ᵗʰ **T17.420** **Food in trachea** causing asphyxiation

√7ᵗʰ **T17.428** **Food in trachea** causing other injury

√6ᵗʰ **T17.49** **Other foreign object in trachea**

√7ᵗʰ **T17.490** **Other foreign object in trachea** causing asphyxiation

√7ᵗʰ **T17.498** **Other foreign object in trachea** causing other injury

√5ᵗʰ **T17.5** **Foreign body in** bronchus

√6ᵗʰ **T17.50** **Unspecified foreign body in bronchus**

√7ᵗʰ **T17.500** **Unspecified foreign body in bronchus** causing asphyxiation

√7ᵗʰ **T17.508** **Unspecified foreign body in bronchus** causing other injury

√6ᵗʰ **T17.51** **Gastric contents in bronchus**

Aspiration of gastric contents into bronchus
Vomitus in bronchus

√7ᵗʰ **T17.510** **Gastric contents in bronchus** causing asphyxiation

√7ᵗʰ **T17.518** **Gastric contents in bronchus** causing other injury

√6ᵗʰ **T17.52** **Food in bronchus**

Bones in bronchus
Seeds in bronchus

√7ᵗʰ **T17.520** **Food in bronchus** causing asphyxiation

√7ᵗʰ **T17.528** **Food in bronchus** causing other injury

√6ᵗʰ **T17.59** **Other foreign object in bronchus**

√7ᵗʰ **T17.590** **Other foreign object in bronchus** causing asphyxiation

√7ᵗʰ **T17.598** **Other foreign object in bronchus** causing other injury

√5ᵗʰ **T17.8** **Foreign body in other parts of respiratory tract**

Foreign body in bronchioles
Foreign body in lung

√6ᵗʰ **T17.80** **Unspecified foreign body in other parts of respiratory tract**

√7ᵗʰ **T17.800** **Unspecified foreign body in other parts of respiratory tract** causing asphyxiation

√7ᵗʰ **T17.808** **Unspecified foreign body in other parts of respiratory tract** causing other injury

√6ᵗʰ **T17.81** **Gastric contents in other parts of respiratory tract**

Aspiration of gastric contents into other parts of respiratory tract
Vomitus in other parts of respiratory tract

√7ᵗʰ **T17.810** **Gastric contents in other parts of respiratory tract** causing asphyxiation

√7ᵗʰ **T17.818** **Gastric contents in other parts of respiratory tract** causing other injury

√6ᵗʰ **T17.82** **Food in other parts of respiratory tract**

Bones in other parts of respiratory tract
Seeds in other parts of respiratory tract

√7ᵗʰ **T17.820** **Food in other parts of respiratory tract** causing asphyxiation

√7ᵗʰ **T17.828** **Food in other parts of respiratory tract** causing other injury

√6ᵗʰ **T17.89** **Other foreign object in other parts of respiratory tract**

√7ᵗʰ **T17.890** **Other foreign object in other parts of respiratory tract** causing asphyxiation

√7ᵗʰ **T17.898** **Other foreign object in other parts of respiratory tract** causing other injury

√5ᵗʰ **T17.9** **Foreign body in respiratory tract, part unspecified**

√6ᵗʰ **T17.90** **Unspecified foreign body in respiratory tract, part unspecified**

√7ᵗʰ **T17.900** **Unspecified foreign body in respiratory tract, part unspecified** causing asphyxiation

√7ᵗʰ **T17.908** **Unspecified foreign body in respiratory tract, part unspecified** causing other injury

√6ᵗʰ **T17.91** **Gastric contents in respiratory tract, part unspecified**

Aspiration of gastric contents into respiratory tract, part unspecified
Vomitus in trachea respiratory tract, part unspecified

√7ᵗʰ **T17.910** **Gastric contents in respiratory tract, part unspecified** causing asphyxiation

√7ᵗʰ **T17.918** **Gastric contents in respiratory tract, part unspecified** causing other injury

√6ᵗʰ **T17.92** **Food in respiratory tract, part unspecified**

Bones in respiratory tract, part unspecified
Seeds in respiratory tract, part unspecified

√7ᵗʰ **T17.920** **Food in respiratory tract, part unspecified** causing asphyxiation

√7ᵗʰ **T17.928** **Food in respiratory tract, part unspecified** causing other injury

√6ᵗʰ **T17.99** **Other foreign object in respiratory tract, part unspecified**

√7ᵗʰ **T17.990** **Other foreign object in respiratory tract, part unspecified in** causing asphyxiation

AHA: 2019,3Q,15

√7ᵗʰ **T17.998** **Other foreign object in respiratory tract, part unspecified** causing other injury

√4ᵗʰ **T18** **Foreign body in alimentary tract**

EXCLUDES 2   foreign body in pharynx (T17.2-)

> The appropriate 7th character is to be added to each code from category T18.
> A   initial encounter
> D   subsequent encounter
> S   sequela

√x7ᵗʰ **T18.0** **Foreign body in** mouth

√5ᵗʰ **T18.1** **Foreign body in** esophagus

EXCLUDES 2   foreign body in respiratory tract (T17.-)

√6ᵗʰ **T18.10** **Unspecified foreign body in esophagus**

√7ᵗʰ **T18.100** **Unspecified foreign body in esophagus** causing compression of trachea

Unspecified foreign body in esophagus causing obstruction of respiration

√7ᵗʰ **T18.108** **Unspecified foreign body in esophagus** causing other injury

√6ᵗʰ **T18.11** **Gastric contents in esophagus**

Vomitus in esophagus

√7ᵗʰ **T18.110** **Gastric contents in esophagus** causing compression of trachea

Gastric contents in esophagus causing obstruction of respiration

√7ᵗʰ **T18.118** **Gastric contents in esophagus** causing other injury

√6ᵗʰ **T18.12** **Food in esophagus**

Bones in esophagus
Seeds in esophagus

√7ᵗʰ **T18.120** **Food in esophagus** causing compression of trachea

Food in esophagus causing obstruction of respiration

√7ᵗʰ **T18.128** **Food in esophagus** causing other injury

√6ᵗʰ **T18.19** **Other foreign object in esophagus**
AHA: 2022,1Q,27; 2015,1Q,23

√7ᵗʰ **T18.190** **Other foreign object in esophagus causing compression of trachea**
Other foreign body in esophagus causing obstruction of respiration
TIP: Any foreign object lodged in the esophagus requires immediate treatment and is considered an injury. Assign this code when there is respiratory compromise or compression. If no respiratory compromise or compression is documented, assign code T18.198-.

√7ᵗʰ **T18.198** **Other foreign object in esophagus causing other injury**
TIP: Any foreign object lodged in the esophagus requires immediate treatment and is considered an injury. Assign this code when there is no respiratory compromise or compression. If respiratory compromise or compression is documented, assign code T18.190-.

√x7ᵗʰ **T18.2** **Foreign body in stomach**

√x7ᵗʰ **T18.3** **Foreign body in small intestine**

√x7ᵗʰ **T18.4** **Foreign body in colon**

√x7ᵗʰ **T18.5** **Foreign body in anus and rectum**
Foreign body in rectosigmoid (junction)

√x7ᵗʰ **T18.8** **Foreign body in other parts of alimentary tract**

√x7ᵗʰ **T18.9** **Foreign body of alimentary tract, part unspecified**
Foreign body in digestive system NOS
Swallowed foreign body NOS

√4ᵗʰ **T19** **Foreign body in genitourinary tract**
EXCLUDES 2   complications due to implanted mesh (T83.7-)
mechanical complications of contraceptive device (intrauterine) (vaginal) (T83.3-)
presence of contraceptive device (intrauterine) (vaginal) (Z97.5)

The appropriate 7th character is to be added to each code from category T19.
A   initial encounter
D   subsequent encounter
S   sequela

√x7ᵗʰ **T19.0** **Foreign body in urethra**

√x7ᵗʰ **T19.1** **Foreign body in bladder**

√x7ᵗʰ **T19.2** **Foreign body in vulva and vagina** ♀

√x7ᵗʰ **T19.3** **Foreign body in uterus** ♀

√x7ᵗʰ **T19.4** **Foreign body in penis** ♂

√x7ᵗʰ **T19.8** **Foreign body in other parts of genitourinary tract**

√x7ᵗʰ **T19.9** **Foreign body in genitourinary tract, part unspecified**

BURNS AND CORROSIONS (T20-T32)

INCLUDES   burns (thermal) from electrical heating appliances
burns (thermal) from electricity
burns (thermal) from flame
burns (thermal) from friction
burns (thermal) from hot air and hot gases
burns (thermal) from hot objects
burns (thermal) from lightning
burns (thermal) from radiation
chemical burn [corrosion] (external) (internal)
scalds
EXCLUDES 2   erythema [dermatitis] ab igne (L59.0)
radiation-related disorders of the skin and subcutaneous tissue (L55-L59)
sunburn (L55.-)
AHA: 2016,2Q,4

Burns and corrosions of external body surface, specified by site (T20-T25)

INCLUDES   burns and corrosions of first degree [erythema]
burns and corrosions of second degree [blisters] [epidermal loss]
burns and corrosions of third degree [deep necrosis of underlying tissue] [full-thickness skin loss]
Use additional code from category T31 or T32 to identify extent of body surface involved

√4ᵗʰ **T20** **Burn and corrosion of head, face, and neck**
EXCLUDES 2   burn and corrosion of ear drum (T28.41, T28.91)
burn and corrosion of eye and adnexa (T26.-)
burn and corrosion of mouth and pharynx (T28.0)
AHA: 2015,1Q,18-19

The appropriate 7th character is to be added to each code from category T20.
A   initial encounter
D   subsequent encounter
S   sequela

√5ᵗʰ **T20.0** **Burn of unspecified degree of head, face, and neck**
Use additional external cause code to identify the source, place and intent of the burn (X00-X19, X75-X77, X96-X98, Y92)

√x7ᵗʰ **T20.00** **Burn of unspecified degree of head, face, and neck, unspecified site**

√6ᵗʰ **T20.01** **Burn of unspecified degree of ear** [any part, except ear drum]
EXCLUDES 2   burn of ear drum (T28.41-)

√7ᵗʰ **T20.011** **Burn of unspecified degree of right ear** [any part, except ear drum]

√7ᵗʰ **T20.012** **Burn of unspecified degree of left ear** [any part, except ear drum]

√7ᵗʰ **T20.019** **Burn of unspecified degree of unspecified ear** [any part, except ear drum]

√x7ᵗʰ **T20.02** **Burn of unspecified degree of lip(s)**

√x7ᵗʰ **T20.03** **Burn of unspecified degree of chin**

√x7ᵗʰ **T20.04** **Burn of unspecified degree of nose** (septum)

√x7ᵗʰ **T20.05** **Burn of unspecified degree of scalp** [any part]

√x7ᵗʰ **T20.06** **Burn of unspecified degree of forehead and cheek**

√x7ᵗʰ **T20.07** **Burn of unspecified degree of neck**

√x7ᵗʰ **T20.09** **Burn of unspecified degree of multiple sites of head, face, and neck**

√5ᵗʰ **T20.1** **Burn of first degree of head, face, and neck**
Use additional external cause code to identify the source, place and intent of the burn (X00-X19, X75-X77, X96-X98, Y92)

√x7ᵗʰ **T20.10** **Burn of first degree of head, face, and neck, unspecified site**

√6ᵗʰ **T20.11** **Burn of first degree of ear** [any part, except ear drum]
EXCLUDES 2   burn of ear drum (T28.41-)

√7ᵗʰ **T20.111** **Burn of first degree of right ear** [any part, except ear drum]

√7ᵗʰ **T20.112** **Burn of first degree of left ear** [any part, except ear drum]

√7ᵗʰ **T20.119** **Burn of first degree of unspecified ear** [any part, except ear drum]

√x7ᵗʰ **T20.12** **Burn of first degree of lip(s)**

√x7ᵗʰ **T20.13** **Burn of first degree of chin**

√x7ᵗʰ **T20.14** **Burn of first degree of nose** (septum)

√x7ᵗʰ **T20.15** **Burn of first degree of scalp** [any part]

√x7ᵗʰ **T20.16** **Burn of first degree of forehead and cheek**

✓x7th **T20.17**   Burn of first degree of neck

✓x7th **T20.19**   Burn of first degree of multiple sites of head, face, and neck

Degree of Burns

Normal   First Degree Burn

Second Degree Burn   Third Degree Burn

burn

Head

neck

face

✓5th **T20.2**   Burn of second degree of head, face, and neck

Use additional external cause code to identify the source, place and intent of the burn (X00-X19, X75-X77, X96-X98, Y92)

✓x7th **T20.20**   Burn of second degree of head, face, and neck, unspecified site

✓6th **T20.21**   Burn of second degree of ear [any part, except ear drum]

> EXCLUDES 2   *burn of ear drum (T28.41-)*

✓7th **T20.211**   Burn of second degree of right ear [any part, except ear drum]

✓7th **T20.212**   Burn of second degree of left ear [any part, except ear drum]

✓7th **T20.219**   Burn of second degree of unspecified ear [any part, except ear drum]

✓x7th **T20.22**   Burn of second degree of lip(s)

✓x7th **T20.23**   Burn of second degree of chin

✓x7th **T20.24**   Burn of second degree of nose (septum)

✓x7th **T20.25**   Burn of second degree of scalp [any part]

✓x7th **T20.26**   Burn of second degree of forehead and cheek

✓x7th **T20.27**   Burn of second degree of neck

✓x7th **T20.29**   Burn of second degree of multiple sites of head, face, and neck

✓5th **T20.3**   Burn of third degree of head, face, and neck

Use additional external cause code to identify the source, place and intent of the burn (X00-X19, X75-X77, X96-X98, Y92)

✓x7th **T20.30**   Burn of third degree of head, face, and neck, unspecified site   COM

✓6th **T20.31**   Burn of third degree of ear [any part, except ear drum]

> EXCLUDES 2   *burn of ear drum (T28.41-)*

AHA: 2015,1Q,18

✓7th **T20.311**   Burn of third degree of right ear [any part, except ear drum]   COM

✓7th **T20.312**   Burn of third degree of left ear [any part, except ear drum]   COM

✓7th **T20.319**   Burn of third degree of unspecified ear [any part, except ear drum]   COM

✓x7th **T20.32**   Burn of third degree of lip(s)   COM

✓x7th **T20.33**   Burn of third degree of chin   COM

✓x7th **T20.34**   Burn of third degree of nose (septum)   COM

✓x7th **T20.35**   Burn of third degree of scalp [any part]   COM

✓x7th **T20.36**   Burn of third degree of forehead and cheek   COM

✓x7th **T20.37**   Burn of third degree of neck   COM

✓x7th **T20.39**   Burn of third degree of multiple sites of head, face, and neck   COM

✓5th **T20.4**   Corrosion of unspecified degree of head, face, and neck

Code first (T51-T65) to identify chemical and intent

Use additional external cause code to identify place (Y92)

✓x7th **T20.40**   Corrosion of unspecified degree of head, face, and neck, unspecified site

✓6th **T20.41**   Corrosion of unspecified degree of ear [any part, except ear drum]

> EXCLUDES 2   *corrosion of ear drum (T28.91-)*

✓7th **T20.411**   Corrosion of unspecified degree of right ear [any part, except ear drum]

✓7th **T20.412**   Corrosion of unspecified degree of left ear [any part, except ear drum]

✓7th **T20.419**   Corrosion of unspecified degree of unspecified ear [any part, except ear drum]

✓x7th **T20.42**   Corrosion of unspecified degree of lip(s)

✓x7th **T20.43**   Corrosion of unspecified degree of chin

✓x7th **T20.44**   Corrosion of unspecified degree of nose (septum)

✓x7th **T20.45**   Corrosion of unspecified degree of scalp [any part]

✓x7th **T20.46**   Corrosion of unspecified degree of forehead and cheek

✓x7th **T20.47**   Corrosion of unspecified degree of neck

✓x7th **T20.49**   Corrosion of unspecified degree of multiple sites of head, face, and neck

✓5th **T20.5**   Corrosion of first degree of head, face, and neck

Code first (T51-T65) to identify chemical and intent

Use additional external cause code to identify place (Y92)

✓x7th **T20.50**   Corrosion of first degree of head, face, and neck, unspecified site

✓6th **T20.51**   Corrosion of first degree of ear [any part, except ear drum]

> EXCLUDES 2   *corrosion of ear drum (T28.91-)*

✓7th **T20.511**   Corrosion of first degree of right ear [any part, except ear drum]

✓7th **T20.512**   Corrosion of first degree of left ear [any part, except ear drum]

✓7th **T20.519**   Corrosion of first degree of unspecified ear [any part, except ear drum]

✓x7th **T20.52**   Corrosion of first degree of lip(s)

✓x7th **T20.53**   Corrosion of first degree of chin

✓x7th **T20.54**   Corrosion of first degree of nose (septum)

✓x7th **T20.55**   Corrosion of first degree of scalp [any part]

✓x7th **T20.56**   Corrosion of first degree of forehead and cheek

✓x7th **T20.57**   Corrosion of first degree of neck

✓x7th **T20.59**   Corrosion of first degree of multiple sites of head, face, and neck

✓5th **T20.6**   Corrosion of second degree of head, face, and neck

Code first (T51-T65) to identify chemical and intent

Use additional external cause code to identify place (Y92)

✓x7th **T20.60**   Corrosion of second degree of head, face, and neck, unspecified site

✓6th **T20.61**   Corrosion of second degree of ear [any part, except ear drum]

> EXCLUDES 2   *corrosion of ear drum (T28.91-)*

✓7th **T20.611**   Corrosion of second degree of right ear [any part, except ear drum]

✓7th **T20.612**   Corrosion of second degree of left ear [any part, except ear drum]

✓7th **T20.619**   Corrosion of second degree of unspecified ear [any part, except ear drum]

✓x7th **T20.62**   Corrosion of second degree of lip(s)

✓x7th **T20.63**   Corrosion of second degree of chin

✓x7th **T20.64**   Corrosion of second degree of nose (septum)

✓x7th **T20.65**   Corrosion of second degree of scalp [any part]

✓x7th **T20.66**   Corrosion of second degree of forehead and cheek

✓x7th **T20.67**   Corrosion of second degree of neck

✓x7th **T20.69**   Corrosion of second degree of multiple sites of head, face, and neck

✓5th **T20.7**   Corrosion of third degree of head, face, and neck

Code first (T51-T65) to identify chemical and intent

Use additional external cause code to identify place (Y92)

✓x7th **T20.70**   Corrosion of third degree of head, face, and neck, unspecified site   COM

√6ᵗʰ **T20.71 Corrosion of third degree of** ear [any part, except ear drum]
> EXCLUDES 2   corrosion of ear drum (T28.91-)

√7ᵗʰ **T20.711 Corrosion of third degree of** right ear [any part, except ear drum] COM

√7ᵗʰ **T20.712 Corrosion of third degree of** left ear [any part, except ear drum] COM

√7ᵗʰ **T20.719 Corrosion of third degree of unspecified ear** [any part, except ear drum] COM

√x7ᵗʰ **T20.72 Corrosion of third degree of** lip(s) COM

√x7ᵗʰ **T20.73 Corrosion of third degree of** chin COM

√x7ᵗʰ **T20.74 Corrosion of third degree of** nose (septum) COM

√x7ᵗʰ **T20.75 Corrosion of third degree of** scalp [any part] COM

√x7ᵗʰ **T20.76 Corrosion of third degree of** forehead and cheek COM

√x7ᵗʰ **T20.77 Corrosion of third degree of** neck COM

√x7ᵗʰ **T20.79 Corrosion of third degree of** multiple sites of head, face, and neck COM

√4ᵗʰ **T21 Burn and corrosion of trunk**

> INCLUDES   burns and corrosion of hip region
> EXCLUDES 2   burns and corrosion of axilla (T22.- with fifth character 4)
> burns and corrosion of scapular region (T22.- with fifth character 6)
> burns and corrosion of shoulder (T22.- with fifth character 5)

> The appropriate 7th character is to be added to each code from category T21.
> A initial encounter
> D subsequent encounter
> S sequela

√5ᵗʰ **T21.0 Burn of unspecified degree of trunk**

> Use additional external cause code to identify the source, place and intent of the burn (X00-X19, X75-X77, X96-X98, Y92)

√x7ᵗʰ **T21.00 Burn of unspecified degree of trunk, unspecified site**

√x7ᵗʰ **T21.01 Burn of unspecified degree of** chest wall
> Burn of unspecified degree of breast

√x7ᵗʰ **T21.02 Burn of unspecified degree of** abdominal wall
> Burn of unspecified degree of flank
> Burn of unspecified degree of groin

√x7ᵗʰ **T21.03 Burn of unspecified degree of** upper back
> Burn of unspecified degree of interscapular region

√x7ᵗʰ **T21.04 Burn of unspecified degree of** lower back

√x7ᵗʰ **T21.05 Burn of unspecified degree of** buttock
> Burn of unspecified degree of anus

√x7ᵗʰ **T21.06 Burn of unspecified degree of** male genital region ♂
> Burn of unspecified degree of penis
> Burn of unspecified degree of scrotum
> Burn of unspecified degree of testis

√x7ᵗʰ **T21.07 Burn of unspecified degree of** female genital region ♀
> Burn of unspecified degree of labium (majus) (minus)
> Burn of unspecified degree of perineum
> Burn of unspecified degree of vulva
> EXCLUDES 2   burn of vagina (T28.3)

√x7ᵗʰ **T21.09 Burn of unspecified degree of other site of trunk**

√5ᵗʰ **T21.1 Burn of** first degree of trunk

> Use additional external cause code to identify the source, place and intent of the burn (X00-X19, X75-X77, X96-X98, Y92)

√x7ᵗʰ **T21.10 Burn of first degree of trunk, unspecified site**

√x7ᵗʰ **T21.11 Burn of first degree of** chest wall
> Burn of first degree of breast

√x7ᵗʰ **T21.12 Burn of first degree of** abdominal wall
> Burn of first degree of flank
> Burn of first degree of groin

√x7ᵗʰ **T21.13 Burn of first degree of** upper back
> Burn of first degree of interscapular region

√x7ᵗʰ **T21.14 Burn of first degree of** lower back

√x7ᵗʰ **T21.15 Burn of first degree of** buttock
> Burn of first degree of anus

√x7ᵗʰ **T21.16 Burn of first degree of** male genital region ♂
> Burn of first degree of penis
> Burn of first degree of scrotum
> Burn of first degree of testis

√x7ᵗʰ **T21.17 Burn of first degree of** female genital region ♀
> Burn of first degree of labium (majus) (minus)
> Burn of first degree of perineum
> Burn of first degree of vulva
> EXCLUDES 2   burn of vagina (T28.3)

√x7ᵗʰ **T21.19 Burn of first degree of other site of trunk**

√5ᵗʰ **T21.2 Burn of** second degree of trunk

> Use additional external cause code to identify the source, place and intent of the burn (X00-X19, X75-X77, X96-X98, Y92)

√x7ᵗʰ **T21.20 Burn of second degree of trunk, unspecified site**

√x7ᵗʰ **T21.21 Burn of second degree of** chest wall
> Burn of second degree of breast

√x7ᵗʰ **T21.22 Burn of second degree of** abdominal wall
> Burn of second degree of flank
> Burn of second degree of groin

√x7ᵗʰ **T21.23 Burn of second degree of** upper back
> Burn of second degree of interscapular region

√x7ᵗʰ **T21.24 Burn of second degree of** lower back

√x7ᵗʰ **T21.25 Burn of second degree of** buttock
> Burn of second degree of anus

√x7ᵗʰ **T21.26 Burn of second degree of** male genital region ♂
> Burn of second degree of penis
> Burn of second degree of scrotum
> Burn of second degree of testis

√x7ᵗʰ **T21.27 Burn of second degree of** female genital region ♀
> Burn of second degree of labium (majus) (minus)
> Burn of second degree of perineum
> Burn of second degree of vulva
> EXCLUDES 2   burn of vagina (T28.3)

√x7ᵗʰ **T21.29 Burn of second degree of other site of trunk**

√5ᵗʰ **T21.3 Burn of** third degree of trunk

> Use additional external cause code to identify the source, place and intent of the burn (X00-X19, X75-X77, X96-X98, Y92)

√x7ᵗʰ **T21.30 Burn of third degree of trunk, unspecified site** COM

√x7ᵗʰ **T21.31 Burn of third degree of** chest wall COM
> Burn of third degree of breast
> **AHA:** 2016,2Q,5

√x7ᵗʰ **T21.32 Burn of third degree of** abdominal wall COM
> Burn of third degree of flank
> Burn of third degree of groin

√x7ᵗʰ **T21.33 Burn of third degree of** upper back COM
> Burn of third degree of interscapular region

√x7ᵗʰ **T21.34 Burn of third degree of** lower back COM

√x7ᵗʰ **T21.35 Burn of third degree of** buttock COM
> Burn of third degree of anus

√x7ᵗʰ **T21.36 Burn of third degree of** male genital region COM ♂
> Burn of third degree of penis
> Burn of third degree of scrotum
> Burn of third degree of testis

√x7ᵗʰ **T21.37 Burn of third degree of** female genital region COM ♀
> Burn of third degree of labium (majus) (minus)
> Burn of third degree of perineum
> Burn of third degree of vulva
> EXCLUDES 2   burn of vagina (T28.3)

√x7ᵗʰ **T21.39 Burn of third degree of other site of trunk** COM

√5ᵗʰ **T21.4 Corrosion of unspecified degree of trunk**

> Code first (T51-T65) to identify chemical and intent
> Use additional external cause code to identify place (Y92)

√x7ᵗʰ **T21.40 Corrosion of unspecified degree of trunk, unspecified site**

√x7ᵗʰ **T21.41 Corrosion of unspecified degree of** chest wall
> Corrosion of unspecified degree of breast

√x7ᵗʰ **T21.42** **Corrosion of unspecified degree of** abdominal wall
Corrosion of unspecified degree of flank
Corrosion of unspecified degree of groin

√x7ᵗʰ **T21.43** **Corrosion of unspecified degree of** upper back
Corrosion of unspecified degree of interscapular region

√x7ᵗʰ **T21.44** **Corrosion of unspecified degree of** lower back

√x7ᵗʰ **T21.45** **Corrosion of unspecified degree of** buttock
Corrosion of unspecified degree of anus

√x7ᵗʰ **T21.46** **Corrosion of unspecified degree of** male genital region ♂
Corrosion of unspecified degree of penis
Corrosion of unspecified degree of scrotum
Corrosion of unspecified degree of testis

√x7ᵗʰ **T21.47** **Corrosion of unspecified degree of** female genital region ♀
Corrosion of unspecified degree of labium (majus) (minus)
Corrosion of unspecified degree of perineum
Corrosion of unspecified degree of vulva
EXCLUDES 2   corrosion of vagina (T28.8)

√x7ᵗʰ **T21.49** **Corrosion of unspecified degree of other site of trunk**

√5ᵗʰ **T21.5** **Corrosion of** first degree of trunk
Code first (T51-T65) to identify chemical and intent
Use additional external cause code to identify place (Y92)

√x7ᵗʰ **T21.50** **Corrosion of first degree of trunk, unspecified site**

√x7ᵗʰ **T21.51** **Corrosion of first degree of** chest wall
Corrosion of first degree of breast

√x7ᵗʰ **T21.52** **Corrosion of first degree of** abdominal wall
Corrosion of first degree of flank
Corrosion of first degree of groin

√x7ᵗʰ **T21.53** **Corrosion of first degree of** upper back
Corrosion of first degree of interscapular region

√x7ᵗʰ **T21.54** **Corrosion of first degree of** lower back

√x7ᵗʰ **T21.55** **Corrosion of first degree of** buttock
Corrosion of first degree of anus

√x7ᵗʰ **T21.56** **Corrosion of first degree of** male genital region ♂
Corrosion of first degree of penis
Corrosion of first degree of scrotum
Corrosion of first degree of testis

√x7ᵗʰ **T21.57** **Corrosion of first degree of** female genital region ♀
Corrosion of first degree of labium (majus) (minus)
Corrosion of first degree of perineum
Corrosion of first degree of vulva
EXCLUDES 2   corrosion of vagina (T28.8)

√x7ᵗʰ **T21.59** **Corrosion of first degree of other site of trunk**

√5ᵗʰ **T21.6** **Corrosion of** second degree of trunk
Code first (T51-T65) to identify chemical and intent
Use additional external cause code to identify place (Y92)

√x7ᵗʰ **T21.60** **Corrosion of second degree of trunk, unspecified site**

√x7ᵗʰ **T21.61** **Corrosion of second degree of** chest wall
Corrosion of second degree of breast

√x7ᵗʰ **T21.62** **Corrosion of second degree of** abdominal wall
Corrosion of second degree of flank
Corrosion of second degree of groin

√x7ᵗʰ **T21.63** **Corrosion of second degree of** upper back
Corrosion of second degree of interscapular region

√x7ᵗʰ **T21.64** **Corrosion of second degree of** lower back

√x7ᵗʰ **T21.65** **Corrosion of second degree of** buttock
Corrosion of second degree of anus

√x7ᵗʰ **T21.66** **Corrosion of second degree of** male genital region ♂
Corrosion of second degree of penis
Corrosion of second degree of scrotum
Corrosion of second degree of testis

√x7ᵗʰ **T21.67** **Corrosion of second degree of** female genital region ♀
Corrosion of second degree of labium (majus) (minus)
Corrosion of second degree of perineum
Corrosion of second degree of vulva
EXCLUDES 2   corrosion of vagina (T28.8)

√x7ᵗʰ **T21.69** **Corrosion of second degree of other site of trunk**

√5ᵗʰ **T21.7** **Corrosion of** third degree of trunk
Code first (T51-T65) to identify chemical and intent
Use additional external cause code to identify place (Y92)

√x7ᵗʰ **T21.70** **Corrosion of third degree of trunk, unspecified site** COM

√x7ᵗʰ **T21.71** **Corrosion of third degree of** chest wall COM
Corrosion of third degree of breast

√x7ᵗʰ **T21.72** **Corrosion of third degree of** abdominal wall COM
Corrosion of third degree of flank
Corrosion of third degree of groin

√x7ᵗʰ **T21.73** **Corrosion of third degree of** upper back COM
Corrosion of third degree of interscapular region

√x7ᵗʰ **T21.74** **Corrosion of third degree of** lower back COM

√x7ᵗʰ **T21.75** **Corrosion of third degree of** buttock COM
Corrosion of third degree of anus

√x7ᵗʰ **T21.76** **Corrosion of third degree of** male genital region COM ♂
Corrosion of third degree of penis
Corrosion of third degree of scrotum
Corrosion of third degree of testis

√x7ᵗʰ **T21.77** **Corrosion of third degree of** female genital region COM ♀
Corrosion of third degree of labium (majus) (minus)
Corrosion of third degree of perineum
Corrosion of third degree of vulva
EXCLUDES 2   corrosion of vagina (T28.8)

√x7ᵗʰ **T21.79** **Corrosion of third degree of other site of trunk** COM

√4ᵗʰ **T22** **Burn and corrosion of shoulder and upper limb, except wrist and hand**
EXCLUDES 2   burn and corrosion of interscapular region (T21.-)
      burn and corrosion of wrist and hand (T23.-)

The appropriate 7th character is to be added to each code from category T22.
A   initial encounter
D   subsequent encounter
S   sequela

√5ᵗʰ **T22.0** **Burn of unspecified degree of shoulder and upper limb, except wrist and hand**
Use additional external cause code to identify the source, place and intent of the burn (X00-X19, X75-X77, X96-X98, Y92)

√x7ᵗʰ **T22.00** **Burn of unspecified degree of shoulder and upper limb, except wrist and hand, unspecified site**

√6ᵗʰ **T22.01** **Burn of unspecified degree of** forearm

√7ᵗʰ **T22.011** **Burn of unspecified degree of** right forearm

√7ᵗʰ **T22.012** **Burn of unspecified degree of** left forearm

√7ᵗʰ **T22.019** **Burn of unspecified degree of unspecified forearm**

√6ᵗʰ **T22.02** **Burn of unspecified degree of** elbow

√7ᵗʰ **T22.021** **Burn of unspecified degree of** right elbow

√7ᵗʰ **T22.022** **Burn of unspecified degree of** left elbow

√7ᵗʰ **T22.029** **Burn of unspecified degree of unspecified elbow**

√6ᵗʰ **T22.03** **Burn of unspecified degree of** upper arm

√7ᵗʰ **T22.031** **Burn of unspecified degree of** right upper arm

√7ᵗʰ **T22.032** **Burn of unspecified degree of** left upper arm

√7ᵗʰ **T22.039** **Burn of unspecified degree of unspecified upper arm**

√6ᵗʰ **T22.04** **Burn of unspecified degree of** axilla

√7ᵗʰ **T22.041** **Burn of unspecified degree of** right axilla

√7ᵗʰ **T22.042** **Burn of unspecified degree of** left axilla

√7ᵗʰ **T22.049** **Burn of unspecified degree of unspecified axilla**

Chapter 19. Injury, Poisoning and Certain Other Consequences of External Causes

T21.42–T22.049

Chapter 19. Injury, Poisoning and Certain Other Consequences of External Causes

T22.05–T22.349

√6ᵗʰ **T22.05** Burn of unspecified degree of shoulder
- √7ᵗʰ **T22.051** Burn of unspecified degree of right shoulder
- √7ᵗʰ **T22.052** Burn of unspecified degree of left shoulder
- √7ᵗʰ **T22.059** Burn of unspecified degree of unspecified shoulder

√6ᵗʰ **T22.06** Burn of unspecified degree of scapular region
- √7ᵗʰ **T22.061** Burn of unspecified degree of right scapular region
- √7ᵗʰ **T22.062** Burn of unspecified degree of left scapular region
- √7ᵗʰ **T22.069** Burn of unspecified degree of unspecified scapular region

√6ᵗʰ **T22.09** Burn of unspecified degree of multiple sites of shoulder and upper limb, except wrist and hand
- √7ᵗʰ **T22.091** Burn of unspecified degree of multiple sites of right shoulder and upper limb, except wrist and hand
- √7ᵗʰ **T22.092** Burn of unspecified degree of multiple sites of left shoulder and upper limb, except wrist and hand
- √7ᵗʰ **T22.099** Burn of unspecified degree of multiple sites of unspecified shoulder and upper limb, except wrist and hand

√5ᵗʰ **T22.1** Burn of first degree of shoulder and upper limb, except wrist and hand
> Use additional external cause code to identify the source, place and intent of the burn (X00-X19, X75-X77, X96-X98, Y92)

√x7ᵗʰ **T22.10** Burn of first degree of shoulder and upper limb, except wrist and hand, unspecified site

√6ᵗʰ **T22.11** Burn of first degree of forearm
- √7ᵗʰ **T22.111** Burn of first degree of right forearm
- √7ᵗʰ **T22.112** Burn of first degree of left forearm
- √7ᵗʰ **T22.119** Burn of first degree of unspecified forearm

√6ᵗʰ **T22.12** Burn of first degree of elbow
- √7ᵗʰ **T22.121** Burn of first degree of right elbow
- √7ᵗʰ **T22.122** Burn of first degree of left elbow
- √7ᵗʰ **T22.129** Burn of first degree of unspecified elbow

√6ᵗʰ **T22.13** Burn of first degree of upper arm
- √7ᵗʰ **T22.131** Burn of first degree of right upper arm
- √7ᵗʰ **T22.132** Burn of first degree of left upper arm
- √7ᵗʰ **T22.139** Burn of first degree of unspecified upper arm

√6ᵗʰ **T22.14** Burn of first degree of axilla
- √7ᵗʰ **T22.141** Burn of first degree of right axilla
- √7ᵗʰ **T22.142** Burn of first degree of left axilla
- √7ᵗʰ **T22.149** Burn of first degree of unspecified axilla

√6ᵗʰ **T22.15** Burn of first degree of shoulder
- √7ᵗʰ **T22.151** Burn of first degree of right shoulder
- √7ᵗʰ **T22.152** Burn of first degree of left shoulder
- √7ᵗʰ **T22.159** Burn of first degree of unspecified shoulder

√6ᵗʰ **T22.16** Burn of first degree of scapular region
- √7ᵗʰ **T22.161** Burn of first degree of right scapular region
- √7ᵗʰ **T22.162** Burn of first degree of left scapular region
- √7ᵗʰ **T22.169** Burn of first degree of unspecified scapular region

√6ᵗʰ **T22.19** Burn of first degree of multiple sites of shoulder and upper limb, except wrist and hand
- √7ᵗʰ **T22.191** Burn of first degree of multiple sites of right shoulder and upper limb, except wrist and hand
- √7ᵗʰ **T22.192** Burn of first degree of multiple sites of left shoulder and upper limb, except wrist and hand
- √7ᵗʰ **T22.199** Burn of first degree of multiple sites of unspecified shoulder and upper limb, except wrist and hand

√5ᵗʰ **T22.2** Burn of second degree of shoulder and upper limb, except wrist and hand
> Use additional external cause code to identify the source, place and intent of the burn (X00-X19, X75-X77, X96-X98, Y92)

√x7ᵗʰ **T22.20** Burn of second degree of shoulder and upper limb, except wrist and hand, unspecified site

√6ᵗʰ **T22.21** Burn of second degree of forearm
- √7ᵗʰ **T22.211** Burn of second degree of right forearm
- √7ᵗʰ **T22.212** Burn of second degree of left forearm
- √7ᵗʰ **T22.219** Burn of second degree of unspecified forearm

√6ᵗʰ **T22.22** Burn of second degree of elbow
- √7ᵗʰ **T22.221** Burn of second degree of right elbow
- √7ᵗʰ **T22.222** Burn of second degree of left elbow
- √7ᵗʰ **T22.229** Burn of second degree of unspecified elbow

√6ᵗʰ **T22.23** Burn of second degree of upper arm
- √7ᵗʰ **T22.231** Burn of second degree of right upper arm
- √7ᵗʰ **T22.232** Burn of second degree of left upper arm
- √7ᵗʰ **T22.239** Burn of second degree of unspecified upper arm

√6ᵗʰ **T22.24** Burn of second degree of axilla
- √7ᵗʰ **T22.241** Burn of second degree of right axilla
- √7ᵗʰ **T22.242** Burn of second degree of left axilla
- √7ᵗʰ **T22.249** Burn of second degree of unspecified axilla

√6ᵗʰ **T22.25** Burn of second degree of shoulder
- √7ᵗʰ **T22.251** Burn of second degree of right shoulder
- √7ᵗʰ **T22.252** Burn of second degree of left shoulder
- √7ᵗʰ **T22.259** Burn of second degree of unspecified shoulder

√6ᵗʰ **T22.26** Burn of second degree of scapular region
- √7ᵗʰ **T22.261** Burn of second degree of right scapular region
- √7ᵗʰ **T22.262** Burn of second degree of left scapular region
- √7ᵗʰ **T22.269** Burn of second degree of unspecified scapular region

√6ᵗʰ **T22.29** Burn of second degree of multiple sites of shoulder and upper limb, except wrist and hand
- √7ᵗʰ **T22.291** Burn of second degree of multiple sites of right shoulder and upper limb, except wrist and hand
- √7ᵗʰ **T22.292** Burn of second degree of multiple sites of left shoulder and upper limb, except wrist and hand
- √7ᵗʰ **T22.299** Burn of second degree of multiple sites of unspecified shoulder and upper limb, except wrist and hand

√5ᵗʰ **T22.3** Burn of third degree of shoulder and upper limb, except wrist and hand
> Use additional external cause code to identify the source, place and intent of the burn (X00-X19, X75-X77, X96-X98, Y92)

√x7ᵗʰ **T22.30** Burn of third degree of shoulder and upper limb, except wrist and hand, unspecified site   COM

√6ᵗʰ **T22.31** Burn of third degree of forearm
- √7ᵗʰ **T22.311** Burn of third degree of right forearm   COM
- √7ᵗʰ **T22.312** Burn of third degree of left forearm   COM
- √7ᵗʰ **T22.319** Burn of third degree of unspecified forearm   COM

√6ᵗʰ **T22.32** Burn of third degree of elbow
- √7ᵗʰ **T22.321** Burn of third degree of right elbow   COM
- √7ᵗʰ **T22.322** Burn of third degree of left elbow   COM
- √7ᵗʰ **T22.329** Burn of third degree of unspecified elbow   COM

√6ᵗʰ **T22.33** Burn of third degree of upper arm
- √7ᵗʰ **T22.331** Burn of third degree of right upper arm   COM
- √7ᵗʰ **T22.332** Burn of third degree of left upper arm   COM
- √7ᵗʰ **T22.339** Burn of third degree of unspecified upper arm   COM

√6ᵗʰ **T22.34** Burn of third degree of axilla
- √7ᵗʰ **T22.341** Burn of third degree of right axilla   COM
- √7ᵗʰ **T22.342** Burn of third degree of left axilla   COM
- √7ᵗʰ **T22.349** Burn of third degree of unspecified axilla   COM

√6ᵗʰ **T22.35** Burn of third degree of shoulder

     √7ᵗʰ **T22.351** Burn of third degree of right shoulder   COM

     √7ᵗʰ **T22.352** Burn of third degree of left shoulder   COM

     √7ᵗʰ **T22.359** Burn of third degree of unspecified shoulder   COM

√6ᵗʰ **T22.36** Burn of third degree of scapular region

     √7ᵗʰ **T22.361** Burn of third degree of right scapular region   COM

     √7ᵗʰ **T22.362** Burn of third degree of left scapular region   COM

     √7ᵗʰ **T22.369** Burn of third degree of unspecified scapular region   COM

√6ᵗʰ **T22.39** Burn of third degree of multiple sites of shoulder and upper limb, except wrist and hand

     √7ᵗʰ **T22.391** Burn of third degree of multiple sites of right shoulder and upper limb, except wrist and hand   COM

     √7ᵗʰ **T22.392** Burn of third degree of multiple sites of left shoulder and upper limb, except wrist and hand   COM

     √7ᵗʰ **T22.399** Burn of third degree of multiple sites of unspecified shoulder and upper limb, except wrist and hand   COM

√5ᵗʰ **T22.4** Corrosion of unspecified degree of shoulder and upper limb, except wrist and hand

     Code first (T51-T65) to identify chemical and intent

     Use additional external cause code to identify place (Y92)

   √x7ᵗʰ **T22.40** Corrosion of unspecified degree of shoulder and upper limb, except wrist and hand, unspecified site

   √6ᵗʰ **T22.41** Corrosion of unspecified degree of forearm

     √7ᵗʰ **T22.411** Corrosion of unspecified degree of right forearm

     √7ᵗʰ **T22.412** Corrosion of unspecified degree of left forearm

     √7ᵗʰ **T22.419** Corrosion of unspecified degree of unspecified forearm

   √6ᵗʰ **T22.42** Corrosion of unspecified degree of elbow

     √7ᵗʰ **T22.421** Corrosion of unspecified degree of right elbow

     √7ᵗʰ **T22.422** Corrosion of unspecified degree of left elbow

     √7ᵗʰ **T22.429** Corrosion of unspecified degree of unspecified elbow

   √6ᵗʰ **T22.43** Corrosion of unspecified degree of upper arm

     √7ᵗʰ **T22.431** Corrosion of unspecified degree of right upper arm

     √7ᵗʰ **T22.432** Corrosion of unspecified degree of left upper arm

     √7ᵗʰ **T22.439** Corrosion of unspecified degree of unspecified upper arm

   √6ᵗʰ **T22.44** Corrosion of unspecified degree of axilla

     √7ᵗʰ **T22.441** Corrosion of unspecified degree of right axilla

     √7ᵗʰ **T22.442** Corrosion of unspecified degree of left axilla

     √7ᵗʰ **T22.449** Corrosion of unspecified degree of unspecified axilla

   √6ᵗʰ **T22.45** Corrosion of unspecified degree of shoulder

     √7ᵗʰ **T22.451** Corrosion of unspecified degree of right shoulder

     √7ᵗʰ **T22.452** Corrosion of unspecified degree of left shoulder

     √7ᵗʰ **T22.459** Corrosion of unspecified degree of unspecified shoulder

   √6ᵗʰ **T22.46** Corrosion of unspecified degree of scapular region

     √7ᵗʰ **T22.461** Corrosion of unspecified degree of right scapular region

     √7ᵗʰ **T22.462** Corrosion of unspecified degree of left scapular region

     √7ᵗʰ **T22.469** Corrosion of unspecified degree of unspecified scapular region

   √6ᵗʰ **T22.49** Corrosion of unspecified degree of multiple sites of shoulder and upper limb, except wrist and hand

     √7ᵗʰ **T22.491** Corrosion of unspecified degree of multiple sites of right shoulder and upper limb, except wrist and hand

     √7ᵗʰ **T22.492** Corrosion of unspecified degree of multiple sites of left shoulder and upper limb, except wrist and hand

     √7ᵗʰ **T22.499** Corrosion of unspecified degree of multiple sites of unspecified shoulder and upper limb, except wrist and hand

√5ᵗʰ **T22.5** Corrosion of first degree of shoulder and upper limb, except wrist and hand

     Code first (T51-T65) to identify chemical and intent

     Use additional external cause code to identify place (Y92)

   √x7ᵗʰ **T22.50** Corrosion of first degree of shoulder and upper limb, except wrist and hand unspecified site

   √6ᵗʰ **T22.51** Corrosion of first degree of forearm

     √7ᵗʰ **T22.511** Corrosion of first degree of right forearm

     √7ᵗʰ **T22.512** Corrosion of first degree of left forearm

     √7ᵗʰ **T22.519** Corrosion of first degree of unspecified forearm

   √6ᵗʰ **T22.52** Corrosion of first degree of elbow

     √7ᵗʰ **T22.521** Corrosion of first degree of right elbow

     √7ᵗʰ **T22.522** Corrosion of first degree of left elbow

     √7ᵗʰ **T22.529** Corrosion of first degree of unspecified elbow

   √6ᵗʰ **T22.53** Corrosion of first degree of upper arm

     √7ᵗʰ **T22.531** Corrosion of first degree of right upper arm

     √7ᵗʰ **T22.532** Corrosion of first degree of left upper arm

     √7ᵗʰ **T22.539** Corrosion of first degree of unspecified upper arm

   √6ᵗʰ **T22.54** Corrosion of first degree of axilla

     √7ᵗʰ **T22.541** Corrosion of first degree of right axilla

     √7ᵗʰ **T22.542** Corrosion of first degree of left axilla

     √7ᵗʰ **T22.549** Corrosion of first degree of unspecified axilla

   √6ᵗʰ **T22.55** Corrosion of first degree of shoulder

     √7ᵗʰ **T22.551** Corrosion of first degree of right shoulder

     √7ᵗʰ **T22.552** Corrosion of first degree of left shoulder

     √7ᵗʰ **T22.559** Corrosion of first degree of unspecified shoulder

   √6ᵗʰ **T22.56** Corrosion of first degree of scapular region

     √7ᵗʰ **T22.561** Corrosion of first degree of right scapular region

     √7ᵗʰ **T22.562** Corrosion of first degree of left scapular region

     √7ᵗʰ **T22.569** Corrosion of first degree of unspecified scapular region

   √6ᵗʰ **T22.59** Corrosion of first degree of multiple sites of shoulder and upper limb, except wrist and hand

     √7ᵗʰ **T22.591** Corrosion of first degree of multiple sites of right shoulder and upper limb, except wrist and hand

     √7ᵗʰ **T22.592** Corrosion of first degree of multiple sites of left shoulder and upper limb, except wrist and hand

     √7ᵗʰ **T22.599** Corrosion of first degree of multiple sites of unspecified shoulder and upper limb, except wrist and hand

√5ᵗʰ **T22.6** Corrosion of second degree of shoulder and upper limb, except wrist and hand

     Code first (T51-T65) to identify chemical and intent

     Use additional external cause code to identify place (Y92)

   √x7ᵗʰ **T22.60** Corrosion of second degree of shoulder and upper limb, except wrist and hand, unspecified site

   √6ᵗʰ **T22.61** Corrosion of second degree of forearm

     √7ᵗʰ **T22.611** Corrosion of second degree of right forearm

     √7ᵗʰ **T22.612** Corrosion of second degree of left forearm

     √7ᵗʰ **T22.619** Corrosion of second degree of unspecified forearm

   √6ᵗʰ **T22.62** Corrosion of second degree of elbow

     √7ᵗʰ **T22.621** Corrosion of second degree of right elbow

     √7ᵗʰ **T22.622** Corrosion of second degree of left elbow

     √7ᵗʰ **T22.629** Corrosion of second degree of unspecified elbow

   √6ᵗʰ **T22.63** Corrosion of second degree of upper arm

     √7ᵗʰ **T22.631** Corrosion of second degree of right upper arm

---

Chapter 19. Injury, Poisoning and Certain Other Consequences of External Causes

T22.632–T23.071

✓7ᵗʰ **T22.632** Corrosion of second degree of left upper arm

✓7ᵗʰ **T22.639** Corrosion of second degree of unspecified upper arm

✓6ᵗʰ **T22.64** Corrosion of second degree of axilla

    ✓7ᵗʰ **T22.641** Corrosion of second degree of right axilla

    ✓7ᵗʰ **T22.642** Corrosion of second degree of left axilla

    ✓7ᵗʰ **T22.649** Corrosion of second degree of unspecified axilla

✓6ᵗʰ **T22.65** Corrosion of second degree of shoulder

    ✓7ᵗʰ **T22.651** Corrosion of second degree of right shoulder

    ✓7ᵗʰ **T22.652** Corrosion of second degree of left shoulder

    ✓7ᵗʰ **T22.659** Corrosion of second degree of unspecified shoulder

✓6ᵗʰ **T22.66** Corrosion of second degree of scapular region

    ✓7ᵗʰ **T22.661** Corrosion of second degree of right scapular region

    ✓7ᵗʰ **T22.662** Corrosion of second degree of left scapular region

    ✓7ᵗʰ **T22.669** Corrosion of second degree of unspecified scapular region

✓6ᵗʰ **T22.69** Corrosion of second degree of multiple sites of shoulder and upper limb, except wrist and hand

    ✓7ᵗʰ **T22.691** Corrosion of second degree of multiple sites of right shoulder and upper limb, except wrist and hand

    ✓7ᵗʰ **T22.692** Corrosion of second degree of multiple sites of left shoulder and upper limb, except wrist and hand

    ✓7ᵗʰ **T22.699** Corrosion of second degree of multiple sites of unspecified shoulder and upper limb, except wrist and hand

✓5ᵗʰ **T22.7** Corrosion of third degree of shoulder and upper limb, except wrist and hand

    Code first (T51-T65) to identify chemical and intent

    Use additional external cause code to identify place (Y92)

✓x7ᵗʰ **T22.70** Corrosion of third degree of shoulder and upper limb, except wrist and hand, unspecified site   COM

✓6ᵗʰ **T22.71** Corrosion of third degree of forearm

    ✓7ᵗʰ **T22.711** Corrosion of third degree of right forearm   COM

    ✓7ᵗʰ **T22.712** Corrosion of third degree of left forearm   COM

    ✓7ᵗʰ **T22.719** Corrosion of third degree of unspecified forearm   COM

✓6ᵗʰ **T22.72** Corrosion of third degree of elbow

    ✓7ᵗʰ **T22.721** Corrosion of third degree of right elbow   COM

    ✓7ᵗʰ **T22.722** Corrosion of third degree of left elbow   COM

    ✓7ᵗʰ **T22.729** Corrosion of third degree of unspecified elbow   COM

✓6ᵗʰ **T22.73** Corrosion of third degree of upper arm

    ✓7ᵗʰ **T22.731** Corrosion of third degree of right upper arm   COM

    ✓7ᵗʰ **T22.732** Corrosion of third degree of left upper arm   COM

    ✓7ᵗʰ **T22.739** Corrosion of third degree of unspecified upper arm   COM

✓6ᵗʰ **T22.74** Corrosion of third degree of axilla

    ✓7ᵗʰ **T22.741** Corrosion of third degree of right axilla   COM

    ✓7ᵗʰ **T22.742** Corrosion of third degree of left axilla   COM

    ✓7ᵗʰ **T22.749** Corrosion of third degree of unspecified axilla   COM

✓6ᵗʰ **T22.75** Corrosion of third degree of shoulder

    ✓7ᵗʰ **T22.751** Corrosion of third degree of right shoulder   COM

    ✓7ᵗʰ **T22.752** Corrosion of third degree of left shoulder   COM

    ✓7ᵗʰ **T22.759** Corrosion of third degree of unspecified shoulder   COM

✓6ᵗʰ **T22.76** Corrosion of third degree of scapular region

    ✓7ᵗʰ **T22.761** Corrosion of third degree of right scapular region   COM

✓7ᵗʰ **T22.762** Corrosion of third degree of left scapular region   COM

✓7ᵗʰ **T22.769** Corrosion of third degree of unspecified scapular region   COM

✓6ᵗʰ **T22.79** Corrosion of third degree of multiple sites of shoulder and upper limb, except wrist and hand

    ✓7ᵗʰ **T22.791** Corrosion of third degree of multiple sites of right shoulder and upper limb, except wrist and hand   COM

    ✓7ᵗʰ **T22.792** Corrosion of third degree of multiple sites of left shoulder and upper limb, except wrist and hand   COM

    ✓7ᵗʰ **T22.799** Corrosion of third degree of multiple sites of unspecified shoulder and upper limb, except wrist and hand   COM

✓4ᵗʰ **T23** **Burn and corrosion of wrist and hand**

    AHA: 2015,1Q,19

    The appropriate 7th character is to be added to each code from category T23.
    A   initial encounter
    D   subsequent encounter
    S   sequela

✓5ᵗʰ **T23.0** Burn of unspecified degree of wrist and hand

    Use additional external cause code to identify the source, place and intent of the burn (X00-X19, X75-X77, X96-X98, Y92)

✓6ᵗʰ **T23.00** Burn of unspecified degree of hand, unspecified site

    ✓7ᵗʰ **T23.001** Burn of unspecified degree of right hand, unspecified site

    ✓7ᵗʰ **T23.002** Burn of unspecified degree of left hand, unspecified site

    ✓7ᵗʰ **T23.009** Burn of unspecified degree of unspecified hand, unspecified site

✓6ᵗʰ **T23.01** Burn of unspecified degree of thumb (nail)

    ✓7ᵗʰ **T23.011** Burn of unspecified degree of right thumb (nail)

    ✓7ᵗʰ **T23.012** Burn of unspecified degree of left thumb (nail)

    ✓7ᵗʰ **T23.019** Burn of unspecified degree of unspecified thumb (nail)

✓6ᵗʰ **T23.02** Burn of unspecified degree of single finger (nail) except thumb

    ✓7ᵗʰ **T23.021** Burn of unspecified degree of single right finger (nail) except thumb

    ✓7ᵗʰ **T23.022** Burn of unspecified degree of single left finger (nail) except thumb

    ✓7ᵗʰ **T23.029** Burn of unspecified degree of unspecified single finger (nail) except thumb

✓6ᵗʰ **T23.03** Burn of unspecified degree of multiple fingers (nail), not including thumb

    ✓7ᵗʰ **T23.031** Burn of unspecified degree of multiple right fingers (nail), not including thumb

    ✓7ᵗʰ **T23.032** Burn of unspecified degree of multiple left fingers (nail), not including thumb

    ✓7ᵗʰ **T23.039** Burn of unspecified degree of unspecified multiple fingers (nail), not including thumb

✓6ᵗʰ **T23.04** Burn of unspecified degree of multiple fingers (nail), including thumb

    ✓7ᵗʰ **T23.041** Burn of unspecified degree of multiple right fingers (nail), including thumb

    ✓7ᵗʰ **T23.042** Burn of unspecified degree of multiple left fingers (nail), including thumb

    ✓7ᵗʰ **T23.049** Burn of unspecified degree of unspecified multiple fingers (nail), including thumb

✓6ᵗʰ **T23.05** Burn of unspecified degree of palm

    ✓7ᵗʰ **T23.051** Burn of unspecified degree of right palm

    ✓7ᵗʰ **T23.052** Burn of unspecified degree of left palm

    ✓7ᵗʰ **T23.059** Burn of unspecified degree of unspecified palm

✓6ᵗʰ **T23.06** Burn of unspecified degree of back of hand

    ✓7ᵗʰ **T23.061** Burn of unspecified degree of back of right hand

    ✓7ᵗʰ **T23.062** Burn of unspecified degree of back of left hand

    ✓7ᵗʰ **T23.069** Burn of unspecified degree of back of unspecified hand

✓6ᵗʰ **T23.07** Burn of unspecified degree of wrist

    ✓7ᵗʰ **T23.071** Burn of unspecified degree of right wrist

✓7ᵗʰ **T23.072** Burn of unspecified degree of left wrist
✓7ᵗʰ **T23.079** Burn of unspecified degree of unspecified wrist
✓6ᵗʰ **T23.09** Burn of unspecified degree of multiple sites of wrist and hand
✓7ᵗʰ **T23.091** Burn of unspecified degree of multiple sites of right wrist and hand
✓7ᵗʰ **T23.092** Burn of unspecified degree of multiple sites of left wrist and hand
✓7ᵗʰ **T23.099** Burn of unspecified degree of multiple sites of unspecified wrist and hand

✓5ᵗʰ **T23.1** Burn of first degree of wrist and hand
Use additional external cause code to identify the source, place and intent of the burn (X00-X19, X75-X77, X96-X98, Y92)

✓6ᵗʰ **T23.10** Burn of first degree of hand, unspecified site
✓7ᵗʰ **T23.101** Burn of first degree of right hand, unspecified site
✓7ᵗʰ **T23.102** Burn of first degree of left hand, unspecified site
✓7ᵗʰ **T23.109** Burn of first degree of unspecified hand, unspecified site
✓6ᵗʰ **T23.11** Burn of first degree of thumb (nail)
✓7ᵗʰ **T23.111** Burn of first degree of right thumb (nail)
✓7ᵗʰ **T23.112** Burn of first degree of left thumb (nail)
✓7ᵗʰ **T23.119** Burn of first degree of unspecified thumb (nail)
✓6ᵗʰ **T23.12** Burn of first degree of single finger (nail) except thumb
✓7ᵗʰ **T23.121** Burn of first degree of single right finger (nail) except thumb
✓7ᵗʰ **T23.122** Burn of first degree of single left finger (nail) except thumb
✓7ᵗʰ **T23.129** Burn of first degree of unspecified single finger (nail) except thumb
✓6ᵗʰ **T23.13** Burn of first degree of multiple fingers (nail), not including thumb
✓7ᵗʰ **T23.131** Burn of first degree of multiple right fingers (nail), not including thumb
✓7ᵗʰ **T23.132** Burn of first degree of multiple left fingers (nail), not including thumb
✓7ᵗʰ **T23.139** Burn of first degree of unspecified multiple fingers (nail), not including thumb
✓6ᵗʰ **T23.14** Burn of first degree of multiple fingers (nail), including thumb
✓7ᵗʰ **T23.141** Burn of first degree of multiple right fingers (nail), including thumb
✓7ᵗʰ **T23.142** Burn of first degree of multiple left fingers (nail), including thumb
✓7ᵗʰ **T23.149** Burn of first degree of unspecified multiple fingers (nail), including thumb
✓6ᵗʰ **T23.15** Burn of first degree of palm
✓7ᵗʰ **T23.151** Burn of first degree of right palm
✓7ᵗʰ **T23.152** Burn of first degree of left palm
✓7ᵗʰ **T23.159** Burn of first degree of unspecified palm
✓6ᵗʰ **T23.16** Burn of first degree of back of hand
✓7ᵗʰ **T23.161** Burn of first degree of back of right hand
✓7ᵗʰ **T23.162** Burn of first degree of back of left hand
✓7ᵗʰ **T23.169** Burn of first degree of back of unspecified hand
✓6ᵗʰ **T23.17** Burn of first degree of wrist
✓7ᵗʰ **T23.171** Burn of first degree of right wrist
✓7ᵗʰ **T23.172** Burn of first degree of left wrist
✓7ᵗʰ **T23.179** Burn of first degree of unspecified wrist
✓6ᵗʰ **T23.19** Burn of first degree of multiple sites of wrist and hand
✓7ᵗʰ **T23.191** Burn of first degree of multiple sites of right wrist and hand
✓7ᵗʰ **T23.192** Burn of first degree of multiple sites of left wrist and hand
✓7ᵗʰ **T23.199** Burn of first degree of multiple sites of unspecified wrist and hand

✓5ᵗʰ **T23.2** Burn of second degree of wrist and hand
Use additional external cause code to identify the source, place and intent of the burn (X00-X19, X75-X77, X96-X98, Y92)

✓6ᵗʰ **T23.20** Burn of second degree of hand, unspecified site
✓7ᵗʰ **T23.201** Burn of second degree of right hand, unspecified site

✓7ᵗʰ **T23.202** Burn of second degree of left hand, unspecified site
✓7ᵗʰ **T23.209** Burn of second degree of unspecified hand, unspecified site
✓6ᵗʰ **T23.21** Burn of second degree of thumb (nail)
✓7ᵗʰ **T23.211** Burn of second degree of right thumb (nail)
✓7ᵗʰ **T23.212** Burn of second degree of left thumb (nail)
✓7ᵗʰ **T23.219** Burn of second degree of unspecified thumb (nail)
✓6ᵗʰ **T23.22** Burn of second degree of single finger (nail) except thumb
✓7ᵗʰ **T23.221** Burn of second degree of single right finger (nail) except thumb
✓7ᵗʰ **T23.222** Burn of second degree of single left finger (nail) except thumb
✓7ᵗʰ **T23.229** Burn of second degree of unspecified single finger (nail) except thumb
✓6ᵗʰ **T23.23** Burn of second degree of multiple fingers (nail), not including thumb
✓7ᵗʰ **T23.231** Burn of second degree of multiple right fingers (nail), not including thumb
✓7ᵗʰ **T23.232** Burn of second degree of multiple left fingers (nail), not including thumb
✓7ᵗʰ **T23.239** Burn of second degree of unspecified multiple fingers (nail), not including thumb
✓6ᵗʰ **T23.24** Burn of second degree of multiple fingers (nail), including thumb
✓7ᵗʰ **T23.241** Burn of second degree of multiple right fingers (nail), including thumb
✓7ᵗʰ **T23.242** Burn of second degree of multiple left fingers (nail), including thumb
✓7ᵗʰ **T23.249** Burn of second degree of unspecified multiple fingers (nail), including thumb
✓6ᵗʰ **T23.25** Burn of second degree of palm
✓7ᵗʰ **T23.251** Burn of second degree of right palm
✓7ᵗʰ **T23.252** Burn of second degree of left palm
✓7ᵗʰ **T23.259** Burn of second degree of unspecified palm
✓6ᵗʰ **T23.26** Burn of second degree of back of hand
✓7ᵗʰ **T23.261** Burn of second degree of back of right hand
✓7ᵗʰ **T23.262** Burn of second degree of back of left hand
✓7ᵗʰ **T23.269** Burn of second degree of back of unspecified hand
✓6ᵗʰ **T23.27** Burn of second degree of wrist
✓7ᵗʰ **T23.271** Burn of second degree of right wrist
✓7ᵗʰ **T23.272** Burn of second degree of left wrist
✓7ᵗʰ **T23.279** Burn of second degree of unspecified wrist
✓6ᵗʰ **T23.29** Burn of second degree of multiple sites of wrist and hand
✓7ᵗʰ **T23.291** Burn of second degree of multiple sites of right wrist and hand
✓7ᵗʰ **T23.292** Burn of second degree of multiple sites of left wrist and hand
✓7ᵗʰ **T23.299** Burn of second degree of multiple sites of unspecified wrist and hand

✓5ᵗʰ **T23.3** Burn of third degree of wrist and hand
Use additional external cause code to identify the source, place and intent of the burn (X00-X19, X75-X77, X96-X98, Y92)

✓6ᵗʰ **T23.30** Burn of third degree of hand, unspecified site
AHA: 2016,2Q,5
✓7ᵗʰ **T23.301** Burn of third degree of right hand, unspecified site COM
✓7ᵗʰ **T23.302** Burn of third degree of left hand, unspecified site COM
✓7ᵗʰ **T23.309** Burn of third degree of unspecified hand, unspecified site COM
✓6ᵗʰ **T23.31** Burn of third degree of thumb (nail)
✓7ᵗʰ **T23.311** Burn of third degree of right thumb (nail) COM
✓7ᵗʰ **T23.312** Burn of third degree of left thumb (nail) COM
✓7ᵗʰ **T23.319** Burn of third degree of unspecified thumb (nail) COM

Additional Character Required   ✓x7ᵗʰ Placeholder Alert   Manifestation   Unspecified Dx   Q QPP   UPD Unacceptable PDx

Chapter 19. Injury, Poisoning and Certain Other Consequences of External Causes

T23.32-T23.531

√6ᵗʰ **T23.32** Burn of third degree of single finger (nail) except thumb
- √7ᵗʰ **T23.321** Burn of third degree of single right finger (nail) except thumb COM
- √7ᵗʰ **T23.322** Burn of third degree of single left finger (nail) except thumb COM
- √7ᵗʰ **T23.329** Burn of third degree of unspecified single finger (nail) except thumb COM

√6ᵗʰ **T23.33** Burn of third degree of multiple fingers (nail), not including thumb
- √7ᵗʰ **T23.331** Burn of third degree of multiple right fingers (nail), not including thumb COM
- √7ᵗʰ **T23.332** Burn of third degree of multiple left fingers (nail), not including thumb COM
- √7ᵗʰ **T23.339** Burn of third degree of unspecified multiple fingers (nail), not including thumb COM

√6ᵗʰ **T23.34** Burn of third degree of multiple fingers (nail), including thumb
- √7ᵗʰ **T23.341** Burn of third degree of multiple right fingers (nail), including thumb COM
- √7ᵗʰ **T23.342** Burn of third degree of multiple left fingers (nail), including thumb COM
- √7ᵗʰ **T23.349** Burn of third degree of unspecified multiple fingers (nail), including thumb COM

√6ᵗʰ **T23.35** Burn of third degree of palm
- √7ᵗʰ **T23.351** Burn of third degree of right palm COM
- √7ᵗʰ **T23.352** Burn of third degree of left palm COM
- √7ᵗʰ **T23.359** Burn of third degree of unspecified palm COM

√6ᵗʰ **T23.36** Burn of third degree of back of hand
- √7ᵗʰ **T23.361** Burn of third degree of back of right hand COM
- √7ᵗʰ **T23.362** Burn of third degree of back of left hand COM
- √7ᵗʰ **T23.369** Burn of third degree of back of unspecified hand COM

√6ᵗʰ **T23.37** Burn of third degree of wrist
- √7ᵗʰ **T23.371** Burn of third degree of right wrist COM
- √7ᵗʰ **T23.372** Burn of third degree of left wrist COM
- √7ᵗʰ **T23.379** Burn of third degree of unspecified wrist COM

√6ᵗʰ **T23.39** Burn of third degree of multiple sites of wrist and hand
- √7ᵗʰ **T23.391** Burn of third degree of multiple sites of right wrist and hand COM
- √7ᵗʰ **T23.392** Burn of third degree of multiple sites of left wrist and hand COM
- √7ᵗʰ **T23.399** Burn of third degree of multiple sites of unspecified wrist and hand COM

√5ᵗʰ **T23.4** Corrosion of unspecified degree of wrist and hand
Code first (T51-T65) to identify chemical and intent
Use additional external cause code to identify place (Y92)

√6ᵗʰ **T23.40** Corrosion of unspecified degree of hand, unspecified site
- √7ᵗʰ **T23.401** Corrosion of unspecified degree of right hand, unspecified site
- √7ᵗʰ **T23.402** Corrosion of unspecified degree of left hand, unspecified site
- √7ᵗʰ **T23.409** Corrosion of unspecified degree of unspecified hand, unspecified site

√6ᵗʰ **T23.41** Corrosion of unspecified degree of thumb (nail)
- √7ᵗʰ **T23.411** Corrosion of unspecified degree of right thumb (nail)
- √7ᵗʰ **T23.412** Corrosion of unspecified degree of left thumb (nail)
- √7ᵗʰ **T23.419** Corrosion of unspecified degree of unspecified thumb (nail)

√6ᵗʰ **T23.42** Corrosion of unspecified degree of single finger (nail) except thumb
- √7ᵗʰ **T23.421** Corrosion of unspecified degree of single right finger (nail) except thumb
- √7ᵗʰ **T23.422** Corrosion of unspecified degree of single left finger (nail) except thumb
- √7ᵗʰ **T23.429** Corrosion of unspecified degree of unspecified single finger (nail) except thumb

√6ᵗʰ **T23.43** Corrosion of unspecified degree of multiple fingers (nail), not including thumb
- √7ᵗʰ **T23.431** Corrosion of unspecified degree of multiple right fingers (nail), not including thumb
- √7ᵗʰ **T23.432** Corrosion of unspecified degree of multiple left fingers (nail), not including thumb
- √7ᵗʰ **T23.439** Corrosion of unspecified degree of unspecified multiple fingers (nail), not including thumb

√6ᵗʰ **T23.44** Corrosion of unspecified degree of multiple fingers (nail), including thumb
- √7ᵗʰ **T23.441** Corrosion of unspecified degree of multiple right fingers (nail), including thumb
- √7ᵗʰ **T23.442** Corrosion of unspecified degree of multiple left fingers (nail), including thumb
- √7ᵗʰ **T23.449** Corrosion of unspecified degree of unspecified multiple fingers (nail), including thumb

√6ᵗʰ **T23.45** Corrosion of unspecified degree of palm
- √7ᵗʰ **T23.451** Corrosion of unspecified degree of right palm
- √7ᵗʰ **T23.452** Corrosion of unspecified degree of left palm
- √7ᵗʰ **T23.459** Corrosion of unspecified degree of unspecified palm

√6ᵗʰ **T23.46** Corrosion of unspecified degree of back of hand
- √7ᵗʰ **T23.461** Corrosion of unspecified degree of back of right hand
- √7ᵗʰ **T23.462** Corrosion of unspecified degree of back of left hand
- √7ᵗʰ **T23.469** Corrosion of unspecified degree of back of unspecified hand

√6ᵗʰ **T23.47** Corrosion of unspecified degree of wrist
- √7ᵗʰ **T23.471** Corrosion of unspecified degree of right wrist
- √7ᵗʰ **T23.472** Corrosion of unspecified degree of left wrist
- √7ᵗʰ **T23.479** Corrosion of unspecified degree of unspecified wrist

√6ᵗʰ **T23.49** Corrosion of unspecified degree of multiple sites of wrist and hand
- √7ᵗʰ **T23.491** Corrosion of unspecified degree of multiple sites of right wrist and hand
- √7ᵗʰ **T23.492** Corrosion of unspecified degree of multiple sites of left wrist and hand
- √7ᵗʰ **T23.499** Corrosion of unspecified degree of multiple sites of unspecified wrist and hand

√5ᵗʰ **T23.5** Corrosion of first degree of wrist and hand
Code first (T51-T65) to identify chemical and intent
Use additional external cause code to identify place (Y92)

√6ᵗʰ **T23.50** Corrosion of first degree of hand, unspecified site
- √7ᵗʰ **T23.501** Corrosion of first degree of right hand, unspecified site
- √7ᵗʰ **T23.502** Corrosion of first degree of left hand, unspecified site
- √7ᵗʰ **T23.509** Corrosion of first degree of unspecified hand, unspecified site

√6ᵗʰ **T23.51** Corrosion of first degree of thumb (nail)
- √7ᵗʰ **T23.511** Corrosion of first degree of right thumb (nail)
- √7ᵗʰ **T23.512** Corrosion of first degree of left thumb (nail)
- √7ᵗʰ **T23.519** Corrosion of first degree of unspecified thumb (nail)

√6ᵗʰ **T23.52** Corrosion of first degree of single finger (nail) except thumb
- √7ᵗʰ **T23.521** Corrosion of first degree of single right finger (nail) except thumb
- √7ᵗʰ **T23.522** Corrosion of first degree of single left finger (nail) except thumb
- √7ᵗʰ **T23.529** Corrosion of first degree of unspecified single finger (nail) except thumb

√6ᵗʰ **T23.53** Corrosion of first degree of multiple fingers (nail), not including thumb
- √7ᵗʰ **T23.531** Corrosion of first degree of multiple right fingers (nail), not including thumb

√7ᵗʰ **T23.532** Corrosion of first degree of multiple left fingers (nail), not including thumb
√7ᵗʰ **T23.539** Corrosion of first degree of unspecified multiple fingers (nail), not including thumb
√6ᵗʰ **T23.54** Corrosion of first degree of multiple fingers (nail), including thumb
√7ᵗʰ **T23.541** Corrosion of first degree of multiple right fingers (nail), including thumb
√7ᵗʰ **T23.542** Corrosion of first degree of multiple left fingers (nail), including thumb
√7ᵗʰ **T23.549** Corrosion of first degree of unspecified multiple fingers (nail), including thumb
√6ᵗʰ **T23.55** Corrosion of first degree of palm
√7ᵗʰ **T23.551** Corrosion of first degree of right palm
√7ᵗʰ **T23.552** Corrosion of first degree of left palm
√7ᵗʰ **T23.559** Corrosion of first degree of unspecified palm
√6ᵗʰ **T23.56** Corrosion of first degree of back of hand
√7ᵗʰ **T23.561** Corrosion of first degree of back of right hand
√7ᵗʰ **T23.562** Corrosion of first degree of back of left hand
√7ᵗʰ **T23.569** Corrosion of first degree of back of unspecified hand
√6ᵗʰ **T23.57** Corrosion of first degree of wrist
√7ᵗʰ **T23.571** Corrosion of first degree of right wrist
√7ᵗʰ **T23.572** Corrosion of first degree of left wrist
√7ᵗʰ **T23.579** Corrosion of first degree of unspecified wrist
√6ᵗʰ **T23.59** Corrosion of first degree of multiple sites of wrist and hand
√7ᵗʰ **T23.591** Corrosion of first degree of multiple sites of right wrist and hand
√7ᵗʰ **T23.592** Corrosion of first degree of multiple sites of left wrist and hand
√7ᵗʰ **T23.599** Corrosion of first degree of multiple sites of unspecified wrist and hand
√5ᵗʰ **T23.6** Corrosion of second degree of wrist and hand
Code first (T51-T65) to identify chemical and intent
Use additional external cause code to identify place (Y92)
√6ᵗʰ **T23.60** Corrosion of second degree of hand, unspecified site
√7ᵗʰ **T23.601** Corrosion of second degree of right hand, unspecified site
√7ᵗʰ **T23.602** Corrosion of second degree of left hand, unspecified site
√7ᵗʰ **T23.609** Corrosion of second degree of unspecified hand, unspecified site
√6ᵗʰ **T23.61** Corrosion of second degree of thumb (nail)
√7ᵗʰ **T23.611** Corrosion of second degree of right thumb (nail)
√7ᵗʰ **T23.612** Corrosion of second degree of left thumb (nail)
√7ᵗʰ **T23.619** Corrosion of second degree of unspecified thumb (nail)
√6ᵗʰ **T23.62** Corrosion of second degree of single finger (nail) except thumb
√7ᵗʰ **T23.621** Corrosion of second degree of single right finger (nail) except thumb
√7ᵗʰ **T23.622** Corrosion of second degree of single left finger (nail) except thumb
√7ᵗʰ **T23.629** Corrosion of second degree of unspecified single finger (nail) except thumb
√6ᵗʰ **T23.63** Corrosion of second degree of multiple fingers (nail), not including thumb
√7ᵗʰ **T23.631** Corrosion of second degree of multiple right fingers (nail), not including thumb
√7ᵗʰ **T23.632** Corrosion of second degree of multiple left fingers (nail), not including thumb
√7ᵗʰ **T23.639** Corrosion of second degree of unspecified multiple fingers (nail), not including thumb
√6ᵗʰ **T23.64** Corrosion of second degree of multiple fingers (nail), including thumb
√7ᵗʰ **T23.641** Corrosion of second degree of multiple right fingers (nail), including thumb
√7ᵗʰ **T23.642** Corrosion of second degree of multiple left fingers (nail), including thumb
√7ᵗʰ **T23.649** Corrosion of second degree of unspecified multiple fingers (nail), including thumb

√6ᵗʰ **T23.65** Corrosion of second degree of palm
√7ᵗʰ **T23.651** Corrosion of second degree of right palm
√7ᵗʰ **T23.652** Corrosion of second degree of left palm
√7ᵗʰ **T23.659** Corrosion of second degree of unspecified palm
√6ᵗʰ **T23.66** Corrosion of second degree of back of hand
√7ᵗʰ **T23.661** Corrosion of second degree back of right hand
√7ᵗʰ **T23.662** Corrosion of second degree back of left hand
√7ᵗʰ **T23.669** Corrosion of second degree back of unspecified hand
√6ᵗʰ **T23.67** Corrosion of second degree of wrist
√7ᵗʰ **T23.671** Corrosion of second degree of right wrist
√7ᵗʰ **T23.672** Corrosion of second degree of left wrist
√7ᵗʰ **T23.679** Corrosion of second degree of unspecified wrist
√6ᵗʰ **T23.69** Corrosion of second degree of multiple sites of wrist and hand
√7ᵗʰ **T23.691** Corrosion of second degree of multiple sites of right wrist and hand
√7ᵗʰ **T23.692** Corrosion of second degree of multiple sites of left wrist and hand
√7ᵗʰ **T23.699** Corrosion of second degree of multiple sites of unspecified wrist and hand
√5ᵗʰ **T23.7** Corrosion of third degree of wrist and hand
Code first (T51-T65) to identify chemical and intent
Use additional external cause code to identify place (Y92)
√6ᵗʰ **T23.70** Corrosion of third degree of hand, unspecified site
√7ᵗʰ **T23.701** Corrosion of third degree of right hand, unspecified site [COM]
√7ᵗʰ **T23.702** Corrosion of third degree of left hand, unspecified site [COM]
√7ᵗʰ **T23.709** Corrosion of third degree of unspecified hand, unspecified site [COM]
√6ᵗʰ **T23.71** Corrosion of third degree of thumb (nail)
√7ᵗʰ **T23.711** Corrosion of third degree of right thumb (nail) [COM]
√7ᵗʰ **T23.712** Corrosion of third degree of left thumb (nail) [COM]
√7ᵗʰ **T23.719** Corrosion of third degree of unspecified thumb (nail) [COM]
√6ᵗʰ **T23.72** Corrosion of third degree of single finger (nail) except thumb
√7ᵗʰ **T23.721** Corrosion of third degree of single right finger (nail) except thumb [COM]
√7ᵗʰ **T23.722** Corrosion of third degree of single left finger (nail) except thumb [COM]
√7ᵗʰ **T23.729** Corrosion of third degree of unspecified single finger (nail) except thumb [COM]
√6ᵗʰ **T23.73** Corrosion of third degree of multiple fingers (nail), not including thumb
√7ᵗʰ **T23.731** Corrosion of third degree of multiple right fingers (nail), not including thumb [COM]
√7ᵗʰ **T23.732** Corrosion of third degree of multiple left fingers (nail), not including thumb [COM]
√7ᵗʰ **T23.739** Corrosion of third degree of unspecified multiple fingers (nail), not including thumb [COM]
√6ᵗʰ **T23.74** Corrosion of third degree of multiple fingers (nail), including thumb
√7ᵗʰ **T23.741** Corrosion of third degree of multiple right fingers (nail), including thumb [COM]
√7ᵗʰ **T23.742** Corrosion of third degree of multiple left fingers (nail), including thumb [COM]
√7ᵗʰ **T23.749** Corrosion of third degree of unspecified multiple fingers (nail), including thumb [COM]
√6ᵗʰ **T23.75** Corrosion of third degree of palm
√7ᵗʰ **T23.751** Corrosion of third degree of right palm [COM]
√7ᵗʰ **T23.752** Corrosion of third degree of left palm [COM]
√7ᵗʰ **T23.759** Corrosion of third degree of unspecified palm [COM]

✔ Additional Character Required   √x7ᵗʰ Placeholder Alert   Manifestation   Unspecified Dx   🄠 QPP   [UPD] Unacceptable PDx

✓6ᵗʰ **T23.76** **Corrosion of third degree of** back of hand

     ✓7ᵗʰ **T23.761** **Corrosion of third degree of back of** right **hand** `COM`

     ✓7ᵗʰ **T23.762** **Corrosion of third degree of back of** left **hand** `COM`

     ✓7ᵗʰ **T23.769** **Corrosion of third degree back of unspecified hand**

✓6ᵗʰ **T23.77** **Corrosion of third degree of** wrist

     ✓7ᵗʰ **T23.771** **Corrosion of third degree of** right **wrist** `COM`

     ✓7ᵗʰ **T23.772** **Corrosion of third degree of** left **wrist** `COM`

     ✓7ᵗʰ **T23.779** **Corrosion of third degree of unspecified wrist** `COM`

✓6ᵗʰ **T23.79** **Corrosion of third degree of** multiple sites **of wrist and hand**

     ✓7ᵗʰ **T23.791** **Corrosion of third degree of multiple sites of** right **wrist and hand** `COM`

     ✓7ᵗʰ **T23.792** **Corrosion of third degree of multiple sites of** left **wrist and hand** `COM`

     ✓7ᵗʰ **T23.799** **Corrosion of third degree of multiple sites of unspecified wrist and hand** `COM`

✓4ᵗʰ **T24** **Burn and corrosion of lower limb, except ankle and foot**

> `EXCLUDES 2`   burn and corrosion of ankle and foot (T25.-)
>   burn and corrosion of hip region (T21.-)

> The appropriate 7th character is to be added to each code from category T24.
> A   initial encounter
> D   subsequent encounter
> S   sequela

✓5ᵗʰ **T24.0** **Burn of unspecified degree of lower limb, except ankle and foot**

     Use additional external cause code to identify the source, place and intent of the burn (X00-X19, X75-X77, X96-X98, Y92)

     ✓6ᵗʰ **T24.00** **Burn of unspecified degree of unspecified site of lower limb, except ankle and foot**

         ✓7ᵗʰ **T24.001** **Burn of unspecified degree of unspecified site of** right **lower limb, except ankle and foot**

         ✓7ᵗʰ **T24.002** **Burn of unspecified degree of unspecified site of** left **lower limb, except ankle and foot**

         ✓7ᵗʰ **T24.009** **Burn of unspecified degree of unspecified site of unspecified lower limb, except ankle and foot**

     ✓6ᵗʰ **T24.01** **Burn of unspecified degree of** thigh

         ✓7ᵗʰ **T24.011** **Burn of unspecified degree of** right **thigh**

         ✓7ᵗʰ **T24.012** **Burn of unspecified degree of** left **thigh**

         ✓7ᵗʰ **T24.019** **Burn of unspecified degree of unspecified thigh**

     ✓6ᵗʰ **T24.02** **Burn of unspecified degree of** knee

         ✓7ᵗʰ **T24.021** **Burn of unspecified degree of** right **knee**

         ✓7ᵗʰ **T24.022** **Burn of unspecified degree of** left **knee**

         ✓7ᵗʰ **T24.029** **Burn of unspecified degree of unspecified knee**

     ✓6ᵗʰ **T24.03** **Burn of unspecified degree of** lower leg

         ✓7ᵗʰ **T24.031** **Burn of unspecified degree of** right **lower leg**

         ✓7ᵗʰ **T24.032** **Burn of unspecified degree of** left **lower leg**

         ✓7ᵗʰ **T24.039** **Burn of unspecified degree of unspecified lower leg**

     ✓6ᵗʰ **T24.09** **Burn of unspecified degree of** multiple sites **of lower limb, except ankle and foot**

         ✓7ᵗʰ **T24.091** **Burn of unspecified degree of multiple sites of** right **lower limb, except ankle and foot**

         ✓7ᵗʰ **T24.092** **Burn of unspecified degree of multiple sites of** left **lower limb, except ankle and foot**

         ✓7ᵗʰ **T24.099** **Burn of unspecified degree of multiple sites of unspecified lower limb, except ankle and foot**

✓5ᵗʰ **T24.1** **Burn of** first degree **of lower limb, except ankle and foot**

     Use additional external cause code to identify the source, place and intent of the burn (X00-X19, X75-X77, X96-X98, Y92)

     ✓6ᵗʰ **T24.10** **Burn of first degree of unspecified site of lower limb, except ankle and foot**

         ✓7ᵗʰ **T24.101** **Burn of first degree of unspecified site of** right **lower limb, except ankle and foot**

         ✓7ᵗʰ **T24.102** **Burn of first degree of unspecified site of** left **lower limb, except ankle and foot**

         ✓7ᵗʰ **T24.109** **Burn of first degree of unspecified site of unspecified lower limb, except ankle and foot**

     ✓6ᵗʰ **T24.11** **Burn of first degree of** thigh

         ✓7ᵗʰ **T24.111** **Burn of first degree of** right **thigh**

         ✓7ᵗʰ **T24.112** **Burn of first degree of** left **thigh**

         ✓7ᵗʰ **T24.119** **Burn of first degree of unspecified thigh**

     ✓6ᵗʰ **T24.12** **Burn of first degree of** knee

         ✓7ᵗʰ **T24.121** **Burn of first degree of** right **knee**

         ✓7ᵗʰ **T24.122** **Burn of first degree of** left **knee**

         ✓7ᵗʰ **T24.129** **Burn of first degree of unspecified knee**

     ✓6ᵗʰ **T24.13** **Burn of first degree of** lower leg

         ✓7ᵗʰ **T24.131** **Burn of first degree of** right **lower leg**

         ✓7ᵗʰ **T24.132** **Burn of first degree of** left **lower leg**

         ✓7ᵗʰ **T24.139** **Burn of first degree of unspecified lower leg**

     ✓6ᵗʰ **T24.19** **Burn of first degree of** multiple sites **of lower limb, except ankle and foot**

         ✓7ᵗʰ **T24.191** **Burn of first degree of multiple sites of** right **lower limb, except ankle and foot**

         ✓7ᵗʰ **T24.192** **Burn of first degree of multiple sites of** left **lower limb, except ankle and foot**

         ✓7ᵗʰ **T24.199** **Burn of first degree of multiple sites of unspecified lower limb, except ankle and foot**

✓5ᵗʰ **T24.2** **Burn of** second degree **of lower limb, except ankle and foot**

     Use additional external cause code to identify the source, place and intent of the burn (X00-X19, X75-X77, X96-X98, Y92)

     ✓6ᵗʰ **T24.20** **Burn of second degree of unspecified site of lower limb, except ankle and foot**

         ✓7ᵗʰ **T24.201** **Burn of second degree of unspecified site of** right **lower limb, except ankle and foot**

         ✓7ᵗʰ **T24.202** **Burn of second degree of unspecified site of** left **lower limb, except ankle and foot**

         ✓7ᵗʰ **T24.209** **Burn of second degree of unspecified site of unspecified lower limb, except ankle and foot**

     ✓6ᵗʰ **T24.21** **Burn of second degree of** thigh

         ✓7ᵗʰ **T24.211** **Burn of second degree of** right **thigh**

         ✓7ᵗʰ **T24.212** **Burn of second degree of** left **thigh**

         ✓7ᵗʰ **T24.219** **Burn of second degree of unspecified thigh**

     ✓6ᵗʰ **T24.22** **Burn of second degree of** knee

         ✓7ᵗʰ **T24.221** **Burn of second degree of** right **knee**

         ✓7ᵗʰ **T24.222** **Burn of second degree of** left **knee**

         ✓7ᵗʰ **T24.229** **Burn of second degree of unspecified knee**

     ✓6ᵗʰ **T24.23** **Burn of second degree of** lower leg

         ✓7ᵗʰ **T24.231** **Burn of second degree of** right **lower leg**

         ✓7ᵗʰ **T24.232** **Burn of second degree of** left **lower leg**

         ✓7ᵗʰ **T24.239** **Burn of second degree of unspecified lower leg**

     ✓6ᵗʰ **T24.29** **Burn of second degree of** multiple sites **of lower limb, except ankle and foot**

         ✓7ᵗʰ **T24.291** **Burn of second degree of multiple sites of** right **lower limb, except ankle and foot**

         ✓7ᵗʰ **T24.292** **Burn of second degree of multiple sites of** left **lower limb, except ankle and foot**

         ✓7ᵗʰ **T24.299** **Burn of second degree of multiple sites of unspecified lower limb, except ankle and foot**

`HCC` CMS-HCC   `Rx` Rx HCC   `ESR` ESRD HCC   `COM` Commercial HCC   `N` Newborn: 0   `P` Pediatric: 0-17   `M` Maternity: 9-64   `A` Adult: 15-124

1126   ICD-10-CM 2023

✓5ᵗʰ **T24.3** **Burn of** third degree **of lower limb, except ankle and foot**

Use additional external cause code to identify the source, place and intent of the burn (X00-X19, X75-X77, X96-X98, Y92)

✓6ᵗʰ **T24.30** **Burn of third degree of unspecified site of lower limb, except ankle and foot**

✓7ᵗʰ **T24.301** **Burn of third degree of unspecified site of** right **lower limb, except ankle and foot** COM

✓7ᵗʰ **T24.302** **Burn of third degree of unspecified site of** left **lower limb, except ankle and foot** COM

✓7ᵗʰ **T24.309** **Burn of third degree of unspecified site of unspecified lower limb, except ankle and foot** COM

✓6ᵗʰ **T24.31** **Burn of third degree of** thigh

✓7ᵗʰ **T24.311** **Burn of third degree of** right **thigh** COM

✓7ᵗʰ **T24.312** **Burn of third degree of** left **thigh** COM

✓7ᵗʰ **T24.319** **Burn of third degree of unspecified thigh** COM

✓6ᵗʰ **T24.32** **Burn of third degree of** knee

✓7ᵗʰ **T24.321** **Burn of third degree of** right **knee** COM

✓7ᵗʰ **T24.322** **Burn of third degree of** left **knee** COM

✓7ᵗʰ **T24.329** **Burn of third degree of unspecified knee** COM

✓6ᵗʰ **T24.33** **Burn of third degree of** lower leg

✓7ᵗʰ **T24.331** **Burn of third degree of** right **lower leg** COM

✓7ᵗʰ **T24.332** **Burn of third degree of** left **lower leg** COM

✓7ᵗʰ **T24.339** **Burn of third degree of unspecified lower leg** COM

✓6ᵗʰ **T24.39** **Burn of third degree of** multiple sites **of lower limb, except ankle and foot**

AHA: 2016,2Q,4

✓7ᵗʰ **T24.391** **Burn of third degree of multiple sites of** right **lower limb, except ankle and foot** COM

✓7ᵗʰ **T24.392** **Burn of third degree of multiple sites of** left **lower limb, except ankle and foot** COM

✓7ᵗʰ **T24.399** **Burn of third degree of multiple sites of unspecified lower limb, except ankle and foot** COM

✓5ᵗʰ **T24.4** **Corrosion of unspecified degree of lower limb, except ankle and foot**

Code first (T51-T65) to identify chemical and intent
Use additional external cause code to identify place (Y92)

✓6ᵗʰ **T24.40** **Corrosion of unspecified degree of unspecified site of lower limb, except ankle and foot**

✓7ᵗʰ **T24.401** **Corrosion of unspecified degree of unspecified site of** right **lower limb, except ankle and foot**

✓7ᵗʰ **T24.402** **Corrosion of unspecified degree of unspecified site of** left **lower limb, except ankle and foot**

✓7ᵗʰ **T24.409** **Corrosion of unspecified degree of unspecified site of unspecified lower limb, except ankle and foot**

✓6ᵗʰ **T24.41** **Corrosion of unspecified degree of** thigh

✓7ᵗʰ **T24.411** **Corrosion of unspecified degree of** right **thigh**

✓7ᵗʰ **T24.412** **Corrosion of unspecified degree of** left **thigh**

✓7ᵗʰ **T24.419** **Corrosion of unspecified degree of unspecified thigh**

✓6ᵗʰ **T24.42** **Corrosion of unspecified degree of** knee

✓7ᵗʰ **T24.421** **Corrosion of unspecified degree of** right **knee**

✓7ᵗʰ **T24.422** **Corrosion of unspecified degree of** left **knee**

✓7ᵗʰ **T24.429** **Corrosion of unspecified degree of unspecified knee**

✓6ᵗʰ **T24.43** **Corrosion of unspecified degree of** lower leg

✓7ᵗʰ **T24.431** **Corrosion of unspecified degree of** right **lower leg**

✓7ᵗʰ **T24.432** **Corrosion of unspecified degree of** left **lower leg**

✓7ᵗʰ **T24.439** **Corrosion of unspecified degree of unspecified lower leg**

✓6ᵗʰ **T24.49** **Corrosion of unspecified degree of** multiple sites **of lower limb, except ankle and foot**

✓7ᵗʰ **T24.491** **Corrosion of unspecified degree of multiple sites of** right **lower limb, except ankle and foot**

✓7ᵗʰ **T24.492** **Corrosion of unspecified degree of multiple sites of** left **lower limb, except ankle and foot**

✓7ᵗʰ **T24.499** **Corrosion of unspecified degree of multiple sites of unspecified lower limb, except ankle and foot**

✓5ᵗʰ **T24.5** **Corrosion of** first degree **of lower limb, except ankle and foot**

Code first (T51-T65) to identify chemical and intent
Use additional external cause code to identify place (Y92)

✓6ᵗʰ **T24.50** **Corrosion of first degree of unspecified site of lower limb, except ankle and foot**

✓7ᵗʰ **T24.501** **Corrosion of first degree of unspecified site of** right **lower limb, except ankle and foot**

✓7ᵗʰ **T24.502** **Corrosion of first degree of unspecified site of** left **lower limb, except ankle and foot**

✓7ᵗʰ **T24.509** **Corrosion of first degree of unspecified site of unspecified lower limb, except ankle and foot**

✓6ᵗʰ **T24.51** **Corrosion of first degree of** thigh

✓7ᵗʰ **T24.511** **Corrosion of first degree of** right **thigh**

✓7ᵗʰ **T24.512** **Corrosion of first degree of** left **thigh**

✓7ᵗʰ **T24.519** **Corrosion of first degree of unspecified thigh**

✓6ᵗʰ **T24.52** **Corrosion of first degree of** knee

✓7ᵗʰ **T24.521** **Corrosion of first degree of** right **knee**

✓7ᵗʰ **T24.522** **Corrosion of first degree of** left **knee**

✓7ᵗʰ **T24.529** **Corrosion of first degree of unspecified knee**

✓6ᵗʰ **T24.53** **Corrosion of first degree of** lower leg

✓7ᵗʰ **T24.531** **Corrosion of first degree of** right **lower leg**

✓7ᵗʰ **T24.532** **Corrosion of first degree of** left **lower leg**

✓7ᵗʰ **T24.539** **Corrosion of first degree of unspecified lower leg**

✓6ᵗʰ **T24.59** **Corrosion of first degree of** multiple sites **of lower limb, except ankle and foot**

✓7ᵗʰ **T24.591** **Corrosion of first degree of multiple sites of** right **lower limb, except ankle and foot**

✓7ᵗʰ **T24.592** **Corrosion of first degree of multiple sites of** left **lower limb, except ankle and foot**

✓7ᵗʰ **T24.599** **Corrosion of first degree of multiple sites of unspecified lower limb, except ankle and foot**

✓5ᵗʰ **T24.6** **Corrosion of** second degree **of lower limb, except ankle and foot**

Code first (T51-T65) to identify chemical and intent
Use additional external cause code to identify place (Y92)

✓6ᵗʰ **T24.60** **Corrosion of second degree of unspecified site of lower limb, except ankle and foot**

✓7ᵗʰ **T24.601** **Corrosion of second degree of unspecified site of** right **lower limb, except ankle and foot**

✓7ᵗʰ **T24.602** **Corrosion of second degree of unspecified site of** left **lower limb, except ankle and foot**

✓7ᵗʰ **T24.609** **Corrosion of second degree of unspecified site of unspecified lower limb, except ankle and foot**

✓6ᵗʰ **T24.61** **Corrosion of second degree of** thigh

✓7ᵗʰ **T24.611** **Corrosion of second degree of** right **thigh**

✓7ᵗʰ **T24.612** **Corrosion of second degree of** left **thigh**

✓7ᵗʰ **T24.619** **Corrosion of second degree of unspecified thigh**

✓6ᵗʰ **T24.62** **Corrosion of second degree of** knee

✓7ᵗʰ **T24.621** **Corrosion of second degree of** right **knee**

✓7ᵗʰ **T24.622** **Corrosion of second degree of** left **knee**

✓7ᵗʰ **T24.629** **Corrosion of second degree of unspecified knee**

✓6ᵗʰ **T24.63** **Corrosion of second degree of** lower leg

✓7ᵗʰ **T24.631** **Corrosion of second degree of** right **lower leg**

Chapter 19. Injury, Poisoning and Certain Other Consequences of External Causes

T24.632–T25.299

✓7ᵗʰ **T24.632** Corrosion of second degree of left lower leg

✓7ᵗʰ **T24.639** Corrosion of second degree of unspecified lower leg

✓6ᵗʰ **T24.69** Corrosion of second degree of multiple sites of lower limb, except ankle and foot

✓7ᵗʰ **T24.691** Corrosion of second degree of multiple sites of right lower limb, except ankle and foot

✓7ᵗʰ **T24.692** Corrosion of second degree of multiple sites of left lower limb, except ankle and foot

✓7ᵗʰ **T24.699** Corrosion of second degree of multiple sites of unspecified lower limb, except ankle and foot

✓5ᵗʰ **T24.7** Corrosion of third degree of lower limb, except ankle and foot

Code first (T51-T65) to identify chemical and intent
Use additional external cause code to identify place (Y92)

✓6ᵗʰ **T24.70** Corrosion of third degree of unspecified site of lower limb, except ankle and foot

✓7ᵗʰ **T24.701** Corrosion of third degree of unspecified site of right lower limb, except ankle and foot `COM`

✓7ᵗʰ **T24.702** Corrosion of third degree of unspecified site of left lower limb, except ankle and foot `COM`

✓7ᵗʰ **T24.709** Corrosion of third degree of unspecified site of unspecified lower limb, except ankle and foot `COM`

✓6ᵗʰ **T24.71** Corrosion of third degree of thigh

✓7ᵗʰ **T24.711** Corrosion of third degree of right thigh `COM`

✓7ᵗʰ **T24.712** Corrosion of third degree of left thigh `COM`

✓7ᵗʰ **T24.719** Corrosion of third degree of unspecified thigh `COM`

✓6ᵗʰ **T24.72** Corrosion of third degree of knee

✓7ᵗʰ **T24.721** Corrosion of third degree of right knee `COM`

✓7ᵗʰ **T24.722** Corrosion of third degree of left knee `COM`

✓7ᵗʰ **T24.729** Corrosion of third degree of unspecified knee `COM`

✓6ᵗʰ **T24.73** Corrosion of third degree of lower leg

✓7ᵗʰ **T24.731** Corrosion of third degree of right lower leg `COM`

✓7ᵗʰ **T24.732** Corrosion of third degree of left lower leg `COM`

✓7ᵗʰ **T24.739** Corrosion of third degree of unspecified lower leg `COM`

✓6ᵗʰ **T24.79** Corrosion of third degree of multiple sites of lower limb, except ankle and foot

✓7ᵗʰ **T24.791** Corrosion of third degree of multiple sites of right lower limb, except ankle and foot `COM`

✓7ᵗʰ **T24.792** Corrosion of third degree of multiple sites of left lower limb, except ankle and foot `COM`

✓7ᵗʰ **T24.799** Corrosion of third degree of multiple sites of unspecified lower limb, except ankle and foot `COM`

✓4ᵗʰ **T25** Burn and corrosion of ankle and foot

The appropriate 7th character is to be added to each code from category T25.
A   initial encounter
D   subsequent encounter
S   sequela

✓5ᵗʰ **T25.0** Burn of unspecified degree of ankle and foot

Use additional external cause code to identify the source, place and intent of the burn (X00-X19, X75-X77, X96-X98, Y92)

✓6ᵗʰ **T25.01** Burn of unspecified degree of ankle

✓7ᵗʰ **T25.011** Burn of unspecified degree of right ankle

✓7ᵗʰ **T25.012** Burn of unspecified degree of left ankle

✓7ᵗʰ **T25.019** Burn of unspecified degree of unspecified ankle

✓6ᵗʰ **T25.02** Burn of unspecified degree of foot

EXCLUDES 2   burn of unspecified degree of toe(s) (nail) (T25.03-)

✓7ᵗʰ **T25.021** Burn of unspecified degree of right foot

✓7ᵗʰ **T25.022** Burn of unspecified degree of left foot

✓7ᵗʰ **T25.029** Burn of unspecified degree of unspecified foot

✓6ᵗʰ **T25.03** Burn of unspecified degree of toe(s) (nail)

✓7ᵗʰ **T25.031** Burn of unspecified degree of right toe(s) (nail)

✓7ᵗʰ **T25.032** Burn of unspecified degree of left toe(s) (nail)

✓7ᵗʰ **T25.039** Burn of unspecified degree of unspecified toe(s) (nail)

✓6ᵗʰ **T25.09** Burn of unspecified degree of multiple sites of ankle and foot

✓7ᵗʰ **T25.091** Burn of unspecified degree of multiple sites of right ankle and foot

✓7ᵗʰ **T25.092** Burn of unspecified degree of multiple sites of left ankle and foot

✓7ᵗʰ **T25.099** Burn of unspecified degree of multiple sites of unspecified ankle and foot

✓5ᵗʰ **T25.1** Burn of first degree of ankle and foot

Use additional external cause code to identify the source, place and intent of the burn (X00-X19, X75-X77, X96-X98, Y92)

✓6ᵗʰ **T25.11** Burn of first degree of ankle

✓7ᵗʰ **T25.111** Burn of first degree of right ankle

✓7ᵗʰ **T25.112** Burn of first degree of left ankle

✓7ᵗʰ **T25.119** Burn of first degree of unspecified ankle

✓6ᵗʰ **T25.12** Burn of first degree of foot

EXCLUDES 2   burn of first degree of toe(s) (nail) (T25.13-)

✓7ᵗʰ **T25.121** Burn of first degree of right foot

✓7ᵗʰ **T25.122** Burn of first degree of left foot

✓7ᵗʰ **T25.129** Burn of first degree of unspecified foot

✓6ᵗʰ **T25.13** Burn of first degree of toe(s) (nail)

✓7ᵗʰ **T25.131** Burn of first degree of right toe(s) (nail)

✓7ᵗʰ **T25.132** Burn of first degree of left toe(s) (nail)

✓7ᵗʰ **T25.139** Burn of first degree of unspecified toe(s) (nail)

✓6ᵗʰ **T25.19** Burn of first degree of multiple sites of ankle and foot

✓7ᵗʰ **T25.191** Burn of first degree of multiple sites of right ankle and foot

✓7ᵗʰ **T25.192** Burn of first degree of multiple sites of left ankle and foot

✓7ᵗʰ **T25.199** Burn of first degree of multiple sites of unspecified ankle and foot

✓5ᵗʰ **T25.2** Burn of second degree of ankle and foot

Use additional external cause code to identify the source, place and intent of the burn (X00-X19, X75-X77, X96-X98, Y92)

✓6ᵗʰ **T25.21** Burn of second degree of ankle

✓7ᵗʰ **T25.211** Burn of second degree of right ankle

✓7ᵗʰ **T25.212** Burn of second degree of left ankle

✓7ᵗʰ **T25.219** Burn of second degree of unspecified ankle

✓6ᵗʰ **T25.22** Burn of second degree of foot

EXCLUDES 2   burn of second degree of toe(s) (nail) (T25.23-)

✓7ᵗʰ **T25.221** Burn of second degree of right foot

✓7ᵗʰ **T25.222** Burn of second degree of left foot

✓7ᵗʰ **T25.229** Burn of second degree of unspecified foot

✓6ᵗʰ **T25.23** Burn of second degree of toe(s) (nail)

✓7ᵗʰ **T25.231** Burn of second degree of right toe(s) (nail)

✓7ᵗʰ **T25.232** Burn of second degree of left toe(s) (nail)

✓7ᵗʰ **T25.239** Burn of second degree of unspecified toe(s) (nail)

✓6ᵗʰ **T25.29** Burn of second degree of multiple sites of ankle and foot

✓7ᵗʰ **T25.291** Burn of second degree of multiple sites of right ankle and foot

✓7ᵗʰ **T25.292** Burn of second degree of multiple sites of left ankle and foot

✓7ᵗʰ **T25.299** Burn of second degree of multiple sites of unspecified ankle and foot

HCC CMS-HCC   **Rx** Rx HCC   **ESR** ESRD HCC   **COM** Commercial HCC   **N** Newborn: 0   **P** Pediatric: 0-17   **M** Maternity: 9-64   **A** Adult: 15-124

1128   ICD-10-CM 2023

√5ᵗʰ **T25.3** **Burn of** third degree **of ankle and foot**

     Use additional external cause code to identify the source, place and intent of the burn (X00-X19, X75-X77, X96-X98, Y92)

√6ᵗʰ   **T25.31**   **Burn of third degree of** ankle

     √7ᵗʰ   **T25.311**   **Burn of third degree of** right **ankle** `COM`

     √7ᵗʰ   **T25.312**   **Burn of third degree of** left **ankle** `COM`

     √7ᵗʰ   **T25.319**   **Burn of third degree of unspecified ankle** `COM`

√6ᵗʰ   **T25.32**   **Burn of third degree of** foot

     `EXCLUDES 2`   burn of third degree of toe(s) (nail) (T25.33-)

     √7ᵗʰ   **T25.321**   **Burn of third degree of** right **foot** `COM`

     √7ᵗʰ   **T25.322**   **Burn of third degree of** left **foot** `COM`

     √7ᵗʰ   **T25.329**   **Burn of third degree of unspecified foot** `COM`

√6ᵗʰ   **T25.33**   **Burn of third degree of** toe(s) (nail)

     √7ᵗʰ   **T25.331**   **Burn of third degree of** right **toe(s) (nail)** `COM`

     √7ᵗʰ   **T25.332**   **Burn of third degree of** left **toe(s) (nail)** `COM`

     √7ᵗʰ   **T25.339**   **Burn of third degree of unspecified toe(s) (nail)** `COM`

√6ᵗʰ   **T25.39**   **Burn of third degree of** multiple sites **of ankle and foot**

     √7ᵗʰ   **T25.391**   **Burn of third degree of multiple sites of** right **ankle and foot** `COM`

     √7ᵗʰ   **T25.392**   **Burn of third degree of multiple sites of** left **ankle and foot** `COM`

     √7ᵗʰ   **T25.399**   **Burn of third degree of multiple sites of unspecified ankle and foot** `COM`

√5ᵗʰ **T25.4** **Corrosion of unspecified degree of ankle and foot**

     Code first (T51-T65) to identify chemical and intent
     Use additional external cause code to identify place (Y92)

√6ᵗʰ   **T25.41**   **Corrosion of unspecified degree of** ankle

     √7ᵗʰ   **T25.411**   **Corrosion of unspecified degree of** right **ankle**

     √7ᵗʰ   **T25.412**   **Corrosion of unspecified degree of** left **ankle**

     √7ᵗʰ   **T25.419**   **Corrosion of unspecified degree of unspecified ankle**

√6ᵗʰ   **T25.42**   **Corrosion of unspecified degree of** foot

     `EXCLUDES 2`   corrosion of unspecified degree of toe(s) (nail) (T25.43-)

     √7ᵗʰ   **T25.421**   **Corrosion of unspecified degree of** right **foot**

     √7ᵗʰ   **T25.422**   **Corrosion of unspecified degree of** left **foot**

     √7ᵗʰ   **T25.429**   **Corrosion of unspecified degree of unspecified foot**

√6ᵗʰ   **T25.43**   **Corrosion of unspecified degree of** toe(s) (nail)

     √7ᵗʰ   **T25.431**   **Corrosion of unspecified degree of** right **toe(s) (nail)**

     √7ᵗʰ   **T25.432**   **Corrosion of unspecified degree of** left **toe(s) (nail)**

     √7ᵗʰ   **T25.439**   **Corrosion of unspecified degree of unspecified toe(s) (nail)**

√6ᵗʰ   **T25.49**   **Corrosion of unspecified degree of** multiple sites **of ankle and foot**

     √7ᵗʰ   **T25.491**   **Corrosion of unspecified degree of multiple sites of** right **ankle and foot**

     √7ᵗʰ   **T25.492**   **Corrosion of unspecified degree of multiple sites of** left **ankle and foot**

     √7ᵗʰ   **T25.499**   **Corrosion of unspecified degree of multiple sites of unspecified ankle and foot**

√5ᵗʰ **T25.5** **Corrosion of** first degree **of ankle and foot**

     Code first (T51-T65) to identify chemical and intent
     Use additional external cause code to identify place (Y92)

√6ᵗʰ   **T25.51**   **Corrosion of first degree of** ankle

     √7ᵗʰ   **T25.511**   **Corrosion of first degree of** right **ankle**

     √7ᵗʰ   **T25.512**   **Corrosion of first degree of** left **ankle**

     √7ᵗʰ   **T25.519**   **Corrosion of first degree of unspecified ankle**

√6ᵗʰ   **T25.52**   **Corrosion of first degree of** foot

     `EXCLUDES 2`   corrosion of first degree of toe(s) (nail) (T25.53-)

     √7ᵗʰ   **T25.521**   **Corrosion of first degree of** right **foot**

√7ᵗʰ   **T25.522**   **Corrosion of first degree of** left **foot**

√7ᵗʰ   **T25.529**   **Corrosion of first degree of unspecified foot**

√6ᵗʰ   **T25.53**   **Corrosion of first degree of** toe(s) (nail)

     √7ᵗʰ   **T25.531**   **Corrosion of first degree of** right **toe(s) (nail)**

     √7ᵗʰ   **T25.532**   **Corrosion of first degree of** left **toe(s) (nail)**

     √7ᵗʰ   **T25.539**   **Corrosion of first degree of unspecified toe(s) (nail)**

√6ᵗʰ   **T25.59**   **Corrosion of first degree of** multiple sites **of ankle and foot**

     √7ᵗʰ   **T25.591**   **Corrosion of first degree of multiple sites of** right **ankle and foot**

     √7ᵗʰ   **T25.592**   **Corrosion of first degree of multiple sites of** left **ankle and foot**

     √7ᵗʰ   **T25.599**   **Corrosion of first degree of multiple sites of unspecified ankle and foot**

√5ᵗʰ **T25.6** **Corrosion of** second degree **of ankle and foot**

     Code first (T51-T65) to identify chemical and intent
     Use additional external cause code to identify place (Y92)

√6ᵗʰ   **T25.61**   **Corrosion of second degree of** ankle

     √7ᵗʰ   **T25.611**   **Corrosion of second degree of** right **ankle**

     √7ᵗʰ   **T25.612**   **Corrosion of second degree of** left **ankle**

     √7ᵗʰ   **T25.619**   **Corrosion of second degree of unspecified ankle**

√6ᵗʰ   **T25.62**   **Corrosion of second degree of** foot

     `EXCLUDES 2`   corrosion of second degree of toe(s) (nail) (T25.63-)

     √7ᵗʰ   **T25.621**   **Corrosion of second degree of** right **foot**

     √7ᵗʰ   **T25.622**   **Corrosion of second degree of** left **foot**

     √7ᵗʰ   **T25.629**   **Corrosion of second degree of unspecified foot**

√6ᵗʰ   **T25.63**   **Corrosion of second degree of** toe(s) (nail)

     √7ᵗʰ   **T25.631**   **Corrosion of second degree of** right **toe(s) (nail)**

     √7ᵗʰ   **T25.632**   **Corrosion of second degree of** left **toe(s) (nail)**

     √7ᵗʰ   **T25.639**   **Corrosion of second degree of unspecified toe(s) (nail)**

√6ᵗʰ   **T25.69**   **Corrosion of second degree of** multiple sites **of ankle and foot**

     √7ᵗʰ   **T25.691**   **Corrosion of second degree of** right **ankle and foot**

     √7ᵗʰ   **T25.692**   **Corrosion of second degree of** left **ankle and foot**

     √7ᵗʰ   **T25.699**   **Corrosion of second degree of unspecified ankle and foot**

√5ᵗʰ **T25.7** **Corrosion of** third degree **of ankle and foot**

     Code first (T51-T65) to identify chemical and intent
     Use additional external cause code to identify place (Y92)

√6ᵗʰ   **T25.71**   **Corrosion of third degree of** ankle

     √7ᵗʰ   **T25.711**   **Corrosion of third degree of** right **ankle** `COM`

     √7ᵗʰ   **T25.712**   **Corrosion of third degree of** left **ankle** `COM`

     √7ᵗʰ   **T25.719**   **Corrosion of third degree of unspecified ankle** `COM`

√6ᵗʰ   **T25.72**   **Corrosion of third degree of** foot

     `EXCLUDES 2`   corrosion of third degree of toe(s) (nail) (T25.73-)

     √7ᵗʰ   **T25.721**   **Corrosion of third degree of** right **foot** `COM`

     √7ᵗʰ   **T25.722**   **Corrosion of third degree of** left **foot** `COM`

     √7ᵗʰ   **T25.729**   **Corrosion of third degree of unspecified foot** `COM`

√6ᵗʰ   **T25.73**   **Corrosion of third degree of** toe(s) (nail)

     √7ᵗʰ   **T25.731**   **Corrosion of third degree of** right **toe(s) (nail)** `COM`

     √7ᵗʰ   **T25.732**   **Corrosion of third degree of** left **toe(s) (nail)** `COM`

     √7ᵗʰ   **T25.739**   **Corrosion of third degree of unspecified toe(s) (nail)** `COM`

√6ᵗʰ   **T25.79**   **Corrosion of third degree of** multiple sites **of ankle and foot**

     √7ᵗʰ   **T25.791**   **Corrosion of third degree of multiple sites of** right **ankle and foot** `COM`

✓7ᵗʰ **T25.792** Corrosion of third degree of multiple sites of left ankle and foot `COM`

✓7ᵗʰ **T25.799** Corrosion of third degree of multiple sites of unspecified ankle and foot `COM`

Burns and corrosions confined to eye and internal organs (T26-T28)

✓4ᵗʰ **T26 Burn and corrosion confined to eye and adnexa**

The appropriate 7th character is to be added to each code from category T26.
A   initial encounter
D   subsequent encounter
S   sequela

✓5ᵗʰ **T26.0 Burn of eyelid and periocular area**

Use additional external cause code to identify the source, place and intent of the burn (X00-X19, X75-X77, X96-X98, Y92)

✓x7ᵗʰ **T26.00** Burn of unspecified eyelid and periocular area
✓x7ᵗʰ **T26.01** Burn of right eyelid and periocular area
✓x7ᵗʰ **T26.02** Burn of left eyelid and periocular area

✓5ᵗʰ **T26.1 Burn of cornea and conjunctival sac**

Use additional external cause code to identify the source, place and intent of the burn (X00-X19, X75-X77, X96-X98, Y92)

✓x7ᵗʰ **T26.10** Burn of cornea and conjunctival sac, unspecified eye
✓x7ᵗʰ **T26.11** Burn of cornea and conjunctival sac, right eye
✓x7ᵗʰ **T26.12** Burn of cornea and conjunctival sac, left eye

✓5ᵗʰ **T26.2 Burn with resulting rupture and destruction of eyeball**

Use additional external cause code to identify the source, place and intent of the burn (X00-X19, X75-X77, X96-X98, Y92)

✓x7ᵗʰ **T26.20** Burn with resulting rupture and destruction of unspecified eyeball
✓x7ᵗʰ **T26.21** Burn with resulting rupture and destruction of right eyeball
✓x7ᵗʰ **T26.22** Burn with resulting rupture and destruction of left eyeball

✓5ᵗʰ **T26.3 Burns of other specified parts of eye and adnexa**

Use additional external cause code to identify the source, place and intent of the burn (X00-X19, X75-X77, X96-X98, Y92)

✓x7ᵗʰ **T26.30** Burns of other specified parts of unspecified eye and adnexa
✓x7ᵗʰ **T26.31** Burns of other specified parts of right eye and adnexa
✓x7ᵗʰ **T26.32** Burns of other specified parts of left eye and adnexa

✓5ᵗʰ **T26.4 Burn of eye and adnexa, part unspecified**

Use additional external cause code to identify the source, place and intent of the burn (X00-X19, X75-X77, X96-X98, Y92)

✓x7ᵗʰ **T26.40** Burn of unspecified eye and adnexa, part unspecified
✓x7ᵗʰ **T26.41** Burn of right eye and adnexa, part unspecified
✓x7ᵗʰ **T26.42** Burn of left eye and adnexa, part unspecified

✓5ᵗʰ **T26.5 Corrosion of eyelid and periocular area**

Code first (T51-T65) to identify chemical and intent
Use additional external cause code to identify place (Y92)

✓x7ᵗʰ **T26.50** Corrosion of unspecified eyelid and periocular area
✓x7ᵗʰ **T26.51** Corrosion of right eyelid and periocular area
✓x7ᵗʰ **T26.52** Corrosion of left eyelid and periocular area

✓5ᵗʰ **T26.6 Corrosion of cornea and conjunctival sac**

Code first (T51-T65) to identify chemical and intent
Use additional external cause code to identify place (Y92)

✓x7ᵗʰ **T26.60** Corrosion of cornea and conjunctival sac, unspecified eye
✓x7ᵗʰ **T26.61** Corrosion of cornea and conjunctival sac, right eye
✓x7ᵗʰ **T26.62** Corrosion of cornea and conjunctival sac, left eye

✓5ᵗʰ **T26.7 Corrosion with resulting rupture and destruction of eyeball**

Code first (T51-T65) to identify chemical and intent
Use additional external cause code to identify place (Y92)

✓x7ᵗʰ **T26.70** Corrosion with resulting rupture and destruction of unspecified eyeball
✓x7ᵗʰ **T26.71** Corrosion with resulting rupture and destruction of right eyeball
✓x7ᵗʰ **T26.72** Corrosion with resulting rupture and destruction of left eyeball

✓5ᵗʰ **T26.8 Corrosions of other specified parts of eye and adnexa**

Code first (T51-T65) to identify chemical and intent
Use additional external cause code to identify place (Y92)

✓x7ᵗʰ **T26.80** Corrosions of other specified parts of unspecified eye and adnexa
✓x7ᵗʰ **T26.81** Corrosions of other specified parts of right eye and adnexa
✓x7ᵗʰ **T26.82** Corrosions of other specified parts of left eye and adnexa

✓5ᵗʰ **T26.9 Corrosion of eye and adnexa, part unspecified**

Code first (T51-T65) to identify chemical and intent
Use additional external cause code to identify place (Y92)

✓x7ᵗʰ **T26.90** Corrosion of unspecified eye and adnexa, part unspecified
✓x7ᵗʰ **T26.91** Corrosion of right eye and adnexa, part unspecified
✓x7ᵗʰ **T26.92** Corrosion of left eye and adnexa, part unspecified

✓4ᵗʰ **T27 Burn and corrosion of respiratory tract**

Use additional external cause code to identify the source and intent of the burn (X00-X19, X75-X77, X96-X98)
Use additional external cause code to identify place (Y92)

The appropriate 7th character is to be added to each code from category T27.
A   initial encounter
D   subsequent encounter
S   sequela

✓x7ᵗʰ **T27.0** Burn of larynx and trachea
✓x7ᵗʰ **T27.1** Burn involving larynx and trachea with lung
✓x7ᵗʰ **T27.2** Burn of other parts of respiratory tract
Burn of thoracic cavity
✓x7ᵗʰ **T27.3** Burn of respiratory tract, part unspecified
✓x7ᵗʰ **T27.4** Corrosion of larynx and trachea
Code first (T51-T65) to identify chemical and intent
✓x7ᵗʰ **T27.5** Corrosion involving larynx and trachea with lung
Code first (T51-T65) to identify chemical and intent
✓x7ᵗʰ **T27.6** Corrosion of other parts of respiratory tract
Code first (T51-T65) to identify chemical and intent
✓x7ᵗʰ **T27.7** Corrosion of respiratory tract, part unspecified
Code first (T51-T65) to identify chemical and intent

✓4ᵗʰ **T28 Burn and corrosion of other internal organs**

Use additional external cause code to identify the source and intent of the burn (X00-X19, X75-X77, X96-X98)
Use additional external cause code to identify place (Y92)

The appropriate 7th character is to be added to each code from category T28.
A   initial encounter
D   subsequent encounter
S   sequela

✓x7ᵗʰ **T28.0** Burn of mouth and pharynx
✓x7ᵗʰ **T28.1** Burn of esophagus
✓x7ᵗʰ **T28.2** Burn of other parts of alimentary tract
✓x7ᵗʰ **T28.3** Burn of internal genitourinary organs
✓5ᵗʰ **T28.4** Burns of other and unspecified internal organs
✓x7ᵗʰ **T28.40** Burn of unspecified internal organ
✓6ᵗʰ **T28.41** Burn of ear drum
✓7ᵗʰ **T28.411** Burn of right ear drum
✓7ᵗʰ **T28.412** Burn of left ear drum
✓7ᵗʰ **T28.419** Burn of unspecified ear drum
✓x7ᵗʰ **T28.49** Burn of other internal organ
✓x7ᵗʰ **T28.5** Corrosion of mouth and pharynx
Code first (T51-T65) to identify chemical and intent
✓x7ᵗʰ **T28.6** Corrosion of esophagus
Code first (T51-T65) to identify chemical and intent
✓x7ᵗʰ **T28.7** Corrosion of other parts of alimentary tract
Code first (T51-T65) to identify chemical and intent
✓x7ᵗʰ **T28.8** Corrosion of internal genitourinary organs
Code first (T51-T65) to identify chemical and intent
✓5ᵗʰ **T28.9** Corrosions of other and unspecified internal organs
Code first (T51-T65) to identify chemical and intent
✓x7ᵗʰ **T28.90** Corrosions of unspecified internal organs

✓6ᵗʰ **T28.91 Corrosions of** ear drum

    ✓7ᵗʰ **T28.911 Corrosions of** right **ear drum**

    ✓7ᵗʰ **T28.912 Corrosions of** left **ear drum**

    ✓7ᵗʰ **T28.919 Corrosions of** unspecified **ear drum**

✓x7ᵗʰ **T28.99 Corrosions of other internal organs**

Burns and corrosions of multiple and unspecified body regions (T30-T32)

✓4ᵗʰ **T30 Burn and corrosion, body region unspecified**

    T30.0 Burn of unspecified body region, unspecified degree
This code is not for inpatient use. Code to specified site and degree of burns
Burn NOS
Multiple burns NOS

    T30.4 Corrosion of unspecified body region, unspecified degree
This code is not for inpatient use. Code to specified site and degree of corrosion
Corrosion NOS
Multiple corrosion NOS

✓4ᵗʰ **T31 Burns classified according to extent of body surface involved**

    NOTE   This category is to be used as the primary code only when the site of the burn is unspecified. It should be used as a supplementary code with categories T20-T25 when the site is specified.

    T31.0 Burns involving less than 10% **of body surface**

✓5ᵗʰ **T31.1 Burns involving** 10-19% **of body surface**

    T31.10 Burns involving 10-19% of body surface with 0% **to 9% third degree burns**   COM
Burns involving 10-19% of body surface NOS

    T31.11 Burns involving 10-19% of body surface with 10-19% third degree burns   HCC ESR COM

✓5ᵗʰ **T31.2 Burns involving** 20-29% **of body surface**

    T31.20 Burns involving 20-29% of body surface with 0% **to 9% third degree burns**   COM
Burns involving 20-29% of body surface NOS

    T31.21 Burns involving 20-29% of body surface with 10-19% third degree burns   HCC ESR COM

    T31.22 Burns involving 20-29% of body surface with 20-29% third degree burns   HCC ESR COM

✓5ᵗʰ **T31.3 Burns involving** 30-39% **of body surface**

    T31.30 Burns involving 30-39% of body surface with 0% **to 9% third degree burns**   COM
Burns involving 30-39% of body surface NOS

    T31.31 Burns involving 30-39% of body surface with 10-19% third degree burns   HCC ESR COM

    T31.32 Burns involving 30-39% of body surface with 20-29% third degree burns   HCC ESR COM

    T31.33 Burns involving 30-39% of body surface with 30-39% third degree burns   HCC ESR COM

✓5ᵗʰ **T31.4 Burns involving** 40-49% **of body surface**

    T31.40 Burns involving 40-49% of body surface with 0% **to 9% third degree burns**   COM
Burns involving 40-49% of body surface NOS

    T31.41 Burns involving 40-49% of body surface with 10-19% third degree burns   HCC ESR COM

    T31.42 Burns involving 40-49% of body surface with 20-29% third degree burns   HCC ESR COM

    T31.43 Burns involving 40-49% of body surface with 30-39% third degree burns   HCC ESR COM

    T31.44 Burns involving 40-49% of body surface with 40-49% third degree burns   HCC ESR COM

✓5ᵗʰ **T31.5 Burns involving** 50-59% **of body surface**

    T31.50 Burns involving 50-59% of body surface with 0% **to 9% third degree burns**   COM
Burns involving 50-59% of body surface NOS

    T31.51 Burns involving 50-59% of body surface with 10-19% third degree burns   HCC ESR COM

    T31.52 Burns involving 50-59% of body surface with 20-29% third degree burns   HCC ESR COM

    T31.53 Burns involving 50-59% of body surface with 30-39% third degree burns   HCC ESR COM

    T31.54 Burns involving 50-59% of body surface with 40-49% third degree burns   HCC ESR COM

    T31.55 Burns involving 50-59% of body surface with 50-59% third degree burns   HCC ESR COM

✓5ᵗʰ **T31.6 Burns involving** 60-69% **of body surface**

    T31.60 Burns involving 60-69% of body surface with 0% **to 9% third degree burns**   COM
Burns involving 60-69% of body surface NOS

    T31.61 Burns involving 60-69% of body surface with 10-19% third degree burns   HCC ESR COM

    T31.62 Burns involving 60-69% of body surface with 20-29% third degree burns   HCC ESR COM

    T31.63 Burns involving 60-69% of body surface with 30-39% third degree burns   HCC ESR COM

    T31.64 Burns involving 60-69% of body surface with 40-49% third degree burns   HCC ESR COM

    T31.65 Burns involving 60-69% of body surface with 50-59% third degree burns   HCC ESR COM

    T31.66 Burns involving 60-69% of body surface with 60-69% third degree burns   HCC ESR COM

✓5ᵗʰ **T31.7 Burns involving** 70-79% **of body surface**

    T31.70 Burns involving 70-79% of body surface with 0% **to 9% third degree burns**   COM
Burns involving 70-79% of body surface NOS

    T31.71 Burns involving 70-79% of body surface with 10-19% third degree burns   HCC ESR COM

    T31.72 Burns involving 70-79% of body surface with 20-29% third degree burns   HCC ESR COM

    T31.73 Burns involving 70-79% of body surface with 30-39% third degree burns   HCC ESR COM

    T31.74 Burns involving 70-79% of body surface with 40-49% third degree burns   HCC ESR COM

    T31.75 Burns involving 70-79% of body surface with 50-59% third degree burns   HCC ESR COM

    T31.76 Burns involving 70-79% of body surface with 60-69% third degree burns   HCC ESR COM

    T31.77 Burns involving 70-79% of body surface with 70-79% third degree burns   HCC ESR COM

✓5ᵗʰ **T31.8 Burns involving** 80-89% **of body surface**

    T31.80 Burns involving 80-89% of body surface with 0% **to 9% third degree burns**   COM
Burns involving 80-89% of body surface NOS

    T31.81 Burns involving 80-89% of body surface with 10-19% third degree burns   HCC ESR COM

    T31.82 Burns involving 80-89% of body surface with 20-29% third degree burns   HCC ESR COM

    T31.83 Burns involving 80-89% of body surface with 30-39% third degree burns   HCC ESR COM

    T31.84 Burns involving 80-89% of body surface with 40-49% third degree burns   HCC ESR COM

    T31.85 Burns involving 80-89% of body surface with 50-59% third degree burns   HCC ESR COM

    T31.86 Burns involving 80-89% of body surface with 60-69% third degree burns   HCC ESR COM

    T31.87 Burns involving 80-89% of body surface with 70-79% third degree burns   HCC ESR COM

    T31.88 Burns involving 80-89% of body surface with 80-89% third degree burns   HCC ESR COM

✓5ᵗʰ **T31.9 Burns involving** 90% or more **of body surface**

    T31.90 Burns involving 90% or more of body surface with 0% to 9% third degree burns   COM
Burns involving 90% or more of body surface NOS

    T31.91 Burns involving 90% or more of body surface with 10-19% third degree burns   HCC ESR COM

    T31.92 Burns involving 90% or more of body surface with 20-29% third degree burns   HCC ESR COM

    T31.93 Burns involving 90% or more of body surface with 30-39% third degree burns   HCC ESR COM

    T31.94 Burns involving 90% or more of body surface with 40-49% third degree burns   HCC ESR COM

    T31.95 Burns involving 90% or more of body surface with 50-59% third degree burns   HCC ESR COM

    T31.96 Burns involving 90% or more of body surface with 60-69% third degree burns   HCC ESR COM

    T31.97 Burns involving 90% or more of body surface with 70-79% third degree burns   HCC ESR COM

    T31.98 Burns involving 90% or more of body surface with 80-89% third degree burns   HCC ESR COM

✔ Additional Character Required   ✓x7ᵗʰ Placeholder Alert   Manifestation   Unspecified Dx   Q QPP   UPD Unacceptable PDx

T31.99   **Burns involving 90% or more of body surface with 90% or more third degree burns** `HCC` `ESR` `COM`

Rule of Nines Estimation of Total Body Surface Burned

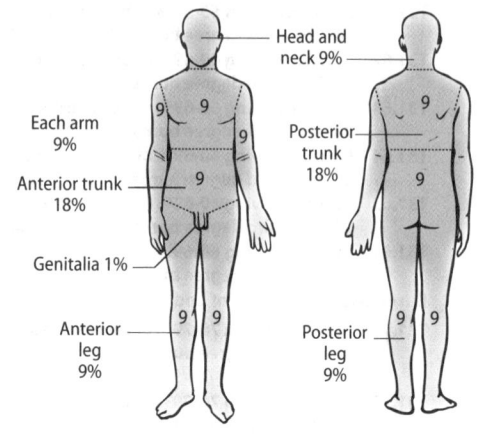

- Head and neck 9%
- Each arm 9%
- Posterior trunk 18%
- Anterior trunk 18%
- Genitalia 1%
- Anterior leg 9%
- Posterior leg 9%

✓4th **T32**   **Corrosions classified according to extent of body surface involved**

> **NOTE**   This category is to be used as the primary code only when the site of the corrosion is unspecified. It may be used as a supplementary code with categories T20-T25 when the site is specified.

T32.0   **Corrosions involving less than 10% of body surface**

✓5th **T32.1**   **Corrosions involving 10-19% of body surface**

     T32.10   **Corrosions involving 10-19% of body surface with 0% to 9% third degree corrosion** `COM`
         Corrosions involving 10-19% of body surface NOS

     T32.11   **Corrosions involving 10-19% of body surface with 10-19% third degree corrosion** `HCC` `ESR` `COM`

✓5th **T32.2**   **Corrosions involving 20-29% of body surface**

     T32.20   **Corrosions involving 20-29% of body surface with 0% to 9% third degree corrosion** `COM`

     T32.21   **Corrosions involving 20-29% of body surface with 10-19% third degree corrosion** `HCC` `ESR` `COM`

     T32.22   **Corrosions involving 20-29% of body surface with 20-29% third degree corrosion** `HCC` `ESR` `COM`

✓5th **T32.3**   **Corrosions involving 30-39% of body surface**

     T32.30   **Corrosions involving 30-39% of body surface with 0% to 9% third degree corrosion** `COM`

     T32.31   **Corrosions involving 30-39% of body surface with 10-19% third degree corrosion** `HCC` `ESR` `COM`

     T32.32   **Corrosions involving 30-39% of body surface with 20-29% third degree corrosion** `HCC` `ESR` `COM`

     T32.33   **Corrosions involving 30-39% of body surface with 30-39% third degree corrosion** `HCC` `ESR` `COM`

✓5th **T32.4**   **Corrosions involving 40-49% of body surface**

     T32.40   **Corrosions involving 40-49% of body surface with 0% to 9% third degree corrosion** `COM`

     T32.41   **Corrosions involving 40-49% of body surface with 10-19% third degree corrosion** `HCC` `ESR` `COM`

     T32.42   **Corrosions involving 40-49% of body surface with 20-29% third degree corrosion** `HCC` `ESR` `COM`

     T32.43   **Corrosions involving 40-49% of body surface with 30-39% third degree corrosion** `HCC` `ESR` `COM`

     T32.44   **Corrosions involving 40-49% of body surface with 40-49% third degree corrosion** `HCC` `ESR` `COM`

✓5th **T32.5**   **Corrosions involving 50-59% of body surface**

     T32.50   **Corrosions involving 50-59% of body surface with 0% to 9% third degree corrosion** `COM`

     T32.51   **Corrosions involving 50-59% of body surface with 10-19% third degree corrosion** `HCC` `ESR` `COM`

     T32.52   **Corrosions involving 50-59% of body surface with 20-29% third degree corrosion** `HCC` `ESR` `COM`

     T32.53   **Corrosions involving 50-59% of body surface with 30-39% third degree corrosion** `HCC` `ESR` `COM`

     T32.54   **Corrosions involving 50-59% of body surface with 40-49% third degree corrosion** `HCC` `ESR` `COM`

     T32.55   **Corrosions involving 50-59% of body surface with 50-59% third degree corrosion** `HCC` `ESR` `COM`

✓5th **T32.6**   **Corrosions involving 60-69% of body surface**

     T32.60   **Corrosions involving 60-69% of body surface with 0% to 9% third degree corrosion** `COM`

     T32.61   **Corrosions involving 60-69% of body surface with 10-19% third degree corrosion** `HCC` `ESR` `COM`

     T32.62   **Corrosions involving 60-69% of body surface with 20-29% third degree corrosion** `HCC` `ESR` `COM`

     T32.63   **Corrosions involving 60-69% of body surface with 30-39% third degree corrosion** `HCC` `ESR` `COM`

     T32.64   **Corrosions involving 60-69% of body surface with 40-49% third degree corrosion** `HCC` `ESR` `COM`

     T32.65   **Corrosions involving 60-69% of body surface with 50-59% third degree corrosion** `HCC` `ESR` `COM`

     T32.66   **Corrosions involving 60-69% of body surface with 60-69% third degree corrosion** `HCC` `ESR` `COM`

✓5th **T32.7**   **Corrosions involving 70-79% of body surface**

     T32.70   **Corrosions involving 70-79% of body surface with 0% to 9% third degree corrosion** `COM`

     T32.71   **Corrosions involving 70-79% of body surface with 10-19% third degree corrosion** `HCC` `ESR` `COM`

     T32.72   **Corrosions involving 70-79% of body surface with 20-29% third degree corrosion** `HCC` `ESR` `COM`

     T32.73   **Corrosions involving 70-79% of body surface with 30-39% third degree corrosion** `HCC` `ESR` `COM`

     T32.74   **Corrosions involving 70-79% of body surface with 40-49% third degree corrosion** `HCC` `ESR` `COM`

     T32.75   **Corrosions involving 70-79% of body surface with 50-59% third degree corrosion** `HCC` `ESR` `COM`

     T32.76   **Corrosions involving 70-79% of body surface with 60-69% third degree corrosion** `HCC` `ESR` `COM`

     T32.77   **Corrosions involving 70-79% of body surface with 70-79% third degree corrosion** `HCC` `ESR` `COM`

✓5th **T32.8**   **Corrosions involving 80-89% of body surface**

     T32.80   **Corrosions involving 80-89% of body surface with 0% to 9% third degree corrosion** `COM`

     T32.81   **Corrosions involving 80-89% of body surface with 10-19% third degree corrosion** `HCC` `ESR` `COM`

     T32.82   **Corrosions involving 80-89% of body surface with 20-29% third degree corrosion** `HCC` `ESR` `COM`

     T32.83   **Corrosions involving 80-89% of body surface with 30-39% third degree corrosion** `HCC` `ESR` `COM`

     T32.84   **Corrosions involving 80-89% of body surface with 40-49% third degree corrosion** `HCC` `ESR` `COM`

     T32.85   **Corrosions involving 80-89% of body surface with 50-59% third degree corrosion** `HCC` `ESR` `COM`

     T32.86   **Corrosions involving 80-89% of body surface with 60-69% third degree corrosion** `HCC` `ESR` `COM`

     T32.87   **Corrosions involving 80-89% of body surface with 70-79% third degree corrosion** `HCC` `ESR` `COM`

     T32.88   **Corrosions involving 80-89% of body surface with 80-89% third degree corrosion** `HCC` `ESR` `COM`

✓5th **T32.9**   **Corrosions involving 90% or more of body surface**

     T32.90   **Corrosions involving 90% or more of body surface with 0% to 9% third degree corrosion** `COM`

     T32.91   **Corrosions involving 90% or more of body surface with 10-19% third degree corrosion** `HCC` `ESR` `COM`

     T32.92   **Corrosions involving 90% or more of body surface with 20-29% third degree corrosion** `HCC` `ESR` `COM`

     T32.93   **Corrosions involving 90% or more of body surface with 30-39% third degree corrosion** `HCC` `ESR` `COM`

     T32.94   **Corrosions involving 90% or more of body surface with 40-49% third degree corrosion** `HCC` `ESR` `COM`

     T32.95   **Corrosions involving 90% or more of body surface with 50-59% third degree corrosion** `HCC` `ESR` `COM`

     T32.96   **Corrosions involving 90% or more of body surface with 60-69% third degree corrosion** `HCC` `ESR` `COM`

     T32.97   **Corrosions involving 90% or more of body surface with 70-79% third degree corrosion** `HCC` `ESR` `COM`

     T32.98   **Corrosions involving 90% or more of body surface with 80-89% third degree corrosion** `HCC` `ESR` `COM`

     T32.99   **Corrosions involving 90% or more of body surface with 90% or more third degree corrosion** `HCC` `ESR` `COM`

`HCC` CMS-HCC   `Rx` Rx HCC   `ESR` ESRD HCC   `COM` Commercial HCC   N Newborn: 0   P Pediatric: 0-17   M Maternity: 9-64   A Adult: 15-124

1132   ICD-10-CM 2023

Frostbite (T33-T34)

EXCLUDES 2   *hypothermia and other effects of reduced temperature (T68, T69.-)*

√4ᵗʰ **T33   Superficial frostbite**

INCLUDES   frostbite with partial thickness skin loss

The appropriate 7th character is to be added to each code from category T33.
A   initial encounter
D   subsequent encounter
S   sequela

√5ᵗʰ **T33.0   Superficial frostbite of** head
  √6ᵗʰ **T33.01   Superficial frostbite of** ear
    √7ᵗʰ **T33.011   Superficial frostbite of** right **ear**
    √7ᵗʰ **T33.012   Superficial frostbite of** left **ear**
    √7ᵗʰ **T33.019   Superficial frostbite of unspecified ear**
  √x7ᵗʰ **T33.02   Superficial frostbite of** nose
  √x7ᵗʰ **T33.09   Superficial frostbite of other part of head**

√x7ᵗʰ **T33.1   Superficial frostbite of** neck
√x7ᵗʰ **T33.2   Superficial frostbite of** thorax
√x7ᵗʰ **T33.3   Superficial frostbite of** abdominal wall, lower back and pelvis

√5ᵗʰ **T33.4   Superficial frostbite of** arm
  EXCLUDES 2   *superficial frostbite of wrist and hand (T33.5-)*
  √x7ᵗʰ **T33.40   Superficial frostbite of unspecified arm**
  √x7ᵗʰ **T33.41   Superficial frostbite of** right **arm**
  √x7ᵗʰ **T33.42   Superficial frostbite of** left **arm**

√5ᵗʰ **T33.5   Superficial frostbite of** wrist, hand, and fingers
  √6ᵗʰ **T33.51   Superficial frostbite of** wrist
    √7ᵗʰ **T33.511   Superficial frostbite of** right **wrist**
    √7ᵗʰ **T33.512   Superficial frostbite of** left **wrist**
    √7ᵗʰ **T33.519   Superficial frostbite of unspecified wrist**
  √6ᵗʰ **T33.52   Superficial frostbite of** hand
    EXCLUDES 2   *superficial frostbite of fingers (T33.53-)*
    √7ᵗʰ **T33.521   Superficial frostbite of** right **hand**
    √7ᵗʰ **T33.522   Superficial frostbite of** left **hand**
    √7ᵗʰ **T33.529   Superficial frostbite of unspecified hand**
  √6ᵗʰ **T33.53   Superficial frostbite of** finger(s)
    √7ᵗʰ **T33.531   Superficial frostbite of** right **finger(s)**
    √7ᵗʰ **T33.532   Superficial frostbite of** left **finger(s)**
    √7ᵗʰ **T33.539   Superficial frostbite of unspecified finger(s)**

√5ᵗʰ **T33.6   Superficial frostbite of** hip and thigh
  √x7ᵗʰ **T33.60   Superficial frostbite of unspecified hip and thigh**
  √x7ᵗʰ **T33.61   Superficial frostbite of** right **hip and thigh**
  √x7ᵗʰ **T33.62   Superficial frostbite of** left **hip and thigh**

√5ᵗʰ **T33.7   Superficial frostbite of** knee and lower leg
  EXCLUDES 2   *superficial frostbite of ankle and foot (T33.8-)*
  √x7ᵗʰ **T33.70   Superficial frostbite of unspecified knee and lower leg**
  √x7ᵗʰ **T33.71   Superficial frostbite of** right **knee and lower leg**
  √x7ᵗʰ **T33.72   Superficial frostbite of** left **knee and lower leg**

√5ᵗʰ **T33.8   Superficial frostbite of** ankle, foot, and toe(s)
  √6ᵗʰ **T33.81   Superficial frostbite of** ankle
    √7ᵗʰ **T33.811   Superficial frostbite of** right **ankle**
    √7ᵗʰ **T33.812   Superficial frostbite of** left **ankle**
    √7ᵗʰ **T33.819   Superficial frostbite of unspecified ankle**
  √6ᵗʰ **T33.82   Superficial frostbite of** foot
    √7ᵗʰ **T33.821   Superficial frostbite of** right **foot**
    √7ᵗʰ **T33.822   Superficial frostbite of** left **foot**
    √7ᵗʰ **T33.829   Superficial frostbite of unspecified foot**
  √6ᵗʰ **T33.83   Superficial frostbite of** toe(s)
    √7ᵗʰ **T33.831   Superficial frostbite of** right **toe(s)**
    √7ᵗʰ **T33.832   Superficial frostbite of** left **toe(s)**
    √7ᵗʰ **T33.839   Superficial frostbite of unspecified toe(s)**

√5ᵗʰ **T33.9   Superficial frostbite of other and unspecified sites**
  √x7ᵗʰ **T33.90   Superficial frostbite of unspecified sites**
    Superficial frostbite NOS

√x7ᵗʰ **T33.99   Superficial frostbite of other sites**
  Superficial frostbite of leg NOS
  Superficial frostbite of trunk NOS

√4ᵗʰ **T34   Frostbite with tissue necrosis**

The appropriate 7th character is to be added to each code from category T34.
A   initial encounter
D   subsequent encounter
S   sequela

√5ᵗʰ **T34.0   Frostbite with tissue necrosis of** head
  √6ᵗʰ **T34.01   Frostbite with tissue necrosis of** ear
    √7ᵗʰ **T34.011   Frostbite with tissue necrosis of** right **ear**   COM
    √7ᵗʰ **T34.012   Frostbite with tissue necrosis of** left **ear**   COM
    √7ᵗʰ **T34.019   Frostbite with tissue necrosis of unspecified ear**   COM
  √x7ᵗʰ **T34.02   Frostbite with tissue necrosis of** nose   COM
  √x7ᵗʰ **T34.09   Frostbite with tissue necrosis of other part of head**   COM

√x7ᵗʰ **T34.1   Frostbite with tissue necrosis of** neck   COM
√x7ᵗʰ **T34.2   Frostbite with tissue necrosis of** thorax   COM
√x7ᵗʰ **T34.3   Frostbite with tissue necrosis of** abdominal wall, lower back and pelvis   COM

√5ᵗʰ **T34.4   Frostbite with tissue necrosis of** arm
  EXCLUDES 2   *frostbite with tissue necrosis of wrist and hand (T34.5-)*
  √x7ᵗʰ **T34.40   Frostbite with tissue necrosis of unspecified arm**   COM
  √x7ᵗʰ **T34.41   Frostbite with tissue necrosis of** right **arm**   COM
  √x7ᵗʰ **T34.42   Frostbite with tissue necrosis of** left **arm**   COM

√5ᵗʰ **T34.5   Frostbite with tissue necrosis of** wrist, hand, and finger(s)
  √6ᵗʰ **T34.51   Frostbite with tissue necrosis of** wrist
    √7ᵗʰ **T34.511   Frostbite with tissue necrosis of** right **wrist**   COM
    √7ᵗʰ **T34.512   Frostbite with tissue necrosis of** left **wrist**   COM
    √7ᵗʰ **T34.519   Frostbite with tissue necrosis of unspecified wrist**   COM
  √6ᵗʰ **T34.52   Frostbite with tissue necrosis of** hand
    EXCLUDES 2   *frostbite with tissue necrosis of finger(s) (T34.53-)*
    √7ᵗʰ **T34.521   Frostbite with tissue necrosis of** right **hand**   COM
    √7ᵗʰ **T34.522   Frostbite with tissue necrosis of** left **hand**   COM
    √7ᵗʰ **T34.529   Frostbite with tissue necrosis of unspecified hand**   COM
  √6ᵗʰ **T34.53   Frostbite with tissue necrosis of** finger(s)
    √7ᵗʰ **T34.531   Frostbite with tissue necrosis of** right **finger(s)**   COM
    √7ᵗʰ **T34.532   Frostbite with tissue necrosis of** left **finger(s)**   COM
    √7ᵗʰ **T34.539   Frostbite with tissue necrosis of unspecified finger(s)**   COM

√5ᵗʰ **T34.6   Frostbite with tissue necrosis of** hip and thigh
  √x7ᵗʰ **T34.60   Frostbite with tissue necrosis of unspecified hip and thigh**
  √x7ᵗʰ **T34.61   Frostbite with tissue necrosis of** right **hip and thigh**
  √x7ᵗʰ **T34.62   Frostbite with tissue necrosis of** left **hip and thigh**   COM

√5ᵗʰ **T34.7   Frostbite with tissue necrosis of** knee and lower leg
  EXCLUDES 2   *frostbite with tissue necrosis of ankle and foot (T34.8-)*
  √x7ᵗʰ **T34.70   Frostbite with tissue necrosis of unspecified knee and lower leg**
  √x7ᵗʰ **T34.71   Frostbite with tissue necrosis of** right **knee and lower leg**   COM
  √x7ᵗʰ **T34.72   Frostbite with tissue necrosis of** left **knee and lower leg**   COM

√5ᵗʰ **T34.8   Frostbite with tissue necrosis of** ankle, foot, and toe(s)
  √6ᵗʰ **T34.81   Frostbite with tissue necrosis of** ankle
    √7ᵗʰ **T34.811   Frostbite with tissue necrosis of** right **ankle**   COM

✔ Additional Character Required   √x7ᵗʰ Placeholder Alert   Manifestation   Unspecified Dx   Q QPP   UPD Unacceptable PDx

√7ᵗʰ **T34.812** Frostbite with tissue necrosis of left ankle COM

√7ᵗʰ **T34.819** Frostbite with tissue necrosis of unspecified ankle COM

√6ᵗʰ **T34.82** Frostbite with tissue necrosis of foot

√7ᵗʰ **T34.821** Frostbite with tissue necrosis of right foot

√7ᵗʰ **T34.822** Frostbite with tissue necrosis of left foot

√7ᵗʰ **T34.829** Frostbite with tissue necrosis of unspecified foot

√6ᵗʰ **T34.83** Frostbite with tissue necrosis of toe(s)

√7ᵗʰ **T34.831** Frostbite with tissue necrosis of right toe(s)

√7ᵗʰ **T34.832** Frostbite with tissue necrosis of left toe(s)

√7ᵗʰ **T34.839** Frostbite with tissue necrosis of unspecified toe(s)

√5ᵗʰ **T34.9** Frostbite with tissue necrosis of other and unspecified sites

√x7ᵗʰ **T34.90** Frostbite with tissue necrosis of unspecified sites

Frostbite with tissue necrosis NOS

√x7ᵗʰ **T34.99** Frostbite with tissue necrosis of other sites

Frostbite with tissue necrosis of leg NOS
Frostbite with tissue necrosis of trunk NOS

Poisoning by, adverse effects of and underdosing of drugs, medicaments and biological substances (T36-T50)

INCLUDES adverse effect of correct substance properly administered
poisoning by overdose of substance
poisoning by wrong substance given or taken in error
underdosing by (inadvertently) (deliberately) taking less substance than prescribed or instructed

Code first, for adverse effects, the nature of the adverse effect, such as:
adverse effect NOS (T88.7)
aspirin gastritis (K29.-)
blood disorders (D56-D76)
contact dermatitis (L23-L25)
dermatitis due to substances taken internally (L27.-)
nephropathy (N14.Ø-N14.2)

taken error
wrong route.

NOTE The drug giving rise to the adverse effect should be identified by use of codes from categories T36-T50 with fifth or sixth character 5.

Use additional code(s) to specify:
manifestations of poisoning
underdosing or failure in dosage during medical and surgical care (Y63.6, Y63.8-Y63.9)
underdosing of medication regimen (Z91.12-, Z91.13-)

EXCLUDES 1 toxic reaction to local anesthesia in pregnancy (O29.3-)

EXCLUDES 2 abuse and dependence of psychoactive substances (F1Ø-F19)
abuse of non-dependence-producing substances (F55.-)
drug reaction and poisoning affecting newborn (PØØ-P96)
immunodeficiency due to drugs (D84.821)
pathological drug intoxication (inebriation) (F1Ø-F19)

AHA: 2018,4Q,71; 2016,2Q,8; 2015,3Q,22

√4ᵗʰ **T36** Poisoning by, adverse effect of and underdosing of systemic antibiotics

EXCLUDES 1 antineoplastic antibiotics (T45.1-)
locally applied antibiotic NEC (T49.Ø)
topically used antibiotic for ear, nose and throat (T49.6)
topically used antibiotic for eye (T49.5)

poisoning

The appropriate 7th character is to be added to each code from category T36.
A initial encounter
D subsequent encounter
S sequela

√5ᵗʰ **T36.Ø** Poisoning by, adverse effect of and underdosing of penicillins

√6ᵗʰ **T36.ØX** Poisoning by, adverse effect of and underdosing of penicillins

√7ᵗʰ **T36.ØX1** Poisoning by penicillins, accidental (unintentional)

Poisoning by penicillins NOS

² √7ᵗʰ **T36.ØX2** Poisoning by penicillins, intentional self-harm HCC Rx ESR COM

√7ᵗʰ **T36.ØX3** Poisoning by penicillins, assault

√7ᵗʰ **T36.ØX4** Poisoning by penicillins, undetermined

√7ᵗʰ **T36.ØX5** Adverse effect of penicillins UPD

√7ᵗʰ **T36.ØX6** Underdosing of penicillins UPD

√5ᵗʰ **T36.1** Poisoning by, adverse effect of and underdosing of cephalosporins and other beta-lactam antibiotics

√6ᵗʰ **T36.1X** Poisoning by, adverse effect of and underdosing of cephalosporins and other beta-lactam antibiotics

√7ᵗʰ **T36.1X1** Poisoning by cephalosporins and other beta-lactam antibiotics, accidental (unintentional)

Poisoning by cephalosporins and other beta-lactam antibiotics NOS

² √7ᵗʰ **T36.1X2** Poisoning by cephalosporins and other beta-lactam antibiotics, intentional self-harm HCC Rx ESR COM

√7ᵗʰ **T36.1X3** Poisoning by cephalosporins and other beta-lactam antibiotics, assault

√7ᵗʰ **T36.1X4** Poisoning by cephalosporins and other beta-lactam antibiotics, undetermined

√7ᵗʰ **T36.1X5** Adverse effect of cephalosporins and other beta-lactam antibiotics UPD

√7ᵗʰ **T36.1X6** Underdosing of cephalosporins and other beta-lactam antibiotics UPD

√5ᵗʰ **T36.2** Poisoning by, adverse effect of and underdosing of chloramphenicol group

√6ᵗʰ **T36.2X** Poisoning by, adverse effect of and underdosing of chloramphenicol group

√7ᵗʰ **T36.2X1** Poisoning by chloramphenicol group, accidental (unintentional)

Poisoning by chloramphenicol group NOS

² √7ᵗʰ **T36.2X2** Poisoning by chloramphenicol group, intentional self-harm HCC Rx ESR COM

√7ᵗʰ **T36.2X3** Poisoning by chloramphenicol group, assault

√7ᵗʰ **T36.2X4** Poisoning by chloramphenicol group, undetermined

√7ᵗʰ **T36.2X5** Adverse effect of chloramphenicol group UPD

√7ᵗʰ **T36.2X6** Underdosing of chloramphenicol group UPD

√5ᵗʰ **T36.3** Poisoning by, adverse effect of and underdosing of macrolides

√6ᵗʰ **T36.3X** Poisoning by, adverse effect of and underdosing of macrolides

√7ᵗʰ **T36.3X1** Poisoning by macrolides, accidental (unintentional)

Poisoning by macrolides NOS

² √7ᵗʰ **T36.3X2** Poisoning by macrolides, intentional self-harm HCC Rx ESR COM

√7ᵗʰ **T36.3X3** Poisoning by macrolides, assault

√7ᵗʰ **T36.3X4** Poisoning by macrolides, undetermined

√7ᵗʰ **T36.3X5** Adverse effect of macrolides UPD

√7ᵗʰ **T36.3X6** Underdosing of macrolides UPD

√5ᵗʰ **T36.4** Poisoning by, adverse effect of and underdosing of tetracyclines

√6ᵗʰ **T36.4X** Poisoning by, adverse effect of and underdosing of tetracyclines

√7ᵗʰ **T36.4X1** Poisoning by tetracyclines, accidental (unintentional)

Poisoning by tetracyclines NOS

² √7ᵗʰ **T36.4X2** Poisoning by tetracyclines, intentional self-harm HCC Rx ESR COM

√7ᵗʰ **T36.4X3** Poisoning by tetracyclines, assault

√7ᵗʰ **T36.4X4** Poisoning by tetracyclines, undetermined

√7ᵗʰ **T36.4X5** Adverse effect of tetracyclines UPD

√7ᵗʰ **T36.4X6** Underdosing of tetracyclines UPD

√5ᵗʰ **T36.5** Poisoning by, adverse effect of and underdosing of aminoglycosides

Poisoning by, adverse effect of and underdosing of streptomycin

√6ᵗʰ **T36.5X** Poisoning by, adverse effect of and underdosing of aminoglycosides

√7ᵗʰ **T36.5X1** Poisoning by aminoglycosides, accidental (unintentional)

Poisoning by aminoglycosides NOS

² √7ᵗʰ **T36.5X2** Poisoning by aminoglycosides, intentional self-harm HCC Rx ESR COM

√7ᵗʰ **T36.5X3** Poisoning by aminoglycosides, assault

√7ᵗʰ **T36.5X4** Poisoning by aminoglycosides, undetermined

√7ᵗʰ **T36.5X5** Adverse effect of aminoglycosides UPD

√7ᵗʰ **T36.5X6** Underdosing of aminoglycosides UPD

✓5ᵗʰ **T36.6 Poisoning by, adverse effect of and underdosing of rifampicin**

  ✓6ᵗʰ **T36.6X Poisoning by, adverse effect of and underdosing of rifampicins**

    ✓7ᵗʰ **T36.6X1 Poisoning by rifampicins, accidental (unintentional)**
         Poisoning by rifampicins NOS

    ² ✓7ᵗʰ **T36.6X2 Poisoning by rifampicins, intentional self-harm** `HCC` `Rx` `ESR` `COM`

    ✓7ᵗʰ **T36.6X3 Poisoning by rifampicins, assault**

    ✓7ᵗʰ **T36.6X4 Poisoning by rifampicins, undetermined**

    ✓7ᵗʰ **T36.6X5 Adverse effect of rifampicins** `UPD`

    ✓7ᵗʰ **T36.6X6 Underdosing of rifampicins** `UPD`

✓5ᵗʰ **T36.7 Poisoning by, adverse effect of and underdosing of antifungal antibiotics, systemically used**

  ✓6ᵗʰ **T36.7X Poisoning by, adverse effect of and underdosing of antifungal antibiotics, systemically used**

    ✓7ᵗʰ **T36.7X1 Poisoning by antifungal antibiotics, systemically used, accidental (unintentional)**
         Poisoning by antifungal antibiotics, systemically used NOS

    ² ✓7ᵗʰ **T36.7X2 Poisoning by antifungal antibiotics, systemically used, intentional self-harm** `HCC` `Rx` `ESR` `COM`

    ✓7ᵗʰ **T36.7X3 Poisoning by antifungal antibiotics, systemically used, assault**

    ✓7ᵗʰ **T36.7X4 Poisoning by antifungal antibiotics, systemically used, undetermined**

    ✓7ᵗʰ **T36.7X5 Adverse effect of antifungal antibiotics, systemically used** `UPD`

    ✓7ᵗʰ **T36.7X6 Underdosing of antifungal antibiotics, systemically used** `UPD`

✓5ᵗʰ **T36.8 Poisoning by, adverse effect of and underdosing of other systemic antibiotics**

  ✓6ᵗʰ **T36.8X Poisoning by, adverse effect of and underdosing of other systemic antibiotics**
     AHA: 2017,1Q,39

    ✓7ᵗʰ **T36.8X1 Poisoning by other systemic antibiotics, accidental (unintentional)**
         Poisoning by other systemic antibiotics NOS

    ² ✓7ᵗʰ **T36.8X2 Poisoning by other systemic antibiotics, intentional self-harm** `HCC` `Rx` `ESR` `COM`

    ✓7ᵗʰ **T36.8X3 Poisoning by other systemic antibiotics, assault**

    ✓7ᵗʰ **T36.8X4 Poisoning by other systemic antibiotics, undetermined**

    ✓7ᵗʰ **T36.8X5 Adverse effect of other systemic antibiotics** `UPD`

    ✓7ᵗʰ **T36.8X6 Underdosing of other systemic antibiotics** `UPD`

✓5ᵗʰ **T36.9 Poisoning by, adverse effect of and underdosing of unspecified systemic antibiotic**

  ✓×7ᵗʰ **T36.91 Poisoning by unspecified systemic antibiotic, accidental (unintentional)**
     Poisoning by systemic antibiotic NOS

  ² ✓×7ᵗʰ **T36.92 Poisoning by unspecified systemic antibiotic, intentional self-harm** `HCC` `Rx` `ESR` `COM`

  ✓×7ᵗʰ **T36.93 Poisoning by unspecified systemic antibiotic, assault**

  ✓×7ᵗʰ **T36.94 Poisoning by unspecified systemic antibiotic, undetermined**

  ✓×7ᵗʰ **T36.95 Adverse effect of unspecified systemic antibiotic** `UPD`

  ✓×7ᵗʰ **T36.96 Underdosing of unspecified systemic antibiotic** `UPD`

✓4ᵗʰ **T37 Poisoning by, adverse effect of and underdosing of other systemic anti-infectives and antiparasitics**

   EXCLUDES 1   *anti-infectives topically used for ear, nose and throat (T49.6-)*
         anti-infectives topically used for eye (T49.5-)
         locally applied anti-infectives NEC (T49.0-)

> The appropriate 7th character is to be added to each code from category T37.
> A   initial encounter
> D   subsequent encounter
> S   sequela

✓5ᵗʰ **T37.0 Poisoning by, adverse effect of and underdosing of sulfonamides**

  ✓6ᵗʰ **T37.0X Poisoning by, adverse effect of and underdosing of sulfonamides**

    ✓7ᵗʰ **T37.0X1 Poisoning by sulfonamides, accidental (unintentional)**
         Poisoning by sulfonamides NOS

    ² ✓7ᵗʰ **T37.0X2 Poisoning by sulfonamides, intentional self-harm** `HCC` `Rx` `ESR` `COM`

    ✓7ᵗʰ **T37.0X3 Poisoning by sulfonamides, assault**

    ✓7ᵗʰ **T37.0X4 Poisoning by sulfonamides, undetermined**

    ✓7ᵗʰ **T37.0X5 Adverse effect of sulfonamides** `UPD`

    ✓7ᵗʰ **T37.0X6 Underdosing of sulfonamides** `UPD`

✓5ᵗʰ **T37.1 Poisoning by, adverse effect of and underdosing of antimycobacterial drugs**

   EXCLUDES 1   *rifampicins (T36.6-)*
         streptomycin (T36.5-)

  ✓6ᵗʰ **T37.1X Poisoning by, adverse effect of and underdosing of antimycobacterial drugs**

    ✓7ᵗʰ **T37.1X1 Poisoning by antimycobacterial drugs, accidental (unintentional)**
         Poisoning by antimycobacterial drugs NOS

    ² ✓7ᵗʰ **T37.1X2 Poisoning by antimycobacterial drugs, intentional self-harm** `HCC` `Rx` `ESR` `COM`

    ✓7ᵗʰ **T37.1X3 Poisoning by antimycobacterial drugs, assault**

    ✓7ᵗʰ **T37.1X4 Poisoning by antimycobacterial drugs, undetermined**

    ✓7ᵗʰ **T37.1X5 Adverse effect of antimycobacterial drugs** `UPD`

    ✓7ᵗʰ **T37.1X6 Underdosing of antimycobacterial drugs** `UPD`

✓5ᵗʰ **T37.2 Poisoning by, adverse effect of and underdosing of antimalarials and drugs acting on other blood protozoa**

   EXCLUDES 1   *hydroxyquinoline derivatives (T37.8-)*

  ✓6ᵗʰ **T37.2X Poisoning by, adverse effect of and underdosing of antimalarials and drugs acting on other blood protozoa**

    ✓7ᵗʰ **T37.2X1 Poisoning by antimalarials and drugs acting on other blood protozoa, accidental (unintentional)**
         Poisoning by antimalarials and drugs acting on other blood protozoa NOS

    ² ✓7ᵗʰ **T37.2X2 Poisoning by antimalarials and drugs acting on other blood protozoa, intentional self-harm** `HCC` `Rx` `ESR` `COM`

    ✓7ᵗʰ **T37.2X3 Poisoning by antimalarials and drugs acting on other blood protozoa, assault**

    ✓7ᵗʰ **T37.2X4 Poisoning by antimalarials and drugs acting on other blood protozoa, undetermined**

    ✓7ᵗʰ **T37.2X5 Adverse effect of antimalarials and drugs acting on other blood protozoa** `UPD`

    ✓7ᵗʰ **T37.2X6 Underdosing of antimalarials and drugs acting on other blood protozoa** `UPD`

✓5ᵗʰ **T37.3 Poisoning by, adverse effect of and underdosing of other antiprotozoal drugs**

  ✓6ᵗʰ **T37.3X Poisoning by, adverse effect of and underdosing of other antiprotozoal drugs**

    ✓7ᵗʰ **T37.3X1 Poisoning by other antiprotozoal drugs, accidental (unintentional)**
         Poisoning by other antiprotozoal drugs NOS

    ² ✓7ᵗʰ **T37.3X2 Poisoning by other antiprotozoal drugs, intentional self-harm** `HCC` `Rx` `ESR` `COM`

    ✓7ᵗʰ **T37.3X3 Poisoning by other antiprotozoal drugs, assault**

    ✓7ᵗʰ **T37.3X4 Poisoning by other antiprotozoal drugs, undetermined**

√7ᵗʰ **T37.3X5** Adverse effect of other antiprotozoal drugs UPD

√7ᵗʰ **T37.3X6** Underdosing of other antiprotozoal drugs UPD

√5ᵗʰ **T37.4** Poisoning by, adverse effect of and underdosing of anthelminthics

√6ᵗʰ **T37.4X** Poisoning by, adverse effect of and underdosing of anthelminthics

√7ᵗʰ **T37.4X1** **Poisoning by anthelminthics,** accidental **(unintentional)**
Poisoning by anthelminthics NOS

² √7ᵗʰ **T37.4X2** **Poisoning by anthelminthics,** intentional **self-harm** HCC Rx ESR COM

√7ᵗʰ **T37.4X3** **Poisoning by anthelminthics,** assault

√7ᵗʰ **T37.4X4** **Poisoning by anthelminthics, undetermined**

√7ᵗʰ **T37.4X5** Adverse effect of anthelminthics UPD

√7ᵗʰ **T37.4X6** Underdosing of anthelminthics UPD

√5ᵗʰ **T37.5** Poisoning by, adverse effect of and underdosing of antiviral drugs

EXCLUDES 1 amantadine (T42.8-)
cytarabine (T45.1-)

√6ᵗʰ **T37.5X** Poisoning by, adverse effect of and underdosing of antiviral drugs

√7ᵗʰ **T37.5X1** **Poisoning by antiviral drugs,** accidental **(unintentional)**
Poisoning by antiviral drugs NOS

² √7ᵗʰ **T37.5X2** **Poisoning by antiviral drugs,** intentional **self-harm** HCC Rx ESR COM

√7ᵗʰ **T37.5X3** **Poisoning by antiviral drugs,** assault

√7ᵗʰ **T37.5X4** **Poisoning by antiviral drugs, undetermined**

√7ᵗʰ **T37.5X5** Adverse effect of antiviral drugs UPD

√7ᵗʰ **T37.5X6** Underdosing of antiviral drugs UPD

√5ᵗʰ **T37.8** Poisoning by, adverse effect of and underdosing of other specified systemic anti-infectives and antiparasitics
Poisoning by, adverse effect of and underdosing of hydroxyquinoline derivatives
EXCLUDES 1 antimalarial drugs (T37.2-)

√6ᵗʰ **T37.8X** Poisoning by, adverse effect of and underdosing of other specified systemic anti-infectives and antiparasitics

√7ᵗʰ **T37.8X1** **Poisoning by other specified systemic anti-infectives and antiparasitics,** accidental **(unintentional)**
Poisoning by other specified systemic anti-infectives and antiparasitics NOS

² √7ᵗʰ **T37.8X2** **Poisoning by other specified systemic anti-infectives and antiparasitics, intentional self-harm** HCC Rx ESR COM

√7ᵗʰ **T37.8X3** **Poisoning by other specified systemic anti-infectives and antiparasitics,** assault

√7ᵗʰ **T37.8X4** **Poisoning by other specified systemic anti-infectives and antiparasitics, undetermined**

√7ᵗʰ **T37.8X5** Adverse effect of other specified systemic anti-infectives and antiparasitics UPD

√7ᵗʰ **T37.8X6** Underdosing of other specified systemic anti-infectives and antiparasitics UPD

√5ᵗʰ **T37.9** Poisoning by, adverse effect of and underdosing of unspecified systemic anti-infective and antiparasitics

√x7ᵗʰ **T37.91** **Poisoning by unspecified systemic anti-infective and antiparasitics,** accidental **(unintentional)**
Poisoning by, adverse effect of and underdosing of systemic anti-infective and antiparasitics NOS

² √x7ᵗʰ **T37.92** **Poisoning by unspecified systemic anti-infective and antiparasitics,** intentional **self-harm** HCC Rx ESR COM

√x7ᵗʰ **T37.93** **Poisoning by unspecified systemic anti-infective and antiparasitics,** assault

√x7ᵗʰ **T37.94** **Poisoning by unspecified systemic anti-infective and antiparasitics, undetermined**

√x7ᵗʰ **T37.95** Adverse effect of unspecified systemic anti-infective and antiparasitic UPD

√x7ᵗʰ **T37.96** Underdosing of unspecified systemic anti-infectives and antiparasitics UPD

√4ᵗʰ **T38** **Poisoning by, adverse effect of and underdosing of hormones and their synthetic substitutes and antagonists, not elsewhere classified**

EXCLUDES 1 mineralocorticoids and their antagonists (T50.0-)
oxytocic hormones (T48.0-)
parathyroid hormones and derivatives (T50.9-)

The appropriate 7th character is to be added to each code from category T38.
A initial encounter
D subsequent encounter
S sequela

√5ᵗʰ **T38.0** Poisoning by, adverse effect of and underdosing of glucocorticoids and synthetic analogues
EXCLUDES 1 glucocorticoids, topically used (T49.-)

√6ᵗʰ **T38.0X** Poisoning by, adverse effect of and underdosing of glucocorticoids and synthetic analogues

√7ᵗʰ **T38.0X1** **Poisoning by glucocorticoids and synthetic analogues,** accidental **(unintentional)**
Poisoning by glucocorticoids and synthetic analogues NOS

² √7ᵗʰ **T38.0X2** **Poisoning by glucocorticoids and synthetic analogues,** intentional **self-harm** HCC Rx ESR COM

√7ᵗʰ **T38.0X3** **Poisoning by glucocorticoids and synthetic analogues,** assault

√7ᵗʰ **T38.0X4** **Poisoning by glucocorticoids and synthetic analogues,** undetermined

√7ᵗʰ **T38.0X5** Adverse effect of glucocorticoids and synthetic analogues UPD

√7ᵗʰ **T38.0X6** Underdosing of glucocorticoids and synthetic analogues UPD

√5ᵗʰ **T38.1** Poisoning by, adverse effect of and underdosing of thyroid hormones and substitutes

√6ᵗʰ **T38.1X** Poisoning by, adverse effect of and underdosing of thyroid hormones and substitutes

√7ᵗʰ **T38.1X1** **Poisoning by thyroid hormones and substitutes,** accidental **(unintentional)**
Poisoning by thyroid hormones and substitutes NOS

² √7ᵗʰ **T38.1X2** **Poisoning by thyroid hormones and substitutes,** intentional **self-harm** HCC Rx ESR COM

√7ᵗʰ **T38.1X3** **Poisoning by thyroid hormones and substitutes,** assault

√7ᵗʰ **T38.1X4** **Poisoning by thyroid hormones and substitutes, undetermined**

√7ᵗʰ **T38.1X5** Adverse effect of thyroid hormones and substitutes UPD

√7ᵗʰ **T38.1X6** Underdosing of thyroid hormones and substitutes UPD

√5ᵗʰ **T38.2** Poisoning by, adverse effect of and underdosing of antithyroid drugs

√6ᵗʰ **T38.2X** Poisoning by, adverse effect of and underdosing of antithyroid drugs

√7ᵗʰ **T38.2X1** **Poisoning by antithyroid drugs,** accidental **(unintentional)**
Poisoning by antithyroid drugs NOS

² √7ᵗʰ **T38.2X2** **Poisoning by antithyroid drugs,** intentional self-harm HCC Rx ESR COM

√7ᵗʰ **T38.2X3** **Poisoning by antithyroid drugs,** assault

√7ᵗʰ **T38.2X4** **Poisoning by antithyroid drugs, undetermined**

√7ᵗʰ **T38.2X5** Adverse effect of antithyroid drugs UPD

√7ᵗʰ **T38.2X6** Underdosing of antithyroid drugs UPD

√5ᵗʰ **T38.3** Poisoning by, adverse effect of and underdosing of insulin and oral hypoglycemic [antidiabetic] drugs

√6ᵗʰ **T38.3X** Poisoning by, adverse effect of and underdosing of insulin and oral hypoglycemic [antidiabetic] drugs

√7ᵗʰ **T38.3X1** **Poisoning by insulin and oral hypoglycemic [antidiabetic] drugs,** accidental **(unintentional)**
Poisoning by insulin and oral hypoglycemic [antidiabetic] drugs NOS

² √7ᵗʰ **T38.3X2** **Poisoning by insulin and oral hypoglycemic [antidiabetic] drugs,** intentional self-harm HCC Rx ESR COM

manifestation first (handwritten note)

✓7ᵗʰ **T38.3X3** Poisoning by insulin and oral hypoglycemic [antidiabetic] drugs, **assault**

✓7ᵗʰ **T38.3X4** Poisoning by insulin and oral hypoglycemic [antidiabetic] drugs, undetermined

✓7ᵗʰ **T38.3X5** Adverse effect of insulin and oral hypoglycemic [antidiabetic] drugs **UPD**

✓7ᵗʰ **T38.3X6** Underdosing of insulin and oral hypoglycemic [antidiabetic] drugs **UPD**

✓5ᵗʰ **T38.4** Poisoning by, adverse effect of and underdosing of oral contraceptives
Poisoning by, adverse effect of and underdosing of multiple- and single-ingredient oral contraceptive preparations

✓6ᵗʰ **T38.4X** Poisoning by, adverse effect of and underdosing of oral contraceptives

  ✓7ᵗʰ **T38.4X1** Poisoning by oral contraceptives, accidental (unintentional)
Poisoning by oral contraceptives NOS

  ² ✓7ᵗʰ **T38.4X2** Poisoning by oral contraceptives, intentional self-harm **HCC Rx ESR COM**

  ✓7ᵗʰ **T38.4X3** Poisoning by oral contraceptives, assault

  ✓7ᵗʰ **T38.4X4** Poisoning by oral contraceptives, undetermined

  ✓7ᵗʰ **T38.4X5** Adverse effect of oral contraceptives **UPD**

  ✓7ᵗʰ **T38.4X6** Underdosing of oral contraceptives **UPD**

✓5ᵗʰ **T38.5** Poisoning by, adverse effect of and underdosing of other estrogens and progestogens
Poisoning by, adverse effect of and underdosing of estrogens and progestogens mixtures and substitutes

✓6ᵗʰ **T38.5X** Poisoning by, adverse effect of and underdosing of other estrogens and progestogens

  ✓7ᵗʰ **T38.5X1** Poisoning by other estrogens and progestogens, accidental (unintentional)
Poisoning by other estrogens and progestogens NOS

  ² ✓7ᵗʰ **T38.5X2** Poisoning by other estrogens and progestogens, intentional self-harm **HCC Rx ESR COM**

  ✓7ᵗʰ **T38.5X3** Poisoning by other estrogens and progestogens, assault

  ✓7ᵗʰ **T38.5X4** Poisoning by other estrogens and progestogens, undetermined

  ✓7ᵗʰ **T38.5X5** Adverse effect of other estrogens and progestogens **UPD**

  ✓7ᵗʰ **T38.5X6** Underdosing of other estrogens and progestogens **UPD**

✓5ᵗʰ **T38.6** Poisoning by, adverse effect of and underdosing of antigonadotrophins, antiestrogens, antiandrogens, not elsewhere classified
Poisoning by, adverse effect of and underdosing of tamoxifen

✓6ᵗʰ **T38.6X** Poisoning by, adverse effect of and underdosing of antigonadotrophins, antiestrogens, antiandrogens, not elsewhere classified

  ✓7ᵗʰ **T38.6X1** Poisoning by antigonadotrophins, antiestrogens, antiandrogens, not elsewhere classified, accidental (unintentional)
Poisoning by antigonadotrophins, antiestrogens, antiandrogens, not elsewhere classified NOS

  ² ✓7ᵗʰ **T38.6X2** Poisoning by antigonadotrophins, antiestrogens, antiandrogens, not elsewhere classified, intentional self-harm **HCC Rx ESR COM**

  ✓7ᵗʰ **T38.6X3** Poisoning by antigonadotrophins, antiestrogens, antiandrogens, not elsewhere classified, assault

  ✓7ᵗʰ **T38.6X4** Poisoning by antigonadotrophins, antiestrogens, antiandrogens, not elsewhere classified, undetermined

  ✓7ᵗʰ **T38.6X5** Adverse effect of antigonadotrophins, antiestrogens, antiandrogens, not elsewhere classified **UPD**

  ✓7ᵗʰ **T38.6X6** Underdosing of antigonadotrophins, antiestrogens, antiandrogens, not elsewhere classified **UPD**

✓5ᵗʰ **T38.7** Poisoning by, adverse effect of and underdosing of androgens and anabolic congeners

✓6ᵗʰ **T38.7X** Poisoning by, adverse effect of and underdosing of androgens and anabolic congeners

  ✓7ᵗʰ **T38.7X1** Poisoning by androgens and anabolic congeners, accidental (unintentional)
Poisoning by androgens and anabolic congeners NOS

  ² ✓7ᵗʰ **T38.7X2** Poisoning by androgens and anabolic congeners, intentional self-harm **HCC Rx ESR COM**

  ✓7ᵗʰ **T38.7X3** Poisoning by androgens and anabolic congeners, assault

  ✓7ᵗʰ **T38.7X4** Poisoning by androgens and anabolic congeners, undetermined

  ✓7ᵗʰ **T38.7X5** Adverse effect of androgens and anabolic congeners **UPD**

  ✓7ᵗʰ **T38.7X6** Underdosing of androgens and anabolic congeners **UPD**

✓5ᵗʰ **T38.8** Poisoning by, adverse effect of and underdosing of other and unspecified hormones and synthetic substitutes

✓6ᵗʰ **T38.80** Poisoning by, adverse effect of and underdosing of unspecified hormones and synthetic substitutes

  ✓7ᵗʰ **T38.801** Poisoning by unspecified hormones and synthetic substitutes, accidental (unintentional)
Poisoning by unspecified hormones and synthetic substitutes NOS

  ² ✓7ᵗʰ **T38.802** Poisoning by unspecified hormones and synthetic substitutes, intentional self-harm **HCC Rx ESR COM**

  ✓7ᵗʰ **T38.803** Poisoning by unspecified hormones and synthetic substitutes, assault

  ✓7ᵗʰ **T38.804** Poisoning by unspecified hormones and synthetic substitutes, undetermined

  ✓7ᵗʰ **T38.805** Adverse effect of unspecified hormones and synthetic substitutes **UPD**

  ✓7ᵗʰ **T38.806** Underdosing of unspecified hormones and synthetic substitutes **UPD**

✓6ᵗʰ **T38.81** Poisoning by, adverse effect of and underdosing of anterior pituitary [adenohypophyseal] hormones

  ✓7ᵗʰ **T38.811** Poisoning by anterior pituitary [adenohypophyseal] hormones, accidental (unintentional)
Poisoning by anterior pituitary [adenohypophyseal] hormones NOS

  ² ✓7ᵗʰ **T38.812** Poisoning by anterior pituitary [adenohypophyseal] hormones, intentional self-harm **HCC Rx ESR COM**

  ✓7ᵗʰ **T38.813** Poisoning by anterior pituitary [adenohypophyseal] hormones, assault

  ✓7ᵗʰ **T38.814** Poisoning by anterior pituitary [adenohypophyseal] hormones, undetermined

  ✓7ᵗʰ **T38.815** Adverse effect of anterior pituitary [adenohypophyseal] hormones **UPD**

  ✓7ᵗʰ **T38.816** Underdosing of anterior pituitary [adenohypophyseal] hormones **UPD**

✓6ᵗʰ **T38.89** Poisoning by, adverse effect of and underdosing of other hormones and synthetic substitutes

  ✓7ᵗʰ **T38.891** Poisoning by other hormones and synthetic substitutes, accidental (unintentional)
Poisoning by other hormones and synthetic substitutes NOS

  ² ✓7ᵗʰ **T38.892** Poisoning by other hormones and synthetic substitutes, intentional self-harm **HCC Rx ESR COM**

  ✓7ᵗʰ **T38.893** Poisoning by other hormones and synthetic substitutes, assault

  ✓7ᵗʰ **T38.894** Poisoning by other hormones and synthetic substitutes, undetermined

  ✓7ᵗʰ **T38.895** Adverse effect of other hormones and synthetic substitutes **UPD**

  ✓7ᵗʰ **T38.896** Underdosing of other hormones and synthetic substitutes **UPD**

✓5ᵗʰ **T38.9** **Poisoning by, adverse effect of and underdosing of other and unspecified hormone antagonists**

  ✓6ᵗʰ **T38.90** **Poisoning by, adverse effect of and underdosing of unspecified hormone antagonists**

    ✓7ᵗʰ **T38.901** **Poisoning by unspecified hormone antagonists, accidental (unintentional)**
      Poisoning by unspecified hormone antagonists NOS

    ² ✓7ᵗʰ **T38.902** **Poisoning by unspecified hormone antagonists, intentional self-harm** HCC Rx ESR COM

    ✓7ᵗʰ **T38.903** **Poisoning by unspecified hormone antagonists, assault**

    ✓7ᵗʰ **T38.904** **Poisoning by unspecified hormone antagonists, undetermined**

    ✓7ᵗʰ **T38.905** **Adverse effect of unspecified hormone antagonists** UPD

    ✓7ᵗʰ **T38.906** **Underdosing of unspecified hormone antagonists** UPD

  ✓6ᵗʰ **T38.99** **Poisoning by, adverse effect of and underdosing of other hormone antagonists**

    ✓7ᵗʰ **T38.991** **Poisoning by other hormone antagonists, accidental (unintentional)**
      Poisoning by other hormone antagonists NOS

    ² ✓7ᵗʰ **T38.992** **Poisoning by other hormone antagonists, intentional self-harm** HCC Rx ESR COM

    ✓7ᵗʰ **T38.993** **Poisoning by other hormone antagonists, assault**

    ✓7ᵗʰ **T38.994** **Poisoning by other hormone antagonists, undetermined**

    ✓7ᵗʰ **T38.995** **Adverse effect of other hormone antagonists** UPD

    ✓7ᵗʰ **T38.996** **Underdosing of other hormone antagonists** UPD

✓4ᵗʰ **T39** **Poisoning by, adverse effect of and underdosing of nonopioid analgesics, antipyretics and antirheumatics**

  The appropriate 7th character is to be added to each code from category T39.
  A initial encounter
  D subsequent encounter
  S sequela

✓5ᵗʰ **T39.0** **Poisoning by, adverse effect of and underdosing of salicylates**

  ✓6ᵗʰ **T39.01** **Poisoning by, adverse effect of and underdosing of aspirin**
    Poisoning by, adverse effect of and underdosing of acetylsalicylic acid

    ✓7ᵗʰ **T39.011** **Poisoning by aspirin, accidental (unintentional)**

    ² ✓7ᵗʰ **T39.012** **Poisoning by aspirin, intentional self-harm** HCC Rx ESR COM

    ✓7ᵗʰ **T39.013** **Poisoning by aspirin, assault**

    ✓7ᵗʰ **T39.014** **Poisoning by aspirin, undetermined**

    ✓7ᵗʰ **T39.015** **Adverse effect of aspirin** UPD
      AHA: 2016,1Q,15

    ✓7ᵗʰ **T39.016** **Underdosing of aspirin** UPD

  ✓6ᵗʰ **T39.09** **Poisoning by, adverse effect of and underdosing of other salicylates**

    ✓7ᵗʰ **T39.091** **Poisoning by salicylates, accidental (unintentional)**
      Poisoning by salicylates NOS

    ² ✓7ᵗʰ **T39.092** **Poisoning by salicylates, intentional self-harm** HCC Rx ESR COM

    ✓7ᵗʰ **T39.093** **Poisoning by salicylates, assault**

    ✓7ᵗʰ **T39.094** **Poisoning by salicylates, undetermined**

    ✓7ᵗʰ **T39.095** **Adverse effect of salicylates** UPD

    ✓7ᵗʰ **T39.096** **Underdosing of salicylates** UPD

✓5ᵗʰ **T39.1** **Poisoning by, adverse effect of and underdosing of 4-Aminophenol derivatives**

  ✓6ᵗʰ **T39.1X** **Poisoning by, adverse effect of and underdosing of 4-Aminophenol derivatives**

    ✓7ᵗʰ **T39.1X1** **Poisoning by 4-Aminophenol derivatives, accidental (unintentional)**
      Poisoning by 4-Aminophenol derivatives NOS

    ² ✓7ᵗʰ **T39.1X2** **Poisoning by 4-Aminophenol derivatives, intentional self-harm** HCC Rx ESR COM

    ✓7ᵗʰ **T39.1X3** **Poisoning by 4-Aminophenol derivatives, assault**

    ✓7ᵗʰ **T39.1X4** **Poisoning by 4-Aminophenol derivatives, undetermined**

    ✓7ᵗʰ **T39.1X5** **Adverse effect of 4-Aminophenol derivatives** UPD

    ✓7ᵗʰ **T39.1X6** **Underdosing of 4-Aminophenol derivatives** UPD

✓5ᵗʰ **T39.2** **Poisoning by, adverse effect of and underdosing of pyrazolone derivatives**

  ✓6ᵗʰ **T39.2X** **Poisoning by, adverse effect of and underdosing of pyrazolone derivatives**

    ✓7ᵗʰ **T39.2X1** **Poisoning by pyrazolone derivatives, accidental (unintentional)**
      Poisoning by pyrazolone derivatives NOS

    ² ✓7ᵗʰ **T39.2X2** **Poisoning by pyrazolone derivatives, intentional self-harm** HCC Rx ESR COM

    ✓7ᵗʰ **T39.2X3** **Poisoning by pyrazolone derivatives, assault**

    ✓7ᵗʰ **T39.2X4** **Poisoning by pyrazolone derivatives, undetermined**

    ✓7ᵗʰ **T39.2X5** **Adverse effect of pyrazolone derivatives** UPD

    ✓7ᵗʰ **T39.2X6** **Underdosing of pyrazolone derivatives** UPD

✓5ᵗʰ **T39.3** **Poisoning by, adverse effect of and underdosing of other nonsteroidal anti-inflammatory drugs [NSAID]**

  ✓6ᵗʰ **T39.31** **Poisoning by, adverse effect of and underdosing of propionic acid derivatives**
    Poisoning by, adverse effect of and underdosing of fenoprofen
    Poisoning by, adverse effect of and underdosing of flurbiprofen
    Poisoning by, adverse effect of and underdosing of ibuprofen
    Poisoning by, adverse effect of and underdosing of ketoprofen
    Poisoning by, adverse effect of and underdosing of naproxen
    Poisoning by, adverse effect of and underdosing of oxaprozin

    ✓7ᵗʰ **T39.311** **Poisoning by propionic acid derivatives, accidental (unintentional)**

    ² ✓7ᵗʰ **T39.312** **Poisoning by propionic acid derivatives, intentional self-harm** HCC Rx ESR COM

    ✓7ᵗʰ **T39.313** **Poisoning by propionic acid derivatives, assault**

    ✓7ᵗʰ **T39.314** **Poisoning by propionic acid derivatives, undetermined**

    ✓7ᵗʰ **T39.315** **Adverse effect of propionic acid derivatives** UPD

    ✓7ᵗʰ **T39.316** **Underdosing of propionic acid derivatives** UPD

  ✓6ᵗʰ **T39.39** **Poisoning by, adverse effect of and underdosing of other nonsteroidal anti-inflammatory drugs [NSAID]**

    ✓7ᵗʰ **T39.391** **Poisoning by other nonsteroidal anti-inflammatory drugs [NSAID], accidental (unintentional)**
      Poisoning by other nonsteroidal anti-inflammatory drugs NOS

    ² ✓7ᵗʰ **T39.392** **Poisoning by other nonsteroidal anti-inflammatory drugs [NSAID], intentional self-harm** HCC Rx ESR COM

    ✓7ᵗʰ **T39.393** **Poisoning by other nonsteroidal anti-inflammatory drugs [NSAID], assault**

    ✓7ᵗʰ **T39.394** **Poisoning by other nonsteroidal anti-inflammatory drugs [NSAID], undetermined**

    ✓7ᵗʰ **T39.395** **Adverse effect of other nonsteroidal anti-inflammatory drugs [NSAID]** UPD

    ✓7ᵗʰ **T39.396** **Underdosing of other nonsteroidal anti-inflammatory drugs [NSAID]** UPD

✓5ᵗʰ **T39.4 Poisoning by, adverse effect of and underdosing of antirheumatics, not elsewhere classified**

     EXCLUDES 1   *poisoning by, adverse effect of and underdosing of glucocorticoids (T38.0-)*

                       poisoning by, adverse effect of and underdosing of salicylates (T39.0-)

   ✓6ᵗʰ **T39.4X Poisoning by, adverse effect of and underdosing of antirheumatics, not elsewhere classified**

     ✓7ᵗʰ **T39.4X1 Poisoning by antirheumatics, not elsewhere classified, accidental (unintentional)**

          Poisoning by antirheumatics, not elsewhere classified NOS

     ² ✓7ᵗʰ **T39.4X2 Poisoning by antirheumatics, not elsewhere classified, intentional self-harm** HCC Rx ESR COM

     ✓7ᵗʰ **T39.4X3 Poisoning by antirheumatics, not elsewhere classified, assault**

     ✓7ᵗʰ **T39.4X4 Poisoning by antirheumatics, not elsewhere classified, undetermined**

     ✓7ᵗʰ **T39.4X5 Adverse effect of antirheumatics, not elsewhere classified** UPD

     ✓7ᵗʰ **T39.4X6 Underdosing of antirheumatics, not elsewhere classified** UPD

✓5ᵗʰ **T39.8 Poisoning by, adverse effect of and underdosing of other nonopioid analgesics and antipyretics, not elsewhere classified**

   ✓6ᵗʰ **T39.8X Poisoning by, adverse effect of and underdosing of other nonopioid analgesics and antipyretics, not elsewhere classified**

     ✓7ᵗʰ **T39.8X1 Poisoning by other nonopioid analgesics and antipyretics, not elsewhere classified, accidental (unintentional)**

          Poisoning by other nonopioid analgesics and antipyretics, not elsewhere classified NOS

     ² ✓7ᵗʰ **T39.8X2 Poisoning by other nonopioid analgesics and antipyretics, not elsewhere classified, intentional self-harm** HCC Rx ESR COM

     ✓7ᵗʰ **T39.8X3 Poisoning by other nonopioid analgesics and antipyretics, not elsewhere classified, assault**

     ✓7ᵗʰ **T39.8X4 Poisoning by other nonopioid analgesics and antipyretics, not elsewhere classified, undetermined**

     ✓7ᵗʰ **T39.8X5 Adverse effect of other nonopioid analgesics and antipyretics, not elsewhere classified** UPD

     ✓7ᵗʰ **T39.8X6 Underdosing of other nonopioid analgesics and antipyretics, not elsewhere classified** UPD

✓5ᵗʰ **T39.9 Poisoning by, adverse effect of and underdosing of unspecified nonopioid analgesic, antipyretic and antirheumatic**

   ✓x7ᵗʰ **T39.91 Poisoning by unspecified nonopioid analgesic, antipyretic and antirheumatic, accidental (unintentional)**

          Poisoning by nonopioid analgesic, antipyretic and antirheumatic NOS

   ² ✓x7ᵗʰ **T39.92 Poisoning by unspecified nonopioid analgesic, antipyretic and antirheumatic, intentional self-harm** HCC Rx ESR COM

   ✓x7ᵗʰ **T39.93 Poisoning by unspecified nonopioid analgesic, antipyretic and antirheumatic, assault**

   ✓x7ᵗʰ **T39.94 Poisoning by unspecified nonopioid analgesic, antipyretic and antirheumatic, undetermined**

   ✓x7ᵗʰ **T39.95 Adverse effect of unspecified nonopioid analgesic, antipyretic and antirheumatic** UPD

   ✓x7ᵗʰ **T39.96 Underdosing of unspecified nonopioid analgesic, antipyretic and antirheumatic** UPD

✓4ᵗʰ **T40 Poisoning by, adverse effect of and underdosing of narcotics and psychodysleptics [hallucinogens]**

     EXCLUDES 2   *drug dependence and related mental and behavioral disorders due to psychoactive substance use (F10.-F19.-)*

   The appropriate 7th character is to be added to each code from category T40.
   A   initial encounter
   D   subsequent encounter
   S   sequela

✓5ᵗʰ **T40.0 Poisoning by, adverse effect of and underdosing of opium**

   ✓6ᵗʰ **T40.0X Poisoning by, adverse effect of and underdosing of opium**

     ¹ ✓7ᵗʰ **T40.0X1 Poisoning by opium, accidental (unintentional)** HCC ESR COM

          Poisoning by opium NOS

     ² ✓7ᵗʰ **T40.0X2 Poisoning by opium, intentional self-harm** HCC Rx ESR COM

     ✓7ᵗʰ **T40.0X3 Poisoning by opium, assault**

     ¹ ✓7ᵗʰ **T40.0X4 Poisoning by opium, undetermined** HCC ESR COM

     ✓7ᵗʰ **T40.0X5 Adverse effect of opium** UPD

     ✓7ᵗʰ **T40.0X6 Underdosing of opium** UPD

✓5ᵗʰ **T40.1 Poisoning by and adverse effect of heroin**

   ✓6ᵗʰ **T40.1X Poisoning by and adverse effect of heroin**

     ¹ ✓7ᵗʰ **T40.1X1 Poisoning by heroin, accidental (unintentional)** HCC ESR COM

          Poisoning by heroin NOS

     ² ✓7ᵗʰ **T40.1X2 Poisoning by heroin, intentional self-harm** HCC Rx ESR COM

     ✓7ᵗʰ **T40.1X3 Poisoning by heroin, assault**

     ¹ ✓7ᵗʰ **T40.1X4 Poisoning by heroin, undetermined** HCC ESR COM

✓5ᵗʰ **T40.2 Poisoning by, adverse effect of and underdosing of other opioids**

   ✓6ᵗʰ **T40.2X Poisoning by, adverse effect of and underdosing of other opioids**

     ¹ ✓7ᵗʰ **T40.2X1 Poisoning by other opioids, accidental (unintentional)** HCC ESR COM

          Poisoning by other opioids NOS

     ² ✓7ᵗʰ **T40.2X2 Poisoning by other opioids, intentional self-harm** HCC Rx ESR COM

     ✓7ᵗʰ **T40.2X3 Poisoning by other opioids, assault**

     ¹ ✓7ᵗʰ **T40.2X4 Poisoning by other opioids, undetermined** HCC ESR COM

     ✓7ᵗʰ **T40.2X5 Adverse effect of other opioids** UPD

          Demerol (handwritten)

          AHA: 2020,2Q,24

     ✓7ᵗʰ **T40.2X6 Underdosing of other opioids** UPD

✓5ᵗʰ **T40.3 Poisoning by, adverse effect of and underdosing of methadone**

   ✓6ᵗʰ **T40.3X Poisoning by, adverse effect of and underdosing of methadone**

     ¹ ✓7ᵗʰ **T40.3X1 Poisoning by methadone, accidental (unintentional)** HCC ESR COM

          Poisoning by methadone NOS

     ² ✓7ᵗʰ **T40.3X2 Poisoning by methadone, intentional self-harm** HCC Rx ESR COM

     ✓7ᵗʰ **T40.3X3 Poisoning by methadone, assault**

     ✓7ᵗʰ **T40.3X4 Poisoning by methadone, undetermined** HCC ESR COM

     ✓7ᵗʰ **T40.3X5 Adverse effect of methadone** UPD

     ✓7ᵗʰ **T40.3X6 Underdosing of methadone** UPD

✓5ᵗʰ **T40.4 Poisoning by, adverse effect of and underdosing of other synthetic narcotics**

     AHA: 2020,4Q,40

   ✓6ᵗʰ **T40.41 Poisoning by, adverse effect of and underdosing of fentanyl or fentanyl analogs**

     ✓7ᵗʰ **T40.411 Poisoning by fentanyl or fentanyl analogs, accidental (unintentional)** HCC ESR COM

     ✓7ᵗʰ **T40.412 Poisoning by fentanyl or fentanyl analogs, intentional self-harm** HCC Rx ESR COM

     ✓7ᵗʰ **T40.413 Poisoning by fentanyl or fentanyl analogs, assault**

     ✓7ᵗʰ **T40.414 Poisoning by fentanyl or fentanyl analogs, undetermined** HCC ESR COM

✓7ᵗʰ **T40.415** Adverse effect of fentanyl or fentanyl analogs `UPD`

✓7ᵗʰ **T40.416** Underdosing of fentanyl or fentanyl analogs `UPD`

✓6ᵗʰ **T40.42** Poisoning by, adverse effect of and underdosing of tramadol

✓7ᵗʰ **T40.421** Poisoning by tramadol, accidental (unintentional) `HCC` `ESR` `COM`

✓7ᵗʰ **T40.422** Poisoning by tramadol, intentional self-harm `HCC` `Rx` `ESR` `COM`

✓7ᵗʰ **T40.423** Poisoning by tramadol, assault

✓7ᵗʰ **T40.424** Poisoning by tramadol, undetermined `HCC` `ESR` `COM`

✓7ᵗʰ **T40.425** Adverse effect of tramadol `UPD`

✓7ᵗʰ **T40.426** Underdosing of tramadol `UPD`

✓6ᵗʰ **T40.49** Poisoning by, adverse effect of and underdosing of other synthetic narcotics

✓7ᵗʰ **T40.491** Poisoning by other synthetic narcotics, accidental (unintentional) `HCC` `ESR` `COM`

✓7ᵗʰ **T40.492** Poisoning by other synthetic narcotics, intentional self-harm `HCC` `Rx` `ESR` `COM`

✓7ᵗʰ **T40.493** Poisoning by other synthetic narcotics, assault

✓7ᵗʰ **T40.494** Poisoning by other synthetic narcotics, undetermined `HCC` `ESR` `COM`

✓7ᵗʰ **T40.495** Adverse effect of other synthetic narcotics `UPD`

✓7ᵗʰ **T40.496** Underdosing of other synthetic narcotics `UPD`

✓5ᵗʰ **T40.5** Poisoning by, adverse effect of and underdosing of cocaine

✓6ᵗʰ **T40.5X** Poisoning by, adverse effect of and underdosing of cocaine

1 ✓7ᵗʰ **T40.5X1** Poisoning by cocaine, accidental (unintentional) `HCC` `ESR` `COM`
Poisoning by cocaine NOS
AHA: 2016,2Q,8

2 ✓7ᵗʰ **T40.5X2** Poisoning by cocaine, intentional self-harm `HCC` `Rx` `ESR` `COM`

✓7ᵗʰ **T40.5X3** Poisoning by cocaine, assault

1 ✓7ᵗʰ **T40.5X4** Poisoning by cocaine, undetermined `HCC` `ESR` `COM`

✓7ᵗʰ **T40.5X5** Adverse effect of cocaine `UPD`

✓7ᵗʰ **T40.5X6** Underdosing of cocaine `UPD`

✓5ᵗʰ **T40.6** Poisoning by, adverse effect of and underdosing of other and unspecified narcotics

✓6ᵗʰ **T40.60** Poisoning by, adverse effect of and underdosing of unspecified narcotics

1 ✓7ᵗʰ **T40.601** Poisoning by unspecified narcotics, accidental (unintentional) `HCC` `ESR` `COM`
Poisoning by narcotics NOS

2 ✓7ᵗʰ **T40.602** Poisoning by unspecified narcotics, intentional self-harm `HCC` `Rx` `ESR` `COM`

✓7ᵗʰ **T40.603** Poisoning by unspecified narcotics, assault

1 ✓7ᵗʰ **T40.604** Poisoning by unspecified narcotics, undetermined `HCC` `ESR` `COM`

✓7ᵗʰ **T40.605** Adverse effect of unspecified narcotics `UPD`

✓7ᵗʰ **T40.606** Underdosing of unspecified narcotics `UPD`

✓6ᵗʰ **T40.69** Poisoning by, adverse effect of and underdosing of other narcotics

1 ✓7ᵗʰ **T40.691** Poisoning by other narcotics, accidental (unintentional) `HCC` `ESR` `COM`
Poisoning by other narcotics NOS

2 ✓7ᵗʰ **T40.692** Poisoning by other narcotics, intentional self-harm `HCC` `Rx` `ESR` `COM`

✓7ᵗʰ **T40.693** Poisoning by other narcotics, assault

1 ✓7ᵗʰ **T40.694** Poisoning by other narcotics, undetermined `HCC` `ESR` `COM`

✓7ᵗʰ **T40.695** Adverse effect of other narcotics `UPD`

✓7ᵗʰ **T40.696** Underdosing of other narcotics `UPD`

✓5ᵗʰ **T40.7** Poisoning by, adverse effect of and underdosing of cannabis (derivatives)

✓6ᵗʰ **T40.71** Poisoning by, adverse effect of and underdosing of cannabis (derivatives)
AHA: 2021,4Q,30

✓7ᵗʰ **T40.711** Poisoning by cannabis, accidental (unintentional)

✓7ᵗʰ **T40.712** Poisoning by cannabis, intentional self-harm `HCC` `Rx` `ESR` `COM`

✓7ᵗʰ **T40.713** Poisoning by cannabis, assault

✓7ᵗʰ **T40.714** Poisoning by cannabis, undetermined

✓7ᵗʰ **T40.715** Adverse effect of cannabis `UPD`

✓7ᵗʰ **T40.716** Underdosing of cannabis `UPD`

✓6ᵗʰ **T40.72** Poisoning by, adverse effect of and underdosing of synthetic cannabinoids
AHA: 2021,4Q,30

✓7ᵗʰ **T40.721** Poisoning by synthetic cannabinoids, accidental (unintentional)

✓7ᵗʰ **T40.722** Poisoning by synthetic cannabinoids, intentional self-harm `HCC` `Rx` `ESR` `COM`

✓7ᵗʰ **T40.723** Poisoning by synthetic cannabinoids, assault

✓7ᵗʰ **T40.724** Poisoning by synthetic cannabinoids, undetermined

✓7ᵗʰ **T40.725** Adverse effect of synthetic cannabinoids `UPD`

✓7ᵗʰ **T40.726** Underdosing of synthetic cannabinoids `UPD`

✓5ᵗʰ **T40.8** Poisoning by and adverse effect of lysergide [LSD]

✓6ᵗʰ **T40.8X** Poisoning by and adverse effect of lysergide [LSD]

1 ✓7ᵗʰ **T40.8X1** Poisoning by lysergide [LSD], accidental (unintentional) `HCC` `ESR` `COM`
Poisoning by lysergide [LSD] NOS

2 ✓7ᵗʰ **T40.8X2** Poisoning by lysergide [LSD], intentional self-harm `HCC` `Rx` `ESR` `COM`

✓7ᵗʰ **T40.8X3** Poisoning by lysergide [LSD], assault

1 ✓7ᵗʰ **T40.8X4** Poisoning by lysergide [LSD], undetermined `HCC` `ESR` `COM`

✓5ᵗʰ **T40.9** Poisoning by, adverse effect of and underdosing of other and unspecified psychodysleptics [hallucinogens]

✓6ᵗʰ **T40.90** Poisoning by, adverse effect of and underdosing of unspecified psychodysleptics [hallucinogens]

1 ✓7ᵗʰ **T40.901** Poisoning by unspecified psychodysleptics [hallucinogens], accidental (unintentional) `HCC` `ESR` `COM`

2 ✓7ᵗʰ **T40.902** Poisoning by unspecified psychodysleptics [hallucinogens], intentional self-harm `HCC` `Rx` `ESR` `COM`

✓7ᵗʰ **T40.903** Poisoning by unspecified psychodysleptics [hallucinogens], assault

1 ✓7ᵗʰ **T40.904** Poisoning by unspecified psychodysleptics [hallucinogens], undetermined `HCC` `ESR` `COM`

✓7ᵗʰ **T40.905** Adverse effect of unspecified psychodysleptics [hallucinogens] `UPD`

✓7ᵗʰ **T40.906** Underdosing of unspecified psychodysleptics [hallucinogens] `UPD`

✓6ᵗʰ **T40.99** Poisoning by, adverse effect of and underdosing of other psychodysleptics [hallucinogens]

1 ✓7ᵗʰ **T40.991** Poisoning by other psychodysleptics [hallucinogens], accidental (unintentional) `HCC` `ESR` `COM`
Poisoning by other psychodysleptics [hallucinogens] NOS

2 ✓7ᵗʰ **T40.992** Poisoning by other psychodysleptics [hallucinogens], intentional self-harm `HCC` `Rx` `ESR` `COM`

✓7ᵗʰ **T40.993** Poisoning by other psychodysleptics [hallucinogens], assault

1 ✓7ᵗʰ **T40.994** Poisoning by other psychodysleptics [hallucinogens], undetermined `HCC` `ESR` `COM`

✓7ᵗʰ **T40.995** Adverse effect of other psychodysleptics [hallucinogens] `UPD`

✓7ᵗʰ **T40.996** Underdosing of other psychodysleptics [hallucinogens] `UPD`

`HCC` CMS-HCC   `Rx` Rx HCC   `ESR` ESRD HCC   `COM` Commercial HCC   N Newborn: 0   P Pediatric: 0-17   M Maternity: 9-64   A Adult: 15-124

1140   ICD-10-CM 2023

✓4ᵗʰ **T41 Poisoning by, adverse effect of and underdosing of anesthetics and therapeutic gases**

EXCLUDES 1 *benzodiazepines (T42.4-)*
cocaine (T40.5-)
complications of anesthesia during labor and delivery (O74.-)
complications of anesthesia during pregnancy (O29.-)
complications of anesthesia during the puerperium (O89.-)
opioids (T40.0-T40.2-)

The appropriate 7th character is to be added to each code from category T41.
A initial encounter
D subsequent encounter
S sequela

✓5ᵗʰ **T41.0 Poisoning by, adverse effect of and underdosing of inhaled anesthetics**

EXCLUDES 1 *oxygen (T41.5-)*

✓6ᵗʰ **T41.0X Poisoning by, adverse effect of and underdosing of** inhaled anesthetics

  ✓7ᵗʰ **T41.0X1 Poisoning by inhaled anesthetics, accidental (unintentional)**
    Poisoning by inhaled anesthetics NOS

  ² ✓7ᵗʰ **T41.0X2 Poisoning by inhaled anesthetics, intentional self-harm** HCC Rx ESR COM

  ✓7ᵗʰ **T41.0X3 Poisoning by inhaled anesthetics, assault**

  ✓7ᵗʰ **T41.0X4 Poisoning by inhaled anesthetics, undetermined**

  ✓7ᵗʰ **T41.0X5 Adverse effect of inhaled anesthetics** UPD

  ✓7ᵗʰ **T41.0X6 Underdosing of inhaled anesthetics** UPD

✓5ᵗʰ **T41.1 Poisoning by, adverse effect of and underdosing of intravenous anesthetics**
  Poisoning by, adverse effect of and underdosing of thiobarbiturates

✓6ᵗʰ **T41.1X Poisoning by, adverse effect of and underdosing of** intravenous anesthetics

  ✓7ᵗʰ **T41.1X1 Poisoning by intravenous anesthetics, accidental (unintentional)**
    Poisoning by intravenous anesthetics NOS

  ² ✓7ᵗʰ **T41.1X2 Poisoning by intravenous anesthetics, intentional self-harm** HCC Rx ESR COM

  ✓7ᵗʰ **T41.1X3 Poisoning by intravenous anesthetics, assault**

  ✓7ᵗʰ **T41.1X4 Poisoning by intravenous anesthetics, undetermined**

  ✓7ᵗʰ **T41.1X5 Adverse effect of intravenous anesthetics** UPD

  ✓7ᵗʰ **T41.1X6 Underdosing of intravenous anesthetics** UPD

✓5ᵗʰ **T41.2 Poisoning by, adverse effect of and underdosing of other and unspecified general anesthetics**

✓6ᵗʰ **T41.20 Poisoning by, adverse effect of and underdosing of unspecified general anesthetics**

  ✓7ᵗʰ **T41.201 Poisoning by unspecified general anesthetics, accidental (unintentional)**
    Poisoning by general anesthetics NOS

  ² ✓7ᵗʰ **T41.202 Poisoning by unspecified general anesthetics, intentional self-harm** HCC Rx ESR COM

  ✓7ᵗʰ **T41.203 Poisoning by unspecified general anesthetics, assault**

  ✓7ᵗʰ **T41.204 Poisoning by unspecified general anesthetics, undetermined**

  ✓7ᵗʰ **T41.205 Adverse effect of unspecified general anesthetics** UPD
    AHA: 2016,4Q,73

  ✓7ᵗʰ **T41.206 Underdosing of unspecified general anesthetics** UPD

✓6ᵗʰ **T41.29 Poisoning by, adverse effect of and underdosing of other general anesthetics**

  ✓7ᵗʰ **T41.291 Poisoning by other general anesthetics, accidental (unintentional)**
    Poisoning by other general anesthetics NOS

  ² ✓7ᵗʰ **T41.292 Poisoning by other general anesthetics, intentional self-harm** HCC Rx ESR COM

  ✓7ᵗʰ **T41.293 Poisoning by other general anesthetics, assault**

  ✓7ᵗʰ **T41.294 Poisoning by other general anesthetics, undetermined**

  ✓7ᵗʰ **T41.295 Adverse effect of other general anesthetics** UPD

  ✓7ᵗʰ **T41.296 Underdosing of other general anesthetics** UPD

✓5ᵗʰ **T41.3 Poisoning by, adverse effect of and underdosing of local anesthetics**
  Cocaine (topical)

EXCLUDES 2 *poisoning by cocaine used as a central nervous system stimulant (T40.5X1-T40.5X4)*

✓6ᵗʰ **T41.3X Poisoning by, adverse effect of and underdosing of** local anesthetics

  ✓7ᵗʰ **T41.3X1 Poisoning by local anesthetics, accidental (unintentional)**
    Poisoning by local anesthetics NOS

  ² ✓7ᵗʰ **T41.3X2 Poisoning by local anesthetics, intentional self-harm** HCC Rx ESR COM

  ✓7ᵗʰ **T41.3X3 Poisoning by local anesthetics, assault**

  ✓7ᵗʰ **T41.3X4 Poisoning by local anesthetics, undetermined**

  ✓7ᵗʰ **T41.3X5 Adverse effect of local anesthetics** UPD

  ✓7ᵗʰ **T41.3X6 Underdosing of local anesthetics** UPD

✓5ᵗʰ **T41.4 Poisoning by, adverse effect of and underdosing of unspecified anesthetic**

  ✓x7ᵗʰ **T41.41 Poisoning by unspecified anesthetic, accidental (unintentional)**
    Poisoning by anesthetic NOS

  ² ✓x7ᵗʰ **T41.42 Poisoning by unspecified anesthetic, intentional self-harm** HCC Rx ESR COM

  ✓x7ᵗʰ **T41.43 Poisoning by unspecified anesthetic, assault**

  ✓x7ᵗʰ **T41.44 Poisoning by unspecified anesthetic, undetermined**

  ✓x7ᵗʰ **T41.45 Adverse effect of unspecified anesthetic** UPD

  ✓x7ᵗʰ **T41.46 Underdosing of unspecified anesthetics** UPD

✓5ᵗʰ **T41.5 Poisoning by, adverse effect of and underdosing of therapeutic gases**

✓6ᵗʰ **T41.5X Poisoning by, adverse effect of and underdosing of** therapeutic gases

  ✓7ᵗʰ **T41.5X1 Poisoning by therapeutic gases, accidental (unintentional)**
    Poisoning by therapeutic gases NOS

  ² ✓7ᵗʰ **T41.5X2 Poisoning by therapeutic gases, intentional self-harm** HCC Rx ESR COM

  ✓7ᵗʰ **T41.5X3 Poisoning by therapeutic gases, assault**

  ✓7ᵗʰ **T41.5X4 Poisoning by therapeutic gases, undetermined**

  ✓7ᵗʰ **T41.5X5 Adverse effect of therapeutic gases** UPD

  ✓7ᵗʰ **T41.5X6 Underdosing of therapeutic gases** UPD

✓4ᵗʰ **T42 Poisoning by, adverse effect of and underdosing of antiepileptic, sedative- hypnotic and antiparkinsonism drugs**

EXCLUDES 2 *drug dependence and related mental and behavioral disorders due to psychoactive substance use (F10.- - F19.-)*

The appropriate 7th character is to be added to each code from category T42.
A initial encounter
D subsequent encounter
S sequela

✓5ᵗʰ **T42.0 Poisoning by, adverse effect of and underdosing of hydantoin derivatives**

✓6ᵗʰ **T42.0X Poisoning by, adverse effect of and underdosing of** hydantoin derivatives

  ✓7ᵗʰ **T42.0X1 Poisoning by hydantoin derivatives, accidental (unintentional)**
    Poisoning by hydantoin derivatives NOS

  ² ✓7ᵗʰ **T42.0X2 Poisoning by hydantoin derivatives, intentional self-harm** HCC Rx ESR COM

  ✓7ᵗʰ **T42.0X3 Poisoning by hydantoin derivatives, assault**

  ✓7ᵗʰ **T42.0X4 Poisoning by hydantoin derivatives, undetermined**

  ✓7ᵗʰ **T42.0X5 Adverse effect of hydantoin derivatives** UPD

  ✓7ᵗʰ **T42.0X6 Underdosing of hydantoin derivatives** UPD

✓5ᵗʰ T42.1 Poisoning by, adverse effect of and underdosing of iminostilbenes

Poisoning by, adverse effect of and underdosing of carbamazepine

     ✓6ᵗʰ T42.1X Poisoning by, adverse effect of and underdosing of iminostilbenes

         ✓7ᵗʰ T42.1X1 Poisoning by iminostilbenes, accidental (unintentional)

             Poisoning by iminostilbenes NOS

         ² **✓7ᵗʰ T42.1X2 Poisoning by iminostilbenes,** intentional self-harm   HCC Rx ESR COM

         ✓7ᵗʰ T42.1X3 Poisoning by iminostilbenes, assault

         ✓7ᵗʰ T42.1X4 Poisoning by iminostilbenes, undetermined

         ✓7ᵗʰ T42.1X5 Adverse effect of iminostilbenes   UPD

         ✓7ᵗʰ T42.1X6 Underdosing of iminostilbenes   UPD

✓5ᵗʰ T42.2 Poisoning by, adverse effect of and underdosing of succinimides and oxazolidinediones

     ✓6ᵗʰ T42.2X Poisoning by, adverse effect of and underdosing of succinimides and oxazolidinediones

         ✓7ᵗʰ T42.2X1 Poisoning by succinimides and oxazolidinediones, accidental (unintentional)

             Poisoning by succinimides and oxazolidinediones NOS

         ² **✓7ᵗʰ T42.2X2 Poisoning by succinimides and oxazolidinediones,** intentional self-harm   HCC Rx ESR COM

         ✓7ᵗʰ T42.2X3 Poisoning by succinimides and oxazolidinediones, assault

         ✓7ᵗʰ T42.2X4 Poisoning by succinimides and oxazolidinediones, undetermined

         ✓7ᵗʰ T42.2X5 Adverse effect of succinimides and oxazolidinediones   UPD

         ✓7ᵗʰ T42.2X6 Underdosing of succinimides and oxazolidinediones   UPD

✓5ᵗʰ T42.3 Poisoning by, adverse effect of and underdosing of barbiturates

     EXCLUDES 1   poisoning by, adverse effect of and underdosing of thiobarbiturates (T41.1-)

     ✓6ᵗʰ T42.3X Poisoning by, adverse effect of and underdosing of barbiturates

         ✓7ᵗʰ T42.3X1 Poisoning by barbiturates, accidental (unintentional)

             Poisoning by barbiturates NOS

         ² **✓7ᵗʰ T42.3X2 Poisoning by barbiturates,** intentional self-harm   HCC Rx ESR COM

         ✓7ᵗʰ T42.3X3 Poisoning by barbiturates, assault

         ✓7ᵗʰ T42.3X4 Poisoning by barbiturates, undetermined

         ✓7ᵗʰ T42.3X5 Adverse effect of barbiturates   UPD

         ✓7ᵗʰ T42.3X6 Underdosing of barbiturates   UPD

✓5ᵗʰ T42.4 Poisoning by, adverse effect of and underdosing of benzodiazepines

     ✓6ᵗʰ T42.4X Poisoning by, adverse effect of and underdosing of benzodiazepines

         ✓7ᵗʰ T42.4X1 Poisoning by benzodiazepines, accidental (unintentional)

Valium pill

             Poisoning by benzodiazepines NOS

         ² **✓7ᵗʰ T42.4X2 Poisoning by benzodiazepines,** intentional self-harm   HCC Rx ESR COM

         ✓7ᵗʰ T42.4X3 Poisoning by benzodiazepines, assault

         ✓7ᵗʰ T42.4X4 Poisoning by benzodiazepines, undetermined

         ✓7ᵗʰ T42.4X5 Adverse effect of benzodiazepines   UPD

         ✓7ᵗʰ T42.4X6 Underdosing of benzodiazepines   UPD

✓5ᵗʰ T42.5 Poisoning by, adverse effect of and underdosing of mixed antiepileptics

     ✓6ᵗʰ T42.5X Poisoning by, adverse effect of and underdosing of antiepileptics

         ✓7ᵗʰ T42.5X1 Poisoning by mixed antiepileptics, accidental (unintentional)

             Poisoning by mixed antiepileptics NOS

         ² **✓7ᵗʰ T42.5X2 Poisoning by mixed antiepileptics,** intentional self-harm   HCC Rx ESR COM

         ✓7ᵗʰ T42.5X3 Poisoning by mixed antiepileptics, assault

         ✓7ᵗʰ T42.5X4 Poisoning by mixed antiepileptics, undetermined

---

         ✓7ᵗʰ T42.5X5 Adverse effect of mixed antiepileptics   UPD

         ✓7ᵗʰ T42.5X6 Underdosing of mixed antiepileptics   UPD

✓5ᵗʰ T42.6 Poisoning by, adverse effect of and underdosing of other antiepileptic and sedative-hypnotic drugs

Poisoning by, adverse effect of and underdosing of methaqualone

Poisoning by, adverse effect of and underdosing of valproic acid

     EXCLUDES 1   poisoning by, adverse effect of and underdosing of carbamazepine (T42.1-)

     ✓6ᵗʰ T42.6X Poisoning by, adverse effect of and underdosing of other antiepileptic and sedative-hypnotic drugs

         ✓7ᵗʰ T42.6X1 Poisoning by other antiepileptic and sedative-hypnotic drugs, accidental (unintentional)

             Poisoning by other antiepileptic and sedative-hypnotic drugs NOS

         ² **✓7ᵗʰ T42.6X2 Poisoning by other antiepileptic and sedative-hypnotic drugs,** intentional self-harm   HCC Rx ESR COM

         ✓7ᵗʰ T42.6X3 Poisoning by other antiepileptic and sedative-hypnotic drugs, assault

         ✓7ᵗʰ T42.6X4 Poisoning by other antiepileptic and sedative-hypnotic drugs, undetermined

         ✓7ᵗʰ T42.6X5 Adverse effect of other antiepileptic and sedative-hypnotic drugs   UPD

         ✓7ᵗʰ T42.6X6 Underdosing of other antiepileptic and sedative-hypnotic drugs   UPD

✓5ᵗʰ T42.7 Poisoning by, adverse effect of and underdosing of unspecified antiepileptic and sedative-hypnotic drugs

     ✓x7ᵗʰ T42.71 Poisoning by unspecified antiepileptic and sedative-hypnotic drugs, accidental (unintentional)

         Poisoning by antiepileptic and sedative-hypnotic drugs NOS

     ² **✓x7ᵗʰ T42.72 Poisoning by unspecified antiepileptic and sedative-hypnotic drugs,** intentional self-harm   HCC Rx ESR COM

     ✓x7ᵗʰ T42.73 Poisoning by unspecified antiepileptic and sedative-hypnotic drugs, assault

     ✓x7ᵗʰ T42.74 Poisoning by unspecified antiepileptic and sedative-hypnotic drugs, undetermined

     ✓x7ᵗʰ T42.75 Adverse effect of unspecified antiepileptic and sedative-hypnotic drugs   UPD

     ✓x7ᵗʰ T42.76 Underdosing of unspecified antiepileptic and sedative-hypnotic drugs   UPD

✓5ᵗʰ T42.8 Poisoning by, adverse effect of and underdosing of antiparkinsonism drugs and other central muscle-tone depressants

Poisoning by, adverse effect of and underdosing of amantadine

     ✓6ᵗʰ T42.8X Poisoning by, adverse effect of and underdosing of antiparkinsonism drugs and other central muscle-tone depressants

         ✓7ᵗʰ T42.8X1 Poisoning by antiparkinsonism drugs and other central muscle-tone depressants, accidental (unintentional)

             Poisoning by antiparkinsonism drugs and other central muscle-tone depressants NOS

         ² **✓7ᵗʰ T42.8X2 Poisoning by antiparkinsonism drugs and other central muscle-tone depressants,** intentional self-harm   HCC Rx ESR COM

         ✓7ᵗʰ T42.8X3 Poisoning by antiparkinsonism drugs and other central muscle-tone depressants, assault

         ✓7ᵗʰ T42.8X4 Poisoning by antiparkinsonism drugs and other central muscle-tone depressants, undetermined

         ✓7ᵗʰ T42.8X5 Adverse effect of antiparkinsonism drugs and other central muscle-tone depressants   UPD

         ✓7ᵗʰ T42.8X6 Underdosing of antiparkinsonism drugs and other central muscle-tone depressants   UPD

✓4ᵗʰ **T43 Poisoning by, adverse effect of and underdosing of psychotropic drugs, not elsewhere classified**

     EXCLUDES 1   appetite depressants (T50.5-)
                  barbiturates (T42.3-)
                  benzodiazepines (T42.4-)
                  methaqualone (T42.6-)
                  psychodysleptics [hallucinogens] (T40.7-T40.9-)
     EXCLUDES 2   drug dependence and related mental and behavioral disorders due to psychoactive substance use (F10.- – F19.-)

> The appropriate 7th character is to be added to each code from category T43.
> A   initial encounter
> D   subsequent encounter
> S   sequela

✓5ᵗʰ **T43.0 Poisoning by, adverse effect of and underdosing of tricyclic and tetracyclic antidepressants**

   ✓6ᵗʰ **T43.01 Poisoning by, adverse effect of and underdosing of tricyclic antidepressants**

     ✓7ᵗʰ **T43.011 Poisoning by tricyclic antidepressants, accidental (unintentional)**
           Poisoning by tricyclic antidepressants NOS

     ² ✓7ᵗʰ **T43.012 Poisoning by tricyclic antidepressants, intentional self-harm** HCC Rx ESR COM

     ✓7ᵗʰ **T43.013 Poisoning by tricyclic antidepressants, assault**

     ✓7ᵗʰ **T43.014 Poisoning by tricyclic antidepressants, undetermined**

     ✓7ᵗʰ **T43.015 Adverse effect of tricyclic antidepressants** UPD

     ✓7ᵗʰ **T43.016 Underdosing of tricyclic antidepressants** UPD

   ✓6ᵗʰ **T43.02 Poisoning by, adverse effect of and underdosing of tetracyclic antidepressants**

     ✓7ᵗʰ **T43.021 Poisoning by tetracyclic antidepressants, accidental (unintentional)**
           Poisoning by tetracyclic antidepressants NOS

     ² ✓7ᵗʰ **T43.022 Poisoning by tetracyclic antidepressants, intentional self-harm** HCC Rx ESR COM

     ✓7ᵗʰ **T43.023 Poisoning by tetracyclic antidepressants, assault**

     ✓7ᵗʰ **T43.024 Poisoning by tetracyclic antidepressants, undetermined**

     ✓7ᵗʰ **T43.025 Adverse effect of tetracyclic antidepressants** UPD

     ✓7ᵗʰ **T43.026 Underdosing of tetracyclic antidepressants** UPD

✓5ᵗʰ **T43.1 Poisoning by, adverse effect of and underdosing of monoamine-oxidase-inhibitor antidepressants**

   ✓6ᵗʰ **T43.1X Poisoning by, adverse effect of and underdosing of monoamine-oxidase-inhibitor antidepressants**

     ✓7ᵗʰ **T43.1X1 Poisoning by monoamine-oxidase-inhibitor antidepressants, accidental (unintentional)**
           Poisoning by monoamine-oxidase-inhibitor antidepressants NOS

     ² ✓7ᵗʰ **T43.1X2 Poisoning by monoamine-oxidase-inhibitor antidepressants, intentional self-harm** HCC Rx ESR COM

     ✓7ᵗʰ **T43.1X3 Poisoning by monoamine-oxidase-inhibitor antidepressants, assault**

     ✓7ᵗʰ **T43.1X4 Poisoning by monoamine-oxidase-inhibitor antidepressants, undetermined**

     ✓7ᵗʰ **T43.1X5 Adverse effect of monoamine-oxidase-inhibitor antidepressants** UPD

     ✓7ᵗʰ **T43.1X6 Underdosing of monoamine-oxidase-inhibitor antidepressants** UPD

✓5ᵗʰ **T43.2 Poisoning by, adverse effect of and underdosing of other and unspecified antidepressants**

   ✓6ᵗʰ **T43.20 Poisoning by, adverse effect of and underdosing of unspecified antidepressants**

     ✓7ᵗʰ **T43.201 Poisoning by unspecified antidepressants, accidental (unintentional)**
           Poisoning by antidepressants NOS

     ² ✓7ᵗʰ **T43.202 Poisoning by unspecified antidepressants, intentional self-harm** HCC Rx ESR COM

     ✓7ᵗʰ **T43.203 Poisoning by unspecified antidepressants, assault**

     ✓7ᵗʰ **T43.204 Poisoning by unspecified antidepressants, undetermined**

     ✓7ᵗʰ **T43.205 Adverse effect of unspecified antidepressants** UPD
           Antidepressant discontinuation syndrome

     ✓7ᵗʰ **T43.206 Underdosing of unspecified antidepressants** UPD

   ✓6ᵗʰ **T43.21 Poisoning by, adverse effect of and underdosing of selective serotonin and norepinephrine reuptake inhibitors**
       Poisoning by, adverse effect of and underdosing of SSNRI antidepressants

     ✓7ᵗʰ **T43.211 Poisoning by selective serotonin and norepinephrine reuptake inhibitors, accidental (unintentional)**

     ² ✓7ᵗʰ **T43.212 Poisoning by selective serotonin and norepinephrine reuptake inhibitors, intentional self-harm** HCC Rx ESR COM

     ✓7ᵗʰ **T43.213 Poisoning by selective serotonin and norepinephrine reuptake inhibitors, assault**

     ✓7ᵗʰ **T43.214 Poisoning by selective serotonin and norepinephrine reuptake inhibitors, undetermined**

     ✓7ᵗʰ **T43.215 Adverse effect of selective serotonin and norepinephrine reuptake inhibitors** UPD

     ✓7ᵗʰ **T43.216 Underdosing of selective serotonin and norepinephrine reuptake inhibitors** UPD

   ✓6ᵗʰ **T43.22 Poisoning by, adverse effect of and underdosing of selective serotonin reuptake inhibitors**
       Poisoning by, adverse effect of and underdosing of SSRI antidepressants

     ✓7ᵗʰ **T43.221 Poisoning by selective serotonin reuptake inhibitors, accidental (unintentional)**

     ² ✓7ᵗʰ **T43.222 Poisoning by selective serotonin reuptake inhibitors, intentional self-harm** HCC Rx ESR COM

     ✓7ᵗʰ **T43.223 Poisoning by selective serotonin reuptake inhibitors, assault**

     ✓7ᵗʰ **T43.224 Poisoning by selective serotonin reuptake inhibitors, undetermined**

     ✓7ᵗʰ **T43.225 Adverse effect of selective serotonin reuptake inhibitors** UPD
           AHA: 2022,2Q,11

     ✓7ᵗʰ **T43.226 Underdosing of selective serotonin reuptake inhibitors** UPD

   ✓6ᵗʰ **T43.29 Poisoning by, adverse effect of and underdosing of other antidepressants**

     ✓7ᵗʰ **T43.291 Poisoning by other antidepressants, accidental (unintentional)**
           Poisoning by other antidepressants NOS

     ² ✓7ᵗʰ **T43.292 Poisoning by other antidepressants, intentional self-harm** HCC Rx ESR COM

     ✓7ᵗʰ **T43.293 Poisoning by other antidepressants, assault**

     ✓7ᵗʰ **T43.294 Poisoning by other antidepressants, undetermined**

     ✓7ᵗʰ **T43.295 Adverse effect of other antidepressants** UPD

     ✓7ᵗʰ **T43.296 Underdosing of other antidepressants** UPD

✓5ᵗʰ T43.3 Poisoning by, adverse effect of and underdosing of phenothiazine antipsychotics and neuroleptics

  ✓6ᵗʰ T43.3X Poisoning by, adverse effect of and underdosing of phenothiazine antipsychotics and neuroleptics

    ✓7ᵗʰ T43.3X1 Poisoning by phenothiazine antipsychotics and neuroleptics, accidental (unintentional)
      Poisoning by phenothiazine antipsychotics and neuroleptics NOS

    ² **✓7ᵗʰ T43.3X2 Poisoning by phenothiazine antipsychotics and neuroleptics, intentional self-harm** HCC Rx ESR COM

    ✓7ᵗʰ T43.3X3 Poisoning by phenothiazine antipsychotics and neuroleptics, assault

    ✓7ᵗʰ T43.3X4 Poisoning by phenothiazine antipsychotics and neuroleptics, undetermined

    ✓7ᵗʰ T43.3X5 Adverse effect of phenothiazine antipsychotics and neuroleptics UPD

    ✓7ᵗʰ T43.3X6 Underdosing of phenothiazine antipsychotics and neuroleptics UPD

✓5ᵗʰ T43.4 Poisoning by, adverse effect of and underdosing of butyrophenone and thiothixene neuroleptics

  ✓6ᵗʰ T43.4X Poisoning by, adverse effect of and underdosing of butyrophenone and thiothixene neuroleptics

    ✓7ᵗʰ T43.4X1 Poisoning by butyrophenone and thiothixene neuroleptics, accidental (unintentional)
      Poisoning by butyrophenone and thiothixene neuroleptics NOS

    ² **✓7ᵗʰ T43.4X2 Poisoning by butyrophenone and thiothixene neuroleptics, intentional self-harm** HCC Rx ESR COM

    ✓7ᵗʰ T43.4X3 Poisoning by butyrophenone and thiothixene neuroleptics, assault

    ✓7ᵗʰ T43.4X4 Poisoning by butyrophenone and thiothixene neuroleptics, undetermined

    ✓7ᵗʰ T43.4X5 Adverse effect of butyrophenone and thiothixene neuroleptics UPD

    ✓7ᵗʰ T43.4X6 Underdosing of butyrophenone and thiothixene neuroleptics UPD

✓5ᵗʰ T43.5 Poisoning by, adverse effect of and underdosing of other and unspecified antipsychotics and neuroleptics

  EXCLUDES 1   poisoning by, adverse effect of and underdosing of rauwolfia (T46.5-)

  ✓6ᵗʰ T43.50 Poisoning by, adverse effect of and underdosing of unspecified antipsychotics and neuroleptics

    ✓7ᵗʰ T43.501 Poisoning by unspecified antipsychotics and neuroleptics, accidental (unintentional)
      Poisoning by antipsychotics and neuroleptics NOS

    ² **✓7ᵗʰ T43.502 Poisoning by unspecified antipsychotics and neuroleptics, intentional self-harm** HCC Rx ESR COM

    ✓7ᵗʰ T43.503 Poisoning by unspecified antipsychotics and neuroleptics, assault

    ✓7ᵗʰ T43.504 Poisoning by unspecified antipsychotics and neuroleptics, undetermined

    ✓7ᵗʰ T43.505 Adverse effect of unspecified antipsychotics and neuroleptics UPD

    ✓7ᵗʰ T43.506 Underdosing of unspecified antipsychotics and neuroleptics UPD

  ✓6ᵗʰ T43.59 Poisoning by, adverse effect of and underdosing of other antipsychotics and neuroleptics
    AHA: 2017,1Q,40

    ✓7ᵗʰ T43.591 Poisoning by other antipsychotics and neuroleptics, accidental (unintentional)
      Poisoning by other antipsychotics and neuroleptics NOS

    ² **✓7ᵗʰ T43.592 Poisoning by other antipsychotics and neuroleptics, intentional self-harm** HCC Rx ESR COM

    ✓7ᵗʰ T43.593 Poisoning by other antipsychotics and neuroleptics, assault

    ✓7ᵗʰ T43.594 Poisoning by other antipsychotics and neuroleptics, undetermined

    ✓7ᵗʰ T43.595 Adverse effect of other antipsychotics and neuroleptics UPD
      AHA: 2022,2Q,11

    ✓7ᵗʰ T43.596 Underdosing of other antipsychotics and neuroleptics UPD

✓5ᵗʰ T43.6 Poisoning by, adverse effect of and underdosing of psychostimulants

  EXCLUDES 1   poisoning by, adverse effect of and underdosing of cocaine (T40.5-)

  ✓6ᵗʰ T43.60 Poisoning by, adverse effect of and underdosing of unspecified psychostimulant

    ¹ **✓7ᵗʰ T43.601 Poisoning by unspecified psychostimulants, accidental (unintentional)** HCC ESR COM
      Poisoning by psychostimulants NOS

    ² **✓7ᵗʰ T43.602 Poisoning by unspecified psychostimulants, intentional self-harm** HCC Rx ESR COM

    ✓7ᵗʰ T43.603 Poisoning by unspecified psychostimulants, assault

    ¹ **✓7ᵗʰ T43.604 Poisoning by unspecified psychostimulants, undetermined** HCC ESR COM

    ✓7ᵗʰ T43.605 Adverse effect of unspecified psychostimulants UPD

    ✓7ᵗʰ T43.606 Underdosing of unspecified psychostimulants UPD

  ✓6ᵗʰ T43.61 Poisoning by, adverse effect of and underdosing of caffeine

    ¹ **✓7ᵗʰ T43.611 Poisoning by caffeine, accidental (unintentional)** HCC ESR COM
      Poisoning by caffeine NOS

    ² **✓7ᵗʰ T43.612 Poisoning by caffeine, intentional self-harm** HCC Rx ESR COM

    ✓7ᵗʰ T43.613 Poisoning by caffeine, assault

    ¹ **✓7ᵗʰ T43.614 Poisoning by caffeine, undetermined** HCC ESR COM

    ✓7ᵗʰ T43.615 Adverse effect of caffeine UPD

    ✓7ᵗʰ T43.616 Underdosing of caffeine UPD

  ✓6ᵗʰ T43.62 Poisoning by, adverse effect of and underdosing of amphetamines
    ~~Poisoning by, adverse effect of and underdosing of methamphetamines~~

    ¹ **✓7ᵗʰ T43.621 Poisoning by amphetamines, accidental (unintentional)** HCC ESR COM
      Poisoning by amphetamines NOS
      AHA: 2021,3Q,8

    ² **✓7ᵗʰ T43.622 Poisoning by amphetamines, intentional self-harm** HCC Rx ESR COM

    ✓7ᵗʰ T43.623 Poisoning by amphetamines, assault

    ¹ **✓7ᵗʰ T43.624 Poisoning by amphetamines, undetermined** HCC ESR COM

    ✓7ᵗʰ T43.625 Adverse effect of amphetamines UPD

    ✓7ᵗʰ T43.626 Underdosing of amphetamines UPD

  ✓6ᵗʰ T43.63 Poisoning by, adverse effect of and underdosing of methylphenidate

    ¹ **✓7ᵗʰ T43.631 Poisoning by methylphenidate, accidental (unintentional)** HCC ESR COM
      Poisoning by methylphenidate NOS

    ² **✓7ᵗʰ T43.632 Poisoning by methylphenidate, intentional self-harm** HCC Rx ESR COM

    ✓7ᵗʰ T43.633 Poisoning by methylphenidate, assault

    ¹ **✓7ᵗʰ T43.634 Poisoning by methylphenidate, undetermined** HCC ESR COM

    ✓7ᵗʰ T43.635 Adverse effect of methylphenidate UPD

    ✓7ᵗʰ T43.636 Underdosing of methylphenidate UPD

  ✓6ᵗʰ T43.64 Poisoning by ecstasy
    Poisoning by MDMA
    Poisoning by 3,4-methylenedioxymethamphetamine
    AHA: 2018,4Q,30-31

    ¹ **✓7ᵗʰ T43.641 Poisoning by ecstasy, accidental (unintentional)** HCC ESR COM
      Poisoning by ecstasy NOS

    ² **✓7ᵗʰ T43.642 Poisoning by ecstasy, intentional self-harm** HCC Rx ESR COM

    ✓7ᵗʰ T43.643 Poisoning by ecstasy, assault

    ¹ **✓7ᵗʰ T43.644 Poisoning by ecstasy, undetermined** HCC ESR COM

HCC CMS-HCC   Rx Rx HCC   ESR ESRD HCC   COM Commercial HCC   N Newborn: 0   P Pediatric: 0-17   M Maternity: 9-64   A Adult: 15-124

- ✓6th **T43.65** **Poisoning by, adverse effect of and underdosing of** methamphetamines
  - ✓7th **T43.651** **Poisoning by methamphetamines accidental (unintentional)**
    Poisoning by methamphetamines NOS
  - ✓7th **T43.652** **Poisoning by methamphetamines intentional self-harm**
  - ✓7th **T43.653** **Poisoning by methamphetamines,** assault
  - ✓7th **T43.654** **Poisoning by methamphetamines, undetermined**
  - ✓7th **T43.655** **Adverse effect of methamphetamines**
  - ✓7th **T43.656** **Underdosing of methamphetamines**

- ✓6th **T43.69** **Poisoning by, adverse effect of and underdosing of other psychostimulants**
  - 1 ✓7th **T43.691** **Poisoning by other psychostimulants, accidental (unintentional)** HCC ESR COM
    Poisoning by other psychostimulants NOS
  - 2 ✓7th **T43.692** **Poisoning by other psychostimulants, intentional self-harm** HCC Rx ESR COM
  - ✓7th **T43.693** **Poisoning by other psychostimulants, assault**
  - 1 ✓7th **T43.694** **Poisoning by other psychostimulants, undetermined** HCC ESR COM
  - ✓7th **T43.695** **Adverse effect of other psychostimulants** UPD
  - ✓7th **T43.696** **Underdosing of other psychostimulants** UPD

- ✓5th **T43.8** **Poisoning by, adverse effect of and underdosing of other psychotropic drugs**
  - ✓6th **T43.8X** **Poisoning by, adverse effect of and underdosing of other psychotropic drugs**
    - ✓7th **T43.8X1** **Poisoning by other psychotropic drugs, accidental (unintentional)**
      Poisoning by other psychotropic drugs NOS
    - 2 ✓7th **T43.8X2** **Poisoning by other psychotropic drugs, intentional self-harm** HCC Rx ESR COM
    - ✓7th **T43.8X3** **Poisoning by other psychotropic drugs, assault**
    - ✓7th **T43.8X4** **Poisoning by other psychotropic drugs, undetermined**
    - ✓7th **T43.8X5** **Adverse effect of other psychotropic drugs** UPD
    - ✓7th **T43.8X6** **Underdosing of other psychotropic drugs** UPD

- ✓5th **T43.9** **Poisoning by, adverse effect of and underdosing of unspecified psychotropic drug**
  - ✓x7th **T43.91** **Poisoning by unspecified psychotropic drug, accidental (unintentional)**
    Poisoning by psychotropic drug NOS
  - 2 ✓x7th **T43.92** **Poisoning by unspecified psychotropic drug, intentional self-harm** HCC Rx ESR COM
  - ✓x7th **T43.93** **Poisoning by unspecified psychotropic drug,** assault
  - ✓x7th **T43.94** **Poisoning by unspecified psychotropic drug, undetermined**
  - ✓x7th **T43.95** **Adverse effect of unspecified psychotropic drug** UPD
  - ✓x7th **T43.96** **Underdosing of unspecified psychotropic drug** UPD

- ✓4th **T44** **Poisoning by, adverse effect of and underdosing of drugs primarily affecting the autonomic nervous system**

  The appropriate 7th character is to be added to each code from category T44.
  A   initial encounter
  D   subsequent encounter
  S   sequela

  - ✓5th **T44.0** **Poisoning by, adverse effect of and underdosing of anticholinesterase agents**
    - ✓6th **T44.0X** **Poisoning by, adverse effect of and underdosing of anticholinesterase agents**
      - ✓7th **T44.0X1** **Poisoning by anticholinesterase agents, accidental (unintentional)**
        Poisoning by anticholinesterase agents NOS
      - 2 ✓7th **T44.0X2** **Poisoning by anticholinesterase agents, intentional self-harm** HCC Rx ESR COM
      - ✓7th **T44.0X3** **Poisoning by anticholinesterase agents, assault**
      - ✓7th **T44.0X4** **Poisoning by anticholinesterase agents, undetermined**

- ✓7th **T44.0X5** **Adverse effect of anticholinesterase agents** UPD
- ✓7th **T44.0X6** **Underdosing of anticholinesterase agents** UPD

- ✓5th **T44.1** **Poisoning by, adverse effect of and underdosing of other parasympathomimetics [cholinergics]**
  - ✓6th **T44.1X** **Poisoning by, adverse effect of and underdosing of other parasympathomimetics [cholinergics]**
    - ✓7th **T44.1X1** **Poisoning by other parasympathomimetics [cholinergics], accidental (unintentional)**
      Poisoning by other parasympathomimetics [cholinergics] NOS
    - 2 ✓7th **T44.1X2** **Poisoning by other parasympathomimetics [cholinergics], intentional self-harm** HCC Rx ESR COM
    - ✓7th **T44.1X3** **Poisoning by other parasympathomimetics [cholinergics], assault**
    - ✓7th **T44.1X4** **Poisoning by other parasympathomimetics [cholinergics], undetermined**
    - ✓7th **T44.1X5** **Adverse effect of other parasympathomimetics [cholinergics]** UPD
    - ✓7th **T44.1X6** **Underdosing of other parasympathomimetics [cholinergics]** UPD

- ✓5th **T44.2** **Poisoning by, adverse effect of and underdosing of ganglionic blocking drugs**
  - ✓6th **T44.2X** **Poisoning by, adverse effect of and underdosing of** ganglionic blocking drugs
    - ✓7th **T44.2X1** **Poisoning by ganglionic blocking drugs, accidental (unintentional)**
      Poisoning by ganglionic blocking drugs NOS
    - 2 ✓7th **T44.2X2** **Poisoning by ganglionic blocking drugs, intentional self-harm** HCC Rx ESR COM
    - ✓7th **T44.2X3** **Poisoning by ganglionic blocking drugs, assault**
    - ✓7th **T44.2X4** **Poisoning by ganglionic blocking drugs, undetermined**
    - ✓7th **T44.2X5** **Adverse effect of ganglionic blocking drugs** UPD
    - ✓7th **T44.2X6** **Underdosing of ganglionic blocking drugs** UPD

- ✓5th **T44.3** **Poisoning by, adverse effect of and underdosing of other parasympatholytics [anticholinergics and antimuscarinics] and spasmolytics**
  Poisoning by, adverse effect of and underdosing of papaverine
  - ✓6th **T44.3X** **Poisoning by, adverse effect of and underdosing of other parasympatholytics [anticholinergics and antimuscarinics] and spasmolytics**
    - ✓7th **T44.3X1** **Poisoning by other parasympatholytics [anticholinergics and antimuscarinics] and spasmolytics, accidental (unintentional)**
      Poisoning by other parasympatholytics [anticholinergics and antimuscarinics] and spasmolytics NOS
    - 2 ✓7th **T44.3X2** **Poisoning by other parasympatholytics [anticholinergics and antimuscarinics] and spasmolytics, intentional self-harm** HCC Rx ESR COM
    - ✓7th **T44.3X3** **Poisoning by other parasympatholytics [anticholinergics and antimuscarinics] and spasmolytics, assault**
    - ✓7th **T44.3X4** **Poisoning by other parasympatholytics [anticholinergics and antimuscarinics] and spasmolytics, undetermined**
    - ✓7th **T44.3X5** **Adverse effect of other parasympatholytics [anticholinergics and antimuscarinics] and spasmolytics** UPD
    - ✓7th **T44.3X6** **Underdosing of other parasympatholytics [anticholinergics and antimuscarinics] and spasmolytics** UPD

✓5ᵗʰ **T44.4** **Poisoning by, adverse effect of and underdosing of predominantly alpha-adrenoreceptor agonists**

Poisoning by, adverse effect of and underdosing of metaraminol

✓6ᵗʰ **T44.4X** **Poisoning by, adverse effect of and underdosing of** predominantly alpha-adrenoreceptor agonists

     ✓7ᵗʰ **T44.4X1** **Poisoning by predominantly alpha-adrenoreceptor agonists, accidental (unintentional)**

         Poisoning by predominantly alpha-adrenoreceptor agonists NOS

     ² ✓7ᵗʰ **T44.4X2** **Poisoning by predominantly alpha-adrenoreceptor agonists, intentional self-harm** `HCC` `Rx` `ESR` `COM`

     ✓7ᵗʰ **T44.4X3** **Poisoning by predominantly alpha-adrenoreceptor agonists, assault**

     ✓7ᵗʰ **T44.4X4** **Poisoning by predominantly alpha-adrenoreceptor agonists, undetermined**

     ✓7ᵗʰ **T44.4X5** **Adverse effect of predominantly alpha-adrenoreceptor agonists** `UPD`

     ✓7ᵗʰ **T44.4X6** **Underdosing of predominantly alpha-adrenoreceptor agonists** `UPD`

✓5ᵗʰ **T44.5** **Poisoning by, adverse effect of and underdosing of predominantly beta-adrenoreceptor agonists**

EXCLUDES 1   *poisoning by, adverse effect of and underdosing of beta-adrenoreceptor agonists used in asthma therapy (T48.6-)*

✓6ᵗʰ **T44.5X** **Poisoning by, adverse effect of and underdosing of** predominantly beta-adrenoreceptor agonists

     ✓7ᵗʰ **T44.5X1** **Poisoning by predominantly beta-adrenoreceptor agonists, accidental (unintentional)**

         Poisoning by predominantly beta-adrenoreceptor agonists NOS

     ² ✓7ᵗʰ **T44.5X2** **Poisoning by predominantly beta-adrenoreceptor agonists, intentional self-harm** `HCC` `Rx` `ESR` `COM`

     ✓7ᵗʰ **T44.5X3** **Poisoning by predominantly beta-adrenoreceptor agonists, assault**

     ✓7ᵗʰ **T44.5X4** **Poisoning by predominantly beta-adrenoreceptor agonists, undetermined**

     ✓7ᵗʰ **T44.5X5** **Adverse effect of predominantly beta-adrenoreceptor agonists** `UPD`

     ✓7ᵗʰ **T44.5X6** **Underdosing of predominantly beta-adrenoreceptor agonists** `UPD`

✓5ᵗʰ **T44.6** **Poisoning by, adverse effect of and underdosing of alpha-adrenoreceptor antagonists**

EXCLUDES 1   *poisoning by, adverse effect of and underdosing of ergot alkaloids (T48.0)*

✓6ᵗʰ **T44.6X** **Poisoning by, adverse effect of and underdosing of** alpha-adrenoreceptor antagonists

     ✓7ᵗʰ **T44.6X1** **Poisoning by alpha-adrenoreceptor antagonists, accidental (unintentional)**

         Poisoning by alpha-adrenoreceptor antagonists NOS

     ² ✓7ᵗʰ **T44.6X2** **Poisoning by alpha-adrenoreceptor antagonists, intentional self-harm** `HCC` `Rx` `ESR` `COM`

     ✓7ᵗʰ **T44.6X3** **Poisoning by alpha-adrenoreceptor antagonists, assault**

     ✓7ᵗʰ **T44.6X4** **Poisoning by alpha-adrenoreceptor antagonists, undetermined**

     ✓7ᵗʰ **T44.6X5** **Adverse effect of alpha-adrenoreceptor antagonists** `UPD`

     ✓7ᵗʰ **T44.6X6** **Underdosing of alpha-adrenoreceptor antagonists** `UPD`

✓5ᵗʰ **T44.7** **Poisoning by, adverse effect of and underdosing of beta-adrenoreceptor antagonists**

✓6ᵗʰ **T44.7X** **Poisoning by, adverse effect of and underdosing of** beta-adrenoreceptor antagonists

     ✓7ᵗʰ **T44.7X1** **Poisoning by beta-adrenoreceptor antagonists, accidental (unintentional)**

         Poisoning by beta-adrenoreceptor antagonists NOS

     ² ✓7ᵗʰ **T44.7X2** **Poisoning by beta-adrenoreceptor antagonists, intentional self-harm** `HCC` `Rx` `ESR` `COM`

     ✓7ᵗʰ **T44.7X3** **Poisoning by beta-adrenoreceptor antagonists, assault**

     ✓7ᵗʰ **T44.7X4** **Poisoning by beta-adrenoreceptor antagonists, undetermined**

     ✓7ᵗʰ **T44.7X5** **Adverse effect of beta-adrenoreceptor antagonists** `UPD`

     ✓7ᵗʰ **T44.7X6** **Underdosing of beta-adrenoreceptor antagonists** `UPD`

✓5ᵗʰ **T44.8** **Poisoning by, adverse effect of and underdosing of centrally-acting and adrenergic-neuron- blocking agents**

EXCLUDES 2   *poisoning by, adverse effect of and underdosing of clonidine (T46.5)*

         poisoning by, adverse effect of and underdosing of guanethidine (T46.5)

✓6ᵗʰ **T44.8X** **Poisoning by, adverse effect of and underdosing of** centrally-acting and adrenergic- neuron-blocking agents

     ✓7ᵗʰ **T44.8X1** **Poisoning by centrally-acting and adrenergic-neuron-blocking agents, accidental (unintentional)**

         Poisoning by centrally-acting and adrenergic-neuron-blocking agents NOS

     ² ✓7ᵗʰ **T44.8X2** **Poisoning by centrally-acting and adrenergic-neuron-blocking agents, intentional self-harm** `HCC` `Rx` `ESR` `COM`

     ✓7ᵗʰ **T44.8X3** **Poisoning by centrally-acting and adrenergic-neuron-blocking agents, assault**

     ✓7ᵗʰ **T44.8X4** **Poisoning by centrally-acting and adrenergic-neuron-blocking agents, undetermined**

     ✓7ᵗʰ **T44.8X5** **Adverse effect of centrally-acting and adrenergic-neuron-blocking agents** `UPD`

     ✓7ᵗʰ **T44.8X6** **Underdosing of centrally-acting and adrenergic-neuron-blocking agents** `UPD`

✓5ᵗʰ **T44.9** **Poisoning by, adverse effect of and underdosing of other and unspecified drugs primarily affecting the autonomic nervous system**

Poisoning by, adverse effect of and underdosing of drug stimulating both alpha and beta-adrenoreceptors

✓6ᵗʰ **T44.90** **Poisoning by, adverse effect of and underdosing of unspecified drugs primarily affecting the autonomic nervous system**

     ✓7ᵗʰ **T44.901** **Poisoning by unspecified drugs primarily affecting the autonomic nervous system, accidental (unintentional)**

         Poisoning by unspecified drugs primarily affecting the autonomic nervous system NOS

     ² ✓7ᵗʰ **T44.902** **Poisoning by unspecified drugs primarily affecting the autonomic nervous system, intentional self-harm** `HCC` `Rx` `ESR` `COM`

     ✓7ᵗʰ **T44.903** **Poisoning by unspecified drugs primarily affecting the autonomic nervous system, assault**

     ✓7ᵗʰ **T44.904** **Poisoning by unspecified drugs primarily affecting the autonomic nervous system, undetermined**

     ✓7ᵗʰ **T44.905** **Adverse effect of unspecified drugs primarily affecting the autonomic nervous system** `UPD`

     ✓7ᵗʰ **T44.906** **Underdosing of unspecified drugs primarily affecting the autonomic nervous system** `UPD`

✓6ᵗʰ **T44.99** **Poisoning by, adverse effect of and underdosing of other drugs primarily affecting the autonomic nervous system**

     ✓7ᵗʰ **T44.991** **Poisoning by other drug primarily affecting the autonomic nervous system, accidental (unintentional)**

         Poisoning by other drugs primarily affecting the autonomic nervous system NOS

     ² ✓7ᵗʰ **T44.992** **Poisoning by other drug primarily affecting the autonomic nervous system, intentional self-harm** `HCC` `Rx` `ESR` `COM`

     ✓7ᵗʰ **T44.993** **Poisoning by other drug primarily affecting the autonomic nervous system, assault**

     ✓7ᵗʰ **T44.994** **Poisoning by other drug primarily affecting the autonomic nervous system, undetermined**

`HCC` CMS-HCC   `Rx` Rx HCC   `ESR` ESRD HCC   `COM` Commercial HCC   N Newborn: 0   P Pediatric: 0-17   M Maternity: 9-64   A Adult: 15-124

√7ᵗʰ **T44.995** Adverse effect of other drug primarily affecting the autonomic nervous system ᴜᴘᴅ

√7ᵗʰ **T44.996** Underdosing of other drug primarily affecting the autonomic nervous system ᴜᴘᴅ

√4ᵗʰ **T45** Poisoning by, adverse effect of and underdosing of primarily systemic and hematological agents, not elsewhere classified

> The appropriate 7th character is to be added to each code from category T45.
> A   initial encounter
> D   subsequent encounter
> S   sequela

√5ᵗʰ **T45.0** Poisoning by, adverse effect of and underdosing of antiallergic and antiemetic drugs

> ᴇxᴄʟᴜᴅᴇs 1   poisoning by, adverse effect of and underdosing of phenothiazine-based neuroleptics (T43.3)

√6ᵗʰ **T45.0X** Poisoning by, adverse effect of and underdosing of antiallergic and antiemetic drugs

√7ᵗʰ **T45.0X1** Poisoning by antiallergic and antiemetic drugs, accidental (unintentional)
> Poisoning by antiallergic and antiemetic drugs NOS

² √7ᵗʰ **T45.0X2** Poisoning by antiallergic and antiemetic drugs, intentional self-harm ʜᴄᴄ ʀx ᴇsʀ ᴄᴏᴍ

√7ᵗʰ **T45.0X3** Poisoning by antiallergic and antiemetic drugs, assault

√7ᵗʰ **T45.0X4** Poisoning by antiallergic and antiemetic drugs, undetermined

√7ᵗʰ **T45.0X5** Adverse effect of antiallergic and antiemetic drugs ᴜᴘᴅ

√7ᵗʰ **T45.0X6** Underdosing of antiallergic and antiemetic drugs ᴜᴘᴅ

√5ᵗʰ **T45.1** Poisoning by, adverse effect of and underdosing of antineoplastic and immunosuppressive drugs

> ᴇxᴄʟᴜᴅᴇs 1   poisoning by, adverse effect of and underdosing of tamoxifen (T38.6)

> **AHA:** 2019,1Q,17,20; 2014,4Q,22

√6ᵗʰ **T45.1X** Poisoning by, adverse effect of and underdosing of antineoplastic and immunosuppressive drugs

√7ᵗʰ **T45.1X1** Poisoning by antineoplastic and immunosuppressive drugs, accidental (unintentional)
> Poisoning by antineoplastic and immunosuppressive drugs NOS

² √7ᵗʰ **T45.1X2** Poisoning by antineoplastic and immunosuppressive drugs, intentional self-harm ʜᴄᴄ ʀx ᴇsʀ ᴄᴏᴍ

√7ᵗʰ **T45.1X3** Poisoning by antineoplastic and immunosuppressive drugs, assault

√7ᵗʰ **T45.1X4** Poisoning by antineoplastic and immunosuppressive drugs, undetermined

√7ᵗʰ **T45.1X5** Adverse effect of antineoplastic and immunosuppressive drugs ᴜᴘᴅ
> **AHA:** 2021,3Q,4; 2020,4Q,11; 2020,3Q,22; 2019,2Q,24,28

√7ᵗʰ **T45.1X6** Underdosing of antineoplastic and immunosuppressive drugs ᴜᴘᴅ

√5ᵗʰ **T45.2** Poisoning by, adverse effect of and underdosing of vitamins

> ᴇxᴄʟᴜᴅᴇs 2   poisoning by, adverse effect of and underdosing of iron (T45.4)
> poisoning by, adverse effect of and underdosing of nicotinic acid (derivatives) (T46.7)
> poisoning by, adverse effect of and underdosing of vitamin K (T45.7)

√6ᵗʰ **T45.2X** Poisoning by, adverse effect of and underdosing of vitamins

√7ᵗʰ **T45.2X1** Poisoning by vitamins, accidental (unintentional)
> Poisoning by vitamins NOS

² √7ᵗʰ **T45.2X2** Poisoning by vitamins, intentional self-harm ʜᴄᴄ ʀx ᴇsʀ ᴄᴏᴍ

√7ᵗʰ **T45.2X3** Poisoning by vitamins, assault

√7ᵗʰ **T45.2X4** Poisoning by vitamins, undetermined

√7ᵗʰ **T45.2X5** Adverse effect of vitamins ᴜᴘᴅ

√7ᵗʰ **T45.2X6** Underdosing of vitamins ᴜᴘᴅ
> ᴇxᴄʟᴜᴅᴇs 1   vitamin deficiencies (E50-E56)

√5ᵗʰ **T45.3** Poisoning by, adverse effect of and underdosing of enzymes

√6ᵗʰ **T45.3X** Poisoning by, adverse effect of and underdosing of enzymes

√7ᵗʰ **T45.3X1** Poisoning by enzymes, accidental (unintentional)
> Poisoning by enzymes NOS

² √7ᵗʰ **T45.3X2** Poisoning by enzymes, intentional self-harm ʜᴄᴄ ʀx ᴇsʀ ᴄᴏᴍ

√7ᵗʰ **T45.3X3** Poisoning by enzymes, assault

√7ᵗʰ **T45.3X4** Poisoning by enzymes, undetermined

√7ᵗʰ **T45.3X5** Adverse effect of enzymes ᴜᴘᴅ

√7ᵗʰ **T45.3X6** Underdosing of enzymes ᴜᴘᴅ

√5ᵗʰ **T45.4** Poisoning by, adverse effect of and underdosing of iron and its compounds

√6ᵗʰ **T45.4X** Poisoning by, adverse effect of and underdosing of iron and its compounds

√7ᵗʰ **T45.4X1** Poisoning by iron and its compounds, accidental (unintentional)
> Poisoning by iron and its compounds NOS

² √7ᵗʰ **T45.4X2** Poisoning by iron and its compounds, intentional self-harm ʜᴄᴄ ʀx ᴇsʀ ᴄᴏᴍ

√7ᵗʰ **T45.4X3** Poisoning by iron and its compounds, assault

√7ᵗʰ **T45.4X4** Poisoning by iron and its compounds, undetermined

√7ᵗʰ **T45.4X5** Adverse effect of iron and its compounds ᴜᴘᴅ

√7ᵗʰ **T45.4X6** Underdosing of iron and its compounds ᴜᴘᴅ
> ᴇxᴄʟᴜᴅᴇs 1   iron deficiency (E61.1)

√5ᵗʰ **T45.5** Poisoning by, adverse effect of and underdosing of anticoagulants and antithrombotic drugs

√6ᵗʰ **T45.51** Poisoning by, adverse effect of and underdosing of anticoagulants

√7ᵗʰ **T45.511** Poisoning by anticoagulants, accidental (unintentional)
> Poisoning by anticoagulants NOS

² √7ᵗʰ **T45.512** Poisoning by anticoagulants, intentional self-harm ʜᴄᴄ ʀx ᴇsʀ ᴄᴏᴍ

√7ᵗʰ **T45.513** Poisoning by anticoagulants, assault

√7ᵗʰ **T45.514** Poisoning by anticoagulants, undetermined

Heparin √7ᵗʰ **T45.515** Adverse effect of anticoagulants ᴜᴘᴅ
> **AHA:** 2021,1Q,4; 2016,1Q,14; 2013,2Q,34

√7ᵗʰ **T45.516** Underdosing of anticoagulants ᴜᴘᴅ

√6ᵗʰ **T45.52** Poisoning by, adverse effect of and underdosing of antithrombotic drugs
> Poisoning by, adverse effect of and underdosing of antiplatelet drugs
> ᴇxᴄʟᴜᴅᴇs 2   poisoning by, adverse effect of and underdosing of aspirin (T39.01-)
> poisoning by, adverse effect of and underdosing of acetylsalicylic acid (T39.01-)

√7ᵗʰ **T45.521** Poisoning by antithrombotic drugs, accidental (unintentional)
> Poisoning by antithrombotic drug NOS

² √7ᵗʰ **T45.522** Poisoning by antithrombotic drugs, intentional self-harm ʜᴄᴄ ʀx ᴇsʀ ᴄᴏᴍ

√7ᵗʰ **T45.523** Poisoning by antithrombotic drugs, assault

√7ᵗʰ **T45.524** Poisoning by antithrombotic drugs, undetermined

√7ᵗʰ **T45.525** Adverse effect of antithrombotic drugs ᴜᴘᴅ
> **AHA:** 2016,1Q,15

√7ᵗʰ **T45.526** Underdosing of antithrombotic drugs ᴜᴘᴅ

Chapter 19. Injury, Poisoning and Certain Other Consequences of External Causes

T45.6–T46.0X1

√5ᵗʰ **T45.6 Poisoning by, adverse effect of and underdosing of fibrinolysis-affecting drugs**

√6ᵗʰ **T45.60 Poisoning by, adverse effect of and underdosing of unspecified fibrinolysis-affecting drugs**

√7ᵗʰ **T45.601 Poisoning by unspecified fibrinolysis-affecting drugs,** accidental (unintentional)

Poisoning by fibrinolysis-affecting drug NOS

² √7ᵗʰ **T45.602 Poisoning by unspecified fibrinolysis-affecting drugs,** intentional self-harm   HCC Rx ESR COM

√7ᵗʰ **T45.603 Poisoning by unspecified fibrinolysis-affecting drugs,** assault

√7ᵗʰ **T45.604 Poisoning by unspecified fibrinolysis-affecting drugs,** undetermined

√7ᵗʰ **T45.605 Adverse effect of unspecified fibrinolysis-affecting drugs**   UPD

√7ᵗʰ **T45.606 Underdosing of unspecified fibrinolysis-affecting drugs**   UPD

√6ᵗʰ **T45.61 Poisoning by, adverse effect of and underdosing of thrombolytic drugs**

√7ᵗʰ **T45.611 Poisoning by thrombolytic drug,** accidental (unintentional)

Poisoning by thrombolytic drug NOS

² √7ᵗʰ **T45.612 Poisoning by thrombolytic drug,** intentional self-harm   HCC Rx ESR COM

√7ᵗʰ **T45.613 Poisoning by thrombolytic drug,** assault

√7ᵗʰ **T45.614 Poisoning by thrombolytic drug,** undetermined

√7ᵗʰ **T45.615 Adverse effect of thrombolytic drugs**   UPD

AHA: 2017,2Q,9

√7ᵗʰ **T45.616 Underdosing of thrombolytic drugs**   UPD

√6ᵗʰ **T45.62 Poisoning by, adverse effect of and underdosing of hemostatic drugs**

√7ᵗʰ **T45.621 Poisoning by hemostatic drug,** accidental (unintentional)

Poisoning by hemostatic drug NOS

² √7ᵗʰ **T45.622 Poisoning by hemostatic drug,** intentional self-harm   HCC Rx ESR COM

√7ᵗʰ **T45.623 Poisoning by hemostatic drug,** assault

√7ᵗʰ **T45.624 Poisoning by hemostatic drug,** undetermined

√7ᵗʰ **T45.625 Adverse effect of hemostatic drug**   UPD

√7ᵗʰ **T45.626 Underdosing of hemostatic drugs**   UPD

√6ᵗʰ **T45.69 Poisoning by, adverse effect of and underdosing of other fibrinolysis-affecting drugs**

√7ᵗʰ **T45.691 Poisoning by other fibrinolysis-affecting drugs,** accidental (unintentional)

Poisoning by other fibrinolysis-affecting drug NOS

² √7ᵗʰ **T45.692 Poisoning by other fibrinolysis-affecting drugs,** intentional self-harm   HCC Rx ESR COM

√7ᵗʰ **T45.693 Poisoning by other fibrinolysis-affecting drugs,** assault

√7ᵗʰ **T45.694 Poisoning by other fibrinolysis-affecting drugs,** undetermined

√7ᵗʰ **T45.695 Adverse effect of other fibrinolysis-affecting drugs**   UPD

√7ᵗʰ **T45.696 Underdosing of other fibrinolysis-affecting drugs**   UPD

√5ᵗʰ **T45.7 Poisoning by, adverse effect of and underdosing of anticoagulant antagonists, vitamin K and other coagulants**

√6ᵗʰ **T45.7X Poisoning by, adverse effect of and underdosing of anticoagulant antagonists, vitamin K and other coagulants**

√7ᵗʰ **T45.7X1 Poisoning by anticoagulant antagonists, vitamin K and other coagulants,** accidental (unintentional)

Poisoning by anticoagulant antagonists, vitamin K and other coagulants NOS

² √7ᵗʰ **T45.7X2 Poisoning by anticoagulant antagonists, vitamin K and other coagulants,** intentional self-harm   HCC Rx ESR COM

√7ᵗʰ **T45.7X3 Poisoning by anticoagulant antagonists, vitamin K and other coagulants,** assault

√7ᵗʰ **T45.7X4 Poisoning by anticoagulant antagonists, vitamin K and other coagulants,** undetermined

√7ᵗʰ **T45.7X5 Adverse effect of anticoagulant antagonists, vitamin K and other coagulants**   UPD

√7ᵗʰ **T45.7X6 Underdosing of anticoagulant antagonist, vitamin K and other coagulants**   UPD

EXCLUDES 1   vitamin K deficiency (E56.1)

√5ᵗʰ **T45.8 Poisoning by, adverse effect of and underdosing of other primarily systemic and hematological agents**

Poisoning by, adverse effect of and underdosing of liver preparations and other antianemic agents

Poisoning by, adverse effect of and underdosing of natural blood and blood products

Poisoning by, adverse effect of and underdosing of plasma substitute

EXCLUDES 2   poisoning by, adverse effect of and underdosing of immunoglobulin (T50.Z1)

poisoning by, adverse effect of and underdosing of iron (T45.4)

transfusion reactions (T80.-)

√6ᵗʰ **T45.8X Poisoning by, adverse effect of and underdosing of other primarily systemic and hematological agents**

√7ᵗʰ **T45.8X1 Poisoning by other primarily systemic and hematological agents,** accidental (unintentional)

Poisoning by other primarily systemic and hematological agents NOS

² √7ᵗʰ **T45.8X2 Poisoning by other primarily systemic and hematological agents,** intentional self-harm   HCC Rx ESR COM

√7ᵗʰ **T45.8X3 Poisoning by other primarily systemic and hematological agents,** assault

√7ᵗʰ **T45.8X4 Poisoning by other primarily systemic and hematological agents,** undetermined

√7ᵗʰ **T45.8X5 Adverse effect of other primarily systemic and hematological agents**   UPD

AHA: 2016,4Q,42

√7ᵗʰ **T45.8X6 Underdosing of other primarily systemic and hematological agents**   UPD

√5ᵗʰ **T45.9 Poisoning by, adverse effect of and underdosing of unspecified primarily systemic and hematological agent**

√x7ᵗʰ **T45.91 Poisoning by unspecified primarily systemic and hematological agent,** accidental (unintentional)

Poisoning by primarily systemic and hematological agent NOS

² √x7ᵗʰ **T45.92 Poisoning by unspecified primarily systemic and hematological agent,** intentional self-harm   HCC Rx ESR COM

√x7ᵗʰ **T45.93 Poisoning by unspecified primarily systemic and hematological agent,** assault

√x7ᵗʰ **T45.94 Poisoning by unspecified primarily systemic and hematological agent,** undetermined

√x7ᵗʰ **T45.95 Adverse effect of unspecified primarily systemic and hematological agent**   UPD

√x7ᵗʰ **T45.96 Underdosing of unspecified primarily systemic and hematological agent**   UPD

√4ᵗʰ **T46 Poisoning by, adverse effect of and underdosing of agents primarily affecting the cardiovascular system**

EXCLUDES 1   poisoning by, adverse effect of and underdosing of metaraminol (T44.4)

The appropriate 7th character is to be added to each code from category T46.

A   initial encounter
D   subsequent encounter
S   sequela

√5ᵗʰ **T46.0 Poisoning by, adverse effect of and underdosing of cardiac-stimulant glycosides and drugs of similar action**

√6ᵗʰ **T46.0X Poisoning by, adverse effect of and underdosing of cardiac-stimulant glycosides and drugs of similar action**

√7ᵗʰ **T46.0X1 Poisoning by cardiac-stimulant glycosides and drugs of similar action,** accidental (unintentional)

Poisoning by cardiac-stimulant glycosides and drugs of similar action NOS

2 √7ᵗʰ **T46.0X2** **Poisoning by cardiac-stimulant glycosides and drugs of similar action,** intentional **self-harm** `HCC` `Rx` `ESR` `COM`

√7ᵗʰ **T46.0X3** **Poisoning by cardiac-stimulant glycosides and drugs of similar action,** assault

√7ᵗʰ **T46.0X4** **Poisoning by cardiac-stimulant glycosides and drugs of similar action,** undetermined

√7ᵗʰ **T46.0X5** Adverse effect **of cardiac-stimulant glycosides and drugs of similar action** `UPD`

√7ᵗʰ **T46.0X6** Underdosing **of cardiac-stimulant glycosides and drugs of similar action** `UPD`

√5ᵗʰ **T46.1** **Poisoning by, adverse effect of and underdosing of calcium-channel blockers**

√6ᵗʰ **T46.1X** **Poisoning by, adverse effect of and underdosing of** calcium-channel blockers

√7ᵗʰ **T46.1X1** **Poisoning by calcium-channel blockers,** accidental (unintentional)
Poisoning by calcium-channel blockers NOS

2 √7ᵗʰ **T46.1X2** **Poisoning by calcium-channel blockers,** intentional self-harm `HCC` `Rx` `ESR` `COM`

√7ᵗʰ **T46.1X3** **Poisoning by calcium-channel blockers,** assault

√7ᵗʰ **T46.1X4** **Poisoning by calcium-channel blockers,** undetermined

√7ᵗʰ **T46.1X5** Adverse effect **of calcium-channel blockers** `UPD`

√7ᵗʰ **T46.1X6** Underdosing **of calcium-channel blockers** `UPD`

√5ᵗʰ **T46.2** **Poisoning by, adverse effect of and underdosing of other antidysrhythmic drugs, not elsewhere classified**
EXCLUDES 1 *poisoning by, adverse effect of and underdosing of beta-adrenoreceptor antagonists (T44.7-)*

√6ᵗʰ **T46.2X** **Poisoning by, adverse effect of and underdosing of other antidysrhythmic drugs**

√7ᵗʰ **T46.2X1** **Poisoning by other antidysrhythmic drugs,** accidental (unintentional)
Poisoning by other antidysrhythmic drugs NOS

2 √7ᵗʰ **T46.2X2** **Poisoning by other antidysrhythmic drugs,** intentional self-harm `HCC` `Rx` `ESR` `COM`

√7ᵗʰ **T46.2X3** **Poisoning by other antidysrhythmic drugs,** assault

√7ᵗʰ **T46.2X4** **Poisoning by other antidysrhythmic drugs,** undetermined

√7ᵗʰ **T46.2X5** Adverse effect **of other antidysrhythmic drugs** `UPD`

√7ᵗʰ **T46.2X6** Underdosing **of other antidysrhythmic drugs** `UPD`

√5ᵗʰ **T46.3** **Poisoning by, adverse effect of and underdosing of coronary vasodilators**
Poisoning by, adverse effect of and underdosing of dipyridamole
EXCLUDES 1 *poisoning by, adverse effect of and underdosing of calcium-channel blockers (T46.1)*

√6ᵗʰ **T46.3X** **Poisoning by, adverse effect of and underdosing of** coronary vasodilators

√7ᵗʰ **T46.3X1** **Poisoning by coronary vasodilators,** accidental (unintentional)
Poisoning by coronary vasodilators NOS

2 √7ᵗʰ **T46.3X2** **Poisoning by coronary vasodilators,** intentional self-harm `HCC` `Rx` `ESR` `COM`

√7ᵗʰ **T46.3X3** **Poisoning by coronary vasodilators,** assault

√7ᵗʰ **T46.3X4** **Poisoning by coronary vasodilators,** undetermined

√7ᵗʰ **T46.3X5** Adverse effect **of coronary vasodilators** `UPD`

√7ᵗʰ **T46.3X6** Underdosing **of coronary vasodilators** `UPD`

√5ᵗʰ **T46.4** **Poisoning by, adverse effect of and underdosing of angiotensin-converting-enzyme inhibitors**

√6ᵗʰ **T46.4X** **Poisoning by, adverse effect of and underdosing of** angiotensin-converting-enzyme inhibitors

√7ᵗʰ **T46.4X1** **Poisoning by angiotensin-converting-enzyme inhibitors,** accidental (unintentional)
Poisoning by angiotensin-converting-enzyme inhibitors NOS

2 √7ᵗʰ **T46.4X2** **Poisoning by angiotensin-converting-enzyme inhibitors,** intentional self-harm `HCC` `Rx` `ESR` `COM`

√7ᵗʰ **T46.4X3** **Poisoning by angiotensin-converting-enzyme inhibitors,** assault

√7ᵗʰ **T46.4X4** **Poisoning by angiotensin-converting-enzyme inhibitors,** undetermined

√7ᵗʰ **T46.4X5** Adverse effect **of angiotensin-converting-enzyme inhibitors** `UPD`

√7ᵗʰ **T46.4X6** Underdosing **of angiotensin-converting-enzyme inhibitors** `UPD`

√5ᵗʰ **T46.5** **Poisoning by, adverse effect of and underdosing of other antihypertensive drugs**
EXCLUDES 2 *poisoning by, adverse effect of and underdosing of beta-adrenoreceptor antagonists (T44.7)*
poisoning by, adverse effect of and underdosing of calcium-channel blockers (T46.1)
poisoning by, adverse effect of and underdosing of diuretics (T50.0-T50.2)

√6ᵗʰ **T46.5X** **Poisoning by, adverse effect of and underdosing of other antihypertensive drugs**

√7ᵗʰ **T46.5X1** **Poisoning by other antihypertensive drugs,** accidental (unintentional)
Poisoning by other antihypertensive drugs NOS

2 √7ᵗʰ **T46.5X2** **Poisoning by other antihypertensive drugs,** intentional self-harm `HCC` `Rx` `ESR` `COM`

√7ᵗʰ **T46.5X3** **Poisoning by other antihypertensive drugs,** assault

√7ᵗʰ **T46.5X4** **Poisoning by other antihypertensive drugs,** undetermined

√7ᵗʰ **T46.5X5** Adverse effect **of other antihypertensive drugs** `UPD`

√7ᵗʰ **T46.5X6** Underdosing **of other antihypertensive drugs** `UPD`
AHA: 2022,1Q,36

√5ᵗʰ **T46.6** **Poisoning by, adverse effect of and underdosing of antihyperlipidemic and antiarteriosclerotic drugs**

√6ᵗʰ **T46.6X** **Poisoning by, adverse effect of and underdosing of** antihyperlipidemic and antiarteriosclerotic drugs

√7ᵗʰ **T46.6X1** **Poisoning by antihyperlipidemic and antiarteriosclerotic drugs,** accidental (unintentional)
Poisoning by antihyperlipidemic and antiarteriosclerotic drugs NOS

2 √7ᵗʰ **T46.6X2** **Poisoning by antihyperlipidemic and antiarteriosclerotic drugs,** intentional self-harm `HCC` `Rx` `ESR` `COM`

√7ᵗʰ **T46.6X3** **Poisoning by antihyperlipidemic and antiarteriosclerotic drugs,** assault

√7ᵗʰ **T46.6X4** **Poisoning by antihyperlipidemic and antiarteriosclerotic drugs,** undetermined

√7ᵗʰ **T46.6X5** Adverse effect **of antihyperlipidemic and antiarteriosclerotic drugs** `UPD`

√7ᵗʰ **T46.6X6** Underdosing **of antihyperlipidemic and antiarteriosclerotic drugs** `UPD`

Chapter 19. Injury, Poisoning and Certain Other Consequences of External Causes

T46.7–T47.3X2

√5ᵗʰ **T46.7 Poisoning by, adverse effect of and underdosing of peripheral vasodilators**
Poisoning by, adverse effect of and underdosing of nicotinic acid (derivatives)
EXCLUDES 1 poisoning by, adverse effect of and underdosing of papaverine (T44.3)

√6ᵗʰ **T46.7X Poisoning by, adverse effect of and underdosing of peripheral vasodilators**
√7ᵗʰ **T46.7X1 Poisoning by peripheral vasodilators, accidental (unintentional)**
Poisoning by peripheral vasodilators NOS
² √7ᵗʰ **T46.7X2 Poisoning by peripheral vasodilators, intentional self-harm** HCC Rx ESR COM
√7ᵗʰ **T46.7X3 Poisoning by peripheral vasodilators, assault**
√7ᵗʰ **T46.7X4 Poisoning by peripheral vasodilators, undetermined**
√7ᵗʰ **T46.7X5 Adverse effect of peripheral vasodilators** UPD
√7ᵗʰ **T46.7X6 Underdosing of peripheral vasodilators** UPD

√5ᵗʰ **T46.8 Poisoning by, adverse effect of and underdosing of antivaricose drugs, including sclerosing agents**
√6ᵗʰ **T46.8X Poisoning by, adverse effect of and underdosing of antivaricose drugs, including sclerosing agents**
√7ᵗʰ **T46.8X1 Poisoning by antivaricose drugs, including sclerosing agents, accidental (unintentional)**
Poisoning by antivaricose drugs, including sclerosing agents NOS
² √7ᵗʰ **T46.8X2 Poisoning by antivaricose drugs, including sclerosing agents, intentional self-harm** HCC Rx ESR COM
√7ᵗʰ **T46.8X3 Poisoning by antivaricose drugs, including sclerosing agents, assault**
√7ᵗʰ **T46.8X4 Poisoning by antivaricose drugs, including sclerosing agents, undetermined**
√7ᵗʰ **T46.8X5 Adverse effect of antivaricose drugs, including sclerosing agents** UPD
√7ᵗʰ **T46.8X6 Underdosing of antivaricose drugs, including sclerosing agents** UPD

√5ᵗʰ **T46.9 Poisoning by, adverse effect of and underdosing of other and unspecified agents primarily affecting the cardiovascular system**
√6ᵗʰ **T46.90 Poisoning by, adverse effect of and underdosing of unspecified agents primarily affecting the cardiovascular system**
√7ᵗʰ **T46.901 Poisoning by unspecified agents primarily affecting the cardiovascular system, accidental (unintentional)**
² √7ᵗʰ **T46.902 Poisoning by unspecified agents primarily affecting the cardiovascular system, intentional self-harm** HCC Rx ESR COM
√7ᵗʰ **T46.903 Poisoning by unspecified agents primarily affecting the cardiovascular system, assault**
√7ᵗʰ **T46.904 Poisoning by unspecified agents primarily affecting the cardiovascular system, undetermined**
√7ᵗʰ **T46.905 Adverse effect of unspecified agents primarily affecting the cardiovascular system** UPD
√7ᵗʰ **T46.906 Underdosing of unspecified agents primarily affecting the cardiovascular system** UPD
√6ᵗʰ **T46.99 Poisoning by, adverse effect of and underdosing of other agents primarily affecting the cardiovascular system**
√7ᵗʰ **T46.991 Poisoning by other agents primarily affecting the cardiovascular system, accidental (unintentional)**
² √7ᵗʰ **T46.992 Poisoning by other agents primarily affecting the cardiovascular system, intentional self-harm** HCC Rx ESR COM
√7ᵗʰ **T46.993 Poisoning by other agents primarily affecting the cardiovascular system, assault**
√7ᵗʰ **T46.994 Poisoning by other agents primarily affecting the cardiovascular system, undetermined**

√7ᵗʰ **T46.995 Adverse effect of other agents primarily affecting the cardiovascular system** UPD
√7ᵗʰ **T46.996 Underdosing of other agents primarily affecting the cardiovascular system** UPD

√4ᵗʰ **T47 Poisoning by, adverse effect of and underdosing of agents primarily affecting the gastrointestinal system**

The appropriate 7th character is to be added to each code from category T47.
A initial encounter
D subsequent encounter
S sequela

√5ᵗʰ **T47.0 Poisoning by, adverse effect of and underdosing of histamine H2-receptor blockers**
√6ᵗʰ **T47.0X Poisoning by, adverse effect of and underdosing of histamine H2-receptor blockers**
√7ᵗʰ **T47.0X1 Poisoning by histamine H2-receptor blockers, accidental (unintentional)**
Poisoning by histamine H2-receptor blockers NOS
² √7ᵗʰ **T47.0X2 Poisoning by histamine H2-receptor blockers, intentional self-harm** HCC Rx ESR COM
√7ᵗʰ **T47.0X3 Poisoning by histamine H2-receptor blockers, assault**
√7ᵗʰ **T47.0X4 Poisoning by histamine H2-receptor blockers, undetermined**
√7ᵗʰ **T47.0X5 Adverse effect of histamine H2-receptor blockers** UPD
√7ᵗʰ **T47.0X6 Underdosing of histamine H2-receptor blockers** UPD

√5ᵗʰ **T47.1 Poisoning by, adverse effect of and underdosing of other antacids and anti-gastric-secretion drugs**
√6ᵗʰ **T47.1X Poisoning by, adverse effect of and underdosing of other antacids and anti-gastric-secretion drugs**
√7ᵗʰ **T47.1X1 Poisoning by other antacids and anti-gastric-secretion drugs, accidental (unintentional)**
Poisoning by other antacids and anti-gastric-secretion drugs NOS
² √7ᵗʰ **T47.1X2 Poisoning by other antacids and anti-gastric-secretion drugs, intentional self-harm** HCC Rx ESR COM
√7ᵗʰ **T47.1X3 Poisoning by other antacids and anti-gastric-secretion drugs, assault**
√7ᵗʰ **T47.1X4 Poisoning by other antacids and anti-gastric-secretion drugs, undetermined**
√7ᵗʰ **T47.1X5 Adverse effect of other antacids and anti-gastric-secretion drugs** UPD
√7ᵗʰ **T47.1X6 Underdosing of other antacids and anti-gastric-secretion drugs** UPD

√5ᵗʰ **T47.2 Poisoning by, adverse effect of and underdosing of stimulant laxatives**
√6ᵗʰ **T47.2X Poisoning by, adverse effect of and underdosing of stimulant laxatives**
√7ᵗʰ **T47.2X1 Poisoning by stimulant laxatives, accidental (unintentional)**
Poisoning by stimulant laxatives NOS
² √7ᵗʰ **T47.2X2 Poisoning by stimulant laxatives, intentional self-harm** HCC Rx ESR COM
√7ᵗʰ **T47.2X3 Poisoning by stimulant laxatives, assault**
√7ᵗʰ **T47.2X4 Poisoning by stimulant laxatives, undetermined**
√7ᵗʰ **T47.2X5 Adverse effect of stimulant laxatives** UPD
√7ᵗʰ **T47.2X6 Underdosing of stimulant laxatives** UPD

√6ᵗʰ **T47.3 Poisoning by, adverse effect of and underdosing of saline and osmotic laxatives**
√6ᵗʰ **T47.3X Poisoning by and adverse effect of saline and osmotic laxatives**
√7ᵗʰ **T47.3X1 Poisoning by saline and osmotic laxatives, accidental (unintentional)**
Poisoning by saline and osmotic laxatives NOS
² √7ᵗʰ **T47.3X2 Poisoning by saline and osmotic laxatives, intentional self-harm** HCC Rx ESR COM

☑7ᵗʰ **T47.3X3** **Poisoning by saline and osmotic laxatives,** assault

☑7ᵗʰ **T47.3X4** **Poisoning by saline and osmotic laxatives,** undetermined

☑7ᵗʰ **T47.3X5** Adverse effect of saline and osmotic laxatives   UPD

☑7ᵗʰ **T47.3X6** Underdosing of saline and osmotic laxatives   UPD

✓5ᵗʰ **T47.4** **Poisoning by, adverse effect of and underdosing of other laxatives**

✓6ᵗʰ **T47.4X** **Poisoning by, adverse effect of and underdosing of other laxatives**

☑7ᵗʰ **T47.4X1** **Poisoning by other laxatives,** accidental **(unintentional)**
Poisoning by other laxatives NOS

² ☑7ᵗʰ **T47.4X2** **Poisoning by other laxatives,** intentional self-harm   HCC Rx ESR COM

☑7ᵗʰ **T47.4X3** **Poisoning by other laxatives,** assault

☑7ᵗʰ **T47.4X4** **Poisoning by other laxatives,** undetermined

☑7ᵗʰ **T47.4X5** Adverse effect of other laxatives   UPD

☑7ᵗʰ **T47.4X6** Underdosing of other laxatives   UPD

✓5ᵗʰ **T47.5** **Poisoning by, adverse effect of and underdosing of digestants**

✓6ᵗʰ **T47.5X** **Poisoning by, adverse effect of and underdosing of digestants**

☑7ᵗʰ **T47.5X1** **Poisoning by digestants,** accidental **(unintentional)**
Poisoning by digestants NOS

² ☑7ᵗʰ **T47.5X2** **Poisoning by digestants,** intentional self-harm   HCC Rx ESR COM

☑7ᵗʰ **T47.5X3** **Poisoning by digestants,** assault

☑7ᵗʰ **T47.5X4** **Poisoning by digestants,** undetermined

☑7ᵗʰ **T47.5X5** Adverse effect of digestants   UPD

☑7ᵗʰ **T47.5X6** Underdosing of digestants   UPD

✓5ᵗʰ **T47.6** **Poisoning by, adverse effect of and underdosing of antidiarrheal drugs**

EXCLUDES 2   poisoning by, adverse effect of and underdosing of systemic antibiotics and other anti-infectives (T36-T37)

✓6ᵗʰ **T47.6X** **Poisoning by, adverse effect of and underdosing of antidiarrheal drugs**

☑7ᵗʰ **T47.6X1** **Poisoning by antidiarrheal drugs,** accidental **(unintentional)**
Poisoning by antidiarrheal drugs NOS

² ☑7ᵗʰ **T47.6X2** **Poisoning by antidiarrheal drugs,** intentional self-harm   HCC Rx ESR COM

☑7ᵗʰ **T47.6X3** **Poisoning by antidiarrheal drugs,** assault

☑7ᵗʰ **T47.6X4** **Poisoning by antidiarrheal drugs,** undetermined

☑7ᵗʰ **T47.6X5** Adverse effect of antidiarrheal drugs   UPD

☑7ᵗʰ **T47.6X6** Underdosing of antidiarrheal drugs   UPD

✓5ᵗʰ **T47.7** **Poisoning by, adverse effect of and underdosing of emetics**

✓6ᵗʰ **T47.7X** **Poisoning by, adverse effect of and underdosing of emetics**

☑7ᵗʰ **T47.7X1** **Poisoning by emetics,** accidental **(unintentional)**
Poisoning by emetics NOS

² ☑7ᵗʰ **T47.7X2** **Poisoning by emetics,** intentional self-harm   HCC Rx ESR COM

☑7ᵗʰ **T47.7X3** **Poisoning by emetics,** assault

☑7ᵗʰ **T47.7X4** **Poisoning by emetics,** undetermined

☑7ᵗʰ **T47.7X5** Adverse effect of emetics   UPD

☑7ᵗʰ **T47.7X6** Underdosing of emetics   UPD

✓5ᵗʰ **T47.8** **Poisoning by, adverse effect of and underdosing of other agents primarily affecting gastrointestinal system**

✓6ᵗʰ **T47.8X** **Poisoning by, adverse effect of and underdosing of other agents primarily affecting gastrointestinal system**

☑7ᵗʰ **T47.8X1** **Poisoning by other agents primarily affecting gastrointestinal system,** accidental **(unintentional)**
Poisoning by other agents primarily affecting gastrointestinal system NOS

² ☑7ᵗʰ **T47.8X2** **Poisoning by other agents primarily affecting gastrointestinal system,** intentional self-harm   HCC Rx ESR COM

☑7ᵗʰ **T47.8X3** **Poisoning by other agents primarily affecting gastrointestinal system,** assault

☑7ᵗʰ **T47.8X4** **Poisoning by other agents primarily affecting gastrointestinal system,** undetermined

☑7ᵗʰ **T47.8X5** Adverse effect of other agents primarily affecting gastrointestinal system   UPD

☑7ᵗʰ **T47.8X6** Underdosing of other agents primarily affecting gastrointestinal system   UPD

✓5ᵗʰ **T47.9** **Poisoning by, adverse effect of and underdosing of unspecified agents primarily affecting the gastrointestinal system**

✓x7ᵗʰ **T47.91** **Poisoning by unspecified agents primarily affecting the gastrointestinal system,** accidental **(unintentional)**
Poisoning by agents primarily affecting the gastrointestinal system NOS

² ✓x7ᵗʰ **T47.92** **Poisoning by unspecified agents primarily affecting the gastrointestinal system,** intentional self-harm   HCC Rx ESR COM

✓x7ᵗʰ **T47.93** **Poisoning by unspecified agents primarily affecting the gastrointestinal system,** assault

✓x7ᵗʰ **T47.94** **Poisoning by unspecified agents primarily affecting the gastrointestinal system,** undetermined

✓x7ᵗʰ **T47.95** Adverse effect of unspecified agents primarily affecting the gastrointestinal system   UPD

✓x7ᵗʰ **T47.96** Underdosing of unspecified agents primarily affecting the gastrointestinal system   UPD

✓4ᵗʰ **T48** **Poisoning by, adverse effect of and underdosing of agents primarily acting on smooth and skeletal muscles and the respiratory system**

The appropriate 7th character is to be added to each code from category T48.
A   initial encounter
D   subsequent encounter
S   sequela

✓5ᵗʰ **T48.0** **Poisoning by, adverse effect of and underdosing of oxytocic drugs**

EXCLUDES 1   poisoning by, adverse effect of and underdosing of estrogens, progestogens and antagonists (T38.4-T38.6)

✓6ᵗʰ **T48.0X** **Poisoning by, adverse effect of and underdosing of oxytocic drugs**

☑7ᵗʰ **T48.0X1** **Poisoning by oxytocic drugs,** accidental **(unintentional)**
Poisoning by oxytocic drugs NOS

² ☑7ᵗʰ **T48.0X2** **Poisoning by oxytocic drugs,** intentional self-harm   HCC Rx ESR COM

☑7ᵗʰ **T48.0X3** **Poisoning by oxytocic drugs,** assault

☑7ᵗʰ **T48.0X4** **Poisoning by oxytocic drugs,** undetermined

☑7ᵗʰ **T48.0X5** Adverse effect of oxytocic drugs   UPD

☑7ᵗʰ **T48.0X6** Underdosing of oxytocic drugs   UPD

✓5ᵗʰ **T48.1** **Poisoning by, adverse effect of and underdosing of skeletal muscle relaxants [neuromuscular blocking agents]**

✓6ᵗʰ **T48.1X** **Poisoning by, adverse effect of and underdosing of skeletal muscle relaxants [neuromuscular blocking agents]**

☑7ᵗʰ **T48.1X1** **Poisoning by skeletal muscle relaxants [neuromuscular blocking agents],** accidental **(unintentional)**
Poisoning by skeletal muscle relaxants [neuromuscular blocking agents] NOS

² ☑7ᵗʰ **T48.1X2** **Poisoning by skeletal muscle relaxants [neuromuscular blocking agents],** intentional self-harm   HCC Rx ESR COM

☑7ᵗʰ **T48.1X3** **Poisoning by skeletal muscle relaxants [neuromuscular blocking agents],** assault

☑7ᵗʰ **T48.1X4** **Poisoning by skeletal muscle relaxants [neuromuscular blocking agents],** undetermined

☑7ᵗʰ **T48.1X5** Adverse effect of skeletal muscle relaxants [neuromuscular blocking agents]   UPD

☑7ᵗʰ **T48.1X6** Underdosing of skeletal muscle relaxants [neuromuscular blocking agents]   UPD

Chapter 19. Injury, Poisoning and Certain Other Consequences of External Causes

T48.2–T48.996

- ☑5ᵗʰ **T48.2 Poisoning by, adverse effect of and underdosing of other and unspecified drugs acting on muscles**
  - ☑6ᵗʰ **T48.20 Poisoning by, adverse effect of and underdosing of unspecified drugs acting on muscles**
    - ☑7ᵗʰ **T48.201 Poisoning by unspecified drugs acting on muscles, accidental (unintentional)**
      Poisoning by unspecified drugs acting on muscles NOS
    - ² ☑7ᵗʰ **T48.202 Poisoning by unspecified drugs acting on muscles, intentional self-harm** HCC Rx ESR COM
    - ☑7ᵗʰ **T48.203 Poisoning by unspecified drugs acting on muscles, assault**
    - ☑7ᵗʰ **T48.204 Poisoning by unspecified drugs acting on muscles, undetermined**
    - ☑7ᵗʰ **T48.205 Adverse effect of unspecified drugs acting on muscles** UPD
    - ☑7ᵗʰ **T48.206 Underdosing of unspecified drugs acting on muscles** UPD
  - ☑6ᵗʰ **T48.29 Poisoning by, adverse effect of and underdosing of other drugs acting on muscles**
    - ☑7ᵗʰ **T48.291 Poisoning by other drugs acting on muscles, accidental (unintentional)**
      Poisoning by other drugs acting on muscles NOS
    - ² ☑7ᵗʰ **T48.292 Poisoning by other drugs acting on muscles, intentional self-harm** HCC Rx ESR COM
    - ☑7ᵗʰ **T48.293 Poisoning by other drugs acting on muscles, assault**
    - ☑7ᵗʰ **T48.294 Poisoning by other drugs acting on muscles, undetermined**
    - ☑7ᵗʰ **T48.295 Adverse effect of other drugs acting on muscles** UPD
    - ☑7ᵗʰ **T48.296 Underdosing of other drugs acting on muscles** UPD
- ☑5ᵗʰ **T48.3 Poisoning by, adverse effect of and underdosing of antitussives**
  - ☑6ᵗʰ **T48.3X Poisoning by, adverse effect of and underdosing of antitussives**
    - ☑7ᵗʰ **T48.3X1 Poisoning by antitussives, accidental (unintentional)**
      Poisoning by antitussives NOS
    - ² ☑7ᵗʰ **T48.3X2 Poisoning by antitussives, intentional self-harm** HCC Rx ESR COM
    - ☑7ᵗʰ **T48.3X3 Poisoning by antitussives, assault**
    - ☑7ᵗʰ **T48.3X4 Poisoning by antitussives, undetermined**
    - ☑7ᵗʰ **T48.3X5 Adverse effect of antitussives** UPD
    - ☑7ᵗʰ **T48.3X6 Underdosing of antitussives** UPD
- ☑5ᵗʰ **T48.4 Poisoning by, adverse effect of and underdosing of expectorants**
  - ☑6ᵗʰ **T48.4X Poisoning by, adverse effect of and underdosing of expectorants**
    - ☑7ᵗʰ **T48.4X1 Poisoning by expectorants, accidental (unintentional)**
      Poisoning by expectorants NOS
    - ² ☑7ᵗʰ **T48.4X2 Poisoning by expectorants, intentional self-harm** HCC Rx ESR COM
    - ☑7ᵗʰ **T48.4X3 Poisoning by expectorants, assault**
    - ☑7ᵗʰ **T48.4X4 Poisoning by expectorants, undetermined**
    - ☑7ᵗʰ **T48.4X5 Adverse effect of expectorants** UPD
    - ☑7ᵗʰ **T48.4X6 Underdosing of expectorants** UPD
- ☑5ᵗʰ **T48.5 Poisoning by, adverse effect of and underdosing of other anti-common-cold drugs**
  Poisoning by, adverse effect of and underdosing of decongestants
  - EXCLUDES 2 *poisoning by, adverse effect of and underdosing of antipyretics, NEC (T39.9-)*
    poisoning by, adverse effect of and underdosing of non-steroidal antiinflammatory drugs (T39.3-)
    poisoning by, adverse effect of and underdosing of salicylates (T39.0-)
  - ☑6ᵗʰ **T48.5X Poisoning by, adverse effect of and underdosing of other anti-common-cold drugs**
    - ☑7ᵗʰ **T48.5X1 Poisoning by other anti-common-cold drugs, accidental (unintentional)**
      Poisoning by other anti-common-cold drugs NOS
    - ² ☑7ᵗʰ **T48.5X2 Poisoning by other anti-common-cold drugs, intentional self-harm** HCC Rx ESR COM
    - ☑7ᵗʰ **T48.5X3 Poisoning by other anti-common-cold drugs, assault**
    - ☑7ᵗʰ **T48.5X4 Poisoning by other anti-common-cold drugs, undetermined**
    - ☑7ᵗʰ **T48.5X5 Adverse effect of other anti-common-cold drugs** UPD
    - ☑7ᵗʰ **T48.5X6 Underdosing of other anti-common-cold drugs** UPD
- ☑5ᵗʰ **T48.6 Poisoning by, adverse effect of and underdosing of antiasthmatics, not elsewhere classified**
  Poisoning by, adverse effect of and underdosing of beta-adrenoreceptor agonists used in asthma therapy
  - EXCLUDES 1 *poisoning by, adverse effect of and underdosing of anterior pituitary [adenohypophyseal] hormones (T38.8)*
    poisoning by, adverse effect of and underdosing of beta-adrenoreceptor agonists not used in asthma therapy (T44.5)
  - ☑6ᵗʰ **T48.6X Poisoning by, adverse effect of and underdosing of antiasthmatics**
    - ☑7ᵗʰ **T48.6X1 Poisoning by antiasthmatics, accidental (unintentional)**
      Poisoning by antiasthmatics NOS
    - ² ☑7ᵗʰ **T48.6X2 Poisoning by antiasthmatics, intentional self-harm** HCC Rx ESR COM
    - ☑7ᵗʰ **T48.6X3 Poisoning by antiasthmatics, assault**
    - ☑7ᵗʰ **T48.6X4 Poisoning by antiasthmatics, undetermined**
    - ☑7ᵗʰ **T48.6X5 Adverse effect of antiasthmatics** UPD
    - ☑7ᵗʰ **T48.6X6 Underdosing of antiasthmatics** UPD
- ☑5ᵗʰ **T48.9 Poisoning by, adverse effect of and underdosing of other and unspecified agents primarily acting on the respiratory system**
  - ☑6ᵗʰ **T48.90 Poisoning by, adverse effect of and underdosing of unspecified agents primarily acting on the respiratory system**
    - ☑7ᵗʰ **T48.901 Poisoning by unspecified agents primarily acting on the respiratory system, accidental (unintentional)**
    - ² ☑7ᵗʰ **T48.902 Poisoning by unspecified agents primarily acting on the respiratory system, intentional self-harm** HCC Rx ESR COM
    - ☑7ᵗʰ **T48.903 Poisoning by unspecified agents primarily acting on the respiratory system, assault**
    - ☑7ᵗʰ **T48.904 Poisoning by unspecified agents primarily acting on the respiratory system, undetermined**
    - ☑7ᵗʰ **T48.905 Adverse effect of unspecified agents primarily acting on the respiratory system** UPD
    - ☑7ᵗʰ **T48.906 Underdosing of unspecified agents primarily acting on the respiratory system** UPD
  - ☑6ᵗʰ **T48.99 Poisoning by, adverse effect of and underdosing of other agents primarily acting on the respiratory system**
    - ☑7ᵗʰ **T48.991 Poisoning by other agents primarily acting on the respiratory system, accidental (unintentional)**
    - ² ☑7ᵗʰ **T48.992 Poisoning by other agents primarily acting on the respiratory system, intentional self-harm** HCC Rx ESR COM
    - ☑7ᵗʰ **T48.993 Poisoning by other agents primarily acting on the respiratory system, assault**
    - ☑7ᵗʰ **T48.994 Poisoning by other agents primarily acting on the respiratory system, undetermined**
    - ☑7ᵗʰ **T48.995 Adverse effect of other agents primarily acting on the respiratory system** UPD
    - ☑7ᵗʰ **T48.996 Underdosing of other agents primarily acting on the respiratory system** UPD

✓4th T49 Poisoning by, adverse effect of and underdosing of topical agents primarily affecting skin and mucous membrane and by ophthalmological, otorhinolaryngological and dental drugs

> INCLUDES poisoning by, adverse effect of and underdosing of glucocorticoids, topically used

> The appropriate 7th character is to be added to each code from category T49.
> A   initial encounter
> D   subsequent encounter
> S   sequela

✓5th T49.0 Poisoning by, adverse effect of and underdosing of local antifungal, anti-infective and anti-inflammatory drugs

  ✓6th T49.0X Poisoning by, adverse effect of and underdosing of local antifungal, anti-infective and anti-inflammatory drugs

    ✓7th T49.0X1 Poisoning by local antifungal, anti-infective and anti-inflammatory drugs, accidental **(unintentional)**
       Poisoning by local antifungal, anti-infective and anti-inflammatory drugs NOS

    2 **✓7th T49.0X2 Poisoning by local antifungal, anti-infective and anti-inflammatory drugs,** intentional **self-harm**   HCC Rx ESR COM

    ✓7th T49.0X3 Poisoning by local antifungal, anti-infective and anti-inflammatory drugs, assault

    ✓7th T49.0X4 Poisoning by local antifungal, anti-infective and anti-inflammatory drugs, undetermined

    ✓7th T49.0X5 Adverse effect of local antifungal, anti-infective and anti-inflammatory drugs   UPD

    ✓7th T49.0X6 Underdosing of local antifungal, anti-infective and anti-inflammatory drugs   UPD

✓5th T49.1 Poisoning by, adverse effect of and underdosing of antipruritics

  ✓6th T49.1X Poisoning by, adverse effect of and underdosing of antipruritics

    ✓7th T49.1X1 Poisoning by antipruritics, accidental **(unintentional)**
       Poisoning by antipruritics NOS

    2 **✓7th T49.1X2 Poisoning by antipruritics,** intentional self-harm   HCC Rx ESR COM

    ✓7th T49.1X3 Poisoning by antipruritics, assault

    ✓7th T49.1X4 Poisoning by antipruritics, undetermined

    ✓7th T49.1X5 Adverse effect of antipruritics   UPD

    ✓7th T49.1X6 Underdosing of antipruritics   UPD

✓5th T49.2 Poisoning by, adverse effect of and underdosing of local astringents and local detergents

  ✓6th T49.2X Poisoning by, adverse effect of and underdosing of local astringents and local detergents

    ✓7th T49.2X1 Poisoning by local astringents and local detergents, accidental **(unintentional)**
       Poisoning by local astringents and local detergents NOS

    2 **✓7th T49.2X2 Poisoning by local astringents and local detergents,** intentional self-harm   HCC Rx ESR COM

    ✓7th T49.2X3 Poisoning by local astringents and local detergents, assault

    ✓7th T49.2X4 Poisoning by local astringents and local detergents, undetermined

    ✓7th T49.2X5 Adverse effect of local astringents and local detergents   UPD

    ✓7th T49.2X6 Underdosing of local astringents and local detergents   UPD

✓5th T49.3 Poisoning by, adverse effect of and underdosing of emollients, demulcents and protectants

  ✓6th T49.3X Poisoning by, adverse effect of and underdosing of emollients, demulcents and protectants

    ✓7th T49.3X1 Poisoning by emollients, demulcents and protectants, accidental **(unintentional)**
       Poisoning by emollients, demulcents and protectants NOS

    2 **✓7th T49.3X2 Poisoning by emollients, demulcents and protectants,** intentional self-harm   HCC Rx ESR COM

    ✓7th T49.3X3 Poisoning by emollients, demulcents and protectants, assault

    ✓7th T49.3X4 Poisoning by emollients, demulcents and protectants, undetermined

    ✓7th T49.3X5 Adverse effect of emollients, demulcents and protectants   UPD

    ✓7th T49.3X6 Underdosing of emollients, demulcents and protectants   UPD

✓5th T49.4 Poisoning by, adverse effect of and underdosing of keratolytics, keratoplastics, and other hair treatment drugs and preparations

  ✓6th T49.4X Poisoning by, adverse effect of and underdosing of keratolytics, keratoplastics, and other hair treatment drugs and preparations

    ✓7th T49.4X1 Poisoning by keratolytics, keratoplastics, and other hair treatment drugs and preparations, accidental **(unintentional)**
       Poisoning by keratolytics, keratoplastics, and other hair treatment drugs and preparations NOS

    2 **✓7th T49.4X2 Poisoning by keratolytics, keratoplastics, and other hair treatment drugs and preparations,** intentional self-harm   HCC Rx ESR COM

    ✓7th T49.4X3 Poisoning by keratolytics, keratoplastics, and other hair treatment drugs and preparations, assault

    ✓7th T49.4X4 Poisoning by keratolytics, keratoplastics, and other hair treatment drugs and preparations, undetermined

    ✓7th T49.4X5 Adverse effect of keratolytics, keratoplastics, and other hair treatment drugs and preparations   UPD

    ✓7th T49.4X6 Underdosing of keratolytics, keratoplastics, and other hair treatment drugs and preparations   UPD

✓5th T49.5 Poisoning by, adverse effect of and underdosing of ophthalmological drugs and preparations

  ✓6th T49.5X Poisoning by, adverse effect of and underdosing of ophthalmological drugs and preparations

    ✓7th T49.5X1 Poisoning by ophthalmological drugs and preparations, accidental **(unintentional)**
       Poisoning by ophthalmological drugs and preparations NOS

    2 **✓7th T49.5X2 Poisoning by ophthalmological drugs and preparations,** intentional self-harm   HCC Rx ESR COM

    ✓7th T49.5X3 Poisoning by ophthalmological drugs and preparations, assault

    ✓7th T49.5X4 Poisoning by ophthalmological drugs and preparations, undetermined

    ✓7th T49.5X5 Adverse effect of ophthalmological drugs and preparations   UPD

    ✓7th T49.5X6 Underdosing of ophthalmological drugs and preparations   UPD

✓5th T49.6 Poisoning by, adverse effect of and underdosing of otorhinolaryngological drugs and preparations

  ✓6th T49.6X Poisoning by, adverse effect of and underdosing of otorhinolaryngological drugs and preparations

    ✓7th T49.6X1 Poisoning by otorhinolaryngological drugs and preparations, accidental **(unintentional)**
       Poisoning by otorhinolaryngological drugs and preparations NOS

    2 **✓7th T49.6X2 Poisoning by otorhinolaryngological drugs and preparations,** intentional self-harm   HCC Rx ESR COM

    ✓7th T49.6X3 Poisoning by otorhinolaryngological drugs and preparations, assault

    ✓7th T49.6X4 Poisoning by otorhinolaryngological drugs and preparations, undetermined

    ✓7th T49.6X5 Adverse effect of otorhinolaryngological drugs and preparations   UPD

    ✓7th T49.6X6 Underdosing of otorhinolaryngological drugs and preparations   UPD

✓5th T49.7 Poisoning by, adverse effect of and underdosing of dental drugs, topically applied

  ✓6th T49.7X Poisoning by, adverse effect of and underdosing of dental drugs, topically applied

    ✓7th T49.7X1 Poisoning by dental drugs, topically applied, accidental **(unintentional)**
       Poisoning by dental drugs, topically applied NOS

Chapter 19. Injury, Poisoning and Certain Other Consequences of External Causes

T49.7X2–T50.4X6

2 ✓7ᵗʰ **T49.7X2** **Poisoning by dental drugs, topically applied,** intentional self-harm   HCC Rx ESR COM

✓7ᵗʰ **T49.7X3** **Poisoning by dental drugs, topically applied,** assault

✓7ᵗʰ **T49.7X4** **Poisoning by dental drugs, topically applied,** undetermined

✓7ᵗʰ **T49.7X5** Adverse effect **of dental drugs, topically applied** UPD

✓7ᵗʰ **T49.7X6** Underdosing **of dental drugs, topically applied** UPD

✓5ᵗʰ **T49.8** **Poisoning by, adverse effect of and underdosing of other topical agents**
Poisoning by, adverse effect of and underdosing of spermicides

✓6ᵗʰ **T49.8X** **Poisoning by, adverse effect of and underdosing of other topical agents**

✓7ᵗʰ **T49.8X1** **Poisoning by other topical agents,** accidental (unintentional)
Poisoning by other topical agents NOS

2 ✓7ᵗʰ **T49.8X2** **Poisoning by other topical agents,** intentional self-harm   HCC Rx ESR COM

✓7ᵗʰ **T49.8X3** **Poisoning by other topical agents,** assault

✓7ᵗʰ **T49.8X4** **Poisoning by other topical agents,** undetermined

✓7ᵗʰ **T49.8X5** Adverse effect **of other topical agents** UPD

✓7ᵗʰ **T49.8X6** Underdosing **of other topical agents** UPD

✓5ᵗʰ **T49.9** **Poisoning by, adverse effect of and underdosing of unspecified topical agent**

✓x7ᵗʰ **T49.91** **Poisoning by unspecified topical agent,** accidental (unintentional)

2 ✓x7ᵗʰ **T49.92** **Poisoning by unspecified topical agent,** intentional self-harm   HCC Rx ESR COM

✓x7ᵗʰ **T49.93** **Poisoning by unspecified topical agent,** assault

✓x7ᵗʰ **T49.94** **Poisoning by unspecified topical agent,** undetermined

✓x7ᵗʰ **T49.95** Adverse effect **of unspecified topical agent** UPD

✓x7ᵗʰ **T49.96** Underdosing **of unspecified topical agent** UPD

✓4ᵗʰ **T50** **Poisoning by, adverse effect of and underdosing of diuretics and other and unspecified drugs, medicaments and biological substances**

> The appropriate 7th character is to be added to each code from category T50.
> A initial encounter
> D subsequent encounter
> S sequela

✓5ᵗʰ **T50.0** **Poisoning by, adverse effect of and underdosing of mineralocorticoids and their antagonists**

✓6ᵗʰ **T50.0X** **Poisoning by, adverse effect of and underdosing of** mineralocorticoids **and their antagonists**

✓7ᵗʰ **T50.0X1** **Poisoning by mineralocorticoids and their antagonists,** accidental (unintentional)
Poisoning by mineralocorticoids and their antagonists NOS

2 ✓7ᵗʰ **T50.0X2** **Poisoning by mineralocorticoids and their antagonists,** intentional self-harm   HCC Rx ESR COM

✓7ᵗʰ **T50.0X3** **Poisoning by mineralocorticoids and their antagonists,** assault

✓7ᵗʰ **T50.0X4** **Poisoning by mineralocorticoids and their antagonists,** undetermined

✓7ᵗʰ **T50.0X5** Adverse effect **of mineralocorticoids and their antagonists** UPD

✓7ᵗʰ **T50.0X6** Underdosing **of mineralocorticoids and their antagonists** UPD

✓5ᵗʰ **T50.1** **Poisoning by, adverse effect of and underdosing of loop [high-ceiling] diuretics**

✓6ᵗʰ **T50.1X** **Poisoning by, adverse effect of and underdosing of** loop [high-ceiling] diuretics

✓7ᵗʰ **T50.1X1** **Poisoning by loop [high-ceiling] diuretics,** accidental (unintentional)
Poisoning by loop [high-ceiling] diuretics NOS

2 ✓7ᵗʰ **T50.1X2** **Poisoning by loop [high-ceiling] diuretics,** intentional self-harm   HCC Rx ESR COM

✓7ᵗʰ **T50.1X3** **Poisoning by loop [high-ceiling] diuretics,** assault

✓7ᵗʰ **T50.1X4** **Poisoning by loop [high-ceiling] diuretics,** undetermined

✓7ᵗʰ **T50.1X5** Adverse effect **of loop [high-ceiling] diuretics** UPD

✓7ᵗʰ **T50.1X6** Underdosing **of loop [high-ceiling] diuretics** UPD

✓5ᵗʰ **T50.2** **Poisoning by, adverse effect of and underdosing of carbonic-anhydrase inhibitors, benzothiadiazides and other diuretics**
Poisoning by, adverse effect of and underdosing of acetazolamide

✓6ᵗʰ **T50.2X** **Poisoning by, adverse effect of and underdosing of** carbonic-anhydrase inhibitors, benzothiadiazides and other diuretics

✓7ᵗʰ **T50.2X1** **Poisoning by carbonic-anhydrase inhibitors, benzothiadiazides and other diuretics,** accidental (unintentional)
Poisoning by carbonic-anhydrase inhibitors, benzothiadiazides and other diuretics NOS

2 ✓7ᵗʰ **T50.2X2** **Poisoning by carbonic-anhydrase inhibitors, benzothiadiazides and other diuretics,** intentional self-harm   HCC Rx ESR COM

✓7ᵗʰ **T50.2X3** **Poisoning by carbonic-anhydrase inhibitors, benzothiadiazides and other diuretics,** assault

✓7ᵗʰ **T50.2X4** **Poisoning by carbonic-anhydrase inhibitors, benzothiadiazides and other diuretics,** undetermined

✓7ᵗʰ **T50.2X5** Adverse effect **of carbonic-anhydrase inhibitors, benzothiadiazides and other diuretics** UPD

✓7ᵗʰ **T50.2X6** Underdosing **of carbonic-anhydrase inhibitors, benzothiadiazides and other diuretics** UPD

✓5ᵗʰ **T50.3** **Poisoning by, adverse effect of and underdosing of electrolytic, caloric and water-balance agents**
Poisoning by, adverse effect of and underdosing of oral rehydration salts

✓6ᵗʰ **T50.3X** **Poisoning by, adverse effect of and underdosing of** electrolytic, caloric and water-balance agents

✓7ᵗʰ **T50.3X1** **Poisoning by electrolytic, caloric and water-balance agents,** accidental (unintentional)
Poisoning by electrolytic, caloric and water-balance agents NOS

2 ✓7ᵗʰ **T50.3X2** **Poisoning by electrolytic, caloric and water-balance agents,** intentional self-harm   HCC Rx ESR COM

✓7ᵗʰ **T50.3X3** **Poisoning by electrolytic, caloric and water-balance agents,** assault

✓7ᵗʰ **T50.3X4** **Poisoning by electrolytic, caloric and water-balance agents,** undetermined

✓7ᵗʰ **T50.3X5** Adverse effect **of electrolytic, caloric and water-balance agents** UPD
AHA: 2022,2Q,10

✓7ᵗʰ **T50.3X6** Underdosing **of electrolytic, caloric and water-balance agents** UPD

✓5ᵗʰ **T50.4** **Poisoning by, adverse effect of and underdosing of drugs affecting uric acid metabolism**

✓6ᵗʰ **T50.4X** **Poisoning by, adverse effect of and underdosing of** drugs affecting uric acid metabolism

✓7ᵗʰ **T50.4X1** **Poisoning by drugs affecting uric acid metabolism,** accidental (unintentional)
Poisoning by drugs affecting uric acid metabolism NOS

2 ✓7ᵗʰ **T50.4X2** **Poisoning by drugs affecting uric acid metabolism,** intentional self-harm   HCC Rx ESR COM

✓7ᵗʰ **T50.4X3** **Poisoning by drugs affecting uric acid metabolism,** assault

✓7ᵗʰ **T50.4X4** **Poisoning by drugs affecting uric acid metabolism,** undetermined

✓7ᵗʰ **T50.4X5** Adverse effect **of drugs affecting uric acid metabolism** UPD

✓7ᵗʰ **T50.4X6** Underdosing **of drugs affecting uric acid metabolism** UPD

√5th T50.5 Poisoning by, adverse effect of and underdosing of appetite depressants
- **√6th T50.5X Poisoning by, adverse effect of and underdosing of** appetite depressants
  - **√7th T50.5X1 Poisoning by appetite depressants, accidental (unintentional)**
    - Poisoning by appetite depressants NOS
  - ² **√7th T50.5X2 Poisoning by appetite depressants, intentional self-harm** `HCC` `Rx` `ESR` `COM`
  - **√7th T50.5X3 Poisoning by appetite depressants, assault**
  - **√7th T50.5X4 Poisoning by appetite depressants, undetermined**
  - **√7th T50.5X5 Adverse effect of appetite depressants** `UPD`
  - **√7th T50.5X6 Underdosing of appetite depressants** `UPD`

√5th T50.6 Poisoning by, adverse effect of and underdosing of antidotes and chelating agents
- Poisoning by, adverse effect of and underdosing of alcohol deterrents
- **√6th T50.6X Poisoning by, adverse effect of and underdosing of** antidotes and chelating agents
  - **√7th T50.6X1 Poisoning by antidotes and chelating agents, accidental (unintentional)**
    - Poisoning by antidotes and chelating agents NOS
  - ² **√7th T50.6X2 Poisoning by antidotes and chelating agents, intentional self-harm** `HCC` `Rx` `ESR` `COM`
  - **√7th T50.6X3 Poisoning by antidotes and chelating agents, assault**
  - **√7th T50.6X4 Poisoning by antidotes and chelating agents, undetermined**
  - **√7th T50.6X5 Adverse effect of antidotes and chelating agents** `UPD`
  - **√7th T50.6X6 Underdosing of antidotes and chelating agents** `UPD`

√5th T50.7 Poisoning by, adverse effect of and underdosing of analeptics and opioid receptor antagonists
- **√6th T50.7X Poisoning by, adverse effect of and underdosing of** analeptics and opioid receptor antagonists
  - **√7th T50.7X1 Poisoning by analeptics and opioid receptor antagonists, accidental (unintentional)**
    - Poisoning by analeptics and opioid receptor antagonists NOS
  - ² **√7th T50.7X2 Poisoning by analeptics and opioid receptor antagonists, intentional self-harm** `HCC` `Rx` `ESR` `COM`
  - **√7th T50.7X3 Poisoning by analeptics and opioid receptor antagonists, assault**
  - **√7th T50.7X4 Poisoning by analeptics and opioid receptor antagonists, undetermined**
  - **√7th T50.7X5 Adverse effect of analeptics and opioid receptor antagonists** `UPD`
  - **√7th T50.7X6 Underdosing of analeptics and opioid receptor antagonists** `UPD`

√5th T50.8 Poisoning by, adverse effect of and underdosing of diagnostic agents
- **√6th T50.8X Poisoning by, adverse effect of and underdosing of** diagnostic agents
  - **√7th T50.8X1 Poisoning by diagnostic agents, accidental (unintentional)**
    - Poisoning by diagnostic agents NOS
  - ² **√7th T50.8X2 Poisoning by diagnostic agents, intentional self-harm** `HCC` `Rx` `ESR` `COM`
  - **√7th T50.8X3 Poisoning by diagnostic agents, assault**
  - **√7th T50.8X4 Poisoning by diagnostic agents, undetermined**
  - **√7th T50.8X5 Adverse effect of diagnostic agents** `UPD`
    - AHA: 2021,3Q,9-10
  - **√7th T50.8X6 Underdosing of diagnostic agents** `UPD`

√5th T50.A Poisoning by, adverse effect of and underdosing of bacterial vaccines
- **√6th T50.A1 Poisoning by, adverse effect of and underdosing of** pertussis vaccine, including combinations with a pertussis component
  - **√7th T50.A11 Poisoning by pertussis vaccine, including combinations with a pertussis component, accidental (unintentional)**
  - ² **√7th T50.A12 Poisoning by pertussis vaccine, including combinations with a pertussis component, intentional self-harm** `HCC` `Rx` `ESR` `COM`
  - **√7th T50.A13 Poisoning by pertussis vaccine, including combinations with a pertussis component, assault**
  - **√7th T50.A14 Poisoning by pertussis vaccine, including combinations with a pertussis component, undetermined**
  - **√7th T50.A15 Adverse effect of pertussis vaccine, including combinations with a pertussis component** `UPD`
  - **√7th T50.A16 Underdosing of pertussis vaccine, including combinations with a pertussis component** `UPD`
- **√6th T50.A2 Poisoning by, adverse effect of and underdosing of** mixed bacterial vaccines without a pertussis component
  - **√7th T50.A21 Poisoning by mixed bacterial vaccines without a pertussis component, accidental (unintentional)**
  - ² **√7th T50.A22 Poisoning by mixed bacterial vaccines without a pertussis component, intentional self-harm** `HCC` `Rx` `ESR` `COM`
  - **√7th T50.A23 Poisoning by mixed bacterial vaccines without a pertussis component, assault**
  - **√7th T50.A24 Poisoning by mixed bacterial vaccines without a pertussis component, undetermined**
  - **√7th T50.A25 Adverse effect of mixed bacterial vaccines without a pertussis component** `UPD`
  - **√7th T50.A26 Underdosing of mixed bacterial vaccines without a pertussis component** `UPD`
- **√6th T50.A9 Poisoning by, adverse effect of and underdosing of other bacterial vaccines**
  - **√7th T50.A91 Poisoning by other bacterial vaccines, accidental (unintentional)**
  - ² **√7th T50.A92 Poisoning by other bacterial vaccines, intentional self-harm** `HCC` `Rx` `ESR` `COM`
  - **√7th T50.A93 Poisoning by other bacterial vaccines, assault**
  - **√7th T50.A94 Poisoning by other bacterial vaccines, undetermined**
  - **√7th T50.A95 Adverse effect of other bacterial vaccines** `UPD`
  - **√7th T50.A96 Underdosing of other bacterial vaccines** `UPD`

√5th T50.B Poisoning by, adverse effect of and underdosing of viral vaccines
- **√6th T50.B1 Poisoning by, adverse effect of and underdosing of** smallpox vaccines
  - **√7th T50.B11 Poisoning by smallpox vaccines, accidental (unintentional)**
  - ² **√7th T50.B12 Poisoning by smallpox vaccines, intentional self-harm** `HCC` `Rx` `ESR` `COM`
  - **√7th T50.B13 Poisoning by smallpox vaccines, assault**
  - **√7th T50.B14 Poisoning by smallpox vaccines, undetermined**
  - **√7th T50.B15 Adverse effect of smallpox vaccines** `UPD`
  - **√7th T50.B16 Underdosing of smallpox vaccines** `UPD`
- **√6th T50.B9 Poisoning by, adverse effect of and underdosing of other viral vaccines**
  - **√7th T50.B91 Poisoning by other viral vaccines, accidental (unintentional)**
  - ² **√7th T50.B92 Poisoning by other viral vaccines, intentional self-harm** `HCC` `Rx` `ESR` `COM`
  - **√7th T50.B93 Poisoning by other viral vaccines, assault**
  - **√7th T50.B94 Poisoning by other viral vaccines, undetermined**
  - **√7th T50.B95 Adverse effect of other viral vaccines** `UPD`
    - AHA: 2021,1Q,43
  - **√7th T50.B96 Underdosing of other viral vaccines** `UPD`

√5th T50.Z Poisoning by, adverse effect of and underdosing of other vaccines and biological substances
- **√6th T50.Z1 Poisoning by, adverse effect of and underdosing of** immunoglobulin
  - **√7th T50.Z11 Poisoning by immunoglobulin, accidental (unintentional)**

Chapter 19. Injury, Poisoning and Certain Other Consequences of External Causes

² ✓7ᵗʰ **T50.Z12** **Poisoning by immunoglobulin,** intentional self-harm   HCC Rx ESR COM

✓7ᵗʰ **T50.Z13** **Poisoning by immunoglobulin,** assault

✓7ᵗʰ **T50.Z14** **Poisoning by immunoglobulin,** undetermined

✓7ᵗʰ **T50.Z15** Adverse effect of immunoglobulin   UPD

✓7ᵗʰ **T50.Z16** Underdosing of immunoglobulin   UPD

✓6ᵗʰ **T50.Z9** **Poisoning by, adverse effect of and underdosing of other vaccines and biological substances**

✓7ᵗʰ **T50.Z91** **Poisoning by other vaccines and biological substances,** accidental (unintentional)

² ✓7ᵗʰ **T50.Z92** **Poisoning by other vaccines and biological substances,** intentional self-harm   HCC Rx ESR COM

✓7ᵗʰ **T50.Z93** **Poisoning by other vaccines and biological substances,** assault

✓7ᵗʰ **T50.Z94** **Poisoning by other vaccines and biological substances,** undetermined

✓7ᵗʰ **T50.Z95** Adverse effect of other vaccines and biological substances   UPD
       AHA: 2020,1Q,18

✓7ᵗʰ **T50.Z96** Underdosing of other vaccines and biological substances   UPD

✓5ᵗʰ **T50.9** **Poisoning by, adverse effect of and underdosing of other and unspecified drugs, medicaments and biological substances**

✓6ᵗʰ **T50.90** **Poisoning by, adverse effect of and underdosing of unspecified drugs, medicaments and biological substances**

✓7ᵗʰ **T50.901** **Poisoning by unspecified drugs, medicaments and biological substances,** accidental (unintentional)

² ✓7ᵗʰ **T50.902** **Poisoning by unspecified drugs, medicaments and biological substances,** intentional self-harm   HCC Rx ESR COM

✓7ᵗʰ **T50.903** **Poisoning by unspecified drugs, medicaments and biological substances,** assault

✓7ᵗʰ **T50.904** **Poisoning by unspecified drugs, medicaments and biological substances,** undetermined

✓7ᵗʰ **T50.905** Adverse effect of unspecified drugs, medicaments and biological substances

✓7ᵗʰ **T50.906** Underdosing of unspecified drugs, medicaments and biological substances

✓6ᵗʰ **T50.91** **Poisoning by, adverse effect of and underdosing of multiple unspecified drugs, medicaments and biological substances**
     Multiple drug ingestion NOS
     Code also any specific drugs, medicaments and biological substances

✓7ᵗʰ **T50.911** **Poisoning by multiple unspecified drugs, medicaments and biological substances,** accidental (unintentional)

² ✓7ᵗʰ **T50.912** **Poisoning by multiple unspecified drugs, medicaments and biological substances,** intentional self-harm   HCC Rx ESR COM

✓7ᵗʰ **T50.913** **Poisoning by multiple unspecified drugs, medicaments and biological substances,** assault

✓7ᵗʰ **T50.914** **Poisoning by multiple unspecified drugs, medicaments and biological substances,** undetermined

✓7ᵗʰ **T50.915** Adverse effect of multiple unspecified drugs, medicaments and biological substances   UPD

✓7ᵗʰ **T50.916** Underdosing of multiple unspecified drugs, medicaments and biological substances   UPD

✓6ᵗʰ **T50.99** **Poisoning by, adverse effect of and underdosing of other drugs, medicaments and biological substances**

✓7ᵗʰ **T50.991** **Poisoning by other drugs, medicaments and biological substances,** accidental (unintentional)

² ✓7ᵗʰ **T50.992** **Poisoning by other drugs, medicaments and biological substances,** intentional self-harm   HCC Rx ESR COM

✓7ᵗʰ **T50.993** **Poisoning by other drugs, medicaments and biological substances,** assault

✓7ᵗʰ **T50.994** **Poisoning by other drugs, medicaments and biological substances,** undetermined

✓7ᵗʰ **T50.995** Adverse effect of other drugs, medicaments and biological substances

✓7ᵗʰ **T50.996** Underdosing of other drugs, medicaments and biological substances

Toxic effects of substances chiefly nonmedicinal as to source (T51-T65)

NOTE   When no intent is indicated code to accidental. Undetermined intent is only for use when there is specific documentation in the record that the intent of the toxic effect cannot be determined.

Use additional code(s) for all associated manifestations of toxic effect, such as:
    personal history of foreign body fully removed (Z87.821)
    respiratory conditions due to external agents (J60-J70)
    to identify any retained foreign body, if applicable (Z18.-)
   EXCLUDES 1   contact with and (suspected) exposure to toxic substances (Z77.-)
AHA: 2017,1Q,39-40

✓4ᵗʰ **T51** **Toxic effect of alcohol**

> The appropriate 7th character is to be added to each code from category T51.
> A   initial encounter
> D   subsequent encounter
> S   sequela

✓5ᵗʰ **T51.0** **Toxic effect of ethanol**
     Toxic effect of ethyl alcohol
     EXCLUDES 2   acute alcohol intoxication or "hangover" effects (F10.129, F10.229, F10.929)
          drunkenness (F10.129, F10.229, F10.929)
          pathological alcohol intoxication (F10.129, F10.229, F10.929)

✓6ᵗʰ **T51.0X** **Toxic effect of** ethanol

¹ ✓7ᵗʰ **T51.0X1** **Toxic effect of ethanol,** accidental (unintentional)   HCC ESR
       Toxic effect of ethanol NOS

² ✓7ᵗʰ **T51.0X2** **Toxic effect of ethanol,** intentional self-harm   HCC Rx ESR COM

✓7ᵗʰ **T51.0X3** **Toxic effect of ethanol,** assault

¹ ✓7ᵗʰ **T51.0X4** **Toxic effect of ethanol,** undetermined   HCC ESR

✓5ᵗʰ **T51.1** **Toxic effect of methanol**
     Toxic effect of methyl alcohol

✓6ᵗʰ **T51.1X** **Toxic effect of** methanol

✓7ᵗʰ **T51.1X1** **Toxic effect of methanol,** accidental (unintentional)
       Toxic effect of methanol NOS

² ✓7ᵗʰ **T51.1X2** **Toxic effect of methanol,** intentional self-harm   HCC Rx ESR COM

✓7ᵗʰ **T51.1X3** **Toxic effect of methanol,** assault

✓7ᵗʰ **T51.1X4** **Toxic effect of methanol,** undetermined

✓5ᵗʰ **T51.2** **Toxic effect of 2-Propanol**
     Toxic effect of isopropyl alcohol

✓6ᵗʰ **T51.2X** **Toxic effect of** 2-Propanol

✓7ᵗʰ **T51.2X1** **Toxic effect of 2-Propanol,** accidental (unintentional)
       Toxic effect of 2-Propanol NOS

² ✓7ᵗʰ **T51.2X2** **Toxic effect of 2-Propanol,** intentional self-harm   HCC Rx ESR COM

✓7ᵗʰ **T51.2X3** **Toxic effect of 2-Propanol,** assault

✓7ᵗʰ **T51.2X4** **Toxic effect of 2-Propanol,** undetermined

✓5ᵗʰ **T51.3** **Toxic effect of fusel oil**
     Toxic effect of amyl alcohol
     Toxic effect of butyl [1-butanol] alcohol
     Toxic effect of propyl [1-propanol] alcohol

✓6ᵗʰ **T51.3X** **Toxic effect of** fusel oil

✓7ᵗʰ **T51.3X1** **Toxic effect of fusel oil,** accidental (unintentional)
       Toxic effect of fusel oil NOS

² ✓7ᵗʰ **T51.3X2** **Toxic effect of fusel oil,** intentional self-harm   HCC Rx ESR COM

✓7ᵗʰ **T51.3X3** **Toxic effect of fusel oil,** assault

✓7ᵗʰ **T51.3X4** **Toxic effect of fusel oil,** undetermined

✓5th **T51.8 Toxic effect of other alcohols**
  ✓6th **T51.8X Toxic effect of other alcohols**
    ✓7th **T51.8X1 Toxic effect of other alcohols, accidental (unintentional)**
      Toxic effect of other alcohols NOS
    2 ✓7th **T51.8X2 Toxic effect of other alcohols, intentional self-harm** HCC Rx ESR COM
    ✓7th **T51.8X3 Toxic effect of other alcohols, assault**
    ✓7th **T51.8X4 Toxic effect of other alcohols, undetermined**
✓5th **T51.9 Toxic effect of unspecified alcohol**
  ✓x7th **T51.91 Toxic effect of unspecified alcohol, accidental (unintentional)**
  2 ✓x7th **T51.92 Toxic effect of unspecified alcohol, intentional self-harm** HCC Rx ESR COM
  ✓x7th **T51.93 Toxic effect of unspecified alcohol, assault**
  ✓x7th **T51.94 Toxic effect of unspecified alcohol, undetermined**

✓4th **T52 Toxic effect of organic solvents**
  EXCLUDES 1   halogen derivatives of aliphatic and aromatic hydrocarbons (T53.-)

> The appropriate 7th character is to be added to each code from category T52.
> A   initial encounter
> D   subsequent encounter
> S   sequela

✓5th **T52.0 Toxic effects of petroleum products**
  Toxic effects of ether petroleum
  Toxic effects of gasoline [petrol]
  Toxic effects of kerosene [paraffin oil]
  Toxic effects of naphtha petroleum
  Toxic effects of paraffin wax
  Toxic effects of spirit petroleum
  ✓6th **T52.0X Toxic effects of petroleum products**
    ✓7th **T52.0X1 Toxic effect of petroleum products, accidental (unintentional)**
      Toxic effects of petroleum products NOS
    2 ✓7th **T52.0X2 Toxic effect of petroleum products, intentional self-harm** HCC Rx ESR COM
    ✓7th **T52.0X3 Toxic effect of petroleum products, assault**
    ✓7th **T52.0X4 Toxic effect of petroleum products, undetermined**
✓5th **T52.1 Toxic effects of benzene**
  EXCLUDES 1   homologues of benzene (T52.2)
       nitroderivatives and aminoderivatives of benzene and its homologues (T65.3)
  ✓6th **T52.1X Toxic effects of benzene**
    ✓7th **T52.1X1 Toxic effect of benzene, accidental (unintentional)**
      Toxic effects of benzene NOS
    2 ✓7th **T52.1X2 Toxic effect of benzene, intentional self-harm** HCC Rx ESR COM
    ✓7th **T52.1X3 Toxic effect of benzene, assault**
    ✓7th **T52.1X4 Toxic effect of benzene, undetermined**
✓5th **T52.2 Toxic effects of homologues of benzene**
  Toxic effects of toluene [methylbenzene]
  Toxic effects of xylene [dimethylbenzene]
  ✓6th **T52.2X Toxic effects of homologues of benzene**
    ✓7th **T52.2X1 Toxic effect of homologues of benzene, accidental (unintentional)**
      Toxic effects of homologues of benzene NOS
    2 ✓7th **T52.2X2 Toxic effect of homologues of benzene, intentional self-harm** HCC Rx ESR COM
    ✓7th **T52.2X3 Toxic effect of homologues of benzene, assault**
    ✓7th **T52.2X4 Toxic effect of homologues of benzene, undetermined**
✓5th **T52.3 Toxic effects of glycols**
  ✓6th **T52.3X Toxic effects of glycols**
    ✓7th **T52.3X1 Toxic effect of glycols, accidental (unintentional)**
      Toxic effects of glycols NOS
    2 ✓7th **T52.3X2 Toxic effect of glycols, intentional self-harm** HCC Rx ESR COM

    ✓7th **T52.3X3 Toxic effect of glycols, assault**
    ✓7th **T52.3X4 Toxic effect of glycols, undetermined**
✓5th **T52.4 Toxic effects of ketones**
  ✓6th **T52.4X Toxic effects of ketones**
    ✓7th **T52.4X1 Toxic effect of ketones, accidental (unintentional)**
      Toxic effects of ketones NOS
    2 ✓7th **T52.4X2 Toxic effect of ketones, intentional self-harm** HCC Rx ESR COM
    ✓7th **T52.4X3 Toxic effect of ketones, assault**
    ✓7th **T52.4X4 Toxic effect of ketones, undetermined**
✓5th **T52.8 Toxic effects of other organic solvents**
  ✓6th **T52.8X Toxic effects of other organic solvents**
    ✓7th **T52.8X1 Toxic effect of other organic solvents, accidental (unintentional)**
      Toxic effects of other organic solvents NOS
    2 ✓7th **T52.8X2 Toxic effect of other organic solvents, intentional self-harm** HCC Rx ESR COM
    ✓7th **T52.8X3 Toxic effect of other organic solvents, assault**
    ✓7th **T52.8X4 Toxic effect of other organic solvents, undetermined**
✓5th **T52.9 Toxic effects of unspecified organic solvent**
  ✓x7th **T52.91 Toxic effect of unspecified organic solvent, accidental (unintentional)**
  2 ✓x7th **T52.92 Toxic effect of unspecified organic solvent, intentional self-harm** HCC Rx ESR COM
  ✓x7th **T52.93 Toxic effect of unspecified organic solvent, assault**
  ✓x7th **T52.94 Toxic effect of unspecified organic solvent, undetermined**

✓4th **T53 Toxic effect of halogen derivatives of aliphatic and aromatic hydrocarbons**

> The appropriate 7th character is to be added to each code from category T53.
> A   initial encounter
> D   subsequent encounter
> S   sequela

✓5th **T53.0 Toxic effects of carbon tetrachloride**
  Toxic effects of tetrachloromethane
  ✓6th **T53.0X Toxic effects of carbon tetrachloride**
    ✓7th **T53.0X1 Toxic effect of carbon tetrachloride, accidental (unintentional)**
      Toxic effects of carbon tetrachloride NOS
    2 ✓7th **T53.0X2 Toxic effect of carbon tetrachloride, intentional self-harm** HCC Rx ESR COM
    ✓7th **T53.0X3 Toxic effect of carbon tetrachloride, assault**
    ✓7th **T53.0X4 Toxic effect of carbon tetrachloride, undetermined**
✓5th **T53.1 Toxic effects of chloroform**
  Toxic effects of trichloromethane
  ✓6th **T53.1X Toxic effects of chloroform**
    ✓7th **T53.1X1 Toxic effect of chloroform, accidental (unintentional)**
      Toxic effects of chloroform NOS
    2 ✓7th **T53.1X2 Toxic effect of chloroform, intentional self-harm** HCC Rx ESR COM
    ✓7th **T53.1X3 Toxic effect of chloroform, assault**
    ✓7th **T53.1X4 Toxic effect of chloroform, undetermined**
✓5th **T53.2 Toxic effects of trichloroethylene**
  Toxic effects of trichloroethene
  ✓6th **T53.2X Toxic effects of trichloroethylene**
    ✓7th **T53.2X1 Toxic effect of trichloroethylene, accidental (unintentional)**
      Toxic effects of trichloroethylene NOS
    2 ✓7th **T53.2X2 Toxic effect of trichloroethylene, intentional self-harm** HCC Rx ESR COM
    ✓7th **T53.2X3 Toxic effect of trichloroethylene, assault**
    ✓7th **T53.2X4 Toxic effect of trichloroethylene, undetermined**

✓ Additional Character Required   ✓x7th Placeholder Alert   Manifestation   Unspecified Dx   ◑ QPP   UPD Unacceptable PDx

Chapter 19. Injury, Poisoning and Certain Other Consequences of External Causes

T53.3–T54.94

√5ᵗʰ **T53.3 Toxic effects of tetrachloroethylene**

Toxic effects of perchloroethylene
Toxic effect of tetrachloroethene

√6ᵗʰ **T53.3X Toxic effects of** tetrachloroethylene

√7ᵗʰ **T53.3X1 Toxic effect of tetrachloroethylene,** accidental (unintentional)
Toxic effects of tetrachloroethylene NOS

² √7ᵗʰ **T53.3X2 Toxic effect of tetrachloroethylene,** intentional self-harm HCC Rx ESR COM

√7ᵗʰ **T53.3X3 Toxic effect of tetrachloroethylene,** assault

√7ᵗʰ **T53.3X4 Toxic effect of tetrachloroethylene,** undetermined

√5ᵗʰ **T53.4 Toxic effects of dichloromethane**

Toxic effects of methylene chloride

√6ᵗʰ **T53.4X Toxic effects of** dichloromethane

√7ᵗʰ **T53.4X1 Toxic effect of dichloromethane,** accidental (unintentional)
Toxic effects of dichloromethane NOS

² √7ᵗʰ **T53.4X2 Toxic effect of dichloromethane,** intentional self-harm HCC Rx ESR COM

√7ᵗʰ **T53.4X3 Toxic effect of dichloromethane, assault**

√7ᵗʰ **T53.4X4 Toxic effect of dichloromethane,** undetermined

√5ᵗʰ **T53.5 Toxic effects of chlorofluorocarbons**

√6ᵗʰ **T53.5X Toxic effects of** chlorofluorocarbons

√7ᵗʰ **T53.5X1 Toxic effect of chlorofluorocarbons,** accidental (unintentional)
Toxic effects of chlorofluorocarbons NOS

² √7ᵗʰ **T53.5X2 Toxic effect of chlorofluorocarbons,** intentional self-harm HCC Rx ESR COM

√7ᵗʰ **T53.5X3 Toxic effect of chlorofluorocarbons,** assault

√7ᵗʰ **T53.5X4 Toxic effect of chlorofluorocarbons,** undetermined

√5ᵗʰ **T53.6 Toxic effects of other halogen derivatives of aliphatic hydrocarbons**

√6ᵗʰ **T53.6X Toxic effects of** other halogen derivatives of aliphatic hydrocarbons

√7ᵗʰ **T53.6X1 Toxic effect of other halogen derivatives of aliphatic hydrocarbons,** accidental (unintentional)
Toxic effects of other halogen derivatives of aliphatic hydrocarbons NOS

² √7ᵗʰ **T53.6X2 Toxic effect of other halogen derivatives of aliphatic hydrocarbons,** intentional self-harm HCC Rx ESR COM

√7ᵗʰ **T53.6X3 Toxic effect of other halogen derivatives of aliphatic hydrocarbons,** assault

√7ᵗʰ **T53.6X4 Toxic effect of other halogen derivatives of aliphatic hydrocarbons,** undetermined

√5ᵗʰ **T53.7 Toxic effects of other halogen derivatives of aromatic hydrocarbons**

√6ᵗʰ **T53.7X Toxic effects of** other halogen derivatives of aromatic hydrocarbons

√7ᵗʰ **T53.7X1 Toxic effect of other halogen derivatives of aromatic hydrocarbons,** accidental (unintentional)
Toxic effects of other halogen derivatives of aromatic hydrocarbons NOS

² √7ᵗʰ **T53.7X2 Toxic effect of other halogen derivatives of aromatic hydrocarbons,** intentional self-harm HCC Rx ESR COM

√7ᵗʰ **T53.7X3 Toxic effect of other halogen derivatives of aromatic hydrocarbons,** assault

√7ᵗʰ **T53.7X4 Toxic effect of other halogen derivatives of aromatic hydrocarbons,** undetermined

√5ᵗʰ **T53.9 Toxic effects of unspecified halogen derivatives of aliphatic and aromatic hydrocarbons**

√x7ᵗʰ **T53.91 Toxic effect of unspecified halogen derivatives of aliphatic and aromatic hydrocarbons, accidental (unintentional)**

² √x7ᵗʰ **T53.92 Toxic effect of unspecified halogen derivatives of aliphatic and aromatic hydrocarbons, intentional self-harm** HCC Rx ESR COM

√x7ᵗʰ **T53.93 Toxic effect of unspecified halogen derivatives of aliphatic and aromatic hydrocarbons, assault**

√x7ᵗʰ **T53.94 Toxic effect of unspecified halogen derivatives of aliphatic and aromatic hydrocarbons, undetermined**

√4ᵗʰ **T54 Toxic effect of corrosive substances**

The appropriate 7th character is to be added to each code from category T54.
A initial encounter
D subsequent encounter
S sequela

√5ᵗʰ **T54.0 Toxic effects of phenol and phenol homologues**

√6ᵗʰ **T54.0X Toxic effects of** phenol and phenol homologues

√7ᵗʰ **T54.0X1 Toxic effect of phenol and phenol homologues,** accidental (unintentional)
Toxic effects of phenol and phenol homologues NOS

² √7ᵗʰ **T54.0X2 Toxic effect of phenol and phenol homologues,** intentional self-harm HCC Rx ESR COM

√7ᵗʰ **T54.0X3 Toxic effect of phenol and phenol homologues,** assault

√7ᵗʰ **T54.0X4 Toxic effect of phenol and phenol homologues,** undetermined

√5ᵗʰ **T54.1 Toxic effects of other corrosive organic compounds**

√6ᵗʰ **T54.1X Toxic effects of other corrosive organic compounds**

√7ᵗʰ **T54.1X1 Toxic effect of other corrosive organic compounds,** accidental (unintentional)
Toxic effects of other corrosive organic compounds NOS

² √7ᵗʰ **T54.1X2 Toxic effect of other corrosive organic compounds,** intentional self-harm HCC Rx ESR COM

√7ᵗʰ **T54.1X3 Toxic effect of other corrosive organic compounds,** assault

√7ᵗʰ **T54.1X4 Toxic effect of other corrosive organic compounds,** undetermined

√5ᵗʰ **T54.2 Toxic effects of corrosive acids and acid-like substances**

Toxic effects of hydrochloric acid
Toxic effects of sulfuric acid

√6ᵗʰ **T54.2X Toxic effects of** corrosive acids and acid-like substances

√7ᵗʰ **T54.2X1 Toxic effect of corrosive acids and acid-like substances,** accidental (unintentional)
Toxic effects of corrosive acids and acid-like substances NOS

² √7ᵗʰ **T54.2X2 Toxic effect of corrosive acids and acid-like substances,** intentional self-harm HCC Rx ESR COM

√7ᵗʰ **T54.2X3 Toxic effect of corrosive acids and acid-like substances,** assault

√7ᵗʰ **T54.2X4 Toxic effect of corrosive acids and acid-like substances,** undetermined

√5ᵗʰ **T54.3 Toxic effects of corrosive alkalis and alkali-like substances**

Toxic effects of potassium hydroxide
Toxic effects of sodium hydroxide

√6ᵗʰ **T54.3X Toxic effects of** corrosive alkalis and alkali-like substances

√7ᵗʰ **T54.3X1 Toxic effect of corrosive alkalis and alkali-like substances,** accidental (unintentional)
Toxic effects of corrosive alkalis and alkali-like substances NOS

² √7ᵗʰ **T54.3X2 Toxic effect of corrosive alkalis and alkali-like substances,** intentional self-harm HCC Rx ESR COM

√7ᵗʰ **T54.3X3 Toxic effect of corrosive alkalis and alkali-like substances,** assault

√7ᵗʰ **T54.3X4 Toxic effect of corrosive alkalis and alkali-like substances,** undetermined

√5ᵗʰ **T54.9 Toxic effects of unspecified corrosive substance**

√x7ᵗʰ **T54.91 Toxic effect of unspecified corrosive substance,** accidental (unintentional)

² √x7ᵗʰ **T54.92 Toxic effect of unspecified corrosive substance,** intentional self-harm HCC Rx ESR COM

√x7ᵗʰ **T54.93 Toxic effect of unspecified corrosive substance,** assault

√x7ᵗʰ **T54.94 Toxic effect of unspecified corrosive substance,** undetermined

✓4ᵗʰ **T55 Toxic effect of soaps and detergents**

> The appropriate 7th character is to be added to each code from category T55.
> A   initial encounter
> D   subsequent encounter
> S   sequela

✓5ᵗʰ **T55.0 Toxic effect of soaps**

✓6ᵗʰ **T55.0X Toxic effect of** soaps

✓7ᵗʰ **T55.0X1 Toxic effect of soaps, accidental (unintentional)**
Toxic effect of soaps NOS

² ✓7ᵗʰ **T55.0X2 Toxic effect of soaps, intentional self-harm** HCC Rx ESR COM

✓7ᵗʰ **T55.0X3 Toxic effect of soaps, assault**

✓7ᵗʰ **T55.0X4 Toxic effect of soaps, undetermined**

✓5ᵗʰ **T55.1 Toxic effect of detergents**

✓6ᵗʰ **T55.1X Toxic effect of** detergents

✓7ᵗʰ **T55.1X1 Toxic effect of detergents, accidental (unintentional)**
Toxic effect of detergents NOS

² ✓7ᵗʰ **T55.1X2 Toxic effect of detergents, intentional self-harm** HCC Rx ESR COM

✓7ᵗʰ **T55.1X3 Toxic effect of detergents, assault**

✓7ᵗʰ **T55.1X4 Toxic effect of detergents, undetermined**

✓4ᵗʰ **T56 Toxic effect of metals**

INCLUDES toxic effects of fumes and vapors of metals
toxic effects of metals from all sources, except medicinal substances
Use additional code to identify any retained metal foreign body, if applicable (Z18.0-, T18.1-)

EXCLUDES 1 arsenic and its compounds (T57.0)
manganese and its compounds (T57.2)

> The appropriate 7th character is to be added to each code from category T56.
> A   initial encounter
> D   subsequent encounter
> S   sequela

✓5ᵗʰ **T56.0 Toxic effects of lead and its compounds**

✓6ᵗʰ **T56.0X Toxic effects of** lead **and its compounds**

✓7ᵗʰ **T56.0X1 Toxic effect of lead and its compounds, accidental (unintentional)**
Toxic effects of lead and its compounds NOS

² ✓7ᵗʰ **T56.0X2 Toxic effect of lead and its compounds, intentional self-harm** HCC Rx ESR COM

✓7ᵗʰ **T56.0X3 Toxic effect of lead and its compounds, assault**

✓7ᵗʰ **T56.0X4 Toxic effect of lead and its compounds, undetermined**

✓5ᵗʰ **T56.1 Toxic effects of mercury and its compounds**

✓6ᵗʰ **T56.1X Toxic effects of** mercury **and its compounds**

✓7ᵗʰ **T56.1X1 Toxic effect of mercury and its compounds, accidental (unintentional)**
Toxic effects of mercury and its compounds NOS

² ✓7ᵗʰ **T56.1X2 Toxic effect of mercury and its compounds, intentional self-harm** HCC Rx ESR COM

✓7ᵗʰ **T56.1X3 Toxic effect of mercury and its compounds, assault**

✓7ᵗʰ **T56.1X4 Toxic effect of mercury and its compounds, undetermined**

✓5ᵗʰ **T56.2 Toxic effects of chromium and its compounds**

✓6ᵗʰ **T56.2X Toxic effects of** chromium **and its compounds**

✓7ᵗʰ **T56.2X1 Toxic effect of chromium and its compounds, accidental (unintentional)**
Toxic effects of chromium and its compounds NOS

² ✓7ᵗʰ **T56.2X2 Toxic effect of chromium and its compounds, intentional self-harm** HCC Rx ESR COM

✓7ᵗʰ **T56.2X3 Toxic effect of chromium and its compounds, assault**

✓7ᵗʰ **T56.2X4 Toxic effect of chromium and its compounds, undetermined**

✓5ᵗʰ **T56.3 Toxic effects of cadmium and its compounds**

✓6ᵗʰ **T56.3X Toxic effects of** cadmium **and its compounds**

✓7ᵗʰ **T56.3X1 Toxic effect of cadmium and its compounds, accidental (unintentional)**
Toxic effects of cadmium and its compounds NOS

² ✓7ᵗʰ **T56.3X2 Toxic effect of cadmium and its compounds, intentional self-harm** HCC Rx ESR COM

✓7ᵗʰ **T56.3X3 Toxic effect of cadmium and its compounds, assault**

✓7ᵗʰ **T56.3X4 Toxic effect of cadmium and its compounds, undetermined**

✓5ᵗʰ **T56.4 Toxic effects of copper and its compounds**

✓6ᵗʰ **T56.4X Toxic effects of** copper **and its compounds**

✓7ᵗʰ **T56.4X1 Toxic effect of copper and its compounds, accidental (unintentional)**
Toxic effects of copper and its compounds NOS

² ✓7ᵗʰ **T56.4X2 Toxic effect of copper and its compounds, intentional self-harm** HCC Rx ESR COM

✓7ᵗʰ **T56.4X3 Toxic effect of copper and its compounds, assault**

✓7ᵗʰ **T56.4X4 Toxic effect of copper and its compounds, undetermined**

✓5ᵗʰ **T56.5 Toxic effects of zinc and its compounds**

✓6ᵗʰ **T56.5X Toxic effects of** zinc **and its compounds**

✓7ᵗʰ **T56.5X1 Toxic effect of zinc and its compounds, accidental (unintentional)**
Toxic effects of zinc and its compounds NOS

² ✓7ᵗʰ **T56.5X2 Toxic effect of zinc and its compounds, intentional self-harm** HCC Rx ESR COM

✓7ᵗʰ **T56.5X3 Toxic effect of zinc and its compounds, assault**

✓7ᵗʰ **T56.5X4 Toxic effect of zinc and its compounds, undetermined**

✓5ᵗʰ **T56.6 Toxic effects of tin and its compounds**

✓6ᵗʰ **T56.6X Toxic effects of** tin **and its compounds**

✓7ᵗʰ **T56.6X1 Toxic effect of tin and its compounds, accidental (unintentional)**
Toxic effects of tin and its compounds NOS

² ✓7ᵗʰ **T56.6X2 Toxic effect of tin and its compounds, intentional self-harm** HCC Rx ESR COM

✓7ᵗʰ **T56.6X3 Toxic effect of tin and its compounds, assault**

✓7ᵗʰ **T56.6X4 Toxic effect of tin and its compounds, undetermined**

✓5ᵗʰ **T56.7 Toxic effects of beryllium and its compounds**

✓6ᵗʰ **T56.7X Toxic effects of** beryllium **and its compounds**

✓7ᵗʰ **T56.7X1 Toxic effect of beryllium and its compounds, accidental (unintentional)**
Toxic effects of beryllium and its compounds NOS

² ✓7ᵗʰ **T56.7X2 Toxic effect of beryllium and its compounds, intentional self-harm** HCC Rx ESR COM

✓7ᵗʰ **T56.7X3 Toxic effect of beryllium and its compounds, assault**

✓7ᵗʰ **T56.7X4 Toxic effect of beryllium and its compounds, undetermined**

✓5ᵗʰ **T56.8 Toxic effects of other metals**

✓6ᵗʰ **T56.81 Toxic effect of** thallium

✓7ᵗʰ **T56.811 Toxic effect of thallium, accidental (unintentional)**
Toxic effect of thallium NOS

² ✓7ᵗʰ **T56.812 Toxic effect of thallium, intentional self-harm** HCC Rx ESR

✓7ᵗʰ **T56.813 Toxic effect of thallium, assault**

✓7ᵗʰ **T56.814 Toxic effect of thallium, undetermined**

✓6ᵗʰ **T56.89 Toxic effects of other metals**

✓7ᵗʰ **T56.891 Toxic effect of other metals, accidental (unintentional)**
Toxic effects of other metals NOS

² ✓7ᵗʰ **T56.892 Toxic effect of other metals, intentional self-harm** HCC Rx ESR COM

✓7ᵗʰ **T56.893 Toxic effect of other metals, assault**

√7ᵗʰ **T56.894** Toxic effect of other metals, undetermined

√5ᵗʰ **T56.9** Toxic effects of unspecified metal

  √x7ᵗʰ **T56.91** Toxic effect of unspecified metal, accidental (unintentional)

  ² √x7ᵗʰ **T56.92** Toxic effect of unspecified metal, intentional self-harm HCC Rx ESR COM

  √x7ᵗʰ **T56.93** Toxic effect of unspecified metal, assault

  √x7ᵗʰ **T56.94** Toxic effect of unspecified metal, undetermined

√4ᵗʰ **T57** Toxic effect of other inorganic substances

> The appropriate 7th character is to be added to each code from category T57.
> A initial encounter
> D subsequent encounter
> S sequela

√5ᵗʰ **T57.0** Toxic effect of arsenic and its compounds

  √6ᵗʰ **T57.0X** Toxic effect of arsenic and its compounds

    √7ᵗʰ **T57.0X1** Toxic effect of arsenic and its compounds, accidental (unintentional)
      Toxic effect of arsenic and its compounds NOS

    ² √7ᵗʰ **T57.0X2** Toxic effect of arsenic and its compounds, intentional self-harm HCC Rx ESR COM

    √7ᵗʰ **T57.0X3** Toxic effect of arsenic and its compounds, assault

    √7ᵗʰ **T57.0X4** Toxic effect of arsenic and its compounds, undetermined

√5ᵗʰ **T57.1** Toxic effect of phosphorus and its compounds

  EXCLUDES 1   organophosphate insecticides (T60.0)

  √6ᵗʰ **T57.1X** Toxic effect of phosphorus and its compounds

    √7ᵗʰ **T57.1X1** Toxic effect of phosphorus and its compounds, accidental (unintentional)
      Toxic effect of phosphorus and its compounds NOS

    ² √7ᵗʰ **T57.1X2** Toxic effect of phosphorus and its compounds, intentional self-harm HCC Rx ESR COM

    √7ᵗʰ **T57.1X3** Toxic effect of phosphorus and its compounds, assault

    √7ᵗʰ **T57.1X4** Toxic effect of phosphorus and its compounds, undetermined

√5ᵗʰ **T57.2** Toxic effect of manganese and its compounds

  √6ᵗʰ **T57.2X** Toxic effect of manganese and its compounds

    √7ᵗʰ **T57.2X1** Toxic effect of manganese and its compounds, accidental (unintentional)
      Toxic effect of manganese and its compounds NOS

    ² √7ᵗʰ **T57.2X2** Toxic effect of manganese and its compounds, intentional self-harm HCC Rx ESR COM

    √7ᵗʰ **T57.2X3** Toxic effect of manganese and its compounds, assault

    √7ᵗʰ **T57.2X4** Toxic effect of manganese and its compounds, undetermined

√5ᵗʰ **T57.3** Toxic effect of hydrogen cyanide

  √6ᵗʰ **T57.3X** Toxic effect of hydrogen cyanide

    √7ᵗʰ **T57.3X1** Toxic effect of hydrogen cyanide, accidental (unintentional)
      Toxic effect of hydrogen cyanide NOS

    ² √7ᵗʰ **T57.3X2** Toxic effect of hydrogen cyanide, intentional self-harm HCC Rx ESR COM

    √7ᵗʰ **T57.3X3** Toxic effect of hydrogen cyanide, assault

    √7ᵗʰ **T57.3X4** Toxic effect of hydrogen cyanide, undetermined

√5ᵗʰ **T57.8** Toxic effect of other specified inorganic substances

  √6ᵗʰ **T57.8X** Toxic effect of other specified inorganic substances

    √7ᵗʰ **T57.8X1** Toxic effect of other specified inorganic substances, accidental (unintentional)
      Toxic effect of other specified inorganic substances NOS

    ² √7ᵗʰ **T57.8X2** Toxic effect of other specified inorganic substances, intentional self-harm HCC Rx ESR COM

    √7ᵗʰ **T57.8X3** Toxic effect of other specified inorganic substances, assault

    √7ᵗʰ **T57.8X4** Toxic effect of other specified inorganic substances, undetermined

√5ᵗʰ **T57.9** Toxic effect of unspecified inorganic substance

  √x7ᵗʰ **T57.91** Toxic effect of unspecified inorganic substance, accidental (unintentional)

  ² √x7ᵗʰ **T57.92** Toxic effect of unspecified inorganic substance, intentional self-harm HCC Rx ESR COM

  √x7ᵗʰ **T57.93** Toxic effect of unspecified inorganic substance, assault

  √x7ᵗʰ **T57.94** Toxic effect of unspecified inorganic substance, undetermined

√4ᵗʰ **T58** Toxic effect of carbon monoxide

> INCLUDES   asphyxiation from carbon monoxide
>   toxic effect of carbon monoxide from all sources

> The appropriate 7th character is to be added to each code from category T58.
> A initial encounter
> D subsequent encounter
> S sequela

√5ᵗʰ **T58.0** Toxic effect of carbon monoxide from motor vehicle exhaust
  Toxic effect of exhaust gas from gas engine
  Toxic effect of exhaust gas from motor pump

  √x7ᵗʰ **T58.01** Toxic effect of carbon monoxide from motor vehicle exhaust, accidental (unintentional)

  ² √x7ᵗʰ **T58.02** Toxic effect of carbon monoxide from motor vehicle exhaust, intentional self-harm HCC Rx ESR COM

  √x7ᵗʰ **T58.03** Toxic effect of carbon monoxide from motor vehicle exhaust, assault

  √x7ᵗʰ **T58.04** Toxic effect of carbon monoxide from motor vehicle exhaust, undetermined

√5ᵗʰ **T58.1** Toxic effect of carbon monoxide from utility gas
  Toxic effect of acetylene
  Toxic effect of gas NOS used for lighting, heating, cooking
  Toxic effect of water gas

CO   √x7ᵗʰ **T58.11** Toxic effect of carbon monoxide from utility gas, accidental (unintentional)

  ² √x7ᵗʰ **T58.12** Toxic effect of carbon monoxide from utility gas, intentional self-harm HCC Rx ESR COM

  √x7ᵗʰ **T58.13** Toxic effect of carbon monoxide from utility gas, assault

  √x7ᵗʰ **T58.14** Toxic effect of carbon monoxide from utility gas, undetermined

√5ᵗʰ **T58.2** Toxic effect of carbon monoxide from incomplete combustion of other domestic fuels
  Toxic effect of carbon monoxide from incomplete combustion of coal, coke, kerosene, wood

  √6ᵗʰ **T58.2X** Toxic effect of carbon monoxide from incomplete combustion of other domestic fuels

    √7ᵗʰ **T58.2X1** Toxic effect of carbon monoxide from incomplete combustion of other domestic fuels, accidental (unintentional)

    ² √7ᵗʰ **T58.2X2** Toxic effect of carbon monoxide from incomplete combustion of other domestic fuels, intentional self-harm HCC Rx ESR COM

    √7ᵗʰ **T58.2X3** Toxic effect of carbon monoxide from incomplete combustion of other domestic fuels, assault

    √7ᵗʰ **T58.2X4** Toxic effect of carbon monoxide from incomplete combustion of other domestic fuels, undetermined

√5ᵗʰ **T58.8** Toxic effect of carbon monoxide from other source
  Toxic effect of carbon monoxide from blast furnace gas
  Toxic effect of carbon monoxide from fuels in industrial use
  Toxic effect of carbon monoxide from kiln vapor

  √6ᵗʰ **T58.8X** Toxic effect of carbon monoxide from other source

    √7ᵗʰ **T58.8X1** Toxic effect of carbon monoxide from other source, accidental (unintentional)

    ² √7ᵗʰ **T58.8X2** Toxic effect of carbon monoxide from other source, intentional self-harm HCC Rx ESR COM

    √7ᵗʰ **T58.8X3** Toxic effect of carbon monoxide from other source, assault

    √7ᵗʰ **T58.8X4** Toxic effect of carbon monoxide from other source, undetermined

√5ᵗʰ **T58.9** Toxic effect of carbon monoxide from unspecified source

  √x7ᵗʰ **T58.91** Toxic effect of carbon monoxide from unspecified source, accidental (unintentional)

  ² √x7ᵗʰ **T58.92** Toxic effect of carbon monoxide from unspecified source, intentional self-harm HCC Rx ESR COM

√x7ʰ **T58.93** Toxic effect of carbon monoxide from unspecified source, assault

√x7ʰ **T58.94** Toxic effect of carbon monoxide from unspecified source, undetermined

✓4ʰ **T59 Toxic effect of other gases, fumes and vapors**

INCLUDES   aerosol propellants

EXCLUDES 1   *chlorofluorocarbons (T53.5)*

The appropriate 7th character is to be added to each code from category T59.
A   initial encounter
D   subsequent encounter
S   sequela

✓5ʰ **T59.0 Toxic effect of nitrogen oxides**

  ✓6ʰ **T59.0X** Toxic effect of nitrogen oxides

    √7ʰ **T59.0X1** Toxic effect of nitrogen oxides, accidental (unintentional)
       Toxic effect of nitrogen oxides NOS

    ² √7ʰ **T59.0X2** Toxic effect of nitrogen oxides, intentional self-harm   HCC Rx ESR COM

    √7ʰ **T59.0X3** Toxic effect of nitrogen oxides, assault

    √7ʰ **T59.0X4** Toxic effect of nitrogen oxides, undetermined

✓5ʰ **T59.1 Toxic effect of sulfur dioxide**

  ✓6ʰ **T59.1X** Toxic effect of sulfur dioxide

    √7ʰ **T59.1X1** Toxic effect of sulfur dioxide, accidental (unintentional)
       Toxic effect of sulfur dioxide NOS

    ² √7ʰ **T59.1X2** Toxic effect of sulfur dioxide, intentional self-harm   HCC Rx ESR COM

    √7ʰ **T59.1X3** Toxic effect of sulfur dioxide, assault

    √7ʰ **T59.1X4** Toxic effect of sulfur dioxide, undetermined

✓5ʰ **T59.2 Toxic effect of formaldehyde**

  ✓6ʰ **T59.2X** Toxic effect of formaldehyde

    √7ʰ **T59.2X1** Toxic effect of formaldehyde, accidental (unintentional)
       Toxic effect of formaldehyde NOS

    ² √7ʰ **T59.2X2** Toxic effect of formaldehyde, intentional self-harm   HCC Rx ESR COM

    √7ʰ **T59.2X3** Toxic effect of formaldehyde, assault

    √7ʰ **T59.2X4** Toxic effect of formaldehyde, undetermined

✓5ʰ **T59.3 Toxic effect of lacrimogenic gas**

   Toxic effect of tear gas

  ✓6ʰ **T59.3X** Toxic effect of lacrimogenic gas

    √7ʰ **T59.3X1** Toxic effect of lacrimogenic gas, accidental (unintentional)
       Toxic effect of lacrimogenic gas NOS

    ² √7ʰ **T59.3X2** Toxic effect of lacrimogenic gas, intentional self-harm   HCC Rx ESR COM

    √7ʰ **T59.3X3** Toxic effect of lacrimogenic gas, assault

    √7ʰ **T59.3X4** Toxic effect of lacrimogenic gas, undetermined

✓5ʰ **T59.4 Toxic effect of chlorine gas**

  ✓6ʰ **T59.4X** Toxic effect of chlorine gas

    √7ʰ **T59.4X1** Toxic effect of chlorine gas, accidental (unintentional)
       Toxic effect of chlorine gas NOS

    ² √7ʰ **T59.4X2** Toxic effect of chlorine gas, intentional self-harm   HCC Rx ESR COM

    √7ʰ **T59.4X3** Toxic effect of chlorine gas, assault

    √7ʰ **T59.4X4** Toxic effect of chlorine gas, undetermined

✓5ʰ **T59.5 Toxic effect of fluorine gas and hydrogen fluoride**

  ✓6ʰ **T59.5X** Toxic effect of fluorine gas and hydrogen fluoride

    √7ʰ **T59.5X1** Toxic effect of fluorine gas and hydrogen fluoride, accidental (unintentional)
       Toxic effect of fluorine gas and hydrogen fluoride NOS

    ² √7ʰ **T59.5X2** Toxic effect of fluorine gas and hydrogen fluoride, intentional self-harm   HCC Rx ESR COM

    √7ʰ **T59.5X3** Toxic effect of fluorine gas and hydrogen fluoride, assault

    √7ʰ **T59.5X4** Toxic effect of fluorine gas and hydrogen fluoride, undetermined

✓5ʰ **T59.6 Toxic effect of hydrogen sulfide**

  ✓6ʰ **T59.6X** Toxic effect of hydrogen sulfide

    √7ʰ **T59.6X1** Toxic effect of hydrogen sulfide, accidental (unintentional)
       Toxic effect of hydrogen sulfide NOS

    ² √7ʰ **T59.6X2** Toxic effect of hydrogen sulfide, intentional self-harm   HCC Rx ESR COM

    √7ʰ **T59.6X3** Toxic effect of hydrogen sulfide, assault

    √7ʰ **T59.6X4** Toxic effect of hydrogen sulfide, undetermined

✓5ʰ **T59.7 Toxic effect of carbon dioxide**

  ✓6ʰ **T59.7X** Toxic effect of carbon dioxide

    √7ʰ **T59.7X1** Toxic effect of carbon dioxide, accidental (unintentional)
       Toxic effect of carbon dioxide NOS

    ² √7ʰ **T59.7X2** Toxic effect of carbon dioxide, intentional self-harm   HCC Rx ESR COM

    √7ʰ **T59.7X3** Toxic effect of carbon dioxide, assault

    √7ʰ **T59.7X4** Toxic effect of carbon dioxide, undetermined

✓5ʰ **T59.8 Toxic effect of other specified gases, fumes and vapors**

  ✓6ʰ **T59.81** Toxic effect of smoke

     Smoke inhalation

     EXCLUDES 2   *toxic effect of cigarette (tobacco) smoke (T65.22-)*

    √7ʰ **T59.811** Toxic effect of smoke, accidental (unintentional)
       Toxic effect of smoke NOS
       AHA: 2013,4Q,121

    ² √7ʰ **T59.812** Toxic effect of smoke, intentional self-harm   HCC Rx ESR COM

    √7ʰ **T59.813** Toxic effect of smoke, assault

    √7ʰ **T59.814** Toxic effect of smoke, undetermined

  ✓6ʰ **T59.89** Toxic effect of other specified gases, fumes and vapors

    √7ʰ **T59.891** Toxic effect of other specified gases, fumes and vapors, accidental (unintentional)

    ² √7ʰ **T59.892** Toxic effect of other specified gases, fumes and vapors, intentional self-harm   HCC Rx ESR COM

    √7ʰ **T59.893** Toxic effect of other specified gases, fumes and vapors, assault

    √7ʰ **T59.894** Toxic effect of other specified gases, fumes and vapors, undetermined

✓5ʰ **T59.9 Toxic effect of unspecified gases, fumes and vapors**

  √x7ʰ **T59.91** Toxic effect of unspecified gases, fumes and vapors, accidental (unintentional)

  ² √x7ʰ **T59.92** Toxic effect of unspecified gases, fumes and vapors, intentional self-harm   HCC Rx ESR COM

  √x7ʰ **T59.93** Toxic effect of unspecified gases, fumes and vapors, assault

  √x7ʰ **T59.94** Toxic effect of unspecified gases, fumes and vapors, undetermined

✓4ʰ **T60 Toxic effect of pesticides**

INCLUDES   toxic effect of wood preservatives

The appropriate 7th character is to be added to each code from category T60.
A   initial encounter
D   subsequent encounter
S   sequela

✓5ʰ **T60.0 Toxic effect of organophosphate and carbamate insecticides**

  ✓6ʰ **T60.0X** Toxic effect of organophosphate and carbamate insecticides

    √7ʰ **T60.0X1** Toxic effect of organophosphate and carbamate insecticides, accidental (unintentional)
       Toxic effect of organophosphate and carbamate insecticides NOS

    ² √7ʰ **T60.0X2** Toxic effect of organophosphate and carbamate insecticides, intentional self-harm   HCC Rx ESR COM

    √7ʰ **T60.0X3** Toxic effect of organophosphate and carbamate insecticides, assault

    √7ʰ **T60.0X4** Toxic effect of organophosphate and carbamate insecticides, undetermined

√5ᵗʰ **T60.1** **Toxic effect of halogenated insecticides**
  EXCLUDES 1 *chlorinated hydrocarbon (T53.-)*
  √6ᵗʰ **T60.1X** **Toxic effect of** halogenated insecticides
    √7ᵗʰ **T60.1X1** **Toxic effect of halogenated insecticides, accidental (unintentional)**
      Toxic effect of halogenated insecticides NOS
    ² √7ᵗʰ **T60.1X2** **Toxic effect of halogenated insecticides, intentional self-harm** HCC Rx ESR COM
    √7ᵗʰ **T60.1X3** **Toxic effect of halogenated insecticides, assault**
    √7ᵗʰ **T60.1X4** **Toxic effect of halogenated insecticides, undetermined**
√5ᵗʰ **T60.2** **Toxic effect of other insecticides**
  √6ᵗʰ **T60.2X** **Toxic effect of** other insecticides
    √7ᵗʰ **T60.2X1** **Toxic effect of other insecticides, accidental (unintentional)**
      Toxic effect of other insecticides NOS
    ² √7ᵗʰ **T60.2X2** **Toxic effect of other insecticides, intentional self-harm** HCC Rx ESR COM
    √7ᵗʰ **T60.2X3** **Toxic effect of other insecticides, assault**
    √7ᵗʰ **T60.2X4** **Toxic effect of other insecticides, undetermined**
√5ᵗʰ **T60.3** **Toxic effect of herbicides and fungicides**
  √6ᵗʰ **T60.3X** **Toxic effect of** herbicides and fungicides
    √7ᵗʰ **T60.3X1** **Toxic effect of herbicides and fungicides, accidental (unintentional)**
      Toxic effect of herbicides and fungicides NOS
    ² √7ᵗʰ **T60.3X2** **Toxic effect of herbicides and fungicides, intentional self-harm** HCC Rx ESR COM
    √7ᵗʰ **T60.3X3** **Toxic effect of herbicides and fungicides, assault**
    √7ᵗʰ **T60.3X4** **Toxic effect of herbicides and fungicides, undetermined**
√5ᵗʰ **T60.4** **Toxic effect of rodenticides**
  EXCLUDES 1 *strychnine and its salts (T65.1)*
    thallium (T56.81-)
  √6ᵗʰ **T60.4X** **Toxic effect of** rodenticides
    √7ᵗʰ **T60.4X1** **Toxic effect of rodenticides, accidental (unintentional)**
      Toxic effect of rodenticides NOS
    ² √7ᵗʰ **T60.4X2** **Toxic effect of rodenticides, intentional self-harm** HCC Rx ESR COM
    √7ᵗʰ **T60.4X3** **Toxic effect of rodenticides, assault**
    √7ᵗʰ **T60.4X4** **Toxic effect of rodenticides, undetermined**
√5ᵗʰ **T60.8** **Toxic effect of other pesticides**
  √6ᵗʰ **T60.8X** **Toxic effect of** other pesticides
    √7ᵗʰ **T60.8X1** **Toxic effect of other pesticides, accidental (unintentional)**
      Toxic effect of other pesticides NOS
    ² √7ᵗʰ **T60.8X2** **Toxic effect of other pesticides, intentional self-harm** HCC Rx ESR COM
    √7ᵗʰ **T60.8X3** **Toxic effect of other pesticides, assault**
    √7ᵗʰ **T60.8X4** **Toxic effect of other pesticides, undetermined**
√5ᵗʰ **T60.9** **Toxic effect of unspecified pesticide**
  √x7ᵗʰ **T60.91** **Toxic effect of unspecified pesticide, accidental (unintentional)**
  ² √x7ᵗʰ **T60.92** **Toxic effect of unspecified pesticide, intentional self-harm** HCC Rx ESR COM
  √x7ᵗʰ **T60.93** **Toxic effect of unspecified pesticide, assault**
  √x7ᵗʰ **T60.94** **Toxic effect of unspecified pesticide, undetermined**

√4ᵗʰ **T61** **Toxic effect of noxious substances eaten as seafood**
  EXCLUDES 1 *allergic reaction to food, such as:*
    anaphylactic reaction or shock due to adverse food reaction (T78.0-)
    bacterial foodborne intoxications (A05.-)
    dermatitis (L23.6, L25.4, L27.2)
    food protein-induced enterocolitis syndrome (K52.21)
    food protein-induced enteropathy (K52.22)
    gastroenteritis (noninfective) (K52.29)
    toxic effect of aflatoxin and other mycotoxins (T64)
    toxic effect of cyanides (T65.0-)
    toxic effect of harmful algae bloom (T65.82-)
    toxic effect of hydrogen cyanide (T57.3-)
    toxic effect of mercury (T56.1-)
    toxic effect of red tide (T65.82-)

  The appropriate 7th character is to be added to each code from category T61.
  A   initial encounter
  D   subsequent encounter
  S   sequela

  √5ᵗʰ **T61.0** Ciguatera fish **poisoning**
    √x7ᵗʰ **T61.01** **Ciguatera fish poisoning,** accidental (unintentional)
    ² √x7ᵗʰ **T61.02** **Ciguatera fish poisoning,** intentional self-harm HCC Rx ESR COM
    √x7ᵗʰ **T61.03** **Ciguatera fish poisoning,** assault
    √x7ᵗʰ **T61.04** **Ciguatera fish poisoning,** undetermined
  √5ᵗʰ **T61.1** Scombroid fish **poisoning**
    Histamine-like syndrome
    √x7ᵗʰ **T61.11** **Scombroid fish poisoning,** accidental (unintentional)
    ² √x7ᵗʰ **T61.12** **Scombroid fish poisoning,** intentional self-harm HCC Rx ESR COM
    √x7ᵗʰ **T61.13** **Scombroid fish poisoning,** assault
    √x7ᵗʰ **T61.14** **Scombroid fish poisoning,** undetermined
  √5ᵗʰ **T61.7** **Other fish and shellfish poisoning**
    √6ᵗʰ **T61.77** **Other** fish **poisoning**
      √7ᵗʰ **T61.771** **Other fish poisoning,** accidental (unintentional)
      ² √7ᵗʰ **T61.772** **Other fish poisoning,** intentional self-harm HCC Rx ESR COM
      √7ᵗʰ **T61.773** **Other fish poisoning,** assault
      √7ᵗʰ **T61.774** **Other fish poisoning,** undetermined
    √6ᵗʰ **T61.78** **Other** shellfish **poisoning**
      √7ᵗʰ **T61.781** **Other shellfish poisoning,** accidental (unintentional)
      ² √7ᵗʰ **T61.782** **Other shellfish poisoning,** intentional self-harm HCC Rx ESR COM
      √7ᵗʰ **T61.783** **Other shellfish poisoning,** assault
      √7ᵗʰ **T61.784** **Other shellfish poisoning,** undetermined
  √5ᵗʰ **T61.8** **Toxic effect of other seafood**
    √6ᵗʰ **T61.8X** **Toxic effect of other seafood**
      √7ᵗʰ **T61.8X1** **Toxic effect of other seafood,** accidental (unintentional)
      ² √7ᵗʰ **T61.8X2** **Toxic effect of other seafood,** intentional self-harm HCC Rx ESR COM
      √7ᵗʰ **T61.8X3** **Toxic effect of other seafood,** assault
      √7ᵗʰ **T61.8X4** **Toxic effect of other seafood,** undetermined
  √5ᵗʰ **T61.9** **Toxic effect of unspecified seafood**
    √x7ᵗʰ **T61.91** **Toxic effect of unspecified seafood,** accidental (unintentional)
    ² √x7ᵗʰ **T61.92** **Toxic effect of unspecified seafood,** intentional self-harm HCC Rx ESR COM
    √x7ᵗʰ **T61.93** **Toxic effect of unspecified seafood,** assault
    √x7ᵗʰ **T61.94** **Toxic effect of unspecified seafood,** undetermined

✓4ᵗʰ **T62 Toxic effect of other noxious substances eaten as food**

EXCLUDES 1   *allergic reaction to food, such as:*
         anaphylactic shock (reaction) due to adverse food reaction
           (T78.0-)
         bacterial food borne intoxications (A05.-)
         dermatitis (L23.6, L25.4, L27.2)
         food protein-induced enterocolitis syndrome (K52.21)
         food protein-induced enteropathy (K52.22)
         gastroenteritis (noninfective) (K52.29)
     toxic effect of aflatoxin and other mycotoxins (T64)
     toxic effect of cyanides (T65.0-)
     toxic effect of hydrogen cyanide (T57.3-)
     toxic effect of mercury (T56.1-)

> The appropriate 7th character is to be added to each code from category T62.
> A   initial encounter
> D   subsequent encounter
> S   sequela

✓5ᵗʰ **T62.0 Toxic effect of ingested mushrooms**

   ✓6ᵗʰ **T62.0X Toxic effect of** ingested mushrooms

     ✓7ᵗʰ **T62.0X1 Toxic effect of ingested mushrooms, accidental (unintentional)**
          Toxic effect of ingested mushrooms NOS

     ² ✓7ᵗʰ **T62.0X2 Toxic effect of ingested mushrooms, intentional self-harm** HCC Rx ESR COM

     ✓7ᵗʰ **T62.0X3 Toxic effect of ingested mushrooms, assault**

     ✓7ᵗʰ **T62.0X4 Toxic effect of ingested mushrooms, undetermined**

✓5ᵗʰ **T62.1 Toxic effect of ingested berries**

   ✓6ᵗʰ **T62.1X Toxic effect of** ingested berries

     ✓7ᵗʰ **T62.1X1 Toxic effect of ingested berries, accidental (unintentional)**
          Toxic effect of ingested berries NOS

     ² ✓7ᵗʰ **T62.1X2 Toxic effect of ingested berries, intentional self-harm** HCC Rx ESR COM

     ✓7ᵗʰ **T62.1X3 Toxic effect of ingested berries, assault**

     ✓7ᵗʰ **T62.1X4 Toxic effect of ingested berries, undetermined**

✓5ᵗʰ **T62.2 Toxic effect of other ingested (parts of) plant(s)**

   ✓6ᵗʰ **T62.2X Toxic effect of** other ingested (parts of) plant(s)

     ✓7ᵗʰ **T62.2X1 Toxic effect of other ingested (parts of) plant(s), accidental (unintentional)**
          Toxic effect of other ingested (parts of) plant(s) NOS

     ² ✓7ᵗʰ **T62.2X2 Toxic effect of other ingested (parts of) plant(s), intentional self-harm** HCC Rx ESR COM

     ✓7ᵗʰ **T62.2X3 Toxic effect of other ingested (parts of) plant(s), assault**

     ✓7ᵗʰ **T62.2X4 Toxic effect of other ingested (parts of) plant(s), undetermined**

✓5ᵗʰ **T62.8 Toxic effect of other specified noxious substances eaten as food**

   ✓6ᵗʰ **T62.8X Toxic effect of other specified noxious substances eaten as food**

     ✓7ᵗʰ **T62.8X1 Toxic effect of other specified noxious substances eaten as food, accidental (unintentional)**
          Toxic effect of other specified noxious substances eaten as food NOS

     ² ✓7ᵗʰ **T62.8X2 Toxic effect of other specified noxious substances eaten as food, intentional self-harm** HCC Rx ESR COM

     ✓7ᵗʰ **T62.8X3 Toxic effect of other specified noxious substances eaten as food, assault**

     ✓7ᵗʰ **T62.8X4 Toxic effect of other specified noxious substances eaten as food, undetermined**

✓5ᵗʰ **T62.9 Toxic effect of unspecified noxious substance eaten as food**

   ✓x7ᵗʰ **T62.91 Toxic effect of unspecified noxious substance eaten as food, accidental (unintentional)**
       Toxic effect of unspecified noxious substance eaten as food NOS

   ² ✓x7ᵗʰ **T62.92 Toxic effect of unspecified noxious substance eaten as food, intentional self-harm** HCC Rx ESR COM

   ✓x7ᵗʰ **T62.93 Toxic effect of unspecified noxious substance eaten as food, assault**

   ✓x7ᵗʰ **T62.94 Toxic effect of unspecified noxious substance eaten as food, undetermined**

✓4ᵗʰ **T63 Toxic effect of contact with venomous animals and plants**

INCLUDES   bite or touch of venomous animal
          pricked or stuck by thorn or leaf
EXCLUDES 2   *ingestion of toxic animal or plant (T61.-, T62.-)*

> The appropriate 7th character is to be added to each code from category T63.
> A   initial encounter
> D   subsequent encounter
> S   sequela

✓5ᵗʰ **T63.0 Toxic effect of** snake venom

   ✓6ᵗʰ **T63.00 Toxic effect of unspecified snake venom**

     ✓7ᵗʰ **T63.001 Toxic effect of unspecified snake venom, accidental (unintentional)**
          Toxic effect of unspecified snake venom NOS

     ² ✓7ᵗʰ **T63.002 Toxic effect of unspecified snake venom, intentional self-harm** HCC Rx ESR COM

     ✓7ᵗʰ **T63.003 Toxic effect of unspecified snake venom, assault**

     ✓7ᵗʰ **T63.004 Toxic effect of unspecified snake venom, undetermined**

   ✓6ᵗʰ **T63.01 Toxic effect of** rattlesnake **venom**

     ✓7ᵗʰ **T63.011 Toxic effect of rattlesnake venom, accidental (unintentional)**
          Toxic effect of rattlesnake venom NOS

     ² ✓7ᵗʰ **T63.012 Toxic effect of rattlesnake venom, intentional self-harm** HCC Rx ESR COM

     ✓7ᵗʰ **T63.013 Toxic effect of rattlesnake venom,** assault

     ✓7ᵗʰ **T63.014 Toxic effect of rattlesnake venom, undetermined**

   ✓6ᵗʰ **T63.02 Toxic effect of** coral snake **venom**

     ✓7ᵗʰ **T63.021 Toxic effect of coral snake venom, accidental (unintentional)**
          Toxic effect of coral snake venom NOS

     ² ✓7ᵗʰ **T63.022 Toxic effect of coral snake venom, intentional self-harm** HCC Rx ESR COM

     ✓7ᵗʰ **T63.023 Toxic effect of coral snake venom,** assault

     ✓7ᵗʰ **T63.024 Toxic effect of coral snake venom, undetermined**

   ✓6ᵗʰ **T63.03 Toxic effect of** taipan **venom**

     ✓7ᵗʰ **T63.031 Toxic effect of taipan venom, accidental (unintentional)**
          Toxic effect of taipan venom NOS

     ² ✓7ᵗʰ **T63.032 Toxic effect of taipan venom, intentional self-harm** HCC Rx ESR COM

     ✓7ᵗʰ **T63.033 Toxic effect of taipan venom, assault**

     ✓7ᵗʰ **T63.034 Toxic effect of taipan venom, undetermined**

   ✓6ᵗʰ **T63.04 Toxic effect of** cobra **venom**

     ✓7ᵗʰ **T63.041 Toxic effect of cobra venom, accidental (unintentional)**
          Toxic effect of cobra venom NOS

     ² ✓7ᵗʰ **T63.042 Toxic effect of cobra venom, intentional self-harm** HCC Rx ESR COM

     ✓7ᵗʰ **T63.043 Toxic effect of cobra venom, assault**

     ✓7ᵗʰ **T63.044 Toxic effect of cobra venom, undetermined**

   ✓6ᵗʰ **T63.06 Toxic effect of venom of** other North and South American snake

     ✓7ᵗʰ **T63.061 Toxic effect of venom of other North and South American snake, accidental (unintentional)**
          Toxic effect of venom of other North and South American snake NOS

     ² ✓7ᵗʰ **T63.062 Toxic effect of venom of other North and South American snake, intentional self-harm** HCC Rx ESR COM

     ✓7ᵗʰ **T63.063 Toxic effect of venom of other North and South American snake, assault**

     ✓7ᵗʰ **T63.064 Toxic effect of venom of other North and South American snake, undetermined**

✅ Additional Character Required   ✓x7ᵗʰ Placeholder Alert   Manifestation   Unspecified Dx   Q QPP   UPD Unacceptable PDx

✓6ᵗʰ **T63.07** **Toxic effect of venom of** other Australian snake

    ✓7ᵗʰ **T63.071** **Toxic effect of venom of other Australian snake, accidental (unintentional)**
       Toxic effect of venom of other Australian snake NOS

    ² ✓7ᵗʰ **T63.072** **Toxic effect of venom of other Australian snake, intentional self-harm** `HCC` `Rx` `ESR` `COM`

    ✓7ᵗʰ **T63.073** **Toxic effect of venom of other Australian snake, assault**

    ✓7ᵗʰ **T63.074** **Toxic effect of venom of other Australian snake, undetermined**

✓6ᵗʰ **T63.08** **Toxic effect of venom of** other African and Asian snake

    ✓7ᵗʰ **T63.081** **Toxic effect of venom of other African and Asian snake, accidental (unintentional)**
       Toxic effect of venom of other African and Asian snake NOS

    ² ✓7ᵗʰ **T63.082** **Toxic effect of venom of other African and Asian snake, intentional self-harm** `HCC` `Rx` `ESR` `COM`

    ✓7ᵗʰ **T63.083** **Toxic effect of venom of other African and Asian snake, assault**

    ✓7ᵗʰ **T63.084** **Toxic effect of venom of other African and Asian snake, undetermined**

✓6ᵗʰ **T63.09** **Toxic effect of venom of** other snake

    ✓7ᵗʰ **T63.091** **Toxic effect of venom of other snake, accidental (unintentional)**
       Toxic effect of venom of other snake NOS

    ² ✓7ᵗʰ **T63.092** **Toxic effect of venom of other snake, intentional self-harm** `HCC` `Rx` `ESR` `COM`

    ✓7ᵗʰ **T63.093** **Toxic effect of venom of other snake, assault**

    ✓7ᵗʰ **T63.094** **Toxic effect of venom of other snake, undetermined**

✓5ᵗʰ **T63.1** **Toxic effect of venom of other reptiles**

   ✓6ᵗʰ **T63.11** **Toxic effect of venom of** gila monster

    ✓7ᵗʰ **T63.111** **Toxic effect of venom of gila monster, accidental (unintentional)**
       Toxic effect of venom of gila monster NOS

    ² ✓7ᵗʰ **T63.112** **Toxic effect of venom of gila monster, intentional self-harm** `HCC` `Rx` `ESR` `COM`

    ✓7ᵗʰ **T63.113** **Toxic effect of venom of gila monster, assault**

    ✓7ᵗʰ **T63.114** **Toxic effect of venom of gila monster, undetermined**

   ✓6ᵗʰ **T63.12** **Toxic effect of venom of other venomous lizard**

    ✓7ᵗʰ **T63.121** **Toxic effect of venom of other venomous lizard, accidental (unintentional)**
       Toxic effect of venom of other venomous lizard NOS

    ² ✓7ᵗʰ **T63.122** **Toxic effect of venom of other venomous lizard, intentional self-harm** `HCC` `Rx` `ESR` `COM`

    ✓7ᵗʰ **T63.123** **Toxic effect of venom of other venomous lizard, assault**

    ✓7ᵗʰ **T63.124** **Toxic effect of venom of other venomous lizard, undetermined**

   ✓6ᵗʰ **T63.19** **Toxic effect of venom of other reptiles**

    ✓7ᵗʰ **T63.191** **Toxic effect of venom of other reptiles, accidental (unintentional)**
       Toxic effect of venom of other reptiles NOS

    ² ✓7ᵗʰ **T63.192** **Toxic effect of venom of other reptiles, intentional self-harm** `HCC` `Rx` `ESR` `COM`

    ✓7ᵗʰ **T63.193** **Toxic effect of venom of other reptiles, assault**

    ✓7ᵗʰ **T63.194** **Toxic effect of venom of other reptiles, undetermined**

✓5ᵗʰ **T63.2** **Toxic effect of venom of scorpion**

   ✓6ᵗʰ **T63.2X** **Toxic effect of** venom of scorpion

    ✓7ᵗʰ **T63.2X1** **Toxic effect of venom of scorpion, accidental (unintentional)**
       Toxic effect of venom of scorpion NOS

    ² ✓7ᵗʰ **T63.2X2** **Toxic effect of venom of scorpion, intentional self-harm** `HCC` `Rx` `ESR` `COM`

    ✓7ᵗʰ **T63.2X3** **Toxic effect of venom of scorpion,** assault

    ✓7ᵗʰ **T63.2X4** **Toxic effect of venom of scorpion, undetermined**

✓5ᵗʰ **T63.3** **Toxic effect of** venom of spider

   ✓6ᵗʰ **T63.30** **Toxic effect of unspecified spider venom**

    ✓7ᵗʰ **T63.301** **Toxic effect of unspecified spider venom, accidental (unintentional)**

    ² ✓7ᵗʰ **T63.302** **Toxic effect of unspecified spider venom, intentional self-harm** `HCC` `Rx` `ESR` `COM`

    ✓7ᵗʰ **T63.303** **Toxic effect of unspecified spider venom, assault**

    ✓7ᵗʰ **T63.304** **Toxic effect of unspecified spider venom, undetermined**

   ✓6ᵗʰ **T63.31** **Toxic effect of venom of** black widow **spider**

    ✓7ᵗʰ **T63.311** **Toxic effect of venom of black widow spider, accidental (unintentional)**

    ² ✓7ᵗʰ **T63.312** **Toxic effect of venom of black widow spider, intentional self-harm** `HCC` `Rx` `ESR` `COM`

    ✓7ᵗʰ **T63.313** **Toxic effect of venom of black widow spider, assault**

    ✓7ᵗʰ **T63.314** **Toxic effect of venom of black widow spider, undetermined**

   ✓6ᵗʰ **T63.32** **Toxic effect of venom of** tarantula

    ✓7ᵗʰ **T63.321** **Toxic effect of venom of tarantula, accidental (unintentional)**

    ² ✓7ᵗʰ **T63.322** **Toxic effect of venom of tarantula, intentional self-harm** `HCC` `Rx` `ESR` `COM`

    ✓7ᵗʰ **T63.323** **Toxic effect of venom of tarantula,** assault

    ✓7ᵗʰ **T63.324** **Toxic effect of venom of tarantula, undetermined**

   ✓6ᵗʰ **T63.33** **Toxic effect of venom of** brown recluse **spider**

    ✓7ᵗʰ **T63.331** **Toxic effect of venom of brown recluse spider, accidental (unintentional)**

    ² ✓7ᵗʰ **T63.332** **Toxic effect of venom of brown recluse spider, intentional self-harm** `HCC` `Rx` `ESR` `COM`

    ✓7ᵗʰ **T63.333** **Toxic effect of venom of brown recluse spider, assault**

    ✓7ᵗʰ **T63.334** **Toxic effect of venom of brown recluse spider, undetermined**

   ✓6ᵗʰ **T63.39** **Toxic effect of venom of other spider**

    ✓7ᵗʰ **T63.391** **Toxic effect of venom of other spider, accidental (unintentional)**

    ² ✓7ᵗʰ **T63.392** **Toxic effect of venom of other spider, intentional self-harm** `HCC` `Rx` `ESR` `COM`

    ✓7ᵗʰ **T63.393** **Toxic effect of venom of other spider, assault**

    ✓7ᵗʰ **T63.394** **Toxic effect of venom of other spider, undetermined**

✓5ᵗʰ **T63.4** **Toxic effect of venom of other arthropods**

   ✓6ᵗʰ **T63.41** **Toxic effect of venom of** centipedes and venomous millipedes

    ✓7ᵗʰ **T63.411** **Toxic effect of venom of centipedes and venomous millipedes, accidental (unintentional)**

    ² ✓7ᵗʰ **T63.412** **Toxic effect of venom of centipedes and venomous millipedes, intentional self-harm** `HCC` `Rx` `ESR` `COM`

    ✓7ᵗʰ **T63.413** **Toxic effect of venom of centipedes and venomous millipedes, assault**

    ✓7ᵗʰ **T63.414** **Toxic effect of venom of centipedes and venomous millipedes, undetermined**

   ✓6ᵗʰ **T63.42** **Toxic effect of venom of** ants

    ✓7ᵗʰ **T63.421** **Toxic effect of venom of ants,** accidental (unintentional)

    ² ✓7ᵗʰ **T63.422** **Toxic effect of venom of ants,** intentional self-harm `HCC` `Rx` `ESR` `COM`

    ✓7ᵗʰ **T63.423** **Toxic effect of venom of ants,** assault

    ✓7ᵗʰ **T63.424** **Toxic effect of venom of ants, undetermined**

   ✓6ᵗʰ **T63.43** **Toxic effect of venom of** caterpillars

    ✓7ᵗʰ **T63.431** **Toxic effect of venom of caterpillars, accidental (unintentional)**

    ² ✓7ᵗʰ **T63.432** **Toxic effect of venom of caterpillars,** intentional self-harm `HCC` `Rx` `ESR` `COM`

    ✓7ᵗʰ **T63.433** **Toxic effect of venom of caterpillars, assault**

    ✓7ᵗʰ **T63.434** **Toxic effect of venom of caterpillars, undetermined**

   ✓6ᵗʰ **T63.44** **Toxic effect of venom of** bees

    ✓7ᵗʰ **T63.441** **Toxic effect of venom of bees,** accidental (unintentional)

`HCC` CMS-HCC   `Rx` Rx HCC   `ESR` ESRD HCC   `COM` Commercial HCC   N Newborn: 0   P Pediatric: 0-17   M Maternity: 9-64   A Adult: 15-124

1164   ICD-10-CM 2023

²√7ᵗʰ **T63.442** **Toxic effect of venom of bees,** intentional self-harm   `HCC` `Rx` `ESR` `COM`

√7ᵗʰ **T63.443** **Toxic effect of venom of bees,** assault

√7ᵗʰ **T63.444** **Toxic effect of venom of bees,** undetermined

√6ᵗʰ **T63.45** **Toxic effect of venom of** hornets

√7ᵗʰ **T63.451** **Toxic effect of venom of hornets,** accidental (unintentional)

²√7ᵗʰ **T63.452** **Toxic effect of venom of hornets,** intentional self-harm   `HCC` `Rx` `ESR` `COM`

√7ᵗʰ **T63.453** **Toxic effect of venom of hornets,** assault

√7ᵗʰ **T63.454** **Toxic effect of venom of hornets,** undetermined

√6ᵗʰ **T63.46** **Toxic effect of venom of** wasps

Toxic effect of yellow jacket

√7ᵗʰ **T63.461** **Toxic effect of venom of wasps,** accidental (unintentional)

²√7ᵗʰ **T63.462** **Toxic effect of venom of wasps,** intentional self-harm   `HCC` `Rx` `ESR` `COM`

√7ᵗʰ **T63.463** **Toxic effect of venom of wasps,** assault

√7ᵗʰ **T63.464** **Toxic effect of venom of wasps,** undetermined

√6ᵗʰ **T63.48** **Toxic effect of venom of other arthropod**

√7ᵗʰ **T63.481** **Toxic effect of venom of other arthropod,** accidental (unintentional)

²√7ᵗʰ **T63.482** **Toxic effect of venom of other arthropod,** intentional self-harm   `HCC` `Rx` `ESR` `COM`

√7ᵗʰ **T63.483** **Toxic effect of venom of other arthropod,** assault

√7ᵗʰ **T63.484** **Toxic effect of venom of other arthropod,** undetermined

√5ᵗʰ **T63.5** **Toxic effect of contact with** venomous fish

EXCLUDES 2   poisoning by ingestion of fish (T61.-)

√6ᵗʰ **T63.51** **Toxic effect of contact with** stingray

√7ᵗʰ **T63.511** **Toxic effect of contact with stingray,** accidental (unintentional)

²√7ᵗʰ **T63.512** **Toxic effect of contact with stingray,** intentional self-harm   `HCC` `Rx` `ESR` `COM`

√7ᵗʰ **T63.513** **Toxic effect of contact with stingray,** assault

√7ᵗʰ **T63.514** **Toxic effect of contact with stingray,** undetermined

√6ᵗʰ **T63.59** **Toxic effect of contact with other venomous fish**

√7ᵗʰ **T63.591** **Toxic effect of contact with other venomous fish,** accidental (unintentional)

²√7ᵗʰ **T63.592** **Toxic effect of contact with other venomous fish,** intentional self-harm   `HCC` `Rx` `ESR` `COM`

√7ᵗʰ **T63.593** **Toxic effect of contact with other venomous fish,** assault

√7ᵗʰ **T63.594** **Toxic effect of contact with other venomous fish,** undetermined

√5ᵗʰ **T63.6** **Toxic effect of contact with other** venomous marine animals

EXCLUDES 1   sea-snake venom (T63.09)

EXCLUDES 2   poisoning by ingestion of shellfish (T61.78-)

√6ᵗʰ **T63.61** **Toxic effect of contact with** Portuguese Man-o-war

Toxic effect of contact with bluebottle

√7ᵗʰ **T63.611** **Toxic effect of contact with Portuguese Man-o-war,** accidental (unintentional)

²√7ᵗʰ **T63.612** **Toxic effect of contact with Portuguese Man-o-war,** intentional self-harm   `HCC` `Rx` `ESR` `COM`

√7ᵗʰ **T63.613** **Toxic effect of contact with Portuguese Man-o-war,** assault

√7ᵗʰ **T63.614** **Toxic effect of contact with Portuguese Man-o-war,** undetermined

√6ᵗʰ **T63.62** **Toxic effect of contact with other jellyfish**

√7ᵗʰ **T63.621** **Toxic effect of contact with other jellyfish,** accidental (unintentional)

²√7ᵗʰ **T63.622** **Toxic effect of contact with other jellyfish,** intentional self-harm   `HCC` `Rx` `ESR` `COM`

√7ᵗʰ **T63.623** **Toxic effect of contact with other jellyfish,** assault

√7ᵗʰ **T63.624** **Toxic effect of contact with other jellyfish,** undetermined

√6ᵗʰ **T63.63** **Toxic effect of contact with** sea anemone

√7ᵗʰ **T63.631** **Toxic effect of contact with sea anemone,** accidental (unintentional)

---

²√7ᵗʰ **T63.632** **Toxic effect of contact with sea anemone,** intentional self-harm   `HCC` `Rx` `ESR` `COM`

√7ᵗʰ **T63.633** **Toxic effect of contact with sea anemone,** assault

√7ᵗʰ **T63.634** **Toxic effect of contact with sea anemone,** undetermined

√6ᵗʰ **T63.69** **Toxic effect of contact with other venomous marine animals**

√7ᵗʰ **T63.691** **Toxic effect of contact with other venomous marine animals,** accidental (unintentional)

²√7ᵗʰ **T63.692** **Toxic effect of contact with other venomous marine animals,** intentional self-harm   `HCC` `Rx` `ESR` `COM`

√7ᵗʰ **T63.693** **Toxic effect of contact with other venomous marine animals,** assault

√7ᵗʰ **T63.694** **Toxic effect of contact with other venomous marine animals,** undetermined

√5ᵗʰ **T63.7** **Toxic effect of contact with** venomous plant

√6ᵗʰ **T63.71** **Toxic effect of contact with venomous** marine plant

√7ᵗʰ **T63.711** **Toxic effect of contact with venomous marine plant,** accidental (unintentional)

²√7ᵗʰ **T63.712** **Toxic effect of contact with venomous marine plant,** intentional self-harm   `HCC` `Rx` `ESR` `COM`

√7ᵗʰ **T63.713** **Toxic effect of contact with venomous marine plant,** assault

√7ᵗʰ **T63.714** **Toxic effect of contact with venomous marine plant,** undetermined

√6ᵗʰ **T63.79** **Toxic effect of contact with other venomous plant**

√7ᵗʰ **T63.791** **Toxic effect of contact with other venomous plant,** accidental (unintentional)

²√7ᵗʰ **T63.792** **Toxic effect of contact with other venomous plant,** intentional self-harm   `HCC` `Rx` `ESR` `COM`

√7ᵗʰ **T63.793** **Toxic effect of contact with other venomous plant,** assault

√7ᵗʰ **T63.794** **Toxic effect of contact with other venomous plant,** undetermined

√5ᵗʰ **T63.8** **Toxic effect of contact with other venomous animals**

√6ᵗʰ **T63.81** **Toxic effect of contact with venomous** frog

EXCLUDES 1   contact with nonvenomous frog (W62.0)

√7ᵗʰ **T63.811** **Toxic effect of contact with venomous frog,** accidental (unintentional)

²√7ᵗʰ **T63.812** **Toxic effect of contact with venomous frog,** intentional self-harm   `HCC` `Rx` `ESR` `COM`

√7ᵗʰ **T63.813** **Toxic effect of contact with venomous frog,** assault

√7ᵗʰ **T63.814** **Toxic effect of contact with venomous frog,** undetermined

√6ᵗʰ **T63.82** **Toxic effect of contact with venomous toad**

EXCLUDES 1   contact with nonvenomous toad (W62.1)

√7ᵗʰ **T63.821** **Toxic effect of contact with venomous toad,** accidental (unintentional)

²√7ᵗʰ **T63.822** **Toxic effect of contact with venomous toad,** intentional self-harm   `HCC` `Rx` `ESR` `COM`

√7ᵗʰ **T63.823** **Toxic effect of contact with venomous toad,** assault

√7ᵗʰ **T63.824** **Toxic effect of contact with venomous toad,** undetermined

√6ᵗʰ **T63.83** **Toxic effect of contact with other venomous amphibian**

EXCLUDES 1   contact with nonvenomous amphibian (W62.9)

√7ᵗʰ **T63.831** **Toxic effect of contact with other venomous amphibian,** accidental (unintentional)

²√7ᵗʰ **T63.832** **Toxic effect of contact with other venomous amphibian,** intentional self-harm   `HCC` `Rx` `ESR` `COM`

√7ᵗʰ **T63.833** **Toxic effect of contact with other venomous amphibian,** assault

√7ᵗʰ **T63.834** **Toxic effect of contact with other venomous amphibian,** undetermined

√6ᵗʰ **T63.89** **Toxic effect of contact with other venomous animals**

√7ᵗʰ **T63.891** **Toxic effect of contact with other venomous animals,** accidental (unintentional)

---

² ✓7ᵗʰ **T63.892 Toxic effect of contact with other venomous animals, intentional self-harm** `HCC` `Rx` `ESR` `COM`

✓7ᵗʰ **T63.893 Toxic effect of contact with other venomous animals, assault**

✓7ᵗʰ **T63.894 Toxic effect of contact with other venomous animals, undetermined**

✓5ᵗʰ **T63.9 Toxic effect of contact with unspecified venomous animal**

✓x7ᵗʰ **T63.91 Toxic effect of contact with unspecified venomous animal, accidental (unintentional)**

² ✓x7ᵗʰ **T63.92 Toxic effect of contact with unspecified venomous animal, intentional self-harm** `HCC` `Rx` `ESR` `COM`

✓x7ᵗʰ **T63.93 Toxic effect of contact with unspecified venomous animal, assault**

✓x7ᵗʰ **T63.94 Toxic effect of contact with unspecified venomous animal, undetermined**

✓4ᵗʰ **T64 Toxic effect of aflatoxin and other mycotoxin food contaminants**

> The appropriate 7th character is to be added to each code from category T64.
> A   initial encounter
> D   subsequent encounter
> S   sequela

✓5ᵗʰ **T64.0 Toxic effect of aflatoxin**

✓x7ᵗʰ **T64.01 Toxic effect of aflatoxin, accidental (unintentional)**

² ✓x7ᵗʰ **T64.02 Toxic effect of aflatoxin, intentional self-harm** `HCC` `Rx` `ESR` `COM`

✓x7ᵗʰ **T64.03 Toxic effect of aflatoxin, assault**

✓x7ᵗʰ **T64.04 Toxic effect of aflatoxin, undetermined**

✓5ᵗʰ **T64.8 Toxic effect of other mycotoxin food contaminants**

✓x7ᵗʰ **T64.81 Toxic effect of other mycotoxin food contaminants, accidental (unintentional)**

² ✓x7ᵗʰ **T64.82 Toxic effect of other mycotoxin food contaminants, intentional self-harm** `HCC` `Rx` `ESR` `COM`

✓x7ᵗʰ **T64.83 Toxic effect of other mycotoxin food contaminants, assault**

✓x7ᵗʰ **T64.84 Toxic effect of other mycotoxin food contaminants, undetermined**

✓4ᵗʰ **T65 Toxic effect of other and unspecified substances**

> The appropriate 7th character is to be added to each code from category T65.
> A   initial encounter
> D   subsequent encounter
> S   sequela

✓5ᵗʰ **T65.0 Toxic effect of cyanides**

    EXCLUDES 1   hydrogen cyanide (T57.3-)

✓6ᵗʰ **T65.0X Toxic effect of cyanides**

✓7ᵗʰ **T65.0X1 Toxic effect of cyanides, accidental (unintentional)**
    Toxic effect of cyanides NOS

² ✓7ᵗʰ **T65.0X2 Toxic effect of cyanides, intentional self-harm** `HCC` `Rx` `ESR` `COM`

✓7ᵗʰ **T65.0X3 Toxic effect of cyanides, assault**

✓7ᵗʰ **T65.0X4 Toxic effect of cyanides, undetermined**

✓5ᵗʰ **T65.1 Toxic effect of strychnine and its salts**

✓6ᵗʰ **T65.1X Toxic effect of strychnine and its salts**

✓7ᵗʰ **T65.1X1 Toxic effect of strychnine and its salts, accidental (unintentional)**
    Toxic effect of strychnine and its salts NOS

² ✓7ᵗʰ **T65.1X2 Toxic effect of strychnine and its salts, intentional self-harm** `HCC` `Rx` `ESR` `COM`

✓7ᵗʰ **T65.1X3 Toxic effect of strychnine and its salts, assault**

✓7ᵗʰ **T65.1X4 Toxic effect of strychnine and its salts, undetermined**

✓5ᵗʰ **T65.2 Toxic effect of tobacco and nicotine**

    EXCLUDES 2   nicotine dependence (F17.-)

✓6ᵗʰ **T65.21 Toxic effect of chewing tobacco**

✓7ᵗʰ **T65.211 Toxic effect of chewing tobacco, accidental (unintentional)**
    Toxic effect of chewing tobacco NOS

² ✓7ᵗʰ **T65.212 Toxic effect of chewing tobacco, intentional self-harm** `HCC` `Rx` `ESR` `COM`

✓7ᵗʰ **T65.213 Toxic effect of chewing tobacco, assault**

✓7ᵗʰ **T65.214 Toxic effect of chewing tobacco, undetermined**

✓6ᵗʰ **T65.22 Toxic effect of tobacco cigarettes**
    Toxic effect of tobacco smoke
    Use additional code for exposure to second hand tobacco smoke (Z57.31, Z77.22)

✓7ᵗʰ **T65.221 Toxic effect of tobacco cigarettes, accidental (unintentional)**
    Toxic effect of tobacco cigarettes NOS

² ✓7ᵗʰ **T65.222 Toxic effect of tobacco cigarettes, intentional self-harm** `HCC` `Rx` `ESR` `COM`

✓7ᵗʰ **T65.223 Toxic effect of tobacco cigarettes, assault**

✓7ᵗʰ **T65.224 Toxic effect of tobacco cigarettes, undetermined**

✓6ᵗʰ **T65.29 Toxic effect of other tobacco and nicotine**

✓7ᵗʰ **T65.291 Toxic effect of other tobacco and nicotine, accidental (unintentional)**
    Toxic effect of other tobacco and nicotine NOS

² ✓7ᵗʰ **T65.292 Toxic effect of other tobacco and nicotine, intentional self-harm** `HCC` `Rx` `ESR` `COM`

✓7ᵗʰ **T65.293 Toxic effect of other tobacco and nicotine, assault**

✓7ᵗʰ **T65.294 Toxic effect of other tobacco and nicotine, undetermined**

✓5ᵗʰ **T65.3 Toxic effect of nitroderivatives and aminoderivatives of benzene and its homologues**
    Toxic effect of anilin [benzenamine]
    Toxic effect of nitrobenzene
    Toxic effect of trinitrotoluene

✓6ᵗʰ **T65.3X Toxic effect of nitroderivatives and aminoderivatives of benzene and its homologues**

✓7ᵗʰ **T65.3X1 Toxic effect of nitroderivatives and aminoderivatives of benzene and its homologues, accidental (unintentional)**
    Toxic effect of nitroderivatives and aminoderivatives of benzene and its homologues NOS

² ✓7ᵗʰ **T65.3X2 Toxic effect of nitroderivatives and aminoderivatives of benzene and its homologues, intentional self-harm** `HCC` `Rx` `ESR` `COM`

✓7ᵗʰ **T65.3X3 Toxic effect of nitroderivatives and aminoderivatives of benzene and its homologues, assault**

✓7ᵗʰ **T65.3X4 Toxic effect of nitroderivatives and aminoderivatives of benzene and its homologues, undetermined**

✓5ᵗʰ **T65.4 Toxic effect of carbon disulfide**

✓6ᵗʰ **T65.4X Toxic effect of carbon disulfide**

✓7ᵗʰ **T65.4X1 Toxic effect of carbon disulfide, accidental (unintentional)**
    Toxic effect of carbon disulfide NOS

² ✓7ᵗʰ **T65.4X2 Toxic effect of carbon disulfide, intentional self-harm** `HCC` `Rx` `ESR` `COM`

✓7ᵗʰ **T65.4X3 Toxic effect of carbon disulfide, assault**

✓7ᵗʰ **T65.4X4 Toxic effect of carbon disulfide, undetermined**

✓5ᵗʰ **T65.5 Toxic effect of nitroglycerin and other nitric acids and esters**
    Toxic effect of 1,2,3-Propanetriol trinitrate

✓6ᵗʰ **T65.5X Toxic effect of nitroglycerin and other nitric acids and esters**

✓7ᵗʰ **T65.5X1 Toxic effect of nitroglycerin and other nitric acids and esters, accidental (unintentional)**
    Toxic effect of nitroglycerin and other nitric acids and esters NOS

² ✓7ᵗʰ **T65.5X2 Toxic effect of nitroglycerin and other nitric acids and esters, intentional self-harm** `HCC` `Rx` `ESR` `COM`

✓7ᵗʰ **T65.5X3 Toxic effect of nitroglycerin and other nitric acids and esters, assault**

✓7ᵗʰ **T65.5X4 Toxic effect of nitroglycerin and other nitric acids and esters, undetermined**

✓5ᵗʰ **T65.6 Toxic effect of paints and dyes, not elsewhere classified**

✓6ᵗʰ **T65.6X Toxic effect of paints and dyes, not elsewhere classified**

✓7ᵗʰ **T65.6X1 Toxic effect of paints and dyes, not elsewhere classified, accidental (unintentional)**
    Toxic effect of paints and dyes NOS

`HCC` CMS-HCC   `Rx` Rx HCC   `ESR` ESRD HCC   `COM` Commercial HCC   N Newborn: 0   P Pediatric: 0-17   M Maternity: 9-64   A Adult: 15-124

1166   ICD-10-CM 2023

² ☑7ᵗʰ **T65.6X2** **Toxic effect of paints and dyes, not elsewhere classified,** intentional self-harm   HCC Rx ESR COM

☑7ᵗʰ **T65.6X3** **Toxic effect of paints and dyes, not elsewhere classified,** assault

☑7ᵗʰ **T65.6X4** **Toxic effect of paints and dyes, not elsewhere classified,** undetermined

☑5ᵗʰ **T65.8** **Toxic effect of other specified substances**

  ☑6ᵗʰ **T65.81** **Toxic effect of** latex

    ☑7ᵗʰ **T65.811** **Toxic effect of latex,** accidental (unintentional)
      Toxic effect of latex NOS

    ² ☑7ᵗʰ **T65.812** **Toxic effect of latex,** intentional self-harm   HCC Rx ESR COM

    ☑7ᵗʰ **T65.813** **Toxic effect of latex,** assault

    ☑7ᵗʰ **T65.814** **Toxic effect of latex,** undetermined

  ☑6ᵗʰ **T65.82** **Toxic effect of harmful** algae and algae toxins
    Toxic effect of (harmful) algae bloom NOS
    Toxic effect of blue-green algae bloom
    Toxic effect of brown tide
    Toxic effect of cyanobacteria bloom
    Toxic effect of Florida red tide
    Toxic effect of pfiesteria piscicida
    Toxic effect of red tide

    ☑7ᵗʰ **T65.821** **Toxic effect of harmful algae and algae toxins,** accidental (unintentional)
      Toxic effect of harmful algae and algae toxins NOS

    ² ☑7ᵗʰ **T65.822** **Toxic effect of harmful algae and algae toxins,** intentional self-harm   HCC Rx ESR COM

    ☑7ᵗʰ **T65.823** **Toxic effect of harmful algae and algae toxins,** assault

    ☑7ᵗʰ **T65.824** **Toxic effect of harmful algae and algae toxins,** undetermined

  ☑6ᵗʰ **T65.83** **Toxic effect of** fiberglass

    ☑7ᵗʰ **T65.831** **Toxic effect of fiberglass,** accidental (unintentional)
      Toxic effect of fiberglass NOS

    ² ☑7ᵗʰ **T65.832** **Toxic effect of fiberglass,** intentional self-harm   HCC Rx ESR COM

    ☑7ᵗʰ **T65.833** **Toxic effect of fiberglass,** assault

    ☑7ᵗʰ **T65.834** **Toxic effect of fiberglass,** undetermined

  ☑6ᵗʰ **T65.89** **Toxic effect of other specified substances**

    ☑7ᵗʰ **T65.891** **Toxic effect of other specified substances,** accidental (unintentional)
      Toxic effect of other specified substances NOS
      AHA: 2018,1Q,5

    ² ☑7ᵗʰ **T65.892** **Toxic effect of other specified substances,** intentional self-harm   HCC Rx ESR COM

    ☑7ᵗʰ **T65.893** **Toxic effect of other specified substances,** assault

    ☑7ᵗʰ **T65.894** **Toxic effect of other specified substances,** undetermined

☑5ᵗʰ **T65.9** **Toxic effect of unspecified substance**

  ☑x7ᵗʰ **T65.91** **Toxic effect of unspecified substance,** accidental (unintentional)
    Poisoning NOS

  ² ☑x7ᵗʰ **T65.92** **Toxic effect of unspecified substance,** intentional self-harm   HCC Rx ESR COM

  ☑x7ᵗʰ **T65.93** **Toxic effect of unspecified substance,** assault

  ☑x7ᵗʰ **T65.94** **Toxic effect of unspecified substance,** undetermined

Other and unspecified effects of external causes (T66-T78)

☑x7ᵗʰ **T66** **Radiation sickness, unspecified**

  EXCLUDES 1   *specified adverse effects of radiation, such as:*
    burns (T20-T31)
    leukemia (C91-C95)
  radiation gastroenteritis and colitis (K52.0)
  radiation pneumonitis (J70.0)
  radiation related disorders of the skin and subcutaneous tissue (L55-L59)
  radiation sunburn (L55.-)

  The appropriate 7th character is to be added to code T66.
  A   initial encounter
  D   subsequent encounter
  S   sequela

☑4ᵗʰ **T67** **Effects of heat and light**

  EXCLUDES 1   *erythema [dermatitis] ab igne (L59.0)*
    malignant hyperpyrexia due to anesthesia (T88.3)
    radiation-related disorders of the skin and subcutaneous tissue (L55-L59)

  EXCLUDES 2   *burns (T20-T31)*
    sunburn (L55.-)
    sweat disorder due to heat (L74-L75)

  The appropriate 7th character is to be added to each code from category T67.
  A   initial encounter
  D   subsequent encounter
  S   sequela

  ☑5ᵗʰ **T67.0** **Heatstroke and sunstroke**
    Use additional code(s) to identify any associated complications of heatstroke, such as:
    coma and stupor (R40.-)
    rhabdomyolysis (M62.82)
    systemic inflammatory response syndrome (R65.1-)
    AHA: 2019,4Q,17-18
    DEF: Headache, vertigo, cramps, and elevated body temperature due to prolonged exposure to high environmental temperatures that requires emergency intervention.

    ☑x7ᵗʰ **T67.01** **Heatstroke and sunstroke**
      Heat apoplexy
      Heat pyrexia
      Siriasis
      Thermoplegia

    ☑x7ᵗʰ **T67.02** **Exertional** heatstroke

    ☑x7ᵗʰ **T67.09** **Other heatstroke and sunstroke**

  ☑x7ᵗʰ **T67.1** **Heat** syncope
    Heat collapse

  ☑x7ᵗʰ **T67.2** **Heat** cramp

  ☑x7ᵗʰ **T67.3** **Heat exhaustion,** anhydrotic
    Heat prostration due to water depletion
    EXCLUDES 1   *heat exhaustion due to salt depletion (T67.4)*

  ☑x7ᵗʰ **T67.4** **Heat exhaustion** due to salt depletion
    Heat prostration due to salt (and water) depletion

  ☑x7ᵗʰ **T67.5** **Heat exhaustion, unspecified**
    Heat prostration NOS

  ☑x7ᵗʰ **T67.6** **Heat** fatigue, transient

  ☑x7ᵗʰ **T67.7** **Heat** edema

  ☑x7ᵗʰ **T67.8** **Other effects of heat and light**

  ☑x7ᵗʰ **T67.9** **Effect of heat and light, unspecified**

☑ Additional Character Required   ☑x7ᵗʰ Placeholder Alert   Manifestation   Unspecified Dx   ◻ QPP   UPD Unacceptable PDx

√x7ᵗʰ T68 Hypothermia

Accidental hypothermia
Hypothermia NOS
Use additional code to identify source of exposure:
  exposure to excessive cold of man-made origin (W93)
  exposure to excessive cold of natural origin (X31)

EXCLUDES 1   *hypothermia following anesthesia (T88.51)*
           hypothermia not associated with low environmental
              temperature (R68.0)
           hypothermia of newborn (P80.-)

EXCLUDES 2   *frostbite (T33-T34)*

> The appropriate 7th character is to be added to code T68.
> A   initial encounter
> D   subsequent encounter
> S   sequela

√4ᵗʰ T69 Other effects of reduced temperature

Use additional code to identify source of exposure:
  exposure to excessive cold of man-made origin (W93)
  exposure to excessive cold of natural origin (X31)

EXCLUDES 2   *frostbite (T33-T34)*

> The appropriate 7th character is to be added to each code from
> category T69.
> A   initial encounter
> D   subsequent encounter
> S   sequela

√5ᵗʰ T69.0 Immersion hand and foot

√6ᵗʰ T69.01 Immersion hand

√7ᵗʰ **T69.011** Immersion hand, right hand
√7ᵗʰ **T69.012** Immersion hand, left hand
√7ᵗʰ **T69.019** Immersion hand, unspecified hand

√6ᵗʰ T69.02 Immersion foot

Trench foot
√7ᵗʰ **T69.021** Immersion foot, right foot
√7ᵗʰ **T69.022** Immersion foot, left foot
√7ᵗʰ **T69.029** Immersion foot, unspecified foot

√x7ᵗʰ T69.1 Chilblains

DEF: Red, swollen, itchy skin primarily affecting the fingers and toes, nose and ears, and legs. Chilblains follows damp-cold exposure, and can also be associated with pruritus and a burning feeling.

√x7ᵗʰ T69.8 Other specified effects of reduced temperature

√x7ᵗʰ T69.9 Effect of reduced temperature, unspecified

√4ᵗʰ T70 Effects of air pressure and water pressure

> The appropriate 7th character is to be added to each code from
> category T70.
> A   initial encounter
> D   subsequent encounter
> S   sequela

√x7ᵗʰ T70.0 Otitic barotrauma

Aero-otitis media
Effects of change in ambient atmospheric pressure or water pressure on ears

√x7ᵗʰ T70.1 Sinus barotrauma

Aerosinusitis
Effects of change in ambient atmospheric pressure on sinuses

√5ᵗʰ T70.2 Other and unspecified effects of high altitude

EXCLUDES 2   *polycythemia due to high altitude (D75.1)*

√x7ᵗʰ T70.20 Unspecified effects of high altitude

√x7ᵗʰ T70.29 Other effects of high altitude

Alpine sickness
Anoxia due to high altitude
Barotrauma NOS
Hypobaropathy
Mountain sickness

√x7ᵗʰ T70.3 Caisson disease [decompression sickness]

Compressed-air disease
Diver's palsy or paralysis
DEF: Rapid reduction in air pressure while breathing compressed air. Symptoms include skin lesions, joint pains, and respiratory and neurological problems.

√x7ᵗʰ T70.4 Effects of high-pressure fluids

Hydraulic jet injection (industrial)
Pneumatic jet injection (industrial)
Traumatic jet injection (industrial)

√x7ᵗʰ T70.8 Other effects of air pressure and water pressure

√x7ᵗʰ T70.9 Effect of air pressure and water pressure, unspecified

√4ᵗʰ T71 Asphyxiation

Mechanical suffocation
Traumatic suffocation

EXCLUDES 1   *acute respiratory distress (syndrome) (J80)*
           anoxia due to high altitude (T70.2)
           asphyxia NOS (R09.01)
           asphyxia from carbon monoxide (T58.-)
           asphyxia from inhalation of food or foreign body (T17.-)
           asphyxia from other gases, fumes and vapors (T59.-)
           respiratory distress (syndrome) in newborn (P22.-)

> The appropriate 7th character is to be added to each code from
> category T71.
> A   initial encounter
> D   subsequent encounter
> S   sequela

√5ᵗʰ T71.1 Asphyxiation due to mechanical threat to breathing

Suffocation due to mechanical threat to breathing

√6ᵗʰ T71.11 Asphyxiation due to smothering under pillow

√7ᵗʰ **T71.111 Asphyxiation due to smothering under pillow, accidental**
     Asphyxiation due to smothering under pillow NOS

² √7ᵗʰ **T71.112 Asphyxiation due to smothering under pillow, intentional self-harm**   HCC Rx ESR COM

√7ᵗʰ **T71.113 Asphyxiation due to smothering under pillow, assault**

√7ᵗʰ **T71.114 Asphyxiation due to smothering under pillow, undetermined**

√6ᵗʰ T71.12 Asphyxiation due to plastic bag

√7ᵗʰ **T71.121 Asphyxiation due to plastic bag, accidental**
     Asphyxiation due to plastic bag NOS

² √7ᵗʰ **T71.122 Asphyxiation due to plastic bag, intentional self-harm**   HCC Rx ESR COM

√7ᵗʰ **T71.123 Asphyxiation due to plastic bag, assault**

√7ᵗʰ **T71.124 Asphyxiation due to plastic bag, undetermined**

√6ᵗʰ T71.13 Asphyxiation due to being trapped in bed linens

√7ᵗʰ **T71.131 Asphyxiation due to being trapped in bed linens, accidental**
     Asphyxiation due to being trapped in bed linens NOS

² √7ᵗʰ **T71.132 Asphyxiation due to being trapped in bed linens, intentional self-harm**   HCC Rx ESR COM

√7ᵗʰ **T71.133 Asphyxiation due to being trapped in bed linens, assault**

√7ᵗʰ **T71.134 Asphyxiation due to being trapped in bed linens, undetermined**

√6ᵗʰ T71.14 Asphyxiation due to smothering under another person's body (in bed)

√7ᵗʰ **T71.141 Asphyxiation due to smothering under another person's body (in bed), accidental**
     Asphyxiation due to smothering under another person's body (in bed) NOS

√7ᵗʰ **T71.143 Asphyxiation due to smothering under another person's body (in bed), assault**

√7ᵗʰ **T71.144 Asphyxiation due to smothering under another person's body (in bed), undetermined**

√6ᵗʰ T71.15 Asphyxiation due to smothering in furniture

√7ᵗʰ **T71.151 Asphyxiation due to smothering in furniture, accidental**
     Asphyxiation due to smothering in furniture NOS

² √7ᵗʰ **T71.152 Asphyxiation due to smothering in furniture, intentional self-harm**   HCC Rx ESR COM

√7ᵗʰ **T71.153 Asphyxiation due to smothering in furniture, assault**

✓7ᵗʰ **T71.154**   **Asphyxiation due to smothering in furniture,** undetermined

✓6ᵗʰ **T71.16**   **Asphyxiation due to** hanging

     Hanging by window shade cord
     Use additional code for any associated injuries, such as:
         crushing injury of neck (S17.-)
         fracture of cervical vertebrae (S12.0-S12.2-)
         open wound of neck (S11.-)

     ✓7ᵗʰ **T71.161**   **Asphyxiation due to hanging,** accidental
         Asphyxiation due to hanging NOS
         Hanging NOS

     ² ✓7ᵗʰ **T71.162**   **Asphyxiation due to hanging,** intentional self-harm   HCC Rx ESR COM

     ✓7ᵗʰ **T71.163**   **Asphyxiation due to hanging,** assault

     ✓7ᵗʰ **T71.164**   **Asphyxiation due to hanging,** undetermined

✓6ᵗʰ **T71.19**   **Asphyxiation due to mechanical threat to breathing due to other causes**

     ✓7ᵗʰ **T71.191**   **Asphyxiation due to mechanical threat to breathing due to other causes,** accidental
         Asphyxiation due to other causes NOS

     ² ✓7ᵗʰ **T71.192**   **Asphyxiation due to mechanical threat to breathing due to other causes,** intentional self-harm   HCC Rx ESR COM

     ✓7ᵗʰ **T71.193**   **Asphyxiation due to mechanical threat to breathing due to other causes,** assault

     ✓7ᵗʰ **T71.194**   **Asphyxiation due to mechanical threat to breathing due to other causes,** undetermined

✓5ᵗʰ **T71.2**   **Asphyxiation due to** systemic oxygen deficiency due to low oxygen content in ambient air

     Suffocation due to systemic oxygen deficiency due to low oxygen content in ambient air

     ✓ₓ7ᵗʰ **T71.20**   **Asphyxiation due to systemic oxygen deficiency due to low oxygen content in ambient air due to unspecified cause**

     ✓ₓ7ᵗʰ **T71.21**   **Asphyxiation due to** cave-in or falling earth
         Use additional code for any associated cataclysm (X34-X38)

✓6ᵗʰ **T71.22**   **Asphyxiation due to** being trapped in a car trunk

     ✓7ᵗʰ **T71.221**   **Asphyxiation due to being trapped in a car trunk,** accidental

     ² ✓7ᵗʰ **T71.222**   **Asphyxiation due to being trapped in a car trunk,** intentional self-harm   HCC Rx ESR COM

     ✓7ᵗʰ **T71.223**   **Asphyxiation due to being trapped in a car trunk,** assault

     ✓7ᵗʰ **T71.224**   **Asphyxiation due to being trapped in a car trunk,** undetermined

✓6ᵗʰ **T71.23**   **Asphyxiation due to being** trapped in a (discarded) refrigerator

     ✓7ᵗʰ **T71.231**   **Asphyxiation due to being trapped in a (discarded) refrigerator,** accidental

     ² ✓7ᵗʰ **T71.232**   **Asphyxiation due to being trapped in a (discarded) refrigerator,** intentional self-harm   HCC Rx ESR COM

     ✓7ᵗʰ **T71.233**   **Asphyxiation due to being trapped in a (discarded) refrigerator,** assault

     ✓7ᵗʰ **T71.234**   **Asphyxiation due to being trapped in a (discarded) refrigerator,** undetermined

     ✓ₓ7ᵗʰ **T71.29**   **Asphyxiation due to being trapped in other low oxygen environment**

✓ₓ7ᵗʰ **T71.9**   **Asphyxiation due to unspecified cause**

     Suffocation (by strangulation) due to unspecified cause
     Suffocation NOS
     Systemic oxygen deficiency due to low oxygen content in ambient air due to unspecified cause
     Systemic oxygen deficiency due to mechanical threat to breathing due to unspecified cause
     Traumatic asphyxia NOS

✓4ᵗʰ **T73**   **Effects of other deprivation**

     The appropriate 7th character is to be added to each code from category T73.
     A   initial encounter
     D   subsequent encounter
     S   sequela

     ✓ₓ7ᵗʰ **T73.0**   **Starvation**
         Deprivation of food

     ✓ₓ7ᵗʰ **T73.1**   **Deprivation of water**

     ✓ₓ7ᵗʰ **T73.2**   **Exhaustion due to exposure**

     ✓ₓ7ᵗʰ **T73.3**   **Exhaustion due to excessive exertion**
         Exhaustion due to overexertion

     ✓ₓ7ᵗʰ **T73.8**   **Other effects of deprivation**

     ✓ₓ7ᵗʰ **T73.9**   **Effect of deprivation, unspecified**

✓4ᵗʰ **T74**   **Adult and child abuse, neglect and other maltreatment,** confirmed

     Use additional code, if applicable, to identify any associated current injury
     Use additional external cause code to identify perpetrator, if known (Y07.-)

     EXCLUDES 1   abuse and maltreatment in pregnancy (O9A.3-, O9A.4-, O9A.5-)
         adult and child maltreatment, suspected (T76.-)

     The appropriate 7th character is to be added to each code from category T74.
     A   initial encounter
     D   subsequent encounter
     S   sequela

     ✓5ᵗʰ **T74.0**   **Neglect or abandonment, confirmed**

     ✓ₓ7ᵗʰ **T74.01**   Adult **neglect or abandonment, confirmed**   A

     ✓ₓ7ᵗʰ **T74.02**   Child **neglect or abandonment, confirmed**   P

     ✓5ᵗʰ **T74.1**   **Physical abuse, confirmed**
         EXCLUDES 2   sexual abuse (T74.2-)

     ✓ₓ7ᵗʰ **T74.11**   Adult **physical abuse, confirmed**   A

     ✓ₓ7ᵗʰ **T74.12**   Child **physical abuse, confirmed**   P
         EXCLUDES 2   shaken infant syndrome (T74.4)

     ✓5ᵗʰ **T74.2**   **Sexual abuse, confirmed**
         Rape, confirmed
         Sexual assault, confirmed

     ✓ₓ7ᵗʰ **T74.21**   Adult **sexual abuse, confirmed**   A

     ✓ₓ7ᵗʰ **T74.22**   Child **sexual abuse, confirmed**   P

     ✓5ᵗʰ **T74.3**   **Psychological abuse, confirmed**
         Bullying and intimidation, confirmed
         Intimidation through social media, confirmed

     ✓ₓ7ᵗʰ **T74.31**   Adult **psychological abuse, confirmed**   A

     ✓ₓ7ᵗʰ **T74.32**   Child **psychological abuse, confirmed**   P

     ✓ₓ7ᵗʰ **T74.4**   **Shaken infant syndrome**   P

     ✓5ᵗʰ **T74.5**   **Forced sexual exploitation, confirmed**
         AHA: 2018,4Q,32-33,65

     ✓ₓ7ᵗʰ **T74.51**   Adult **forced sexual exploitation, confirmed**   A

     ✓ₓ7ᵗʰ **T74.52**   Child **sexual exploitation, confirmed**   P

     ✓5ᵗʰ **T74.6**   **Forced labor exploitation, confirmed**
         AHA: 2018,4Q,32-33,65

     ✓ₓ7ᵗʰ **T74.61**   Adult **forced labor exploitation, confirmed**   A

     ✓ₓ7ᵗʰ **T74.62**   Child **forced labor exploitation, confirmed**   P

     ✓5ᵗʰ **T74.9**   **Unspecified maltreatment, confirmed**

     ✓ₓ7ᵗʰ **T74.91**   Unspecified adult **maltreatment, confirmed**   A

     ✓ₓ7ᵗʰ **T74.92**   Unspecified child **maltreatment, confirmed**   P

✔ Additional Character Required   ✓ₓ7ᵗʰ Placeholder Alert   Manifestation   Unspecified Dx   Q QPP   UPD Unacceptable PDx

T75 Other and unspecified effects of other external causes

EXCLUDES 1 adverse effects NEC (T78.-)
EXCLUDES 2 burns (electric) (T20-T31)

The appropriate 7th character is to be added to each code from category T75.
A initial encounter
D subsequent encounter
S sequela

T75.0 Effects of lightning
Struck by lightning
T75.00 Unspecified effects of lightning
Struck by lightning NOS
T75.01 Shock due to being struck by lightning
T75.09 Other effects of lightning
Use additional code for other effects of lightning

T75.1 Unspecified effects of drowning and nonfatal submersion
Immersion
EXCLUDES 1 specified effects of drowning - code to effects

T75.2 Effects of vibration
T75.20 Unspecified effects of vibration
T75.21 Pneumatic hammer syndrome
T75.22 Traumatic vasospastic syndrome
T75.23 Vertigo from infrasound
EXCLUDES 1 vertigo NOS (R42)
T75.29 Other effects of vibration

T75.3 Motion sickness
Airsickness
Seasickness
Travel sickness
Use additional external cause code to identify vehicle or type of motion (Y92.81-, Y93.5-)

T75.4 Electrocution
Shock from electric current
Shock from electroshock gun (taser)

T75.8 Other specified effects of external causes
T75.81 Effects of abnormal gravitation [G] forces
T75.82 Effects of weightlessness
T75.89 Other specified effects of external causes

T76 Adult and child abuse, neglect and other maltreatment, suspected
Use additional code, if applicable, to identify any associated current injury
EXCLUDES 1 adult and child maltreatment, confirmed (T74.-)
suspected abuse and maltreatment in pregnancy (O9A.3-, O9A.4-, O9A.5-)
suspected adult physical abuse, ruled out (Z04.71)
suspected adult sexual abuse, ruled out (Z04.41)
suspected child physical abuse, ruled out (Z04.72)
suspected child sexual abuse, ruled out (Z04.42)
AHA: 2018,4Q,72

The appropriate 7th character is to be added to each code from category T76.
A initial encounter
D subsequent encounter
S sequela

T76.0 Neglect or abandonment, suspected
T76.01 Adult neglect or abandonment, suspected
T76.02 Child neglect or abandonment, suspected
T76.1 Physical abuse, suspected
T76.11 Adult physical abuse, suspected
T76.12 Child physical abuse, suspected
AHA: 2019,2Q,12
T76.2 Sexual abuse, suspected
Rape, suspected
EXCLUDES 1 alleged abuse, ruled out (Z04.7)
T76.21 Adult sexual abuse, suspected
T76.22 Child sexual abuse, suspected
T76.3 Psychological abuse, suspected
Bullying and intimidation, suspected
Intimidation through social media, suspected
T76.31 Adult psychological abuse, suspected

T76.32 Child psychological abuse, suspected
T76.5 Forced sexual exploitation, suspected
AHA: 2018,4Q,32-33,65
T76.51 Adult forced sexual exploitation, suspected
T76.52 Child sexual exploitation, suspected
T76.6 Forced labor exploitation, suspected
AHA: 2018,4Q,32-33,65
T76.61 Adult forced labor exploitation, suspected
T76.62 Child forced labor exploitation, suspected
T76.9 Unspecified maltreatment, suspected
T76.91 Unspecified adult maltreatment, suspected
T76.92 Unspecified child maltreatment, suspected

T78 Adverse effects, not elsewhere classified
EXCLUDES 2 complications of surgical and medical care NEC (T80-T88)

The appropriate 7th character is to be added to each code from category T78.
A initial encounter
D subsequent encounter
S sequela

T78.0 Anaphylactic reaction due to food
Anaphylactic reaction due to adverse food reaction
Anaphylactic shock or reaction due to nonpoisonous foods
Anaphylactoid reaction due to food
T78.00 Anaphylactic reaction due to unspecified food
T78.01 Anaphylactic reaction due to peanuts
T78.02 Anaphylactic reaction due to shellfish (crustaceans)
T78.03 Anaphylactic reaction due to other fish
T78.04 Anaphylactic reaction due to fruits and vegetables
T78.05 Anaphylactic reaction due to tree nuts and seeds
EXCLUDES 2 anaphylactic reaction due to peanuts (T78.01)
T78.06 Anaphylactic reaction due to food additives
T78.07 Anaphylactic reaction due to milk and dairy products
T78.08 Anaphylactic reaction due to eggs
T78.09 Anaphylactic reaction due to other food products
T78.1 Other adverse food reactions, not elsewhere classified
Use additional code to identify the type of reaction, if applicable
EXCLUDES 1 anaphylactic reaction or shock due to adverse food reaction (T78.0-)
anaphylactic reaction due to food (T78.0-)
bacterial food borne intoxications (A05.-)
EXCLUDES 2 allergic and dietetic gastroenteritis and colitis (K52.29)
allergic rhinitis due to food (J30.5)
dermatitis due to food in contact with skin (L23.6, L24.6, L25.4)
dermatitis due to ingested food (L27.2)
food protein-induced enterocolitis syndrome (K52.21)
food protein-induced enteropathy (K52.22)
T78.2 Anaphylactic shock, unspecified
Allergic shock
Anaphylactic reaction
Anaphylaxis
EXCLUDES 1 anaphylactic reaction or shock due to adverse effect of correct medicinal substance properly administered (T88.6)
anaphylactic reaction or shock due to adverse food reaction (T78.0-)
anaphylactic reaction or shock due to serum (T80.5-)
T78.3 Angioneurotic edema
Allergic angioedema
Giant urticaria
Quincke's edema
EXCLUDES 1 serum urticaria (T80.6-)
urticaria (L50.-)

✓5ᵗʰ **T78.4 Other and unspecified allergy**

EXCLUDES 1   specified types of allergic reaction such as:
   allergic diarrhea (K52.29)
   allergic gastroenteritis and colitis (K52.29)
   dermatitis (L23-L25, L27.-)
   food protein-induced enterocolitis syndrome
      (K52.21)
   food protein-induced enteropathy (K52.22)
   hay fever (J30.1)

✓7ᵗʰ **T78.40 Allergy, unspecified**
   Allergic reaction NOS
   Hypersensitivity NOS

✓7ᵗʰ **T78.41 Arthus phenomenon**
   Arthus reaction

✓7ᵗʰ **T78.49 Other allergy**
   AHA: 2021,1Q,42

✓7ᵗʰ **T78.8 Other adverse effects, not elsewhere classified**

Certain early complications of trauma (T79)

✓4ᵗʰ **T79 Certain early complications of trauma, not elsewhere classified**

EXCLUDES 2   acute respiratory distress syndrome (J80)
   complications occurring during or following medical
      procedures (T80-T88)
   complications of surgical and medical care NEC (T80-T88)
   newborn respiratory distress syndrome (P22.0)

The appropriate 7th character is to be added to each code from
category T79.
A   initial encounter
D   subsequent encounter
S   sequela

1 ✓7ᵗʰ **T79.0 Air embolism (traumatic)**   HCC ESR COM

EXCLUDES 1   air embolism complicating abortion or ectopic or
      molar pregnancy (O00-O07, O08.2)
   air embolism complicating pregnancy, childbirth and
      the puerperium (O88.0)
   air embolism following infusion, transfusion, and
      therapeutic injection (T80.0)
   air embolism following procedure NEC (T81.7-)

DEF: Arterial or venous obstruction due to the introduction of air
bubbles into the blood vessels following surgery or trauma.

1 ✓7ᵗʰ **T79.1 Fat embolism (traumatic)**   HCC ESR COM

EXCLUDES 1   fat embolism complicating:
      abortion or ectopic or molar pregnancy (O00-O07,
         O08.2)
      pregnancy, childbirth and the puerperium (O88.8)

DEF: Arterial blockage due to the entrance of fat into the
circulatory system after a fracture of the large bones or
administration of corticosteroids.

1 ✓7ᵗʰ **T79.2 Traumatic secondary and recurrent hemorrhage and
seroma**   HCC ESR

1 ✓7ᵗʰ **T79.4 Traumatic shock**   HCC ESR COM
   Shock (immediate) (delayed) following injury

EXCLUDES 1   anaphylactic shock due to adverse food reaction
      (T78.0-)
   anaphylactic shock due to correct medicinal
      substance properly administered (T88.6)
   anaphylactic shock due to serum (T80.5-)
   anaphylactic shock NOS (T78.2)
   electric shock (T75.4)
   nontraumatic shock NEC (R57.-)
   obstetric shock (O75.1)
   postprocedural shock (T81.1-)
   septic shock (R65.21)
   shock complicating abortion or ectopic or molar
      pregnancy (O00-O07, O08.3)
   shock due to anesthesia (T88.2)
   shock due to lightning (T75.01)
   shock NOS (R57.9)

1 ✓7ᵗʰ **T79.5 Traumatic anuria**   HCC ESR
   Crush syndrome
   Renal failure following crushing

1 ✓x7ᵗʰ **T79.6 Traumatic ischemia of muscle**   HCC ESR
   Traumatic rhabdomyolysis
   Volkmann's ischemic contracture

EXCLUDES 2   anterior tibial syndrome (M76.8)
   compartment syndrome (traumatic) (T79.A-)
   nontraumatic ischemia of muscle (M62.2-)

AHA: 2019,2Q,12

1 ✓x7ᵗʰ **T79.7 Traumatic subcutaneous emphysema**   HCC ESR

EXCLUDES 2   emphysema NOS (J43)
   emphysema (subcutaneous) resulting from a
      procedure (T81.82)

✓5ᵗʰ **T79.A Traumatic compartment syndrome**

EXCLUDES 1   fibromyalgia (M79.7)
   nontraumatic compartment syndrome (M79.A-)
EXCLUDES 2   traumatic ischemic infarction of muscle (T79.6)

DEF: Compression of nerves and blood vessels within an enclosed
muscle space due to previous trauma, which leads to impaired
blood flow and muscle and nerve damage.

1 ✓x7ᵗʰ **T79.A0 Compartment syndrome, unspecified**   HCC ESR
   Compartment syndrome NOS

✓6ᵗʰ **T79.A1 Traumatic compartment syndrome of upper
extremity**
   Traumatic compartment syndrome of shoulder, arm,
   forearm, wrist, hand, and fingers

1 ✓7ᵗʰ **T79.A11 Traumatic compartment syndrome of
right upper extremity**   HCC ESR

1 ✓7ᵗʰ **T79.A12 Traumatic compartment syndrome of left
upper extremity**   HCC ESR

1 ✓7ᵗʰ **T79.A19 Traumatic compartment syndrome of
unspecified upper extremity**   HCC ESR

✓6ᵗʰ **T79.A2 Traumatic compartment syndrome of lower
extremity**
   Traumatic compartment syndrome of hip, buttock,
   thigh, leg, foot, and toes

1 ✓7ᵗʰ **T79.A21 Traumatic compartment syndrome of
right lower extremity**   HCC ESR

1 ✓7ᵗʰ **T79.A22 Traumatic compartment syndrome of left
lower extremity**   HCC ESR

1 ✓7ᵗʰ **T79.A29 Traumatic compartment syndrome of
unspecified lower extremity**   HCC ESR

1 ✓x7ᵗʰ **T79.A3 Traumatic compartment syndrome of
abdomen**   HCC ESR

1 ✓x7ᵗʰ **T79.A9 Traumatic compartment syndrome of other
sites**   HCC ESR

1 ✓x7ᵗʰ **T79.8 Other early complications of trauma**   HCC ESR

1 ✓x7ᵗʰ **T79.9 Unspecified early complication of trauma**   HCC ESR

Chapter 19. Injury, Poisoning and Certain Other Consequences of External Causes

Complications of surgical and medical care, not elsewhere classified (T80-T88)

Use additional code for adverse effect, if applicable, to identify drug (T36-T50 with fifth or sixth character 5)

Use additional code(s) to identify the specified condition resulting from the complication

Use additional code to identify devices involved and details of circumstances (Y62-Y82)

EXCLUDES 2 *any encounters with medical care for postprocedural conditions in which no complications are present, such as:*
 artificial opening status (Z93.-)
 closure of external stoma (Z43.-)
 fitting and adjustment of external prosthetic device (Z44.-)
 burns and corrosions from local applications and irradiation (T20-T32)
 complications of surgical procedures during pregnancy, childbirth and the puerperium (O00-O9A)
 mechanical complication of respirator [ventilator] (J95.850)
 poisoning and toxic effects of drugs and chemicals (T36-T65 with fifth or sixth character 1-4 or 6)
 postprocedural fever (R50.82)
 specified complications classified elsewhere, such as:
 cerebrospinal fluid leak from spinal puncture (G97.0)
 colostomy malfunction (K94.0-)
 disorders of fluid and electrolyte imbalance (E86-E87)
 functional disturbances following cardiac surgery (I97.0-I97.1)
 intraoperative and postprocedural complications of specified body systems (D78.-, E36.-, E89.-, G97.3-, G97.4, H59.3-, H59.-, H95.2-, H95.3, I97.4-, I97.5, J95.6-, J95.7, K91.6-, L76.-, M96.-, N99.-)
 ostomy complications (J95.0-, K94.-, N99.5-)
 postgastric surgery syndromes (K91.1)
 postlaminectomy syndrome NEC (M96.1)
 postmastectomy lymphedema syndrome (I97.2)
 postsurgical blind-loop syndrome (K91.2)
 ventilator associated pneumonia (J95.851)

AHA: 2015,1Q,15

✓4ᵗʰ T80 Complications following infusion, transfusion and therapeutic injection
 INCLUDES complications following perfusion
 EXCLUDES 2 *bone marrow transplant rejection (T86.01)*
 febrile nonhemolytic transfusion reaction (R50.84)
 fluid overload due to transfusion (E87.71)
 posttransfusion purpura (D69.51)
 transfusion associated circulatory overload (TACO) (E87.71)
 transfusion (red blood cell) associated hemochromatosis (E83.111)
 transfusion related acute lung injury (TRALI) (J95.84)

> The appropriate 7th character is to be added to each code from category T80.
> A   initial encounter
> D   subsequent encounter
> S   sequela

✓x7ᵗʰ T80.0 Air embolism following infusion, transfusion and therapeutic injection

✓x7ᵗʰ T80.1 Vascular complications following infusion, transfusion and therapeutic injection
 Use additional code to identify the vascular complication
 EXCLUDES 2 *extravasation of vesicant agent (T80.81-)*
 infiltration of vesicant agent (T80.81-)
 postprocedural vascular complications (T81.7-)
 vascular complications specified as due to prosthetic devices, implants and grafts (T82.8-, T83.8-, T84.8-, T85.8-)

✓5ᵗʰ T80.2 Infections following infusion, transfusion and therapeutic injection
 Use additional code to identify the specific infection, such as: sepsis (A41.9)
 Use additional code (R65.2-) to identify severe sepsis, if applicable
 EXCLUDES 2 *infections specified as due to prosthetic devices, implants and grafts (T82.6-T82.7, T83.5-T83.6, T84.5-T84.7, T85.7)*
 postprocedural infections (T81.4-)
 AHA: 2018,4Q,62

✓6ᵗʰ T80.21 Infection due to central venous catheter
 Infection due to pulmonary artery catheter (Swan-Ganz catheter)
 AHA: 2019,1Q,13-14
 DEF: Central venous catheter: Catheter positioned in the superior vena cava or right atrium and introduced through a large vein, such as the jugular or subclavian, and used to measure venous pressure or administer fluids or medication.
 TIP: Code assignment is based on the location of the catheter and not how the catheter is being used; for example, for hemodialysis. Infections resulting from catheters that are not central lines should be coded to T82.7-.

✓7ᵗʰ T80.211 Bloodstream infection due to central venous catheter
 Catheter-related bloodstream infection (CRBSI) NOS
 Central line-associated bloodstream infection (CLABSI)
 Bloodstream infection due to Hickman catheter
 Bloodstream infection due to peripherally inserted central catheter (PICC)
 Bloodstream infection due to portacath (port-a-cath)
 Bloodstream infection due to pulmonary artery catheter
 Bloodstream infection due to triple lumen catheter
 Bloodstream infection due to umbilical venous catheter
 AHA: 2019,1Q,13,14; 2018,4Q,89

✓7ᵗʰ T80.212 Local infection due to central venous catheter
 Exit or insertion site infection
 Local infection due to Hickman catheter
 Local infection due to peripherally inserted central catheter (PICC)
 Local infection due to portacath (port-a-cath)
 Local infection due to pulmonary artery catheter
 Local infection due to triple lumen catheter
 Local infection due to umbilical venous catheter
 Port or reservoir infection
 Tunnel infection

✓7ᵗʰ T80.218 Other infection due to central venous catheter
 Other central line-associated infection
 Other infection due to Hickman catheter
 Other infection due to peripherally inserted central catheter (PICC)
 Other infection due to portacath (port-a-cath)
 Other infection due to pulmonary artery catheter
 Other infection due to triple lumen catheter
 Other infection due to umbilical venous catheter

✓7ᵗʰ T80.219 Unspecified infection due to central venous catheter
Central line-associated infection NOS
Unspecified infection due to Hickman catheter
Unspecified infection due to peripherally inserted central catheter (PICC)
Unspecified infection due to portacath (port-a-cath)
Unspecified infection due to pulmonary artery catheter
Unspecified infection due to triple lumen catheter
Unspecified infection due to umbilical venous catheter

✓x7ᵗʰ T80.22 Acute infection following transfusion, infusion, or injection of blood and blood products

✓x7ᵗʰ T80.29 Infection following other infusion, transfusion and therapeutic injection

✓5ᵗʰ T80.3 ABO incompatibility reaction due to transfusion of blood or blood products
EXCLUDES 1   *minor blood group antigens reactions (Duffy) (E) (K) (Kell) (Kidd) (Lewis) (M) (N) (P) (S) (T80.A-)*

✓x7ᵗʰ T80.30 ABO incompatibility reaction due to transfusion of blood or blood products, unspecified
ABO incompatibility blood transfusion NOS
Reaction to ABO incompatibility from transfusion NOS

✓6ᵗʰ T80.31 ABO incompatibility with hemolytic transfusion reaction

✓7ᵗʰ T80.310 ABO incompatibility with acute hemolytic transfusion reaction
ABO incompatibility with hemolytic transfusion reaction less than 24 hours after transfusion
Acute hemolytic transfusion reaction (AHTR) due to ABO incompatibility

✓7ᵗʰ T80.311 ABO incompatibility with delayed hemolytic transfusion reaction
ABO incompatibility with hemolytic transfusion reaction 24 hours or more after transfusion
Delayed hemolytic transfusion reaction (DHTR) due to ABO incompatibility

✓7ᵗʰ T80.319 ABO incompatibility with hemolytic transfusion reaction, unspecified
ABO incompatibility with hemolytic transfusion reaction at unspecified time after transfusion
Hemolytic transfusion reaction (HTR) due to ABO incompatibility NOS

✓x7ᵗʰ T80.39 Other ABO incompatibility reaction due to transfusion of blood or blood products
Delayed serologic transfusion reaction (DSTR) from ABO incompatibility
Other ABO incompatible blood transfusion
Other reaction to ABO incompatible blood transfusion

✓5ᵗʰ T80.4 Rh incompatibility reaction due to transfusion of blood or blood products
Reaction due to incompatibility of Rh antigens (C) (c) (D) (E) (e)

✓x7ᵗʰ T80.40 Rh incompatibility reaction due to transfusion of blood or blood products, unspecified
Reaction due to Rh factor in transfusion NOS
Rh incompatible blood transfusion NOS

✓6ᵗʰ T80.41 Rh incompatibility with hemolytic transfusion reaction

✓7ᵗʰ T80.410 Rh incompatibility with acute hemolytic transfusion reaction
Acute hemolytic transfusion reaction (AHTR) due to Rh incompatibility
Rh incompatibility with hemolytic transfusion reaction less than 24 hours after transfusion

✓7ᵗʰ T80.411 Rh incompatibility with delayed hemolytic transfusion reaction
Delayed hemolytic transfusion reaction (DHTR) due to Rh incompatibility
Rh incompatibility with hemolytic transfusion reaction 24 hours or more after transfusion

✓7ᵗʰ T80.419 Rh incompatibility with hemolytic transfusion reaction, unspecified
Rh incompatibility with hemolytic transfusion reaction at unspecified time after transfusion
Hemolytic transfusion reaction (HTR) due to Rh incompatibility NOS

✓x7ᵗʰ T80.49 Other Rh incompatibility reaction due to transfusion of blood or blood products
Delayed serologic transfusion reaction (DSTR) from Rh incompatibility
Other reaction to Rh incompatible blood transfusion

✓5ᵗʰ T80.A Non-ABO incompatibility reaction due to transfusion of blood or blood products
Reaction due to incompatibility of minor antigens (Duffy) (Kell) (Kidd) (Lewis) (M) (N) (P) (S)

✓x7ᵗʰ T80.A0 Non-ABO incompatibility reaction due to transfusion of blood or blood products, unspecified
Non-ABO antigen incompatibility reaction from transfusion NOS

✓6ᵗʰ T80.A1 Non-ABO incompatibility with hemolytic transfusion reaction

✓7ᵗʰ T80.A10 Non-ABO incompatibility with acute hemolytic transfusion reaction
Acute hemolytic transfusion reaction (AHTR) due to non-ABO incompatibility
Non-ABO incompatibility with hemolytic transfusion reaction less than 24 hours after transfusion

✓7ᵗʰ T80.A11 Non-ABO incompatibility with delayed hemolytic transfusion reaction
Delayed hemolytic transfusion reaction (DHTR) due to non-ABO incompatibility
Non-ABO incompatibility with hemolytic transfusion reaction 24 or more hours after transfusion

✓7ᵗʰ T80.A19 Non-ABO incompatibility with hemolytic transfusion reaction, unspecified
Hemolytic transfusion reaction (HTR) due to non-ABO incompatibility NOS
Non-ABO incompatibility with hemolytic transfusion reaction at unspecified time after transfusion

✓x7ᵗʰ T80.A9 Other non-ABO incompatibility reaction due to transfusion of blood or blood products
Delayed serologic transfusion reaction (DSTR) from non-ABO incompatibility
Other reaction to non-ABO incompatible blood transfusion

✓5ᵗʰ T80.5 Anaphylactic reaction due to serum
Allergic shock due to serum
Anaphylactic shock due to serum
Anaphylactoid reaction due to serum
Anaphylaxis due to serum
EXCLUDES 1   *ABO incompatibility reaction due to transfusion of blood or blood products (T80.3-)*
allergic reaction or shock NOS (T78.2)
anaphylactic reaction or shock NOS (T78.2)
anaphylactic reaction or shock due to adverse effect of correct medicinal substance properly administered (T88.6)
other serum reaction (T80.6-)
DEF: Life-threatening hypersensitivity to a foreign serum causing respiratory distress, vascular collapse, and shock.

✓x7ᵗʰ T80.51 Anaphylactic reaction due to administration of blood and blood products

✓x7ᵗʰ T80.52 Anaphylactic reaction due to vaccination
AHA: 2021,1Q,43

✓x7ᵗʰ T80.59 Anaphylactic reaction due to other serum

✓5ᵗʰ T80.6 Other serum reactions

Intoxication by serum
Protein sickness
Serum rash
Serum sickness
Serum urticaria

> **EXCLUDES 2**   serum hepatitis (B16-B19)

DEF: Serum sickness: Hypersensitivity to a foreign serum that causes fever, hives, swelling, and lymphadenopathy.

✓x7ᵗʰ T80.61 Other serum reaction due to administration of blood and blood products

✓x7ᵗʰ T80.62 Other serum reaction due to vaccination

> **AHA:** 2021,1Q,42

✓x7ᵗʰ T80.69 Other serum reaction due to other serum

> Code also, if applicable, arthropathy in hypersensitivity reactions classified elsewhere (M36.4)

✓5ᵗʰ T80.8 Other complications following infusion, transfusion and therapeutic injection

✓6ᵗʰ T80.81 Extravasation of vesicant agent

> Infiltration of vesicant agent

✓7ᵗʰ T80.810 Extravasation of vesicant antineoplastic chemotherapy

> Infiltration of vesicant antineoplastic chemotherapy

✓7ᵗʰ T80.818 Extravasation of other vesicant agent

> Infiltration of other vesicant agent

✓x7ᵗʰ T80.82 Complication of immune effector cellular therapy

> Complication of chimeric antigen receptor (CAR-T) cell therapy
> Complication of IEC therapy
> Use additional code to identify the specific complication, such as:
> cytokine release syndrome (D89.83-)
> immune effector cell-associated neurotoxicity syndrome (G92.0-)

> **EXCLUDES 2**   complication of bone marrow transplant (T86.0)
> complication of stem cell transplant (T86.5)

> **AHA:** 2021,4Q,31

✓x7ᵗʰ T80.89 Other complications following infusion, transfusion and therapeutic injection

> Delayed serologic transfusion reaction (DSTR), unspecified incompatibility
> Use additional code to identify graft-versus-host reaction, if applicable, (D89.81-)

> **AHA:** 2020,4Q,14

✓5ᵗʰ T80.9 Unspecified complication following infusion, transfusion and therapeutic injection

✓x7ᵗʰ T80.90 Unspecified complication following infusion and therapeutic injection

✓6ᵗʰ T80.91 Hemolytic transfusion reaction, unspecified incompatibility

> **EXCLUDES 1**   ABO incompatibility with hemolytic transfusion reaction (T80.31-)
> non-ABO incompatibility with hemolytic transfusion reaction (T80.A1-)
> Rh incompatibility with hemolytic transfusion reaction (T80.41-)

✓7ᵗʰ T80.910 Acute hemolytic transfusion reaction, unspecified incompatibility

✓7ᵗʰ T80.911 Delayed hemolytic transfusion reaction, unspecified incompatibility

✓7ᵗʰ T80.919 Hemolytic transfusion reaction, unspecified incompatibility, unspecified as acute or delayed

> Hemolytic transfusion reaction NOS

✓x7ᵗʰ T80.92 Unspecified transfusion reaction

> Transfusion reaction NOS

✓4ᵗʰ T81 Complications of procedures, not elsewhere classified

> Use additional code for adverse effect, if applicable, to identify drug (T36-T50 with fifth or sixth character 5)

> **EXCLUDES 2**   complications following immunization (T88.0-T88.1)
> complications following infusion, transfusion and therapeutic injection (T80.-)
> complications of transplanted organs and tissue (T86.-)
> specified complications classified elsewhere, such as:
> complication of prosthetic devices, implants and grafts (T82-T85)
> dermatitis due to drugs and medicaments (L23.3, L24.4, L25.1, L27.0-L27.1)
> endosseous dental implant failure (M27.6-)
> floppy iris syndrome (IFIS) (intraoperative) (H21.81)
> intraoperative and postprocedural complications of specific body system (D78.-, E36.-, E89.-, G97.3-, G97.4, H59.3-, H59.-, H95.2-, H95.3, I97.4-, I97.5, J95, K91.-, L76.-, M96.-, N99.-)
> ostomy complications (J95.0-, K94.-, N99.5-)
> plateau iris syndrome (post-iridectomy) (postprocedural) H21.82
> poisoning and toxic effects of drugs and chemicals (T36-T65 with fifth or sixth character 1-4 or 6)

> **AHA:** 2019,2Q,21

> The appropriate 7th character is to be added to each code from category T81.
> A   initial encounter
> D   subsequent encounter
> S   sequela

✓5ᵗʰ T81.1 Postprocedural shock

> Shock during or resulting from a procedure, not elsewhere classified

> **EXCLUDES 1**   anaphylactic shock due to correct substance properly administered (T88.6)
> anaphylactic shock due to serum (T80.5-)
> anaphylactic shock NOS (T78.2)
> electric shock (T75.4)
> obstetric shock (O75.1)
> septic shock (R65.21)
> shock due to anesthesia (T88.2)
> shock following abortion or ectopic or molar pregnancy (O00-O07, O08.3)
> traumatic shock (T79.4)

> **AHA:** 2021,1Q,13

✓x7ᵗʰ T81.10 Postprocedural shock unspecified

> Collapse NOS during or resulting from a procedure, not elsewhere classified
> Postprocedural failure of peripheral circulation
> Postprocedural shock NOS

¹ **✓x7ᵗʰ T81.11 Postprocedural cardiogenic shock**   `HCC` `ESR`

¹ **✓x7ᵗʰ T81.12 Postprocedural septic shock**   `HCC` `ESR` `UPD`

> Postprocedural endotoxic shock resulting from a procedure, not elsewhere classified
> Postprocedural gram-negative shock resulting from a procedure, not elsewhere classified
> Code first underlying infection
> Use additional code, to identify any associated acute organ dysfunction, if applicable

> **AHA:** 2018,4Q,63

✓x7ᵗʰ T81.19 Other postprocedural shock

> Postprocedural hypovolemic shock

✓5ᵗʰ T81.3 Disruption of wound, not elsewhere classified

> Disruption of any suture materials or other closure methods

> **EXCLUDES 1**   breakdown (mechanical) of permanent sutures (T85.612)
> displacement of permanent sutures (T85.622)
> disruption of cesarean delivery wound (O90.0)
> disruption of perineal obstetric wound (O90.1)
> mechanical complication of permanent sutures NEC (T85.692)

> **AHA:** 2014,1Q,23

✓x7ᵗʰ T81.30 Disruption of wound, unspecified

> Disruption of wound NOS

`HCC` CMS-HCC   `Rx` Rx HCC   `ESR` ESRD HCC   `COM` Commercial HCC   `N` Newborn: 0   `P` Pediatric: 0-17   `M` Maternity: 9-64   `A` Adult: 15-124

1174   ICD-10-CM 2023

✓x7ᵗʰ **T81.31** **Disruption of** external operation **(surgical) wound, not elsewhere classified**

Dehiscence of operation wound NOS

Disruption of operation wound NOS

Disruption or dehiscence of closure of cornea

Disruption or dehiscence of closure of mucosa

Disruption or dehiscence of closure of skin and subcutaneous tissue

Full-thickness skin disruption or dehiscence

Superficial disruption or dehiscence of operation wound

EXCLUDES 1   dehiscence of amputation stump (T87.81)

✓x7ᵗʰ **T81.32** **Disruption of** internal operation **(surgical) wound, not elsewhere classified**

Deep disruption or dehiscence of operation wound NOS

Disruption or dehiscence of closure of internal organ or other internal tissue

Disruption or dehiscence of closure of muscle or muscle flap

Disruption or dehiscence of closure of ribs or rib cage

Disruption or dehiscence of closure of skull or craniotomy

Disruption or dehiscence of closure of sternum or sternotomy

Disruption or dehiscence of closure of tendon or ligament

Disruption or dehiscence of closure of superficial or muscular fascia

AHA: 2020,2Q,22; 2017,3Q,4

✓x7ᵗʰ **T81.33** **Disruption of** traumatic injury **wound** repair

Disruption or dehiscence of closure of traumatic laceration (external) (internal)

✓5ᵗʰ **T81.4** **Infection following a procedure**

Wound abscess following a procedure

Use additional code to identify infection

Use additional code (R65.2-) to identify severe sepsis, if applicable

EXCLUDES 2   bleb associated endophthalmitis (H59.4-)

infection due to infusion, transfusion and therapeutic injection (T80.2-)

infection due to prosthetic devices, implants and grafts (T82.6-T82.7, T83.5-T83.6, T84.5-T84.7, T85.7)

obstetric surgical wound infection (O86.0-)

postprocedural fever NOS (R50.82)

postprocedural retroperitoneal abscess (K68.11)

AHA: 2018,4Q,33-34,62; 2014,1Q,23

✓x7ᵗʰ **T81.40** **Infection following a procedure, unspecified**

✓x7ᵗʰ **T81.41** **Infection following a procedure,** superficial incisional surgical site

Subcutaneous abscess following a procedure

Stitch abscess following a procedure

✓x7ᵗʰ **T81.42** **Infection following a procedure,** deep incisional surgical site

Intra-muscular abscess following a procedure

✓x7ᵗʰ **T81.43** **Infection following a procedure,** organ and space surgical site

Intra-abdominal abscess following a procedure

Subphrenic abscess following a procedure

1 ✓x7ᵗʰ **T81.44** **Sepsis following a procedure** HCC ESR COM

Use additional code to identify the sepsis

✓x7ᵗʰ **T81.49** **Infection following a procedure, other surgical site**

✓5ᵗʰ **T81.5** **Complications of** foreign body accidentally left in body following procedure

AHA: 2014,4Q,24

✓6ᵗʰ **T81.50** **Unspecified complication of foreign body accidentally left in body following procedure**

✓7ᵗʰ **T81.500** **Unspecified complication of foreign body accidentally left in body following** surgical operation

✓7ᵗʰ **T81.501** **Unspecified complication of foreign body accidentally left in body following** infusion or transfusion

✓7ᵗʰ **T81.502** **Unspecified complication of foreign body accidentally left in body following** kidney dialysis HCC Rx ESR

✓7ᵗʰ **T81.503** **Unspecified complication of foreign body accidentally left in body following** injection or immunization

✓7ᵗʰ **T81.504** **Unspecified complication of foreign body accidentally left in body following** endoscopic examination

✓7ᵗʰ **T81.505** **Unspecified complication of foreign body accidentally left in body following** heart catheterization

✓7ᵗʰ **T81.506** **Unspecified complication of foreign body accidentally left in body following** aspiration, puncture or other catheterization

✓7ᵗʰ **T81.507** **Unspecified complication of foreign body accidentally left in body following** removal of catheter or packing

✓7ᵗʰ **T81.508** **Unspecified complication of foreign body accidentally left in body following other procedure**

✓7ᵗʰ **T81.509** **Unspecified complication of foreign body accidentally left in body following** unspecified procedure

✓6ᵗʰ **T81.51** **Adhesions** due to foreign body accidentally left in body following procedure

✓7ᵗʰ **T81.510** **Adhesions due to foreign body accidentally left in body following** surgical operation

✓7ᵗʰ **T81.511** **Adhesions due to foreign body accidentally left in body following** infusion or transfusion

✓7ᵗʰ **T81.512** **Adhesions due to foreign body accidentally left in body following** kidney dialysis HCC Rx ESR

✓7ᵗʰ **T81.513** **Adhesions due to foreign body accidentally left in body following** injection or immunization

✓7ᵗʰ **T81.514** **Adhesions due to foreign body accidentally left in body following** endoscopic examination

✓7ᵗʰ **T81.515** **Adhesions due to foreign body accidentally left in body following** heart catheterization

✓7ᵗʰ **T81.516** **Adhesions due to foreign body accidentally left in body following** aspiration, puncture or other catheterization

✓7ᵗʰ **T81.517** **Adhesions due to foreign body accidentally left in body following** removal of catheter or packing

✓7ᵗʰ **T81.518** **Adhesions due to foreign body accidentally left in body following other procedure**

✓7ᵗʰ **T81.519** **Adhesions due to foreign body accidentally left in body following** unspecified procedure

✓6ᵗʰ **T81.52** **Obstruction** due to foreign body accidentally left in body following procedure

✓7ᵗʰ **T81.520** **Obstruction due to foreign body accidentally left in body following** surgical operation

✓7ᵗʰ **T81.521** **Obstruction due to foreign body accidentally left in body following** infusion or transfusion

✓7ᵗʰ **T81.522** **Obstruction due to foreign body accidentally left in body following** kidney dialysis HCC Rx ESR

✓7ᵗʰ **T81.523** **Obstruction due to foreign body accidentally left in body following** injection or immunization

✓7ᵗʰ **T81.524** **Obstruction due to foreign body accidentally left in body following** endoscopic examination

✓7ᵗʰ **T81.525** **Obstruction due to foreign body accidentally left in body following** heart catheterization

✓7ᵗʰ **T81.526** **Obstruction due to foreign body accidentally left in body following** aspiration, puncture or other catheterization

✓7ᵗʰ **T81.527** **Obstruction due to foreign body accidentally left in body following** removal of catheter or packing

✓7ᵗʰ **T81.528** **Obstruction due to foreign body accidentally left in body following other procedure**

√7ᵗʰ **T81.529** **Obstruction due to foreign body accidentally left in body following unspecified procedure**

√6ᵗʰ **T81.53** Perforation due to foreign body accidentally left in body following procedure

√7ᵗʰ **T81.530** **Perforation due to foreign body accidentally left in body following surgical operation**

√7ᵗʰ **T81.531** **Perforation due to foreign body accidentally left in body following infusion or transfusion**

√7ᵗʰ **T81.532** **Perforation due to foreign body accidentally left in body following** kidney dialysis `HCC` `Rx` `ESR`

√7ᵗʰ **T81.533** **Perforation due to foreign body accidentally left in body following injection or immunization**

√7ᵗʰ **T81.534** **Perforation due to foreign body accidentally left in body following endoscopic examination**

√7ᵗʰ **T81.535** **Perforation due to foreign body accidentally left in body following** heart catheterization

√7ᵗʰ **T81.536** **Perforation due to foreign body accidentally left in body following aspiration, puncture or other catheterization**

√7ᵗʰ **T81.537** **Perforation due to foreign body accidentally left in body following removal of catheter or packing**

√7ᵗʰ **T81.538** **Perforation due to foreign body accidentally left in body following other procedure**

√7ᵗʰ **T81.539** **Perforation due to foreign body accidentally left in body following unspecified procedure**

√6ᵗʰ **T81.59** **Other complications of foreign body accidentally left in body following procedure**
EXCLUDES 2 *obstruction or perforation due to prosthetic devices and implants intentionally left in body (T82.0-T82.5, T83.0-T83.4, T83.7, T84.0-T84.4, T85.0-T85.6)*

√7ᵗʰ **T81.590** **Other complications of foreign body accidentally left in body following surgical operation**

√7ᵗʰ **T81.591** **Other complications of foreign body accidentally left in body following infusion or transfusion**

√7ᵗʰ **T81.592** **Other complications of foreign body accidentally left in body following** kidney dialysis `HCC` `Rx` `ESR`

√7ᵗʰ **T81.593** **Other complications of foreign body accidentally left in body following injection or immunization**

√7ᵗʰ **T81.594** **Other complications of foreign body accidentally left in body following endoscopic examination**

√7ᵗʰ **T81.595** **Other complications of foreign body accidentally left in body following** heart catheterization

√7ᵗʰ **T81.596** **Other complications of foreign body accidentally left in body following aspiration, puncture or other catheterization**

√7ᵗʰ **T81.597** **Other complications of foreign body accidentally left in body following removal of catheter or packing**

√7ᵗʰ **T81.598** **Other complications of foreign body accidentally left in body following other procedure**

√7ᵗʰ **T81.599** **Other complications of foreign body accidentally left in body following unspecified procedure**

√5ᵗʰ **T81.6** **Acute reaction to foreign substance accidentally left during a procedure**
EXCLUDES 2 *complications of foreign body accidentally left in body cavity or operation wound following procedure (T81.5-)*

√x7ᵗʰ **T81.60** **Unspecified acute reaction to foreign substance accidentally left during a procedure**

√x7ᵗʰ **T81.61** Aseptic peritonitis **due to foreign substance accidentally left during a procedure**
Chemical peritonitis

√x7ᵗʰ **T81.69** **Other acute reaction to foreign substance accidentally left during a procedure**

√5ᵗʰ **T81.7** **Vascular complications following a procedure, not elsewhere classified**
Air embolism following procedure NEC
Phlebitis or thrombophlebitis resulting from a procedure
EXCLUDES 1 *embolism complicating abortion or ectopic or molar pregnancy (O00-O07, O08.2)*
embolism complicating pregnancy, childbirth and the puerperium (O88.-)
traumatic embolism (T79.0)
EXCLUDES 2 *embolism due to prosthetic devices, implants and grafts (T82.8-, T83.81, T84.8-, T85.81-)*
embolism following infusion, transfusion and therapeutic injection (T80.0)
AHA: 2019,2Q,22

√6ᵗʰ **T81.71** **Complication of artery following a procedure, not elsewhere classified**

√7ᵗʰ **T81.710** **Complication of** mesenteric **artery following a procedure, not elsewhere classified**

√7ᵗʰ **T81.711** **Complication of** renal **artery following a procedure, not elsewhere classified**

√7ᵗʰ **T81.718** **Complication of other artery following a procedure, not elsewhere classified**
AHA: 2019,2Q,21-22

√7ᵗʰ **T81.719** **Complication of unspecified artery following a procedure, not elsewhere classified**

√x7ᵗʰ **T81.72** **Complication of** vein **following a procedure, not elsewhere classified**

√5ᵗʰ **T81.8** **Other complications of procedures, not elsewhere classified**
EXCLUDES 2 *hypothermia following anesthesia (T88.51)*
malignant hyperpyrexia due to anesthesia (T88.3)

√x7ᵗʰ **T81.81** **Complication of inhalation therapy**

√x7ᵗʰ **T81.82** **Emphysema (subcutaneous) resulting from a procedure**

√x7ᵗʰ **T81.83** **Persistent postprocedural fistula**
AHA: 2017,3Q,3-4

√x7ᵗʰ **T81.89** **Other complications of procedures, not elsewhere classified**
Use additional code to specify complication, such as: postprocedural delirium (F05)
AHA: 2014,1Q,23

√x7ᵗʰ **T81.9** **Unspecified complication of procedure**

√4ᵗʰ **T82** **Complications of cardiac and vascular prosthetic devices, implants and grafts**
EXCLUDES 2 *failure and rejection of transplanted organs and tissue (T86.-)*
AHA: 2020,3Q,36-37

> The appropriate 7th character is to be added to each code from category T82.
> A initial encounter
> D subsequent encounter
> S sequela

√5ᵗʰ **T82.0** **Mechanical complication of** heart valve prosthesis
Mechanical complication of artificial heart valve
EXCLUDES 1 *mechanical complication of biological heart valve graft (T82.22-)*

√x7ᵗʰ **T82.01** Breakdown **(mechanical) of heart valve prosthesis**

√x7ᵗʰ **T82.02** Displacement **of heart valve prosthesis**
Malposition of heart valve prosthesis

√x7ᵗʰ **T82.03** Leakage **of heart valve prosthesis**

√x7ᵗʰ **T82.09** **Other mechanical complication of heart valve prosthesis**
Obstruction (mechanical) of heart valve prosthesis
Perforation of heart valve prosthesis
Protrusion of heart valve prosthesis

√5ᵗʰ **T82.1** **Mechanical complication of** cardiac electronic device

√6ᵗʰ **T82.11** Breakdown **(mechanical) of cardiac electronic device**

√7ᵗʰ **T82.110** **Breakdown (mechanical) of cardiac electrode**

√7ᵗʰ **T82.111** **Breakdown (mechanical) of cardiac** pulse generator (battery)

    ✓7ᵗʰ **T82.118** **Breakdown (mechanical) of other cardiac electronic device**

    ✓7ᵗʰ **T82.119** **Breakdown (mechanical) of unspecified cardiac electronic device**

   ✓6ᵗʰ **T82.12** Displacement of cardiac electronic device

     Malposition of cardiac electronic device

    ✓7ᵗʰ **T82.120** **Displacement of** cardiac electrode

    ✓7ᵗʰ **T82.121** **Displacement of cardiac** pulse generator (battery)

    ✓7ᵗʰ **T82.128** **Displacement of other cardiac electronic device**

    ✓7ᵗʰ **T82.129** **Displacement of unspecified cardiac electronic device**

   ✓6ᵗʰ **T82.19** **Other mechanical complication of cardiac electronic device**

     Leakage of cardiac electronic device

     Obstruction of cardiac electronic device

     Perforation of cardiac electronic device

     Protrusion of cardiac electronic device

    ✓7ᵗʰ **T82.190** **Other mechanical complication of** cardiac electrode

    ✓7ᵗʰ **T82.191** **Other mechanical complication of cardiac pulse generator (battery)**

    ✓7ᵗʰ **T82.198** **Other mechanical complication of other cardiac electronic device**

    ✓7ᵗʰ **T82.199** **Other mechanical complication of unspecified cardiac device**

  ✓5ᵗʰ **T82.2** **Mechanical complication of coronary artery bypass graft and biological heart valve graft**

    EXCLUDES 1   *mechanical complication of artificial heart valve prosthesis (T82.0-)*

   ✓6ᵗʰ **T82.21** **Mechanical complication of** coronary artery bypass graft

    ✓7ᵗʰ **T82.211** **Breakdown (mechanical) of coronary artery bypass graft**

    ✓7ᵗʰ **T82.212** **Displacement of coronary artery bypass graft**

     Malposition of coronary artery bypass graft

    ✓7ᵗʰ **T82.213** **Leakage of coronary artery bypass graft**

    ✓7ᵗʰ **T82.218** **Other mechanical complication of coronary artery bypass graft**

     Obstruction, mechanical of coronary artery bypass graft

     Perforation of coronary artery bypass graft

     Protrusion of coronary artery bypass graft

   ✓6ᵗʰ **T82.22** **Mechanical complication of** biological heart valve graft

    ✓7ᵗʰ **T82.221** **Breakdown (mechanical) of biological heart valve graft**

    ✓7ᵗʰ **T82.222** **Displacement of biological heart valve graft**

     Malposition of biological heart valve graft

    ✓7ᵗʰ **T82.223** **Leakage of biological heart valve graft**

    ✓7ᵗʰ **T82.228** **Other mechanical complication of biological heart valve graft**

     Obstruction of biological heart valve graft

     Perforation of biological heart valve graft

     Protrusion of biological heart valve graft

  ✓5ᵗʰ **T82.3** **Mechanical complication of other vascular grafts**

   ✓6ᵗʰ **T82.31** Breakdown (mechanical) of other vascular grafts

    1 ✓7ᵗʰ **T82.310** **Breakdown (mechanical) of** aortic (bifurcation) graft (replacement)   HCC ESR

     AHA: 2020,3Q,3-8

    1 ✓7ᵗʰ **T82.311** **Breakdown (mechanical) of** carotid arterial graft (bypass)   HCC ESR

    1 ✓7ᵗʰ **T82.312** **Breakdown (mechanical) of** femoral arterial graft (bypass)   HCC ESR

    1 ✓7ᵗʰ **T82.318** **Breakdown (mechanical) of other vascular grafts**   HCC ESR

    1 ✓7ᵗʰ **T82.319** **Breakdown (mechanical) of unspecified vascular grafts**   HCC ESR

   ✓6ᵗʰ **T82.32** Displacement of other vascular grafts

     Malposition of other vascular grafts

    1 ✓7ᵗʰ **T82.320** **Displacement of** aortic (bifurcation) graft (replacement)   HCC ESR

    1 ✓7ᵗʰ **T82.321** **Displacement of** carotid arterial graft (bypass)   HCC ESR

    1 ✓7ᵗʰ **T82.322** **Displacement of** femoral arterial graft (bypass)   HCC ESR

    1 ✓7ᵗʰ **T82.328** **Displacement of other vascular grafts**   HCC ESR

    1 ✓7ᵗʰ **T82.329** **Displacement of unspecified vascular grafts**   HCC ESR

   ✓6ᵗʰ **T82.33** Leakage of other vascular grafts

    1 ✓7ᵗʰ **T82.330** **Leakage of** aortic (bifurcation) graft (replacement)   HCC ESR

     AHA: 2020,3Q,3-8

    1 ✓7ᵗʰ **T82.331** **Leakage of** carotid arterial graft (bypass)   HCC ESR

    1 ✓7ᵗʰ **T82.332** **Leakage of** femoral arterial graft (bypass)   HCC ESR

    1 ✓7ᵗʰ **T82.338** **Leakage of other vascular grafts**   HCC ESR

    1 ✓7ᵗʰ **T82.339** **Leakage of unspecified vascular graft**   HCC ESR

   ✓6ᵗʰ **T82.39** **Other mechanical complication of other vascular grafts**

     Obstruction (mechanical) of other vascular grafts

     Perforation of other vascular grafts

     Protrusion of other vascular grafts

    1 ✓7ᵗʰ **T82.390** **Other mechanical complication of** aortic (bifurcation) graft (replacement)   HCC ESR

     AHA: 2020,3Q,3-5

    1 ✓7ᵗʰ **T82.391** **Other mechanical complication of** carotid arterial graft (bypass)   HCC ESR

    1 ✓7ᵗʰ **T82.392** **Other mechanical complication of** femoral arterial graft (bypass)   HCC ESR

    1 ✓7ᵗʰ **T82.398** **Other mechanical complication of other vascular grafts**   HCC ESR

    1 ✓7ᵗʰ **T82.399** **Other mechanical complication of unspecified vascular grafts**   HCC ESR

  ✓5ᵗʰ **T82.4** **Mechanical complication of** vascular dialysis catheter

     Mechanical complication of hemodialysis catheter

    EXCLUDES 1   *mechanical complication of intraperitoneal dialysis catheter (T85.62)*

   ✓x7ᵗʰ **T82.41** Breakdown (mechanical) of vascular dialysis catheter   HCC Rx ESR

   ✓x7ᵗʰ **T82.42** Displacement of vascular dialysis catheter   HCC Rx ESR

     Malposition of vascular dialysis catheter

   ✓x7ᵗʰ **T82.43** Leakage of vascular dialysis catheter   HCC Rx ESR

   ✓x7ᵗʰ **T82.49** **Other complication of vascular dialysis catheter**   HCC Rx ESR

     Obstruction (mechanical) of vascular dialysis catheter

     Perforation of vascular dialysis catheter

     Protrusion of vascular dialysis catheter

  ✓5ᵗʰ **T82.5** **Mechanical complication of other cardiac and vascular devices and implants**

    EXCLUDES 2   *mechanical complication of epidural and subdural infusion catheter (T85.61)*

   ✓6ᵗʰ **T82.51** Breakdown (mechanical) of other cardiac and vascular devices and implants

    1 ✓7ᵗʰ **T82.510** **Breakdown (mechanical) of** surgically created arteriovenous fistula   HCC ESR

     AHA: 2020,3Q,36

    1 ✓7ᵗʰ **T82.511** **Breakdown (mechanical) of** surgically created arteriovenous shunt   HCC ESR

     AHA: 2020,3Q,37

    ✓7ᵗʰ **T82.512** **Breakdown (mechanical) of** artificial heart

    1 ✓7ᵗʰ **T82.513** **Breakdown (mechanical) of** balloon (counterpulsation) device   HCC ESR

    1 ✓7ᵗʰ **T82.514** **Breakdown (mechanical) of** infusion catheter   HCC ESR

    1 ✓7ᵗʰ **T82.515** **Breakdown (mechanical) of** umbrella device   HCC ESR

    1 ✓7ᵗʰ **T82.518** **Breakdown (mechanical) of other cardiac and vascular devices and implants**   HCC ESR

    ✓7ᵗʰ **T82.519** **Breakdown (mechanical) of unspecified cardiac and vascular devices and implants**

Chapter 19. Injury, Poisoning and Certain Other Consequences of External Causes

✓6ᵗʰ **T82.52** Displacement of other cardiac and vascular devices and implants

Malposition of other cardiac and vascular devices and implants

¹ ✓7ᵗʰ **T82.520** Displacement of surgically created arteriovenous fistula   HCC ESR
AHA: 2020,3Q,36

¹ ✓7ᵗʰ **T82.521** Displacement of surgically created arteriovenous shunt   HCC ESR

✓7ᵗʰ **T82.522** Displacement of artificial heart

¹ ✓7ᵗʰ **T82.523** Displacement of balloon (counterpulsation) device   HCC ESR

¹ ✓7ᵗʰ **T82.524** Displacement of infusion catheter   HCC ESR
AHA: 2020,2Q,21; 2019,3Q,15

¹ ✓7ᵗʰ **T82.525** Displacement of umbrella device   HCC ESR

¹ ✓7ᵗʰ **T82.528** Displacement of other cardiac and vascular devices and implants   HCC ESR

✓7ᵗʰ **T82.529** Displacement of unspecified cardiac and vascular devices and implants

✓6ᵗʰ **T82.53** Leakage of other cardiac and vascular devices and implants

¹ ✓7ᵗʰ **T82.530** Leakage of surgically created arteriovenous fistula   HCC ESR
AHA: 2020,3Q,36

¹ ✓7ᵗʰ **T82.531** Leakage of surgically created arteriovenous shunt   HCC ESR

✓7ᵗʰ **T82.532** Leakage of artificial heart

¹ ✓7ᵗʰ **T82.533** Leakage of balloon (counterpulsation) device   HCC ESR

¹ ✓7ᵗʰ **T82.534** Leakage of infusion catheter   HCC ESR

¹ ✓7ᵗʰ **T82.535** Leakage of umbrella device   HCC ESR

¹ ✓7ᵗʰ **T82.538** Leakage of other cardiac and vascular devices and implants   HCC ESR

✓7ᵗʰ **T82.539** Leakage of unspecified cardiac and vascular devices and implants

✓6ᵗʰ **T82.59** Other mechanical complication of other cardiac and vascular devices and implants

Obstruction (mechanical) of other cardiac and vascular devices and implants

Perforation of other cardiac and vascular devices and implants

Protrusion of other cardiac and vascular devices and implants

¹ ✓7ᵗʰ **T82.590** Other mechanical complication of surgically created arteriovenous fistula   HCC ESR
AHA: 2020,3Q,36

¹ ✓7ᵗʰ **T82.591** Other mechanical complication of surgically created arteriovenous shunt   HCC ESR

✓7ᵗʰ **T82.592** Other mechanical complication of artificial heart

¹ ✓7ᵗʰ **T82.593** Other mechanical complication of balloon (counterpulsation) device   HCC ESR

¹ ✓7ᵗʰ **T82.594** Other mechanical complication of infusion catheter   HCC ESR

¹ ✓7ᵗʰ **T82.595** Other mechanical complication of umbrella device   HCC ESR

¹ ✓7ᵗʰ **T82.598** Other mechanical complication of other cardiac and vascular devices and implants   HCC ESR

✓7ᵗʰ **T82.599** Other mechanical complication of unspecified cardiac and vascular devices and implants

¹ ✓x7ᵗʰ **T82.6** Infection and inflammatory reaction due to cardiac valve prosthesis   HCC ESR

Use additional code to identify infection

¹ ✓x7ᵗʰ **T82.7** Infection and inflammatory reaction due to other cardiac and vascular devices, implants and grafts   HCC ESR

Use additional code to identify infection

AHA: 2019,1Q,13-14

DEF: Midline catheter: Long peripheral catheter introduced via the cephalic, basilic, brachial, or median cubital veins in the upper arm and positioned so that the tip is level or near the level of the axilla and distal to the shoulder. Midline catheters are typically used for IV access, fluid replacement, and medication administration.

TIP: Assign this code for infections and/or cellulitis resulting from catheters that are not centrally placed (e.g., midline catheters).

✓5ᵗʰ **T82.8** Other specified complications of cardiac and vascular prosthetic devices, implants and grafts

AHA: 2016,4Q,70

✓6ᵗʰ **T82.81** Embolism due to cardiac and vascular prosthetic devices, implants and grafts

✓7ᵗʰ **T82.817** Embolism due to cardiac prosthetic devices, implants and grafts

¹ ✓7ᵗʰ **T82.818** Embolism due to vascular prosthetic devices, implants and grafts   HCC ESR

✓6ᵗʰ **T82.82** Fibrosis due to cardiac and vascular prosthetic devices, implants and grafts

✓7ᵗʰ **T82.827** Fibrosis due to cardiac prosthetic devices, implants and grafts

¹ ✓7ᵗʰ **T82.828** Fibrosis due vascular prosthetic devices, implants and grafts   HCC ESR

✓6ᵗʰ **T82.83** Hemorrhage due to cardiac and vascular prosthetic devices, implants and grafts

✓7ᵗʰ **T82.837** Hemorrhage due to cardiac prosthetic devices, implants and grafts

¹ ✓7ᵗʰ **T82.838** Hemorrhage due to vascular prosthetic devices, implants and grafts   HCC ESR
AHA: 2020,3Q,36-37

✓6ᵗʰ **T82.84** Pain due to cardiac and vascular prosthetic devices, implants and grafts

✓7ᵗʰ **T82.847** Pain due to cardiac prosthetic devices, implants and grafts

¹ ✓7ᵗʰ **T82.848** Pain due to vascular prosthetic devices, implants and grafts   HCC ESR

✓6ᵗʰ **T82.85** Stenosis due to cardiac and vascular prosthetic devices, implants and grafts

✓7ᵗʰ **T82.855** Stenosis of coronary artery stent

In-stent stenosis (restenosis) of coronary artery stent

Restenosis of coronary artery stent

AHA: 2021,3Q,6-7

¹ ✓7ᵗʰ **T82.856** Stenosis of peripheral vascular stent   HCC ESR

In-stent stenosis (restenosis) of peripheral vascular stent

Restenosis of peripheral vascular stent

✓7ᵗʰ **T82.857** Stenosis of other cardiac prosthetic devices, implants and grafts

¹ ✓7ᵗʰ **T82.858** Stenosis of other vascular prosthetic devices, implants and grafts   HCC ESR

✓6ᵗʰ **T82.86** Thrombosis of cardiac and vascular prosthetic devices, implants and grafts

✓7ᵗʰ **T82.867** Thrombosis due to cardiac prosthetic devices, implants and grafts

¹ ✓7ᵗʰ **T82.868** Thrombosis due to vascular prosthetic devices, implants and grafts   HCC ESR

✓6ᵗʰ **T82.89** Other specified complication of cardiac and vascular prosthetic devices, implants and grafts

✓7ᵗʰ **T82.897** Other specified complication of cardiac prosthetic devices, implants and grafts
AHA: 2019,2Q,33

¹ ✓7ᵗʰ **T82.898** Other specified complication of vascular prosthetic devices, implants and grafts   HCC ESR
AHA: 2020,3Q,3-5

✓x7ᵗʰ **T82.9** Unspecified complication of cardiac and vascular prosthetic device, implant and graft

√4ᵗʰ **T83** **Complications of genitourinary prosthetic devices, implants and grafts**

> EXCLUDES 2   *failure and rejection of transplanted organs and tissue (T86.-)*

AHA: 2016,4Q,70-71

> The appropriate 7th character is to be added to each code from category T83.
> A   initial encounter
> D   subsequent encounter
> S   sequela

√5ᵗʰ **T83.0** **Mechanical complication of** urinary catheter

> EXCLUDES 2   *complications of stoma of urinary tract (N99.5-)*

√6ᵗʰ   **T83.01**   **Breakdown (mechanical) of urinary catheter**

¹ √7ᵗʰ   **T83.010**   **Breakdown (mechanical) of** cystostomy catheter   HCC ESR

¹ √7ᵗʰ   **T83.011**   **Breakdown (mechanical) of** indwelling urethral catheter   HCC ESR

¹ √7ᵗʰ   **T83.012**   **Breakdown (mechanical) of** nephrostomy catheter   HCC ESR

¹ √7ᵗʰ   **T83.018**   **Breakdown (mechanical) of other urinary catheter**   HCC ESR
> Breakdown (mechanical) of Hopkins catheter
> Breakdown (mechanical) of ileostomy catheter
> Breakdown (mechanical) urostomy catheter

√6ᵗʰ   **T83.02**   **Displacement of urinary catheter**
> Malposition of urinary catheter

¹ √7ᵗʰ   **T83.020**   **Displacement of** cystostomy catheter   HCC ESR

¹ √7ᵗʰ   **T83.021**   **Displacement of** indwelling urethral catheter   HCC ESR

¹ √7ᵗʰ   **T83.022**   **Displacement of** nephrostomy catheter   HCC ESR

¹ √7ᵗʰ   **T83.028**   **Displacement of other urinary catheter**   HCC ESR
> Displacement of Hopkins catheter
> Displacement of ileostomy catheter
> Displacement of urostomy catheter

√6ᵗʰ   **T83.03**   **Leakage of urinary catheter**

¹ √7ᵗʰ   **T83.030**   **Leakage of** cystostomy catheter   HCC ESR
> **AHA:** 2021,4Q,18

¹ √7ᵗʰ   **T83.031**   **Leakage of** indwelling urethral catheter   HCC ESR

¹ √7ᵗʰ   **T83.032**   **Leakage of** nephrostomy catheter   HCC ESR

¹ √7ᵗʰ   **T83.038**   **Leakage of other urinary catheter**   HCC ESR
> Leakage of Hopkins catheter
> Leakage of ileostomy catheter
> Leakage of urostomy catheter

√6ᵗʰ   **T83.09**   **Other mechanical complication of urinary catheter**
> Obstruction (mechanical) of urinary catheter
> Perforation of urinary catheter
> Protrusion of urinary catheter

¹ √7ᵗʰ   **T83.090**   **Other mechanical complication of** cystostomy **catheter**   HCC ESR

¹ √7ᵗʰ   **T83.091**   **Other mechanical complication of** indwelling urethral **catheter**   HCC ESR

¹ √7ᵗʰ   **T83.092**   **Other mechanical complication of** nephrostomy **catheter**   HCC ESR

¹ √7ᵗʰ   **T83.098**   **Other mechanical complication of other urinary catheter**   HCC ESR
> Other mechanical complication of Hopkins catheter
> Other mechanical complication of ileostomy catheter
> Other mechanical complication of urostomy catheter

√5ᵗʰ **T83.1** **Mechanical complication of other urinary devices and implants**

√6ᵗʰ   **T83.11**   **Breakdown (mechanical) of other urinary devices and implants**

¹ √7ᵗʰ   **T83.110**   **Breakdown (mechanical) of urinary electronic stimulator device**   HCC ESR
> EXCLUDES 2   *breakdown (mechanical) of electrode (lead) for sacral nerve neurostimulator (T85.111)*
> *breakdown (mechanical) of implanted electronic sacral neurostimulator, pulse generator or receiver (T85.113)*

¹ √7ᵗʰ   **T83.111**   **Breakdown (mechanical) of** implanted urinary sphincter   HCC ESR

¹ √7ᵗʰ   **T83.112**   **Breakdown (mechanical) of** indwelling ureteral stent   HCC ESR

¹ √7ᵗʰ   **T83.113**   **Breakdown (mechanical) of other urinary stents**   HCC ESR
> Breakdown (mechanical) of ileal conduit stent
> Breakdown (mechanical) of nephroureteral stent

¹ √7ᵗʰ   **T83.118**   **Breakdown (mechanical) of other urinary devices and implants**   HCC ESR

√6ᵗʰ   **T83.12**   **Displacement of other urinary devices and implants**
> Malposition of other urinary devices and implants

¹ √7ᵗʰ   **T83.120**   **Displacement of urinary** electronic stimulator device   HCC ESR
> EXCLUDES 2   *displacement of electrode (lead) for sacral nerve neurostimulator (T85.121)*
> *displacement of implanted electronic sacral neurostimulator, pulse generator or receiver (T85.123)*

¹ √7ᵗʰ   **T83.121**   **Displacement of** implanted urinary sphincter   HCC ESR

¹ √7ᵗʰ   **T83.122**   **Displacement of** indwelling ureteral stent   HCC ESR

¹ √7ᵗʰ   **T83.123**   **Displacement of other urinary stents**   HCC ESR
> Displacement of ileal conduit stent
> Displacement of nephroureteral stent

¹ √7ᵗʰ   **T83.128**   **Displacement of other urinary devices and implants**   HCC ESR

√6ᵗʰ   **T83.19**   **Other mechanical complication of other urinary devices and implants**
> Leakage of other urinary devices and implants
> Obstruction (mechanical) of other urinary devices and implants
> Perforation of other urinary devices and implants
> Protrusion of other urinary devices and implants

¹ √7ᵗʰ   **T83.190**   **Other mechanical complication of urinary electronic stimulator device**   HCC ESR
> EXCLUDES 2   *other mechanical complication of electrode (lead) for sacral nerve neurostimulator (T85.191)*
> *other mechanical complication of implanted electronic sacral neurostimulator, pulse generator or receiver (T85.193)*

¹ √7ᵗʰ   **T83.191**   **Other mechanical complication of** implanted urinary sphincter   HCC ESR

¹ √7ᵗʰ   **T83.192**   **Other mechanical complication of** indwelling ureteral stent   HCC ESR

¹ √7ᵗʰ   **T83.193**   **Other mechanical complication of other urinary stent**   HCC ESR
> Other mechanical complication of ileal conduit stent
> Other mechanical complication of nephroureteral stent

¹ √7ᵗʰ   **T83.198**   **Other mechanical complication of other urinary devices and implants**   HCC ESR

✔ Additional Character Required   √x7ᵗʰ Placeholder Alert   Manifestation   Unspecified Dx   Q QPP   UPD Unacceptable PDx

√5ᵗʰ **T83.2 Mechanical complication of** graft of urinary organ

¹ √x7ᵗʰ **T83.21 Breakdown (mechanical) of graft of urinary organ** [HCC] [ESR]

¹ √x7ᵗʰ **T83.22 Displacement of graft of urinary organ** [HCC] [ESR]
Malposition of graft of urinary organ

¹ √x7ᵗʰ **T83.23 Leakage of graft of urinary organ** [HCC] [ESR]

¹ √x7ᵗʰ **T83.24 Erosion of graft of urinary organ** [HCC] [ESR]

¹ √x7ᵗʰ **T83.25 Exposure of graft of urinary organ** [HCC] [ESR]

¹ √x7ᵗʰ **T83.29 Other mechanical complication of graft of urinary organ** [HCC] [ESR]
Obstruction (mechanical) of graft of urinary organ
Perforation of graft of urinary organ
Protrusion of graft of urinary organ

√5ᵗʰ **T83.3 Mechanical complication of** intrauterine contraceptive device

√x7ᵗʰ **T83.31 Breakdown (mechanical) of intrauterine contraceptive device** ♀

√x7ᵗʰ **T83.32 Displacement of intrauterine contraceptive device** ♀
Malposition of intrauterine contraceptive device
Missing string of intrauterine contraceptive device
AHA: 2018,1Q,5

√x7ᵗʰ **T83.39 Other mechanical complication of intrauterine contraceptive device** ♀
Leakage of intrauterine contraceptive device
Obstruction (mechanical) of intrauterine contraceptive device
Perforation of intrauterine contraceptive device
Protrusion of intrauterine contraceptive device

√5ᵗʰ **T83.4 Mechanical complication of other prosthetic devices, implants and grafts of genital tract**

√6ᵗʰ **T83.41 Breakdown (mechanical) of other prosthetic devices, implants and grafts of genital tract**

¹ √7ᵗʰ **T83.410 Breakdown (mechanical) of** implanted penile prosthesis [HCC] [ESR] ♂
Breakdown (mechanical) of penile prosthesis cylinder
Breakdown (mechanical) of penile prosthesis pump
Breakdown (mechanical) of penile prosthesis reservoir

¹ √7ᵗʰ **T83.411 Breakdown (mechanical) of** implanted testicular prosthesis [HCC] [ESR]

¹ √7ᵗʰ **T83.418 Breakdown (mechanical) of other prosthetic devices, implants and grafts of genital tract** [HCC] [ESR]

√6ᵗʰ **T83.42 Displacement of other prosthetic devices, implants and grafts of genital tract**
Malposition of other prosthetic devices, implants and grafts of genital tract

¹ √7ᵗʰ **T83.420 Displacement of** implanted penile prosthesis [HCC] [ESR] ♂
Displacement of penile prosthesis cylinder
Displacement of penile prosthesis pump
Displacement of penile prosthesis reservoir

¹ √7ᵗʰ **T83.421 Displacement of** implanted testicular prosthesis [HCC] [ESR]

¹ √7ᵗʰ **T83.428 Displacement of other prosthetic devices, implants and grafts of genital tract** [HCC] [ESR]
AHA: 2018,1Q,5

√6ᵗʰ **T83.49 Other mechanical complication of other prosthetic devices, implants and grafts of genital tract**
Leakage of other prosthetic devices, implants and grafts of genital tract
Obstruction, mechanical of other prosthetic devices, implants and grafts of genital tract
Perforation of other prosthetic devices, implants and grafts of genital tract
Protrusion of other prosthetic devices, implants and grafts of genital tract

¹ √7ᵗʰ **T83.490 Other mechanical complication of** implanted penile prosthesis [HCC] [ESR] ♂
Other mechanical complication of penile prosthesis cylinder
Other mechanical complication of penile prosthesis pump
Other mechanical complication of penile prosthesis reservoir

¹ √7ᵗʰ **T83.491 Other mechanical complication of** implanted testicular prosthesis [HCC] [ESR]

¹ √7ᵗʰ **T83.498 Other mechanical complication of other prosthetic devices, implants and grafts of genital tract** [HCC] [ESR]

√5ᵗʰ **T83.5 Infection and inflammatory reaction due to prosthetic device, implant and graft in** urinary system
Use additional code to identify infection

√6ᵗʰ **T83.51 Infection and inflammatory reaction due to** urinary catheter
[EXCLUDES 2]   complications of stoma of urinary tract (N99.5-)
AHA: 2019,3Q,17

¹ √7ᵗʰ **T83.510 Infection and inflammatory reaction due to** cystostomy catheter [HCC] [ESR]

¹ √7ᵗʰ **T83.511 Infection and inflammatory reaction due to** indwelling urethral catheter [HCC] [ESR]
AHA: 2022,2Q,7

¹ √7ᵗʰ **T83.512 Infection and inflammatory reaction due to** nephrostomy catheter [HCC] [ESR]

¹ √7ᵗʰ **T83.518 Infection and inflammatory reaction due to** other urinary catheter [HCC] [ESR]
Infection and inflammatory reaction due to Hopkins catheter
Infection and inflammatory reaction due to ileostomy catheter
Infection and inflammatory reaction due to urostomy catheter

√6ᵗʰ **T83.59 Infection and inflammatory reaction due to** prosthetic device, implant and graft **in urinary system**

¹ √7ᵗʰ **T83.590 Infection and inflammatory reaction due to implanted urinary** neurostimulation device [HCC] [ESR]
[EXCLUDES 2]   infection and inflammatory reaction due to electrode lead of sacral nerve neurostimulator (T85.732)
infection and inflammatory reaction due to pulse generator or receiver of sacral nerve neurostimulator (T85.734)

¹ √7ᵗʰ **T83.591 Infection and inflammatory reaction due to** implanted urinary sphincter [HCC] [ESR]

¹ √7ᵗʰ **T83.592 Infection and inflammatory reaction due to** indwelling ureteral stent [HCC] [ESR]

¹ √7ᵗʰ **T83.593 Infection and inflammatory reaction due to** other urinary stents [HCC] [ESR]
Infection and inflammatory reaction due to ileal conduit stents
Infection and inflammatory reaction due to nephroureteral stent

¹ √7ᵗʰ **T83.598 Infection and inflammatory reaction due to** other prosthetic device, implant and graft in urinary system [HCC] [ESR]
AHA: 2020,3Q,25

[HCC] CMS-HCC   [Rx] Rx HCC   [ESR] ESRD HCC   [COM] Commercial HCC   [N] Newborn: 0   [P] Pediatric: 0-17   [M] Maternity: 9-64   [A] Adult: 15-124

1180   ICD-10-CM 2023

✓5ᵗʰ **T83.6 Infection and inflammatory reaction due to prosthetic device, implant and graft in** genital tract
Use additional code to identify infection

1 ✓x7ᵗʰ **T83.61 Infection and inflammatory reaction due to** implanted penile prosthesis   HCC ESR
Infection and inflammatory reaction due to penile prosthesis cylinder
Infection and inflammatory reaction due to penile prosthesis pump
Infection and inflammatory reaction due to penile prosthesis reservoir

1 ✓x7ᵗʰ **T83.62 Infection and inflammatory reaction due to** implanted testicular prosthesis   HCC ESR

1 ✓x7ᵗʰ **T83.69 Infection and inflammatory reaction due to other prosthetic device, implant and graft in genital tract**   HCC ESR

✓5ᵗʰ **T83.7 Complications due to** implanted mesh and other prosthetic materials

✓6ᵗʰ **T83.71 Erosion of implanted mesh and other prosthetic materials**

1 ✓7ᵗʰ **T83.711 Erosion of implanted** vaginal **mesh to surrounding organ or tissue** HCC ESR ♀
Erosion of implanted vaginal mesh into pelvic floor muscles

1 ✓7ᵗʰ **T83.712 Erosion of implanted** urethral **mesh to surrounding organ or tissue** HCC ESR
Erosion of implanted female urethral sling
Erosion of implanted male urethral sling
Erosion of implanted urethral mesh into pelvic floor muscles

1 ✓7ᵗʰ **T83.713 Erosion of implanted** urethral bulking agent **to surrounding organ or tissue** HCC ESR

1 ✓7ᵗʰ **T83.714 Erosion of implanted** ureteral bulking agent **to surrounding organ or tissue** HCC ESR

1 ✓7ᵗʰ **T83.718 Erosion of other implanted mesh to organ or tissue** HCC ESR

1 ✓7ᵗʰ **T83.719 Erosion of other prosthetic materials to surrounding organ or tissue** HCC ESR

✓6ᵗʰ **T83.72 Exposure of implanted mesh and other prosthetic materials into surrounding organ or tissue**
Extrusion of implanted mesh

1 ✓7ᵗʰ **T83.721 Exposure of implanted** vaginal mesh **into** vagina HCC ESR ♀
Exposure of implanted vaginal mesh through vaginal wall

1 ✓7ᵗʰ **T83.722 Exposure of implanted** urethral mesh **into** urethra HCC ESR
Exposure of implanted female urethral sling
Exposure of implanted male urethral sling
Exposure of implanted urethral mesh through urethral wall

1 ✓7ᵗʰ **T83.723 Exposure of implanted** urethral bulking agent **into** urethra HCC ESR

1 ✓7ᵗʰ **T83.724 Exposure of implanted** ureteral bulking agent **into** ureter HCC ESR

1 ✓7ᵗʰ **T83.728 Exposure of** other implanted mesh **into organ or tissue** HCC ESR

1 ✓7ᵗʰ **T83.729 Exposure of** other prosthetic materials **into organ or tissue** HCC ESR

1 ✓x7ᵗʰ **T83.79 Other specified complications due to other genitourinary prosthetic materials** HCC ESR

✓5ᵗʰ **T83.8 Other specified complications of** genitourinary prosthetic devices, implants and grafts

1 ✓x7ᵗʰ **T83.81 Embolism due to genitourinary prosthetic devices, implants and grafts** HCC ESR

1 ✓x7ᵗʰ **T83.82 Fibrosis due to genitourinary prosthetic devices, implants and grafts** HCC ESR

1 ✓x7ᵗʰ **T83.83 Hemorrhage due to genitourinary prosthetic devices, implants and grafts** HCC ESR

1 ✓x7ᵗʰ **T83.84 Pain due to genitourinary prosthetic devices, implants and grafts** HCC ESR

1 ✓x7ᵗʰ **T83.85 Stenosis due to genitourinary prosthetic devices, implants and grafts** HCC ESR

1 ✓x7ᵗʰ **T83.86 Thrombosis due to genitourinary prosthetic devices, implants and grafts** HCC ESR

1 ✓x7ᵗʰ **T83.89 Other specified complication of genitourinary prosthetic devices, implants and grafts** HCC ESR
AHA: 2016,1Q,19

1 ✓x7ᵗʰ **T83.9 Unspecified complication of genitourinary prosthetic device, implant and graft** HCC ESR

✓4ᵗʰ **T84 Complications of internal orthopedic prosthetic devices, implants and grafts**
EXCLUDES 2 *failure and rejection of transplanted organs and tissues (T86.-)*
fracture of bone following insertion of orthopedic implant, joint prosthesis or bone plate (M96.6)

The appropriate 7th character is to be added to each code from category T84.
A initial encounter
D subsequent encounter
S sequela

✓5ᵗʰ **T84.0 Mechanical complication of** internal joint prosthesis

✓6ᵗʰ **T84.01 Broken internal joint prosthesis**
Breakage (fracture) of prosthetic joint
Broken prosthetic joint implant
EXCLUDES 1 *periprosthetic joint implant fracture (M97.-)*
AHA: 2016,4Q,42

1 ✓7ᵗʰ **T84.010 Broken internal** right hip **prosthesis** HCC ESR

1 ✓7ᵗʰ **T84.011 Broken internal** left hip **prosthesis** HCC ESR

1 ✓7ᵗʰ **T84.012 Broken internal** right knee **prosthesis** HCC ESR

1 ✓7ᵗʰ **T84.013 Broken internal** left knee **prosthesis** HCC ESR

1 ✓7ᵗʰ **T84.018 Broken internal joint prosthesis, other site** HCC ESR
Use additional code to identify the joint (Z96.6-)

1 ✓7ᵗʰ **T84.019 Broken internal joint prosthesis, unspecified site** HCC ESR

✓6ᵗʰ **T84.02 Dislocation of internal joint prosthesis**
Instability of internal joint prosthesis
Subluxation of internal joint prosthesis
AHA: 2019,2Q,27

1 ✓7ᵗʰ **T84.020 Dislocation of internal** right hip **prosthesis** HCC ESR

1 ✓7ᵗʰ **T84.021 Dislocation of internal** left hip **prosthesis** HCC ESR

1 ✓7ᵗʰ **T84.022 Instability of internal** right knee **prosthesis** HCC ESR

1 ✓7ᵗʰ **T84.023 Instability of internal** left knee **prosthesis** HCC ESR

1 ✓7ᵗʰ **T84.028 Dislocation of other internal joint prosthesis** HCC ESR
Use additional code to identify the joint (Z96.6-)

1 ✓7ᵗʰ **T84.029 Dislocation of unspecified internal joint prosthesis** HCC ESR

✓6ᵗʰ **T84.03 Mechanical loosening of internal prosthetic joint**
Aseptic loosening of prosthetic joint

1 ✓7ᵗʰ **T84.030 Mechanical loosening of internal** right hip prosthetic joint HCC ESR

1 ✓7ᵗʰ **T84.031 Mechanical loosening of internal** left hip prosthetic joint HCC ESR

1 ✓7ᵗʰ **T84.032 Mechanical loosening of internal** right knee prosthetic joint HCC ESR

1 ✓7ᵗʰ **T84.033 Mechanical loosening of internal** left knee prosthetic joint HCC ESR

1 ✓7ᵗʰ **T84.038 Mechanical loosening of other internal prosthetic joint** HCC ESR
Use additional code to identify the joint (Z96.6-)

1 ✓7ᵗʰ **T84.039 Mechanical loosening of unspecified internal prosthetic joint** HCC ESR

✓6ᵗʰ **T84.05 Periprosthetic osteolysis of internal prosthetic joint**
Use additional code to identify major osseous defect, if applicable (M89.7-)

1 ✓7ᵗʰ **T84.050 Periprosthetic osteolysis of internal prosthetic** right hip joint HCC ESR

1 ✓7ᵗʰ **T84.051 Periprosthetic osteolysis of internal prosthetic** left hip joint HCC ESR

Chapter 19. Injury, Poisoning and Certain Other Consequences of External Causes

T84.052–T84.220

¹ √7ᵗʰ **T84.052** **Periprosthetic osteolysis of internal prosthetic** right knee joint `HCC` `ESR`

¹ √7ᵗʰ **T84.053** **Periprosthetic osteolysis of internal prosthetic** left knee joint `HCC` `ESR`

¹ √7ᵗʰ **T84.058** **Periprosthetic osteolysis of other internal prosthetic joint** `HCC` `ESR`
  Use additional code to identify the joint (Z96.6-)

¹ √7ᵗʰ **T84.059** **Periprosthetic osteolysis of unspecified internal prosthetic joint** `HCC` `ESR`

√6ᵗʰ **T84.06** **Wear of articular bearing surface of internal prosthetic joint**

¹ √7ᵗʰ **T84.060** **Wear of articular bearing surface of internal prosthetic** right hip joint `HCC` `ESR`

¹ √7ᵗʰ **T84.061** **Wear of articular bearing surface of internal prosthetic** left hip joint `HCC` `ESR`

¹ √7ᵗʰ **T84.062** **Wear of articular bearing surface of internal prosthetic** right knee joint `HCC` `ESR`

¹ √7ᵗʰ **T84.063** **Wear of articular bearing surface of internal prosthetic** left knee joint `HCC` `ESR`

¹ √7ᵗʰ **T84.068** **Wear of articular bearing surface of other internal prosthetic joint** `HCC` `ESR`
  Use additional code to identify the joint (Z96.6-)

¹ √7ᵗʰ **T84.069** **Wear of articular bearing surface of unspecified internal prosthetic joint** `HCC` `ESR`

√6ᵗʰ **T84.09** **Other mechanical complication of internal joint prosthesis**
  Prosthetic joint implant failure NOS
  AHA: 2019,1Q,20

¹ √7ᵗʰ **T84.090** **Other mechanical complication of internal** right hip prosthesis `HCC` `ESR`

¹ √7ᵗʰ **T84.091** **Other mechanical complication of internal** left hip prosthesis `HCC` `ESR`

¹ √7ᵗʰ **T84.092** **Other mechanical complication of internal** right knee prosthesis `HCC` `ESR`

¹ √7ᵗʰ **T84.093** **Other mechanical complication of internal** left knee prosthesis `HCC` `ESR`

¹ √7ᵗʰ **T84.098** **Other mechanical complication of other internal joint prosthesis** `HCC` `ESR`
  Use additional code to identify the joint (Z96.6-)

¹ √7ᵗʰ **T84.099** **Other mechanical complication of unspecified internal joint prosthesis** `HCC` `ESR`

√5ᵗʰ **T84.1** **Mechanical complication of** internal fixation device **of bones of** limb
  `EXCLUDES 2` *mechanical complication of internal fixation device of bones of feet (T84.2-)*
  mechanical complication of internal fixation device of bones of fingers (T84.2-)
  mechanical complication of internal fixation device of bones of hands (T84.2-)
  mechanical complication of internal fixation device of bones of toes (T84.2-)

√6ᵗʰ **T84.11** **Breakdown** (mechanical) **of internal fixation device of bones of limb**

¹ √7ᵗʰ **T84.110** **Breakdown (mechanical) of internal fixation device of** right humerus `HCC` `ESR`

¹ √7ᵗʰ **T84.111** **Breakdown (mechanical) of internal fixation device of** left humerus `HCC` `ESR`

¹ √7ᵗʰ **T84.112** **Breakdown (mechanical) of internal fixation device of bone of** right forearm `HCC` `ESR`

¹ √7ᵗʰ **T84.113** **Breakdown (mechanical) of internal fixation device of bone of** left forearm `HCC` `ESR`

¹ √7ᵗʰ **T84.114** **Breakdown (mechanical) of internal fixation device of** right femur `HCC` `ESR`

¹ √7ᵗʰ **T84.115** **Breakdown (mechanical) of internal fixation device of** left femur `HCC` `ESR`

¹ √7ᵗʰ **T84.116** **Breakdown (mechanical) of internal fixation device of bone of** right lower leg `HCC` `ESR`

¹ √7ᵗʰ **T84.117** **Breakdown (mechanical) of internal fixation device of bone of** left lower leg `HCC` `ESR`

¹ √7ᵗʰ **T84.119** **Breakdown (mechanical) of internal fixation device of unspecified bone of limb** `HCC` `ESR`

√6ᵗʰ **T84.12** **Displacement of internal fixation device of bones of limb**
  Malposition of internal fixation device of bones of limb

¹ √7ᵗʰ **T84.120** **Displacement of internal fixation device of** right humerus `HCC` `ESR`

¹ √7ᵗʰ **T84.121** **Displacement of internal fixation device of** left humerus `HCC` `ESR`

¹ √7ᵗʰ **T84.122** **Displacement of internal fixation device of bone of** right forearm `HCC` `ESR`

¹ √7ᵗʰ **T84.123** **Displacement of internal fixation device of bone of** left forearm `HCC` `ESR`

¹ √7ᵗʰ **T84.124** **Displacement of internal fixation device of** right femur `HCC` `ESR`

¹ √7ᵗʰ **T84.125** **Displacement of internal fixation device of** left femur `HCC` `ESR`

¹ √7ᵗʰ **T84.126** **Displacement of internal fixation device of bone of** right lower leg `HCC` `ESR`

¹ √7ᵗʰ **T84.127** **Displacement of internal fixation device of bone of** left lower leg `HCC` `ESR`

¹ √7ᵗʰ **T84.129** **Displacement of internal fixation device of unspecified bone of limb** `HCC` `ESR`

√6ᵗʰ **T84.19** **Other mechanical complication of internal fixation device of bones of limb**
  Obstruction (mechanical) of internal fixation device of bones of limb
  Perforation of internal fixation device of bones of limb
  Protrusion of internal fixation device of bones of limb

¹ √7ᵗʰ **T84.190** **Other mechanical complication of internal fixation device of** right humerus `HCC` `ESR`

¹ √7ᵗʰ **T84.191** **Other mechanical complication of internal fixation device of** left humerus `HCC` `ESR`

¹ √7ᵗʰ **T84.192** **Other mechanical complication of internal fixation device of bone of** right forearm `HCC` `ESR`

¹ √7ᵗʰ **T84.193** **Other mechanical complication of internal fixation device of bone of** left forearm `HCC` `ESR`

¹ √7ᵗʰ **T84.194** **Other mechanical complication of internal fixation device of** right femur `HCC` `ESR`

¹ √7ᵗʰ **T84.195** **Other mechanical complication of internal fixation device of** left femur `HCC` `ESR`

¹ √7ᵗʰ **T84.196** **Other mechanical complication of internal fixation device of bone of** right lower leg `HCC` `ESR`

¹ √7ᵗʰ **T84.197** **Other mechanical complication of internal fixation device of bone of** left lower leg `HCC` `ESR`

¹ √7ᵗʰ **T84.199** **Other mechanical complication of internal fixation device of unspecified bone of limb** `HCC` `ESR`

√5ᵗʰ **T84.2** **Mechanical complication of** internal fixation device **of** other bones

√6ᵗʰ **T84.21** **Breakdown** (mechanical) **of internal fixation device of other bones**

¹ √7ᵗʰ **T84.210** **Breakdown (mechanical) of internal fixation device of bones of** hand and fingers `HCC` `ESR`

¹ √7ᵗʰ **T84.213** **Breakdown (mechanical) of internal fixation device of bones of** foot and toes `HCC` `ESR`

¹ √7ᵗʰ **T84.216** **Breakdown (mechanical) of internal fixation device of** vertebrae `HCC` `ESR`

¹ √7ᵗʰ **T84.218** **Breakdown (mechanical) of internal fixation device of other bones** `HCC` `ESR`

√6ᵗʰ **T84.22** **Displacement of internal fixation device of other bones**
  Malposition of internal fixation device of other bones

¹ √7ᵗʰ **T84.220** **Displacement of internal fixation device of bones of** hand and fingers `HCC` `ESR`

`HCC` CMS-HCC   `Rx` Rx HCC   `ESR` ESRD HCC   `COM` Commercial HCC   `N` Newborn: 0   `P` Pediatric: 0-17   `M` Maternity: 9-64   `A` Adult: 15-124

1182
ICD–10-CM 2023

¹ √7ᵗʰ **T84.223 Displacement of internal fixation device of bones of** foot and toes `HCC` `ESR`

¹ √7ᵗʰ **T84.226 Displacement of internal fixation device of** vertebrae `HCC` `ESR`

¹ √7ᵗʰ **T84.228 Displacement of internal fixation device of** other bones `HCC` `ESR`

√6ᵗʰ **T84.29 Other mechanical complication of internal fixation device of other bones**

Obstruction (mechanical) of internal fixation device of other bones

Perforation of internal fixation device of other bones

Protrusion of internal fixation device of other bones

¹ √7ᵗʰ **T84.290 Other mechanical complication of internal fixation device of bones of** hand and fingers `HCC` `ESR`

¹ √7ᵗʰ **T84.293 Other mechanical complication of internal fixation device of bones of** foot and toes `HCC` `ESR`

¹ √7ᵗʰ **T84.296 Other mechanical complication of internal fixation device of** vertebrae `HCC` `ESR`

¹ √7ᵗʰ **T84.298 Other mechanical complication of internal fixation device of other bones** `HCC` `ESR`

√5ᵗʰ **T84.3 Mechanical complication of other bone devices, implants and grafts**

> EXCLUDES 2   *other complications of bone graft (T86.83-)*

√6ᵗʰ **T84.31 Breakdown (mechanical) of other bone devices, implants and grafts**

¹ √7ᵗʰ **T84.310 Breakdown (mechanical) of** electronic bone stimulator `HCC` `ESR`

¹ √7ᵗʰ **T84.318 Breakdown (mechanical) of other bone devices, implants and grafts** `HCC` `ESR`

√6ᵗʰ **T84.32 Displacement of other bone devices, implants and grafts**

Malposition of other bone devices, implants and grafts

¹ √7ᵗʰ **T84.320 Displacement of** electronic bone stimulator `HCC` `ESR`

¹ √7ᵗʰ **T84.328 Displacement of other bone devices, implants and grafts** `HCC` `ESR`

> AHA: 2014,4Q,28

√6ᵗʰ **T84.39 Other mechanical complication of other bone devices, implants and grafts**

Obstruction (mechanical) of other bone devices, implants and grafts

Perforation of other bone devices, implants and grafts

Protrusion of other bone devices, implants and grafts

¹ √7ᵗʰ **T84.390 Other mechanical complication of** electronic bone stimulator `HCC` `ESR`

¹ √7ᵗʰ **T84.398 Other mechanical complication of other bone devices, implants and grafts** `HCC` `ESR`

√5ᵗʰ **T84.4 Mechanical complication of other internal orthopedic devices, implants and grafts**

√6ᵗʰ **T84.41 Breakdown (mechanical) of other internal orthopedic devices, implants and grafts**

¹ √7ᵗʰ **T84.410 Breakdown (mechanical) of** muscle and tendon graft `HCC` `ESR`

¹ √7ᵗʰ **T84.418 Breakdown (mechanical) of other internal orthopedic devices, implants and grafts** `HCC` `ESR`

√6ᵗʰ **T84.42 Displacement of other internal orthopedic devices, implants and grafts**

Malposition of other internal orthopedic devices, implants and grafts

¹ √7ᵗʰ **T84.420 Displacement of** muscle and tendon graft `HCC` `ESR`

¹ √7ᵗʰ **T84.428 Displacement of other internal orthopedic devices, implants and grafts** `HCC` `ESR`

√6ᵗʰ **T84.49 Other mechanical complication of other internal orthopedic devices, implants and grafts**

Mechanical complication of other internal orthopedic devices, implants and grafts NOS

Obstruction (mechanical) of other internal orthopedic devices, implants and grafts

Perforation of other internal orthopedic devices, implants and grafts

Protrusion of other internal orthopedic devices, implants and grafts

¹ √7ᵗʰ **T84.490 Other mechanical complication of** muscle and tendon graft `HCC` `ESR`

¹ √7ᵗʰ **T84.498 Other mechanical complication of other internal orthopedic devices, implants and grafts** `HCC` `ESR`

√5ᵗʰ **T84.5 Infection and inflammatory reaction due to** internal joint prosthesis

Use additional code to identify infection

> AHA: 2019,3Q,16; 2015,1Q,16

¹ √x7ᵗʰ **T84.50 Infection and inflammatory reaction due to unspecified internal joint prosthesis** `HCC` `ESR`

¹ √x7ᵗʰ **T84.51 Infection and inflammatory reaction due to internal** right hip **prosthesis** `HCC` `ESR`

¹ √x7ᵗʰ **T84.52 Infection and inflammatory reaction due to internal** left hip **prosthesis** `HCC` `ESR`

¹ √x7ᵗʰ **T84.53 Infection and inflammatory reaction due to internal** right knee **prosthesis** `HCC` `ESR`

¹ √x7ᵗʰ **T84.54 Infection and inflammatory reaction due to internal** left knee **prosthesis** `HCC` `ESR`

¹ √x7ᵗʰ **T84.59 Infection and inflammatory reaction due to other internal joint prosthesis** `HCC` `ESR`

√5ᵗʰ **T84.6 Infection and inflammatory reaction due to** internal fixation device

Use additional code to identify infection

¹ √x7ᵗʰ **T84.60 Infection and inflammatory reaction due to internal fixation device of unspecified site** `HCC` `ESR`

√6ᵗʰ **T84.61 Infection and inflammatory reaction due to internal fixation device of** arm

¹ √7ᵗʰ **T84.610 Infection and inflammatory reaction due to internal fixation device of** right humerus `HCC` `ESR`

¹ √7ᵗʰ **T84.611 Infection and inflammatory reaction due to internal fixation device of** left humerus `HCC` `ESR`

¹ √7ᵗʰ **T84.612 Infection and inflammatory reaction due to internal fixation device of** right radius `HCC` `ESR`

¹ √7ᵗʰ **T84.613 Infection and inflammatory reaction due to internal fixation device of** left radius `HCC` `ESR`

¹ √7ᵗʰ **T84.614 Infection and inflammatory reaction due to internal fixation device of** right ulna `HCC` `ESR`

¹ √7ᵗʰ **T84.615 Infection and inflammatory reaction due to internal fixation device of** left ulna `HCC` `ESR`

¹ √7ᵗʰ **T84.619 Infection and inflammatory reaction due to internal fixation device of unspecified bone of arm** `HCC` `ESR`

√6ᵗʰ **T84.62 Infection and inflammatory reaction due to internal fixation device of** leg

¹ √7ᵗʰ **T84.620 Infection and inflammatory reaction due to internal fixation device of** right femur `HCC` `ESR`

¹ √7ᵗʰ **T84.621 Infection and inflammatory reaction due to internal fixation device of** left femur `HCC` `ESR`

¹ √7ᵗʰ **T84.622 Infection and inflammatory reaction due to internal fixation device of** right tibia `HCC` `ESR`

¹ √7ᵗʰ **T84.623 Infection and inflammatory reaction due to internal fixation device of** left tibia `HCC` `ESR`

¹ √7ᵗʰ **T84.624 Infection and inflammatory reaction due to internal fixation device of** right fibula `HCC` `ESR`

¹ √7ᵗʰ **T84.625 Infection and inflammatory reaction due to internal fixation device of** left fibula `HCC` `ESR`

¹ √x7ᵗʰ **T84.629** Infection and inflammatory reaction due to internal fixation device of unspecified bone of leg `HCC` `ESR`

¹ √x7ᵗʰ **T84.63** Infection and inflammatory reaction due to internal fixation device of spine `HCC` `ESR`

¹ √x7ᵗʰ **T84.69** Infection and inflammatory reaction due to internal fixation device of other site `HCC` `ESR`

¹ √x7ᵗʰ **T84.7** Infection and inflammatory reaction due to other internal orthopedic prosthetic devices, implants and grafts `HCC` `ESR`
     Use additional code to identify infection

√5ᵗʰ **T84.8** Other specified complications of internal orthopedic prosthetic devices, implants and grafts

¹ √x7ᵗʰ **T84.81** Embolism due to internal orthopedic prosthetic devices, implants and grafts `HCC` `ESR`

¹ √x7ᵗʰ **T84.82** Fibrosis due to internal orthopedic prosthetic devices, implants and grafts `HCC` `ESR`

¹ √x7ᵗʰ **T84.83** Hemorrhage due to internal orthopedic prosthetic devices, implants and grafts `HCC` `ESR`

¹ √x7ᵗʰ **T84.84** Pain due to internal orthopedic prosthetic devices, implants and grafts `HCC` `ESR`

¹ √x7ᵗʰ **T84.85** Stenosis due to internal orthopedic prosthetic devices, implants and grafts `HCC` `ESR`

¹ √x7ᵗʰ **T84.86** Thrombosis due to internal orthopedic prosthetic devices, implants and grafts `HCC` `ESR`

¹ √x7ᵗʰ **T84.89** Other specified complication of internal orthopedic prosthetic devices, implants and grafts `HCC` `ESR`

¹ √x7ᵗʰ **T84.9** Unspecified complication of internal orthopedic prosthetic device, implant and graft `HCC` `ESR`

√4ᵗʰ **T85** Complications of other internal prosthetic devices, implants and grafts
> EXCLUDES 2   failure and rejection of transplanted organs and tissue (T86.-)

AHA: 2016,4Q,71-72

> The appropriate 7th character is to be added to each code from category T85.
> A   initial encounter
> D   subsequent encounter
> S   sequela

√5ᵗʰ **T85.0** Mechanical complication of ventricular intracranial (communicating) shunt

¹ √x7ᵗʰ **T85.01** Breakdown (mechanical) of ventricular intracranial (communicating) shunt `HCC` `ESR`

¹ √x7ᵗʰ **T85.02** Displacement of ventricular intracranial (communicating) shunt `HCC` `ESR`
     Malposition of ventricular intracranial (communicating) shunt

¹ √x7ᵗʰ **T85.03** Leakage of ventricular intracranial (communicating) shunt `HCC` `ESR`

¹ √x7ᵗʰ **T85.09** Other mechanical complication of ventricular intracranial (communicating) shunt `HCC` `ESR`
     Obstruction (mechanical) of ventricular intracranial (communicating) shunt
     Perforation of ventricular intracranial (communicating) shunt
     Protrusion of ventricular intracranial (communicating) shunt

√5ᵗʰ **T85.1** Mechanical complication of implanted electronic stimulator of nervous system

√6ᵗʰ **T85.11** Breakdown (mechanical) of implanted electronic stimulator of nervous system

¹ √7ᵗʰ **T85.110** Breakdown (mechanical) of implanted electronic neurostimulator of brain electrode (lead) `HCC` `ESR`

¹ √7ᵗʰ **T85.111** Breakdown (mechanical) of implanted electronic neurostimulator of peripheral nerve electrode (lead) `HCC` `ESR`
     Breakdown of electrode (lead) for cranial nerve neurostimulators
     Breakdown of electrode (lead) for gastric neurostimulator
     Breakdown of electrode (lead) for sacral nerve neurostimulator
     Breakdown of electrode (lead) for vagal nerve neurostimulators

¹ √7ᵗʰ **T85.112** Breakdown (mechanical) of implanted electronic neurostimulator of spinal cord electrode (lead) `HCC` `ESR`

¹ √7ᵗʰ **T85.113** Breakdown (mechanical) of implanted electronic neurostimulator, generator `HCC` `ESR`
     Breakdown (mechanical) of implanted electronic neurostimulator generator, brain, peripheral, gastric, spinal
     Breakdown (mechanical) of implanted electronic sacral neurostimulator, pulse generator or receiver

¹ √7ᵗʰ **T85.118** Breakdown (mechanical) of other implanted electronic stimulator of nervous system `HCC` `ESR`

√6ᵗʰ **T85.12** Displacement of implanted electronic stimulator of nervous system
     Malposition of implanted electronic stimulator of nervous system

¹ √7ᵗʰ **T85.120** Displacement of implanted electronic neurostimulator of brain electrode (lead) `HCC` `ESR`

¹ √7ᵗʰ **T85.121** Displacement of implanted electronic neurostimulator of peripheral nerve electrode (lead) `HCC` `ESR`
     Displacement of electrode (lead) for cranial nerve neurostimulators
     Displacement of electrode (lead) for gastric neurostimulator
     Displacement of electrode (lead) for sacral nerve neurostimulator
     Displacement of electrode (lead) for vagal nerve neurostimulators

¹ √7ᵗʰ **T85.122** Displacement of implanted electronic neurostimulator of spinal cord electrode (lead) `HCC` `ESR`

¹ √7ᵗʰ **T85.123** Displacement of implanted electronic neurostimulator, generator `HCC` `ESR`
     Displacement of implanted electronic neurostimulator generator, brain, peripheral, gastric, spinal
     Displacement of implanted electronic sacral neurostimulator, pulse generator or receiver

¹ √7ᵗʰ **T85.128** Displacement of other implanted electronic stimulator of nervous system `HCC` `ESR`

√6ᵗʰ **T85.19** Other mechanical complication of implanted electronic stimulator of nervous system
     Leakage of implanted electronic stimulator of nervous system
     Obstruction (mechanical) of implanted electronic stimulator of nervous system
     Perforation of implanted electronic stimulator of nervous system
     Protrusion of implanted electronic stimulator of nervous system

¹ √7ᵗʰ **T85.190** Other mechanical complication of implanted electronic neurostimulator of brain electrode (lead) `HCC` `ESR`

¹ √7ᵗʰ **T85.191** Other mechanical complication of implanted electronic neurostimulator of peripheral nerve electrode (lead) `HCC` `ESR`
     Other mechanical complication of electrode (lead) for cranial nerve neurostimulators
     Other mechanical complication of electrode (lead) for gastric neurostimulator
     Other mechanical complication of electrode (lead) for sacral nerve neurostimulator
     Other mechanical complication of electrode (lead) for vagal nerve neurostimulators

¹ √7ᵗʰ **T85.192** Other mechanical complication of implanted electronic neurostimulator of spinal cord electrode (lead) `HCC` `ESR`

`HCC` CMS-HCC   `Rx` Rx HCC   `ESR` ESRD HCC   `COM` Commercial HCC   `N` Newborn: 0   `P` Pediatric: 0-17   `M` Maternity: 9-64   `A` Adult: 15-124

1184   ICD-10-CM 2023

[1] ☑7ᵗʰ **T85.193** **Other mechanical complication of implanted electronic neurostimulator, generator** `HCC` `ESR`

Other mechanical complication of implanted electronic neurostimulator generator, brain, peripheral, gastric, spinal

Other mechanical complication of implanted electronic sacral neurostimulator, pulse generator or receiver

[1] ☑7ᵗʰ **T85.199** **Other mechanical complication of other implanted electronic stimulator of nervous system** `HCC` `ESR`

☑5ᵗʰ **T85.2** **Mechanical complication of** intraocular lens

☑x7ᵗʰ **T85.21** Breakdown (mechanical) of intraocular lens

☑x7ᵗʰ **T85.22** Displacement of intraocular lens

Malposition of intraocular lens

☑x7ᵗʰ **T85.29** **Other mechanical complication of intraocular lens**

Obstruction (mechanical) of intraocular lens
Perforation of intraocular lens
Protrusion of intraocular lens

☑5ᵗʰ **T85.3** **Mechanical complication of other ocular prosthetic devices, implants and grafts**

`EXCLUDES 2` other complications of corneal graft (T86.84-)

☑6ᵗʰ **T85.31** Breakdown (mechanical) of other ocular prosthetic devices, implants and grafts

☑7ᵗʰ **T85.310** **Breakdown (mechanical) of prosthetic orbit of** right eye

☑7ᵗʰ **T85.311** **Breakdown (mechanical) of prosthetic orbit of** left eye

☑7ᵗʰ **T85.318** **Breakdown (mechanical) of other ocular prosthetic devices, implants and grafts**

☑6ᵗʰ **T85.32** Displacement of other ocular prosthetic devices, implants and grafts

Malposition of other ocular prosthetic devices, implants and grafts

☑7ᵗʰ **T85.320** **Displacement of prosthetic orbit of** right eye

☑7ᵗʰ **T85.321** **Displacement of prosthetic orbit of** left eye

☑7ᵗʰ **T85.328** **Displacement of other ocular prosthetic devices, implants and grafts**

☑6ᵗʰ **T85.39** **Other mechanical complication of other ocular prosthetic devices, implants and grafts**

Obstruction (mechanical) of other ocular prosthetic devices, implants and grafts
Perforation of other ocular prosthetic devices, implants and grafts
Protrusion of other ocular prosthetic devices, implants and grafts

☑7ᵗʰ **T85.390** **Other mechanical complication of prosthetic orbit of** right eye

☑7ᵗʰ **T85.391** **Other mechanical complication of prosthetic orbit of** left eye

☑7ᵗʰ **T85.398** **Other mechanical complication of other ocular prosthetic devices, implants and grafts**

☑5ᵗʰ **T85.4** **Mechanical complication of** breast prosthesis and implant

☑x7ᵗʰ **T85.41** Breakdown (mechanical) of breast prosthesis and implant

☑x7ᵗʰ **T85.42** Displacement of breast prosthesis and implant

Malposition of breast prosthesis and implant

☑x7ᵗʰ **T85.43** Leakage of breast prosthesis and implant

☑x7ᵗʰ **T85.44** Capsular contracture of breast implant

☑x7ᵗʰ **T85.49** **Other mechanical complication of breast prosthesis and implant**

Obstruction (mechanical) of breast prosthesis and implant
Perforation of breast prosthesis and implant
Protrusion of breast prosthesis and implant

☑5ᵗʰ **T85.5** **Mechanical complication of** gastrointestinal prosthetic devices, implants and grafts

☑6ᵗʰ **T85.51** Breakdown (mechanical) of gastrointestinal prosthetic devices, implants and grafts

☑7ᵗʰ **T85.510** **Breakdown (mechanical) of** bile duct prosthesis

☑7ᵗʰ **T85.511** **Breakdown (mechanical) of** esophageal anti-reflux device

☑7ᵗʰ **T85.518** **Breakdown (mechanical) of other gastrointestinal prosthetic devices, implants and grafts**

☑6ᵗʰ **T85.52** Displacement of gastrointestinal prosthetic devices, implants and grafts

Malposition of gastrointestinal prosthetic devices, implants and grafts

☑7ᵗʰ **T85.520** **Displacement of** bile duct **prosthesis**

☑7ᵗʰ **T85.521** **Displacement of** esophageal anti-reflux device

☑7ᵗʰ **T85.528** **Displacement of other gastrointestinal prosthetic devices, implants and grafts**

☑6ᵗʰ **T85.59** **Other mechanical complication of gastrointestinal prosthetic devices, implants and**

Obstruction, mechanical of gastrointestinal prosthetic devices, implants and grafts
Perforation of gastrointestinal prosthetic devices, implants and grafts
Protrusion of gastrointestinal prosthetic devices, implants and grafts

☑7ᵗʰ **T85.590** **Other mechanical complication of** bile duct prosthesis

☑7ᵗʰ **T85.591** **Other mechanical complication of** esophageal anti-reflux **device**

☑7ᵗʰ **T85.598** **Other mechanical complication of other gastrointestinal prosthetic devices, implants and grafts**

[handwritten: insulin pump]

[handwritten: failure]

☑5ᵗʰ **T85.6** **Mechanical complication of other specified internal and external prosthetic devices, implants and grafts**

[handwritten: malfunction (first code)]

☑6ᵗʰ **T85.61** Breakdown (mechanical) of other specified internal prosthetic devices, implants and grafts

☑7ᵗʰ **T85.610** **Breakdown (mechanical) of** cranial or spinal infusion catheter

Breakdown (mechanical) of epidural infusion catheter
Breakdown (mechanical) of intrathecal infusion catheter
Breakdown (mechanical) of subarachnoid infusion catheter
Breakdown (mechanical) of subdural infusion catheter

☑7ᵗʰ **T85.611** **Breakdown (mechanical) of** intraperitoneal dialysis catheter `HCC` `Rx` `ESR`

`EXCLUDES 1` mechanical complication of vascular dialysis catheter (T82.4-)

☑7ᵗʰ **T85.612** **Breakdown (mechanical) of** permanent sutures

`EXCLUDES 1` mechanical complication of permanent (wire) suture used in bone repair (T84.1-T84.2)

☑7ᵗʰ **T85.613** **Breakdown (mechanical) of** artificial skin graft and decellularized allodermis

Failure of artificial skin graft and decellularized allodermis
Non-adherence of artificial skin graft and decellularized allodermis
Poor incorporation of artificial skin graft and decellularized allodermis
Shearing of artificial skin graft and decellularized allodermis

☑7ᵗʰ **T85.614** **Breakdown (mechanical) of** insulin pump

[1] ☑7ᵗʰ **T85.615** **Breakdown (mechanical) of other nervous system device, implant or graft** `HCC` `ESR`

Breakdown (mechanical) of intrathecal infusion pump

☑7ᵗʰ **T85.618** **Breakdown (mechanical) of other specified internal prosthetic devices, implants and grafts**

✓6ᵗʰ T85.62 Displacement of other specified internal prosthetic devices, implants and grafts

Malposition of other specified internal prosthetic devices, implants and grafts

✓7ᵗʰ T85.620 Displacement of cranial or spinal infusion catheter

Displacement of epidural infusion catheter

Displacement of intrathecal infusion catheter

Displacement of subarachnoid infusion catheter

Displacement of subdural infusion catheter

✓7ᵗʰ T85.621 Displacement of intraperitoneal dialysis catheter HCC Rx ESR

EXCLUDES 1   *mechanical complication of vascular dialysis catheter (T82.4-)*

✓7ᵗʰ T85.622 Displacement of permanent sutures

EXCLUDES 1   *mechanical complication of permanent (wire) suture used in bone repair (T84.1-T84.2)*

✓7ᵗʰ T85.623 Displacement of artificial skin graft and decellularized allodermis

Dislodgement of artificial skin graft and decellularized allodermis

✓7ᵗʰ T85.624 Displacement of insulin pump

¹ ✓7ᵗʰ T85.625 Displacement of other nervous system device, implant or graft HCC ESR

Displacement of intrathecal infusion pump

✓7ᵗʰ T85.628 Displacement of other specified internal prosthetic devices, implants and grafts

✓6ᵗʰ T85.63 Leakage of other specified internal prosthetic devices, implants and grafts

✓7ᵗʰ T85.630 Leakage of cranial or spinal infusion catheter

Leakage of epidural infusion catheter

Leakage of intrathecal infusion catheter infusion catheter

Leakage of subdural infusion catheter

Leakage of subarachnoid infusion catheter

✓7ᵗʰ T85.631 Leakage of intraperitoneal dialysis catheter HCC Rx ESR

EXCLUDES 1   *mechanical complication of vascular dialysis catheter (T82.4)*

✓7ᵗʰ T85.633 Leakage of insulin pump

¹ ✓7ᵗʰ T85.635 Leakage of other nervous system device, implant or graft HCC ESR

Leakage of intrathecal infusion pump

✓7ᵗʰ T85.638 Leakage of other specified internal prosthetic devices, implants and grafts

✓6ᵗʰ T85.69 Other mechanical complication of other specified internal prosthetic devices, implants and grafts

Obstruction, mechanical of other specified internal prosthetic devices, implants and grafts

Perforation of other specified internal prosthetic devices, implants and grafts

Protrusion of other specified internal prosthetic devices, implants and grafts

✓7ᵗʰ T85.690 Other mechanical complication of cranial or spinal infusion catheter

Other mechanical complication of epidural infusion catheter

Other mechanical complication of intrathecal infusion catheter

Other mechanical complication of subarachnoid infusion catheter

Other mechanical complication of subdural infusion catheter

✓7ᵗʰ T85.691 Other mechanical complication of intraperitoneal dialysis catheter HCC Rx ESR

EXCLUDES 1   *mechanical complication of vascular dialysis catheter (T82.4)*

✓7ᵗʰ T85.692 Other mechanical complication of permanent sutures

EXCLUDES 1   *mechanical complication of permanent (wire) suture used in bone repair (T84.1-T84.2)*

✓7ᵗʰ T85.693 Other mechanical complication of artificial skin graft and decellularized allodermis

✓7ᵗʰ T85.694 Other mechanical complication of insulin pump

¹ ✓7ᵗʰ T85.695 Other mechanical complication of other nervous system device, implant or graft HCC ESR

Other mechanical complication of intrathecal infusion pump

✓7ᵗʰ T85.698 Other mechanical complication of other specified internal prosthetic devices, implants and grafts

Mechanical complication of nonabsorbable surgical material NOS

✓5ᵗʰ T85.7 Infection and inflammatory reaction due to other internal prosthetic devices, implants and grafts

Use additional code to identify infection

✓x7ᵗʰ T85.71 Infection and inflammatory reaction due to peritoneal dialysis catheter HCC Rx ESR

¹ ✓x7ᵗʰ T85.72 Infection and inflammatory reaction due to insulin pump HCC ESR

✓6ᵗʰ T85.73 Infection and inflammatory reaction due to nervous system devices, implants and graft

¹ ✓7ᵗʰ T85.730 Infection and inflammatory reaction due to ventricular intracranial (communicating) shunt HCC ESR

¹ ✓7ᵗʰ T85.731 Infection and inflammatory reaction due to implanted electronic neurostimulator of brain, electrode (lead) HCC ESR

¹ ✓7ᵗʰ T85.732 Infection and inflammatory reaction due to implanted electronic neurostimulator of peripheral nerve, electrode (lead) HCC ESR

Infection and inflammatory reaction due to electrode (lead) for cranial nerve neurostimulators

Infection and inflammatory reaction due to electrode (lead) for gastric neurostimulator

Infection and inflammatory reaction due to electrode (lead) for sacral nerve neurostimulator

Infection and inflammatory reaction due to electrode (lead) for vagal nerve neurostimulators

¹ ✓7ᵗʰ T85.733 Infection and inflammatory reaction due to implanted electronic neurostimulator of spinal cord, electrode (lead) HCC ESR

¹ ✓7ᵗʰ T85.734 Infection and inflammatory reaction due to implanted electronic neurostimulator, generator HCC ESR

Generator pocket infection

¹ ✓7ᵗʰ T85.735 Infection and inflammatory reaction due to cranial or spinal infusion catheter HCC ESR

Infection and inflammatory reaction due to epidural catheter

Infection and inflammatory reaction due to intrathecal infusion catheter

Infection and inflammatory reaction due to subarachnoid catheter

Infection and inflammatory reaction due to subdural catheter

¹ ✓7ᵗʰ T85.738 Infection and inflammatory reaction due to other nervous system device, implant or graft HCC ESR

Infection and inflammatory reaction due to intrathecal infusion pump

¹ ✓x7ᵗʰ T85.79 Infection and inflammatory reaction due to other internal prosthetic devices, implants and grafts HCC ESR

AHA: 2022,2Q,7

Chapter 19. Injury, Poisoning and Certain Other Consequences of External Causes

✓5ᵗʰ T85.8 Other specified complications of internal prosthetic devices, implants and grafts, not elsewhere classified

    ✓6ᵗʰ T85.81 Embolism due to internal prosthetic devices, implants and grafts, not elsewhere classified

        ¹ **✓7ᵗʰ T85.810 Embolism due to nervous system prosthetic devices, implants and grafts** `HCC` `ESR`

        ✓7ᵗʰ T85.818 Embolism due to other internal prosthetic devices, implants and grafts

    ✓6ᵗʰ T85.82 Fibrosis due to internal prosthetic devices, implants and grafts, not elsewhere classified

        ¹ **✓7ᵗʰ T85.820 Fibrosis due to nervous system prosthetic devices, implants and grafts** `HCC` `ESR`

        ✓7ᵗʰ T85.828 Fibrosis due to other internal prosthetic devices, implants and grafts

    ✓6ᵗʰ T85.83 Hemorrhage due to internal prosthetic devices, implants and grafts, not elsewhere classified

        ¹ **✓7ᵗʰ T85.830 Hemorrhage due to nervous system prosthetic devices, implants and grafts** `HCC` `ESR`

        ✓7ᵗʰ T85.838 Hemorrhage due to other internal prosthetic devices, implants and grafts

    ✓6ᵗʰ T85.84 Pain due to internal prosthetic devices, implants and grafts, not elsewhere classified

        ¹ **✓7ᵗʰ T85.840 Pain due to nervous system prosthetic devices, implants and grafts** `HCC` `ESR`

        ✓7ᵗʰ T85.848 Pain due to other internal prosthetic devices, implants and grafts

    ✓6ᵗʰ T85.85 Stenosis due to internal prosthetic devices, implants and grafts, not elsewhere classified

        ¹ **✓7ᵗʰ T85.850 Stenosis due to nervous system prosthetic devices, implants and grafts** `HCC` `ESR`

        ✓7ᵗʰ T85.858 Stenosis due to other internal prosthetic devices, implants and grafts

    ✓6ᵗʰ T85.86 Thrombosis due to internal prosthetic devices, implants and grafts, not elsewhere classified

        ¹ **✓7ᵗʰ T85.860 Thrombosis due to nervous system prosthetic devices, implants and grafts** `HCC` `ESR`

        ✓7ᵗʰ T85.868 Thrombosis due to other internal prosthetic devices, implants and grafts

    ✓6ᵗʰ T85.89 Other specified complication of internal prosthetic devices, implants and grafts, not elsewhere classified
        Erosion or breakdown of subcutaneous device pocket

        ¹ **✓7ᵗʰ T85.890 Other specified complication of nervous system prosthetic devices, implants and grafts** `HCC` `ESR`

        ✓7ᵗʰ T85.898 Other specified complication of other internal prosthetic devices, implants and grafts

✓x7ᵗʰ T85.9 Unspecified complication of internal prosthetic device, implant and graft
    Complication of internal prosthetic device, implant and graft NOS

✓4ᵗʰ T86 Complications of transplanted organs and tissue
    Use additional code to identify other transplant complications, such as:
        graft-versus-host disease (D89.81-)
        malignancy associated with organ transplant (C80.2)
        post-transplant lymphoproliferative disorders (PTLD) (D47.Z1)
    AHA: 2020,1Q,18

    ✓5ᵗʰ T86.0 Complications of bone marrow transplant

        T86.00 Unspecified complication of bone marrow transplant `HCC` `Rx` `ESR` `COM`

        T86.01 Bone marrow transplant rejection `HCC` `Rx` `ESR` `COM`

        T86.02 Bone marrow transplant failure `HCC` `Rx` `ESR` `COM`

        T86.03 Bone marrow transplant infection `HCC` `Rx` `ESR` `COM`

        T86.09 Other complications of bone marrow transplant `HCC` `Rx` `ESR` `COM`

    ✓5ᵗʰ T86.1 Complications of kidney transplant

        T86.10 Unspecified complication of kidney transplant `Rx` `COM`

        T86.11 Kidney transplant rejection `Rx` `COM`

        T86.12 Kidney transplant failure `Rx` `COM`
        AHA: 2013,1Q,24

        T86.13 Kidney transplant infection `Rx` `COM`
        Use additional code to specify infection

        T86.19 Other complication of kidney transplant `Rx` `COM`
        AHA: 2019,2Q,7

    ✓5ᵗʰ T86.2 Complications of heart transplant

        EXCLUDES 1   complication of:
            artificial heart device (T82.5-)
            heart-lung transplant (T86.3-)

        T86.20 Unspecified complication of heart transplant `HCC` `Rx` `ESR` `COM`

        T86.21 Heart transplant rejection `HCC` `Rx` `ESR` `COM`

        T86.22 Heart transplant failure `HCC` `Rx` `ESR` `COM`

        T86.23 Heart transplant infection `HCC` `Rx` `ESR` `COM`
        Use additional code to specify infection

        ✓6ᵗʰ T86.29 Other complications of heart transplant

            T86.290 Cardiac allograft vasculopathy `HCC` `Rx` `ESR` `COM`
                EXCLUDES 1   atherosclerosis of coronary arteries (I25.75-, I25.76-, I25.81-)

            T86.298 Other complications of heart transplant `HCC` `Rx` `ESR` `COM`

    ✓5ᵗʰ T86.3 Complications of heart-lung transplant

        T86.30 Unspecified complication of heart-lung transplant `HCC` `Rx` `ESR` `COM`

        T86.31 Heart-lung transplant rejection `HCC` `Rx` `ESR` `COM`

        T86.32 Heart-lung transplant failure `HCC` `Rx` `ESR` `COM`

        T86.33 Heart-lung transplant infection `HCC` `Rx` `ESR` `COM`
        Use additional code to specify infection

        T86.39 Other complications of heart-lung transplant `HCC` `Rx` `ESR` `COM`

    ✓5ᵗʰ T86.4 Complications of liver transplant

        T86.40 Unspecified complication of liver transplant `HCC` `Rx` `ESR` `COM`

        T86.41 Liver transplant rejection `HCC` `Rx` `ESR` `COM`

        T86.42 Liver transplant failure `HCC` `Rx` `ESR` `COM`

        T86.43 Liver transplant infection `HCC` `Rx` `ESR` `COM`
        Use additional code to identify infection, such as: cytomegalovirus (CMV) infection (B25.-)

        T86.49 Other complications of liver transplant `HCC` `Rx` `ESR` `COM`

    T86.5 Complications of stem cell transplant `HCC` `Rx` `ESR` `COM`
        Complications from stem cells from peripheral blood
        Complications from stem cells from umbilical cord
        AHA: 2020,4Q,14

    ✓5ᵗʰ T86.8 Complications of other transplanted organs and tissues

        ✓6ᵗʰ T86.81 Complications of lung transplant

            EXCLUDES 1   complication of heart-lung transplant (T86.3-)

            T86.810 Lung transplant rejection `HCC` `Rx` `ESR` `COM`

            T86.811 Lung transplant failure `HCC` `Rx` `ESR` `COM`

            T86.812 Lung transplant infection `HCC` `Rx` `ESR` `COM`
            Use additional code to specify infection

            T86.818 Other complications of lung transplant `HCC` `Rx` `ESR` `COM`
            AHA: 2019,2Q,6

            T86.819 Unspecified complication of lung transplant `HCC` `Rx` `ESR` `COM`

        ✓6ᵗʰ T86.82 Complications of skin graft (allograft) (autograft)

            EXCLUDES 2   complication of artificial skin graft (T85.693)

            T86.820 Skin graft (allograft) rejection

            T86.821 Skin graft (allograft) (autograft) failure

            T86.822 Skin graft (allograft) (autograft) infection
            Use additional code to specify infection

            T86.828 Other complications of skin graft (allograft) (autograft)

            T86.829 Unspecified complication of skin graft (allograft) (autograft)

        ✓6ᵗʰ T86.83 Complications of bone graft

            EXCLUDES 2   mechanical complications of bone graft (T84.3-)

            T86.830 Bone graft rejection

            T86.831 Bone graft failure

Chapter 19. Injury, Poisoning and Certain Other Consequences of External Causes

T86.832   **Bone graft** infection
> Use additional code to specify infection

T86.838   **Other complications of bone graft**

T86.839   **Unspecified complication of bone graft**

✓6ᵗʰ **T86.84**   **Complications of** corneal **transplant**
> EXCLUDES 2   *mechanical complications of corneal graft (T85.3-)*
>
> AHA: 2020,4Q,40

✓7ᵗʰ **T86.840**   **Corneal transplant** rejection

    T86.8401   **Corneal transplant rejection, right** eye

    T86.8402   **Corneal transplant rejection, left** eye

    T86.8403   **Corneal transplant rejection, bilateral**

    T86.8409   **Corneal transplant rejection, unspecified eye**

✓7ᵗʰ **T86.841**   **Corneal transplant** failure

    T86.8411   **Corneal transplant failure, right** eye

    T86.8412   **Corneal transplant failure, left** eye

    T86.8413   **Corneal transplant failure, bilateral**

    T86.8419   **Corneal transplant failure, unspecified eye**

✓7ᵗʰ **T86.842**   **Corneal transplant** infection
> Use additional code to specify infection

    T86.8421   **Corneal transplant infection, right** eye   `HCC` `ESR`

    T86.8422   **Corneal transplant infection, left** eye   `HCC` `ESR`

    T86.8423   **Corneal transplant infection, bilateral**   `HCC` `ESR`

    T86.8429   **Corneal transplant infection, unspecified eye**   `HCC` `ESR`

✓7ᵗʰ **T86.848**   **Other complications of corneal transplant**

    T86.8481   **Other complications of corneal transplant, right** eye

    T86.8482   **Other complications of corneal transplant, left** eye

    T86.8483   **Other complications of corneal transplant, bilateral**

    T86.8489   **Other complications of corneal transplant, unspecified eye**

✓7ᵗʰ **T86.849**   **Unspecified complication of corneal transplant**

    T86.8491   **Unspecified complication of corneal transplant, right** eye

    T86.8492   **Unspecified complication of corneal transplant, left** eye

    T86.8493   **Unspecified complication of corneal transplant, bilateral**

    T86.8499   **Unspecified complication of corneal transplant, unspecified eye**

✓6ᵗʰ **T86.85**   **Complication of** intestine **transplant**

T86.850   **Intestine transplant rejection**   `HCC` `Rx` `ESR` `COM`

T86.851   **Intestine transplant failure**   `HCC` `Rx` `ESR` `COM`

T86.852   **Intestine transplant infection**   `HCC` `Rx` `ESR` `COM`
> Use additional code to specify infection

T86.858   **Other complications of intestine transplant**   `HCC` `Rx` `ESR` `COM`

T86.859   **Unspecified complication of intestine transplant**   `HCC` `Rx` `ESR` `COM`

✓6ᵗʰ **T86.89**   **Complications of other transplanted tissue**
> Transplant failure or rejection of pancreas
>
> AHA: 2020,1Q,18

T86.890   **Other transplanted tissue** rejection

T86.891   **Other transplanted tissue** failure

T86.892   **Other transplanted tissue** infection
> Use additional code to specify infection

T86.898   **Other complications of other transplanted tissue**

T86.899   **Unspecified complication of other transplanted tissue**

✓6ᵗʰ **T86.9**   **Complication of unspecified transplanted organ and tissue**

T86.90   **Unspecified complication of unspecified transplanted organ and tissue**

T86.91   **Unspecified transplanted organ and tissue** rejection

T86.92   **Unspecified transplanted organ and tissue** failure

T86.93   **Unspecified transplanted organ and tissue** infection
> Use additional code to specify infection

T86.99   **Other complications of unspecified transplanted organ and tissue**

✓4ᵗʰ **T87**   **Complications peculiar to reattachment and amputation**

✓5ᵗʰ **T87.0**   **Complications of reattached (part of)** upper extremity

✓6ᵗʰ **T87.0X**   **Complications of reattached (part of) upper extremity**

    T87.0X1   **Complications of reattached (part of) right upper extremity**   `HCC` `ESR` `COM`

    T87.0X2   **Complications of reattached (part of)** left **upper extremity**   `HCC` `ESR` `COM`

    T87.0X9   **Complications of reattached (part of) unspecified upper extremity**   `HCC` `ESR` `COM`

✓5ᵗʰ **T87.1**   **Complications of reattached (part of)** lower extremity

✓6ᵗʰ **T87.1X**   **Complications of reattached (part of) lower extremity**

    T87.1X1   **Complications of reattached (part of) right lower extremity**   `HCC` `ESR` `COM`

    T87.1X2   **Complications of reattached (part of)** left **lower extremity**   `HCC` `ESR` `COM`

    T87.1X9   **Complications of reattached (part of) unspecified lower extremity**   `HCC` `ESR` `COM`

T87.2   **Complications of other reattached body part**   `HCC` `ESR`

✓5ᵗʰ **T87.3**   Neuroma **of amputation stump**
> DEF: Non-neoplastic tumor generated at the proximal end of severed, partially transected, or injured nerve following amputation.

T87.30   **Neuroma of amputation stump, unspecified extremity**   `HCC` `ESR` `COM`

T87.31   **Neuroma of amputation stump, right upper extremity**   `HCC` `ESR` `COM`

T87.32   **Neuroma of amputation stump,** left upper **extremity**   `HCC` `ESR` `COM`

T87.33   **Neuroma of amputation stump, right lower extremity**   `HCC` `ESR` `COM`

T87.34   **Neuroma of amputation stump,** left lower **extremity**   `HCC` `ESR` `COM`

✓5ᵗʰ **T87.4**   Infection **of amputation stump**

T87.40   **Infection of amputation stump, unspecified extremity**   `HCC` `ESR` `COM`

T87.41   **Infection of amputation stump, right upper extremity**   `HCC` `ESR` `COM`

T87.42   **Infection of amputation stump,** left upper **extremity**   `HCC` `ESR` `COM`

T87.43   **Infection of amputation stump, right lower extremity**   `HCC` `ESR` `COM`

T87.44   **Infection of amputation stump,** left lower **extremity**   `HCC` `ESR` `COM`

✓5ᵗʰ **T87.5**   Necrosis **of amputation stump**

T87.50   **Necrosis of amputation stump, unspecified extremity**   `HCC` `ESR` `COM`

T87.51   **Necrosis of amputation stump, right upper extremity**   `HCC` `ESR` `COM`

T87.52   **Necrosis of amputation stump,** left upper **extremity**   `HCC` `ESR` `COM`

T87.53   **Necrosis of amputation stump, right lower extremity**   `HCC` `ESR` `COM`

T87.54   **Necrosis of amputation stump,** left lower **extremity**   `HCC` `ESR` `COM`

✓5ᵗʰ **T87.8**   **Other complications of amputation stump**

T87.81   Dehiscence **of amputation stump**   `HCC` `ESR` `COM`

`HCC` CMS-HCC   `Rx` Rx HCC   `ESR` ESRD HCC   `COM` Commercial HCC   N Newborn: 0   P Pediatric: 0-17   M Maternity: 9-64   A Adult: 15-124

1188   ICD-10-CM 2023

T87.89 Other complications of amputation stump `HCC` `ESR` `COM`

Amputation stump contracture
Amputation stump contracture of next proximal joint
Amputation stump flexion
Amputation stump edema
Amputation stump hematoma
EXCLUDES 2   *phantom limb syndrome (G54.6-G54.7)*

T87.9 Unspecified complications of amputation stump `HCC` `ESR` `COM`

☑4ᵗʰ T88 Other complications of surgical and medical care, not elsewhere classified

EXCLUDES 2   *complication following infusion, transfusion and therapeutic injection (T80.-)*
complication following procedure NEC (T81.-)
complications of anesthesia in labor and delivery (O74.-)
complications of anesthesia in pregnancy (O29.-)
complications of anesthesia in puerperium (O89.-)
complications of devices, implants and grafts (T82-T85)
complications of obstetric surgery and procedure (O75.4)
dermatitis due to drugs and medicaments (L23.3, L24.4, L25.1, L27.0-L27.1)
poisoning and toxic effects of drugs and chemicals (T36-T65 with fifth or sixth character 1-4 or 6)
specified complications classified elsewhere

The appropriate 7th character is to be added to each code from category T88.
A   initial encounter
D   subsequent encounter
S   sequela

✓x7ᵗʰ T88.0 Infection following immunization
Sepsis following immunization
AHA: 2018,4Q,62-63

✓x7ᵗʰ T88.1 Other complications following immunization, not elsewhere classified
Generalized vaccinia
Rash following immunization
EXCLUDES 1   *vaccinia not from vaccine (B08.011)*
EXCLUDES 2   *anaphylactic shock due to serum (T80.5-)*
other serum reactions (T80.6-)
postimmunization arthropathy (M02.2)
postimmunization encephalitis (G04.02)
postimmunization fever (R50.83)

✓x7ᵗʰ T88.2 Shock due to anesthesia
Use additional code for adverse effect, if applicable, to identify drug (T41.- with fifth or sixth character 5)
EXCLUDES 1   *complications of anesthesia (in):*
labor and delivery (O74.-)
postprocedural shock NOS (T81.1-)
pregnancy (O29.-)
puerperium (O89.-)

✓x7ᵗʰ T88.3 Malignant hyperthermia due to anesthesia
Use additional code for adverse effect, if applicable, to identify drug (T41.- with fifth or sixth character 5)

✓x7ᵗʰ T88.4 Failed or difficult intubation

☑5ᵗʰ T88.5 Other complications of anesthesia
Use additional code for adverse effect, if applicable, to identify drug (T41.- with fifth or sixth character 5)

✓x7ᵗʰ T88.51 Hypothermia following anesthesia

✓x7ᵗʰ T88.52 Failed moderate sedation during procedure
Failed conscious sedation during procedure
EXCLUDES 2   *personal history of failed moderate sedation (Z92.83)*

✓x7ᵗʰ T88.53 Unintended awareness under general anesthesia during procedure
EXCLUDES 2   *personal history of unintended awareness under general anesthesia (Z92.84)*
AHA: 2016,4Q,72-73

✓x7ᵗʰ T88.59 Other complications of anesthesia

✓x7ᵗʰ T88.6 Anaphylactic reaction due to adverse effect of correct drug or medicament properly administered
Anaphylactic shock due to adverse effect of correct drug or medicament properly administered
Anaphylactoid reaction NOS
Use additional code for adverse effect, if applicable, to identify drug (T36-T50 with fifth or sixth character 5)
EXCLUDES 1   *anaphylactic reaction due to serum (T80.5-)*
anaphylactic shock or reaction due to adverse food reaction (T78.0-)
AHA: 2020,1Q,18

✓x7ᵗʰ T88.7 Unspecified adverse effect of drug or medicament
Drug hypersensitivity NOS
Drug reaction NOS
Use additional code for adverse effect, if applicable, to identify drug (T36-T50 with fifth or sixth character 5)
EXCLUDES 1   *specified adverse effects of drugs and medicaments (A00-R94 and T80-T88.6, T88.8)*

✓x7ᵗʰ T88.8 Other specified complications of surgical and medical care, not elsewhere classified
Use additional code to identify the complication
AHA: 2022,2Q,7

✓x7ᵗʰ T88.9 Complication of surgical and medical care, unspecified

Chapter 20. External Causes of Morbidity (V00–Y99)

Chapter-specific Guidelines with Coding Examples

The chapter-specific guidelines from the ICD-10-CM Official Guidelines for Coding and Reporting have been provided below. Along with these guidelines are coding examples, contained in the shaded boxes, that have been developed to help illustrate the coding and/or sequencing guidance found in these guidelines.

The external causes of morbidity codes should never be sequenced as the first-listed or principal diagnosis.

External cause codes are intended to provide data for injury research and evaluation of injury prevention strategies. These codes capture how the injury or health condition happened (cause), the intent (unintentional or accidental; or intentional, such as suicide or assault), the place where the event occurred the activity of the patient at the time of the event, and the person's status (e.g., civilian, military).

There is no national requirement for mandatory ICD-10-CM external cause code reporting. Unless a provider is subject to a state-based external cause code reporting mandate or these codes are required by a particular payer, reporting of ICD-10-CM codes in Chapter 20, External Causes of Morbidity, is not required. In the absence of a mandatory reporting requirement, providers are encouraged to voluntarily report external cause codes, as they provide valuable data for injury research and evaluation of injury prevention strategies.

a. General external cause coding guidelines

1) Used with any code in the range of A00.0–T88.9, Z00–Z99

An external cause code may be used with any code in the range of A00.0–T88.9, Z00-Z99, classification that represents a health condition due to an external cause. Though they are most applicable to injuries, they are also valid for use with such things as infections or diseases due to an external source, and other health conditions, such as a heart attack that occurs during strenuous physical activity.

Actinic reticuloid due to tanning bed use	
L57.1	**Actinic reticuloid**
W89.1XXA	**Exposure to tanning bed, initial encounter**

Explanation: An external cause code may be used with any code in the range of A00.0–T88.9, Z00–Z99, classifications that describe health conditions due to an external cause. Code W89.1 Exposure to tanning bed requires a seventh character of A to report this initial encounter, with a placeholder X for the fifth and sixth characters.

2) External cause code used for length of treatment

Assign the external cause code, with the appropriate 7th character (initial encounter, subsequent encounter or sequela) for each encounter for which the injury or condition is being treated.

Most categories in chapter 20 have a 7th character requirement for each applicable code. Most categories in this chapter have three 7th character values: A, initial encounter, D, subsequent encounter and S, sequela. While the patient may be seen by a new or different provider over the course of treatment for an injury or condition, assignment of the 7th character for external cause should match the 7th character of the code assigned for the associated injury or condition for the encounter.

3) Use the full range of external cause codes

Use the full range of external cause codes to completely describe the cause, the intent, the place of occurrence, and if applicable, the activity of the patient at the time of the event, and the patient's status, for all injuries, and other health conditions due to an external cause.

4) Assign as many external cause codes as necessary

Assign as many external cause codes as necessary to fully explain each cause. If only one external code can be recorded, assign the code most related to the principal diagnosis.

5) The selection of the appropriate external cause code

The selection of the appropriate external cause code is guided by the Alphabetic Index of External Causes and by Inclusion and Exclusion notes in the Tabular List.

6) External cause code can never be a principal diagnosis

An external cause code can never be a principal (first-listed) diagnosis.

7) Combination external cause codes

Certain of the external cause codes are combination codes that identify sequential events that result in an injury, such as a fall which results in striking against an object. The injury may be due to either event or both.

The combination external cause code used should correspond to the sequence of events regardless of which caused the most serious injury.

Toddler tripped and fell while walking and struck his head on an end table, sustaining a scalp contusion	
S00.03XA	**Contusion of scalp, initial encounter**
W01.190A	**Fall on same level from slipping, tripping and stumbling with subsequent striking against furniture, initial encounter**

Explanation: Combination external cause codes identify sequential events that result in an injury, such as a fall resulting in striking against an object. The injury may be due to either or both events.

8) No external cause code needed in certain circumstances

No external cause code from Chapter 20 is needed if the external cause and intent are included in a code from another chapter (e.g., T36.0X1-, Poisoning by penicillins, accidental (unintentional)).

b. Place of occurrence guideline

Codes from category Y92, Place of occurrence of the external cause, are secondary codes for use after other external cause codes to identify the location of the patient at the time of injury or other condition.

Generally, a place of occurrence code is assigned only once, at the initial encounter for treatment. However, in the rare instance that a new injury occurs during hospitalization, an additional place of occurrence code may be assigned. No 7th characters are used for Y92.

Do not use place of occurrence code Y92.9 if the place is not stated or is not applicable.

A farmer was working in his barn and sustained a foot contusion when the horse stepped on his left foot	
S90.32XA	**Contusion of left foot, initial encounter**
W55.19XA	**Other contact with horse, initial encounter**
Y92.71	**Barn as the place of occurrence of the external cause**

Explanation: A place-of-occurrence code from category Y92 is assigned at the initial encounter to identify the location of the patient at the time the injury occurred.

c. Activity code

Assign a code from category Y93, Activity code, to describe the activity of the patient at the time the injury or other health condition occurred.

An activity code is used only once, at the initial encounter for treatment. Only one code from Y93 should be recorded on a medical record.

The activity codes are not applicable to poisonings, adverse effects, misadventures or sequela.

Do not assign Y93.9, Unspecified activity, if the activity is not stated.

A code from category Y93 is appropriate for use with external cause and intent codes if identifying the activity provides additional information about the event.

Ranch hand who was grooming a horse sustained a foot contusion when the horse stepped on his left foot	
S90.32XA	**Contusion of left foot, initial encounter**
W55.19XA	**Other contact with horse, initial encounter**
Y93.K3	**Activity, grooming and shearing an animal**

Explanation: One activity code from category Y93 is assigned at the initial encounter only to describe the activity of the patient at the time the injury occurred.

d. Place of occurrence, activity, and status codes used with other external cause code

When applicable, place of occurrence, activity, and external cause status codes are sequenced after the main external cause code(s). Regardless of the number of external cause codes assigned, generally there should be only one place of occurrence code, one activity code, and one external cause status code assigned to an encounter. However, in the rare instance that a new injury occurs during hospitalization, an additional place of occurrence code may be assigned.

e. If the reporting format limits the number of external cause codes

If the reporting format limits the number of external cause codes that can be used in reporting clinical data, report the code for the cause/intent most related to the principal diagnosis. If the format permits capture of additional external cause codes, the cause/intent, including medical misadventures, of the additional events should be reported rather than the codes for place, activity, or external status.

f. Multiple external cause coding guidelines

More than one external cause code is required to fully describe the external cause of an illness or injury. The assignment of external cause codes should be sequenced in the following priority:

If two or more events cause separate injuries, an external cause code should be assigned for each cause. The first-listed external cause code will be selected in the following order:

External codes for child and adult abuse take priority over all other external cause codes.

See Section I.C.19., Child and Adult abuse guidelines.

External cause codes for terrorism events take priority over all other external cause codes except child and adult abuse.

External cause codes for cataclysmic events take priority over all other external cause codes except child and adult abuse and terrorism.

External cause codes for transport accidents take priority over all other external cause codes except cataclysmic events, child and adult abuse and terrorism.

Activity and external cause status codes are assigned following all causal (intent) external cause codes.

The first-listed external cause code should correspond to the cause of the most serious diagnosis due to an assault, accident, or self-harm, following the order of hierarchy listed above..

30-year-old man accidentally discharged his hunting rifle, sustaining an open gunshot wound, with no retained bullet fragments, to the right thigh, which caused him to fall down the stairs, resulting in closed displaced comminuted fracture of his left radial shaft	
S71.131A	**Puncture wound without foreign body, right thigh, initial encounter**
W33.02XA	**Accidental discharge of hunting rifle, initial encounter**
S52.352A	**Displaced comminuted fracture of shaft of radius, left arm, initial encounter for closed fracture**
W10.9XXA	**Fall (on) (from) unspecified stairs and steps, initial encounter**

Explanation: If two or more events cause separate injuries, an external cause code should be assigned for each cause.

g. Child and adult abuse guideline

Adult and child abuse, neglect and maltreatment are classified as assault. Any of the assault codes may be used to indicate the external cause of any injury resulting from the confirmed abuse.

For confirmed cases of abuse, neglect and maltreatment, when the perpetrator is known, a code from Y07, Perpetrator of maltreatment and neglect, should accompany any other assault codes.

See Section I.C.19. Adult and child abuse, neglect and other maltreatment

h. Unknown or undetermined intent guideline

If the intent (accident, self-harm, assault) of the cause of an injury or other condition is unknown or unspecified, code the intent as accidental intent. All transport accident categories assume accidental intent.

1) Use of undetermined intent

External cause codes for events of undetermined intent are only for use if the documentation in the record specifies that the intent cannot be determined.

i. Sequelae (late effects) of external cause guidelines

1) Sequelae external cause codes

Sequela are reported using the external cause code with the 7th character "S" for sequela. These codes should be used with any report of a late effect or sequela resulting from a previous injury.

See Section I.B.10. Sequela (Late Effects)

2) Sequela external cause code with a related current injury

A sequela external cause code should never be used with a related current nature of injury code.

3) Use of sequela external cause codes for subsequent visits

Use a late effect external cause code for subsequent visits when a late effect of the initial injury is being treated. Do not use a late effect external cause code for subsequent visits for follow-up care (e.g., to assess healing, to receive rehabilitative therapy) of the injury when no late effect of the injury has been documented.

j. Terrorism guidelines

1) Cause of injury identified by the Federal Government (FBI) as terrorism

When the cause of an injury is identified by the Federal Government (FBI) as terrorism, the first-listed external cause code should be a code from category Y38, Terrorism. The definition of terrorism employed by the FBI is found at the inclusion note at the beginning of category Y38. Use additional code for place of occurrence (Y92.-). More than one Y38 code may be assigned if the injury is the result of more than one mechanism of terrorism.

2) Cause of an injury is suspected to be the result of terrorism

When the cause of an injury is suspected to be the result of terrorism a code from category Y38 should not be assigned. Suspected cases should be classified as assault.

3) Code Y38.9, Terrorism, secondary effects

Assign code Y38.9, Terrorism, secondary effects, for conditions occurring subsequent to the terrorist event. This code should not be assigned for conditions that are due to the initial terrorist act.

It is acceptable to assign code Y38.9 with another code from Y38 if there is an injury due to the initial terrorist event and an injury that is a subsequent result of the terrorist event.

k. External cause status

A code from category Y99, External cause status, should be assigned whenever any other external cause code is assigned for an encounter, including an Activity code, except for the events noted below. Assign a code from category Y99, External cause status, to indicate the work status of the person at the time the event occurred. The status code indicates whether the event occurred during military activity, whether a non-military person was at work, whether an individual including a student or volunteer was involved in a non-work activity at the time of the causal event.

A code from Y99, External cause status, should be assigned, when applicable, with other external cause codes, such as transport accidents and falls. The external cause status codes are not applicable to poisonings, adverse effects, misadventures or late effects.

Do not assign a code from category Y99 if no other external cause codes (cause, activity) are applicable for the encounter.

An external cause status code is used only once, at the initial encounter for treatment. Only one code from Y99 should be recorded on a medical record.

Do not assign code Y99.9, Unspecified external cause status, if the status is not stated.

Chapter 20. External Causes of Morbidity (V00-Y99)

NOTE   This chapter permits the classification of environmental events and circumstances as the cause of injury, and other adverse effects. Where a code from this section is applicable, it is intended that it shall be used secondary to a code from another chapter of the Classification indicating the nature of the condition. Most often, the condition will be classifiable to Chapter 19, Injury, poisoning and certain other consequences of external causes (S00-T88). Other conditions that may be stated to be due to external causes are classified in Chapters I to XVIII. For these conditions, codes from Chapter 20 should be used to provide additional information as to the cause of the condition.

AHA: 2018,4Q,58-60

This chapter contains the following blocks:

V00-X58	Accidents
V00-V99	Transport accidents
V00-V09	Pedestrian injured in transport accident
V10-V19	Pedal cycle rider injured in transport accident
V20-V29	Motorcycle rider injured in transport accident
V30-V39	Occupant of three-wheeled motor vehicle injured in transport accident
V40-V49	Car occupant injured in transport accident
V50-V59	Occupant of pick-up truck or van injured in transport accident
V60-V69	Occupant of heavy transport vehicle injured in transport accident
V70-V79	Bus occupant injured in transport accident
V80-V89	Other land transport accidents
V90-V94	Water transport accidents
V95-V97	Air and space transport accidents
V98-V99	Other and unspecified transport accidents
W00-X58	Other external causes of accidental injury
W00-W19	Slipping, tripping, stumbling and falls
W20-W49	Exposure to inanimate mechanical forces
W50-W64	Exposure to animate mechanical forces
W65-W74	Accidental non-transport drowning and submersion
W85-W99	Exposure to electric current, radiation and extreme ambient air temperature and pressure
X00-X08	Exposure to smoke, fire and flames
X10-X19	Contact with heat and hot substances
X30-X39	Exposure to forces of nature
X50	Overexertion and strenuous or repetitive movements
X52-X58	Accidental exposure to other specified factors
X71-X83	Intentional self-harm
X92-Y09	Assault
Y21-Y33	Event of undetermined intent
Y35-Y38	Legal intervention, operations of war, military operations, and terrorism
Y62-Y84	Complications of medical and surgical care
Y62-Y69	Misadventures to patients during surgical and medical care
Y70-Y82	Medical devices associated with adverse incidents in diagnostic and therapeutic use
Y83-Y84	Surgical and other medical procedures as the cause of abnormal reaction of the patient, or of later complication, without mention of misadventure at the time of the procedure
Y90-Y99	Supplementary factors related to causes of morbidity classified elsewhere

ACCIDENTS (V00-X58)

AHA: 2018,2Q,7-8

Transport accidents (V00-V99)

NOTE   This section is structured in 12 groups. Those relating to land transport accidents (V00-V89) reflect the victim's mode of transport and are subdivided to identify the victim's 'counterpart' or the type of event. The vehicle of which the injured person is an occupant is identified in the first two characters since it is seen as the most important factor to identify for prevention purposes. A transport accident is one in which the vehicle involved must be moving or running or in use for transport purposes at the time of the accident.

Use additional code to identify:
airbag injury (W22.1)
type of street or road (Y92.4-)
use of cellular telephone and other electronic equipment at the time of the transport accident (Y93.C-)

EXCLUDES 1   *agricultural vehicles in stationary use or maintenance (W31.-)*
assault by crashing of motor vehicle (Y03.-)
automobile or motor cycle in stationary use or maintenance - code to type of accident
crashing of motor vehicle, undetermined intent (Y32)
intentional self-harm by crashing of motor vehicle (X82)

EXCLUDES 2   *transport accidents due to cataclysm (X34-X38)*

NOTE   Definitions related to transport accidents:

(a)   A transport accident (V00-V99) is any accident involving a device designed primarily for, or used at the time primarily for, conveying persons or good from one place to another.

(b)   A public highway [trafficway] or street is the entire width between property lines (or other boundary lines) of land open to the public as a matter of right or custom for purposes of moving persons or property from one place to another. A roadway is that part of the public highway designed, improved and customarily used for vehicular traffic.

(c)   A traffic accident is any vehicle accident occurring on the public highway [i.e. originating on, terminating on, or involving a vehicle partially on the highway]. A vehicle accident is assumed to have occurred on the public highway unless another place is specified, except in the case of accidents involving only off-road motor vehicles, which are classified as nontraffic accidents unless the contrary is stated.

(d)   A nontraffic accident is any vehicle accident that occurs entirely in any place other than a public highway.

(e)   A pedestrian is any person involved in an accident who was not at the time of the accident riding in or on a motor vehicle, railway train, streetcar or animal-drawn or other vehicle, or on a pedal cycle or animal. This includes, a person changing a tire, working on a parked car, or a person on foot. It also includes the user of a pedestrian conveyance such as a baby stroller, ice-skates, skis, sled, roller skates, a skateboard, nonmotorized or motorized wheelchair, motorized mobility scooter, or nonmotorized scooter.

(f)   A driver is an occupant of a transport vehicle who is operating or intending to operate it.

(g)   A passenger is any occupant of a transport vehicle other than the driver, except a person traveling on the outside of the vehicle.

(h)   A person on the outside of a vehicle is any person being transported by a vehicle but not occupying the space normally reserved for the driver or passengers, or the space intended for the transport of property. This includes a person travelling on the bodywork, bumper, fender, roof, running board or step of a vehicle, as well as, hanging on the outside of the vehicle.

(i)   A pedal cycle is any land transport vehicle operated solely by nonmotorized pedals including a bicycle or tricycle.

(j)   A pedal cyclist is any person riding a pedal cycle or in a sidecar or trailer attached to a pedal cycle.

(k)   A motorcycle is a two-wheeled motor vehicle with one or two riding saddles and sometimes with a third wheel for the support of a sidecar. The sidecar is considered part of the motorcycle. This includes a moped, motor scooter, or motorized bicycle.

(l)   A motorcycle rider is any person riding a motorcycle or in a sidecar or trailer attached to the motorcycle.

(m)   A three-wheeled motor vehicle is a motorized tricycle designed primarily for on-road use. This includes a motor-driven tricycle, a motorized rickshaw, or a three-wheeled motor car.

(n)   A car [automobile] is a four-wheeled motor vehicle designed primarily for carrying up to 7 persons. A trailer being towed by the car is considered part of the car. It does not include a van or minivan — see definition (o).

(o)   A pick-up truck or van is a four or six-wheeled motor vehicle designed for carrying passengers as well as property or cargo weighing less than the local limit for classification as a heavy goods vehicle, and not requiring a special driver's license. This includes a minivan and a sport-utility vehicle (SUV).

(p)   A heavy transport vehicle is a motor vehicle designed primarily for carrying property, meeting local criteria for classification as a heavy goods vehicle in terms of weight and requiring a special driver's license.

(q)   A bus (coach) is a motor vehicle designed or adapted primarily for carrying more than 10 passengers, and requiring a special driver's license.

(r)   A railway train or railway vehicle is any device, with or without freight or passenger cars couple to it, designed for traffic on a railway track. This includes subterranean (subways) or elevated trains.

(s)   A streetcar, is a device designed and used primarily for transporting passengers within a municipality, running on rails, usually subject to normal traffic control signals, and operated principally on a right-of-way that forms part of the roadway. This includes a tram or trolley that runs on rails. A trailer being towed by a streetcar is considered part of the streetcar.

(t)   A special vehicle mainly used on industrial premises is a motor vehicle designed primarily for use within the buildings and premises of industrial or commercial establishments. This includes battery-powered airport passenger vehicles or baggage/mail trucks, forklifts, coal-cars in a coal mine, logging cars and trucks used in mines or quarries.

(u)   A special vehicle mainly used in agriculture is a motor vehicle designed specifically for use in farming and agriculture (horticulture), to work the land, tend and harvest crops and transport materials on the farm. This includes harvesters, farm machinery and tractor and trailers.

(v) A special construction vehicle is a motor vehicle designed specifically for use on construction and demolition sites. This includes bulldozers, diggers, earth levellers, dump trucks. backhoes, front-end loaders, pavers, and mechanical shovels.

(w) A special all-terrain vehicle is a motor vehicle of special design to enable it to negotiate over rough or soft terrain, snow or sand. Examples of special design are high construction, special wheels and tires, tracks, and support on a cushion of air. This includes snow mobiles, All-terrain vehicles (ATV), and dune buggies. It does not include passenger vehicle designated as Sport Utility Vehicles. (SUV)

(x) A watercraft is any device designed for transporting passengers or goods on water. This includes motor or sailboats, ships, and hovercraft.

(y) An aircraft is any device for transporting passengers or goods in the air. This includes hot-air balloons, gliders, helicopters and airplanes.

(z) A military vehicle is any motorized vehicle operating on a public roadway owned by the military and being operated by a member of the military.

Pedestrian injured in transport accident (V00-V09)

INCLUDES　person changing tire on transport vehicle
person examining engine of vehicle broken down in (on side of) road
EXCLUDES 1　fall due to non-transport collision with other person (W03)
pedestrian on foot falling (slipping) on ice and snow (W00.-)
struck or bumped by another person (W51)

The appropriate 7th character is to be added to each code from categories V00-V09.
A　initial encounter
D　subsequent encounter
S　sequela

✓4ᵗʰ **V00　Pedestrian conveyance accident**

Use additional place of occurrence and activity external cause codes, if known (Y92.-, Y93.-)

EXCLUDES 1　collision with another person without fall (W51)
fall due to person on foot colliding with another person on foot (W03)
fall from non-moving wheelchair, nonmotorized scooter and motorized mobility scooter without collision (W05.-)
pedestrian (conveyance) collision with other land transport vehicle (V01-V09)
pedestrian on foot falling (slipping) on ice and snow (W00.-)

✓5ᵗʰ **V00.0　Pedestrian on foot injured in collision with pedestrian conveyance**

✓x7ᵗʰ　**V00.01　Pedestrian on foot injured in collision with roller-skater**

✓x7ᵗʰ　**V00.02　Pedestrian on foot injured in collision with skateboarder**

✓6ᵗʰ　**V00.03　Pedestrian on foot injured in collision with standing micro-mobility pedestrian conveyance**

✓7ᵗʰ　**V00.031　Pedestrian on foot injured in collision with rider of standing electric scooter**

✓7ᵗʰ　**V00.038　Pedestrian on foot injured in collision with rider of other standing micro-mobility pedestrian conveyance**
Pedestrian on foot injured in collision with rider of hoverboard
Pedestrian on foot injured in collision with rider of segway

✓x7ᵗʰ　**V00.09　Pedestrian on foot injured in collision with other pedestrian conveyance**

✓5ᵗʰ **V00.1　Rolling-type pedestrian conveyance accident**

EXCLUDES 1　accident with baby stroller (V00.82-)
accident with motorized mobility scooter (V00.83-)
accident with wheelchair (powered) (V00.81-)

✓6ᵗʰ　**V00.11　In-line roller-skate accident**

✓7ᵗʰ　**V00.111　Fall from in-line roller-skates**

✓7ᵗʰ　**V00.112　In-line roller-skater colliding with stationary object**

✓7ᵗʰ　**V00.118　Other in-line roller-skate accident**

EXCLUDES 1　roller-skater collision with other land transport vehicle (V01-V09 with 5th character 1)

✓6ᵗʰ　**V00.12　Non-in-line roller-skate accident**

✓7ᵗʰ　**V00.121　Fall from non-in-line roller-skates**

✓7ᵗʰ　**V00.122　Non-in-line roller-skater colliding with stationary object**

✓7ᵗʰ　**V00.128　Other non-in-line roller-skating accident**

EXCLUDES 1　roller-skater collision with other land transport vehicle (V01-V09 with 5th character 1)

✓6ᵗʰ　**V00.13　Skateboard accident**

✓7ᵗʰ　**V00.131　Fall from skateboard**

✓7ᵗʰ　**V00.132　Skateboarder colliding with stationary object**

✓7ᵗʰ　**V00.138　Other skateboard accident**

EXCLUDES 1　skateboarder collision with other land transport vehicle (V01-V09 with 5th character 2)

✓6ᵗʰ　**V00.14　Scooter (nonmotorized) accident**

EXCLUDES 1　motor scooter accident (V20-V29)

✓7ᵗʰ　**V00.141　Fall from scooter (nonmotorized)**

✓7ᵗʰ　**V00.142　Scooter (nonmotorized) colliding with stationary object**

✓7ᵗʰ　**V00.148　Other scooter (nonmotorized) accident**

EXCLUDES 1　scooter (nonmotorized) collision with other land transport vehicle (V01-V09 with fifth character 9)

✓6ᵗʰ　**V00.15　Heelies accident**
Rolling shoe
Wheeled shoe
Wheelies accident

✓7ᵗʰ　**V00.151　Fall from heelies**

✓7ᵗʰ　**V00.152　Heelies colliding with stationary object**

✓7ᵗʰ　**V00.158　Other heelies accident**

✓6ᵗʰ　**V00.18　Accident on other rolling-type pedestrian conveyance**

✓7ᵗʰ　**V00.181　Fall from other rolling-type pedestrian conveyance**

✓7ᵗʰ　**V00.182　Pedestrian on other rolling-type pedestrian conveyance colliding with stationary object**

✓7ᵗʰ　**V00.188　Other accident on other rolling-type pedestrian conveyance**

✓5ᵗʰ **V00.2　Gliding-type pedestrian conveyance accident**

✓6ᵗʰ　**V00.21　Ice-skates accident**

✓7ᵗʰ　**V00.211　Fall from ice-skates**

✓7ᵗʰ　**V00.212　Ice-skater colliding with stationary object**

✓7ᵗʰ　**V00.218　Other ice-skates accident**

EXCLUDES 1　ice-skater collision with other land transport vehicle (V01-V09 with 5th character 9)

✓6ᵗʰ　**V00.22　Sled accident**

✓7ᵗʰ　**V00.221　Fall from sled**

✓7ᵗʰ　**V00.222　Sledder colliding with stationary object**

✓7ᵗʰ　**V00.228　Other sled accident**

EXCLUDES 1　sled collision with other land transport vehicle (V01-V09 with 5th character 9)

✓6ᵗʰ　**V00.28　Other gliding-type pedestrian conveyance accident**

✓7ᵗʰ　**V00.281　Fall from other gliding-type pedestrian conveyance**

✓7ᵗʰ　**V00.282　Pedestrian on other gliding-type pedestrian conveyance colliding with stationary object**

HCC CMS-HCC　　**Rx** Rx HCC　　**ESR** ESRD HCC　　**COM** Commercial HCC　　N Newborn: 0　　P Pediatric: 0-17　　M Maternity: 9-64　　A Adult: 15-124

1194　　　ICD-10-CM 2023

☑7ᵗʰ **V00.288 Other accident on other gliding-type pedestrian conveyance**

    EXCLUDES 1   *gliding-type pedestrian conveyance collision with other land transport vehicle (V01-V09 with 5th character 9)*

☑5ᵗʰ **V00.3 Flat-bottomed pedestrian conveyance accident**

  ☑6ᵗʰ **V00.31 Snowboard accident**

    ☑7ᵗʰ **V00.311 Fall from snowboard**

    ☑7ᵗʰ **V00.312 Snowboarder colliding with stationary object**

    ☑7ᵗʰ **V00.318 Other snowboard accident**

       EXCLUDES 1   *snowboarder collision with other land transport vehicle (V01-V09 with 5th character 9)*

  ☑6ᵗʰ **V00.32 Snow-ski accident**

    ☑7ᵗʰ **V00.321 Fall from snow-skis**

    ☑7ᵗʰ **V00.322 Snow-skier colliding with stationary object**

    ☑7ᵗʰ **V00.328 Other snow-ski accident**

       EXCLUDES 1   *snow-skier collision with other land transport vehicle (V01-V09 with 5th character 9)*

  ☑6ᵗʰ **V00.38 Other flat-bottomed pedestrian conveyance accident**

    ☑7ᵗʰ **V00.381 Fall from other flat-bottomed pedestrian conveyance**

    ☑7ᵗʰ **V00.382 Pedestrian on other flat-bottomed pedestrian conveyance colliding with stationary object**

    ☑7ᵗʰ **V00.388 Other accident on other flat-bottomed pedestrian conveyance**

☑5ᵗʰ **V00.8 Accident on other pedestrian conveyance**

  ☑6ᵗʰ **V00.81 Accident with wheelchair (powered)**

    ☑7ᵗʰ **V00.811 Fall from moving wheelchair (powered)**

       EXCLUDES 1   *fall from non-moving wheelchair (W05.0)*

    ☑7ᵗʰ **V00.812 Wheelchair (powered) colliding with stationary object**

    ☑7ᵗʰ **V00.818 Other accident with wheelchair (powered)**

  ☑6ᵗʰ **V00.82 Accident with baby stroller**

    ☑7ᵗʰ **V00.821 Fall from baby stroller**

    ☑7ᵗʰ **V00.822 Baby stroller colliding with stationary object**

    ☑7ᵗʰ **V00.828 Other accident with baby stroller**

  ☑6ᵗʰ **V00.83 Accident with motorized mobility scooter**

    ☑7ᵗʰ **V00.831 Fall from motorized mobility scooter**

       EXCLUDES 1   *fall from non-moving motorized mobility scooter (W05.2)*

    ☑7ᵗʰ **V00.832 Motorized mobility scooter colliding with stationary object**

    ☑7ᵗʰ **V00.838 Other accident with motorized mobility scooter**

  ☑6ᵗʰ **V00.84 Accident with standing micro-mobility pedestrian conveyance**

    ☑7ᵗʰ **V00.841 Fall from standing electric scooter**

    ☑7ᵗʰ **V00.842 Pedestrian on standing electric scooter colliding with stationary object**

    ☑7ᵗʰ **V00.848 Other accident with standing micro-mobility pedestrian conveyance**

       Accident with hoverboard

       Accident with segway

  ☑6ᵗʰ **V00.89 Accident on other pedestrian conveyance**

    ☑7ᵗʰ **V00.891 Fall from other pedestrian conveyance**

    ☑7ᵗʰ **V00.892 Pedestrian on other pedestrian conveyance colliding with stationary object**

☑7ᵗʰ **V00.898 Other accident on other pedestrian conveyance**

    EXCLUDES 1   *other pedestrian (conveyance) collision with other land transport vehicle (V01-V09 with 5th character 9)*

☑4ᵗʰ **V01 Pedestrian injured in collision with pedal cycle**

  ☑5ᵗʰ **V01.0 Pedestrian injured in collision with pedal cycle in nontraffic accident**

    ☑×7ᵗʰ **V01.00 Pedestrian on foot injured in collision with pedal cycle in nontraffic accident**

       Pedestrian NOS injured in collision with pedal cycle in nontraffic accident

    ☑×7ᵗʰ **V01.01 Pedestrian on roller-skates injured in collision with pedal cycle in nontraffic accident**

    ☑×7ᵗʰ **V01.02 Pedestrian on skateboard injured in collision with pedal cycle in nontraffic accident**

    ☑6ᵗʰ **V01.03 Pedestrian on standing micro-mobility pedestrian conveyance injured in collision with pedal cycle in nontraffic accident**

      ☑7ᵗʰ **V01.031 Pedestrian on standing electric scooter injured in collision with pedal cycle in nontraffic accident**

      ☑7ᵗʰ **V01.038 Pedestrian on other standing micro-mobility pedestrian conveyance injured in collision with pedal cycle in nontraffic accident**

        Pedestrian on hoverboard injured in collision with pedal cycle in nontraffic accident

        Pedestrian on segway injured in collision with pedal cycle in nontraffic accident

    ☑×7ᵗʰ **V01.09 Pedestrian with other conveyance injured in collision with pedal cycle in nontraffic accident**

       Pedestrian with baby stroller injured in collision with pedal cycle in nontraffic accident

       Pedestrian on ice-skates injured in collision with pedal cycle in nontraffic accident

       Pedestrian on nonmotorized scooter injured in collision with pedal cycle in nontraffic accident

       Pedestrian on sled injured in collision with pedal cycle in nontraffic accident

       Pedestrian on snowboard injured in collision with pedal cycle in nontraffic accident

       Pedestrian on snow-skis injured in collision with pedal cycle in nontraffic accident

       Pedestrian in wheelchair (powered) injured in collision with pedal cycle in nontraffic accident

       Pedestrian in motorized mobility scooter injured in collision with pedal cycle in nontraffic accident

  ☑5ᵗʰ **V01.1 Pedestrian injured in collision with pedal cycle in traffic accident**

    ☑×7ᵗʰ **V01.10 Pedestrian on foot injured in collision with pedal cycle in traffic accident**

       Pedestrian NOS injured in collision with pedal cycle in traffic accident

    ☑×7ᵗʰ **V01.11 Pedestrian on roller-skates injured in collision with pedal cycle in traffic accident**

    ☑×7ᵗʰ **V01.12 Pedestrian on skateboard injured in collision with pedal cycle in traffic accident**

    ☑6ᵗʰ **V01.13 Pedestrian on standing micro-mobility pedestrian conveyance injured in collision with pedal cycle in traffic accident**

      ☑7ᵗʰ **V01.131 Pedestrian on standing electric scooter injured in collision with pedal cycle in traffic accident**

      ☑7ᵗʰ **V01.138 Pedestrian on other standing micro-mobility pedestrian conveyance injured in collision with pedal cycle in traffic accident**

        Pedestrian on hoverboard injured in collision with pedal cycle in traffic accident

        Pedestrian on segway injured in collision with pedal cycle in traffic accident

---

☑ Additional Character Required   ☑×7ᵗʰ Placeholder Alert   Manifestation   Unspecified Dx   Ⓠ QPP   UPD Unacceptable PDx

Chapter 20. External Causes of Morbidity

V01.19–V02.131

✓x7ᵗʰ **V01.19 Pedestrian with other conveyance injured in collision with pedal cycle in traffic accident**

Pedestrian with baby stroller injured in collision with pedal cycle in traffic accident

Pedestrian on ice-skates injured in collision with pedal cycle in traffic accident

Pedestrian on nonmotorized scooter injured in collision with pedal cycle in traffic accident

Pedestrian on sled injured in collision with pedal cycle in traffic accident

Pedestrian on snowboard injured in collision with pedal cycle in traffic accident

Pedestrian on snow-skis injured in collision with pedal cycle in traffic accident

Pedestrian in wheelchair (powered) injured in collision with pedal cycle in traffic accident

Pedestrian in motorized mobility scooter injured in collision with pedal cycle in traffic accident

✓5ᵗʰ **V01.9 Pedestrian injured in collision with pedal cycle, unspecified whether traffic or nontraffic accident**

✓x7ᵗʰ **V01.90 Pedestrian on foot injured in collision with pedal cycle, unspecified whether traffic or nontraffic accident**

Pedestrian NOS injured in collision with pedal cycle, unspecified whether traffic or nontraffic accident

✓x7ᵗʰ **V01.91 Pedestrian on roller-skates injured in collision with pedal cycle, unspecified whether traffic or nontraffic accident**

✓x7ᵗʰ **V01.92 Pedestrian on skateboard injured in collision with pedal cycle, unspecified whether traffic or nontraffic accident**

✓6ᵗʰ **V01.93 Pedestrian on standing micro-mobility pedestrian conveyance injured in collision with pedal cycle, unspecified whether traffic or nontraffic accident**

✓7ᵗʰ **V01.931 Pedestrian on standing electric scooter injured in collision with pedal cycle, unspecified whether traffic or nontraffic accident**

✓7ᵗʰ **V01.938 Pedestrian on other standing micro-mobility pedestrian conveyance injured in collision with pedal cycle, unspecified whether traffic or nontraffic accident**

Pedestrian on hoverboard injured in collision with pedal cycle, unspecified whether traffic or nontraffic accident

Pedestrian on segway injured in collision with pedal cycle, unspecified whether traffic or nontraffic accident

✓x7ᵗʰ **V01.99 Pedestrian with other conveyance injured in collision with pedal cycle, unspecified whether traffic or nontraffic accident**

Pedestrian with baby stroller injured in collision with pedal cycle, unspecified whether traffic or nontraffic accident

Pedestrian on ice-skates injured in collision with pedal cycle unspecified, whether traffic or nontraffic accident

Pedestrian on nonmotorized scooter injured in collision with pedal cycle, unspecified whether traffic or nontraffic accident

Pedestrian on sled injured in collision with pedal cycle unspecified, whether traffic or nontraffic accident

Pedestrian on snowboard injured in collision with pedal cycle, unspecified whether traffic or nontraffic accident

Pedestrian on snow-skis injured in collision with pedal cycle, unspecified whether traffic or nontraffic accident

Pedestrian in wheelchair (powered) injured in collision with pedal cycle, unspecified whether traffic or nontraffic accident

Pedestrian in motorized mobility scooter injured in collision with pedal cycle, unspecified whether traffic or nontraffic accident

✓4ᵗʰ **V02 Pedestrian injured in collision with two- or three-wheeled motor vehicle**

✓5ᵗʰ **V02.0 Pedestrian injured in collision with two- or three-wheeled motor vehicle in nontraffic accident**

✓x7ᵗʰ **V02.00 Pedestrian on foot injured in collision with two- or three-wheeled motor vehicle in nontraffic accident**

Pedestrian NOS injured in collision with two- or three-wheeled motor vehicle in nontraffic accident

✓x7ᵗʰ **V02.01 Pedestrian on roller-skates injured in collision with two- or three-wheeled motor vehicle in nontraffic accident**

✓x7ᵗʰ **V02.02 Pedestrian on skateboard injured in collision with two- or three-wheeled motor vehicle in nontraffic accident**

✓6ᵗʰ **V02.03 Pedestrian on standing micro-mobility pedestrian conveyance injured in collision with two- or three-wheeled motor vehicle in nontraffic accident**

✓7ᵗʰ **V02.031 Pedestrian on standing electric scooter injured in collision with two- or three-wheeled motor vehicle in nontraffic accident**

✓7ᵗʰ **V02.038 Pedestrian on other standing micro-mobility pedestrian conveyance injured in collision with two- or three-wheeled motor vehicle in nontraffic accident**

Pedestrian on hoverboard injured in collision with two-or three wheeled motor vehicle in nontraffic accident

Pedestrian on segway injured in collision with two- or three-wheeled motor vehicle in nontraffic accident

✓x7ᵗʰ **V02.09 Pedestrian with other conveyance injured in collision with two- or three-wheeled motor vehicle in nontraffic accident**

Pedestrian with baby stroller injured in collision with two- or three-wheeled motor vehicle in nontraffic accident

Pedestrian on ice-skates injured in collision with two- or three-wheeled motor vehicle in nontraffic accident

Pedestrian on nonmotorized scooter injured in collision with two- or three-wheeled motor vehicle in nontraffic accident

Pedestrian on sled injured in collision with two- or three-wheeled motor vehicle in nontraffic accident

Pedestrian on snowboard injured in collision with two- or three-wheeled motor vehicle in nontraffic accident

Pedestrian on snow-skis injured in collision with two- or three-wheeled motor vehicle in nontraffic accident

Pedestrian in wheelchair (powered) injured in collision with two- or three-wheeled motor vehicle in nontraffic accident

Pedestrian in motorized mobility scooter injured in collision with two- or three-wheeled motor vehicle in nontraffic accident

✓5ᵗʰ **V02.1 Pedestrian injured in collision with two- or three-wheeled motor vehicle in traffic accident**

✓x7ᵗʰ **V02.10 Pedestrian on foot injured in collision with two- or three-wheeled motor vehicle in traffic accident**

Pedestrian NOS injured in collision with two- or three-wheeled motor vehicle in traffic accident

✓x7ᵗʰ **V02.11 Pedestrian on roller-skates injured in collision with two- or three-wheeled motor vehicle in traffic accident**

✓x7ᵗʰ **V02.12 Pedestrian on skateboard injured in collision with two- or three-wheeled motor vehicle in traffic accident**

✓6ᵗʰ **V02.13 Pedestrian on standing micro-mobility pedestrian conveyance injured in collision with two- or three-wheeled motor vehicle in traffic accident**

✓7ᵗʰ **V02.131 Pedestrian on standing electric scooter injured in collision with two- or three-wheeled motor vehicle in traffic accident**

√7ᵗʰ **V02.138 Pedestrian on other standing micro-mobility pedestrian conveyance injured in collision with two- or three-wheeled motor vehicle in traffic accident**

    Pedestrian on hoverboard injured in collision with two-or three wheeled motor vehicle in traffic accident

    Pedestrian on segway injured in collision with two- or three-wheeled motor vehicle in traffic accident

√x7ᵗʰ **V02.19 Pedestrian with other conveyance injured in collision with two- or three-wheeled motor vehicle in traffic accident**

    Pedestrian with baby stroller injured in collision with two- or three-wheeled motor vehicle in traffic accident

    Pedestrian on ice-skates injured in collision with two- or three-wheeled motor vehicle in traffic accident

    Pedestrian on nonmotorized scooter injured in collision with two- or three-wheeled motor vehicle in traffic accident

    Pedestrian on sled injured in collision with two- or three-wheeled motor vehicle in traffic accident

    Pedestrian on snowboard injured in collision with two- or three-wheeled motor vehicle in traffic accident

    Pedestrian on snow-skis injured in collision with two- or three-wheeled motor vehicle in traffic accident

    Pedestrian in wheelchair (powered) injured in collision with two- or three-wheeled motor vehicle in traffic accident

    Pedestrian in motorized mobility scooter injured in collision with two- or three-wheeled motor vehicle in traffic accident

√5ᵗʰ **V02.9 Pedestrian injured in collision with two- or three-wheeled motor vehicle, unspecified whether traffic or nontraffic accident**

√7ᵗʰ **V02.90 Pedestrian on foot injured in collision with two- or three-wheeled motor vehicle, unspecified whether traffic or nontraffic accident**

    Pedestrian NOS injured in collision with two- or three-wheeled motor vehicle, unspecified whether traffic or nontraffic accident

√x7ᵗʰ **V02.91 Pedestrian on roller-skates injured in collision with two- or three-wheeled motor vehicle, unspecified whether traffic or nontraffic accident**

√x7ᵗʰ **V02.92 Pedestrian on skateboard injured in collision with two- or three-wheeled motor vehicle, unspecified whether traffic or nontraffic accident**

√6ᵗʰ **V02.93 Pedestrian on standing micro-mobility pedestrian conveyance injured in collision with two- or three-wheeled motor vehicle, unspecified whether traffic or nontraffic accident**

√7ᵗʰ **V02.931 Pedestrian on standing electric scooter injured in collision with two- or three wheeled motor vehicle, unspecified whether traffic or nontraffic accident**

√7ᵗʰ **V02.938 Pedestrian on other standing micro-mobility pedestrian conveyance injured in collision with two- or three wheeled motor vehicle, unspecified whether traffic or nontraffic accident**

    Pedestrian on hoverboard injured in collision with two-three-wheeled motor vehicle, unspecified whether traffic or nontraffic accident

    Pedestrian on segway injured in collision with two- or three wheeled motor vehicle, unspecified whether traffic or nontraffic accident

√x7ᵗʰ **V02.99 Pedestrian with other conveyance injured in collision with two- or three-wheeled motor vehicle, unspecified whether traffic or nontraffic accident**

    Pedestrian with baby stroller injured in collision with two- or three-wheeled motor vehicle, unspecified whether traffic or nontraffic accident

    Pedestrian on ice-skates injured in collision with two- or three-wheeled motor vehicle, unspecified whether traffic or nontraffic accident

    Pedestrian on nonmotorized scooter injured in collision with two- or three-wheeled motor vehicle, unspecified whether traffic or nontraffic accident

    Pedestrian on sled injured in collision with two- or three-wheeled motor vehicle, unspecified whether traffic or nontraffic accident

    Pedestrian on snowboard injured in collision with two- or three-wheeled motor vehicle, unspecified whether traffic or nontraffic accident

    Pedestrian on snow-skis injured in collision with two- or three-wheeled motor vehicle, unspecified whether traffic or nontraffic accident

    Pedestrian in wheelchair (powered) injured in collision with two- or three-wheeled motor vehicle, unspecified whether traffic or nontraffic accident

    Pedestrian in motorized mobility scooter injured in collision with two- or three wheeled motor vehicle, unspecified whether traffic or nontraffic accident

√4ᵗʰ **V03 Pedestrian injured in collision with car, pick-up truck or van**

√5ᵗʰ **V03.0 Pedestrian injured in collision with car, pick-up truck or van in nontraffic accident**

√x7ᵗʰ **V03.00 Pedestrian on foot injured in collision with car, pick-up truck or van in nontraffic accident**

    Pedestrian NOS injured in collision with car, pick-up truck or van in nontraffic accident

√x7ᵗʰ **V03.01 Pedestrian on roller-skates injured in collision with car, pick-up truck or van in nontraffic accident**

√x7ᵗʰ **V03.02 Pedestrian on skateboard injured in collision with car, pick-up truck or van in nontraffic accident**

√6ᵗʰ **V03.03 Pedestrian on standing micro-mobility pedestrian conveyance injured in collision with car, pick-up or van in nontraffic accident**

√7ᵗʰ **V03.031 Pedestrian on standing electric scooter injured in collision with car, pick-up or van in nontraffic accident**

√7ᵗʰ **V03.038 Pedestrian on other standing micro-mobility pedestrian conveyance injured in collision with car, pick-up or van in nontraffic accident**

    Pedestrian on hoverboard injured in collision with car, pick-up or van in nontraffic accident

    Pedestrian on segway injured in collision with car, pick-up or van in nontraffic accident

√x7ᵗʰ **V03.09 Pedestrian with other conveyance injured in collision with car, pick-up truck or van in nontraffic accident**

    Pedestrian with baby stroller injured in collision with car, pick-up truck or van in nontraffic accident

    Pedestrian on ice-skates injured in collision with car, pick-up truck or van in nontraffic accident

    Pedestrian on nonmotorized scooter injured in collision with car, pick-up truck or van in nontraffic accident

    Pedestrian on sled injured in collision with car, pick-up truck or van in nontraffic accident

    Pedestrian on snowboard injured in collision with car, pick-up truck or van in nontraffic accident

    Pedestrian on snow-skis injured in collision with car, pick-up truck or van in nontraffic accident

    Pedestrian in wheelchair (powered) injured in collision with car, pick-up truck or van in nontraffic accident

    Pedestrian in motorized mobility scooter injured in collision with car, pick-up truck or van in nontraffic accident

---

☑ Additional Character Required   √x7ᵗʰ Placeholder Alert   Manifestation   Unspecified Dx   Q QPP   UPD Unacceptable PDx

☑5ᵗʰ V03.1 Pedestrian injured in collision with car, pick-up truck or van in traffic accident

☑x7ᵗʰ V03.10 Pedestrian on foot injured in collision with car, pick-up truck or van in traffic accident
Pedestrian NOS injured in collision with car, pick-up truck or van in traffic accident

☑x7ᵗʰ V03.11 Pedestrian on roller-skates injured in collision with car, pick-up truck or van in traffic accident

☑x7ᵗʰ V03.12 Pedestrian on skateboard injured in collision with car, pick-up truck or van in traffic accident

☑6ᵗʰ V03.13 Pedestrian on standing micro-mobility pedestrian conveyance injured in collision with car, pick-up or van in traffic accident

☑7ᵗʰ V03.131 Pedestrian on standing electric scooter injured in collision with car, pick-up or van in traffic accident

☑7ᵗʰ V03.138 Pedestrian on other standing micro-mobility pedestrian conveyance injured in collision with car, pick-up or van in traffic accident
Pedestrian on hoverboard injured in collision with car, pick-up or van in traffic accident
Pedestrian on segway injured in collision with car, pick-up or van in traffic accident

☑x7ᵗʰ V03.19 Pedestrian with other conveyance injured in collision with car, pick-up truck or van in traffic accident
Pedestrian with baby stroller injured in collision with car, pick-up truck or van in traffic accident
Pedestrian on ice-skates injured in collision with car, pick-up truck or van in traffic accident
Pedestrian on nonmotorized scooter injured in collision with car, pick-up truck or van in nontraffic accident
Pedestrian on sled injured in collision with car, pick-up truck or van in traffic accident
Pedestrian on snowboard injured in collision with car, pick-up truck or van in traffic accident
Pedestrian on snow-skis injured in collision with car, pick-up truck or van in traffic accident
Pedestrian in wheelchair (powered) injured in collision with car, pick-up truck or van in traffic accident
Pedestrian in motorized mobility scooter injured in collision with car, pick-up truck or van in nontraffic accident

☑5ᵗʰ V03.9 Pedestrian injured in collision with car, pick-up truck or van, unspecified whether traffic or nontraffic accident

☑x7ᵗʰ V03.90 Pedestrian on foot injured in collision with car, pick-up truck or van, unspecified whether traffic or nontraffic accident
Pedestrian NOS injured in collision with car, pick-up truck or van, unspecified whether traffic or nontraffic accident

☑x7ᵗʰ V03.91 Pedestrian on roller-skates injured in collision with car, pick-up truck or van, unspecified whether traffic or nontraffic accident

☑x7ᵗʰ V03.92 Pedestrian on skateboard injured in collision with car, pick-up truck or van, unspecified whether traffic or nontraffic accident

☑6ᵗʰ V03.93 Pedestrian on standing micro-mobility pedestrian conveyance injured in collision with car, pick-up or van, unspecified whether traffic or nontraffic accident

☑7ᵗʰ V03.931 Pedestrian on standing electric scooter injured in collision with car, pick-up or van, unspecified whether traffic or nontraffic accident

☑7ᵗʰ V03.938 Pedestrian on other standing micro-mobility pedestrian conveyance injured in collision with car, pick-up or van, unspecified whether traffic or nontraffic accident
Pedestrian on hoverboard injured in collision with car, pick-up or van, unspecified whether traffic or nontraffic accident
Pedestrian on segway injured in collision with car, pick-up or van, unspecified whether traffic or nontraffic accident

☑x7ᵗʰ V03.99 Pedestrian with other conveyance injured in collision with car, pick-up truck or van, unspecified whether traffic or nontraffic accident
Pedestrian with baby stroller injured in collision with car, pick-up truck or van, unspecified whether traffic or nontraffic accident
Pedestrian on ice-skates injured in collision with car, pick-up truck or van, unspecified whether traffic or nontraffic accident
Pedestrian on nonmotorized scooter injured in collision with car, pick-up truck or van, unspecified whether traffic or nontraffic accident
Pedestrian on sled injured in collision with car, pick-up truck or van in nontraffic accident
Pedestrian on snowboard injured in collision with car, pick-up truck or van, unspecified whether traffic or nontraffic accident
Pedestrian on snow-skis injured in collision with car, pick-up truck or van, unspecified whether traffic or nontraffic accident
Pedestrian in wheelchair (powered) injured in collision with car, pick-up truck or van, unspecified whether traffic or nontraffic accident
Pedestrian in motorized mobility scooter injured in collision with car, pick-up truck or van, unspecified whether traffic or nontraffic accident

☑4ᵗʰ V04 Pedestrian injured in collision with heavy transport vehicle or bus
EXCLUDES 1 pedestrian injured in collision with military vehicle (V09.01, V09.21)

☑5ᵗʰ V04.0 Pedestrian injured in collision with heavy transport vehicle or bus in nontraffic accident

☑x7ᵗʰ V04.00 Pedestrian on foot injured in collision with heavy transport vehicle or bus in nontraffic accident
Pedestrian NOS injured in collision with heavy transport vehicle or bus in nontraffic accident

☑x7ᵗʰ V04.01 Pedestrian on roller-skates injured in collision with heavy transport vehicle or bus in nontraffic accident

☑x7ᵗʰ V04.02 Pedestrian on skateboard injured in collision with heavy transport vehicle or bus in nontraffic accident

☑6ᵗʰ V04.03 Pedestrian on standing micro-mobility pedestrian conveyance injured in collision with heavy transport vehicle or bus in nontraffic accident

☑7ᵗʰ V04.031 Pedestrian on standing electric scooter injured in collision with heavy transport vehicle or bus in nontraffic accident

☑7ᵗʰ V04.038 Pedestrian on other standing micro-mobility pedestrian conveyance injured in collision with heavy transport vehicle or bus in nontraffic accident
Pedestrian on hoverboard injured in collision with heavy transport vehicle or bus in nontraffic accident
Pedestrian on segway injured in collision with heavy transport vehicle or bus in nontraffic accident

☑x7ᵗʰ **V04.09** **Pedestrian with other conveyance injured in collision with heavy transport vehicle or bus in nontraffic accident**

Pedestrian with baby stroller injured in collision with heavy transport vehicle or bus in nontraffic accident

Pedestrian on ice-skates injured in collision with heavy transport vehicle or bus in nontraffic accident

Pedestrian on nonmotorized scooter injured in collision with heavy transport vehicle or bus in nontraffic accident

Pedestrian on sled injured in collision with heavy transport vehicle or bus in nontraffic accident

Pedestrian on snowboard injured in collision with heavy transport vehicle or bus in nontraffic accident

Pedestrian on snow-skis injured in collision with heavy transport vehicle or bus in nontraffic accident

Pedestrian in wheelchair (powered) injured in collision with heavy transport vehicle or bus in nontraffic accident

Pedestrian in motorized mobility scooter injured in collision with heavy transport vehicle or bus in nontraffic accident

☑5ᵗʰ **V04.1** **Pedestrian injured in collision with heavy transport vehicle or bus in traffic accident**

☑x7ᵗʰ **V04.10** **Pedestrian on foot injured in collision with heavy transport vehicle or bus in traffic accident**

Pedestrian NOS injured in collision with heavy transport vehicle or bus in traffic accident

☑x7ᵗʰ **V04.11** **Pedestrian on roller-skates injured in collision with heavy transport vehicle or bus in traffic accident**

☑x7ᵗʰ **V04.12** **Pedestrian on skateboard injured in collision with heavy transport vehicle or bus in traffic accident**

☑6ᵗʰ **V04.13** **Pedestrian on standing micro-mobility pedestrian conveyance injured in collision with heavy transport vehicle or bus in traffic accident**

☑7ᵗʰ **V04.131** **Pedestrian on standing electric scooter injured in collision with heavy transport vehicle or bus in traffic accident**

☑7ᵗʰ **V04.138** **Pedestrian on other standing micro-mobility pedestrian conveyance injured in collision with heavy transport vehicle or bus in traffic accident**

Pedestrian on hoverboard injured in collision with heavy transport vehicle or bus in traffic accident

Pedestrian on segway injured in collision with heavy transport vehicle or bus in traffic accident

☑x7ᵗʰ **V04.19** **Pedestrian with other conveyance injured in collision with heavy transport vehicle or bus in traffic accident**

Pedestrian with baby stroller injured in collision with heavy transport vehicle or bus in traffic accident

Pedestrian on ice-skates injured in collision with heavy transport vehicle or bus in traffic accident

Pedestrian on nonmotorized scooter injured in collision with heavy transport vehicle or bus in traffic accident

Pedestrian on sled injured in collision with heavy transport vehicle or bus in traffic accident

Pedestrian on snowboard injured in collision with heavy transport vehicle or bus in traffic accident

Pedestrian on snow-skis injured in collision with heavy transport vehicle or bus in traffic accident

Pedestrian in wheelchair (powered) injured in collision with heavy transport vehicle or bus in traffic accident

Pedestrian in motorized mobility scooter injured in collision with heavy transport vehicle or bus in traffic accident

☑5ᵗʰ **V04.9** **Pedestrian injured in collision with heavy transport vehicle or bus, unspecified whether traffic or nontraffic accident**

☑x7ᵗʰ **V04.90** **Pedestrian on foot injured in collision with heavy transport vehicle or bus, unspecified whether traffic or nontraffic accident**

Pedestrian NOS injured in collision with heavy transport vehicle or bus, unspecified whether traffic or nontraffic accident

☑x7ᵗʰ **V04.91** **Pedestrian on roller-skates injured in collision with heavy transport vehicle or bus, unspecified whether traffic or nontraffic accident**

☑x7ᵗʰ **V04.92** **Pedestrian on skateboard injured in collision with heavy transport vehicle or bus, unspecified whether traffic or nontraffic accident**

☑6ᵗʰ **V04.93** **Pedestrian on standing micro-mobility pedestrian conveyance injured in collision with heavy transport vehicle or bus, unspecified whether traffic or nontraffic accident**

☑7ᵗʰ **V04.931** **Pedestrian on standing electric scooter injured in collision with heavy transport vehicle or bus, unspecified whether traffic or nontraffic accident**

☑7ᵗʰ **V04.938** **Pedestrian on other standing micro-mobility pedestrian conveyance injured in collision with heavy transport vehicle or bus, unspecified whether traffic or nontraffic accident**

Pedestrian on hoverboard injured in collision with heavy transport vehicle or bus, unspecified whether traffic or nontraffic accident

Pedestrian on segway injured in collision with heavy transport vehicle or bus, unspecified whether traffic or nontraffic accident

☑x7ᵗʰ **V04.99** **Pedestrian with other conveyance injured in collision with heavy transport vehicle or bus, unspecified whether traffic or nontraffic accident**

Pedestrian with baby stroller injured in collision with heavy transport vehicle or bus, unspecified whether traffic or nontraffic accident

Pedestrian on ice-skates injured in collision with heavy transport vehicle or bus, unspecified whether traffic or nontraffic accident

Pedestrian on nonmotorized scooter injured in collision with heavy transport vehicle or bus, unspecified whether traffic or nontraffic accident

Pedestrian on sled injured in collision with heavy transport vehicle or bus, unspecified whether traffic or nontraffic accident

Pedestrian on snowboard injured in collision with heavy transport vehicle or bus, unspecified whether traffic or nontraffic accident

Pedestrian on snow-skis injured in collision with heavy transport vehicle or bus, unspecified whether traffic or nontraffic accident

Pedestrian in wheelchair (powered) injured in collision with heavy transport vehicle or bus, unspecified whether traffic or nontraffic accident

Pedestrian in motorized mobility scooter injured in collision with heavy transport vehicle or bus, unspecified whether traffic or nontraffic accident

☑4ᵗʰ **V05** **Pedestrian injured in collision with railway train or railway vehicle**

☑5ᵗʰ **V05.0** **Pedestrian injured in collision with railway train or railway vehicle in nontraffic accident**

☑x7ᵗʰ **V05.00** **Pedestrian on foot injured in collision with railway train or railway vehicle in nontraffic accident**

Pedestrian NOS injured in collision with railway train or railway vehicle in nontraffic accident

☑x7ᵗʰ **V05.01** **Pedestrian on roller-skates injured in collision with railway train or railway vehicle in nontraffic accident**

☑x7ᵗʰ **V05.02** **Pedestrian on skateboard injured in collision with railway train or railway vehicle in nontraffic accident**

☑6ᵗʰ **V05.03** **Pedestrian on standing micro-mobility pedestrian conveyance injured in collision with railway train or railway vehicle in nontraffic accident**

☑7ᵗʰ **V05.031** **Pedestrian on standing electric scooter injured in collision with railway train or railway vehicle in nontraffic accident**

Chapter 20. External Causes of Morbidity

√7ᵗʰ **V05.038 Pedestrian on other standing micro-mobility pedestrian conveyance injured in collision with railway train or railway vehicle in nontraffic accident**
  Pedestrian on hoverboard injured in collision with railway train or railway vehicle in nontraffic accident
  Pedestrian on segway injured in collision with railway train or railway vehicle in nontraffic accident

√x7ᵗʰ **V05.09 Pedestrian with other conveyance injured in collision with railway train or railway vehicle in nontraffic accident**
  Pedestrian with baby stroller injured in collision with railway train or railway vehicle in nontraffic accident
  Pedestrian on ice-skates injured in collision with railway train or railway vehicle in nontraffic accident
  Pedestrian on nonmotorized scooter injured in collision with railway train or railway vehicle in nontraffic accident
  Pedestrian on sled injured in collision with railway train or railway vehicle in nontraffic accident
  Pedestrian on snowboard injured in collision with railway train or railway vehicle in nontraffic accident
  Pedestrian on snow-skis injured in collision with railway train or railway vehicle in nontraffic accident
  Pedestrian in wheelchair (powered) injured in collision with railway train or railway vehicle in nontraffic accident
  Pedestrian in motorized mobility scooter injured in collision with railway train or railway vehicle in nontraffic accident

√5ᵗʰ **V05.1 Pedestrian injured in collision with railway train or railway vehicle in traffic accident**
  √7ᵗʰ **V05.10 Pedestrian on foot injured in collision with railway train or railway vehicle in traffic accident**
    Pedestrian NOS injured in collision with railway train or railway vehicle in traffic accident
  √x7ᵗʰ **V05.11 Pedestrian on roller-skates injured in collision with railway train or railway vehicle in traffic accident**
  √x7ᵗʰ **V05.12 Pedestrian on skateboard injured in collision with railway train or railway vehicle in traffic accident**
  √6ᵗʰ **V05.13 Pedestrian on standing micro-mobility pedestrian conveyance injured in collision with railway train or railway vehicle in traffic accident**
    √7ᵗʰ **V05.131 Pedestrian on standing electric scooter injured in collision with railway train or railway vehicle in traffic accident**
    √7ᵗʰ **V05.138 Pedestrian on other standing micro-mobility pedestrian conveyance injured in collision with railway train or railway vehicle in traffic accident**
      Pedestrian on hoverboard injured in collision with railway train or railway vehicle in traffic accident
      Pedestrian on segway injured in collision with railway train or railway vehicle in traffic accident

√x7ᵗʰ **V05.19 Pedestrian with other conveyance injured in collision with railway train or railway vehicle in traffic accident**
  Pedestrian with baby stroller injured in collision with railway train or railway vehicle in traffic accident
  Pedestrian on ice-skates injured in collision with railway train or railway vehicle in traffic accident
  Pedestrian on nonmotorized scooter injured in collision with railway train or railway vehicle in traffic accident
  Pedestrian on sled injured in collision with railway train or railway vehicle in traffic accident
  Pedestrian on snowboard injured in collision with railway train or railway vehicle in traffic accident
  Pedestrian on snow-skis injured in collision with railway train or railway vehicle in traffic accident
  Pedestrian in wheelchair (powered) injured in collision with railway train or railway vehicle in traffic accident
  Pedestrian in motorized mobility scooter injured in collision with railway train or railway vehicle in traffic accident

√5ᵗʰ **V05.9 Pedestrian injured in collision with railway train or railway vehicle, unspecified whether traffic or nontraffic accident**
  √x7ᵗʰ **V05.90 Pedestrian on foot injured in collision with railway train or railway vehicle, unspecified whether traffic or nontraffic accident**
    Pedestrian NOS injured in collision with railway train or railway vehicle, unspecified whether traffic or nontraffic accident
  √x7ᵗʰ **V05.91 Pedestrian on roller-skates injured in collision with railway train or railway vehicle, unspecified whether traffic or nontraffic accident**
  √x7ᵗʰ **V05.92 Pedestrian on skateboard injured in collision with railway train or railway vehicle, unspecified whether traffic or nontraffic accident**
  √6ᵗʰ **V05.93 Pedestrian on standing micro-mobility pedestrian conveyance injured in collision with railway train or railway vehicle, unspecified whether traffic or nontraffic accident**
    √7ᵗʰ **V05.931 Pedestrian on standing electric scooter injured in collision with railway train or railway vehicle, unspecified whether traffic or nontraffic accident**
    √7ᵗʰ **V05.938 Pedestrian on other standing micro-mobility pedestrian conveyance injured in collision with railway train or railway vehicle, unspecified whether traffic or nontraffic accident**
      Pedestrian on hoverboard injured in collision with railway train or railway vehicle, unspecified whether traffic or nontraffic accident
      Pedestrian on segway injured in collision with railway train or railway vehicle, unspecified whether traffic or nontraffic accident

√x7ᵗʰ V05.99 Pedestrian with other conveyance injured in collision with railway train or railway vehicle, unspecified whether traffic or nontraffic accident

Pedestrian with baby stroller injured in collision with railway train or railway vehicle, unspecified whether traffic or nontraffic

Pedestrian on ice-skates injured in collision with railway train or railway vehicle, unspecified whether traffic or nontraffic

Pedestrian on nonmotorized scooter injured in collision with railway train or railway vehicle, unspecified whether traffic or nontraffic

Pedestrian on sled injured in collision with railway train or railway vehicle, unspecified whether traffic or nontraffic

Pedestrian on snowboard injured in collision with railway train or railway vehicle, unspecified whether traffic or nontraffic

Pedestrian on snow-skis injured in collision with railway train or railway vehicle, unspecified whether traffic or nontraffic

Pedestrian in wheelchair (powered) injured in collision with railway train or railway vehicle, unspecified whether traffic or nontraffic

Pedestrian in motorized mobility scooter injured in collision with railway train or railway vehicle, unspecified whether traffic or nontraffic

√4ᵗʰ V06 Pedestrian injured in collision with other nonmotor vehicle

> **INCLUDES** collision with animal-drawn vehicle, animal being ridden, nonpowered streetcar
>
> **EXCLUDES 1** *pedestrian injured in collision with pedestrian conveyance (V00.0-)*

√5ᵗʰ V06.0 Pedestrian injured in collision with other nonmotor vehicle in nontraffic accident

√x7ᵗʰ V06.00 Pedestrian on foot injured in collision with other nonmotor vehicle in nontraffic accident

Pedestrian NOS injured in collision with other nonmotor vehicle in nontraffic accident

√x7ᵗʰ V06.01 Pedestrian on roller-skates injured in collision with other nonmotor vehicle in nontraffic accident

√x7ᵗʰ V06.02 Pedestrian on skateboard injured in collision with other nonmotor vehicle in nontraffic accident

√6ᵗʰ V06.03 Pedestrian on standing micro-mobility pedestrian conveyance injured in collision with other nonmotor vehicle in nontraffic accident

√7ᵗʰ V06.031 Pedestrian on standing electric scooter injured in collision with other nonmotor vehicle in nontraffic accident

√7ᵗʰ V06.038 Pedestrian on other standing micro-mobility pedestrian conveyance injured in collision with other nonmotor vehicle in nontraffic accident

Pedestrian on hoverboard injured in collision with other nonmotor vehicle in nontraffic accident

Pedestrian on segway injured in collision with other nonmotor vehicle in nontraffic accident

√x7ᵗʰ V06.09 Pedestrian with other conveyance injured in collision with other nonmotor vehicle in nontraffic accident

Pedestrian with baby stroller injured in collision with other nonmotor vehicle in nontraffic accident

Pedestrian on ice-skates injured in collision with other nonmotor vehicle in nontraffic accident

Pedestrian on nonmotorized scooter injured in collision with other nonmotor vehicle in nontraffic accident

Pedestrian on sled injured in collision with other nonmotor vehicle in nontraffic accident

Pedestrian on snowboard injured in collision with other nonmotor vehicle in nontraffic accident

Pedestrian on snow-skis injured in collision with other nonmotor vehicle in nontraffic accident

Pedestrian in wheelchair (powered) injured in collision with other nonmotor vehicle in nontraffic accident

Pedestrian in motorized mobility scooter injured in collision with other nonmotor vehicle in nontraffic accident

√5ᵗʰ V06.1 Pedestrian injured in collision with other nonmotor vehicle in traffic accident

√x7ᵗʰ V06.10 Pedestrian on foot injured in collision with other nonmotor vehicle in traffic accident

Pedestrian NOS injured in collision with other nonmotor vehicle in traffic accident

√x7ᵗʰ V06.11 Pedestrian on roller-skates injured in collision with other nonmotor vehicle in traffic accident

√x7ᵗʰ V06.12 Pedestrian on skateboard injured in collision with other nonmotor vehicle in traffic accident

√6ᵗʰ V06.13 Pedestrian on standing micro-mobility pedestrian conveyance injured in collision with other nonmotor vehicle in traffic accident

√7ᵗʰ V06.131 Pedestrian on standing electric scooter injured in collision with other nonmotor vehicle in traffic accident

√7ᵗʰ V06.138 Pedestrian on other standing micro-mobility pedestrian conveyance injured in collision with other nonmotor vehicle in traffic accident

Pedestrian on hoverboard injured in collision with other nonmotor vehicle in traffic accident

Pedestrian on segway injured in collision with other nonmotor vehicle in traffic accident

√x7ᵗʰ V06.19 Pedestrian with other conveyance injured in collision with other nonmotor vehicle in traffic accident

Pedestrian with baby stroller injured in collision with other nonmotor vehicle in nontraffic accident

Pedestrian on ice-skates injured in collision with other nonmotor vehicle in traffic accident

Pedestrian on nonmotorized scooter injured in collision with other nonmotor vehicle in traffic accident

Pedestrian on sled injured in collision with other nonmotor vehicle in traffic accident

Pedestrian on snowboard injured in collision with other nonmotor vehicle in traffic accident

Pedestrian on snow-skis injured in collision with other nonmotor vehicle in traffic accident

Pedestrian in wheelchair (powered) injured in collision with other nonmotor vehicle in traffic accident

Pedestrian in motorized mobility scooter injured in collision with other nonmotor vehicle in traffic accident

√5ᵗʰ V06.9 Pedestrian injured in collision with other nonmotor vehicle, unspecified whether traffic or nontraffic accident

√x7ᵗʰ V06.90 Pedestrian on foot injured in collision with other nonmotor vehicle, unspecified whether traffic or nontraffic accident

Pedestrian NOS injured in collision with other nonmotor vehicle, unspecified whether traffic or nontraffic accident

√x7ᵗʰ V06.91 Pedestrian on roller-skates injured in collision with other nonmotor vehicle, unspecified whether traffic or nontraffic accident

Chapter 20. External Causes of Morbidity

✓x7ᵗʰ V06.92 Pedestrian on skateboard injured in collision with other nonmotor vehicle, unspecified whether traffic or nontraffic accident

✓6ᵗʰ V06.93 Pedestrian on standing micro-mobility pedestrian conveyance injured in collision with other nonmotor vehicle, unspecified whether traffic or nontraffic accident

✓7ᵗʰ V06.931 Pedestrian on standing electric scooter injured in collision with other nonmotor vehicle, unspecified whether traffic or nontraffic accident

✓7ᵗʰ V06.938 Pedestrian on other standing micro-mobility pedestrian conveyance injured in collision with other nonmotor vehicle, unspecified whether traffic or nontraffic accident

Pedestrian on hoverboard injured in collision with other nonmotor, unspecified whether traffic or nontraffic accident

Pedestrian on segway injured in collision with other nonmotor vehicle, unspecified whether traffic or nontraffic accident

✓x7ᵗʰ V06.99 Pedestrian with other conveyance injured in collision with other nonmotor vehicle, unspecified whether traffic or nontraffic accident

Pedestrian with baby stroller injured in collision with other nonmotor vehicle, unspecified whether traffic or nontraffic accident

Pedestrian on ice-skates injured in collision with other nonmotor vehicle, unspecified whether traffic or nontraffic accident

Pedestrian on nonmotorized scooter injured in collision with other nonmotor vehicle, unspecified whether traffic or nontraffic accident

Pedestrian on sled injured in collision with other nonmotor vehicle, unspecified whether traffic or nontraffic accident

Pedestrian on snowboard injured in collision with other nonmotor vehicle, unspecified whether traffic or nontraffic accident

Pedestrian on snow-skis injured in collision with other nonmotor vehicle, unspecified whether traffic or nontraffic accident

Pedestrian in wheelchair (powered) injured in collision with other nonmotor vehicle, unspecified whether traffic or nontraffic accident

Pedestrian in motorized mobility scooter injured in collision with other nonmotorized vehicle, unspecified whether traffic or nontraffic accident

✓4ᵗʰ V09 Pedestrian injured in other and unspecified transport accidents

✓5ᵗʰ V09.0 Pedestrian injured in nontraffic accident involving other and unspecified motor vehicles

✓x7ᵗʰ V09.00 Pedestrian injured in nontraffic accident involving unspecified motor vehicles

✓x7ᵗʰ V09.01 Pedestrian injured in nontraffic accident involving military vehicle

✓x7ᵗʰ V09.09 Pedestrian injured in nontraffic accident involving other motor vehicles

Pedestrian injured in nontraffic accident by special vehicle

✓x7ᵗʰ V09.1 Pedestrian injured in unspecified nontraffic accident

✓5ᵗʰ V09.2 Pedestrian injured in traffic accident involving other and unspecified motor vehicles

✓x7ᵗʰ V09.20 Pedestrian injured in traffic accident involving unspecified motor vehicles

✓x7ᵗʰ V09.21 Pedestrian injured in traffic accident involving military vehicle

✓x7ᵗʰ V09.29 Pedestrian injured in traffic accident involving other motor vehicles

✓x7ᵗʰ V09.3 Pedestrian injured in unspecified traffic accident

✓x7ᵗʰ V09.9 Pedestrian injured in unspecified transport accident

Pedal cycle rider injured in transport accident (V10-V19)

INCLUDES any non-motorized vehicle, excluding an animal-drawn vehicle, or a sidecar or trailer attached to the pedal cycle

EXCLUDES 2 rupture of pedal cycle tire (W37.0)

The appropriate 7th character is to be added to each code from categories V10-V19.
A   initial encounter
D   subsequent encounter
S   sequela

✓4ᵗʰ V10 Pedal cycle rider injured in collision with pedestrian or animal

EXCLUDES 1 pedal cycle rider collision with animal-drawn vehicle or animal being ridden (V16.-)

✓x7ᵗʰ V10.0 Pedal cycle driver injured in collision with pedestrian or animal in nontraffic accident

✓x7ᵗʰ V10.1 Pedal cycle passenger injured in collision with pedestrian or animal in nontraffic accident

✓x7ᵗʰ V10.2 Unspecified pedal cyclist injured in collision with pedestrian or animal in nontraffic accident

✓x7ᵗʰ V10.3 Person boarding or alighting a pedal cycle injured in collision with pedestrian or animal

✓x7ᵗʰ V10.4 Pedal cycle driver injured in collision with pedestrian or animal in traffic accident

✓x7ᵗʰ V10.5 Pedal cycle passenger injured in collision with pedestrian or animal in traffic accident

✓x7ᵗʰ V10.9 Unspecified pedal cyclist injured in collision with pedestrian or animal in traffic accident

✓4ᵗʰ V11 Pedal cycle rider injured in collision with other pedal cycle

✓x7ᵗʰ V11.0 Pedal cycle driver injured in collision with other pedal cycle in nontraffic accident

✓x7ᵗʰ V11.1 Pedal cycle passenger injured in collision with other pedal cycle in nontraffic accident

✓x7ᵗʰ V11.2 Unspecified pedal cyclist injured in collision with other pedal cycle in nontraffic accident

✓x7ᵗʰ V11.3 Person boarding or alighting a pedal cycle injured in collision with other pedal cycle

✓x7ᵗʰ V11.4 Pedal cycle driver injured in collision with other pedal cycle in traffic accident

✓x7ᵗʰ V11.5 Pedal cycle passenger injured in collision with other pedal cycle in traffic accident

✓x7ᵗʰ V11.9 Unspecified pedal cyclist injured in collision with other pedal cycle in traffic accident

✓4ᵗʰ V12 Pedal cycle rider injured in collision with two- or three-wheeled motor vehicle

✓x7ᵗʰ V12.0 Pedal cycle driver injured in collision with two- or three-wheeled motor vehicle in nontraffic accident

✓x7ᵗʰ V12.1 Pedal cycle passenger injured in collision with two- or three-wheeled motor vehicle in nontraffic accident

✓x7ᵗʰ V12.2 Unspecified pedal cyclist injured in collision with two- or three-wheeled motor vehicle in nontraffic accident

✓x7ᵗʰ V12.3 Person boarding or alighting a pedal cycle injured in collision with two- or three-wheeled motor vehicle

✓x7ᵗʰ V12.4 Pedal cycle driver injured in collision with two- or three-wheeled motor vehicle in traffic accident

✓x7ᵗʰ V12.5 Pedal cycle passenger injured in collision with two- or three-wheeled motor vehicle in traffic accident

✓x7ᵗʰ V12.9 Unspecified pedal cyclist injured in collision with two- or three-wheeled motor vehicle in traffic accident

✓4ᵗʰ V13 Pedal cycle rider injured in collision with car, pick-up truck or van

✓x7ᵗʰ V13.0 Pedal cycle driver injured in collision with car, pick-up truck or van in nontraffic accident

✓x7ᵗʰ V13.1 Pedal cycle passenger injured in collision with car, pick-up truck or van in nontraffic accident

✓x7ᵗʰ V13.2 Unspecified pedal cyclist injured in collision with car, pick-up truck or van in nontraffic accident

✓x7ᵗʰ V13.3 Person boarding or alighting a pedal cycle injured in collision with car, pick-up truck or van

✓x7ᵗʰ V13.4 Pedal cycle driver injured in collision with car, pick-up truck or van in traffic accident

✓x7ᵗʰ V13.5 Pedal cycle passenger injured in collision with car, pick-up truck or van in traffic accident

✓x7ᵗʰ V13.9 Unspecified pedal cyclist injured in collision with car, pick-up truck or van in traffic accident

✓4ᵗʰ V14 Pedal cycle rider injured in collision with heavy transport vehicle or bus

EXCLUDES 1 pedal cycle rider injured in collision with military vehicle (V19.81)

✓x7ᵗʰ V14.0 Pedal cycle driver injured in collision with heavy transport vehicle or bus in nontraffic accident

HCC CMS-HCC   **Rx** Rx HCC   **ESR** ESRD HCC   **COM** Commercial HCC   **N** Newborn: 0   **P** Pediatric: 0-17   **M** Maternity: 9-64   **A** Adult: 15-124

1202   ICD-10-CM 2023

√x7ᵗʰ **V14.1** Pedal cycle passenger injured in collision with heavy transport vehicle or bus in nontraffic accident

√x7ᵗʰ **V14.2** Unspecified pedal cyclist injured in collision with heavy transport vehicle or bus in nontraffic accident

√x7ᵗʰ **V14.3** Person boarding or alighting a pedal cycle injured in collision with heavy transport vehicle or bus

√x7ᵗʰ **V14.4** Pedal cycle driver injured in collision with heavy transport vehicle or bus in traffic accident

√x7ᵗʰ **V14.5** Pedal cycle passenger injured in collision with heavy transport vehicle or bus in traffic accident

√x7ᵗʰ **V14.9** Unspecified pedal cyclist injured in collision with heavy transport vehicle or bus in traffic accident

√4ᵗʰ **V15** Pedal cycle rider injured in collision with railway train or railway vehicle

√x7ᵗʰ **V15.0** Pedal cycle driver injured in collision with railway train or railway vehicle in nontraffic accident

√x7ᵗʰ **V15.1** Pedal cycle passenger injured in collision with railway train or railway vehicle in nontraffic accident

√x7ᵗʰ **V15.2** Unspecified pedal cyclist injured in collision with railway train or railway vehicle in nontraffic accident

√x7ᵗʰ **V15.3** Person boarding or alighting a pedal cycle injured in collision with railway train or railway vehicle

√x7ᵗʰ **V15.4** Pedal cycle driver injured in collision with railway train or railway vehicle in traffic accident

√x7ᵗʰ **V15.5** Pedal cycle passenger injured in collision with railway train or railway vehicle in traffic accident

√x7ᵗʰ **V15.9** Unspecified pedal cyclist injured in collision with railway train or railway vehicle in traffic accident

√4ᵗʰ **V16** Pedal cycle rider injured in collision with other nonmotor vehicle

 INCLUDES collision with animal-drawn vehicle, animal being ridden, streetcar

√x7ᵗʰ **V16.0** Pedal cycle driver injured in collision with other nonmotor vehicle in nontraffic accident

√x7ᵗʰ **V16.1** Pedal cycle passenger injured in collision with other nonmotor vehicle in nontraffic accident

√x7ᵗʰ **V16.2** Unspecified pedal cyclist injured in collision with other nonmotor vehicle in nontraffic accident

√x7ᵗʰ **V16.3** Person boarding or alighting a pedal cycle injured in collision with other nonmotor vehicle in nontraffic accident

√x7ᵗʰ **V16.4** Pedal cycle driver injured in collision with other nonmotor vehicle in traffic accident

√x7ᵗʰ **V16.5** Pedal cycle passenger injured in collision with other nonmotor vehicle in traffic accident

√x7ᵗʰ **V16.9** Unspecified pedal cyclist injured in collision with other nonmotor vehicle in traffic accident

√4ᵗʰ **V17** Pedal cycle rider injured in collision with fixed or stationary object

√x7ᵗʰ **V17.0** Pedal cycle driver injured in collision with fixed or stationary object in nontraffic accident

√x7ᵗʰ **V17.1** Pedal cycle passenger injured in collision with fixed or stationary object in nontraffic accident

√x7ᵗʰ **V17.2** Unspecified pedal cyclist injured in collision with fixed or stationary object in nontraffic accident

√x7ᵗʰ **V17.3** Person boarding or alighting a pedal cycle injured in collision with fixed or stationary object

√x7ᵗʰ **V17.4** Pedal cycle driver injured in collision with fixed or stationary object in traffic accident

√x7ᵗʰ **V17.5** Pedal cycle passenger injured in collision with fixed or stationary object in traffic accident

√x7ᵗʰ **V17.9** Unspecified pedal cyclist injured in collision with fixed or stationary object in traffic accident

√4ᵗʰ **V18** Pedal cycle rider injured in noncollision transport accident

 INCLUDES fall or thrown from pedal cycle (without antecedent collision)
  overturning pedal cycle NOS
  overturning pedal cycle without collision

√x7ᵗʰ **V18.0** Pedal cycle driver injured in noncollision transport accident in nontraffic accident

√x7ᵗʰ **V18.1** Pedal cycle passenger injured in noncollision transport accident in nontraffic accident

√x7ᵗʰ **V18.2** Unspecified pedal cyclist injured in noncollision transport accident in nontraffic accident

√x7ᵗʰ **V18.3** Person boarding or alighting a pedal cycle injured in noncollision transport accident

√x7ᵗʰ **V18.4** Pedal cycle driver injured in noncollision transport accident in traffic accident

√x7ᵗʰ **V18.5** Pedal cycle passenger injured in noncollision transport accident in traffic accident

√x7ᵗʰ **V18.9** Unspecified pedal cyclist injured in noncollision transport accident in traffic accident

√4ᵗʰ **V19** Pedal cycle rider injured in other and unspecified transport accidents

√5ᵗʰ **V19.0** Pedal cycle driver injured in collision with other and unspecified motor vehicles in nontraffic accident

√x7ᵗʰ **V19.00** Pedal cycle driver injured in collision with unspecified motor vehicles in nontraffic accident

√x7ᵗʰ **V19.09** Pedal cycle driver injured in collision with other motor vehicles in nontraffic accident

√5ᵗʰ **V19.1** Pedal cycle passenger injured in collision with other and unspecified motor vehicles in nontraffic accident

√x7ᵗʰ **V19.10** Pedal cycle passenger injured in collision with unspecified motor vehicles in nontraffic accident

√x7ᵗʰ **V19.19** Pedal cycle passenger injured in collision with other motor vehicles in nontraffic accident

√5ᵗʰ **V19.2** Unspecified pedal cyclist injured in collision with other and unspecified motor vehicles in nontraffic accident

√x7ᵗʰ **V19.20** Unspecified pedal cyclist injured in collision with unspecified motor vehicles in nontraffic accident
  Pedal cycle collision NOS, nontraffic

√x7ᵗʰ **V19.29** Unspecified pedal cyclist injured in collision with other motor vehicles in nontraffic accident

√x7ᵗʰ **V19.3** Pedal cyclist (driver) (passenger) injured in unspecified nontraffic accident
  Pedal cycle accident NOS, nontraffic
  Pedal cyclist injured in nontraffic accident NOS

√5ᵗʰ **V19.4** Pedal cycle driver injured in collision with other and unspecified motor vehicles in traffic accident

√x7ᵗʰ **V19.40** Pedal cycle driver injured in collision with unspecified motor vehicles in traffic accident

√x7ᵗʰ **V19.49** Pedal cycle driver injured in collision with other motor vehicles in traffic accident

√5ᵗʰ **V19.5** Pedal cycle passenger injured in collision with other and unspecified motor vehicles in traffic accident

√x7ᵗʰ **V19.50** Pedal cycle passenger injured in collision with unspecified motor vehicles in traffic accident

√x7ᵗʰ **V19.59** Pedal cycle passenger injured in collision with other motor vehicles in traffic accident

√5ᵗʰ **V19.6** Unspecified pedal cyclist injured in collision with other and unspecified motor vehicles in traffic accident

√x7ᵗʰ **V19.60** Unspecified pedal cyclist injured in collision with unspecified motor vehicles in traffic accident
  Pedal cycle collision NOS (traffic)

√x7ᵗʰ **V19.69** Unspecified pedal cyclist injured in collision with other motor vehicles in traffic accident

√5ᵗʰ **V19.8** Pedal cyclist (driver) (passenger) injured in other specified transport accidents

√x7ᵗʰ **V19.81** Pedal cyclist (driver) (passenger) injured in transport accident with military vehicle

√x7ᵗʰ **V19.88** Pedal cyclist (driver) (passenger) injured in other specified transport accidents

√x7ᵗʰ **V19.9** Pedal cyclist (driver) (passenger) injured in unspecified traffic accident
  Pedal cycle accident NOS

Motorcycle rider injured in transport accident (V20-V29)

INCLUDES ▶electric bicycle◀
  ▶e-bike◀
  ▶e-bicycle◀
  moped
  motorcycle with sidecar
  motorized bicycle
  motor scooter

EXCLUDES 1 three-wheeled motor vehicle (V30-V39)

The appropriate 7th character is to be added to each code from categories V20-V29.
A initial encounter
D subsequent encounter
S sequela

√4ᵗʰ **V20** Motorcycle rider injured in collision with pedestrian or animal

 EXCLUDES 1 motorcycle rider collision with animal-drawn vehicle or animal being ridden (V26.-)

√5ᵗʰ **V20.0** Motorcycle driver injured in collision with pedestrian or animal in nontraffic accident

● √x7ᵗʰ **V20.01** Electric (assisted) bicycle driver injured in collision with pedestrian or animal in nontraffic accident

● √x7ᵗʰ **V20.09** Other motorcycle driver injured in collision with pedestrian or animal in nontraffic accident

✔ Additional Character Required √x7ᵗʰ Placeholder Alert Manifestation Unspecified Dx **Q** QPP **UPD** Unacceptable PDx

ICD-10-CM 2023   **1203**

✓5th **V20.1** Motorcycle passenger **injured in collision with pedestrian or animal** in nontraffic accident

- ✓x7th **V20.11** Electric (assisted) bicycle **passenger injured in collision with pedestrian or animal in nontraffic accident**
- ✓x7th **V20.19** Other motorcycle passenger injured in collision with pedestrian or animal in nontraffic accident

✓5th **V20.2** Unspecified motorcycle rider injured in collision with pedestrian or animal in nontraffic accident

- ✓x7th **V20.21** Unspecified electric (assisted) bicycle **rider injured in collision with pedestrian or animal in nontraffic accident**
- ✓x7th **V20.29** Unspecified rider of other motorcycle injured in collision with pedestrian or animal in nontraffic accident

✓5th **V20.3** Person boarding or alighting a motorcycle injured in collision with pedestrian or animal

- ✓x7th **V20.31** Person boarding or alighting an electric (assisted) bicycle injured in collision with pedestrian or animal
- ✓x7th **V20.39** Person boarding or alighting other motorcycle injured in collision with pedestrian or animal

✓5th **V20.4** Motorcycle driver **injured in collision with pedestrian or animal** in traffic accident

- ✓x7th **V20.41** Electric (assisted) bicycle **driver injured in collision with pedestrian or animal in traffic accident**
- ✓x7th **V20.49** Other motorcycle driver injured in collision with pedestrian or animal in traffic accident

✓5th **V20.5** Motorcycle passenger **injured in collision with pedestrian or animal** in traffic accident

- ✓x7th **V20.51** Electric (assisted) bicycle **passenger injured in collision with pedestrian or animal in traffic accident**
- ✓x7th **V20.59** Other motorcycle passenger injured in collision with pedestrian or animal in traffic accident

✓5th **V20.9** Unspecified motorcycle rider injured in collision with pedestrian or animal in traffic accident

- ✓x7th **V20.91** Unspecified electric (assisted) bicycle **rider injured in collision with pedestrian or animal in traffic accident**
- ✓x7th **V20.99** Unspecified rider of other motorcycle injured in collision with pedestrian or animal in traffic accident

✓4th **V21** Motorcycle rider injured in collision with pedal cycle

✓5th **V21.0** Motorcycle driver **injured in collision with pedal cycle** in nontraffic accident

- ✓x7th **V21.01** Electric (assisted) bicycle **driver injured in collision with pedal cycle in nontraffic accident**
- ✓x7th **V21.09** Other motorcycle driver injured in collision with pedal cycle in nontraffic accident

✓5th **V21.1** Motorcycle passenger **injured in collision with pedal cycle** in nontraffic accident

- ✓x7th **V21.11** Electric (assisted) bicycle **passenger injured in collision with pedal cycle in nontraffic accident**
- ✓x7th **V21.19** Other motorcycle passenger injured in collision with pedal cycle in nontraffic accident

✓5th **V21.2** Unspecified motorcycle rider injured in collision with pedal cycle in nontraffic accident

- ✓x7th **V21.21** Unspecified electric (assisted) bicycle **rider injured in collision with pedal cycle in nontraffic accident**
- ✓x7th **V21.29** Unspecified rider of other motorcycle injured in collision with pedal cycle in nontraffic accident

✓5th **V21.3** Person boarding or alighting a motorcycle injured in collision with pedal cycle

- ✓x7th **V21.31** Person boarding or alighting an electric (assisted) bicycle injured in collision with pedal cycle
- ✓x7th **V21.39** Person boarding or alighting other motorcycle injured in collision with pedal cycle

✓5th **V21.4** Motorcycle driver **injured in collision with pedal cycle** in traffic accident

- ✓x7th **V21.41** Electric (assisted) bicycle **driver injured in collision with pedal cycle in traffic accident**
- ✓x7th **V21.49** Other motorcycle driver injured in collision with pedal cycle in traffic accident

✓5th **V21.5** Motorcycle passenger **injured in collision with pedal cycle** in traffic accident

- ✓x7th **V21.51** Electric (assisted) bicycle **passenger injured in collision with pedal cycle in traffic accident**
- ✓x7th **V21.59** Other motorcycle passenger injured in collision with pedal cycle in traffic accident

✓5th **V21.9** Unspecified motorcycle rider injured in collision with pedal cycle in traffic accident

- ✓x7th **V21.91** Unspecified electric (assisted) bicycle **rider injured in collision with pedal cycle in traffic accident**
- ✓x7th **V21.99** Unspecified rider of other motorcycle injured in collision with pedal cycle in traffic accident

✓4th **V22** Motorcycle rider injured in collision with two- or three-wheeled motor vehicle

✓5th **V22.0** Motorcycle driver **injured in collision with two- or three-wheeled motor vehicle** in nontraffic accident

- ✓x7th **V22.01** Electric (assisted) bicycle **driver injured in collision with two- or three-wheeled motor vehicle in nontraffic accident**
- ✓x7th **V22.09** Other motorcycle driver injured in collision with two- or three-wheeled motor vehicle in nontraffic accident

✓5th **V22.1** Motorcycle passenger **injured in collision with two- or three-wheeled motor vehicle** in nontraffic accident

- ✓x7th **V22.11** Electric (assisted) bicycle **passenger injured in collision with two- or three-wheeled motor vehicle in nontraffic accident**
- ✓x7th **V22.19** Other motorcycle passenger injured in collision with two- or three-wheeled motor vehicle in nontraffic accident

✓5th **V22.2** Unspecified motorcycle rider injured in collision with two- or three-wheeled motor vehicle in nontraffic accident

- ✓x7th **V22.21** Unspecified electric (assisted) bicycle **rider injured in collision with two- or three-wheeled motor vehicle in nontraffic accident**
- ✓x7th **V22.29** Unspecified rider of other motorcycle injured in collision with two- or three-wheeled motor vehicle in nontraffic accident

✓5th **V22.3** Person boarding or alighting a motorcycle injured in collision with two- or three-wheeled motor vehicle

- ✓x7th **V22.31** Person boarding or alighting an electric (assisted) bicycle injured in collision with two- or three-wheeled motor vehicle
- ✓x7th **V22.39** Person boarding or alighting other motorcycle injured in collision with two- or three-wheeled motor vehicle

✓5th **V22.4** Motorcycle driver **injured in collision with two- or three-wheeled motor vehicle** in traffic accident

- ✓x7th **V22.41** Electric (assisted) bicycle **driver injured in collision with two- or three-wheeled motor vehicle in traffic accident**
- ✓x7th **V22.49** Other motorcycle driver injured in collision with two- or three-wheeled motor vehicle in traffic accident

✓5th **V22.5** Motorcycle passenger **injured in collision with two- or three-wheeled motor vehicle** in traffic accident

- ✓x7th **V22.51** Electric (assisted) bicycle **passenger injured in collision with two- or three-wheeled motor vehicle in traffic accident**
- ✓x7th **V22.59** Other motorcycle passenger injured in collision with two- or three-wheeled motor vehicle in traffic accident

✓5th **V22.9** Unspecified motorcycle rider injured in collision with two- or three-wheeled motor vehicle in traffic accident

- ✓x7th **V22.91** Unspecified electric (assisted) bicycle **rider injured in collision with two- or three-wheeled motor vehicle in traffic accident**
- ✓x7th **V22.99** Unspecified rider of other motorcycle injured in collision with two- or three-wheeled motor vehicle in traffic accident

✓4th **V23** Motorcycle rider injured in collision with car, pick-up truck or van

✓5th **V23.0** Motorcycle driver **injured in collision with car, pick-up truck or van** in nontraffic accident

- ✓x7th **V23.01** Electric (assisted) bicycle **driver injured in collision with car, pick-up truck or van in nontraffic accident**
- ✓x7th **V23.09** Other motorcycle driver injured in collision with car, pick-up truck or van in nontraffic accident

✓5th **V23.1** Motorcycle passenger **injured in collision with car, pick-up truck or van** in nontraffic accident

- ✓x7th **V23.11** Electric (assisted) bicycle **passenger injured in collision with car, pick-up truck or van in nontraffic accident**
- ✓x7th **V23.19** Other motorcycle passenger injured in collision with car, pick-up truck or van in nontraffic accident

√5ᵗʰ **V23.2** Unspecified motorcycle rider injured in collision with car, pick-up truck or van in nontraffic accident

- √x7ᵗʰ **V23.21** Unspecified electric (assisted) bicycle rider injured in collision with car, pick-up truck or van in nontraffic accident
- √x7ᵗʰ **V23.29** Unspecified rider of other motorcycle injured in collision with car, pick-up truck or van in nontraffic accident

√5ᵗʰ **V23.3** Person boarding or alighting a motorcycle injured in collision with car, pick-up truck or van

- √x7ᵗʰ **V23.31** Person boarding or alighting an electric (assisted) bicycle injured in collision with car, pick-up truck or van
- √x7ᵗʰ **V23.39** Person boarding or alighting other motorcycle injured in collision with car, pick-up truck or van

√5ᵗʰ **V23.4** Motorcycle driver injured in collision with car, pick-up truck or van in traffic accident

- √x7ᵗʰ **V23.41** Electric (assisted) bicycle driver injured in collision with car, pick-up truck or van in traffic accident
- √x7ᵗʰ **V23.49** Other motorcycle driver injured in collision with car, pick-up truck or van in traffic accident

√5ᵗʰ **V23.5** Motorcycle passenger injured in collision with car, pick-up truck or van in traffic accident

- √x7ᵗʰ **V23.51** Electric (assisted) bicycle passenger injured in collision with car, pick-up truck or van in traffic accident
- √x7ᵗʰ **V23.59** Other motorcycle passenger injured in collision with car, pick-up truck or van in traffic accident

√5ᵗʰ **V23.9** Unspecified motorcycle rider injured in collision with car, pick-up truck or van in traffic accident

- √x7ᵗʰ **V23.91** Unspecified electric (assisted) bicycle rider injured in collision with car, pick-up truck or van in traffic accident
- √x7ᵗʰ **V23.99** Unspecified rider of other motorcycle injured in collision with car, pick-up truck or van in traffic accident

√4ᵗʰ **V24 Motorcycle rider injured in collision with heavy transport vehicle or bus**

EXCLUDES 1   motorcycle rider injured in collision with military vehicle ▶(V29.818)◀

√6ᵗʰ **V24.0** Motorcycle driver injured in collision with heavy transport vehicle or bus in nontraffic accident

- √x7ᵗʰ **V24.01** Electric (assisted) bicycle driver injured in collision with heavy transport vehicle or bus in nontraffic accident
- √x7ᵗʰ **V24.09** Other motorcycle driver injured in collision with heavy transport vehicle or bus in nontraffic accident

√5ᵗʰ **V24.1** Motorcycle passenger injured in collision with heavy transport vehicle or bus in nontraffic accident

- √x7ᵗʰ **V24.11** Electric (assisted) bicycle passenger injured in collision with heavy transport vehicle or bus in nontraffic accident
- √x7ᵗʰ **V24.19** Other motorcycle passenger injured in collision with heavy transport vehicle or bus in nontraffic accident

√5ᵗʰ **V24.2** Unspecified motorcycle rider injured in collision with heavy transport vehicle or bus in nontraffic accident

- √x7ᵗʰ **V24.21** Unspecified electric (assisted) bicycle rider injured in collision with heavy transport vehicle or bus in nontraffic accident
- √x7ᵗʰ **V24.29** Unspecified rider of other motorcycle injured in collision with heavy transport vehicle or bus in nontraffic accident

√5ᵗʰ **V24.3** Person boarding or alighting a motorcycle injured in collision with heavy transport vehicle or bus

- √x7ᵗʰ **V24.31** Person boarding or alighting an electric (assisted) bicycle injured in collision with heavy transport vehicle or bus
- √x7ᵗʰ **V24.39** Person boarding or alighting other motorcycle injured in collision with heavy transport vehicle or bus

√5ᵗʰ **V24.4** Motorcycle driver injured in collision with heavy transport vehicle or bus in traffic accident

- √x7ᵗʰ **V24.41** Electric (assisted) bicycle driver injured in collision with heavy transport vehicle or bus in traffic accident
- √x7ᵗʰ **V24.49** Other motorcycle driver injured in collision with heavy transport vehicle or bus in traffic accident

√5ᵗʰ **V24.5** Motorcycle passenger injured in collision with heavy transport vehicle or bus in traffic accident

- √x7ᵗʰ **V24.51** Electric (assisted) bicycle passenger injured in collision with heavy transport vehicle or bus in traffic accident

- √x7ᵗʰ **V24.59** Other motorcycle passenger injured in collision with heavy transport vehicle or bus in traffic accident

√5ᵗʰ **V24.9** Unspecified motorcycle rider injured in collision with heavy transport vehicle or bus in traffic accident

- √x7ᵗʰ **V24.91** Unspecified electric (assisted) bicycle rider injured in collision with heavy transport vehicle or bus in traffic accident
- √x7ᵗʰ **V24.99** Unspecified rider of other motorcycle injured in collision with heavy transport vehicle or bus in traffic accident

√4ᵗʰ **V25 Motorcycle rider injured in collision with railway train or railway vehicle**

√5ᵗʰ **V25.0** Motorcycle driver injured in collision with railway train or railway vehicle in nontraffic accident

- √x7ᵗʰ **V25.01** Electric (assisted) bicycle driver injured in collision with railway train or railway vehicle in nontraffic accident
- √x7ᵗʰ **V25.09** Other motorcycle driver injured in collision with railway train or railway vehicle in nontraffic accident

√5ᵗʰ **V25.1** Motorcycle passenger injured in collision with railway train or railway vehicle in nontraffic accident

- √x7ᵗʰ **V25.11** Electric (assisted) bicycle passenger injured in collision with railway train or railway vehicle in nontraffic accident
- √x7ᵗʰ **V25.19** Other motorcycle passenger injured in collision with railway train or railway vehicle in nontraffic accident

√5ᵗʰ **V25.2** Unspecified motorcycle rider injured in collision with railway train or railway vehicle in nontraffic accident

- √x7ᵗʰ **V25.21** Unspecified electric (assisted) bicycle rider injured in collision with railway train or railway vehicle in nontraffic accident
- √x7ᵗʰ **V25.29** Unspecified rider of other motorcycle injured in collision with railway train or railway vehicle in nontraffic accident

√5ᵗʰ **V25.3** Person boarding or alighting a motorcycle injured in collision with railway train or railway vehicle

- √x7ᵗʰ **V25.31** Person boarding or alighting an electric (assisted) bicycle injured in collision with railway train or railway vehicle
- √x7ᵗʰ **V25.39** Person boarding or alighting other motorcycle injured in collision with railway train or railway vehicle

√5ᵗʰ **V25.4** Motorcycle driver injured in collision with railway train or railway vehicle in traffic accident

- √x7ᵗʰ **V25.41** Electric (assisted) bicycle driver injured in collision with railway train or railway vehicle in traffic accident
- √x7ᵗʰ **V25.49** Other motorcycle driver injured in collision with railway train or railway vehicle in traffic accident

√5ᵗʰ **V25.5** Motorcycle passenger injured in collision with railway train or railway vehicle in traffic accident

- √x7ᵗʰ **V25.51** Electric (assisted) bicycle passenger injured in collision with railway train or railway vehicle in traffic accident
- √x7ᵗʰ **V25.59** Other motorcycle passenger injured in collision with railway train or railway vehicle in traffic accident

√5ᵗʰ **V25.9** Unspecified motorcycle rider injured in collision with railway train or railway vehicle in traffic accident

- √x7ᵗʰ **V25.91** Unspecified electric (assisted) bicycle rider injured in collision with railway train or railway vehicle in traffic accident
- √x7ᵗʰ **V25.99** Unspecified rider of other motorcycle injured in collision with railway train or railway vehicle in traffic accident

√4ᵗʰ **V26 Motorcycle rider injured in collision with other nonmotor vehicle**

INCLUDES   collision with animal-drawn vehicle, animal being ridden, streetcar

√5ᵗʰ **V26.0** Motorcycle driver injured in collision with other nonmotor vehicle in nontraffic accident

- √x7ᵗʰ **V26.01** Electric (assisted) bicycle driver injured in collision with other nonmotor vehicle in nontraffic accident
- √x7ᵗʰ **V26.09** Other motorcycle driver injured in collision with other nonmotor vehicle in nontraffic accident

√5ᵗʰ **V26.1** Motorcycle passenger injured in collision with other nonmotor vehicle in nontraffic accident

- √x7ᵗʰ **V26.11** Electric (assisted) bicycle passenger injured in collision with other nonmotor vehicle in nontraffic accident

Chapter 20. External Causes of Morbidity

V26.19–V29.Ø98

- ✓x7ᵗʰ **V26.19** Other motorcycle passenger injured in collision with other nonmotor vehicle in nontraffic accident
- ✓5ᵗʰ **V26.2** Unspecified motorcycle rider injured in collision with other nonmotor vehicle in nontraffic accident
  - ✓x7ᵗʰ **V26.21** Unspecified electric (assisted) bicycle rider injured in collision with other nonmotor vehicle in nontraffic accident
  - ✓x7ᵗʰ **V26.29** Unspecified rider of other motorcycle injured in collision with other nonmotor vehicle in nontraffic accident
- ✓5ᵗʰ **V26.3** Person boarding or alighting a motorcycle injured in collision with other nonmotor vehicle
  - ✓x7ᵗʰ **V26.31** Person boarding or alighting an electric (assisted) bicycle injured in collision with other nonmotor vehicle
  - ✓x7ᵗʰ **V26.39** Person boarding or alighting other motorcycle injured in collision with other nonmotor vehicle
- ✓5ᵗʰ **V26.4** Motorcycle driver injured in collision with other nonmotor vehicle in traffic accident
  - ✓x7ᵗʰ **V26.41** Electric (assisted) bicycle driver injured in collision with other nonmotor vehicle in traffic accident
  - ✓x7ᵗʰ **V26.49** Other motorcycle driver injured in collision with other nonmotor vehicle in traffic accident
- ✓5ᵗʰ **V26.5** Motorcycle passenger injured in collision with other nonmotor vehicle in traffic accident
  - ✓x7ᵗʰ **V26.51** Electric (assisted) bicycle passenger injured in collision with other nonmotor vehicle in traffic accident
  - ✓x7ᵗʰ **V26.59** Other motorcycle passenger injured in collision with other nonmotor vehicle in traffic accident
- ✓5ᵗʰ **V26.9** Unspecified motorcycle rider injured in collision with other nonmotor vehicle in traffic accident
  - ✓x7ᵗʰ **V26.91** Unspecified electric (assisted) bicycle rider injured in collision with other nonmotor vehicle in traffic accident
  - ✓x7ᵗʰ **V26.99** Unspecified rider of other motorcycle injured in collision with other nonmotor vehicle in traffic accident

✓4ᵗʰ **V27 Motorcycle rider injured in collision with fixed or stationary object**
- ✓5ᵗʰ **V27.Ø** Motorcycle driver injured in collision with fixed or stationary object in nontraffic accident
  - ✓x7ᵗʰ **V27.Ø1** Electric (assisted) bicycle driver injured in collision with fixed or stationary object in nontraffic accident
  - ✓x7ᵗʰ **V27.Ø9** Other motorcycle driver injured in collision with fixed or stationary object in nontraffic accident
- ✓5ᵗʰ **V27.1** Motorcycle passenger injured in collision with fixed or stationary object in nontraffic accident
  - ✓x7ᵗʰ **V27.11** Electric (assisted) bicycle passenger injured in collision with fixed or stationary object in nontraffic accident
  - ✓x7ᵗʰ **V27.19** Other motorcycle passenger injured in collision with fixed or stationary object in nontraffic accident
- ✓5ᵗʰ **V27.2** Unspecified motorcycle rider injured in collision with fixed or stationary object in nontraffic accident
  - ✓x7ᵗʰ **V27.21** Unspecified electric (assisted) bicycle rider injured in collision with fixed or stationary object in nontraffic accident
  - ✓x7ᵗʰ **V27.29** Unspecified rider of other motorcycle injured in collision with fixed or stationary object in nontraffic accident
- ✓5ᵗʰ **V27.3** Person boarding or alighting a motorcycle injured in collision with fixed or stationary object
  - ✓x7ᵗʰ **V27.31** Person boarding or alighting an electric (assisted) bicycle injured in collision with fixed or stationary object
  - ✓x7ᵗʰ **V27.39** Person boarding or alighting other motorcycle injured in collision with fixed or stationary object
- ✓5ᵗʰ **V27.4** Motorcycle driver injured in collision with fixed or stationary object in traffic accident
  - ✓x7ᵗʰ **V27.41** Electric (assisted) bicycle driver injured in collision with fixed or stationary object in traffic accident
  - ✓x7ᵗʰ **V27.49** Other motorcycle driver injured in collision with fixed or stationary object in traffic accident
- ✓5ᵗʰ **V27.5** Motorcycle passenger injured in collision with fixed or stationary object in traffic accident
  - ✓x7ᵗʰ **V27.51** Electric (assisted) bicycle passenger injured in collision with fixed or stationary object in traffic accident
  - ✓x7ᵗʰ **V27.59** Other motorcycle passenger injured in collision with fixed or stationary object in traffic accident

- ✓5ᵗʰ **V27.9** Unspecified motorcycle rider injured in collision with fixed or stationary object in traffic accident
  - ✓x7ᵗʰ **V27.91** Unspecified electric (assisted) bicycle rider injured in collision with fixed or stationary object in traffic accident
  - ✓x7ᵗʰ **V27.99** Unspecified rider of other motorcycle injured in collision with fixed or stationary object in traffic accident

✓4ᵗʰ **V28 Motorcycle rider injured in noncollision transport accident**
> **INCLUDES** fall or thrown from motorcycle (without antecedent collision)
> overturning motorcycle NOS
> overturning motorcycle without collision

- ✓5ᵗʰ **V28.Ø** Motorcycle driver injured in noncollision transport accident in nontraffic accident
  - ✓x7ᵗʰ **V28.Ø1** Electric (assisted) bicycle driver injured in noncollision transport accident in nontraffic accident
  - ✓x7ᵗʰ **V28.Ø9** Other motorcycle driver injured in noncollision transport accident in nontraffic accident
- ✓5ᵗʰ **V28.1** Motorcycle passenger injured in noncollision transport accident in nontraffic accident
  - ✓x7ᵗʰ **V28.11** Electric (assisted) bicycle passenger injured in noncollision transport accident in nontraffic accident
  - ✓x7ᵗʰ **V28.19** Other motorcycle passenger injured in noncollision transport accident in nontraffic accident
- ✓5ᵗʰ **V28.2** Unspecified motorcycle rider injured in noncollision transport accident in nontraffic accident
  - ✓x7ᵗʰ **V28.21** Unspecified electric (assisted) bicycle rider injured in noncollision transport accident in nontraffic accident
  - ✓x7ᵗʰ **V28.29** Unspecified rider of other motorcycle injured in noncollision transport accident in nontraffic accident
- ✓5ᵗʰ **V28.3** Person boarding or alighting a motorcycle injured in noncollision transport accident
  - ✓x7ᵗʰ **V28.31** Person boarding or alighting an electric (assisted) bicycle injured in noncollision transport accident
  - ✓x7ᵗʰ **V28.39** Person boarding or alighting other motorcycle injured in noncollision transport accident
- ✓5ᵗʰ **V28.4** Motorcycle driver injured in noncollision transport accident in traffic accident
  - ✓x7ᵗʰ **V28.41** Electric (assisted) bicycle driver injured in noncollision transport accident in traffic accident
  - ✓x7ᵗʰ **V28.49** Other motorcycle driver injured in noncollision transport accident in traffic accident
- ✓5ᵗʰ **V28.5** Motorcycle passenger injured in noncollision transport accident in traffic accident
  - ✓x7ᵗʰ **V28.51** Electric (assisted) bicycle passenger injured in noncollision transport accident in traffic accident
  - ✓x7ᵗʰ **V28.59** Other motorcycle passenger injured in noncollision transport accident in traffic accident
- ✓5ᵗʰ **V28.9** Unspecified motorcycle rider injured in noncollision transport accident in traffic accident
  - ✓x7ᵗʰ **V28.91** Unspecified electric (assisted) bicycle rider injured in noncollision transport accident in traffic accident
  - ✓x7ᵗʰ **V28.99** Unspecified rider of other motorcycle injured in noncollision transport accident in traffic accident

✓4ᵗʰ **V29 Motorcycle rider injured in other and unspecified transport accidents**
- ✓5ᵗʰ **V29.Ø** Motorcycle driver injured in collision with other and unspecified motor vehicles in nontraffic accident
  - ✓6ᵗʰ **V29.ØØ** Motorcycle driver injured in collision with unspecified motor vehicles in nontraffic accident
    - ✓7ᵗʰ **V29.ØØ1** Electric (assisted) bicycle driver injured in collision with unspecified motor vehicles in nontraffic accident
    - ✓7ᵗʰ **V29.ØØ8** Other motorcycle driver injured in collision with unspecified motor vehicles in nontraffic accident
  - ✓6ᵗʰ **V29.Ø9** Motorcycle driver injured in collision with other motor vehicles in nontraffic accident
    - ✓7ᵗʰ **V29.Ø91** Electric (assisted) bicycle driver injured in collision with other motor vehicles in nontraffic accident
    - ✓7ᵗʰ **V29.Ø98** Other motorcycle driver injured in collision with other motor vehicles in nontraffic accident

HCC CMS-HCC   **Rx** Rx HCC   **ESR** ESRD HCC   **COM** Commercial HCC   **N** Newborn: 0   **P** Pediatric: 0-17   **M** Maternity: 9-64   **A** Adult: 15-124

1206

ICD-10-CM 2023

☑5ᵗʰ **V29.1** Motorcycle passenger injured in collision with other and unspecified motor vehicles in nontraffic accident

  ☑6ᵗʰ **V29.10** Motorcycle passenger injured in collision with unspecified motor vehicles in nontraffic accident

●   ☑7ᵗʰ **V29.101** Electric (assisted) bicycle passenger injured in collision with unspecified motor vehicles in nontraffic accident

●   ☑7ᵗʰ **V29.108** Other motorcycle passenger injured in collision with unspecified motor vehicles in nontraffic accident

  ☑6ᵗʰ **V29.19** Motorcycle passenger injured in collision with other motor vehicles in nontraffic accident

●   ☑7ᵗʰ **V29.191** Electric (assisted) bicycle passenger injured in collision with other motor vehicles in nontraffic accident

    ☑7ᵗʰ **V29.198** Other motorcycle passenger injured in collision with other motor vehicles in nontraffic accident

☑5ᵗʰ **V29.2** Unspecified motorcycle rider injured in collision with other and unspecified motor vehicles in nontraffic accident

  ☑6ᵗʰ **V29.20** Unspecified motorcycle rider injured in collision with unspecified motor vehicles in nontraffic accident

    Motorcycle collision NOS, nontraffic

●   ☑7ᵗʰ **V29.201** Unspecified electric (assisted) bicycle rider injured in collision with unspecified motor vehicles in nontraffic accident

●   ☑7ᵗʰ **V29.208** Unspecified rider of other motorcycle injured in collision with unspecified motor vehicles in nontraffic accident

    Motorcycle collision NOS, nontraffic

  ☑6ᵗʰ **V29.29** Unspecified motorcycle rider injured in collision with other motor vehicles in nontraffic accident

●   ☑7ᵗʰ **V29.291** Unspecified electric (assisted) bicycle rider injured in collision with other motor vehicles in nontraffic accident

●   ☑7ᵗʰ **V29.298** Unspecified rider of other motorcycle injured in collision with other motor vehicles in nontraffic accident

☑5ᵗʰ **V29.3** Motorcycle rider (driver) (passenger) injured in unspecified nontraffic accident

    Motorcycle accident NOS, nontraffic

    Motorcycle rider injured in nontraffic accident NOS

●   ☑×7ᵗʰ **V29.31** Electric (assisted) bicycle (driver) (passenger) injured in unspecified nontraffic accident

●   ☑×7ᵗʰ **V29.39** Other motorcycle (driver) (passenger) injured in unspecified nontraffic accident

    Motorcycle accident NOS, nontraffic

    Motorcycle rider injured in nontraffic accident NOS

☑5ᵗʰ **V29.4** Motorcycle driver injured in collision with other and unspecified motor vehicles in traffic accident

  ☑6ᵗʰ **V29.40** Motorcycle driver injured in collision with unspecified motor vehicles in traffic accident

●   ☑7ᵗʰ **V29.401** Electric (assisted) bicycle driver injured in collision with unspecified motor vehicles in traffic accident

●   ☑7ᵗʰ **V29.408** Other motorcycle driver injured in collision with unspecified motor vehicles in traffic accident

  ☑6ᵗʰ **V29.49** Motorcycle driver injured in collision with other motor vehicles in traffic accident

●   ☑7ᵗʰ **V29.491** Electric (assisted) bicycle driver injured in collision with other motor vehicles in traffic accident

●   ☑7ᵗʰ **V29.498** Other motorcycle driver injured in collision with other motor vehicles in traffic accident

☑5ᵗʰ **V29.5** Motorcycle passenger injured in collision with other and unspecified motor vehicles in traffic accident

  ☑6ᵗʰ **V29.50** Motorcycle passenger injured in collision with unspecified motor vehicles in traffic accident

●   ☑7ᵗʰ **V29.501** Electric (assisted) bicycle passenger injured in collision with unspecified motor vehicles in traffic accident

●   ☑7ᵗʰ **V29.508** Other motorcycle passenger injured in collision with unspecified motor vehicles in traffic accident

  ☑6ᵗʰ **V29.59** Motorcycle passenger injured in collision with other motor vehicles in traffic accident

●   ☑7ᵗʰ **V29.591** Electric (assisted) bicycle passenger injured in collision with other motor vehicles in traffic accident

●   ☑7ᵗʰ **V29.598** Other motorcycle passenger injured in collision with other motor vehicles in traffic accident

☑5ᵗʰ **V29.6** Unspecified motorcycle rider injured in collision with other and unspecified motor vehicles in traffic accident

  ☑6ᵗʰ **V29.60** Unspecified motorcycle rider injured in collision with unspecified motor vehicles in traffic accident

    Motorcycle collision NOS (traffic)

●   ☑7ᵗʰ **V29.601** Unspecified electric (assisted) bicycle rider injured in collision with unspecified motor vehicles in traffic accident

●   ☑7ᵗʰ **V29.608** Unspecified rider of other motorcycle injured in collision with unspecified motor vehicles in traffic accident

    Motorcycle collision NOS (traffic)

  ☑6ᵗʰ **V29.69** Unspecified motorcycle rider injured in collision with other motor vehicles in traffic accident

●   ☑7ᵗʰ **V29.691** Unspecified electric (assisted) bicycle rider injured in collision with other motor vehicles in traffic accident

●   ☑7ᵗʰ **V29.698** Unspecified rider of other motorcycle injured in collision with other motor vehicles in traffic accident

☑5ᵗʰ **V29.8** Motorcycle rider (driver) (passenger) injured in other specified transport accidents

  ☑6ᵗʰ **V29.81** Motorcycle rider (driver) (passenger) injured in transport accident with military vehicle

    ☑7ᵗʰ **V29.811** Electric (assisted) bicycle rider (driver) (passenger) injured in transport accident with military vehicle

    ☑7ᵗʰ **V29.818** Rider (driver) (passenger) of other motorcycle injured in transport accident with military vehicle

  ☑6ᵗʰ **V29.88** Motorcycle rider (driver) (passenger) injured in other specified transport accidents

●   ☑7ᵗʰ **V29.881** Electric (assisted) bicycle rider (driver) (passenger) injured in other specified transport accidents

●   ☑7ᵗʰ **V29.888** Rider (driver) (passenger) of other motorcycle injured in other specified transport accidents

☑5ᵗʰ **V29.9** Motorcycle rider (driver) (passenger) injured in unspecified traffic accident

    Motorcycle accident NOS

●   ☑×7ᵗʰ **V29.91** Electric (assisted) bicycle rider (driver) (passenger) injured in unspecified traffic accident

  ☑×7ᵗʰ **V29.99** Rider (driver) (passenger) of other motorcycle injured in unspecified traffic accident

    Motorcycle accident NOS

Occupant of three-wheeled motor vehicle injured in transport accident (V30-V39)

INCLUDES   motorized tricycle
               motorized rickshaw
               three-wheeled motor car

EXCLUDES 1   *all-terrain vehicles (V86.-)*
               motorcycle with sidecar (V20-V29)
               vehicle designed primarily for off-road use (V86.-)

The appropriate 7th character is to be added to each code from categories V30-V39.
A   initial encounter
D   subsequent encounter
S   sequela

☑4ᵗʰ **V30** Occupant of three-wheeled motor vehicle injured in collision with pedestrian or animal

    EXCLUDES 1   *three-wheeled motor vehicle collision with animal-drawn vehicle or animal being ridden (V36.-)*

  ☑×7ᵗʰ **V30.0** Driver of three-wheeled motor vehicle injured in collision with pedestrian or animal in nontraffic accident

  ☑×7ᵗʰ **V30.1** Passenger in three-wheeled motor vehicle injured in collision with pedestrian or animal in nontraffic accident

  ☑×7ᵗʰ **V30.2** Person on outside of three-wheeled motor vehicle injured in collision with pedestrian or animal in nontraffic accident

  ☑×7ᵗʰ **V30.3** Unspecified occupant of three-wheeled motor vehicle injured in collision with pedestrian or animal in nontraffic accident

  ☑×7ᵗʰ **V30.4** Person boarding or alighting a three-wheeled motor vehicle injured in collision with pedestrian or animal

  ☑×7ᵗʰ **V30.5** Driver of three-wheeled motor vehicle injured in collision with pedestrian or animal in traffic accident

  ☑×7ᵗʰ **V30.6** Passenger in three-wheeled motor vehicle injured in collision with pedestrian or animal in traffic accident

---

☑ Additional Character Required   ☑×7ᵗʰ Placeholder Alert   Manifestation   Unspecified Dx   🆀 QPP   UPD Unacceptable PDx

√x7ᵗʰ **V30.7** Person on outside of three-wheeled motor vehicle injured in collision with pedestrian or animal in traffic accident

√x7ᵗʰ **V30.9** Unspecified occupant of three-wheeled motor vehicle injured in collision with pedestrian or animal in traffic accident

✓4ᵗʰ **V31** Occupant of three-wheeled motor vehicle injured in collision with pedal cycle

√x7ᵗʰ **V31.0** Driver of three-wheeled motor vehicle injured in collision with pedal cycle in nontraffic accident

√x7ᵗʰ **V31.1** Passenger in three-wheeled motor vehicle injured in collision with pedal cycle in nontraffic accident

√x7ᵗʰ **V31.2** Person on outside of three-wheeled motor vehicle injured in collision with pedal cycle in nontraffic accident

√x7ᵗʰ **V31.3** Unspecified occupant of three-wheeled motor vehicle injured in collision with pedal cycle in nontraffic accident

√x7ᵗʰ **V31.4** Person boarding or alighting a three-wheeled motor vehicle injured in collision with pedal cycle

√x7ᵗʰ **V31.5** Driver of three-wheeled motor vehicle injured in collision with pedal cycle in traffic accident

√x7ᵗʰ **V31.6** Passenger in three-wheeled motor vehicle injured in collision with pedal cycle in traffic accident

√x7ᵗʰ **V31.7** Person on outside of three-wheeled motor vehicle injured in collision with pedal cycle in traffic accident

√x7ᵗʰ **V31.9** Unspecified occupant of three-wheeled motor vehicle injured in collision with pedal cycle in traffic accident

✓4ᵗʰ **V32** Occupant of three-wheeled motor vehicle injured in collision with two- or three-wheeled motor vehicle

√x7ᵗʰ **V32.0** Driver of three-wheeled motor vehicle injured in collision with two- or three-wheeled motor vehicle in nontraffic accident

√x7ᵗʰ **V32.1** Passenger in three-wheeled motor vehicle injured in collision with two- or three-wheeled motor vehicle in nontraffic accident

√x7ᵗʰ **V32.2** Person on outside of three-wheeled motor vehicle injured in collision with two- or three-wheeled motor vehicle in nontraffic accident

√x7ᵗʰ **V32.3** Unspecified occupant of three-wheeled motor vehicle injured in collision with two- or three-wheeled motor vehicle in nontraffic accident

√x7ᵗʰ **V32.4** Person boarding or alighting a three-wheeled motor vehicle injured in collision with two- or three-wheeled motor vehicle

√x7ᵗʰ **V32.5** Driver of three-wheeled motor vehicle injured in collision with two- or three-wheeled motor vehicle in traffic accident

√x7ᵗʰ **V32.6** Passenger in three-wheeled motor vehicle injured in collision with two- or three-wheeled motor vehicle in traffic accident

√x7ᵗʰ **V32.7** Person on outside of three-wheeled motor vehicle injured in collision with two- or three-wheeled motor vehicle in traffic accident

√x7ᵗʰ **V32.9** Unspecified occupant of three-wheeled motor vehicle injured in collision with two- or three-wheeled motor vehicle in traffic accident

✓4ᵗʰ **V33** Occupant of three-wheeled motor vehicle injured in collision with car, pick-up truck or van

√x7ᵗʰ **V33.0** Driver of three-wheeled motor vehicle injured in collision with car, pick-up truck or van in nontraffic accident

√x7ᵗʰ **V33.1** Passenger in three-wheeled motor vehicle injured in collision with car, pick-up truck or van in nontraffic accident

√x7ᵗʰ **V33.2** Person on outside of three-wheeled motor vehicle injured in collision with car, pick-up truck or van in nontraffic accident

√x7ᵗʰ **V33.3** Unspecified occupant of three-wheeled motor vehicle injured in collision with car, pick-up truck or van in nontraffic accident

√x7ᵗʰ **V33.4** Person boarding or alighting a three-wheeled motor vehicle injured in collision with car, pick-up truck or van

√x7ᵗʰ **V33.5** Driver of three-wheeled motor vehicle injured in collision with car, pick-up truck or van in traffic accident

√x7ᵗʰ **V33.6** Passenger in three-wheeled motor vehicle injured in collision with car, pick-up truck or van in traffic accident

√x7ᵗʰ **V33.7** Person on outside of three-wheeled motor vehicle injured in collision with car, pick-up truck or van in traffic accident

√x7ᵗʰ **V33.9** Unspecified occupant of three-wheeled motor vehicle injured in collision with car, pick-up truck or van in traffic accident

✓4ᵗʰ **V34** Occupant of three-wheeled motor vehicle injured in collision with heavy transport vehicle or bus

EXCLUDES 1 *occupant of three-wheeled motor vehicle injured in collision with military vehicle (V39.81)*

√x7ᵗʰ **V34.0** Driver of three-wheeled motor vehicle injured in collision with heavy transport vehicle or bus in nontraffic accident

√x7ᵗʰ **V34.1** Passenger in three-wheeled motor vehicle injured in collision with heavy transport vehicle or bus in nontraffic accident

√x7ᵗʰ **V34.2** Person on outside of three-wheeled motor vehicle injured in collision with heavy transport vehicle or bus in nontraffic accident

√x7ᵗʰ **V34.3** Unspecified occupant of three-wheeled motor vehicle injured in collision with heavy transport vehicle or bus in nontraffic accident

√x7ᵗʰ **V34.4** Person boarding or alighting a three-wheeled motor vehicle injured in collision with heavy transport vehicle or bus

√x7ᵗʰ **V34.5** Driver of three-wheeled motor vehicle injured in collision with heavy transport vehicle or bus in traffic accident

√x7ᵗʰ **V34.6** Passenger in three-wheeled motor vehicle injured in collision with heavy transport vehicle or bus in traffic accident

√x7ᵗʰ **V34.7** Person on outside of three-wheeled motor vehicle injured in collision with heavy transport vehicle or bus in traffic accident

√x7ᵗʰ **V34.9** Unspecified occupant of three-wheeled motor vehicle injured in collision with heavy transport vehicle or bus in traffic accident

✓4ᵗʰ **V35** Occupant of three-wheeled motor vehicle injured in collision with railway train or railway vehicle

√x7ᵗʰ **V35.0** Driver of three-wheeled motor vehicle injured in collision with railway train or railway vehicle in nontraffic accident

√x7ᵗʰ **V35.1** Passenger in three-wheeled motor vehicle injured in collision with railway train or railway vehicle in nontraffic accident

√x7ᵗʰ **V35.2** Person on outside of three-wheeled motor vehicle injured in collision with railway train or railway vehicle in nontraffic accident

√x7ᵗʰ **V35.3** Unspecified occupant of three-wheeled motor vehicle injured in collision with railway train or railway vehicle in nontraffic accident

√x7ᵗʰ **V35.4** Person boarding or alighting a three-wheeled motor vehicle injured in collision with railway train or railway vehicle

√x7ᵗʰ **V35.5** Driver of three-wheeled motor vehicle injured in collision with railway train or railway vehicle in traffic accident

√x7ᵗʰ **V35.6** Passenger in three-wheeled motor vehicle injured in collision with railway train or railway vehicle in traffic accident

√x7ᵗʰ **V35.7** Person on outside of three-wheeled motor vehicle injured in collision with railway train or railway vehicle in traffic accident

√x7ᵗʰ **V35.9** Unspecified occupant of three-wheeled motor vehicle injured in collision with railway train or railway vehicle in traffic accident

✓4ᵗʰ **V36** Occupant of three-wheeled motor vehicle injured in collision with other nonmotor vehicle

INCLUDES collision with animal-drawn vehicle, animal being ridden, streetcar

√x7ᵗʰ **V36.0** Driver of three-wheeled motor vehicle injured in collision with other nonmotor vehicle in nontraffic accident

√x7ᵗʰ **V36.1** Passenger in three-wheeled motor vehicle injured in collision with other nonmotor vehicle in nontraffic accident

√x7ᵗʰ **V36.2** Person on outside of three-wheeled motor vehicle injured in collision with other nonmotor vehicle in nontraffic accident

√x7ᵗʰ **V36.3** Unspecified occupant of three-wheeled motor vehicle injured in collision with other nonmotor vehicle in nontraffic accident

√x7ᵗʰ **V36.4** Person boarding or alighting a three-wheeled motor vehicle injured in collision with other nonmotor vehicle

√x7ᵗʰ **V36.5** Driver of three-wheeled motor vehicle injured in collision with other nonmotor vehicle in traffic accident

√x7ᵗʰ **V36.6** Passenger in three-wheeled motor vehicle injured in collision with other nonmotor vehicle in traffic accident

√x7ᵗʰ **V36.7** Person on outside of three-wheeled motor vehicle injured in collision with other nonmotor vehicle in traffic accident

√x7ᵗʰ **V36.9** Unspecified occupant of three-wheeled motor vehicle injured in collision with other nonmotor vehicle in traffic accident

✓4ᵗʰ **V37** Occupant of three-wheeled motor vehicle injured in collision with fixed or stationary object

√x7ᵗʰ **V37.0** Driver of three-wheeled motor vehicle injured in collision with fixed or stationary object in nontraffic accident

√x7ᵗʰ **V37.1** Passenger in three-wheeled motor vehicle injured in collision with fixed or stationary object in nontraffic accident

√x7ᵗʰ **V37.2** Person on outside of three-wheeled motor vehicle injured in collision with fixed or stationary object in nontraffic accident

√x7ᵗʰ **V37.3** Unspecified occupant of three-wheeled motor vehicle injured in collision with fixed or stationary object in nontraffic accident

√x7ᵗʰ **V37.4** Person boarding or alighting a three-wheeled motor vehicle injured in collision with fixed or stationary object

√x7ᵗʰ **V37.5** Driver of three-wheeled motor vehicle injured in collision with fixed or stationary object in traffic accident

HCC CMS-HCC　　**Rx** Rx HCC　　**ESR** ESRD HCC　　**COM** Commercial HCC　　**N** Newborn: 0　　**P** Pediatric: 0-17　　**M** Maternity: 9-64　　**A** Adult: 15-124

1208　　　　　ICD-10-CM 2023

√x7ᵗʰ **V37.6** Passenger in three-wheeled motor vehicle injured in collision with fixed or stationary object in traffic accident

√x7ᵗʰ **V37.7** Person on outside of three-wheeled motor vehicle injured in collision with fixed or stationary object in traffic accident

√x7ᵗʰ **V37.9** Unspecified occupant of three-wheeled motor vehicle injured in collision with fixed or stationary object in traffic accident

√4ᵗʰ **V38** **Occupant of three-wheeled motor vehicle injured in noncollision transport accident**

     INCLUDES   fall or thrown from three-wheeled motor vehicle
                  overturning of three-wheeled motor vehicle NOS
                  overturning of three-wheeled motor vehicle without collision

√x7ᵗʰ **V38.0** Driver of three-wheeled motor vehicle injured in noncollision transport accident in nontraffic accident

√x7ᵗʰ **V38.1** Passenger in three-wheeled motor vehicle injured in noncollision transport accident in nontraffic accident

√x7ᵗʰ **V38.2** Person on outside of three-wheeled motor vehicle injured in noncollision transport accident in nontraffic accident

√x7ᵗʰ **V38.3** Unspecified occupant of three-wheeled motor vehicle injured in noncollision transport accident in nontraffic accident

√x7ᵗʰ **V38.4** Person boarding or alighting a three-wheeled motor vehicle injured in noncollision transport accident

√x7ᵗʰ **V38.5** Driver of three-wheeled motor vehicle injured in noncollision transport accident in traffic accident

√x7ᵗʰ **V38.6** Passenger in three-wheeled motor vehicle injured in noncollision transport accident in traffic accident

√x7ᵗʰ **V38.7** Person on outside of three-wheeled motor vehicle injured in noncollision transport accident in traffic accident

√x7ᵗʰ **V38.9** Unspecified occupant of three-wheeled motor vehicle injured in noncollision transport accident in traffic accident

√4ᵗʰ **V39** **Occupant of three-wheeled motor vehicle injured in other and unspecified transport accidents**

√5ᵗʰ **V39.0** Driver of three-wheeled motor vehicle injured in collision with other and unspecified motor vehicles in nontraffic accident

     √x7ᵗʰ **V39.00** Driver of three-wheeled motor vehicle injured in collision with unspecified motor vehicles in nontraffic accident

     √x7ᵗʰ **V39.09** Driver of three-wheeled motor vehicle injured in collision with other motor vehicles in nontraffic accident

√5ᵗʰ **V39.1** Passenger in three-wheeled motor vehicle injured in collision with other and unspecified motor vehicles in nontraffic accident

     √x7ᵗʰ **V39.10** Passenger in three-wheeled motor vehicle injured in collision with unspecified motor vehicles in nontraffic accident

     √x7ᵗʰ **V39.19** Passenger in three-wheeled motor vehicle injured in collision with other motor vehicles in nontraffic accident

√5ᵗʰ **V39.2** Unspecified occupant of three-wheeled motor vehicle injured in collision with other and unspecified motor vehicles in nontraffic accident

     √x7ᵗʰ **V39.20** Unspecified occupant of three-wheeled motor vehicle injured in collision with unspecified motor vehicles in nontraffic accident
            Collision NOS involving three-wheeled motor vehicle, nontraffic

     √x7ᵗʰ **V39.29** Unspecified occupant of three-wheeled motor vehicle injured in collision with other motor vehicles in nontraffic accident

√x7ᵗʰ **V39.3** Occupant (driver) (passenger) of three-wheeled motor vehicle injured in unspecified nontraffic accident
         Accident NOS involving three-wheeled motor vehicle, nontraffic
         Occupant of three-wheeled motor vehicle injured in nontraffic accident NOS

√5ᵗʰ **V39.4** Driver of three-wheeled motor vehicle injured in collision with other and unspecified motor vehicles in traffic accident

     √x7ᵗʰ **V39.40** Driver of three-wheeled motor vehicle injured in collision with unspecified motor vehicles in traffic accident

     √x7ᵗʰ **V39.49** Driver of three-wheeled motor vehicle injured in collision with other motor vehicles in traffic accident

√5ᵗʰ **V39.5** Passenger in three-wheeled motor vehicle injured in collision with other and unspecified motor vehicles in traffic accident

     √x7ᵗʰ **V39.50** Passenger in three-wheeled motor vehicle injured in collision with unspecified motor vehicles in traffic accident

     √x7ᵗʰ **V39.59** Passenger in three-wheeled motor vehicle injured in collision with other motor vehicles in traffic accident

√5ᵗʰ **V39.6** Unspecified occupant of three-wheeled motor vehicle injured in collision with other and unspecified motor vehicles in traffic accident

     √x7ᵗʰ **V39.60** Unspecified occupant of three-wheeled motor vehicle injured in collision with unspecified motor vehicles in traffic accident
            Collision NOS involving three-wheeled motor vehicle (traffic)

     √x7ᵗʰ **V39.69** Unspecified occupant of three-wheeled motor vehicle injured in collision with other motor vehicles in traffic accident

√5ᵗʰ **V39.8** Occupant (driver) (passenger) of three-wheeled motor vehicle injured in other specified transport accidents

     √x7ᵗʰ **V39.81** Occupant (driver) (passenger) of three-wheeled motor vehicle injured in transport accident with military vehicle

     √x7ᵗʰ **V39.89** Occupant (driver) (passenger) of three-wheeled motor vehicle injured in other specified transport accidents

√x7ᵗʰ **V39.9** Occupant (driver) (passenger) of three-wheeled motor vehicle injured in unspecified traffic accident
         Accident NOS involving three-wheeled motor vehicle

Car occupant injured in transport accident (V40-V49)

     INCLUDES   a four-wheeled motor vehicle designed primarily for carrying passengers
                  automobile (pulling a trailer or camper)

     EXCLUDES 1   bus (V50-V59)
                  minibus (V50-V59)
                  minivan (V50-V59)
                  motorcoach (V70-V79)
                  pick-up truck (V50-V59)
                  sport utility vehicle (SUV) (V50-V59)

The appropriate 7th character is to be added to each code from categories V40-V49.
A   initial encounter
D   subsequent encounter
S   sequela

√4ᵗʰ **V40** **Car occupant injured in collision with pedestrian or animal**

     EXCLUDES 1   car collision with animal-drawn vehicle or animal being ridden (V46.-)

√x7ᵗʰ **V40.0** Car driver injured in collision with pedestrian or animal in nontraffic accident

√x7ᵗʰ **V40.1** Car passenger injured in collision with pedestrian or animal in nontraffic accident

√x7ᵗʰ **V40.2** Person on outside of car injured in collision with pedestrian or animal in nontraffic accident

√x7ᵗʰ **V40.3** Unspecified car occupant injured in collision with pedestrian or animal in nontraffic accident

√x7ᵗʰ **V40.4** Person boarding or alighting a car injured in collision with pedestrian or animal

√x7ᵗʰ **V40.5** Car driver injured in collision with pedestrian or animal in traffic accident

√x7ᵗʰ **V40.6** Car passenger injured in collision with pedestrian or animal in traffic accident

√x7ᵗʰ **V40.7** Person on outside of car injured in collision with pedestrian or animal in traffic accident

√x7ᵗʰ **V40.9** Unspecified car occupant injured in collision with pedestrian or animal in traffic accident

√4ᵗʰ **V41** **Car occupant injured in collision with pedal cycle**

√x7ᵗʰ **V41.0** Car driver injured in collision with pedal cycle in nontraffic accident

√x7ᵗʰ **V41.1** Car passenger injured in collision with pedal cycle in nontraffic accident

√x7ᵗʰ **V41.2** Person on outside of car injured in collision with pedal cycle in nontraffic accident

√x7ᵗʰ **V41.3** Unspecified car occupant injured in collision with pedal cycle in nontraffic accident

√x7ᵗʰ **V41.4** Person boarding or alighting a car injured in collision with pedal cycle

√x7ᵗʰ **V41.5** Car driver injured in collision with pedal cycle in traffic accident

√x7ᵗʰ **V41.6** Car passenger injured in collision with pedal cycle in traffic accident

√x7ᵗʰ **V41.7** Person on outside of car injured in collision with pedal cycle in traffic accident

√x7ᵗʰ **V41.9** Unspecified car occupant injured in collision with pedal cycle in traffic accident

✓4ᵗʰ **V42 Car occupant injured in collision with two- or three-wheeled motor vehicle**

√x7ᵗʰ **V42.0** Car driver injured in collision with two- or three-wheeled motor vehicle in nontraffic accident

√x7ᵗʰ **V42.1** Car passenger injured in collision with two- or three-wheeled motor vehicle in nontraffic accident

√x7ᵗʰ **V42.2** Person on outside of car injured in collision with two- or three-wheeled motor vehicle in nontraffic accident

√x7ᵗʰ **V42.3** Unspecified car occupant injured in collision with two- or three-wheeled motor vehicle in nontraffic accident

√x7ᵗʰ **V42.4** Person boarding or alighting a car injured in collision with two- or three-wheeled motor vehicle

√x7ᵗʰ **V42.5** Car driver injured in collision with two- or three-wheeled motor vehicle in traffic accident

√x7ᵗʰ **V42.6** Car passenger injured in collision with two- or three-wheeled motor vehicle in traffic accident

√x7ᵗʰ **V42.7** Person on outside of car injured in collision with two- or three-wheeled motor vehicle in traffic accident

√x7ᵗʰ **V42.9** Unspecified car occupant injured in collision with two- or three-wheeled motor vehicle in traffic accident

✓4ᵗʰ **V43 Car occupant injured in collision with car, pick-up truck or van**

√5ᵗʰ **V43.0** Car driver injured in collision with car, pick-up truck or van in nontraffic accident

√x7ᵗʰ **V43.01** Car driver injured in collision with sport utility vehicle in nontraffic accident

√x7ᵗʰ **V43.02** Car driver injured in collision with other type car in nontraffic accident

√x7ᵗʰ **V43.03** Car driver injured in collision with pick-up truck in nontraffic accident

√x7ᵗʰ **V43.04** Car driver injured in collision with van in nontraffic accident

√5ᵗʰ **V43.1** Car passenger injured in collision with car, pick-up truck or van in nontraffic accident

√x7ᵗʰ **V43.11** Car passenger injured in collision with sport utility vehicle in nontraffic accident

√x7ᵗʰ **V43.12** Car passenger injured in collision with other type car in nontraffic accident

√x7ᵗʰ **V43.13** Car passenger injured in collision with pick-up truck in nontraffic accident

√x7ᵗʰ **V43.14** Car passenger injured in collision with van in nontraffic accident

√5ᵗʰ **V43.2** Person on outside of car injured in collision with car, pick-up truck or van in nontraffic accident

√x7ᵗʰ **V43.21** Person on outside of car injured in collision with sport utility vehicle in nontraffic accident

√x7ᵗʰ **V43.22** Person on outside of car injured in collision with other type car in nontraffic accident

√x7ᵗʰ **V43.23** Person on outside of car injured in collision with pick-up truck in nontraffic accident

√x7ᵗʰ **V43.24** Person on outside of car injured in collision with van in nontraffic accident

√5ᵗʰ **V43.3** Unspecified car occupant injured in collision with car, pick-up truck or van in nontraffic accident

√x7ᵗʰ **V43.31** Unspecified car occupant injured in collision with sport utility vehicle in nontraffic accident

√x7ᵗʰ **V43.32** Unspecified car occupant injured in collision with other type car in nontraffic accident

√x7ᵗʰ **V43.33** Unspecified car occupant injured in collision with pick-up truck in nontraffic accident

√x7ᵗʰ **V43.34** Unspecified car occupant injured in collision with van in nontraffic accident

√5ᵗʰ **V43.4** Person boarding or alighting a car injured in collision with car, pick-up truck or van

√x7ᵗʰ **V43.41** Person boarding or alighting a car injured in collision with sport utility vehicle

√x7ᵗʰ **V43.42** Person boarding or alighting a car injured in collision with other type car

√x7ᵗʰ **V43.43** Person boarding or alighting a car injured in collision with pick-up truck

√x7ᵗʰ **V43.44** Person boarding or alighting a car injured in collision with van

√5ᵗʰ **V43.5** Car driver injured in collision with car, pick-up truck or van in traffic accident

√x7ᵗʰ **V43.51** Car driver injured in collision with sport utility vehicle in traffic accident

√x7ᵗʰ **V43.52** Car driver injured in collision with other type car in traffic accident

√x7ᵗʰ **V43.53** Car driver injured in collision with pick-up truck in traffic accident

√x7ᵗʰ **V43.54** Car driver injured in collision with van in traffic accident

√5ᵗʰ **V43.6** Car passenger injured in collision with car, pick-up truck or van in traffic accident

√x7ᵗʰ **V43.61** Car passenger injured in collision with sport utility vehicle in traffic accident

√x7ᵗʰ **V43.62** Car passenger injured in collision with other type car in traffic accident

√x7ᵗʰ **V43.63** Car passenger injured in collision with pick-up truck in traffic accident

√x7ᵗʰ **V43.64** Car passenger injured in collision with van in traffic accident

√5ᵗʰ **V43.7** Person on outside of car injured in collision with car, pick-up truck or van in traffic accident

√x7ᵗʰ **V43.71** Person on outside of car injured in collision with sport utility vehicle in traffic accident

√x7ᵗʰ **V43.72** Person on outside of car injured in collision with other type car in traffic accident

√x7ᵗʰ **V43.73** Person on outside of car injured in collision with pick-up truck in traffic accident

√x7ᵗʰ **V43.74** Person on outside of car injured in collision with van in traffic accident

√5ᵗʰ **V43.9** Unspecified car occupant injured in collision with car, pick-up truck or van in traffic accident

√x7ᵗʰ **V43.91** Unspecified car occupant injured in collision with sport utility vehicle in traffic accident

√x7ᵗʰ **V43.92** Unspecified car occupant injured in collision with other type car in traffic accident

√x7ᵗʰ **V43.93** Unspecified car occupant injured in collision with pick-up truck in traffic accident

√x7ᵗʰ **V43.94** Unspecified car occupant injured in collision with van in traffic accident

✓4ᵗʰ **V44 Car occupant injured in collision with heavy transport vehicle or bus**

> **EXCLUDES 1** car occupant injured in collision with military vehicle (V49.81)

√x7ᵗʰ **V44.0** Car driver injured in collision with heavy transport vehicle or bus in nontraffic accident

√x7ᵗʰ **V44.1** Car passenger injured in collision with heavy transport vehicle or bus in nontraffic accident

√x7ᵗʰ **V44.2** Person on outside of car injured in collision with heavy transport vehicle or bus in nontraffic accident

√x7ᵗʰ **V44.3** Unspecified car occupant injured in collision with heavy transport vehicle or bus in nontraffic accident

√x7ᵗʰ **V44.4** Person boarding or alighting a car injured in collision with heavy transport vehicle or bus

√x7ᵗʰ **V44.5** Car driver injured in collision with heavy transport vehicle or bus in traffic accident

√x7ᵗʰ **V44.6** Car passenger injured in collision with heavy transport vehicle or bus in traffic accident

√x7ᵗʰ **V44.7** Person on outside of car injured in collision with heavy transport vehicle or bus in traffic accident

√x7ᵗʰ **V44.9** Unspecified car occupant injured in collision with heavy transport vehicle or bus in traffic accident

✓4ᵗʰ **V45 Car occupant injured in collision with railway train or railway vehicle**

√x7ᵗʰ **V45.0** Car driver injured in collision with railway train or railway vehicle in nontraffic accident

√x7ᵗʰ **V45.1** Car passenger injured in collision with railway train or railway vehicle in nontraffic accident

√x7ᵗʰ **V45.2** Person on outside of car injured in collision with railway train or railway vehicle in nontraffic accident

√x7ᵗʰ **V45.3** Unspecified car occupant injured in collision with railway train or railway vehicle in nontraffic accident

√x7ᵗʰ **V45.4** Person boarding or alighting a car injured in collision with railway train or railway vehicle

√x7ᵗʰ **V45.5** Car driver injured in collision with railway train or railway vehicle in traffic accident

√x7ᵗʰ **V45.6** Car passenger injured in collision with railway train or railway vehicle in traffic accident

√x7ᵗʰ **V45.7** Person on outside of car injured in collision with railway train or railway vehicle in traffic accident

√x7ᵗʰ **V45.9** Unspecified car occupant injured in collision with railway train or railway vehicle in traffic accident

✓4ᵗʰ **V46 Car occupant injured in collision with other nonmotor vehicle**

> **INCLUDES** collision with animal-drawn vehicle, animal being ridden, streetcar

√x7ᵗʰ **V46.0** Car driver injured in collision with other nonmotor vehicle in nontraffic accident

√x7ᵗʰ **V46.1** Car passenger injured in collision with other nonmotor vehicle in nontraffic accident

√x7ᵗʰ **V46.2** Person on outside of car injured in collision with other nonmotor vehicle in nontraffic accident

HCC CMS-HCC   **Rx** Rx HCC   **ESR** ESRD HCC   **COM** Commercial HCC   **N** Newborn: 0   **P** Pediatric: 0-17   **M** Maternity: 9-64   **A** Adult: 15-124

1210   ICD-10-CM 2023

√x7ᵗʰ **V46.3** Unspecified car occupant injured in collision with other nonmotor vehicle in nontraffic accident

√x7ᵗʰ **V46.4** Person boarding or alighting a car injured in collision with other nonmotor vehicle

√x7ᵗʰ **V46.5** Car driver injured in collision with other nonmotor vehicle in traffic accident

√x7ᵗʰ **V46.6** Car passenger injured in collision with other nonmotor vehicle in traffic accident

√x7ᵗʰ **V46.7** Person on outside of car injured in collision with other nonmotor vehicle in traffic accident

√x7ᵗʰ **V46.9** Unspecified car occupant injured in collision with other nonmotor vehicle in traffic accident

√4ᵗʰ **V47** Car occupant injured in collision with fixed or stationary object
     AHA: 2016,4Q,73

√x7ᵗʰ **V47.0** Car driver injured in collision with fixed or stationary object in nontraffic accident

√x7ᵗʰ **V47.1** Car passenger injured in collision with fixed or stationary object in nontraffic accident

√x7ᵗʰ **V47.2** Person on outside of car injured in collision with fixed or stationary object in nontraffic accident

√x7ᵗʰ **V47.3** Unspecified car occupant injured in collision with fixed or stationary object in nontraffic accident

√x7ᵗʰ **V47.4** Person boarding or alighting a car injured in collision with fixed or stationary object

√x7ᵗʰ **V47.5** Car driver injured in collision with fixed or stationary object in traffic accident

√x7ᵗʰ **V47.6** Car passenger injured in collision with fixed or stationary object in traffic accident

√x7ᵗʰ **V47.7** Person on outside of car injured in collision with fixed or stationary object in traffic accident

√x7ᵗʰ **V47.9** Unspecified car occupant injured in collision with fixed or stationary object in traffic accident

√4ᵗʰ **V48** Car occupant injured in noncollision transport accident
     INCLUDES   overturning car NOS
                    overturning car without collision

√x7ᵗʰ **V48.0** Car driver injured in noncollision transport accident in nontraffic accident

√x7ᵗʰ **V48.1** Car passenger injured in noncollision transport accident in nontraffic accident

√x7ᵗʰ **V48.2** Person on outside of car injured in noncollision transport accident in nontraffic accident

√x7ᵗʰ **V48.3** Unspecified car occupant injured in noncollision transport accident in nontraffic accident

√x7ᵗʰ **V48.4** Person boarding or alighting a car injured in noncollision transport accident

√x7ᵗʰ **V48.5** Car driver injured in noncollision transport accident in traffic accident

√x7ᵗʰ **V48.6** Car passenger injured in noncollision transport accident in traffic accident

√x7ᵗʰ **V48.7** Person on outside of car injured in noncollision transport accident in traffic accident

√x7ᵗʰ **V48.9** Unspecified car occupant injured in noncollision transport accident in traffic accident

√4ᵗʰ **V49** Car occupant injured in other and unspecified transport accidents

√5ᵗʰ **V49.0** Driver injured in collision with other and unspecified motor vehicles in nontraffic accident

√x7ᵗʰ   **V49.00** Driver injured in collision with unspecified motor vehicles in nontraffic accident

√x7ᵗʰ   **V49.09** Driver injured in collision with other motor vehicles in nontraffic accident

√5ᵗʰ **V49.1** Passenger injured in collision with other and unspecified motor vehicles in nontraffic accident

√x7ᵗʰ   **V49.10** Passenger injured in collision with unspecified motor vehicles in nontraffic accident

√x7ᵗʰ   **V49.19** Passenger injured in collision with other motor vehicles in nontraffic accident

√5ᵗʰ **V49.2** Unspecified car occupant injured in collision with other and unspecified motor vehicles in nontraffic accident

√x7ᵗʰ   **V49.20** Unspecified car occupant injured in collision with unspecified motor vehicles in nontraffic accident
             Car collision NOS, nontraffic

√x7ᵗʰ   **V49.29** Unspecified car occupant injured in collision with other motor vehicles in nontraffic accident

√x7ᵗʰ **V49.3** Car occupant (driver) (passenger) injured in unspecified nontraffic accident
     Car accident NOS, nontraffic
     Car occupant injured in nontraffic accident NOS

√5ᵗʰ **V49.4** Driver injured in collision with other and unspecified motor vehicles in traffic accident

√x7ᵗʰ   **V49.40** Driver injured in collision with unspecified motor vehicles in traffic accident

√x7ᵗʰ   **V49.49** Driver injured in collision with other motor vehicles in traffic accident

√5ᵗʰ **V49.5** Passenger injured in collision with other and unspecified motor vehicles in traffic accident

√x7ᵗʰ   **V49.50** Passenger injured in collision with unspecified motor vehicles in traffic accident

√x7ᵗʰ   **V49.59** Passenger injured in collision with other motor vehicles in traffic accident

√5ᵗʰ **V49.6** Unspecified car occupant injured in collision with other and unspecified motor vehicles in traffic accident

√x7ᵗʰ   **V49.60** Unspecified car occupant injured in collision with unspecified motor vehicles in traffic accident
             Car collision NOS (traffic)

√x7ᵗʰ   **V49.69** Unspecified car occupant injured in collision with other motor vehicles in traffic accident

√5ᵗʰ **V49.8** Car occupant (driver) (passenger) injured in other specified transport accidents

√x7ᵗʰ   **V49.81** Car occupant (driver) (passenger) injured in transport accident with military vehicle

√x7ᵗʰ   **V49.88** Car occupant (driver) (passenger) injured in other specified transport accidents

√x7ᵗʰ **V49.9** Car occupant (driver) (passenger) injured in unspecified traffic accident
     Car accident NOS

Occupant of pick-up truck or van injured in transport accident (V50-V59)

INCLUDES   a four or six wheel motor vehicle designed primarily for carrying passengers and property but weighing less than the local limit for classification as a heavy goods vehicle
             minibus
             minivan
             sport utility vehicle (SUV)
             truck
             van

EXCLUDES 1   heavy transport vehicle (V60-V69)

The appropriate 7th character is to be added to each code from categories V50-V59.
A   initial encounter
D   subsequent encounter
S   sequela

√4ᵗʰ **V50** Occupant of pick-up truck or van injured in collision with pedestrian or animal
     EXCLUDES 1   pick-up truck or van collision with animal-drawn vehicle or animal being ridden (V56.-)

√x7ᵗʰ **V50.0** Driver of pick-up truck or van injured in collision with pedestrian or animal in nontraffic accident

√x7ᵗʰ **V50.1** Passenger in pick-up truck or van injured in collision with pedestrian or animal in nontraffic accident

√x7ᵗʰ **V50.2** Person on outside of pick-up truck or van injured in collision with pedestrian or animal in nontraffic accident

√x7ᵗʰ **V50.3** Unspecified occupant of pick-up truck or van injured in collision with pedestrian or animal in nontraffic accident

√x7ᵗʰ **V50.4** Person boarding or alighting a pick-up truck or van injured in collision with pedestrian or animal

√x7ᵗʰ **V50.5** Driver of pick-up truck or van injured in collision with pedestrian or animal in traffic accident

√x7ᵗʰ **V50.6** Passenger in pick-up truck or van injured in collision with pedestrian or animal in traffic accident

√x7ᵗʰ **V50.7** Person on outside of pick-up truck or van injured in collision with pedestrian or animal in traffic accident

√x7ᵗʰ **V50.9** Unspecified occupant of pick-up truck or van injured in collision with pedestrian or animal in traffic accident

√4ᵗʰ **V51** Occupant of pick-up truck or van injured in collision with pedal cycle

√x7ᵗʰ **V51.0** Driver of pick-up truck or van injured in collision with pedal cycle in nontraffic accident

√x7ᵗʰ **V51.1** Passenger in pick-up truck or van injured in collision with pedal cycle in nontraffic accident

√x7ᵗʰ **V51.2** Person on outside of pick-up truck or van injured in collision with pedal cycle in nontraffic accident

√x7ᵗʰ **V51.3** Unspecified occupant of pick-up truck or van injured in collision with pedal cycle in nontraffic accident

√x7ᵗʰ **V51.4** Person boarding or alighting a pick-up truck or van injured in collision with pedal cycle

√x7ᵗʰ **V51.5** Driver of pick-up truck or van injured in collision with pedal cycle in traffic accident

Chapter 20. External Causes of Morbidity

V51.6–V58.9

√x7th **V51.6** Passenger in pick-up truck or van injured in collision with pedal cycle in traffic accident

√x7th **V51.7** Person on outside of pick-up truck or van injured in collision with pedal cycle in traffic accident

√x7th **V51.9** Unspecified occupant of pick-up truck or van injured in collision with pedal cycle in traffic accident

√4th **V52** Occupant of pick-up truck or van injured in collision with two- or three-wheeled motor vehicle

√x7th **V52.0** Driver of pick-up truck or van injured in collision with two- or three-wheeled motor vehicle in nontraffic accident

√x7th **V52.1** Passenger in pick-up truck or van injured in collision with two- or three-wheeled motor vehicle in nontraffic accident

√x7th **V52.2** Person on outside of pick-up truck or van injured in collision with two- or three-wheeled motor vehicle in nontraffic accident

√x7th **V52.3** Unspecified occupant of pick-up truck or van injured in collision with two- or three-wheeled motor vehicle in nontraffic accident

√x7th **V52.4** Person boarding or alighting a pick-up truck or van injured in collision with two- or three-wheeled motor vehicle

√x7th **V52.5** Driver of pick-up truck or van injured in collision with two- or three-wheeled motor vehicle in traffic accident

√x7th **V52.6** Passenger in pick-up truck or van injured in collision with two- or three-wheeled motor vehicle in traffic accident

√x7th **V52.7** Person on outside of pick-up truck or van injured in collision with two- or three-wheeled motor vehicle in traffic accident

√x7th **V52.9** Unspecified occupant of pick-up truck or van injured in collision with two- or three-wheeled motor vehicle in traffic accident

√4th **V53** Occupant of pick-up truck or van injured in collision with car, pick-up truck or van

√x7th **V53.0** Driver of pick-up truck or van injured in collision with car, pick-up truck or van in nontraffic accident

√x7th **V53.1** Passenger in pick-up truck or van injured in collision with car, pick-up truck or van in nontraffic accident

√x7th **V53.2** Person on outside of pick-up truck or van injured in collision with car, pick-up truck or van in nontraffic accident

√x7th **V53.3** Unspecified occupant of pick-up truck or van injured in collision with car, pick-up truck or van in nontraffic accident

√x7th **V53.4** Person boarding or alighting a pick-up truck or van injured in collision with car, pick-up truck or van

√x7th **V53.5** Driver of pick-up truck or van injured in collision with car, pick-up truck or van in traffic accident

√x7th **V53.6** Passenger in pick-up truck or van injured in collision with car, pick-up truck or van in traffic accident

√x7th **V53.7** Person on outside of pick-up truck or van injured in collision with car, pick-up truck or van in traffic accident

√x7th **V53.9** Unspecified occupant of pick-up truck or van injured in collision with car, pick-up truck or van in traffic accident

√4th **V54** Occupant of pick-up truck or van injured in collision with heavy transport vehicle or bus

EXCLUDES 1   occupant of pick-up truck or van injured in collision with military vehicle (V59.81)

√x7th **V54.0** Driver of pick-up truck or van injured in collision with heavy transport vehicle or bus in nontraffic accident

√x7th **V54.1** Passenger in pick-up truck or van injured in collision with heavy transport vehicle or bus in nontraffic accident

√x7th **V54.2** Person on outside of pick-up truck or van injured in collision with heavy transport vehicle or bus in nontraffic accident

√x7th **V54.3** Unspecified occupant of pick-up truck or van injured in collision with heavy transport vehicle or bus in nontraffic accident

√x7th **V54.4** Person boarding or alighting a pick-up truck or van injured in collision with heavy transport vehicle or bus

√x7th **V54.5** Driver of pick-up truck or van injured in collision with heavy transport vehicle or bus in traffic accident

√x7th **V54.6** Passenger in pick-up truck or van injured in collision with heavy transport vehicle or bus in traffic accident

√x7th **V54.7** Person on outside of pick-up truck or van injured in collision with heavy transport vehicle or bus in traffic accident

√x7th **V54.9** Unspecified occupant of pick-up truck or van injured in collision with heavy transport vehicle or bus in traffic accident

√4th **V55** Occupant of pick-up truck or van injured in collision with railway train or railway vehicle

√x7th **V55.0** Driver of pick-up truck or van injured in collision with railway train or railway vehicle in nontraffic accident

√x7th **V55.1** Passenger in pick-up truck or van injured in collision with railway train or railway vehicle in nontraffic accident

√x7th **V55.2** Person on outside of pick-up truck or van injured in collision with railway train or railway vehicle in nontraffic accident

√x7th **V55.3** Unspecified occupant of pick-up truck or van injured in collision with railway train or railway vehicle in nontraffic accident

√x7th **V55.4** Person boarding or alighting a pick-up truck or van injured in collision with railway train or railway vehicle

√x7th **V55.5** Driver of pick-up truck or van injured in collision with railway train or railway vehicle in traffic accident

√x7th **V55.6** Passenger in pick-up truck or van injured in collision with railway train or railway vehicle in traffic accident

√x7th **V55.7** Person on outside of pick-up truck or van injured in collision with railway train or railway vehicle in traffic accident

√x7th **V55.9** Unspecified occupant of pick-up truck or van injured in collision with railway train or railway vehicle in traffic accident

√4th **V56** Occupant of pick-up truck or van injured in collision with other nonmotor vehicle

INCLUDES   collision with animal-drawn vehicle, animal being ridden, streetcar

√x7th **V56.0** Driver of pick-up truck or van injured in collision with other nonmotor vehicle in nontraffic accident

√x7th **V56.1** Passenger in pick-up truck or van injured in collision with other nonmotor vehicle in nontraffic accident

√x7th **V56.2** Person on outside of pick-up truck or van injured in collision with other nonmotor vehicle in nontraffic accident

√x7th **V56.3** Unspecified occupant of pick-up truck or van injured in collision with other nonmotor vehicle in nontraffic accident

√x7th **V56.4** Person boarding or alighting a pick-up truck or van injured in collision with other nonmotor vehicle

√x7th **V56.5** Driver of pick-up truck or van injured in collision with other nonmotor vehicle in traffic accident

√x7th **V56.6** Passenger in pick-up truck or van injured in collision with other nonmotor vehicle in traffic accident

√x7th **V56.7** Person on outside of pick-up truck or van injured in collision with other nonmotor vehicle in traffic accident

√x7th **V56.9** Unspecified occupant of pick-up truck or van injured in collision with other nonmotor vehicle in traffic accident

√4th **V57** Occupant of pick-up truck or van injured in collision with fixed or stationary object

√x7th **V57.0** Driver of pick-up truck or van injured in collision with fixed or stationary object in nontraffic accident

√x7th **V57.1** Passenger in pick-up truck or van injured in collision with fixed or stationary object in nontraffic accident

√x7th **V57.2** Person on outside of pick-up truck or van injured in collision with fixed or stationary object in nontraffic accident

√x7th **V57.3** Unspecified occupant of pick-up truck or van injured in collision with fixed or stationary object in nontraffic accident

√x7th **V57.4** Person boarding or alighting a pick-up truck or van injured in collision with fixed or stationary object

√x7th **V57.5** Driver of pick-up truck or van injured in collision with fixed or stationary object in traffic accident

√x7th **V57.6** Passenger in pick-up truck or van injured in collision with fixed or stationary object in traffic accident

√x7th **V57.7** Person on outside of pick-up truck or van injured in collision with fixed or stationary object in traffic accident

√x7th **V57.9** Unspecified occupant of pick-up truck or van injured in collision with fixed or stationary object in traffic accident

√4th **V58** Occupant of pick-up truck or van injured in noncollision transport accident

INCLUDES   overturning pick-up truck or van NOS
       overturning pick-up truck or van without collision

√x7th **V58.0** Driver of pick-up truck or van injured in noncollision transport accident in nontraffic accident

√x7th **V58.1** Passenger in pick-up truck or van injured in noncollision transport accident in nontraffic accident

√x7th **V58.2** Person on outside of pick-up truck or van injured in noncollision transport accident in nontraffic accident

√x7th **V58.3** Unspecified occupant of pick-up truck or van injured in noncollision transport accident in nontraffic accident

√x7th **V58.4** Person boarding or alighting a pick-up truck or van injured in noncollision transport accident

√x7th **V58.5** Driver of pick-up truck or van injured in noncollision transport accident in traffic accident

√x7th **V58.6** Passenger in pick-up truck or van injured in noncollision transport accident in traffic accident

√x7th **V58.7** Person on outside of pick-up truck or van injured in noncollision transport accident in traffic accident

√x7th **V58.9** Unspecified occupant of pick-up truck or van injured in noncollision transport accident in traffic accident

☑4ᵗʰ **V59 Occupant of pick-up truck or van injured in other and unspecified transport accidents**

   ☑5ᵗʰ **V59.0** Driver of pick-up truck or van injured in collision with other and unspecified motor vehicles in nontraffic accident

     ☑x7ᵗʰ **V59.00** Driver of pick-up truck or van injured in collision with unspecified motor vehicles in nontraffic accident

     ☑x7ᵗʰ **V59.09** Driver of pick-up truck or van injured in collision with other motor vehicles in nontraffic accident

   ☑5ᵗʰ **V59.1** Passenger in pick-up truck or van injured in collision with other and unspecified motor vehicles in nontraffic accident

     ☑x7ᵗʰ **V59.10** Passenger in pick-up truck or van injured in collision with unspecified motor vehicles in nontraffic accident

     ☑x7ᵗʰ **V59.19** Passenger in pick-up truck or van injured in collision with other motor vehicles in nontraffic accident

   ☑5ᵗʰ **V59.2** Unspecified occupant of pick-up truck or van injured in collision with other and unspecified motor vehicles in nontraffic accident

     ☑x7ᵗʰ **V59.20** Unspecified occupant of pick-up truck or van injured in collision with unspecified motor vehicles in nontraffic accident

        Collision NOS involving pick-up truck or van, nontraffic

     ☑x7ᵗʰ **V59.29** Unspecified occupant of pick-up truck or van injured in collision with other motor vehicles in nontraffic accident

   ☑x7ᵗʰ **V59.3** Occupant (driver) (passenger) of pick-up truck or van injured in unspecified nontraffic accident

       Accident NOS involving pick-up truck or van, nontraffic

       Occupant of pick-up truck or van injured in nontraffic accident NOS

   ☑6ᵗʰ **V59.4** Driver of pick-up truck or van injured in collision with other and unspecified motor vehicles in traffic accident

     ☑x7ᵗʰ **V59.40** Driver of pick-up truck or van injured in collision with unspecified motor vehicles in traffic accident

     ☑x7ᵗʰ **V59.49** Driver of pick-up truck or van injured in collision with other motor vehicles in traffic accident

   ☑5ᵗʰ **V59.5** Passenger in pick-up truck or van injured in collision with other and unspecified motor vehicles in traffic accident

     ☑x7ᵗʰ **V59.50** Passenger in pick-up truck or van injured in collision with unspecified motor vehicles in traffic accident

     ☑x7ᵗʰ **V59.59** Passenger in pick-up truck or van injured in collision with other motor vehicles in traffic accident

   ☑5ᵗʰ **V59.6** Unspecified occupant of pick-up truck or van injured in collision with other and unspecified motor vehicles in traffic accident

     ☑x7ᵗʰ **V59.60** Unspecified occupant of pick-up truck or van injured in collision with unspecified motor vehicles in traffic accident

        Collision NOS involving pick-up truck or van (traffic)

     ☑x7ᵗʰ **V59.69** Unspecified occupant of pick-up truck or van injured in collision with other motor vehicles in traffic accident

   ☑5ᵗʰ **V59.8** Occupant (driver) (passenger) of pick-up truck or van injured in other specified transport accidents

     ☑x7ᵗʰ **V59.81** Occupant (driver) (passenger) of pick-up truck or van injured in transport accident with military vehicle

     ☑x7ᵗʰ **V59.88** Occupant (driver) (passenger) of pick-up truck or van injured in other specified transport accidents

   ☑x7ᵗʰ **V59.9** Occupant (driver) (passenger) of pick-up truck or van injured in unspecified traffic accident

       Accident NOS involving pick-up truck or van

Occupant of heavy transport vehicle injured in transport accident (V60-V69)

INCLUDES	18 wheeler
	armored car
	panel truck
EXCLUDES 1	bus
	motorcoach

The appropriate 7th character is to be added to each code from categories V60-V69.
A   initial encounter
D   subsequent encounter
S   sequela

☑4ᵗʰ **V60 Occupant of heavy transport vehicle injured in collision with pedestrian or animal**

     EXCLUDES 1   *heavy transport vehicle collision with animal-drawn vehicle or animal being ridden (V66.-)*

   ☑x7ᵗʰ **V60.0** Driver of heavy transport vehicle injured in collision with pedestrian or animal in nontraffic accident

   ☑x7ᵗʰ **V60.1** Passenger in heavy transport vehicle injured in collision with pedestrian or animal in nontraffic accident

   ☑x7ᵗʰ **V60.2** Person on outside of heavy transport vehicle injured in collision with pedestrian or animal in nontraffic accident

   ☑x7ᵗʰ **V60.3** Unspecified occupant of heavy transport vehicle injured in collision with pedestrian or animal in nontraffic accident

   ☑x7ᵗʰ **V60.4** Person boarding or alighting a heavy transport vehicle injured in collision with pedestrian or animal

   ☑x7ᵗʰ **V60.5** Driver of heavy transport vehicle injured in collision with pedestrian or animal in traffic accident

   ☑x7ᵗʰ **V60.6** Passenger in heavy transport vehicle injured in collision with pedestrian or animal in traffic accident

   ☑x7ᵗʰ **V60.7** Person on outside of heavy transport vehicle injured in collision with pedestrian or animal in traffic accident

   ☑x7ᵗʰ **V60.9** Unspecified occupant of heavy transport vehicle injured in collision with pedestrian or animal in traffic accident

☑4ᵗʰ **V61 Occupant of heavy transport vehicle injured in collision with pedal cycle**

   ☑x7ᵗʰ **V61.0** Driver of heavy transport vehicle injured in collision with pedal cycle in nontraffic accident

   ☑x7ᵗʰ **V61.1** Passenger in heavy transport vehicle injured in collision with pedal cycle in nontraffic accident

   ☑x7ᵗʰ **V61.2** Person on outside of heavy transport vehicle injured in collision with pedal cycle in nontraffic accident

   ☑x7ᵗʰ **V61.3** Unspecified occupant of heavy transport vehicle injured in collision with pedal cycle in nontraffic accident

   ☑x7ᵗʰ **V61.4** Person boarding or alighting a heavy transport vehicle injured in collision with pedal cycle while boarding or alighting

   ☑x7ᵗʰ **V61.5** Driver of heavy transport vehicle injured in collision with pedal cycle in traffic accident

   ☑x7ᵗʰ **V61.6** Passenger in heavy transport vehicle injured in collision with pedal cycle in traffic accident

   ☑x7ᵗʰ **V61.7** Person on outside of heavy transport vehicle injured in collision with pedal cycle in traffic accident

   ☑x7ᵗʰ **V61.9** Unspecified occupant of heavy transport vehicle injured in collision with pedal cycle in traffic accident

☑4ᵗʰ **V62 Occupant of heavy transport vehicle injured in collision with two- or three-wheeled motor vehicle**

   ☑x7ᵗʰ **V62.0** Driver of heavy transport vehicle injured in collision with two- or three-wheeled motor vehicle in nontraffic accident

   ☑x7ᵗʰ **V62.1** Passenger in heavy transport vehicle injured in collision with two- or three-wheeled motor vehicle in nontraffic accident

   ☑x7ᵗʰ **V62.2** Person on outside of heavy transport vehicle injured in collision with two- or three-wheeled motor vehicle in nontraffic accident

   ☑x7ᵗʰ **V62.3** Unspecified occupant of heavy transport vehicle injured in collision with two- or three-wheeled motor vehicle in nontraffic accident

   ☑x7ᵗʰ **V62.4** Person boarding or alighting a heavy transport vehicle injured in collision with two- or three-wheeled motor vehicle

   ☑x7ᵗʰ **V62.5** Driver of heavy transport vehicle injured in collision with two- or three-wheeled motor vehicle in traffic accident

   ☑x7ᵗʰ **V62.6** Passenger in heavy transport vehicle injured in collision with two- or three-wheeled motor vehicle in traffic accident

   ☑x7ᵗʰ **V62.7** Person on outside of heavy transport vehicle injured in collision with two- or three-wheeled motor vehicle in traffic accident

   ☑x7ᵗʰ **V62.9** Unspecified occupant of heavy transport vehicle injured in collision with two- or three-wheeled motor vehicle in traffic accident

Chapter 20. External Causes of Morbidity

V63–V69.20

✓4th **V63** **Occupant of heavy transport vehicle injured in collision with car, pick-up truck or van**

✓x7th **V63.0** Driver of heavy transport vehicle injured in collision with car, pick-up truck or van in nontraffic accident

✓x7th **V63.1** Passenger in heavy transport vehicle injured in collision with car, pick-up truck or van in nontraffic accident

✓x7th **V63.2** Person on outside of heavy transport vehicle injured in collision with car, pick-up truck or van in nontraffic accident

✓x7th **V63.3** Unspecified occupant of heavy transport vehicle injured in collision with car, pick-up truck or van in nontraffic accident

✓x7th **V63.4** Person boarding or alighting a heavy transport vehicle injured in collision with car, pick-up truck or van

✓x7th **V63.5** Driver of heavy transport vehicle injured in collision with car, pick-up truck or van in traffic accident

✓x7th **V63.6** Passenger in heavy transport vehicle injured in collision with car, pick-up truck or van in traffic accident

✓x7th **V63.7** Person on outside of heavy transport vehicle injured in collision with car, pick-up truck or van in traffic accident

✓x7th **V63.9** Unspecified occupant of heavy transport vehicle injured in collision with car, pick-up truck or van in traffic accident

✓4th **V64** **Occupant of heavy transport vehicle injured in collision with heavy transport vehicle or bus**

> EXCLUDES 1   occupant of heavy transport vehicle injured in collision with military vehicle (V69.81)

✓x7th **V64.0** Driver of heavy transport vehicle injured in collision with heavy transport vehicle or bus in nontraffic accident

✓x7th **V64.1** Passenger in heavy transport vehicle injured in collision with heavy transport vehicle or bus in nontraffic accident

✓x7th **V64.2** Person on outside of heavy transport vehicle injured in collision with heavy transport vehicle or bus in nontraffic accident

✓x7th **V64.3** Unspecified occupant of heavy transport vehicle injured in collision with heavy transport vehicle or bus in nontraffic accident

✓x7th **V64.4** Person boarding or alighting a heavy transport vehicle injured in collision with heavy transport vehicle or bus while boarding or alighting

✓x7th **V64.5** Driver of heavy transport vehicle injured in collision with heavy transport vehicle or bus in traffic accident

✓x7th **V64.6** Passenger in heavy transport vehicle injured in collision with heavy transport vehicle or bus in traffic accident

✓x7th **V64.7** Person on outside of heavy transport vehicle injured in collision with heavy transport vehicle or bus in traffic accident

✓x7th **V64.9** Unspecified occupant of heavy transport vehicle injured in collision with heavy transport vehicle or bus in traffic accident

✓4th **V65** **Occupant of heavy transport vehicle injured in collision with railway train or railway vehicle**

✓x7th **V65.0** Driver of heavy transport vehicle injured in collision with railway train or railway vehicle in nontraffic accident

✓x7th **V65.1** Passenger in heavy transport vehicle injured in collision with railway train or railway vehicle in nontraffic accident

✓x7th **V65.2** Person on outside of heavy transport vehicle injured in collision with railway train or railway vehicle in nontraffic accident

✓x7th **V65.3** Unspecified occupant of heavy transport vehicle injured in collision with railway train or railway vehicle in nontraffic accident

✓x7th **V65.4** Person boarding or alighting a heavy transport vehicle injured in collision with railway train or railway vehicle

✓x7th **V65.5** Driver of heavy transport vehicle injured in collision with railway train or railway vehicle in traffic accident

✓x7th **V65.6** Passenger in heavy transport vehicle injured in collision with railway train or railway vehicle in traffic accident

✓x7th **V65.7** Person on outside of heavy transport vehicle injured in collision with railway train or railway vehicle in traffic accident

✓x7th **V65.9** Unspecified occupant of heavy transport vehicle injured in collision with railway train or railway vehicle in traffic accident

✓4th **V66** **Occupant of heavy transport vehicle injured in collision with other nonmotor vehicle**

> INCLUDES   collision with animal-drawn vehicle, animal being ridden, streetcar

✓x7th **V66.0** Driver of heavy transport vehicle injured in collision with other nonmotor vehicle in nontraffic accident

✓x7th **V66.1** Passenger in heavy transport vehicle injured in collision with other nonmotor vehicle in nontraffic accident

✓x7th **V66.2** Person on outside of heavy transport vehicle injured in collision with other nonmotor vehicle in nontraffic accident

✓x7th **V66.3** Unspecified occupant of heavy transport vehicle injured in collision with other nonmotor vehicle in nontraffic accident

✓x7th **V66.4** Person boarding or alighting a heavy transport vehicle injured in collision with other nonmotor vehicle

✓x7th **V66.5** Driver of heavy transport vehicle injured in collision with other nonmotor vehicle in traffic accident

✓x7th **V66.6** Passenger in heavy transport vehicle injured in collision with other nonmotor vehicle in traffic accident

✓x7th **V66.7** Person on outside of heavy transport vehicle injured in collision with other nonmotor vehicle in traffic accident

✓x7th **V66.9** Unspecified occupant of heavy transport vehicle injured in collision with other nonmotor vehicle in traffic accident

✓4th **V67** **Occupant of heavy transport vehicle injured in collision with fixed or stationary object**

✓x7th **V67.0** Driver of heavy transport vehicle injured in collision with fixed or stationary object in nontraffic accident

✓x7th **V67.1** Passenger in heavy transport vehicle injured in collision with fixed or stationary object in nontraffic accident

✓x7th **V67.2** Person on outside of heavy transport vehicle injured in collision with fixed or stationary object in nontraffic accident

✓x7th **V67.3** Unspecified occupant of heavy transport vehicle injured in collision with fixed or stationary object in nontraffic accident

✓x7th **V67.4** Person boarding or alighting a heavy transport vehicle injured in collision with fixed or stationary object

✓x7th **V67.5** Driver of heavy transport vehicle injured in collision with fixed or stationary object in traffic accident

✓x7th **V67.6** Passenger in heavy transport vehicle injured in collision with fixed or stationary object in traffic accident

✓x7th **V67.7** Person on outside of heavy transport vehicle injured in collision with fixed or stationary object in traffic accident

✓x7th **V67.9** Unspecified occupant of heavy transport vehicle injured in collision with fixed or stationary object in traffic accident

✓4th **V68** **Occupant of heavy transport vehicle injured in noncollision transport accident**

> INCLUDES   overturning heavy transport vehicle NOS
> overturning heavy transport vehicle without collision

✓x7th **V68.0** Driver of heavy transport vehicle injured in noncollision transport accident in nontraffic accident

✓x7th **V68.1** Passenger in heavy transport vehicle injured in noncollision transport accident in nontraffic accident

✓x7th **V68.2** Person on outside of heavy transport vehicle injured in noncollision transport accident in nontraffic accident

✓x7th **V68.3** Unspecified occupant of heavy transport vehicle injured in noncollision transport accident in nontraffic accident

✓x7th **V68.4** Person boarding or alighting a heavy transport vehicle injured in noncollision transport accident

✓x7th **V68.5** Driver of heavy transport vehicle injured in noncollision transport accident in traffic accident

✓x7th **V68.6** Passenger in heavy transport vehicle injured in noncollision transport accident in traffic accident

✓x7th **V68.7** Person on outside of heavy transport vehicle injured in noncollision transport accident in traffic accident

✓x7th **V68.9** Unspecified occupant of heavy transport vehicle injured in noncollision transport accident in traffic accident

✓4th **V69** **Occupant of heavy transport vehicle injured in other and unspecified transport accidents**

✓5th **V69.0** Driver of heavy transport vehicle injured in collision with other and unspecified motor vehicles in nontraffic accident

   ✓x7th **V69.00** Driver of heavy transport vehicle injured in collision with unspecified motor vehicles in nontraffic accident

   ✓x7th **V69.09** Driver of heavy transport vehicle injured in collision with other motor vehicles in nontraffic accident

✓5th **V69.1** Passenger in heavy transport vehicle injured in collision with other and unspecified motor vehicles in nontraffic accident

   ✓x7th **V69.10** Passenger in heavy transport vehicle injured in collision with unspecified motor vehicles in nontraffic accident

   ✓x7th **V69.19** Passenger in heavy transport vehicle injured in collision with other motor vehicles in nontraffic accident

✓5th **V69.2** Unspecified occupant of heavy transport vehicle injured in collision with other and unspecified motor vehicles in nontraffic accident

   ✓x7th **V69.20** Unspecified occupant of heavy transport vehicle injured in collision with unspecified motor vehicles in nontraffic accident

     Collision NOS involving heavy transport vehicle, nontraffic

√x7ᵗʰ **V69.29** Unspecified occupant of heavy transport vehicle injured in collision with other motor vehicles in nontraffic accident

√x7ᵗʰ **V69.3** Occupant (driver) (passenger) of heavy transport vehicle injured in unspecified nontraffic accident
> Accident NOS involving heavy transport vehicle, nontraffic
> Occupant of heavy transport vehicle injured in nontraffic accident NOS

√5ᵗʰ **V69.4** Driver of heavy transport vehicle injured in collision with other and unspecified motor vehicles in traffic accident

√x7ᵗʰ **V69.40** Driver of heavy transport vehicle injured in collision with unspecified motor vehicles in traffic accident

√x7ᵗʰ **V69.49** Driver of heavy transport vehicle injured in collision with other motor vehicles in traffic accident

√5ᵗʰ **V69.5** Passenger in heavy transport vehicle injured in collision with other and unspecified motor vehicles in traffic accident

√x7ᵗʰ **V69.50** Passenger in heavy transport vehicle injured in collision with unspecified motor vehicles in traffic accident

√x7ᵗʰ **V69.59** Passenger in heavy transport vehicle injured in collision with other motor vehicles in traffic accident

√5ᵗʰ **V69.6** Unspecified occupant of heavy transport vehicle injured in collision with other and unspecified motor vehicles in traffic accident

√x7ᵗʰ **V69.60** Unspecified occupant of heavy transport vehicle injured in collision with unspecified motor vehicles in traffic accident
> Collision NOS involving heavy transport vehicle (traffic)

√x7ᵗʰ **V69.69** Unspecified occupant of heavy transport vehicle injured in collision with other motor vehicles in traffic accident

√5ᵗʰ **V69.8** Occupant (driver) (passenger) of heavy transport vehicle injured in other specified transport accidents

√x7ᵗʰ **V69.81** Occupant (driver) (passenger) of heavy transport vehicle injured in transport accidents with military vehicle

√x7ᵗʰ **V69.88** Occupant (driver) (passenger) of heavy transport vehicle injured in other specified transport accidents

√x7ᵗʰ **V69.9** Occupant (driver) (passenger) of heavy transport vehicle injured in unspecified traffic accident
> Accident NOS involving heavy transport vehicle

Bus occupant injured in transport accident (V70-V79)

INCLUDES motorcoach
EXCLUDES 1 minibus (V50-V59)

The appropriate 7th character is to be added to each code from categories V70-V79.
A   initial encounter
D   subsequent encounter
S   sequela

√4ᵗʰ **V70** Bus occupant injured in collision with pedestrian or animal
> **EXCLUDES 1** bus collision with animal-drawn vehicle or animal being ridden (V76.-)

√x7ᵗʰ **V70.0** Driver of bus injured in collision with pedestrian or animal in nontraffic accident

√x7ᵗʰ **V70.1** Passenger on bus injured in collision with pedestrian or animal in nontraffic accident

√x7ᵗʰ **V70.2** Person on outside of bus injured in collision with pedestrian or animal in nontraffic accident

√x7ᵗʰ **V70.3** Unspecified occupant of bus injured in collision with pedestrian or animal in nontraffic accident

√x7ᵗʰ **V70.4** Person boarding or alighting from bus injured in collision with pedestrian or animal

√x7ᵗʰ **V70.5** Driver of bus injured in collision with pedestrian or animal in traffic accident

√x7ᵗʰ **V70.6** Passenger on bus injured in collision with pedestrian or animal in traffic accident

√x7ᵗʰ **V70.7** Person on outside of bus injured in collision with pedestrian or animal in traffic accident

√x7ᵗʰ **V70.9** Unspecified occupant of bus injured in collision with pedestrian or animal in traffic accident

√4ᵗʰ **V71** Bus occupant injured in collision with pedal cycle

√x7ᵗʰ **V71.0** Driver of bus injured in collision with pedal cycle in nontraffic accident

√x7ᵗʰ **V71.1** Passenger on bus injured in collision with pedal cycle in nontraffic accident

√x7ᵗʰ **V71.2** Person on outside of bus injured in collision with pedal cycle in nontraffic accident

√x7ᵗʰ **V71.3** Unspecified occupant of bus injured in collision with pedal cycle in nontraffic accident

√x7ᵗʰ **V71.4** Person boarding or alighting from bus injured in collision with pedal cycle

√x7ᵗʰ **V71.5** Driver of bus injured in collision with pedal cycle in traffic accident

√x7ᵗʰ **V71.6** Passenger on bus injured in collision with pedal cycle in traffic accident

√x7ᵗʰ **V71.7** Person on outside of bus injured in collision with pedal cycle in traffic accident

√x7ᵗʰ **V71.9** Unspecified occupant of bus injured in collision with pedal cycle in traffic accident

√4ᵗʰ **V72** Bus occupant injured in collision with two- or three-wheeled motor vehicle

√x7ᵗʰ **V72.0** Driver of bus injured in collision with two- or three-wheeled motor vehicle in nontraffic accident

√x7ᵗʰ **V72.1** Passenger on bus injured in collision with two- or three-wheeled motor vehicle in nontraffic accident

√x7ᵗʰ **V72.2** Person on outside of bus injured in collision with two- or three-wheeled motor vehicle in nontraffic accident

√x7ᵗʰ **V72.3** Unspecified occupant of bus injured in collision with two- or three-wheeled motor vehicle in nontraffic accident

√x7ᵗʰ **V72.4** Person boarding or alighting from bus injured in collision with two- or three-wheeled motor vehicle

√x7ᵗʰ **V72.5** Driver of bus injured in collision with two- or three-wheeled motor vehicle in traffic accident

√x7ᵗʰ **V72.6** Passenger on bus injured in collision with two- or three-wheeled motor vehicle in traffic accident

√x7ᵗʰ **V72.7** Person on outside of bus injured in collision with two- or three-wheeled motor vehicle in traffic accident

√x7ᵗʰ **V72.9** Unspecified occupant of bus injured in collision with two- or three-wheeled motor vehicle in traffic accident

√4ᵗʰ **V73** Bus occupant injured in collision with car, pick-up truck or van

√x7ᵗʰ **V73.0** Driver of bus injured in collision with car, pick-up truck or van in nontraffic accident

√x7ᵗʰ **V73.1** Passenger on bus injured in collision with car, pick-up truck or van in nontraffic accident

√x7ᵗʰ **V73.2** Person on outside of bus injured in collision with car, pick-up truck or van in nontraffic accident

√x7ᵗʰ **V73.3** Unspecified occupant of bus injured in collision with car, pick-up truck or van in nontraffic accident

√x7ᵗʰ **V73.4** Person boarding or alighting from bus injured in collision with car, pick-up truck or van

√x7ᵗʰ **V73.5** Driver of bus injured in collision with car, pick-up truck or van in traffic accident

√x7ᵗʰ **V73.6** Passenger on bus injured in collision with car, pick-up truck or van in traffic accident

√x7ᵗʰ **V73.7** Person on outside of bus injured in collision with car, pick-up truck or van in traffic accident

√x7ᵗʰ **V73.9** Unspecified occupant of bus injured in collision with car, pick-up truck or van in traffic accident

√4ᵗʰ **V74** Bus occupant injured in collision with heavy transport vehicle or bus
> **EXCLUDES 1** bus occupant injured in collision with military vehicle (V79.81)

√x7ᵗʰ **V74.0** Driver of bus injured in collision with heavy transport vehicle or bus in nontraffic accident

√x7ᵗʰ **V74.1** Passenger on bus injured in collision with heavy transport vehicle or bus in nontraffic accident

√x7ᵗʰ **V74.2** Person on outside of bus injured in collision with heavy transport vehicle or bus in nontraffic accident

√x7ᵗʰ **V74.3** Unspecified occupant of bus injured in collision with heavy transport vehicle or bus in nontraffic accident

√x7ᵗʰ **V74.4** Person boarding or alighting from bus injured in collision with heavy transport vehicle or bus

√x7ᵗʰ **V74.5** Driver of bus injured in collision with heavy transport vehicle or bus in traffic accident

√x7ᵗʰ **V74.6** Passenger on bus injured in collision with heavy transport vehicle or bus in traffic accident

√x7ᵗʰ **V74.7** Person on outside of bus injured in collision with heavy transport vehicle or bus in traffic accident

√x7ᵗʰ **V74.9** Unspecified occupant of bus injured in collision with heavy transport vehicle or bus in traffic accident

√4ᵗʰ **V75** Bus occupant injured in collision with railway train or railway vehicle

√x7ᵗʰ **V75.0** Driver of bus injured in collision with railway train or railway vehicle in nontraffic accident

√x7ᵗʰ **V75.1** Passenger on bus injured in collision with railway train or railway vehicle in nontraffic accident

√x7ᵗʰ **V75.2** Person on outside of bus injured in collision with railway train or railway vehicle in nontraffic accident

---

Chapter 20. External Causes of Morbidity

V75.3–V80.12

✓x7ᵗʰ **V75.3** Unspecified occupant of bus injured in collision with railway train or railway vehicle *in nontraffic accident*

✓x7ᵗʰ **V75.4** *Person boarding or alighting* from bus injured in collision with railway train or railway vehicle

✓x7ᵗʰ **V75.5** *Driver* of bus injured in collision with railway train or railway vehicle *in traffic accident*

✓x7ᵗʰ **V75.6** *Passenger* on bus injured in collision with railway train or railway vehicle *in traffic accident*

✓x7ᵗʰ **V75.7** *Person on outside* of bus injured in collision with railway train or railway vehicle *in traffic accident*

✓x7ᵗʰ **V75.9** Unspecified occupant of bus injured in collision with railway train or railway vehicle *in traffic accident*

✓4ᵗʰ **V76** **Bus occupant injured in collision with other nonmotor vehicle**

INCLUDES   collision with animal-drawn vehicle, animal being ridden, streetcar

✓x7ᵗʰ **V76.0** *Driver* of bus injured in collision with other nonmotor vehicle *in nontraffic accident*

✓x7ᵗʰ **V76.1** *Passenger* on bus injured in collision with other nonmotor vehicle *in nontraffic accident*

✓x7ᵗʰ **V76.2** *Person on outside* of bus injured in collision with other nonmotor vehicle *in nontraffic accident*

✓x7ᵗʰ **V76.3** Unspecified occupant of bus injured in collision with other nonmotor vehicle *in nontraffic accident*

✓x7ᵗʰ **V76.4** *Person boarding or alighting* from bus injured in collision with other nonmotor vehicle

✓x7ᵗʰ **V76.5** *Driver* of bus injured in collision with other nonmotor vehicle *in traffic accident*

✓x7ᵗʰ **V76.6** *Passenger* on bus injured in collision with other nonmotor vehicle *in traffic accident*

✓x7ᵗʰ **V76.7** *Person on outside* of bus injured in collision with other nonmotor vehicle *in traffic accident*

✓x7ᵗʰ **V76.9** Unspecified occupant of bus injured in collision with other nonmotor vehicle *in traffic accident*

✓4ᵗʰ **V77** **Bus occupant injured in collision with fixed or stationary object**

✓x7ᵗʰ **V77.0** *Driver* of bus injured in collision with fixed or stationary object *in nontraffic accident*

✓x7ᵗʰ **V77.1** *Passenger* on bus injured in collision with fixed or stationary object *in nontraffic accident*

✓x7ᵗʰ **V77.2** *Person on outside* of bus injured in collision with fixed or stationary object *in nontraffic accident*

✓x7ᵗʰ **V77.3** Unspecified occupant of bus injured in collision with fixed or stationary object *in nontraffic accident*

✓x7ᵗʰ **V77.4** *Person boarding or alighting* from bus injured in collision with fixed or stationary object

✓x7ᵗʰ **V77.5** *Driver* of bus injured in collision with fixed or stationary object *in traffic accident*

✓x7ᵗʰ **V77.6** *Passenger* on bus injured in collision with fixed or stationary object *in traffic accident*

✓x7ᵗʰ **V77.7** *Person on outside* of bus injured in collision with fixed or stationary object *in traffic accident*

✓x7ᵗʰ **V77.9** Unspecified occupant of bus injured in collision with fixed or stationary object *in traffic accident*

✓4ᵗʰ **V78** **Bus occupant injured in noncollision transport accident**

INCLUDES   overturning bus NOS
           overturning bus without collision

✓x7ᵗʰ **V78.0** *Driver* of bus injured in noncollision transport accident *in nontraffic accident*

✓x7ᵗʰ **V78.1** *Passenger* on bus injured in noncollision transport accident *in nontraffic accident*

✓x7ᵗʰ **V78.2** *Person on outside* of bus injured in noncollision transport accident *in nontraffic accident*

✓x7ᵗʰ **V78.3** Unspecified occupant of bus injured in noncollision transport accident *in nontraffic accident*

✓x7ᵗʰ **V78.4** *Person boarding or alighting* from bus injured in noncollision transport accident

✓x7ᵗʰ **V78.5** *Driver* of bus injured in noncollision transport accident *in traffic accident*

✓x7ᵗʰ **V78.6** *Passenger* on bus injured in noncollision transport accident *in traffic accident*

✓x7ᵗʰ **V78.7** *Person on outside* of bus injured in noncollision transport accident *in traffic accident*

✓x7ᵗʰ **V78.9** Unspecified occupant of bus injured in noncollision transport accident *in traffic accident*

✓4ᵗʰ **V79** **Bus occupant injured in other and unspecified transport accidents**

✓5ᵗʰ **V79.0** *Driver* of bus injured in collision with other and unspecified motor vehicles *in nontraffic accident*

✓x7ᵗʰ **V79.00** Driver of bus injured in collision with unspecified motor vehicles in nontraffic accident

✓x7ᵗʰ **V79.09** Driver of bus injured in collision with other motor vehicles in nontraffic accident

✓5ᵗʰ **V79.1** *Passenger* on bus injured in collision with other and unspecified motor vehicles *in nontraffic accident*

✓x7ᵗʰ **V79.10** Passenger on bus injured in collision with unspecified motor vehicles in nontraffic accident

✓x7ᵗʰ **V79.19** Passenger on bus injured in collision with other motor vehicles in nontraffic accident

✓5ᵗʰ **V79.2** Unspecified bus occupant injured in collision with other and unspecified motor vehicles *in nontraffic accident*

✓x7ᵗʰ **V79.20** Unspecified bus occupant injured in collision with unspecified motor vehicles in nontraffic accident
Bus collision NOS, nontraffic

✓x7ᵗʰ **V79.29** Unspecified bus occupant injured in collision with other motor vehicles in nontraffic accident

✓x7ᵗʰ **V79.3** Bus occupant (driver) (passenger) injured in unspecified nontraffic accident
Bus accident NOS, nontraffic
Bus occupant injured in nontraffic accident NOS

✓5ᵗʰ **V79.4** *Driver* of bus injured in collision with other and unspecified motor vehicles *in traffic accident*

✓x7ᵗʰ **V79.40** Driver of bus injured in collision with unspecified motor vehicles in traffic accident

✓x7ᵗʰ **V79.49** Driver of bus injured in collision with other motor vehicles in traffic accident

✓5ᵗʰ **V79.5** *Passenger* on bus injured in collision with other and unspecified motor vehicles *in traffic accident*

✓x7ᵗʰ **V79.50** Passenger on bus injured in collision with unspecified motor vehicles in traffic accident

✓x7ᵗʰ **V79.59** Passenger on bus injured in collision with other motor vehicles in traffic accident

✓5ᵗʰ **V79.6** Unspecified bus occupant injured in collision with other and unspecified motor vehicles *in traffic accident*

✓x7ᵗʰ **V79.60** Unspecified bus occupant injured in collision with unspecified motor vehicles in traffic accident
Bus collision NOS (traffic)

✓x7ᵗʰ **V79.69** Unspecified bus occupant injured in collision with other motor vehicles in traffic accident

✓5ᵗʰ **V79.8** Bus *occupant (driver) (passenger)* injured in other specified transport accidents

✓x7ᵗʰ **V79.81** Bus occupant (driver) (passenger) injured in transport accidents with *military vehicle*

✓x7ᵗʰ **V79.88** Bus occupant (driver) (passenger) injured in other specified transport accidents

✓x7ᵗʰ **V79.9** Bus occupant (driver) (passenger) injured in unspecified traffic accident
Bus accident NOS

Other land transport accidents (V80-V89)

The appropriate 7th character is to be added to each code from categories V80-V89.
A   initial encounter
D   subsequent encounter
S   sequela

✓4ᵗʰ **V80** **Animal-rider or occupant of animal-drawn vehicle injured in transport accident**

✓5ᵗʰ **V80.0** **Animal-rider or occupant of animal drawn vehicle injured by fall from or being thrown from animal or animal-drawn vehicle in** *noncollision accident*

✓6ᵗʰ **V80.01** *Animal-rider* injured by fall from or being thrown from animal in noncollision accident

✓7ᵗʰ **V80.010** Animal-rider injured by fall from or being thrown from *horse* in noncollision accident

✓7ᵗʰ **V80.018** Animal-rider injured by fall from or being thrown from other animal in noncollision accident

✓x7ᵗʰ **V80.02** *Occupant* of animal-drawn vehicle injured by fall from or being thrown from animal-drawn vehicle in noncollision accident
Overturning animal-drawn vehicle NOS
Overturning animal-drawn vehicle without collision

✓5ᵗʰ **V80.1** **Animal-rider or occupant of animal-drawn vehicle injured in collision with** *pedestrian or animal*

EXCLUDES 1   *animal-rider or animal-drawn vehicle collision with animal-drawn vehicle or animal being ridden (V80.7)*

✓x7ᵗʰ **V80.11** *Animal-rider* injured in collision with pedestrian or animal

✓x7ᵗʰ **V80.12** *Occupant* of animal-drawn vehicle injured in collision with pedestrian or animal

✓5ᵗʰ V80.2 Animal-rider or occupant of animal-drawn vehicle injured in collision with pedal cycle
- **✓x7ᵗʰ V80.21** Animal-rider injured in collision with pedal cycle
- **✓x7ᵗʰ V80.22** Occupant of animal-drawn vehicle injured in collision with pedal cycle

✓5ᵗʰ V80.3 Animal-rider or occupant of animal-drawn vehicle injured in collision with two- or three-wheeled motor vehicle
- **✓x7ᵗʰ V80.31** Animal-rider injured in collision with two- or three-wheeled motor vehicle
- **✓x7ᵗʰ V80.32** Occupant of animal-drawn vehicle injured in collision with two- or three-wheeled motor vehicle

✓5ᵗʰ V80.4 Animal-rider or occupant of animal-drawn vehicle injured in collision with car, pick-up truck, van, heavy transport vehicle or bus
- EXCLUDES 1 animal-rider injured in collision with military vehicle (V80.910)
- occupant of animal-drawn vehicle injured in collision with military vehicle (V80.920)
- **✓x7ᵗʰ V80.41** Animal-rider injured in collision with car, pick-up truck, van, heavy transport vehicle or bus
- **✓x7ᵗʰ V80.42** Occupant of animal-drawn vehicle injured in collision with car, pick-up truck, van, heavy transport vehicle or bus

✓5ᵗʰ V80.5 Animal-rider or occupant of animal-drawn vehicle injured in collision with other specified motor vehicle
- **✓x7ᵗʰ V80.51** Animal-rider injured in collision with other specified motor vehicle
- **✓x7ᵗʰ V80.52** Occupant of animal-drawn vehicle injured in collision with other specified motor vehicle

✓5ᵗʰ V80.6 Animal-rider or occupant of animal-drawn vehicle injured in collision with railway train or railway vehicle
- **✓x7ᵗʰ V80.61** Animal-rider injured in collision with railway train or railway vehicle
- **✓x7ᵗʰ V80.62** Occupant of animal-drawn vehicle injured in collision with railway train or railway vehicle

✓5ᵗʰ V80.7 Animal-rider or occupant of animal-drawn vehicle injured in collision with other nonmotor vehicles
- **✓6ᵗʰ V80.71** Animal-rider or occupant of animal-drawn vehicle injured in collision with animal being ridden
  - **✓7ᵗʰ V80.710** Animal-rider injured in collision with other animal being ridden
  - **✓7ᵗʰ V80.711** Occupant of animal-drawn vehicle injured in collision with animal being ridden
- **✓6ᵗʰ V80.72** Animal-rider or occupant of animal-drawn vehicle injured in collision with other animal-drawn vehicle
  - **✓7ᵗʰ V80.720** Animal-rider injured in collision with animal-drawn vehicle
  - **✓7ᵗʰ V80.721** Occupant of animal-drawn vehicle injured in collision with other animal-drawn vehicle
- **✓6ᵗʰ V80.73** Animal-rider or occupant of animal-drawn vehicle injured in collision with streetcar
  - **✓7ᵗʰ V80.730** Animal-rider injured in collision with streetcar
  - **✓7ᵗʰ V80.731** Occupant of animal-drawn vehicle injured in collision with streetcar
- **✓6ᵗʰ V80.79** Animal-rider or occupant of animal-drawn vehicle injured in collision with other nonmotor vehicles
  - **✓7ᵗʰ V80.790** Animal-rider injured in collision with other nonmotor vehicles
  - **✓7ᵗʰ V80.791** Occupant of animal-drawn vehicle injured in collision with other nonmotor vehicles

✓5ᵗʰ V80.8 Animal-rider or occupant of animal-drawn vehicle injured in collision with fixed or stationary object
- **✓x7ᵗʰ V80.81** Animal-rider injured in collision with fixed or stationary object
- **✓x7ᵗʰ V80.82** Occupant of animal-drawn vehicle injured in collision with fixed or stationary object

✓5ᵗʰ V80.9 Animal-rider or occupant of animal-drawn vehicle injured in other and unspecified transport accidents
- **✓6ᵗʰ V80.91** Animal-rider injured in other and unspecified transport accidents
  - **✓7ᵗʰ V80.910** Animal-rider injured in transport accident with military vehicle
  - **✓7ᵗʰ V80.918** Animal-rider injured in other transport accident
  - **✓7ᵗʰ V80.919** Animal-rider injured in unspecified transport accident
    Animal rider accident NOS

- **✓6ᵗʰ V80.92** Occupant of animal-drawn vehicle injured in other and unspecified transport accidents
  - **✓7ᵗʰ V80.920** Occupant of animal-drawn vehicle injured in transport accident with military vehicle
  - **✓7ᵗʰ V80.928** Occupant of animal-drawn vehicle injured in other transport accident
  - **✓7ᵗʰ V80.929** Occupant of animal-drawn vehicle injured in unspecified transport accident
    Animal-drawn vehicle accident NOS

✓4ᵗʰ V81 Occupant of railway train or railway vehicle injured in transport accident
- INCLUDES derailment of railway train or railway vehicle
  person on outside of train
- EXCLUDES 1 streetcar (V82.-)

✓x7ᵗʰ V81.0 Occupant of railway train or railway vehicle injured in collision with motor vehicle in nontraffic accident
- EXCLUDES 1 occupant of railway train or railway vehicle injured due to collision with military vehicle (V81.83)

✓x7ᵗʰ V81.1 Occupant of railway train or railway vehicle injured in collision with motor vehicle in traffic accident
- EXCLUDES 1 occupant of railway train or railway vehicle injured due to collision with military vehicle (V81.83)

✓x7ᵗʰ V81.2 Occupant of railway train or railway vehicle injured in collision with or hit by rolling stock

✓x7ᵗʰ V81.3 Occupant of railway train or railway vehicle injured in collision with other object
Railway collision NOS

✓x7ᵗʰ V81.4 Person injured while boarding or alighting from railway train or railway vehicle

✓x7ᵗʰ V81.5 Occupant of railway train or railway vehicle injured by fall in railway train or railway vehicle

✓x7ᵗʰ V81.6 Occupant of railway train or railway vehicle injured by fall from railway train or railway vehicle

✓x7ᵗʰ V81.7 Occupant of railway train or railway vehicle injured in derailment without antecedent collision

✓5ᵗʰ V81.8 Occupant of railway train or railway vehicle injured in other specified railway accidents
- **✓x7ᵗʰ V81.81** Occupant of railway train or railway vehicle injured due to explosion or fire on train
- **✓x7ᵗʰ V81.82** Occupant of railway train or railway vehicle injured due to object falling onto train
  - Occupant of railway train or railway vehicle injured due to falling earth onto train
  - Occupant of railway train or railway vehicle injured due to falling rocks onto train
  - Occupant of railway train or railway vehicle injured due to falling snow onto train
  - Occupant of railway train or railway vehicle injured due to falling trees onto train
- **✓x7ᵗʰ V81.83** Occupant of railway train or railway vehicle injured due to collision with military vehicle
- **✓x7ᵗʰ V81.89** Occupant of railway train or railway vehicle injured due to other specified railway accident

✓x7ᵗʰ V81.9 Occupant of railway train or railway vehicle injured in unspecified railway accident
Railway accident NOS

✓4ᵗʰ V82 Occupant of powered streetcar injured in transport accident
- INCLUDES interurban electric car
  person on outside of streetcar
  tram (car)
  trolley (car)
- EXCLUDES 1 bus (V70-V79)
  motorcoach (V70-V79)
  nonpowered streetcar (V76.-)
  train (V81.-)

✓x7ᵗʰ V82.0 Occupant of streetcar injured in collision with motor vehicle in nontraffic accident

✓x7ᵗʰ V82.1 Occupant of streetcar injured in collision with motor vehicle in traffic accident

✓x7ᵗʰ V82.2 Occupant of streetcar injured in collision with or hit by rolling stock

✓x7ᵗʰ V82.3 Occupant of streetcar injured in collision with other object
- EXCLUDES 1 collision with animal-drawn vehicle or animal being ridden (V82.8)

✓x7ᵗʰ V82.4 Person injured while boarding or alighting from streetcar

Chapter 20. External Causes of Morbidity

V82.5–V86.24

√x 7ᵗʰ **V82.5** **Occupant of streetcar injured by** fall in streetcar

> EXCLUDES 1   *fall in streetcar:*
> > *while boarding or alighting (V82.4)*
> > *with antecedent collision (V82.0-V82.3)*

√x 7ᵗʰ **V82.6** **Occupant of streetcar injured by** fall from streetcar

> EXCLUDES 1   *fall from streetcar:*
> > *while boarding or alighting (V82.4)*
> > *with antecedent collision (V82.0-V82.3)*

√x 7ᵗʰ **V82.7** **Occupant of streetcar injured in** derailment **without antecedent collision**

> EXCLUDES 1   *occupant of streetcar injured in derailment with antecedent collision (V82.0-V82.3)*

√x 7ᵗʰ **V82.8** **Occupant of streetcar injured in other specified transport accidents**

> Streetcar collision with military vehicle
> Streetcar collision with train or nonmotor vehicles

√x 7ᵗʰ **V82.9** **Occupant of streetcar injured in unspecified traffic accident**

> Streetcar accident NOS

✓4ᵗʰ **V83** **Occupant of special vehicle mainly used on industrial premises injured in transport accident**

> INCLUDES   battery-powered airport passenger vehicle
> > battery-powered truck (baggage) (mail)
> > coal-car in mine
> > forklift (truck)
> > logging car
> > self-propelled industrial truck
> > station baggage truck (powered)
> > tram, truck, or tub (powered) in mine or quarry
>
> EXCLUDES 1   *special construction vehicles (V85.-)*
> > *special industrial vehicle in stationary use or maintenance (W31.-)*

√x 7ᵗʰ **V83.0** **Driver** of special industrial vehicle injured in traffic accident

√x 7ᵗʰ **V83.1** **Passenger** of special industrial vehicle injured in traffic accident

√x 7ᵗʰ **V83.2** **Person on outside** of special industrial vehicle injured in traffic accident

√x 7ᵗʰ **V83.3** **Unspecified occupant of special industrial vehicle injured** in traffic accident

√x 7ᵗʰ **V83.4** **Person injured while** boarding or alighting **from special industrial vehicle**

√x 7ᵗʰ **V83.5** **Driver** of special industrial vehicle injured in nontraffic accident

√x 7ᵗʰ **V83.6** **Passenger** of special industrial vehicle injured in nontraffic accident

√x 7ᵗʰ **V83.7** **Person on outside** of special industrial vehicle injured in nontraffic accident

√x 7ᵗʰ **V83.9** **Unspecified occupant of special industrial vehicle injured** in nontraffic accident

> Special-industrial-vehicle accident NOS

✓4ᵗʰ **V84** **Occupant of special vehicle mainly used in agriculture injured in transport accident**

> INCLUDES   self-propelled farm machinery
> > tractor (and trailer)
>
> EXCLUDES 1   *animal-powered farm machinery accident (W30.8-)*
> > *contact with combine harvester (W30.0)*
> > *special agricultural vehicle in stationary use or maintenance (W30.-)*

√x 7ᵗʰ **V84.0** **Driver** of special agricultural vehicle injured in traffic accident

√x 7ᵗʰ **V84.1** **Passenger** of special agricultural vehicle injured in traffic accident

√x 7ᵗʰ **V84.2** **Person on outside** of special agricultural vehicle injured in traffic accident

√x 7ᵗʰ **V84.3** **Unspecified occupant of special agricultural vehicle injured** in traffic accident

√x 7ᵗʰ **V84.4** **Person injured while** boarding or alighting **from special agricultural vehicle**

√x 7ᵗʰ **V84.5** **Driver** of special agricultural vehicle injured in nontraffic accident

√x 7ᵗʰ **V84.6** **Passenger** of special agricultural vehicle injured in nontraffic accident

√x 7ᵗʰ **V84.7** **Person on outside** of special agricultural vehicle injured in nontraffic accident

√x 7ᵗʰ **V84.9** **Unspecified occupant of special agricultural vehicle injured** in nontraffic accident

> Special-agricultural vehicle accident NOS

✓4ᵗʰ **V85** **Occupant of special construction vehicle injured in transport accident**

> INCLUDES   bulldozer
> > digger
> > dump truck
> > earth-leveller
> > mechanical shovel
> > road-roller
>
> EXCLUDES 1   *special industrial vehicle (V83.-)*
> > *special construction vehicle in stationary use or maintenance (W31.-)*

√x 7ᵗʰ **V85.0** **Driver** of special construction vehicle injured in traffic accident

√x 7ᵗʰ **V85.1** **Passenger** of special construction vehicle injured in traffic accident

√x 7ᵗʰ **V85.2** **Person on outside** of special construction vehicle injured in traffic accident

√x 7ᵗʰ **V85.3** **Unspecified occupant of special construction vehicle injured in traffic accident**

√x 7ᵗʰ **V85.4** **Person injured while** boarding or alighting **from special construction vehicle**

√x 7ᵗʰ **V85.5** **Driver** of special construction vehicle injured in nontraffic accident

√x 7ᵗʰ **V85.6** **Passenger** of special construction vehicle injured in nontraffic accident

√x 7ᵗʰ **V85.7** **Person on outside** of special construction vehicle injured in nontraffic accident

√x 7ᵗʰ **V85.9** **Unspecified occupant of special construction vehicle injured in nontraffic accident**

> Special-construction-vehicle accident NOS

✓4ᵗʰ **V86** **Occupant of special all-terrain or other off-road motor vehicle, injured in transport accident**

> EXCLUDES 1   *special all-terrain vehicle in stationary use or maintenance (W31.-)*
> > *sport-utility vehicle (V50-V59)*
> > *three-wheeled motor vehicle designed for on-road use (V30-V39)*
>
> **AHA:** 2017,4Q,26

√5ᵗʰ **V86.0** **Driver** of special all-terrain or other off-road motor vehicle injured in traffic accident

> √x 7ᵗʰ **V86.01** **Driver of** ambulance or fire engine **injured in traffic accident**
>
> √x 7ᵗʰ **V86.02** **Driver of** snowmobile **injured in traffic accident**
>
> √x 7ᵗʰ **V86.03** **Driver of** dune buggy **injured in traffic accident**
>
> √x 7ᵗʰ **V86.04** **Driver of** military vehicle **injured in traffic accident**
>
> √x 7ᵗʰ **V86.05** **Driver of** 3- or 4- wheeled all-terrain vehicle (ATV) **injured in traffic accident**
>
> √x 7ᵗʰ **V86.06** **Driver of** dirt bike or motor/cross bike **injured in traffic accident**
>
> √x 7ᵗʰ **V86.09** **Driver of other special all-terrain or other off-road motor vehicle injured in traffic accident**
> > Driver of go cart injured in traffic accident
> > Driver of golf cart injured in traffic accident

√5ᵗʰ **V86.1** **Passenger** of special all-terrain or other off-road motor vehicle injured in traffic accident

> √x 7ᵗʰ **V86.11** **Passenger of** ambulance or fire engine **injured in traffic accident**
>
> √x 7ᵗʰ **V86.12** **Passenger of** snowmobile **injured in traffic accident**
>
> √x 7ᵗʰ **V86.13** **Passenger of** dune buggy **injured in traffic accident**
>
> √x 7ᵗʰ **V86.14** **Passenger of** military vehicle **injured in traffic accident**
>
> √x 7ᵗʰ **V86.15** **Passenger of** 3- or 4- wheeled all-terrain vehicle (ATV) **injured in traffic accident**
>
> √x 7ᵗʰ **V86.16** **Passenger of** dirt bike or motor/cross bike **injured in traffic accident**
>
> √x 7ᵗʰ **V86.19** **Passenger of other special all-terrain or other off-road motor vehicle injured in traffic accident**
> > Passenger of go cart injured in traffic accident
> > Passenger of golf cart injured in traffic accident

√5ᵗʰ **V86.2** **Person on outside** of special all-terrain or other off-road motor vehicle injured in traffic accident

> √x 7ᵗʰ **V86.21** **Person on outside of** ambulance or fire engine **injured in traffic accident**
>
> √x 7ᵗʰ **V86.22** **Person on outside of** snowmobile **injured in traffic accident**
>
> √x 7ᵗʰ **V86.23** **Person on outside of** dune buggy **injured in traffic accident**
>
> √x 7ᵗʰ **V86.24** **Person on outside of** military vehicle **injured in traffic accident**

√x7ᵗʰ **V86.25** **Person on outside of** 3- or 4- wheeled all-terrain vehicle (ATV) **injured in traffic accident**

√x7ᵗʰ **V86.26** **Person on outside of** dirt bike or motor/cross bike **injured in traffic accident**

√x7ᵗʰ **V86.29** **Person on outside of other special all-terrain or other off-road motor vehicle injured in traffic accident**

Person on outside of go cart in traffic accident

Person on outside of golf cart injured in traffic accident

√5ᵗʰ **V86.3** **Unspecified occupant of special all-terrain or other off-road motor vehicle injured in traffic accident**

√x7ᵗʰ **V86.31** **Unspecified occupant of** ambulance or fire engine **injured in traffic accident**

√x7ᵗʰ **V86.32** **Unspecified occupant of** snowmobile **injured in traffic accident**

√x7ᵗʰ **V86.33** **Unspecified occupant of** dune buggy **injured in traffic accident**

√x7ᵗʰ **V86.34** **Unspecified occupant of** military vehicle **injured in traffic accident**

√x7ᵗʰ **V86.35** **Unspecified occupant of** 3- or 4- wheeled all-terrain vehicle (ATV) **injured in traffic accident**

√x7ᵗʰ **V86.36** **Unspecified occupant of** dirt bike or motor/cross bike **injured in traffic accident**

√x7ᵗʰ **V86.39** **Unspecified occupant of other special all-terrain or other off-road motor vehicle injured in traffic accident**

Unspecified occupant of go cart injured in traffic accident

Unspecified occupant of golf cart injured in traffic accident

√5ᵗʰ **V86.4** **Person injured while** boarding or alighting **from special all-terrain or other off-road motor vehicle**

√x7ᵗʰ **V86.41** **Person injured while boarding or alighting from** ambulance or fire engine

√x7ᵗʰ **V86.42** **Person injured while boarding or alighting from** snowmobile

√x7ᵗʰ **V86.43** **Person injured while boarding or alighting from** dune buggy

√x7ᵗʰ **V86.44** **Person injured while boarding or alighting from** military vehicle

√x7ᵗʰ **V86.45** **Person injured while boarding or alighting from a** 3- or 4- wheeled all-terrain vehicle (ATV)

√x7ᵗʰ **V86.46** **Person injured while boarding or alighting from a** dirt bike or motor/cross bike

√x7ᵗʰ **V86.49** **Person injured while boarding or alighting from other special all-terrain or other off-road motor vehicle**

Person injured while boarding or alighting from go cart

Person injured while boarding or alighting from golf cart

√5ᵗʰ **V86.5** **Driver of** special all-terrain or other off-road motor vehicle **injured** in nontraffic accident

√x7ᵗʰ **V86.51** **Driver of** ambulance or fire engine **injured in nontraffic accident**

√x7ᵗʰ **V86.52** **Driver of** snowmobile **injured in nontraffic accident**

√x7ᵗʰ **V86.53** **Driver of** dune buggy **injured in nontraffic accident**

√x7ᵗʰ **V86.54** **Driver of** military vehicle **injured in nontraffic accident**

√x7ᵗʰ **V86.55** **Driver of** 3- or 4- wheeled all-terrain vehicle (ATV) **injured in nontraffic accident**

√x7ᵗʰ **V86.56** **Driver of** dirt bike or motor/cross bike **injured in nontraffic accident**

√x7ᵗʰ **V86.59** **Driver of other special all-terrain or other off-road motor vehicle injured in nontraffic accident**

Driver of go cart injured in nontraffic accident

Driver of golf cart injured in nontraffic accident

√5ᵗʰ **V86.6** **Passenger of** special all-terrain or other off-road motor vehicle injured in nontraffic accident

√x7ᵗʰ **V86.61** **Passenger of** ambulance or fire engine **injured in nontraffic accident**

√x7ᵗʰ **V86.62** **Passenger of** snowmobile **injured in nontraffic accident**

√x7ᵗʰ **V86.63** **Passenger of** dune buggy **injured in nontraffic accident**

√x7ᵗʰ **V86.64** **Passenger of** military vehicle **injured in nontraffic accident**

√x7ᵗʰ **V86.65** **Passenger of** 3- or 4- wheeled all-terrain vehicle (ATV) **injured in nontraffic accident**

√x7ᵗʰ **V86.66** **Passenger of** dirt bike or motor/cross bike **injured in nontraffic accident**

√x7ᵗʰ **V86.69** **Passenger of other special all-terrain or other off-road motor vehicle injured in nontraffic accident**

Passenger of go cart injured in nontraffic accident

Passenger of golf cart injured in nontraffic accident

√5ᵗʰ **V86.7** **Person on outside** of special all-terrain or other off-road motor vehicle injured in nontraffic accident

√x7ᵗʰ **V86.71** **Person on outside of** ambulance or fire engine **injured in nontraffic accident**

√x7ᵗʰ **V86.72** **Person on outside of** snowmobile **injured in nontraffic accident**

√x7ᵗʰ **V86.73** **Person on outside of** dune buggy **injured in nontraffic accident**

√x7ᵗʰ **V86.74** **Person on outside of** military vehicle **injured in nontraffic accident**

√x7ᵗʰ **V86.75** **Person on outside of** 3- or 4- wheeled all-terrain vehicle (ATV) **injured in nontraffic accident**

√x7ᵗʰ **V86.76** **Person on outside of** dirt bike or motor/cross bike **injured in nontraffic accident**

√x7ᵗʰ **V86.79** **Person on outside of other special all-terrain or other off-road motor vehicles injured in nontraffic accident**

Person on outside of go cart injured in nontraffic accident

Person on outside of golf cart injured in nontraffic accident

√5ᵗʰ **V86.9** **Unspecified occupant of special all-terrain or other off-road motor vehicle injured** in nontraffic accident

√x7ᵗʰ **V86.91** **Unspecified occupant of** ambulance or fire engine **injured in nontraffic accident**

√x7ᵗʰ **V86.92** **Unspecified occupant of** snowmobile **injured in nontraffic accident**

√x7ᵗʰ **V86.93** **Unspecified occupant of** dune buggy **injured in nontraffic accident**

√x7ᵗʰ **V86.94** **Unspecified occupant of** military vehicle **injured in nontraffic accident**

√x7ᵗʰ **V86.95** **Unspecified occupant of** 3- or 4- wheeled all-terrain vehicle (ATV) **injured in nontraffic accident**

√x7ᵗʰ **V86.96** **Unspecified occupant of** dirt bike or motor/cross bike **injured in nontraffic accident**

√x7ᵗʰ **V86.99** **Unspecified occupant of other special all-terrain or other off-road motor vehicle injured in nontraffic accident**

Off-road motor-vehicle accident NOS

Other motor-vehicle accident NOS

Unspecified occupant of go cart injured in nontraffic accident

Unspecified occupant of golf cart injured in nontraffic accident

√4ᵗʰ **V87** **Traffic accident of specified type but victim's mode of transport unknown**

    EXCLUDES 1 *collision involving:*

pedal cycle (V10-V19)

pedestrian (V01-V09)

√x7ᵗʰ **V87.0** **Person injured in collision between** car and two- or three-wheeled powered vehicle (traffic)

√x7ᵗʰ **V87.1** **Person injured in collision between other** motor vehicle and two- or three-wheeled motor vehicle (traffic)

√x7ᵗʰ **V87.2** **Person injured in collision between** car and pick-up truck or van (traffic)

√x7ᵗʰ **V87.3** **Person injured in collision between** car and bus (traffic)

√x7ᵗʰ **V87.4** **Person injured in collision between** car and heavy transport vehicle (traffic)

√x7ᵗʰ **V87.5** **Person injured in collision between** heavy transport vehicle and bus (traffic)

√x7ᵗʰ **V87.6** **Person injured in collision between** railway train or railway vehicle and car (traffic)

√x7ᵗʰ **V87.7** **Person injured in collision between** other specified motor vehicles (traffic)

√x7ᵗʰ **V87.8** **Person injured in other specified** noncollision transport accidents involving motor vehicle (traffic)

√x7ᵗʰ **V87.9** **Person injured in other specified (collision)(noncollision) transport accidents** involving nonmotor vehicle (traffic)

✓4ᵗʰ **V88** **Nontraffic accident of specified type but victim's mode of transport unknown**

> EXCLUDES 1 *collision involving:*
> *pedal cycle (V10-V19)*
> *pedestrian (V01-V09)*

✓x7ᵗʰ **V88.0** **Person injured in collision between** car and two- or three-wheeled motor vehicle, **nontraffic**

✓x7ᵗʰ **V88.1** **Person injured in collision between other** motor vehicle and two- or three-wheeled motor vehicle, **nontraffic**

✓x7ᵗʰ **V88.2** **Person injured in collision between** car and pick-up truck or van, **nontraffic**

✓x7ᵗʰ **V88.3** **Person injured in collision between** car and bus, **nontraffic**

✓x7ᵗʰ **V88.4** **Person injured in collision between** car and heavy transport vehicle, **nontraffic**

✓x7ᵗʰ **V88.5** **Person injured in collision between** heavy transport vehicle and bus, **nontraffic**

✓x7ᵗʰ **V88.6** **Person injured in collision between** railway train or railway vehicle and car, **nontraffic**

✓x7ᵗʰ **V88.7** **Person injured in collision between other specified motor vehicle, nontraffic**

✓x7ᵗʰ **V88.8** **Person injured in other specified** noncollision **transport accidents** involving motor vehicle, **nontraffic**

✓x7ᵗʰ **V88.9** **Person injured in other specified (collision)(noncollision) transport accidents** involving nonmotor vehicle, **nontraffic**

✓4ᵗʰ **V89** **Motor- or nonmotor-vehicle accident, type of vehicle unspecified**

✓x7ᵗʰ **V89.0** **Person injured in unspecified** motor-vehicle **accident, nontraffic**
> Motor-vehicle accident NOS, nontraffic

✓x7ᵗʰ **V89.1** **Person injured in unspecified** nonmotor-vehicle **accident, nontraffic**
> Nonmotor-vehicle accident NOS (nontraffic)

✓x7ᵗʰ **V89.2** **Person injured in unspecified** motor-vehicle **accident, traffic**
> Motor-vehicle accident [MVA] NOS
> Road (traffic) accident [RTA] NOS

✓x7ᵗʰ **V89.3** **Person injured in unspecified** nonmotor-vehicle **accident, traffic**
> Nonmotor-vehicle traffic accident NOS

✓x7ᵗʰ **V89.9** **Person injured in unspecified vehicle accident**
> Collision NOS

Water transport accidents (V90-V94)

The appropriate 7th character is to be added to each code from categories V90-V94.
A initial encounter
D subsequent encounter
S sequela

✓4ᵗʰ **V90** **Drowning and submersion due to accident to watercraft**

> EXCLUDES 1 *civilian water transport accident involving military watercraft (V94.81-)*
> *fall into water not from watercraft (W16.-)*
> *military watercraft accident in military or war operations (Y36.0-, Y37.0-)*
> *water-transport-related drowning or submersion without accident to watercraft (V92.-)*

✓5ᵗʰ **V90.0** **Drowning and submersion due to** watercraft overturning

✓x7ᵗʰ **V90.00** **Drowning and submersion due to** merchant ship **overturning**

✓x7ᵗʰ **V90.01** **Drowning and submersion due to** passenger ship **overturning**
> Drowning and submersion due to Ferry-boat overturning
> Drowning and submersion due to Liner overturning

✓x7ᵗʰ **V90.02** **Drowning and submersion due to** fishing boat **overturning**

✓x7ᵗʰ **V90.03** **Drowning and submersion due to other** powered **watercraft overturning**
> Drowning and submersion due to Hovercraft (on open water) overturning
> Drowning and submersion due to Jet ski overturning

✓x7ᵗʰ **V90.04** **Drowning and submersion due to** sailboat **overturning**

✓x7ᵗʰ **V90.05** **Drowning and submersion due to** canoe or kayak **overturning**

✓x7ᵗʰ **V90.06** **Drowning and submersion due to (nonpowered)** inflatable craft **overturning**

✓x7ᵗʰ **V90.08** **Drowning and submersion due to other** unpowered **watercraft overturning**
> Drowning and submersion due to windsurfer overturning

✓x7ᵗʰ **V90.09** **Drowning and submersion due to unspecified watercraft overturning**
> Drowning and submersion due to boat NOS overturning
> Drowning and submersion due to ship NOS overturning
> Drowning and submersion due to watercraft NOS overturning

✓5ᵗʰ **V90.1** **Drowning and submersion due to** watercraft sinking

✓x7ᵗʰ **V90.10** **Drowning and submersion due to** merchant ship **sinking**

✓x7ᵗʰ **V90.11** **Drowning and submersion due to** passenger ship **sinking**
> Drowning and submersion due to Ferry-boat sinking
> Drowning and submersion due to Liner sinking

✓x7ᵗʰ **V90.12** **Drowning and submersion due to** fishing boat **sinking**

✓x7ᵗʰ **V90.13** **Drowning and submersion due to other** powered **watercraft sinking**
> Drowning and submersion due to Hovercraft (on open water) sinking
> Drowning and submersion due to Jet ski sinking

✓x7ᵗʰ **V90.14** **Drowning and submersion due to** sailboat **sinking**

✓x7ᵗʰ **V90.15** **Drowning and submersion due to** canoe or kayak **sinking**

✓x7ᵗʰ **V90.16** **Drowning and submersion due to (nonpowered)** inflatable craft **sinking**

✓x7ᵗʰ **V90.18** **Drowning and submersion due to other** unpowered **watercraft sinking**

✓x7ᵗʰ **V90.19** **Drowning and submersion due to unspecified watercraft sinking**
> Drowning and submersion due to boat NOS sinking
> Drowning and submersion due to ship NOS sinking
> Drowning and submersion due to watercraft NOS sinking

✓5ᵗʰ **V90.2** **Drowning and submersion due to** falling or jumping from burning watercraft

✓x7ᵗʰ **V90.20** **Drowning and submersion due to falling or jumping from burning** merchant ship

✓x7ᵗʰ **V90.21** **Drowning and submersion due to falling or jumping from burning** passenger ship
> Drowning and submersion due to falling or jumping from burning Ferry-boat
> Drowning and submersion due to falling or jumping from burning Liner

✓x7ᵗʰ **V90.22** **Drowning and submersion due to falling or jumping from burning** fishing boat

✓x7ᵗʰ **V90.23** **Drowning and submersion due to falling or jumping from other burning** powered **watercraft**
> Drowning and submersion due to falling and jumping from burning Hovercraft (on open water)
> Drowning and submersion due to falling and jumping from burning Jet ski

✓x7ᵗʰ **V90.24** **Drowning and submersion due to falling or jumping from burning** sailboat

✓x7ᵗʰ **V90.25** **Drowning and submersion due to falling or jumping from burning** canoe or kayak

✓x7ᵗʰ **V90.26** **Drowning and submersion due to falling or jumping from burning (nonpowered)** inflatable craft

✓x7ᵗʰ **V90.27** **Drowning and submersion due to falling or jumping from burning** water-skis

✓x7ᵗʰ **V90.28** **Drowning and submersion due to falling or jumping from other burning** unpowered **watercraft**
> Drowning and submersion due to falling and jumping from burning surf-board
> Drowning and submersion due to falling and jumping from burning windsurfer

✓x7ᵗʰ **V90.29** **Drowning and submersion due to falling or jumping from unspecified burning watercraft**
> Drowning and submersion due to falling or jumping from burning boat NOS
> Drowning and submersion due to falling or jumping from burning ship NOS
> Drowning and submersion due to falling or jumping from burning watercraft NOS

√5ᵗʰ **V90.3** **Drowning and submersion due to** falling or jumping from crushed watercraft

√x7ᵗʰ **V90.30** **Drowning and submersion due to falling or jumping from crushed** merchant ship

√x7ᵗʰ **V90.31** **Drowning and submersion due to falling or jumping from crushed** passenger ship
Drowning and submersion due to falling and jumping from crushed Ferry boat
Drowning and submersion due to falling and jumping from crushed Liner

√x7ᵗʰ **V90.32** **Drowning and submersion due to falling or jumping from crushed** fishing boat

√x7ᵗʰ **V90.33** **Drowning and submersion due to falling or jumping from other crushed** powered **watercraft**
Drowning and submersion due to falling and jumping from crushed Hovercraft
Drowning and submersion due to falling and jumping from crushed Jet ski

√x7ᵗʰ **V90.34** **Drowning and submersion due to falling or jumping from crushed** sailboat

√x7ᵗʰ **V90.35** **Drowning and submersion due to falling or jumping from crushed** canoe or kayak

√x7ᵗʰ **V90.36** **Drowning and submersion due to falling or jumping from crushed (nonpowered)** inflatable craft

√x7ᵗʰ **V90.37** **Drowning and submersion due to falling or jumping from crushed** water-skis

√x7ᵗʰ **V90.38** **Drowning and submersion due to falling or jumping from other crushed** unpowered **watercraft**
Drowning and submersion due to falling and jumping from crushed surf-board
Drowning and submersion due to falling and jumping from crushed windsurfer

√x7ᵗʰ **V90.39** **Drowning and submersion due to falling or jumping from crushed unspecified watercraft**
Drowning and submersion due to falling and jumping from crushed boat NOS
Drowning and submersion due to falling and jumping from crushed ship NOS
Drowning and submersion due to falling and jumping from crushed watercraft NOS

√5ᵗʰ **V90.8** **Drowning and submersion due to other accident to watercraft**

√x7ᵗʰ **V90.80** **Drowning and submersion due to other accident to** merchant ship

√x7ᵗʰ **V90.81** **Drowning and submersion due to other accident to** passenger ship
Drowning and submersion due to other accident to Ferry-boat
Drowning and submersion due to other accident to Liner

√x7ᵗʰ **V90.82** **Drowning and submersion due to other accident to** fishing boat

√x7ᵗʰ **V90.83** **Drowning and submersion due to other accident to** powered **watercraft**
Drowning and submersion due to other accident to Hovercraft (on open water)
Drowning and submersion due to other accident to Jet ski

√x7ᵗʰ **V90.84** **Drowning and submersion due to other accident to** sailboat

√x7ᵗʰ **V90.85** **Drowning and submersion due to other accident to** canoe or kayak

√x7ᵗʰ **V90.86** **Drowning and submersion due to other accident to (nonpowered)** inflatable craft

√x7ᵗʰ **V90.87** **Drowning and submersion due to other accident to** water-skis

√x7ᵗʰ **V90.88** **Drowning and submersion due to other accident to other** unpowered **watercraft**
Drowning and submersion due to other accident to surf-board
Drowning and submersion due to other accident to windsurfer

√x7ᵗʰ **V90.89** **Drowning and submersion due to other accident to unspecified watercraft**
Drowning and submersion due to other accident to boat NOS
Drowning and submersion due to other accident to ship NOS
Drowning and submersion due to other accident to watercraft NOS

√4ᵗʰ **V91** **Other injury due to accident to watercraft**

INCLUDES   any injury except drowning and submersion as a result of an accident to watercraft

EXCLUDES 1   *civilian water transport accident involving military watercraft (V94.81-)*
military watercraft accident in military or war operations (Y36, Y37.-)

EXCLUDES 2   *drowning and submersion due to accident to watercraft (V90.-)*

√5ᵗʰ **V91.0** **Burn due to watercraft on fire**

EXCLUDES 1   *burn from localized fire or explosion on board ship without accident to watercraft (V93.-)*

√x7ᵗʰ **V91.00** **Burn due to** merchant ship **on fire**

√x7ᵗʰ **V91.01** **Burn due to** passenger ship **on fire**
Burn due to Ferry-boat on fire
Burn due to Liner on fire

√x7ᵗʰ **V91.02** **Burn due to** fishing boat **on fire**

√x7ᵗʰ **V91.03** **Burn due to other** powered **watercraft on fire**
Burn due to Hovercraft (on open water) on fire
Burn due to Jet ski on fire

√x7ᵗʰ **V91.04** **Burn due to** sailboat **on fire**

√x7ᵗʰ **V91.05** **Burn due to** canoe or kayak **on fire**

√x7ᵗʰ **V91.06** **Burn due to (nonpowered)** inflatable craft **on fire**

√x7ᵗʰ **V91.07** **Burn due to** water-skis **on fire**

√x7ᵗʰ **V91.08** **Burn due to other** unpowered **watercraft on fire**

√x7ᵗʰ **V91.09** **Burn due to unspecified watercraft on fire**
Burn due to boat NOS on fire
Burn due to ship NOS on fire
Burn due to watercraft NOS on fire

√5ᵗʰ **V91.1** **Crushed between watercraft and other watercraft or other object due to collision**
Crushed by lifeboat after abandoning ship in a collision

NOTE   Select the specified type of watercraft that the victim was on at the time of the collision

√x7ᵗʰ **V91.10** **Crushed between** merchant ship **and other watercraft or other object due to collision**

√x7ᵗʰ **V91.11** **Crushed between** passenger ship **and other watercraft or other object due to collision**
Crushed between Ferry-boat and other watercraft or other object due to collision
Crushed between Liner and other watercraft or other object due to collision

√x7ᵗʰ **V91.12** **Crushed between** fishing boat **and other watercraft or other object due to collision**

√x7ᵗʰ **V91.13** **Crushed between other** powered **watercraft and other watercraft or other object due to collision**
Crushed between Hovercraft (on open water) and other watercraft or other object due to collision
Crushed between Jet ski and other watercraft or other object due to collision

√x7ᵗʰ **V91.14** **Crushed between** sailboat **and other watercraft or other object due to collision**

√x7ᵗʰ **V91.15** **Crushed between** canoe or kayak **and other watercraft or other object due to collision**

√x7ᵗʰ **V91.16** **Crushed between (nonpowered)** inflatable craft **and other watercraft or other object due to collision**

√x7ᵗʰ **V91.18** **Crushed between other** unpowered **watercraft and other watercraft or other object due to collision**
Crushed between surfboard and other watercraft or other object due to collision
Crushed between windsurfer and other watercraft or other object due to collision

---

☑ Additional Character Required   √x7ᵗʰ Placeholder Alert   Manifestation   Unspecified Dx   Q QPP   UPD Unacceptable PDx

✓x7ᵗʰ **V91.19** **Crushed between unspecified watercraft and other watercraft or other object due to collision**
    Crushed between boat NOS and other watercraft or other object due to collision
    Crushed between ship NOS and other watercraft or other object due to collision
    Crushed between watercraft NOS and other watercraft or other object due to collision

✓5ᵗʰ **V91.2** **Fall due to collision between watercraft and other watercraft or other object**
    Fall while remaining on watercraft after collision
    NOTE Select the specified type of watercraft that the victim was on at the time of the collision
    EXCLUDES 1 crushed between watercraft and other watercraft and other object due to collision (V91.1-)
        drowning and submersion due to falling from crushed watercraft (V90.3-)

✓x7ᵗʰ **V91.20** **Fall due to collision between merchant ship and other watercraft or other object**

✓x7ᵗʰ **V91.21** **Fall due to collision between passenger ship and other watercraft or other object**
    Fall due to collision between Ferry-boat and other watercraft or other object
    Fall due to collision between Liner and other watercraft or other object

✓x7ᵗʰ **V91.22** **Fall due to collision between fishing boat and other watercraft or other object**

✓x7ᵗʰ **V91.23** **Fall due to collision between other powered watercraft and other watercraft or other object**
    Fall due to collision between Hovercraft (on open water) and other watercraft or other object
    Fall due to collision between Jet ski and other watercraft or other object

✓x7ᵗʰ **V91.24** **Fall due to collision between sailboat and other watercraft or other object**

✓x7ᵗʰ **V91.25** **Fall due to collision between canoe or kayak and other watercraft or other object**

✓x7ᵗʰ **V91.26** **Fall due to collision between (nonpowered) inflatable craft and other watercraft or other object**

✓x7ᵗʰ **V91.29** **Fall due to collision between unspecified watercraft and other watercraft or other object**
    Fall due to collision between boat NOS and other watercraft or other object
    Fall due to collision between ship NOS and other watercraft or other object
    Fall due to collision between watercraft NOS and other watercraft or other object

✓5ᵗʰ **V91.3** **Hit or struck by falling object due to accident to watercraft**
    Hit or struck by falling object (part of damaged watercraft or other object) after falling or jumping from damaged watercraft
    EXCLUDES 2 drowning or submersion due to fall or jumping from damaged watercraft (V90.2-, V90.3-)

✓x7ᵗʰ **V91.30** **Hit or struck by falling object due to accident to merchant ship**

✓x7ᵗʰ **V91.31** **Hit or struck by falling object due to accident to passenger ship**
    Hit or struck by falling object due to accident to Ferry-boat
    Hit or struck by falling object due to accident to Liner

✓x7ᵗʰ **V91.32** **Hit or struck by falling object due to accident to fishing boat**

✓x7ᵗʰ **V91.33** **Hit or struck by falling object due to accident to other powered watercraft**
    Hit or struck by falling object due to accident to Hovercraft (on open water)
    Hit or struck by falling object due to accident to Jet ski

✓x7ᵗʰ **V91.34** **Hit or struck by falling object due to accident to sailboat**

✓x7ᵗʰ **V91.35** **Hit or struck by falling object due to accident to canoe or kayak**

✓x7ᵗʰ **V91.36** **Hit or struck by falling object due to accident to (nonpowered) inflatable craft**

✓x7ᵗʰ **V91.37** **Hit or struck by falling object due to accident to water-skis**
    Hit by water-skis after jumping off of waterskis

✓x7ᵗʰ **V91.38** **Hit or struck by falling object due to accident to other unpowered watercraft**
    Hit or struck by surf-board after falling off damaged surf-board
    Hit or struck by object after falling off damaged windsurfer

✓x7ᵗʰ **V91.39** **Hit or struck by falling object due to accident to unspecified watercraft**
    Hit or struck by falling object due to accident to boat NOS
    Hit or struck by falling object due to accident to ship NOS
    Hit or struck by falling object due to accident to watercraft NOS

✓5ᵗʰ **V91.8** **Other injury due to other accident to watercraft**

✓x7ᵗʰ **V91.80** **Other injury due to other accident to merchant ship**

✓x7ᵗʰ **V91.81** **Other injury due to other accident to passenger ship**
    Other injury due to other accident to Ferry-boat
    Other injury due to other accident to Liner

✓x7ᵗʰ **V91.82** **Other injury due to other accident to fishing boat**

✓x7ᵗʰ **V91.83** **Other injury due to other accident to other powered watercraft**
    Other injury due to other accident to Hovercraft (on open water)
    Other injury due to other accident to Jet ski

✓x7ᵗʰ **V91.84** **Other injury due to other accident to sailboat**

✓x7ᵗʰ **V91.85** **Other injury due to other accident to canoe or kayak**

✓x7ᵗʰ **V91.86** **Other injury due to other accident to (nonpowered) inflatable craft**

✓x7ᵗʰ **V91.87** **Other injury due to other accident to water-skis**

✓x7ᵗʰ **V91.88** **Other injury due to other accident to other unpowered watercraft**
    Other injury due to other accident to surf-board
    Other injury due to other accident to windsurfer

✓x7ᵗʰ **V91.89** **Other injury due to other accident to unspecified watercraft**
    Other injury due to other accident to boat NOS
    Other injury due to other accident to ship NOS
    Other injury due to other accident to watercraft NOS

✓4ᵗʰ **V92** **Drowning and submersion due to accident on board watercraft, without accident to watercraft**
    EXCLUDES 1 civilian water transport accident involving military watercraft (V94.81-)
        drowning or submersion due to accident to watercraft (V90-V91)
        drowning or submersion of diver who voluntarily jumps from boat not involved in an accident (W16.711, W16.721)
        fall into water without watercraft (W16.-)
        military watercraft accident in military or war operations (Y36, Y37)

✓5ᵗʰ **V92.0** **Drowning and submersion due to fall off watercraft**
    Drowning and submersion due to fall from gangplank of watercraft
    Drowning and submersion due to fall overboard watercraft
    EXCLUDES 2 hitting head on object or bottom of body of water due to fall from watercraft (V94.0-)

✓x7ᵗʰ **V92.00** **Drowning and submersion due to fall off merchant ship**

✓x7ᵗʰ **V92.01** **Drowning and submersion due to fall off passenger ship**
    Drowning and submersion due to fall off Ferry-boat
    Drowning and submersion due to fall off Liner

✓x7ᵗʰ **V92.02** **Drowning and submersion due to fall off fishing boat**

✓x7ᵗʰ **V92.03** **Drowning and submersion due to fall off other powered watercraft**
    Drowning and submersion due to fall off Hovercraft (on open water)
    Drowning and submersion due to fall off Jet ski

✓x7ᵗʰ **V92.04** **Drowning and submersion due to fall off sailboat**

✓x7ᵗʰ **V92.05** **Drowning and submersion due to fall off canoe or kayak**

✓x7ᵗʰ **V92.06** **Drowning and submersion due to fall off (nonpowered) inflatable craft**

✓x 7th **V92.07** **Drowning and submersion due to fall off** water-skis

> EXCLUDES 1   *drowning and submersion due to falling off burning water-skis (V90.27)*
> *drowning and submersion due to falling off crushed water-skis (V90.37)*
> *hit by boat while water-skiing NOS (V94.X)*

✓x 7th **V92.08** **Drowning and submersion due to fall off other** unpowered **watercraft**

> Drowning and submersion due to fall off surf-board
> Drowning and submersion due to fall off windsurfer

> EXCLUDES 1   *drowning and submersion due to fall off burning unpowered watercraft (V90.28)*
> *drowning and submersion due to fall off crushed unpowered watercraft (V90.38)*
> *drowning and submersion due to fall off damaged unpowered watercraft (V90.88)*
> *drowning and submersion due to rider of nonpowered watercraft being hit by other watercraft (V94.-)*
> *other injury due to rider of nonpowered watercraft being hit by other watercraft (V94.-)*

✓x 7th **V92.09** **Drowning and submersion due to fall off unspecified watercraft**

> Drowning and submersion due to fall off boat NOS
> Drowning and submersion due to fall off ship
> Drowning and submersion due to fall off watercraft NOS

✓5th **V92.1** **Drowning and submersion due to being** thrown overboard **by motion of watercraft**

> EXCLUDES 1   *drowning and submersion due to fall off surf-board (V92.08)*
> *drowning and submersion due to fall off water-skis (V92.07)*
> *drowning and submersion due to fall off windsurfer (V92.08)*

✓x 7th **V92.10** **Drowning and submersion due to being thrown overboard by motion of** merchant ship

✓x 7th **V92.11** **Drowning and submersion due to being thrown overboard by motion of** passenger ship

> Drowning and submersion due to being thrown overboard by motion of Ferry-boat
> Drowning and submersion due to being thrown overboard by motion of Liner

✓x 7th **V92.12** **Drowning and submersion due to being thrown overboard by motion of** fishing boat

✓x 7th **V92.13** **Drowning and submersion due to being thrown overboard by motion of other** powered **watercraft**

> Drowning and submersion due to being thrown overboard by motion of Hovercraft

✓x 7th **V92.14** **Drowning and submersion due to being thrown overboard by motion of** sailboat

✓x 7th **V92.15** **Drowning and submersion due to being thrown overboard by motion of** canoe or kayak

✓x 7th **V92.16** **Drowning and submersion due to being thrown overboard by motion of (nonpowered)** inflatable craft

✓x 7th **V92.19** **Drowning and submersion due to being thrown overboard by motion of unspecified watercraft**

> Drowning and submersion due to being thrown overboard by motion of boat NOS
> Drowning and submersion due to being thrown overboard by motion of ship NOS
> Drowning and submersion due to being thrown overboard by motion of watercraft NOS

✓5th **V92.2** **Drowning and submersion due to being** washed overboard **from watercraft**

> Code first any associated cataclysm (X37.0-)

✓x 7th **V92.20** **Drowning and submersion due to being washed overboard from** merchant ship

---

✓x 7th **V92.21** **Drowning and submersion due to being washed overboard from** passenger ship

> Drowning and submersion due to being washed overboard from Ferry-boat
> Drowning and submersion due to being washed overboard from Liner

✓x 7th **V92.22** **Drowning and submersion due to being washed overboard from** fishing boat

✓x 7th **V92.23** **Drowning and submersion due to being washed overboard from other** powered **watercraft**

> Drowning and submersion due to being washed overboard from Hovercraft (on open water)
> Drowning and submersion due to being washed overboard from Jet ski

✓x 7th **V92.24** **Drowning and submersion due to being washed overboard from** sailboat

✓x 7th **V92.25** **Drowning and submersion due to being washed overboard from** canoe or kayak

✓x 7th **V92.26** **Drowning and submersion due to being washed overboard from (nonpowered)** inflatable craft

✓x 7th **V92.27** **Drowning and submersion due to being washed overboard from** water-skis

> EXCLUDES 1   *drowning and submersion due to fall off water-skis (V92.07)*

✓x 7th **V92.28** **Drowning and submersion due to being washed overboard from other** unpowered **watercraft**

> Drowning and submersion due to being washed overboard from surf-board
> Drowning and submersion due to being washed overboard from windsurfer

✓x 7th **V92.29** **Drowning and submersion due to being washed overboard from unspecified watercraft**

> Drowning and submersion due to being washed overboard from boat NOS
> Drowning and submersion due to being washed overboard from ship NOS
> Drowning and submersion due to being washed overboard from watercraft NOS

✓4th **V93** **Other injury due to accident on board watercraft, without accident to watercraft**

> EXCLUDES 1   *civilian water transport accident involving military watercraft (V94.81-)*
> *other injury due to accident to watercraft (V91.-)*
> *military watercraft accident in military or war operations (Y36, Y37.-)*

> EXCLUDES 2   *drowning and submersion due to accident on board watercraft, without accident to watercraft (V92.-)*

✓5th **V93.0** **Burn due to localized fire on board watercraft**

> EXCLUDES 1   *burn due to watercraft on fire (V91.0-)*

✓x 7th **V93.00** **Burn due to localized fire on board** merchant vessel

✓x 7th **V93.01** **Burn due to localized fire on board** passenger vessel

> Burn due to localized fire on board Ferry-boat
> Burn due to localized fire on board Liner

✓x 7th **V93.02** **Burn due to localized fire on board** fishing boat

✓x 7th **V93.03** **Burn due to localized fire on board other** powered **watercraft**

> Burn due to localized fire on board Hovercraft
> Burn due to localized fire on board Jet ski

✓x 7th **V93.04** **Burn due to localized fire on board** sailboat

✓x 7th **V93.09** **Burn due to localized fire on board unspecified watercraft**

> Burn due to localized fire on board boat NOS
> Burn due to localized fire on board ship NOS
> Burn due to localized fire on board watercraft NOS

✓5th **V93.1** **Other burn on board watercraft**

> Burn due to source other than fire on board watercraft
> EXCLUDES 1   *burn due to watercraft on fire (V91.0-)*

✓x 7th **V93.10** **Other burn on board** merchant vessel

✓x 7th **V93.11** **Other burn on board** passenger vessel

> Other burn on board Ferry-boat
> Other burn on board Liner

✓x 7th **V93.12** **Other burn on board** fishing boat

✓x 7th **V93.13** **Other burn on board other** powered **watercraft**

> Other burn on board Hovercraft
> Other burn on board Jet ski

✓x 7th **V93.14** **Other burn on board** sailboat

√x7ᵗʰ **V93.19** Other burn on board unspecified watercraft

Other burn on board boat NOS

Other burn on board ship NOS

Other burn on board watercraft NOS

√5ᵗʰ **V93.2 Heat exposure on board watercraft**

EXCLUDES 1 *exposure to man-made heat not aboard watercraft (W92)*

exposure to natural heat while on board watercraft (X30)

exposure to sunlight while on board watercraft (X32)

EXCLUDES 2 *burn due to fire on board watercraft (V93.0-)*

√x7ᵗʰ **V93.20 Heat exposure on board** merchant ship

√x7ᵗʰ **V93.21 Heat exposure on board** passenger ship

Heat exposure on board Ferry-boat

Heat exposure on board Liner

√x7ᵗʰ **V93.22 Heat exposure on board** fishing boat

√x7ᵗʰ **V93.23 Heat exposure on board other** powered **watercraft**

Heat exposure on board hovercraft

√x7ᵗʰ **V93.24 Heat exposure on board** sailboat

√x7ᵗʰ **V93.29 Heat exposure on board unspecified watercraft**

Heat exposure on board boat NOS

Heat exposure on board ship NOS

Heat exposure on board watercraft NOS

√5ᵗʰ **V93.3 Fall on board watercraft**

EXCLUDES 1 *fall due to collision of watercraft (V91.2-)*

√x7ᵗʰ **V93.30 Fall on board** merchant ship

√x7ᵗʰ **V93.31 Fall on board** passenger ship

Fall on board Ferry-boat

Fall on board Liner

√x7ᵗʰ **V93.32 Fall on board** fishing boat

√x7ᵗʰ **V93.33 Fall on board other** powered **watercraft**

Fall on board Hovercraft (on open water)

Fall on board Jet ski

√x7ᵗʰ **V93.34 Fall on board** sailboat

√x7ᵗʰ **V93.35 Fall on board** canoe or kayak

√x7ᵗʰ **V93.36 Fall on board (nonpowered)** inflatable craft

√x7ᵗʰ **V93.38 Fall on board other** unpowered **watercraft**

√x7ᵗʰ **V93.39 Fall on board unspecified watercraft**

Fall on board boat NOS

Fall on board ship NOS

Fall on board watercraft NOS

√5ᵗʰ **V93.4 Struck by falling object on board watercraft**

Hit by falling object on board watercraft

EXCLUDES 1 *struck by falling object due to accident to watercraft (V91.3)*

√x7ᵗʰ **V93.40 Struck by falling object on** merchant ship

√x7ᵗʰ **V93.41 Struck by falling object on** passenger ship

Struck by falling object on Ferry-boat

Struck by falling object on Liner

√x7ᵗʰ **V93.42 Struck by falling object on** fishing boat

√x7ᵗʰ **V93.43 Struck by falling object on other** powered **watercraft**

Struck by falling object on Hovercraft

√x7ᵗʰ **V93.44 Struck by falling object on** sailboat

√x7ᵗʰ **V93.48 Struck by falling object on other** unpowered **watercraft**

√x7ᵗʰ **V93.49 Struck by falling object on unspecified watercraft**

√5ᵗʰ **V93.5 Explosion on board watercraft**

Boiler explosion on steamship

EXCLUDES 2 *fire on board watercraft (V93.0-)*

√x7ᵗʰ **V93.50 Explosion on board** merchant ship

√x7ᵗʰ **V93.51 Explosion on board** passenger ship

Explosion on board Ferry-boat

Explosion on board Liner

√x7ᵗʰ **V93.52 Explosion on board** fishing boat

√x7ᵗʰ **V93.53 Explosion on board other** powered **watercraft**

Explosion on board Hovercraft

Explosion on board Jet ski

√x7ᵗʰ **V93.54 Explosion on board** sailboat

√x7ᵗʰ **V93.59 Explosion on board unspecified watercraft**

Explosion on board boat NOS

Explosion on board ship NOS

Explosion on board watercraft NOS

√5ᵗʰ **V93.6 Machinery accident on board watercraft**

EXCLUDES 1 *machinery explosion on board watercraft (V93.4-)*

machinery fire on board watercraft (V93.0-)

√x7ᵗʰ **V93.60 Machinery accident on board** merchant ship

√x7ᵗʰ **V93.61 Machinery accident on board** passenger ship

Machinery accident on board Ferry-boat

Machinery accident on board Liner

√x7ᵗʰ **V93.62 Machinery accident on board** fishing boat

√x7ᵗʰ **V93.63 Machinery accident on board other** powered **watercraft**

Machinery accident on board Hovercraft

√x7ᵗʰ **V93.64 Machinery accident on board** sailboat

√x7ᵗʰ **V93.69 Machinery accident on board unspecified watercraft**

Machinery accident on board boat NOS

Machinery accident on board ship NOS

Machinery accident on board watercraft NOS

√5ᵗʰ **V93.8 Other injury due to other accident on board watercraft**

Accidental poisoning by gases or fumes on watercraft

√x7ᵗʰ **V93.80 Other injury due to other accident on board** merchant ship

√x7ᵗʰ **V93.81 Other injury due to other accident on board** passenger ship

Other injury due to other accident on board Ferry-boat

Other injury due to other accident on board Liner

√x7ᵗʰ **V93.82 Other injury due to other accident on board** fishing boat

√x7ᵗʰ **V93.83 Other injury due to other accident on board other** powered **watercraft**

Other injury due to other accident on board Hovercraft

Other injury due to other accident on board Jet ski

√x7ᵗʰ **V93.84 Other injury due to other accident on board** sailboat

√x7ᵗʰ **V93.85 Other injury due to other accident on board** canoe or kayak

√x7ᵗʰ **V93.86 Other injury due to other accident on board (nonpowered)** inflatable craft

√x7ᵗʰ **V93.87 Other injury due to other accident on board** water-skis

Hit or struck by object while waterskiing

√x7ᵗʰ **V93.88 Other injury due to other accident on board other** unpowered **watercraft**

Hit or struck by object while surfing

Hit or struck by object while on board windsurfer

√x7ᵗʰ **V93.89 Other injury due to other accident on board unspecified watercraft**

Other injury due to other accident on board boat NOS

Other injury due to other accident on board ship NOS

Other injury due to other accident on board watercraft NOS

√4ᵗʰ **V94 Other and unspecified water transport accidents**

EXCLUDES 1 *military watercraft accidents in military or war operations (Y36, Y37)*

√x7ᵗʰ **V94.0 Hitting object or bottom of body of water due to fall from watercraft**

EXCLUDES 2 *drowning and submersion due to fall from watercraft (V92.0-)*

√5ᵗʰ **V94.1 Bather struck by watercraft**

Swimmer hit by watercraft

√x7ᵗʰ **V94.11 Bather struck by** powered **watercraft**

√x7ᵗʰ **V94.12 Bather struck by** nonpowered **watercraft**

√5ᵗʰ **V94.2 Rider of nonpowered watercraft struck by other watercraft**

√x7ᵗʰ **V94.21 Rider of nonpowered watercraft struck by other** nonpowered **watercraft**

Canoer hit by other nonpowered watercraft

Surfer hit by other nonpowered watercraft

Windsurfer hit by other nonpowered watercraft

√x7ᵗʰ **V94.22 Rider of nonpowered watercraft struck by** powered **watercraft**
    Canoer hit by motorboat
    Surfer hit by motorboat
    Windsurfer hit by motorboat

√5ᵗʰ **V94.3 Injury to rider of (inflatable) watercraft being pulled behind other watercraft**

    √x7ᵗʰ **V94.31 Injury to rider of (inflatable)** recreational **watercraft being pulled behind other watercraft**
        Injury to rider of inner-tube pulled behind motor boat

    √x7ᵗʰ **V94.32 Injury to rider of** non-recreational **watercraft being pulled behind other watercraft**
        Injury to occupant of dingy being pulled behind boat or ship
        Injury to occupant of life-raft being pulled behind boat or ship

√x7ᵗʰ **V94.4 Injury to barefoot water-skier**
    Injury to person being pulled behind boat or ship

√5ᵗʰ **V94.8 Other water transport accident**

    √6ᵗʰ **V94.81 Water transport accident involving military watercraft**

        √7ᵗʰ **V94.810 Civilian watercraft involved in water transport accident with military watercraft**
            Passenger on civilian watercraft injured due to accident with military watercraft

        √7ᵗʰ **V94.811 Civilian in water injured by military watercraft**

        √7ᵗʰ **V94.818 Other water transport accident involving military watercraft**

    √x7ᵗʰ **V94.89 Other water transport accident**

√x7ᵗʰ **V94.9 Unspecified water transport accident**
    Water transport accident NOS

Air and space transport accidents (V95-V97)

EXCLUDES 1   *military aircraft accidents in military or war operations (Y36, Y37)*

The appropriate 7th character is to be added to each code from categories V95-V97.
A   initial encounter
D   subsequent encounter
S   sequela

√4ᵗʰ **V95 Accident to powered aircraft causing injury to occupant**

√5ᵗʰ **V95.0** Helicopter **accident injuring occupant**

    √x7ᵗʰ **V95.00 Unspecified helicopter accident injuring occupant**

    √x7ᵗʰ **V95.01 Helicopter** crash **injuring occupant**

    √x7ᵗʰ **V95.02** Forced landing **of helicopter injuring occupant**

    √x7ᵗʰ **V95.03 Helicopter** collision **injuring occupant**
        Helicopter collision with any object, fixed, movable or moving

    √x7ᵗʰ **V95.04 Helicopter** fire **injuring occupant**

    √x7ᵗʰ **V95.05 Helicopter** explosion **injuring occupant**

    √x7ᵗʰ **V95.09 Other helicopter accident injuring occupant**

√5ᵗʰ **V95.1** Ultralight, microlight or powered-glider **accident injuring occupant**

    √x7ᵗʰ **V95.10 Unspecified ultralight, microlight or powered-glider accident injuring occupant**

    √x7ᵗʰ **V95.11 Ultralight, microlight or powered-glider** crash **injuring occupant**

    √x7ᵗʰ **V95.12** Forced landing **of ultralight, microlight or powered-glider injuring occupant**

    √x7ᵗʰ **V95.13 Ultralight, microlight or powered-glider** collision **injuring occupant**
        Ultralight, microlight or powered-glider collision with any object, fixed, movable or moving

    √x7ᵗʰ **V95.14 Ultralight, microlight or powered-glider** fire **injuring occupant**

    √x7ᵗʰ **V95.15 Ultralight, microlight or powered-glider** explosion **injuring occupant**

    √x7ᵗʰ **V95.19 Other ultralight, microlight or powered-glider accident injuring occupant**

√5ᵗʰ **V95.2 Other private fixed-wing aircraft accident injuring occupant**

    √x7ᵗʰ **V95.20 Unspecified accident to other private fixed-wing aircraft, injuring occupant**

    √x7ᵗʰ **V95.21 Other private fixed-wing aircraft crash injuring occupant**

√x7ᵗʰ **V95.22 Forced landing of other private fixed-wing aircraft injuring occupant**

√x7ᵗʰ **V95.23 Other private fixed-wing aircraft collision injuring occupant**
    Other private fixed-wing aircraft collision with any object, fixed, movable or moving

√x7ᵗʰ **V95.24 Other private fixed-wing aircraft fire injuring occupant**

√x7ᵗʰ **V95.25 Other private fixed-wing aircraft explosion injuring occupant**

√x7ᵗʰ **V95.29 Other accident to other private fixed-wing aircraft injuring occupant**

√5ᵗʰ **V95.3** Commercial fixed-wing **aircraft accident injuring occupant**

    √x7ᵗʰ **V95.30 Unspecified accident to commercial fixed-wing aircraft injuring occupant**

    √x7ᵗʰ **V95.31 Commercial fixed-wing aircraft** crash **injuring occupant**

    √x7ᵗʰ **V95.32** Forced landing **of commercial fixed-wing aircraft injuring occupant**

    √x7ᵗʰ **V95.33 Commercial fixed-wing aircraft** collision **injuring occupant**
        Commercial fixed-wing aircraft collision with any object, fixed, movable or moving

    √x7ᵗʰ **V95.34 Commercial fixed-wing aircraft** fire **injuring occupant**

    √x7ᵗʰ **V95.35 Commercial fixed-wing aircraft** explosion **injuring occupant**

    √x7ᵗʰ **V95.39 Other accident to commercial fixed-wing aircraft injuring occupant**

√5ᵗʰ **V95.4** Spacecraft **accident injuring occupant**

    √x7ᵗʰ **V95.40 Unspecified spacecraft accident injuring occupant**

    √x7ᵗʰ **V95.41 Spacecraft** crash **injuring occupant**

    √x7ᵗʰ **V95.42** Forced landing **of spacecraft injuring occupant**

    √x7ᵗʰ **V95.43 Spacecraft** collision **injuring occupant**
        Spacecraft collision with any object, fixed, moveable or moving

    √x7ᵗʰ **V95.44 Spacecraft** fire **injuring occupant**

    √x7ᵗʰ **V95.45 Spacecraft** explosion **injuring occupant**

    √x7ᵗʰ **V95.49 Other spacecraft accident injuring occupant**

√x7ᵗʰ **V95.8 Other powered aircraft accidents injuring occupant**

√x7ᵗʰ **V95.9 Unspecified aircraft accident injuring occupant**
    Aircraft accident NOS
    Air transport accident NOS

√4ᵗʰ **V96 Accident to nonpowered aircraft causing injury to occupant**

√5ᵗʰ **V96.0** Balloon **accident injuring occupant**

    √x7ᵗʰ **V96.00 Unspecified balloon accident injuring occupant**

    √x7ᵗʰ **V96.01 Balloon** crash **injuring occupant**

    √x7ᵗʰ **V96.02** Forced landing **of balloon injuring occupant**

    √x7ᵗʰ **V96.03 Balloon** collision **injuring occupant**
        Balloon collision with any object, fixed, moveable or moving

    √x7ᵗʰ **V96.04 Balloon** fire **injuring occupant**

    √x7ᵗʰ **V96.05 Balloon** explosion **injuring occupant**

    √x7ᵗʰ **V96.09 Other balloon accident injuring occupant**

√5ᵗʰ **V96.1** Hang-glider **accident injuring occupant**

    √x7ᵗʰ **V96.10 Unspecified hang-glider accident injuring occupant**

    √x7ᵗʰ **V96.11 Hang-glider** crash **injuring occupant**

    √x7ᵗʰ **V96.12** Forced landing **of hang-glider injuring occupant**

    √x7ᵗʰ **V96.13 Hang-glider** collision **injuring occupant**
        Hang-glider collision with any object, fixed, moveable or moving

    √x7ᵗʰ **V96.14 Hang-glider** fire **injuring occupant**

    √x7ᵗʰ **V96.15 Hang-glider** explosion **injuring occupant**

    √x7ᵗʰ **V96.19 Other hang-glider accident injuring occupant**

√6ᵗʰ **V96.2** Glider (nonpowered) **accident injuring occupant**

    √x7ᵗʰ **V96.20 Unspecified glider (nonpowered) accident injuring occupant**

    √x7ᵗʰ **V96.21 Glider (nonpowered) crash injuring occupant**

    √x7ᵗʰ **V96.22** Forced landing **of glider (nonpowered) injuring occupant**

√x7ᵗʰ **V96.23** **Glider (nonpowered) collision injuring occupant**

Glider (nonpowered) collision with any object, fixed, moveable or moving

√x7ᵗʰ **V96.24** **Glider (nonpowered) fire injuring occupant**

√x7ᵗʰ **V96.25** **Glider (nonpowered) explosion injuring occupant**

√x7ᵗʰ **V96.29** **Other glider (nonpowered) accident injuring occupant**

√x7ᵗʰ **V96.8** **Other nonpowered-aircraft accidents injuring occupant**

Kite carrying a person accident injuring occupant

√x7ᵗʰ **V96.9** **Unspecified nonpowered-aircraft accident injuring occupant**

Nonpowered-aircraft accident NOS

√4ᵗʰ **V97** **Other specified air transport accidents**

√x7ᵗʰ **V97.0** **Occupant of aircraft injured in other specified air transport accidents**

Fall in, on or from aircraft in air transport accident

EXCLUDES 1   *accident while boarding or alighting aircraft (V97.1)*

√x7ᵗʰ **V97.1** **Person injured while boarding or alighting from aircraft**

√5ᵗʰ **V97.2** **Parachutist accident**

√x7ᵗʰ **V97.21** **Parachutist entangled in object**

Parachutist landing in tree

√x7ᵗʰ **V97.22** **Parachutist injured on landing**

√x7ᵗʰ **V97.29** **Other parachutist accident**

√5ᵗʰ **V97.3** **Person on ground injured in air transport accident**

√x7ᵗʰ **V97.31** **Hit by object falling from aircraft**

Hit by crashing aircraft
Injured by aircraft hitting house
Injured by aircraft hitting car

√x7ᵗʰ **V97.32** **Injured by rotating propeller**

√x7ᵗʰ **V97.33** **Sucked into jet engine**

√x7ᵗʰ **V97.39** **Other injury to person on ground due to air transport accident**

√5ᵗʰ **V97.8** **Other air transport accidents, not elsewhere classified**

EXCLUDES 1   *aircraft accident NOS (V95.9)*

exposure to changes in air pressure during ascent or descent (W94.-)

√6ᵗʰ **V97.81** **Air transport accident involving military aircraft**

√7ᵗʰ **V97.810** **Civilian aircraft involved in air transport accident with military aircraft**

Passenger in civilian aircraft injured due to accident with military aircraft

√7ᵗʰ **V97.811** **Civilian injured by military aircraft**

√7ᵗʰ **V97.818** **Other air transport accident involving military aircraft**

√x7ᵗʰ **V97.89** **Other air transport accidents, not elsewhere classified**

Injury from machinery on aircraft

Other and unspecified transport accidents (V98-V99)

EXCLUDES 1   *vehicle accident, type of vehicle unspecified (V89.-)*

The appropriate 7th character is to be added to each code from categories V98-V99.
A   initial encounter
D   subsequent encounter
S   sequela

√4ᵗʰ **V98** **Other specified transport accidents**

√x7ᵗʰ **V98.0** **Accident to, on or involving cable-car, not on rails**

Caught or dragged by cable-car, not on rails
Fall or jump from cable-car, not on rails
Object thrown from or in cable-car, not on rails

√x7ᵗʰ **V98.1** **Accident to, on or involving land-yacht**

√x7ᵗʰ **V98.2** **Accident to, on or involving ice yacht**

√x7ᵗʰ **V98.3** **Accident to, on or involving ski lift**

Accident to, on or involving ski chair-lift
Accident to, on or involving ski-lift with gondola

√x7ᵗʰ **V98.8** **Other specified transport accidents**

√x7ᵗʰ **V99** **Unspecified transport accident**

OTHER EXTERNAL CAUSES OF ACCIDENTAL INJURY (W00-X58)

Slipping, tripping, stumbling and falls (W00-W19)

EXCLUDES 1   *assault involving a fall (Y01-Y02)*
fall from animal (V80.-)
fall (in) (from) machinery (in operation) (W28-W31)
fall (in) (from) transport vehicle (V01-V99)
intentional self-harm involving a fall (X80-X81)

EXCLUDES 2   *at risk for fall (history of fall) Z91.81*
fall (in) (from) burning building (X00.-)
fall into fire (X00-X04, X08)

The appropriate 7th character is to be added to each code from categories W00-W19.
A   initial encounter
D   subsequent encounter
S   sequela

√4ᵗʰ **W00** **Fall due to ice and snow**

INCLUDES   pedestrian on foot falling (slipping) on ice and snow

EXCLUDES 1   *fall on (from) ice and snow involving pedestrian conveyance (V00.-)*

fall from stairs and steps not due to ice and snow (W10.-)

AHA: 2016,2Q,4

√x7ᵗʰ **W00.0** **Fall on same level due to ice and snow**

√x7ᵗʰ **W00.1** **Fall from stairs and steps due to ice and snow**

√x7ᵗʰ **W00.2** **Other fall from one level to another due to ice and snow**

√x7ᵗʰ **W00.9** **Unspecified fall due to ice and snow**

√4ᵗʰ **W01** **Fall on same level from slipping, tripping and stumbling**

INCLUDES   fall on moving sidewalk

EXCLUDES 1   *fall due to bumping (striking) against object (W18.0-)*
fall in shower or bathtub (W18.2-)
fall on same level NOS (W18.30)
fall on same level from slipping, tripping and stumbling due to ice or snow (W00.0)
fall off or from toilet (W18.1-)
slipping, tripping and stumbling NOS (W18.40)
slipping, tripping and stumbling without falling (W18.4-)

√x7ᵗʰ **W01.0** **Fall on same level from slipping, tripping and stumbling without subsequent striking against object**

Falling over animal   *[handwritten: slipping on floor]*

[handwritten: W01.0XXA]

√5ᵗʰ **W01.1** **Fall on same level from slipping, tripping and stumbling with subsequent striking against object**

√x7ᵗʰ **W01.10** **Fall on same level from slipping, tripping and stumbling with subsequent striking against unspecified object**

√6ᵗʰ **W01.11** **Fall on same level from slipping, tripping and stumbling with subsequent striking against sharp object**

√7ᵗʰ **W01.110** **Fall on same level from slipping, tripping and stumbling with subsequent striking against sharp glass**

√7ᵗʰ **W01.111** **Fall on same level from slipping, tripping and stumbling with subsequent striking against power tool or machine**

√7ᵗʰ **W01.118** **Fall on same level from slipping, tripping and stumbling with subsequent striking against other sharp object**

√7ᵗʰ **W01.119** **Fall on same level from slipping, tripping and stumbling with subsequent striking against unspecified sharp object**

√6ᵗʰ **W01.19** **Fall on same level from slipping, tripping and stumbling with subsequent striking against other object**

√7ᵗʰ **W01.190** **Fall on same level from slipping, tripping and stumbling with subsequent striking against furniture**

√7ᵗʰ **W01.198** **Fall on same level from slipping, tripping and stumbling with subsequent striking against other object**

√x7ᵗʰ W03 Other fall on same level due to collision with another person
> Fall due to non-transport collision with other person
> > *EXCLUDES 1*   *collision with another person without fall (W51)*
> > *crushed or pushed by a crowd or human stampede (W52)*
> > *fall involving pedestrian conveyance (V00-V09)*
> > *fall due to ice or snow (W00)*
> > *fall on same level NOS (W18.30)*
> **AHA:** 2012,4Q,108

√x7ᵗʰ W04 Fall while being carried or supported by other persons
> Accidentally dropped while being carried

√4ᵗʰ W05 Fall from non-moving wheelchair, nonmotorized scooter and motorized mobility scooter
> > *EXCLUDES 1*   *fall from moving wheelchair (powered) (V00.811)*
> > *fall from moving motorized mobility scooter (V00.831)*
> > *fall from nonmotorized scooter (V00.141)*

> **√x7ᵗʰ W05.0 Fall from non-moving wheelchair**
> > **AHA:** 2019,2Q,27

> **√x7ᵗʰ W05.1 Fall from non-moving nonmotorized scooter**

> **√x7ᵗʰ W05.2 Fall from non-moving motorized mobility scooter**

√x7ᵗʰ W06 Fall from bed

√x7ᵗʰ W07 Fall from chair

√x7ᵗʰ W08 Fall from other furniture
> ▶Fall from stool◀

√4ᵗʰ W09 Fall on and from playground equipment
> > *EXCLUDES 1*   *fall involving recreational machinery (W31)*

> **√x7ᵗʰ W09.0 Fall on or from playground slide**

> **√x7ᵗʰ W09.1 Fall from playground swing**

> **√x7ᵗʰ W09.2 Fall on or from jungle gym**

> **√x7ᵗʰ W09.8 Fall on or from other playground equipment**

√4ᵗʰ W10 Fall on and from stairs and steps
> > *EXCLUDES 1*   *Fall from stairs and steps due to ice and snow (W00.1)*

> **√x7ᵗʰ W10.0 Fall (on)(from) escalator**

> **√x7ᵗʰ W10.1 Fall (on)(from) sidewalk curb**

> **√x7ᵗʰ W10.2 Fall (on)(from) incline**
> > Fall (on) (from) ramp

> **√x7ᵗʰ W10.8 Fall (on) (from) other stairs and steps**

> **√x7ᵗʰ W10.9 Fall (on) (from) unspecified stairs and steps**

√x7ᵗʰ W11 Fall on and from ladder

√x7ᵗʰ W12 Fall on and from scaffolding

√4ᵗʰ W13 Fall from, out of or through building or structure

> **√x7ᵗʰ W13.0 Fall from, out of or through balcony**
> > Fall from, out of or through railing

> **√x7ᵗʰ W13.1 Fall from, out of or through bridge**

> **√x7ᵗʰ W13.2 Fall from, out of or through roof**

> **√x7ᵗʰ W13.3 Fall through floor**

> **√x7ᵗʰ W13.4 Fall from, out of or through window**
> > *EXCLUDES 2*   *fall with subsequent striking against sharp glass (W01.110-)*

> **√x7ᵗʰ W13.8 Fall from, out of or through other building or structure**
> > Fall from, out of or through viaduct
> > Fall from, out of or through wall
> > Fall from, out of or through flag-pole

> **√x7ᵗʰ W13.9 Fall from, out of or through building, not otherwise specified**
> > *EXCLUDES 1*   *collapse of a building or structure (W20.-)*
> > *fall or jump from burning building or structure (X00.-)*

√x7ᵗʰ W14 Fall from tree

√x7ᵗʰ W15 Fall from cliff

√4ᵗʰ W16 Fall, jump or diving into water
> > *EXCLUDES 1*   *accidental non-watercraft drowning and submersion not involving fall (W65-W74)*
> > *effects of air pressure from diving (W94.-)*
> > *fall into water from watercraft (V90-V94)*
> > *hitting an object or against bottom when falling from watercraft (V94.0)*
> > *EXCLUDES 2*   *striking or hitting diving board (W21.4)*

> **√5ᵗʰ W16.0 Fall into swimming pool**
> > Fall into swimming pool NOS
> > > *EXCLUDES 1*   *fall into empty swimming pool (W17.3)*

> > **√6ᵗʰ W16.01 Fall into swimming pool striking water surface**
> > > **√7ᵗʰ W16.011 Fall into swimming pool striking water surface causing drowning and submersion**
> > > > *EXCLUDES 1*   *drowning and submersion while in swimming pool without fall (W67)*

> > > **√7ᵗʰ W16.012 Fall into swimming pool striking water surface causing other injury**

> > **√6ᵗʰ W16.02 Fall into swimming pool striking bottom**
> > > **√7ᵗʰ W16.021 Fall into swimming pool striking bottom causing drowning and submersion**
> > > > *EXCLUDES 1*   *drowning and submersion while in swimming pool without fall (W67)*

> > > **√7ᵗʰ W16.022 Fall into swimming pool striking bottom causing other injury**

> > **√6ᵗʰ W16.03 Fall into swimming pool striking wall**
> > > **√7ᵗʰ W16.031 Fall into swimming pool striking wall causing drowning and submersion**
> > > > *EXCLUDES 1*   *drowning and submersion while in swimming pool without fall (W67)*

> > > **√7ᵗʰ W16.032 Fall into swimming pool striking wall causing other injury**

> **√5ᵗʰ W16.1 Fall into natural body of water**
> > Fall into lake
> > Fall into open sea
> > Fall into river
> > Fall into stream

> > **√6ᵗʰ W16.11 Fall into natural body of water striking water surface**
> > > **√7ᵗʰ W16.111 Fall into natural body of water striking water surface causing drowning and submersion**
> > > > *EXCLUDES 1*   *drowning and submersion while in natural body of water without fall (W69)*

> > > **√7ᵗʰ W16.112 Fall into natural body of water striking water surface causing other injury**

> > **√6ᵗʰ W16.12 Fall into natural body of water striking bottom**
> > > **√7ᵗʰ W16.121 Fall into natural body of water striking bottom causing drowning and submersion**
> > > > *EXCLUDES 1*   *drowning and submersion while in natural body of water without fall (W69)*

> > > **√7ᵗʰ W16.122 Fall into natural body of water striking bottom causing other injury**

> > **√6ᵗʰ W16.13 Fall into natural body of water striking side**
> > > **√7ᵗʰ W16.131 Fall into natural body of water striking side causing drowning and submersion**
> > > > *EXCLUDES 1*   *drowning and submersion while in natural body of water without fall (W69)*

> > > **√7ᵗʰ W16.132 Fall into natural body of water striking side causing other injury**

> **√5ᵗʰ W16.2 Fall in (into) filled bathtub or bucket of water**
> > **√6ᵗʰ W16.21 Fall in (into) filled bathtub**
> > > *EXCLUDES 1*   *fall into empty bathtub (W18.2)*

> > > **√7ᵗʰ W16.211 Fall in (into) filled bathtub causing drowning and submersion**
> > > > *EXCLUDES 1*   *drowning and submersion while in filled bathtub without fall (W65)*

> > > **√7ᵗʰ W16.212 Fall in (into) filled bathtub causing other injury**

✓6ᵗʰ **W16.22**   **Fall in (into)** bucket of water

    ✓7ᵗʰ **W16.221**   **Fall in (into) bucket of water causing** drowning and submersion

    ✓7ᵗʰ **W16.222**   **Fall in (into) bucket of water causing other injury**

✓5ᵗʰ **W16.3**   **Fall into other water**

   Fall into fountain

   Fall into reservoir

   ✓6ᵗʰ **W16.31**   **Fall into other water** striking water surface

    ✓7ᵗʰ **W16.311**   **Fall into other water striking water surface causing** drowning and submersion

      EXCLUDES 1   drowning and submersion while in other water without fall (W73)

    ✓7ᵗʰ **W16.312**   **Fall into other water striking water surface causing other injury**

   ✓6ᵗʰ **W16.32**   **Fall into other water** striking bottom

    ✓7ᵗʰ **W16.321**   **Fall into other water striking bottom causing** drowning and submersion

      EXCLUDES 1   drowning and submersion while in other water without fall (W73)

    ✓7ᵗʰ **W16.322**   **Fall into other water striking bottom causing other injury**

   ✓6ᵗʰ **W16.33**   **Fall into other water** striking wall

    ✓7ᵗʰ **W16.331**   **Fall into other water striking wall causing** drowning and submersion

      EXCLUDES 1   drowning and submersion while in other water without fall (W73)

    ✓7ᵗʰ **W16.332**   **Fall into other water striking wall causing other injury**

✓5ᵗʰ **W16.4**   **Fall into unspecified water**

   ✓x7ᵗʰ **W16.41**   **Fall into unspecified water causing** drowning and submersion

   ✓x7ᵗʰ **W16.42**   **Fall into unspecified water causing other injury**

✓5ᵗʰ **W16.5**   **Jumping or diving into** swimming pool

   ✓6ᵗʰ **W16.51**   **Jumping or diving into swimming pool** striking water surface

    ✓7ᵗʰ **W16.511**   **Jumping or diving into swimming pool striking water surface causing** drowning and submersion

      EXCLUDES 1   drowning and submersion while in swimming pool without jumping or diving (W67)

    ✓7ᵗʰ **W16.512**   **Jumping or diving into swimming pool striking water surface causing other injury**

   ✓6ᵗʰ **W16.52**   **Jumping or diving into swimming pool** striking bottom

    ✓7ᵗʰ **W16.521**   **Jumping or diving into swimming pool striking bottom causing** drowning and submersion

      EXCLUDES 1   drowning and submersion while in swimming pool without jumping or diving (W67)

    ✓7ᵗʰ **W16.522**   **Jumping or diving into swimming pool striking bottom causing other injury**

   ✓6ᵗʰ **W16.53**   **Jumping or diving into swimming pool** striking wall

    ✓7ᵗʰ **W16.531**   **Jumping or diving into swimming pool striking wall causing** drowning and submersion

      EXCLUDES 1   drowning and submersion while in swimming pool without jumping or diving (W67)

    ✓7ᵗʰ **W16.532**   **Jumping or diving into swimming pool striking wall causing other injury**

✓5ᵗʰ **W16.6**   **Jumping or diving into** natural body of water

   Jumping or diving into lake

   Jumping or diving into open sea

   Jumping or diving into river

   Jumping or diving into stream

   ✓6ᵗʰ **W16.61**   **Jumping or diving into natural body of water** striking water surface

    ✓7ᵗʰ **W16.611**   **Jumping or diving into natural body of water striking water surface causing** drowning and submersion

      EXCLUDES 1   drowning and submersion while in natural body of water without jumping or diving (W69)

    ✓7ᵗʰ **W16.612**   **Jumping or diving into natural body of water striking water surface causing other injury**

   ✓6ᵗʰ **W16.62**   **Jumping or diving into natural body of water** striking bottom

    ✓7ᵗʰ **W16.621**   **Jumping or diving into natural body of water striking bottom causing** drowning and submersion

      EXCLUDES 1   drowning and submersion while in natural body of water without jumping or diving (W69)

    ✓7ᵗʰ **W16.622**   **Jumping or diving into natural body of water striking bottom causing other injury**

✓5ᵗʰ **W16.7**   **Jumping or diving** from boat

      EXCLUDES 1   fall from boat into water - see watercraft accident (V90-V94)

   ✓6ᵗʰ **W16.71**   **Jumping or diving from boat** striking water surface

    ✓7ᵗʰ **W16.711**   **Jumping or diving from boat striking water surface causing** drowning and submersion

    ✓7ᵗʰ **W16.712**   **Jumping or diving from boat striking water surface causing other injury**

   ✓6ᵗʰ **W16.72**   **Jumping or diving from boat** striking bottom

    ✓7ᵗʰ **W16.721**   **Jumping or diving from boat striking bottom causing** drowning and submersion

    ✓7ᵗʰ **W16.722**   **Jumping or diving from boat striking bottom causing other injury**

✓5ᵗʰ **W16.8**   **Jumping or diving into other water**

   Jumping or diving into fountain

   Jumping or diving into reservoir

   ✓6ᵗʰ **W16.81**   **Jumping or diving into other water** striking water surface

    ✓7ᵗʰ **W16.811**   **Jumping or diving into other water striking water surface causing** drowning and submersion

      EXCLUDES 1   drowning and submersion while in other water without jumping or diving (W73)

    ✓7ᵗʰ **W16.812**   **Jumping or diving into other water striking water surface causing other injury**

   ✓6ᵗʰ **W16.82**   **Jumping or diving into other water** striking bottom

    ✓7ᵗʰ **W16.821**   **Jumping or diving into other water striking bottom causing** drowning and submersion

      EXCLUDES 1   drowning and submersion while in other water without jumping or diving (W73)

    ✓7ᵗʰ **W16.822**   **Jumping or diving into other water striking bottom causing other injury**

   ✓6ᵗʰ **W16.83**   **Jumping or diving into other water** striking wall

    ✓7ᵗʰ **W16.831**   **Jumping or diving into other water striking wall causing** drowning and submersion

      EXCLUDES 1   drowning and submersion while in other water without jumping or diving (W73)

    ✓7ᵗʰ **W16.832**   **Jumping or diving into other water striking wall causing other injury**

√5ᵗʰ **W16.9**   **Jumping or diving into unspecified water**

    √x7ᵗʰ **W16.91**   **Jumping or diving into unspecified water causing** drowning and submersion

    √x7ᵗʰ **W16.92**   **Jumping or diving into unspecified water causing other injury**

✓4ᵗʰ **W17**   **Other fall from one level to another**

    √x7ᵗʰ **W17.0**   **Fall into well**

    √x7ᵗʰ **W17.1**   **Fall into storm drain or manhole**

    √x7ᵗʰ **W17.2**   **Fall into hole**

       Fall into pit

    √x7ᵗʰ **W17.3**   **Fall into empty swimming pool**

       EXCLUDES 1   *fall into filled swimming pool (W16.0-)*

    √x7ᵗʰ **W17.4**   **Fall from dock**

    √5ᵗʰ **W17.8**   **Other fall from one level to another**

       √x7ᵗʰ **W17.81**   **Fall down embankment (hill)**

       √x7ᵗʰ **W17.82**   **Fall from (out of) grocery cart**

          Fall due to grocery cart tipping over

       √x7ᵗʰ **W17.89**   **Other fall from one level to another**

          Fall from cherry picker

          Fall from lifting device

          Fall from mobile elevated work platform [MEWP]

          Fall from sky lift

          AHA: 2015,2Q,6

✓4ᵗʰ **W18**   **Other slipping, tripping and stumbling and falls**

    √5ᵗʰ **W18.0**   **Fall due to bumping against object**

       Striking against object with subsequent fall

       EXCLUDES 1   *fall on same level due to slipping, tripping, or stumbling with subsequent striking against object (W01.1-)*

       √x7ᵗʰ **W18.00**   **Striking against unspecified object with subsequent fall**

       √x7ᵗʰ **W18.01**   **Striking against** sports equipment **with subsequent fall**

       √x7ᵗʰ **W18.02**   **Striking against** glass **with subsequent fall**

       √x7ᵗʰ **W18.09**   **Striking against other object with subsequent fall**

    √5ᵗʰ **W18.1**   **Fall from or off toilet**

       √x7ᵗʰ **W18.11**   **Fall from or off toilet** without subsequent striking against object

          Fall from (off) toilet NOS

       √x7ᵗʰ **W18.12**   **Fall from or off toilet** with subsequent striking against object

    √x7ᵗʰ **W18.2**   **Fall in (into) shower or empty bathtub**

       EXCLUDES 1   *fall in full bathtub causing drowning or submersion (W16.21-)*

    √5ᵗʰ **W18.3**   **Other and unspecified fall on same level**

       √x7ᵗʰ **W18.30**   **Fall on same level, unspecified**

       √x7ᵗʰ **W18.31**   **Fall on same level due to stepping on an object**

          Fall on same level due to stepping on an animal

          EXCLUDES 1   *slipping, tripping and stumbling without fall due to stepping on animal (W18.41)*

       √x7ᵗʰ **W18.39**   **Other fall on same level**

    √5ᵗʰ **W18.4**   **Slipping, tripping and stumbling without falling**

       EXCLUDES 1   *collision with another person without fall (W51)*

       √x7ᵗʰ **W18.40**   **Slipping, tripping and stumbling without falling, unspecified**

       √x7ᵗʰ **W18.41**   **Slipping, tripping and stumbling without falling due to** stepping on object

          Slipping, tripping and stumbling without falling due to stepping on animal

          EXCLUDES 1   *slipping, tripping and stumbling with fall due to stepping on animal (W18.31)*

       √x7ᵗʰ **W18.42**   **Slipping, tripping and stumbling without falling due to** stepping into hole or opening

       √x7ᵗʰ **W18.43**   **Slipping, tripping and stumbling without falling due to** stepping from one level to another

       √x7ᵗʰ **W18.49**   **Other slipping, tripping and stumbling without falling**

√x7ᵗʰ **W19**   **Unspecified fall**

       Accidental fall NOS

       AHA: 2012,4Q,95

Exposure to inanimate mechanical forces (W20-W49)

   EXCLUDES 1   *assault (X92-Y09)*

               contact or collision with animals or persons (W50-W64)

               exposure to inanimate mechanical forces involving military or war operations (Y36.-, Y37.-)

               intentional self-harm (X71-X83)

The appropriate 7th character is to be added to each code from categories W20-W49.
A   initial encounter
D   subsequent encounter
S   sequela

√4ᵗʰ **W20**   **Struck by thrown, projected or falling object**

       Code first any associated:

       cataclysm (X34-X39)

       lightning strike (T75.00)

       EXCLUDES 1   *falling object in machinery accident (W24, W28-W31)*

               falling object in transport accident (V01-V99)

               object set in motion by explosion (W35-W40)

               object set in motion by firearm (W32-W34)

               struck by thrown sports equipment (W21.-)

    √x7ᵗʰ **W20.0**   **Struck by falling object in cave-in**

       EXCLUDES 2   *asphyxiation due to cave-in (T71.21)*

    √x7ᵗʰ **W20.1**   **Struck by object due to collapse of building**

       EXCLUDES 1   *struck by object due to collapse of burning building (X00.2, X02.2)*

    √x7ᵗʰ **W20.8**   **Other cause of strike by thrown, projected or falling object**

       EXCLUDES 1   *struck by thrown sports equipment (W21.-)*

√4ᵗʰ **W21**   **Striking against or struck by sports equipment**

       EXCLUDES 1   *assault with sports equipment (Y08.0-)*

               striking against or struck by sports equipment with subsequent fall (W18.01)

    √5ᵗʰ **W21.0**   **Struck by** hit or thrown ball

       √x7ᵗʰ **W21.00**   **Struck by hit or thrown ball, unspecified type**

       √x7ᵗʰ **W21.01**   **Struck by** football

       √x7ᵗʰ **W21.02**   **Struck by** soccer ball

       √x7ᵗʰ **W21.03**   **Struck by** baseball

       √x7ᵗʰ **W21.04**   **Struck by** golf ball

       √x7ᵗʰ **W21.05**   **Struck by** basketball

       √x7ᵗʰ **W21.06**   **Struck by** volleyball

       √x7ᵗʰ **W21.07**   **Struck by** softball

       √x7ᵗʰ **W21.09**   **Struck by other hit or thrown ball**

    √5ᵗʰ **W21.1**   **Struck by** bat, racquet or club

       √x7ᵗʰ **W21.11**   **Struck by** baseball bat

       √x7ᵗʰ **W21.12**   **Struck by** tennis racquet

       √x7ᵗʰ **W21.13**   **Struck by** golf club

       √x7ᵗʰ **W21.19**   **Struck by other bat, racquet or club**

    √5ᵗʰ **W21.2**   **Struck by** hockey stick or puck

       √6ᵗʰ **W21.21**   **Struck by** hockey stick

          √7ᵗʰ **W21.210**   **Struck by** ice hockey stick

          √7ᵗʰ **W21.211**   **Struck by** field hockey stick

       √6ᵗʰ **W21.22**   **Struck by** hockey puck

          √7ᵗʰ **W21.220**   **Struck by** ice hockey puck

          √7ᵗʰ **W21.221**   **Struck by** field hockey puck

    √5ᵗʰ **W21.3**   **Struck by** sports foot wear

       √x7ᵗʰ **W21.31**   **Struck by shoe** cleats

          Stepped on by shoe cleats

       √x7ᵗʰ **W21.32**   **Struck by skate** blades

          Skated over by skate blades

       √x7ᵗʰ **W21.39**   **Struck by other sports foot wear**

    √x7ᵗʰ **W21.4**   **Striking against** diving board

       Use additional code for subsequent falling into water, if applicable (W16.-)

    √5ᵗʰ **W21.8**   **Striking against or struck by other sports equipment**

       √x7ᵗʰ **W21.81**   **Striking against or struck by** football helmet

       √x7ᵗʰ **W21.89**   **Striking against or struck by other sports equipment**

    √x7ᵗʰ **W21.9**   **Striking against or struck by unspecified sports equipment**

☑ Additional Character Required   √x7ᵗʰ Placeholder Alert   Manifestation   Unspecified Dx   Q QPP   UPD Unacceptable PDx

✓4ᵗʰ **W22 Striking against or struck by other objects**
> *EXCLUDES 1*   striking against or struck by object with subsequent fall (W18.09)

✓5ᵗʰ **W22.0 Striking against** stationary object
> *EXCLUDES 1*   striking against stationary sports equipment (W21.8)

✓7ᵗʰ **W22.01 Walked into** wall

✓7ᵗʰ **W22.02 Walked into** lamppost

✓7ᵗʰ **W22.03 Walked into** furniture

✓6ᵗʰ **W22.04 Striking against wall of** swimming pool

✓7ᵗʰ **W22.041 Striking against wall of swimming pool causing** drowning and submersion
> *EXCLUDES 1*   drowning and submersion while swimming without striking against wall (W67)

✓7ᵗʰ **W22.042 Striking against wall of swimming pool causing other injury**

✓7ᵗʰ **W22.09 Striking against other stationary object**

✓5ᵗʰ **W22.1 Striking against or struck by** automobile airbag

✓7ᵗʰ **W22.10 Striking against or struck by unspecified automobile airbag**

✓7ᵗʰ **W22.11 Striking against or struck by** driver side **automobile airbag**

✓7ᵗʰ **W22.12 Striking against or struck by** front passenger side **automobile airbag**

✓7ᵗʰ **W22.19 Striking against or struck by other automobile airbag**

✓7ᵗʰ **W22.8 Striking against or struck by other objects**
> Striking against or struck by object NOS
> *EXCLUDES 1*   struck by thrown, projected or falling object (W20.-)

✓4ᵗʰ **W23 Caught, crushed, jammed or pinched in or between objects**
> *EXCLUDES 1*   injury caused by cutting or piercing instruments (W25-W27)
> injury caused by firearms malfunction (W32.1, W33.1-, W34.1-)
> injury caused by lifting and transmission devices (W24.-)
> injury caused by machinery (W28-W31)
> injury caused by nonpowered hand tools (W27.-)
> injury caused by transport vehicle being used as a means of transportation (V01-V99)
> injury caused by struck by thrown, projected or falling object (W20.-)

✓7ᵗʰ **W23.0 Caught, crushed, jammed, or pinched between** moving objects

✓7ᵗʰ **W23.1 Caught, crushed, jammed, or pinched between** stationary objects

● ✓7ᵗʰ **W23.2 Caught, crushed, jammed or pinched between a** moving and stationary object

✓4ᵗʰ **W24 Contact with lifting and transmission devices, not elsewhere classified**
> *EXCLUDES 1*   transport accidents (V01-V99)

✓7ᵗʰ **W24.0 Contact with lifting devices, not elsewhere classified**
> Contact with chain hoist
> Contact with drive belt
> Contact with pulley (block)

✓7ᵗʰ **W24.1 Contact with transmission devices, not elsewhere classified**
> Contact with transmission belt or cable

✓7ᵗʰ **W25 Contact with sharp glass**
> Code first any associated:
> injury due to flying glass from explosion or firearm discharge (W32-W40)
> transport accident (V00-V99)
> *EXCLUDES 1*   fall on same level due to slipping, tripping and stumbling with subsequent striking against sharp glass (W01.110-)
> striking against sharp glass with subsequent fall (W18.02-)
> *EXCLUDES 2*   glass embedded in skin (W45.-)

[handwritten: cut thumb with sharp glass]

✓4ᵗʰ **W26 Contact with other sharp objects**
> *EXCLUDES 2*   sharp object(s) embedded in skin (W45.-)
> **AHA:** 2016,4Q,73

✓7ᵗʰ **W26.0 Contact with knife**
> *EXCLUDES 1*   contact with electric knife (W29.1)

✓7ᵗʰ **W26.1 Contact with sword or dagger**

✓7ᵗʰ **W26.2 Contact with edge of stiff paper**
> Paper cut

✓7ᵗʰ **W26.8 Contact with other sharp object(s), not elsewhere classified**
> Contact with tin can lid

✓7ᵗʰ **W26.9 Contact with unspecified sharp object(s)**

✓4ᵗʰ **W27 Contact with nonpowered hand tool**

✓7ᵗʰ **W27.0 Contact with** workbench tool
> Contact with auger
> Contact with axe
> Contact with chisel
> Contact with handsaw
> Contact with screwdriver

✓7ᵗʰ **W27.1 Contact with** garden tool
> Contact with hoe
> Contact with nonpowered lawn mower
> Contact with pitchfork
> Contact with rake

✓7ᵗʰ **W27.2 Contact with** scissors

✓7ᵗʰ **W27.3 Contact with** needle (sewing)
> *EXCLUDES 1*   contact with hypodermic needle (W46.-)

✓7ᵗʰ **W27.4 Contact with** kitchen utensil
> Contact with fork
> Contact with ice-pick
> Contact with can-opener NOS

✓7ᵗʰ **W27.5 Contact with** paper-cutter

✓7ᵗʰ **W27.8 Contact with other nonpowered hand tool**
> Contact with nonpowered sewing machine
> Contact with shovel

✓7ᵗʰ **W28 Contact with powered lawn mower**
> Powered lawn mower (commercial) (residential)
> *EXCLUDES 1*   contact with nonpowered lawn mower (W27.1)
> *EXCLUDES 2*   exposure to electric current (W86.-)

✓4ᵗʰ **W29 Contact with other powered hand tools and household machinery**
> *EXCLUDES 1*   contact with commercial machinery (W31.82)
> contact with hot household appliance (X15)
> contact with nonpowered hand tool (W27.-)
> exposure to electric current (W86)

✓7ᵗʰ **W29.0 Contact with powered kitchen appliance**
> Contact with blender
> Contact with can-opener
> Contact with garbage disposal
> Contact with mixer

✓7ᵗʰ **W29.1 Contact with electric knife**

✓7ᵗʰ **W29.2 Contact with other powered household machinery**
> Contact with electric fan
> Contact with powered dryer (clothes) (powered) (spin)
> Contact with washing-machine
> Contact with sewing machine

✓7ᵗʰ **W29.3 Contact with powered garden and outdoor hand tools and machinery**
> Contact with chainsaw
> Contact with edger
> Contact with garden cultivator (tiller)
> Contact with hedge trimmer
> Contact with other powered garden tool
> *EXCLUDES 1*   contact with powered lawn mower (W28)

✓7ᵗʰ **W29.4 Contact with nail gun**

✓7ᵗʰ **W29.8 Contact with other powered hand tools and household machinery**
> Contact with do-it-yourself tool NOS

✓4ᵗʰ **W30 Contact with agricultural machinery**
> *INCLUDES*   animal-powered farm machine
> *EXCLUDES 1*   agricultural transport vehicle accident (V01-V99)
> explosion of grain store (W40.8)
> exposure to electric current (W86.-)

✓7ᵗʰ **W30.0 Contact with combine harvester**
> Contact with reaper
> Contact with thresher

✓7ᵗʰ **W30.1 Contact with power take-off devices (PTO)**

✓7ᵗʰ **W30.2 Contact with hay derrick**

√x7ᵗʰ **W30.3** **Contact with grain storage elevator**
> EXCLUDES 1   *explosion of grain store (W40.8)*

√5ᵗʰ **W30.8** **Contact with other specified agricultural machinery**

√x7ᵗʰ **W30.81** **Contact with agricultural transport vehicle in stationary use**
> Contact with agricultural transport vehicle under repair, not on public roadway
> > EXCLUDES 1   *agricultural transport vehicle accident (V01-V99)*

√x7ᵗʰ **W30.89** **Contact with other specified agricultural machinery**

√x7ᵗʰ **W30.9** **Contact with unspecified agricultural machinery**
> Contact with farm machinery NOS

√4ᵗʰ **W31** **Contact with other and unspecified machinery**
> EXCLUDES 1   *contact with agricultural machinery (W30.-)*
> *contact with machinery in transport under own power or being towed by a vehicle (V01-V99)*
> *exposure to electric current (W86)*

√x7ᵗʰ **W31.0** **Contact with mining and earth-drilling machinery**
> Contact with bore or drill (land) (seabed)
> Contact with shaft hoist
> Contact with shaft lift
> Contact with undercutter

√x7ᵗʰ **W31.1** **Contact with metalworking machines**
> Contact with abrasive wheel
> Contact with forging machine
> Contact with lathe
> Contact with mechanical shears
> Contact with metal drilling machine
> Contact with milling machine
> Contact with power press
> Contact with rolling-mill
> Contact with metal sawing machine

√x7ᵗʰ **W31.2** **Contact with powered woodworking and forming machines**
> Contact with band saw
> Contact with bench saw
> Contact with circular saw
> Contact with molding machine
> Contact with overhead plane
> Contact with powered saw
> Contact with radial saw
> Contact with sander
> > EXCLUDES 1   *nonpowered woodworking tools (W27.0)*

√x7ᵗʰ **W31.3** **Contact with prime movers**
> Contact with gas turbine
> Contact with internal combustion engine
> Contact with steam engine
> Contact with water driven turbine

√5ᵗʰ **W31.8** **Contact with other specified machinery**

√x7ᵗʰ **W31.81** **Contact with recreational machinery**
> Contact with roller coaster

√x7ᵗʰ **W31.82** **Contact with other commercial machinery**
> Contact with commercial electric fan
> Contact with commercial kitchen appliances
> Contact with commercial powered dryer (clothes) (powered) (spin)
> Contact with commercial washing-machine
> Contact with commercial sewing machine
> > EXCLUDES 1   *contact with household machinery (W29.-)*
> > *contact with powered lawn mower (W28)*

√x7ᵗʰ **W31.83** **Contact with special construction vehicle in stationary use**
> Contact with special construction vehicle under repair, not on public roadway
> > EXCLUDES 1   *special construction vehicle accident (V01-V99)*

√x7ᵗʰ **W31.89** **Contact with other specified machinery**

√x7ᵗʰ **W31.9** **Contact with unspecified machinery**
> Contact with machinery NOS

√4ᵗʰ **W32** **Accidental handgun discharge and malfunction**
> INCLUDES   accidental discharge and malfunction of gun for single hand use
> accidental discharge and malfunction of pistol
> accidental discharge and malfunction of revolver
> handgun discharge and malfunction NOS
> > EXCLUDES 1   *accidental airgun discharge and malfunction (W34.010, W34.110)*
> > *accidental BB gun discharge and malfunction (W34.010, W34.110)*
> > *accidental pellet gun discharge and malfunction (W34.010, W34.110)*
> > *accidental shotgun discharge and malfunction (W33.01, W33.11)*
> > *assault by handgun discharge (X93)*
> > *handgun discharge involving legal intervention (Y35.0-)*
> > *handgun discharge involving military or war operations (Y36.4-)*
> > *intentional self-harm by handgun discharge (X72)*
> > *Very pistol discharge and malfunction (W34.09, W34.19)*

√x7ᵗʰ **W32.0** **Accidental handgun discharge**

√x7ᵗʰ **W32.1** **Accidental handgun malfunction**
> Injury due to explosion of handgun (parts)
> Injury due to malfunction of mechanism or component of handgun
> Injury due to recoil of handgun
> Powder burn from handgun

√4ᵗʰ **W33** **Accidental rifle, shotgun and larger firearm discharge and malfunction**
> INCLUDES   rifle, shotgun and larger firearm discharge and malfunction NOS
> > EXCLUDES 1   *accidental airgun discharge and malfunction (W34.010, W34.110)*
> > *accidental BB gun discharge and malfunction (W34.010, W34.110)*
> > *accidental handgun discharge and malfunction (W32.-)*
> > *accidental pellet gun discharge and malfunction (W34.010, W34.110)*
> > *assault by rifle, shotgun and larger firearm discharge (X94)*
> > *firearm discharge involving legal intervention (Y35.0-)*
> > *firearm discharge involving military or war operations (Y36.4-)*
> > *intentional self-harm by rifle, shotgun and larger firearm discharge (X73)*

√5ᵗʰ **W33.0** **Accidental rifle, shotgun and larger firearm discharge**

√x7ᵗʰ **W33.00** **Accidental discharge of unspecified larger firearm**
> Discharge of unspecified larger firearm NOS

√x7ᵗʰ **W33.01** **Accidental discharge of shotgun**
> Discharge of shotgun NOS

√x7ᵗʰ **W33.02** **Accidental discharge of hunting rifle**
> Discharge of hunting rifle NOS

√x7ᵗʰ **W33.03** **Accidental discharge of machine gun**
> Discharge of machine gun NOS

√x7ᵗʰ **W33.09** **Accidental discharge of other larger firearm**
> Discharge of other larger firearm NOS

√5ᵗʰ **W33.1** **Accidental rifle, shotgun and larger firearm malfunction**
> Injury due to explosion of rifle, shotgun and larger firearm (parts)
> Injury due to malfunction of mechanism or component of rifle, shotgun and larger firearm
> Injury due to piercing, cutting, crushing or pinching due to (by) slide trigger mechanism, scope or other gun part
> Injury due to recoil of rifle, shotgun and larger firearm
> Powder burn from rifle, shotgun and larger firearm

√x7ᵗʰ **W33.10** **Accidental malfunction of unspecified larger firearm**
> Malfunction of unspecified larger firearm NOS

√x7ᵗʰ **W33.11** **Accidental malfunction of shotgun**
> Malfunction of shotgun NOS

√x7ᵗʰ **W33.12** **Accidental malfunction of hunting rifle**
> Malfunction of hunting rifle NOS

√x7ᵗʰ **W33.13** **Accidental malfunction of machine gun**
> Malfunction of machine gun NOS

Chapter 20. External Causes of Morbidity

√x 7ᵗʰ **W33.19**   **Accidental malfunction of other larger firearm**
     Malfunction of other larger firearm NOS

√4ᵗʰ **W34**   **Accidental discharge and malfunction from other and unspecified firearms and guns**

√5ᵗʰ **W34.0**   **Accidental discharge from other and unspecified firearms and guns**

√x 7ᵗʰ **W34.00**   **Accidental discharge from unspecified firearms or gun**
     Discharge from firearm NOS
     Gunshot wound NOS
     Shot NOS

√6ᵗʰ **W34.01**   **Accidental discharge of gas, air or spring-operated guns**

√7ᵗʰ **W34.010**   **Accidental discharge of airgun**
     Accidental discharge of BB gun
     Accidental discharge of pellet gun

√7ᵗʰ **W34.011**   **Accidental discharge of paintball gun**
     Accidental injury due to paintball discharge

√7ᵗʰ **W34.018**   **Accidental discharge of other gas, air or spring-operated gun**

√x 7ᵗʰ **W34.09**   **Accidental discharge from other specified firearms**
     Accidental discharge from Very pistol [flare]

√5ᵗʰ **W34.1**   **Accidental malfunction from other and unspecified firearms and guns**

√x 7ᵗʰ **W34.10**   **Accidental malfunction from unspecified firearms or gun**
     Firearm malfunction NOS

√6ᵗʰ **W34.11**   **Accidental malfunction of gas, air or spring-operated guns**

√7ᵗʰ **W34.110**   **Accidental malfunction of airgun**
     Accidental malfunction of BB gun
     Accidental malfunction of pellet gun

√7ᵗʰ **W34.111**   **Accidental malfunction of paintball gun**
     Accidental injury due to paintball gun malfunction

√7ᵗʰ **W34.118**   **Accidental malfunction of other gas, air or spring-operated gun**

√x 7ᵗʰ **W34.19**   **Accidental malfunction from other specified firearms**
     Accidental malfunction from Very pistol [flare]

√x 7ᵗʰ **W35**   **Explosion and rupture of boiler**
   EXCLUDES 1   explosion and rupture of boiler on watercraft (V93.4)

√4ᵗʰ **W36**   **Explosion and rupture of gas cylinder**

√x 7ᵗʰ **W36.1**   **Explosion and rupture of aerosol can**

√x 7ᵗʰ **W36.2**   **Explosion and rupture of air tank**

√x 7ᵗʰ **W36.3**   **Explosion and rupture of pressurized-gas tank**

√x 7ᵗʰ **W36.8**   **Explosion and rupture of other gas cylinder**

√x 7ᵗʰ **W36.9**   **Explosion and rupture of unspecified gas cylinder**

√4ᵗʰ **W37**   **Explosion and rupture of pressurized tire, pipe or hose**

√x 7ᵗʰ **W37.0**   **Explosion of bicycle tire**

√x 7ᵗʰ **W37.8**   **Explosion and rupture of other pressurized tire, pipe or hose**

√x 7ᵗʰ **W38**   **Explosion and rupture of other specified pressurized devices**

√x 7ᵗʰ **W39**   **Discharge of firework**

√4ᵗʰ **W40**   **Explosion of other materials**
   EXCLUDES 1   assault by explosive material (X96)
     explosion involving legal intervention (Y35.1-)
     explosion involving military or war operations (Y36.0-, Y36.2-)
     intentional self-harm by explosive material (X75)

√x 7ᵗʰ **W40.0**   **Explosion of blasting material**
     Explosion of blasting cap
     Explosion of detonator
     Explosion of dynamite
     Explosion of explosive (any) used in blasting operations

√x 7ᵗʰ **W40.1**   **Explosion of explosive gases**
     Explosion of acetylene
     Explosion of butane
     Explosion of coal gas
     Explosion in mine NOS
     Explosion of explosive gas
     Explosion of fire damp
     Explosion of gasoline fumes
     Explosion of methane
     Explosion of propane

√x 7ᵗʰ **W40.8**   **Explosion of other specified explosive materials**
     Explosion in dump NOS
     Explosion in factory NOS
     Explosion in grain store
     Explosion in munitions
   EXCLUDES 1   explosion involving legal intervention (Y35.1-)
     explosion involving military or war operations (Y36.0-, Y36.2-)

√x 7ᵗʰ **W40.9**   **Explosion of unspecified explosive materials**
     Explosion NOS

√4ᵗʰ **W42**   **Exposure to noise**

√x 7ᵗʰ **W42.0**   **Exposure to supersonic waves**

√x 7ᵗʰ **W42.9**   **Exposure to other noise**
     Exposure to sound waves NOS

√4ᵗʰ **W45**   **Foreign body or object entering through skin**
   INCLUDES   foreign body or object embedded in skin
     nail embedded in skin
   EXCLUDES 2   contact with hand tools (nonpowered) (powered) (W27-W29)
     contact with other sharp objects (W26.-)
     contact with sharp glass (W25.-)
     struck by objects (W20-W22)

√x 7ᵗʰ **W45.0**   **Nail entering through skin**

√x 7ᵗʰ **W45.8**   **Other foreign body or object entering through skin**
     Splinter in skin NOS

√4ᵗʰ **W46**   **Contact with hypodermic needle**

√x 7ᵗʰ **W46.0**   **Contact with hypodermic needle**
     Hypodermic needle stick NOS

√x 7ᵗʰ **W46.1**   **Contact with contaminated hypodermic needle**

√4ᵗʰ **W49**   **Exposure to other inanimate mechanical forces**
   INCLUDES   exposure to abnormal gravitational [G] forces
     exposure to inanimate mechanical forces NEC
   EXCLUDES 1   exposure to inanimate mechanical forces involving military or war operations (Y36.-, Y37.-)

√5ᵗʰ **W49.0**   **Item causing external constriction**

√x 7ᵗʰ **W49.01**   **Hair causing external constriction**

√x 7ᵗʰ **W49.02**   **String or thread causing external constriction**

√x 7ᵗʰ **W49.03**   **Rubber band causing external constriction**

√x 7ᵗʰ **W49.04**   **Ring or other jewelry causing external constriction**

√x 7ᵗʰ **W49.09**   **Other specified item causing external constriction**

√x 7ᵗʰ **W49.9**   **Exposure to other inanimate mechanical forces**

Exposure to animate mechanical forces (W50-W64)

   EXCLUDES 1   toxic effect of contact with venomous animals and plants (T63.-)

The appropriate 7th character is to be added to each code from categories W50-W64.
A   initial encounter
D   subsequent encounter
S   sequela

√4ᵗʰ **W50**   **Accidental hit, strike, kick, twist, bite or scratch by another person**
   INCLUDES   hit, strike, kick, twist, bite, or scratch by another person NOS
   EXCLUDES 1   assault by bodily force (Y04)
     struck by objects (W20-W22)

√x 7ᵗʰ **W50.0**   **Accidental hit or strike by another person**
     Hit or strike by another person NOS

√x 7ᵗʰ **W50.1**   **Accidental kick by another person**
     Kick by another person NOS

√x 7ᵗʰ **W50.2**   **Accidental twist by another person**
     Twist by another person NOS

☑x7ᵗʰ W50.3　Accidental bite by another person
　　Human bite
　　Bite by another person NOS

☑x7ᵗʰ W50.4　Accidental scratch by another person
　　Scratch by another person NOS

☑x7ᵗʰ W51　Accidental striking against or bumped into by another person
　　EXCLUDES 1　*assault by striking against or bumping into by another person (Y04.2)*
　　　　　　fall due to collision with another person (W03)

☑x7ᵗʰ W52　Crushed, pushed or stepped on by crowd or human stampede
　　Crushed, pushed or stepped on by crowd or human stampede with or without fall

☑4ᵗʰ W53　Contact with rodent
　　INCLUDES　contact with saliva, feces or urine of rodent

☑5ᵗʰ W53.0　Contact with mouse
　　☑x7ᵗʰ W53.01　Bitten by mouse
　　☑x7ᵗʰ W53.09　Other contact with mouse

☑5ᵗʰ W53.1　Contact with rat
　　☑x7ᵗʰ W53.11　Bitten by rat
　　☑x7ᵗʰ W53.19　Other contact with rat

☑5ᵗʰ W53.2　Contact with squirrel
　　☑x7ᵗʰ W53.21　Bitten by squirrel
　　☑x7ᵗʰ W53.29　Other contact with squirrel

☑5ᵗʰ W53.8　Contact with other rodent
　　☑x7ᵗʰ W53.81　Bitten by other rodent
　　☑x7ᵗʰ W53.89　Other contact with other rodent

☑4ᵗʰ W54　Contact with dog
　　INCLUDES　contact with saliva, feces or urine of dog

☑x7ᵗʰ W54.0　Bitten by dog
☑x7ᵗʰ W54.1　Struck by dog
　　Knocked over by dog
☑x7ᵗʰ W54.8　Other contact with dog

☑4ᵗʰ W55　Contact with other mammals
　　INCLUDES　contact with saliva, feces or urine of mammal
　　EXCLUDES 1　*animal being ridden - see transport accidents*
　　　　　　bitten or struck by dog (W54)
　　　　　　bitten or struck by rodent (W53.-)
　　　　　　contact with marine mammals (W56.-)

☑5ᵗʰ W55.0　Contact with cat
　　☑x7ᵗʰ W55.01　Bitten by cat
　　☑x7ᵗʰ W55.03　Scratched by cat
　　☑x7ᵗʰ W55.09　Other contact with cat

☑5ᵗʰ W55.1　Contact with horse
　　☑x7ᵗʰ W55.11　Bitten by horse
　　☑x7ᵗʰ W55.12　Struck by horse
　　☑x7ᵗʰ W55.19　Other contact with horse

☑5ᵗʰ W55.2　Contact with cow
　　Contact with bull
　　☑x7ᵗʰ W55.21　Bitten by cow
　　☑x7ᵗʰ W55.22　Struck by cow
　　　　Gored by bull
　　☑x7ᵗʰ W55.29　Other contact with cow

☑5ᵗʰ W55.3　Contact with other hoof stock
　　Contact with goats
　　Contact with sheep
　　☑x7ᵗʰ W55.31　Bitten by other hoof stock
　　☑x7ᵗʰ W55.32　Struck by other hoof stock
　　　　Gored by goat
　　　　Gored by ram
　　☑x7ᵗʰ W55.39　Other contact with other hoof stock

☑5ᵗʰ W55.4　Contact with pig
　　☑x7ᵗʰ W55.41　Bitten by pig
　　☑x7ᵗʰ W55.42　Struck by pig
　　☑x7ᵗʰ W55.49　Other contact with pig

☑5ᵗʰ W55.5　Contact with raccoon
　　☑x7ᵗʰ W55.51　Bitten by raccoon

　　☑x7ᵗʰ W55.52　Struck by raccoon
　　☑x7ᵗʰ W55.59　Other contact with raccoon

☑5ᵗʰ W55.8　Contact with other mammals
　　☑x7ᵗʰ W55.81　Bitten by other mammals
　　☑x7ᵗʰ W55.82　Struck by other mammals
　　☑x7ᵗʰ W55.89　Other contact with other mammals

☑4ᵗʰ W56　Contact with nonvenomous marine animal
　　EXCLUDES 1　*contact with venomous marine animal (T63.-)*

☑5ᵗʰ W56.0　Contact with dolphin
　　☑x7ᵗʰ W56.01　Bitten by dolphin
　　☑x7ᵗʰ W56.02　Struck by dolphin
　　☑x7ᵗʰ W56.09　Other contact with dolphin

☑5ᵗʰ W56.1　Contact with sea lion
　　☑x7ᵗʰ W56.11　Bitten by sea lion
　　☑x7ᵗʰ W56.12　Struck by sea lion
　　☑x7ᵗʰ W56.19　Other contact with sea lion

☑5ᵗʰ W56.2　Contact with orca
　　Contact with killer whale
　　☑x7ᵗʰ W56.21　Bitten by orca
　　☑x7ᵗʰ W56.22　Struck by orca
　　☑x7ᵗʰ W56.29　Other contact with orca

☑5ᵗʰ W56.3　Contact with other marine mammals
　　☑x7ᵗʰ W56.31　Bitten by other marine mammals
　　☑x7ᵗʰ W56.32　Struck by other marine mammals
　　☑x7ᵗʰ W56.39　Other contact with other marine mammals

☑5ᵗʰ W56.4　Contact with shark
　　☑x7ᵗʰ W56.41　Bitten by shark
　　☑x7ᵗʰ W56.42　Struck by shark
　　☑x7ᵗʰ W56.49　Other contact with shark

☑5ᵗʰ W56.5　Contact with other fish
　　☑x7ᵗʰ W56.51　Bitten by other fish
　　☑x7ᵗʰ W56.52　Struck by other fish
　　☑x7ᵗʰ W56.59　Other contact with other fish

☑5ᵗʰ W56.8　Contact with other nonvenomous marine animals
　　☑x7ᵗʰ W56.81　Bitten by other nonvenomous marine animals
　　☑x7ᵗʰ W56.82　Struck by other nonvenomous marine animals
　　☑x7ᵗʰ W56.89　Other contact with other nonvenomous marine animals

☑x7ᵗʰ W57　Bitten or stung by nonvenomous insect and other nonvenomous arthropods
　　EXCLUDES 1　*contact with venomous insects and arthropods (T63.2-, T63.3-, T63.4-)*

☑4ᵗʰ W58　Contact with crocodile or alligator
☑5ᵗʰ W58.0　Contact with alligator
　　☑x7ᵗʰ W58.01　Bitten by alligator
　　☑x7ᵗʰ W58.02　Struck by alligator
　　☑x7ᵗʰ W58.03　Crushed by alligator
　　☑x7ᵗʰ W58.09　Other contact with alligator

☑5ᵗʰ W58.1　Contact with crocodile
　　☑x7ᵗʰ W58.11　Bitten by crocodile
　　☑x7ᵗʰ W58.12　Struck by crocodile
　　☑x7ᵗʰ W58.13　Crushed by crocodile
　　☑x7ᵗʰ W58.19　Other contact with crocodile

☑4ᵗʰ W59　Contact with other nonvenomous reptiles
　　EXCLUDES 1　*contact with venomous reptile (T63.0-, T63.1-)*

☑5ᵗʰ W59.0　Contact with nonvenomous lizards
　　☑x7ᵗʰ W59.01　Bitten by nonvenomous lizards
　　☑x7ᵗʰ W59.02　Struck by nonvenomous lizards
　　☑x7ᵗʰ W59.09　Other contact with nonvenomous lizards
　　　　Exposure to nonvenomous lizards

☑5ᵗʰ W59.1　Contact with nonvenomous snakes
　　☑x7ᵗʰ W59.11　Bitten by nonvenomous snake
　　☑x7ᵗʰ W59.12　Struck by nonvenomous snake
　　☑x7ᵗʰ W59.13　Crushed by nonvenomous snake
　　☑x7ᵗʰ W59.19　Other contact with nonvenomous snake

✓5ᵗʰ **W59.2** **Contact with** turtles
> EXCLUDES 1 *contact with tortoises (W59.8-)*

✓x7ᵗʰ **W59.21** **Bitten by turtle**

✓x7ᵗʰ **W59.22** **Struck by turtle**

✓x7ᵗʰ **W59.29** **Other contact with turtle**
> Exposure to turtles

✓5ᵗʰ **W59.8** **Contact with other nonvenomous reptiles**

✓x7ᵗʰ **W59.81** **Bitten by other nonvenomous reptiles**

✓x7ᵗʰ **W59.82** **Struck by other nonvenomous reptiles**

✓x7ᵗʰ **W59.83** **Crushed by other nonvenomous reptiles**

✓x7ᵗʰ **W59.89** **Other contact with other nonvenomous reptiles**

✓x7ᵗʰ **W60** **Contact with nonvenomous plant thorns and spines and sharp leaves**
> EXCLUDES 1 *contact with venomous plants (T63.7-)*

✓4ᵗʰ **W61** **Contact with birds (domestic) (wild)**
> INCLUDES contact with excreta of birds

✓5ᵗʰ **W61.0** **Contact with** parrot

✓x7ᵗʰ **W61.01** **Bitten by parrot**

✓x7ᵗʰ **W61.02** **Struck by parrot**

✓x7ᵗʰ **W61.09** **Other contact with parrot**
> Exposure to parrots

✓5ᵗʰ **W61.1** **Contact with** macaw

✓x7ᵗʰ **W61.11** **Bitten by macaw**

✓x7ᵗʰ **W61.12** **Struck by macaw**

✓x7ᵗʰ **W61.19** **Other contact with macaw**
> Exposure to macaws

✓5ᵗʰ **W61.2** **Contact with other** psittacines

✓x7ᵗʰ **W61.21** **Bitten by other psittacines**

✓x7ᵗʰ **W61.22** **Struck by other psittacines**

✓x7ᵗʰ **W61.29** **Other contact with other psittacines**
> Exposure to other psittacines

✓5ᵗʰ **W61.3** **Contact with** chicken

✓x7ᵗʰ **W61.32** **Struck by chicken**

✓x7ᵗʰ **W61.33** **Pecked by chicken**

✓x7ᵗʰ **W61.39** **Other contact with chicken**
> Exposure to chickens

✓5ᵗʰ **W61.4** **Contact with** turkey

✓x7ᵗʰ **W61.42** **Struck by turkey**

✓x7ᵗʰ **W61.43** **Pecked by turkey**

✓x7ᵗʰ **W61.49** **Other contact with turkey**

✓5ᵗʰ **W61.5** **Contact with** goose

✓x7ᵗʰ **W61.51** **Bitten by goose**

✓x7ᵗʰ **W61.52** **Struck by goose**

✓x7ᵗʰ **W61.59** **Other contact with goose**

✓5ᵗʰ **W61.6** **Contact with** duck

✓x7ᵗʰ **W61.61** **Bitten by duck**

✓x7ᵗʰ **W61.62** **Struck by duck**

✓x7ᵗʰ **W61.69** **Other contact with duck**

✓5ᵗʰ **W61.9** **Contact with other birds**

✓x7ᵗʰ **W61.91** **Bitten by other birds**

✓x7ᵗʰ **W61.92** **Struck by other birds**

✓x7ᵗʰ **W61.99** **Other contact with other birds**
> Contact with bird NOS

✓4ᵗʰ **W62** **Contact with nonvenomous amphibians**
> EXCLUDES 1 *contact with venomous amphibians (T63.81-R63.83)*

✓x7ᵗʰ **W62.0** **Contact with nonvenomous** frogs

✓x7ᵗʰ **W62.1** **Contact with nonvenomous** toads

✓x7ᵗʰ **W62.9** **Contact with other nonvenomous amphibians**

✓x7ᵗʰ **W64** **Exposure to other animate mechanical forces**
> INCLUDES exposure to nonvenomous animal NOS
> EXCLUDES 1 *contact with venomous animal (T63.-)*

Accidental non-transport drowning and submersion (W65-W74)

> EXCLUDES 1 *accidental drowning and submersion due to fall into water (W16.-)*
> *accidental drowning and submersion due to water transport accident (V90.-, V92.-)*
> EXCLUDES 2 *accidental drowning and submersion due to cataclysm (X34-X39)*

The appropriate 7th character is to be added to each code from categories W65-W74.
A   initial encounter
D   subsequent encounter
S   sequela

✓x7ᵗʰ **W65** **Accidental drowning and submersion while in** bath-tub
> EXCLUDES 1 *accidental drowning and submersion due to fall in (into) bathtub (W16.211)*

✓x7ᵗʰ **W67** **Accidental drowning and submersion while in** swimming-pool
> EXCLUDES 1 *accidental drowning and submersion due to fall into swimming pool (W16.011, W16.021, W16.031)*
> *accidental drowning and submersion due to striking into wall of swimming pool (W22.041)*

✓x7ᵗʰ **W69** **Accidental drowning and submersion while in** natural water
> Accidental drowning and submersion while in lake
> Accidental drowning and submersion while in open sea
> Accidental drowning and submersion while in river
> Accidental drowning and submersion while in stream
> EXCLUDES 1 *accidental drowning and submersion due to fall into natural body of water (W16.111, W16.121, W16.131)*

✓x7ᵗʰ **W73** **Other specified cause of accidental non-transport drowning and submersion**
> Accidental drowning and submersion while in quenching tank
> Accidental drowning and submersion while in reservoir
> EXCLUDES 1 *accidental drowning and submersion due to fall into other water (W16.311, W16.321, W16.331)*

✓x7ᵗʰ **W74** **Unspecified cause of accidental drowning and submersion**
> Drowning NOS

Exposure to electric current, radiation and extreme ambient air temperature and pressure (W85-W99)

> EXCLUDES 1 *exposure to:*
> *failure in dosage of radiation or temperature during surgical and medical care (Y63.2-Y63.5)*
> *lightning (T75.0-)*
> *natural cold (X31)*
> *natural heat (X30)*
> *natural radiation NOS (X39)*
> *radiological procedure and radiotherapy (Y84.2)*
> *sunlight (X32)*

AHA: 2018,2Q,7-8

The appropriate 7th character is to be added to each code from categories W85-W99.
A   initial encounter
D   subsequent encounter
S   sequela

✓x7ᵗʰ **W85** **Exposure to electric transmission lines**
> Broken power line

✓4ᵗʰ **W86** **Exposure to other specified electric current**

✓x7ᵗʰ **W86.0** **Exposure to domestic wiring and appliances**

✓x7ᵗʰ **W86.1** **Exposure to industrial wiring, appliances and electrical machinery**
> Exposure to conductors
> Exposure to control apparatus
> Exposure to electrical equipment and machinery
> Exposure to transformers

✓x7ᵗʰ **W86.8** **Exposure to other electric current**
> Exposure to wiring and appliances in or on farm (not farmhouse)
> Exposure to wiring and appliances outdoors
> Exposure to wiring and appliances in or on public building
> Exposure to wiring and appliances in or on residential institutions
> Exposure to wiring and appliances in or on schools

✓4ᵗʰ **W88** **Exposure to ionizing radiation**
> EXCLUDES 1 *exposure to sunlight (X32)*

✓x7ᵗʰ **W88.0** **Exposure to** X-rays

✓x7ᵗʰ **W88.1** **Exposure to** radioactive isotopes

√x7ᵗʰ **W88.8 Exposure to other ionizing radiation**

√4ᵗʰ **W89 Exposure to man-made visible and ultraviolet light**

     INCLUDES   exposure to welding light (arc)

     EXCLUDES 2   *exposure to sunlight (X32)*

     √x7ᵗʰ **W89.0 Exposure to welding light (arc)**

     √x7ᵗʰ **W89.1 Exposure to tanning bed**

     √x7ᵗʰ **W89.8 Exposure to other man-made visible and ultraviolet light**

     √x7ᵗʰ **W89.9 Exposure to unspecified man-made visible and ultraviolet light**

√4ᵗʰ **W90 Exposure to other nonionizing radiation**

     EXCLUDES 2   *exposure to sunlight (X32)*

     AHA: 2019,1Q,21

     √x7ᵗʰ **W90.0 Exposure to radiofrequency**

     √x7ᵗʰ **W90.1 Exposure to infrared radiation**

     √x7ᵗʰ **W90.2 Exposure to laser radiation**

     √x7ᵗʰ **W90.8 Exposure to other nonionizing radiation**

√x7ᵗʰ **W92 Exposure to excessive heat of man-made origin**

√4ᵗʰ **W93 Exposure to excessive cold of man-made origin**

     √5ᵗʰ **W93.0 Contact with or inhalation of dry ice**

         √x7ᵗʰ **W93.01 Contact with dry ice**

         √x7ᵗʰ **W93.02 Inhalation of dry ice**

     √5ᵗʰ **W93.1 Contact with or inhalation of liquid air**

         √x7ᵗʰ **W93.11 Contact with liquid air**

             Contact with liquid hydrogen

             Contact with liquid nitrogen

         √x7ᵗʰ **W93.12 Inhalation of liquid air**

             Inhalation of liquid hydrogen

             Inhalation of liquid nitrogen

     √x7ᵗʰ **W93.2 Prolonged exposure in deep freeze unit or refrigerator**

     √x7ᵗʰ **W93.8 Exposure to other excessive cold of man-made origin**

√4ᵗʰ **W94 Exposure to high and low air pressure and changes in air pressure**

     √x7ᵗʰ **W94.0 Exposure to prolonged high air pressure**

     √5ᵗʰ **W94.1 Exposure to prolonged low air pressure**

         √x7ᵗʰ **W94.11 Exposure to residence or prolonged visit at high altitude**

         √x7ᵗʰ **W94.12 Exposure to other prolonged low air pressure**

     √5ᵗʰ **W94.2 Exposure to rapid changes in air pressure during ascent**

         √x7ᵗʰ **W94.21 Exposure to reduction in atmospheric pressure while surfacing from deep-water diving**

         √x7ᵗʰ **W94.22 Exposure to reduction in atmospheric pressure while surfacing from underground**

         √x7ᵗʰ **W94.23 Exposure to sudden change in air pressure in aircraft during ascent**

         √x7ᵗʰ **W94.29 Exposure to other rapid changes in air pressure during ascent**

     √5ᵗʰ **W94.3 Exposure to rapid changes in air pressure during descent**

         √x7ᵗʰ **W94.31 Exposure to sudden change in air pressure in aircraft during descent**

         √x7ᵗʰ **W94.32 Exposure to high air pressure from rapid descent in water**

         √x7ᵗʰ **W94.39 Exposure to other rapid changes in air pressure during descent**

√x7ᵗʰ **W99 Exposure to other man-made environmental factors**

Exposure to smoke, fire and flames (X00-X08)

   EXCLUDES 1   *arson (X97)*

   EXCLUDES 2   *explosions (W35-W40)*

                lightning (T75.0-)

                transport accident (V01-V99)

AHA: 2018,2Q,7-8

> The appropriate 7th character is to be added to each code from categories X00-X08.
> A   initial encounter
> D   subsequent encounter
> S   sequela

√4ᵗʰ **X00 Exposure to uncontrolled fire in building or structure**

     INCLUDES   conflagration in building or structure

     Code first any associated cataclysm

     EXCLUDES 2   *exposure to ignition or melting of nightwear (X05)*

                exposure to ignition or melting of other clothing and apparel (X06.-)

                exposure to other specified smoke, fire and flames (X08.-)

     AHA: 2016,2Q,5

     √x7ᵗʰ **X00.0 Exposure to flames in uncontrolled fire in building or structure**

     √x7ᵗʰ **X00.1 Exposure to smoke in uncontrolled fire in building or structure**

     √x7ᵗʰ **X00.2 Injury due to collapse of burning building or structure in uncontrolled fire**

         EXCLUDES 1   *injury due to collapse of building not on fire (W20.1)*

     √x7ᵗʰ **X00.3 Fall from burning building or structure in uncontrolled fire**

     √x7ᵗʰ **X00.4 Hit by object from burning building or structure in uncontrolled fire**

         AHA: 2016,2Q,4

     √x7ᵗʰ **X00.5 Jump from burning building or structure in uncontrolled fire**

     √x7ᵗʰ **X00.8 Other exposure to uncontrolled fire in building or structure**

√4ᵗʰ **X01 Exposure to uncontrolled fire, not in building or structure**

     INCLUDES   exposure to forest fire

     √x7ᵗʰ **X01.0 Exposure to flames in uncontrolled fire, not in building or structure**

     √x7ᵗʰ **X01.1 Exposure to smoke in uncontrolled fire, not in building or structure**

     √x7ᵗʰ **X01.3 Fall due to uncontrolled fire, not in building or structure**

     √x7ᵗʰ **X01.4 Hit by object due to uncontrolled fire, not in building or structure**

     √x7ᵗʰ **X01.8 Other exposure to uncontrolled fire, not in building or structure**

√4ᵗʰ **X02 Exposure to controlled fire in building or structure**

     INCLUDES   exposure to fire in fireplace

                exposure to fire in stove

     √x7ᵗʰ **X02.0 Exposure to flames in controlled fire in building or structure**

     √x7ᵗʰ **X02.1 Exposure to smoke in controlled fire in building or structure**

     √x7ᵗʰ **X02.2 Injury due to collapse of burning building or structure in controlled fire**

         EXCLUDES 1   *injury due to collapse of building not on fire (W20.1)*

     √x7ᵗʰ **X02.3 Fall from burning building or structure in controlled fire**

     √x7ᵗʰ **X02.4 Hit by object from burning building or structure in controlled fire**

     √x7ᵗʰ **X02.5 Jump from burning building or structure in controlled fire**

     √x7ᵗʰ **X02.8 Other exposure to controlled fire in building or structure**

√4ᵗʰ **X03 Exposure to controlled fire, not in building or structure**

     INCLUDES   exposure to bon fire

                exposure to camp-fire

                exposure to trash fire

     √x7ᵗʰ **X03.0 Exposure to flames in controlled fire, not in building or structure**

     √x7ᵗʰ **X03.1 Exposure to smoke in controlled fire, not in building or structure**

     √x7ᵗʰ **X03.3 Fall due to controlled fire, not in building or structure**

     √x7ᵗʰ **X03.4 Hit by object due to controlled fire, not in building or structure**

     √x7ᵗʰ **X03.8 Other exposure to controlled fire, not in building or structure**

☑ Additional Character Required   √x7ᵗʰ Placeholder Alert   Manifestation   Unspecified Dx   Q QPP   UPD Unacceptable PDx

Chapter 20. External Causes of Morbidity

X04–X32

√x7ᵗʰ **X04 Exposure to ignition of highly flammable material**
  Exposure to ignition of gasoline
  Exposure to ignition of kerosene
  Exposure to ignition of petrol
  EXCLUDES 2   *exposure to ignition or melting of nightwear (X05)*
        exposure to ignition or melting of other clothing and apparel (X06)
  AHA: 2016,2Q,4

√x7ᵗʰ **X05 Exposure to ignition or melting of nightwear**
  EXCLUDES 2   *exposure to uncontrolled fire in building or structure (X00.-)*
        exposure to uncontrolled fire, not in building or structure (X01.-)
        exposure to controlled fire in building or structure (X02.-)
        exposure to controlled fire, not in building or structure (X03.-)
        exposure to ignition of highly flammable materials (X04.-)

√4ᵗʰ **X06 Exposure to ignition or melting of other clothing and apparel**
  EXCLUDES 2   *exposure to uncontrolled fire in building or structure (X00.-)*
        exposure to uncontrolled fire, not in building or structure (X01.-)
        exposure to controlled fire in building or structure (X02.-)
        exposure to controlled fire, not in building or structure (X03.-)
        exposure to ignition of highly flammable materials (X04.-)
  √x7ᵗʰ **X06.0 Exposure to ignition of plastic jewelry**
  √x7ᵗʰ **X06.1 Exposure to melting of plastic jewelry**
  √x7ᵗʰ **X06.2 Exposure to ignition of other clothing and apparel**
  √x7ᵗʰ **X06.3 Exposure to melting of other clothing and apparel**

√4ᵗʰ **X08 Exposure to other specified smoke, fire and flames**
  √5ᵗʰ **X08.0 Exposure to bed fire**
       Exposure to mattress fire
      √x7ᵗʰ **X08.00 Exposure to bed fire due to unspecified burning material**
      √x7ᵗʰ **X08.01 Exposure to bed fire due to burning cigarette**
      √x7ᵗʰ **X08.09 Exposure to bed fire due to other burning material**
  √5ᵗʰ **X08.1 Exposure to sofa fire**
      √x7ᵗʰ **X08.10 Exposure to sofa fire due to unspecified burning material**
      √x7ᵗʰ **X08.11 Exposure to sofa fire due to burning cigarette**
      √x7ᵗʰ **X08.19 Exposure to sofa fire due to other burning material**
  √5ᵗʰ **X08.2 Exposure to other furniture fire**
      √x7ᵗʰ **X08.20 Exposure to other furniture fire due to unspecified burning material**
      √x7ᵗʰ **X08.21 Exposure to other furniture fire due to burning cigarette**
      √x7ᵗʰ **X08.29 Exposure to other furniture fire due to other burning material**
  √x7ᵗʰ **X08.8 Exposure to other specified smoke, fire and flames**

Contact with heat and hot substances (X10-X19)

EXCLUDES 1   *exposure to excessive natural heat (X30)*
      exposure to fire and flames (X00-X08)
AHA: 2018,2Q,7-8

The appropriate 7th character is to be added to each code from categories X10-X19.
A   initial encounter
D   subsequent encounter
S   sequela

√4ᵗʰ **X10 Contact with hot drinks, food, fats and cooking oils**
  √x7ᵗʰ **X10.0 Contact with hot drinks**
  √x7ᵗʰ **X10.1 Contact with hot food**
  √x7ᵗʰ **X10.2 Contact with fats and cooking oils**

√4ᵗʰ **X11 Contact with hot tap-water**
  INCLUDES   contact with boiling tap-water
        contact with boiling water NOS
  EXCLUDES 1   *contact with water heated on stove (X12)*
  √x7ᵗʰ **X11.0 Contact with hot water in bath or tub**
      EXCLUDES 1   *contact with running hot water in bath or tub (X11.1)*
  √x7ᵗʰ **X11.1 Contact with running hot water**
       Contact with hot water running out of hose
       Contact with hot water running out of tap

√x7ᵗʰ **X11.8 Contact with other hot tap-water**
       Contact with hot water in bucket
       Contact with hot tap-water NOS

√x7ᵗʰ **X12 Contact with other hot fluids**
       Contact with water heated on stove
  EXCLUDES 1   *hot (liquid) metals (X18)*

√4ᵗʰ **X13 Contact with steam and other hot vapors**
  √x7ᵗʰ **X13.0 Inhalation of steam and other hot vapors**
  √x7ᵗʰ **X13.1 Other contact with steam and other hot vapors**

√4ᵗʰ **X14 Contact with hot air and other hot gases**
  √x7ᵗʰ **X14.0 Inhalation of hot air and gases**
  √x7ᵗʰ **X14.1 Other contact with hot air and other hot gases**

√4ᵗʰ **X15 Contact with hot household appliances**
  EXCLUDES 1   *contact with heating appliances (X16)*
        contact with powered household appliances (W29.-)
        exposure to controlled fire in building or structure due to household appliance (X02.8)
        exposure to household appliances electrical current (W86.0)
  √x7ᵗʰ **X15.0 Contact with hot stove (kitchen)**
  √x7ᵗʰ **X15.1 Contact with hot toaster**
  √x7ᵗʰ **X15.2 Contact with hotplate**
  √x7ᵗʰ **X15.3 Contact with hot saucepan or skillet**
       ►Contact with hot cooking pan◄
       ►Contact with hot cooking pot◄
  √x7ᵗʰ **X15.8 Contact with other hot household appliances**
       Contact with cooker
       Contact with kettle
       Contact with light bulbs

√x7ᵗʰ **X16 Contact with hot heating appliances, radiators and pipes**
  EXCLUDES 1   *contact with powered appliances (W29.-)*
        exposure to controlled fire in building or structure due to appliance (X02.8)
        exposure to industrial appliances electrical current (W86.1)

√x7ᵗʰ **X17 Contact with hot engines, machinery and tools**
  EXCLUDES 1   *contact with hot heating appliances, radiators and pipes (X16)*
        contact with hot household appliances (X15)

√x7ᵗʰ **X18 Contact with other hot metals**
       Contact with liquid metal

√x7ᵗʰ **X19 Contact with other heat and hot substances**
  EXCLUDES 1   *objects that are not normally hot, e.g., an object made hot by a house fire (X00-X08)*

Exposure to forces of nature (X30-X39)

AHA: 2018,2Q,7-8

The appropriate 7th character is to be added to each code from categories X30-X39.
A   initial encounter
D   subsequent encounter
S   sequela

√x7ᵗʰ **X30 Exposure to excessive natural heat**
       Exposure to excessive heat as the cause of sunstroke
       Exposure to heat NOS
  EXCLUDES 1   *excessive heat of man-made origin (W92)*
        exposure to man-made radiation (W89)
        exposure to sunlight (X32)
        exposure to tanning bed (W89)

√x7ᵗʰ **X31 Exposure to excessive natural cold**
       Excessive cold as the cause of chilblains NOS
       Excessive cold as the cause of immersion foot or hand
       Exposure to cold NOS
       Exposure to weather conditions
  EXCLUDES 1   *cold of man-made origin (W93.-)*
        contact with or inhalation of dry ice (W93.-)
        contact with or inhalation of liquefied gas (W93.-)

√x7ᵗʰ **X32 Exposure to sunlight**
  EXCLUDES 1   *man-made radiation (tanning bed) (W89)*
  EXCLUDES 2   *radiation-related disorders of the skin and subcutaneous tissue (L55-L59)*

☑x7th X34 Earthquake

> EXCLUDES 2   *tidal wave (tsunami) due to earthquake (X37.41)*

☑x7th X35 Volcanic eruption

> EXCLUDES 2   *tidal wave (tsunami) due to volcanic eruption (X37.41)*

☑4th X36 Avalanche, landslide and other earth movements

> INCLUDES   victim of mudslide of cataclysmic nature
> EXCLUDES 1   *earthquake (X34)*
> EXCLUDES 2   *transport accident involving collision with avalanche or landslide not in motion (V01-V99)*

> **☑x7th X36.0 Collapse of dam or man-made structure causing earth movement**

> **☑x7th X36.1 Avalanche, landslide, or mudslide**

☑4th X37 Cataclysmic storm

> **☑x7th X37.0 Hurricane**
> > Storm surge
> > Typhoon

> **☑x7th X37.1 Tornado**
> > Cyclone
> > Twister

> **☑x7th X37.2 Blizzard (snow)(ice)**

> **☑x7th X37.3 Dust storm**

> **☑5th X37.4 Tidalwave**

> > **☑x7th X37.41 Tidal wave due to** earthquake or volcanic eruption
> > > Tidal wave NOS
> > > Tsunami

> > **☑x7th X37.42 Tidal wave due to** storm

> > **☑x7th X37.43 Tidal wave due to** landslide

> **☑x7th X37.8 Other cataclysmic storms**
> > Cloudburst
> > Torrential rain
> > > EXCLUDES 2   *flood (X38)*

> **☑x7th X37.9 Unspecified cataclysmic storm**
> > Storm NOS
> > > EXCLUDES 1   *collapse of dam or man-made structure causing earth movement (X36.0)*

☑x7th X38 Flood

> Flood arising from remote storm
> Flood of cataclysmic nature arising from melting snow
> Flood resulting directly from storm
> > EXCLUDES 1   *collapse of dam or man-made structure causing earth movement (X36.0)*
> > *tidal wave NOS (X37.41)*
> > *tidal wave caused by storm (X37.42)*

☑4th X39 Exposure to other forces of nature

> **☑5th X39.0 Exposure to natural radiation**
> > EXCLUDES 1   *contact with and (suspected) exposure to radon and other naturally occurring radiation (Z77.123)*
> > *exposure to man-made radiation (W88-W90)*
> > *exposure to sunlight (X32)*

> > **☑x7th X39.01 Exposure to radon**

> > **☑x7th X39.08 Exposure to other natural radiation**

> **☑x7th X39.8 Other exposure to forces of nature**

Overexertion and strenuous or repetitive movements (X50)

☑4th X50 Overexertion and strenuous or repetitive movements

> AHA: 2018,2Q,7-8; 2016,4Q,73-74

> The appropriate 7th character is to be added to each code from category X50.
> A   initial encounter
> D   subsequent encounter
> S   sequela

> **☑x7th X50.0 Overexertion from strenuous movement or load**
> > Lifting heavy objects
> > Lifting weights

☑x7th X50.1 Overexertion from prolonged static or awkward postures

> Prolonged bending
> Prolonged kneeling
> Prolonged reaching
> Prolonged sitting
> Prolonged standing
> Prolonged twisting
> Static bending
> Static kneeling
> Static reaching
> Static sitting
> Static standing
> Static twisting

☑x7th X50.3 Overexertion from repetitive movements

> Use of hand as hammer
> > EXCLUDES 2   *overuse from prolonged static or awkward postures (X50.1)*

☑x7th X50.9 Other and unspecified overexertion or strenuous movements or postures

> Contact pressure
> Contact stress

Accidental exposure to other specified factors (X52-X58)

AHA: 2018,2Q,7-8

> The appropriate 7th character is to be added to each code from categories X52-X58.
> A   initial encounter
> D   subsequent encounter
> S   sequela

☑x7th X52 Prolonged stay in weightless environment

> Weightlessness in spacecraft (simulator)

☑x7th X58 Exposure to other specified factors

> Accident NOS
> Exposure NOS

Intentional self-harm (X71-X83)

Purposely self-inflicted injury
Suicide (attempted)

> The appropriate 7th character is to be added to each code from categories X71-X83.
> A   initial encounter
> D   subsequent encounter
> S   sequela

☑4th X71 Intentional self-harm by drowning and submersion

> **☑x7th X71.0 Intentional self-harm by drowning and submersion while in bathtub**   HCC Rx ESR COM

> **☑x7th X71.1 Intentional self-harm by drowning and submersion while in swimming pool**   HCC Rx ESR COM

> **☑x7th X71.2 Intentional self-harm by drowning and submersion** after jump into swimming pool   HCC Rx ESR COM

> **☑x7th X71.3 Intentional self-harm by drowning and submersion in** natural water   HCC Rx ESR COM

> **☑x7th X71.8 Other intentional self-harm by drowning and submersion**   HCC Rx ESR COM

> **☑x7th X71.9 Intentional self-harm by drowning and submersion, unspecified**   HCC Rx ESR COM

☑x7th X72 Intentional self-harm by handgun discharge   HCC Rx ESR COM

> Intentional self-harm by gun for single hand use
> Intentional self-harm by pistol
> Intentional self-harm by revolver
> > EXCLUDES 1   *Very pistol (X74.8)*

☑4th X73 Intentional self-harm by rifle, shotgun and larger firearm discharge

> EXCLUDES 1   *airgun (X74.01)*

> **☑x7th X73.0 Intentional self-harm by** shotgun discharge   HCC Rx ESR COM

> **☑x7th X73.1 Intentional self-harm by** hunting rifle discharge   HCC Rx ESR COM

> **☑x7th X73.2 Intentional self-harm by** machine gun discharge   HCC Rx ESR COM

> **☑x7th X73.8 Intentional self-harm by other larger firearm discharge**   HCC Rx ESR COM

> **☑x7th X73.9 Intentional self-harm by unspecified larger firearm discharge**   HCC Rx ESR COM

✓4ᵗʰ **X74** **Intentional self-harm by other and unspecified firearm and gun discharge**

✓5ᵗʰ **X74.0** **Intentional self-harm by** gas, air or spring-operated guns

✓x7ᵗʰ **X74.01** **Intentional self-harm by** airgun HCC Rx ESR COM
Intentional self-harm by BB gun discharge
Intentional self-harm by pellet gun discharge

✓x7ᵗʰ **X74.02** **Intentional self-harm by** paintball gun HCC Rx ESR COM

✓x7ᵗʰ **X74.09** **Intentional self-harm by other gas, air or spring-operated gun** HCC Rx ESR COM

✓x7ᵗʰ **X74.8** **Intentional self-harm by other firearm discharge** HCC Rx ESR COM
Intentional self-harm by Very pistol [flare] discharge

✓x7ᵗʰ **X74.9** **Intentional self-harm by unspecified firearm discharge** HCC Rx ESR COM

✓x7ᵗʰ **X75** **Intentional self-harm by explosive material** HCC Rx ESR COM

✓x7ᵗʰ **X76** **Intentional self-harm by smoke, fire and flames** HCC Rx ESR COM

✓4ᵗʰ **X77** **Intentional self-harm by steam, hot vapors and hot objects**

✓x7ᵗʰ **X77.0** **Intentional self-harm by** steam or hot vapors HCC Rx ESR COM

✓x7ᵗʰ **X77.1** **Intentional self-harm by hot** tap water HCC Rx ESR COM

✓x7ᵗʰ **X77.2** **Intentional self-harm by other hot fluids** HCC Rx ESR COM

✓x7ᵗʰ **X77.3** **Intentional self-harm by hot** household appliances HCC Rx ESR COM

✓x7ᵗʰ **X77.8** **Intentional self-harm by other hot objects** HCC Rx ESR COM

✓x7ᵗʰ **X77.9** **Intentional self-harm by unspecified hot objects** HCC Rx ESR COM

✓4ᵗʰ **X78** **Intentional self-harm by sharp object**

✓x7ᵗʰ **X78.0** **Intentional self-harm by sharp** glass HCC Rx ESR COM

✓x7ᵗʰ **X78.1** **Intentional self-harm by** knife HCC Rx ESR COM

✓x7ᵗʰ **X78.2** **Intentional self-harm by** sword or dagger HCC Rx ESR COM

✓x7ᵗʰ **X78.8** **Intentional self-harm by other sharp object** HCC Rx ESR COM
AHA: 2022,1Q,27

✓x7ᵗʰ **X78.9** **Intentional self-harm by unspecified sharp object** HCC Rx ESR COM

✓x7ᵗʰ **X79** **Intentional self-harm by blunt object** HCC Rx ESR COM

✓x7ᵗʰ **X80** **Intentional self-harm by jumping from a high place** HCC Rx ESR COM
Intentional fall from one level to another

✓4ᵗʰ **X81** **Intentional self-harm by jumping or lying in front of moving object**

✓x7ᵗʰ **X81.0** **Intentional self-harm by jumping or lying in front of** motor vehicle HCC Rx ESR COM

✓x7ᵗʰ **X81.1** **Intentional self-harm by jumping or lying in front of (subway) train** HCC Rx ESR COM

✓x7ᵗʰ **X81.8** **Intentional self-harm by jumping or lying in front of other moving object** HCC Rx ESR COM

✓4ᵗʰ **X82** **Intentional self-harm by crashing of motor vehicle**

✓x7ᵗʰ **X82.0** **Intentional collision of motor vehicle with other motor vehicle** HCC Rx ESR COM

✓x7ᵗʰ **X82.1** **Intentional collision of motor vehicle with train** HCC Rx ESR COM

✓x7ᵗʰ **X82.2** **Intentional collision of motor vehicle with tree** HCC Rx ESR COM

✓x7ᵗʰ **X82.8** **Other intentional self-harm by crashing of motor vehicle** HCC Rx ESR COM

✓4ᵗʰ **X83** **Intentional self-harm by other specified means**
EXCLUDES 1   *intentional self-harm by poisoning or contact with toxic substance - see Table of Drugs and Chemicals*

✓x7ᵗʰ **X83.0** **Intentional self-harm by** crashing of aircraft HCC Rx ESR COM

✓x7ᵗʰ **X83.1** **Intentional self-harm by** electrocution HCC Rx ESR COM

✓x7ᵗʰ **X83.2** **Intentional self-harm by** exposure to extremes of cold HCC Rx ESR COM

✓x7ᵗʰ **X83.8** **Intentional self-harm by other specified means** HCC Rx ESR COM

Assault (X92-Y09)

INCLUDES   homicide
injuries inflicted by another person with intent to injure or kill, by any means

EXCLUDES 1   *injuries due to legal intervention (Y35.-)*
injuries due to operations of war (Y36.-)
injuries due to terrorism (Y38.-)

The appropriate 7th character is to be added to each code from categories X92-Y04 and Y08.
A   initial encounter
D   subsequent encounter
S   sequela

✓4ᵗʰ **X92** **Assault by drowning and submersion**

✓x7ᵗʰ **X92.0** **Assault by drowning and submersion while in** bathtub

✓x7ᵗʰ **X92.1** **Assault by drowning and submersion while in** swimming pool

✓x7ᵗʰ **X92.2** **Assault by drowning and submersion** after push into swimming pool

✓x7ᵗʰ **X92.3** **Assault by drowning and submersion** in natural water

✓x7ᵗʰ **X92.8** **Other assault by drowning and submersion**

✓x7ᵗʰ **X92.9** **Assault by drowning and submersion, unspecified**

✓x7ᵗʰ **X93** **Assault by** handgun **discharge**
Assault by discharge of gun for single hand use
Assault by discharge of pistol
Assault by discharge of revolver
EXCLUDES 1   *Very pistol (X95.8)*

✓4ᵗʰ **X94** **Assault by** rifle, shotgun and larger firearm **discharge**
EXCLUDES 1   *airgun (X95.01)*

✓x7ᵗʰ **X94.0** **Assault by** shotgun

✓x7ᵗʰ **X94.1** **Assault by** hunting rifle

✓x7ᵗʰ **X94.2** **Assault by** machine gun

✓x7ᵗʰ **X94.8** **Assault by other larger firearm discharge**

✓x7ᵗʰ **X94.9** **Assault by unspecified larger firearm discharge**

✓4ᵗʰ **X95** **Assault by other and unspecified firearm and gun discharge**

✓5ᵗʰ **X95.0** **Assault by** gas, air or spring-operated **guns**

✓x7ᵗʰ **X95.01** **Assault by** airgun **discharge**
Assault by BB gun discharge
Assault by pellet gun discharge

✓x7ᵗʰ **X95.02** **Assault by** paintball gun **discharge**

✓x7ᵗʰ **X95.09** **Assault by other gas, air or spring-operated gun**

✓x7ᵗʰ **X95.8** **Assault by other firearm discharge**
Assault by Very pistol [flare] discharge

✓x7ᵗʰ **X95.9** **Assault by unspecified firearm discharge**

✓4ᵗʰ **X96** **Assault by explosive material**
EXCLUDES 1   *incendiary device (X97)*
terrorism involving explosive material (Y38.2-)

✓x7ᵗʰ **X96.0** **Assault by** antipersonnel **bomb**
EXCLUDES 1   *antipersonnel bomb use in military or war (Y36.2-)*

✓x7ᵗʰ **X96.1** **Assault by** gasoline **bomb**

✓x7ᵗʰ **X96.2** **Assault by** letter **bomb**

✓x7ᵗʰ **X96.3** **Assault by** fertilizer **bomb**

✓x7ᵗʰ **X96.4** **Assault by** pipe **bomb**

✓x7ᵗʰ **X96.8** **Assault by other specified explosive**

✓x7ᵗʰ **X96.9** **Assault by unspecified explosive**

✓x7ᵗʰ **X97** **Assault by smoke, fire and flames**
Assault by arson
Assault by cigarettes
Assault by incendiary device

✓4ᵗʰ **X98** **Assault by steam, hot vapors and hot objects**

✓x7ᵗʰ **X98.0** **Assault by** steam or hot vapors

✓x7ᵗʰ **X98.1** **Assault by hot** tap water

✓x7ᵗʰ **X98.2** **Assault by hot** fluids

✓x7ᵗʰ **X98.3** **Assault by hot** household appliances

✓x7ᵗʰ **X98.8** **Assault by other hot** objects

✓x7ᵗʰ **X98.9** **Assault by unspecified hot objects**

√4ᵗʰ **X99 Assault by sharp object**

> EXCLUDES 1   *assault by strike by sports equipment (Y08.0-)*

√x7ᵗʰ **X99.0 Assault by sharp** glass

√x7ᵗʰ **X99.1 Assault by** knife

√x7ᵗʰ **X99.2 Assault by** sword or dagger

√x7ᵗʰ **X99.8 Assault by other sharp object**

√x7ᵗʰ **X99.9 Assault by unspecified sharp object**
> Assault by stabbing NOS

√x7ᵗʰ **Y00 Assault by blunt object**

> EXCLUDES 1   *assault by strike by sports equipment (Y08.0-)*

√x7ᵗʰ **Y01 Assault by pushing from high place**

√4ᵗʰ **Y02 Assault by pushing or placing victim in front of moving object**

√x7ᵗʰ **Y02.0 Assault by pushing or placing victim in front of** motor vehicle

√x7ᵗʰ **Y02.1 Assault by pushing or placing victim in front of (subway)** train

√x7ᵗʰ **Y02.8 Assault by pushing or placing victim in front of other moving object**

√4ᵗʰ **Y03 Assault by crashing of motor vehicle**

√x7ᵗʰ **Y03.0 Assault by being hit or run over by motor vehicle**

√x7ᵗʰ **Y03.8 Other assault by crashing of motor vehicle**

√4ᵗʰ **Y04 Assault by bodily force**

> EXCLUDES 1   *assault by:*
> *submersion (X92.-)*
> *use of weapon (X93-X95, X99, Y00)*

√x7ᵗʰ **Y04.0 Assault by** unarmed brawl or fight

√x7ᵗʰ **Y04.1 Assault by** human bite

√x7ᵗʰ **Y04.2 Assault by** strike **against or bumped into by another person**

√x7ᵗʰ **Y04.8 Assault by other bodily force**
> Assault by bodily force NOS

√4ᵗʰ **Y07 Perpetrator of assault, maltreatment and neglect**

> NOTE   Codes from this category are for use only in cases of confirmed abuse (T74.-)
>
> Selection of the correct perpetrator code is based on the relationship between the perpetrator and the victim
>
> INCLUDES   perpetrator of abandonment
> perpetrator of emotional neglect
> perpetrator of mental cruelty
> perpetrator of physical abuse
> perpetrator of physical neglect
> perpetrator of sexual abuse
> perpetrator of torture

√5ᵗʰ **Y07.0 Spouse or partner, perpetrator of maltreatment and neglect**
> Spouse or partner, perpetrator of maltreatment and neglect against spouse or partner

Y07.01 Husband, perpetrator of maltreatment and neglect

Y07.02 Wife, perpetrator of maltreatment and neglect

Y07.03 Male partner, perpetrator of maltreatment and neglect

Y07.04 Female partner, perpetrator of maltreatment and neglect

√5ᵗʰ **Y07.1 Parent (adoptive) (biological), perpetrator of maltreatment and neglect**

Y07.11 Biological father, perpetrator of maltreatment and neglect

Y07.12 Biological mother, perpetrator of maltreatment and neglect

Y07.13 Adoptive father, perpetrator of maltreatment and neglect

Y07.14 Adoptive mother, perpetrator of maltreatment and neglect

√5ᵗʰ **Y07.4 Other family member, perpetrator of maltreatment and neglect**

√6ᵗʰ **Y07.41 Sibling, perpetrator of maltreatment and neglect**

> EXCLUDES 1   *stepsibling, perpetrator of maltreatment and neglect (Y07.435, Y07.436)*

Y07.410 Brother, perpetrator of maltreatment and neglect

Y07.411 Sister, perpetrator of maltreatment and neglect

√6ᵗʰ **Y07.42 Foster parent, perpetrator of maltreatment and neglect**

Y07.420 Foster father, perpetrator of maltreatment and neglect

Y07.421 Foster mother, perpetrator of maltreatment and neglect

√6ᵗʰ **Y07.43 Stepparent or stepsibling, perpetrator of maltreatment and neglect**

Y07.430 Stepfather, perpetrator of maltreatment and neglect

Y07.432 Male friend of parent (co-residing in household), perpetrator of maltreatment and neglect

Y07.433 Stepmother, perpetrator of maltreatment and neglect

Y07.434 Female friend of parent (co-residing in household), perpetrator of maltreatment and neglect

Y07.435 Stepbrother, perpetrator or maltreatment and neglect

Y07.436 Stepsister, perpetrator of maltreatment and neglect

√6ᵗʰ **Y07.49 Other family member, perpetrator of maltreatment and neglect**

Y07.490 Male cousin, perpetrator of maltreatment and neglect

Y07.491 Female cousin, perpetrator of maltreatment and neglect

Y07.499 Other family member, perpetrator of maltreatment and neglect

√5ᵗʰ **Y07.5 Non-family member, perpetrator of maltreatment and neglect**

Y07.50 Unspecified non-family member, perpetrator of maltreatment and neglect

√6ᵗʰ **Y07.51 Daycare provider, perpetrator of maltreatment and neglect**

Y07.510 At-home childcare provider, perpetrator of maltreatment and neglect

Y07.511 Daycare center childcare provider, perpetrator of maltreatment and neglect

Y07.512 At-home adultcare provider, perpetrator of maltreatment and neglect

Y07.513 Adultcare center provider, perpetrator of maltreatment and neglect

Y07.519 Unspecified daycare provider, perpetrator of maltreatment and neglect

√6ᵗʰ **Y07.52 Healthcare provider, perpetrator of maltreatment and neglect**

Y07.521 Mental health provider, perpetrator of maltreatment and neglect

Y07.528 Other therapist or healthcare provider, perpetrator of maltreatment and neglect
> Nurse perpetrator of maltreatment and neglect
> Occupational therapist perpetrator of maltreatment and neglect
> Physical therapist perpetrator of maltreatment and neglect
> Speech therapist perpetrator of maltreatment and neglect

Y07.529 Unspecified healthcare provider, perpetrator of maltreatment and neglect

Y07.53 Teacher or instructor, perpetrator of maltreatment and neglect
> Coach, perpetrator of maltreatment and neglect

Y07.59 Other non-family member, perpetrator of maltreatment and neglect

Y07.6 Multiple perpetrators of maltreatment and neglect
> AHA: 2018,4Q,32

Y07.9 Unspecified perpetrator of maltreatment and neglect

√4ᵗʰ **Y08 Assault by other specified means**

√5ᵗʰ **Y08.0 Assault by strike by** sport equipment

√x7ᵗʰ **Y08.01 Assault by strike by** hockey stick

√x7ᵗʰ **Y08.02 Assault by strike by** baseball bat

√x7ᵗʰ **Y08.09 Assault by strike by other specified type of sport equipment**

√5ᵗʰ **Y08.8 Assault by other specified means**

√x7ᵗʰ **Y08.81 Assault by crashing of** aircraft

√x7ᵗʰ **Y08.89 Assault by other specified means**

Y09   **Assault by unspecified means**
Assassination (attempted) NOS
Homicide (attempted) NOS
Manslaughter (attempted) NOS
Murder (attempted) NOS

Event of undetermined intent (Y21-Y33)

Undetermined intent is only for use when there is specific documentation in the record that the intent of the injury cannot be determined. If no such documentation is present, code to accidental (unintentional).

The appropriate 7th character is to be added to each code from categories Y21-Y33.
A   initial encounter
D   subsequent encounter
S   sequela

✓4ᵗʰ **Y21**   **Drowning and submersion, undetermined intent**

✓x7ᵗʰ   **Y21.0**   **Drowning and submersion** while in bathtub, **undetermined intent**

✓x7ᵗʰ   **Y21.1**   **Drowning and submersion** after fall into bathtub, **undetermined intent**

✓x7ᵗʰ   **Y21.2**   **Drowning and submersion** while in swimming pool, **undetermined intent**

✓x7ᵗʰ   **Y21.3**   **Drowning and submersion** after fall into swimming pool, **undetermined intent**

✓x7ᵗʰ   **Y21.4**   **Drowning and submersion** in natural water, **undetermined intent**

✓x7ᵗʰ   **Y21.8**   **Other drowning and submersion, undetermined intent**

✓x7ᵗʰ   **Y21.9**   **Unspecified drowning and submersion, undetermined intent**

✓x7ᵗʰ **Y22**   **Handgun discharge, undetermined intent**
Discharge of gun for single hand use, undetermined intent
Discharge of pistol, undetermined intent
Discharge of revolver, undetermined intent
EXCLUDES 2   Very pistol (Y24.8)

✓4ᵗʰ **Y23**   **Rifle, shotgun and larger firearm discharge, undetermined intent**
EXCLUDES 2   airgun (Y24.0)

✓x7ᵗʰ   **Y23.0**   **Shotgun discharge, undetermined intent**

✓x7ᵗʰ   **Y23.1**   **Hunting rifle discharge, undetermined intent**

✓x7ᵗʰ   **Y23.2**   **Military firearm discharge, undetermined intent**

✓x7ᵗʰ   **Y23.3**   **Machine gun discharge, undetermined intent**

✓x7ᵗʰ   **Y23.8**   **Other larger firearm discharge, undetermined intent**

✓x7ᵗʰ   **Y23.9**   **Unspecified larger firearm discharge, undetermined intent**

✓4ᵗʰ **Y24**   **Other and unspecified firearm discharge, undetermined intent**

✓x7ᵗʰ   **Y24.0**   **Airgun discharge, undetermined intent**
BB gun discharge, undetermined intent
Pellet gun discharge, undetermined intent

✓x7ᵗʰ   **Y24.8**   **Other firearm discharge, undetermined intent**
Paintball gun discharge, undetermined intent
Very pistol [flare] discharge, undetermined intent

✓x7ᵗʰ   **Y24.9**   **Unspecified firearm discharge, undetermined intent**

✓x7ᵗʰ **Y25**   **Contact with explosive material, undetermined intent**

✓x7ᵗʰ **Y26**   **Exposure to smoke, fire and flames, undetermined intent**

✓4ᵗʰ **Y27**   **Contact with steam, hot vapors and hot objects, undetermined intent**

✓x7ᵗʰ   **Y27.0**   **Contact with steam and hot vapors, undetermined intent**

✓x7ᵗʰ   **Y27.1**   **Contact with hot tap water, undetermined intent**

✓x7ᵗʰ   **Y27.2**   **Contact with hot fluids, undetermined intent**

✓x7ᵗʰ   **Y27.3**   **Contact with hot household appliance, undetermined intent**

✓x7ᵗʰ   **Y27.8**   **Contact with other hot objects, undetermined intent**

✓x7ᵗʰ   **Y27.9**   **Contact with unspecified hot objects, undetermined intent**

✓4ᵗʰ **Y28**   **Contact with sharp object, undetermined intent**

✓x7ᵗʰ   **Y28.0**   **Contact with sharp glass, undetermined intent**

✓x7ᵗʰ   **Y28.1**   **Contact with knife, undetermined intent**

✓x7ᵗʰ   **Y28.2**   **Contact with sword or dagger, undetermined intent**

✓x7ᵗʰ   **Y28.8**   **Contact with other sharp object, undetermined intent**

✓x7ᵗʰ   **Y28.9**   **Contact with unspecified sharp object, undetermined intent**

✓x7ᵗʰ **Y29**   **Contact with blunt object, undetermined intent**

✓x7ᵗʰ **Y30**   **Falling, jumping or pushed from a high place, undetermined intent**
Victim falling from one level to another, undetermined intent

✓x7ᵗʰ **Y31**   **Falling, lying or running before or into moving object, undetermined intent**

✓x7ᵗʰ **Y32**   **Crashing of motor vehicle, undetermined intent**

✓x7ᵗʰ **Y33**   **Other specified events, undetermined intent**

Legal intervention, operations of war, military operations, and terrorism (Y35-Y38)

The appropriate 7th character is to be added to each code from categories Y35-Y38.
A   initial encounter
D   subsequent encounter
S   sequela

✓4ᵗʰ **Y35**   **Legal intervention**
INCLUDES   any injury sustained as a result of an encounter with any law enforcement official, serving in any capacity at the time of the encounter, whether on-duty or off-duty. Includes injury to law enforcement official, suspect and bystander
AHA: 2019,4Q,18-19

✓5ᵗʰ   **Y35.0**   **Legal intervention involving firearm discharge**

✓6ᵗʰ   **Y35.00**   **Legal intervention involving unspecified firearm discharge**
Legal intervention involving gunshot wound
Legal intervention involving shot NOS

✓7ᵗʰ   **Y35.001**   **Legal intervention involving unspecified firearm discharge, law enforcement official injured**

✓7ᵗʰ   **Y35.002**   **Legal intervention involving unspecified firearm discharge, bystander injured**

✓7ᵗʰ   **Y35.003**   **Legal intervention involving unspecified firearm discharge, suspect injured**

✓7ᵗʰ   **Y35.009**   **Legal intervention involving unspecified firearm discharge, unspecified person injured**

✓6ᵗʰ   **Y35.01**   **Legal intervention involving injury by machine gun**

✓7ᵗʰ   **Y35.011**   **Legal intervention involving injury by machine gun, law enforcement official injured**

✓7ᵗʰ   **Y35.012**   **Legal intervention involving injury by machine gun, bystander injured**

✓7ᵗʰ   **Y35.013**   **Legal intervention involving injury by machine gun, suspect injured**

✓7ᵗʰ   **Y35.019**   **Legal intervention involving injury by machine gun, unspecified person injured**

✓6ᵗʰ   **Y35.02**   **Legal intervention involving injury by handgun**

✓7ᵗʰ   **Y35.021**   **Legal intervention involving injury by handgun, law enforcement official injured**

✓7ᵗʰ   **Y35.022**   **Legal intervention involving injury by handgun, bystander injured**

✓7ᵗʰ   **Y35.023**   **Legal intervention involving injury by handgun, suspect injured**

✓7ᵗʰ   **Y35.029**   **Legal intervention involving injury by handgun, unspecified person injured**

✓6ᵗʰ   **Y35.03**   **Legal intervention involving injury by rifle pellet**

✓7ᵗʰ   **Y35.031**   **Legal intervention involving injury by rifle pellet, law enforcement official injured**

✓7ᵗʰ   **Y35.032**   **Legal intervention involving injury by rifle pellet, bystander injured**

✓7ᵗʰ   **Y35.033**   **Legal intervention involving injury by rifle pellet, suspect injured**

✓7ᵗʰ   **Y35.039**   **Legal intervention involving injury by rifle pellet, unspecified person injured**

✓6ᵗʰ   **Y35.04**   **Legal intervention involving injury by rubber bullet**

✓7ᵗʰ   **Y35.041**   **Legal intervention involving injury by rubber bullet, law enforcement official injured**

✓7ᵗʰ   **Y35.042**   **Legal intervention involving injury by rubber bullet, bystander injured**

✓7ᵗʰ   **Y35.043**   **Legal intervention involving injury by rubber bullet, suspect injured**

✓7ᵗʰ   **Y35.049**   **Legal intervention involving injury by rubber bullet, unspecified person injured**

✓6ᵗʰ   **Y35.09**   **Legal intervention involving other firearm discharge**

✓7ᵗʰ   **Y35.091**   **Legal intervention involving other firearm discharge, law enforcement official injured**

√7ᵗʰ **Y35.092** Legal intervention involving other firearm discharge, **bystander** injured

√7ᵗʰ **Y35.093** Legal intervention involving other firearm discharge, **suspect** injured

√7ᵗʰ **Y35.099** Legal intervention involving other firearm discharge, unspecified person injured

√5ᵗʰ **Y35.1** Legal intervention involving **explosives**

     √6ᵗʰ **Y35.10** Legal intervention involving unspecified explosives

         √7ᵗʰ **Y35.101** Legal intervention involving unspecified explosives, **law enforcement official** injured

         √7ᵗʰ **Y35.102** Legal intervention involving unspecified explosives, **bystander** injured

         √7ᵗʰ **Y35.103** Legal intervention involving unspecified explosives, **suspect** injured

         √7ᵗʰ **Y35.109** Legal intervention involving unspecified explosives, unspecified person injured

     √6ᵗʰ **Y35.11** Legal intervention involving injury by **dynamite**

         √7ᵗʰ **Y35.111** Legal intervention involving injury by dynamite, **law enforcement official** injured

         √7ᵗʰ **Y35.112** Legal intervention involving injury by dynamite, **bystander** injured

         √7ᵗʰ **Y35.113** Legal intervention involving injury by dynamite, **suspect** injured

         √7ᵗʰ **Y35.119** Legal intervention involving injury by dynamite, unspecified person injured

     √6ᵗʰ **Y35.12** Legal intervention involving injury by **explosive shell**

         √7ᵗʰ **Y35.121** Legal intervention involving injury by explosive shell, **law enforcement official** injured

         √7ᵗʰ **Y35.122** Legal intervention involving injury by explosive shell, **bystander** injured

         √7ᵗʰ **Y35.123** Legal intervention involving injury by explosive shell, **suspect** injured

         √7ᵗʰ **Y35.129** Legal intervention involving injury by explosive shell, unspecified person injured

     √6ᵗʰ **Y35.19** Legal intervention involving other explosives

         Legal intervention involving injury by grenade

         Legal intervention involving injury by mortar bomb

         √7ᵗʰ **Y35.191** Legal intervention involving other explosives, **law enforcement official** injured

         √7ᵗʰ **Y35.192** Legal intervention involving other explosives, **bystander** injured

         √7ᵗʰ **Y35.193** Legal intervention involving other explosives, **suspect** injured

         √7ᵗʰ **Y35.199** Legal intervention involving other explosives, unspecified person injured

√5ᵗʰ **Y35.2** Legal intervention involving **gas**

     Legal intervention involving asphyxiation by gas

     Legal intervention involving poisoning by gas

     √6ᵗʰ **Y35.20** Legal intervention involving unspecified gas

         √7ᵗʰ **Y35.201** Legal intervention involving unspecified gas, **law enforcement official** injured

         √7ᵗʰ **Y35.202** Legal intervention involving unspecified gas, **bystander** injured

         √7ᵗʰ **Y35.203** Legal intervention involving unspecified gas, **suspect** injured

         √7ᵗʰ **Y35.209** Legal intervention involving unspecified gas, unspecified person injured

     √6ᵗʰ **Y35.21** Legal intervention involving injury by **tear gas**

         √7ᵗʰ **Y35.211** Legal intervention involving injury by tear gas, **law enforcement official** injured

         √7ᵗʰ **Y35.212** Legal intervention involving injury by tear gas, **bystander** injured

         √7ᵗʰ **Y35.213** Legal intervention involving injury by tear gas, **suspect** injured

         √7ᵗʰ **Y35.219** Legal intervention involving injury by tear gas, unspecified person injured

     √6ᵗʰ **Y35.29** Legal intervention involving other gas

         √7ᵗʰ **Y35.291** Legal intervention involving other gas, **law enforcement official** injured

         √7ᵗʰ **Y35.292** Legal intervention involving other gas, **bystander** injured

         √7ᵗʰ **Y35.293** Legal intervention involving other gas, **suspect** injured

√7ᵗʰ **Y35.299** Legal intervention involving other gas, unspecified person injured

√5ᵗʰ **Y35.3** Legal intervention involving **blunt objects**

     Legal intervention involving being hit or struck by blunt object

     √6ᵗʰ **Y35.30** Legal intervention involving unspecified blunt objects

         √7ᵗʰ **Y35.301** Legal intervention involving unspecified blunt objects, **law enforcement official** injured

         √7ᵗʰ **Y35.302** Legal intervention involving unspecified blunt objects, **bystander** injured

         √7ᵗʰ **Y35.303** Legal intervention involving unspecified blunt objects, **suspect** injured

         √7ᵗʰ **Y35.309** Legal intervention involving unspecified blunt objects, unspecified person injured

     √6ᵗʰ **Y35.31** Legal intervention involving **baton**

         √7ᵗʰ **Y35.311** Legal intervention involving baton, **law enforcement official** injured

         √7ᵗʰ **Y35.312** Legal intervention involving baton, **bystander** injured

         √7ᵗʰ **Y35.313** Legal intervention involving baton, **suspect** injured

         √7ᵗʰ **Y35.319** Legal intervention involving baton, unspecified person injured

     √6ᵗʰ **Y35.39** Legal intervention involving other blunt objects

         √7ᵗʰ **Y35.391** Legal intervention involving other blunt objects, **law enforcement official** injured

         √7ᵗʰ **Y35.392** Legal intervention involving other blunt objects, **bystander** injured

         √7ᵗʰ **Y35.393** Legal intervention involving other blunt objects, **suspect** injured

         √7ᵗʰ **Y35.399** Legal intervention involving other blunt objects, unspecified person injured

√5ᵗʰ **Y35.4** Legal intervention involving **sharp objects**

     Legal intervention involving being cut by sharp objects

     Legal intervention involving being stabbed by sharp objects

     √6ᵗʰ **Y35.40** Legal intervention involving unspecified sharp objects

         √7ᵗʰ **Y35.401** Legal intervention involving unspecified sharp objects, **law enforcement official** injured

         √7ᵗʰ **Y35.402** Legal intervention involving unspecified sharp objects, **bystander** injured

         √7ᵗʰ **Y35.403** Legal intervention involving unspecified sharp objects, **suspect** injured

         √7ᵗʰ **Y35.409** Legal intervention involving unspecified sharp objects, unspecified person injured

     √6ᵗʰ **Y35.41** Legal intervention involving **bayonet**

         √7ᵗʰ **Y35.411** Legal intervention involving bayonet, **law enforcement official** injured

         √7ᵗʰ **Y35.412** Legal intervention involving bayonet, **bystander** injured

         √7ᵗʰ **Y35.413** Legal intervention involving bayonet, **suspect** injured

         √7ᵗʰ **Y35.419** Legal intervention involving bayonet, unspecified person injured

     √6ᵗʰ **Y35.49** Legal intervention involving other sharp objects

         √7ᵗʰ **Y35.491** Legal intervention involving other sharp objects, **law enforcement official** injured

         √7ᵗʰ **Y35.492** Legal intervention involving other sharp objects, **bystander** injured

         √7ᵗʰ **Y35.493** Legal intervention involving other sharp objects, **suspect** injured

         √7ᵗʰ **Y35.499** Legal intervention involving other sharp objects, unspecified person injured

√5ᵗʰ **Y35.8** Legal intervention involving **other specified means**

     AHA: 2019,4Q,19

     √6ᵗʰ **Y35.81** Legal intervention involving **manhandling**

         √7ᵗʰ **Y35.811** Legal intervention involving manhandling, **law enforcement official** injured

         √7ᵗʰ **Y35.812** Legal intervention involving manhandling, **bystander** injured

         √7ᵗʰ **Y35.813** Legal intervention involving manhandling, **suspect** injured

         √7ᵗʰ **Y35.819** Legal intervention involving manhandling, unspecified person injured

---

☑ Additional Character Required   √x7ᵗʰ Placeholder Alert   Manifestation   Unspecified Dx   ⓠ QPP   UPD Unacceptable PDx

Chapter 20. External Causes of Morbidity

☑6ᵗʰ **Y35.83** **Legal intervention involving a** conducted energy device
Electroshock device (taser)
Stun gun

☑7ᵗʰ **Y35.831** **Legal intervention involving a conducted energy device,** law enforcement official **injured**

☑7ᵗʰ **Y35.832** **Legal intervention involving a conducted energy device,** bystander **injured**

☑7ᵗʰ **Y35.833** **Legal intervention involving a conducted energy device,** suspect **injured**

☑7ᵗʰ **Y35.839** **Legal intervention involving a conducted energy device, unspecified person injured**

☑6ᵗʰ **Y35.89** **Legal intervention involving other specified means**

☑7ᵗʰ **Y35.891** **Legal intervention involving other specified means,** law enforcement official **injured**

☑7ᵗʰ **Y35.892** **Legal intervention involving other specified means,** bystander **injured**

☑7ᵗʰ **Y35.893** **Legal intervention involving other specified means,** suspect **injured**
AHA: 2018,1Q,5

☑7ᵗʰ **Y35.899** **Legal intervention involving other specified means, unspecified person injured**

☑5ᵗʰ **Y35.9** **Legal intervention, means unspecified**

☑x7ᵗʰ **Y35.91** **Legal intervention, means unspecified,** law enforcement official **injured**

☑x7ᵗʰ **Y35.92** **Legal intervention, means unspecified,** bystander **injured**

☑x7ᵗʰ **Y35.93** **Legal intervention, means unspecified,** suspect **injured**

☑x7ᵗʰ **Y35.99** **Legal intervention, means unspecified, unspecified person injured**

☑4ᵗʰ **Y36** **Operations of war**

INCLUDES   injuries to military personnel and civilians caused by war, civil insurrection, and peacekeeping missions

EXCLUDES 1   injury to military personnel occurring during peacetime military operations (Y37.-)
military vehicles involved in transport accidents with non-military vehicle during peacetime ▶(V09.01, V09.21, V19.81, V29.818, V39.81, V49.81, V59.81, V69.81, V79.81)◀

AHA: 2014,3Q,4

☑5ᵗʰ **Y36.0** **War operations involving** explosion of marine weapons

☑6ᵗʰ **Y36.00** **War operations involving explosion of unspecified marine weapon**
War operations involving underwater blast NOS

☑7ᵗʰ **Y36.000** **War operations involving explosion of unspecified marine weapon,** military personnel

☑7ᵗʰ **Y36.001** **War operations involving explosion of unspecified marine weapon,** civilian

☑6ᵗʰ **Y36.01** **War operations involving explosion of** depth-charge

☑7ᵗʰ **Y36.010** **War operations involving explosion of depth-charge,** military personnel

☑7ᵗʰ **Y36.011** **War operations involving explosion of depth-charge,** civilian

☑6ᵗʰ **Y36.02** **War operations involving explosion of** marine mine
War operations involving explosion of marine mine, at sea or in harbor

☑7ᵗʰ **Y36.020** **War operations involving explosion of marine mine,** military personnel

☑7ᵗʰ **Y36.021** **War operations involving explosion of marine mine,** civilian

☑6ᵗʰ **Y36.03** **War operations involving explosion of** sea-based artillery shell

☑7ᵗʰ **Y36.030** **War operations involving explosion of sea-based artillery shell,** military personnel

☑7ᵗʰ **Y36.031** **War operations involving explosion of sea-based artillery shell,** civilian

☑6ᵗʰ **Y36.04** **War operations involving explosion of** torpedo

☑7ᵗʰ **Y36.040** **War operations involving explosion of torpedo,** military personnel

☑7ᵗʰ **Y36.041** **War operations involving explosion of torpedo,** civilian

☑6ᵗʰ **Y36.05** **War operations involving** accidental detonation of onboard marine weapons

☑7ᵗʰ **Y36.050** **War operations involving accidental detonation of onboard marine weapons, military personnel**

☑7ᵗʰ **Y36.051** **War operations involving accidental detonation of onboard marine weapons, civilian**

☑6ᵗʰ **Y36.09** **War operations involving explosion of other marine weapons**

☑7ᵗʰ **Y36.090** **War operations involving explosion of other marine weapons,** military personnel

☑7ᵗʰ **Y36.091** **War operations involving explosion of other marine weapons,** civilian

☑5ᵗʰ **Y36.1** **War operations involving** destruction of aircraft

☑6ᵗʰ **Y36.10** **War operations involving unspecified destruction of aircraft**

☑7ᵗʰ **Y36.100** **War operations involving unspecified destruction of aircraft,** military personnel

☑7ᵗʰ **Y36.101** **War operations involving unspecified destruction of aircraft,** civilian

☑6ᵗʰ **Y36.11** **War operations involving destruction of aircraft due to** enemy fire or explosives
War operations involving destruction of aircraft due to air to air missile
War operations involving destruction of aircraft due to explosive placed on aircraft
War operations involving destruction of aircraft due to rocket propelled grenade [RPG]
War operations involving destruction of aircraft due to small arms fire
War operations involving destruction of aircraft due to surface to air missile

☑7ᵗʰ **Y36.110** **War operations involving destruction of aircraft due to enemy fire or explosives,** military personnel

☑7ᵗʰ **Y36.111** **War operations involving destruction of aircraft due to enemy fire or explosives,** civilian

☑6ᵗʰ **Y36.12** **War operations involving destruction of aircraft due to** collision with other aircraft

☑7ᵗʰ **Y36.120** **War operations involving destruction of aircraft due to collision with other aircraft,** military personnel

☑7ᵗʰ **Y36.121** **War operations involving destruction of aircraft due to collision with other aircraft,** civilian

☑6ᵗʰ **Y36.13** **War operations involving destruction of aircraft due to** onboard fire

☑7ᵗʰ **Y36.130** **War operations involving destruction of aircraft due to onboard fire,** military personnel

☑7ᵗʰ **Y36.131** **War operations involving destruction of aircraft due to onboard fire,** civilian

☑6ᵗʰ **Y36.14** **War operations involving destruction of aircraft due to** accidental detonation of onboard munitions and explosives

☑7ᵗʰ **Y36.140** **War operations involving destruction of aircraft due to accidental detonation of onboard munitions and explosives,** military personnel

☑7ᵗʰ **Y36.141** **War operations involving destruction of aircraft due to accidental detonation of onboard munitions and explosives,** civilian

☑6ᵗʰ **Y36.19** **War operations involving other destruction of aircraft**

☑7ᵗʰ **Y36.190** **War operations involving other destruction of aircraft,** military personnel

☑7ᵗʰ **Y36.191** **War operations involving other destruction of aircraft,** civilian

✓5ᵗʰ **Y36.2** **War operations involving other explosions and fragments**
> EXCLUDES 1 *war operations involving explosion of aircraft (Y36.1-)*
> *war operations involving explosion of marine weapons (Y36.0-)*
> *war operations involving explosion of nuclear weapons (Y36.5-)*
> *war operations involving explosion occurring after cessation of hostilities (Y36.8-)*

✓6ᵗʰ **Y36.20** **War operations involving unspecified explosion and fragments**
> War operations involving air blast NOS
> War operations involving blast NOS
> War operations involving blast fragments NOS
> War operations involving blast wave NOS
> War operations involving blast wind NOS
> War operations involving explosion NOS
> War operations involving explosion of bomb NOS

✓7ᵗʰ **Y36.200** **War operations involving unspecified explosion and fragments, military personnel**

✓7ᵗʰ **Y36.201** **War operations involving unspecified explosion and fragments, civilian**

✓6ᵗʰ **Y36.21** **War operations involving explosion of aerial bomb**

✓7ᵗʰ **Y36.210** **War operations involving explosion of aerial bomb, military personnel**

✓7ᵗʰ **Y36.211** **War operations involving explosion of aerial bomb, civilian**

✓6ᵗʰ **Y36.22** **War operations involving explosion of guided missile**

✓7ᵗʰ **Y36.220** **War operations involving explosion of guided missile, military personnel**

✓7ᵗʰ **Y36.221** **War operations involving explosion of guided missile, civilian**

✓6ᵗʰ **Y36.23** **War operations involving explosion of improvised explosive device [IED]**
> War operations involving explosion of person-borne improvised explosive device [IED]
> War operations involving explosion of vehicle-borne improvised explosive device [IED]
> War operations involving explosion of roadside improvised explosive device [IED]

✓7ᵗʰ **Y36.230** **War operations involving explosion of improvised explosive device [IED], military personnel**

✓7ᵗʰ **Y36.231** **War operations involving explosion of improvised explosive device [IED], civilian**

✓6ᵗʰ **Y36.24** **War operations involving explosion due to accidental detonation and discharge of own munitions or munitions launch device**

✓7ᵗʰ **Y36.240** **War operations involving explosion due to accidental detonation and discharge of own munitions or munitions launch device, military personnel**

✓7ᵗʰ **Y36.241** **War operations involving explosion due to accidental detonation and discharge of own munitions or munitions launch device, civilian**

✓6ᵗʰ **Y36.25** **War operations involving fragments from munitions**

✓7ᵗʰ **Y36.250** **War operations involving fragments from munitions, military personnel**

✓7ᵗʰ **Y36.251** **War operations involving fragments from munitions, civilian**

✓6ᵗʰ **Y36.26** **War operations involving fragments of improvised explosive device [IED]**
> War operations involving fragments of person-borne improvised explosive device [IED]
> War operations involving fragments of vehicle-borne improvised explosive device [IED]
> War operations involving fragments of roadside improvised explosive device [IED]

✓7ᵗʰ **Y36.260** **War operations involving fragments of improvised explosive device [IED], military personnel**

✓7ᵗʰ **Y36.261** **War operations involving fragments of improvised explosive device [IED], civilian**

✓6ᵗʰ **Y36.27** **War operations involving fragments from weapons**

✓7ᵗʰ **Y36.270** **War operations involving fragments from weapons, military personnel**

✓7ᵗʰ **Y36.271** **War operations involving fragments from weapons, civilian**

✓6ᵗʰ **Y36.29** **War operations involving other explosions and fragments**
> War operations involving explosion of grenade
> War operations involving explosions of land mine
> War operations involving shrapnel NOS

✓7ᵗʰ **Y36.290** **War operations involving other explosions and fragments, military personnel**

✓7ᵗʰ **Y36.291** **War operations involving other explosions and fragments, civilian**

✓5ᵗʰ **Y36.3** **War operations involving fires, conflagrations and hot substances**
> War operations involving smoke, fumes, and heat from fires, conflagrations and hot substances
> EXCLUDES 1 *war operations involving fires and conflagrations aboard military aircraft (Y36.1-)*
> *war operations involving fires and conflagrations aboard military watercraft (Y36.0-)*
> *war operations involving fires and conflagrations caused indirectly by conventional weapons (Y36.2-)*
> *war operations involving fires and thermal effects of nuclear weapons (Y36.53-)*

✓6ᵗʰ **Y36.30** **War operations involving unspecified fire, conflagration and hot substance**

✓7ᵗʰ **Y36.300** **War operations involving unspecified fire, conflagration and hot substance, military personnel**

✓7ᵗʰ **Y36.301** **War operations involving unspecified fire, conflagration and hot substance, civilian**

✓6ᵗʰ **Y36.31** **War operations involving gasoline bomb**
> War operations involving incendiary bomb
> War operations involving petrol bomb

✓7ᵗʰ **Y36.310** **War operations involving gasoline bomb, military personnel**

✓7ᵗʰ **Y36.311** **War operations involving gasoline bomb, civilian**

✓6ᵗʰ **Y36.32** **War operations involving incendiary bullet**

✓7ᵗʰ **Y36.320** **War operations involving incendiary bullet, military personnel**

✓7ᵗʰ **Y36.321** **War operations involving incendiary bullet, civilian**

✓6ᵗʰ **Y36.33** **War operations involving flamethrower**

✓7ᵗʰ **Y36.330** **War operations involving flamethrower, military personnel**

✓7ᵗʰ **Y36.331** **War operations involving flamethrower, civilian**

✓6ᵗʰ **Y36.39** **War operations involving other fires, conflagrations and hot substances**

✓7ᵗʰ **Y36.390** **War operations involving other fires, conflagrations and hot substances, military personnel**

✓7ᵗʰ **Y36.391** **War operations involving other fires, conflagrations and hot substances, civilian**

✓5ᵗʰ **Y36.4** **War operations involving firearm discharge and other forms of conventional warfare**

✓6ᵗʰ **Y36.41** **War operations involving rubber bullets**

✓7ᵗʰ **Y36.410** **War operations involving rubber bullets, military personnel**

✓7ᵗʰ **Y36.411** **War operations involving rubber bullets, civilian**

✓6ᵗʰ **Y36.42** **War operations involving firearms pellets**

✓7ᵗʰ **Y36.420** **War operations involving firearms pellets, military personnel**

✓7ᵗʰ **Y36.421** **War operations involving firearms pellets, civilian**

✓6ᵗʰ **Y36.43** **War operations involving other firearms discharge**
> War operations involving bullets NOS
> EXCLUDES 1 *war operations involving munitions fragments (Y36.25-)*
> *war operations involving incendiary bullets (Y36.32-)*

✓7ᵗʰ **Y36.430** **War operations involving other firearms discharge, military personnel**

✓7ᵗʰ **Y36.431** **War operations involving other firearms discharge, civilian**

✓6th **Y36.44 War operations involving** unarmed hand to hand combat

> EXCLUDES 1   *war operations involving combat using blunt or piercing object (Y36.45-)*
> *war operations involving intentional restriction of air and airway (Y36.46-)*
> *war operations involving unintentional restriction of air and airway (Y36.47-)*

✓7th **Y36.440 War operations involving unarmed hand to hand combat, military personnel**

✓7th **Y36.441 War operations involving unarmed hand to hand combat, civilian**

✓6th **Y36.45 War operations involving combat using** blunt or piercing object

✓7th **Y36.450 War operations involving combat using blunt or piercing object, military personnel**

✓7th **Y36.451 War operations involving combat using blunt or piercing object, civilian**

✓6th **Y36.46 War operations involving** intentional restriction of air and airway

✓7th **Y36.460 War operations involving intentional restriction of air and airway, military personnel**

✓7th **Y36.461 War operations involving intentional restriction of air and airway, civilian**

✓6th **Y36.47 War operations involving** unintentional restriction of air and airway

✓7th **Y36.470 War operations involving unintentional restriction of air and airway, military personnel**

✓7th **Y36.471 War operations involving unintentional restriction of air and airway, civilian**

✓6th **Y36.49 War operations involving other forms of conventional warfare**

✓7th **Y36.490 War operations involving other forms of conventional warfare, military personnel**

✓7th **Y36.491 War operations involving other forms of conventional warfare, civilian**

✓5th **Y36.5 War operations involving** nuclear weapons

> War operations involving dirty bomb NOS

✓6th **Y36.50 War operations involving unspecified effect of nuclear weapon**

✓7th **Y36.500 War operations involving unspecified effect of nuclear weapon, military personnel**

✓7th **Y36.501 War operations involving unspecified effect of nuclear weapon, civilian**

✓6th **Y36.51 War operations involving** direct blast **effect of nuclear weapon**

> War operations involving blast pressure of nuclear weapon

✓7th **Y36.510 War operations involving direct blast effect of nuclear weapon, military personnel**

✓7th **Y36.511 War operations involving direct blast effect of nuclear weapon, civilian**

✓6th **Y36.52 War operations involving** indirect blast **effect of nuclear weapon**

> War operations involving being thrown by blast of nuclear weapon
> War operations involving being struck or crushed by blast debris of nuclear weapon

✓7th **Y36.520 War operations involving indirect blast effect of nuclear weapon, military personnel**

✓7th **Y36.521 War operations involving indirect blast effect of nuclear weapon, civilian**

✓6th **Y36.53 War operations involving** thermal radiation **effect of nuclear weapon**

> War operations involving direct heat from nuclear weapon
> War operation involving fireball effects from nuclear weapon

✓7th **Y36.530 War operations involving thermal radiation effect of nuclear weapon, military personnel**

✓7th **Y36.531 War operations involving thermal radiation effect of nuclear weapon, civilian**

✓6th **Y36.54 War operation involving** nuclear radiation **effects of nuclear weapon**

> War operation involving acute radiation exposure from nuclear weapon
> War operation involving exposure to immediate ionizing radiation from nuclear weapon
> War operation involving fallout exposure from nuclear weapon
> War operation involving secondary effects of nuclear weapons

✓7th **Y36.540 War operation involving nuclear radiation effects of nuclear weapon, military personnel**

✓7th **Y36.541 War operation involving nuclear radiation effects of nuclear weapon, civilian**

✓6th **Y36.59 War operation involving other effects of nuclear weapons**

✓7th **Y36.590 War operation involving other effects of nuclear weapons, military personnel**

✓7th **Y36.591 War operation involving other effects of nuclear weapons, civilian**

✓5th **Y36.6 War operations involving biological weapons**

✓6th **Y36.6X War operations involving** biological weapons

✓7th **Y36.6X0 War operations involving biological weapons, military personnel**

✓7th **Y36.6X1 War operations involving biological weapons, civilian**

✓5th **Y36.7 War operations involving chemical weapons and other forms of unconventional warfare**

> EXCLUDES 1   *war operations involving incendiary devices (Y36.3-, Y36.5-)*

✓6th **Y36.7X War operations involving** chemical weapons and other forms of unconventional warfare

✓7th **Y36.7X0 War operations involving chemical weapons and other forms of unconventional warfare, military personnel**

✓7th **Y36.7X1 War operations involving chemical weapons and other forms of unconventional warfare, civilian**

✓5th **Y36.8 War operations occurring** after cessation of hostilities

> War operations classifiable to categories Y36.0-Y36.8 but occurring after cessation of hostilities

✓6th **Y36.81 Explosion of** mine **placed during war operations but exploding after cessation of hostilities**

✓7th **Y36.810 Explosion of mine placed during war operations but exploding after cessation of hostilities, military personnel**

✓7th **Y36.811 Explosion of mine placed during war operations but exploding after cessation of hostilities, civilian**

✓6th **Y36.82 Explosion of** bomb **placed during war operations but exploding after cessation of hostilities**

✓7th **Y36.820 Explosion of bomb placed during war operations but exploding after cessation of hostilities, military personnel**

✓7th **Y36.821 Explosion of bomb placed during war operations but exploding after cessation of hostilities, civilian**

✓6th **Y36.88 Other war operations occurring after cessation of hostilities**

✓7th **Y36.880 Other war operations occurring after cessation of hostilities, military personnel**

✓7th **Y36.881 Other war operations occurring after cessation of hostilities, civilian**

✓6th **Y36.89 Unspecified war operations occurring after cessation of hostilities**

✓7th **Y36.890 Unspecified war operations occurring after cessation of hostilities, military personnel**

✓7th **Y36.891 Unspecified war operations occurring after cessation of hostilities, civilian**

✓5th **Y36.9 Other and unspecified war operations**

✓x7th **Y36.90 War operations, unspecified**

✓x7th **Y36.91 War operations involving unspecified** weapon of mass destruction [WMD]

✓x7th **Y36.92 War operations involving** friendly fire

✓4ᵗʰ **Y37 Military operations**

INCLUDES   injuries to military personnel and civilians occurring during peacetime on military property and during routine military exercises and operations

EXCLUDES 1   military aircraft involved in aircraft accident with civilian aircraft (V97.81-)

military vehicles involved in transport accident with civilian vehicle ▶(V09.01, V09.21, V19.31, V29.818, V39.81, V49.81, V59.81, V69.81, V79.81)◀

military watercraft involved in water transport accident with civilian watercraft (V94.81-)

war operations (Y36.-)

✓5ᵗʰ **Y37.0 Military operations involving** explosion of marine weapons

✓6ᵗʰ **Y37.00 Military operations involving explosion of unspecified marine weapon**

Military operations involving underwater blast NOS

✓7ᵗʰ **Y37.000 Military operations involving explosion of unspecified marine weapon,** military personnel

✓7ᵗʰ **Y37.001 Military operations involving explosion of unspecified marine weapon,** civilian

✓6ᵗʰ **Y37.01 Military operations involving explosion of** depth-charge

✓7ᵗʰ **Y37.010 Military operations involving explosion of depth-charge,** military personnel

✓7ᵗʰ **Y37.011 Military operations involving explosion of depth-charge,** civilian

✓6ᵗʰ **Y37.02 Military operations involving explosion of** marine mine

Military operations involving explosion of marine mine, at sea or in harbor

✓7ᵗʰ **Y37.020 Military operations involving explosion of marine mine,** military personnel

✓7ᵗʰ **Y37.021 Military operations involving explosion of marine mine,** civilian

✓6ᵗʰ **Y37.03 Military operations involving explosion of** sea-based artillery shell

✓7ᵗʰ **Y37.030 Military operations involving explosion of sea-based artillery shell,** military personnel

✓7ᵗʰ **Y37.031 Military operations involving explosion of sea-based artillery shell,** civilian

✓6ᵗʰ **Y37.04 Military operations involving explosion of** torpedo

✓7ᵗʰ **Y37.040 Military operations involving explosion of torpedo,** military personnel

✓7ᵗʰ **Y37.041 Military operations involving explosion of torpedo,** civilian

✓6ᵗʰ **Y37.05 Military operations involving accidental detonation of** onboard marine weapons

✓7ᵗʰ **Y37.050 Military operations involving accidental detonation of onboard marine weapons,** military personnel

✓7ᵗʰ **Y37.051 Military operations involving accidental detonation of onboard marine weapons,** civilian

✓6ᵗʰ **Y37.09 Military operations involving explosion of other marine weapons**

✓7ᵗʰ **Y37.090 Military operations involving explosion of other marine weapons,** military personnel

✓7ᵗʰ **Y37.091 Military operations involving explosion of other marine weapons,** civilian

✓5ᵗʰ **Y37.1 Military operations involving** destruction of aircraft

✓6ᵗʰ **Y37.10 Military operations involving unspecified destruction of aircraft**

✓7ᵗʰ **Y37.100 Military operations involving unspecified destruction of aircraft,** military personnel

✓7ᵗʰ **Y37.101 Military operations involving unspecified destruction of aircraft,** civilian

✓6ᵗʰ **Y37.11 Military operations involving destruction of aircraft** due to enemy fire or explosives

Military operations involving destruction of aircraft due to air to air missile

Military operations involving destruction of aircraft due to explosive placed on aircraft

Military operations involving destruction of aircraft due to rocket propelled grenade [RPG]

Military operations involving destruction of aircraft due to small arms fire

Military operations involving destruction of aircraft due to surface to air missile

✓7ᵗʰ **Y37.110 Military operations involving destruction of aircraft due to enemy fire or explosives,** military personnel

✓7ᵗʰ **Y37.111 Military operations involving destruction of aircraft due to enemy fire or explosives,** civilian

✓6ᵗʰ **Y37.12 Military operations involving destruction of aircraft** due to collision with other aircraft

✓7ᵗʰ **Y37.120 Military operations involving destruction of aircraft due to collision with other aircraft,** military personnel

✓7ᵗʰ **Y37.121 Military operations involving destruction of aircraft due to collision with other aircraft,** civilian

✓6ᵗʰ **Y37.13 Military operations involving destruction of aircraft** due to onboard fire

✓7ᵗʰ **Y37.130 Military operations involving destruction of aircraft due to onboard fire,** military personnel

✓7ᵗʰ **Y37.131 Military operations involving destruction of aircraft due to onboard fire,** civilian

✓6ᵗʰ **Y37.14 Military operations involving destruction of aircraft** due to accidental detonation of onboard munitions and explosives

✓7ᵗʰ **Y37.140 Military operations involving destruction of aircraft due to accidental detonation of onboard munitions and explosives,** military personnel

✓7ᵗʰ **Y37.141 Military operations involving destruction of aircraft due to accidental detonation of onboard munitions and explosives,** civilian

✓6ᵗʰ **Y37.19 Military operations involving other destruction of aircraft**

✓7ᵗʰ **Y37.190 Military operations involving other destruction of aircraft,** military personnel

✓7ᵗʰ **Y37.191 Military operations involving other destruction of aircraft,** civilian

✓5ᵗʰ **Y37.2 Military operations involving** other explosions and fragments

EXCLUDES 1   military operations involving explosion of aircraft (Y37.1-)

military operations involving explosion of marine weapons (Y37.0-)

military operations involving explosion of nuclear weapons (Y37.5-)

✓6ᵗʰ **Y37.20 Military operations involving unspecified explosion and fragments**

Military operations involving air blast NOS

Military operations involving blast NOS

Military operations involving blast fragments NOS

Military operations involving blast wave NOS

Military operations involving blast wind NOS

Military operations involving explosion NOS

Military operations involving explosion of bomb NOS

✓7ᵗʰ **Y37.200 Military operations involving unspecified explosion and fragments,** military personnel

✓7ᵗʰ **Y37.201 Military operations involving unspecified explosion and fragments,** civilian

✓6ᵗʰ **Y37.21 Military operations involving explosion of** aerial bomb

✓7ᵗʰ **Y37.210 Military operations involving explosion of aerial bomb,** military personnel

✓7ᵗʰ **Y37.211 Military operations involving explosion of aerial bomb,** civilian

✓6ᵗʰ **Y37.22 Military operations involving explosion of** guided missile

✓7ᵗʰ **Y37.220 Military operations involving explosion of guided missile,** military personnel

✓7th **Y37.221 Military operations involving explosion of guided missile, civilian**

✓6th **Y37.23 Military operations involving explosion of improvised explosive device [IED]**
Military operations involving explosion of person-borne improvised explosive device [IED]
Military operations involving explosion of vehicle-borne improvised explosive device [IED]
Military operations involving explosion of roadside improvised explosive device [IED]

✓7th **Y37.230 Military operations involving explosion of improvised explosive device [IED], military personnel**

✓7th **Y37.231 Military operations involving explosion of improvised explosive device [IED], civilian**

✓6th **Y37.24 Military operations involving explosion due to accidental detonation and discharge of own munitions or munitions launch device**

✓7th **Y37.240 Military operations involving explosion due to accidental detonation and discharge of own munitions or munitions launch device, military personnel**

✓7th **Y37.241 Military operations involving explosion due to accidental detonation and discharge of own munitions or munitions launch device, civilian**

✓6th **Y37.25 Military operations involving fragments from munitions**

✓7th **Y37.250 Military operations involving fragments from munitions, military personnel**

✓7th **Y37.251 Military operations involving fragments from munitions, civilian**

✓6th **Y37.26 Military operations involving fragments of improvised explosive device [IED]**
Military operations involving fragments of person-borne improvised explosive device [IED]
Military operations involving fragments of vehicle-borne improvised explosive device [IED]
Military operations involving fragments of roadside improvised explosive device [IED]

✓7th **Y37.260 Military operations involving fragments of improvised explosive device [IED], military personnel**

✓7th **Y37.261 Military operations involving fragments of improvised explosive device [IED], civilian**

✓6th **Y37.27 Military operations involving fragments from weapons**

✓7th **Y37.270 Military operations involving fragments from weapons, military personnel**

✓7th **Y37.271 Military operations involving fragments from weapons, civilian**

✓6th **Y37.29 Military operations involving other explosions and fragments**
Military operations involving explosion of grenade
Military operations involving explosions of land mine
Military operations involving shrapnel NOS

✓7th **Y37.290 Military operations involving other explosions and fragments, military personnel**

✓7th **Y37.291 Military operations involving other explosions and fragments, civilian**

✓5th **Y37.3 Military operations involving fires, conflagrations and hot substances**
Military operations involving smoke, fumes, and heat from fires, conflagrations and hot substances
EXCLUDES 1 *military operations involving fires and conflagrations aboard military aircraft (Y37.1-)*
military operations involving fires and conflagrations aboard military watercraft (Y37.0-)
military operations involving fires and conflagrations caused indirectly by conventional weapons (Y37.2-)
military operations involving fires and thermal effects of nuclear weapons (Y36.53-)

✓6th **Y37.30 Military operations involving unspecified fire, conflagration and hot substance**

✓7th **Y37.300 Military operations involving unspecified fire, conflagration and hot substance, military personnel**

✓7th **Y37.301 Military operations involving unspecified fire, conflagration and hot substance, civilian**

✓6th **Y37.31 Military operations involving gasoline bomb**
Military operations involving incendiary bomb
Military operations involving petrol bomb

✓7th **Y37.310 Military operations involving gasoline bomb, military personnel**

✓7th **Y37.311 Military operations involving gasoline bomb, civilian**

✓6th **Y37.32 Military operations involving incendiary bullet**

✓7th **Y37.320 Military operations involving incendiary bullet, military personnel**

✓7th **Y37.321 Military operations involving incendiary bullet, civilian**

✓6th **Y37.33 Military operations involving flamethrower**

✓7th **Y37.330 Military operations involving flamethrower, military personnel**

✓7th **Y37.331 Military operations involving flamethrower, civilian**

✓6th **Y37.39 Military operations involving other fires, conflagrations and hot substances**

✓7th **Y37.390 Military operations involving other fires, conflagrations and hot substances, military personnel**

✓7th **Y37.391 Military operations involving other fires, conflagrations and hot substances, civilian**

✓5th **Y37.4 Military operations involving firearm discharge and other forms of conventional warfare**

✓6th **Y37.41 Military operations involving rubber bullets**

✓7th **Y37.410 Military operations involving rubber bullets, military personnel**

✓7th **Y37.411 Military operations involving rubber bullets, civilian**

✓6th **Y37.42 Military operations involving firearms pellets**

✓7th **Y37.420 Military operations involving firearms pellets, military personnel**

✓7th **Y37.421 Military operations involving firearms pellets, civilian**

✓6th **Y37.43 Military operations involving other firearms discharge**
Military operations involving bullets NOS
EXCLUDES 1 *military operations involving munitions fragments (Y37.25-)*
military operations involving incendiary bullets (Y37.32-)

✓7th **Y37.430 Military operations involving other firearms discharge, military personnel**

✓7th **Y37.431 Military operations involving other firearms discharge, civilian**

✓6th **Y37.44 Military operations involving unarmed hand to hand combat**
EXCLUDES 1 *military operations involving combat using blunt or piercing object (Y37.45-)*
military operations involving intentional restriction of air and airway (Y37.46-)
military operations involving unintentional restriction of air and airway (Y37.47-)

✓7th **Y37.440 Military operations involving unarmed hand to hand combat, military personnel**

✓7th **Y37.441 Military operations involving unarmed hand to hand combat, civilian**

✓6th **Y37.45 Military operations involving combat using blunt or piercing object**

✓7th **Y37.450 Military operations involving combat using blunt or piercing object, military personnel**

✓7th **Y37.451 Military operations involving combat using blunt or piercing object, civilian**

✓6th **Y37.46 Military operations involving intentional restriction of air and airway**

✓7th **Y37.460 Military operations involving intentional restriction of air and airway, military personnel**

✓7th **Y37.461 Military operations involving intentional restriction of air and airway, civilian**

✓6ᵗʰ **Y37.47** **Military operations involving** unintentional restriction of air and airway

✓7ᵗʰ **Y37.470** **Military operations involving unintentional restriction of air and airway,** military personnel

✓7ᵗʰ **Y37.471** **Military operations involving unintentional restriction of air and airway,** civilian

✓6ᵗʰ **Y37.49** **Military operations involving other forms of conventional warfare**

✓7ᵗʰ **Y37.490** **Military operations involving other forms of conventional warfare,** military personnel

✓7ᵗʰ **Y37.491** **Military operations involving other forms of conventional warfare,** civilian

✓5ᵗʰ **Y37.5** **Military operations involving** nuclear weapons

Military operation involving dirty bomb NOS

✓6ᵗʰ **Y37.50** **Military operations involving unspecified effect of nuclear weapon**

✓7ᵗʰ **Y37.500** **Military operations involving unspecified effect of nuclear weapon,** military personnel

✓7ᵗʰ **Y37.501** **Military operations involving unspecified effect of nuclear weapon,** civilian

✓6ᵗʰ **Y37.51** **Military operations involving** direct blast effect **of nuclear weapon**

Military operations involving blast pressure of nuclear weapon

✓7ᵗʰ **Y37.510** **Military operations involving direct blast effect of nuclear weapon,** military personnel

✓7ᵗʰ **Y37.511** **Military operations involving direct blast effect of nuclear weapon,** civilian

✓6ᵗʰ **Y37.52** **Military operations involving** indirect blast effect **of nuclear weapon**

Military operations involving being thrown by blast of nuclear weapon

Military operations involving being struck or crushed by blast debris of nuclear weapon

✓7ᵗʰ **Y37.520** **Military operations involving indirect blast effect of nuclear weapon,** military personnel

✓7ᵗʰ **Y37.521** **Military operations involving indirect blast effect of nuclear weapon,** civilian

✓6ᵗʰ **Y37.53** **Military operations involving** thermal radiation effect **of nuclear weapon**

Military operations involving direct heat from nuclear weapon

Military operation involving fireball effects from nuclear weapon

✓7ᵗʰ **Y37.530** **Military operations involving thermal radiation effect of nuclear weapon,** military personnel

✓7ᵗʰ **Y37.531** **Military operations involving thermal radiation effect of nuclear weapon,** civilian

✓6ᵗʰ **Y37.54** **Military operation involving** nuclear radiation effects of nuclear weapon

Military operation involving acute radiation exposure from nuclear weapon

Military operation involving exposure to immediate ionizing radiation from nuclear weapon

Military operation involving fallout exposure from nuclear weapon

Military operation involving secondary effects of nuclear weapons

✓7ᵗʰ **Y37.540** **Military operation involving nuclear radiation effects of nuclear weapon,** military personnel

✓7ᵗʰ **Y37.541** **Military operation involving nuclear radiation effects of nuclear weapon,** civilian

✓6ᵗʰ **Y37.59** **Military operation involving** other effects of nuclear weapons

✓7ᵗʰ **Y37.590** **Military operation involving other effects of nuclear weapons,** military personnel

✓7ᵗʰ **Y37.591** **Military operation involving other effects of nuclear weapons,** civilian

✓5ᵗʰ **Y37.6** **Military operations involving** biological weapons

✓6ᵗʰ **Y37.6X** **Military operations involving biological weapons**

✓7ᵗʰ **Y37.6X0** **Military operations involving biological weapons,** military personnel

✓7ᵗʰ **Y37.6X1** **Military operations involving biological weapons,** civilian

✓5ᵗʰ **Y37.7** **Military operations involving chemical weapons and other forms of unconventional warfare**

EXCLUDES 1　military operations involving incendiary devices (Y36.3-, Y36.5-)

✓6ᵗʰ **Y37.7X** **Military operations involving** chemical weapons and other forms of unconventional warfare

✓7ᵗʰ **Y37.7X0** **Military operations involving chemical weapons and other forms of unconventional warfare,** military personnel

✓7ᵗʰ **Y37.7X1** **Military operations involving chemical weapons and other forms of unconventional warfare,** civilian

✓5ᵗʰ **Y37.9** **Other and unspecified military operations**

✓x7ᵗʰ **Y37.90** **Military operations, unspecified**

✓x7ᵗʰ **Y37.91** **Military operations involving unspecified** weapon of mass destruction [WMD]

✓x7ᵗʰ **Y37.92** **Military operations involving** friendly fire

✓4ᵗʰ **Y38** **Terrorism**

NOTE　These codes are for use to identify injuries resulting from the unlawful use of force or violence against persons or property to intimidate or coerce a Government, the civilian population, or any segment thereof, in furtherance of political or social objective

Use additional code for place of occurrence (Y92.-)

✓5ᵗʰ **Y38.0** **Terrorism involving explosion of marine weapons**

Terrorism involving depth-charge

Terrorism involving marine mine

Terrorism involving mine NOS, at sea or in harbor

Terrorism involving sea-based artillery shell

Terrorism involving torpedo

Terrorism involving underwater blast

✓6ᵗʰ **Y38.0X** **Terrorism involving explosion of** marine weapons

✓7ᵗʰ **Y38.0X1** **Terrorism involving explosion of marine weapons,** public safety official **injured**

✓7ᵗʰ **Y38.0X2** **Terrorism involving explosion of marine weapons,** civilian **injured**

✓7ᵗʰ **Y38.0X3** **Terrorism involving explosion of marine weapons,** terrorist **injured**

✓5ᵗʰ **Y38.1** **Terrorism involving destruction of aircraft**

Terrorism involving aircraft burned

Terrorism involving aircraft exploded

Terrorism involving aircraft being shot down

Terrorism involving aircraft used as a weapon

✓6ᵗʰ **Y38.1X** **Terrorism involving** destruction of aircraft

✓7ᵗʰ **Y38.1X1** **Terrorism involving destruction of aircraft,** public safety official **injured**

✓7ᵗʰ **Y38.1X2** **Terrorism involving destruction of aircraft,** civilian **injured**

✓7ᵗʰ **Y38.1X3** **Terrorism involving destruction of aircraft,** terrorist **injured**

✓5ᵗʰ **Y38.2** **Terrorism involving other explosions and fragments**

Terrorism involving antipersonnel (fragments) bomb

Terrorism involving blast NOS

Terrorism involving explosion NOS

Terrorism involving explosion of breech block

Terrorism involving explosion of cannon block

Terrorism involving explosion (fragments) of artillery shell

Terrorism involving explosion (fragments) of bomb

Terrorism involving explosion (fragments) of grenade

Terrorism involving explosion (fragments) of guided missile

Terrorism involving explosion (fragments) of land mine

Terrorism involving explosion of mortar bomb

Terrorism involving explosion of munitions

Terrorism involving explosion (fragments) of rocket

Terrorism involving explosion (fragments) of shell

Terrorism involving shrapnel

Terrorism involving mine NOS, on land

EXCLUDES 1　terrorism involving explosion of nuclear weapon (Y38.5)

terrorism involving suicide bomber (Y38.81)

✓6ᵗʰ **Y38.2X** **Terrorism involving other explosions and fragments**

✓7ᵗʰ **Y38.2X1** **Terrorism involving other explosions and fragments,** public safety official **injured**

✓ Additional Character Required　　✓x7ᵗʰ Placeholder Alert　　Manifestation　　Unspecified Dx　　Ⓠ QPP　　ᵁᴾᴰ Unacceptable PDx

√7ᵗʰ **Y38.2X2** **Terrorism involving other explosions and fragments,** civilian **injured**

√7ᵗʰ **Y38.2X3** **Terrorism involving other explosions and fragments,** terrorist **injured**

√5ᵗʰ **Y38.3** **Terrorism involving fires, conflagration and hot substances**

Terrorism involving conflagration NOS

Terrorism involving fire NOS

Terrorism involving petrol bomb

EXCLUDES 1   *terrorism involving fire or heat of nuclear weapon (Y38.5)*

√6ᵗʰ **Y38.3X** **Terrorism involving** fires, conflagration and hot substances

√7ᵗʰ **Y38.3X1** **Terrorism involving fires, conflagration and hot substances,** public safety official **injured**

√7ᵗʰ **Y38.3X2** **Terrorism involving fires, conflagration and hot substances,** civilian **injured**

√7ᵗʰ **Y38.3X3** **Terrorism involving fires, conflagration and hot substances,** terrorist **injured**

√5ᵗʰ **Y38.4** **Terrorism involving firearms**

Terrorism involving carbine bullet

Terrorism involving machine gun bullet

Terrorism involving pellets (shotgun)

Terrorism involving pistol bullet

Terrorism involving rifle bullet

Terrorism involving rubber (rifle) bullet

√6ᵗʰ **Y38.4X** **Terrorism involving** firearms

√7ᵗʰ **Y38.4X1** **Terrorism involving firearms,** public safety official **injured**

√7ᵗʰ **Y38.4X2** **Terrorism involving firearms,** civilian **injured**

√7ᵗʰ **Y38.4X3** **Terrorism involving firearms,** terrorist **injured**

√5ᵗʰ **Y38.5** **Terrorism involving nuclear weapons**

Terrorism involving blast effects of nuclear weapon

Terrorism involving exposure to ionizing radiation from nuclear weapon

Terrorism involving fireball effect of nuclear weapon

Terrorism involving heat from nuclear weapon

√6ᵗʰ **Y38.5X** **Terrorism involving** nuclear weapons

√7ᵗʰ **Y38.5X1** **Terrorism involving nuclear weapons,** public safety official **injured**

√7ᵗʰ **Y38.5X2** **Terrorism involving nuclear weapons,** civilian **injured**

√7ᵗʰ **Y38.5X3** **Terrorism involving nuclear weapons,** terrorist **injured**

√5ᵗʰ **Y38.6** **Terrorism involving biological weapons**

Terrorism involving anthrax

Terrorism involving cholera

Terrorism involving smallpox

√6ᵗʰ **Y38.6X** **Terrorism involving** biological weapons

√7ᵗʰ **Y38.6X1** **Terrorism involving biological weapons,** public safety official **injured**

√7ᵗʰ **Y38.6X2** **Terrorism involving biological weapons,** civilian **injured**

√7ᵗʰ **Y38.6X3** **Terrorism involving biological weapons,** terrorist **injured**

√5ᵗʰ **Y38.7** **Terrorism involving chemical weapons**

Terrorism involving gases, fumes, chemicals

Terrorism involving hydrogen cyanide

Terrorism involving phosgene

Terrorism involving sarin

√6ᵗʰ **Y38.7X** **Terrorism involving** chemical weapons

√7ᵗʰ **Y38.7X1** **Terrorism involving chemical weapons,** public safety official **injured**

√7ᵗʰ **Y38.7X2** **Terrorism involving chemical weapons,** civilian **injured**

√7ᵗʰ **Y38.7X3** **Terrorism involving chemical weapons,** terrorist **injured**

√5ᵗʰ **Y38.8** **Terrorism involving other and unspecified means**

√×7ᵗʰ **Y38.80** **Terrorism involving unspecified means**

Terrorism NOS

√6ᵗʰ **Y38.81** **Terrorism involving** suicide bomber

√7ᵗʰ **Y38.811** **Terrorism involving suicide bomber,** public safety official **injured**

√7ᵗʰ **Y38.812** **Terrorism involving suicide bomber,** civilian **injured**

√6ᵗʰ **Y38.89** **Terrorism involving other means**

Terrorism involving drowning and submersion

Terrorism involving lasers

Terrorism involving piercing or stabbing instruments

√7ᵗʰ **Y38.891** **Terrorism involving other means,** public safety official **injured**

√7ᵗʰ **Y38.892** **Terrorism involving other means,** civilian **injured**

√7ᵗʰ **Y38.893** **Terrorism involving other means,** terrorist **injured**

√5ᵗʰ **Y38.9** **Terrorism, secondary effects**

NOTE   This code is for use to identify conditions occurring subsequent to a terrorist attack not those that are due to the initial terrorist attack

√6ᵗʰ **Y38.9X** **Terrorism,** secondary effects

√7ᵗʰ **Y38.9X1** **Terrorism, secondary effects,** public safety official **injured**

√7ᵗʰ **Y38.9X2** **Terrorism, secondary effects,** civilian **injured**

COMPLICATIONS OF MEDICAL AND SURGICAL CARE (Y62-Y84)

INCLUDES   complications of medical devices

surgical and medical procedures as the cause of abnormal reaction of the patient, or of later complication, without mention of misadventure at the time of the procedure

Misadventures to patients during surgical and medical care (Y62-Y69)

EXCLUDES 1   *surgical and medical procedures as the cause of abnormal reaction of the patient, without mention of misadventure at the time of the procedure (Y83-Y84)*

EXCLUDES 2   *breakdown or malfunctioning of medical device (during procedure) (after implantation) (ongoing use) (Y70-Y82)*

√4ᵗʰ **Y62** **Failure of** sterile precautions **during surgical and medical care**

Y62.0 **Failure of sterile precautions during** surgical operation

Y62.1 **Failure of sterile precautions during** infusion or transfusion

Y62.2 **Failure of sterile precautions during** kidney dialysis and other perfusion   HCC Rx ESR

Y62.3 **Failure of sterile precautions during** injection or immunization

Y62.4 **Failure of sterile precautions during** endoscopic examination

Y62.5 **Failure of sterile precautions during** heart catheterization

Y62.6 **Failure of sterile precautions during** aspiration, puncture and other catheterization

Y62.8 **Failure of sterile precautions during** other surgical and medical care

Y62.9 **Failure of sterile precautions during** unspecified surgical and medical care

√4ᵗʰ **Y63** **Failure in** dosage **during surgical and medical care**

EXCLUDES 2   *accidental overdose of drug or wrong drug given in error (T36-T50)*

Y63.0 **Excessive amount of blood or other fluid given during transfusion or infusion**

Y63.1 **Incorrect dilution of fluid used during infusion**

Y63.2 **Overdose of radiation given during therapy**

Y63.3 **Inadvertent exposure of patient to radiation during medical care**

Y63.4 **Failure in dosage in electroshock or insulin-shock therapy**

Y63.5 **Inappropriate temperature in local application and packing**

Y63.6 **Underdosing and nonadministration of necessary drug, medicament or biological substance**

AHA: 2018,4Q,72

Y63.8 **Failure in dosage during other surgical and medical care**

AHA: 2018,4Q,72

Y63.9 **Failure in dosage during unspecified surgical and medical care**

AHA: 2018,4Q,72

√4ᵗʰ **Y64** **Contaminated** medical or biological **substances**

Y64.0 **Contaminated medical or biological substance,** transfused or infused

Y64.1 **Contaminated medical or biological substance,** injected or used for immunization

Y64.8 **Contaminated medical or biological substance administered by other means**

Chapter 20. External Causes of Morbidity

Y64.9 **Contaminated medical or biological substance administered by unspecified means**
    Administered contaminated medical or biological substance NOS

☑4ᵗʰ Y65 **Other misadventures during surgical and medical care**

  Y65.0 **Mismatched blood in transfusion**

  Y65.1 **Wrong fluid used in infusion**

  Y65.2 **Failure in suture or ligature during surgical operation**

  Y65.3 **Endotracheal tube wrongly placed during anesthetic procedure**

  Y65.4 **Failure to introduce or to remove other tube or instrument**

  ☑5ᵗʰ Y65.5 **Performance of** wrong procedure **(operation)**

    Y65.51 **Performance of wrong procedure (operation) on** correct patient
      Wrong device implanted into correct surgical site
      EXCLUDES 1 *performance of correct procedure (operation) on wrong side or body part (Y65.53)*

    Y65.52 **Performance of procedure (operation) on** patient not scheduled for surgery
      Performance of procedure (operation) intended for another patient
      Performance of procedure (operation) on wrong patient

    Y65.53 **Performance of correct procedure (operation) on** wrong side or body part
      Performance of correct procedure (operation) on wrong side
      Performance of correct procedure (operation) on wrong site

  Y65.8 **Other specified misadventures during surgical and medical care**
    AHA: 2022,1Q,22; 2019,2Q,23-24

Y66 **Nonadministration of surgical and medical care**
  Premature cessation of surgical and medical care
  EXCLUDES 1 *DNR status (Z66)*
    palliative care (Z51.5)

Y69 **Unspecified misadventure during surgical and medical care**

Medical devices associated with adverse incidents in diagnostic and therapeutic use (Y70-Y82)

INCLUDES breakdown or malfunction of medical devices (during use) (after implantation) (ongoing use)

EXCLUDES 2 *later complications following use of medical devices without breakdown or malfunctioning of device (Y83-Y84)*
  misadventure to patients during surgical and medical care, classifiable to (Y62-Y69)
  surgical and other medical procedures as the cause of abnormal reaction of the patient, or of later complication, without mention of misadventure at the time of the procedure (Y83-Y84)

☑4ᵗʰ Y70 **Anesthesiology** devices associated with adverse incidents

  Y70.0 Diagnostic and monitoring **anesthesiology devices associated with adverse incidents**

  Y70.1 Therapeutic **(nonsurgical)** and rehabilitative **anesthesiology devices associated with adverse incidents**

  Y70.2 Prosthetic and other implants, **materials and accessory anesthesiology devices associated with adverse incidents**

  Y70.3 Surgical instruments, **materials and anesthesiology devices (including sutures) associated with adverse incidents**

  Y70.8 Miscellaneous anesthesiology devices associated with adverse incidents, not elsewhere classified

☑4ᵗʰ Y71 Cardiovascular **devices associated with adverse incidents**

  Y71.0 Diagnostic and monitoring **cardiovascular devices associated with adverse incidents**

  Y71.1 Therapeutic **(nonsurgical)** and rehabilitative **cardiovascular devices associated with adverse incidents**

  Y71.2 Prosthetic and other implants, **materials and accessory cardiovascular devices associated with adverse incidents**

  Y71.3 Surgical instruments, **materials and cardiovascular devices (including sutures) associated with adverse incidents**

  Y71.8 Miscellaneous cardiovascular devices associated with adverse incidents, not elsewhere classified

☑4ᵗʰ Y72 Otorhinolaryngological **devices associated with adverse incidents**

  Y72.0 Diagnostic and monitoring **otorhinolaryngological devices associated with adverse incidents**

  Y72.1 Therapeutic **(nonsurgical)** and rehabilitative **otorhinolaryngological devices associated with adverse incidents**

  Y72.2 Prosthetic and other implants, **materials and accessory otorhinolaryngological devices associated with adverse incidents**

  Y72.3 Surgical instruments, **materials and otorhinolaryngological devices (including sutures) associated with adverse incidents**

  Y72.8 Miscellaneous otorhinolaryngological devices associated with adverse incidents, not elsewhere classified

☑4ᵗʰ Y73 Gastroenterology and urology **devices associated with adverse incidents**

  Y73.0 Diagnostic and monitoring **gastroenterology and urology devices associated with adverse incidents**

  Y73.1 Therapeutic **(nonsurgical)** and rehabilitative **gastroenterology and urology devices associated with adverse incidents**

  Y73.2 Prosthetic and other implants, **materials and accessory gastroenterology and urology devices associated with adverse incidents**

  Y73.3 Surgical instruments, **materials and gastroenterology and urology devices (including sutures) associated with adverse incidents**

  Y73.8 Miscellaneous gastroenterology and urology devices associated with adverse incidents, not elsewhere classified

☑4ᵗʰ Y74 General hospital **and personal-use devices associated with adverse incidents**

  Y74.0 Diagnostic and monitoring **general hospital and personal-use devices associated with adverse incidents**

  Y74.1 Therapeutic **(nonsurgical)** and rehabilitative **general hospital and personal-use devices associated with adverse incidents**

  Y74.2 Prosthetic and other implants, **materials and accessory general hospital and personal-use devices associated with adverse incidents**

  Y74.3 Surgical instruments, **materials and general hospital and personal-use devices (including sutures) associated with adverse incidents**

  Y74.8 Miscellaneous general hospital and personal-use devices associated with adverse incidents, not elsewhere classified

☑4ᵗʰ Y75 Neurological **devices associated with adverse incidents**

  Y75.0 Diagnostic and monitoring **neurological devices associated with adverse incidents**

  Y75.1 Therapeutic **(nonsurgical)** and rehabilitative **neurological devices associated with adverse incidents**

  Y75.2 Prosthetic and other implants, **materials and neurological devices associated with adverse incidents**

  Y75.3 Surgical instruments, **materials and neurological devices (including sutures) associated with adverse incidents**

  Y75.8 Miscellaneous neurological devices associated with adverse incidents, not elsewhere classified

☑4ᵗʰ Y76 Obstetric and gynecological **devices associated with adverse incidents**

  Y76.0 Diagnostic and monitoring **obstetric and gynecological devices associated with adverse incidents** ♀

  Y76.1 Therapeutic **(nonsurgical)** and rehabilitative **obstetric and gynecological devices associated with adverse incidents** ♀

  Y76.2 Prosthetic and other implants, **materials and accessory obstetric and gynecological devices associated with adverse incidents** ♀

  Y76.3 Surgical instruments, **materials and obstetric and gynecological devices (including sutures) associated with adverse incidents** ♀

  Y76.8 Miscellaneous obstetric and gynecological devices associated with adverse incidents, not elsewhere classified ♀

☑4ᵗʰ Y77 Ophthalmic **devices associated with adverse incidents**

  Y77.0 Diagnostic and monitoring **ophthalmic devices associated with adverse incidents**

  ☑5ᵗʰ Y77.1 Therapeutic **(nonsurgical)** and rehabilitative **ophthalmic devices associated with adverse incidents**
    AHA: 2020,4Q,41

    Y77.11 Contact lens **associated with adverse incidents**
      Rigid gas permeable contact lens associated with adverse incidents
      Soft (hydrophilic) contact lens associated with adverse incidents

    Y77.19 **Other therapeutic (nonsurgical) and rehabilitative ophthalmic devices associated with adverse incidents**

  Y77.2 Prosthetic and other implants, **materials and accessory ophthalmic devices associated with adverse incidents**

  Y77.3 Surgical instruments, **materials and ophthalmic devices (including sutures) associated with adverse incidents**

Y77.8 Miscellaneous ophthalmic devices associated with adverse incidents, not elsewhere classified

✓4ᵗʰ **Y78** Radiological devices associated with adverse incidents

Y78.0 Diagnostic and monitoring radiological devices associated with adverse incidents

Y78.1 Therapeutic (nonsurgical) and rehabilitative radiological devices associated with adverse incidents

Y78.2 Prosthetic and other implants, materials and accessory radiological devices associated with adverse incidents

Y78.3 Surgical instruments, materials and radiological devices (including sutures) associated with adverse incidents

Y78.8 Miscellaneous radiological devices associated with adverse incidents, not elsewhere classified

✓4ᵗʰ **Y79** Orthopedic devices associated with adverse incidents

Y79.0 Diagnostic and monitoring orthopedic devices associated with adverse incidents

Y79.1 Therapeutic (nonsurgical) and rehabilitative orthopedic devices associated with adverse incidents

Y79.2 Prosthetic and other implants, materials and accessory orthopedic devices associated with adverse incidents

Y79.3 Surgical instruments, materials and orthopedic devices (including sutures) associated with adverse incidents

Y79.8 Miscellaneous orthopedic devices associated with adverse incidents, not elsewhere classified

✓4ᵗʰ **Y80** Physical medicine devices associated with adverse incidents

Y80.0 Diagnostic and monitoring physical medicine devices associated with adverse incidents

Y80.1 Therapeutic (nonsurgical) and rehabilitative physical medicine devices associated with adverse incidents

Y80.2 Prosthetic and other implants, materials and accessory physical medicine devices associated with adverse incidents

Y80.3 Surgical instruments, materials and physical medicine devices (including sutures) associated with adverse incidents

Y80.8 Miscellaneous physical medicine devices associated with adverse incidents, not elsewhere classified

✓4ᵗʰ **Y81** General- and plastic-surgery devices associated with adverse incidents

Y81.0 Diagnostic and monitoring general- and plastic-surgery devices associated with adverse incidents

Y81.1 Therapeutic (nonsurgical) and rehabilitative general- and plastic-surgery devices associated with adverse incidents

Y81.2 Prosthetic and other implants, materials and accessory general- and plastic-surgery devices associated with adverse incidents

Y81.3 Surgical instruments, materials and general- and plastic-surgery devices (including sutures) associated with adverse incidents

Y81.8 Miscellaneous general- and plastic-surgery devices associated with adverse incidents, not elsewhere classified

✓4ᵗʰ **Y82** Other and unspecified medical devices associated with adverse incidents

Y82.8 Other medical devices associated with adverse incidents

Y82.9 Unspecified medical devices associated with adverse incidents

Surgical and other medical procedures as the cause of abnormal reaction of the patient, or of later complication, without mention of misadventure at the time of the procedure (Y83-Y84)

EXCLUDES 1   misadventures to patients during surgical and medical care, classifiable to (Y62-Y69)

EXCLUDES 2   breakdown or malfunctioning of medical device (during procedure) (after implantation) (ongoing use) (Y70-Y82)

✓4ᵗʰ **Y83** Surgical operation and other surgical procedures as the cause of abnormal reaction of the patient, or of later complication, without mention of misadventure at the time of the procedure

Y83.0 Surgical operation with transplant of whole organ as the cause of abnormal reaction of the patient, or of later complication, without mention of misadventure at the time of the procedure

Y83.1 Surgical operation with implant of artificial internal device as the cause of abnormal reaction of the patient, or of later complication, without mention of misadventure at the time of the procedure

Y83.2 Surgical operation with anastomosis, bypass or graft as the cause of abnormal reaction of the patient, or of later complication, without mention of misadventure at the time of the procedure

Y83.3 Surgical operation with formation of external stoma as the cause of abnormal reaction of the patient, or of later complication, without mention of misadventure at the time of the procedure

Y83.4 Other reconstructive surgery as the cause of abnormal reaction of the patient, or of later complication, without mention of misadventure at the time of the procedure

Y83.5 Amputation of limb(s) as the cause of abnormal reaction of the patient, or of later complication, without mention of misadventure at the time of the procedure

Y83.6 Removal of other organ (partial) (total) as the cause of abnormal reaction of the patient, or of later complication, without mention of misadventure at the time of the procedure

Y83.8 Other surgical procedures as the cause of abnormal reaction of the patient, or of later complication, without mention of misadventure at the time of the procedure

Y83.9 Surgical procedure, unspecified as the cause of abnormal reaction of the patient, or of later complication, without mention of misadventure at the time of the procedure

✓4ᵗʰ **Y84** Other medical procedures as the cause of abnormal reaction of the patient, or of later complication, without mention of misadventure at the time of the procedure

Y84.0 Cardiac catheterization as the cause of abnormal reaction of the patient, or of later complication, without mention of misadventure at the time of the procedure

Y84.1 Kidney dialysis as the cause of abnormal reaction of the patient, or of later complication, without mention of misadventure at the time of the procedure

Y84.2 Radiological procedure and radiotherapy as the cause of abnormal reaction of the patient, or of later complication, without mention of misadventure at the time of the procedure
   AHA: 2019,1Q,21; 2017,1Q,33

Y84.3 Shock therapy as the cause of abnormal reaction of the patient, or of later complication, without mention of misadventure at the time of the procedure

Y84.4 Aspiration of fluid as the cause of abnormal reaction of the patient, or of later complication, without mention of misadventure at the time of the procedure

Y84.5 Insertion of gastric or duodenal sound as the cause of abnormal reaction of the patient, or of later complication, without mention of misadventure at the time of the procedure

Y84.6 Urinary catheterization as the cause of abnormal reaction of the patient, or of later complication, without mention of misadventure at the time of the procedure

Y84.7 Blood-sampling as the cause of abnormal reaction of the patient, or of later complication, without mention of misadventure at the time of the procedure

Y84.8 Other medical procedures as the cause of abnormal reaction of the patient, or of later complication, without mention of misadventure at the time of the procedure
   AHA: 2021,1Q,5; 2014,4Q,24

Y84.9 Medical procedure, unspecified as the cause of abnormal reaction of the patient, or of later complication, without mention of misadventure at the time of the procedure

Supplementary factors related to causes of morbidity classified elsewhere (Y90-Y99)

NOTE   These categories may be used to provide supplementary information concerning causes of morbidity. They are not to be used for single-condition coding.

✓4ᵗʰ **Y90** Evidence of alcohol involvement determined by blood alcohol level

Code first any associated alcohol related disorders (F10)

Y90.0 Blood alcohol level of less than 20 mg/100 ml
Y90.1 Blood alcohol level of 20-39 mg/100 ml
Y90.2 Blood alcohol level of 40-59 mg/100 ml
Y90.3 Blood alcohol level of 60-79 mg/100 ml
Y90.4 Blood alcohol level of 80-99 mg/100 ml
Y90.5 Blood alcohol level of 100-119 mg/100 ml
Y90.6 Blood alcohol level of 120-199 mg/100 ml
Y90.7 Blood alcohol level of 200-239 mg/100 ml
Y90.8 Blood alcohol level of 240 mg/100 ml or more
Y90.9 Presence of alcohol in blood, level not specified

✓4th **Y92** **Place of occurrence of the external cause**

> The following category is for use, when relevant, to identify the place of occurrence of the external cause. Use in conjunction with an activity code.
>
> Place of occurrence should be recorded only at the initial encounter for treatment

✓5th **Y92.0** **Non-institutional (private) residence** as the place of occurrence of the external cause

> EXCLUDES 1   *abandoned or derelict house (Y92.89)*
> *home under construction but not yet occupied (Y92.6-)*
> *institutional place of residence (Y92.1-)*

✓6th **Y92.00** **Unspecified non-institutional (private) residence** as the place of occurrence of the external cause

Y92.000 Kitchen of unspecified non-institutional (private) residence as the place of occurrence of the external cause

Y92.001 Dining room of unspecified non-institutional (private) residence as the place of occurrence of the external cause

Y92.002 Bathroom of unspecified non-institutional (private) residence as the place of occurrence of the external cause

Y92.003 Bedroom of unspecified non-institutional (private) residence as the place of occurrence of the external cause

Y92.007 Garden or yard of unspecified non-institutional (private) residence as the place of occurrence of the external cause

Y92.008 Other place in unspecified non-institutional (private) residence as the place of occurrence of the external cause

Y92.009 Unspecified place in unspecified non-institutional (private) residence as the place of occurrence of the external cause

> Home (NOS) as the place of occurrence of the external cause

✓6th **Y92.01** **Single-family non-institutional (private) house** as the place of occurrence of the external cause

> Farmhouse as the place of occurrence of the external cause
>
> EXCLUDES 1   *barn (Y92.71)*
> *chicken coop or hen house (Y92.72)*
> *farm field (Y92.73)*
> *orchard (Y92.74)*
> *single family mobile home or trailer (Y92.02-)*
> *slaughter house (Y92.86)*

Y92.010 Kitchen of single-family (private) house as the place of occurrence of the external cause

Y92.011 Dining room of single-family (private) house as the place of occurrence of the external cause

Y92.012 Bathroom of single-family (private) house as the place of occurrence of the external cause

Y92.013 Bedroom of single-family (private) house as the place of occurrence of the external cause

Y92.014 Private driveway to single-family (private) house as the place of occurrence of the external cause

Y92.015 Private garage of single-family (private) house as the place of occurrence of the external cause

Y92.016 Swimming-pool in single-family (private) house or garden as the place of occurrence of the external cause

Y92.017 Garden or yard in single-family (private) house as the place of occurrence of the external cause

Y92.018 Other place in single-family (private) house as the place of occurrence of the external cause

Y92.019 Unspecified place in single-family (private) house as the place of occurrence of the external cause

✓6th **Y92.02** **Mobile home** as the place of occurrence of the external cause

Y92.020 Kitchen in mobile home as the place of occurrence of the external cause

Y92.021 Dining room in mobile home as the place of occurrence of the external cause

Y92.022 Bathroom in mobile home as the place of occurrence of the external cause

Y92.023 Bedroom in mobile home as the place of occurrence of the external cause

Y92.024 Driveway of mobile home as the place of occurrence of the external cause

Y92.025 Garage of mobile home as the place of occurrence of the external cause

Y92.026 Swimming-pool of mobile home as the place of occurrence of the external cause

Y92.027 Garden or yard of mobile home as the place of occurrence of the external cause

Y92.028 Other place in mobile home as the place of occurrence of the external cause

Y92.029 Unspecified place in mobile home as the place of occurrence of the external cause

✓6th **Y92.03** **Apartment** as the place of occurrence of the external cause

> Condominium as the place of occurrence of the external cause
>
> Co-op apartment as the place of occurrence of the external cause

Y92.030 Kitchen in apartment as the place of occurrence of the external cause

Y92.031 Bathroom in apartment as the place of occurrence of the external cause

Y92.032 Bedroom in apartment as the place of occurrence of the external cause

Y92.038 Other place in apartment as the place of occurrence of the external cause

Y92.039 Unspecified place in apartment as the place of occurrence of the external cause

✓6th **Y92.04** **Boarding-house** as the place of occurrence of the external cause

Y92.040 Kitchen in boarding-house as the place of occurrence of the external cause

Y92.041 Bathroom in boarding-house as the place of occurrence of the external cause

Y92.042 Bedroom in boarding-house as the place of occurrence of the external cause

Y92.043 Driveway of boarding-house as the place of occurrence of the external cause

Y92.044 Garage of boarding-house as the place of occurrence of the external cause

Y92.045 Swimming-pool of boarding-house as the place of occurrence of the external cause

Y92.046 Garden or yard of boarding-house as the place of occurrence of the external cause

Y92.048 Other place in boarding-house as the place of occurrence of the external cause

Y92.049 Unspecified place in boarding-house as the place of occurrence of the external cause

✓6th **Y92.09** **Other non-institutional residence** as the place of occurrence of the external cause

> AHA: 2017,2Q,10

Y92.090 Kitchen in other non-institutional residence as the place of occurrence of the external cause

Y92.091 Bathroom in other non-institutional residence as the place of occurrence of the external cause

Y92.092 Bedroom in other non-institutional residence as the place of occurrence of the external cause

Y92.093 Driveway of other non-institutional residence as the place of occurrence of the external cause

Y92.094 Garage of other non-institutional residence as the place of occurrence of the external cause

Y92.095 Swimming-pool of other non-institutional residence as the place of occurrence of the external cause

Y92.096 Garden or yard of other non-institutional residence as the place of occurrence of the external cause

Y92.Ø98 Other place in other non-institutional residence as the place of occurrence of the external cause

Y92.Ø99 Unspecified place in other non-institutional residence as the place of occurrence of the external cause

✓5ᵗʰ Y92.1 Institutional (nonprivate) residence as the place of occurrence of the external cause

Y92.1Ø Unspecified residential institution as the place of occurrence of the external cause

✓6ᵗʰ Y92.11 Children's home and orphanage as the place of occurrence of the external cause

Y92.11Ø Kitchen in children's home and orphanage as the place of occurrence of the external cause

Y92.111 Bathroom in children's home and orphanage as the place of occurrence of the external cause

Y92.112 Bedroom in children's home and orphanage as the place of occurrence of the external cause

Y92.113 Driveway of children's home and orphanage as the place of occurrence of the external cause

Y92.114 Garage of children's home and orphanage as the place of occurrence of the external cause

Y92.115 Swimming-pool of children's home and orphanage as the place of occurrence of the external cause

Y92.116 Garden or yard of children's home and orphanage as the place of occurrence of the external cause

Y92.118 Other place in children's home and orphanage as the place of occurrence of the external cause

Y92.119 Unspecified place in children's home and orphanage as the place of occurrence of the external cause

✓6ᵗʰ Y92.12 Nursing home as the place of occurrence of the external cause

    Home for the sick as the place of occurrence of the external cause

    Hospice as the place of occurrence of the external cause

AHA: 2017,2Q,10

Y92.12Ø Kitchen in nursing home as the place of occurrence of the external cause

Y92.121 Bathroom in nursing home as the place of occurrence of the external cause

Y92.122 Bedroom in nursing home as the place of occurrence of the external cause

Y92.123 Driveway of nursing home as the place of occurrence of the external cause

Y92.124 Garage of nursing home as the place of occurrence of the external cause

Y92.125 Swimming-pool of nursing home as the place of occurrence of the external cause

Y92.126 Garden or yard of nursing home as the place of occurrence of the external cause

Y92.128 Other place in nursing home as the place of occurrence of the external cause

Y92.129 Unspecified place in nursing home as the place of occurrence of the external cause

✓6ᵗʰ Y92.13 Military base as the place of occurrence of the external cause

    EXCLUDES 1 military training grounds (Y92.84)

Y92.13Ø Kitchen on military base as the place of occurrence of the external cause

Y92.131 Mess hall on military base as the place of occurrence of the external cause

Y92.133 Barracks on military base as the place of occurrence of the external cause

Y92.135 Garage on military base as the place of occurrence of the external cause

Y92.136 Swimming-pool on military base as the place of occurrence of the external cause

Y92.137 Garden or yard on military base as the place of occurrence of the external cause

Y92.138 Other place on military base as the place of occurrence of the external cause

Y92.139 Unspecified place military base as the place of occurrence of the external cause

✓6ᵗʰ Y92.14 Prison as the place of occurrence of the external cause

Y92.14Ø Kitchen in prison as the place of occurrence of the external cause

Y92.141 Dining room in prison as the place of occurrence of the external cause

Y92.142 Bathroom in prison as the place of occurrence of the external cause

Y92.143 Cell of prison as the place of occurrence of the external cause

Y92.146 Swimming-pool of prison as the place of occurrence of the external cause

Y92.147 Courtyard of prison as the place of occurrence of the external cause

Y92.148 Other place in prison as the place of occurrence of the external cause

Y92.149 Unspecified place in prison as the place of occurrence of the external cause

✓6ᵗʰ Y92.15 Reform school as the place of occurrence of the external cause

Y92.15Ø Kitchen in reform school as the place of occurrence of the external cause

Y92.151 Dining room in reform school as the place of occurrence of the external cause

Y92.152 Bathroom in reform school as the place of occurrence of the external cause

Y92.153 Bedroom in reform school as the place of occurrence of the external cause

Y92.154 Driveway of reform school as the place of occurrence of the external cause

Y92.155 Garage of reform school as the place of occurrence of the external cause

Y92.156 Swimming-pool of reform school as the place of occurrence of the external cause

Y92.157 Garden or yard of reform school as the place of occurrence of the external cause

Y92.158 Other place in reform school as the place of occurrence of the external cause

Y92.159 Unspecified place in reform school as the place of occurrence of the external cause

✓6ᵗʰ Y92.16 School dormitory as the place of occurrence of the external cause

    EXCLUDES 1 reform school as the place of occurrence of the external cause (Y92.15-)
          school buildings and grounds as the place of occurrence of the external cause (Y92.2-)
          school sports and athletic areas as the place of occurrence of the external cause (Y92.3-)

Y92.16Ø Kitchen in school dormitory as the place of occurrence of the external cause

Y92.161 Dining room in school dormitory as the place of occurrence of the external cause

Y92.162 Bathroom in school dormitory as the place of occurrence of the external cause

Y92.163 Bedroom in school dormitory as the place of occurrence of the external cause

Y92.168 Other place in school dormitory as the place of occurrence of the external cause

Y92.169 Unspecified place in school dormitory as the place of occurrence of the external cause

✓6ᵗʰ Y92.19 Other specified residential institution as the place of occurrence of the external cause

AHA: 2017,2Q,10

Y92.19Ø Kitchen in other specified residential institution as the place of occurrence of the external cause

Y92.191 Dining room in other specified residential institution as the place of occurrence of the external cause

Y92.192 Bathroom in other specified residential institution as the place of occurrence of the external cause

Y92.193 Bedroom in other specified residential institution as the place of occurrence of the external cause

Y92.194 Driveway of other specified residential institution as the place of occurrence of the external cause

Y92.195 Garage of other specified residential institution as the place of occurrence of the external cause

Y92.196 Pool of other specified residential institution as the place of occurrence of the external cause

Y92.197 Garden or yard of other specified residential institution as the place of occurrence of the external cause

Y92.198 Other place in other specified residential institution as the place of occurrence of the external cause

Y92.199 Unspecified place in other specified residential institution as the place of occurrence of the external cause

✓5ᵗʰ **Y92.2** School, other institution and public administrative area as the place of occurrence of the external cause

Building and adjacent grounds used by the general public or by a particular group of the public

> EXCLUDES 1   *building under construction as the place of occurrence of the external cause (Y92.6)*
>
> *residential institution as the place of occurrence of the external cause (Y92.1)*
>
> *school dormitory as the place of occurrence of the external cause (Y92.16-)*
>
> *sports and athletics area of schools as the place of occurrence of the external cause (Y92.3-)*

✓6ᵗʰ **Y92.21** School (private) (public) (state) as the place of occurrence of the external cause

Y92.210 Daycare center as the place of occurrence of the external cause

Y92.211 Elementary school as the place of occurrence of the external cause

> Kindergarten as the place of occurrence of the external cause

Y92.212 Middle school as the place of occurrence of the external cause

Y92.213 High school as the place of occurrence of the external cause

> AHA: 2012,4Q,108

Y92.214 College as the place of occurrence of the external cause

> University as the place of occurrence of the external cause

Y92.215 Trade school as the place of occurrence of the external cause

Y92.218 Other school as the place of occurrence of the external cause

Y92.219 Unspecified school as the place of occurrence of the external cause

Y92.22 Religious institution as the place of occurrence of the external cause

> Church as the place of occurrence of the external cause
>
> Mosque as the place of occurrence of the external cause
>
> Synagogue as the place of occurrence of the external cause

✓6ᵗʰ **Y92.23** Hospital as the place of occurrence of the external cause

> EXCLUDES 1   *ambulatory (outpatient) health services establishments (Y92.53-)*
>
> *home for the sick as the place of occurrence of the external cause (Y92.12-)*
>
> *hospice as the place of occurrence of the external cause (Y92.12-)*
>
> *nursing home as the place of occurrence of the external cause (Y92.12-)*

Y92.230 Patient room in hospital as the place of occurrence of the external cause

Y92.231 Patient bathroom in hospital as the place of occurrence of the external cause

Y92.232 Corridor of hospital as the place of occurrence of the external cause

Y92.233 Cafeteria of hospital as the place of occurrence of the external cause

Y92.234 Operating room of hospital as the place of occurrence of the external cause

Y92.238 Other place in hospital as the place of occurrence of the external cause

Y92.239 Unspecified place in hospital as the place of occurrence of the external cause

✓6ᵗʰ **Y92.24** Public administrative building as the place of occurrence of the external cause

Y92.240 Courthouse as the place of occurrence of the external cause

Y92.241 Library as the place of occurrence of the external cause

Y92.242 Post office as the place of occurrence of the external cause

Y92.243 City hall as the place of occurrence of the external cause

Y92.248 Other public administrative building as the place of occurrence of the external cause

✓6ᵗʰ **Y92.25** Cultural building as the place of occurrence of the external cause

Y92.250 Art Gallery as the place of occurrence of the external cause

Y92.251 Museum as the place of occurrence of the external cause

Y92.252 Music hall as the place of occurrence of the external cause

Y92.253 Opera house as the place of occurrence of the external cause

Y92.254 Theater (live) as the place of occurrence of the external cause

Y92.258 Other cultural public building as the place of occurrence of the external cause

Y92.26 Movie house or cinema as the place of occurrence of the external cause

Y92.29 Other specified public building as the place of occurrence of the external cause

> Assembly hall as the place of occurrence of the external cause
>
> Clubhouse as the place of occurrence of the external cause

✓5ᵗʰ **Y92.3** Sports and athletics area as the place of occurrence of the external cause

✓6ᵗʰ **Y92.31** Athletic court as the place of occurrence of the external cause

> EXCLUDES 1   *tennis court in private home or garden (Y92.09)*

Y92.310 Basketball court as the place of occurrence of the external cause

Y92.311 Squash court as the place of occurrence of the external cause

Y92.312 Tennis court as the place of occurrence of the external cause

Y92.318 Other athletic court as the place of occurrence of the external cause

✓6ᵗʰ **Y92.32** Athletic field as the place of occurrence of the external cause

Y92.320 Baseball field as the place of occurrence of the external cause

Y92.321 Football field as the place of occurrence of the external cause

Y92.322 Soccer field as the place of occurrence of the external cause

Y92.328 Other athletic field as the place of occurrence of the external cause

> Cricket field as the place of occurrence of the external cause
>
> Hockey field as the place of occurrence of the external cause

✓6ᵗʰ **Y92.33** Skating rink as the place of occurrence of the external cause

Y92.330 Ice skating rink (indoor) (outdoor) as the place of occurrence of the external cause

Y92.331 Roller skating rink as the place of occurrence of the external cause

Y92.34 Swimming pool (public) as the place of occurrence of the external cause

> EXCLUDES 1   *swimming pool in private home or garden (Y92.016)*

✅ Additional Character Required   ✓x7ᵗʰ Placeholder Alert   Manifestation   Unspecified Dx   ᴏ QPP   UPD Unacceptable PDx

Y92.39   **Other specified sports and athletic area as the place of occurrence of the external cause**
  Golf-course as the place of occurrence of the external cause
  Gymnasium as the place of occurrence of the external cause
  Riding-school as the place of occurrence of the external cause
  Stadium as the place of occurrence of the external cause

✓5ᵗʰ **Y92.4**   **Street, highway and other paved roadways as the place of occurrence of the external cause**
  EXCLUDES 1   *private driveway of residence (Y92.014, Y92.024, Y92.043, Y92.093, Y92.113, Y92.123, Y92.154, Y92.194)*

✓6ᵗʰ **Y92.41**   **Street and highway as the place of occurrence of the external cause**

  Y92.410   **Unspecified street and highway as the place of occurrence of the external cause**
    Road NOS as the place of occurrence of the external cause

  Y92.411   **Interstate highway as the place of occurrence of the external cause**
    Freeway as the place of occurrence of the external cause
    Motorway as the place of occurrence of the external cause

  Y92.412   **Parkway as the place of occurrence of the external cause**

  Y92.413   **State road as the place of occurrence of the external cause**

  Y92.414   **Local residential or business street as the place of occurrence of the external cause**

  Y92.415   **Exit ramp or entrance ramp of street or highway as the place of occurrence of the external cause**

✓6ᵗʰ **Y92.48**   **Other paved roadways as the place of occurrence of the external cause**

  Y92.480   **Sidewalk as the place of occurrence of the external cause**

  Y92.481   **Parking lot as the place of occurrence of the external cause**

  Y92.482   **Bike path as the place of occurrence of the external cause**

  Y92.488   **Other paved roadways as the place of occurrence of the external cause**

✓5ᵗʰ **Y92.5**   **Trade and service area as the place of occurrence of the external cause**
  EXCLUDES 1   *garage in private home (Y92.015)*
    schools and other public administration buildings (Y92.2-)

✓6ᵗʰ **Y92.51**   **Private commercial establishments as the place of occurrence of the external cause**

  Y92.510   **Bank as the place of occurrence of the external cause**

  Y92.511   **Restaurant or café as the place of occurrence of the external cause**

  Y92.512   **Supermarket, store or market as the place of occurrence of the external cause**

  Y92.513   **Shop (commercial) as the place of occurrence of the external cause**

✓6ᵗʰ **Y92.52**   **Service areas as the place of occurrence of the external cause**

  Y92.520   **Airport as the place of occurrence of the external cause**

  Y92.521   **Bus station as the place of occurrence of the external cause**

  Y92.522   **Railway station as the place of occurrence of the external cause**

  Y92.523   **Highway rest stop as the place of occurrence of the external cause**

  Y92.524   **Gas station as the place of occurrence of the external cause**
    Petroleum station as the place of occurrence of the external cause
    Service station as the place of occurrence of the external cause

✓6ᵗʰ **Y92.53**   **Ambulatory health services establishments as the place of occurrence of the external cause**

  Y92.530   **Ambulatory surgery center as the place of occurrence of the external cause**
    Outpatient surgery center, including that connected with a hospital as the place of occurrence of the external cause
    Same day surgery center, including that connected with a hospital as the place of occurrence of the external cause

  Y92.531   **Health care provider office as the place of occurrence of the external cause**
    Physician office as the place of occurrence of the external cause

  Y92.532   **Urgent care center as the place of occurrence of the external cause**

  Y92.538   **Other ambulatory health services establishments as the place of occurrence of the external cause**
    AHA: 2019,1Q,21

Y92.59   **Other trade areas as the place of occurrence of the external cause**
  Office building as the place of occurrence of the external cause
  Casino as the place of occurrence of the external cause
  Garage (commercial) as the place of occurrence of the external cause
  Hotel as the place of occurrence of the external cause
  Radio or television station as the place of occurrence of the external cause
  Shopping mall as the place of occurrence of the external cause
  Warehouse as the place of occurrence of the external cause

✓5ᵗʰ **Y92.6**   **Industrial and construction area as the place of occurrence of the external cause**

  Y92.61   **Building [any] under construction as the place of occurrence of the external cause**

  Y92.62   **Dock or shipyard as the place of occurrence of the external cause**
    Dockyard as the place of occurrence of the external cause
    Dry dock as the place of occurrence of the external cause
    Shipyard as the place of occurrence of the external cause

  Y92.63   **Factory as the place of occurrence of the external cause**
    Factory building as the place of occurrence of the external cause
    Factory premises as the place of occurrence of the external cause
    Industrial yard as the place of occurrence of the external cause

  Y92.64   **Mine or pit as the place of occurrence of the external cause**
    Mine as the place of occurrence of the external cause

  Y92.65   **Oil rig as the place of occurrence of the external cause**
    Pit (coal) (gravel) (sand) as the place of occurrence of the external cause

  Y92.69   **Other specified industrial and construction area as the place of occurrence of the external cause**
    Gasworks as the place of occurrence of the external cause
    Power-station (coal) (nuclear) (oil) as the place of occurrence of the external cause
    Tunnel under construction as the place of occurrence of the external cause
    Workshop as the place of occurrence of the external cause

✓5ᵗʰ **Y92.7**   **Farm as the place of occurrence of the external cause**
  Ranch as the place of occurrence of the external cause
  EXCLUDES 1   *farmhouse and home premises of farm (Y92.01-)*

  Y92.71   **Barn as the place of occurrence of the external cause**

Y92.72   **Chicken coop** as the place of occurrence of the external cause

     Hen house as the place of occurrence of the external cause

Y92.73   **Farm field** as the place of occurrence of the external cause

Y92.74   **Orchard** as the place of occurrence of the external cause

Y92.79   **Other farm location** as the place of occurrence of the external cause

✓5ᵗʰ **Y92.8**   **Other places as the place of occurrence of the external cause**

   ✓6ᵗʰ **Y92.81**   **Transport vehicle** as the place of occurrence of the external cause

       EXCLUDES 1   transport accidents (V00-V99)

     Y92.810   **Car** as the place of occurrence of the external cause

     Y92.811   **Bus** as the place of occurrence of the external cause

     Y92.812   **Truck** as the place of occurrence of the external cause

     Y92.813   **Airplane** as the place of occurrence of the external cause

     Y92.814   **Boat** as the place of occurrence of the external cause

     Y92.815   **Train** as the place of occurrence of the external cause

     Y92.816   **Subway** car as the place of occurrence of the external cause

     Y92.818   **Other transport vehicle** as the place of occurrence of the external cause

   ✓6ᵗʰ **Y92.82**   **Wilderness area**

     Y92.820   **Desert** as the place of occurrence of the external cause

     Y92.821   **Forest** as the place of occurrence of the external cause

     Y92.828   **Other wilderness area** as the place of occurrence of the external cause

       Swamp as the place of occurrence of the external cause

       Mountain as the place of occurrence of the external cause

       Marsh as the place of occurrence of the external cause

       Prairie as the place of occurrence of the external cause

   ✓6ᵗʰ **Y92.83**   **Recreation area** as the place of occurrence of the external cause

     Y92.830   **Public park** as the place of occurrence of the external cause

     Y92.831   **Amusement park** as the place of occurrence of the external cause

     Y92.832   **Beach** as the place of occurrence of the external cause

       Seashore as the place of occurrence of the external cause

     Y92.833   **Campsite** as the place of occurrence of the external cause

     Y92.834   **Zoological garden (Zoo)** as the place of occurrence of the external cause

     Y92.838   **Other recreation area** as the place of occurrence of the external cause

   Y92.84   **Military training ground** as the place of occurrence of the external cause

   Y92.85   **Railroad track** as the place of occurrence of the external cause

   Y92.86   **Slaughter house** as the place of occurrence of the external cause

   Y92.89   **Other specified places** as the place of occurrence of the external cause

     Derelict house as the place of occurrence of the external cause

Y92.9   **Unspecified place or not applicable**

✓4ᵗʰ **Y93**   **Activity codes**

   NOTE   Category Y93 is provided for use to indicate the activity of the person seeking healthcare for an injury or health condition, such as a heart attack while shoveling snow, which resulted from, or was contributed to, by the activity. These codes are appropriate for use for both acute injuries, such as those from chapter 19, and conditions that are due to the long-term, cumulative effects of an activity, such as those from chapter 13. They are also appropriate for use with external cause codes for cause and intent if identifying the activity provides additional information on the event. These codes should be used in conjunction with codes for external cause status (Y99) and place of occurrence (Y92).

This section contains the following broad activity categories:

Y93.0   Activities involving walking and running

Y93.1   Activities involving water and water craft

Y93.2   Activities involving ice and snow

Y93.3   Activities involving climbing, rappelling, and jumping off

Y93.4   Activities involving dancing and other rhythmic movement

Y93.5   Activities involving other sports and athletics played individually

Y93.6   Activities involving other sports and athletics played as a team or group

Y93.7   Activities involving other specified sports and athletics

Y93.A   Activities involving other cardiorespiratory exercise

Y93.B   Activities involving other muscle strengthening exercises

Y93.C   Activities involving computer technology and electronic devices

Y93.D   Activities involving arts and handcrafts

Y93.E   Activities involving personal hygiene and interior property and clothing maintenance

Y93.F   Activities involving caregiving

Y93.G   Activities involving food preparation, cooking and grilling

Y93.H   Activities involving exterior property and land maintenance, building and construction

Y93.I   Activities involving roller coasters and other types of external motion

Y93.J   Activities involving playing musical instrument

Y93.K   Activities involving animal care

Y93.8   Activities, other specified

Y93.9   Activity, unspecified   *initial en Guide only*

✓5ᵗʰ **Y93.0**   **Activities involving walking and running**

       EXCLUDES 1   activity, walking an animal (Y93.K1)

                 activity, walking or running on a treadmill (Y93.A1)

   Y93.01   **Activity, walking, marching and hiking**

     Activity, walking, marching and hiking on level or elevated terrain

       EXCLUDES 1   activity, mountain climbing (Y93.31)

   Y93.02   **Activity, running**

✓5ᵗʰ **Y93.1**   **Activities involving water and water craft**

       EXCLUDES 1   activities involving ice (Y93.2-)

   Y93.11   **Activity, swimming**

   Y93.12   **Activity, springboard and platform diving**

   Y93.13   **Activity, water polo**

   Y93.14   **Activity, water aerobics and water exercise**

   Y93.15   **Activity, underwater diving and snorkeling**

     Activity, SCUBA diving

   Y93.16   **Activity, rowing, canoeing, kayaking, rafting and tubing**

     Activity, canoeing, kayaking, rafting and tubing in calm and turbulent water

   Y93.17   **Activity, water skiing and wake boarding**

   Y93.18   **Activity, surfing, windsurfing and boogie boarding**

     Activity, water sliding

   Y93.19   **Activity, other involving water and watercraft**

     Activity involving water NOS

     Activity, parasailing

     Activity, water survival training and testing

✓5ᵗʰ **Y93.2   Activities involving ice and snow**
> EXCLUDES 1   *activity, shoveling ice and snow (Y93.H1)*

Y93.21   Activity, ice skating
Activity, figure skating (singles) (pairs)
Activity, ice dancing
> EXCLUDES 1   *activity, ice hockey (Y93.22)*

Y93.22   Activity, ice hockey

Y93.23   Activity, snow (alpine) (downhill) skiing, snowboarding, sledding, tobogganing and snow tubing
> EXCLUDES 1   *activity, cross country skiing (Y93.24)*

Y93.24   Activity, cross country skiing
Activity, nordic skiing

Y93.29   Activity, other involving ice and snow
Activity involving ice and snow NOS

✓5ᵗʰ **Y93.3   Activities involving climbing, rappelling and jumping off**
> EXCLUDES 1   *activity, hiking on level or elevated terrain (Y93.01)*
> *activity, jumping rope (Y93.56)*
> *activity, trampoline jumping (Y93.44)*

Y93.31   Activity, mountain climbing, rock climbing and wall climbing

Y93.32   Activity, rappelling

Y93.33   Activity, BASE jumping
Activity, Building, Antenna, Span, Earth jumping

Y93.34   Activity, bungee jumping

Y93.35   Activity, hang gliding

Y93.39   Activity, other involving climbing, rappelling and jumping off

✓5ᵗʰ **Y93.4   Activities involving dancing and other rhythmic movement**
> EXCLUDES 1   *activity, martial arts (Y93.75)*

Y93.41   Activity, dancing
AHA: 2012,4Q,108

Y93.42   Activity, yoga

Y93.43   Activity, gymnastics
Activity, rhythmic gymnastics
> EXCLUDES 1   *activity, trampolining (Y93.44)*

Y93.44   Activity, trampolining

Y93.45   Activity, cheerleading

Y93.49   Activity, other involving dancing and other rhythmic movements

✓5ᵗʰ **Y93.5   Activities involving other sports and athletics played individually**
> EXCLUDES 1   *activity, dancing (Y93.41)*
> *activity, gymnastic (Y93.43)*
> *activity, trampolining (Y93.44)*
> *activity, yoga (Y93.42)*

Y93.51   Activity, roller skating (inline) and skateboarding

Y93.52   Activity, horseback riding

Y93.53   Activity, golf

Y93.54   Activity, bowling

Y93.55   Activity, bike riding

Y93.56   Activity, jumping rope

Y93.57   Activity, non-running track and field events
> EXCLUDES 1   *activity, running (any form) (Y93.02)*

Y93.59   Activity, other involving other sports and athletics played individually
> EXCLUDES 1   *activities involving climbing, rappelling, and jumping (Y93.3-)*
> *activities involving ice and snow (Y93.2-)*
> *activities involving walking and running (Y93.0-)*
> *activities involving water and watercraft (Y93.1-)*

✓5ᵗʰ **Y93.6   Activities involving other sports and athletics played as a team or group**
> EXCLUDES 1   *activity, ice hockey (Y93.22)*
> *activity, water polo (Y93.13)*

Y93.61   Activity, American tackle football
Activity, football NOS

Y93.62   Activity, American flag or touch football

Y93.63   Activity, rugby

Y93.64   Activity, baseball
Activity, softball

Y93.65   Activity, lacrosse and field hockey

Y93.66   Activity, soccer

Y93.67   Activity, basketball

Y93.68   Activity, volleyball (beach) (court)

Y93.6A   Activity, physical games generally associated with school recess, summer camp and children
Activity, capture the flag
Activity, dodge ball
Activity, four square
Activity, kickball

Y93.69   Activity, other involving other sports and athletics played as a team or group
Activity, cricket

✓5ᵗʰ **Y93.7   Activities involving other specified sports and athletics**

Y93.71   Activity, boxing

Y93.72   Activity, wrestling

Y93.73   Activity, racquet and hand sports
Activity, handball
Activity, racquetball
Activity, squash
Activity, tennis

Y93.74   Activity, frisbee
Activity, ultimate frisbee

Y93.75   Activity, martial arts
Activity, combatives

Y93.79   Activity, other specified sports and athletics
> EXCLUDES 1   *sports and athletics activities specified in categories Y93.0-Y93.6*

✓5ᵗʰ **Y93.A   Activities involving other cardiorespiratory exercise**
Activities involving physical training

Y93.A1   Activity, exercise machines primarily for cardiorespiratory conditioning
Activity, elliptical and stepper machines
Activity, stationary bike
Activity, treadmill

Y93.A2   Activity, calisthenics
Activity, jumping jacks
Activity, warm up and cool down

Y93.A3   Activity, aerobic and step exercise

Y93.A4   Activity, circuit training

Y93.A5   Activity, obstacle course
Activity, challenge course
Activity, confidence course

Y93.A6   Activity, grass drills
Activity, guerilla drills

Y93.A9   Activity, other involving cardiorespiratory exercise
> EXCLUDES 1   *activities involving cardiorespiratory exercise specified in categories Y93.0-Y93.7*

✓5ᵗʰ **Y93.B   Activities involving other muscle strengthening exercises**

Y93.B1   Activity, exercise machines primarily for muscle strengthening

Y93.B2   Activity, push-ups, pull-ups, sit-ups

Y93.B3   Activity, free weights
Activity, barbells
Activity, dumbbells

Y93.B4   Activity, pilates

Y93.B9   Activity, other involving muscle strengthening exercises
> EXCLUDES 1   *activities involving muscle strengthening specified in categories Y93.0-Y93.A*

✓5ᵗʰ **Y93.C   Activities involving computer technology and electronic devices**
> EXCLUDES 1   *activity, electronic musical keyboard or instruments (Y93.J-)*

Y93.C1   Activity, computer keyboarding
Activity, electronic game playing using keyboard or other stationary device

Y93.C2   Activity, hand held interactive electronic device
Activity, cellular telephone and communication device
Activity, electronic game playing using interactive device
> EXCLUDES 1   *activity, electronic game playing using keyboard or other stationary device (Y93.C1)*

Y93.C9   Activity, other involving computer technology and electronic devices

✓5ᵗʰ **Y93.D   Activities involving arts and handcrafts**
> EXCLUDES 1   *activities involving playing musical instrument (Y93.J-)*

Y93.D1   Activity, knitting and crocheting

Y93.D2   **Activity,** sewing

Y93.D3   **Activity,** furniture building and finishing

            Activity, furniture repair

Y93.D9   **Activity, other involving arts and handcrafts**

✓5ᵗʰ **Y93.E**   **Activities involving personal hygiene and interior property and clothing maintenance**

     EXCLUDES 1   *activities involving cooking and grilling (Y93.G-)*

              activities involving exterior property and land maintenance, building and construction (Y93.H-)

              activities involving caregiving (Y93.F-)

              activity, dishwashing (Y93.G1)

              activity, food preparation (Y93.G1)

              activity, gardening (Y93.H2)

Y93.E1   **Activity,** personal bathing and showering

Y93.E2   **Activity,** laundry

Y93.E3   **Activity,** vacuuming

Y93.E4   **Activity,** ironing

Y93.E5   **Activity,** floor mopping and cleaning

Y93.E6   **Activity,** residential relocation

            Activity, packing up and unpacking involved in moving to a new residence

Y93.E8   **Activity, other personal hygiene**

Y93.E9   **Activity, other interior property and clothing maintenance**

✓5ᵗʰ **Y93.F**   **Activities involving** caregiving

        Activity involving the provider of caregiving

Y93.F1   **Activity, caregiving,** bathing

Y93.F2   **Activity, caregiving,** lifting

Y93.F9   **Activity, other caregiving**

✓5ᵗʰ **Y93.G**   **Activities involving food preparation, cooking and grilling**

Y93.G1   **Activity,** food preparation and clean up

            Activity, dishwashing

Y93.G2   **Activity,** grilling and smoking food

Y93.G3   **Activity,** cooking and baking

            Activity, use of stove, oven and microwave oven

Y93.G9   **Activity, other involving cooking and grilling**

✓5ᵗʰ **Y93.H**   **Activities involving exterior property and land maintenance, building and construction**

Y93.H1   **Activity,** digging, shoveling and raking

            Activity, dirt digging

            Activity, raking leaves

            Activity, snow shoveling

Y93.H2   **Activity,** gardening and landscaping

            Activity, pruning, trimming shrubs, weeding

Y93.H3   **Activity,** building and construction

Y93.H9   **Activity, other involving exterior property and land maintenance, building and construction**

✓5ᵗʰ **Y93.I**   **Activities involving roller coasters and other types of external motion**

Y93.I1   **Activity,** rollercoaster riding

Y93.I9   **Activity, other involving external motion**

✓5ᵗʰ **Y93.J**   **Activities involving playing musical instrument**

        Activity involving playing electric musical instrument

Y93.J1   **Activity,** piano **playing**

            Activity, musical keyboard (electronic) playing

Y93.J2   **Activity,** drum and other percussion instrument **playing**

Y93.J3   **Activity,** string instrument **playing**

Y93.J4   **Activity,** winds and brass instrument **playing**

✓5ᵗʰ **Y93.K**   **Activities involving animal care**

     EXCLUDES 1   *activity, horseback riding (Y93.52)*

Y93.K1   **Activity,** walking **an animal**

Y93.K2   **Activity,** milking **an animal**

Y93.K3   **Activity,** grooming and shearing **an animal**

Y93.K9   **Activity, other involving animal care**

✓5ᵗʰ **Y93.8**   **Activities, other specified**

Y93.81   **Activity,** refereeing **a sports activity**

Y93.82   **Activity,** spectator **at an event**

Y93.83   **Activity,** rough housing and horseplay

Y93.84   **Activity,** sleeping

Y93.85   **Activity,** choking game

            Activity, blackout game

            Activity, fainting game

            Activity, pass out game

            AHA: 2016,4Q,74-76

Y93.89   **Activity, other specified**

Y93.9   **Activity, unspecified**

Y95   **Nosocomial condition**

      AHA: 2013,4Q,119

✓4ᵗʰ **Y99**   **External cause status**

     NOTE   A single code from category Y99 should be used in conjunction with the external cause code(s) assigned to a record to indicate the status of the person at the time the event occurred.

Y99.0   Civilian **activity done for income or pay**

        Civilian activity done for financial or other compensation

     EXCLUDES 1   *military activity (Y99.1)*

             volunteer activity (Y99.2)

Y99.1   Military **activity**

     EXCLUDES 1   *activity of off duty military personnel (Y99.8)*

Y99.2   Volunteer **activity**

     EXCLUDES 1   *activity of child or other family member assisting in compensated work of other family member (Y99.8)*

Y99.8   **Other external cause status**

        Activity NEC

        Activity of child or other family member assisting in compensated work of other family member

        Hobby not done for income

        Leisure activity

        Off-duty activity of military personnel

        Recreation or sport not for income or while a student

        Student activity

     EXCLUDES 1   *civilian activity done for income or compensation (Y99.0)*

             military activity (Y99.1)

        AHA: 2012,4Q,108

Y99.9   **Unspecified external cause status**

Chapter 21. Factors Influencing Health Status and Contact with Health Services (Z00–Z99)

Chapter-specific Guidelines with Coding Examples

The chapter-specific guidelines from the ICD-10-CM Official Guidelines for Coding and Reporting have been provided below. Along with these guidelines are coding examples, contained in the shaded boxes, that have been developed to help illustrate the coding and/or sequencing guidance found in these guidelines.

Note: The chapter-specific guidelines provide additional information about the use of Z codes for specified encounters.

a. Use of Z Codes in any healthcare setting

Z codes are for use in any healthcare setting. Z codes may be used as either a first-listed (principal diagnosis code in the inpatient setting) or secondary code, depending on the circumstances of the encounter. Certain Z codes may only be used as first-listed or principal diagnosis.

Patient with middle lobe lung cancer presents for initiation of chemotherapy

Z51.11   **Encounter for antineoplastic chemotherapy**

C34.2   **Malignant neoplasm of middle lobe, bronchus or lung**

Explanation: A Z code can be used as first-listed in this situation based on guidelines in this chapter as well as chapter 2, "Neoplasms."

Patient has chronic lymphocytic leukemia for which the patient had previous chemotherapy and is now in remission

C91.11   **Chronic lymphocytic leukemia of B-cell type in remission**

Z92.21   **Personal history of antineoplastic chemotherapy**

Explanation: The personal history Z code is used to describe a secondary (supplementary) diagnosis to identify that this patient has had chemotherapy in the past.

---

b. Z Codes indicate a reason for an encounter or provide additional information about a patient encounter

Z codes are not procedure codes. A corresponding procedure code must accompany a Z code to describe any procedure performed.

c. Categories of Z Codes

1) Contact/exposure

Category Z20 indicates contact with, and suspected exposure to, communicable diseases. These codes are for patients who are suspected to have been exposed to a disease by close personal contact with an infected individual or are in an area where a disease is epidemic.

Category Z77, Other contact with and (suspected) exposures hazardous to health, indicates contact with and suspected exposures hazardous to health.

Contact/exposure codes may be used as a first-listed code to explain an encounter for testing, or, more commonly, as a secondary code to identify a potential risk.

2) Inoculations and vaccinations

Code Z23 is for encounters for inoculations and vaccinations. It indicates that a patient is being seen to receive a prophylactic inoculation against a disease. Procedure codes are required to identify the actual administration of the injection and the type(s) of immunizations given. Code Z23 may be used as a secondary code if the inoculation is given as a routine part of preventive health care, such as a well-baby visit.

3) Status

Status codes indicate that a patient is either a carrier of a disease or has the sequelae or residual of a past disease or condition. This includes such things as the presence of prosthetic or mechanical devices resulting from past treatment. A status code is informative, because the status may affect the course of treatment and its outcome. A status code is distinct from a history code. The history code indicates that the patient no longer has the condition.

A status code should not be used with a diagnosis code from one of the body system chapters, if the diagnosis code includes the information provided by the status code. For example, code Z94.1, Heart transplant status, should not be used with a code from subcategory T86.2, Complications of heart transplant. The status code does not provide additional information. The complication code indicates that the patient is a heart transplant patient.

For encounters for weaning from a mechanical ventilator, assign a code from subcategory J96.1, Chronic respiratory failure, followed by code Z99.11, Dependence on respirator [ventilator] status.

The status Z codes/categories are:

Z14   Genetic carrier

     Genetic carrier status indicates that a person carries a gene, associated with a particular disease, which may be passed to offspring who may develop that disease. The person does not have the disease and is not at risk of developing the disease.

Z15   Genetic susceptibility to disease

     Genetic susceptibility indicates that a person has a gene that increases the risk of that person developing the disease.

     Codes from category Z15 should not be used as principal or first-listed codes. If the patient has the condition to which he/she is susceptible, and that condition is the reason for the encounter, the code for the current condition should be sequenced first. If the patient is being seen for follow-up after completed treatment for this condition, and the condition no longer exists, a follow-up code should be sequenced first, followed by the appropriate personal history and genetic susceptibility codes. If the purpose of the encounter is genetic counseling associated with procreative management, code Z31.5, Encounter for genetic counseling, should be assigned as the first-listed code, followed by a code from category Z15. Additional codes should be assigned for any applicable family or personal history.

Z16   Resistance to antimicrobial drugs

     This code indicates that a patient has a condition that is resistant to antimicrobial drug treatment. Sequence the infection code first.

Z17   Estrogen receptor status

Z18   Retained foreign body fragments

Z19   Hormone sensitivity malignancy status

Z21   Asymptomatic HIV infection status

     This code indicates that a patient has tested positive for HIV but has manifested no signs or symptoms of the disease.

Z22   Carrier of infectious disease

     Carrier status indicates that a person harbors the specific organisms of a disease without manifest symptoms and is capable of transmitting the infection.

Z28.3   Underimmunization status

     See Section I.B.14. for underimmunization documentation by clinicians other than the patient's provider.

Z33.1   Pregnant state, incidental

     This code is a secondary code only for use when the pregnancy is in no way complicating the reason for visit. Otherwise, a code from the obstetric chapter is required.

Z66   Do not resuscitate

     This code may be used when it is documented by the provider that a patient is on do not resuscitate status at any time during the stay.

Z67   Blood type

Z68   Body mass index (BMI)

     BMI codes should only be assigned when there is an associated, reportable diagnosis (such as obesity). Do not assign BMI codes during pregnancy.

     See Section I.B.14. for BMI documentation by clinicians other than the patient's provider.

Patient seen today for chest pain, noncardiac in nature. Nurses notes identify a BMI of 20.5.

R07.89   **Other chest pain**

Explanation: Section I.B.14 stipulates that the BMI can be assigned from documentation of someone other than the patient's provider, such as nursing notes, only when the provider has documented that the diagnosis is associated with the BMI. As there is no supporting documentation from the provider linking the BMI to an associated condition, no code is assigned for the BMI.

Z74.Ø1   Bed confinement status

Z76.82   Awaiting organ transplant status

Z78   Other specified health status

Code Z78.1, Physical restraint status, may be used when it is documented by the provider that a patient has been put in restraints during the current encounter. Please note that this code should not be reported when it is documented by the provider that a patient is temporarily restrained during a procedure.

Z79   Long-term (current) drug therapy

Codes from this category indicate a patient's continuous use of a prescribed drug (including such things as aspirin therapy) for the long-term treatment of a condition or for prophylactic use. It is not for use for patients who have addictions to drugs. This subcategory is not for use of medications for detoxification or maintenance programs to prevent withdrawal symptoms (e.g., methadone maintenance for opiate dependence). Assign the appropriate code for the drug use, abuse, or dependence instead.

Assign a code from Z79 if the patient is receiving a medication for an extended period as a prophylactic measure (such as for the prevention of deep vein thrombosis) or as treatment of a chronic condition (such as arthritis) or a disease requiring a lengthy course of treatment (such as cancer). Do not assign a code from category Z79 for medication being administered for a brief period of time to treat an acute illness or injury (such as a course of antibiotics to treat acute bronchitis).

Z88   Allergy status to drugs, medicaments and biological substances

Except: Z88.9, Allergy status to unspecified drugs, medicaments and biological substances status

Z89   Acquired absence of limb

Z90   Acquired absence of organs, not elsewhere classified

Z91.Ø-   Allergy status, other than to drugs and biological substances

Z92.82   Status post administration of tPA (rtPA) in a different facility within the last 24 hours prior to admission to a current facility

Assign code Z92.82, Status post administration of tPA (rtPA) in a different facility within the last 24 hours prior to admission to current facility, as a secondary diagnosis when a patient is received by transfer into a facility and documentation indicates they were administered tissue plasminogen activator (tPA) within the last 24 hours prior to admission to the current facility.

This guideline applies even if the patient is still receiving the tPA at the time they are received into the current facility.

The appropriate code for the condition for which the tPA was administered (such as cerebrovascular disease or myocardial infarction) should be assigned first.

Code Z92.82 is only applicable to the receiving facility record and not to the transferring facility record.

Z93   Artificial opening status

Z94   Transplanted organ and tissue status

Z95   Presence of cardiac and vascular implants and grafts

Z96   Presence of other functional implants

Z97   Presence of other devices

Z98   Other postprocedural states

Assign code Z98.85, Transplanted organ removal status, to indicate that a transplanted organ has been previously removed. This code should not be assigned for the encounter in which the transplanted organ is removed. The complication necessitating removal of the transplant organ should be assigned for that encounter.

See section I.C.19. for information on the coding of organ transplant complications.

Z99   Dependence on enabling machines and devices, not elsewhere classified

Note: Categories Z89-Z9Ø and Z93-Z99 are for use only if there are no complications or malfunctions of the organ or tissue replaced, the amputation site or the equipment on which the patient is dependent.

4) History (of)

There are two types of history Z codes, personal and family. Personal history codes explain a patient's past medical condition that no longer exists and is not receiving any treatment, but that has the potential for recurrence, and therefore may require continued monitoring.

Family history codes are for use when a patient has a family member(s) who has had a particular disease that causes the patient to be at higher risk of also contracting the disease.

Personal history codes may be used in conjunction with follow-up codes and family history codes may be used in conjunction with screening codes to explain the need for a test or procedure. History codes are also acceptable on any medical record regardless of the reason for visit. A history of an illness, even if no longer present, is important information that may alter the type of treatment ordered.

The reason for the encounter (for example, screening or counseling) should be sequenced first and the appropriate personal and/or family history code(s) should be assigned as additional diagnos(es).

The history Z code categories are:

Z8Ø   Family history of primary malignant neoplasm

Z81   Family history of mental and behavioral disorders

Z82   Family history of certain disabilities and chronic diseases (leading to disablement)

Z83   Family history of other specific disorders

Z84   Family history of other conditions

Z85   Personal history of malignant neoplasm

Z86   Personal history of certain other diseases

Z87   Personal history of other diseases and conditions

Z91.4-   Personal history of psychological trauma, not elsewhere classified

Z91.5-   Personal history of self-harm

Z91.81   History of falling

Z91.82   Personal history of military deployment

Z92   Personal history of medical treatment

Except: Z92.Ø, Personal history of contraception

Except: Z92.82, Status post administration of tPA (rtPA) in a different facility within the last 24 hours prior to admission to a current facility

5) Screening

Screening is the testing for disease or disease precursors in seemingly well individuals so that early detection and treatment can be provided for those who test positive for the disease (e.g., screening mammogram).

The testing of a person to rule out or confirm a suspected diagnosis because the patient has some sign or symptom is a diagnostic examination, not a screening. In these cases, the sign or symptom is used to explain the reason for the test.

A screening code may be a first-listed code if the reason for the visit is specifically the screening exam. It may also be used as an additional code if the screening is done during an office visit for other health problems. A screening code is not necessary if the screening is inherent to a routine examination, such as a pap smear done during a routine pelvic examination.

Should a condition be discovered during the screening then the code for the condition may be assigned as an additional diagnosis.

Prostate screening of healthy 5Ø-year-old male patient; PSA noted to be elevated but normal digital rectal exam

Z12.5   **Encounter for screening for malignant neoplasm of prostate**

R97.2Ø   **Elevated prostate specific antigen [PSA]**

Explanation: The patient had no signs or symptoms of any prostate-related illness prior to coming in for the screening. The screening code is appropriately used as the first-listed code to signify that this was for routine screening. The elevated PSA is reported as a secondary diagnosis to reflect that an abnormal lab value was found as a result of the screening procedure(s).

The Z code indicates that a screening exam is planned. A procedure code is required to confirm that the screening was performed.

The screening Z codes/categories:

Z11   Encounter for screening for infectious and parasitic diseases

Z12   Encounter for screening for malignant neoplasms

Z13   Encounter for screening for other diseases and disorders

Except: Z13.9, Encounter for screening, unspecified

Z36   Encounter for antenatal screening for mother

6) Observation

There are three observation Z code categories. They are for use in very limited circumstances when a person is being observed for a suspected condition that is ruled out. The observation codes are not for use if an injury or illness or any signs or symptoms related to the suspected condition are present. In such cases the diagnosis/symptom code is used with the corresponding external cause code.

The observation codes are primarily to be used as a principal/first-listed diagnosis. An observation code may be assigned as a secondary diagnosis code when the patient is being observed for a condition that is ruled out and is unrelated to the principal/first-listed diagnosis. Also, when the principal diagnosis is required to be a code from category Z38, Liveborn infants according to place of birth and type of delivery. Then a code from category Z05, Encounter for observation and evaluation of newborn for suspected diseases and conditions ruled out, is sequenced after the Z38 code. Additional codes may be used in addition to the observation code but only if they are unrelated to the suspected condition being observed.

Codes from subcategory Z03.7, Encounter for suspected maternal and fetal conditions ruled out, may either be used as a first-listed or as an additional code assignment depending on the case. They are for use in very limited circumstances on a maternal record when an encounter is for a suspected maternal or fetal condition that is ruled out during that encounter (for example, a maternal or fetal condition may be suspected due to an abnormal test result). These codes should not be used when the condition is confirmed. In those cases, the confirmed condition should be coded. In addition, these codes are not for use if an illness or any signs or symptoms related to the suspected condition or problem are present. In such cases the diagnosis/symptom code is used.

Additional codes may be used in addition to the code from subcategory Z03.7, but only if they are unrelated to the suspected condition being evaluated.

Codes from subcategory Z03.7 may not be used for encounters for antenatal screening of mother. *See Section I.C.21. Screening.*

For encounters for suspected fetal condition that are inconclusive following testing and evaluation, assign the appropriate code from category O35, O36, O40 or O41.

The observation Z code categories: *[handwritten: Can first listed diagnosis]*

Z03   Encounter for medical observation for suspected diseases and conditions ruled out

Z04   Encounter for examination and observation for other reasons

       Except: Z04.9, Encounter for examination and observation for unspecified reason

Z05   Encounter for observation and evaluation of newborn for suspected diseases and conditions ruled out

7) Aftercare

Aftercare visit codes cover situations when the initial treatment of a disease has been performed and the patient requires continued care during the healing or recovery phase, or for the long-term consequences of the disease. The aftercare Z code should not be used if treatment is directed at a current, acute disease. The diagnosis code is to be used in these cases. Exceptions to this rule are codes Z51.0, Encounter for antineoplastic radiation therapy, and codes from subcategory Z51.1, Encounter for antineoplastic chemotherapy and immunotherapy. These codes are to be first listed, followed by the diagnosis code when a patient's encounter is solely to receive radiation therapy, chemotherapy, or immunotherapy for the treatment of a neoplasm. If the reason for the encounter is more than one type of antineoplastic therapy, code Z51.0 and a code from subcategory Z51.1 may be assigned together, in which case one of these codes would be reported as a secondary diagnosis.

The aftercare Z codes should also not be used for aftercare for injuries. For aftercare of an injury, assign the acute injury code with the appropriate 7th character (for subsequent encounter).

The aftercare codes are generally first listed to explain the specific reason for the encounter. An aftercare code may be used as an additional code when some type of aftercare is provided in addition to the reason for admission and no diagnosis code is applicable. An example of this would be the closure of a colostomy during an encounter for treatment of another condition.

Aftercare codes should be used in conjunction with other aftercare codes or diagnosis codes to provide better detail on the specifics of an aftercare encounter visit, unless otherwise directed by the classification. The sequencing of multiple aftercare codes depends on the circumstances of the encounter.

Patient presents for third round of gemcitabine and first dose of antineoplastic radiation therapy for advanced pancreatic carcinoma

Z51.11	Encounter for antineoplastic chemotherapy
Z51.0	Encounter for antineoplastic radiation therapy
C25.9	Malignant neoplasm of pancreas, unspecified

Explanation: Gemcitabine is an antineoplastic chemotherapy. Since the encounter was solely to administer antineoplastic treatment, both forms of treatment are reported and either code can be the first-listed diagnosis, followed by the neoplastic condition code. Aftercare codes are typically not assigned for current treatment of disease; however, Z51.0 and subcategory Z51.1 are an exception to this standard.

Certain aftercare Z code categories need a secondary diagnosis code to describe the resolving condition or sequelae. For others, the condition is included in the code title.

Additional Z code aftercare category terms include fitting and adjustment, and attention to artificial openings.

Status Z codes may be used with aftercare Z codes to indicate the nature of the aftercare. For example code Z95.1, Presence of aortocoronary bypass graft, may be used with code Z48.812, Encounter for surgical aftercare following surgery on the circulatory system, to indicate the surgery for which the aftercare is being performed. A status code should not be used when the aftercare code indicates the type of status, such as using Z43.0, Encounter for attention to tracheostomy, with Z93.0, Tracheostomy status.

The aftercare Z category/codes:

Z42	Encounter for plastic and reconstructive surgery following medical procedure or healed injury
Z43	Encounter for attention to artificial openings
Z44	Encounter for fitting and adjustment of external prosthetic device
Z45	Encounter for adjustment and management of implanted device
Z46	Encounter for fitting and adjustment of other devices
Z47	Orthopedic aftercare
Z48	Encounter for other postprocedural aftercare
Z49	Encounter for care involving renal dialysis
Z51	Encounter for other aftercare and medical care

8) Follow-up

The follow-up codes are used to explain continuing surveillance following completed treatment of a disease, condition, or injury. They imply that the condition has been fully treated and no longer exists. They should not be confused with aftercare codes, or injury codes with a 7th character for subsequent encounter, that explain ongoing care of a healing condition or its sequelae. Follow-up codes may be used in conjunction with history codes to provide the full picture of the healed condition and its treatment. The follow-up code is sequenced first, followed by the history code.

A follow-up code may be used to explain multiple visits. Should a condition be found to have recurred on the follow-up visit, then the diagnosis code for the condition should be assigned in place of the follow-up code.

The follow-up Z code categories:

Z08	Encounter for follow-up examination after completed treatment for malignant neoplasm
Z09	Encounter for follow-up examination after completed treatment for conditions other than malignant neoplasm
Z39	Encounter for maternal postpartum care and examination

Follow-up for patient several months after completing a regime of IV antibiotics for recurrent pneumonia; lungs are clear and pneumonia is resolved

Z09	Encounter for follow-up examination after completed treatment for conditions other than malignant neoplasm
Z87.01	Personal history of pneumonia (recurrent)

Explanation: Code Z09 identifies the follow-up visit as being unrelated to a malignant neoplasm, and code Z87 describes the condition that has now resolved.

Follow-up for patient several months after completing a regime of IV antibiotics for recurrent pneumonia; pneumonia has recurred, and a new antibiotic regimen has been prescribed

J18.9   Pneumonia, unspecified organism

Explanation: Since the follow-up exam for pneumonia determined that the pneumonia was not resolved or recurred, code Z09 Encounter for follow-up examination after completed treatment for conditions other than malignant neoplasm, no longer applies. Instead the first-listed code describes the pneumonia.

9) Donor

Codes in category Z52, Donors of organs and tissues, are used for living individuals who are donating blood or other body tissue. These codes are for individuals donating for others, as well as for self-donations. They are not used to identify cadaveric donations.

10) Counseling

Counseling Z codes are used when a patient or family member receives assistance in the aftermath of an illness or injury, or when support is required in coping with family or social problems.

The counseling Z codes/categories:

Z30.0-	Encounter for general counseling and advice on contraception
Z31.5	Encounter for procreative genetic counseling
Z31.6-	Encounter for general counseling and advice on procreation
Z32.2	Encounter for childbirth instruction
Z32.3	Encounter for childcare instruction
Z69	Encounter for mental health services for victim and perpetrator of abuse
Z70	Counseling related to sexual attitude, behavior and orientation
Z71	Persons encountering health services for other counseling and medical advice, not elsewhere classified

Note: Code Z71.84, Encounter for health counseling related to travel, is to be used for health risk and safety counseling for future travel purposes.

Code Z71.85, Encounter for immunization safety counseling, is to be used for counseling of the patient or caregiver regarding the safety of a vaccine. This code should not be used for the provision of general information regarding risks and potential side effects during routine encounters for the administration of vaccines.

Code Z71.87, Encounter for pediatric-to-adult transition counseling, should be assigned when pediatric-to-adult transition counseling is the sole reason for the encounter or when this counseling is provided in addition to other services, such as treatment of a chronic condition. If both transition counseling and treatment of a medical condition are provided during the same encounter, the code(s) for the medical condition(s) treated and code Z71.87 should be assigned, with sequencing depending on the circumstances of the encounter.

Z76.81	Expectant mother prebirth pediatrician visit

11) Encounters for obstetrical and reproductive services

See Section I.C.15. Pregnancy, Childbirth, and the Puerperium, for further instruction on the use of these codes.

Z codes for pregnancy are for use in those circumstances when none of the problems or complications included in the codes from the Obstetrics chapter exist (a routine prenatal visit or postpartum care). Codes in category Z34, Encounter for supervision of normal pregnancy, are always first-listed and are not to be used with any other code from the OB chapter.

Codes in category Z3A, Weeks of gestation, may be assigned to provide additional information about the pregnancy. Category Z3A codes should not be assigned for pregnancies with abortive outcomes (categories O00-O08), elective termination of pregnancy (code O33.2), nor for postpartum conditions, as category Z3A is not applicable to these conditions. The date of the admission should be used to determine weeks of gestation for inpatient admissions that encompass more than one gestational week.

The outcome of delivery, category Z37, should be included on all maternal delivery records. It is always a secondary code.

Codes in category Z37 should not be used on the newborn record.

Z codes for family planning (contraceptive) or procreative management and counseling should be included on an obstetric record either during the pregnancy or the postpartum stage, if applicable.

Z codes/categories for obstetrical and reproductive services:

Z30	Encounter for contraceptive management
Z31	Encounter for procreative management
Z32.2	Encounter for childbirth instruction

Z32.3	Encounter for childcare instruction
Z33	Pregnant state
Z34	Encounter for supervision of normal pregnancy
Z36	Encounter for antenatal screening of mother
Z3A	Weeks of gestation
Z37	Outcome of delivery
Z39	Encounter for maternal postpartum care and examination
Z76.81	Expectant mother prebirth pediatrician visit

12) Newborns and infants

See Section I.C.16. Newborn (Perinatal) Guidelines, for further instruction on the use of these codes.

Newborn Z codes/categories:

Z76.1	Encounter for health supervision and care of foundling
Z00.1-	Encounter for routine child health examination
Z38	Liveborn infants according to place of birth and type of delivery

13) Routine and administrative examinations

The Z codes allow for the description of encounters for routine examinations, such as, a general check-up, or, examinations for administrative purposes, such as, a pre-employment physical. The codes are not to be used if the examination is for diagnosis of a suspected condition or for treatment purposes. In such cases the diagnosis code is used. During a routine exam, should a diagnosis or condition be discovered, it should be coded as an additional code. Pre-existing and chronic conditions and history codes may also be included as additional codes as long as the examination is for administrative purposes and not focused on any particular condition.

Some of the codes for routine health examinations distinguish between "with" and "without" abnormal findings. Code assignment depends on the information that is known at the time the encounter is being coded. For example, if no abnormal findings were found during the examination, but the encounter is being coded before test results are back, it is acceptable to assign the code for "without abnormal findings." When assigning a code for "with abnormal findings," additional code(s) should be assigned to identify the specific abnormal finding(s).

12-month-old boy presented for well-child visit; pediatrician notices some eczema on the child's scalp and back of the knees

Z00.121   Encounter for routine child health examination with abnormal findings

L30.9   Dermatitis, unspecified

Explanation: The Z code identifying that this is a routine well-child visit is reported first. Because an abnormal finding (eczema) was documented, a code for this condition may also be appended.

Pre-operative examination and pre-procedural laboratory examination Z codes are for use only in those situations when a patient is being cleared for a procedure or surgery and no treatment is given.

The Z codes/categories for routine and administrative examinations:

Z00	Encounter for general examination without complaint, suspected or reported diagnosis
Z01	Encounter for other special examination without complaint, suspected or reported diagnosis
Z02	Encounter for administrative examination
	Except: Z02.9, Encounter for administrative examinations, unspecified
Z32.0-	Encounter for pregnancy test

14) Miscellaneous Z codes

The miscellaneous Z codes capture a number of other health care encounters that do not fall into one of the other categories. Some of these codes identify the reason for the encounter; others are for use as additional codes that provide useful information on circumstances that may affect a patient's care and treatment.

Prophylactic organ removal

For encounters specifically for prophylactic removal of an organ (such as prophylactic removal of breasts due to a genetic susceptibility to cancer or a family history of cancer), the principal or first-listed code should be a code from category Z40, Encounter for prophylactic surgery, followed by the appropriate codes to identify the associated risk factor (such as genetic susceptibility or family history).

If the patient has a malignancy of one site and is having prophylactic removal at another site to prevent either a new primary malignancy or metastatic disease, a code for the malignancy should also be assigned in addition to a code from subcategory Z40.0, Encounter for prophylactic surgery for risk factors related to malignant neoplasms. A Z40.0 code should not be assigned if the patient is having organ removal for treatment of a malignancy, such as the removal of the testes for the treatment of prostate cancer.

Miscellaneous Z codes/categories:

Z28	Immunization not carried out
	Except: Z28.3-, Underimmunization status
Z29	Encounter for other prophylactic measures
Z40	Encounter for prophylactic surgery
Z41	Encounter for procedures for purposes other than remedying health state
	Except: Z41.9, Encounter for procedure for purposes other than remedying health state, unspecified
Z53	Persons encountering health services for specific procedures and treatment, not carried out
Z72	Problems related to lifestyle
	Note: These codes should be assigned only when the documentation specifies that the patient has an associated problem
Z73	Problems related to life management difficulty
	Note: These codes should be assigned only when the documentation specifies that the patient has an associated problem.
Z74	Problems related to care provider dependency
	Except: Z74.01, Bed confinement status
Z75	Problems related to medical facilities and other health care
Z76.0	Encounter for issue of repeat prescription
Z76.3	Healthy person accompanying sick person
Z76.4	Other boarder to healthcare facility
Z76.5	Malingerer [conscious simulation]
Z91.1-	Patient's noncompliance with medical treatment and regimen
Z91.83	Wandering in diseases classified elsewhere
Z91.84-	Oral health risk factors
Z91.89	Other specified personal risk factors, not elsewhere classified

See Section I.B.14. for Z55-Z65 Persons with potential health hazards related to socioeconomic and psychosocial circumstances, documentation by clinicians other than the patient's provider

15) Nonspecific Z codes

Certain Z codes are so non-specific, or potentially redundant with other codes in the classification, that there can be little justification for their use in the inpatient setting. Their use in the outpatient setting should be limited to those instances when there is no further documentation to permit more precise coding. Otherwise, any sign or symptom or any other reason for visit that is captured in another code should be used.

Nonspecific Z codes/categories:

Z02.9	Encounter for administrative examinations, unspecified
Z04.9	Encounter for examination and observation for unspecified reason
Z13.9	Encounter for screening, unspecified
Z41.9	Encounter for procedure for purposes other than remedying health state, unspecified
Z52.9	Donor of unspecified organ or tissue
Z86.59	Personal history of other mental and behavioral disorders
Z88.9	Allergy status to unspecified drugs, medicaments and biological substances status
Z92.0	Personal history of contraception

16) Z codes that may only be principal/first-listed diagnosis

The following Z codes/categories may only be reported as the principal/first-listed diagnosis, except when there are multiple encounters on the same day and the medical records for the encounters are combined:

Z00	Encounter for general examination without complaint, suspected or reported diagnosis
	Except: Z00.6
Z01	Encounter for other special examination without complaint, suspected or reported diagnosis
Z02	Encounter for administrative examination
Z04	Encounter for examination and observation for other reasons
Z33.2	Encounter for elective termination of pregnancy
Z31.81	Encounter for male factor infertility in female patient
Z31.83	Encounter for assisted reproductive fertility procedure cycle
Z31.84	Encounter for fertility preservation procedure
Z34	Encounter for supervision of normal pregnancy
Z39	Encounter for maternal postpartum care and examination
Z38	Liveborn infants according to place of birth and type of delivery
Z40	Encounter for prophylactic surgery
Z42	Encounter for plastic and reconstructive surgery following medical procedure or healed injury
Z51.0	Encounter for antineoplastic radiation therapy
Z51.1-	Encounter for antineoplastic chemotherapy and immunotherapy
Z52	Donors of organs and tissues
	Except: Z52.9, Donor of unspecified organ or tissue
Z76.1	Encounter for health supervision and care of foundling
Z76.2	Encounter for health supervision and care of other healthy infant and child
Z99.12	Encounter for respirator [ventilator] dependence during power failure

Female patient seen at 32 weeks' gestation to check the progress of her first pregnancy

Z34.03	**Encounter for supervision of normal first pregnancy, third trimester**
Z3A.32	**32 weeks gestation of pregnancy**

Explanation: Category Z34 is appropriate as a first-listed diagnosis. Category Z3A helps to clarify at which point in the pregnancy the patient was provided supervision.

17) Social determinants of health

Codes describing **problems or risk factors related to** social determinants of health (SDOH) should be assigned when this information is documented. **Assign as many SDOH codes as are necessary to describe all of the problems or risk factors. These codes should be assigned only when the documentation specifies that the patient has an associated problem or risk factor. For example, not every individual living alone would be assigned code Z60.2, Problems related to living alone.**

For social determinants of health, such as information found in categories Z55-Z65, Persons with potential health hazards related to socioeconomic and psychosocial circumstances, code assignment may be based on medical record documentation from clinicians involved in the care of the patient who are not the patient's provider since this information represents social information, rather than medical diagnoses.

For example, coding professionals may utilize documentation of social information from social workers, community health workers, case managers, or nurses, if their documentation is included in the official medical record.

Patient self-reported documentation may be used to assign codes for social determinants of health, as long as the patient self-reported information is signed-off by and incorporated into the medical record by either a clinician or provider.

Social determinants of health codes are located primarily in these Z code categories:

Z55	Problems related to education and literacy
Z56	Problems related to employment and unemployment
Z57	Occupational exposure to risk factors
Z58	Problems related to physical environment
Z59	Problems related to housing and economic circumstances
Z60	Problems related to social environment
Z62	Problems related to upbringing
Z63	Other problems related to primary support group, including family circumstances
Z64	Problems related to certain psychosocial circumstances
Z65	Problems related to other psychosocial circumstances

See Section I.B.14. Documentation by Clinicians Other than the Patient's Provider.

Z3A.25 = 25 weeks pregnancy
Z3A.32 = 32 weeks pregnancy

Chapter 21. Factors Influencing Health Status and Contact With Health Services (Z00-Z99)

NOTE   Z codes represent reasons for encounters. A corresponding procedure code must accompany a Z code if a procedure is performed. Categories Z00-Z99 are provided for occasions when circumstances other than a disease, injury or external cause classifiable to categories A00-Y89 are recorded as "diagnoses" or "problems." This can arise in two main ways:

(a) When a person who may or may not be sick encounters the health services for some specific purpose, such as to receive limited care or service for a current condition, to donate an organ or tissue, to receive prophylactic vaccination (immunization), or to discuss a problem which is in itself not a disease or injury.

(b) When some circumstance or problem is present which influences the person's health status but is not in itself a current illness or injury.

AHA: 2018,4Q,60-61

This chapter contains the following blocks:

Z00-Z13	Persons encountering health services for examinations
Z14-Z15	Genetic carrier and genetic susceptibility to disease
Z16	Resistance to antimicrobial drugs
Z17	Estrogen receptor status
Z18	Retained foreign body fragments
Z19	Hormone sensitivity malignancy status
Z20-Z29	Persons with potential health hazards related to communicable diseases
Z30-Z39	Persons encountering health services in circumstances related to reproduction
Z40-Z53	Encounters for other specific health care
Z55-Z65	Persons with potential health hazards related to socioeconomic and psychosocial circumstances
Z66	Do not resuscitate status
Z67	Blood type
Z68	Body mass index (BMI)
Z69-Z76	Persons encountering health services in other circumstances
Z77-Z99	Persons with potential health hazards related to family and personal history and certain conditions influencing health status

Persons encountering health services for examinations (Z00-Z13)

NOTE   Nonspecific abnormal findings disclosed at the time of these examinations are classified to categories R70-R94.

EXCLUDES 1   examinations related to pregnancy and reproduction (Z30-Z36, Z39.-)

✓4ᵗʰ **Z00**   **Encounter for general examination without complaint, suspected or reported diagnosis**

EXCLUDES 1   encounter for examination for administrative purposes (Z02.-)

EXCLUDES 2   encounter for pre-procedural examinations (Z01.81-)
special screening examinations (Z11-Z13)

AHA: 2017,4Q,95

✓5ᵗʰ **Z00.0**   **Encounter for general adult medical examination**

Encounter for adult periodic examination (annual) (physical) and any associated laboratory and radiologic examinations

EXCLUDES 1   encounter for examination of sign or symptom - code to sign or symptom
general health check-up of infant or child (Z00.12.-)

Z00.00   **Encounter for general adult medical examination without abnormal findings** PDx A

[handwritten: Routine X-ray]

Encounter for adult health check-up NOS

AHA: 2016,1Q,36

Z00.01   **Encounter for general adult medical examination with abnormal findings** PDx A

Use additional code to identify abnormal findings

AHA: 2016,1Q,35-36

✓5ᵗʰ **Z00.1**   **Encounter for newborn, infant and child health examinations**

✓6ᵗʰ **Z00.11**   **Newborn health examination**

Health check for child under 29 days old

Use additional code to identify any abnormal findings

EXCLUDES 1   health check for child over 28 days old (Z00.12-)

Z00.110   **Health examination for newborn under 8 days old** PDx N

Health check for newborn under 8 days old

Z00.111   **Health examination for newborn 8 to 28 days old** PDx N

Health check for newborn 8 to 28 days old
Newborn weight check

[handwritten left margin: nonprog 28 weeks 86 ... pregre ?< deeer ...]

✓6ᵗʰ **Z00.12**   **Encounter for routine child health examination**

Health check (routine) for child over 28 days old
Immunizations appropriate for age
Routine developmental screening of infant or child
Routine vison and hearing testing

EXCLUDES 1   health check for child under 29 days old (Z00.11-)
health supervision of foundling or other healthy infant or child (Z76.1-Z76.2)
newborn health examination (Z00.11-)

AHA: 2018,4Q,36

Z00.121   **Encounter for routine child health examination with abnormal findings** PDx P

Use additional code to identify abnormal findings

AHA: 2016,1Q,34-35

Z00.129   **Encounter for routine child health examination without abnormal findings** PDx P

Encounter for routine child health examination NOS

AHA: 2016,1Q,34

Z00.2   **Encounter for examination for period of rapid growth in childhood** PDx P

Z00.3   **Encounter for examination for adolescent development state** PDx P

Encounter for puberty development state

Z00.5   **Encounter for examination of potential donor of organ and tissue** PDx

Z00.6   **Encounter for examination for normal comparison and control in clinical research program**

Examination of participant or control in clinical research program

✓5ᵗʰ **Z00.7**   **Encounter for examination for period of delayed growth in childhood**

Z00.70   **Encounter for examination for period of delayed growth in childhood without abnormal findings** PDx P

Z00.71   **Encounter for examination for period of delayed growth in childhood with abnormal findings** PDx P

Use additional code to identify abnormal findings

Z00.8   **Encounter for other general examination** PDx

Encounter for health examination in population surveys

✓4ᵗʰ **Z01**   **Encounter for other special examination without complaint, suspected or reported diagnosis**

INCLUDES   routine examination of specific system

NOTE   Codes from category Z01 represent the reason for the encounter. A separate procedure code is required to identify any examinations or procedures performed

EXCLUDES 1   encounter for examination for administrative purposes (Z02.-)
encounter for examination for suspected conditions, proven not to exist (Z03.-)
encounter for laboratory and radiologic examinations as a component of general medical examinations (Z00.0-)
encounter for laboratory, radiologic and imaging examinations for sign(s) and symptom(s) - code to the sign(s) or symptom(s)

EXCLUDES 2   screening examinations (Z11-Z13)

✓5ᵗʰ **Z01.0**   **Encounter for examination of eyes and vision**

EXCLUDES 1   examination for driving license (Z02.4)

[handwritten: Primary never additional]

Z01.00   **Encounter for examination of eyes and vision without abnormal findings** PDx

Encounter for examination of eyes and vision NOS

Z01.01   **Encounter for examination of eyes and vision with abnormal findings** PDx

Use additional code to identify abnormal findings

AHA: 2016,4Q,21

HCC CMS-HCC   Rx Rx HCC   ESR ESRD HCC   COM Commercial HCC   PDx Primary Dx Only   N Newborn: 0   P Pediatric: 0-17   M Maternity: 9-64   A Adult: 15-124

1264   ICD-10-CM 2023

☑6ᵗʰ **Z01.02 Encounter for examination of eyes and vision following failed vision screening**
　　EXCLUDES 1　*encounter for examination of eyes and vision with abnormal findings (Z01.01)*
　　encounter for examination of eyes and vision without abnormal findings (Z01.00)
　　AHA: 2019,4Q,20

Z01.020 Encounter for examination of eyes and vision following failed vision screening without abnormal findings PDx

Z01.021 Encounter for examination of eyes and vision following failed vision screening with abnormal findings PDx
　　Use additional code to identify abnormal findings

☑5ᵗʰ **Z01.1 Encounter for examination of ears and hearing**

Z01.10 Encounter for examination of ears and hearing without abnormal findings PDx
　　Encounter for examination of ears and hearing NOS
　　AHA: 2016,4Q,24

☑6ᵗʰ **Z01.11 Encounter for examination of ears and hearing with abnormal findings**
　　AHA: 2016,3Q,17-18

Z01.110 Encounter for hearing examination following failed hearing screening

Z01.118 Encounter for examination of ears and hearing with other abnormal findings PDx
　　Use additional code to identify abnormal findings

Z01.12 Encounter for hearing conservation and treatment PDx

☑5ᵗʰ **Z01.2 Encounter for dental examination and cleaning**

Z01.20 Encounter for dental examination and cleaning without abnormal findings PDx
　　Encounter for dental examination and cleaning NOS

Z01.21 Encounter for dental examination and cleaning with abnormal findings PDx
　　Use additional code to identify abnormal findings

☑5ᵗʰ **Z01.3 Encounter for examination of blood pressure**

Z01.30 Encounter for examination of blood pressure without abnormal findings PDx
　　Encounter for examination of blood pressure NOS

Z01.31 Encounter for examination of blood pressure with abnormal findings PDx
　　Use additional code to identify abnormal findings

☑5ᵗʰ **Z01.4 Encounter for gynecological examination**
　　EXCLUDES 2　*pregnancy examination or test (Z32.0-)*
　　routine examination for contraceptive maintenance (Z30.4-)

☑6ᵗʰ **Z01.41 Encounter for routine gynecological examination**
　　Encounter for general gynecological examination with or without cervical smear
　　Encounter for gynecological examination (general) (routine) NOS
　　Encounter for pelvic examination (annual) (periodic)
　　Use additional code:
　　　for screening for human papillomavirus, if applicable, (Z11.51)
　　　for screening vaginal pap smear, if applicable (Z12.72)
　　　to identify acquired absence of uterus, if applicable (Z90.71-)
　　EXCLUDES 1　*gynecologic examination status-post hysterectomy for malignant condition (Z08)*
　　screening cervical pap smear not a part of a routine gynecological examination (Z12.4)

Z01.411 Encounter for gynecological examination (general) (routine) with abnormal findings PDx ♀
　　Use additional code to identify abnormal findings

Z01.419 Encounter for gynecological examination (general) (routine) without abnormal findings PDx ♀

Z01.42 Encounter for cervical smear to confirm findings of recent normal smear following initial abnormal smear PDx ♀

☑5ᵗʰ **Z01.8 Encounter for other specified special examinations**

☑6ᵗʰ **Z01.81 Encounter for preprocedural examinations**
　　Encounter for preoperative examinations
　　Encounter for radiological and imaging examinations as part of preprocedural examination
　　TIP: Assign a code for the condition necessitating surgery and any findings as additional diagnoses.

Z01.810 Encounter for preprocedural cardiovascular examination PDx

Z01.811 Encounter for preprocedural respiratory examination PDx

Z01.812 Encounter for preprocedural laboratory examination PDx
　　Blood and urine tests prior to treatment or procedure
　　AHA: 2020,3Q,14
　　TIP: During the COVID-19 pandemic, assign this code followed by code Z20.822 Contact with and (suspected) exposure to COVID-19, when COVID-19 testing is being performed as part of preoperative testing.

Z01.818 Encounter for other preprocedural examination PDx
　　Encounter for preprocedural examination NOS
　　Encounter for examinations prior to antineoplastic chemotherapy

Z01.82 Encounter for allergy testing PDx
　　EXCLUDES 1　*encounter for antibody response examination (Z01.84)*

Z01.83 Encounter for blood typing PDx
　　Encounter for Rh typing

Z01.84 Encounter for antibody response examination PDx
　　Encounter for immunity status testing
　　EXCLUDES 1　*encounter for allergy testing (Z01.82)*
　　AHA: 2020,2Q,11

Z01.89 Encounter for other specified special examinations PDx

☑4ᵗʰ **Z02 Encounter for administrative examination**

Z02.0 Encounter for examination for admission to educational institution PDx
　　Encounter for examination for admission to preschool (education)
　　Encounter for examination for re-admission to school following illness or medical treatment

Z02.1 Encounter for pre-employment examination PDx

Z02.2 Encounter for examination for admission to residential institution PDx
　　EXCLUDES 1　*examination for admission to prison (Z02.89)*

Z02.3 Encounter for examination for recruitment to armed forces PDx

Z02.4 Encounter for examination for driving license PDx

Z02.5 Encounter for examination for participation in sport PDx
　　EXCLUDES 1　*blood-alcohol and blood-drug test (Z02.83)*

Z02.6 Encounter for examination for insurance purposes PDx

☑5ᵗʰ **Z02.7 Encounter for issue of medical certificate**
　　EXCLUDES 1　*encounter for general medical examination (Z00-Z01, Z02.0-Z02.6, Z02.8-Z02.9)*

Z02.71 Encounter for disability determination PDx
　　Encounter for issue of medical certificate of incapacity
　　Encounter for issue of medical certificate of invalidity

Z02.79 Encounter for issue of other medical certificate PDx

☑5ᵗʰ **Z02.8 Encounter for other administrative examinations**

Z02.81 Encounter for paternity testing PDx

Z02.82 Encounter for adoption services PDx

Z02.83 **Encounter for blood-alcohol and blood-drug test** `PDx`

Use additional code for findings of alcohol or drugs in blood (R78.-)

Z02.89 **Encounter for other administrative examinations** `PDx`

Encounter for examination for admission to prison

Encounter for examination for admission to summer camp

Encounter for immigration examination

Encounter for naturalization examination

Encounter for premarital examination

> `EXCLUDES 1` health supervision of foundling or other healthy infant or child (Z76.1-Z76.2)

Z02.9 **Encounter for administrative examinations, unspecified** `PDx`

never secondary Dx

√4ᵗʰ **Z03** **Encounter for medical observation for suspected diseases and conditions ruled out**

observation

Ruled out

This category is to be used when a person without a diagnosis is suspected of having an abnormal condition, without signs or symptoms, which requires study, but after examination and observation, is ruled out. This category is also for use for administrative and legal observation status.

> `EXCLUDES 1` contact with and (suspected) exposures hazardous to health (Z77.-)
>
> encounter for observation and evaluation of newborn for suspected diseases and conditions ruled out (Z05.-)
>
> person with feared complaint in whom no diagnosis is made (Z71.1)
>
> signs or symptoms under study - code to signs or symptoms

AHA: 2020,2Q,8; 2018,2Q,7-8; 2017,4Q,27

Z03.6 **Encounter for observation for suspected toxic effect from ingested substance ruled out**

Encounter for observation for suspected adverse effect from drug

Encounter for observation for suspected poisoning

√5ᵗʰ **Z03.7** **Encounter for suspected maternal and fetal conditions ruled out**

Can't use with screening

Encounter for suspected maternal and fetal conditions not found

> `EXCLUDES 1` known or suspected fetal anomalies affecting management of mother, not ruled out (O26.-, O35.-, O36.-, O40.-, O41.-)

Z03.71 **Encounter for suspected problem with amniotic cavity and membrane ruled out** `M` `♀`

Encounter for suspected oligohydramnios ruled out

Encounter for suspected polyhydramnios ruled out

Z03.72 **Encounter for suspected placental problem ruled out** `M` `♀`

Suspected but normal

Z03.73 **Encounter for suspected fetal anomaly ruled out** `M` `♀`

Z03.74 **Encounter for suspected problem with fetal growth ruled out** `M` `♀`

Z03.75 **Encounter for suspected cervical shortening ruled out** `M` `♀`

Z03.79 **Encounter for other suspected maternal and fetal conditions ruled out** `M` `♀`

√5ᵗʰ **Z03.8** **Encounter for observation for other suspected diseases and conditions ruled out**

√6ᵗʰ **Z03.81** **Encounter for observation for suspected exposure to biological agents ruled out**

Z03.810 **Encounter for observation for suspected exposure to anthrax ruled out**

Z03.818 **Encounter for observation for suspected exposure to other biological agents ruled out**

AHA: 2020,2Q,8; 2020,1Q,34-36

TIP: During the COVID-19 pandemic, possible exposure to COVID-19 should be coded using Z20.822 Contact with and (suspected) exposure to COVID-19, even when the COVID-19 infection has been ruled out.

√6ᵗʰ **Z03.82** **Encounter for observation for suspected foreign body ruled out**

> `EXCLUDES 1` retained foreign body (Z18.-)
>
> retained foreign body in eyelid (H02.81)
>
> residual foreign body in soft tissue (M79.5)
>
> `EXCLUDES 2` confirmed foreign body ingestion or aspiration including:
>
> foreign body in alimentary tract (T18)
>
> foreign body in ear (T16)
>
> foreign body on external eye (T15)
>
> foreign body in respiratory tract (T17)

AHA: 2020,4Q,42

Z03.821 **Encounter for observation for suspected ingested foreign body ruled out**

Z03.822 **Encounter for observation for suspected aspirated (inhaled) foreign body ruled out**

Z03.823 **Encounter for observation for suspected inserted (injected) foreign body ruled out**

Encounter for observation for suspected inserted (injected) foreign body in eye ruled out

Encounter for observation for suspected inserted (injected) foreign body in orifice ruled out

Encounter for observation for suspected inserted (injected) foreign body in skin ruled out

Z03.83 **Encounter for observation for suspected conditions related to home physiologic monitoring device ruled out**

Encounter for observation for apnea alarm without findings

Encounter for observation for bradycardia alarm without findings

Encounter for observation for malfunction of home cardiorespiratory monitor

Encounter for observation for non-specific findings home physiologic monitoring device

Encounter for observation for pulse oximeter alarm without findings

> `EXCLUDES 1` apnea NOS (R06.81)
>
> neonatal bradycardia (P29.12)
>
> newborn apnea (P28.4-)
>
> primary sleep apnea of newborn (P28.3-)
>
> sleep apnea (G47.3-)

Z03.89 **Encounter for observation for other suspected diseases and conditions ruled out**

√4ᵗʰ **Z04** **Encounter for examination and observation for other reasons**

primary Dx

> `INCLUDES` encounter for examination for medicolegal reasons

This category is to be used when a person without a diagnosis is suspected of having an abnormal condition, without signs or symptoms, which requires study, but after examination and observation, is ruled-out. This category is also for use for administrative and legal observation status.

AHA: 2018,2Q,7-8

Z04.1 **Encounter for examination and observation following transport accident** `PDx`

> `EXCLUDES 1` encounter for examination and observation following work accident (Z04.2)

AHA: 2019,2Q,11; 2018,2Q,8

Z04.2 **Encounter for examination and observation following work accident** `PDx`

Z04.3 **Encounter for examination and observation following other accident** `PDx`

√5ᵗʰ **Z04.4** **Encounter for examination and observation following alleged rape**

Encounter for examination and observation of victim following alleged rape

Encounter for examination and observation of victim following alleged sexual abuse

Z04.41 **Encounter for examination and observation following alleged adult rape** `PDx` `A`

Suspected adult rape, ruled out

Suspected adult sexual abuse, ruled out

`HCC` CMS-HCC   `Rx` Rx HCC   `ESR` ESRD HCC   `COM` Commercial HCC   `PDx` Primary Dx Only   `N` Newborn: 0   `P` Pediatric: 0-17   `M` Maternity: 9-64   `A` Adult: 15-124

1266   ICD-10-CM 2023

Z04.42   Encounter for examination and observation following alleged **child rape** `PDx` `P`
- Suspected child rape, ruled out
- Suspected child sexual abuse, ruled out

Z04.6   Encounter for **general psychiatric examination, requested by authority** `PDx`

✓5th Z04.7   Encounter for examination and observation following **alleged physical abuse**

     Z04.71   Encounter for examination and observation following alleged **adult physical abuse** `PDx` `A`
- Suspected adult physical abuse, ruled out
  - `EXCLUDES 1`   confirmed case of adult physical abuse (T74.-)
  - encounter for examination and observation following alleged adult sexual abuse (Z04.41)
  - suspected case of adult physical abuse, not ruled out (T76.-)

     Z04.72   Encounter for examination and observation following alleged **child physical abuse** `PDx` `P`
- Suspected child physical abuse, ruled out
  - `EXCLUDES 1`   confirmed case of child physical abuse (T74.-)
  - encounter for examination and observation following alleged child sexual abuse (Z04.42)
  - suspected case of child physical abuse, not ruled out (T76.-)

✓5th Z04.8   Encounter for examination and observation for **other specified reasons**
- Encounter for examination and observation for request for expert evidence
- AHA: 2018,4Q,32,35,72

     Z04.81   Encounter for examination and observation of **victim following forced sexual exploitation** `PDx`

     Z04.82   Encounter for examination and observation of **victim following forced labor exploitation** `PDx`

     Z04.89   Encounter for examination and observation for **other specified reasons** `PDx`

Z04.9   Encounter for examination and observation for unspecified reason `PDx`
- Encounter for observation NOS

✓4th Z05   Encounter for observation and evaluation of newborn for **suspected diseases and conditions ruled out**
- This category is to be used for newborns, within the neonatal period (the first 28 days of life), who are suspected of having an abnormal condition, but without signs or symptoms, and which, after examination and observation, is ruled out.
- AHA: 2022,1Q,17-18; 2017,4Q,27; 2016,4Q,77

     Z05.0   Observation and evaluation of newborn for suspected **cardiac** condition ruled out `N`

     Z05.1   Observation and evaluation of newborn for suspected **infectious** condition ruled out `N`
- AHA: 2019,2Q,10

     Z05.2   Observation and evaluation of newborn for suspected **neurological** condition ruled out `N`

     Z05.3   Observation and evaluation of newborn for suspected **respiratory** condition ruled out `N`

✓5th Z05.4   Observation and evaluation of newborn for suspected **genetic, metabolic or immunologic** condition ruled out

     Z05.41   Observation and evaluation of newborn for suspected **genetic** condition ruled out `N`
- AHA: 2016,4Q,55

     Z05.42   Observation and evaluation of newborn for suspected **metabolic** condition ruled out `N`

     Z05.43   Observation and evaluation of newborn for suspected **immunologic** condition ruled out `N`

     Z05.5   Observation and evaluation of newborn for suspected **gastrointestinal** condition ruled out `N`

     Z05.6   Observation and evaluation of newborn for suspected **genitourinary** condition ruled out `N`

✓5th Z05.7   Observation and evaluation of newborn for suspected **skin, subcutaneous, musculoskeletal and connective tissue** condition ruled out

     Z05.71   Observation and evaluation of newborn for suspected **skin and subcutaneous tissue** condition ruled out `N`

     Z05.72   Observation and evaluation of newborn for suspected **musculoskeletal** condition ruled out `N`

     Z05.73   Observation and evaluation of newborn for suspected **connective tissue** condition ruled out `N`

Z05.8   Observation and evaluation of newborn for other specified suspected condition ruled out `N`
- AHA: 2022,1Q,17-18

Z05.9   Observation and evaluation of newborn for unspecified suspected condition ruled out `N`

Z08   Encounter for **follow-up examination after completed treatment for malignant neoplasm**
- Medical surveillance following completed treatment
- Use additional code to identify any acquired absence of organs (Z90.-)
- Use additional code to identify the personal history of malignant neoplasm (Z85.-)
  - `EXCLUDES 1`   aftercare following medical care (Z43-Z49, Z51)
- AHA: 2020,3Q,30

Z09   Encounter for **follow-up examination after completed treatment for conditions** other **than malignant neoplasm**
- Medical surveillance following completed treatment
- Use additional code to identify any applicable history of disease code (Z86.-, Z87.-)
  - `EXCLUDES 1`   aftercare following medical care (Z43-Z49, Z51)
  - surveillance of contraception (Z30.4-)
  - surveillance of prosthetic and other medical devices (Z44-Z46)
- AHA: 2021,1Q,33; 2020,2Q,10; 2017,1Q,9; 2015,1Q,8

✓4th Z11   Encounter for **screening for infectious and parasitic diseases**
- Screening is the testing for disease or disease precursors in asymptomatic individuals so that early detection and treatment can be provided for those who test positive for the disease.
  - `EXCLUDES 1`   encounter for diagnostic examination - code to sign or symptom

     Z11.0   Encounter for screening for **intestinal infectious diseases**

     Z11.1   Encounter for screening for **respiratory tuberculosis**
- Encounter for screening for active tuberculosis disease

     Z11.2   Encounter for screening for **other bacterial diseases**

     Z11.3   Encounter for screening for infections with a **predominantly sexual mode of transmission**
- `EXCLUDES 2`   encounter for screening for human immunodeficiency virus [HIV] (Z11.4)
- encounter for screening for human papillomavirus (Z11.51)

     Z11.4   Encounter for screening for **human immunodeficiency virus [HIV]**

✓5th Z11.5   Encounter for screening for **other viral diseases**
- `EXCLUDES 2`   encounter for screening for viral intestinal disease (Z11.0)

     Z11.51   Encounter for screening for **human papillomavirus (HPV)**

     Z11.52   Encounter for screening for **COVID-19**
- AHA: 2021,1Q,27,37,41
- TIP: This code is not appropriate for use during the pandemic phase of COVID-19. Use Z20.822 Contact with or (suspected) exposure to COVID-19, instead.

     Z11.59   Encounter for screening for **other viral diseases**
- AHA: 2020,3Q,14

     Z11.6   Encounter for screening for **other protozoal diseases and helminthiases**
- `EXCLUDES 2`   encounter for screening for protozoal intestinal disease (Z11.0)

     Z11.7   Encounter for testing for **latent tuberculosis infection**
- AHA: 2019,4Q,20

     Z11.8   Encounter for screening for **other infectious and parasitic diseases**
- Encounter for screening for chlamydia
- Encounter for screening for rickettsial
- Encounter for screening for spirochetal
- Encounter for screening for mycoses

     Z11.9   Encounter for screening for infectious and parasitic diseases, unspecified

✓4ᵗʰ Z12 Encounter for screening for malignant neoplasms

Screening is the testing for disease or disease precursors in asymptomatic individuals so that early detection and treatment can be provided for those who test positive for the disease.

Use additional code to identify any family history of malignant neoplasm (Z80.-)

> EXCLUDES 1 encounter for diagnostic examination - code to sign or symptom

Z12.Ø Encounter for screening for malignant neoplasm of stomach

✓5ᵗʰ Z12.1 Encounter for screening for malignant neoplasm of intestinal tract

AHA: 2017,1Q,8,9

Z12.1Ø Encounter for screening for malignant neoplasm of intestinal tract, unspecified

Z12.11 Encounter for screening for malignant neoplasm of colon ◨

Encounter for screening colonoscopy NOS

AHA: 2019,1Q,32-33; 2018,1Q,6

TIP: Surveillance colonoscopies are a type of screening exam used to screen for malignancies in those patients with history of polyps and/or cancer (previously removed). If polyps or cancer are removed during the colonoscopy, code the appropriate neoplasm code instead of Z12.11.

Z12.12 Encounter for screening for malignant neoplasm of rectum

AHA: 2018,1Q,6

Z12.13 Encounter for screening for malignant neoplasm of small intestine

Z12.2 Encounter for screening for malignant neoplasm of respiratory organs

✓5ᵗʰ Z12.3 Encounter for screening for malignant neoplasm of breast

Z12.31 Encounter for screening mammogram for malignant neoplasm of breast

> EXCLUDES 1 inconclusive mammogram (R92.2)

AHA: 2015,1Q,24

Z12.39 Encounter for other screening for malignant neoplasm of breast

Z12.4 Encounter for screening for malignant neoplasm of cervix ♀

Encounter for screening pap smear for malignant neoplasm of cervix

> EXCLUDES 1 when screening is part of general gynecological examination (Z01.4-)
>
> EXCLUDES 2 encounter for screening for human papillomavirus (Z11.51)

Z12.5 Encounter for screening for malignant neoplasm of prostate ♂

Z12.6 Encounter for screening for malignant neoplasm of bladder

✓5ᵗʰ Z12.7 Encounter for screening for malignant neoplasm of other genitourinary organs

Z12.71 Encounter for screening for malignant neoplasm of testis ♂

Z12.72 Encounter for screening for malignant neoplasm of vagina ♀

Vaginal pap smear status-post hysterectomy for non-malignant condition

Use additional code to identify acquired absence of uterus (Z90.71-)

> EXCLUDES 1 vaginal pap smear status-post hysterectomy for malignant conditions (Z08)

Z12.73 Encounter for screening for malignant neoplasm of ovary ♀

Z12.79 Encounter for screening for malignant neoplasm of other genitourinary organs

✓5ᵗʰ Z12.8 Encounter for screening for malignant neoplasm of other sites

Z12.81 Encounter for screening for malignant neoplasm of oral cavity

Z12.82 Encounter for screening for malignant neoplasm of nervous system

Z12.83 Encounter for screening for malignant neoplasm of skin

Z12.89 Encounter for screening for malignant neoplasm of other sites

AHA: 2021,1Q,14

Z12.9 Encounter for screening for malignant neoplasm, site unspecified

✓4ᵗʰ Z13 Encounter for screening for other diseases and disorders

Screening is the testing for disease or disease precursors in asymptomatic individuals so that early detection and treatment can be provided for those who test positive for the disease.

> EXCLUDES 1 encounter for diagnostic examination - code to sign or symptom

Z13.Ø Encounter for screening for diseases of the blood and blood-forming organs and certain disorders involving the immune mechanism

Z13.1 Encounter for screening for diabetes mellitus

✓5ᵗʰ Z13.2 Encounter for screening for nutritional, metabolic and other endocrine disorders

Z13.21 Encounter for screening for nutritional disorder

✓6ᵗʰ Z13.22 Encounter for screening for metabolic disorder

Z13.220 Encounter for screening for lipoid disorders

Encounter for screening for cholesterol level

Encounter for screening for hypercholesterolemia

Encounter for screening for hyperlipidemia

Z13.228 Encounter for screening for other metabolic disorders

Z13.29 Encounter for screening for other suspected endocrine disorder

> EXCLUDES 2 encounter for screening for diabetes mellitus (Z13.1)

✓5ᵗʰ Z13.3 Encounter for screening examination for mental health and behavioral disorders

AHA: 2018,4Q,35-36

Z13.3Ø Encounter for screening examination for mental health and behavioral disorders, unspecified

Z13.31 Encounter for screening for depression

Encounter for screening for depression, adult

Encounter for screening for depression for child or adolescent

Z13.32 Encounter for screening for maternal depression ♀

Encounter for screening for perinatal depression

Z13.39 Encounter for screening examination for other mental health and behavioral disorders

Encounter for screening for alcoholism

Encounter for screening for intellectual disabilities

✓5ᵗʰ Z13.4 Encounter for screening for certain developmental disorders in childhood

Encounter for development testing of infant or child

Encounter for screening for developmental handicaps in early childhood

> EXCLUDES 2 encounter for routine child health examination (Z00.12-)

AHA: 2018,4Q,36

Z13.4Ø Encounter for screening for unspecified developmental delays

Z13.41 Encounter for autism screening

Z13.42 Encounter for screening for global developmental delays (milestones)

Encounter for screening for developmental handicaps in early childhood

Z13.49 Encounter for screening for other developmental delays

Z13.5 Encounter for screening for eye and ear disorders

> EXCLUDES 2 encounter for general hearing examination (Z01.1-)
>
> encounter for general vision examination (Z01.0-)

AHA: 2016,3Q,17

Z13.6 Encounter for screening for cardiovascular disorders

✓5ᵗʰ Z13.7 Encounter for screening for genetic and chromosomal anomalies

> EXCLUDES 1 genetic testing for procreative management (Z31.4-)

Z13.71 Encounter for nonprocreative screening for genetic disease carrier status

Z13.79 Encounter for other screening for genetic and chromosomal anomalies

✓5ᵗʰ Z13.8 Encounter for screening for other specified diseases and disorders

> EXCLUDES 2 screening for malignant neoplasms (Z12.-)

✓6ᵗʰ Z13.81 Encounter for screening for digestive system disorders

Z13.81Ø Encounter for screening for upper gastrointestinal disorder

Z13.811 **Encounter for screening for** lower gastrointestinal **disorder**

EXCLUDES 1   *encounter for screening for intestinal infectious disease (Z11.0)*

Z13.818 **Encounter for screening for other digestive system disorders**

√6ᵗʰ Z13.82 **Encounter for screening for** musculoskeletal **disorder**

Z13.820 **Encounter for screening for** osteoporosis

Z13.828 **Encounter for screening for other musculoskeletal disorder**

Z13.83 **Encounter for screening for** respiratory **disorder NEC**

EXCLUDES 1   *encounter for screening for respiratory tuberculosis (Z11.1)*

Z13.84 **Encounter for screening for** dental **disorders**

√6ᵗʰ Z13.85 **Encounter for screening for** nervous system **disorders**

Z13.850 **Encounter for screening for** traumatic brain injury

Z13.858 **Encounter for screening for other nervous system disorders**

Z13.88 **Encounter for screening for disorder** due to exposure to contaminants

EXCLUDES 1   *those exposed to contaminants without suspected disorders (Z57.-, Z77.-)*

Z13.89 **Encounter for screening for other disorder**

Encounter for screening for genitourinary disorders

Z13.9 **Encounter for screening, unspecified**

Genetic carrier and genetic susceptibility to disease (Z14-Z15)

√4ᵗʰ Z14 **Genetic carrier**

DEF: Individuals carrying a gene mutation associated with a certain disease that typically do not develop the disease but are able to pass the mutated genes to offspring.

√5ᵗʰ Z14.0 **Hemophilia A carrier**

Z14.01 **Asymptomatic hemophilia A carrier**

Z14.02 **Symptomatic hemophilia A carrier**

Z14.1 **Cystic fibrosis carrier**

Z14.8 **Genetic carrier of other disease**

√4ᵗʰ Z15 **Genetic susceptibility to disease**

INCLUDES   confirmed abnormal gene

Use additional code, if applicable, for any associated family history of the disease (Z80-Z84)

EXCLUDES 1   *chromosomal anomalies (Q90-Q99)*

√5ᵗʰ Z15.0 **Genetic susceptibility to** malignant neoplasm   *[handwritten: risk 11]*

[handwritten: not primary code]

Code first, if applicable, any current malignant neoplasm (C00-C75, C81-C96)

Use additional code, if applicable, for any personal history of malignant neoplasm (Z85.-)

Z15.01 **Genetic susceptibility to malignant neoplasm of breast**

Z15.02 **Genetic susceptibility to malignant neoplasm of ovary** ♀

Z15.03 **Genetic susceptibility to malignant neoplasm of prostate** ♂

Z15.04 **Genetic susceptibility to malignant neoplasm of endometrium** ♀

Z15.09 **Genetic susceptibility to other malignant neoplasm**

AHA: 2021,1Q,14

√5ᵗʰ Z15.8 **Genetic susceptibility to other disease**

Z15.81 **Genetic susceptibility to** multiple endocrine neoplasia [MEN]

EXCLUDES 1   *multiple endocrine neoplasia [MEN] syndromes (E31.2-)*

DEF: Group of conditions in which several endocrine glands grow excessively (such as in adenomatous hyperplasia) and/or develop benign or malignant tumors. Tumors and hyperplasia associated with MEN often produce excess hormones, which impede normal physiology. There is no comprehensive cure known for MEN syndrome. Treatment is directed at the hyperplasia or tumors in each individual gland. Tumors are usually surgically removed and oral medications or hormonal injections are used to correct hormone imbalances.

Z15.89 **Genetic susceptibility to other disease**

Resistance to antimicrobial drugs (Z16)

√4ᵗʰ Z16 **Resistance to antimicrobial drugs**   *[handwritten: infection code first]*

NOTE   The codes in this category are provided for use as additional codes to identify the resistance and non-responsiveness of a condition to antimicrobial drugs.

Code first the infection

EXCLUDES 1   *Methicillin resistant Staphylococcus aureus infection (A49.02)*
Methicillin resistant Staphylococcus aureus pneumonia (J15.212)
sepsis due to Methicillin resistant Staphylococcus aureus (A41.02)

√5ᵗʰ Z16.1 **Resistance to** beta lactam **antibiotics**

Z16.10 **Resistance to unspecified beta lactam antibiotics**   UPD

Z16.11 **Resistance to** penicillins   UPD

Resistance to amoxicillin
Resistance to ampicillin

Z16.12 **Extended spectrum beta lactamase (ESBL) resistance**   UPD

EXCLUDES 2   *Methicillin resistant Staphylococcus aureus infection in diseases classified elsewhere (B95.62)*

Z16.19 **Resistance to other specified beta lactam antibiotics**   UPD

Resistance to cephalosporins

√5ᵗʰ Z16.2 **Resistance to other antibiotics**

Z16.20 **Resistance to unspecified antibiotic**   UPD

Resistance to antibiotics NOS

Z16.21 **Resistance to** vancomycin   UPD

Z16.22 **Resistance to** vancomycin related **antibiotics**   UPD

Z16.23 **Resistance to** quinolones and fluoroquinolones   UPD

Z16.24 **Resistance to** multiple **antibiotics**   UPD

Z16.29 **Resistance to other single specified antibiotic**   UPD

Resistance to aminoglycosides
Resistance to macrolides
Resistance to sulfonamides
Resistance to tetracyclines

√5ᵗʰ Z16.3 **Resistance to other antimicrobial drugs**

EXCLUDES 1   *resistance to antibiotics (Z16.1-, Z16.2-)*

Z16.30 **Resistance to unspecified antimicrobial drugs**   UPD

Drug resistance NOS

Z16.31 **Resistance to** antiparasitic **drug(s)**   UPD

Resistance to quinine and related compounds

Z16.32 **Resistance to** antifungal **drug(s)**   UPD

Z16.33 **Resistance to** antiviral **drug(s)**   UPD

√6ᵗʰ Z16.34 **Resistance to** antimycobacterial **drug(s)**

Resistance to tuberculostatics

Z16.341 **Resistance to** single **antimycobacterial drug**

Resistance to antimycobacterial drug NOS

Z16.342 **Resistance to** multiple **antimycobacterial drugs**   UPD

Z16.35 **Resistance to** multiple **antimicrobial drugs**   UPD

EXCLUDES 1   *resistance to multiple antibiotics only (Z16.24)*

Z16.39 **Resistance to other specified antimicrobial drug**   UPD

Estrogen receptor status (Z17)

√4ᵗʰ Z17 **Estrogen receptor status**

Code first malignant neoplasm of breast (C50.-)

DEF: Receptor status of breast cancer cells for the hormone estrogen that is used to help determine treatment and evaluate prognosis. ER+ breast cancer responds to hormone therapies while ER- breast cancer does not.

Z17.0 **Estrogen receptor** positive **status [ER+]**   UPD

Z17.1 **Estrogen receptor** negative **status [ER-]**   UPD

Retained foreign body fragments (Z18)

✓4ᵗʰ **Z18 Retained foreign body fragments**

INCLUDES embedded fragment (status)
embedded splinter (status)
retained foreign body status

EXCLUDES 1 artificial joint prosthesis status (Z96.6-)
foreign body accidentally left during a procedure (T81.5-)
foreign body entering through orifice (T15-T19)
in situ cardiac device (Z95.-)
organ or tissue replaced by means other than transplant (Z96.-, Z97.-)
organ or tissue replaced by transplant (Z94.-)
personal history of retained foreign body fully removed Z87.821
superficial foreign body (non-embedded splinter) - code to superficial foreign body, by site

DEF: Embedded or retained fragment, splinter, or foreign body, natural or synthetic that can cause infection.

✓5ᵗʰ **Z18.0 Retained radioactive fragments**

Z18.01 Retained depleted uranium fragments

Z18.09 Other retained radioactive fragments
Other retained depleted isotope fragments
Retained nontherapeutic radioactive fragments

✓5ᵗʰ **Z18.1 Retained metal fragments**

EXCLUDES 1 retained radioactive metal fragments (Z18.01-Z18.09)

Z18.10 Retained metal fragments, unspecified
Retained metal fragment NOS

Z18.11 Retained magnetic metal fragments

Z18.12 Retained nonmagnetic metal fragments

Z18.2 Retained plastic fragments
Acrylics fragments
Diethylhexyl phthalates fragments
Isocyanate fragments

✓5ᵗʰ **Z18.3 Retained organic fragments**

Z18.31 Retained animal quills or spines

Z18.32 Retained tooth

Z18.33 Retained wood fragments

Z18.39 Other retained organic fragments

✓5ᵗʰ **Z18.8 Other specified retained foreign body**

Z18.81 Retained glass fragments

Z18.83 Retained stone or crystalline fragments
Retained concrete or cement fragments

Z18.89 Other specified retained foreign body fragments

Z18.9 Retained foreign body fragments, unspecified material

Hormone sensitivity malignancy status (Z19)

✓4ᵗʰ **Z19 Hormone sensitivity malignancy status**
Code first malignant neoplasm — see Table of Neoplasms, by site, malignant
AHA: 2016,4Q,76

Z19.1 Hormone sensitive malignancy status UPD

Z19.2 Hormone resistant malignancy status UPD
Castrate resistant prostate malignancy status

Persons with potential health hazards related to communicable diseases (Z20-Z29)

✓4ᵗʰ **Z20 Contact with and (suspected) exposure to communicable diseases**

EXCLUDES 1 carrier of infectious disease (Z22.-)
diagnosed current infectious or parasitic disease - see Alphabetic Index

EXCLUDES 2 personal history of infectious and parasitic diseases (Z86.1-)

✓5ᵗʰ **Z20.0 Contact with and (suspected) exposure to intestinal infectious diseases**

Z20.01 Contact with and (suspected) exposure to intestinal infectious diseases due to Escherichia coli (E. coli)

Z20.09 Contact with and (suspected) exposure to other intestinal infectious diseases

Z20.1 Contact with and (suspected) exposure to tuberculosis

Z20.2 Contact with and (suspected) exposure to infections with a predominantly sexual mode of transmission

Z20.3 Contact with and (suspected) exposure to rabies

Z20.4 Contact with and (suspected) exposure to rubella

Z20.5 Contact with and (suspected) exposure to viral hepatitis

Z20.6 Contact with and (suspected) exposure to human immunodeficiency virus [HIV]

EXCLUDES 1 asymptomatic human immunodeficiency virus [HIV] HIV infection status (Z21)

Z20.7 Contact with and (suspected) exposure to pediculosis, acariasis and other infestations

✓5ᵗʰ **Z20.8 Contact with and (suspected) exposure to other communicable diseases**

✓6ᵗʰ **Z20.81 Contact with and (suspected) exposure to other bacterial communicable diseases**

Z20.810 Contact with and (suspected) exposure to anthrax

Z20.811 Contact with and (suspected) exposure to meningococcus

Z20.818 Contact with and (suspected) exposure to other bacterial communicable diseases
AHA: 2019,2Q,10

✓6ᵗʰ **Z20.82 Contact with and (suspected) exposure to other viral communicable diseases**

Z20.820 Contact with and (suspected) exposure to varicella

Z20.821 Contact with and (suspected) exposure to Zika virus
AHA: 2018,4Q,35,64

Z20.822 Contact with and (suspected) exposure to COVID-19
Contact with and (suspected) exposure to SARS-CoV-2
AHA: 2022,2Q,28-29; 2021,4Q,109; 2021,1Q,27-29,37-38,41

Z20.828 Contact with and (suspected) exposure to other viral communicable diseases
AHA: 2021,1Q,37-38; 2020,4Q,99; 2020,3Q,14-15; 2020,2Q,4,8; 2020,1Q,34-36

Z20.89 Contact with and (suspected) exposure to other communicable diseases

Z20.9 Contact with and (suspected) exposure to unspecified communicable disease

Z21 Asymptomatic human immunodeficiency virus [HIV] infection status HCC Rx ESR COM
HIV positive NOS
Code first human immunodeficiency virus [HIV] disease complicating pregnancy, childbirth and the puerperium, if applicable (O98.7-)

EXCLUDES 1 acquired immunodeficiency syndrome (B20)
contact with human immunodeficiency virus [HIV] (Z20.6)
exposure to human immunodeficiency virus [HIV] (Z20.6)
human immunodeficiency virus [HIV] disease (B20)
inconclusive laboratory evidence of human immunodeficiency virus [HIV] (R75)

AHA: 2022,1Q,36; 2019,1Q,8-11
DEF: Phase of human immunodeficiency virus (HIV) infection with no clinical symptoms. This phase may last for 10 years or more.

✓4ᵗʰ **Z22 Carrier of infectious disease**

INCLUDES colonization status
suspected carrier

EXCLUDES 2 carrier of viral hepatitis (B18.-)

Z22.0 Carrier of typhoid

Z22.1 Carrier of other intestinal infectious diseases

Z22.2 Carrier of diphtheria

✓5ᵗʰ **Z22.3 Carrier of other specified bacterial diseases**

Z22.31 Carrier of bacterial disease due to meningococci

✓6ᵗʰ **Z22.32 Carrier of bacterial disease due to staphylococci**

Z22.321 Carrier or suspected carrier of Methicillin susceptible Staphylococcus aureus
MSSA colonization

Z22.322 Carrier or suspected carrier of Methicillin resistant Staphylococcus aureus
MRSA colonization
DEF: Carriers (colonization) of methicillin resistant Staphylococcus aureus (MRSA) have MRSA on their skin or in their body but do not exhibit signs of infection. These individuals are able to pass MRSA on to others who may develop an infection.

HCC CMS-HCC   Rx Rx HCC   ESR ESRD HCC   COM Commercial HCC   PDx Primary Dx Only   N Newborn: 0   P Pediatric: 0-17   M Maternity: 9-64   A Adult: 15-124

1270   ICD-10-CM 2023

Z22.33   Carrier of bacterial disease due to streptococci

     Z22.330   Carrier of Group B streptococcus

         EXCLUDES 1   carrier of streptococcus group B (GBS) complicating pregnancy, childbirth and the puerperium (O99.82-)

     Z22.338   Carrier of other streptococcus

   Z22.39   Carrier of other specified bacterial diseases

Z22.4   Carrier of infections with a predominantly sexual mode of transmission

Z22.6   Carrier of human T-lymphotropic virus type-1 [HTLV-1] infection

Z22.7   Latent tuberculosis

   Latent tuberculosis infection (LTBI)

     EXCLUDES 1   nonspecific reaction to cell mediated immunity measurement of gamma interferon antigen response without active tuberculosis (R76.12)

         nonspecific reaction to tuberculin skin test without active tuberculosis (R76.11)

   AHA: 2019,4Q,19

Z22.8   Carrier of other infectious diseases

Z22.9   Carrier of infectious disease, unspecified

Z23   Encounter for immunization

   NOTE   Procedure codes are required to identify the types of immunizations given

   Code first any routine childhood examination

   Code also, if applicable, encounter for immunization safety counseling (Z71.85)

Z28   Immunization not carried out and underimmunization status

   INCLUDES   vaccination not carried out

   Code also, if applicable, encounter for immunization safety counseling (Z71.85)

Z28.0   Immunization not carried out because of contraindication

   DEF: Contraindication: Situation where a drug, surgery, or other procedure may negatively affect or cause harm to a patient.

     Z28.01   Immunization not carried out because of acute illness of patient

     Z28.02   Immunization not carried out because of chronic illness or condition of patient

     Z28.03   Immunization not carried out because of immune compromised state of patient

     Z28.04   Immunization not carried out because of patient allergy to vaccine or component

     Z28.09   Immunization not carried out because of other contraindication

Z28.1   Immunization not carried out because of patient decision for reasons of belief or group pressure

   Immunization not carried out because of religious belief

Z28.2   Immunization not carried out because of patient decision for other and unspecified reason

     Z28.20   Immunization not carried out because of patient decision for unspecified reason

     Z28.21   Immunization not carried out because of patient refusal

     Z28.29   Immunization not carried out because of patient decision for other reason

Z28.3   Underimmunization status

   Delinquent immunization status

   Lapsed immunization schedule status

   ▶Use additional code, if applicable, to identify:◀

   ▶immunization not carried out because of contraindication (Z28.0-)◀

   ▶immunization not carried out because of patient decision for other and unspecified reason (Z28.2-)◀

   ▶immunization not carried out because of patient decision for reasons of belief or group pressure (Z28.1)◀

   ▶immunization not carried out for other reason (Z28.8-)◀

   AHA: 2022,1Q,4-5

     Z28.31   Underimmunization for COVID-19 status

       NOTE   These codes should not be used for individuals who are not eligible for the COVID-19 vaccines, as determined by the healthcare provider.

       Z28.310   Unvaccinated for COVID-19

       Z28.311   Partially vaccinated for COVID-19

Z28.39   Other underimmunization status

   Delinquent immunization status

   Lapsed immunization schedule status

Z28.8   Immunization not carried out for other reason

   Z28.81   Immunization not carried out due to patient having the disease

   Z28.82   Immunization not carried out because of caregiver refusal

     Immunization not carried out because of guardian refusal

     Immunization not carried out because of parent refusal

     EXCLUDES 1   immunization not carried out because of caregiver refusal because of religious belief (Z28.1)

   Z28.83   Immunization not carried out due to unavailability of vaccine

     Delay in delivery of vaccine

     Lack of availability of vaccine

     Manufacturer delay of vaccine

     AHA: 2018,4Q,36

   Z28.89   Immunization not carried out for other reason

Z28.9   Immunization not carried out for unspecified reason

Z29   Encounter for other prophylactic measures

   EXCLUDES 1   desensitization to allergens (Z51.6)

         prophylactic surgery (Z40.-)

   AHA: 2016,4Q,78-79

Z29.1   Encounter for prophylactic immunotherapy

   Encounter for administration of immunoglobulin

     Z29.11   Encounter for prophylactic immunotherapy for respiratory syncytial virus (RSV)

     Z29.12   Encounter for prophylactic antivenin

     Z29.13   Encounter for prophylactic Rho(D) immune globulin

       AHA: 2019,3Q,5

     Z29.14   Encounter for prophylactic rabies immune globin

Z29.3   Encounter for prophylactic fluoride administration

Z29.8   Encounter for other specified prophylactic measures

   AHA: 2022,2Q,27

Z29.9   Encounter for prophylactic measures, unspecified

Persons encountering health services in circumstances related to reproduction (Z30-Z39)

Z30   Encounter for contraceptive management

   AHA: 2016,4Q,78

   DEF: Contraceptive management to prevent pregnancy. Methods include oral medications, intrauterine devices, and surgical procedures for males and females (sterilization).

Z30.0   Encounter for general counseling and advice on contraception

     Z30.01   Encounter for initial prescription of contraceptives

       EXCLUDES 1   encounter for surveillance of contraceptives (Z30.4-)

       Z30.011   Encounter for initial prescription of contraceptive pills   ♀

       Z30.012   Encounter for prescription of emergency contraception   ♀

         Encounter for postcoital contraception

       Z30.013   Encounter for initial prescription of injectable contraceptive   ♀

       Z30.014   Encounter for initial prescription of intrauterine contraceptive device   ♀

         EXCLUDES 1   encounter for insertion of intrauterine contraceptive device (Z30.430, Z30.432)

       Z30.015   Encounter for initial prescription of vaginal ring hormonal contraceptive   ♀

       Z30.016   Encounter for initial prescription of transdermal patch hormonal contraceptive device

       Z30.017   Encounter for initial prescription of implantable subdermal contraceptive

Z30.018 **Encounter for initial prescription of other contraceptives** ♀
Encounter for initial prescription of barrier contraception
Encounter for initial prescription of diaphragm

Z30.019 **Encounter for initial prescription of contraceptives, unspecified** ♀

Z30.02 **Counseling and instruction in** natural family planning **to avoid pregnancy**

Z30.09 **Encounter for other general counseling and advice on contraception**
Encounter for family planning advice NOS

(handwritten: Sterilization)
Z30.2 **Encounter for** sterilization
AHA: 2021,3Q,13

✓5th Z30.4 **Encounter for** surveillance of contraceptives

Z30.40 **Encounter for surveillance of contraceptives, unspecified**

Z30.41 **Encounter for surveillance of contraceptive pills** ♀
Encounter for repeat prescription for contraceptive pill

Z30.42 **Encounter for surveillance of** injectable contraceptive ♀

✓6th Z30.43 **Encounter for surveillance of** intrauterine contraceptive device *(handwritten: IUD)*

(handwritten: insertion)
Z30.430 **Encounter for** insertion **of intrauterine contraceptive device** ♀

Z30.431 **Encounter for** routine checking **of intrauterine contraceptive device** ♀

(handwritten: Removal)
Z30.432 **Encounter for** removal **of intrauterine contraceptive device** ♀

Z30.433 **Encounter for** removal and reinsertion **of intrauterine contraceptive device** ♀
Encounter for replacement of intrauterine contraceptive device

Z30.44 **Encounter for surveillance of** vaginal ring hormonal **contraceptive device** ♀

Z30.45 **Encounter for surveillance of** transdermal patch hormonal **contraceptive device** ♀

(handwritten: Removal. Nexplanon)
Z30.46 **Encounter for surveillance of** implantable subdermal **contraceptive**
Encounter for checking, reinsertion or removal of implantable subdermal contraceptive

Z30.49 **Encounter for surveillance of other contraceptives** ♀
Encounter for surveillance of barrier contraception
Encounter for surveillance of diaphragm

Z30.8 **Encounter for other contraceptive management**
Encounter for postvasectomy sperm count
Encounter for routine examination for contraceptive maintenance
EXCLUDES 1 sperm count following sterilization reversal (Z31.42)
sperm count for fertility testing (Z31.41)

Z30.9 **Encounter for contraceptive management, unspecified**

✓4th Z31 **Encounter for procreative management**
EXCLUDES 2 complications associated with artificial fertilization (N98.-)
female infertility (N97.-)
male infertility (N46.-)

Z31.0 **Encounter for** reversal of previous sterilization

✓5th Z31.4 **Encounter for** procreative investigation and testing
EXCLUDES 1 postvasectomy sperm count (Z30.8)

Z31.41 **Encounter for** fertility testing
Encounter for fallopian tube patency testing
Encounter for sperm count for fertility testing

Z31.42 **Aftercare following** sterilization reversal
Sperm count following sterilization reversal

✓6th Z31.43 **Encounter for genetic testing of** female **for procreative management**
Use additional code for recurrent pregnancy loss, if applicable (N96, O26.2-)
EXCLUDES 1 nonprocreative genetic testing (Z13.7-)

Z31.430 **Encounter of female for testing for genetic** disease carrier status **for procreative management** ♀

Z31.438 **Encounter for other genetic testing of female for procreative management** ♀

(handwritten: Reproduction Lyf. 085)

✓6th Z31.44 **Encounter for genetic testing of** male **for procreative management**
EXCLUDES 1 nonprocreative genetic testing (Z13.7-)

Z31.440 **Encounter of male for testing for genetic disease carrier status for procreative management** ♂

Z31.441 **Encounter for testing of male partner of patient with** recurrent pregnancy loss Ⓐ♂

Z31.448 **Encounter for other genetic testing of male for procreative management** Ⓐ♂

Z31.49 **Encounter for other procreative investigation and testing**

Z31.5 **Encounter for procreative genetic counseling**
AHA: 2017,4Q,27

(handwritten: Z15)
✓6th Z31.6 **Encounter for general counseling and advice on procreation**

(handwritten: Conseling pro creation)
Z31.61 **Procreative counseling and advice using** natural family planning

Z31.62 **Encounter for** fertility preservation **counseling**
Encounter for fertility preservation counseling prior to cancer therapy
Encounter for fertility preservation counseling prior to surgical removal of gonads

Z31.69 **Encounter for other general counseling and advice on procreation**

Z31.7 **Encounter for procreative management and counseling for gestational carrier**
EXCLUDES 1 pregnant state, gestational carrier (Z33.3)
AHA: 2016,4Q,78

✓5th Z31.8 **Encounter for other procreative management**

(handwritten: primary Dx only for first DA)
Z31.81 **Encounter for** male factor **infertility in female patient** PDx ♀

(handwritten: RH- Rhogam im)
Z31.82 **Encounter for** Rh incompatibility **status** ♀
AHA: 2015,3Q,40; 2014,4Q,17

(handwritten: primary Dx IVF)
Z31.83 **Encounter for** assisted reproductive fertility procedure cycle PDx ♀
Patient undergoing in vitro fertilization cycle
Use additional code to identify the type of infertility
EXCLUDES 1 pre-cycle diagnosis and testing - code to reason for encounter
AHA: 2022,2Q,15-16

(handwritten: Z 46.8 fitthy/adi of device primary Dx)
Z31.84 **Encounter for** fertility preservation **procedure** PDx
Encounter for fertility preservation procedure prior to cancer therapy
Encounter for fertility preservation procedure prior to surgical removal of gonads

Z31.89 **Encounter for other procreative management**

Z31.9 **Encounter for procreative management, unspecified**

✓4th Z32 **Encounter for pregnancy test and childbirth and childcare instruction**

✓5th Z32.0 **Encounter for** pregnancy test

Z32.00 **Encounter for pregnancy test,** result unknown ♀
Encounter for pregnancy test NOS

(handwritten: not in OB pack)
Z32.01 **Encounter for pregnancy test,** result positive COM M ♀

Z32.02 **Encounter for pregnancy test,** result negative ♀

Z32.2 **Encounter for** childbirth instruction

Z32.3 **Encounter for** childcare instruction
Encounter for prenatal or postpartum childcare instruction

✓4th Z33 **Pregnant state** *(handwritten: never be primary · or stand alone)*

(handwritten: Incidental)
Z33.1 **Pregnant state,** incidental COM M ♀
Pregnancy NOS
Pregnant state NOS *(handwritten: cut thumb)*
EXCLUDES 1 complications of pregnancy (O00-O9A)
pregnant state, gestational carrier (Z33.3)

(handwritten: Primary Dx)
(handwritten: cant be Z3A together)
Z33.2 **Encounter for** elective termination of pregnancy PDx M ♀
EXCLUDES 1 early fetal death with retention of dead fetus (O02.1)
late fetal death (O36.4) *(handwritten: elective abortion)*
spontaneous abortion (O03)
AHA: 2022,1Q,20
TIP: Do not assign a code from category Z3A with this code.

(handwritten: liveborn cant use post elective AB complication)

Z33.3 Pregnant state, gestational carrier COM M ♀
> EXCLUDES 1   *encounter for procreative management and counseling for gestational carrier (Z31.7)*
> AHA: 2016,4Q,78

(handwritten: no complication)

✓4ᵗʰ **Z34 Encounter for supervision of normal pregnancy** ★ *(handwritten: can't be use with chapters codes)*
> EXCLUDES 1   *any complication of pregnancy (O00-O9A)*
> *encounter for pregnancy test (Z32.0-)*
> *encounter for supervision of high risk pregnancy (O09.-)*
> AHA: 2019,3Q,5; 2014,4Q,17

✓5ᵗʰ **Z34.0 Encounter for supervision of normal first pregnancy**
(handwritten: no code / 4th character = first pregnancy / 5th character = trimester)

Z34.00 Encounter for supervision of normal first pregnancy, unspecified trimester COM PDx M ♀
Z34.01 Encounter for supervision of normal first pregnancy, first trimester COM PDx M ♀
Z34.02 Encounter for supervision of normal first pregnancy, second trimester COM PDx M ♀
Z34.03 Encounter for supervision of normal first pregnancy, third trimester COM PDx M ♀

✓5ᵗʰ **Z34.8 Encounter for supervision of other normal pregnancy**
Z34.80 Encounter for supervision of other normal pregnancy, unspecified trimester COM PDx M ♀
Z34.81 Encounter for supervision of other normal pregnancy, first trimester COM PDx M ♀
Z34.82 Encounter for supervision of other normal pregnancy, second trimester COM PDx M ♀
Z34.83 Encounter for supervision of other normal pregnancy, third trimester COM PDx M ♀

(handwritten: can't be "code together" / RH)

✓5ᵗʰ **Z34.9 Encounter for supervision of normal pregnancy, unspecified**
Z34.90 Encounter for supervision of normal pregnancy, unspecified, unspecified trimester COM PDx M ♀
Z34.91 Encounter for supervision of normal pregnancy, unspecified, first trimester COM PDx M ♀
Z34.92 Encounter for supervision of normal pregnancy, unspecified, second trimester COM PDx M ♀
Z34.93 Encounter for supervision of normal pregnancy, unspecified, third trimester COM PDx M ♀

✓4ᵗʰ **Z36 Encounter for antenatal screening of mother**

(handwritten: no complication / RH blood type)

> INCLUDES   encounter for placental sample (taken vaginally)
> screening is the testing for disease or disease precursors in asymptomatic individuals so that early detection and treatment can be provided for those who test positive for the disease.
> EXCLUDES 1   *diagnostic examination - code to sign or symptom*
> *encounter for suspected maternal and fetal conditions ruled out (Z03.7-)*
> *suspected fetal condition affecting management of pregnancy - code to condition in Chapter 15*
> EXCLUDES 2   *abnormal findings on antenatal screening of mother (O28.-)*
> *genetic counseling and testing (Z31.43-, Z31.5)*
> *routine prenatal care (Z34)*
> AHA: 2017,4Q,28

Z36.0 Encounter for antenatal screening for chromosomal anomalies COM M ♀
Z36.1 Encounter for antenatal screening for raised alphafetoprotein level COM M ♀
> Encounter for antenatal screening for elevated maternal serum alphafetoprotein level
> DEF: High levels of alpha-fetoprotein (AFP) that may indicate a possibility of spina bifida and other neural tube defects, anencephaly, or omphalocele in the fetus.
Z36.2 Encounter for other antenatal screening follow-up COM M ♀
> Non-visualized anatomy on a previous scan
Z36.3 Encounter for antenatal screening for malformations COM M ♀
> Screening for a suspected anomaly
Z36.4 Encounter for antenatal screening for fetal growth retardation COM M ♀
> Intrauterine growth restriction (IUGR)/small-for-dates
Z36.5 Encounter for antenatal screening for isoimmunization COM M ♀

✓5ᵗʰ **Z36.8 Encounter for other antenatal screening**
Z36.81 Encounter for antenatal screening for hydrops fetalis COM M ♀
(handwritten crossed out: RH blood type)
> DEF: Hydrops fetalis: Abnormal accumulation of fluid in two or more parts of the fetus, such as ascites, effusion of the pleural or pericardial tissues, or edema.
Z36.82 Encounter for antenatal screening for nuchal translucency COM M ♀
Z36.83 Encounter for fetal screening for congenital cardiac abnormalities COM M ♀
Z36.84 Encounter for antenatal screening for fetal lung maturity COM M ♀
Z36.85 Encounter for antenatal screening for Streptococcus B COM M ♀
Z36.86 Encounter for antenatal screening for cervical length COM M ♀
> Screening for risk of pre-term labor
Z36.87 Encounter for antenatal screening for uncertain dates COM M ♀
Z36.88 Encounter for antenatal screening for fetal macrosomia COM M ♀
> Screening for large-for-dates
Z36.89 Encounter for other specified antenatal screening COM M ♀
Z36.8A Encounter for antenatal screening for other genetic defects COM M ♀

Z36.9 Encounter for antenatal screening, unspecified COM M ♀

✓4ᵗʰ **Z3A Weeks of gestation**   *(handwritten: "Mothers chart Only")*
> NOTE   Codes from category Z3A are for use, only on the maternal record, to indicate the weeks of gestation of the pregnancy, if known.
> Code first obstetric condition or encounter for delivery (O09-O60, O80-O82)
> AHA: 2022,2Q,3; 2019,2Q,11; 2016,2Q,34; 2014,3Q,17; 2014,2Q,9; 2013,2Q,33
> TIP: Do not assign a code from this category with codes from categories O00-O08 or code Z33.2.

(handwritten: pregnancy test / with serum)

✓5ᵗʰ **Z3A.0 Weeks of gestation of pregnancy, unspecified or less than 10 weeks**
(handwritten: abortive outcome)
Z3A.00 Weeks of gestation of pregnancy not specified COM UPD M ♀
Z3A.01 Less than 8 weeks gestation of pregnancy COM UPD ♀
Z3A.08 8 weeks gestation of pregnancy COM UPD M ♀
Z3A.09 9 weeks gestation of pregnancy COM UPD M ♀

✓5ᵗʰ **Z3A.1 Weeks of gestation of pregnancy, weeks 10-19**
Z3A.10 10 weeks gestation of pregnancy COM UPD M ♀
Z3A.11 11 weeks gestation of pregnancy COM UPD M ♀
Z3A.12 12 weeks gestation of pregnancy COM UPD M ♀
Z3A.13 13 weeks gestation of pregnancy COM UPD M ♀
Z3A.14 14 weeks gestation of pregnancy COM UPD M ♀
Z3A.15 15 weeks gestation of pregnancy COM UPD M ♀
Z3A.16 16 weeks gestation of pregnancy COM UPD M ♀
Z3A.17 17 weeks gestation of pregnancy COM UPD M ♀
Z3A.18 18 weeks gestation of pregnancy COM UPD M ♀
Z3A.19 19 weeks gestation of pregnancy COM UPD M ♀

✓5ᵗʰ **Z3A.2 Weeks of gestation of pregnancy, weeks 20-29**
Z3A.20 20 weeks gestation of pregnancy COM UPD M ♀
Z3A.21 21 weeks gestation of pregnancy COM UPD M ♀
Z3A.22 22 weeks gestation of pregnancy COM UPD M ♀
Z3A.23 23 weeks gestation of pregnancy COM UPD M ♀
Z3A.24 24 weeks gestation of pregnancy COM UPD M ♀
Z3A.25 25 weeks gestation of pregnancy COM UPD M ♀
Z3A.26 26 weeks gestation of pregnancy COM UPD M ♀
Z3A.27 27 weeks gestation of pregnancy COM UPD M ♀
Z3A.28 28 weeks gestation of pregnancy COM UPD M ♀
Z3A.29 29 weeks gestation of pregnancy COM UPD M ♀

✓5ᵗʰ **Z3A.3 Weeks of gestation of pregnancy, weeks 30-39**
(handwritten: O36.80X / Preg. viability inconclusive.)
Z3A.30 30 weeks gestation of pregnancy COM UPD M ♀
Z3A.31 31 weeks gestation of pregnancy COM UPD M ♀
Z3A.32 32 weeks gestation of pregnancy COM UPD M ♀
Z3A.33 33 weeks gestation of pregnancy COM UPD M ♀
Z3A.34 34 weeks gestation of pregnancy COM UPD ♀
Z3A.35 35 weeks gestation of pregnancy COM UPD M ♀

Z3A.36   **36 weeks gestation** of pregnancy   COM UPD M ♀

Z3A.37   **37 weeks gestation** of pregnancy   COM UPD M ♀

Z3A.38   **38 weeks gestation** of pregnancy   COM UPD M ♀

Z3A.39   **39 weeks gestation** of pregnancy   COM UPD M ♀

√5ᵗʰ **Z3A.4   Weeks of gestation of pregnancy, weeks 40 or greater**

    AHA: 2014,4Q,23

Z3A.40   **40 weeks gestation** of pregnancy   COM UPD M ♀

Z3A.41   **41 weeks gestation** of pregnancy   COM UPD M ♀

Z3A.42   **42 weeks gestation** of pregnancy   COM UPD M ♀

Z3A.49   **Greater than 42 weeks gestation** of pregnancy   COM UPD M ♀

√4ᵗʰ **Z37   Outcome of delivery**   *[handwritten: Delivery Outcome]*

    This category is intended for use as an additional code to identify the outcome of delivery on the mother's record. It is not for use on the newborn record.

    EXCLUDES 1   stillbirth (P95)

Z37.0   **Single live birth**   COM UPD M ♀

      AHA: 2016,2Q,34; 2014,2Q,9

Z37.1   **Single stillbirth**   COM UPD M ♀

Z37.2   **Twins, both liveborn**   COM UPD M ♀

Z37.3   **Twins, one liveborn and one stillborn**   COM UPD M ♀

Z37.4   **Twins, both stillborn**   COM UPD M ♀

√5ᵗʰ Z37.5   **Other multiple births, all liveborn**

    Z37.50   **Multiple births, unspecified, all liveborn**   COM UPD M ♀

    Z37.51   **Triplets, all liveborn**   COM UPD M ♀

    Z37.52   **Quadruplets, all liveborn**   COM UPD M ♀

    Z37.53   **Quintuplets, all liveborn**   COM UPD M ♀

    Z37.54   **Sextuplets, all liveborn**   COM UPD M ♀

    Z37.59   **Other multiple births, all liveborn**   COM UPD M ♀

√5ᵗʰ Z37.6   **Other multiple births, some liveborn**

    Z37.60   **Multiple births, unspecified, some liveborn**   COM UPD M ♀

    Z37.61   **Triplets, some liveborn**   COM UPD M ♀

    Z37.62   **Quadruplets, some liveborn**   COM UPD M ♀

    Z37.63   **Quintuplets, some liveborn**   COM UPD M ♀

    Z37.64   **Sextuplets, some liveborn**   COM UPD M ♀

    Z37.69   **Other multiple births, some liveborn**   COM UPD M ♀

Z37.7   **Other multiple births, all stillborn**   COM UPD M ♀

Z37.9   **Outcome of delivery, unspecified**   COM UPD M ♀

    Multiple birth NOS

    Single birth NOS

√4ᵗʰ **Z38   Liveborn infants according to place of birth and type of delivery**

    [handwritten: observation then Z05]

    This category is for use as the principal code on the initial record of a newborn baby. It is to be used for the initial birth record only. It is not to be used on the mother's record.

    AHA: 2020,2Q,13; 2017,2Q,5-7; 2016,3Q,18; 2015,2Q,15

    TIP: For attending physician services, a code from this category can be reported as first listed every time the physician visits the newborn during the birth admission.

√5ᵗʰ Z38.0   **Single liveborn infant, born in hospital**

    Single liveborn infant, born in birthing center or other health care facility

    Z38.00   **Single liveborn infant, delivered vaginally**   COM PDx N

    Z38.01   **Single liveborn infant, delivered by cesarean**   COM PDx N

Z38.1   **Single liveborn infant, born outside hospital**   COM PDx N

Z38.2   **Single liveborn infant, unspecified as to place of birth**   COM PDx N

    Single liveborn infant NOS

√5ᵗʰ Z38.3   **Twin liveborn infant, born in hospital**

    Z38.30   **Twin liveborn infant, delivered vaginally**   COM PDx N

    Z38.31   **Twin liveborn infant, delivered by cesarean**   COM PDx N

Z38.4   **Twin liveborn infant, born outside hospital**   COM PDx N

Z38.5   **Twin liveborn infant, unspecified as to place of birth**   COM PDx N

√5ᵗʰ Z38.6   **Other multiple liveborn infant, born in hospital**

    Z38.61   **Triplet liveborn infant, delivered vaginally**   COM PDx N

Z38.62   **Triplet liveborn infant, delivered by cesarean**   COM PDx N

Z38.63   **Quadruplet liveborn infant, delivered vaginally**   COM PDx N

Z38.64   **Quadruplet liveborn infant, delivered by cesarean**   COM PDx N

Z38.65   **Quintuplet liveborn infant, delivered vaginally**   COM PDx N

Z38.66   **Quintuplet liveborn infant, delivered by cesarean**   COM PDx N

Z38.68   **Other multiple liveborn infant, delivered vaginally**   COM PDx N

Z38.69   **Other multiple liveborn infant, delivered by cesarean**   COM PDx N

Z38.7   **Other multiple liveborn infant, born outside hospital**   COM PDx N

Z38.8   **Other multiple liveborn infant, unspecified as to place of birth**   COM PDx N

    [handwritten: Principal Dx]

√4ᵗʰ **Z39   Encounter for maternal postpartum care and examination**

Z39.0   **Encounter for care and examination of mother immediately after delivery**   COM PDx M ♀

    [handwritten: post partum outside of hospital delivered]

    Care and observation in uncomplicated cases when the delivery occurs outside a healthcare facility

    EXCLUDES 1   care for postpartum complication - see Alphabetic Index

    AHA: 2021,3Q,13

Z39.1   **Encounter for care and examination of lactating mother**   PDx M ♀

    Encounter for supervision of lactation

    EXCLUDES 1   disorders of lactation (O92.-)

Z39.2   **Encounter for routine postpartum follow-up**   COM PDx M ♀

    [handwritten: if have dx code first]

Encounters for other specific health care (Z40-Z53)

    Categories Z40-Z53 are intended for use to indicate a reason for care. They may be used for patients who have already been treated for a disease or injury, but who are receiving aftercare or prophylactic care, or care to consolidate the treatment, or to deal with a residual state

    EXCLUDES 2   follow-up examination for medical surveillance after treatment (Z08-Z09)

√4ᵗʰ **Z40   Encounter for prophylactic surgery**

    EXCLUDES 1   organ donations (Z52.-)

           therapeutic organ removal - code to condition

    DEF: Treatment measure intended to prevent or ward off a disease or condition.

√5ᵗʰ Z40.0   **Encounter for prophylactic surgery for risk factors related to malignant neoplasms**

    Admission for prophylactic organ removal

    Use additional code to identify risk factor

    AHA: 2017,4Q,28-29

    Z40.00   **Encounter for prophylactic removal of unspecified organ**   PDx

    Z40.01   **Encounter for prophylactic removal of breast**   PDx

    Z40.02   **Encounter for prophylactic removal of ovary(s)**   PDx ♀

       Encounter for prophylactic removal of ovary(s) and fallopian tube(s)

    Z40.03   **Encounter for prophylactic removal of fallopian tube(s)**   PDx ♀

    Z40.09   **Encounter for prophylactic removal of other organ**   PDx

Z40.8   **Encounter for other prophylactic surgery**   PDx

Z40.9   **Encounter for prophylactic surgery, unspecified**   PDx

√4ᵗʰ **Z41   Encounter for procedures for purposes other than remedying health state**

Z41.1   **Encounter for cosmetic surgery**

    Encounter for cosmetic breast implant

    Encounter for cosmetic procedure

    EXCLUDES 1   encounter for plastic and reconstructive surgery following medical procedure or healed injury (Z42.-)

         encounter for post-mastectomy breast implantation (Z42.1)

HCC CMS-HCC   Rx Rx HCC   ESR ESRD HCC   COM Commercial HCC   PDx Primary Dx Only   N Newborn: 0   P Pediatric: 0-17   M Maternity: 9-64   A Adult: 15-124

1274   ICD-10-CM 2023

After Care (handwritten)

Z41.2 Encounter for routine and ritual male circumcision ♂
Circumcision (handwritten)
     AHA: 2018,3Q,15
     TIP: This code should only be reported when the circumcision is elective (unrelated to a specific diagnosis) and was not performed during the birth admission.

Z41.3 Encounter for ear piercing

Z41.8 Encounter for other procedures for purposes other than remedying health state

Z41.9 Encounter for procedure for purposes other than remedying health state, unspecified

Z42 Encounter for plastic and reconstructive surgery following medical procedure or healed injury
after care (handwritten, left margin)
     EXCLUDES 1   encounter for cosmetic plastic surgery (Z41.1)
               encounter for plastic surgery for treatment of current injury - code to relevent injury

Z42.1 Encounter for breast reconstruction following mastectomy   PDx A
     EXCLUDES 1   deformity and disproportion of reconstructed breast (N65.1-)

Z42.8 Encounter for other plastic and reconstructive surgery following medical procedure or healed injury   PDx
     AHA: 2017,1Q,42

Z43 Encounter for attention to artificial openings
     INCLUDES   closure of artificial openings
               passage of sounds or bougies through artificial openings
               reforming artificial openings
               removal of catheter from artificial openings
               toilet or cleansing of artificial openings
     EXCLUDES 1   complications of external stoma (J95.0-, K94.-, N99.5-)
     EXCLUDES 2   fitting and adjustment of prosthetic and other devices (Z44-Z46)
     AHA: 2019,2Q,33

Z43.0 Encounter for attention to tracheostomy   HCC ESR COM

Z43.1 Encounter for attention to gastrostomy   HCC ESR COM
     EXCLUDES 2   artificial opening status only, without need for care (Z93.-)

Z43.2 Encounter for attention to ileostomy   HCC ESR COM

Z43.3 Encounter for attention to colostomy   HCC ESR COM

Z43.4 Encounter for attention to other artificial openings of digestive tract   HCC ESR COM

Z43.5 Encounter for attention to cystostomy   HCC ESR COM

Z43.6 Encounter for attention to other artificial openings of urinary tract   HCC ESR COM
     Encounter for attention to nephrostomy
     Encounter for attention to ureterostomy
     Encounter for attention to urethrostomy

Z43.7 Encounter for attention to artificial vagina

Z43.8 Encounter for attention to other artificial openings   HCC ESR COM

Z43.9 Encounter for attention to unspecified artificial opening   HCC ESR COM

Z44 Encounter for fitting and adjustment of external prosthetic device
     INCLUDES   removal or replacement of external prosthetic device
     EXCLUDES 1   malfunction or other complications of device - see Alphabetical Index
               presence of prosthetic device (Z97.-)

Z44.0 Encounter for fitting and adjustment of artificial arm

     Z44.00 Encounter for fitting and adjustment of unspecified artificial arm
         Z44.001 Encounter for fitting and adjustment of unspecified right artificial arm   COM
         Z44.002 Encounter for fitting and adjustment of unspecified left artificial arm   COM
         Z44.009 Encounter for fitting and adjustment of unspecified artificial arm, unspecified arm   COM

     Z44.01 Encounter for fitting and adjustment of complete artificial arm
         Z44.011 Encounter for fitting and adjustment of complete right artificial arm   COM
         Z44.012 Encounter for fitting and adjustment of complete left artificial arm   COM
         Z44.019 Encounter for fitting and adjustment of complete artificial arm, unspecified arm   COM

after care (handwritten, left margin)

Z44.02 Encounter for fitting and adjustment of partial artificial arm
     Z44.021 Encounter for fitting and adjustment of partial artificial right arm   COM
     Z44.022 Encounter for fitting and adjustment of partial artificial left arm   COM
     Z44.029 Encounter for fitting and adjustment of partial artificial arm, unspecified arm   COM

Z44.1 Encounter for fitting and adjustment of artificial leg

     Z44.10 Encounter for fitting and adjustment of unspecified artificial leg
         Z44.101 Encounter for fitting and adjustment of unspecified right artificial leg   HCC ESR COM
         Z44.102 Encounter for fitting and adjustment of unspecified left artificial leg   HCC ESR COM
         Z44.109 Encounter for fitting and adjustment of unspecified artificial leg, unspecified leg   HCC ESR COM

     Z44.11 Encounter for fitting and adjustment of complete artificial leg
         Z44.111 Encounter for fitting and adjustment of complete right artificial leg   HCC ESR COM
         Z44.112 Encounter for fitting and adjustment of complete left artificial leg   HCC ESR COM
         Z44.119 Encounter for fitting and adjustment of complete artificial leg, unspecified leg   HCC ESR COM

     Z44.12 Encounter for fitting and adjustment of partial artificial leg
         Z44.121 Encounter for fitting and adjustment of partial artificial right leg   HCC ESR COM
         Z44.122 Encounter for fitting and adjustment of partial artificial left leg   HCC ESR COM
         Z44.129 Encounter for fitting and adjustment of partial artificial leg, unspecified leg   HCC ESR COM

Z44.2 Encounter for fitting and adjustment of artificial eye
     EXCLUDES 1   mechanical complication of ocular prosthesis (T85.3)
     Z44.20 Encounter for fitting and adjustment of artificial eye, unspecified
     Z44.21 Encounter for fitting and adjustment of artificial right eye
     Z44.22 Encounter for fitting and adjustment of artificial left eye

Z44.3 Encounter for fitting and adjustment of external breast prosthesis
     EXCLUDES 1   complications of breast implant (T85.4-)
               encounter for adjustment or removal of breast implant (Z45.81-)
               encounter for initial breast implant insertion for cosmetic breast augmentation (Z41.1)
               encounter for breast reconstruction following mastectomy (Z42.1)

     Z44.30 Encounter for fitting and adjustment of external breast prosthesis, unspecified breast
     Z44.31 Encounter for fitting and adjustment of external right breast prosthesis
     Z44.32 Encounter for fitting and adjustment of external left breast prosthesis

Z44.8 Encounter for fitting and adjustment of other external prosthetic devices

Z44.9 Encounter for fitting and adjustment of unspecified external prosthetic device

after Care (handwritten)

✓4ᵗʰ **Z45 Encounter for adjustment and management of implanted device**

INCLUDES   removal or replacement of implanted device

EXCLUDES 1   malfunction or other complications of device - see Alphabetical Index

EXCLUDES 2   encounter for fitting and adjustment of non-implanted device (Z46.-)

✓5ᵗʰ **Z45.0 Encounter for adjustment and management of** cardiac device

TIP: Assign an additional code for the associated condition if that condition requires constant intervention from the device, as in cases of sick sinus syndrome. For conditions that do not require constant intervention from the device, as in cases of ventricular fibrillation, an additional code for the associated condition should be assigned only if the patient is experiencing the condition and the device is firing during the current admission.

✓6ᵗʰ **Z45.01 Encounter for adjustment and management of cardiac** pacemaker

Encounter for adjustment and management of cardiac resynchronization therapy pacemaker (CRT-P)

EXCLUDES 1   encounter for adjustment and management of automatic implantable cardiac defibrillator with synchronous cardiac pacemaker (Z45.02)

Z45.010 Encounter for checking and testing of cardiac pacemaker pulse generator **[battery]**

Encounter for replacing cardiac pacemaker pulse generator [battery]

Z45.018 Encounter for adjustment and management of other part of cardiac pacemaker

EXCLUDES 1   presence of other part of cardiac pacemaker (Z95.0)

EXCLUDES 2   presence of prosthetic and other devices (Z95.1-Z95.5, Z95.811-Z97)

Z45.02 Encounter for adjustment and management of automatic implantable cardiac defibrillator

Encounter for adjustment and management of automatic implantable cardiac defibrillator with synchronous cardiac pacemaker

Encounter for adjustment and management of cardiac resynchronization therapy defibrillator (CRT-D)

Z45.09 Encounter for adjustment and management of other cardiac device

Z45.1 Encounter for adjustment and management of infusion pump

Z45.2 Encounter for adjustment and management of vascular access device

Encounter for adjustment and management of vascular catheters

EXCLUDES 1   encounter for adjustment and management of renal dialysis catheter (Z49.01)

AHA: 2020,2Q,21; 2018,3Q,20

✓5ᵗʰ **Z45.3 Encounter for adjustment and management of implanted** devices of the special senses

Z45.31 Encounter for adjustment and management of implanted visual substitution device

✓6ᵗʰ **Z45.32 Encounter for adjustment and management of implanted** hearing device

EXCLUDES 1   encounter for fitting and adjustment of hearing aide (Z46.1)

Z45.320 Encounter for adjustment and management of bone conduction device

Z45.321 Encounter for adjustment and management of cochlear device

Z45.328 Encounter for adjustment and management of other implanted hearing device

✓5ᵗʰ **Z45.4 Encounter for adjustment and management of implanted** nervous system device

Z45.41 Encounter for adjustment and management of cerebrospinal fluid drainage device

Encounter for adjustment and management of cerebral ventricular (communicating) shunt

Z45.42 Encounter for adjustment and management of neurostimulator

Encounter for adjustment and management of brain neurostimulator

Encounter for adjustment and management of gastric neurostimulator

Encounter for adjustment and management of peripheral nerve neurostimulator

Encounter for adjustment and management of sacral nerve neurostimulator

Encounter for adjustment and management of spinal cord neurostimulator

Encounter for adjustment and management of vagus nerve neurostimulator

Z45.49 Encounter for adjustment and management of other implanted nervous system device

AHA: 2014,3Q,19

✓5ᵗʰ **Z45.8 Encounter for adjustment and management of other implanted devices**

✓6ᵗʰ **Z45.81 Encounter for adjustment or** removal of breast implant

Encounter for elective implant exchange (different material) (different size)

Encounter for removal of tissue expander with or without synchronous insertion of permanent implant

EXCLUDES 1   complications of breast implant (T85.4-)

encounter for initial breast implant insertion for cosmetic breast augmentation (Z41.1)

encounter for breast reconstruction following mastectomy (Z42.1)

Z45.811 Encounter for adjustment or removal of right **breast implant**

Z45.812 Encounter for adjustment or removal of left **breast implant**

Z45.819 Encounter for adjustment or removal of unspecified breast implant

Z45.82 Encounter for adjustment or removal of myringotomy device **(stent) (tube)**

Z45.89 Encounter for adjustment and management of other implanted devices

AHA: 2014,4Q,26-28

Z45.9 Encounter for adjustment and management of unspecified implanted device

✓4ᵗʰ **Z46 Encounter for fitting and adjustment of other devices**

INCLUDES   removal or replacement of other device

EXCLUDES 1   malfunction or other complications of device - see Alphabetical Index

EXCLUDES 2   encounter for fitting and management of implanted devices (Z45.-)

issue of repeat prescription only (Z76.0)

presence of prosthetic and other devices (Z95-Z97)

Z46.0 Encounter for fitting and adjustment of spectacles and contact lenses

Z46.1 Encounter for fitting and adjustment of hearing aid

EXCLUDES 1   encounter for adjustment and management of implanted hearing device (Z45.32-)

Z46.2 Encounter for fitting and adjustment of other devices related to nervous system and special senses

EXCLUDES 2   encounter for adjustment and management of implanted nervous system device (Z45.4-)

encounter for adjustment and management of implanted visual substitution device (Z45.31)

Z46.3 Encounter for fitting and adjustment of dental prosthetic device

Encounter for fitting and adjustment of dentures

Z46.4 Encounter for fitting and adjustment of orthodontic device

✓5ᵗʰ **Z46.5 Encounter for fitting and adjustment of other** gastrointestinal appliance and device

EXCLUDES 1   encounter for attention to artificial openings of digestive tract (Z43.1-Z43.4)

Z46.51 Encounter for fitting and adjustment of gastric lap band

Z46.59 Encounter for fitting and adjustment of other gastrointestinal appliance and device

Z46.6 Encounter for fitting and adjustment of urinary device

> EXCLUDES 2 *attention to artificial openings of urinary tract (Z43.5, Z43.6)*

✓5ᵗʰ **Z46.8 Encounter for fitting and adjustment of other specified devices**

Z46.81 Encounter for fitting and adjustment of insulin pump
> Encounter for insulin pump instruction and training
> Encounter for insulin pump titration

Z46.82 Encounter for fitting and adjustment of non-vascular catheter

Z46.89 Encounter for fitting and adjustment of other specified devices
> Encounter for fitting and adjustment of wheelchair

pessory

Z46.9 Encounter for fitting and adjustment of unspecified device

✓4ᵗʰ **Z47 Orthopedic aftercare**

> EXCLUDES 1 *aftercare for healing fracture - code to fracture with 7th character D*

Z47.1 Aftercare following joint replacement surgery
> Use additional code to identify the joint (Z96.6-)
> **AHA:** 2020,1Q,23

Z47.2 Encounter for removal of internal fixation device

> EXCLUDES 1 *encounter for adjustment of internal fixation device for fracture treatment - code to fracture with appropriate 7th character*
> *encounter for removal of external fixation device - code to fracture with 7th character D*
> *infection or inflammatory reaction to internal fixation device (T84.6-)*
> *mechanical complication of internal fixation device (T84.1-)*

✓5ᵗʰ **Z47.3 Aftercare following explantation of** joint prosthesis
> Aftercare following explantation of joint prosthesis, staged procedure
> Encounter for joint prosthesis insertion following prior explantation of joint prosthesis
> **AHA:** 2020,1Q,23; 2015,1Q,16
> **TIP:** For staged removal of elbow joint prosthesis, assign code Z47.1.

Z47.31 Aftercare following explantation of shoulder **joint prosthesis**
> EXCLUDES 1 *acquired absence of shoulder joint following prior explantation of shoulder joint prosthesis (Z89.23-)*
> *shoulder joint prosthesis explantation status (Z89.23-)*

Z47.32 Aftercare following explantation of hip **joint prosthesis**
> EXCLUDES 1 *acquired absence of hip joint following prior explantation of hip joint prosthesis (Z89.62-)*
> *hip joint prosthesis explantation status (Z89.62-)*

Z47.33 Aftercare following explantation of knee **joint prosthesis**
> EXCLUDES 1 *acquired absence of knee joint following prior explantation of knee prosthesis (Z89.52-)*
> *knee joint prosthesis explantation status (Z89.52-)*

✓5ᵗʰ **Z47.8 Encounter for other orthopedic aftercare**

Z47.81 Encounter for orthopedic aftercare following surgical amputation
> Use additional code to identify the limb amputated (Z89.-)

Z47.82 Encounter for orthopedic aftercare following scoliosis surgery

Z47.89 Encounter for other orthopedic aftercare
> **AHA:** 2015,1Q,8

✓4ᵗʰ **Z48 Encounter for other postprocedural aftercare**

> EXCLUDES 1 *encounter for aftercare following injury - code to Injury, by site, with appropriate 7th character for subsequent encounter*
> *encounter for follow-up examination after completed treatment (Z08-Z09)*

> EXCLUDES 2 *encounter for attention to artificial openings (Z43.-)*
> *encounter for fitting and adjustment of prosthetic and other devices (Z44-Z46)*

AHA: 2015,4Q,38; 2015,1Q,6-7

✓5ᵗʰ **Z48.0 Encounter for** attention to dressings, sutures and drains

> EXCLUDES 1 *encounter for planned postprocedural wound closure (Z48.1)*

Z48.00 Encounter for change or removal of nonsurgical wound dressing
> Encounter for change or removal of wound dressing NOS

Z48.01 Encounter for change or removal of surgical **wound** dressing
> **AHA:** 2019,2Q,33

Z48.02 Encounter for removal of sutures
> Encounter for removal of staples

Suture removal

Z48.03 Encounter for change or removal of drains
> **AHA:** 2019,2Q,33

Z48.1 Encounter for planned postprocedural **wound closure**

> EXCLUDES 1 *encounter for attention to dressings and sutures (Z48.0-)*

✓5ᵗʰ **Z48.2 Encounter for aftercare following** organ transplant

Z48.21 Encounter for aftercare following heart transplant `HCC` `Rx` `ESR` `COM`

Z48.22 Encounter for aftercare following kidney transplant `Rx` `COM`

Z48.23 Encounter for aftercare following liver transplant `HCC` `Rx` `ESR` `COM`

Z48.24 Encounter for aftercare following lung transplant `HCC` `Rx` `ESR` `COM`

✓6ᵗʰ **Z48.28 Encounter for aftercare following** multiple **organ transplant**

Z48.280 Encounter for aftercare following heart-lung transplant `HCC` `Rx` `ESR` `COM`

Z48.288 Encounter for aftercare following multiple **organ transplant**

✓6ᵗʰ **Z48.29 Encounter for aftercare following other organ transplant**

Z48.290 Encounter for aftercare following bone marrow transplant `HCC` `Rx` `ESR` `COM`

Z48.298 Encounter for aftercare following other organ transplant

Z48.3 Aftercare following surgery for neoplasm
> Use additional code to identify the neoplasm

Residual ① Fibroid
endometrial ① Cancer staple remre

✓5ᵗʰ **Z48.8 Encounter for other specified postprocedural aftercare**

✓6ᵗʰ **Z48.81 Encounter for surgical aftercare following** surgery on specified body systems
> These codes identify the body system requiring aftercare. They are for use in conjunction with other aftercare codes to fully explain the aftercare encounter. The condition treated should also be coded if still present.

② C54.1 Cancer
③ status Z 48.02

> EXCLUDES 1 *aftercare for injury - code the injury with 7th character D*
> *aftercare following surgery for neoplasm (Z48.3)*

> EXCLUDES 2 *aftercare following organ transplant (Z48.2-)*
> *orthopedic aftercare (Z47.-)*

AHA: 2015,4Q,38

Z48.810 Encounter for surgical aftercare following surgery on the sense organs

Z48.811 Encounter for surgical aftercare following surgery on the nervous system
> EXCLUDES 2 *encounter for surgical aftercare following surgery on the sense organs (Z48.810)*

Z48.812 Encounter for surgical aftercare following surgery on the circulatory system
> **AHA:** 2012,4Q,96

✅ Additional Character Required ✓x7ᵗʰ Placeholder Alert Manifestation Unspecified Dx 🇶 QPP UPD Unacceptable PDx

Z48.813 Encounter for surgical aftercare following surgery on the **respiratory system**
AHA: 2019,2Q,33

Z48.814 Encounter for surgical aftercare following surgery on the **teeth or oral cavity**

Z48.815 Encounter for surgical aftercare following surgery on the **digestive system**

Z48.816 Encounter for surgical aftercare following surgery on the **genitourinary system**
EXCLUDES 1 *encounter for aftercare following sterilization reversal (Z31.42)*

Z48.817 Encounter for surgical aftercare following surgery on the **skin and subcutaneous tissue**

Z48.89 Encounter for other specified surgical aftercare

✓4th **Z49** **Encounter for care involving renal dialysis**
Code also associated end stage renal disease (N18.6)

✓5th **Z49.0** **Preparatory care for renal dialysis**
Encounter for dialysis instruction and training

Z49.01 **Encounter for fitting and adjustment of extracorporeal dialysis catheter** HCC Rx ESR
Removal or replacement of renal dialysis catheter
Toilet or cleansing of renal dialysis catheter

Continued Care

Z49.02 **Encounter for fitting and adjustment of peritoneal dialysis catheter** HCC Rx ESR

✓5th **Z49.3** **Encounter for adequacy testing for dialysis**

Z49.31 **Encounter for adequacy testing for hemodialysis** HCC Rx ESR

Z49.32 **Encounter for adequacy testing for peritoneal dialysis** HCC Rx ESR
Encounter for peritoneal equilibration test

✓4th **Z51** **Encounter for other aftercare and medical care**
Code also condition requiring care
EXCLUDES 1 *follow-up examination after treatment (Z08-Z09)*

Z51.0 **Encounter for antineoplastic radiation therapy** PDx
AHA: 2017,4Q,103
chiefly
TIP: Do not assign when admission is for insertion/implantation of radioactive elements. Assign a code for the malignancy instead. Any complications related to the radioactive elements should be assigned as secondary diagnoses.

✓5th **Z51.1** **Encounter for antineoplastic chemotherapy and immunotherapy**
EXCLUDES 2 *encounter for chemotherapy and immunotherapy for nonneoplastic condition - code to condition*
after Chemo for ovarian Cancer
Z51.11 **Encounter for antineoplastic chemotherapy** PDx
AHA: 2022,1Q,16; 2015,3Q,19

Z51.12 **Encounter for antineoplastic immunotherapy** PDx

Z51.5 **Encounter for palliative care**
AHA: 2022,1Q,18; 2020,4Q,98; 2017,1Q,48

Z51.6 **Encounter for desensitization to allergens**
AHA: 2016,4Q,77

✓5th **Z51.8** **Encounter for other specified aftercare**
EXCLUDES 1 *holiday relief care (Z75.5)*

Z51.81 **Encounter for therapeutic drug level monitoring**
Code also any long-term (current) drug therapy (Z79.-)
EXCLUDES 1 *encounter for blood-drug test for administrative or medicolegal reasons (Z02.83)*
DEF: Drug monitoring: Measurement of the level of a specific drug in the body or measurement of a specific function to assess effectiveness of a drug.

Z51.89 **Encounter for other specified aftercare**
AHA: 2012,4Q,95-97

✓4th **Z52** **Donors of organs and tissues** *not for cadaver*
INCLUDES autologous and other living donors
EXCLUDES 1 *cadaveric donor - omit code*
examination of potential donor (Z00.5)
AHA: 2012,4Q,99

✓5th **Z52.0** **Blood donor**

✓6th **Z52.00** **Unspecified blood donor**
Z52.000 Unspecified donor, **whole blood** PDx
Z52.001 Unspecified donor, **stem cells** PDx
Z52.008 Unspecified donor, **other blood** PDx

✓6th **Z52.01** **Autologous blood donor**
Z52.010 Autologous donor, **whole blood** PDx
Z52.011 Autologous donor, **stem cells** PDx
Z52.018 Autologous donor, **other blood** PDx

✓6th **Z52.09** **Other blood donor**
Volunteer donor
Z52.090 Other blood donor, **whole blood** PDx
Z52.091 Other blood donor, **stem cells** PDx
Z52.098 Other blood donor, **other blood** PDx

✓5th **Z52.1** **Skin donor**
Z52.10 Skin donor, **unspecified** PDx
Z52.11 Skin donor, **autologous** PDx
Z52.19 Skin donor, **other** PDx

✓6th **Z52.2** **Bone donor**
Z52.20 Bone donor, **unspecified** PDx
Z52.21 Bone donor, **autologous** PDx
Z52.29 Bone donor, **other** PDx

Z52.3 **Bone marrow donor** PDx

Z52.4 **Kidney donor** PDx

Z52.5 **Cornea donor** PDx

Z52.6 **Liver donor** PDx

✓5th **Z52.8** **Donor of other specified organs or tissues**

✓6th **Z52.81** **Egg (Oocyte) donor**
Z52.810 Egg (Oocyte) donor **under age 35, anonymous recipient** PDx ♀
Egg donor under age 35 NOS
Z52.811 Egg (Oocyte) donor **under age 35, designated recipient** PDx ♀
Z52.812 Egg (Oocyte) donor **age 35 and over, anonymous recipient** PDx ♀
Egg donor age 35 and over NOS
Z52.813 Egg (Oocyte) donor **age 35 and over, designated recipient** PDx ♀
Z52.819 Egg (Oocyte) donor, **unspecified** PDx ♀

Z52.89 Donor of other specified organs or tissues PDx

Z52.9 **Donor of unspecified organ or tissue**
Donor NOS

✓4th **Z53** **Persons encountering health services for specific procedures and treatment, not carried out**

✓5th **Z53.0** **Procedure and treatment not carried out because of contraindication**
Z53.01 **Procedure and treatment not carried out due to patient smoking**
Z53.09 **Procedure and treatment not carried out because of other contraindication**

Z53.1 **Procedure and treatment not carried out because of patient's decision for reasons of belief and group pressure**

✓5th **Z53.2** **Procedure and treatment not carried out because of patient's decision for other and unspecified reasons**
Z53.20 **Procedure and treatment not carried out because of patient's decision for unspecified reasons**
Z53.21 **Procedure and treatment not carried out due to patient leaving prior to being seen by health care provider**
Z53.29 **Procedure and treatment not carried out because of patient's decision for other reasons**

✓5th **Z53.3** **Procedure converted to open procedure**
AHA: 2016,4Q,79
Z53.31 **Laparoscopic surgical procedure converted to open procedure** UPD
Z53.32 **Thoracoscopic surgical procedure converted to open procedure** UPD
Z53.33 **Arthroscopic surgical procedure converted to open procedure** UPD
Z53.39 **Other specified procedure converted to open procedure** UPD

Z53.8 Procedure and treatment not carried out for other reasons

Z53.9 Procedure and treatment not carried out, unspecified reason

Persons with potential health hazards related to socioeconomic and psychosocial circumstances (Z55-Z65)

AHA: 2021,4Q,34-37; 2019,4Q,66; 2018,4Q,58,73; 2018,1Q,18

DEF: Social determinants of health: Socioeconomic factors that can affect a person's health, including both environmental and societal conditions such as education and literacy, employment, health behaviors, housing, lack of adequate food or water, occupational exposure to risk factors, social support, transportation, and violence. Tracking social needs that impact patients allows providers to identify population health trends and to promote the personalized care that addresses the medical and social needs of individual patients. *Synonym(s): SDOH.*

TIP: Because codes in these categories represent social information rather than medical diagnoses, they can be assigned based on documentation by nonphysician clinicians involved in the care of these patients as well as self-reported documentation from the patient, as long as the information is approved and incorporated into the medical record by a clinician or provider.

✓4ᵗʰ **Z55 Problems related to education and literacy**

EXCLUDES 1   disorders of psychological development (F80-F89)

moderate

Z55.0 Illiteracy and low-level literacy

Z55.1 Schooling unavailable and unattainable

Z55.2 Failed school examinations

Z55.3 Underachievement in school

Z55.4 Educational maladjustment and discord with teachers and classmates

Z55.5 Less than a high school diploma   UPD
     No general equivalence degree (GED)

Z55.8 Other problems related to education and literacy
     Problems related to inadequate teaching

Z55.9 Problems related to education and literacy, unspecified
     Academic problems NOS

✓4ᵗʰ **Z56 Problems related to employment and unemployment**

EXCLUDES 2   occupational exposure to risk factors (Z57.-)
         problems related to housing and economic circumstances (Z59.-)

Z56.0 Unemployment, unspecified

Z56.1 Change of job   A

Z56.2 Threat of job loss

Z56.3 Stressful work schedule

Z56.4 Discord with boss and workmates

Z56.5 Uncongenial work environment
     Difficult conditions at work

Z56.6 Other physical and mental strain related to work

✓5ᵗʰ **Z56.8 Other problems related to employment**

     Z56.81 Sexual harassment on the job

     Z56.82 Military deployment status
         Individual (civilian or military) currently deployed in theater or in support of military war, peacekeeping and humanitarian operations

     Z56.89 Other problems related to employment

Z56.9 Unspecified problems related to employment
     Occupational problems NOS

✓4ᵗʰ **Z57 Occupational exposure to risk factors**

Z57.0 Occupational exposure to noise

Z57.1 Occupational exposure to radiation

Z57.2 Occupational exposure to dust

✓5ᵗʰ **Z57.3 Occupational exposure to other air contaminants**

     Z57.31 Occupational exposure to environmental tobacco smoke
         EXCLUDES 2   exposure to environmental tobacco smoke (Z77.22)

     Z57.39 Occupational exposure to other air contaminants

Z57.4 Occupational exposure to toxic agents in agriculture
     Occupational exposure to solids, liquids, gases or vapors in agriculture

Z57.5 Occupational exposure to toxic agents in other industries
     Occupational exposure to solids, liquids, gases or vapors in other industries

Z57.6 Occupational exposure to extreme temperature

Z57.7 Occupational exposure to vibration

Z57.8 Occupational exposure to other risk factors

Z57.9 Occupational exposure to unspecified risk factor

✓4ᵗʰ **Z58 Problems related to physical environment**

EXCLUDES 2   occupational exposure (Z57.-)

Z58.6 Inadequate drinking-water supply
     Lack of safe drinking water
     EXCLUDES 2   deprivation of water (T73.1)

✓4ᵗʰ **Z59 Problems related to housing and economic circumstances**

EXCLUDES 2   problems related to upbringing (Z62.-)

✓5ᵗʰ **Z59.0 Homelessness**

     Z59.00 Homelessness unspecified   UPD

     Z59.01 Sheltered homelessness   UPD
         Doubled up
         Living in a shelter such as: motel, scattered site housing, temporary or transitional living situation

     Z59.02 Unsheltered homelessness   UPD
         Residing in place not meant for human habitation such as: abandoned buildings, cars, parks, sidewalk
         Residing on the street

Z59.1 Inadequate housing
     Lack of heating
     Restriction of space
     Technical defects in home preventing adequate care
     Unsatisfactory surroundings
     EXCLUDES 1   problems related to the natural and physical environment (Z77.1-)

Z59.2 Discord with neighbors, lodgers and landlord

Z59.3 Problems related to living in residential institution
     Boarding-school resident
     EXCLUDES 1   institutional upbringing (Z62.2)

✓5ᵗʰ **Z59.4 Lack of adequate food**

     EXCLUDES 2   deprivation of food (T73.0)
         effects of hunger (T73.0)
         inappropriate diet or eating habits (Z72.4)
         malnutrition (E40-E46)

     Z59.41 Food insecurity   UPD

     Z59.48 Other specified lack of adequate food   UPD
         Inadequate food
         Lack of food

Z59.5 Extreme poverty

Z59.6 Low income

Z59.7 Insufficient social insurance and welfare support

✓5ᵗʰ **Z59.8 Other problems related to housing and economic circumstances**

     ✓6ᵗʰ **Z59.81 Housing instability, housed**
         Foreclosure on home loan
         Past due on rent or mortgage
         Unwanted multiple moves in the last 12 months

         Z59.811 Housing instability, housed, with risk of homelessness   UPD
             Imminent risk of homelessness

         Z59.812 Housing instability, housed, homelessness in past 12 months   UPD

         Z59.819 Housing instability, housed unspecified   UPD

     Z59.82 Transportation insecurity
         Excessive transportation time
         Inaccessible transportation
         Inadequate transportation
         Lack of transportation
         Unaffordable transportation
         Unreliable transportation
         Unsafe transportation

Z59.86 Financial insecurity
Bankruptcy
Burdensome debt
Economic strain
Financial strain
Money problems
Running out of money
Unable to make ends meet
EXCLUDES 2   extreme poverty (Z59.5)
low income (Z59.6)
material hardship, not elsewhere classified (Z59.87)

Z59.87 Material hardship
Material deprivation
Unable to obtain adequate childcare
Unable to obtain adequate clothing
Unable to obtain adequate utilities
Unable to obtain basic needs
EXCLUDES 2   extreme poverty (Z59.5)
financial insecurity, not elsewhere classified (Z59.86)
low income (Z59.6)

Z59.89 Other problems related to housing and economic circumstances   UPD
Foreclosure on loan
Isolated dwelling
Problems with creditors

Z59.9 Problem related to housing and economic circumstances, unspecified

Z60 Problems related to social environment

Z60.0 Problems of adjustment to life-cycle transitions
Empty nest syndrome
Phase of life problem
Problem with adjustment to retirement [pension]

Z60.2 Problems related to living alone

Z60.3 Acculturation difficulty
Problem with migration
Problem with social transplantation
DEF: Problem adapting to a different culture or environment not based on any coexisting mental disorder.

Z60.4 Social exclusion and rejection
Exclusion and rejection on the basis of personal characteristics, such as unusual physical appearance, illness or behavior.
EXCLUDES 1   target of adverse discrimination such as for racial or religious reasons (Z60.5)

Z60.5 Target of (perceived) adverse discrimination and persecution
EXCLUDES 1   social exclusion and rejection (Z60.4)

Z60.8 Other problems related to social environment

Z60.9 Problem related to social environment, unspecified

Z62 Problems related to upbringing
INCLUDES   current and past negative life events in childhood
current and past problems of a child related to upbringing
EXCLUDES 2   maltreatment syndrome (T74.-)
problems related to housing and economic circumstances (Z59.-)

Z62.0 Inadequate parental supervision and control

Z62.1 Parental overprotection

Z62.2 Upbringing away from parents
EXCLUDES 1   problems with boarding school (Z59.3)

Z62.21 Child in welfare custody   P
Child in care of non-parental family member
Child in foster care
EXCLUDES 2   problem for parent due to child in welfare custody (Z63.5)

Z62.22 Institutional upbringing
Child living in orphanage or group home

Z62.29 Other upbringing away from parents

Z62.3 Hostility towards and scapegoating of child   P

Z62.6 Inappropriate (excessive) parental pressure

Z62.8 Other specified problems related to upbringing

Z62.81 Personal history of abuse in childhood

Z62.810 Personal history of physical and sexual abuse in childhood
EXCLUDES 1   current child physical abuse (T74.12, T76.12)
current child sexual abuse (T74.22, T76.22)

Z62.811 Personal history of psychological abuse in childhood
EXCLUDES 1   current child psychological abuse (T74.32, T76.32)

Z62.812 Personal history of neglect in childhood
EXCLUDES 1   current child neglect (T74.02, T76.02)

Z62.813 Personal history of forced labor or sexual exploitation in childhood
AHA: 2018,4Q,32,35

Z62.819 Personal history of unspecified abuse in childhood
EXCLUDES 1   current child abuse NOS (T74.92, T76.92)

Z62.82 Parent-child conflict

Z62.820 Parent-biological child conflict
Parent-child problem NOS

Z62.821 Parent-adopted child conflict

Z62.822 Parent-foster child conflict

Z62.89 Other specified problems related to upbringing

Z62.890 Parent-child estrangement NEC

Z62.891 Sibling rivalry

Z62.898 Other specified problems related to upbringing

Z62.9 Problem related to upbringing, unspecified

Z63 Other problems related to primary support group, including family circumstances
EXCLUDES 2   maltreatment syndrome (T74.-, T76)
parent-child problems (Z62.-)
problems related to negative life events in childhood (Z62.-)
problems related to upbringing (Z62.-)

Z63.0 Problems in relationship with spouse or partner
Relationship distress with spouse or intimate partner
EXCLUDES 1   counseling for spousal or partner abuse problems (Z69.1)
counseling related to sexual attitude, behavior, and orientation (Z70.-)

Z63.1 Problems in relationship with in-laws

Z63.3 Absence of family member
EXCLUDES 1   absence of family member due to disappearance and death (Z63.4)
absence of family member due to separation and divorce (Z63.5)

Z63.31 Absence of family member due to military deployment
Individual or family affected by other family member being on military deployment
EXCLUDES 1   family disruption due to return of family member from military deployment (Z63.71)

Z63.32 Other absence of family member

Z63.4 Disappearance and death of family member
Assumed death of family member
Bereavement
AHA: 2014,1Q,25

Z63.5 Disruption of family by separation and divorce
Marital estrangement

Z63.6 Dependent relative needing care at home

Z63.7 Other stressful life events affecting family and household

Z63.71 Stress on family due to return of family member from military deployment
Individual or family affected by family member having returned from military deployment (current or past conflict)

Z63.72 Alcoholism and drug addiction in family

Z63.79   **Other stressful life events affecting family and household**
- Anxiety (normal) about sick person in family
- Health problems within family
- Ill or disturbed family member
- Isolated family

Z63.8   **Other specified problems related to primary support group**
- Family discord NOS
- Family estrangement NOS
- High expressed emotional level within family
- Inadequate family support NOS
- Inadequate or distorted communication within family

Z63.9   **Problem related to primary support group, unspecified**
- Relationship disorder NOS

✓4ᵗʰ **Z64**   **Problems related to certain psychosocial circumstances**

Z64.0   **Problems related to unwanted pregnancy**   ♀

Z64.1   **Problems related to multiparity**   ♀

Z64.4   **Discord with counselors**
- Discord with probation officer
- Discord with social worker

✓4ᵗʰ **Z65**   **Problems related to other psychosocial circumstances**

Z65.0   **Conviction in civil and criminal proceedings without imprisonment**

Z65.1   **Imprisonment and other incarceration**

Z65.2   **Problems related to release from prison**

Z65.3   **Problems related to other legal circumstances**
- Arrest
- Child custody or support proceedings
- Litigation
- Prosecution

Z65.4   **Victim of crime and terrorism**
- Victim of torture

Z65.5   **Exposure to disaster, war and other hostilities**
- EXCLUDES 1   *target of perceived discrimination or persecution (Z60.5)*

Z65.8   **Other specified problems related to psychosocial circumstances**
- Religious or spiritual problem

Z65.9   **Problem related to unspecified psychosocial circumstances**

Do not resuscitate status (Z66)

Z66   **Do not resuscitate**
- DNR status
- **DEF:** Medical order written by a physician that instructs others not to perform cardiopulmonary resuscitation (CPR), intubation, or advanced cardiac life support (ACLS). It prevents unnecessary invasive treatment to prolong life should breathing stop or cardiac arrest occur.

Blood type (Z67)

✓4ᵗʰ **Z67**   **Blood type**
- **AHA:** 2015,3Q,40

✓5ᵗʰ **Z67.1**   **Type A blood**
- **Z67.10**   **Type A blood, Rh positive**
- **Z67.11**   **Type A blood, Rh negative**

✓5ᵗʰ **Z67.2**   **Type B blood**
- **Z67.20**   **Type B blood, Rh positive**
- **Z67.21**   **Type B blood, Rh negative**

✓5ᵗʰ **Z67.3**   **Type AB blood**
- **Z67.30**   **Type AB blood, Rh positive**
- **Z67.31**   **Type AB blood, Rh negative**

✓5ᵗʰ **Z67.4**   **Type O blood**
- **Z67.40**   **Type O blood, Rh positive**
- **Z67.41**   **Type O blood, Rh negative**

✓5ᵗʰ **Z67.9**   **Unspecified blood type**
- **Z67.90**   **Unspecified blood type, Rh positive**   *RH⁺*
- **Z67.91**   **Unspecified blood type, Rh negative**   *RH⁻*

Body mass index [BMI] (Z68)

✓4ᵗʰ **Z68**   **Body mass index [BMI]**   *do not assign for pregnancy*
- Kilograms per meters squared
- **NOTE**   BMI adult codes are for use for persons 20 years of age or older
  - BMI pediatric codes are for use for persons 2-19 years of age.
  - These percentiles are based on the growth charts published by the Centers for Disease Control and Prevention (CDC)
- **AHA:** 2019,4Q,19,57; 2018,4Q,73,77-83; 2017,1Q,39
- **DEF:** Index used to help determine whether an individual is underweight, a healthy weight, overweight, or obese.
- **TIP:** A BMI code may be assigned to support an associated condition based on medical record documentation from clinicians who are not the patient's provider.
- **TIP:** In order to assign a BMI code, the associated condition must meet the definition of a reportable diagnosis for outpatient encounters, per section IV.J of the *ICD-10-CM Official Guidelines for Coding and Reporting.*

Z68.1   **Body mass index [BMI] 19.9 or less, adult**   UPD A

✓5ᵗʰ **Z68.2**   **Body mass index [BMI] 20-29, adult**
- **Z68.20**   **Body mass index [BMI] 20.0-20.9, adult**   UPD A
- **Z68.21**   **Body mass index [BMI] 21.0-21.9, adult**   UPD A
- **Z68.22**   **Body mass index [BMI] 22.0-22.9, adult**   UPD A
- **Z68.23**   **Body mass index [BMI] 23.0-23.9, adult**   UPD A
- **Z68.24**   **Body mass index [BMI] 24.0-24.9, adult**   UPD A
- **Z68.25**   **Body mass index [BMI] 25.0-25.9, adult**   UPD A
- **Z68.26**   **Body mass index [BMI] 26.0-26.9, adult**   UPD A
- **Z68.27**   **Body mass index [BMI] 27.0-27.9, adult**   UPD A
- **Z68.28**   **Body mass index [BMI] 28.0-28.9, adult**   UPD A
- **Z68.29**   **Body mass index [BMI] 29.0-29.9, adult**   UPD A

✓5ᵗʰ **Z68.3**   **Body mass index [BMI] 30-39, adult**
- **Z68.30**   **Body mass index [BMI] 30.0-30.9, adult**   UPD A
- **Z68.31**   **Body mass index [BMI] 31.0-31.9, adult**   UPD A
- **Z68.32**   **Body mass index [BMI] 32.0-32.9, adult**   UPD A
- **Z68.33**   **Body mass index [BMI] 33.0-33.9, adult**   UPD A
- **Z68.34**   **Body mass index [BMI] 34.0-34.9, adult**   UPD A
- **Z68.35**   **Body mass index [BMI] 35.0-35.9, adult**   UPD A
- **Z68.36**   **Body mass index [BMI] 36.0-36.9, adult**   UPD A
- **Z68.37**   **Body mass index [BMI] 37.0-37.9, adult**   UPD A
- **Z68.38**   **Body mass index [BMI] 38.0-38.9, adult**   UPD A
- **Z68.39**   **Body mass index [BMI] 39.0-39.9, adult**   UPD A

✓5ᵗʰ **Z68.4**   **Body mass index [BMI] 40 or greater, adult**
- **Z68.41**   **Body mass index [BMI] 40.0-44.9, adult**   HCC ESR UPD A
- **Z68.42**   **Body mass index [BMI] 45.0-49.9, adult**   HCC ESR UPD A
- **Z68.43**   **Body mass index [BMI] 50.0-59.9, adult**   HCC ESR UPD A
- **Z68.44**   **Body mass index [BMI] 60.0-69.9, adult**   HCC ESR UPD A
- **Z68.45**   **Body mass index [BMI] 70 or greater, adult**   HCC ESR UPD A

✓5ᵗʰ **Z68.5**   **Body mass index [BMI] pediatric**
- **AHA:** 2018,4Q,81-82
- **Z68.51**   **Body mass index [BMI] pediatric, less than 5th percentile for age**   UPD
- **Z68.52**   **Body mass index [BMI] pediatric, 5th percentile to less than 85th percentile for age**   UPD
- **Z68.53**   **Body mass index [BMI] pediatric, 85th percentile to less than 95th percentile for age**   UPD
- **Z68.54**   **Body mass index [BMI] pediatric, greater than or equal to 95th percentile for age**   UPD

Persons encountering health services in other circumstances (Z69-Z76)

✓4ᵗʰ Z69 Encounter for mental health services for victim and perpetrator of abuse

INCLUDES   counseling for victims and perpetrators of abuse

✓5ᵗʰ Z69.0 Encounter for mental health services for child abuse problems

✓6ᵗʰ Z69.01 Encounter for mental health services for parental child abuse

Z69.010 Encounter for mental health services for victim of parental child abuse P

Encounter for mental health services for victim of child abuse by parent

Encounter for mental health services for victim of child neglect by parent

Encounter for mental health services for victim of child psychological abuse by parent

Encounter for mental health services for victim of child sexual abuse by parent

Z69.011 Encounter for mental health services for perpetrator of parental child abuse

Encounter for mental health services for perpetrator of parental child neglect

Encounter for mental health services for perpetrator of parental child psychological abuse

Encounter for mental health services for perpetrator of parental child sexual abuse

EXCLUDES 1   encounter for mental health services for non-parental child abuse (Z69.02-)

✓6ᵗʰ Z69.02 Encounter for mental health services for non-parental child abuse

Z69.020 Encounter for mental health services for victim of non-parental child abuse P

Encounter for mental health services for victim of non-parental child neglect

Encounter for mental health services for victim of non-parental child psychological abuse

Encounter for mental health services for victim of non-parental child sexual abuse

Z69.021 Encounter for mental health services for perpetrator of non-parental child abuse

Encounter for mental health services for perpetrator of non-parental child neglect

Encounter for mental health services for perpetrator of non-parental child psychological abuse

Encounter for mental health services for perpetrator of non-parental child sexual abuse

✓5ᵗʰ Z69.1 Encounter for mental health services for spousal or partner abuse **problems**

Z69.11 Encounter for mental health services for victim of spousal or partner abuse

Encounter for mental health services for victim of spouse or partner neglect

Encounter for mental health services for victim of spouse or partner psychological abuse

Encounter for mental health services for victim of spouse or partner violence, physical

Z69.12 Encounter for mental health services for perpetrator of spousal or partner abuse

Encounter for mental health services for perpetrator of spouse or partner neglect

Encounter for mental health services for perpetrator of spouse or partner psychological abuse

Encounter for mental health services for perpetrator of spouse or partner violence, physical

Encounter for mental health services for perpetrator of spouse or partner violence, sexual

✓5ᵗʰ Z69.8 Encounter for mental health services for victim or perpetrator of other abuse

Z69.81 Encounter for mental health services for victim of other abuse

Encounter for mental health services for victim of non-spousal adult abuse

Encounter for mental health services for victim of spouse or partner violence, sexual

Encounter for rape victim counseling

Z69.82 Encounter for mental health services for perpetrator of **other abuse**

Encounter for mental health services for perpetrator of non-spousal adult abuse

✓4ᵗʰ Z70 Counseling related to sexual attitude, behavior and orientation

INCLUDES   encounter for mental health services for sexual attitude, behavior and orientation

EXCLUDES 2   contraceptive or procreative counseling (Z30-Z31)

Z70.0 Counseling related to sexual attitude

Z70.1 Counseling related to patient's sexual behavior and orientation

Patient concerned regarding impotence

Patient concerned regarding non-responsiveness

Patient concerned regarding promiscuity

Patient concerned regarding sexual orientation

Z70.2 Counseling related to sexual behavior and orientation of third party

Advice sought regarding sexual behavior and orientation of child

Advice sought regarding sexual behavior and orientation of partner

Advice sought regarding sexual behavior and orientation of spouse

Z70.3 Counseling related to combined concerns regarding sexual attitude, behavior and orientation

Z70.8 Other sex counseling

Encounter for sex education

Z70.9 Sex counseling, unspecified

✓4ᵗʰ Z71 Persons encountering health services for other counseling and medical advice, not elsewhere classified

EXCLUDES 2   contraceptive or procreation counseling (Z30-Z31)

sex counseling (Z70.-)

Z71.0 Person encountering health services to consult on behalf of another person

Person encountering health services to seek advice or treatment for non-attending third party

EXCLUDES 2   anxiety (normal) about sick person in family (Z63.7)

expectant (adoptive) parent(s) pre-birth pediatrician visit (Z76.81)

Z71.1 Person with feared health complaint in whom no diagnosis is made

Person encountering health services with feared condition which was not demonstrated

Person encountering health services in which problem was normal state

"Worried well"

EXCLUDES 1   medical observation for suspected diseases and conditions proven not to exist (Z03.-)

Z71.2 Person consulting for explanation of examination or test findings

Z71.3 Dietary counseling and surveillance

Use additional code for any associated underlying medical condition

Use additional code to identify body mass index (BMI), if known (Z68.-)

✓5ᵗʰ Z71.4 Alcohol abuse counseling and surveillance

Use additional code for alcohol abuse or dependence (F10.-)

Z71.41 Alcohol abuse counseling and surveillance of alcoholic

Z71.42 Counseling for family member of alcoholic

Counseling for significant other, partner, or friend of alcoholic

✓5ᵗʰ Z71.5 Drug abuse counseling and surveillance

Use additional code for drug abuse or dependence (F11-F16, F18-F19)

Z71.51 Drug abuse counseling and surveillance of drug abuser

HCC CMS-HCC   Rx Rx HCC   ESR ESRD HCC   COM Commercial HCC   PDx Primary Dx Only   N Newborn: 0   P Pediatric: 0-17   M Maternity: 9-64   A Adult: 15-124

1282   ICD-10-CM 2023

Z71.52 **Counseling for** family member of drug abuser
Counseling for significant other, partner, or friend of drug abuser

Z71.6 Tobacco **abuse counseling**
Use additional code for nicotine dependence (F17.-)

Z71.7 Human immunodeficiency virus [HIV] counseling

✓5ᵗʰ **Z71.8** **Other specified counseling**
EXCLUDES 2   counseling for contraception (Z30.0-)
AHA: 2017,4Q,27

Z71.81 Spiritual or religious **counseling**

Z71.82 Exercise **counseling**

Z71.83 **Encounter for** nonprocreative genetic **counseling**
EXCLUDES 1   counseling for procreative genetics (Z31.5)
counseling for procreative management (Z31.6)

Z71.84 **Encounter for** health counseling related to travel
Encounter for health risk and safety counseling for (international) travel
Code also, if applicable, encounter for immunization (Z23)
EXCLUDES 2   encounter for administrative examination (Z02.-)
encounter for other special examination without complaint, suspected or reported diagnosis (Z01.-)
AHA: 2019,4Q,20,57

Z71.85 **Encounter for** immunization safety counseling
Encounter for vaccine product safety counseling
Code also, if applicable, encounter for immunization (Z23)
Code also, if applicable, immunization not carried out (Z28.-)
EXCLUDES 1   encounter for health counseling related to travel (Z71.84)
AHA: 2021,4Q,34

Z71.87 **Encounter for** pediatric-to-adult transition counseling
Code also chronic condition, if applicable, such as:
autism spectrum disorder (F84.0)
congenital malformations of the circulatory system (Q20-Q28)
cystic fibrosis (E84-)
sickle-cell disorder (D57-)

Z71.88 **Encounter for counseling for** socioeconomic factors

Z71.89 **Other specified counseling**

Z71.9 **Counseling, unspecified**
Encounter for medical advice NOS   *PEP(+) Conseling HPV(+)*

✓4ᵗʰ **Z72** **Problems related to lifestyle**
EXCLUDES 2   problems related to life-management difficulty (Z73.-)
problems related to socioeconomic and psychosocial circumstances (Z55-Z65)

Z72.0 **Tobacco use**
Tobacco use NOS
EXCLUDES 1   history of tobacco dependence (Z87.891)
nicotine dependence (F17.2-)
tobacco dependence (F17.2-)
tobacco use during pregnancy (O99.33-)

Z72.3 **Lack of physical exercise**

Z72.4 **Inappropriate diet and eating habits**
EXCLUDES 1   behavioral eating disorders of infancy or childhood (F98.2-F98.3)
eating disorders (F50.-)
lack of adequate food (Z59.48)
malnutrition and other nutritional deficiencies (E40-E64)

✓5ᵗʰ **Z72.5** High risk sexual behavior
Promiscuity
EXCLUDES 1   paraphilias (F65)

Z72.51 **High risk** heterosexual **behavior**

Z72.52 **High risk** homosexual **behavior**

Z72.53 **High risk** bisexual **behavior**

Z72.6 **Gambling and betting**
EXCLUDES 1   compulsive or pathological gambling (F63.0)

✓5ᵗʰ **Z72.8** **Other problems related to lifestyle**

✓6ᵗʰ **Z72.81** **Antisocial behavior**
EXCLUDES 1   conduct disorders (F91.-)

Z72.810 Child and adolescent antisocial behavior   P
Antisocial behavior (child) (adolescent) without manifest psychiatric disorder
Delinquency NOS
Group delinquency
Offenses in the context of gang membership
Stealing in company with others
Truancy from school

Z72.811 Adult antisocial behavior   A
Adult antisocial behavior without manifest psychiatric disorder

✓6ᵗʰ **Z72.82** **Problems related to sleep**

Z72.820 Sleep deprivation
Lack of adequate sleep
EXCLUDES 1   insomnia (G47.0-)

Z72.821 Inadequate sleep hygiene
Bad sleep habits
Irregular sleep habits
Unhealthy sleep wake schedule
EXCLUDES 1   insomnia (F51.0-, G47.0-)

Z72.823 **Risk of suffocation (smothering) under another while sleeping**
Child-caregiver co-sleeping
Infant bed-sharing

Z72.89 **Other problems related to lifestyle**
Self-damaging behavior

Z72.9 **Problem related to lifestyle, unspecified**

✓4ᵗʰ **Z73** **Problems related to life management difficulty**
EXCLUDES 2   problems related to socioeconomic and psychosocial circumstances (Z55-Z65)
DEF: State of emotional, mental, and physical exhaustion causing difficulties in managing personal, school, or work circumstances. It is usually due to prolonged stress or poor interpersonal relationship skills or parenting skills.

Z73.0 **Burn-out**

Z73.1 **Type A behavior pattern**

Z73.2 **Lack of relaxation and leisure**

Z73.3 **Stress, not elsewhere classified**
Physical and mental strain NOS
EXCLUDES 1   stress related to employment or unemployment (Z56.-)

Z73.4 **Inadequate social skills, not elsewhere classified**

Z73.5 **Social role conflict, not elsewhere classified**

Z73.6 **Limitation of activities due to disability**
EXCLUDES 1   care-provider dependency (Z74.-)

✓5ᵗʰ **Z73.8** **Other problems related to life management difficulty**

✓6ᵗʰ **Z73.81** **Behavioral insomnia of childhood**
DEF: Behaviors on the part of the child or caregivers that cause negative compliance with a child's sleep schedule resulting in lack of adequate sleep.

Z73.810 **Behavioral insomnia of childhood, sleep-onset association type**   P

Z73.811 **Behavioral insomnia of childhood, limit setting type**   P

Z73.812 **Behavioral insomnia of childhood, combined type**   P

Z73.819 **Behavioral insomnia of childhood, unspecified type**   P

Z73.82 **Dual sensory impairment**

Z73.89 **Other problems related to life management difficulty**

Z73.9 **Problem related to life management difficulty, unspecified**

✓4ᵗʰ **Z74** **Problems related to care provider dependency**
EXCLUDES 2   dependence on enabling machines or devices NEC (Z99.-)

✓5ᵗʰ **Z74.0** **Reduced mobility**

Z74.01 **Bed confinement status**
Bedridden

Chapter 21. Factors Influencing Health Status and Contact With Health Services

Z74.09   **Other reduced mobility**
Chair ridden
Reduced mobility NOS
EXCLUDES 2   *wheelchair dependence (Z99.3)*

Z74.1   **Need for assistance with** personal care

Z74.2   **Need for assistance at home and** no other household member able to render care

Z74.3   **Need for** continuous supervision

Z74.8   **Other problems related to care provider dependency**

Z74.9   **Problem related to care provider dependency, unspecified**

✅4ᵗʰ   **Z75   Problems related to medical facilities and other health care**

Z75.0   **Medical services** not available in home
EXCLUDES 1   *no other household member able to render care (Z74.2)*

Z75.1   **Person** awaiting admission **to adequate facility elsewhere**

Z75.2   **Other waiting period for investigation and treatment**

Z75.3   Unavailability **and inaccessibility of** health-care facilities
EXCLUDES 1   *bed unavailable (Z75.1)*

Z75.4   Unavailability **and inaccessibility of other** helping agencies

Z75.5   Holiday relief care

Z75.8   **Other problems related to medical facilities and other health care**

Z75.9   **Unspecified problem related to medical facilities and other health care**

✅4ᵗʰ   **Z76   Persons encountering health services in other circumstances**

Z76.0   **Encounter for issue of repeat prescription**
Encounter for issue of repeat prescription for appliance
Encounter for issue of repeat prescription for medicaments
Encounter for issue of repeat prescription for spectacles
EXCLUDES 2   *issue of medical certificate (Z02.7)*
         repeat prescription for contraceptive (Z30.4-)

Z76.1   **Encounter for health supervision and care of foundling**   PDx

Z76.2   **Encounter for health supervision and care of other healthy infant and child**   PDx P
Encounter for medical or nursing care or supervision of healthy infant under circumstances such as adverse socioeconomic conditions at home
Encounter for medical or nursing care or supervision of healthy infant under circumstances such as awaiting foster or adoptive placement
Encounter for medical or nursing care or supervision of healthy infant under circumstances such as maternal illness
Encounter for medical or nursing care or supervision of healthy infant under circumstances such as number of children at home preventing or interfering with normal care

Z76.3   **Healthy person accompanying sick person**

Z76.4   **Other boarder to healthcare facility**
EXCLUDES 1   *homelessness (Z59.0-)*

Z76.5   **Malingerer [conscious simulation]**
Person feigning illness (with obvious motivation)
EXCLUDES 1   *factitious disorder (F68.1-, F68.A)*
         peregrinating patient (F68.1-)
DEF: Act of intentionally exaggerating an illness or disability in order to receive personal gain or to avoid punishment or responsibility.

✅5ᵗʰ   Z76.8   **Persons encountering health services in other specified circumstances**

Pediatrician   Z76.81   **Expectant parent(s) prebirth pediatrician visit**
Pre-adoption pediatrician visit for adoptive parent(s)

Z76.82   **Awaiting organ transplant status**
Patient waiting for organ availability

Z76.89   **Persons encountering health services in other specified circumstances**
Persons encountering health services NOS
AHA: 2014,2Q,10

Code also any follow-up examination (Z08-Z09)

✅4ᵗʰ   **Z77   Other contact with and (suspected) exposures hazardous to health**
INCLUDES   contact with and (suspected) exposures to potential hazards to health
EXCLUDES 2   *contact with and (suspected) exposure to communicable diseases (Z20.-)*
         exposure to (parental) (environmental) tobacco smoke in the perinatal period (P96.81)
         newborn affected by noxious substances transmitted via placenta or breast milk (P04.-)
         occupational exposure to risk factors (Z57.-)
         retained foreign body (Z18.-)
         retained foreign body fully removed (Z87.821)
         toxic effects of substances chiefly nonmedicinal as to source (T51-T65)

✅5ᵗʰ   Z77.0   **Contact with and (suspected) exposure to** hazardous, chiefly nonmedicinal, chemicals

✅6ᵗʰ   Z77.01   **Contact with and (suspected) exposure to hazardous** metals

Z77.010   **Contact with and (suspected) exposure to** arsenic

Z77.011   **Contact with and (suspected) exposure to** lead

Z77.012   **Contact with and (suspected) exposure to** uranium
EXCLUDES 1   *retained depleted uranium fragments (Z18.01)*

Z77.018   **Contact with and (suspected) exposure to other hazardous metals**
Contact with and (suspected) exposure to chromium compounds
Contact with and (suspected) exposure to nickel dust

✅6ᵗʰ   Z77.02   **Contact with and (suspected) exposure to hazardous** aromatic compounds

Z77.020   **Contact with and (suspected) exposure to** aromatic amines

Z77.021   **Contact with and (suspected) exposure to** benzene

Z77.028   **Contact with and (suspected) exposure to other hazardous aromatic compounds**
Aromatic dyes NOS
Polycyclic aromatic hydrocarbons

✅6ᵗʰ   Z77.09   **Contact with and (suspected) exposure to other hazardous, chiefly** nonmedicinal, chemicals

Z77.090   **Contact with and (suspected) exposure to** asbestos

Z77.098   **Contact with and (suspected) exposure to other hazardous, chiefly nonmedicinal, chemicals**
Dyes NOS

✅5ᵗʰ   Z77.1   **Contact with and (suspected) exposure to** environmental pollution and hazards in the physical environment

✅6ᵗʰ   Z77.11   **Contact with and (suspected) exposure to** environmental pollution

Z77.110   **Contact with and (suspected) exposure to** air pollution

Z77.111   **Contact with and (suspected) exposure to** water pollution

Z77.112   **Contact with and (suspected) exposure to** soil pollution

Z77.118   **Contact with and (suspected) exposure to other environmental pollution**

✅6ᵗʰ   Z77.12   **Contact with and (suspected) exposure to** hazards in the physical environment

Z77.120   **Contact with and (suspected) exposure to** mold **(toxic)**

Z77.121 Contact with and (suspected) exposure to harmful algae and algae toxins
Contact with and (suspected) exposure to (harmful) algae bloom NOS
Contact with and (suspected) exposure to blue-green algae bloom
Contact with and (suspected) exposure to brown tide
Contact with and (suspected) exposure to cyanobacteria bloom
Contact with and (suspected) exposure to Florida red tide
Contact with and (suspected) exposure to pfiesteria piscicida
Contact with and (suspected) exposure to red tide

Z77.122 Contact with and (suspected) exposure to noise

Z77.123 Contact with and (suspected) exposure to radon and other naturally occurring radiation
EXCLUDES 2   radiation exposure as the cause of a confirmed condition (W88-W90, X39.0-)
radiation sickness NOS (T66)

Z77.128 Contact with and (suspected) exposure to other hazards in the physical environment

✓5ᵗʰ **Z77.2 Contact with and (suspected) exposure to other hazardous substances**

Z77.21 Contact with and (suspected) exposure to potentially hazardous body fluids

Z77.22 Contact with and (suspected) exposure to environmental tobacco smoke **(acute) (chronic)**
Exposure to second hand tobacco smoke (acute) (chronic)
Passive smoking (acute) (chronic)
EXCLUDES 1   nicotine dependence (F17.-)
tobacco use (Z72.0)
EXCLUDES 2   occupational exposure to environmental tobacco smoke (Z57.31)

Z77.29 Contact with and (suspected) exposure to other hazardous substances
AHA: 2016,2Q,33

Z77.9 Other contact with and (suspected) exposures hazardous to health

✓4ᵗʰ **Z78 Other specified health status**
EXCLUDES 2   asymptomatic human immunodeficiency virus [HIV] infection status (Z21)
postprocedural status (Z93-Z99)
sex reassignment status (Z87.890)

Z78.0 Asymptomatic menopausal state   A ♀
Menopausal state NOS
Postmenopausal status NOS
EXCLUDES 2   symptomatic menopausal state (N95.1)

Z78.1 Physical restraint status   *not code for temporary restrain*
EXCLUDES 1   physical restraint due to a procedure - omit code
DEF: Application of mechanical restraining devices or manual restraints to limit physical mobility of a patient.

Z78.9 Other specified health status

✓4ᵗʰ **Z79 Long term (current) drug therapy**   *not for acute disease*
INCLUDES   long term (current) drug use for prophylactic purposes   *Brief Tx.*
Code also any therapeutic drug level monitoring (Z51.81)
EXCLUDES 2   drug abuse and dependence (F11-F19)
drug use complicating pregnancy, childbirth, and the puerperium (O99.32-)
AHA: 2021,1Q,12

✓5ᵗʰ **Z79.0 Long term (current) use of anticoagulants and antithrombotics/antiplatelets**
EXCLUDES 2   long term (current) use of aspirin (Z79.82)

Z79.01 Long term (current) use of anticoagulants
AHA: 2022,2Q,17; 2021,1Q,4; 2020,2Q,20

Z79.02 Long term (current) use of antithrombotics/antiplatelets   UPD

Z79.1 Long term (current) use of non-steroidal anti-inflammatories (NSAID)   UPD
EXCLUDES 2   long term (current) use of aspirin (Z79.82)

Z79.2 Long term (current) use of antibiotics   UPD

Z79.3 Long term (current) use of hormonal contraceptives
Long term (current) use of birth control pill or patch

Z79.4 Long term (current) use of insulin   HCC Rx ESR COM
EXCLUDES 2   ▶long-term (current) use of injectable non-insulin antidiabetic drugs (Z79.85)◀
long term (current) use of oral antidiabetic drugs (Z79.84)
long term (current) use of oral hypoglycemic drugs (Z79.84)
AHA: 2020,3Q,31

if not mentioned long or short use long → 024.4

✓5ᵗʰ **Z79.5 Long term (current) use of steroids**

Z79.51 Long term (current) use of inhaled steroids   UPD
Z79.52 Long term (current) use of systemic steroids   UPD

✓5ᵗʰ **Z79.6 Long term (current) use of immunomodulators and immunosuppressants**
EXCLUDES 2   long term (current) use of steroids (Z79.5-)
long term (current) use of agents affecting estrogen receptors and estrogen levels (Z79.81-)

Z79.60 Long term (current) use of unspecified immunomodulators and immunosuppressants

Z79.61 Long term (current) use of immunomodulator
Long term (current) use of apremilast
Long term (current) use of immunomodulatory imide drug
Long term (current) use of lenalidomide
Long term (current) use of pomalidomide

✓6ᵗʰ **Z79.62 Long term (current) use of** immunosuppressant

Z79.620 Long term (current) use of immunosuppressive biologic
Long term (current) use of adalimumab
Long term (current) use of etanercept
Long term (current) use of infliximab
Long term (current) use of monoclonal antibodies

Z79.621 Long term (current) use of calcineurin inhibitor
Long term (current) use of cyclosporine
Long term (current) use of tacrolimus

Z79.622 Long term (current) use of Janus kinase inhibitor
Long term (current) use of tofacitinib

Z79.623 Long term (current) use of mammalian target of rapamycin (mTOR) inhibitor
Long term (current) use of sirolimus

Z79.624 Long term (current) use of inhibitors of nucleotide synthesis
Long term (current) use of azathioprine
Long term (current) use omycophenolate
Long term (current) use of purine synthesis (IMDH) inhibitors

✓6ᵗʰ **Z79.63 Long term (current) use of chemotherapeutic agent**

Z79.630 Long term (current) use of alkylating agent
Long term (current) use of chlorambucil
Long term (current) use of cisplatin
Long term (current) use of cyclophosphamide

Z79.631 Long term (current) use of antimetabolite agent
Long term (current) use of 5-fluorouracil
Long term (current) use of 6-mercaptopurine
Long term (current) use of cytarabine
Long term (current) use of methotrexate

Z79.632 Long term (current) use of antitumor antibiotic
Long term (current) use of bleomycin
Long term (current) use of doxorubicin
Long term (current) use of mitomycin C

Z79.633 Long term (current) use of mitotic inhibitor
Long term (current) use of paclitaxel
Long term (current) use of plant alkaloids
Long term (current) use of vinblastine
Long term (current) use of vincristine

● | **Z79.634** **Long term (current) use of** topoisomerase inhibitor
      Long term (current) use of etoposide
      Long term (current) use of irinotecan
      Long term (current) use of topotecan

● **Z79.64** **Long term (current) use of** myelosuppressive agent
      Long term (current) use of hydroxyurea

● **Z79.69** **Long term (current) use of other immunomodulators and immunosuppressants**

√5ᵗʰ **Z79.8** **Other long term (current) drug therapy**

√6ᵗʰ **Z79.81** **Long term (current) use of agents affecting estrogen receptors and estrogen levels**
      Code first, if applicable:
        malignant neoplasm of breast (C50.-)
        malignant neoplasm of prostate (C61)
      Use additional code, if applicable, to identify:
        estrogen receptor positive status (Z17.0)
        family history of breast cancer (Z80.3)
        genetic susceptibility to malignant neoplasm (cancer) (Z15.0-)
        personal history of breast cancer (Z85.3)
        personal history of prostate cancer (Z85.46)
        postmenopausal status (Z78.0)
      EXCLUDES 1   hormone replacement therapy (Z79.890)

Z79.810 **Long term (current) use of selective estrogen receptor modulators (SERMs)** UPD
      Long term (current) use of raloxifene (Evista)
      Long term (current) use of tamoxifen (Nolvadex)
      Long term (current) use of toremifene (Fareston)

Z79.811 **Long term (current) use of** aromatase inhibitors UPD
      Long term (current) use of anastrozole (Arimidex)
      Long term (current) use of exemestane (Aromasin)
      Long term (current) use of letrozole (Femara)

Z79.818 **Long term (current) use of other agents affecting estrogen receptors and estrogen levels** UPD
      Long term (current) use of estrogen receptor downregulators
      Long term (current) use of fulvestrant (Faslodex)
      Long term (current) use of gonadotropin-releasing hormone (GnRH) agonist
      Long term (current) use of goserelin acetate (Zoladex)
      Long term (current) use of leuprolide acetate (leuprorelin) (Lupron)
      Long term (current) use of megestrol acetate (Megace)

Z79.82 **Long term (current) use of** aspirin

Z79.83 **Long term (current) use of** bisphosphonates UPD
      AHA: 2016,4Q,42

Z79.84 **Long term (current) use of** oral hypoglycemic drugs UPD
      [handwritten: E11 024.4]
      Long term (current) use of oral antidiabetic drugs
      EXCLUDES 2 ▶long-term (current) use of injectable non-insulin antidiabetic drugs (Z79.85)◀
        long term (current) use of insulin (Z79.4)
      AHA: 2020,3Q,31; 2016,4Q,76

● **Z79.85** **Long-term (current) use of** injectable non-insulin antidiabetic drugs
      [handwritten: E11 024.4]
      EXCLUDES 2   long term (current) use of insulin (Z79.4)
        long term (current) use of oral hypoglycemic drugs (Z79.84)

√6ᵗʰ **Z79.89** **Other long term (current) drug therapy**

Z79.890 **Hormone replacement therapy** UPD

Z79.891 **Long term (current) use of** opiate analgesic
      Long term (current) use of methadone for pain management
      EXCLUDES 1   methodone use NOS (F11.9-)
        use of methadone for treatment of heroin addiction (F11.2-)

Z79.899 **Other long term (current) drug therapy** *[handwritten: injectable non-insulin antiDM drugs]*
      AHA: 2020,4Q,11; 2020,3Q,31; 2020,2Q,14; 2015,4Q,34; 2015,3Q,21

√4ᵗʰ **Z80** **Family history of primary malignant neoplasm**

Z80.0 **Family history of malignant neoplasm of** digestive organs UPD
      Conditions classifiable to C15-C26
      AHA: 2018,1Q,6

Z80.1 **Family history of malignant neoplasm of** trachea, bronchus and lung UPD
      Conditions classifiable to C33-C34

Z80.2 **Family history of malignant neoplasm of other respiratory and intrathoracic organs** UPD
      Conditions classifiable to C30-C32, C37-C39

Z80.3 **Family history of malignant neoplasm of** breast UPD
      Conditions classifiable to C50.-

√5ᵗʰ **Z80.4** **Family history of malignant neoplasm of genital organs**   *[handwritten: Family history]*
      Conditions classifiable to C51-C63

Z80.41 **Family history of malignant neoplasm of** ovary UPD

Z80.42 **Family history of malignant neoplasm of** prostate UPD

Z80.43 **Family history of malignant neoplasm of** testis UPD

Z80.49 **Family history of malignant neoplasm of other genital organs**

√5ᵗʰ **Z80.5** **Family history of malignant neoplasm of urinary tract**
      Conditions classifiable to C64-C68

Z80.51 **Family history of malignant neoplasm of** kidney UPD

Z80.52 **Family history of malignant neoplasm of** bladder UPD

Z80.59 **Family history of malignant neoplasm of other urinary tract organ** UPD

Z80.6 **Family history of** leukemia UPD
      Conditions classifiable to C91-C95

Z80.7 **Family history of other malignant neoplasms of** lymphoid, hematopoietic and related tissues UPD
      Conditions classifiable to C81-C90, C96.-

Z80.8 **Family history of malignant neoplasm of other organs or systems** UPD
      Conditions classifiable to C00-C14, C40-C49, C69-C79

Z80.9 **Family history of malignant neoplasm, unspecified** UPD
      Conditions classifiable to C80.1

√4ᵗʰ **Z81** **Family history of mental and behavioral disorders**

Z81.0 **Family history of** intellectual disabilities
      Conditions classifiable to F70-F79

Z81.1 **Family history of** alcohol abuse and dependence
      Conditions classifiable to F10.-

Z81.2 **Family history of** tobacco abuse and dependence
      Conditions classifiable to F17.-

Z81.3 **Family history of other psychoactive substance abuse and dependence**
      Conditions classifiable to F11-F16, F18-F19

Z81.4 **Family history of other substance abuse and dependence**
      Conditions classifiable to F55

Z81.8 **Family history of other mental and behavioral disorders**
      Conditions classifiable elsewhere in F01-F99

√4ᵗʰ **Z82** **Family history of certain disabilities and chronic diseases (leading to disablement)**

Z82.0 **Family history of** epilepsy and other diseases of the nervous system UPD
      Conditions classifiable to G00-G99

Z82.1 **Family history of** blindness and visual loss UPD
      Conditions classifiable to H54.-

Z82.2 **Family history of** deafness and hearing loss UPD
      Conditions classifiable to H90-H91

HCC CMS-HCC   Rx Rx HCC   ESR ESRD HCC   COM Commercial HCC   PDx Primary Dx Only   N Newborn: 0   P Pediatric: 0-17   M Maternity: 9-64   A Adult: 15-124

1286
ICD-10-CM 2023

Z82.3   **Family history of** stroke   `UPD`
    Conditions classifiable to I60-I64

`✓5ᵗʰ` **Z82.4**   **Family history of ischemic heart disease and other diseases of the circulatory system**
    Conditions classifiable to I00-I5A, I65-I99

    Z82.41   **Family history of** sudden cardiac death   `UPD`

    Z82.49   **Family history of** ischemic heart disease **and other diseases of the circulatory system**   `UPD`

Z82.5   **Family history of** asthma **and other chronic lower respiratory diseases**   `UPD`
    Conditions classifiable to J40-J47

    EXCLUDES 2   family history of other diseases of the respiratory system (Z83.6)

`✓5ᵗʰ` **Z82.6**   **Family history of arthritis and other diseases of the musculoskeletal system and connective tissue**
    Conditions classifiable to M00-M99

    Z82.61   **Family history of** arthritis   `UPD`

    Z82.62   **Family history of** osteoporosis   `UPD`

    Z82.69   **Family history of other diseases of the musculoskeletal system and connective tissue**   `UPD`

`✓5ᵗʰ` **Z82.7**   **Family history of congenital malformations, deformations and chromosomal abnormalities**
    Conditions classifiable to Q00-Q99

    Z82.71   **Family history of** polycystic kidney   `UPD`

    Z82.79   **Family history of other congenital malformations, deformations and chromosomal abnormalities**   `UPD`

Z82.8   **Family history of other disabilities and chronic diseases leading to disablement, not elsewhere classified**   `UPD`

`✓4ᵗʰ` **Z83**   **Family history of other specific disorders**

    EXCLUDES 2   contact with and (suspected) exposure to communicable disease in the family (Z20.-)

Z83.0   **Family history of** human immunodeficiency virus [HIV] **disease**   `UPD`
    Conditions classifiable to B20

Z83.1   **Family history of other infectious and parasitic diseases**   `UPD`
    Conditions classifiable to A00-B19, B25-B94, B99

Z83.2   **Family history of diseases of the** blood and blood-forming organs **and certain disorders involving the immune mechanism**   `UPD`
    Conditions classifiable to D50-D89

Z83.3   **Family history of** diabetes mellitus   `UPD`
    Conditions classifiable to E08-E13

`✓5ᵗʰ` **Z83.4**   **Family history of other endocrine, nutritional and metabolic diseases**
    Conditions classifiable to E00-E07, E15-E88

    Z83.41   **Family history of** multiple endocrine neoplasia [MEN] syndrome   `UPD`

    Z83.42   **Family history of** familial hypercholesterolemia   `UPD`
      AHA: 2016,4Q,77

    `✓6ᵗʰ` **Z83.43**   **Family history of other disorder of lipoprotein metabolism and other lipidemias**
      AHA: 2018,4Q,6,35

      Z83.430   **Family history of** elevated lipoprotein(a)   `UPD`
        Family history of elevated Lp(a)

      Z83.438   **Family history of other disorder of lipoprotein metabolism and other lipidemia**   `UPD`
        Family history of familial combined hyperlipidemia

    Z83.49   **Family history of other endocrine, nutritional and metabolic diseases**   `UPD`

`✓5ᵗʰ` **Z83.5**   **Family history of eye and ear disorders**

    `✓6ᵗʰ` **Z83.51**   **Family history of** eye **disorders**
      Conditions classifiable to H00-H53, H55-H59
      EXCLUDES 2   family history of blindness and visual loss (Z82.1)

      Z83.511   **Family history of** glaucoma   `UPD`

      Z83.518   **Family history of other specified eye disorder**   `UPD`

    Z83.52   **Family history of** ear **disorders**   `UPD`
      Conditions classifiable to H60-H83, H92-H95
      EXCLUDES 2   family history of deafness and hearing loss (Z82.2)

Z83.6   **Family history of other diseases of the** respiratory system   `UPD`
    Conditions classifiable to J00-J39, J60-J99
    EXCLUDES 2   family history of asthma and other chronic lower respiratory diseases (Z82.5)

`✓5ᵗʰ` **Z83.7**   **Family history of diseases of the digestive system**
    Conditions classifiable to K00-K93

    Z83.71   **Family history of** colonic polyps   `UPD`
      EXCLUDES 2   family history of malignant neoplasm of digestive organs (Z80.0)
      AHA: 2021,1Q,14

    Z83.79   **Family history of other diseases of the digestive system**   `UPD`

`✓4ᵗʰ` **Z84**   **Family history of other conditions**

Z84.0   **Family history of diseases of the** skin and subcutaneous tissue   `UPD`
    Conditions classifiable to L00-L99

Z84.1   **Family history of disorders of** kidney and ureter   `UPD`
    Conditions classifiable to N00-N29

Z84.2   **Family history of other diseases of the** genitourinary system   `UPD`
    Conditions classifiable to N30-N99

Z84.3   **Family history of** consanguinity   `UPD`

`✓5ᵗʰ` **Z84.8**   **Family history of other specified conditions**

    Z84.81   **Family history of carrier of** genetic disease   `UPD`
      AHA: 2021,1Q,14

    Z84.82   **Family history of** sudden infant death syndrome   `UPD`
      Family history of SIDS
      AHA: 2016,4Q,77

    Z84.89   **Family history of other specified conditions**   `UPD`

`✓4ᵗʰ` **Z85**   **Personal history of malignant neoplasm**   *no longer exist*
    Code first any follow-up examination after treatment of malignant neoplasm (Z08)
    Personal History   Use additional code to identify:
      alcohol use and dependence (F10.-)
      exposure to environmental tobacco smoke (Z77.22)
      history of tobacco dependence (Z87.891)
      occupational exposure to environmental tobacco smoke (Z57.31)
      tobacco dependence (F17.-)
      tobacco use (Z72.0)
    EXCLUDES 2   personal history of benign neoplasm (Z86.01-)
        personal history of carcinoma-in-situ (Z86.00-)
    AHA: 2020,3Q,30; 2018,4Q,64

`✓5ᵗʰ` **Z85.0**   **Personal history of malignant neoplasm of** digestive organs
    AHA: 2017,1Q,9

    Z85.00   **Personal history of malignant neoplasm of unspecified digestive organ**

    Z85.01   **Personal history of malignant neoplasm of esophagus**
      Conditions classifiable to C15   *carcinomas*

    `✓6ᵗʰ` **Z85.02**   **Personal history of malignant neoplasm of** stomach

      Z85.020   **Personal history of malignant** carcinoid **tumor of stomach**
        Conditions classifiable to C7A.092

      Z85.028   **Personal history of other malignant neoplasm of stomach**
        Conditions classifiable to C16

    `✓6ᵗʰ` **Z85.03**   **Personal history of malignant neoplasm of** large intestine   *personal history*

      Z85.030   **Personal history of malignant** carcinoid **tumor of large intestine**
        Conditions classifiable to C7A.022-C7A.025, C7A.029

      Z85.038   **Personal history of other malignant neoplasm of large intestine**
        Conditions classifiable to C18

    `✓6ᵗʰ` **Z85.04**   **Personal history of malignant neoplasm of** rectum, rectosigmoid junction, and anus

      Z85.040   **Personal history of malignant** carcinoid **tumor of rectum**
        Conditions classifiable to C7A.026

Chapter 21. Factors Influencing Health Status and Contact With Health Services

                Z85.048 Personal history of other malignant neoplasm of rectum, rectosigmoid junction, and anus
                    Conditions classifiable to C19-C21

        Z85.05 Personal history of malignant neoplasm of liver
            Conditions classifiable to C22

    ✓6ᵗʰ   **Z85.06 Personal history of malignant neoplasm of small intestine**

                Z85.060 Personal history of malignant carcinoid tumor of small intestine
                    Conditions classifiable to C7A.01-

                Z85.068 Personal history of other malignant neoplasm of small intestine
                    Conditions classifiable to C17

        Z85.07 Personal history of malignant neoplasm of pancreas
            Conditions classifiable to C25

        Z85.09 Personal history of malignant neoplasm of other digestive organs

✓5ᵗʰ   **Z85.1 Personal history of malignant neoplasm of trachea, bronchus and lung**

    ✓6ᵗʰ   **Z85.11 Personal history of malignant neoplasm of bronchus and lung**

                Z85.110 Personal history of malignant carcinoid tumor of bronchus and lung
                    Conditions classifiable to C7A.090

                Z85.118 Personal history of other malignant neoplasm of bronchus and lung
                    Conditions classifiable to C34

        Z85.12 Personal history of malignant neoplasm of trachea
            Conditions classifiable to C33

✓5ᵗʰ   **Z85.2 Personal history of malignant neoplasm of other respiratory and intrathoracic organs**

        Z85.20 Personal history of malignant neoplasm of unspecified respiratory organ

        Z85.21 Personal history of malignant neoplasm of larynx
            Conditions classifiable to C32

        Z85.22 Personal history of malignant neoplasm of nasal cavities, middle ear, and accessory sinuses
            Conditions classifiable to C30-C31

    ✓6ᵗʰ   **Z85.23 Personal history of malignant neoplasm of thymus**

                Z85.230 Personal history of malignant carcinoid tumor of thymus
                    Conditions classifiable to C7A.091

                Z85.238 Personal history of other malignant neoplasm of thymus
                    Conditions classifiable to C37

        Z85.29 Personal history of malignant neoplasm of other respiratory and intrathoracic organs

      Z85.3 Personal history of malignant neoplasm of breast
        Conditions classifiable to C50.-

✓5ᵗʰ   **Z85.4 Personal history of malignant neoplasm of genital organs**
      Conditions classifiable to C51-C63

        Z85.40 Personal history of malignant neoplasm of unspecified female genital organ ♀

        Z85.41 Personal history of malignant neoplasm of cervix uteri ♀

        Z85.42 Personal history of malignant neoplasm of other parts of uterus ♀

        Z85.43 Personal history of malignant neoplasm of ovary ♀

        Z85.44 Personal history of malignant neoplasm of other female genital organs ♀

        Z85.45 Personal history of malignant neoplasm of unspecified male genital organ ♂

        Z85.46 Personal history of malignant neoplasm of prostate ♂

        Z85.47 Personal history of malignant neoplasm of testis ♂

        Z85.48 Personal history of malignant neoplasm of epididymis ♂

        Z85.49 Personal history of malignant neoplasm of other male genital organs ♂

✓5ᵗʰ   **Z85.5 Personal history of malignant neoplasm of urinary tract**
      Conditions classifiable to C64-C68

        Z85.50 Personal history of malignant neoplasm of unspecified urinary tract organ

        Z85.51 Personal history of malignant neoplasm of bladder

    ✓6ᵗʰ   **Z85.52 Personal history of malignant neoplasm of kidney**
            EXCLUDES 1 *personal history of malignant neoplasm of renal pelvis (Z85.53)*

                Z85.520 Personal history of malignant carcinoid tumor of kidney
                    Conditions classifiable to C7A.093

                Z85.528 Personal history of other malignant neoplasm of kidney
                    Conditions classifiable to C64

        Z85.53 Personal history of malignant neoplasm of renal pelvis

        Z85.54 Personal history of malignant neoplasm of ureter

        Z85.59 Personal history of malignant neoplasm of other urinary tract organ

      Z85.6 Personal history of leukemia
        Conditions classifiable to C91-C95
        EXCLUDES 1 *leukemia in remission C91.0-C95.9 with 5th character 1*

✓5ᵗʰ   **Z85.7 Personal history of other malignant neoplasms of lymphoid, hematopoietic and related tissues**

        Z85.71 Personal history of Hodgkin lymphoma
            Conditions classifiable to C81

        Z85.72 Personal history of non-Hodgkin lymphomas
            Conditions classifiable to C82-C85

        Z85.79 Personal history of other malignant neoplasms of lymphoid, hematopoietic and related tissues
            Conditions classifiable to C88-C90, C96
            EXCLUDES 1 *multiple myeloma in remission (C90.01)*
                      plasma cell leukemia in remission (C90.11)
                      plasmacytoma in remission (C90.21)

✓5ᵗʰ   **Z85.8 Personal history of malignant neoplasms of other organs and systems**
      Conditions classifiable to C00-C14, C40-C49, C69-C75, C7A.098, C76-C79

    ✓6ᵗʰ   **Z85.81 Personal history of malignant neoplasm of lip, oral cavity, and pharynx**
            Conditions classifiable to C00-C14

                Z85.810 Personal history of malignant neoplasm of tongue

                Z85.818 Personal history of malignant neoplasm of other sites of lip, oral cavity, and pharynx

                Z85.819 Personal history of malignant neoplasm of unspecified site of lip, oral cavity, and pharynx

    ✓6ᵗʰ   **Z85.82 Personal history of malignant neoplasm of skin**

                Z85.820 Personal history of malignant melanoma of skin
                    Conditions classifiable to C43

                Z85.821 Personal history of Merkel cell carcinoma
                    Conditions classifiable to C4A

                Z85.828 Personal history of other malignant neoplasm of skin
                    Conditions classifiable to C44

    ✓6ᵗʰ   **Z85.83 Personal history of malignant neoplasm of bone and soft tissue**
            Conditions classifiable to C40-C41; C45-C49

                Z85.830 Personal history of malignant neoplasm of bone

                Z85.831 Personal history of malignant neoplasm of soft tissue
                  EXCLUDES 2 *personal history of malignant neoplasm of skin (Z85.82-)*

    ✓6ᵗʰ   **Z85.84 Personal history of malignant neoplasm of eye and nervous tissue**
            Conditions classifiable to C69-C72

                Z85.840 Personal history of malignant neoplasm of eye

                Z85.841 Personal history of malignant neoplasm of brain

                Z85.848 Personal history of malignant neoplasm of other parts of nervous tissue

    ✓6ᵗʰ   **Z85.85 Personal history of malignant neoplasm of endocrine glands**
            Conditions classifiable to C73-C75

                Z85.850 Personal history of malignant neoplasm of thyroid

                Z85.858 Personal history of malignant neoplasm of other endocrine glands

HCC CMS-HCC   Rx Rx HCC   ESRD ESRD HCC   COM Commercial HCC   PDx Primary Dx Only   N Newborn: 0   P Pediatric: 0-17   M Maternity: 9-64   A Adult: 15-124

1288   ICD-10-CM 2023

Z85.89   Personal history of malignant neoplasm of other organs and systems
Conditions classifiable to C7A.098, C76, C77-C79

Z85.9   Personal history of malignant neoplasm, unspecified
Conditions classifiable to C7A.00, C80.1

✓4ᵗʰ **Z86   Personal history of certain other diseases**
Code first any follow-up examination after treatment (Z09)

✓5ᵗʰ **Z86.0   Personal history of in-situ and benign neoplasms and neoplasms of uncertain behavior**
EXCLUDES 2   personal history of malignant neoplasms (Z85.-)
AHA: 2017,1Q,9

✓6ᵗʰ **Z86.00   Personal history of in-situ neoplasm**
Conditions classifiable to D00-D09
AHA: 2019,4Q,20

Z86.000   Personal history of in-situ neoplasm of breast
Conditions classifiable to D05

Z86.001   Personal history of in-situ neoplasm of cervix uteri   ♀
Conditions classifiable to D06
Personal history of cervical intraepithelial neoplasia III [CIN III]

Z86.002   Personal history of in-situ neoplasm of other and unspecified genital organs
Conditions classifiable to D07
Personal history of high-grade prostatic intraepithelial neoplasia III [HGPIN III]
Personal history of vaginal intraepithelial neoplasia III [VAIN III]
Personal history of vulvar intraepithelial neoplasia III [VIN III]

Z86.003   Personal history of in-situ neoplasm of oral cavity, esophagus and stomach
Conditions classifiable to D00

Z86.004   Personal history of in-situ neoplasm of other and unspecified digestive organs
Conditions classifiable to D01
Personal history of anal intraepithelial neoplasia (AIN III)

Z86.005   Personal history of in-situ neoplasm of middle ear and respiratory system
Conditions classifiable to D02

Z86.006   Personal history of melanoma in-situ
Conditions classifiable to D03
EXCLUDES 2   sites other than skin - code to personal history of in-situ neoplasm of the site

Z86.007   Personal history of in-situ neoplasm of skin
Conditions classifiable to D04
Personal history of carcinoma in situ of skin

Z86.008   Personal history of in-situ neoplasm of other site
Conditions classifiable to D09

✓6ᵗʰ **Z86.01   Personal history of benign neoplasm**

Z86.010   Personal history of colonic polyps
AHA: 2021,1Q,14; 2017,1Q,14

Z86.011   Personal history of benign neoplasm of the brain

Z86.012   Personal history of benign carcinoid tumor

Z86.018   Personal history of other benign neoplasm
AHA: 2017,1Q,14

Z86.03   Personal history of neoplasm of uncertain behavior

✓5ᵗʰ **Z86.1   Personal history of infectious and parasitic diseases**
Conditions classifiable to A00-B89, B99
EXCLUDES 1   personal history of infectious diseases specific to a body system
sequelae of infectious and parasitic diseases (B90-B94)

Z86.11   Personal history of tuberculosis

Z86.12   Personal history of poliomyelitis

Z86.13   Personal history of malaria

Z86.14   Personal history of Methicillin resistant Staphylococcus aureus infection
Personal history of MRSA infection

Z86.15   Personal history of latent tuberculosis infection

Z86.16   Personal history of COVID-19   UPD
EXCLUDES 1   post COVID-19 condition (U09.9)
AHA: 2021,4Q,107-108;
2021,1Q,28-29,33-35,40-41,44-45

Z86.19   Personal history of other infectious and parasitic diseases
AHA: 2021,1Q,33-34,40; 2020,3Q,13; 2020,2Q,10,12

Z86.2   Personal history of diseases of the blood and blood-forming organs and certain disorders involving the immune mechanism
Conditions classifiable to D50-D89

✓5ᵗʰ **Z86.3   Personal history of endocrine, nutritional and metabolic diseases**
Conditions classifiable to E00-E88

Z86.31   Personal history of diabetic foot ulcer
EXCLUDES 2   current diabetic foot ulcer (E08.621, E09.621, E10.621, E11.621, E13.621)

Z86.32   Personal history of gestational diabetes   ♀
Personal history of conditions classifiable to O24.4-
EXCLUDES 1   gestational diabetes mellitus in current pregnancy (O24.4-)

Z86.39   Personal history of other endocrine, nutritional and metabolic disease
AHA: 2020,1Q,12

✓5ᵗʰ **Z86.5   Personal history of mental and behavioral disorders**
Conditions classifiable to F40-F59

Z86.51   Personal history of combat and operational stress reaction   A

Z86.59   Personal history of other mental and behavioral disorders

✓5ᵗʰ **Z86.6   Personal history of diseases of the nervous system and sense organs**
Conditions classifiable to G00-G99, H00-H95

Z86.61   Personal history of infections of the central nervous system
Personal history of encephalitis
Personal history of meningitis

Z86.69   Personal history of other diseases of the nervous system and sense organs
AHA: 2016,4Q,24

✓5ᵗʰ **Z86.7   Personal history of diseases of the circulatory system**
Conditions classifiable to I00-I99
EXCLUDES 2   old myocardial infarction (I25.2)
personal history of anaphylactic shock (Z87.892)
postmyocardial infarction syndrome (I24.1)

✓6ᵗʰ **Z86.71   Personal history of venous thrombosis and embolism**

Z86.711   Personal history of pulmonary embolism

Z86.718   Personal history of other venous thrombosis and embolism
AHA: 2020,2Q,20

Z86.72   Personal history of thrombophlebitis

Z86.73   Personal history of transient ischemic attack (TIA), and cerebral infarction without residual deficits
Personal history of prolonged reversible ischemic neurological deficit (PRIND)
Personal history of stroke NOS without residual deficits
EXCLUDES 1   personal history of traumatic brain injury (Z87.820)
sequelae of cerebrovascular disease (I69.-)
AHA: 2012,4Q,92

Z86.74   Personal history of sudden cardiac arrest
Personal history of sudden cardiac death successfully resuscitated

Z86.79   Personal history of other diseases of the circulatory system
AHA: 2022,2Q,14; 2020,1Q,12

✓4ᵗʰ **Z87   Personal history of other diseases and conditions**
Code first any follow-up examination after treatment (Z09)

✓5ᵗʰ **Z87.0   Personal history of diseases of the respiratory system**
Conditions classifiable to J00-J99

Z87.01   Personal history of pneumonia (recurrent)

Z87.09   Personal history of other diseases of the respiratory system

✓5ᵗʰ **Z87.1   Personal history of diseases of the digestive system**
Conditions classifiable to K00-K93

Z87.11   Personal history of peptic ulcer disease

Z87.19   **Personal history of other diseases of the digestive system** *hypoplastic colon polyp.* [handwritten]
rectal polyp. [handwritten]
    AHA: 2017,1Q,14

Z87.2   **Personal history of diseases of the skin and subcutaneous tissue**
    Conditions classifiable to L00-L99
      EXCLUDES 2   *personal history of diabetic foot ulcer (Z86.31)*

☑5ᵗʰ Z87.3   **Personal history of diseases of the musculoskeletal system and connective tissue**
    Conditions classifiable to M00-M99
      EXCLUDES 2   *personal history of (healed) traumatic fracture (Z87.81)*

    ☑6ᵗʰ Z87.31   **Personal history of (healed) nontraumatic fracture**

       Z87.310   **Personal history of (healed) osteoporosis fracture**
         Personal history of (healed) fragility fracture
         Personal history of (healed) collapsed vertebra due to osteoporosis
         TIP: Assign for history of osteoporosis fractures that have resolved, even when a code from category M80 indicating current osteoporosis fracture is also reported.

       Z87.311   **Personal history of (healed) other pathological fracture**
         Personal history of (healed) collapsed vertebra NOS
           EXCLUDES 2   *personal history of osteoporosis fracture (Z87.310)*

       Z87.312   **Personal history of (healed) stress fracture**
         Personal history of (healed) fatigue fracture

    Z87.39   **Personal history of other diseases of the musculoskeletal system and connective tissue**

☑5ᵗʰ Z87.4   **Personal history of diseases of the genitourinary system**
    Conditions classifiable to N00-N99

    ☑6ᵗʰ Z87.41   **Personal history of dysplasia of the female genital tract**
      EXCLUDES 1   *personal history of intraepithelial neoplasia III of female genital tract (Z86.001, Z86.008)*
          personal history of malignant neoplasm of female genital tract (Z85.40-Z85.44)

       Z87.410   **Personal history of cervical dysplasia** ♀

       Z87.411   **Personal history of vaginal dysplasia** ♀

       Z87.412   **Personal history of vulvar dysplasia** ♀

    Z87.42   **Personal history of other diseases of the female genital tract** ♀

ovarian surgery [handwritten]

    ☑6ᵗʰ Z87.43   **Personal history of diseases of the male genital organs**

       Z87.430   **Personal history of prostatic dysplasia** ♂
          EXCLUDES 1   *personal history of malignant neoplasm of prostate (Z85.46)*

       Z87.438   **Personal history of other diseases of male genital organs** ♂

    ☑6ᵗʰ Z87.44   **Personal history of diseases of the urinary system**
      EXCLUDES 1   *personal history of malignant neoplasm of cervix uteri (Z85.41)*

       Z87.440   **Personal history of urinary (tract) infections**

       Z87.441   **Personal history of nephrotic syndrome**

       Z87.442   **Personal history of urinary calculi**
         Personal history of kidney stones

       Z87.448   **Personal history of other diseases of urinary system**

☑5ᵗʰ Z87.5   **Personal history of complications of pregnancy, childbirth and the puerperium**
    Conditions classifiable to O00-O9A
      EXCLUDES 2   *recurrent pregnancy loss (N96)*

    Z87.51   **Personal history of pre-term labor** ♀
      EXCLUDES 1   *current pregnancy with history of pre-term labor (O09.21-)*

Z87.59   **Personal history of other complications of pregnancy, childbirth and the puerperium** ♀
    Personal history of trophoblastic disease

☑5ᵗʰ Z87.6   **Personal history of certain (corrected) conditions arising in the perinatal period**
    Conditions classifiable to P00-P96
      EXCLUDES 1   *personal history of (corrected) congenital malformations (Z87.7-)*

    Z87.61   **Personal history of (corrected) necrotizing enterocolitis of newborn**

    Z87.68   **Personal history of other (corrected) conditions arising in the perinatal period**

☑5ᵗʰ Z87.7   **Personal history of (corrected) congenital malformations**
    Conditions classifiable to Q00-Q89 that have been repaired or corrected
      EXCLUDES 1   ~~*congenital malformations that have been partially corrected or repair but which still require medical treatment - code to condition*~~
      EXCLUDES 2   ▶*congenital malformations that have been partially corrected or repaired but which still require medical treatment - code to condition*◀
         other postprocedural states (Z98.-)
         personal history of medical treatment (Z92.-)
         presence of cardiac and vascular implants and grafts (Z95.-)
         presence of other devices (Z97.-)
         presence of other functional implants (Z96.-)
         transplanted organ and tissue status (Z94.-)

    ☑6ᵗʰ Z87.71   **Personal history of (corrected) congenital malformations of genitourinary system**

       Z87.710   **Personal history of (corrected) hypospadias** ♂

       Z87.718   **Personal history of other specified (corrected) congenital malformations of genitourinary system**

    ☑6ᵗʰ Z87.72   **Personal history of (corrected) congenital malformations of nervous system and sense organs**

       Z87.720   **Personal history of (corrected) congenital malformations of eye**

       Z87.721   **Personal history of (corrected) congenital malformations of ear**

       Z87.728   **Personal history of other specified (corrected) congenital malformations of nervous system and sense organs**

    ☑6ᵗʰ Z87.73   **Personal history of (corrected) congenital malformations of digestive system**

       Z87.730   **Personal history of (corrected) cleft lip and palate**

       Z87.731   **Personal history of (corrected) tracheoesophageal fistula or atresia**

       Z87.732   **Personal history of (corrected) persistent cloaca or cloacal malformations**

       Z87.738   **Personal history of other specified (corrected) congenital malformations of digestive system**

    Z87.74   **Personal history of (corrected) congenital malformations of heart and circulatory system**

    Z87.75   **Personal history of (corrected) congenital malformations of respiratory system**

    ☑6ᵗʰ Z87.76   **Personal history of (corrected) congenital malformations of integument, limbs and musculoskeletal system**

       Z87.760   **Personal history of (corrected) congenital diaphragmatic hernia or other congenital diaphragm malformations**

       Z87.761   **Personal history of (corrected) gastroschisis**

       Z87.762   **Personal history of (corrected) prune belly malformation**

       Z87.763   **Personal history of other (corrected) congenital abdominal wall malformations**

       Z87.768   **Personal history of other specified (corrected) congenital malformations of integument, limbs and musculoskeletal system**

    ☑6ᵗʰ Z87.79   **Personal history of other (corrected) congenital malformations**

       Z87.790   **Personal history of (corrected) congenital malformations of face and neck**

       Z87.798   **Personal history of other (corrected) congenital malformations**

HCC CMS-HCC   **Rx** Rx HCC   **ESR** ESRD HCC   **COM** Commercial HCC   **PDx** Primary Dx Only   **N** Newborn: 0   **P** Pediatric: 0-17   **M** Maternity: 9-64   **A** Adult: 15-124

1290   ICD-10-CM 2023

√5ᵗʰ **Z87.8 Personal history of other specified conditions**
     EXCLUDES 2   *personal history of self harm (Z91.5-)*

   Z87.81 Personal history of (healed) traumatic fracture
       EXCLUDES 2   *personal history of (healed) nontraumatic fracture (Z87.31-)*

   √6ᵗʰ **Z87.82 Personal history of other (healed) physical injury and trauma**
       Conditions classifiable to S00-T88, except traumatic fractures

     Z87.820 Personal history of traumatic brain injury
       EXCLUDES 1   *personal history of transient ischemic attack (TIA), and cerebral infarction without residual deficits (Z86.73)*

     Z87.821 Personal history of retained foreign body fully removed

     Z87.828 Personal history of other (healed) physical injury and trauma

   √6ᵗʰ **Z87.89 Personal history of other specified conditions**

     Z87.890 Personal history of sex reassignment

     Z87.891 Personal history of nicotine dependence
       EXCLUDES 1   *current nicotine dependence (F17.2-)*
       AHA: 2017,2Q,27

     Z87.892 Personal history of anaphylaxis
       Code also allergy status such as:
       allergy status to drugs, medicaments and biological substances (Z88.-)
       allergy status, other than to drugs and biological substances (Z91.0-)

     Z87.898 Personal history of other specified conditions
       AHA: 2013,1Q,21

√4ᵗʰ **Z88 Allergy status to drugs, medicaments and biological substances**
     EXCLUDES 2   *allergy status, other than to drugs and biological substances (Z91.0-)*
     AHA: 2015,3Q,23

   Z88.0 Allergy status to penicillin
   Z88.1 Allergy status to other antibiotic agents
   Z88.2 Allergy status to sulfonamides
   Z88.3 Allergy status to other anti-infective agents
   Z88.4 Allergy status to anesthetic agent
   Z88.5 Allergy status to narcotic agent
   Z88.6 Allergy status to analgesic agent
   Z88.7 Allergy status to serum and vaccine
   Z88.8 Allergy status to other drugs, medicaments and biological substances
   Z88.9 Allergy status to unspecified drugs, medicaments and biological substances
     non allergy drug. [handwritten]

√4ᵗʰ **Z89 Acquired absence of limb**
     INCLUDES   amputation status
       postprocedural loss of limb
       post-traumatic loss of limb
     EXCLUDES 1   *acquired deformities of limbs (M20-M21)*
       congenital absence of limbs (Q71-Q73)

   √5ᵗʰ **Z89.0 Acquired absence of thumb and other finger(s)**

     √6ᵗʰ **Z89.01 Acquired absence of thumb**
       Z89.011 Acquired absence of right thumb
       Z89.012 Acquired absence of left thumb
       Z89.019 Acquired absence of unspecified thumb

     √6ᵗʰ **Z89.02 Acquired absence of other finger(s)**
       EXCLUDES 2   *acquired absence of thumb (Z89.01-)*
       Z89.021 Acquired absence of right finger(s)
       Z89.022 Acquired absence of left finger(s)
       Z89.029 Acquired absence of unspecified finger(s)

   √5ᵗʰ **Z89.1 Acquired absence of hand and wrist**

     √6ᵗʰ **Z89.11 Acquired absence of hand**
       Z89.111 Acquired absence of right hand COM
       Z89.112 Acquired absence of left hand COM
       Z89.119 Acquired absence of unspecified hand COM

     √6ᵗʰ **Z89.12 Acquired absence of wrist**
       Disarticulation at wrist
       Z89.121 Acquired absence of right wrist COM

     Z89.122 Acquired absence of left wrist COM
     Z89.129 Acquired absence of unspecified wrist COM

   √5ᵗʰ **Z89.2 Acquired absence of upper limb above wrist**

     √6ᵗʰ **Z89.20 Acquired absence of upper limb, unspecified level**
       Z89.201 Acquired absence of right upper limb, unspecified level COM
       Z89.202 Acquired absence of left upper limb, unspecified level COM
       Z89.209 Acquired absence of unspecified upper limb, unspecified level COM
       Acquired absence of arm NOS

     √6ᵗʰ **Z89.21 Acquired absence of upper limb below elbow**
       Z89.211 Acquired absence of right upper limb below elbow COM
       Z89.212 Acquired absence of left upper limb below elbow COM
       Z89.219 Acquired absence of unspecified upper limb below elbow COM

     √6ᵗʰ **Z89.22 Acquired absence of upper limb above elbow**
       Disarticulation at elbow
       Z89.221 Acquired absence of right upper limb above elbow COM
       Z89.222 Acquired absence of left upper limb above elbow COM
       Z89.229 Acquired absence of unspecified upper limb above elbow COM

     √6ᵗʰ **Z89.23 Acquired absence of shoulder**
       Acquired absence of shoulder joint following explantation of shoulder joint prosthesis, with or without presence of antibiotic-impregnated cement spacer
       Z89.231 Acquired absence of right shoulder
       Z89.232 Acquired absence of left shoulder
       Z89.239 Acquired absence of unspecified shoulder

   √5ᵗʰ **Z89.4 Acquired absence of toe(s), foot, and ankle**

     √6ᵗʰ **Z89.41 Acquired absence of great toe**
       Z89.411 Acquired absence of right great toe HCC ESR
       Z89.412 Acquired absence of left great toe HCC ESR
       Z89.419 Acquired absence of unspecified great toe HCC ESR

     √6ᵗʰ **Z89.42 Acquired absence of other toe(s)**
       EXCLUDES 2   *acquired absence of great toe (Z89.41-)*
       Z89.421 Acquired absence of other right toe(s) HCC ESR
       Z89.422 Acquired absence of other left toe(s) HCC ESR
       Z89.429 Acquired absence of other toe(s), unspecified side HCC ESR

     √6ᵗʰ **Z89.43 Acquired absence of foot**
       Z89.431 Acquired absence of right foot HCC ESR COM
       Z89.432 Acquired absence of left foot HCC ESR COM
       Z89.439 Acquired absence of unspecified foot HCC ESR COM

     √6ᵗʰ **Z89.44 Acquired absence of ankle**
       Disarticulation of ankle
       Z89.441 Acquired absence of right ankle HCC ESR COM
       Z89.442 Acquired absence of left ankle HCC ESR COM
       Z89.449 Acquired absence of unspecified ankle HCC ESR COM

   √5ᵗʰ **Z89.5 Acquired absence of leg below knee**

     √6ᵗʰ **Z89.51 Acquired absence of leg below knee**
       Z89.511 Acquired absence of right leg below knee HCC ESR COM
       Z89.512 Acquired absence of left leg below knee HCC ESR COM
       Z89.519 Acquired absence of unspecified leg below knee HCC ESR COM

Chapter 21. Factors Influencing Health Status and Contact With Health Services *(left margin)*

√6ᵗʰ **Z89.52 Acquired absence of** knee

Acquired absence of knee joint following explantation of knee joint prosthesis, with or without presence of antibiotic-impregnated cement spacer

Z89.521 Acquired absence of right **knee**

Z89.522 Acquired absence of left **knee**

Z89.529 Acquired absence of unspecified knee

√5ᵗʰ **Z89.6 Acquired absence of leg above knee**

√6ᵗʰ **Z89.61 Acquired absence of** leg above knee

Acquired absence of leg NOS

Disarticulation at knee

Z89.611 Acquired absence of right **leg above knee** `HCC` `ESR` `COM`

Z89.612 Acquired absence of left **leg above knee** `HCC` `ESR` `COM`

Z89.619 Acquired absence of unspecified leg above knee `HCC` `ESR` `COM`

√6ᵗʰ **Z89.62 Acquired absence of** hip

Acquired absence of hip joint following explantation of hip joint prosthesis, with or without presence of antibiotic-impregnated cement spacer

Disarticulation at hip

Z89.621 Acquired absence of right **hip joint**

Z89.622 Acquired absence of left **hip joint**

Z89.629 Acquired absence of unspecified hip joint

Z89.9 Acquired absence of limb, unspecified `COM`

√4ᵗʰ **Z90 Acquired absence of organs, not elsewhere classified** *(handwritten: after hysterectomy)*

`INCLUDES` postprocedural or post-traumatic loss of body part NEC

`EXCLUDES 1` congenital absence - see Alphabetical Index

`EXCLUDES 2` postprocedural absence of endocrine glands (E89.-)

√5ᵗʰ **Z90.0 Acquired absence of part of** head and neck *(handwritten: after mastectomy)*

Z90.01 Acquired absence of eye

Z90.02 Acquired absence of larynx

Z90.09 Acquired absence of other part of head and neck

Acquired absence of nose

`EXCLUDES 2` teeth (K08.1)

√5ᵗʰ **Z90.1 Acquired absence of** breast and nipple

Z90.10 Acquired absence of unspecified breast and nipple

Z90.11 Acquired absence of right **breast and nipple**

Z90.12 Acquired absence of left **breast and nipple**

Z90.13 Acquired absence of bilateral **breasts and nipples**

Z90.2 Acquired absence of lung [part of]

Z90.3 Acquired absence of stomach [part of]

√5ᵗʰ **Z90.4 Acquired absence of other specified parts of digestive tract**

√6ᵗʰ **Z90.41 Acquired absence of** pancreas

Code also exocrine pancreatic insufficiency (K86.81)

Use additional code to identify any associated:

diabetes mellitus, postpancreatectomy (E13.-)

insulin use (Z79.4)

Z90.410 Acquired total absence of pancreas

Acquired absence of pancreas NOS

Z90.411 Acquired partial absence of pancreas

Z90.49 Acquired absence of other specified parts of digestive tract

Z90.5 Acquired absence of kidney

Z90.6 Acquired absence of other parts of urinary tract

Acquired absence of bladder

√5ᵗʰ **Z90.7 Acquired absence of** genital organ(s)

`EXCLUDES 1` personal history of sex reassignment (Z87.890)

`EXCLUDES 2` female genital mutilation status (N90.81-)

√6ᵗʰ **Z90.71 Acquired absence of** cervix and uterus *(handwritten: After hysterectomy)*

Z90.710 Acquired absence of both cervix and uterus ♀

Acquired absence of uterus NOS

Status post total hysterectomy

Z90.711 Acquired absence of uterus with remaining cervical stump ♀

Status post partial hysterectomy with remaining cervical stump

Z90.712 Acquired absence of cervix with remaining uterus ♀

√6ᵗʰ **Z90.72 Acquired absence of** ovaries

Z90.721 Acquired absence of ovaries, unilateral ♀

Z90.722 Acquired absence of ovaries, bilateral ♀

Z90.79 Acquired absence of other genital organ(s)

√5ᵗʰ **Z90.8 Acquired absence of other organs**

Z90.81 Acquired absence of spleen

Z90.89 Acquired absence of other organs

√4ᵗʰ **Z91 Personal risk factors, not elsewhere classified**

`EXCLUDES 2` contact with and (suspected) exposures hazardous to health (Z77.-)

exposure to pollution and other problems related to physical environment (Z77.1-)

female genital mutilation status (N90.81-)

personal history of physical injury and trauma (Z87.81, Z87.82-)

occupational exposure to risk factors (Z57.-)

√5ᵗʰ **Z91.0 Allergy status, other than to drugs and biological substances** *(handwritten: not drug allergy)*

`EXCLUDES 2` allergy status to drugs, medicaments, and biological substances (Z88.-)

√6ᵗʰ **Z91.01 Food allergy status**

`EXCLUDES 2` food additives allergy status (Z91.02)

Z91.010 Allergy to peanuts

Z91.011 Allergy to milk products

`EXCLUDES 1` lactose intolerance (E73.-)

Z91.012 Allergy to eggs

Z91.013 Allergy to seafood

Allergy to shellfish

Allergy to octopus or squid ink

Z91.014 Allergy to mammalian meats

Allergy to beef

Allergy to lamb

Allergy to pork

Allergy to red meats

AHA: 2021,4Q,33

Z91.018 Allergy to other foods

Allergy to nuts other than peanuts

Z91.02 Food additives allergy status

√6ᵗʰ **Z91.03 Insect allergy status**

Z91.030 Bee allergy status

Z91.038 Other insect allergy status

√6ᵗʰ **Z91.04 Nonmedicinal substance allergy status**

Z91.040 Latex allergy status

Latex sensitivity status

Z91.041 Radiographic dye allergy status

Allergy status to contrast media used for diagnostic X-ray procedure

Z91.048 Other nonmedicinal substance allergy status

Z91.09 Other allergy status, other than to drugs and biological substances

√5ᵗʰ **Z91.1 Patient's noncompliance with medical treatment and regimen**

`EXCLUDES 2` ▶caregiver noncompliance with patient's medical treatment and regimen (Z91.A-)◀

√6ᵗʰ **Z91.11 Patient's noncompliance with** dietary regimen ▲

▶Code also, if applicable, food insecurity (Z59.4-)◀

Z91.110 Patient's noncompliance with dietary regimen due to financial hardship ●

Z91.118 Patient's noncompliance with dietary regimen for other reason ●

Inability to comply with dietary regimen

Z91.119 Patient's noncompliance with dietary regimen due to unspecified reason ●

√6ᵗʰ **Z91.12 Patient's** intentional underdosing **of medication regimen**

Code first underdosing of medication (T36-T50) with fifth or sixth character 6

`EXCLUDES 1` adverse effect of prescribed drug taken as directed - code to adverse effect poisoning (overdose) - code to poisoning

AHA: 2018,4Q,72

Z91.120 Patient's intentional underdosing of medication regimen due to financial hardship

Z91.128 Patient's intentional underdosing of medication regimen for other reason

`HCC` CMS-HCC   `Rx` Rx HCC   `ESR` ESRD HCC   `COM` Commercial HCC   `PDx` Primary Dx Only   `N` Newborn: 0   `P` Pediatric: 0-17   `M` Maternity: 9-64   `A` Adult: 15-124

1292   ICD-10-CM 2023

☑6ᵗʰ **Z91.13** **Patient's unintentional underdosing of medication regimen**
Code first underdosing of medication (T36-T50) with fifth or sixth character 6
> **EXCLUDES 1**   adverse effect of prescribed drug taken as directed - code to adverse effect
> poisoning (overdose) - code to poisoning

AHA: 2018,4Q,72

Z91.130 **Patient's unintentional underdosing of medication regimen due to age-related debility**

Z91.138 **Patient's unintentional underdosing of medication regimen for other reason**

Z91.14 **Patient's other noncompliance with medication regimen**
Patient's underdosing of medication NOS
AHA: 2022,1Q,36; 2018,4Q,72

Z91.15 **Patient's noncompliance with renal dialysis** `HCC` `Rx` `ESR`

▲ ☑6ᵗʰ **Z91.19** **Patient's noncompliance with other medical treatment and regimen**
▶Patient's nonadherence to medical treatment◀

● **Z91.190** **Patient's noncompliance with other medical treatment and regimen due to financial hardship**

● **Z91.198** **Patient's noncompliance with other medical treatment and regimen for other reason**

● **Z91.199** **Patient's noncompliance with other medical treatment and regimen due to unspecified reason**

● ☑5ᵗʰ **Z91.A** **Caregiver's noncompliance with patient's medical treatment and regimen**

● ☑6ᵗʰ **Z91.A1** **Caregiver's noncompliance with patient's dietary regimen**
Caregiver's inability to comply with patient's dietary regimen
Code also, if applicable, food insecurity (Z59.4-)

● **Z91.A10** **Caregiver's noncompliance with patient's dietary regimen due to financial hardship**

● **Z91.A18** **Caregiver's noncompliance with patient's dietary regimen for other reason**

● ☑6ᵗʰ **Z91.A2** **Caregiver's intentional underdosing of patient's medication regimen**
Code first underdosing of medication (T36-T50) with fifth or sixth character 6

● **Z91.A20** **Caregiver's intentional underdosing of patient's medication regimen due to financial hardship**

● **Z91.A28** **Caregiver's intentional underdosing of medication regimen for other reason**

● **Z91.A3** **Caregiver's unintentional underdosing of patient's medication regimen**
Code first underdosing of medication (T36-T50) with fifth or sixth character 6

● **Z91.A4** **Caregiver's other noncompliance with patient's medication regimen**
Caregiver's underdosing of patient's medication NOS

Z91.A5 **Caregiver's noncompliance with patient's renal dialysis**

● **Z91.A9** **Caregiver's noncompliance with patient's other medical treatment and regimen**
Caregiver's nonadherence to patient's medical treatment

☑5ᵗʰ **Z91.4** **Personal history of psychological trauma, not elsewhere classified**

☑6ᵗʰ **Z91.41** **Personal history of adult abuse**
> **EXCLUDES 2**   personal history of abuse in childhood (Z62.81-)

Z91.410 **Personal history of adult physical and sexual abuse** `A`
> **EXCLUDES 1**   current adult physical abuse (T74.11, T76.11)
> current adult sexual abuse (T74.21, T76.11)

Z91.411 **Personal history of adult psychological abuse** `A`

Z91.412 **Personal history of adult neglect** `A`
> **EXCLUDES 1**   current adult neglect (T74.01, T76.01)

Z91.419 **Personal history of unspecified adult abuse** `A`

Z91.42 **Personal history of forced labor or sexual exploitation**
AHA: 2018,4Q,32,35

Z91.49 **Other personal history of psychological trauma, not elsewhere classified**

☑5ᵗʰ **Z91.5** **Personal history of self-harm**
Code also mental health disorder, if known
AHA: 2021,4Q,33

Z91.51 **Personal history of suicidal behavior** `UPD`
Personal history of parasuicide
Personal history of self-poisoning
Personal history of suicide attempt

Z91.52 **Personal history of nonsuicidal self-harm** `UPD`
Personal history of nonsuicidal self-injury
Personal history of self-inflicted injury without suicidal intent
Personal history of self-mutilation

☑5ᵗʰ **Z91.8** **Other specified personal risk factors, not elsewhere classified**

Z91.81 **History of falling**
At risk for falling

Z91.82 **Personal history of military deployment** `A`
Individual (civilian or military) with past history of military war, peacekeeping and humanitarian deployment (current or past conflict)
Returned from military deployment

Z91.83 *Wandering in diseases classified elsewhere*
Code first underlying disorder such as:
Alzheimer's disease (G30.-)
autism or pervasive developmental disorder (F84.-)
intellectual disabilities (F70-F79)
unspecified dementia with behavioral disturbance ▶(F03.9-, F03.A-, F03.B-, F03.C-)◀

☑6ᵗʰ **Z91.84** **Oral health risk factors**
AHA: 2017,4Q,29

Z91.841 **Risk for dental caries, low**
Z91.842 **Risk for dental caries, moderate**
Z91.843 **Risk for dental caries, high**
Z91.849 **Unspecified risk for dental caries**

Z91.89 **Other specified personal risk factors, not elsewhere classified**
AHA: 2017,1Q,45

☑4ᵗʰ **Z92** **Personal history of medical treatment**
> **EXCLUDES 2**   postprocedural states (Z98.-)

Z92.0 **Personal history of contraception**
> **EXCLUDES 1**   counseling or management of current contraceptive practices (Z30.-)
> long term (current) use of contraception (Z79.3)
> presence of (intrauterine) contraceptive device (Z97.5)

☑5ᵗʰ **Z92.2** **Personal history of drug therapy**
> **EXCLUDES 2**   long term (current) drug therapy (Z79.-)

Z92.21 **Personal history of antineoplastic chemotherapy**
Z92.22 **Personal history of monoclonal drug therapy**
Z92.23 **Personal history of estrogen therapy**
☑6ᵗʰ **Z92.24** **Personal history of steroid therapy**

Z92.240 **Personal history of inhaled steroid therapy**
Z92.241 **Personal history of systemic steroid therapy**
Personal history of steroid therapy NOS

Z92.25 **Personal history of immunosuppression therapy**
> **EXCLUDES 2**   personal history of steroid therapy (Z92.24)

Z92.29 **Personal history of other drug therapy**

Z92.3 **Personal history of irradiation**
Personal history of exposure to therapeutic radiation
> **EXCLUDES 1**   exposure to radiation in the physical environment (Z77.12)
> occupational exposure to radiation (Z57.1)

☑5ᵗʰ **Z92.8** **Personal history of other medical treatment**

Z92.81 **Personal history of extracorporeal membrane oxygenation (ECMO)**

[handwritten margin note: tPA: plasminogen activator only for receiving facility. not for trans]

Z92.82 Status post administration of tPA (rtPA) in a different facility within the last 24 hours prior to admission to current facility   `UPD`

Code first condition requiring tPA administration, such as:
- acute cerebral infarction (I63.-)
- acute myocardial infarction (I21.-, I22.-)

AHA: 2013,4Q,124

Z92.83 Personal history of failed moderate sedation

Personal history of failed conscious sedation

`EXCLUDES 2`   failed moderate sedation during procedure (T88.52)

Z92.84 Personal history of unintended awareness under general anesthesia

`EXCLUDES 2`   unintended awareness under general anesthesia during procedure (T88.53)

AHA: 2016,4Q,72-73,77

√6ᵗʰ **Z92.85** Personal history of cellular therapy

AHA: 2021,4Q,33-34

    Z92.850 Personal history of Chimeric Antigen Receptor T-cell therapy   `UPD`

       Personal history of CAR T-cell therapy

    Z92.858 Personal history of other cellular therapy   `UPD`

    Z92.859 Personal history of cellular therapy, unspecified   `UPD`

Z92.86 Personal history of gene therapy   `UPD`

AHA: 2021,4Q,33-34

[handwritten margin note: High risk]

Z92.89 Personal history of other medical treatment

AHA: 2020,1Q,18

√4ᵗʰ **Z93** Artificial opening status

`EXCLUDES 1`   artificial openings requiring attention or management (Z43.-)

       complications of external stoma (J95.0-, K94.-, N99.5-)

Z93.0 Tracheostomy status   `HCC` `ESR` `COM`

     AHA: 2013,4Q,129

Z93.1 Gastrostomy status   `HCC` `ESR` `COM`

Z93.2 Ileostomy status   `HCC` `ESR` `COM`

Z93.3 Colostomy status   `HCC` `ESR` `COM`

Z93.4 Other artificial openings of gastrointestinal tract status   `HCC` `ESR` `COM`

√5ᵗʰ **Z93.5** Cystostomy status

    Z93.50 Unspecified cystostomy status   `HCC` `ESR` `COM`

    Z93.51 Cutaneous-vesicostomy status   `HCC` `ESR` `COM`

    Z93.52 Appendico-vesicostomy status   `HCC` `ESR` `COM`

    Z93.59 Other cystostomy status   `HCC` `ESR` `COM`

Z93.6 Other artificial openings of urinary tract status   `HCC` `ESR` `COM`

     Nephrostomy status

     Ureterostomy status

     Urethrostomy status

Z93.8 Other artificial opening status   `HCC` `ESR` `COM`

Z93.9 Artificial opening status, unspecified   `HCC` `ESR` `COM`

√4ᵗʰ **Z94** Transplanted organ and tissue status

`INCLUDES`   organ or tissue replaced by heterogenous or homogenous transplant

`EXCLUDES 1`   complications of transplanted organ or tissue - see Alphabetical Index

`EXCLUDES 2`   presence of vascular grafts (Z95.-)

Z94.0 Kidney transplant status   `Rx` `COM`

Z94.1 Heart transplant status   `HCC` `Rx` `ESR` `COM`

     `EXCLUDES 1`   artificial heart status (Z95.812)

       heart-valve replacement status (Z95.2-Z95.4)

[handwritten margin note: ↓T86.2]

Z94.2 Lung transplant status   `HCC` `Rx` `ESR` `COM`

Z94.3 Heart and lungs transplant status   `HCC` `Rx` `ESR` `COM`

Z94.4 Liver transplant status   `HCC` `Rx` `ESR` `COM`

Z94.5 Skin transplant status

     Autogenous skin transplant status

Z94.6 Bone transplant status

Z94.7 Corneal transplant status

√5ᵗʰ **Z94.8** Other transplanted organ and tissue status

    Z94.81 Bone marrow transplant status   `HCC` `Rx` `ESR` `COM`

    Z94.82 Intestine transplant status   `HCC` `Rx` `ESR` `COM`

    Z94.83 Pancreas transplant status   `HCC` `Rx` `ESR` `COM`

    Z94.84 Stem cells transplant status   `HCC` `Rx` `ESR` `COM`

    Z94.89 Other transplanted organ and tissue status

Z94.9 Transplanted organ and tissue status, unspecified

√4ᵗʰ **Z95** Presence of cardiac and vascular implants and grafts

`EXCLUDES 2`   complications of cardiac and vascular devices, implants and grafts (T82.-)

Z95.0 Presence of cardiac pacemaker

Presence of cardiac resynchronization therapy (CRT-P) pacemaker

`EXCLUDES 1`   adjustment or management of cardiac device (Z45.0-)

       adjustment or management of cardiac pacemaker (Z45.0)

       presence of automatic (implantable) cardiac defibrillator with synchronous cardiac pacemaker (Z95.810)

AHA: 2022,2Q,14; 2019,1Q,33

TIP: Assign an additional code for the associated condition if that condition requires constant intervention from the device, as in cases of sick sinus syndrome. For conditions that do not require constant intervention from the device, as in cases of ventricular fibrillation, an additional code for the associated condition should be assigned only if the patient is experiencing the condition and the device is firing during the current admission.

Z95.1 Presence of aortocoronary bypass graft

Presence of coronary artery bypass graft

Z95.2 Presence of prosthetic heart valve

Presence of heart valve NOS

Z95.3 Presence of xenogenic heart valve

Z95.4 Presence of other heart-valve replacement

Z95.5 Presence of coronary angioplasty implant and graft

`EXCLUDES 1`   coronary angioplasty status without implant and graft (Z98.61)

√5ᵗʰ **Z95.8** Presence of other cardiac and vascular implants and grafts

√6ᵗʰ   **Z95.81** Presence of other cardiac implants and grafts

      Z95.810 Presence of automatic (implantable) cardiac defibrillator

         Presence of automatic (implantable) cardiac defibrillator with synchronous cardiac pacemaker

         Presence of cardiac resynchronization therapy defibrillator (CRT-D)

         Presence of cardioverter-defibrillator (ICD)

         AHA: 2022,2Q,14; 2019,1Q,33

         TIP: Assign an additional code for the associated condition if that condition requires constant intervention from the device, as in cases of sick sinus syndrome. For conditions that do not require constant intervention from the device, as in cases of ventricular fibrillation, an additional code for the associated condition should be assigned only if the patient is experiencing the condition and the device is firing during the current admission.

      Z95.811 Presence of heart assist device   `HCC` `ESR` `COM`

      Z95.812 Presence of fully implantable artificial heart   `HCC` `ESR` `COM`

      Z95.818 Presence of other cardiac implants and grafts

√6ᵗʰ   **Z95.82** Presence of other vascular implants and grafts

      Z95.820 Peripheral vascular angioplasty status with implants and grafts

         `EXCLUDES 1`   peripheral vascular angioplasty without implant and graft (Z98.62)

      Z95.828 Presence of other vascular implants and grafts

         Presence of intravascular prosthesis NEC

Z95.9 Presence of cardiac and vascular implant and graft, unspecified

√4ᵗʰ **Z96** Presence of other functional implants

`EXCLUDES 2`   complications of internal prosthetic devices, implants and grafts (T82-T85)

       fitting and adjustment of prosthetic and other devices (Z44-Z46)

Z96.0 Presence of urogenital implants

`HCC` CMS-HCC   `Rx` Rx HCC   `ESR` ESRD HCC   `COM` Commercial HCC   `PDx` Primary Dx Only   `N` Newborn: 0   `P` Pediatric: 0-17   `M` Maternity: 9-64   `A` Adult: 15-124

1294

ICD-10-CM 2023

Z96.1 **Presence of** intraocular lens
     Presence of pseudophakia
✓5ᵗ Z96.2 **Presence of** otological and audiological **implants**
   Z96.20 **Presence of otological and audiological implant, unspecified**
   Z96.21 **Cochlear implant status**
   Z96.22 **Myringotomy tube(s) status**
   Z96.29 **Presence of other otological and audiological implants**
     Presence of bone-conduction hearing device
     Presence of eustachian tube stent
     Stapes replacement
Z96.3 **Presence of** artificial larynx
✓5ᵗ Z96.4 **Presence of** endocrine **implants**
   Z96.41 **Presence of insulin pump (external) (internal)**
   Z96.49 **Presence of other endocrine implants**
Z96.5 **Presence of** tooth-root and mandibular **implants**
✓5ᵗ Z96.6 **Presence of** orthopedic joint **implants**
   AHA: 2019,3Q,16
   Z96.60 **Presence of unspecified orthopedic joint implant**
  ✓6ᵗ Z96.61 **Presence of** artificial shoulder joint
    Z96.611 **Presence of** right **artificial shoulder joint**
    Z96.612 **Presence of** left **artificial shoulder joint**
    Z96.619 **Presence of unspecified artificial shoulder joint**
  ✓6ᵗ Z96.62 **Presence of** artificial elbow joint
    Z96.621 **Presence of** right **artificial elbow joint**
    Z96.622 **Presence of** left **artificial elbow joint**
    Z96.629 **Presence of unspecified artificial elbow joint**
  ✓6ᵗ Z96.63 **Presence of** artificial wrist joint
    Z96.631 **Presence of** right **artificial wrist joint**
    Z96.632 **Presence of** left **artificial wrist joint**
    Z96.639 **Presence of unspecified artificial wrist joint**
  ✓6ᵗ Z96.64 **Presence of** artificial hip joint
    Hip-joint replacement (partial) (total)
    Z96.641 **Presence of** right **artificial hip joint**
    Z96.642 **Presence of** left **artificial hip joint**
    Z96.643 **Presence of artificial hip joint,** bilateral
    Z96.649 **Presence of unspecified artificial hip joint**
  ✓6ᵗ Z96.65 **Presence of** artificial knee joint
    Z96.651 **Presence of** right **artificial knee joint**
    Z96.652 **Presence of** left **artificial knee joint**
    Z96.653 **Presence of artificial knee joint,** bilateral
    Z96.659 **Presence of unspecified artificial knee joint**
  ✓6ᵗ Z96.66 **Presence of** artificial ankle joint
    Z96.661 **Presence of** right **artificial ankle joint**
    Z96.662 **Presence of** left **artificial ankle joint**
    Z96.669 **Presence of unspecified artificial ankle joint**
  ✓6ᵗ Z96.69 **Presence of other orthopedic joint implants**
    Z96.691 **Finger-joint replacement of** right **hand**
    Z96.692 **Finger-joint replacement of** left **hand**
    Z96.693 **Finger-joint replacement,** bilateral
    Z96.698 **Presence of other orthopedic joint implants**
Z96.7 **Presence of other bone and tendon implants**
     Presence of skull plate
✓5ᵗ Z96.8 **Presence of other specified functional implants**
   Z96.81 **Presence of** artificial skin
   Z96.82 **Presence of** neurostimulator
     Presence of brain neurostimulator
     Presence of gastric neurostimulator
     Presence of peripheral nerve neurostimulator
     Presence of sacral nerve neurostimulator
     Presence of spinal cord neurostimulator
     Presence of vagus nerve neurostimulator
     AHA: 2019,4Q,19
   Z96.89 **Presence of other specified functional implants**
Z96.9 **Presence of functional implant, unspecified**

✓4ᵗ Z97 **Presence of other devices**
  EXCLUDES 1   complications of internal prosthetic devices, implants and grafts (T82-T85)
  EXCLUDES 2   fitting and adjustment of prosthetic and other devices (Z44-Z46)
     presence of cerebrospinal fluid drainage device (Z98.2)
Z97.0 **Presence of** artificial eye
✓5ᵗ Z97.1 **Presence of** artificial limb (complete) (partial)
   Z97.10 **Presence of artificial limb (complete) (partial), unspecified** COM
   Z97.11 **Presence of artificial** right **arm (complete) (partial)** COM
   Z97.12 **Presence of artificial** left **arm (complete) (partial)** COM
   Z97.13 **Presence of artificial** right **leg (complete) (partial)** COM
   Z97.14 **Presence of artificial** left **leg (complete) (partial)** COM
   Z97.15 **Presence of artificial arms, bilateral (complete) (partial)** COM
   Z97.16 **Presence of artificial legs, bilateral (complete) (partial)** COM
Z97.2 **Presence of dental prosthetic device (complete) (partial)**
     Presence of dentures (complete) (partial)
Z97.3 **Presence of spectacles and contact lenses**
Z97.4 **Presence of external hearing-aid**
Z97.5 **Presence of (intrauterine) contraceptive device** ♀
  EXCLUDES 1   checking, reinsertion or removal of implantable subdermal contraceptive (Z30.46)
     checking, reinsertion or removal of intrauterine contraceptive device (Z30.43-)
Z97.8 **Presence of other specified devices**
✓4ᵗ Z98 **Other postprocedural states**
  EXCLUDES 2   aftercare (Z43-Z49, Z51)
     follow-up medical care (Z08-Z09)
     postprocedural complication - see Alphabetical Index
Z98.0 **Intestinal bypass and anastomosis status**
  EXCLUDES 2   bariatric surgery status (Z98.84)
     gastric bypass status (Z98.84)
     obesity surgery status (Z98.84)
Z98.1 **Arthrodesis status**
Z98.2 **Presence of cerebrospinal fluid drainage device**
     Presence of CSF shunt
Z98.3 **Post therapeutic collapse of lung status** UPD
     Code first underlying disease
✓5ᵗ Z98.4 **Cataract extraction status**
     Use additional code to identify intraocular lens implant status (Z96.1)
  EXCLUDES 1   aphakia (H27.0)
   Z98.41 **Cataract extraction status,** right **eye**
   Z98.42 **Cataract extraction status,** left **eye**
   Z98.49 **Cataract extraction status, unspecified eye**
✓5ᵗ Z98.5 **Sterilization status**
  EXCLUDES 1   female infertility (N97.-)
     male infertility (N46.-)
   Z98.51 **Tubal ligation status** ♀
   Z98.52 **Vasectomy status** A ♂
✓5ᵗ Z98.6 **Angioplasty status**
   Z98.61 **Coronary angioplasty status**
    EXCLUDES 1   coronary angioplasty status with implant and graft (Z95.5)
   Z98.62 **Peripheral vascular angioplasty status**
    EXCLUDES 1   peripheral vascular angioplasty status with implant and graft (Z95.820)
✓5ᵗ Z98.8 **Other specified postprocedural states**
  ✓6ᵗ Z98.81 **Dental procedure status**
    Z98.810 **Dental sealant status**
    Z98.811 **Dental restoration status**
     Dental crown status
     Dental fillings status
    Z98.818 **Other dental procedure status**
   Z98.82 **Breast implant status**
    EXCLUDES 1   breast implant removal status (Z98.86)

Z98.83 **Filtering (vitreous) bleb after glaucoma surgery status**

> EXCLUDES 1   *inflammation (infection) of postprocedural bleb (H59.4-)*

> AHA: 2020,3Q,29

Z98.84 **Bariatric surgery status**

> Gastric banding status
> Gastric bypass status for obesity
> Obesity surgery status

> EXCLUDES 1   *bariatric surgery status complicating pregnancy, childbirth, or the puerperium (O99.84)*

> EXCLUDES 2   *intestinal bypass and anastomosis status (Z98.0)*

> AHA: 2020,1Q,12

Z98.85 **Transplanted organ removal status**

after removal

> Transplanted organ previously removed due to complication, failure, rejection or infection

> EXCLUDES 1   *encounter for removal of transplanted organ - code to complication of transplanted organ (T86.-)*

Z98.86 **Personal history of breast implant removal**

√6ᵗʰ **Z98.87** **Personal history of** in utero procedure

Z98.870 **Personal history of in utero procedure during pregnancy**   ♀

> EXCLUDES 2   *complications from in utero procedure for current pregnancy (O35.7)*
> *supervision of current pregnancy with history of in utero procedure during previous pregnancy (O09.82-)*

Z98.871 **Personal history of in utero procedure while a fetus**

√6ᵗʰ **Z98.89** **Other specified postprocedural states**

Z98.890 **Other specified postprocedural states**

> Personal history of surgery, not elsewhere classified

Z98.891 **History of uterine scar from previous surgery**   ♀

> EXCLUDES 1   *maternal care due to uterine scar from previous surgery (O34.2-)*

> AHA: 2016,4Q,51-52,76

√4ᵗʰ **Z99** **Dependence on enabling machines and devices, not elsewhere classified**

> AHA: 2020,1Q,11   *Pt is dependent*

Z99.0 **Dependence on** aspirator

√5ᵗʰ **Z99.1** **Dependence on** respirator   ① Jᴵ96.1 ② Z99.1

> Dependence on ventilator

Z99.11 **Dependence on respirator [ventilator] status**   HCC ESR COM

> AHA: 2015,1Q,21

Z99.12 **Encounter for respirator [ventilator] dependence during power failure**   HCC ESR COM PDx

> EXCLUDES 1   *mechanical complication of respirator [ventilator] (J95.850)*

Z99.2 **Dependence on** renal dialysis   HCC Rx ESR

> Hemodialysis status
> Peritoneal dialysis status
> Presence of arteriovenous shunt for dialysis
> Renal dialysis status NOS

> EXCLUDES 1   *encounter for fitting and adjustment of dialysis catheter (Z49.0-)*

> EXCLUDES 2   *noncompliance with renal dialysis (Z91.15)*

> AHA: 2016,1Q,12; 2013,4Q,125

Z99.3 **Dependence on** wheelchair

> Wheelchair confinement status
> Code first cause of dependence, such as:
> muscular dystrophy (G71.0-)
> obesity (E66.-)

√5ᵗʰ **Z99.8** **Dependence on other enabling machines and devices**

Z99.81 **Dependence on** supplemental oxygen

> Dependence on long-term oxygen

> AHA: 2013,4Q,129

Z99.89 **Dependence on other enabling machines and devices**

> Dependence on machine or device NOS

> AHA: 2020,1Q,11

HCC CMS-HCC   Rx Rx HCC   ESR ESRD HCC   COM Commercial HCC   PDx Primary Dx Only   N Newborn: 0   P Pediatric: 0-17   M Maternity: 9-64   A Adult: 15-124

1296   ICD-10-CM 2023

Chapter 22. Codes for Special Purposes (U00–U85)

Chapter-specific Guidelines

U07.0   Vaping-related disorder (see Section I.C.10.e., Vaping-related disorders)

U07.1   COVID-19 (see Section I.C.1.g.1., COVID-19 infection)

U09.9   Post COVID-19 condition, unspecified (see Section I.C.1.g.1.m.)

Chapter 22. Codes for Special Purposes (U00-U85)

This chapter contains the following blocks:

U00-U49   Provisional assignment of new diseases of uncertain etiology or emergency use

Provisional assignment of new diseases of uncertain etiology or emergency use (U00-U49)

✓4ᵗʰ U07   Emergency use of U07

U07.0   Vaping-related disorder

Dabbing related lung damage

Dabbing related lung injury

E-cigarette, or vaping, product use associated lung injury [EVALI]

Electronic cigarette related lung damage

Electronic cigarette related lung injury

Use additional code, to identify manifestations, such as:

     abdominal pain (R10.84)

     acute respiratory distress syndrome (J80)

     diarrhea (R19.7)

     drug-induced interstitial lung disorder (J70.4)

     lipoid pneumonia (J69.1)

     weight loss (R63.4)

DEF: Respiratory illness or injury caused by harmful aerosolized substances and chemicals produced by electronic cigarettes, vapes, e-pipes, and other battery-powered vaping devices. Symptoms may include shortness of breath and fever, while some patients experience severe, sometimes fatal, lung damage. **Synonym(s):** *e-cigarette and vaping product use-associated lung injury, EVALI.*

U07.1   COVID-19

Use additional code to identify pneumonia or other manifestations, such as:

pneumonia due to COVID-19 (J12.82)

EXCLUDES 2   *coronavirus as the cause of diseases classified elsewhere (B97.2-)*

     coronavirus infection, unspecified (B34.2)

     pneumonia due to SARS-associated coronavirus (J12.81)

AHA: 2022,2Q,28; 2021,4Q,101,107-108; 2021,1Q,25-30,31-49; 2020,4Q,14,99; 2020,3Q,9-16; 2020,2Q,3-13

DEF: First diagnosed in December 2019 in China, coronavirus disease 2019 (COVID-19) is a respiratory infection caused by a newly identified (novel) virus not previously seen in humans, known as severe acute respiratory syndrome coronavirus 2 (SARS-CoV-2). Symptoms of this lower respiratory illness include fever, dry cough, and tiredness that may progress to include difficulty breathing. Older patients and those with high blood pressure, heart problems, and diabetes are more likely to develop serious symptoms of the illness. **Synonym(s):** *SARS-CoV-2, coronavirus disease 2019.*

TIP: Only a confirmed diagnosis of COVID-19 can be coded to U07.1; a positive COVID-19 test result or documentation by the provider that the disease is confirmed is sufficient.

TIP: Assign for asymptomatic individuals who test positive for COVID-19. Even though asymptomatic, the individual is considered to have the COVID-19 infection due to the positive test result.

TIP: Assign appropriate codes for presenting signs/symptoms associated with COVID-19 (cough, fever, shortness of breath), instead of U07.1, if a definitive diagnosis has not been established.

✓4ᵗʰ U09   Post COVID-19 condition

U09.9   Post COVID-19 condition, unspecified

NOTE   This code enables establishment of a link with COVID-19.

This code is not to be used in cases that are still presenting with active COVID-19. However, an exception is made in cases of re-infection with COVID-19, occurring with a condition related to prior COVID-19.

~~Post-acute sequela of COVID-19~~

▶Post-acute sequela of COVID-19◀

Code first the specific condition related to COVID-19 if known, such as:

     chronic respiratory failure (J96.1-)

     loss of smell (R43.8)

     loss of taste (R43.8)

     multisystem inflammatory syndrome (M35.81)

     pulmonary embolism (I26.-)

     pulmonary fibrosis (J84.10)

AHA: 2021,4Q,31-32,102-106

Notes

Notes

Notes

Notes

Appendix A: Valid 3-character ICD-10-CM Codes

A09	Infectious gastroenteritis and colitis, unspecified
A33	Tetanus neonatorum
A34	Obstetrical tetanus
A35	Other tetanus
A46	Erysipelas
A55	Chlamydial lymphogranuloma (venereum)
A57	Chancroid
A58	Granuloma inguinale
A64	Unspecified sexually transmitted disease
A65	Nonvenereal syphilis
A70	Chlamydia psittaci infections
A78	Q fever
A86	Unspecified viral encephalitis
A89	Unspecified viral infection of central nervous system
A90	Dengue fever [classical dengue]
A91	Dengue hemorrhagic fever
A94	Unspecified arthropod-borne viral fever
A99	Unspecified viral hemorrhagic fever
B03	Smallpox
B04	Monkeypox
B09	Unspecified viral infection characterized by skin and mucous membrane lesions
B20	Human immunodeficiency virus [HIV] disease
B49	Unspecified mycosis
B54	Unspecified malaria
B59	Pneumocystosis
B64	Unspecified protozoal disease
B72	Dracunculiasis
B75	Trichinellosis
B79	Trichuriasis
B80	Enterobiasis
B86	Scabies
B89	Unspecified parasitic disease
B91	Sequelae of poliomyelitis
B92	Sequelae of leprosy
C01	Malignant neoplasm of base of tongue
C07	Malignant neoplasm of parotid gland
C12	Malignant neoplasm of pyriform sinus
C19	Malignant neoplasm of rectosigmoid junction
C20	Malignant neoplasm of rectum
C23	Malignant neoplasm of gallbladder
C33	Malignant neoplasm of trachea
C37	Malignant neoplasm of thymus
C52	Malignant neoplasm of vagina
C55	Malignant neoplasm of uterus, part unspecified
C58	Malignant neoplasm of placenta
C61	Malignant neoplasm of prostate
C73	Malignant neoplasm of thyroid gland
D34	Benign neoplasm of thyroid gland
D45	Polycythemia vera
D62	Acute posthemorrhagic anemia
D65	Disseminated intravascular coagulation [defibrination syndrome]
D66	Hereditary factor VIII deficiency
D67	Hereditary factor IX deficiency
D71	Functional disorders of polymorphonuclear neutrophils
D77	Other disorders of blood and blood-forming organs in diseases classified elsewhere
E02	Subclinical iodine-deficiency hypothyroidism
E15	Nondiabetic hypoglycemic coma
E35	Disorders of endocrine glands in diseases classified elsewhere
E40	Kwashiorkor
E41	Nutritional marasmus
E42	Marasmic kwashiorkor
E43	Unspecified severe protein-calorie malnutrition
E45	Retarded development following protein-calorie malnutrition

E46	Unspecified protein-calorie malnutrition
E52	Niacin deficiency [pellagra]
E54	Ascorbic acid deficiency
E58	Dietary calcium deficiency
E59	Dietary selenium deficiency
E60	Dietary zinc deficiency
E65	Localized adiposity
E68	Sequelae of hyperalimentation
F04	Amnestic disorder due to known physiological condition
F05	Delirium due to known physiological condition
F09	Unspecified mental disorder due to known physiological condition
F21	Schizotypal disorder
F22	Delusional disorders
F23	Brief psychotic disorder
F24	Shared psychotic disorder
F28	Other psychotic disorder not due to a substance or known physiological condition
F29	Unspecified psychosis not due to a substance or known physiological condition
F39	Unspecified mood [affective] disorder
F54	Psychological and behavioral factors associated with disorders or diseases classified elsewhere
F59	Unspecified behavioral syndromes associated with physiological disturbances and physical factors
F66	Other sexual disorders
F69	Unspecified disorder of adult personality and behavior
F70	Mild intellectual disabilities
F71	Moderate intellectual disabilities
F72	Severe intellectual disabilities
F73	Profound intellectual disabilities
F79	Unspecified intellectual disabilities
F82	Specific developmental disorder of motor function
F88	Other disorders of psychological development
F89	Unspecified disorder of psychological development
F99	Mental disorder, not otherwise specified
G01	Meningitis in bacterial diseases classified elsewhere
G02	Meningitis in other infectious and parasitic diseases classified elsewhere
G07	Intracranial and intraspinal abscess and granuloma in diseases classified elsewhere
G08	Intracranial and intraspinal phlebitis and thrombophlebitis
G09	Sequelae of inflammatory diseases of central nervous system
G10	Huntington's disease
G14	Postpolio syndrome
G20	Parkinson's disease
G26	Extrapyramidal and movement disorders in diseases classified elsewhere
G35	Multiple sclerosis
G53	Cranial nerve disorders in diseases classified elsewhere
G55	Nerve root and plexus compressions in diseases classified elsewhere
G59	Mononeuropathy in diseases classified elsewhere
G63	Polyneuropathy in diseases classified elsewhere
G64	Other disorders of peripheral nervous system
G94	Other disorders of brain in diseases classified elsewhere
H22	Disorders of iris and ciliary body in diseases classified elsewhere
H28	Cataract in diseases classified elsewhere
H32	Chorioretinal disorders in diseases classified elsewhere
H36	Retinal disorders in diseases classified elsewhere
H42	Glaucoma in diseases classified elsewhere
I00	Rheumatic fever without heart involvement
I10	Essential (primary) hypertension
I32	Pericarditis in diseases classified elsewhere
I38	Endocarditis, valve unspecified
I39	Endocarditis and heart valve disorders in diseases classified elsewhere

I41	Myocarditis in diseases classified elsewhere
I43	Cardiomyopathy in diseases classified elsewhere
I52	Other heart disorders in diseases classified elsewhere
I5A	Non-ischemic myocardial injury (non-traumatic)
I76	Septic arterial embolism
I81	Portal vein thrombosis
I96	Gangrene, not elsewhere classified
J00	Acute nasopharyngitis (common cold)
J13	Pneumonia due to Streptococcus pneumoniae
J14	Pneumonia due to Hemophilus influenzae
J17	Pneumonia in diseases classified elsewhere
J22	Unspecified acute lower respiratory infection
J36	Peritonsillar abscess
J40	Bronchitis, not specified as acute or chronic
J42	Unspecified chronic bronchitis
J60	Coalworker's pneumoconiosis
J61	Pneumoconiosis due to asbestos and other mineral fibers
J64	Unspecified pneumoconiosis
J65	Pneumoconiosis associated with tuberculosis
J80	Acute respiratory distress syndrome
J90	Pleural effusion, not elsewhere classified
J99	Respiratory disorders in diseases classified elsewhere
K23	Disorders of esophagus in diseases classified elsewhere
K30	Functional dyspepsia
K36	Other appendicitis
K37	Unspecified appendicitis
K67	Disorders of peritoneum in infectious diseases classified elsewhere
K77	Liver disorders in diseases classified elsewhere
K87	Disorders of gallbladder, biliary tract and pancreas in diseases classified elsewhere
L00	Staphylococcal scalded skin syndrome
L14	Bullous disorders in diseases classified elsewhere
L22	Diaper dermatitis
L26	Exfoliative dermatitis
L42	Pityriasis rosea
L45	Papulosquamous disorders in diseases classified elsewhere
L52	Erythema nodosum
L54	Erythema in diseases classified elsewhere
L62	Nail disorders in diseases classified elsewhere
L80	Vitiligo
L83	Acanthosis nigricans
L84	Corns and callosities
L86	Keratoderma in diseases classified elsewhere
L88	Pyoderma gangrenosum
L99	Other disorders of skin and subcutaneous tissue in diseases classified elsewhere
N08	Glomerular disorders in diseases classified elsewhere
N10	Acute tubulo-interstitial nephritis
N12	Tubulo-interstitial nephritis, not specified as acute or chronic
N16	Renal tubulo-interstitial disorders in diseases classified elsewhere
N19	Unspecified kidney failure
N22	Calculus of urinary tract in diseases classified elsewhere
N23	Unspecified renal colic
N29	Other disorders of kidney and ureter in diseases classified elsewhere
N33	Bladder disorders in diseases classified elsewhere
N37	Urethral disorders in diseases classified elsewhere
N51	Disorders of male genital organs in diseases classified elsewhere
N62	Hypertrophy of breast
N72	Inflammatory disease of cervix uteri
N74	Female pelvic inflammatory disorders in diseases classified elsewhere
N86	Erosion and ectropion of cervix uteri
N96	Recurrent pregnancy loss
O68	Labor and delivery complicated by abnormality of fetal acid-base balance

O76	Abnormality in fetal heart rate and rhythm complicating labor and delivery
O80	Encounter for full-term uncomplicated delivery
O82	Encounter for cesarean delivery without indication
O85	Puerperal sepsis
O94	Sequelae of complication of pregnancy, childbirth, and the puerperium
P53	Hemorrhagic disease of newborn
P60	Disseminated intravascular coagulation of newborn
P84	Other problems with newborn
P90	Convulsions of newborn
P95	Stillbirth
Q02	Microcephaly
R12	Heartburn
R17	Unspecified jaundice
R21	Rash and other nonspecific skin eruption
R32	Unspecified urinary incontinence
R34	Anuria and oliguria
R37	Sexual dysfunction, unspecified
R42	Dizziness and giddiness
R52	Pain, unspecified
R54	Age-related physical debility
R55	Syncope and collapse
R58	Hemorrhage, not elsewhere classified
R61	Generalized hyperhidrosis
R64	Cachexia
R69	Illness, unspecified
R75	Inconclusive laboratory evidence of human immunodeficiency virus [HIV]
R81	Glycosuria
R99	Ill-defined and unknown cause of mortality
Y09	Assault by unspecified means
Y66	Nonadministration of surgical and medical care
Y69	Unspecified misadventure during surgical and medical care
Y95	Nosocomial condition
Z08	Encounter for follow-up examination after completed treatment for malignant neoplasm
Z09	Encounter for follow-up examination after completed treatment for conditions other than malignant neoplasm
Z21	Asymptomatic human immunodeficiency virus [HIV] infection status
Z23	Encounter for immunization
Z66	Do not resuscitate

Appendix B: Pharmacology List 2023

This section enables the coder to quickly review drugs, drug actions, and indications that are often associated with overlooked or undocumented diagnoses. The coder should review the patient's medication record and know what condition the physician is treating with the prescribed medication based on documentation in the medical record. When documentation is lacking, the coder can reference this section to locate the drug, determine the drug action, confirm drug indications, and when necessary query the physician. When applicable, some of the drugs provided in this resource have also been mapped to their appropriate Z code for long-term drug use.

Drug	Z Code	Drug Action/Classification	Indications
5-fluorouracil (5-FU) [fluorouracil]	Z79.631	Antimetabolite agent	Skin, colorectal, breast, stomach, and pancreas cancer
6-mercaptopurine (6-MP) [mercaptopurine]	Z79.631	Antimetabolite agent	Acute lymphoblastic leukemia
Abilify [aripiprazole]		Antipsychotic	Depression; bipolar disorder; schizophrenia; autism symptoms
Acarbose [acarbose]	Z79.84	Oral hypoglycemic	Diabetes mellitus
Accupril [quinapril hydrochloride]		ACE inhibitor	Congestive heart failure; hypertension
Acetaminophen with codeine [acetaminophen/codeine phosphate]	Z79.891	Analgesic, narcotic	Pain, moderate to severe
Aclasta [zoledronic acid]	Z79.83	Bisphosphonate	Paget's disease; bone loss prevention in postmenopausal women
Actemra [tocilizumab]	Z79.620	Immunosuppressive biologic; monoclonal antibody	Rheumatoid arthritis; systemic sclerosis-associated interstitial lung disease; giant cell arteritis; polyarticular or systemic juvenile idiopathic arthritis; cytokine release syndrome
Actimmune [interferon gamma-1b]	Z79.69	Other immunosuppressant/ immunomodulator	Chronic granulomatous disease; malignant osteopetrosis
Activella [estradiol/norethindrone acetate]	Z79.890	Estrogen therapy	Menopause symptoms; vaginal and vulvar atrophy; osteoporosis prevention
Actonel [risedronate sodium]	Z79.83	Bisphosphonate	Decrease in bone loss in multiple myeloma patients; Paget's disease; hyperparathyroidism; osteoporosis
Actoplus Met [metformin hydrochloride/pioglitazone hydrochloride]	Z79.84	Oral hypoglycemic	Diabetes mellitus
Actos [pioglitazone hydrochloride]	Z79.84	Oral hypoglycemic	Diabetes mellitus
Aczone [dapsone]		Acne agent, topical	Acne vulgaris
Adalat CC [nifedipine]		Calcium channel blocker	Vasospastic angina; chronic stable angina; hypertension
Adderall XR [amphetamine aspartate and sulfate/dextroamphetamine saccharate and sulfate]		CNS stimulant	Attention deficit hyperactivity disorder (ADHD)
Adlarity [donepezil hydrochloride]		Acetylcholinesterase/cholinesterase inhibitors	Dementia due to Alzheimer's
Adlyxin [lixisenatide]	Z79.85	Antidiabetic – non-insulin injectable	Diabetes mellitus
Admelog [insulin lispro]	Z79.4	Insulin	Diabetes mellitus
Advair [fluticasone propionate/salmeterol xinafoate]	Z79.51	Corticosteroid – inhaled; antiasthmatic	Prophylaxis and treatment of asthma and COPD
Advil [ibuprofen]	Z79.1	Nonsteroidal anti-inflammatory drug (NSAID)	Pain or fever relief
Afrezza [human insulin recombinant]	Z79.899	Insulin – inhaled	Diabetes mellitus
Aggrastat [tirofiban hydrochloride]	Z79.02	Antiplatelet	Unstable angina; heart attacks
Aggrenox [aspirin/dipyridamole]	Z79.02	Antiplatelet	Lessening of the chance of heart attack or stroke
Aimovig [erenumab-aooe]	Z79.620	Immunosuppressive biologic; monoclonal antibody	Migraine headache prevention
AirDuo RespiClick [fluticasone propionate/salmeterol xinafoate]	Z79.51	Corticosteroid – inhaled; antiasthmatic	Asthma
Aklief [trifarotene]		Acne agent, topical	Acne vulgaris
Aldactone [spironolactone]		Cardiovascular agent; antihypertensive agent; diuretic; electrolytic and renal agent	Severe heart failure; ascites associated with cirrhosis; hypokalemia
Aleve [naproxen sodium]	Z79.1	Nonsteroidal anti-inflammatory drug (NSAID)	Reduction of temporary aches and pains
Allegra allergy [fexofenadine hydrochloride]		Antihistamine	Seasonal allergic rhinitis
Allopurinol [allopurinol]		Antigout	Gouty arthritis; renal calculus; hyperuricemia; hyperuricemia secondary to leukemia; hyperuricemia secondary to lymphoma

Drug	Z Code	Drug Action/Classification	Indications
Alora [estradiol]	Z79.890	Estrogen therapy	Menopause symptoms
Alphagan P [brimonidine tartrate]		Antiglaucoma agent (ophthalmic); antihypertensive, ocular	Open angle glaucoma or another condition in which pressure in the eye is too high (ocular hypertension)
Alprazolam [alprazolam]		Antianxiety; sedative/hypnotic	Anxiety and panic disorders
Altabax [retapamulin]	Z79.2	Antibiotic, topical	Skin infections
Altace [ramipril]		ACE inhibitor	Congestive heart failure; hypertension
Altavera [ethinyl estradiol/levonorgestrel]	Z79.3	Contraceptive	Prevention of pregnancy
Alvesco [ciclesonide]	Z79.51	Corticosteroid – inhaled; antiasthmatic	Prophylaxis and treatment of asthma
Alyacen [ethinyl estradiol/norethindrone]	Z79.3	Contraceptive	Prevention of pregnancy
Amaryl [glimepiride]	Z79.84	Oral hypoglycemic	Diabetes mellitus
Ambien [zolpidem tartrate]		CNS depressant; anxiolytic/sedative/hypnotic	Insomnia
Amikacin [amikacin sulfate]	Z79.2	Antibiotic	Gram-negative bacterial infections such as Pseudomonas, Escherichia coli (E. coli), Proteus, Klebsiella-Enterobacter-Serratia
Amitriptyline HCl [amitriptyline hydrochloride]		Antidepressant	Depression
Amoxicillin [amoxicillin]	Z79.2	Antibiotic	Treatment of infections with a broad spectrum of bactericidal activity against many gram-positive and gram-negative microorganisms; otitis media, gonorrhea, skin, respiratory, gastrointestinal, and genitourinary infections
Ampicillin [ampicillin sodium]	Z79.2	Antibiotic	Bacterial infections
Ampyra [dalfampridine]		Potassium channel blocker	Improvement in walking in patients with multiple sclerosis
Amrix [cyclobenzaprine hydrochloride]		Muscle relaxant	Adjunct to rest and physical therapy for muscle spasms
Anaprox DS [naproxen sodium]	Z79.1	Nonsteroidal anti-inflammatory drug (NSAID)	Pain, inflammation or fever relief
Anastrozole [anastrozole]	Z79.811	Aromatase inhibitor	Postmenopausal breast cancer
Androderm [testosterone]	Z79.890	Testosterone therapy – topical	Primary hypogonadism; hypogonadotropic hypogonadism
AndroGel [testosterone]	Z79.890	Testosterone therapy – topical	Primary hypogonadism; hypogonadotropic hypogonadism
Angeliq [drospirenone/estradiol]	Z79.890	Estrogen therapy	Menopause symptoms
Angiomax [bivalirudin]	Z79.01	Anticoagulant	Prevention of blood clots
Antabuse [disulfiram]		Alcohol treatment	Alcoholism
Antineoplastic/chemotherapy	Z79.899	Antineoplastic	Cancer
Apidra [insulin glulisine recombinant]	Z79.4	Insulin	Diabetes mellitus
Aranelle [ethinyl estradiol/norethindrone]	Z79.3	Contraceptive	Prevention of pregnancy; acne
Aranesp [darbepoetin alfa]		Erythropoiesis-stimulating agent (ESA)	Treatment of lower than normal blood cells (anemia) from disorders such as CKD and neoplasms
Aredia [pamidronate disodium]	Z79.83	Bisphosphonate	Prevention of thinning of the bones (osteoporosis)
Argatroban [argatroban]	Z79.01	Anticoagulant	Prophylaxis and treatment of venous thrombosis in thrombocytopenia patients
Aricept [donepezil hydrochloride]		Acetylcholinesterase/cholinesterase inhibitors	Dementia due to Alzheimer's
Arimidex [anastrozole]	Z79.811	Aromatase inhibitor	Postmenopausal breast cancer
Aristospan [triamcinolone hexacetonide]	Z79.52	Corticosteroid	Severe inflammation
Arixtra [fondaparinux sodium]	Z79.01	Anticoagulant	Venous thrombosis and pulmonary embolism
Arnuity Ellipta [fluticasone furoate]	Z79.51	Corticosteroid – inhaled; antiasthmatic	Prophylaxis and treatment of asthma
Aromasin [exemestane]	Z79.811	Aromatase inhibitor	Postmenopausal breast cancer
Arthrotec [diclofenac sodium/misoprostol]	Z79.1	Nonsteroidal anti-inflammatory drug (NSAID)-prostaglandin combo	Treatment of patients with arthritis who may develop stomach ulcers from taking nonsteroidal anti-inflammatory drugs (NSAIDs) alone; used to help relieve some symptoms of arthritis, such as inflammation, swelling, stiffness, and joint pain
Asacol HD [mesalamine]		Anti-inflammatory	Ulcerative colitis
Ashlyna [ethinyl estradiol/levonorgestrel]	Z79.3	Contraceptive	Prevention of pregnancy

Drug	Z Code	Drug Action/Classification	Indications
Asmanex [mometasone furoate]	Z79.51	Corticosteroid – inhaled; antiasthmatic	Prophylaxis and treatment of asthma
Astagraf XL [tacrolimus]	Z79.621	Calcineurin inhibitor	Prophylaxis of organ transplant rejection
Atelvia [risedronate sodium]	Z79.83	Bisphosphonate	Prevention of thinning of the bones (osteoporosis)
Atenolol [atenolol]		Beta blocker	Angina pectoris; hypertension; acute myocardial infarction
Ativan [lorazepam]		Antianxiety; sedative/hypnotic	Anxiety disorder associated with depressive symptoms; controls tension, agitation, irritability, and insomnia
Atripla [efavirenz/emtricitabine/tenofovir disoproxil fumarate]	Z79.899	Antiretroviral	HIV
Atrovent HFA [ipratropium bromide]		Antiasthmatic/bronchodilator	Chronic bronchitis, emphysema; bronchial asthma
Augmentin [amoxicillin/clavulanate potassium]	Z79.2	Antibiotic	Middle ear, lower respiratory, sinus, skin and skin structures, and urinary tract infections
Avandia [rosiglitazone maleate]	Z79.84	Oral hypoglycemic	Diabetes mellitus
Avapro [irbesartan]		Antihypertensive	Hypertension
Avelox [moxifloxacin hydrochloride]	Z79.2	Antibiotic	Bacterial infections of the skin, sinuses, lungs, or stomach; plague
Aviane-28 [ethinyl estradiol/levonorgestrel]	Z79.3	Contraceptive	Prevention of pregnancy
Avonex [interferon beta-1a]	Z79.69	Other immunosuppressant/ immunomodulator	Treatment of relapsing multiple sclerosis
Axid AR [nizatidine]		Histamine H2-receptor antagonist	Acid/peptic disorder; gastroesophageal reflux; duodenal, gastric, and peptic ulcers
Ayvakit [avapritinib]		Multikinase inhibitor	Unresectable or metastatic gastrointestinal stromal tumor (GIST); advanced systemic mastocytosis
Azactam [aztreonam]	Z79.2	Antibiotic	Severe bacterial infections
Azithromycin [azithromycin]	Z79.2	Antibiotic	Bacterial infections
Azstarys [serdexmethylphenidate and dexmethylphenidate]		CNS stimulant	Attention deficit hyperactivity disorder (ADHD)
Bactrim [sulfamethoxazole/trimethoprim]	Z79.2	Antibiotic	Treatment of urinary tract infections, acute otitis media, acute exacerbation of chronic bronchitis, shigellosis, and pneumocystis carinii
Bactroban [mupirocin topical]	Z79.2	Antibiotic, topical	Bacterial skin infections
Balziva-28 [ethinyl estradiol/norethindrone]	Z79.3	Contraceptive	Prevention of pregnancy
Basaglar [insulin glargine]	Z79.4	Insulin	Diabetes mellitus
Bayer [acetylsalicylic acid]	Z79.82	Aspirin	Prophylaxis and treatment of heart attacks, angina or strokes; reduction of fever, pain and inflammation
Beconase AQ [beclomethasone dipropionate monohydrate]	Z79.899	Corticosteroid – intranasal	Perennial and seasonal allergies; vasomotor rhinitis
Bekyree [desogestrel/ethinyl estradiol]	Z79.3	Contraceptive	Prevention of pregnancy
Betaseron [interferon beta-1b]	Z79.69	Other immunosuppressant/ immunomodulator	Treatment of relapsing multiple sclerosis
Betoptic [betaxolol hydrochloride]		Beta blocker; ophthalmic glaucoma agent	Lowering of intraocular pressure; also used for treatment of ocular hypertension and chronic open-angle glaucoma
Bevyxxa [betrixaban]	Z79.01	Anticoagulant	Prophylaxis of venous thromboembolism
Beyaz [drospirenone/ethinyl estradiol/levomefolate calcium]	Z79.3	Contraceptive	Prevention of pregnancy; acne
Biaxin XL [clarithromycin]	Z79.2	Antibiotic	Acid/peptic disorder or ulcer; acute exacerbation chronic bronchitis; human immunodeficiency virus; lower and upper respiratory tract infection; sinus infection; prophylaxis mycobacterium avium complex; pharyngitis; pneumonia; tonsillitis
Bijuva [estradiol/progesterone]	Z79.890	Estrogen/progesterone therapy	Menopausal symptoms
Biktarvy [bictegravir sodium/emtricitabine/ tenofovir alafenamide fumarate]	Z79.899	Antiretroviral	HIV
Biltricide [praziquantel]		Antiparasitic	Infections from Schistosoma species and liver flukes
Binosto [alendronate sodium]	Z79.83	Bisphosphonate	Prevention of thinning of the bones (osteoporosis)
Bleomycin [bleomycin]	Z79.632	Antitumor antibiotic	Squamous cell carcinoma; Hodgkin's disease; non-Hodgkin's lymphoma; malignant pleural effusion; testicular cancer

Drug	Z Code	Drug Action/Classification	Indications
Boniva [ibandronate sodium]	Z79.83	Bisphosphonate	Prevention of thinning of the bones (osteoporosis)
Breo Ellipta [fluticasone furoate/vilanterol trifenatate]	Z79.51	Corticosteroid – inhaled; antiasthmatic	Maintenance treatment of asthma and COPD
Brevicon 28-day [ethinyl estradiol/norethindrone]	Z79.3	Contraceptive	Prevention of pregnancy; acne
Brexafemme [ibrexafungerp]		Antifungal	Vulvovaginal candidiasis
Briellyn [ethinyl estradiol/norethindrone]	Z79.3	Contraceptive	Prevention of pregnancy
Brilinta [ticagrelor]	Z79.Ø2	Antiplatelet	Unstable angina; heart attacks; prevention of blood clots
Brisdelle [paroxetine]		Selective serotonin reuptake inhibitor (SSRI)	Vasomotor symptoms related to menopause
Bufferin [aspirin]	Z79.82	Aspirin	Pain, reduce fever or inflammation; prophylaxis and treatment of heart attack, stroke, angina
Buprenex [buprenorphine hydrochloride]	Z79.891	Analgesic, narcotic	Moderate to severe pain
Buprenorphine HCl and Naloxone HCl [buprenorphine hydrochloride/naloxone hydrochloride]	Z79.891	Analgesic, narcotic	Moderate to severe pain
Buspirone HCl [buspirone hydrochloride]		Antianxiety	Generalized anxiety disorder
Busulfex [busulfan]	Z79.63Ø	Chemotherapeutic alkylating agent	Chronic myelogenous leukemia
Butrans [buprenorphine]	Z79.891	Analgesic, narcotic	Chronic pain
Bydureon [exenatide]	Z79.85	Antidiabetic – non-insulin injectable	Diabetes mellitus
Byetta [exenatide]	Z79.85	Antidiabetic – non-insulin injectable	Diabetes mellitus
Calan [verapamil hydrochloride]		Calcium channel blocker	Angina pectoris at rest and chronic stable, arrhythmia, atrial fibrillation, atrial flutter, paroxysmal supraventricular tachycardia, ventricular arrhythmia, hypertension
Caldolor [ibuprofen]	Z79.1	Nonsteroidal anti-inflammatory drug (NSAID)	Pain or fever relief
Cambia [diclofenac potassium]	Z79.1	Nonsteroidal anti-inflammatory drug (NSAID)	Migraine headache
Camila [norethindrone]	Z79.3	Contraceptive	Prevention of pregnancy; menstrual disorders
Camptosar [irinotecan]	Z79.634	Topoisomerase inhibitor	Metastatic colon or rectal cancer
Caplyta [lumateperone]		Antipsychotic	Schizophrenia
Cardizem CD [diltiazem hydrochloride]		Calcium channel blocker	Chronic stable angina, atrial fibrillation, atrial flutter, hypertension, paroxysmal supraventricular tachycardia
Cardura [doxazosin mesylate]		Antihypertensive	Benign prostatic hyperplasia; hypertension
Carmustine [carmustine]	Z79.63Ø	Chemotherapeutic alkylating agent	Brain tumors; Hodgkin's disease; multiple myeloma; non-Hodgkin's lymphoma
Cefazolin sodium [cefazolin sodium]	Z79.2	Antibiotic	Respiratory tract infections due to Streptococcus pneumoniae, Klebsiella species, Haemophilus influenzae (H. influenzae), Staphylococcus aureus, and group A beta-hemolytic streptococci; urinary tract infections due to E. coli, Proteus mirabilis, Klebsiella species, and some strains of Enterobacter and enterococci; skin and skin structure infections, biliary tract infections, bone and joint infections, genital infections, septicemia, and endocarditis
Ceftriaxone [ceftriaxone sodium]	Z79.2	Antibiotic	Bacterial infections
Cefzil [cefprozil]	Z79.2	Antibiotic	Acute exacerbation and chronic bronchitis, lower respiratory tract infection, upper respiratory tract infection, pharyngitis, tonsillitis
Celebrex [celecoxib]	Z79.1	Nonsteroidal anti-inflammatory drug (NSAID)	Relief of symptoms caused by arthritis, such as inflammation, swelling, stiffness, and joint pain
Celestone Soluspan [betamethasone acetate/betamethasone sodium phosphate]	Z79.52	Corticosteroid; antiasthmatic	Asthma; severe inflammation
Celexa [citalopram hydrobromide]		Antidepressant	Depression
CellCept [mycophenolate mofetil]	Z79.624	Inhibitors of nucleotide synthesis	Prophylaxis of organ transplant rejection
Centany [mupirocin]	Z79.2	Antibiotic, topical	Bacterial skin infections
Cephalexin [cephalexin]	Z79.2	Antibiotic	Bacterial infections
Cerubidine [daunorubicin hydrochloride]	Z79.632	Antitumor antibiotic	Leukemia
Chantix [varenicline tartrate]		Smoking cessation aid	Nicotine addiction, smoking

Appendix B: Pharmacology List 2023

Drug	Z Code	Drug Action/Classification	Indications
Chlorambucil [chlorambucil]	Z79.630	Chemotherapeutic alkylating agent	Chronic lymphocytic leukemia; malignant lymphoma
Cibinqo [abrocitinib]	Z79.622	Janus kinase (JAK) inhibitor	Atopic dermatitis
Cimduo [lamivudine/tenofovir disoproxil fumarate]	Z79.899	Antiretroviral	HIV; chronic hepatitis B
Cipro [ciprofloxacin hydrochloride]	Z79.2	Antibiotic	Cystitis; infectious diarrhea; gonorrhea; bone and joint infection; gastrointestinal tract infection; lower and upper respiratory tract infection; sinus infection; urinary tract infection; nosocomial pneumonia; chronic prostatitis
Ciprofloxacin [ciprofloxacin]	Z79.2	Antibiotic	Bacterial infections
Cisplatin [cisplatin]	Z79.630	Chemotherapeutic alkylating agent	Cancer
Clarithromycin [clarithromycin]	Z79.2	Antibiotic	Skin and respiratory bacterial infections
Claritin [loratadine]		Antihistamine	Seasonal allergic rhinitis; chronic idiopathic urticaria
Cleocin [clindamycin phosphate]	Z79.2	Antibiotic	Bacterial infections
Climara [estradiol]	Z79.890	Estrogen therapy	Osteoporosis prevention and to treat menopausal symptoms; vaginal and vulvar atrophy; hypoestrogenism; ovarian failure
Clindamycin [clindamycin phosphate]	Z79.2	Antibiotic	Bacterial infections
Clonazepam [clonazepam]		Anticonvulsant	Absence, akinetic, and myoclonic epilepsy; Lennox-Gastaut syndrome
Clonidine HCl [clonidine hydrochloride]		Antihypertensive	Hypertension
Clopidogrel bisulfate [clopidogrel bisulfate]	Z79.02	Antiplatelet	Unstable angina; heart attacks; prevention of blood clots
Codeine [codeine sulfate]	Z79.891	Analgesic, narcotic	Mild to moderate pain
Cogentin [benztropine mesylate]		Antiparkinsonism	Parkinson's disease
Colace [docusate sodium]		Gastrointestinal agent; laxative, stool softener	Constipation
Colazal [balsalazide]		Anti-inflammatory	Ulcerative colitis
Colocort [hydrocortisone]	Z79.52	Corticosteroid	Inflammation of the colon
CombiPatch [ethinyl estradiol/norethindrone acetate]	Z79.890	Estrogen therapy	Menopause symptoms; vaginal and vulvar atrophy; osteoporosis prevention
Combivent Respimat [ipratropium bromide/albuterol sulfate]		Antiasthmatic/bronchodilator	Chronic bronchitis, emphysema; bronchial asthma
Compro [prochlorperazine]		Antiemetic; antipsychotic	Nausea, vomiting, and manic phase of bipolar syndrome or schizophrenia
Conjupri [levamlodipine maleate]		Antihypertensive	Hypertension
Copaxone [glatiramer acetate]	Z79.69	Other immunosuppressant/ immunomodulator	Treatment of relapsing multiple sclerosis
Coreg [carvedilol]		Beta blocker	Hypertension; chronic heart failure; left ventricular dysfunction following myocardial infarction
Coreg CR [carvedilol phosphate]		Beta blocker	Hypertension; chronic heart failure; left ventricular dysfunction following myocardial infarction
Cortef [hydrocortisone]	Z79.52	Corticosteroid	Severe inflammation
Cortenema [hydrocortisone]	Z79.52	Corticosteroid	Inflammation of the colon
Cortifoam [hydrocortisone acetate]	Z79.52	Corticosteroid	Colon and rectum inflammation
Cortisone acetate [cortisone acetate]	Z79.52	Corticosteroid	Inflammation
Cortisporin [hydrocortisone acetate/neomycin sulfate/polymyxin B sulfate]		Topical anti-infective, topical steroid	Dermatosis
Cosentyx [secukinumab]	Z79.620	Immunosuppressive biologic; monoclonal antibody	Plaque psoriasis; psoriatic arthritis; ankylosing spondylitis
Coumadin [warfarin sodium]	Z79.01	Anticoagulant	Prophylaxis and treatment of venous thrombosis; treatment of atrial fibrillation with embolization (pulmonary embolism), arrhythmias, myocardial infarction, and stroke prevention
Cozaar [losartan potassium]		Antihypertensive	Hypertension
Crestor [rosuvastatin calcium]		HMG-CoA reductase inhibitor (statin)	Hypercholesterolemia; hyperlipidemia; hyperproteinemia
Cryselle [ethinyl estradiol/norgestrel]	Z79.3	Contraceptive	Prevention of pregnancy
Cubicin [daptomycin]	Z79.2	Antibiotic	Bacterial skin infections; Staphylococcus aureus bloodstream infections

Appendix B: Pharmacology List 2023

Drug	Z Code	Drug Action/Classification	Indications
Cyclafem [ethinyl estradiol/norethindrone]	Z79.3	Contraceptive	Prevention of pregnancy
Cyclessa [desogestrel/ethinyl estradiol]	Z79.3	Contraceptive	Prevention of pregnancy
Cyclosporine [cyclosporine]	Z79.621	Calcineurin inhibitor	Prophylaxis of organ transplant rejection
Cyltezo [adalimumab-abdm]	Z79.620	Immunosuppressive biologic; monoclonal antibody	Rheumatoid arthritis; juvenile idiopathic arthritis; psoriatic arthritis; Crohn's disease; ulcerative colitis; plaque psoriasis
Cymbalta [duloxetine hydrochloride]		Antidepressant, serotonin and norepinephrine reuptake inhibitor (SNRI)	Major depressive disorder; general anxiety disorder; fibromyalgia; diabetic peripheral neuropathy; chronic musculoskeletal pain
Cytarabine [cytarabine]	Z79.631	Antimetabolite agent	Leukemia
Cytomel [liothyronine sodium]		Thyroid hormone	Hypothyroidism or prevention of euthyroid goiters
Cytoxan [cyclophosphamide]	Z79.630	Chemotherapeutic alkylating agent	Cancer
Daptomycin [daptomycin]	Z79.2	Antibiotic	Skin and underlying tissue bacterial infections
Dasetta [ethinyl estradiol/norethindrone]	Z79.3	Contraceptive	Prevention of pregnancy
Daypro [oxaprozin]	Z79.1	Nonsteroidal anti-inflammatory drug (NSAID)	Osteoarthritis and rheumatoid arthritis
Daysee [ethinyl estradiol/levonorgestrel]	Z79.3	Contraceptive	Prevention of pregnancy
Delestrogen [estradiol valerate]	Z79.890	Estrogen therapy	Menopause symptoms
Demerol [meperidine hydrochloride]	Z79.891	Analgesic, narcotic	Moderate to severe pain
Depakote [divalproex sodium]		Anticonvulsant	Bipolar affective disorder; complex absence, complex partial and mixed pattern epilepsy; migraine headache
Depo-Medrol [methylprednisolone acetate]	Z79.52	Corticosteroid	Arthritis; joint disorders
Depo-Provera [medroxyprogesterone acetate]	Z79.3, Z79.890	Antineoplastic; contraceptive; progestin	Amenorrhea; carcinoma, endometrium, adjunct; carcinoma, renal; prevention of pregnancy; hemorrhage
Depo-SubQ Provera [medroxyprogesterone acetate]	Z79.3	Contraceptive	Prevention of pregnancy; menstrual disorder pain
Descovy [emtricitabine/tenofovir alafenamide]	Z79.899	Antiretroviral	HIV
Desogen [desogestrel/ethinyl estradiol]	Z79.3	Contraceptive	Prevention of pregnancy
Detrol [tolterodine tartrate]		Muscarinic receptor antagonist	Overactive bladders in patients with urinary frequency, urgency, or urge incontinence
Dexamethasone Intensol [dexamethasone]	Z79.52	Corticosteroid	Arthritis; allergic disorders; breathing disorders; lupus
Dexilant [dexlansoprazole]		Proton pump inhibitor	Healing of erosive esophagitis; relieve of heartburn; treatment of nonerosive gastroesophageal reflux disease
DiaBeta [glyburide]	Z79.84	Oral hypoglycemic	Diabetes mellitus
Diclegis [doxylamine succinate/pyridoxine hydrochloride]		Antiemetic	Nausea/vomiting in pregnancy
Dificid [fidaxomicin]	Z79.2	Antibiotic	Clostridium difficile
Diflucan [fluconazole]		Antifungal	Oropharyngeal and esophageal candidiasis and cryptococcal meningitis in AIDS patients
Digoxin [digoxin]		Cardiotonic glycoside	Heart failure, atrial flutter, atrial fibrillation, and supraventricular tachycardia
Dilantin [phenytoin sodium]		Anticonvulsant	Grand mal and psychomotor seizures
Dilaudid [hydromorphone hydrochloride]	Z79.891	Analgesic, narcotic	Moderate to severe pain
Diovan [valsartan]		Antihypertensive	Hypertension
Diskets [methadone hydrochloride]		Opioid agonist	Treatment of opioid addiction
Divigel [estradiol]	Z79.890	Estrogen therapy – topical	Menopause symptoms
Dolophine HCl [methadone hydrochloride]	Z79.891	Analgesic, narcotic; opioid agonist	Pain; treatment of opioid addiction
Dovato [dolutegravir sodium/lamivudine]	Z79.899	Antiretroviral	HIV; chronic hepatitis B
Doxorubicin [doxorubicin]	Z79.632	Antitumor antibiotic	Hodgkin lymphoma; non-Hodgkin lymphoma; specific types of cancers and leukemias
Doxycycline [doxycycline]	Z79.2	Antibiotic	Bacterial infections; acne

Drug	Z Code	Drug Action/Classification	Indications
Duavee [bazedoxifene acetate/conjugated estrogens]	Z79.890	Estrogen therapy	Menopause symptoms; osteoporosis prevention
Duetact [glimepiride/pioglitazone hydrochloride]	Z79.84	Oral hypoglycemic	Diabetes mellitus
Duexis [famotidine/ibuprofen]	Z79.1	Nonsteroidal anti-inflammatory drug (NSAID)	Symptomatic treatment of osteoarthritis and rheumatoid arthritis; reduce risk of ulcers
Dulera [formoterol fumarate/mometasone furoate]	Z79.51	Corticosteroid – inhaled; antiasthmatic	Prophylaxis and treatment of asthma
Dupixent [dupilumab]	Z79.620	Immunosuppressive biologic; monoclonal antibody	Atopic dermatitis; asthma
Duragesic [fentanyl]	Z79.891	Analgesic, narcotic	Chronic pain
Duramorph PF [morphine sulfate]	Z79.891	Analgesic, narcotic	Moderate to severe pain
Durlaza [aspirin]	Z79.82	Aspirin	Prevention of heart attack, stroke, angina
Dymista [azelastine/fluticasone]	Z79.899	Corticosteroid – intranasal	Seasonal allergies
Dynacin [minocycline hydrochloride]	Z79.2	Antibiotic	Severe acne treatment
E.E.S. [erythromycin ethylsuccinate]	Z79.2	Antibiotic	Bacterial infections
Effexor XR [venlafaxine hydrochloride]		Antidepressant, serotonin and norepinephrine reuptake inhibitors (SNRIs)	Major depressive disorder; social anxiety disorder; panic disorder
Effient [prasugrel hydrochloride]	Z79.02	Antiplatelet	Lessening of the chance of heart attack or stroke
Elestrin [estradiol]	Z79.890	Estrogen therapy	Menopause symptoms
Eligard [leuprolide acetate]	Z79.818	Agents affecting estrogen receptors and estrogen levels	Palliative treatment of prostate cancer symptoms
Elinest [norgestrel/ethinyl estradiol]	Z79.3	Contraceptive	Prevention of pregnancy
Eliquis [apixaban]	Z79.01	Anticoagulant	Venous thrombosis
Elyxyb [celecoxib]	Z79.1	Nonsteroidal anti-inflammatory drug (NSAID)	Migraine headache
Emoquette [ethinyl estradiol/desogestrel]	Z79.3	Contraceptive	Prevention of pregnancy
Emtriva [emtricitabine]	Z79.899	Antiretroviral	HIV
Enbrel [etanercept]	Z79.620	Immunosuppressive biologic	Rheumatoid arthritis; polyarticular juvenile idiopathic arthritis; psoriatic arthritis; ankylosing spondylitis; plaque psoriasis
Enpresse-28 [ethinyl estradiol/levonorgestrel]	Z79.3	Contraceptive	Prevention of pregnancy
Enskyce [desogestrel/ethinyl estradiol]	Z79.3	Contraceptive	Prevention of pregnancy
Entocort EC [budesonide]	Z79.52	Corticosteroid	Crohn's disease; ulcerative colitis
Entresto [sacubitril/valsartan]		Angiotensin II receptor blocker; neprilysin inhibitor	Chronic heart failure
Entyvio [vedolizumab]	Z79.620	Immunosuppressive biologic; monoclonal antibody	Ulcerative colitis; Crohn's disease
Envarsus XR [tacrolimus]	Z79.621	Calcineurin inhibitor	Prophylaxis of organ transplant rejection
Epinephrine [epinephrine]		Bronchodilator, cardiotonic	Most commonly, relief of distress due to bronchospasm and restoration of cardiac rhythm in cardiac arrest
Epivir, Epivir-HBV [lamivudine]	Z79.899	Antiretroviral	HIV; chronic hepatitis B
Erelzi [etanercept-szzs]	Z79.899	Antirheumatic	Rheumatoid arthritis; polyarticular juvenile idiopathic arthritis; psoriatic arthritis; ankylosing spondylitis; plaque psoriasis
Errin [norethindrone]	Z79.3	Contraceptive	Prevention of pregnancy
Ertapenem [ertapenem sodium]	Z79.2	Antibiotic	Stomach, urinary tract, pelvis, skin and lung infections
ERYC [erythromycin]	Z79.2	Antibiotic	Respiratory tract infections
Erygel [erythromycin]	Z79.2	Antibiotic, topical	Bacterial skin infections
EryPed [erythromycin ethylsuccinate]	Z79.2	Antibiotic	Bacterial infections; rheumatic fever attacks
Ery-Tab [erythromycin]	Z79.2	Antibiotic	Bacterial infections
Erythrocin [erythromycin lactobionate]	Z79.2	Antibiotic	Bacterial infections
Erythromycin [erythromycin]	Z79.2	Antibiotic	Respiratory tract infections
Estarylla [ethinyl estradiol/norgestimate]	Z79.3	Contraceptive	Prevention of pregnancy
Estrace [estradiol]	Z79.890	Estrogen therapy	Vaginal cream for treatment of vaginal and vulvar atrophy

Drug	Z Code	Drug Action/Classification	Indications
EstroGel [estradiol]	Z79.890	Estrogen therapy – topical	Menopause symptoms
Estrostep Fe [ethinyl estradiol/norethindrone acetate]	Z79.3	Contraceptive	Prevention of pregnancy
Etoposide [etoposide]	Z79.634	Topoisomerase inhibitor	Small cell lung cancer
Evista [raloxifene hydrochloride]	Z79.810	Selective estrogen receptor modulator (SERM)	Prevention of thinning of the bones (osteoporosis) only in postmenopausal women
Exemestane [exemestane]	Z79.811	Aromatase inhibitor	Postmenopausal breast cancer
Factive [gemifloxacin mesylate]	Z79.2	Antibiotic	Bacterial lung infections
Falmina [ethinyl estradiol/levonorgestrel]	Z79.3	Contraceptive	Prevention of pregnancy
Fareston [toremifene citrate]	Z79.810	Selective estrogen receptor modulator (SERM)	Treatment of metastatic breast cancer in postmenopausal women
Farxiga [dapagliflozin propanediol]	Z79.84	Oral hypoglycemic	Diabetes mellitus
Faslodex [fulvestrant]	Z79.818	Agents affecting estrogen receptors and estrogen levels	Hormone-related breast cancer; metastatic breast cancer
Feldene [piroxicam]	Z79.1	Nonsteroidal anti-inflammatory drug (NSAID)	Treatment of pain and inflammation due to arthritis
Femara [letrozole]	Z79.811	Aromatase inhibitor	Postmenopausal breast cancer
Femhrt [ethinyl estradiol/norethindrone acetate]	Z79.3, Z79.890	Contraceptive; estrogen therapy	Prevention of pregnancy; menopause symptoms; osteoporosis prevention
Femring [estradiol acetate]	Z79.890	Estrogen therapy	Osteoporosis prevention and to treat menopausal symptoms; hypoestrogenism; ovarian failure
Fentanyl citrate [fentanyl citrate]	Z79.891	Analgesic, narcotic	Postprocedural or chronic pain
Fentora [fentanyl citrate]	Z79.891	Analgesic, narcotic	Breakthrough cancer pain
Fetroja [cefiderocol]	Z79.2	Antibiotic	Complicated urinary tract infections; pyelonephritis
Fiasp [insulin aspart]	Z79.4	Insulin	Diabetes mellitus
Fioricet with codeine [acetaminophen/butalbital/caffeine/codeine phosphate]	Z79.891	Analgesic, narcotic	Tension headaches
Firmagon [degarelix]	Z79.890	Hormone therapy	Prostate cancer
Flagyl [metronidazole]	Z79.2	Antibiotic	Bacterial infections
Flavoxate HCl [flavoxate hydrochloride]		Urinary tract spasmolytic	Relief of dysuria, urgency, nocturia, suprapubic pain, frequency, and incontinence associated with cystitis, prostatitis, urethritis, and urethrocystitis/urethrotrigonitis
Flomax [tamsulosin hydrochloride]		Antiadrenergic	Benign prostatic hyperplasia
Flonase allergy relief [fluticasone propionate]	Z79.899	Corticosteroid – intranasal	Perennial and seasonal allergic rhinitis
Flovent HFA [fluticasone propionate]	Z79.51	Corticosteroid – inhaled; antiasthmatic	Asthma
Fortaz [ceftazidime]	Z79.2	Antibiotic	Pneumonia and lower respiratory infections
Fosamax [alendronate sodium]	Z79.83	Bisphosphonate	Osteoporosis; Paget's disease
Fosinopril sodium [fosinopril sodium]		ACE inhibitor	Hypertension
Fosrenol [lanthanum carbonate]		Phosphate binder	End-stage renal disease (ESRD)
Fragmin [dalteparin sodium]	Z79.01	Anticoagulant	Prophylaxis and treatment of blood clots
Garamycin [gentamicin sulfate]	Z79.2	Antibiotic	Severe bacterial infections
Gengraf [cyclosporine]	Z79.621	Calcineurin inhibitor	Prophylaxis of organ transplant rejection
Gentamicin sulfate [gentamicin sulfate]	Z79.2	Antibiotic	Severe bacterial infections
Gildagia [ethinyl estradiol/norethindrone]	Z79.3	Contraceptive	Prevention of pregnancy
Gildess [ethinyl estradiol/norethindrone acetate]	Z79.3	Contraceptive	Prevention of pregnancy
Glimepiride [glimepiride]	Z79.84	Oral hypoglycemic	Diabetes mellitus
Glucotrol [glipizide]	Z79.84	Oral hypoglycemic	Diabetes mellitus
Glumetza [metformin hydrochloride]	Z79.84	Oral hypoglycemic	Diabetes mellitus
Glyburide (micronized) [glyburide]	Z79.84	Oral hypoglycemic	Diabetes mellitus
Glynase [glyburide]	Z79.84	Oral hypoglycemic	Diabetes mellitus
Glyset [miglitol]	Z79.84	Oral hypoglycemic	Diabetes mellitus

Drug	Z Code	Drug Action/Classification	Indications
Harvoni [ledipasvir/sofosbuvir]	Z79.899	Antiviral	Chronic hepatitis C
Heparin sodium [heparin sodium]	Z79.Ø1	Anticoagulant	Prophylaxis and treatment of venous thrombosis, pulmonary embolism; prevention of cerebral thrombosis, and treatment of consumptive coagulopathies
Hiprex [methenamine]	Z79.2	Antibiotic	Recurring bladder infection
Humalog [insulin lispro recombinant]	Z79.4	Insulin	Diabetes mellitus
Humira [adalimumab]	Z79.62Ø	Immunosuppressive biologic; monoclonal antibody	Rheumatoid arthritis; juvenile idiopathic arthritis; psoriatic arthritis; Crohn's disease; ulcerative colitis; plaque psoriasis; hidradenitis suppurativa; uveitis
Humulin R [insulin recombinant]	Z79.4	Insulin	Diabetes mellitus
Hycamtin [topotecan]	Z79.634	Topoisomerase inhibitor	Cancer
Hydrocodone [acetaminophen/hydrocodone bitartrate]	Z79.891	Analgesic, narcotic	Moderate to severe pain
Hydrocodone bitartrate and acetaminophen [acetaminophen/hydrocodone bitartrate]	Z79.891	Analgesic, narcotic	Pain, moderate to severe
Hydrocortisone [hydrocortisone]	Z79.52	Corticosteroid	Addison's disease; arthritis; immune disorders; allergies; breathing problems
Hydromorphone HCl [hydromorphone hydrochloride]	Z79.891	Analgesic, narcotic	Moderate to severe pain
Hydroxyurea [hydroxyurea]	Z79.64	Myelosuppressive agent	Pain related to sickle cell disease; chronic myeloid leukemia; ovarian cancer
Hyrimoz [adalimumab-adaz]	Z79.62Ø	Immunosuppressive biologic; monoclonal antibody	Rheumatoid arthritis; juvenile idiopathic arthritis; psoriatic arthritis; Crohn's disease; ulcerative colitis; plaque psoriasis
Hyzaar [hydrochlorothiazide/ losartan potassium]		Antihypertensive	Hypertension
Ibsrela [tenapanor hydrochloride]		NHE-3 inhibitor	Irritable bowel syndrome with constipation (IBS-C)
Ibuprofen [ibuprofen]	Z79.1	Nonsteroidal anti-inflammatory drug (NSAID)	Pain or fever relief
Imitrex [sumatriptan succinate]		Antimigraine	Migraine headache
Imuran [azathioprine]	Z79.624	Inhibitors of nucleotide synthesis	Rheumatoid arthritis; prophylaxis of organ transplant rejection
Inderal XL [propranolol hydrochloride]		Beta blocker	Angina pectoris; hypertension; cardiac arrhythmias
Indocin [indomethacin]	Z79.1	Nonsteroidal anti-inflammatory drug (NSAID)	Treatment of pain and inflammation
Integrilin [eptifibatide]	Z79.Ø2	Antiplatelet	Unstable angina; heart attacks; prevention of blood clots
Intron A [interferon alfa 2-b]	Z79.69	Other immunosuppressant/ immunomodulator	Cancer; hepatitis
Introvale [levonorgestrel/ethinyl estradiol]	Z79.3	Contraceptive	Prevention of pregnancy
Invanz [ertapenem sodium]	Z79.2	Antibiotic	Stomach, urinary tract, pelvis, skin, and lung infections
Invokamet [canagliflozin/metformin hydrochloride]	Z79.84	Oral hypoglycemic	Diabetes mellitus
Invokana [canagliflozin]	Z79.84	Oral hypoglycemic	Diabetes mellitus
Isoniazid [isoniazid]	Z79.2	Antibiotic	Tuberculosis
Isopto Carpine [pilocarpine hydrochloride]		Cholinergic parasympathomimetic agent	Reduction of intraocular pressure in open-angle glaucoma or ocular hypertension; management of acute angle-closure glaucoma
Isordil Titradose [isosorbide dinitrate]		Smooth muscle relaxant	Acute anginal attacks
Isturisa [osilodrostat]		Cortisol synthesis inhibitor	Cushing's disease in adults
Isuprel [isoproterenol hydrochloride]		Adrenergic agent	Bronchodilator for asthma, chronic pulmonary emphysema, bronchitis, and other conditions accompanied by bronchospasm; can be used in cardiogenic shock cases
Ixempra [ixabepilone]	Z79.633	Mitotic inhibitor	Advanced breast cancer
Jantoven [warfarin sodium]	Z79.Ø1	Anticoagulant	Prophylaxis and treatment of venous thrombosis, pulmonary embolism; prevention of cerebral thrombosis, and treatment of consumptive coagulopathies
Janumet [metformin hydrochloride/sitagliptin phosphate]	Z79.84	Oral hypoglycemic	Diabetes mellitus

Appendix B: Pharmacology List 2023

Drug	Z Code	Drug Action/Classification	Indications
Januvia [sitagliptin phosphate]	Z79.84	Oral hypoglycemic	Diabetes mellitus
Jencycla [norethindrone]	Z79.3	Contraceptive	Prevention of pregnancy
Jentadueto [linagliptin/metformin hydrochloride]]	Z79.84	Oral hypoglycemic	Diabetes mellitus
Junel [ethinyl estradiol/norethindrone acetate]	Z79.3	Contraceptive	Prevention of pregnancy
Kadian [morphine sulfate]	Z79.891	Analgesic, narcotic	Moderate to severe pain
Kariva [desogestrel/ethinyl estradiol]	Z79.3	Contraceptive	Prevention of pregnancy
Katerzia [amlodipine benzoate]		Antihypertensive	Hypertension; coronary artery disease (CAD); chronic stable angina; prinzmetal's angina; variant angina
Kazano [alogliptin benzoate/metformin hydrochloride]	Z79.84	Oral hypoglycemic	Diabetes mellitus
Keflex [cephalexin]	Z79.2	Antibiotic	Bone, middle ear, skin and skin structures, upper respiratory tract and urinary tract infections; acute prostatitis
Kelnor [ethynodiol diacetate/ethinyl estradiol]	Z79.3	Contraceptive	Prevention of pregnancy
Kenalog-10; Kenalog-40 [triamcinolone acetonide]	Z79.52	Corticosteroid	Gouty arthritis; bursitis; tenosynovitis; epicondylitis; rheumatoid arthritis; synovitis; osteoarthritis
Keytruda [pembrolizumab]	Z79.620	Immunosuppressive biologic; monoclonal antibody	Cancer
Kimidess [ethinyl estradiol/desogestrel]	Z79.3	Contraceptive	Prevention of pregnancy
Klaron [sulfacetamide sodium]	Z79.2	Antibiotic, topical	Acne vulgaris
Klonopin [clonazepam]		Anticonvulsant; CNS depressant	Epilepsy; seizures; panic disorder
Klor-Con [potassium chloride]		Replaces potassium and maintains potassium level	Hypokalemia
Kombiglyze [metformin hydrochloride/saxagliptin hydrochloride]	Z79.84	Oral hypoglycemic	Diabetes mellitus
K-Tab [potassium chloride]		Replaces potassium and maintains potassium level	Hypokalemia
Kurvelo [ethinyl estradiol/levonorgestrel]	Z79.3	Contraceptive	Prevention of pregnancy; menstrual disorders
Kyleena [levonorgestrel]	Z79.3	Contraceptive	Prevention of pregnancy
Lamisil [terbinafine hydrochloride]		Antifungal	Tinea cruris (jock itch); T. pedis (athlete's foot); T. corporis (ringworm)
Lanoxin [digoxin]		Cardiotonic glycoside	Congestive heart failure
Lantus [insulin glargine recombinant]	Z79.4	Insulin	Diabetes mellitus
Larin [ethinyl estradiol/norethindrone acetate]	Z79.3	Contraceptive	Prevention of pregnancy
Lasix [furosemide]		Antihypertensive; diuretic	Management of edema associated with congestive heart failure, renal disease, including nephrotic syndrome and hypertension
Lazanda [fentanyl citrate]	Z79.891	Analgesics, narcotic	Breakthrough cancer pain
Lescol XL [fluvastatin sodium]		HMG-CoA reductase inhibitor (statin)	Hypercholesterolemia; hyperlipidemia; hyperlipoproteinemia
Lessina-28 [ethinyl estradiol/levonorgestrel]	Z79.3	Contraceptive	Prevention of pregnancy
Letrozole [letrozole]	Z79.811	Aromatase inhibitor	Postmenopausal breast cancer
Leukeran [chlorambucil]	Z79.630	Chemotherapeutic alkylating agent	Cancer
Levemir [insulin detemir recombinant]	Z79.4	Insulin	Diabetes mellitus
Levonest [levonorgestrel/ethinyl estradiol]	Z79.3	Contraceptive	Prevention of pregnancy; menstrual disorders; acne
Levora [levonorgestrel/ethinyl estradiol]	Z79.3	Contraceptive	Prevention of pregnancy
Levoxyl [levothyroxine sodium]		Thyroid hormone	Euthyroid goiter; hypothyroidism
Lexapro [escitalopram oxalate]		Antidepressant, selective serotonin reuptake inhibitor (SSRI)	Depression; anxiety
Lialda [mesalamine]		Anti-inflammatory	Ulcerative colitis
Lidocaine HCl [lidocaine hydrochloride]		Antiarrhythmic	Management of ventricular arrhythmias or during cardiac manipulation, such as cardiac surgery

Drug	Z Code	Drug Action/Classification	Indications
Liletta [levonorgestrel]	Z79.3	Contraceptive	Intrauterine device to prevent pregnancy
Lincocin [lincocin hydrochloride]	Z79.2	Antibiotic	Severe bacterial infections
Lipitor [atorvastatin calcium]		HMG-CoA reductase inhibitor (statin)	Hypercholesterolemia; hyperlipidemia; hyperproteinemia
Lithium carbonate [lithium carbonate]		Antimanic	Control of manic episodes in bipolar disorders
Livtencity [maribavir]	Z79.899	Antiviral	Post-transplant CMV infection/disease
Lo Loestrin Fe [ethinyl estradiol/norethindrone acetate]	Z79.3	Contraceptive	Prevention of pregnancy
Locoid [hydrocortisone butyrate]	Z79.52	Corticosteroid – topical	Atopic dermatitis; other dermatoses
Loestrin [ethinyl estradiol/norethindrone acetate]	Z79.3	Contraceptive	Prevention of pregnancy
Lomotil [diphenoxylate hydrochloride/atropine sulfate]		Antidiarrheal	Symptoms of chronic and functional diarrhea
Lopid [gemfibrozil]		Lipid regulating agent	Hypercholesterolemia; hyperlipidemia; hyperlipoproteinemia; hypertriglyceridemia
Lopressor [metoprolol tartrate]		Beta blocker	Angina pectoris; hypertension; acute myocardial infarction
Lorazepam [lorazepam]		Antianxiety; sedative/hypnotic	Anxiety disorder associated with depressive symptoms; controls tension, agitation, irritability, and insomnia
Loryna [drospirenone/ethinyl estradiol]	Z79.3	Contraceptive	Prevention of pregnancy
LoSeasonique [ethinyl estradiol/levonorgestrel]	Z79.3	Contraceptive	Prevention of pregnancy
Lotensin [benazepril hydrochloride]		ACE inhibitor	Hypertension
Lotrel [amlodipine besylate/benazepril hydrochloride]		Antihypertensive	Hypertension
Lotrisone [clotrimazole/ betamethasone dipropionate]		Antifungal-corticosteroid	Relief of redness, swelling, itching, and other discomfort of fungus infections
Lovastatin [lovastatin]		HMG-CoA reductase inhibitor (statin)	Hypercholesterolemia; hyperlipidemia; hyperlipoproteinemia
Lovenox [enoxaparin sodium]	Z79.Ø1	Anticoagulant	Prophylaxis and treatment of venous thrombosis and pulmonary embolism
Low-Ogestrel-28 [norgestrel/ethinyl estradiol]	Z79.3	Contraceptive	Prevention of pregnancy
Lupkynis [voclosporin]	Z79.621	Calcineurin inhibitor	Lupus nephritis
Lupron Depot [leuprolide acetate]	Z79.818	Agents affecting estrogen receptors and estrogen levels	Endometriosis symptoms; uterine fibroids
Macrobid [nitrofurantoin]	Z79.2	Antibiotic	Urinary tract infections
Macrodantin [nitrofurantoin]	Z79.2	Antibiotic	Urinary tract infections
Marlissa [ethinyl estradiol/levonorgestrel]	Z79.3	Contraceptive	Prevention of pregnancy
Maxipime [cefepime hydrochloride]	Z79.2	Antibiotic	Bacterial infections
Meclizine hydrochloride [meclizine hydrochloride]		Antihistamine	Nausea and vomiting, and dizziness associated with motion sickness
Medrol [methylprednisolone]	Z79.52	Corticosteroid	Endocrine, rheumatic, hematologic disorders; collagen, dermatological, ophthalmic, respiratory, neoplastic, gastrointestinal, nervous system disorders; allergic and edematous states
Megace ES [megestrol acetate]	Z79.818	Agents affecting estrogen receptors and estrogen levels	Endometrial or advanced breast cancers; weight loss due to AIDS
Menest [esterified estrogens]	Z79.89Ø	Estrogen therapy	Menopause symptoms; ovarian failure
Menostar [estradiol]	Z79.89Ø	Estrogen therapy	Menopause symptoms; osteoporosis prevention
Mepron [atovaquone]	Z79.2	Antibiotic	Pneumonia due to pneumocystis jirovecii
Merrem [meropenem]	Z79.2	Antibiotic	Bacterial infections of skin or stomach; bacterial meningitis
Metformin [metformin hydrochloride]	Z79.84	Oral hypoglycemic	Diabetes mellitus
Methadone HCl [methadone hydrochloride]	Z79.891	Analgesic, narcotic; opioid agonist	Pain; treatment of opioid addiction
Methadose [methadone hydrochloride]	Z79.891	Analgesic, narcotic	Acute and chronic pain
Methergine [methylergonovine maleate]		Oxytocic agent	Routine management of postpartum hemorrhage after delivery of placenta
Methotrexate [methotrexate]	Z79.631	Antimetabolite agent	Cancer

Drug	Z Code	Drug Action/Classification	Indications
Methylprednisolone [methylprednisolone]	Z79.52	Corticosteroid	Inflammatory disorders
Metronidazole [metronidazole]	Z79.2	Antibiotic	Bacterial infections
Miacalcin [calcitonin salmon]		Calcitonin; a peptide hormone	Hypercalcemia; osteoporosis; postmenopausal symptoms; Paget's disease
Microgestin [ethinyl estradiol/norethindrone acetate]	Z79.3	Contraceptive	Prevention of pregnancy
Minastrin [ethinyl estradiol/norethindrone acetate]	Z79.3	Contraceptive	Prevention of pregnancy
Minivelle [estradiol]	Z79.890	Estrogen therapy	Menopause symptoms; osteoporosis prevention
Minocin [minocycline hydrochloride]	Z79.2	Antibiotic	Bacterial infections; acne
Mirena [levonorgestrel]	Z79.3	Contraceptive	Intrauterine device for prevention of pregnancy; menstrual disorders
Mitomycin [mitomycin]	Z79.632	Antitumor antibiotic	Stomach and pancreas cancer
Mobic [meloxicam]	Z79.1	Nonsteroidal anti-inflammatory drug (NSAID)	Treatment of pain and inflammation due to osteoarthritis and rheumatoid arthritis
Monoclonal antibodies	Z79.620	Immunosuppressive biologic	Cancer; prophylaxis of organ transplant rejection
Monodox [doxycycline]	Z79.2	Antibiotic	Bacterial infections; acne
Mono-Linyah [norgestimate/ethinyl estradiol]	Z79.3	Contraceptive	Prevention of pregnancy; menstrual disorders; acne
Monurol [fosfomycin tromethamine]	Z79.2	Antibiotic	Bacterial bladder infections
Morphine sulfate [morphine sulfate]	Z79.891	Analgesic, narcotic	Moderate to severe pain
Motrin IB [ibuprofen]	Z79.1	Nonsteroidal anti-inflammatory drug (NSAID)	Pain or fever relief
MS Contin [morphine sulfate]	Z79.891	Analgesic, narcotic	Moderate to severe pain
Multaq [dronedarone hydrochloride]		Cardiac rhythm regulator	Treatment of patients with recent episodes of atrial fibrillation or atrial flutter
Mycobutin [rifabutin]	Z79.2	Antibiotic	Mycobacterium avium complex (MAC) prophylactic in HIV patients
Mytesi [crofelemer]		Antidiarrheal	Diarrhea occurring in HIV/AIDs patient's on anti-retroviral therapy
Myzilra [ethinyl estradiol/levonorgestrel]	Z79.3	Contraceptive	Prevention of pregnancy
Nabumetone [nabumetone]	Z79.1	Nonsteroidal anti-inflammatory drug (NSAID)	Osteoarthritis and rheumatoid arthritis
Nalfon [fenoprofen calcium]	Z79.1	Nonsteroidal anti-inflammatory drug (NSAID)	Pain or inflammation relief
Namzaric [memantine/donepezil hydrochlorides]		Acetylcholinesterase/cholinesterase inhibitors	Dementia due to Alzheimer's
Naprelan [naproxen sodium]	Z79.1	Nonsteroidal anti-inflammatory drug (NSAID)	Pain or inflammation relief
Naprosyn [naproxen]	Z79.1	Nonsteroidal anti-inflammatory drug (NSAID)	Rheumatoid, gouty arthritis and osteoarthritis; ankylosing spondylitis; bursitis; dysmenorrhea; pain, mild to moderate; tendonitis
Natazia [estradiol valerate/dienogest]	Z79.3	Contraceptive	Prevention of pregnancy; menstrual disorders
Nebupent [pentamidine isethionate]	Z79.2	Antibiotic	Severe bacterial lung infection in high risk patients with HIV
Nefazodone HCl [nefazodone hydrochloride]		Antidepressant	Depression
Nembutal sodium [pentobarbital sodium]		Sedative/hypnotic	Adjunct medication in diagnostic procedures or for emergency use with convulsive disorders
NeoProfen [ibuprofen lysine]	Z79.1	Nonsteroidal anti-inflammatory drug (NSAID)	Pain or fever relief
Neoral [cyclosporine]	Z79.621	Calcineurin inhibitor	Prophylaxis of organ transplant rejection
Neosporin [bacitracin, neomycin]	Z79.2	Antibiotic, topical	Bacterial skin infections
Neurontin [gabapentin]		Anticonvulsant	Epilepsy, partial
Nexium [esomeprazole magnesium]		Proton pump inhibitor	Gastroesophageal reflux disease (GERD), erosive esophagitis
Nexletol [bempedoic acid]	Z79.899	Antihyperlipidemic	Heterozygous familial hypercholesterolemia; established atherosclerotic cardiovascular disease requiring additional lowering of LDL-C
Nexplanon [etonogestrel]	Z79.3	Contraceptive	Implantable device used for prevention of pregnancy

Drug	Z Code	Drug Action/Classification	Indications
Nextstellis [drospirenone and estetrol]	Z79.3	Contraceptive	Prevention of pregnancy
Nitrofurantoin [nitrofurantoin]	Z79.2	Antibiotic	Bacterial urinary tract infections
Nitropress [sodium nitroprusside]		Vasodilator	Potent, rapid action in reducing blood pressure in hypertensive crisis or for controlling bleeding during anesthesia by producing controlled hypotension
Nitrostat [nitroglycerin]		Muscle relaxant; antianginal; antihypertensive; coronary vasodilator	Prophylaxis and treatment of angina pectoris; heart failure associated with myocardial infarction; hypertension, perioperative; surgery, adjunct
Norco [acetaminophen/hydrocodone bitartrate]	Z79.891	Analgesic, narcotic	Moderate to severe pain
Norinyl [mestranol/norethisterone]	Z79.3	Contraceptive	Prevention of pregnancy
Norpace [disopyramide phosphate]		Antiarrhythmic	Coronary artery disease, for prevention, recurrence, and control of unifocal, multifocal, and paired PVCs
Nortrel [ethinyl estradiol/norethindrone]	Z79.3	Contraceptive	Prevention of pregnancy
Norvasc [amlodipine besylate]		Antihypertensive	Hypertension; coronary artery disease (CAD); chronic stable angina; prinzmetal's angina; variant angina
Novolin [insulin recombinant]	Z79.4	Insulin	Diabetes mellitus
Novolog [insulin aspart recombinant]	Z79.4	Insulin	Diabetes mellitus
Nucynta [tapentadol hydrochloride]	Z79.891	Analgesic, narcotic	Moderate to severe pain
NuvaRing [etonogestrel/ethinyl estradiol]	Z79.3	Contraceptive	Vaginal ring to prevent pregnancy
Ogestrel [norgestrel/ethinyl estradiol]	Z79.3	Contraceptive	Prevention of pregnancy
Olumiant [baricitinib]	Z79.622	Janus kinase (JAK) inhibitor	Rheumatoid arthritis
Onglyza [saxagliptin hydrochloride]	Z79.84	Oral hypoglycemic	Diabetes mellitus
Oracea [doxycycline]	Z79.2	Antibiotic	Rosacea
Orapred ODT [prednisolone sodium phosphate]	Z79.52	Corticosteroid	Inflammatory disorders
Orbactiv [oritavancin diphosphate]	Z79.2	Antibiotic	Bacterial skin infections
Orencia [abatacept]	Z79.69	Other immunosuppressant/immunomodulator	Rheumatoid arthritis; polyarticular juvenile idiopathic arthritis; psoriatic arthritis
Orilissa [elagolix]	Z79.890	Hormone therapy	Pain associated with endometriosis
Orphenadrine citrate [orphenadrine citrate]		Muscle relaxant	Acute spasms, tension, and post-trauma cases
Orsythia [ethinyl estradiol/levonorgestrel]	Z79.3	Contraceptive	Prevention of pregnancy
Ortho-Novum [norethindrone/ethinyl estradiol]	Z79.3	Contraceptive	Prevention of pregnancy
Oseni [alogliptin benzoate/pioglitazone hydrochloride]	Z79.84	Oral hypoglycemic	Diabetes mellitus
Osphena [ospemifene]	Z79.810, Z79.890	Selective estrogen receptor modulator (SERM)	Postmenopausal dyspareunia due to vaginal atrophy; osteoporosis prevention and treatment of menopausal symptoms
Otezla [apremilast]	Z79.61	Antirheumatic; immunomodulator	Psoriatic arthritis; plaque psoriasis
Oxazepam [oxazepam]		Antianxiety	Anxiety, tension, and alcohol withdrawal
Oxbryta [voxelotor]		Hemoglobin S polymerization inhibitor	Sickle cell disease
Oxycodone HCl [oxycodone hydrochloride]	Z79.891	Analgesic, narcotic	Moderate to severe pain
OxyContin [oxycodone hydrochloride]	Z79.891	Analgesic, narcotic	Moderate to severe pain
Ozempic [semaglutide]	Z79.85	Antidiabetic – non-insulin injectable	Diabetes mellitus
Paclitaxel [paclitaxel]	Z79.633	Mitotic inhibitor	Cancer
Paxil [paroxetine hydrochloride]		Antidepressant	Anxiety with panic disorder and depression; obsessive-compulsive disorder
PediaPred [prednisolone sodium phosphate]	Z79.52	Corticosteroid	Inflammatory disorders
PegIntron [peginterferon alfa-2b]	Z79.69	Other immunosuppressant/immunomodulator	Hepatitis C

Drug	Z Code	Drug Action/Classification	Indications
Penicillin-VK [penicillin V potassium]	Z79.2	Antibiotic	Chorea, prevention; endocarditis, prevention, secondary to tooth extraction; erysipelas; infections of the skin and skin structures, upper respiratory tract; rheumatic fever, prophylaxis; scarlet fever; Vincent's gingivitis; Vincent's pharyngitis
Pentam [pentamidine isethionate]	Z79.2	Antibiotic	Severe bacterial lung infections
Pentasa [mesalamine]		Anti-inflammatory	Ulcerative colitis and Crohn's disease
Pepcid [famotidine]		Histamine H2-receptor inhibitor	Acid/peptic disorder; adenoma, secretory; gastroesophageal reflux; duodenal and gastric ulcer; Zollinger-Ellison syndrome
Percocet [oxycodone hydrochloride/acetaminophen]	Z79.891	Analgesic, narcotic	Pain, moderate to severe
Persantine [dipyridamole]	Z79.02	Antiplatelet	Therapy for chronic angina pectoris, preventing clots post heart valve surgery
Pfizerpen [penicillin g potassium]	Z79.2	Antibiotic	Severe bacterial infections
Phenobarbital [phenobarbital sodium]		Anticonvulsant	Grand mal epilepsy
Philith [ethinyl estradiol/norethindrone]	Z79.3	Contraceptive	Prevention of pregnancy
Pimtrea [desogestrel/ethinyl estradiol]	Z79.3	Contraceptive	Prevention of pregnancy
Piqray [alpelisib]		Kinase inhibitor	Postmenopausal advanced or metastatic breast cancer that is HR positive, HER2 negative
Pirmella [ethinyl estradiol/norethindrone]	Z79.3	Contraceptive	Prevention of pregnancy
Pitocin [oxytocin]		Uterotonic	Induction or stimulation of labor at term
Plan B One-Step [levonorgestrel]	Z79.3	Contraceptive	Prevention of pregnancy
Plavix [clopidogrel bisulfate]	Z79.02	Antiplatelet	Lessening of the chance of heart attack or stroke
Pluvicto [lutetium Lu 177 vipivotide tetraxetan]		Radioligand therapeutic agent	Metastatic castration-resistant prostate cancer (mCRPC)
Pomalyst [pomalidomide]	Z79.61	Immunomodulator	Multiple myeloma; Kaposi sarcoma
Ponstel [mefenamic acid]	Z79.1	Nonsteroidal anti-inflammatory drug (NSAID)	Treatment of pain
Ponvory [ponesimod]	Z79.69	Other immunosuppressant/ immunomodulator	Relapsing forms of multiple sclerosis (MS)
Portia-28 [ethinyl estradiol/levonorgestrel]	Z79.3	Contraceptive	Prevention of pregnancy
Pradaxa [dabigatran etexilate mesylate]	Z79.01	Anticoagulant	Prophylaxis and treatment of blood clots in patients with atrial fibrillation
Prasugrel [prasugrel hydrochloride]	Z79.02	Antiplatelet	Lessening the chance of heart attack or stroke
Pravachol [pravastatin sodium]		HMG-CoA reductase inhibitor (statin)	Hypercholesterolemia; hyperlipidemia; hyperlipoproteinemia
Prednisolone [prednisolone]	Z79.52	Corticosteroid	Inflammatory disorders
Prednisone [prednisone]	Z79.52	Corticosteroid	Used for its immunosuppressant effects and for relief of inflammation; used in arthritis, polymyositis and other systemic diseases
Pregnyl [chorionic gonadotropin]		Gonadotropic hormone	Prepubertal cryptorchidism; hypogonadism; corpus luteum insufficiency and infertility
Prempro [conjugated estrogens/medroxyprogesterone acetate]	Z79.890	Estrogen/progesterone therapy	Menopause; osteoporosis; atrophic vaginitis
Prevacid [lansoprazole]		Proton pump inhibitor	Acid/peptic disorder; erosive esophagitis; duodenal ulcer; Zollinger-Ellison syndrome
Previfem [ethinyl estradiol/norgestimate]	Z79.3	Contraceptive	Prevention of pregnancy
Prezcobix [darunavir/cobicistat]	Z79.899	Antiretroviral	HIV
Prezista [darunavir]	Z79.899	Antiretroviral	HIV
Priftin [rifapentine]	Z79.2	Antibiotic	Tuberculosis
Prilosec [omeprazole magnesium]		Proton pump inhibitor	Acid/peptic disorder; endocrine adenoma; erosive esophagitis; systemic mastocytosis; gastroesophageal reflux; duodenal, peptic and gastric ulcer; Zollinger-Ellison syndrome
Primaxin [cilastatin sodium/imipenem]	Z79.2	Antibiotic	Skin, stomach, bone, joint, endocarditis, UTI, female reproductive organs or lower respiratory tract infections
Prinivil [lisinopril]		ACE inhibitor	Congestive heart failure; hypertension

Drug	Z Code	Drug Action/Classification	Indications
Pristiq [desvenlafaxine]		Antidepressant; serotonin and norepinephrine reuptake inhibitor (SNRI)	Major depressive disorder
Procardia [nifedipine]		Calcium channel blocker	Management of vasospastic angina and chronic stable angina, hypertension
Prograf [tacrolimus]	Z79.621	Calcineurin inhibitor	Prophylaxis of organ transplant rejection
Prolia [denosumab]	Z79.620	Immunosuppressive biologic; monoclonal antibody	Treatment and prevention of bone resorption and prevention of bone fracture
Promethazine hydrochloride [promethazine hydrochloride]		Anesthesia, adjunct to; antiemetic; antihistamine; antitussive/expectorant; sedative/hypnotic; vertigo/motion sickness/vomiting	Anesthesia; adjunct; angioedema; conjunctivitis; dermographism; hypersensitivity, motion sickness; pain; perennial, seasonal, and allergic rhinitis; sedation, obstetrical; urticaria
Protonix [pantoprazole]		Proton pump inhibitor	Short-term treatment and maintenance therapy of erosive esophagitis associated with gastroesophageal reflux disease (GERD)
Protopic [tacrolimus]	Z79.621	Calcineurin inhibitor	Atomic dermatitis (eczema)
Proventil-HFA [albuterol sulfate]		Antiasthmatic/bronchodilator	Asthma
Provera [medroxyprogesterone acetate]	Z79.3, Z79.890	Antineoplastic; contraceptive; progestin	Amenorrhea; carcinoma, endometrium, adjunct; carcinoma, renal; prevention of pregnancy; hemorrhage
Prozac [fluoxetine hydrochloride]		Selective serotonin reuptake inhibitor (SSRI)	Bulimia nervosa; depression; obsessive-compulsive disorder
Pulmicort [budesonide]	Z79.51	Corticosteroid – inhaled; antiasthmatic	Prophylaxis and treatment of asthma
Qelbree [viloxazine hydrochloride]		Selective norepinephrine reuptake inhibitor	Attention deficit hyperactivity disorder (ADHD)
Qnasl [beclomethasone dipropionate]	Z79.899	Corticosteroid – intranasal	Perennial and seasonal allergies; vasomotor rhinitis
Qtern [dapagliflozin/saxagliptin]	Z79.84	Oral hypoglycemic	Diabetes mellitus
Quartette [levonorgestrel/ethinyl estradiol]	Z79.3	Contraceptive	Prevention of pregnancy
Qulipta [atogepant]		Calcitonin gene-related peptide inhibitor	Migraine headache prevention
Quviviq [daridorexant hydrochloride]		CNS depressant	Insomnia
Qvar Redihaler [beclomethasone dipropionate]	Z79.51	Corticosteroid – inhaled; antiasthmatic	Prophylaxis and treatment of asthma
Raloxifene HCl [raloxifene hydrochloride]	Z79.810	Selective estrogen receptor modulator (SERM)	Prevention of thinning of the bones (osteoporosis) only in postmenopausal women
Rapaflo [silodosin]		Antiadrenergic	Benign prostatic hyperplasia
Rapamune [sirolimus]	Z79.623	Mammalian target of rapamycin (mTOR) inhibitor	Prophylaxis of organ transplant rejection
Rayos [prednisone]	Z79.52	Corticosteroid; antiasthmatic	Arthritis; blood disorders; allergies; asthma
Rebetol [ribavirin]	Z79.899	Antiviral	Chronic hepatitis C
Rebif [interferon beta-1a]	Z79.69	Other immunosuppressant/ immunomodulator	Treatment of relapsing multiple sclerosis
Reclast [zoledronic acid]	Z79.83	Bisphosphonate	Prevention of thinning of the bones (osteoporosis); Paget's disease; bone cancer
Relenza [zanamivir]		Antiviral	Treat and prevent influenza A and B
Remicade [infliximab]	Z79.620	Immunosuppressive biologic; monoclonal antibody	Ankylosing spondylitis; psoriatic arthritis; rheumatoid arthritis; Crohn's disease; ulcerative colitis
Renvela [sevelamer carbonate]		Phosphate binder	Chronic kidney disease (CKD) on dialysis
Repaglinide [repaglinide]	Z79.84	Oral hypoglycemic	Diabetes mellitus
Restasis [cyclosporine ophthalmic emulsion]		Anti-inflammatory, ophthalmic	Ocular inflammation due to keratoconjunctivitis sicca
Restoril [temazepam]		Sedative/hypnotic	Insomnia
Retrovir [zidovudine]	Z79.899	Antiretroviral	HIV
Revlimid [lenalidomide]	Z79.61	Immunomodulator	Multiple myeloma following autologous stem cell transplant; myelodysplastic syndromes; mantle cell lymphoma
Reyvow [lasmiditan]		Antimigraine	Migraine headache
Rifadin [rifampin]	Z79.2	Antibiotic	Tuberculosis
Rimactane [rifampin]	Z79.2	Antibiotic	Tuberculosis
Rinvoq [upadacitinib]	Z79.622	Janus kinase (JAK) inhibitor	Rheumatoid arthritis; psoriatic arthritis; ankylosing spondylitis; ulcerative colitis
Riomet [metformin hydrochloride]	Z79.84	Oral hypoglycemic	Diabetes mellitus

Drug	Z Code	Drug Action/Classification	Indications
Risperdal [risperidone]		Antipsychotic/antimanic	Schizophrenia; bipolar I disorder
Ritalin [methylphenidate hydrochloride]		CNS stimulant	Attention deficit hyperactivity disorder (ADHD); narcolepsy
Rituxan [rituximab]	Z79.620	Immunosuppressive biologic; monoclonal antibody	Non-Hodgkin's lymphoma; chronic lymphocytic leukemia; rheumatoid arthritis; granulomatosis with polyangiitis; pemphigus vulgaris
Roxicet [oxycodone hydrochloride/acetaminophen]	Z79.891	Analgesic, narcotic	Pain, moderate to severe
Roxicodone [oxycodone hydrochloride]	Z79.891	Analgesic, narcotic	Pain relief
Rukobia [fostemsavir tromethamine]	Z79.899	Antiretroviral	HIV
Rybelsus [semaglutide]	Z79.84	Oral hypoglycemic	Diabetes mellitus
Sabril [vigabatrin]		Anticonvulsant	Refractory complex partial seizures
Safyral [drospirenone/ethinyl estradiol/levomefolate calcium]	Z79.3	Contraceptive	Prevention of pregnancy
Sandimmune [cyclosporine]	Z79.621	Calcineurin inhibitor	Prophylaxis of organ transplant rejection
Sarafem [fluoxetine hydrochloride]		Selective serotonin reuptake inhibitor (SSRI)	Premenstrual dysphoric disorder (PMDD)
Savaysa [edoxaban tosylate]	Z79.01	Anticoagulant	Prophylaxis and treatment of venous thrombosis, pulmonary embolism; prevention of blood clots due to atrial fibrillation
Scemblix [asciminib hydrochloride]		Kinase inhibitor	Philadelphia chromosome-positive chronic myeloid leukemia
Seasonale [levonorgestrel/ethinyl estradiol]	Z79.3	Contraceptive	Prevention of pregnancy
Seasonique [ethinyl estradiol/levonorgestrel]	Z79.3	Contraceptive	Prevention of pregnancy
Septra [sulfamethoxazole trimethoprim]	Z79.2	Antibiotic	Urinary tract infections; acute otitis media; acute exacerbations of chronic bronchitis; shigellosis
Serevent [salmeterol xinafoate]		Bronchodilator	Asthma
Seromycin [cycloserine]	Z79.2	Antibiotic	Tuberculosis; urinary tract infections
Seroquel XR [quetiapine fumarate]		Antipsychotic	Schizophrenia; bipolar disorder; major depressive disorder
Setlakin [ethinyl estradiol/levonorgestrel]	Z79.3	Contraceptive	Prevention of pregnancy
Silvadene [silver sulfadiazine]	Z79.2	Antibiotic, topical	Wound sepsis due to second/third degree burns
Simulect [basiliximab]	Z79.620	Immunosuppressive biologic; monoclonal antibody	Prophylaxis of organ transplant rejection
Sinemet [carbidopa/levodopa]		Antiparkinsonism	Parkinson's disease
Singulair [montelukast sodium]		Antiasthmatic	Asthma; exercise-induced bronchoconstriction; perennial and seasonal allergic rhinitis
Sirolimus [sirolimus]	Z79.623	Mammalian target of rapamycin (mTOR) inhibitor	Prophylaxis of organ transplant rejection
Sitagliptin [sitagliptin/metformin hydrochloride]	Z79.84	Oral hypoglycemic	Diabetes mellitus
Sivextro [tedizolid phosphate]	Z79.2	Antibiotic	Skin infections including MRSA
Skyla [levonorgestrel]	Z79.3	Contraceptive	Intrauterine device to prevent pregnancy
Skyrizi [risankizumab]	Z79.620	Immunosuppressive biologic; monoclonal antibody	Plaque psoriasis
Soliqua [insulin glargine/lixisenatide]	Z79.4	Insulin	Diabetes mellitus
Solodyn [minocycline hydrochloride]	Z79.2	Antibiotic	Bacterial infections
Solosec [secnidazole]	Z79.2	Antibiotic	Bacterial vaginal inflammation; trichomoniasis
Soltamox [tamoxifen citrate]	Z79.810	Selective estrogen receptor modulator (SERM)	Breast cancer
Solu-Cortef [hydrocortisone sodium succinate]	Z79.52	Corticosteroid; antiasthmatic	Asthma; severe inflammation; allergic reactions
Solu-Medrol [methylprednisolone sodium succinate]	Z79.52	Corticosteroid	Anti-inflammatory and antiallergenic for shock and ulcerative colitis
Spiriva [tiotropium bromide]		Antiasthmatic/bronchodilator	Chronic obstructive pulmonary disease (COPD); asthma
Sprintec [norgestimate/ethinyl estradiol]	Z79.3	Contraceptive	Prevention of pregnancy
Stelara [ustekinumab]	Z79.620	Immunosuppressive biologic; monoclonal antibody	Plaque psoriasis; psoriatic arthritis; Crohn's disease; ulcerative colitis

Drug	Z Code	Drug Action/Classification	Indications
Strattera [atomoxetine hydrochloride]		CNS stimulant	Severe bacterial infections
Streptomycin sulfate [streptomycin sulfate]	Z79.2	Antibiotic	Treatment of opioid addiction
Suboxone [buprenorphine/naloxone]		Opioid agonist	Precocious puberty
Supprelin LA [histrelin acetate]	Z79.818	Agents affecting estrogen receptors and estrogen levels	Bacterial infections
Suprax [cefixime]	Z79.2	Antibiotic	Various bacterial infections
Sustiva [efavirenz]	Z79.899	Antiretroviral	HIV
Syeda [drospirenone/ethinyl estradiol]	Z79.3	Contraceptive	Prevention of pregnancy
Sylatron [peginterferon alfa-2b]	Z79.69	Other immunosuppressant/ immunomodulator	Prevention of recurrent malignant melanoma
Symbicort [budesonide/formoterol fumarate dihydrate]	Z79.51	Corticosteroid – inhaled; antiasthmatic	Prophylaxis and treatment of asthma and COPD
Symbyax [olanzapine/fluoxetine]		Antidepressant	Acute depressive episodes associated with bipolar I disorder; treatment resistant depression
Symlin [pramlintide]	Z79.85	Antidiabetic – non-insulin injectable	Diabetes mellitus
Symtuza [darunavir/cobicistat/emtricitabine/ tenofovir alafenamide]	Z79.899	Antiretroviral	HIV
Synarel [nafarelin acetate]	Z79.818	Agents affecting estrogen receptors and estrogen levels	Endometriosis symptoms; precocious puberty
Synercid [dalfopristin/quinupristin]	Z79.2	Antibiotic	Severe blood infections
Synjardy [empagliflozin/metformin hydrochloride]	Z79.84	Oral hypoglycemic	Diabetes mellitus
Synthroid [levothyroxine sodium]		Thyroid hormone	Hypothyroidism
Tacrolimus [tacrolimus]	Z79.621	Calcineurin inhibitor	Prophylaxis of organ transplant rejection
Talicia [omeprazole magnesium/ amoxicillin/rifabutin]	Z79.2	Combination antibiotic	Helicobacter pylori infection
Taltz [ixekizumab]	Z79.620	Immunosuppressive biologic; monoclonal antibody	Plaque psoriasis; psoriatic arthritis; ankylosing spondylitis; axial spondyloarthritis
Tamiflu [oseltamivir phosphate]		Antiviral	Treatment and prevention of influenza A and B
Tamoxifen citrate [tamoxifen citrate]	Z79.810	Selective estrogen receptor modulator (SERM)	Metastatic breast cancer in postmenopausal women
Tavneos [avacopan]	Z79.69	Other immunosuppressant/ immunomodulator	ANCA-associated vasculitis
Taxotere [docetaxel]	Z79.633	Mitotic inhibitor	Cancer
Tazicef [ceftazidime]	Z79.2	Antibiotic	Confirmed or suspected bacterial infections
Teflaro [ceftaroline fosamil]	Z79.2	Antibiotic	Bacterial skin infections; pneumonia
Tegretol [carbamazepine]		Anticonvulsant; analgesic	Epilepsy, especially with complex symptomatology; specific analgesic for trigeminal neuralgia
Temozolomide [temozolomide]	Z79.630	Chemotherapeutic alkylating agent	Chronic myelogenous leukemia
Tenormin [atenolol]		Beta blocker	Angina pectoris; hypertension; acute myocardial infarction
Terazosin HCl [terazosin hydrochloride]		Antiadrenergic	Benign prostatic hypertrophy; hypertension
Testim [testosterone]	Z79.890	Testosterone therapy – topical	Primary hypogonadism
Tetracycline [tetracycline]	Z79.2	Antibiotic	Bacterial infections
Thalidomide [thalidomide]	Z79.61	Immunomodulator	Multiple myeloma; erythema nodosum leprosum
Tiazac [diltiazem hydrochloride]		Calcium channel blocker	Chronic stable angina; atrial fibrillation; atrial flutter; hypertension; paroxysmal supraventricular tachycardia
Tivorbex [indomethacin]	Z79.1	Nonsteroidal anti-inflammatory drug (NSAID)	Treatment of pain, inflammation, and joint stiffness
Tobradex [tobramycin/dexamethasone]		Aminoglycoside ocular anti-infective; anti-inflammatory	Infectious conjunctivitis; dermatosis, corticosteroid-responsive with secondary infection; foreign body in eye; corneal inflammation; uveitis
Tobramycin [dexamethasone/tobramycin]	Z79.2	Antibiotic	Bacterial eye infections
Topamax [topiramate]		Anticonvulsant	Epilepsy; primary generalized tonic-clonic seizures; seizures associated with Lennox-Gastaut syndrome; migraine headache

Drug	Z Code	Drug Action/Classification	Indications
Toprol-XL [metoprolol succinate]		Beta blocker	Angina pectoris; hypertension
Toremifene citrate [toremifene citrate]	Z79.810	Selective estrogen receptor modulator (SERM)	Metastatic breast cancer in postmenopausal women
Torisel [temsirolimus]	Z79.623	Mammalian target of rapamycin (mTOR) inhibitor	Renal cell carcinoma
Toujeo Solostar [insulin glargine recombinant]	Z79.4	Insulin	Diabetes mellitus
Tradjenta [linagliptin]	Z79.84	Oral hypoglycemic	Diabetes mellitus
Trazodone HCl [trazodone hydrochloride]		Antidepressant	Depression
Trelegy Ellipta [fluticasone furoate/umeclidinium bromide/vilanterol trifenatate]	Z79.51	Corticosteroid -- inhaled; antiasthmatic	COPD
Trelstar [triptorelin pamoate]	Z79.818	Agents affecting estrogen receptors and estrogen levels	Palliative treatment of prostate cancer symptoms
Tremfya [guselkumab]	Z79.620	Immunosuppressive biologic; monoclonal antibody	Plaque psoriasis
Tresiba [insulin degludec]	Z79.4	Insulin	Diabetes mellitus
Triamterene and hydrochlorothiazide [triamterene/ hydrochlorothiazide]		Antihypertensive; diuretic	Edema; hypertension
Tri-Estarylla [ethinyl estradiol/norgestimate]	Z79.3	Contraceptive	Prevention of pregnancy; acne
Trijardy XR [empagliflozin/linagliptin/metformin hydrochloride]	Z79.84	Oral hypoglycemic	Diabetes mellitus
Tri-Legest [ethinyl estradiol/norethindrone acetate]	Z79.3	Contraceptive	Prevention of pregnancy
Tri-Linyah [ethinyl estradiol/norgestimate]	Z79.3	Contraceptive	Prevention of pregnancy
Tri-Lo-Estarylla [ethinyl estradiol/norgestimate]	Z79.3	Contraceptive	Prevention of pregnancy
Tri-Lo-Sprintec [ethinyl estradiol/norgestimate]	Z79.3	Contraceptive	Prevention of pregnancy
Trimethoprim [trimethoprim]	Z79.2	Antibiotic	Acute exacerbation chronic bronchitis; travelers' diarrhea; infections of the middle, lower respiratory tract, and urinary tract; pneumonia, pneumocystis; shigellosis
Tri-Previfem [ethinyl estradiol/norgestimate]	Z79.3	Contraceptive	Prevention of pregnancy
Triptodur [triptorelin]	Z79.818	Agents affecting estrogen receptors and estrogen levels	Precocious puberty
Tri-Sprintec [ethinyl estradiol/norgestimate]	Z79.3	Contraceptive	Prevention of pregnancy; acne
Trivora-28 [ethinyl estradiol/ levonorgestrel]	Z79.3	Contraceptive	Prevention of pregnancy
Trokendi XR [topiramate]		Anticonvulsant	Epilepsy; primary generalized tonic-clonic seizures; seizures associated with Lennox-Gastaut syndrome; migraine headache
Trulicity [dulaglutide]	Z79.85	Antidiabetic – non-insulin injectable	Diabetes mellitus
Truvada [emtricitabine/tenofovir disoproxil fumarate]	Z79.899	Antiretroviral	HIV
Turalio [pexidartinib]		Kinase inhibitor	Symptomatic tenosynovial giant cell tumor
Tygacil [tigecycline]	Z79.2	Antibiotic	Bacterial skin or digestive system infections; pneumonia
Tylenol with codeine [acetaminophen/codeine phosphate]	Z79.891	Analgesic, narcotic	Pain and cough
Ubrelvy [ubrogepant]		Calcitonin gene-related peptide inhibitor	Migraine headache
Ultram [tramadol hydrochloride]	Z79.891	Analgesic, non-narcotic (opiate, narcotic-like)	Moderate to severe pain
Unasyn [ampicillin sodium/sulbactam sodium]	Z79.2	Antibiotic	Bacterial infections
Vabomere [meropenem; vaborbactam]	Z79.2	Antibiotic	Complicated urinary tract infections; pyelonephritis
Vagifem [estradiol]	Z79.890	Estrogen therapy	Menopause symptoms

Drug	Z Code	Drug Action/Classification	Indications
Valium [diazepam]		Antianxiety; muscle relaxant; anticonvulsant	Anxiety, tension, withdrawal from alcohol, muscle spasms and anticonvulsant therapy; epilepsy, generalized tonic-clonic; status epilepticus; stiff-man syndrome; tetanus
Vancocin HCl [vancomycin hydrochloride]	Z79.2	Antibiotic	Severe bacterial infections
Vancomycin HCl [vancomycin hydrochloride]	Z79.2	Antibiotic	Severe bacterial infections
Vantas [histrelin acetate]	Z79.818	Agents affecting estrogen receptors and estrogen levels	Palliative treatment of prostate cancer symptoms
Vasotec [enalaprilat maleate]		ACE inhibitor	Congestive heart failure; hypertension
Velivet [desogestrel/ethinyl estradiol]	Z79.3	Contraceptive	Prevention of pregnancy
Venlafaxine HCl [venlafaxine hydrochloride]		Antidepressant, serotonin and norepinephrine reuptake inhibitor (SNRI)	Major depressive disorder; social anxiety disorder; panic disorder
Ventolin HFA [albuterol sulfate]		Antiasthmatic/bronchodilator	Asthma
Verapamil HCL [verapamil hydrochloride]		Calcium channel blocker	Angina pectoris; chronic stable angina; atrial fibrillation; atrial flutter; paroxysmal supraventricular tachycardia; ventricular arrhythmia; hypertension
Viagra [sildenafil citrate]		Phosphodiesterase-5 (PDE5) inhibitor	Erectile dysfunction
Vibativ [telavancin hydrochloride]	Z79.2	Antibiotic	Pneumonia; severe bacterial skin infections
Vibramycin [doxycycline calcium]	Z79.2	Antibiotic	Bacterial infections
Victoza [liraglutide]	Z79.85	Antidiabetic – non-insulin injectable	Diabetes mellitus
Vienva [ethinyl estradiol/levonorgestrel]	Z79.3	Contraceptive	Prevention of pregnancy
Vinblastine [vinblastine]	Z79.633	Mitotic inhibitor	Cancer
Vincristine [vincristine]	Z79.633	Mitotic inhibitor	Cancer
Viorele [desogestrel/ethinyl estradiol]	Z79.3	Contraceptive	Prevention of pregnancy
Virazole [ribavirin]	Z79.899	Antiviral	Respiratory syncytial virus (RSV)
Viread [tenofovir disoproxil fumarate]	Z79.899	Antiretroviral	HIV; chronic hepatitis B
Voltaren [diclofenac sodium]	Z79.1	Nonsteroidal anti-inflammatory drug (NSAID)	Treatment of pain, inflammation, and joint stiffness due to arthritis
Vumerity [diroximel fumarate]	Z79.69	Other immunosuppressant/immunomodulator	Relapsing forms of multiple sclerosis (MS)
Vytorin [ezetimibe/simvastatin]		HMG-CoA reductase inhibitor (statin); cholesterol absorption inhibitor	Hyperlipidemia; hypercholesterolemia
Wakix [pitolisant hydrochloride]		CNS stimulant	Narcolepsy
Warfarin [warfarin sodium]	Z79.01	Anticoagulant	Prophylaxis and treatment of venous thrombosis; treatment of atrial fibrillation with embolization (pulmonary embolism), arrhythmias, myocardial infarction, and stroke prevention
Wellbutrin SR, Wellbutrin XL [bupropion hydrochloride]		Antidepressant	Depression
Wera [ethinyl estradiol/norethindrone]	Z79.3	Contraceptive	Prevention of pregnancy
Xalatan [latanoprost]		Prostaglandin F2α analogue	Glaucoma, open-angle; ocular hypertension
Xanax, Xanax XR [alprazolam]		Antianxiety; sedative/hypnotic	Anxiety disorders with panic disorder and depression
Xarelto [rivaroxaban]	Z79.01	Anticoagulant	Prophylaxis and treatment of venous thrombosis, pulmonary embolism; prevention of blood clots due to atrial fibrillation
Xeljanz, Xeljanz XR [tofacitinib]	Z79.622	Janus kinase (JAK) inhibitor	Rheumatoid arthritis; psoriatic arthritis
Xeloda [capecitabine]	Z79.631	Antimetabolite agent	Breast cancer, colon/colorectal cancer
Xelstrym [dextroamphetamine]		CNS stimulant	Attention deficit hyperactivity disorder (ADHD)
Xenleta [lefamulin acetate]	Z79.2	Antibiotic	Community-acquired bacterial pneumonia
Xgeva [denosumab]	Z79.620	Immunosuppressive biologic; monoclonal antibody	Treatment and prevention of bone resorption and prevention of bone fracture
Xifaxan [rifaximin]	Z79.2	Antibiotic	E. coli diarrhea
Xigduo [dapagliflozin propanediol/metformin hydrochloride]	Z79.84	Oral hypoglycemic	Diabetes mellitus
Xpovio [selinexor]	Z79.899	Antineoplastic	Multiple myeloma in adults
Xultophy [insulin degludec/liraglutide]	Z79.4	Insulin	Diabetes mellitus

Drug	Z Code	Drug Action/Classification	Indications
Xyrem [sodium oxybate]		CNS depressant; anxiolytic/sedative/hypnotic	Cataplexy and/or excessive daytime sleepiness in narcolepsy
Xyzal [levocetirizine dihydrochloride]		Antihistamine	Perennial allergic rhinitis; chronic idiopathic urticaria
Yasmin [drospirenone/ethinyl estradiol]	Z79.3	Contraceptive	Prevention of pregnancy
Yaz [drospirenone/ethinyl estradiol]	Z79.3	Contraceptive	Prevention of pregnancy; menstrual disorders
Zerbaxa [ceftolozane sulfate/tazobactam sodium]	Z79.2	Antibiotic	Complicated urinary tract and intra-abdominal infections
Zestoretic [lisinopril/hydrochlorothiazide]		ACE inhibitor	Congestive heart failure; hypertension
Zestril [lisinopril]		ACE inhibitor	Congestive heart failure; hypertension
Zetia [ezetimibe]		Antihyperlipidemic	Hypercholesterolemia; sitosterolemia
Ziac [bisoprolol fumarate/hydrochlorothiazide]		Antihypertensive	Hypertension
Zinacef [cefuroxime sodium]	Z79.2	Antibiotic	Bacterial infections
Zipsor [diclofenac potassium]	Z79.1	Nonsteroidal anti-inflammatory drug (NSAID)	Pain and inflammation relief
Zithromax [azithromycin]	Z79.2	Antibiotic	Infections of the cervix, lower respiratory tract, skin and skin structures, urethra, nongonococcal; mycobacterium avium complex; pharyngitis, streptococcal pneumonia; tonsillitis
Zocor [simvastatin]		HMG-CoA reductase inhibitor (statin)	Hypercholesterolemia; hyperlipidemia; hyperlipoproteinemia; hypertriglyceridemia
Zoladex [goserelin acetate]	Z79.818	Agents affecting estrogen receptors and estrogen levels	Palliative treatment of prostate cancer and breast cancer symptoms; endometriosis
Zoloft [sertraline hydrochloride]		Antidepressant	Anxiety with panic disorder and depression; obsessive-compulsive disorder
Zometa [zoledronic acid]	Z79.83	Bisphosphonate	Multiple myeloma; Paget's disease
Zortress [everolimus]	Z79.623	Mammalian target of rapamycin (mTOR) inhibitor	Prophylaxis of organ transplant rejection
Zorvolex [diclofenac]	Z79.1	Nonsteroidal anti-inflammatory drug (NSAID)	Pain, inflammation or fever relief
Zosyn [piperacillin sodium/tazobactam sodium]	Z79.2	Antibiotic	Bacterial infections
Zovia [ethynodiol diacetate/ethinyl estradiol]	Z79.3	Contraceptive	Prevention of pregnancy
Zovirax [acyclovir]	Z79.899	Antiviral	Genital herpes and herpes zoster infections
Zubsolv [buprenorphine/naloxone]		Opioid agonist	Treatment of opioid addiction
Zyloprim [allopurinol]		Antigout	Gouty arthritis; renal calculus; hyperuricemia; hyperuricemia secondary to leukemia; hyperuricemia secondary to lymphoma
Zyprexa [olanzapine]		Antipsychotic/antimanic	Psychotic disorders; schizophrenia
Zyrtec allergy [cetirizine hydrochloride]		Antihistamine	Perennial and seasonal allergic rhinitis; chronic urticaria
Zyvox [linezolid]	Z79.2	Antibiotic	Severe bacterial infections

Appendix C: Z Codes for Long-Term Drug Use with Associated Drugs

This resource correlates the Z codes that are used to identify current long-term drug use with a list of drugs that are typically categorized to that class of drug. These lists are not all-inclusive, providing only the more commonly used drugs.

Z79.01 **Long term (current) use of anticoagulants**
Angiomax
Argatroban
Arixtra
Bevyxxa
Coumadin
Eliquis
Fragmin
Heparin
Jantoven
Lovenox
Pradaxa
Savaysa
Warfarin
Xarelto

Z79.02 **Long term (current) use of antithrombotics/antiplatelets**
Aggrastat
Aggrenox
Brilinta
Clopidogrel bisulfate
Effient
Integrilin
Persantine
Plavix
Prasugrel

Z79.1 **Long term (current) use of non-steroidal anti-inflammatories (NSAID)**
Advil
Aleve
Anaprox DS
Arthrotec
Caldolor
Cambia
Celebrex
Daypro
Duexis
Elyxyb
Feldene
Ibuprofen
Indocin
Mobic
Motrin IB
Nabumetone
Nalfon
Naprelan
Naprosyn
NeoProfen
Ponstel
Tivorbex
Voltaren
Zipsor
Zorvolex

Z79.2 **Long term (current) use of antibiotics**
Altabax
Amikacin
Amoxicillin
Ampicillin
Augmentin
Avelox
Azactam
Azithromycin

Bactrim
Bactroban
Biaxin XL
Cefazolin sodium
Ceftriaxone
Cefzil
Centany
Cephalexin
Cipro
Ciprofloxacin
Clarithromycin
Cleocin
Clindamycin
Cubicin
Daptomycin
Dificid
Doxycycline
Dynacin
E.E.S.
Ertapenem
ERYC
Erygel
EryPed
Ery-Tab
Erythrocin
Erythromycin
Factive
Fetroja
Flagyl
Fortaz
Garamycin
Gentamicin sulfate
Hiprex
Invanz
Isoniazid
Keflex
Klaron
Lincocin
Macrobid
Macrodantin
Maxipime
Mepron
Merrem
Metronidazole
Minocin
Monodox
Monurol
Mycobutin
Nebupent
Neosporin
Nitrofurantoin
Oracea
Orbactiv
Penicillin-VK
Pentam
Pfizerpen
Priftin
Primaxin
Rifadin
Rimactane
Septra
Seromycin
Silvadene
Sivextro

Solodyn
Solosec
Streptomycin sulfate
Suprax
Synercid
Talicia
Tazicef
Teflaro
Tetracycline
Tobramycin
Trimethoprim
Tygacil
Unasyn
Vabomere
Vancocin HCl
Vancomycin HCl
Vibativ
Vibramycin
Xenleta
Xifaxan
Zerbaxa
Zinacef
Zithromax
Zosyn
Zyvox

Z79.3 **Long term (current) use of hormonal contraceptives**
Altavera
Alyacen
Aranelle
Ashlyna
Aviane-28
Balziva-28
Bekyree
Beyaz
Brevicon 28-day
Briellyn
Camila
Cryselle
Cyclafem
Cyclessa
Dasetta
Daysee
Depo-Provera
Depo-SubQ Provera
Desogen
Elinest
Emoquette
Enpresse-28
Enskyce
Errin
Estarylla
Estrostep Fe
Falmina
Femhrt
Gildagia
Gildess
Introvale
Jencycla
Junel
Kariva
Kelnor
Kimidess
Kurvelo

Kyleena
Larin
Lessina-28
Levonest
Levora
Liletta
Lo Loestrin Fe
Loestrin
Loryna
LoSeasonique
Low-Ogestrel-28
Marlissa
Microgestin
Minastrin
Mirena
Mono-Linyah
Myzilra
Natazia
Nexplanon
Nextstellis
Norinyl
Nortrel
NuvaRing
Ogestrel
Orsythia
Ortho-Novum
Philith
Pimtrea
Pirmella
Plan B One-Step
Portia-28
Previfem
Provera
Quartette
Safyral
Seasonale
Seasonique
Setlakin
Skyla
Sprintec
Syeda
Tri-Estarylla
Tri-Legest
Tri-Linyah
Tri-Lo-Estarylla
Tri-Lo-Sprintec
Tri-Previfem
Tri-Sprintec
Trivora-28
Velivet
Vienva
Viorele
Wera
Yasmin
Yaz
Zovia

Z79.4 Long term (current) use of insulin
Admelog
Apidra
Basaglar
Fiasp
Humalog
Humulin R
Lantus
Levemir
Novolin
Novolog
Soliqua
Toujeo Solostar

Tresiba
Xultophy

Z79.51 Long term (current) use of inhaled steroids
Advair
AirDuo RespiClick
Alvesco
Arnuity Ellipta
Asmanex
Breo Ellipta
Dulera
Flovent HFA
Pulmicort
Qvar Redihaler
Symbicort
Trelegy Ellipta

Z79.52 Long term (current) use of systemic steroids
Aristospan
Celestone Soluspan
Colocort
Cortef
Cortenema
Cortifoam
Cortisone acetate
Depo-Medrol
Dexamethasone Intensol
Entocort EC
Hydrocortisone
Kenalog-10
Kenalog-40
Locoid
Medrol
Methylprednisolone
Orapred ODT
PediaPred
Prednisolone
Prednisone
Rayos
Solu-Cortef
Solu-Medrol

Z79.61 Long term (current) use of immunomodulator
Apremilast
Otezla
Pomalyst
Revlimid
Thalidomide

Z79.620 Long term (current) use of immunosuppressive biologic
Actemra
Aimovig
Cosentyx
Cyltezo
Dupixent
Enbrel
Entyvio
Humira
Hyrimoz
Keytruda
Monoclonal antibodies
Prolia
Remicade
Rituxan
Simulect
Skyrizi
Stelara
Taltz
Tremfya

Xgeva

Z79.621 Long term (current) use of calcineurin inhibitor
Astagraf XL
Cyclosporin
Envarsus XR
Gengraf
Lupkynis
Neoral
Prograf
Protopic
Sandimmune
Tacrolimus

Z79.622 Long term (current) use of Janus kinase inhibitor
Cibinqo
Olumiant
Rinvoq
Xeljanz XR

Z79.623 Long term (current) use of mammalian target of rapamycin (mTOR) inhibitor
Rapamune
Sirolimus
Torisel
Zortress

Z79.624 Long term (current) use of inhibitors of nucleotide synthesis
CellCept
Imuran

Z79.630 Long term (current) use of alkylating agent
Busulfex
Carmustine
Chlorambucil
Cisplatin
Cytoxan
Leukeran
Temozolomide

Z79.631 Long term (current) use of antimetabolite agent
5-fluorouracil (5-FU)
6-mercaptopurine (6-MP)
Cytarabine
Methotrexate
Xeloda

Z79.632 Long term (current) use of antitumor antibiotic
Bleomycin
Cerubidine
Doxorubicin
Mitomycin

Z79.633 Long term (current) use of mitotic inhibitor
Ixempra
Paclitaxel
Taxotere
Vinblastine
Vincristine

Z79.634 Long term (current) use of topoisomerase inhibitor
Camptosar
Etoposide
Hycamtin

Z79.64 Long term (current) use of myelosuppressive agent
Hydroxyurea

Z79.69   Long term (current) use of other immunomodulators and immunosuppressants
Actimmune
Avonex
Betaseron
Copaxone
Intron A
Orencia
PegIntron
Ponvory
Rebif
Sylatron
Tavneos
Vumerity

Z79.810   Long term (current) use of selective estrogen receptor modulators (SERMs)
Evista
Fareston
Osphena
Raloxifene HCl
Soltamox
Tamoxifen citrate
Toremifene citrate

Z79.811   Long term (current) use of aromatase inhibitors
Anastrozole
Arimidex
Aromasin
Exemestane
Femara
Letrozole

Z79.818   Long term (current) use of other agents affecting estrogen receptors and estrogen levels
Eligard
Faslodex
Lupron Depot
Megace ES
Supprelin LA
Synarel
Trelstar
Triptodur
Vantas
Zoladex

Z79.82   Long term (current) use of aspirin
Bayer
Bufferin
Durlaza

Z79.83   Long term (current) use of bisphosphonates
Aclasta
Actonel
Aredia
Atelvia
Binosto
Boniva
Fosamax
Reclast
Zometa

Z79.84   Long term (current) use of oral hypoglycemic drugs
Acarbose
Actoplus Met
Actos

Amaryl
Avandia
DiaBeta
Duetact
Farxiga
Glimepiride
Glucotrol
Glumetza
Glyburide
Glynase
Glyset
Invokamet
Invokana
Janumet
Januvia
Jentadueto
Kazano
Kombiglyze
Metformin
Onglyza
Oseni
Qtern
Repaglinide
Riomet
Rybelsus
Sitagliptin
Synjardy
Tradjenta
Trijardy XR
Xigduo

Z79.85   Long-term (current) use of injectable non-insulin antidiabetic drugs
Adlyxin
Bydureon
Byetta
Ozempic
Symlin
Trulicity
Victoza

Z79.890   Hormone replacement therapy
Activella
Alora
Androderm
AndroGel
Angeliq
Bijuva
Climara
CombiPatch
Delestrogen
Depo-Provera
Divigel
Duavee
Elestrin
Estrace
EstroGel
Femhrt
Femring
Firmagon
Menest
Menostar
Minivelle
Orilissa
Osphena
Prempro
Provera
Testim
Vagifem

Z79.891   Long term (current) use of opiate analgesic
Acetaminophen with codeine
Buprenex
Buprenorphine HCl and Naloxone HCl
Butrans
Codeine
Demerol
Dilaudid
Dolophine HCl
Duragesic
Duramorph PF
Fentanyl citrate
Fentora
Fioricet with codeine
Hydrocodone
Hydrocodone bitartrate and acetaminophen
Hydromorphone HCl
Kadian
Lazanda
Methadone HCl
Methadose
Morphine sulfate
MS Contin
Norco
Nucynta
Oxycodone HCl
OxyContin
Percocet
Roxicet
Roxicodone
Tylenol with codeine
Ultram

Z79.899   Other long term (current) drug therapy
Afrezza
Antineoplastic/chemotherapy
Atripla
Beconase AQ
Biktarvy
Cimduo
Descovy
Dovato
Dymista
Emtriva
Epivir
Epivir-HBV
Erelzi
Flonase
Harvoni
Livtencity
Nexletol
Prezcobix
Prezista
Qnasl
Rebetol
Retrovir
Rukobia
Sustiva
Symtuza
Truvada
Virazole
Viread
Xpovio
Zovirax

Appendix D: Z Codes Only as Principal/First-Listed Diagnosis

Z00.00	Z01.118	Z02.1	Z04.6	Z34.83	Z38.66	Z51.11	Z52.4
Z00.01	Z01.12	Z02.2	Z04.71	Z34.90	Z38.68	Z51.12	Z52.5
Z00.110	Z01.20	Z02.3	Z04.72	Z34.91	Z38.69	Z52.000	Z52.6
Z00.111	Z01.21	Z02.4	Z04.81	Z34.92	Z38.7	Z52.001	Z52.810
Z00.121	Z01.30	Z02.5	Z04.82	Z34.93	Z38.8	Z52.008	Z52.811
Z00.129	Z01.31	Z02.6	Z04.89	Z38.00	Z39.0	Z52.010	Z52.812
Z00.2	Z01.411	Z02.71	Z04.9	Z38.01	Z39.1	Z52.011	Z52.813
Z00.3	Z01.419	Z02.79	Z31.81	Z38.1	Z39.2	Z52.018	Z52.819
Z00.5	Z01.42	Z02.81	Z31.83	Z38.2	Z40.00	Z52.090	Z52.89
Z00.70	Z01.810	Z02.82	Z31.84	Z38.30	Z40.01	Z52.091	Z76.1
Z00.71	Z01.811	Z02.83	Z33.2	Z38.31	Z40.02	Z52.098	Z76.2
Z00.8	Z01.812	Z02.89	Z34.00	Z38.4	Z40.03	Z52.10	Z99.12
Z01.00	Z01.818	Z02.9	Z34.01	Z38.5	Z40.09	Z52.11	
Z01.01	Z01.82	Z04.1	Z34.02	Z38.61	Z40.8	Z52.19	
Z01.020	Z01.83	Z04.2	Z34.03	Z38.62	Z40.9	Z52.20	
Z01.021	Z01.84	Z04.3	Z34.80	Z38.63	Z42.1	Z52.21	
Z01.10	Z01.89	Z04.41	Z34.81	Z38.64	Z42.8	Z52.29	
Z01.110	Z02.0	Z04.42	Z34.82	Z38.65	Z51.0	Z52.3	

Appendix E: Centers for Medicare & Medicaid Services Hierarchical Condition Categories (CMS-HCC)

In the 1970s, Medicare began demonstration projects that contracted with health maintenance organizations (HMOs) to provide care for Medicare beneficiaries in exchange for prospective payments. In 1985, this project changed from demonstration status to a regular part of the Medicare program, Medicare Part C. The Balanced Budget Act (BBA) of 1997 named Medicare's Part C managed care program Medicare+Choice, and the Medicare Modernization Act (MMA) of 2003 again renamed it to Medicare Advantage (MA).

Medicare is one of the world's largest health insurance programs, and about one-third of the beneficiaries on Medicare are enrolled in a MA private health care plan. Due to the great variance in the health status of Medicare beneficiaries, risk adjustment provides a means of adequately compensating those plans with large numbers of seriously ill patients while not overburdening other plans that have healthier individuals. Medicare Advantage (MA) plans have been using the Hierarchical Condition Category (HCC) risk adjustment model since 2004.

The Risk Adjustment Model

The primary purpose of a risk adjustment model is to predict (on average) the future health care costs for specific consortiums enrolled in Medicare Advantage (MA) health plans. CMS is then able to provide capitation payments to these private health plans. Capitation payments are an incentive for health plans to enroll not only healthier individuals but those with chronic conditions or who are more seriously ill by removing some of the financial burden.

The MA risk adjustment model uses HCCs to assess the disease burden of its enrollees. HCC diagnostic groupings were created after examining claims data so that enrollees with similar disease processes, and consequently similar health care expenditures, could be pooled into a larger data set in which an average expenditure rate could be determined. The medical conditions included in HCC categories are those that were determined to most predictably affect the health status and health care costs of any individual. Several important principles to the risk adjustment model and the development of the HCC categories include but are not limited to:

1. The HCC diagnostic categories should be clinically meaningful.
   - Diagnostic categories are well-defined.
   - Clinically specific diseases or medical conditions are grouped to each category.
2. The HCC diagnostic categories should predict medical expenditures.
   - The diagnoses grouped to a specific category should have as close to the same cost burden not only in the current year but also in the future.
3. The HCC diagnostic categories should have adequate sample sizes and discretionary categories excluded to be as accurate and stable in their estimate of costs as possible.
   - A diagnostic category that groups extremely rare diseases or conditions would not be reliably effective in determining current or future costs.
   - Codes that are not credible as cost predictors or may be subject to coding variation should be excluded, when possible.
4. The HCC diagnostic categories should be both hierarchical and additive.
   - Hierarchical measurement is used within a specific disease process.
   - Disease processes that are unrelated to each other are measured additively.
5. The diagnostic classification should encourage specificity and should not reward coding proliferation.
   - More diagnosis codes and vague diagnosis codes do not equal greater disease burden.

More than 10,000 ICD-10-CM diagnosis codes map to 86 HCCs in the current risk adjustment model. Diagnoses are excluded from mapping when they do not predict future cost or are vague or variable in diagnosis, coding, or treatment, such as symptoms or osteoarthritis. Also excluded are diagnosis codes from laboratories, radiology, and home health claims.

Risk Adjustment Factors

The CMS-HCC risk adjustment model uses "risk adjustment factors" to calculate a risk score for each member. This score summarizes that particular patient's expected cost of care relative to other members'. Each member's risk score is based on demographic and health status information and is calculated as the sum of these demographic and health factors weighted by their estimated marginal contributions to total risk. The model also takes into account where the patient resides (community or institutional), Medicaid eligibility (full or partial benefits), the patient's Medicare enrollment status (new or established), age, disability status, whether the patient is frail or has end-stage renal disease (ESRD), and even prescription drug use.

No procedure codes, ICD-10-PCS or CPT, are included in the MA risk adjustment model. The model relies solely on diagnostic and demographic data. Not all ICD-10-CM diagnoses map to an HCC, and there is no specific code sequencing involved. The CMS-HCC model is additive as well as hierarchical. The additive functionality allows a patient to have more than one HCC category assigned, providing a more complete clinical picture and prediction of resource consumption. The hierarchical aspect of the model provides a means of ranking diagnoses that are similar in disease process, by severity. The hierarchy of the condition categories ensures the patient's conditions are classified to the most severe condition within the related group. Less severe conditions within a particular hierarchy are superseded by more severe diagnoses within the same group. The hierarchy and additive relationship permits this model to characterize the person's illness level within each disease process, while still allowing the effects of unrelated disease processes to be counted in the patient's overall score.

Certain combinations of coexisting diagnoses for an individual can increase medical costs. The CMS-HCC model adjusts for these higher costs by the addition of "disease interaction" factors. For each patient, multiple HCCs assigned, along with demographic and disease interaction factors, are used to calculate a single, combined risk adjustment factor (RAF). The RAF score for an individual member represents all of the HCCs that have been submitted from all sources for that member to CMS during the course of an entire calendar year.

There are separate CMS-HCC models for new enrollees and continuing enrollees. The new enrollee model uses demographic factors only, such as age, sex, and disability status, and is used when the enrollee has less than 12 months of medical history. The community model accounts for age, sex, original reason for Medicare entitlement (age or disability), Medicaid eligibility, and clinical conditions as measured by HCCs. In the second step, expected costs are adjusted for outliers based on the member's risk score and whether the patient has ESRD.

Demographic data (age, sex, eligibility) as well as health status (diagnoses codes submitted on claims to CMS) of an MA population are used to determine the reimbursement to the health plan to care for their members.

CMS considers a RAF score of 1.0 as the benchmark to indicate the score of the average healthy patient with the same demographic and diagnostic factors. These patients are expected to use average or lower-than-average resources. When the RAF score is higher than 1.0, CMS considers the patient to be sicker than the average patient with the same criteria and expects greater-than-average resource utilization.

A low RAF score may accurately indicate a healthier patient, but it may also falsely indicate a healthier patient due to incomplete or inaccurate coding, incomplete or insufficient record documentation, or patients who fail to complete an annual assessment.

A high RAF score may accurately indicate a sicker patient, or it may be falsely inflated from overcoding due to diagnoses that are reported but not documented, or from copying and pasting from previous encounters or problem lists of resolved conditions.

Documentation Requirements

Payment is made per HCC category (not per diagnosis code). No matter how many times in the year the diagnosis codes are reported, a single payment is made to the MA plan each year. Each year the list of HCCs and the RAF for each patient is "reset." This means the annual health assessment is extremely important, and adequate documentation is critical. Accurate risk adjustment payment relies on complete medical record documentation and diagnosis coding. CMS requires that all applicable diagnosis codes be reported and that all diagnoses be reported to the highest level of specificity and that these be substantiated by the medical record.

> CMS's Guiding Principle:
>
> The risk adjustment diagnosis must be based on clinical medical record documentation from a face-to-face encounter, coded according to the *ICD-10-CM Guidelines for Coding and Reporting*; assigned based on dates of service within the data collection period, submitted to the MA organization from an appropriate risk adjustment provider type and an appropriate risk adjustment physician data source.

A "face-to-face" health service encounter between a patient and healthcare provider describes an encounter between the patient and the provider (MD, DO), including qualified nonphysician practitioners (NPP) (e.g. nurse practitioner or physician's assistant), which is face-to-face with the patient. CMS provides a current listing of acceptable physician specialty types for risk adjustment data submission within the 2012 Regional Technical Assistance Participant Guide. The only exception to the face-to-face encounter requirement is pathology services (professional component only). Due to the 2019 coronavirus disease (COVID-19) pandemic, CMS is allowing MA organizations to submit diagnoses from telehealth services that meet the risk adjustment face-to-face requirement when the services are provided using interactive audio and video telecommunications systems that permit real-time interactive communication. Currently, CMS does not provide a listing of all services that are considered face-to-face visits for risk adjustment data, but does provide guidance on what types of services are not acceptable for risk adjustment in the Participant Guide. For example, diagnostic radiology does not qualify because diagnostic radiologists typically do not document confirmed diagnoses. Other examples of services that are not acceptable include diagnostic reports that have not been interpreted, such as laboratory reports.

It is essential that the medical record documentation show evidence by provider authentication that the direct face-to-face service was personally furnished by the physician or qualified NPP. Examples of these services include office visits, hospital visits, preoperative anesthesia assessment, and surgical and invasive procedures.

Risk adjustment relies on annual health information. Each enrollee is assigned an individual risk score based on the health status information obtained from the diagnosis codes on the claims. The CMS-HCC model relies on ICD-10-CM coding specificity for accurate risk adjustment by using the most specific code available that is substantiated by the documentation in the medical record. Providers should fully document and accurately code the evaluation and management of all severe and chronic conditions to ensure a full, complete, and accurate clinical record of the patient's condition and reflect the work involved in caring for the patient, particularly those with complex and challenging health issues. All conditions affecting the treatment or management of the patient's health should be documented at least once a year, as applicable to care provided, to accurately describe the true complexity and severity of the patient's health. If the diagnosis coding on the claim is not accurate or complete, the claim may indicate that the provider did much less medical decision-making, evaluation, and management than was actually performed.

Documentation to support or validate risk adjustment conditions may be found anywhere in the note for the face-to-face encounter. It is important to ensure that the note accurately reflects all chronic conditions that affect the health and care of the patient. Each encounter must be unique and reflect only that visit as it occurred. Insufficient documentation influences the assignment of diagnosis codes and directly affects the patient's risk score.

Documentation should properly validate all reported conditions. Each page of progress notes should be properly authenticated and include the patient's name and the date.

Providers should document each clinical diagnosis to the highest degree of specificity per encounter, including all complications and/or manifestations, including clear links to causal conditions. Only confirmed conditions should be documented—no rule-out conditions or abnormal findings without clinical significance. All known conditions, including chronic conditions, that affect the care and treatment of the patient at least once per year should be noted.

Providers should specifically document the condition and clinical significance, and pertinent changes using terminology such as decreased, increased, worsening, improving, or unchanged, or abnormal findings.

Documentation Tips

- Document all cause-and-effect relationships.
- Report the most specific diagnosis code available that is supported by the documentation.
- Include all current diagnoses as part of the current medical decision-making, and document for every visit.
- Identify diagnoses that are current or chronic problems rather than a past medical history or previous resolved condition.
- Document history of heart attack, status codes, etc., that affect the patient's care as "history of" or "PMH" when they no longer exist or are not current conditions.
- Ensure each progress note has the date, signature, and credentials/specialty.
- Document the thought processes used to assess each condition.

- Know high revenue HCCs that are often undiagnosed or undercoded.
- Avoid "unspecified" codes.
- Ensure the codes reported are accurate.
- Ensure each encounter is billed.
- Review rejection reports, and audit reports to assess risks.

Audits

Because reimbursement is by patient, rather than based on an average of the entire population, and is based upon documentation, there is the potential for upcoding. Audits are conducted by the MA plan and CMS recovery auditors.

Initial Validation Audit (IVA)

CMS requires that the MA plan validate HCCs. This is usually performed by an independent auditor working with the plan or a contracted vendor to validate the MA plan's data submitted to CMS.

The MA plan submits the one best medical record that supports each HCC identified for the beneficiary.

Risk Adjustment Data Validation Audit

Risk adjustment data validation (RADV) audits were introduced in 2011 and updated for 2015. They are performed by CMS to validate the integrity and accuracy of risk-adjusted payments by verifying that the diagnosis codes the MA plans submit are supported by the medical record documentation for a member. On March 30, 2020, CMS announced it was suspending RADV activities related to the payment year 2015 audit and will not initiate any additional contract-level audits until after the 2019 coronavirus public health emergency (PHE) has ended, at which time CMS will make an announcement when normal audit activities will resume.

MA plans can be selected by CMS for RADV audits annually and if chosen are required to submit their members' medical records to CMS. Providers are required to assist the MA plan by providing the medical record documentation included in the audit. Even though each diagnosis needs to be reported only once in a calendar year, during a RADV audit up to five dates of service may be submitted to support any one HCC.

To be validated, medical record documentation must meet certain criteria and standards. Even if the diagnosis is documented and coded correctly, any deficiency in the documentation can make the encounter and the HCC invalid. Diagnoses that cannot be validated are considered payment errors. The results of the audit are communicated to the MA plan, which then communicates these results to the provider. Under- and overpayments are subject to payment adjustment. The results of RADV audits can be extrapolated over the MA plan population to calculate potential payment errors and overpayments/recoupments. Regulations include a RADV appeal process, a document dispute process, and a procedure for obtaining physician-signature attestations.

The following items are reviewed during the validation process:

- The record is for the correct enrollee.
- The record is from the correct calendar year for the payment year being audited.
- The record is legible.
- The date of service is present on the records and is for a face-to-face visit.
- The record is from a valid provider type.
- Valid credentials and/or a valid physician specialty are documented on the record.
- The record contains a signature from an acceptable type of physician.
- There is a diagnosis on the record.
- The diagnosis supports an HCC.
- The diagnosis supports the submitted HCC.

Mitigate audit risk by coding each reportable diagnosis each time it meets reporting guidelines. Audit regularly to assess areas of risk and in need of improvement and to capture conditions documented but not coded. Check for additional qualifying HCCs. Ensure claims are submitted and that corrected claims are submitted when indicated. There are three claims submission deadlines: January, March, and September. CMS adjusts each member's risk score twice a year, with the final reconciliation in August of the year after the plan year.

If providers emphasize correct coding and documentation and perform internal audits to determine where the risks are and prepare for audits, incorrect payment is less likely. For additional information on risk adjustment coding, see Optum's *Risk Adjustment Coding and HCC Guide.*

Appendix F: Centers for Medicare & Medicaid Services Quality Payment Program

In 2015, in an effort to repeal the faulty Medicare sustainable growth rate (SGR), focus on quality of patient outcomes, and control Medicare spending, Congress passed the Medicare Access and CHIP Reauthorization Act (MACRA), which included sweeping changes for practitioners who provide services reimbursed under the Medicare physician fee schedule (MPFS). MACRA repealed the Medicare SGR methodology used for updating the MPFS and replaced it with the Quality Payment Program (QPP).

Under the QPP, providers who demonstrate success at controlling costs while providing high-quality care to their patients are eligible to earn increased payments. Clinicians who successfully report on determined criteria receive a larger payment. Those who do not participate at all or do not fulfill the defined requirements receive a negative payment adjustment of 9 percent of Medicare Part B reimbursements based on 2020 performance to be applied in 2022, negative payment adjustment of up to 9 percent of Medicare Part B reimbursements based on 2021 performance to be applied in 2023.

Passage of the Medicare Access and CHIP Reauthorization Act of 2015

The final rule for implementing MACRA was published November 4, 2016. The final rule primarily provided details on how the QPP was to be implemented, including requiring the secretary of Health and Human Services (HHS) to sunset the value-based (VM) modifier incentive program, the Medicare electronic health record (EHR) incentive program, and the Physician Quality Reporting System (PQRS), and incorporated these incentive programs into the QPP.

Replacement of the Sustainable Growth Rate

Under the SGR, if overall physician costs were higher than a targeted Medicare expenditure, payments were reduced across the board. With the SGR method, payments to clinicians would have resulted in substantial cuts.

Because the QPP replaces the SGR methodology, the following revisions were detailed in MACRA:

- Established conversion factor updates:
  - a Medicare physician fee schedule conversion factor adjustment of 0.5 percent in 2016–2019 and a conversion factor adjustment of 0.00 percent for 2020–2025
  - the qualifying participant (QP) alternative payment models (APM) conversion factor of 0.75 percent and a nonqualifying provider APM conversion factor of 0.25 percent for 2026 and each subsequent year

Under the QPP, the Centers for Medicare and Medicaid Services (CMS) aims to:

- Support quality of patient care improvement by focusing on better outcomes for patients, decreasing provider burden, and preserving the independent clinical practice
- Promote the adoption of APMs, which align incentives across healthcare stakeholders
- Advance existing efforts of delivery system reform, including ensuring a smooth transition to a new system that promotes high-quality, efficient care through unification of CMS legacy programs such as the EHR incentive program

Quality Payment Program Established

The MACRA final rule established the Quality Payment Program (QPP) effective January 1, 2017. Within the QPP there are two interrelated pathways: Advanced Alternative Payment Models (APM) and the Merit-based Incentive Payment System (MIPS).

Eligible clinicians (EC) select the track/pathway—MIPS or advanced APMs—they wish to participate in based on the practice size, specialty, location, and patient population. Unlike previous quality initiatives, a provider does not have to enroll in the QPP. However, groups wishing to participate in the MIPS program via the Consumer Assessment of Healthcare Providers and Systems (CAHPS) for MIPS survey measures or CMS Web Interface (WI) must register by June 30 each year. Note that beginning with the 2022 performance period, the CMS WI will no longer be available as a submission or collection type. The CAHPS for MIPS survey is an optional quality measure that groups participating in MIPS can elect to administer.

In the 2020 Physician Fee Schedule Final Rule, CMS finalized a new participation framework to begin in 2021 known as MIPS Value Pathways (MVPs). The MVPs allow for a more cohesive participation experience by connecting activities and measures that are relevant to a specialty, medical condition, or a particular population. Due to the 2019 Coronavirus public health emergency (PHE), CMS postponed the implementation of MVPs as a reporting option for MIPS measures and activities through at least 2021. CMS finalized proposed updates for the criteria, process and MVP implementation, and anticipate the first MVP candidates to be proposed in the CY2022 notice of proposed rule making (NPRM). For additional and updated information on MVPs, see https://qpp.cms.gov/mips/mips-value-pathways.

Merit-based Incentive Payment System

MIPS is the track for clinicians who opt to participate in traditional Medicare as opposed to participating through an advanced APM. In doing so, clinicians may earn a payment adjustment related to evidence-based and practice-specific quality data. As a result, depending on the degree and success of performance in all four categories for CY 2021, clinicians receive one of the following:

- Positive payment adjustment in which additional compensation is received; bonuses are also available for meeting the exceptional performance threshold
- Neutral payment adjustment that neither increases nor reduces Medicare payments
- Negative payment adjustment of up to 9 percent of Medicare payment furnished in calendar year (CY) 2023

Participation in the MIPS track is determined based on the amount billed to Medicare and the number of beneficiaries seen per year. The following provider types are eligible for participation if they meet or exceed at least one of the following criteria:

- Medicare billings are greater than $90,000
- Care is provided for more than 200 covered services
- Care is provided to 200 or more Medicare patients each year

For 2021, the following clinician types are considered ECs:

- Physicians (MD, DO, DDS, DMD, DPM, OD)
- Physician assistants (PA)
- Nurse practitioners (NP)
- Clinical nurse specialists (CNS)
- Certified registered nurse anesthetists (CRNA)
- Physical therapists (PT)
- Occupational therapists (OT)
- Qualified speech-language pathologists
- Qualified audiologists
- Clinical psychologists
- Osteopathic practitioners
- Chiropractor
- Registered dieticians or nutrition professionals
- Any clinician group that includes one of the professionals listed above

Anatomy of MIPS

A measurement-based regime creates a single reporting framework for physicians that comprise four performance categories:

- Quality
- Improvement Activities (IA)—implemented in 2017
- Promoting Interoperability
- Cost

MIPS eligible clinicians may participate in the program as an individual clinician, group, virtual group, or APM entity (applicable for 2021). Each of the four performance categories has been weighted, with greatest emphasis placed on the Quality category. Performance category weights for individuals, groups, and virtual groups placed the Quality category at 40 percent, Promoting Interoperability is second at 25 percent, IA at 15 percent, and Cost at 20 percent. Performance category weights for APM entities reporting traditional MIPS for the 2021 performance period are weighted differently than these participation levels. The emphasis is still on the Quality category at 50 percent, Promoting Interoperability is second at 30 percent, Improvement Activities is third at 20 percent, and Cost is at 0 percent. Beginning with the 2022 performance period regardless of participation level (e.g., individual, group, etc.) the quality and cost performance categories will be equally weighted at 30%.

The 2021 MIPS performance threshold equates to 60 points out of a possible 100 points. Simply put, eligible clinicians are required to score 60 points to avoid the negative 9 percent payment adjustment.

Quality Performance

Under the MIPS Quality performance category, ECs and groups must select six measures from a listing of more than 200 measures, with at least one of the six measures being an outcome measure, high-priority measure (in absences of outcome measure), or complete specialty measure set. Patient outcomes such as mortality, whether a patient is readmitted to the hospital, and the patient's experience are areas that CMS and the healthcare industry seek to improve. An outcome measure is the way CMS can quantify changes in the health of an individual, groups of individuals, and even certain populations that they can attribute back to a specific intervention or series of interventions.

Quality measures are tools for quantifying, or measuring, healthcare processes and patient outcomes and perceptions, as well as organizational structure and/or systems linked to the ability to provide high-quality healthcare. These measures play an important role under the MIPS. Reporting should be done on a minimum of half of the EC's or group practice's Medicare Part B patients. Performance data is reported for 70 percent of the patients who qualify for each measure. Each measure is worth up to 10 points and is compared to a national benchmark.

Improvement Activities

The IA category assesses to what degree a clinician participates in activities designed to improve clinical practices. ECs are required to attest that they have participated in two high-weighted activities, one high-weighted activity and two medium-weighted activities, or four medium-weighted activities. The activities may be selected from an expanded inventory of more than 100 activities across eight subcategories for 90 consecutive days. These eight subcategories include:

- Expanded practice access
- Population management
- Care coordination
- Beneficiary engagement
- Patient safety and practice assessment
- Achieving health equity
- Integrating behavioral and mental health
- Emergency preparedness and response

This category was created with some inherent flexibility; for example, for groups with 15 or fewer participants, nonpatient-facing clinicians (e.g., pathologists), or those ECs in a rural or health professional shortage area (HPSA) receive two times the points when they report activities for at least 90 consecutive days.

Promoting Interoperability

CMS wants to encourage and promote the use of certified EHR technology (CEHRT) among providers and, in particular, the use of interoperability and sharing of information among clinicians and between providers and patients. In response to the 21st Century Cures Act Final Rule, CMS updated the CEHRT requirements to include technology certified to the 2015 Edition Cures Update certification criteria, the current 2015 Edition certification criteria, or a combination of both criteria to collect and report PI data.

Successful reporting of measures in this category require the EC to report measures from the four objectives and measures based exclusively on the 2015 edition of CEHRT and, as applicable, claim an exclusion. Exclusions are reported by submitting a "0" in addition to the exclusion type that applies to the EC because some measures may be associated with more than one exclusion.

The PI performance category contains four objectives:

- E-Prescribing
- Health Information Exchange
- Provider to Patient Exchange
- Public Health and Clinical Data Exchange

Data collected for each of the four objectives must be submitted for the same minimum continuous 90 days (unless an exclusion is applicable).

Cost

In this performance category, CMS determines an EC or group practice's cost score by calculating data from two measures previously included in the value-based payment modifier that involves the total cost of care for attributed beneficiaries and what Medicare spends per beneficiary. This amount is the total of both Medicare Part A and B payments from three days before through 30 days after a beneficiary has had an inpatient hospitalization episode. CMS then determines which ECs and practices have an adequate number of beneficiaries and hospitalizations associated with them. This number is compared with national benchmarks established for the performance period.

There are a total of 20 cost measures:

- Total Per Capita Cost (TPCC)
- Medicare Spending Per Beneficiary Clinician (MSPB Clinician)
- 13 Procedural episode-based measures and 5 acute inpatient medical condition episode-based measures (18 measures)

For procedure episodes, the case minimum established is 10 with credit for the episodes going to the clinician who performs the procedure. For acute inpatient medical condition episodes, the case minimum is set at 20, and credit is assigned to each clinician who bills the inpatient evaluation and management (E/M) claim lines during a triggered inpatient hospitalization under a TIN that furnishes at least 30 percent of the inpatient E/M claim lines during that particular hospitalization.

Clinicians have no additional submission responsibilities associated with this category as the score is determined from Medicare administrative claims data.

The category also has separate benchmarks. The Cost score is determined and compared with those benchmarks with points assigned based on the decile system in a similar manner to the Quality performance category with some differences such as:

- Benchmarks for performance are for the *same* year versus prior year performance.
- Scores are determined once case minimum requirements for each of the two measures in this category have been met.

MIPS Scoring

CMS uses scoring to determine an EC's successful participation in the QPP and thereby determine if the clinician's reimbursement will be negative, neutral, or positive.

The scoring methodology is a unified approach across all performance categories, allowing eligible clinicians to understand what is expected so they can perform successfully in the MIPS. For more information and details on QPP, see https:/qpp.cms.gov.

Illustrations

Chapter 3. Diseases of the Blood and Blood-forming Organs and Certain Disorders Involving the Immune Mechanism (D50–D89)

Red Blood Cells

White Blood Cell

Platelet

Coagulation

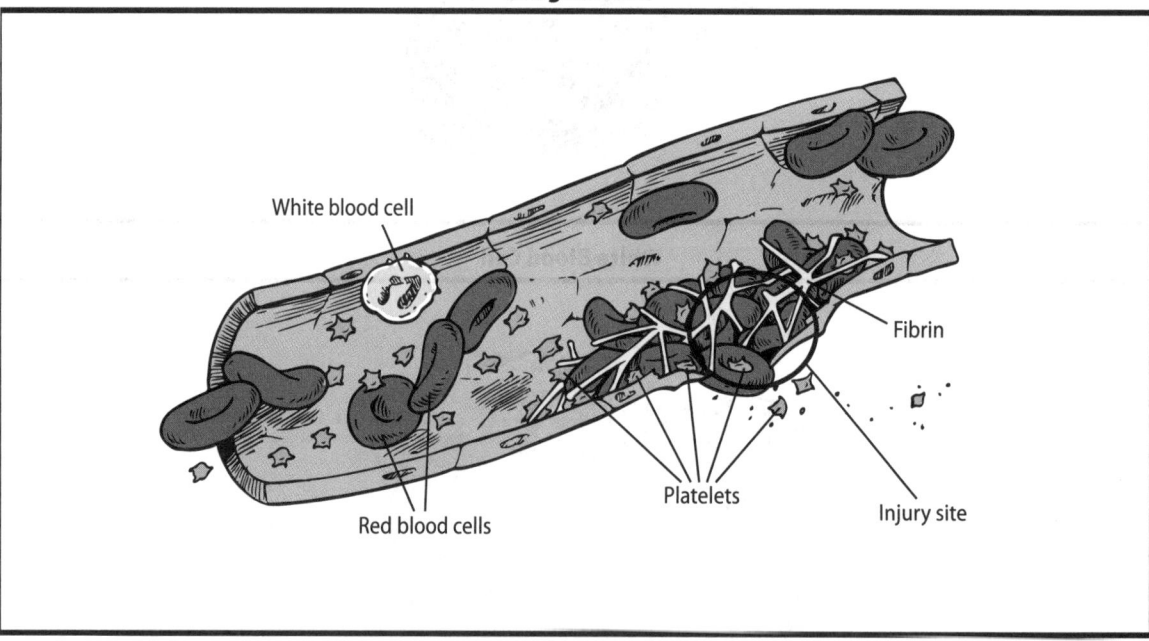

Spleen Anatomical Location and External Structures

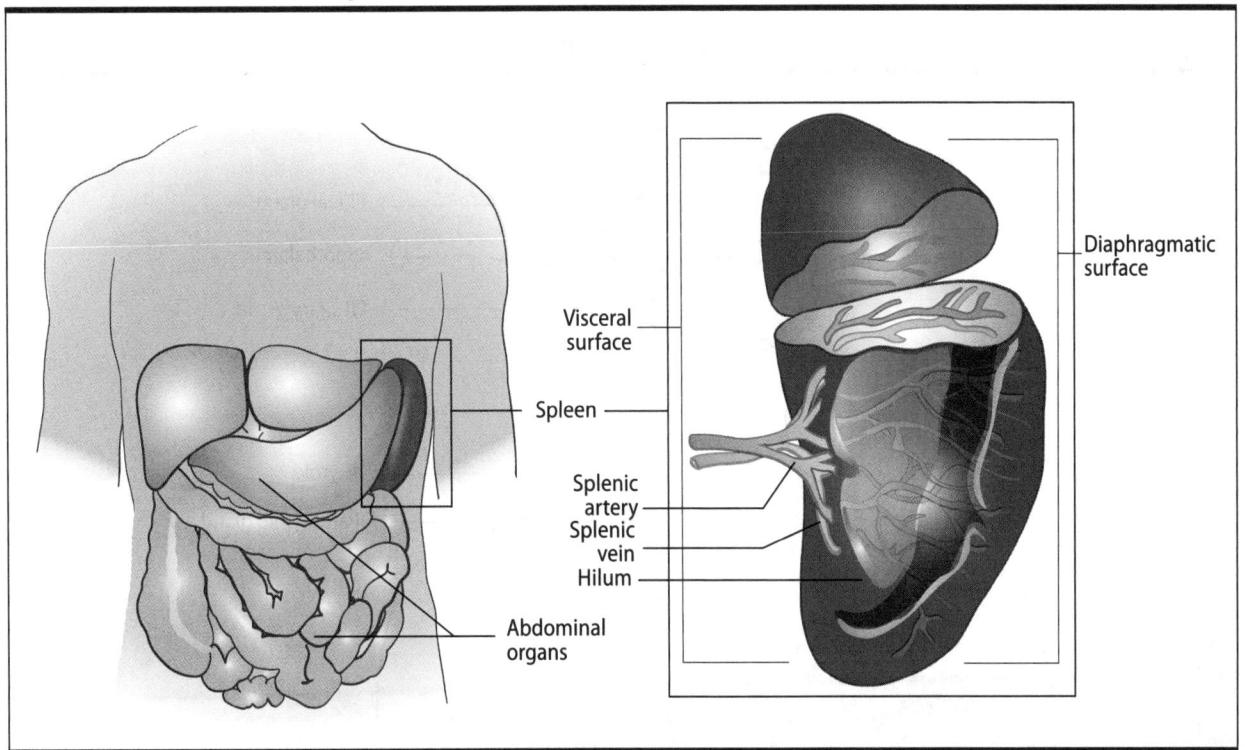

Spleen Interior Structures

Chapter 4. Endocrine, Nutritional and Metabolic Diseases (E00–E89)

Endocrine System

Thyroid

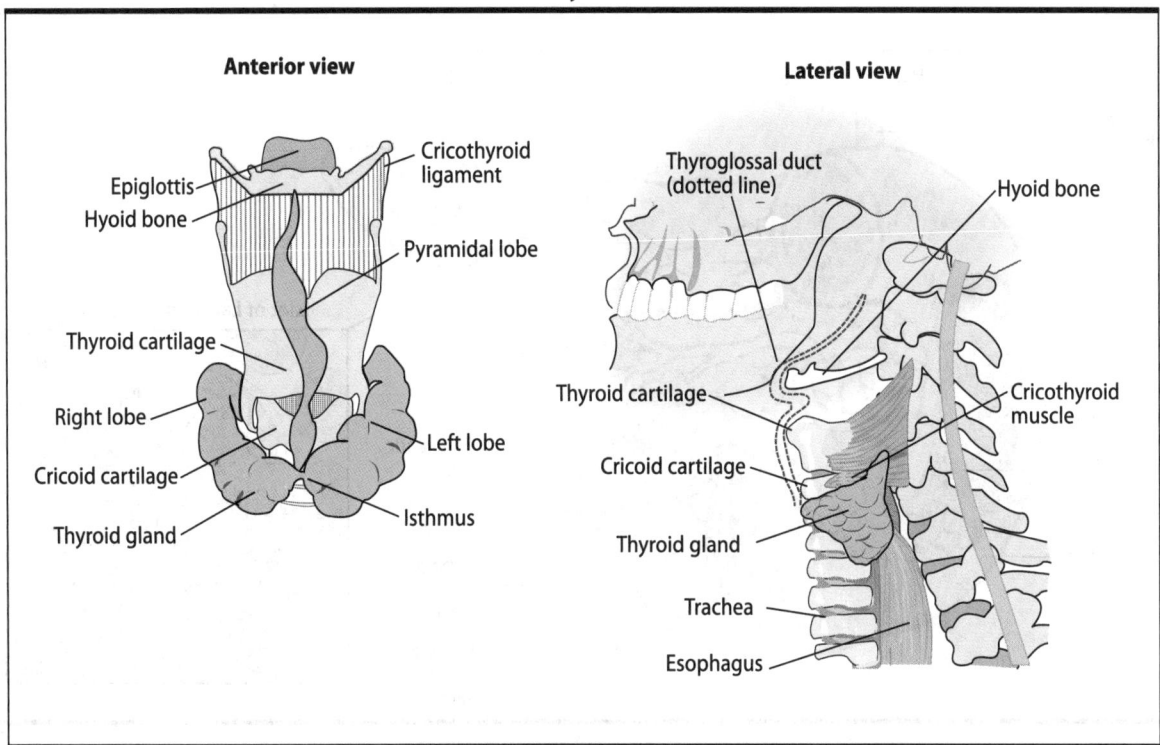

Thyroid and Parathyroid Glands

Pancreas

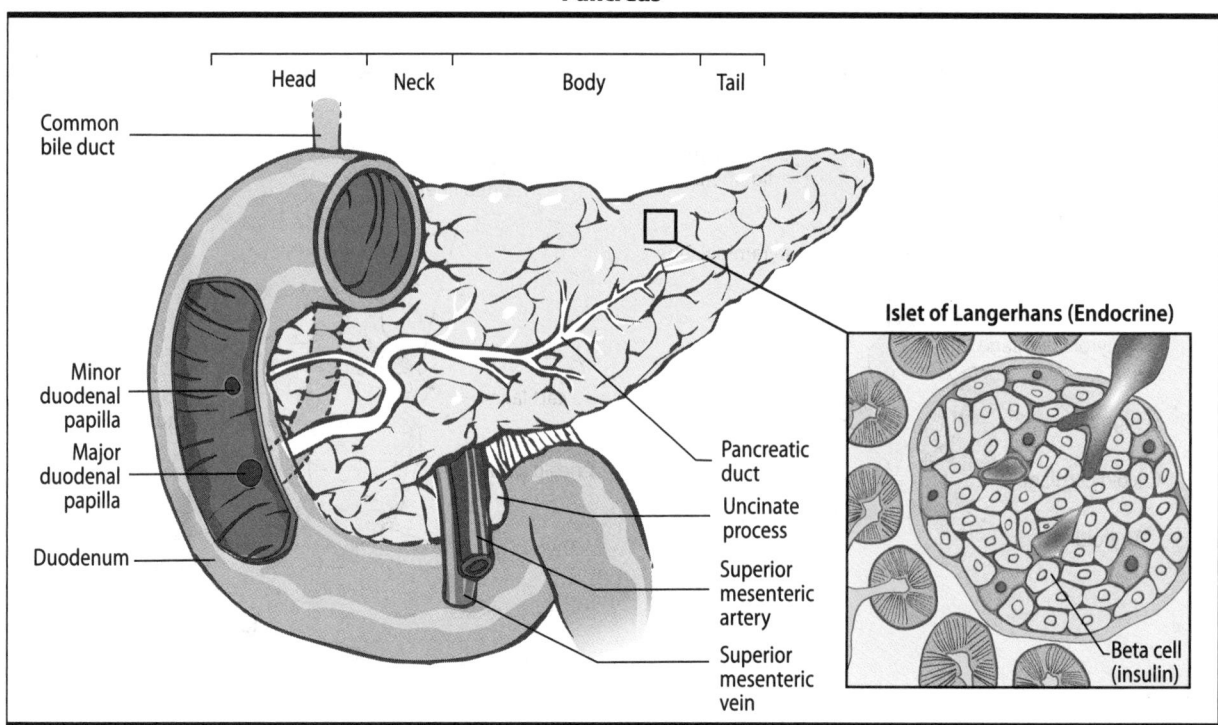

Head   Neck   Body   Tail

Common bile duct

Minor duodenal papilla

Major duodenal papilla

Duodenum

Pancreatic duct

Uncinate process

Superior mesenteric artery

Superior mesenteric vein

Islet of Langerhans (Endocrine)

Beta cell (insulin)

Anatomy of the Adrenal Gland

Adrenal glands

Kidney

Capsule

Cortex

Medulla

Structure of an Ovary

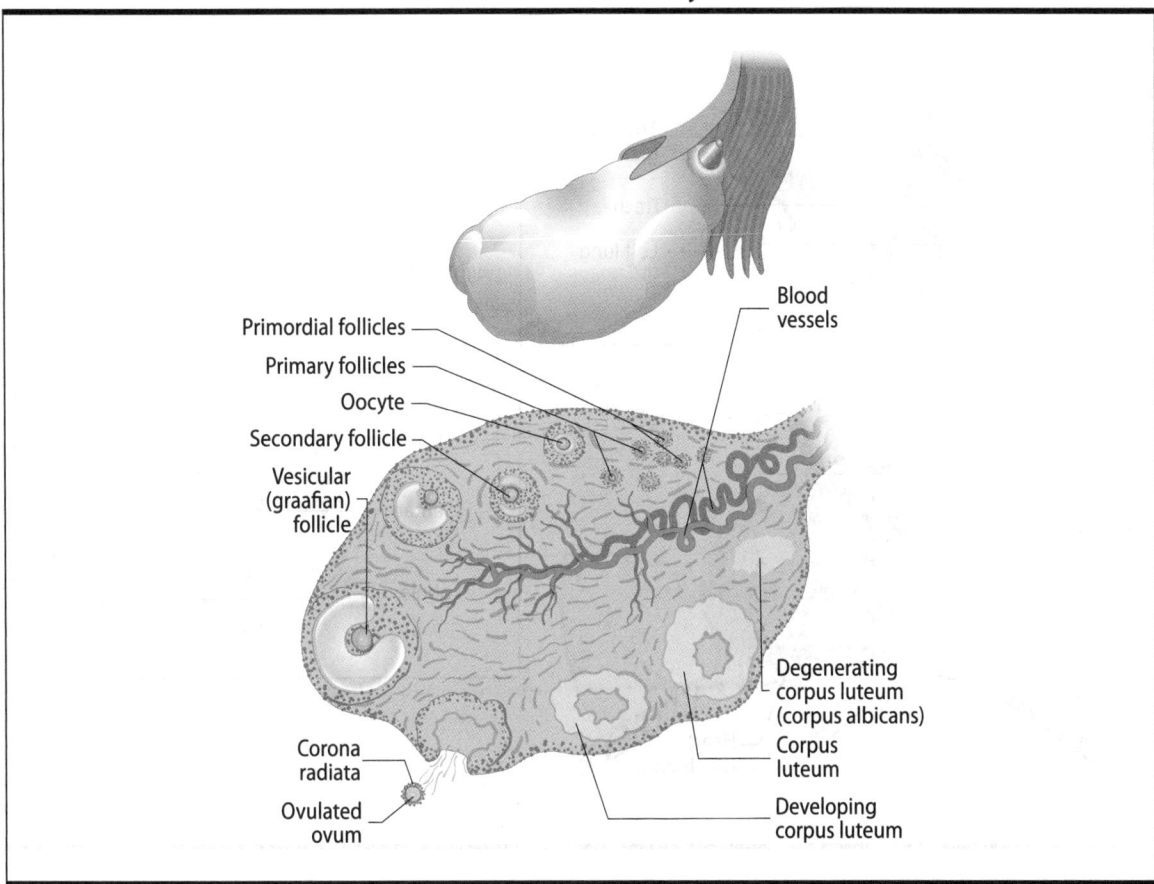

Testis and Associated Structures

Thymus

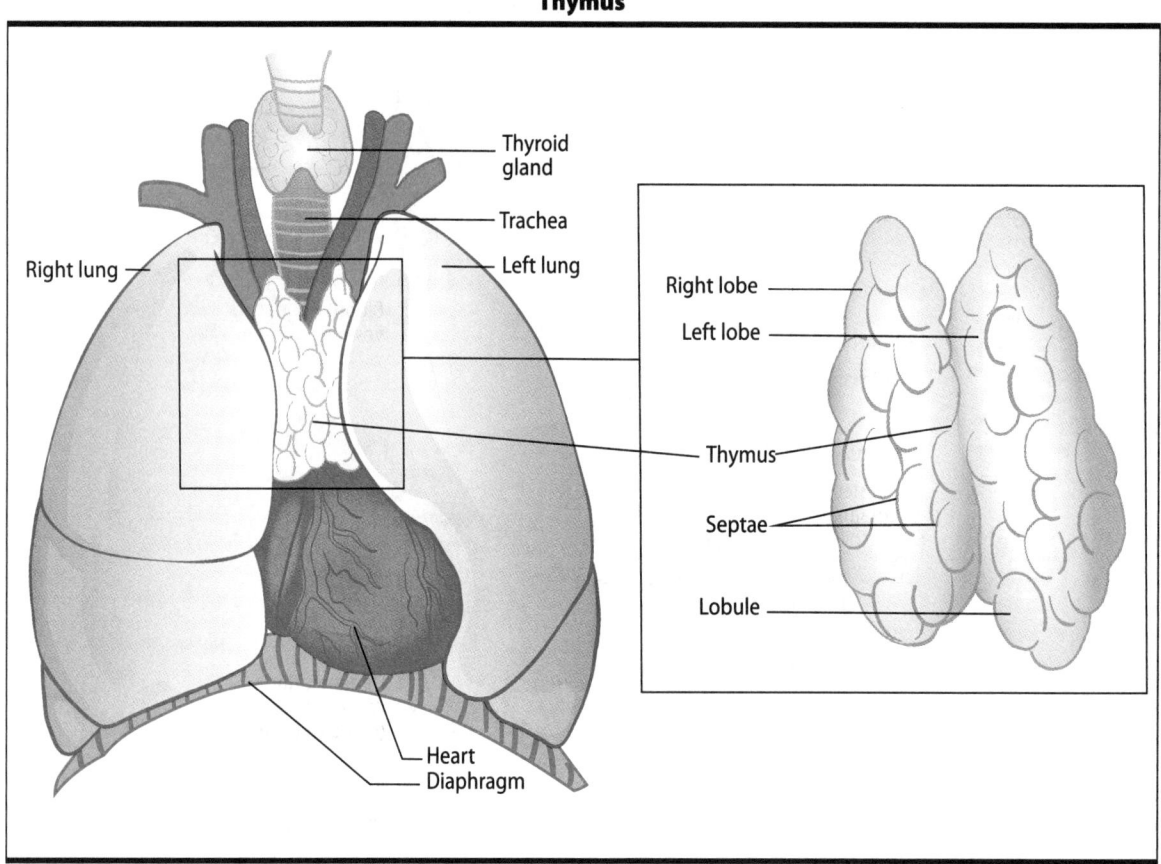

Chapter 6. Diseases of the Nervous System (G00–G99)

Brain

Cranial Nerves

Peripheral Nervous System

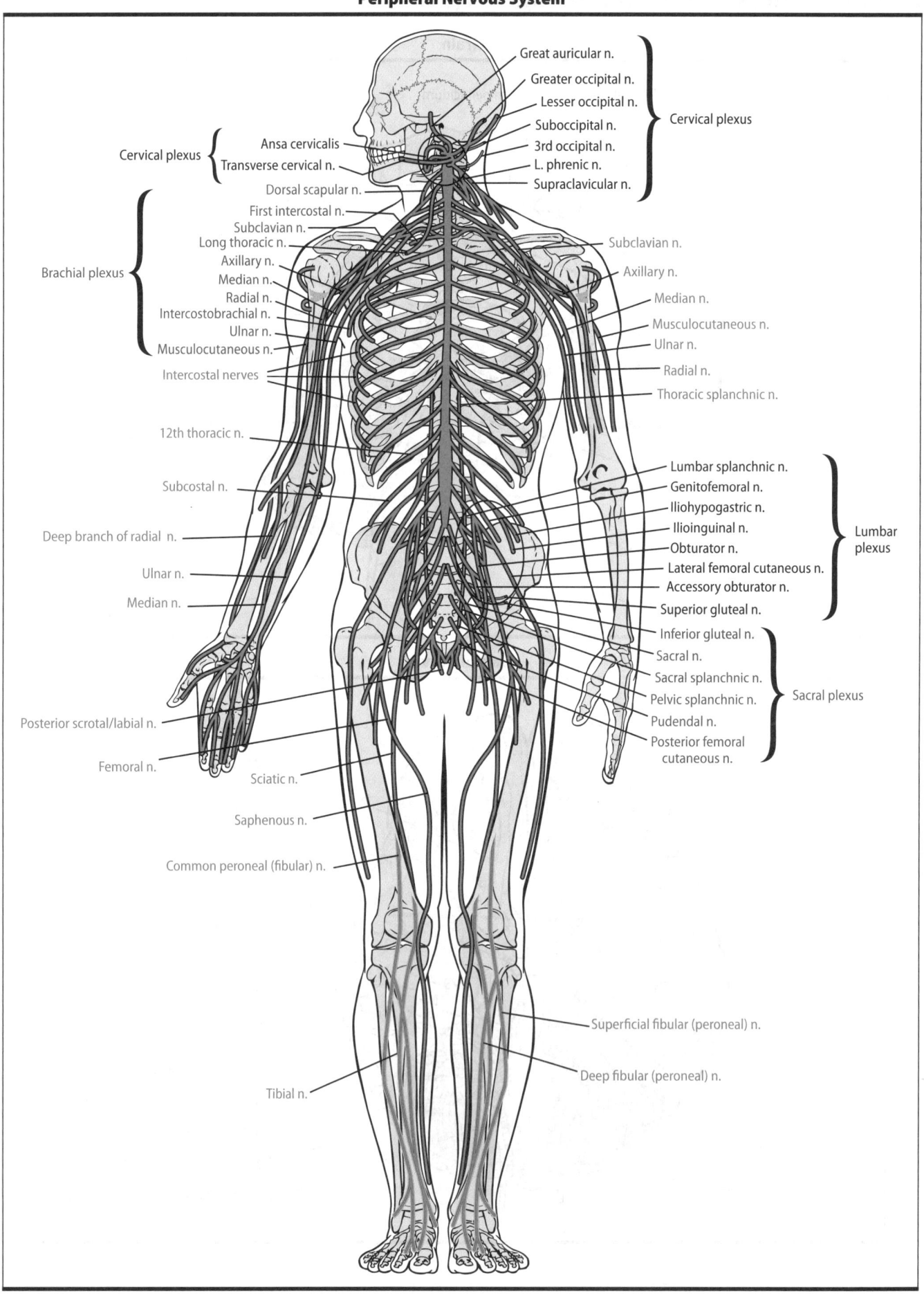

Great auricular n.
Greater occipital n.
Lesser occipital n.
Suboccipital n.
3rd occipital n.
L. phrenic n.
Supraclavicular n.
Cervical plexus

Ansa cervicalis
Transverse cervical n.
Cervical plexus

Dorsal scapular n.
First intercostal n.
Subclavian n.
Long thoracic n.
Axillary n.
Median n.
Radial n.
Intercostobrachial n.
Ulnar n.
Musculocutaneous n.
Intercostal nerves
Brachial plexus

Subclavian n.
Axillary n.
Median n.
Musculocutaneous n.
Ulnar n.
Radial n.
Thoracic splanchnic n.

12th thoracic n.

Subcostal n.

Deep branch of radial n.

Ulnar n.

Median n.

Lumbar splanchnic n.
Genitofemoral n.
Iliohypogastric n.
Ilioinguinal n.
Obturator n.
Lateral femoral cutaneous n.
Accessory obturator n.
Superior gluteal n.
Lumbar plexus

Inferior gluteal n.
Sacral n.
Sacral splanchnic n.
Pelvic splanchnic n.
Pudendal n.
Posterior femoral cutaneous n.
Sacral plexus

Posterior scrotal/labial n.

Femoral n.

Sciatic n.

Saphenous n.

Common peroneal (fibular) n.

Superficial fibular (peroneal) n.

Deep fibular (peroneal) n.

Tibial n.

Spinal Cord and Spinal Nerves

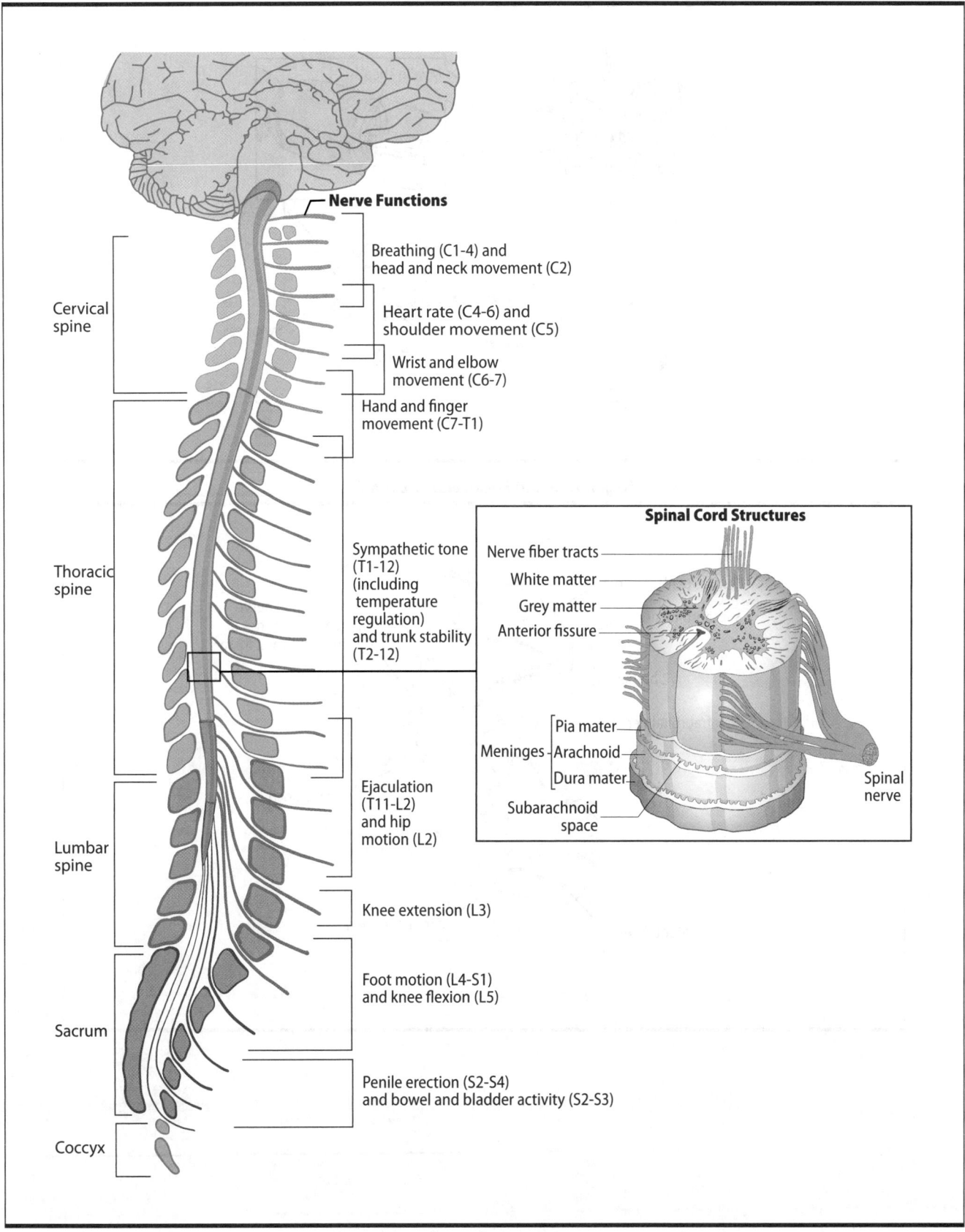

Nerve Functions

Breathing (C1-4) and
head and neck movement (C2)

Heart rate (C4-6) and
shoulder movement (C5)

Wrist and elbow
movement (C6-7)

Hand and finger
movement (C7-T1)

Sympathetic tone
(T1-12)
(including
temperature
regulation)
and trunk stability
(T2-12)

Ejaculation
(T11-L2)
and hip
motion (L2)

Knee extension (L3)

Foot motion (L4-S1)
and knee flexion (L5)

Penile erection (S2-S4)
and bowel and bladder activity (S2-S3)

Cervical spine

Thoracic spine

Lumbar spine

Sacrum

Coccyx

Spinal Cord Structures

Nerve fiber tracts

White matter

Grey matter

Anterior fissure

Pia mater

Meninges — Arachnoid

Dura mater

Subarachnoid space

Spinal nerve

Nerve Cell

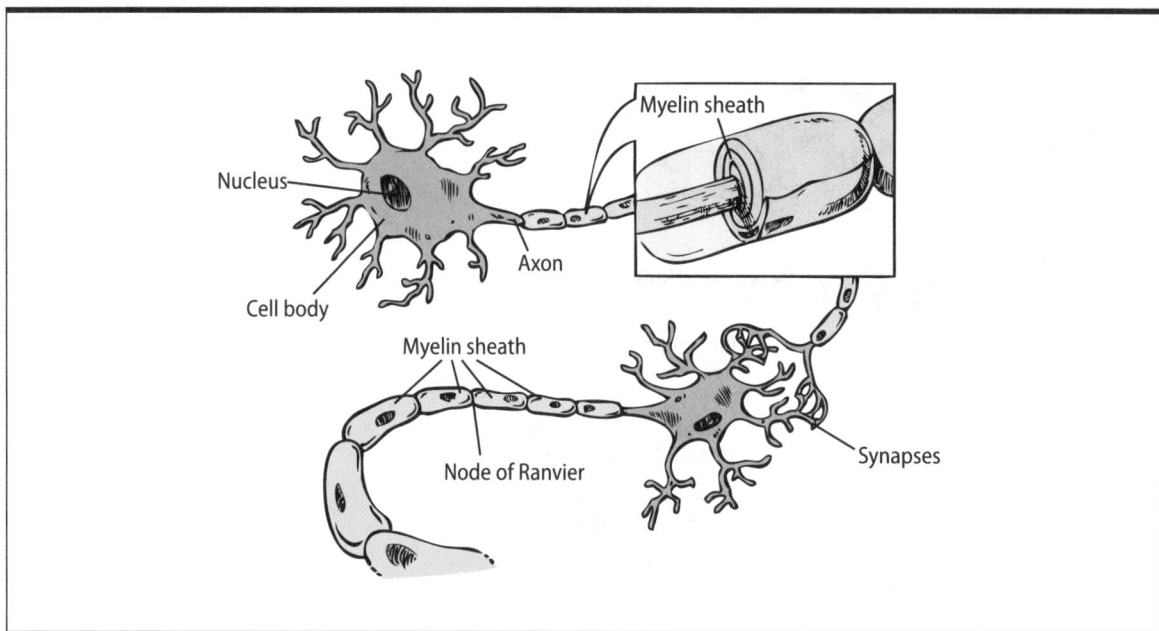

Trigeminal and Facial Nerve Branches

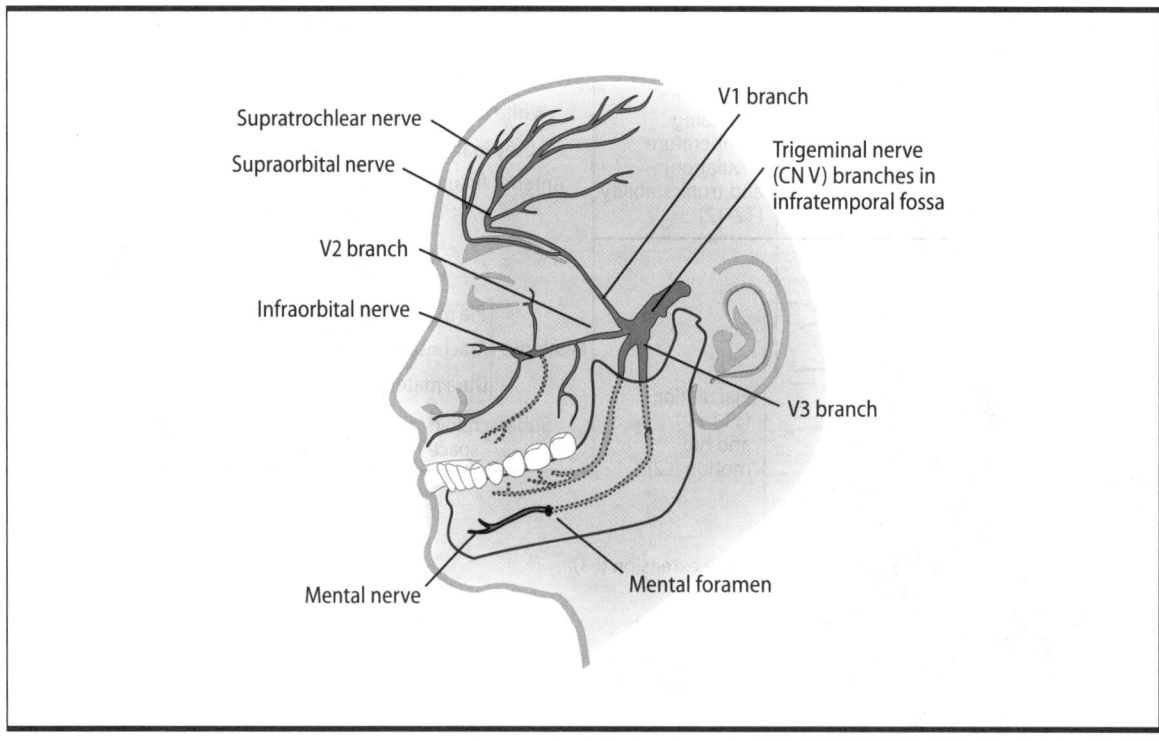

Chapter 7. Diseases of the Eye and Adnexa (H00–H59)

Eye

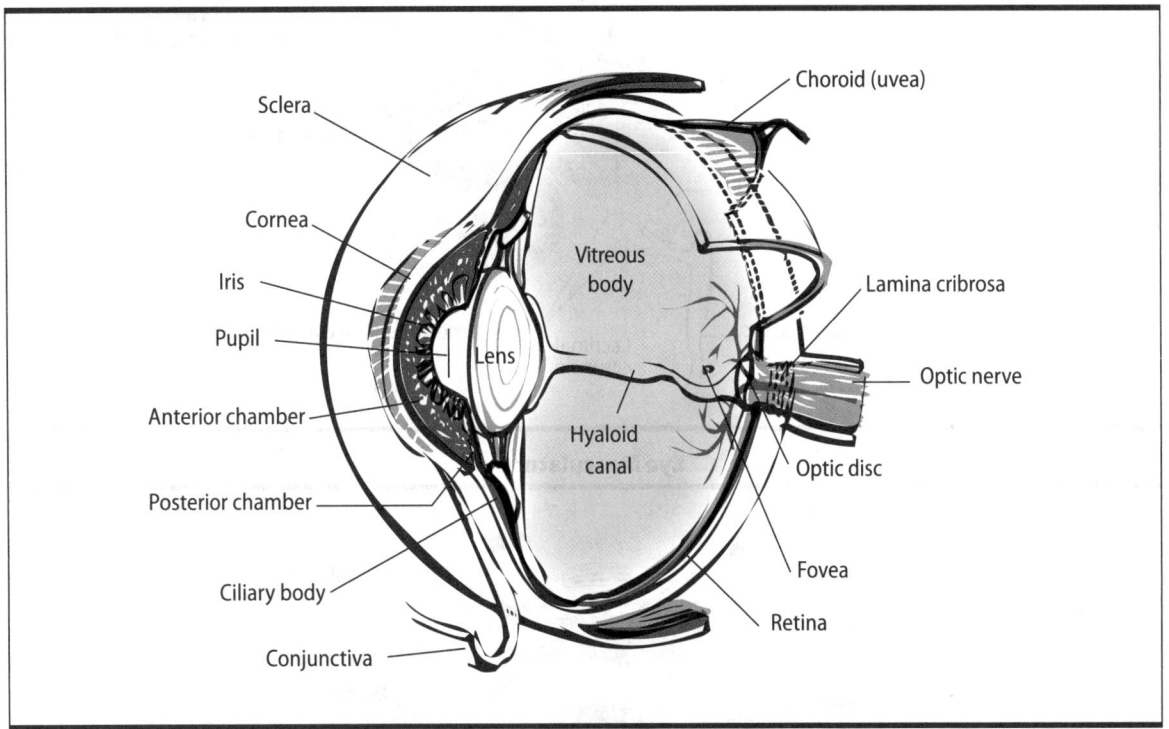

Posterior Pole of Globe/Flow of Aqueous Humor

Lacrimal System

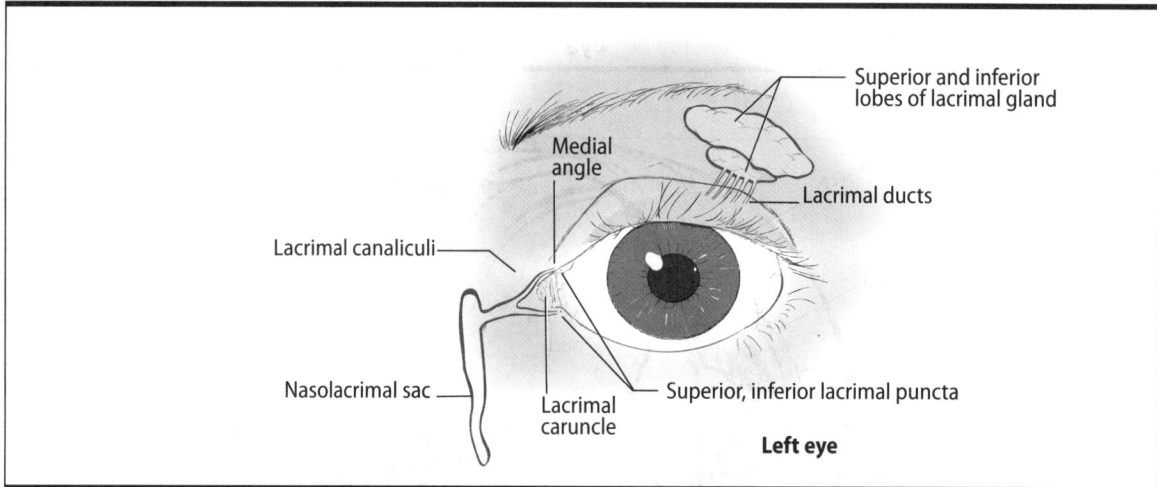

Superior and inferior lobes of lacrimal gland

Medial angle

Lacrimal ducts

Lacrimal canaliculi

Nasolacrimal sac

Lacrimal caruncle

Superior, inferior lacrimal puncta

Left eye

Eye Musculature

Superior rectus

Superior oblique

Lateral rectus

Medial rectus

Inferior rectus

Inferior oblique

Muscles and actions (right eye)

Eyelid Structures

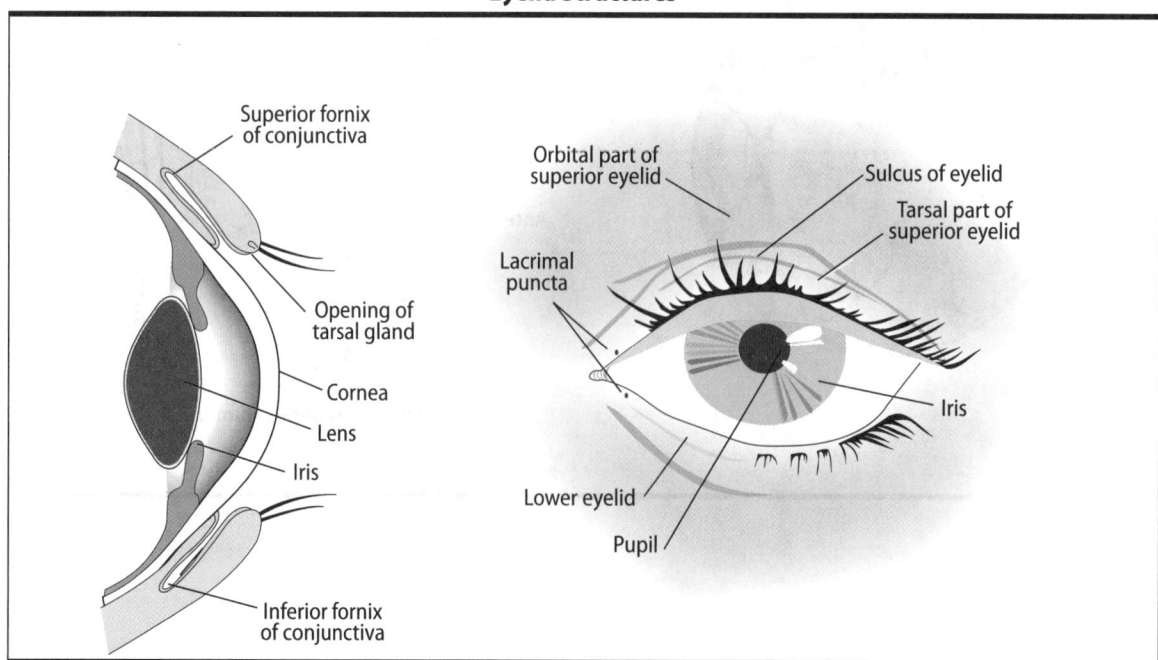

Superior fornix of conjunctiva

Opening of tarsal gland

Cornea

Lens

Iris

Inferior fornix of conjunctiva

Orbital part of superior eyelid

Sulcus of eyelid

Tarsal part of superior eyelid

Lacrimal puncta

Iris

Lower eyelid

Pupil

Chapter 8. Diseases of the Ear and Mastoid Process (H6Ø–H95)

Ear Anatomy

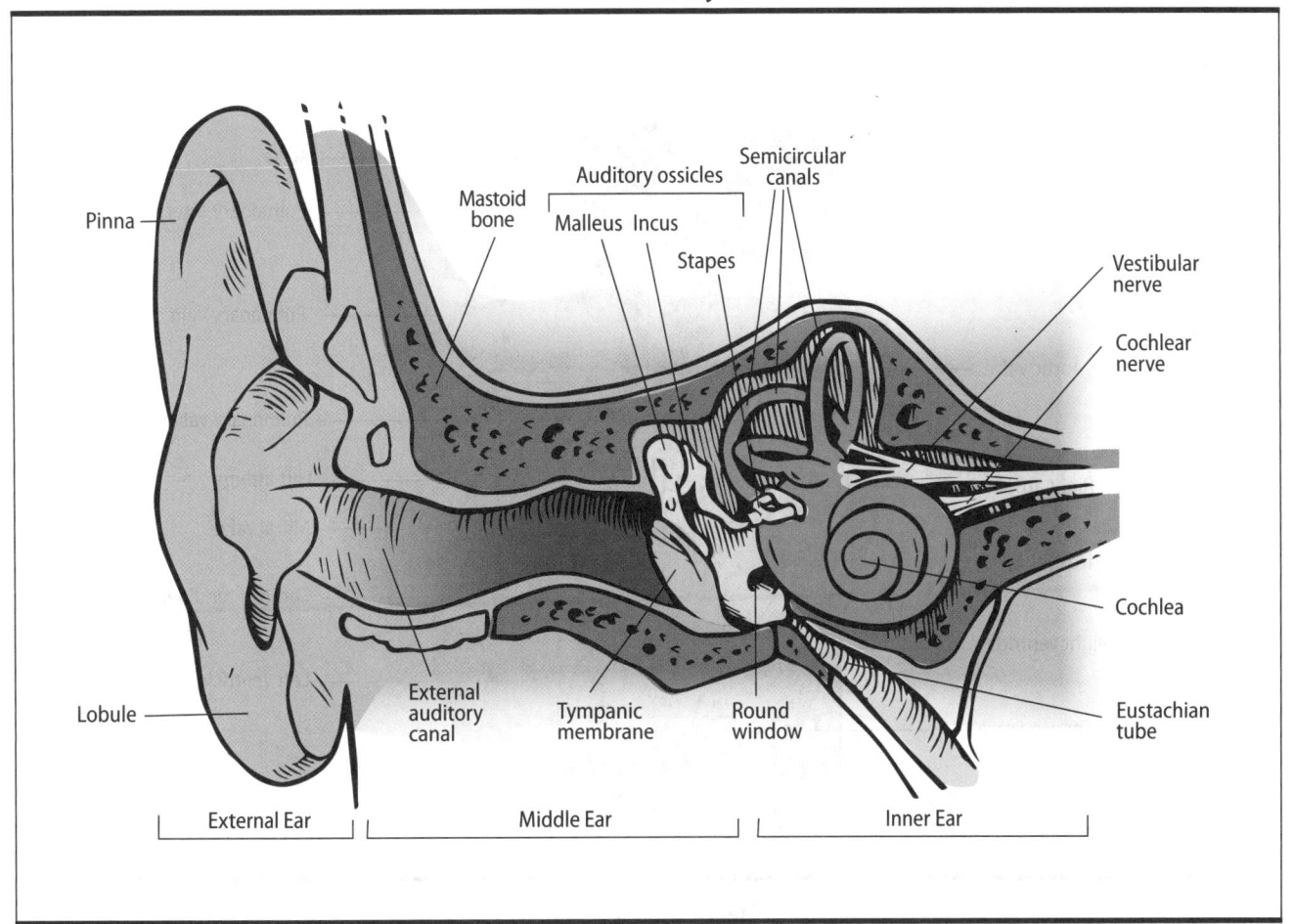

Chapter 9. Diseases of the Circulatory System (I00–I99)

Anatomy of the Heart

Heart Cross Section

Heart Valves

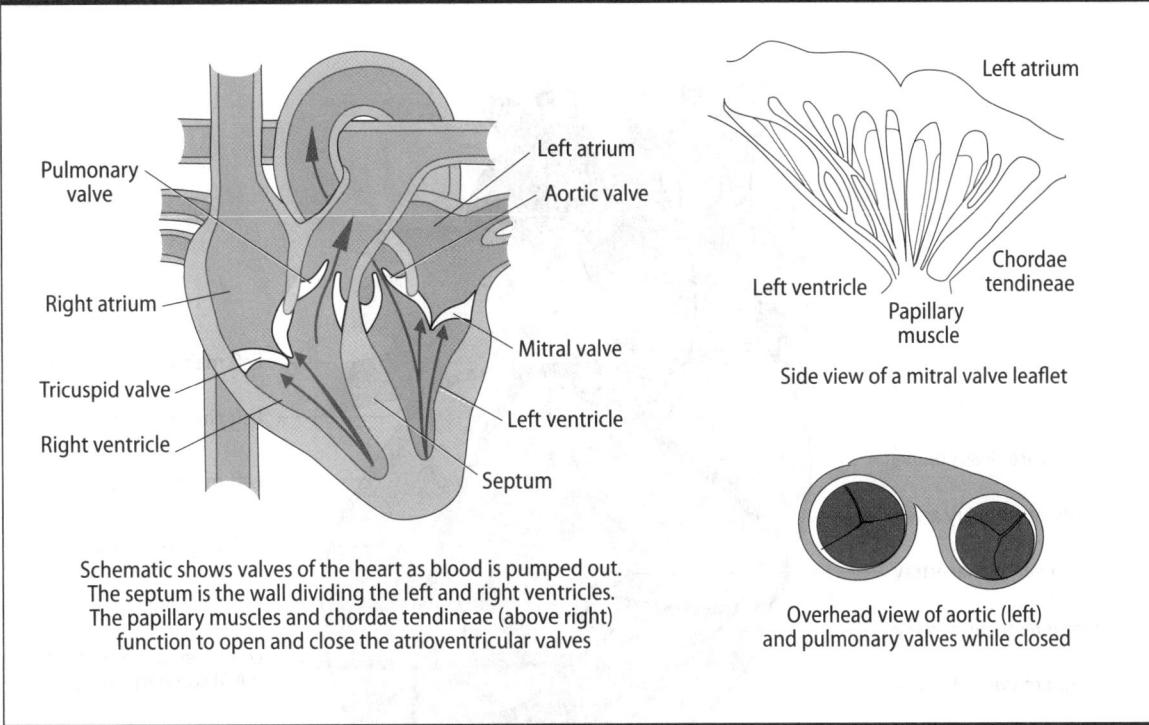

Schematic shows valves of the heart as blood is pumped out.
The septum is the wall dividing the left and right ventricles.
The papillary muscles and chordae tendineae (above right)
function to open and close the atrioventricular valves

Side view of a mitral valve leaflet

Overhead view of aortic (left)
and pulmonary valves while closed

Heart Conduction System

Coronary Arteries

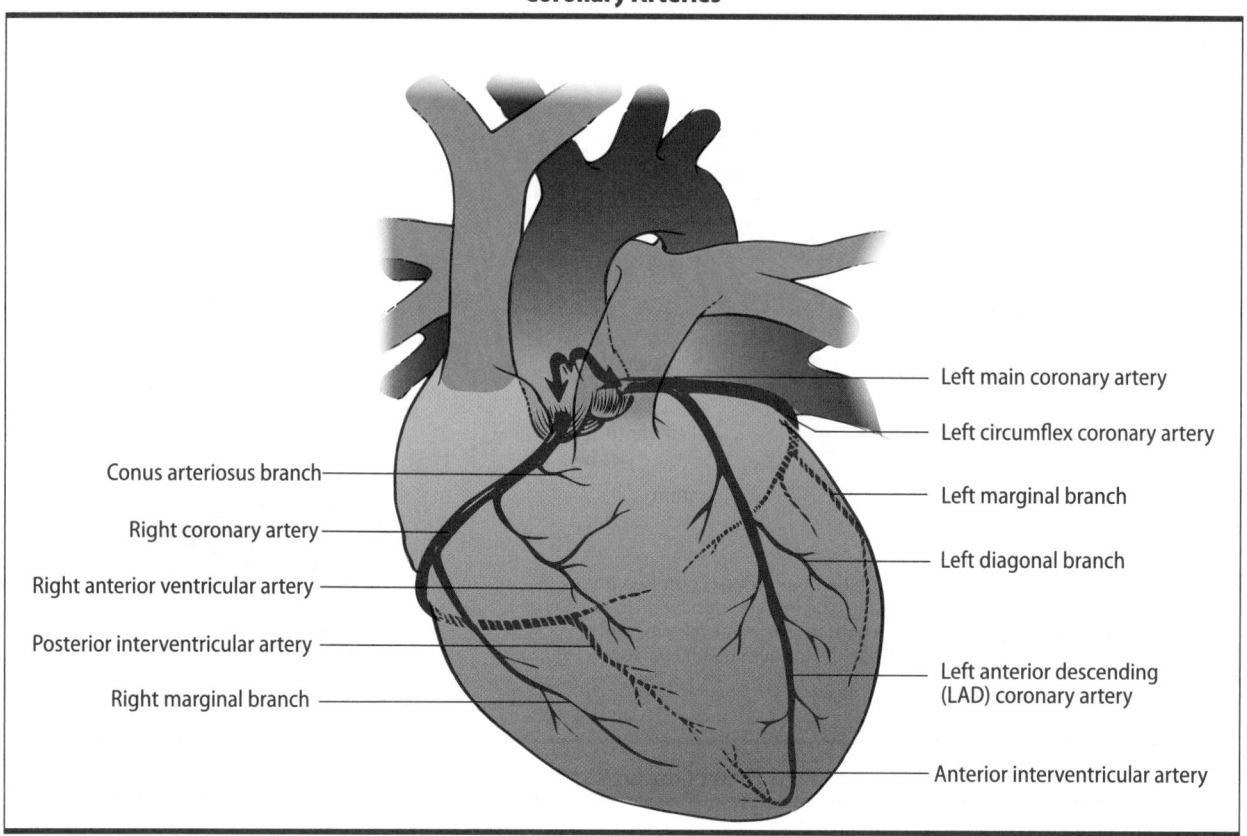

Left main coronary artery

Left circumflex coronary artery

Conus arteriosus branch

Left marginal branch

Right coronary artery

Left diagonal branch

Right anterior ventricular artery

Posterior interventricular artery

Left anterior descending (LAD) coronary artery

Right marginal branch

Anterior interventricular artery

Arteries

Veins

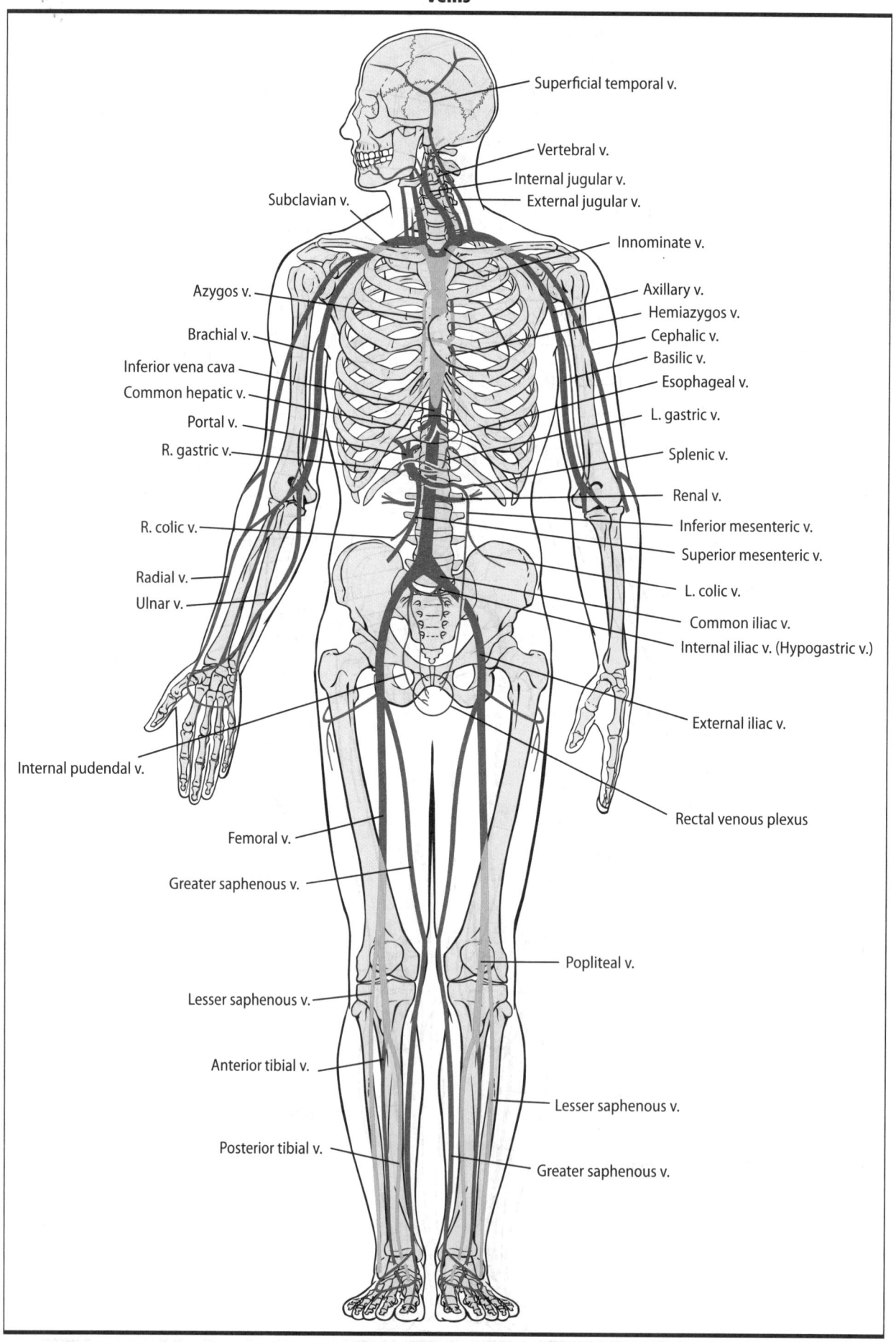

Internal Carotid and Vertebral Arteries and Branches

Side View

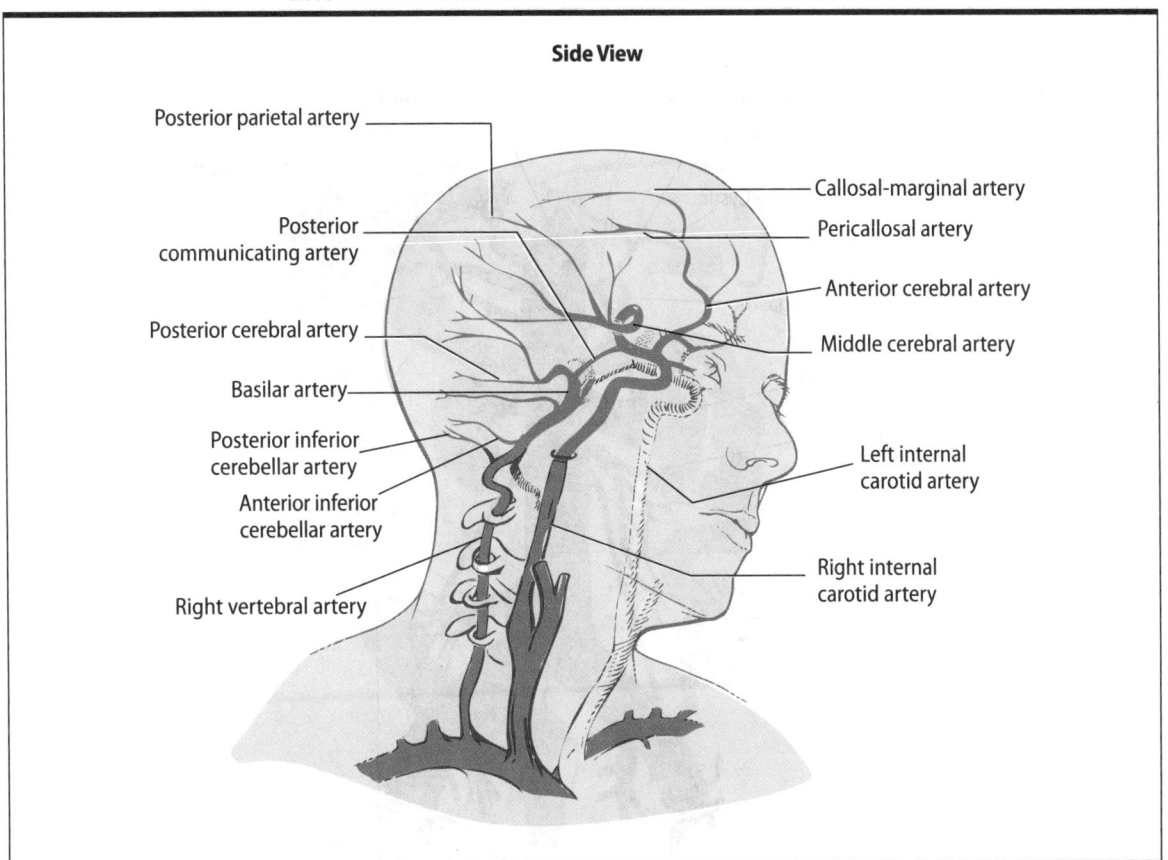

External Carotid Artery and Branches

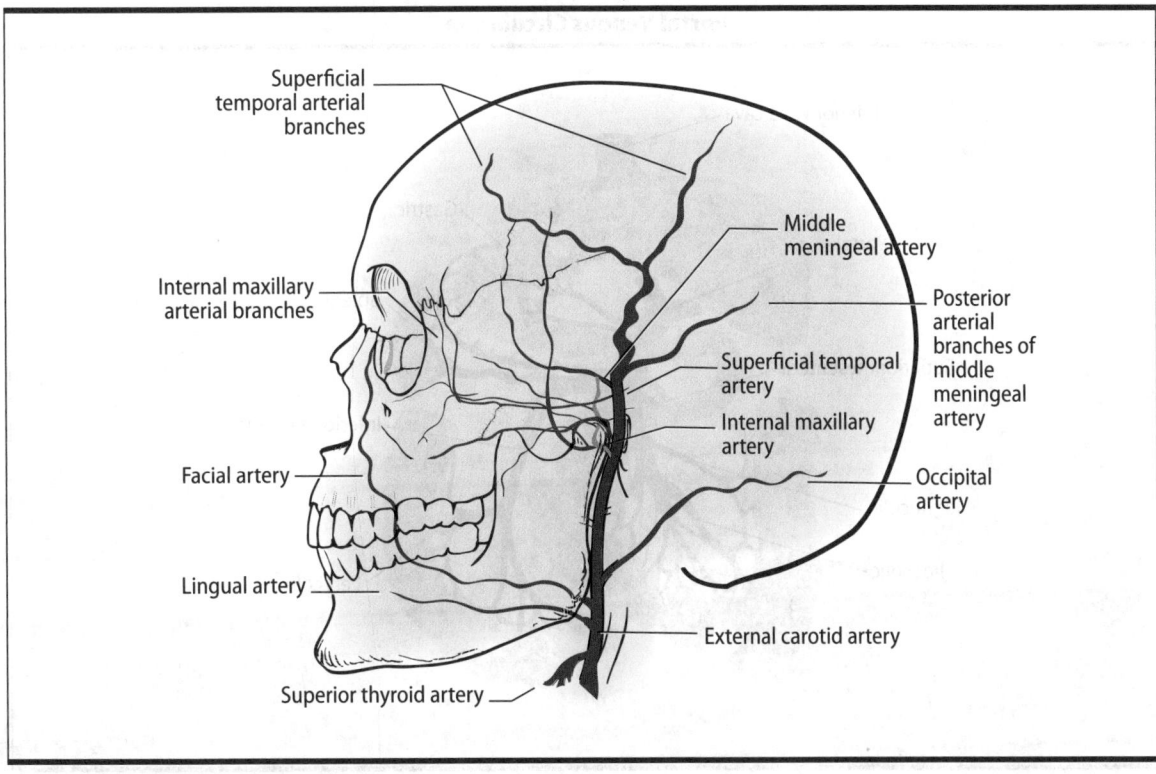

Branches of Abdominal Aorta

Portal Venous Circulation

Lymphatic System

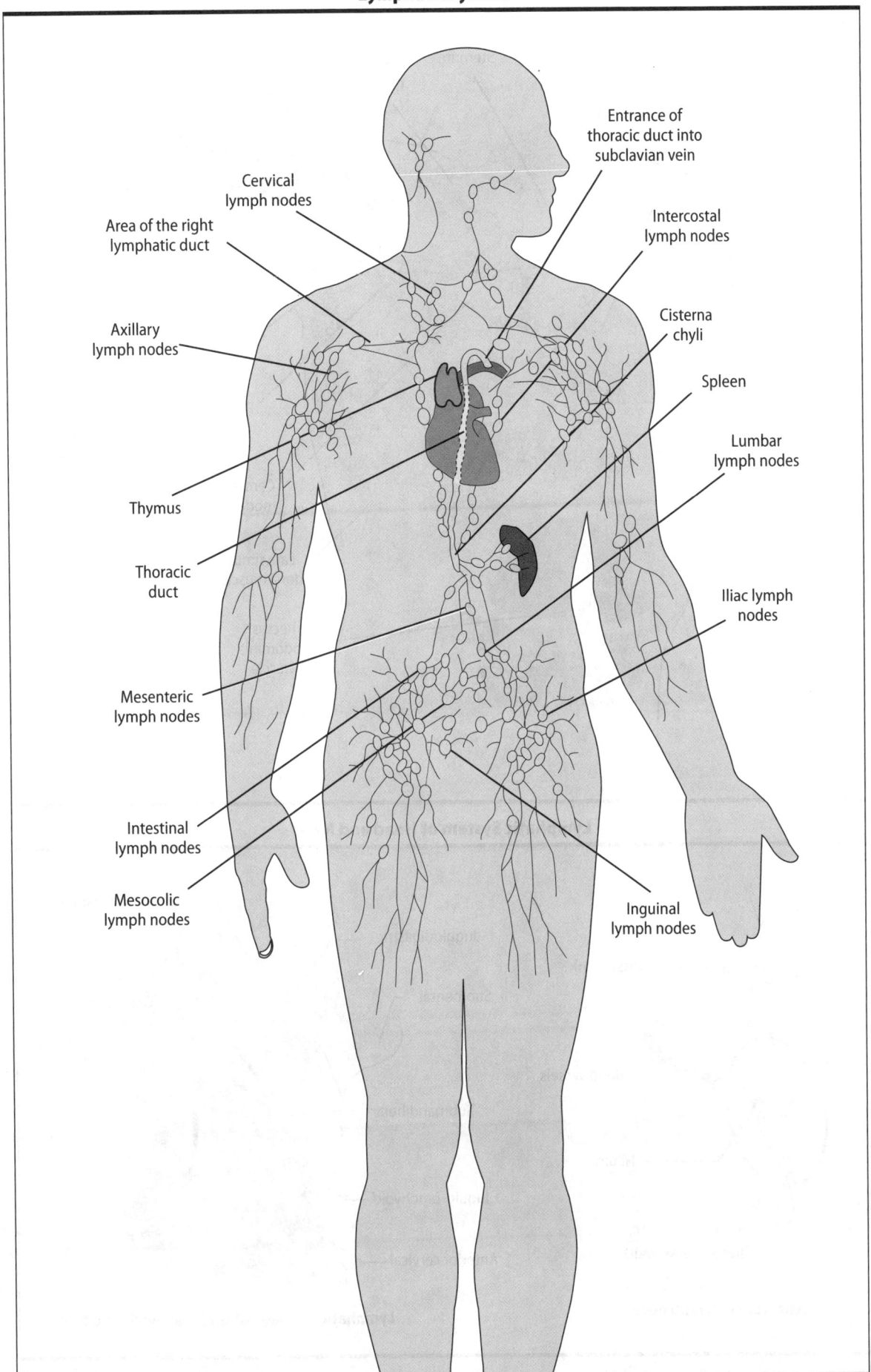

Axillary Lymph Nodes

Sternum

Clavicle

Deltoid muscle

Brachialis muscle

Parasternal nodes

Lateral nodes

Subscapular nodes

Pectoral nodes

Axillary lymph nodes

Central nodes

Latissimus dorsi muscle

Rectus abdominis muscle

Lymphatic System of Head and Neck

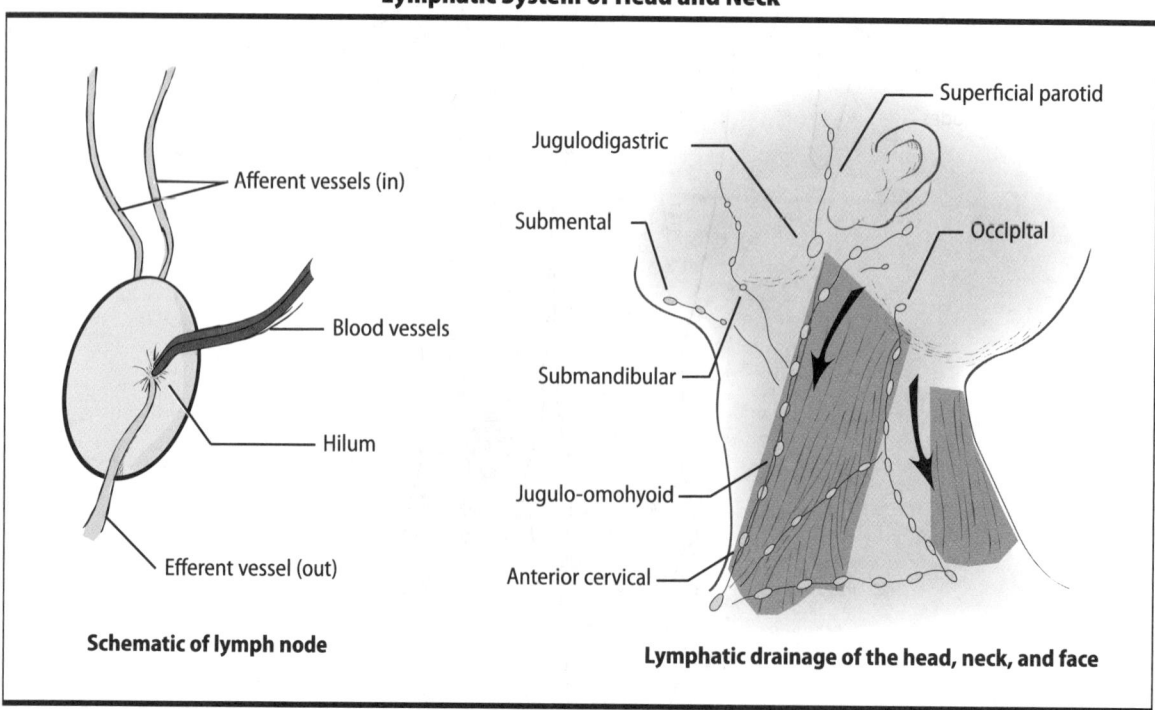

Afferent vessels (in)

Jugulodigastric

Superficial parotid

Submental

Occipital

Blood vessels

Submandibular

Hilum

Jugulo-omohyoid

Efferent vessel (out)

Anterior cervical

Schematic of lymph node

Lymphatic drainage of the head, neck, and face

Lymphatic Capillaries

Schematic of lymphatic capillaries

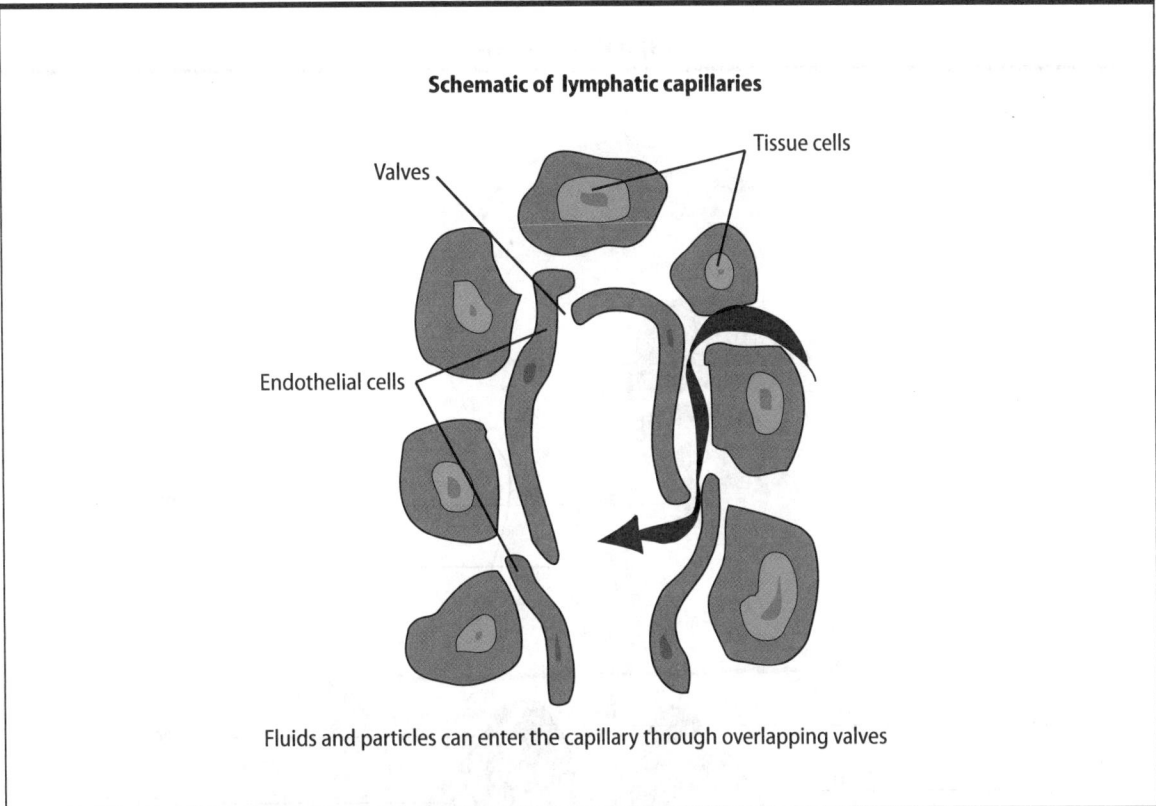

Fluids and particles can enter the capillary through overlapping valves

Lymphatic Drainage

Lymphatic drainage of the colon follows blood supply

Chapter 10. Diseases of the Respiratory System (J00–J99)

Respiratory System

Upper Respiratory System

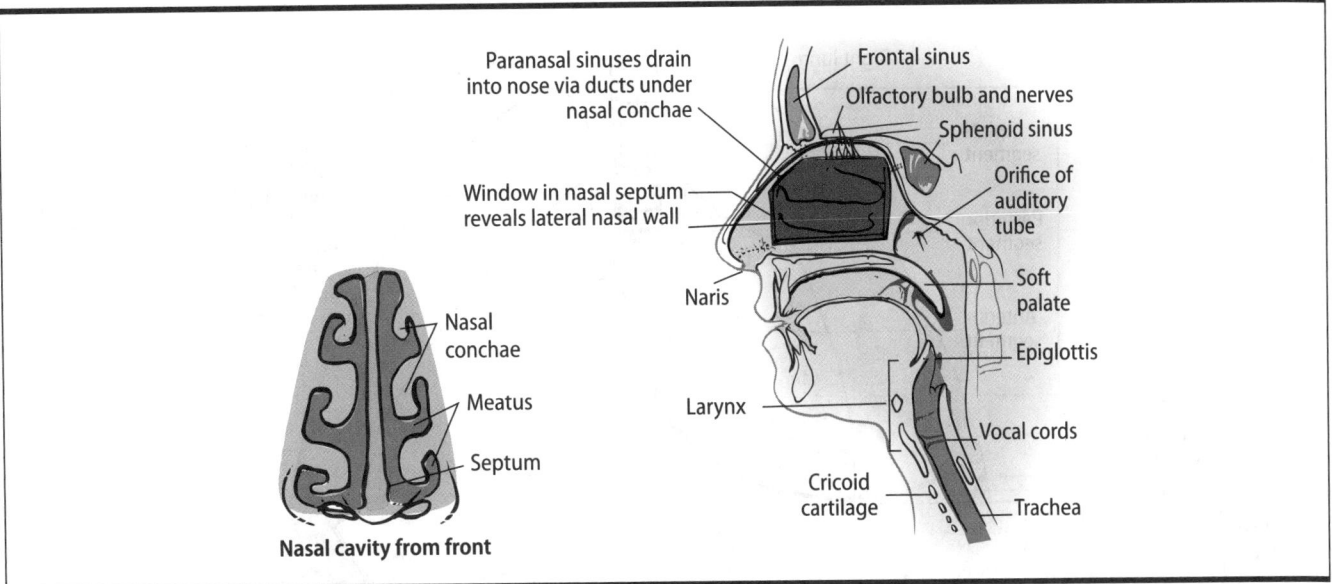

Paranasal sinuses drain into nose via ducts under nasal conchae

Window in nasal septum reveals lateral nasal wall

Naris

Frontal sinus

Olfactory bulb and nerves

Sphenoid sinus

Orifice of auditory tube

Soft palate

Epiglottis

Larynx

Vocal cords

Cricoid cartilage

Trachea

Nasal conchae

Meatus

Septum

Nasal cavity from front

Lower Respiratory System

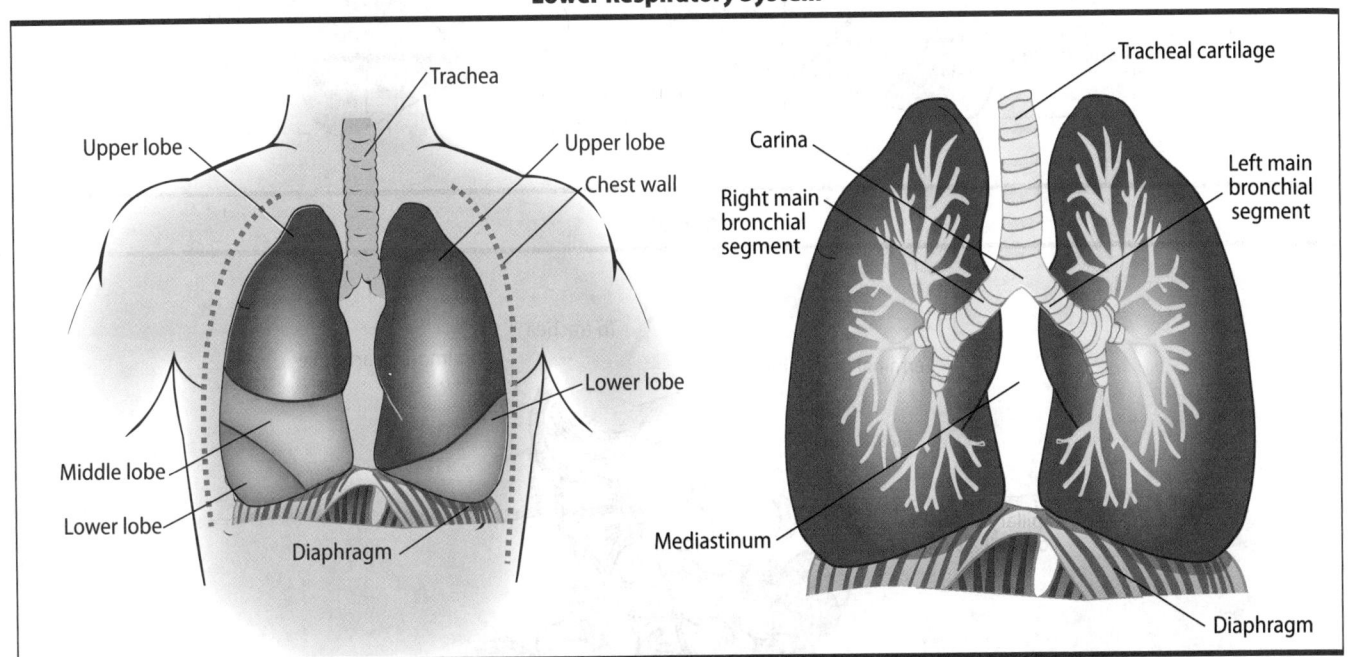

Trachea

Upper lobe

Upper lobe

Chest wall

Lower lobe

Middle lobe

Lower lobe

Diaphragm

Tracheal cartilage

Carina

Right main bronchial segment

Left main bronchial segment

Mediastinum

Diaphragm

Paranasal Sinuses

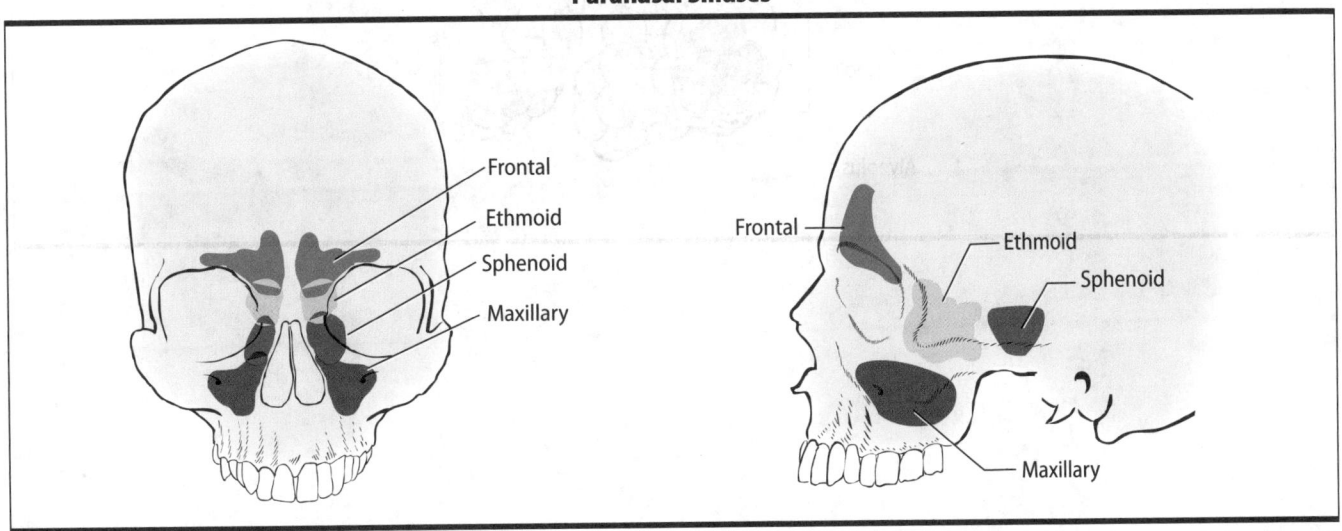

Frontal

Ethmoid

Sphenoid

Maxillary

Frontal

Ethmoid

Sphenoid

Maxillary

Lung Segments

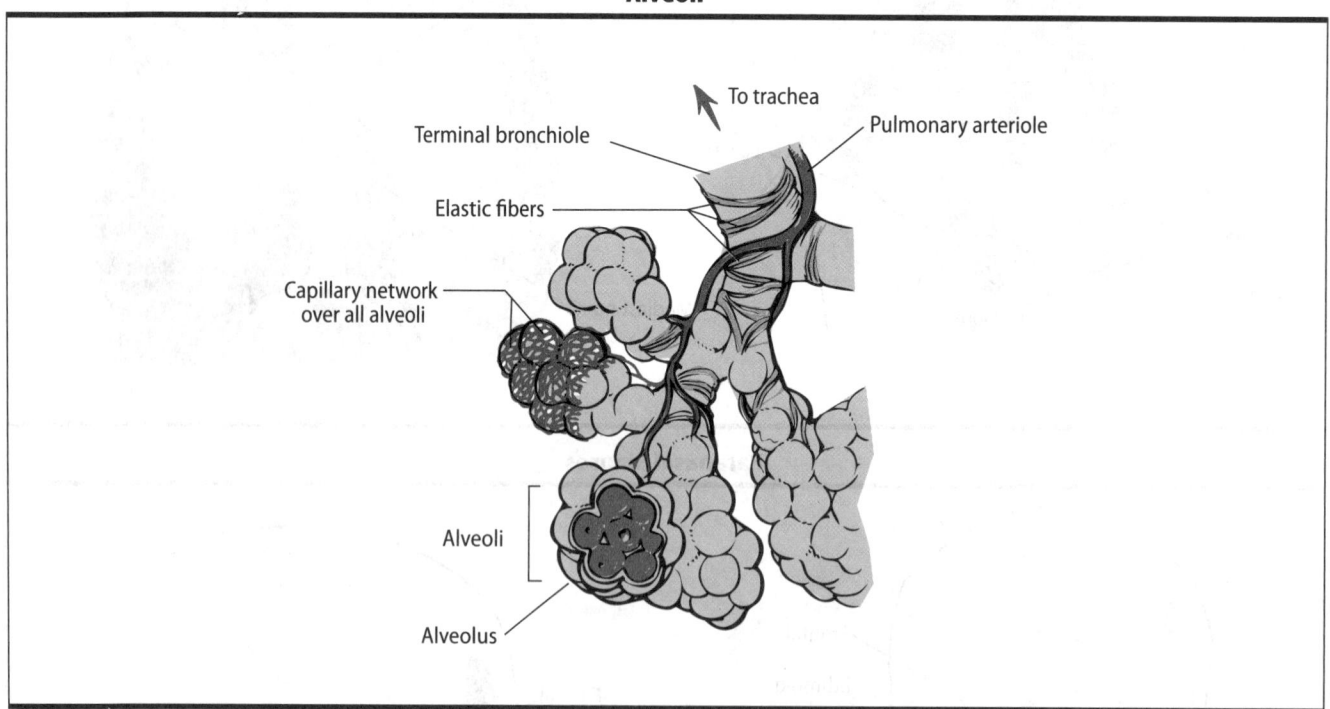

Right lung

Left lung

Apical segment

Apical-posterior segment

Anterior segment

Superior lobe

Posterior segment

Superior lingular segment

Superior lobe

Anterior segment

Inferior lingular segment

Medial basal segment

Superior basal segment

Lateral segment

Lateral basal segment

Middle lobe

Superior segment

Inferior lobe

Inferior lobe

Posterior basal segment

Anterior medial segment

Anterior basal segment

Horizontal fissure

Oblique fissures

Alveoli

To trachea

Terminal bronchiole

Pulmonary arteriole

Elastic fibers

Capillary network over all alveoli

Alveoli

Alveolus

Chapter 11. Diseases of the Digestive System (K00–K95)

Digestive System

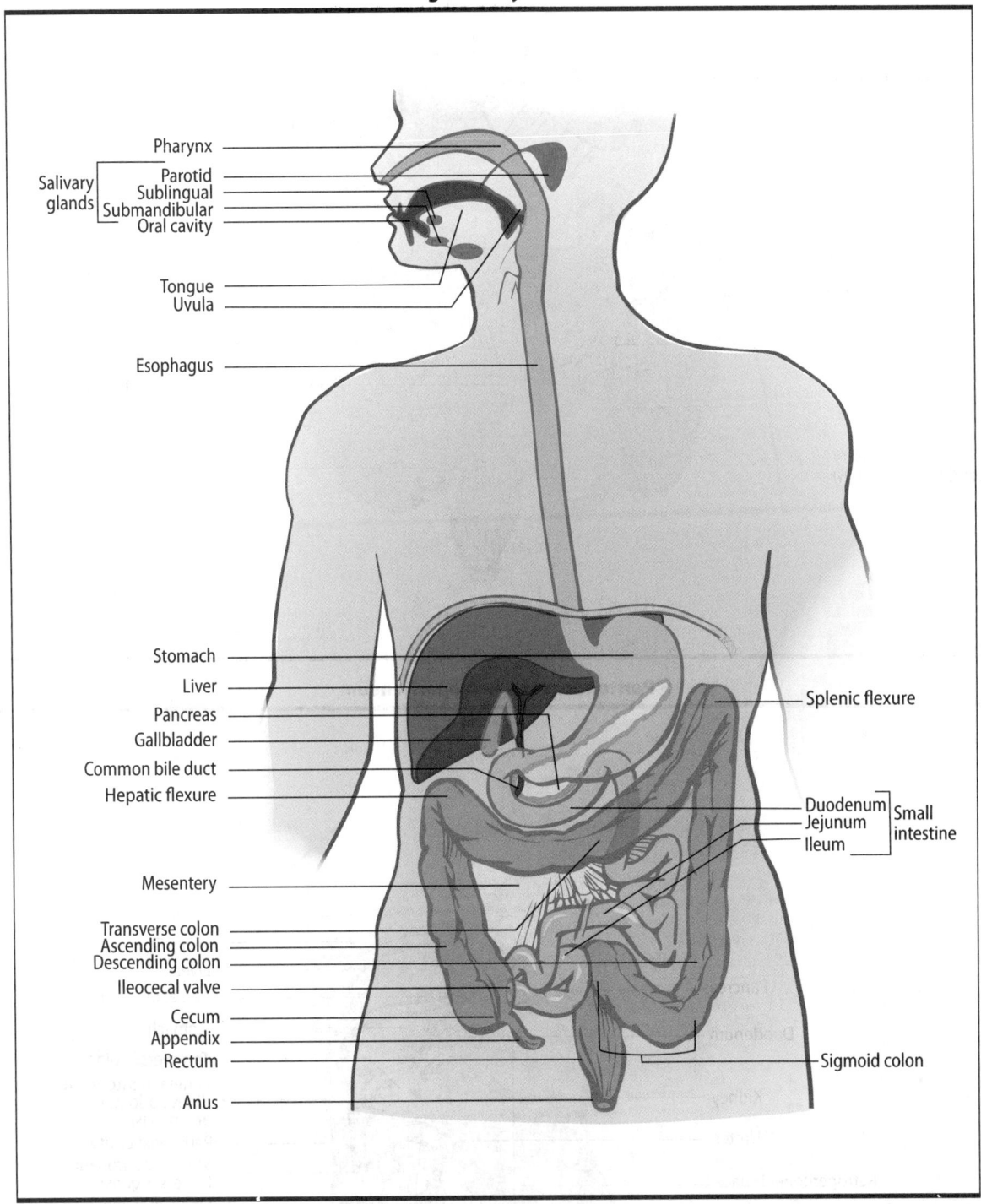

Omentum and Mesentery

Lesser omentum

Greater omentum
(cut edge)

Transverse colon

Ascending colon

Descending
colon

Small intestine

Mesentery
(transverse mesocolon)

Mesentery proper

Mesentery
(descending mesocolon)

Mesentery
(ascending mesocolon)

Sigmoid colon

Peritoneum and Retroperitoneum

Pancreas

Duodenum

Diaphragm

Liver

Lesser omentum

Stomach

Transverse colon

Kidney

Parietal peritoneum
(lines abdomen
and pelvis)

Ureter

Peritoneal cavity

Retroperitoneal space

Visceral peritoneum
(covers organs)

Small intestine

Mesentery

Greater omentum

Sigmoid colon

Bladder

Rectum

Chapter 12. Diseases of the Skin and Subcutaneous Tissue (LØØ–L99)

Nail Anatomy

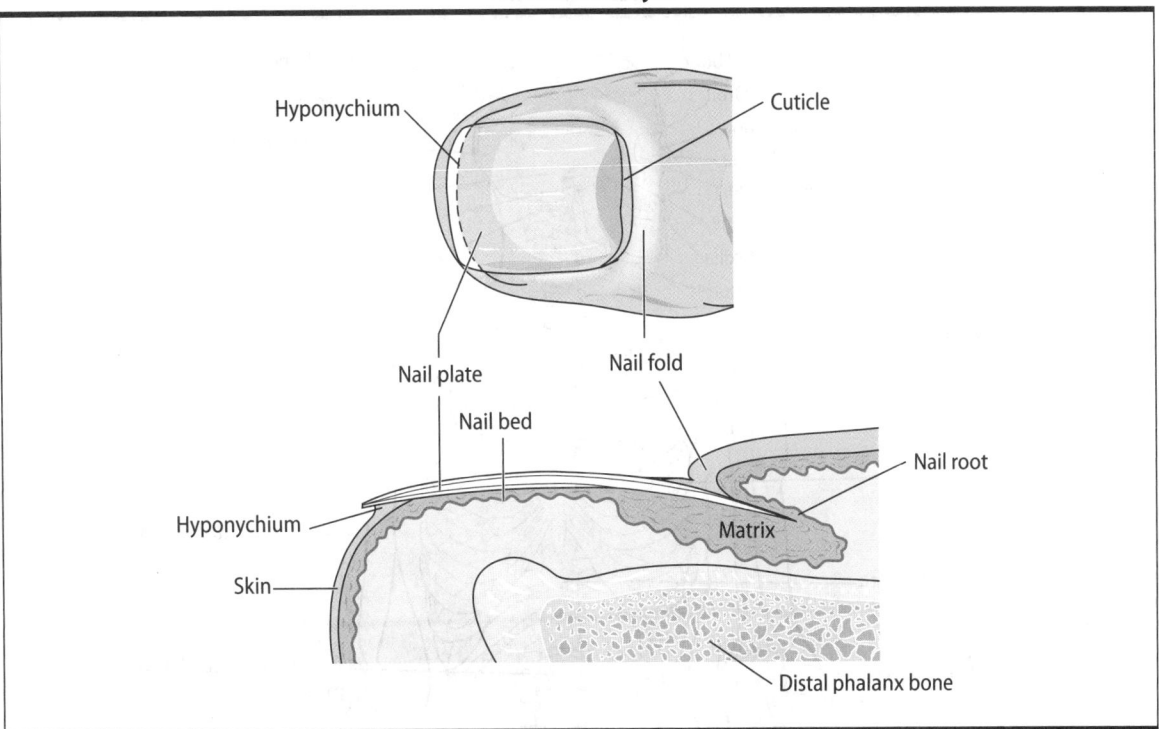

Skin and Subcutaneous Tissue

Chapter 13. Diseases of the Musculoskeletal System and Connective Tissue (MØØ–M99)

Bones and Joints

Shoulder Anterior View

Shoulder Posterior View

Elbow Anterior View

Elbow Posterior View

Hand

Hip Anterior View

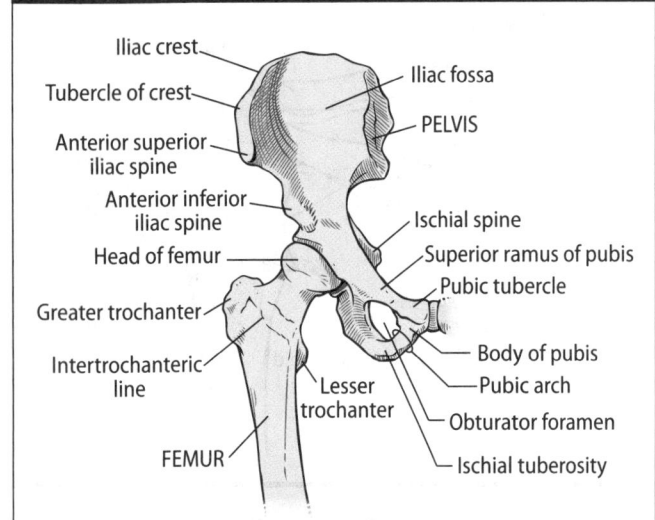

- Iliac crest
- Tubercle of crest
- Anterior superior iliac spine
- Anterior inferior iliac spine
- Head of femur
- Greater trochanter
- Intertrochanteric line
- Lesser trochanter
- FEMUR
- Iliac fossa
- PELVIS
- Ischial spine
- Superior ramus of pubis
- Pubic tubercle
- Body of pubis
- Pubic arch
- Obturator foramen
- Ischial tuberosity

Hip Posterior View

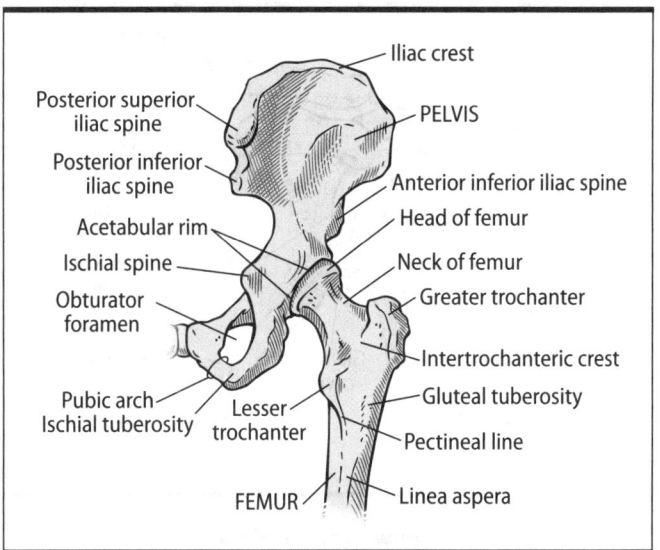

- Posterior superior iliac spine
- Posterior inferior iliac spine
- Acetabular rim
- Ischial spine
- Obturator foramen
- Pubic arch
- Ischial tuberosity
- Lesser trochanter
- Iliac crest
- PELVIS
- Anterior inferior iliac spine
- Head of femur
- Neck of femur
- Greater trochanter
- Intertrochanteric crest
- Gluteal tuberosity
- Pectineal line
- FEMUR
- Linea aspera

Knee Anterior View

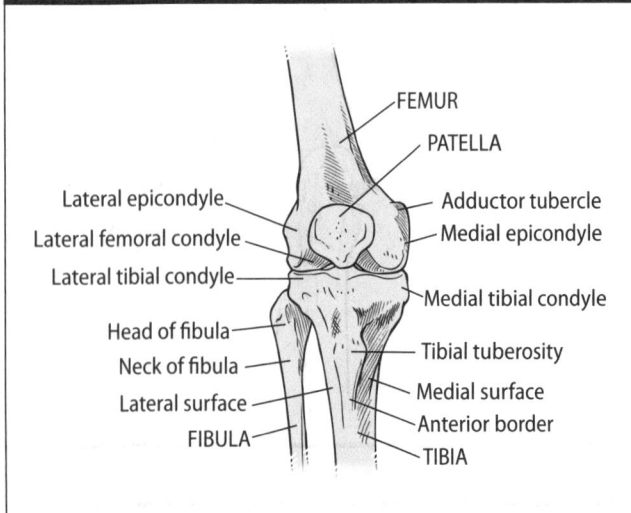

- FEMUR
- PATELLA
- Lateral epicondyle
- Lateral femoral condyle
- Lateral tibial condyle
- Head of fibula
- Neck of fibula
- Lateral surface
- FIBULA
- Adductor tubercle
- Medial epicondyle
- Medial tibial condyle
- Tibial tuberosity
- Medial surface
- Anterior border
- TIBIA

Knee Posterior View

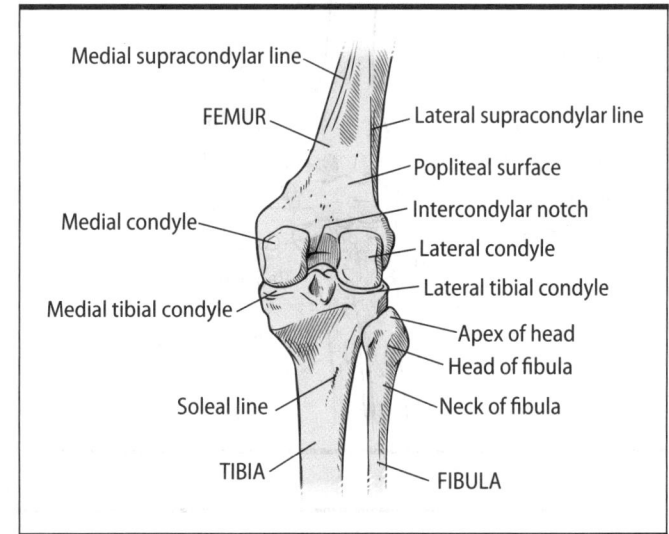

- Medial supracondylar line
- FEMUR
- Medial condyle
- Medial tibial condyle
- Soleal line
- TIBIA
- Lateral supracondylar line
- Popliteal surface
- Intercondylar notch
- Lateral condyle
- Lateral tibial condyle
- Apex of head
- Head of fibula
- Neck of fibula
- FIBULA

Foot

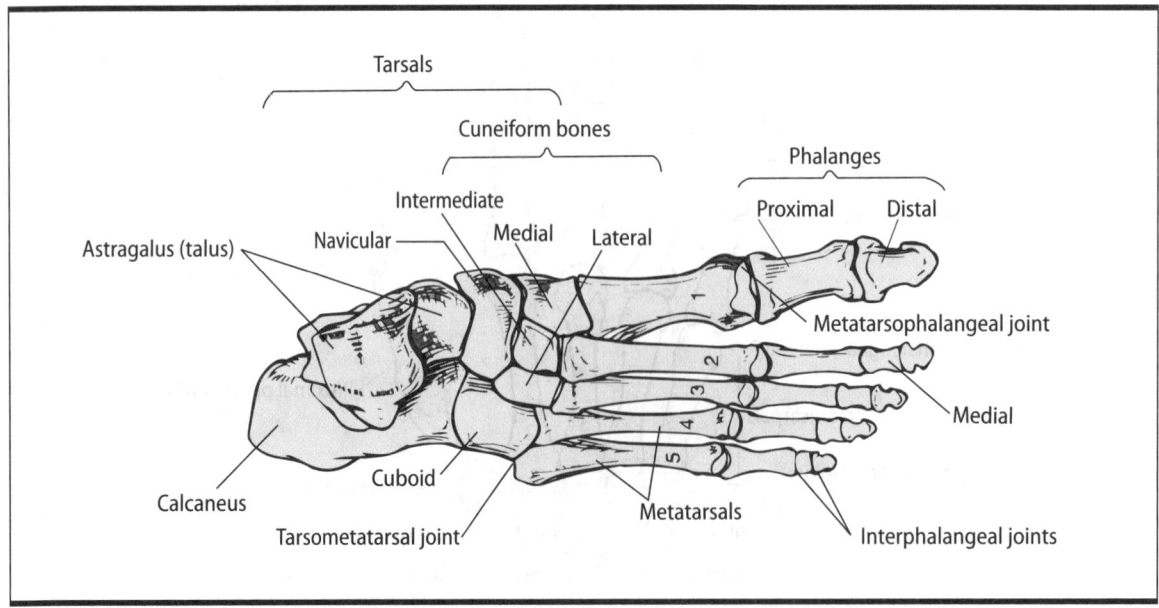

- Tarsals
- Cuneiform bones
- Phalanges
- Intermediate
- Medial
- Lateral
- Proximal
- Distal
- Navicular
- Astragalus (talus)
- Metatarsophalangeal joint
- Medial
- Calcaneus
- Cuboid
- Metatarsals
- Tarsometatarsal joint
- Interphalangeal joints

Muscles

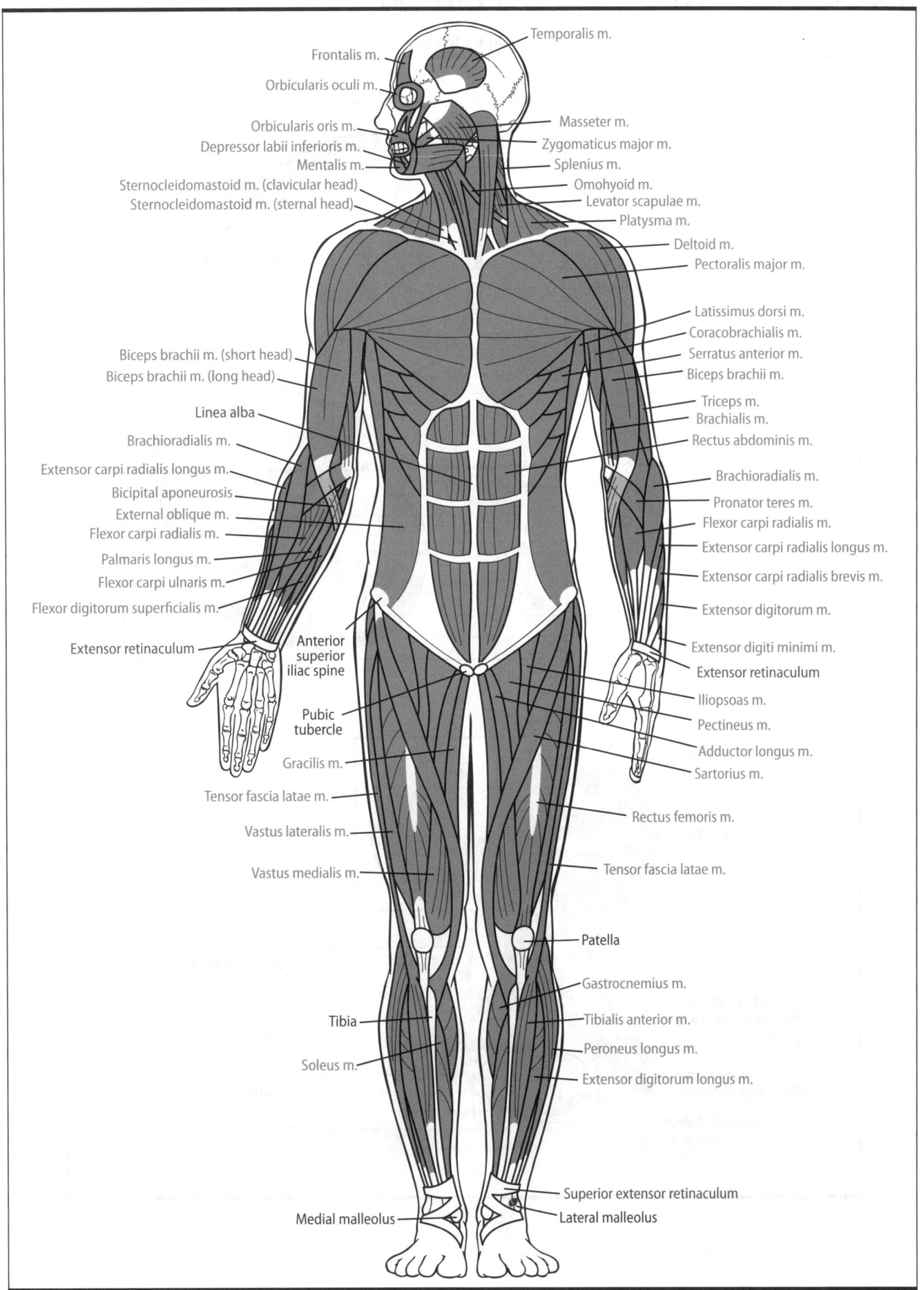

Temporalis m.
Frontalis m.
Orbicularis oculi m.
Orbicularis oris m.
Masseter m.
Depressor labii inferioris m.
Zygomaticus major m.
Mentalis m.
Splenius m.
Sternocleidomastoid m. (clavicular head)
Omohyoid m.
Sternocleidomastoid m. (sternal head)
Levator scapulae m.
Platysma m.
Deltoid m.
Pectoralis major m.
Latissimus dorsi m.
Coracobrachialis m.
Biceps brachii m. (short head)
Serratus anterior m.
Biceps brachii m. (long head)
Biceps brachii m.
Triceps m.
Linea alba
Brachialis m.
Brachioradialis m.
Rectus abdominis m.
Extensor carpi radialis longus m.
Brachioradialis m.
Bicipital aponeurosis
Pronator teres m.
External oblique m.
Flexor carpi radialis m.
Flexor carpi radialis m.
Extensor carpi radialis longus m.
Palmaris longus m.
Extensor carpi radialis brevis m.
Flexor carpi ulnaris m.
Extensor digitorum m.
Flexor digitorum superficialis m.
Extensor digiti minimi m.
Extensor retinaculum
Anterior superior iliac spine
Extensor retinaculum
Iliopsoas m.
Pubic tubercle
Pectineus m.
Adductor longus m.
Gracilis m.
Sartorius m.
Tensor fascia latae m.
Vastus lateralis m.
Rectus femoris m.
Vastus medialis m.
Tensor fascia latae m.
Patella
Gastrocnemius m.
Tibia
Tibialis anterior m.
Peroneus longus m.
Soleus m.
Extensor digitorum longus m.
Superior extensor retinaculum
Medial malleolus
Lateral malleolus

Chapter 14. Diseases of the Genitourinary System (NØØ–N99)

Urinary System

Male Genitourinary System

Female Internal Genitalia

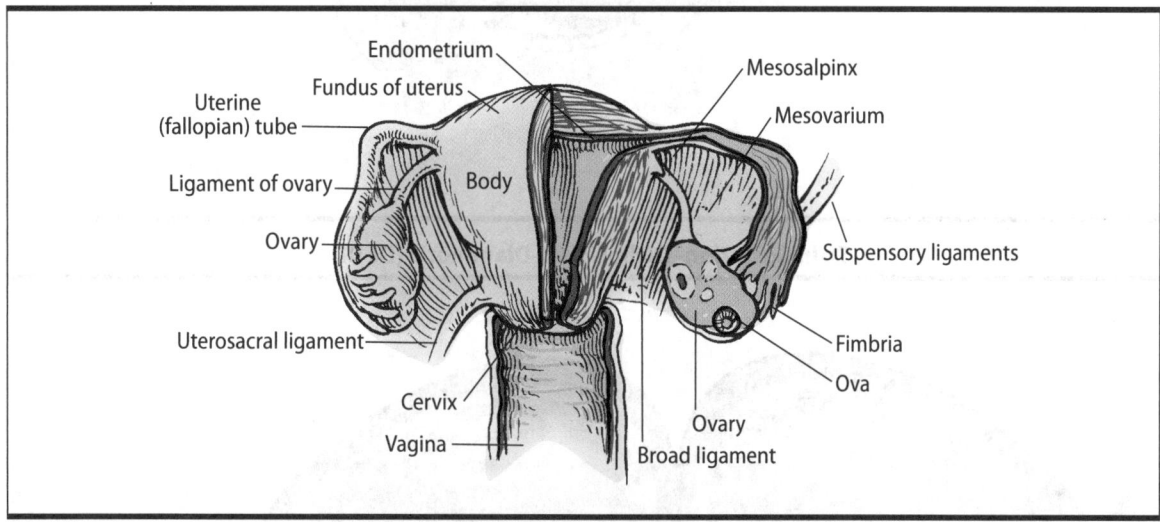

Female Genitourinary Tract Lateral View

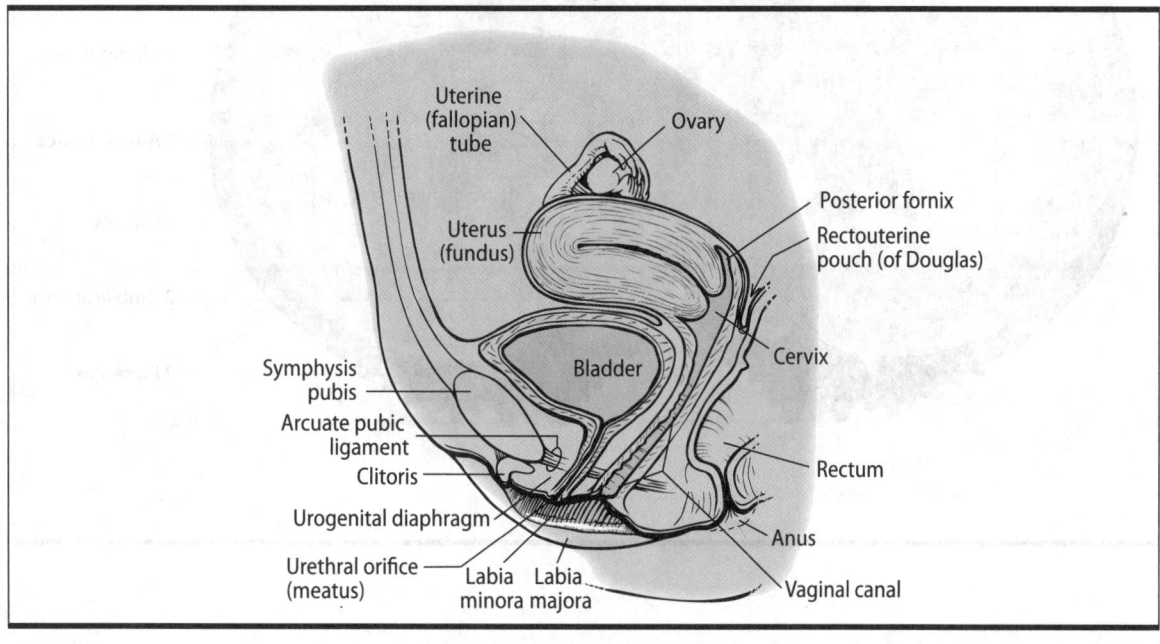

Chapter 15. Pregnancy, Childbirth and the Puerperium (O00–O9A)

Term Pregnancy – Single Gestation

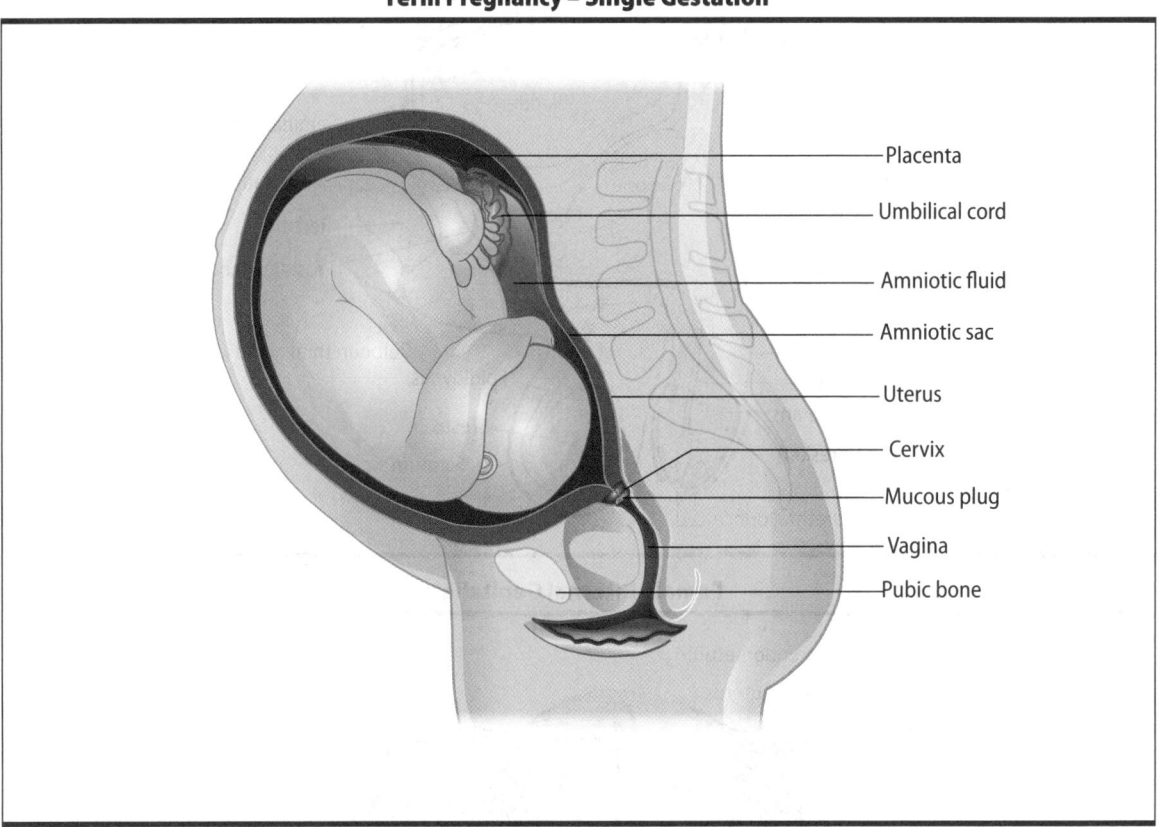

Placenta
Umbilical cord
Amniotic fluid
Amniotic sac
Uterus
Cervix
Mucous plug
Vagina
Pubic bone

Twin Gestation–Dichorionic–Diamniotic (DI-DI)

2 Chorionic sacs
2 Amniotic sacs
2 Fetuses
2 Umbilical cords
2 Placentas

Twin Gestation–Monochorionic–Diamniotic (MO-DI)

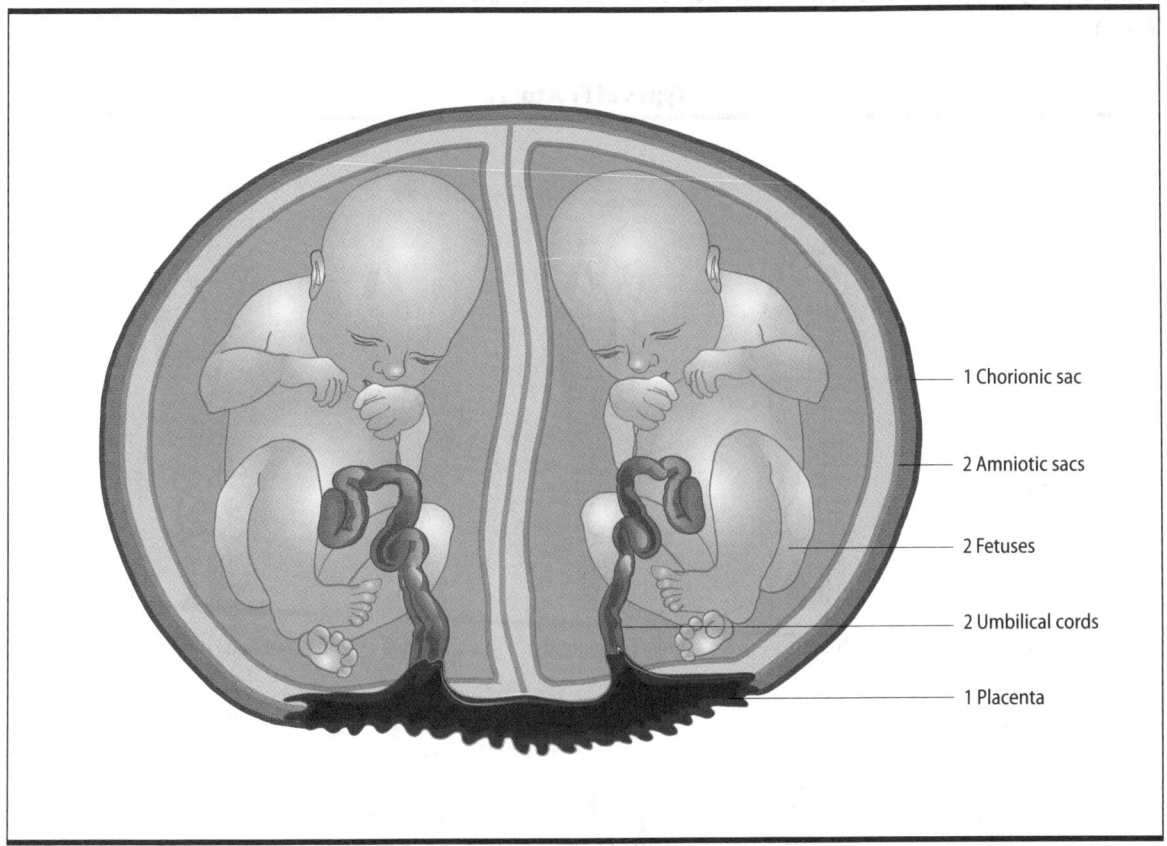

1 Chorionic sac

2 Amniotic sacs

2 Fetuses

2 Umbilical cords

1 Placenta

Twin Gestation–Monochorionic–Monoamniotic (MO-MO)

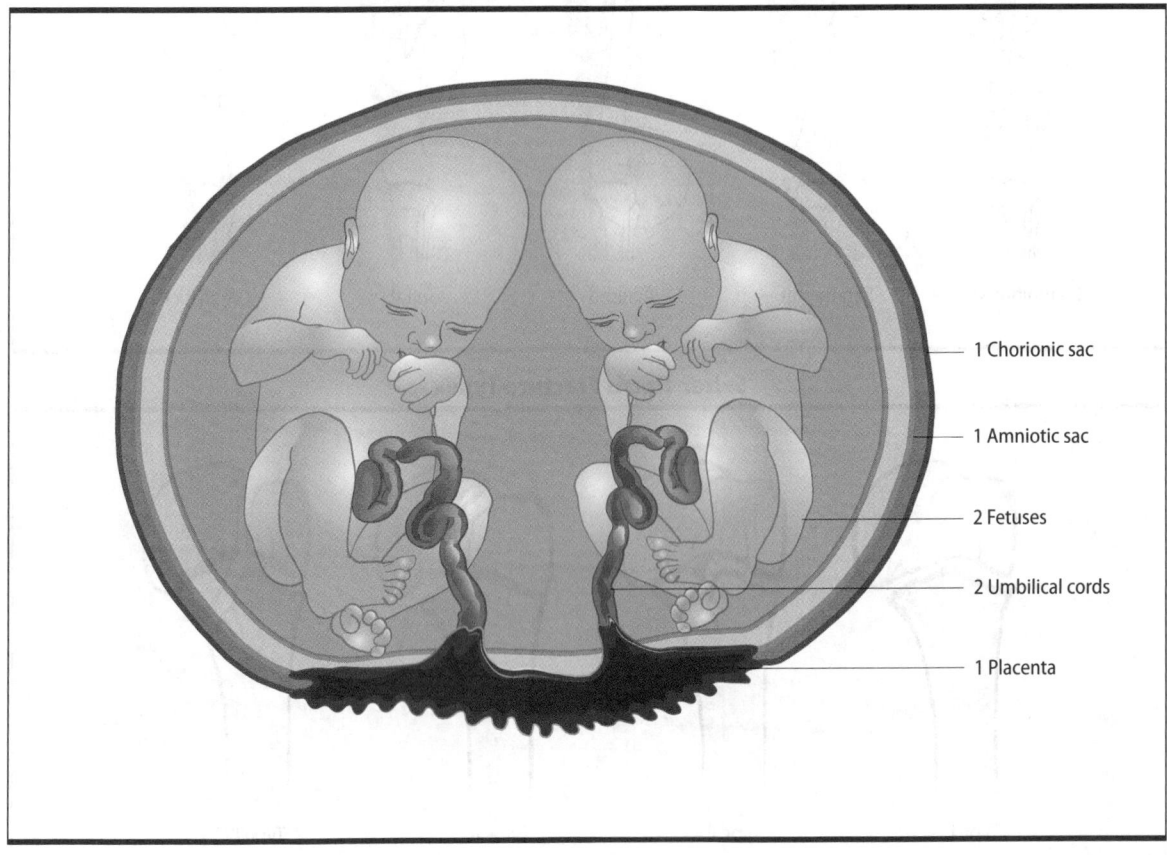

1 Chorionic sac

1 Amniotic sac

2 Fetuses

2 Umbilical cords

1 Placenta

Chapter 19. Injury, Poisoning and Certain Other Consequences of External Causes (S00–T88)

Types of Fractures

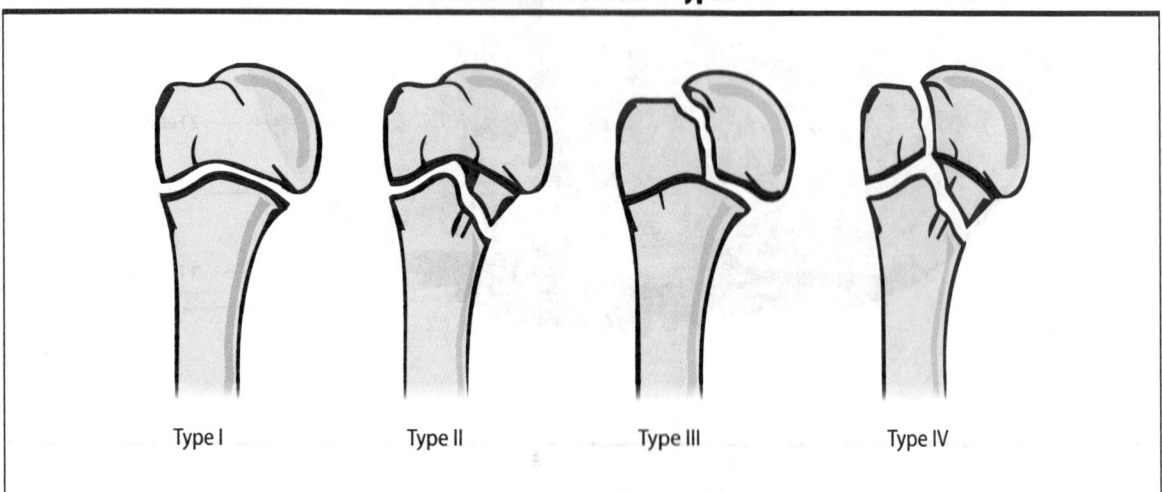

Normal	Transverse	Open/Compound	Oblique	Oblique displaced

Comminuted	Segmental	Avulsed	Spiral	Greenstick

Salter-Harris Fracture Types

Type I	Type II	Type III	Type IV